Shlomo Melmed, MD
Professor of Medicine
Senior Vice President and Dean of the Faculty
Cedars-Sinai Medical Center
Los Angeles, California

Kenneth S. Polonsky, MD
Richard T. Crane Distinguished Service Professor
Dean of the Division of the Biological Sciences
and the Pritzker School of Medicine
Executive Vice President of Medical Affairs
The University of Chicago
Chicago, Illinois

P. Reed Larsen, MD, FACP, FRCP
Professor of Medicine
Harvard Medical School
Senior Physician and Chief
Thyroid Section
Division of Endocrinology, Diabetes, and Metabolism
Brigham and Women's Hospital
Boston, Massachusetts

Henry M. Kronenberg, MD
Professor of Medicine
Harvard Medical School
Chief, Endocrine Unit
Massachusetts General Hospital
Boston, Massachusetts

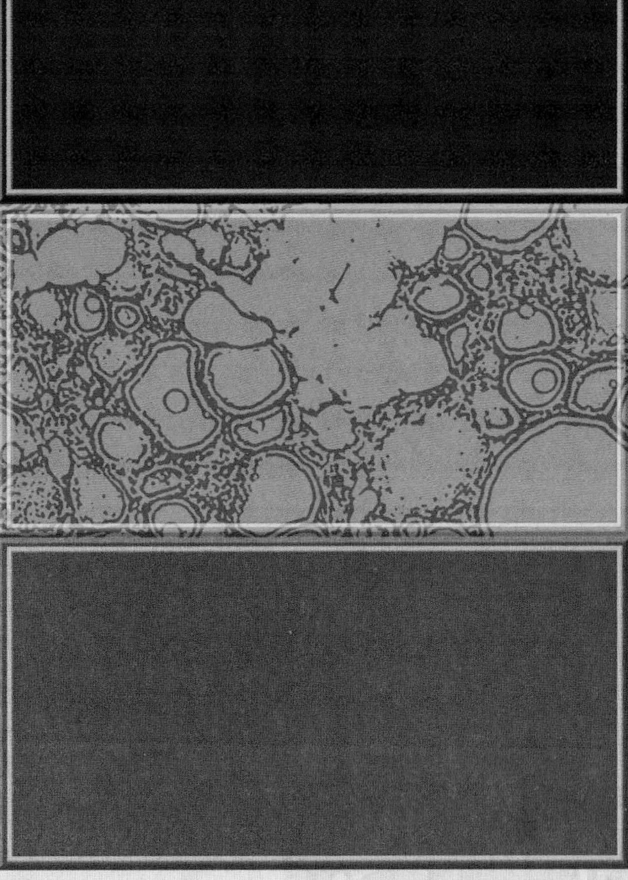

WILLIAMS Textbook of **Endocrinology**

12th EDITION

ELSEVIER
SAUNDERS

ELSEVIER
SAUNDERS

1600 John F. Kennedy Blvd.
Ste 1800
Philadelphia, PA 19103-2899

WILLIAMS TEXTBOOK OF ENDOCRINOLOGY ISBN: 978-1-4377-0324-5

Notices

Knowledge and best practice in this field are constantly changing. As new research and experience broaden our understanding, changes in research methods, professional practices, or medical treatment may become necessary.

Practitioners and researchers must always rely on their own experience and knowledge in evaluating and using any information, methods, compounds, or experiments described herein. In using such information or methods they should be mindful of their own safety and the safety of others, including parties for whom they have a professional responsibility.

With respect to any drug or pharmaceutical products identified, readers are advised to check the most current information provided (i) on procedures featured or (ii) by the manufacturer of each product to be administered, to verify the recommended dose or formula, the method and duration of administration, and contraindications. It is the responsibility of practitioners, relying on their own experience and knowledge of their patients, to make diagnoses, to determine dosages and the best treatment for each individual patient, and to take all appropriate safety precautions.

To the fullest extent of the law, neither the Publisher nor the authors, contributors, or editors, assume any liability for any injury and/or damage to persons or property as a matter of products liability, negligence or otherwise, or from any use or operation of any methods, products, instructions, or ideas contained in the material herein.

Library of Congress Cataloging-in-Publication Data

Williams textbook of endocrinology.—12th ed. / Shlomo Melmed ... [et al.].
p. ; cm.
Textbook of endocrinology
Includes bibliographical references and index.
ISBN 978-1-4377-0324-5 (hardcover : alk. paper) 1. Endocrinology. 2. Endocrine glands—Diseases. I. Melmed, Shlomo. II. Williams, Robert Hardin. III. Title: Textbook of endocrinology.
[DNLM: 1. Endocrine Glands. 2. Endocrine System Diseases. WK 100]
RC648.T46 2011
616.4—dc22

2011004321

Acquisitions Editor: Pamela Hetherington
Developmental Editor: Joan Ryan
Publishing Services Manager: Patricia Tannian
Team Manager: Radhika Pallamparthy
Senior Project Manager: Sharon Corell
Project Manager: Jayavel Radhakrishnan
Design Direction: Louis Forgione

Printed in the United States of America
Last digit is the print number: 9 8 7 6 5 4 3 2 1

CONTRIBUTORS

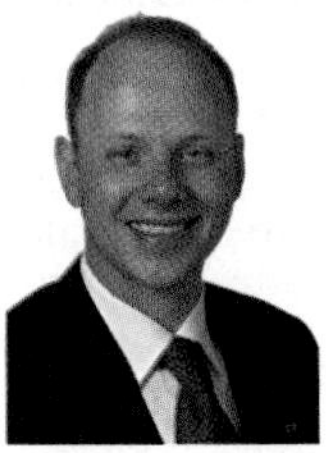

John C. Achermann, MD, PhD
Wellcome Trust Senior Fellow in Clinical Science
UCL Institute of Child Health
Honorary Consultant in Pediatric Endocrinology
Great Ormond Street Hospital NHS Trust
London, UK

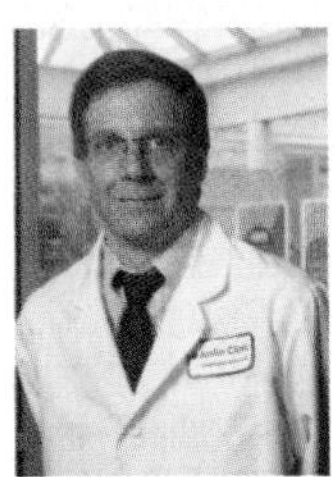

Lloyd P. Aiello, MD, PhD
Associate Professor
Harvard Medical School
Director
Beetham Eye Institute, Joslin Diabetes Center
Boston, Massachusetts, USA

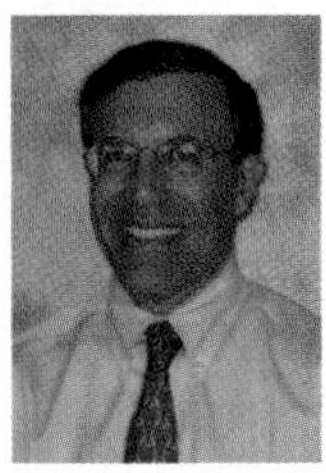

Andrew Arnold, MD
Murray-Heilig Chair in Molecular Medicine
Professor of Medicine
Chief, Division of Endocrinology and Metabolism
University of Connecticut School of Medicine
Farmington, Connecticut, USA

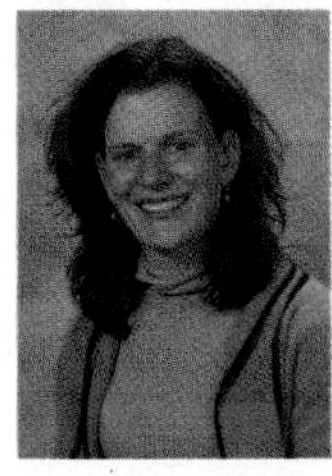

Jennifer M. Barker, MD
Assistant Professor of Pediatrics
University of Colorado Denver
Division of Pediatric Endocrinology
The Children's Hospital
Aurora, Colorado, USA

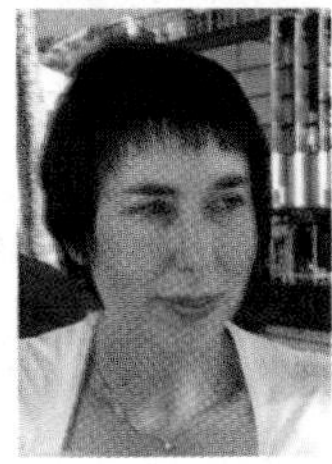

Rosemary Basson, MD, FRCP (UK)
Clinical Professor
Psychiatry
University of British Columbia
Director, Sexual Medicine Program Psychiatry
Vancouver General Hospital
Vancouver, British Columbia, Canada

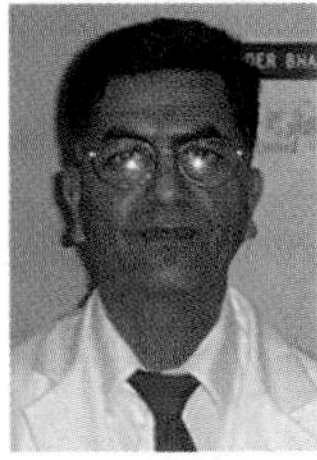

Shalender Bhasin, MD
Boston University School of Medicine
Boston Medical Center
Boston, Massachusetts, USA

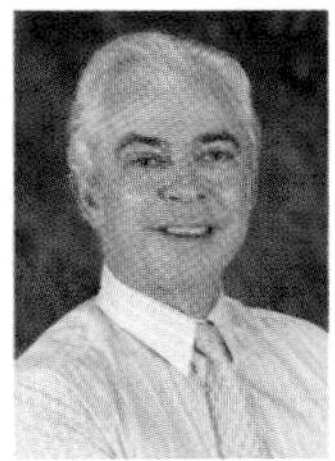

Andrew J.M. Boulton, MD, FRCP
Professor of Medicine
University of Manchester
Consultant Physician
Manchester Royal Infirmary
Manchester, UK

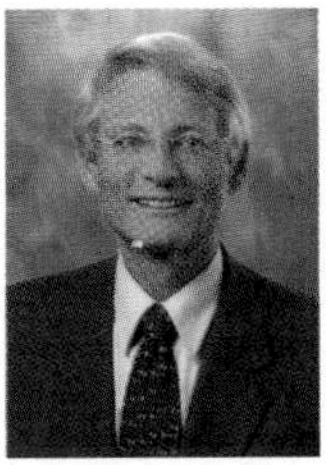

Glenn D. Braunstein, MD
Professor and Chairman
Department of Medicine
The James R. Klinenberg, MD, Chair in Medicine Cedars-Sinai Medical Center
Los Angeles, California, USA

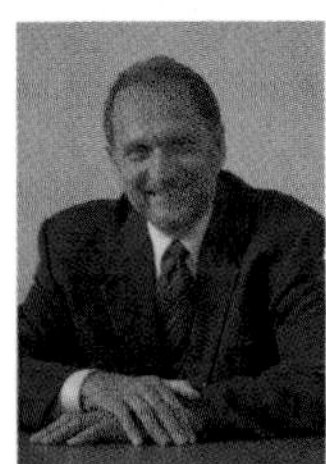

William J. Bremner, MD, PhD
Professor and Chair
Department of Medicine
Robert G. Petersdorf Endowed Chair
University of Washington School of Medicine
Chair
Department of Medicine
University of Washington Medical Center
Seattle, Washington, USA

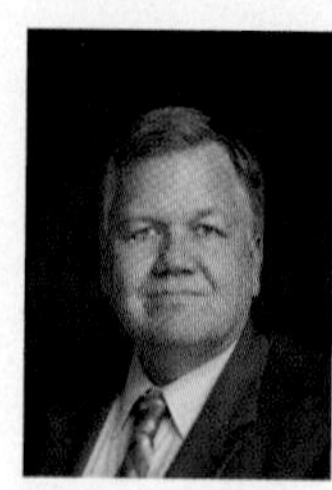

Gregory A. Brent, MD
Professor
Departments of Medicine and Physiology
David Geffen School of Medicine at UCLA
Chair, Department of Medicine
VA Greater Los Angeles Healthcare System
Los Angeles, California, USA

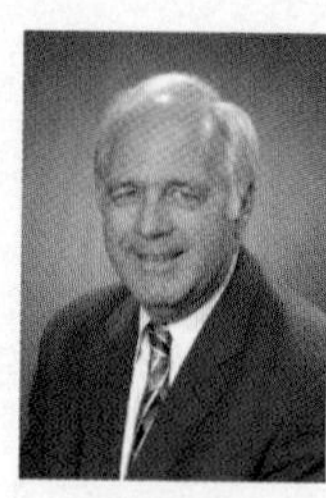

F. Richard Bringhurst, MD
Associate Professor
Medicine
Harvard Medical School
Physician
Medical Service
Massachusetts General Hospital
Boston, Massachusetts, USA

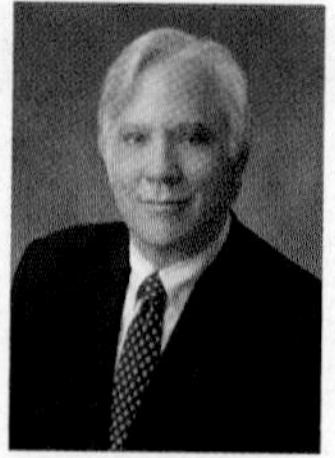

Michael Brownlee, MD
Anita and Jack Saltz Chair in Diabetes Research and Professor
Medicine and Pathology
Associate Director for Biomedical Sciences
Einstein Diabetes Research Center
Albert Einstein College of Medicine
Bronx, New York, USA

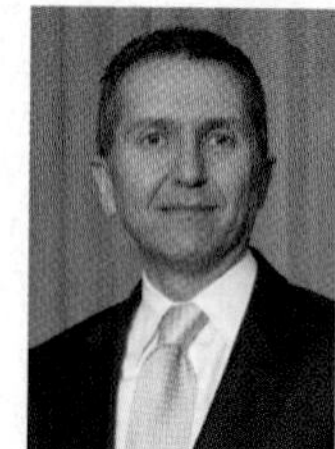

Serdar E. Bulun, MD
Northwestern Memorial Hospital
University of Illinois Hospital
Chicago, Illinois, USA

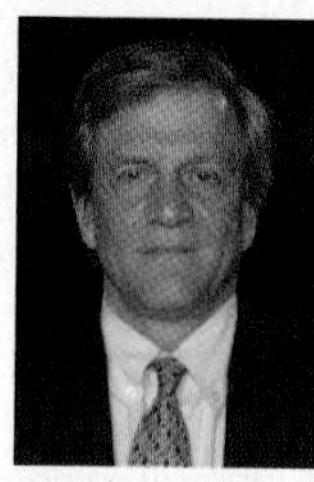

Charles F. Burant, MD, PhD
Professor of Internal Medicine
University of Michigan
Ann Arbor, Michigan, USA

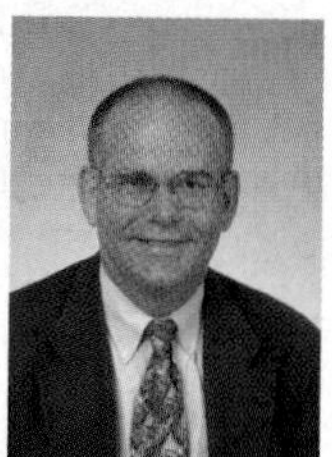

John B. Buse, MD, PhD
Professor of Medicine
Chief, Division of Endocrinology
UNC School of Medicine
Chapel Hill, North Carolina, USA

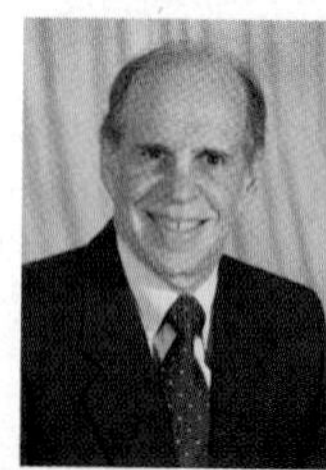

David A. Bushinsky, MD
Professor
Medicine, Pharmacology, and Physiology
University of Rochester School of Medicine
Rochester, New York, USA

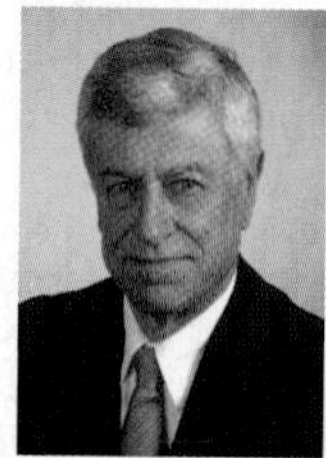

Ernesto Canalis, MD
Professor of Medicine
University of Connecticut School of Medicine
Farmington, Connecticut, USA
Director of Research
St. Francis Hospital and Medical Center
Hartford, Connecticut, USA

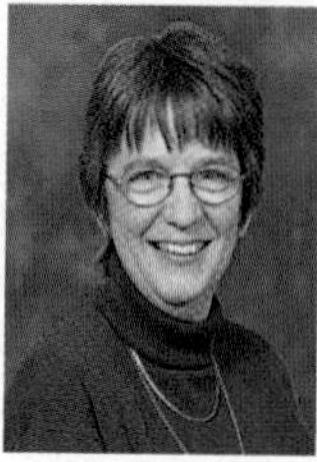

Christin Carter-Su, PhD
Professor
Molecular and Integrative Physiology
University of Michigan Medical School
Associate Director
Michigan Diabetes Research and Training Center
University of Michigan
Ann Arbor, Michigan, USA

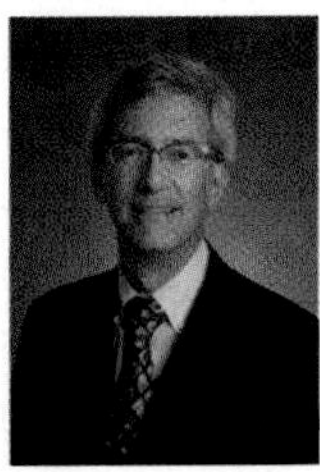

Roger D. Cone, PhD
Professor and Chairman
Molecular Physiology and Biophysics
Vanderbilt University School of Medicine
Nashville, Tennessee, USA

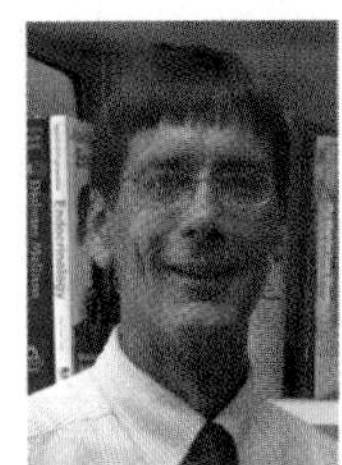

David W. Cooke, MD
Associate Professor
Pediatrics
Johns Hopkins University
School of Medicine
Baltimore, Maryland, USA

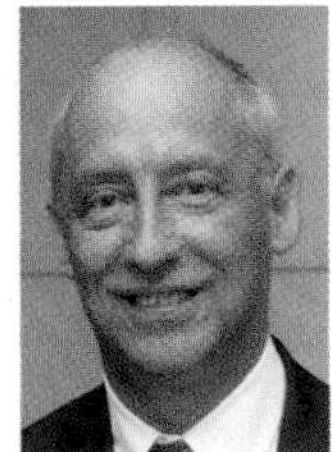

Mark E. Cooper, MB, BS, PhD
Director
JDRF Centre for Diabetic Complications
Professor of Medicine and Immunology
Monash University
Melbourne, Victoria, Australia

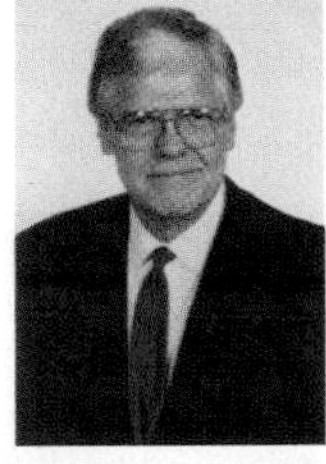

Philip E. Cryer, MD
Irene E. and Michael M. Karl
Professor of Endocrinology and Metabolism in Medicine
Washington University in St. Louis
Physician
Barnes-Jewish Hospital
St. Louis, Missouri, USA

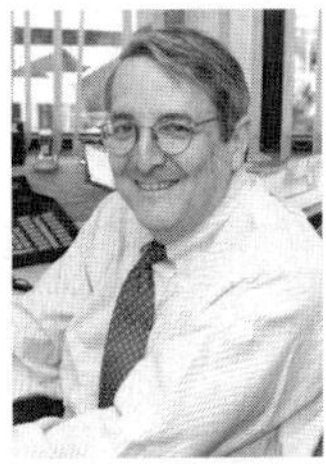

Gilbert H. Daniels, MD
Professor of Medicine
Harvard Medical School
Co-Director Thyroid Clinic
Medical Director Endocrine Tumor Center
Thyroid Unit, Department of Medicine and Cancer Center
Massachusetts General Hospital
Boston, Massachusetts, USA

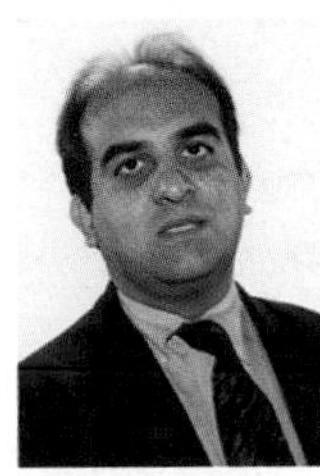

Mehul T. Dattani, FRCPCH, FRCP, MD
Professor and Head of Pediatric Endocrinology
Developmental Endocrinology Research Group, Clinical and Molecular Genetics Unit
UCL Institute of Child Health
Consultant and Lead in Adolescent Endocrinology
University College London Hospitals
London, United Kingdom

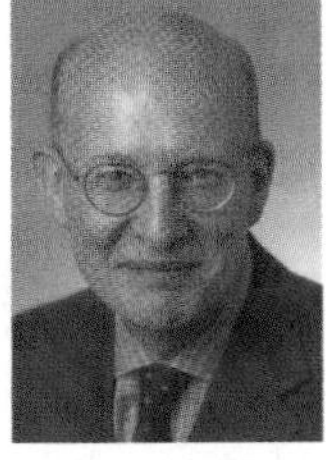

Terry F. Davies, MB.BS, MD, FRCP, FACE
Florence and Theodore Baumritter
Professor of Medicine
Attending Physician
Mount Sinai School of Medicine
New York, New York, USA

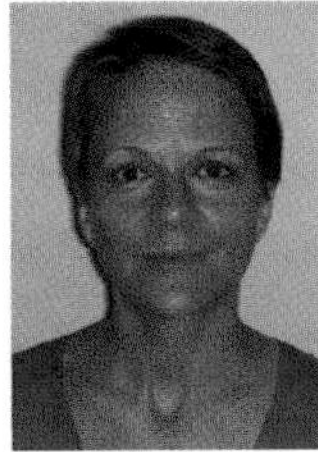

Marie B. Demay, MD
Professor of Medicine
Harvard Medical School
Physician
Endocrine Unit
Department of Medicine
Massachusetts General Hospital
Boston, Massachusetts, USA

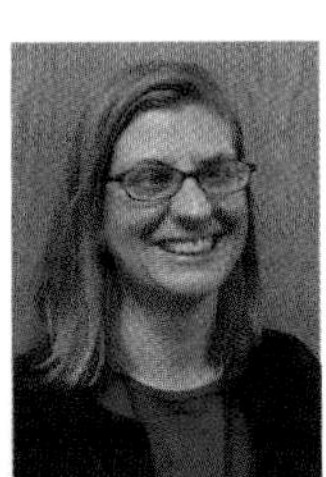

Sara A. DiVall, MD
Assistant Professor
Pediatrics
Johns Hopkins University
Baltimore, Maryland, USA

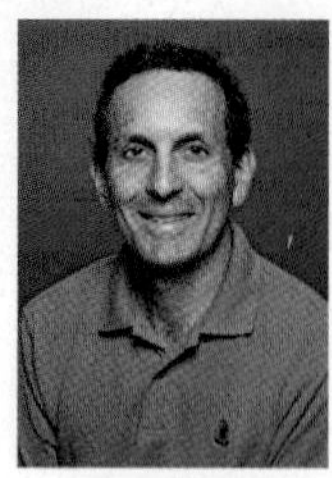

Daniel J. Drucker, MD
Professor of Medicine
University of Toronto
Toronto, Ontario, Canada

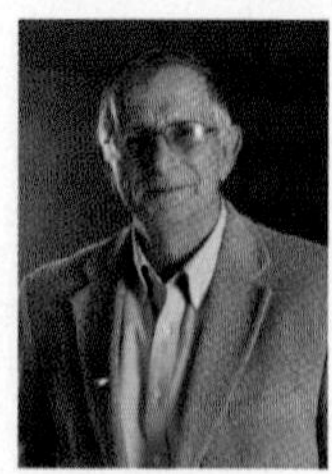

George S. Eisenbarth, MD, PhD
Executive Director
Professor of Pediatrics
Medicine and Immunology
Barbara Davis Center for Childhood Diabetes
University of Colorado at Denver
Professor
University of Colorado Hospital
Professor, Pediatrics
The Children's Hospital
Aurora, Colorado, USA

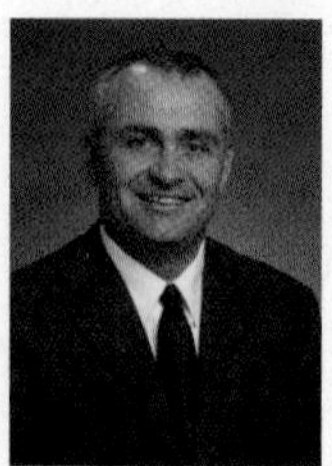

Joel K. Elmquist, DVM, PhD
Professor and Director
Division of Hypothalamic Research
Internal Medicine and Pharmacology
University of Texas
Southwestern Medical
Center at Dallas
Dallas, Texas, USA

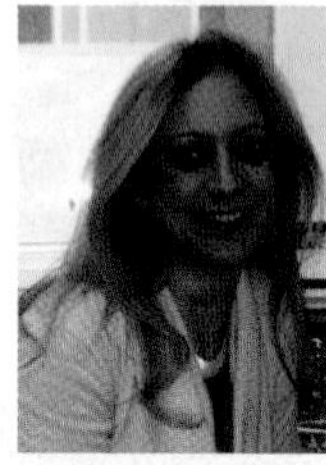

Elisa Fabbrini, MD, PhD
Research Assistant Professor
Center for Human Nutrition
Washington University School of Medicine
St. Louis, Missouri, USA

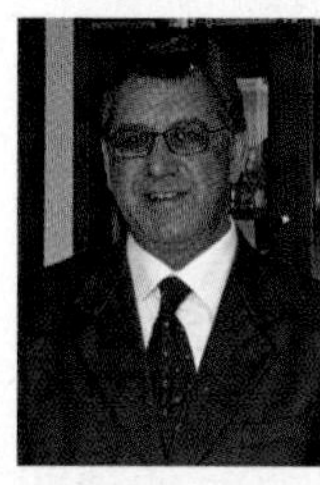

Sebastiano Filetti, MD
Professor of Internal Medicine
Department of Internal Medicine
Sapienza Universita' di Roma
Chief, Internal Medicine
Department of Internal Medicine
Policlinico Umberto I
Rome, Italy

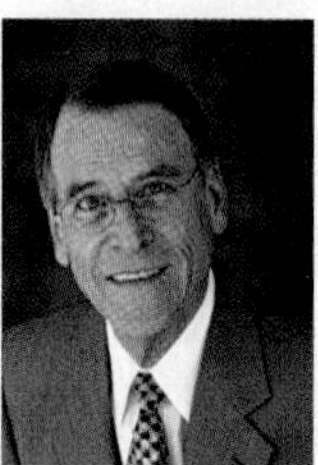

Delbert A. Fisher, MD
Professor Emeritus
Pediatrics and Medicine
David Geffen School of Medicine at UCLA
Los Angeles, California, USA

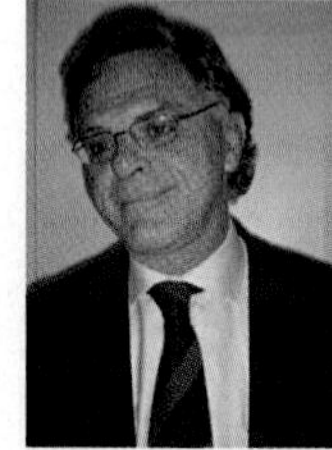

Ezio Ghigo, MD
Professor of Endocrinology
Department of Internal Medicine
University of Turin Faculty of Medicine
Chief, Division of Endocrinology, Diabetology, and Metabolism
Department of Internal Medicine
University Hospital
Turin, Italy

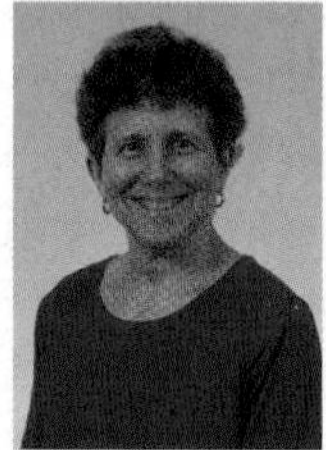

Anne C. Goldberg, MD
Associate Professor of Medicine
Division of Endocrinology, Metabolism, and Lipid Research
Department of Internal Medicine
Washington University School of Medicine
St. Louis, Missouri, USA

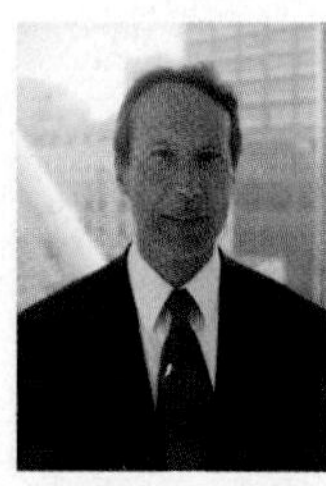

Ira J. Goldberg, MD
Dickinson Richards Jr. Professor
Chief, Division of Preventive Medicine and Nutrition
Columbia University College of Physicians and Surgeons
New York, New York, USA

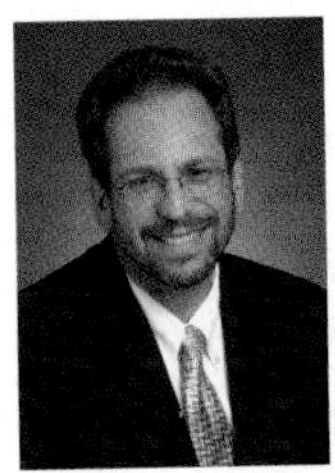

Peter A. Gottlieb, MD
Assistant Professor of Pediatrics and Medicine
The Children's Hospital
University of Colorado Health Science Center
Barbara Davis Center for Childhood Diabetes
Aurora, Colorado, USA

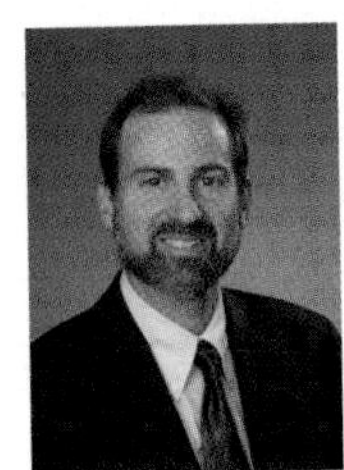

Steven K. Grinspoon, MD
Professor of Medicine
Harvard Medical School
Director
Neuroendocrine Clinical Center
Massachusetts General Hospital
Boston, Massachusetts, USA

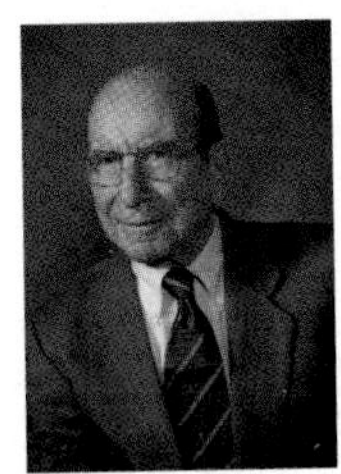

Melvin M. Grumbach, MD, DM
Edward B. Shaw Professor of Pediatrics and Emeritus Chairman
Department of Pediatrics
University of California, San Francisco
Attending Physician
Pediatrics
University of California, San Francisco Medical Center
University of California, San Francisco Children's Hospital
San Francisco, California, USA

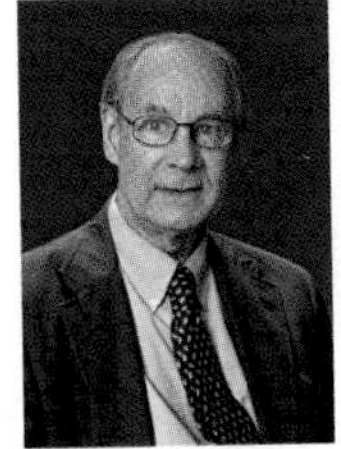

Joel F. Habener, MD
Professor of Medicine
Laboratory of Molecular Endocrinology
Massachusetts General Hospital
Boston, Massachusetts, USA

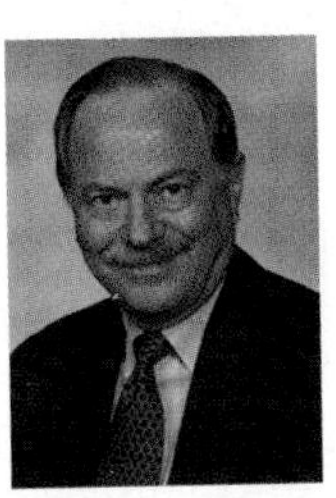

Ian D. Hay, MB, PhD, FACE, FACP, FRCP (E,G & I), FRCPI (Hon)
Professor of Medicine and
Dr. R.F. Emslander Professor of Endocrinology Research
Division of Endocrinology and Internal Medicine
Mayo Clinic College of Medicine
Rochester, Minnesota, USA

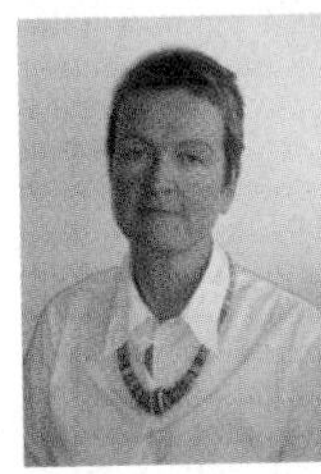

Martha Hickey, BA (Hons), MSc, MBChB, MRCOG, FRANZCOG, MD
Professor of Gynaecology
School of Women's and Infants' Health
University of Western Australia
Perth, Western Australia, Australia

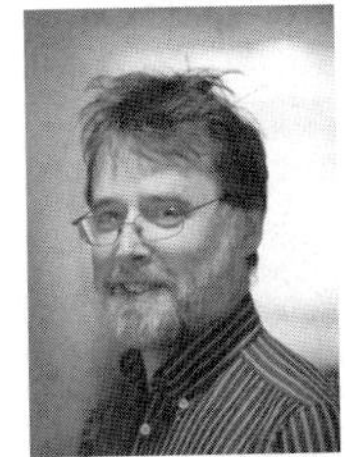

Peter C. Hindmarsh, BSc, MD, FRCP, FRCPCH
Professor of Paediatric Endocrinology
Developmental Endocrinology Research Group
Institute of Child Health
University College, London
Hon. Consultant Paediatric Endocrinologist
Great Ormond Street Hospital for Children
Hon. Consultant Paediatric Endocrinologist
University College London Hospitals
London, United Kingdom

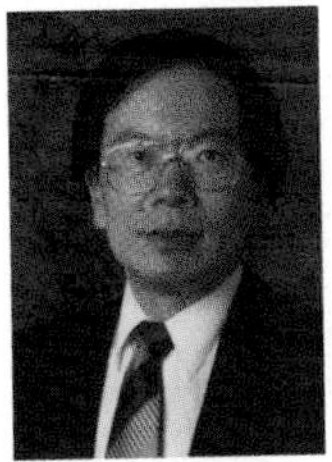

Ken Ho, MD, FRACP, FRCP (UK)
Professor of Medicine
University of Queensland
Chair
Centres for Health Research
Princess Alexandra Hospital
Brisbane, Queensland, Australia

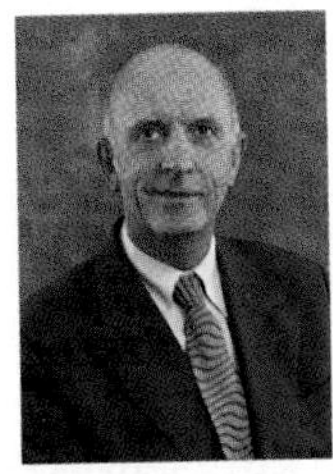

Ieuan A. Hughes, MA, MD, FRCP, FRCP(C), FRCPCH F Med Sci
Professor of Paediatrics
University of Cambridge
Honorary Consultant Paedaitrician
Cambridge University Hospitals NHS Foundation Trust
Cambridge, United Kingdom

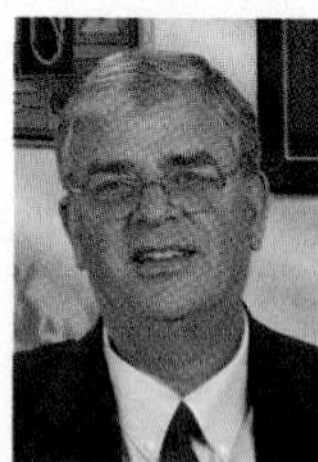

Andrew M. Kaunitz, MD
Professor and Associate Chairman
Obstetrics and Gynecology
University of Florida College of Medicine, Jacksonville
Jacksonville, Florida, USA

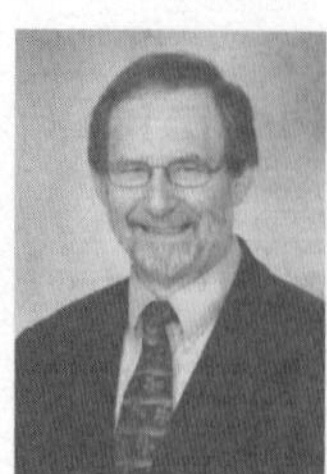

George G. Klee, MD, PhD
Professor of Laboratory Medicine and Pathology
Mayo Clinic College of Medicine
Consultant
Laboratory Medicine and Pathology
Saint Mary's Hospital
Methodist Hospital
Mayo Clinic
Rochester, Minnesota, USA

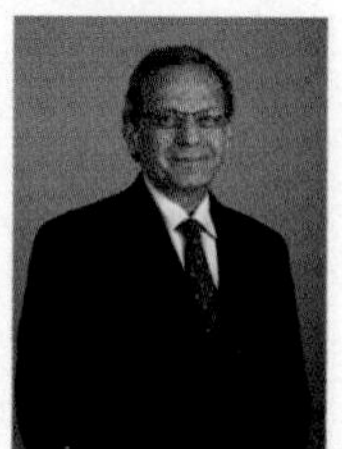

Samuel Klein, MD
William H. Danforth Professor of Medicine and Nutritional Science
Center for Human Nutrition
Washington University School of Medicine
William H. Danforth Professor of Medicine and Nutritional Science
Geriatrics and Nutritional Science
Barnes-Jewish Hospital
St. Louis, Missouri, USA

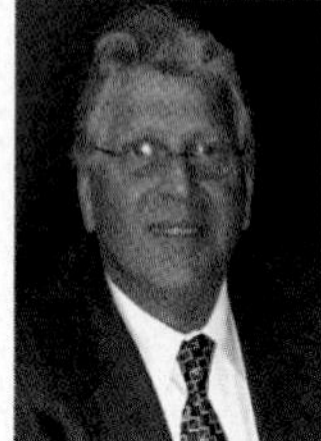

David Kleinberg, MD
Chief of Endocrinology
Veterans Administration Medical Center
Department of Medicine
New York University
New York, New York, USA

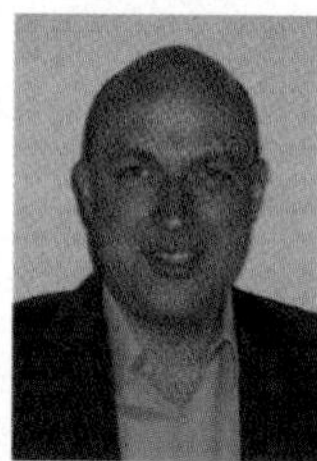

Nils P. Krone, MD
Wellcome Trust Clinician Scientist Fellow
School of Clinical and Experimental Medicine
University of Birmingham
Consultant Paediatric Endocrinologist
Birmingham Children's Hospital
Birmingham, United Kingdom

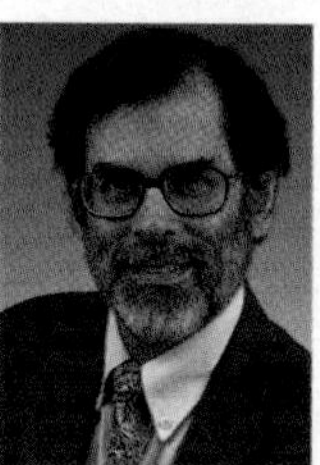

Henry M. Kronenberg, MD
Professor of Medicine
Harvard Medical School
Chief, Endocrine Unit
Massachusetts General Hospital
Boston, Massachusetts, USA

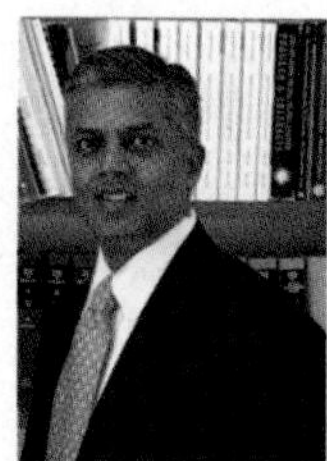

Rohit N. Kulkarni, MD, PhD
Investigator
Cellular and Molecular Physiology
Joslin Diabetes Center
Assistant Professor of Medicine
Department of Medicine
Harvard Medical School
Boston, Massachusetts, USA

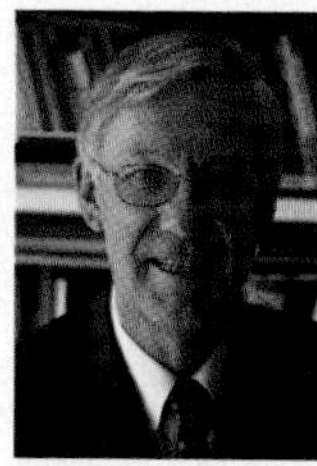

Steven W.J. Lamberts, MD, PhD
Professor
Erasmus Medical Center
Rotterdam, Neatherlands

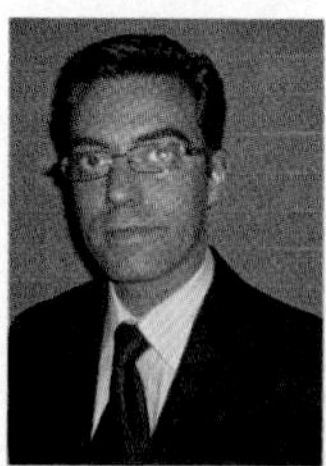

Fabio Lanfranco, MD, PhD
Division of Endocrinology, Diabetology, and Metabolism
Department of Internal Medicine
University of Turin
Turin, Italy

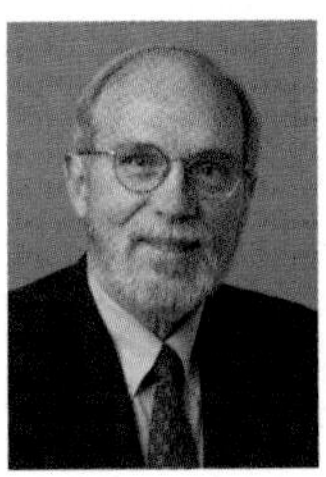

P. Reed Larsen, MD, FACP, FRCP
Professor of Medicine
Harvard Medical School
Senior Physician and Chief
Thyroid Section
Division of Endocrinology, Diabetes, and Metabolism
Brigham and Women's Hospital
Boston, Massachusetts, USA

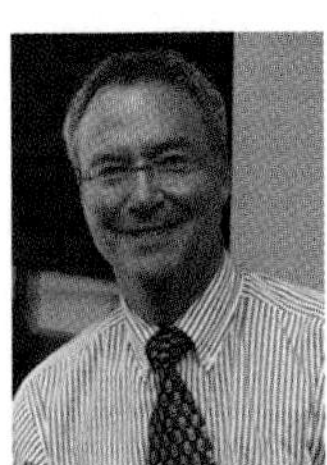

Mitchell A. Lazar, MD, Ph.D.
Professor of Medicine and Genetics
Chief, Division of Endocrinology, Diabetes, and Metabolism
University of Pennsylvania
Philadelphia, Pennsylvania, USA

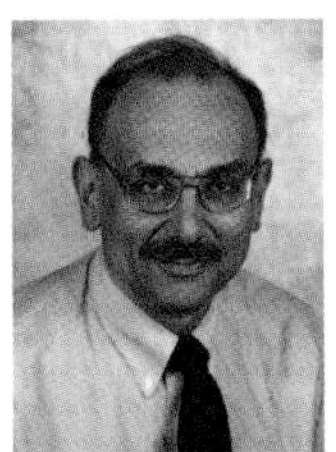

Joseph A. Lorenzo, MD
Professor of Medicine
University of Connecticut Health Center
Attending Physician
John Dempsey Hospital
Farmington, Connecticut, USA

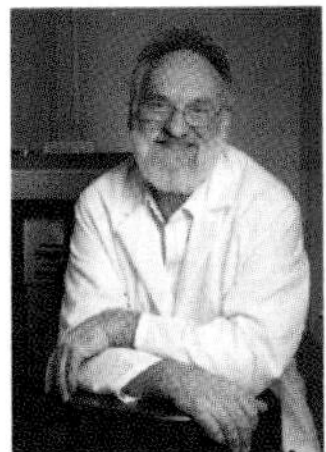

Malcolm J. Low, MD, PhD
Professor of Physiology and Internal Medicine
Department of Molecular and Integrative Physiology
University of Michigan School of Medicine
Ann Arbor, Michigan, USA

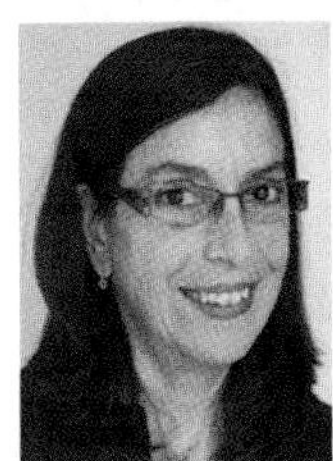

Susan J. Mandel, MD, MPH
Professor of Medicine and Radiology and Associate Chief
Division of Endocrinology, Diabetes, and Metabolism
University of Pennsylvania School of Medicine
Director, Clinical Endocrinology and Diabetes
University of Pennsylvania Health System
Philadelphia, Pennsylvania, USA

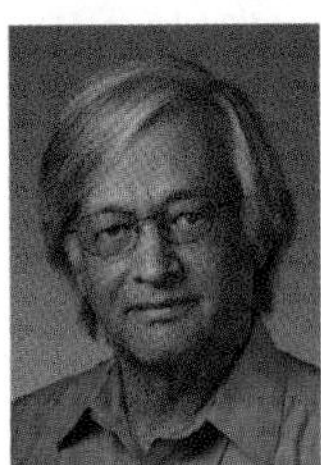

Stephen J. Marx, MD
Branch Chief and Section Chief
Metabolic Diseases Branch
and Genetics and Endocrinology Section
National Institute of Diabetes, Digestive, and Kidney Diseases
Bethesda, Maryland, USA

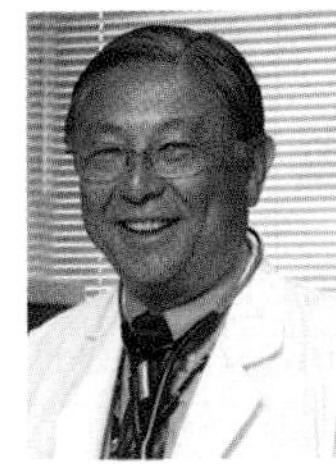

Alvin M. Matsumoto, MD
Professor, Department of Medicine
University of Washington School of Medicine
Associate Director
Geriatric Research, Education, and Clinical Center
Director, Clinical Research Unit
VA Puget Sound Health Care System
Seattle, Washington, USA

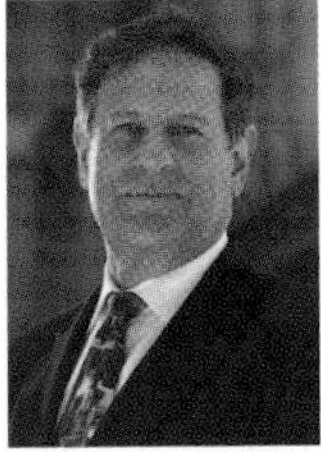

Shlomo Melmed, MD
Professor of Medicine
Senior Vice President and Dean of the Faculty
Cedars-Sinai Medical Center
Los Angeles, California, USA

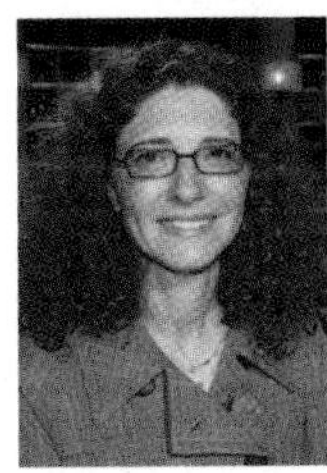

Rebeca D. Monk, MD
Associate Professor of Medicine
Nephrology
Program Director, Nephrology Fellowship
University of Rochester Medical Center
Rochester, New York, USA

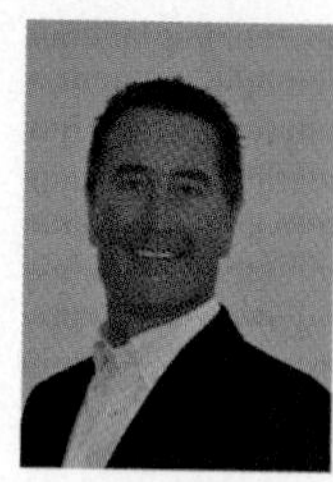

Robert D. Murray, MD
Consultant Endocrinologist and
Honorary Senior Lecturer
Department of Endocrinology
Leads Teaching Hospitals
NHS Trust
Leeds, United Kingdom

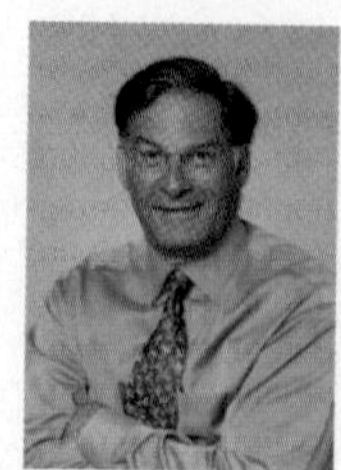

Richard W. Nesto, MD
Northeast Health System
Beverly Hospital
Beverly, Massachusetts, USA
Lahey Clinic
Burlington, Massachusetts, USA

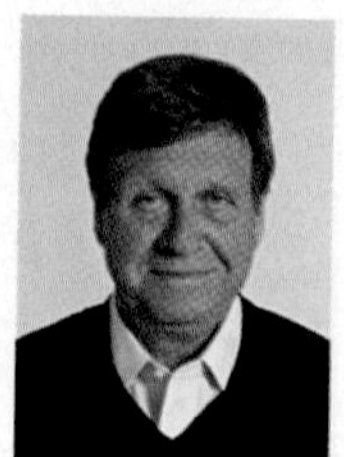

Kjell Oberg, MD, PhD
Professor
Department of Endocrine Oncology
Uppsala University
Uppsala, Sweden

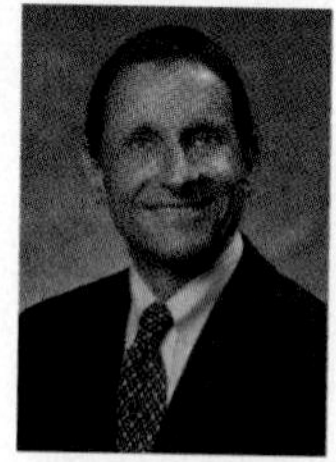

Kenneth S. Polonsky, MD
Richard T. Crane Distinguished
Service Professor
Dean of the Division of the
Biological Sciences and the Pritzker
School of Medicine
Executive Vice President of Medical
Affairs
The University of Chicago
Chicago, Illinois, USA

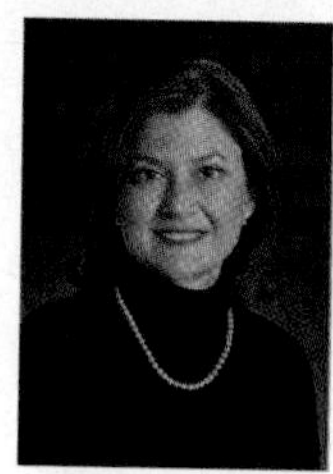

Sally Radovick, MD
Johns Hopkins University School of
Medicine
Johns Hopkins Hospital
Baltimore, Maryland, USA

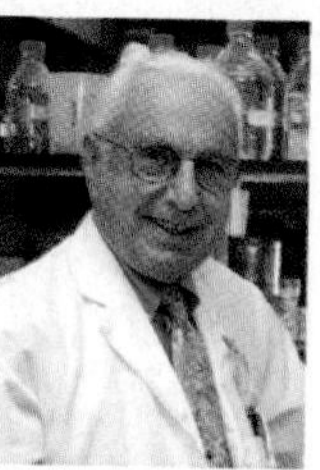

Lawrence G. Raisz, MD
Board of Trustees Distinguished
Professor of Medicine, Emeritus
University of Connecticut
Health Center
Farmington, Connecticut, USA

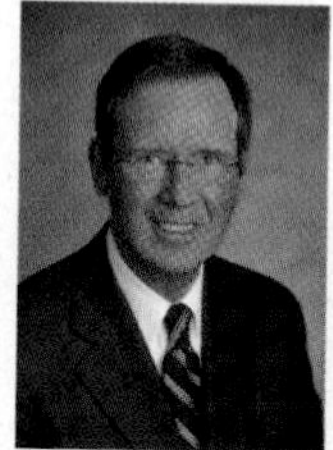

Alan G. Robinson, MD
Associate Vice Chancellor Medical
Sciences, Executive Associate Dean,
and Professor of Medicine
David Geffen School of Medicine
at UCLA
Los Angeles, California, USA

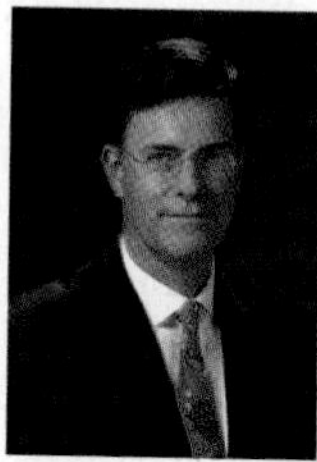

Johannes A. Romijn, MD, PhD
Professor
Endocrinology
Leiden University Medical Center
Leiden, Netherlands

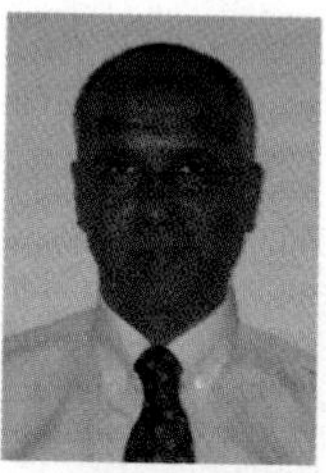

Domenico Salvatore, MD, PhD
Associate Professor of Endocrinology
Department of Molecular and
Clinical Endocrinology and
Oncology
University of Naples "Federico II"
Naples, Italy

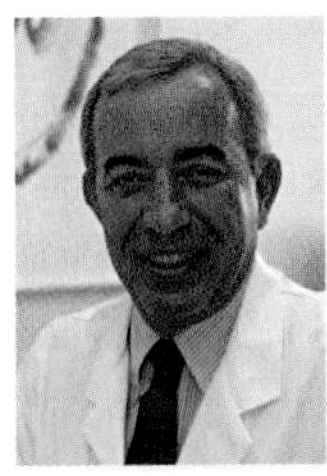

Martin-Jean Schlumberger, MD
Professor of Oncology
Université Paris Sud.
Chair
Nuclear Medicine and Endocrine Oncology
Institut Gustave Roussy
Villejuif, France

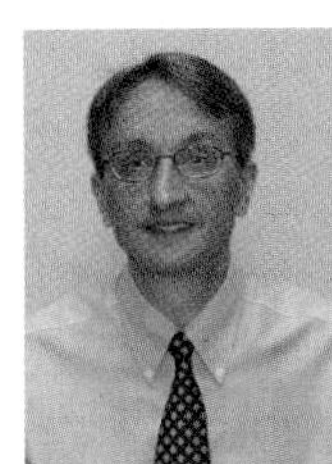

Clay F. Semenkovich, MD
Herbert S. Gasser Professor
Endocrinology, Metabolism, and Lipid Research
Washington University
St. Louis, Missouri, USA

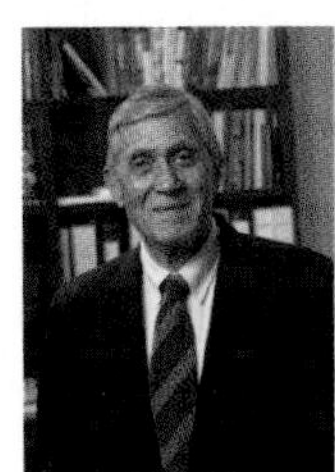

Allen M. Spiegel, MD
The Marilyn and Stanley M. Katz Dean
Albert Einstein College of Medicine
Bronx, New York, USA

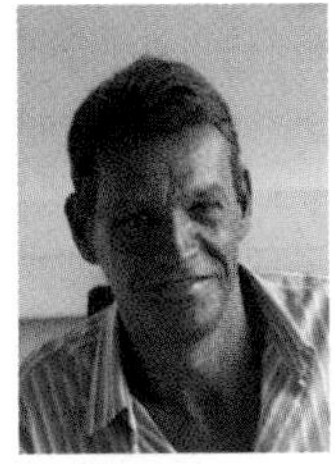

Paul M. Stewart, MD FRCP, FMedSci
Dean of Medicine
University of Birmingham
Consultant Endocrinologist
Queen Elizabeth Hospital
Birmingham, United Kingdom

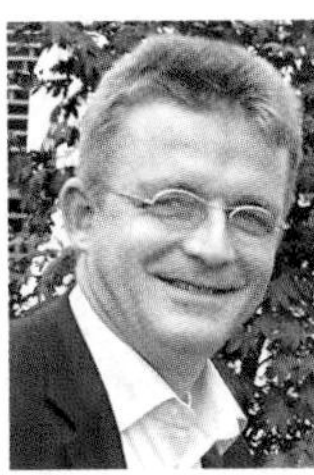

Christian J. Strasburger, MD
Professor of Medicine
Chief
Division of Clinical Endocrinology
Department of Medicine, CCM
Charité Universitätsmedizin
Berlin, Germany

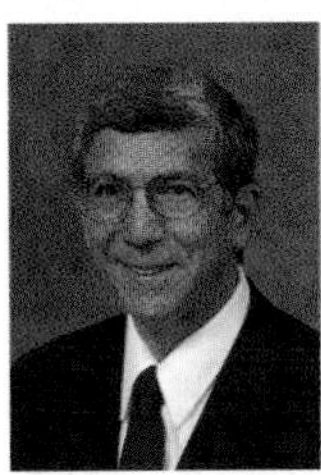

Dennis M. Styne, MD
Professor and Rimsey Chair of Pediatric Endocrinology
University of California Davis
Sacramento, California, USA

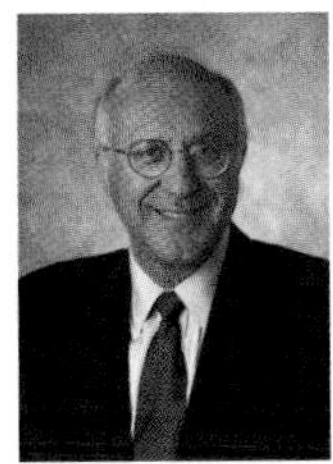

Simeon I. Taylor, MD, PhD
Vice President
Discovery Biology Pharmaceutical Research Institute
Bristol-Myers Squibb
Hopewell, New Jersey, USA

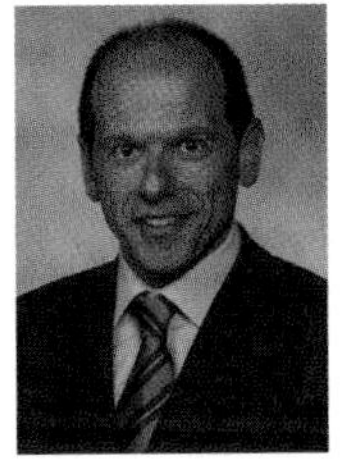

Adrian Vella, MD, FRCP (Edin.)
Professor
Division of Endocrinology & Metabolism
Mayo Clinic
Rochester, Minnesota, USA

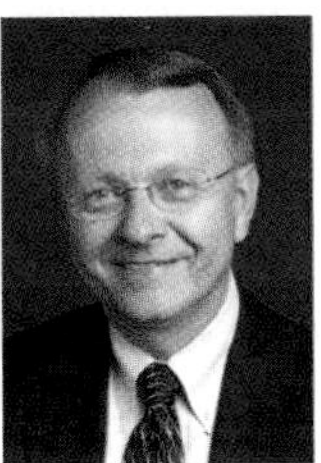

Joseph G. Verbalis, MD
Professor
Medicine and Physiology
Georgetown University
Chief, Endocrinology and Metabolism
Georgetown University Hospital
Washington, DC, USA

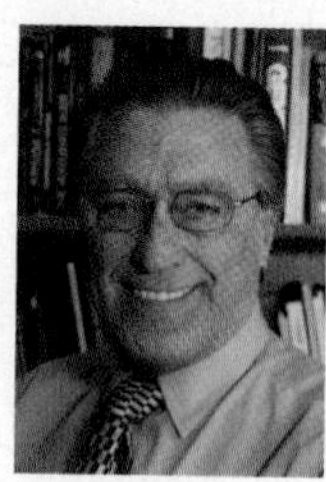

Aaron I. Vinik, MD, PdD
FCP, MACP
Professor of Medicine, Pathology,
Neurobiology
Director of Research and
Neuroendocrine Unit
Eastern Virginia Medical School,
Strelitz Diabetes Center
Norfolk, Virginia, USA

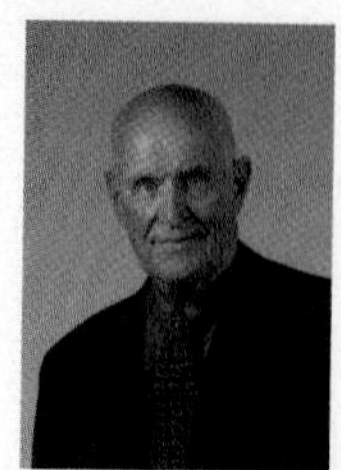

Samuel Wells, Jr., MD
Senior Investigator
Medical Qncology Branch
National Cancer Institute, NIH
Bethesda, Maryland, USA

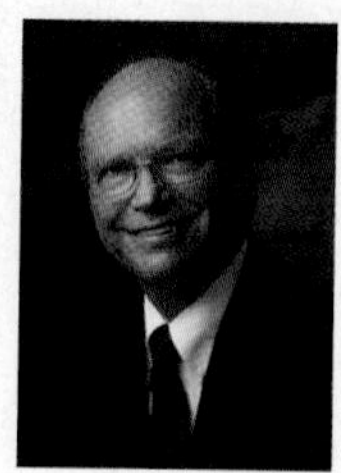

William F. Young, Jr., MD, MSc
Tyson Family Endocrinology Clinical
Professor in Honor of Vahab
Fatourechi, MD
Professor of Medicine
Division of Endocrinology, Diabetes,
Metabolism, and Nutrition
Mayo Clinic
Rochester, Minnesota, USA

PREFACE

Welcome to the twelfth edition of *Williams Textbook of Endocrinology*.

Robert Williams inaugurated this enduring textbook more than 50 years ago, and the goals have remained essentially unchanged (i.e., to publish "a condensed and authoritative discussion of the management of clinical endocrinopathies based upon the application of fundamental information obtained from chemical and physiological investigation"). Of course, today we would add results of cellular and genomic investigation, as well as the wealth of clinical trial data, as aids in clinical management. The immense and often overwhelming body of new information from multiple disciplines, in fact, makes this synthetic endeavor more relevant than ever to help guide endocrinologists in the care of their patients. To encourage the goal of both highest quality scientific rigor and knowledge synthesis, we continue to ask the most distinguished authors to synthesize entire areas of clinical endocrine science. The mandate for concise yet authoritative and comprehensive presentations acknowledges both the time pressures on today's physicians and the desire to make the text affordable and easily navigated.

This edition has involved extensive revisions of the previous text, and 22 new authors have joined our expert faculty. A uniform style facilitates identification and ready use of clinical algorithms.

We express our deep gratitude to the co-workers in our offices: Anita Nichols, Lynn Moulton, Grace Labrado, Louise Ishibashi, and Sherri Turner, whose energetic efforts have made this work possible. We also thank our colleagues at Elsevier—Joan Ryan, Pamela Hetherington, and Dolores Meloni—who skillfully navigated the dynamic world of medical publishing while assuring achievement of our goals. Their efforts have been essential in ensuring the successful publication of this high-quality textbook, which has become the classic text for all professionals engaged in caring for patients with endocrine disorders.

Finally, we would like to recognize and congratulate Dr. Melvin Grumbach for his outstanding contributions to *Williams Textbook of Endocrinology*, beginning with the fourth edition that was published in 1968.

Shlomo Melmed

Kenneth S. Polonsky

P. Reed Larsen

Henry M. Kronenberg

CONTENTS

WILLIAMS Textbook of

Endocrinology

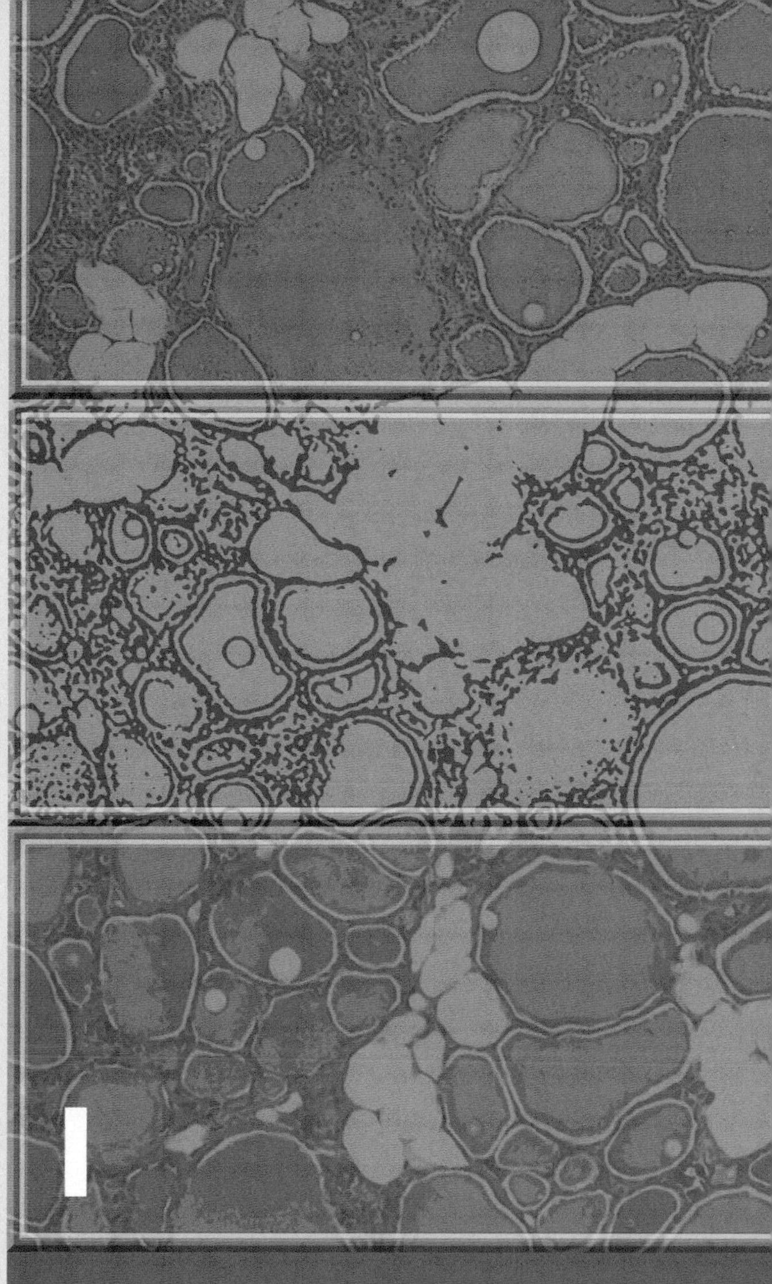

SECTION I

Hormones and Hormone Action

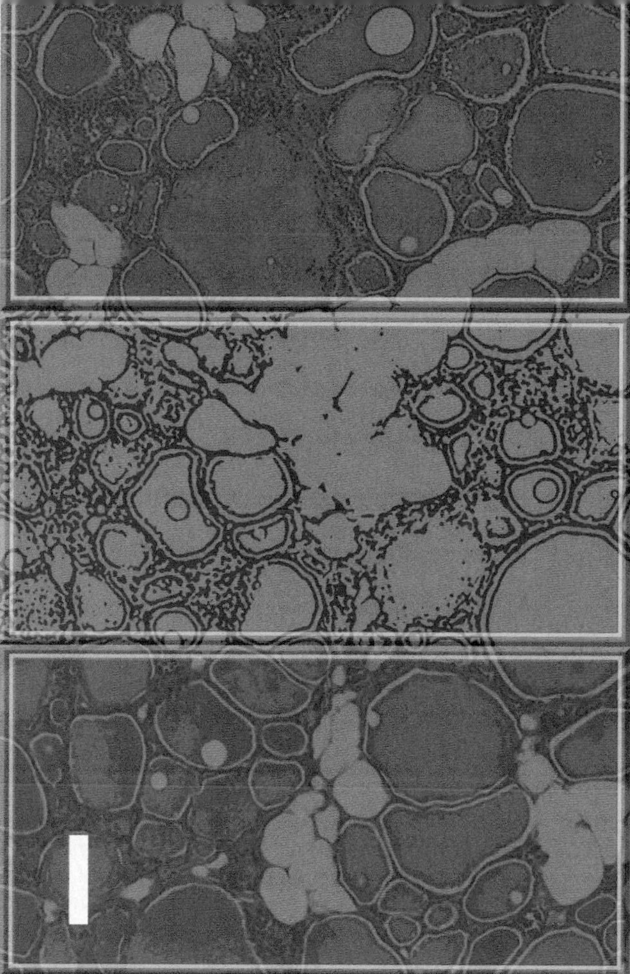

CHAPTER 1

Principles of Endocrinology

HENRY M. KRONENBERG • SHLOMO MELMED • P. REED LARSEN • KENNETH S. POLONSKY

Roughly 100 years ago, Starling coined the term *hormone* to describe secretin, a substance secreted by the small intestine into the bloodstream to stimulate pancreatic secretion. In his Croonian Lectures, Starling considered the endocrine and nervous systems as two distinct mechanisms for coordination and control of organ function. Thus, endocrinology found its first home in the discipline of mammalian physiology.

Work over the next several decades by biochemists, physiologists, and clinical investigators led to the characterization of many hormones secreted into the bloodstream from discrete glands or other organs. Investigations showed that diseases such as hypothyroidism and diabetes could be treated successfully, for the first time, by replacing specific hormones. These initial triumphs formed the foundation of the clinical specialty of endocrinology.

Advances in cell biology, molecular biology, and genetics over the ensuing years began to explain the mechanisms of endocrine diseases and of hormone secretion and action. Even though these advances have embedded endocrinology in the framework of molecular cell biology, they have not changed the essential subject of endocrinology—the signaling mechanisms that coordinate and control the functions of multiple organs and processes. Herein we survey the general themes and principles that underpin the diverse approaches used by clinicians, physiologists, biochemists, cell biologists, and geneticists to understand the endocrine system.

THE EVOLUTIONARY PERSPECTIVE

Hormones can be defined as chemical signals secreted into the bloodstream that act on distant tissues, usually in a regulatory fashion. Hormonal signaling represents a special case of the more general process of signaling between cells. Even unicellular organisms, such as baker's yeast, *Saccharomyces cerevisiae,* secrete short peptide mating factors that act on receptors of other yeast cells to trigger mating between the two cells. These receptors resemble the ubiquitous family of mammalian seven-transmembrane spanning receptors that respond to ligands as diverse as photons and glycoprotein hormones. Because these yeast receptors trigger activation of heterotrimeric G proteins just as mammalian receptors do, this conserved signaling pathway must have been present in the common ancestor of yeast and humans.

Signals from one cell to adjacent cells—so-called paracrine signals—often trigger cellular responses that use the same molecular pathways used by hormonal signals. For example, the sevenless receptor controls the differentiation of retinal cells in the *Drosophila* eye by responding to a membrane-anchored signal from an adjacent cell. Sevenless is a membrane-spanning receptor with an intracellular tyrosine kinase domain that signals in a way that closely resembles the signaling by hormone receptors such as the insulin receptor tyrosine kinase.

Because paracrine factors and hormones can share signaling machinery, it is not surprising that hormones can, in some settings, act as paracrine factors. Testosterone, for example, is secreted into the bloodstream but also acts locally in the testes to control spermatogenesis. Insulin-like growth factor 1 (IGF1) is a polypeptide hormone that is secreted into the bloodstream from the liver and other tissues, but it is also a paracrine factor made locally in most tissues to control cell proliferation.

Furthermore, one receptor can mediate actions of a hormone and a paracrine factor, such as parathyroid hormone (PTH) and parathyroid hormone–related protein. In some cases, the paracrine actions of "hormones" have functions quite unrelated to hormonal functions. For example, macrophages synthesize the active form of vitamin D, 1,25-dihydroxyvitamin D_3 or calcitriol, which can then bind to vitamin D receptors in the same cells and stimulate production of antimicrobial peptides.[1] The vitamin D 1α-hydroxylase responsible for activating 25-hydroxyvitamin D (calcidiol) is synthesized in multiple tissues in which it has functions not apparently related to the calcium homeostatic actions of calcitriol. One can speculate that the hormonal actions of vitamin D might have evolved well after the paracrine vitamin D apparatus provided the raw materials for the hormonal system.

Target cells respond similarly to signals that reach them from the bloodstream (hormones) or from the cell next door (paracrine factors); the cellular response machinery does not distinguish the sites of origin of signals. The shared final common pathways used by hormonal and paracrine signals should not, however, obscure important differences between hormonal and paracrine signaling systems (Fig. 1-1). Paracrine signals do not travel very far; consequently, the specific site of origin of a paracrine factor determines where it will act and provides specificity to that action. When the paracrine factor bone morphogenic protein 4 (BMP4) is secreted by cells in the developing kidney, BMP4 regulates the differentiation of renal cells; when the same factor is secreted by cells in bone, it regulates bone formation. Thus, the site of origin of BMP4 determines its physiologic role. In contrast, because hormones are secreted into the bloodstream, their sites of origin are often divorced from their functions. There is nothing about thyroid hormone function, for example, that requires that the thyroid gland be in the neck.

Because the specificity of paracrine factor action is so dependent on its precise site of origin, elaborate mechanisms have evolved to regulate and constrain the diffusion of paracrine factors. Paracrine factors of the hedgehog family, for example, are covalently bound to cholesterol to constrain the diffusion of these molecules in the

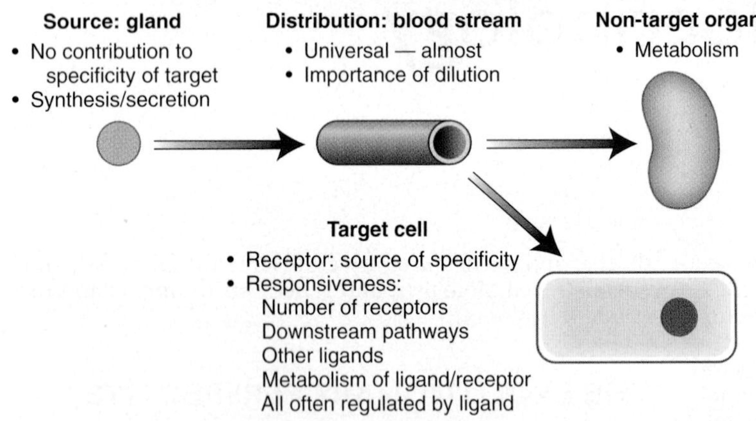

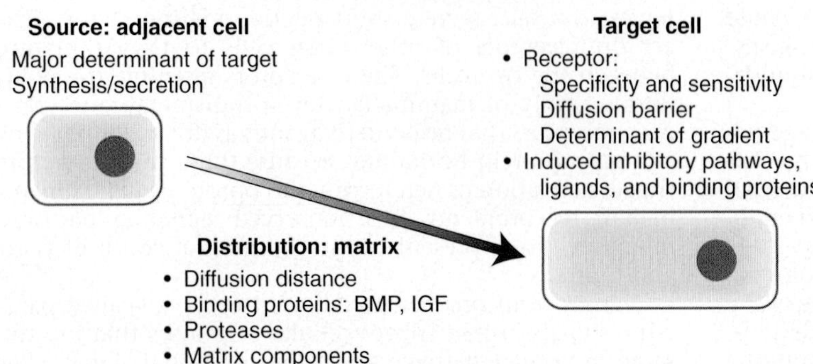

Figure 1-1 Comparison of determinants of endocrine and paracrine signaling.

extracellular milieu. Most paracrine factors interact with binding proteins that block their action and control their diffusion. For example, chordin, noggin, and many other distinct proteins bind to various members of the BMP family to regulate their action. Proteases such as tolloid then destroy the binding proteins at specific sites to liberate BMPs so that they can act on appropriate target cells.

Hormones have rather different constraints. Because they diffuse throughout the body, they must be synthesized in enormous amounts relative to the amounts of paracrine factors needed at specific locations. This synthesis usually occurs in specialized cells designed for that specific purpose. Hormones must then be able to travel in the bloodstream and diffuse in effective concentrations into tissues. Lipophilic hormones, for example, bind to soluble proteins that allow them to travel in the aqueous medium of blood at relatively high concentrations. The ability of hormones to diffuse through the extracellular space means that the local concentration of a hormone at target sites will rapidly decrease when glandular secretion of the hormone stops. Because hormones diffuse throughout extracellular fluid quickly, hormonal metabolism can occur in specialized organs (e.g., liver, kidney) in a manner that determines the effective hormone concentration in other tissues.

In summary, paracrine factors and hormones use several distinct strategies to control their biosynthesis, sites of action, transport, and metabolism. These differing strategies probably explain partly why a hormone such as IGF1, unlike its close relative, insulin, has multiple binding proteins that control its action in tissues. IGF1 exhibits a double life—it is both a hormone and a paracrine factor. Presumably, the local actions of IGF1 mandate an elaborate binding protein apparatus to enable appropriate hormone signaling.

All of the major hormonal signaling programs—G protein–coupled receptors, tyrosine kinase receptors, serine/threonine kinase receptors, ion channels, cytokine receptors, and nuclear receptors—are also used by paracrine factors. In contrast, several paracrine signaling programs appear to be used only by paracrine factors and not by hormones. For example, Notch receptors respond to membrane-based ligands to control cell fate, but no bloodborne ligands are known to use Notch-type signaling. Perhaps the intracellular strategy used by Notch, which involves cleavage of the receptor and subsequent nuclear actions of the receptor's cytoplasmic portion, is too inflexible to serve the purposes of hormones.

The analyses of the complete genomes of multiple bacterial species, the yeast *S. cerevisiae,* the fruit fly *Drosophila melanogaster,* the worm *Caenorhabditis elegans,* the plant *Arabidopsis thaliana,* humans, and many other species have allowed a comprehensive view of the signaling machinery used by various forms of life. As noted earlier, *S. cerevisiae* uses G protein–linked receptors; this organism, however, lacks tyrosine kinase receptors and nuclear receptors that resemble the estrogen/thyroid receptor family. In contrast, the worm and fly share with humans the use of each of these signaling pathways, although with substantial variation in the number of genes committed to each pathway. For example, the *Drosophila* genome encodes 20 nuclear receptors, the *C. elegans* genome 270, and the human genome (tentatively) more than 50. These patterns suggest that ancient multicellular animals must have already established the signaling systems that are the foundation of the endocrine system as we know it in mammals.

Even before the sequencing of the human genome was accomplished, sequence analyses had made clear that many receptor genes are found in mammalian genomes for which no clear ligand or function is known. The analyses of these "orphan" receptors have succeeded in broadening the current understanding of hormonal signaling. For example, the orphan liver X receptor, LXR, was found during searches for unknown nuclear receptors. Subsequent experiments showed that oxygenated derivatives of cholesterol are the ligands for LXR, which regulates genes involved in cholesterol and fatty acid metabolism.[2] LXR and many other examples raise the question of what constitutes a hormone.

The classic view of hormones is that they are synthesized in discrete glands and have no function other than activating receptors on cell membranes or in the nucleus. In contrast, cholesterol, which is converted in cells to oxygenated derivatives that activate the LXR receptor, uses a hormonal strategy to regulate its own metabolism. Other orphan nuclear receptors similarly respond to ligands such as bile acids and fatty acids. These "hormones" have important metabolic roles quite separate from their signaling properties, although the hormone-like signaling serves to allow regulation of the metabolic function. The calcium-sensing receptor is an example from the G protein–linked receptor family that responds to a nonclassic ligand, ionic calcium. Calcium is released into the bloodstream from bone, kidney, and intestine and acts on the calcium-sensing receptors on parathyroid cells, renal tubular cells, and other cells to coordinate cellular responses to calcium. Therefore, many important metabolic factors have taken on hormonal properties as part of a regulatory strategy.

ENDOCRINE GLANDS

Hormone formation may occur either in localized collections of specific cells, the endocrine glands, or in cells that have additional roles. Many protein hormones, such as growth hormone (GH), PTH, prolactin, insulin, and glucagon, are produced in dedicated cells by standard protein synthetic mechanisms common to all cells. These secretory cells usually contain specialized secretory granules designed to store large amounts of hormone and to release the hormone in response to specific signals. Formation of small hormone molecules begins with commonly found precursors, usually located in specific glands such as the adrenals, gonads, or thyroid. In the case of the steroid hormones, the precursor is cholesterol, which is modified by various hydroxylations, methylations, and demethylations to form glucocorticoids, androgens, estrogens, and their biologically active derivatives.

However, not all hormones are formed in dedicated and specialized endocrine glands. For example, the protein hormone, leptin, which regulates appetite and energy expenditure, is formed in adipocytes, providing a specific signal that reflects the nutritional state to the central nervous system. The cholesterol derivative, 7-dehydrocholesterol, the precursor of vitamin D, is produced in skin keratinocytes by a photochemical reaction. In the unique enteroendocrine hormonal system, peptide hormones that regulate metabolic and other responses to oral nutrients are produced and secreted by specialized endocrine cells scattered throughout the intestinal epithelium.

Thyroid hormone synthesis occurs by means of a unique pathway. The thyroid cell synthesizes a 660,000-kd homodimer, thyroglobulin, which is then iodinated at specific iodotyrosines. Certain of these "couple" to form the iodothyronine molecule within thyroglobulin, which is then stored in the lumen of the thyroid follicle. For this to occur, the thyroid cell must concentrate the trace quantities of iodide from the blood and oxidize it via a specific peroxidase. Release of thyroxine (T_4) from the thyroglobulin requires its phagocytosis and cathepsin-catalyzed digestion by the same cells.

Hormones are synthesized in response to biochemical signals generated by various modulating systems. Many of these systems are specific to the effects of the hormone product. For example, PTH synthesis is regulated by the concentration of ionized calcium, and insulin synthesis is regulated by the concentration of glucose. For others, such as gonadal, adrenal, and thyroid hormones, control of hormone synthesis is achieved by the hormonostatic function of the hypothalamic-pituitary axis. Cells in the hypothalamus and pituitary monitor the circulating hormone concentration and secrete tropic hormones, which activate specific pathways for hormone synthesis and release. Typical examples are luteinizing hormone (LH), follicle-stimulating hormone (FSH), thyroid-stimulating hormone (TSH), and adrenocorticotropic hormone (ACTH).

These trophic hormones increase rates of hormone synthesis and secretion, and they may induce target cell division, resulting in enlargement of the various target glands. For example, in hypothyroid individuals living in iodine-deficient areas of the world, TSH secretion causes a marked hyperplasia of thyroid cells. In such regions, the thyroid gland may be 20 to 50 times its normal size. Adrenal hyperplasia occurs in patients with genetic deficiencies in cortisol formation. Hypertrophy and hyperplasia of parathyroid cells, in this case initiated by an intrinsic response to the stress of hypocalcemia, occurs in patients with renal insufficiency or calcium malabsorption.

Hormones may be fully active when they are released into the bloodstream (e.g., GH, insulin), or they may require activation in specific cells to produce their biologic effects. These activation steps are often highly regulated. For example, the T_4 released from the thyroid cell is a prohormone that must undergo a specific deiodination to form the active 3,5,3′-triiodothyronine (T_3). This deiodination reaction can occur in target tissues (e.g., in the central nervous system); in the thyrotrophs, where T_3 provides feedback regulation of TSH production; or in hepatic and renal cells, from which it is released into the circulation for uptake by all tissues. A similar postsecretory activation step, catalyzed by a 5αα-reductase, causes tissue-specific activation of testosterone to dihydrotestosterone in target tissues including the male urogenital tract and genital skin, as well as in liver. Vitamin D undergoes hydroxylation at the 25 position in the liver and at the 1 position in the kidney. Both hydroxylations must occur to produce the active hormone, calcitriol. The activity of 1α-hydroxylase, but not that of 25-hydroxylase, is stimulated by PTH and reduced plasma phosphate but inhibited by calcium, calcitriol, and fibroblast growth factor 23 (FGF23).

Hormones are synthesized as required on a daily, hourly, or minute-to-minute basis with minimal storage, but there are significant exceptions. One is the thyroid gland, which contains enough stored hormone to last for about 2 months. This permits a constant supply despite significant variations in the availability of iodine. However, if iodine deficiency is prolonged, the normal reservoirs of T_4 can be depleted.

The various feedback signaling systems already described enable the hormonal *homeostasis* that is characteristic of virtually all endocrine systems. Regulation may include the central nervous system or local signal recognition mechanisms in the glandular cells, such as the calcium-sensing receptor of the parathyroid cell. Superimposed, centrally programmed increases and decreases in hormone secretion or activation also occur through neuroendocrine pathways. Examples include the circadian variation in secretion of ACTH that directs the synthesis and release of cortisol. The monthly menstrual cycle exemplifies a system with much longer periodicity that requires a complex synergism between central and peripheral axes of the endocrine glands. Disruption of hormonal homeostasis due to glandular or central regulatory system dysfunction has both clinical and laboratory consequences. Recognition and correction of these effects are the essence of clinical endocrinology.

TRANSPORT OF HORMONES IN BLOOD

Protein hormones and some small molecules, such as the catecholamines, are water soluble and readily transported via the circulatory system. Others, such as the steroid and thyroid hormones, are almost insoluble in water, and their distribution presents special problems. Such molecules are bound to 50- to 60-kd carrier plasma glycoproteins such as thyroxine-binding globulin (TBG), sex hormone–binding globulin (SHBG), and corticosteroid-binding globulin, as well as to albumin. The ligand-protein complexes serve as reservoirs of these hormones, ensure ubiquitous distribution of their water-insoluble ligands, and protect the small molecules from rapid inactivation or excretion in the urine or bile. Without these proteins, it is unlikely that hydrophobic molecules would be transported much beyond the veins draining the glands in which they are formed.

The protein-bound hormones exist in rapid equilibrium with the often minute quantities of hormone in the aqueous plasma. It is this "free" fraction of the circulating hormone that is taken up by the cell. For example, if tracer thyroid hormone is injected into the portal vein in a protein-free solution, it becomes bound to hepatocytes at the periphery of the hepatic sinusoid. When the same experiment is repeated with a protein-containing solution, there is a uniform distribution of tracer hormone throughout the hepatic lobule.[3]

Despite the very high affinity of some of the binding proteins for their ligands, a specific protein may not be essential for hormone distribution. For example, in humans with a congenital deficiency of TBG, other proteins, namely transthyretin (TTR) and albumin, subsume its role. Because the affinity of these secondary thyroid hormone transport proteins is several orders of magnitude lower than that of TBG, it is possible for the hypothalamic-pituitary feedback system to maintain free thyroid hormone in the normal range at a much lower total hormone concentration. The fact that the level of "free" hormone concentration is normal in subjects with TBG deficiency indicates that it is this free moiety that is defended by the hypothalamic-pituitary axis and is the active hormone.[4]

The availability of gene targeting techniques has allowed specific tests of the physiologic roles of several hormone-binding proteins. For example, mice with targeted inactivation of the vitamin D–binding protein (DBP) have been generated.[5] Although the absence of DBP markedly reduces the circulating concentration of vitamin D, the mice are otherwise normal. However, they do show enhanced susceptibility to a vitamin D–deficient diet because of the reduced reservoir of this sterol. In addition, the absence of DBP markedly reduces the half-life of calcidiol by accelerating its hepatic uptake, making the mice less susceptible to vitamin D intoxication.

In rodents, TTR carries retinol-binding protein and is also the principal thyroid hormone–binding protein. This protein is synthesized in the liver and in choroid plexus. It is the major thyroid hormone–binding protein in the cerebrospinal fluid of both rodents and humans and was previously thought to possibly serve an important role in thyroid hormone transport into the central nervous system. This hypothesis was later disproved by the fact that mice without TTR have normal concentrations of T_4 in the brain in addition to free T_4 in the plasma.[6,7] To be sure, the serum concentrations of vitamin A and total T_4 are decreased, but the knockout mice have no signs of vitamin A deficiency or hypothyroidism. Such studies suggest that these proteins primarily serve distributive and reservoir functions.

Protein hormones and some small ligands (e.g., catecholamines) produce their effects by interacting with cell surface receptors. Others, such as the steroid and thyroid hormones, must enter the cell to bind to cytosolic or nuclear receptors. In the past, it was thought that much of the transmembrane transport of hormones was passive. Evidence has now demonstrated that specific transporters are involved in cellular uptake of thyroid hormone.[8] This may be found to be the case for other small ligands as well, revealing yet another mechanism for ensuring the distribution of a hormone to its site of action. Studies in mice missing megalin, a large cell surface protein in the low-density lipoprotein (LDL) receptor family, have suggested that estrogen and testosterone uses megalin to enter certain tissues while still bound to SHBG.[9] In this case, therefore, it is the hormone bound to SHBG, rather than the "free" hormone, that is the active moiety that enters cells. It is unclear how generally this apparent exception to the "free hormone" hypothesis occurs.

TARGET CELLS AS ACTIVE PARTICIPANTS

Hormones determine cellular target actions by binding with high specificity to receptor proteins. Whether a peripheral cell is hormonally responsive depends to a large extent on the presence and function of specific and selective hormone receptors. Receptor expression determines which cells will respond as well as the nature of the intracellular effector pathways activated by the hormone signal. Receptor proteins may be localized to the cell membrane, cytoplasm, or nucleus. Broadly, polypeptide hormone receptors are associated with cell membranes, whereas steroid hormones selectively bind soluble intracellular proteins (Fig. 1-2). However, exceptions do occur. For example, epidermal growth factor (EGF) may signal directly to receptors located within the nucleus.

Membrane-associated receptor proteins usually consist of extracellular sequences that recognize and bind ligand, transmembrane anchoring hydrophobic sequences, and intracellular sequences that initiate intracellular signaling. Intracellular signaling is mediated by covalent modification and activation of intracellular signaling molecules

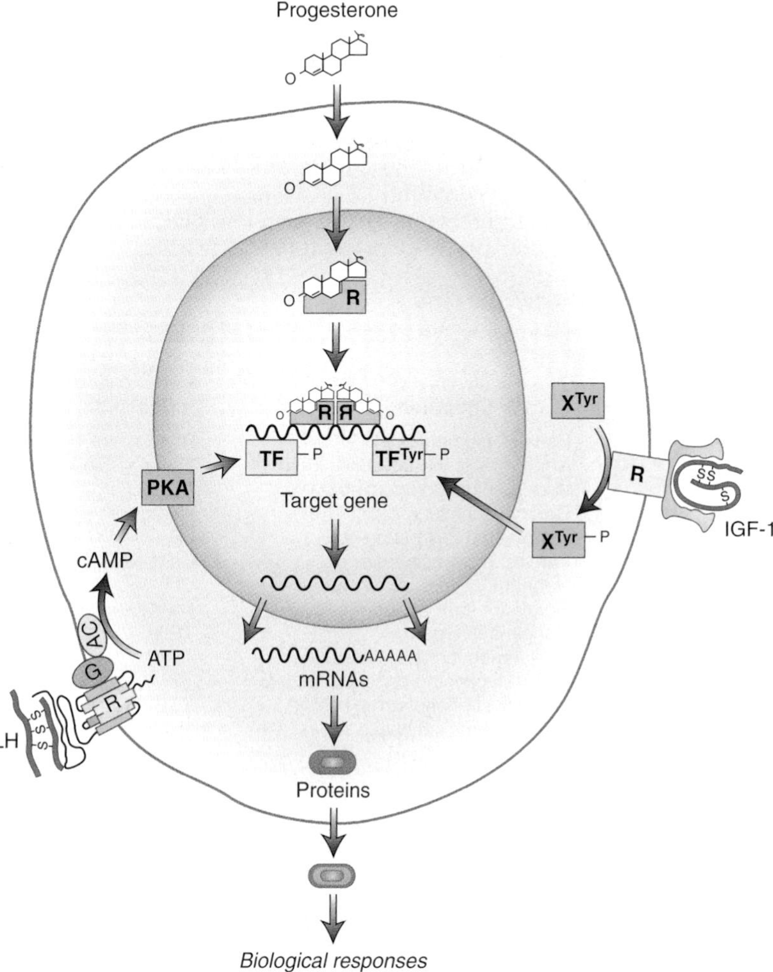

Figure 1-2 Hormonal signaling by cell surface and intracellular receptors. The receptors for the water-soluble polypeptide hormones, luteinizing hormone (LH), and insulin-like growth factor I (IGF-I), are integral membrane proteins located at the cell surface. They bind the hormone-utilizing extracellular sequences and transduce a signal through the generation of second messengers: cyclic adenosine monophosphate (cAMP) for the LH receptor and tyrosine-phosphorylated substrates for the IGF-I receptor. Although effects on gene expression are indicated, direct effects on cellular proteins (e.g., ion channels) are also observed. In contrast, the receptor for the lipophilic steroid hormone, progesterone, resides in the cell nucleus. It binds the hormone and becomes activated and capable of directly modulating target gene transcription.) AC, Adenylate cyclase; G, heterotrimeric G protein; mRNAs, messenger RNAs; PKA, protein kinase A; R, receptor molecule; TF, transcription factor; Tyr, tyrosine found in protein X; X, unknown protein substrate. (Reproduced from Mayo K. Receptors: molecular mediators of hormone action. In: Conn PM, Melmed S, eds. *Endocrinology: Basic and Clinical Principles*. Totowa, NJ: Humana Press, 1997:11.)

(e.g., STAT proteins) or by generation of small molecule second messengers (e.g., cyclic adenosine monophosphate) through activation of heterotrimeric G proteins. The α-, β-, and γ-subunits of these G proteins activate or suppress effector enzymes and ion channels that generate the second messengers. Some of these receptors may in fact exhibit constitutive activity and have been shown to signal in the absence of added ligand.

Several growth factors and hormone receptors (e.g., for insulin) behave as intrinsic tyrosine kinases or activate intracellular protein tyrosine kinases. Ligand activation may cause receptor dimerization (e.g., GH) or heterodimerization (e.g., interleukin-6), followed by activation of intracellular phosphorylation cascades. These activated proteins ultimately determine specific nuclear gene expression.

Both the number of receptors expressed per cell and their responses are regulated, providing a further level of control for hormone action. Several mechanisms account for altered receptor function. Receptor endocytosis causes internalization of cell surface receptors; the hormone-receptor complex is subsequently dissociated, resulting in abrogation of the hormone signal. Receptor trafficking may then result in recycling back to the cell surface (e.g., as for insulin), or the internalized receptor may undergo lysosomal degradation. Both of these mechanisms, triggered by activation of receptors, effectively lead to impaired hormone signaling by downregulation of these receptors. The hormone signaling pathway may also be downregulated by receptor desensitization (e.g., as for epinephrine); ligand-mediated receptor phosphorylation leads to a reversible deactivation of the receptor. Desensitization mechanisms can be activated by a receptor's ligand (homologous desensitization) or by another signal (heterologous desensitization), which attenuates receptor signaling in the continued presence of ligand. Receptor function may also be limited by the action of specific phosphatases (e.g., SHP) or by intracellular negative regulation of the signaling cascade (e.g., suppressor of cytokine signaling [SOCS] proteins inhibiting JAK-STAT signaling).

Mutational changes in receptor structure can also determine hormone action. Constitutive receptor activation may be induced by activating mutations (e.g., TSH receptor) leading to endocrine organ hyperfunction, even in the absence of hormone. Conversely, inactivating receptor mutations may lead to endocrine hypofunction (e.g., testosterone receptor, vasopressin receptor). These syndromes are well characterized and are well described in other chapters of this text (Fig. 1-3).

The functional diversity of receptor signaling also results in overlapping or redundant intracellular pathways. For example, both GH and cytokines activate JAK-STAT signaling, whereas the distal effects of these stimuli clearly differ. Therefore, despite common signaling pathways, hormones elicit highly specific cellular effects. Tissue or cell-type genetic programs or receptor-receptor interactions at the cell surface (e.g., dopamine D_2 hetero-oligomerization with somatotropin release–inhibiting factor [SRIF]) may also confer specific cellular response to a hormone and provide an additive cellular effect.[10]

CONTROL OF HORMONE SECRETION

Anatomically distinct endocrine glands are composed of highly differentiated cells that synthesize, store, and secrete hormones. Circulating hormone concentrations are a function of glandular secretory patterns and hormone clearance rates. Hormone secretion is tightly regulated to attain circulating levels that are most conducive to eliciting the appropriate target tissue response. For example, longitudinal bone growth is initiated and maintained by exquisitely regulated levels of circulating GH: mild GH hypersecretion results in gigantism, and GH deficiency causes growth retardation. Ambient circulating hormone concentrations are not uniform, and the secretion patterns determine appropriate physiologic function. For example, insulin secretion occurs in short pulses elicited by nutrient intake and other signals; gonadotropin secretion is episodic, determined by a hypothalamic pulse generator; and prolactin secretion appears to be relatively continuous with secretory peaks elicited during suckling.

Diseases caused by mutations in G-protein-coupled receptors

Condition	Receptor	Inheritance	Δ Function
Retinitis pigmentosa	Rhodopsin	AD/AR	Loss
Nephrogenic diabetes insipidus	Vasopressin V2	X-linked	Loss
Isolated glucocorticoid deficiency	ACTH	AR	Loss
Color blindness	Red/green opsins	X-linked	Loss
Familial precocious puberty	LH	AD (male)	Gain
Familial hypercalcemia	Ca^{2+} sensing	AD	Loss
Neonatal severe parathyroidism	Ca^{2+} sensing	AR	Loss
Dominant form hypocalcemia	Ca^{2+} sensing	AD	Gain
Congenital hyperthyroidism	TSH	AD	Gain
Resistance to thyroid hormone	TSH	AR (comp het)	Loss
Hyperfunctioning thyroid adenoma	TSH	Somatic	Gain
Metaphyseal chondrodysplasia	PTH-PTHrP	Somatic	Gain
Hirschsprung's disease	Endothelin-B	Multigenic	Loss
Coat color alteration (*E* locus, mice)	MSH	AD/AR	Loss and gain
Dwarfism (*little* locus, mice)	GHRH	AR	Loss

Figure 1-3 Diseases caused by mutations in G-protein–coupled receptors. All are human conditions with the exception of the final two entries, which refer to the mouse. Loss of function refers to inactivating mutations of the receptor, and gain of function to activating mutations. ACTH, adrenocorticotropic hormone; AD, autosomal dominant; AR, autosomal recessive; LH, luteinizing hormone; TSH, thyroid-stimulating hormone; PTH-PTHrP, parathyroid hormone and parathyroid hormone–related peptide; MSH, melanocyte-stimulating hormone; GHRH, growth hormone–releasing hormone; FSH, follicle-stimulating hormone. (Reproduced from Mayo K. Receptors: molecular mediators of hormone action. In Conn PM, Melmed S, eds. *Endocrinology: Basic and Clinical Principles.* Totowa, NJ: Humana Press, 1997:27.)

Hormone secretion also adheres to rhythmic patterns. Circadian rhythms serve as adaptive responses to environmental signals and are controlled by a circadian timing mechanism.[11] Light is the major environmental cue adjusting the endogenous clock. The retinohypothalamic tract entrains circadian pulse generators situated within hypothalamic suprachiasmatic nuclei. These signals subserve timing mechanisms for the sleep-wake cycle and determine patterns of hormone secretion and action. Disturbed circadian timing results in hormonal dysfunction and may also be reflective of entrainment or pulse generator lesions. For example, adult GH deficiency due to a damaged hypothalamus or pituitary is associated with elevations in integrated 24-hour leptin concentrations, decreased leptin pulsatility, and yet preserved circadian rhythm of leptin. GH replacement restores leptin pulsatility, followed by loss of body fat mass.[12] Sleep is also an important cue regulating hormone pulsatility. About 70% of overall GH secretion occurs during slow-wave sleep, and increasing age is associated with declining slow-wave sleep and concomitant decline in GH and elevation of cortisol secretion.[13] Most pituitary hormones are secreted in a circadian (day-night) rhythm, best exemplified by the ACTH peaks that occur before 9 a.m., whereas ovarian steroids follow a 28-day menstrual rhythm. Disrupted episodic rhythms are often a hallmark of endocrine dysfunction. For example, loss of circadian ACTH secretion with high midnight cortisol levels is a feature of Cushing's disease.

Hormone secretion is induced by multiple specific biochemical and neural signals. Integration of these stimuli results in net temporal and quantitative secretion of the hormone (Fig. 1-4). For example, signals elicited by hypothalamic hormones (growth hormone–releasing hormone [GHRH], SRIF), peripheral hormones (IGF1, sex steroids, thyroid hormone), nutrients, adrenergic pathways, stress, and other neuropeptides all converge on the somatotroph cell, resulting in the ultimate pattern and quantity of GH secretion. Networks of reciprocal interactions allow for

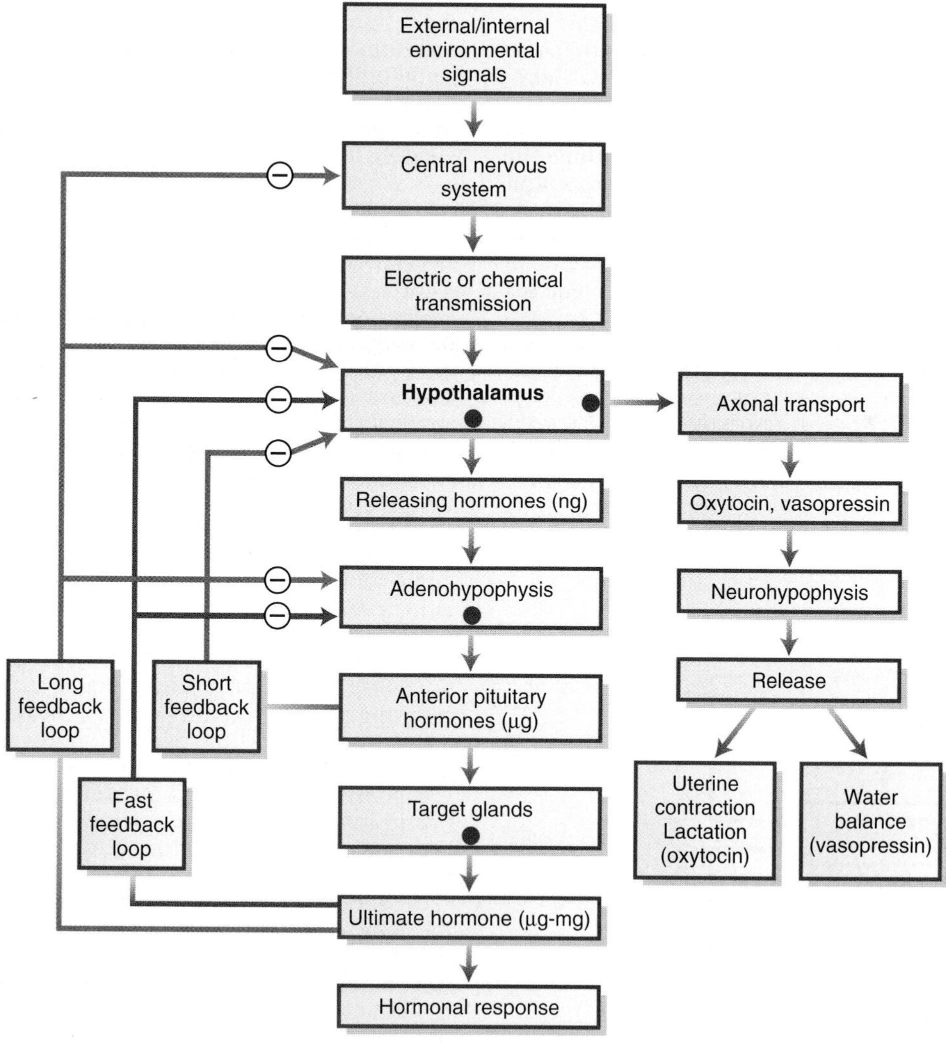

Figure 1-4 Peripheral feedback mechanism and a million-fold amplifying cascade of hormonal signals. Environmental signals are transmitted to the central nervous system, which innervates the hypothalamus, which responds by secreting nanogram amounts of a specific hormone. Releasing hormones are transported down a closed portal system, pass the blood-brain barrier at either end through fenestrations, and bind to specific anterior pituitary cell membrane receptors to elicit secretion of microgram amounts of specific anterior pituitary hormones. These enter the venous circulation through fenestrated local capillaries, bind to specific target gland receptors, trigger release of micrograms to milligrams of daily hormone amounts, and elicit responses by binding to receptors in distal target tissues. Peripheral hormone receptors enable widespread cell signaling by a single initiating environmental signal, thus facilitating intimate homeostatic association with the external environment. *Arrows* with a black dot at their origin indicate a secretory process. (Reproduced from Normal AW, Litwack G. *Hormones*, ed 2. New York, NY: Academic Press, 1997:14.)

dynamic adaptation and shifts in environmental signals. These regulatory systems embrace the hypothalamic pituitary and target endocrine glands as well as the adipocyte and lymphocyte. Peripheral inflammation and stress elicit cytokine signals that interface with the neuroendocrine system, resulting in activation of the hypothalamic-pituitary axis. The parathyroid and pancreatic secreting cells are less tightly controlled by the hypothalamus, but their functions are tightly regulated by the effects they elicit. For example, PTH secretion is induced when serum calcium levels fall, and the signal for sustained PTH secretion is abrogated by rising calcium levels.

Several tiers of control play a part in the ultimate net glandular secretion. First, central nervous system signals, including stress, afferent stimuli, and neuropeptides, signal the synthesis and secretion of hypothalamic hormones and neuropeptides (Fig. 1-5). Four hypothalamic-releasing hormones—GHRH, corticotropin-releasing hormone, thyrotropin-releasing hormone, and gonadotropin-releasing hormone (GnRH)—traverse the hypothalamic portal vessels and impinge upon their respective transmembrane trophic hormone-secreting cell receptors. These distinct cells express GH, ACTH, TSH, and gonadotropins, respectively. In contrast, hypothalamic somatostatin and dopamine suppress secretion of GH, prolactin, and TSH.

Trophic hormones also maintain the structural and functional integrity of endocrine organs, including the thyroid and adrenal glands and the gonads. Target hormones, in turn, serve as powerful negative feedback regulators of their respective trophic hormones; they often also suppress secretion of hypothalamic-releasing hormones. In certain circumstances (e.g., during puberty), peripheral sex steroids may positively induce the hypothalamic-pituitary–target gland axis. LH induces ovarian estrogen secretion, which feeds back positively to induce further LH release. Pituitary hormones themselves, in a short feedback loop, may also regulate their own respective hypothalamic-controlling hormone. Hypothalamic releasing hormones are secreted in nanogram amounts and have short half-lives of a few minutes. Anterior pituitary hormones are produced in microgram amounts and have longer half-lives, whereas peripheral hormones can be produced in up to milligram amounts daily, with much longer half-lives.

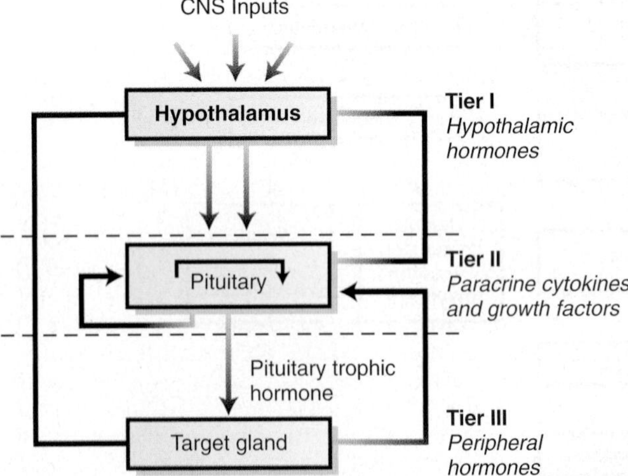

Figure 1-5 Model for regulation of anterior pituitary hormone secretion by three tiers of control. Hypothalamic hormones impinge directly on their respective target cells. Intrapituitary cytokines and growth factors regulate tropic cell function through paracrine (and autocrine) control. Peripheral hormones exert negative feedback inhibition on the synthesis and secretion of their respective pituitary trophic hormones. (Reproduced from Ray D, Melmed S. Pituitary cytokine and growth factor expression and action. *Endocrine Rev.* 1997;18:206-228.)

A further level of secretion control occurs within the gland itself. Intraglandular paracrine or autocrine growth peptides serve to autoregulate pituitary hormone secretion, as exemplified by EGF control of prolactin or IGF1 control of GH secretion. Molecules within the endocrine cell may also subserve an intracellular feedback loop. For example, corticotrope SOCS3 induction by gp130-linked cytokines serves to abrogate the ligand-induced JAK-STAT cascade, blocking transcription of pro-opiomelanocortin and subsequent secretion of ACTH. This rapid on-off regulation of ACTH secretion provides a plastic endocrine response to changes in environmental signaling and serves to maintain homeostatic integrity.[14]

In addition to the central-neuroendocrine interface mediated by hypothalamic chemical signal transduction, the central nervous system directly controls several hormonal secretory processes. Posterior pituitary hormone secretion occurs as direct efferent neural extensions. Postganglionic sympathetic nerves also regulate rapid changes in renin, insulin, and glucagon secretion, and preganglionic sympathetic nerves signal to adrenal medullary cells, eliciting adrenaline release.

HORMONE MEASUREMENT

Endocrine function can be assessed by measuring levels of basal circulating hormone, evoked or suppressed hormone, or hormone-binding proteins. Alternatively, peripheral hormone receptor function can be assessed. Meaningful strategies for timing hormonal measurements vary from system to system. In some cases, circulating hormone concentrations can be measured in randomly collected serum samples. This measurement, when standardized for fasting, environmental stress, age, and gender, is reflective of true hormone concentrations only when levels do not fluctuate appreciably. For example, thyroid hormone, prolactin, and IGF1 levels can be accurately assessed in fasting morning serum samples. If hormone secretion is clearly episodic, timed samples may be required over a defined time course to reflect hormone bioavailability. For example, early morning and late evening cortisol measurements are most appropriate. Sampling over 24 hours for GH measurements, with samples collected every 2, 10, or 20 minutes, is expensive and cumbersome, yet may yield valuable diagnostic information. Random sampling may reflect secretion peaks or nadirs, confounding adequate interpretation of results.

In general, confirmation of failed glandular function is made by attempting to evoke hormone secretion by recognized stimuli. For example, testing of pituitary hormone reserve may be accomplished by injecting appropriate hypothalamic releasing hormones. Injection of trophic hormones, including TSH and ACTH, evokes specific target gland hormone secretion. Pharmacologic stimuli (e.g., metoclopramide for induction of prolactin secretion) may also be useful to test hormone reserve. In contrast, hormone hypersecretion can be diagnosed by suppressing glandular function. For example, failure to appropriately suppress GH levels after a standardized glucose load implies inappropriate GH hypersecretion. The failure to suppress insulin secretion in response to hypoglycemia indicates inappropriate hypersecretion of insulin and should prompt a search for the cause (e.g., an insulin-secreting tumor).

Radioimmunoassays use highly specific antibodies unique to a hormone, or hormone fragment, to quantify hormone levels. Enzyme-linked immunosorbent assays (ELISAs) employ enzymes instead of radioactive hormone markers, and enzyme activity reflects hormone concentration. This sensitive technique has allowed ultrasensitive measurements of physiologic hormone concentrations. Hormone-specific receptors may be employed in place of the antibody in a radioreceptor assay.

ENDOCRINE DISEASES

Endocrine diseases fall into five broad categories: (1) hormone overproduction, (2) hormone underproduction, (3) altered tissue responses to hormones, (4) tumors of endocrine glands, and a relatively new category exemplified in the thyroid axis, (5) hormone deficiency due to its excessive rate of inactivation caused by overexpression of an endogenous enzyme in a tumor.

Hormone Overproduction

Occasionally, hormones are secreted in increased amounts because of genetic abnormalities that cause abnormal regulation of hormone synthesis or release. For example, in glucocorticoid-remediable hyperaldosteronism, an abnormal chromosomal crossover event puts the aldosterone synthetase gene under the control of the ACTH-regulated 11β-hydroxylase gene. More often, diseases of hormone overproduction are associated with an increase in the total number of hormone-producing cells. For example, the hyperthyroidism of Graves' disease, in which antibodies mimic TSH and activate the TSH receptors on thyroid cells, is associated with a dramatic increase in thyroid cell proliferation, as well as increased synthesis and release of thyroid hormone from each thyroid cell. The increase in thyroid cell number represents a polyclonal expansion of thyroid cells in which large numbers of thyroid cells proliferate in response to an abnormal stimulus. However, most endocrine tumors are not polyclonal expansions but instead represent monoclonal expansions of one mutated cell. Pituitary and parathyroid tumors, for example, are usually monoclonal expansions in which somatic mutations in multiple tumor suppressor genes and proto-oncogenes occur. These mutations lead to increased proliferation or survival (or both) of the mutant cells. Sometimes, this proliferation is associated with abnormal secretion of hormone from each tumor cell. For example, mutant G_s α-subunit proteins in somatotrophs can lead to both increased cellular proliferation and increased secretion of GH from each tumor cell.

Hormone Underproduction

Underproduction of hormone can result from a wide variety of processes, ranging from surgical removal of parathyroid glands during neck surgery, to tuberculous destruction of adrenal glands, to iron deposition in beta cells of islets in hemochromatosis. A frequent cause of destruction of hormone-producing cells is autoimmunity. Autoimmune destruction of beta cells in type 1 diabetes mellitus or of thyroid cells in Hashimoto's thyroiditis are two of the most common disorders treated by endocrinologists. More uncommonly, a host of genetic abnormalities can lead to decreased hormone production. These disorders can result from abnormal development of hormone-producing cells (e.g., hypogonadotropic hypogonadism caused by KAL gene mutations), from abnormal synthesis of hormones (e.g., deletion of the GH gene), or from abnormal regulation of hormone secretion (e.g., the hypoparathyroidism associated with activating mutations of the parathyroid cell's calcium-sensing receptor).

Altered Tissue Responses

Resistance to hormones can be caused by a variety of genetic disorders. Examples include mutations in the GH receptor in Laron dwarfism and mutations in the $G_s\alpha$ gene in the hypoparathyroidism of pseudohypoparathyroidism type 1A. The insulin resistance in muscle and liver that is central to the etiology of type 2 diabetes mellitus appears to be polygenic in origin. Type 2 diabetes is also an example of a disease in which end-organ insensitivity is worsened by signals from other organs, in this case by signals originating in fat cells. In other cases, the target organ of hormone action is more directly abnormal, as in the PTH resistance of renal failure.

Increased end-organ function can be caused by mutations in signal reception and propagation. For example, activating mutations in TSH, LH, and PTH receptors can cause increased activity of thyroid cells, Leydig cells, and osteoblasts, even in the absence of ligand. Similarly, activating mutations in the $G_s\alpha$ protein can cause precocious puberty, hyperthyroidism, and acromegaly in McCune-Albright syndrome.

Tumors of Endocrine Glands

Tumors of endocrine glands, as mentioned earlier, often result in hormone overproduction. Some tumors of endocrine glands produce little if any hormone but cause disease through local compressive symptoms or metastatic spread. Examples include so-called nonfunctioning pituitary tumors, which are usually benign but can cause a variety of symptoms due to compression on adjacent structures, and thyroid cancer, which can spread throughout the body without causing hyperthyroidism.

Excessive Hormone Inactivation or Destruction

Although most enzymes important for endocrine systems activate a prohormone or precursor protein, there are also those whose function is to inactivate the hormone in a physiologically regulated fashion. An example is iodothyronine deiodinase type 3 (D3) which inactivates T_3 and T_4 by removing an inner-ring iodine atom from the iodothyronine. The products of these reactions, 3,3′-diiodothyronine and reverse T_3, respectively, are inactive. Several years ago, an infant was identified with hypothyroidism due to a large hepatic hemangioma expressing high amounts of D3. This condition was termed *consumptive hypothyroidism* because it resulted from inactivation of thyroid hormone at a more rapid rate than it could be produced by the infant's normal thyroid gland.[15,16] The condition has now been identified in a number of infants and even in adults with D3-expressing tumors. In theory, accelerated destruction of other hormones could occur from similar processes, but there are no examples reported to date.

THERAPEUTIC STRATEGIES

In general, hormones are employed pharmacologically for their replacement or suppressive effects. Hormones may also be used for diagnostic stimulatory purposes (e.g., hypothalamic hormones) to evoke target organ responses or to diagnose endocrine hyperfunction by suppressing hormone hypersecretion (e.g., T_3). Ablation of endocrine gland function from genetic or acquired causes can be restored by hormone replacement therapy. In general, steroid and thyroid hormones are replaced orally, whereas peptide hormones (e.g., insulin, GH) require injection. Gastrointestinal absorption and first-pass kinetics determine oral hormone dosage and availability. Physiologic replacement can achieve both appropriate hormone levels (e.g., thyroid) and approximate hormone secretory patterns (e.g., GnRH delivered intermittently via a pump).

Hormones can also be used to treat diseases associated with glandular hyperfunction. Long-acting depot preparations of somatostatin analogues suppress GH hypersecretion in acromegaly or 5-hydroxyindoleacetic acid (5-HIAA) hypersecretion in carcinoid syndrome. Estrogen receptor antagonists (e.g., tamoxifen) are useful for some patients with breast cancer, and GnRH analogues may downregulate the gonadotropin axis and benefit patients with prostate cancer.

Novel formulations of receptor-specific hormone ligands are now being clinically developed for more selective therapeutic targeting; examples include estrogen agonists/antagonists and somatostatin receptor subtype ligands. Modes of hormone injection (e.g., for PTH) may also determine therapeutic specificity and efficacy. Improved hormone delivery systems, including computerized minipumps, intranasal sprays (e.g., for desmopressin [DDAVP]), pulmonary inhalations, and depot intramuscular injections, allow added patient compliance and ease of administration. Insulin delivered by inhalation has already been approved for use, and inhaled forms of GH and other hormones are under investigation. Cell-based therapies employing highly programmed pluripotent stem cells expressing a particular hormone or growth factor are also in development These approaches require novel administration systems to allow cell-derived endocrine products to reach their intended target.[17] Novel technologies potentially marked prolongation in the half-life of peptide hormones, which would require less frequent administration. For example, a once-weekly preparation of exenatide, a GLP1 analogue used in the treatment of type 2 diabetes as a twice-daily injection, is undergoing clinical trials.

Despite this tremendous progress, some therapies, such as insulin delivery to rigorously control blood sugar, still require frequent administration by injection and close monitoring by the patient. Novel treatment systems that would link frequent monitoring of glucose levels to appropriate adjustments in the insulin dose promise to substantially reduce the burden of this disease. Hormones are biologically powerful molecules that exert therapeutic benefit and effectively replace pathologic deficits. They should not be prescribed without clearcut indications and should not be administered without careful evaluation by an appropriately qualified medical practitioner.

REFERENCES

1. Liu PT, Stenger S, Li H, et al. Toll-like receptor triggering of a vitamin D-mediated human antimicrobial response. *Science*. 2006;311:1770-1773.
2. Chawla A, Repa JJ, Evans RM, et al. Nuclear receptors and lipid physiology: opening the X-files. *Science*. 2001;294:1866-1870.
3. Mendel CM, Weisiger RA, Jones AL, et al. Thyroid hormone-binding proteins in plasma facilitate uniform distribution of thyroxine within tissues: a perfused rat liver study. *Endocrinology*. 1987;120:1742-1749.
4. Mendel CM. The free hormone hypothesis: physiologically based mathematical model. *Endocr Rev*. 1989;10:232-274.
5. Safadi FF, Thornton P, Magiera H, et al. Osteopathy and resistance to vitamin D toxicity in mice null for vitamin D binding protein. *J Clin Invest*. 1999;103:239-251.
6. Palha JA, Fernandes R, de Escobar GM, et al. Transthyretin regulates thyroid hormone levels in the choroid plexus, but not in the brain parenchyma: study in a transthyretin-null mouse model. *Endocrinology*. 2000;141:3267-3272.
7. Palha JA, Episkopou V, Maeda S, et al. Thyroid hormone metabolism in a transthyretin-null mouse strain. *J Biol Chem*. 1994;269:33135-33139.
8. Visser WE, Friesema EC, Jansen J, et al. Thyroid hormone transport by monocarboxylate transporters. *Best Pract Res Clin Endocrinol Metab*. 2007;21:223-236.
9. Hammes A, Andreassen TK, Spoelgen R, et al. Role of endocytosis in cellular uptake of sex steroids. *Cell*. 2005;122:751-762.
10. Rocheville M, Lange DC, Kumar U, et al. Receptors for dopamine and somatostatin: formation of hetero-oligomers with enhanced functional activity. *Science*. 2000;288:154-157.
11. Moore RY. Circadian rhythms: basic neurobiology and clinical applications. *Ann Rev Med*. 1997;48:253-266.
12. Aftab MA, Guzder R, Wallace AM, et al. Circadian and ultradian rhythm and leptin pulsatility in adult GH deficiency: effects of GH replacement. *J Clin Endocrinol Metab*. 2001;86:3499-3506.
13. Cauter EV, Leproult R, Plat L. Age-related changes in slow wave sleep and REM sleep and relationship with growth hormone and cortisol levels in healthy men. *JAMA*. 2000;284:861-868.
14. Melmed S. The immuno-neuroendocrine interface. *J Clin Invest*. 2001;108:1563-1566.
15. Huang SA, Tu HM, Harney JW, et al. Severe hypothyroidism caused by type 3 iodothyronine deiodinase (D3) in infantile hemangiomas. *N Engl J Med*. 2000;343:185-189.
16. Bianco AC, Salvatore D, Gereben B, et al. Biochemistry, cellular and molecular biology, and physiological roles of the iodothyronine selenodeiodinases. *Endocrine Rev*. 2002;23:38-89.
17. Graf T, Enver T. Forcing cells to change lineages. *Nature*. 2009;462:587-594.

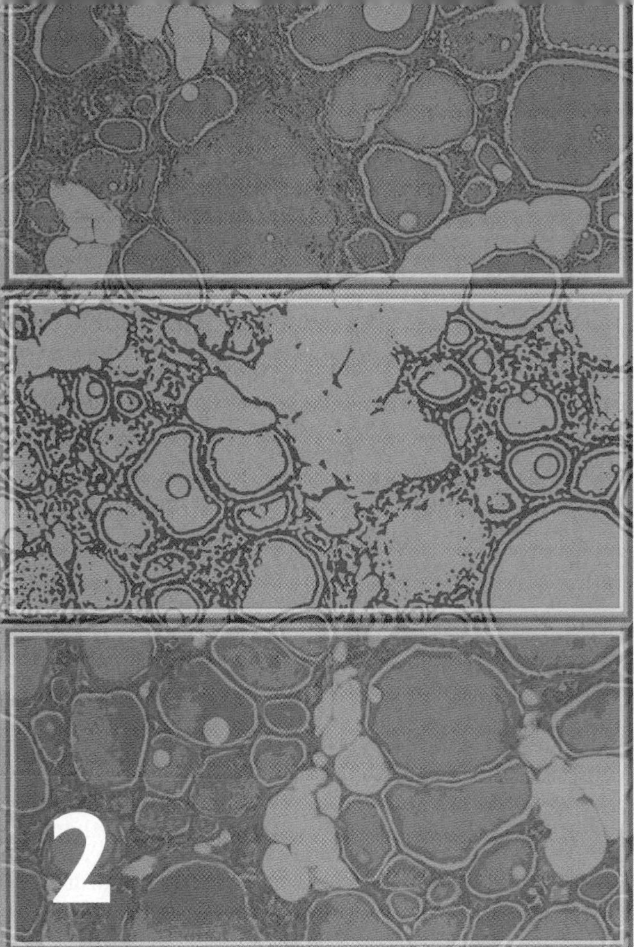

CHAPTER 2

Clinical Endocrinology: A Personal View

GILBERT H. DANIELS

CLINICAL ENDOCRINOLOGY: A RETROSPECTIVE

I love practicing and teaching clinical endocrinology.

As a young physician in the early 1970s, I was drawn to clinical endocrinology by its strong biochemical basis, elegant physiology, relative diagnostic clarity, and dramatic therapeutic efficacy. I liked the fact that clinical endocrinology made intellectual sense, demanded both clinical and laboratory expertise, and could also make patients feel better.

With respect to biochemistry, I found that knowing the steroid hormone biosynthetic pathways was essential to understanding the adrenogenital syndrome. Knowing how catecholamines were metabolized made it possible to understand the diagnostic tests for pheochromocytomas. In other words, I realized that understanding the biochemical basis of an endocrine disorder could eventually lead to its proper diagnosis and treatment.

Understanding the physiologic basis of an endocrine problem was equally critical. Dr. Fuller Albright was the first to describe hormone resistance and the ectopic production of hormones. Albright's physiologic insights also led him to develop the popular arrow drawings detailing the feedback loops between trophic hormones and end organs. Many diseases of hormone excess could be categorized using Albright's reasoning. An exception is destructive thyroiditis, in which hyperthyroidism is caused by the uncoordinated release of stored thyroid hormone. This kind of hormonal excess does not occur in other endocrine organs.

Manipulation of physiology allowed us to distinguish deficiency of growth hormone (GH) or cortisol (i.e., failure of levels to rise after insulin-induced hypoglycemia) from a nadir between pulses of these hormones. Conversely, failure to suppress cortisol after administration of the synthetic glucocorticoid dexamethasone (which does not register in the cortisol assay) was recognized to be a sign of "autonomous" cortisol production rather than a cortisol peak. Dr. Daniel Federman taught generations of endocrinologists to apply two simple rules with respect to pulsatile hormones—"If it's low, stimulate it; if it's high, suppress it"—to determine whether low or high hormone concentrations were physiologic or pathologic.

We found that fitting together all the pieces of an endocrine puzzle could lead to remarkably effective therapies. The administration of deficient hormones (GH for GH deficiency, thyroid hormone for hypothyroidism, cortisol for adrenal insufficiency, insulin for "juvenile" diabetes mellitus, pitressin tannate in oil for diabetes insipidus) was life-altering or even life-saving for patients, as well as immensely gratifying for clinicians. Eliminating excess hormone production produced equally beneficial and often dramatic results. Hyperthyroidism could be treated with medication, with targeted therapy using radioactive iodine, or, less commonly, with surgery. Surgery was required to treat the hormone excesses of Cushing's syndrome, acromegaly, hyperparathyroidism, and pheochromocytoma.

There were also significant limitations to our knowledge of clinical endocrinology in the early 1970s. Our ability to image the thyroid was restricted to radioisotope thyroid scans and the rare ultrasound study. It was almost impossible to image the pituitary or the adrenal glands, because computed tomography (CT scanning) and magnetic resonance imaging (MRI) were not yet available. Thyroid hormone excess was the only type of hormone excess that could be effectively treated nonsurgically. We had a limited knowledge of the spectrum and epidemiology of endocrine diseases (particularly mild functional disease and incidental structural disease) and their diagnostics and therapeutics. There were also endocrine diseases that had yet to be recognized or described, including endocrine disorders precipitated or caused by new therapies for nonendocrine disorders.

Modern Clinical Endocrinology

In the last 40 years, our knowledge of endocrine physiology, pathophysiology, biology, molecular biology, and genetics has dramatically expanded. This new knowledge has changed many of the ways in which we diagnose and treat endocrine disorders. For example, greater understanding of the differential diagnosis and biologic mechanisms of hormone excess has made it possible to distinguish among clinically similar disorders and to identify new disorders.

During the past 40 years, new research has helped explain previously puzzling clinical observations and also opened up entirely new areas of investigation and therapy. Some examples follow.

- The hypokalemia of licorice administration and the hypokalemia of the ectopic adrenocorticotropic hormone (ACTH) syndrome caused by small cell carcinoma of the lung were understood only after the binding of cortisol to the mineralocorticoid receptor and its inactivation by the enzyme, 11β-hydroxysteroid dehydrogenase 2 was described. Inhibition of this enzyme by the licorice component, glycyrrhizic acid, was found to prevent inactivation of cortisol at the mineralocorticoid receptor; the dramatic overproduction of cortisol in the ectopic ACTH syndrome presumably overwhelms this enzyme. Cortisol becomes a potent mineralocorticoid receptor agonist in both situations.[1]
- Molecular biology was necessary to understand glucocorticoid-remediable hyperaldosteronism, in which a genetic crossover allows the ACTH-driven 11β-hydroxylase promoter to drive aldosterone synthesis instead of cortisol synthesis—a rare example of a hormone-overproducing syndrome without an increase in the number of cells making the hormone.
- Defining the role of 5α-reductase in testosterone metabolism led to the understanding of prepubertal "testosterone resistance" in individuals deficient in this enzyme, as well as potential therapies for prostate hypertrophy and androgenic hair loss.
- Familial hypocalciuric hypercalcemia (FHH) was distinguished from primary hyperparathyroidism by means of an extremely low urine calcium excretion (and clearance). Once the calcium sensor was identified, FHH was proven to be caused by an inactivating mutation of that receptor. More recently, an astute endocrine fellow discovered that antibodies inhibiting the calcium sensor caused intermittent primary hyperparathyroidism in a patient with other autoimmune disorders.[2] Conversely, mutations and antibodies that activate the calcium sensor cause hypoparathyroidism.
- New data have emerged about vitamin D. Vitamin D deficiency was identified as a common disorder in adults. The active form of vitamin D (1,25-dihydroxyvitamin D_3, or calcitriol) was characterized as a hormone. It rapidly became an important therapy for hypoparathyroidism and for hereditary syndromes in which it is not produced. Increased production of calcitriol by active granulomas explained the hypercalcemia of sarcoidosis.
- Recognition of hypophosphatemic syndromes such as tumoral osteomalacia was made possible by elucidation of the fibroblast growth factor (FGF23) pathways.
- New therapies were developed for osteoporosis. The well-known industrial chemicals, bisphosphonates, were shown to be effective therapy; the well-described but little known anabolic bone effects of parathyroid hormone (PTH) were exploited in treating osteoporosis; and the recognition that different binders to estrogen receptors could sometimes mimic the action of estradiol and sometimes oppose it led to the use of selective estrogen receptor modulators (SERMs) for treatment of osteoporosis.
- Parathyroid hormone–related protein (PTHrP) was found to be an important cause of the humoral hypercalcemia of malignancy and also to play a major role in bone biology.
- The use of gonadotropin-releasing hormone analogues for the treatment of precocious puberty and for ovulation induction and as therapy for malignancies demonstrated the rewards of careful physiologic studies.
- The observation that more insulin is released after oral glucose than after intravenous glucose administration led to the discovery of incretins as well as the clinical application of glucagon-like peptide-1 (GLP1) agonists for the treatment of diabetes mellitus. It is possible that incretins are responsible for the hypoglycemic syndromes that occur after gastric bypass surgery.[3] Recently, labeled GLP1 agonists have been used to image insulinomas.[4]
- Blood sugar control was shown to be important to prevent the complications of diabetes mellitus.

In addition, the diverse biochemical and physiologic bases of hormone resistance were elucidated, the spectrum of hormone resistance was expanded, and some of this new knowledge led to several important therapies for syndromes of hormone resistance.

- Laron dwarfism is a form of GH resistance caused by a mutation in the GH receptor. Once insulin-like growth factor type 1 (IGF1), the downstream effector of GH, was identified and synthesized, growth could be induced by bypassing the missing step.

- Pseudo–vitamin D deficiency rickets is caused by a deficient enzyme (25-hydroxyvitamin D_3 1α-hydroxylase) and can be treated by administration of calcitriol, the product of that enzyme. However, if the receptor for calcitriol is missing, then true "resistance" is present and cannot be directly overcome.
- Pseudohypoparathyroidism is often caused by mutations in the Gs signaling protein and may be associated with more subtle forms of resistance to hormones other than PTH (e.g., resistance to thyroid-stimulating hormone [TSH]). In pseudohypoparathyroidism type 1A, the renal proximal tubule is resistant to the actions of PTH (because of maternal imprinting in the proximal tubule, where only one allele of the Gs gene is active), but the bones are not resistant. Therefore, resistance may vary among tissues.
- Hormone resistance may be acquired. For example, antibodies to the insulin receptor cause diabetes mellitus with severe insulin resistance requiring thousands of units of insulin daily; obesity worsens the insulin resistance of type 2 diabetes; starvation causes GH resistance; and renal failure causes PTH resistance.
- Hormone resistance at one receptor can result in spillover to other related receptors. For example, insulin resistance leading to elevated insulin can cause hirsutism by stimulating IGF receptors on the ovary.

We now recognize many autoimmune endocrine disorders and are beginning to understand their physiology.

Changing Spectrum of Endocrine Diseases

Most of the endocrine disorders recognized before 1970 were clinically severe and therefore easily diagnosed. In contrast, many of the endocrine disorders identified after 1970 have been clinically more subtle, easy to overlook, and far more prevalent. As a result, the percentage of severe endocrine disorders has declined over the years, whereas the percentage and prevalence of less severe endocrine disorders have risen sharply (Fig. 2-1).

The following are some examples of less severe endocrine disorders that are now commonly diagnosed.

- "Asymptomatic" hyperparathyroidism is often diagnosed through the routine measurement of serum calcium levels with autoanalyzers.

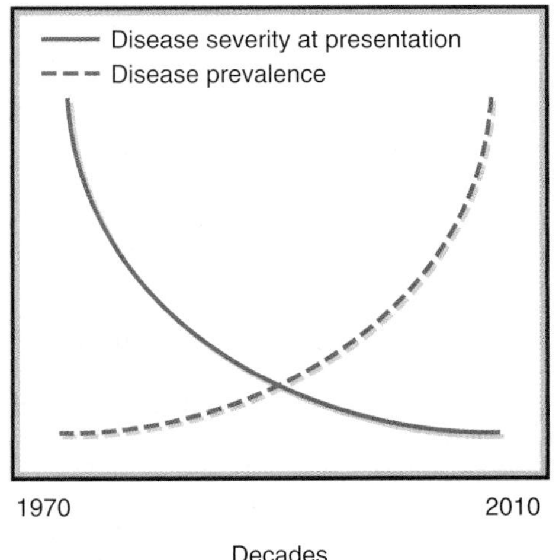

Figure 2-1 Changing pattern of disease severity over time.

- Mild thyroid disease ("subclinical" hyperthyroidism or hypothyroidism) can be detected and studied with the use of readily available sensitive TSH assays.
- "Subclinical" Cushing's syndrome caused by autonomous adrenal nodules can now be detected by appropriate diagnostic testing after the incidental discovery of an adrenal nodule,
- Type 2 diabetes mellitus is now considered to be the most common cause of diabetic microvascular complications and a leading cause of cardiovascular morbidity and mortality.
- Insulin resistance without diabetes mellitus is now considered to be a condition that poses a significant cardiovascular risk.
- Polycystic ovarian disease, once thought to be a rare disease of obese, hirsute women with infertility, has been shown to be a common cause of irregular menses, hirsutism, and insulin resistance.
- The widespread availability of bone densitometry has led to a greater understanding of the spectrum and population consequences of low bone mass.
- Modern diagnostic algorithms have revealed that 8% to 10% of hypertensive patients have primary hyperaldosteronism. Primary aldosteronism may also be associated with cardiovascular morbidity independent of its effect on blood pressure.[5]

Our ability to diagnose ever-milder stages of endocrine disorders has brought with it a variety of challenging new questions for endocrinologists and epidemiologists:

- What constitutes "normal" levels of hormones and metabolites? Are "normal" and "optimal" levels synonymous? Which of these two levels is more physiologically relevant? Is the optimal physiologic level also optimal for disease prevention?
- Is treatment beneficial for patients with mild endocrine disorders? If intervention is beneficial, when should it be done? Does the treatment of mild endocrine and metabolic abnormalities ultimately benefit society?

It is important to keep in mind that there is not yet a general consensus about what defines "normal," "optimal," and "abnormal" levels for any given hormone or metabolite and that these definitions are continuously undergoing revision to reflect the latest research. Some define "normal" in purely statistical terms. Others base their assessment of "optimal" levels on relevant physiologic or pathologic changes. For example, vitamin D deficiency was first recognized as a level of vitamin D so low as to cause rickets and osteomalacia. Investigators then modified the definition of normal to be the level of vitamin D below which PTH levels start to rise. More recently, some have proposed that the optimal level of vitamin D is the one that maximizes bone density in population studies and clinical trials. Diabetologists have used certain glucose concentrations associated with adverse outcomes to define diabetes mellitus, impaired glucose tolerance, and elevated fasting glucose concentrations. The problem is that there is no universally accepted standard for these values.

Radiology and Endocrine Epidemiology

In the 1960s, the great endocrinologist, Dr. George Thorn, reportedly explained in mock exasperation, "Thank goodness we can't feel the adrenal glands!" He was referring to what at the time seemed like an overwhelming number of thyroidectomies being performed to treat palpable goiters. His fear was that once abnormalities became detectable in other glands, the inevitable consequence would be an exponential increase in the number of patients requiring evaluation and treatment.

Forty years later, we have come to realize how prescient Thorn was. Advances in radiology now allow us to scrutinize not only the adrenal gland but every other endocrine gland as well. The use of diagnostic ultrasound, CT scans, and MRIs of the head, neck, and abdomen has led to the clinical discovery of thyroid, pituitary, adrenal, and pancreatic tumors that were previously found only at autopsies or during surgery.

The twin epidemics of these incidentalomas and the mild endocrine diseases discussed earlier has created a new dilemma: there are simply too many patients to be cared for by endocrinologists, even with the help of trained endocrine nurses and assistants. The result is precisely what Thorn had foreseen: all this new radiological information has led to the discovery of numerous "incidentalomas," which in turn has led to a need for diagnostic evaluation and treatment. Part of the endocrinologist's new job description, therefore, should be to educate primary care physicians and nurses in the optimal care of patients with these endocrine disorders.

"New" Endocrine Disorders

One of the most exciting parts of being a clinical endocrinologist is that new or newly recognized endocrine disorders continue to be discovered, and clinicians are often the ones who find them.

The story of one such discovery was often told by the legendary thyroidologist, Dr. Sydney Ingbar. A clinician called Ingbar to discuss a hyperthyroid patient who had a nil radioactive iodine uptake and a painless thyroid. Ingbar led the clinician through the standard differential diagnosis excluding iodine excess, exogenous thyroid hormone, struma ovarii, and painful (DeQuervain's) thyroiditis. Ingbar eventually concluded that there was no such disease. In fact, the patient turned out to have what was subsequently named *painless* or *silent subacute thyroiditis (painless destructive thyroiditis)*. Painless subacute thyroiditis has since been found to occur in 5% to 10% of all women in the postpartum period (postpartum thyroiditis). It had simply been unrecognized. For Ingbar, the story taught an important lesson: when making a diagnosis, the clinician must avoid a rush to judgment and remain open to the possibility of new diseases.

Other endocrine diseases that have been recognized in recent years include the following:

- Endocrine diseases caused by nonendocrine drugs. Many drugs (e.g., amiodarone, lithium, sunitinib) and immune modulators (e.g., denileukin diftitox, interleukin, and interferon in hepatitis C) also cause autoimmune thyroid disorders, and painless subacute thyroiditis in particular. A new B and T lymphocyte–depleting drug for multiple sclerosis (alumtuzemab) induces Graves' disease in 12% of recipients. Etomidate, an anesthetic agent, may produce adrenal insufficiency.
- Somatostatin- and glucagon-secreting tumors of the pancreas
- Maturity-onset diabetes of the young (MODY), which results from a number of different specific biochemical abnormalities
- Lymphocytic hypophysitis, an autoimmune cause of (postpartum) hypopituitarism, possibly related to the postpartum rebound of immune inhibition. This disorder may also be induced during cancer therapy with antibodies targeting cytotoxic T-lymphocyte antigen 4 (CTLA4)
- Human immunodeficiency virus (HIV) infection, the therapy for HIV, and the consequences of acquired immunodeficiency syndrome (AIDS) cause a spectrum of endocrine disorders, particularly ones involving the adrenal and the thyroid.

Although endocrinology has changed fairly dramatically over the last 40 years, the clinical approach to the patient is based on a series of little-changed principles. The following sections present some insights and approaches that I have learned and taught over many years.

THE CLINICAL APPROACH TO THE PATIENT

An endocrinologist should always view the patient's condition as a whole rather than exclusively as an endocrine problem. Skillful questioning, personal interaction, careful deliberation, and sound clinical judgment are essential.

The clinical endocrinologist has to fill many roles at once—radiologist, pharmacologist, physiologist, epidemiologist, public health physician, geneticist, oncologist, and educator. But perhaps the most important role is that of internist, because the endocrine system affects every system of the body. For example, caring for a patient with diabetes mellitus involves monitoring and treating not only blood sugar but also cholesterol levels, blood pressure, kidney function, vision, the cardiovascular system, and the nervous system.

The process of clinical care begins with a carefully performed and recorded history and physical examination. During the history and physical examination, the endocrinologist must consider not only all the possible endocrine causes but also all the possible nonendocrine causes for the patient's symptoms. It is unacceptable to dismiss a patient by saying, "This is not an endocrine problem," without, if possible, suggesting alternative explanations for the symptoms.

- If a patient has neck tightness and intermittent hoarseness, gastroesophageal reflux disease is a more likely etiology than goiter.
- Severe fatigue (possibly in conjunction with hypogonadism, hypertension, and catecholamine excess) might be related to sleep apnea and may be suspected by asking about lack of restful sleep, the presence of snoring, and collar size (a collar size greater than 17 inches is often indicative of sleep apnea). Sleep apnea is a much more likely cause of fatigue than a minimally elevated serum TSH.
- Depression, iron deficiency, and sleeplessness resulting from menopausal hot flashes should also be considered when a patient complains of fatigue.
- A patient with persistent anxiety after treatment of Graves' hyperthyroidism needs more than to be told that there is no endocrine basis for his or her anxiety because the thyroid function is now normal. Based on my observations, these symptoms may be a form of "programmed" anxiety resulting from long-standing hyperthyroidism. These patients often benefit from a clear explanation, cognitive behavioral therapy, and/or anxiolytic therapy.
- Always check the neck veins in a hyperthyroid patient with dyspnea to make sure that the dyspnea is caused by the hyperthyroidism per se rather than by congestive heart failure.

- The "uncontrolled" hypertension of a patient with trivial elevation of urine metanephrines may be explained by a history of extensive use of nonsteroidal anti-inflammatory drugs[6] or by the nonspecific metanephrine elevation of hypertension.
- Weight loss with preserved appetite suggests hyperthyroidism, diabetes mellitus out of control, pheochromocytoma, malabsorption, and possibly anorexia nervosa; weight loss with a poor appetite has other, potentially more serious explanations. However, elderly hyperthyroid individuals may also have anorexia.
- Severe joint pains in a patient with autoimmune thyroid disease may represent rheumatoid arthritis or other nonendocrine autoimmune disorders.
- Vague abdominal pains, unexplained weight loss, or increased requirement for thyroid hormone may be caused by celiac disease, which is more common in patients with autoimmune thyroid disease.

An obvious but often overlooked point is that the patient should be told exactly what the diagnosis means once the clinician makes it. It is important to answer the patient's questions, provide reassurance, and allay any unnecessary fears. For example, many patients with hyperthyroidism and weight loss continue to worry until they hear the key words, "This is *not* cancer."

History and Physical Examination

What can we learn from the initial clinical examination? A careful history and physical examination are the first steps in establishing a diagnosis. All endocrine fellows learn the classic symptoms and signs of hormone excess and deficiency, but learning the characteristic tempo of each disease is equally important. For example, acute onset of Cushing's symptoms or hirsutism suggests a malignancy, and hyperthyroid symptoms lasting longer than 4 months effectively exclude destructive thyroiditis.

The following are several simple but very useful diagnostic tips to keep in mind during the initial clinical examination:

- Regular menses with molimina is the best sign of a normally functioning hypothalamic-pituitary-ovarian axis and essentially precludes the need for hormonal testing for this axis.
- Erectile dysfunction without loss of libido is rarely a symptom of testosterone deficiency.
- Most patients with Cushing's syndrome complain of difficulty falling asleep.
- When a patient with a neck or thyroid mass complains of difficulty swallowing, the first question should be, "Is it difficult to swallow food or saliva?" and not "Which surgeon would you like to see?" Difficulty swallowing saliva is caused by repetitive swallowing when there is nothing to swallow (globus). If the swallowing difficulty occurs with food, then a barium swallow will help determine whether the dysphagia is related to the neck mass.
- Diabetes insipidus is often characterized by the sudden onset of thirst for ice cold water in particular.
- Severe male hypogonadism may be associated with hot flashes.
- Sudden growth of a neck mass in a patient with a history of Hashimoto's thyroiditis raises the specter of a thyroid lymphoma.
- Severe muscle cramps are often caused by severe hypothyroidism, particularly when the onset is acute.

A careful medication history should include ascertainment of prescription medications, over-the-counter medications, vitamins, and supplements, because both prescription and nonprescription medicines can influence endocrine function. Several targeted chemotherapy agents and immunomodulatory drugs may induce endocrine disorders, particularly hyperthyroidism and hypothyroidism. A history of megestrol acetate (Megace) administration, recent intra-articular glucocorticoid injections, or extensive topical glucocorticoid administration may provide the clue to otherwise unexplained suppression of the hypothalamic-pituitary-adrenal axis. High-dose glucocorticoid therapy may explain the slightly low serum TSH in a patient referred for "subclinical hyperthyroidism." A host of drugs have been shown to increase the metabolism of thyroid hormone or cortisol, and knowledge of these drugs and their uses may explain otherwise unexplained worsening of treated or untreated hypothyroidism or Addison's disease. Many drugs and supplements inhibit levothyroxine absorption, and it is important to ask the patient whether any of them are being taken. A hyperthyroid patient with a nil radioactive iodine uptake may be ingesting large amounts of (iodine-containing) kelp or over-the-counter thyroid supplements that contain active hormone. Many drugs are associated with hyperprolactinemia, especially atypical antipsychotics such as risperidone. The use of anticoagulants may be associated with adrenal hemorrhage.

Smokers are at increased risk for severe Graves' ophthalmopathy.

A careful family history is necessary to help diagnose those important endocrine disorders that are genetic or familial. An entirely different approach to diagnosis and therapy is necessary when the patient being evaluated for hyperparathyroidism is found to have a parent or sibling with the same diagnosis. A family history of diabetes mellitus may be an important clue when dealing with atypical hypoglycemia. Surreptitious use of insulin or oral hypoglycemics must be excluded. Remember that insulin is also available without a prescription.

Knowledge of the past medical history and concomitant illnesses may provide important clues to current endocrine problems. A history of head and neck irradiation in childhood necessitates a thyroid ultrasound examination and a higher degree of concern when thyroid nodules are discovered. It also places the patient at increased risk for primary hyperparathyroidism. Infants, children, and fetuses who were exposed to radiation during the power plant meltdown near Chernobyl in 1986 are now at risk for thyroid nodules and thyroid cancer. A history of anti-cardiolipin syndrome may be a clue to the presence of Addison's disease caused by adrenal hemorrhage. A recent CT scan with iodinated contrast may explain the sudden onset of hyperthyroidism in a patient with a long-standing nodular thyroid.

Many helpful clues can be obtained from a careful physical examination. Be sure to look at the patient's skin and hair during the physical examination.

- Early gray hair (1 gray hair before age 30) or vitiligo is a marker of autoimmune disease. A hypopigmented thyroidectomy scar suggests that the surgery was for autoimmune thyroid disease (Graves' disease or Hashimoto's thyroiditis).
- ACTH-driven hyperpigmentation (including the buccal mucosa, extensor surfaces, nipples, and recent scars) may be a sign of Addison's disease, Nelson's syndrome (growth of a corticotroph adenoma after adrenalectomy for Cushing's syndrome), or ectopic

Cushing's syndrome resulting from small cell carcinoma of the lungs. Increased sun tanning may occur in hyperthyroidism (because of hypermetabolism of cortisol with resultant ACTH overproduction). Increased melanin also occurs in hemochromatosis, but in this case it is the iron pigment that stimulates melanin production.

- Angiofibromas and collagenomas are characteristic of multiple endocrine neoplasia (MEN) type 1 and may turn a "simple" case of hyperparathyroidism into a search for this familial syndrome.
- Acanthosis nigricans is common with many disorders of insulin resistance.
- Café-au-lait spots may suggest McCune-Albright syndrome or neurofibromatosis type 1.
- Skin tags may be a clue to the diagnosis of acromegaly (and may predict colonic neoplasms). Shaking hands with an acromegalic has often been likened to shaking hands with the Pillsbury doughboy.

Although neck ultrasound has replaced thyroid examination in many offices, the value of the thyroid examination should not be underestimated. I believe that it is easiest to learn to feel the thyroid when facing the patient; the thyroid is palpated with finger pressure toward the trachea as the patient swallows. If a thyroid bruit is present, hyperthyroidism is almost invariably the result of Graves' disease. If the thyroid remains large when hypothyroidism occurs after radioactive iodine treatment of Graves' disease, the hypothyroidism is likely to be transient ("thyroid stunning"). Careful palpation will distinguish the tender thyroid of painful subacute thyroiditis from general neck tenderness or a painful nodule. Although it is often missed on ultrasound, tracheal deviation is an important physical finding of an asymmetric, possibly substernal thyroid mass.

There are several other points to consider during the physical examination:

- The presence of clitoromegaly directs the differential diagnosis of hirsutism toward more aggressive pathologies (hyperthecosis or androgen-secreting tumor).
- Don't forget to examine the testes, because they may provide the only clue to the diagnosis of Klinefelter's syndrome.
- Anosmia (e.g., inability to smell coffee) may help explain the cause of central hypogonadism (Kallmann's syndrome).
- Feel carefully for an abdominal mass, which will allow you to diagnose an adrenocortical carcinoma (ACC) in a patient with Cushing's syndrome.
- Fawn-like wrinkling around the eyes, failure of the hairline to recede, and a chubby habitus provide almost instant recognition of untreated adult male panhypopituitarism.
- The presence of torus palatinus may be a marker for increased bone density caused by activating mutations of low-density lipoprotein receptor–related protein 5 (LRP5), although this finding is not specific.
- Sudden diastolic hypertension may be caused by hypothyroidism, particularly if it occurs acutely after radioactive iodine therapy. Postural hypotension in a hypertensive patient may be found in patients with pheochromocytomas or primary aldosteronism with hypokalemia. Severe postural hypotension, often resulting from autonomic insufficiency, is an important cause of fatigue in the elderly.
- Filling in of the supraclavicular fat pads may be an early sign of Cushing's syndrome.

Laboratory Testing

Endocrinologists are known among their medical colleagues as physicians who order blood and urine tests. Indeed, one of Dr. Fuller Albright's guiding principles was to "measure something." But it is always important to know what you are measuring, why you are measuring it, and what the advantages and pitfalls of the assay are. Testing for the sake of testing is both foolish and expensive.

Be aware that assays can be misleading. In the 1970s, many malignancies were thought to secrete PTH because the assays used at the time were not specific. We now know that many malignancies produce PTHrP, but very few produce PTH. Although almost all patients with pheochromocytomas have elevated urine metanephrines and/or fractionated catecholamines, minimal elevations above normal limits have little specificity for pheochromocytoma. Learn the cutoffs that provide greater specificity. The 24-hour urine free cortisol level is often falsely elevated at high urine volumes (>4 L/day). Serum gastrin and chromogranin A are usually markedly elevated in patients taking proton pump inhibitors.

Take time to learn about the assays that you use. When serum thyroxine (T_4) was the major thyroid test, we had to learn the causes of falsely high and low T_4 concentrations. More recently, we have learned that most modern free T_4 assays give surprisingly low readings during pregnancy, whereas dialyzable free T_4 is normal or high at that time. A total T_4 measurement may be helpful in this situation.

Even though TSH is a near-perfect thyroid function test in outpatients, the clinician must still have a clear understanding of its physiology and potential pitfalls. A normal serum TSH concentration essentially excludes hyperthyroidism and hypothyroidism if the hypothalamus and pituitary are normal. Use of algorithms that measure only TSH if it is normal but add free T_4 if the TSH is high or triiodothyronine (T_3) and free T_4 if the TSH is low reduces the need for further testing and is more efficient and cost-effective than ordering everything at once or reordering after an isolated abnormal TSH measurement. We also use an algorithm for patients taking levothyroxine that adds free T_4 only if the TSH is less than 0.05 IU/L, because we have determined that information from the free T_4 measurement is useful only when a low TSH is in this range. Almost all patients with a normal TSH and a slightly low free T_4 are euthyroid. The low free T_4 level is likely to be a laboratory aberration (and probably should not have been measured in the first place). Although free T_3 measurements have become popular in diagnosing hyperthyroidism, I find that total T_3 concentrations are sufficient.

Many primary care physicians and some endocrinologists do not understand the exponential relationship between thyroid hormone and TSH and therefore cannot explain it to their patients. A 50% decrease in free T_4 causes a 90-fold increase in TSH. Hence, a doubling of TSH from 5 to 10 mIU/L represents at most a decrease of a few percentage points in thyroid hormone concentration and not a 50% decrease. Once patients understand this simple relationship, their concerns about "wild swings" in their hormones can be allayed.

It should be noted that TSH is less useful and can actually be misleading in patients with pituitary or hypothalamic disease and in acutely ill hospitalized patients. We must always interpret the results in the context of the patient's clinical state. A low TSH (and a low free T_4) may signify central hypothyroidism. A slightly high TSH (with a very low free T_4) occurs in hypothalamic hypothyroidism in which the TSH is biologically inactive. Hyperthyroidism may occur with an elevated TSH (and a high free T_4) if it is caused by a pituitary tumor, but a pituitary tumor also can cause hyperthyroidism with a normal TSH (due to heightened TSH bioactivity). It takes great clinical acumen to suspect hyperthyroidism and order additional thyroid function tests when the TSH is normal. Severe illness ("sick euthyroid") may inhibit TSH release, causing a low serum TSH and, over time, a low serum free T_4.

TSH measurements can be misleading even with an intact hypothalamic-pituitary-thyroid axis in a healthy individual. I recently saw an elderly woman who had become progressively more hyperthyroid because her elevated TSH could not be brought down to normal with supraphysiologic doses of thyroid hormone prescribed by her personal physician. After a brain MRI to exclude a TSH-secreting pituitary tumor, she was sent for consultation to exclude thyroid hormone resistance despite being clinically hyperthyroid. We eventually discovered that she produced heterophilic antibodies that interfered with the TSH assay, resulting in falsely high TSH readings with some TSH assays. TSH measurements in a different laboratory confirmed an undetectable serum TSH until thyroid hormone was stopped and the TSH returned to normal.

Heterophilic antibodies can interfere with other assays as well. Similar to the example just described, a very high prolactin concentration in a woman with regular menses might suggest macroprolactinemia, a false elevation of the serum prolactin level caused by hormone-binding gamma globulins.

Some valuable insights may be gleaned from basic laboratory tests:

- If the TSH remains low and stable over many years (e.g., 0.2 IU/L), nodular disease (toxic nodular goiter) is the likely cause. The mild hyperthyroidism of Graves' disease often waxes and wanes over time.
- Stable hypercalcemia that dates back years is very likely to be caused by hyperparathyroidism.
- If the serum calcium concentration is consistently at the upper range of "normal," it is likely to be abnormal. Although many laboratories consider serum calcium levels lower than 10.5 mg/dL to be normal, most individuals with consistent calcium measurements in the range of 10.2 to 10.5 mg/dL will prove to have an abnormality of calcium metabolism, usually primary hyperparathyroidism.
- The puzzling rise and fall of serum calcium and PTH in patients with primary hyperparathyroidism is caused by the negative feedback of calcium on the abnormal parathyroid glands: the higher the serum calcium, the lower the PTH concentration. When hyperparathyroid patients take in additional calcium, the calcium may rise and the PTH may fall. If calcium intake is decreased or vitamin D deficiency is present, the serum calcium concentration is often lower (or even normal), and the PTH is higher.
- A low serum phosphate level may be a clue to osteomalacia, vitamin D deficiency, hyperparathyroidism, or muscle weakness (phosphate depletion syndrome). However, a low serum phosphate concentration after a meal or during intravenous glucose administration is related to intracellular shifts in phosphate and does not require diagnostic evaluation. After thyroid or parathyroid surgery, a high-normal or elevated serum phosphate concentration suggests hypoparathyroidism. An elevated serum phosphate level may be also found in acromegaly.
- I always check the serum albumin level whenever I check the serum calcium, and I then correct for the albumin concentration. Hemoconcentration (related to use of the tourniquet during phlebotomy) may cause an elevated serum calcium due to an elevated serum albumin level. Hemodilution, often resulting from the administration of intravenous fluids, lowers the serum calcium and albumin concentrations.
- Male hypogonadism is associated with a fall in the hematocrit to the normal female range. Men with appropriate signs and symptoms and a hematocrit in the range of 35% to 40% should be evaluated for hypogonadism.
- An elevated alkaline phosphatase concentration is common in patients with untreated Graves' disease. With treatment, the alkaline phosphatase level usually rises further (as bone heals) and may remain above normal for up to 1 year after the patient is euthyroid.
- A white blood cell count with 1% or 2% eosinophils almost always excludes overt Cushing's syndrome.
- A low neutrophil count may be present in severe Graves' disease before therapy (because of immune destruction of granulocytes by antibodies targeting granulocyte TSH receptors).[7] This is not a contraindication to anti-thyroid drug therapy.
- Hyponatremia without hyperkalemia may be a consequence of glucocorticoid deficiency from central causes.

Learn the appropriate timing for tests and how to interpret their results:

- A low morning cortisol level (<3 μg/dL) suggests adrenal insufficiency, and a low midnight salivary cortisol concentration tends to exclude Cushing's syndrome. A high morning cortisol level (>18 μg/dL) usually excludes adrenal insufficiency.
- Serum prolactin may rise after a meal and therefore should be measured in the fasting state to determine whether minor elevations are abnormal or related to food.
- Although the release of testosterone is pulsatile, testosterone has a diurnal variation, with concentrations being higher in the morning and lower in the evening. As it has been said, only half-jokingly: "If you want to study normal (eugonadal) men, draw a testosterone level in the a.m. If you want to study hypogonadal men, draw a testosterone level in the afternoon." Many patients have been unnecessarily treated with testosterone based on a single afternoon testosterone concentration below the normal range. Be aware that many so-called free testosterone assays report low values even in eugonadal men.
- Once suppressed, the serum TSH may remain undetectable for months, even after the patient is euthyroid. Similarly, the hypothalamic-pituitary-adrenal axis may remain suppressed for 1 year or longer after successful treatment of Cushing's syndrome or weaning from glucocorticoid excess.

Take advantage of clinical serendipity:

- The most useful time to measure serum thyroglobulin in patients with well-differentiated thyroid cancer is when the serum TSH is elevated (after injection of recombinant human TSH or withdrawal of thyroid hormone). If a patient with thyroid cancer is noted to be undertreated with a spontaneously elevated TSH, take advantage of that undertreatment by measuring serum thyroglobulin before increasing the levothyroxine dosage.

- When spontaneous hypoglycemia is reported, try to retrieve the blood sample for an insulin measurement.
- A fully suppressed serum TSH in a patient taking modest doses of levothyroxine suggests thyroid autonomy; a thyroid scan performed when the TSH is low can confirm this suspicion. Note that it is better to perform a "suppression scan" in a patient with a thyroid nodule while the patient is taking thyroid hormone than to stop thyroid hormone before the scan.

Think physiologically:

- A mid-normal or high-normal PTH level in the face of hypercalcemia is inappropriate and hence diagnostic of primary hyperparathyroidism. Similarly, a low PTH level with hypercalcemia excludes hyperparathyroidism. An astute clinical investigator evaluated a critically ill patient with severe hypercalcemia, a low PTH, and a markedly elevated 25-hydroxyvitamin D concentration. Using physiologic reasoning, he concluded that exogenous vitamin D had to be the cause and eventually tracked the source to a miscalculation of the dose of vitamin D added to milk at a specific dairy.[8]
- A "normal" level of follicle-stimulating hormone (FSH) in a postmenopausal woman is inappropriately low and probably indicates a pituitary or hypothalamic problem. Conversely, an elevated postmenopausal FSH is strong (but not conclusive) evidence in favor of normal pituitary function, because loss of gonadotropin function is often an early sign of pituitary failure. Remember that starvation or acute illness can temporarily suppress the serum FSH even when the axis is intact.
- Low levels of plasma cortisol and ACTH in a patient with clinical Cushing's syndrome suggest the use of a potent glucocorticoid (e.g., dexamethasone) that is not measured in the cortisol assay. An alternative explanation is recent administration and withdrawal of supraphysiologic glucocorticoid.

The ability to use the appropriate minimum number of laboratory tests is a hallmark of a thoughtful clinical endocrinologist. Efficient use of tests to *exclude* endocrine diagnoses is particularly important. A normal serum TSH excludes most cases of hyperthyroidism or hypothyroidism. A normal plasma concentration of metanephrines excludes most cases of pheochromocytoma. A normal midnight salivary cortisol or low-dose overnight dexamethasone suppression test effectively excludes most instances of Cushing's syndrome. A normal aldosterone-to-renin ratio effectively excludes primary hyperaldosteronism.

An elevated morning urine osmolality argues against diabetes insipidus. A low GH level after glucose administration or a normal basal IGF1 level effectively excludes acromegaly.

Unfortunately, there is a tendency among some endocrinologists to "check off all the boxes" when ordering tests. Remember, Dr. Albright said to "measure something" not to "measure everything." I see many patients in consultation who have undergone every possible thyroid or adrenal test, sometimes multiple times, even though most of these tests were not needed to make the diagnosis. Take the time to think carefully before ordering laboratory tests and to evaluate the diagnostic value and expense of each test.

- At our institution, the charge for a corticotropin-releasing hormone stimulation test (with eight ACTH measurements) is approximately $3500. A clinician should make sure that expensive tests like this one are absolutely necessary before ordering them.
- It is extremely important to measure thyrotropin receptor antibodies (TRAb) in pregnant patients previously treated with radioactive iodine or surgery for Graves' disease. High-titer TRAb may predict fetal or neonatal Graves' disease. Institution of appropriate therapy in a timely fashion can be life-saving or life-altering for the newborn. Although many endocrinologists routinely (and often unnecessarily) measure TRAb serially in nonpregnant patients with known Graves' disease, they often neglect to measure these antibodies in pregnant women previously "cured" of Graves' disease.
- Although it is relatively inexpensive, a 24-hour urine test for 5-hydroxyindoleacetic acid (5-HIAA) rarely has a true-positive result and is often ordered unnecessarily; most true-positive findings are in patients in whom the diagnosis of carcinoid syndrome can be made clinically.
- Sometimes common sense is superior to standard testing algorithms. If you suspect primary adrenal insufficiency in a hyperpigmented patient, measure the serum cortisol and plasma ACTH. A high ACTH with a low cortisol level is diagnostic of primary adrenal insufficiency. Guidelines are a guide, not gospel.

The role and benefit of screening tests is problematic. Bear in mind that although some screening tests are generally accepted, the value of others remains controversial.

Screening for gestational diabetes is recommended based on data suggesting improved outcomes, but even here the benefits are debated. The value of TSH screening in pregnant women or in the general population is hotly debated. Many European and some North American endocrinologists recommend measurement of serum calcitonin in all patients with thyroid nodules, despite the fact that the relative value of this determination is unknown in terms of benefit (discovery of small medullary thyroid carcinomas) and harm (unnecessary surgery for false-positive calcitonin results or possibly innocent medullary microcarcinomas). In general, the presence of strong feelings on both sides usually indicates that the data suggesting benefit are weak or absent. Although each clinician will decide whether to screen for specific diseases in his or her own practice, major public health decisions about screening need to be supported by compelling data.

Radiology and Interventional Radiology

I was taught to make an endocrine diagnosis before recommending imaging, and adhering to this sequence seems the best way to avoid ordering needless and costly radiologic scans. Imaging of the pituitary in a patient with tests diagnostic of adrenal Cushing's syndrome is unnecessary. Patients who clearly do not have a pheochromocytoma do not need CT scans, MRIs, or ^{131}I-*meta*-iodobenzylguanidine (MIBG) nuclear scans. On the other hand, patients referred for incidentalomas do require hormonal evaluation.

Almost all adrenal nodules are benign. Major radiologic advances with CT and MRI imaging have allowed us to characterize most of these tumors as benign adenomas. Patients with benign adrenal tumors generally require endocrine evaluation for Cushing's syndrome, subclinical Cushing's syndrome, or pheochromocytoma. If the patient is hypertensive, primary aldosteronism should be excluded. Some of these patients with benign adrenal tumors are appropriately referred to surgeons based solely on tumor size.

There is still uncertainty about the adrenal lesions that are characterized radiologically as "not simple adenomas." Most of these lesions turn out to be benign, but all of them require careful follow-up, and some may require surgery. There is an unfortunate misconception among many endocrinologists that needle biopsy can distinguish a benign from a malignant adrenal cortical tumor. In fact, a needle biopsy can diagnose metastasis to the adrenals but only rarely distinguishes adrenocortical adenoma from ACCs. Use of a needle biopsy to diagnose ACC is therefore worthless, not to mention potentially harmful. Most adrenal cancers are large and readily diagnosed by CT or MRI.

Given the clinical epidemic of thyroid nodules, many clinical endocrinologists use ultrasonography to interpret and biopsy thyroid nodules that are incidentally discovered during radiologic imaging for other conditions. Ultrasound can provide guidance about which thyroid nodules need to be biopsied. If multiple nodules are present, newer ultrasound algorithms should be used to help determine which nodules are suspicious, thereby avoiding the need to biopsy all the nodules.

At the same time, keep in mind that simply because an ultrasound machine and a biopsy needle are available does not mean that they have to be used. Always consider the value of the diagnostic information that a biopsy could provide, particularly with ever-smaller thyroid nodules. For example, think about whether there really is an advantage to diagnosing a 5-mm papillary thyroid carcinoma. Likewise, common sense and judgment should lead to treating many nodules more conservatively in the aged. Whereas larger nodules in older patients may be aggressive malignancies, it is reasonable to tell octogenarians who present with five or six thyroid nodules of modest size that even if the risk of malignancy is about 10%, the risk of death from such malignancies is quite remote. These older patients can then decide for themselves whether to undergo one or more biopsies. Choosing not to have a biopsy seems particularly appropriate in this age group, especially when other potentially life-threatening illnesses are present.

When consulted for a case of large multinodular thyroids, most endocrinologists check thyroid function and biopsy all concerning nodules. But in focusing on the individual nodules, they sometimes "miss the forest for the trees" and overlook the fact that the goiter is compressing the trachea or the esophagus. An important part of evaluating large goiters is CT imaging (without contrast) or MRI to exclude compression of local structures.

Until recently, it was standard practice to obtain imaging studies of patients with primary hyperparathyroidism only if they were going to have surgery. But now clinicians sometimes image patients with "asymptomatic" primary hyperparathyroidism to help both the patient and the clinician decide whether surgery may be preferable to observation. For example, the ability to localize an abnormal parathyroid gland by ultrasound and/or sestamibi scanning might lead a clinician to recommend minimally invasive surgery for indications (e.g., unexplained fatigue) that do not meet the guideline criteria or to prevent bone loss in the future. Likewise, some patients will elect surgery rather than observation if they know that a minimally invasive procedure is feasible. But remember that parathyroid imaging should never be performed to establish the diagnosis of primary hyperparathyroidism; that task is solely in the domain of the testing laboratory.

Endocrinologists need to be both mindful of physiology when interpreting radiographic images and judicious in their use of radiology. Some examples may be helpful.

- Pituitary macroadenomas with minimal prolactin elevation should be treated as nonfunctioning tumors rather than prolactinomas. Dopamine agonists are usually ineffective in patients with large tumors and minimal prolactin elevations. The minimal prolactin elevation in pituitary macroadenomas is usually caused by either disinhibition of prolactin production or a tumor that produces prolactin but inefficiently.
- A sellar mass in a patient with diabetes insipidus is unlikely to be a simple pituitary adenoma; it is more likely to be a craniopharyngioma or the result of infiltrative disease.
- Diffuse enlargement of the pituitary after pregnancy is most likely caused by lymphocytic hypophysitis.
- Primary hypothyroidism can cause diffuse reversible pituitary enlargement and mild hyperprolactinemia. Serum TSH should therefore be measured in cases of diffuse pituitary enlargement and as part of an evaluation for hyperprolactinemia.
- A 24-hour radioactive iodine uptake of 5% (normal, 10% to 30%) in the face of an undetectable TSH is characteristic of thyroid autonomy rather than destructive thyroiditis (in which the uptake must be nil). A reason should be sought for low radioiodine uptake (e.g., recent iodine exposure).
- Given the growing concern about possible side effects of radiation from CT imaging, careful thought should be given to the use of repeat CT imaging (e.g., for adrenal nodules).

In certain cases, invasive radiologic procedures are necessary before surgery to localize the specific tumor causing the endocrine hyperfunction. Because incidentalomas are common, a pituitary adenoma seen on MRI in a patient with pituitary Cushing's syndrome or an adrenal nodule seen on CT scanning in a patient with primary aldosteronism cannot be assumed to be the site of hormone overproduction. Even in the presence of MRI- or CT-documented pituitary or adrenal adenomas, pituitary corticotroph adenomas often require localization with bilateral inferior petrosal sinus catheterization; aldosteronomas often require localization or exclusion with bilateral adrenal vein catheterization; and some insulinomas require intra-arterial calcium infusion with venous catheterization. All of these invasive radiologic procedures should be performed at specialized centers with extensive experience and well-established expertise.

Genetic Testing and Family Screening

Endocrinologists are increasingly called upon to discuss genetic testing with their patients. Although it may seem like a straightforward matter of checking a box or ordering a blood test, the clinician should keep in mind that genetic testing has the potential to create profound psychological and practical challenges for patients and their families. We therefore recommend genetic counseling before testing, so that patients are prepared for the various problems they may subsequently encounter. For example, before genetic testing that might possibly identify a family member as a gene carrier for a serious condition, a genetic counselor may recommend the purchase of life insurance, because insurance could be extremely difficult to purchase if the patient is found to have the abnormal gene.

Practical application of clinical tumor genetics began before the advent of gene testing with studies of familial medullary thyroid carcinoma (MEN2). The recognition of this dominantly inherited malignancy led to information about the natural history of the disease, rules for family screening, stimulation tests (pentagastrin and calcium) to diagnose early disease, prophylactic surgery at the first sign of abnormality, and clinical observations that allowed one to predict the risk of developing the disease over time even if the screening test remained normal. The recognition of mutations in the *RET* proto-oncogene made it possible to predict the risk of inheriting MEN2 with greater precision and nuance, and genetic testing replaced endocrine testing as the standard of care for diagnosis of asymptomatic carriers of MEN2. For the first time, individuals in families with known mutations could be excluded as carriers of the disease if their *RET* test was normal. Conversely, carriers of the abnormal gene could be discovered at an early age. As genotype-phenotype correlations improved, recommendations about the appropriate time for testing and prophylactic surgery were modified.

When caring for patients with pheochromocytomas, it is important to realize that a significant minority of these tumors (up to 25%) have a germline mutation that is responsible for the tumor. In fact, the first patient ever diagnosed with pheochromocytoma recently had her pedigree traced to an MEN2 kindred.[9] Although these tumors may be familial, if the patient presents with a de novo mutation, the family history will not be revealing. When a patient with a pheochromocytoma is young, has bilateral disease, or has an extra-adrenal tumor, genetic testing should be strongly considered. Such genetic testing should look for mutations in the von Hippel-Lindau tumor suppressor gene (*VHL*), the gene encoding succinate dehydrogenase complex subunit B (*SDHB*) and also *SDHD* and *SDHC* (newly recognized abnormalities), *RET*, and, less commonly, neurofibromin 1 (*NF1*). Mutations in *SDHB* may predict malignant behavior.

Genetic testing may also be helpful in other circumstances:

- Patients with the cribriform morular variant of papillary thyroid carcinoma often harbor the familial adenomatosis polypi gene (*FAP*). Discovery of this gene may prevent death from colonic cancer when it leads to performance of screening colonoscopies.
- Patients with Cowden's syndrome may have follicular thyroid carcinoma as well as breast cancer. We consider screening younger patients with follicular thyroid carcinoma for Cowden's syndrome, particularly those who have a family history of breast cancer.
- Parathyroid carcinoma is a rare disease that may have a genetic predisposition, particularly when it is associated with jaw tumors and abnormalities of the other parathyroid glands. But a surprisingly high number of patients with apparently sporadic parathyroid cancer harbor familial mutations in *CDC73,* the cell division cycle 73 (parafibromin) gene (formerly called hyperparathyroidism-jaw tumor syndrome 2, or *HRPT2*)—an observation that suggests that genetic testing may be considered for all such patients.
- When patients with hyperparathyroidism are found to have four-gland hyperplasia, we often suggest that other family members be screened for hyperparathyroidism.
- We recommend family screening for individuals with FHH to help family members avoid unnecessary surgery.
- Patients with Zollinger-Ellison syndrome and young patients with hyperparathyroidism or islet cell tumors should be evaluated for possible MEN1. This is also true for patients who have evidence for two possible MEN1 tumors. A careful family history is paramount.

Although gene testing is available for MEN1, mutations may be missed. Even if a mutation is present, careful screening is preferable to prophylactic surgery. With or without genetic testing, both family screening and continued surveillance are important.

Therapeutics

Do all endocrine abnormalities require therapy? According to Sir William Osler, "A desire to take medicine is, perhaps, the great feature which distinguishes man from other animals."[10] To paraphrase Osler, one could say that what distinguishes endocrinologists from other physicians is their desire to replace missing hormones and to take away excess hormones. But as we shall see, logic, a desire to help, and abnormal laboratory tests do not necessarily lead to appropriate therapy.

For many years, estrogen replacement therapy for postmenopausal women seemed to be both therapeutically logical and beneficial: it reduced hot flashes, increased the sense of well-being, and provided a cardiovascular benefit as demonstrated in cross-sectional epidemiologic studies. But appropriately controlled trials not only failed to confirm the cardiovascular benefit but demonstrated that this therapy could actually harm the patient. Additional studies are changing our ideas about postmenopausal hormone replacement therapy still further.

Subclinical hypothyroidism (elevated TSH with a normal free T_4) occurs in up to 20% of the elderly population. It is easily corrected with levothyroxine therapy leading to TSH normalization. But cross-sectional studies of the very elderly (85 years and older) suggest a survival advantage for untreated individuals with subclinical hypothyroidism.[11] Furthermore, a significant minority of patients with subclinical hypothyroidism who are treated with levothyroxine develop subclinical hyperthyroidism, with its potential but unquantified consequences.

Although subclinical hypothyroidism has been implicated in adverse pregnancy outcomes, there are still no controlled trials demonstrating improved outcomes with levothyroxine therapy. Despite this lack of evidence, many excellent endocrinologists demand screening for subclinical hypothyroidism, particularly for women contemplating pregnancy. My own feeling is that screening and therapy for subclinical hypothyroidism (or other mild endocrine disorders) may be reasonable for individual patients, but a recommendation that it become national policy is unwarranted in the absence of appropriate therapeutic trials.

The increasing recognition of subclinical Cushing's syndrome is a consequence of the radiologic detection of adrenal incidentalomas. A diagnosis of subclinical Cushing's syndrome in a patient with an adrenal adenoma is most commonly based on the failure to suppress cortisol after overnight administration of dexamethasone, but the actual criteria for diagnosis vary considerably. There is no consensus about which dose of dexamethasone to use, which dexamethasone-suppressed cortisol value is diagnostic, or, more importantly, when surgical removal of the adrenal is advisable. Some patients clearly benefit from surgery, but the vexing issue for the clinician is that there are no definitive guidelines for recommending surgery.

Endocrine Hormone Replacement Therapy

Endocrine replacement therapy has long been considered to be near-perfect therapy. The dramatic response of the patient with myxedema to sautéed sheep thyroid in the 19th century, the life-saving efficacy of insulin for diabetic ketoacidosis, the use of cortisol for Addison's disease, and HRT for menopausal symptoms are some of the best examples.

But not all endocrine replacement therapy is perfect or even nearly perfect. Indeed, many patients treated with various hormone replacements have decreased quality of life or shortened life expectancy compared with appropriate controls.

- Finger-stick glucose testing, hemoglobin A_{1c} measurements, and a recognition that control of blood sugar is critical have all helped revolutionize diabetes care. Equally important has been the development of "designer" short- and long-acting insulins. But the fact remains that current therapies for type 1 and type 2 diabetes still do not mimic endogenous glucose control. Although excellent glucose control has reduced microvascular complications significantly, only near-perfect glucose control early in the disease appears to prevent macrovascular complications. More rigorous control shows a lack of benefit or even potential harm late in the course of type 2 diabetes or after cardiovascular disease has developed.[12] Hypoglycemia also continues to be a significant problem associated with insulin therapy. Looking ahead, if type 1 diabetes mellitus cannot be prevented, safer and readily available islet cell transplants may be the answer after the immunologic rejection problems are solved. For type 1 and type 2 diabetes mellitus, use of closed-loop glucose monitoring and insulin delivery systems early in the disease, if perfected, may provide near-perfect glucose control. Drugs designed to enhance islet cell regeneration may also turn out to be beneficial.
- Epidemiologic studies suggest that hypothyroid patients receiving replacement therapy do not feel as well as matched controls. Many explanations have been offered. Undertreatment is one possibility, yet the difference remains even when serum TSH is normalized. Whether the lack of well-being reflects inadequate therapy or underlying unrelated symptoms is still unclear. The combination of liothyronine plus levothyroxine was initially hailed as a panacea for symptomatic, treated hypothyroid patients, but it was then rejected. Recent preliminary studies have suggested that only certain individuals (e.g., those with specific type 2 deiodinase polymorphisms) respond favorably to this combination therapy.[13] This possibility raises the general question of pharmacogenetics, wherein patients have variable responses to treatment and require individualized therapies.
- Therapy for Addison's disease is certainly life-saving, but many studies have documented a less favorable quality of life and a possibly decreased life expectancy among treated individuals. It is still difficult to mimic the early-morning cortisol rise with our current therapeutics, but perhaps the newer, slow-release cortisol preparations given at midnight will prove effective. Most adrenal experts favor therapy with hydrocortisone, but I have found that many patients feel better with intermediate-acting glucocorticoids such as prednisone.
- Unfortunately, there is no simple way to monitor glucocorticoid therapy. To prevent excess glucocorticoid administration, we use relatively crude indices such as blood pressure and presence or absence of pigmentation, normal electrolyte levels, and clinical signs of Cushing's syndrome. Multiple daily measurements of cortisol in patients receiving hydrocortisone are used by some investigators but are quite cumbersome.
- The ability to measure bone density easily and reliably ushered in the modern era of diagnosis and treatment of osteoporosis. We continue to debate the appropriate duration and use of therapeutic agents for this condition, particularly when it is apparently mild. The bisphosphonates and other antiresorptives provide an excellent initial therapy for many patients but are far from being a panacea. PTH is anabolic for bone but has minimal effect on cortical bone mass. We await the development of newer safe agents with potent anabolic properties, particularly for cortical bone.
- Currently available therapy for hypoparathyroidism in children often results in hypercalcemia or hypocalcemia. The inconvenience of administering the possibly more effective parenteral PTH will have to be weighed against the benefits, risks, and ease of current oral therapy with calcium and calcitriol.
- Treatment of the adrenogenital syndrome in children must navigate between the Scylla and Charybdis of adrenal insufficiency and glucocorticoid excess. It is debatable whether endoscopic adrenalectomy plus adrenal replacement therapy is a preferable approach.
- Topical testosterone gels provide serum testosterone concentrations that closely mimic mean endogenous testosterone levels. A goal for the future is to find a simple oral treatment that can mimic this pattern. There are no approved testosterone therapies for sexual dysfunction in women, largely because the efficacy of such therapies continues to be debated.
- The use of GH purified from human pituitaries was abandoned after it was associated with the development of Creutzfeldt-Jakob disease. Recombinant human GH has since become the treatment of choice. Guidelines have been established for the diagnosis and treatment of GH deficiency caused by hypothalamic or pituitary disease in children and in adults. But GH deficiency in adults without structural pituitary or hypothalamic disease poses a challenge for clinicians in that they must weigh the uncertain long-term risks and benefits of GH therapy against the high cost of the drug.

Practical Considerations

Several simple points I have learned over the years can make endocrine replacement therapy significantly easier for the patient:

- Levothyroxine has a 7-day half-life. Patients who miss a pill on one day should be instructed to take two on the next. Up to seven pills once weekly may be prescribed. This flexibility often improves overall compliance with levothyroxine therapy. Be aware that some pharmacy handouts incorrectly inform patients not to make up missed doses. The same logic suggests that occasional missed bisphosphonate doses can be made up with mid-week doses (for drugs administered weekly).
- Do not prescribe two different levothyroxine dosages for the same patient. For example, instead of prescribing 0.2 + 0.025 mg of levothyroxine, prescribe two 0.112-mg pills. Prescribing two different doses confuses the patient and also is more expensive because it requires two separate copayments for patients with insurance coverage.
- To decrease or increase the dosage of levothyroxine by 15%, patients may, respectively, skip their medicine on one day per week or add one extra pill per week (e.g., on Sundays). When you are changing to a

new dosage, old prescriptions rarely need to be discarded.
- Given the many interactions between levothyroxine and foods, vitamins, and supplements, patients should be given the option of taking their levothyroxine at night before bedtime. This will not interfere with sleep and may even provide smoother TSH control.
- The treatment of chronic hypoparathyroidism includes calcium and calcitriol. I prefer to limit the dose of calcium to 500 to 600 mg three or four times daily. I adjust the calcitriol up or down to keep calcium within normal limits and avoid hypercalciuria. Some clinicians add hydrochlorothiazide to prevent hypercalciuria. Chlorthalidone is also effective. Hypokalemia caused by chlorthalidone is a common problem, perhaps because of its long duration of action.
- Acute hypoparathyroidism may require higher initial calcium therapy. Calcium should be administered with meals to lower the high phosphate, which often prolongs the hypocalcemia. It is also advisable to avoid dairy products because of their high phosphate content.
- Patients with Addison's disease have certain special needs: they should always wear a necklace or bracelet informing others about their condition (e.g., Medical Alert); they need to be aware that their glucocorticoid dosage will have to be increased in times of stress or illness; and they or their family members should learn how to administer parenteral hydrocortisone sodium succinate in case of an emergency. Those patients who are taking daily hydrocortisone should consider keeping a supply of prednisone to use for extra doses when sick; this is particularly true for older patients, because they are more likely to be intolerant of fluid retention caused by excess hydrocortisone.

In-Patient Therapeutics

Endocrine therapies in hospitalized patients require special attention.

- After years in which a rather casual approach was taken to glucose control in the hospital, controlled trials in intensive care units (ICUs) showed that intensive glucose control increased survival in some ICUs. However, these conclusions have recently been challenged.
- Nurses often become anxious when a non-ICU patient has an extremely high glucose concentration. However, they are quickly reassured once they learn that the situation can easily be brought under control with an intravenous insulin infusion that decreases the glucose by 80 to 100 mg/dL per hour.
- The parathyroid glands may be damaged or removed, either inadvertently during thyroid or parathyroid surgery or intentionally during en bloc surgery for invasive head and neck cancers. The resulting acute hypocalcemia is often difficult to treat properly. Oral calcitriol takes time to work and cannot be administered to patients who are NPO. A simple temporary regimen to maintain normal serum calcium levels in this setting is the constant infusion of calcium. Four or five ampules of calcium gluconate (400 to 500 mg of elemental calcium) in 1000 mL of fluid is infused at a rate of 40 mL/hour. This regimen avoids the frequent peaks and troughs of bolus calcium administration.
- Endocrinologists are often asked to consult on cases of hyponatremia. Appropriate clinical assessment of salt and water balance in these patients is the key to appropriate diagnosis and therapy. Parenteral antidiuretic hormone (ADH) antagonists for the treatment of euvolemic hyponatremia are now available, but it remains unclear how and when these agents should be used.
- Critically ill patients often develop abnormalities of thyroid function, including low T_3, low T_4 and free T_4, and low TSH. These thyroid changes suggest central hypothyroidism. Because it is unclear whether these changes are adaptive or harmful, it is also unclear whether replacement therapy is appropriate for these patients. In the "euthyroid sick" syndrome, the serum TSH is rarely undetectable unless glucocorticoids or dopamine is administered.
- There are new guidelines for treatment of corticosteroid insufficiency in acutely ill patients, based on responses to the ACTH stimulation test. Although these tests may define a population with glucocorticoid-responsive disease, it is difficult for me to categorize patients with very high serum free cortisol concentrations as adrenally insufficient.[14] Whether they have a form of glucocorticoid resistance or another glucocorticoid-responsive illness is unknown.
- Elderly patients with severe hypercalcemia or hyponatremia may be slow to recover their mental function. Do not be discouraged if the mental state remains abnormal for 2 to 7 days after the metabolic abnormality has been corrected.

Treatment of Hormone Excess

As clinicians trained in internal medicine, endocrinologists would like to be able to treat all hormonal overproduction, including tumor-related hormone excess, with medication rather than surgery. The ideal therapy would be a medication given for a limited period that permanently eliminates the tumor as well as the hormone excess. Although medical therapy rarely approaches this ideal, it is often successful in controlling hormone excess.

Graves' hyperthyroidism is the most common condition of hormone excess treated by endocrinologists. Several important clinical points are worthy of consideration.

In the 1930s and 1940s, surgery for Graves' hyperthyroidism was extremely dangerous, and there was no safe way to prepare patients for surgery. As a result, the operative and perioperative mortality rates were high. After radioactive iodine and antithyroid drugs became available in the late 1940s, they rapidly became the treatment of choice. One problem when treating hyperthyroidism is that no regimen has been able to solve the dilemma of rebound weight gain, often to above baseline.

Radioactive iodine has the advantage of treating hyperthyroidism permanently, but it also has certain disadvantages: it usually causes permanent hypothyroidism; it may cause worsening eye disease; it may cause hyperparathyroidism decades later; and, although there is no conclusive evidence, concern has been raised that the radiation may have additional harmful side effects. In selected patients, the addition of potassium iodide after radioactive iodine therapy for Graves' disease accelerates the return to euthyroidism.

Many young patients currently choose anti-thyroid drugs for the initial treatment of Graves' hyperthyroidism. After years of debate, there is now a consensus that methimazole is the anti-thyroid drug of choice, as opposed to propylthiouracil, because of its higher potency, longer duration of action, and lower toxicity. Propylthiouracil is preferred in cases of thyroid storm because of its ability to inhibit the conversion of T_4 to T_3. It is also preferred in early pregnancy and when the patient has a minor allergy to methimazole. Patients must always be informed of the low but significant risk of fatal hepatic necrosis whenever propylthiouracil is prescribed. The 1 in 200 to 1 in 500 risk of agranulocytosis may be somewhat less with lower doses of methimazole.

Hyperthyroid patients who decline both surgery and radioactive iodine therapy are usually given a therapeutic dose of methimazole, which is often tapered over time. There are several other beneficial regimens for treating hyperthyroid patients with methimazole, which endocrinologists should also consider:

- Some patients treated with anti-thyroid drugs develop extremely unpleasant yo-yo swings in thyroid function. They remain hyperthyroid on too little medication, become hypothyroid on too much, and cycle between these two extremes. A block-replace regimen employing a full therapeutic dose of methimazole and the addition of levothyroxine allows stable thyroid function. This approach may also be useful for students going away to school and for patients far removed from laboratories where blood tests can be monitored.
- There are some patients who have repeated relapses after discontinuing anti-thyroid drugs but who continue to decline surgery or radioactive iodine. For many of these patients, therapy with small doses of methimazole (e.g., 5 mg daily) provides long-term stability. Although patients are often told that anti-thyroid drugs can be used for only a limited period, that notion is incorrect, provided that the patient has no long-term toxicity.

Radioactive iodine therapy for a so-called hot nodule (an autonomously producing adenoma) approaches ideal therapy. A single dose of sodium iodide I 131 usually cures the hyperthyroidism. Most patients become euthyroid, and some become hypothyroid. The nodule may persist. It should be noted that some questions have been raised about the potential long-term effects of radiation from radioactive iodine on the remaining normal thyroid gland.

Dopamine agonists are now the therapy of choice for most prolactinomas. In a minority of patients, the tumor disappears and does not recur after the drugs have been withdrawn. The long-acting dopamine agonists (e.g., cabergoline) are easier to administer and have fewer acute side effects than their predecessors. However, some concerns have arisen about cardiac valvular problems with these newer medications.

Primary medical therapy for somatotroph adenomas has become a real possibility with the advent of somatostatin agonists and GH receptor antagonists. The efficacy of these therapies can be monitored by measuring IGF1. Many TSH-secreting pituitary adenomas are also treated successfully with somatostatin analogues. However, GH- and TSH-secreting tumors do not permanently disappear.

Surgery remains the therapy of choice when treatment is needed for primary hyperparathyroidism. Cinacalcet, an activator of the calcium-sensing receptor, is effective in lowering PTH levels in the secondary hyperparathyroidism of renal failure; it also lowers the calcium-phosphate product and is used as part of dialysis treatment. However, although this agent also lowers serum calcium and PTH in primary hyperparathyroidism, it does not improve bone density.

The medical therapy for Cushing's disease is still primitive. Although recurrent Cushing's is often treated with drugs such a ketoconazole, normalization of cortisol is rarely achieved. Treatment of Cushing's syndrome with a glucocorticoid antagonist such as RU-486 (mifepristone) poses a challenge for endocrinologists. The therapeutic effectiveness of this drug must be monitored clinically because it does not lower serum cortisol concentrations.

Surgery, Invasive Radiologic Therapy, and the Endocrinologist

One of the most important tasks for a clinical endocrinologist is to identify and make use of excellent endocrine surgeons. The basic rule to remember about surgeons is that experience is critical. Experienced pituitary surgeons achieve better results with less morbidity than less experienced pituitary surgeons do. Even though approximately half of the thyroid operations in the United States are performed by surgeons who do fewer than 10 thyroid operations per year, experienced thyroid surgeons typically perform more complete surgeries (particularly for cancer) and with lower incidences of hypoparathyroidism and injury to the recurrent laryngeal nerves. Indeed, first-rate endocrine surgeons can remove the thyroid gland safely in Graves' disease, remove the thyroid and perform a central and lateral neck dissection in thyroid cancer, find and remove abnormal parathyroid glands in hyperparathyroidism, safely remove a pheochromocytoma or functioning adrenal adenoma endoscopically, or locate and remove a small corticotroph adenoma.

The following are several do's and don'ts with respect to endocrine surgery:

- Do discuss the various surgical options with your patients, and, when indicated, do help in the management of these cases both preoperatively and postoperatively. Don't be reluctant to let the surgeon know which operation you prefer. Do help the patient and the surgeon decide between a hemithyroidectomy and a total thyroidectomy for a patient with a thyroid nodule.
- Do pre-treat your hyperthyroid patients with antithyroid drugs before thyroidectomy. Do prescribe preoperative iodine drops (to decrease thyroid vascularity) before surgery for Graves' disease, even if the surgeon does not. Do prescribe and adjust the preoperative β-blocker when a hyperthyroid patient who is allergic to anti-thyroid drugs requires a thyroidectomy. Do take responsibility for prescribing and titrating α-blockade (and sometimes β-blockade) before surgery for pheochromocytoma, if indicated.
- Do discuss the role of adrenal-sparing endoscopic surgery with the surgeon in cases of MEN2 patients with pheochromocytomas. Do diagnose and manage secondary adrenal insufficiency after successful surgery for corticotroph adenomas or cortisol-secreting adrenal adenomas, and do monitor the hypothalamic-pituitary-adrenal axis for recovery.
- Do take responsibility for managing postoperative hypoparathyroidism, because endocrinologists usually have the most experience dealing with this condition.

The following are several situations in which I believe surgery is underutilized:

- When amiodarone causes protracted hyperthyroidism or the hyperthyroidism causes major cardiac problems, an expeditious thyroidectomy can be life-saving. We are still uncertain about whether prolonged prednisone therapy for amiodarone-induced destructive thyroiditis is safer than an expeditious operation, but surgery should always be considered as an option.

- In too many cases, unsuccessful surgery for pituitary Cushing's disease is followed by prolonged unsuccessful medical therapy (usually with ketoconazole). The unfortunate result is that patients are exposed to the deleterious effects of glucocorticoid excess for a prolonged period. Bilateral endoscopic adrenalectomy is almost always definitive therapy for hypercortisolemia and results in surgically induced Addison's disease. When hypercortisolemia from ectopic Cushing's syndrome is life-threatening and the primary tumor cannot be excised, a bilateral endoscopic adrenalectomy can dramatically improve the patient's quality of life. On the other hand, if the prognosis from the primary tumor is poor, this is not a reasonable approach.
- Many endocrinologists either do not understand or do not believe that an "indeterminate" thyroid follicular neoplasm (FNA) is actually a "suspicious" FNA with a malignancy risk of 10% to 40% (usually about 20%). If a hot nodule has been excluded by serum TSH measurement or radioiodine scanning, surgery to remove the nodule is the proper treatment.

Some tumors can be treated with interventional radiologic procedures rather than invasive surgery. These procedures include alcohol ablation; radiofrequency ablation (RFA) or laser ablation of hot thyroid nodules; alcohol or laser ablation of parathyroid adenomas; alcohol or RFA ablation of recurrent nodal disease from papillary thyroid carcinoma; arterial ablation of mediastinal parathyroid adenomas; RFA of metastases to the adrenals and, rarely, for functioning adrenal tumors; and alcohol ablation, thermoablation, RFA, or chemoembolization of hepatic metastases from endocrine tumors. Embolization of bony metastases from thyroid cancer, and of spinal metastases in particular, is often performed before surgical resection. In all situations, the potential morbidity of these procedures and the local expertise must be weighed against the morbidity of surgery. For example, in some patients alcohol ablation of parathyroid tumors causes severe pain and scarring, but this may depend on the expertise and experience of the physician. Laser ablation is not currently available in the United States, and it is still not clear when these nonsurgical procedures should be used.

Turning Negatives into Positives

Observant endocrinologists have noted the negative side effects of some drugs and then taken advantage of them for therapy:

- Lithium inhibits the release of thyroid hormone and can cause hypothyroidism. It has occasionally been used to treat Graves' hyperthyroidism.
- Thiazides impair calcium excretion and can elevate the serum calcium level. They have been used to treat the hypercalciuria of primary hyperparathyroidism. The minimal rise in serum calcium may cause a possibly beneficial fall in PTH concentration. It is also of interest that thiazide diuretics are associated with increased bone density in the general population.
- Demeclocycline and lithium can cause mild diabetes insipidus. These drugs have a beneficial effect on chronic hyponatremia resulting from the syndrome of inappropriate secretion of antidiuretic hormone (SIADH).
- Cholestyramine inhibits the absorption of levothyroxine and can worsen hypothyroidism if administered conjointly with levothyroxine. However, hyperthyroidism improves more quickly when cholestyramine is added to the anti-thyroid drug regimen, because it inhibits the enterohepatic circulation of thyroid hormone.
- Amiodarone is the most important cause of drug-induced hyperthyroidism. At the same time, amiodarone is also the most potent currently available inhibitor of T_4-to-T_3 conversion. Because of this property, amiodarone may be added to antithyroid drugs to treat severe hyperthyroidism more quickly.
- The abortifacient RU-486 blocks both the progesterone and the cortisol receptor. It may be useful in the emergency treatment of endogenous Cushing's syndrome or severe glucocorticoid excess.
- Recognition of the downregulation of luteinizing hormone and FSH that occurs after administration of exogenous gonadotropin-releasing hormone (GnRH) has led to the development of GnRH analogues that inhibit gonadotropin release.

THE ENDOCRINOLOGIST AS ONCOLOGIST

Although it is easy to frighten patients, it takes time, patience, and sensitivity to reassure them. For example, the clinician could say to a patient, "Your thyroid (or adrenal) nodule could be a cancer." But for nodules that are obviously not serious malignancies, it would be far better and equally honest to tell the patient, "You have a thyroid nodule. Ninety percent of thyroid nodules are benign, and most thyroid cancers are not life-threatening. We will do a biopsy to help us determine whether surgery is necessary." Although this approach requires a bit of modification for adrenal nodules, it would still be reasonable to say, "The vast majority of adrenal nodules are benign, and adrenal cancers are rare."

With most innocent or nonaggressive thyroid cancers, the rule is to think and act like an endocrinologist. With more aggressive thyroid and other endocrine cancers, a good rule is to think like an oncologist and to refer the patient to one of them if necessary.

In most cases, sensitive tumor markers measured in a simple blood test (thyroglobulin) can tell us whether patients with well-differentiated thyroid cancer are cured. For example, it is relatively common for patients who have undergone total thyroidectomy, with or without nodal dissection for intrathyroidal papillary thyroid carcinoma with nodal metastatic disease, to have persistent, mildly elevated serum thyroglobulin at baseline or after TSH stimulation. But even if these patients are not cured, they should be told that the prognosis is usually excellent. It is important to emphasize to them that an abnormal thyroglobulin concentration is not lethal. Although thyroglobulin persistence is indicative of residual tumor, the remaining tumor is rarely lethal and in many patients never becomes manifest. You might say something like, "We will look for residual disease, and we will remove as much as we can. But even if we do not find anything, you will be fine." Few things cost as little but do as much as a strong dose of reassurance.

Abnormal concentrations of calcitonin and carcinoembryonic antigen after surgery for medullary thyroid carcinoma are of greater concern, because this tumor can have a worse prognosis. Many patients with advanced medullary thyroid carcinoma die of their disease. On the other hand, many patients with persistent modest calcitonin elevations live symptom free for decades despite persistent disease. Although the serum calcitonin concentration roughly correlates with tumor volume, it is not a good indicator of a patient's prognosis. The doubling time of serum calcitonin is a better prognostic indicator: the shorter the doubling time, the worse the prognosis.

Know Your Cancer

It is very important to understand the course, natural history, and manifestations of endocrine malignancies:

- Younger patients with radioactive iodine–refractory papillary or follicular thyroid cancer metastatic to the lungs may have indolent disease that remains unchanged over decades. If these lesions are negative on fluorodeoxyglucose positron emission tomography (FDG-PET) and the patient is asymptomatic, careful observation is often the most appropriate course of action. Surgery cannot cure diffuse pulmonary disease, and current chemotherapy regimens are not indicated for stable or slow-growing disease. Careful observation may also be the best approach in older, asymptomatic patients with slow-growing PET-positive or -negative pulmonary metastases.
- Papillary and follicular thyroid cancers rarely cause pleural effusions even when they are metastatic to the lung. In a patient with well-differentiated thyroid cancer, extensive pleural effusions in the absence of sizable pulmonary metastases suggest the presence of another malignancy or diagnosis.
- In general, most thyroid cancers (with the important exception of anaplastic thyroid carcinoma) do not kill in a systemic way. Even in advanced thyroid cancer, cachexia is rare until the patient is near death. We therefore recommend aggressive local surgery for important lesions, even when removal is not curative. Such resections include both tumors that invade the trachea or esophagus and a limited number of growing pulmonary lesions that threaten the major bronchi. External irradiation may be appropriate for some of these lesions. Growing and symptomatic hepatic metastases may be treated with chemoembolization, alcohol ablation, or RFA even if these procedures are not curative. When treating well-differentiated thyroid cancer, I recommend avoiding whole-brain irradiation for brain metastases whenever possible. Whole-brain irradiation often causes major brain dysfunction within 1 or 2 years. If the patient is expected to live longer than 2 years, whole-brain irradiation seems inappropriate to me. I recommend surgical resection, if possible, and focused irradiation (including proton irradiation) either in addition or as an alternative.
- In some cancer patients, the major cause of morbidity is hormone excess rather than the cancer itself. Cushing's syndrome due to ACTH production by medullary thyroid carcinoma is often not diagnosed even though it is amenable to treatment. Muscle weakness and hypokalemia are important clues to the diagnosis. Hypercalcemia from metastatic parathyroid carcinoma is often refractory to therapy. The best therapy is to try to resect as much tumor as possible. If surgery is not an option or is unsuccessful, cinacalcet in high doses may provide some benefit.
- Anaplastic thyroid carcinoma is almost invariably fatal. Patients must be informed of the prognosis. Although several controlled trials are under way, successful therapy is probably years away.
- Bony metastases from well-differentiated thyroid cancer are invariably lytic before therapy and may be extensive with advanced disease. However, hypercalcemia is rare unless the tumors have shown squamous de-differentiation. Conventional bone scans may be falsely negative in patients with lytic metastases, because these scans measure deposition of isotope-tagged bisphosphonate in bone.
- Hypercalcemia in a patient with medullary thyroid carcinoma is more likely to be related to concomitant hyperparathyroidism (MEN2) than to bony metastases.

Endocrinology-Oncology Collaboration

Radioactive iodine is an effective targeted therapy for well-differentiated thyroid cancer with radioiodine-avid metastatic disease. However, the use of radioiodine as a diagnostic or therapeutic tool is often continued long after it has ceased to be effective.

If the serum thyroglobulin concentration is elevated and a high-dose radioactive iodine scan is not informative, then repeated high-dose scans or low-dose scans will also be futile. Patients are frequently referred to me with metastatic thyroid cancer and elevated serum thyroglobulin levels in whom the only localizing tests have been multiple negative ^{131}I scans. Oncologists know, and endocrinologists need to realize, that conventional imaging is necessary to identify structural disease in this situation. An ultrasound study in skilled hands identifies most neck metastases, and a CT or MRI of the neck identifies almost all of the others. A high-resolution CT of the chest identifies almost all pulmonary metastases and significant intrathoracic nodal disease. If inoperable progressive disease is present, the presence and intensity of FDG uptake may help predict both the lack of ^{131}I efficacy and a worse prognosis. In the case of rapidly progressive or symptomatic radioactive iodine–refractory disease, therapeutic trials or available targeted chemotherapy (currently tyrosine kinase inhibitors) should be considered. Targeted chemotherapy for advanced thyroid cancer using tyrosine kinase inhibitors has had notable but temporary success during the past 5 years.[15]

Patients with pulmonary or other metastases that are refractory to radioactive iodine may or may not need additional therapy. For FDG-PET–negative lesions that are asymptomatic and stable or growing slowly, observation may be best. If the lesion is growing more quickly or is FDG-PET positive, these difficult questions often require the input of an oncologist: What is the likely life expectancy? Is simple observation the appropriate recommendation? Should targeted chemotherapy be considered? If so, when should it start?

There is a growing need for endocrine oncologists or oncologists with expertise in treating endocrine malignancies. Oncologic expertise is essential in the treatment of thyroid lymphomas, anaplastic thyroid carcinoma, advanced well-differentiated and medullary thyroid carcinoma requiring therapy, metastatic ACC, metastatic pheochromocytoma, islet cell malignancies, and parathyroid carcinoma.

It is important for endocrinologists to collaborate with oncologists in treating these endocrine malignancies, because endocrinologists are more familiar with certain endocrine issues that arise during the course of treatment:

- Endocrinologists know that tyrosine kinase inhibitors increase the requirement for thyroid hormone, thus raising the serum TSH (and potentially causing tumor growth) in patients with well-differentiated thyroid cancer.

- Endocrinologists know that mitotane is a potentially important adjunctive therapy for ACC but that it may temporarily or permanently damage the remaining adrenal gland after unilateral adrenalectomy for ACC, and it may accelerate the metabolism of cortisol, thereby causing an increased glucocorticoid requirement and possibly acute adrenal insufficiency.
- Endocrinologists know that the catecholamine excess of metastatic pheochromocytoma often must be treated with α-blockers or inhibitors of catecholamine biosynthesis, either chronically, before surgery, or before therapies associated with release of catecholamines. The metastases themselves require local therapy if they are symptomatic, and they require systemic targeted therapy when resection, radiation therapy, or ablative therapy is not possible or not successful.
- Endocrinologists are skilled at managing the refractory hypoglycemia of insulinomas that are metastatic and unresectable.
- Endocrinologists are most knowledgeable about treating the hypercalcemia of metastatic parathyroid carcinoma with cinacalcet and other agents.

There are many unresolved therapeutic dilemmas concerning endocrine malignancies, particularly when disease is advanced. However, even initial therapeutic decisions can be problematic and might benefit from collaborative efforts with oncologists.

- Pancreatic neuroendocrine tumors are the leading cause of death in MEN1, yet we lack an effective diagnostic and therapeutic approach to these tumors.
- Patients with parathyroid carcinoma require a wide surgical excision and often have a guarded prognosis. However, there is no consensus as to whether prophylactic postoperative external beam irradiation improves the prognosis.
- It is uncertain whether aggressive therapy (local irradiation and chemotherapy) improves the outcome for patients who have ACC without metastatic disease at presentation.

Advances in molecular biology are likely to have an important impact on the evaluation and treatment of endocrine as well as nonendocrine neoplasms. Current evidence suggests that the presence of mutated oncogenes in "follicular neoplasms" may help direct the surgeon toward a bilateral rather than a unilateral thyroidectomy. The presence of *BRAF* proto-oncogene mutations in papillary thyroid carcinoma may predict a worse prognosis and a lack of response to radioactive iodine. Improved ability to predict tumor behavior and to target therapy based on mutated oncogenes is among the goals for the future.

THE ENDOCRINOLOGIST AS EDUCATOR AND STUDENT

Clinical endocrinology requires lifelong learning. The clinician must keep up-to-date with current research, maintain a continuous dialogue with colleagues, know the literature, and take time to think about complicated cases. Only clinicians who understand the subject can teach it clearly and efficiently to students, fellows, colleagues, and patients. If a description or explanation seems fuzzy, it is probably either incomplete or incorrect. Information contained in textbook chapters or on-line textbooks can be helpful, but secondary sources should always be used in conjunction with original data and original publications.

The Internet has both facilitated and complicated patient education. Some Internet information is excellent, some misleading, some sensationalized, and some completely wrong. Clinical endocrinologists must acquire familiarity with the relevant web sites so that they can advise their patients about which ones are most reliable.

All clinical endocrinologists should provide handouts for their patients containing important information about their disease and its treatment. There are some excellent handouts published by professional endocrine societies, but it is often best to explain the material to your patients in your own words.

FUTURE DIRECTIONS AND CONSIDERATIONS

We have come to realize that the body does not act as a single, homogeneous unit with respect to hormone effects, and it may be possible to target additional hormone receptors and pathways for therapeutic purposes.

- When the peripheral conversion of T_4 to T_3 is inhibited, the pituitary remains euthyroid with unchanged TSH production, but the periphery may become hypothyroid (exposed to a low T_3 concentration).
- SERMs permit differential estrogen effects in certain tissues, thereby leading to important therapies for prevention of osteoporosis and breast cancer while avoiding potential negative estrogen effects. Similarly, thyroid hormone analogues have been developed that have very favorable effects on lipid profiles without causing tachycardia. Thyroid analogues capable of TSH suppression without other thyroid hormone actions may be feasible.
- Appropriate targeting of glucocorticoid nuclear activating pathways may eventually be the basis for a therapy that has anti-inflammatory properties without causing immunosuppression.
- If regional Cushing's syndrome resulting from activation of cortisone to cortisol in the liver by 11β-hydroxysteroid dehydrogenase 1 is found to play a role in central obesity and the metabolic syndrome, it is possible that appropriate therapies might follow.
- In Graves' disease, the thyroid gland is an innocent bystander being stimulated by immunoglobulins (TRAb). A magic bullet for Graves' disease would be a therapy that turns off these specific immunoglobulins selectively and safely.
- Therapy for severe Graves' ophthalmopathy (glucocorticoids, orbital radiation, and/or orbital decompression) has been essentially static for decades. New insights and innovations are sorely needed.
- Genome-wide association studies may yet uncover new, unimagined pathways with important diagnostic, preventive, and therapeutic consequences for clinical endocrinology.

Consider for a moment how far we have come in the practice of endocrinology. Forty years ago, we were still debating whether an elevated blood glucose concentration contributes to diabetic complications. Diabetes was monitored by spot urine glucose determinations. It was almost impossible to diagnose subtle endocrine dysfunction. It was thought that ACTH-dependent Cushing's disease was primarily a hypothalamic disorder. The only way to image the pituitary gland itself was to subject the patient to an extremely painful pneumoencephalogram. Immunoassays were still in their infancy: TSH measurements were not yet part of the evaluation for hyperthyroidism, and we could not yet detect serum calcitonin when the concentration was less than 1000 pg/mL. The only treatment for osteoporosis was estrogen or, occasionally, androgens. Thyroid nodules were discovered only by palpation. Only a few major centers offered thyroid biopsies, and these were performed by surgeons with large cutting needles. The promise of molecular biology was precisely that, a promise only. Pituitary hormones were extracted from pituitary glands rather than produced as recombinant human hormones. The concept of oncogenes and tumor suppressor genes was unknown. There was no Internet, and there were no guidelines. Much of the excitement and satisfaction I have experienced in being a clinical endocrinologist during the past 40 years has come from seeing all these changes unfold, integrating them into my own practice, learning this new science and technology, thinking about solutions to complicated clinical problems, and finding new clinical conditions. I can't wait to see what the future holds.

REFERENCES

1. Tomlinson JW, Walker EA, Bujalska IJ, et al. 11Beta-hydroxysteroid dehydrogenase type 1: a tissue-specific regulator of glucocorticoid response. *Endocr Rev*. 2004;25:831-866.
2. Pallais JC, Kifor O, Chen YB, et al. Acquired hypocalciuric hypercalcemia due to autoantibodies against the calcium-sensing receptor. *N Engl J Med*. 2004;351:362-369.
3. Service GJ, Thompson GB, Service FJ, et al. Hyperinsulinemic hypoglycemia with nesidioblastosis after gastric-bypass surgery. *N Engl J Med*. 2005;353:249-254.
4. Christ E, Wild D, Forrer F, et al. Glucagon-like peptide-1 receptor imaging for localization of insulinomas. *J Clin Endocrinol Metab*. 2009;94:4398-4405.
5. Funder JW. The role of aldosterone and mineralocorticoid receptors in cardiovascular disease *Am J Cardiovasc Drugs*. 2007;7:151-157.
6. Pope JE. Hypertension, NSAID, and lessons learned. *J Rheumatol*. 2004;31:1035-1037.
7. Weitzman SA, Stossel TP, Harmon DC, et al. Antineutrophil autoantibodies in Graves' disease: implications of thyrotropin binding to neutrophils. *J Clin Invest*. 1985;75:119-123.
8. Jacobus CH, Holick MF, Shao Q, et al. Hypervitaminosis D associated with drinking milk. *N Engl J Med*. 1992;326:1173-1177.
9. Neumann HP, Vortmeyer A, Schmidt D, et al., Evidence of MEN-2 in the original description of classic pheochromocytoma. *N Engl J Med*. 2007;357:1311-1315.
10. Osler W. Recent advances in medicine. *Science*. 1891;17:170-171.
11. Gussekloo J, van Exel E, de Craen AJ, et al. Thyroid status, disability and cognitive function, and survival in old age. *JAMA*. 2004;292:2591-2599.
12. Park L, Wexler D. Update in diabetes and cardiovascular diseases: synthesizing the evidence from recent trials of glycemic control to prevent cardiovascular disease. *Curr Opin Lipidol*. 2010;21:8-14. Epub 2009 Oct 13.
13. Panicker V, Saravanan P, Vaidya B, et al. Common variation in the DIO2 gene predicts baseline psychological well-being and response to combination thyroxine plus triiodothyronine therapy in hypothyroid patients. *J Clin Endocrinol Metab*. 2009;94:1623-1629.
14. Hamrahian AH, Oseni TS, Arafah BM. Measurements of serum free cortisol in critically ill patients. *N Engl J Med*. 2004;350:1629-1638.
15. Schlumberger M, Sherman SI. Clinical trials for progressive differentiated thyroid cancer: patient selection, study design, and recent advances. *Thyroid*. 2009;19:1393-1400.

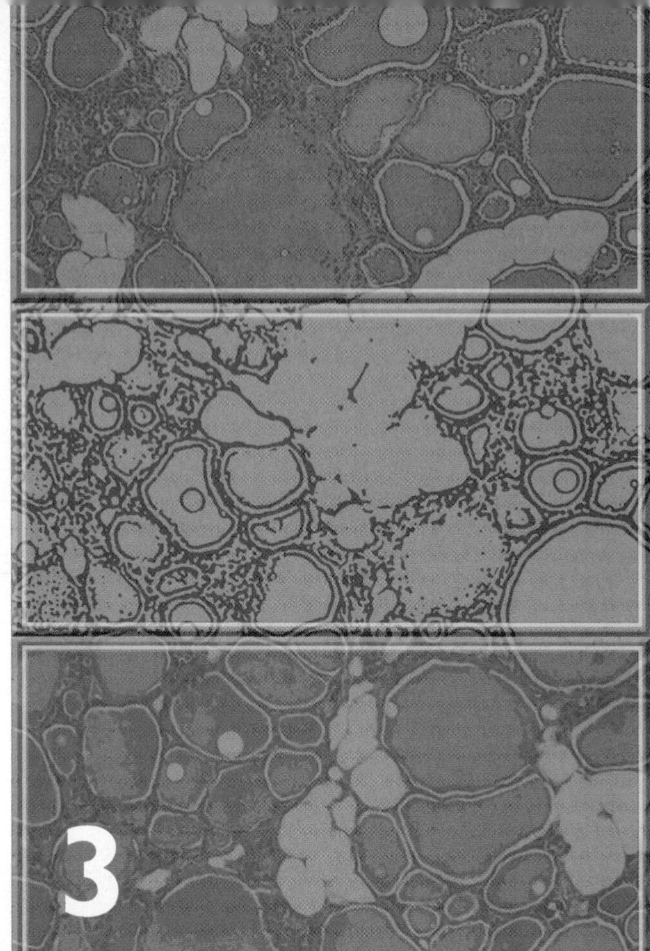

CHAPTER 3

Genetic Control of Peptide Hormone Formation

JOEL F. HABENER

Advances in the fields of molecular and cellular biology have provided insights into the mechanistic workings of cells. Recombinant deoxyribonucleic acid (DNA) technology and sequencing (decoding) of the genomes of human, mouse, and several other species make it possible to analyze the precise structure and function of DNA. Discovery of the unique biochemical and structural properties of DNA provided the conceptual framework with which to begin a systematic investigation of the origins, development, and organization of life forms.[1]

Sequencing of the human and mouse genomes was accomplished in 2003 and 2004, and annotation of the encoded information is nearing completion. A complete blueprint of the structure and organization of all expressed genes has illuminated the basis of genetically determined diseases. Within the next decade, genotyping of individuals shortly after birth likely will be possible and will provide information about the relative risks of developing these diseases. Therapeutic approaches for the correction of genetic defects by techniques of gene replacement are likely to become a reality.

The polypeptide hormones constitute a critically important and diverse set of regulatory molecules encoded by the genome; their functions are to convey specific information among cells and organs. This type of molecular communication arose early in the development of life and evolved into a complex system for the control of growth, development, and reproduction and maintenance of metabolic homeostasis. These hormones, including the many chemokines and cytokines primarily involved in regulation of the immune system, consist of more than 400 small proteins, ranging from as few as 3 amino acids (thyrotropin-releasing hormone [TRH]) to 192 amino acids (growth hormone [GH]). These polypeptides function as hormones, whose actions on distant organs are mediated by way of their transport through the bloodstream, and as local cell-to-cell communicators (Fig. 3-1). The latter function of the polypeptide hormones is exemplified by their elaboration and secretion within neurons of the central, autonomic, and peripheral nervous systems, where they act as neurotransmitters, and in leukocytes, where they modulate immune responses. The multiple modes of expression of the polypeptide hormone genes have aroused great interest in the specific functions of these peptides and the mechanisms of their synthesis and release.

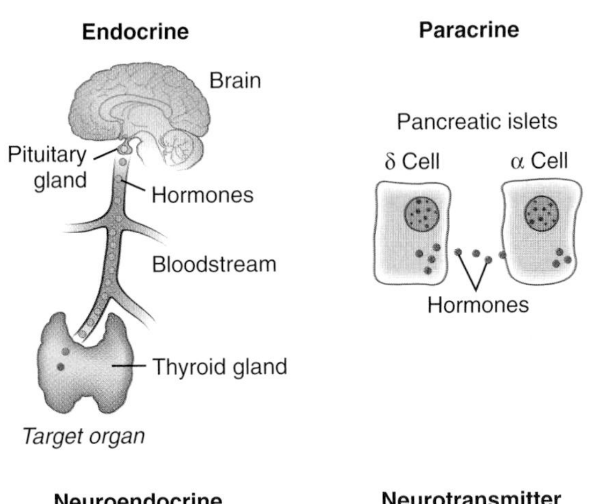

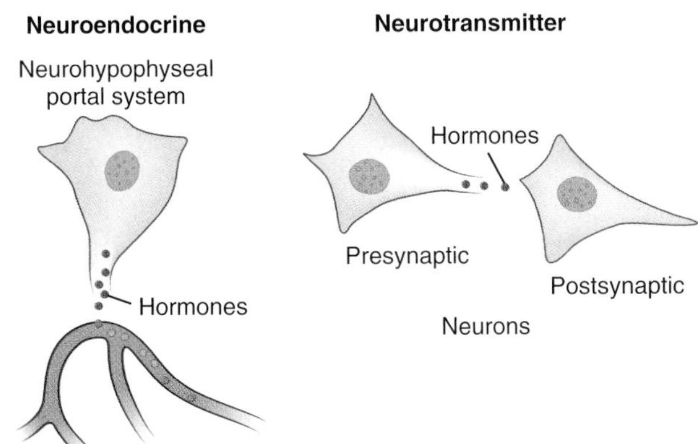

Figure 3-1 Modes of polypeptide hormone expression. The peptide hormones are expressed in at least four ways in fulfilling their functions as cellular messenger molecules: (1) endocrine mode, for purposes of communication among organs (e.g., pituitary-thyroid axis); (2) paracrine mode, for communication among adjacent cells, often located within endocrine organs; (3) neuroendocrine mode, for synthesis and release of peptides from specialized peptidergic neurons for action on distant organs through the bloodstream (e.g., neuroendocrine peptides of hypothalamus); and (4) neurotransmitter mode, for action of peptides in concert with classic amino acid–derived aminergic transmitters in the neuronal communication network. Identical polypeptides are often used in the nervous system as both neuroendocrine hormones and neurotransmitters. In some instances, the same gene product is used in all four modes of expression.

This chapter reviews the diverse structures of genes encoding peptide hormones and the mechanisms that govern their expression. The synthesis of nonpeptide hormones (e.g., catecholamines, thyroid hormones, steroid hormones) involves the action of many enzymes and expression of multiple genes, which are discussed in other chapters of this text.

EVOLUTION OF PEPTIDE HORMONES AND THEIR FUNCTIONS

Peptide hormones arose early in the evolution of life. Polypeptides that are structurally similar to mammalian peptides are present in lower vertebrates, insects, yeasts, and bacteria.[2] An example of the early evolution of regulatory peptides is the α-factor (i.e., mating pheromone) of yeast, which is similar in structure to gonadotropin-releasing hormone (GnRH).[3] The oldest member of the cholecystokinin-gastrin family of peptides appeared at least 500 million years ago in the protochordate *Ciona intestinalis* (sea squirt).[4]

The genes encoding polypeptide hormones, particularly those for regulatory peptides, evolved early in the development of life and initially fulfilled the function of cell-to-cell communication to cope with problems concerning nourishment, growth, development, and reproduction. As specialized organs connected by a circulatory system developed during evolution, similar or identical gene products became hormones for purposes of organ-to-organ communication.

STEPS IN EXPRESSION OF A PROTEIN-ENCODING GENE

The steps involved in transfer of information encoded in the polynucleotide language of DNA to the poly-amino-acid language of biologically active proteins involve gene transcription, post-transcriptional processing of ribonucleic acids (RNAs), translation, and post-translational processing of the proteins. The expression of genes and protein synthesis can be considered in terms of several major processes, any one or more of which may serve as specific control points in the regulation of gene expression (Fig. 3-2).

- *Rearrangements and transpositions of DNA segments.* These processes occur over eons in evolution, with the exception of uncommon mechanisms of somatic gene rearrangements such as rearrangements in the immunoglobulin genes occurring during the lifetime of an individual.
- *Transcription.* Synthesis of RNA results in the formation of RNA copies of the two gene alleles and is catalyzed by the basal RNA polymerase II–associated transcription factors.
- *Post-transcriptional processing.* Specific modifications of RNA include the formation of messenger RNA (mRNA) from the precursor RNA by way of excision and rejoining of RNA segments (introns and exons) and the modification of the 3′ end of the RNA by polyadenylation and of the 5′ end by addition of 7-methylguanine caps.
- *Translation.* Amino acids are assembled by base pairing of the nucleotide triplets (anticodons) of the specific "carrier" amino-acylated transfer RNAs to the corresponding codons of the mRNA bound to polyribosomes and are polymerized into polypeptide chains.
- *Post-translational processing and modification.* Final steps in protein synthesis may involve one or more cleavages of peptide bonds, which result in the conversion of biosynthetic precursors (prohormones) to intermediate or final forms of the protein; derivatization of amino acids (e.g., glycosylation, phosphorylation, acetylation, myristoylation); and folding of the processed polypeptide chain into its native conformation.

Each of the specific steps of gene expression requires the integration of precise enzymatic and other biochemical reactions. These processes have developed to provide high fidelity in reproduction and transmission of the encoded information and to supply control points for genes that direct the expression of the specific phenotype of cells.

Post-translational processing of proteins creates diversity in gene expression through modifications of the protein. Although the functional information contained in a protein is ultimately encoded in the primary amino acid sequence, the specific biologic activities are a consequence of the secondary, tertiary, and quaternary structures of the polypeptide. Given the wide range of possible specific modifications of the amino acids (e.g., glycosylation,

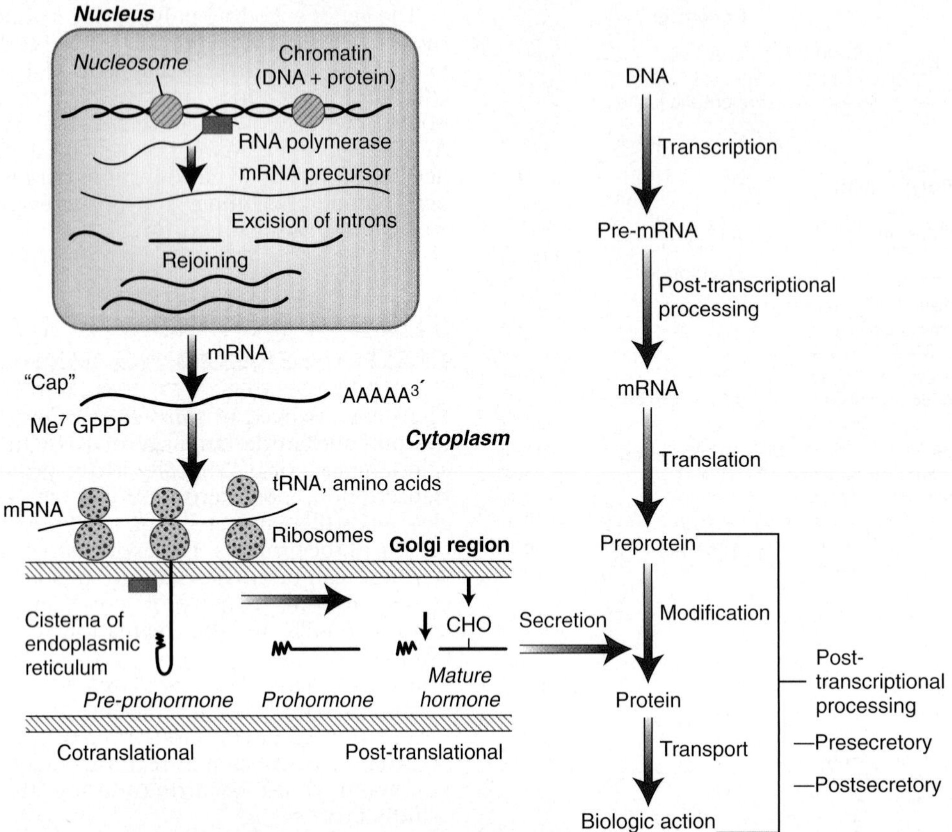

Figure 3-2 Cellular synthesis of polypeptide hormones. Steps that take place within the nucleus include transcription of genetic information into a messenger ribonucleic acid precursor (pre-mRNA) followed by post-transcriptional processing, which includes RNA cleavage, excision of introns, and rejoining of exons, resulting in formation of mRNA. Ends of mRNA are modified by addition of methylguanosine caps at the 5′ end and poly(A) tracts at the 3′ ends. The cytoplasmic mRNA is assembled with ribosomes. Amino acids, carried by amino-acylated transfer RNAs (tRNAs), are then polymerized into a polypeptide chain. The final processess in protein synthesis take place during growth of the nascent polypeptide chain (cotranslational) and after release of the completed chain (post-translational). They include proteolytic cleavages of the polypeptide chain (conversion of pre-prohormones or prohormones to hormones), derivatizations of amino acids (e.g., glycosylation, phosphorylation), and cross-linking and assembly of the polypeptide chain into its conformed structure. Post-translational synthesis and processing of a typical secreted polypeptide require vectorial or unidirectional transport of the polypeptide chain across the membrane bilayer of the endoplasmic reticulum, resulting in sequestration of the polypeptide in the cisterna of the endoplasmic reticulum, a first step in the export of proteins destined for secretion from the cell (see Fig. 3-6). Most translational processing occurs within the cell (presecretory); in some instances, it occurs outside the cell, when further proteolytic cleavages or modifications of the protein take place (postsecretory). CHO, carbohydrate.

phosphorylation, acetylation, amidation, lipidation, sulfation),[5] any one of which may affect the conformation or function of the protein, a single gene may ultimately encode a wide variety of specific proteins as a result of post-translational processes.

Polypeptide hormones are synthesized in the form of larger precursors that appear to fulfill several functions in biologic systems (Fig. 3-3), including intracellular trafficking, by which the cell distinguishes among specific classes of proteins and directs them to their sites of action, and the generation of multiple biologic activities from a common genetically encoded protein by regulated or cell-specific variations in the post-translational modifications (Fig. 3-4).

All peptide hormones and regulatory peptides studied contain signal or leader sequences at the amino-terminus. These hydrophobic, helical sequences recognize specific sites on the membranes of the rough endoplasmic reticulum (ER), which results in the transport of nascent polypeptides into the secretory pathway of the cell (see Figs. 3-2 and 3-3).[6] The consequence of the specialized signal sequences of the precursor proteins is that proteins destined for secretion are selected from a great many other cellular proteins for sequestration and subsequent packaging into secretory granules and export from the cell. Most smaller hormones and regulatory peptides are produced as a consequence of post-translational cleavages of the precursors within the Golgi complex of secretory cells.

SUBCELLULAR STRUCTURE OF CELLS THAT SECRETE PROTEIN HORMONES

Cells whose principal functions are the synthesis and export of proteins contain highly developed, specialized subcellular organelles for translocating secreted proteins and packaging them into secretory granules. The subcellular pathways used in protein secretion were elucidated largely through the early efforts of Palade (reviewed by Jamieson).[7,8] Secretory cells contain an abundance of ER, Golgi apparatus, and secretory granules (Fig. 3-5). The proteins that are to be secreted from the cells are transferred during their synthesis into these subcellular organelles, which transport the proteins to the plasma membrane.

Protein secretion begins with translation of the mRNA encoding the precursor of the protein on the rough ER, which consists of polyribosomes attached to elaborate

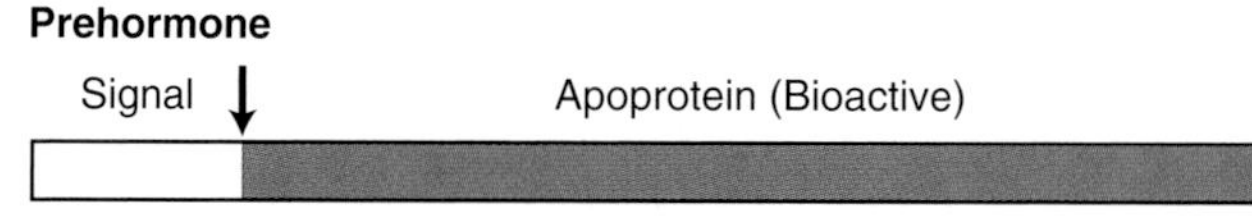

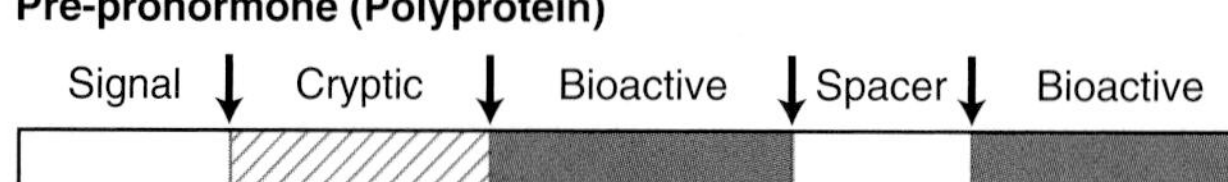

Figure 3-3 Two configurations of precursors of polypeptide hormones. Diagrams represent the polypeptide backbones of protein sequences encoded in messenger RNA (mRNA). One form of precursor consists of the amino-terminal signal, or presequence, followed by the apoprotein portion of the polypeptide that needs no further proteolytic processing for activity. A second form of precursor is a pre-prohormone that consists of the N-terminal signal sequence followed by a polyprotein, or prohormone, sequence made up of two or more peptide domains linked together that are subsequently liberated by cleavages during post-translational processing of the prohormone. The reason for synthesis of polypeptide hormones in the form of precursors is only partly understood. The N-terminal signal sequences function in the early stages of transport of polypeptide into the secretory pathway. Prohormones, or polyproteins, often provide a source of multiple bioactive peptides (see Fig. 3-4). However, many prohormones contain peptide sequences that are removed by cleavage and have no known biologic activity *(cryptic peptides)*. Other peptides may serve as spacer sequences between two bioactive peptides (e.g., the C peptide of proinsulin). When a bioactive peptide is located at the carboxyl-terminus of the prohormone, the N-terminal prohormone sequence may simply facilitate the cotranslational translocation of polypeptide in the endoplasmic reticulum (see Fig. 3-6).

membranous saccules that contain cavities (cisternae). The newly synthesized, nascent proteins are discharged into the cisternae by transport across the lipid bilayer of the membrane. Within the cisternae of the ER, proteins are carried to the Golgi complex by mechanisms that are incompletely understood. The proteins gain access to the Golgi complex by direct transfer from the cisternae, which are in continuity with the membranous channels of the Golgi complex, or by way of shuttling vesicles known as *transition elements* (see Fig. 3-5).

Within the Golgi complex, the proteins are packaged into secretory vesicles or secretory granules that bud from the Golgi stacks in the form of immature granules. Immature granules undergo maturation through condensation of the proteinaceous material and application of a specific coat around the initial Golgi membrane. On receiving the appropriate extracellular stimuli (i.e., regulated pathway of secretion), the granules migrate to the cell surface and fuse to become continuous with the plasma membrane, which results in the release of proteins into the extracellular space, a process known as *exocytosis*.

The second pathway of intracellular transport and secretion involves the transport of proteins contained within secretory vesicles and immature secretory granules (see Fig. 3-5). Although the use of this alternative vesicle-mediated transport pathway remains to be demonstrated conclusively (it is typically considered to be a constitutive, or unregulated, pathway), extracellular stimuli may modulate hormone secretion differently depending on the pathway of secretion. For example, in the parathyroid gland and in the pituitary cell line derived from corticotropic cells (AtT-20), newly synthesized hormone is released more rapidly than hormone synthesized earlier. This finding suggests that the newly synthesized hormone may be transported by way of a vesicle-mediated pathway without incorporation into mature storage granules.

INTRACELLULAR SEGREGATION AND TRANSPORT OF POLYPEPTIDE HORMONES

Specific amino acid sequences encoded in the proteins serve as directional signals for the sorting of proteins within subcellular organelles.[6,9,10] A typical eukaryotic cell synthesizes an estimated 5000 different proteins during its life span. Although these proteins are synthesized by a common pool of polyribosomes, each protein is directed to a specific location within the cell, where its biologic function is expressed. For example, specific groups of proteins are transported into mitochondria, into membranes, into the nucleus, or into other subcellular organelles, where they serve as regulatory proteins, enzymes, or structural proteins. A subset of proteins including immunoglobulins, serum albumin, blood coagulation factors, and protein and

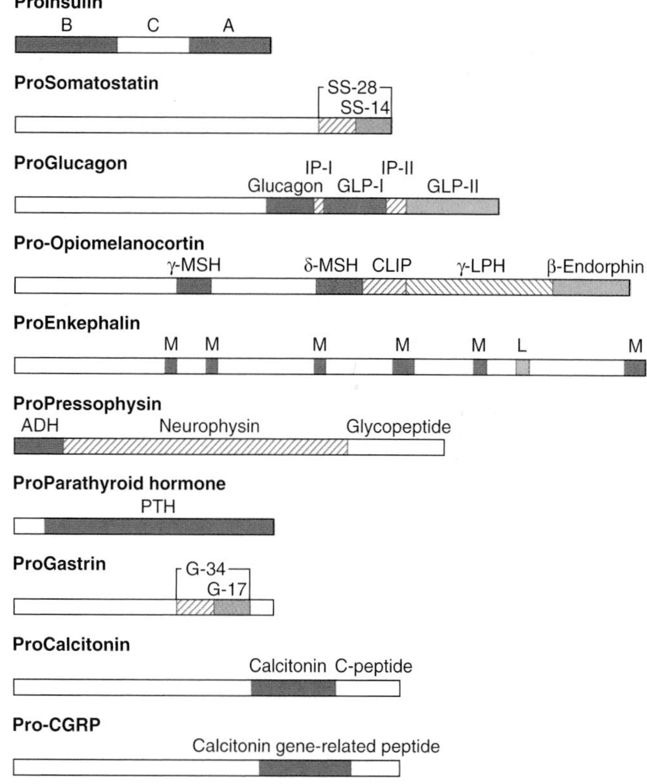

Figure 3-4 Primary structures of some prohormones. The *shaded areas* of prohormones denote regions of sequence that constitute known biologically active peptides after post-translational cleavage from the prohormone. Sequences indicated by *hatching* denote regions of precursor that alter the biologic specificity of that region of precursor. For example, the precursor contains the sequence of γ-melanocyte-stimulating hormone (γ-MSH), but when the latter is covalently attached to the CLIP peptide, it constitutes adrenocorticotropic hormone (ACTH). Somatostatin-28 (SS-28) is an amino-terminally extended form of somatostatin-14 (SS-14) that has higher potency than SS-14 on certain receptors. The neurophysin sequence linked to the carboxyl-terminus of vasopressin (ADH) functions as a carrier protein for the ADH hormone during its transport down the axon of neurons in which it is synthesized. The precursor proenkephalin represents a polyprotein that contains multiple similar peptides within the sequence of met-enkephalin (M) or leu-enkephalin (L). Procalcitonin and procalcitonin gene–related product (CGRP) share identical N-terminal sequences but differ in their C-terminal regions as a result of alternative splicing during post-transcriptional processing of the RNA precursor. γ-LPH, γ-lipotropin; GLP, glucagon-like peptide; IP, intervening peptide.

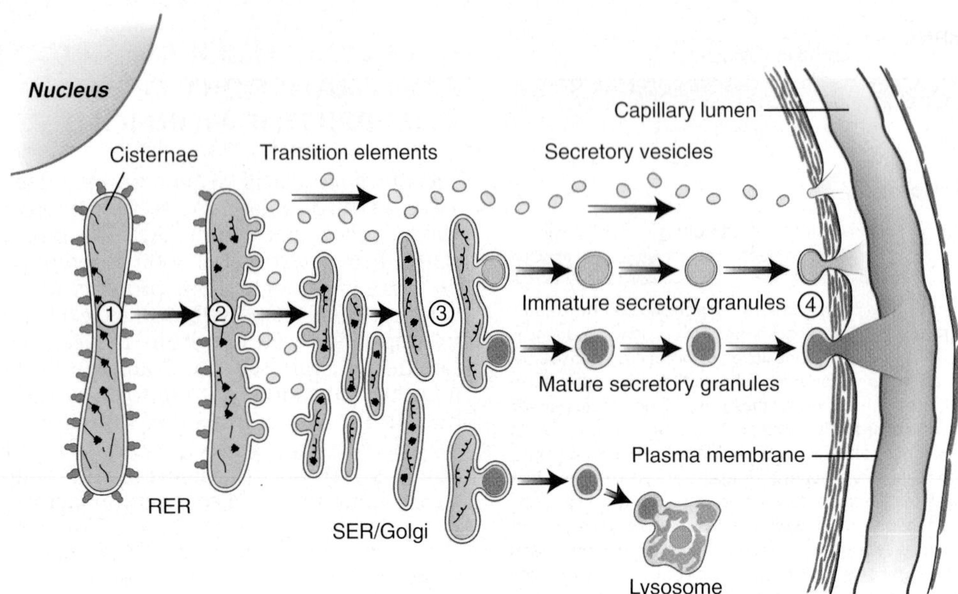

Figure 3-5 Subcellular organelles involved in transport and secretion of polypeptide hormones or other secreted proteins within a protein-secreting cell. (1) Synthesis of proteins on polyribosomes attached to rough endoplasmic reticulum (RER) and vectorial discharge of proteins through the membrane into the cisterna. (2) Formation of shuttling vesicles (transition elements) from endoplasmic reticulum followed by their transport to and incorporation by the Golgi complex. (3) Formation of secretory granules in the Golgi complex. (4) Transport of secretory granules to the plasma membrane, fusion with the plasma membrane, and exocytosis resulting in the release of granule contents into the extracellular space. Notice that secretion may occur by transport of secretory vesicles and immature granules or by transport of mature granules. Some granules are taken up and hydrolyzed by lysosomes (crinophagy). Golgi, Golgi complex; SER, smooth endoplasmic reticulum. (From Habener JF. Hormone biosynthesis and secretion. In: Felig P, Baxter JD, Broadus AE, et al, eds. *Endocrinol Metab.* New York, NY: McGraw-Hill, 1981:29-59.)

polypeptide hormones is specifically designed for export from the cell.

This process of directional transport of proteins involves sophisticated informational signals. Because the information for these translocation processes must reside wholly or in part within the primary structure or in the conformational properties of the protein, sequential post-translational modifications may be crucial for determining the specificity of protein function. Continued investigations of protein sorting and trafficking in cells have revealed increased complexities beyond the simple paradigm illustrated in Figure 3-5.[11] Sequential sorting of proteins to their final destinations, whether they are exported (secreted) from the cells or targeted to a subcellular compartment or organelle, takes place not only in the Golgi apparatus but before then in the ER, and afterward in endosomes and tubulosaccules.[12] Each of the approximately 5000 proteins expressed in a given cell contains a specific targeting signal that is responsible for directing the protein to its final destination. These targeting signals consist of short stretches of amino acids in the proteins that serve as molecular "ZIP codes" to ensure their accurate delivery. Modern approaches using proteomics and bioinformatics can predict localization of proteins in cells based on the characteristics of these targeting signals.[13]

Signal Sequences in Peptide Prohormone Processing and Secretion

The early processes of protein secretion that result in the specific transport of exported proteins into the secretory pathway have become better understood.[6,10-15] Initial clues to this process came from determinations of the amino acid sequences of the proteins programmed by the cell-free translation of mRNAs encoding secreted polypeptides.[16] Secreted proteins are synthesized as precursors that are extended at their N-termini by sequences of 15 to 30 amino acids, called *signal* or *leader sequences*. Signal sequence extensions or their functional equivalents are required for targeting the ribosomal or nascent protein to specific membranes and for vectorial transport of the protein across the membrane of the ER.

On emergence of the signal sequence from the large ribosomal subunit, the ribosomal complex specifically makes contact with the membrane; this results in translocation of the nascent polypeptide across the ER membrane into the cisterna as the first step in its secretory pathway. These observations initially left unanswered the question of how specific polyribosomes that translate mRNAs encoding secretory proteins recognize and attach to the ER (Fig. 3-6). Because microsomal membranes in vitro reproduce the processing activity of intact cells, it was possible to identify the macromolecules responsible for processing precursors and for translocation activities.[17] The ER and the cytoplasm contain an aggregate of molecules, called a *signal recognition particle complex,* that consists of at least 16 proteins, including three guanosine triphosphatases to generate energy[18] and a 7S RNA.[6,10,19,20] This complex, or particle, binds to the polyribosomes involved in the translation of mRNAs encoding secretory polypeptides when the N-terminal signal sequence first emerges from the large subunit of the ribosome.

The specific interaction of the signal recognition particle with the nascent signal sequence and the polyribosome arrests further translation of mRNA. The nascent protein remains in a state of arrested translation until it finds a high-affinity binding protein on the ER, the signal recognition particle receptor or docking protein.[6] On interaction with the specific docking protein, the translational block is released, and protein synthesis resumes. The protein is then transferred across the membrane of the ER through a proteinaceous tunnel called the *translocon.*[20]

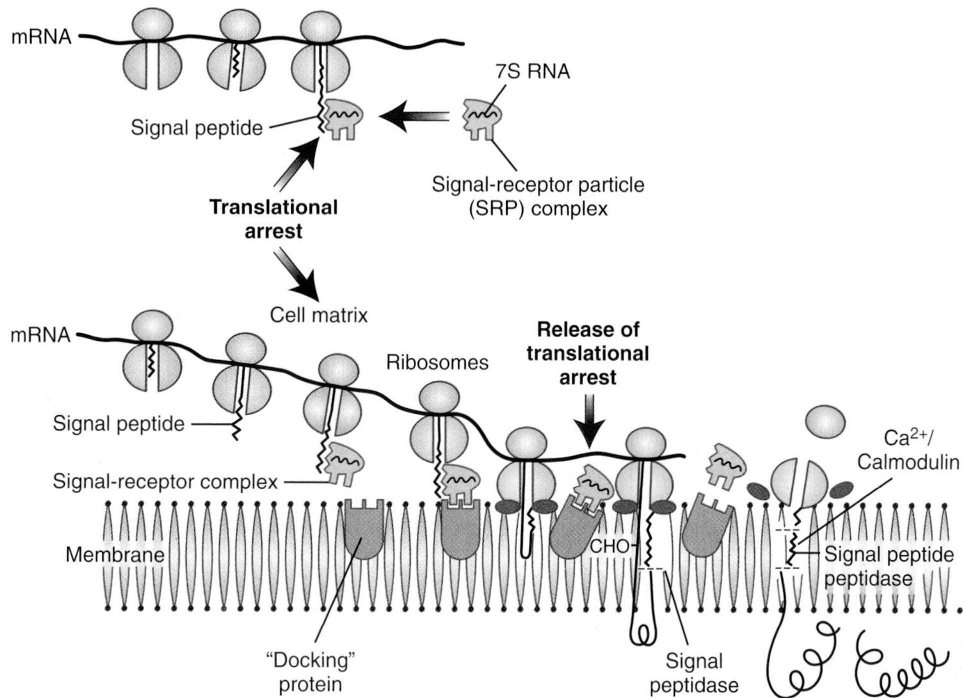

Figure 3-6 Cellular events in the initial stages of synthesis of a polypeptide hormone according to the signal hypothesis. In this schema, a signal recognition particle, consisting of a complex of six proteins and an RNA (7S RNA), interacts with the amino-terminal signal peptide of the nascent polypeptide chain after approximately 70 amino acids are polymerized, arresting further growth of the polypeptide chain. The complex of the signal recognition particle and the polyribosome nascent chain remains in a state of translational arrest until it recognizes and binds to a docking protein, which is a receptor protein located on the cytoplasmic face of the endoplasmic reticular membrane. This interaction of the signal recognition particle complex with the docking protein releases the translational block, and protein synthesis resumes. The nascent polypeptide chain is discharged across the membrane bilayer into the cisterna of the endoplasmic reticulum and is released from the signal peptide by cleavage with a signal peptidase located in the cisternal face of the membrane. In this model, the signal peptide is cleaved from the polypeptide chain by signal peptidase before the chain is completed (i.e., cotranslational cleavage). The configuration of the polypeptide during transport across the membrane and the forces and mechanisms responsible for its translocation are unknown. The loop, or hairpin, configuration of the chain shown here is an arbitrary model; other models are equally possible.

At some point, near the termination of synthesis of the polypeptide chain, the N-terminal signal sequence is cleaved from the polypeptide by a specific signal peptidase located on the cisternal surface of the ER membrane. Removal of the hydrophobic signal sequence frees the protein (prohormone or hormone) so that it may assume its characteristic secondary structure during transport through the ER and the Golgi apparatus. After cleavage from the protein by a signal peptidase, the signal peptide may sometimes be further cleaved in the ER membrane to produce a biologically active peptide. For example, the signal sequence of preprolactin, comprising 30 amino acids, is cleaved by a signal peptide peptidase to yield a charged peptide of 20 amino acids that is released into the cytosol, where it binds to calmodulin and inhibits Ca^{2+}-calmodulin–dependent phosphodiesterase.[21]

This sequence in the directional transport of specific polypeptides ensures optimal cotranslational processing of secretory proteins, even when synthesis commences on free ribosomes. The presence of a cytoplasmic form of the signal recognition particle complex that blocks translation guarantees that the synthesis of the presecretory proteins is not completed in the cytoplasm; the efficient transfer of proteins occurs only after contact has been made with the specific receptor or docking protein on the membrane. Although the presence of signal recognition particles and docking proteins explains the specificity of the binding of ribosomes containing mRNAs encoding the secretory proteins, it does not explain the mode of translocation of the nascent polypeptide chain across the membrane bilayer. Further dissection and analysis of the membrane have identified other macromolecules that are responsible for the transport process.[6]

Cellular Processing of Prohormones

The signal sequences of prehormones and pre-prohormones are involved in the transport of these molecules, but the function of the intermediate hormone precursors (i.e., prohormones) is not fully understood. Conversion of prohormones to their final products begins in the Golgi apparatus. For example, the time that elapses between the synthesis of pre-proparathyroid hormone and the first appearance of parathyroid hormone correlates closely with the time required for radioautographic grains to reach the Golgi apparatus.[22] Similarly, conversion of proinsulin to insulin takes place about 1 hour after the synthesis of proinsulin is complete, and processing of proinsulin to insulin and C peptide takes place during the transport within the secretory granule.[23] The conversion of prohormones to hormones can also be blocked by inhibitors of cellular energy production such as antimycin A and dinitrophenol[24] and by drugs that interfere with the functions of microtubules (e.g., vinblastine, colchicine).[25] Translocation of the prohormone from the rough ER to the Golgi complex depends on metabolic energy and probably involves microtubules.

There is no evidence that sequences specific to the prohormone contribute to or are chemically involved in transport of the newly synthesized protein from the rough ER to the Golgi apparatus, nor that they are involved in the packaging of the hormone in vesicles or granules. Analyses of the structures of the primary products of translation of mRNAs encoding secretory proteins indicate that many of these are not synthesized in the form of prohormone intermediates (see Fig. 3-3). It remains puzzling that some secretory proteins (e.g., parathyroid hormone, insulin, serum albumin) are formed by way of intermediate precursors, whereas others (e.g., GH, prolactin, albumin) are not.

Size constraints may be placed on the length of a secretory polypeptide. When the bioactivity of peptides resides at the carboxyl-termini of the precursors (e.g., somatostatin, calcitonin, gastrin), N-terminal extensions may be required to provide a sufficient "spacer" sequence to allow the signal sequence on the growing nascent polypeptide chain to emerge from the large ribosome subunit for interaction with the signal recognition particle and to provide adequate polypeptide length to span the large ribosomal subunit and the membrane of the ER during vectorial transport of the nascent polypeptide across the membrane (see Fig. 3-6). If the final hormonal product is 100 amino acids long or longer (e.g., GH, prolactin, the α- and β-subunits of the glycoprotein hormones), there may be no requirement for a prohormone intermediate.

Although the exact functions of prohormones remain unknown, certain details of their cleavages have been established. Unlike the situation with prehormones, in which the amino acids at the cleavage site between the signal sequence and the remainder of the molecule (hormone or prohormone) vary from one hormone to the next, the cleavage sites of the prohormone intermediates consist of the basic amino acid lysine or arginine, or both, usually two to three in tandem. This sequence is preferentially cleaved by endopeptidases with trypsin-like activities.

The family of prohormone-converting (PC) enzymes consists of at least eight specific members.[26-28] The most studied of the isozymes are PC2 and PC1/3, which are responsible for the cleavages of proinsulin between the A chain/C peptide and the B chain/C peptide, respectively. A rare patient missing PC1 presented with childhood obesity, hypogonadotropic hypogonadism, and hypercortisolism and was found to have elevated proinsulin levels and presumably widespread abnormalities in neuropeptide modification.[29] Targeted disruption of the PC2 gene in mice resulted in incomplete processing of proinsulin, leaving the A chain and C peptide intact.[30] Proglucagon in the pancreas remained incompletely processed, indicating that PC2 is required for the formation of glucagon. As a consequence of defective PC2 activity and low levels of glucagon, the mice had severe chronic hypoglycemia.

After endopeptidase cleavage, the remaining basic residues are selectively removed by exopeptidases with activity resembling that of carboxypeptidase B. When the C-terminal residue of the peptide hormone is amidated, a process that appears to enhance the stability of a peptide by conferring resistance to carboxypeptidase, specific amidation enzymes (i.e., peptide amidating monooxygenases) in the Golgi complex work in concert with the cleavage enzymes to modify the C-termini of the bioactive peptides.[31,32]

All proproteins and prohormones are cleaved by PC enzymatic processes within the Golgi complex of cells of diverse origins. The significance of specific cleavages of specific prohormones remains incompletely understood, as does the reason for the existence of prohormone intermediates in some but not all secretory proteins. Precursor peptides removed from the prohormones may have intrinsic biologic activities that are still unrecognized.

PROCESSES OF HORMONE SECRETION

Specific extracellular stimuli control the secretion of polypeptide hormones. These stimuli consist of changes in homeostatic balance; the hormonal products released in response to the stimuli act on the respective target organs to reestablish homeostasis (Fig. 3-7). Endocrine systems typically consist of closed-loop feedback mechanisms; if hormones from organ A stimulate organ B, organ B secretes hormones that inhibit the secretion of hormones from organ A. The concerted actions of positive and negative hormonal influences thereby maintain homeostasis. An example of negative feedback regulation is the control of the secretion of adrenocorticotropic hormone (ACTH) by the anterior pituitary gland. An increased ACTH level stimulates the adrenal cortex to produce and secrete cortisol, which suppresses further pituitary secretion of ACTH. These regulatory processes may include feedback loops in which nonhormonal substances controlled by the target organs regulate hormone secretion. For example, an increase in the concentration of plasma electrolytes as a

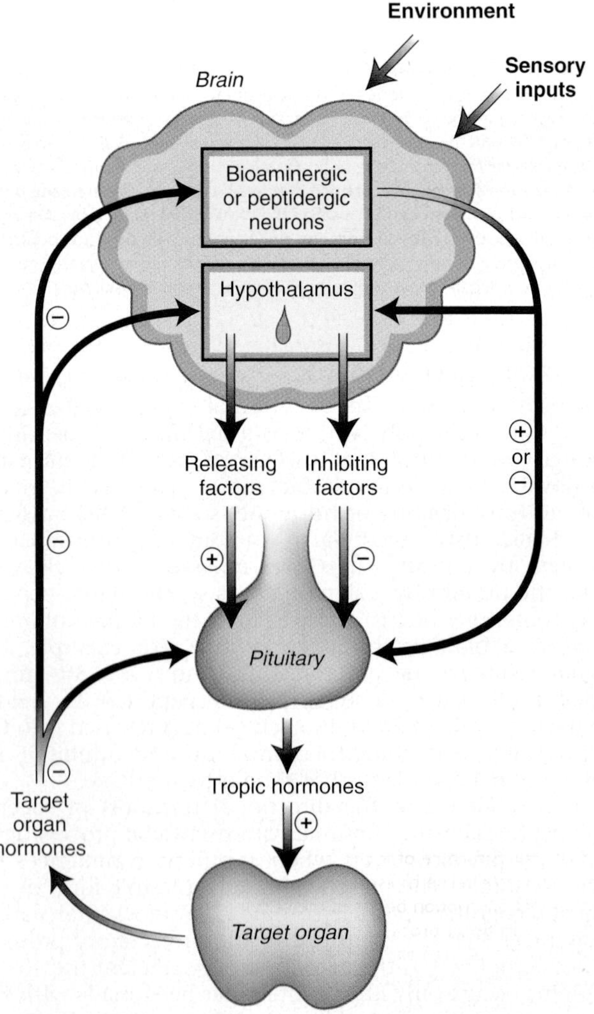

Figure 3-7 Regulatory feedback loops of the hypothalamic-pituitary–target organ axis. As combinations of stimulatory and inhibitory factors, hormones often act in concert to maintain homeostatic balance in the presence of physiologic or pathophysiologic perturbations. The concerted actions of hormones typically establish closed feedback loops by stimulatory and inhibitory effects coupled to maintain homeostasis.

consequence of dehydration stimulates the release of arginine vasopressin (antidiuretic hormone) in the neural lobe of the pituitary gland, and vasopressin in turn acts on the kidney to increase reabsorption of water from the renal tubule, thereby readjusting serum electrolyte concentrations toward normal levels.

In many instances, endocrine regulation is complex and involves the responses of several endocrine glands and their respective target organs. After a meal, the release of a dozen or more hormones is triggered as a result of gastric distention, variations in the pH of the contents of the stomach and duodenum, and increased concentrations of glucose, fatty acids, and amino acids in the blood. The rise in plasma glucose and amino acid levels stimulates the release of insulin and the incretin hormones glucagon-like peptide 1 and glucose-dependent insulinotropic peptide and suppresses the release of glucagon from the pancreas. Both effects promote the net uptake of glucose by the liver: insulin increases cellular transport and uptake of glucose, and the lower blood levels of glucagon decrease the outflow of glucose because of diminished rates of glycogenolysis and gluconeogenesis.

STRUCTURE OF A GENE ENCODING A POLYPEPTIDE HORMONE

Structural analyses of gene sequences have resulted in at least three major discoveries that are important for understanding the expression of peptide-encoding genes. First, sequences of almost all of the known biologically active hormonal peptides are contained within larger precursors that often encode other peptides, many of which are of unknown biologic activity. Second, the transcribed regions of genes (called *exons*) are interrupted by sequences (called *introns*) that are transcribed but subsequently cleaved from the initial RNA transcripts during their nuclear processing and assembly into specific mRNAs. Third, specific regulatory sequences reside in the regions of DNA flanking the structural genes and within introns, and these DNA sequences constitute specific targets for the interactions of DNA-binding proteins that determine the level of expression of the gene.

The DNA of higher organisms is wound around proteins, forming tightly and regularly packed chromosomal structures called *nucleosomes*.[33,34] Nucleosomes are composed of four or five different histone subunits that form a core structure about which approximately 140 base pairs of genomic DNA are wound. The nucleosomes are arranged similarly to beads on a string, and coils of nucleosomes form the fundamental organizational units of the eukaryotic chromosome. The nucleosomal structure serves several purposes. For example, nucleosomes enable the large amount of DNA (approximately 2×10^9 base pairs) included in the genome to be compacted into a small volume. Nucleosomes are involved in the replication of DNA and gene transcription. In addition to histones, other proteins are associated with DNA, and the complex nucleoprotein structure provides specific recognition sites for regulatory proteins and enzymes involved in DNA replication, rearrangements of DNA segments, and gene expression. The processes of acetylation, deacetylation, methylation, and demethylation of histones that are enriched in chromatin are implicated in the regulation of gene transcription (see "Epigenetic Inheritance of Phenotypic Traits").

The histones of open-configured chromatin (i.e., euchromatin) are heavily acetylated and methylated; this loosens their association with DNA and allows the access of transcription factors to the promoter regions of expressed genes. Conversely, the histones of closed chromatin (i.e., heterochromatin) are underacetylated and undermethylated, adhere tightly to DNA, and prevent access of transcription factors to the promoters of transcriptionally silent genes.

A typical protein-encoding gene consists of two functional units (Fig. 3-8). One is a transcriptional region, and the other is a promoter or regulatory region.

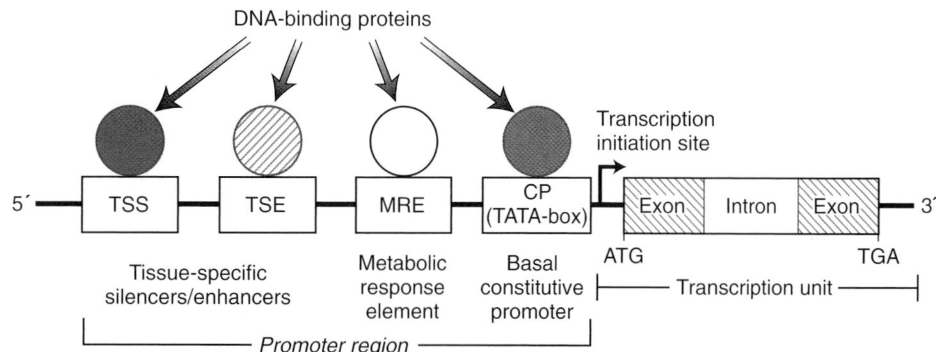

Figure 3-8 Structure of a consensus gene encoding a prototypical polypeptide hormone. A consensus gene typically consists of a promoter region and a transcription unit. The transcription unit is the region of DNA composed of exons and introns that is transcribed into a messenger ribonucleic acid (mRNA) precursor. Transcription begins at the cap site sequence in DNA and extends several hundred bases beyond the poly(A) addition site in the 3′ region. During post-transcriptional processing of the RNA precursor, the 5′ end of mRNA is capped by the addition of methylguanosine residues. The transcript is then cleaved at the poly(A) addition site approximately 20 bases 3′ to the AATAAA signal sequence, and the poly(A) tract is added to the 3′ end of the RNA. Introns are cleaved from the RNA precursor, and exons are joined together. Dinucleotides GT and AG are invariably found at the 5′ and 3′ ends of introns. Translation of mRNA starts with the codon ATG for methionine. Translation is terminated when the polyribosome reaches the stop codon TGA, TAA, or TAG. The promoter region of the gene located 5′ to the cap site contains numerous short regulatory DNA sequences that are targets for interactions with specific DNA-binding proteins. These sequences consist of the basal constitutive promoter (TATA box), metabolic response elements that modulate transcription (e.g., in response to cyclic adenosine monophosphate [cAMP], steroid hormone receptors, or thyroid hormone receptors), and tissue-specific enhancers and silencers that respectively permit or prevent transcription of the gene. The enhancer and silencer elements direct expression of specific subsets of genes to cells of a given phenotype. Whether a gene is or is not expressed in a particular cellular phenotype depends on complex interactions of the various DNA-binding proteins among themselves and, most importantly, with the TATA box proteins of the basal constitutive promoter.

Transcriptional Regions

The transcriptional unit is the segment of the gene that is transcribed into an mRNA precursor. The sequences corresponding to the mature mRNA consist of the exon sequences that are spliced from the primary transcript during cotranscriptional and post-transcriptional processing of the precursor RNA. These exons contain the code for the mRNA sequence that is translated into protein and for untranslated sequences at the 5′ and 3′ flanking regions. The 5′ sequence typically begins with a methylated guanine residue known as the *cap site*. The 3′ untranslated region contains within it a short sequence, AATAAA, that signals the site of cleavage of the 3′ end of the RNA and the addition of a poly(A) tract of 100 to 200 nucleotides located approximately 20 bases from the AATAAA sequence. Although the functions of these modifications of the ends of mRNAs are not completely understood, they appear to provide signals for leaving the nucleus; to enhance stability, perhaps by providing resistance to degradation by exonucleases; and to stimulate initiation of mRNA translation. The protein-coding sequence of the mRNA begins with the codon AUG for methionine and ends with the codon immediately preceding one of the three nonsense, or stop, codons: UGA, UAA, and UAG.

The nature of the enzymatic splicing mechanisms that result in excision of intron-coded sequences and rejoining of exon-coded sequences is incompletely understood. Helpful interpretations of the splicing processes have been provided in recent reviews.[35,36] Short "consensus" sequences of nucleotides reside at the splice junctions; for example, the bases GT and AG at the 5′ and 3′ ends of the introns, respectively, are invariant, and a polypyrimidine stretch is found near the AG.[37] Splicing involves a series of cleavage and ligation steps that remove the introns as a lariat structure, with its 5′ end ligated near the 3′ end of the introns, and ligate the two adjacent exons together. The spliceosome, an elaborate mechanism consisting of five *small nuclear RNAs* (snRNAs) and roughly 50 proteins, directs these steps, guided by base pairing between three of the snRNAs and the mRNA precursor.

Regulatory Regions

The molecular mechanisms involved in regulating the expression of genes that encode polypeptides are becoming understood in some detail. Some experiments have deleted certain 5′ sequence segments that reside upstream from structural genes and then analyzed the expression of those genes after their introduction into cell lines. These regulatory sequences, called *promoter* and *enhancer* regions, consist of short polynucleotide sequences (see Fig. 3-8). They can be divided into at least four groups with respect to their functions and distance from the transcriptional initiation site.

First, the sequence *TATAA* (TATA box or Goldberg-Hogness box) is usually present in the more proximal promoter within 25 to 30 nucleotides upstream from the point of transcriptional initiation. The TATA sequence is required to ensure the accuracy of initiation of transcription at a particular site. The TATA box directs the binding of a complex of several proteins, including RNA polymerase II. The proteins, referred to as *TATA box transcription factors*, number six or more basal factors (IIA, IIB, IID, IIE, IIF, IIH); along with RNA polymerase II, they form the general or basal transcriptional machinery required for the initiation of RNA synthesis.[38-40]

The other three groups of regulatory sequences are the *tissue-specific silencers* (TSSs), which function by binding repressor proteins; the *tissue-specific enhancers* (TSEs), which are activated by the binding of transcriptional activator proteins; and the *metabolic response elements* (MREs), which are regulated by the binding of specialized proteins whose transcriptional (repressor or activator) activities are determined by metabolic signaling that often involves changes in their phosphorylation status.

Introns and Exons

Genes encoding proteins and ribosomal RNAs in eukaryotes are interrupted by intervening DNA sequences (i.e., introns) that separate them into coding blocks (i.e., exons).[35,36,41] In bacterial genes, the nucleotide sequences of the chromosomal genes match precisely the corresponding sequences in the mRNAs. Interruption of the continuity of genetic information appears to be unique to nucleated cells. The reasons for such interruptions are not completely understood, but introns appear to separate exons into functional domains with respect to the proteins that they encode. An example is the gene for proglucagon, a precursor of glucagon in which five introns separate six exons, three of which encode glucagon and the two glucagon-related peptides contained within the precursor (Fig. 3-9).[42] A second example is the GH gene, which is divided into five exons by four introns that separate the promoter region of the gene from the protein-coding region and divide the latter into three partly homologous repeated segments, two of which code for the growth-promoting activity of the hormone and the third for its carbohydrate metabolic functions.[43] As a rule, the genes for the precursors of hormones and regulatory peptides contain introns that are located at or about the region where signal peptides join the apoproteins or prohormones and thus separate the signal sequences from the components of the precursor that are exported from the cell as hormones or peptides.

There are exceptions to the "one exon, one function" theory in mammalian cells. The genes of several precursors of peptide hormones are not interrupted by introns in a manner that corresponds to separation of the functional components of the precursor. For example, the precursor pro-opiomelanocortin (POMC) is cleaved during post-translational processing to produce the peptides ACTH, α-melanocyte–stimulating hormone, and β-endorphin, but the protein-coding region of the *POMC* gene is devoid of introns. Likewise, no introns interrupt the protein-coding region of the gene for the proenkephalin precursor, which contains seven copies of the enkephalin sequences. It is possible that introns separated each of these coding domains in the past and were lost during the course of evolution.

A precedent for the selective loss of introns appears to be exemplified by the rat insulin genes. The rat genome harbors two nonallelic insulin genes, one containing two introns and the other containing a single intron. The most likely explanation is that an ancestral gene containing two introns was transcribed into RNA and spliced, after which that RNA was copied back into DNA by a cellular reverse transcriptase and inserted into the genome at a new site.

REGULATION OF GENE EXPRESSION

Regulation of expression of genes encoding polypeptide hormones can take place at one or more levels in the pathway of hormone biosynthesis[44-46] (Fig. 3-10): DNA synthesis (cell growth and division), transcription,

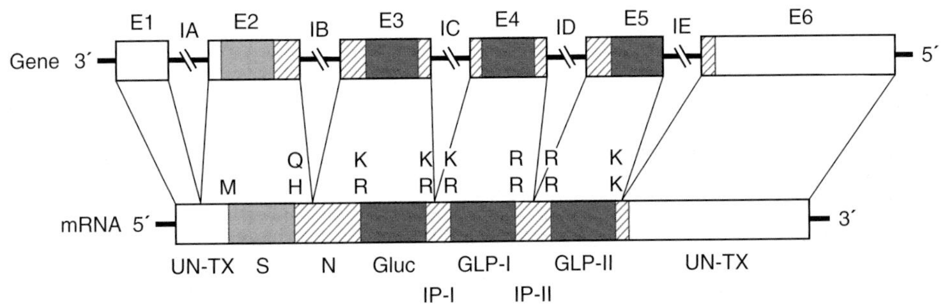

Figure 3-9 The pancreatic glucagon gene and its encoded messenger RNA (mRNA): complementary DNA. In the glucagon gene, exons precisely encode separate functional domains. The gene consists of six exons (E1 through E6) and five introns (1A through 1E). The mRNA encoding pre-proglucagon, the protein precursor of glucagon, consists of 10 specific regions: from left to right, a 5′ untranslated sequence (UN-TX, *open*), a signal sequence (S, *stippled*), an amino-terminal extension sequence (N, *hatched*), glucagon (Gluc, *shaded*), a first intervening peptide (IP-I, *hatched*), a first glucagon-like peptide (GLP-I, *shaded*), a second intervening peptide (IP-II, *hatched*), a second glucagon-like peptide (GLP-II, *shaded*), a dilysyl dipeptide (*hatched*) after the GLP-II sequence, and an untranslated region (UN-TX, *open*). Exons from left to right encode the 5′ untranslated region, signal sequence, glucagon, GLP-I, GLP-II, and 3′ untranslated sequence. Letters shown above the mRNA denote amino acids located at positions in the pre-proglucagon molecule that are cleaved during cellular processing of the precursor. The amino acid methionine (M) marks the initiation of translation of mRNA into pre-proglucagon. H, histidine; K, lysine; Q, glutamine; R, arginine.

post-transcriptional processing of mRNA, translation, or post-translational processing. In different endocrine cells, one or more levels may serve as specific control points for regulation of the production of a hormone (see "Biologic Diversification").

Levels of Gene Control

Newly synthesized prolactin transcripts are formed within minutes after exposure of a prolactin-secreting cell line to TRH.[47] Cortisol has been demonstrated to stimulate GH synthesis in somatotropic cell lines and in pituitary slices through increases in rates of gene transcription and enhancement of the stability of mRNA.[48,49] The time required for cortisol to enhance transcription of the GH gene is 1 to 2 hours, which is considerably longer than the time required for the action of TRH on prolactin gene transcription. Regulation of proinsulin biosynthesis appears to take place primarily at the level of translation.[50,51] Within minutes after the plasma glucose level is raised, the rate of proinsulin biosynthesis increases 5- to 10-fold. Glucose acts directly or indirectly to enhance the efficiency of initiation of translation of proinsulin mRNA.[52]

Rapid metabolic regulation at the level of post-transcriptional processing of mRNA precursors has not been clearly established. However, alternative exon splicing plays a major role in the regulation of the formation of mRNAs during development (see "Biologic Diversification"). For example, the primary RNA transcripts derived from the calcitonin gene are alternatively spliced to provide two or more tissue-specific mRNAs that encode chimeric protein precursors with both common and different amino acid sequences, indicating that regulation takes place at the level of processing of the calcitonin gene transcripts.

In many instances, the level of gene expression under regulatory control is optimal for meeting the secretory and biosynthetic demands of the endocrine organ. For example, after a meal, there is an immediate requirement for the release of large amounts of insulin. This release depletes insulin stores of the pancreatic beta cells within a few minutes, but mechanisms that increase the translational

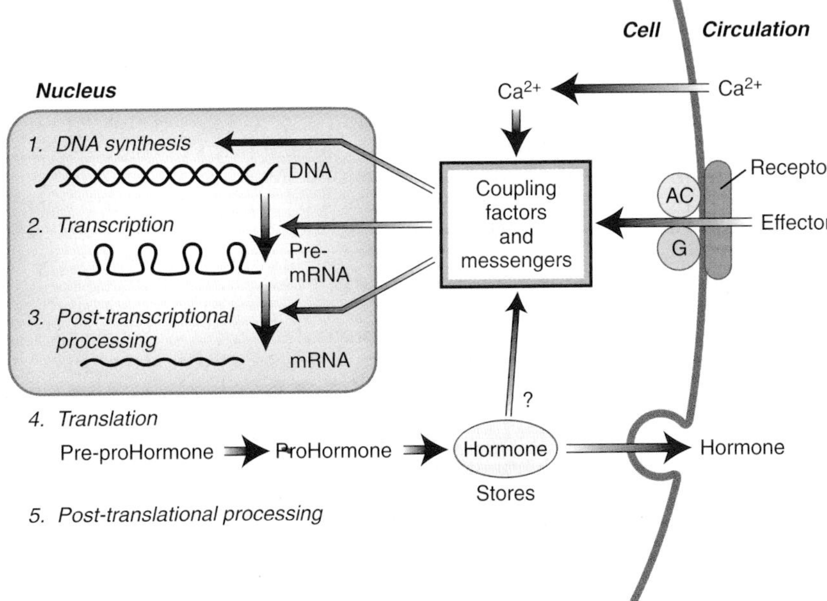

Figure 3-10 Potential control points in an endocrine cell for regulation of gene expression during hormone production. Specific effector substances bind to plasma membrane receptors (peptide effectors) or to cytosolic or nuclear receptors (steroids), which leads to initiation of a series of events that couple the effector signal with gene expression. Peptide effector–receptor complex interactions act initially through activation of adenylate cyclase (AC) coupled with a guanosine triphosphate–binding protein (G). Coupling factors and substances such as glucose, cyclic adenosine monophosphate, and cations activate protein kinases, resulting in a series of phosphorylations of macromolecules. Specific effectors for various endocrine cells appear to act at one or more of the indicated five levels of gene expression (see text for details), with the possible exception of post-translational processing of prohormones, for which no definite examples of metabolic regulation have yet been found.

efficiency of preformed proinsulin mRNA rapidly provide additional hormone.

Tissue-Specific Gene Expression

Differentiated cells have a remarkable capacity for selective expression of specific genes. In one cell type, a single gene may account for a large fraction of the total gene expression, and in another cell type, the same gene may be expressed at undetectable levels.

When a gene can be expressed in a particular cell type, the associated chromatin is loosely arranged; when the same gene is never expressed in a particular cell type, the chromatin organization is more compact. DNA within the chromatin of expressed genes is more susceptible to cleavage by deoxyribonuclease than is the DNA in tissues in which the genes are quiescent.[53-55] Chromatin looseness may facilitate access of RNA polymerase to the gene for purposes of transcription. Inactive genes appear to have a higher content of methylated cytosine residues than the same genes in tissues in which they are expressed.[56,57]

Determinants for the tissue-specific transcriptional expression of genes exist in control sequences that usually reside within 1000 base pairs of the 5′-flanking region of the transcriptional sequence. Enhancer sequences in animal cell genes were first described for immunoglobulin genes, a finding that extended the earlier observations of enhancer control elements in viral genomes.[58] Historically, the first clear demonstrations of these elements directing transcription to cells of distinct phenotypes came from studies of the comparative expression of two model genes, insulin and chymotrypsin, in the endocrine and exocrine pancreas, respectively.[59] The restricted expression of genes in a cell-specific manner is determined by the assembly of specific combinations of DNA-binding proteins on a predetermined array of control elements of the promoter regions of genes to create a transcriptionally active complex of proteins that includes the components of the general or basal transcriptional apparatus.

Epigenetic Inheritance of Phenotypic Traits

Darwinian selection is the generally recognized mechanism by which changes in the nucleotide sequences of genes result in patterns of gene expression that allow the resultant phenotype to better survive in a changing environment. These changes in gene sequences that lead to prosurvival phenotypes occur gradually, over hundreds of generations spanning thousands of years of evolution. However, genomic changes in gene expression in response to environmental changes may occur during development within a single generation by epigenetic mechanisms, independently of any nucleotide sequence changes in the DNA.[60] *Epigenetics* refers to the inheritable phenotypic changes that do not involve alterations in DNA, a nongenetic memory of gene expression functions imparted by environmental cues. Epigenetics defines a nongenetic memory of function that is transmitted from cellular generation to generation.[61] The mechanism of epigenetic memory is beginning to be understood. It involves chromatin modifications—both modifications of cytosines in DNA and post-translational modifications of proteins that collectively define the structure of chromatin.

Broadly speaking, chromatin exists in two configurations that determine whether the involved genes are expressed (active) or are repressed (silent). The two configurations are densely packed *heterochromatin,* in which gene transcription is silent, and *euchromatin,* in which DNA and proteins are loosely gathered, allowing access of transcription factors to DNA promoters of genes and active transcription. The protein components of chromatin consist of histones and nonhistone proteins.

The key to epigenetic memory, the collective state of expressed or repressed genes in the genome, lies with the methylation of DNA and the post-translational modifications of histones, predominantly by acetylation and methylation. These modifications are interpreted by an elaborate series of protein complexes that change the structure of chromatin and the activity of genes.[62] The methylation of cytosines in DNA in the configuration of CpG sequences (*CpG islands*), represses gene transcription by impairing productive interactions of transcription factors with DNA promoter sequences. Histones can be grouped into four major classes: H2A, H2B, H3, and H4. Histones carry a strong positive charge because of their large content of the amino acids lysine and arginine. They bind firmly to negatively charged nucleic acids and phosphates of DNA, form heterochromatin, and thereby repress gene expression. The covalently modified histones bind to specific effector proteins that recognize them. Attachment of hydrophobic side chains to the positively charged lysines (and arginines) of histones reduces the positive charge and loosens binding to DNA. Such side chain modifications include acetylation, methylation, ADP-ribosylation, sumoylation, phosphorylation, and ubiquitination. Acetylation and methylation are predominant mechanisms of histone modification. DNA methylation is regulated by a family of cytosine-directed methylases and demethylases. Methylation and acetylation of histones is mediated by methyl and acetyl transferases, demethylases, and deacetylases.

The effects of DNA methylation and histone acetylation and methylation on gene expression are complex. DNA methylation usually is associated with gene silencing, histone acetylation with gene activation, and histone methylation with either silencing or activation. DNA methylation and histone methylation may bidirectionally regulate each other. For example, DNA methylation induces methylation of lysine 8 of histone 3 (H3K9), and, conversely, methylation of H3K9 enhances DNA methylation. Both DNA methylation and H3K9 methylation repress transcription, so they reinforce each other in silencing genes. These changes in chromatin modifications are durable; they can be passed from parent to daughter cells during cell division and, to some extent, can remain during meiosis. In this way, patterns of gene expression imparted by environmental influences are preserved during cell growth and reproduction.

An example of environmentally induced epigenetic modification of gene expression that is reflected in a modified disease phenotype is the remarkable reprogramming of the genome that takes place in utero in rat embryos subjected to nutrient deprivation by partial ligation of the uterine artery during the last 3 days of gestation (days 19 to 22).[63] The late prenatal, nutrient-deprived pups go on to progressively develop obesity, insulin resistance, severe diabetes, and premature death. Biochemical studies of the affected nutrient-deprived progeny show that key genes involved in insulin secretion and sensitivity are repressed by the transient nutrient deprivation. For example, mRNA levels for the transcription factor PDX1, which is critical for pancreatic beta cell growth and insulin production, is reduced as early as 24 hours after growth retardation, and histone H3 in the chromatin of the PDX1 promoter is hypomethylated on lysine 4 and hypoacetylated on lysine 9, defining a heterochromatin configuration and gene silencing. The growth and functions of beta cells are curtailed by the nutrient deprivation to produce less insulin, because less insulin is needed and excessive insulin would be deleterious to the embryo. Likewise, the histones associated with the promoters of the liver genes *PPARGC1A* (formerly called PGC1A), which is involved in gluconeogenesis, and *CPT1A*, which is involved in fatty acid oxidation, are hyperacetylated, resulting in activation of these genes and loss of insulin regulation of glucose use and oxidation (i.e., insulin resistance).

The mechanisms by which acetylases, methylases, deacetylases, and demethylases are regulated remain unknown. One possibility is that intermediary metabolites formed in response to nutrient deprivation, such as acetyl coenzyme A, nicotinamide adenine dinucleotide, and *S*-adenosyl methionine, may modulate the relative activities of these important enzymes.

Transcription Factors in Developmental Organogenesis of Endocrine Systems

Certain families of transcription factors are critical for organogenesis and the development of the body plan. Among these are the homeodomain proteins[64] and the nuclear receptor proteins.[65-67] The family of homeotic selector, or homeodomain, proteins is highly conserved throughout the animal kingdom from flies to humans. The orchestrated spatial and temporal expression of these proteins and the target genes that they activate determine the orderly development of the body plan of specific tissues, limbs, and organs. Similarly, the actions of families of nuclear receptors (e.g., steroid hormones, thyroid hormones, retinoic acid) are critical for normal development. Inactivating mutations in the genes encoding these essential transcription factors predictably result in loss or impairment of the development of the specific target organ.

This section describes three examples of impaired organogenesis attributable to mutations in essential transcription factors: partial anterior pituitary agenesis (POU1F1), pancreatic agenesis (PDX1), and adrenal and gonadal agenesis (SF1 and NROB1/DAX1).

Partial Pituitary Agenesis

The transcription factor POU1F1, formerly called Pit-1, is a member of the POU family of homeodomain proteins.[68] POU1F1 is a key transcriptional activator of the promoters of the genes that encode GH, prolactin, and thyroid-stimulating hormone-β, which are produced in the anterior pituitary somatotrophs, lactotrophs, and thyrotrophs, respectively. POU1F1 is also the major enhancer activating factor for the promoter of the growth hormone–releasing factor receptor gene.[69] Mutations in POU1F1 that impair its DNA-binding and transcriptional activation functions are responsible for the phenotype of the Jackson and Snell dwarf mice.[68]

Mutations in the *POU1F1* gene have been found in patients with combined pituitary hormone deficiency, a condition in which there is no production of GH, prolactin, or thyroid-stimulating hormone, which results in growth impairment and mental deficiency.[70] In these individuals, hormone production by the other two of the five cell types of the anterior pituitary gland (including production of ACTH and the gonadotropins luteinizing hormone and follicle-stimulating hormone) remains unaffected.[70] The mutated *POU1F1* can bind to its cognate DNA control elements but is defective in *trans*-activating gene transcription. Furthermore, it acts as a dominant negative inhibitor of the actions of *POU1F1* on the unaffected allele.

Pancreatic Agenesis

The homeodomain protein called *pancreas duodenum homeobox 1* or PDX1 (previously referred to as STF1, IDX1, or IPF1) appears to be responsible for the development and growth of the pancreas. Targeted disruption of the *Pdx1* gene in mice resulted in a phenotype of pancreatic agenesis.[71] A child born without a pancreas was shown to be homozygous for inactivating mutations in the *PDX1* gene.[72] Parents and ancestors who are heterozygous for the affected allele have a high incidence of type 2 diabetes mellitus, suggesting that a decrease in gene dosage of *PDX1* may predispose the individual to development of diabetes. The possibility that a mutated *PDX1* allele may be one of several "diabetes genes" is supported by the observation that PDX1 and the helix-loop-helix transcription factors E47 (TCF3) and β2 (TFB2M) appear to be key upregulators of the transcription of the insulin gene.[73]

Agenesis of the Adrenal Gland and Gonads

Two nuclear receptor transcription factors have been identified as critical for the development of the adrenal gland, the gonads, pituitary gonadotrophs, and the ventral medial hypothalamus. These nuclear receptors are SF1 (steroidogenic factor 1)[74] and NROB1 (also called DAX1, for *d*osage-sensitive sex reversal, *a*drenal hypoplasia congenita, *X* chromosome).[75] SF1 binds to half-sites of estrogen response elements that bind estrogen receptors in the promoters of genes. DAX1 binds to retinoic acid receptor (RAR) binding sites in promoters and inhibits RAR actions. Targeted disruption of SF1 in mice results in a phenotype of adrenal and gonadal agenesis. Pituitary gonadotrophs are absent, and the ventral medial hypothalamus is severely underdeveloped.[76,77]

Adrenal hypoplasia congenita is an X-linked developmental disorder of the human adrenal gland that is lethal if untreated. The gene responsible for adrenal hypoplasia congenita was identified by positional cloning and found to encode NROB1/DAX1, a member of the nuclear receptor proteins related to RAR.[75] Several inactivating mutations identified in the gene result in the syndrome of adrenal hypoplasia congenita and hypogonadotropic hypogonadism. Genetically defined and transmitted defects in the genes encoding the transcription factors SF1 and DAX1 result in profound arrest in the development of the target organs regulated by the hypothalamic-pituitary-adrenal axis involved in steroidogenesis: the adrenal gland (e.g., glucocorticoids, mineralocorticoids) and the gonads (e.g., estrogens, androgens).

Coupling of Effector Action to Cellular Response

Another mode of gene control consists of the induction and suppression of genes that are normally expressed in a specific tissue. These processes are at work in the minute-to-minute and day-to-day regulation of rates of production of the specific proteins produced by the cells (e.g., production of polypeptide hormones in response to extracellular stimuli).

At least two classes of signaling pathways—protein phosphorylation and activation of steroid hormone receptors by hormone binding—appear to be involved in the physiologic regulation of hormone gene expression. These two pathways mediate the actions of peptide and steroid hormones, respectively. Peptide ligands bind to receptor complexes on the plasma membrane, which results in enzyme activation, mobilization of calcium, formation of phosphorylated nucleotide intermediates, activation of protein kinases, and phosphorylation of specific regulatory proteins such as transcription factors (see Chapter 5).[77,79]

Because of their hydrophobic composition, steroidal compounds readily diffuse through the plasma membrane, bind to specific receptor proteins, and interact with other macromolecules in the nucleus, including specific domains on the chromatin located in and around the gene that is activated (see Chapter 4).[65-67] Calcium and phosphorylated nucleotides such as cyclic adenosine monophosphate (cAMP), adenosine triphosphate, and guanosine triphosphate appear to have important functions in secretory processes. In particular, fluxes of calcium from the extracellular fluid into the cell and from intracellular organelles (e.g., ER) into the cytosol are closely coupled to secretion.[80,81]

The many cellular signaling pathways that involve protein phosphorylations are complex. They typically consist of sequential phosphorylations and dephosphorylations of molecules, referred to as *protein kinase cascades* or *phosphatase cascades*.[82] These cascades are initiated by hormones, sensor molecules known as *ligands* that bind to and activate receptors located on the surface of cells, resulting in the generation of small second-messenger molecules such as cAMP, diacylglycerol, or calcium ions. These second messengers activate protein kinases that phosphorylate and thereby activate key target proteins (Fig. 3-11). The final step in the signaling pathways is the phosphorylation and activation of important transcription factors resulting in gene expression or repression.

The identities of some phosphoproteins have been elucidated. A specific group of transcription factors, DNA-binding proteins, interacts with cAMP-responsive and phorbol ester–responsive DNA elements to stimulate gene transcription mediated by the cAMP–protein kinase A, diacylglycerol–protein kinase C, and calcium-calmodulin signal transduction pathways (see Fig. 3-11). These proteins are encoded by a complex family of genes and bind to the DNA elements in the form of heterodimers or homodimers through a coiled-coil helical structure known as a *leucine zipper motif*.[83] Phosphorylation of these proteins modulates dimerization, DNA recognition and binding, and transcriptional *trans*-activation activities. Phosphorylation of the protein substrates may change their conformations and activate the proteins, which then interact with coactivator proteins such as the cAMP response element–binding (CREB) protein and the protein components of the basal transcriptional machinery, allowing RNA polymerase to initiate gene transcription.[84]

Second messengers activate serine/threonine kinases, which phosphorylate serine or threonine residues (or both) on proteins, whereas the receptor kinases are tyrosine-specific kinases that phosphorylate tyrosine residues.[82,85] Examples of receptor tyrosine kinases are growth factor receptors such as those for insulin, insulin-like growth factor (IGF), epidermal growth factor, and platelet-derived growth factor. Receptors in the cytokine receptor family, which include leptin, GH, and prolactin, activate associated tyrosine kinases in a variation on the theme.

The different types of signal transduction pathways are described as more or less distinct pathways for semantic purposes. In reality, there is considerable cross-talk among the different pathways that occur developmentally and in cell type–specific settings. An active area of research in endocrine systems is attempting to understand these complex interactions among different signal transduction pathways. Although the growth factor and cytokine receptors are similar in some respects, they differ in other respects. For example, growth factor receptor tyrosine kinases activate transcription factors through cascades that involve both tyrosine phosphorylation and serine/threonine kinases such as mitogen-activated protein kinases, whereas the Janus kinases (JAKs), activated by cytokine receptors, directly tyrosine phosphorylate the signal transducer and activator of transcription (STAT) factors.[85,86]

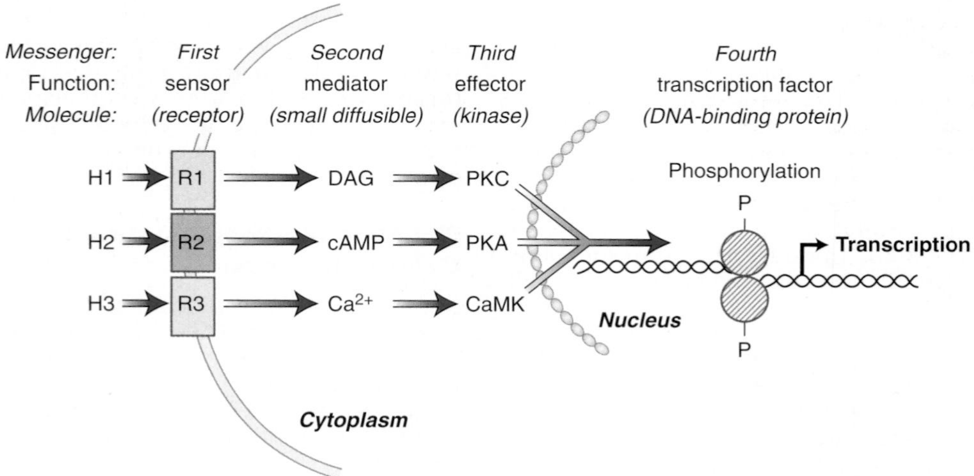

Figure 3-11 Three cell surface receptor–coupled signal transduction pathways involved in the activation of a superfamily of nuclear transcription factors. Peptide hormone molecules (H1, H2, and H3) interact with sensor receptors (R1, R2, and R3) coupled to the diacylglycerol (DAG)–protein kinase C (PKC), cyclic adenosine monophosphate (cAMP)–protein kinase A (PKA), and calcium-calmodulin pathways in which small, diffusible second-messenger molecules are generated (DAG, cAMP, and Ca^{2+}, respectively). The third messengers, or effector protein kinases, are generated and phosphorylate transcription factors such as members of the CREB/ATF and JUN/AP-1 families of DNA-binding proteins to modulate DNA-binding affinities or transcriptional activation, or both. The various proteins bind as dimers determined by a poorly understood code that is not promiscuous (i.e., only certain homodimer or heterodimer combinations are permissible). AP-1, activator protein 1; ATF, activating transcription factor; CaMK, calcium/calmodulin-dependent protein kinase; CREB, cAMP response element–binding protein.

BIOLOGIC DIVERSIFICATION

In addition to providing control points for the regulation of gene expression, the various steps involved in transfer of information encoded in the DNA of the gene to the final bioactive protein are a means for diversification of information stored in the gene (Fig. 3-12). Five steps in gene expression can be arbitrarily described: gene duplication and copy number, transcription, post-transcriptional RNA processing, translation, and post-translational processing.

Gene Duplications

At the level of DNA, diversification of genetic information comes about by way of gene duplication and amplification. Many of the polypeptide hormones are derived from families of multiple, structurally related genes. Examples include the growth hormone family (GH, prolactin, and placental lactogen), the glucagon family (glucagon, vasoactive intestinal peptide, secretin, gastric inhibitory peptide, and growth hormone–releasing hormone), and the glycoprotein hormone family (thyrotropin, luteinizing hormone, follicle-stimulating hormone, and chorionic gonadotropin).

A remarkable example of diversification at the level of gene amplifications is the extraordinarily large number of genes encoding the pheromone and odorant receptors.[87] As many as 1000 of these receptor genes may exist in mouse and rat genomes, each receptive to a particular odorant ligand. Over the course of evolution, an ancestral gene encoding a prototypic polypeptide representative of each of these families was duplicated one or more times, and through mutation and selection, the progeny proteins of the ancestral gene assumed different biologic functions. The exonic-intronic structural organization of the genomes of higher animals lends itself to gene recombination and RNA copying of genetic sequences with subsequent reintegration of DNA reverse-transcribed sequences back into the genome, resulting in rearrangement of transcriptional units and regulatory sequences.[88,89]

Transcription

In addition to duplication of genes and their promoters, another way to create diversity in expression is at the level of gene transcription, by providing genes with alternative promoters[90] and by using a large array of *cis*-regulatory elements in the promoters, governed by complex combinations of transcription factors.

Alternative Promoters

Many of the genes encoding hormones and their receptors use more than one promoter during development or when expressed in different tissue types. Employment of alternative promoters results in the formation of multiple transcripts that are different at their 5′ ends (Fig. 3-13). It is presumed that some genes have multiple promoters because they provide flexibility in the control of expression of the genes. For example, in some cases, expression of genes in more than one tissue or developmental stage requires distinct combinations of tissue-specific transcription factors. This flexibility enables genes in different cell types to respond to the same signal transduction pathways or genes in the same cell type to respond to different signal transduction pathways. A single promoter may not be adequate to respond to a complex array of transcription factors and a changing environment of cellular signals.

The organization of alternative promoters in genes manifests in several patterns within exons or introns in the 5′

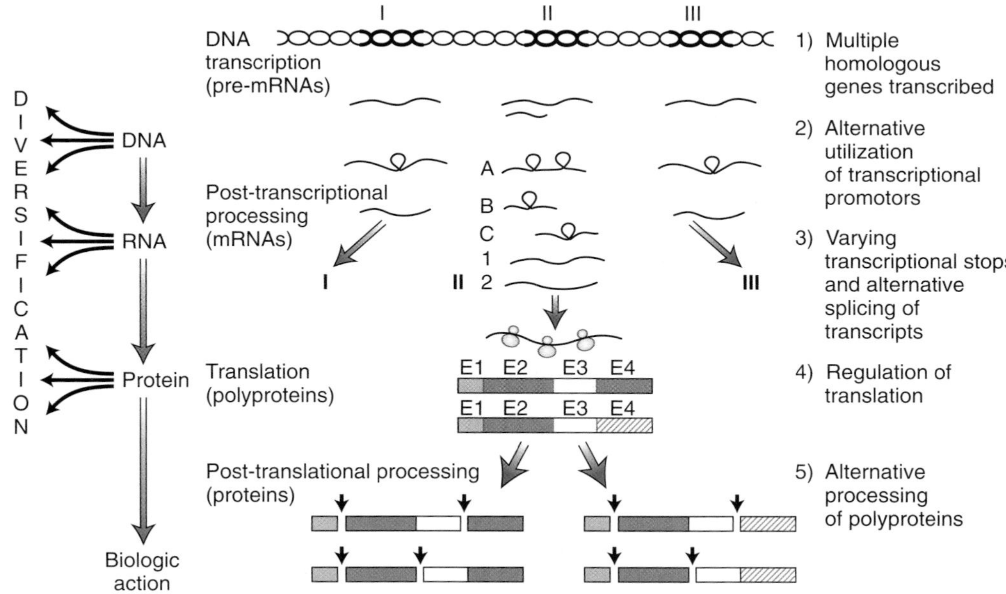

Figure 3-12 Levels in expression of genetic information at which diversification of information encoded in a gene may take place. The three major levels of genetic diversification are (1) gene duplication, a process that occurs in terms of evolutionary time; (2) variation in the processing of ribonucleic acid (RNA) precursors, which results in formation of two or more messenger RNAs (mRNAs) by way of alternative pathways of splicing of transcript (see Figs. 3-13 and 3-14); and (3) use of alternative patterns in processing of protein biosynthetic precursors (polyproteins or prohormones). These mechanisms provide a means for diversification of gene expression at levels of deoxyribonucleic acid (DNA), RNA, or protein. One or a combination of these processes leads to formation of the final biologically active peptide or hormone. Loops depicted in transcripts denote introns; in protein structures, the *stippled, shaded,* and *open* areas denote exons. *A, B, and C* represent splicing intermediates that lead to two distinct transcripts (1, 2) from one precursor. *E1-4* indicate portions of polyproteins cleaved post-translationally as indicated. *I, II, and III* indicate multiple transcribed genes following gene duplication.

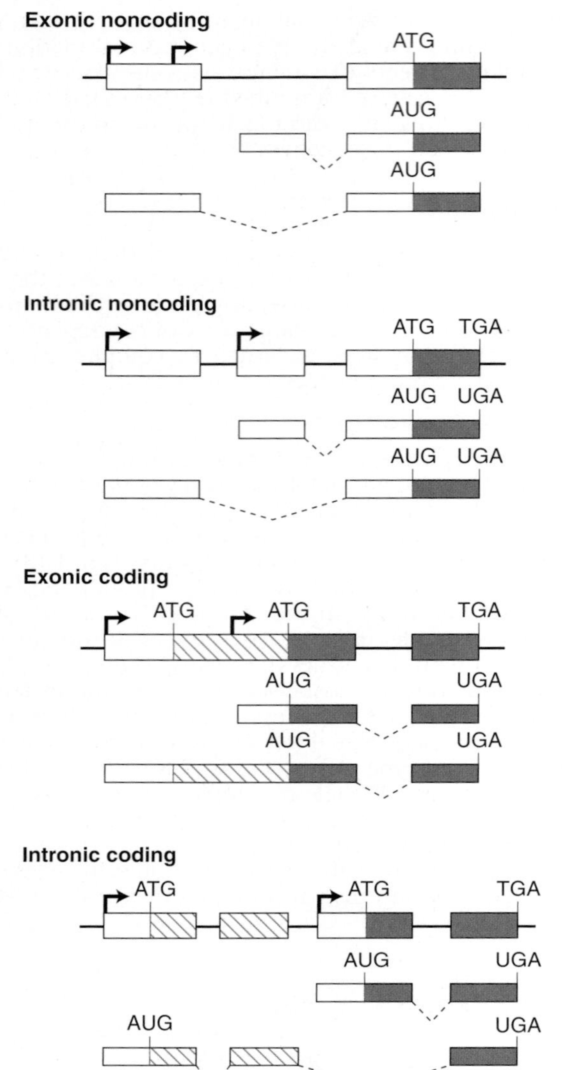

Figure 3-13 Use of alternative promoters in the expression of genes as a means to generate biologic diversification of gene expression. The use of alternative promoters allows a gene to be expressed in a variety of contexts that alter the properties of the messenger ribonucleic acid (mRNA) that is expressed. Alternative promoter use may render the mRNA more or less stable, affect translational efficiencies, or switch the translation of one protein isoform to another. The use of alternative promoters in genes characteristically occurs during development or, after development is completed, to designate tissue-specific patterns of expression of the gene. Exons are shown as boxes whose protein-coding regions are *shaded*. Introns are designated by *horizontal lines*. *Dashed lines* indicate introns that are spliced out. (Adapted from Ayoubi TAY, Van De Ven WJM. Regulation of gene expression by alternative promoters. *FASEB J*. 1996;10:453-460.)

noncoding sequence or the coding sequence (see Fig. 3-13). The most common occurrence of alternative promoters is within the 5′ noncoding or leader exons. Use of different promoters in the 5′ untranslated region of a gene, often accompanied by alternative exon splicing, results in the formation of mRNAs with different 5′ sequences. The alternative use of promoters in 5′ leader exons can affect gene expression and generate diversity in several ways, including developmental stage-specific and temporal expression of genes, tissue-type specificity of expression, levels of expression, responsiveness of gene expression to specific metabolic signals conveyed through signal transduction pathways, stability of the mRNAs, efficiencies of translation, and structures of the N-termini of proteins encoded by the genes.[90]

Examples of genes that use alternative 5′ leader promoters during development are those encoding IGF1, IGF2, the RARs, and glucokinase, all of which are regulated by multiple promoters that are active in a variety of embryonic and adult tissues and are subject to developmental and tissue-specific regulation.[90] During fetal development, promoters P2, P3, and P4 of the *IGF2* gene are active in the liver. These promoters are shut off after birth, at which time the P1 promoter is activated. The P1 and P2 promoters of the *IGF1* gene are differentially responsive to GH; P2 expressed in liver is responsive to GH, whereas P1 expressed in muscle is not.

The RAR exists in alpha, beta, and gamma isoforms (RARA, RARB, and RARG), encoded by separate genes that give rise to at least 17 different mRNAs generated by a combination of multiple promoters and alternative splicing.[91] The RAR isoforms have different specificities for retinoic acid–responsive promoters, different affinities for ligand isoforms, and different *trans*-activating capabilities. The various RAR isoforms are expressed at different times in different tissues during development. It has been proposed that the multiple RAR isoforms provide a means of achieving a diverse set of cellular responses to a single ligand, retinoic acid.[91]

Glucokinase is an example of the alternative use of 5′ leader promoters that have different levels of metabolic responsiveness.[92] Expression of glucokinase in pancreatic beta cells and some other neuroendocrine cells uses an upstream promoter (1β), whereas in liver, a promoter (IL) located 26 kilobases downstream of the 1β promoter is used exclusively. In beta cells, expression of the glucokinase gene is apparently not responsive to hormones. In liver expression mediated by the IL promoter, it is intensely upregulated by insulin and downregulated by glucagon.

The α-amylase gene provides an example in which two alternative promoters in the 5′ noncoding exons expressed in two different tissues have dramatically different strengths of expression.[90] A strong upstream promoter directs expression within the parotid gland, whereas weak expression is directed by an alternative downstream promoter in liver.

Examples of the use of alternative promoters in the coding regions of genes include the progesterone receptor (PR) and the transcription factor, cAMP response element modulator (CREM). In both of these cases, different protein isoforms are produced that have markedly different functional activities. The genes encoding the chicken and human PRs express two isoforms of the receptor.[93] Isoform A initiates translation at a methionine residue located 164 amino acids downstream from the methionine that initiates the translation of the longer form, isoform B. Analyses of the mechanisms responsible for the synthesis of the two isoforms revealed that two promoters exist in the human PR gene, one upstream of the 5′ leader exon and the other in the first protein-coding exon. The two isoforms of the human PR differ markedly in their abilities to *trans*-activate transcription from different progesterone-responsive elements (PREs). Both of the human PR isoforms equivalently activate a canonical PRE. Isoform B is much more efficient than A at activating the PRE in the mouse mammary tumor virus promoter, whereas isoform A, but not B, activates transcription from the ovalbumin promoter.[93]

Use of an alternative intronic promoter within the protein-coding sequence of a gene is exemplified by *CREM*.[94] The *CREM* gene employs a constitutively active, unregulated promoter (P1) that encodes predominantly activator forms of CREM and an internal promoter (P2) located in the fourth intron that is regulated by cAMP signaling and encodes a repressor isoform known as *inducible cAMP early response* (ICER). The remarkable complexity of the alternative mechanisms of expression of the *CREM* and *CREB* genes is discussed later.

Diversity of Transcription Factors

Diversity at the level of gene transcription can be created by the interplay of multiple transcription factors on multiple *cis*-regulatory sequences. The promoters of typical genes may contain 20 to 30 or more *cis*-acting control elements in the form of enhancers or silencers. These control elements may respond to ubiquitous transcription factors found in all cell types and to cell type–specific factors.

Unique patterns of control of gene expression can be affected by several mechanisms acting in concert. The spacing, relative locations, and juxtapositioning of control elements with respect to each other and to the basal transcriptional machinery influence levels of expression. Transcription factors often act in the form of dimers or higher oligomers among factors of the same or different classes. A given transcription factor may act as either an activator or a repressor, according to the existing circumstances. The ambient concentrations of transcription factors within the nucleus, in conjunction with their relative DNA-binding affinities and *trans*-activation potencies, may determine the levels of expression of genes.

Post-transcriptional Processing: Alternative Exon Splicing

Identification of the mosaic structure of transcriptional units encoding polypeptide hormones and other proteins that consist of exons and introns raised the possibility that the use of alternative pathways in RNA splicing could provide informationally distinct molecules. Different proteins could arise by inclusion or exclusion of specific exonic segments or by use of parts of introns in one mRNA as exons in another mRNA. Differences in the splice sites would result in expression of new translational reading frames. Alternative splicing uses two distinct mechanisms (Fig. 3-14). One is *exon skipping*, or switching in or out of exons. The other, known as *intron slippage*, includes use of part of an intron in an exon, splicing out of part of an exon along with the intron, and use of a "coding" intron.

Both mechanisms can generate diversity in endocrine systems. Included among the genes encoding prohormones in which the pre-mRNAs are alternatively spliced by exon skipping or switching are those for procalcitonin/calcitonin gene–related peptide, prosubstance P/K, and the prokininogens. Alternative processing of the RNA transcribed from the calcitonin gene results in production of an mRNA in neural tissues that is distinct from that formed in the C cells of the thyroid gland.[95] The thyroid mRNA encodes a precursor to calcitonin, whereas the mRNA in the neural tissues generates the neuropeptide, calcitonin gene–related peptide. Immunocytochemical analyses of the distribution of the peptide in brain and other tissues suggest functions for the peptide in perception of pain, ingestive behavior, and modulation of the autonomic and endocrine systems.

Splicing of the RNA precursor that encodes substance P can take place in at least two ways.[96] One splicing pattern results in the mRNA that encodes substance P and another peptide called substance K, in a common protein precursor. Other mRNAs are apparently spliced to exclude the coding sequence for substance K. An alternative RNA splicing pattern also occurs in the processing of transcripts arising

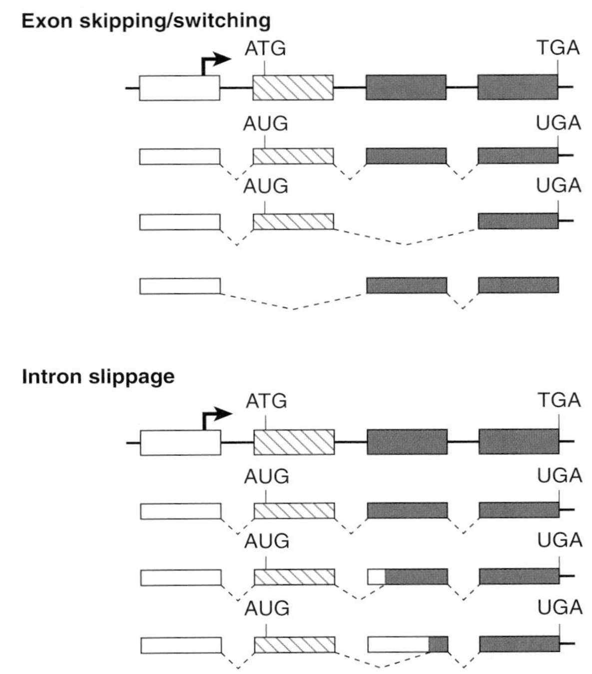

Figure 3-14 Alternative exon splicing provides a means to generate biologic diversification of gene expression. Mechanisms of exon skipping or switching and intron slippage are frequently used in the alternative processing of precursor-messenger ribonucleic acids (mRNAs) to provide unique mRNAs and encoded proteins during development and in a tissue-specific pattern of expression in fully differentiated tissues or organs. Exons are shown as boxes with protein-coding regions *shaded* to designate origin of protein isoforms. Introns are depicted as *horizontal lines. Dashed lines* denote spliced-out introns.

from the gene encoding bradykinin.[97] The high-molecular-weight and low-molecular-weight kininogens are translated from mRNAs that differ in their alternative use of 3′-end exons encoding the C-termini of the prohormones—a situation similar to that found in the transcription of the calcitonin gene.

Other examples of genetic diversification arise from programmed flexibility in the choice of splice acceptor sites within coding regions (i.e., intron slippage), which allows an array of coding sequences (exons) to be put together in a number of useful combinations. For example, the coding sequences of the GH, lutropin-choriogonadotropin,[98] and leptin receptors[99] can be brought together in two different ways, one to include and the other to exclude an exonic coding sequence that specifies the transmembrane-spanning domains of the polypeptide chains that anchor the receptors to the surface of cells. If mRNA splicing excludes the anchor's peptide sequence, a secreted rather than a surface protein is produced.

Translation

The process of translation provides a fourth level for creation of diversity in gene expression. The rate of translational initiation can be regulated, as discussed earlier; this is typified by the proinsulin and prohormone convertase mRNAs, in which translation is augmented by glucose and cAMP. Molecular diversity of translation is generated by the developmentally regulated use of alternative translation initiation (start) codons (i.e., methionine [AUG] codons). The mechanism of translation initiation involves assembly

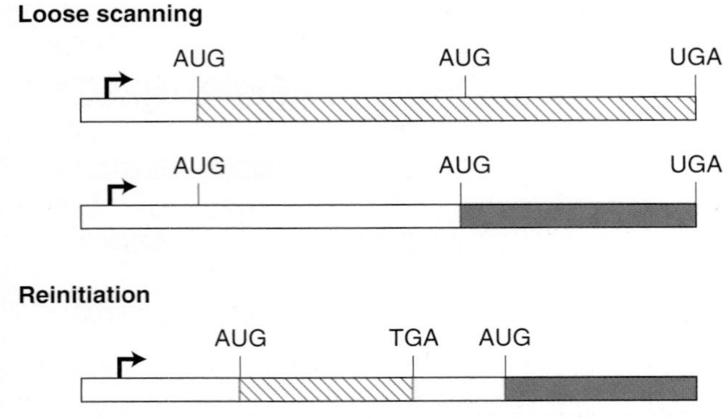

Figure 3-15 Alternative translational initiation sites are used to change the coding sequences of messenger ribonucleic acids to encode different protein isoforms. The two mechanisms shown involve loose scanning and reinitiation of translation (see text for details).

of the 40S ribosome subunit on the 5′ methyl guanosine cap of the mRNA.[100] The ribosome subunit then scans 5′ to 3′ along the mRNA until it encounters an AUG sequence in a context of surrounding nucleotides favorable for initiation of protein synthesis. On encountering a favorable AUG, the subunit pauses and recruits the 60S subunit and a number of other essential translation initiation factors, allowing the polymerization of amino acids.

The use of an alternative downstream start codon for translation can be achieved by the mechanisms of loose scanning and reinitiation (Fig. 3-15).[101] Loose scanning is believed to occur when the most 5′ AUG codon is not in a strongly favorable context; it allows the 40S ribosomal subunit to continue scanning until it encounters a more favorable AUG downstream. In the loose scanning mechanism, both translational start codons are used. In contrast, the mechanism of translational reinitiation involves the termination of translation followed by reinitiation of translation at a downstream start codon. Two proteins are encoded from the same mRNA by a start-and-stop mechanism.

The process of translational reinitiation can occur by continued scanning of the 40S ribosomal subunit after termination of translation followed by reinitiation, as in loose scanning, or by complete dissociation of the ribosomal subunits at the time of termination followed by complete reassembly at a downstream start codon, referred to as an *internal ribosomal entry site* (IRES). This use of alternative translation start codons occurs in mRNAs encoding certain classes of transcription factors, as illustrated by the basic leucine zipper (bZIP) proteins CREB, CREM, and the alpha (CEBPA) and beta (CEBPB) isoforms of CCAAT/enhancer binding proteins (CEBPs). In all four of these DNA-binding proteins, the alternative use of internal start codons results in a switch from activators to repressors.

The *CREB* gene uses translational reinitiation by the somewhat novel mechanism of alternative exon switching that occurs during spermatogenesis.[102] At developmental stages IV and V of the seminiferous tubule of the rat, an exon called *exon W* is spliced into the CREB mRNA. Exon W introduces an in-frame stop codon, thereby terminating translation approximately 40 amino acids upstream of the DNA-binding domain.[103,104] Translation is then reinitiated at each of two downstream start codons, resulting in the synthesis of two repressor or inhibitor isoforms of CREB, called I-CREBs. The I-CREBs are powerful dominant negative inhibitors of activator forms of CREB and CREM because they consist of the DNA-binding domain devoid of any *trans*-activation domains.[102-104] The function of the N-terminal truncated protein consisting of the activation domains devoid of the DNA-binding domain is unknown. It has been postulated that the role of alternative splicing of exon W in the CREB pre-mRNA is to interrupt a forward positive-feedback loop during spermatogenesis.

The CREM, CEBPA, and CEBPB mRNAs use alternative downstream start codons to synthesize repressors during development. Like the I-CREBs, these repressors consist of the DNA-binding domains and lack *trans*-activation domains. The CREM repressor (S-CREM) is expressed during brain development.[94] The CEBPA-30 and CEBPA -20 isoforms are expressed during differentiation of adipoblasts to adipocytes, and the CEBP repressor, liver inhibitory protein, is expressed during the development of the liver.[94]

Post-translational Processing

A fifth level of gene expression at which diversification of biologic information can take place is post-translational processing. Many precursors of polypeptide hormones, particularly those encoding small peptides, contain multiple peptides that are cleaved during post-translational processing of the prohormones.[105] Certain polyprotein precursors, however, contain several copies of the peptide. Examples of prohormones that contain multiple identical peptides are the precursors encoding TRH[106] and the α-factor of yeast,[107] each of which contains four copies of their respective peptide. Polyproteins that contain several distinct peptides include proenkephalins,[108] POMC,[109] and proglucagon.[110]

In many instances, biologic diversification at the level of post-translational processing occurs in a tissue-specific manner. The processing of POMC differs markedly in the anterior and intermediate lobes of the pituitary gland. In the anterior pituitary, the primary peptide products are ACTH and β-endorphin, whereas in the intermediate lobe of the pituitary, one of the primary products is α-melanocyte-stimulating hormone. The smaller peptides produced are extensively modified by acetylation and phosphorylation of amino acid residues.

The processing of proglucagon in the pancreatic alpha cells and in the intestinal L cells is different (see Fig. 3-15).[42] In the pancreatic alpha cells, the predominant bioactive product of the processing of proglucagon is glucagon itself; the two glucagon-like peptides are not processed efficiently from proglucagon in the alpha cells and are biologically inactive by virtue of having N-terminal and C-terminal extensions. In the intestinal L cell, the glucagon immunoreactive product is glicentin, a molecule that consists of the N-terminal extension of the proglucagon plus glucagon and the small C-terminal peptide known as intervening peptide 1. Because glicentin has no glucagon-like biologic activity, the bioactive peptide (or peptides) in the intestinal L cells must be one or both of the glucagon-like peptides. In fact, GLP1(7-37), the 31-amino-acid shortened form of glucagon-like peptide 1, is a potent insulinotropic hormone in its actions of stimulating insulin release from pancreatic beta cells.[111] This peptide is released from the intestines into the bloodstream in response to oral nutrients and appears to be a potent intestinal incretin factor implicated in the augmented release of insulin in response to oral compared with systemic (intravenous) nutrients. The potential for diversification of biologic information provided by the alternative pathways of gene expression is especially impressive because these pathways can occur in multiple combinations.

Small Regulatory RNAs: MicroRNAs and Small Interfering RNAs

The estimated 25,000 protein-coding genes contained in the human genome comprise only 1.25% of transcribed sequences. More than 98% of the transcriptional output of the genome consists of non–protein-coding, potentially regulatory RNAs.[112] The transcription of non–protein-coding RNAs from intronic and intergenic regions of the genome has been recognized for several decades, but it was thought to represent "transcriptional noise," the production of transcripts without function from so-called selfish DNA (i.e., DNA that replicates itself but has no function). In the past few years, however, important functions in development and disease have been identified for the class of small (21 to 25 nucleotides) transcribed RNAs known as *microRNAs* (miRNAs) and *small interfering RNAs* (siRNAs). These small regulatory RNAs negatively regulate gene expression at the post-transcriptional level by antisense hybridization to mRNAs. This process either destabilizes mRNAs or inhibits the translation of mRNAs into proteins. About 1000 miRNAs and several thousand siRNAs have been identified in mammalian cells. Between 1% and 3% of the genome encodes small regulatory RNAs, and they are thought to be involved in the regulation of up to 30% of the protein-coding genes.[113] One miRNA or siRNA can repress the expression of as many as 100 mRNAs. Although it was initially thought that small regulatory RNAs were ubiquitously expressed in tissues, it is now appreciated that their expression is highly regulated and is cell and tissue specific. These small regulatory RNAs play crucial roles in the regulation of gene expression during embryogenesis and organogenesis and in the control of cell proliferation, apoptosis, differentiation, lineage commitment, and metabolism.

The genes encoding miRNAs and siRNAs are transcribed as hairpin-looped RNA precursors (referred to as *primary miRNAs* or pri-miRNAs); these are initially cleaved in the nucleus by Drosha, a ribonuclease that removes a stem loop, thereby producing an intermediate pre-miRNA hairpin of about 70 nucleotides. These duplex pre-miRNA intermediates are exported from the nucleus by the proteins Exportin 5 and RAN-GTP to the cytoplasm, where they are cleaved by the endonuclease Dicer to form the active miRNAs of about 22 nucleotides that become part of the RNA-induced silencing complex (RISC). The duplex miRNAs are bound by the protein argonaute 2 (EIF2C2). One of the strands is eliminated, and the other (antisense) strand is retained as the mature miRNA. MiRNAs function by imperfect base pairing to the 3′ untranslated regions of their target mRNAs, resulting in mRNA degradation or inhibition of translation. MiRNAs are expressed in spatiotemporal patterns to regulate biologic processes at distinct stages of development. As a consequence of their highly specific expression patterns, miRNAs have been implicated in several diseases, including cancer, neurologic disorders, asthma, cardiovascular disorders, viral infections, and diabetes.

MiRNAs may be involved in epigenetic programming of the genome. Convincing evidence indicates that miRNAs in plants and worms have a role in transcriptional gene silencing and do so by contributing to the regulation of histone methylation. A role for miRNAs in gene silencing in mammalian cells is controversial. However, studies suggest that argonaute 2 is required for transcriptional silencing in human cells.[114]

The importance of miRNAs in diseases of endocrine systems has been investigated. Diabetes is a complex endocrine disease involving myriad factors that modulate the growth, survival, and regeneration of the insulin-producing beta cells of the pancreas and the sensitivities of peripheral tissues to the actions of insulin. One revealing study demonstrated the importance of miRNAs in the development of the endocrine cells of the pancreas through knockout of Dicer.[115]

Low Numbers of Expressed Genes in Murine and Human Genomes

Sequencing of the human and mouse genomes revealed that each contain approximately 30,000 genes. This number was viewed as remarkably low because the number of genes in the yeast *(Saccharomyces cerevisiae)*, worm (*Caenorhabditis elegans*), and fly *(Drosophila melanogaster)* genomes is about 20,000. However, tissue-specific alternative exon splicing and alternative promoter use occur much more frequently in humans and mice than in yeast, worms, and flies. The complexities of the mRNAs expressed in humans and mice are exemplified by the growing database of expressed sequence tags, and it seems reasonable to extrapolate that the human genome may express as many as 100,000 to 200,000 mRNAs that encode proteins with distinct, specific functions. This interpretation is based on the observation that alternative exon splicing and promoter are 5 to 10 times more frequent in higher vertebrate mammals than in yeasts and flies.

Genome-Wide Association Studies for Identification of Complex-Trait Disease Genes

Determination of the nucleic sequence of the human genome and mapping of the locations of expressed genes have created opportunities for the identification of genes responsible for complex-trait diseases,[116,117] such as diabetes, obesity, hypertension, asthma, schizophrenia, and bipolar disease. The genetic background of complex-trait diseases consists of multiple genes that collectively account for the disease phenotype. Genome-wide association studies (GWAS) enable identification of marker loci that co-segregate with the disease trait loci and association of the marker with risk for the disease. GWAS do not necessarily reveal the cause of disease, but they can identify gene loci that modify risk for the development of disease.

Association studies are based on the assumption that recombination (rearrangements) of DNA sequences in the genome are relatively slow to occur in the population, so that experimentally detectable marker loci consisting of single-nucleotide polymorphisms (SNPs) remain in place with respect to the disease loci. A large population (1000 to 10,000 individuals) with a high prevalence of the disease trait phenotype can be segregated by the presence or absence of the disease trait into cases and controls, respectively. The DNA from cases is screened for the presence of SNPs by high-output DNA array analyses using common SNPs present in the population genome. There are an estimated 10 million random polymorphisms in the genomes of the general human population (approximately 1 SNP per 100 base pairs of DNA).

Currently available high-density SNP libraries contain up to 770,000 SNPs spanning 74% of the genome, making it possible to identify specific SNPs that lie near the disease locus being studied.[118] Examination of maps of known genes in the region of the associated SNP or SNPs can help to identify potential candidate genes that may be associated with the disease. The polymorphism may represent mutation in the protein-coding region (exons) of the disease gene itself, but more often, the SNPs reside in regions of DNA within the gene (i.e., introns) or flanking the gene.

GWAS have identified many genes potentially associated with disease and have provided insights into pathogenesis and possible drug targets. Because of the limitations of the method—the need for very large study populations and the fact that only alleles associated with common SNPs in the population are identified—only a modest fraction of the genetic contribution to common diseases has been delineated.[119-121]

Type 2 diabetes provides a useful example of what GWAS have accomplished. Screening of large populations in which the prevalence of type 2 diabetes is high (approaching 10%) has uncovered 19 candidate genes to date.[122] One of these genes, the transcription factor TCF7L2, is strongly associated with the existence and predictive development of insulin-deficient type 2 diabetes in multiple populations. Carriers of the *TCF7L2* risk alleles have impaired glucose-stimulated insulin secretion and diminished augmentation of insulin secretion by incretin hormones such as GLP1 and gastric inhibitory polypeptide.[123] TCF7L2 is the predominant DNA-binding protein component of beta-catenin/TCF regulators of gene transcription in beta cells, and beta-catenin/TCF7L2 constitutes the downstream effector of the WNT signaling pathway stimulated by the incretin hormone GLP1 and the chemokine CXCL12 (formerly called SDF1).[124] WNT signaling mediated by GLP1 and CXCL12 is required for beta cell growth and survival, respectively.

ACKNOWLEDGMENTS

I am indebted to the members of the laboratory whose forbearance and helpful discussions of this chapter were invaluable. I thank Apolo Ndyabahika for help in preparation of the manuscript.

REFERENCES

1. Watson JD, Crick FHC. Molecular structure of nucleic acids. *Nature*. 1953;171:737-738.
2. Roth J, LeRoith D, Shiloach J, et al. The evolutionary origins of hormones, neurotransmitters, and other extracellular chemical messengers. *N Engl J Med*. 1982;306:523-527.
3. Loumaye E, Thorner J, Catt KJ. Yeast mating pheromone activates mammalian gonadotrophs: evolutionary conservation of a reproductive hormone? *Science*. 1982;218:1323-1325.
4. Johnsen AH. Phylogeny of the cholecystokinin/gastrin family. *Front Neuroendocrinol*. 1998;19:73-99.
5. Uy R, Wold F. Post-translational covalent modification of proteins. *Science*. 1977;198:890-896.
6. Martoglio B, Dobberstein B. Signal sequences: more than just greasy peptides. *Trends Cell Biol*. 1998;8:410-415.
7. Palade G. Intracellular aspects of the process of protein synthesis. *Science*. 1975;189:347-358.
8. Jamieson JD. The Golgi complex: perspectives and prospectives. *Biochim Biophys Acta*. 1998;1404:3-7.
9. Blobel G. Intracellular protein topogenesis. *Proc Natl Acad Sci U S A*. 1980;77:1496-1500.
10. Hegde RS, Lingappa VR. Regulation of protein biogenesis at the endoplasmic reticulum membrane. *Trends Cell Biol*. 1999;9:132-137.
11. van Vliet C, Thomas EC, Merino-Trigo A, et al. Intracellular sorting and transport of proteins. *Prog Biophys Mol Biol*. 2003;83:1-45.
12. Rodriguez-Boulan E, Musch A. Protein sorting in the Golgi complex: shifting paradigms. *Biochim Biophys Acta*. 2005;1744:455-464.
13. Schneider G, Fechner U. Advances in the prediction of protein targeting signals. *Proteomics*. 2004;4:1571-1580.
14. Nelson DL, Cox MM. *Lehninger's Principles of Biochemistry*. 3rd ed. New York, NY: Worth, 2000.
15. Agarraberes FA, Dice JF. Protein translocation across membranes. *Biochim Biophys Acta*. 2001;1513:1-24.
16. Blobel G, Dobberstein B. Transfer to proteins across membranes: II. Reconstitution of functional rough microsomes from heterologous components. *J Cell Biol*. 1975;67:852-862.
17. Walter P, Blobel F. Signal recognition particle contains a 7S RNA essential for protein translocation across the endoplasmic reticulum. *Nature*. 1982;299:691-698.
18. Bacher G, Pool M, Dobberstein B. The ribosome regulates the GTPase of the beta-subunit of the signal recognition particle receptor. *J Cell Biol*. 1999;146:723-730.
19. Wang L, Dobberstein B. Oligomeric complexes involved in translocation of proteins across the membrane of the endoplasmic reticulum. *FEBS Lett*. 1999;457:316-322.
20. Nagai K, Oubridge C, Kuglstatter A, et al. Structure, function and evolution of the signal recognition particle. *EMBO J*. 2003; 22:3479-3485.
21. Martoglio B, Graf R, Dobberstein B. Signal peptide fragments of preprolactin and NIV-1 p-gp160 interact with calmodulin. *EMBO J*. 1997;16:6636-6645.
22. Habener JF, Amgerdt M, Ravazzola M, et al. Parathyroid hormone biosynthesis. *J Cell Biol*. 1979;80:715-731.
23. Steiner DF, Docherty K, Carroll R. Golgi/granule processing of peptide hormone and neuropeptide precursors: a minireview. *J Cell Biochem*. 1984;24:121-130.
24. Chu LLH, MacGregor RR, Cohn DV. Energy-dependent intracellular translocation of proparathormone. *J Cell Biol*. 1977;72:1-10.
25. Kemper B, Habener JF, Rich A, et al. Microtubules and the intracellular conversion of proparathyroid hormone to parathyroid hormone. *Endocrinology*. 1975;96:902-912.
26. Steiner DF. The proprotein convertases. *Curr Opin Chem Biol*. 1998;2:31-39.
27. Muller L, Lindberg I. The cell biology of the prohormone convertases PC1 and PC2. *Prog Nucleic Acid Res Mol Biol*. 1999;63:69-108.
28. Seidah NG, Chretien M. Proprotein and prohormone convertases: a family of subtilases generating diverse bioactive polypeptides. *Brain Res*. 1999;848:45-62.
29. Jackson RS, Creemers JW, Ohagi S, et al. Obesity and impaired prohormone processing associated with mutations in the human prohormone convertase 1 gene. *Nat Genet*. 1997;16:303-306.
30. Furuta M, Yano H, Zhou A, et al. Defective prohormone processing and altered pancreatic islet morphology in mice lacking active SPC2. *Proc Natl Acad Sci U S A*. 1997;94:6646-6651.
31. Bradbury AF, Smyth DG. Peptide amidation. *Trends Biochem Sci*. 1991;16:112-115.
32. Prigge ST, Mains RE, Eipper BA, et al. New insights into copper monooxygenases and peptide amidation: structure, mechanism and function. *Cell Mol Life Sci*. 2000;57:1236-1259.
33. Kornberg RD. Eukaryotic transcriptional control. *Trends Cell Biol*. 1999;9:M46-M49.
34. Wolffe AP, Kurumizaka H. The nucleosome: a powerful regulator of transcription. *Prog Nucleic Acid Res Mol Biol*. 1998;61:379-422.
35. Blencowe BJ. Alternative splicing: new insights from global analyses. *Cell*. 2006;126:37-47.
36. Roy SW, Gilbert W. The evolution of spliceosomal introns: patterns, puzzles and progress. *Nat Rev Genet*. 2006;7:211-221.
37. Sharp PA. Split genes and RNA splicing. *Cell*. 1994;77:805-815.
38. Albright SR, Tjian R. TAFs revisited: more data reveal new twists and confirm old ideas. *Gene*. 2000;242:1-13.
39. Levine M, Tjian R. Transcription regulation and animal diversity. *Nature*. 2003;424:147-151.
40. Taatjes DJ, Marr MT, Tjian R. Regulatory diversity among metazoan co-activator complexes. *Nat Rev Mol Cell Biol*. 2004;5:403-410.
41. Crick F. Split genes and RNA splicing. *Science*. 1979;204:264-271.
42. Mojsov S, Heinrich G, Wilson IB, et al. Preproglucagon gene expression in pancreas and intestine diversifies at the level of post-translational processing. *J Biol Chem*. 1986;261:11880-11889.
43. Miller W, Eberhardt NL. Structure and evolution of the growth hormone gene family. *Endocr Rev*. 1983;4:97-130.
44. Brown DD. Gene expression in eukaryotes. *Science*. 1981; 211:667-674.
45. Darnell JE. Variety in the level of gene control in eukaryotic cells. *Nature*. 1982;297:365-371.
46. Brivanlou AH, Darnell JE Jr. Signal transduction and the control of gene expression. *Science*. 2002;295:813-818.
47. Murdoch GH, Franco R, Evans RM, et al. Polypeptide hormone regulation of gene expression. *J Biol Chem*. 1983;258:15329-15335.
48. Baxter JD, Ivarie RD. Regulation of gene expression by glucocorticoid hormones: studies of receptors and responses in cultured cells. *Receptors Horm Action*. 1978;2:251-284.
49. Wegnez M, Schachter BS, Baxter JD, et al. Hormonal regulation of growth hormone mRNA. *DNA*. 1982;1:145-153.
50. Itoh N, Okamoto H. Translational control of proinsulin synthesis by glucose. *Nature*. 1980;283:100-102.
51. Skelly RH, Schuppin GT, Ishihara H, et al. Glucose-regulated translational control of proinsulin biosynthesis with that of the proinsulin endopeptidases PC2 and PC3 in the insulin-producing MIN6 cell line. *Diabetes*. 1996;45:37-43.
52. Itoh N, Okamoto H. Translational control of proinsulin synthesis by glucose. *Nature*. 1980;283:100-102.

53. Wu C, Gilbert W. Tissue-specific exposure of chromatin structure at the 5′ terminus of the preproinsulin II gene. *Proc Natl Acad Sci U S A*. 1981;78:1577-1580.
54. Barton MC, Crowe AJ. Chromatin alteration, transcription and replication: what's the opening line to the story? *Oncogene*. 2001; 20:3094-3099.
55. Feil R, Khosla S. Genomic imprinting in mammals: an interplay between chromatin and DNA methylation? *Trends Genet*. 1999;15:431-435.
56. Stallcup MR. Role of protein methylation in chromatin remodeling and transcriptional regulation. *Oncogene*. 2001;20:3014-3020.
57. Wade PA. Methyl CpG binding proteins: coupling chromatin architecture to gene regulation. *Oncogene*. 2001;20:3166-3173.
58. Marx JL. Immunoglobulin genes have enhancers. *Science*. 1983; 221:735-757.
59. Walker MD, Edlund T, Boulet AM, et al. Cell-specific expression controlled by the 5′-flanking region of insulin and chymotrypsin genes. *Nature*. 1983;306:557-561.
60. Godfrey, KM, Lilycrop KA, Burdge GC, et al. Epigenetic mechanisms and the mismatch concept of the developmental origins of health and disease. *Pediatric Research*. 2007;61:5R-10R.
61. Bernstein BE, Meissner A, Lander ES. The mammalian epigenome. *Cell*. 2007;128:669-681.
62. Wu JI, Lessard J, Crabtree GR. Understanding the words of chromatin regulation. *Cell*. 2009;136:200-206.
63. Simmons RA. Developmental origins of beta cell failure in type 2 diabetes: the role of epigenetic mechanisms. *Pediatric Research*. 2007;61:64R-67R.
64. Krumlauf R. Hox genes in vertebrate development. *Cell*. 1994; 78:191-201.
65. Beato M, Klug J. Steroid hormone receptors: an update. *Hum Reprod Update*. 2000;6:225-236.
66. McKenna NJ, Lanz RB, O'Malley BW. Nuclear receptor coregulators: cellular and molecular biology. *Endocr Rev*. 1999;20:321-344.
67. Rosenfeld MG, Glass CK. Coregulator codes of transcriptional regulation by nuclear receptors. *J Biol Chem*. 2001;276:36865-36868.
68. Rosenfeld MG. POU-domain transcription factors: pou-er-ful developmental regulators. *Genes Dev*. 1991;5:897-907.
69. Lin C, Lin S-C, Chang C-P, et al. Pit-1-dependent expression of the receptor for growth hormone releasing factor mediates pituitary cell growth. *Nature*. 1992;360:765-768.
70. Latchman DS. Transcription-factor mutations and disease. *N Engl J Med*. 1996;334:28-33.
71. Jonsson J, Carlsson L, Edlund T, et al. Insulin-promoter-factor 1 is required for pancreas development in mice. *Nature*. 1994; 371:606-609.
72. Stoffers DA, Zinkin NT, Stonojevic V, et al. Pancreatic agenesis attributable to a single nucleotide deletion in the human *IPF1* gene coding sequence. *Nat Genet*. 1996;15:106-110.
73. Peers B, Leonard J, Sharma S, et al. Insulin expression in pancreatic islet cells relies on cooperative interactions between the helix-loop-helix factor E47 and the homeobox factor STF-1. *Mol Endocrinol*. 1994;8:1798-1806.
74. Luo X, Ikeda Y, Parker KL. A cell-specific nuclear receptor is essential for adrenal and gonadal development and sexual differentiation. *Cell*. 1994;77:481-490.
75. Zanaria E, Muscatelli F, Bardoni B, et al. An unusual member of the nuclear hormone receptor superfamily responsible for X-linked adrenal hypoplasia congenita. *Nature*. 1994;372:635-641.
76. Hammer GD, Parker KL, Schimmer BP. Minireview: transcriptional regulation of adrenocortical development. *Endocrinology*. 2005;146:1018-1024.
77. Niakan KK, McCabe ER. DAX1 origin, function, and novel role. *Mol Genet Metab*. 2005;86:70-83.
78. Cohen P. Signal integration at the level of protein kinases, protein phosphatases and their substrates. *Trends Biochem Sci*. 1992;17:408-413.
79. Krebs EG, Graves JD. Interactions between protein kinases and proteases in cellular signaling and regulation. *Adv Enzyme Regul*. 2000; 40:441-470.
80. Berridge MJ. Elementary and global aspects of calcium signalling. *J Physiol (Lond)*. 1997;499:291-306.
81. Bootman MD, Collins TJ, Peppiatt CM, et al. Calcium signalling: an overview. *Semin Cell Dev Biol*. 2001;12:3-10.
82. Hill CS, Treisman R. Transcriptional regulation by extracellular signals: mechanisms and specificity. *Cell*. 1995;80:199-211.
83. Habener JF, Miller CP, Vallejo M. Cyclic AMP-dependent regulation of gene transcription by CREB and CREM. *Vitam Horm*. 1995;51:1-57.
84. Janknecht R, Hunter T. A growing coactivator network. *Nature*. 1996;383:22-23.
85. Cobb MH, Goldsmith EJ. How MAP kinases are regulated. *J Biol Chem*. 1995;270:14843-14846.
86. Schindler C, Darnell JE Jr. Transcriptional responses to polypeptide ligands: the JAK-STAT pathway. *Annu Rev Biochem*. 1995;64:621-651.
87. Axel R. The molecular logic of smell. *Sci Am*. 1995;273(4):154-159.
88. Dover G. Molecular drive: a cohesive mode of species evolution. *Nature*. 1982;299:111-117.
89. Reanney D. Genetic noise in evolution. *Nature*. 1984;307:318-319.
90. Ayoubi TAY, Van De Ven WJM. Regulation of gene expression by alternative promoters. *FASEB J*. 1996;10:453-460.
91. Leid M, Kastner P, Chambon P. Multiplicity generates diversity in the retinoic acid signaling pathways. *Trends Biochem Sci*. 1992; 117:427-433.
92. Davidson EH, Jacobs HT, Britten RJ. Very short repeats and coordinate induction of genes. *Nature*. 1983;301:468-470.
93. Kastner P, Krust A, Turcotte B, et al. Two distinct estrogen-regulated promoters generate transcripts encoding the two functionally different human progesterone receptor forms A and B. *EMBO J*. 1990;9:1603-1614.
94. Foulkes NS, Sassone-Corsi P. More is better: activators and repressors from the same gene. *Cell*. 1992;68:411-414.
95. Rosenfeld MG, Mermod JJ, Amara SG, et al. Production of a novel neuropeptide encoded by the calcitonin gene via tissue-specific RNA processing. *Nature*. 1983;304:129-135.
96. Nawa H, Hirose T, Takashima H, et al. Nucleotide sequences of cloned cDNAs for two types of bovine brain substance P precursor. *Nature*. 1983;306:32-36.
97. Kitamura N, Takagaki Y, Furuto S, et al. A single gene for bovine high molecular weight and low molecular weight kininogens. *Nature*. 1983;305:545-549.
98. Segaloff DL, Ascoli M. The lutropin/choriogonadotropin receptor … 4 years later. *Endocr Rev*. 1993;14:324-347.
99. Lee G-H, Proenca R, Montez JM, et al. Abnormal splicing of the leptin receptor in diabetic mice. *Nature*. 1996;379:632-635.
100. Dreyfuss G, Hentze M, Lamond AI, et al. From transcript to protein. *Cell*. 1996;85:963-972.
101. Kozak M. The scanning model for translation: an update. *J Cell Biol*. 1989;108:229-241.
102. Walker WH, Sanborn BM, Habener JF. An isoform of transcription factor CREM expressed during spermatogenesis lacks the phosphorylation domain and represses cAMP-induced transcription. *Proc Natl Acad Sci U S A*. 1994;91:12423-12427.
103. Walker WH, Girardet C, Habener JF. An alternatively spliced, polycistronic mRNA controls a switch from activator to repressor isoforms of transcription factor CREB during spermatogenesis. *J Biol Chem*. 1996;271:20145-20158.
104. Walker WH, Habener JF. Role of transcription factors CREB and CREM in cAMP-induced regulation of transcription during spermatogenesis. *Trends Endocrinol Metab*. 1996;4:133-138.
105. Neurath H. Proteolytic processing and regulation. *Enzyme*. 1991; 45:239-243.
106. Lechan RM, Wu P, Jackson IME, et al. Thyrotropin-releasing hormone precursor: characterization in rat brain. *Science*. 1986;231:159-161.
107. Kurjan J, Herskowitz I. Structure of a yeast pheromone gene (MF): a putative factor precursor contains four tandem copies of mature factor. *Cell*. 1982;30:933-943.
108. Noda M, Teranishi Y, Yakahashi T, et al. Isolation and structural organization of the human preproenkephalin gene. *Nature*. 1982;297:431-434.
109. Nakanishi S, Inoue A, Kita T, et al. Nucleotide sequence of cloned cDNA for bovine corticotropin-beta-lipotropin precursor. *Nature*. 1979;278:423-427.
110. Heinrich G, Gros P, Lund PK, et al. Pre-proglucagon messenger RNA: nucleotide and encoded amino acid sequences of the rat pancreatic cDNA. *Endocrinology*. 1984;115:2176-2181.
111. Mojsov S, Weir GC, Habener JF. Insulinotropin: glucagon-like peptide I (7-37) coencoded in the glucagon gene is a potent stimulator of insulin release in perfused rat pancreas. *J Clin Invest*. 1987;79:616-619.
112. Matick JS, Makunin IV. Small regulatory RNAs in mammals. *Hum Mol Genet*. 2005;14;R121-R132.
113. Pandey AK, Agarwal P, Kaur K, et al. MicroRNAs in diabetes: tiny players in big disease. *Cell Physiol Biochem*. 2009;23:221-232.
114. Saetrom P, Snove O, Rossi JJ. Epigenetics and microRNAs. *Ped Res*. 2007;61:17R-23R.
115. Lynn FC, Skewes-Cox P, Kosaka Y, et al. MicroRNA expression is required for pancreatic islet cell genesis in the mouse. *Diabetes*. 2007;56:2938-2945.
116. Ioannidis JP, Thomas G, Daly MJ. Validating, augmenting and refining genome-wide association signals. *Nat Rev Genet*. 2007:10;318-329.
117. Rodriquez-Murillo L, Greenberg DA. Genetic association analysis: a primer on how it works, its strengths and its weaknesses. *Int J Androl*. 2008;31:546-556.
118. Evans DM, Cardon LR. Genome-wide association: a promising start to a long race. *Trends Genet*. 2006;22:350-354.
119. Goldstein DB. Common genetic variation and human traits. *N Engl J Med*. 2009;360:1696-1698.
120. Hirschhorn JN. Genomewide association studies: illuminating biologic pathways. *N Engl J Med*. 2009;360:1699-1701.

121. Kraft P, Hunter DJ. Genetic risk prediction: are we there yet? *N Engl J Med*. 2009;360:1701-1703.
122. Zeggini E, Scott LJ, Saxena R, et al. Meta-analysis of genome-wide association data and large-scale replication identifies additional susceptibility loci for type 2 diabetes. *Nat Genet*. 2008;40:638-645.
123. Lyssenko V, Groop L, Genome-wide association study for type 2 diabetes: clinical applications. *Curr Opin Lipidol*. 2009;20:87-91.
124. Liu Z, Habener JF. Wnt signaling in pancreatic islets. *Adv Exp Med Biol*. 2010;654:391-419.

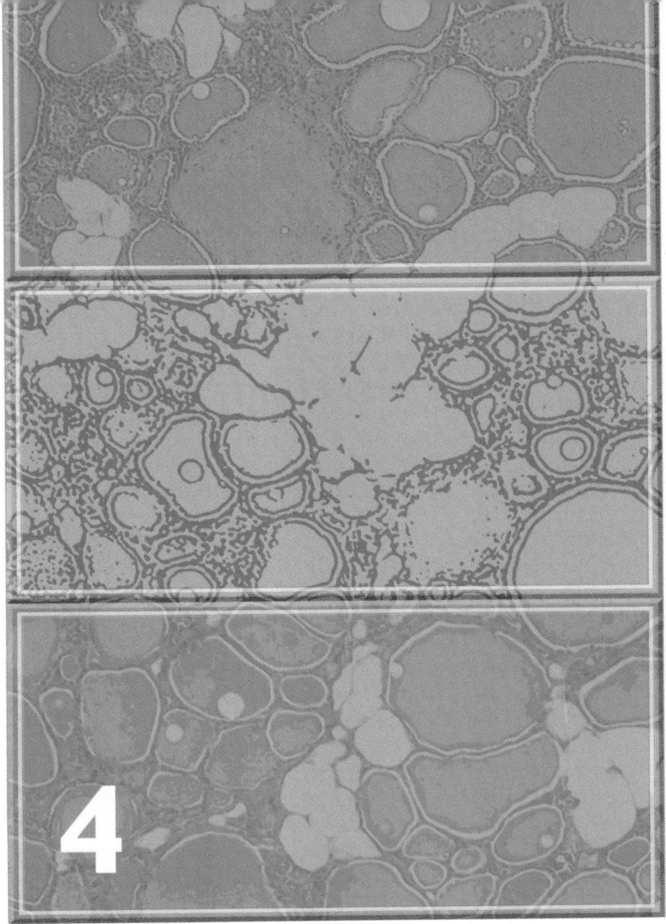

CHAPTER 4

Mechanism of Action of Hormones That Act on Nuclear Receptors

MITCHELL A. LAZAR

Hormones can be divided into two groups on the basis of where they function in a target cell. The first group includes hormones that do not enter cells; instead, they signal by means of second messengers generated by interactions with receptors at the cell surface. All polypeptide hormones (e.g., growth hormone), monoamines (e.g., serotonin), and prostaglandins (e.g., prostaglandin E_2), use cell surface receptors (see Chapter 5). The second group, the focus of this chapter, includes hormones that can enter cells. These hormones bind to intracellular receptors that function in the nucleus of the target cell to regulate gene expression. Classic hormones that use intracellular receptors include thyroid and steroid hormones.

Hormones serve as a major form of communication between different organs and tissues. They allow specialized cells in complex organisms to respond in a coordinated manner to changes in the internal and external environments. Classic endocrine hormones are secreted by endocrine glands and are distributed throughout the body through the bloodstream. These hormones were discovered by purifying the biologically active substances from clearly definable glands.

Numerous other signaling molecules share with thyroid and steroid hormones the ability to function in the nucleus to convey intercellular and environmental signals. Not all of these molecules are produced in glandular tissues. Although some signaling molecules, such as classic endocrine hormones, arrive at target tissues through the bloodstream, others have paracrine functions (i.e., acting on adjacent cells) or autocrine functions (i.e., acting on the cell of origin).

In addition to the classic steroid and thyroid hormones, lipophilic signaling molecules that use nuclear receptors include derivatives of vitamins A and D, endogenous metabolites such as oxysterols and bile acids, and non-natural chemicals encountered in the environment (i.e., xenobiotics). These molecules are referred to as *nuclear receptor ligands*. The nuclear receptors for all of these signaling molecules are structurally related and are collectively referred to as the *nuclear receptor superfamily*.[1-3] The study of these receptors is a rapidly evolving field, and more detailed information can be obtained by visiting the Nuclear Receptor Signaling Atlas web site (http://www.nursa.org [accessed September 2010]).

LIGANDS THAT ACT THROUGH NUCLEAR RECEPTORS

General Features of Nuclear Receptor Ligands

Unlike polypeptide hormones that function through cell surface receptors, no ligands for nuclear receptors are directly encoded in the genome. All nuclear receptor ligands are small (molecular mass <1000 d) and lipophilic, enabling them to enter cells by passive diffusion, although in some cases, a membrane transport protein is involved. For example, several active and specific thyroid hormone transporters have been identified, including monocarboxylate transporter 8 (MCT8), MCT10, and organic anion transporting polypeptide 1C1 (OATP1C1).[4,5] The lipophilicity of nuclear receptor ligands allows them to be absorbed from the gastrointestinal tract, facilitating their use in replacement or pharmacologic therapies for various disease states.

Another common feature of naturally occurring nuclear receptor ligands is that all are derived from dietary, environmental, or metabolic precursors. In this sense, the function of these ligands and their receptors is to translate cues from the external and internal environments into changes in gene expression. Their critical role in maintaining homeostasis in multicellular organisms is highlighted by the fact that nuclear receptors are found in all vertebrates and insects but not in single-cell organisms such as yeast.[6]

Because nuclear receptor ligands are lipophilic, most are readily absorbed from the gastrointestinal tract. This makes nuclear receptors excellent targets for pharmaceutical interventions. In addition to natural ligands, many drugs in clinical use target nuclear receptors, ranging from those used to treat specific hormone deficiencies to those used to treat common multigenic conditions such as inflammation, cancer, and type 2 diabetes.

Subclasses of Nuclear Receptor Ligands

One classification of nuclear receptor ligands is outlined in Table 4-1 and is described in the following paragraphs.

Classic Hormones

The classic hormones that use nuclear receptors for signaling are thyroid hormone and steroid hormones. Steroid hormones include cortisol, aldosterone, estradiol, progesterone, and testosterone. In some cases (e.g., thyroid hormone receptor α and β genes [*THRA* and *THRB*], estrogen receptor α and β genes [*ESR1* and *ESR2*]), there are multiple receptor genes that encode multiple receptors. Multiple receptors for the same hormone can also be derived from a single gene by alternative promoter usage or by alternative splicing (e.g., THRB1 and THRB2).

Some receptors can mediate the signals of multiple hormones. For example, the mineralocorticoid receptor, also known as the aldosterone receptor or nuclear receptor 3C2 (NR3C2), has equal affinity for cortisol[7] and probably functions as a glucocorticoid receptor in some tissues, such as the brain; likewise, the androgen receptor binds and responds to both testosterone and dihydrotestosterone (DHT).[8]

Vitamins

Vitamins are essential constituents of a healthful diet. Two fat-soluble vitamins, A and D, are precursors of important signaling molecules that function as ligands for nuclear receptors.

TABLE 4-1

Nuclear Receptor Ligands and Their Receptors

Ligand	Receptor
Classic Hormones	
Thyroid hormone	Thyroid hormone receptor (TR), subtypes α, β
Estrogen	Estrogen receptor (ER), subtypes α, β
Testosterone	Androgen receptor (AR)
Progesterone	Progesterone receptor (PR)
Aldosterone	Mineralocorticoid receptor (MR)
Cortisol	Glucocorticoid receptor (GR)
Vitamins	
1,25-$(OH)_2$-Vitamin D_3	Vitamin D receptor (VDR)
All-*trans*-retinoic acid	Retinoic acid receptor, subtypes α, β, γ
9-*cis*-Retinoic acid	Retinoid X receptor (RXR), subtypes α, β, γ
Metabolic Intermediates and Products	
Fatty acids	Peroxisome proliferator-activated receptor (PPAR), subtypes α, δ, γ
Oxysterols	Liver X receptor (LXR), subtypes α, β
Bile acids	Bile acid receptor (BAR)
Heme	Rev-Erb subtypes α, β
Xenobiotics	
??	Pregnane X receptor (PXR), constitutive androstane receptor (CAR)

Precursors of vitamin D are synthesized and stored in skin and activated by ultraviolet light; vitamin D can also be derived from dietary sources. Vitamin D is then converted in the liver to 25(OH)D (25-hydroxyvitamin D, calcidiol) and in the kidney to 1,25$(OH)_2$ D_3 (1,25-dihydroxyvitamin D_3, calcitriol), the most potent natural ligand of the vitamin D receptor (VDR). The 1-hydroxylation of calcidiol is tightly regulated, and calcitriol acts as a circulating hormone.

Vitamin A is stored in the liver and is activated by metabolism to all-*trans*-retinoic acid, which is a high-affinity ligand for retinoic acid receptors (RARs).[9] Retinoic acid is likely to function as a signaling molecule in paracrine as well as endocrine pathways. Retinoic acid is also converted to its 9-*cis*-isomer, which is a ligand for another nuclear receptor, the retinoid X receptor (RXR).[10] These retinoids and their receptors are essential for normal development of multiple organs and tissues, and they have pharmaceutical utility for conditions ranging from skin diseases to leukemia.[10]

Metabolic Intermediates and Products

Certain nuclear receptors respond to naturally occurring endogenous metabolic products. The peroxisome proliferator-activated receptors (PPARs) constitute the best defined subfamily of metabolite-sensing nuclear receptors.[11] All three PPAR subtypes are activated by polyunsaturated fatty acids. No single fatty acid has particularly high affinity for any PPAR, and it is possible that these receptors function as integrators of the concentration of a number of fatty acids.

PPARα is expressed primarily in liver; the natural ligand with highest affinity for PPARα is an eicosanoid, 8(*S*)-hydroxyeicosatetraenoic acid,[12,13] although there is evidence that the natural ligand may be a fatty acid derived from lipolysis of circulating triglyceride-rich lipoproteins.[14] The fibrate class of lipid-lowering pharmaceuticals are potent ligands for PPARα, and the very name of this receptor is derived from its ability to induce the proliferation of peroxisomes in the liver.[15] Indeed, stimulation of fatty acid oxidation is an important physiologic role of PPARα.

The other PPARs (δ and γ) are structurally related but are not activated by peroxisome proliferators. PPARδ, also known as PPARβ, is ubiquitous, and its ligands—other than fatty acids—are not well characterized. Activation of PPARδ appears to increase oxidative metabolism in fat and skeletal muscle.[16] PPARγ is expressed primarily in adipocytes and is necessary for differentiation along the adipocyte lineage.[17] PPARγ is also expressed in other cell types, including colonocytes, macrophages, and vascular endothelial cells, where it may play physiologic and pathologic roles. The natural ligand for PPARγ is not known, although prostaglandin J derivatives have been shown to bind and activate the receptor at concentrations in the micromolar range.[13,18,19] PPARγ appears to be the target of thiazolidinedione (TZD) antidiabetic drugs that improve insulin sensitivity.[17,20] These pharmaceutical agents bind to PPARγ with nanomolar affinities, and non-TZD PPARγ ligands are also insulin sensitizers, further implicating PPARγ in this physiologic role.

Another metabolite-responsive nuclear receptor, the liver X receptor (LXR), is activated by oxysterol intermediates in cholesterol biosynthesis. Mice lacking LXRα have a dramatically impaired ability to metabolize cholesterol.[21] A receptor known as farnesyl X receptor (FXR) binds and is activated by bile acids, and it likely plays a role in regulation of bile synthesis and circulation in normal conditions and in disease states.[22]

Xenobiotics

Other nuclear receptors appear to function as integrators of exogenous environmental signals, including natural endobiotics (e.g., medicinal agents and toxins found in plants) and xenobiotics (i.e., compounds that are not naturally occurring). In these cases, the role of the activated nuclear receptor is to induce cytochrome P450 enzymes that facilitate detoxification of potentially dangerous compounds in the liver. Receptors in this class include sterol and xenobiotic receptor (SXR), also known as *pregnane X receptor* (PXR), and constitutive androstane receptor (CAR).[22]

Unlike other nuclear receptors that have high affinity for very specific ligands, xenobiotic receptors have low affinity for a large number of ligands, reflecting their function in defense against a varied and challenging environment. Although these xenobiotic compounds are not hormones in the classic sense, the function of these nuclear receptors is consistent with the general theme of helping the organism to cope with environmental challenges.

Orphan Receptors

The nuclear receptor superfamily is one of the largest families of transcription factors. The hormones and vitamins just described account for the functions of only a fraction of the total number of nuclear receptors. The remaining receptors have been designated as *orphan receptors* because their putative ligands are not known.[23]

From analyses of mice and humans with mutations in various orphan receptors, it is clear that many of them are required for life or for development of specific organs, ranging from brain nuclei to endocrine glands. Some orphan receptors appear to be active in the absence of any ligand (i.e., constitutively active) and may not respond to a natural ligand. Nevertheless, all of the receptors known to respond to metabolites and environmental compounds were originally discovered as orphans. Therefore, future research will likely find that additional orphan receptors function as receptors for physiologic, pharmacologic, or environmental ligands. For example, the nuclear receptor NR1D1 (formerly called Rev-Erbα), which is a regulator of circadian rhythms,[24] has been shown to be a receptor for molecular heme,[25,26] which is involved in the coordination of circadian rhythms and metabolism.

Variant Receptors

The carboxyl-terminus of the nuclear receptors is responsible for hormone binding. In a few nuclear receptors, including THRA and the glucocorticoid receptor, alternative splicing produces variant receptors with unique C-termini that do not bind ligand.[27,28] These variant receptors are normally expressed, but their biologic relevance is uncertain. They may modulate the action of the classic receptor to which they are related by inhibiting its function.

Another type of normally occurring variant nuclear receptors lacks a classic DNA-binding domain (discussed later). These include NROB1 (formerly called DAX1), which is mutated in human disease,[29] and PTPN6 (formerly called SHP1).[30] Their ligands have not been identified, and it is likely that NROB1 and PTPN6 bind to and repress the actions of other receptors.

Rare, naturally occurring mutations of hormone receptors can cause hormone resistance in affected patients.[31] Inheritance of the hormone resistance phenotype is dominant if the mutant receptor inhibits the action of the normal receptor, as occurs with resistance to thyroid hormone or PPARγ ligands.[31] Inheritance is recessive if the mutation results in a complete loss of receptor function, as with the syndrome of hereditary calcitriol-resistant rickets.[32] Inheritance can also be X-linked, as with the mutated androgen receptor in androgen insensitivity syndromes, including testicular feminization.[33]

Regulation of Ligand Levels

Ligand levels can be regulated in several ways (Table 4-2). A dietary precursor may not be available in required amounts (e.g., in hypothyroidism due to iodine deficiency). Pituitary hormones (e.g., thyroid-stimulating hormone) regulate the synthesis and secretion of classic thyroid and steroid hormones. If the glands that synthesize these hormones fail, hormone deficiency can occur.

Many of the nuclear receptor ligands are enzymatically converted from inactive prohormones to biologically active hormones; examples include the 5′ deiodination of thyroxine (T_4) to triiodothyronine (T_3) (see Chapter 11). In other cases, one hormone is a precursor for another, for example, in aromatization of testosterone to estradiol. Biotransformation may occur in a specific tissue that is not the main target of the hormone, as with renal 1-hydroxylation of

TABLE 4-2

Mechanisms Regulating Ligand Levels

Mechanisms Regulating Ligand Levels
Precursor availability
Synthesis
Secretion
Activation (prohormone → active hormone)
Deactivation (active hormone) → inactive hormone)
Elimination (hepatic, renal clearance)

vitamin D (see Chapter 28), or it may occur primarily in target tissues (e.g., 5α-reduction of testosterone to DHT; see Chapter 19). Deficiency or pharmacologic inhibition of an enzyme can also reduce hormone levels.[34]

Hormones can be inactivated by standard hepatic or renal clearance mechanisms or by more specific enzymatic processes. In the latter case, reduction in enzyme activity due to gene mutations or pharmacologic agents can result in symptoms of hormone excess, such as renal deactivation of cortisol by 11β-hydroxysteroid dehydrogenase (11β-HSD). Because cortisol can activate the mineralocorticoid receptor, insufficient 11β-HSD activity due to licorice ingestion, gene mutation, or extremely high cortisol levels causes syndromes of apparent mineralocorticoid excess.[35]

NUCLEAR RECEPTOR SIGNALING MECHANISMS

Nuclear receptors are multifunctional proteins that transduce the signals of their cognate ligands. General features of nuclear receptor signaling are illustrated in Figure 4-1.

For hormone action in the nucleus, the ligand and the nuclear receptor must physically get into the nucleus. The nuclear receptor also must bind its ligand with high affinity. Because a major function of the receptor is to selectively regulate target gene transcription, it must recognize and bind to promoter elements in appropriate target genes. One discriminatory mechanism is dimerization of a receptor with a second copy of itself or with another nuclear receptor. The DNA-bound receptor must work in the context of chromatin to signal the basal transcription machinery to increase or decrease transcription of the target gene. In the regulation of signaling by nuclear receptors, some basic mechanisms are used by many or all members of the nuclear receptor superfamily, whereas other mechanisms impart the specificity that is crucial to the vastly different biologic effects of the many hormones and ligands that use these related receptors.

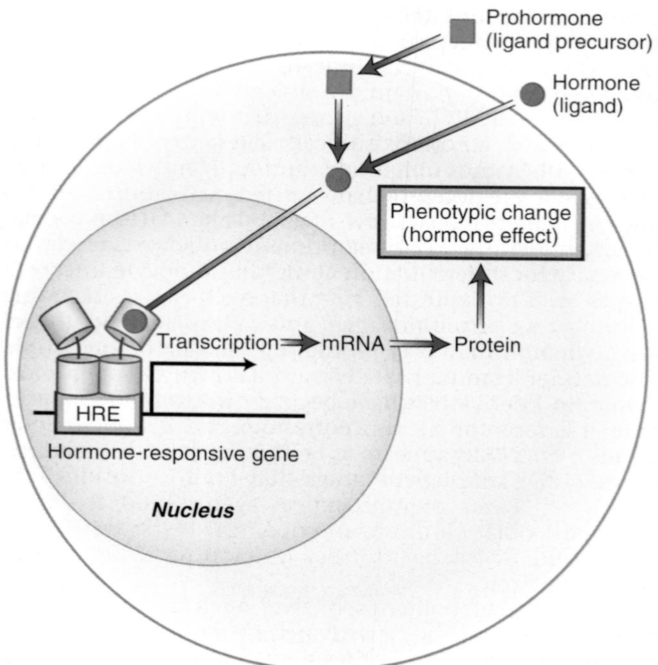

Figure 4-1 Mechanism of signal transduction by hormones and other ligands that act through nuclear receptors. HRE, hormone response element; mRNA, messenger ribonucleic acid.

Domain Structure of Nuclear Receptors

Nuclear receptors are proteins with molecular masses between 50,000 and 100,000 d. They share a common series of domains, referred to as domains A through F (Fig. 4-2). This linear depiction is useful for describing and comparing receptors, but it does not capture the roles of protein folding and tertiary structure in mediating various receptor functions. Investigations have revealed the structures of

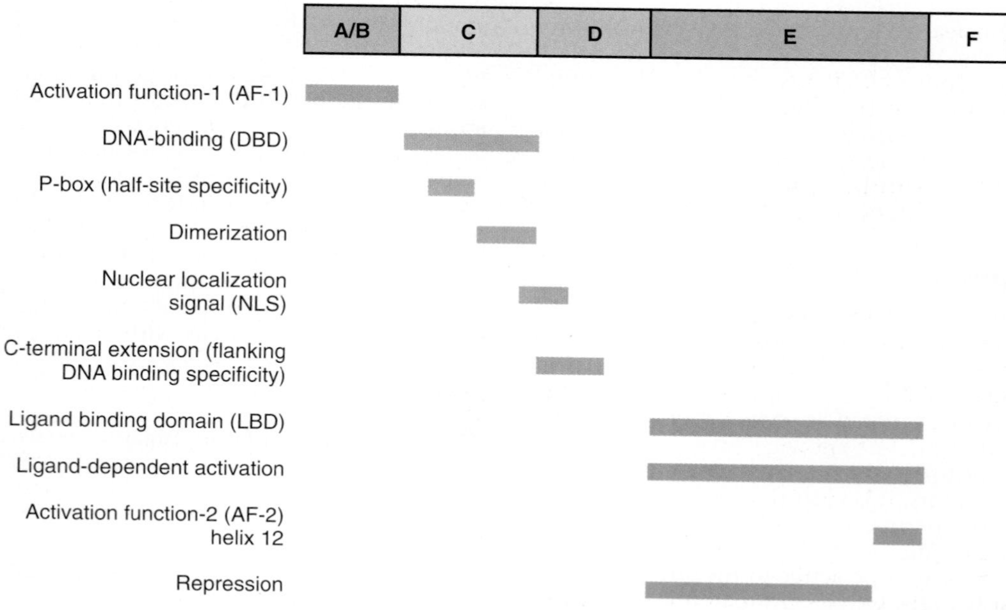

Figure 4-2 Domain structures of nuclear receptors.

individual domains and the first solved structure of a full-length nuclear receptor.

Nuclear Localization

The nuclear receptors, like all cellular proteins, are synthesized on ribosomes that reside outside the nucleus. Import of the nuclear receptors into the nucleus requires the nuclear localization signal (NLS), which is located near the border of the C and D domains (see Fig. 4-2). As a result of their NLSs, most of the nuclear receptors reside in the nucleus, with or without their ligands. A major exception is the glucocorticoid receptor; in the absence of hormone, it is tethered in the cytoplasm to a complex of chaperone molecules, including heat shock proteins (HSPs). Hormone binding to the glucocorticoid receptor induces a conformational change that results in dissociation of the chaperone complex, allowing the hormone-activated glucocorticoid receptor to translocate to the nucleus by means of its NLS.

Hormone Binding

High-affinity binding of a lipophilic ligand is a shared characteristic of many nuclear receptors. This defining function of the receptor is mediated by the C-terminal ligand-binding domain (LBD), domains D and E in Figure 4-2. This region of the receptor has many other functions, including induction of dimerization and transcriptional regulation (see later discussions).

The structure of the LBD has been solved for a number of receptors. All share a similar overall structure consisting of 12 α-helical segments in a highly folded tertiary structure (Fig. 4-3A). The ligand binds within a hydrophobic pocket composed of amino acids in helices 3, 4, and 5 (H3, H4, and H5, respectively). The major structural change induced by ligand binding is an internal folding of the most C-terminal helix (H12), which forms a cap on the ligand-binding pocket (see Fig. 4-3B). Although the overall mechanism of ligand binding is similar for all receptors,

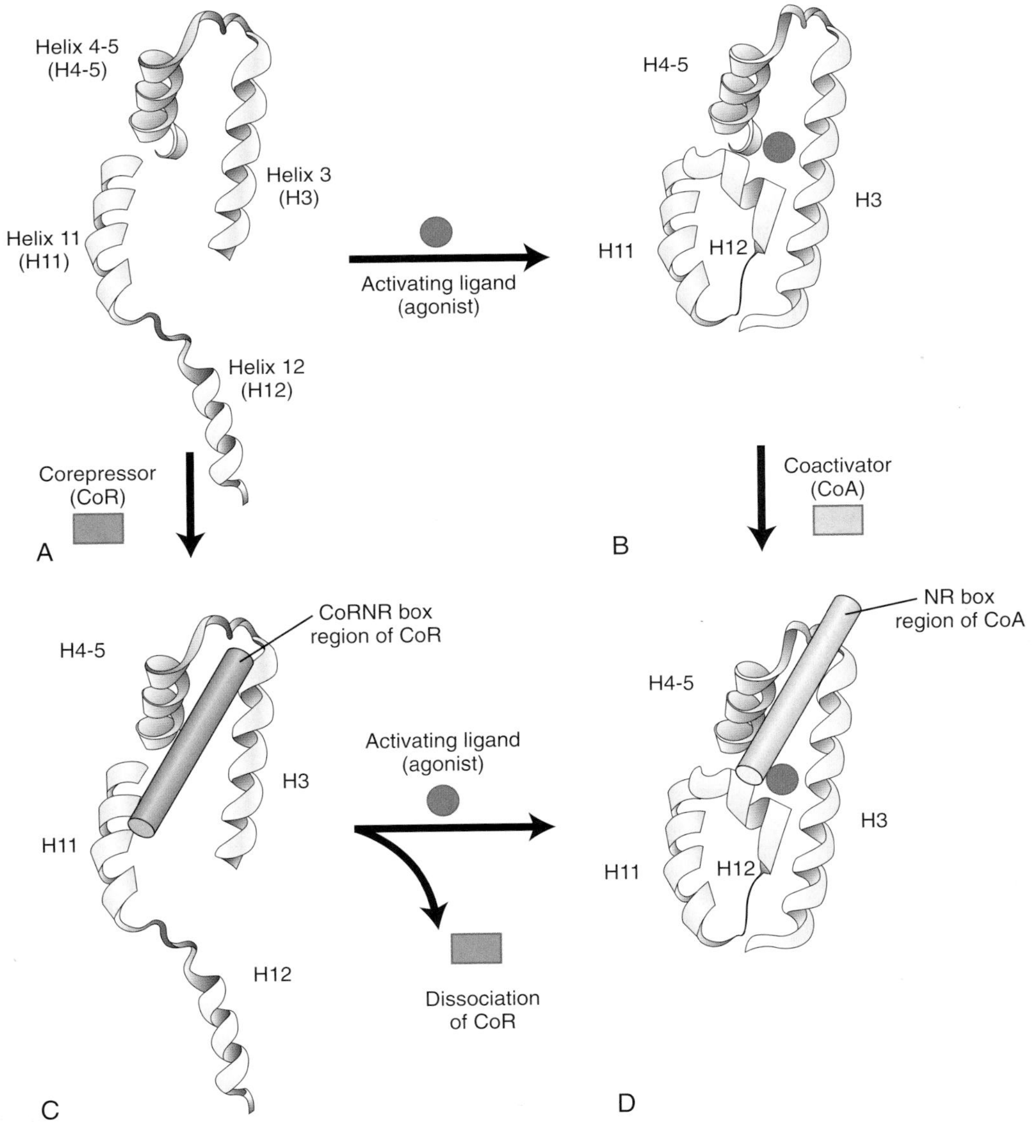

Figure 4-3 Structural basis of nuclear receptor ligand binding and cofactor recruitment. **A** and **B,** Apo-receptor (no ligand bound). **B** and **D,** Ligand-bound receptor. **C** and **D,** Structures showing the positional binding of a corepressor (**C**) or coactivator (**D**). NR, nuclear receptor.

the molecular details are essential for determining ligand specificity.[36,37] Ligand binding is the most critical determinant of receptor specificity.

Target Gene Recognition by Receptors

Another crucial specificity factor for nuclear receptors is their ability to recognize and bind to the subset of genes that is to be regulated by their cognate ligand. Target genes contain specific DNA sequences that are called *hormone response elements* (HREs). Binding to the HRE is mediated by the central C domain of the nuclear receptors (see Fig. 4-2). This region is typically composed of 66 to 68 amino acids, including two subdomains that are called *zinc fingers* because the structure of each subdomain is maintained by four cysteine residues coordinated with a zinc atom.

The first of these zinc-ordered modules contains basic amino acids that contact DNA; as with the LBD, the overall structure of the DNA-binding domain (DBD) is similar for all members of the nuclear receptor superfamily. The specificity of DNA binding is determined by multiple factors (Table 4-3). All steroid hormone receptors, except for the estrogen receptor, bind to the double-stranded DNA sequence AGAACA (Fig. 4-4).

By convention, the double-stranded sequence is described by the sequence of one of its complementary strands, with the bases ordered from the 5′ to the 3′ end. Other nuclear receptors recognize the sequence AGGTCA. The primary determinant of this specificity is a group of amino acid residues in the *P box* of the DBD (see Fig. 4-4). These hexamer DNA sequences are referred to as *half-sites*. The only difference between these hexameric half-sites is the central two base pairs (underlined in Fig. 4-4). For some nuclear receptors, the C-terminal extension of the DBD contributes specificity for extended half-sites containing additional, highly specific DNA sequences 5′ to the hexamer. Another source of specificity for target genes is the spacing and orientation of these half-sites, which in most cases are bound by receptor dimers.

Receptor Dimerization

The nuclear receptor DBD has affinity for the hexameric half-site or for extended half-sites; however, many HREs are composed of repeats of the half-site sequence, and most nuclear receptors bind these HREs as dimers. Steroid receptors, including estrogen receptors, function primarily as homodimers, which preferentially bind to two half-sites oriented toward each other (i.e., inverted repeats [IRs]) with three base pairs in between (IR3) (see Fig. 4-4A). The major dimerization domain in steroid receptors is within the C domain, although the LBD contributes. Ligand binding facilitates dimerization and DNA binding of steroid hormone receptors. Most other receptors, including THR, RAR, PPAR, LXR, and VDR, bind to DNA as heterodimers with RXR (see Fig. 4-4B).

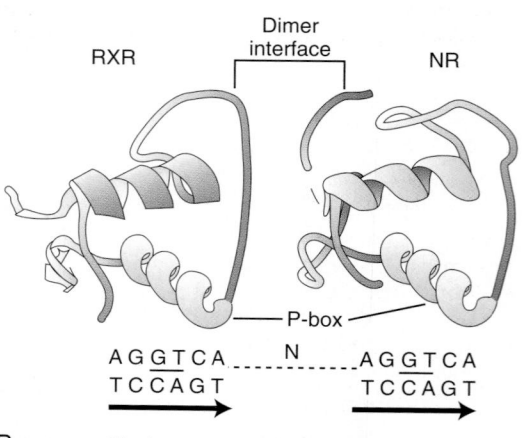

Heterodimerization with RXR is mediated by two distinct interactions, one involving LBDs and the other involving DBDs. The receptor LBD mediates the strongest interaction, which occurs even in the absence of DNA. These receptor heterodimers bind to two half-sites arranged as direct repeats (DRs) with variable numbers of base pairs in between.

The spacing of the half-sites is a major determinant of target gene specificity, and it results from the second receptor-receptor interaction, which involves the DBDs and is highly sensitive to the spacing of the half-sites. For example, VDR/RXR heterodimers bind preferentially to DRs separated by three bases (DR3 sites), TR/RXR binds DR4, and RAR/RXR binds DR5 with highest affinity.[38]

Studies of isolated DBD binding to DNA have shown that these spacing requirements are related to the fact that

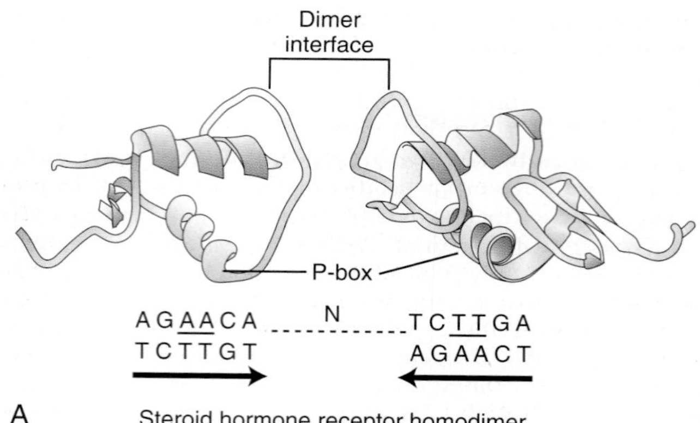

Figure 4-4 Structural basis for nuclear receptor (NR) DNA-binding specificity is shown in the ribbon diagrams of receptor DNA-binding domains (DBDs). **A,** Steroid hormone receptor binding as a homodimer to the inverted repeat *(arrows)* of the AGAACA half-site. The central base pairs are *underlined*. **B,** RXR-NR heterodimer binding to the direct repeat of AGGTCA. The position of the P box, the region of the DBD that makes direct contact with DNA, is shown. N, number of base pairs between the two half-sites; RXR, retinoid X receptor.

TABLE 4-3

Determinants of Target Gene Specificity of Nuclear Receptors

Specificity	Region of Receptor
1. Binding to DNA	DBD (C domain)
2. Binding to specific hexamer	P box in C domain (AGGTCA vs AGAACA)
3. Binding to sequences 5′ to hexamer	C-terminal extension of DBD
4. Binding to hexamer repeats	Dimerization domain (C domain for steroid receptors; D, E, and F for others)
5. Recognition of hexamer spacing	Heterodimerization with RXR (nonsteroid receptors, C domain)

DBD, DNA-binding domain; RXR, retinoid-X receptor.

the RXR binds to the upstream half-site (i.e., farthest from the start of transcription). As a result of the periodicity of the DNA helix, each base pair separating the half-sites leads to a rotation of about 36 degrees of one half-site relative to the other. Subtle differences in the structure of the receptor DBDs make the interactions more or less favorable at different degrees of rotation.[39] Solution of the crystal structure of a nuclear receptor heterodimer (specifically, the PPARγ-RXRα heterodimer) bound to DNA demonstrated that the heterodimer forms a nonsymmetric complex, allowing the LBD of PPARγ to cooperate with both DBDs to enhance response element binding.[40]

The discovery of nuclear receptor binding sites has been largely empiric, based on the finding of binding sites in small numbers of known target genes. Unbiased analysis of thousands of nuclear receptor binding locations in living cells has confirmed the canonical binding sequences for several nuclear receptors, including those of the estrogen receptor,[41,42] the androgen receptor,[43,44] the glucocorticoid receptor,[45] and PPAR/RXR heterodimers.[46,47]

RECEPTOR REGULATION OF GENE TRANSCRIPTION

Nuclear receptors mediate a variety of effects on gene transcription. The most common modes of regulation are ligand-dependent gene activation, ligand-independent repression of transcription, and ligand-dependent negative regulation of transcription (Table 4-4).

Ligand-Dependent Activation

Ligand-dependent activation is the best understood function of nuclear receptors and their ligands. The ligand-bound receptor increases transcription of a target gene to which it is bound. The DBD brings the receptor domains that mediate transcriptional activation to a specific gene. Transcriptional activation itself is mediated primarily by the LBD, which can function in the same way even when it is transferred to a DNA-binding protein that is not related to nuclear receptors. The activation function (AF) of the LBD is referred to as AF-2 (see Fig. 4-2).

Gene transcription is mediated by a large complex of factors that ultimately regulate the activity of ribonucleic acid (RNA) polymerase, the enzyme that uses the chromosomal DNA template to direct the synthesis of messenger RNA. Most mammalian genes are transcribed by RNA polymerase II using a large set of cofactor proteins that include basal transcription factors and associated factors collectively referred to as *general transcription factors* (GTFs). Details about GTFs are of fundamental importance and are available elsewhere.[48]

TABLE 4-4

Regulation of Gene Transcription by Nuclear Receptors

Mode of Regulation	Examples
1. Ligand-dependent gene activation	DNA binding and recruitment of coactivators
2. Ligand-independent gene repression	DNA binding and recruitment of corepressors
3. Ligand-dependent negative regulation of gene expression	DNA binding and recruitment of corepressors or recruitment of coactivators of DNA

TABLE 4-5

Nuclear Receptor Coregulators

Coactivators
Chromatin remodeling
Swi/Snf complex
Histone acetyltransferase
p160 family (SRC-1, GRIP-1, pCIP)
p300/CBP
pCAF (p300/CBP-associated factor)
Activation
TRAP/DRIP
Corepressors
NCoR (nuclear receptor corepressor)
SMRT (silencing mediator for retinoid and thyroid hormone receptors)

CBP, calcium-binding protein; DRIP, vitamin D receptor–interacting proteins; TRAP, thyroid hormone receptor–associated proteins.

The ligand-bound nuclear receptor communicates stimulatory signals to GTFs on the gene to which it is bound. Ligands specifically recruit a set of proteins, collectively called *coregulators*, to the nuclear receptor LBD.[49] Positively acting coregulators, called *coactivators*, specifically recognize the ligand-bound conformation of the LBD and bind to the nuclear receptor on DNA only when an activating (agonist) hormone or ligand is bound.[50] A number of coactivator proteins that bind to liganded nuclear receptors have been described (Table 4-5).[50]

The most important determinant of coactivator binding is the position of H12, which changes dramatically when activating ligands bind receptors (see Fig. 4-3D). Along with H3, H4, and H5, H12 forms a hydrophobic cleft that is bound by short polypeptide regions of the coactivator molecules.[51-53] These polypeptides, called *NR boxes*, have characteristic sequences of LxxLL, in which L is leucine and xx can be any two amino acids.[54]

Coactivators increase the rate of gene transcription. This is accomplished by enzymatic functions, including DNA unwinding in response to histone acetyltransferase (HAT) activity.[55] HAT activity is critically important for activation because chromosomal DNA is tightly wrapped around nucleosomal units composed of core histone proteins; acetylation of lysine tails on histones opens up this chromatin structure.

The best understood class of coactivator proteins is the p160 family, whose name is based on their protein size (approximately 160 kd). The family contains at least three such molecules, and each has many names (see Table 4-5).[56] These factors possess HAT activity and recruit other coactivators, such as calcium-binding protein (CBP) and p300, which are also HATs. A third HAT, p300/CBP-associated factor (PCAF, also designated TAF5L or TAF6L), is also recruited by liganded receptors. These HATs, along with a complex of SMARC molecules (SWI/SNF-related, matrix-associated, actin-dependent regulators of chromatin) that direct adenosine triphosphate (ATP)-dependent DNA unwinding, create a chromatin structure that favors transcription (Fig. 4-5).[57]

Recruitment of multiple HATs may reflect different specificities for core histones and, potentially for some nonhistone proteins. Some HATs also interact directly with GTFs and further enhance their activities. The thyroid hormone receptor–associated protein (TRAP) complex and the vitamin D receptor–interacting protein (DRIP) complex link nuclear receptors to GTFs.[58,59] The HATs and TRAP

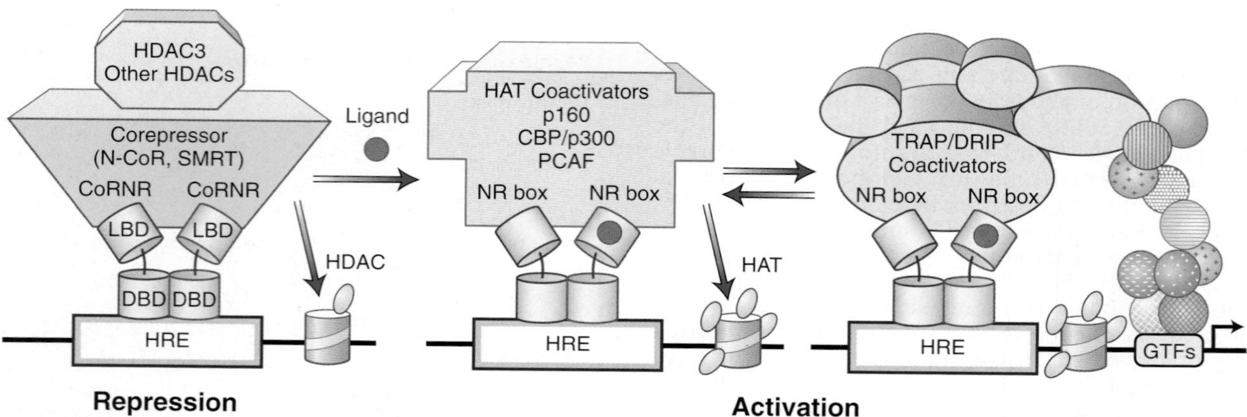

Figure 4-5 Coactivators and corepressors in transcriptional regulation by nuclear receptors. CBP, calcium-binding protein; CoRNR, coreceptor nuclear receptor box; DBD, DNA-binding domain; DRIP, vitamin D receptor–interacting protein; GTFs, general transcription factors; HAT, histone acetyltransferase; HDAC, histone deacetylase; HRE, hormone response element; LBD, ligand-binding domain; N-CoR, nuclear receptor corepressor; NR, nuclear receptor; PCAF, CBP/p300-associated factor; SMRT, silencing mediator of retinoid and thyroid receptors; TRAP, thyroid hormone receptor–associated protein.

factors are recruited to the liganded, target gene–bound receptor in an ordered manner that also involves cycling on and off of receptor gene targets.[60] Although the mechanism is not understood, the cycling may allow multiple coactivators using similar NR boxes to contribute to gene regulation without binding to a single receptor simultaneously.

Repression of Gene Expression by Unliganded Receptor

Although DNA binding is ligand dependent for steroid hormone receptors, other nuclear receptors are bound to DNA even in the absence of their cognate ligand. The unliganded, DNA-bound receptor is not passively waiting for hormone; instead, it actively represses transcription of the target gene. This repression turns off the target gene and amplifies the magnitude of the subsequent activation by hormone or ligand. For instance, if the level of gene transcription in the repressed state is 10% of the basal level in the absence of a receptor, hormone activation to 10-fold above that basal level represents a 100-fold difference of transcription rate between hormone-deficient (repressed) genes and hormone-activated genes (Fig. 4-6).[61]

In many ways, the molecular mechanism of repression is the mirror image of ligand-dependent activation. The unliganded nuclear receptor recruits negatively acting coregulators, called *corepressors*, to the target gene (see Fig. 4-3C). The two major corepressors are large (approximately 270 kd) proteins: nuclear receptor corepressor (NCoR) and silencing mediator for retinoid and thyroid receptors (SMRT).[62] NCoR and SMRT specifically recognize the unliganded conformation of nuclear receptors and use an amphipathic helical sequence similar to the NR box of coactivators to bind to a hydrophobic pocket in the receptor.

For corepressors, the peptide responsible for receptor binding is called the *CoRNR box,* and it contains the sequence (I or L)xx(I or V)I, in which I is isoleucine, L is leucine, V is valine, and xx represents any two amino acids.[63] The receptor uses helices 3 to 5 to form the hydrophobic pocket, as in coactivator binding, but H12 does not promote and even hinders corepressor binding. This negative function of H12 highlights the role of the ligand-dependent change in the position of H12 as the switch that determines repression and activation by nuclear receptors (see Fig. 4-5).[64]

The transcriptional functions of NCoR and SMRT are the opposite of those of the coactivators. The corepressors themselves do not possess enzyme activity but do recruit histone deacetylases (HDACs) to the target gene, thereby reversing the effects of histone acetylation described earlier and leading to a compact, repressed state of chromatin. Although the mammalian genome contains multiple HDACs, several of which may play a role in nuclear receptor function, the main one involved in repression is HDAC3, whose enzyme activity depends on interaction with NCoR or SMRT.[65] The ability of NCoR to bind and activate HDAC3 is required for normal metabolic and circadian physiology.[66] The corepressors interact directly with GTFs to inhibit their transcriptional activities, and they also exist in large, multiprotein complexes whose range of functions is not fully understood.

Ligand-Dependent Negative Regulation of Gene Expression: Transrepression

The ligand-dependent switch between repressed and activated receptor conformations explains how hormones activate gene expression. However, many important gene targets of hormones are turned off in the presence of the ligand. This is referred to as *ligand-dependent negative regulation of transcription*, or *transrepression*, to distinguish it from the repression of basal transcription by unliganded receptors.

The mechanism of negative regulation is less well understood than ligand-dependent activation, and there may be several mechanisms.[67] One mechanism involves nuclear receptor binding to DNA-binding sites that reverse the paradigm of ligand-dependent activation (i.e., negative response elements). For example, when the unliganded thyroid receptor binds to the negative response element of the genes for the β-subunit of thyroid-stimulating hormone or thyroid-stimulating hormone–releasing hormone, transcription is activated.[68] The role and recruitment of coregulators in this process require further investigation. In other cases, negative regulation may result from ligand binding to nuclear receptors that bind to other transcription factors without binding DNA. This interaction leads to removal of coactivators such as p300 and CBP from the other

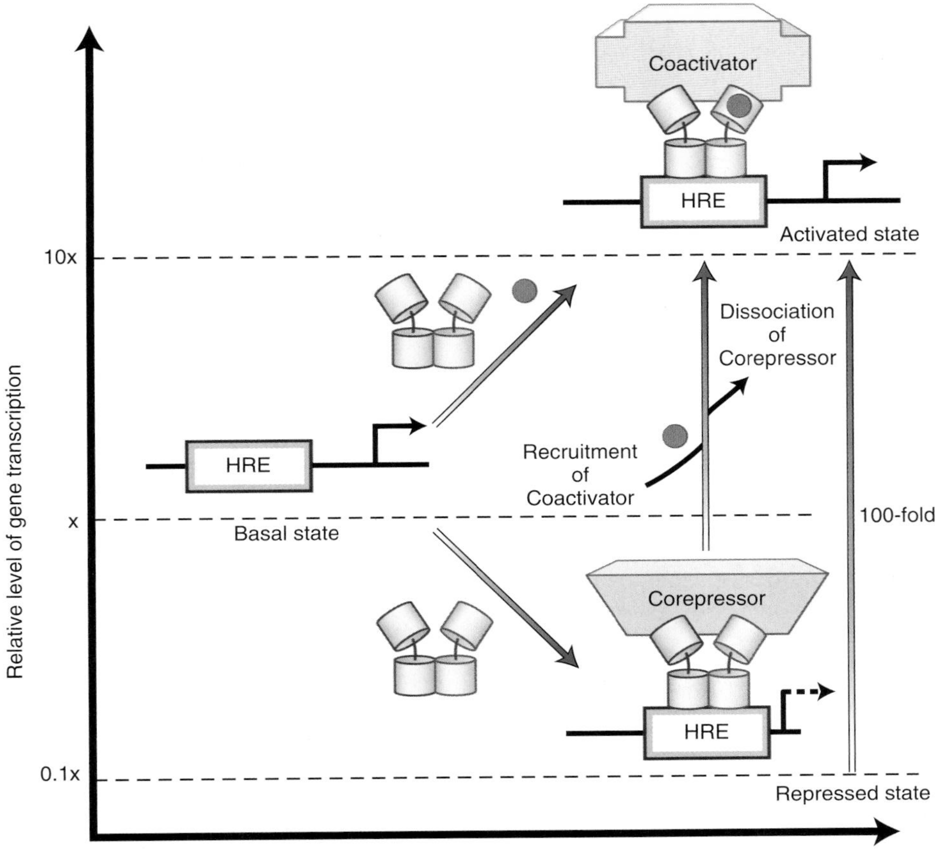

Figure 4-6 Repression and activation functions augment the dynamic range of transcriptional regulation by nuclear receptors. The magnitudes of activation and repression were arbitrarily set at 10-fold for this theoretical example. In cells, these magnitudes vary as a function of coactivator and corepressor concentration and in a target gene–specific manner. HRE, hormone response element.

transcription factors that positively regulate the gene. In this model, inhibition of the activity of the positively acting factors results in the observed negative regulation.

Roles of Other Nuclear Receptor Domains

The amino-terminal A/B domain of the nuclear receptors is the most variable region among all members of the superfamily in terms of length and amino acid sequence. Subtypes of the same receptor often have completely different A/B domains. The function of this domain is the least well defined of any. It is not required for unliganded repression or for ligand-dependent activation. In many receptors, the A/B domain contains positive transcriptional activity, often referred to as activation function 1 (AF-1) (see Fig. 4-2). It is ligand independent but probably interacts with coactivators and may influence the magnitude of activation by agonists or partial agonists. This activation function is tissue specific and tends to be more important for steroid hormone receptors, whose A/B domains are notably longer than those of other members of the superfamily.[69] The F domain of the nuclear receptors is hypervariable in length and sequence, and its function is not known.

Cross-Talk with Other Signaling Pathways

Hormones and cytokines that signal through cell surface receptors also regulate gene transcription, often by activating protein kinases that phosphorylate transcription factors such as cAMP-response element–binding protein (CREB). Such signals can also lead to phosphorylation of nuclear receptors. Multiple signal-dependent kinases can phosphorylate nuclear receptors, leading to conformational changes that regulate function.[70] Phosphorylation can lead to changes in DNA binding, ligand binding, or coactivator binding; these consequences depend on the specific kinase, receptor, and domain of the receptor that is phosphorylated. The properties of coactivators and corepressors are also regulated by phosphorylation.[71]

Receptor Antagonists

Certain ligands function as receptor antagonists by competing with agonists for the ligand-binding site. In the case of steroid hormone receptors, the position of H12 in the antagonist-bound receptor is not identical to that in the unliganded receptor or in the agonist-bound receptor. H12, which has a sequence that resembles the NR box, binds to the coactivator-binding pocket of the receptor and thereby prevents coactivator binding.[72] This antagonist-bound conformation of the receptor also favors corepressor binding to steroid hormone receptors.

Tissue Selectivity of Ligands Interacting with Nuclear Receptors

Many endogenous hormones that act through nuclear receptors do so in a tissue-specific manner. The most

TABLE 4-6

Factors Modulating Receptor Activity in Different Tissues

Concentration of receptor
Cell-specificity
Variation within a given cell type
Post-translational modification of receptor (e.g., phosphorylation)
Regulation of intracellular ligand levels (see Table 4-2)
Pioneer factors determining receptor binding sites (e.g., FOX proteins)
Function of ligand
Agonist
Partial agonist
Antagonist
Concentration and types of coregulators
Coactivators
Corepressors

obvious mechanism is differential expression of the receptors, both in space (e.g., cell-type specificity)[73] and in time (e.g., circadian variation).[74] Ligand levels may be regulated intracellularly (see earlier discussion and Table 4-2), and post-translational modification (e.g., phosphorylation) influences cell-specific receptor function. Although nuclear receptors bind at thousands of sites on genomic DNA, the specific binding sites are regulated in a cell type–specific manner. For example, the estrogen receptor binds to overlapping but clearly different sets of genomic sites in the uterus and in the breast, probably because of the differential actions of so-called pioneer transcription factors, including forkhead box (FOX) proteins.[75]

Some ligands function as antagonists in certain tissues but as full or partial agonists in others. These selective receptor modulators include compounds such as tamoxifen, a selective estrogen receptor modulator (SERM). SERMs are estrogen receptor antagonists with respect to the functions of AF-2, including coregulator binding, and they require the AF-1 for their agonist activity.[76] This agonism, like AF-1 activity, tends to be tissue specific and therefore has great therapeutic utility.[77] Table 4-6 summarizes factors contributing to the tissue specificity of receptor activity.

REFERENCES

1. Chambon P. The nuclear receptor superfamily: a personal retrospect on the first two decades. *Mol Endocrinol.* 2005;19:1418-1428.
2. Evans RM. The nuclear receptor superfamily: a rosetta stone for physiology. *Mol Endocrinol.* 2005;19:1429-1438.
3. O'Malley BW. A life-long search for the molecular pathways of steroid hormone action. *Mol Endocrinol.* 2005;19:1402-1411.
4. Visser WE, Friesema EC, Jansen J, et al. Thyroid hormone transport in and out of cells. *Trends Endocrinol Metab.* 2008;19:50-56.
5. Heuer H, Visser TJ. Minireview: pathophysiological importance of thyroid hormone transporters. *Endocrinology.* 2009;150:1078-1083.
6. Escriva H, Delaunay F, Laudet V. Ligand binding and nuclear receptor evolution. *Bioessays.* 2000;22:717-727.
7. Arriza JL, Weinberger C, Cerelli G, et al. Cloning of human mineralocorticoid receptor complementary cDNA: structure and functional kinship with the glucocorticoid receptor. *Science.* 1987;237:268-275.
8. Roy AK, Tyagi RK, Song CS, et al. Androgen receptor: structural domains and functional dynamics after ligand-receptor interaction. *Ann N Y Acad Sci.* 2001;949:44-57.
9. Germain P, Chambon P, Eichele G, et al. International Union of Pharmacology: LX. Retinoic acid receptors. *Pharmacol Rev.* 2006;58:712-725.
10. Germain P, Chambon P, Eichele G, et al. International Union of Pharmacology: LXIII. Retinoid X receptors. *Pharmacol Rev.* 2006;58:760-772.
11. Michalik L, Auwerx J, Berger JP, et al. International Union of Pharmacology: LXI. Peroxisome proliferator-activated receptors. *Pharmacol Rev.* 2006;58:726-741.
12. Forman BM, Chen J, Evans RM. Hypolipidemic drugs, polyunsaturated fatty acids, and eicosanoids are ligands for peroxisome proliferator-activated receptors alpha and delta. *Proc Natl Acad Sci U S A.* 1997;94:4312-4317.
13. Yu K, Bayonea W, Kallen CB, et al. Differential activation of peroxisome proliferator-activated receptors by eicosanoids. *J Biol Chem.* 1995;270:23975-23983.
14. Ziouzenkova O, Perrey S, Asatryan L, et al. Lipolysis of triglyceride-rich lipoproteins generates PPAR ligands: evidence for an antiinflammatory role for lipoprotein lipase. *Proc Natl Acad Sci U S A.* 2003;100:2730-2735.
15. Issemann I, Green S. Activation of a member of the steroid hormone receptor superfamily by peroxisome proliferators. *Nature.* 1990;347:645-650.
16. Barish GD, Narkar VA, Evans RM. PPAR delta: a dagger in the heart of the metabolic syndrome. *J Clin Invest.* 2006;116:590-597.
17. Rangwala SM, Lazar MA. Peroxisome proliferator-activated receptor gamma in diabetes and metabolism. *Trends Pharmacol Sci.* 2004;25:331-336.
18. Forman BM, Tontonoz P, Chen J, et al. 15-Deoxy, delta 12, 14-prostaglandin J2 is a ligand for the adipocyte determination factor PPARg. *Cell.* 1995;83:803-812.
19. Kliewer SA, Lenhard JM, Willson TM, et al. A prostaglandin J2 metabolite binds peroxisome proliferator-activated receptor gamma and promotes adipocyte differentiation. *Cell.* 1995;83:813-819.
20. Lehmann JM, Moore LB, Smith-Oliver TA, et al. An antidiabetic thiazolidinedione is a high affinity ligand for the nuclear peroxisome proliferator-activated receptor g (PPARg). *J Biol Chem.* 1995;270:12953-12956.
21. Tontonoz P, Mangelsdorf DJ. Liver X receptor signaling pathways in cardiovascular disease. *Mol Endocrinol.* 2003;17:985-993.
22. Moore DD, Kato S, Xie W, et al. International Union of Pharmacology: LXII. The NR1H and NR1I receptors: constitutive androstane receptor, pregnene X receptor, farnesoid X receptor alpha, farnesoid X receptor beta, liver X receptor alpha, liver X receptor beta, and vitamin D receptor. *Pharmacol Rev.* 2006;58:742-759.
23. Benoit G, Cooney A, Giguere V, et al. International Union of Pharmacology: LXVI. Orphan nuclear receptors. *Pharmacol Rev.* 2006;58:798-836.
24. Preitner N, Damiola F, Lopez-Molina L, et al. The orphan nuclear receptor REV-ERBalpha controls circadian transcription within the positive limb of the mammalian circadian oscillator. *Cell.* 2002;110:251-260.
25. Raghuram S, Stayrook KR, Huang P, et al. Identification of heme as the ligand for the orphan nuclear receptors REV-ERBalpha and REV-ERBbeta. *Nat Struct Mol Biol.* 2007;14:1207-1213.
26. Yin L, Wu N, Curtin JC, et al. Rev-erbalpha, a heme sensor that coordinates metabolic and circadian pathways. *Science.* 2007;318:1786-1789.
27. Lu NZ, Cidlowski JA. The origin and functions of multiple human glucocorticoid receptor isoforms. *Ann N Y Acad Sci.* 2004;1024:102-123.
28. Zhang J, Lazar MA. The mechanism of action of thyroid hormone receptors. *Annu Rev Physiol.* 2000;62:439-466.
29. Achermann JC, Jameson JL. Fertility and infertility: genetic contributions from the hypothalamic-pituitary-gonadal axis. *Mol Endocrinol.* 1999;13:812-818.
30. Seol W, Choi HS, Moore DD. An orphan nuclear hormone receptor that lacks a DNA binding domain and heterodimerizes with other receptors. *Science.* 1996;272:1336-1339.
31. Gurnell M, Chatterjee VK. Nuclear receptors in disease: thyroid receptor beta, peroxisome-proliferator-activated receptor gamma and orphan receptors. *Essays Biochem.* 2004;40:169-189.
32. Niu DM, Hwang B, Tiu CM, et al. Contributions of bone maturation measurements to the differential diagnosis of neonatal transient hypothyroidism versus dyshormonogenetic congenital hypothyroidism. *Acta Paediatr.* 2004;93:1301-1306.
33. McPhaul MJ. Molecular defects of the androgen receptor. *Recent Prog Horm Res.* 2002;57:181-194.
34. Palermo M, Quinkler M, Stewart PM. Apparent mineralocorticoid excess syndrome: an overview. *Arq Bras Endocrinol Metabol.* 2004;48:687-696.
35. Stewart PM, Krozowski ZS. 11 Beta-hydroxysteroid dehydrogenase. *Vitam Horm.* 1999;57:249-324.
36. Moras D, Gronemeyer H. The nuclear receptor ligand-binding domain: structure and function. *Curr Opin Cell Biol.* 1998;10:384-391.
37. Weatherman RV, Fletterick RJ, Scanlan TS. Nuclear receptor ligands and ligand-binding domains. *Annu Rev Biochem.* 1999;68:559-581.
38. Umesono K, Murakami KK, Thompson CC, et al. Direct repeats as selective response elements for the thyroid hormone, retinoic acid, and vitamin D3 receptors. *Cell.* 1991;65:1255-1266.
39. Rastinejad F, Perlmann T, Evans RM, et al. Structural determinants of nuclear receptor assembly on DNA direct repeats. *Nature.* 1995;375:203-211.
40. Chandra V, Huang P, Hamuro Y, et al. Structure of the intact PPAR-gamma-RXR-nuclear receptor complex on *DNA*. *Nature.* 2008;456:350-356.

41. Carroll JS, Meyer CA, Song J, et al. Genome-wide analysis of estrogen receptor binding sites. *Nat Genet.* 2006;38:1289-1297.
42. Lin CY, Vega VB, Thomsen JS, et al. Whole-genome cartography of estrogen receptor alpha binding sites. *PLoS Genet.* 2007;3:e87.
43. Bolton EC, So AY, Chaivorapol C, et al. Cell- and gene-specific regulation of primary target genes by the androgen receptor. *Genes Dev.* 2007;21:2005-2017.
44. Wang Q, Li W, Liu XS, et al. A hierarchical network of transcription factors governs androgen receptor-dependent prostate cancer growth. *Mol Cell.* 2007;27:380-392.
45. Wang JC, Derynck MK, Nonaka DF, et al. Chromatin immunoprecipitation (ChIP) scanning identifies primary glucocorticoid receptor target genes. *Proc Natl Acad Sci U S A.* 2004;101:15603-15608.
46. Lefterova MI, Zhang Y, Steger DJ, et al. PPARgamma and C/EBP factors orchestrate adipocyte biology via adjacent binding on a genome-wide scale. *Genes Dev.* 2008;22:2941-2952.
47. Nielsen R, Pedersen TA, Hagenbeek D, et al. Genome-wide profiling of PPARgamma:RXR and RNA polymerase II occupancy reveals temporal activation of distinct metabolic pathways and changes in RXR dimer composition during adipogenesis. *Genes Dev.* 2008;22:2953-2967.
48. Roeder RG. Role of general and gene-specific cofactors in the regulation of eukaryotic transcription. *Cold Spring Harb Symp Quant Biol.* 1998;63:201-218.
49. Halachmi S, Marden E, Martin G, et al. Estrogen receptor-associated proteins: possible mediators of hormone-induced transcription. *Science.* 1994;264:1455-1458.
50. Smith CL, O'Malley BW. Coregulator function: a key to understanding tissue specificity of selective receptor modulators. *Endocr Rev.* 2004;25:45-71.
51. Feng W, Ribieiro RC, Wagner RL, et al. Hormone-dependent coactivator binding to a hydrophobic cleft on nuclear receptors. *Science.* 1998;280:1747-1749.
52. Nolte RT, Wisely GB, Westin S, et al. Ligand binding and co-activator assembly of the peroxisome prolierator-activated receptor-gamma. *Nature.* 1998;395:137-143.
53. Shiau AK, Barstad D, Loria PM, et al. The structural basis of estrogen receptor/coactivator recognition and the antagonism of this interaction by tamoxifen. *Cell.* 1998;95:927-937.
54. Heery DM, Kalkhoven E, Hoare S, et al. A signature motif in transcriptional co-activators mediates binding to nuclear receptors. *Nature.* 1997;387:733-736.
55. Fischle W, Wang Y, Allis CD. Histone and chromatin cross-talk. *Curr Opin Cell Biol.* 2003;15:172-183.
56. Glass CK, Rose DW, Rosenfeld MG. Nuclear receptor coactivators. *Curr Opin Cell Biol.* 1997;9:222-232.
57. Aoyagi S, Trotter KW, Archer TK. ATP-dependent chromatin remodeling complexes and their role in nuclear receptor-dependent transcription in vivo. *Vitam Horm.* 2005;70:281-307.
58. Ito M, Yuan CX, Malik S, et al. Identity between TRAP and SMCC complexes indicates novel pathways for the function of nuclear receptors and diverse mammalian activators. *Mol Cell.* 1999;3:361-370.
59. Rachez C, Suidan Z, Ward J, et al. A novel protein complex that interacts with the vitamin D3 receptor in a ligand-dependent manner and enhances VDR transactivation in a cell-free system. *Genes Dev.* 1998;12:1787-1800.
60. Shang Y, Hu X, DiRenzo J, et al. Cofactor dynamics and sufficiency in estrogen receptor-regulated transcription. *Cell.* 2000;103:843-852.
61. Hu X, Lazar MA. Transcriptional repression by nuclear hormone receptors. *Trends Endocrinol Metab.* 2000;11:6-10.
62. Privalsky ML. The role of corepressors in transcriptional regulation by nuclear hormone receptors. *Annu Rev Physiol.* 2004;66:315-360.
63. Hu X, Lazar MA. The CoRNR motif contols the recruitment of corepressors to nuclear hormone receptors. *Nature.* 1999;402:93-96.
64. Glass CK, Rosenfeld MG. The coregulator exchange in transcriptional functions of nuclear receptors. *Genes Dev.* 2000;14:121-141.
65. Ishizuka T, Lazar MA. The nuclear receptor corepressor deacetylase activating domain is essential for repression by thyroid hormone receptor. *Mol Endocrinol.* 2005;19:1443-1451.
66. Alenghat T, Meyers K, Mullican SE, et al. Nuclear receptor corepressor and histone deacetylase 3 govern circadian metabolic physiology. *Nature.* 2008;456:997-1000.
67. Lazar MA. Thyroid hormone action: a binding contract. *J Clin Invest.* 2003;112:497-499.
68. Chiamolera MI, Wondisford FE. Minireview: thyrotropin-releasing hormone and the thyroid hormone feedback mechanism. *Endocrinology.* 2009;150:1091-1096.
69. Kumar R, Thompson EB. Transactivation functions of the N-terminal domains of nuclear hormone receptors: protein folding and coactivator interactions. *Mol Endocrinol.* 2003;17:1-10.
70. Shao D, Lazar MA. Modulating nuclear receptor function: may the phos be with you. *J Clin Invest.* 1999;103:1617-1618.
71. Han SJ, Lonard DM, O'Malley BW. Multi-modulation of nuclear receptor coactivators through posttranslational modifications. *Trends Endocrinol Metab.* 2009;20:8-15.
72. Gronemeyer H, Gustafsson JA, Laudet V. Principles for modulation of the nuclear receptor superfamily. *Nat Rev Drug Discov.* 2004;3:950-964.
73. Bookout AL, Jeong Y, Downes M, et al. Anatomical profiling of nuclear receptor expression reveals a hierarchical transcriptional network. *Cell.* 2006;126:789-799.
74. Yang X, Downes M, Yu RT, et al. Nuclear receptor expression links the circadian clock to metabolism. *Cell.* 2006;126:801-810.
75. Lupien M, Eeckhoute J, Meyer CA, et al. FoxA1 translates epigenetic signatures into enhancer-driven lineage-specific transcription. *Cell.* 2008;132:958-970.
76. Osborne CK, Zaho H, Fuqua SA. Selective estrogen receptor modulators: structure, function, and clinical use. *J Clin Oncol.* 2000;18:3172-3186.
77. Shang Y, Brown M. Molecular determinants for the tissue specificity of SERMs. *Science.* 2002;295:2465-2468.

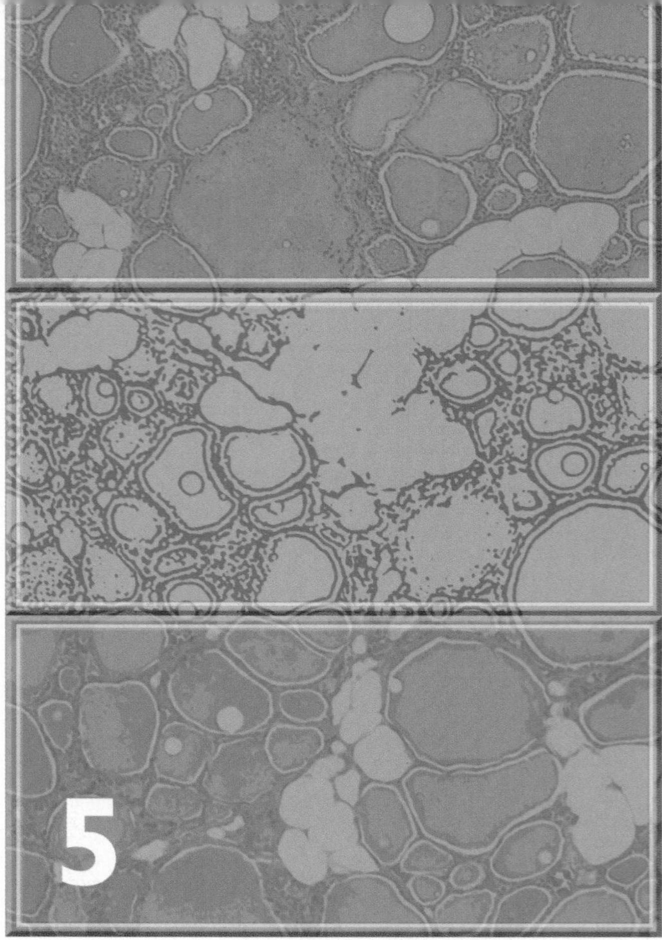

CHAPTER 5

Mechanism of Action of Hormones That Act at the Cell Surface

ALLEN M. SPIEGEL • CHRISTIN CARTER-SU • SIMEON I. TAYLOR • ROHIT N. KULKARNI

Hormones are secreted into the blood and act on target cells at a distance from the secretory gland. To respond to a hormone, a target cell must contain the essential components of a signaling pathway: a receptor to bind the hormone, an effector (e.g., enzymatic activity that is regulated when the hormone binds to its receptor), and appropriate downstream signaling pathways to mediate the physiologic responses to the hormone. This general type of mechanism involving receptors, effectors, and downstream signaling pathways also functions in non-endocrine systems, such as those regulated by neurotransmitters, cytokines, and paracrine and autocrine factors. This chapter reviews several endocrine signaling pathways that begin with activation of receptors located on the surface of target cells and focuses on the molecular mechanisms that function in normal physiology and in pathology.

RECEPTORS

Hormone receptors are defined by their ability to bind hormone and to couple hormone binding to hormone action. Both components of the definition are essential; for example, many hormones bind to binding proteins that are distinct from receptors because the binding proteins do not trigger the signaling pathways that mediate hormone action.

Many classes of receptors are of interest in endocrinology. Some receptors (e.g., receptors for steroid and thyroid hormones) are located within the cell and function as transcription factors. Other receptors (e.g., low-density lipoprotein receptors) are located on the cell surface and function primarily to transport their ligands into the cell by a process referred to as *receptor-mediated endocytosis*. In this chapter, we focus on cell surface receptors that trigger intracellular signaling pathways. These cell surface receptors can be classified according to the molecular mechanisms by which they accomplish signaling:

1. Ligand-gated ion channels (e.g., nicotinic acetylcholine receptors)
2. Receptor tyrosine kinases (e.g., receptors for insulin and insulin-like growth factor 1)
3. Receptor serine/threonine kinases (e.g., receptors for activins and inhibins)
4. Receptor guanylate cyclase (e.g., atrial natriuretic factor receptor)

5. G protein–coupled receptors (e.g., receptors for adrenergic agents, muscarinic cholinergic agents, glycoprotein hormones, glucagon, and parathyroid hormone)
6. Cytokine receptors (e.g., receptors for growth hormone, prolactin, and leptin)

The receptors belonging to classes 1 through 4 are bifunctional molecules that can bind hormone and serve as effectors by functioning as ion channels or as enzymes. The receptors belonging to classes 5 and 6 can bind the hormone but must recruit a separate molecule to catalyze the effector function. For example, G protein–coupled receptors (GPCRs) use G proteins to regulate downstream effector molecules. Similarly, cytokine receptors recruit cytosolic tyrosine kinases (e.g., Janus family tyrosine kinases [JAKs]) as effectors to trigger downstream signaling pathways.

HORMONE BINDING

As predicted by the fact that hormones circulate in relatively low concentrations in the plasma, the binding interaction between a hormone and its receptor is characterized by high binding affinity. Hormone binding has a high degree of specificity, and the receptor usually binds its cognate hormone more tightly than it binds other hormones. However, some receptors bind structurally related hormones with lower affinity. For example, the insulin receptor binds insulin-like growth factors (IGFs) with approximately 100-fold lower affinity than it binds insulin. Similarly, the thyrotropin receptor binds human chorionic gonadotropin with lower affinity than it binds thyrotropin. This phenomenon has been referred to as *specificity spillover,* and it provides an explanation of several pathologic conditions, such as hypoglycemia caused by tumors secreting IGF2 and hyperthyroidism associated with choriocarcinoma.[1]

Binding of a hormone (H) to its receptor (R) can be described mathematically as an equilibrium reaction:

$$\mathrm{H + R \rightleftharpoons HR}$$

At equilibrium,

$$\mathrm{K_a = (HR)/(H)(R)}$$

where K_a is the association constant for the formation of the hormone receptor complex (HR). As was originally shown by Scatchard, it is possible to rearrange this equation in terms of the total concentration of receptor-binding sites, R_0 = (R) + (RH), as follows:

$$\mathrm{K_a = (HP)/\{[R_0 - (HR)](H)\}}$$

$$\mathrm{(HR) = K_a[R_0 - (HR)](H)}$$

$$\mathrm{(HR)/(H) = K_aR_0 - K_a(HR)}$$

A straight line is obtained when (HR)/(H) (i.e., the ratio of bound to free hormone) is plotted as a function of (HR) (the concentration of bound hormone). The slope of the line is $-K_a$, and the line intercepts the horizontal axis at the point where (HR) = R_0 = the total number of binding sites. This type of plot, referred to as a *Scatchard plot,* has been used as a graphic method to estimate the affinity with which a receptor binds its hormone. Although the binding properties of some receptors are described more or less accurately by these simple equations, other receptors exhibit more complex properties. This simple algebraic derivation of the Scatchard equation implicitly assumes that there is only one class of receptors and that the binding sites on the receptors do not interact with one another. If these assumptions do not apply to the interaction of a particular hormone with its receptor, the Scatchard plot may not be linear.

Several molecular mechanisms can contribute to nonlinearity of the Scatchard plot. For example, there may be more than one type of receptor that binds the hormone (e.g., a high-affinity, low-capacity site and a low-affinity, high-capacity site). Some receptors (e.g., insulin receptor) have more than one binding site, and there may be cooperative interactions among the binding sites. The interaction between a G protein and a GPCR may affect the affinity with which the receptor binds its ligand; the effect on binding affinity depends on whether guanosine diphosphate (GDP) or guanosine triphosphate (GTP) is bound to the G protein. A detailed discussion of these complexities is beyond the scope of this chapter.

REGULATION OF HORMONE SENSITIVITY

Early in the history of endocrinology, attention was focused on the regulation of hormone secretion as the most important mechanism for regulating physiology. However, it has become apparent that the target cell is not passive. Many influences can alter the sensitivity of the target cell's response to a given concentration of hormone. For example, the number of receptors can be regulated. All things being equal, hormone sensitivity is directly related to the number of hormone receptors expressed on the cell surface. Posttranslational modifications of the receptor can modify the affinity of hormone binding or the efficiency of coupling to downstream signaling pathways. All of the downstream components in the hormone action pathway are subject to similar types of regulatory influences, which can have a significant impact on the ability of the target cell to respond to hormone.

Just as hormone sensitivity is subject to normal physiologic regulation, pathologic influences can cause disease by targeting components of the hormone action pathway. Multiple etiologic factors can impair the hormone action pathway, such as genetic influences, autoimmune processes, and exogenous toxins. For example, disease mechanisms can alter the functions of cell surface receptors, effectors such as G proteins, and other components of the downstream signaling pathways. Several examples are provided here to illustrate these principles.

RECEPTOR TYROSINE KINASES

Receptor tyrosine kinases have several structural features in common: an extracellular domain containing the ligand-binding site, a single transmembrane domain, and an intracellular portion that includes the tyrosine kinase catalytic domain (Fig. 5-1). Analysis of the human genome suggests that it contains sequences for approximately 100 receptor tyrosine kinases. The tyrosine kinase domain is the most highly conserved sequence among all of the receptors in this family. In contrast, there is considerable variation among the sequences of the extracellular domains. The family of receptor tyrosine kinases has 16 subfamilies, classified primarily on the basis of differences in the structure of the extracellular domain.[2] Receptor tyrosine kinases mediate the biologic actions of a wide variety of ligands, including insulin, epidermal growth factor (EGF),

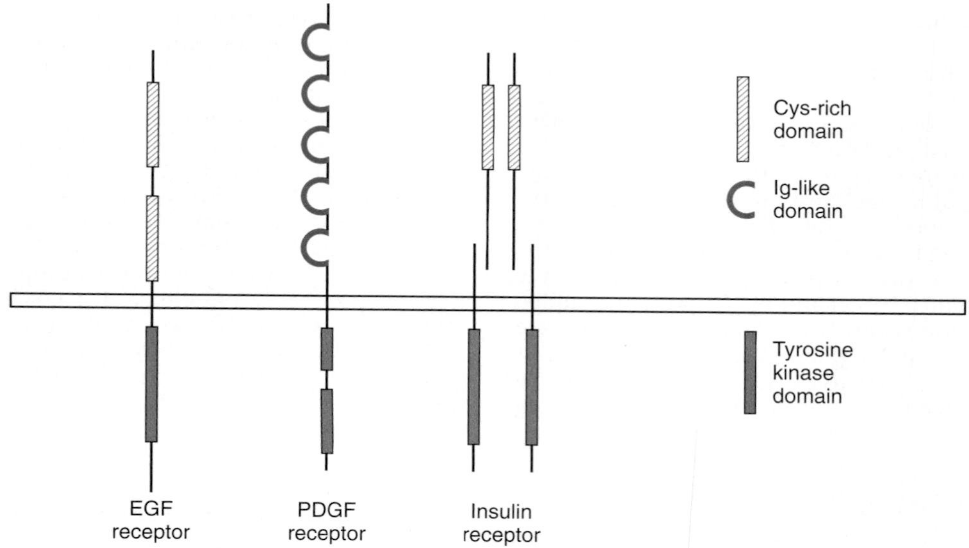

Figure 5-1 Receptor tyrosine kinases. Three of the 16 families of receptor tyrosine kinases are diagrammed.[2,3] All receptor tyrosine kinases possess an extracellular domain containing the ligand-binding site, a single transmembrane domain, and an intracellular portion containing the tyrosine kinase domain. Several structural motifs (i.e., cysteine-rich domain, immunoglobulin (Ig)-like domain, tyrosine kinase domain) in these receptor tyrosine kinases are indicated on the right side of the figure. Cys, cysteine; EGF, epidermal growth factor; PDGF, platelet-derived growth factor.

platelet-derived growth factor (PDGF), and vascular endothelial growth factor (VEGF). The variation in the sequences of the extracellular domains enables the receptors to bind this structurally diverse collection of ligands.

The EGF receptor was the first cell surface receptor demonstrated to possess tyrosine kinase activity,[4] and it was the first receptor tyrosine kinase to be cloned.[5] Like most receptor tyrosine kinases, the EGF receptor exists primarily as a monomer in the absence of ligand. However, binding of ligand induces receptor dimerization. Ligand-induced dimerization is central to the mechanism by which the receptor mediates the biologic activity of EGF. In addition to the ability to form homodimers, the EGF receptor can form heterodimers with other members of the same subfamily of receptor tyrosine kinases. Because a small number of receptors can combine in a large number of pairings, heterodimer formation has the potential to fine-tune the specificity of receptors for ligand binding and downstream signaling.

The insulin receptor is of special interest to endocrinologists because diabetes is among the most common diseases of the endocrine system. The insulin receptor closely resembles the type 1 receptor for IGFs,[6] which mediates the biologic actions of IGF1 and therefore plays an important role in the physiology of growth hormone (GH) in vivo. Although the kinase domains of receptors for insulin and IGF1 closely resemble other receptor tyrosine kinases, at least two distinctive features set them apart. First, the receptors are synthesized as proreceptors that undergo proteolytic cleavage into two subunits (α and β). The α-subunit contains the ligand-binding site; the β-subunit includes the transmembrane and tyrosine kinase domains. Second, both receptors exist as $\alpha_2\beta_2$ heterotetramers that are stabilized by intersubunit disulfide bonds. In contrast to many other receptor tyrosine kinases, which are thought to dimerize in response to ligand binding, the insulin receptor exists as a dimer of $\alpha\beta$ monomers even in the absence of ligand. The remainder of this section reviews the molecular mechanisms by which receptor tyrosine kinases mediate biologic action, with special emphasis on the insulin receptor as an example.

Receptor Activation: Role of Receptor Dimerization

Dimerization plays a central role in the mechanism by which most receptor tyrosine kinases are activated by their cognate ligands.[2,7] Although receptor dimerization is a common theme, the detailed molecular mechanisms vary from receptor to receptor. Three examples of the mechanisms of receptor dimerization are provided[8-12] (Fig. 5-2).

Dimeric Ligand

PDGF and VEGF are examples of dimeric ligands (see Fig. 5-2).[8,9,13] Because each subunit of ligand can bind one receptor molecule, simultaneous binding of two receptor molecules drives receptor dimerization. Direct support for this type of mechanism is provided by the crystal structure of VEGF when bound to its receptor, FLT1.[13]

Two Receptor-Binding Sites on a Monomeric Ligand

The mechanism of two receptor-binding sites on a single ligand is important for many receptor tyrosine kinases, but it was first rigorously demonstrated for the GH receptor, which is not a member of the receptor tyrosine kinase family (see Fig. 5-2).[10-12] The crystal structure of bound GH shows that one molecule of ligand can bind two molecules of receptor. Two distinct receptor-binding sites exist on each GH molecule, and this enables the ligand to bind to receptor dimers and cause the appropriate conformational change to activate the GH receptor–associated tyrosine kinase, JAK2.

This observation has an important implication for pharmacology. By abolishing one of the two receptor-binding sites, it is possible to design mutant ligands that bind to one of the two sites but lack the ability to bind to both. The mutant ligands therefore cannot trigger hormone action but, by binding to receptors, they inhibit the action of the endogenous hormone. Such mutant GH molecules have been developed as therapeutic agents for use in conditions such as acromegaly.

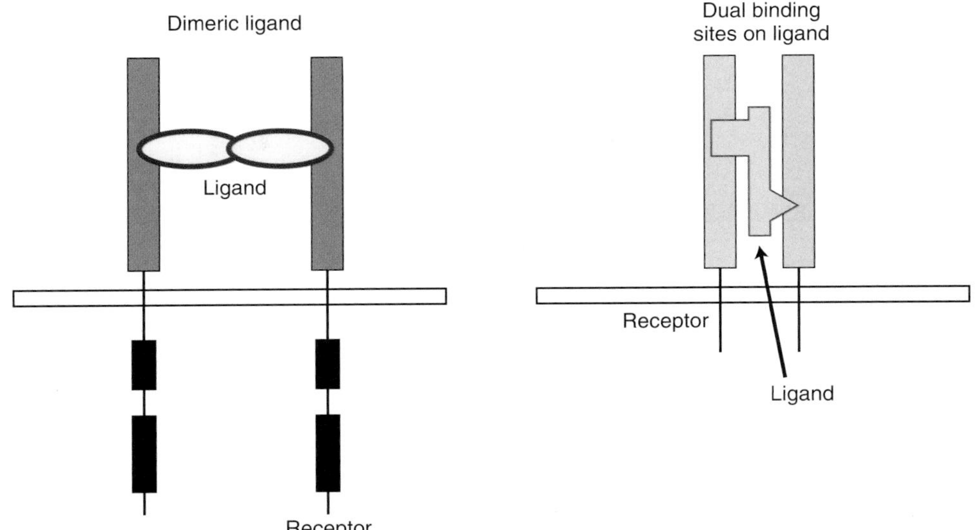

Figure 5-2 Molecular mechanisms of ligand-induced dimerization of receptors. In the example of platelet-derived growth factor *(left)*, the ligand is dimeric and contains two receptor-binding sites.[8,9] In the case of growth hormone *(right)*, a single ligand molecule contains two binding sites so that it can bind simultaneously to two receptor molecules.[10-12]

Preexisting Receptor Dimers

The insulin receptor represents a paradox. Like the GH receptor, the insulin receptor exists as a dimer even in the absence of ligand (i.e., it is an $\alpha_2\beta_2$ heterotetramer, which is a dimer of $\alpha\beta$ monomers). If the receptor is already dimerized, why is it not active? Although the molecular details remain to be elucidated, it seems likely that the two halves of the insulin receptor are not oriented in an optimal way to permit receptor activation in the absence of ligand. Perhaps insulin binding triggers a conformational change that mimics the effects of dimerization in other receptor tyrosine kinases. In any case, several studies have demonstrated that receptor dimerization is necessary for insulin to activate its receptor. For example, $\alpha\beta$ monomers retain the ability to bind insulin but are not activated in response to insulin binding.[14,15] Indirect evidence suggests that a single insulin molecule binds simultaneously to both α-subunits of the insulin receptor,[16,17] and the ability to bind simultaneously to both halves of the dimeric receptor appears to be essential for insulin to activate its receptor.

Receptor Activation: Conformational Changes in the Kinase Domain

When ligand binds to the extracellular domain, it stimulates the tyrosine kinase activity of the intracellular domain. Although the detailed mechanisms of transmembrane signaling are not completely understood, considerable progress has been made in elucidating the molecular mechanisms of receptor activation. Investigations of the three-dimensional structure of the insulin receptor tyrosine kinase domain help to explain why the receptor is maintained in a low-activity state in the absence of insulin (Fig. 5-3).[18-20] In the inactive form of the insulin receptor kinase, Tyr1162 is located in such a position that it blocks protein substrates from binding to the active site. Furthermore, in the inactive state of the tyrosine kinase domain, the active site assumes a conformation that does not accommodate magnesium adenosine triphosphate (ATP). The tyrosine kinase is inactive because the active site cannot bind either of its substrates.

How does insulin activate the receptor? Insulin binding triggers autophosphorylation of three tyrosine residues (Tyr1158, Tyr1162, and Tyr1163) in the activation loop. When these three tyrosine residues become phosphorylated, an important conformational change occurs. As a result of the movement of the activation loop, the active site acquires the ability to bind both ATP and protein substrates. The conformational change induced by autophosphorylation activates the receptor to phosphorylate other substrates.[21,22]

It remains unclear how this process is initiated. Because the inactive state of the tyrosine kinase cannot bind ATP, it seems unlikely that phosphorylation of Tyr1162 proceeds by a true autophosphorylation mechanism. Instead, it is likely that Tyr1162 in one β-subunit is transphosphorylated by the second β-subunit in the $\alpha_2\beta_2$ heterotetramer molecule.[2,23] However, this proposed mechanism poses a chicken-and-egg problem. It requires at least one of the β-subunits to be active before the Tyr residues in the activation loop become phosphorylated. Perhaps the activation loop is somewhat mobile, so that some molecules of unphosphorylated tyrosine kinase can assume an active conformation and initiate a chain reaction of transphosphorylation and receptor activation.

Receptor Tyrosine Kinases Phosphorylate Other Intracellular Proteins

Once activated, tyrosine kinases are capable of phosphorylating other protein substrates. Several factors determine which proteins are phosphorylated under physiologic conditions within the cell.

Amino Acid Sequence Context of Tyr Residue

Tyrosine kinases do not exhibit strict specificity with respect to the amino acid sequence of the phosphorylation site. Nevertheless, most tyrosine phosphorylation sites are located in the vicinity of acidic amino acid residues (i.e., Glu or Asp).[2]

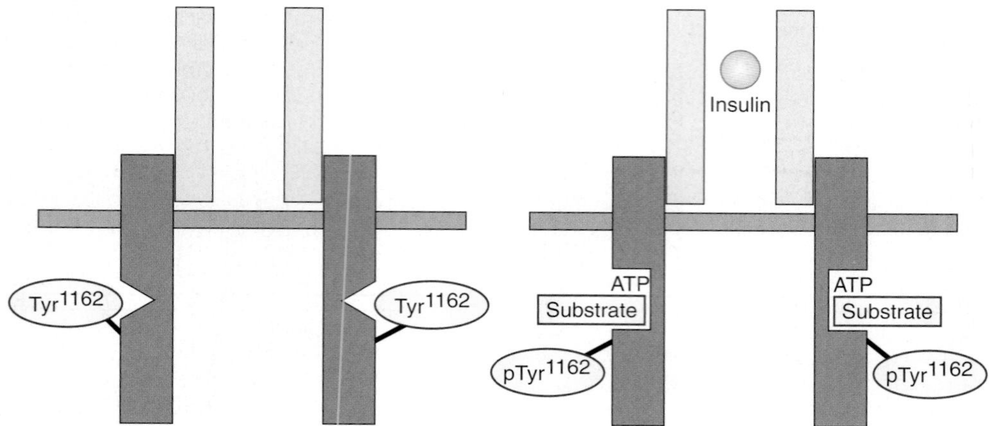

Figure 5-3 Hypothetical mechanism for ligand-stimulated activation of the insulin receptor tyrosine kinase. Phosphorylation of tyrosine residues in the activation loop leads to activation of the insulin receptor tyrosine kinase. The model is based on the three-dimensional structure of the isolated insulin receptor tyrosine kinase as determined by x-ray crystallography.[19,20,23] In the inactive insulin receptor kinase *(left)*, Tyr1162 blocks the active site so that substrates cannot bind. When the tyrosine residues in the activation loop (including Tyr1162) become phosphorylated *(right)*, pTyr1162 moves out of the way; the conformational change allows binding of adenosine triphosphate (ATP) and protein substrate so that the kinase reaction can proceed.

Binding to the Tyrosine Kinase

Some protein substrates bind directly to the intracellular domain of the receptor. The binding interaction brings the substrate close to the kinase, thereby promoting phosphorylation of the substrate. For example, the insulin receptor substrate (IRS) proteins are characterized by a highly conserved phosphotyrosine-binding (PTB) domain that binds to a conserved motif (Asn-Pro-Xaa-pTyr) in the juxtamembrane domain of the insulin receptor.[24-26] Binding of the PTB domain to the insulin receptor requires phosphorylation of the Tyr residue in the Asn-Pro-Xaa-pTyr motif. This provides another mechanism (in addition to activation of the intrinsic receptor tyrosine kinase) by which autophosphorylation of the receptor enhances phosphorylation of IRS proteins.

Similarly, substrates for some tyrosine kinases contain SRC homology 2 (SH2) domains—highly conserved domains that bind phosphotyrosine residues (see "Functional Significance of Tyrosine Phosphorylation"). For example, the activated PDGF receptor contains a phosphotyrosine residue near its carboxyl-terminus that binds the SH2 domain of phospholipase Cγ. This enables the PDGF receptor to phosphorylate and activate phospholipase Cγ.[2,27]

Subcellular Localization

Because receptor tyrosine kinases are located in the plasma membrane, they are close to other plasma membrane proteins. This co-localization has the potential to promote phosphorylation. For example, the insulin receptor has been reported to phosphorylate pp120/hepatocyte antigen 4 (HA4).[28,29] Like the insulin receptor, pp120/HA4 is an integral membrane glycoprotein associated with the plasma membrane of hepatocytes. Similarly, FGF receptor substrate 2 (FRS2), a substrate of the fibroblast growth factor receptor, is targeted to the plasma membrane by an amino-terminal myristoylation site.[30]

Functional Significance of Tyrosine Phosphorylation

Tyrosine phosphorylation regulates protein function by at least two mechanisms. First, tyrosine phosphorylation can induce a conformational change in a protein, altering its function. For example, phosphorylation of the three Tyr residues in the activation loop of the insulin receptor changes the conformation of the active site, facilitating binding of substrates and activating the receptor tyrosine kinase.[18-20] However, most of the effects of tyrosine phosphorylation on protein function are mediated indirectly by regulation of protein-protein interactions. To understand how tyrosine phosphorylation regulates protein-protein interactions, it is useful to review the biochemistry of cellular SRC, the prototype of a nonreceptor tyrosine kinase. When the amino acid sequence of SRC is analyzed, it is apparent that there are three highly conserved domains in the molecule: the kinase catalytic domain and two noncatalytic SRC homology domains that are referred to as SH2 and SH3.

SH2 Domains

SH2 domains consist of conserved sequences (approximately 100 amino acid residues) that are present in many proteins and function in signaling pathways. Functionally, SH2 domains share the ability to bind pTyr residues. However, individual SH2 domains vary with respect to their binding specificity. The binding affinity of an SH2 domain is determined by the three amino acid residues downstream from the pTyr residue. For example, the SH2 domains of phosphatidylinositol 3 kinase (PI3K) exhibit a preference for pTyr-(Met/Xaa)-Xaa-Met, whereas the SH2 domain of growth factor receptor–binding protein 2 (GRB2) prefers to bind pTyr-Xaa-Asn-Xaa. A given SH2 domain binds to a tyrosine-phosphorylated protein if and only if the pTyr residue is located in a context that corresponds to the binding specificity of the SH2 domain.

SH3 Domains

SH3 domains consist of conserved sequences (approximately 50 amino acid residues) that bind to proline-rich sequences. Like SH2 domains, SH3 domains are found in many proteins that function in signaling pathways.

DOWNSTREAM SIGNALING PATHWAYS

Receptor tyrosine kinases mediate the action of many ligands in a wide variety of cell types. The bewildering complexity of the downstream signaling pathways corresponds to the huge number of physiologic processes that are regulated by receptor tyrosine kinases. Although it is beyond the scope of this chapter to attempt an encyclopedic review of all downstream signaling pathways, we have selected examples to illustrate general principles.

As discussed earlier, the activated insulin receptor phosphorylates multiple substrate proteins, including IRS1, IRS2, IRS3L, IRS4,[31] and a newly discovered member, growth factor receptor–binding protein 2–associated binder 1 (GAB1).[32,33] Each of these substrates contains multiple tyrosine phosphorylation sites, many of which correspond to consensus sequences for SH2 domains in important signaling molecules. IRS proteins serve as docking proteins that bind SH2 domain–containing proteins. Among these, two of the most important are PI3K and GRB2. Binding of SH2 domains triggers multiple downstream signaling pathways. It has been suggested that GAB1 serves as a unique intermediate in insulin/IGF1 signaling for induction of early gene expression and stimulation of mitogenesis without direct tyrosine phosphorylation.

Phosphatidylinositol 3 Kinase

The catalytic subunit of PI3K (p110; molecular mass, approximately 110,000 d) is bound to a regulatory subunit. The classic isoforms of the regulatory subunit (p85; molecular mass, approximately 85,000 d) contain two SH2 domains, both of which bind to pTyr in the context of pTyr-(Met/Xaa)-Xaa-Met motifs. Binding of pTyr residues to both SH2 domains of p85 leads to maximal activation of PI3K catalytic activity; submaximal activation can be achieved with occupancy of a single SH2 domain in p85. Because all four IRS molecules (IRS1, IRS2, IRS3L, and IRS4) contain multiple tyrosine phosphorylation sites that conform to the Tyr-(Met/Xaa)-Xaa-Met consensus sequence, insulin-stimulated phosphorylation promotes binding of IRS proteins to the SH2 domains in the regulatory subunit PI3K, thereby increasing the enzymatic activity of the catalytic subunit.[34-37] Activation of PI3K triggers activation of a cascade of downstream kinases, beginning with phosphoinositide-dependent kinases 1 and 2. These kinases phosphorylate and activate multiple downstream protein kinases, including protein kinase B and atypical isoforms of protein kinase C.[38-44]

A large body of evidence demonstrates that the pathways downstream from PI3K mediate the metabolic activities of insulin (e.g., activation of glucose transport into skeletal muscle, activation of glycogen synthesis, inhibition of transcription of the phosphoenolpyruvate carboxykinase gene). Among other lines of evidence, PI3K inhibitors (e.g., LY294002, wortmannin) block the metabolic actions of insulin.[45] Similarly, overexpression of dominant negative mutants of the p85 regulatory subunit of PI3K also inhibits the metabolic actions of insulin.[36] Although it is generally agreed that activation of PI3K is necessary, it is controversial whether it is sufficient to trigger the metabolic actions of insulin. A second parallel pathway may be required, involving tyrosine phosphorylation of CBL, another protein that can be phosphorylated by the insulin receptor in some cell types.[46-48]

GRB2 and the Activation of RAS

GRB2 is a short adaptor molecule that contains an SH2 domain[49] capable of binding to pTyr residues in several signaling molecules such as IRS1 and SHC, another PTB domain–containing protein that is phosphorylated by several receptor tyrosine kinases, including the insulin receptor.[50,51] The SH2 domain of GRB2 is flanked by two SH3 domains,[49] which bind to proline-containing sequences in a mammalian homolog of *Drosophila* son-of-sevenless (mSOS, now designated SOS1 or SOS2).[52] This guanine nucleotide exchange factor can activate RAS, a small G protein that plays an important role in intracellular signaling pathways. The mSOS activates RAS by catalyzing the exchange of GTP for GDP in the guanine nucleotide–binding site of RAS. This, in turn, activates a cascade of serine/threonine-specific protein kinases, including RAF1 kinase, mitogen-activated protein/extracellular signal–regulated kinase (MAP3K), and mitogen-activated protein (MAP) kinase. These pathways downstream from RAS contribute to the ability of tyrosine kinases to promote cell growth and regulate the expression of various genes.

We have focused on the signaling pathways downstream from the insulin receptor because of the importance of insulin and IGF1 in endocrinology (Fig. 5-4). In many ways, the molecular mechanisms closely resemble those downstream from other receptor tyrosine kinases. However, the insulin signaling pathway is atypical in at least one respect: Whereas the insulin receptor phosphorylates docking proteins (e.g., IRS1) that then bind SH2 domain–containing proteins (e.g., PI3K, GRB2), the intracellular domains of most receptor tyrosine kinases contain direct binding sites for SH2 domains. For example, the SH2 domain of GRB2 binds to pTyr716 in the activated PDGF receptor.[2] Similarly, the PDGF receptor contains two Tyr-(Met/Xaa)-Xaa-Met motifs in the kinase insert domain that bind to the two SH2 domains in the p85 subunit of PI3K.[2,53] It is not clear why some tyrosine kinases activate PI3K through a direct binding interaction and others use an indirect mechanism involving docking proteins. However, PDGF receptors are associated with the plasma membrane, whereas IRS proteins appear to be associated with the cytoskeleton.[54] Perhaps this compartmentalization contributes to signaling specificity. Translocation of PI3K to different locations within the cell by two different receptors (e.g., insulin and PDGF receptors) may permit different biologic responses to be elicited by the same signaling molecule (i.e., PI3K).

In addition to being an integral signaling pathway in liver, skeletal muscle, and adipose tissue, most proteins in the insulin/IGF1 signaling pathway are also recognized in pancreatic islet cells[57-59] and in the central nervous system[60-62] (Fig. 5-5). Exogenous insulin can enhance glucose-stimulated insulin secretion in healthy humans.[63] These studies provide insights into the pathogenesis of type 2 diabetes,[64] neurodegenerative diseases, and aging.

OFF SIGNALS: TERMINATION OF HORMONE ACTION

Just as there are complex biochemical pathways that mediate hormone action, there are mechanisms to terminate the biologic response. The necessity for these mechanisms is illustrated by the following example. After we eat a meal, the concentration of plasma glucose increases. This elicits an increase in insulin secretion, which leads to a decrease in plasma glucose levels. If these processes went on unchecked, the level of glucose in the plasma would eventually fall so low that it would lead to symptomatic hypoglycemia. How is insulin action terminated? The answer is not entirely clear, but several mechanisms contribute to turning off the insulin signaling pathway.

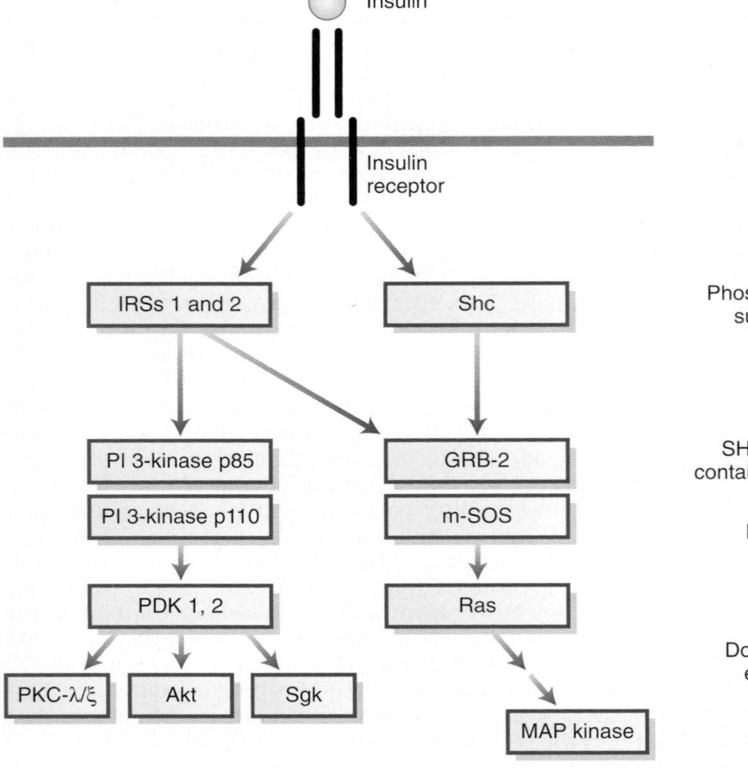

Figure 5-4 Simplified model of signaling pathways downstream from the insulin receptor. Insulin binds to the insulin receptor, activating the receptor tyrosine kinase to phosphorylate tyrosine residues on insulin receptor substrates (IRSs) including IRS1 and IRS2.[31] The phosphotyrosine residues in the IRS molecules bind to SRC homology 2 (SH2) domains in molecules such as growth factor receptor–binding protein 2 (GRB-2) and the p85 regulatory subunit of phosphatidylinositol (PI) 3-kinase (PI3K). These SH2 domain–containing proteins initiate two distinct branches of the signaling pathway. Activation of PI3K leads to activation of phosphoinositide-dependent kinases (PDKs) 1 and 2, which activate multiple protein kinases, including Akt/protein kinase B, atypical protein kinase C (PKC) isoforms, and serum- and glucocorticoid-induced protein kinases (Sgk).[55] GRB2 interacts with mSOS, a guanine nucleotide exchange factor that activates Ras.[56] Activation of Ras triggers a cascade of protein kinases, leading to activation of mitogen-activated protein (MAP) kinase. Shc, SRC homology domain–containing protein.

Receptor-Mediated Endocytosis

Insulin binding to its receptor triggers endocytosis of the receptor. Although most of the internalized receptors are recycled to the plasma membrane, some are transported to lysosomes, where they are degraded.[65,66] As a result, insulin binding accelerates the rate of receptor degradation, down-regulating the number of receptors on the cell surface. Endosomes contain proton pumps that acidify the lumen; the acidic pH within the endosome promotes dissociation of insulin from its receptor, and the insulin is ultimately transported to the lysosome for degradation. Receptor-mediated endocytosis is the principal mechanism by which insulin is cleared from the plasma.[67] Binding of ligands to other receptor tyrosine kinases also triggers receptor-mediated endocytosis by similar mechanisms.

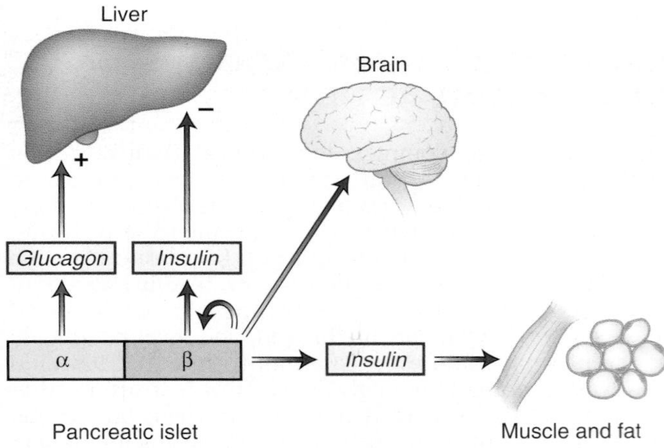

Figure 5-5

Protein Tyrosine Phosphatases

Protein phosphorylation is a dynamic process. Tyrosine kinases catalyze the phosphorylation of tyrosine residues, but there are also protein tyrosine phosphatases (PTPs) to remove the phosphates.[2] PTPs antagonize the action of tyrosine kinases. Studies with knockout mice have demonstrated that the absence of PTP1B is associated with increased insulin sensitivity and protects against weight gain.[68,69] Nevertheless, the human genome encodes a large number of PTPs, and it is an important goal of research to elucidate their physiologic functions. Developing selective inhibitors of the PTPs that oppose the effects of the insulin receptor tyrosine kinase could provide novel therapies for diabetes.

Serine/Threonine Kinases

Most receptor tyrosine kinases, including the insulin receptor, are substrates for phosphorylation by Ser/Thr-specific protein kinases. Ser/Thr phosphorylation appears to inhibit the action of the tyrosine kinase. Other phosphotyrosine-containing proteins are similarly subject to inhibitory influences of Ser/Thr phosphorylation. For example, Ser/Thr phosphorylation of IRS1 may inhibit insulin action, thereby causing insulin resistance.[70-74]

MECHANISMS OF DISEASE

The simplest forms of endocrine disease are caused by a deficiency or an excess of a hormone. Hormone resistance syndromes resulting from defects in the signaling pathways can masquerade as hormone deficiency states, and diseases associated with constitutively activated receptors can mimic states of hormone excess. In some cases, the abnormality in hormone action is genetic in origin, resulting from a mutated gene encoding one of the proteins in the signaling pathway. Similar syndromes also can be caused by other mechanisms; for example, some autoimmune syndromes are caused by autoantibodies directed against cell surface receptors. These clinical syndromes illustrate the principle that understanding the biochemical pathways of hormone action can provide important insights into the pathophysiology of human disease.

Genetic Defects in Receptor Function

At least two major types of genetic defects can cause hormone resistance.[75] First, mutations can lead to a decrease in the number of receptors. In the case of the insulin receptor, mutations have been identified that decrease receptor number by at least three mechanisms: impairing receptor biosynthesis, inhibiting the transport of receptors to their normal location in the plasma membrane, and accelerating the rate of receptor degradation. Second, mutations can impair the intrinsic activities of the receptor. In the case of the insulin receptor, mutations have been reported that decrease the affinity of insulin binding or inhibit receptor tyrosine kinase activity.

Receptor dimerization plays a central role in the mechanisms by which ligands activate many cell surface receptors. This role has been shown most convincingly in the case of the GH receptor (a member of the family of cytokine receptors) but has also been postulated for receptor tyrosine kinases. The syndromes of multiple endocrine neoplasia types 2A and 2B and familial medullary carcinoma of the thyroid are caused by mutations in the gene encoding the RET tyrosine kinase (a subunit of the receptor for glial cell–derived growth factor).[76] Ordinarily, cysteine residues in the extracellular domain of RET participate in the formation of intramolecular disulfide bonds. Mutation of one of the cysteine residues leaves an unpaired cysteine residue that promotes dimerization of RET molecules, thereby activating the RET receptor tyrosine kinase (Fig. 5-6). Activation of the RET tyrosine kinase through this germline mutation converts *RET* into an oncogene.

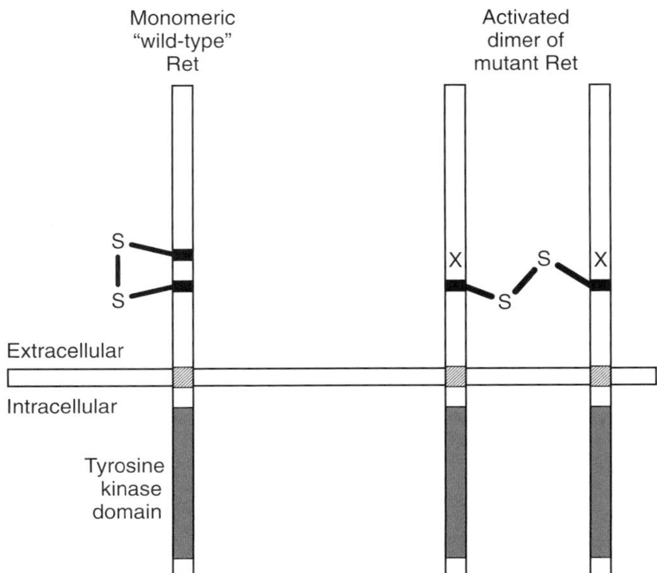

Figure 5-6 Mutations leading to constitutive activation of RET. Wild-type Ret protein has intramolecular disulfide bonds formed by two cysteine residues in the same receptor molecule *(left)*. When one of the two cysteine residues is mutated, the unpaired cysteine residue is available to form an intermolecular disulfide bond with a cysteine residue on another receptor molecule. This leads to receptor dimerization *(right)*, which results in constitutive activation of the receptor tyrosine kinase.[76-78] This type of mutation has been identified in patients with multiple endocrine neoplasia type 2.

Autoantibodies Directed against Cell Surface Receptors

Inhibitory antireceptor autoantibodies were first identified in patients with myasthenia gravis.[79] In this neurologic disease, antibodies to the nicotinic acetylcholine receptor impair neuromuscular transmission, apparently by accelerating receptor degradation. Autoantibodies to the insulin receptor were later shown to block insulin action in the syndrome of type B extreme insulin resistance.[80] Insulin resistance is caused by at least two mechanisms: anti-receptor antibodies inhibit insulin binding to the receptor,[81] and antibodies accelerate receptor degradation.[82]

Graves' disease provided the first example of stimulatory antireceptor autoantibodies.[83] In Graves' disease, autoantibodies are directed against the thyroid-stimulating hormone (TSH) receptor. These antireceptor antibodies activate the TSH receptor, stimulating growth of the thyroid gland and hypersecretion of thyroid hormone. This experiment of nature demonstrates that the receptor can be activated by ligands other than the physiologic ligand and that the normal spectrum of biologic actions can be triggered by this unphysiologic ligand (i.e., the anti-receptor antibody). Similarly, antibodies to the insulin receptor have been demonstrated to activate the insulin receptor by mimicking insulin action. Although it is more common for a patient with anti–insulin receptor autoantibodies to present with insulin resistance, patients with these autoantibodies have also been reported to experience fasting hypoglycemia.[84,85]

RECEPTOR SERINE KINASES

Receptor serine kinases[86] have several features in common with receptor tyrosine kinases. For example, both classes of receptors possess N-terminal extracellular domains that bind ligand; a single transmembrane domain; and C-terminal intracellular domains that possess protein kinase activity. However, the two classes of receptors have different enzymatic specificities. Whereas receptor tyrosine kinases phosphorylate tyrosine residues, receptor serine kinases phosphorylate serine and threonine residues in their protein substrates. There are two types of receptor serine kinases: type I and type II. The human genome contains 12 genes encoding receptor serine kinases—seven type I and five type II receptors—each of which is approximately 500 amino acids long.

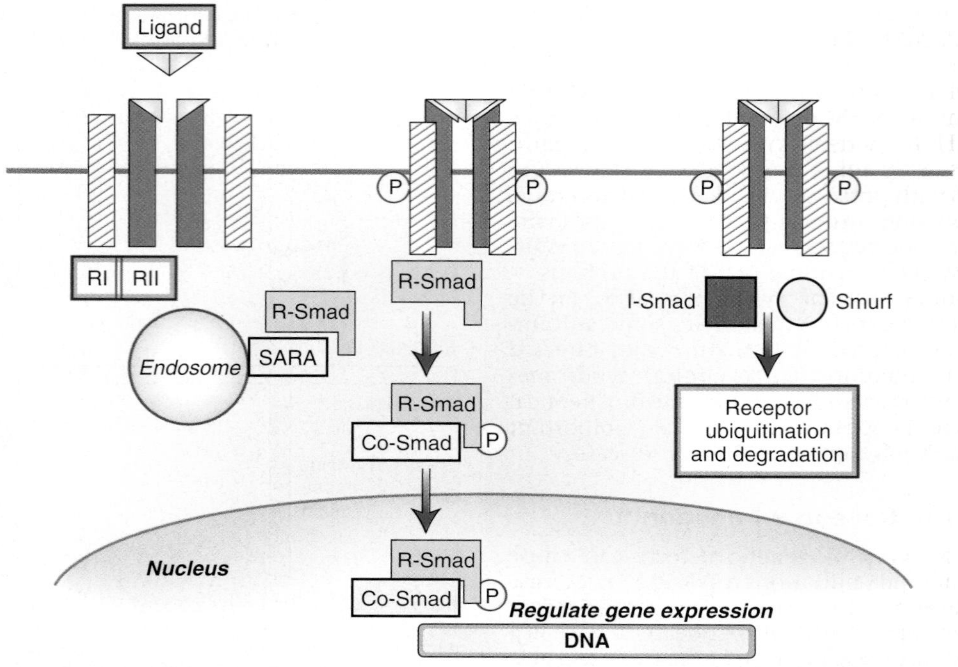

Figure 5-7 Mechanism of action for receptor serine kinases. Binding of dimeric ligand to the type II receptor (RII) subunit triggers assembly of the receptor into the heterotetrameric $[(RI)_2(RII)_2]$ state. RII transphosphorylates the type I receptor (RI), thereby activating phosphorylation of the receptor-regulated SMAD (R-Smad) protein that is bound to the SMAD anchor for receptor activation (SARA) in endosomes. The phosphorylated R-Smad associates with a co-mediator SMAD (Co-Smad). Eventually, the R-Smad is translocated into the nucleus, where it binds to DNA, enabling it to regulate gene transcription. The inhibitory SMAD (I-Smad) also can bind to the activated receptor, promoting ubiquitination and degradation of the receptor. P, phosphorylation; Smurf, SMAD ubiquitination regulatory factor.

Receptor Activation: Role of Receptor Dimerization

Receptor serine kinases mediate the biologic actions (Fig. 5-7) of a single, large family of ligands, the transforming growth factor-β (TGF-β) family, which is characterized by the presence of six conserved cysteine residues.[86] The human genome contains 42 genes encoding cytokines in the TGF-β family, which are divided into two classes: the activin/TGF-β family and the müllerian inhibitory substance (MIS)/bone morphogenic protein (BMP) family. Activin, the related inhibin, and MIS are of particular interest within the field of reproductive endocrinology (see Chapters 8 and 16).

Ligand binding to the receptor serine kinases promotes a physical interaction between the type I receptor (RI) and the type II receptor (RII) (see Fig. 5-7). As a consequence, the RII receptor activates the RI receptor by phosphorylating one or more serine residues in the GS domain (i.e., TTSGSGSG sequence) of the RI receptor.[86] How does the ligand trigger receptor activation? In the case of the MIS/BMP family of cytokines, the ligand binds to the isolated RI receptor with high affinity and to the RII receptor with relatively low affinity. The ligand can bind simultaneously to RI and RII, providing an explanation for its ability to promote a physical interaction between RI and RII. The mechanism is different in the case of the activin/TGF-β family of cytokines. For example, TGF-β binds with high affinity to RII but does not interact directly with RI. However, TGF-β binding appears to induce a conformational change in RII, promoting a direct binding interaction between the intracellular domains of RII and RI. Cytokines such as TGF-β exist as dimers; this permits them to bind simultaneously to two RII molecules, so the activated receptor complex probably exists as a heterotetramer: $(RI)_2(RII)_2$.

An additional level of complexity contributes to the regulation of receptor serine kinases.[86] The biology related to activin provides several examples. Follistatin is a "ligand trap," a soluble protein that binds activin, thereby blocking access to RI and RII. Inhibin is a peptide that inhibits activin signaling by binding to the receptor without activating the phosphorylation of RI. Betaglycan is a membrane-anchored protein that functions as a coreceptor for inhibin by promoting inhibin binding to the activin receptor. Betaglycan itself does not bind activin.

Receptor Serine Kinases Phosphorylate Other Intracellular Proteins

Once activated, receptor serine kinases are capable of phosphorylating other protein substrates. Receptor-regulated SMAD proteins (R-SMADs) function as the immediate downstream effectors of receptor serine kinases (see Fig. 5-7).[86] SMAD proteins are the mammalian homologs of the proteins encoded by the *Drosophila mad* (mothers against decapentaplegic) gene and the *Caenorhabditis elegans Sma* genes. There are five human R-SMAD proteins. SMAD2 and SMAD3 mediate the actions of the activin/TGF-β family of cytokines. SMAD1, SMAD5, and SMAD8 mediate the actions of the MIS/BMP family of cytokines.

The mechanism of action of TGF-β has been studied in considerable detail[81] and provides a prototype for the receptor serine kinases.[86] When RI becomes phosphorylated in its GS domain in response to TGF-β, the binding affinity for R-SMAD proteins such as SMAD2 is increased (see Fig. 5-7). This leads to phosphorylation of the two serine residues in the SSXS sequence at the C-terminus of

SMAD2. Receptor-mediated phosphorylation of SMAD2 takes place when SMAD2 is bound to the SMAD anchor for receptor activation (SARA), which is located in early endosomes. Phosphorylation promotes dissociation of SMAD2 from SARA and binding of SMAD2 to the co-mediator (Co-SMAD), SMAD4. Thus, phosphorylation of the R-SMAD promotes the assembly of heteromeric complexes of R-SMAD molecules with the Co-SMAD. SMADs also contain sites for phosphorylation by other protein kinases, providing an opportunity for regulatory cross-talk with other cellular signaling systems.

SMAD7 is an inhibitory SMAD (I-SMAD). It binds to activated receptors in competition with R-SMADs. Binding of SMAD7 promotes receptor ubiquitination and degradation mediated by E3 ubiquitin ligases and SMAD ubiquitination regulatory factors (SMURFs). These processes represent a negative feedback system that contributes to the termination of TGF-β signaling (see Fig. 5-7).

SMAD Proteins Regulate Gene Expression

Some R-SMADs contain lysine-rich nuclear localization signals (KKLKK) that bind to importin, mediating translocation into the nucleus.[86] Direct binding to components of the nuclear pore complex also may contribute to the mechanism by which SMADs are translocated into the nucleus. Most R-SMADs (with the exception of SMAD2) bind to DNA in a sequence-specific fashion. The minimum SMAD binding element is a 4–base-pair sequence, 5′-AGAC-3′. This sequence is quite short and is not expected to provide a high degree of specificity. Therefore, it seems likely that other factors contribute to the specificity of gene regulation.

RECEPTORS THAT SIGNAL THROUGH ASSOCIATED TYROSINE KINASES

Members of the cytokine family of receptors resemble receptor tyrosine kinases in their mechanism of action, with one important difference. Instead of having a tyrosine kinase that is intrinsic to the receptor, enzymatic activity resides in a protein that associates with the cytokine receptor. As with receptor tyrosine kinases, ligand binding to the cytokine receptor activates the associated kinase. The more than 40 ligands that bind to members of the cytokine receptor family have diverse functions. Three of the ligands are hormones: GH, which is vital for normal body height; prolactin, which is required for reproduction and lactation; and leptin, which suppresses appetite, stimulates energy expenditure, and promotes glucose homeostasis through a variety of mechanisms.[87-89] Other ligands of cytokine receptors, such as erythropoietin, most interleukins, and interferons-α, -β, and -γ, regulate hematopoiesis or the immune response. A number of genetic diseases can be traced to defects in cytokine receptors. For example, Laron dwarfism is caused by autosomal recessive mutations of the GH receptor,[90] and autosomal recessive mutations of the leptin receptor can cause morbid obesity.[91] A gain-of-function mutation of the prolactin receptor has been identified in women with benign breast tumors.[92]

Cytokine Receptors with Multiple Subunits

Members of the cytokine family of receptors share homology in the extracellular and cytoplasmic domains. Some cytokine receptors, including the receptors for GH, prolactin, and leptin, are thought to be composed of dimers of a single receptor subunit (Fig. 5-8). One ligand is thought to bind to both receptor subunits, as discussed earlier for the GH receptor.

Most cytokine receptors are composed of two or more different subunits, with as many as six subunits constituting a single receptor.[93,94] Some of these receptors are thought to bind ligand dimers. One or more receptor subunits are shared by receptors for other cytokines. This phenomenon of mixing and matching receptor subunits is an efficient way for the cell to fine-tune its cellular responses and increase the number of ligands that can be bound by a particular group of receptor subunits. For example, a receptor composed of the gp130 subunit and the leukemia inhibitory factor receptor β-subunit binds leukemia inhibitory factor, a pleiotropic cytokine with multiple functions that appears to serve as a molecular interface between the

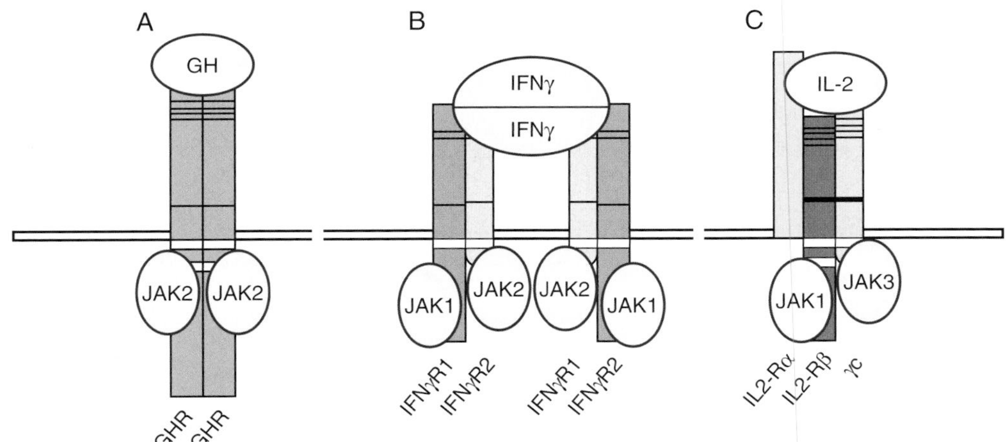

Figure 5-8 Cytokine receptors are composed of multiple subunits and bind to one or more members of the Janus kinase (JAK) family of tyrosine kinases. **A,** Growth hormone (GH), like prolactin and leptin, binds to growth hormone receptor (GHR) homodimers and activates JAK2. **B,** Interferon-γ (IFNγ) homodimers bind to their ligand-binding γR1 subunits. The γR2 subunits are then recruited, leading to activation of JAK1, which binds to the γR1 subunit, and JAK2, which binds to the γR2 subunit. Both subunits and both JAKs are necessary for responses to IFNγ. **C,** Interleukin 2 (IL-2) binds to receptors composed of three subunits: a γc subunit shared with receptors for IL-4, -7, -9, -15, and -21; an IL-2Rβ subunit shared with the IL-15 receptor; and a noncytokine receptor subunit, IL-2Rα. IL-2 activates JAK3, bound to the γc subunit, and JAK1, bound to IL2-Rβ. Extracellular regions of homology are indicated by the black lines and colored patterns. Intracellular regions of homology are indicated by the small *white boxes.* Identical subunits are indicated by *identical colors.*

neuroimmune and endocrine systems.[95] The same receptor subunits, when combined with a ciliary neurotrophic factor receptor subunit, show a preference for ciliary neurotrophic factor, a trophic factor for motor neurons in the ciliary ganglia and spinal cord that is also a potent appetite suppressor.[96] And if two gp130 subunits are combined with an interleukin 6 (IL-6) receptor subunit, the new receptor shows a preference for IL-6, an inducer of the acute phase response with additional anti-inflammatory properties.[97]

Cytokine Receptors Activate Members of the Janus Family of Tyrosine Kinases

Members of the cytokine family of receptors do not themselves exhibit enzymatic activity. Rather, they bind members of the Janus family of tyrosine kinases (JAKs) in a proline-rich region (see Fig. 5-8). There are four known JAKs, designated JAK1, JAK2, JAK3, and TYK2. Like the cytokine receptors themselves, the JAKs mix and match their subunits. Some cytokine receptors show a strong preference for a single JAK, some require two different JAKs, and others appear to activate multiple JAK family members. GH, prolactin, and leptin preferentially activate JAK2; interferon-γ activates JAK1 and JAK2; and IL-2 activates JAK1 and JAK3.[93,98]

Binding of ligand to a cytokine receptor activates the appropriate JAK family member or members. In some cases (e.g., prolactin), the JAKs appear to be constitutively associated with the cytokine receptor, and ligand binding increases their activity.[99] In other cases (e.g., GH receptor), ligand binding appears to increase both the affinity of JAKs for the cytokine receptor and the activity of the associated JAKs.[100] Activation of JAKs requires receptor oligomerization, presumably to bring two or more JAKs sufficiently close to transphosphorylate each other on the activating tyrosine in the kinase domain (see earlier discussion of receptor tyrosine kinases). Both receptor dimerization and ligand-induced changes in receptor conformation appear to be required for receptor activation.[101] Transphosphorylation is thought to cause a conformational change that exposes the ATP-binding or substrate-binding site, or both, and activation is thought to release an autoinhibitory domain.[102] After the JAKs are activated, they phosphorylate themselves and their associated receptor subunits on multiple tyrosines.

JAKs appear to be vital for normal human function. Mutations in the *JAK3* gene have been linked to an autosomal recessive form of severe combined immunodeficiency disease.[103] Targeted disruption of the *JAK2* gene in mice embryos is lethal.[104]

Signaling Pathways Initiated by Cytokine Receptor–JAK Complexes

Phosphorylated tyrosines within the cytokine receptor subunits and their associated JAKs form binding sites for various signaling proteins containing phosphotyrosine-binding domains, such as the SH2 and PTB domains. Each cytokine receptor–JAK complex is expected to have some tyrosine-containing motifs shared with many other cytokine receptor–JAK complexes (e.g., tyrosines within JAKs) and some ligand-specific tyrosine-containing motifs (e.g., tyrosines within a specific combination of receptor subunits). Ligand binding to cytokine receptors is expected to initiate some signaling pathways that are shared by many cytokines and some that are more specialized to a particular cytokine receptor.

The signaling proteins recruited to subsets of cytokine receptor–JAK complexes are generally the same as those recruited to receptor tyrosine kinases. Examples include the IRS proteins, the adaptor proteins SHC and GRB2 that lead to activation of the RAS/MAP kinase pathway, phospholipase Cγ, and PI3K. However, one family of signaling proteins appears to be particularly important for the function of cytokines: the signal transducers and activators of transcription (STATs) (Fig. 5-9).

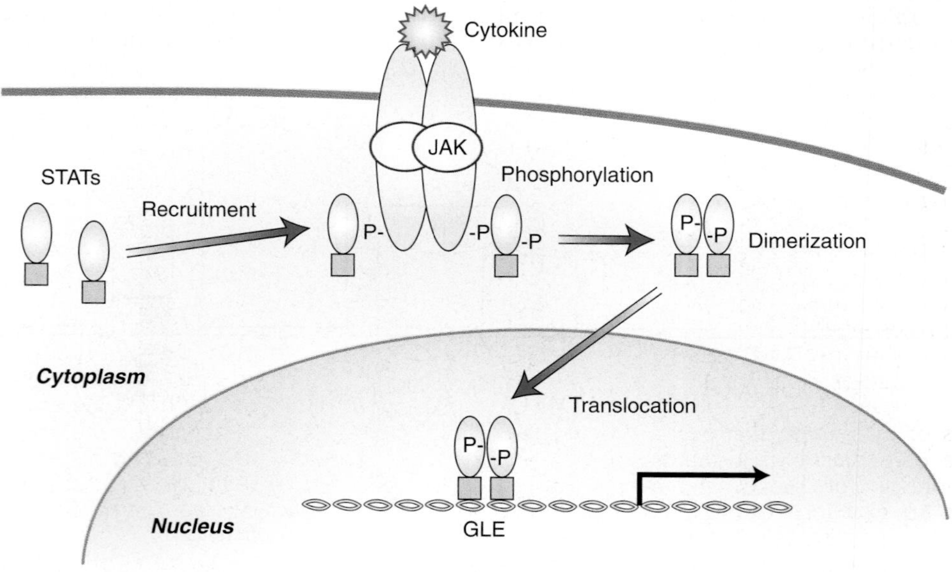

Figure 5-9 Cytokines activate signal transducers and activators of transcription (STATs). STAT proteins are latent cytoplasmic transcription factors. STATs bind through SRC homology 2 (SH2) domains to one or more phosphorylated tyrosines (P) in activated receptor–Janus kinase (JAK) complexes. Once bound, STATs themselves are tyrosyl phosphorylated, presumably by the receptor-associated JAKs. STATs then dissociate from the receptor-JAK complex, homodimerize or heterodimerize with other STAT proteins, move to the nucleus, and bind to gamma-activated sequence-like elements (GLEs) in the promoters of cytokine-responsive genes. P, phosphorylation. (Adapted from J. Herrington, with permission.)

STAT proteins are latent cytoplasmic transcription factors that cycle between the cytoplasm and the nucleus. After ligand activation, inactive STATs in the cytoplasm bind through their SH2 domains to one or more phosphorylated tyrosines in the activated receptor-JAK complexes. Once bound, they are tyrosyl phosphorylated, presumably by the receptor-associated JAKs. STATs then dissociate from the receptor-JAK complexes, homodimerize or heterodimerize with other STAT proteins, move to the nucleus, and bind to gamma-activated sequence-like elements in the promoters of cytokine-responsive genes.[104,105]

The transcriptional response depends on how many STAT binding sites exist in the receptor-JAK complex, with which of the seven known STATs a particular STAT heterodimerizes, to what other proteins a particular STAT binds, other post-translational modifications in the degree of serine or threonine phosphorylation of the STAT, and what other transcription factors are activated. For example, the receptor for leukemia inhibitory factor contains seven STAT3 binding motifs (YxxQ, in which Y is tyrosine, Q is glutamine, and x can be any amino acid [i.e., Tyr-Xaa-Xaa-Gln]), and leukemia inhibitory factor is a particularly potent activator of STAT3.[106] The transcriptional activity of STAT5 is enhanced when it forms a complex with the glucocorticoid, mineralocorticoid, and progesterone receptors but diminished when it forms a complex with the estrogen receptor.[107] The importance of STAT5B for GH signaling is illustrated by the finding that severe growth failure in humans is associated with point mutations in the *STAT5B* gene that result in a defective SH2 domain or an unstable, truncated form of STAT5B.[108,109]

Precise Regulation of Cytokine Receptors Required for Normal Function

Ligand binding to cytokine receptors normally activates JAKs rapidly and transiently. Conversely, constitutively activated JAKs and STATs are associated with cellular transformation. For example, a single acquired activating point mutation in *JAK2* is present in most patients with a myeloproliferative disorder.[110] Constitutively active JAKs and STATs are also a common characteristic of leukemias,[111] and JAK2 and STAT5B have been identified as fusion partners in translocations in leukemias. The TEL-JAK2 fusion protein is constitutively active, leading to constitutively active STAT proteins. Understanding what turns off cytokine receptor signaling is of utmost importance in understanding normal signaling through cytokine receptors.

As with the receptor tyrosine kinases, multiple steps have been hypothesized to serve as points of signal termination for cytokine signaling. They include receptor internalization and degradation (e.g., through a ubiquitination/proteosome and/or lysosomal pathway) and dephosphorylation of tyrosines within the JAK or the receptor (e.g., by a tyrosine phosphatase that binds to receptor-JAK complexes).

The suppressors of cytokine-signaling (SOCS) proteins are thought to be particularly important players in the termination or suppression of cytokine signaling pathways. SOCS proteins are an excellent example of an effective negative feedback loop. They usually are synthesized in response to activation of STAT proteins. The newly synthesized SOCS proteins bind through the SH2 domain to phosphorylated tyrosines within the cytokine receptor–JAK complex and inhibit further cytokine signaling. In some cases (e.g., SOCS1), SOCS proteins are thought to bind to phosphotyrosines in the kinase domain of JAK and inhibit kinase activity.[112] In other cases (e.g., SOCS3), SOCS proteins bind to phosphorylated tyrosines in the receptor and inhibit JAK activity.[113] In some cases (e.g., cytokine-inducible SH2 protein [CIS]), SOCS proteins bind to phosphorylated tyrosines in the receptor and block STAT binding and activation.[114]

SOCS proteins are ubiquitin ligases,[115] and in some cases, they are thought to alternatively or additionally promote receptor-JAK internalization or degradation.[116] SOCS proteins can be synthesized in response to noncytokine receptors, suggesting a mechanism whereby prior exposure to one ligand suppresses subsequent responses to another. For example, SOCS proteins have been implicated in the well-known ability of endotoxin to cause resistance to GH.[117]

Summary of Regulatory Mechanisms

Hormones, growth factors, and cytokines that bind to members of the cytokine family of receptors activate JAK family tyrosine kinases. The activated kinases phosphorylate tyrosines in themselves and in associated receptors. The phosphorylated tyrosines form binding sites for other signaling proteins, including STAT proteins and a variety of other phosphotyrosine-binding proteins. STAT proteins promote the regulation of cytokine-sensitive genes. SOCS proteins that serve a negative feedback function of terminating ligand activation of JAKs or STATs, or both.

This picture of regulation is continuously becoming much more complex. For example, there are reports that members of the SRC family of tyrosine kinases can also be activated by some cytokine receptors (e.g., prolactin receptor),[118] that some JAK-binding proteins (e.g., SH2-B1) are potent activators of specific JAKs,[119] and that other proteins contribute to the downregulation of cytokine-signaling pathways. This last group includes the protein inhibitors of activated STAT (PIAS), proteins that bind to specific STATs and inhibit their transcriptional activity.[120,121] Cytokine receptors, JAKs, STATs, and SOCS proteins also interact with or are components of signaling downstream of some receptor tyrosine kinases (e.g., receptors for insulin, IGF1, EGF) and several GPCRs (e.g., receptors for angiotensin II, serotonin, α-thrombin, luteinizing hormone). In contrast to their essential role in signaling by cytokine receptors, JAKs do not appear to be the primary signaling mediator for either the receptor tyrosine kinases or the GPCRs.

G PROTEIN–COUPLED RECEPTORS

GPCRs are an evolutionarily conserved gene superfamily with members in all eukaryotes from yeast to mammals. They transduce a wide variety of extracellular signals, including photons of light; chemical odorants; divalent cations; monoamine, amino acid, and nucleoside neurotransmitters; lipids; and peptide and protein hormones.[122] All members of the GPCR superfamily share a common structural feature—seven membrane-spanning helices—but various subfamilies diverge in their primary amino acid sequence and in the domains that serve in ligand binding, G protein coupling, and interaction with other effector proteins (Fig. 5-10).

All GPCRs act as guanine nucleotide exchange factors. In their activated (agonist-bound) conformation, they catalyze the exchange of GDP tightly bound to the α-subunit of heterotrimeric G proteins for GTP (Fig. 5-11). This leads to activation of the α-subunit and its dissociation from the G protein βγ dimer. Both G protein subunits are capable of regulating effector activity.[123] Identified G protein–regulated

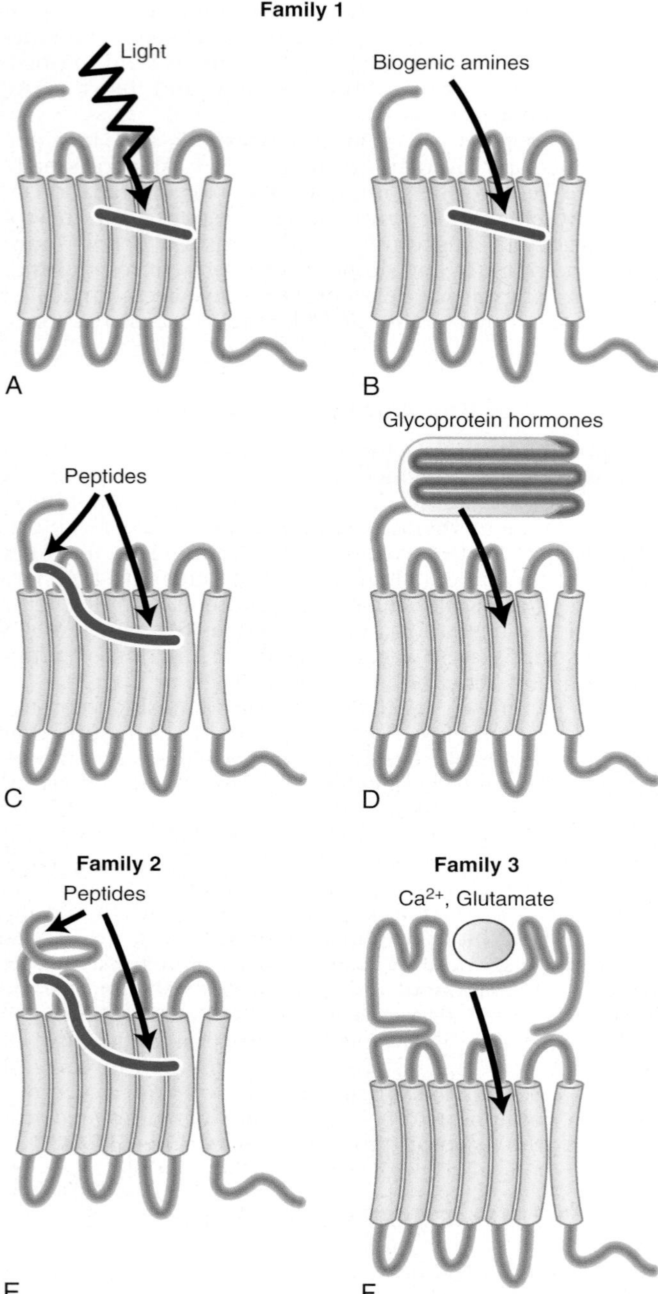

Figure 5-10 The G protein–coupled receptor (GPCR) superfamily: diversity in ligand binding and structure. Each panel depicts members of the GPCR superfamily. The seven-membrane-spanning α-helices are shown as cylinders, with the extracellular amino-terminus and three extracellular loops above them and the intracellular carboxyl-terminus and three intracellular loops below. The superfamily can be divided into three subfamilies on the basis of amino acid sequence conservation within the transmembrane helices. Family 1 includes the opsins, **A,** in which light *(arrow)* causes isomerization of retinal covalently bound within the pocket created by the transmembrane helices *(bar)*; monoamine receptors, **B,** in which agonists *(arrow)* bind noncovalently within the pocket created by the transmembrane helices *(bar)*; receptors for peptides such as vasopressin, **C,** in which agonist binding *(arrow)* may involve parts of the extracellular N-terminus and loops and the transmembrane helices *(bar)*; and glycoprotein hormone receptors, **D,** in which agonists *(oval)* bind to the large extracellular N-terminus, activating the receptor through undefined interactions with the extracellular loops or transmembrane helices *(arrow)*. Family 2, **E,** includes receptors for peptide hormones such as parathyroid hormone and secretin. Agonists *(arrow)* may bind to residues in the extracellular N-terminus and loops and to transmembrane helices *(bar)*. Family 3, **F,** includes the extracellular Ca^{2+}-sensing receptor and metabotropic glutamate receptors. Agonists *(circle)* bind in a cleft of the Venus flytrap–like domain in the large extracellular N-terminus, activating the receptor through undefined interactions with the extracellular loops or transmembrane helices *(arrow)*.

effectors include enzymes of second-messenger metabolism such as adenylyl cyclase and phospholipase Cβ and a variety of ion channels. Agonist binding to GPCRs alters intracellular second-messenger and ion concentrations, with resultant rapid effects on hormone secretion, muscle contraction, and a variety of other physiologic functions. Long-term changes in gene expression result from second messenger–stimulated phosphorylation of transcription factors.

The G protein subunits are encoded by three distinct genes. The α-subunit binds guanine nucleotides with high affinity and specificity and has intrinsic guanosine triphosphatase (GTPase) activity. The β and γ polypeptides are tightly but noncovalently associated in a functional dimer subunit. The three-dimensional structures of the individual and associated subunits have been determined.[123,124] There is considerable diversity in G protein subunits, with multiple genes encoding all three subunits and alternative gene splicing resulting in additional polypeptide products. There are at least 16 distinct α-subunit genes in mammals. These vary widely in range of expression. Some, such as $G_s\alpha$, which couples many GPCRs to stimulation of adenylyl cyclase, are ubiquitous; others, such as $G_{t1}\alpha$, which couples the GPCR rhodopsin to cyclic guanosine monophosphate phosphodiesterase in retinal rod photoreceptor cells, are highly localized.

Because multiple GPCRs, G proteins, and effectors are expressed within a cell, the degree and basis for specificity in G protein coupling to GPCRs and to effectors are major subjects of investigation, with implications for understanding drug actions and disease mechanisms.[12] Since the pioneering work of Rodbell[125] in discovering G proteins and showing that G protein–mediated signal transduction involves three separable components (i.e., receptor, G protein, and effector), additional complexity has emerged.

A large gene family whose members are regulators of G protein signaling (RGS) has been identified. RGS proteins bind to a transition state of the GTP-activated G protein α-subunit and accelerate its GTPase activity, helping to deactivate the α-subunit. RGS domains have also been found in modular proteins with additional functions, in certain cases linking heterotrimeric G protein signaling with the function of low-molecular-weight GTP-binding proteins in the RAS superfamily.[124] Lefkowitz[125] has shown that a family of GPCR kinases and arrestin proteins is involved in GPCR desensitization after agonist binding. GPCRs interact directly with a number of other proteins in addition to G proteins. GPCRs are important targets for treatment of many diseases, and mutations in genes encoding GPCRs have been identified as the cause of several endocrine and non-endocrine disorders.

G Protein–Coupled Receptor Structure and Function

Structure

Hydropathy analysis of the primary sequence of all GPCRs predicts seven membrane-spanning α-helices connected by

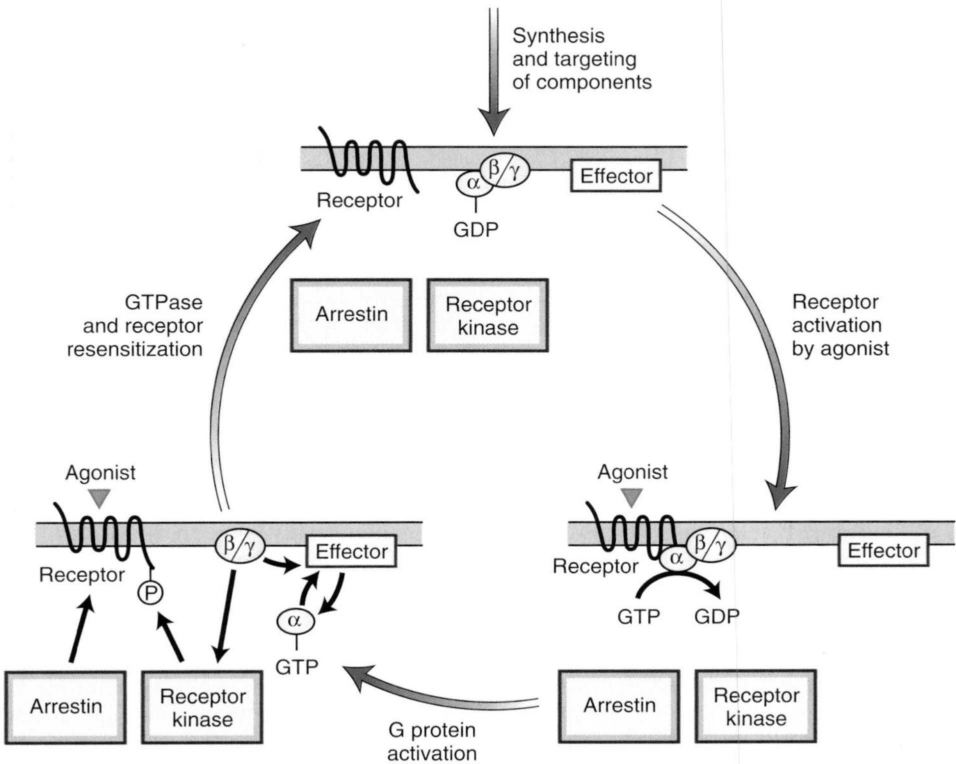

Figure 5-11 The G protein guanosine triphosphatase (GTPase) and G protein–coupled receptor (GPCR) desensitization-resensitization cycle. In each panel, the *shaded area* denotes the plasma membrane, with the extracellular region above and the intracellular region below. In the basal state, the G protein is a heterotrimer with guanosine diphosphate (GDP) tightly bound to the α-subunit. The agonist-activated GPCR catalyzes release of GDP, which permits guanosine triphosphate (GTP) to bind. The GTP-bound α-subunit dissociates from the βγ dimer. *Arrows* from the α-subunit to the effector and from the βγ dimer to the effector indicate regulation of effector activity by the respective subunits. The *arrow* from effector to the α-subunit indicates regulation of its GTPase activity by effector interaction. Under physiologic conditions, effector regulation by G protein subunits is transient and is terminated by the GTPase activity of the α-subunit. The latter converts bound GTP to GDP, thereby returning the α-subunit to its inactivated state with high affinity for the βγ dimer, which reassociates to form the heterotrimer in the basal state. In the basal state, the receptor kinase and arrestin are shown as cytosolic proteins. Dissociation of the GTP-bound α-subunit from the βγ dimer permits the dimer to facilitate binding of receptor kinase to the plasma membrane (*arrow* from βγ dimer to receptor kinase). Plasma membrane binding permits the receptor kinase to phosphorylate the agonist-bound GPCR (P, depicted here as occurring on the carboxyl-terminal tail of the GPCR, although sites on intracellular loops are also possible). GPCR phosphorylation facilitates arrestin binding to the GPCR, resulting in desensitization. Endocytic trafficking of arrestin-bound GPCR and recycling to the plasma membrane during resensitization are not shown.

three intracellular loops and three extracellular loops with an extracellular N-terminus and an intracellular C-terminus (see Fig. 5-10). This basic structure has been verified by x-ray crystallography for rhodopsin, β_1- and β_2-adrenergic, and adenosine A_{2a} receptors.[127] Although there was evidence that visual transduction in the retina and hormone activation of adenylyl cyclase shared common features, the discovery that the β-adrenergic receptor has the same topographic structure as rhodopsin came as a surprise.[126] Cloning of the complementary deoxyribonucleic acids (cDNAs) for a vast number of GPCRs followed elucidation of the primary sequence of the β-adrenergic receptor, and in every case, the same core structure was predicted by hydropathy analysis.

In addition to the predicted core structure, other common features (with exceptions in some subsets of the GPCR superfamily) have been identified[122]:

- A disulfide bridge connecting the first and second extracellular loops
- One or more *N*-linked glycosylation sites, usually in the N-terminus but occasionally in extracellular loops
- Palmitoylation of one or more cysteines in the C-terminus, which effectively creates a fourth intracellular loop
- Potential phosphorylation sites in the C-terminus and occasionally in the third intracellular loop

Glycosylation appears to be important for proper folding and trafficking to the plasma membrane rather than for ligand binding. The disulfide bridge may help in proper arrangement of the transmembrane helices.

Superimposed on the basic structure of GPCRs are a number of variations relevant to differences in ligand binding, G protein coupling, and interaction with other proteins.[122] There are major differences in amino acid sequence among members of the GPCR superfamily. Sequence alignment, especially of the transmembrane helices, allows division of the superfamily into subfamilies (see Fig. 5-10).

Family 1, the largest group, can itself be subdivided. The largest subset includes opsins, odorant receptors, and monoamine, purinergic, and opiate receptors. These are characterized by a short N-terminus. The second subset includes chemokine, protease-activated, and certain peptide hormone receptors characterized by a slightly longer N-terminus. The third subset comprises receptors for the large glycoprotein hormones, TSH, luteinizing hormone, and follicle-stimulating hormone. They have an approximately 400-residue extracellular N-terminus.

Family 2 shows essentially no sequence homology to family 1, even within the transmembrane helices, and it is characterized by an approximately 100-residue N-terminus. Members include receptors for several peptide hormones such as parathyroid hormone (PTH), calcitonin, vasoactive intestinal peptide, and corticotropin-releasing hormone.

Family 3, in addition to having a unique primary sequence, has other distinctive features such as an approximately 200-residue C-terminus and an approximately 600-residue N-terminus. The latter consists of a putative Venus flytrap–like domain and a cysteine-rich domain. Members include the metabotropic glutamate receptors, an extracellular Ca^{2+}-sensing receptor, and putative taste and pheromone receptors.[128] Determination of the three-dimensional crystal structure of part of the extracellular N-terminus of the metabotropic glutamate receptors has verified a two Venus flytrap–like structure linked to the cysteine-rich region by a disulfide bridge.[128]

Ligand Binding

Given the diversity of ligands (>1000) that bind to GPCRs, it is not surprising that considerable diversity is evident in the sequence and structure of presumptive GPCR ligand–binding domains. The opsins are unique among GPCRs in that the ligand, retinal, is covalently bound to a lysine in the seventh transmembrane helix.[127] Ligand binding for other members of family 1 with a short extracellular N-terminus, such as adrenergic and other monoamine receptors, involves a pocket within the transmembrane helices, as has been demonstrated for rhodopsin (see Fig. 5-10). Rhodopsin's N-terminus and extracellular loops form a well-structured domain that occludes the retinal binding site. The hormone receptors have a more open extracellular structure that facilitates ligand entry into the transmembrane domain.[127]

For other family 1 GPCRs, the extracellular N-terminus, perhaps together with extracellular loops and portions of the transmembrane helices, is involved in ligand binding. In the case of the glycoprotein hormone receptors, the large, curved, extracellular N-terminus plays the principal role in hormone binding.[129]

In a model for peptide binding to family 2 receptors, the extracellular N-terminus is responsible for initial binding to the peptide C-terminus, followed by peptide N-terminus binding to the seven-transmembrane domain.[130] For family 3 GPCRs, the three-dimensional structure of the metabotropic glutamate receptor shows that agonist binding occurs within a cleft between the lobes of the Venus flytrap.[128]

G Protein Coupling

Because the number of potential G proteins to which GPCRs couple is much more limited than the number of ligands that bind GPCRs, more conservation of the domains involved in G protein coupling is expected. Although GPCRs can be broadly divided into those that couple to G_s, those that couple to the G_q subfamily, and those that couple to the G_i-G_o subfamily, the situation is probably more complicated.[124] Specificity of coupling to the most recently identified G proteins, G_{12} and G_{13}, is still uncertain. Also, some GPCRs evidently can couple to both G_s and G_q.

Many studies have been performed to define the sites of ligand binding and G protein coupling of GPCRs.[124,131] Considerable evidence points to the third intracellular loop (particularly its membrane-proximal portions) and to the membrane-proximal portion of the C-terminus as key determinants of G protein–coupling specificity. For example, exchanging only the third intracellular loop between different GPCRs confers the G protein–coupling specificity of the exchanged loop on the recipient GPCR.[132] In contrast, the second intracellular loop, although important for G protein coupling, appears to play a role in the activation mechanism rather than in determining specificity of coupling.[132] A tripeptide "DRY" motif (D/E, R, Y/W) at the juncture between the third transmembrane helix and the start of the second intracellular loop that is highly conserved in family 1 GPCRs is critical for G protein activation.[131] The three-dimensional structure of a complex between activated rhodopsin and a C-terminal peptide of the retinal G protein α–subunit shows direct binding of the latter to the arginine of the receptor's DRY motif.[127]

Mechanism of Activation

The precise mechanism of activation after agonist binding has not been defined for most GPCRs, but x-ray crystallographic studies of rhodopsin, β-adrenergic, and adenosine receptors provide the clearest picture available. In the ground state, retinal covalently bound to the seventh transmembrane helix in rhodopsin holds the transmembrane helices in an inactive conformation, at least in part through so-called ion lock created by electrostatic interaction between the arginine at the end of the third transmembrane domain and a glutamate at the end of the sixth transmembrane domain.[127] Isomerization of retinal on absorption of light of the appropriate wavelength converts an antagonist ligand into an agonist. The rhodopsin crystal structure identifies the residues in the transmembrane helices that interact with retinal and suggests a mechanism for movement of the helices, particularly the third and sixth transmembrane domains, on photoactivation of retinal.[127] Movement of the transmembrane helices leads to changes in conformation of cytoplasmic loops that promote G protein activation.

For family 1 receptors related to rhodopsin, determination of their three-dimensional structures validates the idea that a change in conformation of transmembrane helices is the direct result of agonist or antagonist binding to residues within the helices.[127] Molecular modeling by computer on the basis of the rhodopsin structure and experimental testing offers a useful approach to defining critical structural regions of other GPCRs.[133] The availability of three-dimensional structures for β-adrenergic and adenosine receptors also permits *in silico* studies of ligand binding to these receptors.[127]

For other GPCRs whose presumptive site of agonist binding does not solely involve direct contact with transmembrane helices (i.e., families 2 and 3 and the glycoprotein hormone receptors in family 1), much remains to be learned about how agonist binding to the extracellular domain of these GPCRs leads to presumptive changes in conformation of transmembrane helices and receptor activation. Determination of the structure of the extracellular domain of the FSH receptor bound to FSH illustrates the general mechanism of glycoprotein hormone binding to cognate GPCRs and resultant interactions with the seven-transmembrane domain receptor leading to activation.

A hypothesis of GPCR activation postulates that GPCRs are in equilibrium between an activated state and inactive state. These states presumably differ in the disposition of the transmembrane helices and the cytoplasmic domains that determine G protein coupling. According to this ternary complex model, agonists are viewed as stabilizing the activated state. Antagonists may be neutral; that is, they may simply compete with agonists for receptor binding, with their binding having no influence on the equilibrium. Alternatively, they may be inverse agonists, with their binding stabilizing the inactive state of the receptor.[134] Multiple conformational states may exist between the so-called active and inactive conformations, with different ligands capable of promoting a particular conformation. This possibility has important implications for the downstream signaling consequences of a given ligand, a concept called *ligand-directed signaling*[124] or *ligand-biased efficacy*.

Dimerization

Members of the tyrosine kinase receptor family require dimerization as part of their activation mechanism, and many GPCRs form homodimers and heterodimers.[122,124] Residues within transmembrane helix 6 may foster dimerization of small, family 1 GPCRs,[136] and intermolecular disulfide bonds in the extracellular N-terminal domain are involved in homodimerization of most family 3 GPCRs.[128,137,138] A coiled-coil interaction in the C-terminus of γ-aminobutyric acid B receptor subtypes is responsible for heterodimerization, and this is critical for proper receptor function.[139] Modifications of ligand binding, signaling, and receptor sequestration have been demonstrated on heterodimerization of angiotensin with bradykinin receptors, of κ with δ opioid receptors, and of opioid with β-adrenergic receptors, and a role for ligand-independent action of heterodimerized orphan GPCRs (discussed later) has been proposed.[140] Additional studies are needed to elucidate the physiologic relevance of GPCR homodimerization and heterodimerization.

G Protein–Coupled Receptor Desensitization

Pharmacologists have long appreciated that continued exposure to agonist leads to a diminished response, or *desensitization*. This phenomenon has been extensively studied in GPCRs. Two forms are defined: heterologous desensitization, in which binding of agonist to one GPCR leads to a diminished response of a different GPCR to its agonist, and homologous desensitization, in which desensitization occurs only for the GPCR to which agonist is bound. Both forms involve GPCR phosphorylation but by different kinases and at different sites. Stimulation of cyclic adenosine monophosphate formation by agonist binding to a G_s-coupled GPCR leads to activation of protein kinase A, which in turn can phosphorylate and desensitize the GPCR. Phosphorylation may also alter G protein–coupling specificity.[122] Similarly, protein kinase C activation resulting from GPCR coupling to G_q family members may cause protein kinase C–catalyzed phosphorylation of GPCRs with desensitization.

In retinal photoreceptors, a specific rhodopsin kinase and the arrestin protein have been implicated in attenuation of the light response. Just as there are parallels between rhodopsin and GPCR structure, parallels have also been identified in desensitization mechanisms. Rhodopsin kinase is only one member of a family of GPCR kinases and arrestin only one of a family of related proteins that function in desensitization of many members of the GPCR superfamily.[126] GPCR kinases preferentially phosphorylate the agonist-bound form of a GPCR, ensuring homologous desensitization. On GPCR phosphorylation by GPCR kinase, arrestins bind to the third intracellular loop and C-terminal tail of the GPCR, thereby blocking G protein binding (see Fig. 5-11). GPCR kinases and arrestins not only desensitize GPCRs but also mediate other functions, including receptor internalization and interaction with other effectors.

G PROTEIN–COUPLED RECEPTOR INTERACTIONS WITH OTHER PROTEINS

The initial paradigm of GPCR function postulated that G protein activation is the sole outcome of agonist binding to GPCRs. With the identification of GPCR interactions with GPCR kinases and arrestins, this concept was modified to include the proteins involved in GPCR desensitization. Later evidence suggested that GPCR interaction with arrestins may also permit recruitment of other proteins to the GPCR. For example, the SRC tyrosine kinase may interact with the β-adrenergic receptor, with β-arrestin serving as an adaptor.[141] Arrestins may also recruit proteins involved in endocytosis, and GPCR kinases may recruit additional signaling proteins to the GPCR.[141]

Other classes of proteins may interact with specific GPCRs without recruitment by GPCR kinases and arrestins. They include SH2 domain–containing proteins, small GTP-binding proteins, and postsynaptic density protein-95/discs large/zona occludens 1 (PDZ) domain–containing proteins. An examples of the latter is binding of the Na^+/H^+ exchanger regulatory factor to the C-terminus of the β-adrenergic receptor.[141] The long C-terminus of family 3 GPCRs (e.g., metabotropic glutamate receptors) contains polyproline motifs involved in binding members of the Homer family of PDZ proteins, which can facilitate functional interactions with other proteins such as the inositol triphosphate receptor.[142] Receptor activity-modifying proteins (RAMPs), a family of single-transmembrane-domain proteins, appear to heterodimerize with certain GPCRs, assisting them in proper folding and membrane trafficking.[143] This rapidly evolving aspect of GPCR function promises many interesting developments.

G PROTEIN–COUPLED RECEPTORS IN DISEASE PATHOGENESIS AND TREATMENT

Because of their diverse and critical roles in normal physiology, their accessibility on the cell surface, and their ability to synthesize selective agonists and antagonists, GPCRs have been a major target for drug development. One estimate is that about 65% of prescription drugs target GPCRs. Drugs targeting GPCRs may act as agonists, antagonists, or allosteric modulators. For example, calcimimetic drugs inhibit PTH release by binding to the seven-transmembrane domain and acting as positive allosteric modulators of the Ca^{2+}-sensing receptor.[138] With the cloning of GPCR cDNAs, much greater diversity of receptor subclasses became evident than had been anticipated on the basis of pharmacologic studies. For example, five muscarinic receptor subtypes and an even greater number of serotoninergic GPCRs were identified.[130] This information has enabled development of highly specific subtype-selective drugs that have fewer side effects than those produced by previously available agents.

Another result of the cloning of GPCR cDNAs by homology screening and polymerase chain reaction–based approaches is the identification of orphan GPCRs, receptors that have the canonical, predicted seven-transmembrane-domain structure of GPCRs but have no identified physiologic agonists. There have been substantial efforts to identify the relevant ligands for these orphan receptors.[140] For example, the Krebs cycle intermediates, succinate and α-ketoglutarate, were shown to be the physiologically relevant activators of the orphan GPCRs, GPR91, and GPR99, respectively; through binding, they regulate renin release and blood pressure.[144] In addition to revealing novel physiologic and pathophysiologic mechanisms, GPCR "deorphanization" provides novel targets for drug development.

Beyond drug development, defects in GPCRs are an important cause of a variety of human diseases.[145] GPCR mutations can cause loss of function by impairing any of several steps in the normal GPCR-GTPase cycle (see Fig. 5-11), including failure to synthesize the GPCR protein altogether, failure of synthesized GPCR to reach the plasma membrane, failure of GPCR to bind or be activated by agonist, and failure of GPCR to couple to or activate G protein. Because in most cases clinically significant impairment of signal transduction requires loss of both alleles of a GPCR gene, most of these diseases are inherited in autosomal recessive fashion (Table 5-1).

Most diseases manifest as resistance to the action of the normal agonist and mimic deficiency of the agonist. For example, TSH receptor loss-of-function mutations cause a form of hypothyroidism that mimics TSH deficiency, but the serum TSH level is elevated in such cases, reflecting resistance to the hormone's action caused by defective receptor function. Hypogonadotropic hypogonadism may be caused by loss-of-function mutations of the GnRH receptor, the orphan GPR54, or the prokineticin receptor 2 (PROKR2). In the first case, there is resistance to the action of GnRH. In the latter two cases, hypogonadotropic hypogonadism may reflect failure to release GnRH, but the precise mechanism has not been defined.[146,147] Nephrogenic diabetes insipidus (i.e., renal vasopressin resistance) is caused by loss-of-function mutations in the arginine vasopressin receptor 2 gene (*AVPR2*) located on the X chromosome. Males with a single copy of the gene develop the disease when they inherit a mutant gene; most females do not show overt disease because random X inactivation leaves them with an average of 50% of normal gene function. Most *AVPR2* mutations associated with nephrogenic diabetes insipidus cause loss of function by impairing normal synthesis or folding of the receptor, or both. A novel mechanism for receptor loss of function elucidated for an *AVPR2* missense mutation associated with nephrogenic diabetes insipidus involves constitutive arrestin-mediated desensitization.[148]

The extracellular Ca^{2+}-sensing receptor appears to be an interesting exception to the association between GPCR loss-of-function mutations and hormone resistance. Loss-of-function mutations of this receptor mimic a hormone hypersecretion state, primary hyperparathyroidism. Such mutations do cause hormone resistance, but extracellular Ca^{2+} is the hormonal agonist that acts through this receptor to inhibit PTH secretion. A loss-of-function mutation of one copy of the receptor gene typically causes mild resistance to extracellular Ca^{2+}, which manifests as familial hypocalciuric hypercalcemia. If two defective copies are inherited, extreme Ca^{2+} resistance causing neonatal severe primary hyperparathyroidism results (see Table 5-1). In some cases, a heterozygous receptor loss-of-function mutation is associated with neonatal severe primary hyperparathyroidism, perhaps reflecting a dominant negative effect caused by dimerization of wild-type and mutant receptors.[149]

GPCR gain-of-function mutations are an important cause of disease (Table 5-2).[145] Given the dominant nature of activating mutations, most of these diseases are inherited in an autosomal dominant manner. Activating TSH receptor mutations may be inherited in autosomal dominant fashion and cause diffuse thyroid enlargement in familial nonautoimmune hyperthyroidism, or they may occur as somatic mutations causing focal, sporadic, hyperfunctional thyroid nodules.[150] Activating germline LH receptor mutations cause familial male precocious puberty due to LH-independent Leydig cell hyperfunction, and somatic LH receptor mutations may cause focal Leydig cell tumors.[150]

Unlike loss-of-function mutations, which may be missense, nonsense, or frameshift mutations that truncate the normal receptor protein, GPCR gain-of-function mutations are almost always missense mutations. The location and nature of naturally occurring, disease-causing mutations offer important insights into GPCR structure and function. The basis for defective receptor function is clear with mutations that truncate receptor synthesis prematurely. More

TABLE 5-1

Diseases Caused by G Protein–Coupled Receptor Loss-of-Function Mutations

Receptor	Disease	Inheritance
V2 vasopressin	Nephrogenic diabetes insipidus	X-linked
ACTH	Familial ACTH resistance	AR
GHRH	Familial GH deficiency	AR
GnRH	Hypogonadotropic hypogonadism	AR
GPR54	Hypogonadotropic hypogonadism	AR
Prokineticin receptor 2	Hypogonadotropic hypogonadism	AD*
FSH	Hypergonadotropic ovarian dysgenesis	AR
LH	Male pseudohermaphroditism	AR
TSH	Familial hypothyroidism	AR
Ca^{2+} sensing	Familial hypocalciuric hypercalcemia	AD
	Neonatal severe primary hyperparathyroidism	AR
Melanocortin 4	Obesity	AR
PTH/PTHrP	Blomstrand chondrodysplasia	AR

*With incomplete penetrance.

ACTH, adrenocorticotropic hormone; AD, autosomal dominant; AR, autosomal recessive; FSH, follicle-stimulating hormone; GH, growth hormone; GHRH, growth hormone–releasing hormone; GnRH, gonadotropin-releasing hormone; GPR54, orphan G protein–coupled receptor 54; LH, luteinizing hormone; PTH, parathyroid hormone; PTHrP, parathyroid hormone–related protein; TSH, thyroid-stimulating hormone.

TABLE 5-2

Diseases Caused by G Protein–Coupled Receptor Gain-of-Function Mutations

Receptor	Disease	Inheritance
LH	Familial male precocious puberty	AD
TSH	Sporadic hyperfunctional thyroid nodules	Noninherited (somatic)
	Familial nonautoimmune hyperthyroidism	AD
Ca^{2+} sensing	Familial hypocalcemic hypercalciuria	AD
PTH/PTHrP	Jansen's metaphyseal chondrodysplasia	AD
V2 vasopressin	Nephrogenic inappropriate antidiuresis	AD

AD, autosomal dominant; LH, luteinizing hormone; PTH, parathyroid hormone; PTHrP, parathyroid hormone–related protein; TSH, thyroid-stimulating hormone.

subtle missense mutations may impair function if they involve highly conserved residues in transmembrane helices critical for normal protein folding. Activating missense mutations often involve residues within or bordering transmembrane helices and are thought to disrupt normal inhibitory constraints that maintain the receptor in its inactive conformation.[127,151] Mutations disrupting these constraints mimic the effects of agonist binding and shift the equilibrium toward the activated state of the receptor. A striking example is the activating missense mutations in *AVPR2* of arginine 137, part of the DRY motif at the intracellular border of transmembrane helix 3 that is conserved in most family 1 GPCRs, which lead to the syndrome of nephrogenic inappropriate antidiuresis.[152]

Diseases caused by activating GPCR mutations clinically mimic states of agonist excess, but direct measurement shows that agonist concentrations are low, reflecting normal negative feedback mechanisms. The Ca^{2+}-sensing receptor is an apparent exception, with activating mutations causing functional hypoparathyroidism. Although in most GPCRs, disease-associated gain-of-function mutations cause constitutive, agonist-independent activation, such mutations in the Ca^{2+}-sensing receptor, with rare exceptions, cause increased sensitivity to extracellular Ca^{2+} rather than to Ca^{2+}-independent activation.[149]

Naturally occurring animal models of human disease have revealed additional examples of etiologic GPCR mutations. For example, a loss-of-function mutation in the hypocretin (orexin) type 2 receptor gene was identified in canine narcolepsy.[153] Dozens of mouse GPCR gene knockout models have been created, and many have revealed interesting and unexpected phenotypes. Characterization of the phenotype resulting from disruption of a mouse GPCR gene may accurately predict the clinical picture resulting from the corresponding mutation in humans; examples include disruption of the melanocortin 4 receptor gene, which results in obesity[154] and disruption of the PTH/PTH-related protein receptor gene, which impairs normal bone growth and development in mice[155] and in the human disease known as *Blomstrand chondrodysplasia*.[156] Knockouts of orphan GPCR genes can help reveal their physiologic functions. For example, knockout of the mouse gene encoding an orphan GPCR (GPR48) demonstrated its role in regulation of bone formation and remodeling.[157] Studies of a constitutively active GPR3 in the mouse and in *Xenopus* revealed a role in maintaining meiotic arrest in oocytes.[158]

Availability of mouse knockout models of human diseases should facilitate testing of novel therapies, including gene transfer. For example, aminoglycosides, which suppress premature termination codons, were shown to rescue expression and function in mice with nephrogenic diabetes insipidus caused by a nonsense mutant in *AVPR2*.[159] Many disease-causing loss-of-function mutations in GPCRs lead to defective protein folding or protein routing. Novel therapeutic approaches such as use of molecular chaperones and modulation of a cell's quality-control mechanisms have shown promise in in vitro studies.[160]

Screening of GPCR genes for mutations as the potential cause of human disorders may continue to identify more examples, but it is also becoming clear that variations in GPCR gene sequence can have profound consequences beyond causing resistance to or activation independent of the cognate hormone agonist. For example, familial spontaneous ovarian hyperstimulation syndrome occurring in early pregnancy was shown to be caused by missense mutations in the transmembrane helix domain of the FSH receptor.[161] These mutations increase receptor basal activity and permit low-affinity binding of human chorionic gonadotropin to the ectodomain to activate the FSH receptor. Studies are needed to determine whether variable susceptibility to iatrogenic ovarian hyperstimulation occurring in the context of in vitro fertilization may be caused by such variations in FSH receptor sequence.[161]

As more polymorphisms are discovered in the human genome, many examples of variations in the GPCR gene sequence will be found, and the challenge will be to elucidate their possible functional significance.[162] In vitro studies may reveal functional differences but further studies are required to determine whether such differences are important in individual responses to various drugs (i.e., pharmacogenomics) or whether they create other subtle physiologic differences that could confer susceptibility to disease (i.e., complex disease genes). Evidence for an important role of adrenergic receptor polymorphisms in the development and treatment of heart failure supports the need for comparable studies of other GPCR family members.[163] A large proportion of the human genome is devoted to GPCR genes, and studies of this gene superfamily will play a prominent role in the future.

REFERENCES

1. Fradkin JE, Eastman RC, Lesniak MA, et al. Specificity spillover at the hormone receptor—exploring its role in human disease. *N Engl J Med.* 1989;320:640-645.
2. Hunter T. The Croonian Lecture 1997. The phosphorylation of proteins on tyrosine: its role in cell growth and disease. *Philos Trans R Soc Lond B Biol Sci.* 1998;353:583-605.
3. Hanks SK, Hunter T. Protein kinases 6. The eukaryotic protein kinase superfamily: kinase (catalytic) domain structure and classification. *FASEB J.* 1995;9:576-596.
4. Ushiro H, Cohen S. Identification of phosphotyrosine as a product of epidermal growth factor-activated protein kinase in A-431 cell membranes. *J Biol Chem.* 1980;255:8363-8365.
5. Ullrich A, Coussens L, Hayflick JS, et al. Human epidermal growth factor receptor cDNA sequence and aberrant expression of the amplified gene in A431 epidermoid carcinoma cells. *Nature.* 1984;309:418-425.
6. Ullrich A, Gray A, Tam AW, et al. Insulin-like growth factor I receptor primary structure: comparison with insulin receptor suggests structural determinants that define functional specificity. *EMBO J.* 1986;5:2503-2512.
7. Weiss A, Schlessinger J. Switching signals on or off by receptor dimerization. *Cell.* 1998;94:277-280.
8. Westermark B, Claesson-Welsh L, Heldin CH. Structural and functional aspects of the receptors for platelet-derived growth factor. *Prog Growth Factor Res.* 1989;1:253-266.
9. Heldin CH, Ostman A, Ronnstrand L. Signal transduction via platelet-derived growth factor receptors. *Biochim Biophys Acta.* 1998; 1378:F79-F113.
10. Cunningham BC, Ultsch M, De Vos AM, et al. Dimerization of the extracellular domain of the human growth hormone receptor by a single hormone molecule. *Science.* 1991;254:821-825.
11. de Vos AM, Ultsch M, Kossiakoff AA. Human growth hormone and extracellular domain of its receptor: crystal structure of the complex. *Science.* 1992;255:306-312.
12. Wells JA. Binding in the growth hormone receptor complex. *Proc Natl Acad Sci U S A.* 1996;93:1-6.
13. Wiesmann C, Fuh G, Christinger HW, et al. Crystal structure at 1.7 Å resolution of VEGF in complex with domain 2 of the Flt-1 receptor. *Cell.* 1997;91:695-704.
14. Boni-Schnetzler M, Rubin JB, Pilch PF. Structural requirements for the transmembrane activation of the insulin receptor kinase. *J Biol Chem.* 1986;261:15281-15287.
15. Boni-Schnetzler M, Scott W, Waugh SM, et al. The insulin receptor: structural basis for high affinity ligand binding. *J Biol Chem.* 1987;262: 8395-8401.
16. Taouis M, Levy-Toledano R, Roach P, et al. Structural basis by which a recessive mutation in the alpha-subunit of the insulin receptor affects insulin binding. *J Biol Chem.* 1994;269:14912-14918.
17. De Meyts P. The structural basis of insulin and insulin-like growth factor-I receptor binding and negative co-operativity, and its relevance to mitogenic versus metabolic signalling. *Diabetologia.* 1994; 37:S135-S148.
18. Hubbard SR, Wei L, Ellis L, et al. Crystal structure of the tyrosine kinase domain of the human insulin receptor. *Nature.* 1994;372:746-754.

19. Hubbard SR. Crystal structure of the activated insulin receptor tyrosine kinase in complex with peptide substrate and ATP analog. *EMBO J.* 1997;16:5572-5581.
20. Hubbard SR, Mohammadi M, Schlessinger J. Autoregulatory mechanisms in protein-tyrosine kinases. *J Biol Chem.* 1998;273:11987-11990.
21. Herrera R, Rosen OM. Regulation of the protein kinase activity of the human insulin receptor. *J Recept Res.* 1987;7:405-415.
22. Tornqvist HE, Avruch J. Relationship of site-specific beta subunit tyrosine autophosphorylation to insulin activation of the insulin receptor (tyrosine) protein kinase activity. *J Biol Chem.* 1988;263:4593-4601.
23. Ullrich A, Schlessinger J. Signal transduction by receptors with tyrosine kinase activity. *Cell.* 1990;61:202-203.
24. Kavanaugh WM, Williams LT. An alternative to SH2 domains for binding tyrosine-phosphorylated proteins. *Science.* 1994;266:1862-1865.
25. Blaikie P, Immanuel D, Wu J, et al. A region in Shc distinct from the SH2 domain can bind tyrosine-phosphorylated growth factor receptors. *J Biol Chem.* 1994;269:32031-32034.
26. Gustafson TA, He W, Craparo A, et al. Phosphotyrosine-dependent interaction of Shc and insulin receptor substrate 1 with the NPEY motif of the insulin receptor via a novel non-SH2 domain. *Mol Cell Biol.* 1995;15:2500-2508.
27. Anderson D, Koch CA, Grey L, et al. Binding of SH2 domains of phospholipase Cg 1, GAP, and Src to activated growth factor receptors. *Science.* 1990;250:979-982.
28. Perrotti N, Accili D, Marcus-Samuels B, et al. Insulin stimulates phosphorylation of a 120-kDa glycoprotein substrate (pp120) for the receptor-associated protein kinase in intact H-35 hepatoma cells. *Proc Natl Acad Sci U S A.* 1987;84:3137-3140.
29. Najjar SM, Philippe N, Suzuki Y, et al. Insulin-stimulated phosphorylation of recombinant pp120/HA4, an endogenous substrate of the insulin receptor tyrosine kinase. *Biochemistry.* 1995;34:9341-9349.
30. Kouhara H, Hadari YR, Spivak-Kroizman T, et al. A lipid-anchored Grb2-binding protein that links FGF-receptor activation to the Ras/MAPK signaling pathway. *Cell.* 1997;89:692-693.
31. White MF, Yenush L. The IRS-signaling system: a network of docking proteins that mediate insulin and cytokine action. *Curr Top Microbiol Immunol.* 1998;228:178-179.
32. Winnay JN, Brüning JC, Burks DJ, et al. Gab-1-mediated IGF-1 signaling in IRS-1-deficient 3T3 fibroblasts. *J Biol Chem.* 2000;275:10545-10550.
33. Janez A, Worrall DS, Imamura T, et al. The osmotic shock-induced glucose transport pathway in 3T3-L1 adipocytes is mediated by gab-1 and requires Gab-1-associated phosphatidylinositol 3-kinase activity for full activation. *J Biol Chem.* 2000;275:26870-26876.
34. Sun XJ, Rothenberg P, Kahn CR, et al. Structure of the insulin receptor substrate IRS-1 defines a unique signal transduction protein. *Nature.* 1991;352:73-77.
35. Sun XJ, Wang LM, Zhang Y, et al. Role of IRS-2 in insulin and cytokine signaling. *Nature.* 1995;377:173-177.
36. Lavan BE, Lane WS, Lienhard GE. The 60-kDa phosphotyrosine protein in insulin-treated adipocytes is a new member of the insulin receptor substrate family. *J Biol Chem.* 1997;272:11439-11443.
37. Sciacchitano S, Taylor SI. Cloning, tissue expression, and chromosomal localization of the mouse IRS-3 gene. *Endocrinology.* 1997;138:4931-4940.
38. Quon MJ, Chen H, Ing BL, et al. Roles of 1-phosphatidylinositol 3-kinase and ras in regulating translocation of GLUT4 in transfected rat adipose cells. *Mol Cell Biol.* 1995;15:5403-5411.
39. Kohn AD, Summers SA, Birnbaum MJ, et al. Expression of a constitutively active Akt Ser/Thr kinase in 3T3-L1 adipocytes stimulates glucose uptake and glucose transporter 4 translocation. *J Biol Chem.* 1996;271:31372-31378.
40. Cong LN, Chen H, Li Y, et al. Physiological role of Akt in insulin-stimulated translocation of GLUT4 in transfected rat adipose cells. *Mol Endocrinol.* 1997;11:1881-1890.
41. Standaert ML, Galloway L, Karnam P, et al. Protein kinase C-zeta as a downstream effector of phosphatidylinositol 3-kinase during insulin stimulation in rat adipocytes. Potential role in glucose transport. *J Biol Chem.* 1997;272:30075-30082.
42. Kitamura T, Ogawa W, Sakaue H, et al. Requirement for activation of the serine-threonine kinase Akt (protein kinase B) in insulin stimulation of protein synthesis but not of glucose transport. *Mol Cell Biol.* 1998;18:3708-3717.
43. Alessi DR, Deak M, Casamayor A, et al. 3-Phosphoinositide-dependent protein kinase-1 (PDK1): structural and functional homology with the *Drosophila* DSTPK61 kinase. *Curr Biol.* 1997;7:776-779.
44. Alessi DR, Downes CP. The role of PI 3-kinase in insulin action. *Biochim Biophys Acta.* 1998;1436:151-154.
45. Cheatham B, Vlahos CJ, Cheatham L, et al. Phosphatidylinositol 3-kinase activation is required for insulin stimulation of pp70 S6 kinase, DNA synthesis, and glucose transporter translocation. *Mol Cell Biol.* 1994;14:4902-4911.
46. Watson R, Shigematsu S, Chiang S, et al. Lipid raft microdomain compartmentalization of TC10 is required for insulin signaling and GLUT4 translocation. *J Cell Biol.* 2001;154:829-840.
47. Baumann CA, Ribon V, Kanzaki M, et al. CAP defines a second signalling pathway required for insulin-stimulated glucose transport. *Nature.* 2000;407:202-207.
48. Chiang SH, Baumann CA, Kanzaki M, et al. Insulin-stimulated GLUT4 translocation requires the CAP-dependent activation of TC10. *Nature.* 2001;410:944-948.
49. Lowenstein EJ, Daly RJ, Batzer AG, et al. The SH2 and SH3 domain-containing protein GRB2 links receptor tyrosine kinases to ras signaling. *Cell.* 1992;70:431-432.
50. Pronk GJ, McGlade J, Pelicci G, et al. Insulin-induced phosphorylation of the 46- and 52-kDa Shc proteins. *J Biol Chem.* 1993;268:5748-5753.
51. Skolnik EY, Lee CH, Batzer A, et al. The SH2/SH3 domain-containing protein GRB2 interacts with tyrosine-phosphorylated IRS1 and Shc: implications for insulin control of ras signalling. *EMBO J.* 1993;12:1929-1936.
52. Li N, Batzer A, Daly R, et al. Guanine-nucleotide-releasing factor hSos1 binds to Grb2 and links receptor tyrosine kinases to Ras signalling. *Nature.* 1993;363:85-88.
53. Yarden Y, Escobedo JA, Kuang WJ, et al. Structure of the receptor for platelet-derived growth factor helps define a family of closely related growth factor receptors. *Nature.* 1986;323:226-232.
54. Clark SF, Martin S, Carozzi AJ, et al. Intracellular localization of phosphatidylinositide 3-kinase and insulin receptor substrate-1 in adipocytes: potential involvement of a membrane skeleton. *J Cell Biol.* 1998;140:1211-1225.
55. Belham C, Wu S, Avruch J. Intracellular signalling: PDK1-a kinase at the hub of things. *Curr Biol.* 1999;9:R93-R96.
56. Avruch J, Khokhlatchev A, Kyriakis JM, et al. Ras activation of the Raf kinase: tyrosine kinase recruitment of the MAP kinase cascade. *Recent Prog Horm Res.* 2001;56:127-155.
57. Kulkarni RN, Brüning JC, Winnay JN, et al. Tissue-specific knockout of the insulin receptor in pancreatic beta cells creates an insulin secretory defect similar to that in type 2 diabetes. *Cell.* 1999;96:329-339.
58. Withers DJ, Gutierrez JS, Towery H, et al. Disruption of IRS-2 causes type 2 diabetes in mice. *Nature.* 1998;391:900-904.
59. Assmann A, Hinault C, Kulkarni RN. Growth factor control of pancreatic islet regeneration and function. *Pediatr Diabetes.* 2009;10:14-32.
60. Brüning JC, Gautam D, Burks DJ, et al. Role of brain insulin receptor in control of body weight and reproduction. *Science.* 2000;289:2122-2125.
61. Fisher SJ, Brüning JC, Lannon S, et al. Insulin signaling in the central nervous system is critical for the normal sympathoadrenal response to hypoglycemia. *Diabetes.* 2005;54:1447-1451.
62. Taguchi A, Wartschow LM, White MF. Brain IRS2 signaling coordinates life span and nutrient homeostasis. *Science.* 2007;317:369-372.
63. Bouche C, Lopez X, Fleischmann A, et al. Insulin enhances glucose-stimulated insulin secretion in healthy humans. *Proc Natl Acad Sci U S A.* 2010;107:4770-4775.
64. Kahn CR, Brüning JC, Michael MD, et al. Knockout mice challenge our concepts of glucose homeostasis and the pathogenesis of diabetes mellitus. *J Pediatr Endocrinol Metab.* 2000;13(suppl 6):1377-1384.
65 Carpentier JL. Insulin receptor internalization: molecular mechanisms and physiopathological implications. *Diabetologia.* 1994;37:S117-S124.
66. Carpentier JL, Hamer I, Gilbert A, et al. Molecular and cellular mechanisms governing the ligand-specific and non-specific steps of insulin receptor internalization. *Z Gastroenterol.* 1996;34:73-75.
67. Flier JS, Minaker KL, Landsberg L, et al. Impaired in vivo insulin clearance in patients with severe target-cell resistance to insulin. *Diabetes.* 1982;31:132-135.
68. Elchebly M, Payette P, Michaliszyn E, et al. Increased insulin sensitivity and obesity resistance in mice lacking the protein tyrosine phosphatase-1B gene. *Science.* 1999;283:1544-1548.
69. Klaman LD, Boss O, Peroni OD, et al. Increased energy expenditure, decreased adiposity, and tissue-specific insulin sensitivity in protein-tyrosine phosphatase 1B-deficient mice. *Mol Cell Biol.* 2000;20:5479-5489.
70. Hotamisligil GS, Peraldi P, Budavari A, et al. IRS-1-mediated inhibition of insulin receptor tyrosine kinase activity in TNF-alpha-and obesity-induced insulin resistance. *Science.* 1996;271:665-668.
71. De Fea K, Roth RA. Modulation of insulin receptor substrate-1 tyrosine phosphorylation and function by mitogen-activated protein kinase. *J Biol Chem.* 1997;272:31400-31406.
72. Li J, DeFea K, Roth RA. Modulation of insulin receptor substrate-1 tyrosine phosphorylation by an Akt/phosphatidylinositol 3-kinase pathway. *J Biol Chem.* 1999;274:9351-9356.
73. Aguirre V, Uchida T, Yenush L, et al. The c-Jun NH_2 terminal kinase promotes insulin resistance during association with insulin receptor substrate-1 and phosphorylation of Ser(307). *J Biol Chem.* 2000;275:9047-9054.

74. Rui L, Aguirre V, Kim JK, et al. Insulin/IGF-1 and TNF-alpha stimulate phosphorylation of IRS-1 at inhibitory Ser307 via distinct pathways. *J Clin Invest*. 2001;107:181-189.
75. Taylor SI. Lilly lecture: molecular mechanisms of insulin resistance. Lessons from patients with mutations in the insulin-receptor gene. *Diabetes*. 1992;41:1473-1490.
76. Carlomagno F, Salvatore G, Cirafici AM, et al. The different RET-activating capability of mutations of cysteine 620 or cysteine 634 correlates with the multiple endocrine neoplasia type 2 disease phenotype. *Cancer Res*. 1997;57:391-395.
77. Mulligan LM, Kwok JB, Healey CS, et al. Germ-line mutations of the *RET* proto-oncogene in multiple endocrine neoplasia type 2A. *Nature*. 1993;363:458-460.
78. Santoro M, Carlomagno F, Romano A, et al. Activation of *RET* as a dominant transforming gene by germline mutations of *MEN2A* and *MEN2B*. *Science*. 1995;267:381-383.
79. Drachman DB. Myasthenia gravis. *N Engl J Med*. 1994; 330:1797-1810.
80. Kahn CR, Flier JS, Bar RS, et al. The syndromes of insulin resistance and acanthosis nigricans: insulin-receptor disorders in man. *N Engl J Med*. 1976;294:739-745.
81. Flier JS, Kahn CR, Roth J, et al. Antibodies that impair insulin receptor binding in an unusual diabetic syndrome with severe insulin resistance. *Science*. 1975;190:63-65.
82. Taylor SI, Marcus-Samuels B. Anti-receptor antibodies mimic the effect of insulin to down-regulate insulin receptors in cultured human lymphoblastoid (IM-9) cells. *J Clin Endocrinol Metab*. 1984;58: 182-186.
83. Weetman AP. Graves' disease. *N Engl J Med*. 2000;343:1236-1248.
84. Flier JS, Bar RS, Muggeo M, et al. The evolving clinical course of patients with insulin receptor autoantibodies: spontaneous remission or receptor proliferation with hypoglycemia. *J Clin Endocrinol Metab*. 1978;47:985-995.
85. Taylor SI, Grunberger G, Marcus-Samuels B, et al. Hypoglycemia associated with antibodies to the insulin receptor. *N Engl J Med*. 1982;307:1422-1426.
86. Shi Y, Massague J. Mechanisms of TGF-β signaling from cell membrane to the nucleus. *Cell*. 2003;113:685-700.
87. Kulkarni RN, Wang ZL, Wang RM, et al. Leptin rapidly suppresses insulin release from insulinoma cells, rat and human islets and, in vivo, in mice. *J Clin Invest*. 1997;100:2729-2736.
88. Covey SD, Wideman RD, McDonald C, et al. The pancreatic beta cell is a key site for mediating the effects of leptin on glucose homeostasis. *Cell Metab*. 2006;4:291-302.
89. Morioka T, Asilmaz E, Hu J, et al. Disruption of leptin receptor expression in the pancreas directly affects beta cell growth and function in mice. *J Clin Invest*. 2007;117:2860-2868.
90. Amselem S, Duquesnoy P, Attree O, et al. Laron dwarfism and mutations of the growth hormone-receptor gene. *N Engl J Med*. 1989;321:989-995.
91. Clement K, Vaisse C, Lahlou N, et al. A mutation in the human leptin receptor gene causes obesity and pituitary dysfunction. *Nature*. 1998;392:398-401.
92. Bogorad RL, Courtillot C, Mestayer C, et al. Identification of a gain-of-function mutation of the prolactin receptor in women with benign breast tumors. *Proc Natl Acad Sci U S A*. 2008;105:14533-14538.
93. Smit LS, Meyer DJ, Argetsinger LS, et al. Molecular events in growth hormone-receptor interaction and signaling. In: Kostyo JS, Goodman HM, eds. *Handbook of Physiology*. New York, NY: Oxford University Press; 1999:445-480.
94. Bravo J, Heath JK. Receptor recognition by gp130 cytokines. *EMBO J*. 2000;19:2399-2411.
95. Auernhammer CJ, Melmed S. Leukemia-inhibitory factor-neuroimmune modulator of endocrine function. *Endocr Rev*. 2000;21:313-345.
96. Lambert PD, Anderson KD, Sleeman MW, et al. Ciliary neurotrophic factor activates leptin-like pathways and reduces body fat, without cachexia or rebound weight gain, even in leptin-resistant obesity. *Proc Natl Acad Sci U S A*. 2001;98:4652-4657.
97. Opal SM, DePalo VA. Anti-inflammatory cytokines. *Chest*. 2000;117:1162-1172.
98. Heim MH. The JAK-STAT pathway: cytokine signalling from the receptor to the nucleus. *J Recept Signal Transduct Res*. 1999;19:75-120.
99. Campbell GS, Argetsinger LS, Ihle JN, et al. Activation of JAK2 tyrosine kinase by prolactin receptors in Nb2 cells and mouse mammary gland explants. *Proc Natl Acad Sci U S A*. 1994;91:5232-5236.
100. Argetsinger LS, Campbell GS, Yang X, et al. Identification of JAK2 as a growth hormone receptor-associated tyrosine kinase. *Cell*. 1993;74:237-244.
101. Brown RJ, Adams JJ, Pelekanos RA, et al. Model for growth hormone receptor activation based on subunit rotation within a receptor dimer. *Nat Struct Mol Biol*. 2005;12:814-821.
102. Saharinen P, Silvennoinen O. The pseudokinase domain is required for suppression of basal activity of Jak2 and Jak3 tyrosine kinases and for cytokine-inducible activation of signal transduction. *J Biol Chem*. 2002;277:47954-47963.
103. Noguchi M, Yi H, Rosenblatt HM, et al. Interleukin-2 receptor gamma chain mutation results in X-linked severe combined immunodeficiency in humans. *Cell*. 1993;73:147-157.
104. Parganas E, Wang D, Stravopodis D, et al. JAK2 is essential for signaling through a variety of cytokine receptors. *Cell*. 1998;93:385-395.
105. Ihle JN, Thierfelder W, Teglund S, et al. Signaling by the cytokine receptor superfamily. *Ann N Y Acad Sci*. 1998;865:1-9.
106. Stahl N, Boulton TG, Farruggella T, et al. Association and activation of JAK-Tyk kinases by CNTF-LIF-OSM-IL-6 beta receptor components. *Science*. 1994;263:92-95.
107. Stoecklin E, Wissler M, Schaetzle D, et al. Interactions in the transcriptional regulation exerted by STAT5 and by members of the steroid hormone receptor family. *J Steroid Biochem Mol Biol*. 1999;69: 195-204.
108. Kofoed EM, Hwa V, Little B, et al. Growth hormone insensitivity associated with a STAT5b mutation. *N Engl J Med*. 2003;349: 1139-1147.
109. Hwa V, Little B, Adiyaman P, et al. Severe growth hormone insensitivity resulting from total absence of signal transducer and activator of transcription 5b. *J Clin Endocrinol Metab*. 2005;90:4260-4266.
110. Baxter EJ, Scott LM, Campbell PJ, et al. Acquired mutation of the tyrosine kinase JAK2 in human myeloproliferative disorders. *Lancet*. 2005;365:1054-1061.
111. Lin TS, Mahajan S, Frank DA. STAT signaling in the pathogenesis and treatment of leukemias. *Oncogene*. 2000;19:2496-2504.
112. Yasukawa H, Misawa H, Sakamoto H, et al. The JAK-binding protein JAB inhibits Janus tyrosine kinase activity through binding in the activation loop. *EMBO J*. 1999;18:1309-1320.
113. Hansen JA, Lindberg K, Hilton DJ, et al. Mechanism of inhibition of growth hormone receptor signaling by suppressor of cytokine signaling proteins. *Mol Endocrinol*. 1999;13:1832-1843.
114. Ram PA, Waxman DJ. SOCS/CIS protein inhibition of growth hormone-stimulated STAT5 signaling by multiple mechanisms. *J Biol Chem*. 1999;274:35553-35561.
115. Frank SJ, Fuchs SY. Modulation of growth hormone receptor abundance and function: roles for the ubiquitin-proteasome system. *Biochim Biophys Acta*. 2008:784-794.
116. Flores-Morales A, Greenhalgh CJ, Norstedt G, et al. Negative regulation of growth hormone receptor signaling. Mol *Endocrinology*. 2006; 20:241-253.
117. Mao Y, Ling PR, Fitzgibbons TP, et al. Endotoxin-induced inhibition of growth hormone receptor signaling in rat liver in vivo. *Endocrinology*. 1999;140:5505-5515.
118. Clevenger CV, Medaglia MV. The protein tyrosine kinase P59fyn is associated with prolactin (PRL) receptor and is activated by PRL stimulation of T-lymphocytes. *Mol Endocrinol*. 1994;8:674-681.
119. Rui L, Carter-Su C. Identification of SH2-Bbeta as a potent cytoplasmic activator of the tyrosine kinase Janus kinase 2. *Proc Natl Acad Sci U S A*. 1999;96:7172-7177.
120. Shuai K, Liu B. Regulation of gene-activation pathways by PIAS proteins in the immune system. *Nat Rev Immunol*. 2005;5: 593-605.
121. Shuai K. Regulation of cytokine signaling pathways by PIAS proteins. *Cell Res*. 2006;16:196-202.
122. Bockaert J, Pin JP. Molecular tinkering of G protein-coupled receptors: an evolutionary success. *EMBO J*. 1999;18:1723-1729.
123. Neer EJ. Heterotrimeric G proteins: organizers of transmembrane signals. *Cell*. 1995;80:249-257.
124. Oldham WM, Hamm HE. Heterotrimeric G protein activation by G-protein-coupled receptors. *Nature Reviews/Molecular Cell Biology*. 2008;9:60-71.
125. Rodbell M. The role of GTP-binding proteins in signal transduction: from the sublimely simple to the conceptually complex. *Curr Top Cell Regul*. 1992;32:1-47.
126. Lefkowitz RJ. Historical review: a brief history and personal retrospective of seven-transmembrane receptors. *Trends Pharmacol Sci*. 2004;25:413-422.
127. Tate CG, Schertler GFX. Engineering G protein-coupled receptors to facilitate their structure determination. *Curr Opin Struct Biol*. 2009;19:1-10.
128. Muto T, Tsuchiya D, Morikawa K, Jingami H. Structures of the extracellular regions of the group II/III metabotropic glutamate receptors. *Proc Natl Acad Sci*. 2007;104:3759-3764.
129. Fan QR, Hendrickson WA. Structure of the human follicle-stimulating hormone in complex with its receptor. *Nature*. 2005;433:269-277.
130. Hoare SRJ. Mechanisms of peptide and nonpeptide ligand binding to class B G protein-coupled receptors. *Drug Discovery Today*. 2005;10:417-427.
131. Wess J, ed. *Structure-Function Analysis of G Protein-Coupled Receptors*. New York: Wiley-Liss; 1999.
132. Yamashita T, Terakita A, Shichida Y. Distinct roles of the second and third cytoplasmic loops of bovine rhodopsin in G protein activation. *J Biol Chem*. 2000;275:34272-34279.
133. Gershengorn M, Osman R. Insights into G protein-coupled receptor function using molecular models. *Endocrinology*. 2001;142:2-10.

134. Soudijn W, Wijngaarden IV, Ijzerman AP. Structure-activity relationships of inverse agonists for G protein-coupled receptors. *Medicinal Res Rev*. 2005;25:398-426.
135. Audet M, Bouvier M. Insights into signaling from the β_2-adrenergic receptor structure. *Nat Chem Biol*. 2008;4:397-403.
136. Herbert TE, Moffett S, Morello JP, et al. A peptide derived from a β2-adrenergic receptor transmembrane domain inhibits both receptor dimerization and activation. *J Biol Chem*. 1996;271:16384-16392.
137. Ray K, Hauschild BC, Steinbach PJ, et al. Identification of the cysteine residues in the amino-terminal extracellular domain of the human Ca^{2+} receptor critical for dimerization. *J Biol Chem*. 1999;274: 27642-27650.
138. Pin J-P, Kniazeff J, Liu J, et al. Allosteric functioning of dimeric class C G protein-coupled receptors. *FEBS J*. 2005;272:2947-2955.
139. Kaupmann K, Malitschek B, Schuler V, et al. GABA-B receptor subtypes assemble into functional heteromeric complexes. *Nature*. 1998;396: 683-687.
140. Levoye A, Dam J, Ayoub MA, et al. Do orphan G-protein-coupled receptors have ligand-independent functions? New insights from receptor heterodimers. *EMBO J*. 2006;7:1094-1098.
141. Lefkowitz RJ, Shenoy SK. Transduction of receptor signals by β-arrestins. *Science*. 2005;308:512-517.
142. Tu JC, Xiao B, Yuan JP, et al. Homer binds a novel proline-rich motif and links group 1 metabotropic glutamate receptors with IP3 receptors. *Neuron*. 1998;21:717-726.
143. McLatchie L, Fraser N, Main M, et al. RAMPs regulate the transport and ligand specificity of the calcitonin-like receptor. *Nature*. 1998; 393:333-339.
144. Hebert SC. Orphan detectors of metabolism. *Nature*. 2004;429: 143-145.
145. Spiegel AM, Weinstein LS. Inherited diseases involving G proteins and G protein-coupled receptors. *Ann Rev Med*. 2004;55:27-39.
146. Seminara SB, Messager S, Chatzidaki EE, et al. The GPR54 gene as a regulator of puberty. *N Engl J Med*. 2003;349:1614-1627.
147. Cole LW, Sidis Y, Zhang CK, et al. Mutations in *prokineticin 2* and *prokineticin receptor 2* genes in human gonaotrophin-releasing hormone deficiency: molecular genetics and clinical spectrum. *J Clin Endocrinol Metab*. 2008;93:3551-3559.
148. Barak LS, Oakley RH, Laporte SA, et al. Constitutive arrestin-mediated desensitization of a human vasopressin receptor mutant associated with nephrogenic diabetes insipidus. *Proc Natl Acad Sci U S A*. 2001; 98:93-98.
149. Hu J, Spiegel AM. Structure and function of the human calcium-sensing receptor: insights from natural and engineered mutations and allosteric modulators. *J Cellular Molecular Medicine*. 2007;11:908-922.
150. Van Sande J, Parma J, Tonacchera M, et al. Somatic and germline mutations of the TSH receptor gene in thyroid diseases. *J Clin Endocrinol Metab*. 1995;80:2577-2585.
151. Javitch JA, Fu D, Liapakis G, Chen J. Constitutive activation of the β2-adrenergic receptor alters the orientation of its sixth membrane-spanning segment. *J Biol Chem*. 1997;272:18546-18549.
152. Feldman BJ, Rosenthal SM, Vargas GA, et al. Nephrogenic syndrome of inappropriate antidiuresis. *N Engl J Med*. 2005;352: 1884-1890.
153. Lin L, Faraco J, Li R, et al. The sleep disorder canine narcolepsy is caused by a mutation in the hypocretin (orexin) receptor 2 gene. *Cell*. 1999;98:365-376.
154. Farooqi IS, Keough JM, Yeo GS, et al. Clinical spectrum of obesity and mutations in the melanocortin 4 receptor gene. *N Engl J Med*. 2003;348:1085-1095.
155. Lanske B, Karaplis AC, Lee K, et al. PTH/PTHrP receptor in early development and Indian hedgehog-regulated bone growth. *Science*. 1996;273:663-666.
156. Jobert AS, Zhang P, Couvineau A, et al. Absence of functional receptors for parathyroid hormone and parathyroid hormone-related peptide in Blomstrand chondrodysplasia. *J Clin Invest*. 1998;102: 34-40.
157. Luo J, Zhou W, Zhou X, et al. Regulation of bone formation and remodeling by G protein-coupled receptor 48. *Development*. 2009; 136:2747-2756.
158. Deng J, Lang S, Wylie C, Hammes SR. The *Xenopus laevis* isoform of a G protein-coupled receptor 3 (GPR3) is a constitutively active cell surface receptor that participates in maintaining meiotic arrest in *X. laevis* oocytes. *Mol Endocrinol*. 2008;22:1853-1865.
159. Sangkuhl K, Schulz A, Rompler H, et al. Aminoglycoside-mediated rescue of a disease-causing nonsense mutation in the V2 vasopressin receptor gene *in vitro* and *in vivo*. *Hum Mol Gen*. 2004;13:893-903.
160. Castro-Fernandez C, Maya-Nunez G, Conn PM. Beyond the signal sequence: protein routing in health and disease. *Endocr Rev*. 2005;26:479-503.
161. Monanelli L, Delbaere A, Di Carlo C, et al. A mutation in the follicle-stimulating hormone receptor as a cause of familial spontaneous ovarian hyperstimulation syndrome. *J Clin Endocrinol Metab*. 2004;89:1255-1258.
162. Kazius J, Wurdinger K, van Iterson M, et al. GPCR NaVa database: natural variants in human G-protein-coupled receptors. *Human Mutation*. 2008;29:39-44.
163. Dorn GW, Liggett SB. Mechanisms of genetic effects of pharmacogenomic variation within the adrenergic receptor network in heart failure. *Mol Pharm*. 2009;76:466-480.

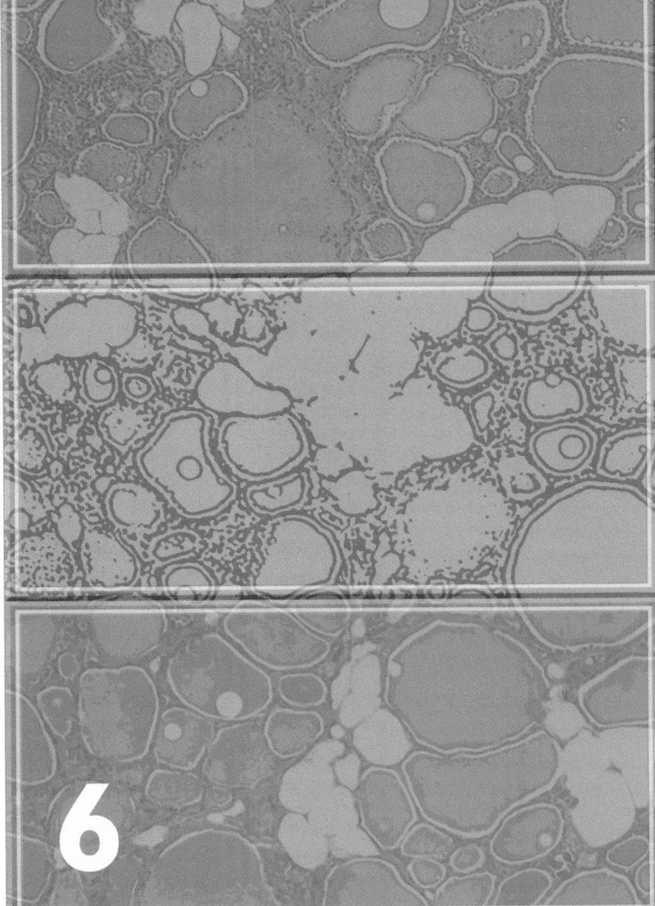

Laboratory Techniques for Recognition of Endocrine Disorders

GEORGE G. KLEE

Endocrinology is a practice of medicine that is highly dependent on accurate laboratory measurements because small changes in hormone levels often may be more specific and more sensitive for early disease than the classic physical signs and symptoms. Most endocrinologists currently do not have facilities to develop and validate laboratory assays; therefore they rely on commercial analytic assays or send a patient's specimen to specialized laboratories. Even most hospital and commercial laboratories have minimal expertise for developing analytic assays. This critical dependence on quality laboratory measurements, combined with minimal information about the performance of these tests, places endocrinologists in a potentially vulnerable position.

This chapter provides an overview of the strengths and weaknesses of the analytic techniques typically used for endocrine measurements in blood and urine. Concentrations of most hormones are much lower than those of general chemistry analytes, and specialized techniques are necessary to measure these low concentrations.

Two major types of assays for measuring hormones are described: immunoassays (both competitive and sandwich) and chromatographic assays with various detection systems including mass spectrometry. Also, a brief overview is provided for selected nucleic acid–based assays for evaluation of genetic alterations.

The analytic performance validation required by the U.S. government for laboratories testing specimens of Medicare patients is outlined, along with explanations of these performance parameters. This information should help endocrinologists better assess the performance of the analytic systems that they are using. Techniques to investigate discordant laboratory test values also are presented to help clinicians work with their specific laboratories to reconcile test values that do not match clinical presentations.

Hormone concentrations are reported in molar units, mass units, or standardized units, such as World Health Organization (WHO) International Units (IU). When these measurements are expressed in molar units, most

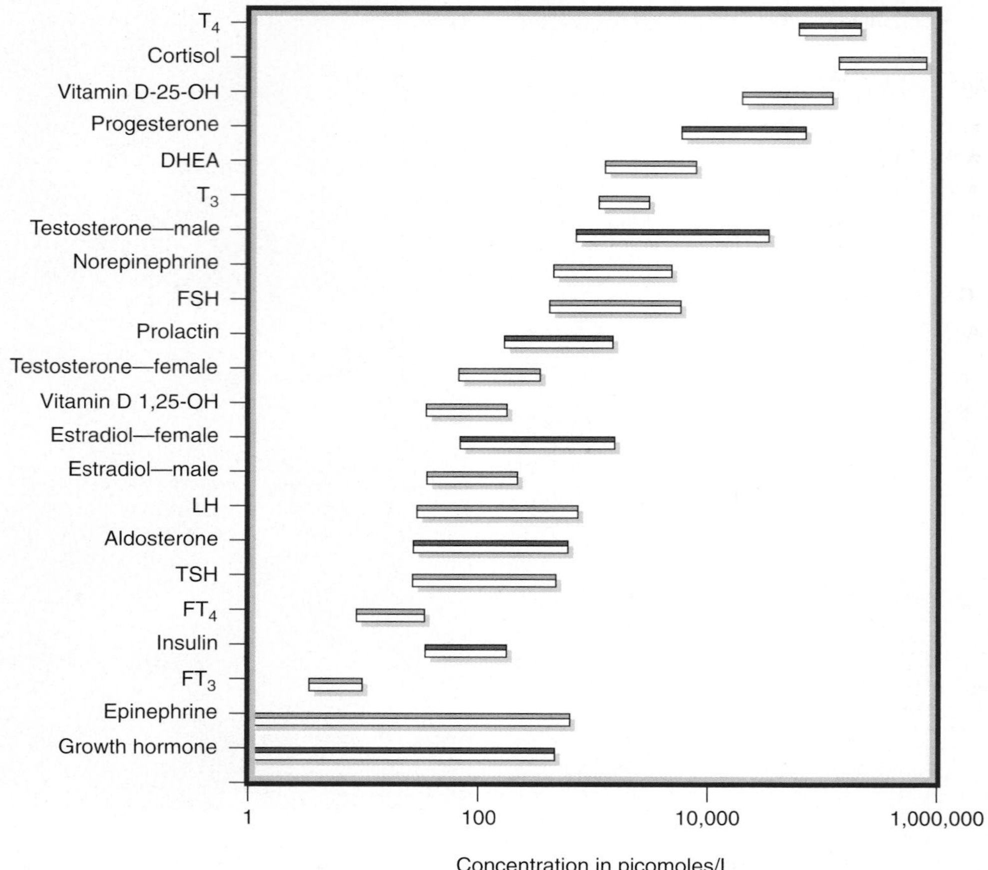

Figure 6-1 Six-logarithm range of normal plasma concentrations in endocrine tests. DHEA, dehydroepiandrosterone; FSH, follicle-stimulating hormone; FT_4, free thyroxine; FT_3, free triiodothyronine; LH, luteinizing hormone; T_3, triiodothyronine; T_4, thyroxine; TSH, thyrotropin.

hormones in blood and urine are present in concentrations of 10^{-6} to 10^{-12} mol/L (Fig. 6-1). The terms used to describe these concentrations are micromolar (10^{-6} mol/L), nanomolar (10^{-9} mol/L), and picomolar (10^{-12} mol/L). The range—from the lowest to the highest concentrations—is more than a million-fold difference. Therefore, laboratory techniques must be targeted to the levels of each given hormone.

The major techniques for measuring the lower picomolar concentrations are immunoassay and mass spectrometry, whereas the higher nanomolar and micromolar concentrations can be measured by these methods or by optical density chromatography and chemical detection systems. Some hormones, such as thyrotropin (thyroid stimulating hormone, or TSH), have very low concentrations, in the femtomolar (10^{-15} mol/L) range, in patients with diseases such as thyrotoxicosis. Exquisitely sensitive immunometric assays are usually used to measure these very low concentrations.[1,2]

TYPES OF ASSAYS

The major techniques used for steroid and protein measurements are (1) antibody-based immunologic assays, of which there are two subcategories—competitive immunoassays and immunometric (sandwich) assays, and (2) chromatographic assays with various detectors including mass spectrometers.

Competitive Immunoassays

The term *competitive radioimmunoassay* refers to a measurement method in which an antigen (e.g., a hormone) in a specimen competes with radiolabeled reagent antigen for a limited number of binding sites on a reagent antibody. The three basic components of a competitive immunoassay are (1) antiserum specific for a unique epitope on a hormone or antigen, (2) labeled antigen that binds to this antiserum, (3) unlabeled antigen in the specimen or standard that is to be measured.[3,4]

The antiserum is diluted to a concentration at which the number of binding sites available on the antibodies is fewer than the number of antigen molecules (labeled and unlabeled) in the reaction mixture. The labeled and unlabeled antigens compete for this limited number of binding sites on the antiserum. The competition is not always equal because the labeled antigen (*tracer*) and the native antigen may react differently with the antibody. This disparity in reactivity may be caused by alteration of the antigen due to the chemical attachment of the label or by differences in the endogenous antigen compared with the form of the antigen used in the reagents. As long as the reactions are reproducible, these differences in reactivity are not important because the reaction can be *calibrated* with standard reference materials having known concentrations.

Figure 6-2 illustrates the concepts of a competitive immunoassay. In the schematic diagram, 8 units of antibody react with 16 units of labeled antigen and 4 units of

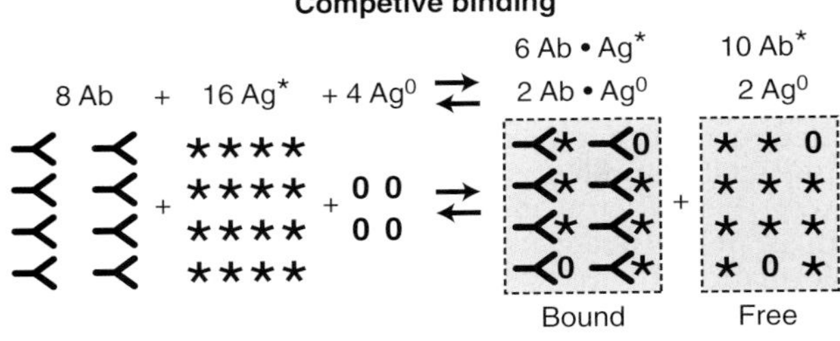

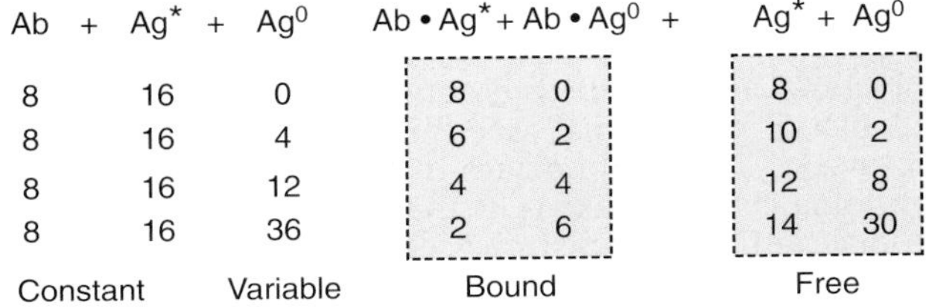

Calibration of standards
Ab + Ag* + Ag0
Ab • Ag* + Ab • Ag0 +
Ag* + Ag0
8 16 0 8 0 8 0
8 16 4 6 2 10 2
8 16 12 4 4 12 8
8 16 36 2 6 14 30
Constant
Variable
Bound
Free
A

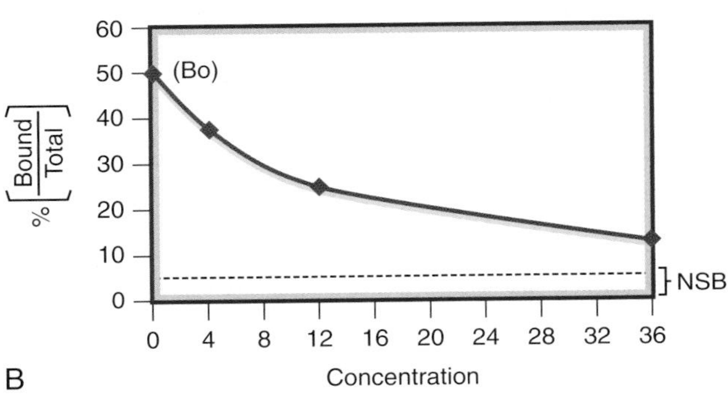

Figure 6-2 **A,** Principles of competitive binding assays. Ab, antibody; Ag*, labeled antigen; AG^0, native antigen. See text for details. **B,** Typical dose-response curve. The point on the curve labeled (B_0) represents the percentage binding of the radiolabeled antigen when zero native antigen is present. The nonspecific binding (NSB) level is the minimal binding level of radiolabeled antigen at high concentrations of native antigen.

native antigen. At equilibrium (assuming equal reactivity), 6 units of label and 2 units of native antigen are bound to the limited supply of antibody. The antigen bound to the antibody is separated from the liquid antigen by any of several methods, and the amount of labeled antigen in the bound portion is quantitated (see Fig. 6-2A). The assay is calibrated by measuring standards with known concentrations and cross-plotting the signal (i.e., counts of the gamma rays emitted from the radioactive label) versus the concentration of the standard to generate a dose-response curve. As the concentration increases, the signal decreases exponentially.

Generally, the antiserum used in a competitive assay is diluted to a titer that binds between 40% and 50% of the labeled antigen when no unlabeled antigen is present. Further dilution of the antiserum increases the analytic sensitivity but decreases both the signal and the range of the assay.

The precision of competitive immunoassays is related to the rate of change of the signal compared with the rate of change of concentration (i.e., the slope of the dose-response curve).[5] In Figure 6-2B, the slope is much lower at higher concentrations, causing the assay precision to be less at higher concentrations. Most competitive immunoassays also have a relatively flat dose-response curve at very low concentrations, causing poor precision at the low end of the assay. Consequently, the precision profile for most immunoassays is U-shaped, having the best coefficients of variation in the center of the dose-response curve.

As shown in Figure 6-2, the higher the concentration of unlabeled antigen, the lower the amount of radiolabeled antigen that binds to the limited amount of antiserum. The signal decreases exponentially, from approximately 50% of total counts at zero concentration to a minimum value at high concentrations. This minimal binding, or *nonspecific binding* (NSB), is a valuable control parameter. Elevations in NSB usually signify impurities in the label that bind to the sides of the tubes and are not competitively displaced. Most assays add surfactants and proteins to minimize the NSB. Monitoring of changes in the NSB provides an early warning of potential assay problems.

Statistical data processing techniques are needed to translate the assay signals into concentrations. As illustrated, these dose-response curves typically are not linear, and numerous curve-fitting algorithms have been developed. Before the introduction of microprocessors, tedious, error-prone, manual calculations were required to mathematically transform the data into linear models. A commonly used model was to cross-plot the logit of the normalized signal versus the logarithm of the concentration and to use linear regression lines to establish the dose-response curve.[5] Today, curve fitting usually is accomplished electronically with the use of programs that automatically test the robustness of fit of multiparameter curves after statistically eliminating discordant data points.[6,7] However, users of these systems must understand their limitations and should pay attention to any warnings presented by the programs during processing of the data.

In radioimmunoassays, radioactive iodine (^{125}I) is usually used to label the antigen. The immune complexes are separated from the unbound molecules by precipitation with centrifugation after reaction with secondary antisera and precipitating reagents (e.g., polyethylene glycol).[8] These radioimmunoassays are labor intensive and may require special handling and licensure to ensure safety of the radioisotopes. Because of the statistical counting errors associated with the relatively low radioactive counts and the poor reproducibility associated with the multiple manual steps, most laboratories perform the measurements in duplicate.[9] Even when the averages of duplicate measurements are used, many manual radioimmunoassays have coefficients of variation between 10% and 15%.

It is important that key quality control parameters for radioimmunoassays be carefully monitored. In addition to NSB, another key quality control parameter is the percentage binding of the radiolabeled when zero native antigen (B_0) is present (i.e., when B represents the signal from tracer bound in the sample). As the label deteriorates, because of aging, the binding often decreases, resulting in a less reliable assay.

Another important quality control parameter is the slope of the dose-response curve. This parameter can be tracked by monitoring the concentration corresponding to half-maximum binding (50% of B/B_0). If this concentration increases significantly, the slope of the response curve decreases and the assay may not be capable of reliably measuring patient specimens at clinically important concentrations.

Many commercial kits and automated immunoassays use nonisotopic signal systems to measure hormone concentrations. These assays often use colorimetric, fluorometric, or chemiluminescent signals rather than radioactivity to quantitate the response. The advantages of these signals are biosafety, longer reagent shelf life, and ease of automation. On the other hand, they are more subject to matrix interferences than radioactive iodine.

Radioactivity is not affected by changes in protein concentration, hemolysis, color, or drugs (except for other radioactive compounds), whereas many of the current signal systems can yield spurious results when such interferences are present. In addition, many automated immunoassays are read kinetically before the reactions reach equilibrium. This early reading accentuates the effects of any matrix differences between the reference standards and patient specimens. Later in this chapter, potential troubleshooting steps are outlined to help clinicians evaluate the integrity of test measurements when spurious results are suspected.

Solid-phase reactions often are used in current immunoassays to facilitate the separation of the bound antibody-antigen complexes from the free reactants.[10] Three frequently used solid-phase materials are microtiter plates, polystyrene beads, and paramagnetic particles.[11] Typically, the antibody is attached to the solid phase, and the separation of the immune complexes from the unbound moieties is accomplished by plate washers, bead washers, or magnetic wash stations, eliminating the need for centrifugation. Another novel way of accomplishing this separation is to attach high-affinity linkers to antiserum, which then can be coupled to a complementary linker on the solid phase.

An excellent pair of linkers is biotin and streptavidin. These compounds bind with affinity constants of approximately 10^{15} L/M.[12] Biotin is a relatively small molecule that can be easily covalently attached to antiserum and used with streptavidin (a 70-kd tetrameric, nonglycosylated protein) conjugated to microtiter plates, beads, or paramagnetic particles to facilitate separation. This technique allows the antibody-antigen reaction to proceed faster with less stearic hindrance than when the antibody is directly coupled to the solid phase.

The antiserum used in these assays is a crucial component. Earlier immunoassays used *polyclonal* antiserum produced in animals. The process of generating these antisera is a combination of art, science, and luck. In general, a relatively pure form of the antigen is conjugated to a carrier protein (especially if the antigen is less than 10 kd), mixed with adjuvant (e.g., Freud's complete adjuvant), and injected intradermally into the host animal. After several boosts with conjugated protein plus Freud's incomplete adjuvant, the host animal recognizes the material as foreign and develops immune responses. The antiserum then is harvested from the animal's blood. Under optimal conditions, moderate quantities of high-affinity antisera that react only with the specific target antigen are developed. The analytic sensitivity of a competitive immunoassay is approximately inversely related to the affinity of the antiserum, such that an antiserum with an affinity constant of 10^9 L/M can be used to measure analytes in the nanomolar concentration range.

The polyclonal antiserum developed by immunizing animals represents a composite of many immunologic clones, with each clone having a different affinity and different immunologic specificity. Most clones have affinities in the 10^7 to 10^8 L/M range, with only rare clones having affinities greater than 10^{12} L/M. Various techniques are used to develop a specific antiserum, including (1) altering the form of the antigen by blocking cross-reacting epitopes and (2) purifying the antiserum by using affinity chromatography to select antibodies directed toward the epitope of interest. Affinity-column purification also can be used for immunoextraction of higher-affinity antisera by selectively eluting antiserum from the column by means of a series of buffers with increasing acidity.[13]

The major disadvantage of a polyclonal antiserum is the limited quantity produced. The large quantities needed by commercial suppliers of immunoassay reagents often require them to use multiple sources of antisera. These changes in antisera can cause significant changes in assay performance. In many instances, laboratories and clinicians are not informed about these changes, a situation that may cause problems in medical decisions.

Monoclonal antisera are used in many current immunoassays. These antisera are made by immunizing animals (usually mice) using techniques similar to those used for polyclonal antisera; instead of harvesting the antisera from the blood, the animal is euthanized and the spleen is removed.[14] The lymphocytes in the spleen are fused with myeloma cells to make cells that will grow in culture and produce antisera. These fused cells are separated into clones by means of serial plating techniques similar to those used in subculturing bacteria. The supernatant of these monoclonal cell lines (or ascites fluid if the cells are transplanted into carrier mice) contains monoclonal antisera. The selection processes used to separate the initial clones can be targeted to identify specific clones, producing antisera with high affinities and low cross-reactivity to related compounds.

The high specificity of monoclonal antisera can cause problems for some endocrine assays. Many hormones circulate in the blood as heterogeneous mixtures of multiple forms. Some of these forms are caused by genetic differences in patients, and others are related to metabolic precursors and degradation products of the hormone. Genetic differences cause some patients to produce variant forms of a hormone such as luteinizing hormone (LH). These genetic differences can cause marked variations in measurements made using assays with specific monoclonal antisera, compared with more uniform measurements made using assays with polyclonal antisera that cross-react with the multiple forms.[15] Well-characterized monoclonal antisera can be mixed together to make an "engineered polyclonal antiserum" with improved sensitivity and specificity.[16] Cross-reactivity with precursor forms of the analytes and with metabolic degradation products can cause major differences in assays. For example, cross-reactivity with six molecular forms of human chorionic gonadotropin (hCG) causes differences in hCG assays, and cross-reactivity with metabolic fragments causes differences in parathyroid hormone (PTH) assays.[17,18] Cortisol is another analyte for which major cross-reactivity with other steroids, such as corticosterone, 11-deoxycortisol, cortisone, and numerous synthetic steroids, causes significant immunoassay interferences.[19] Matrix effects with albumin also can cause major differences in cortisol immunoassays[20] (see "Mass Spectrometry" for a more robust method for measuring steroids).

Extraction of hormones from serum and urine specimens before measurement is a technique that can enhance both the sensitivity and the specificity of immunoassays. Numerous extraction systems have been developed, including organic-aqueous partitioning to remove water-soluble interferences seen with steroids, solid-phase extraction with absorption and selective elution from resins such as silica gels, and immunoaffinity chromatography.[21,22] However, extraction and purification before immunoassay are seldom used in clinical assays; these techniques are difficult to automate and require skills and equipment not available in many clinical laboratories. Although

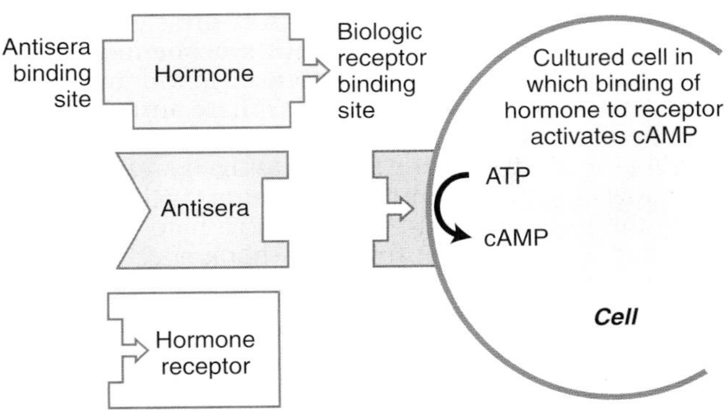

Figure 6-3 Comparison of an immunologic technique for measuring hormone concentration versus a receptor technique for measuring hormone activity. ATP, Adenosine triphosphate; cAMP, cyclic adenosine monophosphate.

commercial assays generally use reagents having adequate sensitivity and specificity to measure *most* patient specimens, some patient specimens may give spurious results, and some disease states may require more analytic sensitivity to ensure sound clinical decisions. In these cases, extraction of specimens before measurement may provide more reliable information.

Immunoassays measure concentrations rather than biologic activity. For most hormones, there is a strong correlation between the concentration of the protein or steroid being measured and the biologic activity, but this is not universally true. The reactive site for most antibodies is relatively small, about 5 to 10 amino acids for linear peptides. Some antiserum reactions are specific for the tertiary structure that corresponds to unique molecular configurations, but immunoassays seldom react with the exact antigenic structure that confers biologic activity.

Figure 6-3 presents a schematic illustration of the difference between the immunologic binding site and the biologic receptor binding site on a hormone. Indirect immunoassays have been developed using cultured cells that synthesize second messengers such as cyclic adenosine monophosphate (cAMP) at rates related to the concentration of hormone in the specimen. An example of this technique is the immunoassay measurement of cAMP produced by osteosarcoma cells to quantitate PTH bioactivity in serum.[23] Unfortunately, these assays are tedious and generally are not reproducible. Techniques using recombinant receptors as immunoassay binders may provide improved specificity with good reliability.[24-26]

Immunometric (Sandwich) Assays

A second immunologic technique used to measure hormones is the immunometric (sandwich) assay. The three basic components of a sandwich assay are (1) an antigen large enough to allow two antibodies to bind concurrently on different binding sites, (2) a *capture* antiserum directed to one of the antigenic sites on the antigen (this antiserum is attached to a solid phase to permit immunologic extraction of the immune complexes), and (3) a *signal* antiserum directed to a second antigenic site on the antigen (this antiserum is attached to an assay signal system).

In contrast to competitive immunoassays, these assays use a large excess of antiserum-binding sites compared with the concentration of antigen. The capture antibody immunoextracts the antigen from the sample, and the signal antibody binds to the capture antibody–antigen complex to form a tertiary complex. As the antigen concentration increases, the signal increases progressively.

Figure 6-4 schematically illustrates these concepts. The capture antiserum (ATB1) is attached to biotin (represented by solid circles). The signal antiserum (ATB2) is labeled with a detection system (asterisks). The ATB1-antigen-ATB2 complexes are immunologically extracted using a streptavidin solid phase (represented by the horizontal cups). After the complex is bound to the solid phase, most of the unbound signal antibody is washed away.

As shown in Figure 6-4B, the signal increases progressively with the concentration. For lower concentrations, the signal increases proportionally to the assay concentrations (after the offset caused by the NSB). At higher concentrations of native antigen, the signal is generally less than proportional, so nonlinear curve-fitting techniques are used to generate the dose-response curves. Again, the relative imprecision, expressed as a coefficient of variation, depends on the slope of the dose-response curve; consequently, the relative precision is less at higher concentrations.

In immunometric assays, the background level of signal is associated with very low concentrations. This background signal is caused by the NSB. The analytic sensitivity of immunometric assays is related to the ratio of the true signal to the NSB signal. Therefore, assays can be made more sensitive by increasing the response signal or by decreasing NSB. Inadvertent increases in NSB caused by

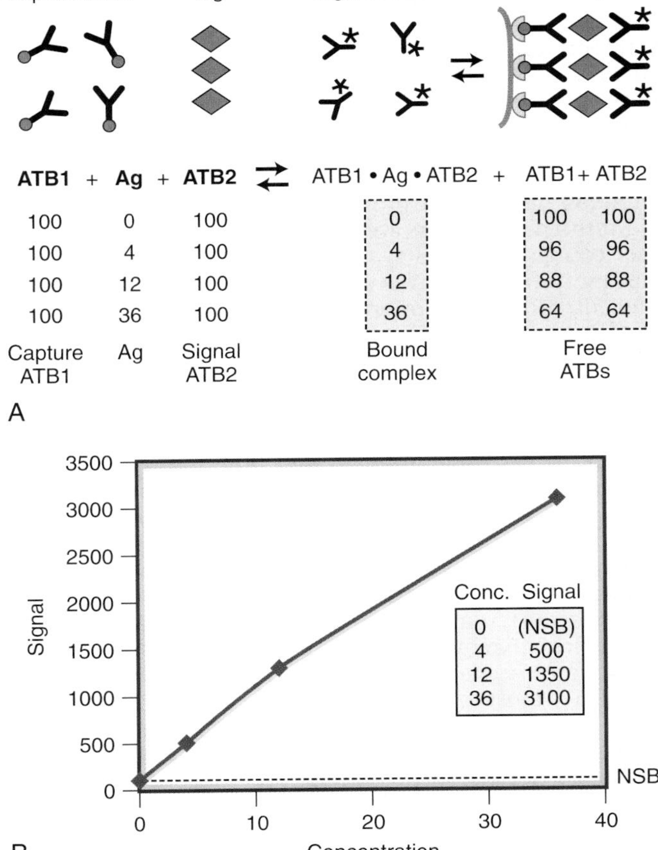

Figure 6-4 **A,** Principles of immunometric assays. Ag, antigen; ATB1, capture antiserum; ATB2, signal antiserum; ATBs, antibodies. See text for details. **B,** Typical dose-response curve. NSB, nonspecific binding level.

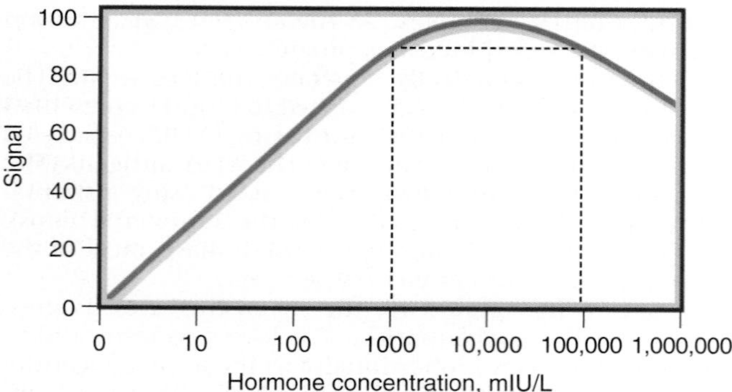

Figure 6-5 Immunometric high-dose hook effect. The response signal reaches a maximum and then decreases when the antigen concentration exceeds the limit of the assay.

specimen interference or reagent deterioration can significantly alter assay performance.

In immunometric assays, it is also important that a large excess of capture antibody be used. As the antigen concentration approaches the effective binding capacity of the capture antibody system, the signal no longer increases. If the antigen concentration exceeds the binding capacity of the capture antibody, the signal may actually decrease.

Figure 6-5 illustrates this *high-dose hook effect* for immunometric assays caused by insufficient amounts of capture or signal antiserum.[27] The signal increases progressively until the hormone concentration exceeds the binding capacity; the signal then decreases, probably as a result of removal of some of the more weakly binding antigen-antibody complexes during the wash cycle on the assay.[28-30] This is a potentially dangerous phenomenon, because the same values might be measured with very high and lower concentrations. If this artifact is suspected, the specimen may be diluted and reanalyzed. If the measured value for the diluted specimen is higher than the original result, a high-dose hook effect probably is present.

Most manufacturers are aware of this potential problem and configure assays with relatively large amounts of capture antibody; however, some patients produce high concentrations of hormones or antigens that may exceed assay limits. Laboratories can detect this phenomenon by analyzing specimens at two dilutions, but this practice generally is not cost-effective. Therefore, feedback to the laboratory about results that are inconsistent with clinical findings is essential.

Another potential problem for immunometric assays is the presence of endogenous heterophile antibodies that cross-react with reagent antiserum.[31] Normally, the signal antibody does not form a "sandwich" with the capture antibody unless the specific antigen is present; however, divalent heterophile antibodies may mimic the antigen by simultaneously binding to the signal and capture reagent antibodies, thereby causing falsely elevated results.[32,33]

Figure 6-6 schematically illustrates this situation. The problem is most common with monoclonal antibodies but may also occur with polyclonal antibodies. Immunoglobulins contain both a *constant* (Fc) region and a *variable* (Fab) region. As implied in the name, the Fc region is constant, or similar, for all immunoglobulins from that species. Therefore, if a patient receives immunotherapy or imaging reagents containing mouse immunoglobulin, he or she is likely to develop human antimouse antibodies (HAMAs) directed to the Fc fragment.[34] Some patients develop heterophile antibodies after exposure to foreign proteins from domestic pets or food contaminants. If these endogenous antibodies are present in a patient's specimen, they may bridge across the reagent antibodies used in immunometric assays and cause falsely high values. These antibodies also may bind to sites on the reagent antibodies, sterically blocking the binding of the specific antigen and leading to falsely low test values. Most manufacturers include nonimmune immunoglobulin in the assays to help block these interferences; as with the high-dose hook effect, however, the amounts added are not always adequate, and some patients with high-titer antibodies may still show in vitro assay interference.[35]

The combined specificity of the two antibodies used in an immunometric assay can produce exquisitely sensitive and specific immunoassays. In the past, a common problem with early competitive immunoassays was cross-reactivity among the structurally similar gonadotropins: LH, follicle-stimulating hormone (FSH), TSH, and hCG. The α-subunits of each of these hormones are almost identical, and the β-subunits have considerable structural homology. Many individual antisera (especially polyclonal antisera) used for measuring one of these hormones may have cross-reactivity for the other gonadotropins. The cross-reactivity of a pair of antibodies is less than the cross-reactivity of each of the individual antibodies because any cross-reacting substance must contain both of the binding epitopes in order to simultaneously bind to both antibodies.

For example, consider two antibodies for LH, each having 1% cross-reactivity with hCG. The cross-reactivity of the pair is less than the product of the two cross-reactivities or, in this case, less than 0.01%. Most current immunoassays for LH have a cross-reactivity of less than 0.01%. This low cross-reactivity is important, because pregnant patients and patients with choriocarcinoma can have very high hCG concentrations that could interfere with measurements of the other gonadotropin hormones.

Most hormones circulate in the blood in multiple forms. Some hormones (e.g., prolactin, growth hormone) circulate with macro forms, which can cause difficulty in their analysis if specimens are not pretreated.[8] For hormones composed of subunits (e.g., the gonadotropins), both the intact and the free subunits circulate in blood. Immunometric assays can be made specific for intact molecules by pairing an antibody specific for the α-β bridge site of the subunits with a second antibody specific for the β-subunit. Assays using these antibody pairs retain the two-antibody, low cross-reactivity needed for measuring gonadotropins and do not react with the free subunit forms of the hormones.

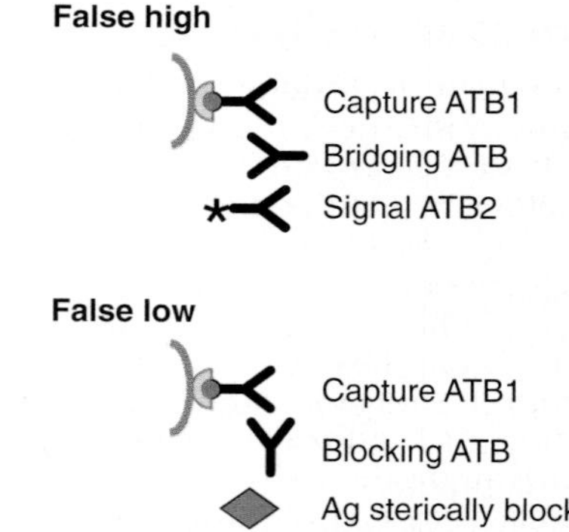

Figure 6-6 Assay interferences caused by heterophile antibodies, which result in either falsely high or falsely low values. Ag, antigen; ATB, antibody; ATB1, capture antiserum; ATB2, signal antiserum.

TABLE 6-1

Effect of Immunoassay Specificity on Calibration of Human Chorionic Gonadotropin (hCG) Assay

	Assay 1	Assay 2	Assay 3
Specificity for intact hCG standard (%)	100	100	100
Cross-reactivity with free β-hCG (%)	0	100	200
Measured values (IU/L)			
Specimen with 0% free β-hCG	10.0	10.0	10.0
Specimen with 10% free β-hCG	9.0	10.0	11.0
Specimen with 50% free β-hCG	5.0	10.0	15.0

The heterogeneous forms of circulating hormones and differences in specificity characteristics of immunoassays for these forms make calibration and harmonization difficult. Two immunoassays calibrated with the same reference preparation can give widely varying measurements on patient specimens. Consider the example of hCG in Table 6-1. The three assays are calibrated with a pure preparation of intact hCG, such as the WHO Third International Reference Preparation.[35] The three assays differ in their cross-reactivity with free β-hCG (0%, 100%, and 200%, respectively). These assays give identical measurements for a specimen containing only intact hCG but progressively disparate values as the percentage of free β-hCG in the specimen increases. In reality, the standardization issue is much more complex, because multiple forms of hormones (i.e., intact hormone, free subunits, nicked forms, glycosylated forms, degradation products) circulate in patients, and each assay has different cross-reactivities for these forms.[17,36]

Free (Unbound) Hormone Assays

Many hormones are tightly bound to specific plasma-binding proteins and loosely bound to albumin. Usually, only the unbound (free) forms and some of the loosely bound forms are biologically active.

Many methods are available to measure these free, unbound forms of a hormone. Theoretically, the best procedure is direct measurement of the free hormone concentration after physical separation of the free hormone from the bound hormone by equilibrium dialysis, ultrafiltration, or gel filtration. However, this method is difficult to perform and therefore is not readily available, and it is subject to technical errors.

The two major clinical applications for free hormone measurements are for thyroid hormones (i.e., thyroxine [T_4] and triiodothyronine [T_3]) and for steroids (testosterone and estradiol). Four techniques are commonly used to estimate free thyroid hormone concentrations: indirect index methods, two-step labeled hormone methods, one-step labeled hormone analogue methods, and labeled antibody methods.

Indirect Index Methods

The *indirect indices* involve two measurements: one for total hormone concentration and another for the thyroxine-binding globulin (TBG), followed by calculation of the ratio or of a normalized free thyroid hormone index (FT_4I or FT_3I). The availability of test results for total T_4 and T_4 binding capacity has the advantage of assessing these two different quantities but the disadvantage that ratios and indices are subject to the combined error of both measurements. These methods correct for routine changes in TBG such as those associated with estrogen levels, but they may produce inappropriately abnormal values in patients with extreme variations in TBG levels, such as those with congenital disorders of the TBG gene, familial dysalbuminemic hyperthyroxinemia, thyroid hormone autoantibodies, or certain nonthyroidal illnesses. Because of the necessity for two measurements and the sensitivity of these methods to interference with drugs, these indirect methods are being used less frequently.

Two-Step Labeled Hormone Methods

The two-step labeled hormone methods immunologically bind the free and loosely bound thyroid hormone to a solid phase. The other serum components are washed away, and the residual binding sites are back-titrated with labeled hormone. When calibrated with appropriate serum standards, these methods are thought to pose fewer problems related to binding protein abnormalities.

One-Step Labeled Hormone Analogue Methods

The one-step labeled hormone analogue methods use synthetic analogues of T_4 and T_3 that bind to the measurement antibody but do not bind to normal TBG. These methods are seldom used because performance has been poor in patients with abnormal albumin concentrations, abnormal free fatty acid concentrations, and all conditions that interfere with the indirect indices.[37]

Labeled Antibody Methods

The labeled antibody methods use kinetic reactions of antibodies with selected affinities that bind preferentially with the free form of the hormone. These methods work best for automated testing instruments and have become popular.

Complexities in Testing

Each of the methods described here works well for correcting for minor changes in TBG levels, but each has problems with some patient sera, especially sera containing interfering substances such as inhibitors and heterophilic antibodies. Most manufacturers have not fully validated their methods in patients with these abnormalities.[38]

Multiple methods are also available for measuring both the free and the biologically active forms of steroid hormones. The preferred method for measurement of free hormones consists of direct physical separation and high-sensitivity assays, similar to those methods recommended for the thyroid hormones. One-step labeled hormone analogue methods also have been developed, but they are associated with interference problems similar to the problems associated with free thyroid hormone assays. The measurement of free testosterone has been problematic. Most immunoassays are unreliable at low concentrations, and the concentration of free testosterone is much lower than that of total testosterone.

Another complexity in regard to steroid hormones is that, in addition to the free hormones, testosterone and estrogen bound to albumin also are biologically active. The concentration of the biologically active forms can be estimated with the use of indirect indices calculated from measurements of the total hormones and sex hormone-binding globulin (SHBG) or by measurement of the residual free and albumin-bound steroids after separation of the SHBG-bound forms after differential precipitation with ammonium sulfate. Recent work with tandem mass spectrometry shows promise as a more reliable test method (see later discussions).

Chromatographic Assays

The second major method of measuring hormone concentrations involves chromatographic separation of the various biochemical forms and quantitation of specific characteristics of the molecules. High-performance liquid chromatography (HPLC) systems use multiple forms of detection, including light absorption, fluorescence, and electrochemical properties.[39,40] Chromatography also is frequently combined with mass spectrometry.

There are two major advantages of these techniques: they can be used to simultaneously measure multiple forms of an analyte, and they are not dependent on unique immunologic reagents. Therefore, harmonization of measurements made with different assays is more feasible. The major disadvantages of these methods are their complexity and their limited availability.

Many chemical separation techniques are based on chromatography, but the two most commonly used for liquid chromatography are *normal-phase* HPLC and *reverse-phase* HPLC.[29] In both systems, a bonded solid-phase column is made that interacts with the analytes as they flow past in a liquid solvent. In normal-phase HPLC, the functional groups of the stationary phase are polar (e.g., amino or nitrile ions) relative to the nonpolar stationary phase (e.g., hexane); in reverse-phase HPLC, a nonpolar stationary phase (e.g., C18 octadecylsilane molecules bonded to silica) is used.

More recently, polymeric packings made of mixed copolymers have been made with C4, C8, and C18 functional groups directly incorporated so that they are more stable over a wide pH range. The mobile and stationary phases are selected to optimize adherence of the analytes to the stationary phase. The adhered molecules can be eluted differentially from the solid phase, after washing to separate specific forms of the analyte from interfering substances. If the composition of the mobile phase remains constant throughout the run, the process is called an *isocratic elution*. If the mobile-phase composition is abruptly changed, a *step elution* occurs. If the composition is gradually changed throughout the run, a *gradient elution* occurs.

The efficiency of separation in a chromatography system is a function of the flow rates of the different substances.[41] The resolution of the system is a measure of the separation of the two solute bands in terms of their relative retention volumes (V_r) and their bandwidths (ω). Resolution (R_s) of solutes A and B is shown as

$$R_s = \frac{2[V_r(B) - V_r(A)]}{\omega(A) + \omega(B)}$$

Values of R_s lower than 0.8 result in inadequate separation, and values greater than 1.25 correspond to baseline separation. The resolution of a chromatography column is a function of flow rates and thermodynamic factors.

Simultaneous measurement of the three catecholamines (epinephrine, norepinephrine, and dopamine) can be performed with reverse-phase HPLC with a C18 column and an electrochemical detection system[42] or fluorometric detection.[43] Prior extraction by absorption on activated alumina and acid elution helps improve specificity. Dihydroxybenzylamine, a molecule similar to endogenous catecholamines, can be used as an internal standard.

Mass Spectrometry

The technique of mass spectrometry involves fragmentation of target molecules, followed by separation and measurement of the mass-to-charge ratio of the components.[41]

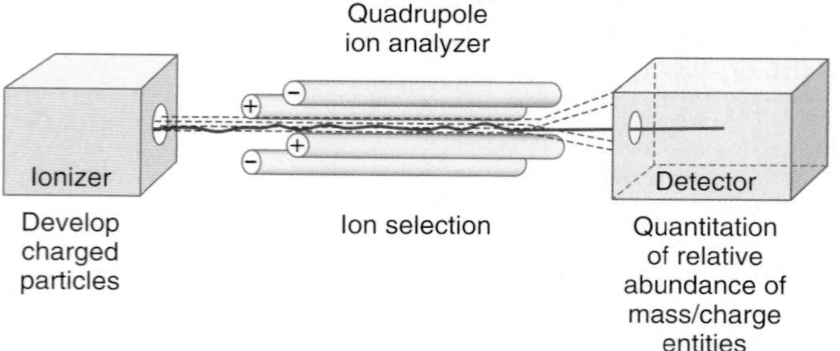

Figure 6-7 Basic components of quadrupole mass spectrometer.

When coupled with liquid chromatography, a mass spectrometer can function as a unique detector to provide structural information about the composition of individual solutes.[44] Inclusion in the specimens of internal standards, which are molecularly similar to the measured compounds, allows precise quantitation of the concentration of the eluting analytes. The measurement of specific mass fragments makes possible the quantitation of multiple specific analytes in complex mixtures.

The basic components of a quadrupole mass spectrometer are an ionizer, an ion analyzer, and a detector (Fig. 6-7). The initial step in mass spectrometry is fragmentation of the target compound into charged ions. Many techniques are used to generate these charged ions, including *chemical ionization* and *electron-impact ionization.*

Chemical ionization uses reagent gas molecules such as methane, ammonia, water, and isobutane to transfer protons. This process produces less fragmentation than other techniques because the process is not highly excited.

The electron impact method bombards gas molecules from the sample with electrons emitted from a heated filament. The process occurs in a vacuum to prevent the filament from burning out. *Electron-spray ionization* is a process in which a solution containing the analyte is introduced into a gas phase and is sprayed across an ionizing potential.[45] The charged droplets are desolvinated and analyzed in a mass spectrometer.

The ion analyzer uses four charged rods to systematically set up a charged field that selects only certain ions with particular mass-to-charge ratios and facilitates their movement along a path to the detector. Regular calibration is necessary to ensure accuracy of the instrument.

A *mass spectrum* is a bar graph in which the heights of the bars correspond to the relative abundance of a particular ion plotted as a function of the mass-to-charge ratio. Modern mass spectrometers can measure molecular masses so accurately and precisely that the elemental composition of a compound can be predicted by comparison with stored spectral libraries. When these systems are used to measure only a few selected compounds with known spectrums, the mass spectrometer can be programmed to focus only on these selected ions.

Stable isotopes of the compounds of interest can be used as internal standards through a technique called *isotope dilution mass spectrometry.* Stable isotopes typically perform the same as the native compounds in terms of extraction, chromatography, and mass spectrometry and therefore are ideal internal standards. However, there must be a sufficient number of isotopic atoms to ensure that their mass is different from that of naturally occurring substances that may be in the specimen.

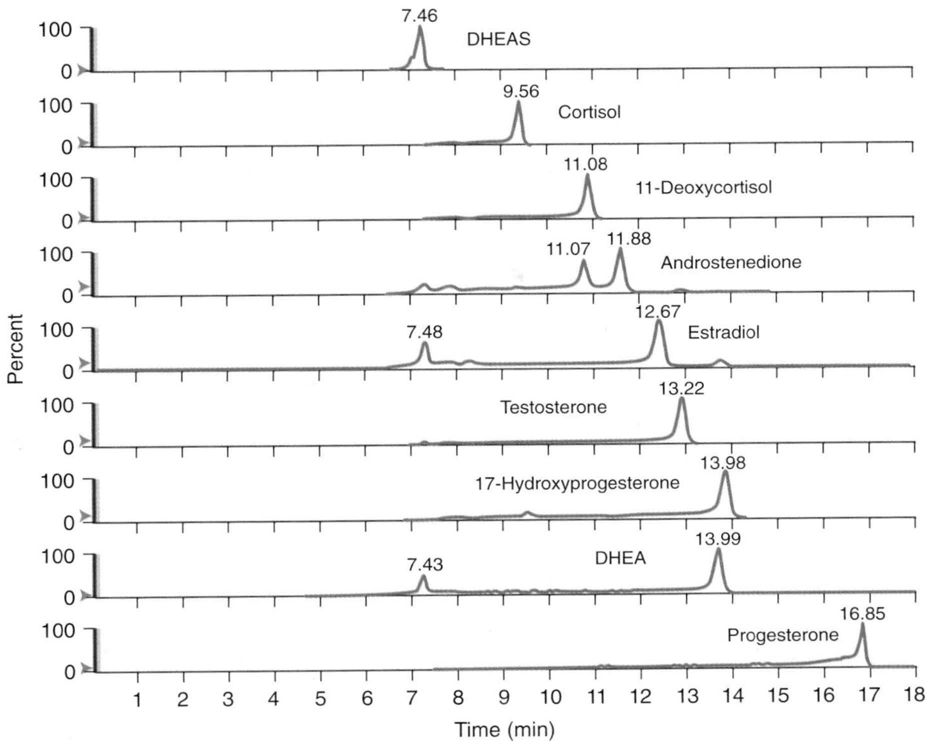

Figure 6-8 **Liquid chromatography–tandem mass spectroscopy profiles of nine steroids.**[49] ***DHEAS*, Dehydroepiandrosterone 3-sulfate; *DHEA*, dehydroepiandrosterone.** (From Guo T, Chan M, Soldin SJ. Steroid profiles using liquid chromatography-tandem mass spectrometry with atmospheric pressure photoionization source. *Arch Pathol Lab Med.* 2004;128:469-475. Reproduced with permission from Archives of Pathology of Laboratory Medicine.)

Tandem mass spectrometry (MS/MS) is a powerful tool consisting of two mass analyzers separated by an ion-activation device.[46,47] The first analyzer is used to isolate and dissociate the ion of interest by activation, and the second mass analyzer to analyze its dissociation products. This technique can be used to provide rapid, definitive measurements of multiple endocrine analytes.[44] For example, liquid chromatography and tandem mass spectrometry can be used to simultaneously quantitate multiple steroid compounds.[48-52] In Figure 6-8, the chromatograph shows well-separated peaks for nine steroids in a standard solution.[48]

Standardization and harmonization of hormone assays have become priorities for quality health care. The National Institute of Standards and Technology (NIST) has developed mass spectrometry reference methods for measuring cortisol, progesterone, estradiol-17β, T_4, and T_3.[51,53-58] The International Federation of Clinical Chemistry (IFCC) has proposed reference measurement procedures for free T_4.[59,60] MS methods also have been developed for insulin, PTH, 17-hydroxyprogesterone, and free T_3, although these are not considered reference methods at this time. Efforts are under way to try to harmonize clinical measurements using these reference methods; however, that will be a difficult task because of the difference inherent in the antibody specificity of the immunoassays used for most measurements.

Nucleic Acid–Based Assays

The decoding of the human genome has set the stage for a large potential increase in nucleic acid–based gene assays. The basic principles of nucleic acid–based assays have been known for several decades, but the identification of specific genes and the mapping of gene defects to clinical disease states have now made these measurements clinically useful.[61] However, as this field has evolved, it has been found that genetic heterogeneity is very common and clinical testing usually is based on strategies to find mutations as efficiently as possible.[62] Four concepts important for nucleic acid measurements are hybridization, amplification, restriction fragment length polymorphisms (RFLPs), and electrophoretic separation.[63] Newer techniques such as comparative genomic hybridization (CGH) and next-generation sequencing offer potential advances for genomic testing.[64-66]

Hybridization

Nucleic acid molecules have a unique ability to fuse with complementary base-pair sequences. When a fragment of a known sequence (probe) is mixed under specific conditions with a specimen containing a complementary sequence, hybridization occurs. This feature is analogous to the antibody-antigen binding used in immunoassays. Many of the formats used for immunoassay have been adopted to nucleic acid assays, including some of the same signal systems (e.g., radioactivity, fluorescence, chemiluminescence) and the same solid-phase capture systems (e.g., magnetic beads, biotin-streptavidin binding). In situ hybridization, which involves the binding of probes to intact tissue and cells, provides information about morphologic localization analogous to that provided by immunohistochemistry.

Amplification

Nucleic acid assays have an advantage in that low concentrations can be amplified in vitro before quantitation. The best-known amplification procedure is the polymerase chain reaction (PCR), first reported by Mullis and Faloona.[67] The three steps in the process (denaturation, annealing, and elongation) occur rapidly at different temperatures. Each cycle of amplification can occur in less than 90 seconds by cycling the temperature. The target double-stranded DNA is denatured at high temperature to make two single-stranded DNA fragments. Oligonucleotide primers, which are specific for the target region, are annealed to the DNA when the temperature is lowered. Addition of DNA polymerase allows the primer DNA to extend across the amplification region, thus doubling the number of DNA copies.

At 85% to 90% efficiency, this process can amplify the DNA by about 250,000-fold in 20 cycles. This huge amplification is subject to major problems with contamination if special precautions are not taken. In one control technique, a psoralen derivative is used to prevent subsequent copying by polymerase during exposure to ultraviolet light.

Restriction Fragment Length Polymorphisms

Some diseases (e.g., sickle cell anemia) are associated with a specific gene mutation; usually, however, a series of deletions and additions of DNA are involved with a particular disease. A number of restriction enzymes that cleave DNA at specific locations have been identified. Changes in the sequence of DNA result in different fragment lengths. The RFLP technique is particularly helpful in family studies for disorders that have a unique *genetic fingerprint*.

Electrophoretic Separation

E. M. Southern invented an electrophoretic separation technique known as *Southern blotting*.[68] Restriction enzymes are used to digest a sample of DNA into fragments, and the product is subjected to electrophoresis. The separated bands of DNA are then transferred to a solid support and hybridized. *Northern blotting* is a similar technique in which RNA is used as the starting material. *Western blotting* refers to electrophoresis and transfer of proteins.

Newer Nucleic Acid Measurement Technologies

Comparative Genome Hybridization

CGH is a molecular-cytogenetic method for analyzing the gains and losses of a given subject's DNA.[64] This technique detects only unbalanced chromosome changes; balanced reciprocal translocations or inversions may not be detected. Currently, this procedure is an adjunct to standard karyotype analysis, but it may provide higher resolution.

Next-Generation Sequencing

Next-generation sequencing uses large numbers of parallel processors to sequence clonally amplified DNA molecules separated in a flow cell.[66] This provides advantages of speed, lower cost, and better accuracy. On the other hand, this technique can rapidly generate large amounts of sequence data, posing challenges to bioinformatic analysis. The interpretation of these data requires linkage with large databases and a good understanding of genomic variations in the targeted regions.

ANALYTIC VALIDATION

Clinicians usually assume that laboratory methods have been validated and that they function correctly. Although this assumption is generally true, it is helpful to understand the level of assay validation performed and the appropriateness of the validation criteria for each clinical application of a test.[69,70]

In the United States, the federal government regulates all laboratories performing complex tests for patients receiving Medicare.[71,72] These regulations, published in the *Federal Register*, outline the validation requirements for Food and Drug Administration (FDA)-approved instruments, kits, and test systems as well as methods developed in house. Laboratories must document analytic accuracy, precision, reportable ranges, and reference ranges for all procedures. The regulations for in-house procedures and modifications of approved commercial procedures are more extensive and require laboratories to further document the analytic sensitivity; analytic specificity, including interfering substances; and other performance characteristics required for testing patient specimens.

Although the details of method validation may be unique to a specific procedure, the following analytic validation studies have proved valuable for most procedures: method comparison, precision, linearity, recovery, detection limit, reportable range, analytic interference, carryover, reference interval, specimen stability, and specimen type. Similar recommendations for validating nucleic acid tests were recently published by the College of American Pathologists.[73] Laboratories should have documentation for each of these performance characteristics, either from the diagnostics manufacturer or from direct studies.

Method Comparison

Ideally, the system should be compared with an established reference method; however, many endocrine tests do not have reference methods, and many laboratories do not have the facilities to perform reference methods when they exist. At a minimum, the assay should be compared with an analytic system that has been clinically validated with specimens from healthy subjects and specimens from patients with the diseases being investigated.[74] The system should be traceable to established reference standards, such as those from the WHO or the NIST.[75-77] Between 100 and 200 different specimens distributed over the assay range are recommended for method comparisons.[78]

A cross-plot portraying the new method on the vertical axis and the established method on the horizontal axis, along with the identity line, reference value lines, and regression statistics, is a useful way of displaying these comparisons. An alternative display method is the Bland-Altman difference plot, in which the difference between the test method and the reference method is plotted against the reference method values.

Although acceptable performance criteria for method comparisons are not well established, some important characteristics to examine are

- Any grossly discordant test values
- The degree of scatter about the regression curve
- The size of the regression offset on the vertical axis
- The number of points crossing between the low, normal, and high reference intervals for the two methods

The European Union has enacted an In Vitro Diagnostics Directive that requires manufacturers marketing in the European Union to establish that their products are "traceable to reference standards and reference procedures of a higher order" when such references exist. Hopefully, medically relevant performance characteristics that define the allowable ranges for differences between a specific assay's test values and the traceable standards will be linked with this traceability requirement.[79] This combination of traceability and allowable error requirements could serve to harmonize many test methods worldwide, because most diagnostic companies market internationally.[80]

Precision

Precision is a measure of the replication of repeated measurements of the same specimen; it is a function of the time between repeats and the concentration of the analyte. Both short-term precision (within a run or within a day) and long-term precision (across calibrations and across batches of reagents) should be documented at clinically appropriate concentration levels.[81]

In general, normal-range, abnormally low-range, and abnormally high-range targets are chosen for precision studies; however, targets focused on critical medical decision limits may be more appropriate for some analytes. Twenty measurements are recommended at each level for both short-term and long-term precision validations. Precision usually is expressed as the coefficient of variation, calculated as 100 times the standard deviation (SD) divided by the average of the replicate measurements.[82]

There is no universal agreement on the performance criteria for analytic precision, although numerous recommendations have been put forth. Two major approaches to defining these criteria have been (1) comparison with biologic variation and (2) expert opinion of clinicians based on their perceived impact of laboratory variation on clinical decisions.

The total variation clinically observed in test measurements is a combination of the analytic and biologic variations. For instance, if the analytic SD is less than one fourth of the biologic SD, the analytic component increases the SD of the total error by less than 3%. If the analytic precision is less than one half of the biologic SD, the total error increases by only 12%. These observations have led to recommendations for maintaining precision of less than one fourth or one half of the biologic variation.

The expert opinion precision recommendations are based on estimates of the magnitude of change of a test value that would cause clinicians to alter their clinical decisions. Table 6-2 lists some precision recommendations for selected endocrine tests.[83-85]

TABLE 6-2

Recommended Analytic Performance Limits*

Analyte	Biologic CVi (%)	Precision (%)	Accuracy (%)
Calcium	1.8	0.9†	0.7
Glucose	4.4	2.2†	1.9
Thyroxine	7.6	3.4†	4.1
Potassium	4.4	2.4†	1.6
Triiodothyronine	8.7†	4.0‡	5.5‡
Thyrotropin	20.2†	8.1‡	8.9‡
Cortisol	15.2†	(7.6)*	
Estradiol	21.7†	(10.9)*	
Follicle-stimulating hormone	30.8†	(15.4)*	
Luteinizing hormone	14.5†	(7.2)*	
Prolactin	40.5†	(20.2)*	
Testosterone	8.3†	(4.1)*	
Insulin	15.2†	(7.6)*	
Dehydroepiandrosterone	5.6†	(2.8)*	
11-Deoxycortisol	21.3†	(10.6)*	

*Numbers in parentheses correspond to one half of within-individual coefficient of variation.

†Data from Fraser CG. Biological variation in clinical chemistry: an update—collated data 1988-1991. *Arch Pathol Lab Med.* 1992;116:916-923.

‡Data from Fraser CG, Petersen PH, Ricos C, et al. Proposed quality specifications for the imprecision and inaccuracy of analytical systems for clinical chemistry. *Eur J Clin Chem Clin Biochem.* 1992;30:311-317.

CVi, intraindividual variation.

Data from Stockl D, Baadenhuijsen H, Fraser CG, et al. Desirable routine analytical goals for quantities assayed in serum. Discussion paper from the members of the External Quality Assessment (EQA) Working Group A on analytical goals in laboratory medicine. *Eur J Clin Chem Clin Biochem.* 1995;33:157-169.

Linearity

Patient specimens commonly contain several different forms of the hormones to be measured, whereas pure forms are contained in the reference standards and calibrators used to establish the assay dose-response curve.[86] When a patient specimen is diluted, the measured value for these dilutions should parallel the dose-response curve and give results proportional to the dilution. Linearity can be evaluated by measuring serial dilutions of patient specimens, with high concentrations diluted in the appropriate assay diluents.[87,88] The product of the measured value multiplied by the dilution factor should be approximately constant. There are no performance standards for linearity, but a reasonable expectation for most hormones is that dilutions are comparable within 10% of the undiluted value.

Recovery

Two methods of assessing the recovery of assays are (1) measuring the increase in test values after the reference analyte is added and (2) measuring the proportional changes caused by mixing high-concentration and low-concentration specimens. Some analytes circulate in the blood in multiple forms, and some of these forms may be bound to carrier proteins. The recovery rate of pure substances added to a specimen may be low if the assay does not measure some of the bound forms. Mixtures of patient specimens may not be measured correctly if one of the specimens contains cross-reacting substances such as autoantibodies. A thorough understanding of the chemical forms of the analyte and their cross-reactivities in the assay is important during assessment of recovery data.

Detection Limit

The minimal analytic detection limit is the smallest concentration that can be statistically differentiated from zero. This concentration is mathematically determined as the upper 95% limit of replicate measurements of the *zero standard,* calculated from the average signal plus 2.0 SD. This minimal detection limit is valid only for the average of multiple replicate measurements. When individual determinations are performed on a specimen having a true concentration exactly at the minimal detection limit, the probability that the measurement is above the noise level of the assay is only about 50%.

A second parameter for the lowest level of reliable measurement for an assay is the *functional detection limit,* or the *limit of quantitation.* For this value to be measured, multiple pools with low concentrations are made and analyzed in the replicate. A cross-plot of the coefficient of variation of the measurements versus concentration allows one to generate a precise profile. The concentration corresponding to a coefficient of variation of 20% is the functional detection limit.[1] This term typically applies to across-assay variation, but it also can be calculated for within-assay variation if one uses the tests to evaluate results measured within one run (e.g., provocative and suppression tests).

Reportable Range

The reportable range of an assay usually spans from the functional detection limit to the concentration of the highest standard. Values above the highest standard may be reported if they are diluted and the measured value is multiplied by the dilution factor. The validity of the analytic range is documented by the linearity and recovery studies. Some laboratories erroneously report the exact values displayed by the test systems even if they are outside the analytic range. It is important for clinicians to understand the limitations of valid measurements and not to inappropriately use meaningless numbers that may be reported.

Another potential source of error is failure of the technologist to multiply the measured value of diluted specimens by the dilution factor to correct for the dilution. In addition, care should be taken to define the number of significant figures used for reporting test values and to establish an appropriate algorithm for rounding test values to the significant number of digits.

Analytic Interference

The cross-reactivity and potential interference of other analytes that may react in a test system should be documented.[84] The choice of potential interfering substances that must be evaluated requires an understanding of the analytic system and the pathophysiology of the analyte being evaluated. In immunoassays, for example, compounds with similar structures, as well as precursor forms and degradation products, should be tested.[89-92] Drugs commonly prescribed for the diseases under evaluation should be assessed for interference, both by addition of the drug to a specimen and by analysis of specimens from patients before and after receiving the drug.[93,94] Most assays also are evaluated for the effects of hemolysis, lipemia, and icterus.

Carryover Studies

Many diagnostic systems use automated sample-handling devices. If a specimen to be tested is preceded by a specimen with a very high concentration, a trace amount remaining from the first specimen may significantly increase the reported concentration in the second specimen. The choice of the concentration that should be tested for carryover depends on the pathophysiology of the disease, but high values may need to be tested because some endocrine disorders can produce high values. A prudent procedure would be to retest all specimens after a specimen with an extraordinarily high value. One also should document that carryover from the sampling probe has not inadvertently contaminated subsequent specimen vials, thereby invalidating subsequently repeated measurements.

Reference Intervals

The development and validation of reference intervals for endocrine tests can be very complex tasks.[95,96] The normal reference interval for most laboratory tests is based on estimates of the central 95-percentile limits of measurements in healthy subjects.[97] A minimum of 120 subjects is needed to reliably define the 2.5 and 97.5 percentiles. The reference intervals for many endocrine tests depend on gender, age, developmental status, and other test values. Formal statistical consultation is recommended to determine the appropriate number of subjects to test and to develop statistical models for defining multivariate reference ranges.

Full evaluation of the adrenal, gonadal, and thyroid axes requires simultaneous measurement of the trophic and target hormones. Bivariate displays of these hormone concentrations along with their multivariate reference intervals facilitate the interpretation.[98] Preanalytic conditions should be well defined and controlled during evaluation of both healthy reference subjects and patients.

Specimen Stability

Analyte stability is a function of storage conditions and specimen type.[99] Although most hormones are relatively stable in serum or urine if they are rapidly frozen and stored in hermetically sealed vials at −70° C, multiple freeze/thaw cycles can damage analytes, and storage in frost-free freezers that repeatedly cycle through thawing temperatures can adversely affect stability. Blood specimens collected in edetate (EDTA) often are more stable than serum or heparinized specimens because edetate chelates calcium and magnesium ions that function as coenzymes for some proteases. The addition of protease inhibitors (e.g., aprotinin) to blood specimens may also improve specimen stability.[100]

Types of Specimens

Most hormones are measured in blood or urine, but alternative testing sources, such as saliva and transdermal membrane monitors, are also used.

Urine Specimens

The 24-hour urine specimen is used for many endocrine tests. Such urine specimens represent a time average that integrates over the multiple pulsatile spikes of hormone secretion occurring throughout the day. The 24-hour urine specimen also has the advantage of better analytic sensitivity for some hormones.[101,102] Urine often contains not only the original hormone but also key metabolites that may or may not have biologic activity.

Drawbacks include the inconvenience of collecting the 24-hour specimen and delays in collection. Another limitation of urine specimens is uncertainty regarding the completeness of the collection. Measurement of urinary creatinine concentrations helps in monitoring collection completeness, especially when this value is compared with the patient's muscle mass. Many urinary hormones are conjugated to carrier proteins before excretion. Therefore, both hepatic function and, to a lesser degree, renal function may alter urinary hormone values.

Blood Specimens

Blood specimens have both the advantage and the limitation of time dependency. The ability to detect rapid changes to a provocative stimulus is a strong advantage, whereas the unsuspected changes resulting from pulsatile secretions may be a major limitation. Most hormones undergo significant biologic variations, including ultradian, diurnal, menstrual, and seasonal changes.[103-105] Many hormones have short half-lives and are rapidly cleared from the blood. The half-life is particularly important when one is attempting to measure the response to a provocative drug, such as the effect of gonadotropin-releasing hormone.[106] The development of rapid intraoperative methods for measuring PTH and growth hormone has highlighted the importance of plasma specimens, which do not require extra waiting time for the blood to clot to make serum.[107,108]

Saliva Specimens

Saliva is becoming an alternative specimen for measuring non–protein-bound hormones and small molecules.[109-113] Small analytes in blood pass into oral fluid by crossing capillary walls and basement membranes and by passing through lipophilic membranes of epithelial cells.[111] This transport involves passive diffusion, ultrafiltration, active transport, or some combination of these processes. The concentration in saliva depends on the concentration of the non–protein-bound analyte in blood, the salivary pH, the acid dissociation constant (pKa) of the analyte, and the size of the analyte. Analytes entering saliva by passive diffusion usually are less than 500 d in size, non–protein bound, and nonionized. Saliva measurements correlate with blood measurements for some hormones such as cortisol, progesterone, estradiol, and testosterone, but they do not correlate well for others (e.g., thyroid and pituitary hormones).[114-116]

Multiple preanalytic variables can affect the salivary measurement. Stimulation of oral fluid production by chewing or by the use of candy or drops that contain stimulants such as citric acid can increase oral fluid volume and stabilize pH but may alter some analyte concentrations. Several commercial devices are available for collection of oral fluid; however, these devices need to be validated for each analyte and each assay system to ensure they adequately recover each of the analytes.

Blood Drops

Blood drops collected on filter paper from punctures of a finger or heel are a convenient system for collecting, transporting, and measuring hormones.[117,118] If standardized collection conditions and extraction techniques are used, these measurements correlate well with serum measurements. Integration of immunochemistry with computer chip technology has also led to immunochips that can measure multiple analytes using a single drop of blood.[119]

Noninvasive Measurements

Noninvasive transcutaneous measurements also have been developed for some endocrine tests.[120] Transcutaneous glucose measurements using near-infrared spectroscopy correlate well with blood measurements.[121] Glycemic control in subjects with diabetes requiring insulin has been shown to improve with continuous real-time transcutaneous glucose monitoring.[122]

QUALITY ASSURANCE

Quality Control Systems

Laboratory quality control programs are intended to ensure that the test procedures are being performed within defined limits. A critical component of control systems is the definition of acceptable performance criteria.[123,124] Such criteria often are not well defined, and many laboratories use floating criteria that change when assays change.[125] Control limits are often set at the mean ± 2 or 3 SDs, where the mean and the SD are arbitrarily assigned based on measurements made in that laboratory. When reagents or equipment changes, new limits are assigned. These types of control systems provide some assurance that the laboratory is functioning at a level of performance similar to that of the recent past, but they provide little assurance that measurements are adequate for clinical decisions.

Statistically, there are two major forms of analytic errors: random and systematic. *Random error* relates to reproducibility; *systematic error* relates to the offset or bias of the test values from the target or reference value. Performance criteria can be defined for each of these parameters, and quality control systems can be programmed to monitor compliance with these criteria. Control systems must have low false-positive rates as well as high statistical power to detect assay deviations. The multirule algorithms developed by Westgard and colleagues[126] use combinations of control rules—such as two consecutive controls outside of *warning limits,* one control outside of *action limits,* or moving average trend analyzers outside of limits—to achieve good statistical error detection characteristics.[127]

Traditionally, quality control programs have focused primarily on precision; however, analytic bias also can cause major clinical problems. If fixed decision levels are used to trigger clinical actions (e.g., therapy, additional investigations), changes in the analytic set point of an assay can cause major changes in the number of follow-up cases.[127] This concept is illustrated in Figure 6-9 for TSH measurements.

Under stable laboratory testing conditions, approximately 122 per 1000 patients tested have TSH values greater than 5.0 mIU/L. If the test shifts upward by 20%, the number of patients with TSH values greater than 5.0 mIU/L increases to 189, which is an increase of more than 50% in the number of patients flagged as abnormal (see Fig. 6-9). These changes in test value distributions often can be sensed by clinicians who encounter multiple patients with unexpectedly elevated test values, causing them to call the laboratory and inquire whether the "test is running high today." Some modern quality control systems use moving averages of patient test values to help monitor changes in analytic bias.[128]

Some medical facilities have linked together into networks to provide more integrated patient care. This crossover of both physicians and patients is increasing the importance of *harmonized* testing systems. For endocrine tests, harmonization is best achieved when all the laboratories in the network use the same test systems. Differences in analytic specificity may cause across-method differences in patient test distributions even when the methods use the same reference standards. Full harmonization of testing requires not only standardization of equipment but also standardization of reagents (including use of the same lot numbers) and standardization of laboratory protocols.

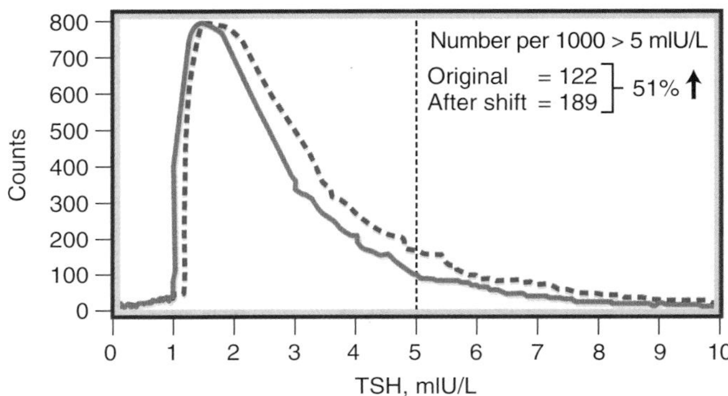

Figure 6-9 Effect of analytic bias, or shift, on the number of patients with elevated levels of thyrotropin (TSH).

Real-time quality control monitors with peer group comparisons across the laboratories in the health care network are necessary to ensure uniformity of testing.

Investigation of Discordant Test Values

The practice of modern endocrinology depends extensively on reliable and accurate test values; even in the best laboratories, however, erroneous results sometimes are reported. Careful correlation of pathophysiology with test values can help to identify values that are "discordant."[98] Some of these discordant test values may be analytically correct, but others may be erroneous. Clinicians can help investigate these suspicious test values by requesting laboratories to perform a few simple validation procedures.

Repeated testing of the same specimen is a valuable first step. If the specimen has been stored under stable conditions, the absolute value of the difference between the initial and the repeated measurements should be less than 3 analytic SDs 95% of the time. Normally, the 95% confidence range is associated with the mean ± 2 SDs; with repeated laboratory tests, however, errors are associated with the first as well as the second measurement. The confidence interval for the uncertainty of the difference between two measurements can be calculated using the statistical rules for propagation of errors.

To better understand this propagation of error, consider

$$D = X_1 - X_2$$

where X_1 is the first measurement, X_2 is the repeated measurement, and D is the difference.

$$\text{Variance}(D) = \text{Variance}(X_1) + \text{Variance}(X_2)$$
$$\text{Variance}(D) = 2\ \text{Variance}(X)$$
$$SD(D) = \sqrt{2\ \text{Variance}(X)}$$
$$SD(D) = \sqrt{2}SD(X)$$

The variance of D is the sum of the variance of X_1 and the variance of X_2. The SD of D is the square root of the variance of D, or the square root of twice the variance of X_1. The SD of D equates to the square root of 2 multiplied by SD(X). Therefore, 95% of the absolute values for D should be within square root of 2 times 2 SD(X), or approximately 3 SD(X). If a repeat measurement exceeds this 3 SD(X) limit, the initial (or reagent) measurement is probably in error.

Linearity and recovery are valuable techniques for evaluating test validity. If the initial test value is elevated, serial dilution of the specimen in the assay diluent and reassay should be considered. If the specimen dilutes nonproportionately, no meaningful value can be reported with that assay. In the example in Figure 6-10, the undiluted specimen reads 22, the twofold dilution multiplies back to 34 (2 × 17), and the fourfold dilution multiplies back to 60 (4 × 15). Therefore, the result depends on the dilution factor, so that no reliable answer can be reported.

If the initial value is low, one may consider adding known quantities of the analyte to part of the specimen. Analyzing these spiked or diluted specimens with the original specimen allows one to evaluate both reproducibility and recovery. It may be helpful to analyze the linearity or recovery of the assay standards at the same time, to provide internal controls of the dilution or spiking procedures and the appropriateness of the diluent and spiking material.

If the replication, dilution, or recovery experiment appears successful, further analytic troubleshooting will

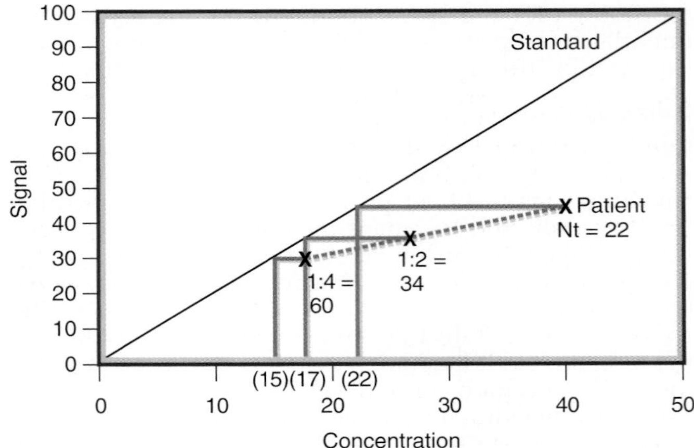

Figure 6-10 Nonproportional dilutions. Discordant values are produced when samples do not dilute linearly. Nt, undiluted (neat).

vary according to the method used. Immunoassays may be affected by interference caused by heterophile antibodies. Addition of nonimmune mouse serum or heterophile antibody-blocking solutions may neutralize these effects.[129,130] Chromatographic assays are usually more robust than immunoassays. Specimens with suspected interference on one type of assay can be reanalyzed by means of an alternative methodology.

Water-soluble interferences have been reported for some direct assays for steroid measurements.[21,22,131] Extraction of the hormones into organic solvents, followed by drying down and reconstitution in the assay zero standard, removes these interferences. Similarly, interferences with cross-reacting drugs and metabolic products can be minimized with selective extraction.

The analytic methods of assessing endocrine problems in patients are continually expanding. The newer systems are often based on analytic techniques similar to those outlined in this chapter, but the configurations are generally more user-friendly. These advances make the systems more convenient, but they also become more of a "black box" that conceals most of the details of the system. The performance validation steps outlined in this chapter become important procedures for ensuring that these systems continue to provide the reliable measurements needed for quality medical care.

REFERENCES

1. Spencer CA, LoPresti JS, Patel A, et al. Applications of a new chemiluminometric thyrotropin assay to subnormal measurement. *J Clin Endocrinol Metab*. 1990;70:453-460.
2. Klee GG, Hay ID. Biochemical testing of thyroid function. *Endocrinol Metab Clin North Am*. 1997;26:763-775.
3. Price CP, Newman DJ, eds. *Principles and Practice of Immunoassay*. New York, NY: Stockton Press; 1996.
4. Thorell JI, Larson SM. *Radioimmunoassay and Related Techniques: Methodology and Clinical Applications*. St. Louis, MO: Mosby; 1978.
5. Rodbard D. Data processing for radioimmunoassays: an overview. In: Natelson S, Pesce AJ, Dietz AA, eds. *Clinical Chemistry and Immunochemistry (AACC): Chemical and Cellular Bases and Applications in Disease*. Washington, DC: AACC; 1978:477-494.
6. Fomenko I, Durst M, Balaban D. Robust regression for high throughput drug screening. *Comput Methods Programs Biomed*. 2006;82:31-37.
7. Gosling JP. A decade of development in immunoassay methodology. *Clin Chem*. 1990;36:1408-1427.
8. Vieira JG, Tachibana TT, Obara LH, et al. Extensive experience and validation of polyethylene glycol precipitation as a screening method for macroprolactinemia. *Clin Chem*. 1998;44:1758-1759.
9. Klee GG, Post G. Effect of counting errors on immunoassay precision. *Clin Chem*. 1989;35:1362-1366.

10. Butler JE, ed. *Immunochemistry of Solid-Phase Immunoassay*. Boston, MA: CRC Press; 1991.
11. Hersh LS, Yaverbaum S. Magnetic solid-phase radioimmunoassay. *Clin Chim Acta*. 1975;63:69-72.
12. Suter M. Streptavidin: production, purification, and use in antibody immobilization. In: Butler JE, ed. *Immunochemistry of Solid-Phase Immunoassay*. Boston, MA: CRC Press; 1991.
13. Hage DS. Survey of recent advances in analytical applications of immunoaffinity chromatography. *J Chromatogr B Biomed Sci Appl*. 1998;715:3-28.
14. Vetterlein D. Monoclonal antibodies: production, purification, and technology. *Adv Clin Chem*. 1989;27:303-354.
15. Pettersson KS, Soderholm JR. Individual differences in lutropin immunoreactivity revealed by monoclonal antibodies. *Clin Chem*. 1991; 37:333-340.
16. Ehrlich PH, Moyle WR. Cooperative immunoassays: ultrasensitive assays with mixed monoclonal antibodies. *Science*. 1983;221: 279-281.
17. Bristow A, Berger P, Midart JM, et al. Establishment, value assignment, and characterization of new WHO reference reagents for six molecular forms of human chorionic gonadotropin. *Clin Chem*. 2005;51:177-182.
18. Gao P, D'Amour P. Evolution of the parathyroid hormone (PTH) assay—importance of circulating PTH immunoheterogeneity and of its regulation. *Clin Lab*. 2005;51:21-29.
19. Roberts RF, Roberts WL. Performance characteristics of five automated serum cortisol immunoassays. *Clin Biochem*. 2004;37:489-493.
20. Barnes SC, Swaminathan R. Effect of albumin concentration on serum cortisol measured by the Bayer Advia Centaur assay. *Ann Clin Biochem*. 2007;44:79-82.
21. Fitzgerald RL, Herold DA. Serum total testosterone: immunoassay compared with negative chemical ionization gas chromatography-mass spectrometry. *Clin Chem*. 1996;42:749-755.
22. Leung YS, Dees K, Cyr R, et al. Falsely increased serum estradiol results reported in direct estradiol assays. *Clin Chem*. 1997;43:1250-1251.
23. Klee GG, Preissner CM, Schloegel IW, et al. Bioassay of parathyrin: analytical characteristics and clinical performance in patients with hypercalcemia. *Clin Chem*. 1988;34:482-488.
24. Di Lorenzo D, Ruggeri G, Iacobello C, et al. Evaluation of a radioreceptor assay to assess exogenous estrogen activity in serum of patients with breast cancer. *Int J Biol Markers*. 1991;6:151-158.
25. Hoare SR, de Vries G, Usdin TB. Measurement of agonist and antagonist ligand-binding parameters at the human parathyroid hormone type 1 receptor: evaluation of receptor states and modulation by guanine nucleotide. *J Pharmacol Exp Ther*. 1999;289:1323-1333.
26. Strasburger CJ, Wu Z, Pflaum CD, et al. Immunofunctional assay of human growth hormone (hGH) in serum: a possible consensus for quantitative hGH measurement. *J Clin Endocrinol Metab*. 1996; 81:2613-2620.
27. Zweig MH, Csako G. High-dose hook effect in a two-site IRMA for measuring thyrotropin. *Ann Clin Biochem*. 1990;27(Pt 5): 494-495.
28. Ooi DS, Escares EA. "High-dose hook effect" in IRMA-Count PSA assay of prostate-specific antigen. *Clin Chem*. 1991;37:771-772.
29. Pesce MA. "High-dose hook effect" with the Centocor CA 125 assay. *Clin Chem*. 1993;39:1347.
30. Wolf E, Brem G. "High-dose hook effect" as a pitfall in quantifying transgene expression in metallothionein-human growth hormone (MT-hGH) transgenic mice. *Clin Chem*. 1991;37:763-765.
31. Ellis MJ, Livesey JH. Techniques for identifying heterophile antibody interference are assay specific: study of seven analytes on two automated immunoassay analyzers. *Clin Chem*. 2005;51:639-641.
32. Klee GG. Human anti-mouse antibodies. *Arch Pathol Lab Med*. 2000;124:921-923.
33. Reinsberg J. Interference by human antibodies with tumor marker assays. *Hybridoma*. 1995;14:205-208.
34. Baum RP, et al. Activating anti-idiotypic human anti-mouse antibodies for immunotherapy of ovarian carcinoma. *Cancer*. 1994;73:1121-1125.
35. Preissner CM, Dodge LA, O'Kane DJ, et al. Prevalence of heterophilic antibody interference in eight automated tumor marker immunoassays. *Clin Chem*. 2005;51:208-210.
36. Cole LA. Immunoassay of human chorionic gonadotropin, its free subunits, and metabolites. *Clin Chem*. 1997;43:2233-2243.
37. Ekins R. Analytic measurements of free thyroxine. *Clin Lab Med*. 1993;13:599-630.
38. Demers LM, Spencer CA. Laboratory medicine practice guidelines: laboratory support for the diagnosis and monitoring of thyroid disease. *Clin Endocrinol (Oxf)*. 2003;58:138-140.
39. Anderson DJ. High-performance liquid chromatography in clinical analysis. *Anal Chem*. 1999;71:314R-327R.
40. Volin P. High-performance liquid chromatographic analysis of corticosteroids. *J Chromatogr B Biomed Appl*. 1995;671:319-340.
41. Ullman MD, Bowers LD, Burtis CA. Chromatography/mass spectrometry. In: Burtis CA, Ashwood R, eds. *Clinical Chemistry*. 3rd ed. Philadelphia, PA: WB Saunders; 1999.
42. Clauson RC. High performance liquid chromatographic separation and determination of catecholamines. In: Marks N, Rodnight R, eds. *Research Methods in Neurochemistry*, vol 6. New York, NY: Plenum; 1985.
43. Willemsen JJ, Ross HA, Jacobs MC, et al. Highly sensitive and specific HPLC with fluorometric detection for determination of plasma epinephrine and norepinephrine applied to kinetic studies in humans. *Clin Chem*. 1995;41:1455-1460.
44. Niessen WM. Advances in instrumentation in liquid chromatography-mass spectrometry and related liquid-introduction techniques. *J Chromatogr A*. 1998;794:407-435.
45. Strege MA. High-performance liquid chromatographic-electrospray ionization mass spectrometric analyses for the integration of natural products with modern high-throughput screening. *J Chromatogr B Biomed Sci Appl*. 1999;725:67-78.
46. Dongre AR, Eng JK, Yates JR 3rd. Emerging tandem-mass-spectrometry techniques for the rapid identification of proteins. *Trends Biotechnol*. 1997;15:418-425.
47. Magera MJ, Lacey JM, Casetta B, et al. Method for the determination of total homocysteine in plasma and urine by stable isotope dilution and electrospray tandem mass spectrometry. *Clin Chem*. 1999; 45:1517-1522.
48. Guo T, Chan M, Soldin SJ. Steroid profiles using liquid chromatography-tandem mass spectrometry with atmospheric pressure photoionization source. *Arch Pathol Lab Med*. 2004;128:469-475.
49. Minutti CZ, Lacey JM, Magera MJ, et al. Steroid profiling by tandem mass spectrometry improves the positive predictive value of newborn screening for congenital adrenal hyperplasia. *J Clin Endocrinol Metab*. 2004;89:3687-3893.
50. Shou WZ, Jiang X, Naidong W. Development and validation of a high-sensitivity liquid chromatography/tandem mass spectrometry (LC/MS/MS) method with chemical derivatization for the determination of ethinyl estradiol in human plasma. *Biomed Chromatogr*. 2004; 18:414-421.
51. Tai SS, Welch MJ. Development and evaluation of a candidate reference method for the determination of total cortisol in human serum using isotope dilution liquid chromatography/mass spectrometry and liquid chromatography/tandem mass spectrometry. *Anal Chem*. 2004;76:1008-1014.
52. Taylor RL, Machacek D, Singh RJ. Validation of a high-throughput liquid chromatography-tandem mass spectrometry method for urinary cortisol and cortisone. *Clin Chem*. 2002;48:1511-1519.
53. National Institute of Standards and Technology. Development of reference methods and reference materials for the determination of hormones in human serum. Available at http://www.nist.gov/cstl/analytical/organic/hormonesinserum.cfm (accessed August 2010).
54. Tai SS, Bunk DM, White ET, et al. Development and evaluation of a reference measurement procedure for the determination of total 3,3′,5-triiodothyronine in human serum using isotope-dilution liquid chromatography-tandem mass spectrometry. *Anal Chem*. 2004; 76:5092-5096.
55. Tai SS, Sniegoski LT, Welch MJ. Candidate reference method for total thyroxine in human serum: use of isotope-dilution liquid chromatography-mass spectrometry with electrospray ionization. *Clin Chem*. 2002;48:637-642.
56. Tai SS, Welch MJ. Development and evaluation of a reference measurement procedure for the determination of estradiol-17beta in human serum using isotope-dilution liquid chromatography-tandem mass spectrometry. *Anal Chem*. 2005;77:6359-6363.
57. Tai SS, Xu B, Welch MJ. Development and evaluation of a candidate reference measurement procedure for the determination of progesterone in human serum using isotope-dilution liquid chromatography/tandem mass spectrometry. *Anal Chem*. 2006;78:6628-6633.
58. Tai SS, Xu B, Welch MJ, et al. Development and evaluation of a candidate reference measurement procedure for the determination of testosterone in human serum using isotope dilution liquid chromatography/tandem mass spectrometry. *Anal Bioanal Chem*. 2007;388:1087-1094.
59. Thienpont LM, Beastall G, Christofides ND, et al. Proposal of a candidate international conventional reference measurement procedure for free thyroxine in serum. *Clin Chem Lab Med*. 2007;45:934-936.
60. Thienpont LM, Beastall G, Christofides ND, et al. Measurement of free thyroxine in laboratory medicine—proposal of measurand definition. *Clin Chem Lab Med*. 2007;45:563-564.
61. Coleman WB, Tsongalis GJ, eds. *Molecular Diagnostics for the Clinical Laboratorian*. Totowa, NJ: Humana Press; 1997.
62. Korf BR. Overview of molecular genetic diagnosis. *Current Protocols in Human Genetics* 0:Unit 9.1. Birmingham, AL: University of Alabama, 2006.
63. Wittwer CT, Kusukawa N. Nucleic acid techniques. In: Burtis CA, Ashwood E, Bruns DE, eds. *Tietz Textbook of Clinical Chemistry and*

Molecular Diagnostics. 4th ed. Philadelphia, PA: Elsevier; 2006: 1407-1449.

64. Edelmann L, Hirschhorn K. Clinical utility of array CGH for the detection of chromosomal imbalances associated with mental retardation and multiple congenital anomalies. *Ann N Y Acad Sci*. 2009;1151: 157-166.
65. Shen Y, Wu BL. Microarray-based genomic DNA profiling technologies in clinical molecular diagnostics. *Clin Chem*. 2009;55:659-669.
66. Voelkerding KV, Dames SA, Durtschi JD. Next-generation sequencing: from basic research to diagnostics. *Clin Chem*. 2009;55:641-658.
67. Mullis KB, Faloona FA. Specific synthesis of DNA in vitro via a polymerase-catalyzed chain reaction. *Methods Enzymol*. 1987;155: 335-350.
68. Southern EM. Detection of specific sequences among DNA fragments separated by gel electrophoresis. *J Mol Biol*. 1975;98:503-517.
69. Carey RN, Garber CC. Evaluation of methods. In: Kaplan LA, Pesce AJ, eds. *Clinical Chemistry: Theory, Practice and Correlation*. 2nd ed. St. Louis, MO: Mosby; 1989:290-310.
70. Clinical Laboratory Standards Institute, National Committee for Clinical Laboratory Standards. *Preliminary Evaluation of Quantitative Clinical Laboratory Methods: Approved Guideline, EP10-A3*. Wayne, PA: CLSI/NCCLS; 2006.
71. Centers for Disease Control and Prevention. Current CLIA Regulations (including all changes through 01/24/2004). Available at http://wwwn.cdc.gov/clia/regs/toc.aspx (accessed August 2010).
72. Rivers PA, Dobalian A, Germinario FA. A review and analysis of the clinical laboratory improvement amendment of 1988: compliance plans and enforcement policy. *Health Care Manage Rev*. 2005;30: 93-102.
73. Jennings L, Van Deerlin VM, Gulley ML. Recommended principles and practices for validating clinical molecular pathology tests. *Arch Pathol Lab Med*. 2009;133:743-755.
74. Clinical Laboratory Standards Institute, National Committee for Clinical Laboratory Standards. *Method Comparison and Bias Estimation Using Patient Samples: Approved Guideline, EP09-A2*. Wayne, PA: CLSI/NCCLS; 2002.
75. Hilleman MR. International biological standardization in historic and contemporary perspective. *Dev Biol Stand*. 1999;100:19-30.
76. Rose MP. Follicle stimulating hormone international standards and reference preparations for the calibration of immunoassays and bioassays. *Clin Chim Acta*. 1998;273:103-117.
77. Taylor BN, Thompson A, eds. *The International System of Units (SI). NIST Special Publication 330*. Washington, DC: National Institute of Standards and Technology, U.S. Department of Commerce; 2008.
78. Linnet K. Necessary sample size for method comparison studies based on regression analysis. *Clin Chem*. 1999;45:882-894.
79. The European Parliament and the Council of the European Union Directive 98/79/EC of the European Parliament and of the Council of October 27, 1998, on in vitro diagnostic medical devices. OJ L 220, 30.8. 1993:23.
80. Powers DM. Regulations and standards: traceability of assay calibrators—the EU's IVD directive raises the bar. *IVD Technol*. 2000:26-33.
81. Fraser CG, Petersen PH. Analytical performance characteristics should be judged against objective quality specifications. *Clin Chem*. 1999; 45:321-323.
82. Clinical Laboratory Standards Institute, National Committee for Clinical Laboratory Standards. *Evaluation of Precision Performance of Quantitative Measurement Methods: Approved Guideline, EP05-A2*. Wayne, PA: CLSI/NCCLS; 2004.
83. Fraser CG. Biological variation in clinical chemistry: an update—collated data, 1988-1991. *Arch Pathol Lab Med*. 1992;116:916-923.
84. Fraser CG, Petersen PH, Ricos C, et al. Proposed quality specifications for the imprecision and inaccuracy of analytical systems for clinical chemistry. *Eur J Clin Chem Clin Biochem*. 1992;30:311-317.
85. Stockl D, Baadenhuijsen H, Fraser CG, et al. Desirable routine analytical goals for quantities assayed in serum. Discussion paper from the members of the External Quality Assessment (EQA) Working Group A on analytical goals in laboratory medicine. *Eur J Clin Chem Clin Biochem*. 1995;33:157-169.
86. Kroll MH, Emancipator K. A theoretical evaluation of linearity. *Clin Chem*. 1993;39:405-413.
87. Clinical Laboratory Standards Institute, National Committee for Clinical Laboratory Standards. *Evaluation of Matrix Effects: Proposed Guideline, EP14-P*. Wayne, PA: CLSI/NCCLS; 1998.
88. Clinical Laboratory Standards Institute, National Committee for Clinical Laboratory Standards. *Evaluation of the Linearity of Quantitative Measurement Procedures—A Statistical Approach: Approved Guideline, EP06-A*. Wayne, PA: CLSI/NCCLS; 2003.
89. Clinical Laboratory Standards Institute, National Committee for Clinical Laboratory Standards. *Interference Testing in Clinical Chemistry: Approved Guideline, EP07-A2*. Wayne, PA: CLSI/NCCLS; 2005.
90. Levine S, Noth R, Loo A, et al. Anomalous serum thyroxin measurements with the Abbott TDx procedure. *Clin Chem*. 1990;36: 1838-1840.
91. Mbuyi-Kalala A, Ehrenstein G. Anomalous effects of hormone fragments on the measurement of parathyroid hormone by radioimmunoassay. *Methods Find Exp Clin Pharmacol*. 1996;18:87-99.
92. Micallef JV, Hayes MM, Latif A, et al. Serum binding of steroid tracers and its possible effects on direct steroid immunoassay. *Ann Clin Biochem*. 1995;32(Pt 6):566-574.
93. Cook NJ, Read GF. Oestradiol measurement in women on oral hormone replacement therapy: the validity of commercial test kits. *Br J Biomed Sci*. 1995;52:97-101.
94. Thomas CM, van den Berg RJ, Segers MF, et al. Inaccurate measurement of 17 beta-estradiol in serum of female volunteers after oral administration of milligram amounts of micronized 17 beta-estradiol. *Clin Chem*. 1993;39:2341-2342.
95. O'Brien PC, Dyck PJ. Procedures for setting normal values. *Neurology*. 1995;45:17-23.
96. Solberg HE. Establishment and use of reference values. In: Burtis CA, Ashwood E, Bruns DE, eds. *Tietz Textbook of Clinical Chemistry and Molecular Diagnostics*. 2nd ed. Philadelphia, PA: Saunders; 1994: 454-484.
97. Clinical Laboratory Standards Institute, National Committee for Clinical Laboratory Standards. *How to Define and Determine Reference Intervals in the Clinical Laboratory: Approved Guideline, C28-A2*. Wayne, PA: CLSI/NCCLS; 2000.
98. Klee GG. Maximizing efficacy of endocrine tests: importance of decision-focused testing strategies and appropriate patient preparation. *Clin Chem*. 1999;45:1323-1330.
99. Heins M, Heil W, Withold W. Storage of serum or whole blood samples? Effects of time and temperature on 22 serum analytes. *Eur J Clin Chem Clin Biochem*. 1995;33:231-238.
100. Tateishi K, Klee GG, Cunningham JM, Lennon VA. Stability of bombesin in serum, plasma, urine, and culture media. *Clin Chem*. 1985;31: 276-278.
101. Demir A, Alfthan H, Stenman UH, Voutilainen R. A clinically useful method for detecting gonadotropins in children: assessment of luteinizing hormone and follicle-stimulating hormone from urine as an alternative to serum by ultrasensitive time-resolved immunofluorometric assays. *Pediatr Res*. 1994;36:221-226.
102. Hourd P, Edwards R. Current methods for the measurement of growth hormone in urine. *Clin Endocrinol (Oxf)*. 1994;40:155-170.
103. Leppaluoto J, Ruskoaho H. Atrial natriuretic peptide, renin activity, aldosterone, urine volume and electrolytes during a 24-h sleep-wake cycle in man. *Acta Physiol Scand*. 1990;139:47-53.
104. Maes M, Mommen K, Hendrickx D, et al. Components of biological variation, including seasonality, in blood concentrations of TSH, TT3, FT4, PRL, cortisol and testosterone in healthy volunteers. *Clin Endocrinol (Oxf)*. 1997;46:587-598.
105. Sebastian-Gambaro MA, Liron-Hernandez FJ, Fuentes-Arderiu X. Intra- and inter-individual biological variability data bank. *Eur J Clin Chem Clin Biochem*. 1997;35:845-852.
106. Demers LM. Pituitary function. In: Burtis CA, Ashwood R, eds. *Tietz Textbook of Clinical Chemistry*. 3rd ed. Philadelphia, PA: WB Saunders; 1999:1470-1475.
107. Abe T, Ludecke DK. Recent primary transnasal surgical outcomes associated with intraoperative growth hormone measurement in acromegaly. *Clin Endocrinol (Oxf)*. 1999;50:27-35.
108. Bergenfelz A, Isaksson A, Lindblom P, et al. Measurement of parathyroid hormone in patients with primary hyperparathyroidism undergoing first and reoperative surgery. *Br J Surg*. 1998;85:1129-1132.
109. Baid SK, Sinaii N, Wade M, et al. Radioimmunoassay and tandem mass spectrometry measurement of bedtime salivary cortisol levels: a comparison of assays to establish hypercortisolism. *J Clin Endocrinol Metab*. 2007;92:3102-3107.
110. Chiu SK, Collier CP, Clark AF, et al. Salivary cortisol on ROCHE Elecsys immunoassay system: pilot biological variation studies. *Clin Biochem*. 2003;36:211-214.
111. Choo RE, Huestis MA. Oral fluid as a diagnostic tool. *Clin Chem Lab Med*. 2004;42:1273-1287.
112. Hansen AM, Garde AH, Christensen JM, et al. Evaluation of a radioimmunoassay and establishment of a reference interval for salivary cortisol in healthy subjects in Denmark. *Scand J Clin Lab Invest*. 2003;63:303-310.
113. Viardot A, Huber P, Puder JJ, et al. Reproducibility of nighttime salivary cortisol and its use in the diagnosis of hypercortisolism compared with urinary free cortisol and overnight dexamethasone suppression test. *J Clin Endocrinol Metab*. 2005;90:5730-5736.
114. Granger DA, Schwartz EB, Booth A, et al. Assessing dehydroepiandrosterone in saliva: a simple radioimmunoassay for use in studies of children, adolescents and adults. *Psychoneuroendocrinology*. 1999; 24:567-579.
115. O'Rorke A, Kane MM, Gosling JP, et al. Development and validation of a monoclonal antibody enzyme immunoassay for measuring progesterone in saliva. *Clin Chem*. 1994;40:454-458.
116. Vining RF, McGinley RA. The measurement of hormones in saliva: possibilities and pitfalls. *J Steroid Biochem*. 1987;27:81-94.

117. Howe CJ, Handelsman DJ. Use of filter paper for sample collection and transport in steroid pharmacology. *Clin Chem*. 1997;43:1408-1415.
118. Worthman CM, Stallings JF. Hormone measures in finger-prick blood spot samples: new field methods for reproductive endocrinology. *Am J Phys Anthropol*. 1997;104:1-21.
119. Kricka LJ. Miniaturization of analytical systems. *Clin Chem*. 1998; 44:2008-2014.
120. Gabriely I, Wozniak R, Mevorach M, et al. Transcutaneous glucose measurement using near-infrared spectroscopy during hypoglycemia. *Diabetes Care*. 1999;22:2026-2032.
121. Tamada JA, Garg S, Jovanovic L, et al. Noninvasive glucose monitoring: comprehensive clinical results. Cygnus Research Team. *JAMA*. 1999;282:1839-1844.
122. Garg S, Zisser H, Schwartz S, et al. Improvement in glycemic excursions with a transcutaneous, real-time continuous glucose sensor: a randomized controlled trial. *Diabetes Care*. 2006;29:44-50.
123. Browning MC. Analytical goals for quantities used to assess thyrometabolic status. *Ann Clin Biochem*. 1989;26(Pt 1):1-12.
124. Westgard JO, Klee GG. Quality management. In: Burtis CA, Ashwood E, Bruns DE, eds. *Tietz Textbook of Clinical Chemistry and Molecular Diagnostics*. 4th ed. Philadelphia, PA: WB Saunders; 2006:485-531.
125. Tietz NW. Accuracy in clinical chemistry—does anybody care? *Clin Chem*. 1994;40:859-861.
126. Westgard JO, Barry PL, Hunt MR, et al. A multi-rule Shewhart chart for quality control in clinical chemistry. *Clin Chem*. 1981;27: 493-501.
127. Klee GG, Schryver PG, Kisabeth RM. Analytic bias specifications based on the analysis of effects on performance of medical guidelines. *Scand J Clin Lab Invest*. 1999;59:509-512.
128. Smith FA, Kroft SH. Optimal procedures for detecting analytic bias using patient samples. *Am J Clin Pathol*. 1997;108:254-268.
129. Nicholson S, Fox M, Epenetos A, et al. Immunoglobulin inhibiting reagent: evaluation of a new method for eliminating spurious elevations in CA125 caused by HAMA. *Int J Biol Markers*. 1996;11: 46-49.
130. Reinsberg J. Different efficacy of various blocking reagents to eliminate interferences by human antimouse antibodies with a two-site immunoassay. *Clin Biochem*. 1996;29:145-148.
131. Wheeler MJ, D'Souza A, Matadeen J, et al. Ciba Corning ACS:180 testosterone assay evaluated. *Clin Chem*. 1996;42:1445-1459.

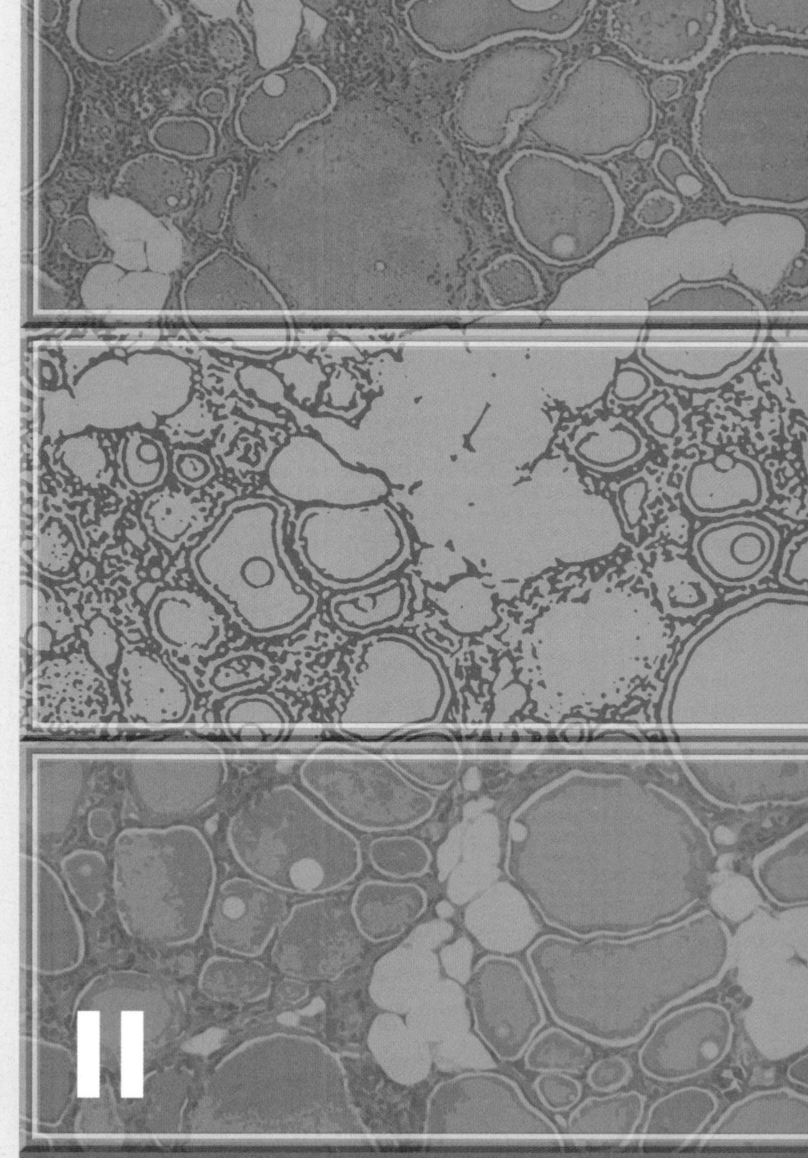

SECTION II

Hypothalamus and Pituitary

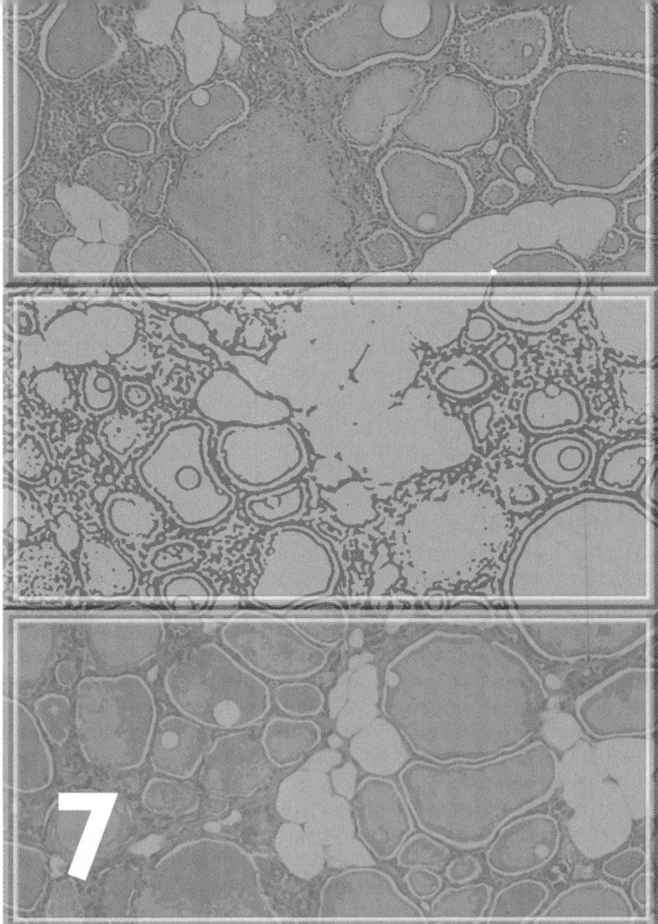

CHAPTER 7

Neuroendocrinology

MALCOLM J. LOW

HISTORICAL PERSPECTIVE

The field of neuroendocrinology has expanded from its original focus on the control of pituitary hormone secretion by the hypothalamus to encompass multiple reciprocal interactions between the central nervous system (CNS) and endocrine systems in the control of homeostasis and physiologic responses to environmental stimuli. Although many of these concepts are relatively recent, the intimate interaction of the hypothalamus and the pituitary gland was recognized more than a century ago. For example, at the end of the 19th century, clinicians including Alfred Fröhlich described an obesity and infertility condition referred to as *adiposogenital dystrophy* in patients with sellar tumors.[1] This condition subsequently became known as *Fröhlich's syndrome* and was most often associated with the accumulation of excessive subcutaneous fat, hypogonadotropic hypogonadism (HH), and growth retardation.

Whether this syndrome was a result of injury to the pituitary gland itself or to the overlying hypothalamus was extremely controversial. Several leaders in the field of endocrinology, including Cushing and his colleagues, argued that the syndrome was caused by disruption of the pituitary gland.[2] However, experimental evidence began to accumulate that the hypothalamus was somehow involved in the control of the pituitary gland. For example, Aschner demonstrated in dogs that precise removal of the pituitary gland without damage to the overlying hypothalamus did not result in obesity.[3] Later, seminal studies by Hetherington and Ranson demonstrated that stereotaxic destruction of the medial basal hypothalamus with electrolytic lesions, sparing the pituitary gland, resulted in morbid obesity and neuroendocrine derangements similar to those of the patients described by Fröhlich.[4] This and subsequent studies clearly established that an intact hypothalamus is required for normal endocrine function. However, the mechanisms by which the hypothalamus was involved in endocrine regulation remained unsettled for years. It is now thought that the phenotypes of Fröhlich's syndrome and of the ventromedial hypothalamic lesion syndrome are caused by dysfunction or destruction of key hypothalamic neurons that regulate pituitary hormone secretion and energy homeostasis.

The field of neuroendocrinology took a major step forward when several groups, especially that of Ernst and Berta Scharrer, recognized that neurons in the hypothalamus are the source of the axons that constitute the neural lobe (see "Neurosecretion"). The hypothalamic control of the anterior pituitary gland remained unclear, however. Popa and Fielding identified the pituitary portal vessels linking the median eminence of the hypothalamus and the anterior pituitary gland.[5] Although they appreciated the fact that this vasculature provided a link between the hypothalamus and the pituitary gland, they initially hypothesized that blood flowed from the pituitary up to the brain. Anatomic studies by Wislocki and King supported the concept that blood flow was from the hypothalamus to the pituitary.[6] Later studies, including the seminal work of Geoffrey Harris, established the flow of blood from the hypothalamus at the median eminence to the anterior pituitary gland.[7] This supported the concept that the hypothalamus controls anterior pituitary gland function indirectly and led to the now accepted hypophyseal-portal chemotransmitter hypothesis.

Subsequently, several important studies, especially those from Schally and colleagues and from the Guillemin group, established that the anterior pituitary is tightly controlled by the hypothalamus.[8,9] Both groups identified several putative peptide hormone-releasing factors (see later sections). These fundamental studies resulted in the awarding of the Nobel Prize in Medicine in 1977 to Andrew Schally and Roger Guillemin.[10,11] We now know that these releasing factors are the fundamental link between the CNS and the control of endocrine function. Furthermore, these neuropeptides are highly conserved across species and are essential for reproduction, growth, and metabolism. The anatomy, physiology, and genetics of these releasing factors constitute a major portion of this chapter.

Over the past 2 decades, work in the field of neuroendocrinology has continued to advance across several fronts. Cloning and characterization of the specific G protein–coupled receptors used by the hypothalamic releasing factors have helped define their signaling mechanisms. Characterization of the distribution of these receptors has universally demonstrated receptor expression in the brain and in peripheral tissues other than the pituitary, arguing for multiple physiologic roles for the neuropeptide-releasing factors. Finally, the last 2 decades have also seen tremendous advances in understanding of regulatory neuronal and humoral inputs to the hypophyseotropic neurons.

The adipostatic hormone leptin, discovered in 1994,[12] is an example of a humoral factor that has profound effects on multiple neuroendocrine circuits. Reduction in circulating leptin is responsible for suppression of the thyroid and reproductive axes during the starvation response. The subsequent discovery of ghrelin,[13] a stomach peptide that regulates appetite and also acts on multiple neuroendocrine axes, demonstrated that much remains to be learned regarding the regulation of the hypothalamic releasing hormones. Traditionally, it has been extremely difficult to study releasing-factor gene expression or the specific regulation of the releasing factor neurons because of their small numbers and, in some cases, diffuse distribution. Transgenic experiments have produced mice in which expression of fluorescent marker proteins is specifically targeted to gonadotropin-releasing hormone (GnRH) neurons[14] and arcuate pro-opiomelanocortin (POMC) neurons,[15] among others. This technology allows detailed study of the electrophysiologic properties of hypothalamic neurons in the more native context of slice preparations or organotypic cultures.

Although much of the field of neuroendocrinology has focused on hypothalamic releasing factors and their influence on reproduction, growth, development, fluid balance, and the stress response through control of pituitary hormone production, the term *neuroendocrinology* has come to mean the study of the interactions of the endocrine and nervous systems in the regulation of homeostasis. The field of neuroendocrinology has been further expanded by input from diverse areas of basic research that has often been fundamental to understanding of the neuroendocrine system. These areas include studies of neuropeptide structure, function, and mechanism of action; neural secretion; hypothalamic neuroanatomy; G protein–coupled receptor structure, function, and signaling; transport of substances into the brain; and the action of hormones on the brain. Moreover, homeostatic systems often involve integrated endocrine, autonomic, and behavioral responses. In many of these systems (e.g., energy homeostasis, immune function), the classic neuroendocrine axes are important but not autonomous pathways, and these subjects are also often studied in the context of neuroendocrinology.

In this chapter, the concepts of neural secretion, the neuroanatomy of the hypothalamic-pituitary unit, and the CNS structures most relevant to control of the neurohypophysis and adenohypophysis are presented. Then, each classic hypothalamic-pituitary axis is described, including a consideration of the immune system and its integration with neuroendocrine function. Finally, the pathophysiology of disorders of neural regulation of endocrine function are reviewed. The neuroendocrinology of energy homeostasis is fully considered in Chapter 35.

NEURAL CONTROL OF ENDOCRINE SECRETION

A fundamental principle of neuroendocrinology encompasses the regulated secretion of hormones, neurotransmitters, or neuromodulators by specialized cells.[16] Endocrine cells and neurons are prototypical secretory cells. Both have electrically excitable plasma membranes and specific ion conductances that regulate exocytosis of their signaling molecules from storage vesicles. Secretory cells are broadly classified by their topographic mechanisms of secretion. For example, *endocrine* cells secrete their contents directly into the bloodstream, allowing these substances to act globally as hormones. Cells classified as *paracrine* secrete their contents into the extracellular space and predominantly affect the function of closely neighboring cells. *Autocrine* secretory cells affect their own function by the local actions of their secretions. In contrast, secretory cells within *exocrine* glands secrete proteinaceous substances, including enzymes, and lipids into the lumen of ductal systems.

Neurosecretion

Neurons are secretory cells that send their axons throughout the nervous system to release their neurotransmitters and neuromodulators predominantly at specialized chemical synapses. Neurohumoral or neurosecretory cells constitute a unique subset of neurons whose axon terminals are not associated with synapses. Two examples of neurosecretory cells are neurohypophyseal and hypophyseotropic cells. The prototypical neurohypophyseal cells are the magnicellular neurons of the paraventricular (PVH) and supraoptic (SON) nuclei in the hypothalamus. Hypophyseotropic cells are neurons that secrete their products into the pituitary portal vessels at the median eminence (Fig. 7-1).

In the most basic sense, neurosecretory cells are neurons that secrete substances directly into the bloodstream to act as hormones. The theory of neurosecretion evolved from the seminal work of Scharrer and Scharrer,[16,17] who used morphologic techniques to identify stained secretory

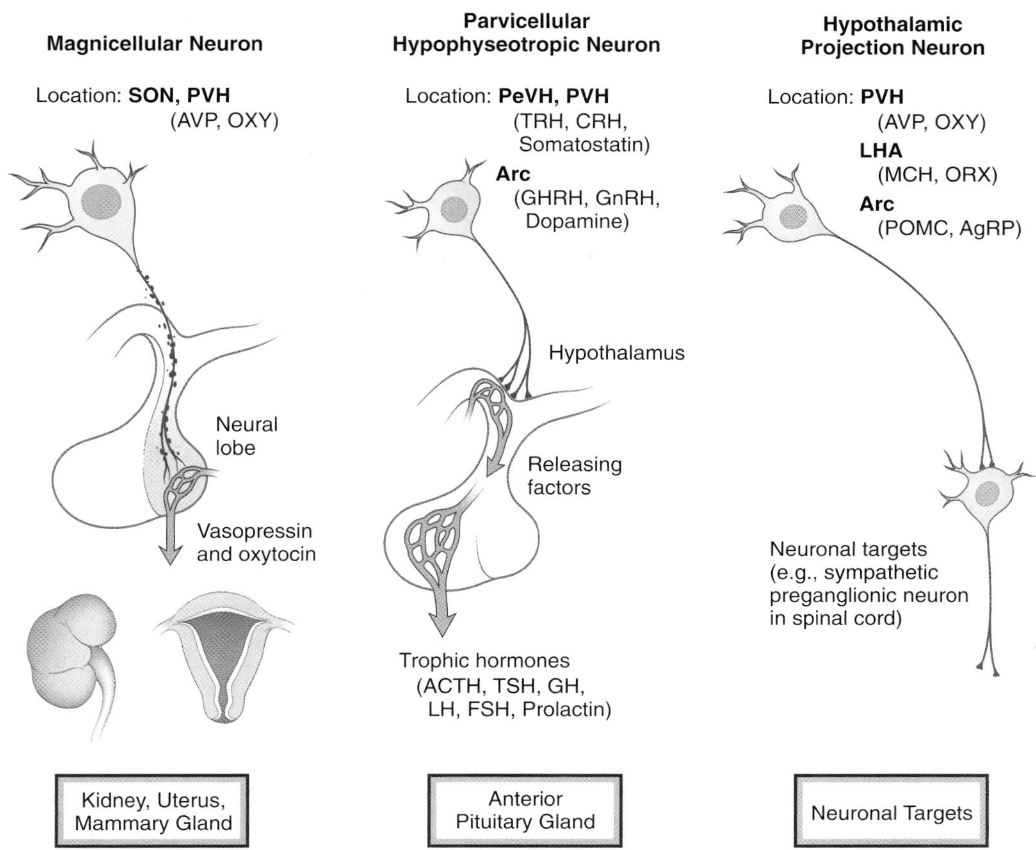

Figure 7-1 Three types of hypothalamic neurosecretory cells. *Left,* A magnicellular neuron that secretes arginine vasopressin (AVP) or oxytocin (OXY). The cell body, which is located in the supraoptic (SON) or paraventricular hypothalamic (PVH) nucleus, projects its neuronal process into the neural lobe, and neurohormone is released from nerve endings. *Center,* Similar peptidergic neurons are located in the medial basal hypothalamus in nuclear groups including the periventricular hypothalamic nucleus (PeVH), the PVH, and the infundibular or arcuate nucleus of the hypothalamus (Arc). The neuropeptides in this case are released into the specialized blood supply to the pituitary to regulate its secretion. *Right,* A third category of hypothalamic peptidergic neurons terminates at chemical synapses on other neurons. These projection neurons are found in sites including the PVH, Arc, and lateral hypothalamic area (LHA) that innervate multiple central nervous system nuclei, including autonomic preganglionic neurons in the brain stem and spinal cord. Such substances act as neurotransmitters or neuromodulators. ACTH, corticotropin; AgRP, agouti-related peptide; CRH, corticotropin-releasing hormone; FSH, follicle-stimulating hormone; GH, growth hormone; GHRH, growth hormone–releasing hormone; GnRH, gonadotropin-releasing hormone; LH, luteinizing hormone; MCH, melanin-concentrating hormone; ORX, orexin/hypocretin; POMC, pro-opiomelanocortin; TRH, thyrotropin-releasing hormone; TSH, thyrotropin.

granules in the SON and PVH neurons. They found that cutting the pituitary stalk led to an accumulation of these granules in the hypothalamus, which led them to hypothesize that hypothalamic neurons were the source of substances secreted by the neural lobe (posterior pituitary). Although this concept initially raised great skepticism among contemporary researchers, it is now known that the axon terminals in the neural lobe arise from the SON and PVH magnicellular neurons that contain oxytocin and the antidiuretic hormone, arginine vasopressin (AVP).

The modern definition of neurosecretion has evolved to include the release of any secretory product from a neuron. Indeed, a fundamental tenet of neuroscience is that all neurons in the CNS, including neurons that secrete AVP and oxytocin in the neural lobe, receive multiple synaptic inputs largely onto their dendrites and cell bodies. In addition, neurons have the basic ability to detect and integrate input from multiple neurons through specific receptors. They in turn fire action potentials that result in the release of neurotransmitters and neuromodulators into synapses formed with postsynaptic neurons. Most communications between neurons are accomplished by the classic fast-acting neurotransmitters (e.g., glutamate, γ-aminobutyric acid [GABA], acetylcholine) and neuromodulators (e.g., neuropeptides) acting at chemical synapses.[11,18] Neurosecretion represents a fundamental concept in understanding the mechanisms used by the nervous system to control behavior and maintain homeostasis.

In the era of the elucidation of the human genome, the importance of these early observations is often not fully appreciated. However, accounts of these early studies are illuminating, and it is not an overstatement that confirmation of the neurosecretion hypothesis represented one of the major advances in the fields of neuroscience and neuroendocrinology. Indeed, these and other early experiments, including the pioneering work of Geoffrey Harris,[7,19] led to the fundamental concept that the hypothalamus releases hormones directly into the bloodstream (neurohypophyseal cells). These observations provided the principles on which the modern discipline of neuroendocrinology is built.

Contribution of the Autonomic Nervous System to Endocrine Control

Another major precept of neuroendocrinology is that the nervous system controls or modifies the function of both endocrine and exocrine glands. The exquisite control of the anterior pituitary gland is accomplished by the action of releasing factor hormones (see "Hypophyseotropic Hormones and Neuroendocrine Axes"). Other endocrine and exocrine organs (e.g., pancreas, adrenal, pineal, salivary glands) are also regulated through direct innervation from the cholinergic and noradrenergic inputs from the autonomic nervous system. Although it is beyond the scope of this chapter, an appreciation of the functional anatomy and pharmacology of the parasympathetic and sympathetic nervous systems is fundamental to understanding of the neural control of endocrine function.

The efferent arms of the autonomic nervous system comprise the sympathetic and parasympathetic systems. These have similar wiring diagrams characterized by a preganglionic neuron that innervates a postganglionic neuron that in turn targets an end organ.[20] Preganglionic and postganglionic parasympathetic neurons are cholinergic. In contrast, preganglionic sympathetic neurons are cholinergic and postganglionic neurons are noradrenergic (except for those innervating sweat glands, which are cholinergic). Another basic concept is that autonomic neurons coexpress several neuropeptides. This coexpression is a common feature of neurons in the central and peripheral nervous systems.[11,18,21] For example, postganglionic noradrenergic neurons coexpress somatostatin and neuropeptide Y (NPY). Postganglionic cholinergic neurons coexpress neuropeptides including vasoactive intestinal polypeptide (VIP) and calcitonin gene–related peptide (CGRP).

Most sympathetic preganglionic neurons lie in the intermediolateral cell column in the thoracolumbar regions of the spinal cord.[20] Most postganglionic sympathetic neurons are located in sympathetic ganglia lying near the vertebral column (e.g., sympathetic chain, superior cervical ganglia). Postganglionic fibers innervate target organs. As a rule, the sympathetic preganglionic fibers are relatively short, and the postganglionic fibers are long. In contrast, the parasympathetic preganglionic neurons lie in the midbrain (perioculomotor area, long misidentified as the Edinger-Westphal nucleus[22]), the medulla oblongata (e.g., dorsal motor nucleus of the vagus, nucleus ambiguus), and the sacral spinal cord. Postganglionic neurons that innervate the eye and salivary glands arise from the ciliary, pterygopalatine, submandibular, and otic ganglia. Postganglionic parasympathetic neurons in the thorax and abdomen typically lie within the target organs, including the gut wall and pancreas.[20] Consequently, the parasympathetic preganglionic fibers are relatively long, and the postganglionic fibers are short.

A dual autonomic innervation of the pancreas illustrates the importance of coordinated neural control of endocrine organs. The endocrine pancreas receives both sympathetic (noradrenergic) and parasympathetic (cholinergic) innervation.[20,23] The latter activity is provided by the vagus nerve (dorsal motor nucleus of the vagus) and is an excellent example of neural modulation, because the cholinergic tone of the beta cells affects their secretion of insulin. For example, vagal input is thought to modulate insulin secretion before (cephalic phase), during, and after ingestion of food.[24] In addition, noradrenergic stimulation of the endocrine pancreas can alter the secretion of glucagon and inhibits insulin release.[23] Of course, a major regulator of insulin secretion is the extracellular concentration of glucose,[25] and glucose can induce insulin secretion in the absence of neural input. However, the exquisite control by the nervous system is illustrated by the fact that populations of neurons in the brain stem and hypothalamus have the ability, like the beta cell, to sense glucose levels in the bloodstream.[26] This information is integrated by the hypothalamus and ultimately results in alterations in the activity of the autonomic nervous system innervating the pancreas. Therefore, neural control of the endocrine pancreas probably contributes to the physiologic control of insulin secretion and may contribute to the pathophysiology of disorders such as diabetes mellitus. Certainly, an increased understanding of this complex interplay between the CNS and endocrine function is necessary to diagnose and clinically manage endocrine disorders.

HYPOTHALAMIC-PITUITARY UNIT

The hypothalamus is one of the most evolutionarily conserved and essential regions of the mammalian brain. Indeed, the hypothalamus is the ultimate brain structure that allows mammals to maintain homeostasis, and destruction of the hypothalamus is not compatible with life. Hypothalamic control of homeostasis stems from the ability of this collection of neurons to orchestrate coordinated endocrine, autonomic, and behavioral responses. A key principle is that the hypothalamus receives sensory inputs from the external environment (e.g., light, nociception, temperature, odorants) and information regarding the internal environment (e.g., blood pressure, blood osmolality, blood glucose levels). Of particular relevance to neuroendocrine control, hormones (e.g., glucocorticoids, estrogen, testosterone, thyroid hormone) exert both negative and positive feedback directly on the hypothalamus.

The hypothalamus integrates diverse sensory and hormonal inputs and provides coordinated responses through motor outputs to key regulatory sites. These include the anterior pituitary gland, posterior pituitary gland, cerebral cortex, premotor and motor neurons in the brain stem and spinal cord, and parasympathetic and sympathetic preganglionic neurons. The patterned hypothalamic outputs to these effector sites ultimately result in coordinated endocrine, behavioral, and autonomic responses that maintain homeostasis. The hypothalamic control of the pituitary gland is an elegant system that underlies the ability of mammals to coordinate endocrine functions that are necessary for survival.

Development and Differentiation of Hypothalamic Nuclei

Tremendous advances in knowledge of the molecular and genetic basis for embryonic development of the hypothalamic-pituitary unit have occurred in the past 2 decades as a result of the genome sequencing projects and use of transgenic model systems.[27] Pituitary development is discussed in detail in Chapter 8, and only a few key points most relevant to the physiology and pathophysiology of the neuroendocrine hypothalamus are presented here.

There has been considerable debate concerning the extent to which developmental studies in the rodent hypothalamic-pituitary system are applicable to the human. However, accumulating data suggest that the similarities outweigh the differences. Ontogenic analyses of the organization of the human hypothalamus using a battery of neurochemical markers have reinforced its homologies to the better-studied rat brain.[28] The cytoarchitectonic boundaries of hypothalamic nuclei are much more easily discerned in fetal human brain than in the adult brain and for the most part correspond to homologous structures in the rat hypothalamus. This finding has important implications for the validity of interspecies comparative analyses.

Two examples further illustrate this point. First, the ventromedial nucleus of the hypothalamic core (ventromedial hypothalamus, or VMH), which plays a role in energy balance and in female sexual behavior, differentiates from neuroblasts in both humans and rodents at a time point that is intermediate between the earlier differentiation of lateral hypothalamic nuclei and later differentiation of the midline nuclei, including the suprachiasmatic nucleus (SCN), the arcuate nucleus, and the PVH.[28,29] Expression of the transcription factor SF1 has been shown to be restricted both temporally and spatially to cells in the VMH, and knockout of the SF1 gene in mice alters VMH development by influencing the migration of cells and their ultimate location.[29] A second example of interspecies homologies in hypothalamic development is the migration of GnRH-secreting neurons from their origins in rostral neuroepithelium to the anterior hypothalamus.[30] As discussed later, spontaneous and inherited mutations in genes that affect the migration of these neurons are an important cause of Kallmann's syndrome or HH associated with anosmia.

In addition to SF1 and the genes associated with Kallmann's syndrome, a growing list of genes primarily encoding transcription factors have been implicated in human neuroendocrine disorders and characterized experimentally in rodent models.[31] This list includes the homeobox transcription factor OTP and the heterodimeric complex formed by the basic helix-loop-helix (bHLH) factors SIM1 and ARNT2. These factors are required for the proper development of the PVH and the SON and for expression of many key hypophyseotropic neuropeptide genes. The physiologic importance of SIM1 is illustrated by the development of an obesity phenotype in both mice and humans with a haploinsufficiency of SIM1 expression.[31] MASH1 and its downstream target GSH1 are both critical for neuron specification and expression of growth hormone–releasing hormone (GHRH).[32]

Two key concepts involved in CNS development, which also apply to the hypothalamus, are the balance between neurogenesis and cell death in the establishment of nuclei and the role of circulating hormones in providing organizational signals that regulate cell number and synaptic remodeling. The most thoroughly characterized examples are the effects of sex steroid hormones on the developing brain, which result in key sexual dimorphisms of functional importance in later reproductive behaviors.[33] This principle has been extended to include organizational effects of other classes of hormones. For example, leptin plays an important role in the development of medial-basal hypothalamic circuits that are important for energy homeostasis by mediating axonal projections between hypothalamic nuclei.[34]

Anatomy of the Hypothalamic-Pituitary Unit

The pituitary gland is regulated by three interacting elements: hypothalamic inputs (releasing factors or hypophyseotropic hormones), feedback effects of circulating hormones, and paracrine and autocrine secretions of the pituitary itself. In humans, the pituitary gland (hypophysis) can be divided into two major parts, the adenohypophysis and the neurohypophysis, which are easily distinguishable on T1-weighted magnetic resonance imaging (MRI) (Fig. 7-2).[35] The adenohypophysis can be subdivided into three distinct lobes: the pars distalis (anterior lobe), pars intermedia (intermediate lobe), and pars tuberalis. Whereas a well-developed intermediate lobe is found in most mammals, only rudimentary vestiges of the intermediate lobe are detectable in adult humans, with the bulk of intermediate lobe cells being dispersed in the anterior and posterior lobes.

The neurohypophysis is composed of the pars nervosa (also known as the neural or posterior lobe), the infundibular stalk, and the median eminence. The infundibular stalk is surrounded by the pars tuberalis, and together they constitute the *hypophyseal stalk*. The pituitary gland lies in the sella turcica ("Turkish saddle") of the sphenoid bone and underlies the base of the hypothalamus. This anatomic location explains the hypothalamic damage described by Fröhlich.[1] In humans, the base of the hypothalamus forms a mound called the *tuber cinereum*, the central region of which gives rise to the median eminence (see Fig. 7-2).[36]

The anterior and intermediate lobes of the pituitary derive from a dorsal invagination of the pharyngeal epithelium, called *Rathke's pouch*, in response to inductive signals from the overlying neuroepithelium of the ventral diencephalon. During development, precursor cells within the pouch undergo steps of organ determination, cell fate commitment to a pituitary phenotype, proliferation, and migration.[27] The intermediate lobe is in direct contact with the neural lobe and is the least prominent of the three lobes. With age, the human intermediate lobe decreases in size to leave a small, residual collection of POMC cells. In nonprimate species, these cells are responsible for secreting the POMC-derived product α-melanocyte–stimulating hormone (α-MSH).[37]

The major component of the neural lobe is a collection of axon terminals arising from magnicellular secretory neurons located in the PVH and SON nuclei of the hypothalamus (Fig. 7-3; see Fig. 7-1). These axon terminals are in close association with a capillary plexus, and they secrete substances including AVP and oxytocin into the hypophyseal veins and thence into the general circulation (Table 7-1). The blood supply to the neurohypophysis arises from the inferior hypophyseal artery (a branch of the internal carotid artery). Glial-like cells called *pituicytes* are scattered among the nerve terminals. As the source of AVP to the general circulation, the PVH and SON nuclei and their axon terminals in the neural lobe are the effector arms for the central regulation of blood osmolality, fluid balance, and blood pressure (see Chapter 10).

The secretion of oxytocin by magnicellular neurons is critical at parturition, resulting in uterine myometrial contraction. In addition, the secretion of oxytocin is regulated by the classic milk let-down reflex.[38] Although the exact neuroanatomic substrate underlying this response is unclear, apparently mechanosensory information from the nipple reaches the magnicellular neurons, directly or indirectly, from the dorsal horn of the spinal cord, resulting in release of oxytocin into the general circulation.[39] Oxytocin acts on receptors on myoepithelial cells in the mammary gland acini, leading to release of milk into the ductal system of the mammary gland.

The Median Eminence and Hypophyseotropic Neuronal System

The median eminence is the functional link between the hypothalamus and the anterior pituitary gland. It lies in the center of the tuber cinereum and is composed of an extensive array of blood vessels and nerve endings (Fig. 7-4; see Fig. 7-2).[17,36,40] Its extremely rich blood supply arises from the superior hypophyseal artery (a branch of the internal carotid artery), which sends off many small branches that form capillary loops. The small capillary loops extend into the internal and external zones of the

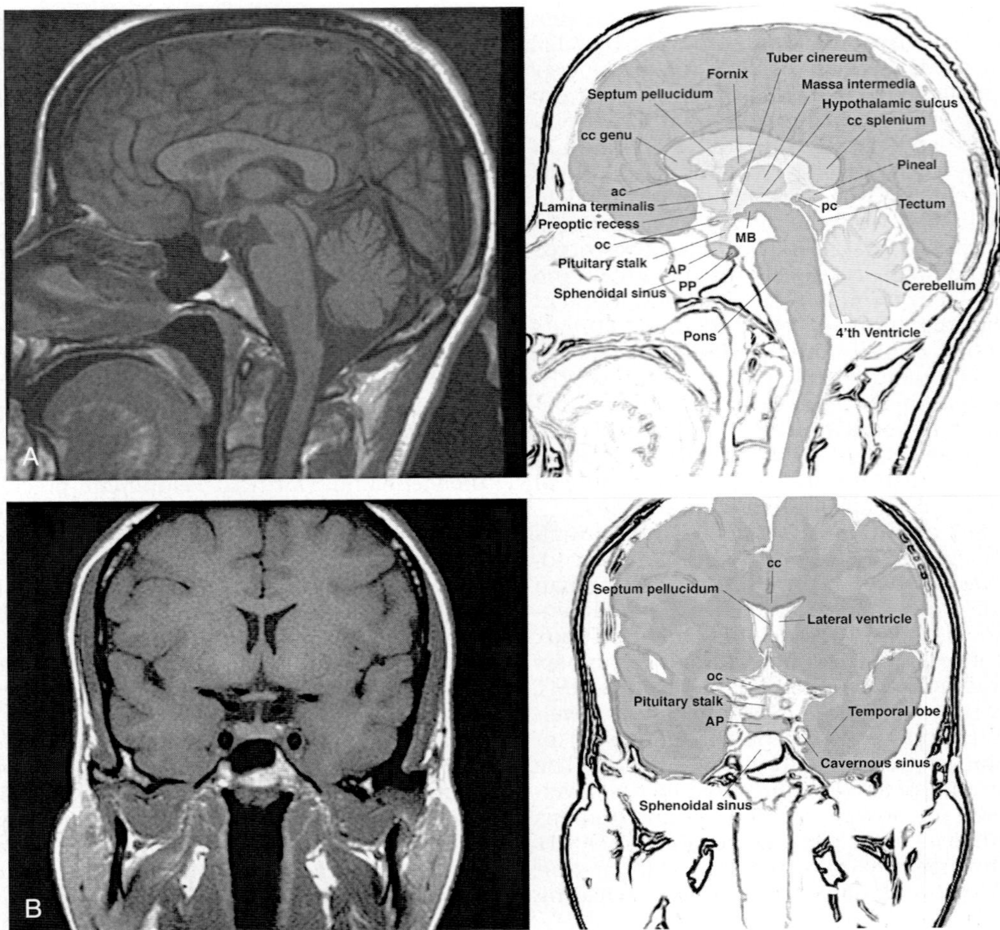

Figure 7-2 Normal anatomy of the human hypothalamic-pituitary unit in sagittal (**A**) and coronal (**B**) planes. Structures that are visible in the T1-weighted magnetic resonance images *(left panels)* are identified in the corresponding diagrams *(right panels)*. The hypothalamus is bounded anteriorly by the optic chiasm, laterally by the sulci formed with the temporal lobes, and posteriorly by the mammillary bodies (in which the mammillary nuclei are located). Dorsally, the hypothalamus is delineated from the thalamus by the hypothalamic sulcus. The smooth, rounded base of the hypothalamus is the tuber cinereum; the pituitary stalk descends from its central region, which is termed the *median eminence*. The median eminence stands out from the rest of the tuber cinereum because of its dense vascularity, which is formed by the primary plexus of the hypophyseal-portal system. The long portal veins run along the ventral surface of the pituitary stalk. Notice the location of the pituitary stalk, the hyperintense signal *(white)* from the posterior pituitary (PP) (panel **A**, *left*), and the anatomic relationships of the pituitary gland to the optic chiasm (oc) and the sphenoidal and cavernous sinuses. ac, anterior commissure; AP, anterior pituitary; cc, corpus callosum; MB, mammillary body; pc, posterior commissure. (Magnetic resonance images courtesy of Dr. D.M. Cook.)

median eminence, form anastomoses, and drain into sinusoids that become the pituitary portal veins that enter the vascular pool of the pituitary gland.[40-42] The flow of blood in these short loops is thought to be predominantly (if not exclusively) in a hypothalamic-to-pituitary direction.[42] This well-developed plexus results in a tremendous increase in the vascular surface area. In addition, the vessels are fenestrated, allowing diffusion of the peptide-releasing factors to their site of action in the anterior pituitary gland. Because this vascular complex in the base of the hypothalamus and its "arteriolized" venous drainage to the pituitary compose a circulatory system analogous to the portal vein system of the liver, it has been termed the *hypophyseal-portal circulation*.

Three distinct compartments of the median eminence are recognized: the innermost ependymal layer, the internal zone, and the external zone (see Fig. 7-4).[40] Ependymal cells form the floor of the third ventricle and are unique in that they have microvilli rather than cilia. Tight junctions at the ventricular pole of the ependymal cells prevent the diffusion of large-molecular-weight substances between the cerebrospinal fluid (CSF) and the extracellular space within the median eminence. The ependymal layer also contains specialized cells, called *tanycytes*, that send processes into the other layers of the median eminence.[43] Tight junctions between tanycytes at the lateral edges of the median eminence likely prevent the diffusion of releasing factors back into the medial basal hypothalamus.

The internal zone of the median eminence is composed of axons of the SON and PVH magnicellular neurons passing en route to the posterior pituitary (see Fig. 7-4C) and axons of the hypophyseotropic neurons destined for the external layer of the median eminence (see Fig. 7-4A and B). In addition, supportive cells populate this layer.

Finally, the external zone of the median eminence represents the exchange point of the hypothalamic releasing factors and the pituitary portal vessels.[40] Two general types of tuberohypophyseal neurons project to the external zone: peptide-secreting (peptidergic) neurons including thyrotropin-releasing hormone (TRH), corticotropin-releasing hormone (CRH), and GnRH (see Fig. 7-1) and neurons containing monoamines (e.g., dopamine,

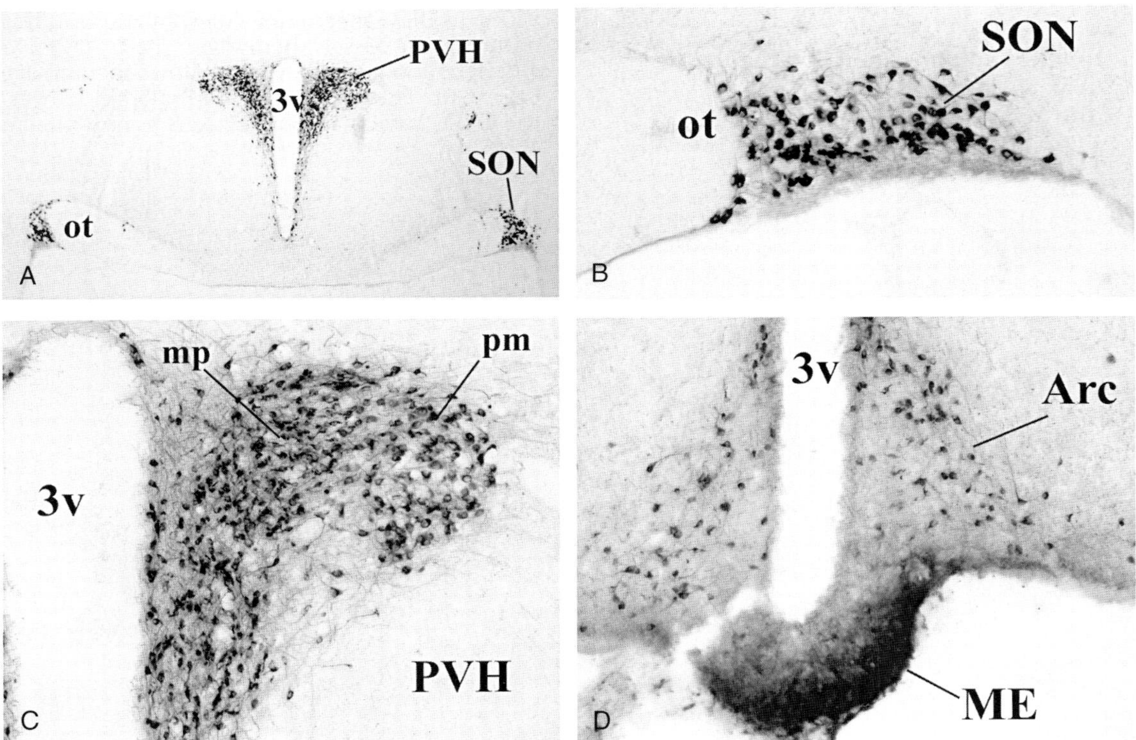

Figure 7-3 The tuberoinfundibular system is revealed by retrograde transport of cholera toxin subunit B (CtB). The location of hypothalamic cell bodies of neurons projecting to the median eminence (ME) and the posterior pituitary are identified by microinjection of a small volume of the retrograde tracer CtB into the median eminence of the rat. **A,** Retrogradely labeled cells can be seen in the paraventricular (PVH) and supraoptic (SON) nuclei of the hypothalamus. **B,** Magnicellular neurons are observed in the SON. **C,** Labeled neurons are found in the posterior magnicellular group (pm) and in the medial parvicellular subdivision (mp). The labeled cells in the PVH include those that contain corticotropin-releasing hormone and thyrotropin-releasing hormone. **D,** Retrogradely labeled cells are also found in the arcuate nucleus of the hypothalamus (Arc). These include neurons that secrete growth hormone–releasing hormone and dopamine. 3v, third ventricle; ot, optic tract. (Photomicrographs courtesy of Dr. R. M. Lechan.)

serotonin). Although the secretion of these substances into the portal circulation is an important control mechanism, some peptides and neurotransmitters in nerve endings are not released into the hypophyseal-portal circulation but instead function to regulate the secretion of other nerve terminals.[44] The anatomic relationships of nerve endings, basement membranes, interstitial spaces, fenestrated (windowed) capillary endothelia, and glia in the median eminence are similar to those in the neural lobe. As in the case of neurohormone secretion from the neurohypophysis, depolarization of hypothalamic cells leads to the release of neuropeptides and monoamines at the median eminence.

Non-neuronal supporting cells in the hypothalamus also play a dynamic role in hypophyseotropic regulation. For example, nerve terminals in the neurohypophysis are enveloped by pituicytes; they surround the nerve endings when the gland is inactive but retract to expose the terminals when AVP secretion is enhanced, as in states of dehydration. Within the median eminence, GnRH nerve endings are enveloped by the tanycytes, which also cover or uncover neurons with changes in functional status.[43,45] Thus, supporting elements, with their own sets of receptors, can change the neuroregulatory milieu within the hypothalamus, median eminence, and pituitary.

The site of production, the genetics, and the regulation of synthesis and release of individual peptide-releasing factors are discussed in detail in later sections. Briefly, there are several cell groups in the medial hypothalamus that contain releasing factors that are secreted into the pituitary portal circulation (Table 7-2).[36,46] These cell groups include the infundibular nucleus (called the *arcuate nucleus* in rodents) (see Fig. 7-3D), the PVH (see Fig. 7-3A and C), and a group of cells in the medial preoptic area near the organum vasculosum of the lamina terminalis (OVLT) (Fig. 7-5). As discussed earlier, magnicellular neurons in the SON and PVH send axons that predominantly traverse the median eminence to terminate in the neural lobe of the pituitary. In addition, a smaller number of magnicellular axons project directly to the external zone of the median eminence, but their functional significance is unknown.

The third structure often grouped as a component of the median eminence is a subdivision of the adenohypophysis called the *pars tuberalis*. It is a thin sheet of glandular tissue that lies around the infundibulum and pituitary stalk. In some animals, the epithelial component makes up as much as 10% of the total glandular tissue of the anterior pituitary. The pars tuberalis contains cells that make pituitary tropic hormones including luteinizing hormone (LH) and thyrotropin (thyroid-stimulating hormone, or TSH). A definitive physiologic function of the pars tuberalis is not established, but melatonin receptors are expressed in the pars tuberalis.

CIRCUMVENTRICULAR ORGANS

A guiding principle of neurophysiology and neuropharmacology is that the brain, including the hypothalamus, resides in an environment that is protected from humoral

TABLE 7-1

Neurotransmitters and Neuromodulators in the Paraventricular Nucleus and the Arcuate Nucleus of the Hypothalamus

Paraventricular Nucleus	Arcuate Nucleus
Magnicellular Division	Acetylcholine
Angiotensin II	γ-Aminobutyric acid (GABA)
Cholecystokinin (CCK)	Agouti-related peptide (AgRP)
Dynorphins	Cocaine- and amphetamine-regulated transcript (CART)
Nitric oxide (NO)	Dopamine
Oxytocin	Dynorphin
Vasopressin (AVP)	Endocannabinoids
Parvicellular Divisions	Enkephalins
γ-Aminobutyric acid (GABA)	Galanin
Angiotensin II	Galanin-like peptide (GALP)
Atrial natriuretic factor (ANF)	Glutamate
Bombesin-like peptides	Gonadotropin-releasing hormone (GnRH)
Cholecystokinin (CCK)	Growth hormone–releasing hormone (GHRH)
Corticotropin-releasing hormone (CRH)	Kisspeptins
Dopamine	Melanocortins (ACTH, α-MSH, β-MSH, γ-MSH)
Endocannabinoids	Neurokinin B (NKB)
Enkephalins	Neuromedin U
Galanin	Neuropeptide Y (NPY)
Glutamate	Neurotensin
Interleukin-1 (IL-1)	Nociceptin/orphanin FQ (OFQ)
Neuropeptide Y (NPY)	Opioids (β-endorphin) peptides
Neurotensin	Pancreatic polypeptide
Nitric oxide (NO)	Prolactin
RFamide–related peptides (RFRP)	Pro-opiomelanocortin
Somatostatin	Pyro-glutamyl-RFamide peptide (QRFP)
Thyrotropin-releasing hormone (TRH)	Somatostatin
Vasopressin (AVP)	Substance P
Vasoactive intestinal peptide (VIP)	

signals.[43,47,48] The exclusion of macromolecules is achieved by the structural vascular specializations that make up the blood-brain barrier. These specializations include tight junctions of brain vascular endothelial cells that preclude the free passage of polarized macromolecules including peptides and hormones. In addition, astrocytic foot processes and perivascular microglial cells contribute to the integrity of the blood-brain barrier.[48] However, to exert homeostatic control, the brain must assess key sensory information from the bloodstream, including levels of hormones, metabolites, and potential toxins. To monitor key signals, the brain has "windows on the circulation" or circumventricular organs (CVOs) that serve as a conduit of peripheral cues into key neuronal cell groups that maintain homeostasis.[47,48]

As the name implies, CVOs are specialized structures that lie on the midline of the brain along the third and fourth ventricles. These structures include the OVLT, subfornical organ (SFO), median eminence, neurohypophysis (posterior pituitary), subcommissural organ (SCO), and area postrema (see Fig. 7-5). Unlike the vasculature in the rest of the brain, the blood vessels in CVOs have fenestrated capillaries that allow relatively free passage of molecules such as proteins and peptide hormones. Thus, neurons and glial cells that reside within the CVOs have access to these macromolecules. In addition to the distinct nature of the vessels themselves, the CVOs have an unusually rich blood supply, which allows them to act as integrators at the interface of the blood-brain barrier. Several of the CVOs have major projections to hypothalamic nuclear

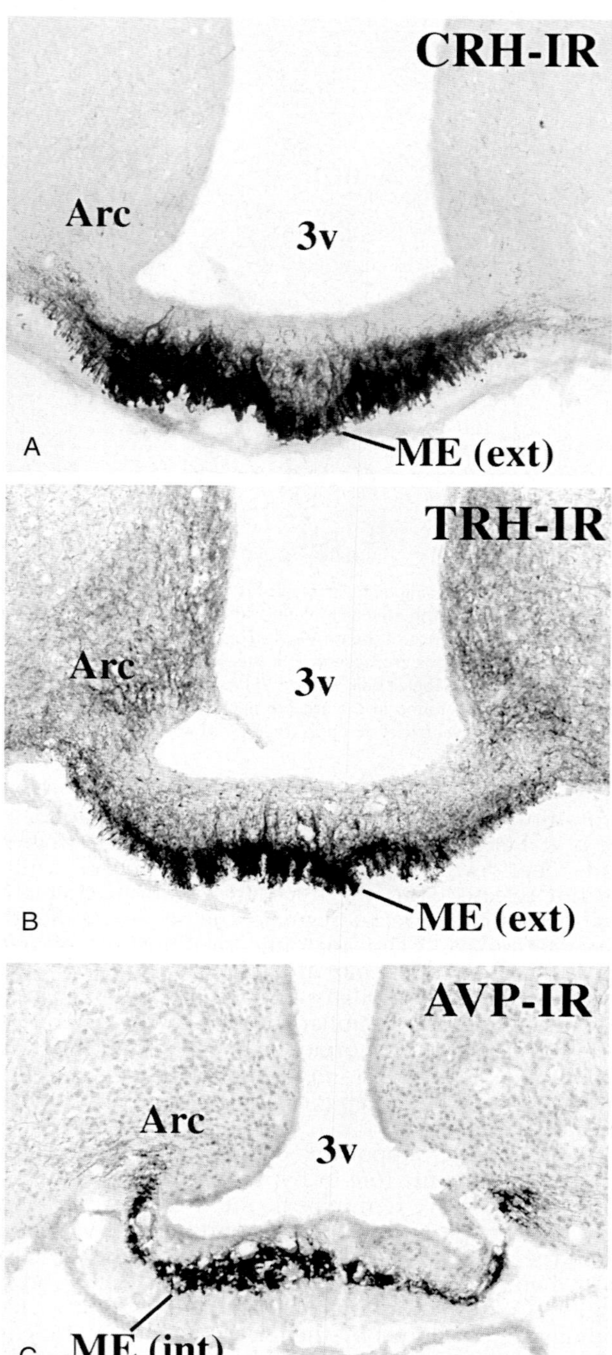

Figure 7-4 The median eminence (ME) is the functional connection between the hypothalamus and the pituitary gland. **A** and **B,** Distribution of corticotropin-releasing hormone (CRH) and thyrotropin-releasing hormone (TRH) immunoreactivity (IR) in the external (ext) layer of the ME of the rat. CRH and TRH cell bodies reside in the medial division of the paraventricular hypothalamic nucleus. **C,** Arginine vasopressin immunoreactivity (AVP-IR) in nerve endings in the internal (int) layer of the ME. Arc, Arcuate nucleus; 3v, third ventricle. (Photomicrographs courtesy of Dr. R.M. Lechan.)

TABLE 7-2

Structural Formulas of Principal Human Hypothalamic Peptides Directly Related to Pituitary Secretion*

Vasopressin
Cys-Tyr-Phe-Gln-Asn-*Cys*-Pro-Arg-Gly-NH_2 (MW = 1084.38)
Oxytocin
Cys-Tyr-Ile-Gln-Asn-*Cys*-Pro-Leu-Gly-NH_2 (MW = 1007.35)
Thyrotropin-Releasing Hormone
pGlu-His-Pro-NH_2 (MW = 362.42)
Gonadotropin-Releasing Hormone
pGlu-His-Trp-Ser-Tyr-Gly-Leu-Arg-Pro-Gly-NH_2 (MW = 1182.39)
Corticotropin-Releasing Hormone
Ser-Glu-Glu-Pro-Pro-Ile-Ser-Leu-Asp-Leu-Thr-Phe-His-Leu-Leu-Arg-Glu-Val-Leu-Glu-Met-Ala-Arg-Ala-Glu-Gln-Leu-Ala-Gln-Gln-Ala-His-Ser-Asn-Arg-Lys-Leu-Met-Glu-Ile-Ile-NH_2 (MW = 4758.14)
Growth Hormone–Releasing Hormone
GHRH(1-40) Tyr-Ala-Asp-Ala-Ile-Phe-Thr-Asn-Ser-Tyr-Arg-Lys-Val-Leu-Gly-Gln-Leu-Ser-Ala-Arg-Lys-Leu-Leu-Gln-Asp-Ile-Met-Ser-Arg-Gln-Gln-Gly-Glu-Ser-Asn-Gln-Glu-Arg-Gly-Ala (MW = 4544.73) *GHRH(1-44)-NH_2* Tyr-Ala-Asp-Ala-Ile-Phe-Thr-Asn-Ser-Tyr-Arg-Lys-Val-Leu-Gly-Gln-Leu-Ser-Ala-Arg-Lys-Leu-Leu-Gln-Asp-Ile-Met-Ser-Arg-Gln-Gln-Gly-Glu-Ser-Asn-Gln-Glu-Arg-Gly-Ala-Arg-Ala-Arg-Leu-NH_2 (MW = 5040.4)
Somatostatin
Ala-Gly-*Cys*-Lys-Asn-Phe-Phe-Trp-Lys-Thr-Phe-Thr-Ser-*Cys* (MW = 1638.12)
Somatostatin-28
SST-28 Ser-Ala-Asn-Ser-Asn-Pro-Ala-Met-Ala-Pro-Arg-Glu-Arg-Lys-Ala-Gly-*Cys*-Lys-Asn-Phe-Phe-Trp-Lys-Thr-Phe-Thr-Ser-*Cys* (MW = 3149.0) *SST-28(1-12)* Ser-Ala-Asn-Ser-Asn-Pro-Ala-Met-Ala-Pro-Arg-Gln (MW = 1244.49)
Vasoactive Intestinal Peptide
His-Ser-Asp-Ala-Val-Phe-Thr-Asp-Asn-Tyr-Thr-Arg-Leu-Arg-Lys-Gln-Met-Ala-Val-Lys-Lys-Tyr-Leu-Asn-Ser-Ile-Leu-Asn-NH_2 (MW = 3326.26)
Prolactin-Releasing Peptide
PrRP31 Ser-Arg-Thr-His-Arg-His-Ser-Met-Glu-Ile-Arg-Thr-Pro-Asp-Ile-Asn-Pro-Ala-Trp-Tyr-Ala-Ser-Arg-Gly-Ile-Arg-Pro-Val-Gly-Arg-Phe-NH_2 (MW = 3665.16) *PrRP20* Thr-Pro-Asp-Ile-Asn-Pro-Ala-Trp-Tyr-Ala-Ser-Arg-Gly-Ile-Arg-Pro-Val-Gly-Arg-Phe-NH_2 (MW = 2273.58)
Ghrelin†
Gly-Ser-Ser-Phe-Leu-Ser-Pro-Glu-His-Gln-Arg-Val-Gln-Gln-Arg-Lys-Glu-Ser-Lys-Lys-Pro-Pro-Ala-Lys-Leu-Gln-Pro-Arg (MW = 3314.9)

*Disulfide bonds between pairs of cystines that produce cyclization of the peptides are indicated by their italicized cognate *Cys* residues.
†The serine at position 3 in ghrelin is *O*-octanoylated.
MW, Molecular weight; pGlu, pyro-glutamyl.

groups that regulate homeostasis (see later discussion). Therefore, the CVOs serve as a critical link between peripheral metabolic cues, hormones, and potential toxins and cell groups within the brain that regulate coordinated endocrine, autonomic, and behavioral responses. Detailed discussion of the physiologic roles of individual CVOs is beyond the scope of this chapter, but several in-depth reviews have assessed the function of each.[47-50]

Median Eminence

The median eminence and neurohypophysis contain the neurosecretory axons that control pituitary function. The role of the median eminence as a link between the hypothalamus and the pituitary gland is detailed in other sections of this chapter (see "Hypothalamic-Pituitary Unit" and Figs. 7-2 and 7-4). The anatomic location of the median eminence places it in a position to serve as an afferent sensory organ as well. Specifically, the median eminence is located adjacent to several neuroendocrine and autonomic regulatory nuclei at the tuberal level of the hypothalamus (see Fig. 7-3). These nuclear groups include the infundibular or arcuate, ventromedial, dorsomedial, and paraventricular nuclei.[36]

A role of the hypothalamic nuclei surrounding the median eminence as afferent sensory centers is supported by several observations. For example, toxins such as monosodium glutamate and gold thioglucose damage neurons in cell groups overlying the median eminence, resulting in obesity and hyperphagia. Experimental evidence suggests that the median eminence is a portal of entry for hormones such as leptin. Indeed, administration of radiolabeled peptides or hormones, such as α-MSH or leptin, led to their

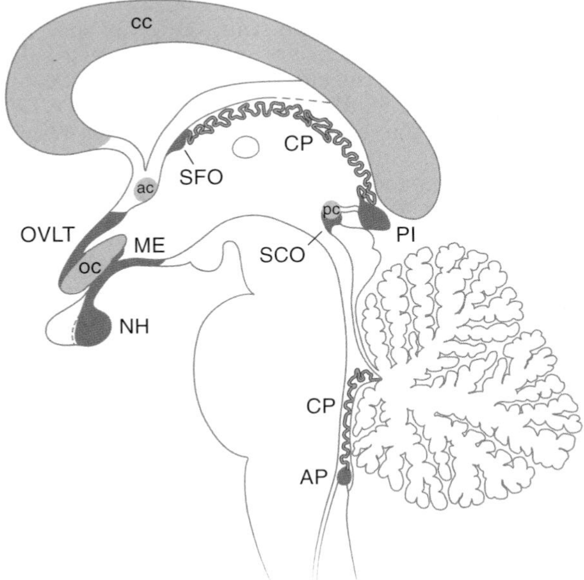

Figure 7-5 Median sagittal section through the human brain shows the circumventricular organs *(dark brown)*. Light brown areas are the optic chiasm (oc), corpus callosum (cc), anterior commissure (ac), and posterior commissure (pc). AP, area postrema; ME, median eminence; NH, neurohypophysis; OVLT, organum vasculosum of the lamina terminalis; PI, pineal gland; SFO, subfornical organ; SCO, subcommissural organ; CP, choroid plexus. (Adapted from Weindl A. Neuroendocrine aspects of circumventricular organs. In: Ganong WF, Martini L, eds. *Frontiers in Neuroendocrinology*, vol 3. New York, NY: Oxford University Press, 1973:3-32.)

accumulation around the median eminence.[51,52] Moreover, leptin receptor messenger ribonucleic acid (mRNA) and leptin-induced gene expression are densely localized in the arcuate, ventromedial, dorsomedial, and ventral premammillary hypothalamic nuclei.[53] Leptin is an established mediator of body weight and neuroendocrine function that acts on several cell groups in the hypothalamus, including POMC neurons that reside in the arcuate nucleus.[15,53,54] Because POMC neurons are also found embedded within the median eminence, it is likely that the median eminence is involved in conveying information from humoral factors such as leptin to key hypothalamic regulatory neurons in the medial basal hypothalamus.[43]

Organum Vasculosum of the Lamina Terminalis and the Subfornical Organ

The OVLT and the SFO are located at the front wall of the third ventricle, the lamina terminalis. The OVLT and SFO lie, respectively, at the ventral and dorsal boundaries of the third ventricle (see Fig. 7-5).[47] Because it lies at the rostral and ventral tip of the third ventricle, the OVLT is surrounded by cell groups of the preoptic region of the hypothalamus. Like other CVOs, the OVLT is composed of neurons, glial cells, and tanycytes. Axon terminals containing several neuropeptides and neurotransmitters including GnRH, somatostatin, angiotensin, dopamine, norepinephrine, serotonin, acetylcholine, oxytocin, AVP, and TRH innervate the OVLT. In the rodent, neurons that contain GnRH surround the OVLT. In addition, the OVLT in the rat brain contains estrogen receptors, and the application of estrogen or electric stimulation at this site is capable of stimulating ovulation through GnRH-containing neurons that project to the median eminence, suggesting that the region regulates sexual behavior in the rat.[45]

The region of the hypothalamus that immediately surrounds the OVLT regulates a diverse array of autonomic processes. However, because the OVLT is potentially involved in the maintenance of so many processes, definitive studies ascribing specific functions to the OVLT are inherently difficult. For example, lesions of the OVLT and surrounding preoptic area led to altered febrile responses after immunologic stimulation and to disruptions in fluid and electrolyte balance, blood pressure, reproduction, and thermoregulation. Large lesions of the OVLT attenuated lipopolysaccharide-induced fever.[55] Consistent with this finding, it was demonstrated that receptors for prostaglandin E_2 are located within and immediately surrounding the OVLT.[56] Because prostaglandin E_2 is thought to be an obligate endogenous pyrogen, the OVLT may be a critical regulator of febrile responses.

The OVLT is also likely to be involved in sensing serum osmolality, because lesions of the OVLT attenuate AVP and oxytocin secretion in response to osmotic stimuli. In addition, hypertonic saline administration in rats induced c-Fos (a marker of neuronal activation) in OVLT neurons.[57] The efferent projections of the OVLT are not well defined because of the fundamental difficulty of injecting this small structure with specific neuroanatomic tracers without contaminating surrounding preoptic nuclei. However, the neurons in the OVLT apparently have a remarkably restricted range of projections that include the PVH and SON nuclei, the dorsomedial hypothalamic nucleus, and the lateral hypothalamic area (J.K. Elmquist, J.E. Sherin, and C.B. Saper, unpublished observations).

The SFO is located in the roof of the third ventricle below the fornix. This CVO critically regulates fluid homeostasis and contributes to blood pressure regulation.[47] Consistent with these functions, the SFO has receptors for angiotensin II and atrial natriuretic peptide.[49,58] In addition to expressing these key receptors, the SFO is thought to regulate fluid homeostasis because of its specific and massive projections to key hypothalamic regulatory sites. Notable among these are the inputs to oxytocin and AVP magnicellular neurons in the SON and PVH. Parvicellular neurons in the PVH concerned with neuroendocrine and autonomic control also receive innervation from the SFO. In addition, the SFO densely innervates the paramedian preoptic region of the hypothalamus (often known as the anteroventral third ventricular region) and other hypothalamic sites including the perifornical area of the lateral hypothalamus. A major cell group within the anteroventral third ventricular region is the median preoptic nucleus, which receives dense innervation from the SFO.[59] Several neuroanatomic studies have demonstrated that the median preoptic nucleus is a major source of afferents to the magnicellular neuroendocrine neurons in the PVH and SON.

In addition to the preceding neuroanatomic findings, physiologic evidence suggests that the SFO is critical in maintaining fluid balance. Simpson and Routtenberg reported that substances such as angiotensin II elicited drinking behavior when microinjected at low doses directly into the SFO.[60] Later studies demonstrated that SFO neurons have electrophysiologic responses to angiotensin II.[49] In addition, stimulation of the SFO elicited AVP secretion. Like the OVLT, the SFO expressed Fos after stimulation by hypertonic saline administration.[57] Therefore, the SFO provides dense direct and indirect innervation to the magnicellular neuroendocrine neurons in the PVH and SON that are critical in the maintenance of fluid balance and blood pressure.

Area Postrema

The area postrema lies at the caudal end of the fourth ventricle, adjacent to the nucleus of the solitary tract (see Fig. 7-5). In experimental animals such as the rat and mouse, it is a midline structure lying above the nucleus of the solitary tract.[48,61] However, in humans, the area postrema is a bilateral structure. Because the area postrema overlies the nucleus of the solitary tract, it also receives direct visceral afferent input from the glossopharyngeal nerve (including the carotid sinus nerve) and the vagus nerve. In addition, the area postrema receives direct input from several hypothalamic nuclei. The efferent projections of the area postrema include projections to the nucleus of the solitary tract, the ventral lateral medulla, and the parabrachial nucleus. Consistent with its role as a sensory organ, the area postrema is enriched with receptors for several neuropeptides, including glucagon-like peptide 1 and cholecystokinin.[62,63] It also contains chemosensory neurons including osmoreceptors.[47] The area postrema is thought to be critical in the detection of potential toxins and can induce vomiting in response to foreign substances. In fact, the area postrema is often referred to as the *chemoreceptor trigger zone*.[61]

The best-described physiologic role of the area postrema is the coordinated control of blood pressure.[47,48] The area postrema contains binding sites for angiotensin II, AVP, and atrial natriuretic peptide. Lesions of the area postrema in rats blunt the rise in blood pressure induced by angiotensin II.[64] Administration of angiotensin II induces the expression of Fos in neurons of the area postrema. This area has also been hypothesized to play a role in responding to inflammatory cytokines during the acute febrile response.

Subcommissural Organ

The SCO is located near the junction of the third ventricle and the cerebral aqueduct, below the posterior commissure and the pineal gland (see Fig. 7-5).[47] It is composed of specialized ependymal cells that secrete a highly glycosylated protein of unknown function. The secretion of this protein leads to aggregation and formation of the so-called Reissner's fibers.[50] The glycoproteins are extruded through the aqueduct, the fourth ventricle, and the spinal cord lumen to terminate in the caudal spinal canal. In humans, intracellular secretory granules are identifiable in the SCO, but Reissner's fibers are absent. The SCO secretion in humans is therefore presumed to be more soluble and to be absorbed directly from the CSF. Compared with other CVOs, the physiologic role of the SCO is largely unknown. Hypothesized roles for the SCO include clearance of substances from the CSF.[50]

PINEAL GLAND

Descartes called the pineal gland the "seat of the soul." A more contemporary, although less colorful, viewpoint is that the pineal integrates information encoded by light into coordinated secretions that underlie biologic rhythmicity.[65,66] The pineal gland is both an endocrine organ and a CVO; it is derived from cells located in the roof of the third ventricle and lies above the posterior commissure near the level of the habenular complex and the sylvian aqueduct. The gland is composed of two cell types, pinealocytes and interstitial (glial-like) cells. Histologic studies suggest that the pineal gland cells are secretory in nature, and indeed the pineal is the principal source of melatonin in mammals.

The pineal is an epithalamic structure and consists of primordial photoreceptive cells. The gland retains its light sensitivity in lower vertebrates such as fish and amphibians but lacks direct photosensitivity in mammals and has evolved as a strictly secretory organ in higher vertebrates. However, neuroanatomic studies have established that light-encoded information is relayed to the pineal by a polysynaptic pathway. This series of synapses ultimately results in innervation of the gland by noradrenergic sympathetic nerve terminals that are critical regulators of melatonin production and release. Specifically, retinal ganglion cells directly innervate the SCN of the hypothalamus through the retinohypothalamic tract.[67] The SCN in turn provides input to the dorsal parvicellular PVH, a key cell group in neuroendocrine and autonomic control. This pathway consists of direct and indirect intrahypothalamic projections.[68,69] The PVH in turn provides direct innervation to sympathetic preganglionic neurons in the intermediolateral cell column of the thoracic regions of the spinal cord.[70] Sympathetic preganglionic neurons innervate postganglionic neurons in the superior cervical ganglion[71] that ultimately supply the noradrenergic innervation to the pineal (see "Hypothalamic-Pituitary Unit"). This rather circuitous pathway represents the anatomic substrate for light to regulate the secretion of melatonin. In the absence of light input, the pineal gland rhythms persist but are not entrained to the external light-dark cycle.

The Pineal Is the Source of Melatonin

The predominant hormone secreted by the pineal gland is melatonin. However, the pineal contains other biogenic amines, peptides, and GABA. Pineal-derived melatonin is synthesized from tryptophan, through serotonin, with the rate-limiting step catalyzed by the enzyme arylalkylamine *N*-acetyltransferase (AANAT) (Fig. 7-6).[72,73] Hydroxyindole-*O*-methyltransferase (HIOMT) catalyzes the final step of melatonin synthesis. These enzymes are expressed in a pineal-specific manner; however, HIOMT is also expressed in the retina and in red blood cells. Melatonin plays a key role in regulating a myriad of circadian rhythms, and a fundamental principle of circadian biology is that the synthesis of melatonin is exquisitely controlled.[65] AANAT mRNA levels, AANAT activity, and melatonin synthesis and release are regulated in a circadian fashion and are entrained by the light-dark cycle, with darkness thought to be the most important signal.[66,72,73] Melatonin and AANAT levels

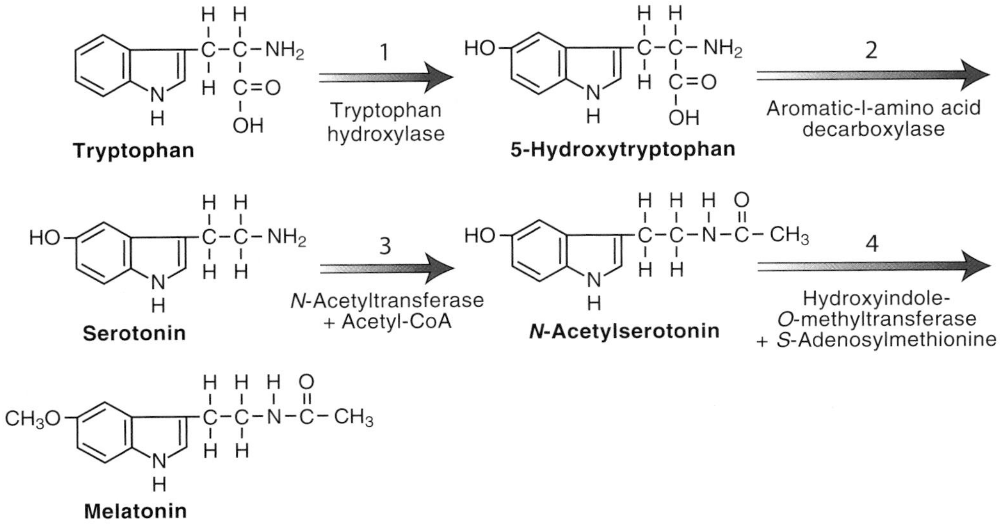

Tryptophan → 1 (Tryptophan hydroxylase) → 5-Hydroxytryptophan → 2 (Aromatic-l-amino acid decarboxylase) → Serotonin → 3 (*N*-Acetyltransferase + Acetyl-CoA) → *N*-Acetylserotonin → 4 (Hydroxyindole-*O*-methyltransferase + *S*-Adenosylmethionine) → Melatonin

Figure 7-6 Biosynthesis of melatonin from tryptophan in the pineal gland. Step 1 is catalyzed by tryptophan hydroxylase, step 2 by aromatic-L-amino acid decarboxylase, step 3 by arylalkylamine *N*-acetyltransferase, and step 4 by hydroxyindole-*O*-methyltransferase. (From Wurtman RJ, Axelrod J, Kelly DE. Biochemistry of the pineal gland. In: Wurtman RJ, Axelrod J, Kelly DE, eds. *The Pineal*. New York, NY: Academic Press, 1968:47-75.)

are highest during the dark and decrease sharply with the onset of light. Melatonin is not stored to any significant degree; it is released into blood or CSF directly after its biosynthesis in proportion to AANAT activity.

CNS control of melatonin secretion during the dark is mediated by the neuroanatomic pathway just outlined. Lack of light ultimately results in the release of norepinephrine from postganglionic sympathetic nerve terminals that act on β-adrenergic receptors in pinealocytes, resulting in an increase in adenylyl cyclase activity and synthesis of cyclic adenosine monophosphate (cAMP) from adenosine triphosphate.[72] Increased levels of intracellular cAMP activate downstream signal transduction cascades, including the catalytic subunits of protein kinase A and phosphorylation of cAMP response element (CRE) binding protein. CREs have been identified in the promoter of AANAT.[72,74] Therefore, light (or lack of it) acting through the sympathetic nervous system induces an increase in cAMP, representing a fundamental regulator of AANAT transcription and melatonin synthesis that ultimately results in a dramatic change of melatonin levels across the day.

Physiologic Roles of Melatonin

One of the best-characterized roles of melatonin is regulation of the reproductive axis, including gonadotropin secretion[75] and the timing and onset of puberty (see "Gonadotropin-Releasing Hormone and Control of the Reproductive Axis"). The potent regulation of the reproductive axis by melatonin is established in rodents and domestic animals such as the sheep. It was observed experimentally with the demonstration that removal of the pineal leads to precocious puberty. In addition, male rats exposed to constant darkness or blinded by enucleation display testicular atrophy and decreased levels of testosterone. These profound effects of gonadal involution are normalized by removal of the pineal gland.[76] The physiologic significance of melatonin is probably most important in species referred to as seasonal breeders. Indeed, the role of melatonin in regulating reproductive capacity in species such as the sheep and the horse is now established. This type of reproductive strategy probably evolved to synchronize the length of day with the gestational period of the species, to ensure that the offspring are born at favorable times of the year and to maximize the viability of the young. Interestingly, although there is a strong and consistent correlation between altered melatonin secretion, day length, and seasonal breeding in diverse species, the valence of the signal can be either positive or negative, depending on the ecologic niche of each species.

Despite the potent effects of day length on reproduction in these species, the exact mechanisms of melatonin regulation of GnRH release are unsettled. However, melatonin inhibits LH release from the rat pars tuberalis.[75] The role of the pineal in human reproduction is even less understood.[77] Earlier onset of menarche in blind women has been reported. In addition, a decline in melatonin at puberty has been described in some but not all studies.

Interspecies comparative studies of melatonin's physiologic function must be tempered by knowledge of key differences between rodent and human melatonin regulation. Significantly more light, as much as 4 log units, is required in humans to produce an equivalent nocturnal suppression of melatonin,[78] and the control of AANAT is largely post-transcriptional in humans, rather than transcriptional.[73]

Melatonin Receptors

Melatonin mediates its effects by acting on a family of G protein–coupled receptors that have been characterized by pharmacologic, neuroanatomic, and molecular approaches.[65,66,73] The first member of the family, MT1 (also called Mel_{1a} or melatonin receptor type 1A [MTNR1A]), is a high-affinity receptor that was isolated originally from *Xenopus* melanophores. The second, MT2 (Mel_{1b} or MTNR1B), has approximately 60% homology with MT1. A third receptor in mammals, MT3, is not a G protein–coupled receptor but instead a high-affinity binding site on the cytosolic enzyme quinone reductase 2 that is involved in cellular detoxification; this might explain some of melatonin's effects as an antioxidant.[66,73]

The mechanisms for melatonin's effects on regulating and entraining circadian rhythms are becoming increasingly understood. For example, melatonin inhibits the activity of neurons in the SCN of the hypothalamus, the master circadian pacemaker in the mammalian brain.[65,79,80] Melatonin can entrain several mammalian circadian rhythms, probably by inhibition of neurons in the SCN. Neuroanatomic evidence suggests that many of the effects of melatonin on circadian rhythms involve actions on MT1 receptors, in that the distribution of MT1 mRNA overlaps with radiolabeled melatonin-binding sites in the relevant brain regions. These sites include the SCN, the retina, and the pars tuberalis of the adenohypophysis. The MT2 receptor is also expressed in retina and brain, particularly in the SCN, but evidently at much lower levels.[65,73,79]

Genetic studies in mice have also helped to illuminate the relative roles of each melatonin receptor in mediating the effects of this hormone. Targeted deletion (knockout) of the MT1 but not the MT2 receptor abolished the ability of melatonin to inhibit the activity of SCN neurons.[80,81] Several studies have suggested that inhibition of SCN neurons by melatonin is of great physiologic significance. For example, Reppert and colleagues proposed that elevations of melatonin at night decrease the responsiveness of the SCN to activity-related stimuli that could result in phase shifts.[80] As noted, light potently inhibits melatonin synthesis and release. Therefore, melatonin may underlie the mechanism by which light induces phase shifts. However, it should be noted that lack of the MT1 gene does not block the ability of melatonin to induce phase shifts. These unexpected and somewhat confusing results have resulted in the hypothesis that MT2 is involved in melatonin-induced phase shifts, because this receptor is expressed in the SCN in human brain.[73]

Melatonin Therapy in Humans

Melatonin is purported to exert multiple beneficial functions that include slowing or reversing the progression of aging, protecting against ischemic damage after vascular reperfusion, and enhancing immune function.[66,73] However, the most studied and established role of melatonin in humans is that of phase shifting and resetting circadian rhythms. In this context, melatonin has been used to treat jet lag and may be effective in treating circadian-based sleep disorders.[82] In addition, melatonin administration has been shown to regulate sleep in humans. Specifically, melatonin has a hypnotic effect at relatively low doses. Melatonin therapy has also been suggested as a way to treat seasonal affective disorders. However, two recent meta-analyses of the published reports on melatonin for treatment of either primary or secondary sleep disorders concluded that there is limited evidence for significant clinical efficacy, although melatonin is safe with short-term use (≤3 months).[83,84] Because melatonin is now available over the counter and without a prescription throughout the United States, it is important that further controlled clinical studies be conducted to assess fully the therapeutic potential and safety of long-term melatonin use in humans.

HYPOPHYSEOTROPIC HORMONES AND NEUROENDOCRINE AXES

With the demonstration by the first half of the 1900s that pituitary secretion is controlled by hypothalamic hormones released into the portal circulation, the race was on to identify the hypothalamic releasing factors. The search for hypothalamic neurohormones with anterior pituitary–regulating properties focused on extracts of stalk median eminence, neural lobe, and hypothalamus from sheep and pigs. To give some idea of the herculean nature of this effort, approximately 250,000 hypothalamic fragments were required to purify and characterize the first such factor, TRH.[9] Such hypophyseotropic substances were initially called *releasing factors* but are now more commonly called *releasing hormones*.

All of the principal hypothalamic-pituitary regulating hormones are peptides, with the notable exception of dopamine, which is a biogenic amine and the major prolactin-inhibiting factor (PIF; see later discussion and Table 7-2). All are available for clinical investigations or diagnostic tests, and therapeutic analogues for dopamine, GnRH, and somatostatin are widely prescribed.

In addition to regulating hormone release, some hypophyseotropic factors control pituitary cell differentiation and proliferation and hormone synthesis. Some act on more than one pituitary hormone. For example, TRH is a potent releaser of prolactin (PRL) and of TSH, and under some circumstances it releases corticotropin (ACTH) and growth hormone (GH). GnRH releases both LH and follicle-stimulating hormone (FSH). Somatostatin inhibits the secretion of GH, TSH, and a wide variety of nonpituitary hormones. The principal inhibitor of PRL secretion, dopamine, also inhibits secretion of TSH, gonadotropin, and, under certain conditions, GH. Dual control is exerted by the interaction of inhibitory and stimulatory hypothalamic hormones. For example, somatostatin interacts with GHRH and TRH to control secretion of GH and TSH, respectively, and dopamine interacts with prolactin-releasing factors (PRFs) to regulate PRL secretion. Some hypothalamic hormones act synergistically; for example, CRH and AVP cooperatively regulate the release of pituitary ACTH.

Secretion of the releasing hormones in turn is regulated by neurotransmitters and neuropeptides released by a complex array of neurons synapsing with hypophyseotropic neurons. Control of secretion is also exerted through feedback control by hormones such as glucocorticoids, gonadal steroids, thyroid hormone, anterior pituitary hormones (short-loop feedback control), and hypophyseotropic factors themselves (ultrashort-loop feedback control).

The distribution of the hypophyseotropic hormones is not limited to the hypothalamus. Most are produced in nonhypophyseotropic hypothalamic neurons, in extrahypothalamic regions of the brain, and in peripheral organs where they mediate functions unrelated to pituitary regulation (e.g., effects on behavior or homeostasis). Most of the peptides, hormones, and neurotransmitters involved in the regulation of hypothalamic-pituitary control transduce their signals through members of the extensive G protein–coupled receptor family (Table 7-3).

Feedback Concepts in Neuroendocrinology

To understand the regulation of each hypothalamic-pituitary–target organ axis, it is important to understand some basic concepts of homeostatic systems. A simplified account of feedback control in relation to neuroendocrine regulation is presented here.[85-87] Hormonal systems form part of a feedback loop in which the controlled variable (usually the blood hormone level or some biochemical surrogate of the hormone) determines the rate of secretion of the hormone. In negative feedback systems, the controlled variable inhibits hormone output, and in positive feedback control systems it increases hormone secretion. Both negative and positive endocrine feedback control systems can be part of a closed loop, in which regulation is entirely restricted to the interacting regulatory glands, or an open loop, in which the nervous system influences the feedback loop. All pituitary feedback systems have nervous system inputs that either alter the set point of the feedback control system or introduce open-loop elements that can influence or override the closed-loop control elements.

In engineering formulations of feedback, three types of controlled variables can be identified: a sensing element that detects the concentration of the controlled variable, a reference input that defines the proper control levels, and an error signal that determines the output of the system. The reference input is the set point of the system.

Hormonal feedback control systems resemble engineering systems in that the concentration of the hormone in the blood (or some function of the hormone) regulates the output of the controlling gland. However, hormonal feedback differs from engineering systems in that the sensor element and the reference input element are not readily distinguishable. The set point of the controlled variable is determined by a complex cascade beginning with the kinetics of binding to a receptor and the activities of successive intermediate messengers. Sophisticated models incorporating control elements, compartmental analysis, and hormone production and clearance rates exist for many systems. This sort of modeling, which is applied to developmental programming, intracellular signaling cascades, and neural circuits in addition to endocrine feedback systems, is commonly referred to as *systems biology*.[88]

Endocrine Rhythms

Virtually all functions of living animals (regardless of their position on the evolutionary scale) are subject to periodic or cyclic changes, many of which are influenced primarily by the nervous system (Table 7-4).[89-92] Most periodic changes are free-running; that is, they are intrinsic to the organism, independent of the environment, and driven by a biologic "clock."

Most free-running rhythms are coordinated (entrained) by external signals (cues), such as light-dark changes, meal patterns, cycles of the lunar periods, or the ratio of day-length to night-length. External signals of this type (*zeitgeber,* or "time givers") do not bring about the rhythm but provide the synchronizing time cue. Many endogenous rhythms have a period of approximately 24 hours. Circadian changes follow an intrinsic program that is about 24 hours long, whereas diurnal rhythms can be either circadian or dependent on shifts in light and dark. Rhythms that occur more frequently than once a day are ultradian. Infradian rhythms have a period longer than 1 day, as in

TABLE 7-3

Receptors for Neurotransmitters and Neuropeptides Involved in Hypothalamic-Pituitary Control and Neuroendocrine Homeostasis

Group and Ligand	Receptor Family	Receptor Protein*	Receptor Gene	Mode of Action†
Classic Neurotransmitters				
Catecholamines (norepinephrine, epinephrine)	α_1-Adrenoreceptors	ADA1A (α1A)	ADRA1A	7-TM, $G_{q/11}$
		ADA1B (α1B)	ADRA1B	7-TM, $G_{q/11}$
		ADA1D (α1D)	ADRA1D	7-TM, $G_{q/11}$
	α_2-Adrenoreceptors	ADA2A (α2A)	ADRA2A	7-TM, $G_{i/o}$
		ADA2B (α2B)	ADRA2B	7-TM, $G_{i/o}$
		ADA2C (α2C)	ADRA2C	7-TM, $G_{i/o}$
	β-Adrenoreceptors	ADRB1 (β1)	ADRB1	7-TM, G_S
		ADRB2 (β2)	ADRB2	7-TM, G_S
		ADRB3 (β3)	ADRB3	7-TM, G_S
Serotonin (5-HT)	5-HT1 receptors	5HT1A (5HT1A-α)	HTR1A	7-TM, $G_{i/o}$
		5HT1B (5HT1D-β)	HTR1B	7-TM, $G_{i/o}$
		5HT1D (5HT1D-α)	HTR1D	7-TM, $G_{i/o}$
		5HT1E	HTR1E	7-TM, $G_{i/o}$
	5-HT2 receptors	5HT2A	HTR2A	7-TM, $G_{q/11}$
		5HT2B	HTR2B	7-TM, $G_{q/11}$
		5HT2C (5HT1C)	HTR2C	7-TM, $G_{q/11}$
	5-HT3 receptors	5HT3	Pentamer	Cation flux
		Subunit genes	HTR3A, HTR3B	
	5-HT4 receptors	5HT4R	HTR4	7-TM, G_S
Dopamine	Dopamine receptors	DRD1 (D1-R, D1A)	DRD1	7-TM, G_S
		DRD2 (D2-R)	DRD2	7-TM, $G_{i/o}$
		DRD3 (D3-R)	DRD3	7-TM, $G_{i/o}$
		DRD4 (D4-R, D2C)	DRD4	7-TM, $G_{i/o}$
		DRD5 (D5-R, D1B)	DRD5	7-TM, G_S
Histamine	Histamine receptors	HRH1 (H1-R)	HRH1	7-TM, $G_{q/11}$
		HRH2 (H2-R)	HRH2	7-TM, G_S
		HRH3 (H3-R)	HRH3	7-TM, $G_{i/o}$
Melatonin	Melatonin receptors	MT1RA (Mel1AR, MT1)	MTNR1A	7-TM, $G_{i/o}$, PLC-β
		MT1RB (Mel1BR, MT2)	MTNR1B	7-TM, $G_{i/o}$, $G_{q/11}$
		MT3 (quinone reductase 2)	NQO2	Cytosolic enzyme
Trace amines	Trace amine receptor	TAAR1 (TaR-1)	TAAR1	7-TM, G_S
Acetylcholine	Muscarinic receptors	ACM1 (M1)	CHRM1	7-TM, $G_{q/11}$
		ACM2 (M2)	CHRM2	7-TM, $G_{q/11}$
		ACM3 (M3)	CHRM3	7-TM, $G_{q/11}$
		ACM4 (M4)	CHRM4	7-TM, $G_{i/o}$
		ACM5 (M5)	CHRM5	7-TM, $G_{q/11}$
	Nicotinic receptors	ACHA-P, ACH1-7	Pentamer	Cation flux
		Subunit genes	CHRNA, CHRNB	
Glutamate	Ionotropic receptors	NMDA (NR1, NR2A-D)	Oligomer	Cation flux
		NMZ1 subunit gene	GRIN1 (NMDAR1)	
		AMPA (GluR1-4)	Oligomer	Cation flux
		GRIA1 subunit gene	GRIA1 (GLUR1)	
		Kainate (GluR5-7, KA-1/2)	Oligomer	Cation flux
		LK1 subunit gene	GRIK1 (GLUR5)	
	Metabotropic receptors	MGR1 (mGluR1)	GRM1	7-TM, $G_{q/11}$
		MGR2 (mGluR2)	GRM2	7-TM, $G_{i/o}$
		MGR3 (mGluR3)	GRM3	7-TM, $G_{i/o}$
		MGR4 (mGluR4)	GRM4	7-TM, $G_{i/o}$
		MGR5 (mGluR5)	GRM5	7-TM, $G_{q/11}$
		MGR6 (mGluR6)	GRM6	7-TM, $G_{i/o}$
		MGR7 (mGluR7)	GRM7	7-TM, $G_{i/o}$
γ-Aminobutyric acid (GABA)	Ionotropic	GAA-E (GABA-A-R)	Pentamer	[Cl^-] ion flux
		GAA1 (α1) subunit gene	GABRA1	
	Heterodimeric	GABR1 (GABA-B-R1)	GABBR1	7-TM, $G_{i/o}$
		GABR2 (GABA-B-R2)	GABBR2	7-TM, $G_{i/o}$

TABLE 7-3

Receptors for Neurotransmitters and Neuropeptides Involved in Hypothalamic-Pituitary Control and Neuroendocrine Homeostasis (Continued)

Group and Ligand	Receptor Family	Receptor Protein*	Receptor Gene	Mode of Action†
Neuropeptides				
Neurohypophyseal hormones				
Vasopressin (AVP)	Vasopressin receptors	V1AR (V1a)	AVPR1A	7-TM, $G_{q/11}$
		V1BR (V1b, V3)	AVPR1B	7-TM, $G_{q/11}$
		V2R (ADH-R)	AVPR2	7-TM, G_S
Oxytocin	Oxytocin receptor	OXYR (OT-R)	OXTR	7-TM, $G_{q/11}$
Hypophyseotropic hormones				
Thyrotropin-releasing hormone (TRH)	TRH receptor	TRFR (TRH-R)	TRHR	7-TM, $G_{q/11}$
Growth hormone–releasing hormone (GHRH)	GHRH receptor	GHRHR (GRFR)	GHRHR	7-TM, G_S
GHRP/Ghrelin	GHS receptor	GHSR (GHRP-R)	GHSR	7-TM, $G_{q/11}$
Gonadotropin-releasing hormone (GnRH)	GnRH receptor	GNRHR (GnRH-R)	GNRHR	7-TM, $G_{q/11}$
Corticotropin-releasing hormone (CRH)/Urocortin	CRH receptors	CRFR1 (CRH-R1)	CRHR1	7-TM, G_S
		CRFR2 (CRH-R2)	CRHR2	7-TM, G_S
Somatostatin/Cortistatin	Somatostatin receptors	SSR1 (SS1R, SRIF-2)	SSTR1	7-TM, $G_{i/o}$
		SSR2 (SS2R, SRIF-1)	SSTR2	7-TM, $G_{i/o}$
		SSR3 (SS3R, SSR-28)	SSTR3	7-TM, $G_{i/o}$
		SSR4 (SS4R)	SSTR4	7-TM, $G_{i/o}$
		SSR5 (SS5R)	SSTR5	7-TM, $G_{i/o}$
Endogenous opioid peptides				
β-Endorphin	Mu opioid receptor	OPRM (μ, MOR-1)	OPRM1	7-TM, $G_{i/o}$
Enkephalin	Delta opioid receptor	OPRD (δ, DOR-1)	OPRD1	7-TM, $G_{i/o}$
Dynorphin	Kappa opioid receptor	OPRK (κ, KOR-1)	OPRK1	7-TM, $G_{i/o}$
Nociceptin/OFQ	OFQ opioid receptor	OPRX (KOR-3)	OPRL1	7-TM, $G_{i/o}$
Melanocortin peptides				
Melanocyte–stimulating hormone (MSH)	MSH receptor	MSHR (MC1-R)	MC1R	7-TM, G_S
Corticotropin (ACTH)	ACTH receptor	ACTHR (MC2-R)	MC2R	7-TM, G_S
γ-MSH, α-MSH	Melanocortin receptor 3	MC3R (MC3-R)	MC3R	7-TM, G_S
α-MSH, β-MSH	Melanocortin receptor 4	MC4R (MC4-R)	MC4R	7-TM, G_S
α-MSH	Melanocortin receptor 5	MC5R (MC5-R)	MC5R	7-TM, G_S
Tachykinins (neurokinins)				
Substance P	Neurokinin receptors	NK1R (SPR)	TACR1	7-TM, $G_{i/o}$
Substance K		NK2R (SKR)	TACR2	7-TM, $G_{i/o}$
Neurokinin B (NKB)		NK3R (NKR)	TACR3	7-TM, $G_{i/o}$
Vasoactive peptides				
Angiotensin II	Angiotensin receptors	AGTR1 (AT1)	AGTR1	7-TM, $G_{q/11}$
		AGTR2 (AT2)	AGTR2	7-TM, $G_{i/o}$
Atrial natriuretic peptide (ANP)	ANP receptors	ANPRA (NPR-A)	NPR1	cGMP, 1-TM
		ANPRB (NPR-B)	NPR2	cGMP, 1-TM
Endothelin	Endothelin receptors	ENDRA (ETA-R)	EDNRA	7-TM, $G_{q/11}$
		ENDRB (ETB-R)	EDNRB	7-TM, $G_{q/11}$
Miscellaneous neuropeptides				
CART	No receptor identified			7-TM, $G_{i/o}$
Orexin/hypocretin	Orexin receptors	OX1R (HCRTR-1)	HCRTR1	7-TM, many
		OX2R (HCRTR-2)	HCRTR2	7-TM, many
Melanin-concentrating hormone (MCH)	MCH receptor	MCHR1 (GPCR24)	MCHR1	7-TM, $G_{i/q}$
Prolactin-releasing peptide (PrRP)	PrRP receptor	PRLHR (GPCR10)	PRLHR	7-TM, $G_{i/o/q}$
Kisspeptins/Metastin	Kisspeptin receptor	KISSR (GPCR54)	KISS1R	7-TM, $G_{q/11}$
Neuromedin U	Neuromedin receptors	NMUR1 (GPCR66)	NMUR1	7-TM, $G_{q/11}$
		NMUR2	NMUR2	7-TM, $G_{q/11}$
Neurotensin	Neurotensin receptor	NTR1 (NTRH)	NTSR1	7-TM, $G_{q/11}$
PACAP	PACAP receptor	PACR (PACAP-R-1)	ADCYAR1R1	7-TM, G_S
Vasoactive intestinal peptide (VIP)	VIP receptors	VIPR1 (PACAP-R-2)	VIPR1	7-TM, G_S
		VIPR2 (PACAP-R-3)	VIPR3	7-TM, G_S
Galanin/GALP	Galanin receptors	GALR1 (GAL1-R)	GALR1	7-TM, $G_{i/o}$
		GALR2 (GAL2-R)	GALR2	7-TM, $G_{i/o}$
		GALR3 (GAL3-R)	GALR3	7-TM, $G_{i/o}$

Table continued on following page

TABLE 7-3

Receptors for Neurotransmitters and Neuropeptides Involved in Hypothalamic-Pituitary Control and Neuroendocrine Homeostasis (Continued)

Group and Ligand	Receptor Family	Receptor Protein*	Receptor Gene	Mode of Action†
Glucagon-like peptide (GLP)	GLP receptor	GLP1R	GLP1R	7-TM, G_S
Cholecystokinin (CCK)/Gastrin	CCK receptors	CCKAR (CCK1-R)	CCKAR	7-TM, $G_{q/11}$
		GASR (CCK2-R)	CCKBR	7-TM, $G_{q/11}$
Neuropeptide Y (NPY)	NPY/PYY/PP receptors	NPY1R (NPY-Y1)	NPY1R	7-TM, $G_{i/o}$
Peptide YY (PYY^{3-32})		NPY2R (NPY-Y2)	NPY2R	7-TM, $G_{i/o}$
Pancreatic polypeptide (PP)		NPY4R (PP1)	PPYR1	7-TM, $G_{i/o}$
Neuropeptide Y		NPY5R (NPY-Y5)	NPY5R	7-TM, $G_{i/o}$
Other				
Cannabinoid	Cannabinoid receptor	CNR1 (CB1)	CNR1	7-TM, $G_{i/o}$

*Receptors cited are human. Swiss-Prot identifiers and alternative names (in parentheses) are provided for each receptor and were obtained with the use of the GPCRDB information system (available at http://www.gpcr.org/7tm/) described in Horn F, Bettler E, Oliveira L, et al. GPCRDB information system for G protein-coupled receptors. *Nucleic Acids Res.* 2003;31:294-297.

†The mode of action designation is oversimplified. It is common for 7-TM GPCRs to interact with multiple different G-protein complexes depending on the specific cell. $G_{i/o}$, GPCR coupled to the $G_{i/o}$ family, inhibits adenylyl cyclase and decreases intracellular cAMP, opens K^+ channels and closes $Ca2^+$ channels; $G_{q/11}$, GPCR coupled to the $G_{q/11}$ family, stimulates the phosphoinositol cascade; G_S, GPCR coupled to the G_S family, stimulates adenylyl cyclase and increases intracellular cAMP; PLC-β, GPCR coupled to G protein that activates phospholipase Cβ (PLC-β); cGMP, guanylate cyclase activity intrinsic to these 1 transmembrane pass receptors.

AMPA, α-amino-3-hydroxy-5-methyl-4-isoxazdeproprionic acid; cAMP, cyclic adenosine monophosphate; CART, cocaine- and amphetamine-responsive transcript; GALP, galanin-like peptide; (GPCR) G protein–coupled receptor; GHS, growth hormone secretagogue; NMDA, *N*-methyl-D-aspartate; OFQ, orphanin FQ; PACAP, pituitary adenylyl cyclase activating peptide; TM, transmembrane.

the approximately 27-day human menstrual cycle and the yearly breeding patterns of some animals.

Most endocrine rhythms are circadian (Fig. 7-7). The secretion of GH and PRL in humans is maximal shortly after the onset of sleep, and that of cortisol is maximal between 2 a.m. and 4 a.m. TSH secretion is lowest in the morning, between 9 a.m. and 12 noon, and maximal between 8 p.m. and midnight. Gonadotropin secretion in adolescents is increased at night. Superimposed on the circadian cycle are ultradian bursts of hormone secretion. LH secretion during adolescence is characterized by rapid, high-amplitude pulsations at night, whereas in sexually mature individuals secretory episodes are lower in amplitude and occur throughout the 24 hours. GH, ACTH, and PRL are also secreted in brief, fairly regular pulses. The short-term fluctuations in hormonal secretion have important functional significance. In the case of LH, the normal endogenous rhythm of pituitary secretion reflects the pulsatile release of GnRH. The period of approximately 90 minutes between LH peaks corresponds to the optimal timing of GnRH pulses to induce maximal pituitary stimulation. Episodic secretion of GH also enhances its biopotency, but for many rhythms, the function is not clear. Most homeostatic activities are rhythmic, including body temperature, water balance, blood volume, sleep, and activity.[93,94]

TABLE 7-4

Terms Used to Describe Cyclic Endocrine Phenomena

Period	Length of the cycle
Circadian	About a day (24 hr)
Diurnal	Exactly a day
Ultradian	Less than a day (i.e., minutes or hours)
Infradian	Longer than a day (i.e., month or year)
Mean	Arithmetic mean of all values within a cycle
Range	Difference between the highest and lowest values
Nadir	Minimal level (inferred from mathematical curve fitting calculations)
Acrophase	Time of maximal levels (inferred from curve fitting)
Zeitgeber	"Time-giver" (German); the external cue, usually the light-dark cycle that synchronizes endogenous rhythms
Entrainment	The process by which an endogenous rhythm is regulated by a zeitgeber
Phase shift	Induced change in an endogenous rhythm
Intrinsic clock	Neural structures that possess intrinsic capacity for spontaneous rhythms; for circadian rhythms, these are located in the suprachiasmatic nucleus

(Adapted from Van Cauter E, Turek FW. Endocrine and other biological rhythms. In DeGroot LJ, ed. *Endocrinology,* 3rd ed. Philadelphia, PA: Saunders, 1995:2497-2548).

Assessment of endocrine function must take into account the variability of hormone levels in the blood. Appropriately obtained samples at different times of day or night may provide useful dynamic indicators of hypothalamic-pituitary function. For example, the loss of diurnal rhythm of GH and ACTH secretion may be an early sign of hypothalamic dysfunction. The optimal timing for administration of glucocorticoids to suppress ACTH secretion (e.g., in therapy for congenital adrenal hyperplasia) must take into account the varying suppressibility of the axis at different times of day.

The best understood neural structures responsible for circadian rhythms are the SCN, paired structures in the anterior hypothalamus above the optic chiasm.[90,94] In addition to the retinohypothalamic projection from the retina described earlier, the SCN receives neuronal input from many nuclei. Individual cells of the SCN have an intrinsic capacity to oscillate in a circadian pattern,[95] and the nucleus is organized to permit many reciprocal neuron-neuron interactions through direct synaptic contacts. It is especially rich in neuropeptides, including somatostatin, VIP, NPY, and neurotensin. Microinjections of pancreatic polypeptide into the SCN reset the timing cycle of some circadian rhythms in hamsters. The SCN also responds to the pineal hormone melatonin through melatonin receptors.[66,73] Studies have indicated that intrinsic pacemaker

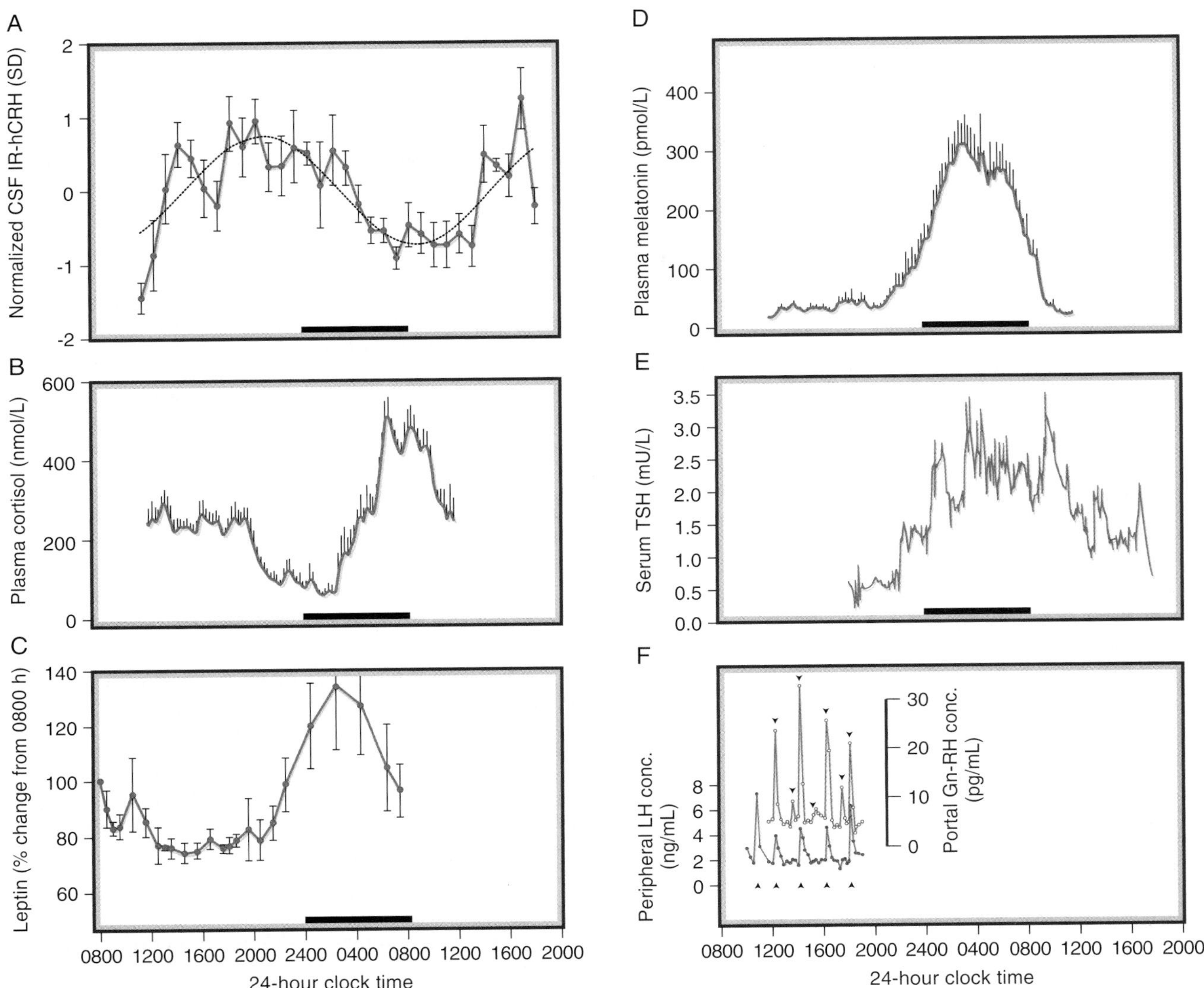

Figure 7-7 Diurnal rhythms of secretion. Secretion of human corticotropin-releasing hormone (hCRH). **A**, Cortisol; **B**, leptin; **C**, melatonin; **D**, and **E**, thyrotropin (TSH). Vertical lines indicate standard deviations (SD). **F**, Relationship between secretion of gonadotropin-releasing hormone (GnRH; *open circles*) and that of luteinizing hormone (LH; *filled circles*) in sheep. CSF, cerebrospinal fluid; IR, immunoreactive. (From Kling MA, DeBellis MD, O'Rourke DK, et al. Diurnal variation of cerebrospinal fluid immunoreactive corticotropin-releasing hormone levels in healthy volunteers. *J Clin Endocrinol Metab.* 1994;79:233-239, Fig. 3; van Coevorden A, Mockel J, Laurent E, et al. Neuroendocrine rhythms and sleep in aging men. *Am J Physiol.* 1991;260:E651-E661, Fig. 1A and C; Sinha MK, Ohannesian JP, Heiman ML, et al. Nocturnal rise of leptin in lean, obese, and non-insulin-dependent diabetes mellitus subjects. *J Clin Invest.* 1996;97:1344-1347, Fig. 2; Brabant G, Prank K, Ranft U, et al. Physiological regulation of circadian and pulsatile thyrotropin secretion in normal man and woman. *J Clin Endocrinol Metab.* 1990;70:403-409, Fig. 2B; and Clarke IJ, Cummins JT. The temporal relationship between gonadotropin releasing hormone [GnRH] and luteinizing hormone [LH] secretion in ovariectomized ewes. *Endocrinology.* 1982;111:1737-1739, Fig. 2A.)

function is not unique to neurons of the SCN; circadian oscillators are also found in many peripheral tissues.[94]

Metabolic changes in the SCN, such as increased uptake of 2-deoxyglucose and an increased level of VIP, accompany circadian rhythms. This nucleus projects to the pineal gland indirectly via the PVH and the autonomic nervous system (see earlier discussion) and regulates its activity.[90] However, the bulk of SCN outflow occurs in a trunk that courses dorsolaterally through the ventral subparaventricular zone and terminates in the dorsal medial hypothalamic nucleus. Polysynaptic pathways involving these latter structures are responsible for the actions of the SCN in producing the circadian rhythms in thermoregulation, glucocorticoid secretion, sleep, arousal, and feeding.[90]

Circadian rhythms during fetal life are regulated by maternal circadian rhythms.[96] Circadian changes can be detected 2 to 3 days before birth, and SCN from fetuses of this age display spontaneous rhythmicity in vitro. Maternal regulation of fetal circadian rhythms may be mediated by circulating melatonin or by cyclic changes in the food intake of the mother. The timing of the circadian pacemaker can be shifted in humans by administration of triazolam (a short-acting benzodiazepine) or melatonin (described earlier) or by altered patterns of intense illumination.[78]

Thyrotropin-Releasing Hormone

Chemistry and Evolution

TRH, the smallest known peptide hypophyseotropic hormone, is the tripeptide pyroGlu-His-Pro-NH_2. Six copies

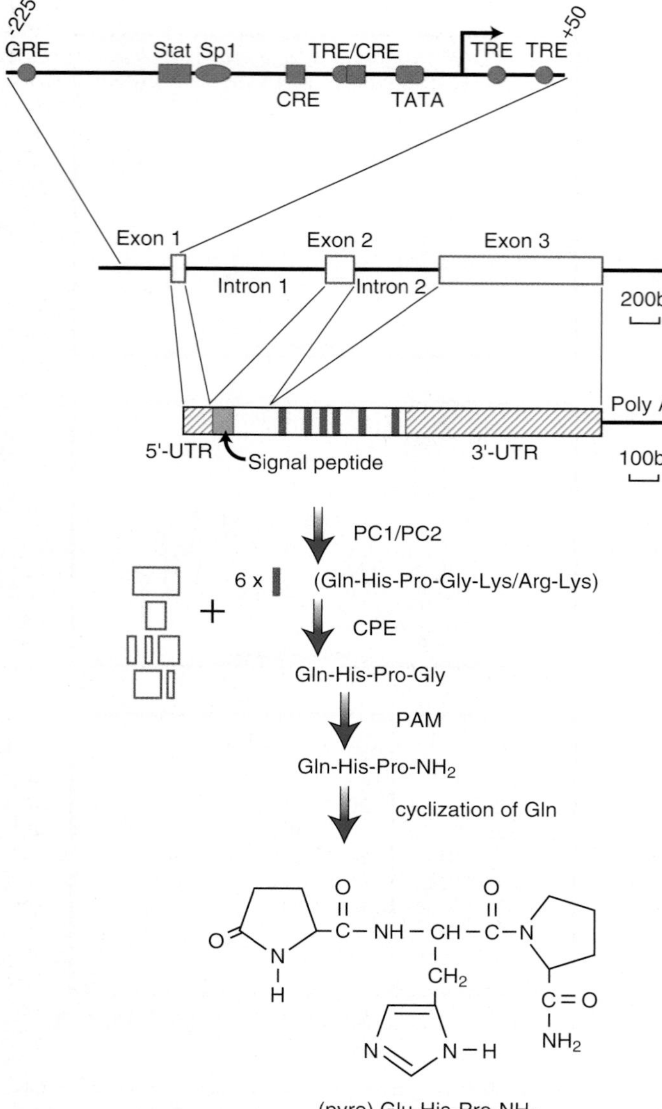

Figure 7-8 Structure of the human thyrotropin-releasing hormone (TRH) gene, complementary DNA, and prohormone, showing six repeats of the TRH peptide sequence encoded within exon 3. CPE, carboxypeptidase E; CRE, cyclic adenosine monophosphate (cAMP) response element; GRE, glucocorticoid response element; PAM, peptidylglycine α-amidating monooxygenase; PC1/PC2, prohormone convertases 1 and 2; Sp1, specificity protein 1 binding sequence; Stat, signal transducer and activator of transcription binding sequence; TATA, Goldstein-Hogness box involved in binding RNA polymerase; TRE, thyroid hormone response element; UTR, untranslated. (Adapted from data in Yamada M, Radovick S, Wondisford FE, et al. Cloning and structure of human genomic DNA and hypothalamic cDNA encoding human preprothyrotropin-releasing hormone. *Mol Endocrinol.* 1990;4:551-556.)

of the TRH peptide sequence are encoded within the human TRH pre-prohormone gene (Fig. 7-8).[97] The rat pro-TRH precursor contains five TRH peptide repeats flanked by dibasic residues (Lys-Arg or Arg-Arg), along with seven or more non-TRH peptides.[98] Two prohormone convertases, PC1 and PC2, cleave the TRH tripeptides at the dibasic residues as the prohormone molecule transits the regulated secretory pathway. Carboxypeptidase E then removes the dibasic residues, leaving the sequence Gln-His-Pro-Gly. This peptide is then amidated at the carboxy terminus by peptidylglycine α-amidating monooxygenase (PAM), with Gly acting as the amide donor. The amino-terminal pyro-glutamate (pyroGlu) residue results from cyclization of the Gln.

TRH is a phylogenetically ancient peptide that has been isolated from primitive vertebrates such as the lamprey and even from invertebrates such as the snail. TRH is widely expressed in both the CNS and periphery in amphibians, reptiles, and fishes but does not stimulate TSH release in these poikilothermic vertebrates. Therefore, TRH has multiple peripheral and central activities and was co-opted as a hypophyseotropic factor midway during the evolution of vertebrates, perhaps specifically as a factor needed for coordinated regulation of temperature homeostasis.

Although the TRH tripeptide is the only established hormone encoded within its large prohormone, rat pro-TRH yields seven additional peptides that have unique tissue distributions.[99] Several biologic activities of these peptides have been observed. The fragment pro-TRH(160-169) may be a hypophyseotropic factor because it is released from hypothalamic slices and potentiates the TSH-releasing effects of TRH. The pro-TRH(178-199) is also released from the median eminence and appears to inhibit ACTH release.

Effects on the Pituitary Gland and Mechanism of Action

After intravenous injection of TRH in humans, serum TSH levels rise within a few minutes,[100] followed by a rise in serum triiodothyronine (T_3) levels. There is an increase in thyroxine (T_4) release as well, but a change in blood levels of T_4 is usually not demonstrable because the pool of circulating T_4 (most of which is bound to carrier proteins) is so large. The clinical applications of TRH testing are covered later in this chapter and in Chapter 11. TRH action on the pituitary is blocked by previous treatment with thyroid hormone, which is a crucial element in the feedback control of pituitary TSH secretion.

TRH is also a potent PRF.[100] The time course of response of blood PRL levels to TRH, the dose-response characteristics, and the suppression by thyroid hormone pretreatment (all of which parallel changes in TSH secretion) suggest that TRH may be involved in the regulation of PRL secretion. Moreover, TRH is present in the hypophyseal-portal blood of lactating rats. However, it is unlikely to be a physiologic regulator of PRL secretion, because the PRL response to nursing in humans is unaccompanied by changes in plasma TSH levels,[101] and mice lacking TRH have normal lactotrophs and normal basal PRL secretion.[102] Nevertheless, TRH may occasionally cause hyperprolactinemia (with or without galactorrhea) in patients with hypothyroidism.

In normal individuals, TRH has no influence on the secretion of pituitary hormones other than TSH and PRL, but it enhances the release of GH in patients with acromegaly and of ACTH in some patients with Cushing's disease. Furthermore, prolonged stimulation of the normal pituitary with GHRH can sensitize it to the GH-releasing effects of TRH. TRH also causes the release of GH in some patients with uremia, hepatic disease, anorexia nervosa, or psychotic depression and in children with hypothyroidism.[100] TRH inhibits sleep-induced GH release through its actions in the CNS (see later discussion).

Stimulatory effects of TRH are initiated by binding of the peptide to specific receptors on the plasma membrane of the thyrotroph.[103] Thyroid hormone and somatostatin antagonize the effects of TRH but do not interfere with its binding. TRH action is mediated mainly through hydrolysis of phosphatidylinositol, with phosphorylation of key protein kinases and an increase in intracellular free calcium (Ca^{2+}) as the crucial steps in postreceptor activation (see Chapter 5).[104] TRH effects can be mimicked by exposure to a Ca^{2+} ionophore and are partially abolished by a Ca^{2+}-free medium. TRH stimulates the formation of mRNAs coding for TSH and PRL, in addition to regulating their secretion and stimulates the mitogenesis of thyrotrophs.

TRH is degraded to acid TRH and to the dipeptide histidylprolineamide, which cyclizes nonenzymatically to histidylproline diketopiperazine (cyclic His-Pro). Acid TRH has some behavioral effects in rats that are similar to those of TRH but no other proven actions. Cyclic His-Pro is reported to act as a PRF and to have other neural effects, including reversal of ethanol-induced sleep (TRH is also effective in this system), elevation of brain cyclic guanosine monophosphate levels, an increase in stereotypical behavior, modification of body temperature, and inhibition of eating behavior. Some of the effects of TRH may be mediated through cyclic His-Pro, but the fact that cyclic His-Pro is abundant in some areas and is not proportional to the amount of TRH suggests that the peptide may not be derived solely from TRH. This latter assertion appears to be confirmed by the detection of substantial amounts of the dipeptide in brains of TRH knockout mice.[102]

Extrapituitary Function

TRH is present in virtually all parts of the brain: cerebral cortex, CVOs, neurohypophysis, pineal gland, and spinal cord.[105] TRH is also found in pancreatic islet cells and in the gastrointestinal tract. Although it exists in low concentration, the total amount in extrahypothalamic tissues exceeds the amount in the hypothalamus.

The extensive extrahypothalamic distribution of TRH, its localization in nerve endings, and the presence of TRH receptors in brain tissue suggest that TRH serves as a neurotransmitter or neuromodulator outside the hypothalamus.[106] TRH is a general stimulant and induces hyperthermia on intracerebroventricular injection, suggesting a role in central thermoregulation.[105] Studies in TRH knockout mice may further clarify the nonhypophyseotropic actions of TRH.[102]

Clinical Applications

The use of TRH for the diagnosis of hyperthyroidism has become less common since the development of ultrasensitive assays for TSH[100] (see Chapter 11). Use of TRH to discriminate between hypothalamic and pituitary causes of TSH deficiency has also declined because of the test's poor specificity,[100] but the application of ultrasensitive assays in conjunction with the TRH test has not been fully evaluated. TRH testing is also not of value in the differential diagnosis of causes of hyperprolactinemia, but it is useful for the demonstration of residual abnormal somatotropin-secreting cells in acromegalic patients who release GH in response to TRH before treatment.

Studies of the effect of TRH on depression have shown inconsistent results, possibly because of poor blood-brain barrier penetration.[105] Intrathecal administration of TRH may improve responses in depressed patients, but its clinical utility is unknown.[107] Although a role for TRH in depression is not established, many depressed patients have a blunted TSH response to TRH, and changes in TRH responsiveness correlate with the clinical course. The mechanism by which blunting occurs is unknown.

TRH has been evaluated for the treatment of diverse neurobiologic disorders (for review, see Gary and colleagues[105]) including spinal muscle atrophy and amyotrophic lateral sclerosis; transient improvement in strength was reported in both disorders, but the combined experience at many centers using a variety of treatment protocols including long-term intrathecal administration failed to confirm efficacy. TRH administration reduces the severity of experimentally induced spinal and ischemic shock; preliminary studies in humans suggest that TRH treatment may improve recovery after spinal cord injury and head trauma. TRH has been used to treat children with neurologic disorders including West's syndrome, Lennox-Gastaut syndrome, early infantile epileptic encephalopathy, and intractable epilepsy.[108] TRH has been proposed to be an analeptic agent. Sleeping or drug-sedated animals were awakened by the administration of TRH, TRH reportedly reversed sedative effects of ethanol in humans, and TRH is said to have awakened a patient with a profound sleep disorder caused by a hypothalamic and midbrain eosinophilic granuloma.[105]

Regulation of Thyrotropin Release

The secretion of TSH is regulated by two interacting elements: negative feedback by thyroid hormone and open-loop neural control by hypothalamic hypophyseotropic factors (Fig. 7-9). TSH secretion is also modified by other hormones, including estrogens, glucocorticoids, and possibly GH, and it is inhibited by cytokines in the pituitary and hypothalamus.[100,109] Aspects of the pituitary-thyroid axis are considered further in Chapter 11.

Feedback Control: Pituitary-Thyroid Axis

In the context of a feedback system, the level of thyroid hormone or of its unbound fraction in blood is the controlled variable, and the set point is the normal resting level of plasma thyroid hormone. Secretion of TSH is inversely regulated by the level of thyroid hormone so that deviations from the set point lead to appropriate changes in the rate of TSH secretion (Fig. 7-10). Factors that determine the rate of TSH secretion required to maintain a given level of thyroid hormone include the rate at which TSH and thyroid hormone disappear from the blood (turnover rate) and the rate at which T_4 is converted to its more active form, T_3.

Thyroid hormones act on both the pituitary and the hypothalamus. Feedback control of the pituitary by thyroid hormone is remarkably precise.[109a,109b] Administration of small doses of T_3 and T_4 inhibited the TSH response to TRH, and barely detectable decreases in plasma thyroid hormone levels were sufficient to sensitize the pituitary to TRH. TRH stimulates TSH secretion within a few minutes through its action on a membrane receptor, whereas thyroid hormone actions, mediated by intranuclear receptors, require several hours to take effect (see Chapter 11).

The secretion of hypothalamic TRH is also regulated by thyroid hormone feedback. Systemic injections of T_3 or implantations of tiny T_3 pellets in the PVH of hypothyroid rats[110] (Fig. 7-11A and B) reduced the concentration of TRH mRNA and TRH prohormone in TRH-secreting cells. Thyroid hormone also suppressed TRH secretion into hypophyseal-portal blood in sheep.

T_4 in the blood gains access to TRH-secreting neurons in the hypothalamus by way of the CSF. The hormone is taken up by epithelial cells of the choroid plexus of the lateral ventricle of the brain, bound within the cell to locally produced transthyretin (T_4-binding prealbumin), and then secreted across the blood-brain barrier.[111] Within the brain, T_4 is converted to T_3 by type II deiodinase, and T_3 interacts with subtypes of the thyroid hormone receptor ($TR\alpha_1$, $TR\beta_1$, and $TR\beta_2$) in the PVH and other brain cells

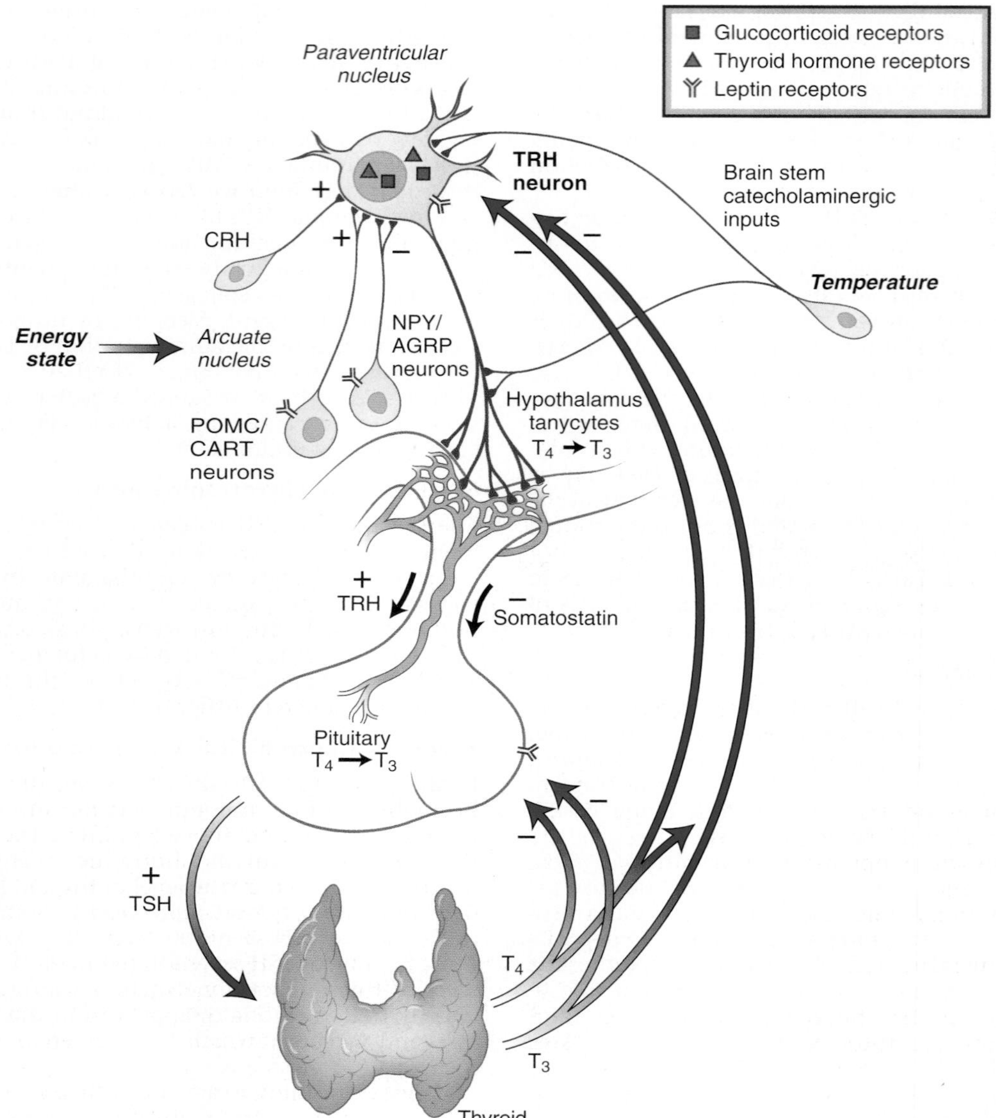

Figure 7-9 Regulation of the hypothalamic-pituitary-thyroid axis. AGRP, agouti-related peptide; CART, cocaine- and amphetamine-regulated transcript; CRH, corticotropin-releasing hormone; NPY, neuropeptide Y; POMC, pro-opiomelanocortin; T_3, triiodothyronine; T_4, thyroxine; TRH, thyrotropin-releasing hormone; TSH, thyrotropin.

(see Chapter 11). In this way, the set point of the pituitary-thyroid axis is determined by thyroid hormone levels within the brain.[112] T_3 in the circulation is not transported into brain in the same manner but presumably gains access to the paraventricular TRH neurons across the blood-brain barrier. The brain T_4 transport and deiodinase system accounts for the fact that higher blood levels of T_3 are required to suppress pituitary-thyroid function after administration of T_3 than after administration of T_4.[112,113]

Transthyretin is present in the brain of early reptiles and in addition is synthesized by the liver in warm-blooded animals.[111] During embryogenesis in mammals, transthyretin is first detected when the blood-brain barrier appears, ensuring thyroid hormone access to the developing nervous system.

Neural Control

The hypothalamus determines the set point of feedback control around which the usual feedback regulatory responses are elicited. Lesions of the thyrotropic area lower basal thyroid hormone levels and make the pituitary more sensitive to inhibition by thyroid hormone, and high doses of TRH raise the levels of TSH and thyroid hormone. Synthesis of TRH in the PVH is regulated by feedback actions of thyroid hormones.[112] The hypothalamus can override normal feedback control through an open-loop mechanism involving neuronal inputs to the hypophyseotropic TRH neurons (see Fig. 7-9). For example, cold exposure causes a sharp increase in TSH release in animals and in human newborns. Circadian changes in TSH secretion are another example of brain-directed changes in the set point of feedback control, but if thyroid hormone levels are sufficiently elevated, as in hyperthyroidism, TRH cannot overcome the inhibition.

Hypothalamic regulation of TSH secretion is also influenced by two inhibitory factors, somatostatin and dopamine. Anti-somatostatin antibodies increase basal TSH levels and potentiate the response to stimuli that normally

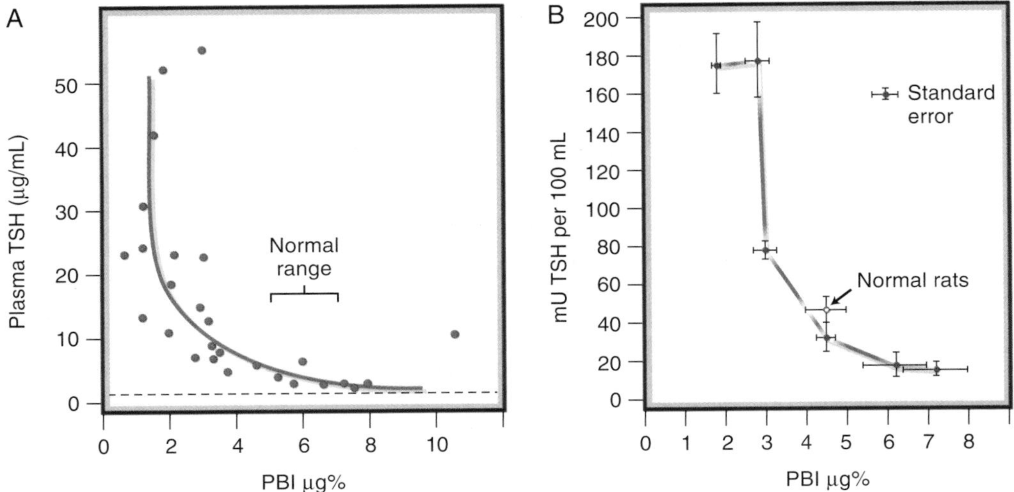

Figure 7-10 Relationship between plasma thyrotropin (TSH) levels and thyroid hormone as determined by measurements of plasma protein-bound iodine (PBI) in humans and rats. These curves illustrate that plasma TSH levels are a curvilinear function of the plasma thyroid hormone level. **A**, Human studies were carried out by giving myxedematous patients successive increments of thyroxine (T_4) at approximately 10-day intervals. Each point represents simultaneous measurements of plasma PBI and plasma TSH at various times in the six patients studied. **B**, The rat studies were performed by treating thyroidectomized animals with various doses of T_4 for 2 weeks before assay of plasma TSH and plasma PBI. These curves illustrate that the secretion of TSH is regulated over the entire range of thyroid hormone levels. At the normal set point for T_4, small changes above and below the control level are followed by appropriate increases or decreases in plasma TSH. (**A** from Reichlin S, Utiger RD. Regulation of the pituitary thyroid axis in man: relationship of TSH concentration to concentration of free and total thyroxine in plasma. *J Clin Endocrinol Metab.* 1967;27:251-255, copyright by The Endocrine Society. **B** from Reichlin S, Martin JB, Boshans RL, et al. Measurement of TSH in plasma and pituitary of the rat by a radioimmunoassay utilizing bovine TSH: effect of thyroidectomy or thyroxine administration on plasma TSH levels. *Endocrinology.* 1970;87:1022-1031, copyright by The Endocrine Society.)

induce TSH release in the rat, such as cold exposure or TRH administration.[114] Thyroid hormone in turn inhibits the release of somatostatin, implying coordinated, reciprocal regulation of TRH and somatostatin by thyroid hormone. GH stimulates hypothalamic somatostatin synthesis and can inhibit TSH secretion. However, the physiologic role of somatostatin in the regulation of TSH secretion in humans is uncertain.

Dopamine has modest effects on TSH secretion, and blockade of dopamine receptors (in the human) stimulates TSH secretion slightly. Changes in the metabolism of thyroid hormone also influence T_3 homeostasis within the brain. In states of thyroid hormone deficiency, brain T_3 levels are maintained by an increase in the deiodinase that converts T_4 to T_3.[43]

The pineal gland has been reported to inhibit thyroid function in some but not all studies. The pineal gland contains TRH, and in the frog its content changes with the season and with light and dark cycles independently of hypothalamic TRH.

Circadian Rhythm

Plasma TSH in humans is characterized by a circadian periodicity, with a maximum between 9 p.m. and 5 a.m. and a minimum between 4 p.m. and 7 p.m. (see Fig. 7-7E).[115] Smaller ultradian TSH peaks occur every 90 to 180 minutes, probably because of bursts of TRH released from the hypothalamus, and are physiologically important in controlling the synthesis and glycosylation of TSH. Glycosylation is a determinant of TSH potency.[116]

Temperature

External cold exposure activates and high ambient temperature inhibits the pituitary-thyroid axis in animals, and analogous changes occur in humans under certain conditions.[117] Exposure of infants to cold at the time of delivery causes an increase in blood TSH levels, possibly because of alterations in the turnover and degradation of the thyroid hormones. Blood thyroid hormone levels are higher in winter than in summer among people living in cold climates but not in other climates. However, it is difficult to show that changes in environmental or body temperature in adults influence TSH secretion. For example, exposure to cold ambient temperature or central hypothalamic cooling does not modify TSH levels in young men. Behavioral changes, activation of the sympathetic nervous system, and shivering appear to be more important than the thyroid response for temperature regulation in adults.

The autonomic nervous system and the thyroid axis work together to maintain temperature homeostasis in mammals, and TRH plays a role in both pathways.[117] Hypothalamic TRH release is rapidly increased (30 to 45 minutes) in rats exposed to cold. Rapid inhibition of somatostatin release in the median eminence has also been documented, and both changes appear to play important roles in the rise in plasma TSH induced by cold exposure. TRH mRNA is elevated within 1 hour of cold exposure (see Fig. 7-11C and D). The regulation of hypophyseotropic TRH release and expression by cold is largely mediated by catecholamines. Noradrenergic and adrenergic fibers, originating in the brain stem, are found in close proximity to TRH nerve endings in the median eminence, and a rapid rise in TRH release was seen after norepinephrine treatment of hypothalamic fragments containing mainly median eminence.[117] Brain stem adrenergic and noradrenergic fibers also make synaptic contacts with TRH neurons in the PVH (see Fig. 7-9),[118] so catecholamines are likely to be involved in the regulation of TRH gene expression by cold. TRH neurons in the PVH are densely innervated by NPY terminals,[119] and a portion of the NPY terminals arising from the C1, C2, C3, and A1 cell groups of the brain stem and projecting to the PVH are known to be catecholaminergic. Somatostatin, dopamine, and serotonin also play a variety of roles in the regulation of TRH.

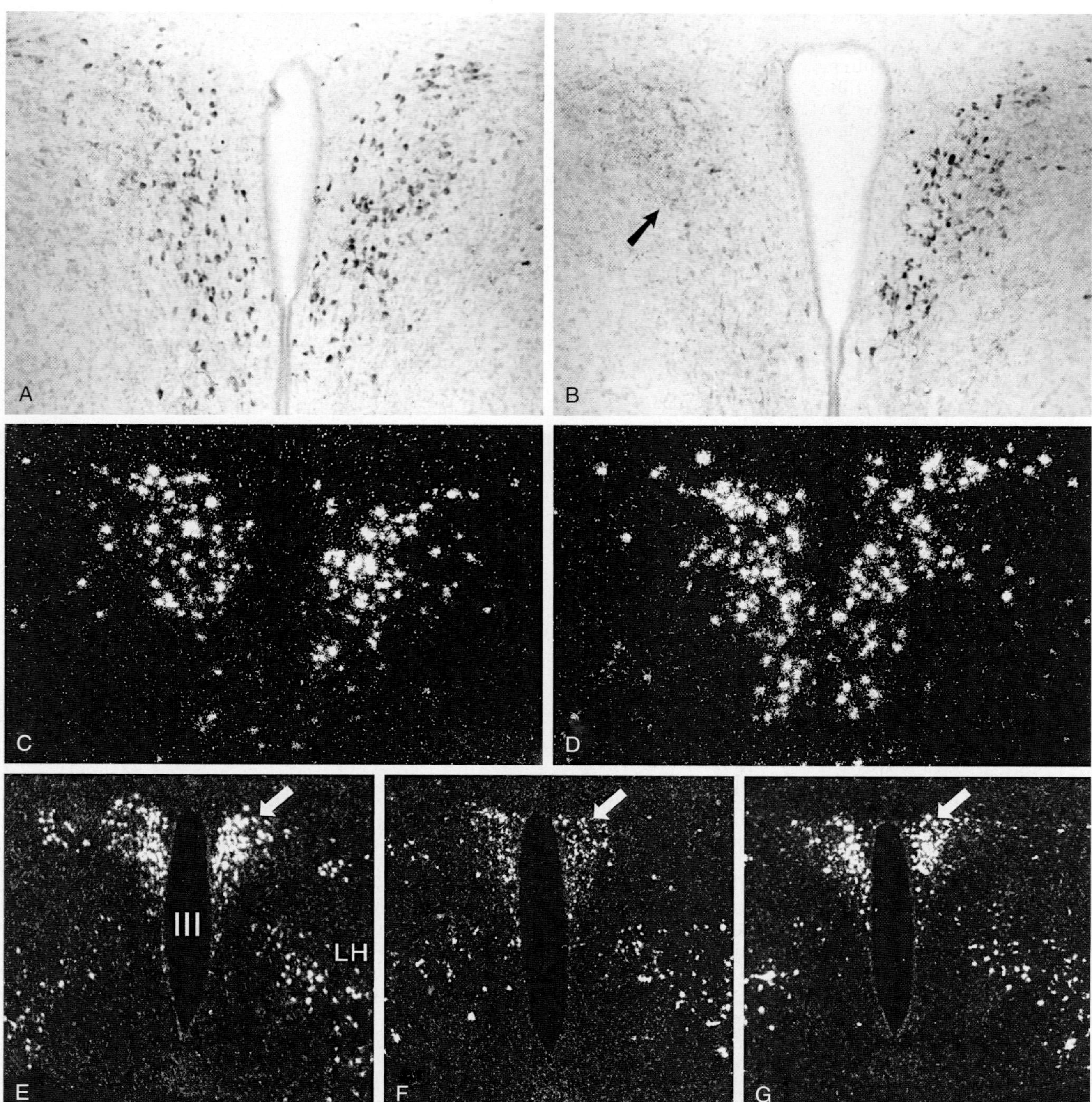

Figure 7-11 Direct effects of triiodothyronine (T_3) on thyrotropin-releasing hormone (TRH) synthesis in the rat hypothalamic paraventricular nucleus (parvicellular division) were shown by immunohistochemical detection of pre-proTRH(25-50) after implantation of a pellet of either inactive diiodotyrosine (T_2) as a control (panel **A**) or T_3 (panel **B**). The T_2 pellet had no effect on the concentration of pre-proTRH, whereas the TRH prohormone concentration was markedly reduced by T_3 (*black arrow* indicates the unilateral pellet implantation). These studies demonstrated that thyroid hormone regulates the hypothalamic component of the pituitary-thyroid axis as well as the pituitary thyrotrope itself. **C** and **D**, Effects on TRH messenger ribonucleic acid (mRNA) levels detected by in situ hybridization before (panel **C**) and after (panel **D**) 1-hour exposure of a rat to 4° C cold. **E** to **G**, Effects on TRH mRNA levels of starvation (**F**) and leptin replacement during starvation (**G**) compared to control levels (**E**). *White arrows* show the location of the paraventricular nucleus. III, third ventricle; LH, lateral hypothalamus. (Photomicrographs in panels **A, B, E, F,** and **G** courtesy of Dr. R. M. Lechan. From Dyess EM, Segerson TP, Liposits Z, et al. Triiodothyronine exerts direct cell-specific regulation of thyrotropin-releasing hormone gene expression in the hypothalamic paraventricular nucleus. *Endocrinology.* 1988;123:2291-2297, copyright by The Endocrine Society; photomicrographs in panels **C** and **D** courtesy of Dr. P. Joseph-Bravo.)

Stress

Stress is another determinant of TSH secretion.[109] In humans, physical stress inhibits TSH release, as indicated by the finding that low levels of T_3 and T_4 in patients with the euthyroid sick syndrome do not cause compensatory increases in TSH secretion as would occur in normal individuals.[120]

A number of observations demonstrate interactions between the thyroid and adrenal axes. Physiologically, the bulk of evidence suggests that glucocorticoids in humans and rodents act to blunt the thyroid axis through actions in the CNS.[121] Some actions may be direct, because the TRH gene (see Fig. 7-8) contains a glucocorticoid response element consensus half-site[98] and hypophyseotropic TRH neurons appear to contain glucocorticoid receptors.[122] The diurnal rhythm of cortisol is opposite that of TSH (see Fig. 7-7), and acute administration of glucocorticoids can block the nocturnal rise in TSH; however, disruption of cortisol synthesis with metyrapone only modestly affects the TSH circadian rhythm.

Nevertheless, several lines of evidence identify conditions in which elevated glucocorticoids are associated with stimulation of the thyroid axis. Human depression is often associated with hypercortisolism and hyperthyroxinemia, and TRH mRNA levels are elevated by glucocorticoids in a number of cell lines as well as in cultured fetal hypothalamic TRH neurons from the rat. Therefore, although glucocorticoids probably stimulate TRH production in TRH neurons, their overall inhibitory effect on the thyroid axis results from indirect glucocorticoid negative feedback on structures such as the hippocampus. Disruption of hippocampal suppression of the hypothalamic-pituitary-adrenal (HPA) axis is proposed to be involved in the hypercortisolemia commonly seen in affective illness, and disruption of hippocampal inputs to the hypothalamus has been shown to produce a rise in hypophyseotropic TRH in the rat.[123]

Starvation

The thyroid axis is depressed during starvation, presumably to help conserve energy by depressing metabolism (Fig. 7-11E to G). In humans, T_3, T_4, and TSH are reduced during starvation or fasting.[124] There are also changes in the thyroid axis in anorexia nervosa, including low blood levels of T_3 and low-normal levels of T_4 (see Chapter 11). Inappropriately low levels of TSH are found, suggesting defective activation of TRH production by low thyroid hormone levels. During starvation in rodents, reduced TRH release into hypophyseal portal blood and reduced pro-TRH mRNA levels are seen, despite lowered thyroid hormone levels.[125] Reduced basal TSH levels are also usually present.

The hypothyroidism seen in fasting or in the leptin-deficient *ob/ob* mouse can be reversed by administration of leptin,[126] and evidence suggests that the mechanism involves leptin's ability to upregulate TRH gene expression in the PVH (see Fig. 7-11E to G).[127] Leptin appears to act both directly through leptin receptors on hypophyseotropic TRH neurons and indirectly through its actions on other hypothalamic cell groups, such as arcuate nucleus POMC and NPY/agouti-related peptide (AgRP) neurons.[128,129] TRH neurons in the PVH receive dense NPY/AgRP and POMC projections from the arcuate and express NPY and melanocortin-4 receptors (MC4R),[130] and α-MSH administration partially prevents the fasting-induced drop in thyroid hormone levels.[128,129] Indeed, the TRH promoter contains a signal transducer and activator of transcription (STAT) response element and a CRE that have been demonstrated to mediate induction of TRH gene expression by leptin and α-MSH, respectively, in a heterologous cell system (see Fig. 7-8).[130] The regulation of TRH by metabolic state is likely to be under redundant control, because leptin-deficient children, unlike rodents, are euthyroid,[131] whereas both rodents and humans with MC4R deficiency are euthyroid.[132]

Infection and Inflammation

The molecular basis of infection- or inflammation-induced TSH suppression is partially established. TSH secretion is inhibited by sterile abscesses; by the injection of interleukin-1β (IL-1β), an endogenous pyrogen and secretory peptide of activated lymphocytes[133]; or by tumor necrosis factor-α (TNF-α). IL-1β stimulates the secretion of somatostatin.[134] TNF-α inhibits TSH secretion directly and induces functional changes in the rat characteristic of the "sick euthyroid" state.[135] It is likely that the TSH inhibition in animal models of the sick euthyroid syndrome results from cytokine-induced changes in hypothalamic and pituitary function.[136] IL-6, IL-1, and TNF-α contribute to the suppression of TSH in the sick euthyroid syndrome.[137]

Corticotropin-Releasing Hormone

Chemistry and Evolution

The HPA axis is the humoral component of an integrated neural and endocrine system that functions to respond to internal and external challenges to homeostasis (stressors). The system comprises the neuronal pathways linked to release of catecholamines from the adrenal medulla (fight-or-flight response) and the hypothalamic-pituitary control of ACTH release through control of glucocorticoid production by the adrenal cortex. Pituitary ACTH release is stimulated primarily by CRH and to a lesser extent by AVP (see Chapter 8). The hypophyseotropic CRH neurons are located in the parvicellular division of the PVH and project to the median eminence (see Figs. 7-3 and 7-4).

In a broader context, the CRH system in the CNS is also vitally important in the behavioral response to stress. This complex system includes not only nonhypophyseotropic CRH neurons but also three CRH-like peptides (urocortin, urocortin 2 or stresscopin-related peptide, and urocortin 3 or stresscopin), at least two cognate receptors (CRH-R1 and CRH-R2), and a high-affinity CRH-binding protein, each with distinct and complex distributions in the CNS.

The Schally and Guillemin laboratories demonstrated in 1955 that extracts from the hypothalamus stimulated ACTH release from the pituitary. The primary active principle, CRH, was purified and characterized from sheep in 1981 by Vale and colleagues.[137a] Human CRH is an amidated 41-amino-acid peptide that is cleaved from the C-terminus of a 196-amino-acid pre-prohormone precursor by PC1 and PC2 (Fig. 7-12).[138] CRH is highly conserved phylogenetically; the human peptide is identical in sequence to the mouse and rat peptides but differs at seven residues from the ovine sequence. Mammalian CRH, the three urocortin peptides, fish urotensin, anuran sauvagine, and the insect diuretic peptides are members of an ancient family of peptides that evolved from an ancestral precursor early in the evolution of metazoans, approximately 500 million years ago.[139] Comparison of peptide sequences in vertebrates suggests a grouping of the peptides into two subfamilies, CRH-urotensin-urocortin-sauvagine and urocortin 2-urocortin 3 (Fig. 7-13).[140] Urocortin and sauvagine appear to represent tetrapod orthologues of fish urotensin. Sauvagine, isolated originally from *Phyllomedusa sauvagei*, is an osmoregulatory

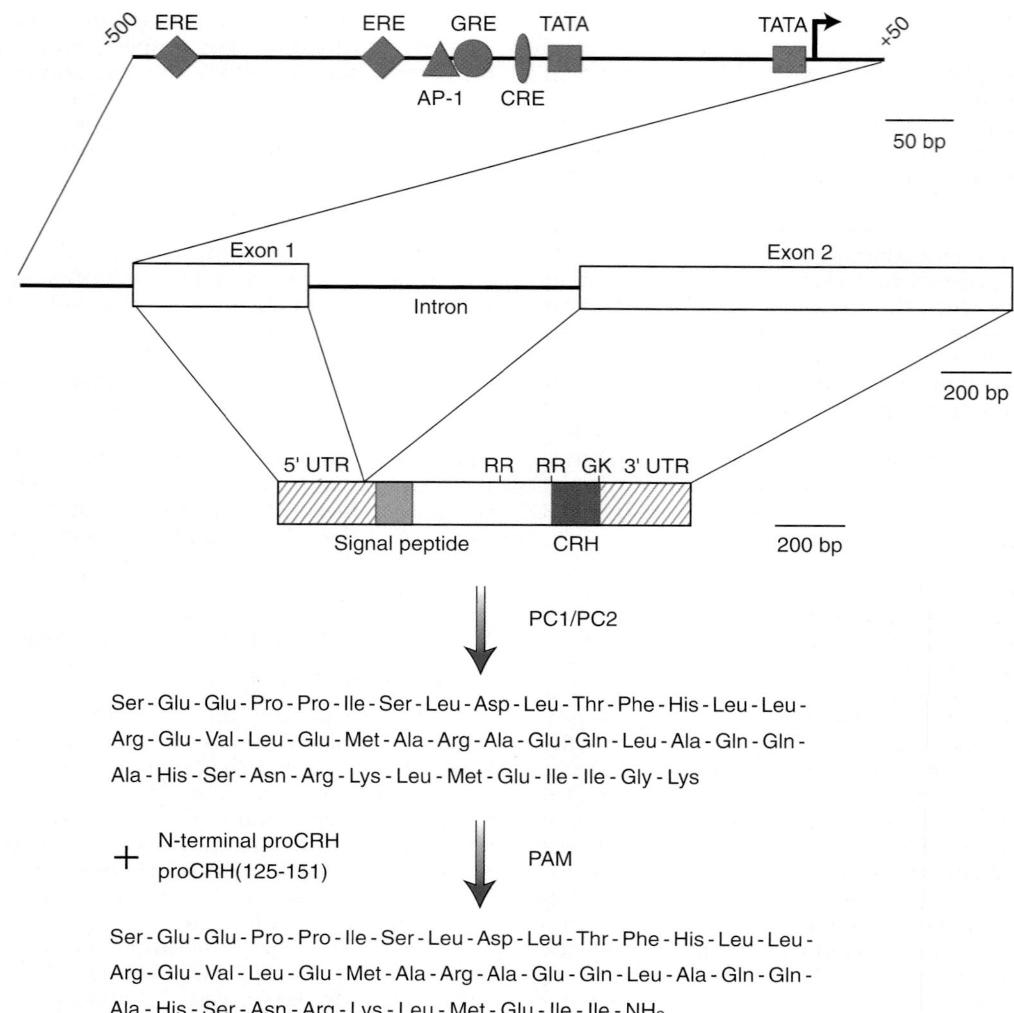

Figure 7-12 Structure of the human corticotropin-releasing hormone (CRH) gene, complementary DNA, and peptide. The sequence encoding CRH occurs at the carboxy-terminus of the prohormone. Dibasic amino acid cleavage sites (RR) and the penultimate Gly and terminal Lys (GK) are shown. AP-1, activator protein-1 binding sequence; CRE, cyclic adenosine monophosphate (cAMP)-response element; ERE, estrogen response element; GRE, glucocorticoid response element; PAM, peptidylglycine α-amidating monooxygenase; PC1/PC2, prohormone convertases 1 and 2; TATA, Goldstein-Hogness box involved in binding RNA polymerase; UTR, untranslated. (Redrawn from data of Shibahara S, Morimoto Y, Furutani Y, et al. Isolation and sequence analysis of the human corticotropin-releasing factor precursor gene. *EMBO J.* 1983;2:775-779.)

peptide produced in the skin of certain frogs; urotensin is an osmoregulatory peptide produced in the caudal neurosecretory system of the fish. Whereas isolation of CRH required 250,000 ovine hypothalami, the "virtual" cloning of urocortin 2 and 3 was accomplished by computer search of the human genome database.[140]

The CRH peptides signal by binding to CRH-R1[141,142] and CRH-R2[143] receptors that couple to the stimulatory G protein (G_s) and activate adenylyl cyclase. Two splice variants of the CRH-R2 receptor that differ in their extracellular N-terminal domain, termed CRH-R2α and CRH-R2β, have been found in both rodents and humans,[144] and a third N-terminal splice variant, CRH-R2γ, has been reported in the human.[145]

CRH, urotensin, and sauvagine are potent agonists of CRH-R1; urocortin is a potent agonist of both receptors; and urocortins 2 and 3 are specific agonists of CRH-R2. CRH-activation of the HPA axis is mediated exclusively

Human CRH	SEE**PPISLDLTF**H**LL**REV**LE**M**AR**AEQLAQ**QA**HS**NR**K**L**M**E**I**I**
Human urocortin	DN**PSLSIDLTF**H**LL**RTL**LE**L**AR**TQSQRER**A**EQ**NR**I**IFDSV**
Human urocortin II(SRP)	HPGSRIV**LSLDV**PIG**LL**QIL**LE**Q**AR**ARAARE**QA**TT**N**AR**I**LAR**V**GHC
Human urocortin III(SCP)	TKFT**LSLDV**PTN**I**MNLLFNI**AK**AKNL**R**A**QA**AA**N**AH**L**MAQ**I**GRRK
Frog sauvagine	QG**PPISIDLS**LE**LL**RKM**IE**IE**K**QEKE**K**Q**QA**AN**NR**L**L**L**D**T**I**
Carp urotensin-I	NDD**PPISIDLTF**H**LL**RNM**IE**M**AR**NENQRE**QA**GL**NR**KYL**D**E**V**

Figure 7-13 Sequence comparison of members of the corticotropin-releasing hormone (CRH) peptide family. Identical or highly conserved amino acids are indicated in bold letters. SCP, stresscopin; SRP, stresscopin-related peptide.

through CRH-R1 expressed in the corticotroph. CRH neurons projecting to the median eminence are found mostly in the PVH, although most hypothalamic nuclei contain some of these neurons (Fig. 7-14A). Some CRH fibers in the PVH also project to the brain stem, and non-hypophyseotropic CRH neurons are abundant elsewhere, primarily in limbic structures involved in processing sensory information and in regulating the autonomic nervous system. Sites include the prefrontal, insular, and cingulate cortices; amygdala; substantia nigra; periaqueductal gray; locus ceruleus; nucleus of the solitary tract; and parabrachial nucleus. In the periphery, CRH is found in human placenta, where it is upregulated 6- to 40-fold during the third trimester, in lymphocytes, in autonomic nerves, and in the gastrointestinal tract. Urocortin is expressed at highest levels in the non-preganglionic Edinger-Westphal nucleus, the lateral superior olive, and the SON nucleus of the rodent brain, with additional sites including the substantia nigra, ventral tegmental area, and dorsal raphe (see Fig. 7-14B). In the human, urocortin is widely distributed, with highest levels in the frontal cortex, temporal cortex, and hypothalamus,[146] and has also been reported in the non-preganglionic Edinger-Westphal nucleus.[22] In the periphery, urocortin is seen in placenta, mucosal inflammatory cells of the gastrointestinal tract, lymphocytes, and cardiomyocytes. Urocortin 2 is expressed in hypothalamic neuroendocrine and stress-related cell groups in the mouse, including the locus ceruleus, whereas urocortin 3 is expressed in hypothalamus and amygdala, and particularly in pancreatic islet beta cells.[147,148]

In addition to its expression in pituitary corticotrophs, CRH-R1 is found in the neocortex and cerebellar cortex, subcortical limbic structures, and amygdala, with little to no expression in the hypothalamus (see Fig. 7-14C). CRH-R1 is also found in a variety of peripheral sites in humans, including ovary, endometrium, and skin. CRH-R2α is found mainly in the brain in rodents, with high levels of expression in the VMH and lateral septum (see Fig. 7-14C)[149]; CRH-R2β is found centrally in cerebral arterioles and peripherally in gastrointestinal tract, heart, and muscle.[143,150] In humans, CRH-R2α is expressed in brain and periphery, whereas the β and γ subtypes are primarily central.[144,145] Little CRH-R2 message is seen in pituitary. Although CRH-R1 appears to be exclusively involved in regulation of pituitary ACTH synthesis and release, both receptors are expressed in the rodent adrenal cortex. Data suggest that this intra-adrenal CRH-ACTH system may be involved in fine-tuning of adrenocortical corticosterone release.

The CRH system is also regulated in both brain and periphery by a 37-kd high-affinity CRH-binding protein.[151-153] This factor was initially postulated from the observation that CRH levels rise dramatically during the second and third trimesters of pregnancy without activating the pituitary-adrenal axis. Among hypophyseotropic factors, CRH is the only one for which a specific binding protein (in addition to the receptor) exists in tissue or blood. The placenta is the principal source of pregnancy-related CRH-binding protein. Human and rat CRH-binding proteins are homologous (85% amino acid identity), but in the rat the protein is expressed only in brain. The binding protein is species specific; bovine CRH, which is almost identical in sequence to rat and human CRH, has a lower affinity of binding to the human binding protein.

The functional significance of the CRH-binding protein is not fully understood. CRH-binding protein does not bind to the CRH receptor but does inhibit CRH action. For this reason, CRH-binding protein probably acts to modulate CRH actions at the cellular level. Corticotroph cells in the anterior pituitary have membrane CRH receptors and intracellular CRH-binding protein; conceivably, the binding protein acts to sequester or terminate the action of membrane-bound CRH. CRH-binding protein is present in many regions of the CNS, including cells that synthesize CRH and cells that receive innervation from CRH-containing neurons. The anatomic distribution of the protein, the variability of its location in relation to the presence of CRH, and its relative sparseness in the CRH tuberohypophyseal neuronal system suggest a control system that is as yet poorly understood. Transgenic mouse models with both overexpression and gene deletion of the CRH-binding protein have been produced with little effect on basal or stress activation of the HPA axis (reviewed by Bale and Vale[154]).

Structure-activity relationship studies have demonstrated that both C-terminal amidation and an α-helical secondary structure are important for biologic activity of CRH. The first CRH antagonist described was termed *α-helical CRH(9-41)*.[155] A second, more potent antagonist, termed *astressin*, has the structure cyclo(30-33)(D-Phe[12], Nle,[12] Glu,[12] Lys[12])hCRH(12-41).[156] Both peptides are somewhat nonspecific, antagonizing both CRH-R1 and CRH-R2. Because of the anxiogenic activity of CRH and urocortin, a number of pharmaceutical companies have developed small-molecule CRH antagonists; several of these are currently in clinical trials for anxiety and depression (see later discussion). Thus far, this structurally diverse group of small-molecule compounds, including antalarmin, CP-154,526, and NBI27914, are potent antagonists of CRH-R1, with little activity at CRH-R2. The efficacy of these compounds across the entire behavioral, neuroendocrine, and autonomic repertoire of response to stress has been demonstrated in a number of laboratory animal studies. For example, oral administration of antalarmin in a social stress model in the primate (introduction of strange males) reduced behavioral measures of anxiety such as lack of exploratory behavior, decreased plasma ACTH and cortisol, and reduced plasma epinephrine and norepinephrine.[157] Other preclinical studies in rhesus monkeys have compared the pharmacologic profiles of astressin B and antalarmin.[158] A peptide antagonist with 100-fold selectivity for the CRH-R2β receptor, (D-Phe[11], His[12])sauvagine 11-40 or anti-sauvagine-30, has also been described.[159]

Effects on the Pituitary and Mechanism of Action

Administration of CRH to humans causes prompt release of ACTH into the blood, followed by secretion of cortisol (Fig. 7-15) and other adrenal steroids including aldosterone. Most studies have used ovine CRH, which is more potent and longer acting than human CRH, but human and porcine CRHs appear to have equal diagnostic value. The effect of CRH is specific to ACTH release and is inhibited by glucocorticoids.

As mentioned earlier, CRH acts on the pituitary corticotroph primarily by binding to CRH-R1 and activating adenylyl cyclase. The concentration of cAMP in the tissue is increased in parallel with the biologic effects and is reduced by glucocorticoids. The rate of transcription of the mRNA that encodes the ACTH prohormone POMC is also enhanced by CRH.

Extrapituitary Functions

CRH and the urocortin peptides have a wide range of biologic activities in addition to the hypophyseotropic role of CRH in regulating ACTH synthesis and release. Centrally, these peptides have behavioral activities in anxiety, mood,

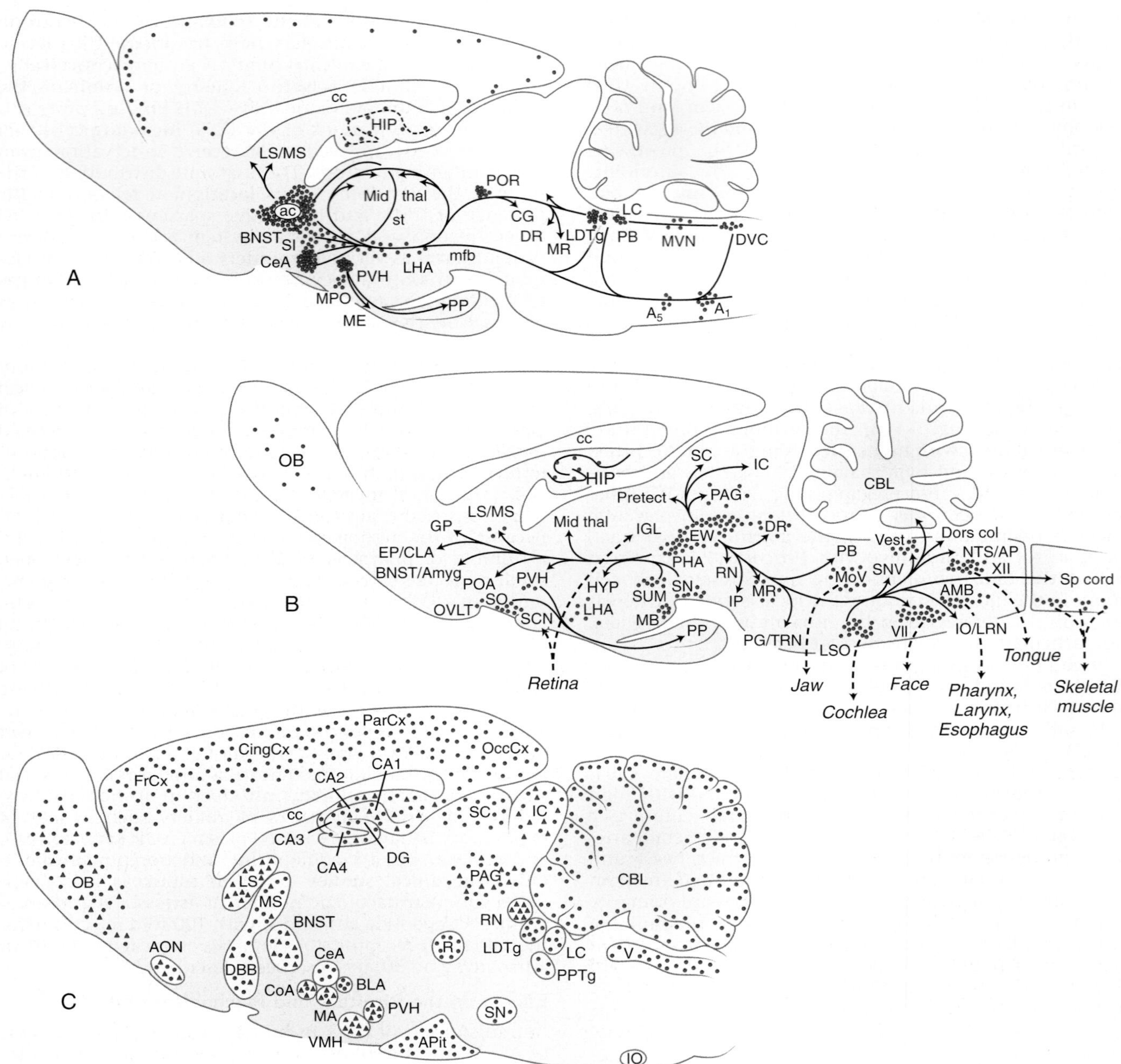

Figure 7-14 Distribution of messenger RNA sequences for corticotropin-releasing hormone (CRH) (**A**), urocortin (**B**), and the CRH receptors CRH-R1 (**C**, *circles*) and CRH-R2 (**C**, *triangles*) in the rat brain. A_1, Noradrenergic cell group 1; A_5, noradrenergic cell group 5; ac, anterior commissure; AMB, nucleus ambiguus; Amyg, amygdala; AON, anterior olfactory nucleus; APit, anterior pituitary; AP, area postrema; BLA, basolateral amygdala; BNST, bed nucleus of the stria terminalis; CA1-4, Fields CA1-4 of Ammon's horn; cc, corpus callosum; CeA, central nucleus amygdala; CBL, cerebellum; CG, central gray; CingCx, cingulate cortex; CoA, cortical nucleus amygdala; DBB, nucleus of the diagonal band; DG, dentate gyrus; Dors col, dorsal column nuclei; DR, dorsal raphe; DVC, dorsal vagal complex; EP/CLa, endopiriform nucleus/clawtrum; EW, Edinger-Westphal nucleus, non-cholinergic; FrCx, frontal cortex; GP, globus pallidus; HIP, hippocampus; HYP, hypothalamus; IC, inferior colliculus; IGL, intergeniculate leaflet; IO, inferior olivary complex; IP interpeduncular nucleus; LC, locus coeruleus; LDTg, laterodorsal tegmental nucleus; LHA, lateral hypothalamic area; LRN, lateral reticular nucleus; LS, lateral septum; LSO, lateral superior olivary nucleus; MA, medial amygdala; MB, mammillary body; ME, median eminence; mfb, medial forebrain bundle; MoV, motor nucleus of the trigeminal nerve; MS, medial septum; Mid Thal, midline thalamic nuclei; mfb, medial forebrain bundle; MPO, medial preoptic area; MR, medial raphe; MVN, medial vestibular nucleus; NTS, nucleus of the tractus solitarius; OB, olfactory bulb; OccCx, occipital cortex; OVLT, organum vasculosum of the lamina terminalis; PAG, periaqueductal gray; ParCx, parietal cortex; PB, parabrachial nucleus; PHA, posterior hypothalamic area; PoA, preoptic hypothalamic area; POR, perioculomotor nucleus; PP, posterior pituitary; PPTg, peripeduncular tegmental nucleus; Pretect, pretectal region; PVH, paraventricular nucleus of the hypothalamus; R, raphe; RN, red nucleus; SC, superior colliculus; SCN, suprachiasmatic nucleas; SI, substantia innominata; SN, substantia nigra; SNV, spinal trigeminal nucleus; SO, supraoptic nucleus; Sp cord, spinal cord; st, stria terminalis; SUM, supramammillary nucleus; V/Vest, vestibular nuclei; VII, facial nucleus; VMH, ventral medial nucleus of the hypothalamus; XII, hypoglossal nucleus. (From Swanson LW, Sawchenko PE, Rivier J, et al. Organization of ovine corticotropin-releasing factor immunoreactive cells and fibers in the rat brain: an immunohistochemical study. *Neuroendocrinology.* 1983;36:165-186; Bittencourt JC, Vaughan J, Arias C, et al. Urocortin expression in rat brain: evidence against a pervasive relationship of urocortin-containing projections with targets bearing type 2 CRF receptors. *J Comp Neurol.* 1999;415:285-312, Fig. 17; Steckler T, Holsboer F. Corticotropin-releasing hormone receptor subtypes and emotion. *Biol Psychol.* 1999;46:1480-1508, Fig. 1.)

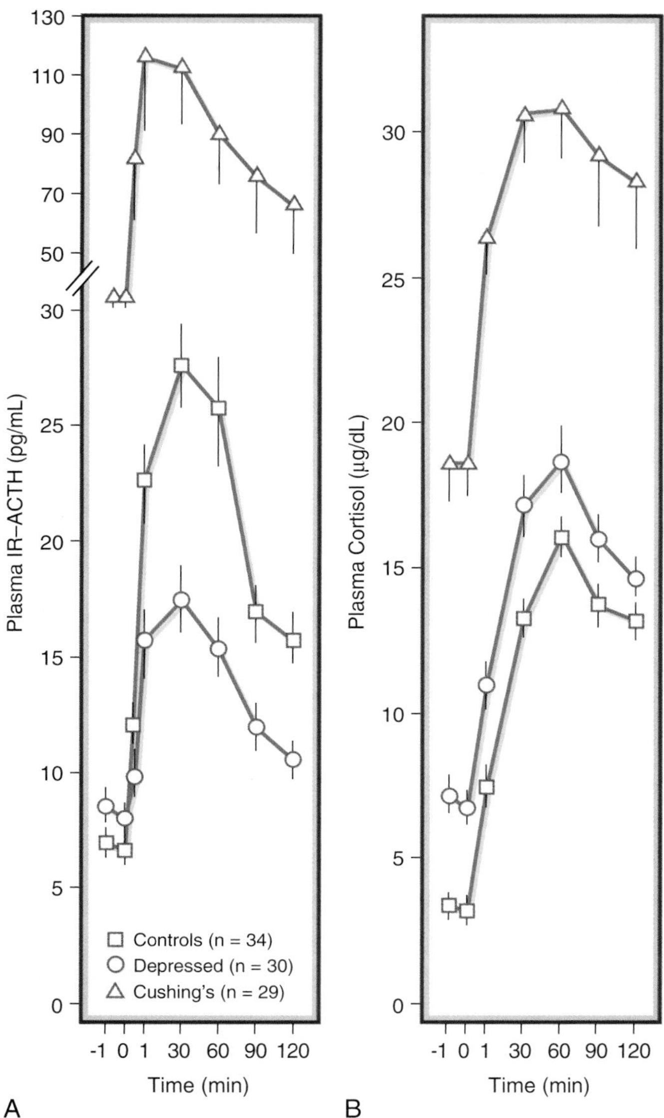

Figure 7-15 Comparison of plasma immunoreactive adrenocorticotropic hormone (IR-ACTH) (**A**) and plasma cortisol (**B**) responses to ovine corticotropin-releasing hormone in control subjects, patients with depression, and patients with Cushing's disease. (From Gold PW, Loriaux DL, Roy A, et al. Responses to corticotropin-releasing hormone in the hypercortisolism of depression and Cushing's disease: pathophysiologic and diagnostic implications. *N Engl J Med.* 1986;314:1329-1335.)

arousal, locomotion, reward, and feeding[160,161] and increase sympathetic activation. Many of the nonhypophyseotropic behavioral and autonomic functions of these peptides can be viewed as complementary to activation of the HPA axis in the maintenance of homeostasis under exposure to stress. In the periphery, activities have been reported in immunity, cardiac function, gastrointestinal function, and reproduction.[162]

The CRH and urocortin peptides have a repertoire of behavioral and autonomic actions after central administration that suggests a role for these pathways in mediating the behavioral-autonomic components of the stress response. Hyperactivity of the HPA axis is a common neuroendocrine finding in affective disorders (see Fig. 7-15).[160,163] Normalization of HPA regulation is highly predictive of successful treatment. Defective dexamethasone suppression of CRH release, implying defective corticosteroid receptor signaling, is seen not only in depressed patients but also in healthy subjects with a family history of depression.[164] Depressed patients also show elevated levels of CRH in the CSF.[165] Extensive behavioral testing in a variety of mutant mouse models with genetically altered expression of the CRH ligands or receptors has generally supported the hypothesis that activation of central CRH pathways is a critical neurobiologic substrate of anxiety and depressive states.[154,161]

Central administration of CRH or urocortin activates neuronal cell groups involved in cardiovascular control and increases blood pressure, heart rate, and cardiac output.[166] However, urocortin is expressed in cardiac myocytes, and intravenous administration of CRH or urocortin decreases blood pressure and increases heart rate in most species, including humans.[166] This hypotensive effect is probably mediated peripherally, because ganglion blockade did not disrupt the hypotensive effects of intravenous urocortin. Furthermore, high levels of CRH-R2β have been seen in the cardiac atria and ventricles,[143,150] and knockout of the CRH-R2 gene in the mouse eliminated the hypotensive effects of intravenous urocortin administration.[167,168]

Cytokines have an important role in extinguishing inflammatory responses through activation of CRH and AVP neurons in the PVH and subsequent elevation of anti-inflammatory glucocorticoids. Interestingly, CRH is generally proinflammatory in the periphery, where it is found in sympathetic efferents, in sensory afferent nerves, in leukocytes, and in macrophages in some species.[162,169] CRH also functions as a paracrine factor in the endometrium, where it may play a role in decidualization and implantation and may act as a uterine vasodilator.[162]

The relative contributions of each of the CRH-urocortin peptides and receptors to the various biologic functions reported has been the topic of considerable analysis, given the receptor-specific antagonists already described and the availability of CRH, CRH-R1, and CRH-R2 knockout mice for study (reviewed by Bale and Vale[154] and Keck and colleagues[161]). Examination of three potent stressors—restraint, ether, and fasting—demonstrated that other ACTH secretagogues, such as AVP, oxytocin, and catecholamines, could not replace CRH in its role in mounting the stress response. In contrast, augmentation of glucocorticoid secretion by a stressor after prolonged stress was not defective in CRH knockout mice, implicating CRH-independent mechanisms.

Although CRH is a potent anxiogenic peptide, CRH knockout mice exhibit normal anxiety behaviors in, for example, conditioned fear paradigms. The nonpeptide CRH-R1–specific antagonist CP-154,526 was anxiolytic in a shock-induced freezing paradigm in both wild-type and CRH knockout mice, suggesting that the anxiogenic activity is a CRH-like peptide acting at the CRH-R1 receptor (see review[154]).

CRH and urocortin peptides also have potent anorexigenic activity, implicating the CRH system in stress-induced inhibition of feeding. However, in CRH knockout mice, stress-induced inhibition of feeding and suppression of the proestrous LH surge by restraint remained intact. Both CRH-R1 and CRH-R2 knockout strains had normal weight and feeding behaviors but were distinctly different from wild-type mice in the anorexigenic response to centrally administered urocortin or CRH. The CRH-R1–deficient mice lacked the acute anorexigenic response (0 to 1.5 hours) to urocortin seen in wild-type mice. Wild-type and CRH-R1 knockout mice exhibited comparable reductions in feeding 3 to 11 hours after administration. In contrast, the late phase of urocortin responsiveness appeared to depend on the presence of CRH-R2. Therefore, signaling through CRH-R1 and CRH-R2 plays a complex role in the acute effects of stress on feeding behavior (see review[154]).

Additional gene knockout studies have suggested that urocortin 2 plays a physiologic role in female mice to dampen basal daily rhythms of the HPA axis and reduce behavioral coping mechanisms in response to chronic stress.[147] Urocortin 3 may have a primary action to augment insulin secretion in response to the metabolic stress of excessive calorie intake.[148]

Clinical Applications

No approved therapeutic application of CRH or CRH-like peptides exists, although the peptide has been demonstrated to have a number of activities in human and primate studies. Intravenous administration was found to stimulate energy expenditure, but CRH is an unlikely pharmaceutical target for inducing weight loss. The development of small-molecule, orally available, CRH-R1 antagonists has produced considerable interest in their potential for treatment of anxiety and depression.[165,170] In particular, the compound R121919 was studied in phase 1 and 2a clinical trials before its discontinuance. These studies of 20 patients demonstrated significant reductions in anxiety and depression scores, using ratings determined by patient or clinician, and also demonstrated the compound's safety and favorable side-effect profile, including a lack of effect on endocrine function or body weight gain.[171]

Feedback Control

The administration of glucocorticoids inhibits ACTH secretion, and, conversely, removal of the adrenals (or administration of drugs that impair secretion of glucocorticoids) leads to increased ACTH release. The set point of pituitary feedback is determined by the hypothalamus acting through hypothalamic releasing hormones CRH and AVP (see Chapter 8).[172-175] Glucocorticoids act on both the pituitary corticotrophs and the hypothalamic neurons that secrete CRH and AVP. These regulatory actions are analogous to the control of the pituitary-thyroid axis. However, whereas TSH becomes completely unresponsive to TRH when thyroid hormone levels are sufficiently high, severe neurogenic stress and large amounts of CRH can break through the feedback inhibition due to glucocorticoids. A still higher level of feedback control is exerted by glucocorticoid-responsive neurons in the hippocampus that project to the hypothalamus; these neurons affect the activity of CRH hypophyseotropic neurons and determine the set point of pituitary responsiveness to glucocorticoids.[175] A comprehensive review of glucocorticoid effects on CRH and AVP and regulation of the HPA axis emphasized the complexity of this control beyond that of a simple closed-loop feedback.[176]

Glucocorticoids are lipid soluble and freely enter the brain through the blood-brain barrier.[174] In brain and pituitary, they can bind to two receptors. Type 1 (encoded by *NR3C2*) is called the *mineralocorticoid receptor* because it binds aldosterone and glucocorticoids with high affinity). Type 2 (*NR3C1*), the glucocorticoid receptor, has low affinity for mineralocorticoids.[173-175] Classic glucocorticoid action involves binding of the steroid-receptor complex to regulator sequences in the genome. MR are saturated by basal levels of glucocorticoids, whereas GR are not saturated under basal conditions but approach saturation during peak phases of the circadian rhythm and during stress. These differences and differences in regional distribution within the brain suggest that MR determine basal activity of the hypothalamic-pituitary axis and GR mediate stress responses.

In the pituitary, glucocorticoids inhibit secretion of ACTH and the synthesis of POMC mRNA; in the hypothalamus, they inhibit the secretion of CRH and AVP and the synthesis of their respective mRNAs, although with distinct temporal patterns.[174-176] Neuron membrane excitability and ion transport properties are suppressed by changes in glucocorticoid-directed synthesis of intracellular protein. Glucocorticoids can exert additional rapid signaling events in neurons, including an endocannabinoid-mediated suppression of synaptic excitation.[177] These rapid events involve membrane-associated complexes and are independent of changes in gene transcription or acute protein translation, but the exact mechanisms and nature of the receptors are still under investigation.[178]

Glucocorticoids block stress-induced ACTH release. The latency of the inhibitory effect is so short (<30 minutes) that it is likely that gene regulation is not the sole basis of the response.[178] Long-term suppression (>1 hour) clearly acts through genomic mechanisms.

Glucocorticoid receptors are also found outside the hypothalamus, in the septum and in the amygdala,[174,175] and these structures are involved in the psychobehavioral changes of hypercortisolism and hypocortisolism. In all of these areas, apart from the CRH neurons of the PVH, glucocorticoids have either a stimulatory or a neutral effect on CRH gene expression.[176] Hippocampal neurons are reduced in number by prolonged elevation of glucocorticoids during chronic stress.[175]

Neural Control

Significant physiologic or psychological stressors evoke an adaptive response that commonly includes activation of both the HPA axis and the sympathoadrenal axis. The end products of these pathways then help to mobilize resources to cope with the physiologic demands in emergency situations, acutely through the fight-or-flight response and over the long term through systemic effects of glucocorticoids on functions such as gluconeogenesis and energy mobilization (see Chapter 15). The HPA axis also has unique stress-specific homeostatic roles, the best example being the role of glucocorticoids in downregulating immune responses after infection and other events that stimulate cytokine production by the immune system.

The PVH is the primary hypothalamic nucleus responsible for providing the integrated whole-animal response to stress.[176,179,180] This nucleus contains within it three major types of effector neurons that are spatially distinct from one another: (1) magnicellular oxytocin and AVP neurons that project to the posterior pituitary and participate in the regulation of blood pressure, fluid homeostasis, lactation, and parturition; (2) neurons projecting to the brain stem and spinal cord that regulate a variety of autonomic responses, including sympathoadrenal activation; and (3) parvicellular CRH neurons that project to the median eminence and regulate ACTH synthesis and release. Many CRH neurons coexpress AVP, which acts as an auxiliary ACTH secretagogue, synergistic with CRH. AVP is regulated quite differently, in parvicellular versus magnicellular neurons, but also somewhat differently from CRH by stressors in parvicellular cells that express both peptides.[176] Different stressors result in different patterns of activation of the three major visceromotor cell groups within the PVH, as measured by the general neuronal activation marker Fos (Fig. 7-16). For example, salt loading

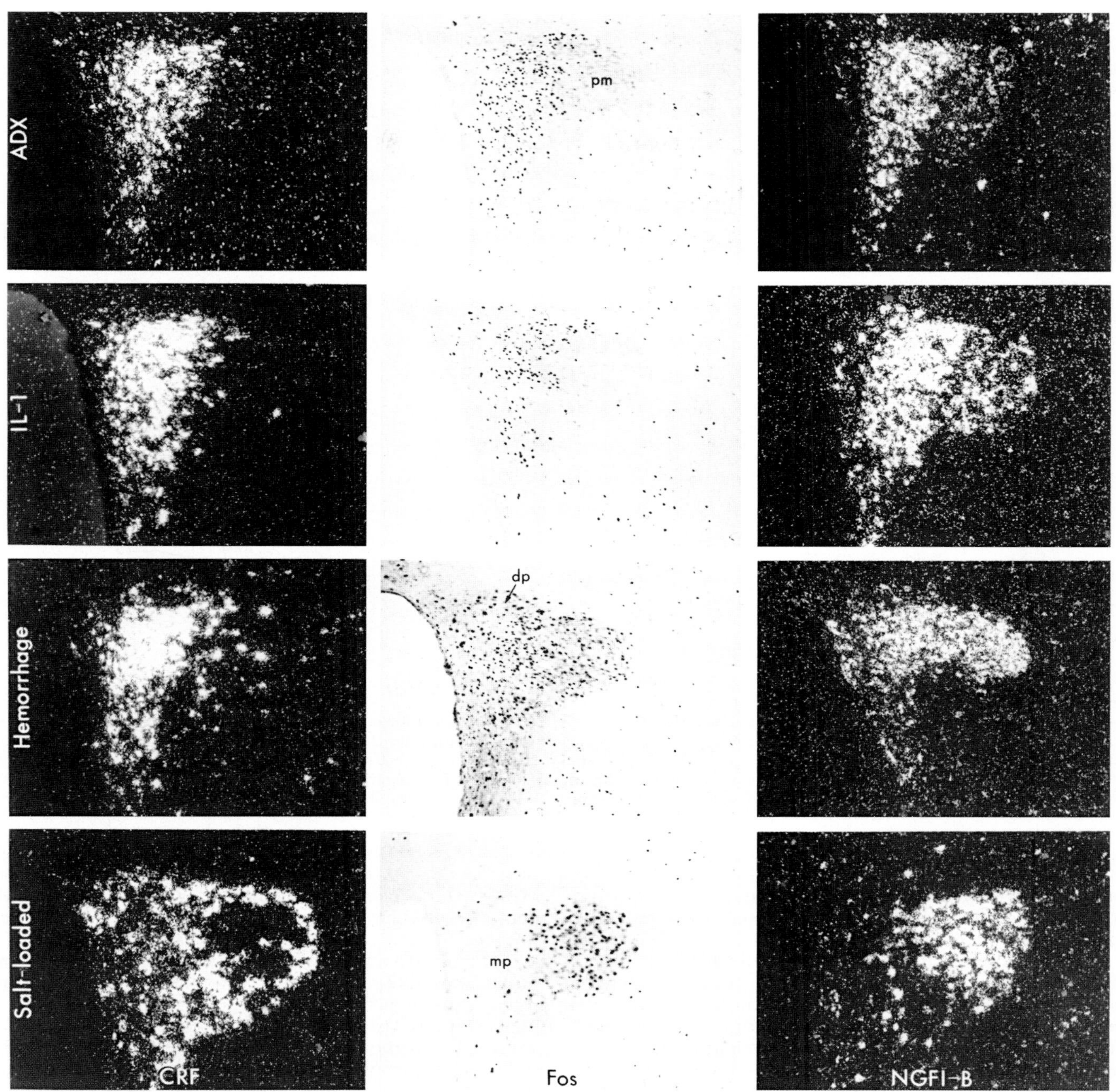

Figure 7-16 Regulation of neurons of the paraventricular nucleus (PVH) by diverse stressors. ADX, adrenalectomy; CRF, corticotropin-releasing factor in situ hybridization (dark-field); dp, dorsal parvicellular; Fos, FOS immunoreactivity (bright-field); IL-1, interleukin-1; pm, posterior magnicellular; NGFI-B, nerve growth factor 1β in situ hybridization (dark-field); mp, medial parvicellular. (From Sawchenko PE, Brown ER, Chan RK, et al. The paraventricular nucleus of the hypothalamus and the functional neuroanatomy of visceromotor responses to stress. *Prog Brain Res.* 1996; 107:201-222.)

downregulates CRH mRNA in parvicellular CRH cells, upregulates CRH in a small number of magnicellular CRH cells, but activates only magnicellular cells. Hemorrhage activates every division of the PVH, whereas cytokine administration primarily activates parvicellular CRH cells, with some minor activation of magnicellular and autonomic divisions.

The synthesis and release of AVP, which regulates renal water absorption and vascular smooth muscle, are controlled mainly by the volume and tonicity of the blood. This information is relayed to the magnicellular AVP cell through the nucleus of the solitary tract and A1 noradrenergic cell group of the ventrolateral medulla and through projections from a triad of CVOs lining the third ventricle: the SFO, the medial preoptic nucleus (MePO), and the OVLT. Oxytocin is primarily involved in reproductive functions, such as parturition, lactation, and milk ejection, although it is cosecreted with AVP in response to osmotic and volume challenges, and oxytocin cells receive direct projections from the nucleus of the solitary tract as well as from the SFO, MePO, and OVLT. In contrast to the neurosecretory neurons functionally defined by the three

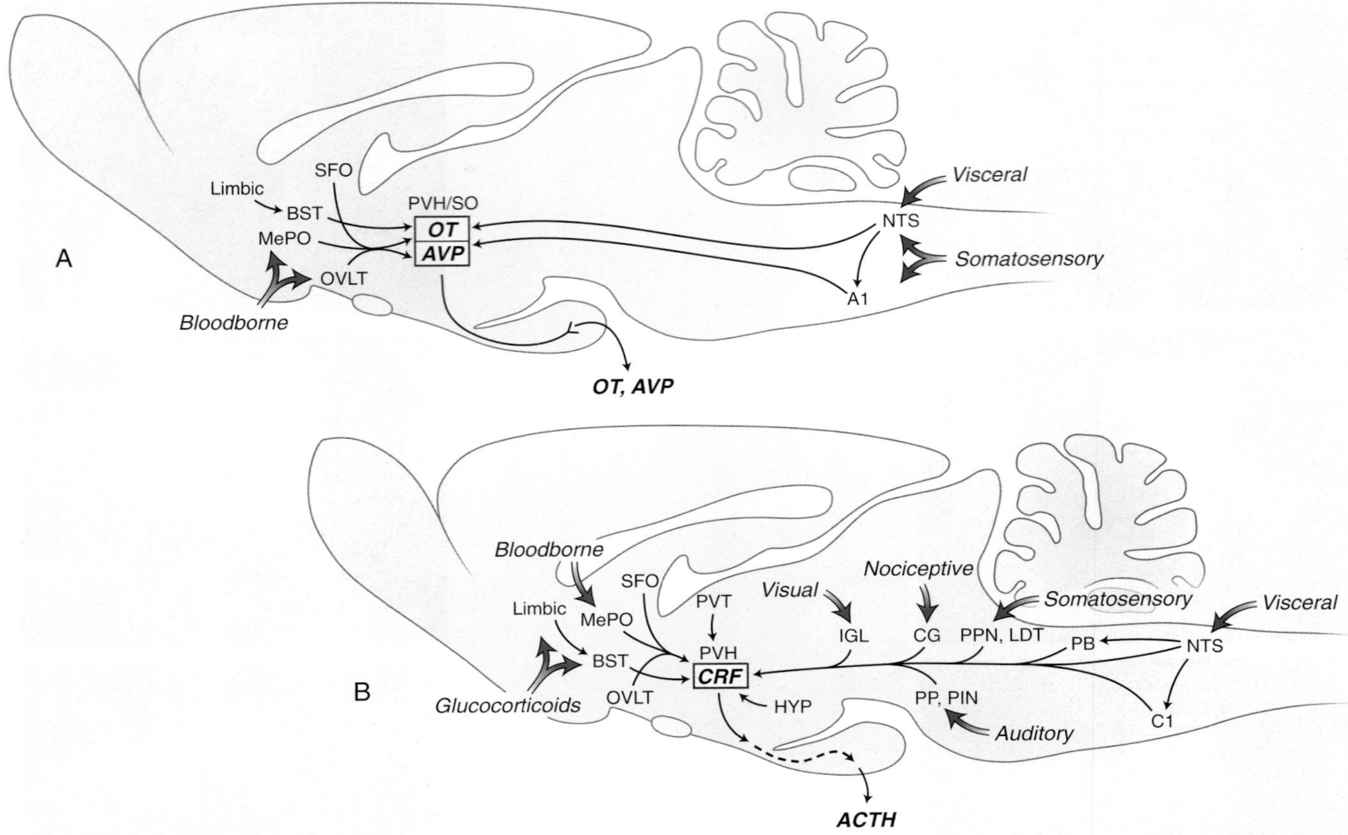

Figure 7-17 **A**, Neuronal inputs to magnicellular and, **B**, parvicellular neurons of the paraventricular nucleus (PVH). ACTH, adrenocorticotropic hormone; A1, A1 noradrenergic cell group; AVP, arginine vasopressin; BST, bed nucleus of the stria terminalis; C1, C1 adrenergic cell group; CG, central gray; CRF, corticotropin-releasing factor; HYP, hypothalamus; IGL, intergeniculate leaflet; LDT, laterodorsal tegmental nucleus; *MePO,* medial preoptic nucleus; NTS, nucleus of the tractus solitarius; OT, oxytocin; OVLT, organum vasculosum of the lamina terminalis; PB, parabrachial nucleus; PIN, posterior intralaminar nucleus; PP, peripeduncular nucleus; PPN, pedunculopontine nucleus; PVT, paraventricular nucleus of the thalamus; SFO, subfornical organ; SO, supraoptic nucleus. (From Sawchenko PE, Brown ER, Chan RK, et al. The paraventricular nucleus of the hypothalamus and the functional neuroanatomy of visceromotor responses to stress. *Prog Brain Res.* 1996;107:201-222.)

peptides CRH, oxytocin, and AVP, PVH neurons projecting to brain stem and spinal cord include neurons expressing each of these peptides.

In the rodent, a wide variety of stressors have been determined to activate parvicellular CRH neurons, including cytokine injection, salt loading, hemorrhage, adrenalectomy, restraint, foot shock, hypoglycemia, fasting, and ether exposure. In contrast to the simplicity of inputs to magnicellular cells (Fig. 7-17A), it is not surprising that parvicellular CRH neurons receive a diverse and complex assortment of inputs (Fig. 7-18; see Fig. 7-17B). These inputs are divided into three major categories: brain stem, limbic forebrain, and hypothalamus. Because the PVH is not known to receive any direct projections from the cerebral cortex or thalamus, stressors relating to emotional or cognitive processing must involve indirect relay to the PVH.

Visceral sensory input to the PVH involves primarily two pathways. The nucleus of the solitary tract, the primary recipient of sensory information from the thoracic and abdominal viscera, sends dense catecholaminergic projections to the PVH, both directly and through relays in the ventrolateral medulla. These brain stem projections account for about half of the NPY fibers present in the PVH. A second major input responsible for transducing signals from bloodborne substances derives from three CVOs adjacent to the third ventricle: the SFO, the OVLT, and the MePO. These pathways account for activation of CRH neurons by what are referred to as *systemic* or *physiologic stressors*.[180]

By contrast, what are termed *neurogenic, emotional*, or *psychological stressors* involve, in addition, nociceptive or somatosensory pathways as well as cognitive and affective brain centers. Using elevation of Fos as an indicator of neuronal activation, detailed studies have compared PVH-projecting neurons activated by IL-1 treatment (systemic stressor) versus foot shock (neurogenic stressor).[180] Only catecholaminergic solitary tract nucleus and ventrolateral medulla neurons were activated by moderate doses of IL-1. In contrast, foot shock activated neurons of the solitary tract nucleus and ventrolateral medulla but also cell groups in the limbic forebrain and hypothalamus. Notably, pharmacologic or mechanical disruption of the ascending catecholaminergic fibers blocked IL-1–mediated activation but not foot shock–mediated activation of the HPA axis. Data suggest that pathways activated by other neurogenic and systemic stressors may overlap significantly with those activated by foot shock and IL-1 treatment, respectively.[179,180]

Except for the catecholaminergic neurons of the nucleus of the solitary tract and ventrolateral medulla, parts of the bed nucleus of the stria terminalis, and the dorsomedial nucleus of the hypothalamus, many inputs to the PVH, such as those deriving from the prefrontal cortex and

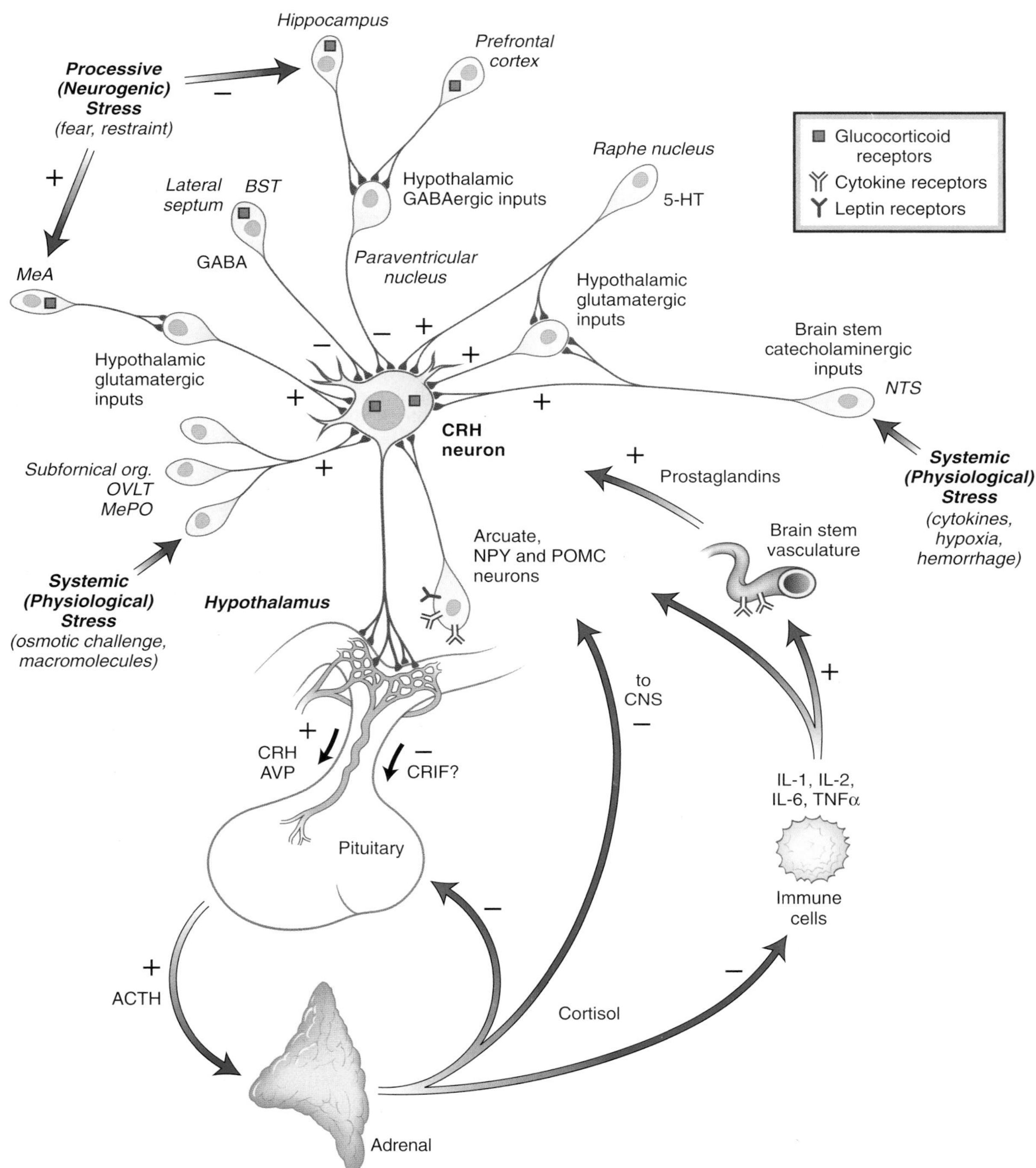

Figure 7-18 Regulation of the hypothalamic-pituitary-adrenal axis. ACTH, adrenocorticotropic hormone; AVP, arginine vasopressin; BST, bed nucleus of the stria terminalis; CNS, central nervous system; CRH, corticotropin-releasing hormone; CRIF, corticotropin release–inhibiting factor; GABA, γ-aminobutyric acid; 5-HT, 5-hydroxytryptamine; IL, interleukin; MeA, medial amygdala; MePO, medial preoptic nucleus; NPY, neuropeptide Y; NTS, nucleus of the tractus solitarius; OVLT, organum vasculosum of the lamina terminalis; POMC, pro-opiomelanocortin; TNFα, tumor necrosis factor-α.

lateral septum, are thought to act indirectly through local hypothalamic glutamatergic[181] and GABAergic neurons[182] with direct synapses to the CRH neurons. The bed nucleus of the stria terminalis is the only limbic region with prominent direct projections to the PVH. With substantial projections from the amygdala, hippocampus, and septal nuclei, this region may serve as a key integrative center for transmission of limbic information to the PVH.[179]

Inflammation and Cytokines

Stimulation of the immune system by foreign pathogens leads to a stereotyped set of responses orchestrated by the CNS. This constellation of stereotyped responses result from the complex interaction of the immune system and the CNS. They are mediated in large part by the hypothalamus and include coordinated autonomic, endocrine, and behavioral components with adapative consequences to restore homeostasis. It is now clear that cytokines produced by peripheral circulating cells of the immune system and central glial cells mediate the CNS responses. Early evidence supporting this hypothesis was provided by the seminal observations that cytokines such as IL-1β can activate the HPA axis.[183-185] Neuroimmunology, the discipline arising from the study of reciprocal interactions between the neuroendocrine and immune systems, and particularly the role of cytokines in mediating cachexia, is covered fully in Chapter 35.

This section focuses on cytokines and activation of the HPA axis. The resultant glucocorticoid secretion acts as a classic negative feedback to the immune system to dampen its response. In general, glucocorticoids inhibit most limbs of the immune response, including lymphocyte proliferation, production of immunoglobulins, cytokines, and cytotoxicity. These inhibitory reactions form the basis of the anti-inflammatory actions of glucocorticoids.

Glucocorticoid feedback on immune responses is regulatory and beneficial because loss of this function makes animals with adrenal insufficiency vulnerable to inflammation. However, this feedback response can have pathophysiologic consequences, because chronic activation of the HPA axis can certainly be detrimental.[186,187] Indeed, it is well established that chronic stress can lead to immunosuppression. The fact that products of inflammation such as IL-1β can activate the HPA axis suggests the operation of a negative feedback control loop to regulate the intensity of inflammation. The role of the hypothalamus in regulating pituitary-adrenal function is an excellent example of neuroimmunomodulation. Proposed models to explain how immune system signals might act on the CNS to modulate homeostatic circuits through integration of vagal input, peripheral cytokine interactions with receptors in the CVOs and cerebral blood vessels, and local production of cytokines within the CNS are explored in Chapter 35.

Other Factors Influencing Secretion of Corticotropin

Circadian Rhythms. Levels of ACTH and cortisol peak in the early morning, fall during the day to reach a nadir at about midnight, and begin to rise between 1 a.m. and 4 a.m. (see Fig. 7-7). Within the circadian cycle, approximately 15 to 18 pulses of ACTH can be discerned, their heights varying with the time of day.[188] The set point of feedback control by glucocorticoids also varies in a circadian pattern. Pituitary-adrenal rhythms are entrained to the light-dark cycle and can be changed over several days by exposure to an altered light schedule. It has long been assumed that the rhythm of ACTH secretion is driven by CRH rhythms, and CRH knockout mice were found to exhibit no circadian rhythm in corticosterone production. Remarkably, however, a diurnal rhythm in corticosterone was restored by a constant infusion of CRH to CRH knockout mice,[189] suggesting that CRH is necessary to permit pituitary or adrenal responsiveness to another diurnal rhythm generator.

Corticotropin Release–Inhibiting Factor. Disconnection of the pituitary from the hypothalamus in several species leads to increased basal levels of ACTH, and certain responses to physical stress (in contrast to psychological stress) are retained in such animals. These observations led several investigators to postulate the existence of an ACTH inhibitory factor, analogous to dopamine in the control of PRL secretion and to somatostatin in the control of GH secretion. Candidate hypothalamic peptides to inhibit ACTH release at the level of the pituitary include somatostatin, atrial natriuretic peptide, activins and inhibins, and peptide sequence 178 to 199 of the TRH prohormone.[190] There is not yet a consensus on the existence or identity of a physiologically relevant ACTH release-inhibiting factor.

Growth Hormone–Releasing Hormone

Chemistry and Evolution

Evidence for neural control of GH secretion came from studies of its regulation in animals with lesions of the hypothalamus[191] and from the demonstration that hypothalamic extracts stimulate the release of GH from the pituitary. After it was shown that GH is released episodically, follows a circadian rhythm, responds rapidly to stress, and is blocked by pituitary stalk section, the concept of neural control of GH secretion became a certainty. However, it was only with the discovery of the paraneoplastic syndrome of ectopic GHRH secretion by pancreatic adenomas in humans that sufficient starting material became available for peptide sequencing and subsequent cloning of a complementary deoxyribonucleic acid (cDNA).[192-195]

Two principal molecular forms of GHRH occur in the human hypothalamus: GHRH(1-44)-NH_2 and GHRH(1-40) (Fig. 7-19).[196] As with other neuropeptides, the various forms of GHRH arise from post-translational modification of a larger prohormone.[192,197] The N-terminal tyrosine of GHRH (or histidine in rodent GHRH) is essential for bioactivity, but a C-terminal NH_2 group is not. Fragments as short as (1-29)-NH_2 are active, but GHRH(1-27)-NH_2 is inactive. A circulating type IV dipeptidylpeptidase potently inactivates GHRH to its principal and more stable metabolite, GHRH(3-44)-NH_2,[198] which accounts for most of the immunoreactive peptide detected in plasma. As in the case of GnRH, there are GHRH differences among species; the peptides from seven species range in sequence homology with the human peptide from 93% in the pig to 67% in the rat.[196] The C-terminal end of GHRH exhibits the most sequence diversity among species, consistent with the exon arrangement of the gene and dispensability of these residues for GHRH receptor binding.

Despite its importance for elucidation of GHRH structure, ectopic secretion of the peptide is a rare cause of acromegaly. Fewer than 1% of acromegalic patients have elevated plasma levels of GHRH (see Chapter 9).[199] Approximately 20% of pancreatic adenomas and 5% of carcinoid tumors contain immunoreactive GHRH, but most are clinically silent.[200]

In addition to expression in the hypothalamus, the GHRH gene is expressed eutopically in human ovary, uterus, and placenta,[201] although its function in these tissues is not known. Studies in rat placenta indicate that an alternative transcriptional start site 10 kilobases upstream from the hypothalamic promoter is used, together with an alternatively spliced exon 1a.[202]

Growth Hormone–Releasing Hormone Receptor

The GHRH receptor is a member of a subfamily of G protein–coupled receptors that includes receptors for VIP, pituitary adenylyl cyclase–activating peptide, secretin, glucagon, glucagon-like peptide 1, calcitonin, parathyroid hormone or parathyroid hormone–related peptide, and gastric inhibitory polypeptide.[203,204] GHRH elevates intracellular cAMP by its receptor coupling to a stimulatory G protein (G_s), which activates adenylyl cyclase, increases

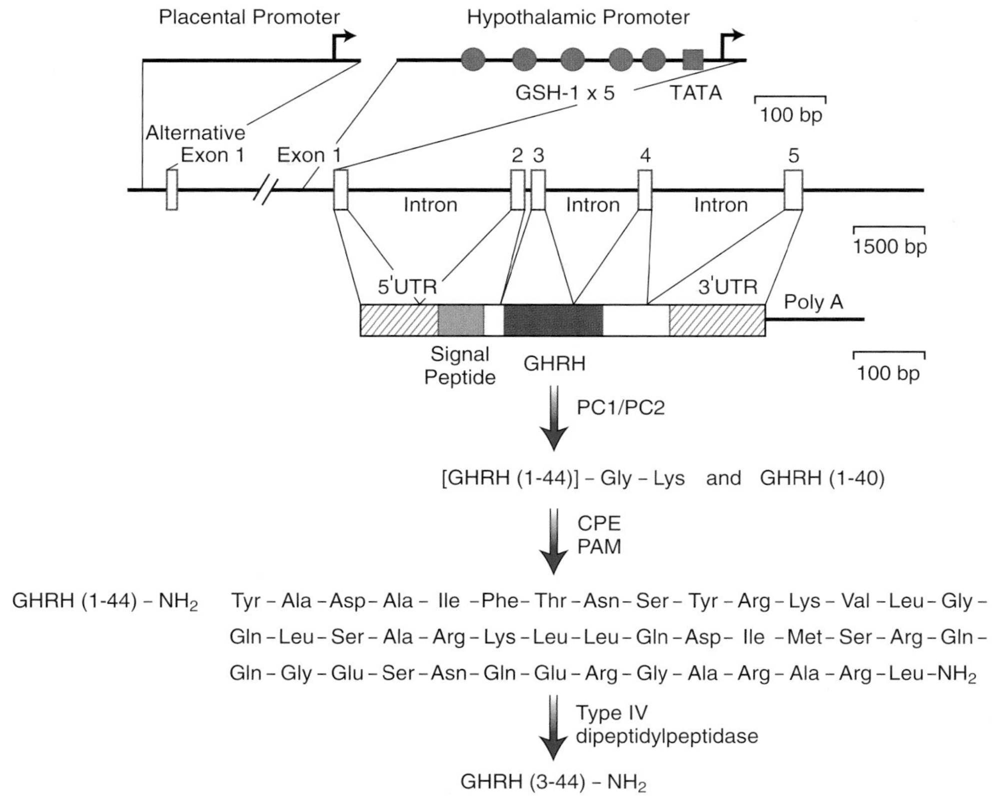

Figure 7-19 Diagram illustrating the genomic organization, messenger RNA structure, and post-translational processing of the human growth hormone–releasing hormone (GHRH) prohormone. The five GSH-1 homeodomain transcription factor binding sites in the proximal promoter have been characterized in the rat gene. All of the amino acid residues required for bioactive GHRH peptides are encoded by exon 3. An amino-terminal exopeptidase that cleaves the Tyr-Ala dipeptide is primarily responsible for inactivation of GHRH peptides in extracellular compartments. CPE, carboxypeptidase E; PAM, peptidylglycine α-amidating monooxygenase; PC1/PC2, prohormone convertases 1 and 2; TATA, Goldstein-Hogness box involved in binding RNA polymerase; UTR, untranslated region. (Compiled from data of Mayo KE, Cerelli GM, Lebo RV, et al. Gene encoding human growth hormone-releasing factor precursor: structure, sequence, and chromosomal assignment. *Proc Natl Acad Sci U S A.* 1985;82:63-67; Frohman LA, Downs TR, Chomczynski P, et al. Growth hormone-releasing hormone: structure, gene expression and molecular heterogeneity. *Acta Paediatr Scand Suppl.* 1990;367:81-86; González-Crespo S, Boronat A. Expression of the rat growth hormone-releasing hormone gene in placenta is directed by an alternative promoter. *Proc Natl Acad Sci U S A.* 1991;88:8749-8753; and Mutsuga N, Iwasaki Y, Morishita M, et al. Homeobox protein Gsh-1-dependent regulation of the rat GHRH gene promoter. *Mol Endocrinol.* 2001;15:2149-2156.)

intracellular free Ca^{2+}, releases preformed GH, and stimulates GH mRNA transcription and new GH synthesis (see Chapter 8).[205] GHRH also increases pituitary phosphatidylinositol turnover. Nonsense mutations in the human GHRH receptor gene are the cause of rare familial forms of GH deficiency[206,207] and indicate that no other gene product can fully compensate for the specific receptor in pituitary.

Effects on the Pituitary and Mechanism of Action

Intravenous administration of GHRH to individuals with normal pituitaries causes a prompt, dose-related increase in serum GH that peaks after 15 and 45 minutes, followed by a return to basal levels by 90 to 120 minutes (Fig. 7-20).[208] A maximally stimulating dose of GHRH is approximately 1 μg/kg, but the response differs considerably among individuals and within the same individual tested on different occasions, presumably because of endogenous cosecretagogue and somatostatin tone that exists at the time of GHRH injection. Repeated bolus administration or sustained infusions of GHRH over several hours cause a modest decrease in the subsequent GH secretory response to acute GHRH administration. However, unlike the marked desensitization of the GnRH receptor and decline in circulating gonadotropins that occur in response to continuous GnRH exposure, pulsatile GH secretion and insulin-like growth factor type 1 (IGF1) production are maintained by constant GHRH in the human.[208] This response suggests the involvement of additional factors that mediate the intrinsic diurnal rhythm of GH, and these factors are addressed in the following sections.

The pituitary effects of a single injection of GHRH are almost completely specific for GH secretion, and there is minimal evidence for any interaction between GHRH and the other classic hypophyseotropic releasing hormones.[208] GHRH has no effect on gut peptide hormone secretion. The GH secretory response to GHRH is enhanced by estrogen administration, glucocorticoids, and starvation. Major factors known to blunt the response to GHRH in humans are somatostatin, obesity, and advancing age.

In addition to its role as a GH secretagogue, GHRH is a physiologically relevant growth factor for somatotrophs. Transgenic mice expressing a GHRH cDNA coupled to a suitable promoter developed diffuse somatotroph hyperplasia and eventually pituitary macroadenomas.[209,210] The intracellular signal transduction pathways mediating the mitogenic action of GHRH are not known with certainty but probably involve an elevation of adenylyl cyclase

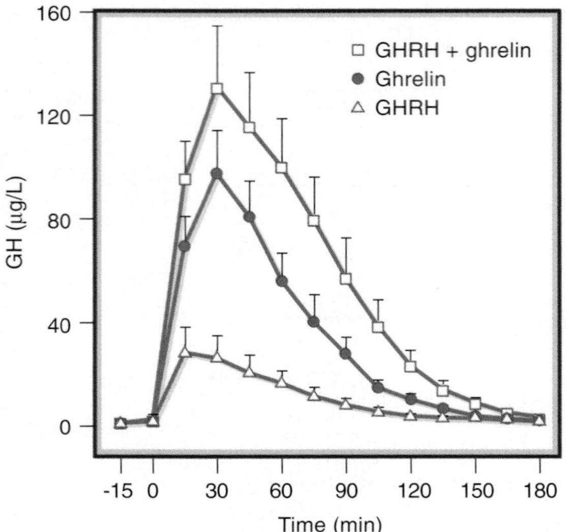

Figure 7-20 Response of normal men to growth hormone–releasing hormone GHRH(1-29) (1 μg/kg), ghrelin (1 μg/kg), or the combination of GHRH(1-29) and ghrelin administered by intravenous injection. Note the prompt release of growth hormone (GH), followed by a rather prolonged fall in hormone level in response to the administered secretagogues. Ghrelin alone was more efficacious than GHRH(1-29), and there was an additive effect when the two peptides were administered simultaneously. (From Arvat E, Macario M, Di Vito L, et al. Endocrine activities of ghrelin, a natural growth hormone secretagogue (GHS), in humans: comparison and interactions with hexarelin, a nonnatural peptidyl GHS, and GH-releasing hormone. *J Clin Endocrinol Metab.* 2001;86:1169-1174.)

activity. Several lines of evidence support this conclusion, including the association of activating mutations of the $G_s\alpha$ polypeptide in many human somatotroph adenomas.[211]

Extrapituitary Functions

GHRH has few known extrapituitary functions. The most important may be its activity as a sleep regulator. The administration of nocturnal GHRH boluses to normal men significantly increased the density of slow-wave sleep, and this has also been shown in other species.[212] Furthermore, there is a striking correlation between the age-related declines in slow-wave sleep and daily integrated GH secretion in healthy men.[213] These and other data suggest that central GHRH secretion is under circadian entrainment, and nocturnal elevations in GHRH pulse amplitude or frequency directly mediate sleep stage and sleep-induced increases in GH secretion.

GHRH has been reported to stimulate food intake in rats and sheep, but the effect is dependent on route of administration, time of administration, and macronutrient composition of the diet.[203] The neuropeptide's physiologic relevance to feeding in humans is unknown, although a study indicated that GHRH stimulated food intake in patients with anorexia nervosa but reduced it in patients with bulimia and in normal female control subjects.[214]

Growth Hormone–Releasing Peptides

In studies of the opioid control of GH secretion, several peptide analogues of met-enkephalin were found to be potent GH secretagogues. These include the GH-releasing peptide GHRP-6 (Fig. 7-21), hexarelin (His-D2MeTrp-Ala-Trp-DPhe-Lys-NH_2), and other more potent analogues including cyclic peptides and modified pentapeptides.[203,215]

GHRP-6: His–DTrp–Ala–Trp–DPhe–Lys–NH_2

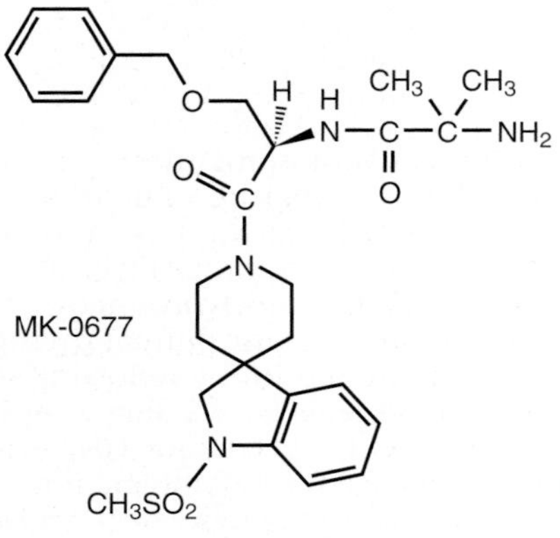

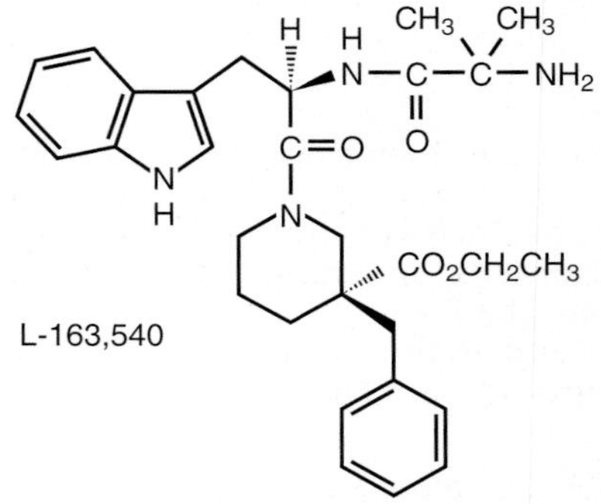

MK-0677

L-163,540

$O = C - (CH_2)_6 - CH_3$

Ghrelin: Gly - Ser - Ser - Phe - Leu - Ser - Pro - Glu - His - Gln - Arg - Val - Gln - Gln - Arg - Lys - Glu - Ser - Lys - Lys - Pro - Pro - Ala - Lys - Leu - Gln - Pro - Arg

Figure 7-21 Structure of a synthetic peptidyl growth hormone (GH) secretagogue (GH-releasing peptide 6, or GHRP-6) and nonpeptidyl GH secretagogue (MK-0677 and L-163,540) and a natural ligand (ghrelin), all of which bind and activate the growth hormone secretagogue (GHS) receptor. Ghrelin is an acylated 28-amino-acid peptide. The *O*-n-octanoylation at Ser3 is essential for biologic activity and is a unique post-translational modification among all known proteins. (Adapted from Smith RG, Feighner S, Prendergast K, et al. A new orphan receptor involved in pulsatile growth hormone release. *Trends Endocrinol Metab.* 1999;10:128-135; Kojima M, Hosoda H, Date Y, et al. Ghrelin is a growth hormone-releasing acylated peptide from stomach. *Nature.* 1999;402:656-660.)

Subsequently, a series of nonpeptidyl GHRP mimetics were synthesized with greater oral bioavailability, including the spiropiperidine MK-0677 and the shorter-acting benzylpiperidine L-163,540 (see Fig. 7-21). Common to all of these compounds, and the basis of their differentiation from GHRH analogues in pharmacologic activity screens, is their activation of phospholipase C and inositol 1,4,5-triphosphate. This property was exploited in a cloning strategy that led to the identification of a G protein–coupled receptor, GHS-R, that is highly selective for the GH secretagogue class of ligands.[216] The GHS-R is unrelated to the GHRH receptor and is highly expressed in the anterior pituitary gland and multiple brain areas, including the medial basal hypothalamus, the hippocampus, and the mesencephalic nuclei that are centers of dopamine and serotonin production.

Peptidyl and nonpeptidyl GHSs are active when administered by intranasal and oral routes, are more potent on a weight basis than GHRH itself, are more effective in vivo than in vitro, synergize with coadministered GHRH and are almost ineffective in the absence of GHRH, and do not suppress somatostatin secretion.[203,208] Prolonged infusions of GHRP amplify pulsatile GH secretion in normal men. GHRP administration, like that of GHRH, facilitates slow-wave sleep. Patients with hypothalamic disease leading to GHRH deficiency have low or no response to hexarelin; similarly, pediatric patients with complete absence of the pituitary stalk have no GH secretory response to hexarelin.[217]

The potent biologic effects of GHRPs and the identification of the GHS-R suggested the existence of a natural ligand for the receptor that is involved in the physiologic regulation of GH secretion. A probable candidate for this ligand is the acylated peptide ghrelin, which is produced and secreted into the circulation from the stomach (Fig. 7-22).[13] The effects of ghrelin on GH secretion in humans are identical to or more potent than those of the non-natural GHRPs (see Fig. 7-20).[218] In addition, ghrelin acutely increases circulating PRL, ACTH, cortisol, and aldosterone levels.[218] There is debate concerning the extent and localization of ghrelin expression in the brain that must be resolved before the implications of gastric-derived ghrelin in the regulation of pituitary hormone secretion are fully understood. A proposed role for ghrelin in appetite and the regulation of food intake is discussed in Chapter 35.

Clinical Applications

GHRH stimulates growth in children with intact pituitaries, but the optimal dosage, route, and frequency of administration, as well as possible usefulness by the nasal route, have not been determined. The availability of recombinant human GH (which requires less frequent injections than GHRH) and the development of the more potent GHSs with improved oral bioavailability have reduced enthusiasm for the clinical use of GHRH or its analogues. GHRH is not useful for the differential diagnosis of hypothalamic and pituitary causes of GH deficiency in children. However, in adults a combined GHRH-GHRP challenge test may be ideal for the diagnosis of GH reserve. GH release in response to the combined secretagogues is not influenced by age, sex, or body mass index, and the test has a wider margin of safety than an insulin tolerance test.[219,220]

The potential clinical applications of GHSs including MK-0677 are still being explored.[203,215] An area of intense interest is the normal decline in GH secretion with age. GH administration in healthy older individuals has been associated with increased lean body mass, increased muscle strength, and decreased fat mass, although there is a high incidence of adverse side effects. The physiologic GH profile induced by MK-0677 may be better tolerated than GH injections. However, in contrast to treatment with GHRH, chronic administration of GHSs leads to significant desensitization of the GHS-R and attenuation of the GH response. The release of pituitary hormones other than GH may also limit the applicability of GHS therapy. Finally, apart from actions on GH secretion, both GHRH and GHSs are being investigated for the treatment of sleep disorders commonly associated with aging.

Neuroendocrine Regulation of Growth Hormone Secretion

GH secretion is regulated by hypothalamic GHRH and somatostatin interacting with circulating hormones and additional modulatory peptides at the level of both the pituitary and the hypothalamus (see Fig. 7-22).[203,208,221] Additional background on somatostatin and its functions other than control of GH secretion are presented in a later section (see "Somatostatin").

Feedback Control

Negative feedback control of GH release is mediated by GH itself and by IGF1, which is synthesized in the liver and other tissues under control of GH. Direct GH effects on the hypothalamus are produced by short-loop feedback, whereas those involving IGF1 and other circulating factors influenced by GH, including free fatty acids and glucose, are long-loop systems analogous to the pituitary-thyroid and pituitary-adrenal axes. Control of GH secretion therefore includes two closed-loop systems (GH and IGF1) and one open-loop regulatory system (neural).

Although most of the evidence for a direct role of GH in its own negative feedback has been derived from animals, an elegant study in normal men demonstrated that GH pretreatment blocks the subsequent GH secretory response to GHRH by a mechanism that is dependent on somatostatin.[222] The mechanism responsible for GH feedback through the hypothalamus has been largely elucidated in rodent models. GH receptors are selectively expressed on somatostatin neurons in the PVH nucleus and on NPY neurons in the arcuate nucleus. Fos gene expression is acutely elevated in both populations of GH receptor–positive neurons by GH administration, indicating an activation of hypothalamic circuitry that includes these neurons. Similarly, GHRH neurons in the arcuate nucleus are acutely activated by MK-0677 because of their selective expression of the GHS-R. Zheng and colleagues[223] showed in the latter group of neurons that Fos induction after MK-0677 administration was blocked by pretreatment of mice with GH (Fig. 7-23). The effect must be indirect, because there are no GH receptors on GHRH neurons. However, type 2 somatostatin receptors are expressed on GHRH neurons, and the somatostatin analogue octreotide also significantly blocked Fos activation in the arcuate nucleus by MK-0677. The inhibitory effects of either GH or octreotide pretreatment were abolished in knockout mice lacking the specific somatostatin receptor (see Fig. 7-23). Together with data from many other experiments, these results strongly support a model of GH-negative feedback regulation that involves the primary activation of periventricular somatostatin neurons by GH. These tuberoinfundibular neurons then inhibit GH secretion directly by release of somatostatin in the median eminence, but they also indirectly inhibit GH secretion by way of collateral axonal projections to the arcuate nucleus that synapse on and inhibit GHRH neurons (see Fig. 7-22). It is probable from evidence in rodents that NPY and

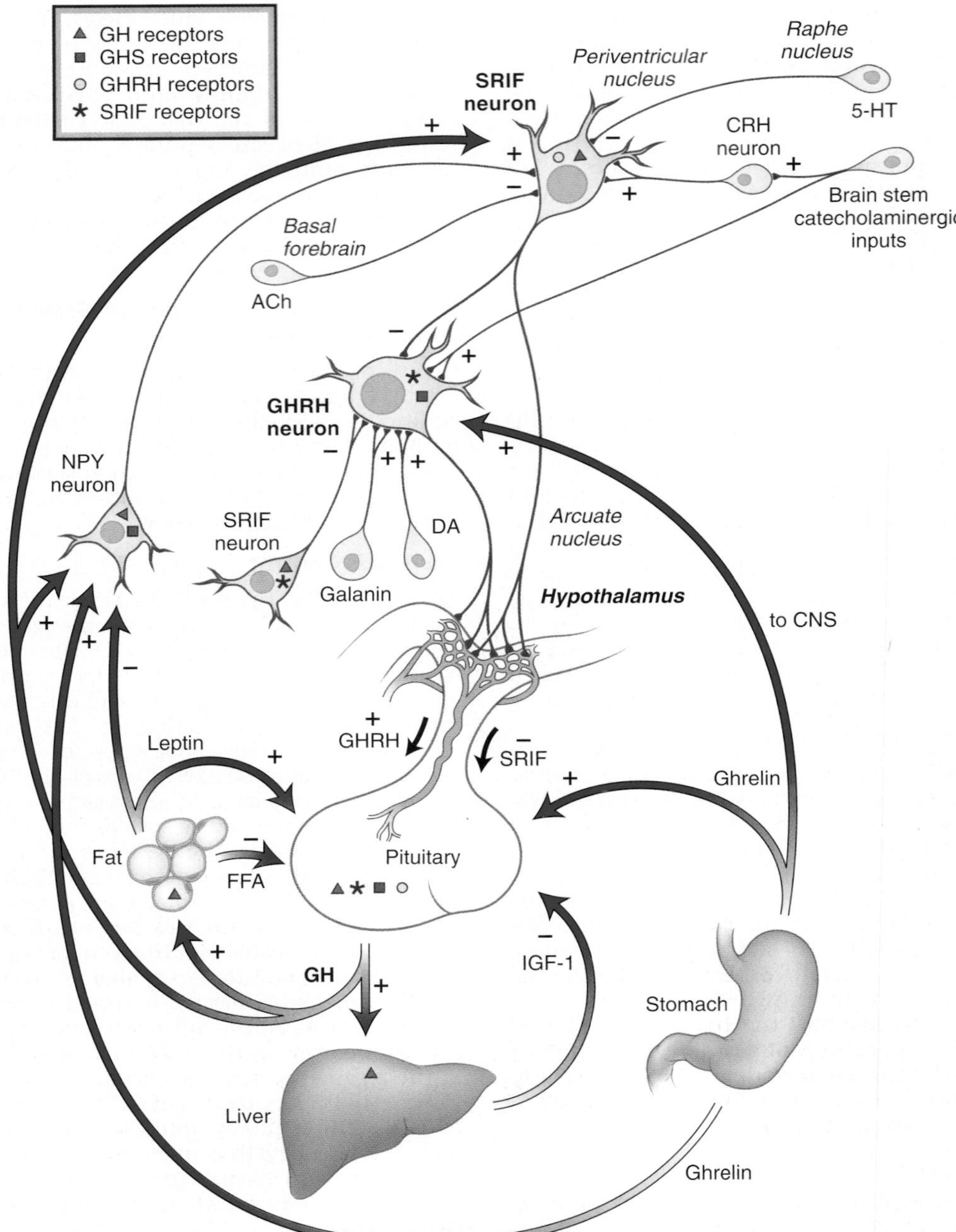

Figure 7-22 Regulation of the hypothalamic-pituitary-growth hormone axis. Growth hormone (GH) secretion by the pituitary is stimulated by growth hormone–releasing hormone (GHRH) and inhibited by somatostatin (SRIF). Negative feedback control of GH secretion is exerted at the pituitary level by insulin-like growth factor type I (IGF-1) and by free fatty acids (FFA). GH itself exerts a short-loop negative feedback through activation of SRIF neurons in the hypothalamic periventricular nucleus. These SRIF neurons directly synapse on arcuate GHRH neurons and project axon collaterals to the median eminence. Neuropeptide Y (NPY) neurons in the arcuate nucleus also indirectly modulate GH secretion by integrating peripheral GH, leptin, and ghrelin signals and projecting to periventricular SRIF neurons. Ghrelin is secreted from the stomach and is a putative natural ligand for the growth hormone secretagogue (GHS) receptor that stimulates GH secretion at both the hypothalamic and pituitary levels. On the basis of indirect pharmacologic data, release of GHRH is stimulated by galanin, γ-aminobutyric acid (GABA), α_2-adrenergic, and dopaminergic inputs and inhibited by somatostatin. Secretion of somatostatin is inhibited by muscarinic acetylcholine (ACh) and 5-HT-1D receptor ligands and increased by β_2-adrenergic stimuli and corticotropin-releasing hormone (CRH). CNS, central nervous system; DA, dopamine; 5-HT, serotonin.

galanin also play a part in the short-loop feedback of GH secretion, but a definitive mechanism in humans is not yet established.

IGF1 has a major inhibitory action on GH secretion at the level of the pituitary gland.[203] IGF1 receptors are expressed on human somatotroph adenoma cells and inhibit both spontaneous and GHRH-stimulated GH release. In addition, gene expression of both GH and the pituitary-specific transcription factor PIT1 is inhibited by IGF1. Conflicting data among species suggest that circulating IGF1 may also regulate GH secretion by actions within the brain. The feedback effects of IGF1 account for the fact that serum GH levels are elevated in conditions in which circulating levels of IGF1 are low, such as anorexia nervosa,

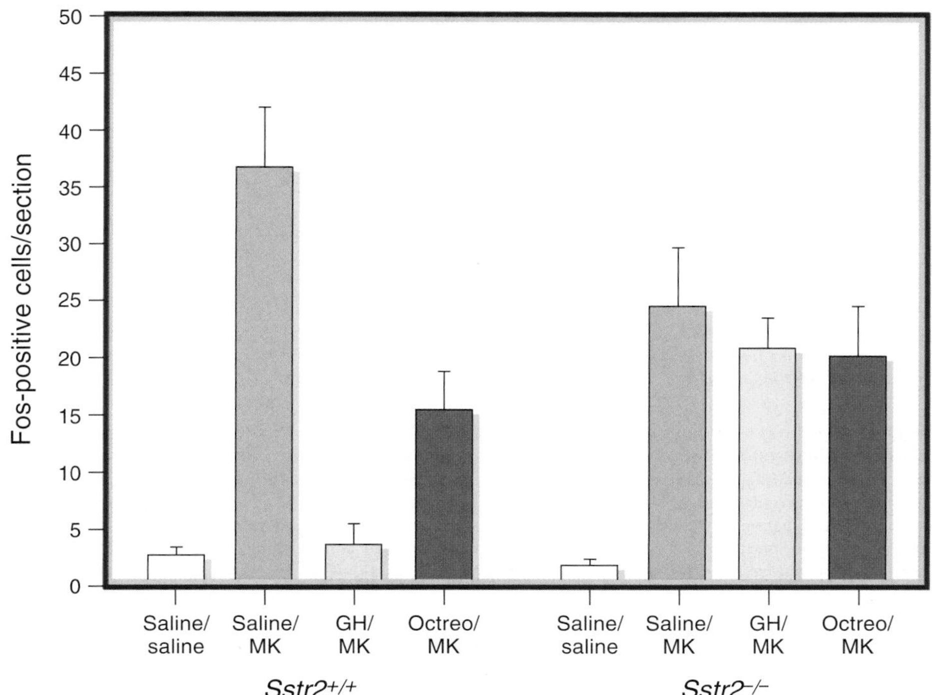

Figure 7-23 Somatostatin and the somatostatin receptor 2 subtype are involved in the short-loop inhibitory feedback of growth hormone (GH) on arcuate neurons. Activation of neurons in the arcuate nucleus was determined by the quantification of immunoreactive Fos-positive cells after administration of the growth hormone secretagogue MK-0677 (MK). Preliminary treatment of wild-type mice (*SstR2+/+*) with either GH or the somatostatin analogue octreotide (Octreo) significantly attenuated the neuronal activation by MK-0677. In contrast, GH and octreotide had no effect on MK-0677 neuronal activation in somatostatin receptor 2-deficient mice (*SstR2−/−*). (Adapted from Zheng H, Bailey A, Jian M-H, et al. Somatostatin receptor subtype 2 knockout mice are refractory to growth hormone-negative feedback on arcuate neurons. *Mol Endocrinol.* 1997;11:1709-1717.)

protein-calorie starvation,[224] and Laron dwarfism (the result of a defect in the GH receptor).

Neural Control

The predominant hypothalamic influence on GH release is stimulatory, and section of the pituitary stalk or lesions of the basal hypothalamus cause reduction of basal and induced GH release.[203] When the somatostatinergic component is inactivated (e.g., by anti-somatostatin antibody injection in rats), basal GH levels and GH responses to the usual provocative stimuli are enhanced.

GHRH-containing nerve fibers that terminate adjacent to portal vessels in the external zone of the median eminence arise principally from within, above, and lateral to the infundibular nucleus in human hypothalamus, corresponding to rodent arcuate and ventromedial nuclei.[225] Perikarya of the tuberoinfundibular somatostatin neurons are located almost completely in the medial periventricular nucleus and the parvicellular component of the anterior PVH. Neuroanatomic and functional evidence suggests a bidirectional synaptic interaction between the two peptidergic systems.[203]

Multiple extrahypothalamic brain regions provide efferent connections to the hypothalamus and regulate GHRH and somatostatin neuronal activity (Fig. 7-24; see Fig. 7-22). Somatosensory and affective information is integrated and filtered through the amygdaloid complex. The basolateral amygdala provides an excitatory input to the hypothalamus, and the central extended amygdala, which includes the central and medial nuclei of the amygdala together with the bed nucleus of the stria terminalis, provides a GABAergic inhibitory input. Many intrinsic neurons of the hypothalamus also release GABA, often with a peptide cotransmitter. Excitatory cholinergic fibers arise to a small extent from forebrain projection nuclei but mostly from hypothalamic cholinergic interneurons, which densely innervate the external zone of the median eminence. Similarly, the origin of dopaminergic and histaminergic neurons is local, with their cell bodies located in the hypothalamic arcuate and tuberomammillary bodies, respectively. Two important ascending pathways to the medial basal hypothalamus regulate GH secretion and originate from serotoninergic neurons in the raphe nuclei and adrenergic neurons in the nucleus of the tractus solitarius and ventral lateral nucleus of the medulla.

Both GHRH and somatostatin neurons express presynaptic and postsynaptic receptors for multiple neurotransmitters and peptides (Table 7-5). The α_2-adrenoreceptor agonist clonidine reliably stimulates GH release, and for this reason a clonidine test was a standard diagnostic tool in pediatric endocrinology. The stimulatory effect is blocked by the specific α_2-antagonist yohimbine and appears to involve a dual mechanism of action—inhibition of somatostatin neurons and activation of GHRH neurons. In addition, partial attenuation of the effects of clonidine by mixed serotonin 5-HT1 and 5-HT2 antagonists suggests that some of the relevant α_2-receptors are located presynaptically on serotoninergic nerve terminals and increase serotonin release. Both norepinephrine and epinephrine play physiologic roles in the adrenergic stimulation of GH secretion. The α_1-agonists have no effect on GH secretion in humans, but β_2-agonists such as the bronchodilator salbutamol inhibit GH secretion by stimulating the release of somatostatin from nerve terminals in the median

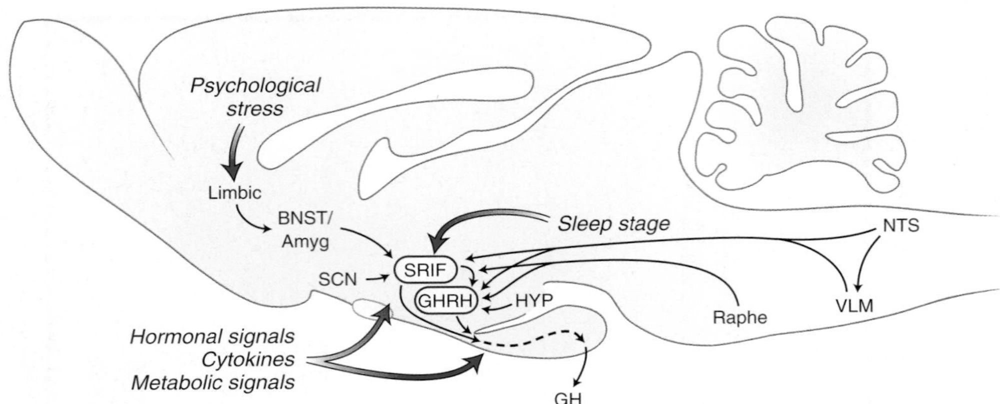

Figure 7-24 Neural pathways involved in growth hormone (GH) regulation. This diagram illustrates the varied pathways by which impulses from the limbic system and brain stem ultimately impinge on the hypothalamic periventricular and arcuate nuclei to stimulate GH release through the mediation of somatostatin (SRIF) and growth hormone–releasing hormone (GHRH). Psychological stress modulates hypothalamic function indirectly through the bed nucleus of the stria terminalis (BNST) and the amygdalar complex (Amyg). Circadian rhythms are entrained in part by projections from the suprachiasmatic nucleus (SCN). Complex reciprocal interactions between sleep stage and GHRH release involve cortex and subcortical nuclei, but the detailed mechanisms are not known. Dopaminergic and histaminergic input are from neurons located in the arcuate and mammillary nuclei, respectively, of the hypothalamus (HYP). Ascending catecholaminergic projections arise in both the nucleus of the tractus solitarius (NTS) and the ventral lateral medulla (VLM). Serotoninergic (5-HT) afferents are from the raphe nuclei. In addition to these neural pathways, a variety of peripheral hormonal and metabolic signals and cytokines influence GH secretion by actions within the medial basal hypothalamus and pituitary gland.

eminence. These effects are blocked by propranolol, a nonspecific β-antagonist. Dopamine generally has a net effect of stimulation of GH secretion, but the mechanism is not clear because of multiple dopamine receptor subtypes and the apparent activation of both GHRH and somatostatin neurons.

Serotonin's effect on GH release in humans was difficult to decipher because of the large number of receptor subtypes. However, clinical studies with the receptor-selective agonist sumatriptan clearly implicated the 5-HT1D receptor subtype in the stimulation of basal GH levels.[226] The drug also potentiates the effect of a maximal dose of GHRH, suggesting the recurring theme of GH disinhibition by inhibition of hypothalamic somatostatin neurons in its mechanism of action. Histaminergic pathways acting through H_1 receptors play only a minor, conditional stimulatory role in GH secretion in humans.

Acetylcholine appears to be an important physiologic regulator of GH secretion.[227] Blockade of muscarinic acetylcholine receptors reduces or abolishes GH secretory responses to GHRH, glucagon and arginine, morphine, and exercise. In contrast, drugs that potentiate cholinergic transmission increase basal GH levels and enhance the GH response to GHRH in normal individuals and in subjects with obesity or Cushing's disease. In vitro acetylcholine inhibits somatostatin release from hypothalamic fragments, and acetylcholine can act directly on the pituitary to inhibit GH release. There may even be a paracrine cholinergic control system within the pituitary. However, the sum of evidence suggests that the primary mechanism of action of muscarinic M1 agonists is inhibition of somatostatin neuronal activity or release of peptide from somatostatinergic terminals. Short-term cholinergic blockade with the M1 muscarinic receptor antagonist pirenzepine reduced the GH excess in patients with poorly controlled diabetes mellitus.[228] However, in the long term, cholinergic blockade did not prevent complications associated with the hypersomatotropic state.

Many neuropeptides in addition to GHRH and somatostatin are involved in the modulation of GH secretion in humans (see Table 7-5).[203,208] Among these, the evidence is most compelling for a stimulatory role of galanin acting in the human hypothalamus by a GHRH-dependent mechanism.[229] Many GHRH neurons are immunopositive for galanin as well as neurotensin and tyrosine hydroxylase. Galanin's actions may be explained, in part, by presynaptic facilitation of catecholamine release from nerve terminals and subsequent direct adrenergic stimulation of GHRH release.[230] Opioid peptides also stimulate GH release, probably by disinhibition of GHRH neurons, but under normal circumstances, endogenous opioid tone in the hypothalamus is presumed to be low because opioid antagonists have little acute effect on GH secretion.

A larger number of neuropeptides are known or suspected to inhibit GH secretion in humans, at least under certain circumstances.[208] The list includes NPY, CRH, calcitonin, oxytocin, neurotensin, VIP, and TRH. Inhibitory actions of NPY are well established in the rat. The effect on GH secretion is secondary to stimulation of somatostatin neurons and is of particular interest because of the presumed role in GH autofeedback (discussed earlier) and the integration of GH secretion with regulation of energy intake and expenditure (see "External and Metabolic Signals"). Finally, TRH has the well-established paradoxical effect of increasing GH secretion in patients with acromegaly, type 1 diabetes mellitus, hypothyroidism, or hepatic or renal failure.

Other Factors Influencing Secretion of Growth Hormone

Human Growth Hormone Rhythms. The deciphering of rhythmic GH secretion has relied on a combination of technical innovations in sampling and GH assay and sophisticated mathematical modeling, including deconvolution analysis and the calculation of approximate entropy as a measure of orderliness or regularity in minute-to-minute secretory patterns.[208] At least three distinct categories of GH rhythms, which differ markedly in their time scales, can be considered here.

TABLE 7-5

Factors That Change Growth Hormone (GH) Secretion in Humans

Physiologic	Hormones and Neurotransmitters	Pathologic
Stimulatory Factors		
Episodic, spontaneous release	Insulin hypoglycemia	Acromegaly
Exercise	2-Deoxyglucose	TRH
Stress	Amino acid infusions	GnRH
Physical	Arginine, lysine	Glucose
Psychological	Neuropeptides	Arginine
Slow-wave sleep	GHRH	Interleukins 1, 2, 6
Postprandial glucose decline	Ghrelin	Protein depletion
Fasting	Galanin	Starvation
	Opioids (μ-receptors)	Anorexia nervosa
	Melatonin	Renal failure
	Classic neurotransmitters	Liver cirrhosis
	α_2-Adrenergic agonists	Type 1 diabetes mellitus
	β-Adrenergic antagonists	
	M1 cholinergic agonists	
	5-HT1D-serotonin agonists	
	H1-histamine agonists	
	GABA (basal levels)	
	Dopamine (? D2 receptor)	
	Estrogen	
	Testosterone	
	Glucocorticoids (acute)	
Inhibitory Factors*		
Postprandial hyperglycemia	Glucose infusion	Acromegaly
Elevated free fatty acids	Neuropeptides	L-Dopa
Elevated GH levels	Somatostatin	D2R DA agonists
Elevated IGF1 (pituitary)	Calcitonin	Phentolamine
REM sleep	Neuropeptide Y (NPY†)	Galanin
Senescence, aging	CRH†	Obesity
	Classic neurotransmitters	Hypothyroidism
	$\alpha_{1/2}$-Adrenergic antagonists	Hyperthyroidism
	β_2-Adrenergic agonists	
	H1 histamine antagonists	
	Serotonin antagonist	
	Nicotinic cholinergic agonists	
	Glucocorticoids (chronic)	

*In many instances, the inhibition can be demonstrated only as a suppression of GH release induced by a pharmacologic stimulus.

†The inhibitory actions of NPY and CRH on GH secretion are firmly established in the rodent and are secondary to increased somatostatin tone. Contradictory evidence exists in the human for both peptides, and further studies are required.

CRH, Corticotropin-releasing hormone; DA, dopamine; GHRH, growth hormone–releasing hormone; GnRH, gonadotropin-releasing hormone; IGF1, insulin-like growth factor type 1; REM, rapid eye movement; TRH, thyrotropin-releasing hormone.

The daily GH secretion rate varies over 2 orders of magnitude, from a maximum of almost 2.0 mg/day in late puberty to a minimum of 20 μg/day in older or obese adults. The neonatal period is characterized by markedly amplified GH secretory bursts followed by a prepubertal decade of stable, moderate GH secretion of 200 to 600 μg/day. There is a marked increase in daily GH secretion during puberty that is accompanied by a commensurate rise in plasma IGF1 to levels that constitute a state of physiologic hypersomatotropism. This pubertal increase in GH secretion is the result of increased GH mass per secretory burst rather than increased pulse frequency. Although the changes are clearly related to the increases in gonadal steroid hormones and can be mimicked by administration of estrogen or testosterone to hypogonadal children, the underlying neuroendocrine mechanisms are not fully understood. One hypothesis is that decreased sensitivity of the hypothalamic-pituitary axis to negative feedback from GH and IGF1 leads to increased GHRH release and action. Young adults have a return of daily GH secretion to prepubertal levels despite continued gonadal steroid elevation. The so-called somatopause is defined by an exponential decline in GH secretory rate with a half-life of 7 years starting in the third decade of life.

GH secretion in young adults exhibits a true circadian rhythm over a 24-hour period, characterized by a greater nocturnal secretory mass that is independent of sleep onset.[231] However, as discussed earlier, GH release is further facilitated when slow-wave sleep coincides with the normal circadian peak. Under basal conditions, GH levels are low most of the time, with an ultradian rhythm of about 10 secretory pulses per 24 hours in men (20 in women), as calculated by deconvolution analysis.[232] Both sexes have an increased pulse frequency during the nighttime hours, but the fraction of total daily GH secretion associated with nocturnal pulses is much greater in men. Overall, women have more continuous GH secretion and more frequent GH pulses that are of more uniform size than in men.[232] A complementary study using approximate entropy analysis concluded that the nonpulsatile regularity of GH secretion is also significantly different in men and women.[233] These sexually dimorphic patterns in the human are actually quite similar to those in the rat, although the sex differences are not as extreme in humans.[208,233]

The neuroendocrine basis for sex differences in the ultradian rhythm of GH secretion is not fully understood. Gonadal sex steroids play both an organizational role during development of the hypothalamus and an activational role in the adult, regulating expression of the genes for many of the peptides and receptors central to GH regulation.[203,208] In the human, unlike the rat, the hypothalamic actions of testosterone appear to result predominantly from its aromatization to 17β-estradiol and interaction with estrogen receptors. Hypothalamic somatostatin appears to play a more prominent role in men than in women in the regulation of pulsatile GH secretion, and this difference is postulated to be a key factor in producing the sexual dimorphism.[232,234,235]

External and Metabolic Signals. The various peripheral signals that modulate GH secretion in humans are summarized in Table 7-5 (also see Figs. 7-22 and 7-24). Of particular importance are factors related to energy intake and metabolism, because they provide a common signal between the peripheral tissues and hypothalamic centers regulating nonendocrine homeostatic pathways in addition to the classic hypophyseotropic neurons. It is also in this complex arena that species-specific regulatory responses are particularly prominent, making extrapolations between rodent experimental models and human GH regulation less reliable.[203,208]

Important triggers of GH release include the normal decrease in blood glucose concentration after intake of a carbohydrate-rich meal, absolute hypoglycemia, exercise, physical and emotional stress, and high intake of protein (mediated by amino acids). Some of the pathologic causes of elevated GH represent extremes of these physiologic signals and include protein-calorie starvation, anorexia nervosa, liver failure, and type 1 diabetes mellitus. A critical concept is that many of these GH triggers work through the same final common mechanism of somatostatin withdrawal and consequent disinhibition of GH secretion. In contrast, postprandial hyperglycemia, glucose infusion, elevated plasma free fatty acids, type 2 diabetes mellitus (with obesity and insulin resistance), and obesity are all associated with inhibition of GH secretion. The role of leptin in mediating increases or decreases in GH release is complicated by its multiple sites of action and coexistent secretory environment. Similarly, other members of the cytokine family including IL-1, IL-2, IL-6, and endotoxin have been inconsistently shown to stimulate GH in humans.

The actions of steroid hormones on GH secretion are complex because of their multiple loci of action within the proximal hypothalamic-pituitary components in addition to secondary effects on other neural and endocrine systems. Glucocorticoids in particular produce opposite responses that are dependent on the chronicity of administration. Moreover, glucocorticoid effects follow an inverted U-shaped dose-response curve. Both low and high glucocorticoid levels reduce GH secretion, the former because of decreased GH gene expression and somatotroph responsiveness to GHRH and the latter because of increased hypothalamic somatostatin tone and decreased GHRH. Similarly, physiologic levels of thyroid hormones are necessary to maintain GH secretion and promote GH gene expression. Excessive thyroid hormone is also inhibitory to the GH axis, and the mechanism is speculated to be a combination of increased hypothalamic somatostatin tone, GHRH deficiency, and suppressed pituitary GH production.

Somatostatin

Chemistry and Evolution

A factor that potently inhibits GH release from pituitary in vitro was unexpectedly identified during early efforts to isolate GHRH from hypothalamic extracts.[236] Somatostatin, the peptide responsible for this inhibition of GH secretion and the inhibition of insulin secretion by a pancreatic islet extract, was eventually isolated from hypothalamus and sequenced by Brazeau and colleagues in 1973.[237] The term *somatostatin* was originally applied to a cyclic peptide containing 14 amino acids, called somatostatin-14 (SST-14) (Fig. 7-25). Subsequently, a second form, known as N-terminal extended somatostatin-28 (SST-28), was identified as a secretory product. Both forms of somatostatin are derived through independent cleavage of a common prohormone by prohormone convertases.[238] In addition, the isolation of SST-28(1-12) in some tissues suggests that SST-14 can be secondarily processed from SST-28. SST-14 is the predominant form in the brain (including the hypothalamus), whereas SST-28 is the major form in the gastrointestinal tract, especially the duodenum and jejunum.

The name *somatostatin* is descriptively inadequate because the molecule also inhibits TSH secretion from the pituitary and has nonpituitary roles including activity as a neurotransmitter or neuromodulator in the central and peripheral nervous systems and as a regulatory peptide in gut and pancreas. As a pituitary regulator, somatostatin is a true neurohormone—that is, a neuronal secretory product that enters the blood (hypophyseal-portal circulation) to affect cell function at remote sites. In the gut, somatostatin is present in the myenteric plexus, where it acts as a neurotransmitter, and in epithelial cells, where it influences the function of adjacent cells as a paracrine secretion. Somatostatin can influence its own secretion from delta cells (an autocrine function) in addition to acting as a paracrine factor in pancreatic islets. Gut exocrine secretion can be modulated by intraluminal action, so it is also a lumone. Because of its wide distribution, broad spectrum of regulatory effects, and evolutionary history, this peptide can be regarded as an archetypical pansystem modulator.

The genes that encode somatostatin in humans[239] (see Fig. 7-25) and a number of other species exhibit striking sequence homology, even in primitive fish such as the anglerfish. Furthermore, the amino acid sequence of SST-14 is identical in all vertebrates. Formerly, it was accepted that all tetrapods have a single gene encoding both SST-14 and SST-28 and that teleost fish have two nonallelic pre-prosomatostatin genes (*PPSI* and *PPSII*), each of which encodes only one form of the mature somatostatin peptides. This situation implied that a common ancestral gene underwent a duplication event after the split of teleosts from the descendants of tetrapods.

However, both lampreys and amphibians, which predate and postdate the teleost evolutionary divergence, respectively, have now been shown to have at least two PPS genes.[240] A more distantly related gene has been identified in mammals that encodes cortistatin, a somatostatin-like peptide that is highly expressed in cortex and hippocampus.[241,242] Cortistatin-14 differs from SST-14 by three amino acid residues but has high affinity for all known subtypes of somatostatin receptors (see later discussion). The human gene sequence predicts a tripeptide-extended cortistatin-17 and a further N-terminal extended cortistatin-29.[243] A revised evolutionary concept of the somatostatin gene family is that a primordial gene underwent duplication at or before the advent of chordates, and the two resulting genes underwent mutation at different rates to produce the distinct pre-prosomatostatin and pre-procortistatin genes in mammals.[240] A second gene duplication probably occurred in teleosts to generate *PPSI* and *PPSII* from the ancestral somatostatin gene.

Apart from its expression in neurons of the PVH and the arcuate hypothalamic nucleus and its involvement in GH secretion (discussed earlier), somatostatin is highly expressed in the cortex, lateral septum, extended amygdala, reticular nucleus of the thalamus, hippocampus, and many brain stem nuclei. Cortistatin is present in the brain, at a small fraction of the level of somatostatin and in a more limited distribution, primarily confined to cortex and hippocampus. The molecular mechanisms underlying the developmental and hormonal regulation of somatostatin gene transcription have been most extensively studied in pancreatic islet cells.[244-246] Less is known concerning the regulation of somatostatin gene expression in neurons, except that activation is strongly controlled by binding of the phosphorylated transcription factor CRE-binding protein to its cognate CRE contained in the promoter sequence.[247,248] Enhancer elements in the somatostatin gene promoter that bind complexes of homeodomain-containing transcription factors (PAX6, PBX, PREP1) and upregulate gene expression in pancreatic islets may actually represent gene silencer elements in neurons (see Fig. 7-25, promoter elements TSE_{II} and UE-A).[246] Conversely,

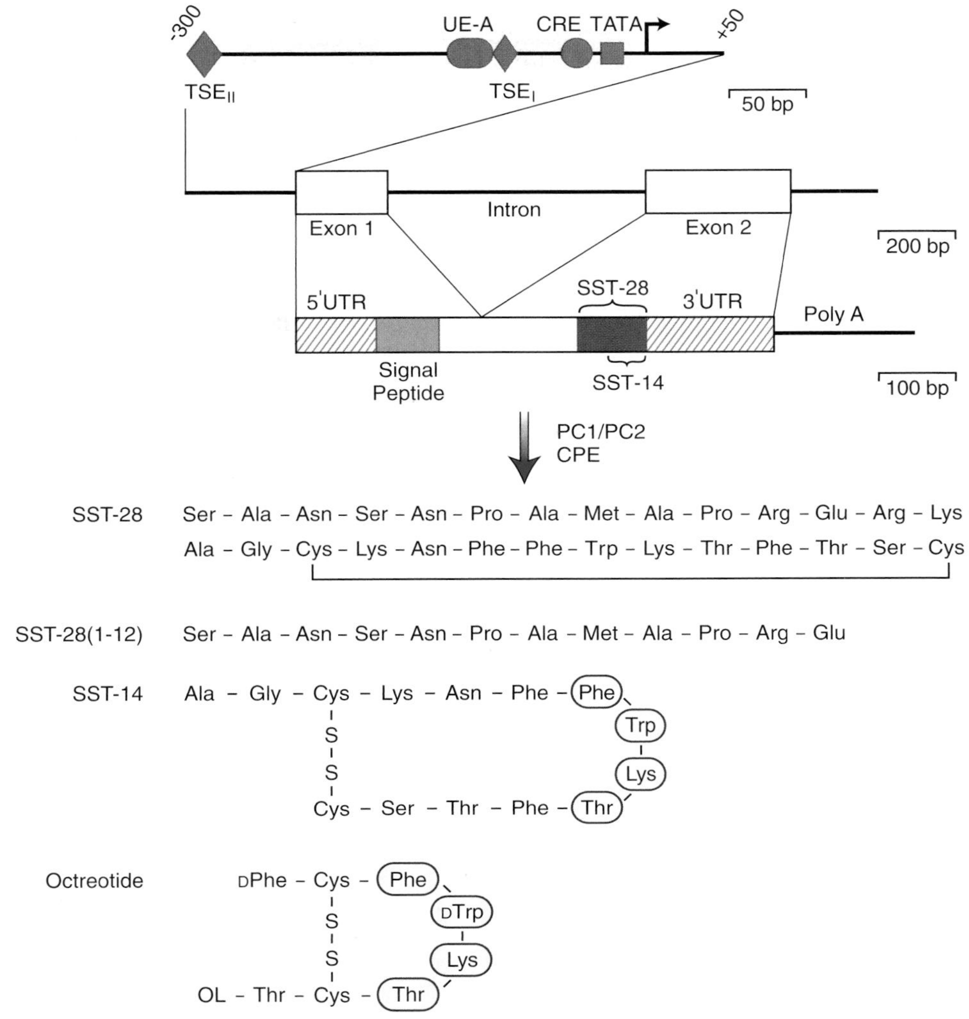

Figure 7-25 Diagram illustrating the genomic organization, messenger RNA structure, and post-translational processing of the human somatostatin prohormone. Transcriptional regulation of the somatostatin gene has been studied extensively in pancreatic islet cell lines. Binding sites for specific factors, including tissue-specific elements (TSE), upstream elements (UE), and the cyclic adenosine monophosphate (cAMP) response element (CRE), have been identified. It is not known whether all or some of these factors are also involved in the neural-specific expression of somatostatin. SST-28 and SST-14 are cyclic peptides that contain a single covalent disulfide bond between a pair of Cys residues. A β-turn containing the tetrapeptide Phe-Trp-Lys-Thr is stabilized by hydrogen bonds to produce the core receptor binding epitope. This minimal structure has been the model for conformationally restrained analogues of somatostatin including octreotide. CPE, carboxypeptidase E; PC1/PC2, prohormone convertases 1 and 2; SST, somatostatin; TATA, Goldstein-Hogness box involved in binding RNA polymerase; UTR, untranslated region. (Compiled from data by Shen LP, Rutter WJ. Sequence of the human somatostatin I gene. *Science.* 1984;224:168-171; Goudet G, Delhalle S, Biemar F, et al. Functional and cooperative interactions between the homeodomain PDX1, Pbx, and Prep1 factors on the somatostatin promoter. *J Biol Chem.* 1999;274:4067-4073; and Milner-White EJ. Predicting the biologically active conformations of short polypeptides. *Trends Pharmacol Sci.* 1989;10:70-74.)

another related *cis* element in the somatostatin gene (see Fig. 7-25, promoter element TSE$_I$) apparently binds a homeodomain transcription factor PDX1 (also called *STF1*, *IDX1*, or *IPF1*) that is common to developing brain, pancreas, and foregut and regulates gene expression in both the CNS and the gut.[249]

The function of somatostatin in GH and TSH regulation was considered earlier in this chapter. Its actions in the extrahypothalamic brain and diagnostic and therapeutic roles are considered in the remainder of this section and in Chapter 8. An additional function of somatostatin in pancreatic islet cell regulation is described in Chapter 34, and the manifestations of somatostatin excess (as in somatostatinoma) are described in Chapter 39.

Somatostatin Receptors

Five somatostatin receptor subtypes (SSTR1 to SSTR5) have been identified by gene cloning techniques, and one of these (SSTR2) is expressed in two alternatively spliced forms.[250] These subtypes are encoded by separate genes located on different chromosomes; they are expressed in unique or partially overlapping distributions in multiple target organs; and they differ in their coupling to second-messenger signaling molecules and therefore in their range and mechanism of intracellular actions.[250,251] The subtypes also differ in their binding affinity to specific somatostatin analogues. Certain of these differences have important implications for the use of somatostatin analogues in therapy and in diagnostic imaging.

TABLE 7-6

Biologic Actions of Somatostatin Outside the Central Nervous System

Hormone Secretion Inhibited (by Gland)	Other Gastrointestinal and Extragastrointestinal Actions Inhibited
Pituitary gland	Gastric acid secretion
GH, thyrotropin, ACTH, prolactin	Gastric and jejunal fluid secretion
Gastrointestinal tract	Gastric emptying
Gastrin	Pancreatic bicarbonate secretion
Secretin	Pancreatic enzyme secretion
Gastrointestinal polypeptide	Stimulates intestinal absorption of water and electrolytes
Motilin	
Glicentin (enteroglucagon)	Gastrointestinal blood flow
Vasoactive intestinal peptide	AVP-stimulated water transport
Pancreas	Bile flow
Insulin	
Glucagon	*Extragastrointestinal Actions*
Somatostatin	Inhibits the function of activated immune cells
Genitourinary tract	Inhibition of tumor growth
Renin	

ACTH, adrenocorticotropic hormone; AVP, arginine vasopressin; GH, growth hormone.

All SSTR subtypes are coupled to pertussis toxin–sensitive G proteins and bind SST-14 and SST-28 with high affinity in the low nanomolar range, although SST-28 has a uniquely high affinity for SSTR5. SSTR1 and SSTR2 are the two most abundant subtypes in brain; they probably function as presynaptic autoreceptors in the hypothalamus and limbic forebrain, respectively, in addition to their postsynaptic actions. SSTR4 is most prominent in hippocampus. All the subtypes are expressed in pituitary, but SSTR2 and SSTR5 are the most abundant subtypes on somatotrophs. They are also the most physiologically important subtypes in pancreatic islets, with SSTR5 responsible for inhibition of insulin secretion from beta cells and SSTR2 responsible for inhibition of glucagon from alpha cells.[252]

Binding of somatostatin to its receptor leads to activation of one or more plasma membrane–bound inhibitory G proteins ($G_{i/o}$), which in turn inhibit adenylyl cyclase activity and lower intracellular cAMP. Other G protein–mediated actions common to all SSTRs are activation of a vanadate-sensitive phosphotyrosine phosphatase and modulation of mitogen-activated protein kinase (MAPK). Different subsets of SSTRs are also coupled to inwardly rectifying K^+ channels, voltage-dependent Ca^{2+} channels, an Na^+/H^+ exchanger, α-amino-3-hydroxy-5-methyl-4-isoxazole proprionic acid (AMPA)-kainate glutamate receptors, phospholipase C, and phospholipase A_2.[250] The lowering of intracellular cAMP and Ca^{2+} is the most important mechanism for inhibition of hormone secretion, and actions on phosphotyrosine phosphatase and MAPK are postulated to play a role in somatostatin's antiproliferative effect on tumor cells.

Effects on Target Tissues and Mechanisms of Action

In the pituitary, somatostatin inhibits secretion of GH, TSH, and, under certain conditions, PRL and ACTH. It exerts inhibitory effects on virtually all endocrine and exocrine secretions of the pancreas, gut, and gallbladder (Table 7-6). Somatostatin inhibits secretion by the salivary glands and, under some conditions, secretion of parathyroid hormone and calcitonin. Somatostatin blocks hormone release in many endocrine-secreting tumors, including insulinomas, glucagonomas, VIPomas, carcinoid tumors, and some gastrinomas.

The physiologic actions of somatostatin in extrahypothalamic brain remain the subject of investigation.[253] In the striatum, somatostatin increases the release of dopamine from nerve terminals by a glutamate-dependent mechanism. It is widely expressed in GABAergic interneurons of limbic cortex and hippocampus, where it modulates the excitability of pyramidal neurons. Temporal lobe epilepsy is associated with a marked reduction in somatostatin-expressing neurons in the hippocampus, consistent with a putative inhibitory action on seizures.[254] A wealth of correlative data has linked reduced forebrain and CSF concentrations of somatostatin with Alzheimer's disease, major depression, and other neuropsychiatric disorders, raising speculation about the role of somatostatin in modulating neural circuits underlying cognitive and affective behaviors. A study using both genetic and pharmacologic methods to induce somatostatin deficiency in mice bolstered the hypothesis that the neuropeptide plays a physiologic role in the acquisition of contextual fear memory, possibly by altering long-term potentiation in hippocampal circuits.[255]

Clinical Applications of Somatostatin Analogues

An extensive pharmaceutical discovery program has produced somatostatin analogues with receptor subtype selectivity and improved pharmacokinetics and oral bioavailability compared with the native peptide. Initial efforts focused on the rational design of constrained cyclic peptides incorporating D-amino acid residues and including the Trp^8-Lys^9 dipeptide of somatostatin, which was shown by structure-function studies to be necessary for high-affinity binding to the somatostatin receptor (see Fig. 7-25). Many such analogues have been studied in clinical trials, including octreotide, lanreotide, vapreotide, and the hexapeptide MK-678. These compounds are agonists with similar high-affinity binding to SSTR2 and SSTR5, moderate binding to SSTR3, and no (or low) binding to SSTR1 and SSTR4. A combinatorial chemistry approach has now led to a new generation of nonpeptidyl somatostatin agonists that bind selectively and with subnanomolar affinity to each of the five SSTR subtypes.[256,257] In contrast to the marked success in development of potent and selective somatostatin agonists, there is a relative paucity of useful antagonists.[250]

The actions of octreotide (SMS 201-995 or Sandostatin) illustrate the general therapeutic potential of somatostatin analogues.[258,259] Octreotide controls excess secretion of GH in acromegaly in most patients and shrinks tumor size in about one third. It is also indicated for the treatment of recurrent TSH-secreting adenomas after surgery. It is used to treat other functioning metastatic neuroendocrine tumors, including carcinoid, VIPoma, glucagonoma, and insulinoma, but is seldom of use for the treatment of gastrinoma. Octreotide is also useful in the management of many forms of diarrhea (acting on salt and water excretion mechanisms in the gut) and in reducing external secretions in pancreatic fistulas (thus permitting healing). A decrease in blood flow to the gastrointestinal tract is the basis for its use in bleeding esophageal varices, but it is not effective in the treatment of bleeding from a peptic ulcer.

The only major undesirable side effect of octreotide is reduction of bile production and of gallbladder contractility, which leads to "sludging" of bile and an increased incidence of gallstones. Other common adverse effects,

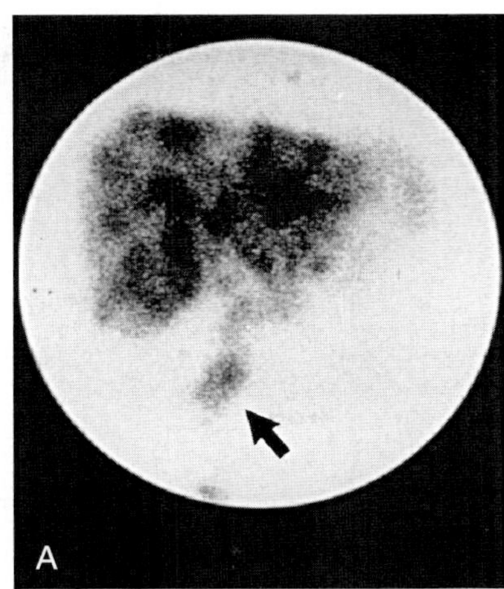

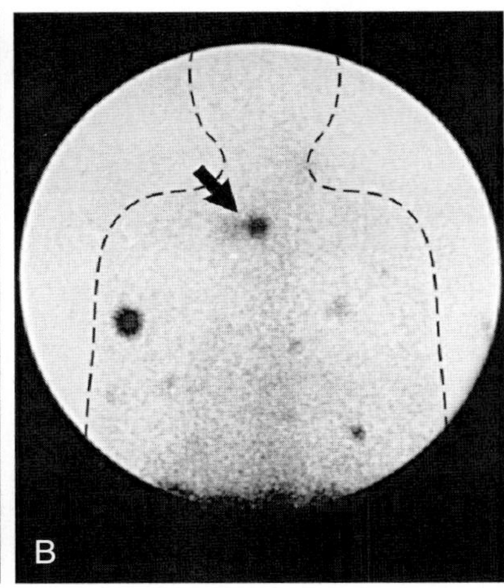

Figure 7-26 The use of ^{111}In-labeled diethylenetriaminepentaacetic acid (DTPA)-octreotide (radioactive somatostatin analogue) and external imaging techniques to localize a carcinoid tumor expressing somatostatin receptors. Scans were obtained 24 hours after administration of labeled tracer. **A,** Anterior view of the abdomen showing nodular metastases in an enlarged liver and the primary carcinoid tumor *(arrow)* in the wall of the jejunum of a patient with severe flushing and diarrhea. **B,** Posterior view of the chest and neck showing a metastasis in a lymph node on the left side of the neck *(arrow)* and multiple metastases in the ribs and pleura. (Reprinted with modifications from Lamberts SWJ, Krenning EP, Reubi J-C. The role of somatostatin and its analogs in the diagnosis and treatment of tumors. *Endocrine Rev.* 1991;12:450-482. Copyright 1991, The Endocrine Society.)

including nausea, abdominal cramps, diarrhea secondary to malabsorption of fat, and flatulence, usually subside spontaneously within 2 weeks of continued treatment. Impaired glucose tolerance is not associated with long-term octreotide therapy, despite an inhibitory effect on insulin secretion, because of compensating reductions in carbohydrate absorption and GH and glucagon secretion that are caused by the drug.

Somatostatin analogues labeled with a radioactive tracer have been used as external imaging agents for a wide range of disorders.[258,259] An indium 111 (^{111}In)-labeled analogue of octreotide (OctreoScan) has been approved for clinical use in the United States and several other countries (Fig. 7-26). The majority of neuroendocrine tumors and many pituitary tumors that express somatostatin receptors are visualized by external imaging techniques after administration of this agent; a variety of nonendocrine tumors and inflammatory lesions are also visualized, all of which have in common the expression of somatostatin receptors. Such tumors include non–small cell cancer of the lung (100%), meningioma (100%), breast cancer (74%), and astrocytomas (67%). Because activated T cells of the immune system display somatostatin receptors, inflammatory lesions that take up the tracer include sarcoidosis, Wegener's granulomatosis, tuberculosis, and many cases of Hodgkin's disease and non-Hodgkin's lymphoma. Although the tracer lacks specificity in differential diagnosis, its ability to identify the presence of abnormality and the extent of the lesion provides important information for management, including tumor staging. The use of a small, hand-held radiation detector in the operating room makes it possible to ensure the completeness of removal of medullary thyroid carcinoma metastases.[260] New developments in the synthesis of tracers chelated to octreotide for positron emission tomography have allowed the sensitive detection of meningiomas only 7 mm in diameter and located beneath osseous structures at the base of the skull.[261]

The ability of somatostatin to inhibit the growth of normal and some neoplastic cell lines and to reduce the growth of experimentally induced tumors in animal models has stimulated interest in somatostatin analogues for the treatment of cancer. Somatostatin's tumoristatic effects may be a combination of direct actions on tumor cells related to inhibition of growth factor receptor expression, inhibition of MAPK, and stimulation of phosphotyrosine phosphatase. SSTR1, SSTR2, SSTR4, and SSTR5 can all promote cell cycle arrest associated with induction of the tumor suppressor retinoblastoma (Rb) and p21 (CDKN1A), and SSTR3 can trigger apoptosis accompanied by induction of the tumor suppressor TP53 and the proapoptotic protein Bax.[250] In addition, somatostatin has indirect effects on tumor growth through inhibition of circulating, paracrine, and autocrine tumor growth–promoting factors, and it can modulate the activity of immune cells and influence tumor blood supply. Despite this promise, the therapeutic utility of octreotide as an antineoplastic agent remains controversial.

Two new treatment approaches in preclinical trials may yet effectively utilize somatostatin receptors in the arrest of cancer cells.[258] The first is receptor-targeted radionuclide therapy using octreotide chelated to a variety of β- or γ-emitting radioisotopes. Theoretical calculations and empiric data suggest that radiolabeled somatostatin analogues can deliver a tumoricidal radiotherapeutic dose to some tumors after receptor-mediated endocytosis. A variation on this theme is the chelation of a cytotoxic chemotherapeutic agent, such as doxorubicin, to a somatostatin analogue. A second approach involves somatic cell gene therapy to transfect SSTR-negative pancreatic cancer cells with an SSTR gene.[262] Therapeutic results can be obtained with the creation of autocrine or paracrine inhibitory growth effects or the addition of targeted radionuclide treatments.

Prolactin-Regulating Factors

Dopamine

It is well known that PRL secretion, unlike the secretion of other pituitary hormones, is primarily under tonic inhibitory control by the hypothalamus (Fig. 7-27).[263] Destruction of the stalk median eminence or transplantation of the pituitary gland to ectopic sites causes a marked constitutive increase in PRL secretion, in contrast to a decrease in the release of GH, TSH, ACTH, and the gonadotropins. Many lines of evidence indicate that dopamine is the principal physiologic PIF released from the hypothalamus.[264] Dopamine is present in hypophyseal–portal vessel blood in sufficient concentration to inhibit PRL release[265]; dopamine inhibits PRL secretion from lactotrophs both in vivo and in vitro[266]; and dopamine D_2 receptors are expressed on the plasma membrane of lactotrophs.[267,268] Mutant mice with a targeted disruption of the D_2 receptor gene (*Drd2*) uniformly developed lactotroph hyperplasia, hyperprolactinemia, and eventually lactotroph adenomas, further emphasizing the importance of dopamine in the

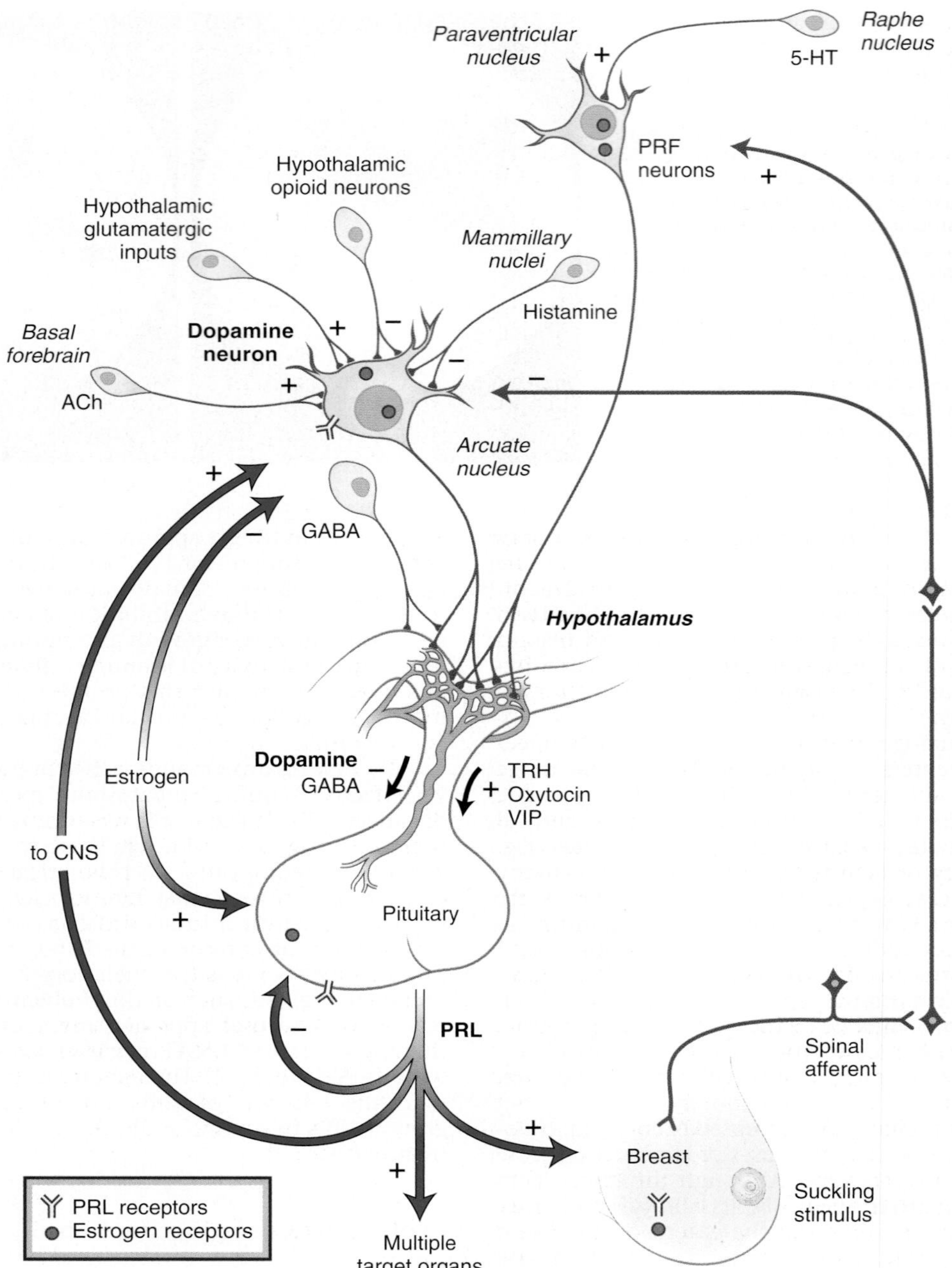

Figure 7-27 Regulation of the hypothalamic-pituitary-prolactin (PRL) axis. The predominant effect of the hypothalamus is inhibitory, an effect mediated principally by the tuberohypophyseal dopaminergic neuron system and dopamine D_2 receptors on lactotrophs. The dopamine neurons are stimulated by acetylcholine (ACh) and glutamate and inhibited by histamine and opioid peptides. One or more prolactin-releasing factors (PRFs) probably mediate acute release of PRL (e.g., in suckling, during stress). There are several candidate PRFs, including thyrotropin-releasing hormone (TRH), vasoactive intestinal polypeptide (VIP), and oxytocin. PRF neurons are activated by serotonin (5-HT). Estrogen sensitizes the pituitary to release PRL, which feeds back on the pituitary to regulate its own secretion (ultrashort-loop feedback) and also influences gonadotropin secretion by suppressing the release of luteinizing hormone–releasing hormone (LHRH). Short-loop feedback is also mediated indirectly by PRL receptor regulation of hypothalamic dopamine synthesis, secretion, and turnover. CNS, central nervous system; GABA, γ-aminobutyric acid.

physiologic regulation of lactotroph proliferation in addition to hormone secretion.[269]

The intrinsic dopamine neurons of the medial-basal hypothalamus constitute a dopaminergic population with regulatory properties that are distinct from those in other areas of the brain. Notably, they lack D_2 autoreceptors but express PRL receptors, which are essential for positive feedback control (discussed in detail later). In the rat, these neurons are subdivided by location into the A12 group within the arcuate nucleus and the A14 group in the anterior PVH. The caudal A12 dopamine neurons are further described as tuberoinfundibular (TIDA) because of their axonal projections to the external zone of the median eminence. Tuberohypophyseal (THDA) neuronal soma are located more rostrally in the arcuate nucleus and project to both the neural lobe and the intermediate lobe through axon collaterals that are found in the internal zone of the median eminence. Finally, the A14 periventricular hypophyseal (PHDA) neurons send their axons only to the intermediate lobe of the pituitary gland.

Although the TIDA neurons are considered to be the major source of dopamine to the anterior lobe through the long portal vessels originating in the median eminence, dopamine can also reach the anterior lobe from the neural and intermediate lobes by the interconnecting short portal veins.[270] Consistent with this pathway for dopamine access to the anterior lobe, surgical removal of the neurointermediate lobe in rats caused a significant increase in basal PRL levels.[271] In addition to direct actions of dopamine on lactotrophs, central dopamine can indirectly affect PRL secretion by altering the activity of inhibitory interneurons that synapse on the TIDA neurons. These effects are complicated by opposing intracellular signaling pathways linked to D_1 and D_2 receptors located on different populations of interneurons.[272]

The binding of dopamine or selective agonists such as bromocriptine to the D_2 receptor has multiple effects on lactotroph function. D_2 receptors are coupled to pertussis toxin–sensitive G proteins and inhibit adenylyl cyclase and decrease intracellular cAMP levels. Other effects include activation of an inwardly rectifying K^+ channel, increase of voltage-activated K^+ currents, decrease of voltage-activated Ca^{2+} currents, and inhibition of inositol phosphate production. Together, this spectrum of intracellular signaling events decreases free Ca^{2+} concentrations and inhibits exocytosis of PRL secretory granules.[273] Dopamine also has a modest effect on thyrotrophs to inhibit the secretion of TSH.

There is continuing debate concerning the mechanism by which D_2 receptor activation inhibits transcription of the PRL gene. Likely pathways involve inhibition of MAPK or protein kinase C, with a resultant reduction in the phosphorylation of Ets family transcription factors. Ets factors are important for the stimulatory responses of TRH, insulin, and epidermal growth factor on PRL expression,[274-276] and they interact cooperatively with the pituitary-specific protein PIT1 (a member of the POU domain family of transcription factors), which is essential for cAMP-mediated PRL gene expression.[277]

The second-messenger pathways used by the D_2 receptor to inhibit lactotroph cell division are also unsettled. A study using primary pituitary cultures from rats demonstrated that forskolin treatment, which activates protein kinase A and elevates intracellular cAMP, or insulin treatment, which activates a potent receptor tyrosine kinase, were both effective mitogenic stimuli for lactotrophs. Bromocriptine competitively antagonized the proliferative response caused by elevated cAMP. Furthermore, inhibition of MAPK signaling by PD98059 markedly suppressed the mitogenic action of both insulin and forskolin, suggesting an interaction of MAPK and protein kinase A signaling.[278]

Another line of study has implicated the stimulation of phopholipase D activity by a Rho A–dependent, pertussis toxin–insensitive pathway in the antiproliferative effects of D_2 receptor activation in both GH4C1 pituitary cells and NCI-H69 small cell lung cancer cells.[279] Therefore, it is clear that dopamine actions on lactotrophs involve multiple different intracellular signaling pathways linked to activation of the D_2 receptor, but different combinations of these pathways are relevant for the inhibitory effects on PRL secretion, PRL gene transcription, and lactotroph proliferation.

The other major action of dopamine in the pituitary is inhibition of hormone secretion from the POMC-expressing cells of the intermediate lobe—although, as noted earlier, the adult human differs from most other mammals in the rudimentary nature of this lobe. THDA and PHDA axon terminals provide a dense plexus of synaptic-like contacts on melanotrophs. Dopamine release from these terminals is inversely correlated with serum MSH levels[280] and also regulates POMC gene expression and melanotroph proliferation.[281]

Other hypothalamic factors probably play a role secondary to that of dopamine as additional PIFs.[263] The primary reason to conjecture the existence of these PIFs is the frequent inconsistency between portal dopamine levels and circulating PRL in different rat models. GABA is the strongest candidate and most likely acts through $GABA_A$ ionotropic receptors in the anterior pituitary. Melanotrophs, like lactotrophs, are inhibited by both dopamine and GABA but with the principal involvement of G protein–coupled, metabotropic $GABA_B$ receptors.[282] Because basal dopamine tone is high, the measurable inhibitory effects of GABA on PRL release are generally small under normal circumstances. Other putative PIFs include somatostatin and calcitonin.

Prolactin-Releasing Factors

Although tonic suppression of PRL release by dopamine is the dominant effect of the hypothalamus on PRL secretion, a number of stimuli promote PRL release, not merely by disinhibition of PIF effects but by causing release of one or more neurohormonal PRFs (see Fig. 7-27). The most important of the putative PRFs are TRH, oxytocin, and VIP, but AVP, angiotensin II, NPY, galanin, substance P, bombesin-like peptides, and neurotensin can also trigger PRL release under different physiologic circumstances.[263] TRH has already been discussed. In humans, there is an imperfect correlation between pulsatile PRL and TSH release, suggesting that TRH cannot be the sole physiologic PRF under basal conditions.[283]

Like TRH, oxytocin, AVP, and VIP fulfill all the basic criteria for a PRF. They are produced in PVH neurons that project to the median eminence. Concentrations of the hormones in portal blood are much higher than in the peripheral circulation and are sufficient to stimulate PRL secretion in vitro. Moreover, there are functional receptors for each of the neurohormones in the anterior pituitary gland, and either pharmacologic antagonism or passive immunization against each hormone can decrease PRL secretion, at least under certain circumstances.[284-288]

AVP is released during stress and hypovolemic shock, as is PRL, suggesting a specific role for AVP as a PRF in these contexts. Similarly, another candidate PRF, peptide histidine isoleucine, may be specifically involved in the secretion of PRL in response to stress. Peptide histidine isoleucine and the human homologue PHM are structurally related to VIP and are synthesized from the same prohormone precursor in their respective species.[289] Both peptides are coexpressed with CRH in parvicellular PVH neurons, and presumably they are released by the same stimuli that cause release of CRH into the hypophyseal-portal vessels.[290]

There is evidence suggesting that dopamine itself may also act as a PRF, in contrast to its predominant function as a PIF.[263] At concentrations 3 orders of magnitude lower than that associated with maximal inhibition of PRL secretion, dopamine was shown to be capable of stimulating secretion from primary cultures of rat pituitary cells.[291] These studies were extended to an in vivo model by Arey and colleagues,[292] who demonstrated that low-dose dopamine infusion in cannulated rats caused a further increase in circulating PRL above the already elevated baseline produced by pharmacologic blockade of endogenous dopamine biosynthesis. The physiologic relevance of these findings to humans has yet to be established.

Finally, reports of newly recognized PRFs continue to be published. Much excitement was generated by the isolation of a mammalian RFamide peptide from bovine hypothalamus named *prolactin-releasing peptide* (PrRP).[293,294] PrRP binds with high affinity to its G protein–coupled receptor GPR10, expressed in human pituitary; it selectively stimulates PRL release from rat pituitary cells with a potency lower than that of TRH by itself, but synergistically in combination with TRH. However, PrRP is expressed predominantly in a subpopulation of noradrenergic neurons in the medulla and a small population of non-neurosecretory neurons of the VMH, raising the serious question about whether PrRP reaches the anterior pituitary and actually causes PRL secretion. Subsequent studies found no direct evidence for release of PrRP in the arcuate nucleus or median eminence, further suggesting that the peptide is not a hypophyseotropic neurohormone. PrRP probably does function as a neuromodulator within the CNS at sites expressing its receptor and probably is involved in the neural circuitry mediating stress responses and satiety.[294,295]

Intrapituitary Regulation of Prolactin Secretion

Probably more than that of any other pituitary hormone, the secretion of PRL is regulated by autocrine-paracrine factors within the anterior lobe and by neurointermediate lobe factors that gain access to venous sinusoids of the anterior lobe by way of the short portal vessels. The wealth of local regulatory mechanisms within the anterior lobe has been reviewed extensively[263,296] and is also discussed in Chapter 8. Galanin, VIP, endothelin-like peptides, angiotensin II, epidermal growth factor, basic fibroblast growth factor, GnRH, and the cytokine IL-6 are among the most potent local stimulators of PRL secretion. Locally produced inhibitors include PRL itself, acetylcholine, transforming growth factor-β, and calcitonin. Although none of these stimulatory or inhibitory factors plays a dominant role in the regulation of lactotroph function and much of the research in this area has not been directly confirmed in human pituitary, it seems apparent that the local milieu of autocrine and paracrine factors plays an essential modulatory role in determining the responsiveness of lactotrophs to hypothalamic factors in different physiologic states.

As noted earlier, a proportion of the inhibitory dopamine tone affecting the anterior lobe lactotrophs is derived from the neurointermediate lobe. It was therefore unanticipated that surgical removal of this structure in rats would block suckling-induced PRL release over the moderate basal increase attributed to partial dopamine disinhibition.[297] Further studies showed that exposure of the anterior pituitary to intermediate-lobe extracts (devoid of VIP, AVP, and other known PRFs) stimulated PRL secretion. At least two kinds of PRF activity have been isolated from intermediate-lobe tumors of the mouse, but the specific molecules involved have yet to be identified.[298] Other researchers have suggested a more passive role for the neurointermediate lobe in the regulation of PRL secretion. Melanotroph-derived *N*-acetylated MSH appears to act as a lactotroph responsiveness factor by recruiting nonsecretory cells to an active state and sensitizing secreting lactotrophs to the actions of other direct PRFs.[299] However, the relevance of the neurointermediate lobe for PRL regulation in primates (including humans) is not clear because of its attenuated structure in these species.

Neuroendocrine Regulation of Prolactin Secretion

Secretion of PRL, like that of other anterior pituitary hormones, is regulated by hormonal feedback and neural influences from the hypothalamus.[263,264,300] Feedback is exerted by PRL itself at the level of the hypothalamus. PRL secretion is regulated by many physiologic states including the estrous and menstrual cycles, pregnancy, and lactation. PRL is stimulated by several exteroceptive stimuli including light, ultrasonic vocalization of pups (in rodents), olfactory cues, and various modalities of stress. Expression and secretion of PRL are also influenced strongly by estrogens at the level of both the lactotrophs and the TIDA neurons[301] (see Fig. 7-27) and by paracrine regulators within the pituitary such as galanin and VIP.

Feedback Control

Negative feedback control of PRL secretion is mediated by a unique short-loop mechanism within the hypothalamus.[302] PRL activates PRL receptors, which are expressed on all three subpopulations of A12 and A14 dopamine neurons, leading to increased tyrosine hydroxylase expression and increased dopamine synthesis and release.[301,303] Ames dwarf mice that secrete virtually no PRL, GH, or TSH have decreased numbers of arcuate dopamine neurons, and this hypoplasia can be reversed by neonatal administration of PRL, suggesting a trophic action on the neurons.[304] However, another mouse model of isolated PRL deficiency generated by gene targeting appears to have normal numbers of hypofunctioning dopamine neurons secondary to the loss of PRL feedback.[305]

Neural Control

Lactotrophs have spontaneously high secretory activity, and therefore the predominant effect of the hypothalamus on PRL secretion is tonic suppression, which is mediated by regulatory hormones synthesized by tuberohypophyseal neurons. Secretory bursts of PRL are caused by the acute withdrawal of dopamine inhibition, stimulation by PRFs, or combinations of both events. At any given moment, locally produced autocrine and paracrine regulators further modulate the responsiveness of individual lactotrophs to neurohormonal PIFs and PRFs.

Multiple neurotransmitter systems impinge on the hypothalamic dopamine and PRF neurons to regulate their neurosecretion (see Fig. 7-27).[263] Nicotinic cholinergic and glutamatergic afferents activate TIDA neurons, whereas histamine, acting predominantly through H_2 receptors, inhibits these neurons. An inhibitory peptidergic input to TIDA neurons of major physiologic significance is that associated with the endogenous opioid peptides enkephalin and dynorphin and their cognate μ- and κ-receptor subtypes.[306] Opioid inhibition of dopamine release has been associated with increased PRL secretion under virtually all physiologic conditions, including the basal state, different phases of the estrous cycle, lactation, and stress.

Ascending serotoninergic inputs from the dorsal raphe nucleus are the major activator of PRF neurons in the PVH.[307] There is still debate concerning the identity of the specific 5-HT receptors involved in this activation.

The PRL regulatory system and its monoaminergic control have been scrutinized in detail because of the frequent occurrence of syndromes of PRL hypersecretion (see Chapter 8). Both the pituitary and the hypothalamus have dopamine receptors, and the response to dopamine receptor stimulation and blockade does not distinguish between central and peripheral actions of the drug. Many commonly used neuroleptic drugs influence PRL secretion. Reserpine (a catecholamine depletor) and phenothiazines such as chlorpromazine and haloperidol enhance PRL release by disinhibition of dopamine action on the pituitary, and the PRL response is an excellent predictor of the antipsychotic effects of phenothiazines because of its correlation with D_2 receptor binding and activation.[308] The major antipsychotic neuroleptic agents act on brain dopamine receptors in the mesolimbic system and in the pituitary-regulating tuberoinfundibular system. Consequently, treatment of such patients with dopamine agonists such as bromocriptine can reverse the psychiatric benefits of these drugs. A report of three patients with psychosis and concomitant prolactinomas recommended the combination of clozapine and quinagolide as the treatment of choice to manage both diseases simultaneously.[309]

Factors Influencing Secretion

Circadian Rhythm. PRL is detectable in plasma at all times during the day but is secreted in discrete pulses superimposed on basal secretion, exhibiting a diurnal rhythm with peak values in the early morning hours.[310] In humans, this is a true circadian rhythm, because it is maintained in a constant environment independently of the sleep rhythm.[311] The combined body of data examining TIDA neuronal activity, dopamine concentrations in the median eminence, and manipulations of the SCN suggests that endogenous diurnal alterations in dopamine tone that are entrained by light constitute the major neuroendocrine mechanism underlying the circadian rhythm of PRL secretion.

External Stimuli. The suckling stimulus is the most important physiologic regulator of PRL secretion. PRL levels rise within 1 to 3 minutes after nipple stimulation, and they remain elevated for 10 to 20 minutes.[312] This reflex is distinct from the milk let-down, which involves oxytocin release from the neurohypophysis and contraction of mammary alveolar myoepithelial cells. These reflexes provide a mechanism by which the infant regulates both the production and the delivery of milk. The nocturnal rise in PRL secretion in nursing and non-nursing women may have evolved as a mechanism of milk maintenance during prolonged nonsuckling periods at night.

Pathways involved in the suckling reflex arise in the nerves innervating the nipple, enter the spinal cord by way of spinal afferent neurons, ascend the spinal cord through spinothalamic tracts to the midbrain, and enter the hypothalamus by way of the median forebrain bundle (see Fig. 7-27). Neurons regulating the oxytocin-dependent milk let-down response accompany those involved in PRL regulation throughout most of this pathway and then separate at the level of the PVH nuclei. The suckling reflex brings about an inhibition of PIF activity and a release of PRFs, although an undisputed suckling-induced PRF has not been identified.

Although their significance for PRL regulation in humans is not certain, environmental stimuli arising from seasonal changes in light duration and auditory and olfactory cues are clearly of great importance to many mammalian species.[263] Seasonal breeders, such as sheep, exhibit a reduction in PRL secretion in response to shortened days. The specific ultrasound vocalization of rodent pups is among the most potent stimuli for PRL secretion in lactating and virgin female rats. Olfactory stimuli from pheromones also have potent actions in rodents. A prime example is the Bruce effect, or spontaneous abortion induced by exposure of a pregnant female rat to an unfamiliar male. It is mediated by a well-studied neural circuitry involving the vomeronasal nerves, the corticomedial amygdala, and the medial preoptic area of the hypothalamus, which results in activation of TIDA neurons and a reduction in circulating PRL that is essential for maintenance of luteal function in the first half of pregnancy.

Stress in many forms dramatically affects PRL secretion, although the teleologic significance is uncertain. It may be related to actions of PRL on cells of the immune system or some other aspect of homeostasis. Different stressors are associated with either a reduction or an increase in PRL secretion, depending on the local regulatory environment at the time of the stress. However, whereas well-documented changes in PRL are associated with relatively severe forms of stress in laboratory animal models, a study of academic stress in college students failed to show any significant correlation of diurnal PRL levels with the time periods before, during, or after final examinations.[313]

Gonadotropin-Releasing Hormone and Control of the Reproductive Axis

Chemistry and Evolution

GnRH is the 10-amino-acid hypothalamic neuropeptide that controls the function of the reproductive axis. It is synthesized as part of a larger precursor molecule that is enzymatically cleaved to remove a signal peptide from the N-terminus and GnRH-associated peptide (GAP) from the C-terminus (Fig. 7-28).[314] All forms of the decapeptide have a pyroGlu at the N-terminus and Gly-amide at the C-terminus, indicating the functional importance of the terminal residues throughout evolution.

Two genes encoding GnRH have been identified within mammals.[315,316] The first, *GNRH1,* encodes a 92-amino-acid precursor protein. This is the form of GnRH that is found in hypothalamic neurons and serves as a releasing factor to regulate pituitary gonadotroph function.[317] The second GnRH gene, *GNRH2,* encodes a decapeptide that differs from the first by three amino acids.[318] This form of GnRH is found in the midbrain region and serves as a neurotransmitter rather than as a pituitary releasing factor. Both GnRH-I and GnRH-II are found in phylogenetically diverse species, from fish to mammals, suggesting that these multiple forms of GnRH diverged from one another early in vertebrate evolution.[317] A third form of GnRH, GnRH-III, has been identified in neurons of the telencephalon in teleost fish. GnRH is also found in cells outside the brain. The roles of GnRH peptides produced outside the brain are not well understood but are an area of current investigation.

All GnRH genes have the same basic structure, with the pre-prohormone mRNA encoded in four exons. Exon 1 contains the 5′ untranslated region of the gene; exon 2 contains the signal peptide, GnRH, and the N-terminus of GAP; exon 3 contains the central portion of GAP; and exon 4 contains the C-terminus of GAP and the 3′ untranslated region (see Fig. 7-28).[317] Among species, the nucleotide sequences encoding the GnRH decapeptide are highly homologous. This chapter focuses on the hypothalamic GnRH that is derived from *GNRH1* mRNA and plays an important role in the regulation of the hypothalamic-pituitary-gonadal axis.

Two transcriptional start sites have been identified in the rat *Gnrh1* gene, at the +1 and −579 positions, with the +1 promoter being active in hypothalamic neurons and the other promoter active in placenta. The first 173 base pairs of the promoter are highly conserved among species. In the rat, this promoter region has been shown to contain

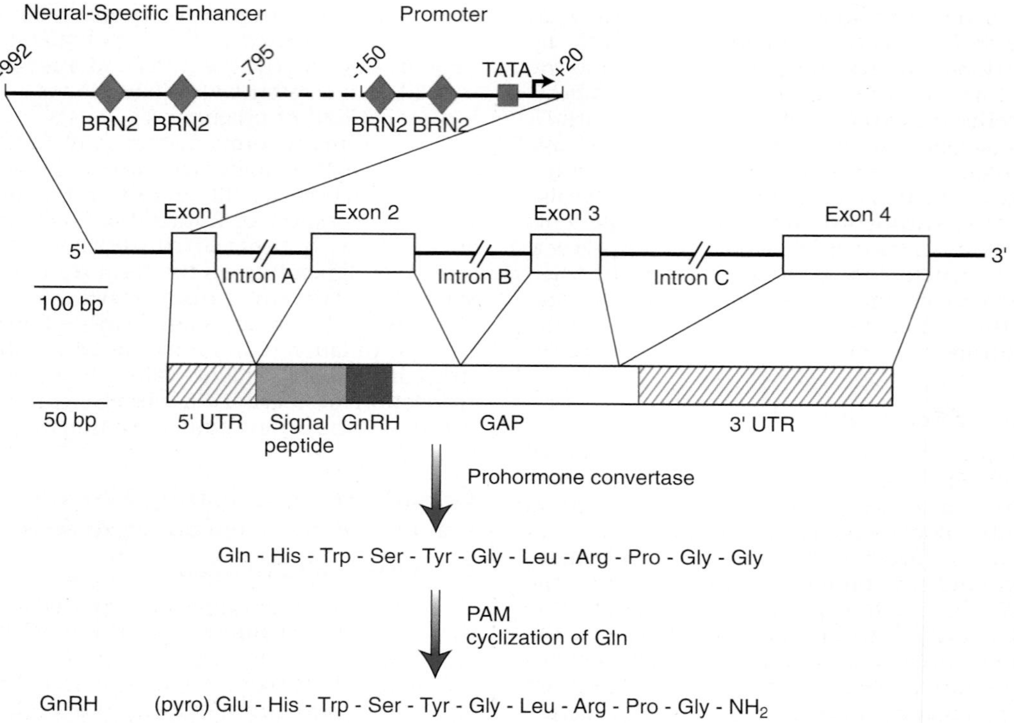

Figure 7-28 Schematic diagram of the human gene for gonadotropin-releasing hormone I (***GNRH1***), the hypothalamic complementary DNA (cDNA), and post-translational processing of the GnRH peptide. A cluster of binding sites for the homeodomain transcription factor BRN2 is present in both the proximal promoter and a distal enhancer region and is important for neuron-specific expression of the gene. Phylogenetically conserved homologous regions have been identified in the rat GnRH-I gene, but in that species the OCT1 transcription factor has been implicated in neuron-specific expression. The cDNA for GnRH-I isolated from human placenta has a longer 5′ untranslated region (UTR) because of differential splicing of the heterogeneous nuclear RNA (hnRNA) and inclusion of intron A sequences. GAP, GnRH-associated peptide; PAM, peptidylglycine α-amidating monooxygenase; TATA, Goldstein-Hogness box involved in binding RNA polymerase. (Compiled from data of Cheng CK, Leung PCK. Molecular biology of gonadotropin-releasing hormone (GnRH)-I, GnRH-II, and their receptors in humans. *Endocr Rev.* 2005;26:283-306; Wolfe A, Kim HH, Tobet S, et al. Identification of a discrete promoter region of the human GnRH gene that is sufficient for directing neuron-specific expression: a role for POU homeodomain transcription factors. *Mol Endocrinol.* 2002;16:435-449.)

two Oct1 binding sites; three regions that bind the POU domain family of transcription factors (Scip, Oct6, and Tst1); and three regions that can bind the progesterone receptor.[319] In addition, a variety of hormones and second messengers have been shown to regulate GnRH gene expression, and the majority of the *cis*-acting elements that have been characterized for hormonal control of GnRH transcription are located in the proximal promoter region.[320,321] The 5′ flanking region of the rodent and human GnRH-I genes also contain a distal 300-base-pair enhancer region that is 1.8 or 0.9 kb, respectively, upstream of the transcription start site.[321,322] Studies have implicated the homeodomain transcription factors OCT1, MSX, and DLX in the specification of neuron expression and developmental activation.[322,323]

Anatomic Distribution

GnRH neurons are small, diffusely located cells that are not concentrated in a discrete nucleus. They are generally bipolar and fusiform in shape, with slender axons projecting predominantly to the median eminence and infundibular stalk. The location of hypothalamic GnRH neurons is species dependent. In the rat, hypothalamic GnRH neurons are concentrated in rostral areas, including the medial preoptic area, the diagonal band of Broca, the septal areas, and the anterior hypothalamus. In humans and nonhuman primates, the majority of hypothalamic GnRH neurons are located more dorsally in the medial basal hypothalamus, the infundibulum, and the periventricular region. Throughout the hypothalamus, neurohypophyseal GnRH neurons are interspersed with non-neuroendocrine GnRH neurons that extend their axons to other regions of the brain including other hypothalamic regions and various regions of the cortex. GnRH secreted from non-neuroendocrine neurons has been implicated in the control of sexual behavior in rodents but not in higher primates.[324]

Embryonic Development

GnRH neuroendocrine neurons are an unusual neuronal population in that they originate outside the CNS, from the epithelial tissue of the nasal placode.[325] During embryonic development, GnRH neurons migrate across the surface of the brain and into the hypothalamus, with the final hypothalamic location differing somewhat among species. Migration is dependent on a scaffolding of neurons and glial cells along which the GnRH neurons move, with neural cell adhesion molecules playing a critical role in guiding the migration process. In contrast to this widely accepted view of GnRH development, more recent data have suggested an alternative embryonic origin of GnRH neurons from the anterior pituitary placode and cranial neural crest.[30]

Failure of GnRH neurons to migrate properly leads to a clinical condition, Kallmann's syndrome, in which GnRH neuroendocrine neurons do not reach their final destination and therefore do not stimulate pituitary gonadotropin secretion.[326] Patients with Kallmann's syndrome do not enter puberty spontaneously. The X-linked form of Kallmann's syndrome results from a deficiency of the *KAL1* gene, which encodes the extracellular glycoprotein termed *anosmin-1*. Loss-of-function mutations in the fibroblast growth factor receptor type 1 gene (*FGFR1*) produce an autosomal dominant form of Kallmann's syndrome. This, together with other known genetic mutations in FGF8, prokinectin receptor 2 (PROKR2), and prokinectin 2 (PROK2), still account for only 30% of cases, and other lesions are yet to be characterized.[327] Administration of exogenous GnRH effectively treats this form of hypothalamic hypogonadism. Patients with Kallmann's syndrome often have other congenital midline defects, including anosmia, which results from hypoplasia of the olfactory bulb and tracts.

Action at the Pituitary

Receptors. GnRH binds to a membrane receptor on pituitary gonadotrophs and stimulates synthesis and secretion of both LH and FSH. The GnRH receptor is a seven-transmembrane-domain G protein–coupled receptor, but it lacks a typical intracellular C-terminal cytoplasmic domain.[321] Under physiologic conditions, GnRH receptor number varies and is usually directly correlated with the gonadotropin secretory capacity of pituitary gonadotrophs. For example, across the rat estrous cycle, a rise in GnRH receptors is seen just before the surge of gonadotropins that occurs on the afternoon of proestrus. GnRH receptor message levels are regulated by a variety of hormones and second messengers, including steroid hormones (estradiol can both suppress and stimulate; progesterone suppresses), gonadotropins (which suppress), and calcium and protein kinase C (which stimulate).[321]

$G_{q/11}$ is the primary guanosine triphosphate–binding protein mediating GnRH responses; however, there is evidence that GnRH receptors can couple to other G proteins, including G_s and G_i.[321] With activation, the GnRH receptor couples to a phosphoinositide-specific phospholipase C, which leads to increases in calcium transport into gonadotrophs and calcium release from internal stores through a diacylglycerol-protein kinase C pathway. Increased calcium entry is a critical step in GnRH-stimulated release of gonadotropin secretion. However, GnRH also stimulates the MAPK cascade.

When there is a decline in GnRH stimulation to the pituitary, as occurs in a variety of physiologic conditions including states of lactation, undernutrition, or seasonal periods of reproductive quiescence, the number of GnRH receptors on pituitary gonadotrophs declines dramatically. Subsequent exposure of the pituitary to pulses of GnRH restores receptor number by a Ca^{2+}-dependent mechanism that requires protein synthesis.[328] The effect of GnRH to induce its own receptor is termed *upregulation* or *self-priming*. Only certain physiologic frequencies of pulsatile GnRH can augment GnRH receptor production, and these frequencies appear to differ among species.[329] Upregulation of GnRH receptors after a period of low GnRH stimulation to the pituitary can take hours to days of exposure to pulsatile GnRH, depending on the duration and extent of the prior decrease in GnRH. The self-priming effect of GnRH to upregulate its own receptors also plays a crucial role in the production of the gonadotropin surge that occurs at midcycle in females of spontaneously ovulating species and triggers ovulation. Just before the gonadotropin surge, two factors—the increased frequency of pulsatile GnRH release and a sensitization of the pituitary gonadotrophs by rising levels of estradiol—make the pituitary exquisitely sensitive to GnRH and allow an output of LH that is an order of magnitude greater than the release seen during the rest of the female reproductive cycle. This surge of LH triggers the ovulatory process at the ovary.

In contrast to upregulation of GnRH receptors by pulsatile regimens of GnRH, continuous exposure to GnRH leads to downregulation of GnRH receptors and an accompanying decrease in LH and FSH synthesis and secretion, termed *desensitization*.[330] Downregulation does not require calcium mobilization or gonadotropin secretion. It involves a rapid uncoupling of receptor from G proteins and sequestration of the receptors from the plasma membrane, followed by internalization and proteolytic degradation of the receptors.

The concept of downregulation has a number of clinical applications. For example, the most common current therapy for precocious puberty of hypothalamic origin (i.e., precocious GnRH secretion) is to treat it with a long-acting GnRH "superagonist" that downregulates pituitary GnRH receptors and effectively turns off the reproductive axis.[329,331] Children with precocious puberty can be maintained with long-acting GnRH agonists for years to suppress the premature activation of the reproductive axis, and at the normal age of puberty agonist treatment can be withdrawn, allowing reactivation of pituitary gonadotrophs and a downstream increase in gonadal steroid hormone production (also see Chapter 25). Long-acting GnRH agonists are also used in the treatment of forms of breast cancer that are estrogen dependent and of other gonadal steroid-dependent cancers.[329] Long-acting antagonists of GnRH have been developed that can also be used for these therapies.[332] Antagonists have the advantage of not having a flare effect; that is, an acute stimulation of gonadotropin secretion that is seen during the initial treatment of individuals with superagonists.

Pulsatile Gonadotropin-Releasing Hormone Stimulation. Because a single pulse of GnRH stimulates the release of both LH and FSH and chronic exposure of the pituitary to pulsatile GnRH supports the synthesis of both LH and FSH, it is generally believed that there is only one releasing factor regulating the synthesis and secretion of LH and FSH. However, because there are divergent patterns of LH and FSH secretion in a number of physiologic conditions, a second FSH-releasing peptide has been proposed, but such a peptide has not been isolated to date. Other mechanisms, discussed in more detail later, are likely to account for the differential regulation of LH and FSH release.

The ensemble of GnRH neurons in the hypothalamus that send axons to the portal blood system in the median eminence fire in a coordinated, repetitive, episodic manner, producing distinct pulses of GnRH in the portal bloodstream.[333] The pulsatile nature of GnRH stimulation of the pituitary leads to the release of distinct pulses of LH into the peripheral circulation. In experimental animals, in which it is possible to collect blood samples simultaneously from the portal and peripheral blood, GnRH and LH pulses have been found to correspond in an approximately 1:1 ratio at most physiologic rates of secretion.[334] Because the portal blood stream is generally inaccessible in humans, the collection of frequent peripheral venous blood samples is used to define the pulsatile nature of LH secretion (i.e., frequency and amplitude of LH pulses), and pulsatile LH is used as an indirect measure of the activity of the GnRH secretory system. Indirect assessment of GnRH secretion by monitoring the rate of pulsatile LH secretion is also used in many animal studies examining the factors that govern the regulation of the pulsatile activity of the reproductive neuroendocrine axis. Unlike LH secretion, FSH secretion is not always pulsatile, and even when it is pulsatile, there is only partial concordance between LH and FSH pulses.

It is possible to place multiple-unit recording electrodes in the medial basal hypothalamus of monkeys and other species and find spikes of electrical activity that are concordant with the pulsatile secretion of LH secretion.[335] However, it is unknown whether these bursts of electrical activity reflect the activity of GnRH neurons themselves or the activity of neurons that impinge on GnRH neurons and govern their firing. With the development of mice in which the gene for green fluorescent protein has been put under the regulation of the GnRH promoter, it has been possible to identify GnRH neurons in hypothalamic tissue slices using fluorescence microscopy and to record from them intracellularly.[14] These studies have shown that many, but not all, GnRH neurons show a bursting pattern of electrical activity. A central, unsolved question in the field of reproductive neuroendocrinology is what causes GnRH neurons to pulse in a coordinated manner. Studies using a line of clonal GnRH neurons have shown that these neurons grown in culture can release GnRH in a pulsatile pattern, suggesting that the pulse-generating capacity of GnRH neurons is intrinsic.[336] The term *GnRH pulse generator* is often used to acknowledge the fact that GnRH secretion occurs in pulses and to refer to the central mechanisms responsible for pulsatile GnRH release.

A critical factor governing LH and FSH secretion is the rate of pulsatile GnRH stimulation of the gonadotrophs. Experimental studies in which the hypothalamus was lesioned and GnRH was replaced by pulsatile administration of exogenous GnRH showed that different frequencies of GnRH can lead to different ratios of LH to FSH secretion from the pituitary. Figure 7-29 shows that in a monkey with a hypothalamic lesion, replacement of one pulse of GnRH per hour led to a relatively low ratio of FSH to LH secretion. Subsequent institution of a slower pulse frequency (one pulse of GnRH every 3 hours) led to a decrease in LH secretion but an increase in FSH secretion, so that the ratio of FSH to LH secretion was greatly elevated. It is likely that this effect of pulse frequency on the ratio of FSH to LH secretion accounts, at least in part, for the clinical finding that at times when the GnRH pulse generator is just turning on, such as at the onset of puberty and during recovery from chronic undernutrition, the ratio of FSH to LH is higher than when it is measured in adults experiencing regular reproductive function. As discussed later, steroid hormones act at both the hypothalamus and the pituitary to influence strongly the rate of pulsatile GnRH release and the amount of LH and FSH secreted from the pituitary.

GnRH pulse frequency not only influences the rate of pulsatile gonadotropin release and the ratio of FSH to LH secretion but also plays an important role in modulating the structural makeup of the gonadotropins. LH and FSH are structurally similar glycoprotein hormones. Each of these hormones is made up of an α and a β subunit. LH, FSH, and TSH share a common α-subunit, and each has a unique β subunit that conveys receptor specificity to the intact hormone. Before secretion of gonadotropins, terminal sugars are attached to each gonadotropin molecule.[116] The sugars include sialic acid, galactose, *N*-acetylglucosamine, and mannose, but the most important is sialic acid. The extent of glycosylation of LH and FSH is important for the physiologic function of these hormones.[116] Forms of gonadotropin with more sialic acid have a longer half-life because they are protected from degradation by the liver. Forms of gonadotropin with less sialic acid can have more potent effects at their biologic receptors. Both the rate of GnRH stimulation and ovarian hormone feedback at the level of the pituitary regulate the degree of LH and FSH glycosylation. For example, slow frequencies of GnRH release, seen during follicular development, are associated with greater degrees of FSH glycosylation, which would provide sustained FSH support to growing follicles. In contrast, faster frequencies of GnRH release, seen just before the midcycle gonadotropin surge, are associated with lesser degrees of FSH glycosylation, providing a more potent but shorter-lasting form of FSH at the time of ovulation.[337]

Regulatory Systems

Many neurotransmitter systems from the brain stem, limbic system, and other areas of the hypothalamus convey information to GnRH neurons (Fig. 7-30). These afferent systems include neurons that contain norepinephrine, dopamine, serotonin, GABA, glutamate, endogenous opiate peptides, NPY, galanin, and a number of other peptide neurotransmitters. Glutamate and norepinephrine play important roles in providing stimulatory drive to the

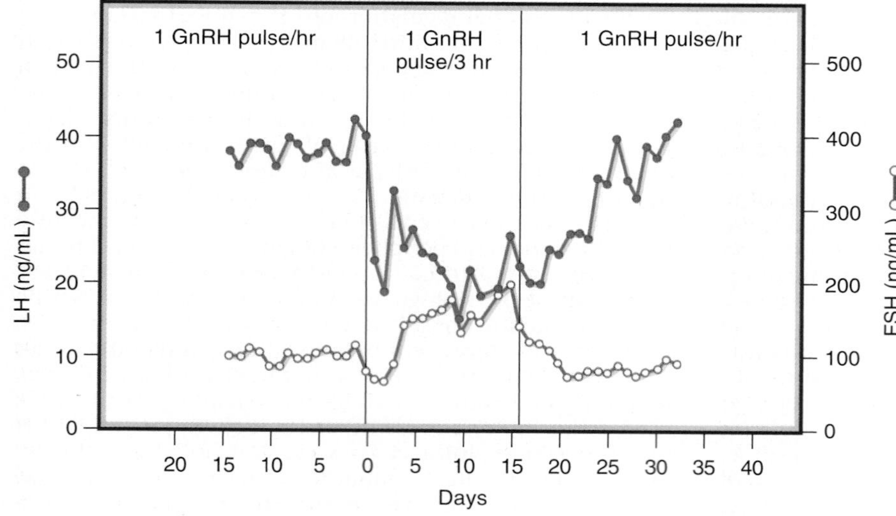

Figure 7-29 The influence of gonadotropin-releasing hormone (GnRH) pulse frequency on luteinizing hormone (LH) and follicle-stimulating hormone (FSH) secretion in a female rhesus monkey with an arcuate nucleus lesion ablating endogenous GnRH support of the pituitary. Decreasing the GnRH pulse frequency from 1 pulse every hour to 1 pulse every 3 hours led to a decrease in plasma LH concentrations but an increase in plasma FSH concentrations. (Redrawn from Wildt L, Haulser A, Marshall G, et al. Frequency and amplitude of gonadotropin-releasing hormone stimulation and gonadotropin secretion in the rhesus monkey. *Endocrinology.* 1981;109:376-385.)

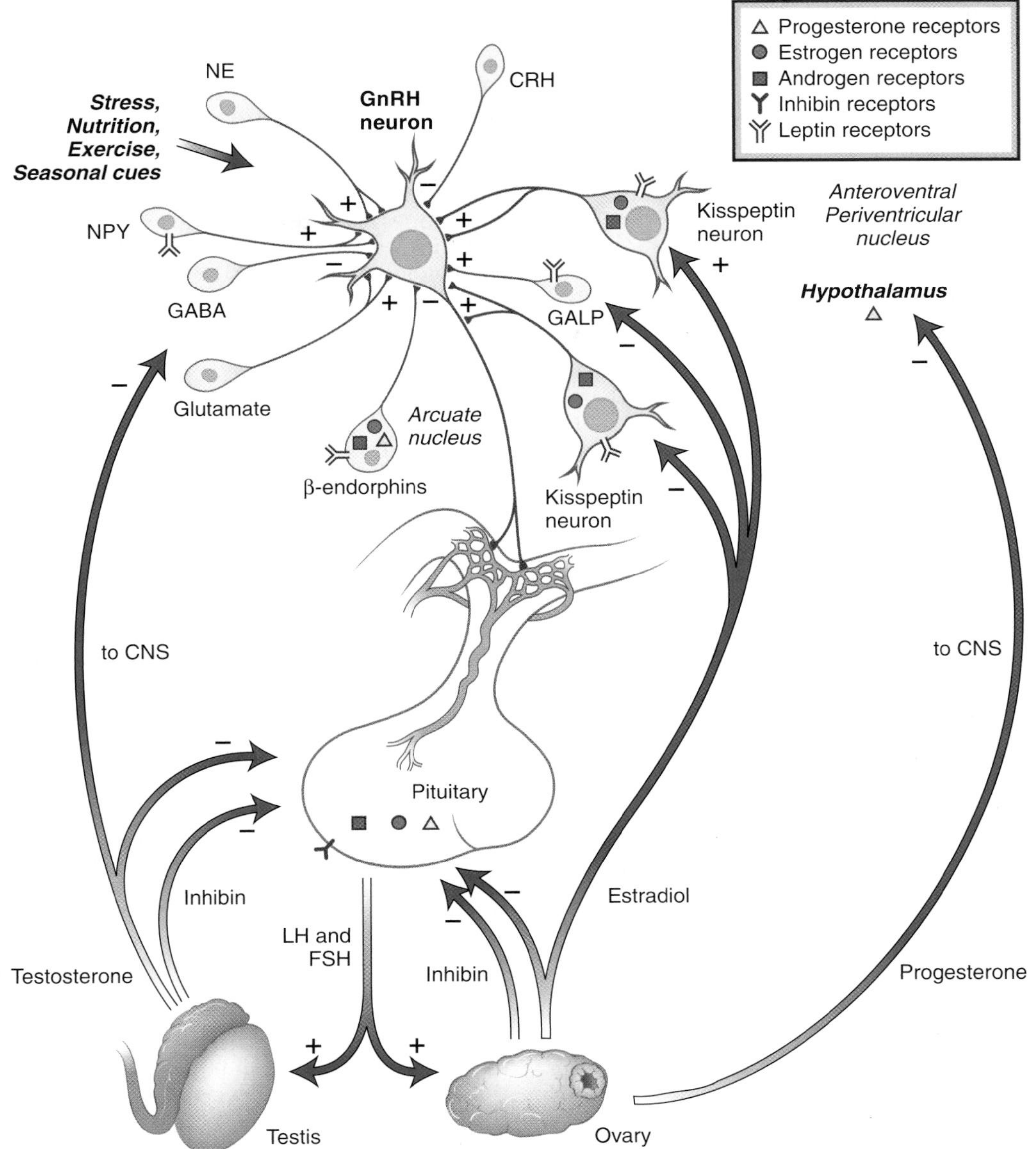

Figure 7-30 Regulation of the hypothalamic-pituitary-gonadal axis. Schematic diagram of the hypothalamic-pituitary-gonadal axis showing neural systems that regulate gonadotropin-releasing hormone (GnRH) secretion and feedback of gonadal steroid hormones at the level of the hypothalamus and pituitary. CNS, central nervous system; CRH, corticotropin-releasing hormone; FSH, follicle-stimulating hormone; GABA, γ-aminobutyric acid; GALP, galanin-like peptide; LH, luteinizing hormone; NE, norepinephrine; NPY, neuropeptide Y.

reproductive axis, whereas GABA and endogenous opioid peptides provide a substantial portion of the inhibitory drive to GnRH neurons. Influences of specific neurotransmitter systems are discussed where appropriate in the following sections, which cover the physiologic regulation of GnRH neurons.

GnRH neurons are surrounded by glial processes, and only a small percentage of their surface area is available to receive dendritic contacts from afferent neurons. Changes in the steroid hormone milieu influence the degree of glial sheathing and may play important roles in regulating afferent input to GnRH neurons by this mechanism.[43,45] Some glial cells also secrete substances including transforming growth factor-α and prostaglandin E_2 that can modulate the activity of GnRH neurons.

Feedback Regulation

Steroid hormone receptors are abundant in the hypothalamus and in many neural systems that impinge on GnRH neurons, including noradrenergic, serotoninergic, β-endorphin–containing, and NPY neurons. Early studies identifying regions of the brain that bind labeled estrogens showed that in rodents the preoptic area and the VMH had the highest concentrations of estrogen receptors in the brain. Further localization studies, identifying estrogen receptors by immunocytochemistry or in situ hybridization, confirmed the strong presence of estrogen receptors in the hypothalamus and in brain areas with abundant connections to the hypothalamus, including the amygdala, septal nuclei, bed nucleus of the stria terminalis, medial part of the nucleus of the solitary tract, and lateral portion of the parabrachial nucleus.[338] In 1986, a new member of the steroid hormone receptor superfamily with high sequence homology to the classic estrogen receptor (now referred to as *estrogen receptor-α*) was isolated from rat prostate and named *estrogen receptor-β*. This novel estrogen receptor was shown to bind estradiol and to activate transcription by binding to estrogen response elements.[339]

In situ hybridization studies examining the localization of estrogen receptor-β mRNA have shown that these receptors are present throughout the rostral-caudal extent of the brain, with a high level of expression in the preoptic area, bed nucleus of the stria terminalis, PVH and SON nuclei, amygdala, and laminae II to VI of the cerebral cortex.[340] Specific receptors for progesterone are induced by estrogen in hypothalamic regions of the brain, including the preoptic area, the ventromedial and ventrolateral nuclei, and the infundibular-arcuate nucleus, although there is also evidence for constitutive expression of progesterone receptors in some regions.[341] Androgen receptor mapping studies have shown considerable overlap in the distribution of androgen and estrogen receptors throughout the brain. The highest density of androgen receptors was found in hypothalamic nuclei known to participate in the control of reproduction and sexual behaviors, including the arcuate nucleus, PVH, medial preoptic nucleus, ventromedial nucleus, and brain regions with strong connections to the hypothalamus including the amygdala, nuclei of the septal region, bed nucleus of the stria terminalis, nucleus of the solitary tract, and lateral division of the parabrachial nucleus.[338] The anterior pituitary also contains receptors for all of the gonadal steroid hormones.

Steroid hormones can dramatically alter the pattern of pulsatile release of GnRH and of the gonadotropins through actions at both the hypothalamus and the pituitary. At the hypothalamus, estradiol, progesterone, and testosterone can all act to slow the frequency of GnRH release into the portal bloodstream as part of a closed negative feedback loop.[342] Because GnRH neurons have generally been shown to lack steroid hormone receptors, it is likely that the effects of steroid hormones on the firing rate of GnRH neurons are mediated by steroid hormone actions on other neural systems that provide afferent input to GnRH neurons. For example, progesterone-mediated negative feedback on GnRH secretion in primates appears to be regulated by β-endorphin–containing neurons in the hypothalamus, acting primarily through μ-opioid receptors. If a μ-receptor antagonist, such as naloxone, is administered along with progesterone, the negative feedback action of progesterone on GnRH secretion can be blocked.

Negative feedback of steroid hormones can also occur directly at the level of the pituitary. For example, estradiol has been shown to be capable of binding to the pituitary, decreasing LH and FSH synthesis and release, and decreasing the sensitivity of pituitary gonadotrophs to the actions of GnRH so that less LH and FSH are released when a pulse of GnRH stimulates the pituitary. Evidence for such a direct pituitary action of estradiol came from studies with rhesus monkeys that had been rendered deficient in endogenous GnRH by a lesion in the arcuate nucleus and showed a decline in endogenous gonadotropin secretion. When these monkeys received a pulsatile regimen of GnRH gonadotropin secretion, subsequent estradiol infusions dramatically suppressed the responsiveness of the pituitary to GnRH and suppressed the gonadotropin secretion that was being driven by the pulsatile administration of GnRH.[343] Similarly, in a compound mutant mouse model on a GnRH-deficient (*hpg*) genetic background, expression of a human FSH-β transgene was inhibited by testosterone directly at the pituitary level.[344] In primate species including humans, there is considerable feedback of estradiol at the pituitary, but most of the progesterone- and testosterone-negative feedback occurs at the level of the hypothalamus.[342]

Most of the time, the hypothalamic-pituitary axis is under the negative feedback influence of gonadal steroid hormones. If the gonads are removed surgically or their normal secretion of steroid hormones is suppressed pharmacologically, there is a dramatic increase (10-fold to 20-fold) in circulating levels of LH and FSH secretion.[342] This type of "castration response" occurs normally at menopause in women, when ovarian follicular development and, therefore, ovarian production of large quantities of estradiol and progesterone decrease and eventually cease.

In addition to negative feedback, estradiol can have a positive feedback action at the level of the hypothalamus and pituitary leading to a massive release of LH and FSH from the pituitary. This massive release of gonadotropins occurs once each menstrual cycle and is referred to as the *LH-FSH surge*. The positive feedback action of estradiol occurs as a response to the rising tide of estradiol that is produced during the process of dominant follicle development in the late follicular phase of the menstrual cycle. In women, elevated estradiol levels are typically maintained at about 300 to 500 pg/mL for approximately 36 hours before the stimulation of the gonadotropin surge.

Experiments have shown that both a critical concentration and a critical duration of elevated estradiol are necessary to achieve positive feedback and a resulting gonadotropin surge. If supraphysiologic doses of estradiol are administered, the surge can occur as early as 18 hours after their administration. Because the ovary is responsible for the production of estradiol and the time course and magnitude of estradiol release control the rate of positive feedback, the ovary has been referred to as the *zeitgeber* of the menstrual cycle. The dependence of the positive feedback system on the magnitude of estradiol production helps explain the fact that the portion of the menstrual cycle that varies most in length is the follicular phase. Production of higher levels of estradiol by a dominant follicle in one cycle leads to a more rapid positive feedback action, with earlier ovulation and therefore a shorter follicular phase, compared with a cycle in which the dominant follicle produced lower levels of estradiol.

As with negative feedback in response to estradiol, the positive feedback actions of estradiol occur both at the hypothalamus, to increase GnRH secretion, and at the pituitary, to greatly enhance pituitary responsiveness to GnRH. Estradiol increases pituitary sensitivity to GnRH by increasing the synthesis of new GnRH receptors and by enhancing the responsiveness to GnRH at a postreceptor site of action. At the level of the hypothalamus in rodent species, estradiol appears to act at a "surge center" to induce the ovulatory surge of GnRH. Lesions in areas adjacent to the medial preoptic area, near the anterior commissure and septal complex, block the ability of estradiol to induce a surge in these species without blocking negative feedback effects of estradiol.[345] In primate species, there does not appear to be a separate surge center mediating the positive feedback actions of estradiol.

Cellular mechanisms that mediate the switch from negative to positive feedback of estrogen are not fully understood, but there is support for the concept that estrogen induction of various transcription factors and receptors (notably progesterone receptors) may play an important role in mediating this switch.[346] The recent isolation of a novel mammalian RFamide peptide, named *kisspeptin* or *metastin*, that is the natural ligand for the former orphan G protein–coupled receptor GPR54 has shed considerable light on this area.[294] Loss-of-function mutations in GPR54 (now termed *KISSR*) cause HH. Kisspeptin is expressed in subpopulations of arcuate and anteroventral periventricular (AVPV) neurons that project to GnRH neurons. Kisspeptin expression is regulated by estradiol and testosterone and is upregulated at the time of puberty, and intracerebroventricular administration of kisspeptin causes the secretion of GnRH and gonadotropins.[347,348] Furthermore, kisspeptin expression in the AVPV, but not in the arcuate nucleus, is sexually diergic, with a much greater number of kisspeptin neurons in the female. This particular subpopulation of kisspeptin neurons is activated in an estrogen-dependent manner immediately preceding the GnRH surge, as detected by Fos expression, and is postulated to play a key role in the positive feedback effects of estradiol on GnRH release.[349]

Regulation of the Ovarian Cycle

Cyclic activity in the ovary is controlled by an interplay between steroid hormones produced by the ovary and the hypothalamic-pituitary neuroendocrine components of the reproductive axis. The duration of each phase of the ovarian cycle is species dependent, but the general mechanisms controlling the cycle are similar in all species that have spontaneous ovarian cycles. In the human menstrual cycle, day 1 is designated as the first day of menstrual bleeding. At this time, small and medium-sized follicles are present in the ovaries and only small amounts of estradiol are being produced by the follicular cells. As a result, there is a low level of negative feedback to the hypothalamic-pituitary axis, LH pulse frequency is relatively fast (one pulse about every 60 minutes), and FSH concentrations are slightly elevated compared with much of the rest of the cycle (Fig. 7-31). FSH acts at the level of the ovarian follicles to stimulate development and causes an increase in follicular estradiol production, which in turn provides increased negative feedback to the hypothalamic-pituitary unit.

A result of the increased negative feedback is a slowing of pulsatile LH secretion over the course of the follicular phase, to a rate of about one pulse every 90 minutes. However, as the growing follicle (or follicles, depending on the species) secretes more estradiol, a positive feedback action of estradiol is triggered and leads to an increase in GnRH release and a surge release of LH and FSH. The surge of gonadotropins acts at the fully developed follicle to stimulate dissolution of the follicular wall, leading to ovulation of the matured ovum into the nearby fallopian tube, where fertilization takes place if sperm are present. Ovulation results in a reorganization of the cells of the follicular wall, which undergo hypertrophy and hyperplasia and start to secrete large amounts of progesterone and some

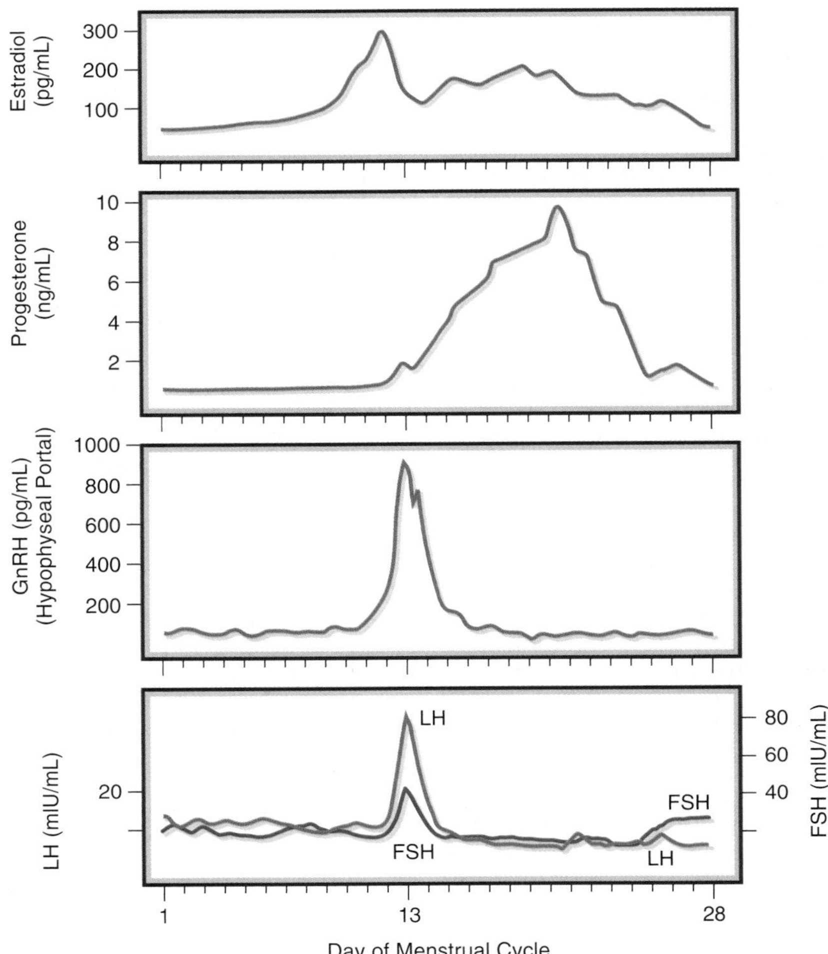

Figure 7-31 Diagrammatic representation of changes in plasma levels of estradiol, progesterone, luteinizing hormone (LH), and follicle-stimulating hormone (FSH) and in portal levels of gonadotropin-releasing hormone (GnRH) over the human menstrual cycle.

estradiol. Progesterone and estradiol have a negative feedback effect at the level of the hypothalamus and pituitary, so the LH pulse frequency becomes very slow during the luteal phase of the menstrual cycle. The corpus luteum has a fixed life span, and without additional stimulation in the form of chorionic gonadotropin from a developing embryo, the corpus luteum regresses spontaneously after about 14 days and secretion of progesterone and estradiol diminishes. This reduces the negative feedback signals to the hypothalamus and pituitary and allows an increase in FSH and LH secretion. The fall in progesterone is also a withdrawal of steroid hormone support to the endometrial lining of the uterus; as a result, the endometrium is shed as menses, and a new cycle begins.

In other species, the interplay between the neuroendocrine and ovarian hormones is similar but the timing of events is different and other factors, such as circadian and seasonal regulatory factors, play a role in regulating the cycle. The rat has a 4- or 5-day ovarian cycle with no menses (the endometrial lining is absorbed rather than shed). The rat also shows strong circadian rhythmicity in the timing of the LH-FSH surge, with the surge always occurring in the afternoon of the day of proestrus. The sheep is an example of a species that has a strongly seasonal pattern of ovarian cyclicity. During the breeding season, sheep have 15-day cycles, with a very short follicular phase and an extended luteal phase; during the nonbreeding season, signals relaying information about day length through the visual system, pineal, and SCN cause a dramatic suppression of GnRH neuronal activity, and cyclic ovarian function is prevented by a decrease in trophic hormonal support from the pituitary.

Early Development and Puberty

Neuroendocrine stimulation of the reproductive axis is initiated during fetal development, and in primates in midgestation circulating levels of LH and FSH reach values similar to those in castrated adults.[350] Later in gestational development, gonadotropin levels decline, restrained by rising levels of circulating gonadal steroids. The steroids that have this effect are probably placental in origin, because after parturition there is a rise in circulating gonadotropin levels that is apparent for a variable period in the first year of life, depending on the species.[351] The decline in reproductive hormone secretion in the postnatal period appears to be caused by a decrease in GnRH stimulation of the reproductive axis because it occurs even in the castrate state and because gonadotropin and gonadal steroid secretion can be supported by administration of pulses of GnRH.[352]

Pubertal reawakening of the reproductive axis occurs in late childhood and is marked initially by nighttime elevations in gonadotropin and gonadal steroid hormone levels.[352,353] The mechanisms controlling the pubertal reawakening of the GnRH pulse generator have been an area of intense investigation for more than 2 decades.[352] Although the mechanisms are not fully understood, significant progress has been made in identifying central changes in the hypothalamus that appear to play a role in this process. At puberty, there is both a decrease in transsynaptic inhibition to the GnRH neuronal system and an increase in stimulatory input to GnRH neurons.[352] One of the major inhibitory inputs to the GnRH system is provided by GABAergic neurons. Studies in rhesus monkeys have shown that hypothalamic levels of GABA decrease during early puberty and that blocking the GABAergic input before puberty, by intrahypothalamic administration of antisense oligodeoxynucleotides against the enzymes responsible for GABA synthesis, results in premature activation of the GnRH neuronal system.

It has been suggested, on the basis of findings that a subset of glutamate receptors (i.e., kainate receptors) increase in the hypothalamus at puberty, that the pubertal decrease in GABA tone may be caused by an increase in glutamatergic transmission. Further evidence pointing to a role for glutamate comes from studies showing that administration of *N*-methyl-D-aspartic acid (NMDA) to prepubertal rhesus monkeys can drive the reawakening of the reproductive axis.[354] Increased stimulatory drive to the GnRH neuronal system also appears to come from increases in norepinephrine and NPY at the time of puberty.[352] Furthermore, as discussed earlier, there is evidence that growth factors act through release of prostaglandin from glial cells at puberty to play a role in stimulating GnRH neurons.[355]

Despite an increased understanding of the neural changes occurring at puberty, the question of what signals trigger the pubertal awakening of the reproductive axis is unanswered at this time.[356] However, the kisspeptin neuron system (described earlier) has become a prime integrative candidate for this function.[349] Also relevant to pubertal onset was the discovery of galanin-like peptide (GALP), which is expressed specifically in the arcuate nucleus and binds with high affinity to galanin receptors. GALP is a potent central stimulator of gonadotropin release and sexual behavior in the rat and can reverse the decreased reproductive function associated with diabetes mellitus and hypoinsulinemia.[357] Both kisspeptin and GALP neurons are targets of leptin and are hypothesized to be involved in the well-known modulation of puberty and reproductive function by food availability and nutritional status (described in the next section).

Reproductive Function and Stress

Many forms of physical stresses, such as energy restriction, exercise, temperature stress, infection, pain, and injury, as well as psychological stresses, such as being subordinate in a dominance hierarchy or being acutely psychologically stressed, can suppress the activity of the reproductive axis.[358] If the stress exposure is brief, there may be acute suppression of circulating gonadotropins and gonadal steroid hormones; in females, normal menstrual cyclicity may be disrupted, but fertility is unlikely to be impaired.[358] In contrast, prolonged periods of significant stress exposure can lead to complete impairment of reproductive function, also characterized by low circulating levels of gonadotropins and gonadal steroids. Stress appears to decrease the activity of the reproductive axis by decreasing GnRH drive to the pituitary, because in all cases in which it has been examined, administration of exogenous GnRH can reverse the effects of the stress-induced decline in reproductive hormone secretion. Although the neural circuits through which many forms of stress suppress GnRH neuronal activity are not known, some forms of stress-induced suppression of reproductive function are better understood.

In the case of foot-shock stress in rats[359] or immune stress (i.e., injection of IL-1α) in primates,[360] the suppression of gonadotropin secretion that occurs was shown to be reversible by administration of a CRH antagonist, implying that endogenous CRH secretion mediates the effects of these stresses on GnRH neurons. In other studies, naloxone, a μ-opioid receptor antagonist, was shown to be capable of reversing restraint stress–induced suppression of gonadotropin secretion in monkeys; however, naloxone was ineffective in reversing the suppression of gonadotropin secretion that occurs during insulin-induced hypoglycemia.[361,362] In the case of metabolic stresses, multiple regulators appear to mediate changes in the neural drive to the reproductive axis.

Various metabolic fuels including glucose and fatty acids can regulate the function of the reproductive axis, and blocking cellular utilization of these fuels can lead to suppression of gonadotropin secretion and decreased gonadal activity. Leptin, a hormone produced by fat cells, can also modulate the activity of the reproductive axis. Mutant *ob/ob* mice that are deficient in leptin or leptin receptors are infertile, and fertility can be restored by administration of leptin.[363] Moreover, leptin administration has been shown to reverse the suppressive effects of undernutrition on the reproductive axis in some situations.[364] Leptin receptors are found in several cell populations that are known to have a strong influence on the reproductive axis, particularly NPY and kisspeptin neurons.[349]

In summary, it appears that a number of neural circuits can mediate effects of stress on the GnRH neuronal system and that the neural systems involved are at least somewhat specific to the type of stress that is experienced.

NEUROENDOCRINE DISEASE

Disease of the hypothalamus can cause pituitary dysfunction, neuropsychiatric and behavioral disorders, and disturbances of autonomic and metabolic regulation. In the diagnosis and treatment of suspected hypothalamic or pituitary disease, four issues must be considered: the extent of the lesion, the physiologic impact, the specific cause, and the psychosocial setting. The etiology of hypothalamic neuroendocrine disorders categorized by age and syndrome is summarized in Tables 7-7 and 7-8.

Manifestations of pituitary insufficiency secondary to hypothalamic or pituitary stalk damage are not identical to those of primary pituitary insufficiency. Hypothalamic injury causes decreased secretion of most pituitary

TABLE 7-7

Etiology of Hypothalamic Disease by Age

Age	Etiology
Premature Infants and Neonates	Intraventricular hemorrhage Meningitis: bacterial Tumors: glioma, hemangioma Trauma Hydrocephalus, kernicterus

1 mo to 2 yr	Tumors
	  Glioma, especially optic glioma
	  Histiocytosis X
	  Hemangioma
	Hydrocephalus
	Meningitis
	Familial disorders
	  Laurence-Moon-Biedl syndrome
	  Prader-Willi syndrome

2 to 10 yr	Neoplasms
	  Craniopharyngioma
	  Glioma, dysgerminoma, hamartoma
	  Histiocytosis X, leukemia
	  Ganglioneuroma, ependymoma
	  Medulloblastoma
	Meningitis
	  Bacterial meningitis
	  Tuberculous meningitis
	Encephalitis
	  Viral
	  Exanthematous demyelinating
	Familial
	  Diabetes insipidus
	Radiation therapy
	Diabetic ketoacidosis
	Moyamoya disease, circle of Willis

10 to 25 yr	Tumors
	  Craniopharyngioma
	  Glioma, hamartoma, dysgerminoma
	  Histiocytosis X, leukemia
	  Dermoid, lipoma, neuroblastoma
	Trauma
	Vascular
	  Subarachnoid hemorrhage
	  Aneurysm
	  Arteriovenous malformation
	Inflammatory disease
	  Meningitis
	  Encephalitis
	  Sarcoidosis
	  Tuberculosis
	Structural brain defect
	  Chronic hydrocephalus
	  Increased intracranial pressure

25 to 50 yr	Nutritional: Wernicke's disease
	Tumors
	  Glioma, lymphoma, meningioma
	  Craniopharyngioma, pituitary tumors
	  Angioma, plasmacytoma, colloid cysts
	  Ependymoma, sarcoma, histiocytosis X
	Inflammatory disease
	  Sarcoidosis
	  Tuberculosis, viral encephalitis
	Vascular
	  Aneurysm, subarachnoid hemorrhage
	  Arteriovenous malformation
	Damage from pituitary radiation therapy

50 yr and Older	Nutritional: Wernicke's disease
	Tumors: pituitary tumors, sarcoma, glioblastoma, ependymoma, meningioma, colloid cysts, lymphoma
	Vascular disease
	  Infarct, subarachnoid hemorrhage
	  Pituitary apoplexy
	Inflammatory disease: encephalitis, sarcoidosis, meningitis
	Damage from radiation therapy for ear-nose-throat carcinoma, pituitary tumors

Adapted from Plum F, Van Uitert R. Nonendocrine diseases and disorders of the hypothalamus. In: Reichlin S, Baldessarini RJ, Martin JB, eds. *The Hypothalamus,* vol 56. New York, NY: Raven Press, 1978:415-473.

TABLE 7-8

Etiology of Endocrine Syndromes of Hypothalamic Origin

Hypophyseotropic Hormone Deficiency
Surgical pituitary stalk section
Inflammatory disease: basilar meningitis and granuloma, sarcoidosis, tuberculosis, sphenoid osteomyelitis, eosinophilic granuloma
Craniopharyngioma
Hypothalamic tumor: infundibuloma; teratoma (ectopic pinealoma); neuroglial tumor, particularly astrocytoma
Maternal deprivation syndrome, psychosocial dwarfism
Isolated GHRH deficiency
Hypothalamic hypothyroidism
Panhypophyseotropic failure
Disorders of Regulation of GnRH Secretion
Female
Precocious puberty: GnRH-secreting hamartoma, hCG-secreting germinoma
Delayed puberty
Neurogenic amenorrhea
Pseudocyesis
Anorexia nervosa
"Functional" amenorrhea and oligomenorrhea
Drug-induced amenorrhea
Male
Precocious puberty
Fröhlich's syndrome
Olfactory-genital dysplasia (Kallmann's syndrome)
Disorders of Regulation of Prolactin-Regulating Factors
Tumor
Sarcoidosis
Drug-induced
Reflex
Herpes zoster of chest wall
Post-thoracotomy
Nipple manipulation
Spinal cord tumor
"Psychogenic"
Hypothyroidism
Carbon dioxide narcosis
Disorders of Regulation of CRH
Paroxysmal corticotropin discharge (Wolff's syndrome)
Loss of circadian variation
Depression
CRH-secreting gangliocytoma

CRH, corticotropin-releasing hormone; hCG, human chorionic gonadotropin; GHRH, growth hormone–releasing hormone; GnRH, gonadotropin-releasing hormone.

hormones but can cause hypersecretion of hormones that are normally under inhibitory control by the hypothalamus, as in hypersecretion of PRL after damage to the pituitary stalk and precocious puberty caused by loss of the normal restraint over gonadotropin maturation. Impairment of inhibitory control of the neurohypophysis can lead to the syndrome of inappropriate vasopressin secretion (SIADH) (see Chapter 10). More subtle abnormalities in secretion can result from impairment of the control system. For example, loss of the normal circadian rhythm of ACTH secretion may occur before loss of pituitary-adrenal secretory reserve, and responses to physiologic stimuli may be paradoxical. Because hypophyseotropic hormone levels cannot be measured directly and pituitary hormone secretion is regulated by complex, multilayered controls, assay of pituitary hormones in blood does not necessarily give a meaningful picture of events at hypothalamic and higher levels. Rarely, tumors secrete excessive amounts of releasing peptides and cause hypersecretion of hormones from the pituitary.

Disorders of the hypothalamic-pituitary unit can result from lesions at several levels. Defects can arise from destruction of the pituitary (as by tumor, infarct, inflammation, or autoimmune disease) or from a hereditary deficiency of a particular hormone (as in rare cases of isolated FSH, GH, or POMC deficiency). Selective loss of thyroid hormone receptors in the pituitary can give rise to increased TSH secretion and thyrotoxicosis. Furthermore, disorders can arise through disruption of the contact zone of the stalk and median eminence, the stalk itself, or the nerve terminals of the tuberohypophyseal system; such disruption occurs after surgical stalk section, with tumors involving the stalk, and in some inflammatory diseases. At a higher level, tonic inhibitory and excitatory inputs can be lost; this is manifested by absence of circadian rhythms or by the development of precocious puberty. Physical stress, cytokine products of inflammatory cells, toxins, and reflex inputs from peripheral homeostatic monitors also impinge on the tuberoinfundibular system. At the highest level of control, emotional stress and psychological disorders can activate the pituitary-adrenal stress response and suppress gonadotropin secretion (e.g., psychogenic amenorrhea) or inhibit GH secretion (e.g., psychosocial dwarfism) (see Chapter 17). Intrinsic disease of the anterior pituitary is reviewed in Chapter 8, and disturbances in neurohypophyseal function are discussed in Chapter 10. This chapter considers primarily diseases of the hypothalamic-pituitary unit.

Pituitary Isolation Syndrome

Destructive lesions of the pituitary stalk, such as may occur with head injury, surgical transection, tumor, or granuloma, produce a characteristic pattern of pituitary dysfunction.[365-367] Central diabetes insipidus (DI) develops in a large percentage of patients, depending on the level at which the stalk has been sectioned. If the cut is close to the hypothalamus, DI is almost always produced, but if the section is low on the stalk, the incidence is lower. The extent to which nerve terminals in the upper stalk are preserved determines the clinical course. The classic triphasic syndrome of initial polyuria followed by normal water control and then by AVP deficiency over a period of 1 week to 10 days occurs in fewer than half of the patients. The sequence is attributed to an initial loss of neurogenic control of the neural lobe, followed by autolysis of the neural lobe with release of AVP into the circulation and finally by complete loss of AVP. However, full expression of polyuria requires adequate cortisol levels; if cortisol is deficient, AVP deficiency may be present with only minimal polyuria. DI can also develop after stalk injury without an overt transitional phase. When DI occurs after head injury or operative trauma, varying degrees of recovery can be seen even after months or years. Sprouting of nerve terminals in the stump of the pituitary stalk may give rise to sufficient functioning tissue to maintain water balance. In contrast to the effects of stalk section, nondestructive injury to the neurohypophysis or stalk, such as during surgical resection of optic chiasmatic astrocytomas, can sometimes give rise to transient SIADH.[368]

Although head injury, granulomas, and tumors are the most common causes of acquired DI, other cases develop in the absence of a clearcut cause.[369] Autoimmune disease of the hypothalamus may be the cause in some instances, as was suggested by the finding of autoantibodies to neurohypophyseal cells in one third of patients with "idiopathic" DI in one series.[370] However, autoantibodies were also frequently found in association with histiocytosis X. Later reports suggested the importance of continued vigilance in cases of idiopathic DI. A definite cause is frequently uncovered in time, including a high proportion of occult germinomas, whose detection by MRI may be preceded by elevated levels of human chorionic gonadotropin (hCG) in CSF.[371,372] Congenital DI can be part of a hereditary disease. DI in the Brattleboro rat is caused by an autosomal recessive genetic defect that impairs production of AVP but not of oxytocin. In contrast, inherited forms of DI in humans have been attributed to mutations in the vasopressin V_2 receptor gene or, less frequently, in the aquaporin or the AVP gene.[373-376]

Menstrual cycles cease after stalk section, although gonadotropins may still be detectable, unlike the situation after hypophysectomy. Plasma glucocorticoid levels and urinary excretion of cortisol and 17-hydroxycorticoids decline after hypophysectomy and stalk section, but the change is slower after stalk section. A transient increase in cortisol secretion after stalk section is believed to result from the release of ACTH from preformed stores. The ACTH response to the lowering of blood cortisol is markedly reduced, but ACTH release after stress may be normal, possibly because of CRH-independent mechanisms. Reduction in thyroid function after stalk section is similar to that seen with hypophysectomy. The fall in GH secretion is said to be the most sensitive indication of damage to the stalk; however, the insidious nature of this endocrinologic change in adults who have suffered traumatic brain injury may cause it to be overlooked and therefore contribute to delayed rehabilitation.[377]

Humans with stalk sections or tumors of the stalk region have widely varying levels of hyperprolactinemia and may have galactorrhea.[378] PRL responses to hypoglycemia and to TRH are blunted, in part because of loss of neural connections with the hypothalamus. PRL responses to dopamine agonists and antagonists in patients with pituitary isolation syndrome are similar to those in patients with prolactinomas. Interestingly, PRL secretion continues to show a diurnal variation in patients with either hypothalamopituitary disconnection or microprolactinoma.[310] Both forms of hyperprolactinemia are characterized by a similarly increased frequency of PRL pulses and a marked rise in nonpulsatile or basal PRL secretion, although the disruption is greater in the tumoral hyperprolactinemia.

An incomplete pituitary isolation syndrome may occur with the empty sella syndrome, intrasellar cysts, or pituitary adenomas.[379-381] Anterior pituitary failure after stalk section is in part due to loss of specific neural and vascular links to the hypothalamus and in part to pituitary infarction.

Hypophyseotropic Hormone Deficiency

Selective pituitary failure can be caused by a deficiency of specific pituitary cell types or a deficiency of one or more hypothalamic hormones. Isolated GnRH deficiency is the most common hypophyseotropic hormone deficiency. In Kallmann's syndrome (gonadotropin deficiency commonly associated with hyposmia),[326] hereditary agenesis of the olfactory lobe may be demonstrable by MRI.[382] Abnormal development of the GnRH system is a result of defective migration of the GnRH-containing neurons from the olfactory nasal epithelium in early embryologic life (see earlier discussion). Other malformations of the cranial midline structures, such as absence of the septum pellucidum in septo-optic dysplasia (De Morsier's syndrome), can cause HH or, less commonly, precocious puberty. A surprisingly large percentage of children with septo-optic dysplasia who otherwise have multiple hypothalamic-pituitary abnormalities actually retain normal gonadotropin function and enter puberty spontaneously.[383] The genetic basis of HH, including Kallmann's syndrome, has now been established in approximately 15% of patients.[327,384] Mutations in *KAL1,* the Kallmann's syndrome gene, and in *NROB1* (formerly *AHC* or *DAX1*), the gene that causes adrenal hypoplasia congenita with hypogonadotropic hypogonadism, produce X-linked recessive disease. Autosomal recessive HH has been associated with mutations in the genes encoding the GnRH receptor, KISS1 (metastin) receptor, leptin, leptin receptor, FSH, LH, PROP1 (combined pituitary deficiency), and HESX1 (septo-optic dysplasia), and deficient FGFR1 function causes an autosomal dominant form of HH. Mutations in *PROK2* and *PROKR2,* which encode prokineticin 2 and its receptor, have been associated with heterozygous, homozygous, compound heterozygous, and oligogenic patterns of genetic penetrance.

The GnRH response test is of little value in the differential diagnosis of HH. Most patients with GnRH deficiency show little or no response to an initial test dose but normal responses after repeated injection. This slow response has been attributed to downregulation of GnRH receptors in response to prolonged GnRH deficiency. In patients with intrinsic pituitary disease, the response to GnRH may be absent or normal. Consequently, it is not possible to distinguish between hypothalamic and pituitary disease with a single injection of GnRH. Prolonged infusions or repeated administration of GnRH agonists after hormone replacement therapy priming may aid in the diagnosis or provide therapeutic options for women with Kallmann's syndrome who wish to become pregnant.[385,386]

Deficiency of TRH secretion gives rise to hypothalamic hypothyroidism, also called *tertiary hypothyroidism,* which can occur in hypothalamic disease or, more rarely, as an isolated defect.[387] Molecular genetic analyses have revealed infrequent autosomal recessive mutations in the TRH and TRH receptor genes in the etiology of central hypothyroidism.[388] Hypothalamic and pituitary causes of TSH deficiency are most readily distinguished by imaging methods. Although it is theoretically reasonable to use the TRH stimulation test for the differentiation of hypothalamic disease from pituitary disease, it is of limited value. The typical pituitary response to TRH administration in patients with TRH deficiency is an enhanced and somewhat delayed peak, whereas the response with pituitary failure is subnormal or absent. The hypothalamic type of response has been attributed to an associated GH deficiency that sensitizes the pituitary to TRH (possibly through suppression of somatostatin secretion), but GH also affects T_4 metabolism and may alter pituitary responses as well.[389] In practice, the responses to TRH in hypothalamic and pituitary disease overlap so much that this test cannot be used reliably for a differential diagnosis. Persistent failure to demonstrate responses to TRH is good evidence for the presence of intrinsic pituitary disease, but the presence of a response does not mean that the pituitary is normal. Deficient TRH secretion leads to altered TSH biosynthesis by the pituitary, including impaired glycosylation. Poorly glycosylated TSH has low biologic activity, and dissociation of bioactive and immunoreactive TSH can lead to the paradox of normal or elevated levels of TSH in hypothalamic hypothyroidism.[387,390]

GHRH deficiency appears to be the principal cause of hGH deficiency in children with idiopathic dwarfism.[391]

This condition is frequently associated with abnormal electroencephalograms, a history of birth trauma, and breech delivery, although a cause-and-effect relationship has not been established. MRI scans show that most children with isolated, idiopathic hGH deficiency have a normal sized or only slightly reduced anterior pituitary; less common findings are ectopic posterior pituitary, anterior pituitary hypoplasia, or empty sella.[392] In contrast, children with idiopathic combined pituitary hormone deficiency are significantly more likely to have evidence of moderate to severe anterior pituitary hypoplasia, ectopic posterior pituitary, complete agenesis of the pituitary stalk (both nervous and vascular components), and a variety of associated midline cerebral malformations.[392] Human GH is the most vulnerable of the anterior pituitary hormones when the pituitary stalk is damaged. It can be difficult to differentiate between primary pituitary disease and GHRH deficiency by standard tests of GH reserve. However, a substantial GH secretory response to a single administration of hexarelin occurs only in the presence of at least a partially intact vascular stalk (Fig. 7-32).[217]

In many children with dwarfism, the anatomic abnormalities of the intrasellar contents and pituitary stalk, together with the frequent occurrence of other midline defects, such as those observed in septo-optic dysplasia, are consistent with the alternative hypothesis of a developmental defect occurring in embryogenesis.[392] There has been a remarkable advance in understanding of the molecular ontogeny of the hypothalamic-pituitary unit, much of it based on mutant mouse models.[27] Parallel genetic analyses have been conducted in children with isolated GH deficiency or combined pituitary hormone deficiencies. These studies have identified autosomal recessive mutations in structural and regulatory genes including the genes encoding the GHRH receptor, PIT1, PROP1, HESX1, LHX3, and LHX4 that are responsible for a sizable proportion of congenital hypothalamic-pituitary disorders once considered idiopathic.[206,207,391,392]

Adrenal insufficiency is another manifestation of hypothalamic disease and rarely is caused by CRH deficiency.[393] Isolated ACTH deficiency is uncommon, but there is suggestive evidence in at least one family of genetic linkage to the *CRH* gene locus.[394] More recent investigations have revealed mutations in *TBX19,* the gene encoding TPIT, a T-box transcription factor expressed only in pituitary corticotrophs and melanotrophs, which is associated with the majority of cases of isolated ACTH deficiency in neonates.[395] The CRH stimulation test does not reliably distinguish hypothalamic from pituitary failure as a cause of ACTH deficiency.[396]

Apart from intrinsic diseases of the hypothalamus such as tumors and granulomas, two environmental causes of central hypophyseotropic deficiencies are of increasing clinical importance: trauma to the brain,[366,367,377] particularly from motor vehicle accidents, and the sequelae of chemotherapy and radiation therapy for intracranial lesions in children and adults.[390,397,398] Improved short-term survival from head injuries associated with coma and CNS malignancies has greatly increased the prevalence of long-term neuroendocrine consequences.

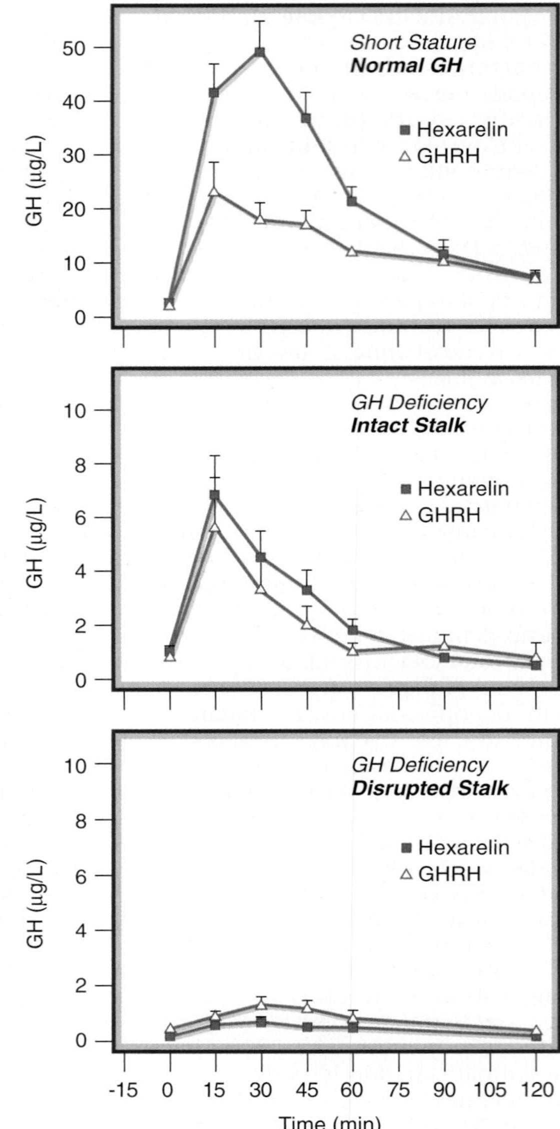

Figure 7-32 Effect of hypothalamic-pituitary disconnection on the growth hormone (GH) secretory responses to growth hormone–releasing hormone (GHRH) (1 µg/kg) and hexarelin (2 µg/kg) administered intravenously to children with GH deficiency. *Top,* Mean responses in a group of 24 prepubertal children with short stature secondary to familial short stature or constitutional growth delay are shown. *Middle,* Children with GH deficiency and an intact vascular pituitary stalk as visualized by dynamic magnetic resonance imaging exhibited a clear, but blunted, GH response to both secretagogues. *Bottom,* In contrast, children with pituitary stalk agenesis (both vascular and neural components) had no response or a markedly attenuated response to both peptides. (From Maghnie M, Spica-Russotto V, Cappa M, et al. The growth hormone response to hexarelin in patients with different hypothalamic-pituitary abnormalities. *J Clin Endocrinol Metab.* 1998;83: 3886-3889.)

Craniopharyngioma

Craniopharyngioma is the most common pediatric tumor occurring in the sellar and parasellar area (see Table 7-7). Because of their location, these benign neoplasms frequently cause significant neuroendocrine dysfunction. The more common adamantinomatous tumors in children usually contain both a cystic component filled with a turbid, cholesterol-rich fluid and a solid component characterized by organized epithelial cells.[399] Roughly 25% of craniopharyngiomas are diagnosed in patients after the age of 25 years, and this subset of tumors is more typically papillary in nature, solid, and less likely to be calcified or cystic.[399] Both forms of craniopharyngioma probably result from metaplastic changes in vestigial epithelial cell rests that originate in Rathke's pouch and the craniopharyngeal duct during fetal development.

Common presenting symptoms are those resulting from a mass intracranial lesion and increased intracranial pressure. Visual field defects, papilledema, and optic atrophy can occur from compression of the optic chiasm or nerves. Between 80% and 90% of affected children have signs and symptoms of endocrine dysfunction, although these are not usually the chief complaint. The most frequent hormone deficiencies are GH and gonadotropins. The latter is almost universal in adolescents and adults and probably is also present, but undetected, in prepubertal children with craniopharyngioma. TSH and ACTH deficiencies are also common. Even if not present at initial diagnosis, endocrine dysfunction often occurs subsequent to treatment and necessitates long-term follow-up and retesting.[400]

MRI is the imaging modality of choice in cases of suspected craniopharyngioma.[401] A recommended examination includes T1-weighted thin sagittal and coronal sections, obtained before and after contrast administration, through the sella and suprasellar regions. T2-weighted and fluid attenuation inversion recovery (FLAIR) images are useful to further delineate cysts and are hyperintense. Computed tomography scans can be useful to determine the presence of calcification.

Hypophyseotropic Hormone Hypersecretion

Pituitary hypersecretion is occasionally caused by tumors of the hypothalamus. GnRH-secreting hamartomas can cause precocious puberty.[402] CRH-secreting gangliocytomas can cause Cushing's syndrome,[403] and GHRH-secreting gangliocytomas of the hypothalamus can cause acromegaly.[404] Although they do not arise from the hypothalamus, paraneoplastic syndromes can also cause pituitary hypersecretion, as with CRH-secreting tumors and GHRH-secreting tumors of the bronchi and pancreas. Bronchial carcinoids and pituitary islet cell tumors are the usual causes of this phenomenon.

Neuroendocrine Disorders of Gonadotropin Regulation

Precocious Puberty

The term *precocious puberty* is used when physiologically normal pituitary-gonadal function appears at an early age (see also Chapter 25).[405] By convention, it is defined as the onset of androgen secretion and spermatogenesis before the age of 9 or 10 years in boys or the onset of estrogen secretion and cyclic ovarian activity before age 7 or 8 in girls.[406,407] Central precocious puberty is caused by disturbed CNS function, which may or may not have an identifiable structural basis. The term *pseudoprecocious puberty* refers to premature sexual development resulting from excessive secretion of androgens, estrogens, or hCG; it is caused by tumors (both gonadal and extragonadal), administration of exogenous gonadal steroids, or genetically determined activation of gonadotropin receptors (see Chapter 25). Central precocious puberty with neurogenic causes and pineal gland disease are discussed in this chapter.

Idiopathic Sexual Precocity. Familial occurrence of idiopathic sexual precocity is uncommon, but there is a hereditary form that is largely confined to boys. Abnormal electroencephalograms and behavioral disturbances, suggesting the presence of brain damage, have been reported occasionally in girls with idiopathic precocious puberty. The pathogenesis may be related to the rate of hypothalamic development or other, undetermined nutritional, environmental, or psychosocial factors. Many cases previously thought to be idiopathic are caused by small hypothalamic hamartomas (see later discussion). It has been argued that localized activation of discrete cellular subsets connected to GnRH neurons may be sufficient to initiate puberty.[408]

Neurogenic Precocious Puberty. Approximately two thirds of hypothalamic lesions that influence the timing of human puberty are located in the posterior hypothalamus, but in the subset of patients who come to autopsy, damage is extensive. Specific lesions known to cause precocity include craniopharyngioma (although delayed puberty is far more common with these lesions), astrocytoma, pineal tumors, subarachnoid cysts, encephalitis, miliary tuberculosis, tuberous sclerosis or neurofibromatosis type 1, the Sturge-Weber syndrome, porencephaly, craniostenosis, microcephaly, hydrocephalus, empty sella syndrome, and Tay-Sachs disease.[409,410]

Hamartoma of the hypothalamus is an exception to the generalization that tumors of the brain cause precocious puberty by impairment of gonadotropin secretion (although hamartomas on occasion cause hypothalamic damage). A hamartoma is a tumor-like collection of normal-appearing nerve tissue lodged in an abnormal location. The parahypothalamic type consists of an encapsulated nodule of nerve tissue attached to the floor of the third ventricle or suspended from the floor by a peduncle; it is typically less than 1 cm in diameter. The intrahypothalamic or sessile type is enveloped by the posterior hypothalamus and can distort the third ventricle. These hamartomas tend to be larger than the pedunculated variety; they grow in the interpeduncular cistern and are frequently accompanied by seizures, mental retardation, and developmental delays. They result in precocious puberty with about half the incidence observed with the parahypothalamic lesions.[411,412] Before the development of high-resolution scanning techniques, this tumor was considered rare, but small ones can now be visualized. Miniature hamartomas of the tuber cinereum are commonly discovered at autopsy. Precocious puberty occurs when the hamartoma makes connections with the median eminence and thus serves as an accessory hypothalamus. Peptidergic nerve terminals containing GnRH have been found in these tumors.[402] Early pubertal development is presumably caused by unrestrained GnRH secretion, although the hamartomas almost certainly have an intrinsic pulse generator of GnRH secretion, because pulsatility is required for stimulation of gonadotropin secretion (see earlier discussion).

Manifestations of premature puberty in patients with hamartomas are similar to those associated with other central causes of precocity. Hamartomas occur in both sexes and may be present as early as age 3 months. In the past, most cases were thought to be fatal by age 20 years, but many hamartomas cause no brain damage and need not be excised.[411] The interpeduncular fossa of the brain is difficult to approach, and surgical experience is somewhat limited. Early in the course of illness, epilepsy manifested as "brief, repetitive, stereotyped attacks of laughter"[413] may provide a clue to the disease. Late in the course, hypothalamic damage can cause severe neurologic defects and intractable seizures.

Hypothyroidism. Hypothyroidism can cause precocious puberty in girls that is reversible with thyroid therapy. Hyperprolactinemia and galactorrhea may be present. One possibility is that elevated TSH levels (in children with thyroid failure) cross-react with the FSH receptor.[414] Alternatively, low levels of thyroid hormone might simultaneously activate release of LH, FSH, and TSH. A third possibility is that hypothyroidism causes hypothalamic encephalopathy that impairs the normal tonic suppression of gonadotropin release by the hypothalamus. The high PRL levels that sometimes accompany this disorder may result from a deficiency in PIF secretion, increased secretion of TRH, or increased sensitivity of the lactotrophs to TRH secretion.

Tumors of the Pineal Gland. Pineal gland tumors account for only a small percentage of intracranial neoplasms. They occur as a central midline mass with an enhancing lesion on MRI frequently accompanied by hydrocephalus. Pinealomas cause a variety of neurologic abnormalities. Parinaud's syndrome, which consists of paralysis of upward gaze, pupillary areflexia (to light), paralysis of convergence, and a wide-based gait, occurs with about half of patients with pinealomas. Gait disturbances can also occur because of brain stem or cerebellar compression. Additional neurologic signs occurring with moderate frequency include spasticity, ataxia, nystagmus, syncope, vertigo, cranial nerve palsies other than VI and VIII, intention tremor, scotoma, and tinnitus.

Several discrete cytopathologic entities account for mass lesions in the pineal region (Table 7-9).[415] The most common non-neoplastic conditions are degenerative pineal cysts, arachnoid cysts, and cavernous hemangioma. Pinealocytes give rise to primitive neuroectodermal tumors, the so-called *small blue-cell tumors* that are immunopositive for the neuronal marker synaptophysin and negative for the lymphocyte marker CD45. True pinealomas can be relatively well differentiated pineocytomas, intermediate mixed forms, or the less differentiated pineoblastomas,[415,416] the latter of which are essentially identical to medulloblastomas, neuroblastomas, and oat cell carcinomas of the lung.

The most common tumors of the pineal gland are actually germinomas (a form of teratoma), so designated because of their presumed origin in germ cells. Germinomas may also occur in the anterior hypothalamus or the floor of the third ventricle, where they are often associated with the clinical triad of DI, pituitary insufficiency, and visual abnormalities.[410] Identical tumors can be found in the testis and anterior mediastinum. Intracranial germinomas have a tendency to spread locally, infiltrate the hypothalamus, and metastasize to the spinal cord and CSF. Extracranial metastases (to skin, lung, or liver) are rare. Teratomas derived from two or more germ cell layers also occur in the pineal region. Chorionic tissue in teratomas and germinomas may secrete hCG in sufficient amounts to cause gonadal maturation, and some of these tumors have histologic and functional characteristics of choriocarcinomas. Diagnosis is confirmed by the combination of a mass lesion, cytologic analysis of CSF, and radioimmunoassay detection of hCG in the CSF.

Precocious puberty is a relatively unusual manifestation of pineal gland disease. When it occurs, neuroanatomic studies suggest that the cause is secondary to pressure or destructive effects of the pineal tumor on the function of the adjacent hypothalamus, or to the secretion of hCG. Most patients have other evidence of hypothalamic involvement, such as DI, polyphagia, somnolence, obesity, or behavioral disturbance. Choriocarcinoma of the pineal gland is associated with high plasma levels of hCG. The hCG can stimulate testosterone secretion from the testis but not estrogen secretion by the ovary; it therefore causes premature puberty almost exclusively in boys. The prevalence of elevated hCG levels in children with premature puberty related to tumors in the pineal region is unknown, but the fact that this phenomenon occurs further challenges the theory that nonparenchymal tumors cause precocious puberty by damaging the normal pineal gland. Rarely, pinealomas cause delayed puberty, raising speculation about a role of melatonin in inhibiting gonadotropin secretion in these cases.

Management of tumors in the pineal region is not straightforward.[415,417] Operative mortality rates can be high, but the rationale for an aggressive approach is based on the need to make a histologic diagnosis, the variety of lesions found in this region, the possibility of cure of an encapsulated lesion, and the effectiveness of chemotherapeutic agents for germinomas and choriocarcinoma. Stereotaxic biopsy of the pineal region provided diagnosis in 33 of 34 cases in one series, suggesting that this is a useful alternative to open surgical exploration for diagnostic purposes.[418] Long-term palliation or cure of many pineal region tumors is possible through combinations of surgery, radiation, gamma knife, or chemotherapy, depending on the nature of the lesion.[419]

TABLE 7-9

Classification of Tumors of the Pineal Region

A. *Germ Cell Tumors*
1. Germinoma
a. Posterior third ventricle and pineal lesions
b. Anterior third ventricle, suprasellar, or intrasellar lesions
c. Combined lesions in anterior and posterior third ventricle, apparently noncontiguous, with or without foci of cystic or solid teratoma
2. Teratoma
a. Evidencing growth along two or three germ lines in varying degrees of differentiation
b. Dermoid and epidermoid cysts with or without solid foci of teratoma
c. Histologically malignant forms with or without differentiated foci of benign, solid, or cystic teratoma-teratocarcinoma, chorioepithelioma, embryonal carcinoma (endodermal–sinus tumor or yolk-sac carcinoma); combinations of these with or without foci of germinoma, chemodectoma
B. *Pineal Parenchymal Tumors*
1. Pinealocytes
a. Pineocytoma
b. Pineoblastoma
c. Ganglioglioma and chemodectoma
d. Mixed forms exhibiting transitions between these
2. Glia
a. Astrocytoma
b. Ependymoma
c. Mixed forms and other less frequent gliomas (e.g., glioblastoma, oligodendroglioma)
C. *Tumors of Supporting or Adjacent Structures*
1. Meningioma
2. Hemangiopericytoma
D. *Nonneoplastic Conditions of Neurosurgical Importance*
1. "Degenerative" cysts of pineal gland lined by fibrillary astrocytes
2. Arachnoid cysts
3. Cavernous hemangioma

From DeGirolami U. Pathology of tumors of the pineal region. In: Schmidek HH, ed. *Pineal Tumors*. New York, NY: Masson; 1977:1-19.

Approach to the Patient with Precocious Puberty. Several groups have reviewed the diagnostic approach to suspected central precocious puberty (see Chapter 25).[420,421] Although guidelines differ, the index of suspicion is clearly inversely proportional to the age of the patient. A GnRH stimulation test to assess gonadotropin release and thereby differentiate between primed and inactive gonadotrophs is probably the single most important endocrinologic measure. If LH and FSH levels are not stimulated and there is no evidence of gonadal germ cell maturation, the cause of precocious puberty lies outside the hypothalamic-pituitary axis, and the diagnostic process should focus on the adrenal glands and gonads (see Chapters 15 and 25). MRI studies are central to the workup for exclusion or characterization of organic lesions in the areas of the sella, optic chiasm, suprasellar hypothalamus, and interpeduncular cistern.[422]

Management of Sexual Precocity. Structural lesions of the hypothalamus are treated by surgery, radiation, chemotherapy, or combinations of these treatments, as indicated by the pathologic diagnosis and extent of disease. Endocrinologic manifestations of precocious puberty are best treated by GnRH agonists with the therapeutic goals of delaying sexual maturation to a more appropriate age and achieving optimal linear growth and bone mass, possibly with the combined use of GH treatment.[423,424] Other approaches include the use of cyproterone acetate, testolactone, or spironolactone to antagonize or inhibit gonadal steroid biosynthesis.[425,426] Precocious puberty is stressful to both the child and the parents, and it is essential that psychological support be provided.

Psychogenic Amenorrhea

Menstrual cycles can cease in young nonpregnant women with no demonstrable abnormalities of the brain, pituitary, or ovary in several situations,[427,428] including pseudocyesis (false pregnancy), anorexia nervosa, excessive exercise, psychogenic disorders, and hyperprolactinemic states (see Chapter 17). Psychogenic amenorrhea, the most common cause of secondary amenorrhea except for pregnancy, can occur with major psychopathology or minor psychic stress and is often temporary. Psychogenic amenorrhea is probably mediated by excessive endogenous opioid activity, because naloxone or naltrexone (both opiate receptor blockers) can induce ovulation in some patients with this disorder.[428]

Exercise-induced amenorrhea may be a variant of psychogenic amenorrhea, or it may result from loss of body fat.[427,429] The syndrome is associated with intense and prolonged physical exertion such as running, swimming, or ballet dancing. Affected women are always at less than ideal body weight and have low stores of fat. If the activity is begun before puberty, normal sexual maturation can be delayed for many years. Fat mass may be a regulator of gonadotropin secretion, with adipocyte-derived leptin as the principal mediator between peripheral energy stores and hypothalamic regulatory centers.[430] Studies in nonhuman primates showed a direct role of caloric intake in the pathogenesis of amenorrhea associated with long-distance running.[431] Exercise and psychogenic amenorrhea can have adverse effects because of the associated estrogen deficiency and accompanying osteopenia (also see Chapter 28).[432]

Neurogenic Hypogonadism in Males

A discussion of neurogenic hypogonadism in males should begin with an account of Fröhlich's syndrome (adiposogenital dystrophy), which was originally characterized as delayed puberty, hypogonadism, and obesity associated with a tumor that impinges on the hypothalamus.[1] It was later recognized that either hypothalamic or pituitary dysfunction can induce hypogonadism, and the presence of obesity indicates that the appetite-regulating regions of the hypothalamus have been damaged. Several organic lesions of the hypothalamus can cause this syndrome, including tumors, encephalitis, microcephaly, Friedreich's ataxia, and demyelinating diseases. Other important causes of HH are Kallmann's syndrome, a disorder caused by failure of GnRH-containing neurons to migrate normally (see earlier discussions of GnRH and hypophyseotropic hormone deficiency), and a subset of the Prader-Willi syndrome.[433]

However, most males with delayed sexual development do not have serious neurologic conditions. Furthermore, most obese boys with delayed sexual development have no structural damage to the hypothalamus but have constitutional delayed puberty, which is commonly associated with obesity. It is not known whether there is a functional disorder of the hypothalamus in this condition. It is thought that psychosexual development of brain maturation depends on the presence of androgens within a critical developmental window corresponding to puberty; therefore, hypogonadism in boys (regardless of cause) should be treated by the middle teen years (15 years of age at the latest).

In adult men, hypogonadism (including reduced spermatogenesis) can be induced by emotional stress or severe exercise,[434] but this abnormality is seldom diagnosed because the symptoms are more subtle than menstrual cycle changes in similarly stressed women. Prolonged physical stress and sleep and energy deficiencies can also decrease testosterone and gonadotropin levels.[435] Chronic intrathecal administration of opiates for the control of intractable pain syndromes is strongly associated with HH, and to a lesser extent with hypocorticism and GH deficiency, in both men and women.[436] Finally, critical illness with multiple causes is well known to be associated with hypogonadism and ineffectual altered pulsation of GnRH.[437]

Neurogenic Disorders of Prolactin Regulation

Neurogenic causes of hyperprolactinemia include irritative lesions of the chest wall (e.g., herpes zoster, thoracotomy), excessive tactile stimulation of the nipple, and lesions within the spinal cord (e.g., ependymoma).[438] Prolonged mechanical stimulation of the nipples by suckling or the use of a breast pump can initiate lactation in some women who are not pregnant, and neurologic lesions that interrupt the hypothalamic-pituitary connection can cause hyperprolactinemia, as discussed earlier. Hyperprolactinemia also occurs after certain forms of epileptic seizures. In one series, six of eight patients with temporal lobe seizures had a marked increase in PRL, whereas only one of eight patients with frontal lobe seizures led to hyperprolactinemia.[439] Agents that block D_2-like dopamine receptors (e.g., phenothiazines, later-generation atypical antipsychotics) or prevent dopamine release (e.g., reserpine, methyldopa) must be excluded in all cases.

Because the nervous system exerts such profound effects on PRL secretion, patients with hyperprolactinemia (including those with adenomas) may have a deficit of PIF or an excess of PRF activity. In studies of PRL secretion in patients apparently cured of hyperprolactinemia by removal of a pituitary microadenoma, regulatory abnormalities persisted in some but not all patients. Regulatory abnormalities may persist because of incomplete removal of tumor, abnormal function of the remaining part of the gland, or underlying hypothalamic abnormalities.[440]

Neurogenic Disorders of Growth Hormone Secretion

Hypothalamic Growth Failure

Loss of the normal nocturnal increase in GH secretion and loss of GH secretory responses to provocative stimuli occur early in the course of hypothalamic disease and may be the most sensitive endocrine indicator of hypothalamic dysfunction. As described earlier, anatomic malformations of midline cerebral structures are associated with abnormal GH secretion, presumably related to failure of the development of normal GH regulatory mechanisms. Such disorders include optic nerve dysplasia and midline prosencephalic malformations (absence of the septum pellucidum, abnormal third ventricle, and abnormal lamina terminalis). Certain complex genetic disorders including Prader-Willi syndrome also commonly involve reduced GH secretory capacity.[441] Idiopathic hypopituitarism with GH deficiency was considered earlier.

Maternal Deprivation Syndrome and Psychosocial Dwarfism

Infant neglect or abuse can impair growth and cause failure to thrive (the maternal deprivation syndrome). Malnutrition interacts with psychological factors to cause growth failure in these children, and each case should be carefully evaluated from this point of view. Older children with growth failure in a setting of abuse or severe emotional disturbance (termed *psychosocial dwarfism*) may also have abnormal circadian rhythms and deficient hGH release after insulin-induced hypoglycemia or arginine infusion (see Chapter 24).[442] Deficient release of ACTH and gonadotropins may also be present. A new variant, termed *hyperphagic short stature,* has been identified.[443] These disorders can be reversed by placing the child in a supportive milieu; growth and neuroendocrine hGH responses rapidly return to normal.[444] The pathogenesis of altered GH secretion in children in response to deprivation is unknown. Furthermore, in the adult human, physical or emotional stress usually causes an increase in hGH secretion (see earlier discussion).

Neuroregulatory Growth Hormone Deficiency

The availability of biosynthetic hGH for treatment of short stature has brought into focus a group of patients who grow at low rates (<3rd percentile) and have low levels of serum IGF1 but a normal hGH secretory reserve. Studies of 24-hour hGH secretion profiles indicate that many of these children do not have normal spontaneous hGH secretion (i.e., abnormal ultradian and circadian rhythms or decreased number or amplitude of secretory bursts, or both). These children with idiopathic short stature may have a functional regulatory disturbance of the hypothalamus and appear to grow normally when given exogenous hGH.[445]

There is considerable uncertainty about the criteria for diagnosis of neuroregulatory hGH deficiency. Many normally growing children have profiles of hGH secretion that are indistinguishable from those of children with the postulated syndrome.[446] Patterns of hGH secretion do not predict which child will benefit from therapy, and there is a poor correlation between hGH secretion and growth. Furthermore, the results of repeated tests in children show considerable variability. It has been suggested that specific genetic defects may underlie the pathogenesis of a subset of children with this heterogeneous syndrome of growth failure.[447] The prevalence of an hGH neuroregulatory deficiency syndrome is therefore unclear, and the decision to treat short children with hGH should be made cautiously.[448,449]

Neurogenic Hypersecretion of Growth Hormone

Diencephalic Syndrome. Children and infants with tumors in and around the third ventricle frequently become cachectic, which is often associated with elevated hGH levels and paradoxical GH secretory responses to glucose and insulin.[450] GH hypersecretion may be caused by a hypothalamic abnormality or by malnutrition. Deficits of pituitary-adrenal regulation are less common. A striking feature is an alert appearance and seeming euphoria despite the profound emaciation. A variety of associated neurologic abnormalities may be present, including nystagmus, irritability, hydrocephalus, optic atrophy, tremor, and excessive sweating. CSF abnormalities include increased protein and the presence of abnormal cells. Most cases are caused by chiasmatic-hypothalamic gliomas, with the majority classified as astrocytomas.[450] Treatment options include surgical resection, radiation therapy, and chemotherapy.[451]

Growth Hormone Hypersecretion Associated with Metabolic Disturbances. Apparently inappropriate hGH hypersecretion occurs with uncontrolled diabetes mellitus, hepatic failure, uremia, anorexia nervosa, and protein-calorie malnutrition. Nutritional factors are probably important in this response, because in normal persons obesity inhibits and fasting stimulates episodic GH hypersecretion.[452] In diabetes mellitus, cholinergic blockers reverse the abnormality,[228] possibly by inhibiting hypothalamic somatostatin secretion (see earlier discussion). Loss of inhibition of GH secretion by IGF1 may also play a role, because most disorders in which this syndrome occurs are associated with low IGF1 levels.

Neurogenic Disorders of Corticotropin Regulation

Hypothalamic CRH hypersecretion is the likely cause of sustained pituitary-adrenal hyperfunction in at least two situations: Cushing's syndrome caused by rare CRH-secreting gangliocytomas of the hypothalamus[453] and severe depression. Severe depression is associated with pituitary-adrenal abnormalities, including inappropriately elevated ACTH levels, abnormal cortisol circadian rhythms, and resistance to dexamethasone suppression.[160,164,165,454] The dexamethasone suppression test has, in fact, been used as an aid to the diagnosis of depressive illness. Another possible example of disordered neurogenic control of CRH associated with stress is the dysmetabolic syndrome.[455,456] This syndrome is characterized by mild hypercortisolism, blunted dexamethasone suppression of the HPA axis, visceral obesity, and hypertension and is strongly associated with greater risks for cardiovascular disease and stroke.

A unique syndrome of ACTH hypersecretion, termed *periodic hypothalamic discharge* (Wolff's syndrome), has been described in one young man. The patient had a recurring cyclic disorder characterized by high fever, paroxysms of glucocorticoid hypersecretion, and electroencephalographic abnormalities.[457]

Nonendocrine Manifestations of Hypothalamic Disease

The hypothalamus is involved in the regulation of diverse functions and behaviors (Table 7-10). Psychological

TABLE 7-10

Neurologic Manifestations of Nonendocrine Hypothalamic Disease

Disorders of Temperature Regulation
Hyperthermia Hypothermia Poikilothermia
Disorders of Food Intake
Hyperphagia (bulimia) Anorexia nervosa, aphagia Cachexia
Disorders of Water Intake
Compulsive water drinking Adipsia Essential hypernatremia
Disorders of Sleep and Consciousness
Narcolepsy/cataplexy Somnolence Sleep rhythm reversal Akinetic mutism Coma Delirium
Periodic Disease of Hypothalamic Origin
Diencephalic epilepsy Kleine-Levin syndrome Periodic discharge syndrome of Wolff
Disorders of Psychic Function
Rage behavior Hallucinations Hypersexuality
Disorders of the Autonomic Nervous System
Pulmonary edema Cardiac arrhythmias Sphincter disturbance
Congenital Hypothalamic Disease
Prader-Willi syndrome Laurence-Moon-Biedl syndrome
Miscellaneous
Diencephalic syndrome of infancy Cerebral gigantism

abnormalities in hypothalamic disease include antisocial behavior; attacks of rage, laughing, or crying; disturbed sleep patterns; excessive sexuality; and hallucinations. Both somnolence (with posterior lesions) and pathologic wakefulness (with anterior lesions) occur, as do bulimia and profound anorexia. The abnormal eating patterns are analogous to the syndromes of hyperphagia produced in rats by destruction of the VMH or connections to the PVH. Lateral hypothalamic damage causes profound anorexia. A more complete discussion of imbalance in energy homeostasis (obesity and cachexia) associated with hypothalamic dysfunction and neuropeptides is presented in Chapter 35.

Patients with hypothalamic damage may experience hyperthermia, hypothermia, unexplained fluctuations in body temperature, and poikilothermy. Disturbances of sweating, acrocyanosis, loss of sphincter control, and diencephalic epilepsy are occasional manifestations. Hypothalamic damage also causes loss of recent memory, believed to result from damage of the mammillothalamic pathways. Severe memory loss, obesity, and personality changes (apathy, loss of ability to concentrate, aggressive antisocial behavior, severe food craving, inability to work or attend school) may occur with suprasellar extension of pituitary tumors, hypothalamic irradiation, or damage incurred from surgical removal of parasellar tumors. Hypothalamic tumors grow slowly and may reach a large size while producing minimal disturbance of behavior or visceral homeostasis, whereas surgery of limited extent can produce striking functional abnormalities. Presumably, this is because slowly growing lesions permit compensatory responses to develop. These potential consequences should be weighed carefully with the neurosurgeon, patient, and patient's family in planning the therapeutic approach. Adverse effects of treatment have led to more conservative surgical guidelines for the treatment of craniopharyngioma. A recent review from the University of Pittsburgh summarizes their individualized treatment program, which includes microsurgical tumor resection, intracavitary ^{32}P radiotherapy, and gamma knife stereotactic radiosurgery to produce maximal benefit with minimal morbidity.[458]

Narcolepsy

A convergence of functional genomics from two animal species, the dog and mouse, has dramatically refocused attention on neuropeptide circuits of the hypothalamus in the control of sleep and wakefulness. Positional cloning was used to identify mutations in the hypocretin-orexin receptor 2 as a cause of canine narcolepsy.[459] Subsequently knockout of the gene encoding the hypocretin-orexin peptide precursor produced an equivalent narcoleptic syndrome in mice,[460] further establishing this neuropeptide system as a major component of sleep-modulating neural circuits. The additional role of hypocretin-orexin in coordinating arousal states and feeding behavior is discussed in Chapter 35. These new discoveries add to the list of other hypothalamic neuropeptides, including GHRH, somatostatin, cortistatin, CRH, galanin, ghrelin, and NPY, that have established functions in modulation of the sleep cycle.

Histaminergic neurons of the tuberomammillary nucleus express both forms of the orexin receptor and make reciprocal synaptic connections with orexin neurons in the lateral hypothalamus. Furthermore, orexin is an excitatory transmitter for the histamine neurons, suggesting that the two populations cooperate in the regulation of rapid eye movement sleep.[461] A recent study suggested that the two populations of neurons also play complementary but distinct roles in the maintenance of wakefulness.[462] Targeted ablation of orexin neurons in the lateral hypothalamus of rats by means of a hypocretin receptor 2-saporin conjugate produced narcoleptic-like sleep behavior,[463] closely paralleling the clinical findings and profound reduction in numbers of hypocretin-orexin neurons in the lateral hypothalamus of humans with narcolepsy.[464]

In summary, most cases of spontaneous narcolepsy with cataplexy result from a degenerative hypothalamic disorder, most likely autoimmune in pathogenesis, that produces a selective destruction of neuropeptidergic neurons. The absence of immunoreactive hypocretin-orexin in CSF is a sensitive diagnostic test for the disease. Future development of bioavailable, hypocretin-orexin receptor–selective compounds may provide a specific treatment alternative or adjunct to the stimulant and antidepressant drugs currently used for the management of symptoms. More generally, these discoveries suggest the possibility that other cryptic hypothalamic disorders could be caused by selective disturbances in other neuropeptidergic circuits.

343. Nakai Y, Plant TM, Hess DL, et al. On the sites of the negative and positive feedback actions of estradiol in the control of gonadotropin secretion in the rhesus monkey. *Endocrinology*. 1978;102:1008-1014.
344. Kumar TR, Low MJ. Hormonal regulation of human follicle-stimulating hormone-beta subunit gene expression: GnRH stimulation and GnRH-independent androgen inhibition. *Neuroendocrinology*. 1995;61:628-637.
345. Bishop W, Kalra PS, Fawcett CP, et al. The effects of hypothalamic lesions on the release of gonadotropins and prolactin in response to estrogen and progesterone treatment in female rats. *Endocrinology*. 1972;91:1404-1410.
346. Levine JE, Chappell PE, Schneider JS, et al. Progesterone receptors as neuroendocrine integrators. *Front Neuroendocrinol*. 2001;22:69-106.
347. Seminara SB. Metastin and its G protein-coupled receptor, GPR54: critical pathway modulating GnRH secretion. *Front Neuroendocrinol*. 2005;26:131-138.
348. Dungan HM, Clifton DK, Steiner RA. Minireview: kisspeptin neurons as central processors in the regulation of gonadotropin-releasing hormone secretion. *Endocrinology*. 2006;147:1154-1158.
349. Popa SM, Clifton DK, Steiner RA. The role of kisspeptins and GPR54 in the neuroendocrine regulation of reproduction. *Annu Rev Physiol*. 2008;70:213-238.
350. Kaplan SL, Grumbach MM, Aubert ML. The ontogenesis of pituitary hormones and hypothalamic factors in the human fetus: maturation of central nervous system regulation of anterior pituitary function. *Recent Prog Horm Res*. 1976;32:161-243.
351. Winter JS, Faiman C, Hobson WC, et al. Pituitary-gonadal relations in infancy: I. Patterns of serum gonadotropin concentrations from birth to four years of age in man and chimpanzee. *J Clin Endocrinol Metab*. 1975;40:545-551.
352. Plant TM. Neurobiological bases underlying the control of the onset of puberty in the rhesus monkey: a representative higher primate. *Front Neuroendocrinol*. 2001;22:107-139.
353. Boyar RM, Rosenfeld RS, Kapen S, et al. Human puberty: simultaneous augmented secretion of luteinizing hormone and testosterone during sleep. *J Clin Invest*. 1974;54:609-618.
354. Gay VL, Plant TM. Sustained intermittent release of gonadotropin-releasing hormone in the prepubertal male rhesus monkey induced by N-methyl-DL-aspartic acid. *Neuroendocrinology*. 1988;48:147-152.
355. Ojeda SR, Ma YJ, Lee BJ, et al. Glia-to-neuron signaling and the neuroendocrine control of female puberty. *Recent Prog Horm Res*. 2000;55:197-223; discussion 223-224.
356. Ebling FJ. The neuroendocrine timing of puberty. *Reproduction*. 2005;129:675-683.
357. Stoyanovitch AG, Johnson MA, Clifton DK, et al. Galanin-like peptide rescues reproductive function in the diabetic rat. *Diabetes*. 2005;54:2471-2476.
358. Cameron JL. Stress and behaviorally induced reproductive dysfunction in primates. *Semin Reprod Endocrinol*. 1997;15:37-45.
359. Rivier C, Rivier J, Vale W. Stress-induced inhibition of reproductive functions: role of endogenous corticotropin-releasing factor. *Science*. 1986;231:607-609.
360. Feng YJ, Shalts E, Xia LN, et al. An inhibitory effect of interleukin-1a on basal gonadotropin release in the ovariectomized rhesus monkey: reversal by a corticotropin-releasing factor antagonist. *Endocrinology*. 1991;128:2077-2082.
361. Chen MD, O'Byrne KT, Chiappini SE, et al. Hypoglycemic "stress" and gonadotropin-releasing hormone pulse generator activity in the rhesus monkey: role of the ovary. *Neuroendocrinology*. 1992;56:666-673.
362. Norman RL, Smith CJ. Restraint inhibits luteinizing hormone and testosterone secretion in intact male rhesus macaques: effects of concurrent naloxone administration. *Neuroendocrinology*. 1992;55:405-415.
363. Chehab FF, Lim ME, Lu R. Correction of the sterility defect in homozygous obese female mice by treatment with the human recombinant leptin. *Nat Genet*. 1996;12:318-320.
364. Schneider JE, Zhou D, Blum RM. Leptin and metabolic control of reproduction. *Horm Behav*. 2000;37:306-326.
365. Honegger J, Buchfelder M, Fahlbusch R. Surgical treatment of craniopharyngiomas: endocrinological results. *J Neurosurg*. 1999;90:251-257.
366. Yuan XQ, Wade CE. Neuroendocrine abnormalities in patients with traumatic brain injury. *Front Neuroendocrinol*. 1991;12:209-230.
367. Benvenga S, Campenni A, Ruggeri RM, et al. Clinical review 113: hypopituitarism secondary to head trauma. *J Clin Endocrinol Metab*. 2000;85:1353-1361.
368. Daaboul J, Steinbok P. Abnormalities of water metabolism after surgery for optic/chiasmatic astrocytomas in children. *Pediatr Neurosurg*. 1998;28:181-185.
369. Maghnie M, Cosi G, Genovese E, et al. Central diabetes insipidus in children and young adults. *N Engl J Med*. 2000;343:998-1007.
370. Scherbaum WA, Wass JA, Besser GM, et al. Autoimmune cranial diabetes insipidus: its association with other endocrine diseases and with histiocytosis X. *Clin Endocrinol (Oxf)*. 1986;25:411-420.
371. Al-Agha AE, Thomsett MJ, Ratcliffe JF, et al. Acquired central diabetes insipidus in children: a 12-year Brisbane experience. *J Paediatr Child Health*. 2001;37:172-175.
372. Mootha SL, Barkovich AJ, Grumbach MM, et al. Idiopathic hypothalamic diabetes insipidus, pituitary stalk thickening, and the occult intracranial germinoma in children and adolescents. *J Clin Endocrinol Metab*. 1997;82:1362-1367.
373. Nagasaki H, Ito M, Yuasa H, et al. Two novel mutations in the coding region for neurophysin-II associated with familial central diabetes insipidus. *J Clin Endocrinol Metab*. 1995;80:1352-1356.
374. Morello JP, Bichet DG. Nephrogenic diabetes insipidus. *Annu Rev Physiol*. 2001;63:607-630.
375. Birnbaumer M. The V2 vasopressin receptor mutations and fluid homeostasis. *Cardiovasc Res*. 2001;51:409-415.
376. Nielsen S, Frokiaer J, Marples D, et al. Aquaporins in the kidney: from molecules to medicine. *Physiol Rev*. 2002;82:205-244.
377. Lieberman SA, Oberoi AL, Gilkison CR, et al. Prevalence of neuroendocrine dysfunction in patients recovering from traumatic brain injury. *J Clin Endocrinol Metab*. 2001;86:2752-2756.
378. Smith MV, Laws ER Jr. Magnetic resonance imaging measurements of pituitary stalk compression and deviation in patients with nonprolactin-secreting intrasellar and parasellar tumors: lack of correlation with serum prolactin levels. *Neurosurgery*. 1994;34:834-839; discussion 839.
379. Voelker JL, Campbell RL, Muller J. Clinical, radiographic, and pathological features of symptomatic Rathke's cleft cysts. *J Neurosurg*. 1991;74:535-544.
380. Zucchini S, Ambrosetto P, Carla G, et al. Primary empty sella: differences and similarities between children and adults. *Acta Paediatr*. 1995;84:1382-1385.
381. Bjerre P. The empty sella: a reappraisal of etiology and pathogenesis. *Acta Neurol Scand Suppl*. 1990;130:1-25.
382. Klingmuller D, Dewes W, Krahe T, et al. Magnetic resonance imaging of the brain in patients with anosmia and hypothalamic hypogonadism (Kallmann's syndrome). *J Clin Endocrinol Metab*. 1987;65:581-584.
383. Nanduri VR, Stanhope R. Why is the retention of gonadotrophin secretion common in children with panhypopituitarism due to septo-optic dysplasia? *Eur J Endocrinol*. 1999;140:48-50.
384. Bhagavath B, Podolsky RH, Ozata M, et al. Clinical and molecular characterization of a large sample of patients with hypogonadotropic hypogonadism. *Fertil Steril*. 2006;85:706-713.
385. Chryssikopoulos A, Gregoriou O, Vitoratos N, et al. The predictive value of double Gn-RH provocation test in unprimed Gn-RH-primed and steroid-primed female patients with Kallmann's syndrome. *Int J Fertil Womens Med*. 1998;43:291-299.
386. Hayes FJ, Seminara SB, Crowley WF Jr. Hypogonadotropic hypogonadism. *Endocrinol Metab Clin North Am*. 1998;27:739-763, vii.
387. Samuels MH, Ridgway EC. Central hypothyroidism. *Endocrinol Metab Clin North Am*. 1992;21:903-919.
388. Winter WE, Signorino MR. Review: molecular thyroidology. *Ann Clin Lab Sci*. 2001;31:221-244.
389. Jorgensen JO, Pedersen SA, Laurberg P, et al. Effects of growth hormone therapy on thyroid function of growth hormone-deficient adults with and without concomitant thyroxine-substituted central hypothyroidism. *J Clin Endocrinol Metab*. 1989;69:1127-1132.
390. Rose SR. Cranial irradiation and central hypothyroidism. *Trends Endocrinol Metab*. 2001;12:97-104.
391. Argente J, Abusrewil SA, Bona G, et al. Isolated growth hormone deficiency in children and adolescents. *J Pediatr Endocrinol Metab*. 2001;14(suppl 2):1003-1008.
392. Maghnie M, Ghirardello S, Genovese E. Magnetic resonance imaging of the hypothalamus-pituitary unit in children suspected of hypopituitarism: who, how and when to investigate. *J Endocrinol Invest*. 2004;27:496-509.
393. Nishihara E, Kimura H, Ishimaru T, et al. A case of adrenal insufficiency due to acquired hypothalamic CRH deficiency. *Endocr J*. 1997;44:121-126.
394. Kyllo JH, Collins MM, Vetter KL, et al. Linkage of congenital isolated adrenocorticotropic hormone deficiency to the corticotropin releasing hormone locus using simple sequence repeat polymorphisms. *Am J Med Genet*. 1996;62:262-267.
395. Vallette-Kasic S, Brue T, Pulichino AM, et al. Congenital isolated adrenocorticotropin deficiency: an underestimated cause of neonatal death, explained by TPIT gene mutations. *J Clin Endocrinol Metab*. 2005;90:1323-1331.
396. Fukata J, Shimizu N, Imura H, et al. Human corticotropin-releasing hormone test in patients with hypothalamopituitary-adrenocortical disorders. *Endocr J*. 1993;40:597-606.
397. Gleeson HK, Shalet SM. Endocrine complications of neoplastic diseases in children and adolescents. *Curr Opin Pediatr*. 2001;13:346-351.
398. Arlt W, Hove U, Muller B, et al. Frequent and frequently overlooked: treatment-induced endocrine dysfunction in adult long-term survivors of primary brain tumors. *Neurology*. 1997;49:498-506.
399. Prabhu VC, Brown HG. The pathogenesis of craniopharyngiomas. *Childs Nerv Syst*. 2005;21:622-627.

400. Halac I, Zimmerman D. Endocrine manifestations of craniopharyngioma. *Childs Nerv Syst.* 2005;21:640-648.
401. Curran JG, O'Connor E. Imaging of craniopharyngioma. *Childs Nerv Syst.* 2005;21:635-639.
402. Hochman HI, Judge DM, Reichlin S. Precocious puberty and hypothalamic hamartoma. *Pediatrics.* 1981;67:236-244.
403. Asa SL, Kovacs K, Tindall GT, et al. Cushing's disease associated with an intrasellar gangliocytoma producing corticotrophin-releasing factor. *Ann Intern Med.* 1984;101:789-793.
404. Asa SL, Scheithauer BW, Bilbao JM, et al. A case for hypothalamic acromegaly: a clinicopathological study of six patients with hypothalamic gangliocytomas producing growth hormone-releasing factor. *J Clin Endocrinol Metab.* 1984;58:796-803.
405. Lee PA. Central precocious puberty: an overview of diagnosis, treatment, and outcome. *Endocrinol Metab Clin North Am.* 1999;28:901-918, xi.
406. De Sanctis V, Corrias A, Rizzo V, et al. Etiology of central precocious puberty in males: the results of the Italian Study Group for Physiopathology of Puberty. *J Pediatr Endocrinol Metab.* 2000;13(suppl 1): 687-693.
407. Cisternino M, Arrigo T, Pasquino AM, et al. Etiology and age incidence of precocious puberty in girls: a multicentric study. *J Pediatr Endocrinol Metab.* 2000;13(suppl 1):695-701.
408. Ojeda SR, Heger S. New thoughts on female precocious puberty. *J Pediatr Endocrinol Metab.* 2001;14:245-256.
409. Virdis R, Sigorini M, Laiolo A, et al. Neurofibromatosis type 1 and precocious puberty. *J Pediatr Endocrinol Metab.* 2000;13(suppl 1):841-844.
410. Rivarola MA, Belgorosky A, Mendilaharzu H, et al. Precocious puberty in children with tumours of the suprasellar and pineal areas: organic central precocious puberty. *Acta Paediatr.* 2001;90:751-756.
411. Arita K, Ikawa F, Kurisu K, et al. The relationship between magnetic resonance imaging findings and clinical manifestations of hypothalamic hamartoma. *J Neurosurg.* 1999;91:212-220.
412. Debeneix C, Bourgeois M, Trivin C, et al. Hypothalamic hamartoma: comparison of clinical presentation and magnetic resonance images. *Horm Res.* 2001;56:12-18.
413. Berkovic SF, Andermann F, Melanson D, et al. Hypothalamic hamartomas and ictal laughter: evolution of a characteristic epileptic syndrome and diagnostic value of magnetic resonance imaging. *Ann Neurol.* 1988;23:429-439.
414. Anasti JN, Flack MR, Froehlich J, et al. A potential novel mechanism for precocious puberty in juvenile hypothyroidism. *J Clin Endocrinol Metab.* 1995;80:276-279.
415. Fauchon F, Jouvet A, Paquis P, et al. Parenchymal pineal tumors: a clinicopathological study of 76 cases. *Int J Radiat Oncol Biol Phys.* 2000;46:959-968.
416. Jouvet A, Saint-Pierre G, Fauchon F, et al. Pineal parenchymal tumors: a correlation of histological features with prognosis in 66 cases. *Brain Pathol.* 2000;10:49-60.
417. Baumgartner JE, Edwards MS. Pineal tumors. *Neurosurg Clin North Am.* 1992;3:853-862.
418. Popovic EA, Kelly PJ. Stereotactic procedures for lesions of the pineal region. *Mayo Clin Proc.* 1993;68:965-970.
419. Dahlborg SA, Petrillo A, Crossen JR, et al. The potential for complete and durable response in nonglial primary brain tumors in children and young adults with enhanced chemotherapy delivery. *Cancer J Sci Am.* 1998;4:110-124.
420. Chalumeau M, Chemaitilly W, Trivin C, et al. Central precocious puberty in girls: an evidence-based diagnosis tree to predict central nervous system abnormalities. *Pediatrics.* 2002;109:61-67.
421. Iughetti L, Predieri B, Ferrari M, et al. Diagnosis of central precocious puberty: endocrine assessment. *J Pediatr Endocrinol Metab.* 2000;13(suppl 1):709-715.
422. Argyropoulou MI, Kiortsis DN. MRI of the hypothalamic-pituitary axis in children. *Pediatr Radiol.* 2005;35:1045-1055.
423. Klein KO, Barnes KM, Jones JV, et al. Increased final height in precocious puberty after long-term treatment with LHRH agonists: the National Institutes of Health experience. *J Clin Endocrinol Metab.* 2001;86:4711-4716.
424. Tato L, Savage MO, Antoniazzi F, et al. Optimal therapy of pubertal disorders in precocious/early puberty. *J Pediatr Endocrinol Metab.* 2001;14(suppl 2):985-995.
425. Laron Z, Kauli R. Experience with cyproterone acetate in the treatment of precocious puberty. *J Pediatr Endocrinol Metab.* 2000;13(suppl 1):805-810.
426. Feuillan P, Merke D, Leschek EW, et al. Use of aromatase inhibitors in precocious puberty. *Endocr Relat Cancer.* 1999;6:303-306.
427. Warren MP, Fried JL. Hypothalamic amenorrhea: the effects of environmental stresses on the reproductive system—a central effect of the central nervous system. *Endocrinol Metab Clin North Am.* 2001; 30:611-629.
428. Yen SS. Female hypogonadotropic hypogonadism: hypothalamic amenorrhea syndrome. *Endocrinol Metab Clin North Am.* 1993;22: 29-58.
429. Cannavo S, Curto L, Trimarchi F. Exercise-related female reproductive dysfunction. *J Endocrinol Invest.* 2001;24:823-832.
430. Moschos S, Chan JL, Mantzoros CS. Leptin and reproduction: a review. *Fertil Steril.* 2002;77:433-444.
431. Williams NI, Helmreich DL, Parfitt DB, et al. Evidence for a causal role of low energy availability in the induction of menstrual cycle disturbances during strenuous exercise training. *J Clin Endocrinol Metab.* 2001;86:5184-5193.
432. Hobart JA, Smucker DR. The female athlete triad. *Am Fam Physician.* 2000;61:3357-3364, 3367.
433. Goldstone AP. Prader-Willi syndrome: advances in genetics, pathophysiology and treatment. *Trends Endocrinol Metab.* 2004;15: 12-20.
434. Hackney AC. Endurance exercise training and reproductive endocrine dysfunction in men: alterations in the hypothalamic-pituitary-testicular axis. *Curr Pharm Des.* 2001;7:261-273.
435. Opstad K. Circadian rhythm of hormones is extinguished during prolonged physical stress, sleep and energy deficiency in young men. *Eur J Endocrinol.* 1994;131:56-66.
436. Abs R, Verhelst J, Maeyaert J, et al. Endocrine consequences of long-term intrathecal administration of opioids. *J Clin Endocrinol Metab.* 2000;85:2215-2222.
437. Vanhorebeek I, Van den Berghe G. The neuroendocrine response to critical illness is a dynamic process. *Crit Care Clin.* 2006;22: 1-15, v.
438. Biller BM, Luciano A, Crosignani PG, et al. Guidelines for the diagnosis and treatment of hyperprolactinemia. *J Reprod Med.* 1999;44: 1075-1084.
439. Meierkord H, Shorvon S, Lightman S, et al. Comparison of the effects of frontal and temporal lobe partial seizures on prolactin levels. *Arch Neurol.* 1992;49:225-230.
440. Molitch ME. Diagnosis and treatment of prolactinomas. *Adv Intern Med.* 1999;44:117-153.
441. Burman P, Ritzen EM, Lindgren AC. Endocrine dysfunction in Prader-Willi syndrome: a review with special reference to GH. *Endocr Rev.* 2001;22:787-799.
442. Gohlke BC, Khadilkar VV, Skuse D, et al. Recognition of children with psychosocial short stature: a spectrum of presentation. *J Pediatr Endocrinol Metab.* 1998;11:509-517.
443. Gilmour J, Skuse D. A case-comparison study of the characteristics of children with a short stature syndrome induced by stress (hyperphagic short stature) and a consecutive series of unaffected "stressed" children. *J Child Psychol Psychiatry.* 1999;40:969-978.
444. Albanese A, Hamill G, Jones J, et al. Reversibility of physiological growth hormone secretion in children with psychosocial dwarfism. *Clin Endocrinol (Oxf).* 1994;40:687-692.
445. Bercu BB, Diamond FB Jr. Growth hormone neurosecretory dysfunction. *Clin Endocrinol Metab.* 1986;15:537-590.
446. Lin TH, Kirkland RT, Sherman BM, et al. Growth hormone testing in short children and their response to growth hormone therapy. *J Pediatr.* 1989;115:57-63.
447. Attie KM. Genetic studies in idiopathic short stature. *Curr Opin Pediatr.* 2000;12:400-404.
448. Voss LD. Short normal stature and psychosocial disadvantage: a critical review of the evidence. *J Pediatr Endocrinol Metab.* 2001;14: 701-711.
449. Mehta A, Hindmarsh PC. The use of somatropin (recombinant growth hormone) in children of short stature. *Paediatr Drugs.* 2002;4: 37-47.
450. Poussaint TY, Barnes PD, Nichols K, et al. Diencephalic syndrome: clinical features and imaging findings. *AJNR Am J Neuroradiol.* 1997;18:1499-1505.
451. Gropman AL, Packer RJ, Nicholson HS, et al. Treatment of diencephalic syndrome with chemotherapy: growth, tumor response, and long term control. *Cancer.* 1998;83:166-172.
452. Ho KY, Veldhuis JD, Johnson ML, et al. Fasting enhances growth hormone secretion and amplifies the complex rhythms of growth hormone secretion in man. *J Clin Invest.* 1988;81:968-975.
453. Saeger W, Puchner MJ, Ludecke DK. Combined sellar gangliocytoma and pituitary adenoma in acromegaly or Cushing's disease: a report of 3 cases. *Virchows Arch.* 1994;425:93-99.
454. Posener JA, DeBattista C, Williams GH, et al. 24-Hour monitoring of cortisol and corticotropin secretion in psychotic and nonpsychotic major depression. *Arch Gen Psychiatry.* 2000;57:755-760.
455. Chrousos GP. The role of stress and the hypothalamic-pituitary-adrenal axis in the pathogenesis of the metabolic syndrome: neuro-endocrine and target tissue-related causes. *Int J Obes Relat Metab Disord.* 2000;24(Suppl 2):S50-S55.
456. Bjorntorp P, Rosmond R. The metabolic syndrome: a neuroendocrine disorder? *Br J Nutr.* 2000;83(suppl 1):S49-S57.
457. Wolff S, Adler R, Buskirk E, et al. A syndrome of periodic hypothalamic discharge. *Am J Med.* 1964;36:956-967.
458. Albright AL, Hadjipanayis CG, Lunsford LD, et al. Individualized treatment of pediatric craniopharyngiomas. *Childs Nerv Syst.* 2005; 21:649-654.

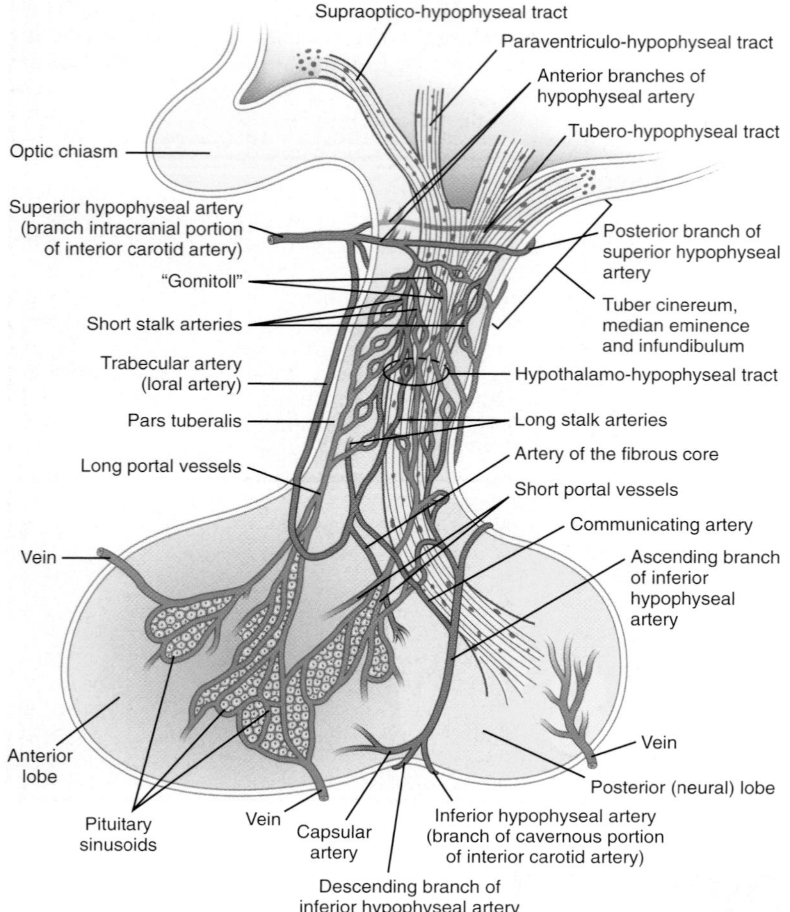

Figure 8-1 Schematic representation of the blood supply of the hypothalamus and pituitary. (Reproduced from Scheithauer BW. The hypothalamus and neurohypophysis. In: Kovacs K, Asa SL, eds. *Functional Endocrine Pathology*. Oxford, UK: Blackwell Scientific; 1991.)

turcica and is overlain by the dural diaphragma sella, through which the stalk connects to the median eminence of the hypothalamus. The adult pituitary weighs approximately 600 mg (range, 400 to 900 mg) and measures approximately 13 mm in the longest transverse diameter, 6 to 9 mm in vertical height, and about 9 mm anteroposteriorly. Structural variation may occur in multiparous women, and gland volume also changes with the menstrual cycle. During pregnancy, size may be increased in any dimension, and pituitary weight increases up to 1 g. Pituitary hypertrophy without evidence for the presence of an adenoma was described in 7 eugonadal women with pituitary height greater than 9 mm and a convex upper gland boundary observed on magnetic resonance imaging (MRI).[6]

The sella turcica, located at the base of the skull, forms the thin, bony roof of the sphenoid sinus. The lateral walls are made up of bony and dural tissue and surround the cavernous sinuses, which are traversed by the third, fourth, and sixth cranial nerves and the internal carotid arteries. The cavernous sinus contents are vulnerable to intrasellar expansion. The dural roofing protects the gland from compression by fluctuant cerebrospinal fluid pressure. The optic chiasm, located anterior to the pituitary stalk, is directly above the diaphragma sella. The optic tracts and central structures are vulnerable to pressure effects from an expanding pituitary mass, which is likely to follow the path of least tissue resistance by lifting the diaphragma sella. The intimate relationship between the pituitary and the chiasm is borne out in optic chiasmic hypoplasia associated with developmental pituitary dysfunction, seen in patients with septo-optic dysplasia.

The posterior pituitary gland, in contrast to the anterior pituitary, is directly innervated by supraopticohypophyseal and tuberohypophyseal nerve tracts of the posterior stalk. Hypothalamic neuronal lesions, stalk disruption, or direct systemically derived metastases are often associated with attenuated secretion of vasopressin (diabetes insipidus) or oxytocin or both.

The hypothalamus contains nerve cell bodies that synthesize hypophysiotropic releasing and inhibiting hormones as well as the neurohypophyseal hormones of the posterior pituitary (vasopressin and oxytocin). Five distinct hormone-secreting cell types are present in the mature anterior pituitary gland:

- Corticotroph cells express pro-opiomelanocortin (POMC) peptides including adrenocorticotropic hormone (ACTH, also called *corticotropin*).
- Somatotroph cells express growth hormone (GH, also called *somatotropin*).
- Thyrotroph cells express the common glycoprotein α-subunit (αGSU) and the specific β-subunit of thyroid-stimulating hormone (TSH, also called *thyrotropin*).
- Gonadotrophs express the α- and β-subunits for both follicle-stimulating hormone (FSH) and luteinizing hormone (LH).
- Lactotrophs expresses prolactin (PRL).

Each cell type is under highly specific signal controls that regulate its differentiated gene expression.

Pituitary Blood Supply

The pituitary gland enjoys an abundant blood supply derived from several sources (see Fig. 8-1). The superior hypophyseal arteries branch from the internal carotid arteries to supply the hypothalamus, where they form a capillary network in the median eminence, external to the blood-brain barrier. The long and short hypophyseal portal vessels originate, respectively, from infundibular plexuses and from the pituitary stalk. These vessels form the hypophyseal-portal circulation, the predominant blood supply to the anterior pituitary gland. They deliver hypothalamic releasing and inhibiting hormones to the trophic hormone–producing cells of the adenohypophysis without significant systemic dilution, allowing the pituitary cells to be sensitively regulated by timed hypothalamic hormone secretion. Vascular transport of hypothalamic hormones is also locally regulated by a contractile internal capillary plexus (*gomitoli*) derived from stalk branches of the superior hypophysial arteries.[7]

Retrograde blood flow toward the median eminence also occurs, facilitating bidirectional functional hypothalamic-pituitary interactions.[8] Systemic arterial blood supply is maintained by inferior hypophysial arterial branches that predominantly supply the posterior pituitary. Disruption of stalk integrity may lead to compromised pituitary portal blood flow, depriving the anterior pituitary cells of hypothalamic hormone access.

Pituitary Development

The pituitary gland arises from within the rostral neural plate. Rathke's pouch, a primitive ectodermal invagination anterior to the roof of the oral cavity, is formed by the 4th or 5th week of gestation[9] and gives rise to the anterior pituitary gland (Fig. 8-2).[10,11] The pouch is directly connected to the stalk and hypothalamic infundibulum and ultimately becomes distinct from the oral cavity and nasopharynx. Rathke's pouch proliferates toward the third ventricle, where it fuses with the diverticulum and subsequently obliterates its lumen, which may persist as Rathke's cleft. The anterior lobe is formed from Rathke's pouch, whereas the diverticulum gives rise to the adjacent posterior lobe. Remnants of pituitary tissue may persist in the nasopharyngeal midline and may rarely give rise to functional ectopic hormone-secreting tumors in the nasopharynx. The neurohypophysis arises from neural ectoderm associated with third ventricle development.[12]

Functional development of the anterior pituitary cell types involves complex spatiotemporal regulation of cell lineage–specific transcription factors expressed in pluripotential pituitary stem cells and dynamic gradients of locally acting soluble factors.[13-16] Critical neuroectodermal signals for organizing the dorsal gradient of pituitary morphogenesis include infundibular bone morphogenetic protein 4 (BMP4), which is required for initial pouch invagination[11]; fibroblast growth factor 8 (FGF8), Wnt5, and Wnt4. Subsequent ventral developmental patterning and transcription factor expression are determined by spatial and graded expression of factors including BMP2 and sonic hedgehog protein (Shh), which appears to be critical for directing early patterns of cell proliferation.[17]

The human fetal Rathke's pouch is evident at 3 weeks of gestation, and the pituitary grows rapidly in utero. By 7 weeks, the anterior pituitary vasculature begins to develop, and by 20 weeks, the entire hypophyseal portal system is already established. The anterior pituitary undergoes major cellular differentiation during the first 12 weeks, by which time all of the major secretory cell compartments are structurally and functionally intact, except for lactotrophs. Totipotential pituitary stem cells give rise to acidophilic (somatotroph, and lactotroph) and basophilic (corticotroph, thyrotroph, and gonadotroph) differentiated pituitary cell types, which appear at clearly demarcated developmental stages.

At 6 weeks, corticotroph cells are morphologically identifiable, and immunoreactive ACTH is detectable by 7 weeks. At 8 weeks, somatotroph cells are evident with abundant immunoreactive cytoplasmic GH expression. Glycoprotein hormone–secreting cells express αGSU, and at 12 weeks, differentiated thyrotrophs and gonadotrophs express immunoreactive β-subunits for TSH and for LH and FSH, respectively. In females, LH- and FSH-expressing gonadotrophs are equally distributed, whereas in the male fetus, LH-expressing gonadotrophs predominate.[18] Fully differentiated PRL-expressing lactotrophs become evident late in gestation (after 24 weeks). Before that time, immunoreactive PRL is detectable only in mixed mammosomatotrophs, which also express GH, reflecting the common genetic origin of these two hormones.[19]

Pituitary Transcription Factors

Determination of anterior pituitary cell type lineages results from a temporally regulated cascade of homeodomain transcription factors.[13] Although most pituitary developmental information has been acquired from murine models,[20] histologic and pathogenetic observations in human subjects largely corroborate these developmental mechanisms (see Fig. 8-2). Early cell differentiation requires intracellular Rpx (*HESX1*) and Ptx (*PITX*) expression. Rathke's pouch expresses several transcription factors of the LIM homeodomain family, including Lhx3, Lhx4, and IsI-1,[20] which are early determinants of functional pituitary development and are required for progenitor cell survival and proliferation. Ptx1 is expressed in the oral ectoderm, and subsequently in all pituitary cell types, particularly those arising ventrally.[21] Rieger's syndrome, which is characterized by defective eye, tooth, umbilical cord, and pituitary development, is caused by mutations in Ptx2.[22]

Ptx behaves as a universal pituitary regulator and activates transcription of αGSU, POMC, LHβ (Ptx1), and GH (Ptx2). Lhx3 determines GH-, PRL-, and TSH-cell differentiation. PROP1 behaves as a prerequisite for POU1F1, which activates GH, PRL, TSH, and growth hormone–releasing hormone (GHRH) receptor transcription. TSH and gonadotropin-expressing cells share αGSU expression under developmental control of *GATA2*.[23] FOXL2, a forkhead transcription factor, regulates differentiation of cell types expressing the αGSU, including gonadotrophs and thyrotrophs.[24] In contrast, activated *Notch2* acts to delay murine gonadotroph differentiation,[25] underscoring the role of Notch signaling pathways, including *Hesx1* in the developmental cascade. Diversity of pituitary cell type determination is mediated by binary Wnt/β-catenin signaling that leads to induction of PROP1 and suppression of *Hesx1*.[26] These specific anterior pituitary transcription factors participate in a highly orchestrated cascade that results in commitment of the five differentiated cell types (see Fig. 8-4). The major proximal determinant of pituitary cell lineage is PROP1 expression, which determines subsequent development of POU1F1-dependent and gonadotroph cell lineages.[27,28]

POU1F1 encodes a POU-homeodomain transcription factor (also called Pit-1) that determines development and appropriate temporal and spatial expression of cells

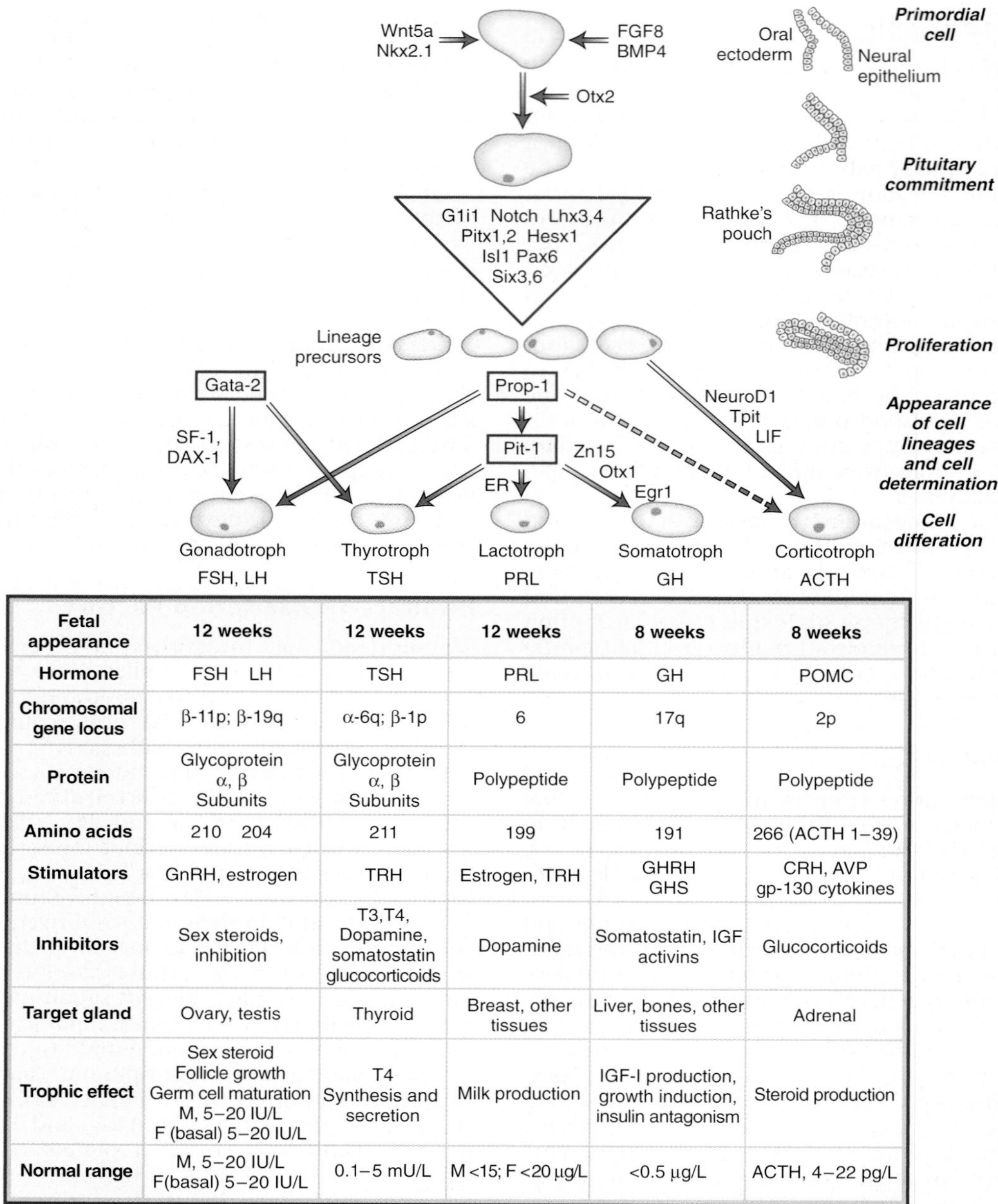

Fetal appearance	12 weeks	12 weeks	12 weeks	8 weeks	8 weeks
Hormone	FSH LH	TSH	PRL	GH	POMC
Chromosomal gene locus	β-11p; β-19q	α-6q; β-1p	6	17q	2p
Protein	Glycoprotein α, β Subunits	Glycoprotein α, β Subunits	Polypeptide	Polypeptide	Polypeptide
Amino acids	210 204	211	199	191	266 (ACTH 1–39)
Stimulators	GnRH, estrogen	TRH	Estrogen, TRH	GHRH GHS	CRH, AVP gp-130 cytokines
Inhibitors	Sex steroids, inhibition	T3,T4, Dopamine, somatostatin glucocorticoids	Dopamine	Somatostatin, IGF activins	Glucocorticoids
Target gland	Ovary, testis	Thyroid	Breast, other tissues	Liver, bones, other tissues	Adrenal
Trophic effect	Sex steroid Follicle growth Germ cell maturation M, 5–20 IU/L F (basal) 5–20 IU/L	T4 Synthesis and secretion	Milk production	IGF-I production, growth induction, insulin antagonism	Steroid production
Normal range	M, 5–20 IU/L F(basal) 5–20 IU/L	0.1–5 mU/L	M <15; F <20 μg/L	<0.5 μg/L	ACTH, 4–22 pg/L

Figure 8-2 Model for development of the human anterior pituitary gland and cell lineage determination by a cascade of transcription factors. Trophic cells are depicted with transcription factors known to determine cell-specific human or murine gene expression. ACTH, corticotropin; AVP, arginine vasopressin; CRH, corticotropin-releasing hormone; ER, estrogen receptor; F, female; FSH, follicle-stimulating hormone; GH, growth hormone; GHRH, growth hormone–releasing hormone; GHS, growth hormone secretagogue; GnRH, gonadotropin-releasing hormone; IGF, insulin-like growth factor; LH, luteinizing hormone; M, male; POMC, pro-opiomelanocortin; PRL, prolactin; T_3, triiodothyronine; T_4, thyroxine; TRH, thyrotropin-releasing hormone; TSH, thyrotropin. (Adapted from Shimon I, Melmed S. Anterior Pituitary Hormones. In: Conn P, Melmed S, eds. *Scientific Basis of Endocrinology.* Totowa, NJ: Humana Press, 1996; and Amselem S. Perspectives on the molecular basis of developmental defects in the human pituitary region. In Rappaport R, Amselem S, eds. *Hypothalamic-Pituitary Development.* Basel, Switzerland: Karger; 2001; and Dasen JS, O'Connell SM, Flynn SE, et al. Reciprocal interactions of Pit1 and GATA2 mediate signaling gradient–induced determination of pituitary cell types. *Cell.* 1999;97:587-598.)

committed to GH, PRL, TSH, and GHRH receptor expression. POU1F1 binds to specific DNA motifs to activate and regulate somatotroph, lactotroph, and thyrotroph development and mature secretory function. Signal-dependent coactivating factors also cooperate with POU1F1 to determine specific hormone expression. For example, in POU1F1-containing cells, high estrogen receptor levels induce a commitment to express PRL, whereas thyrotroph embryonic factor (TEF) favors TSH expression. Selective pituitary cell-type specificity is also perpetuated by binding of POU1F1 to its own DNA regulatory elements as well as those contained within the GH, PRL, and TSH genes. Steroidogenic factor (SF1) and DAX1 (encoded by *NROB1*) determine subsequent gonadotroph development.[29,30] Corticotroph cell commitment occurs earliest during fetal development but is independent of POU1F1-determined lineages. TPIT protein (encoded by *TBX19*) is a prerequisite for POMC expression.[31] Hereditary mutations arising within these transcription factors may result in isolated or combined pituitary hormone failure syndromes (discussed later).[32]

Pituitary Stem Cells

The adult pituitary gland exhibits plastic and regenerative trophic properties that allow maintenance of homeostatic functions.[33] This characteristic is exemplified by pituitary lactotroph expansion during pregnancy and by pituitary trophic hormone cell hyperplasia occurring after target organ ablation. Mechanisms underlying adult pituitary cell renewal and expansion are as yet unclear and may include intrinsic pituitary transdifferentiation, differentiation of previously uncommitted "null" cells, or expansion of already differentiated cells.

Several lines of evidence support the existence of cells with stem or progenitor characteristics in the adult pituitary gland.[34-36] Pituitary progenitor cells exhibit several characteristics of a stem cell phenotype, including an undifferentiated gene profile, clonality, and expression of known stem cell markers such as Scal and CD133. Other markers, including Notch, Wnt, and Shh, are essential transcription factors for cell-type determination and expansion of pituitary cell lineages. SOX2-expressing pituitary progenitor cells exhibit properties for multipotent pituitary cell differentiation, and a population of nestin-expressing murine pituitary cells was found to fulfill criteria consistent with organ-specific multipotent stem cells.[36] These cells form differentiated pituitary-expressing progeny and contribute to a distinct adult pituitary stem cell population distinct from embryonic precursor cells. Factors regulating expansion of these putative adult pituitary stem cells remain to be determined.

Pituitary Control

Three levels of control regulate anterior pituitary hormone secretion (Fig. 8-3). Hypothalamic control is mediated by adenohypophysiotropic hormones secreted into the portal system that impinge directly on anterior pituitary cell surface receptors. G protein–linked cell surface membrane binding sites are highly selective and specific for each of the hypothalamic hormones; they elicit positive or negative signals that mediate pituitary hormone gene transcription and secretion. Peripheral hormones also participate in mediation of pituitary cell function, predominantly through negative feedback regulation of trophic hormones by their respective target hormones. Intrapituitary paracrine and autocrine soluble growth factors and cytokines act to locally regulate neighboring cell development and function.

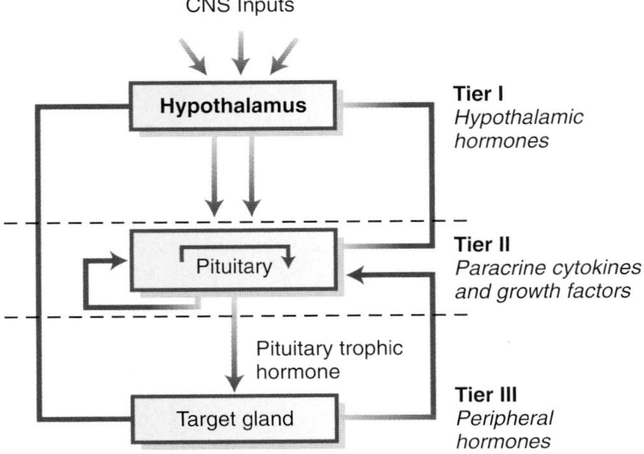

Figure 8-3 Model for regulation of anterior pituitary hormone secretion by three tiers of control. Hypothalamic hormones traverse the portal system and impinge directly on their respective target cells. Intrapituitary cytokines and growth factors regulate tropic cell function by paracrine (and autocrine) control. Peripheral hormones exert negative feedback inhibition of respective pituitary trophic hormone synthesis and secretion. CNS, central nervous system. (Reproduced from Ray D, Melmed S. Pituitary cytokine and growth factor expression and action. *Endocr Rev.* 1997;18:206-228.)

The net result of these three tiers of complex intracellular signals is the controlled pulsatile secretion of the six pituitary trophic hormones (i.e., ACTH, GH, PRL, TSH, FSH, and LH) through the cavernous sinus, the petrosal veins, and, ultimately, the systemic circulation via the superior vena cava (Fig. 8-4). Temporal and quantitative control of pituitary hormone secretion is critical for physiologic integration of peripheral hormonal systems such as the menstrual cycle, which relies on complex and precisely regulated pulse control.

PHYSIOLOGY AND DISORDERS OF PITUITARY HORMONE AXES

Prolactin

Physiology

Until 1970, the identification of PRL in humans was elusive because human GH is highly lactogenic and active in bioassays used to isolate and measure PRL[37] and because GH is present in human pituitary glands in much higher concentrations (5 to 10 mg) than PRL (approximately 100 μg).[38] To distinguish human PRL from GH, lactogenic activity was neutralized with GH antiserum; sera from postpartum women and patients with galactorrhea had high lactogenic activity in the presence of GH antibodies.[39,40] Human PRL, bioassayed by stimulation of pregnant mouse mammary milk production,[41] was elevated in patients with nonpuerperal galactorrhea due to pituitary tumors, exposure to phenothiazines, or withdrawal from oral contraceptives. Purification and isolation of PRL by Friesen and development of a specific radioimmunoassay (RIA) underscored the utility of PRL measurements in understanding human disease.[42,43]

Lactotroph Cells. Lactotroph cells comprise 15% to 25% of functioning anterior pituitary cells (Fig. 8-5). Their absolute number does not change with age, but lactotroph hyperplasia occurs during pregnancy and lactation[44] and resolves within several months after delivery (Fig. 8-6). Most PRL-expressing cells appear to arise from GH-producing cells. Ablation of somatotrophs by expression of GH–diphtheria toxin and GH–thymidine kinase fusion genes inserted into the germline of transgenic mice eliminates most lactotrophs, suggesting that the majority of PRL-producing cells arise from postmitotic somatotrophs.[45] Two cell forms expressing the PRL gene are the large, polyhedral cells found throughout the gland and the smaller, angulated or elongated cells clustered mainly in the lateral wings and median wedge. Large PRL secretory granules (250 to 800 nm) are present in the evenly distributed cells, whereas the laterally localized cells are sparsely populated by smaller granules (200 to 350 nm) (Fig. 8-7). Occasional mammosomatotroph cells may also cosecrete both PRL and GH, often storing both hormones within the same

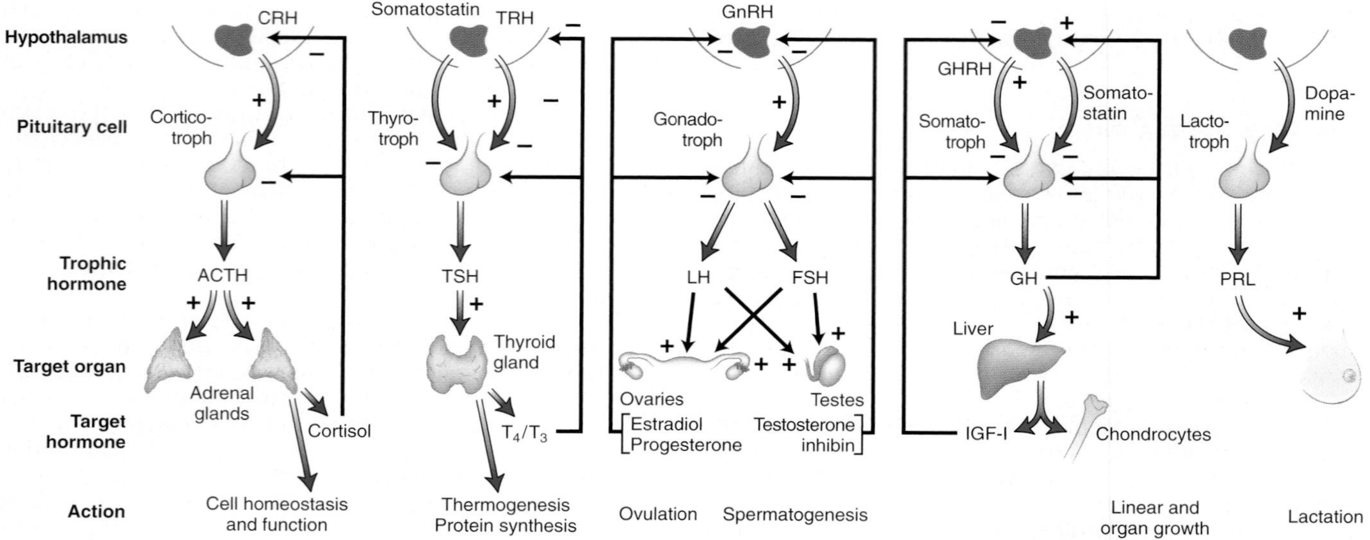

Figure 8-4 Control of hypothalamic-pituitary target organ axes. ACTH, adrenocorticotropic hormone; CRH, corticotropin-releasing hormone; FSH, follicle-stimulating hormone; GH, growth hormone; GHRH, growth hormone–releasing hormone; GnRH, gonadotropin-releasing hormone; IGF, insulin-like growth factor; LH, luteinizing hormone; PFL, prolactin; T_3, triiodothyronine; T_4, thyroxine; TRH, thyrotropin-releasing hormone; TSH, thyroid-stimulating hormone. (Adapted from Melmed S. Mechanisms for pituitary tumorigenesis: the plastic pituitary. *J Clin Invest.* 2003;112:1603-1618.)

granule (Fig. 8-8). In animal models, lactotroph cell function is heterogeneous. For example, responsiveness of dopamine or thyrotropin-releasing hormone (TRH) and shifting proportions of PRL- versus GH-secreting cells may depend on cell location within the pituitary and on the surrounding hormonal milieu, especially that of estrogen.[46]

Prolactin Structure. The human PRL gene, located on chromosome 6,[47] apparently arose from a single common ancestral gene giving rise to the relatively homologous PRL, GH, and placental lactogen-related proteins.[48] Several factors influence PRL gene expression, including estrogen, dopamine, TRH, and thyroid hormones.[49] PRL is

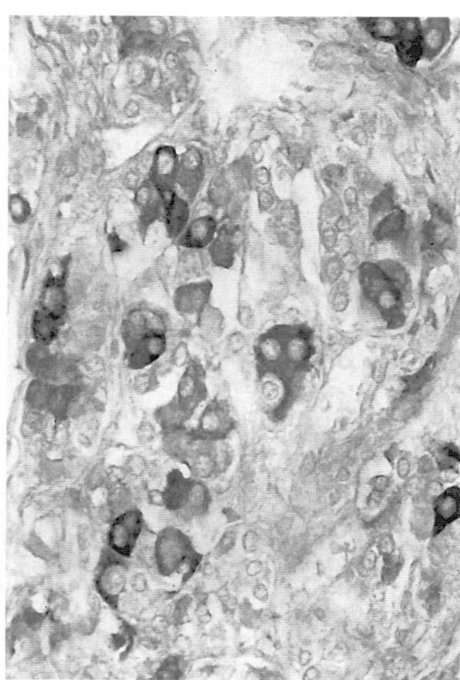

Figure 8-5 Lactotroph cell. Normal prolactin-secreting cells express strong positivity for prolactin within the cytoplasm of polyhedral cells with elongated cell processes. Some processes surround adjacent immunonegative cells that correspond to gonadotrophs. (From Asa SL. Tumors of the pituitary gland. In: Rosai J, ed. *Atlas of Tumor Pathology*, Series III, Fascicle 22. Washington, DC: Armed Forces Institute of Pathology, 1997:15.)

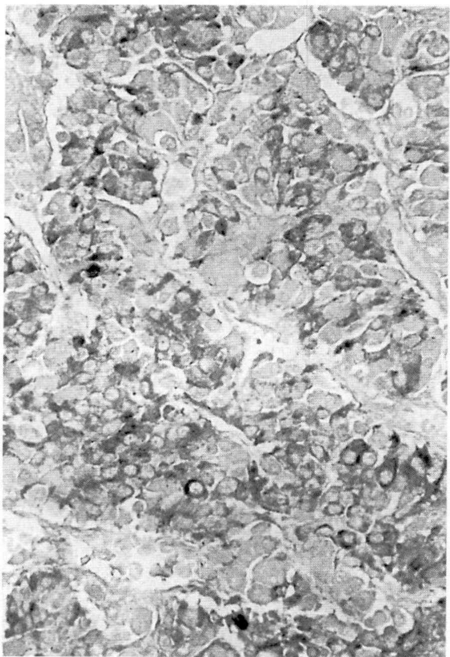

Figure 8-6 Prolactin cell hyperplasia. In the third trimester of pregnancy, hyperplasia of prolactin cells occurs. Cells containing immunoreactive prolactin comprise almost 50% of the cell population of the gland. (From Asa SL. Tumors of the pituitary gland. In: Rosai J, ed. *Atlas of Tumor Pathology*, Series III, Fascicle 22. Washington, DC: Armed Forces Institute of Pathology, 1997:15.)

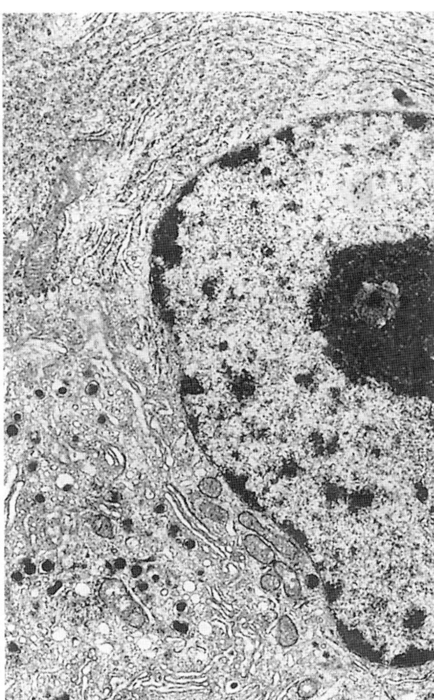

Figure 8-7 Electron micrograph of a normal lactotroph shows a well-developed rough endoplasmic reticulum that forms concentric whorls. A prominent Golgi complex is seen in a juxtanuclear location and harbors forming pleomorphic secretory granules. The cytoplasm is otherwise sparsely granulated. (From Asa SL. Tumors of the pituitary gland. In: Rosai J, ed. *Atlas of Tumor Pathology*, Series III, Fascicle 22. Washington, DC: Armed Forces Institute of Pathology, 1997:16.)

a 199-amino-acid polypeptide containing three intramolecular disulfide bonds. It circulates in blood in various sizes, including the 23-kd monomeric PRL ("little prolactin"), 48- to 56-kd dimeric PRL ("big prolactin"), and polymeric forms larger than 100 kd ("big, big prolactin").[50-52] The monomeric form is the most bioactive PRL. In response to TRH, the proportion of the more active monomeric form increases.

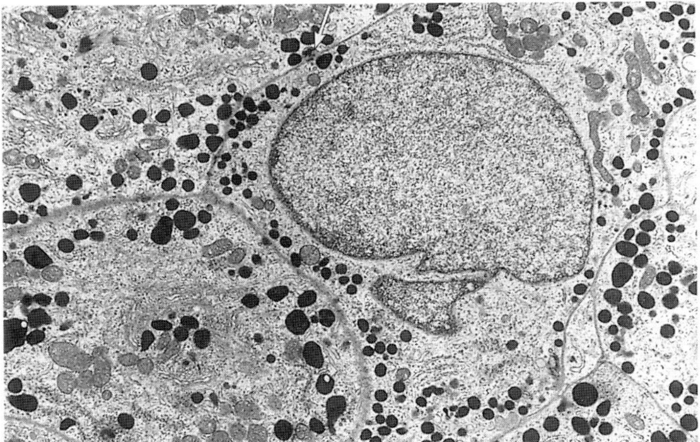

Figure 8-8 Normal mammosomatotroph. Occasional cells resembling densely granulated somatotrophs exhibit atypical features consistent with prolactin secretion: the secretory granules are highly pleomorphic, and there is misplaced exocytosis (i.e., extrusion of secretory material along the lateral cell border), as indicated by the *arrow*. (From Asa SL. Tumors of the Pituitary Gland. In: Rosai J, ed. *Atlas of Tumor Pathology*, Series III, Fascicle 22. Washington, DC: Armed Forces Institute of Pathology, 1997:17.)

A glycosylated form of PRL identified in pituitary extracts is less biologically active than "little prolactin."[53] Monomeric PRL is cleaved into 8- and 16-kd forms,[54] and the 16-kd variant is antiangiogenic.[55,56] A circulating PRL-binding protein corresponds to the extracellular domain of the PRL receptor.[57]

Regulation

PRL secretion is under the inhibitory control of dopamine, which is largely produced by the tuberoinfundibular cells and the hypothalamic tuberohypophyseal dopaminergic system.[58,59] Dopamine reaches the lactotrophs via the hypothalamic pituitary portal system and inhibits PRL secretion by binding to the type 2 dopamine (D_2) receptors on pituitary lactotrophs.[60] PRL participates in negative feedback to control its release by increasing tyrosine hydroxylase activity in the tuberoinfundibular neurons.[59] In PRL-deficient animals, dopamine is decreased in the median eminence.[61] Mice lacking the D_2 receptor develop hyperprolactinemia and lactotroph proliferation.[60] Factors other than dopamine inhibit PRL secretion, including endothelin-1 and transforming growth factor-β1, which act as paracrine PRL inhibitors,[62,63] and calcitonin, which may be derived from the hypothalamus.[64]

Several substances act as PRL-releasing factors. Basic FGF and epidermal growth factor induce PRL synthesis and secretion. Vasoactive intestinal polypeptide (VIP) stimulates PRL synthesis via cyclic adenosine monophosphate (cAMP).[65] A hypothalamic prolactin-releasing peptide (PrRP) acts through a specific receptor[66] in normal pituitary glands and in a subset of PRL-secreting tumors.[67] Oxytocin and pituitary adenylate cyclase–activating protein also release PRL.[59] TRH stimulates PRL[68] but probably does not play an important role in PRL secretion. Estrogen stimulates PRL gene transcription and secretion,[69] explaining why women have higher PRL levels and why cycling women have a higher PRL pulse frequency than do postmenopausal women and men.[70] Galanin is synthesized in both the pituitary and the hypothalamus and may act as a PRL-releasing factor.[71] The physiologic roles of γ-aminobutyric acid (GABA), neurotensin, substance P, bombesin, and cholecystokinin in regulating human PRL secretion are unresolved.[59]

Serotonin may be additive with VIP in releasing PRL, and infusion of 5-hydroxytryptophan (5-HTP), a serotonin precursor, elicits PRL release. Nocturnal PRL secretion is attenuated by cyproheptadine. Serotonin may mediate nocturnal PRL secretion and may also participate with VIP in the suckling reflex. Opiates acutely induce PRL release, although naloxone does not consistently suppress PRL levels. GHRH, when administered at high doses, moderately induces PRL secretion, and patients harboring ectopic GHRH-producing tumors have mild to moderate hyperprolactinemia. GnRH also stimulates PRL in women, especially during the periovulatory menstrual phase. Although posterior pituitary hormones have been shown to regulate rat PRL secretion,[72] the roles of vasopressin, oxytocin, and other neurohypophyseal molecules in regulating human PRL remain unresolved. Histamine may act on the hypothalamus to regulate PRL, and H_2 blockers induce PRL secretion.

A short-loop feedback of PRL has been proposed, and transgenic mice with deleted PRL have decreased hypothalamic dopamine content.[73] In humans, the existence of this regulatory loop has been difficult to prove.

Prolactin Secretion

The calculated production rate of PRL ranges from 200 to 536 μg/day per square meter of body surface area, and the metabolic clearance rate ranges from 40 to 71 mL/min per m^2.[74] PRL is cleared rapidly, with a calculated disappearance half-life ranging from 26 to 47 minutes. PRL secretion occurs episodically; between 4 and 14 secretory pulses occur over 24 hours, each lasting between 67 and 76 minutes.[75,76] PRL is secreted episodically during the day, with highest levels achieved during sleep and lowest occurring between 10 a.m. and noon.[77] The nocturnal elevation is sleep entrained; a temporal relationship exists between rapid-eye-movement (REM) and non-REM sleep cycles,[78] and PRL may cause periods of REM. PRL levels fall with age in both men and women. In older men, less PRL is produced with each secretory burst than in younger men.[79] Likewise, postmenopausal women have lower mean serum PRL levels and lower PRL pulse frequency than do premenopausal women or men, suggesting a stimulatory effect of estrogen on both parameters.[70]

Prolactin Action

The prolactin receptor gene (*PRLR*) is a member of the cytokine receptor superfamily,[80] localizes to chromosome 5p13, and comprises 10 exons. The receptor gene has two 5′ promoters that direct transcription of a 598-amino-acid peptide[81] comprising an extracellular domain, a hydrophobic transmembrane domain, and an intracytoplasmic region homologous to the GH receptor (Fig. 8-9).[82] PRLR dimerization occurs with or without ligand binding and results ultimately in phosphorylation of intracellular JAK/STAT molecules. Two binding sites, encompassing helices 1 and 4 and helices 1 and 3 on the PRL molecule, are critical for formation of the trimeric ligand-receptor complex and subsequent signaling.[83-85] PRLR induces protein tyrosine phosphorylation and activation of JAK2 kinase and signal transducing activators of transcription proteins (STATs) 1 through 5.[86,87] STAT5 phosphorylation mediates transcriptional activation of the β-casein gene.[88]

PRLRs are expressed in breast, pituitary, liver, adrenal cortex, kidneys, prostate, ovary, testes, intestine, epidermis, pancreatic islets, lung, myocardium, brain and lymphocytes. Estrogen also induces liver PRLR expression.[83] Regulation of milk production occurs via a cascade of intracellular events, and homozygous mice in which the PRLR has been inactivated are infertile.[83] A gain-of-function mutation conferring constitutive activity of the PRLR is present in a subset of patients with multiple breast fibroadenomas.[89] PRLR receptor antagonists have been developed for targeting the receptor in PRL-sensitive disturbances, including resistant prolactinomas and breast and prostate tumors.[85,90]

Function of Prolactin. PRL is essential for human species survival, because it is required for milk production during pregnancy and lactation. Additional biologic functions ascribed to PRL include reproductive and metabolic effects, mammary development, pigeon crop sac activity, freshwater survival, melanin synthesis, water-seeking behavior of newts, molting, and parental behavior.[91] Although PRL and its receptor are clearly crucial in lower animals,[92] the impact of PRL on maternal behavior in humans has not been fully delineated.

Mammary Gland Development and Lactation

Puberty. PRL is not essential for pubertal mammary development, which appears to require GH, the action of which is mediated by insulin-like growth factor 1 (IGF1).[93-95] At birth, the rodent mammary gland consists of a fat pad with small areas of ductal anlagen that differentiate into pubertal mammary glandular elements under the influence of estrogen, GH, and IGF1. At puberty, a surge of

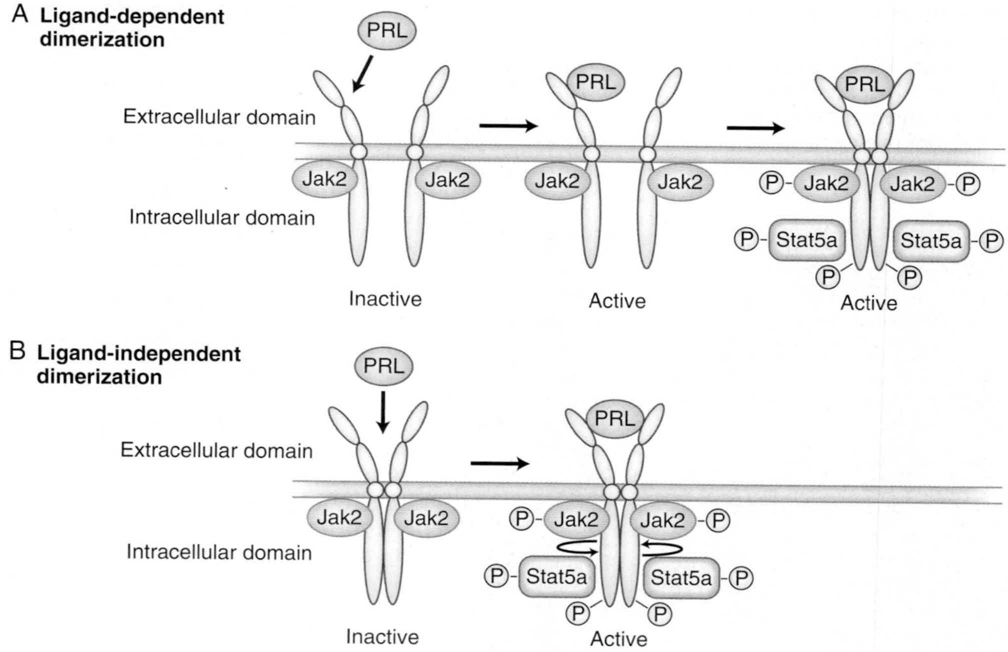

Figure 8-9 Ligand-dependent and -independent dimerization of the prolactin (PRL) receptor (PRLr). **A,** Ligand-dependent dimerization model. PRLr is in monomeric form at the cell membrane. One molecule of PRL first binds to one PRLr monomer via binding site 1, and this 1:1 complex then recruits the second PRLr via binding site 2. Dimerization of the two PRLrs leads to activating changes in the intracellular domain, resulting in PRL signal transduction, such as phosphorylation (P) of the Jak2 kinase, phosphorylation of the PRLr, and recruitment and phosphorylation of Stat5a. **B,** Ligand-independent model. PRLr exists in dimeric form at the cell membrane in the absence of ligand. The receptors are held in an inactive form until binding of PRL to this preformed complex induces activating changes in the intracellular domain, leading to phosphorylation of the Jak2 kinase, phosphorylation of the PRLr, and recruitment and phosphorylation of Stat5a. (From Clevenger C, Gadd SL, Zheng J. New mechanisms for PRLr action in breast cancer. *Trends Endocrinol Metab.* 2009;20:223.)

estrogen begins the process. Terminal end buds form and lead the process of mammary development by branching and extending into the substance of the mammary fat pad, leaving in their wake a network of ducts that virtually fill the mouse mammary fat pad.[96,97] GH acts on the mammary stromal compartment to produce IGF1, which, in turn, stimulates formation of the terminal end buds and ducts in synergy with estrogen.[95,98] Parathyroid hormone–related protein is essential for fetal mammary development,[99] and epidermal growth factor is essential for pubertal mammary development.[100] Progesterone, possibly in association with GH and PRL, causes formation of lobular "decorations" along ducts, which are precursors to true glands; progestins have similar effects.[101] Pubertal mammary development begins in girls between the ages of 8 and 13 (see Chapter 23). Once fully developed, the pubertal mammary gland remains quiescent until pregnancy, although cyclic changes do occur during the menstrual cycle.

In pregnancy, alveolar elements proliferate and begin to produce milk proteins and colostrum. At 3 to 4 weeks of gestation, terminal ductal sprouting occurs, followed by lobular-alveolar formation, and true alveoli form at the end of the first trimester. Glandular elements proliferate further, and secretory products appear in the alveolar lumina. During the third trimester, fat droplets are seen within alveolar cells, and the glands fill with colostrum.[102] A combination of estrogen, PRL, progesterone, and possibly IGF1 and placental hormones are largely responsible for this phase of mammary development.[103] In the absence of PRL, formation of alveolar structures is impaired, as was demonstrated in mice with targeted disruption of the PRL gene.[60] Likewise, women with isolated PRL deficiency are unable to lactate.[104]

Alveolar formation and milk production also require progesterone, and lobular-alveolar formation does not occur in mice lacking the progesterone receptor.[105] Only a minority of women have expressible milk during pregnancy, most likely due to inhibitory effects of estradiol[106] and progesterone[107] on PRL-induced milk production. Hormone perturbations during pregnancy also act on the fetal mammary gland, causing prominent neonatal nipples and secretion of "witch's milk."

Lactation. Mechanisms of milk production are similar in all mammals, but milk composition differs.[108] Active lactation is due in part to attenuation of estrogen and progesterone levels and elevation of PRL levels after delivery. Suckling increases milk production after parturition, and suckling is essential for continued lactation because of its distal effect on pituitary hormone production and because it empties the mammary gland of milk.[109] Milk accumulation further inhibits milk synthesis, explaining why a certain level of nursing activity is necessary for successful breast-feeding. In the absence of suckling, PRL concentrations, which rise throughout gestation, return to normal by 7 days after delivery.[110] Whereas PRL is essential for milk production, the milk yield does not closely correlate with serum PRL levels.[111]

Suckling also stimulates release of oxytocin from the posterior pituitary. In contrast to PRL, oxytocin responses to suckling do not decline as nursing continues for up to 6 months. Mothers who breast-fed exclusively had mean stimulated oxytocin levels significantly higher during late versus early lactation.[112] Oxytocin induces myoepithelial cell contraction, thereby causing milk ejection.[113] Oxytocin also has important effects on alveolar proliferation.[114] Mice that are deficient in oxytocin are unable to nurse their young, and oxytocin replacement permits these dams to nurse.

Lactational Amenorrhea. Lactational amenorrhea results in secondary infertility, and this natural form of contraception depends on the frequency and duration of breast-feeding. Infants of Kung hunter-gatherer women are suckled approximately four times per hour and at will during the night; these women bear a mean of 4.7 children during their reproductive years.[115] In contrast, the Hutterites of North America bear a mean of 10.6 children during their lifetimes, presumably because they nurse according to a rigid schedule, use supplemental feedings, and wean at 1 year. In Edinburgh, resumption of anovulatory menses occurs within 28 weeks after delivery, and the first ovulation occurs at a mean of 34 weeks due to persistently abnormal LH pulsatile secretion.[116]

Immune Function. Previously, evidence had indicated that PRL stimulates immune responsiveness,[117] and PRL was shown to stimulate immune cell functions in immunosuppressed mice.[118] However, more recent evidence[119] indicates that PRL may not be important for immune function, because innate immunity is not altered in mice that lack either the PRLR (*PRLR*$^{-/-}$) or the PRL gene (*PRL*$^{-/-}$).[60,120,121]

Reproductive Function. In mice with disrupted PRLR expression, both ovulation and the number of primary follicles are reduced.[83] These findings underscore the luteotrophic function of PRL but do not explain the suppressed gonadal function observed in patients with hyperprolactinemia,[122] which include short luteal phase, reduced central FSH and LH levels, decreased granulosa cells, decreased estradiol levels, and, ultimately, amenorrhea (Fig. 8-10). Clearly, attenuated gonadotropin secretion is

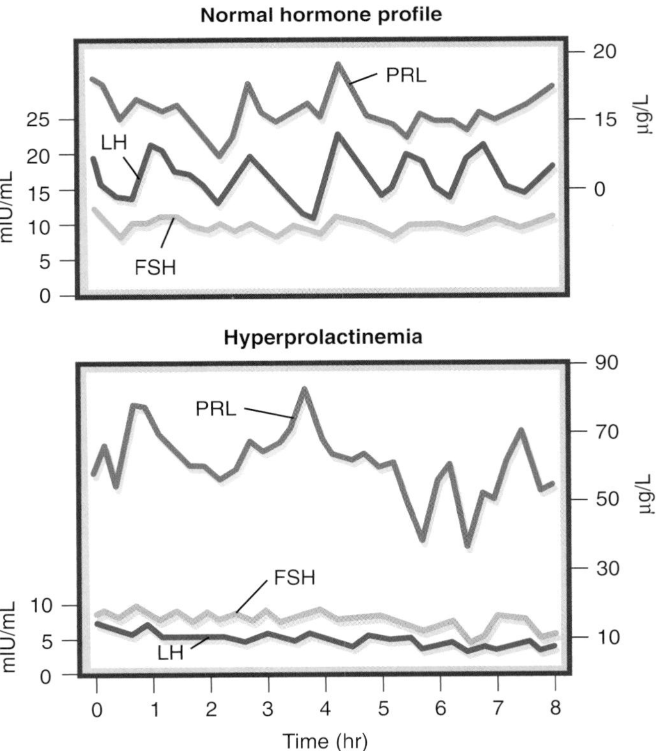

Figure 8-10 Effect of hyperprolactinemia on FSH and LH secretory patterns leading to hypogonadotropism in a female patient. FSH, follicle-stimulating hormone; LH, luteinizing hormone; PRL, prolactin. (Adapted from Tolis G. Prolactin: physiology and pathology. *Hosp Pract.* 1980;15:85-95.)

also a major determinant of ovarian dysfunction in these patients.

Male mice with disrupted PRLRs are fertile with low gonadotropin and normal testosterone levels. In human male subjects with hyperprolactinemia, LH and FSH pulsatility is attenuated, testosterone levels are suppressed, and sperm counts and motility are low.

Prolactin Assays

The PRL RIA is highly specific and clearly distinguishes PRL from GH. PRL measurements are standardized; reference preparations are provided by the National Institute for Biological Standards and Control in London and by the National Hormone and Pituitary Program in the United States. Improved assay efficiency and turnaround time, reproducibility, and sensitivity have been achieved by immunoradiometric (IRMA) and chemiluminescent (ICMA) PRL assays. Because these samples are usually assayed at a single dilution, extremely high PRL concentrations may saturate the ability of these assays to detect the correct level, resulting in a falsely low value being reported.[123] This "hook effect" may result in misdiagnosis of PRL-secreting macroadenomas as clinically nonfunctioning adenomas, with "normal" PRL levels reported in about 5% of the patients. Therefore, for patients harboring macroadenomas with clearcut clinical features of hyperprolactinemia, serum samples should be subjected to dilution of at least 1:100 before assay.

Hyperprolactinemia

The causes of hyperprolactinemia may be physiologic, pathologic, or drug induced (Table 8-1).[124,125]

Physiologic Causes

Pregnancy. During pregnancy, the normal pituitary gland may increase in size by twofold or more[44]; this is the result of a marked increase in the number of PRL-producing cells and a relative decrease in other hormone-secreting cells. Serum PRL concentrations rise to a mean of 207 μg/L during pregnancy,[110] and amniotic fluid PRL concentrations are 100 times those of maternal or fetal blood.[110]

Suckling increases serum PRL levels approximately 8.5-fold in actively nursing mothers,[126,127] and the milk let-down phenomenon is not associated with increased PRL. As nursing continues, PRL concentrations fall, but each suckling episode continues to cause a subsequent episodic rise in serum PRL. Mean serum concentrations were 162 μg/L at 2 to 4 weeks postpartum, 130 μg/L at 5 to 14 weeks, and 77 μg/L at 15 to 24 weeks.[112] It is unclear why active milk production continues despite progressively lower PRL levels after parturition.

Idiopathic Hyperprolactinemia. An elevated circulating PRL level in patients in whom no cause is identified is considered idiopathic, and these cases are relatively resistant to dopamine therapy. Mean serum PRL levels in patients with idiopathic hyperprolactinemia is usually less than 100 μg/L.[128]

Macroprolactinemia. PRL is a 23-kd, single-chain polypeptide, but it may also circulate in higher-molecular-weight forms (50 and 150 kd). High-molecular-weight PRL variants (see earlier discussion) may represent 85% or more of total PRL, but under usual circumstances the 22-kd variety predominates. Macroprolactinemia reflects these larger circulating PRL molecules (particularly the 150-kd variety), which exhibit markedly reduced bioactivity. Few of the expected clinical abnormalities usually associated with hyperprolactinemia (sexual dysfunction, galactorrhea, osteoporosis) occur in patients with macroprolactinemia.[129] Screening for macroprolactinemia can be accomplished by polyethylene glycol precipitation of serum samples. In one survey, macroprolactinemia was detected in 22% of 2089 hyperprolactinemia samples.[130]

Pathologic Causes. Pathologic causes include prolactinomas and pituitary or sellar tumors that inhibit dopamine because of pressure on the pituitary stalk or interruption of the vascular connections between the pituitary and hypothalamus. In a large series of histologically confirmed cases, a serum PRL level greater than 2000 mU/L (approximately 100 μg/L) was almost never encountered as a result of stalk dysfunction.[131] However, prolactinomas can manifest with any level of PRL elevation.

Breast stimulation has only a minimal effect on serum PRL levels. In 18 normal women, serum PRL levels rose from a mean of 10 μg/L to 15 μg/L during breast pump stimulation.[126] Up to 20% of patients with hypothyroidism have elevated PRL levels.[132] Treatment of hypothyroidism with thyroid hormone normalizes serum PRL if the hyperprolactinemia is caused by thyroid hormone deprivation.

PRL is moderately elevated (mean, 28 μg/L) in patients with chronic renal failure and in those being treated with dialysis.[133] The increase is largely a result of an increase in "little prolactin," due in part to decreased glomerular filtration rate. Sexual dysfunction is common in men on dialysis. Reducing PRL with dopamine agonists improves sexual function in patients on chronic hemodialysis[134] but does not normalize menses.[135] Side effects of dopamine agonists in patients with renal failure may be exacerbated because of fluid shifts and multiple medication interactions.

PRL levels rise in response to stress, correlate with the degree of stress, and typically return to normal as stress abates. The mean peak serum PRL level in 19 women undergoing general anesthesia was 39 μg/L immediately before surgery and 173 μg/L at surgery; PRL was still elevated 24 hours after surgery (mean, 47 μg/L).[136]

Severe head trauma also results in hyperprolactinemia, often accompanied by diabetes insipidus or the syndrome of inappropriate antidiuretic hormone secretion (SIADH) and other anterior pituitary hormone deficiencies. Fifty percent of patients develop moderate hyperprolactinemia after cranial and hypothalamic radiation.[137]

Pharmacologic Causes. A variety of medications cause minimal or moderate PRL elevations and may cause galactorrhea, amenorrhea, or reduced male sexual function. Neuroleptic drugs elevate PRL because of their dopamine antagonist properties. Chlorpromazine stimulates PRL, as do neuroleptics, which act by antagonizing both serotonin and dopamine receptors. Risperidone is a potent PRL stimulator.[138]

Unless patients exhibit sexual dysfunction, related osteoporosis, or troublesome galactorrhea, no treatment of drug-induced hyperprolactinemia may be advised.[139] It should not always be assumed that hyperprolactinemia in patients who are taking drugs known to elevate PRL is, in fact, caused by those medications. Prolactinoma, other sellar lesions,[140] hypothyroidism, or renal failure should be considered as causes of hyperprolactinemia requiring active management.

In patients taking neuroleptic medications, if the clinical situation permits, temporary drug withdrawal may be considered to determine whether PRL levels will normalize. If PRL levels do not normalize, a pituitary MRI should be performed. If neuroleptics are elevating PRL levels, switching to olanzapine may be attempted, because it does not

TABLE 8-1

Causes of Hyperprolactinemia

PHYSIOLOGIC	PHARMACOLOGIC (cont'd)
Pregnancy Lactation Stress Sleep Coitus Exercise	***Cholinergic Agonist*** Physostigmine ***Antihypertensives*** Labetalol Reserpine Verapamil
PATHOLOGIC	***H2 Antihistamines*** Cimetidine Ranitidine
Hypothalamic-Pituitary Stalk Damage Tumors: craniopharyngioma, suprasellar pituitary mass extension, meningioma, dysgerminoma, hypothalamic metastases Granulomas Infiltrations Rathke's cyst Irradiation Trauma: pituitary stalk section, sellar surgery, head trauma	***Estrogens*** Oral contraceptives Oral contraceptive withdrawal ***Anticonvulsant*** Phenytoin ***Anesthetics***
Pituitary Prolactinoma Acromegaly Macroadenoma (compressive) Idiopathic Plurihormonal adenoma Lymphocytic hypophysitis or parasellar mass Macroprolactinemia	***Neuroleptics*** Chlorpromazine Risperidone Promazine Promethazine Trifluoperazine Fluphenazine Butaperazine Perphenazine Thiethylperazine Thioridazine Haloperidol Pimozide Thiothixene Molindone
Systemic Disorders Chronic renal failure Polycystic ovary syndrome Cirrhosis Pseudocyesis Epileptic seizures Cranial irradiation Chest: neurogenic chest wall trauma, surgery, herpes zoster	
PHARMACOLOGIC	***Opiates and Opiate Antagonists*** Heroin Methadone Apomorphine Morphine
Neuropeptide Thyrotropin-releasing hormone	***Antidepressants*** Tricyclic antidepressants: chlorimipramine, amitriptyline Selective serotonin reuptake inhibitors: fluoxetine
Drug-Induced Hypersecretion *Dopamine Receptor Blockers* Phenothiazines: chlorpromazine, perphenazine Butyrophenones: haloperidol Thioxanthenes Metoclopramide *Dopamine Synthesis Inhibitors* α-Methyldopa *Catecholamine Depletors* Reserpine	

elevate PRL levels. In determining whether to discontinue a drug or whether to use an alternative medication,[141] the benefits should be weighed against the risks of drug replacement or cessation. Although combined use of dopamine antagonists and dopamine agonists is not usually advised because of increased risk of side effects (e.g., postural hypotension) and exacerbation of underlying psychosis, some advocate the use of both formulations simultaneously.[142]

Clinical Features of Hyperprolactinemia. Galactorrhea and reproductive dysfunction are the hallmarks of nonphysiologic hyperprolactinemia. Women present with galactorrhea associated with a range of menstrual disturbances including oligomenorrhea and amenorrhea, whereas men present with symptoms of hypogonadism and tumor mass effects, although galactorrhea also occurs infrequently in men.

Galactorrhea and amenorrhea were reported in the 19th century by Chiari and Frommel.[143] The Chiari-Frommel syndrome comprises postpartum galactorrhea, amenorrhea, and "utero-ovarian atrophy" in patients not nursing. This disorder is usually self-limited, and fertility eventually returns spontaneously, sometimes without an intervening menstrual period. Patients with postpartum amenorrhea, hyperprolactinemia, and galactorrhea have also been found to harbor prolactinomas. In the 1950s, Argonz[144] and

Forbes[145] and their colleagues associated galactorrhea and amenorrhea with pituitary tumors. In a report of 18 such patients, galactorrhea and amenorrhea were present for up to 11 years after parturition, and the patients had a mean PRL level of 45 μg/L.[132]

Galactorrhea. Inappropriate nipple secretion of milk-like substances[146] may persist after childbirth or discontinuation of nursing for as long as 6 months. After that time, continued milk production is considered abnormal, and other causes for galactorrhea should be investigated. Galactorrhea can occur in women or men; it can be unilateral or bilateral, profuse or sparse, and it can vary in color and thickness. If blood is present in the galactorrhea fluid, it could be the harbinger of an underlying pathologic process (such as a ductal papilloma or carcinoma), and mammography or sonography is indicated.

Twenty-nine of 48 patients with pituitary tumors and galactorrhea had PRL concentrations lower than 200 μg/L, most likely on the basis of stalk compression, suggesting that they harbored pituitary tumors other than prolactinomas.[132] It is likely that most patients with so-called idiopathic galactorrhea with amenorrhea harbor microprolactinomas. Fifty percent of patients with acromegaly also have hyperprolactinemia, because human GH is a potent lactogen and can cause galactorrhea when elevated.[147]

Normoprolactinemic galactorrhea with regular menses represents the largest single cause of galactorrhea. In two thirds of patients, postpartum galactorrhea persists despite the resumption of menses, and this probably does not represent a pathologic entity. Normal PRL levels may still permit milk production, and treatment of such patients with dopamine agonists alleviates galactorrhea. Galactorrhea may also develop transiently after surgical procedures to the chest wall, including mammoplasty. The secretion may be copious and may arise from neural reflex intercostal nerve stimulation.[148]

The management of galactorrhea should be determined by identifying and treating the underlying cause. Regardless of the etiology, galactorrhea associated with hyperprolactinemia responds to correction of the hyperprolactinemia.

Growth Hormone

Physiology

Somatotroph Cells. Mammosomatroph cells expressing both PRL and GH arise from the acidophilic stem cell and immunostain mainly for PRL. Somatotrophs are located predominantly in the lateral wings of the anterior pituitary gland and comprise between 35% and 45% of pituitary cells (Fig. 8-11). These ovoid cells contain prominent secretory granules up to 700 μm in diameter. Juxtanuclear Golgi structures are particularly prominent, with secretory granules in formation. The gland contains a total of 5 to 15 mg of GH.[149]

Biosynthesis. The human GH locus spans approximately 66 kilobases (kb) on the long arm of chromosome 17q22-24.[150] It contains a cluster of five highly conserved genes, each consisting of five exons separated by four introns,[151] that encode the various forms of human growth hormone (hGH) and human chorionic somatomammotropin (hCS):

- hGH-N is encoded by *GH1* (growth hormone 1)
- hCS-L is encoded by *CSHL1* (chorionic somatomammotropin-like 1)

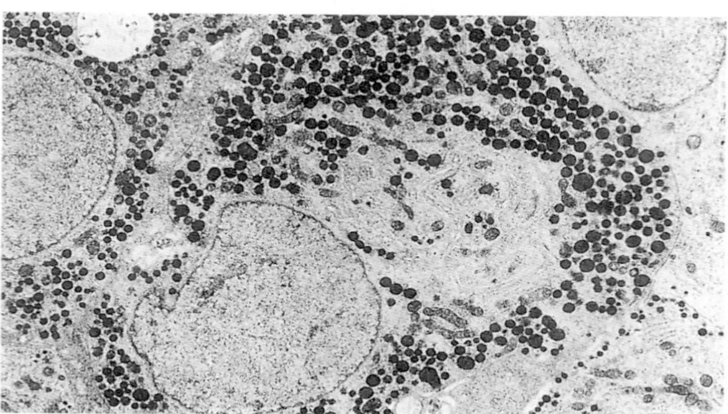

Figure 8-11 Normal somatotroph. A somatotroph in the nontumorous pituitary is large and round to ovoid. It contains numerous electron-dense secretory granules that range from 250 to 700 μm in diameter. Short profiles of rough endoplasmic reticulum are scattered throughout the cytoplasm. The juxtanuclear Golgi complex is prominent and harbors forming secretory granules. (From Asa SL. Tumors of the pituitary gland. In: Rosai J, ed. *Atlas of Tumor Pathology*, Series III, Fascicle 22. Washington, DC: Armed Forces Institute of Pathology, 1997:14.)

- hCS-A is encoded by *CSH1* (chorionic somatomammotropin hormone 1)
- hGH-V is encoded by *GH2* (growth hormone 2)
- hCS-B is encoded by *CSH2* (chorionic somatomammotropin hormone 2)

The hGH-N gene codes for a 22-kd (191-amino-acid) protein and is selectively transcribed in pituitary somatotrophs[152] (see later discussion). Other genes of the hGH/hCS cluster are expressed in the placenta. The hCS-A and hCS-B genes are expressed in placental trophoblasts.[153] hCS-L is found in placental villi but has been considered a pseudogene. hGH-V, expressed in placental syncytiotrophoblasts, encodes a 22-kd protein that can be detected in maternal circulation from midgestation, as well as a minor form called hGH-V2. Elevated maternal hGH-V serum concentrations are accompanied by a decline in hGH-N, suggesting feedback regulation of the maternal hypothalamic pituitary axis. After delivery, circulating hGH-V levels drop rapidly and are undetectable after 1 hour.[154]

The GH1 *hGH* promoter region contains *cis*-elements that mediate both pituitary-specific and hormone-specific signaling. The transcription factor POU1F1 confers tissue-specific GH expression, and a second, ubiquitous factor binds to a distal POU1F1 site containing a consensus sequence for the Sp1 transcription factor. POU1F1 and Sp1 both contribute to GH promoter activation, because mutation of the Sp1 binding site leads to attenuation of promoter activity.[155] Deoxyribonuclease-hypersensitive sites of a locus control region (LCR) of the hGH gene determine somatotroph and lactotroph GH expression, and the LCR is involved in regulation of a chromatin domain in these pituitary cells.[150] GH synthesis and release are under the control of a variety of hormonal agents, including GHRH, somatostatin, ghrelin, IGF1, thyroid hormone, and glucocorticoids. GHRH stimulates GH synthesis and release, mediated by cAMP. cAMP response element (CREB)-binding protein, known as *CREBBP* or *CBP*, is phosphorylated by protein kinase A and is a cofactor for POU1F1-dependent human GH activation. IGF1 attenuates basal and stimulated GH gene expression.

The GH1 molecule, a single-chain polypeptide hormone consisting of 191 amino acids, is synthesized, stored, and secreted by somatotroph cells. The crystal structure of human GH reveals four α-helices.[156] Circulating GH molecules comprise several heterogeneous forms: 22- and 20-kd monomers, an acetylated 22-kd form, and two desamino GH molecules. The 22-kd peptide is the major physiologic GH component, accounting for 75% of pituitary GH secretion. Amino acids 32 through 46 are deleted by alternative splicing of the GH gene to yield 20-kd GH, which accounts for about 10% of pituitary GH. The 20-kd GH has a slower metabolic clearance time,[157] accounting for the fact that plasma ratio of the 20- and 22-kd forms is higher than in the pituitary gland.

Regulation

Neuropeptides, neurotransmitters, and opiates impinge on the hypothalamus and modulate release of GHRH and somatostatin (somatotropin release–inhibiting factor, or SRIF). Integrated effects of these complex neurogenic influences determine the final secretory pattern of GH. Apomorphine, a central dopamine receptor agonist, stimulates GH secretion,[158] as does levodopa (L-dopa). Oral L-dopa administration evokes a brisk serum GH response within 1 hour in healthy young subjects. Norepinephrine increases GH secretion via α-adrenergic pathways and inhibits GH release via β-adrenergic pathways. Insulin-induced hypoglycemia, clonidine, arginine administration, exercise, and L-dopa facilitate GH secretion by α-adrenergic effects.[159] β-Adrenergic blockade increases GHRH-induced GH release, possibly by a direct pituitary action or by decreasing hypothalamic somatostatin release. Endorphins and enkephalins stimulate GH and may account for GH release during severe physical stress and extreme exercise.[159] Galanin, a 29-amino-acid neuropeptide, induces GH release and responses to GHRH. Cholinergic and serotoninergic neurons and several neuropeptides stimulate GH, including neurotensin, VIP, motilin, cholecystokinin, and glucagon.

Interaction of GHRH and SRIF. The somatotroph cell expresses specific receptors for GHRH,[160] growth hormone secretagogues (GHS), and SRIF receptor subtypes 2 and 5, which mediate GH secretion.[161,162] GHRH selectively induces GH gene transcription and hormone release.[163] GHRH administered to normal adults elicits a prompt rise in serum GH levels, with higher levels occurring in female subjects.[164] SRIF suppresses both basal and GHRH-stimulated GH pulse amplitude and frequency but does not affect GH biosynthesis.

Hypothalamic SRIF and GHRH are secreted in independent waves and interact together with additional GH secretagogues to generate pulsatile GH release. The rat hypothalamus releases GHRH and SRIF 180 degrees out of phase every 3 to 4 hours, resulting in pulsatile GH levels. SRIF antibody administration elevates GH levels, but the intervening GH pulses remain intact,[165] implying that hypothalamic SRIF secretion generates GH troughs. GHRH antibodies eliminate spontaneous GH surges. In humans, GH pulsatility persists when GHRH is tonically elevated, as in ectopic tumor GHRH production or during GHRH infusion,[166] suggesting that hypothalamic SRIF is largely responsible for GH pulsatility. Preexposure to SRIF enhances somatotroph sensitivity to GHRH stimulation. Therefore, during a normal GH trough period, the high SRIF level probably primes the somatotroph to respond maximally to a subsequent GHRH pulse, thus optimizing GH release. SRIF also inhibits central GHRH release via direct synaptic connections with hypothalamic SRIF-containing neurons.

Chronic GHRH stimulation, by continuous infusion or repeated bolus administration, eventually desensitizes GH release in vitro and in vivo, possibly due to depletion of a GHRH-sensitive pool of GH. GHRH pretreatment also decreases somatotroph GHRH binding sites.[167] GH stimulates hypothalamic SRIF, GHRH and SRIF autoregulate their own respective secretion, and GHRH also stimulates SRIF release.[168,169] GH secretion is further regulated by its target growth factor, IGF1, which participates in a hypothalamic-pituitary peripheral regulatory feedback system.[170,171] IGF1 stimulates hypothalamic SRIF release and inhibits pituitary GH gene transcription and secretion.

Growth Hormone Secretagogues and Ghrelin. The isolation of ghrelin implicated an additional control system for regulation of GH secretion (see Chapter 7). Ghrelin is a 28-amino-acid peptide that binds the GHS receptor[172] to induce hypothalamic GHRH and pituitary GH.[173] A unique *n*-octanoylated serine 3 residue confers GH-releasing activity to the molecule. Ghrelin is synthesized in peripheral tissues, especially in gastric mucosal neuroendocrine cells, as well as centrally in the hypothalamus. Ghrelin administration dose-dependently evokes GH release and also induces food intake (Fig. 8-12). Hypothalamic ghrelin

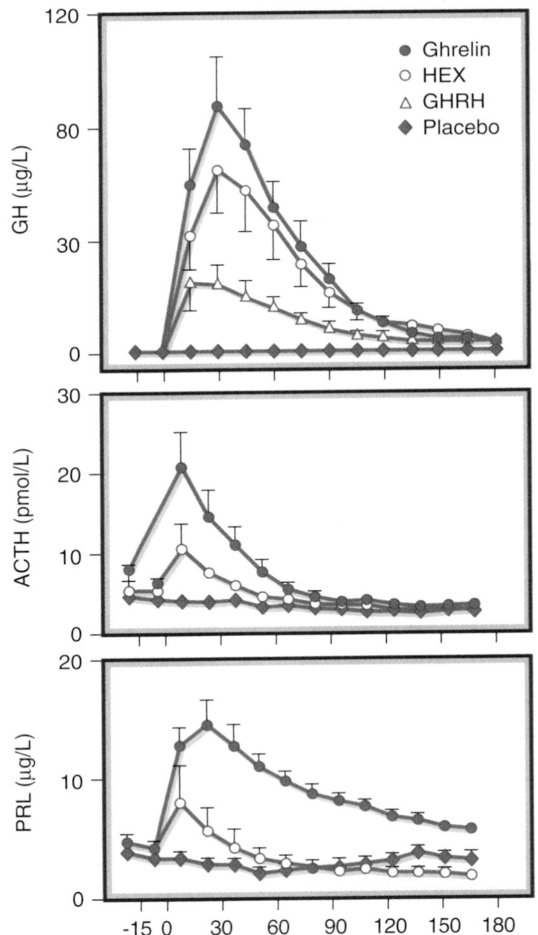

Figure 8-12 Effect of growth hormone (GH) secretagogues on secretion of GH, corticotropin (ACTH), and prolactin (PRL) in healthy subjects. Mean (± standard error of the mean [SEM]) curve responses after administration of ghrelin (1.0 µg/kg), hexarelin (HEX, 1.0 µg/kg), growth hormone–releasing hormone (GHRH, 1.0 µg/kg), or placebo. (Adapted from Arvat E, Maccario M, Di Vito L, et al. Endocrine activities of ghrelin, a natural growth hormone secretagogue [GHS], in humans: comparison and interactions with hexarelin, a nonnatural peptidyl GHS, and GH-releasing hormone. *J Clin Endocrinol Metab.* 2001;86:1169-1174.)

likely controls GH secretion, whereas peripheral sources exhibit additional complex nutritional effects (see Chapter 7). Plasma ghrelin levels are suppressed after gastric bypass surgery,[174] and mice with disrupted ghrelin or GHS receptors are resistant to diet-induced obesity.[175] Accumulating evidence indicates that ghrelin subserves both GH secretion and control of appetite.[176] Control of GH secretion requires hypothalamic GHRH and SRIF as well as ghrelin.[177]

Synthetic hexapeptides (artificial GHSs) recognize the GHS (ghrelin) receptor, induce potent and reproducible GH release, and are useful for the diagnosis of GH deficiency (GHD).[178] GHSs stimulate GH secretion, and GHRH and GHS act through distinct receptors and via different intracellular signaling pathways on somatotroph subpopulations.[179] However, GHRH also acts as an allosteric coagonist for the ghrelin receptor.[180] Ghrelin agonists require the presence of a functional hypothalamus to evoke GH release, as evidenced in patients with intact pituitary but disordered hypothalamic function, in whom GHS does not induce GH.[181] GHS agonists also potentiate GH release in response to a maximal stimulating dose of exogenous GHRH.[182] After a saturating dose of GHRH, subsequent GHRH administration is ineffective, whereas GHS agonists remain effective.[183]

GHSs are now used as pharmacologic tools in the diagnosis of adult GHD. An advantage of GHS testing relates to their lack of side effects, unlike the insulin tolerance test. Modest PRL and ACTH/cortisol increases have been reported with some GHSs, leading to the development of novel GHSs with more selective somatotroph actions.[176]

Secretion. GH secretion is normally episodic and exhibits a diurnal rhythm with approximately two thirds of the total daily GH secretion produced at night, triggered by the onset of slow-wave sleep. Major GH secretory pulses accounting for up to 70% of daily GH secretion occur with the first episode of slow-wave sleep.[184] Normal GH secretion is characterized by secretary episodes separated by troughs of minimal basal secretion during which GH is undetectable.

GH concentration is high in the fetal circulation, peaking at approximately 150 μg/L during midgestation. Neonatal levels are lower (approximately 30 μg/L), possibly reflecting negative feedback control by rising levels of circulating IGF. GH output falls to a stable level during childhood, then rises at the onset of puberty to peak at a twofold to threefold higher level at late puberty. GH output declines exponentially in both sexes at the young adulthood transition, declining to one quarter of the values achieved in late puberty.[159] The decline in GH status occurs by a change in pulse amplitude rather than frequency. On average, the daily production of GH in the prepubertal state is 200 to 600 μg, rising to 1000 to 1800 μg at the pubertal peak.[159] In adulthood, production rates range from approximately 200 to 600 μg/day, with higher rates in women than in men.[159,185] Adiposity that accompanies the aging process accounts for a significant component of declining GH output with increasing age (Table 8-2).[186]

The ultradian rhythm of GH secretion is generated by coordinated interaction of many factors (Fig. 8-13). "Jet lag" increases GH peak amplitude, resulting in a transient increase of 24-hour GH secretion. Exercise and physical stress, including trauma with hypovolemic shock and sepsis, increase GH levels.[187] Emotional deprivation is associated with suppressed GH secretion, and attenuated GH responses to provocative stimuli occur in endogenous depression.[188]

TABLE 8-2

Secretion of Growth Hormone in Adults*

Interval	Young Adult	Fasting	Obesity	Middle Age
24-hr Secretion (μg/24 hr)	540 ± 44	2171 ± 333	77 ± 20	196 ± 65
Secretory bursts (no. in 24 hr)	12 ± 1	32 ± 2	3 ± 0.5	10 ± 1
GH burst (μg)	45 ± 4	64 ± 9	24 ± 5	10 ± 6

*Deconvolution analysis of growth hormone (GH) secretion in adult males.
From Thorner MO, Vance ML, Horvath E, et al. The anterior pituitary. In: Wilson JD, Foster D, eds. *Williams Textbook of Endocrinology*, 8th ed. Philadelphia, PA: Saunders; 1992:221-310.[508,509]

Nutrition plays a major role in GH regulation. Chronic malnutrition and prolonged fasting increase GH pulse frequency and amplitude (Fig. 8-14).[189] Obesity decreases basal and stimulated GH secretion, insulin-induced hypoglycemia stimulates GH, and hyperglycemia inhibits GH secretion. However, chronic hyperglycemia is not associated with low GH levels, and, in fact, poorly controlled diabetes is associated with increased basal and

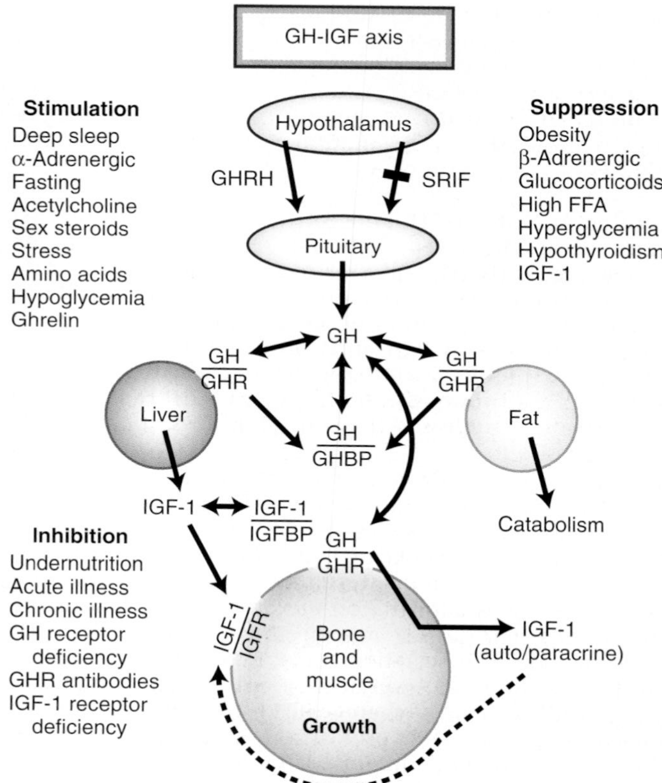

Figure 8-13 The growth hormone (GH) axis. Simplified diagram of the GH–insulin-like growth factor I (IGF-I) axis involving hypophysiotropic hormones controlling pituitary GH release, circulating GH-binding protein (GHBP) and its GH receptor (GHR) source, IGF-I and its largely GH-dependent binding proteins (IGFBP), and cellular responsiveness to GH and IGF-I interacting with their specific receptors. GHRH, growth hormone–releasing hormone; IGFR, IGF-I receptor; FFA, free fatty acids; SRIF, somatostatin. (Reproduced from Rosenbloom A: Growth hormone insensitivity: physiologic and genetic basis, phenotype and treatment. *J Pediatr.* 1999;135:280-289.)

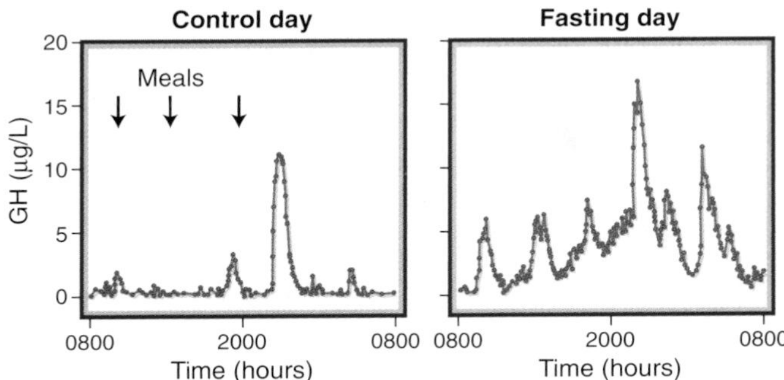

Figure 8-14 Effect of fasting on growth hormone (GH) secretion patterns in a healthy male subject. (Reproduced from Hartman ML, Veldhuis JD, Johnson ML, et al. Augmented growth hormone [GH] secretory burst frequency and amplitude mediate enhanced GH secretion during a two-day fast in normal men. *J Clin Endocrinol Metab.* 1992;74:757-765.)

exercise-induced GH levels.[190] Central glucoreceptors appear to sense glucose fluctuations, rather than absolute levels. High-protein meals and intravenous administration of single amino acids (including arginine and leucine) stimulate GH secretion. Increased serum free fatty acids blunt the effects of arginine infusion, sleep, L-dopa, and exercise on GHRH-stimulated GH release.[191] Leptin plays a key role in regulation of body fat mass,[192] regulating food intake and energy expenditure, and may act as a metabolic signal to regulate GH secretion. Leptin- and neuropeptide Y–producing hypothalamic neurons synapse with somatostatin neurons, and antisera to neuropeptide Y and somatostatin reverse starvation-induced GH release.[193] In GH-deficient hypopituitary adults, leptin concentrations are higher than would be expected from their body fat mass.[194]

Interaction with Other Hormone Axes. There are complex and sometimes opposing interactions between GH and other pituitary hormone axes. Acute glucocorticoid administration stimulates GH secretion, whereas chronic steroid treatment inhibits GH. GH levels rise 3 hours after acute glucocorticoid administration, and they remain elevated for 2 hours.[195] However, supraphysiologic glucocorticoid exposure retards growth, and Cushing's disease is also associated with growth retardation, decreased serum GH, and decreased pituitary GH content surrounding the adenoma.[196] Glucocorticoids administered to normal subjects dose-dependently inhibit GHRH-simulated GH secretion, similar to what is seen in Cushing's syndrome.[195]

There are also complex interactions with the thyroid system. In hyperthyroid patients, GH levels are decreased, but levels normalize when patients are rendered euthyroid. However, thyroid hormones are necessary to evoke normal GH responses to stimulation testing and to achieve optimal responsiveness.[197]

Gonadal steroids regulate GH secretion and GH action by different mechanisms. Testosterone stimulates GH secretion centrally, an effect that is dependent on prior aromatization to estrogen.[198] Estrogen stimulates GH secretion, but this is evident only with oral, not parenteral administration, because of first-pass hepatic inhibition of IGF1 production with oral administration.[199] Therefore, the stimulatory effect on GH secretion by estrogen is indirect and is facilitated by reduction in IGF1 feedback inhibition. Whether estrogen stimulates GH secretion centrally in women is unresolved.[199]

Growth Hormone–Binding Proteins. Circulating growth hormone–binding proteins (GHBPs) include a 20-kd low-affinity GHBP and a 60-kd high-affinity GHBP. The latter corresponds to the extracellular domain of the hepatic GH receptor and binds half of the circulating 22-kd form of GH.[200,201] The high-affinity GHBP in humans is generated by proteolytic cleavage through the action of tumor necrosis factor-α (TNF-α)-converting enzyme, a metalloprotease.[202] The 20-kd GH binds preferentially to the low-affinity BP, which is unrelated to the GH receptor.

The GHBPs function to dampen acute oscillations in serum GH levels associated with pulsatile pituitary GH secretion, and plasma GH half-life is prolonged by decreased renal GH clearance of bound GH. The high-affinity BP also competes with GH for binding to surface GH receptors and, as such, alters GH pharmacokinetics and distribution.

GHBP concentrations are normal in hypopituitarism and acromegaly.[203] Some patients with Laron dwarfism have absent or reduced levels of GHBP, reflecting mutations that result in translation of the GH receptor or the extracellular domain.[204] Serum concentrations of GHBP are low in some children with idiopathic short stature[205] and in African pygmies, suggesting abnormalities in the gene for the GH receptor.[206] GHBP levels are increased in obesity, in pregnancy, and in subjects undergoing refeeding[206] and reduced in individuals with malnutrition, cirrhosis, or hypothyroidism. GHBP levels are reduced by glucocorticoids and androgens[207] and increased by oral estrogen administration.[208]

Action

GH acts to mediate growth and metabolic functions (Fig. 8-15).

Signaling. GH elicits intracellular signaling though a peripheral receptor and initiates a phosphorylation cascade involving the JAK/STAT pathway.[209] The liver contains abundant GH receptors, and several peripheral tissues also express modest amounts of receptor, including muscle and fat (Fig. 8-16).[210] The GH receptor is a 620-amino-acid, 70-kd protein of the class I cytokine/hematopoietin receptor superfamily that consists of an extracellular ligand-binding domain, a single membrane-spanning domain, and a cytoplasmic signaling component.[211] The GH receptor superfamily is homologous with receptors for PRL, interleukin 2 (IL-2) through IL-7, erythropoietin, interferon, and colony-stimulating factor.

GH complexes with two predimerized GH receptor components to induce a conformational rotation that triggers signaling (see Fig. 8-16).[210,212] This is characterized by rapid JAK2 tyrosine kinase activation leading to phosphorylation of intracellular signaling molecules including STAT1, STAT3, and STAT5), critical signaling components for GH action.[213] Phosphorylated STAT proteins are directly translocated to the cell nucleus, where they elicit GH-specific target gene expression by binding to nuclear DNA. STAT1 and STAT5 may also interact directly with the GH receptor molecule.[213] GH also induces c-fos (FOS) induction, insulin receptor substrate 1 (IRS1) phosphorylation, and insulin synthesis. Additional intracellular signaling pathways induced by GH include mitogen-activated protein kinase (MAP kinase), protein kinase C, SH2-β, SHP2 (now called PTPN11), signal regulatory protein-α (SIRPA), SHC, FAK (PTK2), Crk-II, and SRC. How these seemingly overlapping pathways converge to integrate the net cellular effects of GH is at present unclear.

Intracellular GH signaling is abrogated by suppressor of cytokine signaling (SOCS) proteins, which disrupt the JAK/

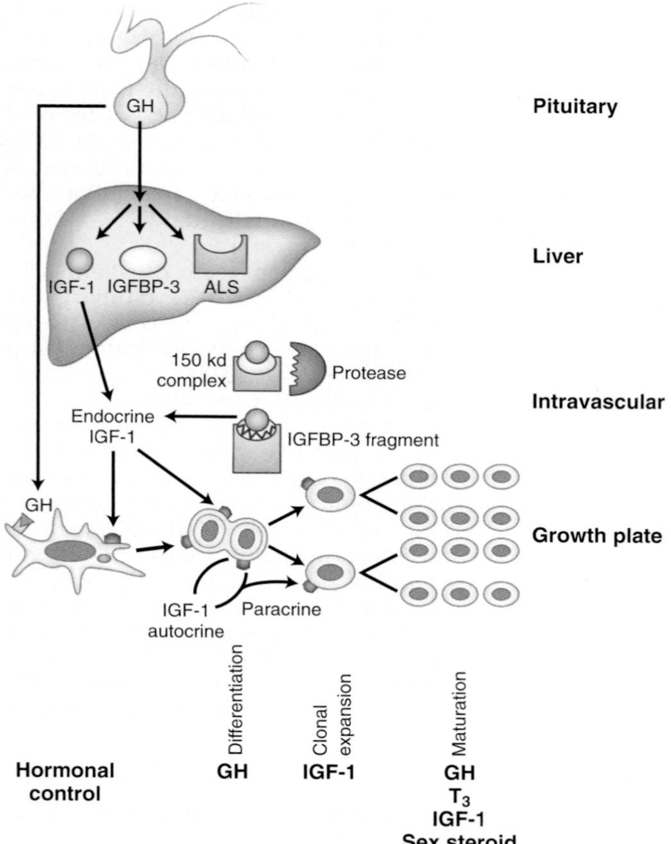

Figure 8-15 Integrated model of the GH-IGFBP-IGF axis in the growth process. Three mechanisms are proposed. In the first hypothesis, growth hormone (GH) stimulates production of insulin-like growth factor I (IGF-I); circulating IGF-I (endocrine IGF-I) then acts at the growth plate. In the second hypothesis, GH regulates hepatic production of IGF-binding protein 3 (IGFBP-3) and the acid-labile subunit (ALS) of the IGFBP complex; IGF-I binds to IGFBP-3 and with ALS, forming the 150-kd ternary complex. Proteases then cleave this complex into fragments that release IGFBP-3 and IGF-I in the intravascular space and at the growth plate. In the third hypothesis, GH induces differentiation and local IGF-I production, and IGF-I acts via autocrine and paracrine mechanisms to stimulate cell division. T_3, triiodothyronine. (From Spagnol A, Rosenfeld RG. The mechanism by which GH brings about growth: the relative contributions of GH and insulin-like growth factors. *Endocrinol Metab Clin North Am.* 1996;25:615-631; and Clemmons DR, Van Wyk JJ, Ridgway EC, et al. Evaluation of acromegaly by radioimmunoassay of somatomedin-C. *N Engl J Med.* 1979;301:1138-1142.)

STAT pathway and thus disrupt GH action.[214] In transgenic mice with deletion of SOCS2, gigantism develops, presumably due to unrestrained GH action. Because SOCS proteins are also induced by pro-inflammatory cytokines, critically ill patients and those with renal failure may develop GH resistance due to cytokine-induced SOCS.[215] Unraveling of the STAT/SOCS regulation in syndromes associated with disordered GH signaling will likely yield mechanistic insights for dysregulated GH action.

The pattern of GH secretion determines tissue responses to GH in addition to the absolute amount of circulating hormone. Gender-specific patterns of GH secretion profiles determine sex-specific expression of cytochrome P450 enzymes. In turn, circulating steroids regulate neuroendocrine release of GH. SRIF, by suppressing interpulse GH levels, serves to masculinize the ultradian GH rhythm. In mice harboring a disrupted SRIF gene, plasma GH secretory patterns are elevated and liver enzyme induction loses its gender-specific dimorphism, but these animals retain sexually dimorphic growth patterns.[216] Linear growth patterns and liver enzyme induction are phenotypically gender-specific due to higher GH pulse frequency rates and also show gender-specific STAT5B activity.[217] Sexually dimorphic patterns of GH secretion and tissue targeting appear to be determined by STAT5B, which is sensitive to repeated pulses of injected GH,[218] unlike other GH-induced responses, which are desensitized by repeated GH administration. Disruption of STAT5B in transgenic mice causes impaired male-pattern body growth[219] associated with female-pattern levels of IGF1 and testosterone. Appropriate GH pulsatility is also required to determine body growth mediated by STAT5B[220,221] but not for metabolic effects of GH on carbohydrate metabolism. A STAT mutation has been described as a cause of short stature.[222]

IGF1 mediates growth-promoting activities of GH[170] in an endocrine or paracrine manner.[223] In mice, paracrine IGF1 produced in extrahepatic tissues appears to be critical for growth, which persists even when hepatic IGF1 is deleted.[224] GH receptor mutations are associated with partial or complete GH insensitivity and growth failure. These syndromes are associated with normal or high circulating GH levels, decreased circulating GHBP levels, and low levels of circulating IGF1. Multiple homozygous or heterozygous exonic and intronic GH receptor mutations have been described. These occur mostly in the extracellular ligand-binding receptor domain (see Chapter 24).

Metabolic Action. GH functions as a major metabolic hormone in the adult by optimizing body composition and physical function and regulating energy and substrate metabolism. Metabolic actions of GH also closely interact with those of insulin in the control of fat, glucose, and protein metabolism during fasted and fed states.

GH promotes fat metabolism by enhancing lipolysis and fatty acid oxidation. This function is particularly important during the fasted state, when GH secretion is enhanced, resulting in the partitioning of fuel utilization toward fat and the sparing of protein. Stimulation of lipolysis occurs indirectly through potentiation of the activity of hormone-sensitive lipase by β-adrenergic stimulation. GH also regulates lipoprotein metabolism by enhancing clearance of low-density lipoprotein (LDL) through activating expression of hepatic LDL receptors.[225,226] The atherogenic profile of lipoproteins is increased in GHD and reduced by GH therapy.[227]

GH exerts profound effects on glucose metabolism both directly and by antagonizing insulin action. GH enhances glucose uptake and utilization in cells; this is referred to as its *insulin-like* effects.[228] At the whole-body level, GH suppresses glucose oxidation and utilization while enhancing hepatic glucose production,[229] potentially for increased use of glucose that is nonoxidative in nature. The target tissues and the biochemical fate of this glucose surplus are unclear. Because GH is an important counterregulatory hormone, it is conceivable that this function protects against hypoglycemia.

Protein anabolism is a signature property of GH that reduces urea synthesis, blood urea concentration, and urinary urea excretion. The conventional view is that GH-induced protein anabolism is mediated by IGF1. However, GH also acutely stimulates amino acid uptake and incorporation into protein in vitro.[230] Arteriovenous measurements in the forearm showed an acute increase in protein synthesis over a few hours after GH infusion, suggesting a direct effect.[231] Whole-body studies in humans using isotopes have consistently shown that GH reduces

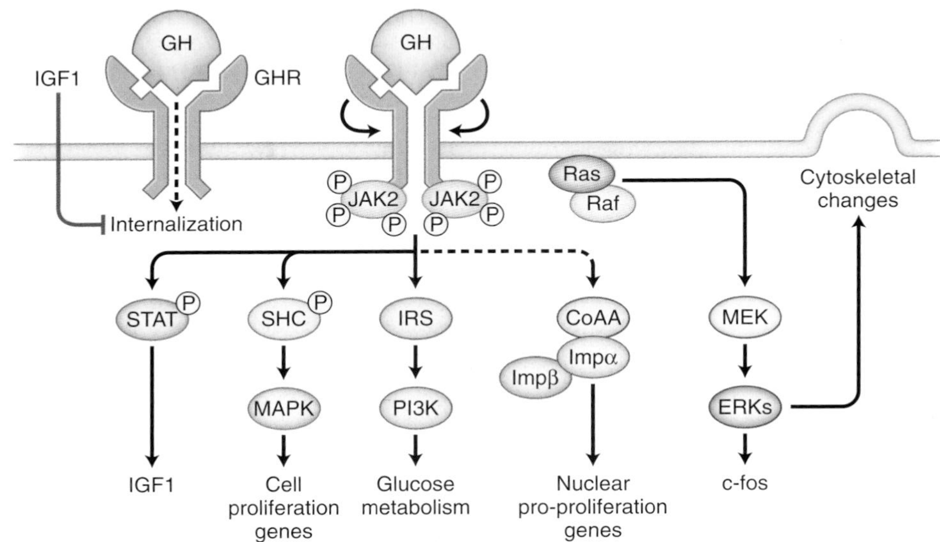

Figure 8-16 Action of growth hormone (GH). GH binds to the growth hormone receptor (GHR) dimer, which undergoes internal rotation, resulting in Jak2 phosphorylation (P) and subsequent signal transduction. Ligand binding to a preformed GHR dimer results in internal rotation and subsequent phosphorylation cascades. GH signaling is mediated by Jak2 phosphorylation of depicted signaling including Src/ERK pathways. STAT, SHC, and IRS cascades. GH targets include insulin-like growth factor I (IGF1), c-fos, cell proliferation genes, glucose metabolism, and cytoskeletal proteins. GHR internalization and translocation *(dotted lines)* induce nuclear proproliferation genes via importin α/β (Impα/Impβ) coactivator (CoAA) signaling. IGF1 may also block GHR internalization, acting in a feedback loop. ERK, extracellular signal-related kinase; IRS, insulin receptor substrate; JAK 2, Janus kinase 2; MEK, dual specifying mitogen-activated kinase 2. (From Lupu F, Terwilliger JD, Lee K, et al. Roles of growth hormone and insulin-like growth factor 1 in mouse postnatal growth. *Dev Biol.* 2001;229:141; and Melmed S. Acromegaly pathogenesis and treatment. *J Clin Invest.* 2009;119:3189-3202.)

protein oxidation and stimulates protein synthesis.[130] The protein-sparing effect of GH is coupled to the availability and increased parallel utilization of free fatty acids, whereas pharmacologic reduction of free fatty acids during fasting augments the rate of protein breakdown.[229]

Growth Hormone Deficiency

GH is the most abundant hormone in the adult pituitary gland, and it plays an important role in maintaining the metabolic process and the integrity of many tissues. GHD in adults is recognized as a distinct entity (Table 8-3).[232-234] GHD has negative effects on body composition, cardiovascular risk, quality of life, and physical functioning.[233,235,236] Life expectancy is reduced in hypopituitary patients with GHD,[237-239] largely as a consequence of cardiovascular and cerebrovascular events, especially in female subjects.[240] Neither estrogen nor thyroid deficiency accounts for this increased risk and reduced survival, and it is not yet rigorously confirmed that the observed increased mortality and morbidity occur solely as a result of GHD.

Pathophysiology. Adult GHD may be acquired or congenital. Of the acquired causes, 50% arise from pituitary tumors, 20% from extrapituitary tumors, and 5% from inflammatory or infiltrative lesions, with up to 15% of cases being idiopathic.[241] Surgical or radiation treatment of pituitary and parasellar tumors is the most common cause of GHD, accounting for almost two thirds of cases.

The frequency of causes is different in childhood-onset versus adult-onset GHD.[241,242] Idiopathic causes are most common in childhood-onset GHD and likely represent a heterogeneous collection of congenital developmental abnormalities, including mutations of *PROP1* and *POU1F1* genes, that cause GHD and other pituitary hormone deficiencies.[243] Isolated GHD may be complete or partial, and

TABLE 8-3

Adult Somatotropin Deficiency

Clinical Consequence	Effect of GH Replacement
Body Composition	
General and central adiposity	Decrease
Reduced lean mass	Increase
Reduced bone mass	Increase
Function	
Reduced exercise capacity	Improve
Muscle weakness	Increase
Impaired cardiac function	Improve
Hypohidrosis	Increase
Quality of Life	
Low mood	Improve
Fatigue	Improve
Low motivation	Improve
Reduced satisfaction	Improve
Cardiovascular Risk Profile	
Abnormal lipid profile	Improve
Insulin resistance	No change
Increased inflammatory markers	Decrease
Intimal media thickening	Decrease
Laboratory	
Blunted peak GH to stimulation (see Table 8-4)	Increase
Low IGF1	Increase
Hyperinsulinemia	Improve
High LDL- and low HDL-cholesterol	Improve

GH, growth hormone; HDL, high-density lipoprotein; IGF1, insulin-like growth factor 1; LDL, low-density lipoprotein.

up to 67% of children initially diagnosed with idiopathic GHD had normal GH responses when subsequently retested as adults for GHD after cessation of GH treatment.[244] Therefore, children with GHD should be retested before GH treatment is continued into adulthood unless they have clearly documented panhypopituitarism or a defined genetic or developmental abnormality that causes complete and irreversible GHD.

Mutations in the GH[245] and GHRH receptor genes[246] and GH insensitivity as a result of primary GH receptor dysfunction[247] result in GHD.

Presentation. Symptoms of GHD are nonspecific and include fatigue, lack of energy, social isolation, low mood, poor concentration, and reduced physical capacity.[232] The signs are also nonspecific and include general and central adiposity, reduced lean tissue, and bone mineral density along with unfavorable biochemical changes such as hyperlipidemia[248,249] and glucose intolerance.[232] Some patients have established evidence of macrovascular disease, such as increased carotid intimal thickness.[250,251] GHD may also be associated with heart abnormalities including reduced left ventricular mass.[252-255] Cardiovascular risk abnormalities are often less pronounced in adults with childhood-onset GHD than in those with GHD acquired during adulthood, who have more pronounced disorders of quality of life, lipids, and body composition.[252,256,257]

Although the features of GHD are recognizable, they are not particularly distinct, and they mimic body compositional and biochemical changes of the aging process. Therefore, clinical suspicion must be confirmed by accurate biochemical diagnosis to ensure that GH-deficient patients are accurately identified and treated.

Evaluation. GHD is diagnosed biochemically within an appropriate clinical context. Biochemical testing for GHD should be considered in patients with a high probability of hypothalamic-pituitary disease manifesting the clinical features of the syndrome.[233,234] These include patients with a history of organic hypothalamic-pituitary dysfunction, cranial irradiation, known childhood-onset GHD, or traumatic brain injury.

Provocative Testing. The diagnosis of adult GHD is established by provocative testing of GH secretion (Table 8-4). Patients should receive adequate replacement for other pituitary hormonal deficits before testing. Provocative tests include the insulin tolerance test (ITT), arginine, glucagon, clonidine, growth hormone–releasing peptide (GHRP), (GURP), and GHRH, alone or in combination with arginine or pyridostigmine. GHRPs are synthetic analogs of ghrelin. Because provocative tests vary in their ability to evoke GH release, a single value cannot be applied as a diagnostic threshold across different tests (Fig. 8-17).[258] ITT is a more potent stimulator of GH release than arginine, clonidine, or L-dopa, and combinations such as arginine plus GHRH, or GHRP plus GHRH are more potent than ITT alone.[178,259,260]

The ITT is the gold standard test for GHD. Normal subjects respond to insulin-induced hypoglycemia with peak GH concentrations of more than 5 µg/L (Fig. 8-18).[261] Severe GHD is defined by a peak GH response to hypoglycemia of less than 3 µg/L.[235] These cutoff values have been defined with the use of GH assays employing polyclonal competitive RIAs.[235] The test is contraindicated in patients with a history or electrocardiographic evidence of ischemic heart disease and in patients with seizure disorders.

Alternative tests that have been validated for the diagnosis of GHD are GHRH plus arginine,[260] GHRH plus GHRP,[178,262] and glucagon.[263] The diagnostic thresholds for these tests are shown in Table 8-4. The ITT evaluates the integrity of the hypothalamic-pituitary axis and has the added advantage of stimulating ACTH secretion. Diagnostic tests employing GHRH or GHRP, both of which directly stimulate GH release from the pituitary gland, may not effectively diagnose GHD caused by hypothalamic disease.[264] This is exemplified by studies in patients treated with cranial irradiation, for whom the ITT showed the greatest sensitivity and specificity within the first 5 years after irradiation.[265] If peak GH levels are normal during a GHRH plus arginine test in a patient who has received radiation therapy, then an ITT should also be performed. In irradiated patients and in those with inflammatory/infiltrative parasellar lesions, GHD may develop many years after the initial insult. This group of patients should undergo long-term monitoring, with repeat testing as clinically indicated. Obesity is a potential confounder in the diagnostic testing of GHD because it is associated with blunted peak GH responses.[266] Reference ranges adjusted for body mass index are available for validating results of the combined arginine-GHRH test.[267]

Growth Hormone–Responsive Markers. Growth hormone–responsive markers include IGF1, IGF binding protein 3 (IGFBP3), and the acid-labile subunit of the IGFBP complex. Serum IGF1 concentrations are useful for diagnosis only when age-adjusted normal ranges are used. Although IGF1 levels are reduced in adult GHD, a normal concentration does not exclude the diagnosis.[261] A subnormal IGF1 level in an adult patient with coexisting pituitary hormone deficits is strongly suggestive of GHD, particularly in the absence of conditions known to reduce IGF1 levels, such as malnutrition, liver disease, poorly controlled diabetes mellitus, and hypothyroidism. The separation of IGF1 values between GH-deficient and normal subjects is greatest in the young. As IGF1 levels decline with aging in normal subjects, IGF1 measurements become less reliable as a biochemical marker of GHD, and in patients older than 50 years, the values merge with those of normal age-matched subjects.[268] Measurement of IGFBP3 or the acid-labile subunit does not offer any advantage over that of IGF1.[233,234]

In patients with organic hypothalamic-pituitary disease, the prevalence of GHD is strongly linked to the number of pituitary hormone deficits, ranging from approximately 25% to 40% in those with no other deficit to 95% to 100% when more than three pituitary hormone deficiencies are present.[269] Patients with three or more pituitary hormone

TABLE 8-4

Validated Stimulation Tests for the Diagnosis of GH Deficiency in Adults

Test	No. Subjects (Normal/ Deficient)	GH Threshold (µg/L)	Reference No.
Insulin-induced hypoglycemia*	35/23	<5	261
Arginine-GHRH*	74/49	<9	260
GHRP6-GHRH*	125/125	<15	178
GHRP2-GHRH*	30/36	<17	262
GHRP2	77/58	<15	510
Glucagon*	46/73	<3	263

*Recommended by the Growth Hormone Research Society and the Endocrine Society.

GH, growth hormone; GHRH, growth hormone–releasing hormone; GHRP, growth hormone–releasing peptide.

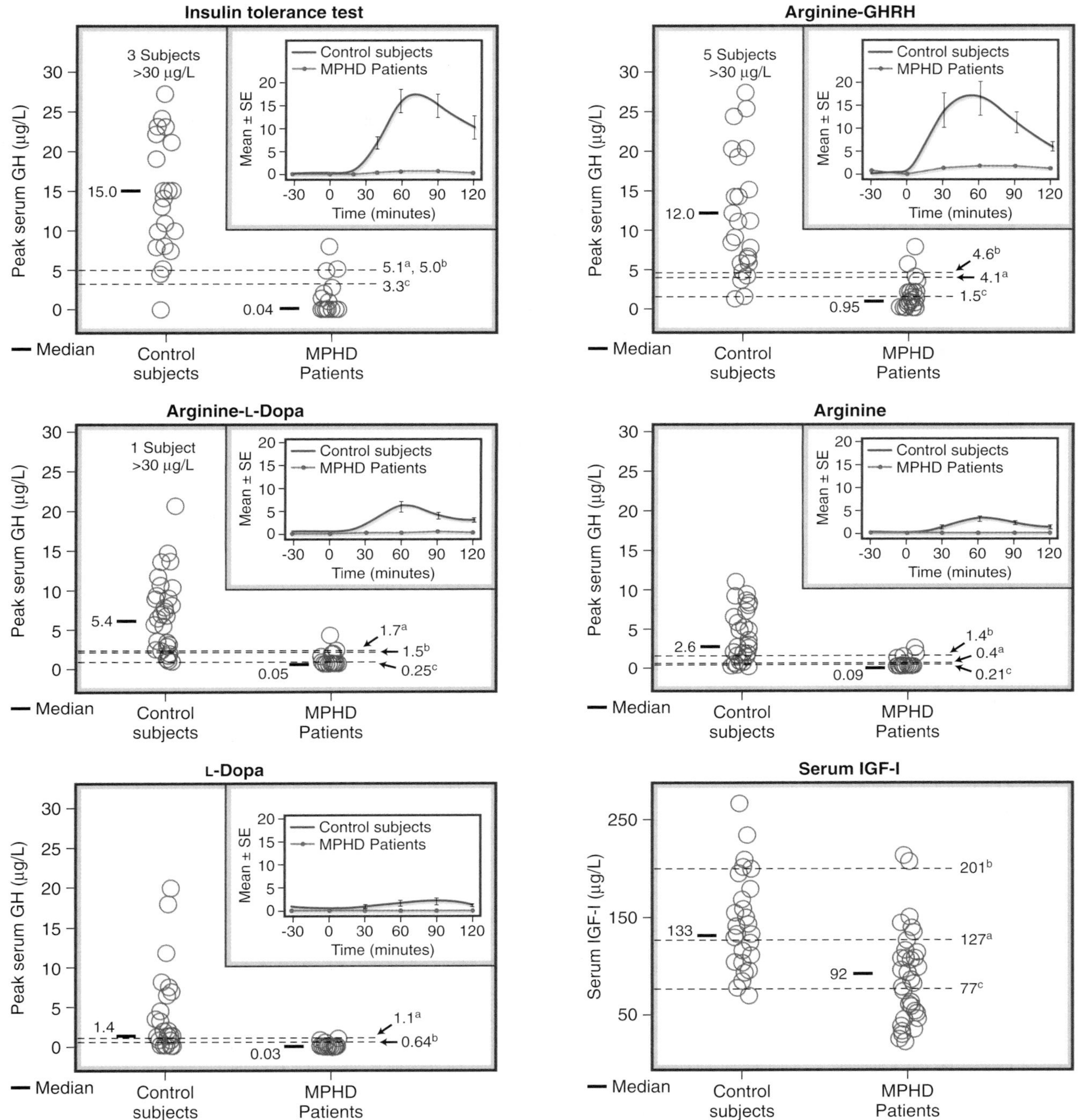

Figure 8-17 Effect of various growth hormone (GH) secretagogues on GH in patients with 0 or 1 deficiency in a pituitary hormone. GHRH, growth hormone–releasing hormone; IGF-1, insulin-like growth factor 1; MPHD, multiple pituitary hormone deficiency. (Reprinted with permission from Biller MK, Samuels MH, Zagar A, et al. Sensitivity and specificity of six tests for the diagnosis of growth hormone deficiency. *J Clin Endocrinol Metab.* 2002;87:2067, 2002.)

deficiencies and an IGF1 level lower than the reference range have a greater than 97% chance of being GH deficient (see Fig. 8-17)[270] and therefore do not require GH stimulation testing.[233,234]

Spontaneous Secretion of Growth Hormone. Because pituitary GH secretion occurs episodically, accurate quantification of integrated GH secretion requires continuous measurement of secretion over 24 hours. This procedure requires insertion of a continuous withdrawal pump or a patent indwelling catheter for frequent sampling with unrestricted food intake and physical activity. Although it is cumbersome and expensive, this method eliminates the error of isolated peak or trough measurements that might otherwise be obtained by single or multiple random GH samplings. Continuous 24-hour GH measurement in the diagnosis of GHD is not superior to provocative testing (see Fig. 8-18).[261]

Urinary Growth Hormone Measurement. Immunoassay methods for urinary GH measurement do not reliably reflect pharmacologic GH testing and do not adequately discriminate between normal and abnormal GH secretion.[271]

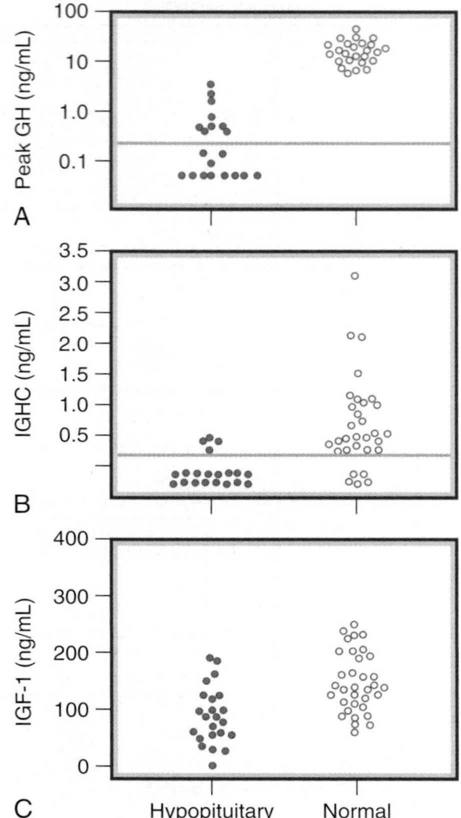

Figure 8-18 **A,** Comparison of peak growth hormone (GH) concentration obtained during an insulin tolerance test, **B,** integrated GH concentration (IGHC) obtained from blood samples withdrawn every 20 minutes over 24 hours, and, **C,** insulin-like growth factor I (IGF-1) concentrations in patients with organic hypopituitarism and sex-matched normal subjects. The horizontal lines represent the limit of reading. (Modified from Hoffman DM, O'Sullivan AJ, Baxter RC, et al. Diagnosis of growth hormone deficiency in adults. *Lancet.* 1994;343:1064-1068.)

Growth Hormone Assays. Plasma GH is measured by RIA (polyclonal or monoclonal) or by IRMA (dual monoclonal), but comparative GH measurements obtained using 11 commercial immunoassays varied by a factor of 3.[272] Measured GH concentrations are antibody dependent, and different antibodies bind to a heterogeneous spectrum of GH isoforms.[273] Furthermore, GH isoform patterns vary among individuals, and all circulating GH forms are not routinely detectable in GH assays, adding further difficulty to comparison of results from different GH immunoassays. Monomeric 22-kd GH1, the most abundant circulating form, is the only GH standard of sufficient purity and quantity, and it is used as the basis for GH measurement; however, it accounts for only about 25% of circulating immunoreactivity.[274] Other GH forms are recognized to varying to largely unknown degrees. Polyclonal antibodies, used in earlier RIAs, recognized several molecular forms of GH; newer immunometric assays employ highly specific monoclonal antibodies.[275]

GH standards also affect comparison of GH values. In 1994, the first World Health Organization (WHO) International Standard for Somatotropin (IRP 88/624)[276] used recombinant technology, in contrast to previous standards prepared from pituitary extracts. GHBPs may also interfere because approximately 50% of GH is complexed to GHBP. Noncompetitive immunometric assays may lead to low estimates of GH. In competitive assays employing antibodies directed against GH molecular epitopes that bind GHBP, spuriously high GH values may be reported.[277] The heterogeneity of GH immunoassay results poses a challenge in the definition of accepted standards for diagnosis of GHD. However, the RIA is now infrequently used, and clinicians should be aware of the nature of the GH assay employed and how values compare to those previously obtained by polyclonal RIA. New GH assays based on measurement of GH bioactivity have been developed, including the eluted stain assay (ESTA) and the immunofunctional assay (IFA). The growth hormone exclusion assay (GHEA) also measures circulating GH isoforms.[275]

Growth Hormone Replacement Therapy. The effects of GH replacement were first reported in 1989; since then, studies lasting up to 10 years have reported sustained benefits on substrate metabolism, body composition, and physical function.[278,279]

GH replacement induces profound effects on protein, fat, and energy metabolism, resulting in increased lean body mass and decreased fat mass without a significant change in body weight (Figs. 8-19 through 8-23).[280] The greatest reduction of body fat occurs in abdominal and

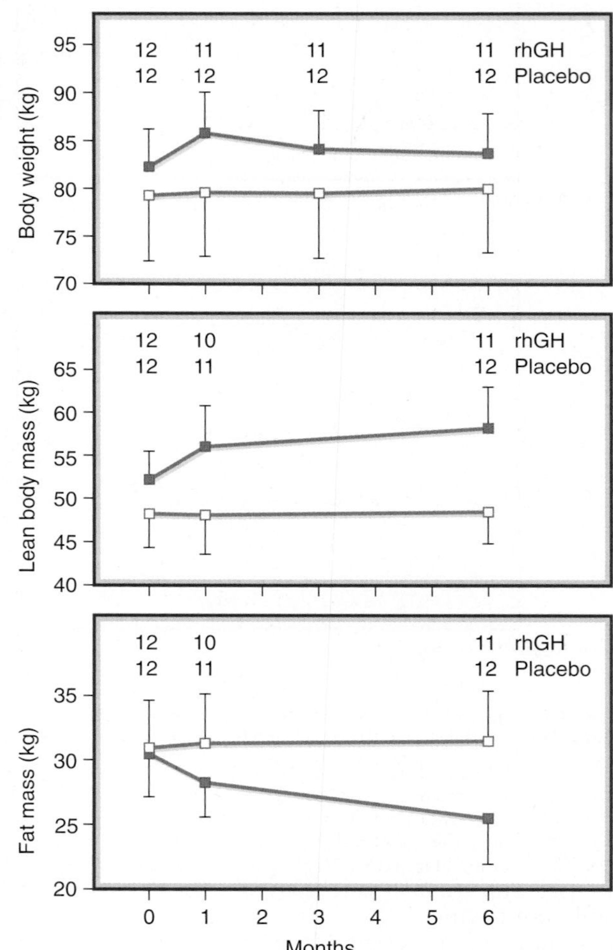

Figure 8-19 Effects of recombinant human growth hormone (rhGH) replacement on lean body mass and fat mass in adults with GH deficiency. (Reproduced with permission from Salomon F, Cuneo RC, Hesp R, et al. The effects of treatment with recombinant human growth hormone on body composition and metabolism in adults with growth hormone deficiency. *N Engl J Med.* 1989;321:1797-1803.)

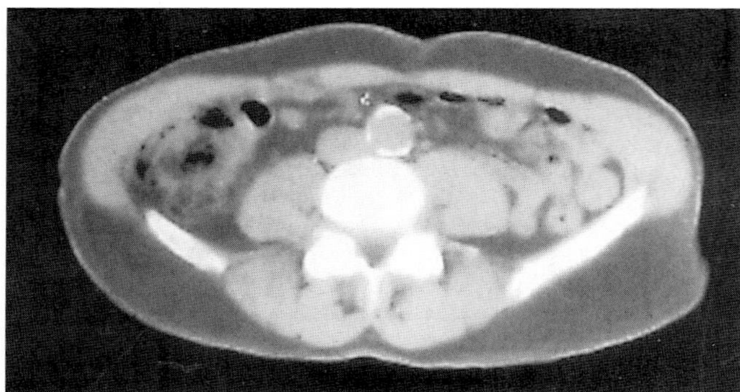

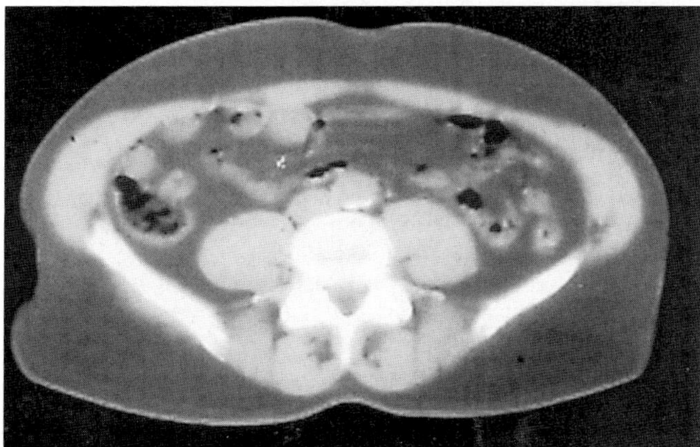

Figure 8-20 Computed tomographic scan through the abdomen before *(top)* and after treatment with human growth hormone (hGH) *(bottom)* in a GH-deficient patient. (Figures provided by B.A. Bengtsson.)

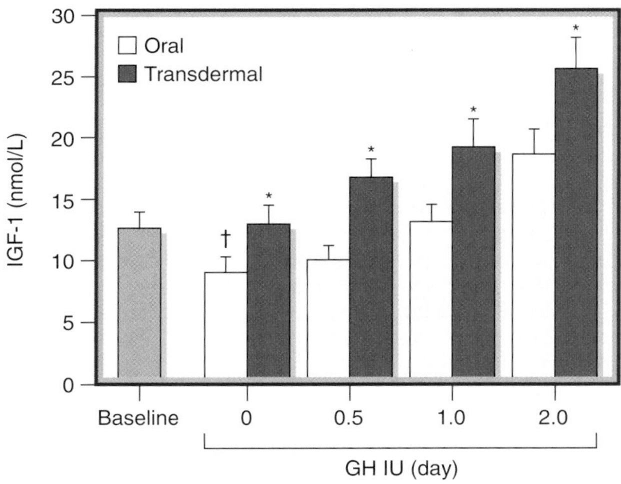

Figure 8-21 Mean concentrations of insulin-like growth factor I (IGF-I) before and during incremental doses of growth hormone (GH)—0.5, 1.0, and 2.0 IU/day, equivalent to approximately 0.25 to 1.0 mg daily—during oral and transdermal estrogen therapy in eight GH-deficient women. (From Wolthers T, Hoffman DM, Nugent AG, et al. Oral estrogen therapy impairs the metabolic effects of growth hormone (GH) in GH deficient women. *Am J Physiol.* 2001;281:E1191-E1196.)

visceral adipose tissue.[281] Significant increases in extracellular water also occur as a consequence of the dose-dependent antinatriuretic properties of GH.[282] GH replacement increases bone density,[283] which is accompanied by activation of both bone formation and bone resorption.[284] Initial studies reporting changes in bone mineral density (BMD) during 6 to 12 months of treatment yielded conflicting results. However, studies reporting long-term results have shown a progressive increase in BMD beyond 12 to 18 months of treatment,[283] reaching a plateau after 3 years. GH-induced reduction in abdominal and visceral fat is accompanied by a significant shift of lipoprotein metabolism to a less atherogenic profile. Most studies report an improvement in cholesterol levels and in HDL-cholesterol ratio with little or no change in triglycerides.[227] The favorable effects of improving the lipoprotein profile are more evident after treatment for more than a year. GH treatment reduces intimal media thickness of the carotid arteries.[250] Pro-inflammatory factors such as C-reactive protein and IL-6, strongly implicated in the pathogenesis of vascular disease, fall significantly with GH treatment.[248]

GH replacement improves exercise capacity and performance in parallel with an increase in maximal oxygen uptake[285,286] and in cardiac output and diastolic function.[287,288] Several but not all studies have reported improved muscle strength. Quadriceps or hip muscle strength improves significantly after 6 months of treatment,[285] but muscle strength normalized after 2 years, without further significant change at 5 years.[289]

The effects on quality of life are less clear. Some[290] but not all studies have reported improved energy, mood, and quality of life. Discrepant results may relate to the varying study tools used, including generic health questionnaires on perceived health status and subjective well-being and those developed specifically for patients with GHD. Disease-specific tools have reported unequivocal improvement in measures of life satisfaction after GH treatment.[290] A large survey in 304 patients showed improved quality of life and also significant reduction in the numbers of sick leave and doctor visits during 12 months of GH therapy.[291] A latency period up to 3 months is required before patients recognize benefits of hGH replacement, and these benefits are most obvious in those patients with the most profound symptoms and signs of GHD.[292]

Growth Hormone Administration

GH secretion is greater in the young, and greater in women than in men. It is recommended that the starting dose of GH should be 0.2 mg/day in young men, 0.3 mg/day in young women, and 0.1 mg/day in older individuals[234]; these doses are then titrated according to serum IGF1 concentrations and at a rate that minimizes side effects (see Fig. 8-23).[293] If side effects occur, the dose should be reduced, and if no side effects are reported, the therapeutic goal is to maintain IGF1 levels in the normal age- and gender-matched range while avoiding levels in the upper quintile or above. Dose determination based on body weight is not recommended due to large interindividual variation in absorption, insensitivity to GH, and lack of evidence that a larger replacement is required for heavier adults.[233] GH is administered by nightly subcutaneous injection to mimic the greater secretion of GH at night. Side effects of GH in children are considerably fewer than those observed in adults.

Women with GHD require higher doses of hGH if they are also receiving oral (rather than transdermal) estrogen[294-296] because of the first-pass hepatic effect. Fifty percent more GH was required during oral estrogen treatment to maintain an IGF1 level equivalent to that achieved during transdermal estrogen administration (see Fig.

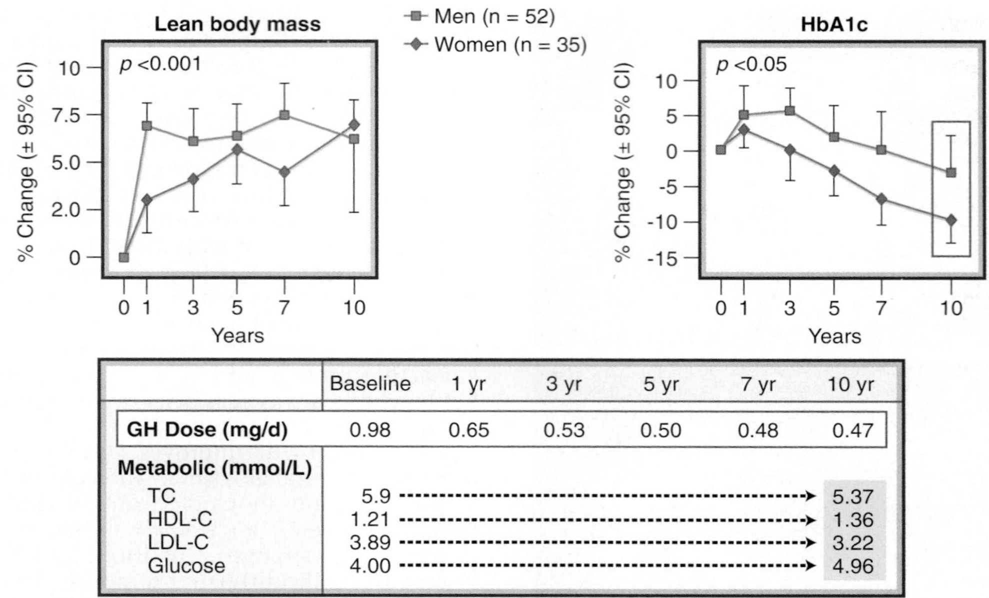

	Baseline	1 yr	3 yr	5 yr	7 yr	10 yr
GH Dose (mg/d)	0.98	0.65	0.53	0.50	0.48	0.47
Metabolic (mmol/L)						
TC	5.9					5.37
HDL-C	1.21					1.36
LDL-C	3.89					3.22
Glucose	4.00					4.96

Figure 8-22 Ten-year growth hormone (GH) therapy in 87 GH-deficient adults.[279] CI, confidence interval; HbA1c, hemoglobin A_{1c}; HDL-C, high-density lipoprotein-cholesterol; LDL-C, low-density lipoprotein-cholesterol; TC, total cholesterol. (Modified from Melmed S. Update in pituitary disease. *J Clin Endocrinol Metab.* 2008;93:331-338.)

8-21).[294] In contrast, androgens enhance metabolic effects of GH.[130] The divergent effects of estrogens and androgens on GH action are a likely explanation for the observation that women are less responsive than men to GH.[297]

Precautions and Caveats of Treating with Human Growth Hormone

The most common side effects of hGH replacement include edema, arthralgias, and myalgias (Table 8-5). However, these symptoms are mild and dose related, and they resolve in most patients spontaneously or with dosage reduction.[293] Although GH antagonizes insulin action, the risk of developing hyperglycemia is very low (see Fig. 8-22). None of 166 patients developed diabetes in an Australian study,[298] and insulin sensitivity did not change after 7 years of GH treatment.[299] A meta-analysis of 13 placebo-controlled trials involving 511 patients found a mean elevation in fasting blood glucose of 0.22 mmol/L compared with placebo levels.[227] Nevertheless, glucose should be monitored, especially in patients who are also being treated for diabetes.

Patients with active malignancies should not be treated with GH. The possibility that hGH might initiate new cancers or stimulate growth of preexisting benign tumors is an important theoretical issue. An epidemiologic association between higher, albeit normal, IGF1 levels and later risk of developing prostate cancer in men,[300] breast cancer in premenopausal women,[301] and colon and lung cancer[302] has been reported. In contrast, patients with acromegaly, who have very high serum levels of IGF1, do not have an increased incidence of breast or prostate cancer or of cancer in general. In fact, the overall risk for cancer in acromegaly is lower than expected. However, these patients have a significantly increased mortality from colon cancer.[303-305]

Analysis of the extensive pediatric experience shows no convincing evidence for a causal link between GH treatment and tumor recurrence or the development of neoplasm including leukemia.[306,307] When comparing the relative risk of brain tumor recurrence in 180 children treated with hGH versus 891 who did not receive hGH, the risk of recurrence after a mean of 6.4 years was lower in the treated group than in those not receiving hGH.[308] GH treatment does, however, increases the risk of radiation-induced second tumor, especially meningiomas.[309] Nevertheless, long-term surveillance with adequate control groups and avoidance of high IGF1 levels in adults being treated for adult GHD are required to ensure that adult GH replacement does not increase the incidence of new cancers or growth of existing benign tumors.

Investigational Uses of Growth Hormone

Catabolic States. The well-recognized anabolic actions of GH have prompted its use in catabolic states including surgery, trauma, burns, parenteral nutrition, and organ failure. These potential indications for GH are not approved in the United States. The negative nitrogen balance in critically ill patients is partly attributable to GH resistance and decreased IGF1 production and action.[310] GH administered to postsurgical patients and to normal subjects receiving hypocaloric intravenous alimentation resulted in reversion to positive nitrogen balance.

Beneficial effects of GH have been reported in patients with extensive burns, in those receiving chronic high-dose glucocorticoid treatment, in those with chronic obstructive pulmonary disease, in cancer patients, and in patients with cardiac failure. Nevertheless, published end points for these studies have not been definitive. When GH was administered to elderly malnourished patients, it was found to be an effective adjuvant for dietary augmentation.[311] A study in which critically ill patients received very high doses of GH (up to 7 mg/day) was prematurely terminated due to enhanced unexplained mortality.[312] It has been suggested that GH may have had an adverse effect on acute phase protein synthesis in these patients.[313] Caution is advised for nonapproved uses of GH in adults.[314]

Osteoporosis. GH has been administered to otherwise healthy subjects with idiopathic osteoporosis in an attempt to decrease bone loss. A 2-year study in osteoporotic women

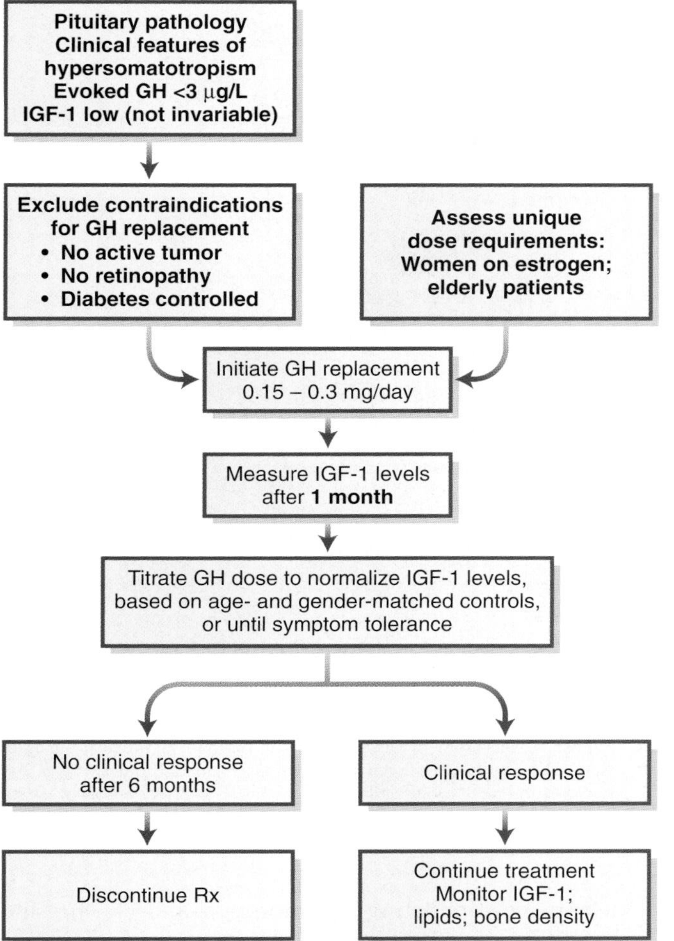

Figure 8-23 Management of somatotropin deficiency in adults. Patients older than 60 years require lower maintenance doses. Women receiving transdermal estrogen require lower doses than those receiving oral estrogen preparations. GH, growth hormone; IGF-1, insulin-like growth factor 1; Rx, treatment.

showed that GH together with calcitonin increased spine and total hip bone mineral density,[315] although the response was less marked than that observed with estrogen or bisphosphonate therapy. A double-blind, placebo-controlled treatment study for 18 months observed improvements in bone mineral content at the lumbar spine, in the femoral neck, and of the whole skeleton by up to 14%, and these improvements were sustained at 4 years.[316] There was a delayed, extended, and dose-dependent effect of GH. These striking findings provide evidence for consideration of GH as a therapeutic option for osteoporosis in the menopause. Unclear long-term side effects and lack of comparative studies with other beneficial therapies for osteoporosis necessitate the need for further study of potential use of GH in treating osteoporosis.

TABLE 8-5

Side Effects of Adult GH Treatment

Edema
Arthralgias
Myalgias
Muscle stiffness
Paresthesias
Carpal tunnel syndrome
Atrial fibrillation
Headache
Benign intracranial hypertension
Increase in melanocytic nevi
Hyperglycemia
Iatrogenic acromegaly

Human Immunodeficiency Virus Infection. GH is approved by the U.S. Food and Drug Administration for adult patients with HIV-associated cachexia, and treatment results in positive nitrogen balance, increased lean body mass, decreased body fat, and improved work output.[317] Ten HIV-infected subjects with fat redistribution syndrome associated with protease inhibitor therapy received GH 6 mg/day subcutaneously for 12 weeks and showed decreased weight-hip ratios and enhanced midthigh circumference.[318,319] One large study using supraphysiologic GH doses of 4 mg/day reported impairment in glucose tolerance.[320] A more recent study using a physiologic dosing approach to maintain IGF1 in the high-normal range reported body compositional changes of lesser magnitude, no changes in HDL or LDL cholesterol, and no adverse changes in fasting glucose or insulin.[321] However, long-term beneficial effects of GH on survival and quality of life in HIV infection have not yet been reported.

Sports. The public policy issues regarding GH abuse in competitive sports have received much attention. GH has been widely abused by athletes to enhance performance.[322] Whether persistent GH use is accompanied by increased muscle strength is unclear. A systematic review concluded that claims of GH enhancement of physical performance are not supported by the scientific literature evaluating effects on aerobic capacity, strength, and power[323] and that more research is needed to conclusively determine the effects of GH on athletic performance. A recent double-blind, placebo-controlled study reported that GH enhances sprint capacity, but not aerobic capacity, strength, or power, in recreational athletes.[324]

Aging. There has been considerable interest in the use of GH as an anti-aging hormone to prevent the body composition changes and physical decline of the aging process that superficially recapitulate features of adults with organic GHD for which beneficial effects of GH replacement have been demonstrated. A systematic review of literature published on randomized, controlled trials in healthy elderly subjects indicated that GH supplementation is associated with small changes in body composition, no functional benefit, and increased rates of adverse events. On the basis of the evidence, GH cannot be recommended as an anti-aging therapy.[325] GH is increasingly marketed and distributed for anti-aging therapy under "off-label" use. Off-label marketing of GH as anti-aging therapy is not approved by the FDA in the United States.[314]

Adrenocorticotropic Hormone

Physiology

The hypothalamic-pituitary-adrenal (HPA) axis plays a critical role in maintaining homeostasis and in mounting an appropriate response to stress. Key components of the stress response are aimed at providing adequate amounts of glucocorticoids that exert vital pleiotropic effects on energy supply, fuel metabolism, immunity, and cardiovascular function.

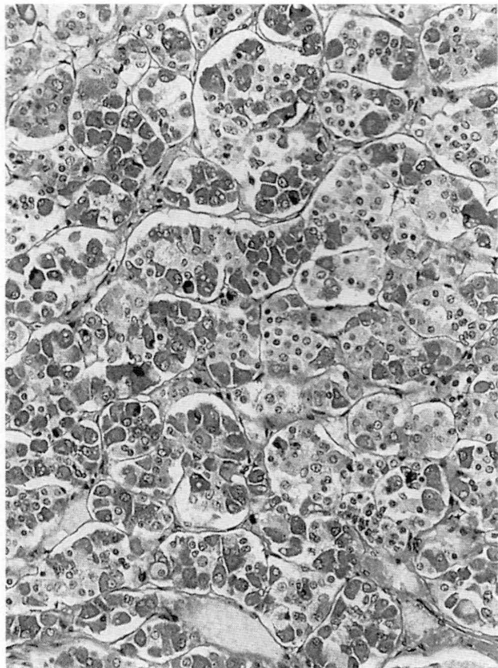

Figure 8-24 Corticotroph cell. The periodic acid–Schiff stain documents the presence of corticotrophs in the normal pituitary, reflecting glycosylation of the ACTH peptide. Some cells have clear cytoplasmic vacuoles corresponding to the so-called enigmatic body. ACTH, corticotropin. (From Asa SL. Tumors of the pituitary gland. In: Rosai J, ed. *Atlas of Tumor Pathology*, Series III, Fascicle 22. Washington, DC: Armed Forces Institute of Pathology, 1997:21.)

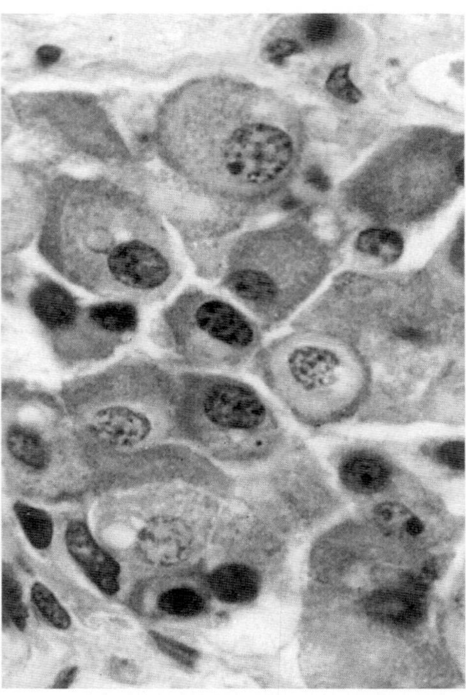

Figure 8-25 Crooke's hyalinization. Pituitary corticotrophs subjected to glucocorticoid excess develop cytoplasmic hyalinization that displaces ACTH-positive secretory material to the cell periphery. The clear vacuoles correspond to complex lysosomes known as enigmatic bodies. (From Asa SL. Tumors of the pituitary gland. In: Rosai J, ed. *Atlas of Tumor Pathology*, Series III, Fascicle 22. Washington, DC: Armed Forces Institute of Pathology, 1997:23.)

Corticotroph Cells. Corticotroph cells comprise about 20% of functional anterior pituitary cells and are the earliest detectable human fetal pituitary cell type, appearing by the 8th week of gestation. Corticotrophs are clustered mainly in the central median pituitary wedge. They are large, irregular cells, and their ultrastructural features include prominent neurosecretory granules (150-400 nm), endoplasmic reticulum, and Golgi bodies (Fig. 8-24).[326] These cells produce the POMC gene products, including ACTH(1-39), β-lipotropin, and endorphins. Because of the rich carbohydrate moiety of these molecules, the cells are strongly positive for periodic acid–Schiff (PAS) staining. In the presence of excess glucocorticoid, characteristic hyaline deposits develop (Fig. 8-25). In normal human pituitary, POMC is expressed only in corticotroph cells. Most mammals possess an intermediate lobe comprising POMC-expressing melanotroph cells, but this lobe is not developed in adult humans. TPIT has been identified[31] as a critical transcriptional factor for corticotroph cell differentiation during pituitary development and for transcription of the POMC gene.

Structure. POMC is the precursor for ACTH, which acts on the adrenal glands to induce synthesis and secretion of adrenal steroids. The primary translation product of POMC is a 266-amino-acid pre-prohormone molecule encoding corticotrophic, opioid, and melanotrophic peptides. The peptide contains a leader sequence and multiple dibasic proteolytic cleavage sites for glycosylation, acetylation, and amidation. Products of this processing include ACTH(1-39) and β-lipotropin, which in turn give rise to α-lipotropin and β-endorphin, also containing metenkephalin. ACTH itself may also be cleaved to a form of α-melanocyte-stimulating hormone, α-MSH(1-13), and corticotropin-like intermediate lobe peptide, CLIP(18-39).

The 8-kb human POMC gene, located on chromosome 2p23,[31,327] consists of three exons interspersed with two intervening introns (Fig. 8-26). The first exon encodes a leader sequence, the second exon encodes the signal initiation sequence and the N-terminal portion of the POMC peptide, and the third exon encodes most of the mature peptide sequences, including ACTH and β-lipotropin.[328] The POMC gene is expressed in pituitary and nonpituitary tissues including brain, skin, placenta, gonads, gastrointestinal tissues, liver, kidney, adrenal medulla, lung, and lymphocytes.

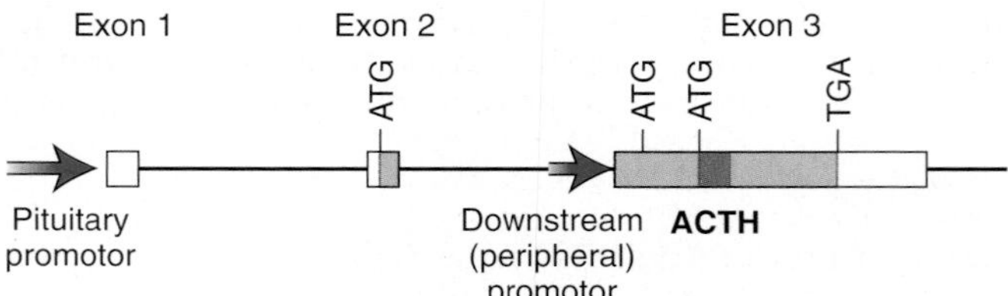

Figure 8-26 Structure of the POMC gene. Exon 1 encodes the RNA leader sequence. Exon 2 encodes the initiator methionine (ATG), the signal peptide, and several amino-terminal residues of the precursor peptide, the remainder of which is encoded by exon 3. Corticotroph expression is determined by the upstream "pituitary" promoter *(longer arrowhead)*, whereas peripheral expression of the short POMC mRNA is determined by the "downstream" promoter *(shorter arrowhead)*. Translation of these shorter transcripts initiates from the initiator methionines (ATG) indicated in exon 3. The precursor peptide coding region is lightly shaded, and the ACTH coding region is darkly shaded. (Reproduced from Adrian JL, Clark AJL, Swords FM. Molecular pathology of corticotroph function. In Rappaport R, Amselem S, eds. *Hypothalamic-Pituitary Development*. Basel, Switzerland: Karger; 2001.)

In corticotroph cells, a pituitary-selective promoter region for POMC generates a POMC messenger RNA (mRNA) transcript of approximately 1200 nucleotides. The 800 nucleotides of the coding region are translated into a pre-POMC molecule that includes a 26-amino-acid signal peptide that is rapidly cleaved. The parent POMC protein of 241 amino acids enters the secretory pathway for subsequent processing (see later discussion).

In extrapituitary tissues, POMC gene expression is quantitatively and qualitatively different from that in the pituitary. An upstream promoter generates a longer transcript (approximately 1350 nucleotides). A downstream promoter generates short truncated transcripts of approximately 800 nucleotides that arise from the 5′ end of exon 3. In the brain, however, neurons in the arcuate nucleus express POMC mRNA that is identical to that of the pituitary.[329] In these neurons, POMC serve as a precursor to brain β-endorphin, α-MSH, and other peptides that have important brain functions including a major role in energy homeostasis.

Transcriptional Regulation

Elements of the promoter regions mediate POMC regulation by glucocorticoids, cAMP, AP1, and STAT signaling molecules.[330]

Multiple signals act in synergy to activate POMC gene expression, including corticotropin-releasing hormone (CRH), cytokines, vasopressin, catecholamines, and VIP. Glucocorticoids inhibit POMC gene expression. The CRH type 1 receptor (CRH-R1) is predominantly expressed on the corticotroph,[331] and its activation increases cAMP, protein kinase A, and CREB induction of CRH-binding protein (CRHBP) to the promoter, leading to POMC transcription.[332]

CRH also activates an AP1 site within the first exon by a MAP kinase–mediated pathway. In addition to mediating ACTH secretion, this receptor also appears to be critical for fear and anxiety responses, possibly through a related ligand, urocortin.[333]

The CRH-R2 is predominantly important for cardiovascular function.[334] Leukemia inhibitory factor (LIF), a proinflammatory cytokine that is expressed in the pituitary and hypothalamus, signals via the JAK/STAT pathway and acts in synergy with CRH to potentiate POMC expression.[335] This mechanism of immunoneuroendocrine interfacing facilitates stimulation of ACTH secretion by inflammation-derived STAT-inducing cytokines.

Glucocorticoid receptor activation leads to transcriptional suppression via two cooperative binding sites. The intracellular glucocorticoid receptor binds directly to 5′-regulatory elements to suppress POMC transcription.[329] CRH action is also potentiated by vasopressin (acting via phospholipase C) and β-adrenergic catecholamines, which enhance POMC mRNA levels, increase ACTH secretion, or both. The net effect of these intracellular signals is the regulation of POMC gene transcription, peptide synthesis, and ACTH secretion for mediating appropriate neuroendocrine responses.[330]

POMC Processing. Several post-translational POMC modification steps are required for polypeptide hormone secretion (Fig. 8-27). First, the N-terminal signal sequence is removed, and this is followed by glycosylation via an *O*-linkage to Thr45 and *N*-linkage to Asn65.[336] Serine-phosphorylation then occurs within the Golgi apparatus. After being transported to secretory vesicles, the constituent peptides are cleaved at dibasic amino acid residues, and ACTH-related peptides are stored in dense secretory granules for ultimate regulated release. Some POMC products also undergo C-terminal amidation mediated by peptidylglycine-amidating monooxygenase (PAM) and peptidylhydroxyglycine-amidating lyase (PAL),[337] and N-terminal acetylation.

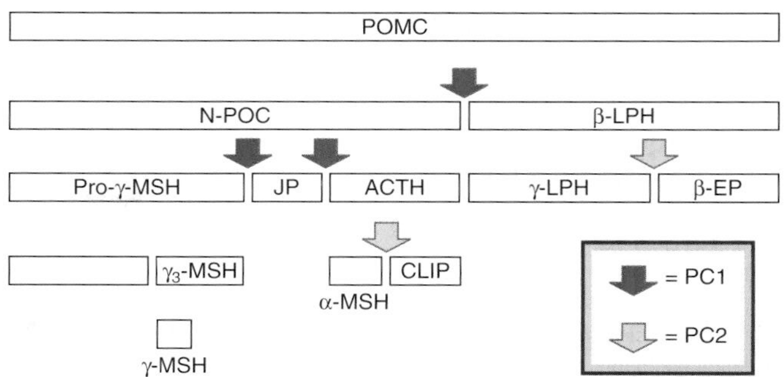

Figure 8-27 Processing and cleavage of pro-opiomelanocortin (POMC). The mature POMC precursor peptide is sequentially cleaved by prohormone convertase 1 (PC1) in the anterior pituitary corticotroph. In the neurointermediate lobe and other cell types, cleavage by PC2 allows release of β-MSH or β-endorphin (β-EP) or both. Carboxypeptidase H (not shown) removes residual basic amino acids at cleavage sites. ACTH, adrenocorticotropic hormone; CLIP, corticotropin-like intermediate lobe peptide; JP, joining peptide; EP, endorphin; LPH, lipotropin; MSH, melanocyte-stimulating hormone; N-POC, N-terminal pro-POMC fragment. (Reproduced from Clark AJL, Swords FM, Molecular pathology of corticotroph function. In: Rappaport R, Amselem S, eds. *Hypothalamic-pituitary development.* Basel, Switzerland: Karger; 2001.)

POMC proteolytic processing occurs at Lys-Arg or Arg-Arg residues by enzymes called *prohormone convertases* (PCs), which are a superfamily of subtilisin/kexin proteinases. They play a critical role in determining the manifestation and function of the peptides at the tissue level through site-specific cleavages. PC1 is most abundant in the pituitary and hypothalamus, whereas PC2 is present in the central nervous system, skin, and pancreatic islets but is absent in the pituitary. In corticotrophs, PC1 expression results in cleavage limited to four sites, with ACTH being a major end product (see Fig. 8-27). In the hypothalamus and central nervous system, the presence of both PC1 and PC2 allows coordinated proteolysis, resulting in the generation of smaller fragments such as α-, β-, and γ-MSH and CLIP. Heterozygous mutations of the PC1 gene have been associated with childhood obesity, adrenal insufficiency, hyperproinsulinemia, and postprandial hypoglycemia[338] with elevated levels of plasma ACTH precursors.

Biologic Actions of POMC-Derived Peptides

POMC products in blood are derived from corticotrophs and are secreted in equimolar amounts. However, circulating concentrations differ in accordance with the half-life of each molecule.

Adrenal Action. Full-length ACTH is the only POMC-derived peptide with adrenocorticotroph function, and it is the ligand of the melanocortin receptor type 2 receptor (MC2R). MC2R activation results in production of adrenal glucocorticoids, androgenic steroids, and, to a lesser extent, mineralocorticoids. There is evidence that the N-terminal peptide, POMC(1-28), exerts an independent mitogenic and growth-sustaining effect on the adrenal gland.[339]

Skin Pigmentation. Melanocyte stimulation occurs through activation of MC1R. ACTH, β-lipotropin (β-LPH), and γ-LPH produced from the corticotroph share a common heptapeptide sequence (Met-Glu-His-Phe-Arg-Trp-Gly) that is required to activate MC1R. These peptides are responsible for inducing skin pigmentation in Addison's disease because the other melanostimulating peptides, α-MSH and β-MSH, are not produced in the pituitary. There is also evidence for a paracrine system regulating skin pigmentation. Local production of ACTH and α-MSH occurs in melanocytes and keratinocytes and is stimulated by cytokines and ultraviolet irradiation in parallel with PC1 and PC2 expression.[340]

Appetite Regulation. POMC-derived peptides, and in particular α-MSH, play a critical role in the central regulation of appetite. The melanocortin system mediates feedback suppression of appetite by leptin through activation of MC3R and MC4R by α-MSH in the hypothalamus. Genetic and pharmacologic abrogation of the melanocortin system causes profound obesity. POMC-deficient mice and humans are hyperphagic, whereas intraventricular infusion of α-MSH or synthetic agonists induces weight loss.[341,342]

Immune Modulation. α-MSH influences the inflammatory process by modulating the function of antigen-presenting cells and T cells. It suppresses fever induced by IL-6 and inhibits macrophage function and leukocyte migration.[343]

Analgesia. β-Endorphin is produced by corticotrophs, and circulating concentrations may be high in Addison's disease. The peptide exerts a potent analgesic effect through opiate receptors. These are unlikely to be of physiologic significance because the peptide does not cross the blood-brain barrier.

Placenta-Derived POMC Peptides. Full-length pituitary-like POMC mRNA is expressed in human placenta along with ACTH, LPH, endorphin, and α-MSH. Intact POMC is not detectable in the nonpregnant state but becomes measurable in early gestation, rising 3- to 10-fold in the second trimester, plateauing thereafter, and returning to prepregnancy levels within 3 days after delivery.[344] The physiologic function of this placental molecule is unknown, and blood levels do not correlate with those of ACTH or cortisol, both of which also increase during pregnancy.

Ectopic Synthesis of ACTH

POMC is also expressed in the gonads, lung, skin, gastrointestinal and adrenal medullary neuroendocrine cells, and white blood cells. Nevertheless, the overwhelming source of circulating ACTH is derived from the anterior pituitary or from neuroendocrine tumor ectopic production. Nonpituitary tumors demonstrate a spectrum of altered POMC gene expression and processing. The ectopic ACTH syndrome occurs in tumors capable of generating high amounts of the pituitary-like 1072-nucleotide mRNA. Processing may not occur because of the lack of PC enzyme or may be abnormal, resulting in preferential generation of smaller fragments such as CLIP and β-MSH.[344] Small cell lung cancers preferentially release intact POMC, whereas carcinoid tumors tend to overprocess the precursor, releasing ACTH and smaller peptides.[344] Defective POMC processing indicates an impaired state of neuroendocrine differentiation in poorly differentiated tumors.

Extrapituitary neuroendocrine tumors associated with ectopic ACTH secretion do not process the prohormone efficiently because of a general defect in PC expression. Because ACTH is synthesized in nontumorous neuroendocrine cells, ectopic tumor hormone production may in fact reflect inappropriate ACTH processing. These patients also exhibit a higher ratio of circulating ACTH precursors and smaller peptides, including CLIP.

ACTH Regulation

The complex control of ACTH secretion patterns is critical for maintenance of adrenal cortex function and reflects the integrated neuroendocrine control of stress homeostasis. Essential metabolic and endocrine functions require a sensitively controlled, nonstress pattern of HPA axis function. This baseline pattern allows the axis to mount an appropriate stress response and to maintain a well-buffered reserve capacity to counteract life-threatening insults.

As with other anterior pituitary hormones, ACTH regulation is subserved by at least three tiers of control. First, the brain and hypothalamus release regulatory molecules (including CRH, vasopressin, and other peptides) that traverse the portal system and directly signal to corticotroph secretory and mitotic activity. Second, intrapituitary cytokines and growth factors act locally to regulate ACTH, either in concert with hypothalamic factors or independently. These paracrine controls often overlap and are redundant, and they have been shown to induce sensitive intracellular molecules that limit the ACTH response and prevent chronic ACTH hypersecretion.[344] Third, glucocorticoids maintain a potent feedback inhibition control of corticotroph secretion and replication. The HPA axis is inhibited by a long feedback inhibition, whereby cortisol rapidly inhibits hypothalamic CRH and pituitary ACTH. These effects may also be delayed 30 to 60 minutes by inhibition of ACTH release rather than synthesis,[345] especially after a single glucocorticoid bolus. After chronic glucocorticoid exposure (>24 hours), HPA suppression may persist for days or longer. In a short feedback loop, pituitary ACTH inhibits hypothalamic CRH, and in an ultrashort loop it may also suppress the corticotroph itself.

Stress Response. Both exogenous and endogenous stress stimuli activate the HPA axis to produce sufficient glucocorticoid in an attempt to counteract the insult. The HPA stress response occurs in the context of a wide variety of peripheral and central adaptors to stress, including vasovagal and catecholamine activation and cytokine secretion and action. A tightly controlled immuno-neuroendocrine interface regulates the ACTH response to peripheral stressors, which include pain, infection, inflammation, hemorrhage, hypovolemia, trauma, psychological stress, and hypoglycemia. These signals vary in their ability to generate ACTH secretion and to sensitize the glucocorticoid response to ACTH. In addition to CRH, peripheral and centrally released pro-inflammatory cytokines potently induce POMC transcription and ACTH secretion.[330] Sensitive intracellular signals within the corticotroph also serve to override the ACTH response to stress, thus preventing persistent and chronic hypercortisolemia.

Cytokines such as IL-6 and LIF activate the HPA axis and enhance glucocorticoid production, thus protecting the organism against lethality by constraining the inflammatory response.[335] Mice with inactivated CRH or LIF genes mount an inadequate neuroendocrine response to stress, inflammation, or endotoxins. During stress, glucocorticoid inhibition of ACTH is also prevented by activation of nuclear factor κB, which interferes with pituitary glucocorticoid receptor function, further exaggerating enhanced ACTH secretion.[346]

Exercise is a physiologic stimulus of ACTH release. Exercising to 90% of maximum oxygen capacity causes a significant elevation of ACTH, similar to levels observed during surgery or hypoglycemia.[347] Levels may remain elevated for up to 6 minutes after the cessation of exercise. Although lower-intensity exercise does not evoke ACTH,[348] well-trained athletes exhibit hypercortisolism, possibly because of decreased adrenal ACTH sensitivity.

Secretion. ACTH is secreted with both circadian periodicity and ultradian pulsatility under the control of the suprachiasmatic nucleus. This centrally controlled pattern is influenced by peripheral corticosteroids. The circadian pattern of ACTH secretion typically begins at about 4 a.m., peaking before 7 a.m., and both ACTH and adrenal steroid levels reach their nadir between 11 p.m. and 3 a.m. Within this overall 24-hour diurnal cycle, periodic ACTH secretory bursts occur at a frequency of 40 pulses per 24 hours; amplitude rather than frequency modulation contributes to diurnal changes in ACTH profile.[349,350]

ACTH circadian rhythm is entrained by visual cues and the light-dark cycle, and it is centrally controlled by CRH and other factors.[351] The mode of CRH signal determines ACTH response, with a continuous signal desensitizing the ACTH response and a pulsatile CRH signal restoring cortisol secretion without depleting the pituitary ACTH pool.[352] Daily ACTH but not cortisol secretion is higher in males, who also exhibit higher pulse frequency and higher peak amplitudes than females,[353] possibly reflecting gender-specific set points for cortisol feedback or a relative male adrenal insensitivity to ACTH. Endogenous and exogenous stress, including hypoglycemia, act centrally to increase ACTH pulse amplitude, whereas corticosteroids directly suppress basal or stimulated ACTH pulse amplitude.[354]

Action. ACTH is a polypeptide of 39 amino acids with a molecular weight of 4.5 kd. The highly conserved 12 N-terminal amino acid residues are critical for adrenal gland steroid synthesis. The primary action of ACTH is to maintain adrenal gland size, structure, and function; ACTH induces adrenal steroidogenesis by activating ACTH receptors situated on the adrenal cortex cell surface. ACTH signals via adenyl cyclase to regulate cytochrome P450 enzyme transcription, cortisol aldosterone (10%), 17-hydroxyprogesterone, and, to a lesser extent, synthesis and secretion of adrenal androgens.[355] ACTH stimulates mitochondrial cholesterol transport and regulates the rate-limiting side-chain cleavage of cholesterol to pregnenolone.[356] Secretory cortisol pulses follow ACTH pulses within 5 to 10 minutes, with a linear dose dependency that is especially evident after physiologic CRH stimulation.[357]

Adrenal cortisol response to ACTH is sensitive to the background ambient ACTH milieu. In states of chronic ACTH deficiency, adrenal reserve is compromised; during ongoing ACTH hypersecretion, the gland is primed such that a given ACTH bolus elicits a higher cortisol response. Both basal and stimulated (e.g., by CRH) ACTH secretion are blunted by glucocorticoids. Conversely, low or absent circulating glucocorticoids (e.g., after adrenalectomy) result in exaggerated ACTH secretion[358,359] and in corticotroph cell hyperplasia.[360]

Disorders of ACTH Secretion

ACTH Deficiency

Causes. Congenital ACTH deficiency may occur as an isolated pituitary defect or as a component of a wider spectrum of multiple pituitary hormone deficiencies. A mutation of TPIT, a transcription factor involved in corticotroph differentiation, has been identified as a cause of isolated ACTH deficiency.[31] Mutations of transcription factors involved in early stages of pituitary cell differentiation or midline brain development may also give rise to ACTH deficiency as a component of multiple hormone deficiencies. These include Lhx4 and HESX1 (Table 8-6). Secondary causes include pituitary tumors, sellar mass lesions, trauma, irradiation, and lymphocytic hypophysitis, which may be associated with other autoimmune manifestations (Table 8-7).

Clinical Features. The manifestations of ACTH deficiency are clinically indistinguishable from those of glucocorticoid deficiency from any cause. Glucocorticoids exert pleiotropic effects on metabolism, appetite, cardiovascular function, fluid homeostasis, and inflammation. The clinical features are dependent on the severity, time of onset, and clinical context. In the newborn, ACTH deficiency may manifest as hypoglycemia and failure to thrive. In the adult, there is slowly progressive weight and appetite loss, anorexia, and generalized fatigue mimicking a wasting syndrome. Because adrenal mineralocorticoid secretion is largely unimpaired, salt wasting, volume contraction, and hyperkalemia—features commonly encountered in Addison's disease—are not manifest. Hyperpigmentation, usually associated with exuberant ACTH-related peptide secretion in the face of adrenal damage, does not occur.

Evaluation. Diagnostic evaluation of adrenal insufficiency involves assessment of glucocorticoid status with concurrent measurement of ACTH. Morning serum cortisol levels lower than 3 µg/dL suggest ACTH deficiency, whereas basal morning cortisol levels greater than 18 µg/dL usually indicate normal ACTH reserve. Patients with ACTH deficiency have low to normal serum cortisol levels and low to normal plasma ACTH levels. Blunted responses to provocative tests such as insulin-induced hypoglycemia or metyrapone are required to document a partial deficiency. Fluctuating levels of cortisol-binding globulin (CBG) may confound interpretation of cortisol values. Cirrhosis and hyperthyroidism lower CBG and cortisol levels, whereas estrogens elevate CBG concentrations.

ACTH Excess

Causes. Excessive ACTH production can arise from a corticotroph adenoma or from an extrapituitary ectopic source. Small cell lung carcinomas, bronchial carcinoids, and neuroendocrine tumors are common causes of ectopic ACTH production.

Clinical Features. ACTH-induced adrenal hyperfunction causes a syndrome of hypercortisolism and androgen excess in women. Manifestations arise from appetite stimulation (weight gain), altered fat distribution (moon facies, buffalo hump, central obesity), catabolism (skin thinning, muscle wasting), mood disturbance (depression, anxiety), sodium retention (hypertension), and androgen excess (menstrual irregularity, hirsutism, acne, and oily skin). The evaluation and management of patients with Cushing's disease is fully described in Chapter 15.

Measurement of ACTH

RIA and IRMA assays employ antisera specifically directed against intact ACTH(1-39) or other POMC fragments. In general, the IRMA is more sensitive, reproducible, and rapid.[361] Most IRMAs have a sensitivity of less than 0.5 ng/L with precise variations of less than 10%. Intact ACTH or POMC precursor peptides are detectable, depending on the sequence specificity of the assay employed. Awareness of the assay peptide specificity may be especially critical when evaluating ectopic POMC products secreted by lung tumors. ACTH precursors are assessed by specific IRMA employing unique monoclonal antibodies to ACTH, N-POMC, β-LPH, or β-endorphin.[362]

Ideally, nonstressed resting subjects should have venous blood withdrawn between 6 a.m. and 9 a.m. Because ACTH is relatively unstable at room temperature and has a propensity to adhere to glass, plasma samples should immediately be separated in iced siliconized glass tubes containing

TABLE 8-6

Hereditary Pituitary Deficiency Caused by Transcription Factor Mutations*

Gene	Chromosome	Pituitary Deficiency	MRI Findings	Associated Malformations	Inheritance Mode
POU1F1†	3p11	GH, PRL, ± TSH	Normal or hypoplastic anterior pituitary		Recessive, dominant
PROP1‡	5q35	GH, PRL, TSH, LH, FSH, ± ACTH	Normal, hypoplastic, hyperplastic, or cystic anterior pituitary		Recessive
HESX1§	3p21	GH, PRL, TSH, LH, FSH, ACTH, posterior defects	Hypoplastic or hyperplastic anterior pituitary	Septo-optic dysplasia	Recessive
PITX2	4q25	GH, PRL, TSH, FSH, LH	Normal or ectopic posterior pituitary	Rieger syndrome	Dominant
LHX3	9q34	GH, PRL, TSH, LH, FSH	Hypoplastic or hyperplastic anterior pituitary	Stubby neck with rigid cervical spine	Recessive
LHX4	1q25	GH, TSH, ACTH	Hypoplastic anterior pituitary, ectopic posterior pituitary		Dominant
TPIT	1q23	ACTH	Normal		Recessive
OTX2		GH, TSH, ACTH	Hypoplastic anterior pituitary, ectopic posterior pituitary	Eye malformations	Dominant/Negative
SIX6	14q22		Hypoplastic pituitary, absent chiasm	Brachio-otorenal and oculoauriculo-vertebral syndromes	Haplo-insufficiency
SOX2	3q26	GH, FSH, LH	Anterior pituitary hypoplasia, midbrain defects	Anophthalmia, esophageal atresia	
SOX3	Xq27	GH, TSH, ACTH, FSH, LH	Anterior pituitary hypoplasia, ectopic posterior pituitary		X-linked recessive

*Genes involved in pituitary development or in maintaining the integrity of the hypothalamic-pituitary axis. Functional defects include missense mutations or frameshifts leading to truncated or deleted protein, DNA binding abnormality, inactivated protein, or impaired coactivation.

†POU1F1 mutations result in varying phenotypes of early growth failure with or without hypothyroidism.

‡PROP1 mutations may be fully manifest only in adulthood.

§HESX1 is critical for corpus development and is associated with structural brain defects.

ACTH, adrenocorticotropic hormone; FSH, follicle-stimulating hormone; GH, growth hormone; LH, luteinizing hormone; PRL, prolactin; TSH, thyroid-stimulating hormone.

(Adapted from Netchine I, Léger J, Rappaport R. Magnetic resonance imaging of the hypothalamic-pituitary region in nontumoral hypopituitarism. In: Rappaport R, Amselem S, eds. *Hypothalamic Pituitary Development.* Basel, Switzerland: Karger; 2001:94-108; and Romero CJ. Molecular basis of hypopituitarism. *Trends Endocrinol Metab.* 2009;20:506.)

ethylenediaminetetra-acetic acid (EDTA) and stored below –20° C for transport. Morning (8 a.m.) plasma ACTH levels range from 8 to 25 ng/L as measured by IRMA. Episodic secretion and short plasma half-life result in wide and rapid fluctuation of plasma measurements. Cortisol values at 4 p.m. are about half those of morning levels, and at 11 p.m. levels are usually less than 5 μg/dL.

Random ACTH values do not on their own provide an accurate assessment of HPA function unless concurrent cortisol levels are obtained. Therefore, an integrated assessment of both hormone levels is required for interpreting the significance of an appropriately obtained ACTH value. Often, measurement of the cortisol level alone provides a useful surrogate end point for assessing ACTH action and HPA axis integrity. Plasma ACTH levels fluctuate broadly within the same individual and are highly sensitive to stress, time of collection, and gender. Pregnant women have higher ambient ACTH levels, possibly because of placental CRH secretion.[363]

Dynamic Testing for ACTH Reserve

Hypothalamic Testing. Insulin hypoglycemia is a potent endogenous stressor that evokes ACTH secretion.[222] Insulin (0.1 to 0.15 U/kg) is injected intravenously after an overnight fast to achieve symptomatic hypoglycemia and a blood glucose level of less than 40 mg/dL. This test must be performed under supervision. A normal HPA response to this stressor evokes cortisol levels higher than 20 μg/dL. Because hypoglycemia acts centrally, a normal response implies integrity of all three tiers of HPA axis control. Up to 20% of patients may require greater amounts of insulin (0.3 U/kg or more) to achieve symptoms of glucopenia, including sweating, hunger, palpitations, and tremors.[364] Venous samples are collected at –15, 0, 15, 30, 45, 60, 90, and 120 minutes for measurement of glucose, ACTH, and cortisol levels. GH can also be measured. After the test, oral glucose should be administered. Intraindividual variations in blood glucose levels attained after a given dose of insulin, as well as fluctuations in central sensitivity to glucose and activation of catecholamines, can lead to difficulties in reproducibility. The test is contraindicated in subjects with a history of seizures, active coronary or cerebral ischemia, and pregnancy. If pronounced adrenal insufficiency is likely, insulin injection may provoke an adrenal crisis due to inadequate adrenal reserve, and hydrocortisone (100 mg) should be available for urgent intravenous use, if required.

Metyrapone blocks cortisol synthesis by inhibiting adrenal 11β-hydroxylase. The drug releases the HPA axis from negative feedback by cortisol, which normally results in an ACTH surge and elevated levels of 11-deoxycortisol (compound S). A single oral dose (2 to 3 g) is given at midnight, and serum levels of ACTH, 11-deoxycortisol, and cortisol are measured at 8 a.m. the following morning. The test is only valid in the face of documented suppressed cortisol levels lower than 10 μg/dL. In normal subjects, peak ACTH values higher than 200 ng/L are achieved. Side effects include nausea, gastrointestinal upset, and insomnia.[365] False-positive results may be obtained when phenytoin is being administered because the drug prevents adequate enzymatic blockade. This test should be performed under observation in the hospital because acute adrenal insufficiency may ensue.

TABLE 8-7

Causes of Acquired Pituitary Insufficiency

TRAUMATIC
Surgical resection
Radiation damage
Traumatic brain injury

INFILTRATIVE/INFLAMMATORY
Primary hypophysitis
Lymphocytic
Granulomatous
Xanthomatous
Secondary hypophysitis
Sarcoidosis
Histiocytosis X
Infections
Wegener's granulomatosis
Takayasu's disease
Hemochromatosis
Circulating Pit1 antibody**

INFECTION-RELATED
Tuberculosis
Pneumocystis jiroveci
Fungal (histoplasmosis, aspergillosis)
Parasites (toxoplasmosis)
Viral (*Cytomegalovirus*)

VASCULAR
Pregnancy-related
Aneurysm
Apoplexy
Diabetes
Hypotension
Arteritis
Sickle cell disease

NEOPLASTIC
Pituitary adenoma
Parasellar mass
Rathke's cyst
Dermoid cyst
Meningioma
Germinoma
Ependymoma
Glioma
Craniopharyngioma
Hypothalamic hamartoma, gangliocytoma
Pituitary metastatic deposits
Hematologic malignancy
Leukemia
Lymphoma

FUNCTIONAL
Nutritional
Caloric restriction
Malnutrition
Excessive exercise
Critical illness
Acute illness
Chronic renal failure
Chronic liver failure
Hormonal
Hyperprolactinemia
Hypothyroidism
Drugs
Anabolic steroids
Glucocorticoid excess
GnRH agonists
Estrogen
Dopamine
Somatostatin analog
Thyroid hormone excess

CAUSES OF ACQUIRED GHD IN 1034 ADULT PATIENTS WITH HYPOPITUITARISM
Pituitary tumor (53.9%)
Craniopharyngioma (12.3%)
Idiopathic (10.2%)
CNS tumor (4.4%)
Empty sella syndrome (4.2%)
Sheehan's syndrome (3.1%)
Head trauma (2.4%)
Hypophysitis (1.6%)
Surgery* (1.5%)
Granulomatous diseases (1.3%)
Irradiation* (1.1%)
CNS malformation (1.0%)
Perinatal trauma or infection (0.5%)
Other (2.5%)

*Other than for pituitary treatment.

**Yamamoto M. et al. Adult combinod GH, prolactin, and TSH deficency associated with circulating Pit 1 antibody in humans. *J Clin Inv.* 2011;121:113-119.

CNS, central nervous system; GnRH, gonadotropin-releasing hormone.

From Abs R, Bengtsson BA, Hernberg-Stahl E, et al. GH replacement in 1034 growth hormone deficient hypopituitary adults: demographic and clinical characteristics, dosing and safety. *Clin Endocrinol (Oxf).* 1999;50:703-713.)

Pituitary Stimulation. Pituitary ACTH secretion may be evoked by injecting CRH or vasopressin. Ovine or human CRH (100 μg or 1 μg/kg) is administered intravenously, and cortisol and ACTH are measured at −5, −1, 0, 15, 30, 60, 90, and 120 minutes. Normally, maximal ACTH responses (twofold to fourfold above baseline) are evoked at 30 minutes,[366] whereas cortisol levels peak (>20 μg/dL) at 60 minutes or increase more than 10 μg/dL above baseline. Although CRH readily induces ACTH secretion and may demonstrate corticotroph ACTH deficiency or ACTH excess, the wide variation of responses observed has limited the utility of this test. The CRH test is usefully applied in making the diagnosis of Cushing's disease with or without dexamethasone pretreatment and in the context of petrosal venous sampling for diagnosing the presence of an ACTH-secreting pituitary adenoma. CRH injection allows a sensitive and specific arteriovenous ACTH gradient to be established, which effectively distinguishes peripheral from pituitary sources of excess ACTH secretion.[367]

Because of the suppressive impact of circulating glucocorticoids on pituitary CRH responsiveness, it may be difficult to distinguish a corticotroph adenoma from pseudo-Cushing's disease, because hypercortisolism is associated with both conditions. In such circumstances, combining the CRH test with dexamethasone suppression may be useful. In the combined dexamethasone-CRH test, dexamethasone 0.5 mg is administered every 6 hours for 48 hours starting at noon and ending at 6 a.m., after which CRH is administered intravenously at 8 a.m.[368] In normal subjects and those with pseudo-Cushing's disorder, cortisol levels do not rise and are lower than 1.4 μg/dL. If cortisol levels elicited at 15 minutes exceed 4 μg/dL, the presence of an ACTH-secreting pituitary tumor is established, with 100% sensitivity and specificity.[368] CRH responsiveness (≥35% cortisol rise) is usually retained in ACTH-secreting adenomas but is not apparent in more than 90% of ectopic ACTH-producing tumors, in which ACTH increases of less than 35% above baseline are usually encountered. The test does not distinguish ACTH-secreting adenomas from a pseudo-Cushing's disorder.[369]

Adrenal Stimulation. The acute response of the adrenal gland to a bolus ACTH injection reflects ambient ACTH concentrations to which the gland has been exposed. The cortisol response to an acute ACTH injection will be blunted if the subject has experienced chronic pituitary ACTH hyposecretion with resultant adrenal atrophy and diminished cortisol reserve. Conversely, persistently elevated ACTH levels lead to adrenal hypertrophy and augmented cortisol responses.[370] A dose of 250 μg ACTH(1-24) (Cortrosyn) is injected intramuscularly or intravenously, and cortisol levels are measured at 0, 30, and 60 minutes. The normal adrenal reserve response is a cortisol value greater than 20 μg/dL or a doubling of the baseline value.

Basal cortisol levels correlate inversely with the incremental response to ACTH.[373] Low-dose stimulation with 1 μg Synacthen evokes maximal serum cortisol levels at 30 minutes, and these correlate well with values observed after insulin or high-dose ACTH administration.[372] A cutoff value of 500 nmol/L provides almost 100% sensitivity and a specificity of 80% to 100%.[374] Failure to respond to low-dose ACTH should be corroborated by use of a standard dose of insulin or ACTH stimulation.

The utility of this test in diagnosing diminished pituitary ACTH reserve has been challenged on the basis that the commonly employed dose of Cortrosyn or Synacthen is pharmacologic and may evoke a "normal" cortisol response in subjects with hypopituitarism. An unacceptably high false-negative rate (approximately 65%) was reported in a large series,[371] although peak cortisol levels at 30 minutes have been shown to correlate well with peak responses to ITT.[372]

Adrenal Steroid Replacement

Hydrocortisone is widely used for glucocorticoid replacement. The normal secretory rate of cortisol is 15 to 20 mg/day, and this is the recommended total daily dose for correcting hypoadrenalism and maintaining blood pressure. Because the plasma circulating half-life of cortisol is less than 2 hours, three-times-daily dosing of a total daily requirement of 10 to 20 mg (5 to 10 mg in the morning, 2.5 to 5 mg at noon, and 2.5 to 5 mg in the evening) is recommended.[375] However, conventional regimens cannot provide the physiologic pattern of cortisol release, and this may explain the high prevalence of poor quality of life in these patients.[376] There is no consensus for monitoring of treatment, although salivary, plasma, and urinary measurements have been advocated.

Doses must be increased during stress and before operative procedures. Cortisone acetate is metabolized to cortisol and has a slower onset of action and longer biologic activity than hydrocortisone. Other synthetic glucocorticoids, including prednisolone (2.5 to 5 mg/day) and dexamethasone (0.25 to 0.5 mg/day), are suitable alternatives. Because of their longer half-lives, they can be administered once daily, but they are less useful because they are difficult to monitor biochemically. Even modest cortisol overreplacement can result in bone mineral loss.[377]

Central diabetes insipidus may rarely be unmasked after initial glucocorticoid replacement. Mineralocorticoid replacement is not required for treatment of secondary hypoadrenalism. Adrenal androgen replacement with dehydroepiandrosterone (DHEA) at doses of 25 mg/day may improve the sense of well-being, fatigue, and sexual function in patients with primary and secondary adrenal insufficiency.[378,379]

Gonadotropins

Physiology

Gonadotrophs. Gonadotroph cells secreting FSH and LH comprise 10% to 15% of the functional anterior pituitary cells. Two classes of electrodense secretory granules are evident: large (350 to 450 nm) and small (150 to 250 nm). The granules are packaged in vesicles (Figs. 8-28 and 8-29). They contain large, round cell bodies with prominent rough endoplasmic reticulum and Golgi apparatus. LH secretory granules often accumulate peripherally, and their Golgi structures may be less prominent. SF1 and DAX1 orphan nuclear receptor determine gonadotroph-specific gene expression.

Structure of Gonadotropins. FSH and LH function to regulate gonadal steroid hormone biosynthesis and to initiate and maintain germ cell development, in concert with peripheral hormones and paracrine soluble factors. The four glycoprotein hormones—LH, FSH, TSH, and human chorionic gonadotropin (hCG)—share structural homology, having evolved from a common ancestral gene. Although the homologous LH and FSH molecules are cosecreted by the gonadotroph cell, their regulatory mechanisms are not uniformly concordant. The α- and β-subunits are encoded by different genes, located on chromosomes

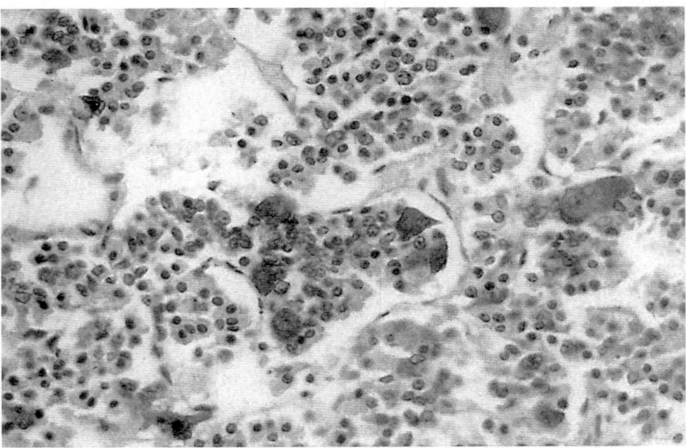

Figure 8-28 Normal gonadotroph cells contain immunoreactive β-follicle-stimulating hormone scattered throughout acini of the nontumorous pituitary. These round cells have evenly dispersed cytoplasmic immunoreactivity for α and β gonadotrophic subunits. (From Asa SL. Tumors of the pituitary gland. In: Rosai J, ed. *Atlas of Tumor Pathology*, Series III, Fascicle 22. Washington, DC: Armed Forces Institute of Pathology, 1997:26.)

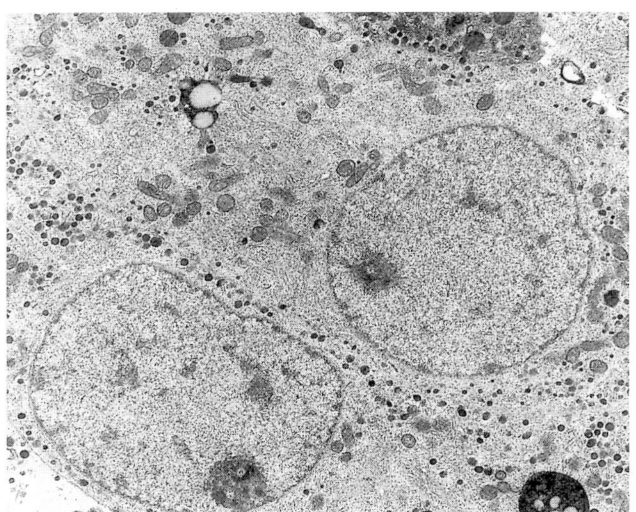

Figure 8-29 Electron micrograph of gonadotroph cell shows large, round to elongated cells with ovoid nuclei with occasional nucleoli. Short profiles of rough endoplasmic reticulum are scattered throughout the cytoplasm; they are dilated and frequently contain electron-lucent material. The Golgi complex is usually well developed and in a juxtanuclear location. Secretory granules are highly variable in size, shape, and electron density, and lysosomes are prominent. (From Asa SL. Tumors of the pituitary gland. In: Rosai J, ed. *Atlas of Tumor Pathology*, Series III, Fascicle 22. Washington, DC: Armed Forces Institute of Pathology, 1997:26.)

6, 11, and 19 respectively (Fig. 8-30). The heterodimeric structure of the common αGSU and unique β subunit is essential for biologic activity of the glycoprotein hormones. Disulfide linkages maintain noncovalent subunit linkage, which determines the ultrastructure of the mature folded molecule.[380] After processing of hormonal protein precursors, glycosylation occurs by transfer of oligosaccharide complexes to asparaginyl residues.[381] Post-translational processing of carbohydrate side chains is critical for hormone signaling; it may be species specific and is not uniformly similar for human LH and FSH.

The complex human LHβ gene cluster comprises seven CG-like genes, one of which encodes LHβ, whose promoter and transcriptional start site differ from that of hCG.[382,383] The three exons and two introns encode a 24-amino-acid leader peptide and a 121-amino-acid mature protein. Unlike LHβ, hCG is present only in primate and equine species, and the hCG peptide product contains a 24-amino-acid C-terminal extension.[384] Cell-specific LH gene expression and GnRH responsiveness of LH are subserved by different transcriptional mechanisms.[385,386] GnRH induces LHβ transcription, as does SF1.[387] The rat LHβ promoter contains an estrogen-responsive motif and an NF-Y binding site that appears to be important for basal, but not GnRH-mediated, trancription.[385] The FSHβ gene comprises three exons and two introns located on chromosome 11.[388] The gene promoter is dissimilar from that of LHβ, and the structure-function mechanisms for transcriptional regulation of the human gene by GnRH and sex steroids are not well clarified.[389]

Regulation

Hypothalamic GnRH neurons represent the pivotal integrator of peripheral signals in the regulation of the pituitary-gonadal axis. Considerable insight has been gained into the process controlling the development, migration from the olfactory placode, and regulation of the GnRH neuron. Kisspeptin peptides and their cognate receptor, orphan G protein–coupled receptor 54 (GPR54), were identified in 2004 as key regulators of GnRH neuronal function.[390] Kisspeptins are a family of peptides encoded by the KISS1 gene whose products also suppress the metastatic potential of breast cancer and melanomas. Loss-of-function mutations of GPR54 lead to hypogonadotropic hypogonadism, whereas administration of kisspeptin stimulates the hypothalamic-pituitary-gonadal axis in animal models.[391] Acute administration of kisspeptin to normal men increases FSH, LH, and testosterone concentrations; in normal women, the peptide stimulates gonadotropin release most potently during the preovulatory surge.[392] There is strong evidence that kisspeptin acts as the endogenous GnRH secretagogue across many species, including humans.

Leptin, a product of peripheral adipose tissue, is a positive regulator of the hypothalamic-pituitary-gonadal axis. This adipokine enables a pivotal link between body fat and reproduction, signaling energy availability centrally.[393] Leptin receptors are expressed specifically on GnRH-secreting neurons, and leptin accelerates GnRH pulsatility.[394] The concentration of leptin in blood is tightly related to body fat mass, and a threshold level is required to activate the hypothalamic-pituitary-gonadal axis. Delayed sexual maturation of food-restricted female rats can be accelerated by central leptin administration, despite decreased body weight. Increasing serum leptin levels during weight gain in treated patients with anorexia nervosa correlate positively with changes in LH, FSH, testosterone, and gonadal steroids.[395]

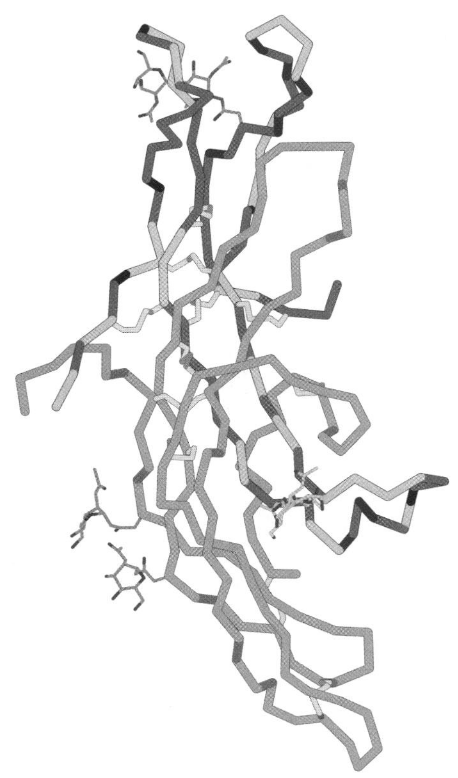

Figure 8-30 Schematic depiction of the subunit structure and glycosylation sites of the four glycoprotein hormone heterodimers (α-subunit, *blue*; β-subunit, *green*). (From the University of Glasgow protein crystallography website, Available at: http://www.chem.gla.ac.uk/protein/glyco/GPH.html [accessed September 2010]).

Secretion of Follicle-Stimulating Hormone and Luteinizing Hormone. FSH and LH secretion patterns reflect the integration of sensitive and complex hypothalamic, pituitary, and peripheral signals. GnRH pulse amplitude and frequency determine the physiologic patterns of LH and FSH secretion (Fig. 8-31).[396] In patients with hypothalamic GnRH deficiency, intravenous GnRH injections (25 ng/kg) that achieve GnRH levels similar to those present in primate hypophyseal-portal blood replicate the physiologic pattern of LH secretion.[397] The magnitude of the LH response exceeds that of FSH. Decreasing GnRH pulse frequency enhances LH pulse amplitudes, whereas increasing GnRH pulse frequency to more than every 2 hours downregulates the subsequent LH response. The interpulse LH secretory interval is 55 minutes, and the pulse amplitude is approximately 40% of basal tonic secretion. Changes in gonadotropin secretion during infancy, childhood, puberty, and aging are described in Chapter 25. A log-linear relationship is evident between the GnRH dose and the quantity of pituitary secretion of LH, FSH, and free α-subunit.

Both pituitary and hypothalamic targets for testosterone signals mediate FSH and LH regulation, and in males, testosterone attenuates gonadotropin secretion (Fig. 8-32). After castration, elevated gonadotropin levels can be partially overcome by testosterone replacement. Mechanisms for these observations are complex, because testosterone also exerts a stimulatory effect on FSHβ mRNA levels. Although estrogen administration decreases LH pulse amplitude in normal and GnRH-deficient male subjects,[398,399] depending on the clinical situation, estrogen may either stimulate or inhibit pituitary gonadotropin synthesis and secretion, and it also can inhibit GnRH synthesis or action. This pattern is manifest in the cyclic control of gonadotropin secretion during the menstrual cycle and during puberty. LH, FSH, free α-subunit, and testosterone pulses are usually concordant in male subjects.[400] Deconvolution pulse analysis allows estimation of "real-time" hormone secretion rates, with an assumed disappearance rate constant. The characteristic secretory episodes characterized for LH and FSH indicate daily production rates of 1000 IU and 200 IU, respectively, and a disappearance half-life of 90 and 500 minutes for each respective β-subunit.[401]

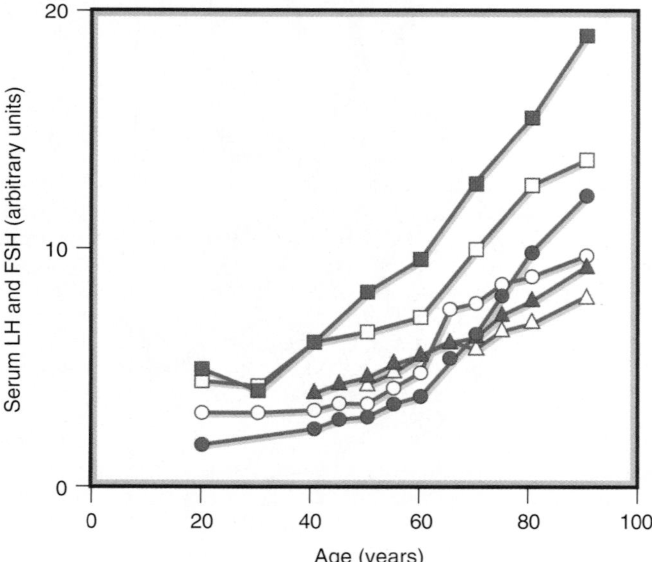

Figure 8-31 Serum luteinizing hormone (LH) levels *(open symbols)* and follicle-stimulating hormone (FSH) levels *(solid symbols)* in men as a function of age from three studies. (From Tenover JL. Male hormone replacement therapy including "andropause." *Endocrinol Metab Clin North Am.* 1998;27:969-987; and Bhasin S, Fisher CE, Sverdloff RS. Follicle-stimulating hormone and luteinizing hormone. In: Melmed, ed. *The Pituitary,* 2nd ed. Malden, MA: Blackwell Scientific, 2002.)

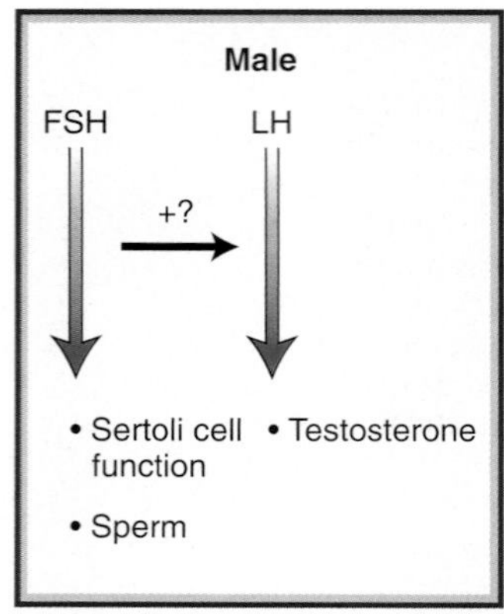

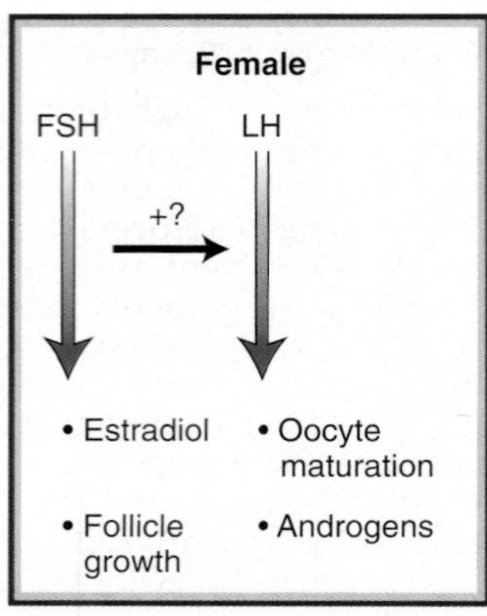

Figure 8-32 Functions of follicle-stimulating hormone (FSH) in human males and females. The plus signs and horizontal arrows indicate potentially unrecognized new functions of FSH since the discovery of FSHβ gene mutations. LH, luteinizing hormone. (Modified from Layman LC. Genetics of human hypogonadotropic hypogonadism. *Am J Med Genet [Semin Med Genet].* 1999;89:240-248; and Bhasin S, Fisher CE, Sverdloff RS. Follicle-stimulating hormone and luteinizing hormone. In: Melmed S, ed. *The Pituitary,* 2nd ed. Malden, MA: Blackwell Science; 2002:216-278.)

Gonadal Peptides. Pituitary gonadotropin secretion is regulated by gonadal peptides including inhibin A, an α:βA heterodimer; inhibin B, an α:βB heterodimer; and follistatin peptides. The activin A βA– and activin AB (βB) homodimers stimulate in vitro FSH secretion.[402] These proteins, which are related to transforming growth factor-β and müllerian-inhibiting factor, are fully described in Chapter 22.

Actions of Follicle-Stimulating Hormone and Luteinizing Hormone

Female. Luteal cell LH receptors signal to enhance cAMP levels and induce cholesterol availability for ovarian steroidogenesis. The steroidogenic acute regulatory (StAR) protein[403] is induced by LH and mediates cholesterol delivery to the inner membrane. LH enhances cytochrome P450–linked enzyme activity in the synthesis of pregnenolone and induces 3β-hydroxysteroid dehydrogenase, 17α-hydroxylase, and 17,20-ylase synthesis.

The FSH receptor, a G protein–linked seven-transmembrane molecule, shares 50% extracellular domain and 80% transmembrane homology with the LH receptor.[404] FSH regulates ovarian estrogen synthesis by inducing 17β-hydroxysteroid dehydrogenase and aromatase and also induces follicular growth. Estrogens are also permissive for FSH action and enhance FSH-induced cAMP levels.[405]

Male. Leydig cell LH receptor signaling induces intratesticular testosterone synthesis mediated by enhanced cAMP production. FSH function in male subjects is not readily apparent but probably mediates the development of spermatozoa from spermatids in concert with testosterone, especially because failed spermatogenesis leads to elevated FSH levels.

Gonadotropin Assays

Because of the high homology of the glycoprotein hormones, development of highly specific assays, especially distinguishing free αGSU from intact hormones, has been challenging. Heterogeneity of circulating LH and FSH molecules; insufficient assay sensitivity, especially for normal healthy measurements; and lack of rigorously pure reference preparations have hampered assay development. Immunofluorometric assays detect LH with a sensitivity of 0.1 mIU/mL.[406] Differences in carbohydrate moieties result in isoelectric charge heterogeneity for LH, accounting for some of the disparities in biologic and immunoreactive LH ratios observed after GnRH agonist treatment, in acute critical illness, or with aging.

LH bioassays include assessment of testosterone generation by cell culture,[407] and FSH bioassays include measurement of granulosa cell or Sertoli cell aromatase generation.[408] Because only intact molecules, not free α- or β-subunits, are biologically active, these assays, although cumbersome, are useful for measuring bioactive hormone without the potential cross-reaction of free subunits.

α-Subunit Secretion

Both GnRH and TRH increase circulating levels of free α-subunit derived from gonadotrophs or thyrotrophs, especially in patients with hypothyroidism, after castration and during menopause. GnRH agonist treatment, TSH-secreting tumors, and nonfunctioning pituitary adenomas may result in discordant ratios due to free α-subunit secretion.

Gonadotropin Deficiency

Causes. Gonadotropin deficiency may be congenital or acquired and may arise from hypothalamic or pituitary lesions. Congenital causes include gene mutations governing the processes of migration and function of GnRH neurons and development of the gonadotroph. Hypogonadotropic hypogonadism may arise from functional or organic disorders. Functional causes are frequently encountered and include stress, malnutrition, chronic illness, depression, excessive exercise, and low body weight. Several centrally acting drugs, including opiates, tranquilizers, antidepressants, and antipsychotic medications, suppress gonadotropin secretion directly or indirectly via induction of hyperprolactinemia. Organic causes include malignant disease, developmental tumors, infiltrative disease, and hypothalamic or pituitary damage from surgery or radiotherapy. Acquired and congenital causes of central hypogonadism are considered fully in Chapter 20.

Isolated Hypogonadotropic Hypogonadism. The genetic basis of isolated hypogonadotropic hypogonadism (IHH) was recognized more than 60 years ago with the description by Kallmann of hypogonadism and anosmia in two families. It was not until 1991 that anosmin, a glycoprotein encoded by the KAL1 gene, was identified.[409] The realization that *KAL1* defects account for only a small proportion of patients with Kallmann's syndrome led to genotype-phenotype studies that provided important insights into the molecular genetics underlying IHH occurring with and without anosmia (Table 8-8). Gene mutations affecting olfactory bulb and GnRH neuronal migration tend to give rise to the Kallmann phenotype, whereas defects in the regulation of GnRH are usually associated with normosmia.

TABLE 8-8

Genetics of Isolated Hypogonadotropic Hypogonadism

Phenotype	Gene and Ref. No.	Inheritance	Function
Kallmann's syndrome	KAL1[409]	X-linked	Anosmin required for cell surface signaling, adhesion, and migration
	FGFR1[511]	AD	Role in axonal development and guidance
	FGF8[512]	AD	Endogenous ligand of FGFR1
	PROK2[513] PROK2R[513]	AD, AR	Development of olfactory bulb and migration of GnRH neurons
	NELF[514]	?	Encoding nasal embryonic LHRH factor
Normosmic IHH	GNRHR[515]	AR	—
	GNRH1[516]	AR	—
	KISS1R[515]	AR	GPR54, receptor for kisspeptins essential for GnRH neuron function

AD, autosomal dominant; AR, autosomal recessive; FGF, fibroblast growth factor; GNRH, gonadotropin-releasing hormone; GPR, orphan G protein–coupled receptor; IHH, isolated hypogonadotropic hypogonadism; KAL, Kallmann's syndrome; KISS, KiSS metastasis suppressor; LHRH, luteinizing hormone–releasing hormone; NELF, nasal embryonic LHRH factor; PROK, prokineticin.

Clinical Features. Gonadotropin deficiency causes hypogonadism with decreased sex steroid production of varying degree, depending on the severity of the insult (Table 8-9). This disorder may occur at any stage of life. In its complete form (e.g., panhypopituitarism; Kallmann's syndrome), primary amenorrhea or total failure of male sexual development may occur. Later in life, a varying spectrum of sexual dysfunction develops, ranging from luteal abnormalities or oligomenorrhea to amenorrhea in women, or to absence of libido, potency, and fertility in men. Women exhibit secondary amenorrhea, vaginal dryness, hot flushes, decreased bone density, decreased breast tissue, and infertility. Men have impotence, testicular hypoplasia or atrophy, decreased libido, low energy, infertility, loss of secondary sexual characteristics, decreased muscle strength and mass, decreased bone mass, decreased body hair growth, and fine facial wrinkling. In both men and women, serum gonadotropin levels are inappropriately low in the face of decreased sex steroids and sexual dysfunction. In women with amenorrhea or oligomenorrhea, serum levels of LH, FSH, and estradiol should be measured. Endogenous estrogen sufficiency can also be assessed by the response to a progesterone challenge (100 mg intramuscularly, or 10 mg/day Provera orally for 5 days). Men should have serum gonadotropin and testosterone levels measured.

Because FSH is required for normal spermatogenesis, isolated FSH deficiency is associated with oligospermia or azoospermia in normally androgenized men in the face of normal testosterone and LH levels.[410] Isolated LH deficiency may manifest with eunuchoid body proportions as a result of low testosterone levels. Low LH levels in these patients lead to low intratesticular testosterone concentrations with resultant decreased spermatogenesis.[411] Serum testosterone levels are restored in this "fertile eunuch" syndrome by hCG administration. IHH[412] occurring after

TABLE 8-9

Clinical Features of Hypogonadotropism

PREPUBERTAL ONSET
High-pitched voice
Terminal facial hair
Decreased or absent body hair
Eunuchoidal body proportions
Female escutcheon
Testicular volume <6 cm^3, hypoplastic
Testicular length <2.5 cm
Penile length <5 cm
Smooth scrotum with no rugae
Small prostate
POSTPUBERTAL ONSET
Decreased libido
Slow beard growth
Decreased body hair
Testes atrophic if long-standing
Normal voice pitch
Decreased muscle and bone mass
Normal
Skeletal proportions
Penis length
Scrotal rugae
Prostate size

apparently normal puberty manifests with relatively mature secondary sex characteristics or even secondary infertility. These patients have abundant gonadotropin responses to pulsatile GRH therapy, which restores reproductive function and fertility.

Management

Evaluation. In evaluating hypogonadal patients without an obvious pituitary or gonadal disorder, the primary diagnostic challenge is to distinguish constitutional pubertal delay from other causes of hypogonadotropism.[413] If puberty is delayed beyond 14 years of age, a primary developmental disorder, hypogonadotropic hypogonadism, should be considered in the absence of acquired causes. No single test clearly distinguishes constitutional delayed puberty from true hypogononadotropism, and expectant follow-up is often helpful because many patients enter puberty spontaneously. To enable androgenization, testosterone replacement should be intermittently provided until age 18 years, with periodic interruptions to unmask physiologic pubertal advance.

Sex Steroid Replacement Therapy. Estrogen or testosterone replacement is required to induce and maintain primary and secondary sexual functions, to minimize cardiovascular risk factors, and to maintain normal body composition and integrity of bone mineral density and muscle mass. For patients not desirous of fertility, sex steroid therapy is warranted to correct central hypogonadism. However, monitoring of LH and FSH responses does not accurately reflect adequate steroid hormonal replacement, because basal gonadotropin levels are already low or undetectable.

Estrogens are available in tablet, patch, gel, and implant forms. For premenopausal women with pituitary deficiency, conjugated equine estrogens (0.625 mg) or estradiol valerate (2 mg) provide relatively physiologic steroid replenishment. Estrogen patches or transcutaneous gels usually enable daily absorption of 50 to 100 μg estradiol. Estrogens in the form of oral contraceptive formulations are to be avoided, because the doses are pharmacologic and can potentially impair hepatic metabolic function. Concomitant cyclic progesterone therapy (e.g., medroxyprogesterone acetate 5 mg or dydrogesterone 10 mg) is indicated for women with an intact uterus to prevent unopposed endometrial proliferation and bleeding.

Although early replacement lessens the risk of developing osteoporosis, effects of estrogen replacement on cardiovascular function are unresolved. In patients with hypopituitarism, estrogen replacement should be maintained at least until 50 years of age, after which continuation should be determined on an individual basis by assessing risks and benefits, especially in terms of bone mineral integrity, cardiovascular function, and cancer risk. In women with ovarian deficiency, addition of androgen may improve libido and sexual function. Estrogen treatment may be associated with thromboembolic disease, breast tenderness, and possibly enhanced risk for breast cancer.

For men, androgen replacement preparations are available in intramuscular gel, patch, and oral forms. Intramuscular injection of testosterone undeconate, 1000 mg, provides satisfactory long-term replacement for 3 to 4 months. The improved pharmacokinetic profile reduces fluctuations in sexual potency, energy level, and mood that are often seen with shorter-acting testosterone 17α-hydroxyl esters (testosterone enanthate and testosterone cypionate), which are usually administered in 200-mg doses every 2 or 3 weeks.[414] Administration of lower doses on a more frequent basis (e.g., 100 mg weekly or 150 mg every 14 days) may also stabilize fluctuations of hormone levels. Elderly men require lower doses, as do boys with delayed puberty. Transdermal testosterone patch and gel systems deliver 4 to 6 mg and sustain testosterone profiles. Patch sites may develop skin irritation, blisters, or vesicles in about 25% of patients.[415] Some patients require combined patches and low-dose injections to maintain adequate potency and energy levels.[416,417] There is no apparent cost-benefit advantage of patch delivery over intramuscular injection. Oral androgen replacement therapy with 17α-hydroxyl ester testosterone undecenoate requires frequent dosing (two to four times daily), and, because absorption is not uniform, testosterone levels may not be adequately maintained. Oral 17α-methyltestosterone is not recommended because of hepatotoxicity.

Testosterone may cause acne, gynecomastia, urinary retention due to prostatic obstruction (rarely), and polycythemia. Although there is no compelling evidence that testosterone replacement causes prostate cancer, benign prostatic hypertrophy could be exacerbated, especially in elderly patients. Testosterone replacement should not be administered to men with diagnosed prostate cancer.

Fertility. In patients with hypogonadotropic hypogonadism, fertility may be achieved with gonadotropin or GnRH therapy. In male patients, coexistence of primary testicular dysfunction precludes the success of direct gonadotropin replacement or GnRH; however, the relatively low sperm counts induced by gonadotropin or GnRH may be adequate for impregnation. Because testosterone therapy may suppress spermatogenesis, the steroid should be discontinued before treatment is initiated. hCG is administered subcutaneously or intramuscularly (1000 to 2000 IU two to three times weekly) to induce spermatogenesis. Lower doses may also be effective.[418] If necessary, after 6 months, human menopausal gonadotropin (hMG) or purified FSH (75 IU three times weekly) should be added to improve sperm quantity, and doses may be doubled after a further 6 months. If testosterone levels are increased, subsequent conversion to estradiol may be enhanced, resulting in gynecomastia. Gonadotropin therapy may also cause androgenized oily skin and acne. Therefore, both testosterone and estradiol levels should be monitored.

Pulsatile GnRH therapy is indicated for patients with normal pituitary function (i.e., those with idiopathic hypogonadotropic hypogonadism or Kallmann's syndrome). GnRH is infused subcutaneously by continuous mini-pump (5 mg every 2 hours); the dose is titrated to maintain normal gonadotropin and testosterone levels and may be marginally more effective and cause less gynecomastia. These approaches require strong patient commitment, because adequate spermatogenesis may not be attained for 2 years or longer despite normalized testosterone levels. Aliquots of successfully generated sperm samples should be frozen for future impregnation.

In women with central hypogonadism, fertility may be effectively achieved by GnRH or gonadotropin therapy (see Chapter 17). Although ovulation is often induced and pregnancy achieved by gonadotropin treatment, a high rate of development of multiple follicles remains a concern. A pregnancy rate of 83% was achieved in 77 patients with hypogonadotropic hypogonadism who were treated with gonadotropins or pulsatile GnRH.[419] If residual pituitary gonadotroph reserve is sufficiently robust, GnRH therapy is more likely to result in ovulation of a single rather than multiple follicles, thereby reducing the chances of multiple gestation.[420] The beneficial role of adding GH to these treatments remains unresolved,[421] except for those women with known hypopituitarism and GHD (see Chapter 17).

Gonadotropin-Releasing Hormone Stimulation Test. A single bolus of GnRH (25 to 100 μg) dose-dependently evokes serum LH and FSH levels within 20 to 30 minutes. LH rises more abundantly than FSH, and peak values range from 8 to 34 mIU/mL; patients with low testosterone levels exhibit more exuberant responses.[422] In contrast, patients with hypogonadotropic hypogonadism and no demonstrable hypothalamic-pituitary lesion have blunted LH responses and reversal of the LH/FSH ratio. The test cannot adequately distinguish hypothalamic from pituitary lesions, and similar patterns are observed in patients with anorexia nervosa. Repetitive GnRH pulses may in fact normalize responses, as would be expected from an intact hypothalamic-pituitary unit. GnRH responses may vary during the stages of puberty, reflecting altered pituitary sensitivity.

Clomiphene (100 mg), administered daily for up to 4 weeks, usually doubles LH levels, whereas FSH increases about 50% over baseline. Because an abnormal or absent response does not distinguish hypothalamic from pituitary lesions, the utility of this test is limited.

Thyroid-Stimulating Hormone

Physiology

The hypothalamic-pituitary-thyroid system plays a critical role in development, growth, and cellular metabolism, with thyroid hormone availability and action controlled by complex mechanisms at the tissue level.

Thyrotrophs. Thyrotroph cells comprise approximately 5% of the functional anterior pituitary cells and are situated predominantly in the anteromedial areas of the gland. They are smaller than the other cell types. They are irregularly shaped, with flattened nuclei and relatively small secretory granules ranging from 120 to 150 μm (Figs. 8-33 and 8-34).

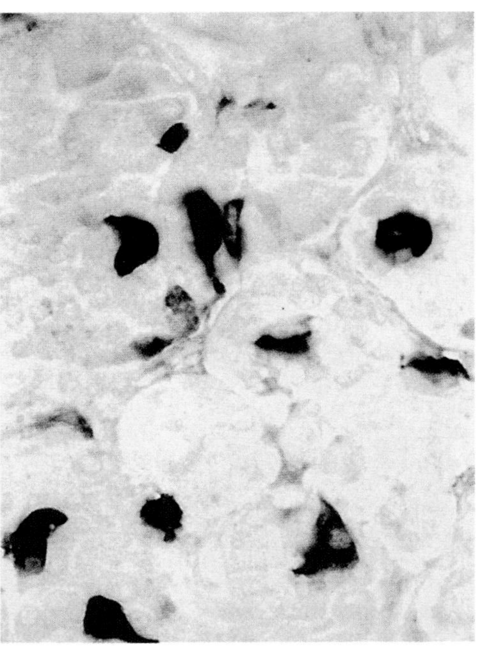

Figure 8-33 Normal thyrotrophs have angular cell bodies with elongated processes. (From Asa SL. Tumors of the pituitary gland. In: Rosai J, ed. *Atlas of Tumor Pathology*, Series III, Fascicle 22. Washington, DC: Armed Forces Institute of Pathology, 1997:19.)

Structure. TSH is a glycoprotein hormone comprising a heterodimer of noncovalently linked α- and β-subunits.[423] The αGSU is common to TSH, LH, FSH, and hCG, whereas the β-subunit is unique and confers specificity of action.[424] The αGSU is the earliest hormone gene expressed embryonically; activation of the β-subunit gene occurs later,

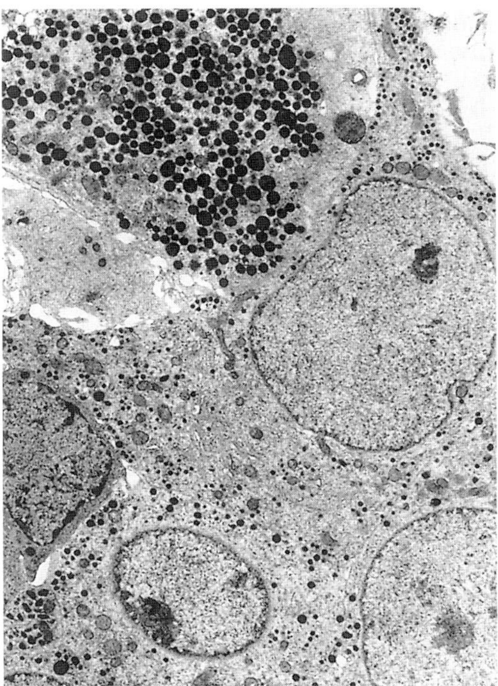

Figure 8-34 Electron micrograph of normal thyrotrophs shows angular cell bodies with elongated processes. (From Asa SL. Tumors of the pituitary gland. In: Rosai J, ed. *Atlas of Tumor Pathology*, Series III, Fascicle 22. Washington, DC: Armed Forces Institute of Pathology, 1997:19.)

under the influence of GATA2 and POU1F1.[425] The 13.5-kb αGSU gene is located on chromosome 6 and consists of four exons and three introns.[426] Although the αGSU gene is expressed in thyrotroph, gonadotroph, and placental cells, its regulation is uniquely cell specific. The downstream promoter region (−200 and further) is required for placental expression, intermediate sequences are required for gonadotroph expression, and upstream promoter elements are required for thyrotroph-specific expression.[427]

α-GSU transcription is inhibited by triiodothyronine (T_3) at regions close to the transcriptional initiation site, in concert with other nuclear corepressors.[428] The 4.9-kb TSH β-subunit gene, located on chromosome 1, comprises three exons and two introns.[429] POU1F1 binds directly to the gene promoter to confer tissue-specific expression.[430] TSH-β gene transcription is suppressed by the thyroid hormone receptor acting directly on exon 1.[431] This potent suppression is evident within 30 minutes after T_3 exposure and is a critical determinant of TSH synthesis and secretion. TSH α- and β-subunit gene transcription is induced by TRH, and depletion of cAMP by dopamine leads to suppressed gene transcription.[432] Intrapituitary TSH is stored in secretory granules, and the mature hormone (molecular weight, 28 kd) is released into the venous circulation, primarily in response to hypothalamic TRH. The predicted structural model of the TSH molecule is that of a cystine knot growth factor. The tertiary TSH structure comprises three hairpin loops separated by central disulfide bonds, with the longest loop straddling one side.[433,434]

Production of the mature heterodimeric TSH molecule requires complex cotranslational glycosylation and folding of nascent α- and β-subunits.[424] After subunit translation and signal peptide cleavage, glycosylation occurs at Asn23 on the β-subunit and at Asn52 and Asn78 on the α-subunit.[435] Appropriate glycosylation is required for accurate molecular folding and subsequent combination of α- and β-subunits within the rough endoplasmic reticulum and Golgi apparatus. Both TRH and T_3 regulate TSH glycosylation, albeit in opposite directions. TRH administration (e.g., in hypothyroidism) or T_3 deprivation (e.g., in T_3 resistance) enhances oligosaccharide addition to the TSH molecule.[436]

Secretion

Daily TSH production is approximately 100 to 400 mU,[437] with a calculated circulating half-life of approximately 50 minutes. Secretion rates are enhanced up to 15-fold in hypothyroid subjects and are suppressed in states of hyperthyroidism. The degree of TSH glycosylation determines the metabolic clearance rate and the bioactivity; in hypothyroidism, the molecule appears to be highly sialylated, enhancing bioactivity.[435] Immunoreactive fetal pituitary TSH is detectable by 12 weeks.

Immediately after full-term birth, there is a brisk rise in TSH, which remains elevated for up to 5 days before stabilizing at adult levels.[438] Although TSH secretion is pulsatile, the low pulse amplitudes and long TSH half-life result in modest circulating variances. Secretory pulses every 2 to 3 hours are interspersed with periods of tonic, nonpulsatile TSH secretion.[439] Circadian TSH secretion peaks between 11 p.m. and 5 a.m., mainly due to increased pulse amplitude, which does not appear to be sleep-entrained.[440] Pulsatile and circadian TSH secretory patterns are largely determined by ambient thyroid hormone levels and TRH release. Thyroid hormones suppress tonic TSH secretion and pulse amplitude. Within hours after T_3 administration, basal TSH levels fall and TRH-evoked TSH levels are attenuated. Primary hypothyroidism is associated with enhanced TSH pulse amplitudes occurring throughout the day, and nocturnal TSH surges are abrogated in patients with critical illness.[441]

Regulation

The TRH neuron plays a central role in determining the set point of the hypothalamic-pituitary-thyroid axis by regulating pituitary TSH release. Located in the paraventricular nucleus, TRH neurons receive direct projections from the leptin system that regulates energy homeostasis, the POMC system that promotes weight loss, and the neuropeptide Y (NPY)/agouti-related protein (AgRP) system that promotes weight gain.[442] Fasting results in reduction of TRH expression, mediated by suppression of the POMC system and stimulation of the NPY/AgRP system.

Feedback regulation of TRH and TSH by thyroid hormones is elaborated through a complex system of local paracrine control. In the hypothalamus, deiodinase 2 (D2), which converts thyroxine (T_4) to triiodothyronine (T_3), is expressed in surrounding glial cells.[443] In contrast, the TRH neuron expresses thyroid hormone receptors, thyroid hormone transporters, and D3, which inactivates T_3, indicating the existence of a level of TRH regulation at the cellular level. T_3 suppresses hypothalamic TRH synthesis and decreases the number of pituitary TRH receptors.

In the anterior pituitary gland, immunoreactive D2 and thyroid hormone transporters are found in folliculo-stellate cells, whereas immunoreactive thyroid hormone receptors and D3 are expressed in thyrotrophs.[443] These findings indicate an important role for glial and folliculo-stellate cells in processing and activating T_4. Production and action of local T_3 occur in separate cell types of the hypothalamus and anterior pituitary gland, setting the level of TSH output.

Other Factors. SRIF inhibits TSH pulse amplitude and blocks the nocturnal TSH surge[444] directly at the pituitary level; it may also suppress TRH release and possibly TRH receptor abundance.[445] Although SRIF analogs are used to treat TSH-secreting pituitary adenomas (see later discussion), long-term SRIF treatment for acromegaly does not lead to hypothyroidism in adult subjects, although T_4 levels may be lowered within the normal range.[446] Dopamine inhibits TSH β-subunit gene expression, and dopamine infusions suppress TSH pulse amplitude by 70% and abrogate the nocturnal TSH surge.[447] Prolonged use of dopamine agonists, however, does not result in hypothyroidism. Glucocorticoids suppress TSH secretion, and in patients with adrenal failure without autoimmune thyroid damage, TSH levels may be elevated. Sex steroids and cytokines alter TSH secretion in animal models, but their contribution to human TSH physiology is as yet unclear. Nonsteroidal anti-inflammatory agents, especially meclofenamate and fenclofenac, decrease serum TSH levels, albeit still within the normal range. The mechanism for this observation may involve displacement of thyroid hormone ligands from their binding proteins or direct inhibition of pituitary TSH.[448]

Action of TSH

TSH acts on the thyroid gland to induce thyroid hormone synthesis and release and to maintain trophic thyroid cell integrity.[449] The TSH G protein–coupled receptor is located on the thyrocyte plasma membrane and is encoded by a gene on chromosome 11q31. Its regulation is comprehensively described in Chapter 11.

Disorders of TSH Secretion

TSH Deficiency

Causes. Congenital isolated TSH deficiency may arise from mutational defects of the TSH or TRH receptor gene. Genetic disorders of pituitary gland development involved in cell differentiation give rise to TSH deficiency as a component of multiple pituitary hormone deficiencies. These include mutations of LHX3, PROP1, and POU1F1 (see Table 8-6). Pituitary damage may result in functional TSH deficiency, often without a clearly demonstrable reduction in serum TSH levels.

Clinical Features. The consequences of TSH deficiency are those of thyroid hormone deficiency, which causes mental or growth retardation, or both, in children and in adults is associated with a broad spectrum of clinical features including hypothermia, fluid retention, voice and skin changes, and, ultimately if untreated, frank myxedema and death.

Thyroid-Stimulating Hormone Assays. Because feedback control of TSH secretion by peripheral thyroid hormones is sensitive, most thyrotroph disorders can be diagnosed by measuring basal TSH and thyroid hormone levels.

The challenge of a clinically compelling robust TSH assay is to readily distinguish circulating TSH levels in euthyroid subjects from levels in both hyperthyroid and hypothyroid patients. The development of immunoradiometric TSH assays has provided high specificity with little or no cross-reactivity with other glycoprotein hormones. These assays detect quantifiable TSH levels in euthyroid control subjects with no overlap with the low values associated with hyperthyroidism.[450,451] The most sensitive commercially available third-generation assays have a functional sensitivity of 0.01 to 0.02 mU/L, and newer fourth-generation assays portend greatly enhanced sensitivity (0.001 to 0.002 mU/L). Levels of free α-subunit (normal range, 0.1 to 1.6 μg/L) are elevated in patients harboring TSH-secreting or nonfunctional pituitary adenomas, in choriocarcinoma, and in several malignancies.

TSH measurement is not helpful in diagnosing central hypothyroidism, which is identified by concurrent measurement of thyroid hormone levels. Only about one third of patients with secondary hypothyroidism have abnormally low basal TSH levels.[452] TSH deficiency is therefore associated with low T_4 levels concomitant with low, normal, or even minimally elevated TSH levels. Importantly, this biochemical profile may also be encountered in critically ill patients with low TSH and T_4 levels but no evidence of pituitary disease.

However, evoked dynamic TSH measurements elicited by TRH may be required to fully assess the integrity of the hypothalamic-pituitary-thyroid axis.[453] TRH (200 to 500 μg) is administered intravenously, and TSH levels are measured at −15, 0, 15, 30, 60, and 120 minutes after injection. In euthyroid subjects, peak TSH levels (up to 22-fold higher than basal concentrations) are observed after 30 minutes.[451] Because feedback suppression of elevated thyroid hormone levels on TSH overrides positive hypothalamic signals, hyperthyroid subjects have undetectable basal TSH levels that do not respond to TRH. In subjects with secondary thyroid failure due to pituitary disease, TSH levels do not change in response to TRH. Within hours after T_3 administration, basal TSH levels fall and TRH-evoked TSH levels are attenuated. Thyroid hormones suppress tonic TSH secretion and pulse amplitude but do not appear to regulate TSH pulse frequency.

Treatment. L-Thyroxine is used for replacement therapy, and dosing variables are similar to those required for treatment of primary hypothyroidism. Hypothyroid features are effectively ameliorated by administration of T_4 (0.075 to 0.25 mg/day). The molecule is converted peripherally into the active T_3 and has a 7-day half-life with stable blood levels. The dose of levothyroxine in hypopituitary patients is titrated to achieve mid-normal clinically euthyroid serum free T_4 levels, because serum TSH levels are low or undetectable in patients with damaged pituitary function. Measurement of TSH levels is not useful in determining thyroid hormone replacement because the damaged thyrotroph is unlikely to adequately reflect appropriate feedback suppression.

Many women with pituitary failure are also receiving estrogen replacement, and in these patients measurement of free T_4 levels is required due to increased levels of thyroxine-binding globulin (TBG). T_4 overdosing may lead to osteopenia and cardiac arrhythmias. Some patients have associated ACTH deficiency, and thyroid hormone replacement should not be initiated until adrenal reserve has been evaluated and, if necessary, treated. Thyroid hormone replacement may also accelerate cortisol metabolism or requirements and may therefore exacerbate primary hypoadrenalism or precipitate adrenal crisis in patients with perturbed adrenal function.

DEVELOPMENTAL AND GENETIC CAUSES OF PITUITARY FAILURE

Developmental Pituitary Dysfunction

Congenital absence of the pituitary gland (aplasia), partial hypoplasia, or ectopic tissue rudiments are rarely encountered. Pituitary development follows midline cell migration from Rathke's pouch, and impaired midline anomalies, including failed forebrain cleavage and anterior commissure and corpus callosum defects, lead to structural pituitary anomalies. Craniofacial developmental anomalies, including anencephaly, result in cleft lip and palate, basal encephalocele, hypertelorism, and optic nerve hypoplasia with varying degrees of pituitary dysplasia and aplasia. If these infants survive, lifelong appropriate pituitary hormone replacement is required. Children with mild forms of midline anomalies are also more prone to GHD.

With sensitive MRI techniques for pituitary visualization, several anatomic features characteristic of hypopituitarism are now apparent. Evidence for acquired pituitary gland damage or destruction is often clearly visible on MRI, whereas patients presenting with hypopituitarism of undetermined etiology may exhibit decreased gland volume, partial or complete empty sella, disturbed sella turcica architecture, absent or transected pituitary stalk, and an absent or ectopic posterior pituitary bright intensity signal.[454] An absent infundibulum noted on MRI is associated with pituitary hormone deficits, and approximately 40% of patients with GHD of unclear cause show imaging evidence of mild stalk defects, reflecting a midline developmental anomaly. Congenital basal encephalocele may result in herniation of the pituitary through the sphenoid sinus roof, resulting in pituitary failure and diabetes insipidus.

Heritable Disorders of Pituitary Failure

Mutations at each level of pituitary function, including hormones, receptors, and transcription factors that determine anterior pituitary development, may lead to pituitary deficiency syndromes (see Tables 8-10 and 8-6).[455] Furthermore, mutations in specific pituitary genes, including those for GH, GHRH receptor, POMC, TSH, LH, and FSH, all lead to single-hormone deficiencies, fully described in Chapter 24). Patients heretofore diagnosed with idiopathic isolated or polyhormonal pituitary failure may in fact harbor a mutation. As the genetic control of pituitary development is further clarified, increasing numbers of mutant genes have become apparent.

PROP1

PROP1 (Online Mendelian Inheritance in Man [OMIM] 601538) gene expression is required for subsequent POU1F1 activation. The gene, located on chromosome 5q, encodes a 223-amino-acid protein expressed in GH-, PRL-, and TSH-secreting cells.[456] The Ames dwarf mouse harbors a missense PROP1 mutation (Ser83Pro) and exhibits a hypoplastic pituitary gland with combined GH, PRL, and TSH deficiency. This mutation abrogates POU1F1 activation and results in failed development of POU1F1-dependent cell lineages.[457] Several human mutations have been associated with GH, PRL, TSH, and gonadotropin deficiencies. The most commonly encountered mutation is a 2-base-pair deletion (301-302delAG) that results in early translational termination and a nonfunctional protein product. The clinical spectrum of combined pituitary hormone deficiency associated with PROP1 mutations is variable and temporal. The phenotype varies with both the type of mutation and the age of the patient.[458]

Human PROP1 mutations are associated with deficiencies in POU1F1-dependent lineages (GH, PRL, and TSH) and impaired FSH, LH, and ACTH reserve function.[243] Because development and mature function of these latter cell types are not POU1F1 dependent, it appears that additional critical developmental factors are disrupted in these patients, leading to the clinical phenotype. Heterogeneous patients with PROP1 mutations leading to combined pituitary hormone deficiency have been described since the original report in 1996,[459] and this disorder appears to be the most common heritable cause of combined pituitary hormone deficiency.

TABLE 8-10

Etiology of Inherited Pituitary Deficiency*

Mutation	Hormone Deficit
Genetic	
Kallmann's syndromes	FSH, LH
Prader-Willi syndrome	FSH, LH
Lawrence-Moon-Biedl syndrome	FSH, LH
Receptor	
GHRH receptor	GH
CRH receptor and CRH	ACTH
GnRH receptor	FSH, LH
GPR54	LH, FSH
TRH receptor	TSH
Leptin receptor	LH, FSH
Structural	
Pituitary aplasia	Any
Pituitary hypoplasia	Any
CNS masses, encephalocele	Any
Transcription Factor Defect	
PITX2	
PROP1	GH, PRL, TSH, LH, FSH, ± ACTH
POU1F1 (PIT1)	PRL, GH, TSH
HESX1	GH, PRL, TSH, LH, FSH, ACTH
LHX3/4	GH, PRL, TSH, LH, FSH
NR0B1 (DAX1)	Adrenal, LH, FSH
TBX19 (TPIT)	ACTH
Hormone Mutation	
GH1	GH
Bioinactive GH	GH
FSHβ	FSH
LHβ	LH
POMC	ACTH
POMC processing defect	ACTH
TSHβ	TSH
Leptin	LH, FSH
PC1	ACTH, FSH, LH
Kisspeptin	LH, FSH

*Developmental deficits may be hypothalamic or pituitary or both.

ACTH, adrenocorticotropic hormone; CNS, central nervous system; CRH, corticotropin-releasing hormone; FSH, follicle-stimulating hormone; GH, growth hormone; GHRH, growth hormone–releasing hormone; GnRH, gonadotropin-releasing hormone; GPR, orphan G protein–coupled receptor; LH, luteinizing hormone; POMC, pro-opiomelanocortin; PRL, prolactin; TSH, thyroid-stimulating hormone; TRH, thyrotropin-releasing hormone.

Molecular Analysis. Inheritance modes of PROP1 mutations usually reflect autosomal recessive patterns. Patients are usually homozygous for either deletion or missense frameshift mutations leading to truncated PROP1 protein products devoid of functional activity.[243,460] A hot spot in PROP1 has been identified at a GA repeat in exon 2. Combination of a GA or AG deletion in this repeat results in a coding frameshift and premature termination at codon 109. Nonafflicted siblings are either heterozygous or bear a normal PROP1 sequence on both alleles. Mutations in the transactivation domain at codon 582 lead to features of hypogonadism as the presenting phenotype.[461]

Clinical Features. The frequency of PROP1 gene mutations in patients with combined pituitary hormone deficiency is high, 30% to 50% of affected subjects.[462] However, in families with multiple affected members, PROP1 mutations account for almost all affected individuals. Patients harboring PROP1 mutations exhibit a predominantly hypogonadal phenotype. Puberty is often delayed or absent, with markedly attenuated LH and FSH responses to GnRH stimulation.[155] Some patients enter puberty spontaneously and subsequently features of central hypogonadism, akin to an acquired presentation.[460] A broad spectrum with variable time of onset and degree of pituitary loss is characteristic of the syndrome. Some older patients also exhibit blunted cortisol responses to Cortrosyn administration, and others present with panhypopituitarism.[463] Although the size of the pituitary gland usually is small or normal, patients have been described with grossly hyperplastic pituitary glands with cystic changes and development of a secondary empty sella.

Slowing of linear growth usually becomes apparent after the age of 3 years, and these patients typically do not enter puberty. Height standard deviation score (SDS) may be severely impaired and may range to −10 with eunuchoid proportions and reduced upper/lower body ratios. Affected adults are short and have infantile external genitalia. The onset of clinically evident pituitary failure usually is with GHD (about 80%) or thyroid failure (TSH deficiency, about 20%), followed by hypogonadism and later subclinical or overt adrenal insufficiency.[464] PROP1 excess has been described in a mouse model.[465] These animals have hypothyroidism, hypogonadism, persistent Rathke's cleft cysts, and, after 1 year, pituitary adenomas.

Pituitary Size. Heterogeneous changes in pituitary size may reflect a combination of apoptotic signals for the POU1F1 lineage, compensatory cystic expansion of nonaffected pituitary cell types with subsequent autoinfarction, and the absence of other unknown factors required for mature pituitary function.[466]

Evaluation. Combined hypothalamic hormone stimulation (GnRH, TRH, CRH, and GHRH) or insulin-evoked hypoglycemia reveals blunted responses consistent with varying degrees of pituitary hormone deficiencies. Serum IGF1 and IGFBP3 levels are usually low, and peripheral thyroid hormone levels are low or at the lower limits of normal ranges. In the face of low or absent TSH responses, these findings are consistent with secondary hypothyroidism. Most older patients also exhibit blunted cortisol responses to CRH or ACTH (or both) or insulin stimulation.[461]

POU1F1

The POU1F1 gene is located on chromosome 3p11 (OMIM 173110) and encodes a 290-amino-acid protein. The N-terminal POU-specific domain activates gene transcription, whereas two DNA-binding domains recognize a TATNCAT consensus sequence that is present in GH, PRL, and TSH hormones and in the GHRH receptor gene.[467] The POU1F1 nuclear protein activates transcription of the GH, PRL, TSH, and GHRH receptor genes and also partners with coactivators including thyroid hormone, estrogen, and retinoic acid receptors and with other transcription factors (e.g., CREB, P-LIM, Ptx1, HESX1, and Zn15). POU1F1 autoregulates its own expression, rendering POU1F1 critical for maintaining appropriate POU1F1 expression. Because of the absolute requirement of POU1F1 for GH, PRL, and TSH cell development and specific gene expression, inactivating mutations of the gene result in a spectrum of pituitary hormone deficiencies.[468] Two dwarf mouse strains harbor *Pou1f1* gene mutations. The Snell dwarf mouse harbors a tryptophan → cysteine missense mutation (Trp261Cys).[469] The Jackson mouse, although also a dwarf, harbors a truncated Pou1f1 protein with defective DNA binding.

Several POU1F1 mutations exhibit characteristic clinical phenotypes.[470] Arg172Tyr mutants are associated with neonatal hypothyroidism and GH and PRL deficiency. Both sporadic patients and multiplex families with multiple pituitary hormone defects have been described, with at least 10 recessive and 3 dominant POU1F1 mutations identified so far. Recessive mutations result in a varied spectrum of loss of DNA binding or transcriptional activation of TSH, GH, or PRL. Impaired retinoic acid activation of the POU1F1 distal enhancer has been described for a POU1F1 Lys-261Glu mutation. This mutant protein also behaves as a dominant negative inhibitor of POU1F1 activation. A sporadic mutation (Arg271Try) binds well to DNA but dominantly inhibits pituitary gene transcription. Compound heterozygosity for a single-base-pair deletion (747delA) and a missense mutation (Trp193Arg) cause defective DNA binding and transcriptional activation with severe combined GH, PRL, and TSH deficiencies.[291] Both p300/CBP1 protein recruitment and POU1F1 dimerization are required for appropriate POU1F1 activation of target hormone genes.[471] Lhx4 appears to activate POU1F1, and mutations of Lhx4 also lead to growth retardation.[472]

HESX1

HESX1 (Rpx) is one of the earliest transcriptional markers of the primitive pituitary, with expression restricted to Rathke's pouch.[473] Coincidentally with the appearance of specific pituitary cell types, *HESX1* expression declines and is extinguished in the mature anterior pituitary,[474] leading to PROP1 activation. The gene is located on chromosome 3p212, encodes an 185-amino-acid protein, and competes with PROP1 for DNA binding. The heterogeneous syndrome of septo-optic dysplasia (hypoplastic optic nerves, absent corpus callosum and septum pellucidum, and panhypopituitarism) is associated with 14 mutations.[475] Although the mutant molecule exhibits reduced DNA binding, panhypopituitarism may also occur secondarily to profound anatomic defects in midline development.

Lhx3

Missense and deletion mutations of LHX3 are associated with panhypopituitarism except for intact ACTH reserve.[476] These patients also exhibit defective neck rotation ability due to a rigid cervical spine.[477]

Lhx4

Patients with LHX4 mutations are unable to activate both PROP1 and POU1F1, and the result is pituitary failure.[472]

Ptx2

Ptx2 Rieger's syndrome (anterior eye, teeth, and umbilical maldevelopment) may be associated with GHD and haploinsufficiency of the *RIEG* (*PITX2*) homeobox gene.[478]

TPIT

TPIT mutations result in early-onset isolated ACTH deficiency and hypocortisolism.[31] Associated phenotypes include those for POMC deficiency—obesity, red hair pigmentation, and other associated pituitary deficiencies.

Heritable pituitary hormone deficiencies caused by transcription factor defects are rare. Among them, PROP1 mutations appear to be the most prevalent cause, accounting for well over 50% of patients in retrospective reports and more than 90% of those with more than one affected sibling. POU1F1 mutations are less commonly encountered.[479] Patients with a family history of pituitary dysfunction and those who exhibit blunted hormonal response to TRH, GHRH, or GnRH stimulation should be subjected to molecular screening for PROP1 or POU1F1 defects (Fig. 8-35).[32] The pronounced clinical phenotype of HESX1 mutations determines the need for further molecular analysis. Approaches to patients harboring rare SOX2,[480] Six6, or Otx2 mutations (see Table 8-6) are described in Chapters 23 and 24.

Lawrence-Moon-Biedl Syndrome. Lawrence-Moon-Biedl syndrome is an autosomal recessive disorder characterized by hypogonadotropic hypogonadism, mental retardation, obesity, retinitis pigmentosa, and hexadactyly, brachydactyly, or syndactyly. By 30 years of age, most patients are blind.[481] Although most patients have evidence of GnRH deficiency, about 25% of afflicted males have primary testicular failure.

Prader-Willi Syndrome. Patients with Prader-Willi syndrome have marked hyperphagia and obesity with retarded mental development, muscle hypotonia, and diabetes mellitus. Related conditions include micrognathia, absent auricular cartilage, and acromicria.[482] The condition has been ascribed to deletion or translocation of chromosome

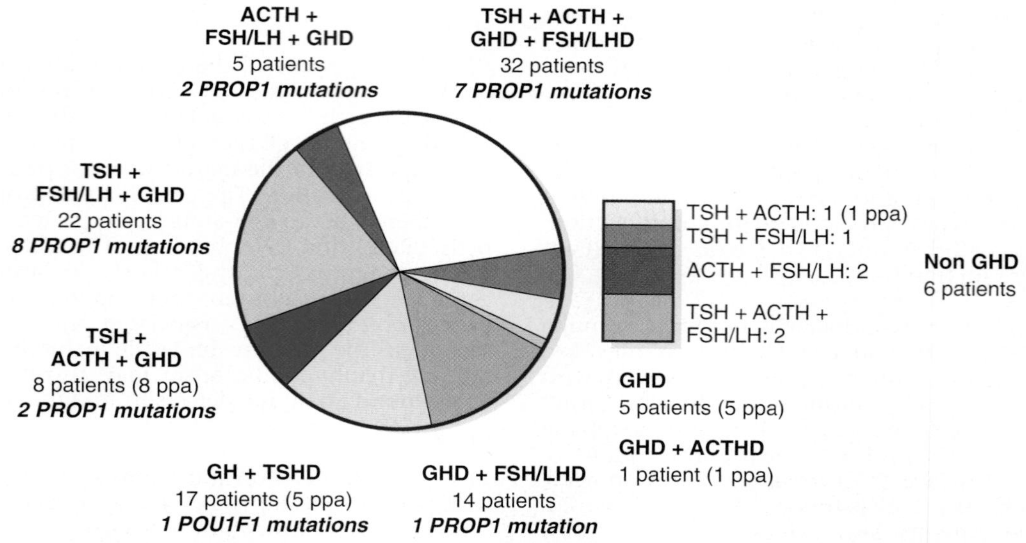

Figure 8-35 Partitioning of pituitary hormone deficiencies in 110 unrelated patients affected by congenital pituitary deficiency without stalk pituitary interruption or septal optic displasia (SOD). Patients were studied for mutations in *PROP1*, *POU1F1*, and *LHX3* according to hormonal deficit (D) phenotype. Twenty mutations of *PROP1* and one mutation of *POU1F1* were found. Gonadotroph function was unavailable for prepubertal-age patients (ppa). ACTH, adrenocorticotropic hormone; FSH, follicle-stimulating hormone; GH, growth hormone; LH, luteinizing hormone; TSH, thyroid-stimulating hormone. (From Reynaud R, Gueydan M, Saveanu A, et al. Genetic screening of combined pituitary hormone deficiency: experience in 195 patients. *J Clin Endocrinol Metab.* 2006;91:3329-3326.)

15. In hypogonadal patients, bilateral cryptorchidism and absent scrotal folds are accompanied by evidence of attenuated GnRH secretion.[483] LH and FSH levels have been restored in some patients with chronic GnRH treatment. Defective oxytocin and vasopressin synthesis have also been reported.

Kallmann's Syndrome

Kallmann's syndrome consists of defective GnRH synthesis with olfactory nerve agenesis or hypoplasia and variable anosmia. Associated developmental disorders include optic atrophy, color blindness, cranial nerve VIII deafness, cleft palate, renal agenesis, cryptorchidism, and movement disorders.[484] This X-linked recessive disorder has been ascribed to a defective *KAL* gene located on chromosome Xp22.3.[485] The KAL protein mediates hypothalamic migration of GnRH cells from the primitive olfactory placode, and its absence leads to defective GnRH synthesis and anosmia.[486,487] Both autosomal recessive and autosomal dominant forms of the disorder have been described, indicating the involvement of FGF1 receptor mutations in the pathogenesis of the disorder.[488]

Clinical Features. Patients with Kallmann's syndrome are exposed to low or absent sex steroids from birth. Consequently, females are tall and present with primary amenorrhea and absent secondary sexual development, and males have delayed puberty and micropenis.[489]

Laboratory. Absent GnRH secretory pulses result in characteristically low LH and FSH levels in the face of very low concentrations of estradiol or testosterone. Because the nonprimed normal pituitary may not respond initially to GnRH stimulation (25 to 100 μg intravenously), this test is of little value in distinguishing the hypothalamic defect. In some patients, repetitive GnRH priming elicits normal pituitary LH and FSH responses, indicating a hypothalamic defect in GnRH secretion.

The differential diagnosis of congenital hypogonadotropic hypogonadism includes Kallmann's syndrome (*KAL* gene mutation), congenital adrenal hypoplasia (DAX1/NROB1 mutation),[490] GnRH receptor mutations, leptin and leptin receptor mutations, *PROP1* gene mutations, and mutations of the LH or FSH molecules. These conditions are characterized by absent or low GnRH-mediated LH secretory patterns in the presence of a structurally normal pituitary gland. The cause of hypogonadotropic hypogonadism remains elusive in more than 80% of patients. In the absence of a structural pituitary defect, genetic evaluation of these patients should be undertaken.[455,479]

Acquired Pituitary Failure

Causes

In the absence of demonstrable hypothalamic-pituitary anatomic damage, and after exclusion of genetic and syndromic causes of pituitary insufficiencies, acquired (often transient) causes of pituitary failure should be considered (see Table 8-7). Causes of pituitary insufficiency discussed earlier include pituitary tumors, parasellar masses, hypophysitis, aneurysms, and pituitary apoplexy (Fig. 8-36).

Hypothalamic damage reflected by the presence of a large parasellar mass leading to decreased GnRH production is associated with hyperphagia, obesity, and central hypogonadism with low levels of FSH and LH (Frohlich's syndrome). Marked caloric restriction, anorexia,[491,492] weight loss of other etiologies, and strenuous exercise may also attenuate GnRH secretion or action. Hypogonadotropic hypogonadism occurs in both men and women (see Chapter 20). Exogenous anabolic steroid and glucocorticoid therapies suppress the reproductive and adrenal axes, respectively. Patients with severe critical illnesses or chronic debilitating disease (including cirrhosis) may have impaired GH-IGF1, adrenal, and gonadal axes. Hyperprolactinemia causes sexual dysfunction by inhibiting GnRH pulsatility via a short feedback loop. Hypothyroidism, hypoadrenalism, or hypogonadism causes hyperplasia of specific trophic cells due to lack of negative feedback and sometimes actual pituitary tumor formation.[493]

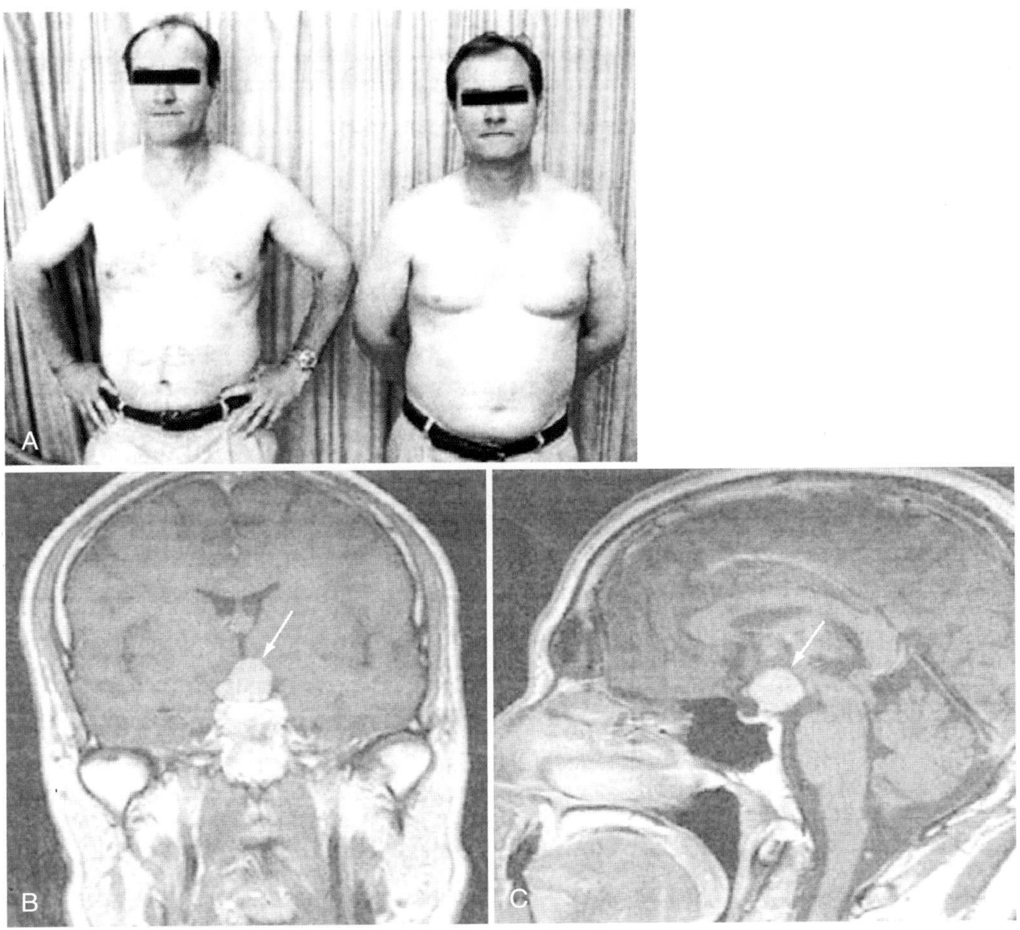

Figure 8-36 Features of hypopituitarism and hypogonadism, including central adiposity, proximal muscle wasting, loss of body hair, and gynecomastia. Notice the contrast between the hypogonadal patient (**A,** *right side*) and his unaffected identical twin *(left side)*. Laboratory tests confirmed secondary hypogonadism, with a testosterone level of 0.4 ng/mL (normal range, 2.9 to 8.0 ng/mL), a follicle-stimulating hormone level of 2.8 IU/L (normal, 1.5 to 12.4 IU/L), and a luteinizing hormone level of 1.5 IU/L (normal, 1.7 to 8.6 IU/L). Coronal **(B)** and sagittal **(C)** Magnetic resonance images showed a lobulated, contrast-enhancing suprasellar mass *(arrow)*. Pathologic analysis confirmed the diagnosis of pituicytoma. (From Newnham HH, Rivera-Woll LM. Images in clinical medicine: hypogonadism due to pituicytoma in an identical twin. *N Engl J Med.* 2008;359:2824.)

AIDS is associated with suppressed pituitary function independent of other associated infections.[494] Drugs such as estrogens, which suppress FSH and LH, and GnRH analogs used for treatment of prostate cancer inhibit gonadotropin action. In addition to pituitary apoplexy, other vascular accidents such as aneurysms, strokes, cavernous sinus thrombosis, and arteritis can cause pituitary hormone insufficiency. Isolated pituitary hormone deficiencies may also occur as a manifestation of vascular abnormalities, including arteritis, or subarachnoid hemorrhage (Table 8-11).

Head Trauma. The pituitary may be partially or totally damaged by birth trauma, cranial hemorrhage, fetal asphyxia, or breech delivery. Head trauma may lead to direct pituitary damage from a sella turcica fracture, pituitary stalk section, trauma-induced vasospasm, or ischemic infarction after blunt trauma.[495] The most common traumatic cause of compromised pituitary function in the adult is iatrogenic neurosurgical trauma. Pituitary manipulation or damage during surgery leads to transient or permanent diabetes insipidus and varying degrees of anterior pituitary dysfunction.

Although hypopituitarism after head trauma is usually manifest within 1 year after the insult, some patients only develop overtly manifest signs of pituitary failure after several decades. Seventy-five percent of patients with post-traumatic pituitary failure are young men (<40 years) who were involved in a motor vehicle accident within 1 year before diagnosis. Almost all patients with subsequent pituitary failure have a history of loss of consciousness after trauma, and half of all such patients have documented skull fracture.[495] One third of these patients have demonstrable signs of hypothalamic or posterior pituitary hemorrhage or anterior lobe infarction on MRI. Diabetes insipidus is the most common endocrine disorder, encountered in about 30% of these patients. Gonadotropin failure, amenorrhea, and hyperprolactinemia may occur in the months following head trauma or may manifest even years later.[496,497]

Pituitary testing performed within the first 48 hours after hospital admission shows that approximately 75% of patients have evidence of hypopituitarism,[498] and the degree of pituitary failure correlates with the severity of head trauma (Table 8-12). Prospective studies of patients retested after 12 months have documented worsening of

TABLE 8-11

Hypopituitarism after Subarachnoid Hemorrhage

Reference	N	Any Degree of Hypopituitarism	Multiple Deficiencies	GH	LH/FSH	ACTH	TSH
Kelly et al., 2000[518]	2	2	0	2	0	0	0
Brandt et al., 2004[519]	10	5	0	1	4	0	0
Aimaretti et al., 2004[520]	40	15	4	10	5	1*	3
Kreitschmann-Andermahr et al., 2004[521]	40	22	3	8	0	16	1
Dimopoulou et al., 2004[522]	30	14	4	11†	4	3	2
Total (%)	122 (100)	58 (48)	11 (9)	32 (26)	13 (11)	20 (16)	6 (5)

*No stimulation test for ACTH.
†No stimulation test for GH (11 patients had low IGF1).
ACTH, adrenocorticotropic hormone; GH, growth hormone; LH, luteinizing hormone; FSH, follicle-stimulating hormone; TSH, thyroid-stimulating hormone.
Modified from Schneider H, Aimaretti G, Kreitschmann-Andermahr I, et al. Hypopituitarism. *Lancet.* 2007;369:1461-1470.

pituitary function despite improvement in some trophic hormone axes. About 20% of patients developed posterior pituitary dysfunction (either diabetes insipidus or SIADH) after traumatic brain injury.[499]

Irradiation. Pituitary irradiation, usually indicated for pituitary adenoma therapy, directly causes atrophy of the gland, in addition to the damaging impact of irradiation on hypothalamic synthesis of hypophysiotropic hormones.[500] Pituitary function in children and adolescents is particularly sensitive to head and neck therapeutic irradiation.[501] Radiation dose exposure, time interval after completion of radiotherapy, and distance of the pituitary or hypothalamus from the central energy field correlate with development of pituitary hormone deficits (Figs. 8-37 and 8-38).

After a median dose of 5000 rads directed at the skull base, nasopharynx, or cranium, up to 75% of patients develop pituitary insufficiency within 10 years.[502] Later manifestations of pituitary failure usually reflect hypothalamic damage rather than atrophy of irradiated pituitary cells. Although the degree of hormone loss after radiation therapy is variable, the pattern of loss usually occurs sequentially: GH, then FSH and LH, followed by ACTH and TSH.[503] Evidence for secondary thyroid or adrenal failure usually implies that the GH and gonadotropin axes are also compromised. Stereotactic radiosurgery directed to the pituitary gland also results in pituitary deficits within 48 to 96 months in 23% of patients.[504] Previously irradiated patients should undergo lifelong periodic anterior pituitary hormone testing. Ideally, rigorous long-term screening will unmask incipient pituitary failure before the onset of morbidity.[505]

Empty Sella Syndrome. Damage to the sellar diaphragm may lead to arachnoid herniation into the sellar space. An empty sella may develop as a consequence of a primary congenital weakness of the diaphragm in those patients in whom no secondary cause is evident. Up to 50% of patients with primary empty sella have associated benign intracranial hypertension.[506] A secondary empty sella may develop subsequent to infarction of a pituitary adenoma or as a result of surgical or radiation-induced damage to the sellar diaphragm. On MRI, these patients usually exhibit demonstrable pituitary tissue compressed against the sellar floor, with lateral stalk deviation. Although an empty sella is usually an incidental finding, pituitary failure occurs if more than 90% of pituitary tissue is compressed or

TABLE 8-12

Hypopituitarism in the Chronic Phase after Traumatic Brain Injury

Reference	N	Any Degree of Hypopituitarism	Multiple Deficiencies	GH	LH/FSH	ACTH	TSH
Kelly et al., 2000[518]	22	8	3	4	4	1	1
Lieberman et al., 2001[523]	70	48	12	7	2	32*	15
Bondanelli et al., 2004[524]	50	27	6	4	7	0†	5
Agha et al., 2004[497]	102	29	6	11	12	13	1
Popovic et al., 2004[525]	67	23	7	10	6	5	3
Aimaretti et al., 2005[498]	70	16	7	14	8	4†	5
Leal-Cerro et al., 2005[526]	170	42	15	6	29	11‡	10
Schneider et al., 2006[496]	70	25	3	7	14	6	2
Tanriverdi et al., 2006[527]	52	26	5	17	4	10	3
Herrmann et al., 2006[528]	76	18	5	6	13	2	2
Total (%)	749 (100)	262 (35)	69 (9)	86 (11)	99 (13)	84 (11)	47 (6)

*Thirty-two patients had low morning cortisol; only 5 patients had cortisol <500 nmol/L after ACTH stimulation.
†No stimulation test for ACTH.
‡Endocrine testing was done only if there was clinical suspicion of hypopituitarism (n = 99).
Modified from Schneider H, Aimaretti G, Kreitschmann-Andermahr I, et al. Hypopituitarism. *Lancet.* 2007;369:1461-1470.

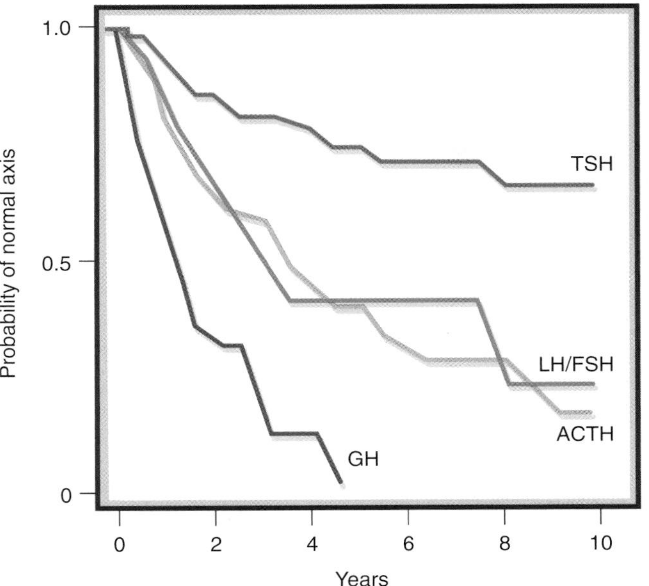

Figure 8-37 Life-table analysis indicating probabilities of initially normal hypothalamic-pituitary-target gland axes remaining normal after radiotherapy (3750 to 4250 cGy). Of the anterior pituitary hormones, growth hormone (GH) secretion is the most sensitive, and thyroid-stimulating hormone (TSH) secretion is the most resistant. In two thirds of patients, gonadotropin deficiency develops before adrenocorticotropic hormone (ACTH) deficiency; the reverse occurs in the remaining third. (From Littley MD, Shalet SM, Beardwell CG, et al. Hypopituitarism following external radiotherapy for pituitary tumors in adults. *QJM*. 1989;70:145-160.)

atrophied. About 10% of patients develop small GH- or PRL-secreting adenomas within the rim of compressed pituitary tissue.

Clinical Features of Hypopituitarism

Patients with pituitary failure, regardless of course, have been found to have excess mortality primarily due to respiratory and vascular disease.[239] Age at diagnosis, female gender, and history of craniopharyngioma were the most striking determinants of increased mortality. The spectrum of clinical features of pituitary insufficiency depends on several factors. In acquired pituitary insufficiency, the clinical spectrum depends on the degree of hormone deficiency, the number of hormones impaired, and the rapidity of onset.[517] In congenital forms, the earlier the age at onset, the greater the severity of thyroid, gonadal, adrenal, growth, or water disturbances. Patients with heritable genetic disorders invariably exhibit the most severe phenotypic changes, although later changes may also occur in these disorders (e.g., with PROP1 mutations).

The resilience of the individual pituitary cell lineages to compressive, inflammatory, vascular, radiation, and invasive insults also varies. The lactotroph cell is often hyperfunctional as a result of decreased tonic inhibitory signals. Therefore, PRL deficiency is exceedingly rare, except that resulting from complete pituitary destruction or genetic syndromes. The order of diminished trophic hormone reserve function related to pituitary compression usually is as follows: GH > FSH > LH > TSH > ACTH. The corticotroph cell appears to be particularly resistant to hypothalamic or pituitary destruction, and it is usually the last cell to lose function.

The qualitative phenotypic manifestations of pituitary failure are determined by which specific trophic hormones are lost (see earlier descriptions of individual hormone deficiencies).

Screening for Pituitary Failure

Because the onset of hypopituitarism can be extremely slow, subclinical pituitary failure is often not apparent to the patient or physician. Screening for pituitary dysfunction should be undertaken in patients with hypothalamic or pituitary mass lesions, developmental craniofacial abnormalities, inflammatory disorders, brain granulomatous disease, prior head or neck irradiation, head trauma, prior skull base surgery, newly discovered empty sella, or previous pregnancy-associated hemorrhage or blood pressure changes[507,510] (Table 8-13).

PRL should be measured, because many patients with hypopituitarism also present with secondary hyperprolactinemia. Up to two thirds of patients harboring pituitary macroadenomas, craniopharyngiomas, or other parasellar lesions have compromised pituitary reserve function. Less commonly, patients with intrasellar aneurysms, pituitary metastases, parasellar meningiomas, optic gliomas, or hypothalamic astrocytomas also have pituitary failure.

Although about one third of patients with hypopituitarism undergoing pituitary surgery recover function after decompression, about 25% experience further loss of pituitary function after surgery and require annual screening. Treatment of pituitary failure is described in Table 8-14.

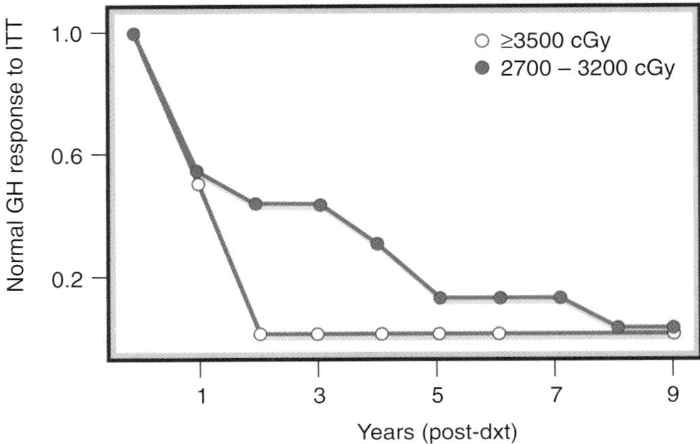

Figure 8-38 The incidence of growth hormone (GH) deficiency in children receiving 27 to 32 Gy or 35 Gy of cranial irradiation for a brain tumor, in relation to time from irradiation (dxt). The speed at which individual pituitary hormone deficits develop is dose dependent: the higher the radiation dose, the earlier GH deficiency occurs. (Courtesy of the Department of Medical Illustrations, Wilkington Hospital, Manchester, England. From Shalet S. Pituitary failure. In: DeGroot LJ, Jameson JL, eds. *Endocrinology*. Philadelphia, PA: Saunders, 2001.)

TABLE 8-13

Assessment of Anterior Pituitary Function

Test	Dose	Normal Response	Side Effects
ACTH			
Insulin tolerance	0.1-0.15 U/kg IV	Peak cortisol response >18 μg/dL, or ↑ ≥5 μg/dL	Sweating, palpitation, tremor
Metyrapone	30 mg/kg PO at 11 p.m.	Peak 11-DOC ≥ 7 μg/dL Peak cortisol ≤7 μg/dL Peak ACTH >75 pg/mL	Nausea, insomnia, adrenal crisis
CRH stimulation	100 μg IV	Peak ACTH ≥2-4-fold Peak cortisol ≥20 μg/dL or ↑ ≥7 μg/dL	Flushing
ACTH stimulation	250 μg IV or IM, or 1 μg IV	Peak cortisol ≥20 μg/dL	Rare
TSH			
Serum T_4 (free T_4) Total T_3 TSH—third generation TRH stimulation	200-500 μg IV	Peak TSH ≥2.5-fold, or ↑ ≥5-6 mU/L (females) or ≥2-3 mU/L (males)	Flushing, nausea, urge to micturate
PRL			
Serum PRL TRH stimulation	200-500 μg IV	PRL ↑ ≥2.5-fold	Flushing, nausea, urge to micturate
LH/FSH			
Serum LH and FSH Serum testosterone GnRH Stimulation	100 μg IV	Elevated in menopause and in men with primary testicular failure (otherwise normal) 300-900 ng/mL LH ≥2-3-fold, or ↑ by 10 IU/L FSH ≥1.5-2-fold, or ↑ ≥2 IU/L	Rare
GH			
Insulin tolerance	0.1-0.15 U/kg	GH peak >5 μg/L	Sweating, palpitation, tremor
L-Arginine	Arginine 0.5 g/kg (maximum, 30 g) IV over 30-120 min	GH peak >0.4 μg/L	Nausea
plus			
GHRH	GHRH 1-5 μg/kg	GH peak >4 μg/L	Flushing

ACTH, adrenocorticotropic hormone; CRH, corticotropin-releasing hormone; 11-DOC, 11-deoxycorticosterone; FSH, follicle-stimulating hormone; GH, growth hormone; GHRH, growth hormone–releasing hormone; GnRH, gonadotropin-releasing hormone; LH, luteinizing hormone; PRL, prolactin; T_3, triiodothyronine; T_4, thyroxine; TSH, thyroid-stimulating hormone; TRH, thyrotropin-releasing hormone.

TABLE 8-14

Replacement Therapy for Adult Hypopituitarism*

Deficient Hormone	Treatment	Remarks
ACTH	Hydrocortisone: 10-20 mg/day in divided doses Cortisone acetate: 15-25 mg/day in divided doses	
TSH	L-Thyroxine: 0.05-0.2 mg/day according to T_4 levels	
FSH/LH (in males)	Testosterone enanthate: 200 mg IM q2-3 wk Testosterone skin patch: 2.5-5.0 mg/day (or up to 7.5 mg/day) Testosterone gel: 3-6 g/day	*For fertility:* hCG three times weekly, or hCG + either FSH or menopausal gonadotropin or GnRH
FSH/LH (in females)	Conjugated estrogen: 0.3-0.625 mg/day Micronized estradiol: 1 mg/day Estradiol valerate: 2 mg Piperazine estrone sulfate: 1.25 mg Estradiol skin patch: 4-8 mg twice weekly	All of the estrogens are administered with progesterone or progestin sequentially or in combination if uterus is present *For fertility:* Menopausal gonadotropin, and hCG, or GnRH
Growth hormone	Somatotropin (in adults): 0.2-1.0 mg/day SC Somatotropin (in children): 0.02-0.05 mg/kg per day	
Vasopressin	Intranasal desmopressin: 10-20 μg bid Oral DDAVP: 300-600 μg/day, usually in divided doses	

*Doses shown should be individualized and reassessed during stress, surgery, or pregnancy. Male and female fertility management are fully discussed in Chapter 20.

ACTH, adrenocorticotropic hormone; DDAVP, desmopressin acetate; FSH, follicle-stimulating hormone; GnRH, gonadotropin-releasing hormone; hCG, human chorionic gonadotropin; LH, luteinizing hormone; T_4, thyroxine; TSH, thyroid-stimulating hormone.

REFERENCES

1. Bernard C. Physiologie; chiens rendus diabetiques. *C R Soc Biol.* 1849;1:60.
2. Marie P. On two cases of acromegaly: marked hypertrophy of the upper and lower limbs and the head. *Rev Med.* 1886;6:297-333.
3. Cushing H. Partial hypophysectomy for acromegaly: with remarks on the function of the hypophysis. *Ann Surg.* 1909;50:1002-1017.
4. Cushing H. Surgical experiences with pituitary disorders. *JAMA.* 1914;63:1515-1525.
5. Harris GW. Neural control of pituitary gland. *Physiol Rev.* 1948;28: 139-179.
6. Chanson P, Daujat F, Young J, et al. Normal pituitary hypertrophy as a frequent cause of pituitary incidentaloma: a follow-up study. *J Clin Endocrinol Metab.* 2001;86:3009-3015.
7. Stanfield JP. The blood supply of the human pituitary gland. *J Anat.* 1960;94:257-273.
8. Bergland RM, Page RB. Pituitary-brain vascular relations: a new paradigm. *Science.* 1979;204:18-24.
9. Rathke H. Ueber die Entsehung der glandula. *Arch Anat Physio Wissened.* 1838;482-485.
10. Etchevers HC, Vincent C, Le Douarin NM, et al. The cephalic neural crest provides pericytes and smooth muscle cells to all blood vessels of the face and forebrain. *Development.* 2001;128:1059-1068.
11. Takuma N, Sheng HZ, Furuta Y, et al. Formation of Rathke's pouch requires dual induction from the diencephalon. *Development.* 1998;125:4835-4840.
12. Gleiberman AS, Fedtsova NG, Rosenfeld MG. Tissue interactions in the induction of anterior pituitary: role of the ventral diencephalon, mesenchyme, and notochord. *Dev Biol.* 1999;213:340-353.
13. Scully KM, Rosenfeld MG. Pituitary development: regulatory codes in mammalian organogenesis. *Science.* 2002;295:2231-2235.
14. Zhu X, Wang J, Ju BG, et al. Signaling and epigenetic regulation of pituitary development. *Curr Opin Cell Biol.* 2007;19:605-611.
15. Pulichino AM, Lamolet B, Vallette-Kasic S, et al. Tpit-/-NeuroD1-/- mice reveal novel aspects of corticotroph development. *Endocr Res.* 2004;30:551-552.
16. Ward RD, Stone BM, Raetzman LT, et al. Cell proliferation and vascularization in mouse models of pituitary hormone deficiency. *Mol Endocrinol.* 2006;20:1378-1390.
17. Treier M, Gleiberman AS, O'Connell SM, et al. Multistep signaling requirements for pituitary organogenesis in vivo. *Genes Dev.* 1998;12:1691-1704.
18. Asa SL, Kovacs K, Laszlo FA, et al. Human fetal adenohypophysis: histologic and immunocytochemical analysis. *Neuroendocrinology.* 1986;43:308-316.
19. Dubois PM, Hemming FJ. Fetal development and regulation of pituitary cell types. *J Electron Microsc Tech.* 1991;19:2-20.
20. Zhu X, Lin CR, Prefontaine GG, et al. Genetic control of pituitary development and hypopituitarism. *Curr Opin Genet Dev.* 2005;15: 332-340.
21. Lanctot C, Gauthier Y, Drouin J. Pituitary homeobox 1 (Ptx1) is differentially expressed during pituitary development. *Endocrinology.* 1999;140:1416-1422.
22. Lu MF, Pressman C, Dyer R, et al. Function of Rieger syndrome gene in left-right asymmetry and craniofacial development. *Nature.* 1999;401:276-278.
23. Charles MA, Saunders TL, Wood WM, Pituitary-specific Gata2 knockout: effects on gonadotrope and thyrotrope function. *Mol Endocrinol.* 2006;20:1366-1377.
24. Ellsworth BS, Egashira N, Haller JL, et al. FOXL2 in the pituitary: molecular, genetic, and developmental analysis. *Mol Endocrinol.* 2006;20:2796-2805.
25. Raetzman LT, Wheeler BS, Ross SA, et al. Persistent expression of Notch2 delays gonadotrope differentiation. *Mol Endocrinol.* 2006;20: 2898-2908.
26. Olson LE, Tollkuhn J, Scafoglio C, et al. Homeodomain-mediated beta-catenin-dependent switching events dictate cell-lineage determination. *Cell.* 2006;125:593-605.
27. Carriere C, Gleiberman A, Lin CR, et al. From panhypopituitarism to combined pituitary deficiencies: do we need the anterior pituitary? *Rev Endocr Metab Disord.* 2004;5:5-13.
28. Pulichino A-M, Vallette-Kasic S, Drouin J. Transcriptional regulation of pituitary gland development: binary choices for cell differentiation. *Curr Opin Endocrinol Metab.* 2004;11:13-17.
29. Muscatelli F, Strom TM, Walker AP, et al. Mutations in the DAX-1 gene give rise to both X-linked adrenal hypoplasia congenita and hypogonadotropic hypogonadism. *Nature.* 1994;372:672-676.
30. Tabarin A, Achermann JC, Recan D, et al. A novel mutation in DAX1 causes delayed-onset adrenal insufficiency and incomplete hypogonadotropic hypogonadism. *J Clin Invest.* 2000;105:321-328.
31. Lamolet B, Pulichino AM, Lamonerie T, et al. A pituitary cell-restricted T box factor, Tpit, activates POMC transcription in cooperation with Pitx homeoproteins. *Cell.* 2001;104:849-859.
32. Reynaud R, Gueydan M, Saveanu A, et al. Genetic screening of combined pituitary hormone deficiency: experience in 195 patients. *J Clin Endocrinol Metab.* 2006;91:3329-3336.
33. Melmed S. Mechanisms for pituitary tumorigenesis: the plastic pituitary. *J Clin Invest.* 2003;112:1603-1618.
34. Fauquier T, Rizzoti K, Dattani M, et al. SOX2-expressing progenitor cells generate all of the major cell types in the adult mouse pituitary gland. *Proc Natl Acad Sci U S A.* 2008;105:2907-2912.
35. Chen J, Crabbe A, Van Duppen V, et al. The notch signaling system is present in the postnatal pituitary: marked expression and regulatory activity in the newly discovered side population. *Mol Endocrinol.* 2006;20:3293-3307.
36. Gleiberman AS, Michurina T, Encinas JM, et al. Genetic approaches identify adult pituitary stem cells. *Proc Natl Acad Sci U S A.* 2008;105:6332-6637.
37. Wilhelmi AE. Fractionation of human pituitary glands. *Can J Bichem.* 1961;39:1659-1668.
38. Suganuma N, Seo H, Yamamoto N, et al. Ontogenesis of pituitary prolactin in the human fetus. *J Clin Endocrinol Metab.* 1986;63: 156-161.
39. Kleinberg DL, Frantz AG. A sensitive in vitro assay for prolactin. Program of the 51st Meeting of the Endocrine Society. 1969 Abstract 32.
40. Frantz AG, Kleinberg DL. Prolactin: evidence that it is separate from growth hormone in human blood. *Science.* 1970;170:745-747.
41. Kleinberg DL, Frantz AG. Human prolactin: measurement in plasma by in vitro bioassay. *J Clin Invest.* 1971;50:1557-1568.
42. Hwang P, Guyda H, Friesen H. A radioimmunoassay for human prolactin. *Proceedings of the National Academy of Science USA.* 1971;68:1902-1906.
43. Friesen HG. The discovery of human prolactin: a very personal account. *Clin Invest Med.* 1995;18:66-72.
44. Scheithauer BW, Sano T, Kovacs KT, et al. The pituitary gland in pregnancy: a clinicopathologic and immunohistochemical study of 69 cases. *Mayo Clin Proc.* 1990;65:461-474.
45. Burrows HL, Birkmeier TS, Seasholtz AF, et al. Targeted ablation of cells in the pituitary primordia of transgenic mice. *Mol Endocrinol.* 1996;10:1467-1477.
46. Boockfor FR, Hoeffler JP, Frawley LS. Estradiol induces a shift in cultured cells that release prolactin or growth hormone. *Am J Physiol.* 1986;250(1 Pt 1):E103-E105.
47. Owerbach D, Rutter WJ, Cooke NE, et al. The prolactin gene is located on chromosome 6 in humans. *Science.* 1981;212:815-816.
48. Cooke NE, Coit D, Weiner RI, et al. Structure of cloned DNA complementary to rat prolactin messenger RNA. *J Biol Chem.* 1980;255: 6502-6510.
49. Lamberts SW, Macleod RM. Regulation of prolactin secretion at the level of the lactotroph. *Physiol Rev.* 1990;70:279-318.
50. Farkouh NH, Packer MG, Frantz AG. Large molecular size prolactin with reduced receptor activity in human serum: high proportion in basal state and reduction after thyrotropin-releasing hormone. *J Clin Endocrinol Metab.* 1979;48:1026-1032.
51. Sinha YN. Structural variants of prolactin: occurrence and physiological significance. *Endocr Rev.* 1995;16:354-369.
52. Suh HK, Frantz AG. Size heterogeneity of human prolactin in plasma and pituitary extracts. *J Clin Endocrinol Metab.* 1974;39:928-935.
53. Lewis UJ, Singh RN, Sinha YN, et al. Glycosylated human prolactin. *Endocrinology.* 1985;116:359-363.
54. Mittra I. A novel "cleaved prolactin" in the rat pituitary: part I—Biosynthesis, characterization and regulatory control. *Biochem Biophys Res Commun.* 1980;95:1750-1759.
55. Lee H, Struman I, Clapp C, et al. Inhibition of urokinase activity by the antiangiogenic factor 16K prolactin: activation of plasminogen activator inhibitor 1 expression. *Endocrinology.* 1998;139:3696-3703.
56. Ferrara N, Clapp C, Weiner R. The 16K fragment of prolactin specifically inhibits basal or fibroblast growth factor stimulated growth of capillary endothelial cells. *Endocrinology.* 1991;129:896-900.
57. Kline JB, Clevenger CV. Identification and characterization of the prolactin-binding protein in human serum and milk. *J Biol Chem.* 2001;276:24760-24766.
58. Liu JW, Ben Jonathan N. Prolactin-releasing activity of neurohypophysial hormones: structure-function relationship. *Endocrinology.* 1994;134:114-118.
59. Horseman ND. Prolactin. In: DeGroot LJ, Jameson JL, eds. *Endocrinology,* 4th ed. Philadelphia, PA: Saunders; 2001:209-220.
60. Horseman ND, Zhao W, Montecino-Rodriguez E, et al. Defective mammopoiesis, but normal hematopoiesis, in mice with targeted disruption of the prolactin gene. *EMBO J.* 1997;16:6926-6935.
61. Steger RW, Chandrashekar V, Zhao W, et al. Neuroendocrine and reproductive functions in male mice with targeted disruption of the prolactin gene. *Endocrinology.* 1998;139:3691-3695.
62. Kanyicska B, Lerant A, Freeman ME. Endothelin is an autocrine regulator of prolactin secretion. *Endocrinology.* 1998;139:5164-5173.
63. Sarkar DK, Kim KH, Minami S. Transforming growth factor-beta 1 messenger RNA and protein expression in the pituitary gland: its

action on prolactin secretion and lactotropic growth. *Mol Endocrinol.* 1992;6:1825-1833.
64. Shah GV, Pedchenko V, Stanley S, et al. Calcitonin is a physiological inhibitor of prolactin secretion in ovariectomized female rats. *Endocrinology.* 1996;137:1814-1822.
65. Ben Jonathan N. Regulation of prolactin secretion. In: Imura H, ed. *The Pituitary Gland.* 2nd ed. New York, NY: Raven Press; 1994: 261-283.
66. Hinuma S, Habata Y, Fujii R, et al. A prolactin-releasing peptide in the brain [see comments] [published erratum appears in Nature 1998; 394:302]. *Nature.* 1998;393:272-276.
67. Rubinek T, Hadani M, Barkai G, et al. Prolactin (PRL)-releasing peptide stimulates PRL secretion from human fetal pituitary cultures and growth hormone release from cultured pituitary adenomas. *J Clin Endocrinol Metab.* 2001;86:2826-2830.
68. Reichlin S. TRH: historical aspects. *Ann NYAcad Sci.* 1989;553:1-6.
69. Cooke NE. Prolactin: normal synthesis, regulation, and actions. In: DeGroot LJ, Besser GM, Cahill GFJ, eds. *Endocrinology.* Philadelphia, PA: Saunders; 1989:384-407.
70. Katznelson L, Riskind PN, Saxe VC, et al. Prolactin pulsatile characteristics in postmenopausal women. *J Clin Endocrinol Metab.* 1998;83: 761-764.
71. Bredow S, Kacsoh B, Obal F Jr, et al. Increase of prolactin mRNA in the rat hypothalamus after intracerebroventricular injection of VIP or PACAP. *Brain Res.* 1994;660:301-308.
72. Peters LL, Hoefer MT, Ben Jonathan N. The posterior pituitary: regulation of anterior pituitary prolactin secretion. *Science.* 1981;213: 659-661.
73. Asa SL, Kelly MA, Grandy DK, et al. Pituitary lactotroph adenomas develop after prolonged lactotroph hyperplasia in dopamine D2 receptor-deficient mice. *Endocrinology.* 1999;140:5348-5355.
74. Cooper DS, Ridgway EC, Kliman B, et al. Metabolic clearance and production rates of prolactin in man. *J Clin Invest.* 1979;64: 1669-1680.
75. Veldhuis JD, Johnson ML. Operating characteristics of the hypothalamo-pituitary-gonadal axis in men: circadian, ultradian, and pulsatile release of prolactin and its temporal coupling with luteinizing hormone. *J Clin Endocrinol Metab.* 1988;67:116-123.
76. Greenspan SL, Klibanski A, Rowe JW, et al. Age alters pulsatile prolactin release: influence of dopaminergic inhibition. *Am J Physiol.* 1990;258(5 Pt 1):E799-E804.
77. Sassin JF, Frantz AG, Weitzman ED, et al. Human prolactin: 24-hour pattern with increased release during sleep. *Science.* 1972;177: 1205-1207.
78. Parker DC, Rossman LG, Vanderlaan EF. Relation of sleep-entrained human prolactin release to REM-nonREM cycles. *J Clin Endocrinol Metab.* 1974;38:646-651.
79. Iranmanesh A, Mulligan T, Veldhuis JD. Mechanisms subserving the physiological nocturnal relative hypoprolactinemia of healthy older men: dual decline in prolactin secretory burst mass and basal release with preservation of pulse duration, frequency, and interpulse interval—a General Clinical Research Center study. *J Clin Endocrinol Metab.* 1999;84:1083-1090.
80. Bazan JF. Structural design and molecular evolution of a cytokine receptor superfamily. *Proc Natl Acad Sci USA* 1990;87:6934-6938.
81. Arden KC, Boutin JM, Djiane J, et al. The receptors for prolactin and growth hormone are localized in the same region of human chromosome 5. *Cytogenet Cell Genet.* 1990;53:161-165.
82. Hu ZZ, Zhuang L, Meng J, et al. The human prolactin receptor gene structure and alternative promoter utilization: the generic promoter hPIII and a novel human promoter hP(N). *J Clin Endocrinol Metab.* 1999;84:1153-1156.
83. Bole-Feysot C, Goffin V, Edery M, et al. Prolactin (PRL) and its receptor: actions, signal transduction pathways and phenotypes observed in PRL receptor knockout mice. *Endocr Rev.* 1998;19:225-268.
84. de Vos AM, Ultsch M, Kossiakoff AA. Human growth hormone and extracellular domain of its receptor: crystal structure of the complex. *Science.* 1992;255:306-312.
85. Clevenger CV, Gadd SL, Zheng J. New mechanisms for PRLr action in breast cancer. *Trends Endocrinol Metab.* 2009;20:223-229.
86. Gao J, Hughes JP, Auperin B, et al. Interactions among JANUS kinases and the prolactin (PRL) receptor in the regulatation of a PRL response element. *Mol Endocrinol.* 1996;10:847-856.
87. Hynes NE, Cella N, Wartmann M. Prolactin mediated intracellular signaling in mammary epithelial cells. *J Mammary Gland Biol Neopl.* 1997;2:19-27.
88. Goffin V, Kelly PA. The prolactin/growth hormone receptor family: structure/function relationships. *J Mammary Gland Biol Neopl.* 1997;2:7-17.
89. Bogorad RL, Courtillot C, Mestayer C, et al. Identification of a gain-of-function mutation of the prolactin receptor in women with benign breast tumors. *Proc Natl Acad Sci U S A.* 2008;105:14533-14538.
90. Jomain JB, Tallet E, Broutin I, et al. Structural and thermodynamic bases for the design of pure prolactin receptor antagonists, x-ray structure of Del1-9-G129R-hPRL. *J Biol Chem.* 2007;282:33118-33131.
91. Riddle O. Prolactin in vertebrate function and organization. *J Nat Cancer Inst.* 1963;31:1039-1110.
92. Lucas BK, Ormandy CJ, Binart N, et al. Null mutation of the prolactin receptor gene produces a defect in maternal behavior. *Endocrinology.* 1998;139:4102-4107.
93. Kleinberg DL, Ruan W, Catanese V, et al. Non-lactogenic effects of growth hormone on growth and insulin-like growth factor-I messenger ribonucleic acid of rat mammary gland [published erratum appears in *Endocrinology* 1990;127:1977]. *Endocrinology.* 1990;126: 3274-3276.
94. Feldman M, Ruan WF, Cunningham BC, et al. Evidence that the growth hormone receptor mediates differentiation and development of the mammary gland. *Endocrinology.* 1993;133:1602-1608.
95. Ruan W, Catanese V, Wieczorek R, et al. Estradiol enhances the stimulatory effect of insulin-like growth factor-I (IGF-I) on mammary development and growth hormone-induced IGF-I messenger ribonucleic acid. *Endocrinology.* 1995;136:1296-1302.
96. Cunha GR. Role of mesenchymal-epithelial interactions in normal and abnormal development of the mammary gland and prostate. [Review]. *Cancer.* 1994;74:1030-1044.
97. Ruan W, Monaco ME, Kleinberg DL. Progesterone stimulates mammary gland ductal morphogenesis by synergizing with and enhancing insulin-like growth factor-I action. *Endocrinology.* 2005;146: 1170-1178.
98. Walden PD, Ruan W, Feldman M, et al. Evidence that growth hormone acts on stromal tissue to stimulate pubertal mammary gland development. Program of the 79th Annual Meeting of the Endocrine Society. 1997:Abstract P1-120.
99. Wysolmerski JJ, Stewart AF. The physiology of parathyroid hormone-related protein: an emerging role as a developmental factor. *Annu Rev Physiol.* 1998;60:431-460.
100. Wiesen JF, Young P, Werb Z, et al. Signaling through the stromal epidermal growth factor receptor is necessary for mammary ductal development. *Development.* 1999;126:335-344.
101. Anderson TJ, Battersby S, King RJB, et al. Oral contraceptive use influences resting breast proliferation. *Hum Pathol.* 1989;20:1139-1144.
102. Vorherr H. Hormonal and biochemical changes of pituitary and breast during pregnancy. *Semin Perinat.* 1979;3:193-198.
103. Richert MM, Wood TL. The insulin-like growth factors (IGF) and the IGF type I receptor during postnatal growth of the murine mammary gland: sites of messenger ribonucleic acid expression and potential functions. *Endocrinology.* 1999;140:454-461.
104. Falk RJ. Isolated prolactin deficiency: a case report. *Fertil Steril.* 1992;58:1060-1062.
105. Humphreys RC, Lydon J, O'Malley BW, et al. Mammary gland development is mediated by both stromal and epithelial progesterone receptors. *Mol Endocrinol.* 1997;11:801-811.
106. Kleinberg DL, Boyd AE II, Wardlaw S, et al. Pergolide for the treatment of pituitary tumors secreting prolactin or growth hormone. *N Engl J Med.* 1983;309:704-709.
107. Graham JD, Clarke CL. Physiological action of progesterone in target tissues. *Endocrine Rev.* 1997;18:502-519.
108. Neville MC. Mammary gland biology and lactation: a short course. Presented at the annual meeting of the International Society for Research on Human Milk and Lactation, Plymouth, MA, October 1997.
109. Vorherr H. Galactopoiesis, galactosecretion, and onset of lactation. In: Vorherr H, ed. *The Breast.* New York, NY: Academic Press; 1974:71-127.
110. Tyson JE, Hwang P, Guyda H. Studies of prolactin secretion in human pregnancy. *Am J Obstet Gynecol.* 1972;113:14-20.
111. Howie PW, McNeilly AS, McArdle T, et al. The relationship between suckling-induced prolactin response and lactogenesis. *J Clin Endocrinol Metab.* 1980;50:670-673.
112. Johnston JM, Amico JA. A prospective longitudinal study of the release of oxytocin and prolactin in response to infant suckling in long term lactation. *J Clin Endocrinol Metab.* 1986;62:653-657.
113. Leite V, Cowden EA, Friesen HG. Endocrinology of lactation and nursing: disorders of lactation. In: DeGroot LJ, ed. *Endocrinology.* 3rd ed. Philadelphia, PA: WB Saunders; 1995:2224-2233.
114. Wagner KU, Young WS, Liu X, et al. Oxytocin and milk removal are required for post partum mammary-gland development. *Genes Funct.* 1997;1:233-244.
115. Short RV. Breast feeding. *Sci Am.* 1984;250:35-41.
116. Glasier A, McNeilly AS. Physiology of lactation. *Bailliere's Clin Endocrinol Metab.* 1990;4:379-395.
117. Walker SE, Allen SH, McMurray RW. Prolactin and autoimmune disease. *Trends Endocrinol Metab.* 1993;4:147-151.
118. Zellweger R, Zhu XH, Wichmann MW, et al. Prolactin administration following hemorrhagic shock improves macrophage cytokine release capacity and decreases mortality from subsequent sepsis. *J Immunol.* 1996;157:5748-5754.
119. Richards SM, Murphy WJ. Use of human prolactin as a therapeutic protein to potentiate immunohematopoietic function. *J Neuroimmunol.* 2000;109:56-62.

120. Dorshkind K, Horseman ND. The roles of prolactin, growth hormone, insulin-like growth factor-I, and thyroid hormones in lymphocyte development and function: insights from genetic models of hormone and hormone receptor deficiency. *Endocr Rev.* 2000;21:292-312.
121. Ormandy CJ, Camus A, Barra J, et al. Null mutation of the prolactin receptor gene produces multiple reproductive defects in the mouse. *Genes Dev.* 1997;11:167-178.
122. Demura R, Ono M, Demura H, et al. Prolactin directly inhibits basal as well as gonadotropin-stimulated secretion of progesterone and 17 beta-estradiol in the human ovary. *J Clin Endocrinol Metab.* 1982;54:1246-1250.
123. Barkan AL, Chandler WF. Giant pituitary prolactinoma with falsely low serum prolactin: the pitfall of the "high-dose hook effect." Case report. *Neurosurgery.* 1998;42:913-915.
124. Chahal J, Schlechte J. Hyperprolactinemia. *Pituitary.* 2008;11:141-146.
125. Molitch ME. Pathologic hyperprolactinemia. *Endocrinol Metab Clin North Am.* 1992;21:877-901.
126. Noel GL, Suh HK, Frantz AG. Prolactin release during nursing and breast stimulation in postpartum and nonpostpartum subjects. *J Clin Endocrinol Metab.* 1974;38:413-423.
127. Diaz S, Seron-Ferre M, Cardenas H, et al. Circadian variation of basal plasma prolactin, prolactin response to suckling, and length of amenorrhea in nursing women. *J Clin Endocrinol Metab.* 1989;68:946-955.
128. Berinder K, Stackenas I, Akre O, et al. Hyperprolactinaemia in 271 women: up to three decades of clinical follow-up. *Clin Endocrinol (Oxf).* 2005;63:450-455.
129. McKenna TJ. Should macroprolactin be measured in all hyperprolactinaemic sera? *Clin Endocrinol (Oxf).* 2009;71:466-469.
130. Gibney J, Smith TP, McKenna TJ. The impact on clinical practice of routine screening for macroprolactin. *J Clin Endocrinol Metab.* 2005;90:3927-3932.
131. Karavitaki N, Thanabalasingham G, Shore HC, et al. Do the limits of serum prolactin in disconnection hyperprolactinaemia need re-definition? A study of 226 patients with histologically verified non-functioning pituitary macroadenoma. *Clin Endocrinol (Oxf).* 2006;65:524-529.
132. Kleinberg DL, Noel GL, Frantz AG. Galactorrhea: a study of 235 cases, including 48 with pituitary tumors. *N Engl J Med.* 1977; 296:589-600.
133. Travaglini P, Moriondo P, Togni E, et al. Effect of oral zinc administration on prolactin and thymulin circulating levels in patients with chronic renal failure. *J Clin Endocrinol Metab.* 1989;68:186-190.
134. Ramirez G, Butcher DE, Newton JL, et al. Bromocriptine and the hypothalamic hypophyseal function in patients with chronic renal failure on chronic hemodialysis. *Am J Kidney Dis.* 1985; 6:111-118.
135. Lim VS, Henriquez C, Sievertsen G, et al. Ovarian function in chronic renal failure: evidence suggesting hypothalamic anovulation. *Ann Intern Med.* 1980;93:21-27.
136. Noel GL, Suh HK, Stone JG, et al. Human prolactin and growth hormone release during surgery and other conditions of stress. *J Clin Endocrinol Metab.* 1972;35:840-851.
137. Agha A, Sherlock M, Brennan S, et al. Hypothalamic-pituitary dysfunction after irradiation of nonpituitary brain tumors in adults. *J Clin Endocrinol Metab.* 2005;90:6355-6360.
138. Szarfman A, Tonning JM, Levine JG, et al. Atypical antipsychotics and pituitary tumors: a pharmacovigilance study. *Pharmacotherapy.* 2006;26:748-758.
139. Misra M, Papakostas GI, Klibanski A. Effects of psychiatric disorders and psychotropic medications on prolactin and bone metabolism. *J Clin Psychiatry.* 2004;65:1607-1618; quiz 590, 760-761.
140. Bonert VS, Melmed S. Acromegaly with moderate hyperprolactinemia caused by an intrasellar macroadenoma. *Nat Clin Pract Endocrinol Metab.* 2006;2:408-412; quiz following 412.
141. Johnsen E, Kroken RA, Abaza M, et al. Antipsychotic-induced hyperprolactinemia: a cross-sectional survey. *J Clin Psychopharmacol.* 2008;28:686-690.
142. Tollin SR. Use of the dopamine agonists bromocriptine and cabergoline in the management of risperidone-induced hyperprolactinemia in patients with psychotic disorders. *J Endocrinol Invest.* 2000; 23:765-770.
143. Sharp EA. Historical review of a syndrome embracing utero-ovarian atrophy with persistent lactation (Frommel's disease). *Am J Obstet Gynecol.* 1935;30:411-414.
144. Argonz J, del Castillo EB. A syndrome characterized by estrogenic insufficiency, galactorrhea and decreased urinary gonadotropin. *J Clin Endocrinol Metab.* 1953;13:79-87.
145. Forbes AP, Henneman PH, Griswold GC, et al. Syndrome characterized by galactorrhea, amenorrhea and low urinary FSH: comparison with acromegaly and normal lactation. *J Clin Endocrinol Metab.* 1954;14:265-271.
146. Kleinberg DL. Endocrinology of mammary development, lactation and galactorrhea. In: DeGroot LJ, Jameson JL, eds. *Endocrinology*, 4th ed. Philadelphia, PA: WB Saunders; 2000:2464-2475.
147. Kleinberg DL, Lieberman A, Todd J, et al. Pergolide mesylate: a potent day-long inhibitor of prolactin in rhesus monkeys and patients with Parkinson's disease. *J Clin Endocrinol Metab.* 1980;51:152-154.
148. MacFarlane IA, Rosin MD. Galactorrhoea following surgical procedures to the chest wall: the role of prolactin. *Postgrad Med J.* 1980; 56:23-25.
149. Frohman LA, Burek L, Stachura MA. Characterization of growth hormone of different molecular weights in rat, dog and human pituitaries. *Endocrinology.* 1972;91:262-269.
150. Ho Y, Liebhaber SA, Cooke NE. Activation of the human GH gene cluster: roles for targeted chromatin modification. *Trends Endocrinol Metab.* 2004;15:40-45.
151. Miller WL, Eberhardt NL. Structure and evolution of the growth hormone gene family. *Endocr Rev.* 1983;4:97-130.
152. Ho Y, Elefant F, Liebhaber SA, et al. Locus control region transcription plays an active role in long-range gene activation. *Mol Cell.* 2006;23:365-375.
153. Kimura AP, Sizova D, Handwerger S, et al. Epigenetic activation of the human growth hormone gene cluster during placental cytotrophoblast differentiation. *Mol Cell Biol.* 2007;27:6555-6568.
154. Frankenne F, Closset J, Gomez F, et al. The physiology of growth hormones (GHs) in pregnant women and partial characterization of the placental GH variant. *J Clin Endocrinol Metab.* 1988;66:1171-1180.
155. Parks JS, Brown MR, Hurley DL, et al. Heritable disorders of pituitary development. *J Clin Endocrinol Metab.* 1999;84:4362-4370.
156. Cunningham BC, Ultsch M, De Vos AM, et al. Dimerization of the extracellular domain of the human growth hormone receptor by a single hormone molecule. *Science.* 1991;254:821-825.
157. Baumann G, MacCart JG, Amburn K. The molecular nature of circulating growth hormone in normal and acromegalic man: evidence for principal and minor monomeric forms. *J Clin Endocrinol Metab.* 1983;56:946-952.
158. Lal S, Martin JB, De la Vega CE, et al. Comparison of the effect of apomorphine and L-DOPA on serum growth hormone levels in normal men. *Clin Endocrinol (Oxf).* 1975;4:277-285.
159. Giustina A, Veldhuis JD. Pathophysiology of the neuroregulation of growth hormone secretion in experimental animals and the human. *Endocr Rev.* 1998;19:717-797.
160. Mayo KE, Miller T, DeAlmeida V, et al. Regulation of the pituitary somatotroph cell by GHRH and its receptor. *Recent Prog Horm Res.* 2000;55:237-266.
161. Shimon I, Taylor JE, Dong JZ, et al. Somatostatin receptor subtype specificity in human fetal pituitary cultures: differential role of SSTR2 and SSTR5 for growth hormone, thyroid-stimulating hormone, and prolactin regulation. *J Clin Invest.* 1997;99:789-798.
162. Shimon I, Yan X, Taylor JE, et al. Somatostatin receptor (SSTR) subtype-selective analogues differentially suppress in vitro growth hormone and prolactin in human pituitary adenomas: novel potential therapy for functional pituitary tumors. *J Clin Invest.* 1997;100:2386-2392.
163. Barinaga M, Yamonoto G, Rivier C, et al. Transcriptional regulation of growth hormone gene expression by growth hormone-releasing factor. *Nature.* 1983;306:84-85.
164. Gelato MC, Pescovitz O, Cassorla F, et al. Effects of a growth hormone releasing factor in man. *J Clin Endocrinol Metab.* 1983;57:674-676.
165. Tannenbaum GS, Ling N. The interrelationship of growth hormone (GH)-releasing factor and somatostatin in generation of the ultradian rhythm of GH secretion. *Endocrinology.* 1984;115:1952-1957.
166. Vance ML, Cragun JR, Reimnitz C, et al. CV205-502 treatment of hyperprolactinemia. *J Clin Endocrinol Metab.* 1989;68:336-339.
167. Bilezikjian LM, Seifert H, Vale W. Desensitization to growth hormone-releasing factor (GRF) is associated with down-regulation of GRF-binding sites. *Endocrinology.* 1986;118:2045-2052.
168. Kineman RD, Teixeira LT, Amargo GV, et al. The effect of GHRH on somatotrope hyperplasia and tumor formation in the presence and absence of GH signaling. *Endocrinology.* 2001;142:3764-3773.
169. Gaykema RP, Compaan JC, Nyakas C, et al. Long-term effects of cholinergic basal forebrain lesions on neuropeptide Y and somatostatin immunoreactivity in rat neocortex. *Brain Res.* 1989;489:392-396.
170. LeRoith D, Buler A. What is the role of circulating IGF-I? *Trends Endocrinol Metab.* 2001;12:48-52.
171. Yamashita S, Melmed S. Insulin regulation of rat growth hormone gene transcription. *J Clin Invest.* 1986;78:1008-1014.
172. Howard AD, Feighner SD, Cully DF, et al. A receptor in pituitary and hypothalamus that functions in growth hormone release. *Science.* 1996;273:974-977.
173. Kojima M, Hosoda H, Date Y, et al. Ghrelin is a growth-hormone-releasing acylated peptide from stomach. *Nature.* 1999;402: 656-660.
174. Cummings DE, Weigle DS, Frayo RS, et al. Plasma ghrelin levels after diet-induced weight loss or gastric bypass surgery. *N Engl J Med.* 2002;346:1623-1630.
175. Grove KL, Cowley MA. Is ghrelin a signal for the development of metabolic systems? *J Clin Invest.* 2005;115:3393-3397.
176. Smith RG, Jiang H, Sun Y. Developments in ghrelin biology and potential clinical relevance. *Trends Endocrinol Metab.* 2005;16:436-442.

177. Tannenbaum GS, Epelbaum J, Bowers CY. Interrelationship between the novel peptide ghrelin and somatostatin/growth hormone-releasing hormone in regulation of pulsatile growth hormone secretion. *Endocrinology*. 2003;144:967-974.
178. Popovic V, Leal A, Micic D, et al. GH-releasing hormone and GH-releasing peptide-6 for diagnostic testing in GH-deficient adults. *Lancet*. 2000;356:1137-1142.
179. Chang CH, Rickes EL, McGuire L, et al. Growth hormone (GH) and insulin-like growth factor I responses after treatments with an orally active GH secretagogue L-163,255 in swine. *Endocrinology*. 1996;137:4851-4856.
180. Casanueva FF, Camina JP, Carreira MC, et al. Growth hormone-releasing hormone as an agonist of the ghrelin receptor GHS-R1a. *Proc Natl Acad Sci U S A*. 2008;105:20452-20457.
181. Popovic V, Damjanovic S, Micic D, et al. Blocked growth hormone-releasing peptide (GHRP-6)-induced GH secretion and absence of the synergic action of GHRP-6 plus GH-releasing hormone in patients with hypothalamopituitary disconnection: evidence that GHRP-6 main action is exerted at the hypothalamic level. *J Clin Endocrinol Metab*. 1995;80:942-947.
182. Penalva A, Pombo M, Carballo A, et al. Influence of sex, age and adrenergic pathways on the growth hormone response to GHRP-6. *Clin Endocrinol (Oxf)*. 1993;38:87-91.
183. Jaffe CA, Friberg RD, Barkan AL. Suppression of growth hormone (GH) secretion by a selective GH-releasing hormone (GHRH) antagonist: direct evidence for involvement of endogenous GHRH in the generation of GH pulses. *J Clin Invest*. 1993;92:695-701.
184. Van Cauter E, Plat L, Copinschi G. Interrelations between sleep and the somatotropic axis. *Sleep*. 1998;21:553-566.
185. Taylor AL, Finster JL, Mintz DH. Metabolic clearance and production rates of human growth hormone. *J Clin Invest*. 1969;48:2349-2358.
186. Vahl N, Jorgensen JO, Jurik AG, et al. Abdominal sdiposity and physical fitness are major determinants of the age associated decline in stimulated GH secretion in healthy adults. *J Clin Endocrinol Metab*. 1996;81:2209-2215.
187. Vigas M, Malatinsky J, Nemeth S, et al. Alpha-adrenergic control of growth hormone release during surgical stress in man. *Metabolism*. 1977;26:399-402.
188. Sachar EJ, Mushrush G, Perlow M, et al. Growth hormone responses to L-dopa in depressed patients. *Science*. 1972;178:1304-1305.
189. Ho KY, Veldhuis JD, Johnson ML, et al. Fasting enhances growth hormone secretion and amplifies the complex rhythms of growth hormone secretion in man. *J Clin Invest*. 1988;81:968-975.
190. Vigneri R, Squatrito S, Pezzino V, et al. Growth hormone levels in diabetes: correlation with the clinical control of the disease. *Diabetes*. 1976;25:167-172.
191. Casanueva FF, Dieguez C. Neuroendocrine regulation and actions of leptin. *Front Neuroendocrinol*. 1999;20:317-363.
192. Carro E, Senaris R, Considine RV, et al. Regulation of in vivo growth hormone secretion by leptin. *Endocrinology*. 1997;138:2203-2206.
193. Okada K, Sugihara H, Minami S, et al. Effect of parenteral administration of selected nutrients and central injection of gamma-globulin from antiserum to neuropeptide Y on growth hormone secretory pattern in food-deprived rats. *Neuroendocrinology*. 1993;57:678-686.
194. al-Shoumer KA, Anyaoku V, Richmond W, et al. Elevated leptin concentrations in growth hormone-deficient hypopituitary adults. *Clin Endocrinol (Oxf)*. 1997;47:153-159.
195. Casanueva FF, Burguera B, Muruais C, et al. Acute administration of corticoids: a new and peculiar stimulus of growth hormone secretion in man. *J Clin Endocrinol Metab*. 1990;70:234-237.
196. Suda T, Demura H, Demura R, et al. Anterior pituitary hormones in plasma and pituitaries from patients with Cushing's disease. *J Clin Endocrinol Metab*. 1980;51:1048-1053.
197. Williams T, Maxon H, Thorner MO, et al. Blunted growth hormone (GH) response to GH-releasing hormone in hypothyroidism resolves in the euthyroid state. *J Clin Endocrinol Metab*. 1985;61:454-456.
198. Weissberger AJ, Ho KKY. Activation of the somatotropic axis by testosterone in adult males: evidence for the role of aromatization. *J Clin Endocrinol Metab*. 1993;76:1407-1412.
199. Meinhardt UJ, Ho KK. Modulation of growth hormone action by sex steroids. *Clin Endocrinol (Oxf)*. 2006;65:413-422.
200. Herington AC, Ymer S, Stevenson J. Identification and characterization of specific binding proteins for growth hormone in normal human sera. *J Clin Invest*. 1986;77:1817-1823.
201. Leung DW, Spencer SA, Cachianes G, et al. Growth hormone receptor and serum binding protein: purification, cloning and expression. *Nature*. 1987;330:537-543.
202. Schantl JA, Roza M, Van Kerkhof P, et al. The growth hormone receptor interacts with its sheddase, the tumour necrosis factor-alpha-converting enzyme (TACE). *Biochem J*. 2004;377(Pt 2):379-384.
203. Ho KY, Valiontis E, Waters MJ, et al. Regulation of growth hormone binding protein in man: comparison of gel chromatography and immunoprecipitation methods. *J Clin Endocrinol Metab*. 1993;76:302-308.
204. Daughaday W, Trivedi B. Absence of serum growth hormone binding protein in patients with growth hormone receptor deficiency (Laron dwarfism). *Proc Natl Acad Sci USA*. 1987;84:4636-4640.
205. Goddard AD, Covello R, Luoh SM, et al. Mutations of the growth hormone receptor in children with idiopathic short stature. The Growth Hormone Insensitivity Study Group. *N Engl J Med*. 1995;333:1093-1098.
206. Baumann G, Shaw MA, Merimee TJ. Low levels of high-affinity growth hormone binding protein in African pigmies. *N Engl J Med*. 1989;320:1705-1709.
207. Ip TP, Hoffman DM, Leung KC, et al. Do androgens regulate growth hormone binding protein in man? *J Clin Endocrinol Metab*. 1995;80:1278-1282.
208. Rajkovic IA, Valiontis E, Ho KKY. Direct quantitation of growth hormone binding protein in human serum by a ligand immunofunctional assay: comparison with immunoprecipitation and chromatography methods. *J Clin Endocrinol Metab*. 1994;78:772-777.
209. Lunning NJ, Carter-Su C. Recent advances in growth homone signaling. *Rev Endocr Netub Disord*. 2006;7:225-235.
210. Brooks AJ, Waters MJ. The growth homone receptor: mechamism of activation and clinical implications. *Nat Rev Edocrinol*. 2010;6:515-525.
211. Leung KC, Waters MJ, Markus I, et al. Insulin and insulin-like growth factor-I acutely inhibit surface translocation of growth hormone receptors in osteoblasts: a novel mechanism of growth hormone receptor regulation. *Proc Natl Acad Sci U S A*. 1997;94:11381-11386.
212. Brooks AJ, Wooh JW, Tunny KA, et al. Growth hormone receptor: mechanism of action. *Int J Biochem Cell Biol*. 2008;40:1984-1989.
213. Xu BC, Wang X, Darus CJ, et al. Growth hormone promotes the association of transcription factor STAT5 with the growth hormone receptor. *J Biol Chem*. 1996;271:19768-19773.
214. Starr R, Hilton DJ. SOCS: suppressors of cytokine signalling. *Int J Biochem Cell Biol*. 1998;30:1081-1085.
215. Greenhalgh CJ, Rico-Bautista E, Lorentzon M, et al. SOCS2 negatively regulates growth hormone action in vitro and in vivo. *J Clin Invest*. 2005;115:397-406.
216. Low MJ, Otero-Corchon V, Parlow AF, et al. Somatostatin is required for masculinization of growth hormone-regulated hepatic gene expression but not of somatic growth. *J Clin Invest*. 2001;107:1571-1580.
217. Udy GB, Towers RP, Snell RG, et al. Requirement of STAT5b for sexual dimorphism of body growth rates and liver gene expression. *Proc Natl Acad Sci U S A*. 1997;94:7239-7244.
218. Ram PA, Park SH, Choi HK, et al. Growth hormone activation of Stat 1, Stat 3, and Stat 5 in rat liver: differential kinetics of hormone desensitization and growth hormone stimulation of both tyrosine phosphorylation and serine/threonine phosphorylation. *J Biol Chem*. 1996;271:5929-5940.
219. Teglund S, McKay C, Schuetz E, et al. Stat5a and Stat5b proteins have essential and nonessential, or redundant, roles in cytokine responses. *Cell*. 1998;93:841-850.
220. Davey HW, Park SH, Grattan DR, et al. STAT5b-deficient mice are growth hormone pulse-resistant: role of STAT5b in sex-specific liver p450 expression. *J Biol Chem*. 1999;274:35331-35336.
221. Park SH, Liu X, Hennighausen L, et al. Distinctive roles of STAT5a and STAT5b in sexual dimorphism of hepatic P450 gene expression: impact of STAT5a gene disruption. *J Biol Chem*. 1999;274:7421-7430.
222. Eugster EA, Pescovitz OH. New revelations about the role of STATs in stature. *N Engl J Med*. 2003;349:1110-1112.
223. LeRoith D, Bondy C, Yakar S, et al. The somatomedin hypothesis: 2001. *Endocr Rev*. 2001;22:53-74.
224. Yakar S, Liu JL, Stannard B, et al. Normal growth and development in the absence of hepatic insulin-like growth factor I. *Proc Natl Acad Sci U S A*. 1999;96:7324-7329.
225. Rudling M, Norstedt G, Olivecrona H, et al. Importance of growth hormone for the induction of hepatic low density lipoprotein receptors. *Proc Natl Acad Sci U S A*. 1992;89:6983-6987.
226. Rudling M, Olivecrona H, Eggertsen G, et al. Regulation of rat hepatic low density lipoprotein receptors: in vivo stimulation by growth hormone is not mediated by insulin-like growth factor I. *J Clin Invest*. 1996;97:292-299.
227. Maison P, Griffin S, Nicoue-Beglah M, et al. Impact of growth hormone (GH) treatment on cardiovascular risk factors in GH-deficient adults: a metaanalysis of blinded, randomized, placebo-controlled trials. *J Clin Endocrinol Metab*. 2004;89:2192-2199.
228. Press M. Growth hormone and metabolism. *Diabetes Metab Rev*. 1988;4:391-414.
229. Moller N, Jorgensen JO. Effects of growth hormone on glucose, lipid, and protein metabolism in human subjects. *Endocr Rev*. 2009;30:152-177.
230. Cameron CM, Kostyo JL, Adamafio NA, et al. The acute effects of growth hormone on amino acid transport and protein synthesis are due to its insulin-like action. *Endocrinology*. 1988;122:471-474.
231. Fryburg DA, Barrett EJ. Growth hormone acutely stimulates skeletal muscle but not whole-body protein synthesis in humans. *Metabolism*. 1993;42:1223-1227.

232. Carroll PV, Christ ER, Bengtsson BA, et al. Growth hormone deficiency in adulthood and the effects of growth hormone replacement: a review. *J Clin Endocrinol Metab.* 1998;83:382-395.
233. Molitch ME, Clemmons DR, Malozowski S, et al. Evaluation and treatment of adult growth hormone deficiency: an Endocrine Society Clinical Practice Guideline. *J Clin Endocrinol Metab.* 2006;91:1621-1634.
234. Ho KK. Consensus guidelines for the diagnosis and treatment of adults with GH deficiency II: a statement of the GH Research Society in association with the European Society for Pediatric Endocrinology, Lawson Wilkins Society, European Society of Endocrinology, Japan Endocrine Society, and Endocrine Society of Australia. *Eur J Endocrinol.* 2007;157:695-700.
235. Growth Hormone Research Society Workshop on Adult Growth Hormone Deficiency. Consensus guidelines for the diagnosis and treatment of adults with growth hormone deficiency: summary statement. *J Clin Endocrinol Metab.* 1998;83:379-381.
236. de Boer H, Blok GJ, van der Veen EA. Clinical aspects of growth hormone deficiency in adults. *Endocr Rev.* 1995;16:63-86.
237. Rosen T, Bengtsson BA. Premature mortality due to cardiovascular disease in hypopituitarism. *Lancet.* 1990;336:285-288.
238. Bates AS, Van't Hoff W, Jones PJ, et al. The effect of hypopituitarism on life expectancy. *J Clin Endocrinol Metab.* 1996;81:1169-1172.
239. Tomlinson JW, Holden N, Hills RK, et al. Association between premature mortality and hypopituitarism. West Midlands Prospective Hypopituitary Study Group. *Lancet.* 2001;357:425-431.
240. Bulow B, Hagmar L, Eskilsson J, et al. Hypopituitary females have a high incidence of cardiovascular morbidity and increased prevalence of cardiovascular risk factors. *J Clin Endocrinol Metab.* 2000;85: 574-584.
241. Ho KKY. Growth hormone deficiency in adults. In: DeGroot LJ, Jameson JL, eds. *De Groot's Textbook of Endocrinology*, 5th ed. Philadelphia, PA: WB Saunders; 2004:550-558.
242. Webb SM, Strasburger CJ, Mo D, et al. Changing patterns of the adult growth hormone deficiency diagnosis documented in a decade-long global surveillance database. *J Clin Endocrinol Metab.* 2009;94: 392-399.
243. Wu W, Cogan JD, Pfaffle RW, et al. Mutations in PROP1 cause familial combined pituitary hormone deficiency. *Nature Gen.* 1998;18: 147-149.
244. Tauber M, Moulin P, Pienkowski C, et al. Growth hormone retesting and auxological data in 131 GH-deficient patients after completion of treatment. *J Clin Endocrinol Metab.* 1997;82:352-356.
245. Cogan JD, Phillips JA, Schenkman SS, et al. Familial growth hormone deficiency: a model of dominant and recessive mutations affecting a monomeric protein. *J Clin Endocrinol Metab.* 1994;79:1261-1265.
246. Baumann G. Mutations in the growth hormone releasing hormone receptor: a new form of dwarfism in humans. *Growth Horm IGF Res.* 1999;9(suppl B):24-29; discussion 29-30.
247. Rosenfeld RG, Rosenbloom AL, Guevara-Aguirre J. Growth hormone (GH) insensitivity due to primary GH receptor deficiency. *EndocrRev.* 1994;15:369-390.
248. Sesmilo G, Biller BM, Llevadot J, et al. Effects of growth hormone administration on inflammatory and other cardiovascular risk markers in men with growth hormone deficiency: a randomized, controlled clinical trial. *Ann Intern Med.* 2000;133:111-122.
249. Attanasio AF, Lamberts SWJ, Matranga AMC, et al. Adult growth hormone (GH)-deficient patients demonstrate heterogeneity between childhood onset and adult onset before and during human GH treatment. *J Clin Endocrinol Metab.* 1997;82:82-88.
250. Pfeifer M, Verhovec R, Zizek B, et al. Growth hormone (GH) treatment reverses early atherosclerotic changes in GH-deficient adults [see comments]. *J Clin Endocrinol Metab.* 1999;84:453-457.
251. Borson-Chazot F, Serusclat A, Kalfallah Y, et al. Decrease in carotid intima-media thickness after one year growth hormone (GH) treatment in adults with GH deficiency. *J Clin Endocrinol Metab.* 1999;84:1329-1333.
252. Newman CB, Kleinberg DL. Adult growth hormone deficiency. *The Endocrinologist.* 1998;8:178-186.
253. Merola B, Cittadini A, Colao A, et al. Cardiac structural and functional abnormalities in adult patients with growth hormone deficiency. *J Clin Endocrinol Metab.* 1993;77:1658-1661.
254. Amato G, Carella C, Fazio S, et al. Body composition, bone metabolism, and heart structure and function in growth hormone (GH)–deficient adults before and after GH replacement therapy at low doses. *J Clin Endocrinol Metab.* 1993;77:1671-1676.
255. Klibanski A. Growth hormone and cardiovascular risk markers. *Growth Horm IGF Res.* 2003;13(suppl A):S109-S115.
256. Aimaretti G, Colao A, Corneli G, et al. The study of spontaneous GH secretion after 36-h fasting distinguishes between GH-deficient and normal adults. *Clin Endocrinol (Oxf).* 1999;51:771-777.
257. Murray RD, Skillicorn CJ, Howell SJ, et al. Dose titration and patient selection increases the efficacy of GH replacement in severely GH deficient adults. *Clin Endocrinol (Oxf).* 1999;50:749-757.
258. Biller MK, Samuels MH, Zagar A, et al. Sensitiviy and specificity of six tests for the diagnosis of adult GH deficiency. *J Clin Endocrinol Metab.* 2002;87:2067-2079.
259. Rahim A, Toogood AA, Shalet SM. The assessment of growth hormone status in normal young adult males using a variety of provocative agents. *Clin Endocrinol.* 1996;45:557-562.
260. Aimaretti G, Cornelli G, Razzore P, et al. Comparison between insulin-induced hypoglycemia and the growth hormone (GH) releasing hormone + arginine as provocative tests for the diagnosis of GH deficiency. *J Clin Endocrinol Metab.* 1998;83:1615-1618.
261. Hoffman DM, O'Sullivan AJ, Baxter RC, Ho KKY. Diagnosis of growth hormone deficiency in adults. *Lancet.* 1994;343:1064-1068.
262. Mahajan T, Lightman SL. A simple test for growth hormone deficiency in adults. *J Clin Endocrinol Metab.* 2000;85:1473-1476.
263. Gomez JM, Espadero RM, Escobar-Jimenez F, et al. Growth hormone release after glucagon as a reliable test of growth hormone assessment in adults. *Clin Endocrinol (Oxf).* 2002;56:329-334.
264. Leal-Cerro A, Garcia E, Astorga R, et al. Growth hormone (GH) responses to the combined administration of GH-releasing peptide 6 in adults with GH deficiency. *Eur J Endocrinol.* 1995;132:712-715.
265. Darzy KH, Aimaretti G, Wieringa G, et al. The usefulness of the combined growth hormone (GH)-releasing hormone and arginine stimulation test in the diagnosis of radiation-induced GH deficiency is dependent on the post-irradiation time interval. *J Clin Endocrinol Metab.* 2003;88:95-102.
266. Bonert VS, Elashoff JD, Barnett P, et al. Body mass index determines evoked growth hormone (GH) responsiveness in normal healthy male subjects: diagnostic caveat for adult GH deficiency. *J Clin Endocrinol Metab.* 2004;89:3397-3401.
267. Corneli G, Di Somma C, Baldelli R, et al. The cut-off limits of the GH response to GH-releasing hormone-arginine test related to body mass index. *Eur J Endocrinol.* 2005;153:257-264.
268. Ghigo E, Aimaretti G, Gianotti L, et al. New approach to the diagnosis of growth hormone deficiency in adults. *Eur J Endocrinol.* 1996; 134:352-356.
269. Toogood AA, Beardwell C, Shalet SM. The severity of growth hormone deficiency in adults with pituitary disease is related to the degree of hypopituitarism. *Clin Endocrinol.* 1994;41:511-516.
270. Hartman ML, Crowe BJ, Biller BM, et al. Which patients do not require a GH stimulation test for the diagnosis of adult GH deficiency? *J Clin Endocrinol Metab.* 2002;87:477-485.
271. Rosenfeld RG, Albertsson-Wikland K, Cassorla F, et al. Diagnostic controversy: the diagnosis of childhood growth hormone deficiency revisited. *J Clin Endocrinol Metab.* 1995;80:1532-1540.
272. Granada ML, Sanmarti A, Lucas A, et al. Assay-dependent results of immunoassayable spontaneous 24-hour growth hormone secretion in short children. *Acta Paediatr Scand Suppl.* 1990;370:63-70.
273. Reiter EO, Morris AH, MacGillivray MH, et al. Variable estimates of serum growth hormone concentrations by different radioassay systems. *J Clin Endocrinol Metab.* 1988;66:68-71.
274. Baumann G, Shaw M, Amburn K, et al. Heterogeneity of circulating growth hormone. *Nucl Med Biol.* 1994;21:369-379.
275. Strasburger CJ, Dattani MT. New growth hormone assays: potential benefits. *Acta Paediatr Suppl.* 1997;423:5-11.
276. Bristow AF, Gaines-Das R, Jeffcoate SL, et al. The First International Standard for Somatropin: report of an international collaborative study. *Growth Regul.* 1995;5:133-141.
277. Fisker S, Orskov H. Factors modifying growth hormone estimates in immunoassays. *Horm Res.* 1996;46:183-187.
278. Gibney J, Wallace JD, Spinks T, et al. The effect of 10 years of recombinant human growth hormone (GH) in adult GH-deficient patients. *J Clin Endocrinol Metab.* 1999;84:2596-2602.
279. Gotherstrom G, Bengtsson BA, Bosaeus I, et al. A 10-year, prospective study of the metabolic effects of growth hormone replacement in adults. *J Clin Endocrinol Metab.* 2007;92:1442-1445.
280. Salomon F, Cuneo RC, Hesp R, et al. The effects of treatment with recombinant human growth hormone on body composition and metabolism in adults with growth hormone deficiency. *N Engl J Med.* 1989;321:1797-1803.
281. Bengtsson B-A, Eden S, Lonn L, et al. Treatment of adults with growth hormone (GH) deficiency with recombinant human GH. *J Clin Endocrinol Metab.* 1993;76:309-317.
282. Hoffman DM, Crampton L, Sernia C, et al. Short term growth hormone (GH) treatment of GH deficient adults increases body sodium and extracellular water but not blood pressure. *J Clin Endocrinol Metab.* 1996;81:1123-1128.
283. Baum HB, Biller BM, Finkelstein JS, et al. Effects of physiologic growth hormone therapy on bone density and body composition in patients with adult-onset growth hormone deficiency: a randomized, placebo-controlled trial. *Ann Intern Med.* 1996;125:883-890.
284. Kotzmann H, Riedl M, Bernecker P, et al. Effect of long-term growth-hormone substitution therapy on bone mineral density and parameters of bone metabolism in adult patients with growth hormone deficiency. *Calcif Tissue Int.* 1998;62:40-46.

285. Cuneo RC, Salomon F, Wiles CM, et al. Growth hormone treatment of growth hormone deficient adults: II. Effects on exercise performance. *J Appl Physiol*. 1991;70:695-700.
286. Nass R, Huber RM, Klauss V, et al. Effect of growth hormone (hGH) replacement therapy on physical work capacity and cardiac and pulmonary function in patients with hGH deficiency acquired in adulthood. *J Clin Endocrinol Metab*. 1995;80:552-557.
287. Boger RH, Skamira C, Bode-Boger SM, et al. Nitric oxide may mediate the hemodynamic effects of recombinant growth hormone in patients with acquired growth hormone deficiency: a double-blind, placebo-controlled study. *J Clin Invest*. 1996;98:2706-2713.
288. Colao A, Marzullo P, Di Somma C, et al. Growth hormone and the heart. *Clin Endocrinol (Oxf)*. 2001;54:137-154.
289. Koranyi J, Svensson J, Gotherstrom G, et al. Baseline characteristics and the effects of five years of GH replacement therapy in adults with GH deficiency of childhood or adulthood onset: a comparative, prospective study. *J Clin Endocrinol Metab*. 2001;86:4693-4699.
290. Rosilio M, Blum WF, Edwards DJ, et al. Long-term improvement of quality of life during growth hormone (GH) replacement therapy in adults with GH deficiency, as measured by questions on life satisfaction-hypopituitarism (QLS-H). *J Clin Endocrinol Metab*. 2004;89:1684-1693.
291. Hernberg-Stahl E, Luger A, Abs R, et al. Healthcare consumption decreases in parallel with improvements in quality of life during GH replacement in hypopituitary adults with GH deficiency. *J Clin Endocrinol Metab*. 2001;86:5277-5281.
292. Drake WM, Howell SJ, Monson JP, et al. Optimizing GH therapy in adults and children. *Endocr Rev*. 2001;22:425-450.
293. de Boer H, Blok GJ, Popp-Snijders C, et al. Monitoring of growth hormone replacement therapy in adults, based on measurement of serum markers. *J Clin Endocrinol Metab*. 1996;81:1371-1377.
294. Wolthers T, Hoffman DM, Nugent AG, et al. Oral estrogen therapy impairs the metabolic effects of growth hormone (GH) in GH deficient women. *Am J Physiol*. 2001;281:E1191-E1196.
295. Cook DM, Ludlam WH, Cook MB. Route of estrogen administration helps to determine growth hormone (GH) replacement dose in GH-deficient adults. *J Clin Endocrinol Metab*. 1999;84:3956-3960.
296. Hoffman DM, Pallasser R, Duncan M, et al. How is whole body protein turnover perturbed in growth hormone-deficient adults? *J Clin Endocrinol Metab*. 1998;83:4344-4349.
297. Gotherstrom G, Svensson J, Koranyi J, et al. A prospective study of 5 years of GH replacement therapy in GH-deficient adults: sustained effects on body composition, bone mass and metabolic indices. *J Clin Endocrinol Metab*. 2001;86:4657-4665.
298. Cuneo RC, Judd S, Wallace JD, et al. The Australian multicentre trial of growth hormone treatment in GH-deficient adults. *J Clin Endocrinol Metab*. 1998;83:107-116.
299. Svensson J, Fowelin J, Landin K, et al. Effects of seven years of GH-replacement therapy on insulin sensitivity in GH-deficient adults. *J Clin Endocrinol Metab*. 2002;87:2121-2127.
300. Chan JM, Stampfer MJ, Giovannucci E, et al. Plasma insulin-like growth factor-I and prostate cancer risk: a prospective study. *Science*. 1998;279:563-566.
301. Hankinson SE, Willett WC, Colditz GA, et al. Circulating concentrations of insulin-like growth factor-I and risk of breast cancer. *Lancet*. 1998;351:1393-1396.
302. Yu H, Rohan T. Role of the insulin-like growth factor family in cancer development and progression. *J Natl Cancer Inst*. 2000;92:1472-1489.
303. Orme S, McNally RJQ, Cartwright RA, et al. Mortality and cancer incidence in acromegaly: a retrospective cohort study. *J Clin Endocrinol Metab*. 1998;83:2730-2734.
304. Melmed S. Acromegaly and cancer: not a problem? *J Clin Endocrinol Metab*. 2001;86:2929-2934.
305. Renehan AG, Bhaskar P, Painter JE, et al. The prevalence and characteristics of colorectal neoplasia in acromegaly. *J Clin Endocrinol Metab*. 2000;85:3417-3424.
306. Allen D. National cooperative growth study safety symposium: safety of human growth hormone therapy. *J Pediatr*. 1996;128:S8-S13.
307. Sklar C. Paying the price for cure-treating cancer survivors with growth hormone. *J Clin Endocrinol Metab*. 2000;85:4441-4443.
308. Swerdlow AJ, Reddingius RE, Higgins CD, et al. Growth hormone treatment of children with brain tumors and risk of tumor recurrence. *J Clin Endocrinol Metab*. 2000;85:4444-4449.
309. Ergun-Longmire B, Mertens AC, Mitby P, et al. Growth hormone treatment and risk of second neoplasms in the childhood cancer survivor. *J Clin Endocrinol Metab*. 2006;91:3494-3498.
310. Jenkins RC, Ross RJ. Growth hormone therapy for protein catabolism. *QJM*. 1996;89:813-819.
311. Chu LW, Lam KS, Tam SC, et al. A randomized controlled trial of low-dose recombinant human growth hormone in the treatment of malnourished elderly medical patients. *J Clin Endocrinol Metab*. 2001;86:1913-1920.
312. Takala J, Ruokonen E, Webster NR, et al. Increased mortality associated with growth hormone treatment in critically ill adults. *N Engl J Med*. 1999;341:785-792.
313. Hoiden-Guthenberg I, Flores-Morales A, Norstedt G, et al. Anabolic actions of growth hormone in catabolic states: analysis of differential gene expression in rats treated with GH and LPS using cDNA microarrays. 83rd Annual Meeting of the Endocrine Society, 2001: Abstract P2-601. Denver, CO: The Endocrine Society; 2001:423.
314. Perls TT, Reisman NR, Olshansky SJ. Provision or distribution of growth hormone for "antiaging": clinical and legal issues. *JAMA*. 2005;294:2086-2090.
315. Holloway L, Kohlmeier L, Kent K, et al. Skeletal effects of cyclic recombinant human growth hormone and salmon calcitonin in osteopenic postmenopausal women. *J Clin Endocrinol Metab*. 1997;82:1111-1117.
316. Landin-Wilhelmsen K, Nilsson A, Bosaeus I, et al. Growth hormone increases bone mineral content in postmenopausal osteoporosis: a randomized placebo-controlled trial. *J Bone Miner Res*. 2003; 18:393-405.
317. Schambelan M, Mulligan K, Grunfeld C, et al. Recombinant human growth hormone in patients with HIV-associated wasting: a randomized, placebo-controlled trial. Serostim Study Group. *Ann Intern Med*. 1996;125:873-882.
318. Grinspoon S, Carr A. Cardiovascular risk and body-fat abnormalities in HIV-infected adults. *N Engl J Med*. 2005;352:48-62.
319. Lo JC, Mulligan K, Noor MA, et al. The effects of recombinant human growth hormone on body composition and glucose metabolism in HIV-infected patients with fat accumulation. *J Clin Endocrinol Metab*. 2001;86:3480-3487.
320. Grunfeld C, Thompson M, Brown SJ, et al. Recombinant human growth hormone to treat HIV-associated adipose redistribution syndrome: 12 week induction and 24-week maintenance therapy. *J Acquir Immune Defic Syndr*. 2007;45:286-297.
321. Lo J, You SM, Canavan B, et al. Low-dose physiological growth hormone in patients with HIV and abdominal fat accumulation: a randomized controlled trial. *JAMA*. 2008;300:509-519.
322. Nelson AE, Ho KK. Abuse of growth hormone by athletes. *Nat Clin Pract Endocrinol Metab*. 2007;3:198-199.
323. Liu H, Bravata DM, Olkin I, et al. Systematic review: the effects of growth hormone on athletic performance. *Ann Intern Med*. 2008;148:747-758.
324. Meinhardt U, Nelson A, Hansen J, et al. The effects of growth hormone on body composition and physical performance in recreational athletes: a placebo-controlled trial. *Ann Intern Med*. 2010;152: 568-577.
325. Liu H, Bravata DM, Olkin I, et al. Systematic review: the safety and efficacy of growth hormone in the healthy elderly. *Ann Intern Med*. 2007;146:104-115.
326. Scheithauer BW, Horvath E, Lloyd RV, et al. Pathology of pituitary adenomas and pituitary hyperplasia. In: Thapar K, Kovacs K, Scheithauer BW, et al, eds. *Diagnosis and Management of Pituitary Tumors*. Totowa, NJ: Humana Press; 2001:91-154.
327. Zabel BU, Naylor SL, Sakaguchi AY, et al. High-resolution chromosomal localization of human genes for amylase, proopiomelanocortin, somatostatin, and a DNA fragment (D3S1) by in situ hybridization. *Proc Natl Acad Sci U S A*. 1983;80:6932-6936.
328. Cochet M, Chang AC, Cohen SN. Characterization of the structural gene and putative 5′-regulatory sequences for human proopiomelanocortin. *Nature*. 1982;297:335-339.
329. Gee CE, Chen CL, Roberts JL, et al. Identification of proopiomelanocortin neurones in rat hypothalamus by in situ cDNA-mRNA hybridization. *Nature*. 1983;306:374-376.
330. Jenks BG. Regulation of proopiomelanocortin gene expression: an overview of the signaling cascades, transcription factors, and responsive elements involved. *Ann N Y Acad Sci*. 2009;1163:17-30.
331. Arai M, Assil IQ, Abou-Samra AB. Characterization of three corticotropin-releasing factor receptors in catfish: a novel third receptor is predominantly expressed in pituitary and urophysis. *Endocrinology*. 2001;142:446-454.
332. Jin WD, Boutillier AL, Glucksman MJ, et al. Characterization of a corticotropin-releasing hormone–responsive element in the rat proopiomelanocortin gene promoter and molecular cloning of its binding protein. *Mol Endocrinol*. 1994;8:1377-1388.
333. Weninger SC, Dunn AJ, Muglia LJ, et al. Stress-induced behaviors require the corticotropin-releasing hormone (CRH) receptor, but not CRH. *Proc Natl Acad Sci U S A*. 1999;96:8283-8288.
334. Coste SC, Kesterson RA, Heldwein KA, et al. Abnormal adaptations to stress and impaired cardiovascular function in mice lacking corticotropin-releasing hormone receptor-2. *Nat Genet*. 2000;24: 403-409.
335. Bousquet C, Zatelli MC, Melmed S. Direct regulation of pituitary proopiomelanocortin by STAT3 provides a novel mechanism for immunoneuroendocrine interfacing. *J Clin Invest*. 2000;106:1417-1425.
336. Seidah NG, Chretien M. Complete amino acid sequence of a human pituitary glycopeptide: an important maturation product of proopiomelanocortin. *Proc Natl Acad Sci U S A*. 1981;78:4236-4240.
337. Fenger M, Johnsen AH. Alpha-amidated peptides derived from proopiomelanocortin in normal human pituitary. *Biochem J*. 1988; 250:781-788.

338. Jackson RS, Creemers JW, Ohagi S, et al. Obesity and impaired prohormone processing associated with mutations in the human prohormone convertase 1 gene. *Nat Genet.* 1997;16:303-306.
339. Bicknell AB, Lomthaisong K, Woods RJ, et al. Characterization of a serine protease that cleaves pro-gamma-melanotropin at the adrenal to stimulate growth. *Cell.* 2001;105:903-912.
340. Scholzen TE, Kalden DH, Brzoska T, et al. Expression of proopiomelanocortin peptides in human dermal microvascular endothelial cells: evidence for a regulation by ultraviolet light and interleukin-1. *J Invest Dermatol.* 2000;115:1021-1028.
341. Krude H, Biebermann H, Luck W, et al. Severe early-onset obesity, adrenal insufficiency and red hair pigmentation caused by POMC mutations in humans. *Nat Genet.* 1998;19:155-157.
342. Yaswen L, Diehl N, Brennan MB, et al. Obesity in the mouse model of pro-opiomelanocortin deficiency responds to peripheral melanocortin. *Nat Med.* 1999;5:1066-1070.
343. Catania A, Delgado R, Airaghi L, et al. Alpha-MSH in systemic inflammation: central and peripheral actions. *Ann N Y Acad Sci.* 1999; 885:183-187.
344. Raffin-Sanson ML, de Keyzer Y, Bertagna X. Proopiomelanocortin, a polypeptide precursor with multiple functions: from physiology to pathological conditions. *Eur J Endocrinol.* 2003;149:79-90.
345. Keller-Wood ME, Dallman MF. Corticosteroid inhibition of ACTH secretion. *Endocr Rev.* 1984;5:1-24.
346. Clark AR. Anti-inflammatory functions of glucocorticoid-induced genes. *Mol Cell Endocrinol.* 2007;275:79-97.
347. Kanaley JA, Weltman JY, Pieper KS, et al. Cortisol and growth hormone responses to exercise at different times of day. *J Clin Endocrinol Metab.* 2001;86:2881-2889.
348. Luger A, Deuster PA, Kyle SB, et al. Acute hypothalamic-pituitary-adrenal responses to the stress of treadmill exercise: physiologic adaptations to physical training. *N Engl J Med.* 1987;316:1309-1315.
349. Veldhuis JD, Iranmanesh A, Johnson ML, et al. Twenty-four-hour rhythms in plasma concentrations of adenohypophyseal hormones are generated by distinct amplitude and/or frequency modulation of underlying pituitary secretory bursts. *J Clin Endocrinol Metab.* 1990;71:1616-1623.
350. Veldhuis JD, Iranmanesh A, Johnson ML, et al. Amplitude, but not frequency, modulation of adrenocorticotropin secretory bursts gives rise to the nyctohemeral rhythm of the corticotropic axis in man. *J Clin Endocrinol Metab.* 1990;71:452-463.
351. Gomez MT, Magiakou MA, Mastorakos G, et al. The pituitary corticotroph is not the rate limiting step in the postoperative recovery of the hypothalamic-pituitary-adrenal axis in patients with Cushing syndrome. *J Clin Endocrinol Metab.* 1993;77:173-177.
352. Desir D, Van Cauter E, Beyloos M, et al. Prolonged pulsatile administration of ovine corticotropin-releasing hormone in normal man. *J Clin Endocrinol Metab.* 1986;63:1292-1299.
353. Horrocks PM, Jones AF, Ratcliffe WA, et al. Patterns of ACTH and cortisol pulsatility over twenty-four hours in normal males and females. *Clin Endocrinol (Oxf).* 1990;32:127-134.
354. Dorin RI, Ferries LM, Roberts B, et al. Assessment of stimulated and spontaneous adrenocorticotropin secretory dynamics identifies distinct components of cortisol feedback inhibition in healthy humans. *J Clin Endocrinol Metab.* 1996;81:3883-3891.
355. Keeney DS, Waterman MR. Regulation of steroid hydroxylase gene expression: importance to physiology and disease. *Pharmacol Ther.* 1993;58:301-317.
356. Ilvesmaki V, Voutilainen R. Interaction of phorbol ester and adrenocorticotropin in the regulation of steroidogenic P450 genes in human fetal and adult adrenal cell cultures. *Endocrinology.* 1991;128:1450-1458.
357. Orth DN. Corticotropin-releasing hormone in humans. *Endocr Rev.* 1992;13:164-191.
358. Debold CR, Jackson RV, Kamilaris TC, et al. Effects of ovine corticotropin-releasing hormone on adrenocorticotropin secretion in the absence of glucocorticoid feedback inhibition in man. *J Clin Endocrinol Metab.* 1989;68:431-437.
359. Sonino N, Zielezny M, Fava GA, et al. Risk factors and long-term outcome in pituitary-dependent Cushing's disease. *J Clin Endocrinol Metab.* 1996;81:2647-2652.
360. Kubota T, Hayashi M, Kabuto M, et al. Corticotroph cell hyperplasia in a patient with Addison disease: case report. *Surg Neurol.* 1992;37:441-447.
361. White A, Smith H, Hoadley M, et al. Clinical evaluation of a two-site immunoradiometric assay for adrenocorticotrophin in unextracted human plasma using monoclonal antibodies. *Clin Endocrinol (Oxf).* 1987;26:41-51.
362. Crosby SR, Stewart MF, Ratcliffe JG, et al. Direct measurement of the precursors of adrenocorticotropin in human plasma by two-site immunoradiometric assay. *J Clin Endocrinol Metab.* 1988;67:1272-1277.
363. Allolio B, Gunther RW, Benker G, et al. A multihormonal response to corticotropin-releasing hormone in inferior petrosal sinus blood of patients with Cushing's disease. *J Clin Endocrinol Metab.* 1990;71: 1195-1201.
364. Abdu TA, Elhadd TA, Neary R, et al. Comparison of the low dose short synacthen test (1 microg), the conventional dose short synacthen test (250 microg), and the insulin tolerance test for assessment of the hypothalamo-pituitary-adrenal axis in patients with pituitary disease. *J Clin Endocrinol Metab.* 1999;84:838-843.
365. Hartzband PI, Van Herle AJ, Sorger L, et al. Assessment of hypothalamic-pituitary-adrenal (HPA) axis dysfunction: comparison of ACTH stimulation, insulin-hypoglycemia and metyrapone. *J Endocrinol Invest.* 1988;11:769-776.
366. Streeten DH, Anderson GH Jr, Dalakos TG, et al. Normal and abnormal function of the hypothalamic-pituitary-adrenocortical system in man. *Endocr Rev.* 1984;5:371-394.
367. Oldfield EH, Doppman JL, Nieman LK, et al. Petrosal sinus sampling with and without corticotropin-releasing hormone for the differential diagnosis of Cushing's syndrome. *N Engl J Med.* 1991;325:897-905.
368. Yanovski JA, Cutler GB Jr, Chrousos GP, et al. Corticotropin-releasing hormone stimulation following low-dose dexamethasone administration: a new test to distinguish Cushing's syndrome from pseudo-Cushing's states. *JAMA.* 1993;269:2232-2238.
369. Nieman LK, Oldfield EH, Wesley R, et al. A simplified morning ovine corticotropin-releasing hormone stimulation test for the differential diagnosis of adrenocorticotropin-dependent Cushing's syndrome. *J Clin Endocrinol Metab.* 1993;77:1308-1312.
370. l'Allemand D, Penhoat A, Lebrethon MC, et al. Insulin-like growth factors enhance steroidogenic enzyme and corticotropin receptor messenger ribonucleic acid levels and corticotropin steroidogenic responsiveness in cultured human adrenocortical cells. *J Clin Endocrinol Metab.* 1996;81:3892-3897.
371. Hurel SJ, Thompson CJ, Watson MJ, et al. The short Synacthen and insulin stress tests in the assessment of the hypothalamic-pituitary-adrenal axis. *Clin Endocrinol (Oxf).* 1996;44:141-146.
372. Rasmuson S, Olsson T, Hagg E. A low dose ACTH test to assess the function of the hypothalamic-pituitary-adrenal axis. *Clin Endocrinol (Oxf).* 1996;44:151-156.
373. Kukreja SC, Williams GA. Corticotrophin stimulation test: inverse correlation between basal serum cortisol and its response to corticotrophin. *Acta Endocrinol (Copenh).* 1981;97:522-524.
374. Shankar RR, Jakacki RI, Haider A, et al. Testing the hypothalamic-pituitary-adrenal axis in survivors of childhood brain and skull-based tumors. *J Clin Endocrinol Metab.* 1997;82:1995-1998.
375. Howlett TA. An assessment of optimal hydrocortisone replacement therapy. *Clin Endocrinol (Oxf).* 1997;46:263-268.
376. Hahner S, Loeffler M, Fassnacht M, et al. Impaired subjective health status in 256 patients with adrenal insufficiency on standard therapy based on cross-sectional analysis. *J Clin Endocrinol Metab.* 2007; 92:3912-3922.
377. Peacey SR, Guo CY, Robinson AM, et al. Glucocorticoid replacement therapy: are patients over treated and does it matter? *Clin Endocrinol (Oxf).* 1997;46:255-261.
378. Arlt W, Callies F, van Vlijmen JC, Koehler I, et al. Dehydroepiandrosterone replacement in women with adrenal insufficiency. *N Engl J Med.* 1999;341:1013-1020.
379. Johannsson G, Burman P, Wiren L, et al. Low dose dehydroepiandrosterone affects behavior in hypopituitary androgen-deficient women: a placebo-controlled trial. *J Clin Endocrinol Metab.* 2002;87:2046-2052.
380. Gharib SD, Wierman ME, Shupnik MA, et al. Molecular biology of the pituitary gonadotropins. *Endocr Rev.* 1990;11:177-199.
381. Sairam MR, Bhargavi GN. A role for glycosylation of the alpha subunit in transduction of biological signal in glycoprotein hormones. *Science.* 1985;229:65-67.
382. Albanese C, Colin IM, Crowley WF, et al. The gonadotropin genes: evolution of distinct mechanisms for hormonal control. *Recent Prog Horm Res.* 1996;51:23-58.
383. Shupnik MA. Gonadotropin gene modulation by steroids and gonadotropin-releasing hormone. *Biol Reprod.* 1996;54:279-286.
384. Ezashi T, Hirai T, Kato T, et al. The gene for the beta subunit of porcine LH: clusters of GC boxes and CACCC elements. *J Mol Endocrinol.* 1990;5:137-146.
385. Keri RA, Bachmann DJ, Behrooz A, et al. An NF-Y binding site is important for basal, but not gonadotropin-releasing hormone–stimulated, expression of the luteinizing hormone beta subunit gene. *J Biol Chem.* 2000;275:13082-13088.
386. Duan WR, Shin JL, Jameson JL. Estradiol suppresses phosphorylation of cyclic adenosine 3′,5′-monophosphate response element binding protein (CREB) in the pituitary: evidence for indirect action via gonadotropin-releasing hormone. *Mol Endocrinol.* 1999;13: 1338-1352.
387. Halvorson LM, Ito M, Jameson JL, et al. Steroidogenic factor-1 and early growth response protein 1 act through two composite DNA binding sites to regulate luteinizing hormone beta-subunit gene expression. *J Biol Chem.* 1998;273:14712-14720.
388. Glaser T, Lewis WH, Bruns GA, et al. The beta-subunit of follicle-stimulating hormone is deleted in patients with aniridia and Wilms' tumour, allowing a further definition of the WAGR locus. *Nature.* 1986;321:882-887.

389. Brown P, McNeilly AS. Transcriptional regulation of pituitary gonadotropin subunit genes. *Rev Reprod*. 1999;4:117-124.
390. Messager S, Chatzidaki EE, Ma D, et al. Kisspeptin directly stimulates gonadotropin-releasing hormone release via G protein-coupled receptor 54. *Proc Natl Acad Sci U S A*. 2005;102:1761-1766.
391. Smith JT, Clifton DK, Steiner RA. Regulation of the neuroendocrine reproductive axis by kisspeptin-GPR54 signaling. *Reproduction*. 2006; 131:623-630.
392. Dhillo WS, Chaudhri OB, Thompson EL, et al. Kisspeptin-54 stimulates gonadotropin release most potently during the preovulatory phase of the menstrual cycle in women. *J Clin Endocrinol Metab*. 2007;92: 3958-3966.
393. Moschos S, Chan JL, Mantzoros CS. Leptin and reproduction: a review. *Fertil Steril*. 2002;77:433-444.
394. Cunningham MJ, Clifton DK, Steiner RA. Leptin's actions on the reproductive axis: perspectives and mechanisms. *Biol Reprod*. 1999;60: 216-222.
395. Wabitsch M, Ballauff A, Holl R, et al. Serum leptin, gonadotropin, and testosterone concentrations in male patients with anorexia nervosa during weight gain. *J Clin Endocrinol Metab*. 2001;86:2982-2988.
396. Knobil E. The neuroendocrine control of the menstrual cycle. *Recent Prog Horm Res*. 1980;36:53-88.
397. Crowley WF Jr, Whitcomb RW, Jameson JL, et al. Neuroendocrine control of human reproduction in the male. *Recent Prog Horm Res*. 1991;47:27-62.
398. Finkelstein JS, O'Dea LS, Whitcomb RW, et al. Sex steroid control of gonadotropin secretion in the human male: II. Effects of estradiol administration in normal and gonadotropin-releasing hormone-deficient men. *J Clin Endocrinol Metab*. 1991;73:621-628.
399. Finkelstein JS, Whitcomb RW, O'Dea LS, et al. Sex steroid control of gonadotropin secretion in the human male: I. Effects of testosterone administration in normal and gonadotropin-releasing hormone-deficient men. *J Clin Endocrinol Metab*. 1991;73:609-620.
400. Litman HJ, Bhasin S, Link CL, et al. Serum androgen levels in black, Hispanic, and white men. *J Clin Endocrinol Metab*. 2006;91: 4326-4334.
401. Veldhuis JD, Pincus SM, Garcia-Rudaz MC, et al. Disruption of the synchronous secretion of leptin, LH, and ovarian androgens in non-obese adolescents with the polycystic ovarian syndrome. *J Clin Endocrinol Metab*. 2001;86:3772-3778.
402. Vale W, Rivier C, Hsueh A, et al. Chemical and biological characterization of the inhibin family of protein hormones. *Recent Prog Horm Res*. 1988;44:1-34.
403. Stocco DM. Tracking the role of a star in the sky of the new millennium. *Mol Endocrinol*. 2001;15:1245-1254.
404. Sprengel R, Braun T, Nikolics K, et al. The testicular receptor for follicle stimulating hormone: structure and functional expression of cloned cDNA. *Mol Endocrinol*. 1990;4:525-530.
405. Hsueh AJ, Adashi EY, Jones PB, et al. Hormonal regulation of the differentiation of cultured ovarian granulosa cells. *Endocr Rev*. 1984; 5:76-127.
406. Jaakkola T, Ding YQ, Kellokumpu-Lehtinen P, et al. The ratios of serum bioactive/immunoreactive luteinizing hormone and follicle-stimulating hormone in various clinical conditions with increased and decreased gonadotropin secretion: reevaluation by a highly sensitive immunometric assay. *J Clin Endocrinol Metab*. 1990;70:1496-1505.
407. Lucky AW, Rich BH, Rosenfield RL, et al. LH bioactivity increases more than immunoreactivity during puberty. *J Pediatr*. 1980;97:205-213.
408. Jia XC, Hsueh AJ. Granulosa cell aromatase bioassay for follicle-stimulating hormone: validation and application of the method. *Endocrinology*. 1986;119:1570-1577.
409. Franco B, Guioli S, Pragliola A, et al. A gene deleted in Kallmann's syndrome shares homology with neural cell adhesion and axonal path-finding molecules. *Nature*. 1991;353:529-536.
410. Zirkin BR, Awoniyi C, Griswold MD, et al. Is FSH required for adult spermatogenesis? *J Androl*. 1994;15:273-276.
411. McCullagh DR. Dual endocrine activity of the testes. *Science*. 1932;76:19-23.
412. Nachtigall LB, Boepple PA, Pralong FP, et al. Adult-onset idiopathic hypogonadotropic hypogonadism: a treatable form of male infertility. *N Engl J Med*. 1997;336:410-415.
413. Anawalt BD, Bremner WJ. Diagnosis and treatment of male gonadotropin insufficiency. In: Lamberts SW, ed. *The Diagnosis and Treatment of Pituitary Insufficiency*. Bristol, UK: BioScientifica Ltd.; 1997: 163-207.
414. Snyder PJ, Lawrence DA. Treatment of male hypogonadism with testosterone enanthate. *J Clin Endocrinol Metab*. 1980;51:1335-1339.
415. Handelsman DJ, Conway AJ, Boylan LM. Pharmacokinetics and pharmacodynamics of testosterone pellets in man. *J Clin Endocrinol Metab*. 1990;71:216-222.
416. Whitsel EA, Boyko EJ, Matsumoto AM, et al. Intramuscular testosterone esters and plasma lipids in hypogonadal men: a meta-analysis. *Am J Med*. 2001;111:261-269.
417. Anawalt BD, Bebb RA, Bremner WJ, et al. A lower dosage levonorgestrel and testosterone combination effectively suppresses spermatogenesis and circulating gonadotropin levels with fewer metabolic effects than higher dosage combinations. *J Androl*. 1999;20:407-414.
418. Bhasin S, Salehian B. Gonadotropin therapy of men with hypogonadotropic hypogonadism. *Curr Ther Endocrinol Metab*. 1997;6:349-352.
419. Balen AH, Braat DD, West C, et al. Cumulative conception and live birth rates after the treatment of anovulatory infertility: safety and efficacy of ovulation induction in 200 patients. *Hum Reprod*. 1994;9: 1563-1570.
420. Martin KA, Hall JE, Adams JM, et al. Comparison of exogenous gonadotropins and pulsatile gonadotropin-releasing hormone for induction of ovulation in hypogonadotropic amenorrhea. *J Clin Endocrinol Metab*. 1993;77:125-129.
421. Suikkari A, MacLachlan V, Koistinen R, et al. Double-blind placebo controlled study: human biosynthetic growth hormone for assisted reproductive technology. *Fertil Steril*. 1996;65:800-805.
422. Mortimer CH, Besser GM, McNeilly AS, et al. Luteinizing hormone and follicle stimulating hormone-releasing hormone test in patients with hypothalamic-pituitary-gonadal dysfunction. *Br Med J*. 1973; 4:73-77.
423. Pierce JG, Parsons TF. Glycoprotein hormones: structure and function. *Annu Rev Biochem*. 1981;50:465-495.
424. Grossmann M, Weintraub BD, Szkudlinski MW. Novel insights into the molecular mechanisms of human thyrotropin action: structural, physiological, and therapeutic implications for the glycoprotein hormone family. *Endocr Rev*. 1997;18:476-501.
425. Dasen JS, O'Connell SM, Flynn SE, et al. Reciprocal interactions of Pit1 and GATA2 mediate signaling gradient–induced determination of pituitary cell types. *Cell*. 1999;97:587-598.
426. Fiddes JC, Goodman HM. The gene encoding the common alpha subunit of the four human glycoprotein hormones. *J Mol Appl Genet*. 1981;1:3-18.
427. Sarapura VD, Strouth HL, Wood WM, et al. Activation of the glycoprotein hormone alpha-subunit gene promoter in thyrotropes. *Mol Cell Endocrinol*. 1998;146:77-86.
428. Tagami T, Madison LD, Nagaya T, et al. Nuclear receptor corepressors activate rather than suppress basal transcription of genes that are negatively regulated by thyroid hormone. *Mol Cell Biol*. 1997; 17:2642-2648.
429. Wondisford FE, Radovick S, Moates JM, et al. Isolation and characterization of the human thyrotropin beta-subunit gene: differences in gene structure and promoter function from murine species. *J Biol Chem*. 1988;263:12538-12542.
430. Steinfelder HJ, Hauser P, Nakayama Y, et al. Thyrotropin-releasing hormone regulation of human TSHB expression: role of a pituitary-specific transcription factor (Pit-1/GHF-1) and potential interaction with a thyroid hormone-inhibitory element. *Proc Natl Acad Sci U S A*. 1991;88:3130-3134.
431. Bodenner DL, Mroczynski MA, Weintraub BD, et al. A detailed functional and structural analysis of a major thyroid hormone inhibitory element in the human thyrotropin beta-subunit gene. *J Biol Chem*. 1991;266:21666-21673.
432. Ross DS, Downing MF, Chin WW, et al. Changes in tissue concentrations of thyrotropin, free thyrotropin beta, and alpha-subunits after thyroxine administration: comparison of mouse hypothyroid pituitary and thyrotropic tumors. *Endocrinology*. 1983;112:2050-2053.
433. Abel ED, Kaulbach HC, Campos-Barros A, et al. Novel insight from transgenic mice into thyroid hormone resistance and the regulation of thyrotropin. *J Clin Invest*. 1999;103:271-279.
434. Beck-Peccoz P, Persani L. Variable biological activity of thyroid-stimulating hormone. *Eur J Endocrinol*. 1994;131:331-340.
435. Lania A, Persani L, Ballare E, et al. Constitutively active Gs alpha is associated with an increased phosphodiesterase activity in human growth hormone-secreting adenomas. *J Clin Endocrinol Metab*. 1998;83:1624-1628.
436. Papandreou MJ, Persani L, Asteria C, et al. Variable carbohydrate structures of circulating thyrotropin as studied by lectin affinity chromatography in different clinical conditions. *J Clin Endocrinol Metab*. 1993;77:393-398.
437. Ridgway EC, Weintraub BD, Maloof F. Metabolic clearance and production rates of human thyrotropin. *J Clin Invest*. 1974;53:895-903.
438. Vanhole C, Aerssens P, Naulaers G, et al. L-Thyroxine treatment of preterm newborns: clinical and endocrine effects. *Pediatr Res*. 1997;42:87-92.
439. Samuels MH, Henry P, Kleinschmidt-DeMasters BK, et al. Pulsatile glycoprotein hormone secretion in glycoprotein-producing pituitary tumors. *J Clin Endocrinol Metab*. 1991;73:1281-1288.
440. Goichot B, Weibel L, Chapotot F, et al. Effect of the shift of the sleep-wake cycle on three robust endocrine markers of the circadian clock. *Am J Physiol*. 1998;275(2 Pt 1):E243-E248.
441. Van den Berghe G, de Zegher F, Veldhuis JD, et al. Thyrotrophin and prolactin release in prolonged critical illness: dynamics of spontaneous secretion and effects of growth hormone-secretagogues. *Clin Endocrinol (Oxf)*. 1997;47:599-612.

442. Lechan RM, Fekete C. The TRH neurone: a hypothalamic integrator of energy metabolism. *Prog Brain Res*. 2006;153:209-235.
443. Fliers E, Unmehope UA, Alkemade A. Functional neuroanatomy of thyroid hormone feedback in the human hypothalamus and pituitary gland. *Mol Cell Endocrinol*. 2006;251:1-8.
444. Samuels MH, Henry P, Ridgway EC. Effects of dopamine and somatostatin on pulsatile pituitary glycoprotein secretion. *J Clin Endocrinol Metab*. 1992;74:217-222.
445. Siler TM, Yen SC, Vale W, et al. Inhibition by somatostatin on the release of TSH induced in man by thyrotropin-releasing factor. *J Clin Endocrinol Metab*. 1974;38:742-745.
446. Newman CB, Melmed S, Snyder PJ, et al. Safety and efficacy of long-term octreotide therapy of acromegaly: results of a multicenter trial in 103 patients—a clinical research center study. *J Clin Endocrinol Metab*. 1995;80:2768-2775.
447. Cooper DS, Klibanski A, Ridgway EC. Dopaminergic modulation of TSH and its subunits: in vivo and in vitro studies. *Clin Endocrinol (Oxf)*. 1983;18:265-275.
448. Wang R, Nelson JC, Wilcox RB. Salsalate administration: a potential pharmacological model of the sick euthyroid syndrome. *J Clin Endocrinol Metab*. 1998;83:3095-3099.
449. Rapoport B, Chazenbalk GD, Jaume JC, et al. The thyrotropin (TSH) receptor: interaction with TSH and autoantibodies. *Endocr Rev*. 1998;19:673-716.
450. Nicoloff JT, Spencer CA. Clinical review 12: the use and misuse of the sensitive thyrotropin assays. *J Clin Endocrinol Metab*. 1990;71: 553-558.
451. Spencer CA, Schwarzbein D, Guttler RB, et al. Thyrotropin (TSH)-releasing hormone stimulation test responses employing third and fourth generation TSH assays. *J Clin Endocrinol Metab*. 1993;76: 494-498.
452. Beck-Peccoz P, Persani L. TSH-producing adenomas. In: DeGroot LJ, Jameson JL, eds. *Endocrinology*, 5th ed. Philadelphia, PA: Elsevier Saunders; 2006:475-484.
453. Faglia G. The clinical impact of the thyrotropin-releasing hormone test. *Thyroid*. 1998;8:903-908.
454. Root AW. Neonatal screening for 21-hydroxylase deficient congenital adrenal hyperplasia: the role of CYP21 analysis. *J Clin Endocrinol Metab*. 1999;84:1503-1504.
455. Mehta A, Dattani MT. Developmental disorders of the hypothalamus and pituitary gland associated with congenital hypopituitarism. *Best Pract Res Clin Endocrinol Metab*. 2008;22:191-206.
456. Duquesnoy P, Roy A, Dastot F, et al. Human Prop-1: cloning, mapping, genomic structure. Mutations in familial combined pituitary hormone deficiency. *FEBS Lett*. 1998;437:216-220.
457. Sornson MW, Wu W, Dasen JS, et al. Pituitary lineage determination by the Prophet of Pit-1 homeodomain factor defective in Ames dwarfism. *Nature*. 1996;384:327-333.
458. Fofanova O, Takamura N, Kinoshita E, et al. Compound heterozygous deletion of the PROP-1 gene in children with combined pituitary hormone deficiency. *J Clin Endocrinol Metab*. 1998;83:2601-2604.
459. Cohen LE, Radovick S. Molecular basis of combined pituitary hormone deficiencies. *Endocr Rev*. 2002;23:431-442.
460. Deladoey J, Fluck C, Buyukgebiz A, et al. "Hot spot" in the PROP1 gene responsible for combined pituitary hormone deficiency. *J Clin Endocrinol Metab*. 1999;84:1645-1650.
461. Reynaud R, Barlier A, Vallette-Kasic S, et al. An uncommon phenotype with familial central hypogonadism caused by a novel PROP1 gene mutant truncated in the transactivation domain. *J Clin Endocrinol Metab*. 2005;90:4880-4887.
462. Turton JP, Mehta A, Raza J, et al. Mutations within the transcription factor PROP1 are rare in a cohort of patients with sporadic combined pituitary hormone deficiency (CPHD). *Clin Endocrinol (Oxf)*. 2005;63: 10-18.
463. Agarwal G, Bhatia V, Cook S, et al. Adrenocorticotropin deficiency in combined pituitary hormone deficiency patients homozygous for a novel PROP1 deletion. *J Clin Endocrinol Metab*. 2000;85: 4556-4561.
464. Rosenbloom AL, Almonte AS, Brown MR, et al. Clinical and biochemical phenotype of familial anterior hypopituitarism from mutation of the PROP1 gene. *J Clin Endocrinol Metab*. 1999;84:50-57.
465. Cushman LJ, Watkins-Chow DE, Brinkmeier ML, et al. Persistent Prop1 expression delays gonadotrope differentiation and enhances pituitary tumor susceptibility. *Hum Mol Genet*. 2001;10:1141-1153.
466. Reynaud R, Saveanu A, Barlier A, et al. Pituitary hormone deficiencies due to transcription factor gene alterations. *Growth Horm IGF Res*. 2004;14:442-448.
467. Voss JW, Rosenfeld MG. Anterior pituitary development: short tales from dwarf mice. *Cell*. 1992;70:527-530.
468. Andersen B, Rosenfeld MG. POU domain factors in the neuroendocrine system: lessons from developmental biology provide insights into human disease. *Endocr Rev*. 2001;22:2-35.
469. Li S, Crenshaw EB 3rd, Rawson EJ, et al. Dwarf locus mutants lacking three pituitary cell types result from mutations in the POU-domain gene pit-1. *Nature*. 1990;347:528-533.
470. Turton JP, Reynaud R, Mehta A, et al. Novel mutations within the POU1F1 gene associated with variable combined pituitary hormone deficiency. *J Clin Endocrinol Metab*. 2005;90:4762-4770.
471. Cohen RN, Brue T, Naik K, et al. The role of CBP/p300 interactions and Pit-1 dimerization in the pathophysiological mechanism of combined pituitary hormone deficiency. *J Clin Endocrinol Metab*. 2006;91:239-247.
472. Machinis K, Amselem S. Functional relationship between LHX4 and POU1F1 in light of the LHX4 mutation identified in patients with pituitary defects. *J Clin Endocrinol Metab*. 2005;90:5456-5462.
473. Dattani MT, Martinez-Barbera JP, Thomas PQ, et al. Mutations in the homeobox gene HESX1/Hesx1 associated with septo-optic dysplasia in human and mouse. *Nat Genet*. 1998;19:125-133.
474. Thomas PQ, Dattani MT, Brickman JM, et al. Heterozygous HESX1 mutations associated with isolated congenital pituitary hypoplasia and septo-optic dysplasia. *Hum Mol Genet*. 2001;10:39-45.
475. Sobrier ML, Maghnie M, Vie-Luton MP, et al. Novel HESX1 mutations associated with a life-threatening neonatal phenotype, pituitary aplasia, but normally located posterior pituitary and no optic nerve abnormalities. *J Clin Endocrinol Metab*. 2006;91:4528-4536.
476. Kristrom B, Zdunek AM, Rydh A, et al. A novel mutation in the LIM homeobox 3 gene is responsible for combined pituitary hormone deficiency, hearing impairment, and vertebral malformations. *J Clin Endocrinol Metab*. 200;94:1154-1161.
477. Netchine I, Sobrier ML, Krude H, et al. Mutations in LHX3 result in a new syndrome revealed by combined pituitary hormone deficiency. *Nat Genet*. 2000;25:182-186.
478. Saadi I, Semina EV, Amendt BA, et al. Identification of a dominant negative homeodomain mutation in Rieger syndrome. *J Biol Chem*. 2001;276:23034-23041.
479. Romero CJ, Nesi-Franca S, Radovick S. The molecular basis of hypopituitarism. *Trends Endocrinol Metab*. 2009;20:506-516.
480. Kelberman D, Rizzoti K, Avilion A, et al. Mutations within Sox2/SOX2 are associated with abnormalities in the hypothalamo-pituitary-gonadal axis in mice and humans. *J Clin Invest*. 2006;116:2442-2455.
481. Green JS, Parfrey PS, Harnett JD, et al. The cardinal manifestations of Bardet-Biedl syndrome, a form of Laurence-Moon-Biedl syndrome. *N Engl J Med*. 1989;321:1002-1009.
482. Bray GA, Dahms WT, Swerdloff RS, et al. The Prader-Willi syndrome: a study of 40 patients and a review of the literature. *Medicine (Baltimore)*. 1983;62:59-80.
483. Ledbetter DH, Mascarello JT, Riccardi VM, et al. Chromosome 15 abnormalities and the Prader-Willi syndrome: a follow-up report of 40 cases. *Am J Hum Genet*. 1982;34:278-285.
484. Kallmann F, Schonfeld WA., Barrera WS. Genetic aspects of primary eunuchoidism. *Am J Ment Defic*. 1944;48:203.
485. Rugarli EI, Ballabio A. Kallmann syndrome: from genetics to neurobiology. *JAMA*. 1993;270:2713-2716.
486. Hardelin JP, Levilliers J, Young J, et al. Xp22.3 deletions in isolated familial Kallmann's syndrome. *J Clin Endocrinol Metab*. 1993;76: 827-831.
487. Prager D, Braunstein GD. X-chromosome-linked Kallmann's syndrome: pathology at the molecular level. *J Clin Endocrinol Metab*. 1993;76:824-826.
488. Pitteloud N, Acierno JS Jr, Meysing A, et al. Mutations in fibroblast growth factor receptor 1 cause both Kallmann syndrome and normosmic idiopathic hypogonadotropic hypogonadism. *Proc Natl Acad Sci U S A*. 2006;103:6281-6286.
489. Lieblich JM, Rogol AD, White BJ, et al. Syndrome of anosmia with hypogonadotropic hypogonadism (Kallmann syndrome): clinical and laboratory studies in 23 cases. *Am J Med*. 1982;73:506-519.
490. Zhang YH, Guo W, Wagner RL, et al. DAX1 mutations map to putative structural domains in a deduced three-dimensional model. *Am J Hum Genet*. 1998;62:855-864.
491. Stoving RK, Hangaard J, Hansen-Nord M, et al. A review of endocrine changes in anorexia nervosa. *J Psychiatr Res*. 1999;33: 139-152.
492. Stoving RK, Veldhuis JD, Flyvbjerg A, et al. Jointly amplified basal and pulsatile growth hormone (GH) secretion and increased process irregularity in women with anorexia nervosa: indirect evidence for disruption of feedback regulation within the GH-insulin-like growth factor I axis. *J Clin Endocrinol Metab*. 1999;84:2056-2063.
493. Kleinberg DL. Pituitary tumors and failure of endocrine target organs. *Arch Intern Med*. 1979;139:969-970.
494. Mulroney SE, McDonnell KJ, Pert CB, et al. HIV gp120 inhibits the somatotropic axis: a possible GH-releasing hormone receptor mechanism for the pathogenesis of AIDS wasting. *Proc Natl Acad Sci U S A*. 1998;95:1927-1932.
495. Benvenga S, Campenni A, Ruggeri RM, et al. Clinical review 113: hypopituitarism secondary to head trauma. *J Clin Endocrinol Metab*. 2000;85:1353-1361.
496. Schneider HJ, Schneider M, Saller B, et al. Prevalence of anterior pituitary insufficiency 3 and 12 months after traumatic brain injury. *Eur J Endocrinol*. 2006;154:259-265.

497. Agha A, Rogers B, Sherlock M, et al. Anterior pituitary dysfunction in survivors of traumatic brain injury. *J Clin Endocrinol Metab*. 2004;89: 4929-4936.
498. Aimaretti G, Ambrosio MR, Di Somma C, et al. Residual pituitary function after brain injury-induced hypopituitarism: a prospective 12-month study. *J Clin Endocrinol Metab*. 2005;90:6085-6092.
499. Agha A, Thornton E, O'Kelly P, et al. Posterior pituitary dysfunction after traumatic brain injury. *J Clin Endocrinol Metab*. 2004;89: 5987-5992.
500. Brada M, Jankowska P. Radiotherapy for pituitary adenomas. *Endocrinol Metab Clin North Am*. 2008;37:263-275, xi.
501. Constine LS, Woolf PD, Cann D, et al. Hypothalamic-pituitary dysfunction after radiation for brain tumors. *N Engl J Med*. 1993;328: 87-94.
502. Clayton PE, Shalet SM. Dose dependency of time of onset of radiation-induced growth hormone deficiency. *J Pediatr*. 1991;118:226-228.
503. Rose SR, Lustig RH, Pitukcheewanont P, et al. Diagnosis of hidden central hypothyroidism in survivors of childhood cancer. *J Clin Endocrinol Metab*. 1999;84:4472-4479.
504. Castinetti F, Nagai M, Morange I, et al. Long-term results of stereotactic radiosurgery in secretory pituitary adenomas. *J Clin Endocrinol Metab*. 2009;94:3400-3407.
505. Toogood AA. Endocrine consequences of brain irradiation. *Growth Horm IGF Res*. 2004;14(suppl A):S118-S124.
506. De Marinis L, Bonadonna S, Bianchi A, et al. Primary empty sella. *J Clin Endocrinol Metab*. 2005;90:5471-5477.
507. Prabhakar VK, Shalet SM. Aetiology, diagnosis, and management of hypopituitarism in adult life. *Postgrad Med J*. 2006;82:259-266.
508. Hartman ML, Veldhuis JD, Johnson ML, et al. Augmented growth hormone (GH) secretory burst frequency and amplitude mediate enhanced GH secretion during a two-day fast in normal men. *J Clin Endocrinol Metab*. 1992;74:757-765.
509. Thorner MO, Vance ML, Horvath E, et al. The anterior pituitary. In: Wilson JD, Foster D, eds. *Williams Textbook of Endocrinology*. Philadelphia, PA: WB Saunders; 1992:221-310.
510. Alatzoglou KS, Dattani MT. Genetic causes of and treatment of isolated growth hormone deficiency—an update. *Nat Rev Endocrinol*. 2010:6: 562-576.
511. Dode C, Levilliers J, Dupont JM, et al. Loss-of-function mutations in FGFR1 cause autosomal dominant Kallmann syndrome. *Nat Genet*. 2003;33:463-465.
512. Falardeau J, Chung WC, Beenken A, et al. Decreased FGF8 signaling causes deficiency of gonadotropin-releasing hormone in humans and mice. *J Clin Invest*. 2008;118:2822-2831.
513. Dode C, Teixeira L, Levilliers J, et al. Kallmann syndrome: mutations in the genes encoding prokineticin-2 and prokineticin receptor-2. *PLoS Genet*. 2006;2:e175.
514. Miura K, Acierno JS Jr, Seminara SB. Characterization of the human nasal embryonic LHRH factor gene, NELF, and a mutation screening among 65 patients with idiopathic hypogonadotropic hypogonadism (IHH). *J Hum Genet*. 2004;49:265-268.
515. de Roux N, Genin E, Carel JC, et al. Hypogonadotropic hypogonadism due to loss of function of the KiSS1-derived peptide receptor GPR54. *Proc Natl Acad Sci U S A*. 2003;100:10972-10976.
516. Bouligand J, Ghervan C, Tello JA, et al. Isolated familial hypogonadotropic hypogonadism and a GNRH1 mutation. *N Engl J Med*. 2009;360:2742-2748.
517. Abs R, Bengtsson BA, Hernberg-Stahl E, et al. GH replacement in 1034 growth hormone deficient hypopituitary adults: demographic and clinical characteristics, dosing and safety. *Clin Endocrinol (Oxf)*. 1999;50:703-713.
518. Kelly DF, Gonzalo IT, Cohan P, et al. Hypopituitarism following traumatic brain injury and aneurysmal subarachnoid hemorrhage: a preliminary report. *J Neurosurg*. 2000;93:743-752.
519. Brandt L, Saveland H, Valdemarsson S, et al. Fatigue after aneurysmal subarachnoid hemorrhage evaluated by pituitary function and 3D-CBF. *Acta Neurol Scand*. 2004;109:91-96.
520. Aimaretti G, Ambrosio MR, Di Somma C, et al. Traumatic brain injury and subarachnoid haemorrhage are conditions at high risk for hypopituitarism: screening study at 3 months after the brain injury. *Clin Endocrinol (Oxf)*. 2004;61:320-326.
521. Kreitschmann-Andermahr I, Hoff C, Saller B, et al. Prevalence of pituitary deficiency in patients after aneurysmal subarachnoid hemorrhage. *J Clin Endocrinol Metab*. 2004;89:4986-4992.
522. Dimopoulou I, Kouyialis AT, Tzanella M, et al. High incidence of neuroendocrine dysfunction in long-term survivors of aneurysmal subarachnoid hemorrhage. *Stroke*. 2004;35:2884-2889.
523. Lieberman SA, Oberoi AL, Gilkison CR, et al. Prevalence of neuroendocrine dysfunction in patients recovering from traumatic brain injury. *J Clin Endocrinol Metab*. 2001;86:2752-2756.
524. Bondanelli M, De Marinis L, Ambrosio MR, et al. Occurrence of pituitary dysfunction following traumatic brain injury. *J Neurotrauma*. 2004;21:685-696.
525. Popovic V, Pekic S, Pavlovic D, et al. Hypopituitarism as a consequence of traumatic brain injury (TBI) and its possible relation with cognitive disabilities and mental distress. *J Endocrinol Invest*. 2004;27:1048-1054.
526. Leal-Cerro A, Flores JM, Rincon M, et al. Prevalence of hypopituitarism and growth hormone deficiency in adults long-term after severe traumatic brain injury. *Clin Endocrinol (Oxf)*. 2005;62:525-532.
527. Tanriverdi F, Senyurek H, Unluhizarci K, et al. High risk of hypopituitarism after traumatic brain injury: a prospective investigation of anterior pituitary function in the acute phase and 12 months after trauma. *J Clin Endocrinol Metab*. 2006;91:2105-2111.
528. Herrmann BL, Rehder J, Kahlke S, et al. Hypopituitarism following severe traumatic brain injury. *Exp Clin Endocrinol Diabetes*. 2006; 114:316-321.

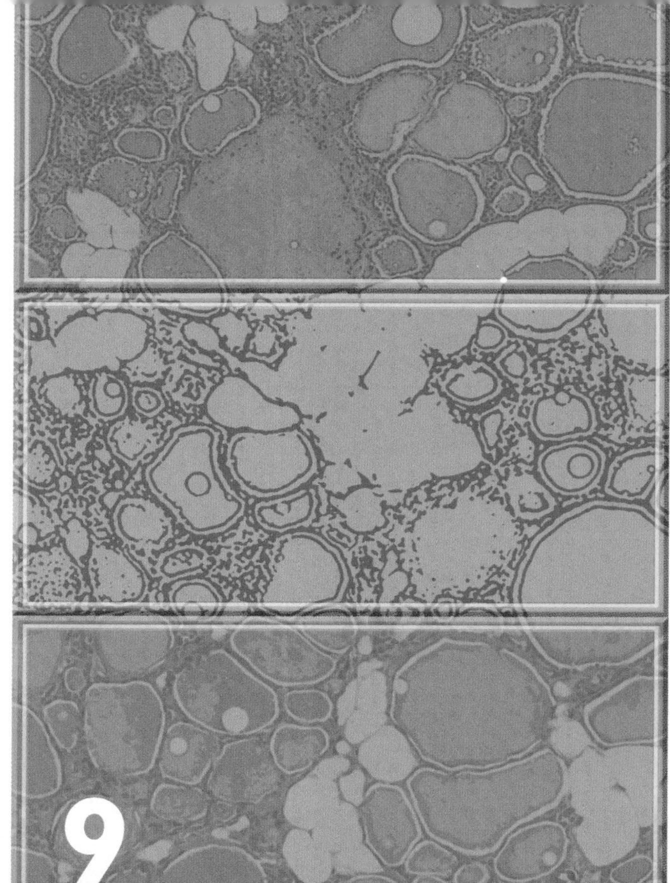

CHAPTER 9

Pituitary Masses and Tumors

SHLOMO MELMED • DAVID KLEINBERG

PITUITARY MASSES

Pituitary Mass Effects

An expanding pituitary mass may inexorably alter the sellar size and shape through bony erosion and remodeling (Fig. 9-1). Although the exact time course for this process is unknown, it appears to be slowly progressive over years or decades. The tumor may invade soft tissue, and the dorsal sellar roof presents the least resistance to expansion from within the confines of the bony sella. Nevertheless, both suprasellar and parasellar compression and invasion may occur with an enlarging mass, with resultant clinical manifestations (Table 9-1).

As tumors impinge on the optic chiasm, they interfere with vision. Because of the anatomy of the chiasm, pressure from below affects temporal visual fields, starting superiorly and ultimately extending to the entire temporal field. Continued growth and pressure on the optic apparatus can extend visual loss to the nasal field and may result in blindness. Long-standing optic chiasmal pressure results in optic disc pallor. Extension of pituitary lesions laterally may impinge on or invade the dural wall of the cavernous sinus. Despite invasion, they only rarely affect the function of the third, fourth, and sixth cranial nerves and the ophthalmic and maxillary branches of the fifth cranial nerve. Although tumors in the cavernous sinus often surround the internal carotid artery, vascular clinical sequelae are rare. Varying degrees of diplopia, ptosis, ophthalmoplegia, and decreased facial sensation may occur infrequently, depending on the extent of the neural involvement by the cavernous sinus mass.

In contrast to cavernous invasion by slow tumor progression, sudden insults to the cavernous sinus caused by hemorrhage or infarction of a pituitary tumor may affect nerves coursing through the sinus. Downward extension into the sphenoid sinus indicates that the parasellar mass has eroded the bony sellar floor. Aggressive tumors may invade the roof of the palate and cause nasopharyngeal obstruction, infection, and leakage of cerebrospinal fluid (CSF). Infrequently, temporal or frontal lobes are invaded, causing uncinate seizures, personality disorders, and anosmia. In addition to the anatomic lesions caused by the expanding mass, direct hypothalamic involvement by the encroaching mass may lead to important metabolic sequelae (see Chapter 7).

Intrasellar tumors commonly manifest with headaches, even in the absence of demonstrable suprasellar extension. Small changes in intrasellar pressure caused by a microadenoma within the confined sella are sufficient to stretch

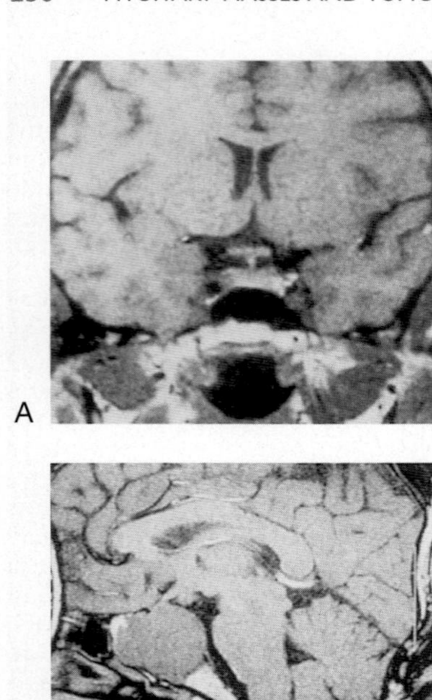

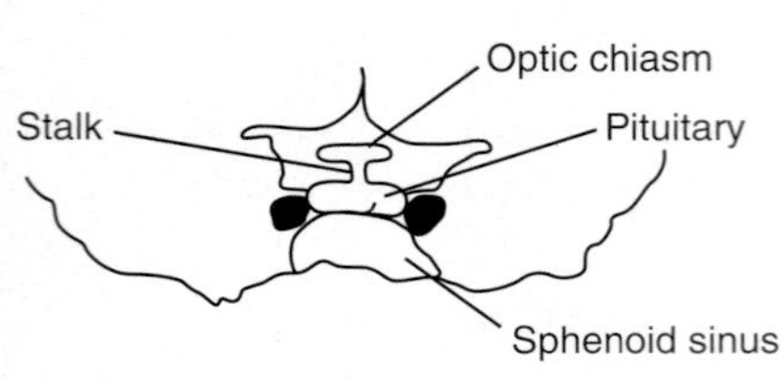

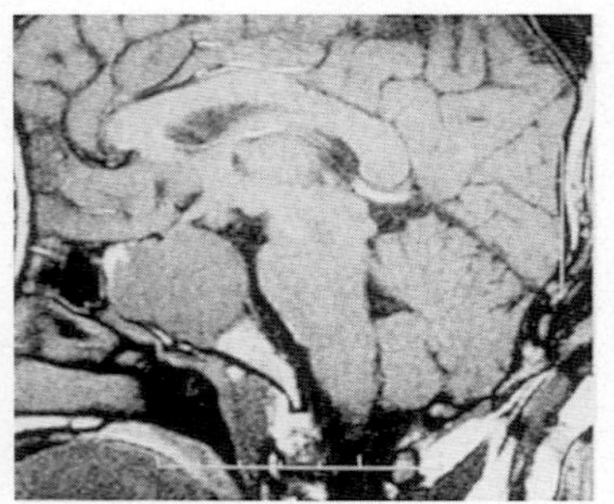

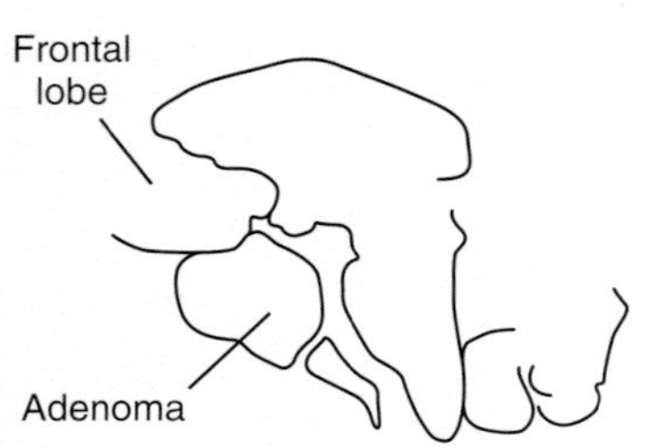

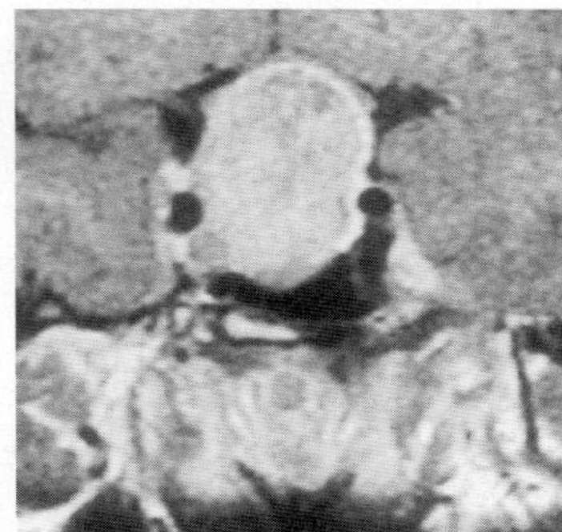

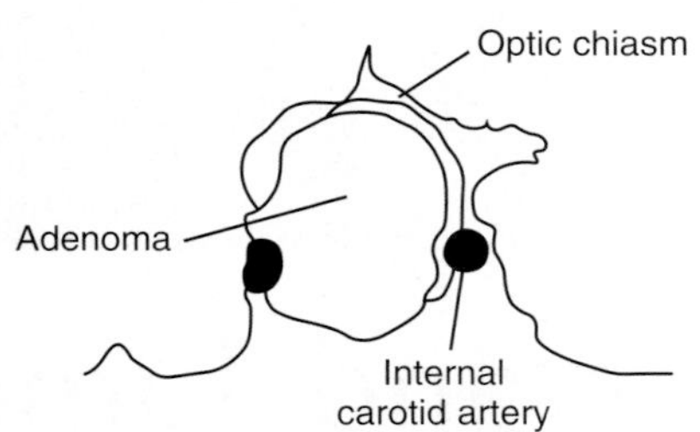

Figure 9-1 Magnetic resonance images of the pituitary. **A,** Coronal section of a normal pituitary gland. **B,** Sagittal view of a large pituitary adenoma lifting and distorting the optic chiasm, invading the sphenoid sinus, and impinging on the frontal lobe. **C,** Coronal view of a large macroadenoma elevating the optic chiasm and invading the right cavernous sinus.

the dural plate with resultant headache. Headache severity does not correlate with the size of the adenoma or the presence of suprasellar extension.[1] Relatively minor diaphragmatic distortions or dural impingement may be associated with persistent headache. Successful medical management of small functional pituitary tumors with dopamine agonists or somatostatin analogues is often accompanied by remarkable headache improvement. In a retrospective assessment of transsphenoidal surgery for microadenomas, headaches resolved or disappeared in 90% of patients with nonfunctioning tumors and in 56% of those with functioning tumors.[2]

Regardless of their etiology or size, pituitary masses, including adenomas, may be associated with compression of surrounding healthy tissue and resultant hypopituitarism. In 49 patients undergoing transsphenoidal resection of pituitary adenomas, mean intrasellar pressure was elevated twofold to threefold in patients with pituitary failure. Furthermore, prevalence of headache and elevated levels of prolactin (PRL) correlated positively with intrasellar pressure levels,[3] suggesting interrupted portal delivery of hypothalamic hormones. Therefore, surgical decompression of a sellar mass may lead to recovery of compromised anterior pituitary function. In patients who do not recover pituitary function postoperatively, ischemic necrosis is likely to have occurred. Stalk compression may result in pituitary failure caused by encroachment on the portal vessels that normally provide pituitary access to the hypothalamic hormones. Stalk compression also usually leads to hyperprolactinemia and concomitant failure of other pituitary trophic hormones.

Evaluation of Pituitary Masses

Approach to the Patient Harboring a Pituitary Mass

Ninety-one percent of 1120 patients undergoing transsphenoidal surgery for sellar masses were diagnosed as harboring pituitary adenomas.[4] Therefore, the differential diagnosis of a pituitary mass should be aimed at excluding the diagnosis of a pituitary adenoma before other rare sellar lesions are considered. Pituitary adenomas arise from differentiated cells secreting trophic hormones including growth hormone (GH), PRL, adrenocorticotropic hormone (corticotropin, or ACTH), thyroid-stimulating hormone (TSH), and gonadotropins. Tumors that immunostain for gonadotropins or, less frequently, ACTH may hypersecrete their respective hormones, or they may be clinically nonsecreting (Fig. 9-2).

The management and prognosis of anterior pituitary adenomas differ markedly from those of other

TABLE 9-1

Local Effects of an Expanding Pituitary, Parasellar, or Hypothalamic Mass

Impacted Structure	Clinical Effect
Pituitary	Growth failure, adult hyposomatotropism, hypogonadism, hypothyroidism, hypoadrenalism
Optic tract	Loss of red perception, bitemporal hemianopsia, superior or bitemporal field defect, scotoma, blindness
Hypothalamus	Temperature dysregulation, obesity, diabetes insipidus; thirst, sleep; appetite, behavioral and autonomic nervous system dysfunctions
Cavernous sinus	Ptosis, diplopia, ophthalmoplegia, facial numbness
Temporal lobe	Uncinate seizures
Frontal lobe	Personality disorder; anosmia
Central	Headache, hydrocephalus, psychosis, dementia, laughing seizures
Neuro-ophthalmologic tract	*Field Defects:*
	Bitemporal hemianopia (50%), amaurosis with hemianopia (12%), contralateral or monocular hemianopia (7%)
	Scotomas—junctional; monocular central, arcuate, altitudinal; hemianopic
	Homonymous hemianopia
	Acuity Loss:
	Snellen
	Contrast sensitivity
	Color vision
	Visual evoked potential
	Pupillary Abnormality:
	Impaired light reactivity
	Afferent defect
	Optic Atrophy:
	Papilledema
	Cranial nerve palsy—oculomotor, trochlear, abducens, sensory trigeminal
	Nystagmus
	Visual hallucinations
	Postfixation blindness

Adapted from Snyder P, Melmed S. In: DeGroot L, Jameson JL. Clinically nonfunctioning sellor masses. *Endocrinology*, 5th ed. Philadelphia: Elsevier; 2010:312-323, and Arnold A. In: Melmed S. *The Pituitary*. Blackwell; 2002.

nonpituitary masses, and an important diagnostic challenge is to effectively distinguish a pituitary adenoma from other parasellar masses. Several physiologic states are associated with pituitary enlargement. Lactotroph hyperplasia occurs during pregnancy, and thyrotroph, gonadotroph, or, rarely, corticotroph hyperplasia occurs in the presence of long-standing primary thyroid, gonadal, or adrenal failure, respectively.[5] Pituitary enlargement may also occur as a result of ectopic secretion of growth hormone–releasing hormone (GHRH) or corticotropin-releasing hormone from carcinoid tumors or hypothalamic gangliocytomas, with resultant hyperplasia of somatotroph or corticotroph cells.

Autopsy series show that up to 20% of individuals harbor an incidental clinically silent pituitary adenoma (incidentaloma). With the widespread use of sensitive imaging techniques for nonpituitary indications including head trauma, chronic sinusitis, and headaches, previously inapparent pituitary lesions are being identified with increasing frequency. Incidental pituitary cysts, hemorrhages, and infarctions are also discovered at autopsy. Pituitary abnormalities compatible with the diagnosis of microadenoma are detectable in about 10% of the normal adult population undergoing magnetic resonance imaging (MRI).[6] Because about 90% of observed pituitary lesions represent pituitary adenomas, initial assessment should determine whether the mass is hormonally functional and whether local mass effects are apparent at the time of diagnosis or likely to develop in the future.

The onset of clinical features associated with disordered hormone secretion is insidious and may be unnoticed for years or decades; therefore, endocrine function should always be tested (Table 9-2). Clinical evaluation for changes compatible with hypersecretion or hyposecretion of GH, gonadotropins, PRL, or ACTH may reveal unique long-term sequelae requiring distinct therapies. In the absence of clinical features of a humoral hypersecretory syndrome, cost-effective laboratory screening should be performed. Serum PRL levels greater than 200 μg/L strongly suggest the presence of a microprolactinoma or macroprolactinoma. Any elevation in serum PRL from minimal to high can occur when a microadenoma is present. A minimal to moderate elevation can also indicate secondary stalk interruption by a pituitary mass (usually a nonfunctioning macroadenoma). A PRL level greater than 500 ng/mL in a nonpregnant individual is considered to be pathognomonic of a prolactinoma, although significant PRL elevations can be caused by drugs such as Risprida.[7]

Elevated concentrations of insulin-like growth factor type 1 (IGF1) for the patient's age and gender indicate the presence of a GH-secreting adenoma, and a high 24-hour urinary free cortisol level or an elevated nighttime salivary cortisol level[8] is an effective screen for most patients with Cushing's disease. Nevertheless, the incidence of functional

TABLE 9-2

Screening Tests for Functional Pituitary Adenomas

Disorder	Test	Comments
Acromegaly	IGF1 OGTT with GH obtained at 0, 30, and 60 min	Interpret IGF1 relative to age- and gender-matched controls. Normal subjects should suppress GH to <1 μg/L.
Prolactinoma	Serum PRL level	A level >500 μg/L is pathognomonic for macroprolactinoma. If >200 μg/L, prolactinoma is likely.*
Cushing's disease	24-hr UFC Nighttime salivary cortisol Dexamethasone (1 mg) at 11 p.m. and fasting plasma cortisol measured at 8 a.m. ACTH assay	Ensure that urine collection is total and accurate by measuring urinary creatinine. Free salivary cortisol reflects circadian rhythm and elevated levels may indicate Cushing's disease. Normal subjects suppress to <1.8 μg/dL. Distinguishes adrenal adenoma from ectopic ACTH or Cushing's disease.
TSH-secreting tumor	TSH measurement Free T_4 by dialysis Total T_3	If T_4 or T_3 is elevated and TSH is measurable or elevated, a TSH-secreting tumor may be present.

*Risperidol may result in prolactin levels >200 μg/L.

ACTH, adrenocorticotropic hormone; GH, growth hormone; IGF1, insulin-like growth factor type 1; OGTT, oral glucose tolerance test; PRL, prolactin; T_3, triiodothyronine; T_4, thyroxine; TSH, thyroid-stimulating hormone; UFC, urinary free cortisol.

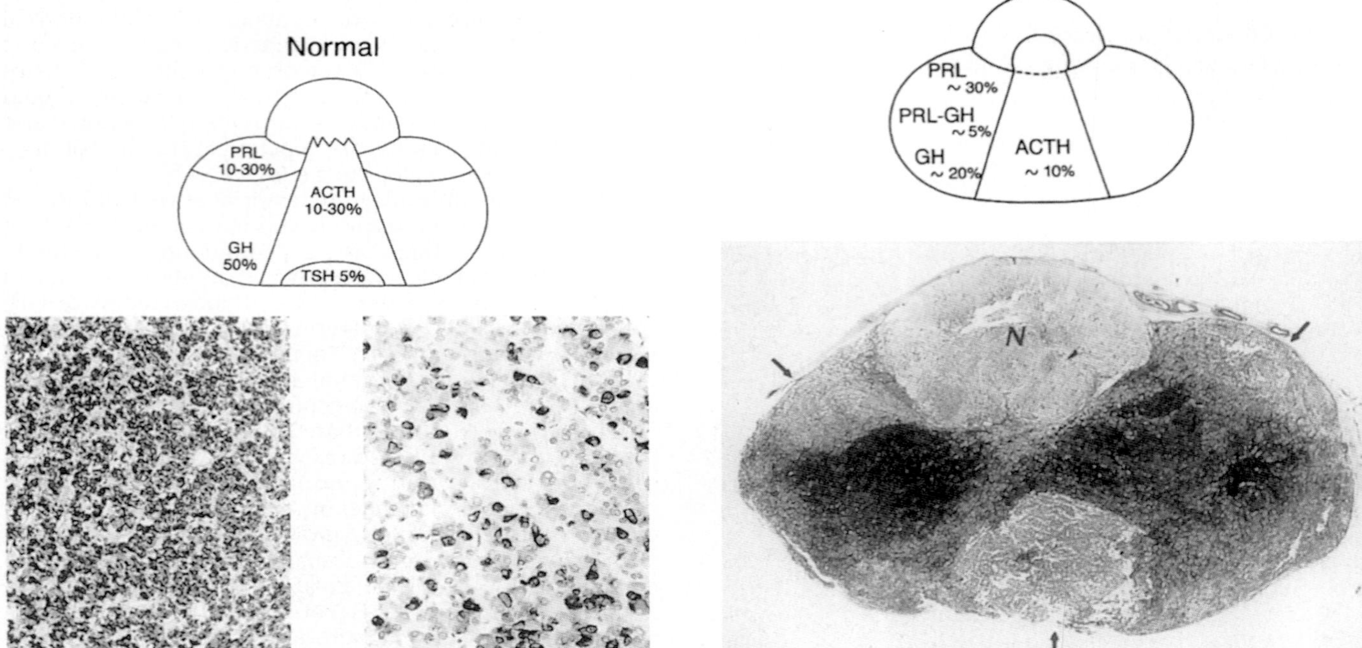

Figure 9-2 Distribution of normal adenohypophyseal cells is reflected in pituitary adenomas. Left panels, normal pituitary with GH cells in lateral wings (*lower left*) and also diseased (*lower right*). Right panels depict adenoma distribution with multiple incidental adenomas shown by arrows. Nonfunctioning tumors, on the other hand, are typically macroadenomas that efface pituitary landmarks. The localization and frequency of functioning microadenomas reflect the maximal concentration of their corresponding normal pituitary cells. ACTH, adrenocorticotropic hormone; GH, growth hormone; N, neurohypophysis; PRL, prolactin; TSH, thyroid-stimulating hormone. (Reproduced from Scheithauer BW, Horvath E, Lloyd RV, et al. Pathology of pituitary adenomas and pituitary hyperplasia. In: Thapar K, Kovacs K, Scheithauer BW, et al., eds. *Diagnosis and Management of Pituitary Tumors.* Totowa, NJ: Humana Press; 2001:91-154.)

hormone-secreting tumors in asymptomatic subjects with incidentally discovered pituitary masses is low.

The presence of, or the potential for, local compressive effects must also be considered. Because the risk for progression of a microadenoma to a compressive macroadenoma is low, no direct intervention may be warranted. For parasellar masses of uncertain origin, histologic tissue examination may be the best approach to yield an accurate diagnosis. Clearly, the benefits and risks of surgery should be considered in such cases, especially for lesions that are not growing or not causing a functional deficit. Although MRI or computed tomographic (CT) imaging features may be helpful in diagnosing the cause of a nonpituitary sellar mass, the final diagnosis may remain elusive until pathologic confirmation is obtained.

Parasellar masses include neoplastic and non-neoplastic lesions and are manifested clinically by local compression of surrounding vital structures or metabolic or hormonal derangements. Rarely, sellar masses or infiltrative processes may be the presenting feature of a previously undiagnosed systemic disorder such as lymphoma, tuberculosis, sarcoidosis,[9] or histiocytosis.[10] Fever with or without associated sterile or septic meningitis may rarely be caused by fluid leakage into the subarachnoid space from Rathke's cleft, dermoid or epidermoid cysts, craniopharyngioma, or apoplexy.[11-13]

Pituitary masses may manifest with hemorrhage and infarction, especially during pregnancy (see earlier discussion), when there is a pituitary tumor, or when an elderly individual with an unsuspected pituitary tumor becomes hypotensive because of another illness. Rarely, these adenomas manifest with CSF leakage, which may predispose to meningitis. Pituitary masses may also undergo silent infarction, leading to the development of a partial or totally empty pituitary sella with normal pituitary reserve, implying that the surrounding rim of pituitary tissue is fully functional. Large sellar cysts may be mistaken for an empty sella.

Rarely, functional pituitary adenomas arise within the remnant pituitary tissue, and these tumors may not be visible on sensitive MRI (i.e., <2 mm in diameter) despite their endocrine hyperactivity. More than one kind of tumor may be found in the same patient, such as a pituitary tumor and a meningioma[14] or a pituitary adenoma with a craniopharyngioma component.[15] Acute or chronic infection with abscess formation may rarely occur within the mass. Compromised pituitary hormone hyposecretion may result from direct pressure effects of the expanding mass on hormone-secreting cells or from parasellar pressure effects that attenuate synthesis or secretion of hypothalamic hormones, with resultant pituitary failure.

Imaging

Tumors of the pituitary gland are best diagnosed with MRI, because this technique has better resolution than other radiologic modalities for identifying soft tissue changes (see Fig. 9-1). If a pituitary tumor or other parasellar mass is suspected, an MRI specifically focused on the pituitary should be requested, because the more widely spaced cuts made during a routine brain MRI are often inadequate to visualize relatively small pituitary tumors.[16,17] This technique permits high-contrast, detailed visualization of tumor mass effects on neighboring soft tissue structures, including the cavernous sinus[18] and optic chiasm. A pituitary MRI includes images of the optic chiasm, hypothalamus, pituitary stalk, and cavernous and sphenoid sinuses.[19,20] High-resolution T1-weighted sections in the coronal and sagittal planes, obtained both before and after gadolinium pentetic acid contrast administration, will distinguish most pituitary masses.[21] Slice thickness should be less than 3 mm to obtain a pixel of 1 mm. Contiguous sections are required to diagnose lesions of 1 to 3 mm.[22] If necessary, especially for diagnosis of high-signaling hemorrhage, T2-weighted images will provide additional diagnostic information.

MRI clearly delineates the pituitary gland, stalk, optic tracts, and surrounding soft tissues. The gland may be concave, convex, or flat. The posterior pituitary lobe exhibits a discrete bright spot of high signal intensity on T1-weighted images, which declines with age and is absent in diabetes insipidus and in most posterior pituitary lesions. This T1 shortening may reflect the presence of antidiuretic hormone (ADH) localized within neurosecetory vesicle phospholipid.[23] The pituitary gland may transiently enlarge during adolescence, pregnancy, and the postpartum period, with teenage girls exhibiting increasing gland convexity during the menstrual cycle.[24] During pregnancy, the gland should normally not exceed 10 to 12 mm, and the stalk should not exceed 4 mm in diameter. Pregnant women may rarely develop visual field deficits due to an enlarging pituitary gland even in the absence of a pituitary tumor. A thickened stalk may indicate the presence of hypophysitis, granuloma, or chordoma.

After administration of gadolinium, microadenomas usually appear hypodense compared with the normal gland, especially when multiple thin-section echo sequences are examined during the first few minutes after contrast injection. It has been suggested that this hypointensity may reflect a compromised microadenoma vasculature.[25] Microadenomas can also cause gland asymmetry or stalk deviation. In contrast, macroadenomas, which are significantly more vascular than microadenomas, have a higher affinity for gadolinium. They often enlarge the sella turcica by remodeling the bony fossa, suggesting a gradual, long-term process. These tumors can grow upward toward the optic apparatus and cause draping of the nerves over the tumor, often accompanied by visual field abnormalities. Tumors can also extend into the sphenoid sinus, and not infrequently they invade the connective tissue separating the pituitary from the cavernous sinus.

Radiologically, visible tumor tissue surrounding the carotid artery confirms cavernous sinus invasion. Infrequently, these patients develop palsies of the third, fourth, or sixth cranial nerve. MRI can readily distinguish pituitary adenomas from other masses, including hyperplasias, craniopharyngiomas, meningiomas, chordomas, cysts, and metastatic lesions. Visualization of a distinct pituitary gland adjacent to a parasellar mass (Fig. 9-3), suggests that the mass is not of pituitary origin.[26] Secondary distinguishing features such as visualization of noninvolved pituitary tissue, mass consistency, calcification, hemorrhage, and suprasellar involvement usually allow an imaging diagnosis of these masses, but often this can be confirmed only by direct tissue histology. Preoperative localization of carotid artery aneurysms can also be confirmed by MRI or magnetic resonance angiography. Administration of gadolinium may be contraindicated in patients with impaired renal function because it can cause acute renal failure or be associated with nephrogenic systemic fibrosis.[27,28]

Pituitary CT allows visualization of bony structures, including the sellar floor and clinoid processes, and identification of bony invasion. CT also recognizes calcifications that characterize craniopharyngiomas, meningiomas, and, rarely, aneurysms that are not evident on MRI. Rarely, pituitary adenomas may calcify. Pituitary CT is indicated for discovery of hemorrhagic lesions, metastatic deposits, chordomas, and evidence of calcification.

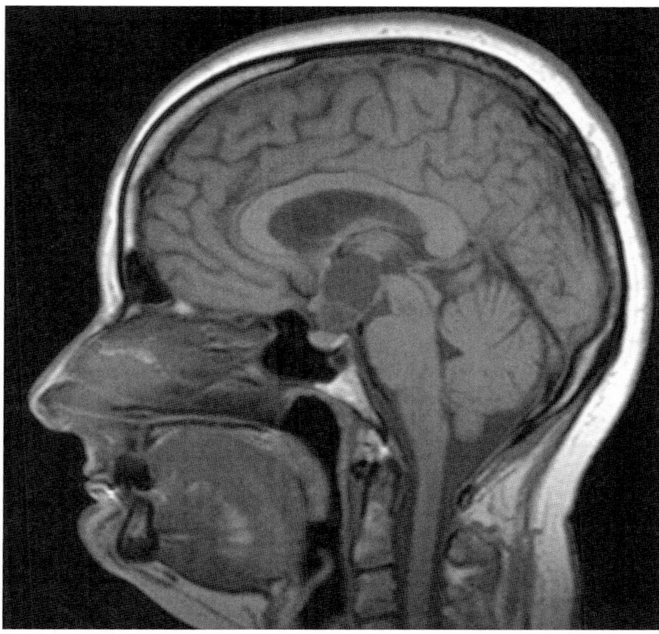

Figure 9-3 Sagittal magnetic resonance image of a craniopharyngioma with cystic and solid components. The tumor is in the suprasellar area, sitting above a normal pituitary gland. The presence of a separate pituitary gland indicates that the suprasellar tumor is not of pituitary origin. (Courtesy of Nikki Karavitaki Oxford University, UK.)

Receptor Imaging. Because prolactinomas express dopamine 2 (D_2) receptors, they can be imaged with a radiolabeled D_2 receptor antagonist (^{123}I-iodobenzamine) using single-photon emission computed tomography (SPECT). Failure to visualize nonfunctioning tumors by this technique has led some to advocate its use to distinguish the two tumor types.[29] Radiolabelled indium pentetreotide has been used for in vivo tumor imaging. Most pituitary adenomas express somatostatin receptor subtypes to a varying degree, thus limiting the specificity of the procedure. Because the sensitivity of SPECT is about 1 cm, and because it also detects normal pituitary tissue receptor expression, its utility is limited for pituitary tumor detection, but it may be helpful for imaging ectopic ACTH-secreting tumors.

Neuro-Ophthalmologic Assessment of Pituitary Masses

The optic tracts are particularly vulnerable to compression by expanding pituitary masses. Accurate neuro-ophthalmologic evaluation is helpful for diagnosing tumors, determining pretreatment baseline visual status for posttreatment monitoring, and detecting mass recurrence.[30] The relationship of the optic chiasm and intracranial components of the optic nerves to the pituitary gland and surrounding vessels is depicted in Figure 9-4. A 10-mm, posteriorly angled gap separates the optic chiasm and the diaphragma sellae (Fig. 9-5). Therefore, extensive suprasellar mass extension is required before visual function becomes compromised. Decussation of neural fibers originating from the nasal half of each retina occurs at the chiasm, whereas those fibers originating from the temporal retinal halves are situated ipsilaterally.[31] Fibers from the superior and inferior retinal aspects are segregated in the corresponding chiasmal regions. Local vascular compromise or chiasmal stretching contributes to the

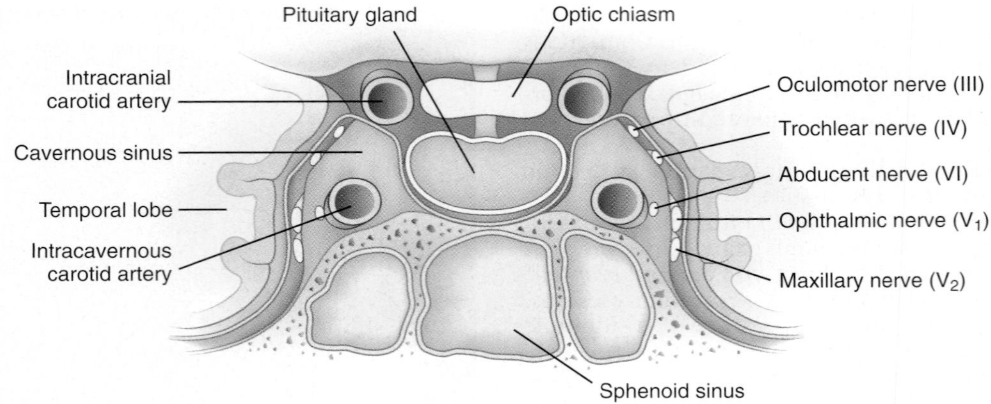

Figure 9-4 **Coronal section of the sellar structures and cavernous sinus, showing the relationship of the oculomotor (III) and trochlear (IV) cranial nerves to the pituitary gland.** (From Silver SI, Sharpe JA. Neuro-ophthalmologic evaluation of pituitary tumors. In: Thapar K, Kovacs K, Scheithauer BW, et al., eds. *Diagnosis and Management of Pituitary Tumor.* Totowa, NJ: Humana Press; 2001:173-200.)

pathogenesis of selective visual compromise. Reversibility of visual effects may correlate inversely with the acuteness of the compressive insult.

Visual Symptoms. An abnormal visual examination may unmask the presence of a pituitary mass in an asymptomatic patient. Before sophisticated assay and imaging techniques became available, almost all pituitary masses manifested with visual loss. Currently, fewer than 10% of patients present with visual loss.[32] These usually have nonfunctioning macroadenomas. Unilateral or bilateral temporal or central visual loss is usually asymmetric and may be quite insidious, remitting or recurring. Rarely, sudden visual loss occurs in a previously asymptomatic patient. Other symptoms include diplopia, impaired depth perception, and, very rarely, visual hallucinations (Fig. 9-6).[33]

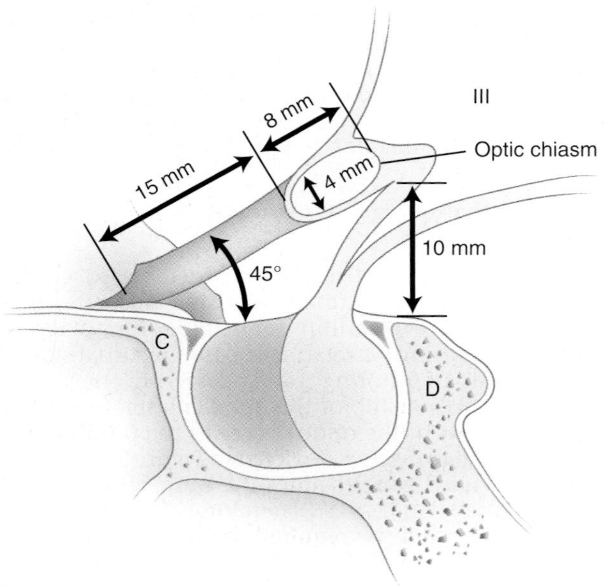

Figure 9-5 Relationship of the pituitary gland to the optic chiasm. The intracranial optic nerve/chiasmal complex lies up to 10 mm above the diaphragma sellae. C, Anterior clinoid process; D, dorsum of the sella turcica. (From Miller NR. *Walsh and Hoyt's Clinical Neuro-Ophthalmology,* 4th ed, vol 1. Baltimore: Williams and Wilkins; 1985:60-69.)

Clinical Signs. Impingement of the inferior crossing chiasmal fibers leads to bitemporal visual loss, especially in the superior field portions, accounting for most pituitary-related visual defects. Rarely, tumors can compress the optic chiasm from above and cause inferior temporal compromise. As damage to the optic chiasm becomes more extreme, field cuts can extend into the nasal field and can also cause optic atrophy. Isolated impairment of nasal visual fields is seen mostly in patients with glaucoma. Pituitary-related defects preferentially marginate at the vertical field midline,[30] in contrast to other causes of bitemporal defects, which tend to occur away from the midline (Fig. 9-7). Despite prominent field defects, many of which can be directly correlated with defined tumor location by MRI, visual acuity in the remaining fields is normal in more than 95% of patients.[34] Anterior tumor extension may damage central visual acuity, and this is detected with the use of the Snellen chart or by loss of color discrimination, especially in the red-green spectrum. Rarely, pupillary abnormalities, optic atrophy, papilledema, cranial nerve palsies, and nystagmus may be encountered. Visual fields are assessed by bedside confrontational testing, Goldmann perimetry, the Amsler grid, and automated quantitative perimetry. Because red vision is lost before white, a small pin (<10 mm in diameter) with the two colors can be employed. The patient should be asked to cover one eye so that the examiner can evaluate both temporal and nasal fields without compromise.

Management of Pituitary Masses

The goals of therapy for masses are to alleviate local compressive mass effects and to suppress hormone hypersecretion or relieve hormone hyposecretion while maintaining intact pituitary trophic function. Three modes of therapy are available: surgical, radiotherapeutic, and medical approaches. In general, the benefits of each therapy should be weighed against the respective risks, and comprehensive physician and patient awareness is required to individualize treatment approaches.

Surgical Management of Pituitary Tumors and Sellar Masses

Pituitary surgery is indicated for excision of mass lesions causing central pressure effects including visual compromise, for primary correction of hormonal hypersecretion,

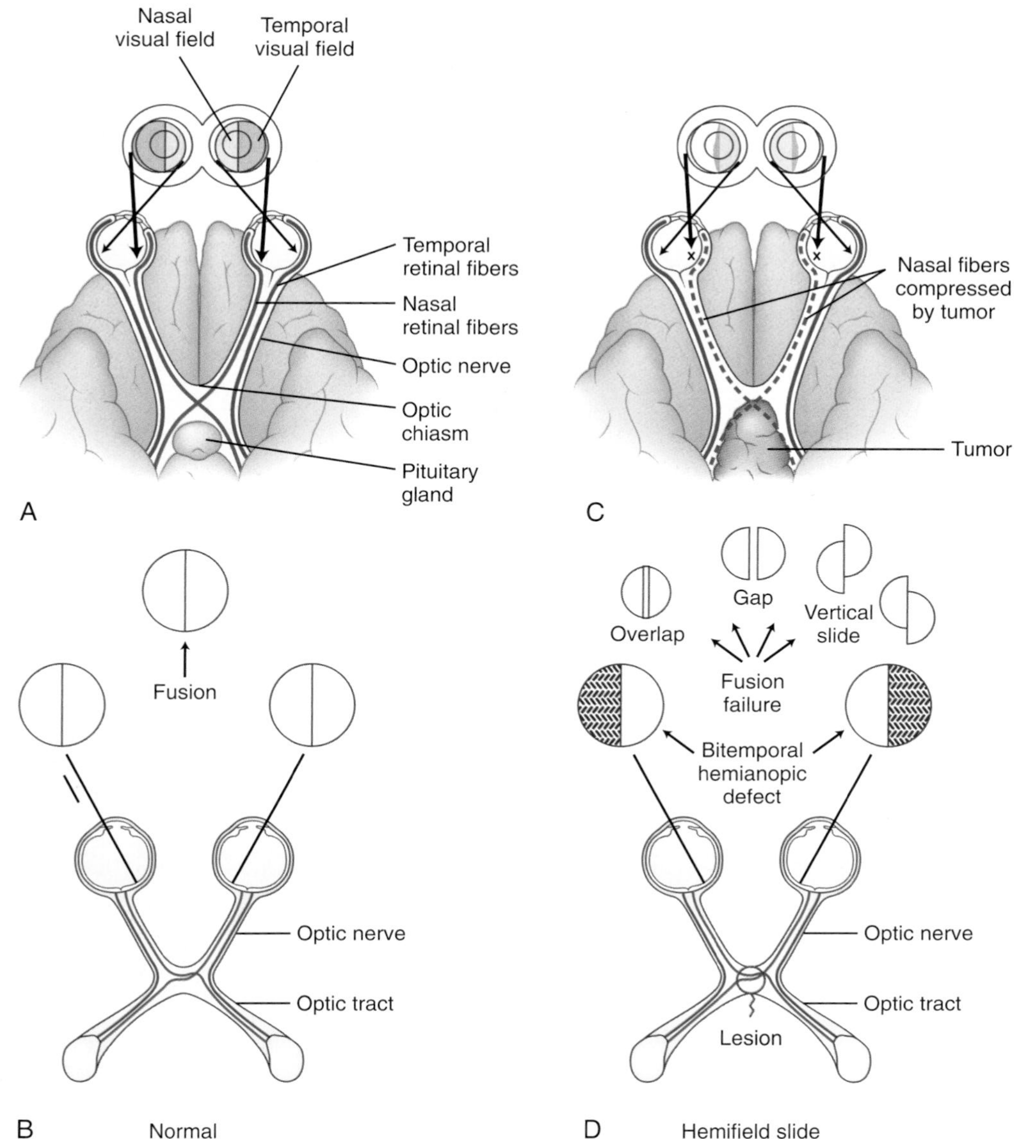

Figure 9-6 Local effects of an expanding pituitary tumor causing visual field defects. **A,** Normal vision; **C,** bitemporal hemianopia. **B** and **D,** Hemifield slide phenomena arising in the setting of bitemporal hemianopia from fusion instability. The nasal and temporal fields lose their linkage, resulting in overlap of the preserved visual fields. (**A** and **C** Reproduced from Newell-Price J. Endocrine assessment. In: Sheaves R, Jenkins PJ, Wass JAH, eds. *Clinical Endocrinology Oncology.* Boston: Blackwell Science; 1997:152-157.) (**B** and **D** Reproduced from Stiver SI, Sharpe JA. Neuro-ophthalmologic Evaluation of Pituitary Tumors. In: Thapar K, Kovacs K, Scheithauer BW, et al., eds. *Diagnosis and Management of Pituitary Tumors.* Totowa, NJ: Humana Press; 2001:173-200. © The Mayo Clinic 2000.)

and for resection of functional tumors that are resistant or not immediately responsive to medical treatment. Unusual sellar lesions may require diagnostic tissue evaluation, and in rare instances, primary or secondary parasellar malignancies require wide excision.

In 1904, Horsley reported the surgical resection of a pituitary tumor by means of a lateral middle fossa approach.[35] The first successful transsphenoidal approach for pituitary tumor resection was reported by Schloffer in 1907[36] and subsequently refined by Cushing, who between 1910 and 1925 operated on 231 patients harboring pituitary tumors with a remarkably low mortality rate of 5.6%.[35,37] Cushing used a sublabial incision to enable an endonasal approach for removal of the septum and improved visualization by using Kanavel's headlight. Hardy later improved the technique by using the operating microscope and intraoperative fluoroscopy, resulting in markedly reduced morbidity and mortality compared with that usually encountered with craniotomy, and this became the mainstay surgical technique for resecting these tumors.

The transsphenoidal approach precludes invasion of the cranial cavity and removes the need for brain tissue manipulation, as is required during a subfrontal surgical approach (Fig. 9-8). A ventral sphenoid approach for resection of pituitary masses likewise does not violate the cranial fossa. Transsphenoidal surgery is associated with minimal morbidity and mortality; most patients are ambulatory within 6 to 9 hours, and the hospital stay is usually about 3 days. Furthermore, the transsphenoidal approach allows for a clearly visible operative field with high magnification and internal illumination. Normal pituitary can be clearly distinguished from tumor tissue, facilitating microdissection

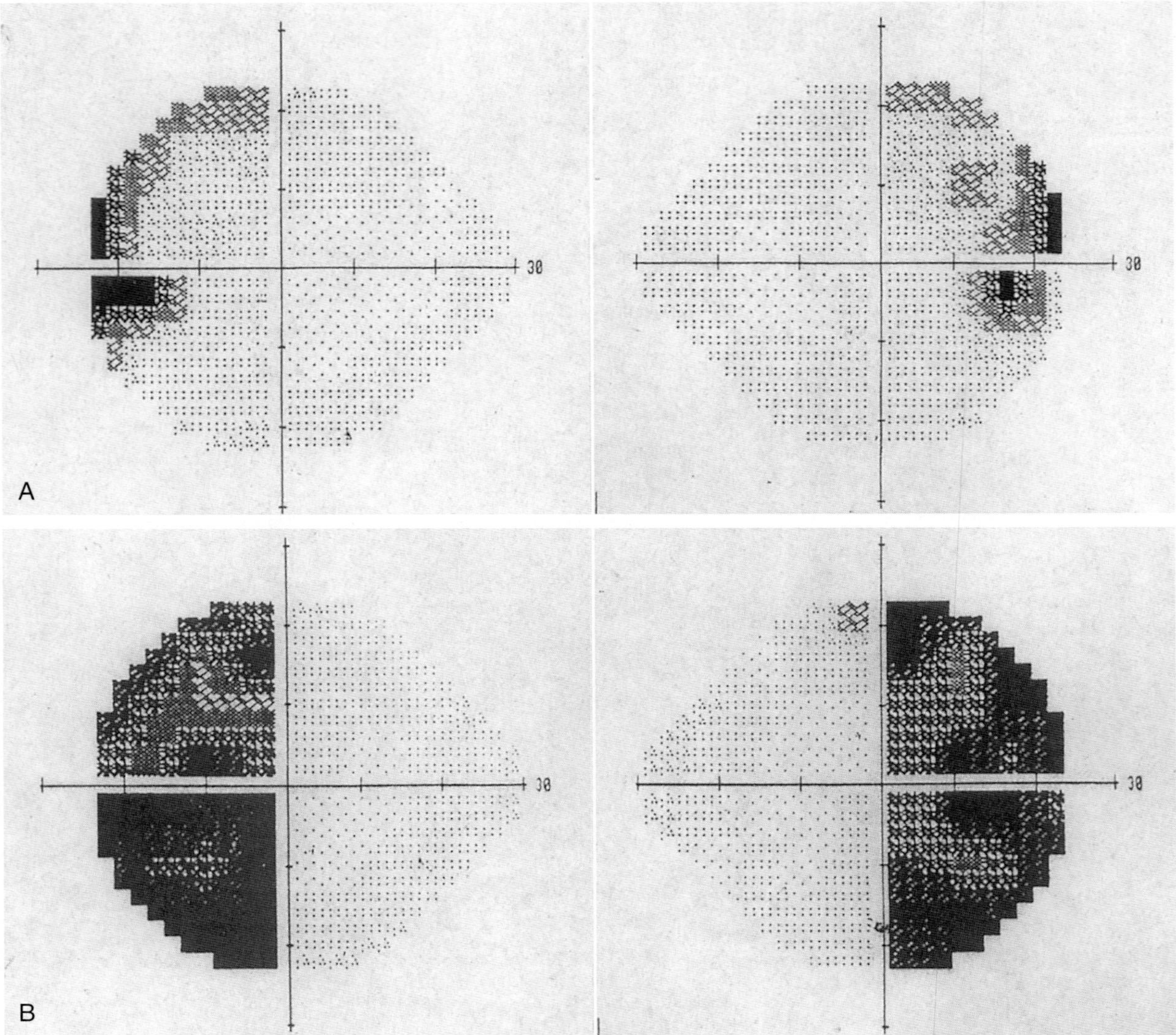

Figure 9-7 Threshold field test showing superior bitemporal hemianopsia in a patient with a pituitary tumor compressing the optic chiasma (**A**), which later advanced to bitemporal hemianopsia (**B**).

and resection of small tumors (Fig. 9-9). The utility of the transsphenoidal approach has been greatly enhanced by several technologic advances, including head immobilization techniques, microinstrumentation, and novel-angled endoscopes. Enhanced MRI sensitivity and precision, as well as the use of intraoperative MRI, allow for clear delineation of tumor location, size, and invasiveness—all critical determinants of surgical success.

The endoscopic surgical technique has enabled an approach to both intrapituitary and some extrasellar masses. Most approaches are endonasal,[38] but some are via the cranial base,[39] and suprasellar lesions are reached by transposing the pituitary to access the lesion.[40] In experienced hands, the endoscopic technique results in complication rates and outcomes, similar to those of the traditional transsphenoidal approach.[41,42]

Craniotomy is indicated for the rare invasive suprasellar mass extending into the frontal or middle cranial fossa or optic nerve and for extensive posterior clival invasion. Suprasellar extension contained by a small diaphragmatic aperture (hourglass configuration) may also require a transcranial approach. Rarely, tumors that are too solid to be removed transsphenoidally may require a combination of transsphenoidal and intracranial surgery.

Goals of Surgery. The goal of pituitary surgery is for total resection limited to the lesion without compromise of postoperative endogenous pituitary function. Careful selective mass resection may be difficult in cases of poorly encapsulated lesions, those embedded deeply within the gland body, those extending into the wall or the body of the cavernous sinuses, and suprasellar lesions. However, suprasellar tumors (e.g., craniopharyngiomas) may also be successfully removed via a transnasal approach. Poor operative field visibility also limits precise resection. Excision of normal pituitary tissue and intraoperative manipulation of the gland should be avoided unless critical for effective tumor dissection. Occasionally, hemihypophysectomy or even nonselective total gland resection may be indicated for multifocal tumors, if the surrounding normal gland is necrotic, or if no mass lesion is discernible despite an accurate clinical and biochemical diagnosis (especially for ACTH-cell tumors). Successful surgery should decompress central visual defects and compromised trophic hormone secretion.

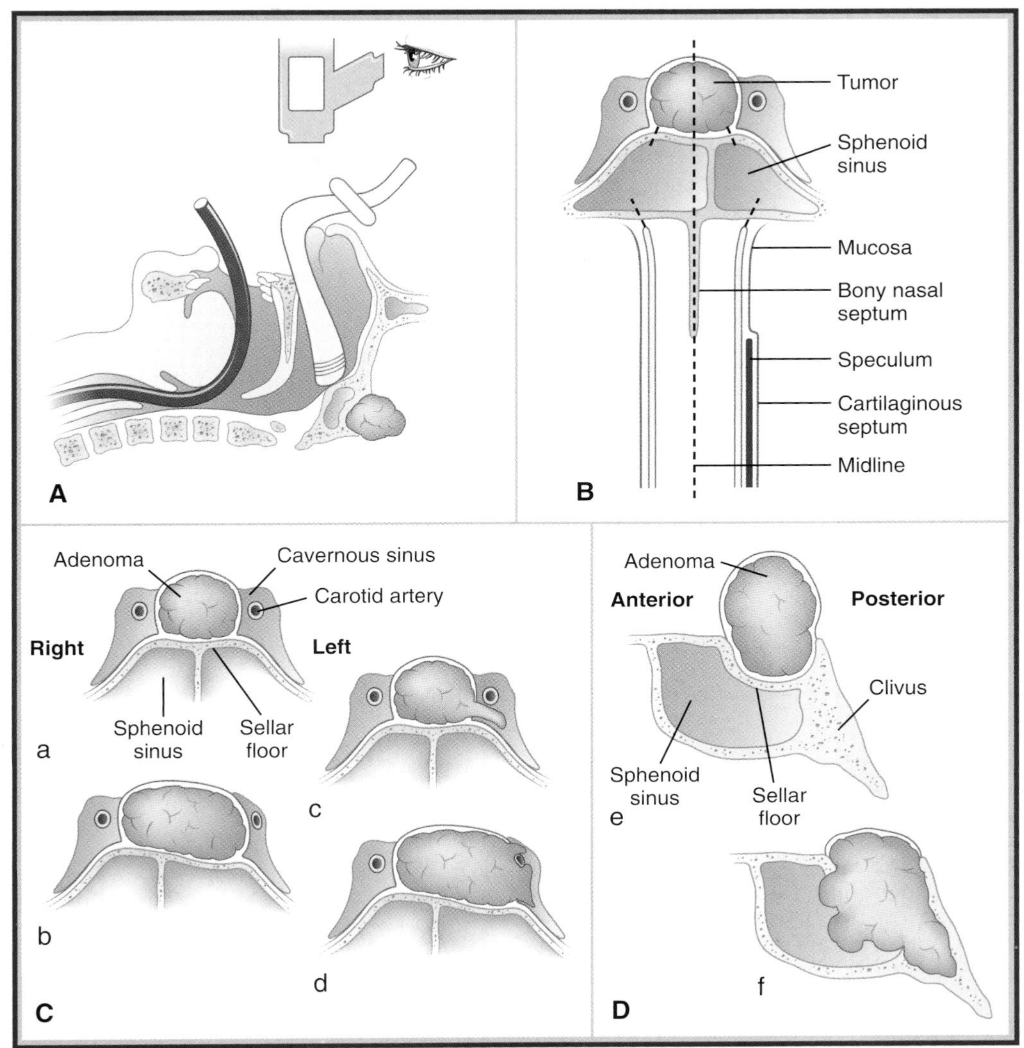

Figure 9-8 Transsphenoidal pituitary surgery. **A,** The route of the transsphenoidal approach (lateral view) and the surgical corridor and positioning of the retractor. **B,** The extent of removal of bone structures including the nasal septum and sphenoid sinus floor and roof is indicated *(gray areas)*. **C,** Parasellar extensions of pituitary adenomas (coronal sections) are shown: a, intrasellar adenoma; b, displacement of the cavernous sinus; c, focal invasion of the cavernous sinus; and d, diffuse invasion of the cavernous sinus by the adenoma. **D,** Extensions of a pituitary adenoma (sagittal sections): e, suprasellar extension; f, invasion of the sphenoid sinus and of the clivus. (Adapted from Honegger J, Buchfelder M, Fahlbusch R. Surgery for pituitary tumors. In: Sheaves R, Jenkins PJ, Wass JAH, eds. *Clinical Endocrinology Oncology.* Boston: Blackwell Science; 1997:176-184.)

For children and young adults, the need for adequate normal tissue for subsequent growth patterns and reproductive function is an important determinant for intraoperative decision-making. Nevertheless, especially for functional tumors, small residual remnants attached to the dura are difficult to access and remain hypersecretory with persistent clinical progression. Therefore, the skilled neurosurgeon carefully balances maximally effective tumor removal with the requirement to preserve nontumorous pituitary trophic function.

Recent advances have enabled improved surgical results, although long-term outcomes using new techniques have not yet been rigorously compared with the results of standard operations performed by skilled surgeons.[43] Image-guided approaches enable intraoperative surgical neuronavigation by three-dimensional imaging. Intraoperative ultrasound and MRI technologies allow for real-time assessment of the dimensions and extent of the pituitary mass and the progress of surgery. Intraoperative MRI is performed while the surgical field is still open; this allows the surgeon to directly assess the need for further dissection and also provides an excellent baseline for postoperative follow-up.[44] If there is suspicion of a vascular lesion, carotid and intracranial angiography is indicated before surgery. In contrast, postoperative image stabilization may not be evident for months after surgery, and MRI may be useful only after 1 year or longer, especially after resection of secretory tumors with measurable serum biomarkers.[45]

Endonasal transsphenoidal endoscopy avoids the use of a retractor or speculum, does not require nasal packing, and sometimes leads to a shorter operating time, allowing for improved postoperative morbidity and a shorter hospital stay (Fig. 9-10). The advantages of the technique include a clear panoramic view of bony landmarks and the ability to access suprasellar and parasellar tumor extensions into the cavernous sinuses.[42] Disadvantages of this approach include perioperative intrasellar bleeding and CSF leaks. Combining both techniques may allow the advantages of both approaches.

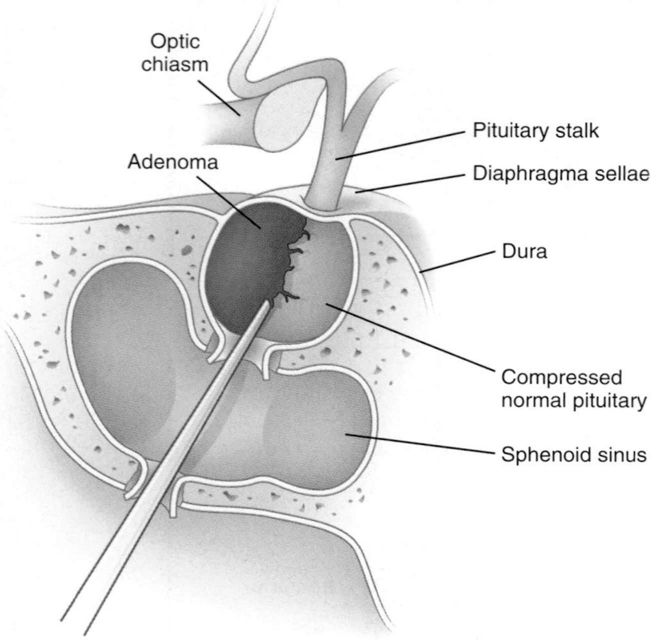

Figure 9-9 Transsphenoidal resection of pituitary adenoma.

Indications for Transsphenoidal Surgery. A pituitary mass that may or may not be compressing local vital structures should be evaluated for surgical resection (Table 9-3). Although surgical resection offers rapid resolution of hormone hypersecretion and many of the resultant clinical features of functioning adenomas, indications for the procedure differ depending on tumor type (see later discussion). In general, patients who are intolerant or resistant to medical therapy require surgery. Surgery is primarily indicated for patients with well-circumscribed GH-secreting adenomas, TSH-secreting adenomas, all ACTH-secreting tumors, and nonfunctioning macroadenomas that require surgery. Surgery may also be indicated when tissue histology is required for diagnosis of the nature of an enigmatic sellar mass. Progressive compressive features such as visual field loss, compromised pituitary function, and other central nervous system (CNS) functional changes are indications for surgical debulking and sellar decompression. Hemorrhage into the encased bony sella turcica, usually occurring within a known or previously unknown

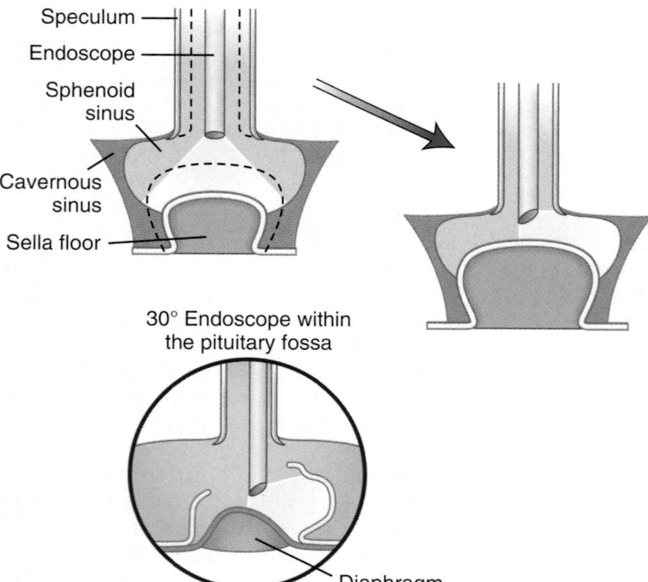

Figure 9-10 Endoscope-assisted microsurgery provides a panoramic view of the sphenoid sinus. Using a 30-degree endoscope, a view "around the corner" is possible. Parasellar structures can be visualized and residual tumor detected and resected. (Reproduced from Fahlbusch R, Buchfelder M, Kreutzer J, et al. Surgical management of acromegaly. In: Wass J, ed. *Handbook of Acromegaly.* Bristol, UK: BioScientifica; 2001.)

TABLE 9-3

Transsphenoidal Pituitary Surgery
Primary Indications
General
Visual tract or central nervous compression arising from within sella
Relief of compressive hypopituitarism by presenting, residual, or recurrent tumor tissue
Tumor recurrence after surgery or irradiation
Pituitary hemorrhage
Cerebrospinal fluid leak
Resistance to medical therapy
Intolerance of medical therapy
Personal choice
Desire for immediate pregnancy with macroadenoma
Requirement for diagnostic tissue histology
Specific
Acromegaly
Cushing's disease
Clinically nonfunctioning macroadenoma
Prolactinoma
Nelson's syndrome
TSH-secreting adenoma
Side Effects
Transient
Diabetes insipidus
Cerebrospinal fluid leak and rhinorrhea
Inappropriate ADH secretion
Arachnoiditis
Meningitis
Postoperative psychosis
Local hematoma
Arterial wall damage
Epistaxis
Local abscess
Pulmonary embolism
Narcolepsy
Permanent (up to 10%)
Diabetes insipidus
Total or partial hypopituitarism
Visual loss
Inappropriate ADH secretion
Vascular occlusion
CNS damage—oculomotor palsy, hemiparesis, encephalopathy
Nasal septum perforation
Surgery-Related Mortality (up to 1%)
Brain, hypothalamic injury
Vascular damage
Postoperative meningitis
Cerebrospinal fluid leak
Pneumocephalus
Acute cardiopulmonary disease
Anesthesia-related
Seizure

ADH, antidiuretic hormone; CNS, central nervous system; TSH, thyroid-stimulating hormone.

adenoma, may require immediate surgical decompression. Urgent surgical decompression is required for acute pituitary hemorrhage, especially in patients who have developed sudden visual field compromise.

Hypopituitarism resulting from increased portal vessel pressure may resolve shortly after decompressive surgery.[46] When pituitary function after surgery was assessed in 234 patients, 52 were found to have developed new trophic hormone dysfunction, whereas 45 of 93 patients with preoperative evidence for hypopituitarism had recovered between one and three previously suppressed axes. Significant factors determining restoration of postoperative pituitary function were no visible tumor remnants as assessed by MRI and no tumor invasion as determined both by the neurosurgeon and by pathologic examination of surrounding tissue.[47] Therefore, because some patients with preoperative pituitary failure recover function, depending on the clinical circumstance, patients should be considered for retesting of pituitary reserve before postoperative substitution therapy is initiated (except for adrenal steroid replacement, which requires greater caution). Indications for a second surgery in the same patient include tumor recurrence, persistent hormonal hypersecretion by tumor remnants, and repair of a CSF leak.

After surgery, patients should be kept on bedrest at an angle of 30 to 45 degrees, with urine and serum osmolality and serum electrolytes measured every 6 hours. Indications for postoperative vasopressin replacement include polyuria, especially with elevated serum sodium and osmolality and inappropriately low urine osmolality. Postoperative polyuria alone is not an indication for vasopressin replacement, unless it is a reflection of compromised posterior pituitary function. Excess fluid given intraoperatively may also result in postoperative polyuria. Requirements for fluid replacement should take into consideration both fluid intake and urine output.

Side Effects. The success of surgery is largely determined by the skill and experience of the neurosurgeon. Higher-volume pituitary centers and experienced surgeons report superior postoperative outcomes and shorter hospital stays.[48,49] Tumor size, degree of invasiveness, preoperative hormone levels, and previous pituitary surgery are all determinants of surgical outcome. CSF leakage, transient diabetes insipidus, and the syndrome of inappropriate antidiuretic hormone secretion (SIADH) are the most commonly encountered transient side effects, occurring in up to 20% of patients (see Table 9-3). Local damage may also result in arachnoiditis, vascular bleeding, hematoma formation, and epistaxis. Rarely, pulmonary embolism, narcolepsy, and local abscess have been reported. Iatrogenic hypopituitarism, diabetes insipidus, or SIADH is reported in up to 10% of patients. Rarely, the CNS may be permanently damaged, resulting in hemiparesis, cranial nerve palsies, or encephalopathy.

A triphasic course of postoperative diabetes insipidus has been described in which the transient disorder is followed by an interphase on days 6 through 11 with no polydipsia or polyuria. During this latter phase, hyponatremia with features of SIADH have been reported even in patients who show no signs and symptoms of diabetes insipidus after surgery.[50,51] The third phase is return of polyuria and polydipsia. Cognitive dysfunction, including anterograde memory deficits and deficits in executive function, were reported in several retrospective studies after transsphenoidal surgery.[52,53] Mortality has been reported in up to 1% of patients undergoing pituitary surgery and may be related to direct hypothalamic or cerebrovascular damage, meningitis, pneumocephalus formation, or complications of anesthesia. Surgical failure may result from a non–pituitary-related event such as an anesthesia-related complication or bleeding disorder. Incomplete tumor removal may also result from inaccurate preoperative MRI localization or identification. Rarely, a previously undiagnosed functioning pituitary tumor or ectopic source of ACTH may be unmasked after initially unsuccessful pituitary surgery.

Pituitary Irradiation

Principles. High-energy ionizing radiation can be delivered to deep tissues by megavoltage techniques. The challenge of this approach is to provide maximal localized necrotizing irradiation to the pituitary lesion while minimally exposing surrounding normal structures to radiation damage. Several advances have improved both efficacy and safety, including highly precise tumor localization, a high-voltage (6 to 15 MeV) linear accelerator, and accurate simulation models with isocentric rotational arcing that allow repeated head positioning at exactly the same points for each recurrent patient visit. Up to a maximum of 5000 rads is administered in 180-rad daily fractions for 5 to 6 weeks.

High-precision techniques such as stereotactic conformal radiotherapy,[54] gamma knife,[24] and proton beam procedures[55] allow delivery of high energy to the pituitary lesion while minimizing the mass of normal brain exposed to radiation (Fig. 9-11).

Indications. The use of radiation for treatment of pituitary tumors is highly individualized and depends on the expertise of the treating center, the conviction of the treating physician in weighing the potential benefits and risks of the procedure, and patient preference based on informed choice (Table 9-4). In general, radiation techniques are indicated for persistent hormone hypersecretion or residual mass effects after surgery, or when surgical resection of a compressive mass is contraindicated. Because GH-secreting and PRL-secreting tumors are generally amenable to

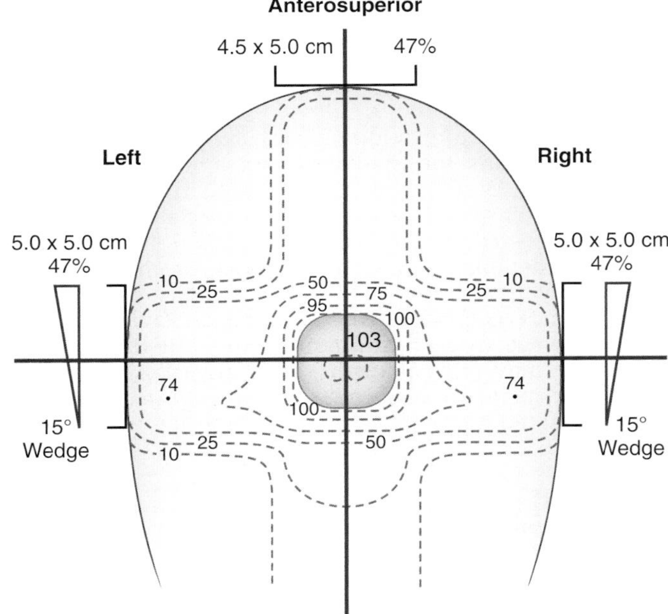

Figure 9-11 Pituitary radiotherapy. An 8-mV X-ray isodosimetric plan is used. The three fields restrict high-dose volume to the target. Numbered areas reflect radiation exposure. (Plowman PN. Pituitary radiotherapy: Techniques and potential complications. In: Sheaves R, Jenkins PJ, Wass JAH, eds. *Clinical Endocrinology Oncology.* Boston: Blackwell Science; 1997:185-188.)

TABLE 9-4

Pituitary Irradiation

INDICATIONS					
Pituitary adenoma—acromegaly, Cushing's disease, nonfunctioning adenoma, prolactinoma					
Craniopharyngioma					
Nelson's syndrome					
Nonadenomatous invasive sellar mass					
Tumor recurrence					
Hormone hypersecretion recurrence					
SIDE EFFECTS					
Hypopituitarism—deficient growth hormone, gonadotropin, TSH, and ACTH reserve					
Eye—visual loss, optic neuritis					
Brain—brain necrosis, temporal lobe deficits, cognitive dysfunction					
RELATIVE RISK OF SECOND BRAIN TUMOR					
Second Tumor	**Observed Incidence**	**Expected Incidence**	**SIR**	**95% CI**	**References**
Astrocytoma (2) Meningioma (1) Meningeal sarcoma (1)	5	0.53	9.4	3.05-21.98	Brada 1992
Gliomas	4	0.25	16	4.4-41	Tsang 1993
Astrocytoma (2) Meningioma (1)	3	1.13	2.7	0.55-7.76	Erfurth 2001*
Meta-analysis	12	1.96	6.1	3.16-10.69	

*Excludes patients with acromegaly.

ACTH, adrenocorticotropic hormone; CI, confidence interval; SIR, standardized incidence ratio for person-years at risk; TSH, thyroid-stimulating hormone.

Adapted from Erfurth EM, Bulow B, Mikoczy Z, et al. Incidence of a second tumor in hypopituitary patients operated for pituitary tumors. *J Clin Endocrinol Metab.* 2001;86:659-662; Brada M, Ford D, Ashley S, et al. Risk of second brain tumour after conservative surgery and radiotherapy for pituitary adenoma. *BMJ* 1992;304:1343-1346; Tsang RW, Laperriere NJ, Simpson WJ, et al. Glioma arising after radiation therapy for pituitary adenoma. A report of four patients and estimation of risk. *Cancer* 1993;72:2227-2233.

medical therapy, indications for their irradiation are rare. Most indications for irradiation are adjuvant to either surgical or medical treatment. Radiation therapy may be indicated after resection of a potentially recurring or inadequately resected pituitary mass, such as a nonfunctioning pituitary adenoma, craniopharyngioma, or chordoma. In acromegaly, the use of irradiation as primary treatment is generally not recommended,[56] but for aggressively growing prolactinomas that are resistant to medical therapy, the procedure may prevent further local invasion. Recurrent pituitary-dependent Cushing's disease appears to be particularly suited for radiation therapy, especially in younger patients.

Side Effects

Hypopituitarism. Pituitary failure occurs commonly in patients who have received pituitary irradiation. Within 10 years after radiation treatment, up to 80% of patients have gonadotroph, somatotroph, thyrotroph, or corticotroph deficits.[56-58] The mechanism for hypopituitarism appears to involve damage to hypothalamic hormone-releasing cells as well as direct pituitary damage. These patients require lifelong endocrine follow-up for pituitary reserve testing and hormone replacement when appropriate.

Second Brain Tumors. Glioma may occur after conventional pituitary irradiation for adenoma or craniopharyngioma with a mean latency period of 11.5 years (see Table 9-4).[59] Among patients receiving radiotherapy for pituitary tumors, it appears that the standardized incidence ratio (SIR) for a second brain tumor is approximately 6 (confidence interval, 3.16 to 10.69), with a latency of 6 to 24 years in separate cohorts.[60-63] Because patients harboring pituitary tumors are more likely to undergo routine brain imaging during follow-up, it is not entirely clear whether observed meningiomas are coincidental findings. However, children undergoing radiation therapy for brain tumors have a higher incidence of postradiation meningioma.[64] This complication, which occurs in fewer than 5% of patients, also appears to be dose-related, so fractionated doses not exceeding 5000 rads should be given. Use of confocal radiation techniques to irradiate a smaller tissue volume, including radiosurgery, fractionated stereotactic radiotherapy, and proton beam therapy, may minimize this adverse effect, but prospectively controlled surveillance studies are required to rigorously evaluate this critical question.

Cerebrovascular Disease. Mortality from cerebrovascular disease appears to be higher among previously irradiated pituitary-deficient patients.[65-68] The direct causality of this relationship is unclear, but direct effects on cerebral vasculature, including atherosclerotic occlusive lesions, have been reported.[69]

Visual Damage. Approximately 2% of patients develop impaired vision due to optic nerve damage after radiotherapy for pituitary tumors.[70] The risk of visual damage is minimized by fractionating dosages to less than 200 rads per treatment session. Although consequent blindness was reported in 2 patients who received 4500 rads in 180-rad fractions,[71] the incidence of reported visual damage in patients undergoing radiosurgery is negligible.[24]

Brain Necrosis. Dose-related radiation-induced brain necrosis was documented by MRI in 14 of 45 patients, with temporal lobe atrophy and cystic and diffuse cerebral atrophy.[72] Cognitive dysfunction, especially memory loss, has also been reported.[73]

Radiosurgery. Proton beam therapy, gamma knife using focused cobalt-60 emissions, and linear accelerators deliver high-dose radiation while sparing surrounding tissue (Fig. 9-12). The delivery of high energy by gamma knife directly targeted at the pituitary tumor minimizes radiation exposure to surrounding tissues.[74] This procedure is best suited for intrasellar and cavernous lesions distant from the optic nerves. Intermediate review of 1621 patients undergoing radiosurgery reported from 35 independent centers emphasized the heterogeneous efficacy rates and the need for controlled prospective comparative trials, especially to assess efficacy and safety in comparison with surgery and medical therapy.[24] In a long-term study of 76 patients with a mean follow-up of 96 months, about half were in remission, 23% developed new-onset hypopituitarism, and 3 patients developed oculomotor palsies.[74] Therefore, there is no current evidence that stereotactic radiosurgery exhibits superior efficacy or safety compared with fractionated treatments.[75]

Medical Management

Pituitary tumors often express receptors mediating hypothalamic control of hormone secretion, and appropriate therapeutic ligands for the D_2 receptor and the somatotropin release–inhibiting factor (SRIF) receptor subtype 2 (SSTR2) are employed to effectively suppress PRL, GH, and/

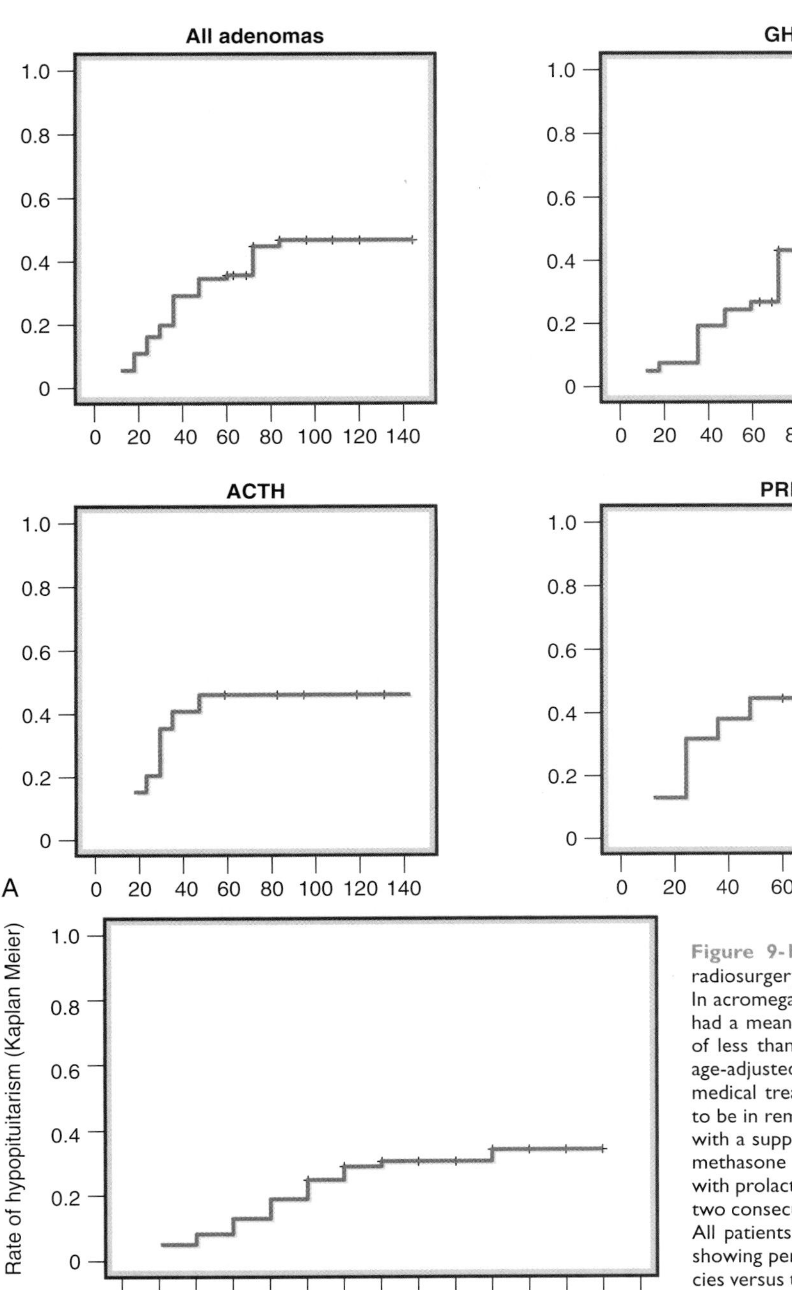

Figure 9-12 **A,** Kaplan-Meier analysis according to time (months) after radiosurgery for adenomas (acromegaly, Cushing's disease, and prolactinomas). In acromegaly *(upper right)*, patients were considered to be in remission if they had a mean growth hormone (GH) level of less than 2 μg/mL or a GH level of less than 1 ng/mL after a glucose tolerance test (or both) and a normal age-adjusted concentration of insulin-like growth factor type 1 (IGF1) without medical treatment. In Cushing's disease *(lower left)*, patients were considered to be in remission if they had a normalized 24-hour urinary free cortisol value with a suppressible plasma cortisol level (<50 nmol/L) after a low-dose dexamethasone suppression test (ACTH, adrenocorticotropic hormone). Patients with prolactinomas *(lower right)* were considered to be in remission if they had two consecutive samplings of prolactin (PRL) in the normal range (<20 ng/mL). All patients had a follow-up of at least 60 months. **B,** Kaplan-Meier analysis showing percentage of patients with new anterior pituitary hormone deficiencies versus time after radiosurgery. x-axis = monthly; y-axis = rate of remission. (Reproduced from Castinetti F, Nagai M, Morange I, et al. Long-term results of stereotactic radiosurgery in secretory pituitary adenomas. *J Clin Endocrinol Metab.* 2009;94:3400-3407.)

or TSH hypersecretion, to block tumor growth, and often to shrink tumor size. A peripheral receptor antagonist blocks GH action and IGF1 generation without targeting the pituitary tumor source. Medical ablation of target glands, including the thyroid and adrenal glands, may also be useful in mitigating the deleterious impact of pituitary tumor hypersecretion. Each of these medical approaches is fully considered later in this chapter.

PARASELLAR MASSES

Hypothalamic masses are fully described in Chapter 7, and parasellar masses are depicted in Table 9-5.[76]

Types of Parasellar Masses

Rathke's Cyst

The anterior and intermediate lobes of the pituitary gland arise embryologically from Rathke's pouch. Inadequate pouch obliteration results in cysts or cystic remnants at the interface between the anterior and posterior pituitary lobes, found in about 20% of pituitary glands at autopsy (Fig. 9-13).[77] Pituitary adenomas may also occasionally contain small cleft cysts,[78] which are lined by cuboidal or columnar ciliated epithelium surrounding mucoid cyst fluid. They arise from midline rudiments of failed Rathke's cyst invagination and account for about 3% of pituitary mass lesions.[79] In contrast, pituitary epidermoid cysts are

TABLE 9-5

Parasellar Masses

Genetic
Transcription factor mutations (e.g., PROP1)
Cysts
Rathke's Arachnoid Epidermoid Dermoid
Tumors
Hormone-secreting or nonfunctional pituitary adenoma Granular cell tumor Craniopharyngioma (cystic components) Chordoma Meningioma Sarcomas Glioma Schwannoma Germ cell tumor Vascular tumor Solid or hematological metastases
Malformation and Hamartomas
Ectopic pituitary, neurohypophyseal, or salivary tissue Hypothalamic hamartoma Gangliocytoma
Miscellaneous Lesions
Aneurysms Hypophysitis Infections Sarcoidosis Giant cell granuloma Histiocytosis X

PROP1, prophet of Pit1 (paired-like homeodomain transcription factor).

lined by squamous epithelium which may rarely become malignant.

Rathke's cysts vary in size and may also extend to the suprasellar region. These lesions have heterogeneous MRI characteristics and may rarely manifest with panhypopituitarism with or without diabetes insipidus.[80] Most, however, are not symptomatic and should be observed expectantly. The extent of headache or visual disturbance is determined by the size and location of the cyst. Cyst formation is associated with sellar enlargement. MRI reveals hyperdense or hypodense masses on either T1- or T2-weighted images, whereas CT scans show homogeneous hypodense areas that may be distinguished from pituitary adenomas.[80] These patients should all be evaluated for hypopituitarism. After surgical resection or drainage, MRI should be performed during long-term follow-up for signs of cyst recurrence.[77,79]

Arachnoid, epidermoid, and dermoid cysts develop mainly in the cerebellopontine angle, but they may also arise in the suprasellar region. Dermoid cysts containing greasy sebaceous products or hair follicles are rarely encountered in the pituitary, and the cyst lining may be calcified. Acquired pituitary cysts may arise secondarily to intrapituitary hemorrhage, usually associated with an underlying adenoma, and these rarely cause pituitary failure.[81] Cyst compression causes internal hydrocephalus, visual disturbances, GH or ACTH deficiency, hyperprolactinemia, and diabetes insipidus. Rarely, squamous cell carcinoma arises in the cyst.[82]

Granular Cell Tumors

Pituitary choristomas, or schwannomas, usually manifest only after the age of 20 years. Their abundant cytoplasmic granules do not contain pituitary hormones, but these lesions may manifest with diabetes insipidus. Pituitary adenomas are occasionally coincidentally associated with these tumors.[83]

Chordomas

Chordomas are slow-growing, cartilaginous tumors that arise from midline notochord remnants; they are locally invasive and may metastasize.[84] Most arise from the vertebrae, although about one third involve the clivus region. Chordomas contain a mucin-rich matrix that allows diagnosis by fine-needle aspiration. They manifest with headaches, asymmetric visual disturbances, hormone deficiency, and, occasionally, nasopharyngeal obstruction. The tumor mass is associated with osteolytic bony erosion and calcification, and MRI may allow the normal pituitary gland to be distinguished from the very heterogeneous and often flocculent tumor mass. At surgery, the tumors are rough, heterogeneous, and lobular. Markers for epithelial cells, including cytokeratin and vimentin, are present. Recurrences commonly occur after surgical excision, with a mean patient survival time of about 5 years. Rarely, chordomas undergo sarcomatous transformation with an aggressive natural history and require extensive surgical dissection.[85] Because of their anatomic location, the endoscopic endonasal approach may be preferable for surgical resection of chordomas.[86]

Craniopharyngiomas

Craniopharyngiomas are parasellar tumors that constitute about 3% of all intracranial tumors and up to 10% of childhood brain tumors. The tumors are commonly diagnosed during childhood and adolescence. However, they show a bimodal age distribution, with peaks occurring in children

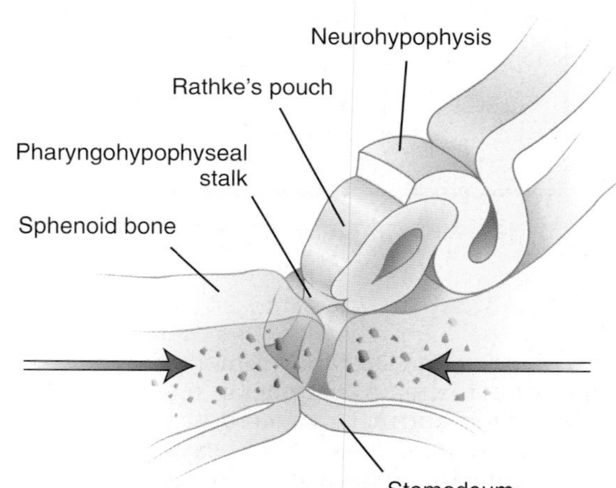

Figure 9-13 Pathogenesis of Rathke's cysts. Schematic diagram of the embryologic progenitors of sellar and parasellar structures. Rathke's pouch arises from an outpocketing of stomodeum (ectoderm) and gives rise to the adenohypophysis. The pharyngohypophyseal stalk, which connects the stomadeum and Rathke's pouch, is divided by the sphenoid bone as it grows together *(arrows)*, isolating Rathke's pouch and the neurohypophysis within the sella. (Reproduced from Harrison MJ, Morgello S., Post KD. Epithelial cystic lesions of the sellar and parasellar region: a continuum of ectodermal derivates? *J Neurosurg*. 1994;80:1018-1025.)

between 5 and 14 years of age and in adults from 50 to 74 years.[87] The tumors arise from embryonic squamous remnants of Rathke's pouch extending dorsally toward the diencephalon. They may be large (>10 cm in diameter) and may invade the third ventricle and associated brain structures. More than 60% arise from within the sella, and others arise from parasellar cell rests.[88-90] When intrasellar, they can often be distinguished from pituitary adenomas by the presence of a separate rim of normal pituitary tissue visible on MRI (see Fig. 9-1A).

The cystic mass is usually filled with a cholesterol-rich viscous fluid that may leak into the CSF, causing aseptic meningitis. The tumor may also contain calcifications and immunoreactive human chorionic gonadotropin. Histologic analysis shows that these tumors comprise two cell populations: cysts are lined with a squamous epithelium containing islands characterized by columnar cells, and a mixed inflammatory reaction may also occur with calcification. Although large craniopharyngiomas may obstruct CSF flow, they rarely undergo malignant transformation. Increased intracranial pressure results in headache, projectile vomiting, papilledema, and somnolence, especially in children. Only about one third of patients are older than 40 years of age, and they commonly present with asymmetric visual disturbances, including papilledema, optic atrophy, and field deficits. If cavernous sinus invasion is present, other cranial nerves may also be involved.

On CT imaging, most children and about half of affected adults exhibit characteristic flocculent or convex calcifications. Rarely, however, pituitary adenomas, other parasellar tumors, and vascular lesions within the sella are also calcified. Although pituitary adenomas rarely cause diabetes insipidus, it is often the earliest feature of craniopharyngioma. These patients may also develop partial or complete pituitary deficiency. GH deficiency, with short stature, diabetes insipidus, and gonadal failure, is common. Pituitary stalk compression or damage to hypothalamic dopaminergic neurons results in hyperprolactinemia. Therefore, craniopharyngioma may mimic a prolactinoma on intrapituitary imaging, by the presence of hyperprolactinemia, and by a favorable biochemical response to dopamine agonists.

Treatment of primary or recurrent craniopharyngioma may involve radical surgery, radiotherapy, or a combination of these modalities.[87,90,91] Recent studies have indicated that postoperative irradiation improves outcome. Although transsphenoidal surgery has been successfully employed for intrasellar craniopharyngiomas,[92,93] the expanded endoscopic transnasal approach has been successfully crafted to approach suprasellar tumors.[94] Stereotactic irradiation has also successfully been employed. A detailed discussion of the neurosurgical management of this disorder is beyond the scope of this text. However, regardless of the form of therapy chosen, ablation of the mass invariably results in anterior and/or posterior pituitary hormone deficits.

Postoperative recurrence may occur in about 20% of patients undergoing radical surgical excision, and there is no difference in outcome when a subtotal surgical excision is followed by radiotherapy. Pure papillary squamous cellular elements in the tumor may portend a higher surgical recurrence rate. Long-term effects of childhood irradiation for these tumors are considered elsewhere (see Chapter 24).

Meningiomas

Meningiomas arise from arachnoid and meningioendothelial cells, and those occurring in the sellar and parasellar region account for about one fifth of all meningiomas.[95] Sellar meningiomas are usually well circumscribed and do not attain the size of craniopharyngiomas. Suprasellar meningiomas may invade the pituitary ventrally, and intrasellar tumor origins are rare.[96] Coexisting functional pituitary adenomas have been described in patients with parasellar meningiomas. Secondary hyperprolactinemia occurs in up to half of patients, who usually present with local mass effects including headache and progressive visual disturbances accompanied by optic atrophy.

The differential distinction of a suprasellar meningioma with downward extension from an upwardly extending pituitary adenoma can be difficult. On MRI, meningiomas are isodense on both T1 and T2 imaging, in contrast to other parasellar lesions, which are usually hyperdense on T2 imaging. Dural calcification may be evident on CT scanning. Because of their rich vascularization, these tumors pose an intraoperative risk for hemorrhage and a resultant higher surgical mortality rate than is usually encountered during resection of pituitary adenomas.

Gliomas

Optic gliomas and low-grade astrocytomas arise from within the optic chiasm or optic tract, often infiltrating the optic nerve; fewer than one third are intraorbital. Von Recklinghausen's disease is the underlying cause in about one third of these patients, and occasionally these tumors are associated with growth retardation and delayed or precocious puberty and with mass effects including visual disturbances, diencephalic syndrome, diabetes insipidus, and hydrocephalus. Rarely, gliomas arise within the sella in association with hyperprolactinemia and should be considered in the uncommon differential diagnosis of a PRL-secreting pituitary adenoma.[97] Important distinguishing features include the young age of these patients (80% are <10 years old), the relatively intact pituitary function, gross visual disturbances, and localization of the mass as visualized on MRI. Gliomas, unlike hamartomas, usually enhance after contrast injection.

Mucocele

Mucoceles are expanding accumulations of fluid within the sphenoid sinus and may compress parasellar structures. Headaches, visual disturbances (usually unilateral), and exophthalmos are characteristic features. On MRI, the homogenous sphenoid mass may be quite prominent but distinguishable from the pituitary gland dorsally.

Parasellar Aneurysms

A parasellar aneurysm may mimic a pituitary adenoma, and intraoperative rupture can be catastrophic, underscoring the absolute need for preoperative diagnosis. Differentiating features of aneurysms from other pituitary masses may be subtle and include eye pain, very intense headaches, and relatively sudden onset of cranial nerve palsies (Fig. 9-14). Although imaging techniques usually distinguish blood and hemorrhage from solid tumor or tissue, a highly vascular meningioma may be confused with an aneurysm.

Pituitary Infections

Acute pituitary abscesses and parasellar arachnoiditis are encountered with sinus infections, especially after transsphenoidal surgery. Pituitary abscesses may develop from hematogenous or direct local spread of infectious agents,[98] or they may arise within a preexisting pituitary adenoma. They can be difficult to distinguish from an adenoma, because these patients may not have fever or signs of

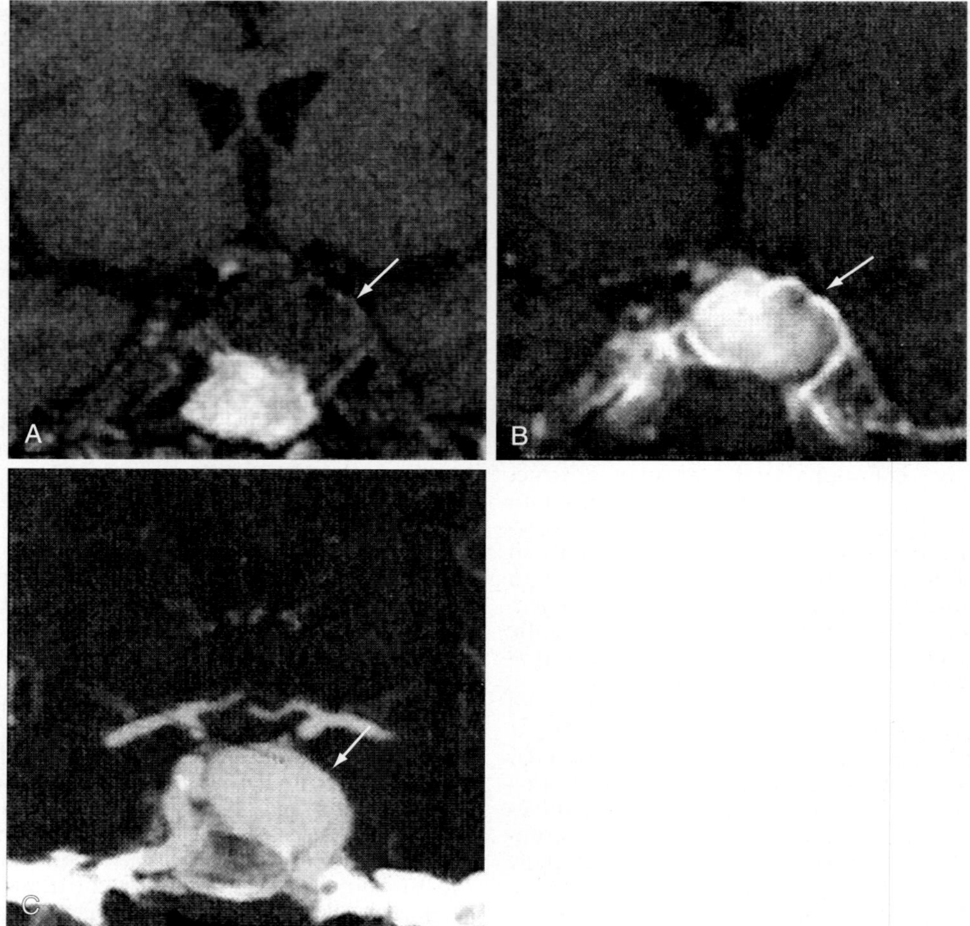

Figure 9-14 **A,** Coronal T1-weighted magnetic resonance image (MRI) without intravenous contrast. A mildly hypointense mass within the sella and left cavernous sinus is shown. **B,** Coronal T1-weighted MRI after gadolinium contrast. The mass enhances heterogeneously. **C,** Computed tomographic angiogram with maximum-intensity projection reconstruction. The arrow in each image indicates the origin of a left internal carotid artery giant cavernous aneurysm. (Reproduced from Lawson EA, Buchbinder BR, Daniels GH. Image in endocrinology: hypopituitarism associated with a giant aneurysm of the internal carotid artery. *J Clin Endocrinol Metab.* 2008;93:4616.)

meningitis. Patients often present with diabetes insipidus and headache, and some have pituitary insufficiency.[99,100] On MRI imaging, an isointense central cavity with surrounding ring enhancement is characteristic of an abscess.[4]

Gram-positive streptococci or staphylococci may originate from nasopharyngeal passages and infect the pituitary.[101] Disseminated *Entamoeba histolytica, Pneumocystis jiroveci* (formerly *Pneumocystis carinii*), or *Klebsiella* can also seed to the pituitary.[102,103] Immunosuppressed patients may develop pituitary infections including cytomegalovirus infection, toxoplasmosis, aspergillosis, histoplasmosis, and coccidiosis. Syphilitic gumma can also lead to pituitary damage and insufficiency. Common viral infections, including influenza, measles, mumps, and herpes, are rarely associated with pituitary damage and insufficiency. Although tuberculosis is rarely confined to the pituitary gland, most of the fewer than 20 reported patients exhibited suprasellar extension of the pituitary mass, compromised pituitary function, and visual defects. Although systemic tuberculosis was usually present, isolated sellar tuberculomas have been described.[104]

Hematologic Malignancies

Primary CNS lymphomas are usually B-cell non-Hodgkin's types, and fewer than 20 patients with pituitary lymphoma have been described.[105-107] The pituitary mass may be an isolated presentation of the underlying disease. The disorder is usually diagnosed by histologic study of tissue obtained by excision biopsy. In one report, six of nine patients had headache, and five had cranial nerve abnormalities with varying degrees of hypopituitarism. MRI reveals cavernous sinus invasion and isodense T1- and T2-weighted images that enhance after gadolinium administration. Patients with solitary pituitary plasmacytoma may or may not develop classic multiple myeloma.[108] Acute lymphoblastic leukemia may be associated with periglandular pituitary infiltrates with minimal pituitary dysfunction.

Pituicytoma

Pituicytoma is a rare, benign suprasellar glial cell tumor that manifests with mass effects or hypopituitarism.[109,110] The tumor arises from cells in the neurohypophysis and stains for vimentin, S100 protein, and glial fibrillar acidic protein.[111]

Sarcoidosis

Hypothalamic granulomatous involvement is commonly encountered in patients with CNS sarcoidosis and may be the sole manifestation of the disease.[112] These patients may present with varying degrees of anterior pituitary failure with or without diabetes insipidus.[113] The hypothalamus, pituitary stalk, and posterior pituitary are diffusely invaded by noncaseating granulomas consisting of giant cells, macrophages, and lymphocytes.[114] Sarcoidosis may be progressive and may eventually result in pituitary damage and even an empty sella. Onset of diabetes insipidus with no obvious features of a pituitary disorder should alert the physician to exclude hypothalamic sarcoid deposits, especially if there is a thickened stalk on MRI.[115] Systemic steroids have been used to treat CNS sarcoid, and cladribine may reverse diabetes insipidus caused by sarcoid.[116]

Hand-Schüller-Christian Disease (Histiocytosis X)

Sleep disorders, adipsia, and morbid obesity are components of Hand-Schüller-Christian disease, also known as histiocytosis X. Other features of granulomatous involvement include axillary skin rash, history of recurrent pneumothorax, classic bony lesions, and new-onset diabetes insipidus.[117] The disorder may be associated with granulomatous damage to the hypothalamus and/or posterior pituitary, resulting in characteristic diabetes insipidus.[118] Pituitary lesions are composed of dendritic Langerhans cells, and pituitary MRI may reveal stalk thickening or a diminished posterior pituitary bright spot. Adults with the disorder should be carefully evaluated for anterior pituitary hormone deficits, and these should be appropriately replaced. Multisystem Langerhans-cell histiocytosis causes long-term morbidity extending into adulthood.[119] Whereas surgery and irradiation have been, for many years, the mainstay treatments for this disorder, a novel chemotherapeutic approach using cladribine has been successful in some patients.[120]

Metastases to the Pituitary Region

Pituitary metastases are found in up to 3.5% of cancer patients,[121,122] especially in older patients with diffuse malignant disease. Because the vascular supply to the posterior pituitary is derived directly from the systemic circulation via the internal carotid arteries, the posterior pituitary is the preferred site for bloodborne metastatic spread. Carcinomas that metastasize to the pituitary include breast, lung, and gastrointestinal tract lesions. Up to one quarter of patients with metastatic breast cancer have pituitary metastases. Symptomatic pituitary metastases (usually diabetes insipidus) may be the presenting sign of occult malignancy and of malignancy of unknown origin. Rarely, isolated metastatic stalk deposits also manifest with pituitary failure. If extensive bony erosion is present and disease onset is rapid, the diagnosis is more readily apparent. However, pituitary imaging may not clearly distinguish metastatic deposits from a pituitary adenoma; these lesions may masquerade as adenomas, with the diagnosis made only by histologic study of the resected specimen.[122] When the diagnosis is clearcut in the presence of a primary cancer, relatively low-dose pituitary irradiation may be sufficient to shrink the metastasis and improve morbidity.

Iron storage diseases, including hemochromatosis and hemosiderosis, result in predominantly gonadotroph cell damage. Idiopathic retroperitoneal fibrosis may also be associated with a suprasellar mass and hypothalamic panhypopituitarism.[123]

Primary Hypophysitis

Pituitary mass lesions comprising inflammatory cells may arise as primary disorders of the anterior and posterior pituitary glands or the neurohypophysis.[124,125] At least three clinicopathologic forms have been described.

Lymphocytic Hypophysitis

Lymphocytic hypophysitis is an apparently autoimmune inflammatory disorder that occurs during or shortly after parturition[126] but has also been reported after menopause[125] and in males (approximately 15% of reported cases).[127] Of the 57% of patients who develop the disorder in association with pregnancy, most do so during the last month of pregnancy or the first 2 months after delivery.[125]

The disorder is characterized by a lymphocytic and plasma cell pituitary infiltrate that may be isolated or associated with other recognized endocrinopathies. Circulating anti-pituitary antibodies have occasionally been reported, and the presence of isolated pituitary hormone deficiency may imply an autoimmune process selectively targeted to pituitary cell types. Although the natural history is often short, the few comprehensive pathologic evaluations that have been performed suggest that secondary adenohypophyseal cell atrophy, with a resultant empty sella, is a frequent outcome.

Pathologic criteria for diagnosis include islands of anterior pituitary cells surrounded by diffuse lymphocytic (T- and B-cell) infiltrates. More than 268 histologically confirmed cases have been reported. The defining feature is lymphocytic infiltration comprising T and B lymphocytes. In a recent review, Caturegli and colleagues reported that plasma cells were found in 53%, eosinophils in 12%, and macrophage histiocytes and neutrophils in 6% of patients.[125] Mast cells have also been identified in hypophysitis.[128]

Clinical Features. More than half of the patients with lymphocytic hypophysitis present with headache, visual field impairment, and hyperprolactinemia[125]; pituitary deficiency accounts for the remaining cases (Table 9-6). Fifty-six percent of patients have secondary hypoadrenalism, followed in frequency by hypothyroidism, hypogonadism, and GH or PRL deficiency. This contrasts with hypopituitarism caused by pituitary adenomas. Hypothyroidism and hyperthyroidism may occur later, even after 9 months. MRI reveals a pituitary mass, often indistinguishable from an adenoma. Associated partially empty sella and contrast enhancement of the pituitary mass may be helpful distinguishing features on MRI.[129]

The inflammatory process often resolves with time, and initially abnormal pituitary function may be restored or may remain chronically compromised. Limited numbers of patients have been reported with histologically proven lymphocytic hypophysitis and documented spontaneous regression of the pituitary mass on follow-up imaging. There can be intrasellar and suprasellar pituitary enlargement, and the pituitary stalk may be thickened, especially when diabetes insipidus is present.[124] In two patients with

TABLE 9-6

Features of Lymphocytic Hypophysitis

Feature	Percentage
Pituitary enlargement	80-95
Headache, visual disturbances	55-70
Hypopituitarism	63-68
Hyperprolactinemia	20-38
Associated autoimmune disease	30
Diabetes insipidus	14-19

histologically proven hypophysitis, spontaneous resolution of the pituitary mass was followed by successful pregnancies.[130,131] Diabetes insipidus is encountered in up to 20% of patients and may be attributed to posterior pituitary or stalk infiltration.[132] In one third of patients, other autoimmune conditions, such as thyroiditis, hypoadrenalism, parathyroid failure, atrophic gastritis, systemic lupus erythematosus, or Sjögren's syndrome, are also present.[133] The differential diagnosis includes prolactinoma and other sellar masses. A careful history and demonstrated loss of the posterior pituitary bright spot on MRI are useful for supporting the diagnosis.

Laboratory Findings. The erythrocyte sedimentation rate is often elevated. Antibodies to a 49-kd cytosolic protein were detected in 70% of patients with histologically confirmed lymphocytic hypophysitis and in 10% of controls.[134] Although the presence of this and two additional antibodies (to 68- and 43-kd human pituitary membrane antigens) has high specificity, all three were detected in only 5 of 13 patients with lymphocytic hypophysitis and 1 of 12 patients with infundibuloneurohypophysitis.[135] Similar results were obtained with the use of radioligand assays for pituitary proteins.[125] PRL levels are usually elevated in both female and male patients. Hyperprolactinemia is expected during pregnancy and the early postpartum period, and the mass effect of the infiltrate may also contribute to stalk compression and secondary hyperprolactinemia. GH and ACTH responses to hypothalamic hormone challenges may be blunted. Rarely, isolated ACTH or TSH deficiencies have been reported.[136]

Management. If the diagnosis is convincingly supported, and in the absence of compressive visual field disturbances, surgical therapy should be withheld, pituitary hormone deficits appropriately replaced, and spontaneous resolution of the inflammatory mass expectantly monitored. Treatment with adrenal steroids is advocated, and it often resolves the sellar mass and improves endocrine dysfunction. Steroids are also indicated if the adrenal reserve is compromised. Transsphenoidal surgery may be required to confirm a tissue diagnosis and may also relieve symptoms of compression,[137] but the degree of surgical resection should be constrained by the need to conserve viable pituitary tissue, particularly in view of frequent spontaneous resolutions.

Granulomatous Hypophysitis

Granulomatous hypophysitis is not usually associated with pregnancy and has an equal incidence in female and male patients. Rarely, the condition may coexist with lymphocytic hypophysitis in the same gland.[137] Pituitary histology shows histiocytes, multinucleated giant cells, and other features of chronic inflammation and granuloma.[138] Patients present with headache and may have aseptic meningitis. MRI studies can reveal a thickened pituitary stalk or a characteristic tongue-shaped extension of the lesion under the hypothalamus. Granulomatous hypophysitis may reflect an underlying systemic disorder such as sarcoidosis[139] or Takayasu's disease.[140]

Xanthomatous Hypophysitis

Xanthomatous hypophysitis, the least common primary pituitary inflammatory process, occurs at equal frequency in both sexes and consists of lipid-laden macrophages resembling postinfectious cell debris. MRI often reveals a highly cystic lesion, leading to the suggestion that this entity reflects an inflammatory response to a damaged or ruptured pituitary cyst.[141]

Hemorrhage and Infarction

Intrapituitary hemorrhage and infarction is usually caused by ischemic damage to the hypophyseal-portal system and can be catastrophic. These acute events cause significant damage to the pituitary gland, and small, clinically silent microinfarcts are found in up to 5% of unselected autopsies. Pituitary cells are relatively resilient to vascular insult, and pituitary insufficiency is clinically apparent only after approximately 75% of the gland is chemically damaged. Ten percent residual functional pituitary cell mass appears sufficient to mask complete pituitary failure. Ischemic damage is limited to the anterior lobe, and posterior pituitary function usually remains intact, reflecting the predominant neural control of oxytocin and ADH secretion. Acute intrapituitary hemorrhage can cause significant life-threatening damage to the pituitary and its surrounding vital structures.[12]

Postpartum Pituitary Infarction

During pregnancy, the pituitary gland normally enlarges in response to estrogen stimulation. The hypervascular gland is particularly vulnerable to arterial pressure changes and prone to hemorrhage. Sheehan's syndrome, classically described after severe postpartum hemorrhage, is less commonly encountered since the advent of modern obstetric care,[142] but it occurs much more frequently in developing countries.[143] The presentation varies from the development of hypovolemic shock resulting in adenohypophyseal vessel vasospasm and pituitary necrosis[144] to the gradual onset of partial to complete pituitary insufficiency over months to years. Most prominent among the symptoms are inability to nurse and postpartum amenorrhea.[143] Pituitary autoimmunity has been implicated in gland failure after postpartum hemorrhage.[145]

Pituitary Apoplexy

Pituitary apoplexy may result from spontaneous hemorrhage into a pituitary adenoma (pituitary tumor apoplexy), or it may occur after head trauma or skull base fracture or in association with hypertension and diabetes mellitus, sickle cell anemia, or acute hypovolemic shock.[146] Precipitating factors include major surgery, pregnancy, gamma knife irradiation, anticoagulant therapy, coagulopathy secondary to liver failure,[147] and administration of thyrotropin-releasing hormone (TRH), gonadotropin-releasing hormone (GnRH) agonists, bromocriptine, or cabergoline.[148-150]

Clinical Features. Pituitary apoplexy is often an endocrine emergency.[13] The condition may evolve over 1 to 2 days, and patients usually present with severe headache and ocular palsies or visual field defects. Cardiovascular collapse, change in consciousness, neck stiffness, and sometimes hypoglycemia may occur. Acute adrenal insufficiency is a frequent occurrence caused by loss of ACTH; it may also be superimposed as a result of disordered intravascular clotting disorders, heparin administration, or acute effects of CNS hemorrhage. Pituitary imaging without contrast (CT or MRI) usually reveals signs of intrapituitary or intra-adenoma hemorrhage, stalk deviation, and compression of normal pituitary tissue, as well as signs of parasellar hemorrhage in severe cases.[151] In a study of 13 consecutive patients with pituitary apoplexy, the baseline serum cortisol level was lower than 5 μg/dL in 7, between 5 and 15 μg/dL in 4, and higher than 15 μg/dL in 2 patients. Five patients also had low levels of thyroxine (T_4), and all 13 had evidence of gonadal dysfunction. Therefore, these patients with underlying pituitary tumors most likely had

TABLE 9-7

Features of Pituitary Apoplexy

Feature	Bills DC et al. (1993)	Randeva HS et al. (1999)	Lubina et al. (2005)
No. patients	37	35	40
No. males/females	25/12	21/14	27/13
Mean age (yr)	56.6	49.8	51.2
No. not operated	1	4	6
Symptoms			
Headache (%)	95	97	63
Visual defects (%)	64	71	61
Ophthalmoplegia (%)	78	69	40
Adenoma Type			
NFPA (%)	52	61	63
PRL-cell (%)	17	6.6	31
Visual fields improvement (%)		76	81
Ocular palsy improvement (%)		91	71
Hormone Deficiency			
Central hypocortisol (%)	82	58	40
Central hypothyroid (%)	89	45	54
Hypogonadism (%)	64	43	79
Diabetes insipidus (%)	11	6	8

NFPA, nonfunctioning pituitary adenoma; PRL, prolactin.

Data from Bills DC, Meyer FB, Laws ER Jr, et al. A retrospective analysis of pituitary apoplexy. *Neurosurgery.* 1993;33:602-608; discussion 608-609; Randeva HS. 1999. *Classical pituitary apoplexy: clinical features, management and outcome.* Randeva HS, Schoebel J, Byrne J, et al. *Clin Endocrinol (Oxf).* 1999 Aug;51(2):181-188; Lubina A, Olchovsky D, Berezin M, et al. Management of pituitary apoplexy: clinical experience with 40 patients. *Acta Neurochir (Wien).* 2005;147:151-157; discussion 157.

preexisting pituitary insufficiency.[152] Apoplexy, like Sheehan's syndrome, is one of the few pituitary tumor presentations in which hyperprolactinemia is not a feature (unless the infarction occurs within a prolactinoma). Patient characteristics, signs and symptoms, and outcomes of 112 patients in three series are shown in Table 9-7.[13]

Management. Patients with visual field compromise require emergency transsphenoidal surgery. Others may recover spontaneously but may develop long-term pituitary insufficiency. Patients who are fully alert and conscious with no visual symptoms may be observed. The decision to initiate therapy with high-dose glucocorticoids depends on the clinical status,[12] but the high incidence of adrenal dysfunction either before or after treatment indicates a need for replacement or stress doses of cortisone in most cases.

Ophthalmoplegia, which is common, may resolve spontaneously over time.[12] Postoperative recovery of visual function correlates inversely with the time elapsed since the acute hemorrhage.[153] Cranial nerve palsies, however, often improve regardless of whether surgery is undertaken. Pituitary function does not commonly recover after resolution of the acute hemorrhage, and patients require adrenal, thyroid, and/or gonadal steroid hormone replacement.[154] The subsequent atrophy of infarcted pituitary tissue often results in development of a complete or partially empty sella evident on MRI.

Pituitary Adenomas

Pathogenesis

Pituitary tumors account for about 15% of all intracranial neoplasms and are commonly encountered at autopsy. The Brain Tumor Registry of Japan reported that 15.8% of 28,424 cases were histologically confirmed pituitary adenomas.[155,156] The prevalence of pituitary tumors in Belgium was 1 in 1064 inhabitants,[157] and in Banbury, United Kingdom, 63 pituitary tumors were noted among 89,334 inhabitants (i.e., a population prevalence of about 77 cases per 100,000). Of these, 57% were prolactinomas, 28% were nonfunctioning adenomas, 11% were GH-secreting adenomas, and 2% were Cushing's adenomas. The median age at onset was 37 years, but nonfunctioning tumors were most commonly encountered in patients older than 60 years of age.[158]

These benign monoclonal adenomas may express and secrete hormones autonomously, leading to hyperprolactinemia, acromegaly, Cushing's disease, and hyperthyroidism, or they may be functionally silent and initially diagnosed as a sellar mass. Although they are almost invariably benign, the neoplastic features of these adenomas represent a unique tumor biology that is reflected in their important local and systemic manifestations. These neoplasms have a slow doubling time and rarely resolve spontaneously. Nevertheless, they can be aggressive and locally invasive or compressive to vital central structures (Fig. 9-15). Pituitary adenomas usually express a single gene product; polyhormonal expression may reflect a primitive stem cell or mature bimorphous cellular origin.

Pituitary Trophic Activity

Benign Adenomas. Several transgenic animal models have been described in which pituitary growth factors or genes were overexpressed or deleted to recapitulate both functional and nonfunctional pituitary adenomas (Table 9-8). Benign human monoclonal pituitary adenomas arise from differentiated pituitary cells (see Fig. 9-2). The pituitary gland responds to central and peripheral signals that regulate both hormone production and cell proliferation. For example, during pregnancy, hypothalamic and peripheral hormones act to regulate pituitary trophic activity, resulting in increased pituitary volume, whereas prolonged target gland failure (e.g., hypothyroidism) causes pituitary hyperplasia. There is, however, no compelling direct evidence in humans that pituitary hyperplasia is a prerequisite for tumor development. Therefore, lactotroph hyperplasia occurring with pregnancy and lactation does not result in increased frequency of prolactinomas. Oral contraception use is also not associated with pituitary adenoma development, and somatotroph hyperplasia caused by ectopic GHRH production[159] is not commonly associated with true adenoma formation. Adenohypophyseal tissue surrounding pituitary tumors is usually not hyperplastic, supporting the notion that hypothalamic hormones, pituitary growth factors, and sex steroid hormones enable a permissive environment that potentiates cell mutation and subsequent tumor growth. Pituitary trophic signals may enhance or restrain expansion of a monoclonal tumor cell population by regulating the intrapituitary milieu.[160]

Malignant Pituitary Tumors. Very rarely, pituitary tumors metastasize either outside the CNS or as a separate focus within the brain.[161] Because no cell markers clearly distinguish aggressive invasiveness from malignancy, demonstration of extracranial metastasis is a prerequisite for the diagnosis of pituitary malignancy. When they occur, these cancers most often secrete either ACTH or PRL.

RAS family mutations are rare in pituitary adenomas. *HRAS* gene mutations have been identified in invasive prolactinoma[162] and in distant metastatic pituitary

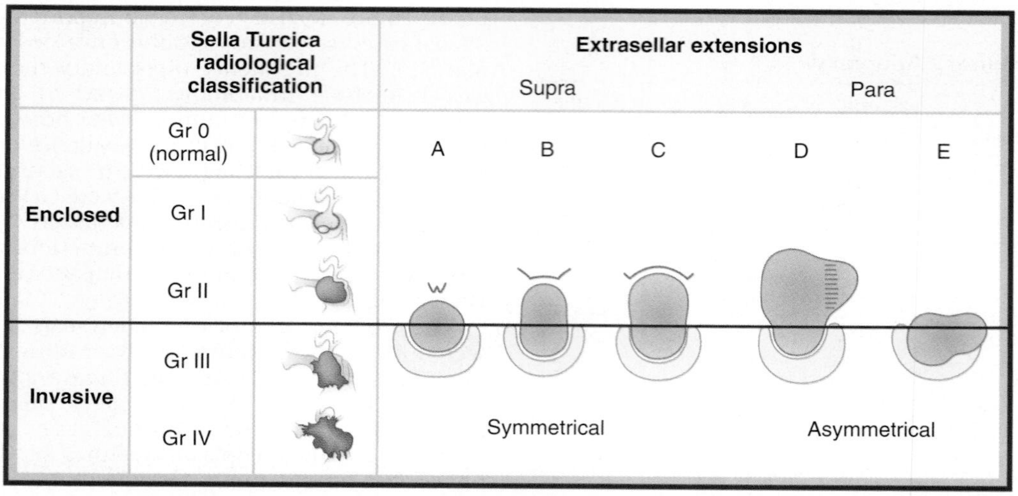

	Sella Turcica radiological classification		Extrasellar extensions				
			Supra			Para	
	Gr 0 (normal)		A	B	C	D	E
Enclosed	Gr I						
	Gr II						
Invasive	Gr III						
	Gr IV		Symmetrical			Asymmetrical	

Hardy classification of pituitary tumors			Extrasellar extensions
Radiologic	**Anatomic**	**Surgical**	***Suprasellar*** *(symmetrical)* A Supresellar cistern B Recesses of III ventricle C Whole anterior III ventricle
Grade 0	Intact, normal contour	Micro enclosed	***Parasellar*** *(asymmetrical)*
Grade I	Intact, focal bulging	Micro enclosed	D Intracranial intradural
Grade II	Intact, enlarged	Macro enclosed	Anterior
Grade III	Destroyed, partially	Macro invasive	Midline
Grade IV	Destroyed, totally	Macro invasive	Posterior
Grade V	Distant spread via CSF or blood	Macro carcinoma	E Extracranial extradural (lateral cavernous sinus)

Figure 9-15 Classification of pituitary tumors. CSF, cerebrospinal fluid; Gr, grade. (Adapted from Thapar K, Laws ER. Growth hormone-secreting pituitary tumors: operative management. In: Krisht AF, Tindall GT, eds. *Pituitary Disorders.* Philadelphia: Lippincott Williams & Wilkins; 1999:243-258; and Asa SL. Tumors of the pituitary gland: pituitary adenomas. In: *Atlas of Tumor Pathology,* series 3, vol 22. Washington, DC: Armed Forces Institute of Pathology; 1998:51.)

carcinomas, but not in their respective primary pituitary tumors, nor in noninvasive adenomas.[163,164] Therefore, *RAS* genetic alterations may be important in the very rare progression to metastatic formation and growth.

Hormonal Factors. Hypothalamic factors may have a specific role in the pathogenesis of pituitary tumors, in addition to regulating pituitary hormone gene expression and secretion (Table 9-9). Ectopic GHRH-secreting tumors (bronchial carcinoids, pancreatic islet-cell tumors, and small-cell lung carcinomas) result in GH hypersecretion, acromegaly, somatotroph hyperplasia, and, rarely, somatotroph adenoma formation.[159,165] In transgenic mice overexpressing a GHRH transgene, the pituitary size increases dramatically due to somatotroph hyperplasia, and older mice develop GH-secreting adenomas.[166] However, adenomatous hormone secretion is usually independent of physiologic hypothalamic control, and the surgical resection of small, well-defined adenomas usually results in definitive cure of hormone hypersecretion. Such observations imply that these tumors do not arise because of excessive polyclonal pituitary cell proliferation resulting from generalized hypothalamic stimulation. However, hypothalamic factors may promote and maintain the growth of already transformed adenomatous pituitary cells.

Normal and hyperplastic pituitary tissues are polyclonal, and pituitary adenomas arise as the result of monoclonal pituitary cell proliferation. X-chromosome inactivation analysis was used to confirm the monoclonal origin of GH-, PRL-,[167] and ACTH-secreting adenomas[168,169] and nonfunctioning pituitary tumors in female patients heterozygous for variant alleles of the X-linked genes hypoxanthine phosphoribosyl transferase (*HPRT* or *CDC73*) and phosphoglycerate kinase (*PGK*). Therefore, an intrinsic somatic pituitary cell genetic alteration likely gives rise to clonal expansion of a single cell, resulting in adenoma formation (Table 9-10).

Genetic Factors. Activating mutations of the stimulatory G protein (G_s) are present in up to 40% of human GH-secreting adenomas.[170-172] These are somatic heterozygous activating point mutations of the portion of the *GNAS* complex locus that encodes the G_s α-subunit ($G_s\alpha$) and involve either arginine 201 (replaced by cysteine or histidine) or glutamine 227 (replaced by arginine or leucine). These mutations constitutively activate the $G_s\alpha$ protein, resulting in the so-called *GSP* oncogene. This G-protein activation increases levels of cyclic adenosine monophosphate (cAMP) and activates protein kinase A, which in turn phosphorylates the cAMP response element–binding protein (CREB) and leads to sustained constitutive GH hypersecretion and cell proliferation.

GSP-bearing adenomas are smaller, have mildly lower GH levels and enhanced intratumoral cAMP, do not

TABLE 9-8

Transgenic Mouse Models for Pituitary Tumors

Genes	Hyperplasia/Adenoma*
Gene Overexpression†	
CMV.**HMGA1**	GH, PRL
CMV.**HMGA2**	GH, PRL
Ubiquitin C.**hCG**	PRL
αGSU.**bLH**	Pit1 lineage
GH.**galanin**	GH, PRL
PRL.**galanin**	PRL‡
PRL.**TGFα**	PRL
αGSU.**PTTG1**	LH, GH, TSH
αGSU.**Prop1**	Nonfunctioning
PRL.**pdt-FGFR4**	PRL
Gene Inactivation	
p27/Kip1 −/−	ACTH, αMSH
p18/INK4c −/−	ACTH, αMSH
Rb +/−	ACTH, αMSH αGSU, GH, βTSH
D2R-deficient	PRL
Men1 +/−	PRL
PRL −/−	Nonfunctioning

*Hormone immunoreactivity/secreting profile.
†Genes are listed in bold and are preceded by the promoter that determines transcriptional control.
‡Pituitary hyperplasia, with no tumor formation.
ACTH, adrenocorticotropic hormone; bLH, bovine active luteinizing hormone; CMV, cytomegalovirus; D2R, dopamine 2 receptor; GH, growth hormone; αGSU, glycoprotein α-subunit; hCG, human chorionic gonadotropin; HMGA, high mobility group A; pdt-FGFR4, pituitary tumor-derived fibroblast growth factor receptor 4; Men1, multiple endocrine neoplasia type 1; MSH, melanocyte-stimulating hormone; p18/INK4c, cyclin-dependent kinase inhibitor 2C; p27/Kip1, cyclin-dependent kinase inhibitor 1B; PRL, prolactin; Prop1, prophet of Pit1 (paired-like homeodomain transcription factor; PTTG, pituitary tumor-transforming gene; Rb, retinoblastoma; TGF, transforming growth factor; TSH, thyroid-stimulating hormone.
(Modified from Melmed S. Pathogenesis of pituitary tumors. *Nat Rev Endocrinol.* 2011.)

respond briskly to GHRH, and are sensitive to the inhibitory effect of somatostatin.[173] *GSP* activating mutations do not occur in PRL-secreting and TSH-producing adenomas and are rarely present in nonfunctioning pituitary tumors and ACTH-secreting tumors (<10%). Similar early postzygotic somatic mutations in codon 201 of the gene encoding $G_s\alpha$ were identified in tissues derived from patients with McCune-Albright syndrome.[174] Transgenic mice overexpressing an inactive pituitary CREB mutant exhibited a dwarf phenotype and somatotroph hypoplasia.[175] Therefore, cAMP likely stimulates somatotroph proliferation mediated by CREB phosphorylation. This hypothesis was borne out by the observation that 15 human GH-secreting pituitary adenomas expressed elevated levels of phosphorylated CREB.[176] However, only four of these tumors also contained the mutant *GSP* oncogene, and CREB phosphorylation was also demonstrated in adenomas overexpressing wild-type $G_s\alpha$ protein, suggesting a trophic role of CREB independent of G-protein actions.

Other signaling pathways overexpressed in pituitary tumors include those for the serine/threonine kinase AKT and mitogen-activated protein kinase (MAPK).[160]

Pituitary tumor-transforming gene (*PTTG*) was isolated from experimental pituitary tumors and shown to be highly abundant in all pituitary tumor types, especially prolactinomas.[177,178] The PTTG protein, a mammalian securin homologue, also induces production of fibroblast growth factor (FGF) and angiogenesis and is upregulated by estrogen.[179] PTTG overexpression may lead to dysregulated chromatid separation and cell aneuploidy,[180,181] and pituitary-targeted *PTTG* transgene expression leads to functional adenomas secreting luteinizing hormone (LH), GH, or TSH.[182] *PTTG* mutations have not been identified in pituitary tumors.

Mice with heterozygous inactivation of the retinoblastoma *Rb1* gene develop pituitary tumors with high penetrance, whereas mice with deregulated pituitary E2f transcription factor activity develop tissue hyperplasia without progression to tumor formation, most likely because sustained E2f activity ultimately triggers premature

TABLE 9-9

Factors Involved in Pituitary Tumor Pathogenesis

Hereditary
MEN1 Transcription factor defect (e.g., PROP1 excess) Carney complex AIP mutations
Hypothalamic
Excess GHRH or CRH production Receptor activation Dopamine deprivation
Pituitary
Signal transduction mutations or constitutive activation (e.g., GSP, CREB, McCune-Albright syndrome) Disrupted paracrine growth factor or cytokine action (e.g., FGF2, FGF4, LIF, BMP, EGF) Activated oncogene or cell cycle disruption (e.g., PTTG; RAS; P27; HMG) Intrapituitary paracrine hypothalamic hormone action (e.g., GHRH, TRH) Loss of tumor suppressor gene function with LOH (11q13, 13, GADD45γ)
Environmental
Estrogens Irradiation
Peripheral
Target failure (ovary, thyroid, adrenal) Ectopic hypothalamic hormone secretion
Evidence for an Intrinsic Pituitary Defect in the Pathogenesis of Pituitary Tumors
Pituitary adenomas are monoclonal. There is no hyperplasia surrounding the adenomas. Surgical resection of well-circumscribed small adenomas leads to control in ~75% of patients. Unrestrained pituitary hormonal hypersecretion persists independently of feedback regulation by elevated target hormones. Hormonal pulsatility pattern is often restored after adenoma resection.

AIP, aryl hydrocarbon receptor–interacting protein; BMP, bone morphogenetic protein; CREB, cyclic adenosine monophosphate response element–binding protein; CRH, corticotropin-releasing hormone; EGF, epidermal growth factor; FGF, fibroblast growth factor; GADD45γ, growth arrest and DNA damage–inducible gamma gene; GHRH, growth hormone–releasing hormone; GSP, stimulatory G protein α-subunit oncogene; HMG, high mobility group; LIF, leukemia inhibitory factor; LOH, loss of heterozygosity; MEN1, multiple endocrine neoplasia type 1; P27, cyclin-dependent kinase inhibitor 1B; PROP1, prophet of Pit1 (paired-like homeodomain transcription factor); PTTG, pituitary tumor-transforming gene; RAS, RAS family of oncogenes; TRH, thyrotropin-releasing hormone.
(Modified from Melmed S. Acromegaly Pathogenesis and Treatment, *J Clin Inv.* 2009; and Melmed S. Pathogenesis of pituitary tumors. *Nat Rev Endocrinol*, 2011.)

TABLE 9-10

Selected Molecular Events Related to Human Pituitary Tumorigenesis

Protein or Gene	Tumor Type	Mechanism of Activation/Inactivation
Activating		
GSP	GH-secreting adenomas	Activating mutation
CREB	GH-secreting adenomas	Increased Ser-phosphorylated CREB promoted by GSP overexpression
Cyclin B2 (*CCNB2*)	All tumor types examined	Overexpression
Cyclin D1 (*CCND1*)	Nonfunctioning	Overexpression
EGF/EGFR	Nonfunctioning	Overexpression
PTTG	All tumor types examined	Overexpression
Gal-3	Prolactinomas ACTH-secreting adenomas	Overexpression
HMGA2	Nonfunctioning ACTH-secreting adenomas Prolactinomas	Overexpression
FGF4	Prolactinomas	Overexpression
Inactivating		
RB1	Negative pRB in ~25% of GH-secreting adenomas	Promoter methylation
13q14	Aggressive tumors	13q14 loss of heterozygosity
AIP	15% of FIPA 2% of sporadic GH-secreting adenomas	Inactivating mutation
MEN1	Prolactinomas in familial MEN1	Inactivating mutation
P16INK4a (*CDKN2A*)	All tumor types examined	Promoter methylation
P27KIP1 (*CDKN1B*)	All tumor types examined	Reduced expression
MEG3a	Nonfunctioning GH-secreting adenomas	Promoter methylation
GADD45-γ	Nonfunctioning GH-secreting adenomas Prolactinomas	Promoter methylation

ACTH, adrenocorticotropic hormone; FIPA, familial isolated pituitary adenomas; GH, growth hormone; MEN1, multiple endocrine neoplasia type 1; pRB, retinoblastoma protein.

(Reproduced from Donangelo I, Melmed S. Molecular pathogenisis of pituitary tumors. In Oxford Textbook of Endocrinology and Diabetes. Wass J, Stewart P [eds], 2010.)

senescence in an Rb-, p16-, and p19-dependent manner.[183] Loss of heterozygosity (LOH) in chromosomes 11q13, 13, and 9 is present in about 15% of spontaneous pituitary adenomas in humans, often correlating with tumor size and invasiveness. Although highly invasive pituitary tumors and pituitary metastases exhibit LOH in region 13q14 (the *RB1* locus), no distinct tumor suppressor gene has been identified for sporadic pituitary tumors,[184] suggesting that another suppressor gene may be located adjacent to the *RB1* locus. Nevertheless, approximately 25% of GH-secreting adenomas do exhibit loss of RB expression, most likely associated with promoter hypermethylation.[185] *TP53* gene mutations have not been detected in pituitary adenomas, nor in pituitary carcinomas or their metastases.[164]

Cyclin D1, D2, and D3 are upregulated when quiescent cells (G_0 phase) enter the proliferative cell cycle, and complexes of cyclin with cyclin-dependent kinase (CDK) lead to RB phosphorylation, releasing E2F to promote cell cycle progression. Allelic imbalance at the *CCND1* locus encoding cyclin D1 is frequently observed in invasive, nonfunctioning pituitary adenomas.[186] The CDK4 and CDK6 inhibitor p16INK4a, encoded by the *CDKN2A* gene, maintains RB in the unphosphorylated state. In nonfunctioning pituitary tumors, the p16INK4a promoter is hypermethylated and consequently not expressed; less frequently, the *CDKN2B* gene, which encodes p15INK4b, is also silenced. Mice that are deficient in p18INK4c develop features of gigantism with intermediate-lobe pituitary hyperplasia and tumors.[187] When the CDK1 and CDK2 inhibitor, p27Kip1 (CDKN1B), is knocked out in mice, multiorgan hyperplasia occurs with development of intermediate-lobe pro-opiomelanocortin–secreting POMC-cell pituitary tumors.[188]

Basic FGF (FGF2) is abundantly expressed in the pituitary, and pituitary expression of PTTG and FGF2 is increased in a time- and dose-dependent manner in estrogen-treated rats.[179] A truncated FGF receptor isoform is expressed in prolactinomas and induces PRL secretion from normal and pituitary adenoma cells.[189] Human prolactinomas express FGF4, and transfected FGF4 enhances PRL secretion and tumor vascularity.[190]

Epidermal growth factor (EGF) exhibits potent mitogenic activity in pituitary cells, and both EGF and its receptor, EGFR, are overexpressed in pituitary tumors, particularly in nonfunctioning adenomas. Both of the receptors ERBB2 and ERBB3 are expressed in aggressive, recurrent prolactionomas.[191] Gefitinib, the EGFR antagonist, decreases experimental prolactinoma cell proliferation and PRL secretion in vitro and in vivo and is associated with abrogated EGFR/ERK signaling.[192] Whether ERBB receptors participate in pituitary tumor cell transformation is unclear.

The growth arrest and DNA damage–inducible protein γ (GADD45G), a tumor growth suppressor, is absent in most pituitary adenomas, as well as in immortalized pituitary cell lines. Pituitary tumor GADD45-γ silencing probably occurs through methylation of CpG islands in the gene promoter.[171] An isoform of maternally expressed gene 3 containing an extra exon (*MEG3A*) is undetectable in both nonfunctioning and GH-secreting pituitary adenomas, conferring a tumor growth advantage, probably as a result of hypermethylation of the promoter region.[193]

Transgenic overexpression of the high mobility group genes *HMGA1* and *HMGA2* causes murine GH-secreting adenomas and prolactinomas, whereas trisomy of chromosome 12, the locus for *HMGA2*, is frequently encountered in human PRL-secreting pituitary adenomas. *HMGA2* was overexpressed in 38 (39%) of 98 pituitary adenomas, in 15 (68%) of 22 adenomas secreting follicle-stimulating hormone (FSH) and/or LH, in 5 (31%) of 15 prolactinomas, and in 12 (67%) of 18 ACTH-secreting adenomas, but it was rarely detected in GH-secreting adenomas.[194] HMGA2 levels correlated with tumor size, invasiveness, and proliferation markers. *HMGA2* tumorigenic effects may also be mediated by induction of cyclin B2 expression[195] and activation of the E2F pathway. HMGA2 is suppressed by *Let-7* (*MIRLET7A1*) microRNA, and expressions of *HMGA2* and *Let-7* are inversely correlated in human pituitary adenoma samples.[194]

Pituitary Senescence

Cellular senescence, or cell growth arrest, is induced by age-linked telomere shortening, DNA damage, oxidative stress, chemotherapy, and oncogene activation.

Oncogene-induced premature cell cycle arrest is protective of the cellular response to oncogenic events, is largely irreversible, and is mediated through upregulation of cell cycle inhibitors including p16INK4a, p15INK4b, p21Cip1 (CDKN1A), and TP53. p21CIP1 induction and senescence markers were elevated in all of 38 GH-secreting adenomas tested. In contrast, p21 was undetectable in GH-producing pituitary carcinomas, nonsecreting pituitary oncocytomas, and null cell adenomas.[196] Activity of senescence-associated β-galactosidase (SA-β-gal), a marker of senescence, is also strongly positive in GH-secreting adenomas (Fig. 9-16). Cellular senescence is protective for malignant transformation,[197] and this process may underlie the invariably benign nature of pituitary adenomas.

Familial Syndromes

The rare familial syndromes are summarized in Table 9-11.

Multiple Endocrine Neoplasia Type 1

Multiple endocrine neoplasia type 1 (MEN1) is an autosomal dominant hereditary disorder that is characterized by tumor formation or hyperfunction of parathyroid, pancreatic islets, anterior pituitary, and, less commonly, carcinoid, thyroid, and adrenal tumors.[198,199] The MEN1 syndrome (fully described in Chapter 41) is associated with germ cell inactivation of the *MEN1* gene (also called *MENIN*) located on chromosome 11q13.[200] Unlike pituitary tumors comprising the MEN1 syndrome, *MEN1* gene mutations were not identified in non-MEN1 familial pituitary adenomas.[201] Mutations of other genes may also confer an MEN1 clinical syndrome. Approximately 20% of patients with a clinical diagnosis of MEN1 do not exhibit identifiable *MEN1* mutations. Rarely, the gene for p27Kip1 (*CDKN1B*) is mutated in patients with clinical features of MEN1 but with no *MEN1* mutations.[202]

Familial Isolated Pituitary Adenomas

Fewer than 5% of prolactinomas and GH-secreting tumors are inherited on a familial basis.[203] In familial acromegaly, about 25% of afflicted individuals are diagnosed as teenagers or young adults, usually with gigantism. These patients have been linked to LOH at the 11q13.1-11q13.3 locus.[204] Germline mutations of the gene encoding aryl hydrocarbon receptor–interacting protein (AIP) were found to predispose to familial pituitary tumors.[205,206] Eleven of 73 families with familial isolated pituitary adenomas were found to have 10 germline aryl hydrocarbon receptor-interacting protein (*AIP*) gene mutations associated with GH- and PRL-secreting tumors,[207,208] and one *AIP* mutation was found in 41 patients with sporadic tumors.[209]

Carney Complex

Carney complex is an autosomal dominant disorder comprising benign mesenchymal tumors including cardiac myxomas, schwannomas, and thyroid and pituitary adenomas associated with spotty skin pigmentation.[210] The disorder has been mapped to chromosome 17q24 and results from a mutated type 1α regulatory subunit of the cAMP-dependent protein kinase A (PRKAR1A).[211] These patients may have elevated levels of GH, IGF1, or PRL, and 10% exhibit clinical acromegaly with GH-secreting tumor formation associated with inactivating mutations of *PRKAR1A*, leading to constitutive protein kinase A catalytic subunit activation. In some patients, the wild-type *PRKAR1A* allele is retained in tumor tissue, and haploinsufficiency may be sufficient for tumorigenesis.

McCune-Albright Syndrome

McCune-Albright syndrome is discussed in detail later in this chapter. In summary, multifactorial mechanisms subserve the multistep pathogenetic process of pituitary adenoma formation, including early initiation of chromosomal mutations that result in mutated pituitary stem or progenitor cells (see Table 9-9). The transformed pituitary cell is subjected to signals facilitating clonal expansion. Permissive factors including hypothalamic hormone receptor signals, intrapituitary growth factors, and disordered cell cycle regulation may determine the ultimate biologic fate of the tumor. Autonomous anterior pituitary hormone production and secretion and cell proliferation, which are the hallmarks of pituitary adenomas, result. However, proximal subcellular events initiating the formation of

TABLE 9-11

Genetic Syndromes Involving Pituitary Tumors

Syndrome	Clinical Features	Chromosome Location	Gene	Protein	Proposed Function
Multiple endocrine neoplasia type 1 (MEN1)	Parathyroid, endocrine pancreas, and pituitary (mostly prolactinomas) tumors	11q13	*MEN1*	MEN1	Nuclear tumor suppressor protein, interacts with JunD and TGFB
Carney syndrome	Skin and cardiac myxomas, adrenal Cushing's syndrome, GH-secreting adenomas	17q24 and 2p16	*PRKAR1A and ?*	PRKAR1A, the regulatory subunit isoform 1A of PKA	Tumor suppressor; inactivating *PRKAR1A* mutation results in constitutive activation of PKA catalytic subunit
Familial isolated pituitary adenomas (FIPA)	Two or more members in a family harboring anterior pituitary tumors without evidence of MEN1 or Carney complex	11q13	*AIP*	AIP	Cytoplasmic tumor suppressor protein; binds to AHR transcription factor
McCune-Albright syndrome	Polyostotic fibrous dysplasia, large café-au-lait spots, precocious puberty, GH excess (may be due to GH-secreting adenomas)	20q13	*GNAS1*	Gsα	Signal transduction activation; constitutive Gsα activation results in elevated cAMP independent of GHRH

AHR, aryl hydrocarbon receptor; AIP, aryl hydrocarbon receptor–interacting protein; cAMP, cyclic adenosine monophosphate; GH, growth hormone; GHRH, growth hormone–releasing hormone; GNAS, stimulatory G protein α-subunit; PKA, protein kinase A; PRKAR1A, cAMP-dependent protein kinase type 1α regulatory subunit; TGFB, transforming growth factor-β.

(Reproduced from Donangelo I, Melmed S. Molecular Pathogenesis of pituitary tumors. In Oxford Textbook of Endocrinology and Diabetes. Wass J., Stewart P. [eds], 2010.)

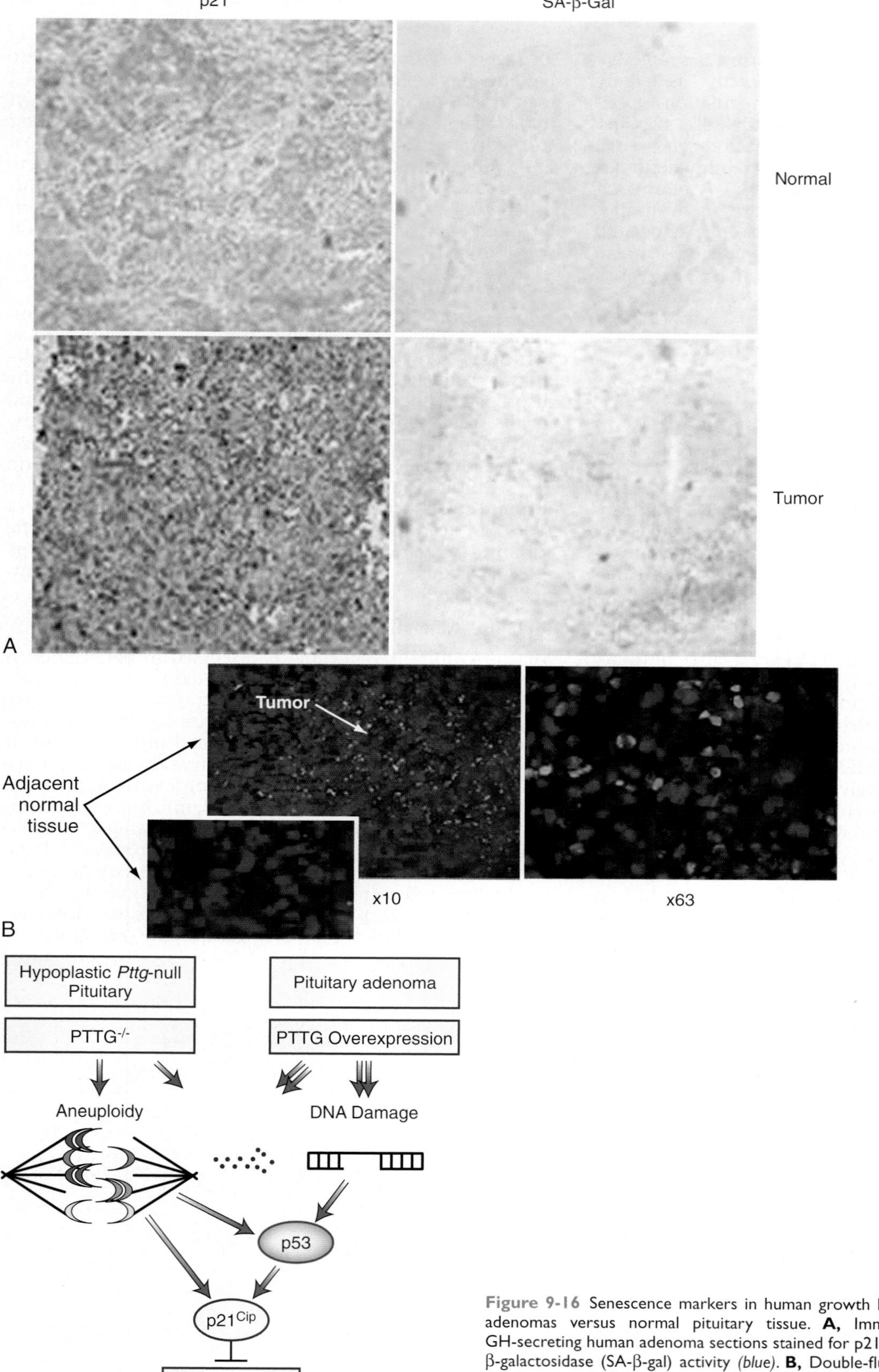

Figure 9-16 Senescence markers in human growth hormone (GH)-producing pituitary adenomas versus normal pituitary tissue. **A,** Immunohistochemistry of the same GH-secreting human adenoma sections stained for p21 *(brown)* and senescence-associated β-galactosidase (SA-β-gal) activity *(blue)*. **B,** Double-fluorescence immunohistochemistry. Confocal image shows coexpression of P21 *(green)* and β-galactosidase *(red)* protein in human pituitary adenomatous tissue but not in normal adjacent tissue *(left)*. High-resolution (×63) image of the same slide is shown on the right. **C,** Proposed model for p21 (Cip)-induced senescence in the hypoplastic PTTG-null pituitary gland and in PTTG-overexpressing pituitary adenomas. Arrows depict proposed pathways. G1 and S are phases of the cell cycle cyclin E-Cdk2. E-Cdk2, cyclin E/cyclin-dependent kinase 2; PTTG, pituitary tumor-transforming gene. (Reproduced from Chesnokova V, Zonis S, Kovacs K, et al. p21Cip1 restrains pituitary tumor growth. *Proc Natl Acad Sci USA.* 2008;105:17498-17503.)

most sporadic pituitary adenomas have not yet been elucidated.[156]

CLASSIFICATION OF PITUITARY TUMORS

Pituitary tumors arise from hormone-secreting adenohypophyseal cells, and their secretory products depend on the cell of origin (Table 9-12). Previously clinically inapparent pituitary adenomas are found in about 11% of autopsies (Table 9-13). They localize to unique areas of the gland, reflecting relative cell type abundance and intragland distribution (see Fig. 9-2). Although 46% of a subset of these lesions immunostain for PRL,[212] expectant management may still be indicated.[213] In a study of 100 normal volunteers, 10 were found to have focal abnormalities on MRI consistent with microadenomas; the lesions measured from 3 to 6 mm in diameter.[6,214,215] Such tumors have been called *incidentalomas*. In a survey of incidentalomas in 506 patients, 20% were found to be nonfunctioning; of these, 20% increased in size during a mean follow-up period of 50 months.[215] When larger, particularly nonfunctioning, tumors are encountered inadvertently, pituitary function should be assessed, including measurements of PRL, IGF1, LH, FSH, and sex steroids. A 24-hour urinary free cortisol or salivary cortisol concentration may help exclude Cushing's disease.[216] In a study of 52 macroadenomas incidentally discovered by CT or MRI, 22 were gonadotroph cell adenomas, 21 were null cell adenomas, and 9 were clinically nonfunctioning but immunostained for various pituitary hormones.[217] Radiologic and surgical classifications are based on tumor localization, size, and degree of invasiveness (see Fig. 9-15). Microadenomas are intrasellar and usually less than 10 mm in widest diameter. Macroadenomas are 10 mm or larger and usually impinge upon adjacent sellar structures.

Specific tumor types for each respective cell type are considered in the following sections. Immunocytochemistry detects pituitary cell gene products at both the light and electron microscopic level and allows classification of pituitary tumors based on their function. Unlike the corticotroph, somatotroph, lactotroph, and thyrotroph cell tumors which hypersecrete their respective hormones,[218] gonadotroph cell tumors are usually clinically silent and do not efficiently secrete their gene products.[219] Double immunostaining identifies mixed tumors expressing combinations of hormones; these are often macroadenomas secreting GH concomitantly with PRL or TSH or ACTH. In general, immunohistochemical identification of pituitary hormones correlates with tumor-specific messenger RNA (mRNA) markers measured either in whole tissue extracts by Northern analysis or at the single cell level by in situ hybridization techniques.[220] With the exception of the glycoprotein α-subunit, immunohistochemical positivity in greater than 5% of cells comprising the tumor is usually reflective of peripheral circulating hormone levels.

Quantification of immunostaining intensity is subjective, and a scale of intensity should also include a description of the extent of staining, such as whether staining was occasional and scattered or whether most tumor cells expressed the immunodetectable protein. Electron microscopy is useful for assessing the ultrastructure of hormone secretory granules, their size, and their distribution. Other subcellular features important for diagnosis include visualization of large mitochondria in nonfunctioning oncocytomas and the secretory nature of Golgi and endoplasmic reticulum, especially for prolactinomas. Peroxidase or colloid gold particles of different diameters are also sensitive electron microscopic markers for identifying and localizing intracellular hormone signals. Because even invasive pituitary tumors are slow growing, the use of mitotic markers such as proliferating cell nuclear antigen (PCNA) and Ki-67 is of limited utility.[221]

PROLACTIN-SECRETING ADENOMAS

Prolactinomas are the most frequently encountered secretory pituitary tumor, occurring with an annual incidence of approximately 30 per 100,000 persons.[158] This incidence would be much higher if the estimate included microadenomas, discovered in approximately 11% of pituitaries at autopsy, 46% of which immunostain positively for PRL.[215] The female-to-male ratio for microprolactinomas is 20:1, whereas for macroadenomas it is roughly 1:1. PRL levels and tumor size usually remain stable, although in some patients the PRL level falls over time. Microadenomas may disappear after discontinuation of dopamine agonist therapy, but 7% to 14% of microadenomas continue to grow.[222]

Macroprolactinomas have a greater propensity to grow, and tumor size correlates with serum PRL levels (Fig. 9-17), so that a PRL level of greater than 200 ng/mL is strongly indicative of a PRL-secreting pituitary tumor. Although prolactinomas account for more than 75% of all female pituitary adenomas,[158] men tend to harbor larger tumors. Among 45 men and 51 women with prolactinomas, the mean serum PRL levels were 2789 ± 572 ng/mL and 292 ± 74 ng/mL, respectively. Tumor size was larger in men than in women (26 ± 2 mm versus 10 ± 1 mm), and the tumors were more invasive and showed histologic evidence of more rapid growth.[223]

PRL levels greater than 200 ng/mL are not always indicative of a prolactinoma and may reflect use of a drug such as Risperdal, whereas levels greater than 500 ng/mL are exclusively observed in patients with prolactinomas.[224] In contrast, a PRL concentration of less than 200 ng/mL in a patient harboring a macroadenoma indicates that the tumor is probably not producing PRL; hyperprolactinemia occurs as a result of mass pressure on the pituitary stalk or portal circulation, which most likely interrupts inhibitory control by dopamine.[225] Importantly, microprolactinomas can be associated with PRL levels ranging from minimal elevations to hundreds of nanograms per milliliter. However, when a patient with a small macroadenoma and a PRL level of approximately 200 ng/mL is first encountered, it is prudent to first treat medically. If the tumor is indeed a prolactinoma, dopamine agonist treatment should lower PRL levels and shrink the tumor. If the tumor does not shrink, the mass is probably not secretory, and hyperprolactinoma is caused by compressive stalk effect.

Pathology and Pathogenesis

Although more than 99% of prolactinomas are benign and are often sharply demarcated without evidence of invasion, about half invade local structures (Fig. 9-18).[226] Invasive tumors may have higher mitotic activity and are more cellular and more pleomorphic than noninvasive types. Invasion into adjacent dura, bone, or venous structures may represent an intermediate form of prolactinoma between the sharply demarcated benign variety and the exceedingly rare malignant tumor. Invasive tumors that do not metastasize are considered benign.[227] Immunostaining for PRL

TABLE 9-12

Clinical and Pathologic Characteristics of Pituitary Adenomas

Adenoma Type	Incidence: *Pathologic (%)*	Incidence: *Clinical (%)*	Incidence: *Annual Incidence (New Cases/10^6)*	Prevalence (Total Cases/10^6)	Messenger RNA Expression	Immunohistochemistry	Electron Microscopic Secretory Granules (nm)	Clinical Syndrome
Lactotroph		29	6-10	60-100				
Sparsely granulated	28				PRL	PRL	150-500	Hypogonadism, galactorrhea
Densely granulated	1				PRL	PRL	400-1200	
Somatotroph		15	4-6	40-60				
Sparsely granulated	5				GH	GH	100-250	Acromegaly or gigantism
Densely granulated	5				GH	GH	300-700	
Combined GH/PRL cell		8						
Mixed GH/PRL	5				GH/PRL	GH/PRL	100-600	
Mammosomatotroph	1				GH/PRL	GH/PRL	350-2000	Hypogonadism, acromegaly, galactorrhea
Acidophil stem cell	3				GH/PRL	GH/PRL	50-300	
Corticotroph			2-3	20-30				
Cushing's disease	10	10			POMC	ACTH	250-700	Cushing's disease
Silent corticotroph	3	6			POMC	ACTH	Variable	None
Nelson's syndrome	2				POMC	ACTH	250-700	Local signs
Thyrotroph	1	0.9			TSH	TSH	50-250	Hyperthyroidism
Plurihormonal	10	4			GH/PRL	GH/PRL/glycoprotein	Mixed	Mixed
Nonfunctioning/Null Cell/Gonadotroph		27	7-9	70-90				
Non-oncocytic	14				FSH/LHα	Glycoprotein	<25% of cells 100-250	Silent or pituitary failure
Oncocytic	6				FSH/LHα	Glycoprotein	<25% of cells 100-250, many mitochondria	Silent or pituitary failure
Gonadotroph	7-15				FSH/LH	FSH/LH	50-200	Silent or pituitary failure

ACTH, adrenocorticotropic hormone; FSH, follicle-stimulating hormone; GH, growth hormone; LHα, luteinizing hormone α-subunit; PRL, prolactin; TSH, thyroid-stimulating hormone.

Data derived from Clayton RN. Sporadic pituitary tumours: from epidemiology to use of databases. *Best Pract Res Clin Endocrinol Metab.* 1999;13:451 (study of a relatively stable 1 million catchment population surrounding Stoke-on-Trent, UK) and from Kovacs & Horvath 1986; Scheithauer 1994; Minderman & Wilson 1994; Asa SL 1993.

TABLE 9-13

Frequency of Pituitary Adenomas Found at Autopsy

Study	No. Pituitaries Examined	No. Adenomas Found	Frequency (%)
Susman	260	23	9
Costello	1,000	225	23
Sommers	400	26	7
McCormick	1,600	140	9
Kovacs	152	20	13
Landolt	100	13	13
Mosca	100	24	24
Burrow	120	32	27
Parent	500	42	8
Muhr	205	3	2
Schwezinger	5,100	485	9
Coulon	100	10	10
Chambers	100	14	14
Siqueira	450	39	9
El-Hamid	486	97	20
Scheithauer	251	41	16
Marin	210	35	16
Mosca	111	13	11
Sano	166	15	9
Teramoto	1,000	51	5
Buurman	3,048	334	11
Total	15,459	1,742	11

Modified from Molitch ME. Pituitary incidentalomas. In: de Herder WW, ed. *Functional and Morphological Imaging of the Endocrine System.* Norwell, MA: Kluwer Academic; 2000:59-70; and Buurman H, Saeger W. Subclinical adenomas in postmortem pituitaries: classification and correlations to clinical data. *Eur J Endocrinol.* 2006;154:753-758.

confirms the diagnosis of prolactinoma; the lesion is usually distinct from the adjacent normal pituitary, but it is not truly encapsulated. These tumors have a "pseudocapsule" composed of compressed adenohypophyseal cells and a reticulin fiber network.[227] For a prolactinoma to be considered malignant, a distant extracranial metastasis must be demonstrated.[228]

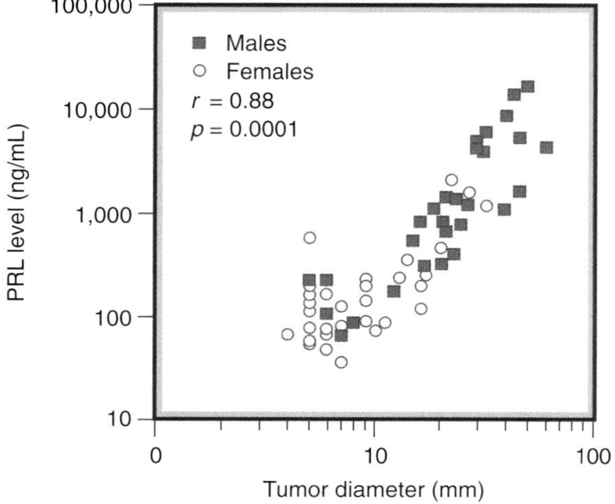

Figure 9-17 Prolactin (PRL)-secreting tumors are more often macroadenomas in men ($n = 31$) than in women ($n = 45$). Serum PRL levels highly correlate with tumor size. (Adapted from Danila DC, Klibanski A. Prolactin secreting pituitary tumors in men. *The Endocrinologist.* 2001;11:105-111.)

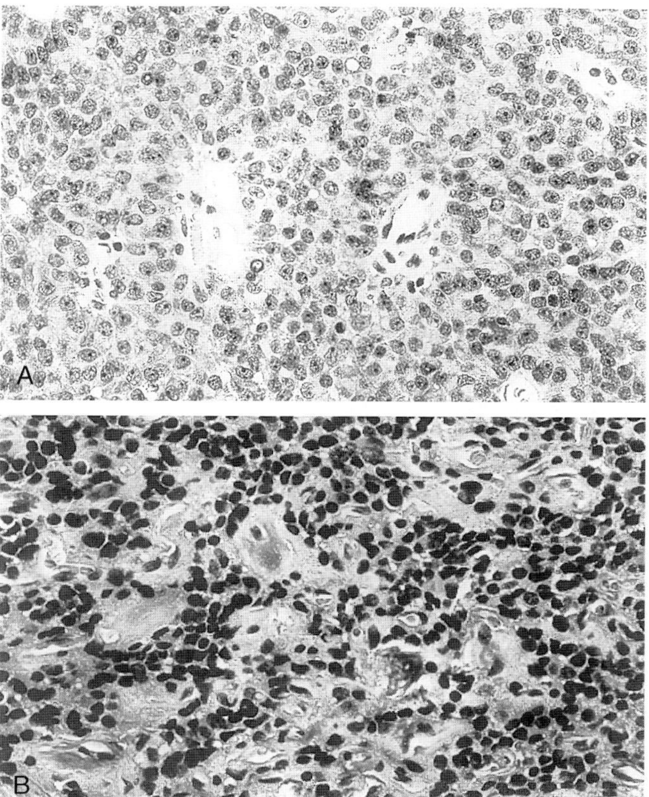

Figure 9-18 **A,** Resected prolactinomas tissue with no dopamine agonist pretreatment. **B,** Prolactin-producing pituitary adenoma removed by surgery from a patient treated with dopamine agonist in the preoperative period. The adenoma cells are small, possessing dark nuclei and a narrow rim of cytoplasm. Mild accumulation of interstitial connective tissue is apparent. (Hematoxylin-eosin stain; original magnification ×400.) (Photomicrograph kindly provided by Kalman Kovacs. University of Toronto, Toronto, Canada.)

Prolactinomas are mostly slow growing, arise sporadically, usually occur singly, and are monoclonal.[167] Infrequently, more than one prolactinoma arises within the gland.[229] Prolactinomas are the pituitary tumors most commonly associated with MEN1, occurring in approximately 20% of one large kindred,[230] although prolactinoma occurrence is not evenly distributed. Familial prolactinomas have been described in patients with no other features of MEN1.[231]

Clinical Features

Prolactinomas usually come to attention because of symptoms or signs associated with either hyperprolactinemia or tumor size or invasiveness (Table 9-14).

Hyperprolactinemia

Both large and small PRL-secreting tumors can manifest with signs and symptoms of hyperprolactinemia. Menstrual irregularities, sexual dysfunction, galactorrhea,[232] and osteopenia[233] are attributable to elevated PRL levels. Elevated PRL causes sexual dysfunction via a short-loop feedback effect on gonadotropin pulsatility that presumably inhibits GnRH[234] as well as LH pulse frequency and amplitude. High PRL also directly inhibits ovarian and testicular function. Women with prolactinomas may present with primary or secondary amenorrhea, oligomenorrhea, menorrhagia, delayed menarche, or regular menses with a short

TABLE 9-14

Signs and Symptoms of Prolactinomas

Signs and Symptoms Associated with Tumor Mass	Signs and Symptoms Associated with Hyperprolactinemia
Visual field abnormalities	Amenorrhea, oligomenorrhea, infertility
Blurred vision or decreased visual acuity	Decreased libido, impotence, premature ejaculation, erectile dysfunction, oligospermia
Symptoms of hypopituitarism	Galactorrhea
Headaches	Osteoporosis
Cranial nerve palsies	
Pituitary apoplexy	
Seizures (temporal lobe)	
Hydrocephalus (rare)	
Unilateral exophthalmos (rare)	

luteal phase that may result in infertility. Patients may also report changes in libido and vaginal dryness. Sexual dysfunction in men usually manifests as loss or decrease in libido, impotence, premature ejaculation or intracoital erection loss, oligospermia, or azospermia.[235]

Up to 50% of women and 35% of men with prolactinomas have galactorrhea.[236] This gender difference may occur because male mammary tissue is less susceptible to lactogenic effects of hyperprolactinemia.[237] Galactorrhea can be overlooked unless actively elicited. Bone density may decrease in both men and women as a result of hyperprolactinemia-induced sex steroid deficiency.[238]

Tumor Mass Effects

Prolactinomas may manifest with signs and symptoms resulting from tumor size or invasiveness. Microadenomas range from entirely asymptomatic tumors found at autopsy that are as small as 2 to 3 mm to larger ones that are still less than 10 mm in diameter. These tumors can be invasive despite their small size. In contrast, macroadenomas range in size from noninvasive or diffuse tumors approximately 1 cm in diameter to huge tumors that may impinge on parasellar structures.

Signs and symptoms caused by large or invasive tumors are often related to compressive effects on visual structures. The most frequent ophthalmic complaint in a series of 1000 patients with tumors was loss of vision.[239] The most frequent objective findings were bitemporal hemianopsia, superior bitemporal defects, and decreased visual acuity. Headaches are common, but seizures (a result of extension into the temporal lobe) and hydrocephalus[240] are rare, as is unilateral exophthalmos. Many tumors invade the cavernous sinuses, yet cranial nerve palsies are only rarely encountered. A sudden insult, such as pituitary apoplexy, is the more common cause of such palsies and may be a presenting symptom. Prolactinomas can also be found inadvertently on an MRI or CT scan performed for another purpose.

Evaluation

All patients with pituitary tumors should have serum PRL levels measured. Conversely, patients with elevated serum PRL levels not fully explicable by an obvious cause (such as pregnancy or exposure to neuroleptic medications) should be evaluated for the presence of a pituitary tumor. Prolactinomas may also coexist with another cause of hyperprolactinemia, such as neuroleptic drug administration (see Chapter 8).[243] Even minimal to moderate PRL elevations are important to investigate, because they may indicate the presence of a large pituitary tumor that does not secrete PRL. PRL levels correlate strongly with tumor size and are usually higher in male patients. Occasionally, a patient with a very high serum PRL level can have a "normal" result reported if serum dilutions are not assayed—a phenomenon called the high-dose hook effect.[241] In contrast, serum PRL may be elevated by the presence of high-molecular-weight PRL, which is a weaker lactogen than the monomeric PRL molecule.

Although they are usually clinically inactive, pituitary tumors also can result in macroprolactinemia. Pituitary adenomas were diagnosed in approximately 20% of patients with macroprolactinemia, and some were associated with galactorrhea, oligomenorrhea or amenorrhea, or erectile dysfunction and decreased libido.[242] Therefore, assessment of macroprolactinemia by polyethylene glycol precipitation should be performed in patients with reported high levels of PRL and few or absent clinical features of hyperprolactinemia.[243]

A careful history often unmasks symptoms or signs of a space-related mass, such as visual field abnormalities, impaired visual acuity, blurred or double vision, CSF rhinorrhea, headaches, diabetes insipidus, rare hydrocephalus,[240] and hypopituitarism. Patients should also be questioned carefully about their sexual history, including onset of menarche, regularity of menses, fertility, libido, potency, and ability to maintain an erection. A history of galactorrhea should also be ascertained. The coexistence of galactorrhea and amenorrhea suggests a diagnosis of pituitary adenoma until otherwise proven.

PRL is elevated in up to 50% of patients with acromegaly.[232] Patients in the early stages of acromegaly and those who have mild disease or harbor acidophil stem cell adenomas may have few obvious signs of GH excess. Because the human GH molecule exhibits lactogenic properties similar to those of PRL,[244] signs and symptoms of a prolactinoma may be mimicked by a purely GH-secreting tumor, and serum IGF1 should be measured. Elevated PRL levels are occasionally encountered in patients with TSH-secreting tumors. Other pituitary hormone functions should be ascertained to determine the presence of hypopituitarism. An MRI is required to establish a definitive diagnosis of prolactinoma.

Treatment

Optimal treatment outcomes for a prolactinoma include normalization of PRL levels (and associated signs and symptoms) and complete tumor removal or shrinkage with a reversal of tumor-mass effects (Table 9-15). Specifically, previously abnormal sexual function and fertility should be restored, galactorrhea stopped, impaired bone density improved, tumor eliminated or reduced in size without impairing pituitary or hypothalamic function, and vision normalized, if impaired.[245]

Medical Treatment

Medical management of prolactinomas with dopamine agonist drugs has been widely recommended as the treatment of choice.

Bromocriptine. Bromocriptine, a semisynthetic ergot alkaloid dopamine agonist, lowers elevated PRL levels, restores abnormal menstrual function in 80% to 90% of patients,[246] shrinks prolactinomas, restores impaired sexual function, and improves galactorrhea.[247] Improvement in

TABLE 9-15

Dopamine Agonist Treatment of Prolactinomas (% of Patients)*

Outcome	Bromocriptine (2.5-7.5 mg/day)	Cabergoline (0.5-1 mg twice weekly)
Microadenomas		
PRL normalized	70	80
Menses resumed	70	80
Macroadenomas		
PRL normalized	65	70
Menses resumed	85	80
Tumor shrinkage:		
None	20	20
≤50%	40	55
≥50%	40	25
Visual field improvement	90	70
Drug intolerance	15	5

*Long-acting cabergoline has improved patient compliance and fewer gastrointestinal side effects. For fertility, bromocriptine is preferred because it is short-acting and can be discontinued immediately on pregnancy confirmation.

PRL, prolactin.

Values derived from Webster J, Piscatelli G, Polli A, et al. A comparison of cabergoline and bromocriptine in the treatment hyperprolactinemic amenorrhea. Cabergoline Comparative Study Group. *N Engl J Med.* 1994;331:904-909; and Verhelst J, Abs R, Maiter D, et al. Cabergoline in the treatment of hyperprolactinemia: a study in 455 patients. *J Clin Endocrinol Metab.* 1999;84:2518-2522.

visual field abnormalities occurs in approximately 90% of affected patients.[248,249] Drug withdrawal can result in rapid tumor expansion.[250] In contrast, tumors that have shrunken during bromocriptine therapy occasionally do not enlarge after drug withdrawal.[251] In a subset of patients, hyperprolactinemia disappears spontaneously after long-term observation.[252] Very occasionally, bromocriptine lowers PRL despite continued tumor expansion,[253] although when tumors grow during dopamine agonist therapy there is usually a simultaneous PRL elevation.

Some patients have lesions that are entirely or partially resistant to the effects of bromocriptine even at high doses, as well as those of cabergoline.[254] Not infrequently, it is difficult to completely normalize the PRL concentration in patients with initially very high levels, although they may respond to treatment with impressive tumor shrinkage and sometimes with improved sexual function. Although use of higher doses or a change in the form of dopamine agonist has been reported to further PRL normalization in some cases,[255] many such patients continue to have elevated PRL concentrations regardless of the treatment employed. Resistance to dopamine agonists may reflect reduced D_2 receptor binding site[256] or receptor gene polymorphisms.[257]

Bromocriptine shrinks prolactinomas by shrinking tumor cell size, including cytoplasmic, nuclear, and nucleolar areas.[258,259] Histologic sections appear very dense as a result of small cell size and clumping of nuclei (see Fig. 9-18). PRL mRNA and PRL synthesis are inhibited, exocytoses are reduced, PRL secretory granules decrease, and structures of the rough endoplasmic reticulum and Golgi apparatus involute. The net effect is reduced cell volume. Tumor necrosis may also occur.[260]

Perivascular fibrosis noted in prolactinomas derived from patients treated with bromocriptine[261] has been attributed to difficulty in tumor removal. However, others found no effect of prior treatment with bromocriptine on surgical success rates.[262] In contrast, bromocriptine was a helpful adjunct to transsphenoidal microsurgery for macroprolactinomas.[263] Even the largest tumors and those with the highest PRL levels respond well to treatment with 2.5 mg bromocriptine three times daily. Higher doses are often not more effective.[236] Once positive effects on tumor size and amenorrhea and galactorrhea are established, some patients can be satisfactorily maintained with smaller doses,[264] but rarely without medication.

Cabergoline. Cabergoline has a longer duration of action than bromocriptine and is usually administered once or twice weekly. Since its introduction, it has surpassed bromocriptine as the first-line therapeutic choice for most patients, unless pregnancy is desired.[265] The long half-life of cabergoline is a result of its high affinity for lactotroph D_2 receptors on lactotrophs and a greater propensity of the drug to remain in pituitary tissue.[266] In pharmacokinetic studies, cabergoline lowered PRL in a dose-related manner.[267] PRL levels were normalized in 83% of 459 women with hyperprolactinemia treated with cabergoline (0.5 to 1 mg twice weekly) and in 52% of women treated with bromocriptine (2.5 to 5 mg twice daily). Cabergoline was also more effective than bromocriptine in restoring ovulatory cycles and fertility (72% versus 52%; $P < .001$), was better tolerated than bromocriptine, and caused fewer but similar side effects (Fig. 9-19). Tumor size decreased in 11 of 15 patients with macroadenomas, and menses resumed in 3 of 4 premenopausal women.[268] Among 85 patients with macroprolactinomas treated with cabergoline (0.25 to 10.5 mg/week), PRL concentrations were normalized in 61% of patients and decreased by at least 75% in an additional 24 patients, and tumor size decreased in 66% of patients (see Table 9-15). Nine patients were resistant to cabergoline despite doses of up to 7 mg/week.[255,269] Despite the continued experience that a subset of hyperprolactinemic patients are resistant to dopamine agonists, cabergoline normalized PRL in 15 of 19 patients with macroprolactinomas previously resistant to other dopamine agonists.[270] Cabergoline also may result in dramatic improvement of prolactinoma-associated headache.[271]

Prolactinomas completely or substantially resistant to medication are infrequently encountered. Most "resistant" patients have only partial resistance (i.e., tumors shrink and PRL levels are lowered but do not normalize). With the

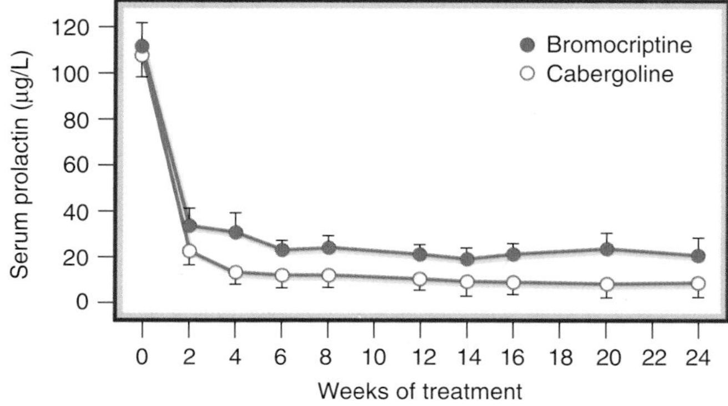

Figure 9-19 Comparison of bromocriptine and cabergoline in suppressing prolactin levels in women with hyperprolactinemia. (Reproduced from Webster J, Piscitelli G, Polli A, et al. A comparison of cabergoline and bromocriptine in the treatment of hyperprolactinemic amenorrhea. *N Engl J Med.* 1996;331-904-909.)

tumor growth controlled on treatment, persistently elevated PRL levels should be addressed by evaluation and treatment of specific disorders caused by hyperprolactinemia.

Administration. Attention to the mode of dopamine agonist administration may avoid or minimize potential adverse effects (Fig. 9-20). Usual starting doses are 1.25 mg bromocriptine (daily), or 0.25 mg cabergoline (weekly). Doses of medication are either increased gradually, as tolerated, or decreased depending on tolerability, and therapy should begin with a small dose taken with food before bedtime. Patients should initially avoid activities that cause peripheral vasodilatation (e.g., hot baths), to decrease the risk of postural hypotension. If side effects are troublesome, the subsequent dose should be halved and doses increased gradually thereafter to achieve effective levels. Switching from one medication to another may be beneficial.[272] Intravaginal bromocriptine administration has been used to alleviate adverse gastrointestinal events.[273]

Adverse Effects of Dopamine Agonists. Side effects of dopamine agonists are common. Nausea occurs in up to 50% of patients. Nasal stuffiness, depression, and digital vasospasm occur, the latter more frequently with higher doses, as seen in patients with Parkinson's disease. Postural hypotension can cause loss of consciousness, occurs infrequently, and is usually avoided by careful dosing. Signs and symptoms of psychosis or exacerbation of preexisting psychosis are encountered in up to 1.3% of patients receiving bromocriptine.[274] In our personal experience, psychosis also occurs with other dopamine agonists, including cabergoline. A history of psychotic symptoms should raise concerns about the use of these medications. If psychosis occurs in a patient in whom dopamine agonists are clearly the treatment of choice, the judicious combination of this agent and antipsychotic medication can be effective. A neuroleptic that is not a potent PRL stimulator, such as olanzapine, is preferred. CSF rhinorrhea occurred during dopamine agonist treatment in up to 6.1% of patients with macroadenomas, some of which were more resistant to

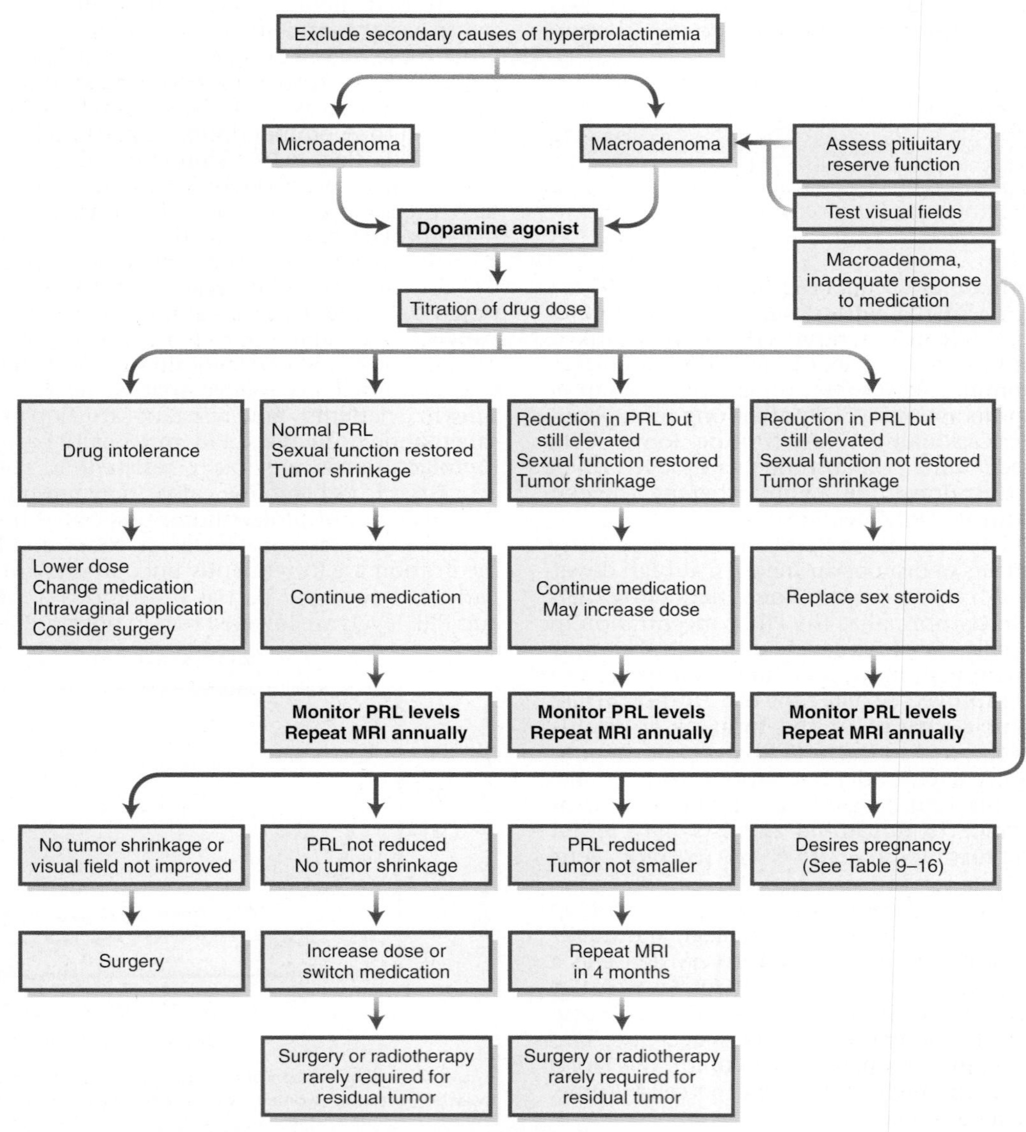

Figure 9-20 Management of prolactinomas. After secondary causes of hyperprolactinemia have been excluded, subsequent management decisions are based on clinical imaging and biochemical criteria. MRI, magnetic resonance imaging; PRL, prolactin.

dopamine agonists.[275,276] Other, rarely reported serious side effects include hepatic dysfunction and cardiac arrythmias.[244,276] Retroperitoneal fibrosis, pleural effusions, and thickening and restrictive mitral regurgitation have been reported in patients taking high doses of bromocriptine.[277,278]

High doses of dopamine agonists with serotoninergic properties were associated with a risk for heart valve regurgitation[279] in 155 patients with Parkinson's disease taking high doses of ergot-derived dopamine agonists. Clinically, significant heart valve regurgitation (moderate to severe, grade 3 to 4) was observed in patients taking pergolide (23.4%) or cabergoline (28.6%) but not in patients taking non–ergot-derived dopamine agonists (0%); valvular regurgitation was noted in 5.6% of control subjects.[280] These observations in patients with Parkinson's disease receiving high ergot doses raise concern for patients with pituitary tumors who mostly take far lower drug doses. Although one study showed an increase in mild tricuspid regurgitation among patients receiving cabergoline for hyperprolactinemia,[281] most reports have shown no evidence to indicate that low doses of cabergoline place patients at risk for significant valve disease.[282-285] A randomized controlled trial will be helpful in firmly establishing the safety of low-dose cabergoline.

Radiation Therapy

Linear accelerator radiotherapy is effective in controlling or reducing the size of prolactinomas. However, this therapy takes years to achieve maximal effect. The usual recommended radiation dose is 4500 to 4600 centigray (cGy), and normalization of PRL was achieved in 18 of 36 patients at a mean of 7.3 years after such treatment.[286] Hypopituitarism occurs as a side effect of irradiation. Five years after radiotherapy (3750 to 4250 cGy)[287] in 165 patients, all were GH deficient, 91% were gonadotrophin deficient, 77% were ACTH deficient, and 42% were TSH deficient. Of 36 patients with prolactinomas, of whom 83% had normal GH responses to insulin-induced hypoglycemia before therapy, 34 were GH deficient at 9 to 12 years after radiotherapy.[286] Therefore, although radiotherapy is useful in the control of tumor growth, it is not as effective as dopamine agonists. Although stereotactic confocal radiotherapy with a linear accelerator can provide greater tumor focus and a smaller radiation field,[54] there are as yet no large-scale results of prolactinoma treatment with gamma knife radiotherapy.

Surgery

The success rate of pituitary surgery correlates inversely with tumor size and serum PRL concentration.[262] In a compilation of results from 31 published surgical series, serum PRL was normalized in 71% of 1224 patients with microprolactinomas. Although surgical cure rates for microprolactinomas are high, the rate of hyperprolactinemia recurrence is also relatively high,[288] occurring in an estimated 17% of patients initially considered cured.[289] In contrast, complete resection of macroprolactinomas, especially large invasive ones, is difficult to achieve, and postoperative serum PRL levels are normalized in only 32% of patients, with a 19% recurrence rate. The experience of the surgeon is of major importance, because the cure rate is not as favorable in the hands of neurosurgeons who perform a limited number of procedures.

Although results of medical therapy are superior to those of surgery, there remains a role for surgery in these patients. Patients with prolactinomas that are resistant to dopamine agonist therapy are particularly well suited for surgery. If tumor removal is only partial, adjunctive radiation therapy should be considered. Prophylactic transsphenoidal surgery should also be considered in women whose prolactinomas are large enough to potentially threaten vision during pregnancy. A subset of patients cannot tolerate available dopamine agonists, and others prefer surgery and refuse medication.

Chemotherapy

There has been growing interest in the use of chemotherapeutic agents for aggressive PRL-secreting tumors unresponsive to other therapies. Temozolomide, an alkylating compound that readily crosses the blood-brain barrier, may control tumor growth in individual patients.[290-292] The response to temozolomide may be predicted by low tumor staining for O^6-methylguanine-DNA-methyltransferase (MGMT).[293]

Pregnancy

The normal pituitary enlarges during pregnancy, and prolactinomas may also increase in size during pregnancy.[212] The incidence of pregnancy-associated tumor enlargement, as determined by development of abnormal visual fields, has been estimated at 1.4% of women with microadenomas and 16% of women with macroadenomas.[294] In other reports, the risk for macroadenoma enlargement has been estimated to be as high as 36%. In a prospective analysis in which 57 patients with microprolactinomas were monitored by formal visual field examinations during pregnancy, none developed visual disturbances. In contrast, six of eight primiparous women with macroadenomas developed visual loss.[295] The results for the patients with macroadenomas were likely skewed, because these patients had been recommended for surgery before pregnancy.

Although dopamine agonists have been used during pregnancy to prevent tumor growth (Fig. 9-21),[296] it seems prudent to reduce fetal exposure to medication if possible. It is recommended that menstrual periods be allowed to occur naturally for a period of time (3 to 4 months), long enough to predict that a missed period might be a result of pregnancy (Table 9-16). Barrier contraception is recommended during this period. Within several days to 1 week after a positive human chorionic gonadotropin test is obtained, medication should be discontinued. In a study

TABLE 9-16

Management of Prolactinomas in Patients Planning Pregnancies

Microadenoma	Macroadenoma
Discontinue dopamine agonist when pregnancy test is positive	Consider surgery before pregnancy
Periodic visual field examinations during pregnancy	Ensure bromocriptine sensitivity before pregnancy
Postpartum MRI after 6 wk*	Monitor visual fields expectantly and frequently
	Administer bromocriptine if vision becomes compromised
	Or, continue bromocriptine throughout pregnancy if tumor previously affected vision
	Consider high-dose steroids or surgery during pregnancy if vision is threatened or adenoma hemorrhage occurs
	Postpartum MRI after 6 wk

*Pituitary MRI may be required during pregnancy if deemed necessary.

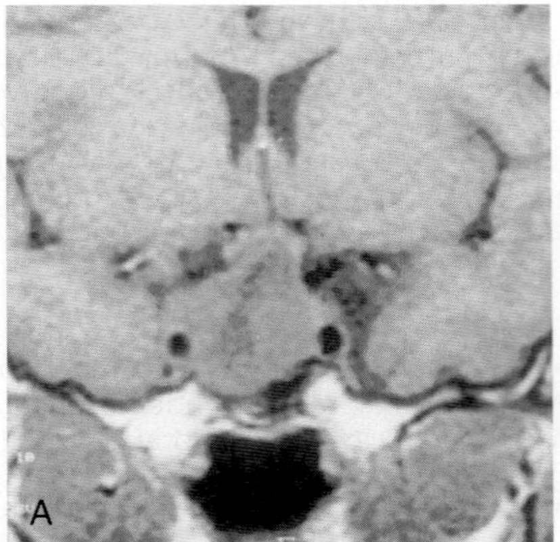

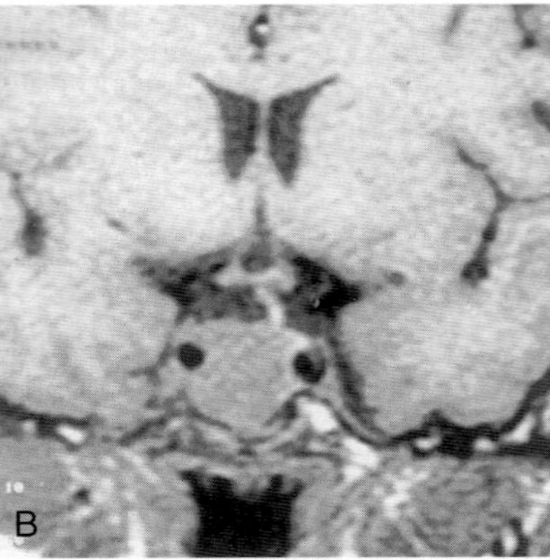

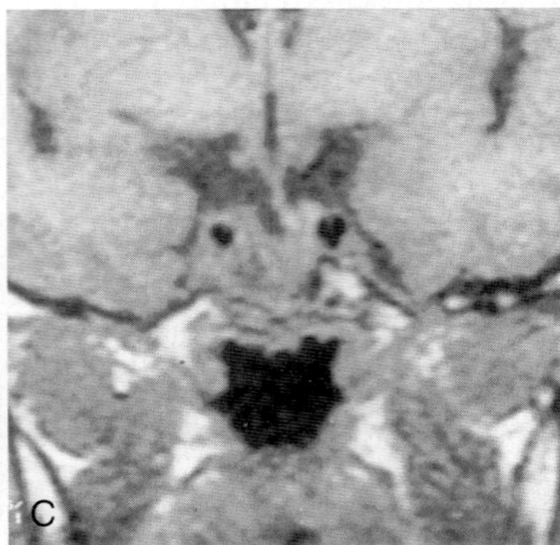

Figure 9-21 Shrinkage of macroadenoma by treatment with cabergoline in a woman harboring a macroadenoma at 22 weeks' gestation (**A**), when the prolactin concentration was 488 μg/L (**B**), and with further reduction at 3 weeks after delivery (**C**). (Reproduced from Liu C, Tyrrell JB. Successful treatment of large macroprolactinoma with cabergoline during pregnancy. *Pituitary.* 2001;4:179-185.)

of 6239 pregnancies in patients managed in this manner, bromocriptine therapy was not associated with increased abortions or terminations, prematurity, multiple births, or infant malformations beyond the incidence expected in the control population. There is no evidence that other dopamine agonists are less safe, but pregnancy exposure to the other agonist forms is less comprehensively documented.

Treatment options for patients harboring prolactinomas whose vision becomes impaired during pregnancy include administration of bromocriptine, use of high-dose steroids, and surgical resection.[294] Of 53 pregnant women receiving bromocriptine, mean offspring birth weight was normal, congenital abnormalities occurred in 4 babies, and physical and intellectual development of children was normal for up to 9 years. In an observational report on 380 pregnancies in women treated with cabergoline, early fetal exposure did not increase the risk of miscarriage or fetal malformation.[297]

To avoid neurologic complications of tumor enlargement during pregnancy, it is recommended that women with prolactinomas be tested for sensitivity to dopamine agonists before proceeding with a pregnancy. If tumors are insensitive to dopamine agonists (i.e., do not respond with tumor shrinkage), prophylactic surgery could be appropriate. If the tumor is a macroadenoma approximating the optic chiasm, the likelihood of visual difficulties is greater, and it could be prudent to undertake surgery before the patient becomes pregnant.[298]

GONADOTROPIN-PRODUCING (CLINICALLY NONFUNCTIONING) PITUITARY TUMORS

Nonfunctioning pituitary tumors comprise 25% to 35% of pituitary tumors.[299] Most arise from gonadotroph cells, and they are monoclonal[167,169] and usually chromophobic. Although they most frequently manifest as clinically nonfunctioning masses and are not associated with elevated serum gonadotrophins, they produce sufficient gonadotrophin subunits to be detectable by immunohistochemistry. In one study, 13 of 14 nonfunctioning gonadotroph tumors produced gonadotrophic hormone subunits detected by immunohistochemistry.[300] In another series of nonfunctioning adenomas, 42% of tumors immunostained for the TSH β-subunit, 83% for the LH β-subunit, 75% for the FSH β-subunit, and 92% for the α-subunit[301]; some also expressed chromogranin A.[302] Although LH, FSH, and/or α-subunit are released from these nonfunctioning tumors when they are maintained in culture, production is usually not sufficient to elevate blood levels.[219] In the past, when immunochemistry was unavailable, these tumors were often classified as null cell adenomas, which do not express glycoprotein subunits.[303] A small subset of tumors secrete sufficient hormone to elevate serum gonadotrophin or α-subunit levels, occasionally resulting in clinical syndromes.

Presentation

Clinically Nonfunctioning Gonadotroph Tumors

Clinically nonfunctioning tumors usually come to attention because of their large size or are detected incidentally (incidentaloma) (Table 9-17).[304] Of 506 incidentally discovered pituitary masses, 324 were clinically nonfunctioning tumors, and the remainder were cystic or parasellar masses.[305] A gradual visual deficit arising from optic chiasmal compression is common, and patients are often unaware of the disturbance. Recognition of visual field deficits is often delayed because formal visual fields are not routinely evaluated unless a defect is suspected clinically. In the absence of associated space-occupying or hormonal disorders, these large tumors may go unrecognized for many years and then be inadvertently detected on scans or x-ray studies performed for other purposes (incidentaloma). Sinusitis evaluation, pituitary apoplexy, or a brain

TABLE 9-17

Presentation of Gonadotroph Adenomas

Common	Uncommon
Clinically nonfunctioning macroadenoma	Intact gonadotrophin overproduction
Immunostain for gonadotrophin subunits (usually more than one)	Immunostain for subunits or intact hormone being hypersecreted
Usually discovered because of space-occupying effects, or inadvertently	Usually discovered because of space-occupying effects, or inadvertently
Pituitary deficiency	May cause clinical syndrome due to hormone overproduction
	Other pituitary hormones may be deficient

MRI performed for an unrelated indication (e.g., head trauma) may bring these tumors to clinical attention.

Although it is not often the initial presenting complaint, these patients are commonly deficient in one or more pituitary hormones (e.g., in two thirds of 56 patients with nonfunctioning macroadenomas[47]). Although the most commonly encountered endocrine symptoms are related to gonadotrophin deficiency, quality of life may be decreased[306] or not altered,[307] and daytime somnolence has also been reported.[308]

Functioning Gonadotroph Tumors

The small subset of gonadotroph adenomas that produce elevated serum FSH, LH, and/or α-subunit concentrations are considered to be functioning adenomas but are not often associated with specific endocrine syndromes. High serum FSH, usually with low LH levels, is generally the only sign that a pituitary tumor is secreting FSH. Paradoxically, these patients may present with hypogonadism due to gonadal downregulation. However, female patients with such tumors may present with pelvic pain due to ovarian hyperstimulation.[309] High gonadotrophin levels associated with menopause or testicular failure may complicate the interpretation of gonadotrophin levels, but both LH and FSH are high in cases of primary gonadal failure. LH-producing tumors are exceedingly rare and in males cause elevations in serum testosterone with acne and skin oiliness.

Evaluation

MRI, visual field examination, and pituitary hormone concentrations should be evaluated, the latter not only to detect hypopituitarism but also to exclude hormone overproduction that may not be clinically apparent. LH, FSH, α-subunit, PRL, T_4, triiodothyronine (T_3), TSH, cortisol, and IGF1 levels should be measured. A serum cortisol measurement at 8 a.m., cortisol response to cosyntropin, or an insulin tolerance test can be helpful in excluding secondary adrenal insufficiency. The extent of hormonal evaluation requires clinical judgment.

If LH or FSH is elevated, the values must be interpreted in light of the patient's physiologic state. An elevated serum FSH value would be interpreted differently in a woman with regular menstrual cycles and in a menopausal patient. Gonadotrophin elevations in patients with primary gonadal failure are not typically limited to one hormone, and circulating α-subunit elevation is consistent with a pituitary tumor but not with gonadal failure. TRH stimulation may differentiate elevated gonadotropin levels ascribed to end-organ failure from those due to independent tumor production. In patients harboring gonadotroph adenomas, increased levels of FSH, LH, LH β-subunit, or α-subunit are evoked in response to TRH.[310] Calculating the molar ratio of LH or FSH to α-subunit may assist in the diagnosis.

Treatment

Clinical judgment should be used in determining the appropriate therapy: surgery, surgery followed by radiotherapy, radiotherapy alone, or expectant observation (Fig. 9-22). No reliable tumor marker is predictive of mass growth or recurrence.

Surgery and Radiotherapy

If a patient's tumor threatens vision or is a macroadenoma whose size threatens vital structures, transsphenoidal surgery is recommended. Vision improves in approximately 75% of patients with impaired vision.[311,312] Among 100 patients undergoing transsphenoidal surgery, 72 had visual disturbances, 61 had hypopituitarism, and 36 had headache. Vision improved in 53 of 72 patients after surgery, and headache improved in all.[313] Expectant follow-up of 65 patients after pituitary surgery for nonfunctioning adenoma showed that 32% of patients not receiving postoperative radiotherapy exhibited tumor regrowth (mean follow-up, 76 months).[314] Similar recurrence rates were observed in a retrospective follow-up study of 212 patients.[315] In another study, tumor recurrence or regrowth occurred in 6% to 46% of patients not receiving radiotherapy after transsphenoidal surgery, whereas patients who underwent radiotherapy had a recurrence rate of 0% to 36%.[316]

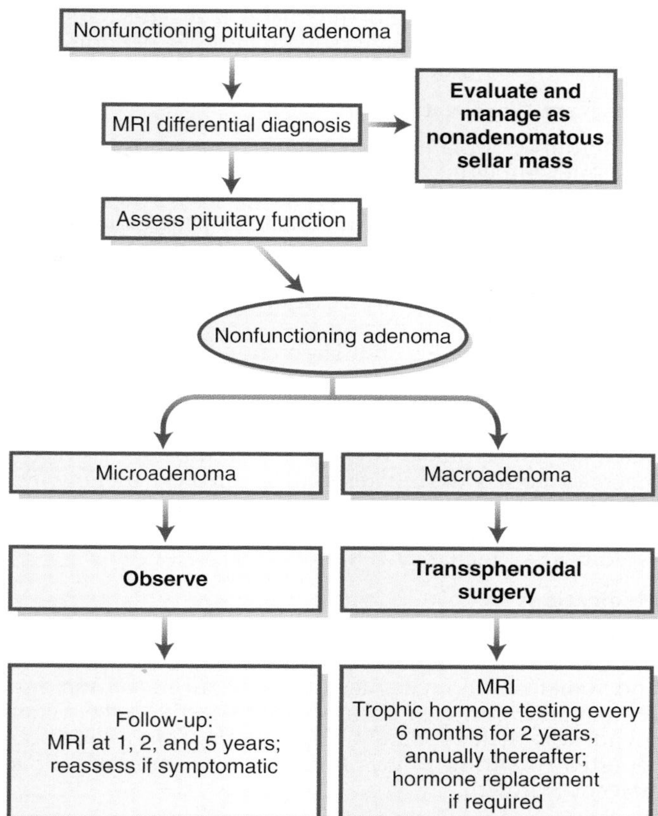

Figure 9-22 Management of nonfunctioning pituitary adenomas. Skilled interpretation of magnetic resonance images (MRI) is crucial to diagnose a nonadenomatous mass such as a meningioma, aneurysm, or other sellar lesion.

Nevertheless, despite the relatively high incidence of postoperative tumor regrowth even after apparently complete resection, many neurosurgeons avoid routine postoperative radiation therapy. This approach requires advising careful follow-up, with periodic annual MRIs and visual evaluations, and encouraging patients to maintain medical follow-up. Radiation can be offered if the tumor mass re-expands.[311]

The role of gamma knife radiosurgery versus fractionated radiotherapy remains unclear.[317] In a retrospective study of 62 patients with nonfunctioning pituitary tumors treated with gamma knife radiosurgery, 60% experienced decreased tumor size, and 37% of tumors remained unchanged. However, the risk of developing new anterior pituitary hormone deficits at 5 years was 32%.[318] Because patients experience tumor regrowth even after radiation therapy, all radiated patients should undergo periodic post-treatment MRIs, albeit less frequently.[319]

Expectant Observation

For nonfunctioning microadenomas or small macroadenomas (incidentalomas), patients may be observed expectantly.[320] Some tumors do not grow over years or even decades.[305] However, regular MRI follow-up is obligatory, especially for those patients with postoperative remnants or tumors that immunostain positively for ACTH (silent corticotroph adenomas).[321] Nonfunctioning adenomas may grow insidiously after surgery and are usually asymptomatic until they become large enough to affect vision. Periodic, but less frequent, endocrine evaluation is also suggested according to the clinical situation. Microadenomas only very rarely impair vision during pregnancy; macroadenomas do so with greater frequency.[322] Because macroadenomas do not respond to medical therapy, the risk of visual impairment arising during a pregnancy must be weighed carefully, and tumor resection may be indicated before pregnancy is undertaken.

Medications

Medications are not usually effective in reducing tumor size and visual compromise. Although GnRH antagonists and somatostatin analogues modestly shrink tumors in a few patients, they are not sufficiently effective to be recommended as therapy. Rarely, dopamine agonists have been reported to shrink some nonfunctioning tumors[323] or to prevent regrowth.[324]

ACROMEGALY

In 1886, Pierre Marie published the first clinical description of disordered somatic growth and proportion and proposed the name "acromegaly." He also recognized cases previously described by others.[325] After the relation of this syndrome to a pituitary tumor was recognized, Benda showed in 1900 that these tumors comprise mainly adenohypophyseal eosinophilic cells, which he proposed to be hyperfunctioning.[326] Cushing, Davidoff, and Bailey documented the clinicopathologic features of acromegaly and demonstrated clinical remission of soft tissue signs after adenoma resection.[327] Evans and Long induced gigantism in rats injected with anterior pituitary extracts, confirming the association of a pituitary factor with somatic growth.[328] Establishment of the unequivocal pathophysiologic link between hyperfunctioning adenoma and acromegaly made this the earliest example of a clinically and pathologically recognized pituitary disorder to be appropriately managed by surgical excision of a hypersecreting source.

Incidence

The prevalence of acromegaly is estimated to range from 38 to 80 cases per million population, and the annual incidence of new patients is 3 to 4 cases per million.[158,329-331] Based on these findings, it is apparent that more than 1000 new cases of acromegaly are diagnosed annually in the United States.

Pathogenesis

GH and IGF1 act both independently and dependently to induce features of hypersomatotropism. Acromegaly is caused by pituitary tumors that secrete GH or, very rarely, by extrapituitary disorders (Fig. 9-23).[332] Regardless of the etiology, the disease is characterized by elevated levels of GH and IGF1 with resultant signs and symptoms of hypersomatotropism.

Pituitary Acromegaly

More than 95% of patients with acromegaly harbor a GH-secreting pituitary adenoma (Table 9-18). Pure GH-cell adenomas contain either densely or sparsely staining cytoplasmic GH granules, and these two variants are slow and rapidly growing, respectively.[333] The former arise insidiously and manifest during or after middle age, whereas the latter arise in younger subjects with more florid disease.

Mixed GH-cell and PRL-cell adenomas are composed of distinct somatotrophs expressing GH and lactotrophs expressing PRL. Monomorphous acidophil stem cell adenomas arise from the common GH and PRL stem cell and also often contain giant mitochondria and misplaced GH granule exocytosis. They grow rapidly, are invasive, and manifest with predominant features of hyperprolactinemia.[334] Monomorphous mammosomatotroph adenomas express both GH and PRL from a single cell, whereas plurihormonal tumors may express GH with any combination of PRL, TSH, ACTH, or α-subunit.[335] These patients present with clinical features of acromegaly as well as hyperprolactinemia, Cushing's disease, or, rarely, hyperthyroxinemia. Somatotroph hyperplasia is difficult to distinguish from a GH-cell adenoma, and silver staining displays a well preserved reticulin network without a surrounding pseudocapsule. The rigorous morphologic diagnosis of GH-cell hyperplasia is usually associated with stimulation by ectopic GHRH derived from an extrapituitary tumor causing acromegaly.

So-called silent somatotroph adenomas immunostain positively for GH and are apparently clinically nonfunctional, although GH and/or PRL levels may be modestly elevated in more than half of these patients.

Pathogenesis of Somatotroph Cell Adenomas. Both pituitary and hypothalamic factors influence pituitary tumor pathogenesis.[336,337] Even when exhibiting marked nuclear pleomorphism, mitotic activity, and invasiveness, these tumors are usually benign.

Disordered GHRH Secretion or Action. Adenomas express receptors for GHRH, ghrelin,[338] and SRIF, but no activating mutations of the GHRH or SRIF receptor have been reported. GHRH directly stimulates GH gene expression and also induces somatotroph mitotic activity. Transgenic GHRH expression causes somatotroph hyperplasia and, ultimately, adenoma. Clinically, GHRH production by hypothalamic, abdominal, or chest neuroendocrine tumors causes somatotroph hyperplasia and, rarely, adenoma, with resultant unrestrained GH secretion and acromegaly.[165] However, histologic examination of most pituitary GH-cell adenoma tissue specimens does not show hyperplastic somatotroph tissue surrounding the adenoma, implying no generalized hypothalamic overstimulation.

Failure to downregulate GH secretion during prolonged GHRH stimulation also points to a role for GHRH in maintaining persistent GH hypersecretion. Furthermore, a GHRH antagonist was found to reduce production of human growth hormone (hGH) in 50 patients with acromegaly, suggesting a role for endogenous GHRH.[339] Expression of intra-adenomatous GHRH correlates with tumor size and activity, implying a paracrine role for GHRH in mediating adenoma pathogenesis.[340] GHRH modestly stimulates PRL secretion, and up to 40% of patients with acromegaly also have hyperprolactinemia.

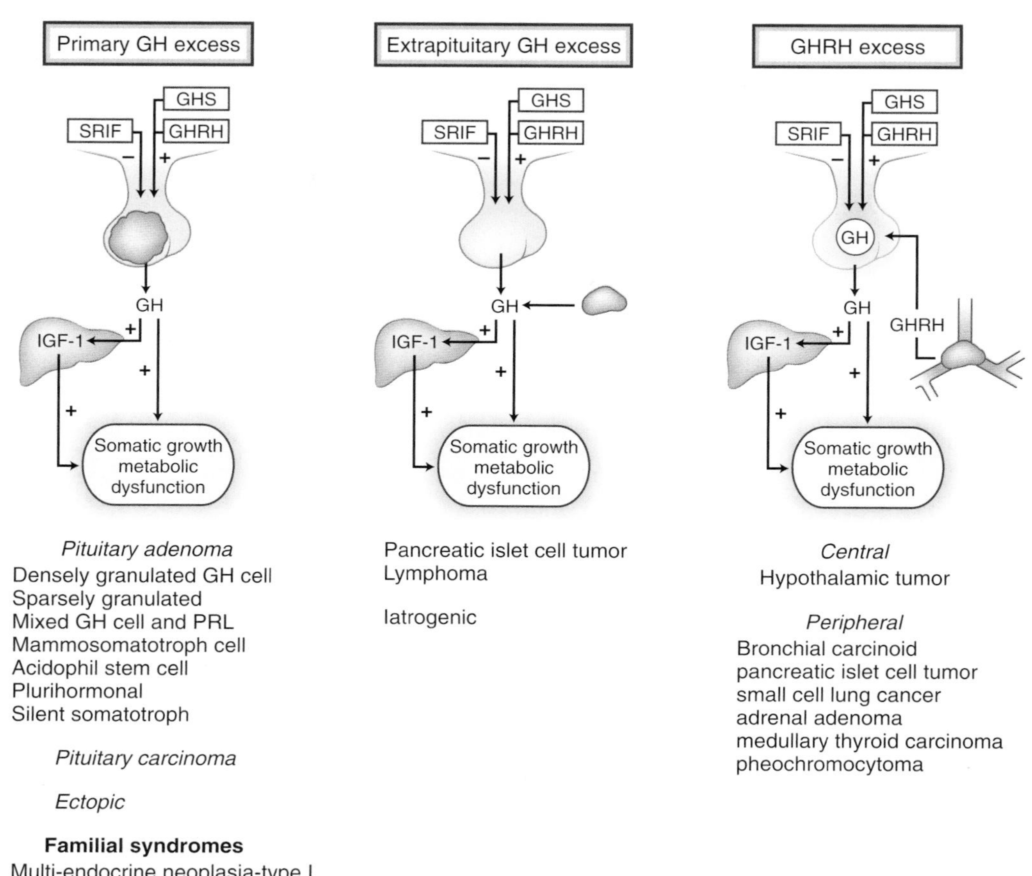

Figure 9-23 Pathogenesis of acromegaly. GH, growth hormone; GHRH, growth hormone–releasing hormone; GHS, growth hormone secretagogue; IGF-1, insulin-like growth factor type 1; PRL, prolactin; SRIF, somatostatin. (Reproduced from Melmed S. Acromegaly. *N Engl J Med.* 2006;355:2558-2573.)

Complete surgical resection of well-defined GH-secreting microadenomas usually results in a definitive cure of excess hormone secretion with very low postoperative tumor recurrence rates, strongly suggesting intact hypothalamic function in these patients. Although basal GH levels are usually high in acromegaly, the episodic pulsatile pattern of GH release is intact, and the nocturnal GH surge is usually preserved.[341] Patients treated with SRIF analogues also retain GH pulsatility, and GH pulse amplitude and sensitivity to GHRH appear to remain intact.

Disordered Somatotroph Cell Function. A somatotroph mutation may be a prerequisite for the abnormal growth response to disordered GHRH secretion or action (see earlier discussion). The monoclonal origin of somatotroph adenomas was determined by X-chromosome inactivation analysis of somatotroph tumor DNA.[167] An altered $G_s(\alpha)$ protein identified in a subset of GH-secreting pituitary adenomas leads to high levels of intracellular cAMP and GH hypersecretion.[173] Point mutations in two critical sites, Arg201, the site for adenosine diphosphate ribosylation, and Gly227, the guanosine triphosphate (GTP)-binding domain of $G_s(\alpha)$, prevent GTPase activity and result in constitutive adenyl cyclase activation. This dominant *GSP* mutant mimics GHRH effects results in elevated cAMP levels and is present in about 30% of GH-secreting tumors. Germline inactivating mutations of *AIP* were found in a subset of familial somatotropinomas,[208,342] especially in younger patients with acromegaly or gigantism. This mutation may have been inherited from an ancestor 57 to 66 generations earlier. AIP mutation is pituitary adenomal. However, no defined tumor suppressor gene has been isolated for sporadic nonfamilial GH-secreting tumors.

The sequence of events leading to somatotroph clonal expansions appears to be multifactorial. An activated oncogene may be required for initiation of tumorigenesis, whereas promotion of tumor growth may require stimulation of GHRH and other growth factors. The cellular mutation may not be sufficient to provide a growth advantage for a GH-secreting adenoma without additional disordered hypothalamic or paracrine growth factor signaling.

Extrapituitary Acromegaly

The source of excess GH secretion in acromegaly may not necessarily be pituitary in origin.[343] Because management of ectopic acromegaly differs from that for pituitary GH hypersecretion, rigorous clinical and biochemical criteria should be fulfilled to confirm the diagnosis of ectopic acromegaly.[344] These include demonstration of elevated circulating GHRH or GH levels in the absence of a primary pituitary lesion, a significant arteriovenous hormone gradient across the ectopic tumor source, biochemical and clinical cure of acromegaly after resection of the ectopic hormone-producing tumor, and normalization of the GHRH-GH-IGF1 axis. Finally, GHRH or GH gene product expression should be shown. Patients with nonconclusive imaging, biochemical, or clinical features of pituitary

TABLE 9-18

Causes of Acromegaly

Cause	Prevalence (%)	Hormonal Products	Clinical Features	Pathologic Characteristics
Excess GH Secretion				
Pituitary	98			
Densely granulated GH-cell adenoma	30	GH	Slow-growing, clinically insidious	Resemble normal somatotrophs, numerous large secretory granules
Sparsely granulated adenoma	30	GH	Rapidly growing, often invasive	Cellular pleomorphism, characteristic ultrastructure
Mixed GH-cell and PRL-cell adenoma	25	GH and PRL	Variable	Densely granulated somatotrophs, sparsely granulated lactotrophs
Mammosomatotroph cell adenoma	10	GH and PRL	Common in children; gigantism, mild hyperprolactinemia	Both GH and PRL in same cell, often same secretory granule
Acidophil stem cell adenoma		PRL and GH	Rapidly growing, invasive, hyperprolactinemia dominant	Distinctive ultrastructure, giant mitochondria
Plurihormonal adenoma		GH (PRL with αGSU, FSH/LH, TSH, or ACTH	Often secondary hormonal products are clinically silent	Variable; either monomorphous or plurimorphous
GH-cell carcinoma or metastases		GH	Usually aggressive	Documented metastasis
MEN1 (adenoma)		GH or PRL	Pancreatic, parathyroid, or pituitary tumors	Adenoma
McCune-Albright syndrome		GH, PRL	Classic triad	Hyperplasia
Ectopic sphenoid or parapharyngeal sinus pituitary adenoma		GH	Ectopic mass	Adenoma
Familial acromegaly		GH	Young patients	Large adenomas
Carney syndrome		GH	Classic syndrome	Adenoma
Extrapituitary Tumor				
Pancreatic islet-cell tumor	<1			Small pituitary
Excess GHRH Secretion				
Central—hypothalamic hamartoma, choristoma, ganglioneuroma	<1		Hypothalamic mass	Somatotroph hyperplasia
Peripheral—bronchial carcinoid, pancreatic islet-cell tumor, small cell lung cancer, adrenal adenoma, medullary thyroid carcinoma, pheochromocytoma	1	GH, PRL	Systemic features	Somatotroph hyperplasia, rarely adenoma

ACTH, adrenocorticotropic hormone; FSH, follicle-stimulating hormone; GH, growth hormone; GHRH, growth hormone–releasing hormone; αGSU, glycoprotein α-subunit; LH, luteinizing hormone; MEN1, multiple endocrine neoplasia type 1; PRL, prolactin; TSH, thyroid-stimulating hormone.

Adapted from Melmed S. Acromegaly. *N Engl J Med.* 2006;355:2558-2573; and Melmed S, Braunstein GD, Horvath E, et al. Pathophysiology of acromegaly. *Endocr Rev.* 1983;4:271-290.

acromegaly may inadvertently be diagnosed as harboring a nonpituitary source of excess GH secretion and be inappropriately treated.

GHRH Hypersecretion. Hypothalamic tumors, including hamartomas, choristomas, gliomas, and gangliocytomas, may produce GHRH with subsequent somatotroph hyperplasia or even a pituitary GH-cell adenoma and resultant acromegaly (see Fig. 9-23).[165] Primary mammosomatotroph hyperplasia with no evidence for pituitary adenoma or an extrapituitary tumor source of GHRH has been described in gigantism.[345] In fact, the structure of hypothalamic GHRH was elucidated from material extracted from pancreatic GHRH-secreting tumors in patients with acromegaly.[159] GHRH immunoreactivity is detectable in about 25% of carcinoid tumor samples, and bronchial carcinoids comprise most tumors associated with ectopic GHRH secretion.[346] However, acromegaly in patients with carcinoid is uncommon. In a retrospective survey of 177 patients with acromegaly, only a single patient was identified with elevated plasma GHRH levels.[347] Rare pancreatic cell tumors, small-cell lung cancers, adrenal adenomas, pheochromocytomas, and medullary thyroid, endometrial, and breast cancers express GHRH and may cause acromegaly.[348,349] Surgical resection of the tumor secreting ectopic GHRH should reverse the GH hypersecretion, and pituitary surgery is not required in these patients. Carcinoid syndrome with ectopic GHRH secretion can also be managed with somatostatin analogues, which lower GH and IGF1 levels and also suppress ectopic tumor elaboration of GHRH.[350]

Ectopic Pituitary Adenomas. GH-secreting adenomas may arise from ectopic pituitary remnants in the sphenoid sinus, petrous temporal bone, or nasopharyngeal cavity.[351] Very rarely, pituitary carcinoma may spread to the meninges, CSF, or cervical lymph nodes, resulting in functional GH-secreting metastases that may be diagnosed by radiolabelled octreotide imaging (Octreoscan).[352]

Peripheral Growth Hormone–Secreting Tumors. Lung adenocarcinoma, breast cancer, and ovarian tissues can contain immunoreactive GH without clinical evidence of acromegaly. Rarely, a GH-secreting intramesenteric pancreatic islet cell tumor[344] or a non-Hodgkin's lymphoma[353] causes acromegaly. These patients have a normal-sized or small pituitary gland on MRI, no GH response to TRH injection, and normal levels of circulating plasma GHRH.

Acromegaloidism. Rarely, patients who exhibit soft tissue and skin changes usually associated with acromegaly but normal baseline and dynamic GH and IGF1 with no demonstrable pituitary or extrapituitary tumor have been termed *acromegaloid*. Pachydermoperiostosis should be considered in the differential diagnosis. Insulin resistance and defective IGF1 binding have been demonstrated in cells derived from some patients with acanthosis nigricans, and treatment is symptomatic.

McCune-Albright Syndrome. The rare hypersecretory syndrome known as McCune-Albright syndrome consists of polyostotic fibrous dysplasia, cutaneous pigmentation, sexual precocity, hyperthyroidism, hypercortisolism, hyperprolactinemia, and acromegaly due to somatotroph hyperplasia.[354] Although few patients have definitive evidence for a pituitary adenoma, $G_s\alpha$ mutations have been detected in both endocrine and nonendocrine tissues.[174] GH hypersecretion can be controlled by somatostatin analogues or pituitary irradiation.

Multiple Endocrine Neoplasia. GH-cell pituitary adenoma is a well-documented component of the autosomal dominant multiple endocrine neoplasia type 1 (MEN1) syndrome, which also includes parathyroid and pancreatic tumors (see Chapter 41). MEN1, associated with germ cell inactivation of the *MENIN* tumor suppressor gene,[200] appears to be intact in sporadic GH-cell adenomas. Rarely, functional pancreatic tumors in patients with MEN1 also express GHRH.

Clinical Features

Manifestations of acromegaly are caused by either central pressure effects of the pituitary mass or peripheral actions of excess GH and IGF1. Central features of the expanding pituitary mass are common to all pituitary masses[355] and have already been described. In acromegaly, headache is often severe and debilitating. Local signs are especially important presenting features, because a higher preponderance of macroadenomas (>65%) is encountered in acromegaly, compared with mostly microadenomas for PRL-secreting tumors.[356]

Gigantism

Tall stature may be caused by a GH-secreting pituitary tumor or hyperplasia.[357] About 20% of patients with gigantism have the McCune-Albright syndrome, with somatotroph hyperplasia or, rarely, pituitary adenoma. Somatotroph hyperplasia and acidophilic stem cell adenomas may rarely cause gigantism during infancy or early childhood, suggesting early hypersecretion of GHRH or disordered pituicyte cell differentiation.[345,358] Pituitary gigantism should be considered in children who are more than 3 standard deviations above normal mean height for age or more than 2 standard deviations over their adjusted mean parental height. The biochemical diagnosis is similar to that for acromegaly: GH levels are in excess of 1 μg/L after a glucose load, and serum IGF1 concentrations are elevated. In children undergoing pubertal growth spurts, GH responses to glucose may be paradoxical, and serum IGF1 concentrations are often physiologically elevated. Therefore, the diagnosis requires clearcut MRI evidence for a pituitary lesion. The differential diagnosis includes familial tall stature, redundancy of Y chromosomes, Marfan's syndrome, and homocystinuria.

Clinical Features of Acromegaly

Effects of hypersomatotropism on acral and soft tissue growth and on metabolic function occur insidiously over several years (Table 9-19; Figs. 9-24 and 9-25).[359] The slow onset and elusive symptomatology often result in delayed diagnosis ranging from 6.6 to 10.2 years, with a mean delay of almost 9 years.[360] Patients may seek care for dental, orthopedic, rheumatologic, or cardiac disorders. Only 13% of 256 patients diagnosed during a 20-year period presented with primary symptoms of altered facial appearance or enlarged extremities.[361] In a review of several hundred patients presenting with acromegaly worldwide, 98% had acral enlargement, and hyperhidrosis was prominent in

TABLE 9-19

Clinical Features of Acromegaly*

Local Tumor Effects	Endocrine-Metabolic Effects
Pituitary enlargement Visual field defects Cranial nerve palsy Headache	*Reproductive* Menstrual abnormalities Galactorrhea Decreased libido, impotence, low sex hormone–blinding globulin
Somatic Effects	*Multiple Endocrine Neoplasia Type I (MENI)*
Acral Enlargement Thickness of hand and feet soft tissue	Hyperparathyroidism Pancreatic islet cell tumors
Musculoskeletal Gigantism Prognathism Jaw malocclusion Arthralgias and arthritis Carpal tunnel syndrome Acroparesthesia Proximal myopathy Hypertrophy of frontal bones	*Carbohydrates* Impaired glucose tolerance Insulin resistance and hyperinsulinemia Diabetes mellitus *Lipids* Hypertriglyceridemia
Skin Hyperhidrosis Oily Skin tags	*Minerals* Hypercalciuria, increased 1,25-hydroxy vitamin D3 Urinary hydroxyproline
Colon Polyps	*Electrolytes* Low renin Increased aldosterone
Cardiovascular Left-ventricular hypertrophy Asymmetric septal hypertrophy Cardiomyopathy Hypertension Congestive heart failure	*Thyroid* Low thyroxine-binding globulin Goiter
Pulmonary Sleep disturbances Sleep apnea—central and obstructive Narcolepsy	
Visceromegaly Tongue Thyroid Salivary gland Liver Spleen Kidney Prostate	

*Most soft tissue and metabolic changes are reversible by tight hormonal control. Bony changes, hypertension, and central sleep apnea are generally not reversible.

Modified from Bonert V, Melmed S. Acromegaly. In: Bar S, ed. *Contemporary Endocrinology.* Totowa, NJ: Humana Press; 2002:201-228.

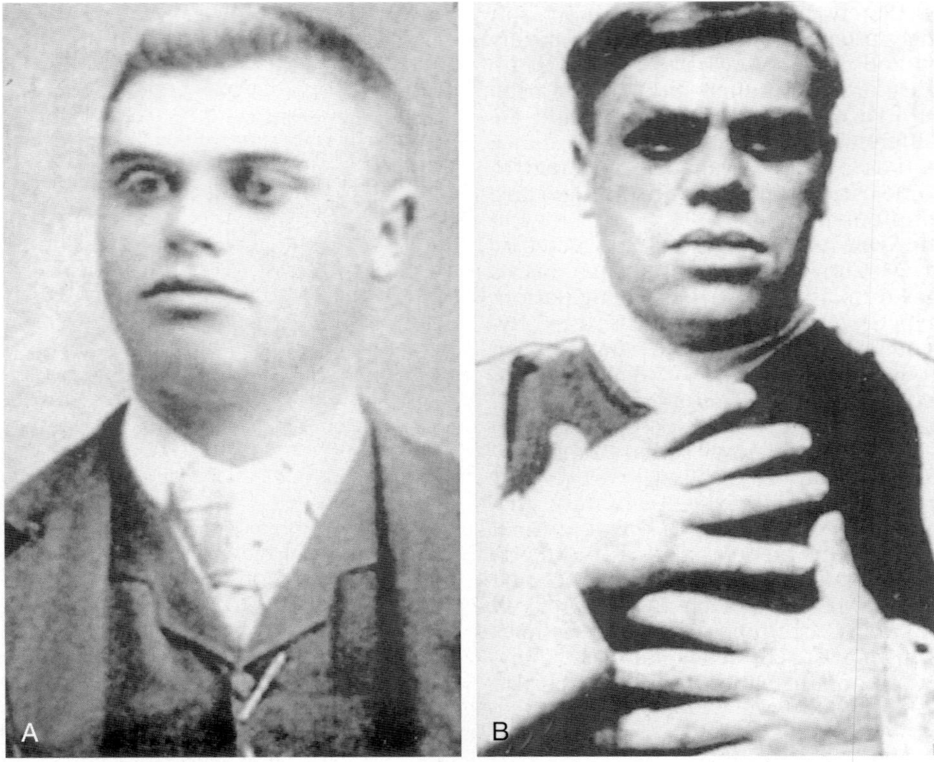

Figure 9-24 Harvey Cushing's first acromegaly patient, some years before presentation (**A**) and at admission (**B**). (Reproduced from Jane JA, Laws ER. History of acromegaly. In: Wass J, ed. *Handbook of Acromegaly.* Bristol, UK: BioScientifica; 2001:3-15.)

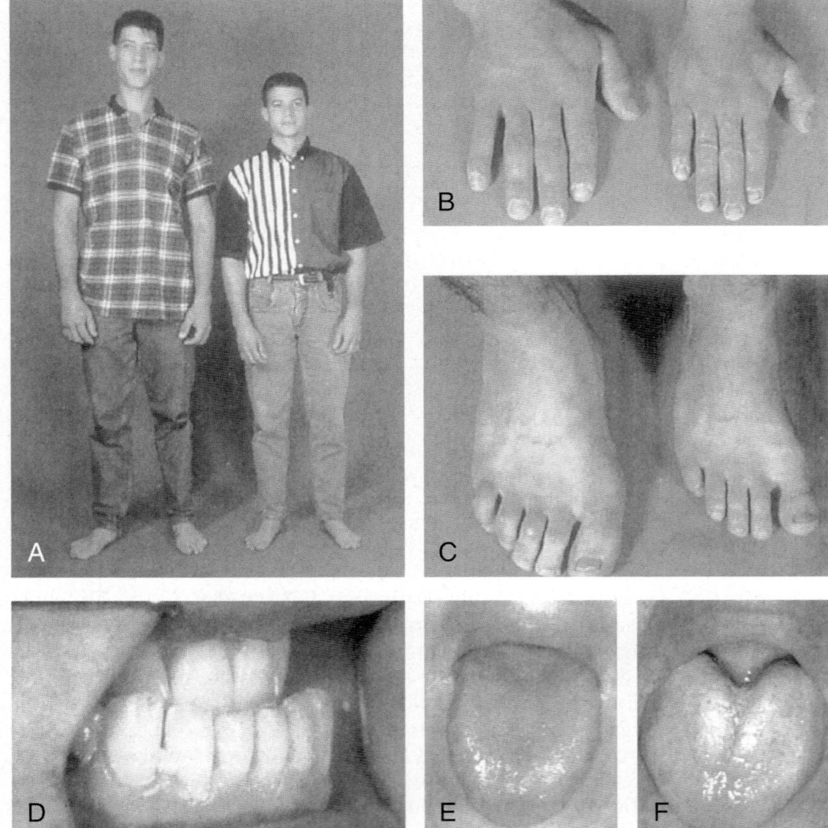

Figure 9-25 Clinical features of acromegaly. Features of acromegaly/gigantism in identical twins whose clinical features began to diverge at the age of approximately 13 years. A 22-year-old man with gigantism due to excess growth hormone is shown to the left of his identical twin. The increased height and prognathism (**A**) and enlarged hand (**B**) and foot (**C**) of the affected twin are apparent. (Reproduced from Gagel R, McCutcheon IE. Images in clinical medicine: pituitary gigantism. *N Engl J Med.* 1999;324:524, with permission.) **D,** Increased incisor spacing and prognathism in patient with acromegaly. **E.** Macroglossia; **F,** a normal tongue. (Reproduced from Turner HE. Clinical features, investigation and complications of acromegaly. In: Wass J, ed. *Handbook of Acromegaly.* Bristol, UK: BioScientifica; 2001; 24-25.)

70%.[359] When patients present early, facial and peripheral features are usually not obvious; serial review of old photographs often accentuates the progress of subtle physical changes. Characteristic features include large fleshy lips and nose, spade-like hands, frontal skull bossing, and cranial ridges. Enlarged tongue, bones, salivary glands, thyroid, heart, liver, and spleen are the effects of generalized visceromegaly. Clinically apparent hepatosplenomegaly, however, is rare. Increase in shoe, ring, or hat size is commonly reported.

Progressive acral changes may lead to facial coarsening and skeletal disfigurement, especially if excess GH secretion begins before epiphyseal closure.[362] These changes include mandibular overgrowth with prognathism, maxillary widening, teeth separation, jaw malocclusion overbite, and a large nose and coarse, oily skin with large pores.[248] Sonorous voice deepening occurs in association with laryngeal hypertrophy and enlarged paranasal sinuses. Up to half of patients experience joint symptoms severe enough to limit daily activities. Arthropathy occurs in about 70% of patients, most of whom exhibit joint swelling, hypermobility, and cartilaginous thickening.[363] These signs often persist after complete remission.[364] Local periarticular fibrous tissue thickening may cause joint stiffening or deformities and nerve entrapment. Knees, hips, shoulders, lumbosacral joints, elbows, and ankles are affected as monoarticular or polyarticular arthritides, but joint effusions rarely develop.[365] Spinal involvement includes osteophytosis, disc space widening, and increased anteroposterior vertebral length that may result in dorsal kyphosis.

Neural enlargement and wrist tissue swelling may lead to carpal tunnel syndrome in up to half of all patients. Median and ulnar nerve cross-sectional areas increase, and nerve conduction is abnormal.[366,367] Chondrocyte proliferation with increased joint space occurs early, and ulcerations and fissures of weight-bearing cartilage areas are often accompanied by new bone formation. Debilitating osteoarthritis may result in bone remodeling, osteophyte formation, subchondral cysts, narrowed joint spaces, and lax periarticular ligaments. Osteophytes commonly occur at the phalangeal tufts and over the anterior aspects of spinal vertebrae. Ligaments may ossify, and periarticular calcium pyrophosphate deposition occurs. Although the duration of hypersomatotropism correlates with clinical severity of the joint changes, it is unclear whether higher GH levels correlate with increased articular disease activity. Therapeutic responses usually depend on the degree of irreversible bony changes already in place. Hyperhidrosis and malodorous oily skin are common early signs, occurring in up to 70% of patients. Facial skin wrinkles, nasolabial folds and heel pads thicken, and body hair may become coarsened[368]; these changes are attributed to glycosaminoglycan deposition and increased connective tissue collagen production.[369] Skin tags are common and may be markers for the adenomatous colonic polyps.[370] Raynaud's phenomenon is reported in up to one third of patients.

Symptomatic cardiac disease is present in about 20% of patients and is a major cause of morbidity and mortality.[371] Hypertension is present in about 50% of patients with active acromegaly, and half of them have evidence of left ventricular dysfunction.[372] Left ventricular hypertrophy is also observed in about half of normotensive patients with acromegaly. Asymmetric septal hypertrophy is common, and cardiac failure with increased ventricular ejection fraction may occur with early or mild cardiomegaly. Subclinical left ventricular diastolic dysfunction results from myocardial hypertrophy, interstitial fibrosis, and lymphocytic myocardial infiltrates. Resting electrocardiograms are abnormal in about 50% of patients, with S-T segment depression, T-wave abnormalities, conduction defects, and arrhythmias. Plasma renin levels are suppressed, and endogenous plasma digitalis-like activity with chronic volume expansion has been identified in acromegaly.[373] Renal sodium channel activity is induced by GH at the aldosterone-sensitive distal nephron.[374] The presence of cardiovascular disease at the time of diagnosis portends a high risk of mortality despite improved cardiac function after effective GH and IGF1 control.[375]

Prognathism, thick lips, macroglossia, and hypertrophied nasal structures may obstruct aiways.[248] Irregular laryngeal mucosa, cartilage hypertrophy, tracheal calcification, and cricoarytenoid joint arthropathy lead to unilateral or bilateral vocal cord fixation or laryngeal stenosis with voice changes. Tracheal intubation may be particularly difficult in patients undergoing anesthesia, and tracheostomy may be required. Both central respiratory depression and airway obstruction lead to paroxysmal daytime sleep (narcolepsy), sleep apnea, and habitual excessive snoring. Obstructive sleep apnea, characterized by excessive daytime sleepiness with at least five episodes of apnea per hour of sleep, causes daytime somnolence, especially in men with acromegaly who also have a ventilation-perfusion defect with hypoxemia. Sleep apnea may also be central in origin and associated with higher GH and IGF1 levels.[376]

Synovial edema leads to hyperplastic wrist ligaments and tendons that contribute to painful median nerve compression. Peripheral acroparesthesias and symmetric peripheral neuropathy should be distinguished from diabetic neuropathy, which may occur secondarily to acromegaly.[377] Proximal myopathy may also be accompanied by myalgias, cramps, and nonspecific myopathic changes on electromyography. Exophthalmos may be present but may be masked by frontal bossing. Hypertrophied tissue surrounding the canal of Schlemm may impede aqueous filtration, leading to open-angle glaucoma. Progressive facial and bodily disfigurement often leads to lowered self-esteem. Depression and mood swings may occur secondarily to physical deformity.[378] Quality of life is also impaired.[379]

Growth Hormone and Tumor Formation

The early practice of hypophysectomy for management of metastatic carcinoma was based on evidence implicating GH as a factor in tumor development. GH and IGF1 exhibit direct and indirect mitogenic effects on mammalian cells and act as permissive growth stimulators of cells previously exposed to other growth factors.[380] The IGF binding protein 3 IGFBP3, also induced by GH (see Chapter 8), inhibits cell proliferation and promotes apoptosis.[381] Therefore, the ultimate impact of elevated GH levels on cell proliferation reflects a balance of apoptotic versus growth-promoting signals.[382]

A compelling cause-and-effect relationship between acromegaly and cancer has not been established.[383-386] Benign colon polyps were reported in 45% of 678 patients in 12 prospective studies (Table 9-20). The presence of more than three skin tags in patients older than 50 years of age may be a peripheral marker for adenomatous colon polyps, unrelated to GH or IGF1 serum levels.[387] Hypertrophic mucosal folds and colonic hypertrophy are commonly present, and dolichomegacolon may be visualized by CT colonography.[388] Although elevated IGF1 levels may correlate with colon polyp prevalence when patients are retested,[383] a recent controlled, prospective study of 161 patients showed no increased incidence of colon polyps in acromegaly.[382,389] Colonoscopy is warranted every 3 to 5

TABLE 9-20

Colon Polyps in Acromegaly*

No. Patients	No. Males/ Females	Mean Age (yr)	Adenoma	Hyperplastic	Total	Carcinoma	Reference
17	10/7	49	5	3	8	2	Klein 1982
12	11/11	56	2	1	3	2	Ituarte 1984
29	n.a.	n.a.	4	0	4	2	Brunner 1990
23	12/11	47	8	1	9	0	Ezzat 1991
54	26/28	47	5	11	19	0	Ladas 1994
50	25/25	25-70	11	12	23	1	Colao 1997
49	30/19	54	11	5	16	0	Vasen 1994
31	11/20	52	11	8	16	0	Terzolo 1994
103	49/54	51	23	25	48	0	Delhougne 1995
129	68/60	57	33	42	75	6	Jenkins 1997
115	63/69	54.8‡	27	18	45	3	Renehan 2000
66†	n.a.	32.7	25	18	43	1	Jenkins 2000
678			**165 (24%)**	**144 (21%)**	**309 (45%)**	**17 (2.5%)**	

*Incidence of colonic lesions in 678 patients prospectively evaluated in 12 studies. Of note, up to 45% of asymptomatic males age >50 yr harbored colon adenomas.

†Repeat colonoscopy.

‡Median age.

From Lieberman DA. Use of colonoscopy to screen asymptomatic adults for colorectal cancer. *N Engl J Med.* 2000;343:162-168; derived from Melmed S. Acromegaly and cancer: not a problem? *J Clin Endocrinol Metab.* 2001;86:2929-2934.

years after diagnosis, depending on the presence of other risk factors.

Increased mortality from colon cancer is largely related to uncontrolled GH levels, rather than an enhanced incidence of the disease in acromegaly (Table 9-21). Analysis of nine retrospective reports (1956-1998) encompassing 21,470 person-years at risk yielded no significant overall increased cancer incidence.[382] Cancer incidence was in fact lower than expected in 1362 patients with acromegaly in the United Kingdom, and the enhanced colon cancer mortality observed in that study correlated with GH levels.[385] In contrast, a nationwide study in Finland on cancer incidence in patients with acromegaly found an increased incidence of thyroid, bladder, and kidney cancers.[390] Therefore, although disordered cell proliferation and an increased risk for promotion of coexisting neoplasms could be anticipated from elevated GH and IGF1 levels, a significantly enhanced cancer incidence has not consistently been reported in acromegaly (Table 9-22). Colon cancer appears to be of particular concern, and a screening colonoscopy should be performed at diagnosis in all patients. Because patients are now living longer due to improved biochemical control, long-term prospective, controlled studies are required to resolve this question in an aging population.

TABLE 9-21

Post-Treatment Growth Hormone (GH) Levels and Mortality in Acromegaly*

	Post-Treatment GH (ng/mL)			
Mortality % (Range)	*<2.5* (n = *541*)	*2.5-9.9* (n = *493*)	*>10* (n = *207*)	Probability Value
Overall	1.10 (0.89-1.15)	1.41 (1.16-1.69)	2.12 (1.70-2.62)	.0001
Cancer-related	0.96 (0.63-1.41)	0.81 (0.50-1.24)	1.81 (1.13-2.74)	<.05

*Post-treatment GH levels correlate with mortality in acromegaly. Standardized mortality ratios are depicted for overall mortality and for cancer-related mortality.

Adapted from Orme S, McNally RJQ, Cartwright RA, et al. Mortality and cancer incidence in acromegaly: a retrospective cohort study. *J Clin Endocrinol Metab.* 1998;83:2730-2734.

Endocrine Complications

About 30% of patients exhibit elevated serum PRL levels (up to 100 μg/L or more), with or without galactorrhea.[391] Functional pituitary stalk compression by a pituitary mass prevents access of hypothalamic dopamine to the lactotroph, releasing the cell from tonic hypothalamic inhibition. GH-secreting adenoma subtypes may also concomitantly secrete PRL. Because GH behaves as an agonist for breast PRL-binding sites, the tumor may cause galactorrhea in the face of normal PRL levels. Tumor mass compressing surrounding normal pituitary tissue may also cause hypopituitarism. More than half of all patients have

TABLE 9-22

Acromegaly and Cancer Incidence: Multicenter Analysis

Study	No. Patients	Person-Years at Risk	Cancers *Observed*	*O/E*	Probability Value
Mustacchi, 1957*					
Females	95	1351	8	1.33	NS
Males	128	1630	5	1.30	NS
Total	223	2981	13	1.3	
Orme, 1998†	4822	21,740	178	0.76-3.4	NA

*Multicenter analysis of cancer incidence in patients with acromegaly ranging in age from 1-79 years. Adapted from Mustacchi P, Shimkin MB. Occurrence of cancer in acromegaly and in hypopituitarism. Cancer 1957;10:100-104.

†Analysis of retrospective published reports (1956-1998) of cancer incidence in patients with acromegaly. Included are data from Wright 1970; Alexander 1980; Nabarro 1987; Bengtsson 1988; Cheung 1997; Popovic 1998; Barzilay 1991; Mustacchi 1956; and Ron 1991. From Orme S, McNally RJQ, Cartwright RA, et al. Mortality and cancer incidence in acromegaly: a retrospective cohort study. *J Clin Endocrinol Metab.* 1998;83:2730-2734.

NA, not applicable; NS, not significant; O/E, observed/expected ratio.

amenorrhea or impotence,[356,392] and secondary thyroid or adrenal failure is present in about 20% of patients. Gonadal dysfunction may result in reduced bone.

The direct anti-insulin effects of GH cause carbohydrate intolerance, and patients may also develop insulin-requiring diabetes mellitus. Carbohydrate intolerance and insulin requirements improve rapidly when GH is lowered after surgery or somatostatin analogue therapy. Hypertriglyceridemia (type IV), hypercalciuria, and hypercalcemia also occur. Thyroid dysfunction in acromegaly may be caused by diffuse or nodular, toxic or nontoxic goiter or by Graves' disease, especially because IGF1 is a major determinant of thyroid cell growth.[393] Associated MEN1 features may be present in affected individuals, including hypercalcemia with hyperparathyroidism or pancreatic tumors. Benign prostatic hypertrophy has been documented in acromegaly with no apparent increase in prostate cancer rates.[394]

Morbidity and Mortality

In a meta-analysis of 16 studies, overall mortality was reported to be increased in acromegaly, with a standardized mortality ratio (SMR) of 1.72. Higher mortality rates were observed before 1993, most likely reflecting the positive impact of the introduction of somatostatin analogues, improved surgical technique, and enhanced cardiac therapies after that date.[395] Cardiovascular disease, respiratory disorders, and diabetes contribute to a threefold enhanced mortality rate in acromegaly.[396-401] Cardiovascular disease is the leading cause of death, followed by respiratory causes (18%) and cerebrovascular disease (14%). Diabetes mellitus, occurring in 20% of patients, is associated with 2.5 times the predicted mortality, and hypertension is present in about half of all patients (Fig. 9-26).[401]

The most significant mortality determinants are GH levels greater than 2.5 μg/L, elevated IGF1 levels, the presence of coexisting hypertension and cardiac disease, older age, a history of pituitary irradiation, and inadequately replaced ACTH-dependent adrenal insufficiency.[68] Importantly, overtreatment of adrenal insufficiency with doses of hydrocortisone greater than 25 mg/day also is predictive of mortality.[68] Moreover, control of GH levels to less than 2.5 μg/L and normal IGF1 levels after surgical or medical treatments significantly reduce both morbidity and mortality (see Fig. 9-26).[402]

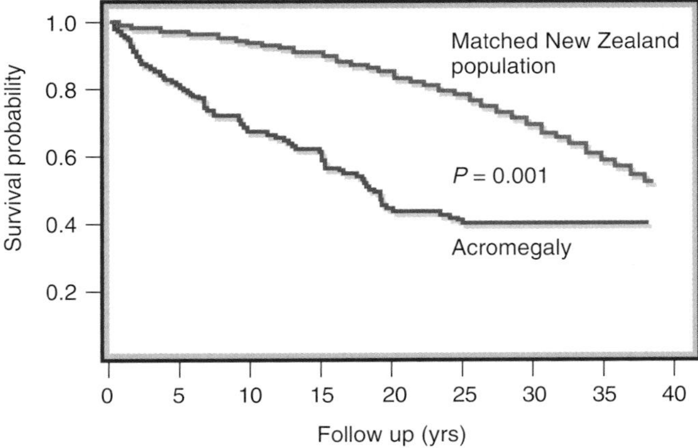

Figure 9-26 Mortality in acromegaly. Mortality outcome in acromegaly. (Data integrated from Holdaway IM, Rajasoorya RC, Wong J, et al. The natural history of treated functional pituitary adenomas. In: Webb S, ed. *Pituitary Tumors*. Bristol, UK: BioScientifica; 1998:31-42.)

Diagnosis

Measurement of Growth Hormone Levels

The diagnosis of acromegaly requires measurement of a GH nadir during oral glucose tolerance testing that is greater than 0.4 μg/L or 1 μg/L (depending on GH standards employed) together with elevation of age-adjusted IGF-1 levels.[403-405] In healthy subjects, serum GH levels initially fall after oral glucose administration and subsequently increase as plasma glucose declines. However, in patients with acromegaly, oral glucose fails to suppress GH, and GH levels are equally likely to increase, remain unchanged, or fall modestly.

Basal morning (a.m.) and random GH levels are usually elevated in acromegaly. Because of the episodic nature of GH secretion, however, serum concentrations may normally fluctuate from "undetectable" up to 30 μg/L. Unlike the largely undetectable nadir GH levels in normal subjects, patients with acromegaly from whom samples were obtained over 24 hours had detectable levels of GH (>2 μg/L).[406] Evoked GH responses to GHRH administration are not of diagnostic utility. A higher episodic GH pulse frequency occurs, which often persists after surgical adenoma resection. Random GH levels measured with sensitive assays in acromegaly may be as low as 0.37 μg/L with persistently elevated postoperative concentrations of IGF1.[400]

Serum IGF1 levels are high[407] and correlate with the log of serum GH determinations. IGF1 elevations (compared with age- and gender-matched subjects) may persist for several months after GH levels become biochemically controlled in response to treatment.[408] Increased IGF1 levels are also encountered during pregnancy and late puberty. A high IGF1 level is therefore highly specific for acromegaly and correlates with clinical indices of disease activity. IGFBP3 levels are also elevated but provide little added diagnostic value. GH-secreting adenomas exhibit discordant GH responses to TRH and GnRH administration in up to 50% of patients, but these adjunctive tests are rarely required to confirm the diagnosis.

Differential Diagnosis of Acromegaly

The overwhelming majority of patients with acromegaly harbor a GH-cell pituitary adenoma; rarely, extrapituitary acromegaly should be considered. Nevertheless, distinguishing pituitary from extrapituitary acromegaly is important for planning effective management. Regardless of the cause of unrestrained GH secretion, IGF1 levels are invariably elevated and GH levels are not suppressed (i.e., to <1 μg/L) after an oral glucose load.[405] When clinical features of acromegaly are associated with normal GH and IGF1 levels, "burned out" or "silent" acromegaly associated with an infarcted pituitary adenoma, often with a secondary empty sella, should be considered.[409] About 5% of consecutive patients with proven GH-cell adenomas have normal GH and increased IGF1 levels. It is likely that improved GH assay sensitivity will unmask abnormal GH secretion in these patients.

Dynamic pituitary testing (response to TRH and dopamine) does not distinguish patients with pituitary adenomas from those harboring extrapituitary tumors. Plasma GHRH levels are invariably elevated in patients with peripheral GHRH-secreting tumors but are normal or low in patients with pituitary adenomas.[410] GHRH plasma level measurement is precise and cost-effective for diagnosis of ectopic acromegaly. Peripheral GHRH levels are not elevated in patients with hypothalamic GHRH-secreting tumors, presumably because eutopic hypothalamic GHRH secretion into the hypophyseal portal system does not appreciably enter the systemic circulation.

The presence of unique or unexpected clinical features, such as respiratory wheezing or dyspnea, facial flushing, peptic ulcers, or renal stones, sometimes indicates the diagnosis of a nonpituitary endocrine tumor. Hypoglycemia, hyperinsulinemia, hypergastrinemia, and, rarely, hypercortisolism—all not usually encountered in pituitary acromegaly—should justify an evaluation for an extrapituitary source of GH excess. MRI and CT scanning may be employed to localize pituitary or extrapituitary tumors. Routine abdominal or chest imaging of all patients yields a very low incidence of true-positive cases of ectopic tumor, and such screening is not recommended as cost-effective. The presence of a normal or small-sized pituitary gland, or of clinical and biochemical features of other tumors known to be associated with extrapituitary acromegaly and elevated circulating GHRH levels, is an indication for extrapituitary imaging. However, an enlarged pituitary is often present in patients with peripheral GHRH-secreting tumors, and the radiologic diagnosis of a pituitary adenoma can be difficult to exclude. The McCune-Albright syndrome should be considered after definitive exclusion of pituitary and extrapituitary tumors.

Treatment

Aims

A comprehensive strategy for treatment of acromegaly should aim to manage the pituitary mass, suppress GH and IGF1 hypersecretion, and prevent long-term clinical sequelae of hypersomatotropism while maintaining normal anterior pituitary function.[403,405] An elevated GH level per se is associated with a threefold increased morbidity rate and is the single most important determinant of mortality.[396,398-401] It is important to reverse the mortality rate to that of age-matched healthy subjects by aiming for tight GH control.[411] Serum GH levels should be suppressed to at least 1 μg/L (or lower) after an oral glucose load, and IGF1 levels should be normalized for age and gender. With good control, there should also be a normal 24-hour integrated secretion of GH (<2.5 μg/L). GH may not be measurable for most of the day, yet the tumor may still be hypersecreting, as reflected by increased levels of IGF1. Current therapeutic modes for acromegaly management, including surgery, irradiation, and medical treatment, do not uniformly fulfill these goals.

Surgical Management

Well-circumscribed somatotroph-cell adenomas should preferably be resected by transsphenoidal surgery.[412-414] Successful resection alleviates preoperative compression effects and compromised trophic hormone secretion and, in the hands of a skilled surgeon, balances the extent of maximal tumor tissue removal with preservation of anterior pituitary function. Within 2 hours after successful resection, metabolic dysfunction and soft tissue swelling start improving, and GH levels are sometimes controlled within 1 hour. Surgical outcome correlates well with adenoma size, with preoperative serum GH levels, and particularly with the experience of the surgeon. Smaller tumors (<5 mm), tumor totally confined within the sella, and preoperative serum GH levels lower than 40 μg/L portend a favorable surgical outcome.

Up to 90% of patients with microadenomas achieve postoperative GH levels lower than 2.5 μg/L, whereas fewer than 50% of patients with macroadenomas of any size had postoperative GH levels lower than 2 μg/L after glucose administration.[415] Fewer than one third of all patients achieve control after resection of adenomas larger than 10 mm, but about 75% of patients with preoperative GH levels lower than 5 μg/L have normalized IGF1. Overall, in 17 studies of 1284 patients published between 1995 and 1999, 82% of patients harboring microadenomas had normalized IGF1 levels and 47% of those with macroadenomas achieved control (Table 9-23). A study of 2665 patients from a single center showed that 72% of patients with microadenomas and 50% of those with macroadenomas achieved GH levels lower than 1.0 μg/L during glucose loading and normal serum IGF1 levels.[416] Eight percent of these patients experienced a recurrence after 10 years.

Endoscopic transnasal surgery offers promise as a less invasive procedure for resection of pituitary tumors[417] and for accessing a cavernous sinus tumor mass, although long-term comparative results are not yet available.

TABLE 9-23

Results of Primary Transsphenoidal Surgery for Growth Hormone–Secreting Pituitary Adenomas

Study	No. Cases	Total Cure Rate (%)	Microadenomas	Macroadenomas	Criteria for Remission
Fahlbusch 1992	222	57	72	49	GH < 2 μg/L OGTT
		71	81	65	GH < 5 μg/L
Sheaves 1996	100	42	61	23	GH ≤ 2.5 μg/L
Abosch 1998	254	76	75	71	GH < 5 μg/L
Freda 1998	115	61	88	53	GH < 2 μg/L (OGTT) or normal IGF1
Swearingen 1998	149	70	91	48	GH < 2.5 μg/L (OGTT), normal IGF1
Laws 2000	117	67	87	50.5	GH ≤ 2.5 μg/L, GH ≤ 1 μg/L (OGTT), normal IGF1
Kreutzer 2001	57	70	N/A	N/A	GH ≤ 2.5 μg/L, GH < 1 μg/L (OGTT), normal IGF1
Shimon 2001	98	74	84	64	GH < 2 μg/L (OGTT), normal IGF1
De 2003	90	54	72	50	GH ≤ 2.5 μg/L, GH < 1 μg/L (OGTT), normal IGF1
Krieger 2003	181	56	80	31	Random GH <2 μg/L
Beauregard 2003	103	65	82	47	GH < 1 μg/L (OGTT), normal IGF1
Mortini 2005	320	59	83	53	GH < 1 μg/L (OGTT), normal IGF1
Nomikos 2005	490	56	78	50	Basal GH ≤ 2.5 μg/L, GH ≤ 1 μg/L (OGTT), normal IGF1

GH, growth hormone; IGF1, insulin-like growth factor type 1; OGTT, oral glucose tolerance test.
Modified from Wass, JAH, ed. *Acromegaly: A Handbook of History, Current Therapy and Future Prospects*. Bristol, UK: BioScientifica; 2009:142.

Difficulties in endotracheal intubation resulting from macroglossia or severe kyphosis may necessitate tracheostomy for anesthesia.

Side Effects. Although they are often transient, surgical complications may require lifelong pituitary hormone replacement. New hypopituitarism develops in up to 20% of patients, reflecting operative damage to the surrounding normal pituitary tissue.[418] Permanent diabetes insipidus, CSF leaks, hemorrhage, and meningitis occur in up to 10% of patients (see Table 9-3). The extent and prevalence of local complications depend on tumor size and invasiveness. Experienced pituitary surgeons report more favorable postoperative complication rates.[49] Biochemical or anatomic recurrence (approximately 7% over 10 years) or postoperative tumor persistence may indicate incomplete resection of adenomatous tissue, surgically inaccessible cavernous sinus tissue, or nesting of functional tumor tissue within the dura.

Radiation Therapy

Primary or adjuvant irradiation of GH-secreting tumors may be achieved by conventional external deep x-ray therapy or by heavy-particle (proton beam)[56,419-421] or gamma knife radiosurgery.[422] Maximal tumor irradiation should ideally be attained with minimal soft tissue damage. Precise MRI localization, accurate simulation, isocentral rotational techniques, and high-voltage (6 to 15 MeV) delivery have improved the efficacy of radiation therapy. Radiotherapy is a highly individualized choice, depending on the expertise and experience of the treating radiotherapist as well as physician and patient choice, considering the benefits of therapy weighed against potential risks. Up to 5000 rads is administered in split doses of 180-rad fractions divided over 6 weeks.

Radiation arrests tumor growth, and most pituitary adenomas ultimately shrink.[421] GH levels fall gradually during the first year after treatment, and levels are lower than 10 μg/L in 70% of patients after 10 years. Radiation therapy effectively shrinks GH-cell adenomas and lowers GH levels over 20 years in more than 90% of patients (Fig. 9-27).[423] However, when pretreatment GH levels were greater than 100 μg/L, only 60% of patients had GH levels lower than 5 μg/L after 18 years. During the first 7 years after irradiation, IGF1 levels were normalized in fewer than 5% of patients with acromegaly in one report,[419] whereas in another study, approximately 70% of patients exhibited normal levels when tested during longer follow-up.[420] Radiotherapy does not normalize GH secretory patterns, and this probably accounts for persistently elevated IGF1 levels in the face of apparently controlled GH levels.[424] Therefore, during the initial years after irradiation, most patients are still exposed to unacceptably high levels of circulating GH and IGF1.

Stereotactic pituitary tumor ablation by the gamma knife has been reported,[425] and 82% of those treated had normal serum IGF1 levels; some of these patients were being treated simultaneously with somatostatin analogues.[426] About 50% of patients achieved glucose-induced GH suppression to less than 1 ng/mL and normal IGF1 levels within 66 months after treatment.[422]

Side Effects. After 10 years, about half of all patients receiving radiotherapy have signs of pituitary trophic hormone disruption, and this prevalence increases annually thereafter, necessitating replacement of gonadal steroids, thyroid hormone, and/or cortisone. Side effects of conventional irradiation, including hair loss, cranial nerve

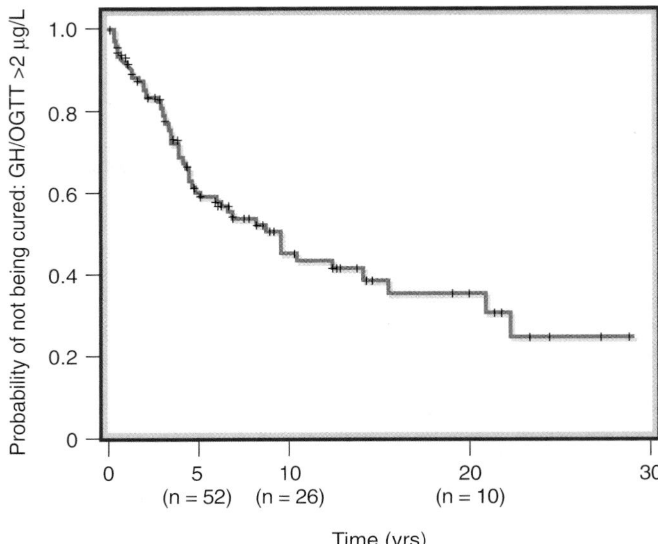

Figure 9-27 Radiation treatment of acromegaly. Long-term effects of radiation therapy on secretion of growth hormone (GH), using a GH nadir after oral glucose load (OGTT) of 2 μg/L or less as the cure criterion, and the probability of not being cured with time after radiotherapy. The number of patients not cured at 5, 10, and 20 years after pituitary irradiation are indicated in parentheses. Each step represents one cure; each cross (+) denotes a patient not cured at the latest follow-up. (Reproduced from Barrande G, Pittino-Lungo M, Coste J, et al. Hormonal and metabolic effects of radiotherapy in acromegaly: long term results in 128 patients followed in a single center. *J Clin Endocrinol Metab.* 2000;85:3779-3785.)

palsies, tumor necrosis with hemorrhage, and, rarely, loss of vision or pituitary apoplexy, have been documented in up to 2% of patients.[427] Lethargy, impaired memory, and personality changes may also occur.[397] The incidence and extent of local complications have been markedly diminished by the use of highly reproducible simulators, precise rotational isocentric arc capability, and doses of less than 5000 rads. The use of Bragg-peak proton beam therapy is contraindicated in patients with suprasellar tumor extension because of unacceptable optic tract exposure to the radiation field. The rare development of second brain tumors in these patients has been reported at a cumulative risk frequency of 1.9% over 20 years.[62,63] In a 10-year follow-up study of 35 patients treated with gamma knife radiosurgery, half the patients developed pituitary hormone deficiencies (40% hypoadrenalism, 11% hypothyroidism, 13% hypogonadism, and 6% GH deficiency).[426]

GH deficiency may result from radiation therapy.[428] Importantly, even patients treated with surgery alone can become GH deficient,[429] and in these patients, quality of life is reduced.[430] Because of side effects, radiation therapy should be employed as an adjuvant when control is not achieved by surgery or medical management and for patients who refuse these other therapies.

Medical Management

Dopamine Agonists. Because dopamine attenuates GH secretion in about one third of patients with acromegaly, D_2 receptor agonists, including bromocriptine and cabergoline, have been used as primary or adjuvant therapy for acromegaly.[270] Usually, up to 20 mg/day of bromocriptine lowers GH—a dose that is higher than that required to suppress PRL in patients harboring prolactinomas. Approximately 15% of patients worldwide have been reported to have suppressed GH levels (<5 μg/L) when taking the medication (7.5 to 80 mg/day),[431] and IGF1 is normalized in fewer than 10% of patients. Dopamine agonist efficacy appears to be independent of PRL concentration.[432] The drug causes minimal tumor shrinkage, but some patients experience subjective clinical improvement despite persistently elevated serum GH or IGF1 levels.

Side effects of bromocriptine are more marked than those of cabergoline, especially because high doses are required. These side effects include gastrointestinal upset, transient nausea and vomiting, headache, transient postural hypotension with dizziness, nasal stuffiness, and, rarely, cold-induced peripheral vasospasm (see earlier discussion). In an open study, cabergoline was reported to suppress GH to less than 2 µg/L and to normalize IGF1 in up to one third of patients with acromegaly.[433] Side effects included gastrointestinal symptoms, dizziness, headache, and mood disorders.

SRIF Receptor Ligands. Of the five SRIF receptor subtypes, SSTR2 and SSTR5 are preferentially expressed on somatotroph and thyrotroph cell surfaces and mediate suppression of GH and TSH secretion.[269,434] Several SRIF receptor ligands (SRLs) have been employed as approved or investigational drugs for acromegaly (Fig. 9-28). For more than 20 years, these analogues have proved safe and effective for controlling acromegaly. Octreotide (D-Phe-Cys-Phe-D-Trp-Lys-Thr-Cys-Thr-OH), an octapeptide SRIF analogue, binds predominantly to SSTR2 and less avidly to SSTR5[435] and inhibits GH secretion with a potency 45 times greater than that of native SRIF, but its potency for inhibiting insulin release is only 1.3-fold that of SRIF. The in vivo half-life of the analogue is prolonged (up to 2 hours) because of its relative resistance to enzymatic degradation. Rebound GH hypersecretion, seen after SRIF infusion, does not occur after octreotide injection. These properties are highly advantageous for long-term use of somatostatin analogues in acromegaly.[436] In vivo Octreoscan imaging

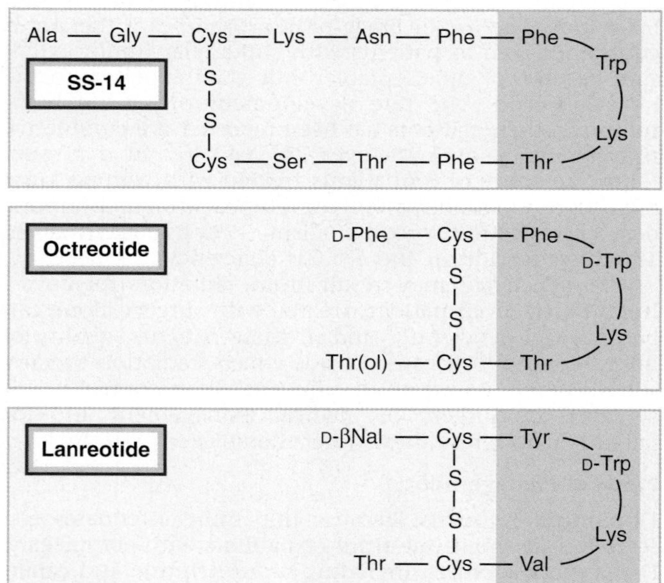

Figure 9-28 Amino acid sequences of somatotropin release–inhibiting factor (SRIF) receptor ligands. Amino acid sequences of the two available somatostatin analogues are shown compared with endogenous somatostatin-14 (SS-14). Color overlay depicts ligand-binding regions. (Reproduced from van der Lely AJ, Lamberts SWJ. Medical therapy for acromegaly. In: Wass J, ed. *Handbook of Acromegaly*. Bristol, UK: BioScientifica; 2001:49-64.)

with visualization of SRIF receptors demonstrates that GH responsiveness directly correlates with the abundance of pituitary receptors, and patients who are resistant to octreotide do not have visible in vivo receptor binding sites.[437] Transfection of the *SSTR2* gene to somatotrophs enhances responsiveness to somatostatin analogues.[438]

A single subcutaneous administration of octreotide (50 or 100 µg) suppresses GH secretion for up to 5 hours. In a double-blind, placebo-controlled trial, octreotide (injections every 8 hours) significantly attenuated GH and IGF1 levels overall in more than 90% of patients.[439] In patients with microadenomas, integrated GH and IGF1 levels are almost invariably normalized, whereas the response in those with larger tumors is less pronounced. A combination of octreotide and bromocriptine or cabergoline may provide added efficacy. Efficacy of octreotide action is determined by the frequency of drug administration, total daily dose, tumor size, presence of densely granulated tumors,[440] and pretreatment GH levels. Increasing the frequency of administration more effectively suppresses GH levels, and continuous subcutaneous infusion (up to 600 µg/day) provides sustained GH control.[441] Total daily octreotide doses of 300 to 1500 µg subcutaneously are optimal, and further dose increases usually are not beneficial for patients with resistant tumors. Elderly male patients are particularly sensitive to the GH-lowering effects of octreotide, and in the long term, desensitization does not occur.[442]

Long-acting somatostatin analogue formulations are convenient, enhance compliance, and allow sustained biochemical control (Fig. 9-29). Serum levels of a long-acting release (LAR) octreotide depot preparation (octreotide LAR, 20 to 30 mg intramuscularly)[443] peak at 28 days after a single injection, with integrated GH levels effectively suppressed for up to 49 days. Monthly injections for 9 years were shown to reduce integrated serum GH levels to less than 2 µg/L in more than 75% of patients.[444] Overall, IGF1 levels are normalized in 60% to 70% of patients,[445] and increasing the monthly dose of octreotide (Sandostatin LAR) to as high as 40 to 60 mg may improve efficacy.[446]

Lanreotide is a slow-release (SR), long-acting depot SRL that is administered as a fixed, 30-mg injectable dose every 7, 10, or 14 days. GH levels lower than 2.5 µg/L were achieved in 60% of 56 patients treated for 48 weeks, and suppression to less than 2.5 µg/L was achieved in about one third of 22 patients treated for up to 3 years, whereas IGF1 levels were normalized in almost two thirds of patients.[447] A longer-acting preparation of lanreotide (lanreotide Autogel, Somatuline Depot) is administered by monthly deep subcutaneous injection. In a randomized, placebo-controlled, multicenter study with a 52-week open extension, serum GH levels decreased by more than 50% from baseline in 63% of patients receiving lanreotide Autogel, compared with 0% of controls, and the medication was effective throughout the trial.[448] In one study, use of either of these SRL formulations was found to control GH levels in 100% and IGF1 levels in 97.8% of patients.[281]

In a critical analysis, octreotide LAR and Somatuline Depot were shown to be equivalent in the control of acromegaly symptoms and biochemical markers (Fig. 9-30).[449] In 166 patients with acromegaly, results of oral glucose tolerance tests were concordant for appropriate diagnosis and to establish efficacy of surgery and radiotherapy but were not helpful to evaluate effectiveness of medical SRL therapy. Measurement of serum IGF1 levels was sufficient to assess the effectiveness of SRL therapy.[450]

Effects of SRLs on Pituitary Adenoma. Tumors rarely grow while patients are receiving depot preparations of

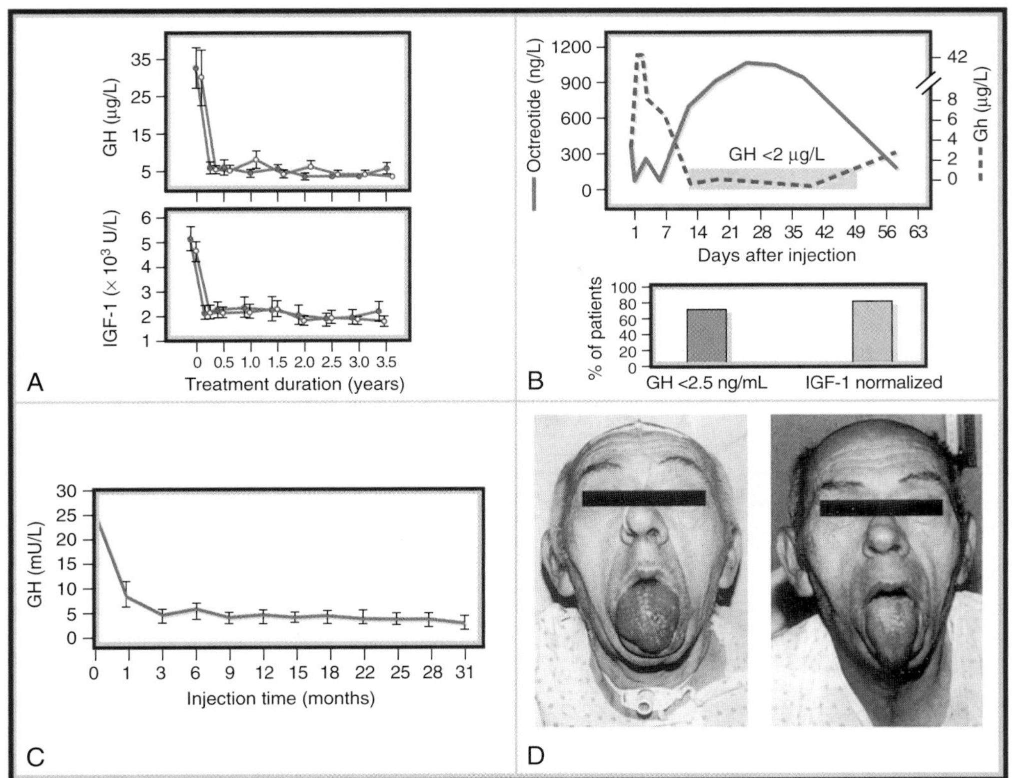

Figure 9-29 **A,** Growth hormone (GH) and insulin-like growth factor I (IGF-1) concentrations with long-term octreotide treatment. Comparison of primary octreotide treatment in 25 previously untreated patients (*open circles*) and in 80 patients who had previously undergone surgical resection or irradiation or both (*filled circles*). (From Newman C, Melmed S, George A, et al. Octreotide as primary therapy for acromegaly. *J Clin Endocrinol Metab.* 1998;83:3034-3040.) **B,** Pharmacodynamics of octreotide long-acting release (LAR). Twelve-hour mean serum octreotide and GH concentrations in a representative patient treated with a single 30-mg injection of Sandostatin LAR and monitored for 60 days. After injection, drug levels peaked at 28 days, and nadir GH levels were sustained for 4 weeks. (Adapted from Lancranjan I, Bruns C, Grass P, et al. Sandostatin LAR: a promising therapeutic tool in the management of acromegalic patients. *Metabolism.* 1996;45[8 suppl 1]:67-71.) **C,** Mean GH concentrations in patients with acromegaly after long-term treatment with octreotide LAR. Serum GH levels after monthly injections in 12 patients for 12 months and in 8 patients for 31 months. (From Davies PH, Stewart SE, Lancranjan I, et al: Long-term therapy with long-acting octreotide [Sandostatin-LAR] for the management of acromegaly. *Clin Endocrinol.* 1998;48:311-316.) **D,** Clinical impact of octreotide in reducing soft tissue swelling in a patient with acromegaly and obstructive sleep apnea before octreotide treatment (*left*). Note the macroglossia, tracheotomy for airway obstruction, and intranasal feeding tube. After 6 months of treatment with octreotide (*right*), tongue size was reduced by half, the tracheotomy and nasal tube were removed, and sleep apnea had resolved. (Courtesy of Seymous Reichlin University of Arizona, Treson.)

SRIF analogues. Significant tumor size decrease was reported in 52% of patients on primary therapy.[451] A critical analysis of 14 studies reported that 37% of patients treated primarily by SRL experienced significant tumor shrinkage.[452] Tumor shrinkage was reported in 75% and 78% of patients receiving octreotide LAR or Somatuline Depot, respectively, for up to 5 years.[281] In a systematic review of the effects of lanreotide SR and lanreotide Autogel, about one third of patients experienced tumor shrinkage (ranging from 10% to 77%).[453] Fifty-nine patients undergoing pituitary surgery were randomly assigned to treatment arms, and the 22 patients who received preoperative octreotide for 3 to 6 months demonstrated improved postoperative outcomes.[454-456]

Effects on Clinical Features. More than 70% of patients experience improved general well-being, and soft tissue swelling dissipates within several days after treatment. Headache, a common symptom in acromegaly, usually resolves within minutes after injection of octreotide,[457] most likely reflecting a specific central analgesic effect. Short-acting octreotide is preferable to long-acting formulations for acute headache resolution. Asymptomatic patients experience significant decreases in blood pressure, heart rate, and left ventricular wall thickness.[458] In patients with cardiac failure, octreotide reversibly reduces systemic arterial resistance, oxygen consumption, and fluid volume and restores functional activity. In 30 patients, improved left ventricular ejection fraction, with unchanged diastolic filling, was associated with octreotide-induced GH suppression to less than 2.5 μg/L. Control of IGF1 and GH levels was associated with improved left ventricular ejection function, but cardiac performance worsened in those who did not achieve such control.[459] Joint function and crepitus improved, there was ultrasound evidence of bone or cartilage repair, and, after several months, sleep apnea improved.[248]

Side Effects. SRLs are generally safe and well tolerated. Gastrointestinal side effects predominate; they include transient loose stools, nausea, mild malabsorption, and flatulence and are reported in about one third of patients. Hypoglycemia and hyperglycemia are not commonly encountered, and insulin requirements in diabetic patients with acromegaly are dramatically reduced within hours after receipt of octreotide, concomitant with GH lowering. Overall, SRLs do not cause major effects on glucose homeostasis, and hyperglycemia is likely associated with uncontrolled underlying disease.[460] The drug attenuates gallbladder contractility, delays emptying, and leads to reversible sludge formation evidenced by ultrasonography in up to 25% of patients.[461] Frank cholecystitis is very rarely reported

Comparing Octreotide LAR and Lanreotide ATG

	SRIF Analog	n	GH <2.5 µg/L (n)	Normal IGF-I (n)	Normal IGF-I GH <2.5 µg/L	Mean dose (mg/4 wks)
Alexopoulou 2004	OCT	25	16	13	9	25
	LAN	25	12	13	8	108
Ashwell 2004	OCT	10	9	6	6	20
	LAN	10	9	8	8	93
Van Thiel 2004	OCT	7	4	3	3	24
	LAN	7	3	3	3	111
Andries 2007	OCT	10	10	5	5	—
	LAN	10	7	6	5	—
Ronchi 2007	OCT	23	10	8	4	24
	LAN	22	13	9	7	96

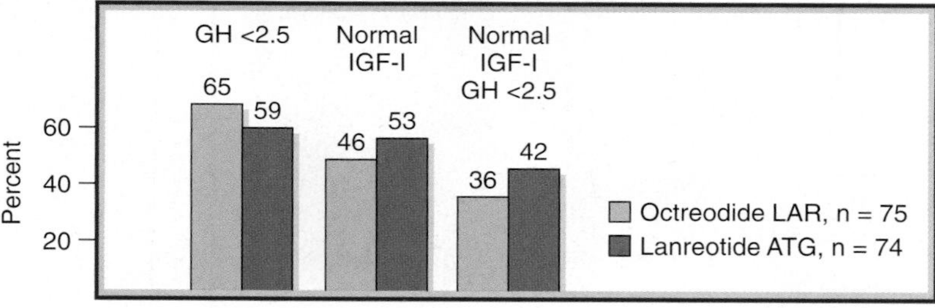

Figure 9-30 Summary of biochemical end points of studies comparing the efficacy of octreotide long-acting release (LAR) versus lanreotide Autogel (ATG). GH, growth hormone; IGF-1, insulin-like growth factor type 1; LAN, lanreotide ATG; OCT, octreotide LAR; SRIF, somatotropin release–inhibiting factor. (Adapted from Murray R, Melmed S. A critical analysis of clinically available somatostatin analog formulations for therapy of acromegaly. *J Clin Endocrinol Metab.* 2008;93:2957-2968.)

in these patients. The incidence of gallbladder sludge or stones is geographically variable, with higher rates reported in China, Australia, and the United Kingdom than elsewhere. In the United States, up to 30% of patients have demonstrable evidence of echogenic gallbladder deposits within the first 18 months after treatment. Thereafter, further sludge formation is not usually encountered.[443]

Octreotide may interact with several drugs, including cyclosporine, enhancing the risk of transplant rejection. SRL dose adjustments should be carefully titrated in patients who require insulin or oral hypoglycemic agents, calcium channel blockers, or β-blockers. Asymptomatic sinus bradycardia has also been recognized.

Growth Hormone Receptor Antagonist. GH action through the surface membrane GH receptor is mediated by ligand-induced receptor signaling.[462] The postreceptor GH signal is not elicited if the receptor is bound (Fig. 9-31) by pegvisomant, a GH-receptor antagonist, which blocks subsequent generation of IGF1.[462] The pegylated molecule also binds to the GH receptor dimer and interacts with growth hormone binding protein.[463] In earlier studies, daily injections of pegvisomant (20 mg) normalized IGF1 levels in more than 90% of patients and dose-dependently improved fatigue, decreased soft tissue swelling as assessed by ring size, and diminished perspiration.[462]

More recently, median 15-mg and mean 16.4-mg daily doses of pegvisomant were shown to normalize IGF1 in 55% of 273 patients in a national database at 6 months and in 71% of 202 patients after 24 months of treatment.[464] However, in a 91-month follow-up study (median follow-up, 18 months), IGF1 levels were controlled in 95% of patients treated in two centers.[465] The drug is particularly useful for patients whose tumors are resistant to SRL therapy because it effectively normalizes IGF1 levels in these patients.[466,467] However, rebound tumor enlargement after discontinuation of somatostatin analogues and tumor growth while receiving pegvisomant should be carefully monitored.[468]

Side Effects. Elevated hepatic transaminases have been reported,[469] and liver enzymes should be measured every 6 months. In one study analyzing liver function in 273 patients treated with pegvisomant, there were abnormalities in 20 patients, and 3 developed hepatobiliary failure.[464] Local injection site inflammation and lipodystrophy have been reported. Long-term impact of the drug on pituitary tumor growth is not yet evident, and MRIs should be performed periodically. Levels of GH rise as the IGF1 negative feedback on the pituitary is lost, and IGF1 should be monitored in these patients.[470]

SRIF Receptor Ligand and Growth Hormone Receptor Antagonist Combination. Combination treatment for acromegaly is most effective for patients in whom treatment with a somatostatin analogue has led to tumor shrinkage with reduction, albeit inadequate, in GH or IGF1 levels (Fig. 9-32). In 11 such uncontrolled patients, dual blockade of the GH axis with pegvisomant and SRLs was shown to exhibit greater efficacy than treatment with either drug alone.[471] Monthly doses of long-acting somatostatin analogue have been successfully combined with weekly doses of pegvisomant.[472] A study of 63 patients showed that 4 years of combination treatment was safe; however, 23 patients developed elevated liver enzymes, particularly if they were diabetic.[473]

Choice of Therapy

Although challenging, tight control of GH secretion and normalization of IGF1 levels should be sought, because adverse mortality rates correlate strongly with GH levels. If GH and IGF1 results after treatment are discordant, the respective assays should be repeated by a reputable laboratory using rigorous assay standardizations and appropriate sensitivity cutoffs.[474] Assessment of clinical activity may

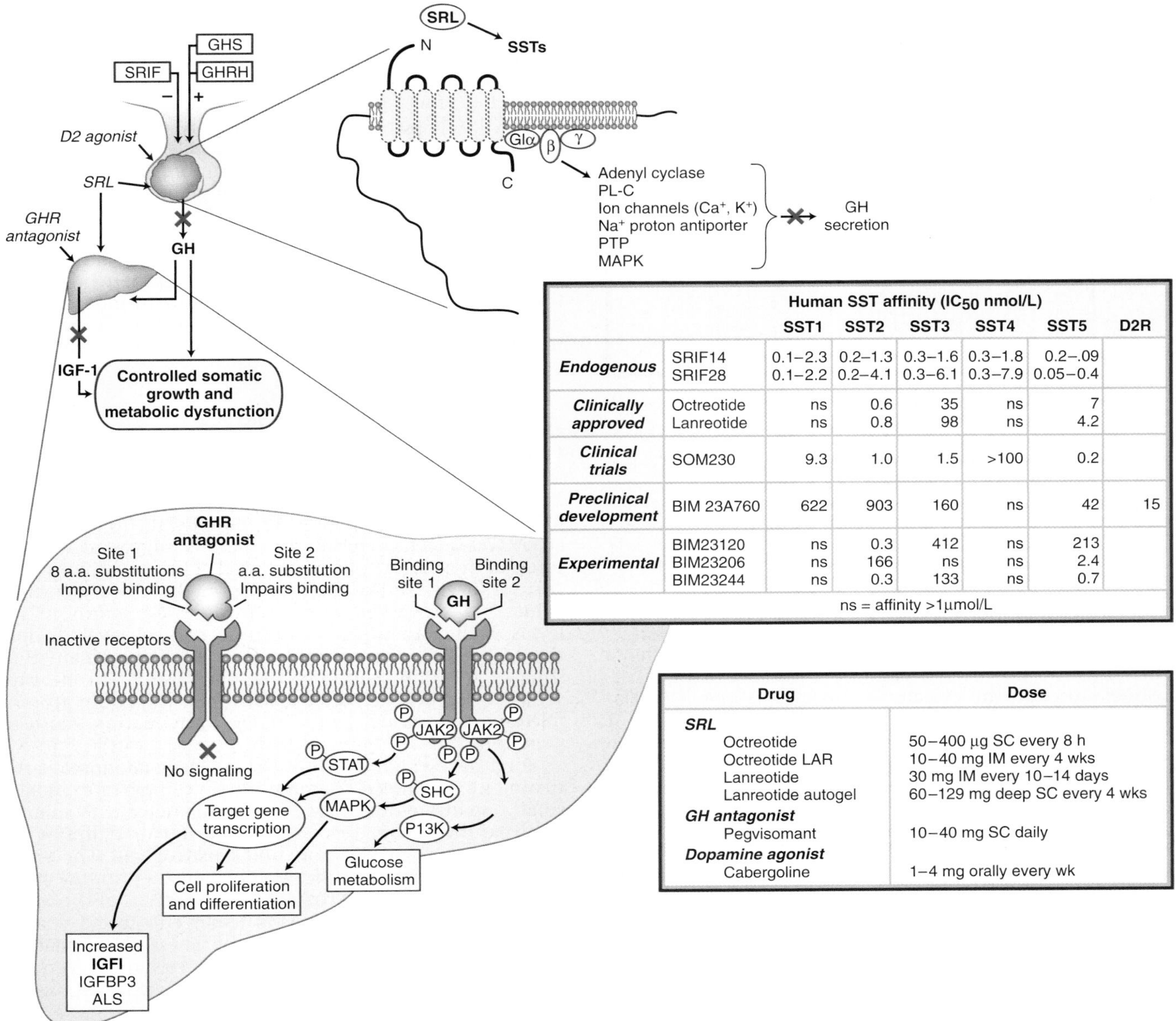

		Human SST affinity (IC_{50} nmol/L)					
		SST1	SST2	SST3	SST4	SST5	D2R
Endogenous	SRIF14 SRIF28	0.1–2.3 0.1–2.2	0.2–1.3 0.2–4.1	0.3–1.6 0.3–6.1	0.3–1.8 0.3–7.9	0.2–.09 0.05–0.4	
Clinically approved	Octreotide Lanreotide	ns ns	0.6 0.8	35 98	ns ns	7 4.2	
Clinical trials	SOM230	9.3	1.0	1.5	>100	0.2	
Preclinical development	BIM 23A760	622	903	160	ns	42	15
Experimental	BIM23120 BIM23206 BIM23244	ns ns ns	0.3 166 0.3	412 ns 133	ns ns ns	213 2.4 0.7	
ns = affinity >1 μmol/L							

Drug	Dose
SRL	
Octreotide	50–400 μg SC every 8 h
Octreotide LAR	10–40 mg IM every 4 wks
Lanreotide	30 mg IM every 10–14 days
Lanreotide autogel	60–129 mg deep SC every 4 wks
GH antagonist	
Pegvisomant	10–40 mg SC daily
Dopamine agonist	
Cabergoline	1–4 mg orally every wk

Figure 9-31 Action of growth hormone receptor (GHR) antagonist, somatostatin receptor ligands (SRLs), and dopamine (D2) agonists. Normally a single molecule of growth hormone (GH) binds two GH receptors through sites 1 and 2, and the GH signal transduction pathway is activated. Pegvisomant increases binding of GH receptor to site 1 and blocks binding at site 2 to prevent functional GH-receptor signaling, initiation of GH action, and induction of insulin-like growth factor type 1 (IGF1) synthesis and secretion. The peripheral effects of excess GH are antagonized at the cellular level, independent of the presence of somatostatin (SST) or D2 receptors on the pituitary tumor. SRLs inhibit GH secretion and IGF1 synthesis and suppress pituitary tumor growth. GH-secreting adenomas express predominantly somatostatin (SST) receptors 2 and 5. The figure depicts affinities for SST receptor subtypes and for the D2 receptor. a.a., amino acid; ALS, acid-labile subunit; C, carboxyl terminal; GHRH, gonadotropin hormone–releasing hormone; GHS, gonadotropin hormone secretagogue; IC_{50}, 50% inhibitory concentration; IGFBP3, insulin-like growth factor–binding protein 3; JAK2, Janus kinase 2 tyrosine kinase; MAPK, mitogen-activated protein kinase; N, amino terminal; ns, not significant; P, elemental phosphorus; PI3K, phosphoinositide 3 kinase; PL-C, phospholipase C; PTP, protein tyrosine phosphatase; SHC, Src homology–containing protein; SRIF, somatotropin release–inhibiting factor (somatostatin); STAT, signal transducer and activator or transcription. (Adapted from Melmed S. Acromegaly. *N Engl J Med.* 2006;355:2558-2573; and Heaney AP, Melmed S. Molecular targets in pituitary tumours. *Nat Rev Cancer.* 2004;4:285-295.)

indicate mild disease with suppressed GH and residual elevated IGF1 levels. Alternatively, normal or low IGF1 levels may be encountered in cases of systemic disease or malnutrition, with GH elevations reflecting persistent disease activity. Each treatment modality has advantages and disadvantages that must be weighed to individualize patient care (Fig. 9-33; Table 9-24).

Selective surgical excision of a well-defined pituitary mass is recommended for most patients with microadenomas. Remission rates are unacceptably low for patients with macroadenomas and locally invasive tumors. Attempted medical debulking of the sellar mass before surgery is desirable, and early controlled, prospective studies have confirmed the validity of this approach to improve surgical morbidity and possibly enhance subsequent postoperative outcomes, especially for patients with surgically inaccessible tumor tissue and cavernous sinus invasion. Debulking may improve subsequent

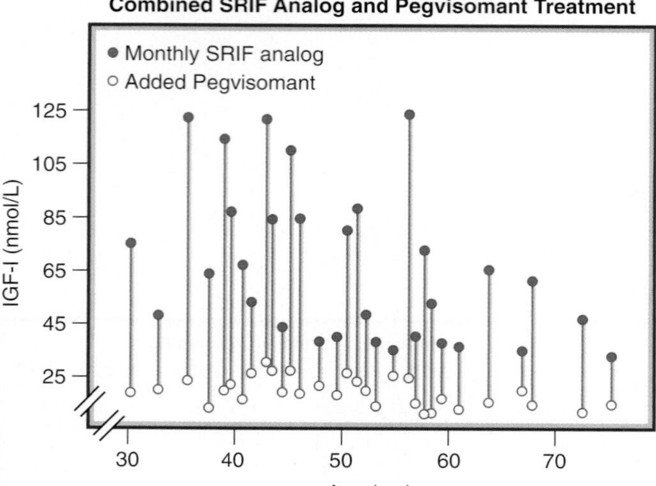

Figure 9-32 Concentrations of insulin-like growth factor type I (IGF-1) in serum of 31 patients with acromegaly before (•) and after (○) 138 weeks (range, 35 to 149 weeks) of combined therapy. Shaded area indicates age-dependent normal range for IGF1. SRIF, somatostatin. (Reproduced from Neggers S, van Aken M, et al. Long-term efficacy and safety of combined treatment of somatostatin analogs and pegvisomant in acromegaly. *J Clin Endocrinol Metab.* 2007;92:4598-4601.)

responsiveness to SRL therapy.[475] Postoperatively, patients with uncontrolled disease can also be treated with cabergoline; although the efficacy of this drug is low, it is relatively inexpensive and free of major side effects. A long-acting SRIF analogue should be administered, because the utility of an initial test dose of short-acting octreotide has been questioned.[476] Some patients may benefit by the addition of bromocriptine or cabergoline to the SRL.

Gallbladder ultrasonography should be performed only in symptomatic patients, and those with demonstrable sludge or gallstones may require prophylactic anticholelithogenic agents or laparoscopic cholecystectomy if symptomatic. Primary therapy with SRLs may be offered to those patients in whom complete tumor removal is not likely and to those who refuse surgery or in whom the risks of surgery or anesthesia are unacceptable. Invasive macroadenomas invariably hypersecrete GH postoperatively and require SRL treatment. In patients whose pituitary lesion does not compress vital structures, primary medical management may therefore be an appropriate therapeutic option.[281,477-479] Preoperative SRL treatment may also enhance subsequent surgical outcomes, especially for macroadenomas.[456] Pegvisomant, either alone or in combination with an SRL, should be offered to patients with resistant disease. Radiation should be administered to patients who are resistant to or cannot tolerate medications, prefer not to receive long-term injections, or cannot afford medication. After irradiation, medications are required for several years until GH levels are effectively controlled.

Tumors that recur despite medical therapy or irradiation may rarely require reoperation. Although tight GH control is critical, these patients also require counseling for anxiety engendered by disfigurements and interpretation of laboratory test results. Patients should be monitored quarterly until biochemical control is achieved. Thereafter, hormone evaluation is performed semiannually. For those patients who are in biochemical remission and have no residual tumor tissue, MRI should be repeated every 1 to 2 years. Follow-up evaluation includes documentation and treatment of new skin tag and lipoma growths, nerve entrapments, and jaw overbites; rheumatologic, dental, and cardiac evaluations; and metabolic assessments. Visual field perimetry (for macroadenomas) and pituitary reserve testing should be repeated semiannually, and pituitary MRI should be performed annually, especially for patients who have residual tumor or require hormone replacement or medical treatment. Mammography and colonoscopy should be performed as clinically indicated for patients older than 50 years of age and for those harboring polyps. Maximal and sustained long-term GH and IGF1 control should ameliorate the deleterious effects of these hormones through judicious use of available treatment modalities. A recent guideline for the approach to treatment has been recommended by the Acromegaly Consensus Group.[405]

ACTH-SECRETING TUMORS (CUSHING'S DISEASE)

The evaluation and management of Cushing's disease is fully described in Chapter 15. Briefly, the diagnosis of an ACTH-secreting pituitary tumor is suggested by features of hypercortisolism, elevated 24-hour urinary free cortisol levels, and/or elevated late-night salivary cortisol values,[480-482] together with nonsuppressed serum ACTH levels. Failure to suppress morning cortisol levels to less than 1.8 μg/dL after administration of 1 mg dexamethasone at 11 p.m. supports the diagnosis.[482] In healthy subjects, glucocorticoid feedback suppresses corticotropin-releasing hormone and ACTH, attenuating cortisol secretion.

Surgical resection of an ACTH-secreting adenoma is the treatment of choice. Because these tumors are usually small, sometimes less than 2 mm in diameter, they may be localized incorrectly, or not at all, by venous sampling for ACTH (see earlier discussion) and sensitive MRI. Therefore, these tumors pose a significant challenge even for the experienced surgeon. Furthermore, the disorder is also characterized by venous hypertension leading to turgid venous sinuses,[483] requiring control by the anesthetist. Bilateral petrosal venous sampling for ACTH levels and cavernous sinus venography should ideally be performed before surgery. However, if sellar venous sinus drainage is predominately unilateral, left-right ACTH gradients may not reliably lateralize the lesion. Hemihypophysectomy may be curative in 80% of patients with clearly defined biochemical features of ACTH-dependent Cushing's disease in whom an ACTH gradient is indeed detected and venous drainage patterns are normal. Meticulous surgical exploration of both anterior and posterior lobes is required for these tiny tumors, which are often off-white and speckled by petechiae and may be inadvertently suctioned. Even carefully performed preoperative lateralization is not infallible, and the so-called normal side should also be carefully explored.

Assessment of Surgical Outcome

Transsphenoidal resection is the preferred treatment for these adenomas.[484] After selective adenomectomy of a clearly identifiable adenoma, remission was achieved in 75% of 295 patients. However, partial hypophysectomy in 31 patients in whom an adenoma could not be identified resulted in biochemical remission in only 10 patients.[89] On the third postoperative day, 1 mg dexamethasone may be given at 10 p.m. and cortisol levels measured the following

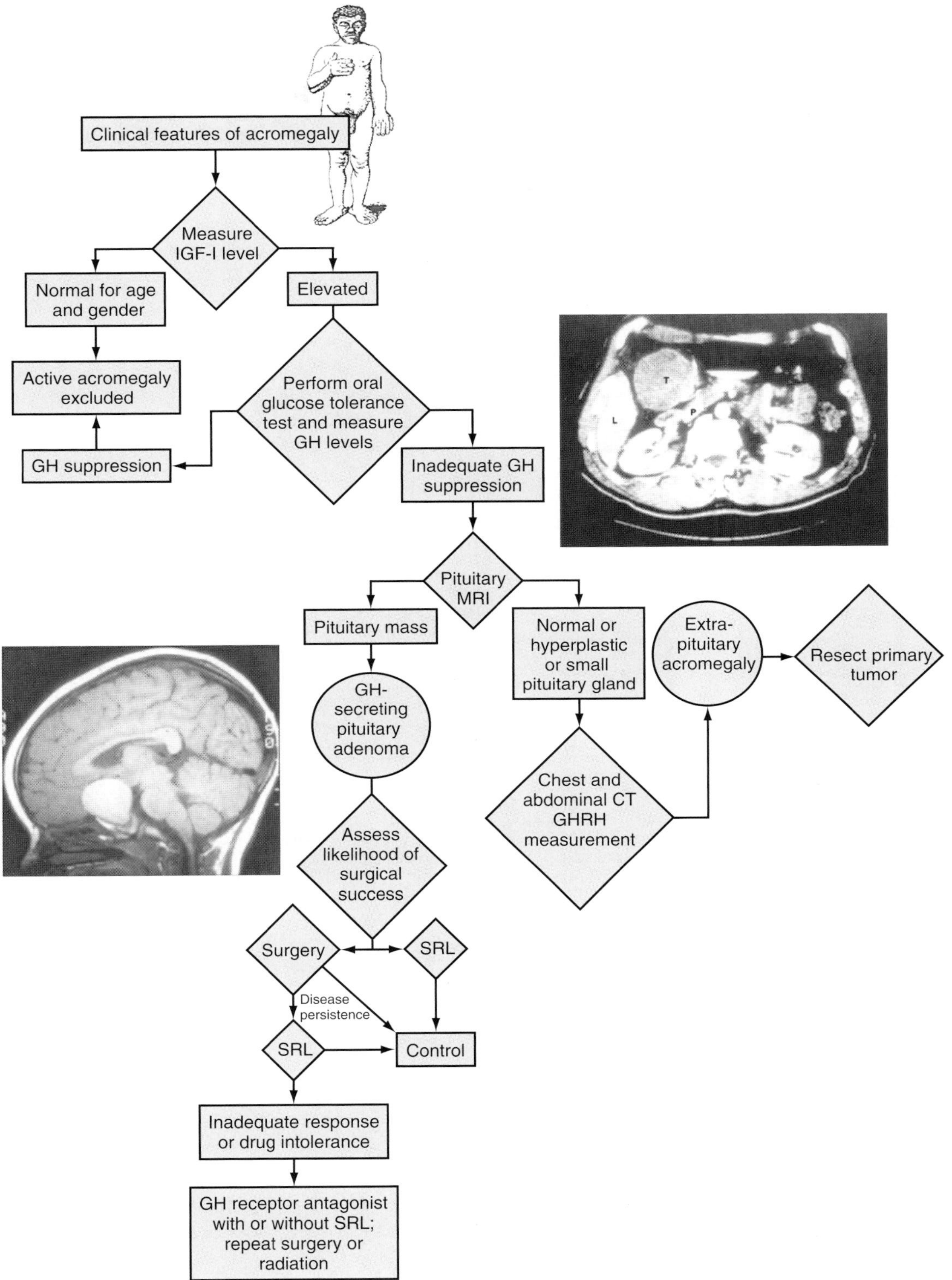

Figure 9-33 Diagnosis and treatment of acromegaly. An oral glucose tolerance test (OGTT) is performed with administration of 75 g glucose and measurements of growth hormone (GH) during the following 2 hours. Disease control implies a nadir GH level of less than 1 µg/L after OGTT with an age- and gender-normal level of insulin-like growth factor type 1 (IGF-1). CT, computed tomography; GHRH, growth hormone–releasing hormone; MRI, magnetic resonance imaging; SRL, somatostatin receptor ligand. Inset on the right shows extrapituitary acromegaly. L, liver; P, pancreas; T, tumor secreting GH. (From Melmed S. Acromegaly. *N Engl J Med.* 2006;355:2558-2573. Clinical features figure is reproduced from Minkowski O. Ueber einen Fal von Akromegalie Berliner. Klin Wochenschr 1887;21:371-374.)

TABLE 9-24
Management of Acromegaly

GOALS					
Control GH and IGF1 secretion Control tumor growth Relieve central compressive effects, if present Preserve or restore pituitary trophic hormone function Treat comorbidities (hypertension, cardiac failure, hyperglycemia, sleep apnea, arthritis) Normalize mortality rates Prevent biochemical recurrence					
TREATMENTS					
Characteristic	**Surgery**	**Radiotherapy**	**SRL**	**GHR Antagonist**	**Dopamine Agonist**
Advantages					
Mode	Transsphenoidal resection	Noninvasive	Monthly injection	Daily injection	Oral
Biochemical Control					
GH < 2.5 μg/L	Macroadenomas, <50% Microadenomas, >80%	~35% in 10 yr	~80%	Increases	<15%
IGF1 normalized		<30%	~70%	>90%	<15%
Onset	Rapid	Slow (years)	Rapid	Rapid	Slow (weeks)
Patient compliance	Onetime consent	Good	Must be sustained	Must be sustained	Good
Tumor mass	Debulked or resected	Ablated	Growth constrained or shrinks ~50%	Unknown	Unchanged
Disadvantages					
Cost	One-time	One-time	Ongoing	Ongoing	Ongoing
Hypopituitarism	~10%	>50%	None	Very low IGF1 if overtreated	None
Other	Tumor persistence or recurrence, 6% Diabetes insipidus, 3% Local complications, 5%	Local nerve damage Second brain tumor Visual and CNS disorders, ~2% Cerebrovascular risk	Gallstones, 20% Nausea, diarrhea	Elevated liver enzymes (rare)	Nausea, ~30% Sinusitis High dose required

OUTCOMES		
Feature	**Evaluation**	**Treatment**
Safe Biochemical Activity		
Nadir GH < 0.4 μg/L Age-matched normal IGF1 Asymptomatic No comorbidities	Assess GH/IGF1 axis Evaluate adrenal, thyroid and gonadal axes Periodic but less frequent MRI	None or no change in current treatment
Unsafe Biochemical Activity		
Nadir GH > 0.4 μg/L Elevated IGF1 Discordant GH and IGF1 Asymptomatic No comorbidities	Assess GH/IGF1 axis Evaluate pituitary function Periodic MRI	Weigh treatment benefit vs risks Consider new treatment if being treated
Unsafe Biochemical and Clinical Activity		
Nadir GH > 1 μg/L Elevated IGF1 Clinically active tumor growing	Assess GH/IGF1 axis Evaluate pituitary function Assess cardiovascular, metabolic, and tumoral comorbidity Periodic MRI	Actively treat or change treatment

GH, growth hormone; GHR, growth hormone receptor; IGF1, insulin-like growth factor type 1; MRI, magnetic resonance imaging; SRL, somatostatin receptor ligand.
Modified from Melmed S. Acromegaly. *N Engl J Med.* 2006;355:2558-2573.

morning, before initiation of hydrocortisone therapy. If the immediate postoperative cortisol level is lower than 3 μg/dL, a 95% 5-year remission rate can be expected. In 21 of 27 patients tested before glucocorticoid administration, postoperative cortisol levels lower than 10 mcg/dL, or lower than those obtained from preoperative midnight sampling, were predictive of remission.[485]

Silent Corticotroph Adenoma

The basophilic tumors known as silent corticotroph adenomas are usually nonfunctional and yet exhibit POMC product immunoreactivity. ACTH secretion is unaltered, and there are no associated clinical or biochemical features of hypercortisolism, although these tumors are morphologically indistinguishable from adenomas associated with Cushing's disease. They may represent up to 7% of all surgically removed adenomas[486] and are usually hemorrhagic and invariably macroadenomas. In contrast to Cushing's disease, they have a 2:1 male preponderance, often present with mass effects, and show preoperative evidence for pituitary insufficiency in about one third of cases. About half of these tumors exhibit cavernous sinus or bony invasion, hemorrhage, necrosis, and cyst formation. These tumors often recur, and postoperative irradiation and reoperation are required to eradicate tumor regrowth or residual mass.[487] Unless appropriate immunostaining is performed, many of these tumors remain undiagnosed and are classified as recurrent nonfunctioning macroadenomas.

THYROTROPIN (TSH)-SECRETING TUMORS

TSH-producing pituitary tumors are rare. During the period 1979 to 1992, Mindermann and Wilson analyzed tumor type by immunohistochemistry and found that the overall prevalence of TSH-secreting tumors was 0.85% (19/2225). Between 1989 and 1991, the same group found a prevalence of 2.8%.[488] It is not clear whether the incidence of this tumor type is increasing or whether tumors are now more readily recognized, perhaps as a result of the development of high-sensitivity TSH assays that can distinguish between frankly low values and those that are apparently normal but in fact inappropriately elevated in relation to thyroid hormone levels in some patients with TSH-producing tumors. TSH-secreting tumors can also cosecrete other hormones, including GH, PRL, and, rarely, ACTH,[489] and they can cause elevated serum IGF1 or PRL levels.[490]

Pathology

These tumors are invasive but for the most part benign, and distant metastases are extremely rare. The secretory pattern is determined by a panel of immunoreactive antibodies to TSH-β, α-subunit, GH, PRL, and ACTH. Twenty-four-hour sampling indicates that the pulse frequency of TSH is increased and the diurnal rhythm is preserved at a higher mean hormone level.[491] TSH-secreting tumors exhibit positive immunostaining for α-subunit and TSH-β in 20% to 75% of cells, as well as for the pituitary-specific transcription factor, Pit-1.[492] These tumors express SSTR2 mRNA and, in some cases, SSTR3 and SSTR5 mRNA.[493]

Presentation

Patients with TSH-secreting tumors present with symptoms resulting from tumor growth (including visual field abnormalities, cranial nerve palsies, and headache) or from hormone overproduction. Signs and symptoms of hyperthyroidism including palpitations, arrhythmias, weight loss, tremor and nervousness, or goiter are common. A case of periodic paralysis has been reported.[494] Serum TSH is often, but not invariably, elevated, and the combination of abnormally high thyroid hormone and a TSH value within the normal range points to a TSH-producing pituitary tumor. A relatively long period of hyperthyroidism, initially thought to be Graves' disease and treated accordingly, often predates the realization that the hyperthyroidism is caused by a TSH-secreting pituitary tumor. Alternatively, thyroid hormone insensitivity can manifest with similar laboratory profiles.[495] TSH-secreting tumors are usually large: 88% are macroadenomas, and 12% are microadenomas. More than 60% are also locally invasive.[496] From an analysis of 10 reports involving a total of 164 patients, it appears that TSH was frankly elevated in 58% of patients (see Table 9-25), with the remainder having normal, albeit inappropriately elevated, TSH levels. Patients previously treated with radioactive iodine for presumed Graves' disease had significantly higher TSH levels at presentation than did patients who had not undergone radioablation (mean concentration, 56 versus 9 mU/L, respectively).[497] An ectopic TSH-producing tumor has also been reported.[498] Serum T_4 is high in the majority of patients, as is the glycoprotein hormone α-subunit. Approximately two thirds[497] of patients with TSH-producing pituitary tumors have a goiter with elevated radioactive iodine uptake. Signs or symptoms of acromegaly or hyperprolactinemia may also be presenting complaints, reflecting a mixed tumor type.

Evaluation

Serum T_4, T_3, TSH (by high-sensitivity assay), and α-subunit should be measured. The combination of high T_4, T_3, and α-subunit; high or inappropriately normal TSH; and a pituitary tumor strongly confirms the diagnosis of a TSH-producing pituitary adenoma. TRH stimulation differentiates between TSH overproduction by a TSH-secreting tumor and thyroid hormone insensitivity. In TSH-secreting tumors, the TSH response elicited by TRH is blunted. In contrast, TSH usually rises in response to TRH in patients with thyroid hormone insensitivity and in normal subjects. Concomitant measurement of α-subunit at each point during the TRH test is helpful because the molar ratio of α-subunit to TRH is high (>1) in almost 85% of patients with TSH-secreting tumors. A T_3 suppression test is helpful in that complete inhibition of TSH does not occur in patients with TSH-secreting tumors. This test can also identify subclinical hypothyroidism in patients who were previously treated with radioactive iodine for hyperthyroidism but later found to have an incidental pituitary tumor.

TSH elevation may also result from inadequate thyroid hormone replacement. A pituitary MRI should be performed, and IGF1 and PRL levels should be determined to exclude acromegaly and hyperprolactinemia. The presence of other pituitary hormones in immunostained histologic sections does not necessarily imply elevated serum levels. Importantly, the degree of hyperthyroidism should be assessed to determine whether control of these signs and symptoms should be undertaken before further evaluation or treatment of the pituitary tumor. Hyperthyroidism in this condition was characterized as being severe in 14 of 25 patients and was judged to have been present in most patients for years before the diagnosis was made.[496] Perioperative deaths in patients with TSH-secreting tumors have been reported, which might possibly be attributed to poorly controlled hyperthyroidism.

Management

Surgery

Surgery has been recommended as first-line treatment, but surgical cures occur in fewer than 40% of patients (Table 9-25; Fig. 9-34).[499,500] However, the rarity of this tumor type has precluded large controlled studies. Fourteen of 22 patients had cavernous or sphenoid sinus invasion and tumors were fibrous and unusually hard; 8 of these patients were considered cured after surgery.[489] In another study, surgery normalized T_4 levels in 15 and normalized parameters of cure in 7 of 17 patients. More than half of the

TABLE 9-25

Management of Thyroid-Stimulating Hormone (TSH)-Secreting Tumors

Study	No. Patients	Microadenoma	Macroadenoma	Extrasellar Extension	Visual Field Deficit	Cured by Surgery	Histology Stain	Radiation Therapy	Cured by Radiation
Grisoli 1987	6	0/6	6/6	4/6	3/6	2/5	4/4 TSH 2/4 TSH, PRL	3/6	1/3
Gesundheit 1989	9	2/9	7/9			3/5	5/7 TSH 3/7 α-subunit	3/8	0/3
McCutcheon 1990	8	1/8	7/8	6/7	4/8	4/8	6/7 TSH 2/7 PRL	3/8	0/3
Beckers 1991	7	1/7	6/7			3/4	2/7 pure TSH 1/7 TSH, PRL 1/7 TSH, PRL, GH		
Chanson 1992	37	2/37	35/37					8/37	0/8
Chanson 1993	52							9/52	0/9
Mindermann 1993	19	0/19	19/19	12/19	6/19	NA	6/14 pure TSH 4/14 TSH, GH, PRL, ACTH 1/14 TSH, GH, PRL 1/14 TSH, PRL 1/14 TSH, GH 1 /14 TSH, ACTH	9/19 E	NA
Losa 1996	17	3/17	14/17	10/14	3/17	7/17	14 TSH 2 GH 3 PRL 1 LH 13/14 α-subunit		
Brucker-Davis 1999	25	2/25	23/25	20/25	7/18	8/22	5/25 GH 4/25 PRL 3/25 FSH	11	
Kuhn 2000	16	5/16	11/16	8/11					
Total	164	15/136 (11%)	121/136 (89%)	60/82 (73%)	23/66 (35%)	24/56 (43%)			

ACTH, adrenocorticotropic hormone; FSH, follicle-stimulating hormone; GH, growth hormone; LH, luteinizing hormone; PRL, prolactin; TSH, thyroid-stimulating hormone.

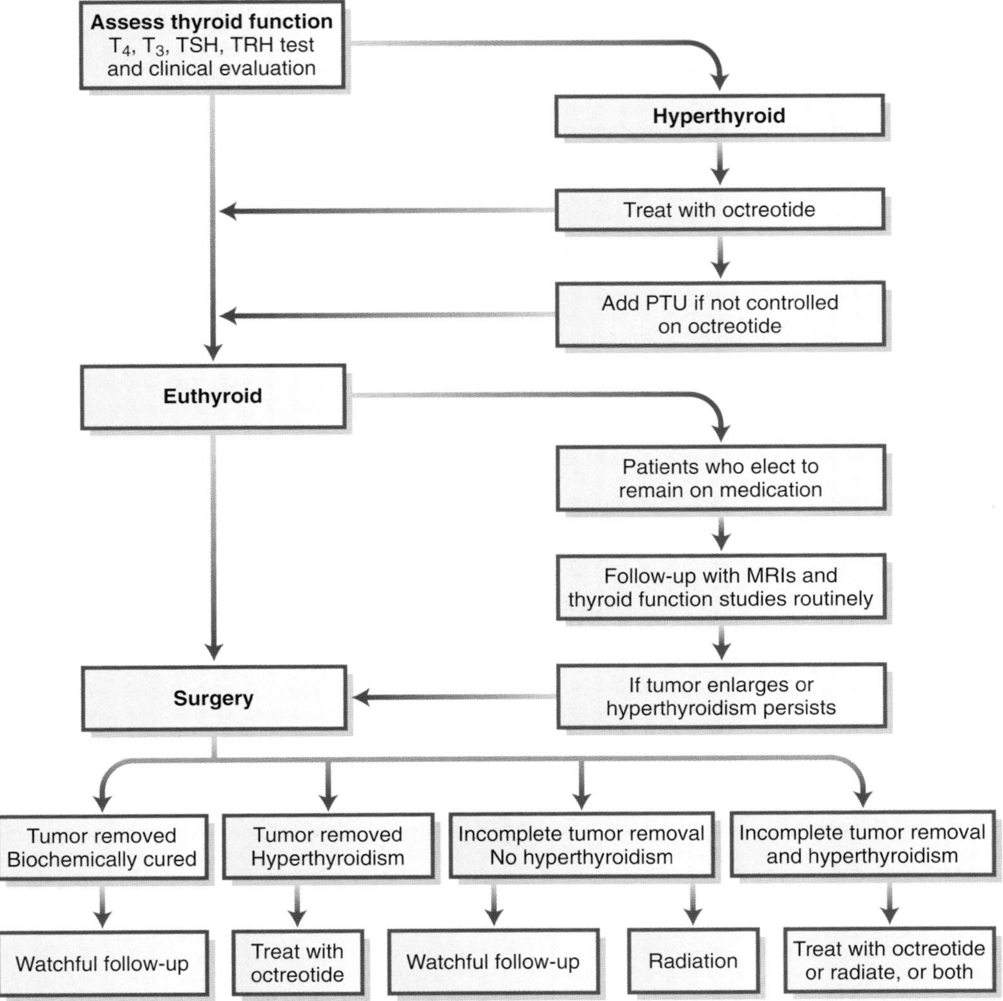

Figure 9-34 Management of thyroid-stimulating hormone (TSH)-secreting pituitary tumors. MRI, magnetic resonance imaging; PTU, propylthiouracil; T_3, triiodothyronine; T_4, thyroxine; TRH, thyrotrophin-releasing hormone.

patients exhibited evidence of residual tumor when assessed by MRI at 6 months after surgery.[501]

Radiation Therapy

There are no large series reporting treatment of TSH-secreting tumors with radiotherapy alone. Radiation has mostly been employed as adjunctive therapy to surgery, especially when the latter was not curative.

Somatostatin Analogues

Octreotide, used as either primary or adjunctive treatment, normalizes T_4 and T_3 and reduces TSH levels by half.[502] Overall, tumor shrinkage occurs in about one third of patients. In 18 patients with TSH-secreting adenomas, lanreotide (30 mg every 10 or 14 days) significantly decreased TSH levels (from 2.72 to 1.89 mU/L) and decreased T_4 levels but did not shrink tumors. Responsiveness to octreotide LAR (up to 30 mg monthly) appeared similar to that observed for the subcutaneous preparation in 7 patients.[503] Octreotide suppressed TSH in 90% of patients with TSH-secreting tumors and reduced tumor size in 50% of these patients.[504]

Unless vision is threatened, patients should be evaluated to determine whether clinical signs of hyperthyroidism warrant immediate treatment (see Table 9-25). Propranolol, thyroid ablation with radioactive iodine, thyroidectomy, anti-thyroid medications including Tapazole and propylthiouracil, and somatostatin analogues are employed.[505] Both radioactive iodine and anti-thyroid medications are targeted to the thyroid gland rather than the pituitary seat of the disorder. This approach also inhibits the remaining negative feedback of T_3 on TSH and leads to increased tumor TSH production.[502] Surgery and somatostatin analogues simultaneously treat hyperthyroidism and tumor TSH hypersecretion. Somatostatin analogues lower TSH, α-subunit, and T_4 and are recommended as first-line drugs in the initial control of hyperthyroidism caused by TSH-secreting tumors, because their onset of action is faster than that of other therapeutic approaches and tumor shrinkage occurs in up to 40% of patients.

No single treatment is expected to cure patients with TSH-secreting adenomas. Surgery is curative in only a minority of patients, and although tumor debulking may normalize thyroid function when invasive tumor tissue persists, patients continue to have abnormal TSH responses to TRH and require somatostatin analogue therapy. The relative rarity of TSH-secreting tumors renders large-scale studies difficult, but there is growing evidence for successful treatment of these tumors with somatostatin analogues as first-line therapy.

REFERENCES

1. Musolino NR, Marino R Jr, Bronstein MD. Headache in acromegaly: dramatic improvement with the somatostatin analogue SMS 201-995. *Clin J Pain*. 1990;6:243-245.
2. Fleseriu M, Yedinak C, Campbell C, et al. Significant headache improvement after transsphenoidal surgery in patients with small sellar lesions. *J Neurosurg*. 2009;110:354-358.
3. Arafah BM, Prunty D, Ybarra J, et al. The dominant role of increased intrasellar pressure in the pathogenesis of hypopituitarism, hyperprolactinemia, and headaches in patients with pituitary adenomas. *J Clin Endocrinol Metab*. 2000;85:1789-1793.
4. Freda PU, Post KD. Differential diagnosis of sellar masses. *Endocrinol Metab Clin North Am*. 1999;28:81-117, vi.
5. Kleinberg DL. Pituitary tumors and failure of endocrine target organs. *Arch Intern Med*. 1979;139:969-970.
6. Hall WA, Luciano MG, Doppman JL, et al. Pituitary magnetic resonance imaging in normal human volunteers: occult adenomas in the general population. *Ann Intern Med*. 1994;120:817-820.
7. Karavitaki N, Thanabalasingham G, Shore HC, et al. Do the limits of serum prolactin in disconnection hyperprolactinaemia need redefinition? A study of 226 patients with histologically verified nonfunctioning pituitary macroadenoma. *Clin Endocrinol (Oxf)*. 2006; 65:524-529.
8. Yaneva M, Mosnier-Pudar H, Dugue MA, et al. Midnight salivary cortisol for the initial diagnosis of Cushing's syndrome of various causes. *J Clin Endocrinol Metab*. 2004;89:3345-3351.
9. Lam KS, Sham MM, Tam SC, et al. Hypopituitarism after tuberculous meningitis in childhood. *Ann Intern Med*. 1993;118:701-706.
10. Makras P, Alexandraki KI, Chrousos GP, et al. Endocrine manifestations in Langerhans cell histiocytosis. *Trends Endocrinol Metab*. 2007;18: 252-257.
11. Bills DC, Meyer FB, Laws ER Jr, et al. A retrospective analysis of pituitary apoplexy. *Neurosurgery*. 1993;33:602-608; discussion 608-609.
12. Maccagnan P, Macedo CL, Kayath MJ, et al. Conservative management of pituitary apoplexy: a prospective study. *J Clin Endocrinol Metab*. 1995;80:2190-2197.
13. Lubina A, Olchovsky D, Berezin M, et al. Management of pituitary apoplexy: clinical experience with 40 patients. *Acta Neurochir (Wien)*. 2005;147:151-157; discussion 157.
14. Rehman HU, Atkin SL. Growth hormone-secreting pituitary macroadenoma and meningioma in a woman: a case report and review of the literature. *The Endocrinologist*. 2001;11:335-337.
15. Gokden M, Mrak RE. Pituitary adenoma with craniopharyngioma component. *Hum Pathol*. 2009;40:1189-1193.
16. Macpherson P, Hadley DM, Teasdale E, Teasdale G. Pituitary microadenomas: does gadolinium enhance their demonstration? *Neuroradiology*. 1989;31:293-298.
17. Witte RJ, Mark LP, Daniels DL, et al. Radiographic evaluation of the pituitary and anterior hypothalamus. In DeGroot LJ, Jameson JL, eds. *Endocrinology*. 4th ed. Philadelphia: Saunders; 2001. 257-268.
18. Kucharczyk W, Peck WW, Kelly WM, et al. Rathke cleft cysts: CT, MR imaging, and pathologic features. *Radiology*. 1987;165:491-495.
19. Elster AD, Chen MY, Williams DW III, et al. Pituitary gland: MR imaging of physiologic hypertrophy in adolescence [see comments]. *Radiology*. 1990;174(3 Pt 1):681-685.
20. Wolpert SM, Molitch ME, Goldman JA, et al. Size, shape, and appearance of the normal female pituitary gland. *AJR Am J Roentgenol*. 1984;143:377-381.
21. Fitzpatrick M, Tartaglino LM, Hollander MD, et al. Imaging of sellar and parasellar pathology. *Radiol Clin North Am*. 1999;37:101-121, x.
22. Pressman BD. Pituitary imaging. In Melmed S, ed. *The Pituitary*, 2nd ed. Boston: Blackwell Science; 2002:663-686.
23. Kucharczyk W, Lenkinski RE, Kucharczyk J, et al. The effect of phospholipid vesicles on the NMR relaxation of water: an explanation for the MR appearance of the neurohypophysis? *AJNR Am J Neuroradiol*. 1990;11:693-700.
24. Sheehan JP, Niranjan A, Sheehan JM, et al. Stereotactic radiosurgery for pituitary adenomas: an intermediate review of its safety, efficacy, and role in the neurosurgical treatment armamentarium. *J Neurosurg*. 2005;102:678-691.
25. Turner HE, Nagy Z, Gatter KC, et al. Angiogenesis in pituitary adenomas and the normal pituitary gland. *J Clin Endocrinol Metab*. 2000;85:1159-1162.
26. Rao VJ, James RA, Mitra D. Imaging characteristics of common suprasellar lesions with emphasis on MRI findings. *Clin Radiol*. 2008;63:939-947.
27. Venkatanarasimha N, Parrish RW. Case 148. Thoracic epidural lipomatosis. *Radiology*. 2009;252:618-622.
28. Issa N, Poggio ED, Fatica RA, et al. Nephrogenic systemic fibrosis and its association with gadolinium exposure during MRI. *Cleve Clin J Med*. 2008;75:95-97, 103-104, 6 passim.
29. de Herder WW, Reijs AE, Kwekkeboom DJ, et al. In vivo imaging of pituitary tumours using a radiolabelled dopamine D2 receptor radioligand. *Clin Endocrinol (Oxf)*. 1996;45:755-767.
30. Arnold A. Neuroophthalmologic evaluation of pituitary disorders. In Melmed S, ed. *The Pituitary*. Boston: Blackwell, 1995:687-707.
31. Hoyt WF. Correlative functional anatomy of the optic chiasm, 1969. *Clin Neurosurg*. 1970;17:189-208.
32. Anderson D, Faber P, Marcovitz S, et al. Pituitary tumors and the ophthalmologist. *Ophthalmology*. 1983;90:1265-1270.
33. Poon A, McNeill P, Harper A, et al. Patterns of visual loss associated with pituitary macroadenomas. *Aust N Z J Ophthalmol*. 1995; 23:107-115.
34. Ikeda H, Yoshimoto T. Visual disturbances in patients with pituitary adenoma. *Acta Neurol Scand*. 1995;92:157-160.
35. Cushing H. Surgical experiences with pituitary disorders. *JAMA*. 1914;63:1515-1525.
36. Schloffer H. Erfolgreiche operation eines hypohysentumors auf nasalem wege: Wein *Klin Wochenschr*; 1907.
37. Henderson WR. The pituitary adenomata: a follow-up study of the surgical results in 338 cases. *Br J Surg*. 1939;26:811-921.
38. Gondim JA, Schops M, de Almeida JP, et al. Endoscopic endonasal transsphenoidal surgery: surgical results of 228 pituitary adenomas treated in a pituitary center. *Pituitary*. 2010;13:68-77. Epub 2009 Aug 21.
39. Schwartz TH, Fraser JF, Brown S, et al. Endoscopic cranial base surgery: classification of operative approaches. *Neurosurgery*. 2008;62:991-1002; discussion 1005.
40. Kassam AB, Prevedello DM, Thomas A, et al. Endoscopic endonasal pituitary transposition for a transdorsum sellae approach to the interpeduncular cistern. *Neurosurgery*. 2008;62(3 Suppl 1):57-72; discussion 74.
41. O'Malley BW Jr, Grady MS, Gabel BC, et al. Comparison of endoscopic and microscopic removal of pituitary adenomas: single-surgeon experience and the learning curve. *Neurosurg Focus*. 2008;25:E10.
42. Tabaee A, Anand VK, Barron Y, et al. Endoscopic pituitary surgery: a systematic review and meta-analysis. *J Neurosurg*. 2009;111:545-554.
43. Laws ER. Surgery for acromegaly: evolution of the techniques and outcomes. *Rev Endocr Metab Disord*. 2008;9:67-70.
44. Steinmeier R, Fahlbusch R, Ganslandt O, et al. Intraoperative magnetic resonance imaging with the magnetom open scanner: concepts, neurosurgical indications, and procedures. A preliminary report. *Neurosurgery*. 1998;43:739-747; discussion 747-748.
45. Zirkzee EJ, Corssmit EP, Biermasz NR, et al. Pituitary magnetic resonance imaging is not required in the postoperative follow-up of acromegalic patients with long-term biochemical cure after transsphenoidal surgery. *J Clin Endocrinol Metab*. 2004;89:4320-4324.
46. Arafah BM, Kailani SH, Nekl KE, et al. Immediate recovery of pituitary function after transsphenoidal resection of pituitary macroadenomas. *J Clin Endocrinol Metab*. 1994;79:348-354.
47. Webb SM, Rigla M, Wagner A, et al. Recovery of hypopituitarism after neurosurgical treatment of pituitary adenomas. *J Clin Endocrinol Metab*. 1999;84:3696-3700.
48. Barker FG 2nd, Klibanski A, Swearingen B. Transsphenoidal surgery for pituitary tumors in the United States, 1996-2000: mortality, morbidity, and the effects of hospital and surgeon volume. *J Clin Endocrinol Metab*. 2003;88:4709-4719.
49. Gittoes NJ, Sheppard MC, Johnson AP, et al. Outcome of surgery for acromegaly—the experience of a dedicated pituitary surgeon. *Q J Med*. 1999;92:741-745.
50. Jane JA Jr, Dumont AS, Sheehan JP, et al. Surgical techniques in transsphenoidal surgery: what is the standard of care in pituitary adenomas surgery? *Curr Opin Endocrinol Diabetes*. 2004;14:264-270.
51. Nemergut EC, Dumont AS, Barry UT, et al. Perioperative management of patients undergoing transsphenoidal pituitary surgery. *Anesth Analg*. 2005;101:1170-1181.
52. Guinan EM, Lowy C, Stanhope N, et al. Cognitive effects of pituitary tumours and their treatments: two case studies and an investigation of 90 patients. *J Neurol Neurosurg Psychiatry*. 1998;65:870-876.
53. Peace KA, Orme SM, Padayatty SJ, et al. Cognitive dysfunction in patients with pituitary tumour who have been treated with transfrontal or transsphenoidal surgery or medication. *Clin Endocrinol (Oxf)*. 1998;49:391-396.
54. Jalali R, Brada M, Perks JR, et al. Stereotactic conformal radiotherapy for pituitary adenomas: technique and preliminary experience. *Clin Endocrinol (Oxf)*. 2000;52:695-702.
55. Petit JH, Biller B, Yock TI, et al. Proton stereotactic radiotherapy for presistent adrenocorticotropin-producing adenomas. *J Clin Endocrinol Metab*. 2008;93:393-399.
56. Barrande G, Pittino-Lungo M, Coste J, et al. Hormonal and metabolic effects of radiotherapy in acromegaly: long-term results in 128 patients followed in a single center. *J Clin Endocrinol Metab*. 2000;85:3779-3785.
57. McCord MW, Buatti JM, Fennell EM, et al. Radiotherapy for pituitary adenoma: long-term outcome and sequelae. *Int J Radiat Oncol Biol Physiol*. 1997;39:437-444.
58. Biermasz NR, van Dulken H, Roelfsema F. Ten-year follow-up results of transsphenoidal microsurgery in acromegaly. *J Clin Endocrinol Metab*. 2000;85:4596-4602.

59. Simmons NE, Laws ER Jr. Glioma occurrence after sellar irradiation: case report and review. *Neurosurgery*. 1998;42:172-178.
60. Erfurth EM, Bulow B, Mikoczy Z, et al. Incidence of a second tumor in hypopituitary patients operated for pituitary tumors. *J Clin Endocrinol Metab*. 2001;86:659-662.
61. Brada M, Ford D, Ashley S, et al. Risk of second brain tumour after conservative surgery and radiotherapy for pituitary adenoma. *BMJ*. 1992;304:1343-1346.
62. Tsang RW, Laperriere NJ, Simpson WJ, et al. Glioma arising after radiation therapy for pituitary adenoma: a report of four patients and estimation of risk. *Cancer*. 1993;72:2227-2233.
63. Minniti G, Traish D, Ashley S, et al. Risk of second brain tumor after conservative surgery and radiotherapy for pituitary adenoma: update after an additional 10 years. *J Clin Endocrinol Metab*. 2005; 90:800-804.
64. Sklar CA, Mertens AC, Mitby P, et al. Risk of disease recurrence and second neoplasms in survivors of childhood cancer treated with growth hormone: a report from the Childhood Cancer Survivor Study. *J Clin Endocrinol Metab*. 2002;87:3136-3141.
65. Tomlinson JW, Holden N, Hills RK, et al. Association between premature mortality and hypopituitarism. West Midlands Prospective Hypopituitary Study Group. *Lancet*. 2001;357:425-431.
66. Erfurth EM, Bulow B, Svahn-Tapper G, et al. Risk factors for cerebrovascular deaths in patients operated and irradiated for pituitary tumors. *J Clin Endocrinol Metab*. 2002;87:4892-4899.
67. Ayuk J, Clayton RN, Holder G, et al. Growth hormone and pituitary radiotherapy, but not serum insulin-like growth factor-I concentrations, predict excess mortality in patients with acromegaly. *J Clin Endocrinol Metab*. 2004;89:1613-1617.
68. Sherlock M, Reulen RC, Alonso AA, et al. ACTH deficiency, higher doses of hydrocortisone replacement, and radiotherapy are independent predictors of mortality in patients with acromegaly. *J Clin Endocrinol Metab*. 2009;94:4216-4223.
69. O'Connor MM, Mayberg MR. Effects of radiation on cerebral vasculature: a review. *Neurosurgery*. 2000;46:138-149; discussion 150-151.
70. Millar JL, Spry NA, Lamb DS, et al. Blindness in patients after external beam irradiation for pituitary adenomas: two cases occurring after small daily fractional doses. *Clin Oncol (R Coll Radiol)*. 1991; 3:291-294.
71. Jones JI, D'Ercole AJ, Camacho-Hubner C, et al. Phosphorylation of insulin-like growth factor (IGF)-binding protein 1 in cell culture and in vivo: effects on affinity for IGF-I. *Proc Natl Acad Sci USA*. 1991; 88:7481-7485.
72. al-Mefty O, Kersh JE, Routh A, et al. The long-term side effects of radiation therapy for benign brain tumors in adults. *J Neurosurg*. 1990;73:502-512.
73. Peace KA, Orme SM, Sebastian JP, et al. The effect of treatment variables on mood and social adjustment in adult patients with pituitary disease. *Clin Endocrinol (Oxf)*. 1997;46:445-450.
74. Castinetti F, Nagai M, Morange I, et al. Long-term results of stereotactic radiosurgery in secretory pituitary adenomas. *J Clin Endocrinol Metab*. 2009;94:3400-3407.
75. Minniti G, Gilbert DC, Brada M. Modern techniques for pituitary radiotherapy. *Rev Endocr Metab Disord*. 2009;10:135-144.
76. Saeki N, Tamaki, K., Murai, H., et al. Long-term outcome of endocrine function in patients with neurohypophyseal germinomas. *Endocr J*. 2000;47:83-89.
77. el-Mahdy W, Powell M. Transsphenoidal management of 28 symptomatic Rathke's cleft cysts, with special reference to visual and hormonal recovery. *Neurosurgery*. 1998;42:7-16; discussion 17.
78. Noh SJ, Ahn JY, Lee KS, et al. Pituitary adenoma and concomitant Rathke's cleft cyst. *Acta Neurochir (Wien)*. 2007;149:1223-1228.
79. Freda PU, Wardlaw SL, Post KD. Unusual causes of sellar/parasellar masses in a large transsphenoidal surgical series. *J Clin Endocrinol Metab*. 1996;81:3455-3459.
80. Mukherjee JJ, Islam N, Kaltsas G, et al. Clinical, radiological and pathological features of patients with Rathke's cleft cysts: tumors that may recur. *J Clin Endocrinol Metab*. 1997;82:2357-2362.
81. Cohen JE, Abdallah JA, Garrote M. Massive rupture of suprasellar dermoid cyst into ventricles: case illustration. *J Neurosurg*. 1997;87:963.
82. Lewis AJ, Cooper PW, Kassel EE, et al. Squamous cell carcinoma arising in a suprasellar epidermoid cyst: case report. *J Neurosurg*. 1983; 59:538-541.
83. Schaller B, Kirsch E, Tolnay M, et al. Symptomatic granular cell tumor of the pituitary gland: case report and review of the literature. *Neurosurgery*. 1998;42:166-170; discussion 170-171.
84. Volpe R, Mazabraud A. A clinicopathologic review of 25 cases of chordoma (a pleomorphic and metastasizing neoplasm). *Am J Surg Pathol*. 1983;7:161-170.
85. Rosenberg AE, Nielsen GP, Keel SB, et al. Chondrosarcoma of the base of the skull: a clinicopathologic study of 200 cases with emphasis on its distinction from chordoma. *Am J Surg Pathol*. 1999;23:1370-1378.
86. Stippler M, Gardner PA, Snyderman CH, et al. Endoscopic endonasal approach for clival chordomas. *Neurosurgery*. 2009;64:268-277; discussion 277-278.
87. Karavitaki N, Wass JA. Craniopharyngiomas. *Endocrinol Metab Clin North Am*. 2008;37:173-193, ix-x.
88. Karavitaki N, Brufani C, Warner JT, et al. Craniopharyngiomas in children and adults: systematic analysis of 121 cases with long-term follow-up. *Clin Endocrinol (Oxf)*. 2005;62:397-409.
89. Fahlbusch R, Thapar K. New developments in pituitary surgical techniques. *Baillieres Best Pract Res Clin Endocrinol Metab*. 1999; 13:471-484.
90. Honegger J, Buchfelder M, Fahlbusch R. Surgical treatment of craniopharyngiomas: endocrinological results. *J Neurosurg*. 1999;90:251-257.
91. Elliott RE, Moshel YA, Wisoff JH. Surgical treatment of ectopic recurrence of craniopharyngioma: report of 4 cases. *J Neurosurg Pediatr*. 2009;4:105-112.
92. Maira G, Anile C, Albanese A, et al. The role of transsphenoidal surgery in the treatment of craniopharyngiomas. *J Neurosurg*. 2004; 100:445-451.
93. Honegger J, Tatagiba M. Craniopharyngioma surgery. *Pituitary*. 2008;11:361-373.
94. Kassam AB, Gardner PA, Snyderman CH, et al. Expanded endonasal approach, a fully endoscopic transnasal approach for the resection of midline suprasellar craniopharyngiomas: a new classification based on the infundibulum. *J Neurosurg*. 2008;108:715-728.
95. Nozaki K, Nagata I, Yoshida K, et al. Intrasellar meningioma: case report and review of the literature. *Surg Neurol*. 1997;47:447-452; discussion 452-454.
96. Beems T, Grotenhuis JA, Wesseling P. Meningioma of the pituitary stalk without dural attachment: case report and review of the literature. *Neurosurgery*. 1999;45:1474-1477.
97. Collet-Solberg PF, Sernyak H, Satin-Smith M, et al. Endocrine outcome in long-term survivors of low-grade hypothalamic/chiasmatic glioma. *Clin Endocrinol (Oxf)*. 1997;47:79-85.
98. Gokalp HZ, Deda H, Baskaya MK, et al. Pituitary abscesses: report of three cases. *Neurosurg Rev*. 1994;17:199-203.
99. Ciappetta P, Calace A, D'Urso PI, et al. Endoscopic treatment of pituitary abscess: two case reports and literature review. *Neurosurg Rev*. 2008;31:237-246; discussion 246.
100. Dalan R, Leow MK. Pituitary abscess: our experience with a case and a review of the literature. *Pituitary*. 2008;11:299-306.
101. Jain KC, Varma A, Mahapatra AK. Pituitary abscess: a series of six cases. *Br J Neurosurg*. 1997;11:139-143.
102. Telzak EE, Cote RJ, Gold JW, et al. Extrapulmonary *Pneumocystis carinii* infections. *Rev Infect Dis*. 1990;12:380-386.
103. Danilowicz K, Sanz CF, Manavela M, et al. Pituitary abscess: a report of two cases. *Pituitary*. 2008;11:89-92.
104. Freda PU. Tuberculosis of the pituitary and sellar region. *Pituitary*. 2002;5:147-148.
105. Capra M, Wherrett D, Weitzman S, et al. Pituitary stalk thickening and primary central nervous system lymphoma. *J Neurooncol*. 2004;67:227-231.
106. Giustina A, Gola M, Doga M, et al. Clinical review 136. Primary lymphoma of the pituitary: an emerging clinical entity. *J Clin Endocrinol Metab*. 2001;86:4567-4575.
107. Moshkin O, Muller P, Scheithauer BW, et al. Primary pituitary lymphoma: a histological, immunohistochemical, and ultrastructural study with literature review. *Endocr Pathol*. 2009;20:46-49.
108. Yaman E, Benekli M, Coskun U, et al. Intrasellar plasmacytoma: an unusual presentation of multiple myeloma. *Acta Neurochir (Wien)*. 2008;150:921-924; discussion 924.
109. Brat DJ, Scheithauer BW, Staugaitis SM, et al. Pituicytoma: a distinctive low-grade glioma of the neurohypophysis. *Am J Surg Pathol*. 2000;24:362-368.
110. Figarella-Branger D, Dufour H, Fernandez C, et al. Pituicytomas, a misdiagnosed benign tumor of the neurohypophysis: report of three cases. *Acta Neuropathol (Berl)*. 2002;104:313-319.
111. Chen KT. Crush cytology of pituicytoma. *Diagn Cytopathol*. 2005;33:255-257.
112. Bell NH. Endocrine complications of sarcoidosis. *Endocrinol Metab Clin North Am*. 1991;20:645-654.
113. Newman LS, Rose CS, Maier LA. Sarcoidosis. *N Engl J Med*. 1997;336:1224-1234.
114. Sharma OP. Neurosarcoidosis: a personal perspective based on the study of 37 patients. *Chest*. 1997;112:220-228.
115. Pitale SU, Camacho PM, Gordon DL. Central nervous system involvement in sarcoidosis presenting as a recurrent pituitary mass. *The Endocrinologist*. 2000;10:429-431.
116. Tikoo RK, Kupersmith MJ, Finlay JL. Treatment of refractory neurosarcoidosis with cladribine. *N Engl J Med*. 2004;350:1798-1799.
117. Kaltsas GA, Powles TB, Evanson J, et al. Hypothalamo-pituitary abnormalities in adult patients with Langerhans cell histiocytosis: clinical, endocrinological, and radiological features and response to treatment. *J Clin Endocrinol Metab*. 2000;85:1370-1376.
118. Braunstein GD, Kohler PO. Pituitary function in Hand-Schuller-Christian disease. Evidence for deficient growth-hormone release in patients with short stature. *N Engl J Med*. 1972;286:1225-1229.

119. Nanduri VR, Pritchard J, Levitt G, et al. Long term morbidity and health related quality of life after multi-system Langerhans cell histiocytosis. *Eur J Cancer*. 2006;42:2563-2569.
120. Dhall G, Finlay JL, Dunkel IJ, et al. Analysis of outcome for patients with mass lesions of the central nervous system due to Langerhans cell histiocytosis treated with 2-chlorodeoxyadenosine. *Pediatr Blood Cancer*. 2008;50:72-79.
121. Komninos J, Vlassopoulou V, Protopapa D, et al. Tumors metastatic to the pituitary gland: case report and literature review. *J Clin Endocrinol Metab*. 2004;89:574-580.
122. Schubiger O, Haller D. Metastases to the pituitary–hypothalamic axis: an MR study of 7 symptomatic patients. *Neuroradiology*. 1992; 34:131-134.
123. Braun J, Schuldes H, Berkefeld J, et al. Panhypopituitarism associated with severe retroperitoneal fibrosis. *Clin Endocrinol (Oxf)*. 2001; 54:273-276.
124. Rivera JA. Lymphocytic hypophysitis: disease spectrum and approach to diagnosis and therapy. *Pituitary*. 2006;9:35-45.
125. Caturegli P, Newschaffer C, Olivi A, et al. Autoimmune hypophysitis. *Endocr Rev*. 2005;26:599-614.
126. Leung GK, Lopes MB, Thorner MO, et al. Primary hypophysitis: a single-center experience in 16 cases. *J Neurosurg*. 2004;101:262-271.
127. Bellastella A, Bizzarro A, Coronella C, et al. Lymphocytic hypophysitis: a rare or underestimated disease? *Eur J Endocrinol*. 2003;149:363-376.
128. Vidal S, Rotondo F, Horvath E, et al. Immunocytochemical localization of mast cells in lymphocytic hypophysitis. *Am J Clin Pathol*. 2002;117:478-483.
129. Unluhizarci K, Bayram F, Colak R, et al. Distinct radiological and clinical appearance of lymphocytic hypophysitis. *J Clin Endocrinol Metab*. 2001;86:1861-1864.
130. Gagneja H, Arafah B, Taylor HC. Histologically proven lymphocytic hypophysitis: spontaneous resolution and subsequent pregnancy. *Mayo Clin Proc*. 1999;74:150-154.
131. Ishihara T, Hino M, Kurahachi H, et al. Long-term clinical course of two cases of lymphocytic adenohypophysitis. *Endocr J*. 1996;43: 433-440.
132. Lee YJ, Lin JC, Shen EY, et al. Loss of visibility of the neurohypophysis as a sign of central diabetes insipidus. *Eur J Radiol*. 1996;21:233-235.
133. Muir A, Maclaren NK. Autoimmune diseases of the adrenal glands, parathyroid glands, gonads, and hypothalamic-pituitary axis. *Endocrinol Metab Clin North Am*. 1991;20:619-644.
134. Crock PA. Cytosolic autoantigens in lymphocytic hypophysitis. *J Clin Endocrinol Metab*. 1998;83:609-618.
135. Nishiki M, Murakami Y, Ozawa Y, et al. Serum antibodies to human pituitary membrane antigens in patients with autoimmune lymphocytic hypophysitis and infundibuloneurohypophysitis. *Clin Endocrinol (Oxf)*. 2001;54:327-333.
136. Burke CW, Moore RA, Rees LH, et al. Isolated ACTH deficiency and TSH deficiency in the adult. *J R Soc Med*. 1979;72:328-335.
137. Honegger J, Fahlbusch R, Bornemann A, et al. Lymphocytic and granulomatous hypophysitis: experience with nine cases. *Neurosurgery*. 1997;40:713-722; discussion 722-723.
138. Shimizu C, Kubo M, Kijima H, et al. Giant cell granulamatous hypophysitis with remarkable uptake on gallium-67 scintigraphy. *Clin Endocrinol (Oxf)*. 1998;49:131-134.
139. Hayashi H, Yamada K, Kuroki T, et al. Lymphocytic hypophysitis and pulmonary sarcoidosis: report of a case. *Am J Clin Pathol*. 1991;95:506-511.
140. Toth M, Szabo P, Racz K, et al. Granulomatous hypophysitis associated with Takayasu's disease. *Clin Endocrinol (Oxf)*. 1996;45:499-503.
141. Tauber JP, Babin T, Tauber MT, et al. Long term effects of continuous subcutaneous infusion of the somatostatin analog octreotide in the treatment of acromegaly. *J Clin Endocrinol Metab*. 1989;68:917-924.
142. Kovacs K. Sheehan syndrome. *Lancet*. 2003;361:520-522.
143. Kelestimur F. Sheehan's syndrome. *Pituitary*. 2003;6:181-188.
144. Yen SSC. *Chronic anovulation due to CNS-hypothalamic dysfunction*. Philadelphia: Saunders; 1991.
145. Goswami R, Kochupillai N, Crock PA, et al. Pituitary autoimmunity in patients with Sheehan's syndrome. *J Clin Endocrinol Metab*. 2002;87:4137-4141.
146. Arafah BM, Harrington JF, Madhoun ZT, et al. Improvement of pituitary function after surgical decompression for pituitary tumor apoplexy. *J Clin Endocrinol Metab*. 1990;71:323-328.
147. Semple PL, Jane JA Jr, Laws ER Jr. Clinical relevance of precipitating factors in pituitary apoplexy. *Neurosurgery*. 2007;61:956-961; discussion 961-962.
148. Hands KE, Alvarez A, Bruder JM. Gonadotropin-releasing hormone agonist-induced pituitary apoplexy in treatment of prostate cancer: case report and review of literature. *Endocr Pract*. 2007;13:642-646.
149. Wang HF, Huang CC, Chen YF, et al. Pituitary apoplexy after thyrotropin-releasing hormone stimulation test in a patient with pituitary macroadenoma. *J Chin Med Assoc*. 2007;70:392-395.
150. Balarini Lima GA, Machado Ede O, et al. Pituitary apoplexy during treatment of cystic macroprolactinomas with cabergoline. *Pituitary*. 2008;11:287-292.
151. Elsasser Imboden PN, De Tribolet N, Lobrinus A, et al. Apoplexy in pituitary macroadenoma: eight patients presenting in 12 months. *Medicine (Baltimore)*. 2005;84:188-196.
152. Zayour DH, Selman WR, Arafah BM. Extreme elevation of intrasellar pressure in patients with pituitary tumor apoplexy: relation to pituitary function. *J Clin Endocrinol Metab*. 2004;89:5649-5654.
153. Rajasekarant S, Wuss J. UK guidelines for management of pituitary apoplexy. *Clin Endo*. 2011;74:9-20.
154. Turgut M. Spinal congenital dermal sinus associated with thoracic meningocele. *Neurosurg Focus*. 2004;16(6):1-ECP1.
155. Sano K. Incidence of primary tumors (1969-1983). In Brain Tumor Registry of Japan. *Neurologia Medico-Chirurgica*. 1992;37(Special Issue): 391-441.
156. Melmed S. Mechanisms for pituitary tumorigenesis: the plastic pituitary. *J Clin Invest*. 2003;112:1603-1618.
157. Daly AF, Rixhon M, Adam C, et al. High prevalence of pituitary adenomas: a cross-sectional study in the province of Liege, Belgium. *J Clin Endocrinol Metab*. 2006;91:4769-4775.
158. Fernandez A, Karavitaki N, Wass JA. Prevalence of pituitary adenomas: a community-based, cross-sectional study in Banbury (Oxfordshire, UK). *Clin Endocrinol (Oxf)*. Epub 2009 Jul 24.
159. Thorner MO, Perryman RL, Cronin MJ, et al. Somatotroph hyperplasia: Successful treatment of acromegaly by removal of a pancreatic islet tumor secreting a growth hormone-releasing factor. *J Clin Invest*. 1982;70:965-977.
160. Grossman AB. The molecular biology of pituitary tumors: a personal perspective. *Pituitary*. 2009;12:265-270.
161. Kaltsas GA, Nomikos P, Kontogeorgos G, et al. Clinical review: diagnosis and management of pituitary carcinomas. *J Clin Endocrinol Metab*. 2005;90:3089-3099.
162. Karga HJ, Alexander JM, Hedley-Whyte ET, et al. Ras mutations in human pituitary tumors. *J Clin Endocrinol Metab*. 1992;74:914-919.
163. Pei L, Melmed S, Scheithauer B, et al. H-ras mutations in human pituitary carcinoma metastases. *J Clin Endocrinol Metab*. 1994;78: 842-846.
164. Herman V, Drazin NZ, Gonsky R, et al. Molecular screening of pituitary adenomas for gene mutations and rearrangements. *J Clin Endocrinol Metab*. 1993;77:50-55.
165. Sano T, Asa SL, Kovacs K. Growth hormone-releasing hormone-producing tumors: clinical, biochemical, and morphological manifestations. *Endocr Rev*. 1988;9:357-373.
166. Mayo KE, Hammer RE, Swanson LW, et al. Dramatic pituitary hyperplasia in transgenic mice expressing a human growth hormone-releasing factor gene. *Mol Endocrinol*. 1988;2:606-612.
167. Herman I, Gonsky R, Fagin J. Clonal origin of secretory and non-secretory pituitary tumors. *Clin Res*. 1990;38:296A (Abstract).
168. Schulte HM, Oldfield EH, Allolio B, et al. Clonal composition of pituitary adenomas in patients with Cushing's disease: determination by X-chromosome inactivation analysis. *J Clin Endocrinol Metab*. 1991;73:1302-1308.
169. Alexander JM, Biller BM, Bikkal H, et al. Clinically nonfunctioning pituitary tumors are monoclonal in origin. *J Clin Invest*. 1990; 86:336-340.
170. Spada A, Vallar L. G-protein oncogenes in acromegaly. *Horm Res*. 1992;38:90-93.
171. Zhang X, Sun H, Danila DC, et al. Loss of expression of GADD45 gamma, a growth inhibitory gene, in human pituitary adenomas: implications for tumorigenesis. *J Clin Endocrinol Metab*. 2002; 87:1262-1267.
172. Levy A, Lightman S. Molecular defects in the pathogenesis of pituitary tumours. *Front Neuroendocrinol*. 2003;24:94-127.
173. Landis CA, Harsh G, Lyons J, et al. Clinical characteristics of acromegalic patients whose pituitary tumors contain mutant Gs protein. *J Clin Endocrinol Metab*. 1990;71:1416-1420.
174. Weinstein LS, Shenker A, Gejman PV, et al. Activating mutations of the stimulatory G protein in the McCune-Albright syndrome. *N Engl J Med*. 1991;325:1688-1695.
175. Struthers RS, Vale WW, Arias C, et al. Somatotroph hypoplasia and dwarfism in transgenic mice expressing a non-phosphorylatable CREB mutant. *Nature*. 1991;350:622-624.
176. Bertherat J, Chanson P, Montminy M. The cyclic adenosine 3′,5′-monophosphate-responsive factor CREB is constitutively activated in human somatotroph adenomas. *Mol Endocrinol*. 1995;9: 777-783.
177. Pei L, Melmed S. Isolation and characterization of a pituitary tumor-transforming gene (PTTG). *Mol Endocrinol*. 1997;11:433-441.
178. Zhang X, Horwitz GA, Heaney AP, et al. Pituitary tumor transforming gene (PTTG) expression in pituitary adenomas. *J Clin Endocrinol Metab*. 1999;84:761-767.
179. Heaney AP, Horwitz GA, Wang Z, et al. Early involvement of estrogen-induced pituitary tumor transforming gene and fibroblast growth factor expression in prolactinoma pathogenesis. *Nat Med*. 1999;5:1317-1321.
180. Zou H, McGarry TJ, Bernal T, Kirschner MW. Identification of a vertebrate sister-chromatid separation inhibitor involved in transformation and tumorigenesis. *Science*. 1999;285:418-422.

181. Yu R, Heaney AP, Lu W, et al. Pituitary tumor transforming gene causes aneuploidy and p53-dependent and p53-independent apoptosis. *J Biol Chem.* 2000;275:36502-36505.
182. Abbud R, Ichiro T, Baker EM, et al. Early multipotential pituitary focal hyperplasia in αGSU-driven pituitary tumor transforming gene (PTTG) transgenic mice. *Mol Endocrinol.* 2005;19:1383-1391. Epub 2005 Jan 27.
183. Lazzerini Denchi E, Attwooll C, Pasini D, et al. Deregulated E2F activity induces hyperplasia and senescence-like features in the mouse pituitary gland. *Mol Cell Biol.* 2005;25:2660-2672.
184. Pei L, Melmed S, Scheithauer B, et al. Frequent loss of heterozygosity at the retinoblastoma susceptibility gene (RB) locus in aggressive pituitary tumors: evidence for a chromosome 13 tumor suppressor gene other than RB. *Cancer Res.* 1995;55:1613-1616.
185. Simpson DJ, Hibberts NA, McNicol AM, et al. Loss of pRb expression in pituitary adenomas is associated with methylation of the RB1 CpG island. *Cancer Res.* 2000;60:1211-1216.
186. Hibberts NA, Simpson DJ, Bicknell JE, et al. Analysis of cyclin D1 (CCND1) allelic imbalance and overexpression in sporadic human pituitary tumors. *Clin Cancer Res.* 1999;5:2133-2139.
187. Franklin DS, Godfrey VL, Lee H, et al. CDK inhibitors p18 (INK4c) and p27 (Kip1) mediate two separate pathways to collaboratively suppress pituitary tumorigenesis. *Genes Dev.* 1998;12:2899-2911.
188. Kiyokawa H, Kineman RD, Manova-Todorova KO, et al. Enhanced growth of mice lacking the cyclin-dependent kinase inhibitor function of p27 (Kip1). *Cell.* 1996;85:721-732.
189. Ezzat S, Zheng L, Zhu XF, et al. Targeted expression of a human pituitary tumor-derived isoform of FGF receptor-4 recapitulates pituitary tumorigenesis. *J Clin Invest.* 2002;109:69-78.
190. Shimon I, Huttner A, Said J, et al. Heparin-binding secretory transforming gene (hst) facilitates rat lactotrope cell tumorigenesis and induces prolactin gene transcription. *J Clin Invest.* 1996;97:187-195.
191. Vlotides G, Cooper O, Chen YH, et al. Heregulin regulates prolactinoma gene expression. *Cancer Res.* 2009;69:4209-4216.
192. Vlotides G, Siegel E, Donangelo I, et al. Rat prolactinoma cell growth regulation by epidermal growth factor receptor ligands. *Cancer Res.* 2008;68:6377-6386.
193. Gejman R, Batista DL, Zhong Y, et al. Selective loss of MEG3 expression and intergenic differentially methylated region hypermethylation in the MEG3/DLK1 locus in human clinically nonfunctioning pituitary adenomas. *J Clin Endocrinol Metab.* 2008;93:4119-4125.
194. Qian ZR, Asa SL, Siomi H, et al. Overexpression of HMGA2 relates to reduction of the let-7 and its relationship to clinicopathological features in pituitary adenomas. *Mod Pathol.* 2009;22:431-441.
195. De Martino I, Visone R, Wierinckx A, et al. HMGA proteins up-regulate CCNB2 gene in mouse and human pituitary adenomas. *Cancer Res.* 2009;69:1844-1850.
196. Chesnokova V, Zonis S, Kovacs K, et al. p21 (Cip1) restrains pituitary tumor growth. *Proc Natl Acad Sci U S A.* 2008;105:17498-17503.
197. Kuilman T, Michaloglou C, Vredeveld LC, et al. Oncogene-induced senescence relayed by an interleukin-dependent inflammatory network. *Cell.* 2008;133:1019-1031.
198. Brandi ML, Gagel RF, Angeli A, et al. Guidelines for diagnosis and therapy of MEN type 1 and type 2. *J Clin Endocrinol Metab.* 2001;86:5658-5671.
199. Trouillas J, Labat-Moleur F, Sturm N, et al. Pituitary tumors and hyperplasia in multiple endocrine neoplasia type 1 syndrome (MEN1): a case-control study in a series of 77 patients versus 2509 non-MEN1 patients. *Am J Surg Pathol.* 2008;32:534-543.
200. Chandrasekharappa SC, Guru SC, Manickam P, et al. Positional cloning of the gene for multiple endocrine neoplasia-type 1. *Science.* 1997; 276:404-407.
201. Tanaka C, Kimura T, Yang P, et al. Analysis of loss of heterozygosity on chromosome 11 and infrequent inactivation of the MEN1 gene in sporadic pituitary adenomas. *J Clin Endocrinol Metab.* 1998;83:2631-2634.
202. Pellegata NS, Quintanilla-Martinez L, Siggelkow H, et al. Germ-line mutations in p27Kip1 cause a multiple endocrine neoplasia syndrome in rats and humans. *Proc Natl Acad Sci U S A.* 2006;103:15558-15563.
203. Beckers A, Daly AF. The clinical, pathological, and genetic features of familial isolated pituitary adenomas. *Eur J Endocrinol.* 2007;157: 371-382.
204. Gadelha MR, Une KN, Rohde K, et al. Isolated familial somatotropinomas: establishment of linkage to chromosome 11q13.1-11q13.3 and evidence for a potential second locus at chromosome 2p16-12. *J Clin Endocrinol Metab.* 2000;85:707-714.
205. Georgitsi M, Raitila A, Karhu A, et al. Molecular diagnosis of pituitary adenoma predisposition caused by aryl hydrocarbon receptor-interacting protein gene mutations. *Proc Natl Acad Sci U S A.* 2007;104:4101-4105.
206. Vierimaa O, Georgitsi M, Lehtonen R, et al. Pituitary adenoma predisposition caused by germline mutations in the AIP gene. *Science.* 2006;312:1228-1230.
207. Daly AF, Vanbellinghen JF, Khoo SK, et al. Aryl hydrocarbon receptor-interacting protein gene mutations in familial isolated pituitary adenomas: analysis in 73 families. *J Clin Endocrinol Metab.* 2007;92:1891-1896.
208. Leontiou CA, Gueorguiev M, van der Spuy J, et al. The role of the aryl hydrocarbon receptor-interacting protein gene in familial and sporadic pituitary adenomas. *J Clin Endocrinol Metab.* 2008;93:2390-2401.
209. Barbieri F, Bajetto A, Stumm R, et al. Overexpression of stromal cell-derived factor 1 and its receptor CXCR4 induces autocrine/paracrine cell proliferation in human pituitary adenomas. *Clin Cancer Res.* 2008;14:5022-5032.
210. Casey M, Vaughan CJ, He J, et al. Mutations in the protein kinase A R1alpha regulatory subunit cause familial cardiac myxomas and Carney complex. *J Clin Invest.* 2000;106:R31-R38.
211. Kirschner LS, Carney JA, Pack SD, et al. Mutations of the gene encoding the protein kinase A type I-alpha regulatory subunit in patients with the Carney complex. *Nat Genet.* 2000;26:89-92.
212. Molitch ME, Thorner MO, Wilson C. Management of prolactinomas. *J Clin Endocrinol Metab.* 1997;82:996-1000.
213. Chanson P, Young J. Pituitary incidentalomas. *The Endocrinologist.* 2003;13:124-135.
214. Howlett TA, Como J, Aron DC. Management of pituitary incidentalomas: a survey of British and American endocrinologists. *Endocrinol Metab Clin North Am.* 2000;29:223-230, xi.
215. Molitch ME. Nonfunctioning pituitary tumors and pituitary incidentalomas. *Endocrinol Metab Clin North Am.* 2008;37:151-171, xi.
216. Sam S, Molitch ME. The pituitary mass: diagnosis and management. *Rev Endocr Metab Disord.* 2005;6:55-62.
217. Suzuki M, Minematsu T, Oyama K, et al. Expression of proliferation markers in human pituitary incidentalomas. *Endocr Pathol.* 2006;17: 263-275.
218. Kovacs K, Horvath E, Stefaneanu L, et al. Pituitary adenoma producing growth hormone and adrenocorticotropin: a histological, immunocytochemical, electron microscopic, and in situ hybridization study. Case report. *J Neurosurg.* 1998;88:1111-1115.
219. Saccomanno K, Bassetti M, Lania A, et al. Immunodetection of glycoprotein hormone subunits in nonfunctioning and glycoprotein hormone-secreting pituitary adenomas. *J Endocrinol Invest.* 1997;20: 59-64.
220. Al-Shraim M, Asa SL. The 2004 World Health Organization classification of pituitary tumors: what is new? *Acta Neuropathol.* 2006; 111:1-7.
221. Osamura RY, Kajiya H, Takei M, et al. Pathology of the human pituitary adenomas. *Histochem Cell Biol.* 2008;130:495-507.
222. Colao A, Di Sarno A, Cappabianca P, et al. Withdrawal of long-term cabergoline therapy for tumoral and nontumoral hyperprolactinemia. *N Engl J Med.* 2003;349:2023-2033.
223. Delgrange E, Trouillas J, Maiter D, et al. Sex-related difference in the growth of prolactinomas: a clinical and proliferation marker study. *J Clin Endocrinol Metab.* 1997;82:2102-2107.
224. Vilar L, Freitas MC, Naves LA, et al. Diagnosis and management of hyperprolactinemia: results of a Brazilian multicenter study with 1234 patients. *J Endocrinol Invest.* 2008;31:436-444.
225. Arafah BM, Nekl KE, Gold RS, Selman WR. Dynamics of prolactin secretion in patients with hypopituitarism and pituitary macroadenomas. *J Clin Endocrinol Metab.* 1995;80:3507-3512.
226. Kovacs K, Horvath E. Pathology of pituitary tumors. *Endocrinol Metab Clin North Am.* 1987;16:529-551.
227. Scheithauer BW, Kovacs KT, Laws ER Jr, et al. Pathology of invasive pituitary tumors with special reference to functional classification. *J Neurosurg.* 1986;65:733-744.
228. Hurel SJ, Harris PE, McNicol AM, et al. Metastatic prolactinoma: effect of octreotide, cabergoline, carboplatin and etoposide—immunocytochemical analysis of proto-oncogene expression. *J Clin Endocrinol Metab.* 1997;82:2962-2965.
229. Kontogeorgos G, Kovacs K, Horvath E, et al. Multiple adenomas of the human pituitary: a retrospective autopsy study with clinical implications. *J Neurosurg.* 1991;74:243-247.
230. Burgess JR, Shepherd JJ, Parameswaran V, et al. Prolactinomas in a large kindred with multiple endocrine neoplasia type 1: clinical features and inheritance pattern. *J Clin Endocrinol Metab.* 1996;81:1841-1845.
231. Berezin M, Karasik A. Familial prolactinoma. *Clin Endocrinol (Oxf).* 1995;42:483-486.
232. Kleinberg DL, Noel GL, Frantz AG. Galactorrhea: a study of 235 cases including 48 with pituitary tumors. *N Engl J Med.* 1977;296:589-600.
233. Klibanski A, Neer RM, Beitins IZ, et al. Decreased bone density in hyperprolactinemic women. *N Engl J Med.* 1980;303:1511-1514.
234. Milenkovic L, D'Angelo G, Kelly PA, Weiner RI. Inhibition of gonadotropin hormone-releasing hormone release by prolactin from GT1 neuronal cell lines through prolactin receptors. *Proc Natl Acad Sci USA.* 1994;91:1244-1247.
235. Ciccarelli A, Guerra E, De Rosa M, et al. PRL secreting adenomas in male patients. *Pituitary.* 2005;8:39-42.
236. Thorner MO, Vance ML, Laws ER Jr, et al. The anterior pituitary. In Wilson JD, Foster DW, eds. *Williams Textbook of Endocrinology.* 9th ed. Philadelphia: Saunders; 1998. 249-340.

237. Kleinberg DL. Endocrinology of mammary development, lactation and galactorrhea. In DeGroot LJ, Jameson JL, eds. *Endocrinology*. 4th ed. Philadelphia: Saunders; 2000. 2464-2475.
238. Klibanski A, Biller BMK, Rosenthal DI, Saxe V. Effects of prolactin and estrogen deficiency in amenorrheic bone loss. *J Clin Endocrinol Metab*. 1988;67:124-130.
239. Hollenhorst RW, Younge BR. Ocular manifestations produced by adenomas of the pituitary gland: analysis of 1000 cases. In Kohler PO, Ross GT, eds. *Diagnosis and Treatment of Pituitary Tumors*. New York: American Elsevier; 1973. 53-64.
240. Zikel OM, Atkinson JL, Hurley DL. Prolactinoma manifesting with symptomatic hydrocephalus. *Mayo Clin Proc*. 1999;74:475-477.
241. Barkan AL, Chandler WF. Giant pituitary prolactinoma with falsely low serum prolactin: the pitfall of the "High-Dose Hook Effect": case report. *Neurosurgery*. 1998;42:913-915.
242. Donadio F, Barbieri A, Angioni R, et al. Patients with macroprolactinaemia: clinical and radiological features. *Eur J Clin Invest*. 2007; 37:552-557.
243. Melmed S, et al. Diagnosis and treatment of hyperprolactinemia: an Endocrine Society Clinical Practical Guideline. *J Clin Endocrinol Metab*. 2011.
244. Kleinberg DL, Todd J. Evidence that human growth hormone is a potent lactogen in primates. *J Clin Endocrinol Metab*. 1980;51:1009-1015.
245. De Rosa M, Ciccarelli A, Zarrilli S, et al. The treatment with cabergoline for 24 month normalizes the quality of seminal fluid in hyperprolactinaemic males. *Clin Endocrinol (Oxf)*. 2006;64:307-313.
246. Thorner MO, Martin WH, Rogol AD, et al. Rapid regression of pituitary prolactinomas during bromocriptine treatment. *J Clin Endocrinol Metab*. 1980;51:438-445.
247. Shimon I, Melmed S. Management of pituitary tumors. *Ann Intern Med*. 1998;129:472-483.
248. Colao A, Ferone D, Marzullo P, et al. Systemic complications of acromegaly: epidemiology, pathogenesis, and management. *Endocr Rev*. 2004;25:102-152.
249. Vance ML, Evans WS, Thorner MO. Drugs five years later: bromocriptine. *Ann Intern Med*. 1984;100:78-91.
250. Thorner MO, Perryman RL, Rogol AD, et al. Rapid changes of prolactinoma volume after withdrawal and reinstitution of bromocriptine. *J Clin Endocrinol Metab*. 1981;53:480-483.
251. Kovacs K, Stefaneanu L, Horvath E, et al. Effect of dopamine agonist medication on prolactin producing pituitary adenomas: a morphological study including immunocytochemistry, electron microscopy and in situ hybridization. *Virchows Arch A Pathol Anat Histopathol*. 1991;418:439-446.
252. Jeffcoate WJ, Pound N, Sturrock ND, et al. Long-term follow-up of patients with hyperprolactinaemia. *Clin Endocrinol (Oxf)*. 1996; 45:299-303.
253. Kupersmith MJ, Kleinberg DL, Warren A, et al. Growth of prolcactinoma despite lowering of serum prolactin by bromocriptine. *Neurosurgery*. 1989;24:417-423.
254. Molitch ME. Pharmacologic resistance in prolactinoma patients. *Pituitary*. 2005;8:43-52.
255. Colao A, Di Sarno A, Landi ML, et al. Long-term and low-dose treatment with cabergoline induces macroprolactinoma shrinkage. *J Clin Endocrinol Metab*. 1997;82:3574-3579.
256. Fusco A, Gunz G, Jaquet P, et al. Somatostatinergic ligands in dopamine-sensitive and resistant prolactinomas. *Eur J Endocrinol*. 2008;158:595-603.
257. Filopanti M, Barbieri AM, Angioni AR, et al. Dopamine D2 receptor gene polymorphisms and response to cabergloine therapy in patients with prolactin secreting pituitary adenomas. *PharmacogenetGenomics*. 2008;8:357-363.
258. Bassetti M, Spada A, Pezzo G, Giannattasio G. Bromocriptine treatment reduces the cell size in human macroprolactinomas: a morphometric study. *J Clin Endocrinol Metab*. 1984;58:268-273.
259. Saitoh Y, Mori S, Arita N, et al. Cytosuppressive effect of bromocriptine on human prolactinomas: stereological analysis of ultrastructural alterations with special reference to secretory granules. *Cancer Res*. 1986;46:1507-1512.
260. Hallenga B, Saeger W, Ludecke DK. Necroses of prolactin-secreting pituitary adenomas under treatment with dopamine agonists: light microscopical and morphometric studies. *Exp Clin Endocrinol*. 1988;92:59-68.
261. Landolt AM, Osterwalder V. Perivascular fibrosis in prolactinomas: is it increased by bromocriptine? *J Clin Endocrinol Metab*. 1984; 58:1179-1183.
262. Tyrrell JB, Lamborn KR, Hannegan LT, et al. Transsphenoidal microsurgical therapy of prolactinomas: initial outcomes and long-term results. *Neurosurgery*. 1999;44:254-261.
263. Fahlbusch R, Buchfelder M, Schrell U. Short-term preoperative treatment of macroprolactinomas by dopamine agonists. *J Neurosurg*. 1987;67:807-815.
264. Biswas M, Smith J, Jadon D, et al. Long-term remission following withdrawal of dopamine agonist therapy in subjects with microprolactinomas. *Clin Endocrinol (Oxf)*. 2005;63:26-31.
265. Cook DM. Long-term management of prolactinomas: use of long-acting dopamine agonists. *Rev Endocr Metab Disord*. 2005;6: 15-21.
266. DiSalle E, Ornati G, Giudici D. A comparison of the in vivo and in vitro duration of prolactin lowering effect in rats of FCE 21336, pergolide and bromocriptine. *J Endocrinol Invest*. 1984;7(suppl 1):32.
267. Webster J, Piscitelli G, Polli A, et al. A comparison of cabergoline and bromocriptine in the treatment of hyperprolactinemic amenorrhea. *N Engl J Med*. 1994;331:904-909.
268. Biller BM, Molitch ME, Vance ML, et al. Treatment of prolactin-secreting macroadenomas with the once-weekly dopamine agonist cabergoline. *J Clin Endocrinol Metab*. 1996;81:2338-2343.
269. Shimon I, Hinton DR, Weiss MH, Melmed S. Prolactinomas express human heparin-binding secretory transforming gene (hst) protein product: marker of tumour invasiveness. *Clin Endocrinol (Oxf)*. 1998;48:23-29.
270. Colao A, Ferone D, Marzullo P, et al. Effect of different dopaminergic agents in the treatment of acromegaly. *J Clin Endocrinol Metab*. 1997;82:518-523.
271. Negoro K, Kawai M, Tada Y, et al. A case of postprandial cluster-like headache with prolactinoma: dramatic response to cabergoline. *Headache*. 2005;45:604-606.
272. Kleinberg DL, Lieberman A, Todd J, et al. Pergolide mesylate: a potent day-long inhibitor of prolactin in rhesus monkeys and patients with Parkinson's disease. *J Clin Endocrinol Metab*. 1980;51:152-154.
273. Kletzky OA, Vermesh M. Effectiveness of vaginal bromocriptine in treating women with hyperprolactinemia. *Fertil Steril*. 1989;51: 269-272.
274. Turner TH, Cookson JC, Wass JA, et al. Psychotic reactions during treatment of pituitary tumours with dopamine agonists. *Br Med J (Clin Res Ed)*. 1984;289:1101-1103.
275. Suliman SG, Gurlek A, Byrne JV, et al. Nonsurgical cerebrospinal fluid rhinorrhea in invasive macroprolactinoma: incidence, radiological, and clinicopathological features. *J Clin Endocrinol Metab*. 2007;92: 3829-3835.
276. Leong KS, Foy PM, Swift AC, et al. CSF rhinorrhoea following treatment with dopamine agonists for massive invasive prolactinomas. *Clin Endocrinol (Oxf)*. 2000;52:43-49.
277. Melmed S, Braunstein GD. Bromocriptine and pleuropulmonary disease. *Arch Intern Med*. 1989;149:258-259.
278. Pinero A, Marcos-Alberca P, Fortes J. Cabergoline-related severe restrictive mitral regurgitation. *N Engl J Med*. 2005;353:1976-1977.
279. Schade R, Andersohn F, Suissa S, et al. Dopamine agonists and the risk of cardiac-valve regurgitation. *N Engl J Med*. 2007;356:29-38.
280. Zanettini R, Antonini A, Gatto G, et al. Valvular heart disease and the use of dopamine agonists for Parkinson's disease. *N Engl J Med*. 2007;356:39-46.
281. Colao A, Auriemma RS, Galdiero M, et al. Effects of initial therapy for five years with somatostatin analogs for acromegaly on growth hormone and insulin-like growth factor-I levels, tumor shrinkage, and cardiovascular disease: a prospective study. *J Clin Endocrinol Metab*. 2009;94:3746-3756.
282. Devin JK, Lakhani VT, Byrd BF III, et al. Prevalence of valvular heart disease in a cohort of patients taking cabergoline for management of hyperprolactinemia. *Endocrinol Pract*. 2008;14:672-677.
283. Wakil A, Rigby AS, Clark AL, et al. Low dose cabergoline for hyperprolactinaemia is not associated with clinically significant valvular heart disease. *Eur J Endocrinol*. 2008;159:R11-R14.
284. Lancellotti P, Livadariu E, Markov M, et al. Cabergoline and the risk of valvular lesions in endocrine disease. *Eur J Endocrinol*. 2008; 159:1-5.
285. Vallette S, Serri K, Rivera J, et al. Long-term cabergoline therapy is not associated with valvular heart disease in patients with prolactinomas. *Pituitary*. 2009;12:153-157.
286. Tsagarakis S, Grossman A, Plowman PN, et al. Megavoltage pituitary irradiation in the management of prolactinomas: long-term follow-up. *Clin Endocrinol (Oxf)*. 1991;34:399-406.
287. Littley MD, Shalet SM, Beardwell CG, et al. Hypopituitarism following external radiotherapy for pituitary tumours in adults. *Q J Med*. 1989;70:145-160.
288. Serri O, Rasio E, Beauregard H, et al. Recurrence of hyperprolactinemia after selective transsphenoidal adenomectomy in women with prolactinoma. *N Engl J Med*. 1983;309:280-283.
289. Molitch ME. Management of prolactinomas. *Annu Rev Med*. 1989;40:225-232.
290. Kovacs K, Horvath E, Syro LV, et al. Temozolomide therapy in a man with an aggressive prolactin-secreting pituitary neoplasm: morphological findings. *Hum Pathol*. 2007;38:185-189.
291. Fadul CE, Kominsky AL, Meyer LP, et al. Long-term response of pituitary carcinoma to temozolomide: report of two cases. *J Neurosurg*. 2006;105:621-626.

292. Neff LM, Weil M, Cole A, et al. Temozolomide in the treatment of an invasive prolactinoma resistant to dopamine agonists. *Pituitary*. 2007;10:81-86.
293. McCormack AI, McDonald KL, Gill AJ, et al. Low O6-methylguanine-DNA methyltransferase (MGMT) expression and response to temozolomide in aggressive pituitary tumours. *Clin Endocrinol (Oxf)*. 2009;71:226-233.
294. Molitch ME. Pregnancy and the hyperprolactinemic woman. *N Engl J Med*. 1985;312:1364-1370.
295. Kupersmith MJ, Rosenberg C, Kleinberg D. Visual loss in pregnant women with pituitary adenomas. *Ann Intern Med*. 1994;121: 473-477.
296. Liu C, Tyrrell JB. Successful treatment of a large macroprolactinoma with cabergoline during pregnancy. *Pituitary*. 2001;4:179-185.
297. Colao A, Abs R, Barcena DG, et al. Pregnancy outcomes following cabergoline treatment: extended results from a 12-year observational study. *Clin Endocrinol (Oxf)*. 2008;68:66-71.
298. Laws ER Jr, Fode NC, Randall RV, et al. Pregnancy following transsphenoidal resection of prolactin-secreting pituitary tumors. *J Neurosurg*. 1983;58:685-688.
299. Horvath E, Kovacs K. Ultrastructural diagnosis of human pituitary adenomas. *Microsc Res Tech*. 1992;20:107-135.
300. Jameson JL, Klibanski A, Black PM, et al. Glycoprotein hormone genes are expressed in clinically nonfunctioning pituitary adenomas. *J Clin Invest*. 1987;80:1472-1478.
301. Samuels MH, Henry P, Kleinschmidt-DeMasters BK, et al. Pulsatile glycoprotein hormone secretion in glycoprotein-producing pituitary tumors. *J Clin Endocrinol Metab*. 1991;73:1281-1288.
302. Nobels FR, Kwekkeboom DJ, Coopmans W, et al. A comparison between the diagnostic value of gonadotropins, alpha-subunit, and chromogranin-A and their response to thyrotropin-releasing hormone in clinically nonfunctioning, alpha-subunit-secreting, and gonadotroph pituitary adenomas. *J Clin Endocrinol Metab*. 1993;77:784-789.
303. Kovacs K, Horvath E, Ryan N, et al. Null cell adenoma of the human pituitary. *Virchows Arch Pathol Anat*. 1980;387:165-174.
304. Chaidarun SS, Klibanski A. Gonadotropinomas. *Semin Reprod Med*. 2002;20:339-348.
305. Sanno N, Teramoto A, Osamura RY, et al. Pathology of pituitary tumors. *Neurosurg Clin North Am*. 2003;14:25-39, vi.
306. Dekkers OM, van der Klaauw AA, Pereira AM, et al. Quality of life is decreased after treatment for nonfunctioning pituitary macroadenoma. *J Clin Endocrinol Metab*. 2006;91:3364-3369.
307. Nielsen EH, Lindholm J, Laurberg P, et al. Nonfunctioning pituitary adenoma: incidence, causes of death and quality of life in relation to pituitary function. *Pituitary*. 2007;10:67-73.
308. van der Klaauw AA, Dekkers OM, Pereira AM, et al. Increased daytime somnolence despite normal sleep patterns in patients treated for nonfunctioning pituitary macroadenoma. *J Clin Endocrinol Metab*. 2007;92:3898-3903.
309. Cooper O, Geller JL, Melmed S. Ovarian hyperstimulation syndrome caused by an FSH secreting pituitary adenoma. *Natl Clin Pract Endocrinol Metab*. 2008;4:234-238.
310. Daneshdoost L, Gennarelli TA, Bashey HM, et al. Recognition of gonadotroph adenomas in women. *N Engl J Med*. 1991;324: 589-594.
311. Boelaert K, Gittoes NJ. Radiotherapy for non-functioning pituitary adenomas. *Eur J Endocrinol*. 2001;144:569-575.
312. Minniti G, Traish D, Ashley S, Gonsalves A, et al. Fractionated stereotactic conformal radiotherapy for secreting and nonsecreting pituitary adenomas. *Clin Endocrinol (Oxf)*. 2006;64:542-548.
313. Ebersold MJ, Quast LM, Laws ER Jr, et al. Long-term results in transsphenoidal removal of nonfunctioning pituitary adenomas. *J Neurosurg*. 1986;64:713-719.
314. Turner HE, Stratton IM, Byrne JV, et al. Audit of selected patients with nonfunctioning pituitary adenomas treated without irradiation: a follow-up study. *Clin Endocrinol (Oxf)*. 1999;51:281-284.
315. O'Sullivan EP, Woods C, Glynn N, et al. The natural history of surgically treated but radiotherapy-naive nonfunctioning pituitary adenomas. *Clin Endocrinol (Oxf)*. 2009;71:709-714.
316. Dekkers OM, Pereira AM, Romijn JA. Treatment and follow-up of clinically nonfunctioning pituitary macroadenomas. *J Clin Endocrinol Metab*. 2008;93:3717-3726.
317. Losa M, Valle M, Mortini P, et al. Gamma knife surgery for treatment of residual nonfunctioning pituitary adenomas after surgical debulking. *J Neurosurg*. 2004;100:438-444.
318. Pollock BE, Cochran J, Natt N, et al. Gamma knife radiosurgery for patients with nonfunctioning pituitary adenomas: results from a 15-year experience. *Int J Radiat Oncol Biol Phys*. 2008;70:1325-1329.
319. Dekkers OM, Pereira AM, Roelfsema F, et al. Observation alone after transsphenoidal surgery for nonfunctioning pituitary macroadenoma. *J Clin Endocrinol Metab*. 2006;91:1796-1801.
320. Greenman Y, Stern N. How should a nonfunctioning pituitary macroadenoma be monitored after debulking surgery? *Clin Endocrinol (Oxf)*. 2009;70:829-832.
321. Erickson D, Scheithauer B, Atkinson J, et al. Silent subtype 3 pituitary adenoma: a clinicopathologic analysis of the Mayo Clinic experience. *Clin Endocrinol (Oxf)*. 2009;71:92-99.
322. Wass JA, Karavitaki N. Nonfunctioning pituitary adenomas: the Oxford experience. *Nat Rev Endocrinol*. 2009;5:519-522.
323. Pivonello R, Ferone D, de Herder WW, et al. Dopamine receptor expression and function in corticotroph pituitary tumors. *J Clin Endocrinol Metab*. 2004;89:2452-2462.
324. Greenman Y. Dopaminergic treatment of nonfunctioning pituitary adenomas. *Natl Clin Pract Endocrinol Metab*. 2007;3:554-555.
325. Marie P. On two cases of acromegaly: marked hypertrophy of the upper and lower limbs and the head. *Rev Med*. 1886;6:297-333.
326. Benda C. Beitrage zur normalen und pathologischen histologic der menschhchen hypophysis cerebri. *Klin Wochenschr*. 1900;36: 1205.
327. Cushing H. Partial hypophysectomy for acromegaly: with remarks on the function of the hypophysis. *Ann Surg*. 1909;50:1002-1017.
328. Evans HM, Long JA. The effect of the anterior lobe of the pituitary administered intra-peritoneally upon growth, maturity and oestrus cycle of the rat. *Anat Rev*. 1921;21:62.
329. Alexander L, Appleton D, Hall R, et al. Epidemiology of acromegaly in the Newcastle region. *Clin Endocrinol (Oxf)*. 1980;12:71-79.
330. Bengtsson BA, Eden S, Ernest I, et al. Epidemiology and long-term survival in acromegaly: a study of 166 cases diagnosed between 1955 and 1984. *Acta Med Scand*. 1988;223:327-335.
331. Ritchie CM, Atkinson AB, Kennedy AL, et al. Ascertainment and natural history of treated acromegaly in Northern Ireland. *Ulster Med J*. 1990;59:55-62.
332. Melmed S. Acromegaly [see comments]. *N Engl J Med*. 1990;322: 966-977.
333. Asa SL, Kovacs K. Pituitary pathology in acromegaly. *Endocrinol Metab Clin North Am*. 1992;21:553-574.
334. Maheshwari HG, Prezant TR, Herman-Bonert V, et al. Long-acting peptidomimergic control of gigantism caused by pituitary acidophilic stem cell adenoma. *J Clin Endocrinol Metab*. 2000;85:3409-3416.
335. Kovacs K, Horvath E, Asa SL, et al. Pituitary cells producing more than one hormone. *Trends Endocrinol Metab*. 1989;1:104-108.
336. Melmed S. Pituitary function and neoplasia. In Jameson JL, ed. *Principles of Molecular Medicine*. Totowa, NJ: Humana Press; 1998: 443-449.
337. Heaney AP, Fernando M, Melmed S. Functional role of estrogen in pituitary tumor pathogenesis. *J Clin Invest*. 2002;109:277-283.
338. Howard AD, Feighner SD, Cully DF, et al. A receptor in pituitary and hypothalamus that functions in growth hormone release. *Science*. 1996;273:974-977.
339. Dimaraki EV, Chandler WF, Brown MB, et al. The role of endogenous growth hormone-releasing hormone in acromegaly. *J Clin Endocrinol Metab*. 2006;91:2185-2190.
340. Thapar K, Kovacs K, Stefaneanu L, et al. Overexpression of the growth-hormone-releasing hormone gene in acromegaly-associated pituitary tumors: an event associated with neoplastic progression and aggressive behavior. *Am J Pathol*. 1997;151:769-784.
341. Ho KY, Veldhuis JD, Johnson ML, et al. Fasting enhances growth hormone secretion and amplifies the complex rhythms of growth hormone secretion in man. *J Clin Invest*. 1988;81:968-975.
342. Cazabat L, Libe R, Perlemoine K, et al. Germline inactivating mutations of the aryl hydrocarbon receptor-interacting protein gene in a large cohort of sporadic acromegaly: mutations are found in a subset of young patients with macroadenomas. *Eur J Endocrinol*. 2007;157: 1-8.
343. Frohman LA, Jansson JO. Growth hormone-releasing hormone. *Endocr Rev*. 1986;7:223-253.
344. Melmed S, Ezrin C, Kovacs K, et al. Acromegaly due to secretion of growth hormone by an ectopic pancreatic islet-cell tumor. *N Engl J Med*. 1985;312:9-17.
345. Moran A, Asa SL, Kovacs K, et al. Gigantism due to pituitary mammosomatotroph hyperplasia. *N Engl J Med*. 1990;323:322-327.
346. Verrua E, Ronchi CL, Ferrante E, et al. Acromegaly secondary to an incidentally discovered growth-hormone-releasing hormone secreting bronchial carcinoid tumour associated to a pituitary incidentaloma. *Pituitary*. Epub 2008 Oct 23.
347. Thorner MO, Frohman LA, Leong DA, et al. Extrahypothalamic growth-hormone-releasing factor (GRF) secretion is a rare cause of acromegaly: plasma GRF levels in 177 acromegalic patients. *J Clin Endocrinol Metab*. 1984;59:846-849.
348. Frohman LA, Szabo M, Berelowitz M, et al. Partial purification and characterization of a peptide with growth hormone-releasing activity from extrapituitary tumors in patients with acromegaly. *J Clin Invest*. 1980;65:43-54.
349. Vieira NL, Taboada GF, Correa LL, et al. Acromegaly secondary to growth hormone-releasing hormone secreted by an incidentally discovered pheochromocytoma. *Endocrinol Pathol*. 2007;18:46-52.
350. Drange MR, Melmed S. Long-acting lanreotide induces clinical and biochemical remission of acromegaly caused by disseminated growth

hormone-releasing hormone-secreting carcinoid [see comments]. *J Clin Endocrinol Metab*. 1998;83:3104-3109.
351. Madonna D, Kendler A, Soliman AM. Ectopic growth hormone-secreting pituitary adenoma in the sphenoid sinus. *Ann Otol Rhinol Laryngol*. 2001;110:99-101.
352. Greenman Y, Melmed S. Diagnosis and management of nonfunctioning pituitary tumors. *Annu Rev Med*. 1996;47:95-106.
353. Beuschlein F, Strasburger CJ, Siegerstetter V, et al. Acromegaly caused by secretion of growth hormone by a non-Hodgkin's lymphoma. *N Engl J Med*. 2000;342:1871-1876.
354. Misaki M, Shima T, Ikoma J, et al. Acromegaly and hyperthyroidism associated with McCune-Albright syndrome. *Horm Res*. 1988; 30:26-27.
355. Melmed S, Braunstein GD, Chang RJ, et al. Pituitary tumors secreting growth hormone and prolactin. Clinical conference. *Ann Intern Med*. 1986;105:238-253.
356. Drange MR, Fram NR, Herman-Bonert V, et al. Pituitary tumor registry: a novel clinical resource. *J Clin Endocrinol Metab*. 2000;85:168-174.
357. de Herder WW. Acromegaly and gigantism in the medical literature: case descriptions in the era before and the early years after the initial publication of Pierre Marie (1886). *Pituitary*. 2009;12:236-244.
358. Daughaday WH. Pituitary gigantism. *Endocrinol Metab Clin North Am*. 1992;21:633-647.
359. Molitch ME. Clinical manifestations of acromegaly. *Endocrinol Metab Clin North Am*. 1992;21:597-614.
360. Jadresic A, Banks LM, Child DF, et al. The acromegaly syndrome: relation between clinical features, growth hormone values and radiological characteristics of the pituitary tumours. *Q J Med*. 1982; 51:189-204.
361. Nabarro JD. Acromegaly. *Clin Endocrinol (Oxf)*. 1987;26:481-512.
362. Colao A, Marzullo P, Ferone D, et al. Prostatic hyperplasia: an unknown feature of acromegaly. *J Clin Endocrinol Metab*. 1998;83:775-779.
363. Lieberman SA, Bjorkengren AG, Hoffman AR. Rheumatologic and skeletal changes in acromegaly. *Endocrinol Metab Clin North Am*. 1992;21:615-631.
364. Biermasz NR, Pereira AM, Smit JW, et al. Morbidity after long-term remission for acromegaly: persisting joint-related complaints cause reduced quality of life. *J Clin Endocrinol Metab*. 2005;90:2731-2739.
365. Dons RF, Rosselet P, Pastakia B, et al. Arthropathy in acromegalic patients before and after treatment: a long-term follow-up study. *Clin Endocrinol (Oxf)*. 1988;28:515-524.
366. Tagliafico A, Resmini E, Nizzo R, et al. Ultrasound measurement of median and ulnar nerve cross-sectional area in acromeagly. *J Clin Endocrinol Metab*. 2008;93:905-909.
367. Resmini E, Tagliafico A, Nizzo R, et al. Ultrasound of peripheral nerves in acromegaly: changes at 1-year follow-up. *Clin Endocrinol (Oxf)*. 2009;71:220-225.
368. Ben-Shlomo A, Melmed S. Skin manifestations in acromegaly. *Clin Dermatol*. 2006;24:256-259.
369. Verde GG, Santi I, Chiodini P, et al. Serum type III procollagen propeptide levels in acromegalic patients. *J Clin Endocrinol Metab*. 1986;63:1406-1410.
370. Leavitt J, Klein I, Kendricks F, et al. Skin tags: a cutaneous marker for colonic polyps. *Ann Intern Med*. 1983;98:928-930.
371. Colao A, Cuocolo A, Marzullo P, et al. Impact of patient's age and disease duration on cardiac performance in acromegaly: a radionuclide angiography study. *J Clin Endocrinol Metab*. 1999;84:1518-1523.
372. Lopez-Velasco R, Escobar-Morreale HF, Vega B, et al. Cardiac involvement in acromegaly: specific myocardiopathy or consequence of systemic hypertension? *J Clin Endocrinol Metab*. 1997;82:1047-1053.
373. Deray G, Rieu M, Devynck MA, et al. Evidence of an endogenous digitalis-like factor in the plasma of patients with acromegaly. *N Engl J Med*. 1987;316:575-580.
374. Kamenicky P, Viengchareun S, Blanchard A, et al. Epithelial sodium channel is a key mediator of growth hormone-induced sodium retention in acromegaly. *Endocrinology*. 2008;149:3294-3305.
375. Colao A, Ferone D, Cappabianca P, et al. Effect of octreotide pretreatment on surgical outcome in acromegaly. *J Clin Endocrinol Metab*. 1997;82:3308-3314.
376. Grunstein RR, Ho KK, Sullivan CE. Effect of octreotide, a somatostatin analog, on sleep apnea in patients with acromegaly. *Ann Intern Med*. 1994;121:478-483.
377. Jenkins PJ, Sohaib SA, Akker S, et al. The pathology of median neuropathy in acromegaly. *Ann Intern Med*. 2000;133:197-201.
378. Furman K, Ezzat S. Psychological features of acromegaly. *Psychother Psychosom*. 1998;67:147-153.
379. Santos A, Resmini E, Martinez MA, et al. Quality of life in patients with pituitary tumors. *Curr Opin Endocrinol Diabetes Obes*. 2009;16: 299-303.
380. Stewart CE, Rotwein P. Growth, differentiation, and survival: multiple physiological functions for insulin-like growth factors. *Physiol Rev*. 1996;76:1005-1026.
381. Cohen P, Peehl DM, Graves HC, Rosenfeld RG. Biological effects of prostate specific antigen as an insulin-like growth factor binding protein-3 protease. *J Endocrinol*. 1994;142:407-415.
382. Melmed S. Acromegaly and cancer: not a problem? *J Clin Endocrinol Metab*. 2001;86:2929-2934.
383. Jenkins PJ, Frajese V, Jones AM, et al. Insulin-like growth factor I and the development of colorectal neoplasia in acromegaly. *J Clin Endocrinol Metab*. 2000;85:3218-3221.
384. Delhougne B, Deneux C, Abs R, et al. The prevalence of colonic polyps in acromegaly: a colonoscopic and pathological study in 103 patients. *J Clin Endocrinol Metab*. 1995;80:3223-3226.
385. Orme S, McNally RJQ, Cartwright RA, et al. Mortality and cancer incidence in acromegaly: a retrospective cohort study. *J Clin Endo Metab*. 1998;83:2730-2734.
386. Ladas SD, Thalassinos NC, Ioannides G, Raptis SA. Does acromegaly really predispose to an increased prevalence of gastrointestinal tumours? *Clin Endocrinol (Oxf)*. 1994;41:597-601.
387. Ezzat S, Strom C, Melmed S. Colon polyps in acromegaly. *Ann Intern Med*. 1991;114:754-755.
388. Resmini E, Tagliafico A, Bacigalupo L, et al. Computed tomography colonography in acromegaly. *J Clin Endocrinol Metab*. 2009;94: 218-222.
389. Renehan AG, Bhaskar P, Painter JE, et al. The prevalence and characteristics of colorectal neoplasia in acromegaly. *J Clin Endocrinol Metab*. 2000;85:3417-3424.
390. Kauppinen-Makelin R, Sane T, Valimaki MJ, et al. Increased cancer incidence in acromegaly: a nationwide survey. *Clin Endocrinol (Oxf)*. 2010;72:278-279. Epub 2009 Apr 30.
391. Barkan AL, Stred SE, Reno K, et al. Increased growth hormone pulse frequency in acromegaly. *J Clin Endocrinol Metab*. 1989;69: 1225-1233.
392. Katznelson L, Kleinberg D, Vance ML, et al. Hypogonadism in patients with acromegaly: data from the multi-centre acromegaly registry pilot study. *Clin Endocrinol (Oxf)*. 2001;54:183-188.
393. Kasagi K, Shimatsu A, Miyamoto S, et al. Goiter associated with acromegaly: sonographic and scintigraphic findings of the thyroid gland. *Thyroid*. 1999;9:791-796.
394. Colao A, Cuocolo A, Marzullo P, et al. Effects of 1-year treatment with octreotide on cardiac performance in patients with acromegaly. *J Clin Endocrinol Metab*. 1999;84:17-23.
395. Dekkers OM, Biermasz NR, Pereira AM, et al. Mortality in acromegaly: a metaanalysis. *J Clin Endocrinol Metab*. 2008;93:61-67.
396. Rajasoorya C, Holdaway IM, Wrightson P, et al. Determinants of clinical outcome and survival in acromegaly. *Clin Endocrinol (Oxf)*. 1994;41:95-102.
397. Alexander MJ, DeSalles AA, Tomiyasu U. Multiple radiation-induced intracranial lesions after treatment for pituitary adenoma: case report. *J Neurosurg*. 1998;88:111-115.
398. Swearingen B, Barker FG, Katznelson L, et al. Long-term mortality after transsphenoidal surgery and adjunctive therapy for acromegaly. *J Clin Endocrinol Metab*. 1998;83:3419-3426.
399. Abosch A, Tyrrell JB, Lamborn KR, et al. Transsphenoidal microsurgery for growth hormone-secreting pituitary adenomas: initial outcome and long-term results. *J Clin Endocrinol Metab*. 1998;83:3411-3418.
400. Freda PU, Post KD, Powell JS, et al. Evaluation of disease status with sensitive measures of growth hormone secretion in 60 postoperative patients with acromegaly. *J Clin Endocrinol Metab*. 1998;83:3808-3816.
401. Holdaway IM, Rajasoorya RC, Gamble GD. Factors influencing mortality in acromegaly. *J Clin Endocrinol Metab*. 2004;89:667-674.
402. Holdaway IM, Bolland MJ, Gamble GD. A meta-analysis of the effect of lowering serum levels of GH and IGF-I on mortality in acromegaly. *Eur J Endocrinol*. 2008;159:89-95.
403. Giustina A, Barkan A, Casanueva FF, et al. Criteria for cure of acromegaly: a consensus statement. *J Clin Endocrinol Metab*. 2000; 85:526-529.
404. Freda PU, Reyes CM, Nuruzzaman AT, et al. Basal and glucose-suppressed GH levels less than 1 microg/L in newly diagnosed acromegaly. *Pituitary*. 2003;6:175-180.
405. Melmed S, Colao A, Barkan A, et al. Guidelines for acromegaly management: an update. *J Clin Endocrinol Metab*. 2009;94:1509-1517.
406. Duncan E, Wass JA. Investigation protocol: acromegaly and its investigation. *Clin Endocrinol (Oxf)*. 1999;50:285-293.
407. Clemmons DR, Van Wyk JJ, Ridgway EC, et al. Evaluation of acromegaly by radioimmunoassay of somatomedin-C. *N Engl J Med*. 1979;301:1138-1142.
408. Costa AC, Rossi A, Martinelli CE Jr, et al. Assessment of disease activity in treated acromegalic patients using a sensitive GH assay: should we achieve strict normal GH levels for a biochemical cure? *J Clin Endocrinol Metab*. 2002;87:3142-3147.
409. Dimaraki EV, Jaffe CA, DeMott-Friberg R, et al. Acromegaly with apparently normal GH secretion: implications for diagnosis and follow-up. *J Clin Endocrinol Metab*. 2002;87:3537-3542.
410. Frohman LA. Ectopic hormone production by tumors. *Clin Neuroendocr Perspect*. 1984;3:201-224.
411. Melmed S. Tight control of growth hormone: an attainable outcome for acromegaly treatment. *J Clin Endocrinol Metab*. 1998;83:3409-3410.

412. Lissett CA, Peacey SR, Laing I, et al. The outcome of surgery for acromegaly: the need for a specialist pituitary surgeon for all types of growth hormone (GH) secreting adenoma. *Clin Endocrinol (Oxf)*. 1998;49:653-657.
413. Ahmed S, Elsheikh M, Stratton IM, et al. Outcome of transphenoidal surgery for acromegaly and its relationship to surgical experience. *Clin Endocrinol (Oxf)*. 1999;50:561-567.
414. Laws ER, Thapar K. Pituitary surgery. *Endocrinol Metab Clin North Am*. 1999;28:119-131.
415. Fahlbusch R, Honegger J, Buchfelder M. Surgical management of acromegaly. *Endocrinol Metab Clin North Am*. 1992;21:669-692.
416. Shimon I, Cohen ZR, Ram Z, et al. Transsphenoidal surgery for acromegaly: endocrinological follow-up of 98 patients. *Neurosurgery*. 2001;48:1239-1243; discussion 1244-1245.
417. Cappabianca P, de Divitiis E. Image guided endoscopic transnasal removal of recurrent pituitary adenomas. *Neurosurgery*. 2003;52:483-484; author reply 484.
418. Kreutzer J, Vance ML, Lopes MB, et al. Surgical management of GH-secreting pituitary adenomas: an outcome study using modern remission criteria. *J Clin Endocrinol Metab*. 2001;86:4072-4077.
419. Barkan AL, Halasz I, Dornfeld KJ, et al. Pituitary irradiation is ineffective in normalizing plasma insulin-like growth factor I in patients with acromegaly. *J Clin Endocrinol Metab*. 1997;82:3187-3191.
420. Powell JS, Wardlaw SL, Post KD, et al. Outcome of radiotherapy for acromegaly using normalization of insulin-like growth factor I to define cure. *J Clin Endocrinol Metab*. 2000;85:2068-2071.
421. Biermasz NR, van Dulken H, Roelfsema F. Long-term follow-up results of postoperative radiotherapy in 36 patients with acromegaly. *J Clin Endocrinol Metab*. 2000;85:2476-2482.
422. Jezkova J, Marek J, Hana V, et al. Gamma knife radiosurgery for acromegaly: long-term experience. *Clin Endocrinol (Oxf)*. 2006;64:588-595.
423. Jenkins PJ, Bates P, Carson MN, et al. Conventional pituitary irradiation is effective in lowering serum growth hormone and insulin-like growth factor-I in patients with acromegaly. *J Clin Endocrinol Metab*. 2006;91:1239-1245.
424. Peacey SR, Toogood AA, Veldhuis JD, et al. The relationship between 24-hour growth hormone secretion and insulin-like growth factor I in patients with successfully treated acromegaly: impact of surgery or radiotherapy. *J Clin Endocrinol Metab*. 2001;86:259-266.
425. Castinetti F, Taieb D, Kuhn JM, et al. Outcome of gamma knife radiosurgery in 82 patients with acromegaly: correlation with initial hypersecretion. *J Clin Endocrinol Metab*. 2005;90:4483-4488.
426. Ronchi CL, Attanasio R, Verrua E, et al. Efficacy and tolerability of gamma knife radiosurgery in acromegaly: a 10-year follow-up study. *Clin Endocrinol (Oxf)*. Epub 2009 Mar 28.
427. van der Lely AJ, de Herder WW, Lamberts SW. The role of radiotherapy in acromegaly. *J Clin Endocrinol Metab*. 1997;82:3185-3186.
428. Murray RD, Darzy KH, Gleeson HK, et al. GH-deficient survivors of childhood cancer: GH replacement during adult life. *J Clin Endocrinol Metab*. 2002;87:129-135.
429. Ronchi CL, Giavoli C, Ferrante E, et al. Prevalence of GH deficiency in cured acromegalic patients: impact of different previous treatments. *Eur J Endocrinol*. 2009;161:37-42.
430. Wexler T, Gunnell L, Omer Z, et al. Growth hormone deficiency is associated with decreased quality of life in patients with prior acromegaly. *J Clin Endocrinol Metab*. 2009;94:2471-2477.
431. Jaffe CA, Barkan AL. Treatment of acromegaly with dopamine agonists. *Endocrinol Metab Clin North Am*. 1992;21:713-735.
432. Sherlock M, Fernandez-Rodriguez E, Alonso AA, et al. Medical therapy in patients with acromegaly: predictors of response and comparison of efficacy of dopamine agonists and somatostatin analogues. *J Clin Endocrinol Metab*. 2009;94:1255-1263.
433. Abs R, Verhelst J, Maiter D, et al. Cabergoline in the treatment of acromegaly: a study in 64 patients. *J Clin Endocrinol Metab*. 1998;83:374-378.
434. Weckbecker G, Lewis I, Albert R, et al. Opportunities in somatostatin research: biological, chemical and therapeutic aspects. *Nat Rev Drug Discov*. 2003;2:999-1017.
435. Lamberts SW, van der Lely AJ, de Herder WW, et al. Octreotide. *N Engl J Med*. 1996;334:246-254.
436. Lamberts SW, Uitterlinden P, Verschoor L, et al. Long-term treatment of acromegaly with the somatostatin analogue SMS 201-995. *N Engl J Med*. 1985;313:1576-1580.
437. Ur E, Mather SJ, Bomanji J, et al. Pituitary imaging using a labelled somatostatin analogue in acromegaly. *Clin Endocrinol (Oxf)*. 1992;36:147-150.
438. Acunzo J, Thirion S, Roche C, et al. Somatostatin receptor sst2 decreases cell viability and hormonal hypersecretion and reverses octreotide resistance of human pituitary adenomas. *Cancer Res*. 2008;68:10163-10170.
439. Ezzat S, Snyder PJ, Young WF, et al. Octreotide treatment of acromegaly: a randomized, multicenter study. *Ann Intern Med*. 1992;117:711-718.
440. Bhayana S, Booth GL, Asa SL, et al. The implication of somatotroph adenoma phenotype to somatostatin analog responsiveness in acromegaly. *J Clin Endocrinol Metab*. 2005;90:6290-6295.
441. Wang C, Lam KS, Arceo E, et al. Comparison of the effectiveness of 2-hourly versus 8-hourly subcutaneous injections of a somatostatin analog (SMS 201-995) in the treatment of acromegaly. *J Clin Endocrinol Metab*. 1989;69:670-677.
442. Newman CB, Melmed S, Snyder PJ, et al. Safety and efficacy of long-term octreotide therapy of acromegaly: results of a multicenter trial in 103 patients. A clinical research center study. *J Clin Endocrinol Metab*. 1995;80:2768-2775.
443. Gillis JC, Noble S, Goa KL. Octreotide long-acting release (LAR): a review of its pharmacological properties and therapeutic use in the management of acromegaly. *Drugs*. 1997;53:681-699.
444. Cozzi R, Montini M, Attanasio R, et al. Primary treatment of acromegaly with octreotide LAR: a long-term (up to nine years) prospective study of its efficacy in the control of disease activity and tumor shrinkage. *J Clin Endocrinol Metab*. 2006;91:1397-1403.
445. Colao A, Ferone D, Marzullo P, et al. Long-term effects of depot long-acting somatostatin analog octreotide on hormone levels and tumor mass in acromegaly. *J Clin Endocrinol Metab*. 2001;86:2779-2786.
446. Giustina A, Bonadonna S, Bugari G, et al. High-dose intramuscular octreotide in patients with acromegaly inadequately controlled on conventional somatostatin analogue therapy: a randomised controlled trial. *Eur J Endocrinol*. 2009;161:331-338.
447. Caron P, Morange-Ramos I, Cogne M, et al. Three year follow-up of acromegalic patients treated with intramuscular slow-release lanreotide. *J Clin Endocrinol Metab*. 1997;82:18-22.
448. Melmed S, Cook D, Schopohl J, et al. Rapid and sustained reduction of serum growth hormone and insulin-like growth factor-1 in patients with acromegaly receiving lanreotide Autogel((R)) therapy: a randomized, placebo-controlled, multicenter study with a 52 week open extension. *Pituitary*. Epub 2009 Jul 29.
449. Murray RD, Melmed S. A critical analysis of clinically available somatostatin analog formulations for therapy of acromegaly. *J Clin Endocrinol Metab*. 2008;93:2957-2968.
450. Carmichael JD, Bonert V, Mirocha JM, et al. The utility of oral glucose tolerance testing for diagnosis and assessment of treatment outcomes in 166 patients with acromegaly. *J Clin Endocrinol Metab*. 2009;94:523-527.
451. Bevan JS. Clinical review: the antitumoral effects of somatostatin analog therapy in acromegaly. *J Clin Endocrinol Metab*. 2005;90:1856-1863.
452. Melmed S, Sternberg R, Cook D, et al. A critical analysis of pituitary tumor shrinkage during primary medical therapy in acromegaly. *J Clin Endocrinol Metab*. 2005;90:4405-4410.
453. Mazziotti G, Giustina A. Effects of lanreotide SR and Autogel on tumor mass in patients with acromegaly: a systematic review. *Pituitary*. Epub 2009 Feb 3.
454. Colao A, Auriemma RS, Rebora A, et al. Significant tumour shrinkage after 12 months of lanreotide Autogel-120 mg treatment given first-line in acromegaly. *Clin Endocrinol (Oxf)*. 2009;71:237-245.
455. Biermasz NR, van Dulken H, Roelfsema F. Direct postoperative and follow-up results of transsphenoidal surgery in 19 acromegalic patients pretreated with octreotide compared to those in untreated matched controls. *J Clin Endocrinol Metab*. 1999;84:3551-3555.
456. Carlsen SM, Lund-Johansen M, Schreiner T, et al. Preoperative octreotide treatment in newly diagnosed acromegalic patients with macroadenomas increases cure short-term postoperative rates: a prospective, randomized trial. *J Clin Endocrinol Metab*. 2008;93:2984-2990.
457. Pascual J, Freijanes J, Berciano J, et al. Analgesic effect of octreotide in headache associated with acromegaly is not mediated by opioid mechanisms: case report. *Pain*. 1991;47:341-344.
458. Colao A, Marzullo P, Ferone D, et al. Cardiovascular effects of depot long-acting somatostatin analog Sandostatin LAR in acromegaly. *J Clin Endocrinol Metab*. 2000;85:3132-3140.
459. Colao A, Cuocolo A, Marzullo P, et al. Is the acromegalic cardiomyopathy reversible? Effect of 5-year normalization of growth hormone and insulin-like growth factor I levels on cardiac performance. *J Clin Endocrinol Metab*. 2001;86:1551-1557.
460. Mazziotti G, Floriani I, Bonadonna S, et al. Effects of somatostatin analogs on glucose homeostasis: a metaanalysis of acromegaly studies. *J Clin Endocrinol Metab*. 2009;94:1500-1508.
461. Melmed S, Dowling RH, Frohman L, et al. Consensus statement: benefits vs. risks of medical therapy for acromegaly. *Am J Med*. 1994;97:468-473.
462. Trainer PJ, Drake WM, Katznelson L, et al. Treatment of acromegaly with the growth hormone-receptor antagonist pegvisomant. *N Engl J Med*. 2000;342:1171-1177.
463. Ross RJ, Leung KC, Maamra M, et al. Binding and functional studies with the growth hormone receptor antagonist, B2036-PEG (pegvisomant), reveal effects of pegylation and evidence that it binds to a receptor dimer. *J Clin Endocrinol Metab*. 2001;86:1716-1723.
464. Buchfelder M, Schlaffer S, Droste M, et al. The German ACROSTUDY: Past and Present. *Eur J Endocrinol*. 2009;161:53.

465. Higham CE, Chung TT, Lawrance J, et al. Long-term experience of pegvisomant therapy as a treatment for acromegaly. *Clin Endocrinol (Oxf)*. 2009;71:86-91.
466. Herman-Bonert VS, Zib K, Scarlett JA, et al. Growth hormone receptor antagonist therapy in acromegalic patients resistant to somatostatin analogs. *J Clin Endocrinol Metab*. 2000;85:2958-2961.
467. Trainer PJ, Ezzat S, D'Souza GA, et al. A randomized, controlled, multicentre trial comparing pegvisomant alone with combination therapy of pegvisomant and long-acting octreotide in patients with acromegaly. *Clin Endocrinol (Oxf)*. 2009;71:549-557.
468. Colao A, Pivonello R, Auriemma RS, et al. Efficacy of 12-month treatment with the GH receptor antagonist pegvisomant in patients with acromegaly resistant to long-term, high-dose somatostatin analog treatment: effect on IGF-I levels, tumor mass, hypertension and glucose tolerance. *Eur J Endocrinol*. 2006;154:467-477.
469. Biering H, Saller B, Bauditz J, et al. Elevated transaminases during medical treatment of acromegaly: a review of the German pegvisomant surveillance experience and a report of a patient with histologically proven chronic mild active hepatitis. *Eur J Endocrinol*. 2006;154:213-220.
470. van der Lely AJ, Muller A, Janssen JA, et al. Control of tumor size and disease activity during cotreatment with octreotide and the growth hormone receptor antagonist pegvisomant in an acromegalic patient. *J Clin Endocrinol Metab*. 2001;86:478-481.
471. Jorgensen JO, Feldt-Rasmussen U, Frystyk J, et al. Cotreatment of acromegaly with a somatostatin analog and a growth hormone receptor antagonist. *J Clin Endocrinol Metab*. 2005;90:5627-5631.
472. Feenstra J, de Herder WW, ten Have SM, et al. Combined therapy with somatostatin analogues and weekly pegvisomant in active acromegaly. *Lancet*. 2005;365:1644-1646.
473. Neggers SJ, de Herder WW, Janssen JA, et al. Combined treatment for acromegaly with long-acting somatostatin analogs and pegvisomant: long-term safety for up to 4.5 years (median 2.2 years) of follow-up in 86 patients. *Eur J Endocrinol*. 2009;160:529-533.
474. Freda PU. Monitoring of acromegaly: what should be performed when GH and IGF-1 levels are discrepant? *Clin Endocrinol (Oxf)*. 2009;71:166-170.
475. Karavitaki N, Turner HE, Adams CB, et al. Surgical debulking of pituitary macroadenomas causing acromegaly improves control by lanreotide. *Clin Endocrinol (Oxf)*. 2008;68:970-975.
476. de Herder WW, Taal HR, Uitterlinden P, et al. Limited predictive value of an acute test with subcutaneous octreotide for long-term IGF-I normalization with Sandostatin LAR in acromegaly. *Eur J Endocrinol*. 2005;153:67-71.
477. Newman CB, Melmed S, George A, et al. Octreotide as primary therapy for acromegaly. *J Clin Endocrinol Metab*. 1998;83:3034-3040.
478. Mercado M, Borges F, Bouterfa H, et al. A prospective, multicentre study to investigate the efficacy, safety and tolerability of octreotide LAR (long-acting repeatable octreotide) in the primary therapy of patients with acromegaly. *Clin Endocrinol (Oxf)*. 2007;66:859-868.
479. Maiza JC, Vezzosi D, Matta M, et al. Long-term (up to 18 years) effects on GH/IGF-1 hypersecretion and tumour size of primary somatostatin analogue (SSTa) therapy in patients with GH-secreting pituitary adenoma responsive to SSTa. *Clin Endocrinol (Oxf)*. 2007;67:282-289.
480. Nunes ML, Vattaut S, Corcuff JB, et al. Late-night salivary cortisol for diagnosis of overt and subclinical Cushing's syndrome in hospitalized and ambulatory patients. *J Clin Endocrinol Metab*. 2009;94:456-462.
481. Raff H. Utility of salivary cortisol measurements in Cushing's syndrome and adrenal insufficiency. *J Clin Endocrinol Metab*. 2009;94:3647-3655.
482. Nieman LK, Biller BM, Findling JW, et al. The diagnosis of Cushing's syndrome: an Endocrine Society Clinical Practice Guideline. *J Clin Endocrinol Metab*. 2008;93:1526-1540.
483. Wilson CB. Surgical management of pituitary tumors. *J Clin Endocrinol Metab*. 1997;82:2381-2385.
484. Biller BM, Grossman AB, Stewart PM, et al. Treatment of adrenocorticotropin-dependent Cushing's syndrome: a consensus statement. *J Clin Endocrinol Metab*. 2008;93:2454-2462.
485. Simmons NE, Alden TD, Thorner MO, et al. Serum cortisol response to transsphenoidal surgery for Cushing disease. *J Neurosurg*. 2001;95:1-8.
486. Scheithauer BW, Horvath E, Lloyd RV, et al. Pathology of pituitary adenomas and pituitary hyperplasia. In Thapar K, Kovacs K, Scheithauer BW, Lloyd RV, ed. *Diagnosis and Management of Pituitary Tumors*. Totowa, NJ: Humana Press; 2001:91-154.
487. Baldeweg SE, Pollock JR, Powell M, Ahlquist J. A spectrum of behaviour in silent corticotroph pituitary adenomas. *Br J Neurosurg*. 2005;19:38-42.
488. Mindermann T, Wilson CB. Thyrotropin-producing pituitary adenomas. *J Neurosurg*. 1993;79:521-527.
489. McCutcheon IE, Weintraub BD, Oldfield EH. Surgical treatment of thyrotropin-secreting pituitary adenomas. *J Neurosurg*. 1990;73:674-683.
490. Roelfsema F, Kok S, Kok P, et al. Pituitary-hormone secretion by thyrotropinomas. *Pituitary*. 2009;12:200-210.
491. Roelfsema F, Pereira AM, Keenan DM, et al. Thyrotropin secretion by thyrotropinomas is characterized by increased pulse frequency, delayed diurnal rhythm, enhanced basal secretion, spikiness, and disorderliness. *J Clin Endocrinol Metab*. 2008;93:4052-4057.
492. Sanno N, Teramoto A, Matsuno A, et al. GH and PRL gene expression by nonradioisotopic in situ hybridization in TSH-secreting pituitary adenomas. *J Clin Endocrinol Metab*. 1995;80:2518-2522.
493. Yoshihara A, Isozaki O, Hizuka N, et al. Expression of type 5 somatostatin receptor in TSH-secreting pituitary adenomas: a possible marker for predicting long-term response to octreotide therapy. *Endocr J*. 2007;54:133-138.
494. Alings AM, Fliers E, de Herder WW, et al. A thyrotropin-secreting pituitary adenoma as a cause of thyrotoxic periodic paralysis. *J Endocrinol Invest*. 1998;21:703-706.
495. Beck-Peccoz P, Brucker-Davis F, Persani L, Thyrotropin-secreting pituitary tumors. *Endocr Rev*. 1996;17:610-638.
496. Brucker-Davis F, Oldfield EH, Skarulis MC, et al. Thyrotropin-secreting pituitary tumors: diagnostic criteria, thyroid hormone sensitivity, and treatment outcome in 25 patients followed at the National Institutes of Health. *J Clin Endocrinol Metab*. 1999;84:476-486.
497. Beck-Peccoz P, Persani L. TSH-producing adenomas. In DeGroot LJ, Jameson JL, eds. *Endocrinology*. 4th ed. Philadelphia: Saunders; 2001. 321-328.
498. Cooper DS, Wenig BM. Hyperthyroidism caused by an ectopic TSH-secreting pituitary tumor. *Thyroid*. 1996;6:337-343.
499. Beckers A, Abs R, Mahler C, et al. Thyrotropin-secreting pituitary adenomas: report of seven cases. *J Clin Endocrinol Metab*. 1991;72:477-483.
500. Chanson P, Weintraub BD, Harris AG. Octreotide therapy for thyroid-stimulating hormone-secreting pituitary adenomas: a follow-up of 52 patients. *Ann Intern Med*. 1993;119:236-240.
501. Losa M, Giovanelli M, Persani L, et al. Criteria of cure and follow-up of central hyperthyroidism due to thyrotropin-secreting pituitary adenomas. *J Clin Endocrinol Metab*. 1996;81:3084-3090.
502. Beck-Peccoz P, Mariotti S, Guillausseau PJ, et al. Treatment of hyperthyroidism due to inappropriate secretion of thyrotropin with the somatostatin analog SMS 201-995. *J Clin Endocrinol Metab*. 1989;68:208-214.
503. Caron P, Arlot S, Bauters C, et al. Efficacy of the long-acting octreotide formulation (octreotide-LAR) in patients with thyrotropin-secreting pituitary adenomas. *J Clin Endocrinol Metab*. 2001;86:2849-2853.
504. Colao A, Pivonello R, Di Somma C, et al. Medical therapy of pituitary adenomas: effects on tumor shrinkage. *Rev Endocr Metab Disord*. 2009;10:111-123.
505. Samuels MH, Wood WM, Gordon DF, et al. Clinical and molecular studies of a thyrotropin-secreting pituitary adenoma. *J Clin Endocrinol Metab*. 1989;68:1211-1215.

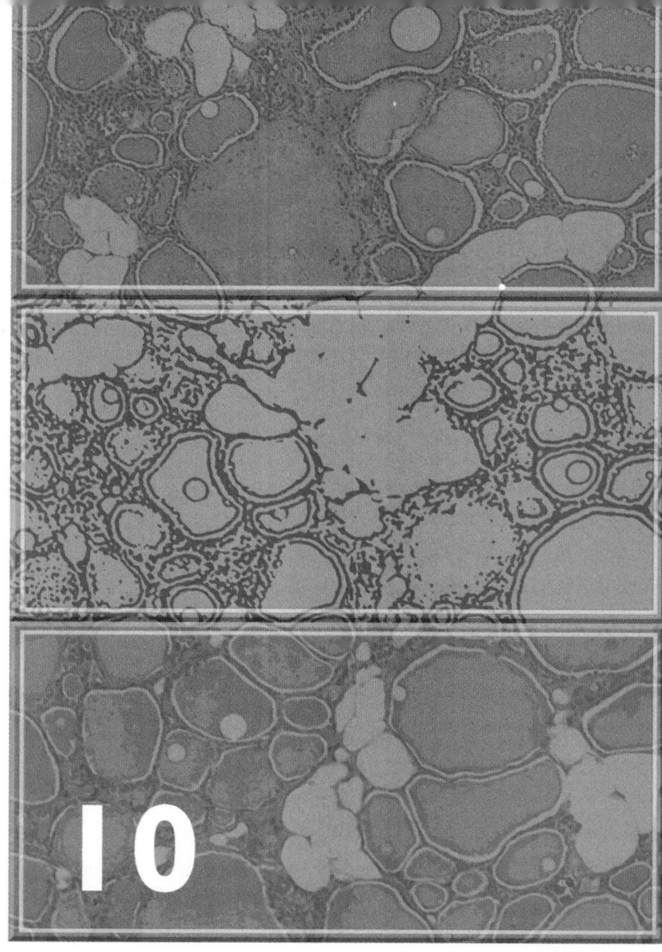

CHAPTER 10

Posterior Pituitary

ALAN G. ROBINSON • JOSEPH G. VERBALIS

ANATOMY

Normal Anatomy

The posterior pituitary is neural tissue and consists only of the distal axons of the hypothalamic magnocellular neurons that make up the neurohypophysis. The perikarya (cell bodies) of these axons are located in paired paraventricular and supraoptic nuclei of the hypothalamus. During embryogenesis,[1] neuroepithelial cells of the lining of the third ventricle mature into magnocellular neurons while migrating laterally to and above the optic chiasm to form the supraoptic nucleus and to the walls of the third ventricle to form the paraventricular nuclei. In the posterior pituitary, the axon terminals of the magnocellular neurons contain neurosecretory granules, membrane-bound packets of hormones stored for subsequent release. The blood for the anterior pituitary is supplied via the hypothalamic-pituitary portal system, but the posterior pituitary blood supply is directly from the inferior hypophyseal arteries, which are branches of the posterior communicating and internal carotid arteries. The drainage is into the cavernous sinus and internal jugular vein.

The hormones of the posterior pituitary, oxytocin and vasopressin, are synthesized in individual hormone-specific magnocellular neurons. The supraoptic nucleus is relatively simple, with 80% to 90% of the neurons producing vasopressin[2] and virtually all axons projecting to the posterior pituitary.[1] The organization of the paraventricular nuclei is much more complex and varies among species. In the human, there are five subnuclei[2] and parvocellular (smaller cells) divisions that synthesize other peptides, such as corticotropin-releasing hormone (CRH), thyrotropin-releasing hormone, somatostatin,[3] and opioids.[4] The parvocellular neurons project to the median eminence, brain stem, and spinal cord,[5] where they take part in a variety of neuroendocrine autonomic functions. The suprachiasmatic nucleus, which is located in the midline at the base of and anterior to the third ventricle, also synthesizes vasopressin and controls circadian and seasonal rhythms.[2]

The major stimulatory neurotransmitter in the neurohypophysis is glutamate; noradrenergic stimulatory inputs act by stimulating glutamate.[6,7] Glutamate receptors account for 25% of synapsis on magnocellular neurons.[6] The major inhibitory input is γ-aminobutyric acid (GABA), which accounts for 20% to 40% of the synaptic input to the magnocellular neurons.[8] Steroid hormone actions on the magnocellular neurons are mediated by GABA or glutamate receptors.[9]

One of the most remarkable aspects of the magnocellular system is the plasticity of the system in response to prolonged stimulation. Plasticity is demonstrated in animals by prolonged osmotic stimulation with hypertonic saline, but it is probably most often of import in humans during parturition and lactation.[8] During prolonged stimulation, the perikarya themselves enlarge and the glia retract, diminishing astrocyte coverage of the neurons and increasing extracellular space between cells so that neurotransmitters can spread among cells. These two events interact to increase the contact between cells, which enhances the synchrony and the pulsatile secretion, which for oxytocin is especially important during parturition and milk letdown of lactation. Secretion of oxytocin by dendrites of the neurons produces a positive feedback in a paracrine/autocrine fashion to enhance the further secretion of the hormone; vasopressin release similarly produces a positive feedback enhancement. Neurotransmitter receptors may increase on the neuron and the astrocytes themselves and contribute to the plasticity, not just by altering their shape but because they function to clear neurotransmitters from the extracellular space and release active substances themselves. This structural plasticity during stimulation is enabled by the continued presence in the supraoptic and paraventricular nuclei of cytoskeleton proteins and cell adhesion molecules that are present elsewhere in the brain only during embryogenesis.[10]

Ectopic Posterior Pituitary

With the development of magnetic resonance imaging of the brain, it was discovered that T1-weighted images with MRI produced a bright signal in the posterior pituitary.[11] This new diagnostic imaging technology (described in detail later) allowed the identification of children with abnormal anatomy of the posterior pituitary in whom the "bright spot" was recognized in the base of the hypothalamus. These cases are referred to as *ectopic posterior pituitary* or *ectopic posterior lobe*. Etiologies include traumatic delivery (these patients have a higher incidence of breech delivery and perinatal injuries) and genetic abnormalities of the transcription factors that regulate pituitary embryogenesis.[12] Cases are recognized in children with growth retardation and anterior pituitary deficiency rather than posterior pituitary deficiency. The degree of anterior pituitary deficit depends on the persistence of a pituitary stalk and a retained portal vasculature from the hypothalamus to the anterior pituitary.[13-15] Deficiency of adrenocorticotropic hormone (ACTH) is common and should be investigated, because the patients may not respond appropriately to stress.[12]

SYNTHESIS AND RELEASE OF NEUROHYPOPHYSEAL HORMONES

Vasopressin and oxytocin are nonapeptides consisting of a 6-amino-acid ring with a cysteine-to-cysteine bridge and a 3-amino-acid tail (Fig. 10-1). All mammals have arginine vasopressin and oxytocin, as illustrated in Figure 10-1, with the exception of the pig. In the pig, a lysine is substituted for arginine in position 8 of vasopressin, producing lysine vasopressin. Both genes are found on chromosome 20,[16] although they are situated in a tail-to-tail position and transcribed in opposite directions.[17] The hormones are each synthesized as part of a precursor molecule consisting of the nonapeptide and a hormone-specific neurophysin and for vasopressin only an additional glycopeptide.[18] The precursor is packaged in neurosecretory granules and cleaved to the products during transport to the posterior pituitary.

A Arginine vasopressin

Phe^3 — Gln^4
Tyr^2 | Asn^5
H_2N — Cys^1 - S-S - Cys^6 — Pro^7 — L Arg^8 — Gly^9 — NH_2

B Oxytocin

Ile^3 — Gln^4
Tyr^2 | Asn^5
H_2N — Cys^1 - S-S - Cys^6 — Pro^7 — Leu^8 — Gly^9 — NH_2

C Desmopressin

Phe^3 — Gln^4
Tyr^2 | Asn^5
H — Cys^1 - S-S - Cys^6 — Pro^7 — D Arg^8 — Gly^9 — NH_2

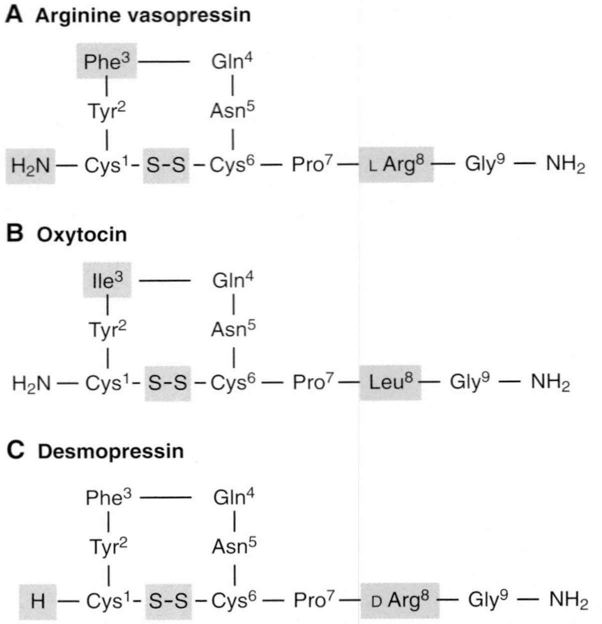

Figure 10-1 Comparison of the chemical structures of, **A,** arginine vasopressin, **B,** oxytocin, and, **C,** desmopressin. The differences are illustrated by the shaded areas. Oxytocin differs from vasopressin in position 3 (Ile for Phe) and position 8 (Leu for Arg). Desmopressin differs from arginine vasopressin in that the terminal cystine is deaminated and the arginine in position 8 is a D rather than an L isomer. (From A. G. Robinson, University of California at Los Angeles, CA, with permission.)

When a stimulus for secretion of vasopressin or oxytocin acts on the appropriate magnocellular cell body, an action potential is generated and propagates down the long axon to the posterior pituitary. The action potential causes an influx of calcium, which induces neurosecretory granules to fuse with the cell membrane and extrude their entire contents into the perivascular space and subsequently into the capillary system of the posterior pituitary. At the physiologic pH of plasma, there is no binding of these hormones (vasopressin or oxytocin) to their respective neurophysins, so each peptide circulates independently in the bloodstream.

The control of hormone synthesis is at the level of transcription. Stimuli for secretion of vasopressin or oxytocin also stimulate transcription and increase the messenger RNA (mRNA) content in the magnocellular neurons. This has been studied in most detail in rats, where dehydration[19] accelerates transcription and increases the levels of vasopressin (and oxytocin) mRNA[20-22] and where hypoosmolality produces a decrease in the content of vasopressin mRNA.[23]

The transport of neurosecretory vesicles from the site of synthesis to the posterior pituitary along microtubule tracks[24] is also regulated. When synthesis is turned off, transport stops, and when synthesis is increased, transport is upregulated.[24] Thus, there is coordination of stimulated release of hormone, transport of hormone, and synthesis of new hormone. There is, however, asynchrony in the timing of these events. The asynchrony is demonstrated by changes in the content of vasopressin stored in the posterior pituitary. The absolute content varies considerably among species but is a remarkable store, generally equivalent to the amount of hormone required to sustain basal release for 30 to 50 days or maximum release for 5 to 10 days.[25] In animals, prolonged and intense stimulation of vasopressin release (e.g., in dehydration or salt-loading) produces a depletion of stored hormone in the posterior pituitary.[22,26,27] When the animals are returned to normal water intake, there is within 7 to 14 days a gradual recovery of pituitary content back to baseline (or higher) levels. This phenomenon was modeled by Fitzsimmons,[28] who provided experimental evidence that a long half-life of the vasopressin message (approximately 2 days) is, from a minimalist point of view, a plausible explanation of the events. When a strong or sustained stimulus releases vasopressin, there is an immediate stimulus for transcription of new mRNA. Because it requires several days for the peak level of mRNA to be reached, translation increases slowly. When the stimulus is removed, the elevated mRNA slowly declines while synthesizing hormone that repletes the store in the posterior pituitary to the previous baseline level.

PHYSIOLOGY OF SECRETION OF VASOPRESSIN AND THIRST

The physiologic regulation of vasopressin synthesis and secretion involves two systems: osmotic and pressure/volume (Fig. 10-2). Functions of these two systems are so distinct that historically it was thought there were two hormones—an antidiuretic hormone (ADH) and a vasopressor hormone (AVP). Hence, the two names are used interchangeably for (8-arginine) vasopressin. There are separate systems at the level of the receptors on the end organs of response. The V_{1a} receptors on blood vessels are distinct from V_2 receptors on renal collecting duct epithelia. A third receptor, V_3 or V_{1b}, is responsible for the nontraditional biologic action of vasopressin to stimulate ACTH secretion from the anterior pituitary. V_2 receptors also regulate the nontraditional action of vasopressin to stimulate production of factor VIII and von Willebrand factor.

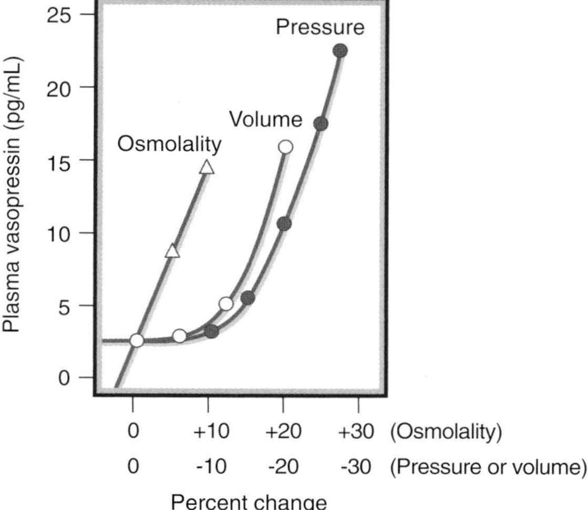

Figure 10-2 Comparison in humans of the release of vasopressin in response to increased osmolality (*open triangles*) or to decreased blood pressure (*filled circles*) or blood volume (*open circles*). Plasma vasopressin is much more sensitive to change in osmolality, responding to as little as a 1% increase, whereas a change of 10% to 15% or greater in volume or pressure is required to stimulate release of vasopressin. (Redrawn from Robertson GL, Berl T. Water metabolism. In: Brenner B, Rector F Jr, eds. *The Kidney*, 3rd ed., vol 1. Philadelphia, PA: Elsevier; 1986:385. Figure by A. G. Robinson, University of California at Los Angeles, CA, with permission.)

Vasopressin is the main hormone involved in the regulation of water homeostasis and osmolality, whereas the renin-angiotensin-aldosterone system (RAAS) is mainly responsible for regulation of blood pressure and volume. Pathologic disorders of the neurohypophysis are primarily expressed as abnormalities of osmolality produced by abnormal excretion or retention of water. In the case of osmoregulation, vasopressin secretion is relatively uncomplicated, with small increases in osmolality producing a parallel increase in vasopressin secretion and small decreases in osmolality causing a parallel decrease in vasopressin secretion. The regulation of volume and blood pressure is significantly more complicated (see review by Thrasher[29]), and experimental models of vasopressin and baroreceptor regulation in animals often involve inhibiting or measuring other concurrent sympathetic inputs to the system, or both, to ascertain direct effects of any stimulus on secretion of vasopressin (see Fig. 10-2). Other influences on vasopressin secretion, such as the inhibiting influence of glucocorticoids and the potent stimulus of nausea and vomiting, are less important as physiologic regulators of vasopressin but may be important in pathologic situations.

Volume and Pressure Regulation

High-pressure arterial baroreceptors are located in the carotid sinus and aortic arch, and low-pressure volume receptors are located in the atria and pulmonary venous system.[29] The afferent signals from these receptors are carried from the chest to the brain stem through cranial nerves IX and X. Interruption of the vagal input by vagotomy or vagal cold block in dogs[30-32] or destruction of the A1 area of the medulla (which receives input from nerves IX and X) in rabbits[33-35] results in an increase in vasopressin secretion. These and other data led to the concept that baroreceptors and volume receptors normally inhibit the magnocellular neurons and that decreases in this tonic inhibition result in release of vasopressin. Arterial and venous constriction induced by vasopressin action on V_{1a} receptors contracts the vessels around the existing plasma volume to effectively "increase" plasma volume and reestablish the inhibition of secretion of vasopressin.

Vasopressin's action at the kidney to retain water does help replace volume, but the major hormonal regulation to control volume is the RAAS, which stimulates sodium reabsorption in the kidney (see Chapter 15). The concept of tonic inhibition of vasopressin secretion by baroreceptors has been questioned,[29,36] but there is agreement that the volume receptor and baroreceptor responses that lead to increased vasopressin release in humans are much less sensitive than the osmoreceptors (see Fig. 10-2). This lesser response has been attributed to the fact that changes in blood volume and central venous pressure have little effect to increase vasopressin in humans as long as arterial pressure can be maintained by alternative regulatory mechanisms such as RAAS and sympathetic reflexes.[29] When the hypovolemia is sufficient to cause a decrease in blood pressure, there is a sudden and exponential increase in the level of vasopressin in plasma (see Fig. 10-2).[29,37] There is also agreement that changes in volume or pressure that are insufficient to cause direct increases in vasopressin can nonetheless modify the response of the vasopressin system to osmoregulatory inputs.[37,38]

Increases in pressure or central volume decrease the secretion of vasopressin,[39] but again, the response of the RAAS to cause sodium excretion is much more sensitive to increases of pressure and volume than is the response to decrease secretion of vasopressin.[29] Consequently, changes in blood pressure and volume involve both excitatory and inhibitory influences from the brain stem to magnocellular neurons, with the dominant influence depending on the physiologic circumstances.

Osmotic Regulation

The primary receptors for sensing changes in osmolality are located in the brain. Most of the brain is within the blood-brain barrier, which is generally impermeable to polar solutes. The osmostat is insensitive to urea and glucose, which readily cross cellular membranes but not the blood-brain barrier; this provides evidence that the osmoreceptors must be outside the blood-brain barrier. Experimental brain lesions in animals have strongly implicated cells in the organum vasculosum of the lamina terminalis (OVLT) and in areas of the adjacent anterior hypothalamus near the anterior wall of the third cerebral ventricle as the primary osmoreceptors. Because these and other circumventricular organs are perfused by fenestrated capillaries, they are outside the blood-brain barrier. Surgical destruction of the OVLT abolishes vasopressin secretion and thirst responses to hyperosmolality but not responses to hypovolemia.[40] Essentially the same occurs in humans with brain damage that destroys the region around the OVLT, and these patients cannot maintain normal plasma osmolalities even under basal conditions.[41] In contrast, destruction of the magnocellular neurons of the supraoptic and paraventricular nuclei eliminates dehydration-induced secretion of vasopressin but does not alter thirst, clearly indicating that osmotically stimulated thirst must be generated at a site proximal to the magnocellular cells.

Extracellular fluid (ECF) osmolality (predominantly determined by the sodium concentration, [Na^+]) varies from 280 to 295 mOsm/kg H_2O in normal subjects, but in any individual it is maintained within a narrower range. The ability to maintain this narrow range depends on the sensitive response of plasma vasopressin to changes in plasma osmolality; the sensitive response of urine osmolality to changes in plasma vasopressin; and then the gain in the system achieved by the response of urine volume to changes in plasma vasopressin (Fig. 10-3). Basal plasma vasopressin is in the range of 0.5 to 2 pg/mL. As little as a 1% increase or decrease in plasma osmolality causes a rapid increase or decrease of vasopressin released from the store of hormone in the posterior pituitary.[37] Rapid metabolism of vasopressin is also characteristic of the hormone, which circulates in plasma with a half-life of approximately 15 minutes, allowing rapid changes in levels of vasopressin in plasma. In this way, small increases in osmolality produce a concentrated urine, and small decreases in osmolality produce a water diuresis.

Figure 10-3 illustrates the linear relationship between plasma osmolality and plasma vasopressin that has been described in humans.[37] This linear relationship persists well above the normal excursion of osmolalities, as demonstrated when the increase is induced by infusion of hypertonic saline or is observed during dehydration of patients with nephrogenic diabetes insipidus.[42] Similarly, Figure 10-3 illustrates that there is a sensitive and linear relationship between the level of vasopressin in plasma and the induced osmolality of the urine. Although plasma vasopressin may increase above the normal physiologic range, the urine osmolality plateaus at approximately 1000 to 1200 mOsm/kg H_2O because the maximum concentration that can be reached by the fluid in the renal collecting duct is the osmolality of the inner medulla.

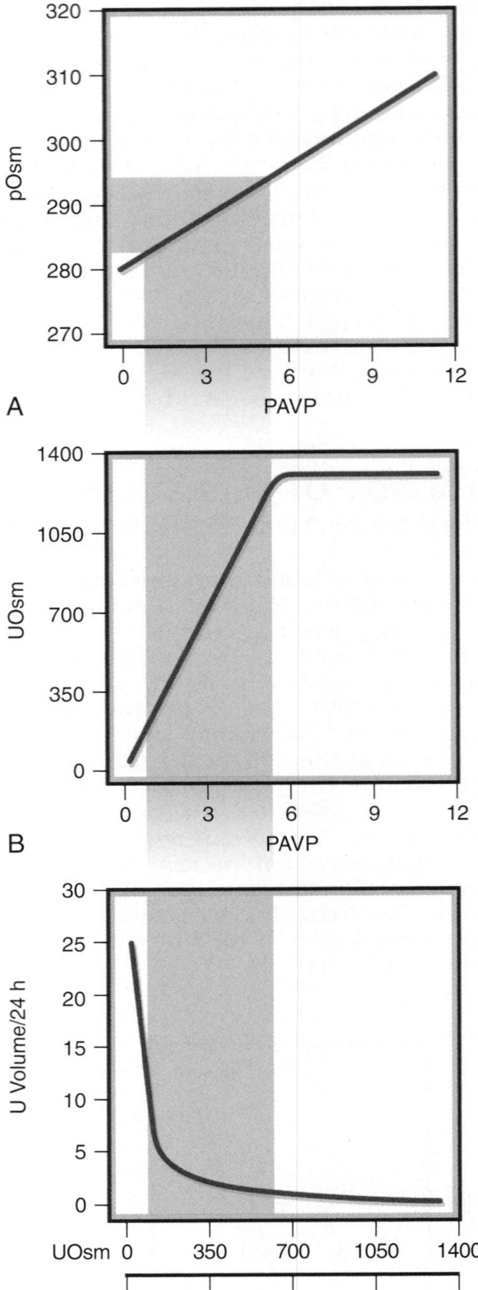

Figure 10-3 Effect of change in plasma osmolality (pOsm, in mOsm/kg of H_2O) on plasma arginine vasopressin (PAVP, in pg/mL) and consequent effects on urine osmolality (UOsm, in mOsm/kg of H_2O) and urine volume (L/day). The shaded area represents the normal range. **A,** Small changes in pOsm induce changes in PAVP, typically between less than 0.5 and 5 to 6 pg/mL. **B,** Changes in PVAP induce changes in UOsm through the full range, from maximally dilute to maximally concentrated urine. Although PAVP can rise to higher levels than 6 pg/mL, this does not translate into increased UOsm, which has a maximum determined by the osmolality of an inner medulla of the kidney. **C,** The relationship of urine volume to UOsm is logarithmic, assuming a constant osmolar load and the urine volume that would excrete that osmolar load at the UOsm indicated. As a result, urine volume changes relatively little with small changes in the other parameters until there is almost complete absence of PAVP, after which the urine volume increases dramatically. (Calculated from a formula presented in Robertson G, Shelton R, Athar S. The osmoregulation of vasopressin. *Kidney Int.* 1976;10:25-37. Figure by A. G. Robinson, University of Los Angeles, CA, with permission of Macmillan Publishers, Ltd.)

Figure 10-3 also shows the relationship of plasma vasopressin to urine volume. This is a calculated relationship based on the urine volume necessary to excrete a fixed quantity of osmolytes (800 milliosmoles) at the urine osmolality produced by the change in plasma vasopressin. These graphs demonstrate the gain in the system that can be observed when the changes in urine volume relative to plasma vasopressin are considered. If vasopressin is absent, 18 to 20 L/day of urine is excreted, but with an increase in vasopressin of as little as 0.5 to 1 pg/mL, urine volume is reduced to less than 4 L/day. This illustrates the important point that small changes at low plasma levels of vasopressin are much larger determinants of polyuria than are greater changes at higher plasma levels.

In the kidney, water is conserved by the combined functions of the loop of Henle and the collecting duct. The loop of Henle generates a high osmolality in the renal medulla by means of the countercurrent multiplier system. Vasopressin acts in the collecting duct to increase its permeability to water (and urea), thereby allowing osmotic equilibration between the urine and the hypertonic medullary interstitium. The net effect of this process is to extract water from the urine (which is removed from the medulla by interstitial blood vessels, vasa recta), resulting in increased urine concentration and decreased urine volume (antidiuresis).

Vasopressin produces antidiuresis by binding to V_2 receptors on the epithelial principal cells of the renal collecting tubule. Binding activates adenylate cyclase, increasing the level of cyclic adenosine monophosphate (cAMP), which then stimulates protein kinase A and leads to insertion of aquaporin 2 into the luminal membrane.[43] Aquaporin 2 is one of the widely expressed family of water channels that mediate rapid water transport across cell membranes.[44] In the kidney, water moves from the collecting duct into the hypertonic inner medulla, producing a concentrated urine.[45] Aquaporins 3 and 4 are constitutively synthesized and are expressed at high levels in the basolateral plasma membranes of principal cells, where they are responsible for the high water permeability of the basolateral plasma membrane.[44,45] Dissociation of vasopressin from the V_2 receptor allows intracellular cAMP levels to decrease, and the water channels are then reinternalized into the intracytoplasmic vesicles, terminating the increased water permeability. The aquaporin-containing vesicles remain just below the apical membrane and can be quickly "shuttled" into and out of the membrane in response to changes in intracellular cAMP levels. This mechanism allows minute-to-minute regulation of renal water excretion in response to changes in ambient levels of vasopressin in plasma.

There is also long-term regulation of collecting duct water permeability in response to prolonged high levels of circulating vasopressin. Chronically high levels of vasopressin induce increased synthesis of aquaporin 2 and aquaporin 3 water channels in the collecting duct principal cells and hence high levels of those proteins. This response requires at least 24 hours and is not as rapidly reversible. Increased numbers of aquaporin 2 and 3 water channels, combined with the short-term effect of vasopressin to insert aquaporin 2 into the apical plasma membrane, allows the collecting ducts to achieve extremely high water permeabilities and water conservation during prolonged dehydration.[44,45] Hypertonicity per se may augment aquaporin 2 expression. A variety of accessory proteins that regulate fusion attachment to membranes as well as factors that control remodeling of the cytoskeleton have also been described as controlling movement of aquaporins.[46]

Thirst

Urine volume can be reduced to a minimum but not completely eliminated, and insensible water loss is a continuous unregulated process. To maintain water homeostasis, water must be consumed to replace the obligate urinary and insensible fluid losses. This is regulated by thirst. As with vasopressin, thirst can be stimulated by increases in osmolality of the ECF or by decreases in intravascular volume. Furthermore, there is evidence that the receptors are similar; that is, osmoreceptors in the anterior hypothalamus and low- and high-pressure baroreceptors in the chest mediate the thirst stimulus (with a likely contribution from circulating angiotensin II to stimulate thirst during more severe degrees of intravascular hypovolemia and hypotension).[47] Studies in humans using quantitative estimates of subjective symptoms of thirst have confirmed that increases in plasma osmolality of 2% to 3% are necessary to produce an unequivocal sensation described as "thirst."[41] As with vasopressin secretion, the threshold for producing thirst by hypovolemia is significantly higher.

Although osmotic changes clearly are effective stimulants of thirst, most humans consume the bulk of their ingested water as a result of the relatively unregulated components of fluid intake. Beverages are consumed with food for reasons of palatability or taken for desired secondary effects (e.g., caffeine) or for social or habitual reasons (e.g., sodas, alcoholic beverages). As a result, humans typically ingest volumes in excess of what can be considered to be an actual "need" for fluid. Consistent with this observation is the fact that, under most conditions, plasma osmolalities in humans remain within 1% to 2% of basal levels—levels thought to be below the threshold levels that stimulate thirst. This suggests that, despite the obvious vital importance of thirst during pathologic situations of hyperosmolality and hypovolemia, under normal physiologic conditions water balance in humans is accomplished more by free water excretion regulated by vasopressin than by water intake regulated by thirst. This also explains why water intake must be consciously restricted in cases of persistent unregulated secretion of vasopressin (see later discussion of SIADH).

Clinical Consequences of Osmotic and Volume Regulation

In most physiologic situations, there is concurrence and synergy between the effect of increased osmolality and that of decreased volume to stimulate release of vasopressin. For example, with dehydration, osmolality increases and volume decreases, and each of these changes stimulates the release of vasopressin. Furthermore, there is good evidence that a decrease in volume shifts the plasma vasopressin/plasma osmolality response curve to the left, resulting in a greater release of vasopressin at any given osmolality.[29,48] Similarly, excess of fluid produces a decrease in osmolality and an increase in volume, both of which cause a decrease in vasopressin secretion.

The physiology of the relationships among plasma osmolality, plasma vasopressin, and, most importantly, urine volume determine some of the pathophysiologic features of decreased or increased secretion of vasopressin. As shown in Figure 10-3, a regular loss of vasopressin neurons that might decrease the secretory capacity of the neurohypophysis from a level that is able to produce a blood vasopressin concentration of 10 to 20 pg/mL one that is only sufficient to maintain a blood level 5 pg/mL would not cause any significant change in the ability to attain a maximum urine osmolality. Below 5 pg/mL, there is a linear decrease in the ability to maximally concentrate the urine. However, from the volume curve it can be seen that this results in only a modest increase in urine volume. It is only when the last few vasopressinergic neurons are lost and the maximum vasopressin concentration that can be maintained drops from 1 to 0.5 pg/mL that there is a large increase in urine volume. These responses, therefore, allow water conservation even with minimal ability to secrete vasopressin, and they may explain why patients with diabetes insipidus that has persisted for a relatively long period (e.g., after surgery or head injury) may eventually be able to discontinue treatment with vasopressin. The number of vasopressinergic neurons that need to recover to maintain an asymptomatic urine *volume* is small. The same pathophysiology is important in considering the syndrome of inappropriate secretion of antidiuretic hormone (SIADH). For example, a patient who is unable to suppress vasopressin to less than 1 pg/mL can excrete 2 L/day at a standard osmolar load, but if fluid intake increases to greater than that which can be excreted with the fixed level of vasopressin (1 pg/mL), then fluid will be retained and the sequence of events that causes hyponatremia in SIADH will be initiated.

An analysis of what is presently known about the regulation of thirst and secretion of vasopressin in humans demonstrates a simple but elegant system to maintain water balance. Under normal physiologic conditions, the sensitivity of the osmoregulatory system for secretion of vasopressin accounts for maintenance of plasma osmolality within narrow limits by adjusting renal water excretion in response to small changes in osmolality. Stimulated thirst does not represent a major regulatory mechanism under these conditions, because unregulated fluid ingestion and water from metabolized food supplies water in excess of true "need." However, when unregulated water intake does not supply body needs even with maximal antidiuresis, plasma osmolality rises to levels that stimulate thirst, producing water intake proportional to the elevation in osmolality. This arrangement has the advantage of freeing animals and humans from frequent episodes of thirst and water-seeking behavior when the water deficiency is sufficiently mild to be compensated for by renal water conservation yet it does stimulate water ingestion when water deficiency reaches a potentially harmful level.

Reset Osmostat during Pregnancy

Major shifts of fluid during normal pregnancy produce a decreased plasma osmolality of about 10 mmol/kg and an increase in plasma volume[49] and is the best example of a true resetting of the osmostat. The shift in osmotic threshold appears at about 5 to 8 weeks of gestation and persists throughout pregnancy, returning to normal by 2 weeks after delivery.[49] The physiology of the reset osmostat has been considered in relation to the expanded plasma volume. Total body water in pregnant women is increased by 7 to 8 L due to profound vasodilatation.[50] This volume is sensed as normal, and vasopressin responds appropriately to decreases and increases of the expanded volume.[49,51] Both the changes in volume and the changes in osmolality have been reproduced by infusion of relaxin, a normal hormone of pregnancy that is a member of the insulin-like growth factor (IGF) family, into virgin female and normal rats,[52,53] and they have been reversed in pregnant rats by immunoneutralization of relaxin,[54] so relaxin is the accepted mediator of the effect.

In women, the placenta produces an enzyme, cysteine aminopeptidase, that is released into the plasma and is known as oxytocinase.[49,55] However, this enzyme degrades vasopressin with equal potency. The activity of oxytocinase (vasopressinase) increases markedly at about 20 weeks of gestation and increases further to 40 weeks, returning slowly to normal over a few weeks after delivery.[56] The potential pathology produced by this condition is described later (see "Diabetes Insipidus").

Osmotic Regulation in Aging

Numerous studies have reported that elderly humans are at risk for both hypernatremia and hyponatremia.[57,58] In older subjects, there is a decrease in glomerular filtration rate (GFR),[57] and the collecting duct in the aged kidney may be less responsive to vasopressin-stimulated increases in aquaporin 2 water channels, thus limiting the ability to excrete free water.[59] Elderly subjects are reported to have a lower nocturnal plasma level of arginine vasopressin and a prolonged effect of administered desmopressin.[60] Many other abnormalities of fluid and electrolyte balance in the elderly result from comorbid conditions or the numerous pharmacologic agents these patients are often taking. Studies of responses to dehydration, osmolar stimulation, or volume stimulation in the elderly are complicated by the fact that, by age 75 to 80 years, there is a decline in total body water to 50% of the level seen in normal young adults.[61] The elderly have a decreased thirst with dehydration and a lesser fluid intake during recovery from dehydration.[62-64] At the other end of the spectrum, elderly patients have been found to excrete a water load less well than younger subjects and at least part of this is due to decreased suppression of vasopressin.[65]

In summary, there are age-related changes in body volumes and renal function that predispose the elderly to abnormalities in water and electrolyte balance. Diseases that are more common in the elderly aggravate this condition, and the therapies for these diseases also affect water balance. Healthy elderly humans probably have at least a normal (or increased) ability to secrete vasopressin but a decreased appreciation for thirst and a decreased ability to achieve either a maximum concentration of urine to retain water or maximum dilution of urine to excrete water. This demonstrates the necessity of paying attention to fluid balance problems in the elderly, because undetected hypernatremia or hyponatremia can lead to increased morbidity and mortality.[66]

DIABETES INSIPIDUS

Diabetes insipidus (DI) is a disorder in which the patient secretes a large volume of urine ("diabetes") that is hypotonic, dilute, and tasteless ("insipid"). This is opposed to the hypertonic and sweet urine of *diabetes mellitus* ("honey"). DI is caused by absence of the hormone vasopressin or inadequate response to vasopressin. The four syndromes of DI—primary polydipsia, hypothalamic DI, DI of pregnancy, and nephrogenic DI—can be explained by the pathophysiology of excess intake of water, decreased synthesis or secretion of vasopressin, accelerated metabolism of vasopressin, or lack of appropriate response to vasopressin by the kidney. The absence of vasopressin produces pathology related only to water, not blood pressure. Most patients have an intact thirst mechanism, so they do not become dehydrated but present with polyuria and polydipsia. Patients with DI who have inadequate thirst can rapidly become dehydrated and develop severe hypernatremia with devastating effects on the central nervous system (CNS). Hypertonic encephalopathy with obtundation, coma, and seizures may be produced by brain shrinkage. A decreased volume of the brain in the skull may lead to subarachnoid hemorrhage, intracerebral bleeding, or petechial hemorrhage.[67] However, the problems associated with severe hypernatremia usually are not observed in patients with DI because of intact thirst. Hypernatremic encephalopathy is a risk only when the patient is unable to respond to thirst because of age or level of consciousness (see later discussion).

To determine whether there is a large volume of urine, one can measure a 24-hour urine volume, but it is easier for an adult patient to keep a diary for 24 hours, recording the volume and time of each voided urine. Simultaneously, there is a determination of whether polyuria is caused by an osmotic agent (e.g., glucose) or intrinsic renal disease. Usually, routine laboratory studies and the clinical setting distinguish these disorders from DI. There is universal agreement that the diagnosis of DI is made when there is some dehydration to stimulate the normal release of vasopressin, but with a less than normal concentration of the urine. The gold standard is a dehydration test in a controlled environment followed by measurement of vasopressin in plasma and of response to administered vasopressin or its analogue, desmopressin. The description that follows is for adults. Special attention is required in children, and testing should be done only by a pediatrician; it should not be done in infants.[43] In children, care should be taken to prevent hyponatremia after administration of desmopressin.[43,68]

If the adult patient has mild polyuria, the test may begin in the evening, with the majority of dehydration carried out overnight. If the patient gives a history of large volumes of urine during the night, it is best to perform the test during the day, when the patient can be observed. The patient voids at the beginning of the test, and the starting weight is recorded. A sample for measurement of serum [Na^+] is obtained, and nothing is allowed by mouth (certainly no fluid) during the test. Each voided urine is then recorded, and the corresponding urine osmolality is measured. The patient is weighed after each liter of urine is passed. When two consecutive measurements of urine osmolality differ by no more than 10% and the patient has lost 2% of body weight, a plasma sample for [Na^+], osmolality, and vasopressin level is drawn, and the patient is given 2 µg of desmopressin intravenously or intramuscularly. Urine output and osmolality are recorded hourly for an additional 2 hours.[69,70] The dehydration is stopped and measurements are taken if the patient loses greater than 3% of body weight or at any time if the [Na^+] becomes elevated above the normal range. The duration of the test varies among patients. Patients with complete diabetes insipidus reach a maximum but low urine osmolality within a few hours, whereas patients with other disorders may take up to 18 hours.

There is no difficulty determining the diagnosis in severe hypothalamic DI or severe nephrogenic DI. In the former, urine is minimally concentrated despite dehydration and there is a marked increase in urine osmolality in response to administered desmopressin—at least a 50% increase but often 200% to 400%. At the end of the test, these patients will have undetectable vasopressin in plasma. In patients with nephrogenic DI, there will similarly be little concentration of the urine despite dehydration, but the urine osmolality will also show little or no increase in response to administered desmopressin. Patients with nephrogenic DI are unequivocally distinguished from those with hypothalamic DI by high levels of vasopressin in plasma at the end of the dehydration, often greater than 5 pg/µL.

There may be difficulty in differentiating patients with partial hypothalamic DI from those with primary polydipsia. With dehydration, both have some concentration of the urine, often beyond the degree of plasma osmolality, but the urine osmolality does not approach the level of 800 to 1200 mOsm/kg that is characteristic of normal subjects. In response to the administered desmopressin, patients with partial hypothalamic DI usually have a further concentration of the urine, by at least 10%, whereas patients with primary polydipsia have no further increase. The reliability of the response to desmopressin is debated, however. Some patients with primary polydipsia achieve a plateau level in urine osmolality before reaching their maximum urine osmolality and therefore respond to desmopressin. On the other hand, some patients with partial hypothalamic DI secrete sufficient vasopressin in severe dehydration to achieve the maximum attainable urine osmolality and do not have a further increase in response to administered desmopressin. Investigators who have a highly sensitive radioimmunoassay for vasopressin are able to distinguish between partial hypothalamic DI and primary polydipsia by measuring vasopressin at the end of the dehydration test[71,72]; they also report that these disorders may be confused on the basis of the standard dehydration test. However, a longitudinal clinical study of patients with autoimmune hypothalamic DI reported good correlation between results of the dehydration test and measured vasopressin to diagnose partial DI.[73] If the diagnosis is in doubt, patients should have adequate follow-up to ensure that a good therapeutic response to desmopressin is obtained and that the patients do not develop hyponatremia. This clinical follow-up and response are a continuation of the diagnosis with the trial of desmopressin as a test agent. If on follow-up desmopressin is found to produce a decrease in polyuria, a decrease in thirst, and a normal [Na^+], the patient almost certainly has partial hypothalamic DI. However, if the polydipsia does not improve and the patient develops hyponatremia, the patient has some abnormality of thirst and primary polydipsia.[71,74]

The clinical presentation is often helpful in the differential diagnosis. In a patient with onset of polyuria or polydipsia immediately after surgery in the hypothalamic-pituitary area or after head trauma (especially with skull fracture and loss of consciousness), the diagnosis of hypothalamic DI is highly likely. Patients with hypothalamic DI often have a sudden onset of symptoms and persistent thirst throughout the day and night associated with a desire for cold liquids.[75] Patients with DI usually have serum [Na^+] in the high range of normal, whereas patients with primary polydipsia have serum [Na^+] in the low range of normal. The blood urea nitrogen concentration is often low in both hypothalamic DI and primary polydipsia because of the high renal clearance, but there is a difference in serum uric acid concentrations. Serum uric acid is elevated in hypothalamic DI because of the modest volume contraction and the absence of the normal action of vasopressin on V_1 receptors in the kidney to increase urate clearance. A serum uric acid value greater than 5 µg/dL was reported to separate hypothalamic DI from primary polydipsia. Presumably in patients with primary polydipsia, there is modest volume expansion and intermittent secretion of vasopressin to act on V_1 receptors to clear serum urate.[76] Urine volume greater than 18 L is highly suggestive of primary polydipsia because it exceeds the amount of

267. Faull CM, Rooke P, Baylis PH. The effect of a highly specific serotonin agonist on osmoregulated vasopressin secretion in healthy man. *Clin Endocrinol (Oxf)*. 1991;35:423-430.
268. Wilkinson TJ, Begg EJ, Winter AC, et al. Incidence and risk factors for hyponatraemia following treatment with fluoxetine or paroxetine in elderly people. *Br J Clin Pharmacol*. 1999;47:211-217.
269. Burgess C, O'Donohoe A, Gill M. Agony and ecstasy: a review of MDMA effects and toxicity. *Eur Psychiatry*. 2000;15:287-294.
270. Kelestimur H, Leach RM, Ward JP, et al. Vasopressin and oxytocin release during prolonged environmental hypoxia in the rat. *Thorax*. 1997;52:84-88.
271. Tang WW, Kaptein EM, Feinstein EI, et al. Hyponatremia in hospitalized patients with the acquired immunodeficiency syndrome (AIDS) and the AIDS-related complex. *Am J Med*. 1993;94:169-174.
272. Yeung KT, Chan M, Chan CK. The safety of i.v. pentamidine administered in an ambulatory setting. *Chest*. 1996;110:136-140.
273. Miller M, Hecker MS, Friedlander DA, et al. Apparent idiopathic hyponatremia in an ambulatory geriatric population. *J Am Geriatr Soc*. 1996;44:404-408.
274. Hirshberg B, Ben-Yehuda A. The syndrome of inappropriate antidiuretic hormone secretion in the elderly. *Am J Med*. 1997;103: 270-273.
275. Ishikawa S, Kuratomi Y, Saito T. A case of oat cell carcinoma of the lung associated with ectopic production of ADH, neurophysin and ACTH. *Endocrinol Jpn*. 1980;27:257-263.
276. Robertson GL, Athar S. The interaction of blood osmolality and blood volume in regulating plasma vasopressin in man. *J Clin Endocrinol Metab*. 1976;42:613-620.
277. Kamoi K. Syndrome of inappropriate antidiuresis without involving inappropriate secretion of vasopressin in an elderly woman: effect of intravenous administration of the nonpeptide vasopressin V2 receptor antagonist OPC-31260. *Nephron*. 1997;76:111-115.
278. Feldman BJ, Rosenthal SM, Vargas GA, et al. Nephrogenic syndrome of inappropriate antidiuresis. *N Engl J Med*. 2005;352:1884-1890.
279. Leaf A, Bartter FC, Santos RF, et al. Evidence in man that urinary electrolyte loss induced by pitressin is a function of water retention. *J Clin Invest*. 1953;32:868-878.
280. Peters JP, Welt LG, Sims EA, et al. A salt-wasting syndrome associated with cerebral disease. *Trans Assoc Am Physicians*. 1950;63:57-64.
281. Nelson PB, Seif S, Gutai J, et al. Hyponatremia and natriuresis following subarachnoid hemorrhage in a monkey model. *J Neurosurg*. 1984;60:233-237.
282. Wijdicks EF, Ropper AH, Hunnicutt EJ, et al. Atrial natriuretic factor and salt wasting after aneurysmal subarachnoid hemorrhage. *Stroke*. 1991;22:1519-1524.
283. Oh MS, Carroll HJ. Cerebral salt-wasting syndrome: we need better proof of its existence. *Nephron*. 1999;82:110-114.
284. Maesaka JK, Gupta S, Fishbane S. Cerebral salt-wasting syndrome: does it exist? *Nephron*. 1999;82:100-109.
285. Diringer MN, Lim JS, Kirsch JR, et al. Suprasellar and intraventricular blood predict elevated plasma atrial natriuretic factor in subarachnoid hemorrhage. *Stroke*. 1991;22:577-581.
286. Diringer MN, Wu KC, Verbalis JG, et al. Hypervolemic therapy prevents volume contraction but not hyponatremia following subarachnoid hemorrhage. *Ann Neurol*. 1992;31:543-550.
287. Cerda-Esteve M, Cuadrado-Godia E, Chillaron JJ, et al. Cerebral salt wasting syndrome: review. *Eur J Intern Med*. 2008;19:249-254.
288. Palmer BF. Hyponatremia in patients with central nervous system disease: SIADH versus CSW. *Trends Endocrinol Metab*. 2003; 14:182-187.
289. Berger TM, Kistler W, Berendes E, et al. Hyponatremia in a pediatric stroke patient: syndrome of inappropriate antidiuretic hormone secretion or cerebral salt wasting? *Crit Care Med*. 2002;30:792-795.
290. Berkenbosch JW, Lentz CW, Jimenez DF, et al. Cerebral salt wasting syndrome following brain injury in three pediatric patients: suggestions for rapid diagnosis and therapy. *Pediatr Neurosurg*. 2002; 36:75-79.
291. Kinik ST, Kandemir N, Baykan A, et al. Fludrocortisone treatment in a child with severe cerebral salt wasting. *Pediatr Neurosurg*. 2001; 35:216-219.
292. von Bismarck P, Ankermann T, Eggert P, et al. Diagnosis and management of cerebral salt wasting (CSW) in children: the role of atrial natriuretic peptide (ANP) and brain natriuretic peptide (BNP). *Childs Nerv Syst*. 2006;22:1275-1281.
293. Taplin CE, Cowell CT, Silink M, et al. Fludrocortisone therapy in cerebral salt wasting. *Pediatrics*. 2006;118:e1904-1908.
294. Tian Y, Sandberg K, Murase T, et al. Vasopressin V2 receptor binding is down-regulated during renal escape from vasopressin-induced antidiuresis. *Endocrinology*. 2000;141:307-314.
295. Verbalis JG, Murase T, Ecelbarger CA, et al. Studies of renal aquaporin-2 expression during renal escape from vasopressin-induced antidiuresis. *Adv Exp Med Biol*. 1998;449:395-406.
296. Fraser CL, Arieff AI. Epidemiology, pathophysiology, and management of hyponatremic encephalopathy. *Am J Med*. 1997;102:67-77.
297. Daggett P, Deanfield J, Moss F. Neurological aspects of hyponatraemia. *Postgrad Med J*. 1982;58:737-740.
298. Ayus JC, Wheeler JM, Arieff AI. Postoperative hyponatremic encephalopathy in menstruant women. *Ann Intern Med*. 1992;117:891-897.
299. Wijdicks EF, Sharbrough FW. New-onset seizures in critically ill patients. *Neurology*. 1993;43:1042-1044.
300. Vexler ZS, Ayus JC, Roberts TP, et al. Hypoxic and ischemic hypoxia exacerbate brain injury associated with metabolic encephalopathy in laboratory animals. *J Clin Invest*. 1994;93:256-264.
301. Ayus JC, Arieff AI. Pulmonary complications of hyponatremic encephalopathy: noncardiogenic pulmonary edema and hypercapnic respiratory failure. *Chest*. 1995;107:517-521.
302. Ayus JC, Varon J, Arieff AI. Hyponatremia, cerebral edema, and noncardiogenic pulmonary edema in marathon runners. *Ann Intern Med*. 2000;132:711-714.
303. Arieff AI, Ayus JC, Fraser CL. Hyponatraemia and death or permanent brain damage in healthy children. *BMJ*. 1992;304:1218-1222.
304. Wattad A, Chiang ML, Hill LL. Hyponatremia in hospitalized children. *Clin Pediatr (Phila)*. 1992;31:153-157.
305. Wijdicks EF, Larson TS. Absence of postoperative hyponatremia syndrome in young, healthy females. *Ann Neurol*. 1994;35:626-628.
306. Carroll PB, McHenry L, Verbalis JG. Isolated adrenocorticotrophic hormone deficiency presenting as chronic hyponatremia. *N Y State J Med*. 1990;90:210-213.
307. Wright DG, Laureno R, Victor M. Pontine and extrapontine myelinolysis. *Brain*. 1979;102:361-385.
308. Verbalis JG, Martinez AJ. Neurological and neuropathological sequelae of correction of chronic hyponatremia. *Kidney Int*. 1991;39: 1274-1282.
309. Sterns RH, Thomas DJ, Herndon RM. Brain dehydration and neurologic deterioration after rapid correction of hyponatremia. *Kidney Int*. 1989;35:69-75.
310. Verbalis JG, Baldwin EF, Robinson AG. Osmotic regulation of plasma vasopressin and oxytocin after sustained hyponatremia. *Am J Physiol*. 1986;250(3 Pt 2):R444-R451.
311. Adler S, Martinez J, Williams DS, et al. Positive association between blood brain barrier disruption and osmotically-induced demyelination. *Mult Scler*. 2000;6:24-31.
312. Baker EA, Tian Y, Adler S, et al. Blood-brain barrier disruption and complement activation in the brain following rapid correction of chronic hyponatremia. *Exp Neurol*. 2000;165:221-230.
313. Sterns RH. The management of symptomatic hyponatremia. *Semin Nephrol*. 1990;10:503-514.
314. Soupart A, Penninckx R, Stenuit A, et al. Treatment of chronic hyponatremia in rats by intravenous saline: comparison of rate versus magnitude of correction. *Kidney Int*. 1992;41:1662-1667.
315. Ayus JC, Krothapalli RK, Arieff AI. Treatment of symptomatic hyponatremia and its relation to brain damage: a prospective study. *N Engl J Med*. 1987;317:1190-1195.
316. Sterns RH, Cappuccio JD, Silver SM, et al. Neurologic sequelae after treatment of severe hyponatremia: a multicenter perspective. *J Am Soc Nephrol*. 1994;4:1522-1530.
317. Ellis SJ. Extrapontine myelinolysis after correction of chronic hyponatraemia with isotonic saline. *Br J Clin Pract*. 1995;49:49-50.
318. Verbalis JG. Hyponatremia endocrinologic causes and consequences of therapy. *Trends Endocrinol Metab*. 1992;3:1-7.
319. Cheng JC, Zikos D, Skopicki HA, et al. Long-term neurologic outcome in psychogenic water drinkers with severe symptomatic hyponatremia: the effect of rapid correction. *Am J Med*. 1990;88:561-566.
320. Adams RD, Victor M, Mancall EL. Central pontine myelinolysis: a hitherto undescribed disease occurring in alcoholic and malnourished patients. *AMA Arch Neurol Psychiatry*. 1959;81:154-172.
321. Kelly J, Wassif W, Mitchard J, et al. Severe hyponatraemia secondary to beer potomania complicated by central pontine myelinolysis. *Int J Clin Pract*. 1998;52:585-587.
322. Soupart A, Penninckx R, Stenuit A, et al. Azotemia (48 h) decreases the risk of brain damage in rats after correction of chronic hyponatremia. *Brain Res*. 2000;852:167-172.
323. Brunner JE, Redmond JM, Haggar AM, et al. Central pontine myelinolysis and pontine lesions after rapid correction of hyponatremia: a prospective magnetic resonance imaging study. *Ann Neurol*. 1990;27:61-66.
324. Kumar SR, Mone AP, Gray LC, et al. Central pontine myelinolysis: delayed changes on neuroimaging. *J Neuroimaging*. 2000;10: 169-172.
325. Soupart A, Penninckx R, Stenuit A, et al. Reinduction of hyponatremia improves survival in rats with myelinolysis-related neurologic symptoms. *J Neuropathol Exp Neurol*. 1996;55:594-601.
326. McComb RD, Pfeiffer RF, Casey JH, et al. Lateral pontine and extrapontine myelinolysis associated with hypernatremia and hyperglycemia. *Clin Neuropathol*. 1989;8:284-288.
327. Berl T. Treating hyponatremia: damned if we do and damned if we don't. *Kidney Int*. 1990;37:1006-1018.
328. Ayus JC, Arieff AI. Brain damage and postoperative hyponatremia: the role of gender. *Neurology*. 1996;46:323-328.

329. Verbalis JG. Adaptation to acute and chronic hyponatremia: implications for symptomatology, diagnosis, and therapy. *Semin Nephrol.* 1998;18:3-19.
330. Hantman D, Rossier B, Zohlman R, et al. Rapid correction of hyponatremia in the syndrome of inappropriate secretion of antidiuretic hormone: an alternative treatment to hypertonic saline. *Ann Intern Med.* 1973;78:870-875.
331. Tanneau RS, Henry A, Rouhart F, et al. High incidence of neurologic complications following rapid correction of severe hyponatremia in polydipsic patients. *J Clin Psychiatry.* 1994;55:349-354.
332. Sugimura Y, Murase T, Takefuji S, et al. Protective effect of dexamethasone on osmotic-induced demyelination in rats. *Exp Neurol.* 2005;192:178-183.
333. Brooks DP, Valente M, Petrone G, et al. Comparison of the water diuretic activity of kappa receptor agonists and a vasopressin receptor antagonist in dogs. *J Pharmacol Exp Ther.* 1997;280:1176-1183.
334. Gadano A, Moreau R, Pessione F, et al. Aquaretic effects of niravoline, a kappa-opioid agonist, in patients with cirrhosis. *J Hepatol.* 2000;32:38-42.
335. Decaux G, Mols P, Cauchi P, et al. Use of urea for treatment of water retention in hyponatraemic cirrhosis with ascites resistant to diuretics. *Br Med J (Clin Res Ed).* 1985;290:1782-1783.
336. De Troyer A. Demeclocycline: treatment for syndrome of inappropriate antidiuretic hormone secretion. *JAMA.* 1977;237:2723-2726.
337. Miller PD, Linas SL, Schrier RW. Plasma demeclocycline levels and nephrotoxicity: correlation in hyponatremic cirrhotic patients. *JAMA.* 1980;243:2513-2515.
338. Forrest JN Jr, Cox M, Hong C, et al. Superiority of demeclocycline over lithium in the treatment of chronic syndrome of inappropriate secretion of antidiuretic hormone. *N Engl J Med.* 1978;298:173-177.
339. Serradeil-Le Gal C, Lacour C, Valette G, et al. Characterization of SR 121463A, a highly potent and selective, orally active vasopressin V2 receptor antagonist. *J Clin Invest.* 1996;98:2729-2738.
340. Tahara A, Tomura Y, Wada KI, et al. Pharmacological profile of YM087, a novel potent nonpeptide vasopressin V1A and V2 receptor antagonist, in vitro and in vivo. *J Pharmacol Exp Ther.* 1997;282:301-308.
341. Yamamura Y, Ogawa H, Yamashita H, et al. Characterization of a novel aquaretic agent, OPC-31260, as an orally effective, nonpeptide vasopressin V2 receptor antagonist. *Br J Pharmacol.* 1992;105:787-791.
342. Greenberg A, Verbalis JG. Vasopressin receptor antagonists. *Kidney Int.* 2006;69:2124-2130.
343. Verbalis J, Martinez A. Determinants of brain myelinolysis following correction of chronic hyponatremia in rats. In: Jard S, Jamison R, eds. *Vasopressin.* Paris: John Libbey; 1991:539-547.
344. Insel TR, Gingrich BS, Young LJ. Oxytocin: who needs it? *Prog Brain Res.* 2001;133:59-66.
345. Glasier A, McNeilly AS. Physiology of lactation. *Baillieres Clin Endocrinol Metab.* 1990;4:379-395.
346. Crowley WR, Armstrong WE. Neurochemical regulation of oxytocin secretion in lactation. *Endocr Rev.* 1992;13:33-65.
347. Giraldi A, Enevoldsen AS, Wagner G. Oxytocin and the initiation of parturition: a review. *Dan Med Bull.* 1990;37:377-383.
348. Uvnas-Moberg K, Eriksson M. Breastfeeding: physiological, endocrine and behavioural adaptations caused by oxytocin and local neurogenic activity in the nipple and mammary gland. *Acta Paediatr.* 1996; 85:525-530.
349. Brown D, Moos F. Onset of bursting in oxytocin cells in suckled rats. *J Physiol.* 1997;503(Pt 3):625-634.
350. McKenzie DN, Leng G, Dyball RE. Electrophysiological evidence for mutual excitation of oxytocin cells in the supraoptic nucleus of the rat hypothalamus. *J Physiol.* 1995;485(Pt 2):485-492.
351. Higuchi T, Okere CO. Role of the supraoptic nucleus in regulation of parturition and milk ejection revisited. *Microsc Res Tech.* 2002;56: 113-121.
352. Wagner KU, Young WS 3rd, Liu X, et al. Oxytocin and milk removal are required for post-partum mammary-gland development. *Genes Funct.* 1997;1:233-244.
353. Young WS 3rd, Shepard E, DeVries AC, et al. Targeted reduction of oxytocin expression provides insights into its physiological roles. *Adv Exp Med Biol.* 1998;449:231-240.
354. Renfrew MJ, Lang S, Woolridge M. Oxytocin for promoting successful lactation. Cochrane Database Syst Rev. 2000;(2):CD000156.
355. Crowley WR, Parker SL, Armstrong WE, et al. Neurotransmitter and neurohormonal regulation of oxytocin secretion in lactation. *Ann N Y Acad Sci.* 1992;652:286-302.
356. Jenkins JS, Nussey SS. The role of oxytocin: present concepts. *Clin Endocrinol (Oxf).* 1991;34:515-525.
357. Lindow SW, Hendricks MS, Nugent FA, et al. Morphine suppresses the oxytocin response in breast-feeding women. *Gynecol Obstet Invest.* 1999;48:33-37.
358. Yokoyama Y, Ueda T, Irahara M, et al. Releases of oxytocin and prolactin during breast massage and suckling in puerperal women. *Eur J Obstet Gynecol Reprod Biol.* 1994;53:17-20.
359. McNeilly AS, Tay CC, Glasier A. Physiological mechanisms underlying lactational amenorrhea. *Ann N Y Acad Sci.* 1994;709:145-155.
360. Wang H, Ward AR, Morris JF. Oestradiol acutely stimulates exocytosis of oxytocin and vasopressin from dendrites and somata of hypothalamic magnocellular neurons. *Neuroscience.* 1995;68:1179-1188.
361. Thomas A, Crowley RS, Amico JA. Effect of progesterone on hypothalamic oxytocin messenger ribonucleic acid levels in the lactating rat. *Endocrinology.* 1995;136:4188-4194.
362. Leng G. Steroidal influences on oxytocin neurones. *J Physiol.* 2000;524(Pt 2):315.
363. Johnston JM, Amico JA. A prospective longitudinal study of the release of oxytocin and prolactin in response to infant suckling in long term lactation. *J Clin Endocrinol Metab.* 1986;62:653-657.
364. De Coopman J. Breastfeeding after pituitary resection: support for a theory of autocrine control of milk supply? *J Hum Lact.* 1993; 9:35-40.
365. Robinson A, Amico J. Remarks on the history of oxytocin. In: Robinson A, Amico J, eds. *Oxytocin: Clinical and Laboratory Studies: Proceedings of the Second International Conference on Oxytocin, Lac Beauport, Quebec, Canada.* Amsterdam: Excerpta Medica; 1985: xvii-xxiv.
366. Lockwood CJ. The initiation of parturition at term. *Obstet Gynecol Clin North Am.* 2004;31:935-947, xii.
367. Smith R. Parturition. *N Engl J Med.* 2007;356:271-283.
368. Terzidou V. Preterm labour: biochemical and endocrinological preparation for parturition. *Best Pract Res Clin Obstet Gynaecol.* 2007;21: 729-756.
369. Mitchell BF, Schmid B. Oxytocin and its receptor in the process of parturition. *J Soc Gynecol Investig.* 2001;8:122-133.
370. Evans JJ. Oxytocin in the human: regulation of derivations and destinations. *Eur J Endocrinol.* 1997;137:559-571.
371. Hertelendy F, Zakar T. Prostaglandins and the myometrium and cervix. *Prostaglandins Leukot Essent Fatty Acids.* 2004;70:207-222.
372. Olson DM, Mijovic JE, Sadowsky DW. Control of human parturition. *Semin Perinatol.* 1995;19:52-63.
373. Moran DJ, McGarrigle HH, Lachelin GC. Lack of normal increase in saliva estriol/progesterone ratio in women with labor induced at 42 weeks' gestation. *Am J Obstet Gynecol.* 1992;167:1563-1564.
374. Smith JG, Merrill DC. Oxytocin for induction of labor. *Clin Obstet Gynecol.* 2006;49:594-608.
375. Mousa HA, Alfirevic Z. Treatment for primary postpartum haemorrhage. Cochrane Database Syst Rev. 2003;(1):CD003249.
376. Su LL, Chong YS, Samuel M. Oxytocin agonists for preventing postpartum haemorrhage. Cochrane Database Syst Rev. 2007;(3): CD005457.
377. Nathanielsz PW. A time to be born: implications of animal studies in maternal-fetal medicine. *Birth.* 1994;21:163-169.
378. Robinson AG, Archer DF, Tolstoi LF. Neurophysin in women during oxytocin-related events. *J Clin Endocrinol Metab.* 1973;37:645-652.
379. Campbell A. Attachment, aggression and affiliation: the role of oxytocin in female social behavior. *Biol Psychol.* 2008;77:1-10.
380. Hammock EA, Young LJ. Oxytocin, vasopressin and pair bonding: implications for autism. *Philos Trans R Soc Lond B Biol Sci.* 2006; 361:2187-2198.
381. Douglas AJ, Johnstone LE, Leng G. Neuroendocrine mechanisms of change in food intake during pregnancy: a potential role for brain oxytocin. *Physiol Behav.* 2007;91:352-365.
382. Frank E, Landgraf R. The vasopressin system: from antidiuresis to psychopathology. *Eur J Pharmacol.* 2008;583:226-242.
383. Marazziti D, Catena Dell'osso M. The role of oxytocin in neuropsychiatric disorders. *Curr Med Chem.* 2008;15:698-704.

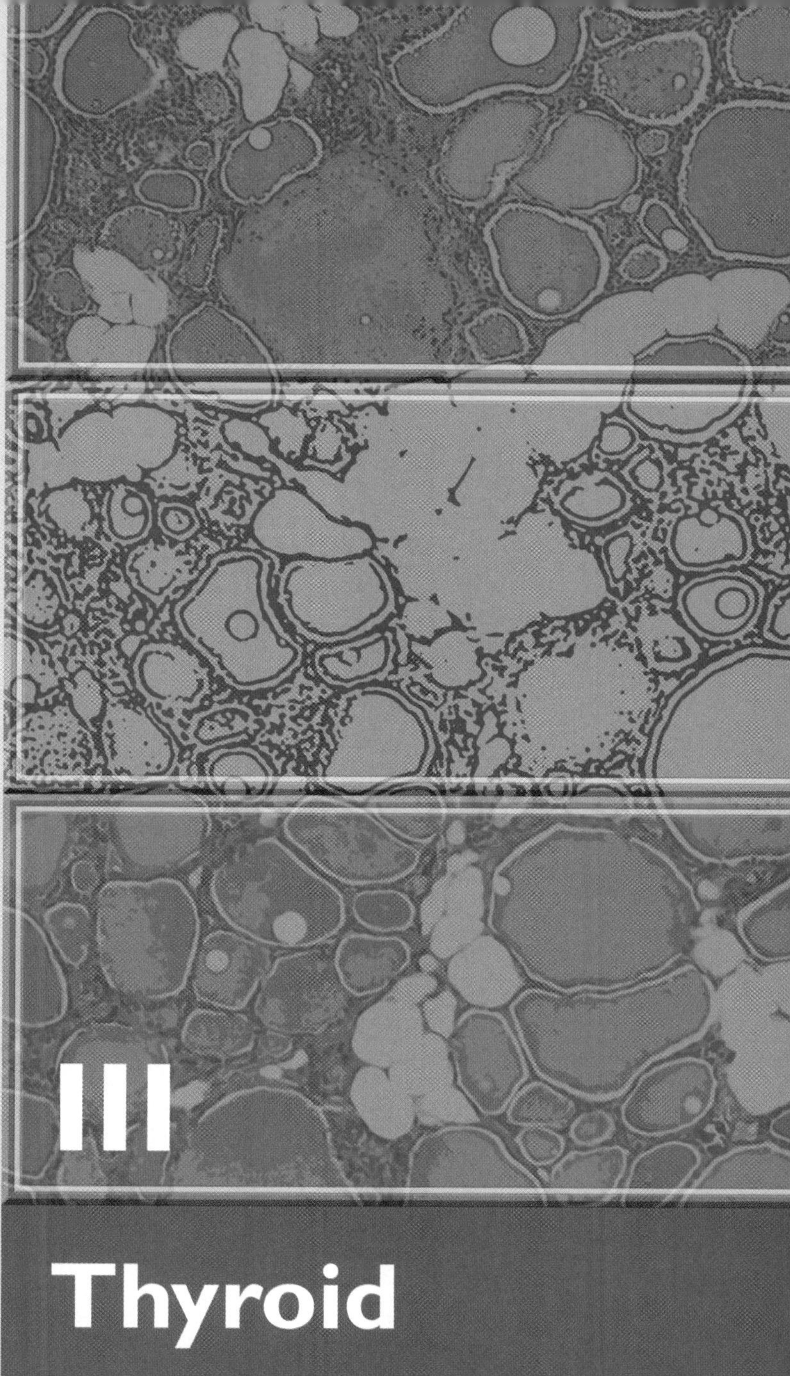

SECTION III

Thyroid

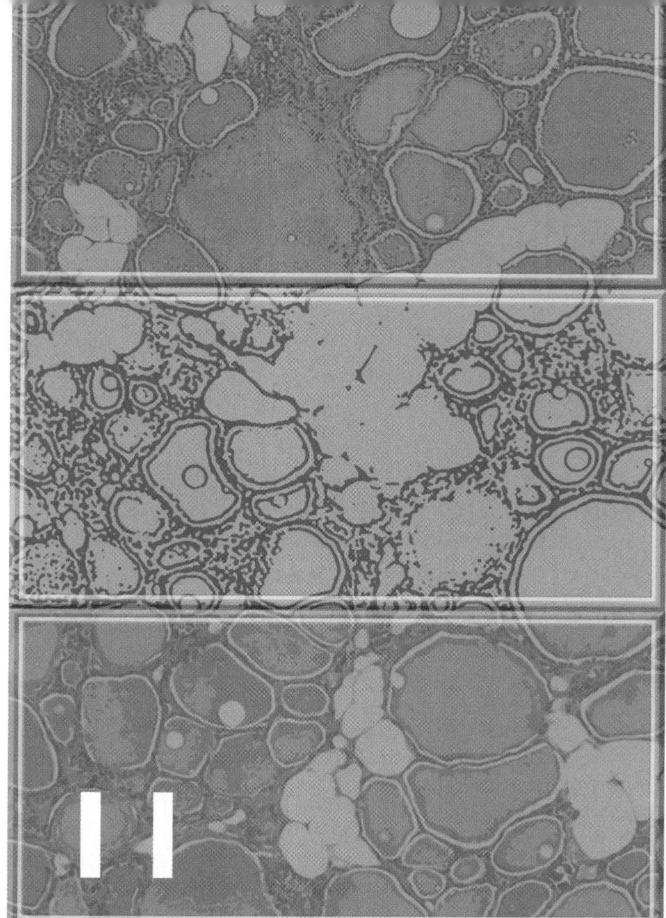

CHAPTER 11

Thyroid Physiology and Diagnostic Evaluation of Patients with Thyroid Disorders

DOMENICO SALVATORE • TERRY F. DAVIES • MARTIN-JEAN SCHLUMBERGER • IAN D. HAY • P. REED LARSEN

Dysfunction and anatomic abnormalities of the thyroid are among the most common diseases of the endocrine glands. This chapter provides the physiologic and biochemical background and describes the various tests for evaluating patients with suspected thyroid disease based on the pathophysiology of these conditions.

PHYLOGENY, EMBRYOLOGY, AND ONTOGENY

Phylogeny

The phylogeny, embryogenesis, and certain aspects of thyroid function are closely interlinked with the gastrointestinal tract. The capacity of the thyroid to metabolize iodine and incorporate it into a variety of organic compounds occurs widely throughout the animal and plant kingdoms. However, the anatomy of the thyroid gland differs considerably among the vertebrate classes. Monoiodotyrosine (3′-monoiodo-L-tyrosine [MIT]) and diiodotyrosine (3,5-diiodo-L-tyrosine [DIT]) are present in a variety of invertebrate species, including mollusks, crustaceans, coelenterates, annelids, insects, and certain marine algae. However, no recognizable thyroid tissue is present in these lower forms. Thyroid tissue is confined to vertebrates, and is present in all vertebrates. A close link to the thyroid of higher vertebrates is evident in the ammocoete, the larval form of the lamprey, where the ventral part of the pharynx is the origin of a structure present only during larval life, the endostyle. The epithelium of the endostyle is capable of carrying out iodinations, and these cells are fated to become follicular cells only after metamorphosis, when they form classic thyroid follicles.[1]

The phylogenetic association of the thyroid gland and the gastrointestinal tract is evident in several functions.

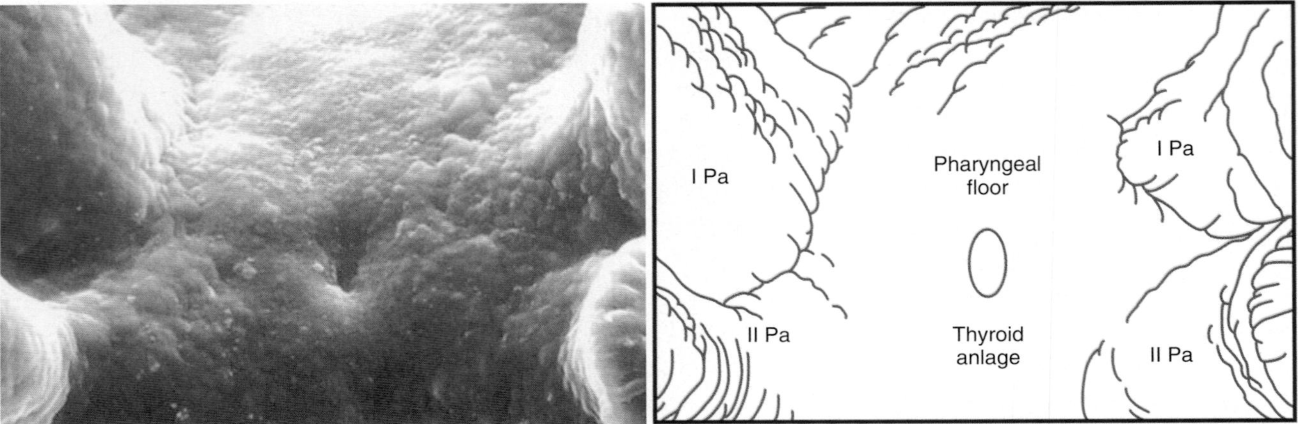

Figure 11-1 The thyroid anlage. *Left*, Scanning electron micrograph of a mouse embryo at embryonic day 9, showing the area where the thyroid bud has invaginated, leaving behind the foramen cecum. The cranial direction is *up*. *Right*, A schematic view of the pharyngeal region of an embryo at the same stage. Pa, pharyngeal arch. (From De Felice M, Di Lauro R. Thyroid development and its disorders: genetic and molecular mechanisms. *Endocr Rev.* 2004;25:722-746. Copyright 2004 by the Endocrine Society.)

The salivary and gastric glands, like the thyroid, are capable of concentrating iodide in their secretions, although iodide transport in these sites is not responsive to stimulation by thyrotropin (thyroid-stimulating hormone [TSH]). The salivary gland contains enzymes that are capable of iodinating tyrosine in the presence of hydrogen peroxide, although it forms insignificant quantities of iodoproteins under normal circumstances.

Structural Embryology

The morphogenesis of the thyroid gland, the anterior-most organ that buds from the gut tube, begins with a thickening of the endodermal epithelium in the foregut, which is referred to as thyroid anlage. The human thyroid anlage is first recognizable at embryonic day 16 or 17. This median thickening deepens and forms first a small pit and then an outpouching of the endoderm adjacent to the developing myocardial cells (Fig. 11-1). With continuing development, the median diverticulum is displaced caudally, following the myocardial cells in their descent. The primitive stalk connecting the primordium with the pharyngeal floor elongates into the thyroglossal duct. During its caudal displacement, the primordium assumes a bilobate shape, coming into contact and fusing with the ventral aspect of the fourth pharyngeal pouch when it reaches its final position at about embryonic day 50.

Normally, the thyroglossal duct undergoes dissolution and fragmentation by about the second month after conception, leaving at its point of origin a small dimple at the junction of the middle and posterior thirds of the tongue, the *foramen caecum*. Cells of the lower portion of the duct differentiate into thyroid tissue, forming the pyramidal lobe of the gland. At the same time, the lobes contact the ultimobranchial glands, leading to incorporation of C cells into the thyroid. Concomitantly, histologic alterations occur throughout the gland. Complex, interconnecting, cord-like arrangements of cells interspersed with vascular connective tissue replace the solid epithelial mass and become tubule-like structures at about the third month of fetal life; shortly thereafter, follicular arrangements devoid of colloid appear, and by 13 to 14 weeks the follicles begin to fill with colloid.

Investigations of thyroid gland development in mice using gene-targeting techniques are beginning to identify the critical factors that are required for normal thyroid gland development.[2,3] The roles of these various proteins are currently being evaluated with respect to the potential for defects in the synthesis or formation of the thyroid gland (see Chapter 13).

Functional Ontogeny

The ontogeny of thyroid function and its regulation in the human fetus are fairly well defined.[4] Future follicular cells acquire the capacity to form thyroglobulin (Tg) as early as the 29th day of gestation, whereas the capacities to concentrate iodide and synthesize thyroxine (T_4) are delayed until about the 11th week. Radioactive iodine inadvertently given to the mother would be accumulated by the fetal thyroid soon thereafter. Early growth and development of the thyroid do not seem to be TSH-dependent, because the capacity of the pituitary to synthesize and secrete TSH is not apparent until the 14th week. Subsequently, rapid changes in pituitary and thyroid function take place. Probably as a consequence of hypothalamic maturation and increasing secretion of thyrotropin-releasing hormone (TRH), the serum TSH concentration increases between 18 and 26 weeks' gestation, after which levels remain higher than those in the mother.[4] The higher levels may reflect a higher set point of the negative feedback control of TSH secretion during fetal life than at maturity. Thyroxine-binding globulin (TBG), the major thyroid hormone–binding protein in plasma, is detectable in the serum by the 10th gestational week and increases in concentration progressively to term. This increase in TBG concentration accounts in part for the progressive increase in the serum T_4 concentration during the second and third trimesters, but increased secretion of T_4 must also play a role, because the concentration of free T_4 also rises.

Several aspects of thyroid development are of note from the clinical standpoint. Rarely, thyroid tissue may develop from remnants of the thyroglossal duct near the base of the tongue. Such lingual thyroid tissue may be the sole functioning thyroid present; if so, its surgical removal will lead to hypothyroidism. More commonly, elements of the thyroglossal duct persist and later give rise to thyroglossal duct cysts, and ectopic thyroid tissue may be present at any location in the mediastinum or, rarely, in the heart.

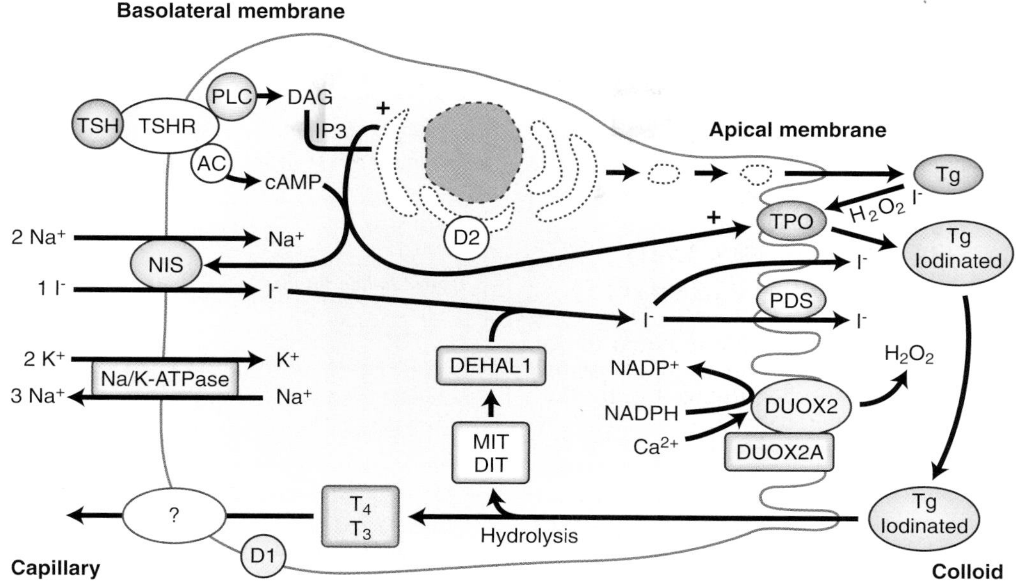

Figure 11-2 Schematic illustration of a follicular cell showing the key aspects of thyroid iodine transport and thyroid hormone synthesis. AC, Adenyl cyclase; ATPase, adenosine triphosphatase; cAMP, cyclic adenosine monophosphate; D1, thyroidal deiodinase type 1; D2, thyroidal deiodinase type 2; DAG, diacylglycerol; DEHAL1, iodotyrosine dehalogenase 1 (IYD); DIT, diiodotyrosine; DUOX, dual oxidase; IP3, inositol triphosphate; MIT, monoiodotyrosine; $NADP^+$, oxidized form of nicotinamide adenosine dinucleotide phosphate; NADPH, reduced nicotinamide adenosine dinucleotide phosphate; NIS, sodium-iodide symporter; PDS, pendrin (SLC26A4); PLC, phospholipase C; T_3, triiodothyronine; T_4, thyroxine; Tg, thyroglobulin; TPO, thyroid peroxidase TSHR, thyrotropin receptor.

ANATOMY AND HISTOLOGY

The thyroid is one of the largest of the endocrine organs, weighing approximately 15 to 20 g in North American adults. Moreover, the potential of the thyroid for growth is tremendous. The enlarged thyroid, commonly termed a *goiter,* can weigh many hundreds of grams. The normal thyroid is made up of two lobes joined by a thin band of tissue, the isthmus, which is approximately 0.5 cm thick, 2 cm wide, and 1 to 2 cm high. The individual lobes normally have a pointed superior pole and a poorly defined, blunt inferior pole that merges medially with the isthmus. Each lobe is approximately 2.0 to 2.5 cm in thickness and width at its largest diameter, and it is approximately 4.0 cm in length. Occasionally, and especially if the remainder of the gland is enlarged, a pyramidal lobe is discernible as a finger-like projection directed upward from the isthmus, usually on the left, just lateral to the midline.

The right lobe is normally more vascular than the left; it is often the larger of the two and tends to enlarge more in disorders associated with a diffuse increase in gland size. Two pairs of vessels constitute the major arterial blood supply: the superior thyroid artery, which arises from the external carotid artery, and the inferior thyroid artery, which arises from the subclavian artery. Estimates of thyroid blood flow range from 4 to 6 mL/minute per gram, well in excess of the blood flow to the kidney (3 mL/minute per gram). In diffuse toxic goiter resulting from Graves' disease, blood flow may exceed 1 L/minute and may be associated with an audible bruit or even a palpable thrill.

The gland is composed of closely packed, spherical units termed *follicles,* which are invested with a rich capillary network. The interior of the follicle is filled with the clear, proteinaceous colloid that normally is the major constituent of the total thyroid mass. On cross-section, thyroid tissue appears as closely packed, ring-shaped structures consisting of a single layer of thyroid cells surrounding a lumen. The diameter of the follicles varies considerably, even within a single gland, but averages about 200 nm. The follicular cells vary in height with the degree of glandular stimulation, becoming columnar when active and cuboidal when inactive. The epithelium rests on a basement membrane that is rich with glycoproteins and separates the follicular cells from the surrounding capillaries. Between 20 and 40 follicles are demarcated by connective tissue septa to form a lobule supplied by a single artery. The function of a given lobule may differ from that of its neighbors.

On electron microscopy, the thyroid follicular epithelium has many features in common with other secretory cells and some that are peculiar to the thyroid. From the apex of the follicular cell, numerous microvilli extend into the colloid. It is at or near this surface of the cell that iodination, exocytosis, and the initial phase of hormone secretion (i.e., colloid resorption) occur (Fig. 11-2). The nucleus has no distinctive features, and the cytoplasm contains an extensive endoplasmic reticulum (ER) laden with microsomes. The ER is composed of a network of wide, irregular tubules that contain the precursor of Tg. The carbohydrate component of Tg is added to this precursor in the Golgi apparatus, which is located apically. Lysosomes and mitochondria are scattered throughout the cytoplasm. Stimulation by TSH results in enlargement of the Golgi apparatus, formation of pseudopodia at the apical surface, and the appearance in the apical portion of the cell of many droplets that contain colloid taken up from the follicular lumen (see Fig. 11-2).

The thyroid also contains parafollicular cells, or C cells, that bilaterally migrate from the neural crest and are the source of calcitonin. These cells originate during embryonic development from the last pair of pharyngeal pouches but ultimately come to rest among the cells of the follicular epithelium or in the thyroid interstitium. They differ from the cells of the follicular epithelium in that they never border on the follicular lumen and they are rich in mitochondria. The C cells undergo hyperplasia early in the syndrome of familial medullary carcinoma of the thyroid (multiple endocrine neoplasia type 2) and give rise to this tumor in both its familial and its sporadic forms (see Chapter 41).

IODINE AND THE SYNTHESIS AND SECRETION OF THYROID HORMONES

The function of the thyroid is to generate the quantity of thyroid hormone necessary to meet the demands of the peripheral tissues. This requires iodide uptake by the thyroidal sodium-iodide symporter (NIS), its transfer to the colloid, and its oxidation by thyroid peroxidase (TPO). The result is the daily synthesis of approximately 110 nmol/L (85 μg) of T_4, which is 65% iodine by weight. This requires the synthesis of Tg, a glycoprotein with a molecular weight of approximately 330 kd. Specific tyrosine residues of Tg homodimers are then iodinated at the apical border of the thyroid cell to form MIT and DIT (see Fig. 11-2). This requires formation of hydrogen peroxide by dual oxidase 1 (DUOX1) and DUOX2 and of TPO, which catalyzes the oxidation of iodide and its transfer to tyrosine. TPO also catalyzes the coupling of two molecules of DIT or one of DIT and one of MIT, leading to formation of T_4 and T_3, respectively (see later discussion). These products are then stored within the colloid, still as part of the Tg molecule. Pinocytosis of stored colloid leads to the formation of phagolysosomes, the colloid droplets in which Tg is digested by specific proteases to release T_4, T_3, DIT, and MIT as the droplet is translocated toward the basal portion of the cell. T_4 and T_3 are transported out of the phagolysosomes and across the basolateral cell membrane, exit the cell, and enter circulation; DIT and MIT are deiodinated by the iodotyrosine dehalogenase to allow recycling of the iodide.

The synthesis of thyroid hormones requires the expression of a number of thyroid cell–specific proteins. In addition to Tg and TPO, the TSH receptor (TSHR) is also required to transduce the effects of extracellular TSH for efficient hormone synthesis. In addition to TSH, a number of transcription factors, including NKX2-1 (TTF-1), Pax8, FOXE1 (TTF-2), and FOXM1 (HNF-3) are necessary to achieve functional differentiation of the thyroid follicular cells and the onset of hormonogenesis.[1,3] Although the biochemical details of these processes are beyond the scope of this discussion, those aspects with clinical relevance are reviewed in greater detail in the following sections.

Dietary Iodine

Formation of normal quantities of thyroid hormone requires the availability of adequate quantities of exogenous iodine to allow thyroidal uptake of approximately 60 to 75 μg daily, taking into account fecal losses of about 10 to 20 μg iodine of iodothyronines as glucuronides and about 100 to 150 μg as urinary iodine in iodine-sufficient populations.[5] Plasma iodide (I^-), the form of the element in biologic solutions, is completely filterable, with 60% to 70% of the filtered load reabsorbed passively. At least 100 μg of iodine per day is required to eliminate all signs of iodine deficiency (Table 11-1). In healthy adults, the absorption of iodide is greater than 90%. In North America, the daily dietary iodine intake is in the range of 150 to 300 μg, largely owing to the iodination of salt; in Japan, where large quantities of foods rich in iodine are consumed, intakes may be as high as several milligrams per day. Notably, iodine intake in the United States is decreasing due to a reduction in salt consumption, with a median urinary iodine of 160 μg/L but a low urinary iodine content (<5 μg/dL) in 11% of the population.[6]

TABLE 11-1

Recommended and Typical Values for Dietary Iodine Intake

	μg/day
Recommended Daily Intake	
Adults	150
During pregnancy	200
Children	90-120
Typical Iodine Intakes	
North America	75-300
Chile	<50-150
Belgium	50-60
Germany	20-70
Switzerland	130-160

The daily dietary intake of iodine varies widely throughout the world, depending on the iodine content of soil and water and on dietary practice (see Table 11-1). Even in a single area, iodine intake varies among different individuals and in the same individual from day to day. Iodine may also enter the body via medications, diagnostic agents, dietary supplements, and food additives. As discussed more extensively later, iodine deficiency is common, especially in mountainous and formerly glaciated regions of the earth.[7] An estimated 1 billion individuals live in iodine-deficient areas of the world, and they often develop TSH-induced compensatory enlargement of the thyroid *(endemic goiter)*. If iodine deficiency is severe during pregnancy, fetal thyroid hormone production falls, causing irreparable damage to the developing central nervous system (CNS). This is manifested by varying degrees of mental retardation and is termed *endemic cretinism*. Iodine-deficiency disorders, including endemic goiter and cretinism, are the most common thyroid-related human illnesses and, indeed, the most common endocrine disorders worldwide.

Plasma iodide is partly replenished by that lost from the thyroid into the blood and by iodide liberated through deiodination of iodothyronines in peripheral tissues. Ultimately, however, the diet is its most important source. Iodine is ingested in both inorganic and organically bound forms. Iodide per se is rapidly and efficiently absorbed from the gastrointestinal tract (within 30 minutes), and little is lost in the stool. In the body, iodide is confined largely to the extracellular fluid. It is also found in red blood cells and is concentrated in the intraluminal fluids of the gastrointestinal tract, notably the saliva and gastric juice, from which it is reabsorbed, thereby re-entering the extracellular fluid. Iodide is also concentrated in milk. Until it is oxidized and bound to tyrosyl residues in Tg, iodide entering the thyroid by active transport is in rapid equilibrium with the main iodide pool. The concentration of iodide in the extracellular fluid is normally 10 to 15 μg/L (approximately 10^{-7} mol/L), and the content of the peripheral pool is approximately 250 μg. The thyroid contains the largest pool of body iodine, under normal circumstances approximately 8000 μg, most of which is in the form of DIT and

MIT. Normally, this pool of iodine turns over slowly (about 1% per day).

Iodide Metabolism by the Thyroid Cell

Because the concentration of iodide in plasma is so low, a mechanism is required for the thyroid cell to concentrate the required amounts of this element. This process, iodide trapping, is accomplished by a membrane protein, the *sodium-iodide symporter (NIS)*, encoded by the gene *SLC5A5*. Human NIS is a 643-amino-acid glycoprotein with 13 membrane-spanning domains. The transport of iodide is an active process that depends on the presence of a sodium gradient across the basal membrane of the thyroid cell such that downhill transport of 2 Na^+ ions results in the entry of one iodide atom against an electrochemical gradient (see Fig. 11-2). In addition to being expressed in the basolateral membrane of the thyroid cell, NIS has also been identified in other iodide-concentrating cells, including salivary and lactating mammary glands, choroid plexus, and gastric mucosa, and in the cytotrophoblast and syncytiotrophoblast.[8,9] In the lactating mammary gland, NIS plays an important role by concentrating iodide in the milk, thereby supplying newborns with iodide for thyroid hormone synthesis.

The iodide transport system generates an iodide gradient of 20 to 40 over the cell membrane, and NIS will also transport pertechnetate (TcO_4^-), perchlorate (ClO_4^-), and thiocyanate (SCN^-), accounting for the utility of radioactive TcO_4^- as a thyroid scanning tool and the capacity of $KClO_4^-$ to block iodide uptake.[10,11] On the other hand, the affinity of NIS for iodide is much higher than it is for the other inorganic anions, such as bromide and chloride, accounting for the selectivity of the thyroid transport mechanism. Transcription of the NIS gene is increased by TSH, and TSH also prolongs NIS protein half-life and targets the protein to the cell membrane. That the iodide-concentrating mechanism is required for normal thyroid function has been known for decades; its absence is associated with congenital hypothyroidism and goiter unless large quantities of inorganic iodide are provided.[12] A number of families have now been identified in which various mutations in the NIS gene are associated with congenital hypothyroidism and an iodide transport defect. Importantly, several studies have documented decreases in NIS expression in human thyroid adenomas and carcinomas that contribute to the loss of iodine uptake in neoplastic thyroid cells which, therefore, present as "cold" nodules on radioisotopic imaging.[12] However, changes in the subcellular location of NIS may also explain this phenomenon.

Pendrin is a highly hydrophobic membrane glycoprotein that is located at the apical membrane of thyrocytes, where it could function as an apical iodide transporter in thyroid cells.[13] Pendrin is also expressed in the kidney and in the inner ear.[14] In the kidney, pendrin plays an important role in acid-base metabolism as a chloride/bicarbonate exchanger.[15] In the inner ear, pendrin is important for generation of the endocochlear potential.[12] Pendrin belongs to the SLC26A family and is encoded by *SLC26A4*. Mutations in *SLC26A4* lead to Pendred syndrome, an autosomal recessive disorder characterized by sensorineural deafness, goiter, and a partial defect in iodide organification.[16,17] Deafness or hearing impairment is the major phenotypic manifestation in Pendred syndrome, and goiter usually develops during childhood. However, there is substantial variation within and between families and among different geographic regions. Curiously, targeted inactivation of *SLC26A4* does not result in thyroid dysfunction in mice. This argues against a rate-limiting role for this protein for apical follicular transport, at least in this animal.

Other proteins (SLC5A8 and chloride channel 5, CLCN5) have been proposed to mediate apical iodide efflux.[18] Functional studies performed in *Xenopus* oocytes and polarized cells of the Madin-Darby canine kidney (MDCK) line clearly demonstrate that SLC5A8, originally designated as human apical iodide transporter (hAIT),[18] does not mediate iodide uptake or efflux.[19] Localization of the CLCN5 protein at the apical membrane of thyrocytes and a thyroidal phenotype of the *ClCn5*-deficient mice that is reminiscent of Pendred syndrome suggest that CLCN5 could be involved in mediating apical iodide efflux or iodide/chloride exchange, possibly in conjunction with other chloride channels.[20]

In addition to active transport of iodide from the extracellular fluid, intracellular iodide is also generated by the action of the enzyme, iodotyrosine dehalogenase 1 (DEHAL1), also called iodotyrosine deiodinase (IYD). IYD transcription is stimulated by cyclic adenosine monophosphate (cAMP) and encodes a membrane protein concentrated at the apical cell surface that catalyzes the reduced nicotinamide adenosine dinucleotide phosphate (NADPH)-dependent deiodination of MIT and DIT, with greater activity against MIT.[21] The iodide thereby released is immediately reconjugated to newly synthesized Tg after exiting the apical membrane of the cell. This process is interrupted by the thiourea class of antithyroid drugs, including methimazole, carbimazole, and propylthiouracil (PTU), which inhibit TPO, resulting in intrathyroidal iodine deficiency in patients receiving these agents.[22] Mutations in homozygosity in the *IYD* gene have been identified in patients with hypothyroidism, goiter, and an elevated DIT level.[23] Functional studies revealed that the mutations abolished the capacity of IYD to deiodinate MIT and DIT.

Iodide Oxidation and Organification

Within the thyroid, iodide participates in a series of reactions that lead to synthesis of the active thyroid hormones. The first of these involves oxidation of iodide and incorporation of the resulting intermediate into the hormonally inactive iodotyrosines, MIT and DIT, a process termed *organification*. Iodide is normally oxidized rapidly, immediately appearing in organic combination in Tg. The iodinations that lead to formation of iodotyrosines occur within Tg, rather than on the free amino acids. Oxidation of thyroidal iodide is mediated by the heme-containing protein TPO and requires the H_2O_2 generated by the calcium-dependent DUOX1 and DUOX2 enzymes. The protein contains a membrane-spanning region near the carboxy terminus, and it is oriented in the apical membrane of the thyroid cell, with residues 1 through 844 in the follicular lumen where iodination occurs (see Fig. 11-2). TPO is the major thyroid microsomal antigen, and recombinant human TPO is now used for the detection of antithyroid microsomal antibodies commonly present in the serum of patients with Hashimoto's thyroiditis. The evanescent product of the peroxidation of iodide (i.e., the active iodinating form) may be free hypoiodous acid, I_2, or iodinium (I^+).[24]

The *DUOX1* and *DUOX2* genes (also termed *THOX1* and *THOX2*) encode glycoflavoproteins predominantly expressed at the apical thyrocyte membrane, where they constitute the catalytic core of the H_2O_2 generator required for thyroid hormone synthesis (see Fig. 11-2).[25] These calcium- and NADPH-dependent oxidases catalyze the formation of the H_2O_2 required for TPO-catalyzed Tg iodination. Dual oxidase maturation factor 2 (DUOXA2), a resident ER protein, is required for the maturation and plasma membrane localization of DUOX2 and for H_2O_2 generation.[26] Iodide excess inhibits DUOX2 glycosylation, which may be an additional mechanism for the Wolff-Chaikoff effect. DUOX-catalyzed generation of H_2O_2 has been found to be an early event of the wound response in zebrafish larvae that is required for rapid recruitment of leukocytes to the wound.[27]

The rate of organic iodination is dependent on the degree of thyroid stimulation by TSH (see later discussion). Congenital defects in the organic binding mechanism cause goitrous congenital hypothyroidism or, if less severe, goiter without hypothyroidism. In some families, thyroidal TPO is absent.[28] Homozygous nonsense mutations in the *DUOX2* gene, as well as heterozygous mutations that prematurely truncate the protein, have been found in patients with mild transient congenital hypothyroidism and a partial iodide organification defect.[29,30] Furthermore, a mutation in the *DUOXA2* gene was found in a patient with congenital hypothyroidism and partial iodine organification defect (see Chapter 13).[31,32]

Iodothyronine Synthesis

MIT and DIT are precursors of the hormonally active iodothyronines, T_4 and T_3. Synthesis of T_4 from DIT requires the TPO-catalyzed fusion of two DIT molecules to yield a structure with two diiodinated rings linked by an ether bridge (the coupling reaction). Concomitantly, a residual dehydroalanine is formed at the site of the DIT residue, contributing the phenolic hydroxyl group.

Efficient synthesis of T_4 and T_3 in the thyroid requires Tg. The Tg messenger RNA (mRNA) is approximately 8.5 kb in length and encodes a 330-kd (12S) subunit that is 10% carbohydrate by weight. There are 134 tyrosyl residues in the 660-kd homodimer. Only 25 to 30 of these are iodinated; only residues 5, 1290, and 2553 form T_4 and residue 2746, T_3.[33] The T_4-forming, readily iodinated, and iodothyronine-forming acceptor residues of Tg from different species are in a Glu/AspTyr or a Thr/SerTyrSer sequence, suggesting an important role of primary sequence in these reactions. There are three to four T_4 molecules in each molecule of human Tg under conditions of normal iodination (25 atoms per Tg molecule, approximately 0.5% iodine by weight), but only about one in five molecules of human Tg contains a T_3 residue. In Tg from patients with untreated Graves' disease, the content of T_4 residues remains approximately the same, but the number of T_3 residues doubles to an average of 0.4 per molecule. This difference is independent of the iodination state of the Tg and is a consequence of thyroidal stimulation. Because the coupling reaction is catalyzed by TPO, virtually all agents that inhibit organic binding (e.g., the thiourea drugs) also inhibit coupling.

Storage and Release of Thyroid Hormone

The thyroid is unique among the endocrine glands because of the large store of hormone it contains and the low rate at which the hormone turns over (1% per day). This aspect of thyroid hormone economy has homeostatic value in that the reservoir provides prolonged protection against depletion of circulating hormone if synthesis ceases. In normal humans, the administration of antithyroid agents for as long as 2 weeks has little effect on serum T_4 concentrations. There is approximately 250 μg T_4 per gram of wet weight in normal human thyroid, or about 5000 μg in a 20-g gland.[22] This is sufficient to maintain a euthyroid state for at least 50 days. When it is released rapidly in an uncontrolled fashion during subacute or painless thyroiditis, this quantity of T_4 will cause significant transient thyrotoxicosis. Tg is present in the plasma of normal individuals at concentrations up to 80 ng/mL, and it probably leaves the thyroid through the lymphatics. However, peripheral hydrolysis of Tg does not contribute significantly to the thyroid hormones in the circulation, even during thyroiditis when large quantities of this protein are present.

The first step in thyroid hormone release is the endocytosis of colloid from the follicular lumen, which is accomplished through two processes: macropinocytosis by pseudopods formed at the apical membrane and micropinocytosis by small coated vesicles that form at the apical surface (see Fig. 11-2). Both processes are stimulated by TSH, but the relative importance of the two pathways varies among species, with micropinocytosis thought to predominate in humans. After endocytosis, endocytotic vesicles fuse with lysosomes, and proteolysis is catalyzed by cathepsin D and D-like thiol proteases, all of which are active at the acidic pH of the lysosome. The iodotyrosines released from Tg are rapidly deiodinated by the NADPH-dependent IYD, and the released iodine is recycled. Thyroid hormones are released from Tg in the lysosome, but it is not clear how their transfer into the cytosol and subsequently into the plasma is effected. Given the expression of the thyroid hormone transporter MCT8 in the thyroid gland (see later discussion), it is possible that this transporter could be involved in the exit of T_4 or T_3, or both, from the phagolysosome or thyroid cell. It has been shown that T_4 can be released from Tg within the thyroid cell with minimal disruption of its molecular weight. This presumably is a consequence of selective proteolysis, which is facilitated by the fact that the major hormonogenic peptides of the Tg molecule are located at the amino-terminus and the C-terminus of the Tg monomer.

Presumably, the T_4 becomes accessible to the thyroidal type 1 and 2 deiodinases (D1 and D2, respectively), because basal and TSH-stimulated conversion of T_4 to T_3 is readily demonstrated in the perfused dog thyroid. Because this conversion is inhibited by PTU, it is catalyzed by D1. The contribution of thyroidal T_4 deiodination to T_3 secretion in humans under physiologic conditions is not known. The fact that the ratio of T_4 to T_3 in human Tg is 15:1, whereas estimates of the molar ratio of T_4 to T_3 in thyroid secretion is approximately 10:1, suggests that this does occur. Stimulation of D1- and D2-catalyzed 5′-deiodination of T_4 in the thyroid of patients with Graves' disease may enhance that pathway and contribute to the marked increase in the ratio of T_3 to T_4 production in that condition.[34] Inhibition of the D1-catalyzed T_4-to-T_3 conversion may contribute to the rapid effect of PTU in reducing circulating T_3 in the patient with Graves' disease (see Chapter 12).[34,35] That deiodinases in thyroid-derived cells can modulate the systemic conversion of T_4 to T_3 has been shown in several patients with metastatic thyroid carcinoma. The high expression of D2 in one large mediastinal tumor mass was associated with a high-normal T_3 with reduced T_4 and a normal TSH. Removal of the tumor reversed these abnormalities.[36]

T_4 release from thyroid cells is inhibited by several agents, the most important of which is iodide. Inhibition of hormone release is responsible for the rapid improvement that iodide causes in hyperthyroid patients. The mechanism by which this effect is mediated is uncertain, but iodide inhibits the stimulation of thyroid adenylate cyclase by TSH and by the stimulatory immunoglobulins produced in Graves' disease. Increasing the iodination of Tg also increases its resistance to hydrolysis by acid proteases in the lysosomes. Lithium inhibits thyroid hormone release, although its mechanism of action is poorly understood and may differ from that of iodide.[37]

Role and Mechanism of Thyrotropin Effects

All steps in the formation and release of thyroid hormones are stimulated by TSH secreted by pituitary thyrotrophs (see Chapter 8). Thyroid cells express the TSHR, a member of the glycoprotein G protein–coupled receptor family. This protein contains a large extracellular N-terminal domain, seven membrane-spanning domains, and an intracellular domain that transduces the signal by promoting exchange of guanosine diphosphate for guanosine triphosphate on the α-subunit of G proteins.[1,3,38] In fact, the TSHR has been reported to couple to 11 different G protein α-subunits in vitro, so much remains to be learned about signaling through it. Although the TSHR mainly couples to the stimulatory protein, G_s, when activated by high concentrations of TSH (100 times the physiologic level), it couples also to G_q/G_{11}, activating the inositol-phosphate diacylglycerol cascade. The induction of signal via the phospholipase C (PLC) and intracellular Ca^{2+} pathways regulates iodide efflux, H_2O_2 production, and Tg iodination, whereas the signal via the protein kinase A (PKA) pathway mediated by cAMP regulates iodine uptake and transcription of Tg, TPO, and NIS mRNAs, leading to thyroid hormone production (Table 11-2).[39,40]

Despite the discovery that mutations in various regions of the TSHR molecule resulted in its intrinsic activation and the identification of important domains for intramolecular TSHR signal transduction (see Chapter 12), the precise mechanisms of receptor activation and the early events of TSHR signal transduction are not fully understood.[38] Studies using mutational analyses suggested that the interactions between the ectodomain and the extracellular loops of the transmembrane domains in the TSHR may be critical for the maintenance of an inactive state with no constitutive activity. When these constraints are removed, an open conformation ensues. Therefore, it has been proposed that the TSHR exists in both a closed (inactive) and an open (active) format. This model predicts that only the open format of the receptor is able to bind ligand and become activated. Further support for this model comes from the development of constitutive activation when the TSHR ectodomain is truncated, suggesting that its presence dampens a constitutively active α-subunit.

The TSHR, in addition to TSH, also binds TSHR-stimulating antibody, thyroid-blocking antibodies, and neutral antibodies to the TSHR (see Chapter 12). The closely related luteinizing hormone (LH) and human chorionic gonadotropin (hCG) also bind to and activate TSHR signaling.[38] The latter accounts for the physiologic hyperthyroidism of early pregnancy.

Besides the thyrocyte, TSHR is also expressed in a variety of tissues such as osteoclasts, fibroblasts, and adipocytes, as well as retroorbital adipocytes and skin.[38,41] As discussed earlier, certain activating and inactivating mutations, either germline or somatic, have been identified in the membrane-spanning and intracellular portions of the TSHR molecule that cause generalized or nodular hyperfunction and congenital hypofunction.[38,42]

TABLE 11-2

Thyroid Cell Functions Stimulated by Thyrotropin

Function Affected	General Mechanism
Iodide Metabolism	
Increase I^- in follicular lumen	PLC
Delayed increased in NIS expression	cAMP
Increase thyroid blood flow	↑ NO synthesis (↓ cellular iodide)
Increase in I^- efflux from thyroid cell	?
Thyroid Hormone Synthesis	
↑ Hydrogen peroxide	PLC
↑ Thyroglobulin and TPO synthesis	cAMP
↑ NADPH via pentose-phosphate pathway	?
Thyroid Hormone Secretion	
↑ Pinocytosis of thyroglobulin	cAMP
↑ Release of thyroglobulin into plasma via the basolateral membrane	cAMP (?)
Mitogenesis	cAMP; PLC; IGFI^- and FGF-mediated kinase activation

cAMP, cyclic adenosine monophosphate; FGF, follicular growth factor; IGFI^-, insulin-like growth factor I^-, plasma iodide; NADPH, reduced nicotinamide adenosine dinucleotide phosphate; S, sodium-iodide symporter; NO, nitric oxide; PLC, phospholipase C; TPO, thyroid peroxidase.

THYROID HORMONES IN PERIPHERAL TISSUES

Plasma Transport

The metabolic transformations of thyroid hormones in peripheral tissues determine their biologic potency and regulate their biologic effects. Consequently, an understanding of thyroid physiopathology requires knowledge of the pathways of thyroid hormone metabolism. A wide variety of iodothyronines and their metabolic derivatives exist in plasma. Of these, T_4 is highest in concentration and the only one that arises solely from direct secretion by the thyroid gland. In normal humans, T_3 is also released from the thyroid, but approximately 80% is derived from the peripheral tissues by enzymatic removal of a single 5′ iodine atom from T_4 (outer ring or 5′ monodeiodination).[43] The remaining iodothyronines and their derivatives are generated in the peripheral tissues from T_4 and T_3. Principal among them are 3,3′,5′-triiodothyronine (reverse T_3, or rT_3) and 3,3′-diiodo-L-thyronine (3,3′-T_2) (Fig. 11-3). Trace concentrations of other diiodothyronines and monoiodothyronines and their conjugates with glucuronic or sulfuric acid are also present.[44,45] Deaminated derivatives of T_4 and T_3 that bear an acetic acid rather than an alanine side chain (tetrac and triac) are also present in low concentrations (see Fig. 11-3). The major iodothyronines are poorly soluble in water and therefore bind reversibly to plasma proteins. The plasma proteins with which T_4 is mainly associated are TBG, transthyretin (TTR, formerly termed T_4-binding prealbumin [TBPA]), and albumin (Table 11-3). About 75% to 80% of T_3 is bound by TBG, and the remainder by TTR and albumin.

Thyroxine-Binding Globulin

TBG is a glycoprotein with a molecular mass of about 54 kd, about 20% of which is carbohydrate, that is encoded by a 3.8-kb transcript located on the X chromosome.[46] The protein sequence of TBG resembles that of the serpin family of serine antiproteases. Because there is one

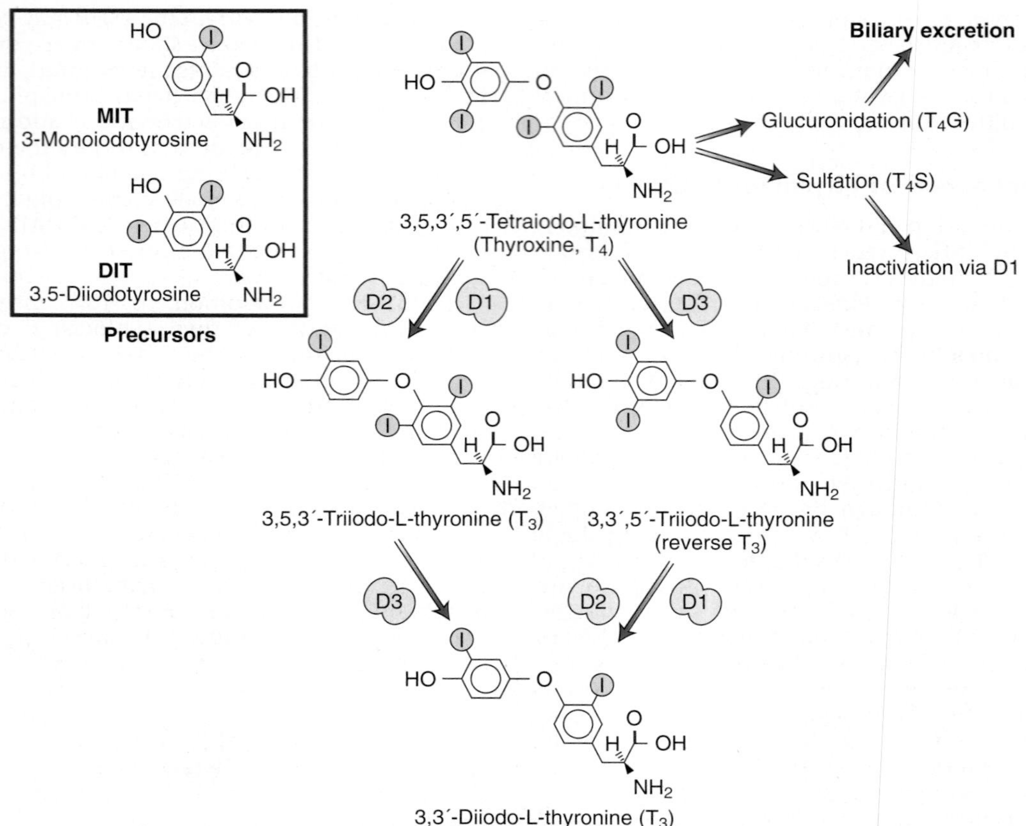

Figure 11-3 Major deiodinative and nondeiodinative pathways of thyroid hormone metabolism. *Arrows* indicate monodeiodination of the outer or inner ring of the iodothyronine nucleus, termed 5′ or 5 by convention, by D1, D2, or D3 (type 1, 2, or 3 deiodinase, respectively). Thyroxine (T_4) is activated by monodeiodination of the phenolic thyronine ring by D1 or D2 to form triiodothyronine (T_3). Deiodination of the tyrosyl ring by D1 or D3 inactivates T_4 and T_3, respectively. This inactivation pathway is markedly favored by sulfation of the phenolic hydroxyl to form T_4SO_4 (T_4S) or T_3SO_4 (T_3S). Glucuronidated T_4 (T_4G) and T_3 (T_3G) are excreted into the bile but may be partially reabsorbed after deglucuronidation in the intestine.

iodothyronine binding site per TBG molecule, the T_4 or T_3 binding capacity of TBG in normal human serum is equivalent to its concentration, which is approximately 270 nmol/L (1.5 μg/dL). The half-life of the protein in plasma is about 5 days. A congenital deficiency of TBG is common, occurring in 1 of every 5000 newborns, and is associated with the complete absence of the protein in males. L-Asparaginase blocks the synthesis of TBG, which accounts for the low T_4 concentrations in patients receiving this agent.

The glycosylation of TBG influences its clearance from the plasma and its behavior during isoelectric focusing. In estrogen-treated patients, there is an increase in the prevalence of the more acidic bands of TBG. The more highly sialylated TBG is cleared more slowly from plasma than the more positively charged TBG, because sialylation inhibits the hepatic uptake of glycoproteins. Sera from pregnant patients, women receiving oral contraceptives, and patients with acute hepatitis have increased fractions of acidic TBG. Patients with inherited TBG excess have normal amounts of highly sialylated TBG, as do men and nonpregnant women. Because TBG is the principal T_4- and T_3-binding protein, changes in TBG or its binding are paralleled by changes in total plasma T_4 and T_3 even though T_4 and T_3 production is little changed.

Another post-translational modification affecting TBG occurs in septic patients or after cardiopulmonary bypass surgery.[47] TBG is subjected to cleavage by a serine protease released from polymorphonuclear leukocytes; this results in the release of a 5-kd C-terminal loop with a consequent decrease in affinity for T_4. An analogous reaction has been described for cortisol-binding globulin, which releases cortisol at the site of inflammation.[48] It has been postulated that the released T_4 plays a critical role in the response to injury, perhaps by providing a supply of iodine for antibacterial purposes.[47] The cleaved TBG of approximately 49 kd circulates and, because it binds T_4 with lower avidity, may account for the increased ratio of free to bound T_4 in acute illness, even when TBG saturation studies or immunoassays indicate that the TBG concentration is normal (see "Thyroid Function during Fasting or Illness").

Transthyretin

TTR exists in part as a complex with retinol (vitamin A)-binding protein, hence its name. It consists of four identical polypeptide chains with a total molecular mass of approximately 55 kd, and it is not glycosylated. Its concentration in plasma is approximately 4 mmol/L (250 μg/mL). Each mole of TTR binds 1 mole of T_4 with high affinity, and a second T_4 molecule is bound with lower affinity at high concentrations of T_4. The half-life of TTR in plasma is normally about 2 days but is less during illness. TTR is expressed in the choroid plexus, and it is the major thyroid hormone–binding protein in the cerebrospinal fluid.[49] Targeted TTR gene disruption in mice shows that there is no impairment of uptake of T_4 into the brain, leaving the role

TABLE 11-3

Comparison of the Major Human Thyroid Hormone–Binding Proteins

Parameter	Thyroxine-Binding Globulin	Transthyretin	Albumin
Molecular weight of holoprotein (kd)	54,000	54,000 (4 subunits)	66,000
Plasma concentrations (μmol/L)	0.27	4.6	640
T_4 binding capacity as μg T_4/dL	21	350	50,000
Association constants of the major binding site (L/M)			
T_4	1×10^{10}	7×10^7	7×10^5
T_3	5×10^8	1.4×10^7	1×10^5
Fraction of sites occupied by T_4 in euthyroid plasma	0.31	0.02	<0.001
Distribution volume (L)	7	5.7	7.8
Turnover rate (% day)	13	59	5
Distribution of iodothyronines (% protein)			
T_4	68	11	20
T_3	80	9	11

L/M, Liters/Mol; T_3, triiodothyronine; T_4, thyroxine.

of TTR in cerebrospinal fluid undefined in regard to thyroid physiology.[50,51]

Variant forms of TTR are associated with familial amyloidotic polyneuropathy.[52,53] In affected families, the TTR monomer has one of several different point mutations, and TTR accumulates in the amyloid tissue deposits. Neither thyroid dysfunction nor altered vitamin A metabolism has been reported, although there is altered affinity of some of the mutant proteins for T_4. Families with high-affinity TTR and a few with increased TTR levels have been reported.

Competition for T_4 and T_3 Binding to TBG and TTR by Therapeutic Agents

The TBG binding site has an affinity for T_3 that is about 20-fold less than that for T_4 (see Table 11-3). Binding of T_4 and T_3 by TBG is inhibited by phenytoin,[54] salicylate,[55] salsalate, furosemide, fenclofenac, and mitotane. The affinity of these compounds for TBG is much weaker than that of the iodothyronines, but their concentration in plasma is sufficiently high to compete with T_4 and T_3 binding and reduce total hormone levels (although free T_4 remains normal). Because all methods used for estimating the free fractions of T_4 and T_3 in human serum except ultrafiltration dilute the serum, euthyroid patients receiving these drugs may appear to have low total and free T_4 or T_3 concentrations even though the free fraction is normal in vivo.

Albumin

The affinity of albumin for T_4 and T_3 binding is much lower than that of either TBG or TTR, but because of its high concentration this protein binds 10% of the plasma thyroid hormones (see Table 11-3). Changes in albumin concentration per se have little influence on total hormone levels unless accompanied by alterations in TBG and TTR, all three of which are synthesized in the liver. Hepatic failure or nephrotic syndrome leads to decreases in the plasma concentration of all three, and the serum albumin concentration in patients with these illnesses may serve as a surrogate for estimating TBG concentrations.

The role of albumin in thyroid physiology becomes clinically important in patients with familial dysalbuminemic hyperthyroxinemia.[56,57] In this autosomal dominant disorder, the plasma contains high amounts of a usually minor albumin variant that binds T_4 (but not T_3) with increased avidity. This increases total T_4, but free T_4 and total and free T_3 remain normal in an otherwise euthyroid patient. However, such patients may have a confusing pattern of test results, especially when analogue methods or labeled T_3 is used to estimate the free T_4 or T_3 (see Chapter 6).

Other Plasma Thyroid Hormone–Binding Proteins

Between 3% and 6% of plasma T_4 and T_3 are bound to lipoproteins. The T_4-binding lipoprotein is a 27-kd homodimer with an affinity for T_4 that is lower than that of TBG. This binding is of uncertain physiologic significance but could play a role in targeting T_4 delivery to specific tissues.

Free Thyroid Hormones

Because most of the circulating T_4 and T_3 is bound to TBG, the concentration and degree of saturation of TBG are the major determinants of the free fraction of T_4. Binding of the thyroid hormones to plasma proteins alters their metabolism. The negligible urinary excretion of T_3 and T_4 is due to the limited filterability of the hormone-protein complexes at the glomerulus. In vitro, the interaction between thyroid hormones and their binding proteins conforms to a reversible binding equilibrium that can be expressed by conventional equilibrium equations. For the formulations that follow, T_4 is used as the prototype, with the understanding that similar interactions apply in the case of T_3. The interaction between T_4 and TBG can be expressed as follows:

$$T_4 + TBG \xrightarrow{k_a} T_4 \cdot TBG$$

where TBG represents the *unoccupied* binding protein, k_a is the equilibrium association constant for the interaction, T_4 is the concentration of *free* T_4, and $T_4 \cdot TBG$ is T_4 bound to TBG (approximately 68% of total T_4 is bound to TBG).

The relationship can be expressed as follows:

$$\frac{T_4 \cdot TBG}{(T_4)(TBG)} = k_a$$

$$\frac{T_4}{T_4 \cdot TBG} = \frac{1}{(TBG)k_a}$$

Thus, the free fraction of T_4 (i.e., $T_4/T_4 \cdot TBG$) is inversely proportional to the concentration of *unoccupied* TBG binding sites. Estimates of the free T_4 concentration in serum can be generated by direct or indirect assays. In normal serum, the free T_4 is approximately 0.02% of the total (about 20 pmol/L, or 1.5 ng/dL). The approximately 20-fold lower affinity of TBG for T_3 results in a higher proportion of unbound T_3 (0.30%) (see Table 11-3).

It is the free hormone that is available to the tissues for intracellular transport and feedback regulation, that

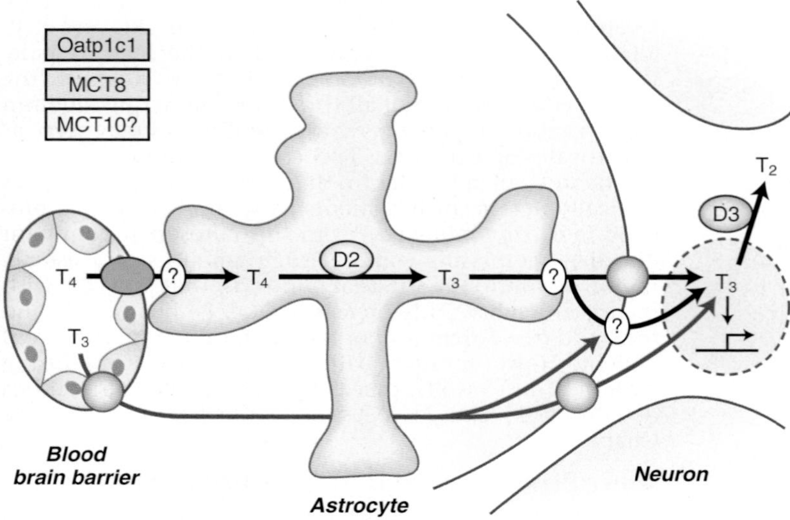

Figure 11-4 Potential pathways for entry of triiodothyronine (T_3) into the central nervous system. Thyroid hormones are transported through the blood-brain barrier via the action of an organic anion transporting polypeptide (OATP) or through the blood-CSF barrier via OATP and monocarboxylate transporter 8 (MCT8). In the astrocytes and tanycytes, thyroxine (T_4) is converted to T_3, which then enters the neurons, possibly via MCT8. In the neurons, both T_4 and T_3 are degraded by type 3 deiodinase (D3). T_3 from the tanycytes may reach the portal vessels in the median eminence. Other transporters may be present on the astrocyte or tanycyte membranes. In most cases, transport could be bidirectional, although only one direction is shown. CSF, cerebrospinal fluid; D2, type 2 iodothyronine deiodinase; MCT10, monocarboxylate transporter 10; T_2, diiodothyronine.

induces its metabolic effects, and that undergoes deiodination or degradation. The bound hormone acts merely as a reservoir. It follows that the concentration of the free hormone is the determinant of the metabolic state, and it is this concentration that is defended by homeostatic mechanisms. If a change in TBG occurs, the free T_4 and T_3 concentrations can be maintained at normal levels only if the bound hormone changes in the same direction. For example, if TBG concentrations are increased by administration of estrogen, the reduction in free T_4 lessens T_4 clearance, allowing an increase in the plasma total T_4 concentration. This is an iterative process that eventually normalizes the free T_4 at a new equilibrium without a change in T_4 secretion rate. The transient decrease in free thyroid hormones also slightly reduces the negative feedback on the hypothalamic-pituitary-thyroid axis, which causes an increase in thyroid hormone production as an additional compensation.[58]

The formulation just described is termed the *free thyroid hormone hypothesis*.[59,60] The question then arises: If it is the free hormone that is available for cellular entry, what is the role, if any, of the hormone-binding proteins? Protein binding facilitates the distribution of the hydrophobic thyroid hormones throughout the vascular system. For example, if a protein-free solution containing tracer T_3 is perfused through rat liver via the portal vein, there is a steep concentration gradient with a decreasing quantity of T_3 in the solution as the distance from the center of the portal lobule increases. In fact, almost all of the T_3 is taken up by the first cells to be contacted by the bolus. In contrast, if albumin is added to the perfusate, the distribution of tracer is uniform throughout the lobule. Both influx and efflux of thyroid hormone from tissues is rapid. Therefore, intracellular free T_3 and T_4 are in equilibrium with the free hormone pool in plasma, although transporter activity and metabolism will influence the magnitude of the ratio. In the steady state, it is the rate of T_3 and T_4 metabolism, not the dissociation rate from plasma proteins, that is rate-limiting in the exit of hormones from the plasma.

T_4 and T_3 Transport across Cell Membranes and Intracellular T_3 Binding

Although it was assumed for a long time that transport of iodothyronines across the plasma membrane occurs by passive diffusion, it is has become increasingly clear that cellular uptake and efflux of thyroid hormone is mediated by transporter proteins.[61] Several specific thyroid hormone transporters have been identified, including monocarboxylate transporter 8 (MCT8, encoded by *SLC16A2*), MCT10 (encoded by *SLC16A10*), and organic anion transporting polypeptide 1C1 (OATP1C1, encoded by *SLCO1C1*). MCT8 and MCT10 are expressed in multiple tissues where they facilitate transport of T_3, T_4, rT_3, and T_2 across cell membranes; OATP1C1 is expressed predominantly in the brain and transports preferentially T_4.

A defect in a single thyroid hormone transporter molecule, MCT8, has been shown to cause a severe developmental neurologic phenotype.[61,62] The Allan-Herndon-Dudley syndrome is an X-linked condition characterized by severe mental retardation, dysarthria, athetoid movements, muscle hypoplasia, and spastic paraplegia associated with an elevated serum T_3 concentration. All patients with this syndrome who were tested were found to have mutations in the MCT8 gene.[58,62] More than 40 different mutations have been identified, including loss of one or more exons; frameshift deletions; single-amino-acid substitutions, insertions, or deletions; and nonsense mutations resulting in truncation of the MCT8 protein. Although most of these mutations result in complete functional inactivation of the MCT8 protein, significant residual activity has been observed with a number of MCT8 mutations, some of which are associated with a milder clinical phenotype.[63] MCT8-null mice, despite the presence of markedly increased T_3 levels, lack any overt neurologic abnormalities, a rather unexpected finding in light of the severe human phenotype.[64,65] Animal studies show high expression of this protein in the choroid plexus, cerebral cortex, hippocampus, and medulla, with a distribution suggesting that the protein is expressed in neurons rather than glial cells.[66]

OATP1C1 is expressed in capillaries throughout the brain and may be involved in the transport of T_4 across the blood-brain barrier.[61] This suggests that the supply of T_3 to neurons may occur according to the schema shown in Figure 11-4[67]: T_4 is transferred into the choroid plexus or into tanycytes by the action of OATP1C1, which is negatively regulated in brain capillaries by thyroid hormone. In the tanycyte or astrocyte, T_4 is converted to T_3 by D2 and exits the cell, possibly via the MCT8/MCT10 transporters,

TABLE 11-4

Human Iodothyronine Selenodeiodinases

Parameter	Type 1 (Outer and Inner Ring)	Type 2 (Outer Ring)	Type 3 (Inner Ring)
Physiologic role	rT_3 and T_3S degradation; source of plasma T_3 in thyrotoxic patients	Provide intracellular T_3 in specific tissues, a source of plasma T_3	Inactivate T_3 and T_4
Tissue location	Liver, kidney, thyroid, pituitary(?); not CNS	CNS, pituitary, BAT, placenta, thyroid, skeletal muscle, heart	Placenta, CNS, hemangiomas, fetal or adult liver, skeletal muscle
Subcellular location	Plasma membrane	Endoplasmic reticulum	Plasma membrane
Preferred substrates (position deiodinated)	rT_3 (5′), T_3S	T_4, rT_3 (5′)	T_3, T_4
K_m	rT_3, 10^{-7}; T_4, 10^{-6}	10^{-9}	10^{-9}
Susceptibility to PTU	High	Absent	Absent
Response to increased T_4	↑	↓	↑

BAT, brown adipose tissue; CNS, central nervous system; K_m, Michaelis-Menten constant; PTU, 6-n propylthiouracil; rT_3, reverse triiodothyronine; T_3, triiodothyronine; T_3S, T_3SO_4; T_4, thyroxine.

where it becomes available for neuronal uptake, also via MCT8.[68,69] Neurons express the D3, which prevents activation of T_4 and catalyzes degradation of T_3 (see "Iodothyronine Deiodination"). This would provide a logical explanation of the association of the mutations in MCT8 with the attention deficit-hyperactivity disorder, although it still remains puzzling why the neurologic manifestations of this condition are so different from those seen in patients with untreated congenital hypothyroidism or severe iodine deficiency (see Chapter 13).

The transport field has become more complex as evidence accumulates of tissue-specific and generalized iodothyronine transporters belonging to a number of different transporter protein families. Each of these has many members with small variations in structure that alter the specificity of the target substance. A thorough review of this topic is beyond the scope of this chapter, and the interested reader is referred to excellent reviews for further information.[61]

In most cells, about 90% of the intracellular T_3 is located in the cytosol. The known exception is in the pituitary, where approximately 50% of the intracellular T_3 is present in the nucleus. The mechanisms determining this distribution are still unknown, but it would not be surprising if thyroid hormones were actively transported in and out of the nucleus and other intracellular compartments. An intracellular T_3-binding protein (mu crystallin) has been identified and is expressed at high levels in human brain and heart, although it is widely distributed. This or similar proteins may also play a role in the subcellular localization of the active hormone.

Iodothyronine Deiodination

The most important pathway for T_4 metabolism is its outer ring (5′) monodeiodination to the active thyroid hormone, T_3. This reaction is catalyzed by D1 and D2 and is the source of more than 80% of the circulating T_3 in humans. Inner ring deiodination, an inactivating step, is catalyzed primarily by D3, which inactivates T_3 and prevents activation of T_4 by converting it to rT_3 (see Fig. 11-3).[43,70] The structures of the three human deiodinases are similar. They are all homodimers and integral membrane proteins, and they contain the rare amino acid selenocysteine in the active catalytic center (Table 11-4). Selenocysteine has nucleophilic properties that make it ideal for catalysis of oxidoreductive reactions such as iodothyronine deiodination and the reduction of H_2O_2 by another family of selenoenzymes, the glutathione peroxidases.[71,72] Selenium is thought to be the iodine acceptor during deiodination reactions. Mutagenesis of selenocysteine in D1 to cysteine (i.e., replacement of selenium with sulfur) reduces the enzyme velocity approximately 200-fold.

The presence of selenocysteine has implications beyond catalytic activity, considering that the cellular processes for synthesizing selenoproteins are complex and inefficient.[43] A specific structural feature, the selenocysteine insertion sequence (SECIS) element, is present in the 3′ untranslated region of the mRNAs encoding these proteins and works together with a specific group of selenocysteine-incorporating gene products. All of these elements are required for the complex cellular function by which the normal "STOP" codon UGA is recognized as the specific codon for insertion of the selenocysteine residue during protein translation.[73]

Enzymology and Regulation of the Selenodeiodinases

Although both D1 and D2 activate T_4, they have several important differences (see Table 11-4). D1 catalyzes both 5′ and 5 deiodination of T_4 to form T_3 and rT_3, respectively, although the Michaelis-Menten constant (K_m) for these reactions is approximately 3 orders of magnitude greater than that of D2 and D3 for this substrate. In fact, the preferred substrates of D1 are rT_3 (5′ deiodination) and T_3SO_4 (5 deiodination). D1 is inhibited by PTU, unlike D2 and D3. D1 also differs from D2 in being markedly increased by excess thyroid hormone through increased gene transcription, whereas D2 mRNA and protein are reduced by thyroid hormones. D2 has a half-life of only 20 to 30 minutes, whereas that of D1 and D3 is more than 12 hours. This is due to the rapid ubiquitination of D2, a process that is accelerated by interaction with its substrate T_4 or rT_3. D1 and D3 are not thought to be ubiquitinated.

The cellular location of D2 close to the nucleus gives the T_3 formed by its catalytic action better access to the nucleus than that formed by D1.[74] The T_3 produced by D2 is especially effective in entering the nucleus and binding to thyroid hormone receptors, a property explained by its location in the ER. D1, on the other hand, is located in the plasma membrane, and the T_3 produced by this enzyme preferentially enters the plasma pool.[43] Therefore, D2 serves the special purpose of providing nuclear T_3 from intracellular T_4 in a cell-specific fashion. This makes D2 especially important for regulating the hypothalamic-pituitary-thyroid axis, where its activity increases in response to a decrease in serum T_4 concentrations (e.g., iodine deficiency, early autoimmune thyroid disease) well before the serum T_3 falls. If the decrease in plasma T_4 is too great to be compensated for by the increase in D2 activity in the hypothalamic-pituitary feedback sensors, an increase in TRH and TSH will occur to stimulate the thyroid. For this reason, D2 has been thought of mainly as an enzyme that provides intracellular T_3, although there is increasing evidence that D2 could also contribute to plasma T_3. On the other hand, in thyrotoxicosis, the threefold to fourfold increase in D1, particularly in the thyroid, and the reduced D2 make D1 the major extrathyroidal source of T_3. This can explain why PTU causes a much more rapid fall in circulating T_3 than does methimazole in the patient with Graves' disease.[34,35]

D3 is the foremost thyroid hormone–inactivating enzyme that functions by deiodinating the inner ring of both T_3 andT_4.[75,76] D3 activity has been identified in only a limited number of postnatal tissues, including placenta and uterine endometrium, the CNS (where it is primarily in neurons), and skin. Much higher D3 expression has been demonstrated in various fetal tissues such as liver, brain, placenta, uterus, and the umbilical arteries and vein. In the adult, D3 has been identified in some malignant cell lines and in a number of human tumors, including astrocytomas, oligodendromas, gliosarcomas, glioblastomas, TSH-secreting pituitary adenomas, and in basal cell carcinomas.[77] Tumoral D3 activity can be robust, and the highest D3 activity reported so far in any human tissue has been in infantile hemangiomas. In infants with extensive hepatic lesions, D3 may overwhelm the secretory capacity of the infant's thyroid, causing hypothyroidism, a syndrome termed *consumptive hypothyroidism*.[78] D3 expression is increased by thyroid hormone at a transcriptional level.[79]

Gene targeting studies have begun to provide further insights into the physiologic roles of the deidodinases in mammals.[80] Inactivation of the D2 gene (*Dio2*) results in a phenotypically normal mouse with an elevated serum T_4, normal serum T_3, and elevated serum TSH.[70,81] These animals have hypothalamic-pituitary resistance to T_4, impaired auditory function, impaired thermogenesis in response to cold stress, and relatively subtle defects in neurologic function, all consistent with the expectations based on earlier studies indicating an especially important role for D2 in brown fat cell function, cochlear maturation, and neurologic development. Mice with targeted inactivation of *Dio1* are phenotypically normal; they also have an elevated serum T_4 and a normal serum T_3, but TSH is normal.[82] The most striking finding in the D1-deficient mouse is a marked shift in the T_4 clearance pathway, from deiodination to biliary/fecal clearance. Interestingly, mice lacking both of the activating deiodinases D1 and D2 are still able (by increasing TSH and thyroidal T_3 secretion) to maintain normal T_3 concentrations in serum and do not suffer from systemic hypothyroidism, indicating that thyroidal T_3 production can guarantee T_3 homeostasis, at least in rodents.[70,81] Mice with inactivation of *Dio3* show profound abnormalities. They have impaired fertility and develop central hypothyroidism in adult life, presumably due to hypothalamic thyrotoxicosis during developmental programming.[83] These problems have precluded more extensive studies at this time.

TABLE 11-5

Comparison of Triiodothyronine (T_3) and Thyroxine (T_4) in Humans*

Parameter	T_3	T_4
Production rate (nmol/day)	50	110
Fraction from thyroid	0.2	1.0
Relative metabolic potency	1.0	0.3
Serum concentration		
Total (nmol/L)	1.8	100.
Free (pmol/L)	5	20
Fraction of total hormone in free form ($\times 10^{-2}$)	0.3	0.02
Distribution volume (L)	40	10
Fraction intracellular	0.64	0.15
Half-life (days)	0.75	6.7

*To convert T_4 from nmol/L to μg/dL (total) or from pmol/L to ng/dL (free), divide by 12.87; to convert T_3 from nmol/L to ng/dL (total) or from pmol/L to pg/dL (free), multiply by 65.1.

Quantitative and Qualitative Aspects of Thyroid Hormone Metabolism

Thyroid Hormone Turnover

In the normal adult, T_4 has a distribution volume of approximately 10 L (Table 11-5). The concentration of total T_4 in plasma is approximately 100 nmol/L (8 μg/dL), and the extrathyroidal T_4 pool is approximately 1 nmol (800 μg). In the adult, the fractional rate of turnover of T_4 in the periphery is about 10% per day (half-life, 6.7 days). Therefore, about 1.1 L of the peripheral T_4 distribution space is cleared of hormone daily, a volume containing approximately 110 nmol (85 μg) of T_4.

The kinetics of T_3 metabolism differ from those of T_4, partly because of its 10- to 15-fold lower affinity for TBG. The volume of distribution of T_3 in the normal adult is about 40 L, four times that of T_4, and its fractional turnover rate is approximately 60% per day. At a mean normal serum T_3 concentration of 1.8 nmol/L (120 ng/dL), 50-fold lower than T_4, the daily production of T_3 is approximately 50 nmol (33 μg), or about 46% that of T_4 (see Table 11-5). The rapid metabolic clearance rate of the product of inner-ring T_4 deiodination, rT_3, and the low concentration in plasma (0.25 nmol/L, or 15 ng/dL) combine to yield daily production rates for rT_3 of about 45 nmol. Therefore, 80% to 85% of T_3 and 100% of rT_3 production in humans can be accounted for by peripheral deiodination of T_4, findings consonant with the high ratio of T_4 to T_3 (15:1) and T_4 to rT_3 (100:1) in human Tg. Of the T_3 generated via T_4 5′ deiodination in euthyroid humans, only 20% to 25% is inhibited by PTU, consistent with a significant contribution of D2-dependent T_3 production.[84] Although much of the T_3 and rT_3 produced from T_4 in peripheral tissues exits those tissues and enters the blood, an uncertain fraction of each is degraded intracellularly before exit. As discussed later, in some D2-containing tissues such as the pituitary, a significant fraction of T_3 in the cell nucleus is derived from deiodination of intracellular T_4 to T_3, rather than from the plasma. This is particularly true in the thyrotroph.[85]

Other pathways are also involved in T_4 and T_3 metabolism. In humans, T_4 undergoes glucuronidation of the phenolic hydroxyl group by the uridine diphosphate glucuronyl transferases (UDPGT), but only minimal amounts of T_3 undergo this process (see Fig. 11-3). This pathway is clinically significant because certain pharmacotherapeutic agents enhance glucuronide conjugation through induction of UDPGT, leading to biliary excretion of T_4-glucuronide into the intestine.[86] These agents include phenobarbital, phenytoin, rifampin, and, possibly, certain synaptosomal serotonin reuptake inhibitors such as sertraline. Because T_4-glucuronide is not easily reabsorbed from intestinal contents, the significance of this pathway is that therapy with such agents generally increases levothyroxine requirements. In patients with an intact thyroid, this will not be apparent because internal adjustments will increase the T_4 production rate to compensate for the accelerated biliary excretion. In patients with hypothyroidism, however, an increase in levothyroxine dosage will often be required. Deamination and decarboxylation reactions that produce tetrac and triac and sulfation of T_4 and T_3 at the phenolic hydroxyl group account for an as yet unidentified fraction of T_4 and T_3 metabolism in humans.

Sources of Intracellular T_3

In view of the differential tissue distribution of the various deiodinases and their different K_m values and differential regulation, it is not surprising that tissues may derive intracellular T_3 via different pathways (Fig. 11-5). In several rat tissues, including tissues expressing D1 such as kidney and liver, most of the nuclear T_3 is derived from plasma T_3. In D2-containing tissues, such as rat cerebral cortex, pituitary, brown fat, and possibly skeletal muscle, D2 functions as an additional intracellular source of T_3, such that the nuclear T_3 concentration is higher because of the combination of T_3 from plasma and T_3 that is locally converted from T_4. In these tissues, half or more of intracellular T_3 is generated locally from T_4 within the tissue. In the CNS, the D2-generated T_3 in neurons is likely to derive from paracrine sources in tanycytes and astrocytes (see Fig. 11-4). In the rat, the tissues that depend on D2 for nuclear T_3 are those in which a constant supply of thyroid hormone is critical for normal development (cerebral cortex), thyroid gland regulation (pituitary), or survival during cold stress (brown adipose tissue). These tissues are also characterized by a high degree of saturation of the nuclear T_3 receptors, compared with to tissues such as liver and kidney, in which

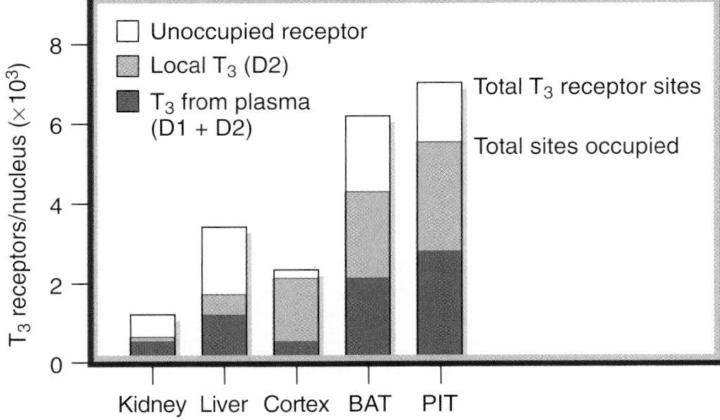

Figure 11-5 Schematic diagram of the origin of the specifically bound nuclear triiodothyronine (T_3) in various rat tissues. Data were derived from studies in which the sources of specifically bound nuclear T_3 in rat tissues were estimated using double-isotope labeling techniques. In tissues in which receptor saturation was significantly greater than 50%, the additional T_3 was provided by type 2 iodothyronine deiodinase (D2)-catalyzed conversion of thyroxine (T_4) to T_3. Approximately 40% of T_3 in rat plasma is derived from thyroid secretion, with the remainder from D1- and D2-catalyzed T_4-to-T_3 conversion. BAT, brown adipose tissue; PIT, pituitary.

nuclear T_3 receptor sites are only about 50% occupied at normal serum T_3 concentrations (see Fig. 11-5).

Intracellular D2-catalyzed T_3 production has important implications for thyroid hormone physiology. First, because the T_3 produced from T_4 occupies a significant fraction of the receptors in those tissues, changes in serum T_4 or T_3 can change receptor occupancy. However, a fall in T_4 will also increase the D2 protein half-life by decreasing the rates of ubiquitination and proteasomal degradation, and the consequent rise in D2 activity will mitigate the impact of the reduction of serum T_4 in D2-expressing tissues, helping to maintain T_3 homeostasis.[43] The requirement for both T_3 and T_4 for normal saturation of pituitary and CNS T_3 receptors permits a response of the hypothalamic-pituitary axis to a reduction in plasma T_4, which is the earliest manifestation of iodine deficiency or primary hypothyroidism (see "Regulation of Thyroid Function"). Because the D2 gene is positively regulated by cAMP, D2 activity and T_3 production increase rapidly in brown adipose tissue under stimulation by the sympathetic nervous system. This response is critical to adaptive thermogenesis during cold exposure in the human neonate and lifelong in the rodent.[87]

Tissues expressing D3 have lower T_3 concentrations than would be expected from the plasma contribution and a gene expression profile similar to that of hypothyroid cells. This is explained by the inactivation of T_3 and T_4 that takes place immediately after these hormones enter the cell. The D3-mediated reduction in T_3 levels likely occurs in several physiologic settings (e.g., development, regeneration) or pathologic conditions (e.g., cancer cells, inflammation, myocardial infarction) in which D3 is upregulated.[88]

Pharmacologic Agents That Inhibit Thyroid Hormone Deiodination

A number of commonly used pharmacologic agents have significant effects on thyroid hormone deiodination. Propylthiouracil inhibition of D1 was mentioned earlier. The antiarrhythmic drug amiodarone shares sufficient structural similarity with T_4 that it can inhibit deiodination of T_4 and rT_3 by D1 and possibly by D2 (Fig. 11-6). This causes an increase in plasma T_4 to maintain serum T_3 in the normal range. There is also an increase in TSH within the first weeks of therapy, which gradually returns to normal as the thyroid axis re-equilibrates.[89] The T_4 and rT_3 metabolic clearance rates are reduced by 20% to 25%, and the fractional T_4-to-T_3 conversion rate is reduced by about 50%. Amiodarone also inhibits the active transport of T_4 and T_3 into hepatocytes, and the drug or one of its products may interfere with T_3 binding to thyroid hormone receptors.

The effects of amiodarone resemble those observed with the iodoaniline derivatives formerly used for gallbladder visualization (see Fig. 11-6). Iopanoic and iopodipic acid inhibit the deiodinases by competing with the iodothyronine substrates.[43] This makes them useful in the acute treatment of severe hyperthyroidism, although these agents are no longer available for clinical use in the United States.

High dosages of glucocorticoids (10 times replacement) will acutely reduce the ratio of T_3 to T_4 in plasma, suggesting that T_4-to-T_3 conversion is blocked. The ratio of rT_3 to T_4 increases, raising the possibility that D3 action is also increased.[90] These effects resolve during long-term therapy such that thyroid function is little affected and thyroid hormone requirements are not increased by chronic glucocorticoid therapy.

Recombinant growth hormone increases the ratio of circulating T_3 to T_4. Growth hormone deficiency is associated with a decrease in the ratio of T_3 to T_4 in serum,

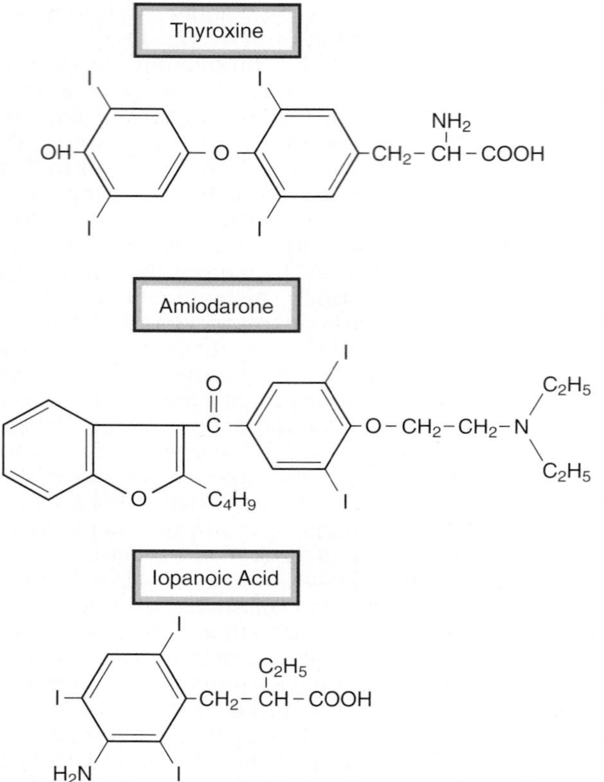

Figure 11-6 Comparison of the chemical structure of thyroxine (T_4) with that of two agents that block the deiodination of the iodothyronines. The inhibition of T_4-to-T_3 conversion that occurs in patients receiving amiodarone may be caused by the drug itself or by a metabolic product. Iopanoic acid and related iodoanilines are competitive inhibitors of all three iodothyronine deiodinases. T3, triiodothyronine.

possibly associated with a decrease in outer ring deiodination. As expected, dietary selenium deficiency also inhibits the synthesis of D1 in humans.[91]

Mechanism of Thyroid Hormone Action

Thyroid hormone acts by binding to a specific nuclear thyroid hormone receptor (TR), which, in turn, binds to DNA, usually as a heterodimer with retinoid X receptor (RXR) at specific sequences called thyroid hormone response elements, or TREs; these sites are dictated by the DNA binding-site preferences of the RXR-TR (or TR-TR) complex (Fig. 11-7). The general mechanism by which nuclear receptor–activating ligands such as T_3 produce their effects is discussed in Chapter 4. T_3 has a 15-fold higher binding affinity for TRs than does T_4, explaining its function as the active thyroid hormone. In humans, there are two TR genes, α and β, that are found on different chromosomes (chromosomes 17 and 3, respectively). There are several alternatively spliced gene products from each of these genes forming both active and inactive gene products. The active proteins are $TR\alpha_1$, $TR\beta_1$, $TR\beta_2$, and $TR\beta_3$.[92] The protein structure of TRs includes three major functional domains—one binding DNA, one binding ligand, and a major transcriptional activation domain in the C-terminus.

There are tissue-specific preferences in expression of the various TRs, suggesting that they serve different functions in different tissues.[93] In general, TRα, particularly $TR\alpha_2$, is thought to be important in the hypothalamus and pituitary where regulation of thyroid function occurs.[94] In addition to differences in the N-terminus between $TR\beta_1$ and $TR\beta_2$, the two proteins are under the regulation of different promoters that can function in tissue-specific patterns. $TR\beta_2$ is downregulated by T_3, whereas $TR\alpha_1$ mRNA expression is not affected by T_3.[95] $TR\beta_2$ is also expressed in the cochlea. $TR\alpha_1$ is expressed in all tissues, although its mRNA is especially highly expressed in the kidney, liver,

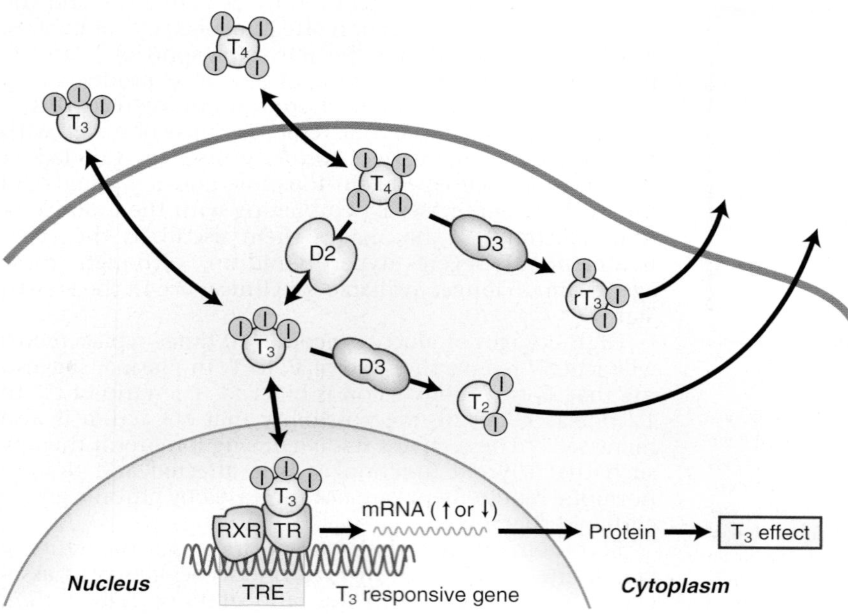

Figure 11-7 Schematic diagram of thyroid hormone activation and inactivation in a cell expressing the iodothyronine deiodinases D2 and D3. The triiodothyronine (T_3) that enters the cell can be deiodinated to 3,3′-diiodothyronine (T_2), or it can enter the nucleus and bind to the thyroid hormone receptor (TR). An additional source of T_3 is that generated by outer ring deiodination of thyroxine (T_4) within the cell. The interaction of T_3 with the TR that is bound as a heterodimer with retinoid X receptor (RXR) to the thyroid hormone response element (TRE), often in the 5′ flanking region of a T_3-responsive gene, causes either an increase or a decrease in the transcription of that gene. This leads to parallel changes in the concentrations of critical proteins, thus producing the thyroid hormone response characteristic of a given cell. mRNA, messenger RNA; rT_3, reverse T_3.

brain, and heart. TRα_1 mRNA is expressed in the brain, in brown adipose tissue, and, at lower levels, in skeletal muscle, lungs, and heart. TRβ_3 mRNA is expressed at very low levels but is more abundant in the liver, kidneys, and lungs than in other tissues.

Experiments with inactivation of TRα and TRβ have illuminated their different physiologic roles. Disruption of the TRβ gene (both TRβ_1 and TRβ_2) in mice causes deafness, a marked reduction in feedback sensitivity of the hypothalamic-pituitary-thyroid axis, and a decrease in hepatic D1. These mice have marked elevations in both TSH and thyroid hormones, similar to those observed in human families with *resistance to thyroid hormone*, a condition in which TRβ mutations markedly reduce the binding affinity of TRβ for T_3. This binding defect produces a TRβ_1 or TRβ_2 protein that acts as a dominant negative inhibitor of the intact TRβ proteins encoded by the normal allele (see Chapters 4 and 13). Despite evidence of impaired feedback regulation, there is relatively little abnormality in the brain and heart of TRβ-deficient mice. The effect of a TRα_1 disruption in the mouse is quite different. The predominant phenotypic effects are modest bradycardia and hypothermia.

These studies have led to the generalization that feedback regulation of thyroid hormone effects and cochlear development are functions of TRβ, whereas cardiac function and energy metabolism are more likely to be regulated by TRα. It is likely that small differences in the ligand-binding domains of TRα and TRβ will allow design of thyroid hormone analogues selective for one or the other of these receptors. This may result in agents that could, for example, suppress TSH in patients with thyroid cancer, without inducing tachycardia, such as GC-1; another example is KB141, a potential treatment for obesity via stimulation of metabolic rate and oxygen consumption.[96]

Other potential mechanisms for thyroid hormone action by interaction with the membrane are under investigation. These nongenomic effects are most likely mediated by cellular binding proteins other than TRs. Integrin $\alpha_V\beta_3$, has been identified as a putative plasma membrane thyroid hormone–binding site. Previously, T_4, but not T_3, was shown to promote actin polymerization and integrin interaction with laminin in neural cells.[97] Continuing investigations have shown that T_4 and thyroid hormone analogues such as GC-1 can activate mitogen-activated protein kinase (MAPK) and can have proangiogenic effects.[98] The MAPK signal results in serine phosphorylation of several nuclear proteins and occurs within minutes after exposure, analogous to the effects of 17β-estradiol. The physiologic relevance of these effects are not well characterized. The proteins include plasma membrane–associated T_3 transporters, calcium adenosine triphosphatase, adenylate cyclase, and glucose transporters; an ER-associated protein called prolyl hydroxylase; and monomeric pyruvate kinase. The effect of T_4 itself in initiating the ubiquitination of D2 is perhaps the most important nongenomic effect at physiologic concentrations of free T_4.[43]

REGULATION OF THYROID FUNCTION

The Hypothalamic-Pituitary-Thyroid Axis

The thyroid participates with the hypothalamus and pituitary in a classic feedback control loop (Fig. 11-8). In addition, there is an inverse relationship between the iodine level in the thyroid and the fractional rate of hormone formation. Such autoregulatory mechanisms stabilize the rate of hormone synthesis despite fluctuations in the availability of iodine. Stability in hormone production is achieved in part because the large intraglandular store of hormone buffers the effect of acute increases or decreases in hormone synthesis. Autoregulatory mechanisms within the gland, in turn, tend to maintain a constant thyroid hormone pool. Finally, the hypothalamic-pituitary feedback mechanism senses variations in the availability of free thyroid hormones, however small, and acts to correct them. There is a close relationship among the hypothalamus, the anterior pituitary, the thyroid gland, and still higher centers in the brain, the function of the entire complex being modified in a typical negative-feedback manner by the availability of the thyroid hormones. In addition, other hormones and neuropeptides also influence this axis (see Chapters 7 and 8).

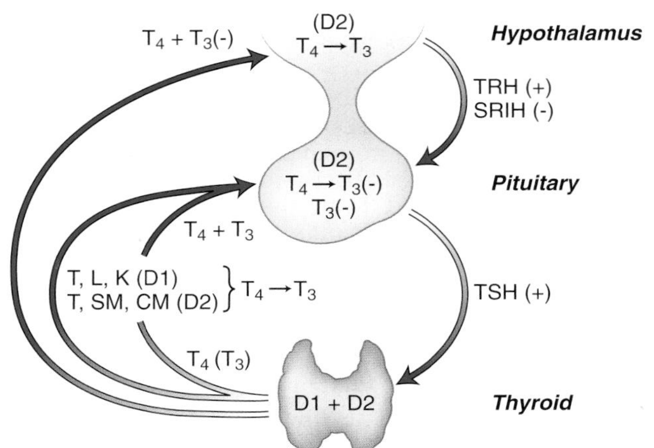

Figure 11-8 Roles of thyroxine (T_4) and triiodothyronine (T_3) in the feedback regulation of secretion of thyrotropin-releasing hormone (TRH) and thyroid-stimulating hormone (TSH). Secreted T_4 must be converted to T_3 to produce its effects. This conversion may take place in tissues such as the liver (L), kidney (K), and thyroid (T) catalyzed by the type I iodothyronine deiodinase, D1. Type 2 (D2) is present in human thyroid (T), skeletal muscle (SM), possibly cardiac muscle (CM), and the pituitary and hypothalamus. SRIH, somatotropin release-inhibiting factor (somatostatin hormone).

Thyrotropin-Releasing Hormone Synthesis and Secretion

TRH, a modified tripeptide (pyroglutamyl-histidyl-proline-amide), is derived from a large pre-proTRH molecule of 29 kd that contains five progenitor sequences. The TRH peptides are released from the pre-proTRH molecule by a peptidase that acts at flanking lysine/arginine residues. TRH is expressed in the hypothalamus, the brain, the C cells of the thyroid gland, the beta cells of the pancreas, the myocardium, the reproductive organs (including prostate and testis), and the spinal cord. The parvocellular region of the paraventricular nuclei of the hypothalamus is the source of the TRH that regulates TSH secretion. The 5′ flanking region of the gene encoding TRH has sequences for mediating responses to glucocorticoids and cAMP. In addition, at least two elements in this region are responsible for the negative regulation of this gene by thyroid hormone.[99] TRH travels in the axons of the peptidergic neurons through the median eminence and is released close to the hypothalamic-pituitary portal plexus. The neuron bodies producing TRH are innervated by catecholamine, leptin agouti-related peptide, neuropeptide Y or melanocyte-stimulating hormone (MSH), and somatostatin-containing axons, all of which potentially influence the rate of synthesis of the pre-proTRH molecule (see Chapter 7).

T_3 suppresses the levels of pre-proTRH mRNA in the hypothalamus,[100,101] but normal feedback regulation of pre-proTRH mRNA synthesis by thyroid hormone requires a combination of T_3 and T_4 in the circulation, the latter giving rise to T_3 via T_4 5′ deiodination in the CNS in astrocytes and tanycytes (see Fig. 11-4). This regulation is observed in vivo exclusively in the parvocellular division of the paraventricular nuclei; in tissues outside the CNS expressing the TRH gene, negative regulation by thyroid hormone is absent. Therefore, part of the negative feedback induced by T_4 may be generated at the median eminence/arcuate nucleus at a point where neuropeptides and T_3 enter the pituitary portal system.[102] In addition to inhibiting the synthesis of pre-proTRH mRNA, thyroid hormone also blocks the capacity of TRH to stimulate TSH release from the thyrotroph.

TRH is rapidly inactivated within the CNS by a cell-surface peptidase called TRH-degrading ectoenzyme (TRH-DE) or protein peptidase II. TRH-DE is very specific: no other ectopeptidase is known to be capable of degrading TRH, and TRH is the only known substrate of this unique enzyme.[103]

Thyrotropin Synthesis and Secretion

Thyrotropin (TSH) is the major regulator of the morphologic and functional states of the thyroid. It is a glycoprotein secreted by the thyrotrophs in the anteromedial portion of the adenohypophysis (see Chapter 8). TSH is composed of an α-subunit of 14 kd (92 amino acids) that is common to LH, follicle-stimulating hormone (FSH), hCG, and a specific β-subunit of 112 amino acids that is synthesized in thyrotrophs. In normal thyrotrophs and in thyrotroph tumors, synthesis of α-subunit is in excess, indicating that the quantity of β-subunit is rate-limiting for TSH secretion. Levels of α-subunit in serum range from 0.5 to 5 μg/L but are increased in postmenopausal women and in patients with pituitary tumors. TRH increases, and thyroid hormone suppresses, the transcription of both subunits, and these are the two most important influences on TSH synthesis.

The pretranslational regulation of TSH synthesis and secretion is a complex process. The physiologic glycosylation of TSH involves several post-translational steps, including excision of signal peptides from both subunits and cotranslational glycosylation with high-mannose oligosaccharides.[104] The glycosylation of the subunits protects them from intracellular degradation and permits normal folding of the protein chains so that internal disulfide linkages are correctly formed. Glycosylation is required for full biologic activity.[105,106] TRH is required for this process, as illustrated by the inappropriately low biologic activity of the TSH in the serum of patients with pituitary tumors or hypothalamic disorders, compared with the level of immunologic activity resulting from TRH deficiency.

In normal serum, TSH is present at concentrations between 0.4 and 4.2 mU/L. The level is increased in primary hypothyroidism and reduced in thyrotoxicosis. The plasma TSH half-life is about 30 minutes, and production rates in humans are 40 to 150 mU/day. Circulating TSH displays both pulsatile and circadian variations. The former are characterized by fluctuations at 1- to 2-hour intervals. The magnitude of TSH pulsations is decreased during fasting or illness and after surgery. There is an acute reduction of TSH in fasted humans; this is associated with a fall in leptin levels and is caused by a decrease in the amplitude of the TSH pulses.[107] The circadian variation is characterized by a nocturnal surge that precedes the onset of sleep and appears to be independent of the cortisol rhythm and of fluctuations in serum T_4 and T_3 concentrations.[108] When the onset of sleep is delayed, the nocturnal TSH surge is enhanced and prolonged; early onset of sleep results in a surge of lesser magnitude and shorter duration.

The degree of thyroid hypofunction after destruction of the hypothalamus is less severe than that which follows hypophysectomy, and residual thyroid function in the former circumstance can be altered by raising or lowering the concentration of thyroid hormones in the blood. Therefore, both T_4 and T_3 mediate the feedback regulation of TSH secretion, and TRH determines its set point (see Fig. 11-8). There is a linear inverse relationship between the serum free T_4 concentration and the log of the TSH (Fig. 11-9), making the serum TSH concentration an exquisitely sensitive indicator of the thyroid state of patients with an intact hypothalamic-pituitary axis. Gene targeting studies show that TRH secretion is probably the dominant factor mediating the thyroid hormone feedback regulation of TSH secretion, because the markedly elevated TSH secretion of mice with inactivation of TRβ cannot be sustained in mice lacking the TRH gene.[109] This is somewhat surprising given the less severe hypothyroidism associated with hypothalamic (as opposed to primary) hypothyroidism, but it may be explained by the absolute nature of the TRH deficiency achieved by genetic manipulation compared with the clinical situation in humans with central hypothyroidism, in whom the TRH deficiency is not likely to be complete.

Somatostatin (somatotropin release-inhibiting factor [SRIF]), acting through inhibitory G protein (G_i), decreases TSH secretion in vitro and in vivo, but prolonged treatment with a somatostatin analogue does not cause hypothyroidism.[110,111] Similar acute effects occur during dopamine infusion and the administration of bromocriptine, a dopamine agonist; both of these agents inhibit adenylate cyclase. Conversely, blockade of the dopamine receptor by metoclopramide increases the basal serum TSH concentration in both euthyroid and hypothyroid patients. These findings indicate that dopamine is a regulator of TSH secretion, but chronic administration of dopamine agonists (e.g., for the treatment of prolactinoma) does not cause central hypothyroidism, indicating that compensatory mechanisms negate these acute effects.[112]

A number of drugs or hormones may suppress or stimulate TSH secretion (Table 11-6). Glucocorticoids given in high doses transiently suppress TSH secretion, although prolonged therapy is not associated with central hypothyroidism.[110] Patients with Cushing's disease have subnormal TSH production but with minimal effects on T_4 production.[110] Bexarotene, an RXR agonist used for treatment of T-cell lymphoma, suppresses TSH sufficiently to cause central hypothyroidism, presumably by reducing transcription of the TSH β-subunit gene.[113,114]

Neurotransmitters are important direct and indirect modulators in TSH synthesis and secretion. A complex network of neurotransmitter neurons terminates on the cell bodies of hypophysiotropic neurons, and several neurotransmitters (e.g., dopamine) are directly released into hypophyseal portal blood, exerting direct effects on anterior pituitary cells. Furthermore, many dopaminergic, serotoninergic, histaminergic, catecholaminergic, opioidergic, and GABAergic systems project from hypothalamic or other brain regions to the hypophysiotropic neurons involved in TSH regulation. These projections are

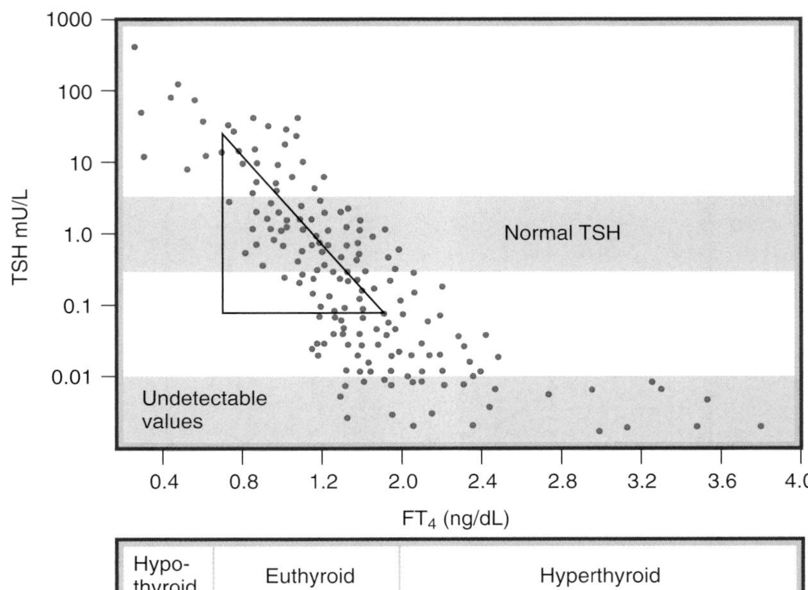

Figure 11-9 The log/linear relationship between thyroid-stimulating hormone (TSH) and the concentration of free T_4 (FT_4) in serum. Typical FT_4 concentrations in hypothyroid, euthyroid, and hyperthyroid patients are shown.

important for maintenance of a normal TSH circadian rhythm and normal response to stress and cold exposure, whereas basal TSH secretion is mainly regulated by intrinsic hypothalamic activity.

Thyrostimulin, a noncovalent heterodimer of two glycoprotein hormone-like proteins (alpha2 and beta5), is an agonist of the TSHR. It is synthesized in the corticotrophs and in placenta, has high affinity for TSHRs, and increases the levels of thyroid hormones in rats with a suppressed TSH.[115] It is ineffective in activating LH or FSH receptors but is expressed in oocytes, where it acts as a paracrine regulator to activate the TSHR expressed in ovary.[116] Thyrostimulin, which evolved before the appearance of gonadotropins, is considered to be the most ancestral glycoprotein hormone. Studies are currently under way to determine whether this protein is present in the circulation and how it is regulated.

TABLE 11-6

Endogenous and Exogenous Agents That May Stimulate or Inhibit Thyrotropin Secretion

Stimulatory Agents	Inhibitory Agents
Thyrotropin-releasing hormone (TRH)	Thyroid hormones and analogues
Prostaglandins (?)	Dopamine and dopamine agonists
α-Adrenergic agonists (? via TRH)	Gastrin
Opioids (humans)	Opioids (rat)
Arginine vasopressin (AVP)	Glucocorticoids (in vivo, high dose)
Glucagon-like peptide 1 (GLP1)	Serotonin
Galanin	Cholecystokinin (CCK)
Leptin	Gastrin-releasing peptide (GRP)
Glucocorticoids (in vitro)	Vasopressin (AVP)
	Neuropeptide Y
	Interleukin 1β (IL-1β) and IL-6
	Tumor necrosis factor α
	Bexarotene (retinoid X receptor agonist)
	Phenytoin
	Somatostatin and somatostatin analogues

Iodine Deficiency

The response of vertebrates to iodine deficiency is designed to conserve this limited resource and to improve the efficiency of its utilization. The adjustments occur at the hypothalamic, pituitary, thyroid, and peripheral tissue levels. Removal of iodine from the diet causes a rapid decrease in the serum T_4 concentration and a simultaneous increase in serum TSH (Fig. 11-10).[117] No detectable decrease in T_3 occurs, suggesting that the signal to increase TSH must derive from a decrease in the T_3 generated intracellularly from T_4 in the pituitary, the hypothalamus, or both. TSH increases NIS, Tg, and TPO synthesis; iodine organification; and Tg turnover (see Fig. 11-2). Because of the decrease in iodide supply and in the ratio of DIT to MIT, the ratio of T_4 to T_3 in Tg decreases, and the rate of thyroidal T_3 secretion may increase despite a fall in T_4 secretion. TSH also stimulates cell division, leading to goiter. In the rat model, the fall in plasma T_4 increases the level of D2 from 5- to 20-fold in the CNS, hypothalamus, and pituitary, increasing the efficiency of T_4 conversion to T_3. With moderately severe iodine deficiency, D3 in the CNS is also reduced, prolonging the mean residence time of T_3 in that organ.[118] This permits serum T_3 to remain normal and the CNS T_3 to be only moderately reduced despite decreases of up to 10-fold in circulating T_4. Supporting an important role for D2 in humans is the positive association between mental retardation in an iodine-deficient region of China and two common single-nucleotide polymorphisms in the D2 gene.[119]

Despite the TSH elevation and the almost undetectable level of serum T_4 in acutely iodine-deficient rodents, growth, oxygen consumption, and thermal homeostasis can be maintained.[120] However, if iodine deficiency is prolonged and severe, hypothyroidism will supervene. In humans, these compensatory alterations in thyroid function come into operation when total iodine intake falls to

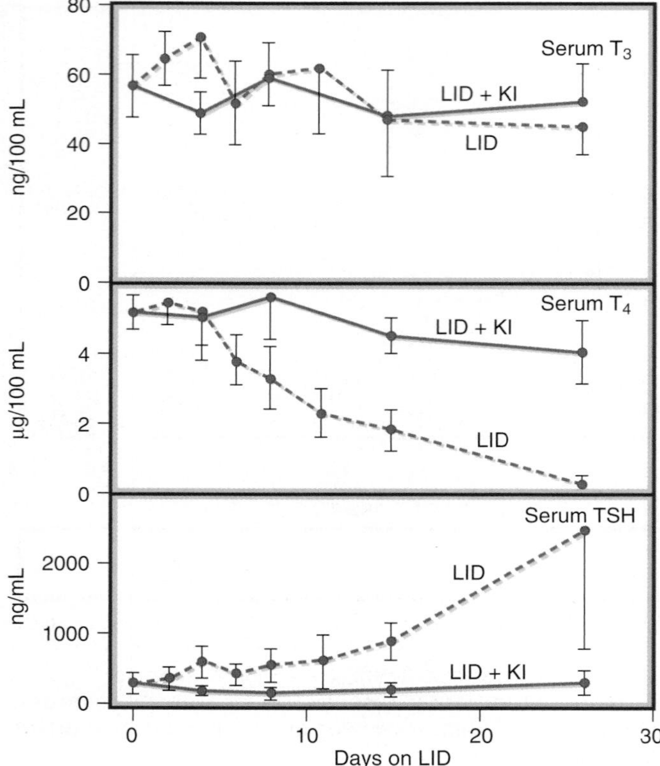

Figure 11-10 Effects of acute depletion of dietary iodine on serum levels of triiodothyronine (T_3), thyroxine (T_4), and thyroid-stimulating hormone (TSH) in rats. Animals received a low-iodine diet (LID) without or with supplementation of potassium iodide (KI) in drinking water. (From Riesco G, Taurog A, Larsen PR, et al. Acute and chronic responses to iodine deficiency in rats. *Endocrinology.* 1977;100:303-313.)

less than 75 μg/day (see Table 11-1). This situation can occur in some countries in Europe and South America and affects several hundred million individuals in China, India, Indonesia, and Africa.[121,122]

Changes in serum hormones seen in experimental animals have been well documented in humans in areas of iodine deficiency and in patients with NIS mutations.[11] However, they may not be seen in older members of the population, in whom thyroid autonomy often develops. The physiologic response to iodine deficiency is similar to that which occurs during the development of primary hypothyroidism in humans. It is also reproduced when the efficiency of iodide trapping and organification is reduced in Hashimoto's disease or in patients with Graves' disease who are receiving thiourea drugs.[22] The physiologic effects of this series of events are clear. T_3 has approximately 10 times the potency of the prohormone T_4 and contains only three iodine atoms. This results in a more efficient use of the iodine atom. Maintenance of normal circulating T_3 independent of serum T_4 concentrations should provide hormone for those tissues in which the nuclear T_3 is completely derived from the plasma, such as liver and kidney (see Fig. 11-5).

Iodine Excess

The thyroid is also protected against an excess of iodide that might otherwise lead to hyperthyroidism. As with the response to iodine deficiency, there are multiple levels of defense against this eventuality. The usual source of excess iodine is pharmaceutical, with radiographic dyes, amiodarone, and povidone-iodine being the most common sources (Table 11-7).

Effects of Increased Iodine Intake on Thyroid Hormone Synthesis

The quantity of iodine organified in Tg, which includes T_4 and T_3, displays a biphasic response to increasing doses of iodide, at first increasing and then decreasing as a result of a relative blockade of organic binding. This decreasing yield of organic iodine from increasing doses of iodide, termed the *Wolff-Chaikoff effect,* results from a high concentration of inorganic iodide within the thyroid cell.[123] Susceptibility to the Wolff-Chaikoff effect can be increased by stimulation of iodide trapping (e.g., in patients with Graves' disease) or during persistent TSH stimulation, by impairment of iodine organification in the human fetus, in patients with Hashimoto's disease, or in thyroids previously irradiated by either iodine 131 (^{131}I) or external beam radiotherapy. In such situations, goiter and hypothyroidism (iodide myxedema) can develop if excess iodide is given for long periods. The mechanism for organification inhibition may involve inhibitory effects of high iodide concentrations on TPO and DUOX2.

In normal subjects given iodide, the inhibition of iodothyronine formation is reduced over time. This escape or adaptation phenomenon occurs because iodide transport activity decreases, probably through a decrease in NIS expression. Consequently, thyroidal iodide falls to levels insufficient to maintain the full Wolff-Chaikoff effect.[12,124] Importantly, this adaptation does not occur in the third-trimester fetus. As a result, chronic high iodine intake during pregnancy must be avoided because it will cause fetal hypothyroidism and compensatory, potentially obstructive goiter (Fig. 11-11).

Effects on Thyroid Hormone Release

An important practical effect of pharmacologic doses of iodine is the prompt inhibition of thyroid hormone release. This occurs to some extent normally but is especially apparent in patients with Graves' disease or toxic nodules (see Chapter 12). The mechanism is unknown, but the effect is mediated at the level of the thyroid cell, rather

TABLE 11-7

Iodine Content of Various Iodinated Pharmaceutical Agents*

Agent	Iodine Content
Saturated solution of potassium iodide	38 mg/drop
Lugol's solution	6 mg/drop
Iodized salt (1 part KI in 10,000 parts NaCl)	760 μg/10 g
Amiodarone	75-200 mg/tablet
Iopanoate, ipodate	350 mg/tablet
Angiographic and CT dyes	400-4000 mg/dose
Povidone-iodine	10 mg/mL
Kelp tablets	150 μg/tablet
Prenatal vitamins	150 μg/tablet
Iodinated glycerol	25 mg/mL
Quantity of iodine required to suppress radioactive iodine to <2%	>30 mg/day

CT, computed tomography; KI, potassium iodide; NaCl, sodium chloride.
*Typical iodide intake in the United States is 100 to 400 μg/day.

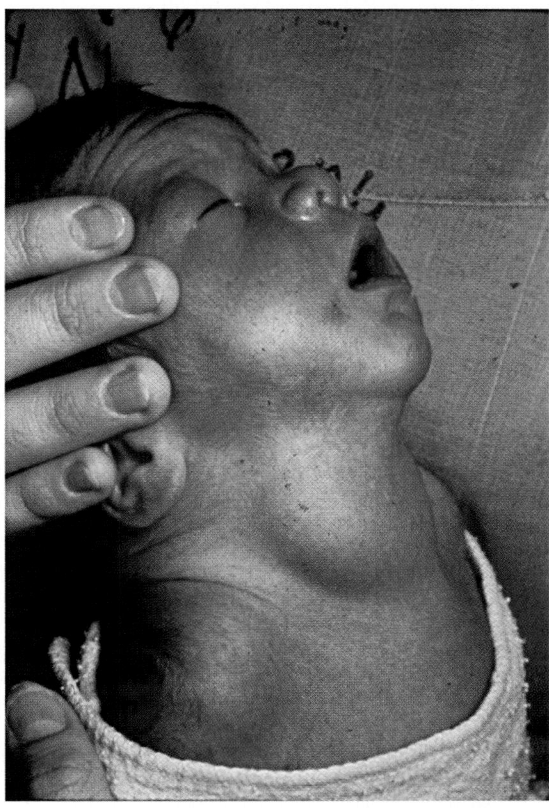

Figure 11-11 Newborn infant with iodide-induced goiter due to treatment of the mother with Lugol's solution during the third trimester. This illustrates the danger of chronic excess iodide administration during pregnancy.

than through an action on TSH. Iodine also diminishes the hypervascularity and hyperplasia that characterize the diffuse toxic goiter of Graves' disease. This effect facilitates surgical therapy for the disorder.

Thyroid Function in Pregnancy and in the Fetus and Newborn

Pregnancy affects virtually all aspects of thyroid hormone economy (Table 11-8).[5,125,126] The total serum T_4 and T_3 concentrations rise to levels about 1.5 times those of nonpregnant women owing to the increase in TBG concentration in the first trimester (Fig. 11-12). The markedly increased TBG extracellular pool must steadily be filled with increasing amounts of T_4 until a new equilibrium is reached. During normal pregnancy, the direct stimulatory effect of hCG on thyrocytes induces a small and transient increase in free T_4 levels near the end of the first trimester (peak circulating hCG), resulting in a partial TSH suppression. When tested in bioassays, normal hCG is only about 1/100 as potent as TSH. This weak thyrotropic activity explains why, in normal conditions, the effects of hCG remain largely unnoticed.[127] In addition to the increase in serum TBG, there is also an increased plasma volume as well as accelerated inactivation of T_3 and T_4 by D3 expression in the fetal-placental-uterine unit.[128] Based on the changes in requirements for levothyroxine during gestation in women with primary hypothyroidism, the estimated increase in T_4 production required during this period is 20% to 40%.

TABLE 11-8

Effects of Pregnancy on Thyroid Physiology

Physiologic Change	Thyroid-Related Consequences
↑ Serum thyroxine-binding globulin	↑ Total T_4 and T_3; ↑ T_4 production
↑ Plasma volume	↑ T_4 and T_3 pool size; ↑ T_4 production; ↑ cardiac output
D3 expression in placenta and (?) uterus	↑ T_4 production
First-trimester ↑ in hCG	↑ Free T_4; ↓ basal thyrotropin; ↑ T_4 production
↑ Renal I^- clearance	↑ Iodine requirements
↑ T_4 production; fetal T_4 synthesis during second and third trimesters	
↑ Oxygen consumption by fetoplacental unit, gravid uterus, and mother	↑ Basal metabolic rate; ↑ cardiac output

D3, type 3 iodothyronine deiodinase; I^-, plasma iodide; hCG, human chorionic gonadotropin; T_3, triiodothyronine; T_4, thyroxine.

The requirement for increased T_4 secretion increases iodine requirements during pregnancy.[129] This need is compounded by the fact that the higher glomerular filtration rate during gestation enhances renal iodide clearance, leading to higher fractional urinary excretion of circulating iodide. In addition, maternal iodine intake must be increased to supply the requirements of the fetal thyroid during the second and third trimesters (see Table 11-8). If these increased requirements for iodide are not met, serum T_4 falls and TSH rises. This series of events is well documented in areas of endemic iodine deficiency or borderline iodine supply, such as Brussels, Belgium.[5] In that city, 70% of pregnant women carefully monitored throughout pregnancy had a 20% or greater increase in thyroid volume during gestation due to increased TSH. After delivery, the

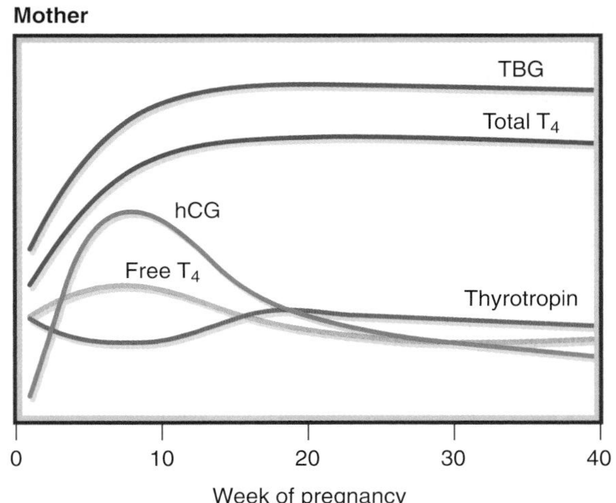

Figure 11-12 Changes in various critical components of the thyroid-pituitary axis during pregnancy. Notice the early increase in free thyroxine (T_4), which is probably a result of thyroidal stimulation by human chorionic gonadotropin (hCG), which causes a reciprocal modest suppression of serum thyroid-stimulating hormone (TSH) during the late first trimester. TBG, thyroxine-binding globulin. (From Burrow GN, Fisher DA, Larsen PR. Mechanisms of disease: maternal and fetal thyroid function. *N Engl J Med.* 1994;331:1072-1078.)

changes in thyroid function gradually return to normal, and serum TBG values reach normal levels within 6 to 8 weeks.

During pregnancy, autoimmunity is suppressed, affecting patients with Graves' or Hashimoto's disease (see Chapters 12 and 13). In general, TSHR-stimulating antibody–mediated thyroid stimulation in the patient with Graves' disease is exacerbated during the first trimester and attenuated during the second and third trimesters, only to exacerbate in the first several months after delivery. Thyroid autoantibody titers fall during gestation in patients with Hashimoto's disease, then rise sharply after delivery, in association with a phase of acute T cell–mediated thyroid cell destruction (postpartum thyroid disease), which occurs in about 30% of patients with Hashimoto's disease and significant residual thyroid tissue.[130]

The basal metabolic rate increases during the second trimester owing to the increase in the total mass of body tissue resulting from the pregnancy. The changes of pregnancy, together with the decreased peripheral vascular resistance, vasodilatation, and modest tachycardia, may suggest thyrotoxicosis (see Table 11-8). It is important to appreciate that such changes are physiologic in pregnancy, especially when managing hyperthyroidism in a pregnant patient.

Fetal Thyroid Function

The peripheral metabolism of T_4 in the human fetus differs markedly from that in the adult, both quantitatively and qualitatively. Overall, rates of production and degradation of T_4 in terms of units per body mass exceed those in the adult by 10-fold. In addition, D1 catalysis is reduced and D3 is enhanced, favoring formation of the inactive rT_3 already introduced at the expense of T_3. D3 is highly expressed in fetal tissues including the liver, skin, tracheobronchial, urothelial, and gastrointestinal epithelia.[128] This results in a persistently subnormal serum T_3 concentration and an elevated serum rT_3. This permits the highly regulatable T_4-to-T_3 conversion by D2 to be the major pathway for generating tissue T_3.[131]

Fetal thyroid function begins at about the end of the first trimester. Thereafter, there are steady increases in fetal TBG and total T_4 and T_3.[5,126] Throughout gestation, the serum TSH values are greater than those in the maternal circulation and higher than would be expected in adults with normal thyroid function. This indicates that there is increasing hypothalamic-pituitary resistance to T_4 during fetal development which is speculated to be a consequence of increased TRH secretion.[132] Despite the low circulating T_3, the fetal concentration of free T_4 approximates that in the maternal circulation from gestational age 28 weeks onward.

Maternal-Fetal Interactions

The fetal pituitary-thyroid axis functions as a unit that is essentially independent from the mother.[4,132] Transplacental passage of TSH from mother to fetus is negligible, but the same is not true of maternal T_4. In infants with congenital hypothyroidism caused by genetic TPO deficiency or by athyreosis, serum concentrations of T_4 in cord blood are usually one third to one half of normal.[28] Therefore, at least when the maternal-fetal concentration gradient is high, transfer of maternal T_4 to the fetal circulation can occur. This transfer may be significant, given the capacity of the fetal brain to increase the efficiency of T_4-to-T_3 conversion. Furthermore, T_4 can be found in coelomic and amniotic fluids before the onset of thyroid function.[133] The major factor limiting T_4 and T_3 transfer from mother to fetus is the D3 expressed in the uterus, placenta, and fetal epithelium.

Thyroid Function in the Newborn

The mean total T_4 level in cord serum is 150 nmol/L (12 μg/dL). Serum TBG concentrations are elevated, but not as high as in the maternal serum. At term, free T_4 concentrations are slightly lower than those in the mother. Cord serum T_3 concentrations are low (0.8 nmol/L or 50 ng/dL), and rT_3 and T_3SO_4 are elevated.[4,134,135] After delivery, the serum TSH level in the neonate increases rapidly to a peak at about 2 to 4 hours after birth, returning to its initial value within 48 hours.[134] Levels greater than 60 mU/L are typical. This neonatal TSH surge is thought to occur because of the rapid reduction in environmental temperature after delivery. In response, the serum T_4, T_3, and Tg concentrations increase rapidly during the first few hours after delivery and are in the hyperthyroid range within 24 hours.[136] The TSH surge doubtless contributes to the increase in serum T_3 concentration, but enhancement of extrathyroidal conversion of T_4 to T_3 by D1 or D2 is thought to be a major factor as well.[43] Adrenergic stimulation of the D2 gene and reactivation of D2 by its deubiquitination in brown adipose tissue are likely to be important contributors to this increase.[137]

Premature infants have an immature hypothalamic-pituitary-thyroid axis with low T_4, T_3, and TSH.[134,138] Serum T_4, TBG, and free T_4 all tend to correlate with gestational age. Preterm infants also have an attenuated TSH surge after delivery. In addition, when prematurity is accompanied by complications such as respiratory distress syndrome or nutritional problems, serum T_4, and especially T_3, may fall to low levels due to a combination of reduced TBG production, immaturity of the thyroid gland, suppression of the hypothalamic-pituitary axis by illness, impairment of T_4-to-T_3 conversion, and increases in D3 activity.[139,140] These changes are, in many respects, similar to those in adults with severe illness. All of these issues need to be taken into account when evaluating the thyroid status of the preterm infant, particularly given the increased prevalence of congenital hypothyroidism in this age group.[138]

Thyroid hormone production rates are higher per unit of body weight in neonatal infants and children than in adults. The daily levothyroxine requirement is about 10 μg/kg in the newborn and decreases progressively to about 1.6 μg/kg in the adult.[138]

Aging and the Thyroid

The thyroid gland undergoes several anatomic changes with age. There are reductions in the weight of the gland, in the size of follicles, and in the content of colloid. There is increased fibrosis, often with marked lymphocytic infiltration. However, these changes do not correlate with thyroid function.[141] In the healthy elderly patient, there is a normal level of free T_4, but serum T_3 may be lower, although studies of selected healthy people indicated that T_3 levels are unaffected by aging.[142] TSH may increase or decrease with age in relation to the iodine intake[143]; however, very elderly persons (≥80 years of age) may have a mild TSH decrease, suggesting the presence of an altered set point of the hypothalamic-pituitary-thyroid axis.[144] The requirement for complete levothyroxine replacement is reduced approximately 20% by the eighth decade.

TABLE 11-9

Changes in Thyroid Hormone Levels during Illness

Severity of Illness	Free T_3	Free T_4	Reverse T_3	TSH	Probable Cause
Mild	↓	N	↑	N	↓ D2, D1
Moderate	↓↓	N, ↑↓	↑↑	N, ↓	↓↓ D2, D1, ?↑ D3
Severe	↓↓↓	↓	↑	↓↓	↓↓ D2, D1, ↑D3
Recovery	↓	↓	↑	↑	?

D1 through D3, iodothyronine deiodinases; N, no change; T_3, triiodothyronine; T_4, thyroxine; TSH, thyroid-stimulating hormone.

Thyroid Function during Fasting or Illness

A number of changes take place in thyroid function during nutritional deprivation or illness. These consist of a central reduction in TSH secretion, decreased plasma T_3 levels, and decreased T_4 and T_3 binding in serum. This constellation of findings is termed the *low T_3 syndrome,* the *euthyroid sick syndrome,* or *nonthyroid illness*. The pattern of changes in circulating thyroid hormones and TSH during fasting and during illness are similar. During fasting, there is a reduction of 50% or more in serum T_3 and an increase in serum rT_3, without initial changes in serum total T_4 or free T_4 (Table 11-9).[107,145] Although the role of specific deiodinases in causing these changes has not been documented at a tissue level in humans during fasting, several lines of evidence suggest that decreases in peripheral T_4-to-T_3 conversion by D1 and D2 and reduced clearance of rT_3 by D1 do contribute to this process.

Whereas the reduction in D1- and D2-catalyzed deiodination could explain the low T_3 and high rT_3 concentrations, the inactivating enzyme, D3, was found to be present in liver and skeletal muscle of patients dying in an intensive care unit, suggesting that a D3-mediated increased catabolism also occurs as part of this process. The finding of normal T_3 plasma levels in mice with the genetic absence of both D1 and D2 enzymes suggests that thyroid by itself is able to compensate for impaired peripheral conversion to normalize serum T_3. This implies that very powerful mechanisms are in place to maintain serum T_3 levels within the normal range, except when it is not meant to be in that range—that is, during fasting or illness. In these circumstances, by a mechanism probably regulated by the hypothalamus, all compensatory mechanisms are reduced, and serum T_3 drops almost to undetectable levels.[74] Deiodination by D3 increases the generation of rT_3 from T_4 and converts T_3 to 3,3′ diiodothyronine (see Fig. 11-3), which would exaggerate the changes resulting from the decrease in outer ring deiodination. The finding that D3 null mice can develop the low T_3 syndrome suggests that D3 upregulation is not the only event occurring in this clinical state. It is not yet known whether such an increase in D3 also occurs during caloric restriction. The attenuation of TSH secretion despite a fall in serum T_3 levels during fasting was discussed earlier (see "The Hypothalamic-Pituitary-Thyroid Axis").

During fasting, basal oxygen consumption and heart rate decline, and nitrogen balance, initially negative, returns toward normal.[146] In some studies, these changes in overall metabolism are partially reversed by replacement of exogenous T_3 as fasting continues. Therefore, the decrease in T_3 during fasting (and presumably during illness) can be viewed as a beneficial energy- and nitrogen-sparing adaptation. Chronic malnutrition, such as occurs in anorexia nervosa, is also associated with a reduction in serum T_3 and, rarely, in free T_4.[147] TSH concentrations remain in the normal range, although again they are inappropriately low in the context of the reductions in circulating T_3. In contrast, overfeeding, particularly with carbohydrate, increases T_3 production rates and the serum T_3 concentration, reduces serum rT_3, and increases basal thermogenesis.[148]

During illness, decreases in T_3 and pulsatile TSH release and increases in rT_3 also occur.[149] If illness progresses, the hypothalamic-pituitary-thyroid axis is even further suppressed with a consequent reduction in the free T_4. The reduction in free T_4 corresponds to the gradual development of a more complex syndrome and worsening of clinical outcome for these patients, and a marked decrease in serum T_4 is associated with a high probability of death. This syndrome is associated with a decrease in TRH mRNA in the human paraventricular nuclei.[150] An increase in T_3 production by D2-catalyzed T_4-to-T_3 conversion in the tanycytes lining the third ventricle may contribute to the blunted response of TSH to the reduced serum T_3, particularly during infections.[151] Cytokines, such as interleukin-6, also increase during illness, coincident with the decrease in circulating T_3, although it is not clear whether this is the cause of the hypothalamic changes.[152] These endogenous changes may be further exaggerated by agents such as dopamine or glucocorticoids, which suppress the TRH-TSH axis, at least transiently.[153]

The changes in thyroid function are a continuum, with the abnormalities becoming progressively more severe in parallel with the patient's clinical condition (see Table 11-9). Mild to moderate changes are observed in patients with illnesses such as mild myocardial infarction, in those undergoing elective surgical procedures, and during infections such as pyelonephritis or pneumonia in otherwise healthy individuals. In these circumstances, the serum free T_3 is reduced by as much as 50%, and the total rT_3 concentration is increased twofold to threefold. The total serum T_4 concentration remains normal, as does TSH. During prolonged critical illness, serum free T_4 and TSH are markedly reduced, and T_3 is reduced in plasma and in tissues to barely detectable levels.[153] Postmortem studies of patients with prolonged critical illness show that hepatic D1 activity is reduced by about 50%, skeletal muscle D2 is absent, and D3 is present in liver and skeletal muscle.[154] Tissue T_3 is reduced in these individuals in parallel with the decrease in the serum hormone concentration. No differences have been found in the T_3 transporter MCT8 in skeletal muscle or liver, and possible abnormalities in other thyroid hormone transporters have not been evaluated.

The same global pattern of changes observed during acute medical illness has also been described in patients with primary hypothyroidism who are receiving levothyroxine.[155] In such patients, serum T_4, T_3, and TSH concentrations fell by about 50% over the first 3 days, presumably due to a disruption of T_4 binding resulting from decreased TBG, TTR, and albumin and to blockade of T_4-protein interactions caused by endogenous interfering substances. A contributing factor may be the translational modification of TBG caused by the serpin-catalyzed release of a C-terminal fragment of TBG in inflamed tissues (see "Thyroxine-Binding Globulin").

Therapies have been introduced to ameliorate certain of the illness-related central abnormalities in the hypothalamic-pituitary axis (including decreases in growth hormone and gonadotropins). One of these, infusions of growth hormone–releasing peptide 2 (GHRP2) combined with TRH, resulted in increases in TSH, T_3, and T_4, as well as insulin-like growth factor 1 (IGF1), insulin, and IGF binding proteins 1, 3, and 5.[156] Although the biochemical improvements were significant, the clinical state did not change. Neither T_3 nor T_4 administration improves the outcomes in sick patients, and insulin-mediated improvements in hyperglycemia have not altered the abnormalities in thyroid-related parameters in critically ill patients.[157]

Although serum TSH concentrations in severely ill patients are reduced, an increase in TSH above the normal range may appear during recovery, with the elevation in TSH concentration persisting until circulating free T_4 and T_3 levels return to normal.[158] This pattern can be confusing if the elevated TSH concentration is found in association with the still-reduced concentrations of free T4. Such patients meet all laboratory criteria for primary hypothyroidism with the exception of the clinical context. Follow-up usually reveals a normalization of TSH and T_4 within 1 to 2 months (see Table 11-9).

Despite the severity of the abnormalities, particularly in serum T_3, there is still disagreement as to whether therapeutic intervention should be initiated even in the most severely ill patients. This is because most controlled studies have not shown beneficial effects of T_4 or T_3 supplementation in such individuals.[157] The one exception is the possible beneficial effect of T_3 therapy after coronary artery bypass grafting, with one study showing a positive effect and a second showing no beneficial effect.[159,160]

The Thyroid Axis and Neuropsychiatric Illness

Patients with neuropsychiatric disease can present with any of a number of abnormalities in thyroid function. Patients with bipolar disorders may show slight elevations in serum TSH and reductions in free T_4, whereas patients with severe depression have slight elevation in serum T_4 and reduced serum TSH. Other acutely psychotic patients may have either high or low serum TSH concentrations and tend to have elevations in free T_4.[161] The etiology of these minor abnormalities is not clear, but such patients may have thyroid function test results resembling those in patients with primary thyroid disease, from whom they must be differentiated.

Effects of Hormones on Thyroid Function

Glucocorticoids

The acute administration of pharmacologic doses of glucocorticoid eliminates pulsatile release of serum TSH in normal patients, presumably by reducing TRH release. With continued administration, there is an escape from this suppression (Table 11-10). Pharmacologic doses of glucocorticoid decrease the serum T_3 concentration in normal and hyperthyroid patients, as well as in hypothyroid patients maintained on levothyroxine. The latter finding and the accompanying increase in rT_3 production suggest that glucocorticoids may increase D3 activity.[90]

Primary adrenal insufficiency may be associated with reduced serum T_4 and elevated serum TSH concentrations, suggesting the coexistence of primary hypothyroidism. However, treatment of the adrenal insufficiency can lead to complete resolution of these abnormalities, suggesting that in some patients they are a consequence of glucocorticoid deficiency rather than primary thyroid disease.[162] Nevertheless, the prevalence of primary hypothyroidism is increased in patients with autoimmune hypoadrenalism, so the two causes must be differentiated (see Chapter 15). Likewise, patients successfully treated for Cushing's disease can develop thyroid autoimmunity.

TABLE 11-10

Effects of Hormones on Thyroid Function

Glucocorticoids
Excess
Decreased TSH, TBG, TTR (high-dose)
Decreased serum T_3/T_4 ratio, increased rT_3/T_4 ratio
Increased rT_3 production (? ↑ D3)
Decreased T_4 and T_3 secretion in Graves' disease
Deficiency
Increased TSH
Estrogen
Increased TBG sialylation and increased half-life in serum
Increased TSH in postmenopausal women
Increased T_4 requirement in hypothyroid patients
Androgen
Decreased TBG
Decreased T_4 turnover in women, reduced T_4 requirement in hypothyroid patients
Growth Hormone
Decreased D3 activity

D3, type 3 deiodinase; rT_3, reverse T_3; T_3, triiodothyronine; T_4, thyroxine; TBG, thyroxine-binding globulin; TSH, thyrotropin; TTR, transthyretin.

Gonadal Steroids

Estrogen increases TBG by mechanisms already mentioned.[163] Estrogen administration to postmenopausal women causes an increase of 15% to 20% in TSH.[164] Presumably, this increases T_4 secretion, in that total T_4 increases and free T_4 is unchanged. Estrogen also increases the levothyroxine requirement in patients with primary hypothyroidism.[58] In contrast, administration of androgens to women decreases TBG and decreases T_4 turnover and levothyroxine requirements in patients with primary hypothyroidism.[165]

Growth Hormone

Growth hormone increases the serum free T_3 and decreases free T_4 in both levothyroxine-treated and normal individuals, suggesting either suppression of D3 activity or increased T_4-to-T_3 conversion.

PHYSICAL EVALUATION OF THE THYROID GLAND

Manifestations of thyroid disease are usually caused by excessive or insufficient production of thyroid hormone, local symptoms in the neck (principally goiter, but occasionally pain or compression of adjacent structures), or, in the case of Graves' disease, ophthalmopathy or dermopathy. A functional diagnosis of thyroid disease is based on a carefully taken history, a thorough search for the physical signs of hypothyroidism or thyrotoxicosis, and an appraisal of the results of laboratory tests. Although conditioned by the functional diagnosis, the anatomic diagnosis depends largely on the physical examination of the thyroid gland itself. The typical symptoms of an excess or a deficiency of thyroid hormone are discussed in Chapters 12 and 13.

Examination of the neck is best accomplished with the patient seated in good light with the neck relaxed. The patient should be provided with a cup of water to facilitate swallowing. The physician should first inspect the neck, especially while the patient swallows, with the neck slightly extended. The presence of old surgical scars, distended veins, and redness or fixation of the overlying skin should be noted. The position of the trachea should be noted. If a mass is present, a determination should be made as to whether it moves with swallowing. A midline mass high in the neck that rises further when the patient extends the tongue is typical of a thyroglossal duct remnant or cyst. Movement on swallowing is a characteristic of the thyroid gland because it is ensheathed in the pretracheal fascia; this feature distinguishes a goiter from most other neck masses. However, if the thyroid is so large that it occupies all the available space in the neck, movement on swallowing may be lost. The physician should also inspect the posterior dorsum of the tongue, which is the origin of the thyroglossal duct and the location of lingual thyroid tissue.

Except when thyroid enlargement is extreme, the thyroid examination can be readily performed with the physician facing the seated patient. The physician should use gentle pressure with his or her thumb to locate the thyroid isthmus just caudal to the cricoid cartilage. This provides a convenient starting point for palpation of the lobes of the gland, but an increase in thickness or a firm texture of the isthmus will already suggest the presence of some generalized thyroid enlargement. To examine the right lobe, the right thumb is moved laterally, without release of gentle pressure, to locate the lobe of the thyroid by pressing it against the trachea as the patient swallows sips of water. In this strategy, the palpating thumb laterally displaces the medial border of the sternocleidomastoid muscle, allowing direct access to the entire thyroid lobe. As the patient swallows with the thumb pressing the lobe against the trachea with sufficient tension to displace it slightly over the midline, the trachea will slide up and down under the ball of the thumb. This permits an appreciation of the size and texture of the gland as well as the presence or absence of nodules. A similar strategy with the left thumb is employed for the left lobe. The thyroid may also be examined with the physician standing behind the seated patient and palpating with the fingertips of both hands.

The examiner should note the shape of the gland, its size in relation to normal, and its consistency, which is usually slightly greater than adipose tissue but less than muscle. The normal thyroid lobe has approximately the same size in frontal projection as the terminal phalanx of the patient's thumb. Whereas a diffuse goiter and the hyperplastic gland in a hyperthyroid patient with Graves' disease may be softer than normal, the gland of a patient with Hashimoto's disease is usually firm. Irregularities of the surface, variations in consistency, and tender areas should be noted. If nodules are palpated, their shape, size, position, translucency, and consistency in relation to the surrounding tissue should be determined. It may seem counterintuitive, but a firm nodule is more likely to be a cyst than a malignancy. A search should be made for the pyramidal lobe; this is a thin band of tissue extending upward from the isthmus to the thyroid cartilage to the right or left of the midline. A hypertrophied pyramidal lobe may be mistaken for a pretracheal lymph node that sometimes accompanies thyroid carcinoma or thyroiditis. It is usually palpable in patients with generalized thyroid disease (e.g., Hashimoto's disease, Graves' disease). During palpation, a vascular thrill may be felt; in the absence of cardiac disease, this is suggestive of hyperthyroidism. Finally, palpation should always include examination of the regional lymph nodes along the jugular vein, posterior to the sternocleidomastoids, and in the supraclavicular region.

Auscultation of the neck may confirm the increased vascularity of an enlarged, hyperactive gland, suggesting Graves' disease. A systolic or continuous bruit is sometimes heard over a hyperplastic gland. Care should be taken to distinguish a thyroid bruit from a murmur transmitted from the base of the heart or from a venous hum that can be obliterated by gentle compression of the external jugular vein or by turning the head. A venous hum is typically found in younger patients with high cardiac output, such as occurs in Graves' disease or with severe anemia.

An arm-raising test is useful when a retrosternal goiter is suspected. The basis for this maneuver is that the size of the thoracic inlet is already reduced by such a goiter. Raising both arms until they touch the sides of the head further narrows the thoracic inlet and causes congestion and venous engorgement of the face and sometimes respiratory distress *(Pemberton's sign)* or even (rarely) syncope.

In addition to examination of the thyroid gland and regional lymph nodes, evidence of compression or displacement of adjacent structures should be sought. Hoarseness may indicate compression of the recurrent laryngeal nerve, usually by a malignant thyroid neoplasm, and this should be confirmed by laryngoscopy. Displacement of the trachea may be evident and is usually associated with a large nodule or nodules; inspiratory stridor may indicate its compression.

It is likely that an ultrasound device will become an ubiquitous instrument in the endocrinologist's office or clinic in the coming years because of its superior sensitivity for the detection of thyroid nodules. This should enhance, not replace, physical examination of the thyroid, the only endocrine gland that is accessible to physical examination.

LABORATORY ASSESSMENT OF THYROID STATUS

In considering the laboratory assessment of known or suspected thyroid disease, the physician should seek to arrive at both a functional and, when appropriate, an anatomic diagnosis. Laboratory determinations will confirm whether there is an excess, normal, or insufficient supply of thyroid hormone to verify the inferences from the clinical history and physical examination. Laboratory tests can be divided into five major categories: (1) those that assess the state of the hypothalamic-pituitary-thyroid axis; (2) estimates of T_4 and T_3 concentrations in the serum; (3) tests that reflect the impact of thyroid hormone on tissues; (4) tests for the presence of autoimmune thyroid disease; and (5) tests that provide information about thyroidal iodine metabolism. The use of iodine and other isotopes for scintiscanning is discussed in Chapter 14.

Tests of the Hypothalamic-Pituitary-Thyroid Axis

Thyroid-Stimulating Hormone

Although they represent an inherently indirect reflection of thyroid hormone supply, tests that assess the state of the hypothalamic-pituitary-thyroid axis play a critical role in the diagnosis of thyroid disease. This is because the rate of

TSH secretion is exquisitely sensitive to the plasma concentrations of free thyroid hormones, thus providing a precise and specific barometer of the thyroid status of the patient (see Figs. 11-8 and 11-9). The rare exceptions to this rule are discussed later. Immunometric assay technology now makes it possible to define the normal range for serum TSH and to ascertain when thyroid function is inadequate or the hormone supply is excessive (see Chapter 6). This assay uses the TSH molecule to link a TSH antibody bound to an inert surface (e.g., particles, the side of a test tube) to a second antibody (directed against a different TSH epitope) that is labeled with a detectable marker such as ^{125}I, an enzyme, or a chemiluminescent reagent. The signal generated is proportional to the concentration of TSH in the serum. This technique is more specific, sensitive, and rapid than radioimmunoassay.

The normal range of the serum TSH concentration by immunometric assay varies slightly in different laboratories but is most commonly 0.4 to 4.2 mU/L. There has been discussion of adopting an even lower upper limit for the normal range, but the value of 4.2 mU/L includes 96% of the disease- and risk-free population.[166,167] The lower limit of 0.4 is too high for a pregnant patient because of hCG-induced hyperthyroidism, as discussed earlier.[127] It should be kept in mind that there is a diurnal variation of TSH secretion, with peak values in the early evening and a nadir in the afternoon. A borderline abnormal value should always be repeated within a week or so to be certain that it is representative. A minimally suitable TSH assay should be able to quantitate concentrations of TSH as small as 0.1 mU/L with a coefficient of variation of less than 20%. Potential artifacts of these assays are discussed in Chapter 6.

The free α-subunit common to TSH, FSH, LH, and hCG is usually detectable in serum, with a normal range of 1 to 5 μg/L, but the TSH β-subunit is not. When FSH and LH production are increased, as in postmenopausal women, or when TSH production is increased, as in primary hypothyroidism, the free α-subunit level is also increased. The α-subunit concentration may also be increased in patients with glycoprotein-producing tumors of the anterior pituitary (see Chapter 9). Its measurement may be useful in the rare patient with hyperthyroidism and a normal or elevated TSH, to differentiate between neoplastic and non-neoplastic causes of TSH excess.[168,169]

TSH in Patients with Thyroid Dysfunction

Patients with hyperthyroidism (excess thyroid hormone secretion) or thyrotoxicosis (excess thyroid hormone from any cause), or both, will virtually always have a subnormal level of TSH. The values fall into two general categories: those between the lower limit of normal and 0.1 mU/L, and those lower than 0.1 mU/L. Individuals in the former category are often asymptomatic *(subclinical hyperthyroidism),* whereas those in the latter group usually have symptomatic thyrotoxicosis and a significant elevation in free T_4.

Patients with hypothalamic or pituitary hypothyroidism often have normal or even slightly elevated serum TSH values. The circulating TSH typically has reduced biologic activity due to abnormal glycosylation, reflecting the impaired access of TRH to the thyrotroph.[105,106] Patients with primary hypothyroidism have serum TSH concentrations that range from minimally elevated to 1000 mU/L. In general, the degree of TSH elevation correlates with the clinical severity of the hypothyroidism. Patients with serum TSH values in the range of 5 to 15 mU/L have few, if any, symptoms; the serum free T_4 or free T_4 index (FT_4I) is typically low-normal, whereas the serum free T_3 concentration is normal. Such individuals with modest TSH elevation are said to have *subclinical hypothyroidism* if the serum free T_4 is in the normal range. These findings indicate minor thyroidal failure with a compensatory increase in TSH secretion.

A detailed discussion of the various conditions associated with abnormal serum TSH concentrations is presented later. Elevation in both serum TSH and free T_4 is unusual and indicates either autonomous TSH production, as with a TSH-secreting pituitary tumor; resistance to thyroid hormone; or hyperthyroidism with an artifactual elevation in TSH. Differentiating among these diagnoses may require magnetic resonance imaging (MRI) of the hypothalamic-pituitary region or consultation with the clinical chemistry laboratory to rule out an assay artifact (see Chapter 6).

QUANTITATION OF SERUM THYROID HORMONE CONCENTRATIONS

Total T_4 and T_3

Quantitation of the circulating thyroid hormone concentrations is essential to confirm that the thyroid status abnormality suggested by an abnormal TSH result is accurate and to document its severity. Sensitive and specific radioimmunoassays are available for measuring the total concentrations of T_4 and T_3 and some of their metabolic byproducts (see Chapter 6). Because the thyroid status correlates with the free, rather than the total, hormone concentration, the physician must also obtain some estimate of free hormone (see later discussion). The degree of abnormality in the free T_4 level generally correlates with the severity of the hormone excess or deficiency, whereas the serum TSH concentration is an indication of the impact of this abnormality in that specific patient. The normal range for total T_4 in healthy, euthyroid adults with a normal circulating TBG concentration is 64 to 142 nmol/L (5 to 11 μg/dL). Normal serum T_3 concentrations are 1.1 to 2.9 nmol/L (70 to 190 ng/dL). At birth (cord serum), T_3 concentrations are about 50% of those in normal adults, but within a few hours T_3 rises abruptly, peaking within about 24 hours at concentrations in the low thyrotoxic range for adults.

Radioimmunoassays for rT_3, T_3SO_4, triac, tetrac, and the diiodothyronines are of primary interest in the research setting, because these iodothyronines are derived from the circulating T_4 or T_3, both of which can be easily quantitated. An exception may be the so-called compound W, an as yet unidentified product of T_4 metabolism in the fetal circulation that appears in maternal sera.[86] If validated, measurements of compound W could serve as a much-needed index of the effects of maternal antithyroid drug therapy on fetal thyroid function.

Concentrations of Free T_4 and T_3

The most accurate and direct measurements of the concentrations of free T_4 and free T_3 in serum are performed by assay of these hormones in a dialysate or ultrafiltrate of serum. This is not practical for clinical purposes, and alternative strategies have been developed to estimate free thyroid hormone concentrations. In one method, serum is enriched with tracer amounts of the labeled hormone, and the concentration of the isotope in the dialysate or ultrafiltrate is expressed as a fraction of that in undiluted serum. The absolute concentration of free hormone is the product of the total hormone concentration and the fraction that is dialyzable or ultrafiltrable. About 0.02% of T_4 and 0.3% of T_3 is free or unbound (see Table 11-5). The normal ranges for free T_4 is 9 to 30 pmol/L (0.7 to 2.5 ng/dL), and for free T_3 is 3 to 8 pmol/L (0.2 to 0.5 ng/dL).

Because T_4 is the major secretory product of the thyroid and correlates most closely with the serum TSH, in most situations a free T_4 estimate is all that is required to ascertain the state of thyroid secretion or supply. An array of methods is used to quantitate free T_4 (or T_3) in whole serum using automated methods. Even though many such automated tests imply that they quantitate free T_4 directly, they do not, and in general the results in sera with abnormal binding proteins are not absolute.[170] There are two categories of methods: comparative free T_4 methods and FT_4I methods. Three general approaches are used: (1) two-step labeled hormone methods, (2) one-step labeled analogue methods, and (3) labeled antibody approaches (see Chapter 6). The two-step labeled hormone back-titration methods are less subject to artifacts caused by abnormal binding proteins, changes in albumin, TBG, or increased free fatty acids, compared with the one-step hormone analogue methods.[171,172] All of the approaches are subject to artifacts from endogenous antibodies to T_4, abnormal binding proteins, or illness.[170,173] Therefore, the clinician must be wary if the free T_4 result obtained by any method does not agree with the clinical state and the TSH. In such cases, another method should be used to estimate the free T_4, the FT_4I should be measured, or the result should be ignored. For pregnant or severely ill patients, the automated methods typically give falsely low results, particularly if one-step procedures are used. A reasonable alternative for pregnancy is to multiply the normal range for the serum T_4 concentration by 1.5 in lieu of an automated free T_4 assay.[125,174]

The Free T_4 Index

It is particularly useful in estimating the free T_4 in severely ill patients to determine the thyroid hormone–binding ratio (THBR) and multiply that result by the total T_4 (or T_3) to obtain a free hormone index (FT_4I or FT_3I). In this test, a tracer quantity of labeled T_4 (or T_3) is added to serum, which is then exposed to a solid phase matrix coated with T_4 or T_3 antibody or to an inert matrix that binds the iodothyronine irreversibly. The proportion of labeled T_4 or T_3 bound by the solid phase is then quantitated. This value, like the free fraction of T_4 quantitated directly in a dialysate, varies inversely with the concentration of unoccupied TBG sites in the serum. If tracer T_3 is used, its binding to TBG is determined by the ratio of T_4 (not T_3) to TBG. T_4 is present in 50- to 60-fold higher concentrations than T_3, has a much higher affinity for TBG than does T_3, and therefore determines the ratio of unoccupied to occupied TBG.

The results of such assays are normalized by comparing them with results obtained simultaneously for standard control sera with normal TBG and serum T_4 concentrations. This is usually done by dividing the result for the unknown sample by that obtained for control sera in the same assay. The quotient is the THBR, which typically has a normal range of 0.85 to 1.10. Because the THBR is proportional to the free fraction of the endogenous thyroid hormones in the serum, it can be multiplied by the total T_4 (or T_3) concentration to estimate the free thyroid hormone concentration, termed the FT_4I or FT_3I. Because the normal THBR is 1.0, the FT_4I has a normal range in units that is identical to that of the total T_4 (or T_3)—for example, 64 to 142 in SI units and 5 to 11 in gravimetric terms. A schematic demonstration of the relationships among total and free T_4, occupied and unoccupied TBG binding sites, and the THBR is shown in Figure 11-13 for

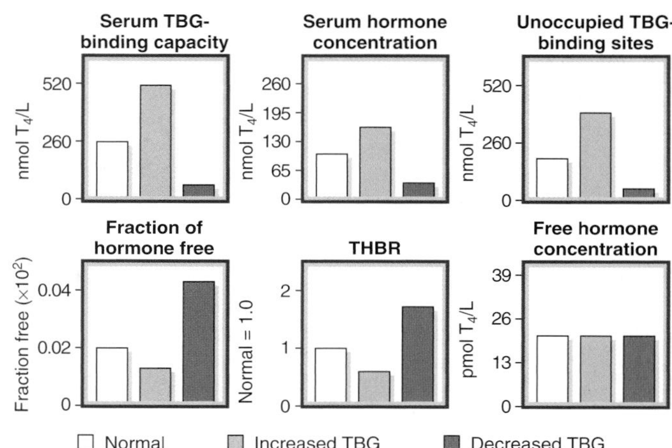

Figure 11-13 Patterns of changes in total serum thyroxine (T_4) concentration and thyroid hormone–binding ratio (THBR) in euthyroid patients with alterations in the circulating concentrations of thyroxine-binding globulin (TBG). To convert T_4 from nmol/L to µg/dL (total) or pmol/L (free), divide by 12.87.

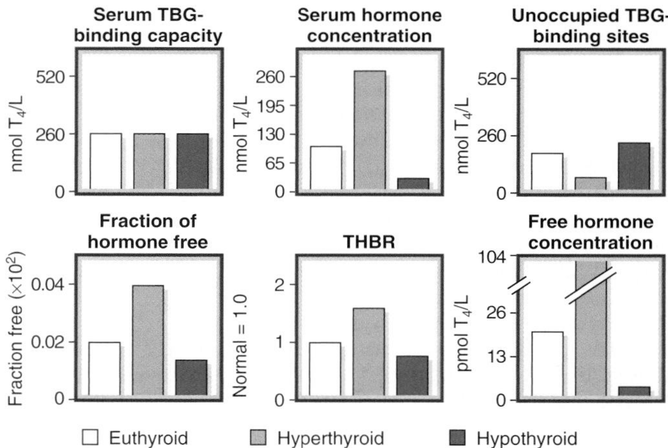

Figure 11-14 Patterns of changes in total serum thyroxine (T_4) concentration and thyroid hormone–binding ratio (THBR) in patients with hyperthyroidism or hypothyroidism with normal concentrations of serum thyroxine-binding globulin (TBG).

euthyroid individuals with variations in TBG concentrations and in Figure 11-14 for subjects with a constant TBG and alterations in serum thyroid hormone production rates.

Estrogen, pregnancy, and severe illness are more common causes of changes in total T_4 than are hyperthyroidism and hypothyroidism (Table 11-11). In the euthyroid person, only about one third of the available binding sites on TBG are occupied by T_4, and the free T_4 fraction is 2×10^{-4} of the total. During pregnancy, the TBG binding capacity, the serum T_4, and the number of unoccupied TBG binding sites approximately double, leading to an approximately 50% reduction in the free T_4 fraction. This is reflected in a reduced THBR. If the reduced THBR (or free fraction) is multiplied by the increased total T_4, the FT_4I estimate will be found to be normal, an accurate reflection of the free T_4 concentration. In patients in whom the serum T_4 concentration is reduced owing to a low TBG, the concentration of unoccupied binding sites is reduced to an

TABLE 11-11

Circumstances Associated with Altered Binding of Thyroxine by Thyroxine-Binding Globulin

Increased Binding	Decreased Binding
Pregnancy	Androgens
Neonatal state	Large doses of glucocorticoids
Estrogens and hyperestrogenemic states	Active acromegaly
Tamoxifen	Nephrotic syndrome
Oral contraceptives	Major systemic illness
Acute intermittent porphyria	Genetic factors
Infectious and chronic active hepatitis	Asparaginase
Biliary cirrhosis	
Genetic factors	
Perphenazine	
Human immunodeficiency virus infection	

even greater extent. This reduction leads to an increase in the free T_4 (and T_3) fractions and the THBR, and both the free T_4 and the FT_4I remain in the normal range.

There is one caution when calculating the FT_4I using the product of the total T_4 and the THBR. The THBR is not linearly related to the free fraction of thyroid hormones at the extremes of its range. Therefore, it is important to consider both the calculated FT_4I and the pattern of the deviations of total hormone and THBR from normal to derive the maximum information. When concentrations of TBG are altered, the deviation of the total T_4 measurement from normal is in the opposite direction to that of the THBR (see Fig. 11-13, central panels). On the other hand, when the T_4 level is elevated due to increased T_4 secretion or overreplacement, the concentration of unoccupied TBG binding sites is reduced, and both the free fraction and the total T_4 are altered in the same direction (see Fig. 11-14). In hypothyroidism, these changes are both in the opposite direction, although of lower magnitude. The reduced FT_4I of hypothyroidism is caused predominantly by the decrease in T_4 rather than a decrease in its free fraction.

Simultaneous abnormalities in both TBG and thyroid hormone production may also occur. Hyperthyroidism should be suspected in a pregnant patient if the T_4 concentration is very high and the THBR is not subnormal. Likewise, a serum T_4 concentration in the lower normal range for a nonpregnant individual, accompanied by a significant reduction in the THBR, indicates hypothyroidism. For pregnant patients, the best strategy may be to use the normal range of total T_4 for the assay being used, multiplied by 1.5.

Several caveats should be kept in mind when interpreting the results of these tests. The use of labeled T_3 in some assays can produce difficulties in three situations: in cases of familial dysalbuminemic hyperthyroxinemia; in the presence of endogenous antibodies directed against T_3; and in sick patients, as discussed earlier. In cases of familial dysalbuminemic hyperthyroxinemia, the abnormal albumin binds T_4, but not T_3, with increased avidity. Therefore, these patients have an elevated total T_4 and a reduced free fraction of T_4, but not of T_3.[56]

An alternative approach to assessing the FT_4I is to measure TBG by saturation analysis or radioimmunoassay. Normal concentrations of TBG on radioimmunoassay are about 270 nmol/L (1.0 to 1.5 mg/dL); levels are only slightly higher in women than in men. However, it should be recalled (see earlier discussion) that the elastase released from leukocytes during infection may reduce the binding affinity of TBG for T_4 (and T_3) but does not change its immunoreactivity or its binding capacity.[175] In such patients, the gravimetric TBG concentration is not paralleled by its binding affinity for T_4 or T_3. With this proviso, the serum TBG concentration result can be employed in one of two ways. First, normalization of the T_4/TBG (or T_3/TBG) ratio yields values that correlate reasonably well with the FT_4I or FT_3I. Second, an FT_4I can be derived from the concentrations of TBG and total T_4 and the association constant for the interaction between the two. In most instances, values calculated in this manner correlate with the FT_4I determined by other techniques, although the T_4/TBG ratio suggests a subnormal FT_4I in some euthyroid patients who have an elevated TBG.[172]

Causes of Abnormal TSH or Thyroid Hormone Concentrations

Several causes of an abnormal TSH should be considered by the clinician (Table 11-12). The clinical status and free T_4 or FT_4I results allow assignment of the etiology. Assay of the FT_3I is rarely required but is included here for completeness.

Causes of a Suppressed TSH. The most common cause of a reduction in serum TSH is an excess supply of thyroid hormone resulting from either increased endogenous thyroid hormone production or excessive exogenous thyroid hormone. Because the concentration of TSH is inversely proportional to the degree of thyroid hormone excess, patients with clinical symptoms almost invariably have serum TSH concentrations lower than 0.1 mU/L. Such patients almost always have an increase in the serum free T_4. In rare patients with low iodine intake and clinical thyrotoxicosis, the FT_4I is only high-normal despite a suppressed TSH. An FT_3I is required in those patients to establish a diagnosis of T_3 thyrotoxicosis. If the thyroid hormone supply is only slightly in excess of the requirement for that patient, serum TSH is suppressed, but clinical manifestations are subtle or absent and the FT_4I (and FT_3I) are in the high-normal range. Such minimal changes can occur with "euthyroid" Graves' disease, autonomous thyroid hormone–producing adenomas, multinodular goiters, subacute or painless thyroiditis, and the ingestion of an amount of exogenous thyroid hormone slightly greater than that required for metabolic needs. This condition is termed *subclinical hyperthyroidism*.

The hypothalamic-pituitary axis may remain suppressed for up to 3 months after complete resolution of the thyrotoxic state.[176] The best test for assessing the physiologic state in such patients is the free T_4 or FT_4I. A common scenario for this pattern is during follow-up of patients receiving antithyroid drugs or ^{131}I for Graves' disease. With time, the TSH feedback regulatory loop normalizes and TSH secretion returns and becomes appropriate for the circulating free thyroid hormone concentration.

In patients with severe illnesses, with or without dopamine infusion or excess glucocorticoid, TSH is suppressed, making assessment of thyroid functional status difficult (see earlier discussion). Because the FT_4I may also be reduced in such patients, astute clinical judgment is required to assign thyroid status.

Because hCG can activate the TSHR, the TSH concentration is often suppressed in conditions in which hCG is elevated, such as in the first trimester of pregnancy, with twin pregnancies, during severe *hyperemesis gravidarum*, and in patients with hydatidiform mole or choriocarcinoma.[127] TSH returns to normal in the second and third

TABLE 11-12

Thyroid Status and Free Thyroid Hormone Levels in Clinical States Associated with Abnormal Serum Thyrotropin (TSH) Concentrations*

	Expected TSH (mU/L)	Clinical Thyroid Status	Free T_4 Index	Free T_3 Index
Thyrotropin Reduced				
Hyperthyroidism of any cause	<0.1	↑	↑	↑
"Euthyroid" Graves' disease	0.2-0.5	N, (↑)	N	N, (↑)
Autonomous nodule or multinodular goiter	0.2-0.5	N, (↑)	N	↑
Exogenous thyroid hormone excess	<0.1-0.5	N, ↑	N, ↑	↑
Thyroiditis (subacute or painless)	<0.1-0.5	N, ↑	N, ↑	↑, (N)
Recent thyrotoxicosis due to any cause	<0.1-0.5	↑, N, ↓	N, ↓	N, ↓
Illness with or without dopamine infusion	<0.1-5.0	N	↑, N, ↓	↓
First trimester of pregnancy	0.2-0.5	N, (↑)	N, (↑)	↑
Hyperemesis gravidarum	0.2-0.5	N, (↑)	↑, (N)	↑
Hydatidiform mole	0.1-0.4	↑	↑	↑
Acute psychosis or depression (rare)	0.4-10	N	N, (↑)	N, (↓ or ↑)
Elderly (small fraction)	0.2-0.5	N	N	N
Glucocorticoids (acute, high dose)	0.1-0.5	N	N	↓
Congenital TSH deficiency				
Pit-1 deficiency	0	↓	↓	↓
CAGYC mutant	0	↓	↓	↓
Thyrotropin Elevated				
Primary hypothyroidism	6-500	↓	↓	N, ↓
Recovery from severe illness	5-30	N, (?)	N, ↓	N, ↓
Iodine deficiency	6-150	N, ↓	↓	N
Thyroid hormone resistance	1-20	↑, N, ↓	↑	↑
Thyrotroph tumor	0.5-50	↑	↑	↑
Hypothalamic-pituitary disease	1-20	↓	↓	N, ↓
Psychiatric illnesses	0.4-10	N	N	N, ↓
Adrenal insufficiency	5-30	N	N	N, ↓
Artifact (endogenous antimouse γ-globulin antibodies)	10-500	N	N	N

*Arrows indicate the nature of the abnormality in the T_4 or T_3 index. Parentheses indicate that such a result is unusual but may occur.

trimesters in the euthyroid patient. A persistently suppressed TSH (<0.1 mU/L) in a pregnant patient after the first trimester suggests that the hyperthyroidism is caused by autonomous thyroid function.

Changes in thyroid test results in patients with psychosis or depression, in the geriatric population, and with the use of long-term glucocorticoids were discussed earlier.

If the serum TSH is suppressed and the serum free T_4 is low, ingestion of liothyronine (triiodothyronine) should be suspected. Desiccated thyroid also has a high T_3/T_4 ratio and, if given in excess, may cause a similar abnormality.[177]

Causes of an Elevated TSH. Elevated TSH values almost always imply a reduction in the supply of T_4 or T_3, which may be permanent or transient. Primary hypothyroidism is by far the most common explanation. Other causes include acute illness (e.g., renal insufficiency[178]) and the asynchronous return of the hypothalamic-pituitary and thyroid axes to normal as patients recover from critical illness.[179] Iodine deficiency is the most common cause of an elevation in TSH worldwide, but this is not the case in North America. The rare patient with resistance to thyroid hormone may be clinically hyperthyroid, euthyroid, or hypothyroid. The most common laboratory pattern is a serum TSH that is normal in absolute terms but inappropriately high for the elevated free T_4. Individuals with a more marked "pituitary" than "general" resistance to thyroid hormone (sometimes termed pituitary resistance to thyroid hormone or PRTH) have symptoms suggesting hyperthyroidism, an elevated FT_4I, and a normal or even elevated serum TSH.[180,181] They must be differentiated from patients with a thyrotroph tumor in whom the persistent secretion of TSH causes hyperthyroidism (see Chapters 9 and 12).[168]

Patients with hypothalamic-pituitary dysfunction may have clinical and chemical hypothyroidism but low, normal, or even elevated serum TSH concentrations. The explanation for this paradox is that the biologic effectiveness of the circulating TSH is impaired due to abnormal glycosylation secondary to reduced TRH stimulation of the thyrotrophs. Nonetheless, the abnormal TSH is a suitable antigen in the immunometric assay. In adrenal insufficiency, TSH may be modestly elevated but returns to normal with glucocorticoid replacement.[162] This may reflect glucocorticoid-mediated amelioration of Hashimoto's thyroiditis.

Despite the utility and general efficacy of the serum TSH measurement alone as a screening tool for identifying patients with thyroid dysfunction, a patient should not receive treatment for this dysfunction solely on the basis of an abnormal TSH. The TSH assay is an indirect reflection of thyroid hormone supply and does not, by itself, permit a conclusive diagnosis of a specific disorder of thyroid hormone production. Accordingly, the TSH abnormality must be confirmed and an alteration in thyroid hormone concentrations verified before treatment is initiated.

Tests That Assess the Metabolic Impact of Thyroid Hormones

Abnormalities in the supply of thyroid hormone to peripheral tissues are associated with alterations in a number of metabolic processes that can be quantitated. Some of these may be useful in rare patients in whom serum TSH is not an accurate barometer of thyroid status, such as those with resistance to thyroid hormone. These tests may be the sole means of evaluating the metabolic response of the peripheral tissues to thyroid hormones in such patients.

Basal Metabolic Rate. Thyroid hormones increase energy expenditure and heat production, as manifested by weight loss, increased caloric requirement, and heat intolerance. Because it is impractical to measure heat production directly, the based metabolic rate (BMR) measures oxygen consumption under specified conditions of fasting, rest, and tranquil surroundings. Under these conditions, the energy equivalent of 1 L of oxygen is 4.83 kcal.

Under basal conditions, energy expenditure in visceral organs (including the liver, kidneys, and heart) accounts for approximately 25% of oxygen consumption; that in the brain for 25%; respiratory activity for 10%; and skeletal muscle activity for the remainder. Because energy expenditure is related to functioning tissue mass, oxygen consumption is related to some index thereof, most often body surface area. Calculated in this way, basal oxygen consumption (resting energy expenditure) is higher in men than in women, and it declines rapidly from infancy to the third decade and more slowly thereafter. Values in patients, calculated as a percentage of established normal mean for gender and age, typically range from −15% to +5%. In severely hypothyroid patients, values may be as low as −40%, and in thyrotoxic patients they may reach +25% to +50%. Abnormal (usually elevated) values are seen during recovery in burn patients and in systemic disorders such as febrile illnesses, pheochromocytoma, myeloproliferative disorders, anxiety, and disorders associated with involuntary muscular activity. Resting energy expenditure correlates very well with the free T_4 and TSH levels in hypothyroid patients given varying doses of exogenous levothyroxine.[182]

Biochemical Markers of Altered Thyroid Status. Occasionally, a diagnosis of thyroid dysfunction is first suspected because of an abnormality in a laboratory result performed during an evaluation for an unrelated medical problem. Classic examples are a markedly elevated creatine kinase MM isoenzyme or low-density lipoprotein (LDL) cholesterol leading to the recognition of hypothyroidism.[183] Other similar markers are listed in Table 11-13. These tests are not useful in the diagnosis of thyroid disease, but some, such as sex hormone–binding globulin, ferritin, or LDL cholesterol, have been used as end points in clinical studies of the responsivity of the liver to thyroid hormone in patients with thyroid hormone resistance.

TABLE 11-13

Biochemical Markers of Thyroid Status

Thyrotoxicosis
Increased
Osteocalcin
Urine pyridinium collagen cross-links
Alkaline phosphatase (bone or liver)
Atrial natriuretic hormone
Sex hormone-binding globulin
Ferritin
von Willebrand's factor
Decreased
Low-density-lipoprotein cholesterol
Lipoprotein(a)
Hypothyroidism
Increased
Creatine kinase (MM isoform)
Low-density-lipoprotein cholesterol
Lipoprotein(a)
Plasma norepinephrine
Decreased
Vasopressin

Serum Thyroglobulin

The functional sensitivity of most Tg assays is 1 ng/mL or less.[184] The results can be artifactually altered by serum anti-Tg antibodies (Tg-Ab), and serum should be screened for Tg-Ab with a sensitive immunoassay. In immunoradiometric assays, interferences lead to underestimations of Tg or false-negative values.

Tg is normally present in the serum, the concentration ranging up to 90 pmol/L (50 ng/mL); mean normal values vary with the assay used but are on the order of 30 pmol/L (20 ng/mL).[185] Concentrations are somewhat higher in women than in men and are several-fold elevated in pregnant women and newborns. Levels are elevated in three types of thyroid disorders: goiter and thyroid hyperfunction, inflammatory or physical injury to the thyroid, and differentiated follicular cell–derived thyroid tumors. Values are elevated in both endemic and sporadic nontoxic goiter, and the degree of elevation correlates with thyroid size. Transient elevations occur in patients with subacute thyroiditis and as a result of trauma to the gland during thyroid surgery or after ^{131}I therapy. Subnormal or undetectable concentrations are found in patients with thyrotoxicosis factitia and aid in differentiating this disorder from other causes of thyrotoxicosis with a low thyroid radioiodine uptake (RAIU).

A major clinical value of measuring the level of serum Tg is in the management, but not in the diagnosis, of differentiated thyroid carcinoma.[184,186] Serum Tg concentrations are increased in both benign and differentiated malignant follicular cell–derived tumors of the thyroid and do not serve to distinguish between the two. After total thyroid ablation for papillary or follicular thyroid carcinoma, Tg should not be detectable, and its subsequent appearance signifies the presence of persistent disease.[186] The serum Tg level is related to the volume of neoplastic tissue and may be undetectable in patients with small lymph node metastases that can be detected on neck ultrasonography (see Chapter 14). Secretion of Tg is TSH dependent. Therefore, the serum Tg level may rise when suppressive therapy is withdrawn or after injections of recombinant human TSH, which increases the sensitivity of the marker for detection of persistent or recurrent thyroid carcinoma, even when ^{131}I scans are negative (see Chapter 14). Supersensitive assays of Tg with a functional sensitivity of less than 0.1 ng/mL improve the sensitivity

TABLE 11-14

Prevalence of Thyroid Autoantibodies (Ab)

Group	TSHR-Ab (%)	hTg-Ab (%)	hTPO-Ab (%)
General population	0	5-20	8-27
Graves' disease	80-95	50-70	50-80
Autoimmune thyroiditis	10-20	80-90	90-100
Relatives of patients	0	40-50	40-50
Patients with IDDM	0	40	40
Pregnant women	0	14	14

IDDM, insulin-dependent diabetes mellitus; hTg-Ab, human thyroglobulin antibody; hTPO-Ab, human thyroid peroxidase antibody; TSHR-Ab, thyroid-stimulating hormone receptor antibody.

during thyroid hormone treatment but at the expense of a decreased specificity.[187,188] Whether the use of these modern assays will allow one to avoid TSH stimulation in the follow-up of some thyroid cancer patients needs further studies. In the hypothyroid newborn, serum Tg is undetectable in patients with thyroid agenesis and is usually elevated in those with ectopic thyroid tissue or goiter.

Tests for Thyroid Autoantibodies

Graves' disease and Hashimoto's thyroiditis are well-characterized and interrelated *autoimmune thyroid disorders* with a variety of clinical manifestations. The diagnostic hallmark of the autoimmune thyroid disorders is the presence, in most patients, of circulating antibodies and reactive T cells against one or another thyroid antigen.[189] Three varieties of thyroid autoantibodies are in common use and widely available in clinical diagnostic laboratories (Table 11-14). In this section, antibodies to Tg and TPO are discussed. Antibodies directed against the TSHR, the cause of hyperthyroidism in patients with Graves' disease, are covered in detail in Chapter 12.

Autoantibodies to Thyroid Peroxidase and Thyroglobulin

Modern assay techniques for thyroid autoantibodies have good precision because they depend on direct measurement of the interaction between autoantibody and autoantigen (i.e., the interaction between labeled thyroid antigen and the patient's serum). In general, the more sensitive an assay, the more precise and antigen-specific it is. However, many euthyroid individuals exhibit low levels of autoantibodies; in this situation, the specificity of the more sensitive tests is reduced and the absolute concentration becomes more important. The higher the concentration of autoantibody, the greater the clinical specificity (see Table 11-14).[190]

So that comparisons of thyroid antibody concentrations can be made from one office visit to the next, among different patients, and among laboratories, assays for thyroid autoantibodies have been standardized, with results expressed as standard units per milliliter. Of course, the actual standard serum preparation cannot be included in every assay. Instead, a serum pool is usually compared and normalized to the original standard. Nevertheless, autoantibodies differ considerably in their affinity and epitope recognition of antigen. As a result, despite this attempt at standardization, assay results from different commercial assays may still vary considerably. Hence, when monitoring antibody titers (e.g., after the treatment of thyroid cancer), it is important to use the same autoantibody assay consistently.

Do Thyroglobulin and Thyroid Peroxidase Antibodies Have a Pathogenic Role?

Tg-Ab and TPO autoantibodies (TPO-Ab) appear to be a secondary response to thyroid injury and are not thought to cause disease themselves, although they may contribute to its development and chronicity. Both types of antibodies are polyclonal, and although they are of the immunoglobulin G class, they are not restricted to one particular immunoglobulin G subclass. Polyclonality mitigates against a primary role in disease pathogenesis.[191,192] For example, these thyroid antibodies cannot transfer disease from mother to fetus or between animals even though they can pass across the placenta. Both antibodies may contribute to disease mechanisms, however. For example, TPO-Ab on the surface of B cells may be involved in antigen presentation, thus activating thyroid-specific T cells.[193] Others may have complement-fixing cytotoxic activity. TPO-Ab, in particular, correlate well with thyroidal damage and lymphocytic infiltration.

Thyroid Autoantibodies in Hashimoto's Thyroiditis and Graves' Disease

The disease most widely associated with Tg-Ab and TPO-Ab is *autoimmune thyroiditis,* or Hashimoto's disease (terms that embrace both goitrous thyroiditis, as first described by Hashimoto, and atrophic thyroid failure, previously referred to as *primary myxedema*). Both Tg-Ab and TPO-Ab are found in almost 100% of such patients, but TPO-Ab has higher affinity and occurs in higher concentrations, so testing for TPO-Ab is the best choice if only a single test is ordered.

Tg-Ab and TPO-Ab are also detectable in 50% to 90% of patients with Graves' disease, indicative of the associated thyroiditis that is evident histologically as a heterogeneous lymphocytic infiltration. Although the presence of such autoantibodies favors an autoimmune cause for the hyperthyroidism over other causes, the tests are neither sensitive nor specific in this setting and are interpretable only as part of the clinical scenario. Testing for TSHR antibodies remains the test of choice in such patients.

Thyroid Autoantibodies in Nonautoimmune Thyroid Disorders

Tg-Ab and TPO-Ab are more common in patients with sporadic goiter, multinodular goiter, or isolated thyroid nodules and cancer than in the general population. This finding usually represents an associated thyroiditis on histologic examination. Low levels of thyroid autoantibodies may occur transiently in patients with subacute (de Quervain's) thyroiditis but correlate poorly with disease course and are probably a nonspecific response to thyroid injury. There is also a higher prevalence of thyroid autoantibodies in other autoimmune diseases, particularly insulin-dependent diabetes mellitus.

The "Normal" Population

Although the prevalence of thyroid autoantibodies depends on the technique used for detection, Tg-Ab and TPO-Ab are common in the general population (see Table 11-14). At all ages, these antibodies are almost five times more common in women than in men.[190] Selected groups at risk include younger women and relatives of patients with an autoimmune thyroid disorder, in whom the incidence is higher.

The low levels of TPO-Ab and Tg-Ab found in many individuals are of uncertain significance in the presence of normal thyroid function; however, they remain a significant risk factor in families with autoimmune thyroid disorders.[194]

Radioiodine Uptake

The only direct test of thyroid function employs a radioactive isotope of iodine as a tag for the body's stable form of iodine, ^{127}I. Most often, the test involves measurement of the fractional uptake by the thyroid of a tracer (chemically inconsequential) dose of radioiodine. However, several factors make this test less frequently used than in the past, including improvements in indirect methods for assessing thyroid status. The normal values for thyroid RAIU have decreased consequent to the widespread increase in daily dietary iodine intake, and this has also reduced the utility of the test in the diagnosis of thyroid disorders.

^{131}I (half-life, 8.1 days) and ^{123}I (half-life, 0.55 day) emit gamma radiation, which permits their external detection and quantitation at sites of accumulation, such as the thyroid. These isotopes (abbreviated I* hereafter) are physiologically indistinguishable, not only from one another but also from the naturally occurring ^{127}I, permitting their use as valid tracers. The shorter half-life of ^{123}I is preferable because the radiation delivered to the thyroid per amount of administered ^{123}I is only about 1% of that delivered by ^{131}I.

Physiologic Basis

When tracer quantities of inorganic radioiodine are administered orally or intravenously, the isotope quickly mixes with the endogenous stable iodide in the extracellular fluid and begins to be removed at the two major sites of clearance, the thyroid and the kidneys. As this process continues, the plasma level of tracer iodide I* decreases exponentially. Low levels are reached by 24 hours, and inorganic I* is virtually undetectable in the plasma 72 hours after its administration. The thyroid content of I* increases rapidly during the early hours, then at a decreasing rate until a plateau is approached. The proportion of administered I* ultimately accumulated by the thyroid is a function of the clearance of iodide by the thyroid and kidneys. The relation is simply expressed as follows:

$$\text{RAIU at plateau} = \frac{C_T}{C_T + C_K}$$

where C_T represents the thyroid iodide clearance rate and C_K is the renal iodide clearance rate. The normal thyroid iodide clearance rate is approximately 0.4 L/hour, and the renal rate is 2.0 L/hour, so uptake of I* normally approximates 20% of the administered dose.

Measurements of RAIU are typically made at 24 hours, both as a matter of convenience and because the value at 24 hours is usually near the plateau, but it can be measured at 6 hours with appropriate determination of a normal range. The RAIU usually indicates the rate of thyroid hormone synthesis and, by inference, the rate of thyroid hormone release into the blood.

Radioactive Iodine Uptake

Little difference will be noted if the uptake is measured at any time during the day following that on which the isotope was administered. For calculation of therapeutic radioiodine doses in the treatment of thyrotoxic Graves' disease, an early uptake at 3 to 6 hours may produce results comparable to those found at 20 to 28 hours.[195] With the use of this modified early RAIU measurement, diagnosis and treatment of thyrotoxic Graves' disease can be accomplished on the same day. The range of normal values in North America is approximately 5% to 25%. Higher values are found in iodine-deficient regions and in patients with thyroid hyperfunction, but, as with other procedures, patients with mild hyperthyroidism may display values at or just above the upper limit of the normal range (Table 11-15).

TABLE 11-15

Factors That Influence 24-Hour Thyroid Iodide Uptake

Factors That Increase Uptake
Increased Hormone Synthesis
Hyperthyroidism
Response to glandular hormone depletion
Recovery from thyroid suppression
Recovery from subacute thyroiditis
Antithyroid agents
Excessive hormone losses
Nephrotic syndrome
Chronic diarrheal states
Soybean ingestion
Normal Hormone Synthesis
Iodine deficiency
Dietary insufficiency
Excessive loss (dehalogenase defect, pregnancy)
Hormone biosynthetic defects
Factors That Decrease Uptake
Decreased Hormone Synthesis
Primary hypofunction
Primary hypothyroidism
Antithyroid agents
Hormone biosynthetic defects
Hashimoto's disease
Subacute thyroiditis
Secondary hypofunction
Exogenous thyroid hormones
Not Reflecting Decreased Hormone Synthesis
Increased availability of iodine
Diet or drugs
Cardiac or renal insufficiency
Increased hormone release
Very severe hyperthyroidism (rare)

The Perchlorate Discharge Test

In normal individuals, more than 90% of thyroidal radioiodine is present as iodotyrosine and iodothyronine within minutes of its entry into the thyroid. It is then no longer in the intracellular iodide pool. In patients with Pendred syndrome or other disorders that inhibit the iodination of tyrosine, such as Hashimoto's thyroiditis, and in those receiving thiourea drugs, this process is delayed, as was shown by the exit (discharge) of more than 10% of thyroidal radioiodine within 2 hours after administration of 500 mg of $KClO_4$.[8] Perchlorate inhibits NIS function by competing with iodide for NIS, eliminating the iodide gradient that is required for maintaining the radioiodide in the gland. This illustrates that both iodide transport by NIS at the basal pole of the thyrocyte and its efflux across the apical membrane mediated by pendrin are required for thyroid hormone synthesis.

States Associated with Increased RAIU

Hyperthyroidism. Hyperthyroidism causes increased RAIU unless body iodide stores are increased. Such increases in uptake are always evident except in patients with severe thyrotoxicosis, in whom release of hormone can be so rapid that the thyroid content of I* has decreased to the normal range by the time the measurement is made. This condition is rare and is usually associated with obvious thyrotoxicosis.

Aberrant Hormone Synthesis. RAIU can be increased in the absence of hyperthyroidism in disorders in which iodine accumulation is normal but the secretion of hormone is impaired, such as abnormal Tg synthesis.[196] The magnitude of the increase in uptake and the time at which the plateau is achieved vary with the nature and severity of the disorder. Differentiation of these states from hyperthyroidism is usually not difficult, because the clinical findings and laboratory evidence of hyperthyroidism are lacking, and indeed hypothyroidism may be present.

Iodine Deficiency. RAIU is increased in acute or chronic iodine deficiency, as demonstrated by measurement of urinary iodine excretion, with urinary iodine values lower than 100 μg/day indicating deficiency. Chronic iodine deficiency is usually the result of inadequate content of iodine in the food and water (endemic iodine deficiency). Patients with cardiac, renal, or hepatic disease may develop iodine deficiency if given diets severely restricted in salt, especially if diuretic agents are administered.

Response to Thyroid Hormone Depletion. Rebound increases in RAIU are seen after withdrawal of antithyroid therapy, after subsidence of transient or subacute thyroiditis, and after recovery from prolonged suppression of thyroid function by exogenous hormone. A striking increase in uptake occurs in patients with iodide-induced myxedema after cessation of iodide administration. The duration of the rebound depends on the time required to replenish thyroid hormone stores.

Excessive Hormone Losses. In nephrotic syndrome, excessive losses of hormone in the urine, occurring in association with urinary loss of binding protein, cause a compensatory increase in hormone synthesis and RAIU. A similar sequence may occur when losses of hormone via the gastrointestinal tract are abnormal, as in chronic diarrheal states or during ingestion of agents, such as soybean protein and cholestyramine, that bind T_4 in the gut.

States Associated with Decreased RAIU

A general increase in iodine intake has made values of the RAIU in hypothyroidism indistinguishable from those at the lower end of the normal range. Therefore, the major indication for measurement of RAIU is to establish whether thyrotoxicosis is due to hyperthyroidism (high RAIU) or thyroiditis (low RAIU).

Exogenous Thyroid Hormone: Thyrotoxicosis Factitia. Except in disorders in which homeostatic control is disrupted or overridden (e.g., Graves' disease, autonomously functioning thyroid nodules), administration of exogenous thyroid hormone suppresses TSH secretion and reduces the RAIU, usually to values lower than 5%.

Low values of the RAIU in a patient who is clinically thyrotoxic may also indicate the presence of *thyrotoxicosis factitia,* the syndrome produced by ingestion of excess thyroid hormone. The unmeasurably low level of Tg in serum differentiates thyrotoxicosis factitia from other causes of thyrotoxicosis with decreased RAIU.[197]

Disorders of Hormone Storage. The RAIU is usually low in the early phase of subacute thyroiditis and in chronic thyroiditis with transient hyperthyroidism. Here, inflammatory follicular disruption leads to loss of the normal storage function of the gland and leakage of hormone into the blood. In the early stage of subacute thyroiditis, leakage of hormone is usually sufficient to suppress TSH secretion and the RAIU. Transient hypothyroidism often occurs late in both diseases, when stores of preformed hormone are depleted; the RAIU may return to normal or increased values at that time.

Exposure to Excessive Iodine. Exposure to excessive iodine is a common cause of a subnormal RAIU. Such decreases are spurious in the clinical sense because they do not indicate decreased absolute iodine uptake or decreased hormone production but can be produced by the introduction of excessive iodine in any form—inorganic, organic, or elemental. Common offenders are organic iodinated dyes used as x-ray contrast media and amiodarone (see Table 11-7). The duration of suppression of the uptake varies among individuals and with the compound administered. In general, dyes used for pyelography or computed tomographic scanning are cleared within a few months, whereas amiodarone may influence the uptake for up to 12 months due to its storage in fat. A single large dose of inorganic iodide can decrease uptake for several days, and chronic ingestion of iodide may depress the uptake for many weeks. Excessive quantities of iodine may also be present in vitamin and mineral preparations, vaginal or rectal suppositories, and iodinated antiseptics such as povidone (see Table 11-7).

The measurement of urinary iodine excretion is an invaluable means of establishing or excluding the existence of excessive body iodide stores; the 24-hour iodine excretion can be roughly extrapolated from the iodide-to-creatinine ratio in a random urine sample. Values in excess of 2 mg/day can account for a low RAIU value, whereas values lower than 1 mg/day suggest that one of the other disorders discussed in this section is the cause of a low RAIU.

REFERENCES

1. De Felice M, Di Lauro R. Murine models for the study of thyroid gland development. *Endocr Dev*. 2007;10:1-14.
2. Kratzsch J, Pulzer F. Thyroid gland development and defects. *Best Pract Res Clin Endocrinol Metab*. 2008;22:57-75.
3. Park SM, Chatterjee VK. Genetics of congenital hypothyroidism. *J Med Genet*. 2005;42:379-389.
4. Burrow GN, Fisher DA, Larsen PR. Mechanisms of disease: maternal and fetal thyroid function. *N Engl J Med*. 1994;331:1072-1078.
5. Glinoer D. Clinical and biological consequences of iodine deficiency during pregnancy. *Endocr Dev*. 2007;10:62-85.
6. Caldwell KL, Miller GA, Wang RY, et al. Iodine status of the U.S. population: National Health and Nutrition Examination Survey 2003-2004. *Thyroid*. 2008;18:1207-1214.
7. Dohan O, De la Vieja A, Paroder V, et al. The sodium/iodide symporter (NIS): characterization, regulation, and medical significance. *Endocr Rev*. 2003;24:48-77.
8. Wolff J. Perchlorate and the thyroid gland. *Pharmacol Rev*. 1998;50:89-105.
9. De La Vieja A, Dohan O, Levy O, et al. Molecular analysis of the sodium/iodide symporter: impact on thyroid and extrathyroid pathophysiology. *Physiol Rev*. 2000;80:1083-1105.
10. Van Sande J, Massart C, Beauwens R, et al. Anion selectivity by the sodium iodide symporter. *Endocrinology*. 2003;144:247-252.
11. Wolff J. Congenital goiter with defective iodide transport. *Endocr Rev*. 1983;4:240-254.

12. Bizhanova A, Kopp P. Minireview: the sodium-iodide symporter NIS and pendrin in iodide homeostasis of the thyroid. *Endocrinology*. 2009;150:1084-1090.
13. Everett LA, Morsli H, Wu DK, et al. Expression pattern of the mouse ortholog of the Pendred's syndrome gene (Pds) suggests a key role for pendrin in the inner ear. *Proc Natl Acad Sci U S A*. 1999;96: 9727-9732.
14. Everett LA, Green ED. A family of mammalian anion transporters and their involvement in human genetic diseases. *Hum Mol Genet*. 1999;8:1883-1891.
15. Royaux IE, Wall SM, Karniski LP, et al. Pendrin, encoded by the Pendred syndrome gene, resides in the apical region of renal intercalated cells and mediates bicarbonate secretion. *Proc Natl Acad Sci U S A*. 2001;98:4221-4226.
16. Morgans ME, Trotter WR. Association of congenital deafness with goitre: the nature of the thyroid defect. *Lancet*. 1958;1:607-609.
17. Kopp P, Pesce L, Solis SJ. Pendred syndrome and iodide transport in the thyroid. *Trends Endocrinol Metab*. 2008;19:260-268.
18. Rodriguez AM, Perron B, Lacroix L, et al. Identification and characterization of a putative human iodide transporter located at the apical membrane of thyrocytes. *J Clin Endocrinol Metab*. 2002;87:3500-3503.
19. Paroder V, Spencer SR, Paroder M, et al. Na(+)/monocarboxylate transport (SMCT) protein expression correlates with survival in colon cancer: molecular characterization of SMCT. *Proc Natl Acad Sci U S A*. 2006;103:7270-7275.
20. van den Hove MF, Croizet-Berger K, Jouret F, et al. The loss of the chloride channel, ClC-5, delays apical iodide efflux and induces a euthyroid goiter in the mouse thyroid gland. *Endocrinology*. 2006;147: 1287-1296.
21. Gnidehou S, Caillou B, Talbot M, et al. Iodotyrosine dehalogenase 1 (DEHAL1) is a transmembrane protein involved in the recycling of iodide close to the thyroglobulin iodination site. *FASEB J*. 2004;18:1574-1576.
22. Larsen PR. Thyroidal triiodothyronine and thyroxine in Graves' disease: correlation with presurgical treatment, thyroid status, and iodine content. *J Clin Endocrinol Metab*. 1975;41:1098-1104.
23. Moreno JC, Klootwijk W, van Toor H, et al. Mutations in the iodotyrosine deiodinase gene and hypothyroidism. *N Engl J Med*. 2008; 358:1811-1818.
24. Taurog A, Dorris ML, Doerge DR. Mechanism of simultaneous iodination and coupling catalyzed by thyroid peroxidase. *Arch Biochem Biophys*. 1996;330:24-32.
25. Ris-Stalpers C. Physiology and pathophysiology of the DUOXes. *Antioxid Redox Signal*. 2006;8:1563-1572.
26. Grasberger H, Refetoff S. Identification of the maturation factor for dual oxidase: evolution of an eukaryotic operon equivalent. *J Biol Chem*. 2006;281:18269-18272.
27. Niethammer P, Grabher C, Look AT, et al. A tissue-scale gradient of hydrogen peroxide mediates rapid wound detection in zebrafish. *Nature*. 2009;459:996-999.
28. Vulsma T, Gons MH, DeVijlder JMM. Maternal fetal transfer of thyroxine in congenital hypothyroidism due to a total organification defect of thyroid dysgenesis. *N Engl J Med*. 1989;321:13-16.
29. Moreno JC, Bikker H, Kempers MJ, et al. Inactivating mutations in the gene for thyroid oxidase 2 (THOX2) and congenital hypothyroidism. *N Engl J Med*. 2002;347:95-102.
30. Zamproni I, Grasberger H, Cortinovis F, et al. Biallelic inactivation of the dual oxidase maturation factor 2 (DUOXA2) gene as a novel cause of congenital hypothyroidism. *J Clin Endocrinol Metab*. 2008;93: 605-610.
31. Bakker B, Bikker H, Vulsma T, et al. Two decades of screening for congenital hypothyroidism in The Netherlands: TPO gene mutations in total iodide organification defects (an update). *J Clin Endocrinol Metab*. 2000;85:3708-3712.
32. Gerard AC, Daumerie C, Mestdagh C, et al. Correlation between the loss of thyroglobulin iodination and the expression of thyroid-specific proteins involved in iodine metabolism in thyroid carcinomas. *J Clin Endocrinol Metab*. 2003;88:4977-4983.
33. Dunn AD, Corsi CM, Myers HE, et al. Tyrosine 130 is an important outer ring donor for thyroxine formation in thyroglobulin. *J Biol Chem*. 1998;273:25223-25229.
34. Abuid J, Larsen PR. Triiodothyronine and thyroxine in hyperthyroidism: comparison of the acute changes during therapy with antithyroid agents. *J Clin Invest*. 1974;54:201-208.
35. Bahn RS, Burch HS, Cooper DS, et al. The role of propylthiouracil in the management of Graves' disease in adults: report of a meeting jointly sponsored by the American Thyroid Association and the Food and Drug Administration. *Thyroid*. 2009;19:673-674.
36. Kim BW, Daniels GH, Harrison BJ, et al. Overexpression of type 2 iodothyronine deiodinase in follicular carcinoma as a cause of low circulating free thyroxine levels. *J Clin Endocrinol Metab*. 2003;88: 594-598.
37. Lazarus JH. The effects of lithium therapy on thyroid and thyrotropin-releasing hormone. *Thyroid*. 1998;8:909-913.
38. Davies TF, Ando T, Lin RY, et al. Thyrotropin receptor-associated diseases: from adenomata to Graves disease. *J Clin Invest*. 2005; 115:1972-1983.
39. Corvilain B, Van Sande J, Dumont JE, et al. Somatic and germline mutations of the TSH receptor and thyroid diseases. *Clin Endocrinol (Oxf)*. 2001;55:143-158.
40. Saavedra AP, Tsygankova OM, Prendergast GV, et al. Role of cAMP, PKA and Rap1A in thyroid follicular cell survival. *Oncogene*. 2002; 21:778-788.
41. Cianfarani F, Baldini E, Cavalli A, et al. TSH receptor and thyroid-specific gene expression in human skin. *J Invest Dermatol*. 2010; 130:93-101.
42. Tonacchera M, Van Sande J, Parma J, et al. TSH receptor and disease. *Clin Endocrinol (Oxf)*. 1996;44:621-633.
43. Bianco AC, Salvatore D, Gereben B, et al. Biochemistry, cellular and molecular biology and physiological roles of the iodothyronine selenodeiodinases. *Endocrine Rev*. 2002;23:38-89.
44. Haugen BR. Drugs that suppress TSH or cause central hypothyroidism. *Best Pract Res Clin Endocrinol Metab*. 2009;23:793-800.
45. Findlay KA, Kaptein E, Visser TJ, et al. Characterization of the uridine diphosphate-glucuronosyltransferase-catalyzing thyroid hormone glucuronidation in man. *J Clin Endocrinol Metab*. 2000;85:2879-2883.
46. Schussler GC. The thyroxine-binding proteins. *Thyroid*. 2000;10: 141-149.
47. Jirasakuldech B, Schussler GC, Yap MG, et al. A characteristic serpin cleavage product of thyroxine-binding globulin appears in sepsis sera. *J Clin Endocrinol Metab*. 2000;85:3996-3999.
48. Pemberton PA, Stein PE, Pepys MB, et al. Hormone binding globulins undergo serpin conformational change in inflammation. *Nature*. 1988;336:257-258.
49. Dickson PW, Aldred AR, Marley PD, et al. Rat choroid plexus specializes in the synthesis and secretion of transthyretin (prealbumin). *J Biol Chem*. 1986;261:3475-3478.
50. Palha JA, Episkopou V, Maeda S, et al. Thyroid hormone metabolism in a transthyretin-null mouse strain. *J Biol Chem*. 1994;269: 33135-33139.
51. Palha JA, Fernandes R, de Escobar GM, et al. Transthyretin regulates thyroid hormone levels in the choroid plexus, but not in the brain parenchyma: study in a transthyretin-null mouse model. *Endocrinology*. 2000;141:3267-3272.
52. Bartalena L. Recent achievements in studies on thyroid hormone-binding proteins. *Endocr Rev*. 1990;11:47-64.
53. Bartalena L. Thyroid hormone-binding proteins: update 1994. *Endocr Rev*. 1994;3:140-142.
54. Chin W, Schussler GC. Decreased serum free thyroxine concentration in patients treated with diphenylhydantoin. *J Clin Endocrinol*. 1968; 28:181-186.
55. Larsen PR. Salicylate-induced increases in free triiodothyronine in human serum. Evidence of inhibition of triiodothyronine binding to thyroxine-binding globulin and thyroxine-binding prealbumin. *J Clin Invest*. 1972;51:1125-1134.
56. Docter R, Bos G, Krenning EP, et al. Inherited thyroxine excess: a serum abnormality due to an increased affinity for modified albumin. *Clin Endocrinol*. 1981;15:363-371.
57. Mendel CM, Cavalieri RR. Thyroxine distribution and metabolism in familial dysalbuminemic hyperthyroxinemia. *J Clin Endocrinol Metab*. 1984;59:499-504.
58. Arafah BM. Increased need for thyroxine in women with hypothyroidism during estrogen therapy. *N Engl J Med*. 2001;344:1743-1749.
59. Robbins J, Rall JE. The interaction of thyroid hormones and protein in biological fluids. *Recent Prog Horm Res*. 1957;13:161-202; discussion 202-208.
60. Mendel CM. The free hormone hypothesis: a physiologically based mathematical model. *Endocr Rev*. 1989;10:232-274.
61. Heuer H, Visser TJ. Minireview: pathophysiological importance of thyroid hormone transporters. *Endocrinology*. 2009;150:1078-1083.
62. Mendel CM, Weisiger RA, Jones AL, et al. Thyroid hormone-binding proteins in plasma facilitate uniform distribution of thyroxine withing tissues: a perfused rat liver study. *Endocrinology*. 1987;120:1742-1749.
63. Visser WE, Friesema EC, Jansen J, et al. Thyroid hormone transport in and out of cells. *Trends Endocrinol Metab*. 2008;19:50-56.
64. Dumitrescu AM, Liao XH, Weiss RE, et al. Tissue-specific thyroid hormone deprivation and excess in monocarboxylate transporter (mct) 8-deficient mice. *Endocrinology*. 2006;147:4036-4043.
65. Trajkovic M, Visser TJ, Mittag J, et al. Abnormal thyroid hormone metabolism in mice lacking the monocarboxylate transporter 8. *J Clin Invest*. 2007;117:627-635.
66. Heuer H, Maier MK, Iden S, et al. The monocarboxylate transporter 8 linked to human psychomotor retardation is highly expressed in thyroid hormone-sensitive neuron populations. *Endocrinology*. 2005;146:1701-1706.
67. Bernal J. The significance of thyroid hormone transporters in the brain. *Endocrinology*. 2005;146:1698-1700.
68. Tu HM, Kim SW, Salvatore D, et al. Regional distribution of type 2 thyroxine deiodinase messenger ribonucleic acid in rat hypothalamus

and pituitary and its regulation by thyroid hormone. *Endocrinology*. 1997;138:3359-3368.

69. Guadano-Ferraz A, Escamez MJ, Rausell E, et al. Expression of type 2 iodothyronine deiodinase in hypothyroid rat brain indicates an important role of thyroid hormone in the development of specific primary sensory systems. *J Neurosci*. 1999;19:3430-3439.
70. St Germain DL, Galton VA, Hernandez A. Minireview: defining the roles of the iodothyronine deiodinases—current concepts and challenges. *Endocrinology*. 2009;150:1097-1107.
71. Berry MJ, Banu L, Larsen PR. Type I iodothyronine deiodinase is a selenocysteine-containing enzyme. *Nature*. 1991;349:438-440.
72. Berry MJ, Larsen PR. The role of selenium in thyroid hormone action. *Endocr Rev*. 1992;13:207-219.
73. Berry MJ, Banu L, Chen YY, et al. Recognition of UGA as a selenocysteine codon in type I deiodinase requires sequences in the 3′ untranslated region. *Nature*. 1991;353:273-276.
74. Gereben B, Zavacki AM, Ribich S, et al. Cellular and molecular basis of deiodinase-regulated thyroid hormone signaling. *Endocr Rev*. 2008;29:898-938.
75. Huang SA. Physiology and pathophysiology of type 3 deiodinase in humans. *Thyroid*. 2005;15:875-881.
76. Salvatore D, Low SC, Berry M, et al. Type 3 lodothyronine deiodinase: cloning, in vitro expression, and functional analysis of the placental selenoenzyme. *J Clin Invest*. 1995;96:2421-2430.
77. Dentice M, Ambrosio R, Salvatore D. Role of type 3 deiodinase in cancer. *Expert Opin Ther Targets*. 2009;13:1363-1373.
78. Huang SA, Tu HM, Harney JW, et al. Severe hypothyroidism caused by type 3 iodothyronine deiodinase in infantile hemangiomas. *N Engl J Med*. 2000;343:185-189.
79. Hernandez A. Structure and function of the type 3 deiodinase gene. *Thyroid*. 2005;15:865-874.
80. St Germain DL, Hernandez A, Schneider MJ, et al. Insights into the role of deiodinases from studies of genetically modified animals. *Thyroid*. 2005;15:905-916.
81. Galton VA, Schneider MJ, Clark AS, et al. Life without thyroxine to 3,5,3′-triiodothyronine conversion: studies in mice devoid of the 5′-deiodinases. *Endocrinology*. 2009;150:2957-2963.
82. Schneider MJ, Fiering SN, Thai B, et al. Targeted disruption of the type 1 selenodeiodinase gene (dio1) results in marked changes in thyroid hormone economy in mice. *Endocrinology*. 2006;147:580-589.
83. Hernandez A, Martinez ME, Fiering S, et al. Type 3 deiodinase is critical for the maturation and function of the thyroid axis. *J Clin Invest*. 2006;116:476-484.
84. Saberi M, Sterling FH, Utiger RD. Reduction in extrathyroidal triiodothyronine production by propylthiouracil in man. *J Clin Invest*. 1975;55:218-223.
85. Christoffolete MA, Ribeiro R, Singru P, et al. Atypical expression of type 2 iodothyronine deiodinase in thyrotrophs explains the thyroxine-mediated pituitary TSH feedback mechanism. *Endocrinology*. 2006; 147:1735-1743.
86. Wu SY, Green WL, Huang WS, et al. Alternate pathways of thyroid hormone metabolism. *Thyroid*. 2005;15:943-958.
87. Ribeiro MO, Carvalho SD, Schultz JJ, et al. Thyroid hormone-sympathetic interaction and adaptive thermogenesis are thyroid hormone receptor isoform-specific. *J Clin Invest*. 2001;108:97-105.
88. Huang SA, Bianco AC. Reawakened interest in type III iodothyronine deiodinase in critical illness and injury. *Nat Clin Pract Endocrinol Metab*. 2008;4:148-155.
89. Martino E, Bartalena L, Bogazzi F, et al. The effects of amiodarone on the thyroid. *Endocr Rev*. 2001;22:240-254.
90. LoPresti JS, Eigen A, Kaptein E, et al. Alterations in 3,3′,5′-triiodothyronine metabolism in response to propylthiouracil, dexamethasone, and thyroxine administration in man. *J Clin Invest*. 1989;84: 1650-1656.
91. Schomburg L, Kohrle J. On the importance of selenium and iodine metabolism for thyroid hormone biosynthesis and human health. *Mol Nutr Food Res*. 2008;52:1235-1246.
92. Lazar MA. Thyroid hormone action: a binding contract. *J Clin Invest*. 2003;112:497-499.
93. Amma LL, Campos-Barros A, Wang Z, et al. Distinct tissue-specific roles for thyroid hormone receptors beta and alpha1 in regulation of type 1 deiodinase expression. *Mol Endocrinol*. 2001;15:467-475.
94. Abel ED, Kaulbach HC, Campos-Barros A, et al. Novel insight from transgenic mice into thyroid hormone resistance and the regulation of thyrotropin. *J Clin Invest*. 1999;103:271-279.
95. Forrest D, Golarai G, Connor J, et al. Genetic analysis of thyroid hormone receptors in development and disease. *Recent Prog Horm Res*. 1996;51:1-22.
96. Togashi M, Borngraeber S, Sandler B, et al. Conformational adaptation of nuclear receptor ligand binding domains to agonists: potential for novel approaches to ligand design. *J Steroid Biochem Mol Biol*. 2005; 93:127-137.
97. Bassett JH, Harvey CB, Williams GR. Mechanisms of thyroid hormone receptor-specific nuclear and extra nuclear actions. *Mol Cell Endocrinol*. 2003;213:1-11.
98. Mousa SA, O'Connor LJ, Bergh JJ, et al. The proangiogenic action of thyroid hormone analogue GC-1 is initiated at an integrin. *J Cardiovasc Pharmacol*. 2005;46:356-360.
99. Hollenberg AN, Monden T, Flynn TR, et al. The human thyrotropin-releasing hormone gene is regulated by thyroid hormone through two distinct classes of negative thyroid hormone response elements. *Mol Endocrinol*. 1995;9:540-550.
100. Segerson TP, Kauer J, Wolfe H, et al. Thyroid hormone regulates TRH biosynthesis in the paraventricular nucleus of the rat hypothalamus. *Science*. 1987;238:78-80.
101. Dyess EM, Segerson TP, Liposits Z, et al. Triiodothyronine exerts direct cell-specific regulation of thyrotropin-releasing hormone gene expression in the hypothalamic paraventricular nucleus. *Endocrinology*. 1988;123:2291-2297.
102. Lechan RM, Fekete C. Role of thyroid hormone deiodination in the hypothalamus. *Thyroid*. 2005;15:883-897.
103. Heuer H, Schafer MK, Bauer K. The thyrotropin-releasing hormone-degrading ectoenzyme: the third element of the thyrotropin-releasing hormone-signaling system. *Thyroid*. 1998;8:915-920.
104. Magner JA. Thyroid-stimulating hormone: biosynthesis, cell biology and bioactivity. *Endocr Rev*. 1990;11:354-385.
105. Gesundheit N, Petrick PA, Nissim M, et al. Thyrotropin-secreting pituitary adenomas: clinical and biochemical heterogeneity. *Ann Intern Med*. 1989;11:827-835.
106. Beck-Peccoz P, Amir S, Menezes-Ferreira MM, et al. Decreased receptor binding of biologically inactive thyrotropin in central hypothyroidism: effect of treatment with thyrotropin-releasing hormone. *N Engl J Med*. 1985;312:1085-1090.
107. Chan JL, Heist K, DePaoli AM, et al. The role of falling leptin levels in the neuroendocrine and metabolic adaptation to short-term starvation in healthy men. *J Clin Invest*. 2003;111:1409-1421.
108. Brabant G, Frank K, Ranft U. Physiological regulation of circadian and pulsatile thyrotropin secretion in normal man and woman. *J Clin Endocrinol Metab*. 1990;70:403-409.
109. Nikrodhanond AA, Ortiga-Carvalho TM, Shibusawa N, et al. Dominant role of thyrotropin-releasing hormone in the hypothalamic-pituitary-thyroid axis. *J Biol Chem*. 2006;281:5000-5007.
110. Chiamolera MI, Wondisford FE. Minireview: thyrotropin-releasing hormone and the thyroid hormone feedback mechanism. *Endocrinology*. 2009;150:1091-1096.
111. Beck-Peccoz P, Brucker-Davis F, Persani L, et al. Thyrotropin-secreting pituitary tumors. *Endocr Rev*. 1996;17:610-638.
112. Biller BM, Molitch ME, Vance ML, et al. Treatment of prolactin-secreting macroadenomas with the once-weekly dopamine agonist cabergoline. *J Clin Endocrinol Metab*. 1996;81:2338-2343.
113. Sherman SI, Gopal J, Haugen BR, et al. Central hypothyroidism associated with retinoid X receptor-selective ligands. *N Engl J Med*. 1999;340:1075-1079.
114. Sharma V, Hays WR, Wood WM, et al. Effects of rexinoids on thyrotrope function and the hypothalamic-pituitary-thyroid axis. *Endocrinology*. 2006;147:1438-1451.
115. Nakabayashi K, Matsumi H, Bhalla A, et al. Thyrostimulin, a heterodimer of two new human glycoprotein hormone subunits, activates the thyroid-stimulating hormone receptor. *J Clin Invest*. 2002;109: 1445-1452.
116. Sun SC, Hsu PJ, Wu FJ, et al. Thyrostimulin, but not thyroid-stimulating hormone, acts as a paracrine regulator to activate thyroid-stimulating hormone receptor in the mammalian ovary. *J Biol Chem*. 2010; 285:3758-3765.
117. Riesco G, Taurog A, Larsen R, et al. Acute and chronic responses to iodine deficiency in rats. *Endocrinology*. 1977;100:303-313.
118. Peeters R, Fekete C, Goncalves C, et al. Regional physiological adaptation of the central nervous system deiodinases to iodine deficiency. *Am J Physiol Endocrinol Metab*. 2001;281:E54-E61.
119. Guo TW, Zhang FC, Yang MS, et al. Positive association of the DIO2 (deiodinase type 2) gene with mental retardation in the iodine-deficient areas of China. *J Med Genet*. 2004;41:585-590.
120. Pazos-Moura CC, Moura EG, Dorris ML, et al. Effect of iodine deficiency and cold exposure on thyroxine 5′-deiodinase activity in various rat tissues. *Am J Physiol*. 1991;260:E175-E182.
121. Zimmermann MB. Iodine deficiency. *Endocr Rev*. 2009;30:376-408.
122. Delange F. The disorders induced by iodine deficiency. *Thyroid*. 1994;4:107-128.
123. Wolff J, Chaikoff IL. Plasma inorganic iodide as a homeostatic regulator of thyroid function. *J Biol Chem*. 1948;174:555-564.
124. Eng PH, Cardona GR, Fang SL, et al. Escape from the acute Wolff-Chaikoff effect is associated with a decrease in thyroid sodium/iodide symporter messenger ribonucleic acid and protein. *Endocrinology*. 1999;140:3404-3410.
125. LeBeau SO, Mandel SJ. Thyroid disorders during pregnancy. *Endocrinol Metab Clin North Am*. 2006;35:117-136, vii.
126. Glinoer D. The regulation of thyroid function during normal pregnancy: importance of the iodine nutrition status. *Best Pract Res Clin Endocrinol Metab*. 2004;18:133-152.

127. Dashe JS, Casey BM, Wells CE, et al. Thyroid-stimulating hormone in singleton and twin pregnancy: importance of gestational age-specific reference ranges. *Obstet Gynecol*. 2005;106:753-757.
128. Huang SA, Dorfman DM, Genest DR, et al. Type 3 Iodothyronine deiodinase is highly expressed in the human uteroplacental unit and in fetal epithelium. *J Clin Endocrinol and Metabolism*. 2003;88: 1384-1388.
129. Alexander EK, Marqusee E, Lawrence J, et al. Timing and magnitude of increases in levothyroxine requirements during pregnancy in women with hypothyroidism. *N Engl J Med*. 2004;351:241-249.
130. Weetman AP. Autoimmune thyroid disease. *Autoimmunity*. 2004; 37:337-340.
131. Dentice M, Bandyopadhyay A, Gereben B, et al. The Hedgehog-inducible ubiquitin ligase subunit WSB-1 modulates thyroid hormone activation and PTHrP secretion in the developing growth plate. *Nat Cell Biol*. 2005;7:698-705.
132. Fisher DA, Schoen EJ, La Franchi S, et al. The hypothalamic-pituitary-thyroid negative feedback control axis in children with treated congenital hypothyroidism. *J Clin Endocrinol Metab*. 2000;85:2722-2727.
133. Contempre B, Jauniaux E, Calvo R, et al. . Detection of thyroid hormones in human embryonic cavities during the first trimester of pregnancy. *J Clin Endocrinol Metab*. 1993;77:1719-1722.
134. Stagnaro-Green A. Maternal thyroid disease and preterm delivery. *J Clin Endocrinol Metab*. 2009;94:21-25.
135. Fisher DA, Nelson JC, Carlton EI, et al. Maturation of human hypothalamic-pituitary-thyroid function and control. *Thyroid*. 2000; 10:229-234.
136. Abuid J, Stinson DA, Larsen PR. Serum triiodothyronine and thyroxine in the neonate and the acute increases in these hormones following delivery. *J Clin Invest*. 1973;52:1195-1199.
137. de Jesus LA, Carvalho SD, Ribeiro MO, et al. The type 2 iodothyronine deiodinase is essential for adaptive thermogenesis in brown adipose tissue. *J Clin Invest*. 2001;108:1379-1385.
138. Fisher DA. Thyroid system immaturities in very low birth weight premature infants. *Semin Perinatol*. 2008;32:387-397.
139. Fisher DA. Thyroid function and dysfunction in premature infants. *Pediatr Endocrinol Rev*. 2007;4:317-328.
140. Shih JL, Agus MS. Thyroid function in the critically ill newborn and child. *Curr Opin Pediatr*. 2009;21:536-540.
141. Mariotti S, Franceschi C, Cossarizza A, et al. The aging thyroid. *Endocr Rev*. 1995;16:686-715.
142. Hershman JM, Pekary AE, Berg L, et al. Serum thyrotropin and thyroid hormone levels in elderly and middle-aged euthyroid persons. *J Am Geriatr Soc*. 1993;41:823-828.
143. Hoogendoorn EH, Hermus AR, de Vegt F, et al. Thyroid function and prevalence of anti-thyroperoxidase antibodies in a population with borderline sufficient iodine intake: influences of age and sex. *Clin Chem*. 2006;52:104-111.
144. Lewis GF, Alessi CA, Imperial JG, et al. Low serum free thyroxine index in ambulating elderly is due to a resetting of the threshold of thyrotropin feedback suppression. *J Clin Endocrinol Metab*. 1991;73: 843-849.
145. Chan JL, Bullen J, Stoyneva V, Depaoli AM, et al. Recombinant methionyl human leptin administration to achieve high physiologic or pharmacologic leptin levels does not alter circulating inflammatory marker levels in humans with leptin sufficiency or excess. *J Clin Endocrinol Metab*. 2005;90:1618-1624.
146. Byerley LO, Heber D. Metabolic effects of triiodothyronine replacement during fasting in obese subjects. *J Clin Endocrinol Metab*. 1996;81:968-976.
147. Onur S, Haas V, Bosy-Westphal A, et al. L-tri-iodothyronine is a major determinant of resting energy expenditure in underweight patients with anorexia nervosa and during weight gain. *Eur J Endocrinol*. 2005;152:179-184.
148. Danforth JE, Horton ES, O'Connell M, et al. Dietary-induced alterations in thyroid hormone metabolism during overnutrition. *J Clin Invest*. 1979;64:1336-1347.
149. Van den Berghe G. Novel insights into the neuroendocrinology of critical illness. *Eur J Endocrinol*. 2000;143:1-13.
150. Alkemade A, Friesema EC, Unmehopa UA, et al. Neuroanatomical pathways for thyroid hormone feedback in the human hypothalamus. *J Clin Endocrinol Metab*. 2005;90:4322-4334.
151. Fekete C, Sarkar S, Christoffolete MA, et al. Bacterial lipopolysaccharide (LPS)-induced type 2 iodothyronine deiodinase (D2) activation in the mediobasal hypothalamus (MBH) is independent of the LPS-induced fall in serum thyroid hormone levels. *Brain Res*. 2005;1056: 97-99.
152. Boelen A, Platvoet-Ter Schiphorst MC, Wiersinga WM. Association between serum interleukin-6 and serum 3,5,3′-triiodothyronine in nonthyroidal illness. *J Clin Endocrinol Metab*. 1993;77:1695-1699.
153. Koenig RJ. Modeling the nonthyroidal illness syndrome. *Curr Opin Endocrinol Diabetes Obes*. 2008;15:466-469.
154. Peeters RP, Wouters PJ, Kaptein E, et al. Reduced activation and increased inactivation of thyroid hormone in tissues of critically ill patients. *J Clin Endocrinol Metab*. 2003;88:3202-3211.
155. Wadwekar D, Kabadi UM. Thyroid hormone indices during illness in six hypothyroid subjects rendered euthyroid with levothyroxine therapy. *Exp Clin Endocrinol Diabetes*. 2004;112:373-377.
156. Van den Berghe G, Wouters P, Weekers F, et al. Reactivation of pituitary hormone release and metabolic improvement by infusion of growth hormone-releasing peptide and thyrotropin-releasing hormone in patients with protracted critical illness. *J Clin Endocrinol Metab*. 1999;84:1311-1323.
157. Brent GA, Hershman JM. Thyroxine therapy in patients with severe nonthyroidal illness and low serum thyroxine concentrations. *J Clin Endocrinol Metab*. 1986;63:1-8.
158. Hamblin PS, Dyer SA, Mohr VS, et al. Relationship between thyrotropin and thyroxine changes during the recovery from severe hypothyroxinemia of critical illness. *J Clin Endocrinol Metab*. 1986;62: 717-722.
159. Bennett-Guerrero E, Jimenez JL, White WD, et al. Cardiovascular effects of intravenous triiodothyronine in patients undergoing coronary artery bypass graft surgery: a randomized, double-blind, placebo-controlled trial. Duke T3 study group. *JAMA*. 1996;275:687-692.
160. Klein I, Danzi S. Thyroid disease and the heart. *Circulation*. 2007; 116:1725-1735.
161. Jackson IM. The thyroid axis and depression. *Thyroid*. 1998;8: 951-956.
162. Topliss DJ, White EL, Stockigt JR. Significance of thyrotropin excess in untreated primary adrenal insufficiency. *J Clin Endocrinol Metab*. 1980;50:52-56.
163. Ain KB, Mori Y, Refetoff S. Reduced clearance rate of thyroxine-binding globulin (TBG) with increased sialylation: a mechanism for estrogen-induced elevation of serum TBG concentration. *J Clin Endocrinol Metab*. 1987;65:689-696.
164. Marqusee E, Braverman LE, Lawrence JE, et al. The effect of droloxifene and estrogen on thyroid function in postmenopausal women. *J Clin Endocrinol Metab*. 2000;85:4407-4410.
165. Arafah BM. Decreased levothyroxine requirement in women with hypothyroidism during androgen therapy for breast cancer. *Ann Intern Med*. 1994;121:247-251.
166. Surks MI, Goswami G, Daniels GH. The thyrotropin reference range should remain unchanged. *J Clin Endocrinol Metab*. 2005;90:5489-5496.
167. Wartofsky L, Dickey RA. The evidence for a narrower thyrotropin reference range is compelling. *J Clin Endocrinol Metab*. 2005;90:5483-5488.
168. Brucker-Davis F, Oldfield EH, Skarulis MC, et al. Thyrotropin-secreting pituitary tumors: diagnostic criteria, thyroid hormone sensitivity, and treatment outcome in 25 patients followed at the National Institutes of Health. *J Clin Endocrinol Metab*. 1999;84:476-486.
169. Kuzuya N, Kinji I, Ishibashi M. Endocrine and immunohistochemical studies on thyrotropin (TSH)-secreting pituitary adenomas: responses of TSH, α-subunit, and growth hormone to hypothalamic releasing hormones and their distribution in adenoma cells. *J Clin Endocrinol Metab*. 1990;71:1103-1111.
170. Wang R, Nelson JC, Weiss RM, et al. Accuracy of free thyroxine measurements across natural ranges of thyroxine binding to serum proteins. *Thyroid*. 2000;10:31-39.
171. Nelson JC, Weiss RM, Wilcox RB. Underestimates of serum free thyroxine (T_4) concentrations by free T_4 immunoassays. *J Clin Endocrinol Metab*. 1994;79:76-79.
172. Faix JD, Rosen HN, Velazquez FR. Indirect estimation of thyroid hormone-binding proteins to calculate free thyroxine index: comparison of nonisotopic methods that use labeled thyroxine ("T-uptake"). *Clin Chem*. 1995;41:41-47.
173. Nelson JC, Weiss RM. The effect of serum dilution on free thyroxine (T_4) concentrations in the low T_4 syndrome of nonthyroidal illness. *J Clin Endocrinol Metab*. 1985;61:239-246.
174. Demers LM, Spencer CA. Laboratory medicine practice guidelines: laboratory support for the diagnosis and monitoring of thyroid disease. *Clin Endocrinol (Oxf)*. 2003;58:138-140.
175. Afandi B, Vera R, Schussler GC, et al. Concordant decreases of thyroxine and thyroxine binding protein concentrations during sepsis. *Metabolism*. 2000;49:753-754.
176. Toft AD, Irvine WJ, Hunter WM, et al. Anomalous plasma TSH levels in patients developing hypothyroidism in the early months after ^{131}I therapy for thyrotoxicosis. *J Clin Endocrinol Metab*. 1974;39:607-609.
177. Rees-Jones RW, Larsen PR. Triiodothyronine and thyroxine content of desiccated thyroid tablets. *Metabolism*. 1977;26:1213-1218.
178. Kaptein EM. Thyroid hormone metabolism and thyroid diseases in chronic renal failure. *Endocr Rev*. 1996;17:45-63.
179. Bacci V, Schussler GC, Kaplan TB. The relationship between serum triiodothyronine and thyrotropin during systemic illness. *J Clin Endocrinol Metab*. 1982;54:1229-1235.
180. Weiss RE, Refetoff S. Treatment of resistance to thyroid hormone—primum non nocere. *J Clin Endocrinol Metab*. 1999;84:401-404.
181. Refetoff S, Weiss RE, Usala SJ. The syndromes of resistance to thyroid hormone. *Endocr Rev*. 1993;14:348-399.

182. al-Adsani H, Hoffer LJ, Silva JE. Resting energy expenditure is sensitive to small dose changes in patients on chronic thyroid hormone replacement. *J Clin Endocrinol Metab.* 1997;82:1118-1125.
183. Becker C. Hypothyroidism and atherosclerotic heart disease: pathogenesis, medical management, and the role of coronary artery bypass surgery. *Endocr Rev.* 1985;6:432-440.
184. Mazzaferri EL, Robbins RJ, Spencer CA, et al. A consensus report of the role of serum thyroglobulin as a monitoring method for low-risk patients with papillary thyroid carcinoma. *J Clin Endocrinol Metab.* 2003;88:1433-1441.
185. Francis Z, Schlumberger M. Serum thyroglobulin determination in thyroid cancer patients. *Best Pract Res Clin Endocrinol Metab.* 2008;22:1039-1046.
186. Spencer CA, Lopresti JS. Measuring thyroglobulin and thyroglobulin autoantibody in patients with differentiated thyroid cancer. *Nat Clin Pract Endocrinol Metab.* 2008;4:223-233.
187. Schlumberger M, Hitzel A, Toubert ME, et al. Comparison of seven serum thyroglobulin assays in the follow-up of papillary and follicular thyroid cancer patients. *J Clin Endocrinol Metab.* 2007;92:2487-2495.
188. Snozek CL, Chambers EP, Reading CC, et al. Serum thyroglobulin, high-resolution ultrasound, and lymph node thyroglobulin in diagnosis of differentiated thyroid carcinoma nodal metastases. *J Clin Endocrinol Metab.* 2007;92:4278-4281.
189. Rapoport B, McLachlan SM. Thyroid autoimmunity. *J Clin Invest.* 2001;108:1253-1259.
190. Hollowell JG, Staehling NW, Flanders WD, et al. Serum TSH, T(4), and thyroid antibodies in the United States population (1988 to 1994): National Health and Nutrition Examination Survey (NHANES III). *J Clin Endocrinol Metab.* 2002;87:489-499.
191. Martin A, Barbesino G, Davies TF. T-cell receptors and autoimmune thyroid disease—signposts for T-cell-antigen driven diseases. *Int Rev Immunol.* 1999;18:111-140.
192. Latrofa F, Pichurin P, Guo J, et al. Thyroglobulin-thyroperoxidase autoantibodies are polyreactive, not bispecific: analysis using human monoclonal autoantibodies. *J Clin Endocrinol Metab.* 2003;88:371-378.
193. Guo J, Wang Y, Rapoport B, et al. Evidence for antigen presentation to sensitized T cells by thyroid peroxidase (TPO)-specific B cells in mice injected with fibroblasts co-expressing TPO and MHC class II. *Clin Exp Immunol.* 2000;119:38-46.
194. Vanderpump MPJ, Tunbridge WMG, French JM, et al. The incidence of thyroid disorders in the community: a twenty-year follow-up of the Whickham survey. *Clin Endocrinol.* 1995;43:55-68.
195. Hayes AA, Akre CM, Gorman CA. Iodine-131 treatment of Graves' disease using modified early iodine-131 uptake measurements in therapy dose calculations. *J Nucl Med.* 1990;31:519-522.
196. Medeiros-Neto G, Kim PS, Vono J, et al. Congenital hypothyroid goiter with deficient thyroglobulin. *J Clin Invest* 1996;98:2838-2844.
197. Mariotti S, Martino E, Cupini C, et al. Low serum thyroblobulin as a clue to the diagnosis of thyrotoxicosis factitia. *N Engl J Med.* 1982;307:410-412.

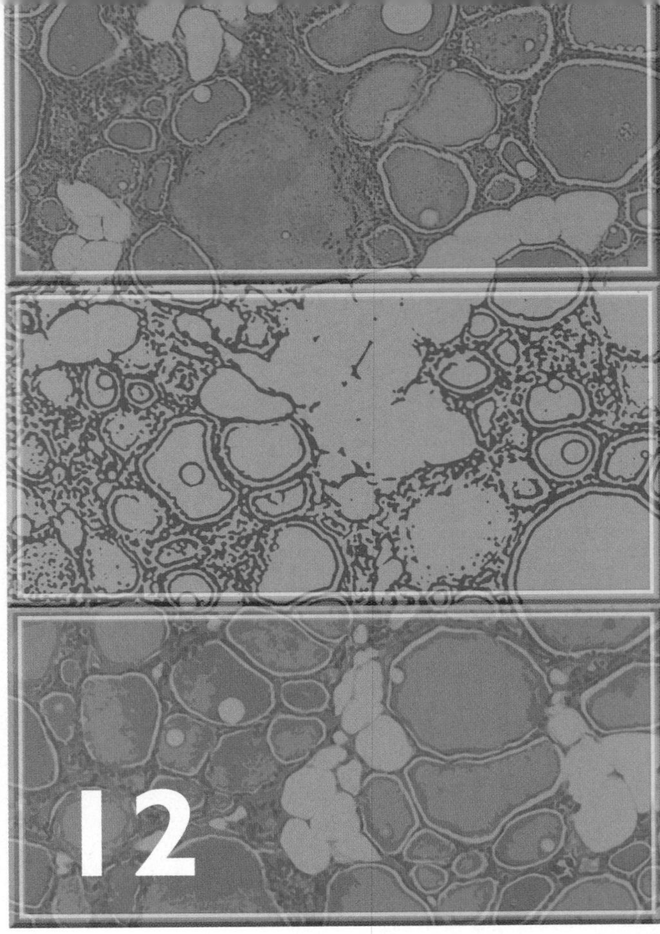

CHAPTER 12

Thyrotoxicosis

SUSAN J. MANDEL • P. REED LARSEN • TERRY F. DAVIES

The term *thyrotoxicosis* refers to the classic physiologic manifestations of excessive quantities of the thyroid hormones that are so characteristic of this condition. The term *thyrotoxicosis,* rather than *hyperthyroidism,* should be used for this disorder because it need not be associated with hyperfunction of the thyroid gland. The term *hyperthyroidism* is reserved for disorders that result from sustained overproduction and release of hormone by the thyroid itself, Graves' disease being the most common example (Table 12-1). The other common conditions causing thyrotoxicosis are inflammation of the thyroid gland (called *thyroiditis*), which is usually autoimmune or viral related, and autonomous nodules.

Hyperthyroidism and thyroiditis must be differentiated from thyrotoxicosis caused by exogenous thyroid hormone, whether iatrogenic or self-administered. For most patients with thyrotoxicosis, it is the symptoms or signs caused by an excess of the thyroid hormone, regardless of source, that lead to medical attention. Other patients have surprisingly few symptoms and are referred because of a suppressed level of thyroid-stimulating hormone (TSH).

This chapter begins with a brief review of the symptoms and signs of thyrotoxicosis and their pathophysiologic basis. The appropriate use of the laboratory tests described in Chapter 11 is then presented to show how these can focus the search for a diagnosis.

CLINICAL MANIFESTATIONS OF THYROTOXICOSIS

One very important clinical clue to the cause of a patient's thyrotoxicosis is the duration of the symptoms. Patients with hyperthyroidism typically have had manifestations for many months before presentation, but because the week-to-week increases in thyroid hormones are so small they may become rather extreme before they are noticed by the patient. In addition, patients often attribute these symptoms to other causes—their fatigue to family or work responsibilities, their heat intolerance to the weather, their weight loss to an effective diet, and their dyspnea and palpitations to a lack of regular exercise.

On the other hand, patients with thyrotoxicosis due to thyroiditis can often date the onset of their symptoms precisely, and they usually seek medical attention within a month or so after onset, as might be expected considering the effects of the release of the equivalent of 30 to 60 days' supply of thyroid hormone into the circulation over a few days to weeks.

Therefore, ascertaining the chronology as well as the spectrum of symptoms is a critical goal of the interview process. Another general characteristic is that the symptoms and signs of thyrotoxicosis are more readily recognized in young than in older patients.[1] The term *masked*

TABLE 12-1

Causes of Thyrotoxicosis

Sustained Hormone Overproduction (Hyperthyroidism)
Low TSH, High RAIU
Graves' disease (von Basedow's disease)
Toxic multinodular goiter
Toxic adenoma
Chorionic gonadotropin-induced
Gestational hyperthyroidism
Physiologic hyperthyroidism of pregnancy
Familial gestational hyperthyroidism due to TSH receptor mutations
Trophoblastic tumors
Inherited nonimmune hyperthyroidism associated with TSH receptor or G protein mutations
Low TSH, Low RAIU
Iodide-induced hyperthyroidism (Jod-Basedow effect)
Amiodarone-associated hyperthyroidism due to iodide release
Struma Ovarii
Metastatic functioning thyroid carcinoma
Normal or Elevated TSH
TSH-secreting pituitary tumors
Thyroid hormone resistance with pituitary predominance
Transient Hormone Excess (Thyrotoxicosis)
Low TSH, Low RAIU
Thyroiditis
Autoimmune
Lymphocytic thyroiditis (silent thyroiditis, painless thyroiditis, postpartum thyroiditis)
Acute exacerbation of Hashimoto's disease
Viral or postviral
Subacute (granulomatous, painful, postviral) thyroiditis
Drug-induced or associated thyroiditis
Amiodarone
Lithium, interferon-α, interleukin-2, GM-CSF
Infectious thyroiditis
Exogenous Thyroid Hormone
Iatrogenic overreplacement
Thyrotoxicosis factitia
Ingestion of natural products containing thyroid hormone
"Hamburger" thyrotoxicosis
Natural foodstuffs
Thyromimetic compounds (e.g., tiratricol PLB)
Occupational exposure to thyroid hormone (e.g., pill manufacturing, veterinary occupations)

GM-CSF, granulocyte-macrophage colony-stimulating factor; RAIU, radioactive iodine uptake; TSH, thyroid-stimulating hormone.

or *apathetic* thyrotoxicosis is used to describe the syndrome sometimes seen in elderly persons, which may manifest as congestive heart failure with arrhythmia or as unexplained weight loss without the increased appetite that is typical in the younger patient.

At present, the ready availability of sensitive serum TSH assays, a reliable indicator of excess thyroid hormone in the ambulatory patient (see Chapter 11), has made the more classic and severe manifestations of long-standing thyrotoxicosis less prevalent. In fact, a current area of controversy is how aggressively to treat the condition termed *subclinical* or *mild* hyperthyroidism, a biochemical diagnosis in which a subnormal serum TSH level is accompanied by normal free thyroid hormone concentrations. Nonetheless, the classic presentation is still common, and it serves to illustrate the pleiotropic physiologic effects of excess thyroid hormones.

If not recognized, hyperthyroidism can progress to life-threatening severity despite the fact that it is a benign condition. The following sections review the pathophysiology of the most important manifestations of excess thyroid hormone.

Cardiovascular System

Alterations in cardiovascular function in the thyrotoxic patient are in part due to increased circulatory demands that result from the hypermetabolism and the need to dissipate the excess heat produced.[2] At rest, peripheral vascular resistance is decreased and cardiac output is increased as a result of an increase, first, in heart rate, and with more severe disease, in stroke volume. Thyroid hormones in excess also have a direct inotropic effect on cardiac contraction mediated by an increase in the ratio of α- to β-myosin heavy chain expression. Tachycardia is almost always present due to a combination of increased sympathetic and decreased vagal tone.[3] Widening of the pulse pressure results from the increase in systolic and decrease in diastolic pressure due to reduced resistance.[4,5] The decreased resistance is caused by increased nitric oxide production.[6]

The increased systolic force is often felt by the patient as a "palpitation" and is evident on inspection or palpation of the precordium. Because of the diffuse and forceful nature of the apex beat, the heart may seem enlarged, and echocardiography may show an increased ventricular mass. In addition, the pre-ejection period is shortened, and the ratio of pre-ejection period to left ventricular ejection time is decreased.[5] The heart sounds are enhanced, particularly S_1, and a scratchy systolic sound along the left sternal border, resembling a pleuropericardial friction rub (*Means-Lerman scratch*), may also be heard. These manifestations abate when a normal metabolic state is restored.

Mitral valve prolapse occurs more frequently in Graves' or Hashimoto's disease than in the normal population.[7,8] Cardiac arrhythmias are almost invariably supraventricular, especially in younger patients.[9] Between 2% and 20% of patients with thyrotoxicosis have atrial fibrillation, and about 15% of patients with otherwise unexplained atrial fibrillation are thyrotoxic.[2] In the Framingham cohort, individuals older than 60 years of age with a suppressed TSH level had a 2.8-fold increased risk of developing atrial fibrillation, compared to those with a normal serum TSH value.[10] This finding was confirmed in the Cardiovascular Health Study.[11]

The increased cardiovascular cost of a standard workload or metabolic challenge is adequately met if the thyrotoxic patient is not, or has not previously been, in heart failure. That is, cardiac competence is maintained in most patients without underlying heart disease. Mild peripheral edema may occur in the absence of heart failure. Heart failure per se usually occurs in patients with preexisting heart disease, and therefore typically in the elderly, but it may not be possible to determine whether underlying heart disease is present until after thyrotoxicosis is relieved.

Atrial fibrillation decreases the efficiency of the cardiac response to any increased circulatory demand and may play a role in causing cardiac failure.[12] Attempts to convert atrial fibrillation to sinus rhythm are not indicated while thyrotoxicosis is present, and about 60% of patients revert spontaneously to sinus rhythm after treatment, usually within 4 months.[13] For this reason and because thromboembolism is rare in patients younger than 50 years of age with thyrotoxicosis, routine anticoagulation is not recommended for younger patients who are without a history of underlying heart disease or prior thrombotic disorder.[14,15] Medical or electrical cardioversion of patients with thyrotoxicosis-induced atrial fibrillation is often successful even after a year has passed.[16]

Protein, Carbohydrate, and Lipid Metabolism

The stimulation of metabolism and heat production in patients with thyrotoxicosis is reflected in an increased basal metabolic rate (BMR), increased appetite, and heat intolerance, but only rarely is the basal body temperature elevated.[17] Despite increased food intake, a state of chronic caloric and nutritional inadequacy often ensues, depending on the degree of increased metabolism. Both synthesis and degradation rates of proteins are increased, the latter to a greater extent than the former, with the result that in severe thyrotoxicosis there is a net decrease in tissue protein, as indicated by loss of weight, muscle wasting, proximal muscle weakness, and even mild hypoalbuminemia. Preexisting diabetes mellitus may be aggravated, one cause being accelerated turnover of insulin. Both lipogenesis and lipolysis are increased in thyrotoxicosis, but the net effect is lipolysis, as reflected by an increase in the plasma concentration of free fatty acids and glycerol and a decrease in the serum cholesterol level; triglyceride levels are usually slightly decreased. The enhanced mobilization and oxidation of free fatty acids in response to fasting or catecholamines is a result of enhancement of lipolytic pathways by thyroid hormones.[17]

Sympathetic Nervous System and Catecholamines

Many of the manifestations of thyrotoxicosis and those of sympathetic nervous system activation are similar. However, plasma concentrations of epinephrine and norepinephrine, as well as their urinary excretion and that of their metabolites, is not increased in patients with thyrotoxicosis, and thyroid hormones exert effects separate from, but similar and additive to, those of the catecholamines.[18]

The improvement in cardiac function with β-blockade in patients with hyperthyroidism has led to the concept that there is increased sympathetic tone or increased cardiac sensitivity to the sympathetic nervous system in these patients.[19] Support for the latter was provided by experiments using transgenic mice in which overexpression of type 2 iodothyronine deiodinase (D2) in the heart increased myocardial triiodothyronine (T_3) and the cyclic adenosine monophosphate (cAMP) response to norepinephrine in cardiac myocytes due to alterations in G proteins.[20,21] In addition, adipocytes from thyrotoxic patients have exhibited 3-fold increases in norepinephrine-induced lipolysis, 15-fold increases in response to β_2-adrenergic receptor agonists, and 3-fold increases in response to forskolin or cAMP.[22] Therefore, thyroid hormones increase sensitivity to catecholamines in both cardiomyocytes and adipocytes by a variety of mechanisms.

Nervous System

Alterations in the function of the nervous system in thyrotoxicosis are manifested by nervousness, emotional lability, and hyperkinesia. Fatigue may be caused by both muscle weakness and insomnia, which is commonly present. Emotional lability is common, and in rare cases mental disturbance may be severe; manic depressive, schizoid, or paranoid reactions may emerge. The hyperkinesia of the thyrotoxic patient is characteristic. During the interview the patient shifts positions frequently, and movements are quick, jerky, exaggerated, and often purposeless. In children, in whom such manifestations tend to be more severe, inability to focus may lead to deterioration of school performance, suggesting attention deficit–hyperactivity disorder. A fine tremor of the hands, tongue, or lightly closed eyelids may appear and mimic that of Parkinsonism. The electroencephalogram reveals an increase in fast-wave activity, and in patients with convulsive disorders, the frequency of seizures is increased.

Muscle

Weakness and fatigability usually are not accompanied by objective evidence of muscle disease, save for the generalized wasting associated with weight loss. The weakness is most prominent in the proximal muscles of the limbs, causing difficulty in climbing stairs or fatigue from minimal exertion, such as using a blowdryer or lifting an infant. Proximal muscle wasting may be out of proportion to the overall loss of weight (*thyrotoxic myopathy*). Myopathy affects men with thyrotoxicosis more commonly than women and may overshadow the other manifestations of the syndrome. In the most severe forms, the myopathy may involve the more distal muscles of the extremities and the muscles of the trunk and face. Although myopathy of ocular muscles is unusual, the disorder may mimic myasthenia gravis or ophthalmic myasthenia.[23] Muscular strength returns to normal when a normal metabolic state is restored, but muscle mass takes longer to recover.

Graves' disease occurs in about 3% to 5% of patients with myasthenia gravis, and about 1% of the patients with Graves' disease develop myasthenia gravis. Antibodies and T cells specific for the TSH and acetylcholine receptors are involved in the pathogenesis of the two diseases.[24] Unlike thyrotoxic myopathy, the association of myasthenia gravis with Graves' disease has a distinct female preponderance. The effect of thyrotoxicosis and its alleviation on the course of myasthenia gravis is variable, but in most instances, myasthenia is accentuated during the thyrotoxic state and improves after a normal metabolic state is restored. A form of myasthenia affecting mainly the orbital muscles may also occur more commonly in patients with Graves' disease and needs to be distinguished from Graves' orbitopathy by the prominence of bilateral ptosis of a variable degree.[23]

Periodic paralysis of the hypokalemic type may occur together with thyrotoxicosis, and its severity is accentuated by the latter disorder. The coincidence of the two disorders is particularly common in Asian and Latino men.[25-27]

Eyes

Retraction of the upper or lower eyelids, or both, is evident as the presence of a rim of sclera between the lid and the limbus and is a common manifestation in all forms of thyrotoxicosis, regardless of the underlying cause; it is responsible for the typical "stare" of these patient. Also common is lid lag, a phenomenon in which the upper lid lags behind the globe when the patient is asked to shift the gaze slowly downward, or globe lag, which becomes evident when the eye lags behind the upper lid when the patient looks up. These ocular manifestations appear to be the result of increased adrenergic tone. It is important to differentiate these signs, which may occur in any form of thyrotoxicosis, from those of infiltrative autoimmune orbitopathy, which are associated with Graves' disease and are described later.

Skin and Hair

The most characteristic change in patients with long-standing thyrotoxicosis is the warm, moist feel of the skin that results from cutaneous vasodilation and excessive sweating. The elbows may be smooth and pink, the complexion is rosy, and the patient blushes readily. Palmar erythema may resemble "liver palms," and telangiectasia may be present. The hair is fine and friable, and hair loss may increase. The nails are often soft and friable. A characteristic but uncommon finding is *Plummer's nails*, or onycholysis, typically involving the fourth and fifth fingers. Vitiligo, another autoimmune disease, is more common in patients with autoimmune thyroid disease.

Respiratory System

Dyspnea is common in severe thyrotoxicosis, and several factors may contribute to this condition. Vital capacity is commonly reduced, mainly from weakness of the respiratory muscles. During exercise, ventilation is increased out of proportion to the increase in oxygen uptake, but the diffusing capacity of the lung is normal.

Alimentary System

An increase in appetite is common but usually is not seen in patients with mild disease. In more severe disease, the increased intake of food is inadequate to meet the increased caloric requirements, and weight is lost at a variable rate. More often, the patient reports a gratifying success after previously frustrated attempts at weight control. The frequency of bowel movements is increased, but diarrhea is rare. The increased gastric emptying and intestinal motility in thyrotoxicosis appear to be responsible for slight malabsorption of fat; these functions return to normal after a normal metabolic state has been restored. Celiac and Graves' diseases may coexist, and there is an increased prevalence of pernicious anemia.

Hepatic dysfunction occurs, particularly when thyrotoxicosis is severe; hypoproteinemia and increases in serum alanine aminotransferase (ALT) occur, and bone or liver alkaline phosphatase levels may be elevated.[28] Hepatomegaly and jaundice can develop with severe, prolonged disease, and liver failure was a cause of death before the development of successful treatment for patients with Graves' disease. Splanchnic oxygen consumption is increased in proportion to the metabolic rate, but splanchnic blood flow is not proportionately increased. As a result, the arteriovenous oxygen difference across the splanchnic bed is increased, and hypoxia may contribute to hepatic dysfunction.[29] A reduction in cardiac output by pulse rate reduction due to β-adrenergic blockade may exacerbate that process, because it does not reduce the hepatic hypermetabolism.

Skeletal System: Calcium and Phosphorus Metabolism

Thyrotoxicosis is generally associated with increased excretion of calcium and phosphorus in urine and stool; with demineralization of bone, as demonstrated by routine bone densitometry; and occasionally with pathologic fractures, especially in elderly women.[30-33] In such instances, the pathologic changes are variable and may include osteitis fibrosa, osteomalacia, or osteoporosis. Urinary excretion of collagen breakdown products is increased in thyrotoxicosis. Kinetic studies indicate an increase in the exchangeable calcium pool and acceleration of both bone resorption and accretion, particularly the former. Thyroid hormone (T_3) has been shown to accelerate activity of the osteoclasts and helps to explain these widespread changes.[34,35] Indeed, data indicate that TSH itself may have a local action that normally helps balance thyroid hormone action on osteoclasts and enhance osteoblast activity.[36,37] Such an action by TSH would be absent in hyperthyroidism, allowing accentuation of the thyroid hormone effects.

These changes in hyperthyroidism lead to decreased bone density in many patients. As the thyrotoxicosis is treated, bone density may normalize in many younger patients, but not in all.[38] Postmenopausal women may have an accelerated reduction in bone density that requires treatment (see Chapter 27). Much controversy has existed regarding the induction of decreased bone density by TSH-suppression therapy in patients with thyroid cancer. Suffice it to say that postmenopausal, but not premenopausal, women given a TSH-suppressive dosage of thyroid hormones are at risk for osteopenia and require prophylaxis with calcium and vitamin D or more aggressive approaches.[39,40] The decision to relax TSH suppression in low-risk patients may be influenced by their bone status.

For all the same reasons, hypercalcemia may occur in patients with severe thyrotoxicosis. The total serum calcium concentration is increased in as many as 27% of patients, and the ionized serum calcium is elevated in 47%. The concentrations of heat-labile serum alkaline phosphatase and osteocalcin are also frequently elevated. These findings resemble those of primary hyperparathyroidism, but the concentration of parathyroid hormone in serum is low-normal in most cases.[41] True primary hyperparathyroidism and thyrotoxicosis sometimes coexist. Plasma 25-hydroxycholecalciferol levels are decreased in thyrotoxic patients, and this alteration could contribute to the decreased intestinal absorption of calcium and osteomalacia observed in some patients.

Renal Function: Water and Electrolyte Metabolism

Thyrotoxicosis produces no symptoms referable to the urinary tract save for mild polyuria, which may lead to nocturia. Nevertheless, renal blood flow, glomerular filtration, and tubular reabsorptive and secretory maxima are increased. Total exchangeable potassium is decreased, possibly due to a decrease in lean body mass, but electrolytes are normal except when hypokalemic periodic paralysis occurs.

Hematopoietic System

The red blood cells are usually normal, as judged by the usual indices, but red blood cell mass is increased. The increase in erythropoiesis results from both a direct effect of thyroid hormones on the erythroid marrow and increased production of erythropoietin. A parallel increase in plasma volume also occurs, with the result that the hematocrit is normal.

Approximately 3% of patients with Graves' disease have pernicious anemia, and a further 3% have antibodies to intrinsic factor but normal absorption of vitamin B_{12}. Autoantibodies against gastric parietal cells may also be present in patients with Graves' disease, and the requirements for vitamin B_{12} and folic acid appear to be increased. The total white blood cell count is often low because of a decrease in the number of neutrophils. The absolute lymphocyte count is normal or increased, leading to a relative lymphocytosis. The numbers of monocytes and eosinophils may also be increased. Splenic enlargement occurs in about 10% of the patients, and enlargement of the thymus and lymph nodes is common. The latter may manifest as a mediastinal mass. Thymic hyperplasia is also sometimes seen in patients with thyroid cancer receiving excess exogenous thyroxine for TSH suppression.[42,43]

Platelet levels and the intrinsic clotting mechanism are normal, but the concentration of factor VIII is often increased, returning to normal after the thyrotoxicosis is treated. Despite this increase, there is an enhanced sensitivity to warfarin because of accelerated clearance of the vitamin K–dependent clotting factors. Therefore, the dosage of warfarin needs to be reduced in thyrotoxic patients.[44] This must be kept in mind if anticoagulant treatment for atrial fibrillation is being initiated.[45] Coincidental autoimmune thrombocytopenia may also occur.

Pituitary and Adrenocortical Function

The thyrotoxic state imposes several challenges on pituitary and adrenocortical function. The hepatic inactivation of cortisol is accelerated with increased levels of $5\alpha/5\beta$-reductases. As a result of these changes, the disposal of cortisol is accelerated, but its rate of secretion is also increased, so the plasma cortisol concentration remains normal. The concentration of corticosteroid-binding globulin in plasma is also normal. The urinary excretion of free cortisol is normal or slightly increased (see Chapter 15).[46]

Reproductive Function

Thyrotoxicosis in early life may cause delayed sexual maturation, although physical development is normal and skeletal growth may be accelerated. Thyrotoxicosis after puberty influences reproductive function, especially in women. The intermenstrual interval may be prolonged or shortened; menstrual flow is initially diminished and ultimately ceases. Fertility may be reduced, and if conception takes place, there is an increased risk of miscarriage.[47,48] In some patients, menstrual cycles are predominantly anovulatory with oligomenorrhea, but ovulation occurs in most, as indicated by a secretory endometrium. In those with anovulatory cycles, a subnormal midcycle surge of luteinizing hormone (LH) may be responsible. In premenopausal women with thyrotoxicosis, basal plasma concentrations of LH and follicle-stimulating hormone (FSH) are reportedly normal but may display enhanced responsiveness to gonadotropin-releasing hormone (GnRH).

Thyrotoxicosis, whether spontaneous or induced by exogenous hormone, is accompanied by an increase in the concentration of sex hormone–binding globulin (SHBG) in plasma.[49] As a result, the plasma concentrations of total testosterone, dihydrotestosterone, and estradiol are increased, but their unbound fractions are normal or transiently decreased. Increased binding in plasma may be responsible for the decreased metabolic clearance rate of testosterone and dihydrotestosterone. In the case of estradiol, however, the metabolic clearance rate is normal, suggesting that tissue metabolism of the hormone is increased. Conversion rates of androstenedione to testosterone, estrone, and estradiol and of testosterone to dihydrotestosterone are increased.[50] The increased rate of conversion of androgens to estrogenic byproducts may be the mechanism for gynecomastia and erectile dysfunction in some 10% of thyrotoxic men and one mechanism for menstrual irregularities in women. Another likely mechanism for menstrual changes is the disruption in amplitude and frequency of LH/FSH pulses caused by thyroid hormone influences on GnRH signaling.

LABORATORY DIAGNOSIS

The effects of thyrotoxicosis on the major organ systems are the same regardless of the underlying etiology, but the frequency and intensity of these effects and the other findings with which they are associated are influenced by the cause of the excess thyroid hormone. To a large extent, the same is true of laboratory test results. However, the patient with thyrotoxic symptoms will almost always have a serum TSH concentration of less than 0.1 mU/L and an elevated concentration of serum-free thyroxine (T_4). In general, when thyrotoxicosis is caused by hyperthyroidism, serum free T_3 is more elevated than the free T_4 is, but this measurement is rarely required for an accurate diagnosis.

If the possibility of exogenous thyroid hormone can be eliminated, the primary differential is between hyperthyroidism and thyroiditis (Fig. 12-1). Often, this differentiation can be made on the basis of the history and physical examination. Laboratory findings, including an increased sedimentation rate and a high serum thyroglobulin level, may favor thyroiditis, but the most critical differentiating test is the radioactive iodine uptake (RAIU), which is elevated or inappropriately high-normal given the suppressed serum TSH level in hyperthyroidism and very low (<5%) in patients with thyroiditis. However, the RAIU may be low in a hyperthyroid patient who has recently received an iodine load, usually iodinated contrast for a computed tomographic (CT) scan or for angiography. A 24-hour urine iodine measurement can confirm this.

If the physical examination or thyroid ultrasonography indicates the presence of a nodular thyroid, scintigraphy can confirm nodular hyperfunction. The association of thyrotoxicosis with an elevated TSH is rare and suggests a TSH-producing pituitary tumor (see Fig. 12-1). The possibility of an artifactually elevated TSH level in a patient with Graves' disease should be ruled out by repetition of the assay by a different method in another laboratory (see Chapter 6). Exceptions to these general guidelines are discussed later, within the appropriate subsection.

GRAVES' DISEASE

Robert Graves' disease, although first described by Parry in 1825,[51] is best known as Graves' disease in the English-speaking world and as von Basedow's disease on the continent of Europe because of the prominence of the disease reports by these eminent physicians. It is the most enigmatic and, in areas of iodine abundance, one of the most common thyroid diseases, representing 50% to 80% of all cases of thyrotoxicosis.

Presentation

Graves' disease is characterized by diffuse goiter and thyrotoxicosis; it may be accompanied by an infiltrative orbitopathy and ophthalmopathy and occasionally by infiltrative dermopathy. In an individual patient, thyroid

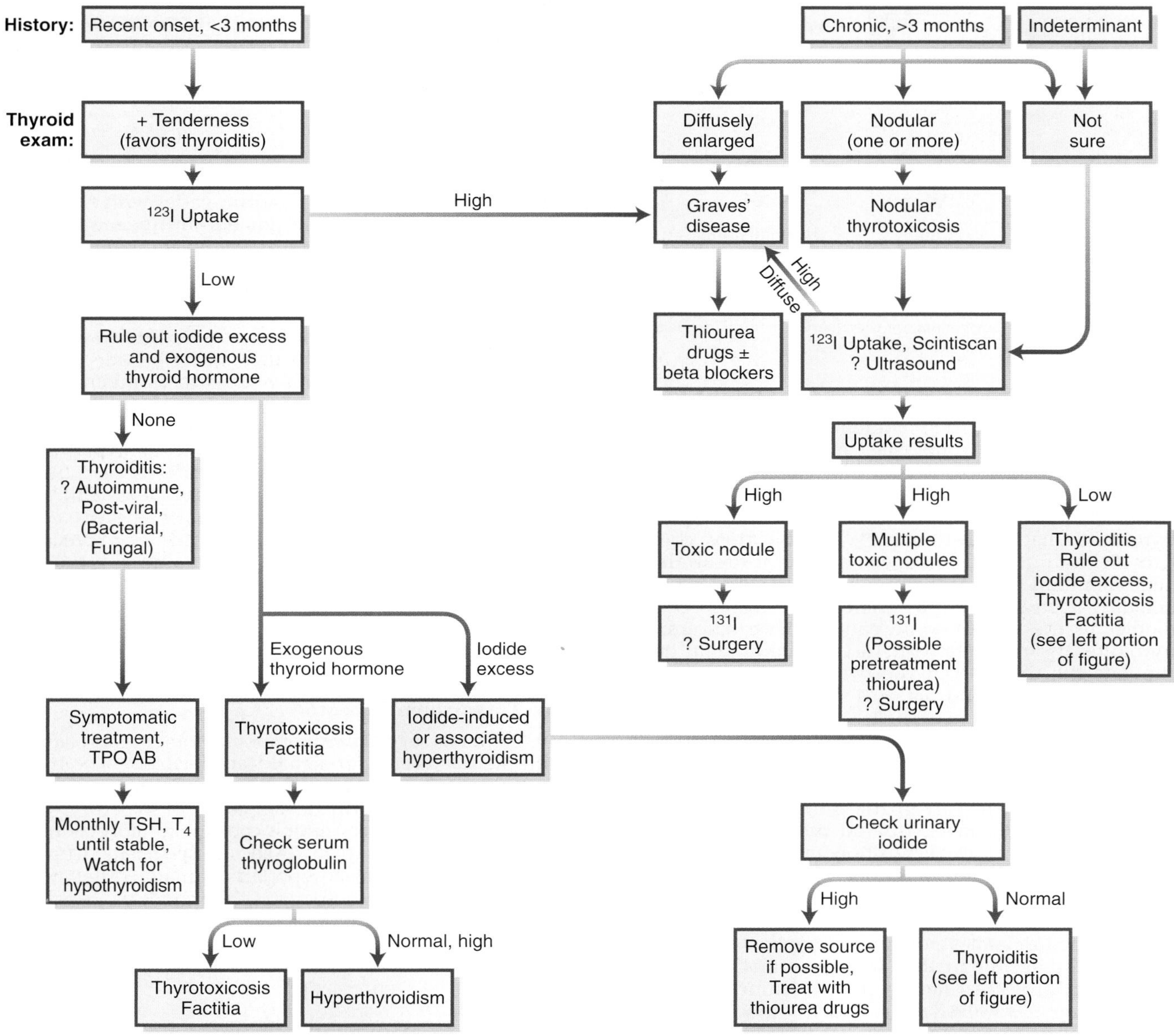

Figure 12-1 Algorithm for determining the cause of thyrotropin-independent thyrotoxicosis. T_3, triiodothyronine; T_4, thyroxine; TPO AB, thyroid peroxidase antibody; TSH, thyroid-stimulating hormone (thyrotropin).

disease and the infiltrative phenomena may occur singly or together, but their courses are largely independent. The thyroid histology is closely related to autoimmune thyroiditis with the presence of lymphocytic infiltrate. In Graves' disease, hyperthyroidism occurs in the presence of some degree of chronic thyroiditis and may ultimately be replaced, in the long term, by thyroid hypofunction. Conversely, hyperthyroidism may occasionally supervene in patients with preexisting Hashimoto's thyroiditis. Both of these diseases may occur within the same family.

Autoimmune Characteristics

Autoimmune thyroid disease is characterized by the occurrence in the serum of antibodies against thyroid peroxidase (TPO) (still incorrectly called the "microsomal" antigen by many physicians), thyroglobulin (Tg), and the TSH receptor (TSHR). T cell–mediated autoimmunity can also be demonstrated against the three primary thyroid antigens, as judged by a variety of criteria, including the ability of the T cells to elaborate various cytokines and to exhibit a mitogenic response when exposed to thyroid antigens or peptide sequences from the antigens.[52] Autoimmune thyroid disease is also characterized by lymphocytic infiltration of the thyroid gland—intense in autoimmune thyroiditis and heterogeneous in Graves' disease. In patients and their relatives, there is an increased frequency of other disorders of autoimmune origin, such as insulin-dependent diabetes mellitus, pernicious anemia, myasthenia gravis, Addison's disease, Sjögren's syndrome,

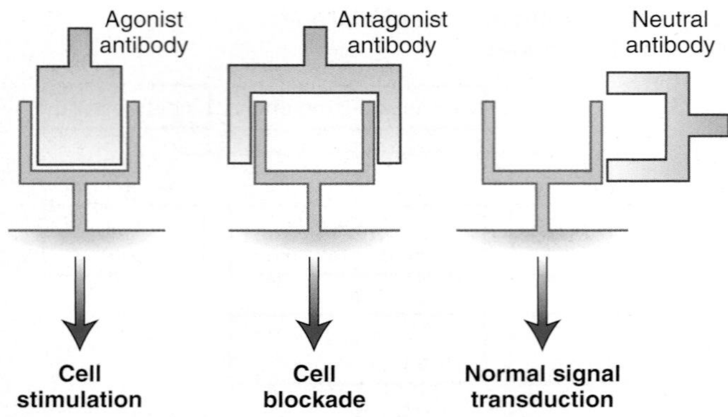

Figure 12-2 Schematic diagram of thyroid cell stimulation and blockade by antibodies to the thyroid-stimulating hormone receptor. Such autoantibodies may act as agonists or antagonists, or they may be neutral, depending on how they interact within the extracellular domain.

lupus erythematosus, rheumatoid arthritis, and idiopathic thrombocytopenic purpura (see Chapter 42).

The circulating autoantibodies specific to hyperthyroid Graves' disease are directed against the TSHR and are called thyrotropin receptor antibodies (TRAbs). They behave as thyroid-stimulating antibodies[53] because they compete with TSH for binding to its specific receptor site in the cell membrane and can activate multiple signaling pathways including adenylate cyclase.[54] Similar but distinct autoantibodies in the sera of some patients with autoimmune thyroiditis also compete with TSH for binding but do not stimulate the thyroid cell very well; they may block the ligand-binding site and act as TSH antagonists or weak agonists. Others are neutral in their influence on TSH binding but may also act as weak agonists (Fig. 12-2).

The thyroid gland itself is the major site of thyroid autoantibody secretion in autoimmune thyroid disease via the B cells that form part of the intrathyroidal infiltrate. Transplantation of Graves' thyroid tissue into T cell– and B cell–deficient mice with severe combined immunodeficiency (SCID mice) results in the appearance of human thyroid autoantibodies, including TRAbs, in the serum.[55] Additional evidence for a role of the thyroid itself in antibody production comes from animal models of thyroiditis and from the decline in thyroid autoantibody levels after anti-thyroid drug treatment,[56] thyroidectomy, or radioiodine ablation.[57] However, some patients shown no loss of autoantibody secretion after thyroidectomy or radioiodine treatment, which suggests extrathyroidal sources of continued production. The role of the TSHR expressed in extrathyroidal tissues in perpetuating this response remains uncertain.

Pathology

In patients with Graves' disease, the thyroid gland is characterized by a nonhomogeneous lymphocytic infiltration with an absence of easily found follicular destruction, although areas of apoptosis can be discerned by specific staining (Fig. 12-3).[58] Anti-thyroid drug treatment may reduce the degree of infiltration, influencing the observed histology.

Although the intrathyroidal lymphocyte population is mixed, most are T lymphocytes (both Th1 and Th2 types, along with CD25+ regulatory T cells); B-cell germinal centers are much less common than in autoimmune thyroiditis. However, both intraepithelial T cells and plasma cells can be seen in peripolesis within the thyroid follicles. Follicular epithelial cell size correlates with the intensity of the local infiltrate, suggesting local thyroid cell stimulation by TRAbs. Memory T cells may predominate within the T-cell population, but this finding can vary from patient to patient. Activated B-cell and T-cell markers are more frequent in intrathyroidal lymphocyte cultures than in peripheral blood cultures.

Prevalence

The prevalence of hyperthyroidism varies with the degree of iodine sufficiency in the population under study. The National Health and Nutrition Examination Survey (NHANES III) data[59] from the United States and a detailed epidemiologic survey in the United Kingdom[60] demonstrated the female preponderance among thyroid patients and the lower prevalence of hyperthyroidism compared to hypothyroidism. The results indicated a prevalence of 1% to 2% in women and about one tenth as much in men. Overall, the incidence in women was estimated to be 1 case per 1000 per year over a 20-year follow-up. Graves' disease is the most common cause of spontaneous hyperthyroidism in patients younger than 40 years of age, and the hazard rate does not change with age. The overall prevalence of autoimmune thyroid disease (i.e., Graves' disease and autoimmune thyroiditis) approaches or exceeds that of diabetes mellitus; when mild thyroid disease is included, the prevalence may be very much higher.

Pathogenesis

The Major Antigen of Graves' Disease: The Thyrotropin Receptor

The TSHR has seven transmembrane domains and employs multiple G proteins for signal transduction.[61] The human TSHR (hTSHR) is the primary autoantigen of Graves' disease, as shown by the development of hyperthyroidism in mice and hamsters after exposure to normal hTSHR antigen.[62-64] Extrathyroidal TSHR messenger RNA (mRNA) and protein have been reported in many other tissues, including fibrocytes, adipocytes, lymphocytes, osteoclasts and osteoblasts, and pituitary cells. Although the physiologic role of TSHRs in these sites is slowly being revealed, their role in autoimmune thyroid disease remains mostly unclear.

Molecular Structure of the Human Thyrotropin Receptor

Cloning of human TSHR complementary DNA (cDNA) made it possible to begin to define the structure of the hTSHR gene; its chromosomal location (14q31) and its crystallographic structure have now been revealed.[65] Seven hydrophobic transmembrane spanning regions in the hTSHR indicate that it is a member of the G protein–coupled receptor gene superfamily, and those receptors with large extracellular domains have been designated subgroup B. The TSH holoreceptor consists of a 100-kd, glycosylated, 744-amino-acid sequence and a 20-amino-acid signal peptide. The TSHR holoreceptor is cleaved into two subunits, designated α (or A) and β (or B), which are linked by disulfide bonds to form the physiologic receptor (Fig. 12-4). The 50-kd α-subunit is water soluble and has TSH-binding activity. TSH and TRAbs bind to the leucine-rich repeat (LRR) regions of the α-subunit.[66,67] The 30-kd β-subunit is water insoluble, contains the membrane-spanning domain with its three extracellular loops and

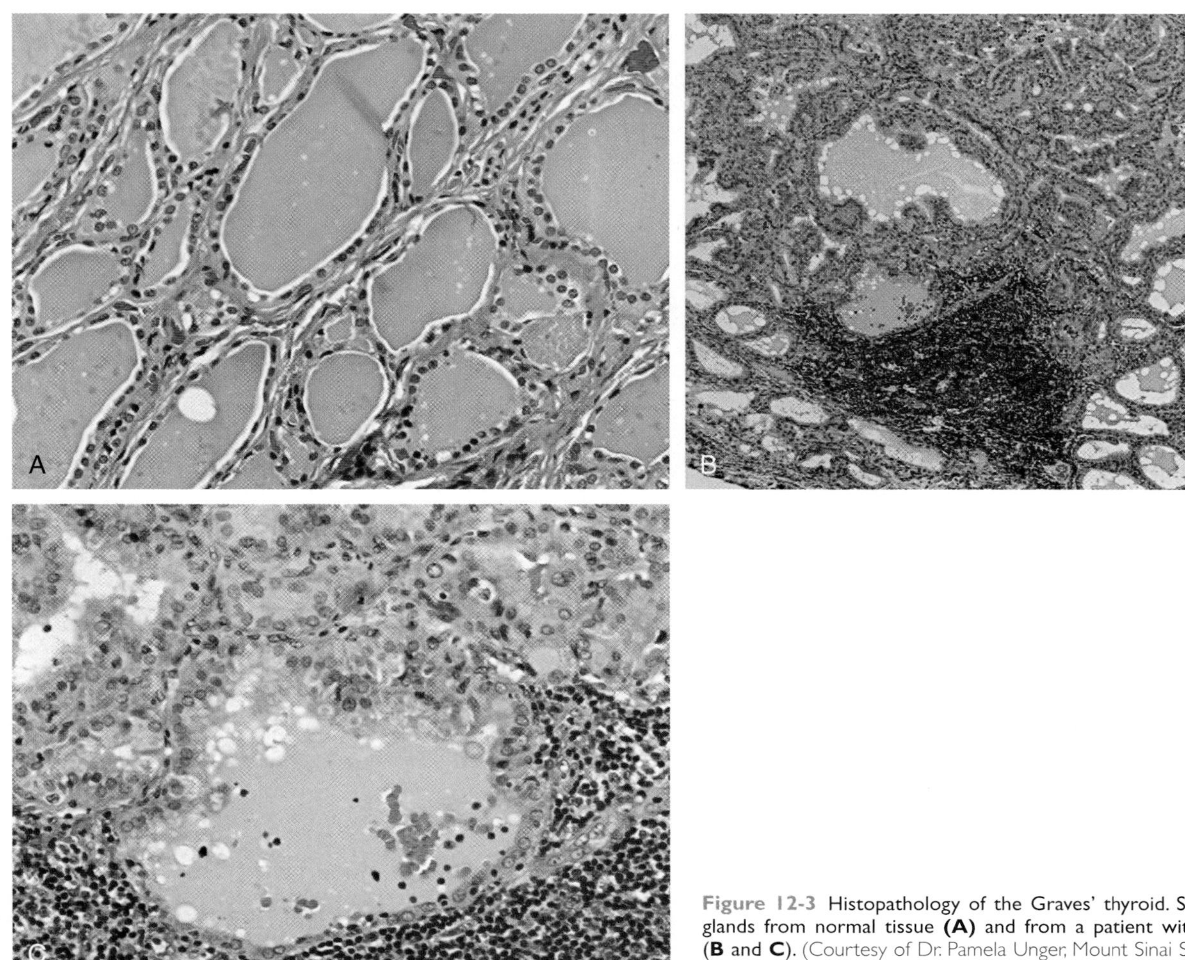

Figure 12-3 Histopathology of the Graves' thyroid. Sections of thyroid glands from normal tissue **(A)** and from a patient with Graves' disease **(B** and **C)**. (Courtesy of Dr. Pamela Unger, Mount Sinai School of Medicine, New York, NY.)

three cytoplasmic loops, and is 70% to 75% homologous with the LH/human chorionic gonadotropin (hCG) receptor. Shedding of the α-subunit has been shown in vitro, and this has been suggested to also occur in vivo. The TSHR forms dimers and multimeric complexes on the thyroid-cell surface, which appears to enhance the stability of the receptor.[53]

Autoantibodies to the Thyrotropin Receptor

In Graves' disease, TRAbs, discovered by Adams and Purves,[68,69] bind to the TSHR and activate $G_s\alpha$ and G_q signaling complexes; this ultimately induces thyroid growth, increases vascularity, and causes an increased rate of thyroid hormone production and secretion. As mentioned earlier, TRAbs in patients with Graves' disease are referred to as thyroid-stimulating antibodies. Other varieties of TRAbs may also be present, and all antibodies that bind to the TSHR appear to have the capacity for signal transduction to varying degrees.[54] Receptor antibodies that act as TSH antagonists are referred to as *blocking* TRAbs, although they may still initiate some signaling. In the same way, *neutral* antibodies may also signal to varying degrees. These different types of TRAbs may co-occur with the stimulating type, and they may predominate in certain patients after treatment with radioiodine, anti-thyroid drugs, or surgery (see Fig. 12-2). Blocking TRAbs can also be found in 15% of patients with autoimmune thyroiditis, particularly in patients without a goiter (the atrophic variety).[70] TRAbs are not detectable in the normal population with the use of currently available methods.

Bioactivity of Thyrotropin Receptor Autoantibodies

The self-infusion of sera from patients with Graves' disease caused thyroid stimulation and was the first demonstration of the role of TRAbs in the induction of human hyperthyroidism.[71] Another example of the in vivo effects of TRAbs came from studies in neonates demonstrating transplacental stimulation of the fetal thyroid in mothers with high titers of TRAbs.[72] TRAbs show light-chain restriction in many patients with Graves' disease, and TRAbs that exhibit TSH agonist bioactivity are in the immunoglobulin G1 (IgG1) subclass; both observations suggest oligoclonality.[73,74]

Prevalence of Thyrotropin Receptor Autoantibodies in Graves' Disease

The fact that TRAbs are detectable only in patients with autoimmune thyroid disease indicates that the autoantibodies are disease specific, in contrast to the high

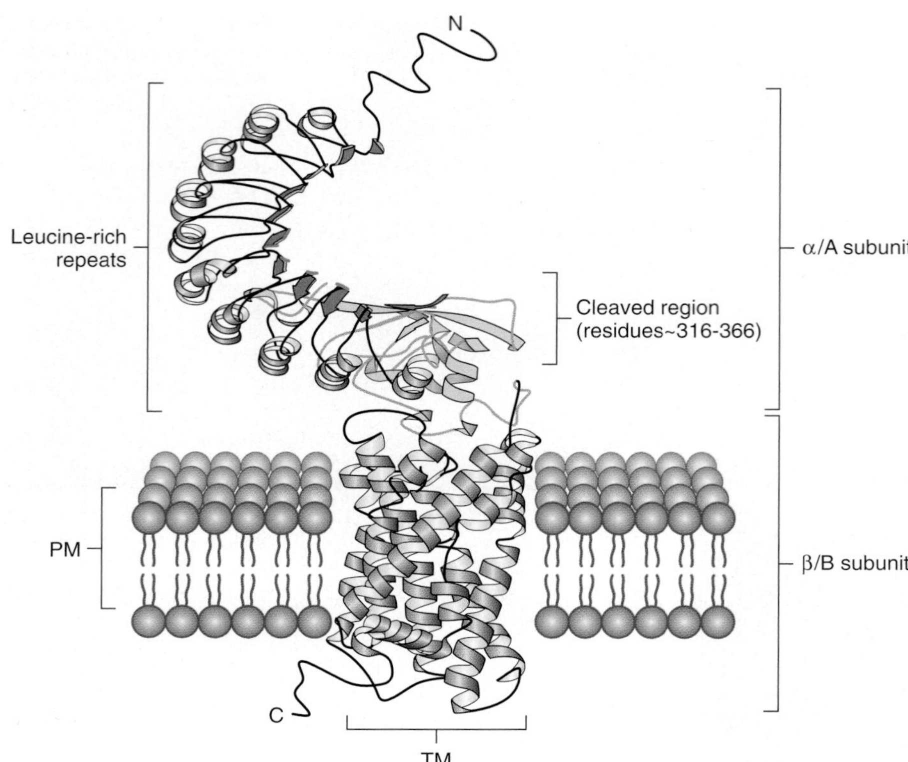

Figure 12-4 Structure of the human thyroid-stimulating hormone receptor (TSHR). The TSHR has seven transmembrane domains, a large extracellular domain, and a small intracellular domain. The receptor is cleaved, probably after activation, into α (or A) and β (or B) subunits. The α-subunit is thought to be shed from the cell surface. C, carboxyterminus; N, aminoterminus; PM, plasma membrane; TM, transmembrane domain. (Adapted from Nunez MR, Sanders J, Jeffreys J, et al. Analysis of the thyrotropin receptor-thyrotropin interaction by comparative modeling. *Thyroid.* 2004;14:991-1011.)

prevalence of Tg antibodies (Tg-Ab) and TPO antibodies (TPO-Ab) in the population. Furthermore, TRAbs are unique human autoantibodies and do not occur in natural animal disease. A total of 90% to 100% of untreated hyperthyroid patients with Graves' disease have detectable TRAbs with thyroid-stimulating activity when measured by a sensitive assay.[75-77] The levels of TRAbs are decreased by treatment of the disease and, when they persist, may predict recurrence.[78-80] With time, TSHR-blocking autoantibodies may become the more prevalent type after treatment of Graves' disease causing hypothyroidism.

Intrathyroidal T Cells

T cells in patients with autoimmune thyroid disease are reactive to thyroid antigens and to peptides derived from these antigens[81,82] and are oligoclonal. About 10% of activated T cells infiltrating the thyroid gland in patients with autoimmune thyroid disease proliferate in response to thyroid-cell antigens. Intrathyroidal T cells from patients with Graves' disease exhibit characteristics of both helper T cell subset 1 (Th1), which are recognized by their secretion of interleukin-2 (IL-2) and interferon-γ, and helper T cell subset 2 (Th2), which are recognized by their secretion of IL-4.[83] The presence of Treg cells and Th17 cells in situ in Graves' thyroid tissue awaits characterization.

Regulation of the Immune Response in Autoimmune Thyroid Disease

Although thyroid hormone excess itself may give rise to changes in T-cell numbers and function, the immune system continues to exert its overall peripheral control. This is achieved by secretion of T-cell cytokines, by the suppressive influence of "anergized" T cells, and by the presence of regulatory cells that are a subset of CD4+ T cells (D25+Fox3p+) and have now been extensively characterized.[84] Such regulatory cells can suppress experimental thyroiditis in a variety of models,[67,85] although their characterization in hyperthyroid patients with Graves' disease has not shown major disruption.[86] Studies of Th17, a new subset of T cells thought to be important in the initiation of autoimmune disease, are awaited.

In addition to these potential regulatory influences, another important mechanism of control is central tolerance caused by positive and negative selection of T cells and B cells in the thymus, where thyroid antigens, including the TSHR, are expressed.[87,88] Here, the role of the *AIRE* gene has been clarified as important in self-antigen presentation, including presentation of thyroid antigens.[89] Failure of such mechanisms may lead to the development of pathology but must be distinguished from those risk factors that allow the initiation of disease, which are discussed separately.

Mechanisms in the Development of Autoimmune Thyroid Disease

The Consequences of an Insult

Initiation of autoimmune thyroid disease is thought to occur with an insult that leads to an immune response (Fig. 12-5). This may take the form of a direct insult to the thyroid gland by a viral infection or another external influence (e.g., trauma) leading to activation of T cells,[90,91] currently presumed to be of the Th17 variety. Alternatively, it may be initiated elsewhere in the body. In the latter case, the arrival of activated T cells in the thyroid gland starts the process. Such an arrival may be nonspecific, because the same T cells may arrive in many glands, but the patient has a particular susceptibility to autoimmune thyroid disease. Initiation of disease may be mediated by bystander

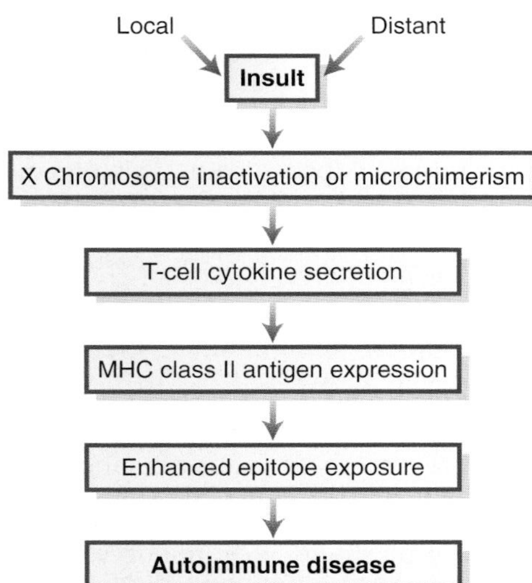

Figure 12-5 An overview of the most likely mechanisms involved in the cause and precipitation of Graves' disease. MHC, major histocompatibility complex.

activation, molecular mimicry, or cryptic antigen presentation, as described in the following sections, but the importance of these different mechanisms in Graves' disease remains uncertain.

Mechanism #1—Bystander Activation

Evidence has mounted that bystander activation of local resident antigen-specific and nonspecific T cells may initiate autoimmunity.[92,93] The presence of activated T cells within the thyroid gland after an insult may induce, via cytokine secretion, the activation of local thyroid-specific and non–thyroid-specific T cells, as demonstrated in animal models of thyroiditis.[94] This series of events can occur only in a susceptible individual with the right immune repertoire. Bystander activation could arise from any T cells within the thyroid gland, which could be activated by many different infections and antigens unrelated to the thyroid gland itself. The attractiveness of this model is that many different types of infection could lead to the same clinical disease phenotype. There is much evidence for residual thyroid-resident T cells and dendritic cells in the glands of patients with Graves' disease that could have been activated by this mechanism at the time of disease onset.[95]

Mechanism #2—Molecular Mimicry (Specificity Crossover)

In addition to the effects of the direct release of cytokines from T cells activated elsewhere via the bystander effect, intrathyroidal T cells may become activated in another nonspecific way. Structural or conformational similarity (i.e., sequence, shape, or both) between different antigens can lead to specificity crossover (or molecular mimicry).[96] Antigenic similarity between bacteria or viruses and human proteins is common, and in one study 4% of monoclonal antibodies raised against a variety of viruses cross-reacted with antigens in tissues.[97] Furthermore, mice infected with reovirus type 1 developed an autoimmune polyendocrinopathy with autoantibodies directed against normal pancreas, pituitary, thyroid, and gastric mucosa, suggesting molecular mimicry between a reoviral antigen and a common tissue antigen.[98] Molecular mimicry has also been reported between *Yersinia enterocolitica* and the TSHR based on the observed cross-reaction between sera from patients with *Yersinia* infection and sera from patients with Graves' disease.[99,100] Similar evidence has been presented on the basis of structural similarities between borellia or retroviral sequences and the TSHR.[101]

Mechanism #3—Thyroid Cell Involvement by Aberrant Expression of Class II HLA Antigens

Normal thyroid epithelial cells do not express human leukocyte antigen (HLA) class II antigens, but they are markedly expressed in thyroid glands from patients with autoimmune thyroid disease (Fig. 12-6).[102] A local insult, whether trauma or infection of the thyroid gland, can cause an inflammatory infiltrate and the production of interferons or other cytokines in the thyroid gland that are able to induce HLA class II antigen expression. HLA class II antigens are used to present antigen to the immune system (discussed earlier), and overexpression on the thyroid cell would lead to enhanced presentation of thyroid autoantigens and activation of local autoreactive thyroid-specific T cells in a susceptible individual. Support for this concept comes from the in vivo induction of such molecules on mouse thyrocytes by interferon-α that also induced autoimmune thyroiditis[103] and from the demonstration of the necessity for major histocompatibility complex (MHC) molecules on TSHR-expressing fibroblasts used in the induction of Graves' disease in mice.[62] A number of viruses may also induce thyroid-cell expression of such antigens independent of immune-cell cytokine secretion; these include reovirus types 1 and 3 and cytomegalovirus.

Mechanism #4—Cryptic Antigens

T-cell tolerance depends on visualization of self-antigens by the immune system in sufficient amounts to initiate continuous T-cell deletion, anergy induction, and regulatory T-cell activation. However, some antigens and antigenic epitopes are not seen in sufficient concentrations to cause the removal of T cells that react to them. These molecules contain what are sometimes called cryptic epitopes.[104] T cells specific for these cryptic epitopes may be

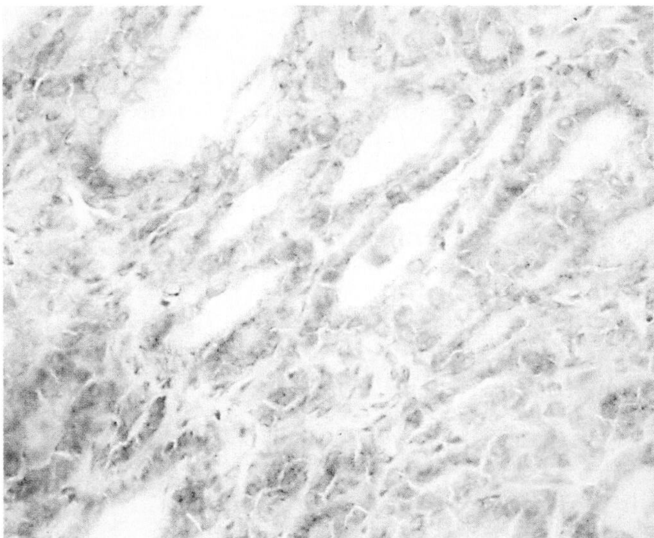

Figure 12-6 Photomicrograph of Graves' thyroid tissue stained for human leukocyte antigen (HLA) class II (DR) antigen expression using the immunoperoxidase technique. Notice the brown thyroid epithelial cells indicating the presence of DR antigen. Notice also the relative lack of lymphocytic infiltration in this region.

present in the immune repertoire, and they may induce autoaggressive T cells if such an epitope is uncovered or increased in concentration by a local insult. HLA class II antigen expression in a situation in which it normally does not occur (e.g., on the thyroid epithelial cell) would then allow the presentation of these normally cryptic thyroid antigens to local autoreactive T cells if they are present. To date, however, such potential cryptic thyroid antigens have not been characterized.

Potential Risk Factors for Graves' Disease

Risk Factor #1—Genetic Susceptibility

The development and course of Graves' disease are greatly influenced by heredity.[105] The role of hereditary factors is evidenced by the increased incidence of other autoimmune disorders in families of these patients, such as Graves' disease, Hashimoto's disease, insulin-dependent diabetes (type 1), or pernicious anemia. Additionally, autoantibodies against endocrine tissues, gastric parietal cells, and intrinsic factor in some families suggest a hereditary influence. Siblings have a high risk of being affected, as shown by a sibling recurrence risk (λs) of 11.6.[106] In addition, monozygotic twins have a higher concordance rate for Graves' disease than do dizygotic twins,[107] despite the rearrangement of B-cell and T-cell V genes that cause the immune repertoires of identical twins to differ (see Chapter 42), thus implicating non-V genes in susceptibility. Nevertheless, the propensity for development of thyroid autoantibodies appears to be an autosomal dominant trait linked to the cytotoxic T-lymphocyte antigen 4 (CTLA4) gene that codes for a modulator of the second signal to T cells.[108]

Because a number of genetic loci may contribute to Graves' disease susceptibility, it is referred to as a polygenic or complex disorder.[109] To date, these genes and gene regions account for only a small part of the calculated genetic susceptibility, so much more remains to be understood. There is a much-investigated association with the HLA gene region (e.g., increased frequency of the HLA DR3 and DQA10501 haplotypes in Caucasians), but this region provides less than 5% of the genetic susceptibility and yields a risk ratio of only twofold to fourfold (Table 12-2).[110,111] Additional nonspecific genetic susceptibility, after the HLA and CTLA4 contributions, includes the genes for lymphoid tyrosine phosphatase (*PTPN22*), the signaling molecule CD40, the IL-2 receptor-α, and the orphan Fc receptor L3, which may all be involved in providing a background autoimmunity susceptibility.

The search for thyroid-specific genetic susceptibility has revealed small influences exerted by polymorphisms in the Tg gene and the TSHR gene but no major thyroid antigen–specific contribution. More remains to be learned about how thyroid disease specificity is engineered into the genetic susceptibility to Graves' disease.

TABLE 12-2

Confirmed Genes Associated with Graves' Disease

Gene	Chromosome	SNPs	Odds Ratio
HLA	6p21		2.0-4.0
CTLA4	2q33	60	1.5-2.2
PTPN22	1p13	250	1.4-1.9
CD40	20q11	125	1.3-1.8
IL2RA	10p15	594	1.1-1.4
FCRL3	1q23	99	1.1-1.3
Tg	8q24	1698	1.3-1.6
TSHR	14q31	984	1.4-2.6

CD40, cluster of differentiation 40; CTLA4, cytotoxic T-lymphocyte antigen 4; FCRL3, Fc receptor L3; HLA, human leukocyte antigen; IL2RA, interleukin 2 receptor-α; PTPN22, protein tyrosine phosphatase nonreceptor type 22; SNPs, single-nucleotide polymorphisms; Tg, thyroglobulin; TSHR, thyroid-stimulating hormone receptor.

Risk Factor #2—Infection

Much has been written about the possible role of infection in the development of autoimmunity acting via bystander effects or molecular mimicry.[112,113] There is no evidence that a specific infection initiates Graves' disease.[90] An identifiable agent should be present in most patients, and transfer of the agent to susceptible recipients should transfer the disease. As discussed earlier, it has been long suggested that Graves' disease is associated with infectious agents (e.g., *Y. enterocolitica*), but no studies meet the necessary criteria to prove this. Infections of the thyroid gland itself (e.g., subacute thyroiditis, congenital rubella, hepatitis C) may be associated with thyroid autoimmune phenomena.[90,114] Nevertheless, a causative role of infectious agents has not been definitively demonstrated in Graves' disease, despite the observation that thyroid disease can be induced in experimental animals by certain viral infections.[115] Reports of retroviral sequences in the thyroid glands of patients with Graves' disease have failed to be reproduced. Clinical infection with human T-cell lymphotropic virus 1 (HTLV-1) has been reported to be associated with the development of autoimmune thyroid disease but most likely as a result of immune-cell changes rather than thyroid infection.[116]

Risk Factor #3—Stress

Commonly, Graves' disease appears to become evident after severe emotional stress (e.g., actual or threatened separation from a loved one) or after an acute fright (e.g., an automobile accident). There are many clinical experiences and reports associating major stress with the onset of Graves' disease, including data on the high incidence of thyrotoxicosis among refugees from Nazi prison camps, which may have been more directly related to iodine status. Some data suggest that stress induces an overall state of immune suppression by nonspecific mechanisms,[117,118] perhaps secondary to the effects of cortisol and the action of corticotropin-releasing hormone at the level of the immune cell. Compared with control groups, more patients with Graves' disease give a history of major stress in the 12 months before disease onset.

After acute immune suppression by stress, there is presumably an overcompensation by the immune system when the suppression is released. This could precipitate autoimmune thyroid disease, similar to the development of thyroiditis or Graves' disease after release from the immunosuppression of pregnancy.[119] The rebound phenomenon would result in greater immune activity than normal and would initiate disease only if the individual were genetically susceptible.

Risk Factor #4—Gender

Graves' disease is more common in women than in men (7:1 to 10:1), and it tends to become more prevalent after puberty. The female preponderance and the fact that the disorder is uncommon before puberty suggest that female sex steroids may be responsible for this difference. Indeed, androgens may actually suppress autoimmune thyroiditis.[120,121] In contrast, estrogen has been shown to influence the immune system, particularly the B-cell repertoire, and

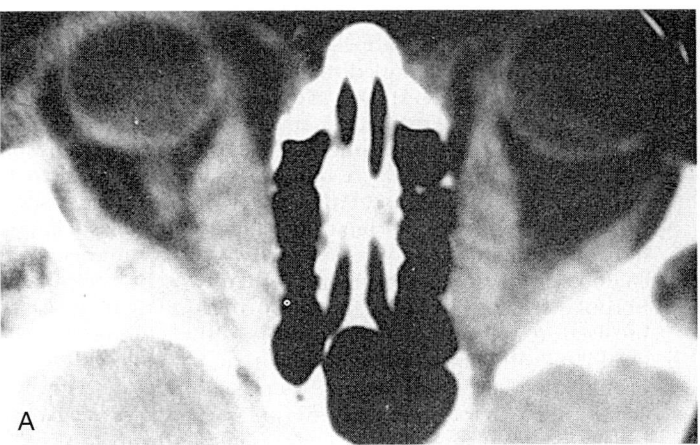

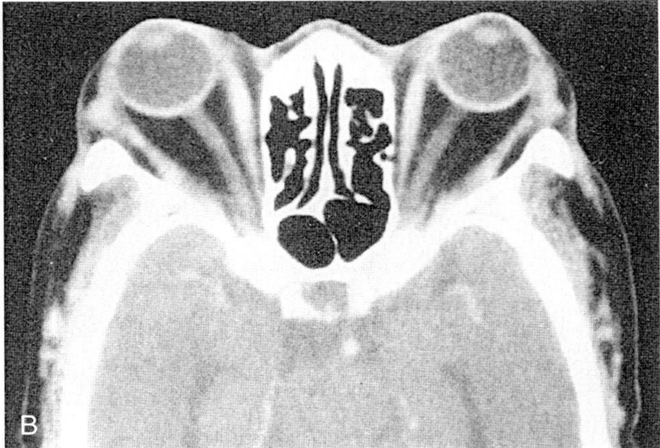

Figure 12-7 Computed tomographic scans of orbits in two patients with Graves' orbitopathy. **A**, Notice the obviously grossly swollen medial rectus extraocular muscles in both orbits and the resulting proptosis. **B**, The patient shows considerable proptosis with only minimal muscle enlargement, suggesting the presence of a large amount of retroorbital fat. (Courtesy of Dr. Peter Som, New York, NY.)

has often been suggested as the reason for female susceptibility. However, Graves' disease continues to occur after the menopause and is seen in many men. When the disease develops in men, it tends to occur at a later age, to be more severe, and to be accompanied more often by ophthalmopathy. Such observations suggest that the X chromosome, rather than sex steroids, may be the responsible element in female susceptibility. Women have two X chromosomes and, therefore, receive twice the gene dose. Genetic studies identified a locus on the X chromosome linked to Graves' disease, but this has not been confirmed in larger studies.[122] The phenomenon of X-chromosome inactivation has also been invoked in autoimmune disease.[123] Female cells may inactivate different X chromosomes to different degrees in different tissues, leading to potentially different immune responses. Evidence for the importance of X-chromosome inactivation has been repeatedly described in Graves' disease.[124-126]

Risk Factor #5—Pregnancy

Severe Graves' disease is uncommon during pregnancy, because hyperthyroidism is associated with reduced fertility. For those women with milder disease who successfully conceive, hyperthyroidism endows an increased risk of pregnancy loss and complications in established pregnancy,[127,128] as exemplified by the influence of high thyroid hormone levels in normal pregnancy in patients with thyroid hormone resistance.[129] Such data indicate that excess thyroid hormone has a direct toxic effect on the fetus. However, pregnancy is a time of immunosuppression, so that the disease tends to improve as pregnancy progresses. Both T-cell and B-cell functions are diminished as pregnancy progresses, under the influence of local placental factors and regulatory T cells (see later discussion).[130] Rebound from this immunosuppression after delivery may contribute to the development of postpartum thyroid disease.[131] As many as 30% of young female patients give a history of pregnancy in the 12 months before the onset of Graves' disease,[132] indicating that postpartum Graves' disease is a surprisingly common presentation and that pregnancy is a major risk factor for development of the disease in susceptible women (see later discussion). Consistent with this observation is the higher rate of Graves' disease relapse occurring after delivery in women who were previously in remission.[133]

Risk Factor #6—Iodine and Drugs

Iodine, iodine-containing drugs (e.g., amiodarone), and iodine-containing contrast media may precipitate Graves' disease or its recurrence in a susceptible individual.[134,135] Iodine is most likely to precipitate thyrotoxicosis in an iodine-deficient population, simply by allowing TRAbs to effectively stimulate the formation of more thyroid hormone. Whether there is any other precipitating event is unclear. Iodine may also damage thyroid cells directly, releasing thyroid antigens to the immune system.

Risk Factor #7—Irradiation

There is no evidence that radiation exposure itself is a risk factor for Graves' disease, although Graves' disease is well known to be precipitated in some patients treated with radioactive iodine for multinodular goiter.[136,137] There is also evidence that thyroid autoantibodies are more prevalent in a radiation-exposed population, and claims of increased autoimmune thyroiditis in such populations have been made.[138-140] In addition, radioactive iodine treatment may cause the onset or worsening of clinical ophthalmopathy, but often this is transient (see later discussion).[141]

Pathogenesis of Graves' Orbitopathy and Dermopathy

The pathogenesis of the orbitopathy and dermopathy is now better understood than ever before. The extraocular muscle and adipose tissue are swollen by the accumulation in the extracellular matrix of glycosaminoglycans that are secreted by fibroblasts under the influence of cytokines such as interferon-γ from local lymphocytes (Fig. 12-7; see also Fig. 12-6).[142] This accumulation of glycosaminoglycans disrupts and impairs the function of muscle. As the disease runs its course and inflammation decreases, the damaged muscles become fibrosed. Histologic examination of the extraocular muscles shows disrupted muscle fibrils and a patchy lymphocytic infiltrate, predominantly of T cells, and some muscle cells exhibit HLA class II antigen as seen within the thyroid gland. Such T cells react in vitro with retroorbital tissue.[143,144] Transplantation of extraocular muscle into mice deficient in B cells and T cells (SCID/SCID mice) causes TRAbs to appear in the murine serum, showing accumulation of TSHR-reactive cells within the muscle samples.[145] Evidence of TSHR expression in retroorbital and pretibial tissues such as fibrocytes and adipocytes has strengthened the notion that it is the TSHR itself that is responsible for the immune response.[142] Retroorbital fibrocytes may be derived from circulating marrow fibrocytes, and they express more TSHR than is seen at other sites, which also supports the TSHRs as the primary antigen of Graves' orbitopathy.[146] Studies on the role of the insulin-like growth factor 1 (IGF1) receptor as a retroorbital antigen and the role of serum IGF1 and IGF1 receptor antibodies may shed further light on the propensity for the eyes and skin to be involved in Graves' disease by acting synergistically with TSHR antibodies.[147,148]

In keeping with the hypothesis that the TSHR is the primary antigen, patients with the most severe orbitopathy have the highest titers of TRAbs, and the level of TRAbs often correlates with the severity of the eye disease. There is currently no convincing evidence that specific antibodies against orbital tissue contents play a primary pathogenic role. More likely, antigen-specific T cells have the major role in initiating the disorder, perhaps augmented by TSHR antibodies providing additional signaling at the target cells. However, non–eye-specific antibodies may serve as markers of extraocular muscle inflammation, including the recently described antibodies to the IGF1 receptor.[149]

Risk Factors for Graves' Orbitopathy and Dermopathy

Although there have been many claims, there is still no reproducible evidence that a separate and distinct genetic risk can be ascribed to severe ophthalmic Graves' disease; this suggests that it is mainly environmental factors that lead to the enhanced retroorbital inflammation in some patients.[150] All of the same risk factors (e.g., infection, stress, gender and gonadal steroids, pregnancy, drugs, irradiation) apply to the onset of both thyroid and eye involvement in Graves' disease.

There are, however, three additional distinct risk factors that deserve attention. The first is smoking, which has increased the risk for ophthalmic involvement in many studies, perhaps by causing anoxia or simply by direct inflammation.[151] The second is radioiodine, which in controlled clinical trials accentuates ophthalmic Graves' disease.[141] However, this worsening is related to the severity of the baseline ophthalmopathy, which may be mild and transient, and it may be ameliorated with corticosteroid treatment lasting 3 to 4 months. Many physicians are reluctant to prescribe radioiodine to patients with moderate or severe eye disease unless they are receiving corticosteroids. Third, the role of trauma in the initiation of thyroid and retroorbital inflammation is well recognized.[88,91,150]

Natural History and Course of Graves' Disease

The course of the thyrotoxic component of Graves' disease is variable. In some patients, thyrotoxicosis persists, although it may vary in severity. In others, the course is cyclic, exhibiting remissions of varying frequency, intensity, and duration. This cyclic feature has an important bearing on treatment. With the passage of months or years, thyrotoxicosis tends to give way to euthyroidism. Approximately one third of patients become hypothyroid within 20 years after treatment with anti-thyroid agents.[152]

The orbitopathy may or may not commence together with the thyrotoxic component. Thyrotoxic patients may initially be free from eye disease but become affected by it months or years later or not at all. Conversely, orbitopathy may be the first manifestation of future Graves' disease, with hyperthyroidism developing later. In euthyroid patients with orbitopathy, evidence of a thyroid abnormality may be manifested only by the presence of TRAbs and other thyroid autoantibodies. Some of these patients become hypothyroid within a few years, some become hyperthyroid, and a few remain euthyroid. However, many such euthyroid patients do have evidence of chronic thyroiditis. The course of thyroid function in many of these patients is therefore unpredictable.

Histopathology

Thyroid Gland

The older designation for Graves' disease, *diffuse toxic goiter,* reflected the fact that the gland is both enlarged and uniformly affected. The gland may vary in consistency, from softer than normal to firm and rubbery, depending on the degree of thyroiditis. The outer surface is usually smooth but may be somewhat lobular; less commonly, the gland is grossly nodular before treatment. The cut surface is red and glistening. Microscopically, the follicles are small and lined with hyperplastic columnar epithelium and contain scant colloid that displays much marginal scalloping and vacuolization (see Fig. 12-3). Nuclei are vesicular and basally located and exhibit occasional mitoses. Papillary projections of the hyperplastic epithelium extend into the lumina of the follicles. Vascularity is increased, and there is a varying heterogeneous infiltration by lymphocytes and plasma cells that collect in aggregates and may form infrequent germinal centers. In such regions, thyroid epithelial cells express HLA class II antigens, a phenomenon not seen in normal thyroid glands, and are large, perhaps due to local stimulation by TRAbs.

When the patient is given iodine or anti-thyroid drugs, the thyroid gland may undergo involution if TRAbs decrease. Then hyperplasia and vascularity regress, papillary projections recede, and follicles enlarge and become filled with colloid once again.

Eyes

In patients with infiltrative orbitopathy, the volume of orbital contents is enlarged because of increases in retrobulbar connective tissue and adipose tissue and in the total extraocular muscle mass (see Fig. 12-7). Some of the increase in muscle mass is due to edema resulting from accumulation in the ground substance of hyaluronic acid and chondroitin sulfates, which are hydrophilic; this is thought to be the result of cytokine action. The extraocular muscles are swollen, and some fibers exhibit loss of striation, fragmentation, and lymphocytic infiltration. The lacrimal glands may also be involved. Ultimately, the tissues fibrose (Fig. 12-8).

Skin

The most uncommon element of the Graves' triad, dermopathy (Fig. 12-9) is usually a late manifestation, and 99% of patients with infiltrative dermopathy have Graves' orbitopathy. The content of hyaluronic acid and chondroitin sulfates in the dermis is increased, probably secondary to cytokine activation of fibroblasts. This causes compression of the dermal lymphatics and nonpitting edema: the collagen fibers are separated and fragmented, and

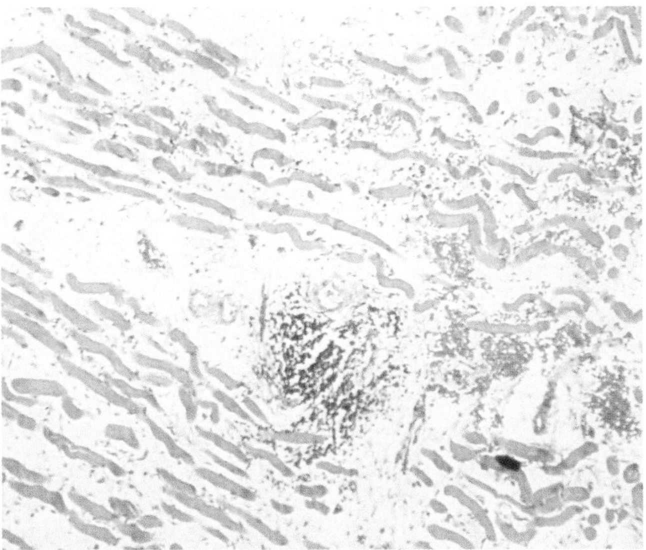

Figure 12-8 Section of extraocular muscle from a biopsy taken from a patient with severe Graves' orbitopathy. Notice the patch of lymphocytic infiltration within the muscle fibers. (Courtesy of Dr. D. Kendler, University of British Columbia, Vancouver, Canada.)

early lesions contain a lymphocytic infiltrate. As discussed earlier, TSHR expression can be demonstrated in fibroblasts and adipocytes,[142] and TRAbs are very high in such patients. Nodule and plaque formation may occur in chronic lesions.

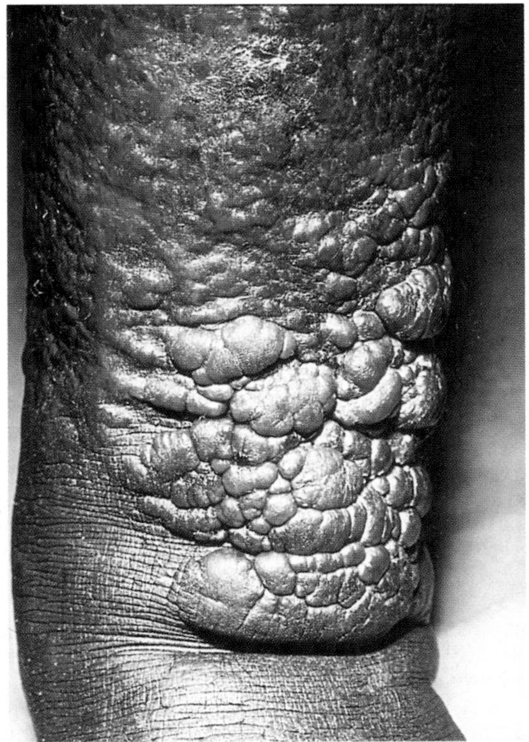

Figure 12-9 Chronic pretibial myxedema in a patient with Graves' disease and orbitopathy. The lesions are firm and nonpitting, with a clear edge to feel. (Courtesy of Dr. Andrew Werner, New York, NY.)

Pathophysiology

In Graves' disease, normal pituitary regulatory mechanisms are overridden by the action of TRAbs of the stimulating variety. The resulting hyperfunction of the thyroid gland leads to suppression of TSH secretion that is reflected in undetectable serum TSH. In this context, the term "functional autonomy" is often misused when the intent is to imply that thyroid function is independent of TSH stimulation. True functional autonomy occurs when the thyroid gland is capable of functioning at a normal or an increased pace in the absence of both TSH and any other circulating thyroid stimulator (e.g., in congenital hyperthyroidism secondary to constitutively activated TSHRs). In Graves' disease, the thyroid gland is controlled by an abnormal stimulator, the TRAbs; in molar pregnancy, hCG is responsible. When the abnormal stimulator is withdrawn (i.e., when the disease enters remission), hyperfunction subsides, and the nonautonomous nature of thyroid function becomes evident in the re-emergence of normal TSH secretion and control of thyroid function.

The molar ratio of T_3 to T_4 in Tg is about twice normal, reflecting chronic hyperstimulation of the gland. The major product of glandular secretion is still T_4, but the ratio of T_3 to T_4 in the thyroid secretion is increased in proportion to the overproduction of T_3. In some instances, especially where there is iodine deficiency, T_3 appears to be the major secretory product, so that the serum T_3 level is increased while serum T_4 concentration is within the normal range (*T_3 thyrotoxicosis*). The proportion of total plasma T_4 and T_3 in the free (or unbound) state is increased because of a decrease in the concentration of thyroxine-binding globulin (TBG) and an increase in the concentration of T_4.

Clinical Picture

The Thyroid Gland

Graves' disease is most common in the third and fourth decades of life; it is rare before age 10 years but still occurs in the elderly, sometimes in an "apathetic" form. The features include diffuse goiter, thyrotoxicosis, infiltrative orbitopathy, and, occasionally, infiltrative dermopathy. Because the orbitopathy and dermopathy can occur independently of other manifestations, they are discussed separately. In other respects, the symptoms and signs of thyrotoxicosis are the same in Graves' disease as in other causes of hyperthyroidism.

In most patients, the thyroid gland is enlarged. However, hyperthyroidism in Graves' disease occurs in a gland of normal size in a minority of patients, and goiter is absent in 20% of elderly patients. The size of the thyroid gland is most often two or three times normal but may be massively enlarged. The consistency varies from soft to firm and rubbery. The enlargement is usually symmetric. The surface is generally smooth but may feel lobular. In severe cases, a thrill can be felt, usually over the upper or lower poles, where the superior and inferior thyroid arteries, respectively, enter the gland. A thrill is always accompanied by an audible bruit. However, the bruit, which occurs in systole, may be difficult to auscultate if the patient is very tachycardic. The bruit should not be confused with a venous hum or murmur arising from the base of the heart. To differentiate a true bruit from a transmitted cardiac flow murmur, the auscultated bruit should be louder over the thyroid than in the upper left sternal area. In addition,

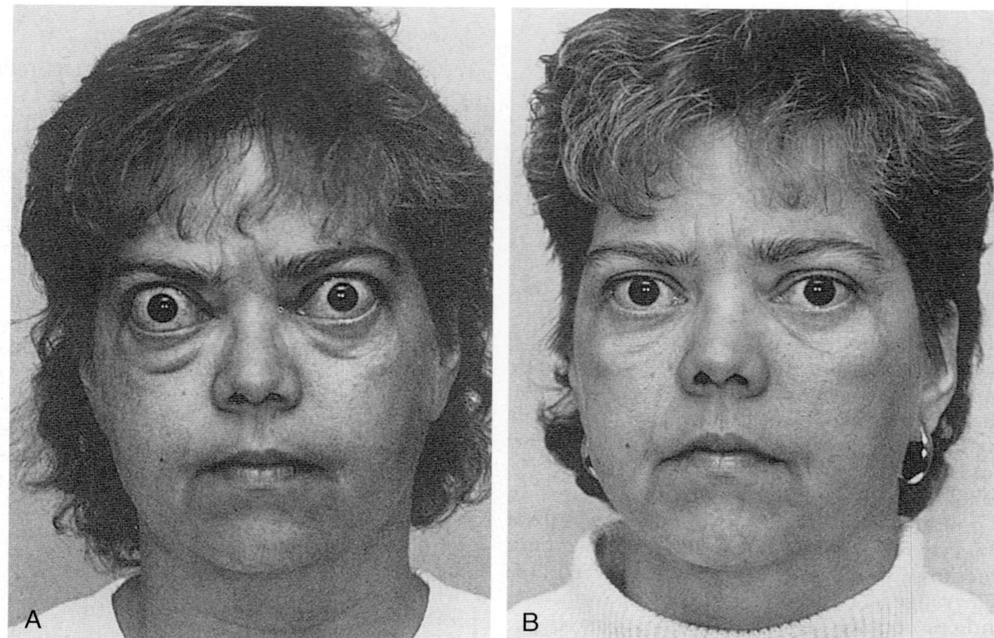

Figure 12-10 Characteristic signs of Graves' orbitopathy (**A**) subsequently corrected by orbital decompression surgery (**B**). Note the thyroid stare, the asymmetry, the proptosis, and the periorbital edema prior to correction. (Courtesy of Dr. Jack Rootman, University of British Colombia, Vancouver, Canada.)

mitral valve prolapse is more common than in the normal population and may account for a cardiac murmur.[153]

Manifestations of Infiltrative Orbitopathy and Dermopathy

Graves' ophthalmopathy is so named because most cases occur in patients with active or past Graves' disease. However, this entity is also termed *thyroid eye disease* or *thyroid-associated orbitopathy,* reflecting its association with any autoimmune thyroid disease.[154] Infiltrative orbitopathy may follow an independent course from the thyrotoxic manifestations and is often uninfluenced by their treatment. The natural history is characterized by rapid onset and deterioration followed by gradual improvement.

Infiltrative orbitopathy is evident in about 25% of patients with Graves' disease. However, ultrasonography[155] CT, or magnetic resonance imaging (MRI) of the orbits reveals changes, such as swelling of extraocular muscles and increased retroorbital fat, in a large majority of the patients, including those in whom the clinical changes are minimal or absent.

Signs and Symptoms. Spasm and retraction of the eyelids lead to widening of the palpebral fissures so that the sclera are exposed above the superior margin of the limbus (Fig. 12-10). Lid retraction may be asymmetric. When the patient looks downward, the upper lid lags behind the globe, exposing more sclera. When the patient gazes upward, often with difficulty, the globe lags behind the lid (lid lag and globe lag). The movements of the lids are jerky and spasmodic, and the lightly closed lids may show a tremor. Simple lid retraction and globe and lid lag are often a manifestation of the thyrotoxicosis per se and frequently abate after the thyrotoxicosis is relieved. On the other hand, significant swelling and inflammation of the muscles and orbital contents (so-called infiltrative orbitopathy) may occur.

The disease symptoms and signs of infiltrative ophthalmopathy appear in varying combinations. Early symptoms and signs include a sense of irritation in the eyes, resembling that caused by a foreign body, and excessive tearing that is often made worse by exposure to air or wind, especially if exophthalmos is present. The conjunctivae may be injected. Exophthalmos is frequently asymmetric and may cause a feeling of pressure behind the globes. If exophthalmos is pronounced, the eyes may not close during sleep, a condition termed lagophthalmos. Exophthalmos may be masked by periorbital edema, which is a common accompaniment and source of complaint. Patients frequently describe blurred vision and easy tiring of the eyes. Double vision may occur in combination with the foregoing symptoms or alone. In severe cases, color vision, and then visual acuity, may be decreased or lost, and the corneas may ulcerate or become infected.

The manifestations of extreme orbitopathy can be catastrophic and can include subluxation of the globe. Blindness may result from ulceration or infection of the cornea secondary to incomplete apposition of the lids or to optic nerve ischemia due to reduced blood flow caused by increased intraocular and intraorbital pressure. In the most severe cases, which should now be unusual, ophthalmoscopic examination reveals venous congestion and papilledema, which may be accompanied by visual field defects.

Objective Assessment of Eye Disease. The American Thyroid Association and the European Group on Graves' Orbitopathy (EUGOGO) recommend that the eye changes of Graves' disease be assessed with the use of an overall activity score, shown in Table 12-3.[156]

Infiltrative Dermopathy. Dermopathy now occurs in fewer than 5% of patients with Graves' disease, and it is almost always accompanied by infiltrative orbitopathy, usually of a severe degree. These lesions cause hyperpigmented, nonpitting induration of the skin of the legs, commonly over the pretibial area (pretibial myxedema) and the dorsa of the feet, sometimes in the form of individual nodules and plaques or becoming confluent with a

TABLE 12-3

Clinical Assessment of the Patient with Graves' Ophthalmopathy

Activity Measures*
Spontaneous retrobulbar pain Pain on attempted up or down gaze Redness of the eyelids Redness of the conjunctiva Swelling of the eyelids Inflammation of the caruncle and/or plica Conjunctival edema
Severity Measures
Lid aperture: distance between lid margins in millimeters with the patient looking in the primary position, sitting relaxed, and with distant fixation Swelling of the eyelids (absent/equivocal, moderate, severe) Redness of the eyelids (absent/present) Redness of the conjunctivae (absent/present) Conjunctival edema (absent, present) Inflammation of the caruncle or plica (absent, present) Exophthalmos: measured in millimeters using the same Hertel exophthalmometer and the same intercanthal distance for an individual patient Subjective diplopia score† Eye muscle involvement (ductions in degrees) Corneal involvement (absent/punctate keratopathy/ulcer) Optic nerve involvement: best-corrected visual acuity, color vision, optic disk, relative afferent pupillary defect (absent/present), plus visual fields if optic nerve compression is suspected

*Based on the seven classic features of inflammation in Graves' ophthalmopathy. The clinical activity score (CAS) is the total number of items present; a CAS ≥3 indicates active ophthalmopathy.

†Subjective diplopia score: 0 = no diplopia; 1 = intermittent (i.e., diplopia in primary position of gaze, when tired, or when first awakening); 2 = inconstant (i.e., diplopia at extremes of gaze); 3 = constant (i.e., continuous diplopia in primary or reading position).

smooth, characteristic edge or shoulder (see Fig. 12-9). Rarely, lesions develop on the face, elbows, or dorsa of the hands. The cause of the characteristic pretibial location of the dermopathy is unclear but most likely depends on trauma to the exposed areas. Indeed, surgical trauma to such tissues aggravates the disease dramatically.[91] Clubbing of the digits is occasionally associated with long-standing thyrotoxicosis (thyroid acropachy), which is now uncommon with early treatment (Fig. 12-11).

Laboratory Tests

In moderate or severe Graves' disease, laboratory findings are consistent with the pathophysiology previously discussed. The serum TSH level, when measured by a sensitive immunoassay, is almost totally suppressed, and serum T_4 and T_3 levels are elevated (see Chapter 11 and Fig. 12-1). The free T_4 and T_3 levels are increased more than are the total T_4 and T_3 levels. The serum T_3 concentration may be proportionally more elevated than the serum T_4 level. The increase in thyroid iodide uptake and clearance rates is often, but not always, reflected in the increased RAIU, which is usually measured at 24 hours. The RAIU may be inappropriately normal in a patient with milder disease given the suppressed serum TSH level. However, in patients with severe accompanying illness, conversion of T_4 to T_3 is impaired, permitting return to normal of the free T_3 concentration but usually not the free T_4 (i.e., *T_4 thyrotoxicosis*). Occasionally, usually in iodine deficiency, the discrepancy between T_4 and T_3 levels is exaggerated, the serum T_4 concentration being normal and only the serum T_3 concentration being elevated (*T_3 thyrotoxicosis*).

Because there are other causes of suppressed serum TSH, such as depression and hypothalamic-pituitary disease (see Table 11-12 in Chapter 11), and to exclude the possibility that an increase in serum T_4 concentration is the result of an increase in hormone binding in the blood, the free T_4 concentration should also be measured.

Determining the RAIU is not useful in the diagnosis when the clinical presentation is compatible with straightforward Graves' disease, but it is appropriate in excluding thyrotoxicosis not caused by hyperthyroidism. Very low values of RAIU in association with thyrotoxicosis signal the presence of (1) thyroiditis (painless, subacute, acute or drug-induced); (2) factitious thyrotoxicosis; (3) ectopic thyroid tissue; or (4) iodine contamination by recent administration of iodinated radiographic contrast, such as for a CT examination or amiodarone administration (see Fig. 12-1).

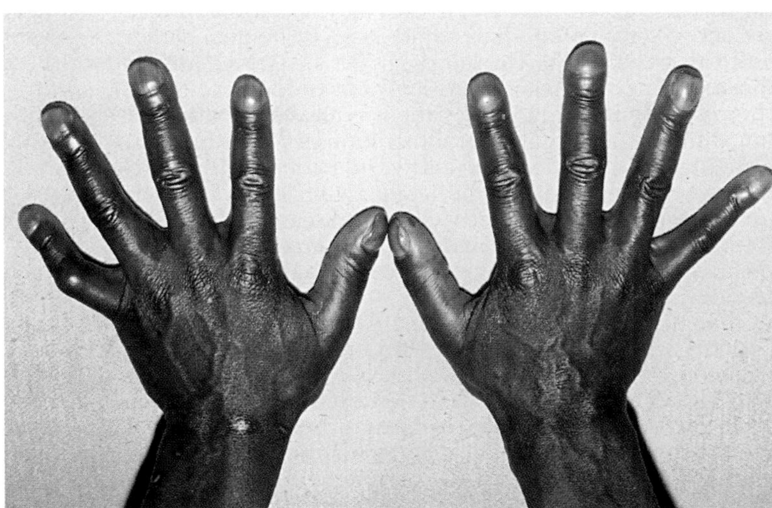

Figure 12-11 Rare thyroid acropachy in a patient with Graves' disease. The hypermetabolic state leads to axial bone destruction, presumably secondary to enhanced osteoclast activity. Acropachy should not be confused with clubbing, which is usually painless. (Courtesy of Dr. Andrew Werner, New York, NY.)

Mild (Subclinical) Graves' Disease

In subtle or mild cases of thyrotoxicosis, laboratory tests are most important, particularly if values are only slightly abnormal. A TSH concentration lower than 0.1 mU/L (normal range, 0.4 to 4.0 mU/L) may be associated with symptoms of an excessive thyroid hormone supply. A value between 0.1 and 0.4 mU/L suggests a supranormal exposure to thyroid hormones but not a condition likely to be associated with severe clinical manifestations. Treatment of such mild (subclinical) thyrotoxicosis is discussed later in this chapter.

Measuring Thyrotropin Receptor Autoantibodies

Two types of tests are usually employed for the detection of TRAbs, and both are available commercially. The first test assesses the capacity of patient serum or IgG to inhibit the binding of labeled TSH to solubilized TSHRs or to compete with a monoclonal antibody to the TSH-binding site on the TSH receptor. These protein-binding inhibition assays are of low cost and good precision, and the frequency of positive results in patients with active and untreated disease has increased as the sensitivity of the assay has improved and is now greater than 90%.

The second type of test is a bioassay that assesses the capacity of the patient's serum or IgG to stimulate adenylate cyclase in thyroid epithelial cells or mammalian cells expressing recombinant TSHR. Tests of this type, which measure the biologic action of the antibodies, are much more expensive, have relatively poor precision, and are positive in 80% to 90% of patients with active untreated Graves' disease. Because of the proliferation of acronyms describing these antibodies, we encourage designation of the specific assay used.

Standardization. As with all autoantibody tests, it is important to use an internationally accepted standard to allow comparison of results from different laboratories. A TRAb standard from the Medical Research Council (MRC) is often employed and reported in MRC units. Alternatively, results have been reported in terms of equivalent TSH units. However, the hTRAbs from different patients may not give parallel results with the MRC standards or TSH standards when measured in different dilutions. This means that the conversion of hTRAb data into MRC units or TSH units can be erroneous.

Indications for Measuring Thyrotropin Receptor Autoantibodies. Quantitation of TRAbs may be a useful indicator of the degree of disease activity in an individual patient and can confirm the clinical diagnosis of Graves' disease in a scientific manner. A bioassay is not needed in a hyperthyroid patient, because the patient is already demonstrating antibody bioactivity. Demonstration of TRAbs may also be of diagnostic value in the euthyroid patient with exophthalmos, especially if it is unilateral. High levels of TRAbs in a pregnant woman with Graves' disease increase the likelihood that fetal or neonatal thyrotoxicosis will be present in her offspring, and in this situation a bioassay late in pregnancy is preferred.

Another use of TRAb testing is in the prognosis of patients with Graves' disease who are treated with antithyroid agents. A persisting high level of TRAbs is a useful predictor of relapse on cessation of the drug.[79,157] In patients with low or negative titers, the test is much less helpful. The presence of iodine deficiency may interrupt the development of hyperthyroidism despite the presence of TRAbs.[158]

Differential Diagnosis

The patient with major manifestations of Graves' disease (namely thyrotoxicosis, goiter with an accompanying bruit or thrill, and infiltrative orbitopathy) does not pose a diagnostic problem. In some patients, however, one of the major manifestations dominates the clinical picture or is present alone, and the disorder may mimic another disease. All of these issues can be resolved by appropriate laboratory testing.

Thyroid Differential

The diffuse goiter of Graves' disease in a patient with severe hyperthyroidism may rarely be confused with that of other thyroid diseases. In subacute thyroiditis, asymmetry of the gland, tenderness on palpation, and systemic evidence of inflammation assist in the diagnosis. If Graves' disease is in a latent or inactive phase and thyrotoxicosis is absent and in patients with extremely mild hyperthyroidism, the goiter may require differentiation from Hashimoto's thyroiditis or simple nontoxic goiter as possible diagnoses. The goiter of Hashimoto's disease is somewhat lobulated and feels firmer and rubbery compared with that of Graves' disease. Serum levels of thyroid antibodies are generally higher in Hashimoto's disease but may not be helpful in distinguishing individual patients. The very low RAIU distinguishes thyrotoxicosis caused by painless or subacute thyroiditis from Graves' disease in the absence of iodine excess (see Fig. 12-1).

Eye Disease Differential

The orbitopathy of Graves' disease, if bilateral and associated with thyrotoxicosis past or present, does not require differentiation from exophthalmos of any other origin, such as is seen in morbid obesity. However, unilateral exophthalmos, even when associated with thyrotoxicosis, should alert the physician to the possibility of a local cause. Rare diseases that may produce unilateral or bilateral exophthalmos include orbital neoplasms, carotid-cavernous sinus fistulas, cavernous sinus thrombosis, infiltrative disorders affecting the orbit, and pseudotumor of the orbit. Mild bilateral exophthalmos, without infiltrative signs, is seen commonly in morbid obesity and is occasionally present on a familial basis; it also sometimes occurs in patients with Cushing's syndrome, cirrhosis, uremia, chronic obstructive pulmonary disease, or superior vena cava syndrome.

Ophthalmoplegia as the sole manifestation of the orbitopathy of Graves' disease requires exclusion of diabetes mellitus and other disorders affecting the brainstem and its connections. The demonstration of swelling of the extraocular muscles by orbital ultrasonography, CT, or MRI is diagnostic of Graves' orbitopathy, as is the detection of TRAbs in serum or the demonstration of a suppressed TSH level.

Treatment

It is not possible to treat the basic pathogenetic factors in Graves' disease in a risk-free way. Existing therapies for the thyrotoxic and ophthalmic manifestations all have significant side effects. The lack of general agreement as to which therapy is the best is due to the fact that none is ideal.[159] Because the therapeutic problems posed by thyrotoxicosis and orbitopathy differ, and because they run independent courses, their treatments are discussed separately.

Treatment of thyrotoxicosis is designed to impose restraint on hormone secretion by means of chemical agents that inhibit hormone synthesis or release or by reducing the quantity of thyroid tissue. There are three effective therapeutic options, and physician and patient preference often dictate the choice. Radioiodine is a popular therapy in the United States, whereas in Europe and Japan the preference is for anti-thyroid drug therapy or surgery.[160]

Anti-Thyroid Agents

Thionamides. The major agents for treating thyrotoxicosis are drugs of the thionamide class, most commonly methimazole, propylthiouracil, and carbimazole (10 mg of carbimazole is metabolized to approximately 6 mg of methimazole).[161] These agents inhibit the oxidation and organic binding of thyroid iodide and therefore produce intrathyroidal iodine deficiency that further increases the ratio of T_3 to T_4 in the thyroid secretion, as reflected in the high T_3/T_4 ratio in the serum. In addition, large doses of propylthiouracil (600 mg), but not methimazole, impair the conversion of T_4 to T_3 by type 1 deiodinase (D1) in the thyroid and peripheral tissues.[162] The propylthiouracil-sensitive D1 is the major source of peripheral T_3 production in the hyperthyroid patient.[163] Because of this additional action, large doses of propylthiouracil may provide rapid alleviation of severe thyrotoxicosis.[164]

The half-life in plasma of methimazole is about 6 hours, whereas that of propylthiouracil is about 1.5 hours, and both drugs are accumulated by the thyroid gland.[161] A single dose of methimazole may exert an anti-thyroid effect for longer than 24 hours. This provides a rational basis for the single-daily-dose regimen of methimazole for mild or moderate thyrotoxicosis. Both of these drugs cross the placenta and can inhibit thyroid function in the fetus, but both drugs have been used highly effectively in pregnant patients (see later discussion).

Immunosuppressive Action of Thionamides. Thionamide drugs may also directly influence the immune response in patients with autoimmune thyroid disease.[56] This action occurs within the thyroid gland, where the drugs are concentrated. The action on the thyroid cells themselves decreases thyroid antigen expression and decreases prostaglandin and cytokine release from thyroid cells. Thionamides also inhibit the generation of oxygen radicals in T cells, B cells, and particularly antigen-presenting cells and hence may cause a further decline in antigen presentation. It has also been shown that methimazole induces the expression of Fas ligand on thyroid epithelial cell, thereby inducing apoptosis of infiltrating lymphocytes such as T cells that express FasL and decreasing the lymphocytic infiltration.[165,166] The clinical importance of immunosuppression and induction of apoptosis compared with inhibition of thyroid hormone formation is unclear. However, the decrease in immune infiltration seen in patients taking such drugs and the fall in autoantibody levels after initiation of such therapy is powerful evidence of their effect.

Use of Thionamides. Based on its half-life, methimazole can be prescribed on a once-daily basis. However, the initial dose of methimazole commonly employed in moderate thyrotoxicosis is 20 to 30 mg/day (or the equivalent of carbimazole) until the patient is euthyroid, followed by a maintenance dose of 5 to 10 mg/day. For significantly hyperthyroid patients, a randomized, controlled trial reported that normalization of free T_4 at 3 months occurred more frequently among patients taking higher-dose methimazole (30 mg/day) than among those taking lower doses (15 mg/day).[167]

Because of propylthiouracil's well-known rare but serious side effect of hepatic failure, sometimes requiring liver transplantation, in June 2009 the U.S. Food and Drug Administration (FDA) issued an advisory that propylthiouracil should not be used as a first-line agent for hyperthyroidism in adults or children. Its use is still recommended in the first trimester of pregnancy and in life-threatening thyrotoxicosis or thyroid storm to take advantage of its ability to inhibit peripheral conversion of T_4 to T_3, and also for those who are intolerant of methimazole.[168] If prescribed, its shorter duration of action requires an equivalent initial propylthiouracil dose of 100-200 mg every 8 hours, depending on the severity of hyperthyroidism, with reduction to a maintenance dose of 50 to 100 mg given two to three times daily as hyperthyroidism ameliorates. When large amounts are required, propylthiouracil should be administered at 4- to 6-hour intervals, although this agent is available only in a 50-mg tablet.

The therapeutic response to effective anti-thyroid therapy invariably occurs after a latent period, because the agents inhibit the synthesis but not the release of hormone; reduction in the supply of hormone to the tissues does not occur until glandular hormone stores are depleted. Although propylthiouracil differs from methimazole in having the additional effect of inhibiting the peripheral conversion of T_4 to T_3, there appears to be little difference in duration of the latent period for these agents when either is employed alone in the usual dosage. This is because the extrathyroidal effect of propylthiouracil on conversion of T_4 to T_3 is more apparent at dosages greater than 600 mg/day. This effect may be an advantage in the acute treatment of severe hyperthyroidism.[162,169] In general, improvement within the first 2 weeks includes decreased nervousness and palpitations, increased strength, and weight gain. Usually, the metabolic state becomes normal within about 6 weeks. At that time, the dosage can often be reduced substantially to maintain a normal metabolic state.

During treatment, the size of the thyroid gland decreases in one third to one half of the patients. In the remainder, it may remain unchanged or even enlarge. In the latter situation, the change signals either an intensification of the disease process, which often requires that the dosage of drug be increased, or the onset of hypothyroidism and increased TSH secretion as a result of excessive treatment. It is important to differentiate between these causes. Clinical criteria are not the main guidelines by which adequacy of treatment can be judged. Adequacy of therapy is assessed by measurement of free T_4 in the first several months, when the serum TSH level usually remains suppressed, and then subsequently by TSH assessment. Mild thyrotoxicosis may persist despite a serum T_4 concentration in the normal range because the serum T_3 concentration remains elevated, typically because of intrathyroidal iodine deficiency[170] and the increased T_3/T_4 ratio in Graves' Tg.[171] The latter phenomenon may also account for maintenance of a normal metabolic state in the setting of a subnormal serum T_4 level. Importantly, the serum TSH concentration may remain subnormal for many months, perhaps secondary to accelerated conversion of T_4 to T_3 in the pituitary thyrotrophs. An enlarging thyroid gland in a treated patient with Graves' disease may also indicate the presence of a neoplasm and should be investigated appropriately.

Anti-thyroid agents can cause hypothyroidism if given in excessive amounts over long periods. When this occurs, the patient often complains of gain in weight, sluggishness, and fatigue, and signs of mild hypothyroidism may be present. As suggested earlier, one major sign of incipient hypothyroidism is enlargement of the thyroid gland secondary to increased TSH. The hypothyroidism can be reversed by reducing the dosage of the anti-thyroid drug or by administering supplemental thyroid hormone.

Block-and-Replace Regimens. The logic behind prescribing a full dose of a thionamide drug and adding T_4 supplements to prevent the patient from becoming hypothyroid is twofold. First, in a few patients, the euthyroid state is difficult to maintain with thionamide therapy alone, and a block-and-replace regimen can be helpful and requires fewer office visits. Second, the immunosuppressive action of the thionamides may be helpful in attenuating the natural history of the autoimmune thyroid diseases directly.

Although an initial report found the relapse rate after the block-and-replace approach to be much reduced,[172] subsequent studies found no such difference.[173,174] One explanation for such disparities may be the iodine status of the various patient groups. In addition, this regimen is associated with a higher rate of side effects.[175]

Predicting the Response to Drug Withdrawal. A central question in the treatment of Graves' disease with anti-thyroid drugs is how to determine the appropriate duration of anti-thyroid drug treatment. As discussed earlier, anti-thyroid therapy may alter the course of the underlying autoimmune process, but remission after withdrawal of treatment will persist only if the disorder has entered an inactive phase. This latter transition and the natural decline in levels of TRAbs are more likely to occur the longer the course of treatment. This reasoning is the basis for the traditional practice of continuing anti-thyroid treatment for at least 12 months.

Remission rates are reported to be lower in men, older patients, smokers, and those with more active Graves' disease (including those with higher titers of TRAbs and larger goiters).[176] Factors preventing a recurrence also include (1) a change from stimulating TRAbs to blocking antibodies, which occurs rarely; (2) progression of concomitant autoimmune thyroiditis; and (3) iodine deficiency itself, which may prevent the recurrence of Graves' disease. The persistence of high levels of circulating TRAbs during treatment of Graves' disease portends recurrence after withdrawal of anti-thyroid drugs. Whether this is helpful in the management of the individual patient remains controversial,[177] and some have been unable to confirm the predictive value of TRAb measurement in areas of iodine deficiency.

However, most patients do not have persisting high levels of TRAb, and predicting their outcome is even more difficult. Genetic typing, for example using HLA, is still not helpful for such predictions in the individual patient. However, the results of combining HLA with Tg haplotyping are beginning to look impressive in a small number of patients.[178]

Anti-thyroid drug therapy usually should be continued for 12 to 18 months and then withdrawn if the serum TSH level returns to normal. Therapeutic duration longer than 18 months does not increase remission rates, according to a meta-analysis.[175] The average rate of remission, as defined by a normal serum TSH level after withdrawal of anti-thyroid therapy, is 30% to 50%; in other words, about 50% of patients relapse or are unable to stop therapy.[161,179]

About 75% of relapses occur during the first 3 months after withdrawal of therapy, and most of the remainder occur during the subsequent 6 months. Suppression of the TSH concentration below normal levels is the first signal of relapse, even in the presence of a normal serum T_4 level. Nevertheless, about one third of patients experience a lasting remission. This fact alone indicates that anti-thyroid agents have a significant role as the sole therapy in the initial treatment of thyrotoxicosis.

TABLE 12-4

Incidence of Major Toxic Reactions to Anti-Thyroid Drugs in Adults

Side Effect	Frequency (%)	Comments
Polyarthritis	1-2	—
ANCA+ vasculitis	Rare	Mostly PTU
Agranulocytosis	0.1-0.5	May be more common with PTU
Hepatitis	0.1-0.2	PTU only
Cholestasis	Rare	Methimazole only

ANCA+, antineutrophil cytoplasmic antibody–positive; *PTU*, propylthiouracil.
Adapted from Cooper DS. Antithyroid drugs. *N Engl J Med.* 2005;352:905-917.

Adverse Reactions. Adverse reactions occur in only a small number of patients taking thionamide drugs, although some can be very severe if left uncared for (Table 12-4). Among the more serious side effects, the one that elicits the most concern is agranulocytosis, which occurs in 0.1% to 0.3% of patients, usually within the first few weeks or months of treatment. Older patients and those taking higher anti-thyroid doses are at higher risk.

Agranulocytosis is accompanied by fever and sore throat.[161] When therapy with a thionamide is begun, the patient should be instructed to discontinue the drug and notify the physician immediately should these symptoms develop. This precaution is more important than frequent measurement of white blood cell counts, because agranulocytosis can develop within a day or two. Because of the high frequency of lymphopenia in hyperthyroidism itself, a complete blood count with differential is recommended before anti-thyroid drug therapy is started. If the absolute neutrophil count falls to less than 1500 cells/μL, the drug should be withdrawn. Similarly, if agranulocytosis occurs, the drug should be discontinued immediately and the patient treated with antibiotics as appropriate. Granulocyte colony-stimulating factor may speed the recovery that invariably takes place. Lymphocytes of patients who have developed agranulocytosis while taking propylthiouracil undergo blast transformation when exposed in vitro to propylthiouracil or methimazole; consequently, these patients should not be given a thionamide drug again.

Granulocytopenia occurs during anti-thyroid therapy and is sometimes a forerunner of agranulocytosis, but it can also be a manifestation of thyrotoxicosis itself. Granulocytopenia that develops during the first few weeks of therapy may be difficult to interpret. In this circumstance, serial measurements of the leukocyte count should be made. If they display a downward trend, the anti-thyroid drugs should be discontinued. If serial measurements of the white blood cell count remain constant or return to normal, treatment need not be interrupted.

Propylthiouracil has in rare instances been associated with fulminant hepatic necrosis, and it is the third most common cause of drug-related liver failure, accounting for 10% of all drug-related liver transplantations. Cessation of the treatment results in recovery in most cases. This propylthiouracil-associated liver failure may occur at any time during therapy, so routine monitoring of liver function may not be helpful.[180] Methimazole is associated with cholestasis rather than hepatic necrosis, and the risk is increased with higher doses administered in older patients.[181] There are no reported cases of liver transplantation attributed to methimazole toxicity.

Mild side effects occur in up to 20% of patients and include skin reactions, arthralgias, gastrointestinal symptoms, an abnormal sense of taste, and, occasionally, sialadenitis. Other effects include thrombocytopenia, enlargement of lymph nodes, a lupus-like syndrome including the development of antineutrophil cytoplasmic antibody (ANCA)-positive vasculitis,[182] and toxic psychoses. The mechanisms underlying these reactions are not known, although some reactions disappear with continuance of treatment.

It is recommended that patients be informed in writing about the possible side effects and stop the medication and inform their physician if they develop pruritic rash, jaundice, acholic stools or dark urine, arthralgias, abdominal pain, nausea, fever, or pharyngitis. In addition, all patients should have a baseline complete blood count with differential white blood count and liver function tests including transaminases, bilirubin, and alkaline phosphatase. We believe that suspicion of any serious manifestation should be an indication for abandonment of anti-thyroid therapy and recourse to surgery or treatment with iodine 131 (^{131}I).

Iodide Transport Inhibitors. Both thiocyanate and perchlorate inhibit thyroid iodide transport. Theoretical and practical disadvantages, such as frequent side effects, preclude their use except in special circumstances.

Iodine and Iodine-Containing Agents. Iodine may be administered directly or contained in contrast media used therapeutically. However, iodine is now rarely used as a sole therapy. The mechanism of action of iodine in relieving thyrotoxicosis differs from that of the thionamides. Although quantities of iodine in excess of several milligrams can acutely inhibit organic binding (acute Wolff-Chaikoff effect), this transient phenomenon probably does not contribute to the therapeutic effect. Instead, the major action of iodine is to inhibit hormone release. Administration of iodine increases glandular stores of organic iodine, but the beneficial effect of iodine is evident more quickly than the effects of even large doses of agents that inhibit hormone synthesis. In patients with Graves' disease, iodine acutely retards the rate of secretion of T_4, an effect that is rapidly lost when iodine is withdrawn.

These features of iodine action provide both disadvantages and advantages. The enrichment of glandular organic iodine stores that occurs when this agent is given alone may retard the clinical response to subsequently administered thionamide, and the decrease in RAIU produced by iodine prevents the use of radioiodine as treatment for several weeks. Furthermore, if iodine is withdrawn, resumption of accelerated release of hormone from an enriched glandular hormone pool may exacerbate the disorder.

Another reason for not using iodine alone is that the therapeutic response on occasion is incomplete or absent. Even if iodine treatment is initially effective, it may lose its effect with time. This phenomenon, which has been termed *iodine escape*, should not be confused with the escape from the acute Wolff-Chaikoff effect (see Chapter 11).[183] Nevertheless, the rapid slowing of hormone release with iodine treatment makes it more effective than the thionamide drugs when prompt relief of thyrotoxicosis is mandatory.

Aside from its use in preparation for thyroid surgery, iodine is useful mainly in patients with actual or impending thyrotoxic crisis, severe thyrocardiac disease, or acute surgical emergencies. If iodide is used in these circumstances, it should be administered with large doses of a thionamide. The dose of iodine required for control of thyrotoxicosis is approximately 6 mg/day, a quantity much less than that usually given. Six milligrams of iodine is present in one eighth of a drop of saturated solution of potassium iodide (SSKI) or approximately 1 drop of Lugol's solution; many physicians, however, prescribe 5 to 10 drops of one of these agents three times daily. Although it is advisable to administer amounts larger than the suggested minimal effective dose, huge quantities of iodine are more likely to produce adverse reactions, including iodide myxedema. We recommend the use of a maximum of 2 to 3 drops of SSKI twice daily.

For patients who are so ill that medications cannot be taken by mouth, anti-thyroid agents may be triturated and administered by stomach tube; iodine may be given by the same route, or it can be absorbed through the oral mucosa. If use of a stomach tube is contraindicated, thionamide drugs cannot be administered, because no parenteral preparations are available. In such cases, the disadvantages attendant on administration of iodine may be accepted if the clinical situation is sufficiently serious. Iodine appears to be particularly effective after administration of a therapeutic dose of ^{131}I for the rapid alleviation of thyrotoxicosis.

Reactions to Iodine. Adverse reactions to iodine are unusual and usually are not serious but may include rash (which may be acneiform), drug fever, sialadenitis, conjunctivitis and rhinitis, vasculitis, and a leukemoid eosinophilic granulocytosis. Sialadenitis may respond to reduction of dosage and the addition of lemon/lime candies to increase salivary flow; if any of the other reactions occur, iodine should be stopped.

Other Anti-Thyroid Agents

Cholecystographic Agents. In doses of 1 g daily, the iodine-containing cholecystographic contrast agent sodium ipodate (or iopanoate) causes a prompt decrease in serum T_4 and serum T_3 concentrations in patients with hyperthyroidism.[184] These effects result from both the release of iodine and the ability of the agent to inhibit peripheral T_3 production from T_4—a combination that can be useful in the seriously ill patient. As with iodine itself, however, withdrawal of the drug carries the risk of an exacerbation. Supplies of this and related agents are no longer available in the United States.

Lithium. Lithium carbonate also inhibits thyroid hormone secretion but, unlike iodine, it does not interfere with the accumulation of radioiodine. Lithium, 300 to 450 mg every 8 hours, is employed only to provide temporary control of thyrotoxicosis in patients who are allergic to both thionamide and iodide. This is because the blocking effect is often lost with time. The goal is to maintain a serum lithium concentration of 1 mEq/L.[185] Another short-term use for lithium has been as an adjunct to radioiodine therapy, because the drug slows the release of iodine from the thyroid.

Dexamethasone. Dexamethasone, 2 mg every 6 hours, inhibits the peripheral conversion of T_4 to T_3 and has well-known immunosuppressive effects.[186] The inhibitory effect of dexamethasone on conversion of T_4 to T_3 is additive to that of propylthiouracil, suggesting a different mechanism of action. Concurrent administration of propylthiouracil, SSKI, and dexamethasone to a patient with severe, life-threatening thyrotoxicosis effects a rapid reduction in serum T_3 concentration, often to the normal range within 24 to 48 hours.[157]

β-Blocking Agents. Drugs that block the response to catecholamines at the receptor site (e.g., propranolol) ameliorate some of the manifestations of thyrotoxicosis and are often used as adjuncts in management. Tremulousness, palpitations, excessive sweating, eyelid retraction, and heart rate decrease; effects are rapidly manifested and appear to be mediated largely through modulation of the increased sensitivity to the sympathetic nervous system induced by excess thyroid hormone (described earlier).[20,22] Propranolol. but not other β-adrenergic blockers, may also weakly block the conversion of T_4 to T_3 via a mechanism independent of its effect on catecholamine signaling.

Adrenergic antagonists are most useful in the interval before the response to thionamide or radioiodine therapy occurs. They are of limited usefulness in patients with mild to moderate disease but are useful in those with thyrotoxic symptoms and in those with impending or actual thyrotoxic crisis (see "Thyroid Storm"). Adrenergic antagonists are especially useful when tachycardia is contributing to cardiac insufficiency. However, the fact that β-adrenergic blockade can reduce cardiac output without altering oxygen consumption can have adverse effects in some organs, such as the liver, where the arteriovenous oxygen difference is already elevated in the hyperthyroid state.[29] Moreover, thyroid hormone also has a direct stimulatory effect on the myocardium independent of the adrenergic nervous system.

Propranolol is the most widely used agent because it is relatively free from adverse effects and has a short half-life, allowing for easy control. It can be given orally in a dose of 20 to 40 mg every 6 or 8 hours. For intravenous use, a shorter-acting agent may be preferable (see "Thyroid Storm"). Propranolol may be contraindicated in patients with asthma or chronic obstructive pulmonary disease because it aggravates bronchospasm. Because of its myocardial depressant action, it is also contraindicated in patients with heart block and in patients with congestive failure, unless severe tachycardia is a contributory factor. β-Blocking agents such as atenolol or metoprolol are longer-acting drugs that allow a once-daily regimen when treatment is likely to be prolonged.

Surgery

Because of the occasional recurrence of hyperthyroidism after subtotal thyroidectomy, the current surgical procedure of choice for treatment of Graves' disease is a near-total thyroidectomy.

Complications of Surgery. The hazards of thyroidectomy are inversely related to the experience and skill of the surgical team[187,188]; in experienced hands, the frequency of complications such as permanent hypoparathyroidism and damage to the recurrent laryngeal nerve is low (Table 12-5). Unless circumstances are otherwise compelling, thyroidectomy should not be performed by surgeons who do the operation only occasionally. Bleeding into the operative site, the most serious postoperative complication, can rapidly produce death by asphyxia and requires immediate evacuation of the blood and ligation of the bleeding vessel. Even with subtotal surgery, the recurrent laryngeal nerve can be damaged. If such damage is unilateral, it causes dysphonia that usually improves in a few weeks but may leave the patient slightly hoarse, especially an older patient.

Hypoparathyroidism can be either transient or permanent. Transient hypoparathyroidism results from inadvertent removal of some parathyroids and impairment of blood supply to those that remain. Depending on the severity of these insults, symptoms and signs of hypocalcemia appear, usually within 1 to 7 days after surgery. Severe hypoparathyroidism should be treated with intravenous calcium gluconate. Milder cases can be treated with oral calcium carbonate and calcitrol in doses of 0.25-0.50, one to three times daily.

TABLE 12-5

Complications of Surgery in 322 Patients with Graves' Hyperthyroidism in Experienced Hands (1986-1995)

Complication	%
Recurrent hyperthyroidism	2.0
Vocal cord paralysis	
Transient	2.5
Permanent	0.3
Prolonged postoperative hypocalcemia (>7 days)	3.7
Permanent hypoparathyroidism	0.6

Adapted from Werga-Kjellman P, Zedenius J, Tallstedt L, et al. Surgical treatment of hyperthyroidism: a ten-year experience. *Thyroid.* 2001;11:187-192.

However, the hypocalcemia that occurs immediately after surgery for thyrotoxicosis may not be caused by transient hypoparathyroidism, because it occurs more frequently in patients with Graves' disease than in those with other thyroid disorders. Instead, it may be caused by "hungry bones," resulting from the demineralization of bone that occurs in hyperthyroidism. This begins to be reversed after cure of the hyperthyroid state and may contribute to the modest elevation in alkaline phosphatase during recovery unless the patient has been rendered euthyroid for some time before surgery. The treatment of hypoparathyroidism is discussed in Chapter 28, but many surgeons who fear that they have caused damage to the parathyroid glands during a total thyroidectomy may reimplant the apparent parathyroid tissue into local muscles.

Preparation for Surgery. Preoperative use of anti-thyroid agents has greatly decreased the morbidity and mortality rates of surgery for Graves' disease, because these drugs deplete glandular hormone stores and restore the metabolic state to normal. However, these agents do not improve the hyperplasia and hypervascularity of the gland in the short term unless TRAb levels fall. Iodine, however, is reported to cause a decrease in height of the follicular cells, enlargement of follicles with retention of colloid, and reduction of hypervascularity. Hence, the aim of preoperative management is to restore the metabolic state to normal with anti-thyroid agents and then to induce involution of the gland with iodine.[189,190]

Patients who are to undergo thyroidectomy are first given anti-thyroid therapy in the manner described earlier. Often, relatively large doses are given to hasten the clinical response and because surgical candidates frequently have severe disease or large goiters. In addition, iodide (SSKI, 2 to 3 drops twice daily) should be initiated at least 7 to 10 days before surgery, as iodide decreases thyroid blood flow and vascularity and, hence, intraoperative blood loss during thyroidectomy.[191] During this period, a preexisting bruit or thrill may decrease in intensity or disappear entirely, and the gland may become firm.

Several cautions should be observed. No date for surgery should be set until a normal metabolic state has been restored. Much too often, the operation is planned well in advance and the patient is given a standardized regimen independent of clinical progress. Therapy with iodide should not be started until a normal metabolic state has been restored; iodine should not be relied on to complete an incomplete response to anti-thyroid therapy, because iodide enriches glandular hormone stores if the anti-thyroid drug is not entirely effective. Anti-thyroid agents should not be withdrawn when iodine therapy is begun.

β-Blockade Alone before Thyroid Surgery. Propranolol may be a useful adjunct in controlling signs and symptoms (see earlier discussion) while the patient is being prepared for surgery. However, propranolol has been used alone in preoperative preparation of patients in whom surgery is to be undertaken.[192] Although this mode of therapy is probably safe and effective in many patients with mild disease, thyroid crises can still occur when patients receive propranolol alone. However, there is no compelling indication for the use of propranolol alone. Restoration of the patient to a eumetabolic state, as outlined earlier, is appropriate before subjecting the patient to the stress of surgery.

Radioiodine Therapy

Radioiodine produces thyroid ablation without the complications of surgery. There has been concern that this form of therapy might produce thyroid carcinoma, leukemia, or an increase in thyroid cell mutation rates. However, during the half-century in which radioiodine has been in use, no increased prevalence of thyroid or other carcinoma in treated adults has been noted.[193] The prevalence of leukemia is also no greater in adults treated with radioiodine, and the frequency of genetic damage in the offspring of patients with prior radioiodine therapy does not appear to be increased. As long as hypothyroidism is treated appropriately, there is no increase in mortality.[194]

In view of the lack of evidence of serious toxicity from radioiodine in doses typically employed for treatment of hyperthyroidism in adults, the age limit for use of radioiodine has been lowered progressively by some physicians, from the initial lower limit of 40 years to age 10 or less.[195] However, in childhood, anti-thyroid drugs continue to be the first treatment of choice, and the use of radioiodine in women of reproductive age remains unpopular. Radioiodine use is contraindicated during pregnancy, and fetuses exposed to ^{131}I after 10 weeks of gestation may be born athyreotic.[196] In addition, ^{131}I should not be administered for at least 8 weeks after cessation of lactation because it is concentrated in breast milk.

Preparation before Radioiodine Therapy. The use of anti-thyroid drugs before radioiodine treatment is widely used to theoretically decrease a post-treatment increase in thyroid hormone release. This is considered especially dangerous in older patients with ischemic heart disease, in whom cardiac deaths have been reported. Anti-thyroid drugs may also prevent the increase in thyroid autoantibodies that occurs after radioiodine therapy and may affect ophthalmopathy.[197] Normally, such drugs are withdrawn 3 to 7 days before treatment; if needed, they can be reintroduced 7 days after treatment.

Radioiodine Dosing. Attempts have been made to standardize the radiation delivered to the thyroid gland by varying the dose of radioiodine according to the size of the gland, the uptake of ^{131}I, and its subsequent rate of release (dosimetry). However, such calculations do not provide uniform results, probably because of variations in individual sensitivity, determined perhaps by stimulating TRAbs. A dose of 20 mCi achieves thyroid ablation in almost all patients and results in hypothyroidism in 75% to 90% of treated patients.[198] Some physicians have settled on an arbitrary dose calculated to result in the delivery of 300 MBq (approximately 8 mCi) of ^{131}I to the thyroid gland 24 hours after administration.[199] Others aim to deliver 50 to 100 Gy (5000 to 10,000 rad) to the gland. No data support an advantage of dosimetry over a fixed-dose regimen.[200]

Drug-induced radioresistance has been the subject of much discussion, particularly in relation to propylthiouracil, but it is not a major issue.[198,201] A meta-analysis reported that methimazole therapy may also be associated with a similar decreased efficacy of radioiodine therapy.[202]

^{131}I administration is contraindicated during pregnancy. A pregnancy test should be carried out in women of childbearing age before ^{131}I therapy is initiated if there is any possibility of pregnancy.[203]

Treatment after Radioiodine Therapy. Treatment with anti-thyroid drugs after radioiodine therapy should be avoided for approximately 1 week because they also reduce the success of treatment, particularly if nonablative doses are used, via their acceleration of ^{131}I release.[204] Although exacerbation of thyrotoxicosis after radioiodine therapy is rare,[205] methimazole use should be considered for patients with severe hyperthyroidism and other comorbidities. Clearly, it is important to monitor serum FT_4 and T_3 levels in at-risk patients and to consider β-adrenergic blockade, whether or not anti-thyroid drugs are used before or after RAI treatment. Patients are seen at 4-week intervals after ^{131}I administration and monitored by measurements of serum T_4 and TSH levels; hypothyroidism is treated if it appears.

Women who are planning to become pregnant are advised to wait for an arbitrary period of 4 to 6 months after ^{131}I therapy to allow for resolution of any transient effects of gonadal irradiation and for stabilization of thyroid function.

If, after 6 months, hyperthyroidism is still present and the patient is symptomatic, the treatment is repeated, usually with about 1.5 times the initial dose of ^{131}I or an ablative amount.

Complications of Radioiodine Therapy

#1—Thyroid Cancer from Low-Level Exposure. There is no increase in thyroid cancer or any other cancer after diagnostic or therapeutic use of radioiodine in hyperthyroid adults,[206] in accord with earlier reports.[193] However, concerns remain about a potentially increased prevalence of thyroid carcinoma in patients treated with low amounts of radiation in childhood or adolescence, as exemplified by the increased prevalence of thyroid cancer among children exposed to the radiation during the Chernobyl incident.[207,208] In the Chernobyl case, exposure for most of the children who developed thyroid carcinoma was to relatively low doses of radiation rather than the thyrodestructive doses prescribed in hyperthyroidism.[209] Nevertheless, many physicians think that the use of radioactivity in children should be avoided whenever possible.

#2—Mortality after Radioiodine. Patients treated with radioiodine for hyperthyroidism had increased mortality compared with age- and period-specific mortality rates in the background population.[194] This effect was not seen in patients rendered hypothyroid. The findings support the idea of treating hyperthyroidism with doses of radioiodine that are sufficient to induce overt hypothyroidism. An association was seen in this study with mortality from ischemic heart disease in patients with subclinical

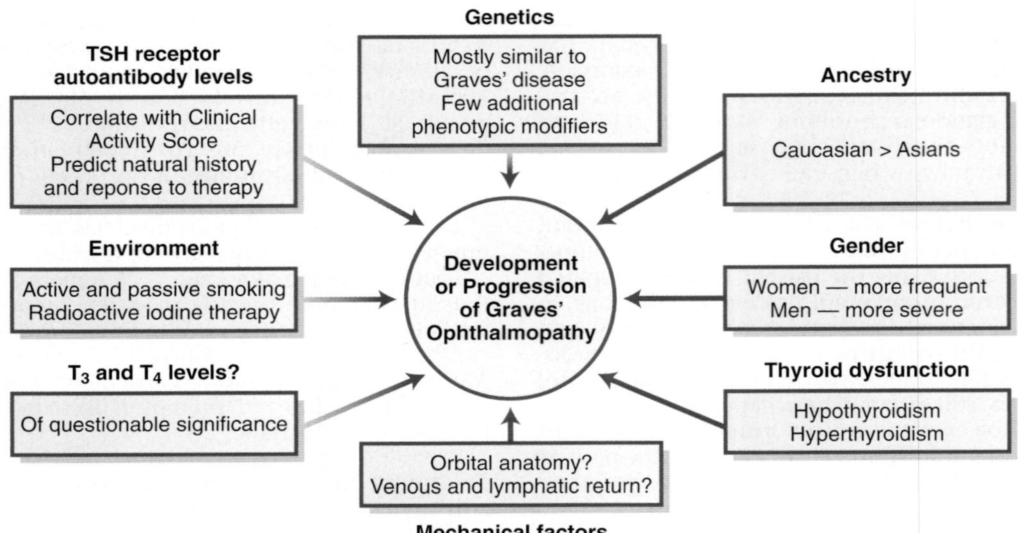

Figure 12-12 Probability of the development or worsening of orbitopathy in patients with Graves' disease. T_3, triiodothyronine; T_4, thyroxine; TSH, thyroid-stimulating hormone. (From Stan MN, Bahn RS. Risk factors for development or deterioration of Graves' ophthalmopathy. *Thyroid.* 2010;20:777-783.)[216]

hypothyroidism, suggesting that T_4 replacement should be considered if this biochemical abnormality develops after radioiodine therapy.

#3—Hypothyroidism after Radioiodine. In theory, the therapeutic goal of ^{131}I administration is to induce euthyroidism so that Graves' disease cannot recur. However, the incidence of hypothyroidism is significant during the first year or two after treatment with radioiodine, regardless of how the dose is calculated. The rate continues to increase by approximately 5% per year thereafter, and this actual incidence does depend on the dose of radioiodine prescribed by dosimetry or based on a standard dose.[200,210] If the dose delivered is sufficient for ablation, permanent hypothyroidism will ensue in more than 80% of patients by 6 months. Many physicians prefer the certainty of induced hypothyroidism rather than the "wait and see" approach.

#4—Radiation Thyroiditis. The early euthyroidism and later hypothyroidism are both consequences of radiation-induced destruction of thyroid parenchyma. With larger doses of radioactive iodine, a tender radiation thyroiditis may develop within the first week after treatment, as evidenced by epithelial swelling and necrosis, disruption of follicular architecture, edema, and infiltration with mononuclear cells. Resolution of the acute phase is followed by fibrosis, vascular narrowing, and further lymphocytic infiltration. These changes account for the early response to radioiodine, whether favorable or excessive.

Radiation thyroiditis may lead to an exacerbation of thyrotoxicosis 10 to 14 days after administration of radioiodine; this occasionally has serious consequences, including precipitation of a thyrotoxic crisis and aggravation of severe thyrotoxicosis or cardiac insufficiency. In patients with thyrocardiac disease, therefore, anti-thyroid drugs should always be given for several months before radioiodine, to deplete glandular hormone stores, and an β-adrenergic blocking regimen should be initiated to limit any potential arrhythmias, if this is appropriate. Anti-thyroid drugs prevent an outpouring of hormone if severe radiation thyroiditis should occur. The anti-thyroid agent should be withdrawn 3 to 7 days before administration of the radioiodine; if the clinical condition warrants, the agent can be started again 1 week later.

#5—Orbitopathy and Radioiodine. As discussed earlier, Graves' orbitopathy is probably the result of a cross-over specificity between retroorbital and thyroid antigens, including the TSHR itself. Therefore, any worsening of the autoimmune thyroid response might worsen the orbital immune response. After radioiodine therapy, the levels of circulating TRAbs are strikingly elevated,[57,211] perhaps secondary to impairment of immune restraint caused by the intrathyroidal irradiation that renders regulatory cells more sensitive. This change is in keeping with exacerbation of pretibial myxedema after radioiodine administration.[212] Similarly, carefully conducted studies indicate that significant eye disease worsens in about 10% of patients with Graves' orbitopathy who are treated with radioiodine (Fig. 12-12),[213,214] although this may not apply in mild disease.[215] Deterioration, if any, is usually mild and temporary but on occasion can involve a dramatic worsening.

Some physicians advocate the use of glucocorticoids at the time of radioiodine treatment to prevent such effects.[141,217] One regimen involves prednisone, 0.4 to 0.5 mg/kg given 1 month before ^{131}I treatment, with a gradual tapering over 3 to 4 months. However, maneuvers such as careful control of thyroid function before and after therapy and cessation of smoking by the patient may also help minimize ocular changes. We do not advocate the use of radioiodine in patients with severe Graves' ophthalmopathy unless steroid therapy is provided.

#6—Other Side Effects of Radioiodine. Additional hazards may attend the use of radioiodine, particularly in large doses. The parathyroid glands are exposed to radiation in patients treated with radioiodine. Although parathyroid reserve may be diminished in some patients, development of overt hypoparathyroidism is rare. The effect of radioiodine on other tissues that concentrate iodide (e.g., salivary glands, gastric glands, breasts) has often had attention but is not likely to be a problem with the relatively low doses prescribed for Graves' disease compared with the treatment of thyroid cancer.

Choice of Therapy

The choice of therapy for thyrotoxicosis is influenced by the experience of the treating clinician, emotional attitudes, economic considerations, and family and personal issues. Our choice of therapy takes into account the natural history of the disease, the advantages and disadvantages of the available therapies, and the features of the patient's population group. Apart from direct request by the patient, surgery is recommended only when the shortcomings of other modes of therapy are of particular importance, such as in patients with allergy to anti-thyroid drugs, a coincident cold nodule, a very large goiter, or need for a rapid return to normal. Occasionally, in young adults, it is necessary to remove a diffuse toxic goiter because of obstructive symptoms or cosmetic disfigurement. Nevertheless, in the United States, only a small percentage of patients with Graves' disease are now recommended for surgery. The choice, therefore, is among anti-thyroid drugs, radioiodine therapy, or a mixture of both.

In one common approach to therapy in adults, the physician initiates treatment with anti-thyroid drugs in all patients to produce a euthyroid state before reaching a final decision regarding a definitive therapeutic strategy. This allows the patient to return to a euthyroid status as rapidly as possible and provides an estimate of the anti-thyroid drug dose requirement. The magnitude of the drug requirement and the size of the thyroid gland are two of a number of factors considered in the evaluation of the patient with regard to the likelihood of a remission. The options for treatment are explained to the patient during these first months of contact, and individual recommendations are then formulated. This approach allows the establishment of a workable physician-patient relationship, which is especially important in addressing anxieties about the use of radioiodine. Such concerns lead many patients, especially those younger than 50 years of age, to elect a prolonged trial of anti-thyroid drugs before definitive therapy with ^{131}I.

Anti-thyroid drug therapy may be especially preferable in patients predicted to have a higher rate of remission. Patients with a large thyroid gland, a maintenance thionamide dose requirement of more than 10 mg of methimazole (or carbimazole equivalent), or high titers of TRAbs are likely to require prolonged anti-thyroid treatment and should be advised that the chance of spontaneous remission is less than 30%. A therapeutic trial is usually pursued for 12 months if long-term thionamide therapy is selected. One can, in theory, treat forever unless side effects occur.

When a decision in favor of radioiodine is made, ^{131}I may be prescribed at a dose designed to result in the retention of about 300 MBq (8 mCi) ^{131}I in the thyroid gland at 24 hours, or an ablative dose (20 mCi) may be prescribed. Radioiodine therapy may be used in young women desiring pregnancy, but they should wait 4 to 6 months after ^{131}I administration to become pregnant. Because of the possibility of exacerbation of Graves' disease following pregnancy and the transplacental passage of anti-thyroid drugs, it is preferable to ablate the thyroid before conception and to adjust levothyroxine dosages during pregnancy.

Hypothyroidism in the Recently Hyperthyroid Patient

The early onset of hypothyroidism may cause distinct symptoms in the previously thyrotoxic patient after ^{131}I or surgical treatment or even after high doses of thionamide drugs. Such patients may develop severe muscle cramps, often in large muscle groups such as the trapezius or latissimus dorsi or the proximal muscles of the extremities. Such symptoms can develop even when the serum hormone levels are only low-normal or slightly decreased and before the serum TSH concentration has risen. It is possible to mistake a symptom such as back or hip pain for an unrelated illness, and the patient should be warned in advance. It is also not unusual for patients to complain of hypothyroid symptoms when thyroid function test results return to the normal range. Such patients appear to have trouble adjusting to normal thyroid hormone levels after being exposed to excessive amounts for long periods. Weight gain is a frequent complaint after recovery from chronic thyrotoxicosis, and patients should be cautioned regarding their diet.[218]

Treatment of Infiltrative Orbitopathy or Infiltrative Dermopathy

Infiltrative orbitopathy varies in severity from the common mild form to a severe form that threatens vision. The latter type is rare and remains difficult to treat, especially if not seen early after disease onset. The natural course of the disorder, which is variable and characterized by exacerbations and remissions, makes conclusions about the efficacy of any treatment difficult.[219-221] A further source of confusion is the variable terminology used to describe the manifestations of orbitopathy and the lack of rigid criteria for defining their severity. Use of a clinical activity score is strongly recommended for everyday clinical practice (see Table 12-3).

Effect of Treatment of the Thyroid Gland on Orbitopathy. The first question that arises is whether different treatments for thyrotoxicosis affect the course of the eye disease differently. Most researchers have found that subtotal or total thyroidectomy and thionamide drug therapy do not influence ophthalmopathy unless they lead to the development of hypothyroidism.[222,223] However, some experienced investigators have found that total thyroidectomy with thyroid ablation of any remnant favors a better long-term outcome for this disorder.[224] However, hypothyroidism has an adverse effect on the disorder and should be treated fully when it occurs. As discussed earlier, controlled studies suggest that radioiodine treatment can lead to a slight but significant worsening of orbitopathy, and it may be best to avoid radioiodine in patients with severe eye disease. Alternatively, concurrent glucocorticoid therapy may prevent deterioration of orbitopathy after radioiodine therapy, but glucocorticoid therapy may itself cause significant side effects.[225]

Symptomatic Treatment. Treatment modalities can be largely symptomatic (useful mainly in the mild form of orbitopathy), or they can attempt to arrest or reverse the progression of the disorder. With milder forms, little treatment is required. The patient who experiences photophobia and sensitivity to wind or cold air can benefit by wearing dark glasses, which also afford protection from foreign bodies. Elevation of the head of the bed at night and instillation of lubricants, such as 1% methylcellulose, may be helpful if the eyelids do not appose completely during sleep. Artificial tears may be used during the day. Because the ophthalmic manifestations tend to be self-limited and progression to a more severe form is uncommon, such measures usually suffice to tide the patient over until the disorder regresses spontaneously.

Glucocorticoids. The appearance of increasing proptosis with inability to appose the eyelids or of severe infiltrative manifestations such as chemosis warrants the use of more vigorous therapeutic measures. Such changes, even when severe, may respond favorably and rapidly to glucocorticoids. Some physicians use large doses of prednisone (100 mg/day). If improvement occurs, the dose is decreased to the lowest level at which improvement is maintained. The latter dose is still likely to be large, but it is hoped that a halt to the progression or actual regression of the disease will occur before untoward effects make withdrawal of the drug necessary. Other physicians find that much smaller doses of prednisone (20 to 30 mg/day) can be highly effective with rapid reduction to a longer-term maintenance dose (10 to 15 mg/day).

Intravenous methylprednisolone pulse therapy (such as 500 mg initially, then 250 mg weekly for 6 weeks) has been shown to have fewer side effects than high doses of oral prednisone and to have a more rapid onset of effectiveness.[226,227] However, liver damage has been reported when used doses are excessive (>10 g total), and this approach has not been widely used in the United States.

It is important to protect the patient's bones during corticosteroid treatment, especially with a postmenopausal woman, and this can be achieved with a bisphosphonate drug such as alendronate, 70 mg once a week, in combination with calcium/vitamin D supplements.

External Radiation. The value of external radiation to the retroorbits has been established in some, but not all, clinical trials.[228-231] This treatment is steroid-sparing rather than steroid-replacing therapy, and it is said by some to work best in combination with steroids, especially early in the onset of the disorder.[141] Whether it is even more effective than prednisone therapy is unclear. Side effects of retroorbital irradiation have included the development of retinal angiogenesis, and the presence of diabetes mellitus is a clear contraindication to this approach. The safe administration of highly collimated supervoltage radiation to the retroorbital space requires experienced personnel and should, in our opinion, be reserved for the early treatment of severe disease. Although periorbital edema may be helped, exophthalmos and ophthalmoparesis are usually minimally affected. There is a clear need for a reliable disease marker to monitor the effects of such treatment.

Orbital Decompression. If glucocorticoid therapy or external radiation (or both) does not halt progression of the disease, or if loss of vision is threatened by ulceration or infection of the cornea or by changes in the retina or optic nerve, orbital decompression can be performed by a variety of techniques.[232,233] In some patients, desire for a nearly complete cosmetic correction may be such that decompression surgery is the only satisfactory route. This procedure usually involves removal of either the lateral wall or the roof of the orbit or resection of the lateral wall of the ethmoid sinus and the roof of the maxillary sinus. However, the operation often causes or worsens diplopia, and even in the best of hands corrective muscle surgery is necessary later. However, overall results are usually good in 95% of patients, and a reduction of up to 5 mm in proptosis can be achieved. Whenever possible, such surgery should be delayed until the disease becomes less active for fear of further inflammatory activity after the surgery.

Newer Treatments for Graves' Orbitopathy. The search for an immunosuppressive approach to Graves' orbitopathy has been long and tortuous. Without knowing the precise immunopathology, such an approach cannot be disease specific. However, use of an anti–B cell monoclonal antibody (rituximab) has produced some impressive early results after single-dose treatments.[234,235] Side effects of this therapy may occur, including the transient induction of retroorbital swelling, which in some patients may threaten vision. Carefully controlled trials will decide whether this approach is suitable for general clinical use.

An Approach to the Treatment of Orbitopathy. We recommend a trial of oral or intravenous glucocorticoid therapy for patients with severe or progressive orbitopathy. If a positive effect is not seen within a few weeks, a course of external irradiation may be attempted in suitable patients if edema predominates. However, oral glucocorticoid therapy may provide an opportune time to treat with radioiodine or to remove the goiter.

Along with these major forms of treatment, local measures should be employed. Ulceration and infection of the cornea should be treated with antibiotics, lubricants, and protective shields. An attempt to appose the eyelids by means of sutures (tarsorrhaphy) should be performed only by an experienced ophthalmologist, because sutures can tear loose and cause scarring.

The management of severe orbitopathy should never be undertaken by the endocrinologist or by the ophthalmologist acting alone. Close, coordinated observation of the effects of medical therapy and the progress of the disease is necessary to determine whether and when surgery is appropriate. Surgery almost invariably halts the progress of the disease and preserves vision if it is performed in time. This decision is influenced by the ability of the available surgical team, because the degree of success of such procedures is proportional to experience.

Treatment of Infiltrative Dermopathy. Treatment of infiltrative dermopathy is necessary as soon as the condition is recognized. The application of a topical, high-potency glucocorticoid preparation with an occlusive dressing may cause regression or disappearance of the lesion.[236,237] Long-standing untreated dermopathy is more resistant to treatment.

Thyroid Storm (Accelerated Hyperthyroidism)

Thyroid storm or *accelerated hyperthyroidism* is an extreme accentuation of thyrotoxicosis. It is an uncommon but serious complication, usually occurring in association with Graves' disease but sometimes with toxic multinodular goiter in the elderly patient.

Presentation

Thyroid storm is usually of abrupt onset and occurs in patients in whom preexisting thyrotoxicosis has been treated incompletely or not at all. The condition is usually precipitated by infection, trauma, surgical emergencies, or planned operations or, less commonly, by radiation thyroiditis, diabetic ketoacidosis, toxemia of pregnancy, or parturition. The mechanisms by which such factors worsen thyrotoxicosis may be related to cytokine release and acute immunologic disturbance caused by the precipitating condition. The serum thyroid hormone levels in crisis are not appreciably greater than those in severe uncomplicated thyrotoxicosis, but the patient can no longer adapt to the metabolic stress. The clinical picture is one of severe hypermetabolism. Fever is almost invariable and may be severe; sweating is profuse. Marked tachycardia of sinus or ectopic origin and arrhythmias may be accompanied by

TABLE 12-6

Diagnostic Criteria for Thyroid Storm

Diagnostic Parameter	Points*
Temperature (° F)	
99-99.9	5
100-100.9	10
101-101.9	15
102-102.9	20
103-103.9	25
≥104.0	30
Central Nervous System Effects	
Absent	0
Mild (agitation)	10
Moderate (delirium, psychosis, extreme lethargy)	20
Severe (seizures, coma)	30
Gastrointestinal-Hepatic Dysfunction	
Absent	0
Moderate (diarrhea, nausea/vomiting, abdominal pain)	10
Severe (unexplained jaundice)	20
Cardiovascular Dysfunction	
Tachycardia (beats/min)	
90-109	5
110-119	10
120-129	15
130-139	20
≥140	25
Congestive Heart Failure	
Absent	0
Mild (pedal edema)	5
Moderate (bibasilar rales)	10
Severe (pulmonary edema)	15
Atrial Fibrillation	
Absent	0
Present	10
Precipitating Event	
Absent	0
Present	10

*Scoring system: A score of 45 or greater is highly suggestive of thyroid storm; 25-44 is suggestive of impending storm, and <25 is unlikely to represent thyroid storm.

Adapted from Burch HB, Wartofsky L. Life-threatening thyrotoxicosis: thyroid storm. *Endocrinol Metab Clin North Am.* 1993;22:263-277.

pulmonary edema or congestive heart failure. Tremulousness and restlessness are present; delirium or frank psychosis may supervene. Nausea, vomiting, and abdominal pain may occur early in the course. As the disorder progresses, apathy, stupor, and coma may supervene, and hypotension can develop. If unrecognized, the condition can be fatal. This clinical picture in a patient with a history of preexisting thyrotoxicosis or with goiter or exophthalmos (or both) is sufficient to establish the diagnosis, and emergency treatment should not await laboratory confirmation. A clinical score (Table 12-6) may be used to help confirm the diagnosis.[238]

Even with this approach, there are no foolproof criteria by which severe thyrotoxicosis complicated by some other serious disease can be distinguished from thyrotoxic crisis induced by that disease. In any event, the differentiation between these alternatives is of no great significance, because treatment is the same in either case.

Treatment of Thyroid Storm

Treatment aims to correct both the severe thyrotoxicosis and the precipitating illness and to provide general support. There are no clinical trials of treatment for accelerated thyrotoxicosis, and opinions vary to some degree on the details, in particular the doses of anti-thyroid drugs that should be used. However, all agree that the patient thought to have thyroid storm should be monitored in a medical intensive care unit during the initial phases of therapy. The therapy itself is designed to inhibit hormone synthesis and release, to antagonize the increased sensitivity to adrenergic stimulation mediated by severe thyrotoxicosis, and to combat the hyperpyrexia.

Large doses of an anti-thyroid agent (up to 400 mg of propylthiouracil every 4 to 6 hours) are given by mouth, by stomach tube, or, if necessary, per rectum. Propylthiouracil is preferable to methimazole because it has the additional action of inhibiting the peripheral as well as the thyroidal generation of T_3 from T_4 by D1, which is the major source of the T_3.[162,163,169,239] Administration of propylthiouracil initiates therapy for the postcrisis period and prevents enrichment of glandular hormone stores by iodide, whose administration is of more immediate importance. The latter, administered either as SSKI (3 drops twice daily) or the equivalent as Lugol's solution (10 drops twice daily) (see earlier discussion), acutely retards the release of preformed hormone from the thyroid gland.

Theoretically, propylthiouracil should be administered before iodine to inhibit the synthesis of additional thyroid hormone from the administered iodine. However, because iodide and blocks its own organification through the Wolff-Chaikoff effect, its administration should not be delayed (until the availability of a thionamide) or omitted in the severely toxic patient in the absence of known allergy to iodide per se.

Large doses of dexamethasone (8 mg orally once daily) or hydrocortisone (100 mg every 8 hours) should be given to support the response to stress and to inhibit both the release of hormone from the gland (in conjunction with iodide) and possibly the peripheral generation of T_3 from T_4 (synergizing with propylthiouracil). The combined use of propylthiouracil, iodide, and glucocorticoids can restore the concentration of T_3 to normal within 24 to 48 hours.[240,241] In the absence of cardiac insufficiency or asthma, a β-adrenergic blocking agent should be given to ameliorate the hyperadrenergic state. Most experience has been with propranolol given at a dose of 40 to 80 mg orally every 6 hours, but a very-short-acting β-adrenergic blocker such as labetalol or esmolol may be safer than propranolol in this situation. High-output congestive heart failure can develop in patients with severe thyrotoxicosis, and a β-adrenergic antagonist may further reduce cardiac output. If β-adrenergic blocking agents are contraindicated, a calcium channel blocker (diltiazem) may be used to slow the heart rate.

Supportive measures include correction of dehydration and hypernatremia, if present, and administration of glucose. Hyperpyrexia should be treated vigorously, and the administration of a wide-spectrum antibiotic is appropriate after blood and urine cultures have been taken. In mild cases, acetaminophen may help, but a cold blanket or ice packs may be required. Salicylates should be avoided because they compete with T_3 and T_4 for binding to TBG and transthyretin (TTR) and therefore increase the free hormone levels.[242] In addition, high doses of salicylates increase the metabolic rate. If heart failure or pulmonary congestion is present, appropriate use of diuretics is

TABLE 12-7

Complications of Hyperthyroidism in Pregnancy

Increased and recurrent pregnancy loss
Preterm delivery
Preeclampsia
Fetal growth restriction
Fetal thyroid hyperfunction or hypofunction caused by TRAbs
Fetal goiter from excessive anti-thyroid drug treatment
Neonatal thyrotoxicosis
Increased perinatal and maternal mortality
Potential for decreased IQ of offspring because of excessive use of anti-thyroid drugs

TRAbs, thyrotropin receptor antibodies.

indicated. In patients with atrial fibrillation, the rapid ventricular response requires appropriate blockade of atrioventricular node conduction.

When treatment is successful, improvement is usually manifested within 1 or 2 days and recovery occurs within 1 week. At that time, the dexamethasone can be tapered and plans for long-term management made.

Graves' Disease during Pregnancy and the Postpartum Period

Although it is seen regularly in clinical practice, a truly overactive thyroid gland is uncommon in established pregnancy, affecting approximately 0.2% of pregnant women. This rate is low because fertility is reduced in thyrotoxicosis. Autoimmune responses tend to be suppressed during pregnancy, and Graves' disease, an autoimmune disorder, is the most common cause of thyrotoxicosis in young women.[130,243] Furthermore, while thyrotoxicosis has a variety of negative influences on fertility itself, it is also associated with increased pregnancy loss and serious medical complications for both the mother and the infant if it should persist[48,244,245] (Table 12-7). More commonly, a woman who is already under treatment for hyperthyroidism becomes pregnant. Whatever the sequence, pregnancy complicates the diagnosis and treatment of hyperthyroidism in Graves' disease and influences its severity and course.

Influence of Pregnancy on the Immune System

The development of pregnancy and growth of the placenta have profound influences on the immune system, as discussed earlier (see Risk Factor #5). The overall suppression of autoimmune responses that occurs is designed to allow the fetus, with its 50% paternal antigens, to survive immune assault.[243,246] The mechanisms invoked in pregnancy are multiple and include peripheral tolerance mechanisms that deplete fetal reactive cells and inhibition of pathways capable of causing damage after immune activation (Table 12-8). These changes promote maternal-fetal tolerance, but the role of regulatory T cells (which increase in number in pregnancy) and their suppression of maternal responses to the fetus appears to be predominant and long lived.[247] It has been shown that a major shift in such T-cell control reduces the effectiveness of all inflammatory T cells.

Fetal Microchimerism

In normal pregnancy, cells pass from mother to child and from child to mother. The presence of fetal microchimerism in parous women has been shown to persist for longer than 20 years,[248] indicating complete tolerance for the fetal cells. This is an exaggerated and long-lasting form of the immunosuppression of pregnancy described earlier. Whether such cells can ever stimulate an immune response as tolerance fades has been the subject of much speculation, fueled by the apparent accumulation of fetal cells at sites of inflammation including the thyroid, but the concept remains unproven.[249] However, fetal microchimerism has been associated with Graves' disease–susceptible HLA haplotypes,[250] and a failure of fetal tolerance remains a likely contributing mechanism to postpartum thyroid disease.[251]

Thyroid Antibodies in Pregnant Patients with Graves' Disease

The hallmark of the immune effects initiated by the placenta is the fall in secretion of thyroid autoantibodies (TPO-Ab, Tg-Ab, and TRAbs) that is seen in almost all patients as pregnancy progresses.[252] This is now considered to be secondary to enhanced regulatory T-cell activity,[253] and it is followed by a rapid increase in autoantibody levels after the immunosuppression is lost in the postpartum period. Assays for TRAbs in the serum of pregnant women with Graves' disease may be of clinical value in selected cases, because a failure of this immunosuppression may indicate potential fetal problems.[72,254-256]

Because maternal antibodies cross the placenta, there is a correlation between the maternal level of stimulatory TRAbs and the development of fetal thyrotoxicosis. Fetal and neonatal thyrotoxicosis occurs in only 1% of infants of mothers with Graves' disease, and high levels of TRAbs, usually greater than three times the upper normal limit, are correlated with fetal thyroid stimulation.[128] Pregnant women who are at risk for failure to suppress thyroid autoantibodies include those with more severe hyperthyroidism and those with significant Graves' orbitopathy or infiltrative dermopathy. In addition, prior ablative treatment of the mother with either surgery or radioiodine may not always be accompanied by a reduction in TRAbs. In such cases, the fetus of a treated patient with Graves' disease may still be at risk for development of fetal or neonatal thyrotoxicosis, and the mother may need anti-thyroid drug treatment. The fetus may require monitoring by umbilical cord blood testing and ultrasonography.[257]

Differential Diagnosis

When mild thyrotoxicosis is present during early pregnancy, it may be a gestational thyrotoxicosis (GTT) that occurs secondary to hCG stimulation of the thyroid gland (see later discussion).[258-260] When it is more severe, it is usually due to Graves' disease, because toxic multinodular goiters and hot nodules are uncommon in this age group.

TABLE 12-8

Mechanisms of Immunosuppression in Pregnancy Leading to Immune Privilege

Maternal Peripheral Immune System
Regulatory T cells suppress fetal-reactive immune cells.
Sex steroids affect the immune system and negatively regulate B cells.
Maternal-Fetal Interface (Trophoblast–Immune Cell Interaction)
Apoptosis is induced in activated T cells by Fas expression on trophoblast cells.
T-cell proliferation is inhibited by local cytokines and chemokines.
Natural killer cells are inhibited by expression of human leukocyte antigen G (HLA-G).
Complement system is inactivated.

Diagnosis

Pregnancy and hyperthyroidism are both accompanied by thyroid stimulation, a hyperdynamic circulation, and hypermetabolism. Amenorrhea may occur in thyrotoxicosis not associated with pregnancy. In pregnancy, serum TBG levels are increased by estrogen-induced changes in glycosylation that lengthen the half-life. Therefore, in both conditions, the total serum T_4 and T_3 levels are elevated so that the upper limit of the normal range during gestation is about 1.5 times the upper nonpregnant reference limit.[128] However, serum free T_4 levels, as measured by both analog and equilibrium dialysis methodologies, may actually decrease as pregnancy progresses, and the normal third-trimester reference range for a given assay is significantly less than its nonpregnant reference range.[128] Serum TSH levels also decrease during normal pregnancy, reaching a nadir between the 8th and 14th gestational week because of stimulation of the thyroid gland by hCG during this interval (GTT), as discussed earlier.

The lower limits for serum TSH levels (95% confidence interval) are 0.06, 0.3, and 0.3 mIU/L, respectively, for the first, second, and third trimesters.[261] Biochemically, the diagnosis of thyrotoxicosis is confirmed if the serum TSH level is lower than the trimester-specific lower limit and the total or free T_4 level is higher than the normative range for pregnancy (see Fig. 11-12 in Chapter 11). Detection of TRAbs can confirm the diagnosis of Graves' disease, which may or may not be obvious from the clinical history and examination.

Treatment during Pregnancy

Mild hyperthyroidism in pregnancy does not lead to a significant increase in risk for mother or fetus, whereas severe thyrotoxicosis can lead to many complications and endanger both lives. However, the management of hyperthyroidism during pregnancy can be an even greater problem than its diagnosis. Graves' disease can worsen in the first trimester, but the subsequent trimesters have an attenuating influence on the hyperthyroid state because of the immunosuppression associated with pregnancy. Pregnancy is also one of the few clinical situations in which an assay of the biologic activity of the TRAbs is helpful in predicting its potential effect on the newborn.

Anti-Thyroid Drugs. Medical therapy is the method of choice in pregnancy. Because of the usual improvement in the disease, the dosage of anti-thyroid drug required to control the disease in the later phases of pregnancy is usually much less than that which would be required in the same patient were she not pregnant. Overtreatment of the hyperthyroid pregnant woman remains a common but avoidable clinical problem with potentially severe consequences for the fetus, and mild undertreatment should be preferred to hypothyroidism.[257,262-264] It is imperative for the clinician to understand the therapeutic targets for titrating anti-thyroid drug dosages during pregnancy.[265]

Certain aspects of placental physiology are relevant to the use of anti-thyroid drugs. Propylthiouracil and methimazole cross the placenta readily and equally well, and they are concentrated in the fetal thyroid. In excess quantity, these agents can cause goitrous hypothyroidism in the fetus.[266] Maternal T_4 crosses the placenta (as evidenced by infants born with significant circulating serum T_4 concentrations despite congenital hypothyroidism), and this is the major source of fetal thyroid hormone before functional development of the hypothalamic-pituitary axis in the fetus is complete (at about 20 weeks' gestation). Transplacental passage of maternal TRAbs in the latter half of pregnancy can result in fetal thyroid stimulation. Therefore, the fetal thyroid is subject to the same factors that influence maternal thyroid hormone production.

Until recently, the anti-thyroid drug of choice throughout pregnancy in the United States was propylthiouracil because of the rare embryopathy (including aplasia cutis and choanal atresia) thought to be associated with methimazole.[262,267-269] However, because of the rare but serious side effect of hepatic failure, in June 2009 the FDA issued an advisory that propylthiouracil should be reserved for the first trimester of pregnancy, while organogenesis is occurring.[168] Subsequently, methimazole should be prescribed. One must keep in mind that the therapeutic anti-thyroid potency ratio of methimazole to propylthiouracil is at least 15:1. A patient who requires only 50 mg of propylthiouracil in the first trimester may not even require a thionamide during the remainder of pregnancy.

The therapeutic target for a pregnant Graves' patients is a healthy infant, meaning one with subclinical hyperthyroidism analogous to the normal gestational physiology of the first trimester.[265] This is associated with the lowest impact on fetal thyroid function and the highest rate of normal neonatal thyroid hormone levels.[270] The maternal serum free T_4 level should be maintained at or just above the upper normal *nonpregnant* range, and no attempt should be made to normalize the serum TSH concentration. However, it is the clinical status of the patient that is the most important indication for treatment or increases in dosage. A modest tachycardia is a physiologic response to the increased metabolic demands of pregnancy, and pulse rates of 90 to 100 are well tolerated without evidence of myocardial decompensation during delivery. The natural amelioration of Graves' disease in the third trimester should be kept in mind. Repeated attempts should be made to reduce or discontinue the thionamide as the delivery date approaches to avoid TSH-induced goiter in the newborn, which could cause asphyxia (see Fig. 11-11 in Chapter 11). A block-and-replace strategy is therefore not appropriate for thionamide therapy in the pregnant patient. The serum TSH concentration should be monitored monthly, more to avoid inadvertant overtreatment rather than as the target for normalization.

All pregnant patients with significant Graves' disease should be managed in close cooperation with obstetricians who are experienced with modern techniques for monitoring the fetus for intrauterine thyroid dysfunction. These techniques include fetal heart rate monitoring and ultrasonographic assessment of fetal growth rate. With advanced ultrasonography, it is usually possible to examine the fetus for the presence of goiter. Convincing evidence of fetal hyperthyroidism may be an indication to consider another approach. In a compliant patient, a dose requirement in excess of 300 mg/day of propylthiouracil is a reasonable threshold for considering subtotal thyroidectomy, preferably in the second trimester. However, transplacental passage of TRAbs may also cause fetal enlargement, although 50 to 100 mg of propylthiouracil is usually sufficient to treat this condition because it is transferred transplacentally.[271]

Iodide and β-Blockers. Obviously, therapeutic radioiodine is contraindicated in pregnancy, although no harm has been found after diagnostic doses of ^{123}I.[203] Iodide itself should also not be used as therapy for longer than 2 to 3 weeks in the pregnant woman, because it readily crosses the placenta and can induce a large goiter that could cause airway obstruction in the newborn (see Fig. 11-11 in

Chapter 11). Large amounts of iodide are contraindicated in the last month of pregnancy but can be used at earlier times in emergent situations. Whether propranolol or other β-blockers should be used in the pregnant woman with hyperthyroidism has been a matter of debate. In the experience of some, it can cause intrauterine growth retardation, delayed lung development, and neonatal hypoglycemia or depression,[272] but large studies have suggested that it can be employed with safety for short periods or at very low doses.[273] Low doses of iodine have been used in pregnancy but only when all other approaches are contraindicated.[274]

Surgery. Surgery during the first and third trimesters is not desirable because of the possible induction of early pregnancy loss or later premature labor, respectively. Surgery may be successful during the second trimester, but it is best to avoid major surgery during pregnancy if possible. Nevertheless, if anti-thyroid drug requirements are very high or cannot be used, surgery may be indicated. Iodide can be given for 7 to 10 days to aid in patient preparation for those with large and highly vascular thyroid glands.

Consequences of Overtreatment. The influence of maternal hypothyroidism on fetal brain development and the subsequently reduced IQ of the children of hypothyroid mothers is discussed elsewhere (see Chapter 13).[275] Overuse of anti-thyroid drugs in pregnancy could potentially lead to the same consequences. There is considerable evidence that many pregnant patients with Graves' disease are overtreated as far as the fetus is concerned, as evidenced by transiently elevated serum TSH levels on newborn screening tests.[276] This is another reason why one should accept a slightly hyperthyroid rather than a slightly hypothyroid maternal status.

Graves' Disease in the Postpartum Period

Postpartum thyroiditis with transient thyrotoxicosis due to thyroid-cell destruction may occur in 5% to 10% of patients during the first 4 to 12 months after delivery.[277] Rapid return of hyperthyroidism is less common.

Changes in the Immune Response in the Postpartum Period. As discussed earlier, pregnancy induces a variety of immune changes that are responses to the paternal foreign antigens so that the fetus is not rejected. These changes include enhanced regulatory T-cell influences and a T-cell shift from Th1 to Th2. They result in an overall decrease in all autoimmune responses, as evidenced by marked decreases in thyroid autoantibodies. After delivery, these immune changes are slowly lost, and a return to normal is observed, but only after a period of exacerbated autoimmune reactivity in which large increases in T-cell and autoantibody activity occur. It is at this time—3 to 12 months postpartum—that new-onset or recurrent thyroid thyrotoxicosis is seen. Such thyroid dysfunction may be transient or permanent.

Presentation of Postpartum Graves' Disease. A high percentage of women in the 20- to 35-year age group give a history of pregnancy in the 12 months before the onset of Graves' disease.[132,278] Pregnancy and the postpartum state also apparently influence the course of preexisting Graves' disease. Patients who are in clinical remission during pregnancy are prone to postpartum relapse. Seventy-eight percent of 41 pregnancies in 35 patients in remission were followed by development of thyrotoxicosis during the postpartum period. The patients with Graves' disease and postpartum thyrotoxicosis were classified into three categories. Some had persistent recurrent hyperthyroidism with an elevated RAIU (classic Graves' disease). Some had a transient disorder associated with a normal or an elevated RAIU (transient Graves' disease). Some patients, especially those with the highest titers of TPO-Ab, experienced a transient thyrotoxicosis with a decreased RAIU (the thyrotoxic phase of postpartum thyroiditis). This phase, in turn, may be followed by a hypothyroid phase.[119]

The Desire for Pregnancy. A special problem related to hyperthyroidism and pregnancy is presented by the patient who wishes to conceive in the near future and is in early remission after a course of anti-thyroid drug treatment or is being treated with anti-thyroid agents for active Graves' disease. In the first scenario, anti-thyroid drugs can be reintroduced, if required, during pregnancy to treat recurrence of symptomatic thyrotoxicosis. In the second situation, definitive therapy (radioiodine or surgery) should be considered to forestall the complexities of managing hyperthyroidism during pregnancy. As with the treatment of Graves' disease in general, such decisions must involve education of the patient so that the risks and benefits of the various alternatives are clearly appreciated.

Nursing and Anti-Thyroid Drugs. Older studies suggested that relatively more methimazole than propylthiouracil appeared in breast milk of women receiving these drugs, but more recent evidence showed little difference between them.[266,279] However, women who take anti-thyroid drugs are advised not to nurse their infants because of the difficulty in monitoring thyroid function in infants. No serious drug side effects have been reported in neonates whose mothers were taking anti-thyroid drugs, although periodic tests of neonatal thyroid function may be appropriate in women taking very high doses.[280]

INHERITED NONIMMUNE HYPERTHYROIDISM

Toxic diffuse thyroid hyperplasia without the pathologic characteristics of autoimmune disease has been reported in families and appears to be inherited as an autosomal dominant condition.[53,281,282] Polymorphic genomic mutations in the TSHR gene have been reported to cause constitutively activated TSHRs differing from family to family. Recessive mutations on both chromosomes have also been described as causing hyperthyroidism while the parents remained euthyroid. These gain-of-function mutations, mostly in the transmembrane regions of the TSHR, are similar to those somatic mutations seen in toxic adenomas but are in the germline.[283] Treatment is by radioiodine ablation or thyroidectomy, depending on the age of the patient.

TOXIC MULTINODULAR GOITER

Toxic multinodular goiter is a disorder in which hyperthyroidism arises in a multinodular goiter, usually one of long standing. It is the result of one of several pathogenetic factors.[284]

Pathogenesis

The pathogenesis of toxic multinodular goiter cannot be considered apart from that of its invariable forerunner, nontoxic multinodular goiter, from which it emerges slowly and insidiously. Two hallmarks of the disorder, structural and functional heterogeneity and functional autonomy, evolve over time. The increase in the extent of autonomous function causes the disease to move from the nontoxic to the toxic phase, but the mechanisms of this change in all cases are uncertain. The somatic mutations in the TSHR gene demonstrated in toxic adenomas have been demonstrated in some cases of toxic multinodular goiter and appear to differ from nodule to nodule.[285] However, only about 60% of toxic nodules have TSHR mutations, and only a very few have G-protein mutations. Hence, there are many nodules with autonomy of undetermined cause.[286]

Radioiodine scintiscans show localization of isotope in one or more discrete nodules, whereas iodine accumulation in the remainder of the gland is usually suppressed. No further suppression is produced by exogenous thyroid hormone, but TSH stimulates iodine uptake in the previously inactive areas, indicating that the suppression is due to lack of TSH. Histopathologically, the functioning areas resemble adenomas in that they are reasonably well demarcated from surrounding tissue. They usually consist of large follicles, sometimes with hyperplastic epithelium, but here, too, architecture correlates poorly with functional state. The remaining tissue appears to be inactive, and zones of degeneration are present in both functioning and nonfunctioning areas. Therefore, from the pathophysiologic standpoint, these thyroids harbor multiple solitary hyperfunctioning and hypofunctioning adenomas interspersed by suppressed normal thyroid tissue.

Clinical Presentation

The overproduction of thyroid hormone in toxic multinodular goiter is usually less than that in Graves' disease. First, the clinical manifestations of thyrotoxicosis are rarely flagrant. Second, the serum T_4 and T_3 concentrations may be only marginally increased, and a suppressed TSH may be the major abnormality. Finally, the total RAIU is only slightly increased or within the normal range. The mildness of the hyperthyroidism is consistent with either of its presumed pathogenetic origins.

Toxic multinodular goiter is a common complication of nontoxic multinodular goiter, but its precise incidence is unknown. Toxic multinodular goiter usually occurs after the age of 50 in patients who have had nontoxic multinodular goiter for many years; such patients often live in regions of iodine deficiency.[287] Like its forerunner, toxic multinodular goiter is many times more common in women than in men. Sometimes, hyperthyroidism develops abruptly, usually after exposure to increased quantities of iodine, which permits autonomous foci to increase hormone secretion to excessive levels and which may simply exacerbate already established mild hyperthyroidism (see "Iodine-Induced Hyperthyroidism"). In addition, Graves' disease may manifest or develop in a multinodular gland, as confirmed by the presence of TRAbs of the stimulating variety. Toxic multinodular goiter is almost never accompanied by infiltrative ophthalmopathy; when the two do coexist, it represents the emergence of Graves' disease.

Cardiovascular manifestations tend to predominate, possibly because of the age of the patients, and include atrial fibrillation or tachycardia with or without heart failure. Weakness and muscle wasting are common—the so-called apathetic or masked thyrotoxicosis. The nervous manifestations are less prominent than in younger patients with thyrotoxicosis, but emotional lability may be pronounced. Because of the physical characteristics of the thyroid gland and its frequent retrosternal extension, obstructive symptoms are more common than in Graves' disease. On palpation, the characteristics of the goiter are the same as those of the more common nontoxic multinodular goiter. In as many as 20% of elderly patients with thyrotoxicosis, the thyroid gland is firm and irregular but not distinctly enlarged. Ultrasound examination will confirm the diagnosis as toxic multinodular goiter rather than a single toxic adenoma or Graves' disease.

Laboratory Tests and Differential Diagnosis

All patients with a multinodular goiter should be screened annually by measurement of serum TSH. If TSH is suppressed, the free T_4 (or if TSH is normal, the free T_3) should be determined. Serum TSH levels intermediate between 0.1 and 0.4 mU/L are not usually associated with significant symptoms. Such patients have thyroid autonomy but are not thyrotoxic (see "Subclinical Hyperthyroidism"). For patients with established thyrotoxicosis, an RAIU scintiscan study will help in gauging the dose of ^{131}I to be administered and will identify the autonomously functioning nodules. The latter can then be treated with ^{131}I.

Treatment

Radioiodine may be the treatment of choice for patients with toxic multinodular goiter despite disagreement about the size and number of doses required to achieve a therapeutic response.[284,288] We attempt to deposit about 12 to 14 mCi into the gland at 24 hours, based on a pretreatment RAIU. In the United States, iodine intake is higher than in many regions in Europe, so that 24-hour RAIU values of 20% to 30% are not unusual. Such patients require 50 mCi or more to restore a euthyroid state and may even require a second treatment.

Because a number of patients with this disorder have underlying heart disease, the administration of radioiodine should be preceded by a course of anti-thyroid therapy with methimazole until a eumetabolic state is achieved. Medication is then discontinued for at least for 4 to 7 days before radioiodine is administered. One week later, the anti-thyroid drug is reinstituted, so that the thyrotoxicosis will be controlled until radioiodine takes effect, which typically requires 3 to 4 months. A decrease in size of the hyperfunctioning nodules is a positive sign. After that occurs, the anti-thyroid drug can be tapered, but if the TSH level remains lower than 0.1 mU/L after 6 months, a second dose may be considered.

Surgical therapy is often recommended after adequate preoperative preparation in patients with obstructive manifestations. In these patients, a CT or MRI study is recommended to define the extent of the goiter and the adequacy of the tracheal walls. Respiratory function studies may also be helpful in assessing the need for surgery. Patients with fixed, especially partially retrosternal, goiter should be considered for therapy because of the risk of more complete obstruction should hemorrhage into a nodule occur. However, if surgery is contraindicated, even significant obstructive symptoms can be relieved by adequate radioiodine therapy.[289]

TOXIC ADENOMA

A third, less common form of hyperthyroidism is caused by one or more autonomous adenomas of the thyroid gland. As used here, the term *toxic adenoma* refers to a tumor in a thyroid that is otherwise intrinsically normal. The disorder is usually caused by a single adenoma that is either palpable or seen on ultrasound as a solitary nodule; hence, it is sometimes referred to as *hyperfunctioning solitary nodule* or *toxic nodule*. Occasionally, two or three adenomas of similar character are present.

Pathogenesis

Toxic adenomas are true follicular adenomas (for histopathologic characteristics, see Chapter 14). The basic pathogenesis in many cases is one of several somatic point mutations in the TSHR gene, commonly in the third transmembrane loop. These single-nucleotide substitutions cause amino acid changes that lead to constitutive activation of the TSHR in the absence of TSH.[290] The TSHR appears to be "tripped" from an "off" state to an "on" state. Similarly, loss-of-function rather than gain-of-function mutations may occur in the TSHR gene and cause hypothyroidism (see later discussion). A small number of autonomous adenomas have mutations in G-protein genes that lead to a similar state of constitutive activation.[286]

Clinical Presentation

The toxic adenoma often manifests as a nodule in a patient with a suppressed TSH; on ultrasonography, it appears as a single hypoechogenic nodule. A radioiodine thyroid scan shows a localized area of increased radioiodine accumulation (Fig. 12-13). This condition occurs in a younger age group than does toxic multinodular goiter, typically in patients in their 30s or 40s.

Frequently there is a history of a long-standing, slowly growing lump in the neck. It is unusual for adenomas to produce thyrotoxicosis until they have achieved a diameter greater than 3 cm.[284] Up to that point, patients have subclinical hyperthyroidism. The adenoma can undergo central necrosis and hemorrhage, spontaneously relieving the thyrotoxicosis, and the remainder of the thyroid may resume its function. Calcification in the area of hemorrhage may take place and may be evident on sonographic examination. Such calcification is usually macroscopic and irregular and does not resemble the finely stippled calcification that is suggestive of papillary cancers. The peripheral clinical manifestations of a toxic adenoma are usually milder than those of Graves' disease and are notable for the absence of infiltrative orbitopathy and myopathy, although cardiovascular manifestations may occur.

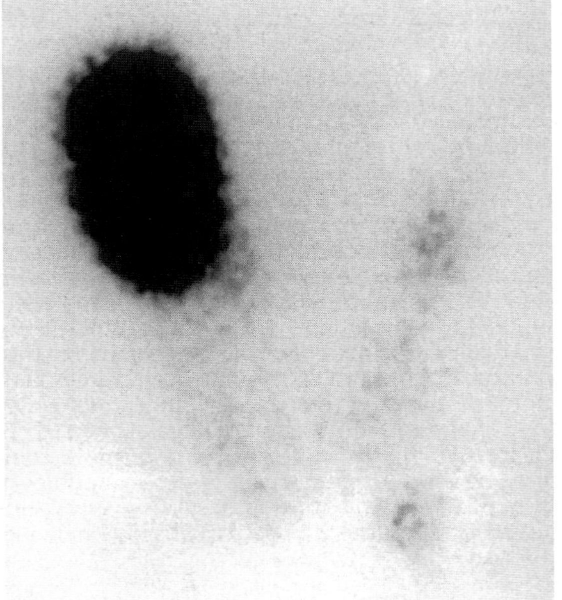

Figure 12-13 Radioiodine (^{123}I) thyroid scan shows a hyperfunctioning hot nodule corresponding to physical examination findings with a faint outline of the remaining suppressed gland. In this unusual case, Graves' disease developed a few months later after an oral contrast agent load. (From Soule J, Mayfield R. Graves' disease after ^{131}I therapy for toxic nodule. *Thyroid*. 2001;11:91-92.)

Laboratory Tests

The results of laboratory tests depend on the stage and function of the adenoma. At first, serum thyroid hormone concentrations are normal except for borderline suppression of the serum TSH. This finding, together with ultrasound examination to exclude multiple nodules, confirms the diagnosis. Later, a thyroid scan may show localization of radioisotope in the palpated nodule, but this does not occur until TSH secretion is suppressed. If the nodule continues to grow, frank hyperthyroidism develops, accompanied by elevation of serum thyroid hormone levels. Occasionally, the serum free T_4 concentration is normal and only the serum T_3 level is increased (T_3 thyrotoxicosis). Incidental thyroid carcinoma may rarely coexist within a gland exhibiting a hyperfunctioning adenoma, although autonomous malignant nodules causing functional hyperthyroidism are very rare.

Treatment

Hyperfunctioning adenomas may eventually cause clinical hyperthyroidism, but many do so slowly, and others not at all.[284] Therefore, treatment of asymptomatic patients with functional adenomas is decided on an individual basis. Clinically euthyroid subjects who wish to avoid both surgery and radioiodine therapy may be monitored with annual TSH measurements. However, suppression of TSH below normal, particularly to less than 0.1 mU/L, indicates hyperthyroidism, and therapy may be warranted. Two definitive therapies are available: radioiodine and surgery.

Radioiodine

In terms of the specificity of treatment, functioning thyroid nodules are good candidates for radioiodine therapy. In theory, the radiation should be directed almost exclusively to the diseased tissue, because TSH is suppressed and the normal thyroid tissue surrounding the nodule does not take up radioiodine. However, this suppression may be incomplete, and a significant fraction of patients receiving ^{131}I develop thyroid failure. For the patient older than 18 years of age with a nodule 5 cm in diameter or smaller, ^{131}I is an appropriate treatment if the risk of eventual hypothyroidism is acceptable to the patient. For such lesions, doses of radioiodine are given sufficient to result in the presence of 300 to 370 MBq (8 to 10 mCi) in the nodule at 24 hours based on the uptake.[284] Because of the potential for hypothyroidism, prolonged follow-up is mandatory.

Surgery

Toxic nodules are readily treated by surgical excision. A hemithyroidectomy may avoid the long-term development of hypothyroidism, and with modern surgical procedures it can be performed on an outpatient basis or even with the use of local anesthesia. Surgical excision may be preferable in patients who are younger than 18 years of age because it avoids the long-term consequences of irradiation, including effects on perinodular tissue. Because toxic adenoma is not diffusely hypervascular, preoperative preparation with iodine is not required. In the patient with overt thyrotoxicosis, however, a normal metabolic state should be restored with the use of an anti-thyroid drug before surgery.

SUBCLINICAL HYPERTHYROIDISM

Definition

As mentioned in Chapter 11, the availability of sensitive assays for TSH has allowed recognition of a syndrome, *subclinical hyperthyroidism,* in which there are no signs or symptoms of thyrotoxicosis but the serum TSH is subnormal despite normal serum free thyroid hormone concentrations. Although the term is somewhat of a misnomer because it is defined by biochemical characteristics, all endocrinologists have a concept of what it means. Nonetheless, the classification of a patient as having subclinical hyperthyroidism may simply reflect the fact that the detection of physiologic evidence of excess thyroid hormone on a chronic basis is less sensitive than measurements of TSH. The situation is further complicated by the fact that the hypothalamic-pituitary axis is sensitive to both serum free T_4 and T_3, whereas the peripheral tissues (e.g., heart) primarily sense the free T_3 (see Chapter 11).[291,292]

Given the wide normal range for free thyroid hormone concentrations, it is easy to assume that an individual with a low-normal free T_4 set point for TSH secretion would have a reduced TSH level if that set-point concentration were exceeded by 50% but still remained within the normal range. In fact, in patients with primary hypothyroidism and normal TSH, small additional quantities of levothyroxine decrease TSH below normal without producing a supranormal free T_4.[291] On the other hand, in the now classic studies in the Framingham population of patients older than 60 years of age, the cumulative incidence of atrial fibrillation over 10 years was 28% in patients with a serum TSH concentration of 0.1 mU/L or less but only 11% in those with serum TSH concentrations between 0.1 and 0.4 mU/L—just slightly higher than the incidence in the normal population.[10,11] Other studies have shown similar results.[293,294]

Bone density is another end point for such studies, because it is well known that thyroid hormone causes a net resorption of cortical bone. Several studies have demonstrated lower bone density in patients with *subclinical thyrotoxicosis,* although others have not.[40] These results illustrate the conundrum of the term "subclinical," because, by definition, such patients should not have any clinical abnormalities associated with thyrotoxicosis.[295]

This is a subject of considerable interest, because the condition is much more common than overt thyrotoxicosis (e.g., 0.7% of the population in NHANES III) and has broad implications with respect to the cost of diagnosis, treatment, and follow-up.[59] In general, normalization of thyroid function in postmenopausal women with subclinical hyperthyroidism seems to improve bone density and certain aspects of cardiac function.[296-298] These data would generally favor treatment in the older population, but there are no large, long-term, randomized studies to allow evidence-based conclusions as to the risk/benefit ratio.

TABLE 12-9

Indications for Treatment of Persistent Subclinical Hyperthyroidism

Postmenopausal osteoporosis
Rheumatic valvular disease with left atrial enlargement or atrial fibrillation
Recent-onset atrial fibrillation or recurrent cardiac arrhythmias
Congestive heart failure
Angina pectoris
Infertility or menstrual disorders
Nonspecific symptoms such as fatigue, nervousness, depression, or gastrointestinal disorders, especially in patients older than 60 years of age (consider therapeutic trial)

Diagnosis

The diagnosis of subclinical hyperthyroidism requires tests revealing several subnormal TSH concentration results spaced months apart in the presence of normal free T_3 and T_4 concentrations. Several studies have shown that suppressed TSH can normalize spontaneously over several years, particularly in patients without nodular goiter.[299,300] As with overt thyrotoxicosis, there are two sources of excess thyroid hormones: endogenous and exogenous. In a study of more than 25,000 individuals attending health fairs in Colorado, 58% of those with a TSH level lower than 0.3 mU/L were receiving thyroid hormones.[301] If thyroid hormones are not being administered intentionally for treatment of persistent thyroid carcinoma, thyroid hormone excess is easily treated by more careful monitoring of the levothyroxine dosage using serum TSH concentrations. Endogenous subclinical thyrotoxicosis has the same causes as in overt thyrotoxicosis (see earlier discussion). In the population older than 60 years of age, multinodular goiter is a more likely cause of hyperthyroidism than it is in younger individuals.

Treatment

There are insufficient data to conclude that individuals with serum TSH concentrations greater than 0.1 mU/L due to hyperthyroidism will benefit from treatment.[302] In considering the decision for or against treatment of persistently subnormal TSH concentrations (i.e., <0.1 mU/L with normal free thyroid hormone concentrations), an evaluation should be made for conditions that may benefit from treatment (Table 12-9) as well as to determine the cause of the hyperthyroidism. In elderly persons, postmenopausal osteoporosis and various cardiac diseases are the primary indications for which treatment should be considered. Infertility and menstrual disorders are important in young women.

Identifying the cause of the hyperthyroidism allows assessment of the potential risks of treatment. At one extreme, the treatment of mild Graves' disease with radioiodine usually causes hypothyroidism, whereas this typically does not occur in patients with multinodular toxic goiter. Therefore, in an asymptomatic patient with mild Graves' disease, watchful waiting for a possible spontaneous remission for several years may be the best course of action.[300] On the other hand, patients with subclinical hyperthyroidism due to toxic nodular goiter or a solitary hyperfunctioning adenoma can often be treated with a single dose of radioactive iodine with a relatively low risk of subsequent hypothyroidism. Therefore, the threshold for treatment of such patients is lower. As always, the rationale for treatment and its risks and benefits should be carefully discussed with the patient, and one should be guided by common sense and not by the principle of simply treating an abnormal test result.[303-305]

IODIDE-INDUCED HYPERTHYROIDISM

Administration of supplemental iodine to subjects with endemic iodine deficiency goiter can result in iodine-induced Graves' disease. This response, termed *iodide-induced hyperthyroidism* or the *Jod-Basedow* effect (*Jod* is derived from the German word for "iodine"), occurs in only a small fraction of individuals at risk. The term jod-Basedow specifically refers to iodine-induced von Basedow's (Graves') disease but is often used to refer to iodine-induced hyperthyroidism of any type.

There are two major patterns of the underlying thyroid disorder.[306] In the first, which is common in older individuals, a nodular goiter with areas of autonomous function is present, and TRAbs are not detectable in the blood. The second pattern occurs in younger individuals with diffuse goiter, in whom stimulating TRAbs are often present. These findings indicate that jod-Basedow occurs in thyroid glands in which thyroid function is independent of TSH stimulation. The occurrence of jod-Basedow is not a contraindication to treatment of endemic iodine deficiency. Apart from the many other benefits that accrue from iodine treatment and prophylaxis, over the long run the frequency of spontaneous hyperthyroidism due to toxic nodular goiter is diminished.[287]

Iodide-induced hyperthyroidism is an important disorder in areas of the world in which dietary iodine intake is high.[307] In regions in which iodine intake is marginal but overt iodine deficiency is absent, moderate increments in iodine intake may induce hyperthyroidism in patients with autonomous thyroid nodules. Consequently. the physician must be alert to the possibility of inducing hyperthyroidism when administering iodine in expectorants, x-ray contrast media, medications containing iodine (e.g., amiodarone), povidone iodine, or any other form to patients with nodular goiter.[308,309] Because nodular goiter is generally a disease of the elderly, induction of the jod-Basedow phenomenon can have serious consequences, because enrichment of the thyroid with iodine forestalls administration of ^{131}I and delays the response to antithyroid agents. Prevention of an acute exacerbation may be achieved by pretreatment of at-risk subjects with methimazole starting before exposure and for several weeks afterward.[310,311]

Although the jod-Basedow phenomenon can occur only when the thyroid is partially autonomous, patients with iodine-induced hyperthyroidism have been reported in whom thyroid function was normal and normally suppressible after iodine was withdrawn and a euthyroid state restored. The mechanism by which iodine induces thyrotoxicosis in such instances is unknown. The treatment in these cases can be difficult. Even after discontinuation of exogenous iodide, the uptake of ^{131}I by the thyroid gland may remain low, not adequate for conventional doses of radioiodine. The elevated thyroid hormone content secondary to the iodide level also makes thionamide drugs less effective. It may be necessary to treat such individuals for prolonged periods (6 to 9 months) before administering radioiodine. On the other hand, if uptake is detectable, larger doses of radioiodine may be given to destroy thyroid tissue, or the use of recombinant TSH may be entertained.

Amiodarone

The drug most commonly associated with iodine-induced thyrotoxicosis is amiodarone. This iodine-rich drug has become increasingly popular because of its effectiveness in combating severe cardiac arrhythmias. However, its use has been limited by toxicity due to its high fat solubility and high iodine content inducing thyroid disease and by pulmonary fibrosis and liver disease.

Amiodarone has complex effects on the thyroid, although the majority of patients (about 80%) remain euthyroid.[312] Structurally, the drug resembles T_4 (see Fig. 11-6 in Chapter 11) and contains 37% iodine by weight. Of the 75 mg of iodine present in a 200-mg tablet, about 6 mg of iodide is released per day. In contrast, the typical daily iodine supply in North America is about 150 to 200 μg. Amiodarone has a half-life of 50 to 60 days and therefore remains available for a long period even after drug withdrawal. In addition to providing huge amounts of iodide, amiodarone inhibits the D1 and probably D2 deiodinases and may compete with T_3 for binding to the thyroid hormone receptor. Amiodarone also has a direct cytotoxic effect on thyroid cells via induction of apoptosis.[313] In addition, the iodine load, the drug, or its metabolites may precipitate autoimmune thyroid disease in susceptible individuals.

A new drug, dronedarone, is a benzofuran derivative related to amiodarone. In dronedarone, the iodine moieties have been removed to reduce the toxic effects on the thyroid and other organs; and a methylsulfonamide group has been added to reduce solubility in fats. Dronedarone continues to display amiodarone-like class III antiarrhythmic activity in vitro and in clinical trials.[314] Whether it will supercede amiodarone in clinical practice remains to be seen.

Clinical Presentation

In all patients receiving amiodarone, its effects, particularly the inhibition of the deiodinases, cause a compensatory increase in TSH secretion. This increases serum free T_4 by 30% to 50%, with the serum T_3 and TSH concentrations remaining normal after equilibrium is established.[315,316] This pattern is identical to that observed in mouse models with low D1 activity due to *Dio1* gene inactivation or genetic D1 deficiency and should not be confused with that of thyrotoxicosis in which TSH is suppressed.[317,318] The pathologic effects on the thyroid may result in iodide-induced hypothyroidism (the most common thyroid complication in iodine-sufficient regions; see Chapter 13), or in hyperthyroidism in susceptible individuals due to the jod-Basedow effect and development of Graves' disease in iodine-deficient regions, or in the direct cytotoxic effect of thyroiditis-type damage to the thyroid gland induced by iodine. The iodine-induced hyperthyroidism and thyroiditis-like syndromes have also been referred to as type I and type II amiodarone-induced thyrotoxicosis, respectively.[260,319]

Amiodarone-induced thyrotoxicosis may develop at the outset of exposure or not until after several years of treatment. It commonly manifests as an exacerbation of the underlying cardiac pathology that was the initial indication for its use. This serious complication can sometimes be anticipated by early recognition of a progressive decrease in serum TSH levels. Monitoring of serum TSH throughout amiodarone treatment on a regular basis, such as every 6 months, should be undertaken by the supervising cardiologist or internist. This is especially important in areas of borderline or deficient iodine supply.

Diagnosis

All patients with amiodarone-induced thyrotoxicosis have a suppressed TSH level, with the degree of suppression proportional to the clinical severity. Serum free T_4 is elevated, but the elevation in serum free T_3 is less than that observed in typical thyrotoxic states due to the blockade of T_4-to-T_3 conversion by the drug. Distinction between the two causes of thyrotoxicosis may not be possible, although many strategies have been suggested. In North America, the cause of thyrotoxicosis is almost always thyroiditis because of the lack of iodine deficiency; a more evenly divided mix of the two causes occurs in Europe.[312,320,321] Doppler-flow ultrasonography showing hypervascularity accompanied by an enlarged gland favors iodine-induced hyperthyroidism, whereas a normal-sized gland and "normal" or reduced vascularity favor thyroiditis, although results can be equivocal.[312,320] RAIU values are almost always low except in areas of low iodine intake.

Treatment

If possible, amiodarone should be discontinued, but this is not absolutely necessary. In patients with thyroiditis, a spontaneous resolution may occur, but in most patients a combination of methimazole or carbimazole (20 to 40 mg/day) and prednisolone/prednisone 20 to 40 mg/day is given to cover both diagnostic possibilities.[322] The latter may be tapered after 3 months to determine whether a remission has occurred. In patients with iodine-induced hyperthyroidism, perchlorate (500 mg twice daily for 1 to 2 weeks) may accelerate the resolution of the condition, although this agent has potentially significant renal and bone marrow toxicities precluding long-term use.[312,323]

For those patients who remain unstable or whose cardiac condition is likely to require lifelong amiodarone therapy, surgery is appropriate. The current consensus is that amiodarone can be restarted in patients who have recovered from thyroiditis, and most patients remain euthyroid if this is done.[260,324]

HYPERTHYROIDISM DUE TO THYROTROPIN SECRETION

Excess thyrotropin is an exceedingly rare cause of hyperthyroidism. However, pituitary thyrotroph tumors cause this condition and may manifest as a Graves'-like syndrome with diffuse goiter and substantial thyrotoxicosis. Laboratory studies demonstrating an inappropriately detectable or somewhat elevated TSH in the presence of thyrotoxic symptoms alert the clinician to this as the most likely possibility once assay artifacts are eliminated. This condition, discussed in depth in Chapter 9, must be differentiated from the rare *familial resistance to thyroid hormone* (*RTH*).[325-327]

Thyroid Hormone Resistance

In some patients with familial RTH due to mutations in the β-isoform of the thyroid hormone receptor, the hypothalamic-pituitary feedback mechanism is more resistant to the effects of thyroid hormone than are peripheral tissues such as the heart, which expresses the thyroid receptor α-isoform.[325-327] These patients may present with a hyperthyroid appearance with tachycardia, nervousness, and goiter associated with an elevated concentration of free T_4. However, because the thyroid hormone hyperproduction is TSH driven, serum TSH concentrations are detectable (>0.1 mU/L) or even elevated inappropriately for the high serum thyroid hormone levels. In general, the manifestations are due not to excessive but, rather, to inadequate thyroid hormone action, and these individuals may require treatment with thyroid hormone (or thyroid hormone analogs) or β-adrenergic receptor-blocking agents, or both, rather than anti-thyroid drugs (see Chapter 13 for a more extensive discussion of RTH). The critical historical point in such patients is a family history, because RTH is inherited in an autosomal dominant pattern.

CHORIONIC GONADOTROPIN–INDUCED HYPERTHYROIDISM

Human chorionic gonadotropin is a glycoprotein heterodimer composed of an α-subunit (identical to that of TSH, LH, and FSH) and a specific β-subunit that has similarity to TSH. This glycoprotein binds and stimulates the human TSHR,[328] with an in vitro potency of about 0.7 μU of human TSH equivalent for every 1 U of hCG. In high concentrations, it causes hyperthyroidism characterized by a diffuse goiter, elevated free T_4, and suppressed TSH. This is readily recognized in the late first trimester of normal pregnancy, a time at which a physiologic mild transient gestational thyrotoxicosis or hyperthyroidism occurs (see Chapter 11).

Transient Gestational Thyrotoxicosis

The syndrome of transient gestational thyrotoxicosis is an exaggeration of the physiologic increase in thyroid stimulation that occurs during the first trimester of pregnancy. It is associated with high levels of hCG (100,000 to 200,000 U/L), similar to those found in twin pregnancies, and is often accompanied by hyperemesis.[329,330] In most patients, the condition is self-limited, but in rare circumstances, low doses of methimazole (≤10 mg/day) may be required for a few weeks until the hCG falls spontaneously. It may be difficult to separate this syndrome from early Graves' disease, and a TRAb test may be helpful.

Two patients have been reported with an inherited variant of gestational thyrotoxicosis in which a mutation in the TSHR gene resulted in a receptor protein with an increase in its responsiveness to hCG.[331] Such patients develop hyperthyroidism with each pregnancy due to physiologic serum hCG concentrations.

Hyperthyroidism Associated with Trophoblastic Tumors

Thyroid hyperfunction may accompany hydatidiform mole, choriocarcinoma, or metastatic embryonal carcinoma of the testis.[260] Such neoplasms, particularly hydatidiform mole, elaborate differentially glycosylated hCG molecules that also exhibit crossover specificity for binding to the TSHR and can induce variable degrees of thyroid overactivity.[332] Some patients have clinically overt thyrotoxicosis; however, clinical manifestations usually are not prominent, and goiter is absent or minimal despite laboratory evidence of a hyperthyroid state. The levels of free T_4 or free T_3 or both are increased, and TSH values are suppressed. The reason for the discordance between the clinical and the laboratory indices is not known, but it may be related to the relatively short duration of thyroid hormone excess. The possibility of a molar pregnancy should be considered in a young woman with hyperthyroidism and amenorrhea, because the appropriate therapy is evacuation of the uterus.

TRANSIENT THYROTOXICOSIS

Overview

As mentioned at the outset of this chapter, transient thyrotoxicosis must be differentiated from the sustained hyperthyroidism of Graves' disease and other causes of hyperthyroidism. Transient thyrotoxicosis is caused by thyroid-cell breakdown, and the hyperthyroid symptoms are of abrupt onset and short duration. This process may be followed by recovery of thyroid function or the development of transient or permanent thyroid failure. The discussion in this chapter focuses on thyroiditis as the most common cause of transient thyrotoxicosis. This disorder is covered more completely in Chapter 13, because Hashimoto's disease most commonly causes hypothyroidism after the initial phase of transient hyperthyroidism.

Transient thyrotoxicosis has a confusing nomenclature that can be clarified as follows:

- In the autoimmune forms *(Hashimoto's thyroiditis)*, there are typically no local symptoms of thyroid inflammation. This has led to the equivalent terms *silent* or *painless thyroiditis, lymphocytic thyroiditis,* and *Hashitoxicosis*. This condition may also manifest with thyroid tenderness.
- In the form of postviral thyroiditis (also termed *subacute, de Quervain's,* or *granulomatous thyroiditis*), thyroid tenderness may be the most prominent symptom. Thyrotoxicosis is rare and typically self-limited, although this form may rarely also be painless.
- Acute thyroiditis resulting from bacterial or fungal infection is only rarely accompanied by thyrotoxicosis, and the local symptoms predominate (see Chapter 13).
- Thyroiditis may also be drug induced, the principal offenders being amiodarone and lithium. Some of the new, small-molecule kinase inhibitors (e.g., sunitinib) may also cause this form of thyroiditis, resulting eventually in hypothyroidism.[333]

Transient Thyrotoxicosis Due to Autoimmune (Hashimoto's) Thyroiditis

As described earlier, Hashimoto's disease causes two different thyrotoxicosis-associated transient syndromes. The more common one is the painless form, in which the symptoms of thyrotoxicosis, usually mild, predominate; the more uncommon form has a painful type of presentation, probably secondary to a more acute onset. Histopathology in such patients with thyroiditis shows diffuse or local lymphocytic infiltration, varying degrees of fibrosis, and disruption of the follicular architecture (Fig. 12-14).

Thyrotoxicosis from Painless Autoimmune Thyroiditis. This presentation may occur in the postpartum period or spontaneously. Postpartum thyroiditis is the most common example, and its pathophysiology, postpartum enhancement of thyroid-directed autoimmunity (Hashimoto's disease), is analogous to the postpartum exacerbation of Graves' disease (see earlier discussion). The incidence of postpartum thyroiditis varies, but it may occur in as many as 10% of women, in more than 30% of those with positive TPO-Ab, and in even a larger fraction of patients with type 1 diabetes mellitus.[245] In women found to be TPO antibody–positive prenatally, postpartum assessment of thyroid function is recommended at 3, 6, and 12 months. As expected, there is a strong association with the HLA DR3 and DR5 haplotypes, which are associated with autoimmune thyroid disease.[334]

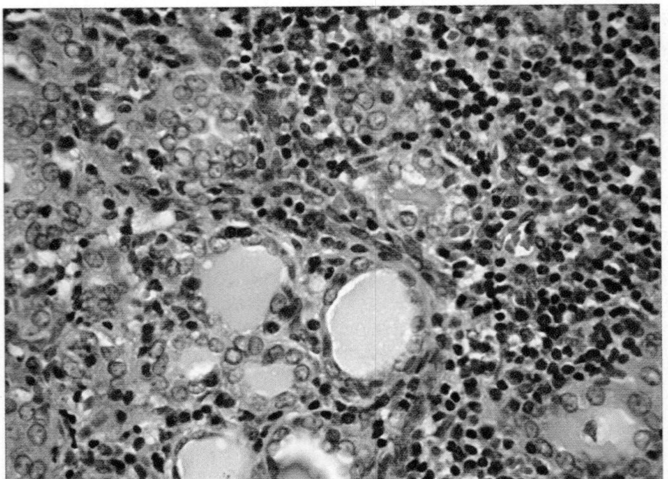

Figure 12-14 Lymphocytic thyroiditis in a patient with transient thyrotoxicosis (painless thyroiditis) secondary to autoimmune (Hashimoto's) thyroiditis. Notice the diffuse lymphocytic invasion of the tissue, including the follicular epithelium, and the loss of follicles. Multinucleated giant cells may also be seen in the follicular lumen. (Courtesy of Dr. Vania Nosé, Brigham and Women's Hospital, Boston, MA.)

Thyrotoxicosis from spontaneous autoimmune thyroiditis has all the same characteristics as postpartum thyroiditis and is seen in patients early in their development of classic Hashimoto's disease and before the onset of hypothyroidism.

Thyrotoxicosis from Painful Autoimmune Thyroiditis. Some patients with thyrotoxicosis due to painful autoimmune thyroiditis present with local thyroid tenderness, but this is uncommon. Such tender episodes, which can be unilateral, may recur until the thyroid gland is completely destroyed by the disease process. Only rarely does the pain persist, sometimes requiring surgical intervention.

Clinical Presentation of Transient Autoimmune Thyrotoxicosis

More than 75% of patients are women who present with acute onset of symptoms of thyrotoxicosis, usually nervousness, palpitations, and irritability; they can often pinpoint the time of recent onset. In the postpartum syndrome, symptoms manifest 3 to 6 months after delivery but may be mild and overlooked amid the myriad of events involved in the care of the newborn. After 1 to 2 months, the thyrotoxic symptoms fade, but they are often replaced by those suggesting hypothyroidism (Fig. 12-15).

In a significant number of postpartum patients, the thyrotoxic phase is too mild to be noticed, and the patient presents somewhat later after delivery with hypothyroid symptoms. The physical examination shows mild signs of thyrotoxicosis, tachycardia being the most prominent, without the specific eye signs or dermopathy associated with Graves' disease. The thyroid gland is normal in size but may be firm if the Hashimoto's disease is chronic.

Diagnosis

Thyrotoxicosis is usually mild, and this is reflected in the degree of suppression of the serum TSH level and the elevation of the serum free T_4. Significant elevation of the TPO-Ab is typical. Systemic manifestations of

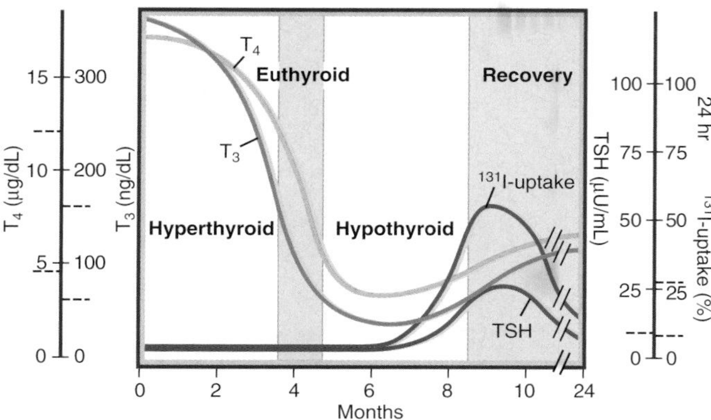

Figure 12-15 The typical course in patients with autoimmune thyroiditis who present with transient thyrotoxicosis. The duration of each phase may vary, and some patients do not experience a discernible hyperthyroid or hypothyroid phase. TSH, thyroid-stimulating hormone. (From Woolf PD. Transient painless thyroiditis with hyperthyroidism: a variant of lymphocytic thyroiditis? *Endocr Rev.* 1980;1:411-420. ©1980, The Endocrine Society.)

inflammation are lacking, and the erythrocyte sedimentation rate is normal or almost normal, but ultrasonography may indicate the heterogeneity of an inflamed gland. If true hyperthyroidism cannot be eliminated as a diagnosis on clinical grounds, the RAIU should be measured unless the patient is nursing. The classic decreased RAIU is due partly to feedback suppression of TSH secretion but also to thyroid follicular-cell destruction. The tendency of the disorder to pass through a hypothyroid phase is not surprising in view of the extensive depletion of Tg, which is processed to thyroxine and not replaced by the dysfunctional cells.

Natural History

The duration of the thyrotoxic phase, which is typically not severe enough to require treatment, averages 1 to 2 months. About one half of the patients return to a euthyroid phase and remain well in the short term. In the remaining half, a hypothyroid phase may follow and may last for 2 to 9 months. In most patients, there is eventual restoration of euthyroidism, but some develop permanent hypothyroidism years later.[335] About one third retain a goiter, usually with persistence of thyroid autoantibodies in the serum. The opposite sequela, recurrence of thyrotoxicosis, may also appear months or years after restoration of a euthyroid state, particularly after pregnancy.

Treatment

The thyrotoxic phase may require alleviation of the peripheral manifestations through the use of β-blockers. Prednisone (20 to 40 mg/day) may decrease the duration of the thyrotoxic phase, but it is typically not needed except when the painful form of the disease is present. If the hypothyroid phase is mild and brief, it also may not require treatment. If treatment with levothyroxine is required, it should be withdrawn slowly approximately 6 months later, because the hypothyroidism is often not permanent.

Subacute Thyroiditis

Subacute thyroiditis (also termed *granulomatous, giant cell,* or *de Quervain's thyroiditis*) is thought to be caused directly or indirectly by a viral infection of the thyroid gland and often follows an upper respiratory illness. A tendency to appear in the spring in the Northern latitudes has been noted, and again there is a female predominance. The mumps virus has been implicated in some cases, and Coxsackie, influenza, echo, and adenoviruses may also be etiologic agents. Positive TPO-Ab are present transiently during the active phase of the disease, although some patients retain evidence of thyroid autoimmunity for many years. A small number of patients eventually develop autoimmune thyroid disease. Subacute thyroiditis is uncommon, but mild cases may be mistakenly diagnosed as pharyngitis.

Pathology

The histopathologic changes are different from those observed in Hashimoto's disease. The lesions are patchy in distribution and vary in their stage of development from area to area. Affected follicles are infiltrated predominantly with mononuclear cells and show disruption of epithelium, partial or complete loss of colloid, and fragmentation and duplication of the basement membrane (Fig. 12-16).

To this extent, the histopathologic appearance may resemble that of Hashimoto's disease. A characteristic feature is the well-developed follicular lesion that consists of a central core of colloid surrounded by the multinucleated giant cells, hence the designation *giant cell thyroiditis*. Colloid may be found in the interstitium or within the giant cells. The follicular changes progress to form granulomas. Interfollicular fibrosis and an interstitial inflammatory reaction are present to varying degrees. After the disease subsides, an essentially normal histologic appearance is restored.

Pathophysiology

Apoptosis of follicular epithelium and loss of follicular integrity are the primary events in the pathophysiology of giant cell thyroiditis. Tg, T_4, and iodinated Tg fragments are released into the circulation, often in quantities sufficient to elevate not just the serum Tg but also the serum free T_4, producing clinical thyrotoxicosis and suppressing TSH secretion. As a result, the RAIU decreases to low levels, and hormone synthesis ceases. Later in the disease, after stores of preformed hormone are depleted, serum T_4 and T_3 concentrations decline, sometimes into the hypothyroid range, and the serum TSH level rises, often to elevated values, exactly as occurs in silent thyroiditis (Fig. 12-17).

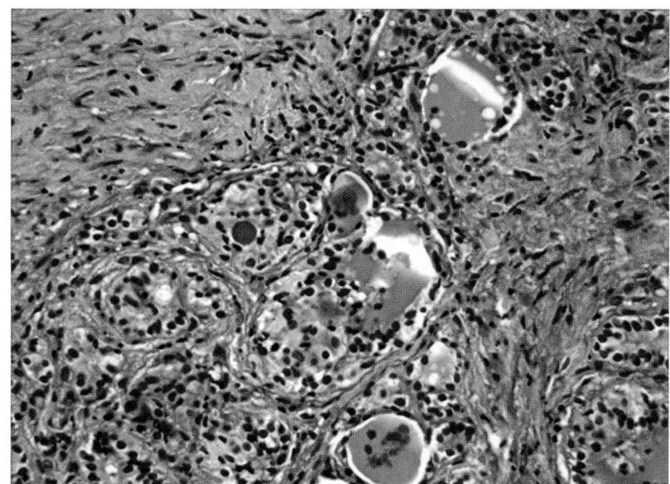

Figure 12-16 Subacute (viral or postviral) thyroiditis. Diffuse neutrophilic invasion with active destruction of follicles and a multinucleated giant cell. Fibrosis and near-complete loss of follicles have occurred. (Courtesy of Dr. Vania Nose, Brigham and Women's Hospital, Boston, MA.)

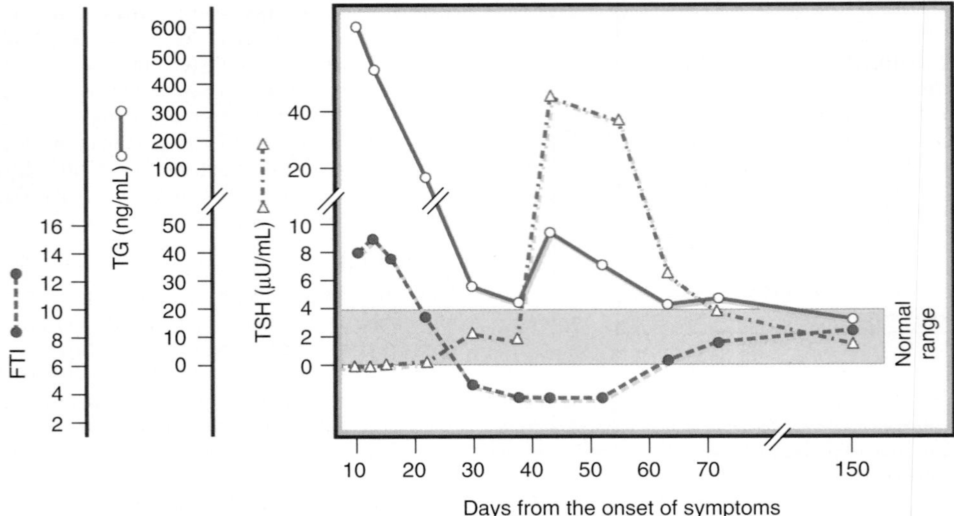

Figure 12-17 Thyroid function in a patient during the course of subacute (viral or postviral) thyroiditis. During the thyrotoxic phase (days 10 to 20), the serum thyroglobulin (TG) concentration was greatly elevated, the free thyroxine index (FTI) was high, and the thyroid-stimulating hormone (TSH) was suppressed; the erythrocyte sedimentation rate was 86 mm/hour, and the thyroidal radioactive iodine uptake (RAIU) was 2%. The Tg level and the FTI declined in parallel. During the phase of hypothyroidism (days 30 to 63), when the FTI was below normal, a modest transient increase in serum Tg occurred in parallel with the increase in serum TSH. All parameters of thyroid function were normal by day 150, 5 months after the onset of symptoms. (From DeGroot LJ, Larsen PR, Hennemann G. Acute and subacute thyroiditis. In: DeGroot LJ, Larsen PR, Hennemann G: *The Thyroid and Its Diseases*, 6th ed. New York, NY: Churchill Livingstone; 1996:705.)

As the disease becomes inactive, the RAIU may be greater than normal for a time as hormone stores are repleted. Ultimately, after hormone secretion resumes, serum T_4 and T_3 concentrations rise, and the serum TSH concentration decreases to normal values.

Clinical Picture

The characteristic feature is the gradual or sudden appearance of pain in the region of the thyroid gland with or without fever. The pain, which is aggravated by turning the head or swallowing, characteristically radiates to the ear, jaw, or occiput and may mimic disorders arising in these areas. The absence of pain does not exclude the diagnosis, because biopsy-proven painless subacute thyroiditis does occur, but it must be distinguished from acute autoimmune thyroiditis. Hoarseness and dysphagia may be present, and patients may complain of palpitation, nervousness, and lassitude. The latter symptoms can be extreme, considering the local nature of the disease, and may suggest a systemic component. Although acute manifestations are present in severe cases, symptoms in milder disease may be present and overlooked for months.

On palpation, at least part of the thyroid is slightly to moderately enlarged, firm, often nodular, and usually exquisitely tender. One lobe is frequently being more severely affected than the other, and the symptoms may be truly unilateral. The overlying skin may be warm and erythematous. Occasionally, the locus of maximal involvement migrates over the course of a few weeks to other parts of the gland. The disease usually subsides within a few months, leaving no residual deficiency of thyroid function in 90% of patients. In rare patients, the disease smolders, with repeated exacerbations over many months, and hypothyroidism is sometimes the final result.

Diagnosis

The laboratory findings vary with the phase of the disease. During the active phase, the erythrocyte sedimentation rate is increased, often to a remarkable extent (>100 mm/hour). Indeed, a diagnosis of active subacute thyroiditis is hardly tenable when the sedimentation rate is normal. The white blood cell count is normal or, at most, moderately increased. The serum Tg level is characteristically high, in keeping with the degree of thyroid destruction.

Subacute thyroiditis must be differentiated from acute hemorrhagic degeneration in a preexisting thyroid nodule, Hashimoto's disease with painful recurrence (discussed earlier), acute pyogenic or fungal thyroiditis, and the rare thyroid malignancy with painful nodules. Acute painful exacerbations of Hashimoto's disease may be difficult to distinguish from subacute thyroiditis. Lack of elevation of the erythrocyte sedimentation rate and high titers of thyroid autoantibodies strongly suggest the former condition. Acute pyogenic thyroiditis is distinguished by the presence of a septic focus elsewhere, by a greater inflammatory reaction in the tissues adjacent to the thyroid, and by much greater leukocytic and febrile responses (see Chapter 13). The RAIU and thyroid function are usually preserved in acute pyogenic thyroiditis. Rarely, widespread infiltrating cancer of the thyroid can manifest with a clinical and laboratory picture almost indistinguishable from that of subacute thyroiditis.[336] Ultrasonography and fine-needle aspiration should be performed if this is a consideration.

Treatment

In mild cases, aspirin, nonsteroidal anti-inflammatory drugs, or cyclooxygenase 2 (COX2) inhibitors may control the symptoms. With more severe pain, glucocorticoids (e.g., prednisone up to 40 mg/day) are the only solution for the extreme discomfort. This treatment may be required for several months and should then be withdrawn gradually. If the TSH is not suppressed, TSH-suppressive therapy with levothyroxine may decrease the size of the gland, relieving the pressure on the thyroid capsule. TSH is needed for thyroid-cell regeneration, so such therapy should be decreased as the symptoms subside.

Drug-Associated Thyroiditis

Thyroiditis is an uncommon complication of pharmacotherapy. Amiodarone is an important exception and was discussed earlier in this chapter. Most cases of thyroiditis associated with various therapeutic agents appear to be caused by drug-induced exacerbation of underlying autoimmune disease. This is understandable with those agents that are specifically administered to modify the immune system, including IL-2, interferon-α, and granulocyte/macrophage colony-stimulating factor (GM-CSF), any of which can precipitate silent thyroiditis.[114,337] This complication has also been described with lithium, and the GnRH agonist leuprolide, but the pathophysiology is obscure.[338-340]

Thyroiditis has been found in association with the use of a multitargeting kinase inhibitor, sunitinib, in patients with gastrointestinal stromal tumors or renal cell carcinoma. This may manifest as subacute thyroiditis, with a suppressed TSH level being the major manifestation in the early phase, followed by progression to destruction of the gland through an unclear mechanism. Although imatinib has been associated with an increase in levothyroxine requirements in hypothyroid patients (analogous to the effects of phenytoin, carbamazepine, and rifampin), those changes are independent of thyroid function.[341]

OTHER CAUSES OF THYROTOXICOSIS WITH A LOW RADIOIODINE UPTAKE

In addition to silent and subacute thyroiditis, several other entities should be considered if a patient with thyrotoxicosis has a thyroid gland that is either not palpable or not enlarged and has biochemical findings of thyrotoxicosis accompanied by a low RAIU.

Thyrotoxicosis Factitia

Thyrotoxicosis that arises from the ingestion, usually chronic, of excessive quantities of thyroid hormone occurs typically in individuals with underlying psychiatric disease, especially in paramedical personnel who have access to thyroid hormone or in patients for whom thyroid hormone medication has been prescribed in the past. Usually, the patient is aware of taking thyroid hormone but may adamantly deny it. In other instances, large doses of thyroid hormone or other thyroactive material may be given without the knowledge of the patient, usually as part of a regimen for weight reduction. Some "natural" products for weight reduction stated not to contain thyroid hormone nonetheless do. Symptoms are typical of thyrotoxicosis and may be severe.

In the absence of preexisting disease of the thyroid, the diagnosis is made from the combination of typical thyrotoxic manifestations together with thyroid atrophy and hypofunction. Infiltrative ophthalmopathy never occurs, but lid lag, stare, and other "thyrotoxic" eye signs may be present. TSH levels are suppressed. Serum T_4 concentrations are increased unless the patient is taking T_3, in which case they are subnormal. Serum T_3 concentrations are increased in either case. Hypofunction of the thyroid gland is evidenced by the subnormal values of RAIU. The presence of low, rather than elevated, values of serum Tg is a clear indication that the thyrotoxicosis results from exogenous hormone rather than thyroid hyperfunction.

This disorder may be confused with other varieties of thyrotoxicosis associated with a subnormal RAIU and absence of goiter, including silent thyroiditis, ectopic thyroid tissue, and hyperfunctioning metastatic follicular carcinoma. Evidence for the last two disorders can be obtained by demonstration of the ectopic focus or foci through external radioiodine scanning or by the presence of normal to elevated serum Tg concentrations. Differentiation from silent thyroiditis may be difficult. The presence of TPO-Ab points to painless chronic autoimmune thyroiditis, whereas a firm thyroid and brief history suggest the painless variant of subacute thyroiditis. Treatment of thyrotoxicosis factitia consists of withdrawal of the offending medication. Psychiatric consultation is often required.

Hamburger Thyrotoxicosis

An unusual form of exogenous thyrotoxicosis occurred in the midwestern portion of the United States in 1984 and 1985. The source was the inclusion of large quantities of bovine thyroid in ground beef preparations.[342] When the slaughtering practices were changed, this condition disappeared. Such a possibility, although remote, should be considered, especially if one is confronted with epidemic exogenous thyrotoxicosis.

Thyrotoxicosis Due to Extrathyroidal Tissue

Struma Ovarii. Thyroid tissue is present in 5% to 10% of teratomas, and occasionally such foci are hyperfunctional.[343,344] About 5% to 10% of these tumors are bilateral. Whereas thyrotoxicosis is unusual, it may occur in as many as 8% to 10% of patients. Rarely, males with germ-cell tumors may develop hCG-induced hyperthyroidism.[345]

Clinical Presentation. Patients present with variable degrees of thyrotoxicosis but without goiter and usually have lower abdominal symptomatology such as a pain or a mass. Rarely, ascites is present. Laboratory studies show reduced TSH and increased free T_4 of a variable degree, but the RAIU is low. The Tg may be elevated, particularly if the teratoma is malignant and has metastasized to the peritoneum. Abdominal CT or MRI shows a multilocular ovarian mass or masses. Rarely, a struma ovarii is accompanied by Graves' disease.[346]

Treatment. The patient should be rendered euthyroid if thyrotoxicosis is significant, after which the involved ovary or ovaries should be removed. Therapeutic radioiodine will be required for metastatic disease after ablation of the normal thyroid gland.[347,348]

Thyrotoxicosis Due to Metastatic Thyroid Carcinoma

In general, thyroid carcinomas are made up of poorly functioning tissue. On occasion, follicular thyroid carcinomas have sufficient function when combined with the total mass of the metastases to result in an elevation in serum free T_4 or T_3. Typically, such a course is a complication of a previously diagnosed lesion (see Chapter 14).[349] The symptoms of thyrotoxicosis are variable, and the metastatic disease is usually obvious from radiologic studies. On occasion, the presentation may be confusing if the patient is receiving TSH-suppressive therapy, and diagnosis will require its discontinuation; TSH will remain suppressed and the serum free T_4 will be elevated. Treatment of this condition is typical for that of thyroid carcinoma and is described in Chapter 14. In patients with thyrotoxicosis due to metastatic tumor, serum Tg is quite elevated, indicating that the thyrotoxicosis is caused by thyroidal tissue that is not located in the neck. An RAIU during the thyrotoxic phase will show no neck uptake due to TSH suppression even if the thyroid is still present.

REFERENCES

1. Davis PJ, Davis FB. Hyperthyroidism in patients over the age of 60 years: clinical features in 85 patients. *Medicine (Baltimore)*. 1974; 53:161-181.
2. Kahaly GJ, Dillmann WH. Thyroid hormone action in the heart. *Endocr Rev*. 2005;26:704-728.
3. Burggraaf J, Tulen JH, Lalezari S, et al. Sympathovagal imbalance in hyperthyroidism. *Am J Physiol Endocrinol Metab*. 2001;281:E190-E195.
4. Kahaly GJ, Wagner S, Nieswandt J, et al. Stress echocardiography in hyperthyroidism. *J Clin Endocrinol Metab*. 1999;84:2308-2313.
5. Fazio S, Palmieri EA, Lombardi G, et al. Effects of thyroid hormone on the cardiovascular system. *Recent Prog Horm Res*. 2004;59:31-50.
6. Napoli R, Biondi B, Guardasole V, et al. Impact of hyperthyroidism and its correction on vascular reactivity in humans. *Circulation* 2001;104:3076-3080.
7. Brauman A, Rosenberg T, Gilboa Y, et al. Prevalence of mitral valve prolapse in chronic lymphocytic thyroiditis and nongoitrous hypothyroidism. *Cardiology*. 1988;75:269-273.
8. Alvarado A, Ribeiro JP, Freitas FM, et al. Lack of association between thyroid function and mitral valve prolapse in Graves' disease. *Braz J Med Biol Res*. 1990;23:133-139.
9. Northcote RJ, MacFarlane P, Kesson CM, et al. Continuous 24-hour electrocardiography in thyrotoxicosis before and after treatment. *Am Heart J*. 1986;112:339-344.
10. Sawin CT, Geller A, Wolf PA, et al. Low serum thyrotropin concentrations as a risk factor for atrial fibrillation in older persons. *N Engl J Med*. 1994;331:1249-1252.
11. Cappola AR, Fried LP, Arnold AM, et al. Thyroid status, cardiovascular risk, and mortality in older adults. *JAMA*. 2006;295:1033-1041.
12. Trivalle C, Doucet J, Chassagne P, et al. Differences in the signs and symptoms of hyperthyroidism in older and younger patients. *J Am Geriatr Soc*. 1996;44:50-53.
13. Nakazawa HK, Sakurai K, Hamada N, et al. Management of atrial fibrillation in the post-thyrotoxic state. *Am J Med*. 1982;72:903-906.
14. Kahaly GJ, Nieswandt J, Mohr-Kahaly S. Cardiac risks of hyperthyroidism in the elderly. *Thyroid*. 1998;8:1165-1169.
15. Petersen P, Hansen JM. Stroke in thyrotoxicosis with atrial fibrillation. *Stroke*. 1988;19:15-18.
16. Nakazawa H, Lythall DA, Noh J, et al. Is there a place for the late cardioversion of atrial fibrillation? A long-term follow-up study of patients with post-thyrotoxic atrial fibrillation. *Eur Heart J*. 2000;21: 327-333.
17. Silva JE. The thermogenic effect of thyroid hormone and its clinical implications. *Ann Intern Med*. 2003;139:205-213.
18. Coulombe P, Dussault JH, Walker P. Plasma catecholamine concentrations in hyperthyroidism and hypothyroidism. *Metabolism*. 1976; 25:973-979.
19. Palmieri EA, Fazio S, Palmieri V, et al. Myocardial contractility and total arterial stiffness in patients with overt hyperthyroidism: acute effects of beta1-adrenergic blockade. *Eur J Endocrinol*. 2004;150: 757-762.
20. Carvalho-Bianco SD, Kim B, Harney JW, et al. Chronic cardiac-specific thyrotoxicosis increases myocardial beta-adrenergic responsiveness. *Mol Endocrinol*. 2004;18:1840-1849.
21. Ojamaa K, Klein I, Sabet A, et al. Changes in adenylyl cyclase isoforms as a mechanism for thyroid hormone modulation of cardiac beta-adrenergic receptor responsiveness. *Metabolism*. 2000;49:275-279.
22. Hellstrom L, Wahrenberg H, Reynisdottir S, et al. Catecholamine-induced adipocyte lipolysis in human hyperthyroidism. *J Clin Endocrinol Metab*. 1997;82:159-166.
23. Marino M, Barbesino G, Pinchera A, et al. Increased frequency of euthyroid ophthalmopathy in patients with Graves' disease associated with myasthenia gravis. *Thyroid*. 2000;10:799-802.
24. Yu Wai Man CY, Chinnery PF, Griffiths PG. Extraocular muscles have fundamentally distinct properties that make them selectively vulnerable to certain disorders. *Neuromuscul Disord*. 2005;15:17-23.
25. Ober KP. Thyrotoxic periodic paralysis in the United States: report of 7 cases and review of the literature. *Medicine (Baltimore)*. 1992;71: 109-120.
26. Kodali VR, Jeffcote B, Clague RB. Thyrotoxic periodic paralysis: a case report and review of the literature. *J Emerg Med*. 1999;17:43-45.
27. Dias Da Silva MR, Cerutti JM, Arnaldi LA, et al. A mutation in the KCNE3 potassium channel gene is associated with susceptibility to thyrotoxic hypokalemic periodic paralysis. *J Clin Endocrinol Metab*. 2002;87:4881-4884.
28. Gurlek A, Cobankara V, Bayraktar M. Liver tests in hyperthyroidism: effect of antithyroid therapy. *J Clin Gastroenterol*. 1997;24:180-183.
29. Myers JD, Brannon ES, Holland BC. A correlative study of the cardiac output and the hepatic circulation in hyperthyroidism. *J Clin Invest*. 1950;29:1069-1077.
30. Wakasugi M, Wakao R, Tawata M, et al. Bone mineral density in patients with hyperthyroidism measured by dual energy X-ray absorptiometry. *Clin Endocrinol (Oxf)*. 1993;38:283-286.
31. Wakasugi M, Wakao R, Tawata M, et al. Change in bone mineral density in patients with hyperthyroidism after attainment of euthyroidism by dual energy X-ray absorptiometry. *Thyroid*. 1994;4: 179-182.
32. Bassett JH, Williams GR. The molecular actions of thyroid hormone in bone. *Trends Endocrinol Metab*. 2003;14:356-364.
33. Mohan HK, Groves AM, Fogelman I, et al. Thyroid hormone and parathyroid hormone competing to maintain calcium levels in the presence of vitamin D deficiency. *Thyroid*. 2004;14:789-791.
34. Mundy GR, Shapiro JL, Bandelin JG, et al. Direct stimulation of bone resorption by thyroid hormones. *J Clin Invest*. 1976;58:529-534.
35. Schiller C, Gruber R, Ho GM, et al. Interaction of triiodothyronine with 1alpha,25-dihydroxyvitamin D3 on interleukin-6-dependent osteoclast-like cell formation in mouse bone marrow cell cultures. *Bone*. 1998;22:341-346.
36. Abe E, Marians RC, Yu W, et al. TSH is a negative regulator of skeletal remodeling. *Cell*. 2003;115:151-162.
37. Zaidi M, Davies TF, Zallone A, et al. Thyroid-stimulating hormone, thyroid hormones, and bone loss. *Curr Osteoporos Rep*. 2009;7:47-52.
38. Wejda B, Hintze G, Katschinski B, et al. Hip fractures and the thyroid: a case-control study. *J Intern Med*. 1995;237:241-247.
39. Faber J, Galloe AM. Changes in bone mass during prolonged subclinical hyperthyroidism due to L-thyroxine treatment: a meta-analysis. *Eur J Endocrinol*. 1994;130:350-356.
40. Bauer DC, Ettinger B, Nevitt MC, et al. Risk for fracture in women with low serum levels of thyroid-stimulating hormone. *Ann Intern Med*. 2001;134:561-568.
41. Iqbal AA, Burgess EH, Gallina DL, et al. Hypercalcemia in hyperthyroidism: patterns of serum calcium, parathyroid hormone, and 1,25-dihydroxyvitamin D3 levels during management of thyrotoxicosis. *Endocr Pract*. 2003;9:517-521.
42. Godart V, Weynand B, Coche E, et al. Intense 18-fluorodeoxyglucose uptake by the thymus on PET scan does not necessarily herald recurrence of thyroid carcinoma. *J Endocrinol Invest*. 2005;28:1024-1028.
43. Montella L, Caraglia M, Abbruzzese A, et al. Mediastinal images resembling thymus following 131-I treatment for thyroid cancer. *Monaldi Arch Chest Dis*. 2005;63:114-117.
44. Erem C, Ersoz HO, Karti SS, et al. Blood coagulation and fibrinolysis in patients with hyperthyroidism. *J Endocrinol Invest*. 2002;25: 345-350.
45. Kurnik D, Loebstein R, Farfel Z, et al. Complex drug-drug-disease interactions between amiodarone, warfarin, and the thyroid gland. *Medicine (Baltimore)*. 2004;83:107-113.
46. Taniyama M, Honma K, Ban Y. Urinary cortisol metabolites in the assessment of peripheral thyroid hormone action: application for diagnosis of resistance to thyroid hormone. *Thyroid*. 1993;3:229-233.
47. Stagnaro-Green A, Roman SH, Cobin RH, et al. Detection of at-risk pregnancy by means of highly sensitive assays for thyroid autoantibodies. *JAMA*. 1990;264:1422-1425.
48. Stagnaro-Green A, Glinoer D. Thyroid autoimmunity and the risk of miscarriage. *Best Pract Res Clin Endocrinol Metab*. 2004;18:167-181.
49. Meikle AW. The interrelationships between thyroid dysfunction and hypogonadism in men and boys. *Thyroid*. 2004;14(suppl 1):S17-S25.
50. Tagawa N, Takano T, Fukata S, et al. Serum concentration of androstenediol and androstenediol sulfate in patients with hyperthyroidism and hypothyroidism. *Endocr J*. 2001;48:345-354.
51. Parry CH. Diseases of the heart: enlargement of the thyroid gland in connection with enlargement or palpitation of the heart. In: *Collections from the Unpublished Medical Writings of the Late Caleb Hillier Parry*. London: Underwoods, Fleet-Street; 1825.
52. Rapoport B, McLachlan SM. Thyroid autoimmunity. *J Clin Invest*. 2001;108:1253-1259.
53. Davies TF, Ando T, Lin RY, et al. Thyrotropin receptor-associated diseases: from adenomata to Graves disease. *J Clin Invest*. 2005;115: 1972-1983.
54. Morshed SA, Latif R, Davies TF. Characterization of thyrotropin receptor antibody-induced signaling cascades. *Endocrinology*. 2009;150: 519-529.
55. Martin A, Valentine M, Unger P, et al. Engraftment of human lymphocytes and thyroid tissue into Scid and Rag2-deficient mice: absent progression of lymphocytic infiltration. *J Clin Endocrinol Metab*. 1994;79:716-723.
56. Weetman AP. The immunomodulatory effects of antithyroid drugs. *Thyroid*. 1994;4:145-146.
57. McGregor AM, Petersen MM, Capiferri R, et al. Effects of radioiodine on thyrotrophin binding inhibiting immunoglobulins in Graves' disease. *Clin Endocrinol*. 1979;11:437-444.
58. Hiromatsu Y, Hoshino T, Yagita H, et al. Functional Fas ligand expression in thyrocytes from patients with Graves' disease. *J Clin Endocrinol Metab*. 1999;84:2896-2902.
59. Hollowell JG, Staehling NW, Flanders WD, et al. Serum TSH, T_4, and thyroid antibodies in the United States population (1988 to 1994): National Health and Nutrition Examination Survey (NHANES III). *J Clin Endocrinol Metab*. 2002;87:489-499.

60. Vanderpump MPJ, Tunbridge WMG, French JM, et al. The incidence of thyroid disorders in the community: a twenty-year follow-up of the Whickham survey. *Clin Endocrinol.* 1995;43:55-68.
61. Latif R, Morshed SA, Zaidi M, et al. The thyroid-stimulating hormone receptor: impact of thyroid-stimulating hormone and thyroid-stimulating hormone receptor antibodies on multimerization, cleavage, and signaling. *Endocrinol Metab Clin North Am.* 2009;38:319-341, viii.
62. Shimojo N, Kohno Y, Yamaguchi K, et al. Induction of Graves-like disease in mice by immunization with fibroblasts transfected with the thyrotropin receptor and a class II molecule. *Proc Natl Acad Sci U S A.* 1996;93:11074-11079.
63. Kita M, Ahmad L, Marians RC, et al. Regulation and transfer of a murine model of thyrotropin receptor antibody mediated Graves' disease. *Endocrinology.* 1999;140:1392-1398.
64. Nagayama Y, Kita-Furuyama M, Ando T, et al. A novel murine model of Graves' hyperthyroidism with intramuscular injection of adenovirus expressing the thyrotropin receptor. *J Immunol.* 2002;168: 2789-2794.
65. Sanders J, Chirgadze DY, Sanders P, et al. Crystal structure of the TSH receptor in complex with a thyroid-stimulating autoantibody. *Thyroid.* 2007;17:395-410.
66. Costagliola S, Bonomi M, Morgenthaler NG, et al. Delineation of the discontinuous-conformational epitope of a monoclonal antibody displaying full in vitro and in vivo thyrotropin activity. *Mol Endocrinol.* 2004;18:3020-3034.
67. Nunez MR, Sanders J, Jeffreys J, et al. Analysis of the thyrotropin receptor-thyrotropin interaction by comparative modeling. *Thyroid.* 2004;14:991-1011.
68. Adams DD, Purves HD. Abnormal responses in the assay of thyrotropin. *Proceedings of the University of Otago Medical School.* 1956; 34:11-12.
69. Adams DD. The presence of an abnormal thyroid-stimulating hormone in the serum of some thyrotoxic patients. *J Clin Endocrinol Metab.* 1958;18:699-712.
70. Kraiem Z, Lahat N, Glaser B, et al. Thyrotropin receptor blocking antibodies: incidence, characterization and in-vitro synthesis. *Clin Endocrinol.* 1987;27:409-421.
71. Adams DD, Fastier FN, Howie JB, et al. Stimulation of the human thyroid by infusions of plasma containing LATS protector. *J Clin Endocrinol Metab.* 1974;39:826-832.
72. Munro DS, Dirmikis SM, Humphries H, et al. The role of thyroid-stimulating immunoglobulins of Graves' disease in neonatal thyrotoxicosis. *Br J Obstet Gynaecol.* 1978;85:837-843.
73. Zakarija MJ. Immunochemical characterization of the thyroid-stimulating antibody (TSab) of Graves' disease: evidence for restricted heterogeneity. *J Clin Lab Immunol.* 1983;10:77-85.
74. Weetman AP, Yateman ME, Ealey PA, et al. Thyroid-stimulating antibody activity between different immunoglobulin G subclasses. *J Clin Invest.* 1990;86:723-727.
75. Bolton J, Sanders J, Oda Y, et al. Measurement of thyroid-stimulating hormone receptor autoantibodies by ELISA. *Clin Chem.* 1999;45: 2285-2287.
76. Costagliola S, Morgenthaler NG, Hoermann R, et al. Second generation assay for thyrotropin receptor antibodies has superior diagnostic sensitivity for Graves' disease. *J Clin Endocrinol Metab.* 1999;84:90-97.
77. Smith BR, Bolton J, Young S, et al. A new assay for thyrotropin receptor autoantibodies. *Thyroid.* 2004;14:830-835.
78. Davies TF, Yeo PP, Evered DC, et al. Value of thyroid-stimulating-antibody determinations in predicting short-term thyrotoxic relapse in Graves' disease. *Lancet.* 1977;1:1181-1182.
79. Davies TF. Thyroid-stimulating antibodies predict hyperthyroidism. *J Clin Endocrinol Metab.* 1998;83:3777-3781.
80. Davies TF, Roti E, Braverman LE, et al. Thyroid controversy-stimulating antibodies. *J Clin Endocrinol Metab.* 1998;83:3777-3785.
81. Mackenzie WA, Schwartz AE, Friedman EW, et al. Intrathyroidal T cell clones from patients with autoimmune thyroid disease. *J Clin Endocrinol Metab.* 1987;64:818-824.
82. Dayan CM, Londei M, Corcoran AE, et al. Autoantigen recognition by thyroid-infiltrating T cells in Graves disease. *Proc Natl Acad Sci USA.* 1991;88:7415-7419.
83. Grubeck Loebenstein B, Turner M, Pirich K, et al. CD4+ T-cell clones from autoimmune thyroid tissue cannot be classified according to their lymphokine production. *Scand J Immunol.* 1990;32:433-440.
84. Valmori D, Merlo A, Souleimanian NE, et al. A peripheral circulating compartment of natural naive CD4 Tregs. *J Clin Invest.* 2005;115: 1953-1962.
85. Verginis P, Li HS, Carayanniotis G. Tolerogenic semimature dendritic cells suppress experimental autoimmune thyroiditis by activation of thyroglobulin-specific CD4+CD25+ T cells. *J Immunol.* 2005;174: 7433-7749.
86. Pan D, Shin YH, Gopalakrishnan G, et al. Regulatory T cells in Graves' disease. *Clin Endocrinol (Oxf).* 2009;71:587-593.
87. Li HS, Carayanniotis G. Detection of thyroglobulin mRNA as truncated isoform(s) in mouse thymus. *Immunology.* 2005;115:85-89.
88. Murakami M, Hosoi Y, Negishi T, et al. Thymic hyperplasia in patients with Graves' disease: identification of thyrotropin receptors in human thymus. *J Clin Invest.* 1996;98:2228-2234.
89. McLachlan SM, Nagayama Y, Pichurin PN, et al. The link between Graves' disease and Hashimoto's thyroiditis: a role for regulatory T cells. *Endocrinology.* 2007;148:5724-5733.
90. Tomer Y, Davies TF. Infection, thyroid disease and autoimmunity. *Endocr Rev.* 1993;14:107-120.
91. Rapoport B, Aalsabeh R, Aftergood D, et al. Elephantiasic pretibial myxedema: insight into (and a hypothesis regarding) the pathogenesis of the extrathyroidal manifestations of Graves' disease. *Thyroid.* 2000;10:685-692.
92. Horwitz MS, Bradley LM, Harbertson J, et al. Diabetes induced by Coxsackie virus: initiation by bystander damage and not molecular mimicry [see comments]. *Nat Med.* 1998;4:781-785.
93. Wen L, Wong FS. How can the innate immune system influence autoimmunity in type 1 diabetes and other autoimmune disorders? *Crit Rev Immunol.* 2005;25:225-250.
94. Arata N, Ando T, Unger P, et al. By-stander activation in autoimmune thyroiditis: studies on experimental autoimmune thyroiditis in the GFP+ fluorescent mouse. *Clin Immunol.* 2006;121:108-117.
95. De Riu A, Martin A, Valentine M, et al. Graves' disease thyroid transplants in Scid mice: persistent selectivity in hTcR V alpha gene family use. *Autoimmunity.* 1994;19:271-277.
96. Wickham S, Carr DJ. Molecular mimicry versus bystander activation: herpetic stromal keratitis. *Autoimmunity.* 2004;37:393-397.
97. Srinivasappa J, Saegusa J, Prabhakar BS, et al. Molecular mimicry: frequency of reactivity of monoclonal antiviral antibodies with normal tissues. *J Virol.* 1986;57:397-401.
98. Haspel MV, Onodrera T, Prabhakar BS, et al. Multiple organ-reactive monoclonal autoantibodies. *Nature.* 1983;304:73-76.
99. Wenzel BE, Strieder TM, Gaspar E, et al. Chronic infection with *Yersinia enterocolitica i*n patients with clinical or latent hyperthyroidism. *Adv Exp Med Biol.* 2003;529:463-466.
100. Gangi E, Kapatral V, El-Azami El-Idrissi M, et al. Characterization of a recombinant *Yersinia enterocolitica* lipoprotein; implications for its role in autoimmune response against thyrotropin receptor. *Autoimmunity.* 2004;37:515-520.
101. Benvenga S, Guarneri F, Vaccaro M, et al. Homologies between proteins of *Borrelia burgdorferi* and thyroid autoantigens. *Thyroid.* 2004;14: 964-966.
102. Mirakian R, Hammond LJ, Bottazzo GF. Pathogenesis of thyroid autoimmunity: the Bottazzo-Feldmann hypothesis. *Immunol Today.* 1998;19:97-98.
103. Kawakami Y, Kuzuya N, Watanabe T, et al. Induction of experimental thyroiditis in mice by recombinant interferon gamma administration. *Acta Endocrinol (Copenh).* 1990;122:41-48.
104. Moudgil KD, Sercarz EE. Understanding crypticity is the key to revealing the pathogenesis of autoimmunity. *Trends Immunol.* 2005;26: 355-359.
105. Davies TF, Greenberg D, Tomer Y. The genetics of the autoimmune thyroid diseases. *Ann Endocrinol (Paris).* 2003;64:28-30.
106. Villanueva R, Greenberg DA, Davies TF, et al. Sibling recurrence risk in autoimmune thyroid disease. *Thyroid.* 2003;13:761-764.
107. Brix TH, Christensen K, Holm NV, et al. A population-based study of Graves' disease in Danish twins. *Clin Endocrinol.* 1998;48:397-400.
108. Tomer Y, Greenberg DA, Barbesino G, et al. CTLA-4 and not CD28 is a susceptibility gene for thyroid autoantibody production. *J Clin Endocrinol Metab.* 2001;86:1687-1693.
109. Davies TF, Latif R, Yin X. Inheriting autoimmune thyroid disease. *Endocr Pract.* 2009;15:63-66.
110. Barbesino G, Tomer Y, Concepcion ES, et al. Linkage analysis of candidate genes in autoimmune thyroid disease: 1. Selected immunoregulatory genes. *J Clin Endocrinol Metab.* 1998;83:1580-1584.
111. Ban Y, Concepcion ES, Villanueva R, et al. Analysis of immune regulatory genes in familial and sporadic Graves' disease. *J Clin Endocrinol Metab.* 2004;89:4562-4568.
112. Samarkos M, Vaiopoulos G. The role of infections in the pathogenesis of autoimmune diseases. *Curr Drug Targets Inflamm Allergy.* 2005; 4:99-103.
113. Olson JK, Croxford JL, Miller SD. Virus-induced autoimmunity: potential role of viruses in initiation, perpetuation, and progression of T-cell-mediated autoimmune disease. *Viral Immunol.* 2001;14:227-250.
114. Tomer Y. Hepatitis C and interferon induced thyroiditis. *J Autoimmun.* 2010;34:J322-J326.
115. Carter JK, Smith RE. Rapid induction of hypothyroidism by an avian leukosis virus. *Infect Immun.* 1983;40:795-805.
116. Matsuda T, Tomita M, Uchihara JN, et al. Human T cell leukemia virus type I-infected patients with Hashimoto's thyroiditis and Graves' disease. *J Clin Endocrinol Metab.* 2005;90:5704-5710.
117. Irwin M. Stress-induced immune suppression: role of brain corticotropin releasing hormone and autonomic nervous system mechanisms. *Adv Neuroimmunol.* 1994;4:29-47.

118. Marshall GD. Neuroendocrine mechanisms of immune dysregulation: applications to allergy and asthma. *Ann Allergy Asthma Immunol*. 2004;93:S11-S17.
119. Amino N, Tada H, Hidaka Y, et al. Therapeutic controversy: screening for postpartum thyroiditis. *J Clin Endocrinol Metab*. 1999;84:1813-1821.
120. Ansar AS, Young PR, Penhale WJ. Beneficial effect of testosterone in the treatment of chronic autoimmune thyroiditis in rats. *J Immunol*. 1986;136:143-147.
121. Fassler R, Dietrich H, Kromer G, et al. The role of testosterone in spontaneous autoimmune thyroiditis of Obese strain (OS) chickens. *J Autoimmun*. 1988;1:97-108.
122. Tomer Y, Davies TF. Searching for the autoimmune thyroid disease susceptibility genes: from gene mapping to gene function. *Endocrine Rev*. 2003;24:694-717.
123. Chow JC, Yen Z, Ziesche SM, et al. Silencing of the mammalian X chromosome. *Annu Rev Genomics Hum Genet*. 2005;6:69-92.
124. Brix TH, Knudsen GP, Kristiansen M, et al. High frequency of skewed X chromosome inactivation in females with autoimmune thyroid disease: a possible explanation for the female predisposition to thyroid autoimmunity. *J Clin Endocrinol Metab*. 2005;90:5949-5953.
125. Reference deleted in proofs.
126. Yin X, Latif R, Tomer Y, et al. Thyroid epigenetics: X chromosome inactivation in patients with autoimmune thyroid disease. *Ann N Y Acad Sci*. 2007;1110:193-200.
127. Mestman JH. Hyperthyroidism in pregnancy. *Endocrinol Metab Clin North Am*. 1998;27:127-149.
128. Chan GW, Mandel SJ. Therapy insight: management of Graves' disease during pregnancy. *Nat Clin Pract Endocrinol Metab*. 2007;3:470-478.
129. Anselmo J, Cao D, Karrison T, et al. Fetal loss associated with excess thyroid hormone exposure. *JAMA*. 2004;292:691-695.
130. Aluvihare VR, Kallikourdis M, Betz AG. Tolerance, suppression and the fetal allograft. *J Mol Med*. 2005;83:88-96.
131. Stagnaro-Green A, Roman SH, Cobin RH, et al. A prospective study of lymphocyte-initiated immunosuppression in normal pregnancy: evidence of a T-cell etiology for postpartum thyroid dysfunction. *J Clin Endocrinol Metab*. 1992;74:645-653.
132. Jansson R, Dahlberg PA, Winsa B, et al. The postpartum period constitutes an important risk for the development of clinical Graves' disease in young women. *Acta Endocrinol*. 1987;116:321-325.
133. Rotondi M, Cappelli C, Pirali B, et al. The effect of pregnancy on subsequent relapse from Graves' disease after a successful course of antithyroid drug therapy. *J Clin Endocrinol Metab*. 2008;93:3985-3988.
134. Bartalena L, Bogazzi F, Martino E. Amiodarone-induced thyrotoxicosis: a difficult diagnostic and therapeutic challenge. *Clin Endocrinol (Oxf)*. 2002;56:23-24.
135. Basaria S, Cooper DS. Amiodarone and the thyroid. *Am J Med*. 2005;118:706-714.
136. DeGroot L. Effects of irradiation on the thyroid gland. *Endocrinol Metab Clin North Am*. 1993;22:607-615.
137. Huysmans D, Hermus A, Edelbrook M, et al. Autoimmune hyperthyroidism occurring late after radioiodine treatment for volume reduction of large multinodular goiters. *Thyroid*. 1997;7:535-539.
138. Pacini F, Vorontsova T, Molinaro E, et al. Prevalence of thyroid autoantibodies in children and adolescents from Belarus exposed to the Chernobyl radioactive fallout. *Lancet*. 1998;352:763-766.
139. Vermiglio F, Castagna MG, Volnova E, et al. Post-Chernobyl increased prevalence of humoral thyroid autoimmunity in children and adolescents from a moderately iodine-deficient area in Russia. *Thyroid*. 1999;9:781-786.
140. Vykhovanets EV, Chernyshov VP, Slukvin I, et al. 131-I dose-dependent thyroid autoimmune disorders in children living around Chernobyl. *Clin Immunol Immunopathol*. 1997;84:251-259.
141. Bartalena L, Marcocci C, Tanda ML, et al. An update on medical management of Graves' ophthalmopathy. *J Endocrinol Invest*. 2005;28:469-478.
142. Prabhakar BS, Bahn RS, Smith TJ. Current perspective on the pathogenesis of Graves' disease and ophthalmopathy. *Endocr Rev*. 2003; 24:802-835.
143. Feldon SE, Park DJ, O'Loughlin CW, et al. Autologous T-lymphocytes stimulate proliferation of orbital fibroblasts derived from patients with Graves' ophthalmopathy. *Invest Ophthalmol Vis Sci*. 2005;46:3913-3921.
144. Grubeck-Loebenstein B, Trieb K, Holter W, et al. Retrobulbar T cells from patients with Graves' ophthalmopathy are CD8+ and specifically autologous fibroblasts. *J Clin Invest*. 1993;93:2738-2743.
145. Mori S, Yoshikawa N, Tokoro T, et al. Studies of retroorbital tissue xenografts from patients with Graves' ophthalmopathy in severe combined immunodeficient (SCID) mice: detection of thyroid-stimulating antibody. *Thyroid*. 1996;6:275-281.
146. Douglas RS, Afifiyan NF, Hwang CJ, et al. Increased generation of fibrocytes in thyroid-associated ophthalmopathy. *J Clin Endocrinol Metab*. 2010;95:430-438.
147. Weightman DR, Perros P, Sherif IH, et al. Autoantibodies to IGF-1 binding sites in thyroid associated ophthalmopathy. *Autoimmunity*. 1993;16:251-257.
148. Smith TJ, Tsai CC, Shih MJ, et al. Unique attributes of orbital fibroblasts and global alterations in IGF-1 receptor signaling could explain thyroid-associated ophthalmopathy. *Thyroid*. 2008;18:983-988.
149. Gianoukakis AG, Douglas RS, King CS, et al. IgG from patients with Graves' disease induces IL-16 and RANTES expression in cultured human thyrocytes: a putative mechanism for T cell infiltration of the thyroid in autoimmune disease. *Endocrinology*. 2006; 147:1941-1949.
150. Villanueva R, Inzerillo AM, Tomer Y, et al. Limited genetic susceptibility to severe Graves' ophthalmopathy: no role for CTLA-4 but evidence for an environmental etiology. *Thyroid*. 2000;10:791-798.
151. Bertelsen JB, Hegedus L. Cigarette smoking and the thyroid. *Thyroid*. 1994;4:327-331.
152. Wood LC, Ingbar SH. Hypothyroidism as a late sequela in patients with Graves' disease treated with antithyroid agents. *J Clin Invest*. 1979;64:1429-1436.
153. Marks AD, Bertram BJ, Channick J, et al. Chronic thyroiditis and mitral valve prolapse. *Ann Intern Med*. 1995;102:479-483.
154. Bahn RS. Clinical review 157. Pathophysiology of Graves' ophthalmopathy: the cycle of disease. *J Clin Endocrinol Metab*. 2003;88:1939-1946.
155. Fledelius HC, Zimmermann-Belsing T, Feldt-Rasmussen U. Ultrasonically measured horizontal eye muscle thickness in thyroid associated orbitopathy: cross-sectional and longitudinal aspects in a Danish series. *Acta Ophthalmol Scand*. 2003;81:143-150.
156. Mourits MP, Prummel MF, Wiersinga WM, et al. Clinical activity score as a guide in the management of patients with Graves' ophthalmopathy. *Clin Endocrinol (Oxf)*. 1997;47:9-14.
157. Mechanick JI, Davies TF. Medical management of hyperthyroidism: theoretical and practical aspects. In: Falk SA, ed. *Thyroid Disease: Endocrinolgy, Surgery, Nuclear Medicine and Tadiotherapy*. 2nd ed. New York, NY: Lippincott-Raven; 1997:253-296.
158. Feldt-Rasmussen U, Schleusner H, Carayon P. Meta-analysis evaluation of the impact of thyrotropin receptor antibodies on long term remission after medical therapy of Graves' disease. *J Clin Endocrinol Metab*. 1994;78:98-102.
159. Singer PA, Cooper DS, Levy E, et al. Treatment guidelines for patients with hyperthyroidism and hypothyroidism. *JAMA*. 1995;273:808-812.
160. Wartofsky L, Glinoer D, Solomon B, et al. Differences and similarities in the diagnosis and treatment of Graves' disease in Europe, Japan, and the United States. *Thyroid*. 1991;1:129-135.
161. Cooper DS. Antithyroid drugs. *N Engl J Med*. 2005;352:905-917.
162. Abuid J, Larsen PR. Triiodothyronine and thyroxine in hyperthyroidism: comparison of the acute changes during therapy with antithyroid agents. *J Clin Invest*. 1974;54:201-208.
163. Maia AL, Kim BW, Huang SA, et al. Type 2 iodothyronine deiodinase is the major source of plasma T3 in euthyroid humans. *J Clin Invest*. 2005;115:2524-2533.
164. Laurberg P, Vestergaard H, Nielsen S, et al. Sources of circulating 3,5,3'-triiodothyronine in hyperthyroidism estimated after blocking of type 1 and type 2 iodothyronine deiodinases. *J Clin Endocrinol Metab*. 2007;92:2149-2156.
165. Stassi G, Zeuner A, Di Liberto D, et al. Fas-FasL in Hashimoto's thyroiditis. *J Clin Immunol*. 2001;21:19-23.
166. Mitsiades N, Poulaki V, Tseleni-Balafouta S, et al. Fas ligand expression in thyroid follicular cells from patients with thionamide-treated Graves' disease. *Thyroid*. 2000;10:527-532.
167. Nakamura H, Noh JY, Itoh K, et al. Comparison of methimazole and propylthiouracil in patients with hyperthyroidism caused by Graves' disease. *J Clin Endocrinol Metab*. 2007;92:2157-2162.
168. Bahn RS, Burch HS, Cooper DS, et al. The role of propylthiouracil in the management of Graves' disease in adults: report of a meeting jointly sponsored by the American Thyroid Association and the Food and Drug Administration. *Thyroid*. 2009;19:673-674.
169. Laurberg P, Torring J, Weeke J. A comparison of the effects of propylthiouracil and methimazol on circulating thyroid hormones and various measures of peripheral thyroid hormone effects in thyrotoxic patients. *Acta Endocrinol (Copenh)*. 1985;108:51-54.
170. Larsen PR. Thyroidal triiodothyronine and thyroxine in Graves' disease: correlation with presurgical treatment, thyroid status, and iodine content. *J Clin Endocrinol Metab*. 1975;41:1098-1104.
171. Izumi M, Larsen PR. Triiodothyronine, thyroxine, and iodine in purified thyroglobulin from patients with Graves' disease. *J Clin Invest*. 1977;59:1105-1112.
172. Romaldini JH, Bromberg N, Werner RS, et al. Comparison of effects of high and low dosage regimens of antithyroid drugs in the management of Graves' hyperthyroidism. *J Clin Endocrinol Metab*. 1983;57:563-570.
173. McIver B, Rae P, Beckett G, et al. Lack of effect of thyroxine in patients with Graves' hyperthyroidism who are treated with an antithyroid drug. *N Engl J Med*. 1996;334:220-224.

174. Rittmaster RS, Abbott EC, Douglas R, et al. Effect of methimazole, with or without L-thyroxine, on remission rates in Graves' disease. *J Clin Endocrinol Metab*. 1998;83:814-818.
175. Abraham P, Avenell A, Park CM, et al. A systematic review of drug therapy for Graves' hyperthyroidism. *Eur J Endocrinol*. 2005;153: 489-498.
176. Allahabadia A, Daykin J, Holder RL, et al. Age and gender predict the outcome of treatment for Graves' hyperthyroidism. *J Clin Endocrinol Metab*. 2000;85:1038-1042.
177. Reference deleted in proofs.
178. Ban Y, Greenberg DA, Concepcion E, et al. Amino acid substitutions in the thyroglobulin gene are associated with susceptibility to human and murine autoimmune thyroid disease. *Proc Natl Acad Sci U S A*. 2003;100:15119-15124.
179. Brent GA. Clinical practice: Graves' disease. *N Engl J Med*. 2008; 358:2594-2605.
180. Cooper DS, Rivkees SA. Putting propylthiouracil in perspective. *J Clin Endocrinol Metab*. 2009;94:1881-1882.
181. Woeber KA. Methimazole-induced hepatotoxicity. *Endocr Pract*. 2002;8:222-224.
182. Harper L, Chin L, Daykin J, et al. Propylthiouracil and carbimazole associated-antineutrophil cytoplasmic antibodies (ANCA) in patients with Graves' disease. *Clin Endocrinol (Oxf)*. 2004;60:671-675.
183. Emerson CH, Anderson AJ, Howard WJ, et al. Serum thyroxine and triiodothyronine concentrations during iodide treatment of hyperthyroidism. *J Clin Endocrinol Metab*. 1975;40:33-36.
184. Braga M, Cooper DS. Clinical review 129. Oral cholecystographic agents and the thyroid. *J Clin Endocrinol Metab*. 2001;86:1853-1860.
185. Lazarus JH, Richards AR, Addison GM, et al. Treatment of thyrotoxicosis with lithium carbonate. *Lancet*. 1974;2:1160-1163.
186. Vigneri R, Pezzino V, Filetti S, et al. Effect of dexamethasone on thyroid hormone response to TSH. *Metabolism*. 1975;24:1209-1213.
187. Werga-Kjellman P, Zedenius J, Tallstedt L, et al. Surgical treatment of hyperthyroidism: a ten-year experience. *Thyroid*. 2001;11:187-192.
188. Sosa JA, Bowman HM, Tielsch JM, et al. The importance of surgeon experience for clinical and economic outcomes from thyroidectomy. *Ann Surg*. 1998;228:320-330.
189. Chang DC, Wheeler MH, Woodcock JP, et al. The effect of preoperative Lugol's iodine on thyroid blood flow in patients with Graves' hyperthyroidism. *Surgery*. 1987;102:1055-1061.
190. Rangaswamy M, Padhy AK, Gopinath PG, et al. Effect of Lugol's iodine on the vascularity of thyroid gland in hyperthyroidism. *Nucl Med Commun*. 1989;10:679-684.
191. Erbil Y, Ozluk Y, Giris M, et al. Effect of Lugol solution on thyroid gland blood flow and microvessel density in the patients with Graves' disease. *J Clin Endocrinol Metab*. 2007;92:2182-2189.
192. Toft AD, Irvine WJ, Sinclair I, et al. Thyroid function after surgical treatment of thyrotoxicosis: a report of 100 cases treated with propranolol before operation. *N Engl J Med*. 1978;298:643-647.
193. Franklyn JA, Maisonneuve P, Sheppard M, et al. Cancer incidence and mortality after radioiodine treatment for hyperthyroidism: a population-based cohort study. *Lancet*. 1999;353:2111-2115.
194. Franklyn JA, Sheppard MC, Maisonneuve P. Thyroid function and mortality in patients treated for hyperthyroidism. *JAMA*. 2005; 294:71-80.
195. Cheetham TD, Wraight P, Hughes IA, et al. Radioiodine treatment of Graves' disease in young people. *Horm Res*. 1998;49:258-262.
196. Berg GE, Nystrom EH, Jacobsson L, et al. Radioiodine treatment of hyperthyroidism in a pregnant women. *J Nucl Med*. 1998;39: 357-361.
197. Nakazato N, Yoshida K, Mori K, et al. Antithyroid drugs inhibit radioiodine-induced increases in thyroid autoantibodies in hyperthyroid Graves' disease. *Thyroid*. 1999;9:775-779.
198. Razvi S, Basu A, McIntyre EA, et al. Low failure rate of fixed administered activity of 400 MBq 131I with pre-treatment with carbimazole for thyrotoxicosis: the Gateshead Protocol. *Nucl Med Commun*. 2004;25:675-682.
199. Alexander EK, Larsen PR. High dose of 1^{311} therapy for the treatment of hyperthyroidism caused by Graves' disease. *J Clin Endocrinol Metab*. 2002;87:1073-1077.
200. Leslie WD, Ward L, Salamon EA, et al. A randomized comparison of radioiodine doses in Graves' hyperthyroidism. *J Clin Endocrinol Metab*. 2003;88:978-983.
201. Tuttle RM, Patience T, Budd S. Treatment with propylthiouracil before radioactive iodine therapy is associated with a higher treatment failure rate than therapy with radioactive iodine alone in Graves' disease. *Thyroid*. 1995;5:243-247.
202. Walter MA, Briel M, Christ-Crain M, et al. Effects of antithyroid drugs on radioiodine treatment: systematic review and meta-analysis of randomised controlled trials. *BMJ*. 2007;334:514.
203. Gorman CA. Radioiodine and pregnancy. *Thyroid*. 1999;9:721-726.
204. Sabri O, Zimny M, Schreckenberger M, et al. Radioiodine therapy in Graves' disease patients with large diffuse goiters treated with or without carbimazole at the time of radioiodine therapy. *Thyroid*. 1999;9:1181-1198.
205. Andrade VA, Gross JL, Maia AL. Effect of methimazole pretreatment on serum thyroid hormone levels after radioactive treatment in Graves' hyperthyroidism. *J Clin Endocrinol Metab*. 1999;84:4012-4016.
206. Dickman PW, Holm LE, Lundell G, et al. Thyroid cancer risk after thyroid examination with 131I: a population-based cohort study in Sweden. *Int J Cancer*. 2003;106:580-587.
207. Moysich KB, Menezes RJ, Michalek AM. Chernobyl-related ionising radiation exposure and cancer risk: an epidemiological review. *Lancet Oncol*. 2002;3:269-279.
208. Nikiforov Y, Heffess C, Korzenko A, et al. Characteristics of follicular tumors and nonneoplastic thyroid lesions in children and adolescents exposed to radiation as a result of the Chernobyl disaster. *Cancer*. 1995;76:900-909.
209. Gavrilin Y, Khrouch V, Shinkarev S, et al. Individual thyroid dose estimation for a case-control study of Chernobyl-related thyroid cancer among children of Belarus: part I. I-131, short-lived radioiodines (I-132, I-133, I-135), and short-lived radiotelluriums (Te-131M and Te-132). *Health Physics*. 2004;86:565-585.
210. Metso S, Jaatinen P, Huhtala H, et al. Long-term follow-up study of radioiodine treatment of hyperthyroidism. *Clin Endocrinol (Oxf)*. 2004;61:641-648.
211. Rubio IG, Perone BH, Silva MN, et al. Human recombinant TSH preceding a therapeutic dose of radioiodine for multinodular goiters has no significant effect in the surge of TSH-receptor and TPO antibodies. *Thyroid*. 2005;15:134-139.
212. Harvey RD, Metclafe RA, Morteo C, et al. Acute pre-tibial myxedema following radioiodine therapy for thyrotoxic Graves' disease. *Clin Endocrinol*. 1995;42:657-660.
213. Bartalena L, Marcocci C, Bogazzi F, et al. Use of corticosteroids to prevent progression of Graves' ophthalmopathy after radioiodine therapy for hyperthyroidism. *N Engl J Med*. 1989;321:1349-1352.
214. Tallestedt L, Lundell G, Torring O, et al. Occurrence of ophthalmopathy after treatment for Graves' disease. *N Engl J Med*. 1992;326: 1733-1738.
215. Gorman CA. Therapeutic controversies: radioiodine therapy does not aggravate Graves' ophthalmopathy. *J Clin Endocrinol Metab*. 1995;80: 340-342.
216. Stan MN, Bahn RS. Risk factors for development or deterioration of Graves' ophthalmopathy. *Thyroid*. 2010;20:777-783.
217. Wartofsky L. Therapeutic controversies: summation, commentary, and overview. Concerns over aggravation of Graves' ophthalmopathy by radioactive iodine treatment and the use of retrobulbar radiation therapy. *J Clin Endocrinol Metab*. 1995;80:347-349.
218. Dale J, Daykin J, Holder R, et al. Weight gain following treatment of hyperthyroidism. *Clin Endocrinol (Oxf)*. 2001;55:233-239.
219. Wiersinga WM, Bartalena L. Epidemiology and prevention of Graves' ophthalmopathy. *Thyroid*. 2002;12:855-860.
220. Perros P, Crombie AL, Kendall-Taylor P. Natural history of thyroid associated ophthalmopathy. *Clin Endocrinol*. 1995;42:45-50.
221. Bartley GB, Fatourechi V, Kadrmas EF, et al. Chronology of Graves' ophthalmopathy in an incidence cohort. *Am J Ophthalmol*. 1996;121: 426-434.
222. Sridama V, DeGroot LJ. Treatment of Graves' disease and the course of ophthalmopathy. *Am J Med*. 1989;87:70-73.
223. Jarhult J, Rudberg C, Larsson E, et al. Graves' disease with moderate-severe endocrine ophthalmopathy—long term results of a prospective, randomized study of total or subtotal thyroid resection. *Thyroid*. 2005;15:1157-1164.
224. Menconi F, Marino M, Pinchera A, et al. Effects of total thyroid ablation versus near-total thyroidectomy alone on mild to moderate Graves' orbitopathy treated with intravenous glucocorticoids. *J Clin Endocrinol Metab*. 2007;92:1653-1658.
225. Wiersinga WM, Prummel MF. An evidence-based approach to the treatment of Graves' ophthalmopathy. *Endocrinol Metab Clin North Am*. 2000;29:297-319, vi-vii.
226. Bartalena L, Baldeschi L, Dickinson A, et al. Consensus statement of the European Group on Graves' orbitopathy (EUGOGO) on management of GO. *Eur J Endocrinol*. 2008;158:273-285.
227. Perros P, Baldeschi L, Boboridis K, et al. A questionnaire survey on the management of Graves' orbitopathy in Europe. *Eur J Endocrinol*. 2006;155:207-211.
228. Beckendorf V, Maalouf T, George JL, et al. Place of radiotherapy in the treatment of Graves' orbitopathy. *Int J Radiat Oncol Biol Phys*. 1999;43:805-815.
229. Perros P, Krassas GE. Orbital irradiation for thyroid-associated orbitopathy: conventional dose, low dose or no dose? *Clin Endocrinol (Oxf)*. 2002;56:689-691.
230. Gorman CA, Garrity JA, Fatourechi V, et al. The aftermath of orbital radiotherapy for graves' ophthalmopathy. *Ophthalmology*. 2002;109: 2100-2107.
231. Gorman CA, Garrity JA, Fatourechi V, et al. A prospective, randomized, double-blind, placebo-controlled study of orbital radiotherapy for Graves' ophthalmopathy. *Ophthalmology*. 2001;108:1523-1534.

232. Rose JG Jr, Burkat CN, Boxrud CA. Diagnosis and management of thyroid orbitopathy. *Otolaryngol Clin North Am.* 2005;38:1043-1074.
233. Boulos PR, Hardy I. Thyroid-associated orbitopathy: a clinicopathologic and therapeutic review. *Curr Opin Ophthalmol.* 2004;15:389-400.
234. Salvi M, Vannucchi G, Campi I, et al. Rituximab in the treatment of thyroid eye disease: science fiction? *Orbit.* 2009;28:251-255.
235. Hegedus L, Smith TJ, Douglas RS, et al. Targeted biological therapies for Graves' disease and thyroid associated ophthalmopathy: focus on B cell depletion with Rituximab. *Clin Endocrinol (Oxf).* 2010 Apr 23 [Epub ahead of print].
236. Fatourechi V. Pretibial myxedema: pathophysiology and treatment options. *Am J Clin Dermatol.* 2005;6:295-309.
237. Chung-Leddon J. Pretibial myxedema. *Dermatol Online J.* 2001;7:18.
238. Burch HB, Wartofsky L. Graves' ophthalmopathy: current concepts regarding pathogenesis and management. *Endocr Rev.* 1993;14:747-793.
239. Bianco AC, Salvatore D, Gereben B, et al. Biochemistry, cellular and molecular biology and physiological roles of the iodothyronine selenodeiodinases. *Endocrine Rev.* 2002;23:38-89.
240. Misaki T, Tramontano D, Ingbar SH. Effects of rat gamma- and non-gamma-interferons on the expression of Ia antigen, growth, and differentiated functions of FRTL5 cells. *Endocrinology.* 1988;123:2849-2857.
241. Croxson MS, Hall TD, Nicoloff JT. Combination drug therapy for treatment of hyperthyroid Graves' disease. *J Clin Endocrinol Metab.* 1977;45:623-630.
242. Larsen PR. Salicylate-induced increases in free triiodothyronine in human serum: evidence of inhibition of triiodothyronine binding to thyroxine-binding globulin and thyroxine-binding prealbumin. *J Clin Invest.* 1972;51:1125-1134.
243. Davies TF. The thyroid immunology of the postpartum period. *Thyroid.* 1999;9:675-684.
244. Galofre JC, Davies TF. Autoimmune thyroid disease in pregnancy: a review. *J Womens Health (Larchmt).* 2009;18:1847-1856.
245. Lazarus JH. Thyroid disease in pregnancy and childhood. *Minerva Endocrinol.* 2005;30:71-87.
246. Weetman AP. Immunity, thyroid function and pregnancy: molecular mechanisms. *Nat Rev Endocrinol.* 2010;6:311-318.
247. Somerset DA, Zheng Y, Kilby MD, et al. Normal human pregnancy is associated with an elevation in the immune suppressive CD25+ CD4+ regulatory T-cell subset. *Immunology.* 2004;112:38-43.
248. Evans PC, Lambert N, Maloney S, et al. Long-term fetal microchimerism in peripheral blood mononuclear cell subsets in healthy women and women with scleroderma. *Blood.* 1999;93:2033-2037.
249. Ando T, Davies TF. Clinical review 160. Postpartum autoimmune thyroid disease: the potential role of fetal microchimerism. *J Clin Endocrinol Metab.* 2003;88:2965-2971.
250. Lambert NC, Evans PC, Hashizumi TL, et al. Cutting edge: persistent fetal microchimerism in T lymphocytes is associated with HLA-DQA1*0501: implications in autoimmunity. *J Immunol.* 2000;164:5545-5548.
251. Ando T, Davies TF. Self-recognition and the role of fetal microchimerism. *Best Pract Res Clin Endocrinol Metab.* 2004;18:197-211.
252. Amino N, Kuro R, Tanizawa O, et al. Changes of serum antithyroid antibodies during and after pregnancy in autoimmune thyroid diseases. *Clin Exp Immunol.* 1978;31:30-37.
253. Aluvihare VR, Kallikourdis M, Betz AG. Regulatory T cells mediate maternal tolerance to the fetus. *Nat Immunol.* 2004;5:266-271.
254. Zakarija M, McKenzie JM. Pregnancy-associated changes in thyroid-stimulating antibody of Graves' disease and the relationship to neonatal hyperthyroidism. *J Clin Endocrinol Metab.* 1983;57:1036-1040.
255. Mejias-Heredia A, Litchfield WR, Zurakowski D. Assessing the risk of neonatal Graves' disease using TSI measurements (abstract P3). 77th Meeting of the Endocrine Society. 1995:460.
256. Tamaki H, Amino N, Aozasa M, et al. Universal predictive criteria for neonatal overt thyroxicosis requiring treatment. *Am J Perinatol.* 1988;5:152-158.
257. Luton D, Le Gac I, Vuillard E, et al. Management of Graves' disease during pregnancy: the key role of fetal thyroid gland monitoring. *J Clin Endocrinol Metab.* 2005;90:6093-6098.
258. Glinoer D, De Nayer P, Bourdoux P, et al. Regulation of maternal thyroid during pregnancy. *J Clin Endocrinol Metab.* 1990;71:276-287.
259. Amino N, Tanizawa O, Mori H, et al. Aggravation of thyrotoxicosis in early pregnancy and after delivery in Graves' disease. *J Clin Endocrinol Metab.* 1982;55:108-112.
260. Hershman JM. Human chorionic gonadotropin and the thyroid: hyperemesis gravidarum and trophoblastic tumors. *Thyroid.* 1999;9:653-657.
261. Stricker R, Echenard M, Eberhart R, et al. Evaluation of maternal thyroid function during pregnancy: the importance of using gestational age-specific reference intervals. *Eur J Endocrinol.* 2007;157:509-514.
262. LeBeau SO, Mandel SJ. Thyroid disorders during pregnancy. *Endocrinol Metab Clin North Am.* 2006;35:117-136, vii.
263. Cheron RG, Kaplan M, Reed Larsen P, et al. Neonatal thyroid function after propylthiouracil therapy for maternal Graves' disease. *N Engl J Med.* 1981;304:525-528.
264. Ochoa-Maya MR, Frates MC, Lee-Parritz A, et al. Resolution of fetal goiter after discontinuation of propylthiouracil in a pregnant woman with Graves' hyperthyroidism. *Thyroid.* 1999;9:1111-1114.
265. Abalovich M, Amino N, Barbour LA, et al. Management of thyroid dysfunction during pregnancy and postpartum: an Endocrine Society Clinical Practice Guideline. *J Clin Endocrinol Metab.* 2007;92:S1-S47.
266. Mortimer RH, Cannell GR, Addison RS, et al. Methimazole and propylthiouracil equally cross the perfused human term placental lobule. *J Clin Endocrinol Metab.* 1997;82:3099-3102.
267. Barbero P, Valdez R, Rodriguez H, et al. Choanal atresia associated with maternal hyperthyroidism treated with methimazole: a case-control study. *Am J Med Genet A.* 2008;146A:2390-2395.
268. Milham S Jr. Scalp defects in infants of mothers treated for hyperthyroidism with methimazole or carbimazole during pregnancy. *Teratology.* 1985;32:321.
269. Foulds N, Walpole I, Elmslie F, et al. Carbimazole embryopathy: an emerging phenotype. *Am J Med Genet A.* 2005;132:130-135.
270. Momotani N, Noh J, Oyanagi H, et al. Antithyroid drug therapy for Graves' disease during pregnancy: optimal regimen for fetal thyroid status. *N Engl J Med.* 1986;315:24-28.
271. Fisher DA. Fetal thyroid function: diagnosis and management of fetal thyroid disorders. *Clin Obstet Gynecol.* 1997;40:16-31.
272. Petit KP, Nielsen HC. Chronic in utero beta-blockade alters fetal lung development. *Dev Pharmacol Ther.* 1992;19:131-140.
273. Ray JG, Vermeulen MJ, Burrows EA, et al. Use of antihypertensive medications in pregnancy and the risk of adverse perinatal outcomes: McMaster Outcome Study of Hypertension In Pregnancy 2 (MOS HIP 2). *BMC Pregnancy Childbirth.* 2001;1:6.
274. Momotani N, Hisaoka T, Noh J, et al. Effects of iodine on thyroid status of fetus versus mother in treatment of Graves' disease complicated by pregnancy. *J Clin Endocrinol Metab.* 1992;75:738-744.
275. Klein RZ, Sargent JD, Larsen PR, et al. Relation of severity of maternal hypothyroidism to cognitive development of offspring. *J Med Screen.* 2001;8:18-20.
276. Lamberg BA, Konen EI, Teramo K, et al. Treatment of maternal hyperthyroidism with antithyroid agents and changes in thyrotropin and thyroxine in the newborn. *Acta Endocrinol.* 1981;97:186-195.
277. Stagnaro-Green A. Recognizing, understanding, and treating postpartum thyroiditis. *Endocrinol Metab Clin North Am.* 2000;29:417-430, ix.
278. Rochester DB, Davies TF. Increased risk of Graves' disease after pregnancy. *Thyroid.* 2005;15:1287-1290.
279. Mandel SJ, Cooper DS. The use of antithyroid drugs in pregnancy and lactation. *J Clin Endocrinol Metab.* 2001;86:2354-2359.
280. Momotani N, Yamashita R, Makino F, et al. Thyroid function in wholly breast-feeding infants whose mothers take high doses of propylthiouracil. *Clin Endocrinol (Oxf).* 2000;53:177-181.
281. Refetoff S. Resistance to thyrotropin. *J Endocrinol Invest.* 2003;26:770-779.
282. Duprez L, Parma J, Van Sande J, et al. Germline mutations in the thyrotropin receptor gene cause non-autoimmune autosomal dominant hyperthyroidism. *Nat Genet.* 1994;7:396-401.
283. Parma J, Duprez L, Van Sande J, et al. Somatic mutations of the thyrotropin receptor gene cause hyperfunctioning thyroid adenomas. *Nature.* 1993;365:649-651.
284. Hegedus L, Bonnema SJ, Bennedbaek FN. Management of simple nodular goiter: current status and future perspectives. *Endocr Rev.* 2003;24:102-132.
285. Tonacchera M, Agretti P, Chiovato L, et al. Activating thyrotropin receptor mutations are present in nonadenomatous hyperfunctioning nodules of toxic or autonomous multinodular goiter. *J Clin Endocrinol Metab.* 2000;85:2270-2274.
286. Krohn K, Fuhrer D, Bayer Y, et al. Molecular pathogenesis of euthyroid and toxic multinodular goiter. *Endocr Rev.* 2005;26:504-524.
287. Baltisberger BL, Minder CE, Burgi H. Decrease of incidence of toxic nodular goitre in a region of Switzerland after full correction of mild iodine deficiency. *Eur J Endocrinol.* 1995;132:546-549.
288. Nygaard B, Hegedus L, Nielsen KG, et al. Long-term effect of radioactive iodine on thyroid function and size in patients with solitary autonomously functioning toxic thyroid nodules. *Clin Endocrinol (Oxf).* 1999;50:197-202.
289. Huysmans DAKC, Hermus RMM, Corstens FHM, et al. Large, compressive, goiters treated with radioiodine. *Ann Intern Med.* 1994;121:757-762.
290. Tonacchera M, Agretti P, Rosellini V, et al. Sporadic nonautoimmune congenital hyperthyroidism due to a strong activating mutation of the thyrotropin receptor gene. *Thyroid.* 2000;10:859-863.
291. Carr K, Mcleod DT, Parry G, et al. Fine adjustment of thyroxine replacement dosage: comparison of the thyrotrophin releasing hormone tests using a sensitive thyrotrophin assay with measurement

of free thyroid hormones and clinical assessment. *Clin Endocrinol.* 1988;28:325-333.
292. Bell GM, Sawers JSA, Forfar JC, et al. The effect of minor increments in plasma thyroxine on heart rate and urinary sodium excretion. *Clin Endocrinol.* 1983;18:511-516.
293. Tenerz A, Forberg R, Jansson R. Is a more active attitude warranted in patients with subclinical thyrotoxicosis? *J Intern Med.* 1990; 228:229-233.
294. Monreal M, Lafoz E, Foz M, et al. Occult thyrotoxicosis in patients with atrial fibrillation and an acute arterial embolism. *Angiology.* 1988;39:981-985.
295. Biondi B, Palmieri EA, Klain M, et al. Subclinical hyperthyroidism: clinical features and treatment options. *Eur J Endocrinol.* 2005; 152:1-9.
296. Faber J, Jensen IW, Petersen L, et al. Normalization of serum thyrotrophin by means of radioiodine treatment in subclinical hyperthyroidism: effect on bone loss in postmenopausal women. *Clin Endocrinol (Oxf).* 1998;48:285-290.
297. Sgarbi JA, Villaca FG, Garbeline B, et al. The effects of early antithyroid therapy for endogenous subclinical hyperthyroidism in clinical and heart abnormalities. *J Clin Endocrinol Metab.* 2003;88:1672-1677.
298. Faber J, Wiinberg N, Schifter S, et al. Haemodynamic changes following treatment of subclinical and overt hyperthyroidism. *Eur J Endocrinol.* 2001;145:391-396.
299. Sawin CT, Geller A, Kaplan MM, et al. Low serum thyrotropin (thyroid-stimulating hormone) in older persons without hyperthyroidism. *Arch Intern Med.* 1991;151:165-168.
300. Woeber KA. Observations concerning the natural history of subclinical hyperthyroidism. *Thyroid.* 2005;15:687-691.
301. Canaris GJ, Manowitz NR, Mayor G, et al. The Colorado thyroid disease prevalence study. *Arch Intern Med.* 2000;160:526-534.
302. Surks MI, Ortiz E, Daniels GH, et al. Subclinical thyroid disease: scientific review and guidelines for diagnosis and management. *JAMA.* 2004;291:228-238.
303. Marqusee E, Haden ST, Utiger RD. Subclinical thyrotoxicosis. *Endocrinol Metab Clin North Am.* 1998;27:37-49.
304. Toft AD. Clinical practice. Subclinical hyperthyroidism. *N Engl J Med.* 2001;345:512-516.
305. Col NF, Surks MI, Daniels GH. Subclinical thyroid disease: clinical applications. *JAMA.* 2004;291:239-243.
306. Roti E, Uberti ED. Iodine excess and hyperthyroidism. *Thyroid.* 2001;11:493-500.
307. Fradkin JE, Wolff J. Iodide-induced thyrotoxicosis. *Medicine (Baltimore).* 1983;62:1-20.
308. Martin FIR, Tress BW, Colman PG, et al. Iodine-induced hyperthyroidism due to nonionic contrast radiography in the elderly. *Am J Med.* 1993;95:78-82.
309. Conn JJ, Sebastian MJ, Deam D, et al. A prospective study of the effect of nonionic contrast media on thyroid function. *Thyroid.* 1996;6: 107-110.
310. Nolte W, Muller R, Siggelkow H, et al. Prophylactic application of thyrostatic drugs during excessive iodine exposure in euthyroid patients with thyroid autonomy: a randomized study. *Eur J Endocrinol.* 1996;134:337-341.
311. Lawrence JE, Lamm SH, Braverman LE. The use of perchlorate for the prevention of thyrotoxicosis in patients given iodine rich contrast agents. *J Endocrinol Invest.* 1999;22:405-407.
312. Martino E, Bartalena L, Bogazzi F, et al. The effects of amiodarone on the thyroid. *Endocr Rev.* 2001;22:240-254.
313. Smyrk TC, Goellner JR, Brennan MD, et al. Pathology of the thyroid in amiodarone-associated thyrotoxicosis. *Am J Surg Pathol.* 1987; 11:197-204.
314. Han TS, Williams GR, Vanderpump MP. Benzofuran derivatives and the thyroid. *Clin Endocrinol (Oxf).* 2009;70:2-13.
315. Melmed S, Nademanee K, Reed AW, et al. Hyperthyroxinemia with bradycardia and normal thyrotropin secretion after chronic amiodarone administration. *J Clin Endocrinol Metab.* 1981;53:997-1001.
316. Bedikian AY, Valdivieso M, Heilbrun LK, et al. Glycerol: an alternative to dexamethasone for patients receiving brain irradiation for metastatic disease. *South Med J.* 1980;73:1210-1214.
317. Berry MJ, Grieco D, Taylor BA, et al. Physiological and genetic analyses of inbred mouse strains with a type I iodothyronine 5′ deiodinase deficiency. *J Clin Invest.* 1993;92:1517-1528.
318. St. Germain DL, Hernandez A, Schneider MJ, et al. Insights into the role of deiodinases from studies of genetically modified animals. *Thyroid.* 2005;15:905-916.
319. Cohen-Lehman J, Dahl P, Danzi S, et al. Effects of amiodarone therapy on thyroid function. *Nat Rev Endocrinol.* 2010;6:34-41.
320. Eaton SE, Euinton HA, Newman CM, et al. Clinical experience of amiodarone-induced thyrotoxicosis over a 3-year period: role of colour-flow Doppler sonography. *Clin Endocrinol (Oxf).* 2002;56:33-38.
321. Osman F, Franklyn JA, Sheppard MC, et al. Successful treatment of amiodarone-induced thyrotoxicosis. *Circulation.* 2002;105:1275-1277.
322. Pearce EN, Farwell AP, Braverman LE. Thyroiditis. *N Engl J Med.* 2003;348:2646-2655.
323. Daniels GH. Amiodarone-induced thyrotoxicosis. *J Clin Endocrinol Metab.* 2001;86:3-8.
324. Ryan LE, Braverman LE, Cooper DS, et al. Can amiodarone be restarted after amiodarone-induced thyrotoxicosis? *Thyroid.* 2004;14:149-153.
325. Refetoff S, Weiss RE, Usala SJ. The syndromes of resistance to thyroid hormone. *Endocr Rev.* 1993;14:348-399.
326. Refetoff S, Weiss RE, Usala SJ, et al. The syndromes of resistance to thyroid hormone: update 1994. *Endocr Rev.* 1994;3:336-342.
327. Beck-Peccoz P, Mannavola D, Persani L. Syndromes of thyroid hormone resistance. *Ann Endocrinol (Paris).* 2005;66:264-269.
328. Hershman JM. Physiological and pathological aspects of the effect of human chorionic gonadotropin on the thyroid. *Best Pract Res Clin Endocrinol Metab.* 2004;18:249-265.
329. Grun JP, Meuris S, De Nayer P, et al. The thyrotrophic role of human chorionic gonadotrophin (hCG) in the early stages of twin (versus single) pregnancies. *Clin Endocrinol (Oxf).* 1997;46:719-725.
330. Goodwin TM, Montoro M, Mestman JH, et al. The role of chorionic gonadotropin in transient hyperthyroidism of hyperemesis gravidarum. *J Clin Endocrinol Metab.* 1992;75:1333-1337.
331. Rodien P, Bremont C, Sanson ML, et al. Familial gestational hyperthyroidism caused by a mutant thyrotropin receptor hypersensitive to human chorionic gonadotropin. *N Engl J Med.* 1998;339:1823-1826.
332. Pekary AE, Jackson IM, Goodwin TM, et al. Increased in vitro thyrotropic activity of partially sialated human chorionic gonadotropin extracted from hydatidiform moles of patients with hyperthyroidism. *J Clin Endocrinol Metab.* 1993;76:70-74.
333. Desai J, Yassa L, Marqusee E, et al. Hypothyroidism after sunitinib treatment for patients with gastrointestinal stromal tumors. *Ann Intern Med.* 2006;145:660-664.
334. Tachi J, Amino N, Tamaki H, et al. Long term followup and HLA association in patients with postpartum hyperthyroidism. *J Clin Endocrinol Metab.* 1988;66:480-484.
335. Sarvghadi F, Hedayati M, Mehrabi Y, et al. Follow up of patients with postpartum thyroiditis: a population-based study. *Endocrine.* 2005;27: 279-282.
336. Rosen IB, Strawbridge HG, Walfish PG, et al. Malignant pseudothyroiditis: a new clinical entity. *Am J Surg.* 1978;136:445-449.
337. Koh LK, Greenspan FS, Yeo PP. Interferon-alpha induced thyroid dysfunction: three clinical presentations and a review of the literature. *Thyroid.* 1997;7:891-896.
338. Doi F, Kakizaki S, Takagi H, et al. Long-term outcome of interferon-alpha-induced autoimmune thyroid disorders in chronic hepatitis C. *Liver Int.* 2005;25:242-246.
339. Miller KK, Daniels GH. Association between lithium use and thyrotoxicosis caused by silent thyroiditis. *Clin Endocrinol (Oxf).* 2001; 55:501-508.
340. Baethge C, Blumentritt H, Berghofer A, et al. Long-term lithium treatment and thyroid antibodies: a controlled study. *J Psychiatry Neurosci.* 2005;30:423-427.
341. de Groot JW, Zonnenberg BA, Plukker JT, et al. Imatinib induces hypothyroidism in patients receiving levothyroxine. *Clin Pharmacol Ther.* 2005;78:433-438.
342. Hedberg CW, Fishbein DB, Janssen RS, et al. An outbreak of thyrotoxicosis caused by the consumption of bovine thyroid gland in ground beef. *N Engl J Med.* 1987;316:993-998.
343. DeSimone CP, Lele SM, Modesitt SC. Malignant struma ovarii: a case report and analysis of cases reported in the literature with focus on survival and I131 therapy. *Gynecol Oncol.* 2003;89:543-548.
344. Dunzendorfer T, deLas Morenas A, Kalir T, et al. Struma ovarii and hyperthyroidism. *Thyroid.* 1999;9:499-502.
345. Giralt SA, Dexeus F, Amato R, et al. Hyperthyroidism in men with germ cell tumors and high levels of beta-human chorionic gonadotropin. *Cancer.* 1992;69:1286-1290.
346. Bayot MR, Chopra IJ. Coexistence of struma ovarii and Graves' disease. *Thyroid.* 1995;5:469-471.
347. Berghella V, Ngadiman S, Rosenberg H, et al. Malignant struma ovarii: a case report and review of the literature. *Gynecol Obstet Invest.* 1997;43:68-72.
348. Volpi E, Ferrero A, Nasi PG, et al. Malignant struma ovarii: a case report of laparoscopic management. *Gynecol Oncol.* 2003;90:191-194.
349. Als C, Gedeon P, Rosler H, et al. Survival analysis of 19 patients with toxic thyroid carcinoma. *J Clin Endocrinol Metab.* 2002;87:4122-4127.

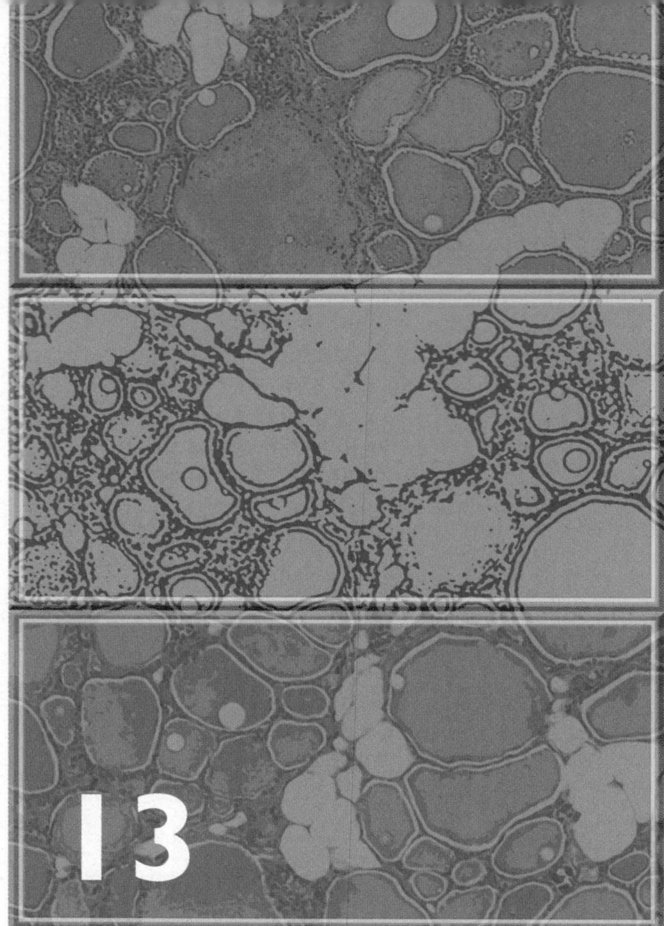

CHAPTER 13

Hypothyroidism and Thyroiditis

GREGORY A. BRENT • TERRY F. DAVIES

HYPOTHYROIDISM

Reduced production of thyroid hormone is the central feature of the clinical state termed *hypothyroidism*.[1,2] Permanent loss or destruction of the thyroid, through processes such as autoimmune destruction or irradiation injury, is described as *primary hypothyroidism* (Table 13-1). Hypothyroidism due to transient or progressive impairment of hormone biosynthesis is typically associated with compensatory thyroid enlargement. Central or secondary hypothyroidism, caused by insufficient stimulation of a normal gland, is the result of hypothalamic or pituitary disease or defects in the thyroid-stimulating hormone (TSH) molecule. Transient or temporary hypothyroidism can be observed as a phase of subacute thyroiditis. Primary hypothyroidism is the etiology in approximately 99% of cases of hypothyroidism. Central hypothyroidism is discussed in Chapters 7 and 9.

Reduced action of thyroid hormone at the tissue level in the face of normal or increased thyroid hormone production from the thyroid gland can also be associated with clinical hypothyroidism. Conditions associated with reduced thyroid hormone action are rare and include abnormalities of thyroid hormone metabolism and defects in nuclear signaling. Consumptive hypothyroidism, identified in an increasing number of clinical settings, is the result of accelerated inactivation of thyroid hormone by the type 3 iodothyronine deiodinase (D3). Defects of activation of the prohormone, thyroxine (T_4), to the active form, triiodothyronine (T_3), have also been identified. Polymorphisms in genes regulating thyroid hormone production and activation may influence thyroid hormone action in some tissues.[3] Resistance to thyroid hormone (RTH), the result of defects in the thyroid hormone nuclear receptor or nuclear cofactors, is associated with elevated circulating levels of thyroid hormone (see later discussion). Some tissues, depending on the level of expression of the mutant receptor and other forms of local compensation, have evidence of reduced thyroid hormone action.

Estimates of the incidence of hypothyroidism vary depending on the population studied.[4,5] In the United States, 0.3% of the population have overt hypothyroidism, defined as an elevated serum TSH concentration and reduced free thyroxine concentration (fT_4), and 4.3% have what has been described as subclinical or mild hypothyroidism.[5] Although a number of clinical manifestations have been associated with this early or mild phase of hypothyroidism, the term *subclinical* is used here to describe this group, as in most clinical studies. Subclinical hypothyroidism is defined as an elevated serum TSH level with a normal serum fT_4 concentration.[6] Subclinical hypothyroidism can progress to overt hypothyroidism,[7] and it can be associated

TABLE 13-1

Causes of Hypothyroidism

Primary Hypothyroidism
Acquired
Hashimoto's thyroiditis
Iodine deficiency (endemic goiter)
Drugs blocking synthesis or release of T_4 (e.g., lithium, ethionamide, sulfonamides, iodide)
Goitrogens in foodstuffs or as endemic substances or pollutants
Cytokines (interferon-γ, interleukin-2)
Thyroid infiltration (amyloidosis, hemochromatosis, sarcoidosis, Riedel's struma, cystinosis, scleroderma)
Postablative thyroiditis due to ^{131}I surgery or therapeutic irradiation for nonthyroidal malignancy
Congenital
Iodide transport or utilization defect (NIS or pendrin mutations)
Iodotyrosine dehalogenase deficiency
Organification disorders (TPO deficiency or dysfunction)
Defects in thyroglobulin synthesis or processing
Thyroid agenesis or dysplasia
TSH receptor defects
Thyroidal G_s protein abnormalities (pseudohypoparathyroidism type 1a)
Idiopathic TSH unresponsiveness
Transient (Post-Thyroiditis) Hypothyroidism
Following subacute, painless, or postpartum thyroiditis
Consumptive Hypothyroidism
Rapid destruction of thyroid hormone due to D3 expression in large hemangiomas or hemangioendotheliomas
Defects of Thyroxine-to-Triiodothyronine Conversion
Selenocysteine insertion sequence–binding protein 2 (SBP2) defect
Drug-Induced Thyroid Destruction
Tyrosine kinase inhibitor (e.g., sunitinib)
Central Hypothyroidism
Acquired
Pituitary origin (secondary)
Hypothalamic disorders (tertiary)
Bexarotene (retinoid X receptor agonist)
Dopamine and/or severe illness
Congenital
TSH deficiency or structural abnormality
TSH receptor defect
Resistance to Thyroid Hormone
Generalized
"Pituitary" dominant

D3, type 3 deiodinase; G_s, stimulatory G protein; NIS, sodium-iodide symporter; TPO, thyroid peroxidase; TSH, thyroid-stimulating hormone.

with manifestations that, in some patients, can be improved with treatment.[6-9] The incidence of hypothyroidism is higher among women, the elderly, and in some racial and ethnic groups.[5] Neonatal screening programs identify hypothyroidism (almost all primary cases) in almost 1 of every 3500 newborns.[10]

CLINICAL PRESENTATION

Hypothyroidism can affect all organ systems. These manifestations are largely independent of the underlying disorder but are a function of the degree of hormone deficiency. The following sections discuss the pathophysiology of each organ system at various levels of thyroid hormone deficiency, from mild to severe. The term *myxedema,* formerly used as a synonym for hypothyroidism, refers to the appearance of the skin and subcutaneous tissues in the patient who is in a severely hypothyroid state (Fig. 13-1). Hypothyroidism of this severity is rarely seen today, and the term should be reserved for description of the physical signs.

Skin and Appendages

Hypothyroidism causes an accumulation of hyaluronic acid that alters the composition of the ground substance in the dermis and other tissues.[11] This material is hygroscopic, producing the mucinous edema that is responsible for the thickened features and puffy appearance (myxedema) observed in patients with full-blown hypothyroidism. Myxedematous tissue is characteristically boggy and nonpitting and is apparent around the eyes, on the dorsa of the hands and feet, and in the supraclavicular fossae (see Fig. 13-1). It causes enlargement of the tongue and thickening of the pharyngeal and laryngeal mucous membranes.

A histologically similar deposit may occur in patients with Graves' disease, usually over the pretibial area (infiltrative dermopathy or pretibial myxedema). In addition to having a puffy appearance, the skin is pale and cool as a result of cutaneous vasoconstriction. Anemia may contribute to the pallor; hypercarotenemia gives the skin a yellow tint but does not cause scleral icterus (see Fig. 13-1). The secretions of the sweat glands and sebaceous glands are reduced, leading to dryness and coarseness of the skin, which in extreme cases may resemble that observed in patients with ichthyosis.

Wounds of the skin tend to heal slowly. Easy bruising occurs because of an increase in capillary fragility. Head and body hair is dry and brittle, lacks luster, and tends to fall out. Hair may be lost from the temporal aspects of the eyebrows, although this feature is not specific for hypothyroidism (see Fig. 13-1B). Growth of hair is retarded, so that haircuts and shaves are required less often. The nails are brittle and grow slowly. Topical T_3 has been shown to accelerate wound healing and stimulate hair growth in a euthyroid mouse model, demonstrating a role for thyroid hormone in these processes.[12]

Histopathologic examination of the skin reveals hyperkeratosis with plugging of hair follicles and sweat glands. The dermis is edematous, and the connective tissue fibers are separated by an increased amount of metachromatically staining, periodic acid–Schiff (PAS)-positive mucinous material. This material consists of protein complexed with two mucopolysaccharides: hyaluronic acid and chondroitin sulfate B. The hygroscopic glycosaminoglycans are mobilized early during treatment with thyroid hormone, leading to an increase in urinary excretion of nitrogen and hexosamine as well as tissue water.[11]

Patients with hypothyroidism due to Hashimoto's thyroiditis may also have skin lesions with loss of pigmentation characteristic of the autoimmune skin condition called *vitiligo*. This is not a manifestation of reduced thyroid hormone action but reflects the common association of autoimmune endocrine disease and this skin condition, which is recognized as a component of autoimmune polyendocrine syndromes.[13]

Cardiovascular System

The cardiac output at rest is decreased because of reduction in both stroke volume and heart rate, reflecting loss of the

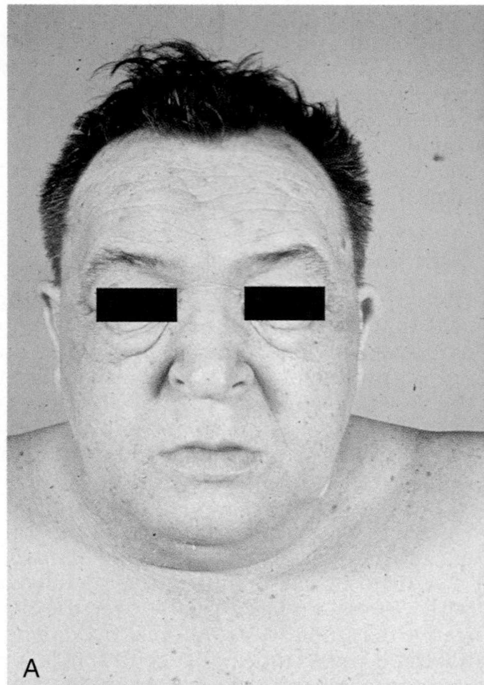

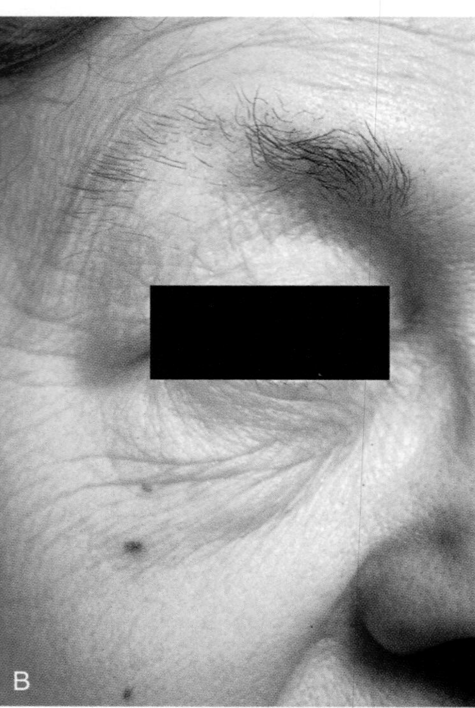

Figure 13-1 **A** and **B,** Typical appearance of patients with moderately severe primary hypothyroidism or myxedema. Notice the dry skin and sallow complexion; absence of scleral pigmentation differentiates the carotenemia from jaundice. Both individuals demonstrate periorbital myxedema. The patient in **B** illustrates the loss of the lateral aspect of the eyebrow, sometimes termed *Queen Anne's sign.* That finding is not unusual in the age group that is commonly affected by severe hypothyroidism and should not be considered to be a specific sign of the condition.

inotropic and chronotropic effects of thyroid hormones. Peripheral vascular resistance at rest is increased, and blood volume is reduced. These hemodynamic alterations cause narrowing of pulse pressure, prolongation of circulation time, and decrease in blood flow to the tissues.[14-17] The reduction in cutaneous circulation is responsible for the coolness and pallor of the skin and the sensitivity to cold. In most tissues, the decrease in blood flow is proportional to the decrease in oxygen consumption, so the arteriovenous oxygen difference remains normal. The hemodynamic alterations at rest resemble those of congestive heart failure. However, in hypothyroidism, cardiac output increases and peripheral vascular resistance decreases normally in response to exercise, unless the hypothyroid state is severe and of long standing.

In severe primary hypothyroidism, the cardiac silhouette is enlarged (Fig. 13-2), and the heart sounds are diminished in intensity.[18] These findings are largely the result of the effusion into the pericardial sac of fluid rich in protein and glycosaminoglycans, but the myocardium may also be dilated. Pericardial effusion is rarely of sufficient magnitude to cause tamponade.

Angina pectoris may first appear or worsen during treatment of the hypothyroid state with thyroid hormone, although most patients with hypothyroidism and coronary artery disease have no change, or improvement, in anginal symptoms with T_4 treatment.[19] Electrocardiographic changes include sinus bradycardia, prolongation of the PR interval, low amplitude of the P wave and QRS complex, alterations of the ST segment, and flattened or inverted T waves. Pericardial effusion is probably responsible for the low amplitude in severe hypothyroidism. Systolic time intervals are altered; the preejection period is prolonged, and the ratio of preejection period to left ventricular ejection time is increased. Echocardiographic studies have revealed resting left ventricular diastolic dysfunction in overt hypothyroidism and, in some studies, subclinical hypothyroidism.[17] These findings normalize when the hypothyroidism is treated.

Serum levels of homocysteine, creatine kinase, aspartate aminotransferase, and lactate dehydrogenase may be increased in hypothyroidism.[14,20] Typically, the isoenzyme patterns suggest that the source of the increased creatine kinase and lactate dehydrogenase is skeletal muscle, not cardiac muscle. All levels return to normal with therapy. Sequential cardiac biopsies in a hypothyroid patient with heart failure showed that messenger RNA (mRNA) levels from genes regulated by thyroid hormone that are important for the strength of myocardial contraction were normalized after T_4 treatment.[21]

The combination of large heart, hemodynamic and electrocardiographic alterations, and the described serum enzyme changes has been termed *myxedema heart*. In the absence of coexisting organic heart disease, treatment with thyroid hormone corrects the hemodynamic, electrocardiographic, and serum enzyme alterations of myxedema heart and restores heart size to normal (see Fig. 13-2).

Hypothyroidism is consistently associated with elevations of total and low-density lipoprotein (LDL) cholesterol, which improve with T_4 replacement.[22] In a study of a cohort from the Framingham population with short-term hypothyroidism, serum TSH in women was positively correlated with total cholesterol and LDL, but the elevation was from the less atherogenic large LDL particles.[23] The higher the original serum TSH concentration and elevation of serum LDL, the greater the magnitude of reduction in LDL cholesterol after T_4 therapy. A subset of younger (<50 years) male hypothyroid patients have elevated

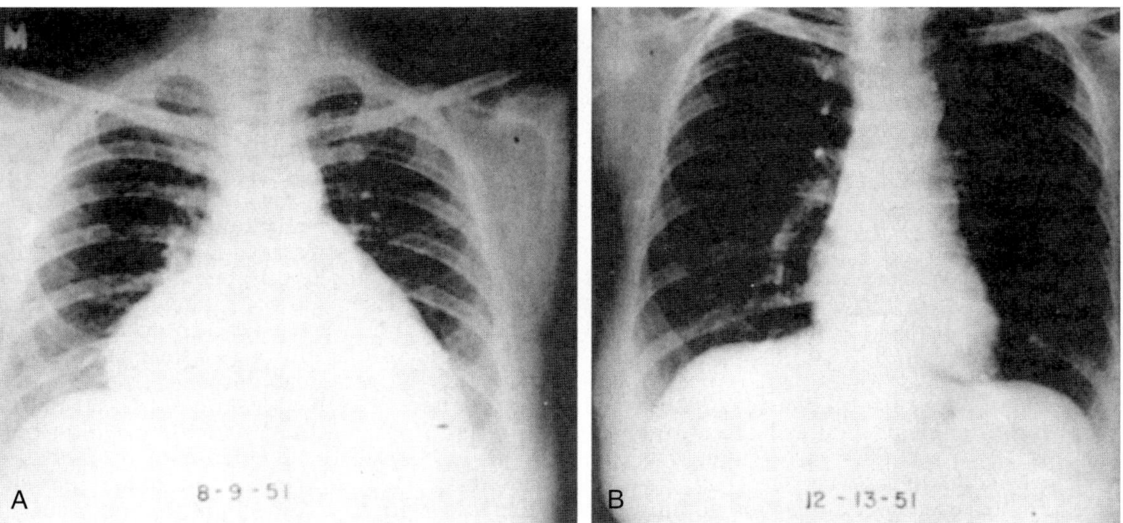

Figure 13-2 **A** and **B,** Chest roentgenograms in a patient with myxedema heart disease. The patient had signs of severe congestive heart failure and was given thyroid hormone alone. Within 4 months, the heart had returned to normal size **(B)**, and there was no evidence of underlying heart disease.

concentrations of serum triglycerides and C-reactive protein that improve with T_4 treatment.[24] Most studies have shown that serum high-density lipoprotein (HDL) levels are not influenced by thyroid status.

Hypothyroidism has been shown to be a risk factor for atherosclerosis and cardiovascular disease in several studies, although others have not shown this association. A prospective study from Japan showed an increased risk of ischemic heart disease in men, but not in women, with subclinical hypothyroidism.[25] The Whickham study showed no increase in cardiovascular mortality among patients with subclinical hypothyroidism who were followed up for more than 20 years.[4] A prospective study in the United States that monitored men and women age 65 or older for more than 10 years showed no influence of hypothyroidism (overt or subclinical) on cardiovascular outcome or mortality.[26] Cardiovascular outcome studies suggest that improvement from treatment of hypothyroidism, especially subclinical hypothyroidism, occurs primarily among those patients who are in middle age and not in older individuals (>65 years of age).[22]

Respiratory System

Pleural effusions usually are evident only on radiologic examination, but in rare instances they may cause dyspnea. Lung volumes are usually normal, but maximal breathing capacity and diffusing capacity are reduced. In severe hypothyroidism, myxedematous involvement of respiratory muscles and depression of both the hypoxic and the hypercapnic ventilatory drives can cause alveolar hypoventilation and carbon dioxide retention, which in turn can contribute to the development of myxedema coma. Obstructive sleep apnea is common but is reversible with restoration of a euthyroid state.

Alimentary System

Although most patients experience a modest gain in weight, appetite is usually reduced. The weight gain that occurs is caused partly by retention of fluid by the hydrophilic glycoprotein deposits in the tissues and does not exceed 10% of body weight. Peristaltic activity is decreased and, together with the decreased food intake, is responsible for the frequent complaint of constipation. The latter may lead to fecal impaction (myxedema megacolon). Gaseous distention of the abdomen (myxedema ileus), if accompanied by colicky pain and vomiting, can mimic mechanical ileus.[27]

Elevations in the serum level of carcinoembryonic antigen, which may occur on the basis of hypothyroidism alone, add to the impression that an obstruction is present. Ascites in the absence of another cause is unusual in hypothyroidism, but it can occur, usually in association with pleural and pericardial effusions. Like pericardial and pleural effusions, the ascitic fluid is rich in protein and glycosaminoglycans.

Achlorhydria after maximal histamine stimulation may be present in patients with primary hypothyroidism. Circulating antibodies against gastric parietal cells have been found in about one third of patients with primary hypothyroidism and may be secondary to atrophy of the gastric mucosa. Hypothyroid patients with positive parietal cell antibodies have a higher T_4 requirement compared with antibody-negative patients.[28] Among Swedish patients with celiac disease, there was a 4.4-fold increased risk for hypothyroidism, compared to the general population.[29] Overt pernicious anemia is reported in about 12% of patients with primary hypothyroidism. The coexistence of pernicious anemia and other autoimmune diseases with primary hypothyroidism reflects the fact that autoimmunity plays the central role in the pathogenesis of these diseases (see Chapter 42).

Hypothyroidism has complex effects on intestinal absorption. Although the rates of absorption for many substances are decreased, the total amount absorbed may be normal or even increased because the decreased bowel motility allows more time for absorption. Malabsorption is occasionally overt.

Liver function test results are usually normal, but levels of aminotransaminases may be elevated, probably because of impaired clearance.[30] The gallbladder contracts sluggishly and may be distended. In a population study of patients without diagnosed thyroid disease, men, but not women, with an elevated TSH had a 3.8-fold increased risk of cholelithiasis.[31]

Atrophy of the gastric and intestinal mucosa and myxedematous infiltration of the bowel wall may be demonstrated on histologic examination. The colon may be greatly distended, and the volume of fluid in the peritoneal cavity is usually increased. The liver and pancreas are normal.

Central and Peripheral Nervous Systems

Thyroid hormone is essential for the development of the central nervous system.[10,32] Deficiency in fetal life or at birth leads to impaired neurologic development, including hypoplasia of cortical neurons with poor development of cellular processes, retarded myelination, and reduced vascularity.[10,29] If the deficiency is not corrected in early postnatal life, the damage is irreversible. Deficiency of thyroid hormone beginning in adult life causes less severe manifestations that usually respond to treatment with the hormone. Cerebral blood flow is reduced, but cerebral oxygen consumption is usually normal; this finding is in accord with the conclusion that the oxygen consumption of isolated brain tissue in vitro, unlike that of most other tissues, is not stimulated by administration of thyroid hormones. In severe cases, decreased cerebral blood flow may lead to cerebral hypoxia.

All intellectual functions, including speech, are slowed in thyroid hormone deficiency.[33] Loss of initiative is present, and memory defects are common; lethargy and somnolence are prominent, and dementia in elderly patients may be mistaken for senile dementia. Positron emission tomography (PET) brain scans of hypothyroid patients before and after T_4 therapy demonstrate reversible reduced glucose uptake in specific brain areas, such as the limbic system, which also correlates with behavioral and psychiatric symptoms.[34] Psychiatric disorders are common and are usually of the paranoid or depressive type and may induce agitation (myxedema madness).[33] Headaches are frequent. Cerebral hypoxia due to circulatory alterations may predispose to confusional attacks and syncope, which may be prolonged and can lead to stupor or coma. Other factors predisposing to coma in hypothyroidism include exposure to severe cold, infection, trauma, hypoventilation with carbon dioxide retention, and depressant drugs.

Epileptic seizures have been reported and tend to occur in myxedema coma. Night blindness is caused by deficient synthesis of the pigment required for dark adaptation. Hearing loss of the perceptive type is frequent due to myxedema of the eighth cranial nerve and serous otitis media. Perceptive deafness may also occur in association with a defect in the organic binding of thyroidal iodide (Pendred's syndrome) (see Chapter 11), but in these instances it is not a result of hypothyroidism per se.

Thick, slurred speech and hoarseness are caused by myxedematous infiltration of the tongue and larynx, respectively. Body movements are slow and clumsy, and cerebellar ataxia may occur. Numbness and tingling of the extremities are frequent; in the fingers, these symptoms may be caused by compression from glycosaminoglycan deposits in and around the median nerve in the carpal tunnel (carpal tunnel syndrome).[35] The tendon reflexes are slow, especially during the relaxation phase, producing the characteristic "hung-up reflexes"; this phenomenon is caused by a decrease in the rate of muscle contraction and relaxation rather than a delay in nerve conduction.

The presence of extensor plantar responses or diminished vibration sense should alert the physician to the possibility of coexisting pernicious anemia with combined systemic disease. Electroencephalographic changes include slow alpha-wave activity and general loss of amplitude. The concentration of protein in the cerebrospinal fluid is often increased, but cerebrospinal pressure is normal.

Histopathologic examination of the brain in patients with untreated hypothyroidism reveals that the nervous system is edematous with mucinous deposits in and around nerve fibers. In patients with cerebellar ataxia, neural myxedematous infiltrates of glycogen and mucinous material are present in the cerebellum. There may be foci of degeneration and an increase in glial tissue. The cerebral vessels may show atherosclerosis, but this is much more common if the patient has had coexistent hypertension.

Hypothyroidism has been associated with several neurologic conditions, although a strong etiologic link has not been established. Epidemiologic studies have shown an association between Alzheimer's disease and hypothyroidism.[36] It is difficult to convincingly demonstrate this association, because the incidence of thyroid disease in the elderly population is high and, like that of dementia, increases with age. A mechanistic link is suggested by the observation of amyloid deposition in Down syndrome, a condition that is associated with an increased incidence of Hashimoto's disease, and the fact that thyroid hormone regulates amyloid gene processing in a number of cellular and animal models. However, subclinical hyperthyroidism has also been associated with Alzheimer's disease.[37] There is an increase in the cerebrospinal fluid concentration of reverse T_3 in Alzheimer's disease patients who have normal circulating thyroid hormone levels, suggesting the potential for altered thyroid hormone metabolism in the brain.[38] However, the impact of normalizing T_3 levels in the brain is not known. A corticosteroid-responsive encephalopathy is associated with chronic Hashimoto's thyroiditis but may be linked to autoimmunity rather than a process mediated specifically by low thyroid hormone levels or thyroid autoantibodies.[39]

Muscular System

Stiffness and aching of muscles are common and are worsened by cold temperatures. Delayed muscle contraction and relaxation cause the slowness of movement and delayed tendon jerks. Muscle mass may be reduced or enlarged due to interstitial myxedema. Muscle mass may be slightly increased, and the muscles tend to be firm. Rarely, a profound increase in muscle mass with slowness of muscular activity may be the predominant manifestation (*Kocher-Debré-Sémélaigne syndrome* or *Hoffmann syndrome*). Myoclonus may be present. The electromyogram may be normal, or it may exhibit disordered discharge, hyperirritability, and polyphasic action potentials.

On histopathologic examination, the muscles appear pale and swollen. The muscle fibers may show swelling, loss of normal striations, and separation by mucinous deposits. Type I muscle fibers tend to predominate.

Skeletal System: Calcium and Phosphorus Metabolism

Thyroid hormone is essential for normal growth and maturation of the skeleton. Growth failure in thyroid deficiency is caused by impaired general protein synthesis, reduced growth hormone, and especially reduced insulin-like growth factor 1 (Fig. 13-3).[40] The thyroid hormone receptor isoforms α and β have specific roles in bone maturation. Before puberty, thyroid hormone plays a major role in the maturation of bone. Deficiency of thyroid hormone in early life leads to both a delay in development and an abnormal,

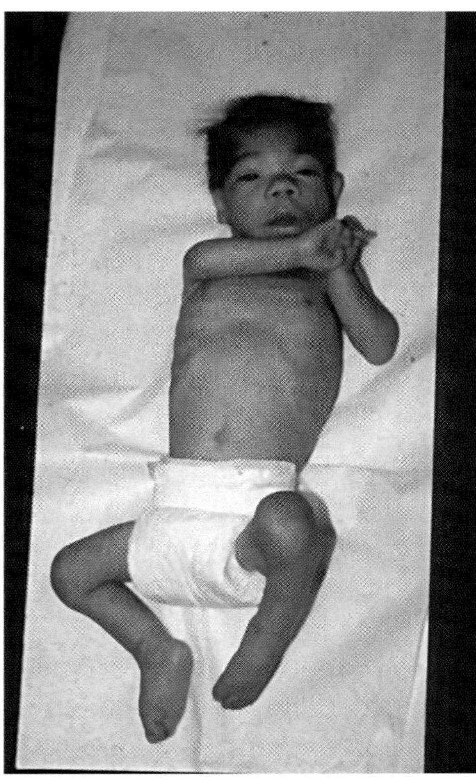

Figure 13-3 The consequences of untreated congenital hypothyroidism are demonstrated in this 17-year-old girl. Her condition was diagnosed at birth but, through a series of misunderstandings, was not treated with thyroid hormone. Notice her size, the poorly developed nasal bridge, the wide-set eyes, and the ears, which are larger than are appropriate for head size. Her tongue is enlarged, and her extremities are inappropriately short in relation to her trunk. (Courtesy of Dr. Ronald B. Stein.)

stippled appearance of the epiphyseal centers of ossification (epiphyseal dysgenesis) (Fig. 13-4). Impairment of linear growth leads to dwarfism in which the limbs are disproportionately short in relation to the trunk but cartilage growth is unaffected (see Fig. 13-3). Children with prolonged hypothyroidism, even after adequate treatment, do not reach predicted height based on midparental height calculations.[41]

Urinary excretion of calcium is decreased, as is the glomerular filtration rate, whereas fecal excretion of calcium and urinary and fecal excretion of phosphorus are variable. Calcium balance is also variable, and any changes are slight. The exchangeable pool of calcium and its rate of turnover are reduced, reflecting decreased bone formation and resorption. Because levels of parathyroid hormone are often slightly increased, some degree of resistance to its action may be present; levels of $1,25(OH)_2D$ (dihydroxyvitamin D) are also increased.

Levels of calcium and phosphorus in serum are usually normal, but calcium may be slightly elevated. The alkaline phosphatase level is usually below normal in infantile and juvenile hypothyroidism. Bone density may be increased. The radiologic appearance of the skeleton in cretinism and juvenile hypothyroidism are discussed later.

Renal Function: Water and Electrolyte Metabolism

Renal blood flow, glomerular filtration rate, and tubular reabsorptive and secretory maxima are reduced. Blood urea nitrogen and serum creatinine levels are normal, but uric acid levels may be increased. Urine flow is reduced, and delay in the excretion of a water load may result in reversal of the normal diurnal pattern of urine excretion. The delay in water excretion appears to be due to decreased volume delivery to the distal diluting segment of the nephron as a result of the diminished renal perfusion; evidence supporting inappropriate secretion of vasopressin (syndrome of inappropriate antidiuretic hormone secretion) is less compelling.[42] These changes are reversed by treatment with

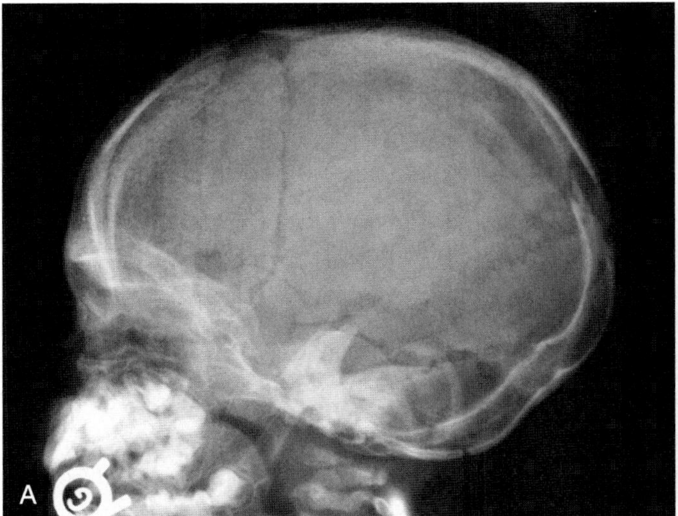

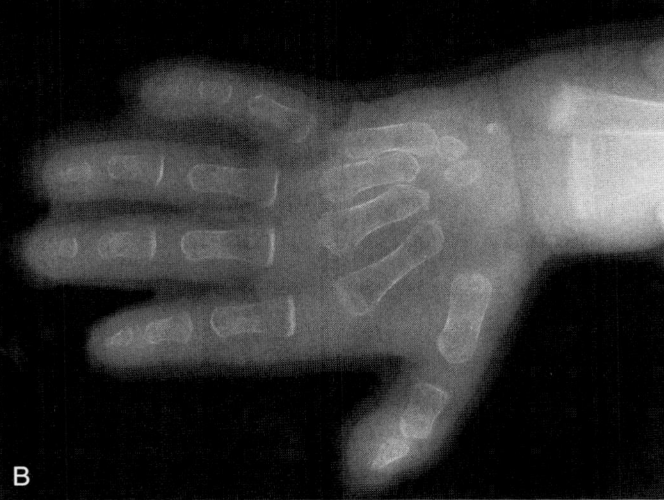

Figure 13-4 X-ray films of the skull and hand of the 17-year-old patient illustrated in Figure 13-3. **A,** Skull film showing that the posterior and anterior fontanelles are open and that the sutures are not fused. The deciduous and permanent teeth are present. **B,** Radiograph of the wrist and hand showing the delayed appearance of the epiphyseal centers of the bones of the hand and the absence of the distal radial epiphysis. The estimated bone age is 9 months. (Courtesy of Dr. Ronald B. Stein.)

thyroid hormone. The ability to concentrate urine may be slightly impaired. Mild proteinuria may occur.

The impaired renal excretion of water and the retention of water by the hydrophilic deposits in the tissues result in an increase in total body water, even though plasma volume is reduced. This increase accounts for the hyponatremia in some patients, because the level of exchangeable sodium is increased. The amount of exchangeable potassium is usually normal in relation to lean body mass. Serum magnesium concentration may be increased, but exchangeable magnesium levels and urinary magnesium excretion are decreased.

Hematopoietic System

In response to the diminished oxygen requirements and decreased production of erythropoietin, the red blood cell mass is decreased; this is evident in the mild normocytic, normochromic anemia that often occurs. Less commonly, the anemia is macrocytic, sometimes from deficiency of vitamin B_{12}. Reference has already been made to the high incidence of pernicious anemia (and of achlorhydria and vitamin B_{12} deficiency without overt anemia) in primary hypothyroidism (see Chapter 42). Conversely, overt and subclinical hypothyroidism is present in 12% and 15% of patients, respectively, with pernicious anemia. Folate deficiency from malabsorption or dietary inadequacy may also cause macrocytic anemia. The frequent menorrhagia and the defective absorption of iron resulting from achlorhydria may contribute to a microcytic, hypochromic anemia.

The total and differential white blood cell counts are usually normal, and platelets are adequate, although platelet adhesiveness may be impaired. If pernicious anemia or significant folate deficiency is present, the characteristic changes in peripheral blood and bone marrow will be found. The intrinsic clotting mechanism may be defective because of decreased concentrations in plasma of factors VIII and IX, and this, together with an increase in capillary fragility and the decrease in platelet adhesiveness, may account for the bleeding tendency that sometimes occurs.[27,43]

Pituitary and Adrenocortical Function

In long-standing primary hypothyroidism, hyperplasia of the thyrotropes may cause the pituitary gland to be enlarged. This feature can be detected radiologically as an increase in the volume of the pituitary fossa.[44] Rarely, the pituitary enlargement compromises the function of other pituitary cells and causes pituitary insufficiency or visual field defects. Patients with severe hypothyroidism may have increased serum prolactin levels, stimulated by the elevation in thyrotropin-releasing hormone (TRH) and proportional to the level of serum TSH elevation, and galactorrhea may develop in some patients. Treatment with thyroid hormone normalizes the serum prolactin and TSH levels and causes disappearance of galactorrhea, if present.

In rodents, thyroid hormone directly regulates growth hormone synthesis. Growth hormone is not directly regulated by thyroid hormone in humans, but thyroid status influences the growth hormone axis.[45] Hypothyroid children have delayed growth, and the response of growth hormone to provocative stimuli may be subnormal.

As a result of the decreased rate of turnover of cortisol due to decreased hepatic 11β-hydroxysteroid dehydrogenase type 1 (HSD11B1), the 24-hour urinary excretion of cortisol and 17-hydroxycorticosteroids is decreased, but the plasma cortisol level is usually normal (see Chapter 15). The response of urinary 17-hydroxycorticosteroid to exogenous adrenocorticotropic hormone is usually normal but may be decreased. The response of plasma cortisol to insulin-induced hypoglycemia may be impaired.

In severe, long-standing primary hypothyroidism, pituitary and adrenal function may be secondarily decreased, and adrenal insufficiency may be precipitated by stress or by rapid replacement therapy with thyroid hormone.[45] The rate of turnover of aldosterone is decreased, but the plasma level is normal. Plasma renin activity is decreased, and sensitivity to angiotensin II is increased, which may contribute to the association of hypertension with hypothyroidism (see Chapter 16).[46]

Reproductive Function

In both sexes, thyroid hormones influence sexual development and reproductive function.[47] Infantile hypothyroidism, if untreated, leads to sexual immaturity, and juvenile hypothyroidism causes a delay in the onset of puberty followed by anovulatory cycles. Paradoxically, primary hypothyroidism may also rarely cause precocious sexual development and galactorrhea, presumably due to "spill-over" of elevated TSH stimulating the luteinizing hormone (LH) receptor[48] and elevated TRH initiating excess prolactin release.

In adult women, severe hypothyroidism may be associated with diminished libido and failure of ovulation. Secretion of progesterone is inadequate, and endometrial proliferation persists, resulting in excessive and irregular breakthrough menstrual bleeding. These changes may be due to deficient secretion of LH or pulse frequency and amplitude, or both. Rarely, in primary hypothyroidism, secondary depression of pituitary function may lead to ovarian atrophy and amenorrhea. Fertility is reduced, and there is an increase in spontaneous abortion and preterm delivery, although many pregnancies are successful.[49] Pregnancy complications are associated with both overt and subclinical hypothyroidism, although the impact has varied among different studies.[50] A randomized prospective study of levothyroxine treatment in pregnant women with thyroid peroxidase (TPO) antibody positivity and normal-range TSH showed that the increased incidences of preterm delivery and spontaneous abortion were reversed by treatment, although this finding remains to be confirmed.[51] Primary ovarian failure can also be seen in patients with Hashimoto's thyroiditis as part of an autoimmune polyendocrine syndrome.[13] Hypothyroidism in men may cause diminished libido, erectile dysfunction, and oligospermia. A significant fraction of men with hypothyroidism or hyperthyroidism have moderate to severe erectile dysfunction that improves with treatment of the thyroid disease.[52]

Values for plasma gonadotropins are usually in the normal range in primary hypothyroidism. Among postmenopausal women, levels are usually somewhat lower than in euthyroid women of the same age but are nevertheless within the menopausal range. This provides a valuable means of differentiating primary from secondary hypothyroidism.

The metabolism of both androgens and estrogens is altered in hypothyroidism. Secretion of androgens is decreased, and the metabolism of testosterone is shifted toward etiocholanolone rather than androsterone. With respect to estradiol and estrone, hypothyroidism favors metabolism of these steroids via 16α-hydroxylation rather than 2-oxygenation, with the result that formation of estriol is increased and that of 2-hydroxyestrone and its derivative, 2-methoxyestrone, is decreased. The sex hormone–binding globulin in plasma is decreased, with the result that plasma concentrations of both testosterone and estradiol are decreased, but the unbound fractions are increased. The alterations in steroid metabolism are corrected by restoration of the euthyroid state.[53]

Catecholamines

The plasma cyclic adenosine monophosphate (cAMP) response to epinephrine is decreased in hypothyroidism, suggesting a state of decreased adrenergic responsiveness. The fact that the responses of plasma cAMP to glucagon and parathyroid hormone are also decreased suggests that thyroid hormones have a general modulating influence on cAMP generation.[54] The reduced adrenergic responsiveness associated with hypothyroidism has been linked to all steps of catecholamine signaling, including receptor and postreceptor actions, resulting in an impaired cAMP response. Direct measurement of norepinephrine in abdominal fat of hypothyroid patients shows reduced levels, and there is reduced production of glycerol in response to adrenergic agonist stimulation.[55] Augmentation of α_2-receptor signaling has also been proposed as a factor reducing catecholamine responsiveness.

Energy Metabolism: Protein, Carbohydrate, and Lipid Metabolism

The decrease in energy metabolism and heat production is reflected in the low basal metabolic rate, decreased appetite, cold intolerance, and slightly low basal body temperature.[56] Both the synthesis and the degradation of protein are decreased, the latter especially so, with the result that nitrogen balance is usually slightly positive. The decrease in protein synthesis is reflected in retardation of both skeletal and soft tissue growth.

Permeability of capillaries to protein is increased, accounting for the high levels of protein in effusions and in cerebrospinal fluid. In addition, the albumin pool is increased because of the greater decrease in albumin degradation compared with albumin synthesis. A greater than normal fraction of exchangeable albumin is in the extravascular space. The total concentration of serum proteins may be increased.

Hypothyroidism is associated with a reduction in the disposition of glucose to skeletal muscle and adipose tissue.[57] Thyroid hormone has been shown to stimulate expression of the insulin-sensitive glucose transporter (GLUT4), and the levels of this transporter are reduced in hypothyroidism. However, hypothyroidism is also associated with reduced gluconeogenesis, and the net effect of these influences is usually a minimal effect of hypothyroidism on serum glucose levels. Thyroid hormone downregulates expression of prohormone processing enzymes, which, therefore, have increased activity in hypothyroidism. Degradation of insulin is slowed, and the sensitivity to exogenous insulin may be increased. In a patient with preexisting diabetes mellitus who develops hypothyroidism, insulin requirements may be reduced. A further influence on glucose uptake may occur at the tissue level. Polymorphisms in the 5′-deiodinase type 2 (D2) gene, which may affect local T_3 production, have shown to be associated with impaired glucose disposal.[58]

Both the synthesis and the degradation of lipid are depressed in hypothyroidism. However, degradation is reduced to a greater extent, with a net effect of accumulation of LDL and triglycerides.[56] The decrease in the lipid degradation rate may reflect the decrease in postheparin lipolytic activity as well as reduced LDL receptors. Plasma free fatty acid levels are decreased, and the mobilization of free fatty acids in response to fasting, catecholamines, and growth hormone is impaired. Impaired lipolysis of white fat in hypothyroid patients at baseline and in response to catecholamine reflects impaired free fatty acid mobilization.[54,55] All of these abnormalities are relieved by treatment.

A correlation was shown between total cholesterol and serum TSH levels in hypothyroid individuals identified from among 25,862 participants in a health fair, including those not aware of being hypothyroid and those on T_4 replacement.[59] An elevation in serum LDL-cholesterol has been associated, in most studies, with overt and subclinical hypothyroidism.[22] According to most studies, serum HDL and triglycerides levels are not influenced by hypothyroidism.[22,56] The reduction in LDL with T_4 therapy is generally related to the original magnitude of LDL and TSH elevation: the higher the initial levels, the greater the observed reduction in LDL.[22] A typical reduction in LDL is 5% to 10% of the original level.

The role of adipocytokines such as leptin, adiponectin, and resistin in metabolic regulation has been increasingly recognized, as well as their potential for interaction with thyroid hormone.[56] Rodent studies have shown that leptin regulates central adaptation between the starved and fed state, and that falling leptin levels, associated with starvation, lead to a suppression of the thyroid axis. Hypothyroidism in rodents is associated with reduced leptin and increased resistin levels. Leptin infusion into the cerebral ventricles reverses some of the metabolic changes seen with hypothyroidism, improving glucose disposal and reducing skeletal muscle fat.[60] However, human studies have not shown consistent changes in adipocytokines in hypothyroidism.[61]

CURRENT CLINICAL PICTURE

In adults, the onset of hypothyroidism is usually so insidious that the typical manifestations may take months or years to appear and may go unnoticed by family and friends. The gradual development of the hypothyroid state is the result of slow progression of thyroid hypofunction and of the clinical manifestations after thyroid failure is complete. This course is in contrast with the more rapid development of the hypothyroid state when replacement therapy is discontinued in a patient with treated primary hypothyroidism or when the thyroid gland of a normal subject is surgically removed. In such patients, manifestations of frank hypothyroidism are usually present by 6 weeks, and myxedema appears by 3 months.

Hypothyroidism continues to be diagnosed at earlier stages. Based on the most recent data, subclinical or early hypothyroidism is seen approximately 14 times more commonly than overt hypothyroidism. Scales for assessment of clinical symptoms that suggest hypothyroidism have been developed, reflecting the more typical earlier identification (Fig. 13-5).[62] Early symptoms are variable and relatively nonspecific. The reason for the increased prevalence of hypothyroid patients presenting with minimal symptoms is largely the availability of sensitive and specific laboratory tests that allow recognition of the primary form of the disease long before severe symptoms have developed. Therefore, there should be a low threshold to test patients for suspected primary hypothyroidism with a serum TSH determination. Patients with significant biochemical

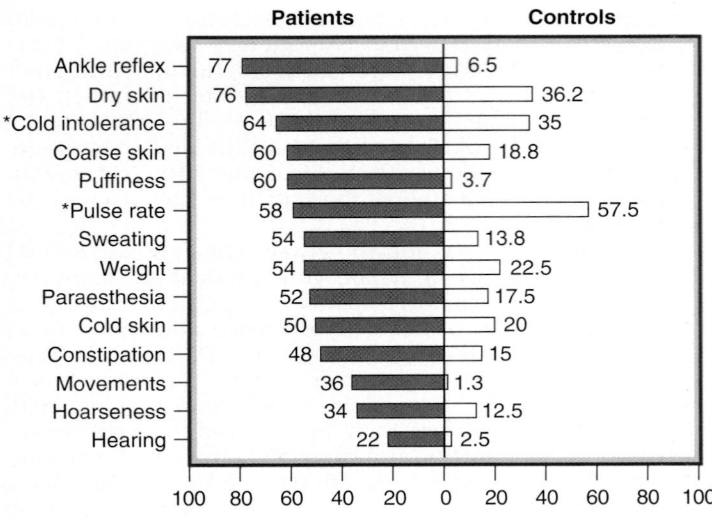

Figure 13-5 Frequency of hypothyroid symptoms and signs (%) in 50 patients with overt hypothyroidism and in 80 euthyroid controls. Two symptoms (pulse rate and cold intolerance, marked by asterisks) showed positive and negative predictive values of less than 70% and therefore were excluded from the new score. (From Zulewski H, Müller B, Exer P, et al. Estimation of tissue hypothyroidism by a new clinical score: evaluation of patients with various grades of hypothyroidism and controls. *J Clin Endocrinol Metab.* 1997;82:771-776.)

abnormalities of hypothyroidism may not score high on indices of symptoms and signs.[62]

With respect to physical signs of hypothyroidism, the presence of coarse skin, periorbital puffiness that obscures the curve of the malar bone (see Fig. 13-1), cold skin, and delayed ankle reflex relaxation phase are all signs that should lead to appropriate diagnostic tests.

Acute hypothyroidism in the previously hyperthyroid patient after radioiodine therapy is characterized by painful cramping of large muscle groups (see Chapter 12).

Hypothyroidism in Infants and Children

Severe hypothyroidism is seldom apparent at birth, hence the requirement for systematic screening for congenital hypothyroidism.[10] Congenital hypothyroidism can be caused by complete thyroid agenesis, ectopic thyroid, or incomplete thyroid development. Mutations in genes important for thyroid development have been identified in a number of patients and in some cases may explain associated abnormalities in development of other structures (e.g., heart) because of their spatial association during development. The age at which symptoms appear depends on the degree of impairment of thyroid function (see Figs. 13-3 and 13-4). Severe hypothyroidism in infancy is termed *cretinism*. As the age at onset increases, the clinical picture of cretinism merges imperceptibly with that of juvenile hypothyroidism. Retardation of mental development and growth, the hallmark of cretinism, becomes manifest only in later infancy, and the mental retardation is largely irreversible. Consequently, early recognition is crucial and has been achieved by universal population screening in the developed world through measurement of the serum T_4 or TSH concentration routinely in blood spots taken from neonates.

During the first few months of life, symptoms and signs of hypothyroidism include feeding problems, failure to thrive, constipation, a hoarse cry, somnolence, and jaundice. In succeeding months, especially in severe cases, protuberance of the abdomen, dry skin, poor growth of hair and nails, and delayed eruption of the deciduous teeth become evident. Retardation of mental and physical development is manifested by delay in reaching the normal milestones of development, such as holding up the head, sitting, walking, and talking.

Thyroid hormone plays a major role in bone development, and thyroid hormone receptors are expressed in osteoclasts and osteoblasts.[40] The primary targets of thyroid hormone have been identified in the epiphyseal plates. Impairment of linear growth in congenital hypothyroidism results in dwarfism, with the limbs disproportionately short in relation to the trunk (see Fig. 13-3). Delayed closure of the fontanelles causes the head to be large in relation to the body. The naso-orbital configuration remains infantile. Maldevelopment of the femoral epiphyses results in a waddling gait. The teeth are malformed and susceptible to caries. The characteristic appearance includes a broad, flat nose; widely set eyes; periorbital puffiness; large protruding tongue; sparse hair; rough skin; short neck; and protuberant abdomen with an umbilical hernia. Mental deficiency is usually severe.

Radiologic examination of the skeleton is diagnostic. The skull shows a poorly developed base; delayed closure of the fontanelles; widely set orbits; and a short, flat nasal bone. The pituitary fossa may be enlarged. Shedding of deciduous teeth and eruption of permanent teeth are delayed (see Fig. 13-4).

The radiologic picture of epiphyseal dysgenesis is pathognomonic of hypothyroidism in infancy and childhood and may involve any center of endochondral ossification, depending on the age at onset of the hypothyroid state; it is usually best seen in the femoral and humeral heads and the navicular bone of the foot. The centers of ossification appear late, so bone age is retarded in relation to chronologic age, and when they eventually appear, instead of a single center, multiple small centers are scattered through a misshapen epiphysis (see Fig. 13-4). These small centers of ossification eventually coalesce and form a single center with an irregular outline and a stippled appearance (stippled epiphysis). Epiphyseal dysgenesis is evident only in centers that normally ossify at a time after the onset of the hypothyroidism. After a normal metabolic state is restored by treatment, centers destined to ossify at a later age develop normally.

Hypothyroidism that begins in childhood is usually Hashimoto's disease and can be transient in this age group. Subclinical hypothyroidism is also seen in children and adolescents, and in one study those affected were more likely to be obese and to have a family history of thyroid disease.[63] The clinical manifestations of hypothyroidism in

TABLE 13-2

Laboratory Evaluation of Patients with Suspected Hypothyroidism or Thyroid Enlargement*

Free T_4 Value	TPO-Ab	Diagnosis
TSH > 10 mU/L		
Low	+	Primary hypothyroidism due to autoimmune thyroid disease
Low-normal	+	Primary "subclinical" hypothyroidism (autoimmune)
Low or low-normal	−	Recovery from systemic illness
		External irradiation, drug-induced, congenital hypothyroidism
		Iodine deficiency
		Seronegative autoimmune thyroid disease
		Rare thyroid disorders (e.g., amyloidosis, sarcoidosis)
		Recovery from subacute granulomatous thyroiditis
Normal	+, −	Consider TSH or T_4 assay artifacts
Elevated	−	Thyroid hormone resistance
		Blockade of T_4 to T_3 conversion (amiodarone) or a congenital 5′-deiodinase deficiency
		Consider assay artifacts
TSH 5-10 mU/L		
Low, low-normal	+	Early primary autoimmune hypothyroidism
Low, low-normal	−	Milder forms of non-autoimmune hypothyroidism (see above)
		Central hypothyroidism with impaired TSH bioactivity
Elevated	−	Consider thyroid hormone resistance
		T_4-to-T_3 conversion blockade (e.g., amiodarone)
TSH 0.5-5 mU/L		
Low, low-normal	−	Central hypothyroidism
		Salicylate or phenytoin therapy
		Desiccated thyroid or T_3 replacement
TSH < 0.5 μU/L		
Low, low-normal	−	"Post-hyperthyroid" hypothyroidism (^{131}I or surgery)
		Central hypothyroidism
		T_3 or desiccated thyroid excess
		Post excess levothyroxine withdrawal

*Initial tests: serum TSH, serum free T_4, TPO-Ab, or Tg-Ab.

T_3, triiodothyronine; T_4, thyroxine; Tg-Ab, anti-thyroglobulin antibody; TPO-Ab, thyroid peroxidase autoantibody; TSH, thyroid-stimulating hormone; +, present; −, not present.

children are intermediate between those of infantile and adult hypothyroidism, in that the developmental retardation is not as severe as that of cretinism and the manifestations of full-blown adult myxedema are rarely seen. Growth and sexual development are affected predominantly. If the hypothyroidism is left untreated, linear growth is severely retarded, and sexual maturation and the onset of puberty are delayed.[40,41] On radiologic examination, epiphyseal dysgenesis may be present, and epiphyseal union is always delayed, resulting in a bone age that is younger relative to the chronologic age.

LABORATORY EVALUATION

Primary and Central Hypothyroidism

A decrease in secretion of the thyroid hormones is common to all varieties of hypothyroidism, except for disorders of thyroid hormone metabolism or action such as *consumptive hypothyroidism* and *RTH* (see later discussion). In patients with primary thyroid disease, the cause of hypothyroidism in more than 99% of the patients, there is a significant increase in basal serum TSH concentration. A strategy for evaluating the patient with suspected hypothyroidism involves a TSH determination (Table 13-2). If the suspicion of hypothyroidism is strong, if a goiter is present, or if central hypothyroidism is part of the differential diagnosis, an fT_4 assay should be included (see Chapter 11). If hypothyroidism is thought to be unlikely but must be excluded, only a TSH determination is required, because primary hypothyroidism is almost always the cause. If TSH is elevated, an fT_4 assay can be added to the same determination (Fig. 13-6). As hypothyroidism progresses, the serum TSH increases further, the serum fT_4 falls, and finally, at the most severe stage, serum T_3 concentrations may become subnormal (see Table 13-2). The persistence of a normal serum T_3 is, in part, due to preferential synthesis and secretion of T_3 by residual functioning thyroid tissue under the influence of the increased plasma TSH. In addition, the efficiency of conversion of T_4 to T_3 by D2 is increased as the serum T_4 level falls.[64] Consequently, the serum T_3 concentration may remain within the normal range.

The principal differential diagnosis is between primary and central hypothyroidism (see Chapter 9). The serum TSH concentration is the critical laboratory determination that, in general, allows recognition of the cause of the disease when the serum fT_4 is reduced. An exception is the individual with a recent history of thyrotoxicosis (and suppressed TSH) in whom a low fT_4 level may be associated with a reduced TSH level for several months after treatment of the thyrotoxicosis. In patients with primary hypothyroidism, the absence of thyroid peroxidase antibodies (TPO-Ab) raises a possible diagnosis of transient

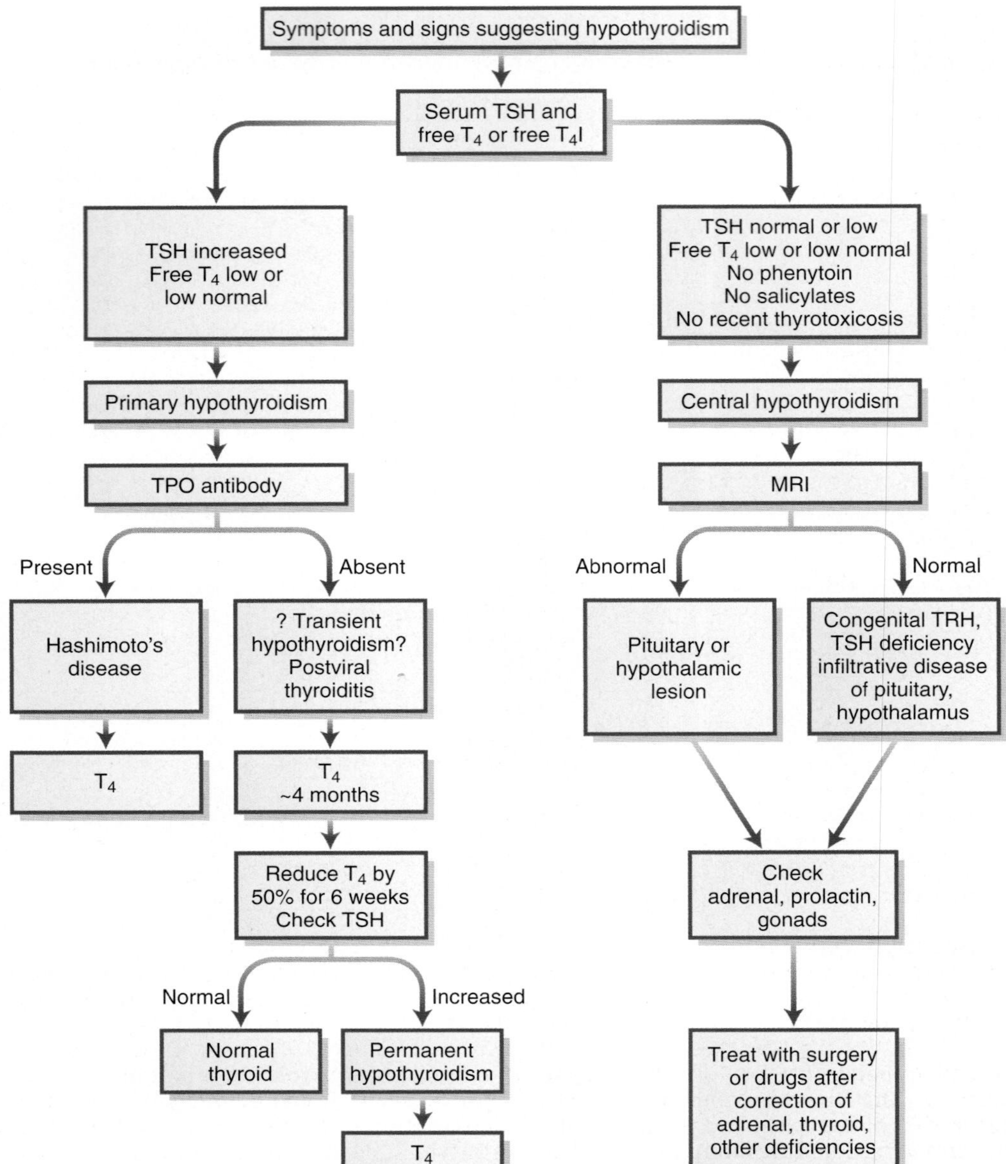

Figure 13-6 Strategy for the laboratory evaluation of patients with suspected hypothyroidism. The principal differential diagnosis is between primary and central hypothyroidism (see Chapter 9). The serum thyrotropin (TSH) concentration is the critical laboratory determination that, in general, allows recognition of the cause of the disease. An exception is the individual with a recent history of thyrotoxicosis (and suppressed TSH), in whom a low free thyroxine (T_4) level may be associated with a reduced TSH level for several months after relief of the thyrotoxicosis. In patients with primary hypothyroidism, the absence of thyroid peroxidase (TPO) antibodies raises a possible diagnosis of transient hypothyroidism after an undiagnosed episode of subacute or postviral thyroiditis. In such patients, a trial of levothyroxine in reduced dosage after 4 months may reveal recovery of thyroid function, thus avoiding permanent levothyroxine replacement. MRI, magnetic resonance imaging; TRH, thyrotropin-releasing hormone.

hypothyroidism after an undiagnosed episode of subacute or postviral thyroiditis.

The differentiation of hypothyroidism due to intrinsic thyroid failure from hypothyroidism due to diminished TSH secretion resulting from hypothalamic or pituitary disease (central or secondary hypothyroidism) is the most critical decision point in this pathway (see Fig. 13-6). A low thyroid hormone level with a normal or low TSH level should lead to an evaluation for the possibility of failure of other endocrine systems that require trophic pituitary hormones for normal function (see Table 13-1 and Chapters 8 and 9). The only exception is the early stages of *posthyperthyroid* hypothyroidism, in which TSH levels may remain suppressed for several months even though hypothyroidism, as revealed by a low fT_4 level, has been induced by ^{131}I therapy, surgery, or anti-thyroid drugs (see Table 13-2). In some patients with central hypothyroidism, the basal serum TSH concentration (and the response to TRH) may even be somewhat elevated, but the TSH has reduced biologic potency even though it is immunologically reactive.[65]

In patients with an elevated TSH level and a reduced fT_4 level, the presence or absence of TPO-Ab should be ascertained (see Fig. 13-6). The presence of TPO-Ab usually points to autoimmune thyroid disease (Hashimoto's disease) as the cause of the hypothyroidism. On the other hand, the absence of TPO-Ab requires a search for less common causes of hypothyroidism, such as transient hypothyroidism, infiltrative thyroid disorders, and external irradiation, as discussed later (see Table 13-1). Nevertheless, approximately 10% of patients with Hashimoto's disease do not have detectable TPO-Ab.

Measurement of radioactive iodine uptake (RAIU) is rarely required in the evaluation of hypothyroidism. Tests that employ radioiodine to assess the function of the thyroid gland display a variable pattern, depending on the underlying thyroid disorder. The diagnostic value of a low RAIU is limited because of the relatively high dietary iodine intake in North America, which reduces uptake of the tracer dose of radioiodine, and variation in iodine intake from day to day in the same individual. National surveys of dietary iodine intake showed a progressive reduction in iodine intake over the last several decades,[66] but the intake has now stablized.[67] The RAIU may be normal or even increased if hypothyroidism results primarily from a biochemical defect in thyroid hormone synthesis rather than thyroid cell destruction, leading to compensatory thyroid enlargement. Specific functional patterns in relation to the causes of hypothyroidism are discussed later. Nonetheless, measurement of RAIU is almost never required in the diagnostic evaluation of the hypothyroid patient.

Differential Diagnosis

The clinical picture of fully developed hypothyroidism is quite characteristic, but the abnormalities can be overlooked, even by experienced clinicians, if the diagnosis is not considered. Despite the availability of inexpensive and specific tests, it is still surprising how often what is retrospectively obvious, severe, primary hypothyroidism is not recognized. A high index of suspicion is required to avoid this oversight.

For the milder forms of hypothyroidism, the clinical presentation overlaps to a significant extent with other conditions. The fact that these disorders often occur in older patients is partly responsible for the diagnostic uncertainty.[64] In some cases, slowing of mental and physical activity, dry skin, and loss of hair may mimic similar findings in hypothyroidism. Furthermore, older people often become hypothermic with cold exposure.

In patients with chronic renal insufficiency, anorexia, torpor, periorbital puffiness, sallow complexion, and anemia (e.g., see Fig. 13-1) may suggest hypothyroidism and may call for specific testing. Distinguishing nephrotic states from hypothyroidism by clinical examination alone can be even more difficult. In this disorder, waxy pallor, edema, hypercholesterolemia, and hypometabolism may suggest hypothyroidism. In addition, the total serum T_4 concentration may be decreased if significant thyroxine-binding globulin is lost in the urine, but the fT_4 and TSH are normal.

In those patients with pernicious anemia, psychiatric abnormalities, pallor, and numbness and tingling of the extremities may mimic similar findings in hypothyroidism. Although there is a clinical and immunologic overlap between primary hypothyroidism and pernicious anemia, this association is not invariable (see Chapter 42). The presence of hypothyroidism is often suspected in patients who are severely ill, especially in the elderly.[22,68] In such patients, the total T_4 concentration may be decreased, often markedly so, but the fT_4 is typically normal unless the patient is severely ill (see Chapter 11). These features, together with the absence of an elevation of serum TSH, usually serve to differentiate the ill euthyroid patient from one with primary hypothyroidism. However, the serum TSH can be transiently increased (up to 20 mU/L) during recovery from severe illness.

Hypothyroidism may develop because of some extrinsic factor or acquired condition or because of a congenital defect that impairs thyroid hormone biosynthesis (see Table 13-1). Inadequate synthesis of hormone leads to hypersecretion of TSH, which in turn produces both goiter and stimulation of all steps in hormone biosynthesis capable of response. In some instances, the compensatory TSH response overcomes the impairment in hormone biosynthesis, and the patient is euthyroid with a goiter. The latter condition (simple or nontoxic goiter) is discussed in Chapter 14. Less commonly, hypothyroidism is associated with an atrophic gland or, in the case of a congenital abnormality, one that never developed properly. Hypothyroidism can also occur after surgical lobectomy, especially in areas of iodine insufficiency or with underlying thyroid TPO-Ab.[69]

CLASSIFICATION

Acquired Causes

Hashimoto's Thyroiditis

Hashimoto's disease is the most common cause of hypothyroidism in areas of the world in which dietary iodine is sufficient. Until it was possible to demonstrate circulating thyroid antigen–specific T cells and thyroid autoantibodies, a diagnosis of Hashimoto's disease could be confirmed only by biopsy of the thyroid. Even now, the terminology used to classify the *autoimmune thyroid diseases* does not reflect current understanding of the pathophysiology of these disorders and suggests that Hashimoto's disease and Graves' disease are distinct entities, which they are certainly not. In pathologic terms, the word *thyroiditis* has implied both the presence of a mononuclear cell infiltrate and destruction of thyroid follicles. However, these are arbitrary criteria. The term *chronic thyroiditis* is more appropriately defined simply as evidence of "intrathyroidal lymphocytic infiltration" without the necessity of follicular damage—which may, however, develop later. By this definition, patients with either Graves' disease or Hashimoto's disease have thyroiditis, and this allows a simple classification for autoimmune thyroid disease into destructive and nondestructive pathologies.[70] However, most classification systems still use the term *autoimmune thyroiditis* as synonymous with either transient or chronic inflammation, associated with follicular destruction.[1,2]

Blockade by autoantibodies to the TSH receptor that act as TSH antagonists may be the cause of some cases of the atrophic form of Hashimoto's disease (in the past referred to as "primary myxedema"), but classic Hashimoto's thyroiditis is associated with goiter formation from the marked lymphocytic infiltration.[71] Both Graves' disease and Hashimoto's disease can occur within the same families, and they may share human leukocyte antigen (HLA) and other genetic susceptibility haplotypes.[71,72] Furthermore, thyroid failure occurs in some patients with Graves' disease, and hyperthyroidism and even orbitopathy may develop in some patients with Hashimoto's disease. Both types of patients can have autoantibodies to thyroglobulin (Tg), TPO, and the TSH receptor. Therefore, the two diseases must be closely related, and autoimmune thyroid disease can be viewed as a spectrum from hyperthyroidism to hypothyroidism.

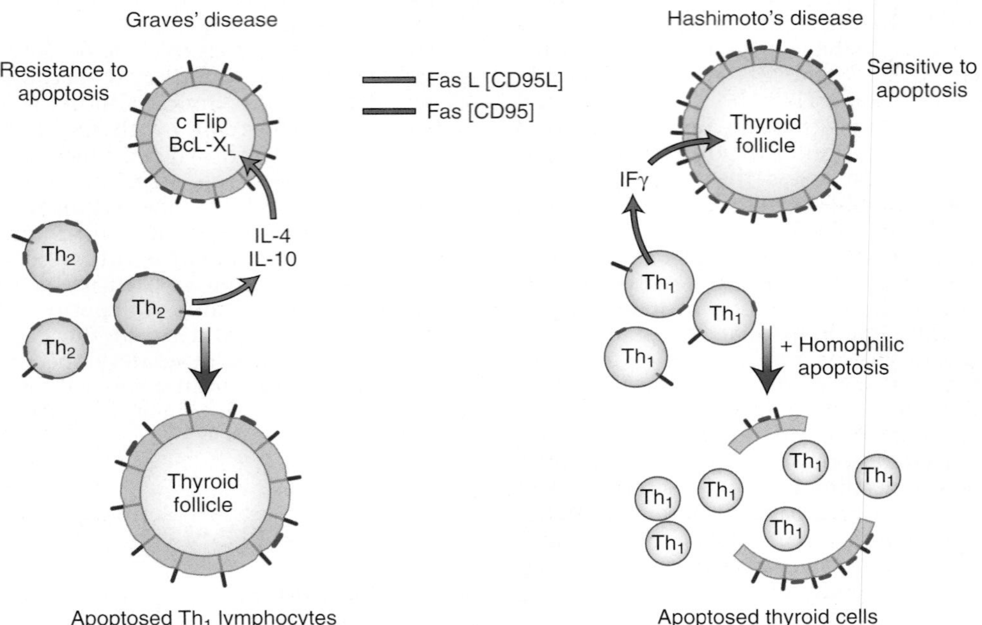

Figure 13-7 Possible involvement of Fas-Fas L in the apoptosis of Hashimoto's thyroiditis. Presence of Fas molecules is indicated by red color; blue color indicates Fas ligand (Fas L). In Graves' disease, the thyroid follicles thrive because the thyroid cells do not express many functional Fas molecules and therefore are resistant to the Fas L, both on the thyroid cells themselves and on the Th_2 T cells. Further apoptotic resistance may be driven by Th_2 cytokines, such as interleukin-4 (IL-4) and IL-10. However, the Th_2 cells express Fas and may themselves be deleted by the Fas L constitutively expressed on the thyroid cells. The result is thyroid cell survival with T-cell destruction. In contrast, in Hashimoto's disease, the thyroid cell expresses many functional Fas molecules, perhaps induced by interferon-γ (IFγ) from the Th_1 type T cells associated with this disease. The expression of thyroid-cell Fas may lead to self (homophilic) apoptosis via thyroid-cell Fas L, or apoptosis may result from attack by the Fas L–armed Th_1 cells. The result is thyroid follicle destruction and T-cell proliferation. BcL-X_L, Mitochondral protein involved in Fas-L signal transduction; CFlip, a protase-deficient caspase homolog that acts as an apoptosis inhibitor.

Hashimoto's disease is common and may be increasing in frequency. The mean incidence in women is approximately 3.5 cases per 1000 people per year, and in men it is 0.8 per 1000.[4,5] No age group is exempt, although the prevalence increases with age in both women and men. Hashimoto's disease is by far the most common cause of goitrous hypothyroidism in areas of iodine sufficiency.

Pathophysiology. Hormone synthesis is impaired due to apoptotic destruction of the thyroid cells. The sick cells exhibit a defect in organic binding of thyroid iodide, as evidenced by a positive perchlorate discharge test (see Chapter 11). In addition, release of iodoproteins, mostly Tg, is enhanced by cell lysis. Approximately 90% of the thyroid gland may be destroyed before clinical hypothyroidism develops. The presence of lymphocytic infiltration of the thyroid (the basis for the older term, *lymphocytic thyroiditis*), circulating thyroid autoantibodies, and clinical or immunologic overlap with other diseases with autoimmune components indicate that Hashimoto's disease is an autoimmune thyroid disorder.

The current understanding of autoimmune mechanisms is discussed in Chapter 12. However, autoimmune thyroiditis is characterized by thyroid cell apoptosis leading to destruction of follicles, rather than the thyroid stimulation and thyroid cell hyperplasia seen in Graves' disease. Although both TPO-Ab) and autoantibodies to thyroglobulin (Tg-Ab) are complement fixing and cytotoxic, the thyroid gland is infiltrated by both B cells and T cells; the latter are armed with Fas ligand and capable of destroying thyroid cells expressing Fas via apoptosis (Fig. 13-7).[73,74] In addition, other cell death pathways may be involved.[75] Fas expression on thyroid cells may be secondary to elaboration of a variety of cytokines from T cells that undergo blast transformation when exposed to thyroid antigens (thyrotropin receptor, TPO, and Tg), suggesting that cell-mediated autoimmune mechanisms are pathogenetically involved.[76]

These manifestations of autoimmunity in Hashimoto's disease and other autoimmune thyroid disorders reflect a hereditary susceptibility to thyroid disease that allows the survival and persistence of B cells and T cells directed against thyroid antigens.[77] The fact that infusion of interleukin-2 (IL-2) and lymphokine-activated killer cells causes progression or development of hypothyroidism in patients with detectable TPO-Ab is additional evidence of the autoimmune nature of this disease.[77] Animal models and increasing use of interferon-α in chronic liver disease have demonstrated a role for cytokines in initiating thyroid destruction in the setting of lymphocytic infiltration of the thyroid.[78,79]

Histopathology. The thyroid gland is pale and firm and has a rubbery texture (Fig. 13-8A). Histopathologic changes vary in type and extent but usually consist of diffuse lymphocytic infiltration with germinal center formation and obliteration of thyroid follicles by widespread apoptosis (see Fig. 13-8B). In most cases, there is destruction of epithelial cells and degeneration and fragmentation of the follicular basement membrane. The remaining epithelial cells may be larger and show oxyphilic changes in the cytoplasm; these so-called Askanazy cells are virtually pathognomonic for Hashimoto's disease. In some cases,

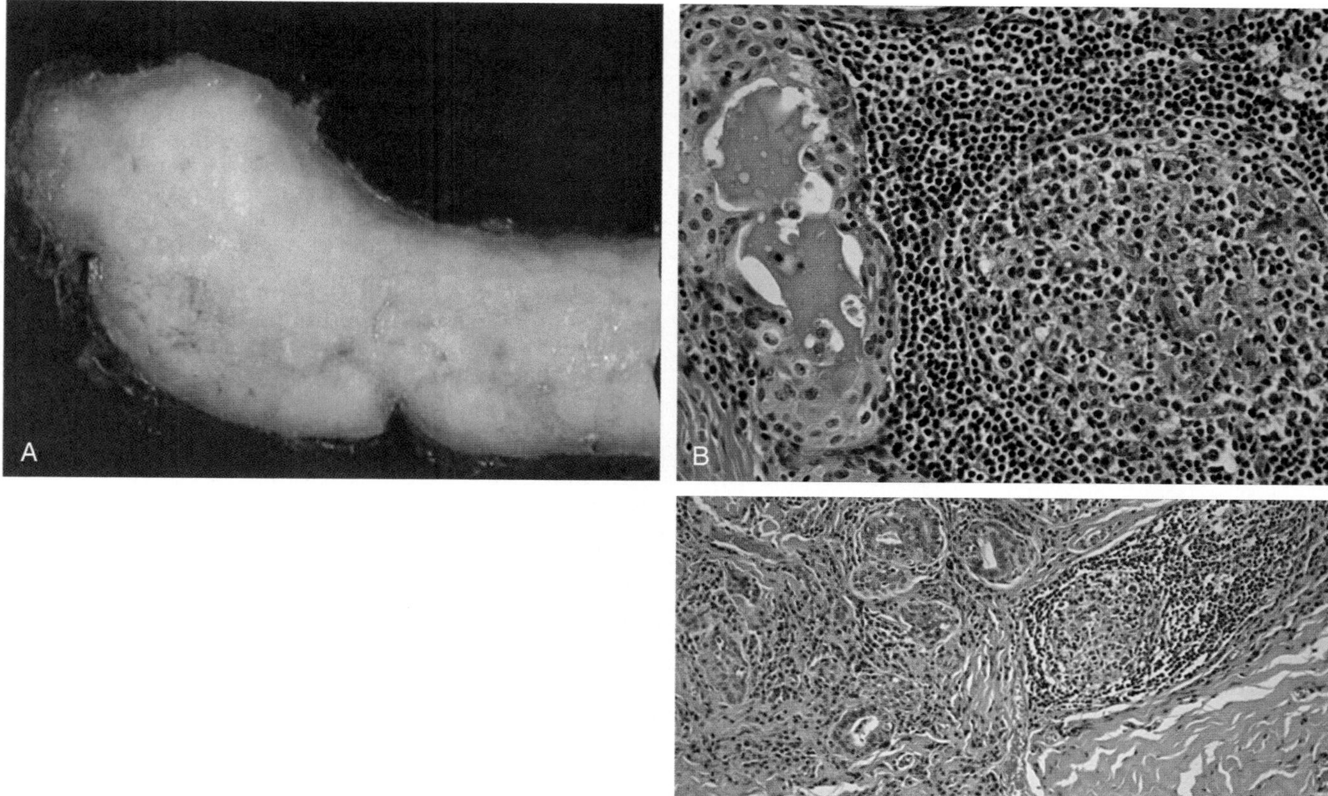

Figure 13-8 Hashimoto's thyroiditis. **A,** Gross appearance of a cut section of the thyroid lobe demonstrating the pale color of the tissue that results from lymphocytic infiltration, fibrosis, and loss of follicles. **B,** Typical histologic appearance illustrating a germinal center, heavy lymphocytic infiltration, and a partially disrupted thyroid follicle. **C,** Fibrous variant showing extensive fibrosis and loss of follicles. (Courtesy of Dr. Vania Nosé, Department of Pathology, Brigham and Women's Hospital, Boston, MA.)

colloid is sparse. Fibrosis is usually present in the more long-standing tissues but not to the extent seen in the variant referred to as Riedel's thyroiditis (see Fig. 13-8C).

In the past, the diagnosis of Hashimoto's disease required the presence of Askanazy cells or lymphoid follicles, but now the primary observation should be follicular destruction, often with mononuclear cell invasion of the follicular spaces. The degree of lymphocytic infiltration usually correlates with the levels of circulating thyroid autoantibodies. In Graves' disease, the heterogeneous lymphocytic infiltration and associated antibodies may favor the development of hypothyroidism in the long term.

Risk Factors

Genetic Susceptibility. We have already referred to the familial predisposition to autoimmune disease in patients with autoimmune thyroid disease. As with Graves' disease, there is a significant but weak association between Hashimoto's disease and HLA DR3 and DR5 haplotypes and certain DQ alleles best correlated with an arginine residue at position 74 of the HLA-DR binding pocket.[71,72] Unlike the situation in diabetes mellitus, formal linkage of specific histocompatibility antigens with autoimmune thyroid disease has been difficult to demonstrate.

The fact that thyroid cells can express HLA-DR antigens, at least as a secondary phenomenon, indicates the potential role of these cells in perpetuating the immune response and may be related to the propensity of autoimmune disease for certain HLA-DR subgroups. Hashimoto's disease almost certainly is associated with a polygenetic susceptibility, HLA being only one of the genes involved. Efforts are under way to identify non-HLA susceptibility genes in families with autoimmune thyroid disease, and a number of such genes have been shown to have weak associations with this disease.[80] Of particular interest has been polymorphisms in the *CTLA4* gene, which codes for a regulatory protein inhibiting T-cell reactivity; such polymorphisms have been consistently linked to the propensity to secrete thyroid autoantibodies and are an important risk factor for the disease itself.[71] To date, the only thyroid-specific gene association with Hashimoto's thyroiditis has been that for Tg.[81]

Nongenetic Risk Factors. Many of the factors that have been identified as increasing the risk for Graves' disease—pregnancy, drugs, age and gender, infection, and irradiation—apply equally to autoimmune thyroiditis. These are detailed in Chapter 12 and are briefly considered here.

Pregnancy. The recognition of transient postpartum thyroiditis as an important clinical entity has also provided an example of the immune manipulation of thyroid disease with a predictable onset and recovery (see Chapter 12). Maternal microchimerism may be an important component of this risk analysis.[82] The disease is essentially postpartum Hashimoto's disease except for its transient nature. Data suggest that 8% to 10% of women experience thyroiditis in the postpartum period with a variety of consequences (see later discussion).[83] Pregnancy is, therefore, an important risk factor, with transient postpartum thyroiditis developing in some patients and thyroid failure developing permanently or in the early years after pregnancy in a significant proportion.

Iodine and Drugs. Iodine and iodine-containing drugs (e.g., amiodarone) precipitate autoimmune thyroiditis in susceptible populations.[84,85] This form should be distinguished from direct blockade and destruction of the thyroid gland by iodine. The mechanism is unknown, but much evidence accumulated in animal models suggests that increased iodination of Tg enhances its immunoreactivity.[86]

Cytokines. Treatment of patients with IL-2 or interferon-α may precipitate the appearance of autoimmune thyroid disease in the form of Hashimoto's thyroiditis or Graves' disease.[78] Destructive thyrotoxicosis may appear suddenly and needs to be distinguished from persistent Graves' disease, which may also develop in such patients. Autoimmune thyroid disease is more common in patients with preexisting TPO-Ab.

Irradiation. Radiation exposure has been shown to induce thyroid autoantibodies and autoimmune thyroid disease in a number of studies. These exposures have arisen from the atomic bomb detonation in Japan,[87] the Chernobyl disaster,[88] and therapeutic irradiation for Hodgkin's, disease.[89] Hodgkin's disease survivors have a 17-fold relative risk of developing hypothyroidism.[89] A long-term follow-up of Japanese atomic bomb survivors after more than 55 years showed a persistent increased risk of thyroid nodules but not thyroid autoantibodies.[90] It is postulated that the specific effect of radiation on thyroid autoantibody expression may diminish with longer-term follow-up, because the incidence of autoimmune thyroid disease in the general population increases with age.

Age. Because autoimmune thyroid failure continues to occur throughout adult life, the prevalence of the disease increases markedly with age.[4-6,68] This is similar to other markers of autoimmunity and may reflect an increasing loss of tolerance to self.

Infection. There is no direct evidence that infection causes classic autoimmune thyroiditis in humans, although there is suggestive evidence that the hepatitis C virus may enter thyroid cells and precipitate thyroid disease in susceptible patients.[78] A number of viral infections in animals also can precipitate thyroid autoimmunity.[91] In addition, persisting signs of thyroid autoimmune disease have been found during long-term follow-up of patients with subacute thyroiditis thought to be a reaction to a viral infection (see later discussion). Infection remains a likely cause of the local or distant insult that is considered to be needed to precipitate autoimmune disease in susceptible individuals (see Chapter 12).

Clinical Picture. Goiter, the hallmark of classic Hashimoto's disease, usually develops gradually and may be found during routine examination or by ultrasonography. On occasion, the thyroid gland enlarges rapidly and, when accompanied by pain and tenderness, may mimic de Quervain's or subacute thyroiditis (see Chapter 12). Some patients, particularly those with the fibrous variant, are hypothyroid when first seen. The goiter is usually moderate in size and firm in consistency and moves freely on swallowing. The surface is either smooth or bumpy, but well-defined nodules are unusual. Both lobes are enlarged, but the gland may be asymmetric. The pyramidal lobe may also be enlarged, and adjacent structures, such as the trachea, esophagus, and recurrent laryngeal nerves, may be compressed. Enlargement of regional lymph nodes is unusual.

Other patients with hypothyroidism present without a goiter (atrophic hypothyroidism, discussed later), and this is thought to represent the end result of autoimmune destruction of the thyroid. Progression of goitrous Hashimoto's disease to the atrophied state is not commonly seen in the individual patient. The atrophic thyroid most likely reflects rapid large-scale apoptosis early in the onset of Hashimoto's disease combined with TSH receptor antibodies of the blocking variety. The general histopathologic picture tends to remain rather static except for an increase in fibrous tissue. A study of thyroid volume by ultrasonography in patients with newly diagnosed autoimmune hypothyroidism found that there was a continuum of thyroid size, with atrophy and goiter representing extremes of the distribution rather than distinct entities.[92]

Clinically, the untreated goiter remains unchanged or enlarges gradually over many years. The manifestations of hypothyroidism may develop over several years in patients who are initially euthyroid. Thyroid lymphoma occurs almost exclusively in patients with underlying Hashimoto's disease and should be suspected if there is rapid, usually painful, enlargement of the thyroid gland.[93] The presence of coexistent Hashimoto's disease may be a favorable prognostic factor in patients with papillary carcinoma.[94]

Occasionally, hyperthyroidism due to Graves' disease develops in patients with Hashimoto's disease. In other patients with early autoimmune thyroiditis, transitory thyrotoxicosis (painless or silent thyroiditis with thyrotoxicosis) occurs as the result of thyroid cell destruction. In such cases, evidence of ongoing thyroid hyperfunction is lacking because the thyroid RAIU is depressed. As described earlier, a phase of transient hypothyroidism begins 3 to 6 months after delivery in 30% of pregnant women with autoimmune thyroiditis, as evidenced by the presence of TPO-Ab.[83] The history may suggest earlier, mild thyrotoxicosis (see the discussion of syndromes associated with transient hyperthyroidism in Chapter 12).

Laboratory Tests. Results of the common tests of thyroid function depend on stage of disease (see Table 13-2). Rarely, the tests suggest thyroid hyperfunction with a suppressed TSH but without overproduction of hormone. The RAIU may be increased in these rare patients, but serum T_4 and T_3 levels remain normal. At this stage, the patient may be eumetabolic. As the TSH level rises, the glandular response at first compensates for the impairment of hormone biosynthesis. With time, the ability of the thyroid to respond to TSH diminishes, and the RAIU and serum T_4 level decline to subnormal values. The serum T_3 concentration remains normal, probably reflecting maximal stimulation of the failing thyroid by the increased serum TSH. The early phases of the foregoing sequence, when the serum TSH is increased but T_4 and T_3 are still normal, is termed *subclinical hypothyroidism* (see Table 13-2).

The diagnosis of Hashimoto's disease is confirmed by the presence of thyroid autoantibodies in the serum, usually in high levels. TPO-Ab are more common and are present in higher concentrations than Tg-Ab, probably because circulating serum Tg absorbs the anti-Tg molecules. Sometimes part of a gland with autoimmune thyroiditis may look and feel like a firm thyroid nodule, and ultrasonography or even aspiration biopsy should be performed to resolve the issue.

Differential Diagnosis. Differentiation of Hashimoto's disease from other uncomplicated disorders of the thyroid is facilitated by the demonstration that high levels of thyroid autoantibodies occur more commonly in Hashimoto's disease than in other thyroid disorders. The frequent coexistence of hypothyroidism and Hashimoto's disease serves to distinguish this disease from nontoxic goiter and thyroid neoplasia.

Differentiation of euthyroid Hashimoto's disease from a multinodular goiter is often difficult without sonography, whereas diffuse nontoxic goiter tends to be softer than in Hashimoto's disease. Ultrasound examination may reveal the heterogeneous echotexture characteristic of Hashimoto's disease. In adolescents, differentiation of Hashimoto's disease from diffuse nontoxic goiter is more difficult, because in this age group Hashimoto's disease may not be accompanied by such high levels of thyroid autoantibodies. The presence of well-defined nodules usually distinguishes nontoxic multinodular goiter from Hashimoto's disease.

Differentiation between euthyroid Hashimoto's disease and thyroid carcinoma can sometimes be made on clinical grounds and ultrasonography. Thyroid carcinoma is usually nodular and firm or hard, and the gland may be fixed to adjacent structures. Compression of the recurrent laryngeal nerve with hoarseness is virtually pathognomonic of thyroid neoplasia but occurs late in the disease progression. A history of a recent enlargement of the goiter is more common in thyroid malignancies (carcinoma or lymphoma) than in Hashimoto's disease. Enlargement of regional lymph nodes also suggests thyroid malignancy. In thyroid carcinoma, ultrasound examination or radioiodine scanning of the thyroid may reveal only the isolated lesion. In Hashimoto's disease, activity is usually heterogeneous.

Treatment. In many patients, no treatment is required because the goiter is small and the disease is asymptomatic, with the TSH level remaining in the normal range. In other patients, treatment with thyroid hormone is directed at alleviating goiter, hypothyroidism, or both.

Levothyroxine treatment is indicated in patients who have a goiter that presses on adjacent structures or is unsightly, and it is most effective with goiters of recent onset. In long-standing goiter, treatment with thyroid hormone is usually ineffective, possibly because of fibrosis.

Glucocorticoids can cause regression of the goiter and decrease autoantibody levels, but these agents are not recommended in most patients because of untoward side effects and the return of activity after treatment is withdrawn.

Full-replacement doses of thyroid hormone should be given when hypothyroidism is present. Surgery is justified if pressure symptoms or unsightly enlargement persists after a trial of suppressive therapy. Administration of levothyroxine should be continued after surgery, because hypothyroidism is inevitable. The importance of maintaining the serum TSH level within the normal range is discussed later.

Iodine Deficiency (Endemic Goiter)

The term *endemic goiter* denotes any goiter that occurs in a region where goiter is prevalent.[84,95] As mentioned, endemic goiter almost always occurs in areas of environmental iodine deficiency. Although this condition is estimated to affect more than 200 million people throughout the world and is of major public health significance, it is most common in mountainous areas, such as the Alps, Himalayas, and Andes, or in the Great Lakes and Mississippi Valley regions of the United States, owing to the depletion of iodine consequent to the persistent glacial run-off in these regions.

The causative role of iodine deficiency in the genesis of endemic goiter is supported by several lines of evidence: the inverse correlation between the iodine content of soil and water and the incidence of goiter, the kinetics of iodine metabolism in patients with the disorder, and a decrease in incidence after iodine prophylaxis. The last finding accounts for the general absence of endemic goiter in the population residing in the Great Plains region of the United States.

The occurrence of endemic goiter can vary, even within an area of known iodine deficiency; the role of dietary minerals or naturally occurring goitrogens and of pollution of water supplies has been suggested in instances of this type.[84] For example, in the Cauca Valley of Colombia, waterborne goitrogens have been implicated, and in many areas of endemic iodine deficiency, consumption of cassava meal, which gives rise to thiocyanate, aggravates the iodine-deficient state by inhibiting thyroid iodide transport. Familial clustering of goiters within iodine-insufficient areas, usually with an autosomal dominant inheritance, suggests an important genetic component.[96]

Most abnormalities in iodine metabolism in patients with endemic goiter are consistent with the expected effects of iodine deficiency (see Chapter 11). Thyroid iodide clearance rates and RAIU are increased in proportion to the decrease in urinary excretion of stable iodine. The absolute iodine uptake is normal or low. In areas of moderate iodine deficiency, the serum T_4 concentration is usually in the lower range of normal; in areas of severe deficiency, values are decreased. Nevertheless, most patients in these areas do not appear to be in a hypothyroid state because of an increase in the synthesis of T_3 at the expense of T_4 and because of an increase in the activity of thyroidal D1 and D2.[64] TSH levels are typically in the upper range of normal.

The incidence and severity of endemic goiter and the metabolic state of the goitrous patient depend mainly on the degree of iodine deficiency. In the absence of hypothyroidism, the effects of the goiter are mainly cosmetic. However, if the goiter becomes nodular, hemorrhage into a nodule may cause acute pain and swelling, mimicking subacute thyroiditis or neoplasia. The goiter may also compress adjacent structures, such as the trachea, esophagus, and recurrent laryngeal nerves. The borderline nature of the iodine supply in many countries of Western Europe is exemplified by the development in Belgium of compensatory maternal and fetal goiter during pregnancy in response to the increased requirement for thyroid hormone during gestation.[97]

The incidence of endemic goiter has been greatly reduced in many areas by the introduction of iodized salt.[84] In the United States, table salt is enriched with potassium iodide to a concentration of 0.01%, which, if the intake of salt is average, would provide an iodine intake of approximately 150 to 300 μg/day, the desired amount in an adult (see Table 11-1 in Chapter 11). The use of iodine-containing flour in bread products and iodized salt in commercially produced food has been markedly reduced.[98] Iodine content of bread and infant formula is variable within a given product and often does not match the measured content.[98] As mentioned, iodine intake in the United States has been decreasing in recent decades, probably because of reduced use of iodine in commercial food products, although iodine intake has now stabilized.[67] A significant fraction of pregnant women in Boston, based on urinary iodine excretion, have iodine intake below the recommended level for pregnancy.[99] Most prescription prenatal vitamins do not contain iodine.[100] An annual injection of iodized oil is another effective means of administering iodine, and endemic goiter can be treated by the addition of iodine to communal drinking water.

Administration of iodine has little, if any, effect on a long-standing endemic goiter, but it causes the early endemic hyperplastic goiter of iodine deficiency to regress.[101] Similarly, thyroid hormone usually has no effect on long-standing goiter or on established mental or skeletal changes, but it should be given in full-replacement doses if there is evidence of hypothyroidism. This is of paramount importance in pregnant women. Surgical treatment is indicated if the adjacent structures are compressed or if the goiter is either very large or enlarging rapidly.

Endemic Cretinism

Endemic cretinism is a developmental disorder that occurs in regions of severe endemic goiter.[84] Both parents of an endemic cretin are usually goitrous, and, in addition to the features of sporadic cretinism described earlier, endemic cretins often have deaf-mutism, spasticity, motor dysfunction, and abnormalities in the basal ganglia demonstrable by magnetic resonance imaging.

Three types of cretins can be discerned: hypothyroid cretins, neurologic cretins, and cretins with combined features of the two. The pathogenesis of neurologic cretinism is obscure but may be the result of severe thyroid hormone deficiency during a critical early phase of central nervous system development in utero.[32] Some cretins are goitrous, but in others the thyroid is atrophic, possibly as a consequence of exhaustion atrophy from continuous overstimulation or lack of iodine.

Iodide Excess

Goiter and hypothyroidism, either alone or in combination, are sometimes induced by chronic administration of large doses of iodine in organic or inorganic form (see Table 11-7 in Chapter 11).[84,85,102] Iodide-induced goiter was formerly seen in patients with chronic respiratory disease who were given potassium iodide as an expectorant. The development of iodide goiter has also been reported after a single administration of radiographic contrast medium, from which iodide is released slowly over a long period, and it may also occur during amiodarone administration. Iodide goiter without hypothyroidism may occur endemically, such as on the island of Hokkaido, Japan, where seaweed products are consumed in large quantities.

From an analysis of reported cases and from the fact that only a small percentage of patients who receive iodides chronically develop goiter, it appears that the disorder evolves on a background of underlying thyroid dysfunction. Categories of susceptible individuals include patients with Hashimoto's disease; patients with Graves' disease, especially after its treatment with radioiodine; and patients with cystic fibrosis. Among these groups, many individuals display a positive iodide-perchlorate discharge test, indicating a defect in the thyroidal organic iodine-binding mechanism (see Chapter 11). However, intrinsic thyroid disease need not be present, because a propensity to develop iodide goiter and hypothyroidism has also been demonstrated in patients who have undergone hemithyroidectomy for a solitary thyroid nodule, in whom the remaining lobe was histologically normal.[69] In these patients, as in those with Hashimoto's disease or Graves' disease studied prospectively, individuals with the highest basal serum TSH concentrations, even within the normal range, were those who developed iodide goiter. Iodinated contrast material, amiodarone, and povidone-iodine are common sources.[101]

Goiter and hypothyroidism commonly occur in newborn infants born to women given large quantities of iodine during pregnancy, and death from neonatal asphyxia has been reported (see Fig. 11-11 in Chapter 11). In such cases, the mother is usually free from goiter. Pregnant women should not receive large doses of iodine (≥1 mg/day) over prolonged periods (>10 days), especially near term. Maternal amiodarone therapy causes thyroidal dysfunction in up to 20% of newborns.[84] It is not known whether iodide goiter in newborns results from an inherent hypersensitivity of the fetal thyroid or from the fact that the placenta concentrates iodide several-fold, or both.

As discussed in Chapter 11, large doses of iodine cause an acute inhibition of organic binding that abates in the normal individual despite continued iodine administration (acute Wolff-Chaikoff effect and escape).[103] Iodide goiter appears to result from a more pronounced inhibition of organic binding and failure of the escape phenomenon. Decreased hormone synthesis and the consequent increase in TSH result in enhanced iodide transport. Because inhibition of organic binding is a function of the intrathyroidal concentration of iodide, a vicious circle, augmented by this increase in serum TSH, is set in motion.

The disorder usually appears as a goiter with or without hypothyroidism, although in rare instances iodine may produce hypothyroidism unaccompanied by goiter. Usually, the thyroid gland is firm and diffusely enlarged, often greatly so. Histopathologic examination reveals intense hyperplasia. The fT_4 concentration is low, the TSH concentration is increased, and the 24-hour urinary iodine excretion and serum inorganic iodide concentration are increased. The disorder regresses after iodine is withdrawn. Thyroid hormone may also be given to relieve severe symptoms.

Drugs That Block Thyroid Hormone Synthesis or Release, Causing Goiter Formation

Ingestion of compounds that block thyroid hormone synthesis or release may cause goiter with or without hypothyroidism. Apart from the agents used in the treatment of hyperthyroidism, anti-thyroid agents may be encountered as drugs for the treatment of disorders unrelated to the thyroid gland or as natural agents in foodstuffs.[83]

Goiter with or without hypothyroidism can occur in patients given lithium, usually for bipolar manic-depressive psychosis.[83] Like iodide, lithium inhibits thyroid hormone release, and in high concentrations it can inhibit organic binding reactions. In the latter respect, iodide and lithium act synergistically, at least acutely. The mechanisms underlying the several effects of lithium are uncertain; what differentiates patients who develop goiter during lithium therapy from those who do not is also unclear. Underlying autoimmune thyroiditis may be at least one factor, because many patients with this combination have autoimmune thyroid disease.

Other drugs that occasionally produce goitrous hypothyroidism include para-aminosalicylic acid, phenylbutazone, aminoglutethimide, and ethionamide. Like the thionamides, these drugs interfere with both the organic binding of iodine and, perhaps in later steps, hormone biosynthesis. Although soybean flour is not an anti-thyroid agent, soybean products in feeding formulas formerly resulted in goiter in infants by enhancing fecal loss of hormone, which, together with the low iodine content of soybean products, produced a state of iodine deficiency. Feeding formulas containing soybean products are now enriched with iodine.

Cigarette smoking increases the risk of hypothyroidism in patients with underlying autoimmune thyroid disease. Although the mechanism is unclear, certain components of cigarette smoke, including thiocyanate, hydroxypyridine, and benzopyrene derivatives, may be responsible. These components of smoke may also interfere with thyroid hormone action.[104]

Both the goiter and the hypothyroidism usually subside after the anti-thyroid agent is withdrawn. If continued administration of pharmacologic goitrogens is required, replacement therapy with thyroid hormone causes the goiter to regress.

Goitrogens in Foodstuffs or as Endemic Substances or Pollutants

Anti-thyroid agents also occur naturally in foods. These are widely distributed in the Cruciferae and Brassicaceae families, particularly in the genus *Brassica,* including cabbages, turnips, kale, kohlrabi, rutabaga, mustard, and various plants that are not eaten by humans but serve as animal fodder. It is likely that some thiocyanate is present in such plants (particularly cabbage). Cassava meal, a dietary staple in many regions of the world, contains linamarin, a cyanogenic glycoside, the preparation of which leads to the formation of thiocyanate. Ingestion of cassava can accentuate goiter formation in areas of endemic iodine deficiency. Except for thiocyanate, dietary goitrogens influence thyroid iodine metabolism in the same manner as do the thionamides, which they resemble chemically; their role in the induction of disease in humans is uncertain. Waterborne, sulfur-containing goitrogens of mineral origin are believed to contribute to the development of endemic goiter in certain areas of Colombia.

A number of synthetic chemical pollutants have been implicated as a cause of goitrous hypothyroidism, including polychlorinated biphenyls and resorcinol derivatives.[105,106] Perchlorate has also been noted in high concentrations in geographic regions in which explosives and rocket fuel were made.[107] Perchlorate has been detected in water, food, and breast milk, although the amount does not appear to be sufficient to disrupt thyroid function.[103] In an area of Chile with a high level of natural perchlorate contamination in the water, thyroid function in pregnant women was not different from that in a region with no perchlorate, although iodine intake was quite high in that area.[108]

Cytokines

Patients with chronic hepatitis C or various malignancies may be given interferon-α or IL-2.[78] Such patients may experience hypothyroidism, which is usually transient but may persist. These agents activate the immune system and can induce a clinical picture suggesting an exacerbation of underlying autoimmune disease such as occurs during postpartum thyroiditis (see Chapter 12). Graves' disease with hyperthyroidism may also develop, and ablative therapy may be required to treat this condition. Patients with preexisting evidence of autoimmune thyroid disease who have positive TPO-Ab are probably at higher risk for this complication and should be monitored carefully during and after a course of treatment with either of these cytokines.

Congenital Causes of Goiter

Inherited defects in hormone biosynthesis are rare causes of goitrous hypothyroidism and account for only about 10% to 15% of the 1 in 3500 newborns with congenital hypothyroidism.[10] In most instances, the defect appears to be transmitted as an autosomal recessive trait. Individuals with goitrous hypothyroidism are believed to be homozygous for the abnormal gene, whereas euthyroid relatives with slightly enlarged thyroids are presumably heterozygous. In the latter group, appropriate functional testing may disclose a mild abnormality of the same biosynthetic step that is defective in the homozygous individual. In contrast with nontoxic goiter, which is more common in females than in males, these defects, as a group, affect females only slightly more commonly than males.

Although goiter may be present at birth, it usually does not appear until several years later. Therefore, the absence of goiter in a child with functioning thyroid tissue does not exclude the presence of hypothyroidism. The goiter is initially diffusely hyperplastic, often intensely so, suggesting papillary carcinoma, but it eventually becomes nodular. In general, the more severe the biosynthetic defect, the earlier the goiter appears, the larger it is, and the greater the likelihood of early development of hypothyroidism or even cretinism. Five specific defects in the pathways of hormone synthesis have been identified.

Iodide Transport Defect. An iodide transport defect, resulting from impaired iodide transport by the sodium-iodide symporter (NIS) protein mechanism, is rare and is reflected in defective iodide transport in the thyroid, salivary gland, and gastric mucosa.[109] Some mutations in such patients produce reduced activity, and others completely inactivate NIS by preventing the protein from being transported and inserted into the membrane. With the milder NIS mutations, administration of iodide raises the plasma and intrathyroidal iodide concentration, permitting the synthesis of normal quantities of hormone.

Defects in Expression or Function of Thyroid Peroxidase. TPO is a protein that is required for normal synthesis of iodothyronines. Quantitative or qualitative abnormalities of TPO were identified in 1 of every 66,000 infants in the Netherlands.[110] The most common of the 16 mutations identified in 35 families was a GGCC insertion in exon 8, leading to a premature stop codon.

Pendred's Syndrome. The most common presentation in patients with Pendred's syndrome is a defect in iodine organification accompanied by sensory nerve deafness.[111] The abnormality is in the *PDS* gene encoding pendrin, which is involved in the apical secretion of iodide into the follicular lumen (see Fig. 11-2 in Chapter 11). Thyroid function is only mildly impaired in this disorder.

Defects in Thyroglobulin Synthesis. Defects in the synthesis of Tg due to genetic causes are rare, having been identified only in a small number of families with congenital hypothyroidism.[112] Some defects lead to premature termination of translation, whereas another causes deficiency in endoplasmic reticulum processing of the Tg molecule. The complex regulation and huge size of this gene makes screening for mutations a difficult task, and considerable work is still required to unravel the extent of the defects in this gene.

Iodotyrosine Dehalogenase Defect. The pathogenesis of goiter and hypothyroidism in the iodotyrosine dehalogenase defect is complex. The major abnormality is an impairment of both intrathyroidal and peripheral deiodination of iodotyrosines, presumably because of the dysfunction of the iodotyrosine *Dehal1b* gene (see Chapter 11).[113] As a consequence of intense thyroid stimulation and lack of intrathyroidal recycling of iodide derived from dehalogenation, iodide is rapidly accumulated by the thyroid gland and is rapidly released; monoiodotyrosine (MIT) and diiodotyrosine (DIT) are elevated in plasma and, together with their deaminated derivatives, in the urine. Hypothyroidism is presumed to result from the loss of large quantities of MIT and DIT in the urine and from secondary iodine deficiency. The goiter and hypothyroidism are relieved by administration of high doses of iodine.

Thyroid Infiltration Causing Hypothyroidism and Goiter

A number of infiltrative or fibrosing conditions can cause hypothyroidism. Some are often associated with goiter, such as Riedel's struma (see later discussion).[114] Others, such as amyloidosis,[115] hemochromatosis,[116] or scleroderma,[117] may not be. Although the other manifestations of these conditions are usually obvious and hypothyroidism is only a complication, the presence of significant hypothyroidism without evidence of autoimmune thyroiditis should lead to a consideration of these rare causes of this condition.

Postablative Hypothyroidism

Postablative hypothyroidism is a common cause of thyroid failure in adults. One type occurs after total thyroidectomy usually performed for thyroid carcinoma. Although functioning remnants may be present, as indicated by foci of radioiodine accumulation, hypothyroidism invariably develops. Another etiologic mechanism is subtotal resection of the diffuse goiter of Graves' disease or multinodular goiter. Its frequency depends on the amount of tissue remaining, but continued autoimmune destruction of the thyroid remnant in patients with Graves' disease may be a factor, because some studies suggest a correlation between the presence of circulating thyroid autoantibodies in thyrotoxicosis and the development of hypothyroidism after surgery.[118] Hypothyroidism can be manifested during the first year after surgery, but, as with postradioiodine hypothyroidism, the incidence increases with time to approach 100%. In some patients, mild hypothyroidism appears during the early postoperative period and then remits, as also occurs after radioiodine treatment.

Hypothyroidism after destruction of thyroid tissue with radioiodine is common and is the one established disadvantage of this form of treatment for hyperthyroidism in adults. Its frequency is determined in large part by the dose of radioiodine and radioiodine uptake, but it is also influenced by other factors, including age, thyroid gland size, magnitude of thyroid hormone elevations, and use of antithyroid drugs.[119] The incidence of postradioiodine hypothyroidism increases with time, approaching 100%. Although the fT_4 is low in patients with postablative hypothyroidism, serum TSH levels may be anomalously low for several months after surgical or ^{131}I-induced hypothyroidism if TSH synthesis has been suppressed for a long period before treatment.

Primary atrophic thyroid failure may also develop in patients with Hodgkin's disease after treatment with mantle irradiation or after high-dose neck irradiation for other forms of lymphoma or carcinoma.[88,89] Surgical, radioiodine, or external-beam therapy may also lead to a state of subclinical hypothyroidism (see Table 13-2).

Congenital Causes

Thyroid Agenesis or Dysplasia

Developmental defects of the thyroid are often responsible for the hypothyroidism that occurs in 1 of every 3500 newborns.[10] These defects may take the form of complete absence of thyroid tissue or failure of the thyroid to descend properly during embryologic development. Thyroid tissue may then be found anywhere along its normal route of descent, from the foramen cecum at the junction of the anterior two thirds and posterior third of the tongue (lingual thyroid) to the normal site or below. Absence of thyroid tissue or its ectopic location can be ascertained by scintiscanning.

As indicated, a number of proteins are known to be crucial for normal thyroid gland development.[10] These include the thyroid-specific transcription factor PAX8 and thyroid transcription factors 1 and 2 (TTF1 and TTF2). It might be anticipated that defects in one or more of these proteins could explain abnormalities in thyroidal development. These have been identified in several patients with *PAX8* mutations, and a mutation in the human *TTF2* gene was associated with thyroid agenesis, cleft palate, and choanal atresia. Despite a specific search, no mutations have been found in the *TTF1* gene in infants with congenital hypothyroidism.

Thyroid Aplasia Due to Thyrotropin Receptor Unresponsiveness

Several families exist in which thyroid hypoplasia, high TSH concentrations, and a low fT_4 level are associated with loss-of-function mutations in the TSH receptor.[120] The thyroid glands were in the normal location but did not trap pertechnetate (TCO_4^-). Somewhat surprisingly, Tg levels were still detectable. The molecular details of these patients are still under study.

A second type of abnormality that could cause TSH unresponsiveness is a mutation in the G_s protein that occurs in pseudohypoparathyroidism type 1A. These patients have inactivating mutations in the α-subunit of the G_s protein and, consequently, mild hypothyroidism.[121] Other patients have been reported to have elevated TSH levels and hypothyroidism in which the molecular nature of the defect has not yet been defined.[122]

Transient Hypothyroidism

Transient hypothyroidism is defined as a period of reduced fT_4 with suppressed, normal, or elevated TSH levels that is eventually followed by a euthyroid state. This form of hypothyroidism usually occurs in the clinical context of a patient with subacute (postviral), lymphocytic (painless), or postpartum thyroiditis. These conditions are reviewed in detail in Chapter 12.

The patient reports mild to moderate symptoms of hypothyroidism of short duration, and serum TSH concentrations are typically elevated, although not greatly so. The patient often has a preceding episode of symptoms consistent with mild or moderate thyrotoxicosis. If these symptoms cannot be elucidated from the history, it may be difficult to distinguish such patients from those with a permanent form of hypothyroidism. In the early phases of post-thyroiditis hypothyroidism, TSH concentrations may still be suppressed even though the fT_4 is low because of the delayed recovery of pituitary TSH synthesis, such as in patients with Graves' disease or with toxic nodules who have undergone surgery and who have experienced rapid relief of hyperthyroidism (see Table 13-2). In the latter situation, the TSH response to hypothyroidism may be suppressed for many months; in post-thyroiditis hypothyroidism, this period is rarely longer than 3 to 4 weeks.

A significant fraction (approximately 33%) of women with autoimmune thyroiditis but normal thyroid function have episodes of hypothyroidism during the postpartum period.[81] In some, the preceding hyperthyroidism was relatively asymptomatic, which can make an accurate clinical diagnosis difficult. Patients who have had an episode of typical subacute postviral thyroiditis with pain, tenderness, and hyperthyroidism are not difficult to recognize.

Diagnostic evaluation should include a determination of TSH, fT_4, and TPO-Ab. Negative or low antibodies argue strongly for a nonautoimmune cause. This is significant, in that it may be possible for the patient to be treated only temporarily for hypothyroidism. In such patients, a trial of a lower levothyroxine dosage after 3 to 6 months may reveal that thyroid function has recovered (see Fig. 13-6). This may also occur in patients with hypothyroidism that follows acute autoimmune thyroiditis (e.g., in the postpartum period), but it is somewhat less likely to occur because of the underlying progressive nature of the autoimmune thyroiditis.

In patients with hypothyroidism due to postviral thyroiditis, the thyroid gland is usually relatively small and atrophic. In patients with hypothyroidism that follows an episode of subacute thyroiditis, the gland is usually slightly enlarged and somewhat firm, reflecting the underlying scarring and infiltration associated with that condition.

Consumptive Hypothyroidism

Consumptive hypothyroidism is the term given to an unusual cause of hypothyroidism that has been identified in infants with visceral hemangiomas or related tumors.[123,124] The first patient reported with this syndrome presented with abdominal distention caused by a large hepatic hemangioma and respiratory compromise secondary to upward displacement of the diaphragm. However, clinical signs suggested hypothyroidism, which was confirmed by finding a markedly elevated TSH level and undetectable T_4 and T_3 levels. The infant's response to an initial intravenous infusion of liothyronine (T_3) was transient, leading to the decision to use parenteral thyroid hormone replacement to relieve the clinical hypothyroidism. The accelerated degradation of thyroid hormone was apparent from the fact that it required 96 μg of liothyronine plus 50 μg of levothyroxine to normalize the TSH level. The equivalent dosage as levothyroxine alone is roughly nine times that ordinarily required for treatment of infants with congenital hypothyroidism. The infant succumbed to complications of the hemangioma, and a postmortem tumor biopsy showed D3 activity in the tumor at levels eightfold higher than those normally present in term placenta. The serum reverse T_3 was extremely elevated (400 ng/dL), and the serum Tg was greater than 1000 ng/mL, indicating the presence of a highly stimulated thyroid gland.

Retrospective search revealed two other patients with similar pathophysiology in whom the cause of the hypothyroidism had not been recognized. Significant D3 expression has now been identified in all proliferating cutaneous hemangiomas studied to date. The cutaneous hemangiomas of infancy, although they express D3, are not associated with hypothyroidism owing to their small size. Because a significant fraction of hemangiomas remit with glucocorticoid and interferon-α therapy, it is important to treat such patients with adequate doses of thyroid hormone, to prevent the permanent neurologic complications associated with untreated hypothyroidism during the critical phase of neurologic development. A similar syndrome has been identified in adults, including an epithelioid hemangioendothelioma and an individual with a fibrous tumor.[124]

Defects in Activation of Thyroxine to Triiodothyronine

The enzymes that convert the precursor T_4 to the active form, T_3, are the 5′-deiodinases, D1 and D2, both of which contain selenocysteine in their active site.[64] A stem loop structure in the 3′-untranslated region of the mRNA, termed the *SECIS element,* directs insertion of selenocysteine at the UGA codon, rather then allowing it to function as a stop codon. Defects in a SECIS-binding protein (SECISBP2) were found in two families with elevated fT_4, reduced T_3, and elevated TSH levels.[125] Affected individuals have growth retardation, compared with unaffected family members.

Polymorphisms in genes associated with thyroid hormone metabolism have been associated with patterns of thyroid function studies as well as obesity. The D2 polymorphism that substitutes an alanine for a threonine at codon 92 (Thr92Ala) has been associated with obesity, reduced glucose disposal, and lower D2 activity in skeletal muscle.[126] This polymorphism also has a higher frequency in groups with a high incidence of obesity and type 2 diabetes (i.e., Mexican Americans and Pima Indians).[126]

Hypothyroidism Due to Drug-Induced Thyroid Destruction

Thyroid inflammation or activation of autoimmune thyroid destruction has been associated with a number of drugs.[83] However, the tyrosine kinase inhibitors (e.g., sunitinib) are associated with a high incidence of hypothyroidism due to thyroid destruction.[127] Sunitinib is used to treat renal cell carcinoma and gastrointestinal stromal tumors; it inhibits multiple cellular pathways including KIT, PDGF, VEGF, and RET. An abnormal TSH was found in 62% of patients taking sunitinib after 37 weeks of follow-up.[128] Patients studied by ultrasonography demonstrated no thyroid tissue. Although 40% of hypothyroid patients initially had a suppressed TSH, suggesting thyroiditis, the long-term course was most consistent with sunitinib-induced follicular-cell apoptosis. These findings indicate that it is important to monitor thyroid function in patients taking tyrosine kinase inhibitors. These agents have now been show to slow disease progression in advanced thyroid cancers that are unresponsive to radioiodine.[129]

Central Hypothyroidism

Central hypothyroidism is the result of TSH deficiency caused by acquired or congenital hypothalamic or pituitary gland disorders. TSH deficiency caused by pituitary dysfunction is called *secondary* hypothyroidism, and that of hypothalamic origin is called *tertiary* hypothyroidism; however, this distinction is not necessary in the initial separation of primary from central hypothyroidism.

In many cases, hyposecretion of TSH is accompanied by decreased secretion of other pituitary hormones, with the result that evidence of somatotroph, gonadotroph, and corticotroph failure is also present. Hyposecretion of TSH as the sole demonstrable abnormality (monotropic deficiency) is less common but does occur in both acquired and congenital forms. Hypothyroidism due to pituitary insufficiency varies in severity from instances in which it is mild and overshadowed by features of gonadal and adrenocortical failure to those in which the features of the hypothyroid state are predominant. Because a small but significant fraction of thyroid gland function (10% to 15%) is independent of TSH, hypothyroidism due to central causes is less severe than primary hypothyroidism.

The causes of central hypothyroidism are both acquired and congenital. The general subject is discussed in Chapters 8 and 9, and those causes with relatively specific thyroid-related deficiencies are mentioned here for completeness. In addition to pituitary tumors, hypothalamic disorders, and the like, an unusual cause of secondary hypothyroidism occurs in individuals given bexarotene (a retinoid X receptor [RXR] agonist) for T-cell lymphoma.[130] This drug suppresses the activity of the human TSH β-subunit promoter in vitro. Serum T_4 concentrations are reduced by about 50%, and patients experience clinical benefit from thyroid hormone replacement. Dopamine, dobutamine, high-dose glucocorticoids, and severe illness may suppress TSH release transiently, leading to a pattern of thyroid hormone abnormalities suggesting central hypothyroidism.[130] As discussed in Chapter 11, this severe state of hypothalamic-pituitary-thyroid suppression is a manifestation of stage 3 illness (see Table 11-9 in Chapter 11). Although these agents might be expected to have similar effects when given for long periods, they do not; nor does somatostatin have a similar effect when given for acromegaly, although it does block the response of TSH to TRH and it has been administered to patients with thyrotropin-secreting pituitary adenomas.[131]

Congenital defects in stimulation or synthesis of TSH or in its structure have been identified as rare causes of congenital hypothyroidism.[10] These include defects in several of the homeobox genes, including *POU1F1* (formerly termed *Pit-1*), *PROP1*, and *HESX1*. The last gene encodes a factor that is necessary for development of the hypothalamus, pituitary, and olfactory portions of the brain. Defects in *POU1F1* and *PROP1* cause hereditary hypothyroidism, usually accompanied by deficiencies in growth hormone and prolactin.[132] One patient has been identified with a familial defect in the TRH receptor gene.[133] All of these conditions are associated with the typical pattern of central hypothyroidism, a reduced fT_4 and TSH.

Structural defects in TSH have also been described. These include a mutation in the CAGYC peptide sequence of the β-subunit, which is thought to be necessary for its association with the α-subunit,[134] and defects that produce premature termination of the TSH β-subunit gene.[135] Some of these abnormalities may be associated with elevations in TSH, suggesting the diagnosis of primary hypothyroidism, but the TSH molecule is immunologically, but not biologically, intact.

Resistance to Thyroid Hormone

The clinical manifestations of RTH depend on the nature of the mutation.[136,137] Most patients with RTH have a mutation in the gene encoding the thyroid hormone receptor β-subunit (TRβ) that interferes with the capacity of that receptor to respond normally to T_3, usually by reducing its T_3-binding affinity (see Fig. 11-7 in Chapter 11). Alternatively, patients with RTH may have hyperthyroidism if the resistance is more severe in the hypothalamic-pituitary axis than in the remainder of the tissues. In clinical terms, patients in the former group are said to have *generalized RTH*, whereas those in the latter group are said to have *pituitary RTH*. The mutations in the TRβ gene (called *THRB*) that cause RTH cluster in three areas of the thyroid hormone receptor have been recognized to have important contacts with the hydrophobic ligand-binding domain cavity of the receptor, as recognized from its crystal structure. The mutations do not interfere with the function of the DNA-binding domain or its region of heterodimerization with RXR.

RTH is probably produced by heterodimerization of the mutant TRβ with RXR or homodimerization with a normal TRβ or TRα. These mutant TRβ–containing dimers compete with wild-type dimers for binding to the thyroid hormone response elements (TREs) of thyroid hormone-dependent genes.[136] Because these complexes bind corepressor molecules that cannot be released in the absence of T_3 binding, genes containing these TREs are more repressed than they would be normally at the prevailing concentrations of circulating thyroid hormones. Receptors that contain mutations in the activation domain may have a combination of both decreased affinity for T_3 and impaired activating potential.

The mutant TRβ complex can interfere with the function of the wild-type TRs, producing a pattern termed *dominant negative inhibition* with an autosomal dominant pattern of inheritance. At least 400 families have been identified with this condition, and there are probably many more unreported cases. The gene frequency estimate is about 1 in every 50,000 persons, and study of the function of the mutant receptors in this disorder has provided valuable insights into the mechanism of thyroid hormone action.[136,137]

Patients with RTH usually are recognized because of thyroid enlargement, which is present in about two thirds of these individuals. Patients usually report a mixture of symptoms of hyperthyroidism and hypothyroidism. With respect to the heart, palpitations and tachycardia are more common than a reduced heart rate; however, patients may also demonstrate growth retardation and retarded skeletal maturation.[138] This has been attributed to the primary dependence of thyroid hormone effects in the heart on TRα rather than TRβ; in contrast, the hypothalamic-pituitary axis is primarily regulated through TRβ.

Abnormalities in neuropsychological development exist, with an increased prevalence of attention deficit-hyperactivity disorder, which is found in approximately 10% of people with RTH.[139] Other neuropsychological abnormalities have also been described.[140] Deafness in patients with RTH reflects the important role of TRβ and thyroid hormone in the normal development of auditory function. The mixture of symptoms, some suggesting hypothyroidism and others suggesting hyperthyroidism, may differ in individuals within the same family, despite the identical mutation, further confusing the clinical picture.

Because patients may present with symptoms suggesting hyperthyroidism, it is important to keep this diagnosis in mind in a patient with tachycardia, goiter, and elevated thyroid hormones. RTH is discussed here because a reduced response to thyroid hormone is the biochemical basis for the condition. However, the laboratory results may be the first clear evidence that a patient, otherwise thought to have hyperthyroidism, has RTH. These tests show the unusual combination of an increased fT_4 accompanied by normal or slightly increased TSH levels (see Table 13-2). Therefore, the principal differential diagnosis is between a TSH-secreting pituitary tumor causing hyperthyroidism and RTH.[140,141]

Factors that may assist in the differential diagnosis include absence of a family history in patients with

TSH-producing tumors, normal thyroid hormone levels in family members of individuals with TSH-induced hyperthyroidism due to pituitary tumor, and the presence of an elevated glycoprotein α-subunit in patients with pituitary tumor but not in those with RTH.

A definitive diagnosis requires sequencing of the *THRB* gene demonstrating the abnormality. Mutations in this gene are found in about 90% of individuals with a clinical diagnosis. In a few patients this is not the case, suggesting that there may be mutations in coactivator proteins or in one of the RXR receptors, leading to a similar presentation.[142]

Treatment is difficult because thyroid hormone analogues that are designed to suppress TSH and thereby relieve the hyperthyroxinemia may lead to worsening of the cardiovascular manifestations of the condition.[143] Therapy with 3,5,3′-triiodothyroacetic acid (TRIAC) has been used in several patients.[144] The development of analogues of thyroid hormone with TRβ (as opposed to mixed or TRα) preferential effects and analogues that selectively bind mutant TRs may eventually prove useful in treatment.[145]

TREATMENT

Hypothyroidism, either primary or central, is gratifying to treat because of the ease and completeness with which it responds to thyroid hormone. Treatment is almost always with levothyroxine, and the proper use of this medication has been reviewed extensively.[146-148] A primary advantage of levothyroxine therapy is that the peripheral deiodination mechanisms can continue to produce the amount of T_3 required in tissues under the normal physiologic control.[64] If one accepts the principle that replicating the natural state is the goal of hormone replacement, it is logical to provide the prohormone and allow the peripheral tissues to activate it by physiologically regulated mechanisms.

Pharmacologic and Physiologic Considerations

Levothyroxine has a 7-day half-life. About 80% of the hormone is absorbed relatively slowly and equilibrates rapidly in its distribution volume, so large postabsorptive perturbations in fT_4 levels are avoided. Because of its long half-life, omission of a single day's tablet has no significant effect, and the patient may safely take an omitted tablet on the following day. In fact, the levothyroxine dosage can be calculated almost as satisfactorily on a weekly as on a daily basis. Although T_4 is well absorbed and does not require fasting, regular ingestion of levothyroxine on an empty stomach results in the least variation in serum TSH concentration.[149]

The U.S. Food and Drug Administration (FDA) has issued standards for single-dose bioequivalence studies in normal volunteers to assess and compare T_4 products in the United States.[150] The area under the curve (AUC) confidence interval must fall within 80% to 125% of the comparison product for a preparation to be considered equivalent. The desirability of a pharmacotherapeutic measurement such as TSH as an end point has been suggested by many professional organizations.[150] Recent regulations have narrowed the guidelines for measured T_4 content, from between 90% and 110% to between 95% and 105% of the stated tablet dose, with that content maintained for the entire shelf-life.[151] The availability in many countries of a multiplicity of tablet strengths with content ranging from 25 to 300 μg allows precise titration of the daily levothyroxine dosage for most patients with a single daily tablet, improving compliance significantly.

The typical dose of levothyroxine, approximately 1.6 to 1.8 μg per kilogram of ideal body weight per day (0.7 to 0.8 μg/pound), usually results in the prescription of 75 to 112 μg/day for women and 125 to 200 μg/day for men. Replacement doses need not be adjusted upward in obese patients and should be based on lean body mass.[152] This dosage is about 20% greater than the T_4 production rate because of incomplete absorption of the levothyroxine. In patients with primary hypothyroidism, these amounts usually result in serum TSH concentrations that are within the normal range. Because of the 7-day half-life, approximately 6 weeks is required before there is complete equilibration of the fT_4 and the biologic effects of levothyroxine. Accordingly, with rare exceptions (e.g., pregnancy), assessments of the adequacy of a given dose or of the effects of a change in dosage should not be made until this interval has passed.

By and large, levothyroxine products are clinically equivalent, although problems do occur.[153] The variation in tablet content permitted by the FDA can result in slight variations in serum TSH in patients with primary hypothyroidism, even when the same brand is used. Using levothyroxine from a single manufacturer reduces variability that may be relevant for patients in whom close titration is required, such as the elderly, pregnant women, and thyroid cancer patients.[154] Although the serum TSH level is an indirect reflection of the levothyroxine effect in patients with primary hypothyroidism, it is superior to any other readily available method of assessing the adequacy of therapy. Return of the serum TSH level to normal is therefore the goal of levothyroxine therapy in patients with primary hypothyroidism. Some patients require slightly higher or lower doses than are generally used, owing to individual variations in absorption, and a number of conditions or associated medications may change levothyroxine requirements in patients with established hypothyroidism (see later discussion).

In decades past, desiccated thyroid was successfully employed for the treatment of hypothyroidism, and it still accounts for a small fraction of the prescriptions written for thyroid replacement in the United States. Although this approach was successful, desiccated thyroid preparations contain thyroid hormone derived from animal thyroid glands that have significantly higher ratios of T_3 to T_4 than the 1:11 value in normal human thyroid gland.[155] Accordingly, these unnatural preparations may lead to supraphysiologic levels of T_3 in the immediate postabsorptive period (2 to 4 hours) due to the rapid release of T_3 from Tg, its immediate and almost complete absorption, and the 1-day period required for T_3 to equilibrate with its 40-L volume of distribution (see Table 11-5 in Chapter 11).[156]

Mixtures of liothyronine and levothyroxine (*liotrix*) contain in a 1-grain (64-mg) equivalent tablet (Thyrolar-1 in the United States) the amounts of T_3 (approximately 12.5 μg) and T_4 (approximately 50 μg) present in the most popular desiccated thyroid tablet.[157] The levothyroxine equivalency of a 1-grain desiccated thyroid tablet or its liotrix equivalent can be estimated as follows. The 12.5 μg of liothyronine (T_3) is completely absorbed from desiccated thyroid or from liotrix tablets.[156] Levothyroxine is approximately 80% absorbed,[158] and about 36% of the 40 μg of levothyroxine absorbed is converted to T_3, with the molecular weight of T_3 (651) being 84% that of T_4 (777). Accordingly, a 1-grain tablet should provide about 25 μg of T_3, which would be approximately equivalent to that obtained from 100 μg of levothyroxine. This equivalency ratio can be used as an initial guide when switching patients from desiccated thyroid or liotrix to levothyroxine. Although levothyroxine is absorbed in the stomach and small intestine, normal gastric acid secretion is required for complete absorption.[159] Patients with impaired acid secretion on levothyroxine therapy require a 22% to 34% higher dose of levothyroxine to maintain the desired serum TSH. In those patients in whom acid secretion was normalized therapeutically, the levothyroxine dose returned to baseline.[159]

As indicated earlier, the use of levothyroxine for thyroid hormone replacement is a compromise with the normal pathway of T_3 production, in which about 80% of T_3 is derived from T_4 5′-monodeiodination and approximately 20% (about 6 μg) is secreted directly from the thyroid gland.[64] Studies in thyroidectomized rats, for example, show that it is not possible to normalize T_3 simultaneously in all tissues by an intravenous infusion of T_4.[160] However, it should be recalled from the earlier discussion of T_4 deiodination that the ratio of T_3/T_4 in the human thyroid gland is about 0.09, but in the rat thyroid gland it is 0.17.[64] Therefore, about 40% of the rat's daily T_3 production is derived from the thyroid, compared with about 20% in humans.[64] Accordingly, the demonstration that T_4 alone cannot provide normal levels of T_3 in all tissues in the rat is of interest but is not strictly applicable to thyroid hormone replacement in humans. Nonetheless, the ratio of T_3 to T_4 in the serum of a patient receiving levothyroxine as the only source of T_3 must be about 20% lower than that in a normal individual.

Similarly, the quantity of levothyroxine required to normalize TSH in an athyreotic patient results in a slightly higher serum fT_4 concentration than is present in normal individuals. This was shown in a comparison of thyroid function in before and after thyroidectomy in the same patient.[161] Although serum T_3 was the same level before and after thyroidectomy, a higher serum T_4 concentration was necessary when the patient was on T_4 replacement to maintain the same serum T_3 level.[161] Although this may, to some extent, compensate for the lack of T_3 secretion, the fact that T_4 has an independent mechanism for TSH suppression, owing to the intracellular generation of T_3 in the hypothalamic-pituitary-thyroid axis, means that a portion of the feedback regulation is independent of the plasma T_3 concentration.

Although the concept of combined T_4/T_3 therapy has been recognized for many years, a positive study published in 1999 generated a great deal of interest in this approach.[162] Patients received 12.5 μg of T_3 as a substitution for 50 μg of their levothyroxine preparation and scored, on average, somewhat higher on tests of mood than when they were taking levothyroxine alone. The dosage of thyroid hormone used in these studies was excessive, as judged by the fact that 20% of the group had serum TSH values below normal on either regimen, and the test period was only a few months. Since this report, a large number of studies using a wide range of replacement strategies and relative T_4/T_3 content have been performed in different populations, and none has shown an advantage for combination therapy over T_4 alone.[163]

On the other hand, another study showed that the fT_4 index correlated as closely as TSH levels with the resting energy expenditure in a group of patients in whom small supplements or decrements in their ideal replacement levothyroxine dosage were made.[164] The correlation with serum T_3 was not statistically significant, suggesting that in humans, perhaps because of differences in peripheral metabolism of T_4 compared with rodents, the fT_4 index may be as accurate as the TSH value as an index of satisfactory thyroid hormone replacement. The practical difficulty with the design of tablets providing combinations of T_3 and T_4 is that the approximate dose of 6 μg of T_3 provided would need to be released in a sustained fashion over 24 hours, which is quite different from the rapid absorption of T_3 (with a peak at 2 to 4 hours) when given in its conventional form. Therefore, it appears that the current approach to thyroid replacement using levothyroxine alone, although not a perfect replication of the normal physiology, is satisfactory for most patients. A sustained-release T_3 preparation has been developed and produces more stable levels of serum T_3.[165] The clinical consequence of this more "physiologic" replacement profile is not known.

Institution of Replacement Therapy

The initial dose of levothyroxine prescribed depends on the degree of hypothyroidism and the age and general health of the patient. Patients who are young or middle age and otherwise healthy with no associated cardiovascular or other abnormalities and mild to moderate hypothyroidism (TSH concentrations, 5 to 50 mU/L) can be given an initial complete replacement dose of about 1.7 μg per kilogram of ideal body weight. The resulting increase in serum T_4 concentration to normal requires 5 to 6 weeks, and the biologic effects of T_3 are sufficiently delayed so that these patients do not experience adverse effects. At the other extreme, an elderly patient who has heart disease, particularly angina pectoris, without reversible coronary lesions should be given a small initial dose of levothyroxine (25 μg/day), and the dosage should be increased in 12.5-μg increments at 2- to 3-month intervals with careful clinical and laboratory evaluation.

The goal in the patient with primary hypothyroidism is to return serum TSH concentrations to normal, reflecting normalization of that patient's thyroid hormone supply. This usually results in a midnormal to high-normal serum fT_4 concentration. The serum TSH should be evaluated 6 weeks after a theoretically complete replacement dose has been instituted, followed by minor adjustments to optimize the individual dose.[166] In patients with central hypothyroidism, serum TSH is not a reliable index of adequate replacement and the serum fT_4 should be restored to a concentration in the upper half of the normal range. T_4 dosing based on body weight and a serum fT_4 in the upper reference range was found to improve markers of thyroid hormone action and was superior to replacement with a combination of T_4/T_3.[167] Patients with central hypothyroidism should also be evaluated and treated for glucocorticoid deficiency, if necessary, before institution of thyroid replacement (see Chapter 9).

Although the adverse effects of the rapid institution of therapy are unusual, pseudotumor cerebri has been reported in profoundly hypothyroid juveniles (8 and 12 years of age) who were given even modest initial levothyroxine replacement.[168] This complication appears 1 to 10 months after initiation of treatment and responds to treatment with acetazolamide and dexamethasone.

The interval between initiation of treatment and the first evidence of improvement depends on the strength of dose given and the degree of the deficit. An early clinical response in moderate to severe hypothyroidism is a diuresis of 2 to 4 kg. The serum sodium level increases even sooner if hyponatremia was present initially. Thereafter, pulse rate and pulse pressure increase, appetite improves, and constipation may disappear. Later, psychomotor activity increases and the delay in the deep tendon reflex disappears. Hoarseness abates slowly, and changes in skin and hair do not disappear for several months. In individuals started on a complete replacement dose, the serum fT_4 level should normalize after 6 weeks; a somewhat longer period may be necessary for serum TSH levels to return to normal, perhaps up to 3 months.

In some cases, it is clinically appropriate to alleviate hypothyroidism rapidly. For example, patients with severe hypothyroidism withstand acute infections or other serious illnesses poorly, and myxedema coma (discussed later) may develop as a complication. In such circumstances, rapid near-repletion of the peripheral hormone pool in the average adult can be accomplished by a single intravenous dose of 500 μg levothyroxine. Alternatively, because of its rapid onset of action, liothyronine (25 μg orally every 12 hours) may be administered if the patient can take medication by mouth. With both approaches, an initial biologic effect is achieved within 24 hours. Parenteral therapy with levothyroxine is then continued with a dose that is 80% of the appropriate oral dose but not in excess of 1.4 μg/kg of ideal body weight. Because of the possibility that rapid increases in metabolic rate will overtax the existing pituitary-adrenocortical reserve, supplemental glucocorticoid (intravenous hydrocortisone, 5 mg/hour) should also be given to patients with severe hypothyroidism who are receiving high initial doses of thyroid hormones. Finally, in view of the tendency of hypothyroid patients to retain free water, intravenous fluids containing only dextrose should not be given.

When replacement therapy is withdrawn for short periods (4 to 6 weeks) for the purpose of evaluating therapy for thyroid cancer, rapid reinstitution of levothyroxine using a loading dose of three times the daily replacement dose for 3 days can usually be given, unless other complicating medical illnesses are present.

When hypothyroidism results from administration of iodine-containing or anti-thyroid drugs, withdrawal of the offending agent usually relieves both the hypothyroidism and the accompanying goiter, although it is appropriate to provide interim replacement until the gland recovers its function. This is especially true for amiodarone, which can remain in tissues for up to 1 year.

Therapy in Infants and Children

In infants with congenital hypothyroidism, the determining factor for eventual intellectual attainment is the age at which adequate treatment with thyroid hormone is begun.[10,169] The therapy in infants with congenital hypothyroidism should consist initially of raising the serum T_4 level to more than 130 nmol/L (10 μg/dL) as rapidly as possible and maintaining it at that level for the first 3 to 4 years of life. This is usually accomplished by administering an initial levothyroxine dose of 50 μg/day, which is higher than the adult dose on a weight basis and in keeping with the higher metabolic clearance of the hormone in the infant. The serum TSH concentration may not return to normal even with this high dose because of residual reset of the pituitary feedback mechanism. After 2 years of age, a TSH level in the normal range is an index of optimal therapy, as it is in adults.[170]

Monitoring Replacement Therapy

Monitoring the adequacy of, and compliance with, thyroid hormone therapy in patients with primary hypothyroidism is easily done by measuring serum TSH. This value should be within the normal range when determined by an assay that is sufficiently sensitive to measure, with confidence, the lower limit of the normal range. The normal serum TSH concentration varies between 0.5 and 4.0 mU/L in most second- and third-generation assays, and results within this range are associated with elimination of all clinical and biochemical manifestations of primary hypothyroidism, except in patients with RTH. Based on analysis of the National Health and Nutrition Examination Surveys III (NHANES III) reference group,[5] a reference TSH range with an upper limit of 2.5 mU/L has been suggested. However, this adjustment would identify a large number of individuals as having abnormal thyroid function without providing a clear indication of the clinical significance of TSH levels in this range.[171] A more recent analysis, based on age-specific references ranges, indicated that older adults without thyroid autoantibodies have an increased upper-limit TSH value (>4.5 mU/L) that is not associated with thyroid disease.[172] In related studies, this progressive shift with age to higher levels of TSH was associated with extreme longevity in several populations.[173]

After the first 6 months of therapy, the dose should be reassessed, because restoration of euthyroidism increases the metabolic clearance of T_4. A dose that was adequate during the early phases of therapy may not be adequate when the same patient is euthyroid owing to an acceleration in the clearance of thyroid hormone.

Under usual circumstances, the finding of a normal serum TSH level on an annual basis is adequate to ensure that the proper levothyroxine dose is being taken by the patient. If the serum TSH level is above the normal range and noncompliance is not the explanation, small adjustments, usually in 12-μg increments, can be made, with reassessment of TSH concentrations after the 6 weeks required for full equilibration have passed. In North America, this strategy is simplified by the availability of multiple tablet strengths, many of which differ by only 12 μg. Most patients can receive the same dose until they reach the seventh or eighth decade, at which point a downward adjustment of 20% to 30% is indicated because thyroid hormone clearance decreases in the elderly.

Thyroid hormone requirements may be altered in several situations (Table 13-3). A reduction in replacement dosage may be required in women who are receiving androgen therapy for adjuvant treatment of breast carcinoma.[174] Most other conditions or medications increase the levothyroxine requirement in patients receiving maintenance therapy. During pregnancy, the levothyroxine requirement is increased by 25% to 50% in most hypothyroid women,[175] and prospective study has demonstrated that the increased requirement occurs early in the first trimester.[176] The increment of increase is higher in athyreotic patients compared to those with autoimmune hypothyroidism.[177] Athyreotic patients who are planning a pregnancy should be advised to increase their dose by about 30% as soon as the diagnosis is confirmed, because the change in requirement appears soon after implantation. The increased requirement probably results from a combination of factors, including increases in T_4-binding globulin and the volume of distribution of T_4, an increase in body mass, and an increase in D3 in placenta and perhaps in the uterus.[64,124] The increased requirement persists throughout pregnancy but returns to normal within a few weeks after delivery. Therefore, the dose should be reduced to the original, prepregnancy level at the time of delivery. Maternal T_4 is critically important to the athyreotic fetus and to the normal fetus in the first trimester,

TABLE 13-3

Conditions That Alter Levothyroxine Requirements

Increased Levothyroxine Requirements
Pregnancy
Gastrointestinal Disorders
Mucosal diseases of the small bowel (e.g., sprue)
After jejunoileal bypass and small-bowel resection
Impaired gastric acid secretion (e.g., atrophic gastritis)
Diabetic diarrhea
Drugs That Interfere with Levothyroxine Absorption
Cholestyramine
Sucralfate
Aluminum hydroxide
Calcium carbonate
Ferrous sulfate
Drugs That Increase the Cytochrome P450 Enzyme (CYP3A4) Activity
Rifampin
Carbamazepine
Estrogen
Phenytoin
Sertraline
Drugs That Block T_4-to-T_3 Conversion
Amiodarone
Conditions That May Block Deiodinase Synthesis
Selenium deficiency
Cirrhosis
Decreased Levothyroxine Requirements
Aging (≥65 yr)
Androgen therapy in women

T_4, Thyroxine; T_3, triiodothyronine.

before the thyroid gland develops.[178] Maternal hypothyroidism has been associated with fetal loss, preterm delivery, and intellectual deficit in the offspring.[49-51,97] These findings are not seen in hypothyroid women on T_4 replacement sufficient to normalize their TSH, suggesting that these associations are directly related to maternal thyroid hormone status. A randomized, prospective study in pregnant women with TPO-Ab and normal-range TSH demonstrated the benefit of levothyroxine treatment to prevent these complications.[51]

Other conditions in which levothyroxine requirements are increased (see Table 13-3) include malabsorption due to bowel disease, impaired gastric acid secretion,[159] and adsorption of levothyroxine to coadministered medications such as sucralfate, aluminum hydroxide, and calcium carbonate,[179] ferrous sulfate,[180] lovastatin,[181] or various resins.[182] Certain medications, notably rifampin,[183] carbamazepine,[184] phenytoin,[185] and sertraline,[186] increase the clearance of levothyroxine by inducing cytochrome P450 isoenzyme 3A4 (CYP3A4) in the liver. Estrogen given to postmenopausal women may act in the same way, although the changes in Tg and distribution volume make exact resolution of the cause of the increased levothyroxine requirement uncertain.[187] Soy protein and soybean isoflavones have been proposed to interfere directly with thyroid hormone action as well as synthetic T_4 absorption.[188] There is no evidence that soy interferes with thyroid function in euthyroid individuals who are iodine sufficient, and the effect of soy on T_4 absorption in hypothyroid patients is modest.[188] Amiodarone increases levothyroxine requirements by blocking conversion of T_4 to T_3 and perhaps by interfering with T_3–thyroid hormone receptor binding.[189] Selenium deficiency is rare, but because it is rate-limiting in the synthesis of D1 (see Fig. 11-6 in Chapter 11),[64] a deficiency, such as may occur in patients receiving diets restricted in protein, may increase levothyroxine requirements.[190]

Occasionally in patients who have been treated with radioactive iodine for Graves' disease or toxic nodular goiter, some degree of thyroid hormone secretion persists; although it is insufficient to sustain normal thyroid hormone levels, it is autonomous. Such patients may have a suppressed TSH despite what otherwise would be considered a replacement dose of levothyroxine. The levothyroxine dose in these individuals should be reduced until TSH levels rise to normal, keeping in mind that several months may be required before TSH secretion recovers after its prolonged suppression. Because of either the delayed effects of radioiodine or the natural history of Graves' disease per se, this autonomous T_4 secretion may decrease with time, leading to an increase in levothyroxine requirements in subsequent years. Rarely, the opposite occurs; that is, a patient treated with radioiodine develops an increased TSH level, but after several months of therapy, the requirement for replacement is reduced or eliminated. This may reflect transient impairment of thyroid function by a combination of pre-irradiation anti-thyroid drug therapy and immediate but transient effects of irradiation on the thyroid. In such patients, frequent monitoring of levothyroxine replacement is required to avoid overreplacement.

In North America, based on the recent changes in assessment of levothyroxine bioequivalence (see earlier discussion), the possibility of a difference in tablet levothyroxine content should be considered if a new preparation changes the biologic or biochemical effects of the same dosage. Although the difference in preparation is unlikely to cause a significant difference in most patients, the change in manufacturer introduces another potential source of variability.[154]

Adverse Effects of Levothyroxine Therapy

Although the administration of excessive doses of levothyroxine causes accelerated bone loss in postmenopausal patients, most authorities believe that returning thyroid status to normal does not have adverse effects on bone density.[191] Administration of excessive doses also increases cardiac wall thickness and contractility, and in elderly patients it increases the risk of atrial fibrillation.[14,17]

In some patients, TSH levels remain elevated despite the prescription of adequate replacement doses. This is most often a consequence of poor adherence. The combination of normal or even elevated serum fT_4 values and elevated TSH levels can occur if the patient does not take levothyroxine regularly but ingests several pills the day before testing. The integrated dose of levothyroxine over prior weeks is best reflected in the serum TSH level, and nonadherent patients require careful education as to the rationale for treatment. Subtle changes in dietary habits, such as increased ingestion of bran-containing products, soy, or calcium, may decrease levothyroxine absorption, and their recognition requires a careful history.[179,188]

Patients with Hypothyroid Symptoms Despite Restitution of Normal Thyroid Function

Symptoms consistent with hypothyroidism may persist in patients taking levothyroxine replacement who have a normal-range serum TSH concentration. In a survey asking patients about symptoms that might be associated with thyroid hormone deficiency,[192] such symptoms were reported by both control patients and those on levothyroxine replacement with normal-range serum TSH, but by a greater fraction of patients in the latter group. Such patients should be educated about the symptoms of hypothyroidism and the role of thyroid hormone in relieving them, and other causes should be sought for the symptomatology. In rare cases, hypothyroid symptoms are associated with hypometabolism despite normal levels of serum thyroid hormones and TSH.[193] These patients may have RTH in peripheral but not central tissues, a situation that has been documented only rarely.

SPECIAL ASPECTS OF HYPOTHYROIDISM

Subclinical Hypothyroidism

The term *subclinical hypothyroidism* was originally used to describe the patient with a low-normal fT_4 but a slightly elevated serum TSH level. Other terms for this condition are *mild hypothyroidism, early thyroid failure, preclinical hypothyroidism,* and *decreased thyroid reserve* (see Table 13-2). The TSH elevation in such patients is modest, with values typically between 4 and 15 mU/L, although those patients with a TSH greater than 10 mU/L more often have a reduced fT_4 and may have some hypothyroid symptoms. The definition of this syndrome depends significantly on the reference range for a normal TSH concentration. The syndrome is most often seen in patients with early Hashimoto's disease and is a common phenomenon, occurring in 7% to 10% of older women.[4-6]

A number of studies on the effects of thyroid hormone treatment in such patients have used physiologic end points (e.g., measurements of various serum enzymes, systolic time intervals, serum lipids, psychometric testing), and results have been variable. In the most carefully controlled studies, one or another of the parameters has returned to normal in 25% to 50% of patients.[6,22] In general, fT_4 and TSH levels normalize, but free T_3, usually normal at the outset, does not change. In one study that employed a double-blind, crossover approach, the 4 of 17 women who improved could be differentiated from the remainder only by a somewhat lower serum free T_3 at the start of the study.[194] Modest improvements in cardiac indices and lipid profiles have been noted in most but not all studies.[6,22] Association of mild hypothyroidism with an increased risk for atherosclerotic heart disease has been shown by some but not other studies.[6,22] The impact of treatment to reduce the risk of atherosclerotic heart disease, other than reduction in risk factors such as cholesterol and C-reactive protein, have not yet been studied.

One factor favoring a decision to recommend levothyroxine therapy is the likelihood of development of overt hypothyroidism. The risk of progression from *subclinical* to *overt* hypothyroidism (i.e., with elevated serum TSH and reduced serum fT_4 concentrations) is most closely related to the magnitude of serum TSH elevation and the presence of TPO-Ab. Prospective studies of women with subclinical hypothyroidism have shown rates of progression ranging from approximately 3% to 8% per year, with the higher rates seen in individuals with initial TSH concentrations greater than 10 mU/L and in those with positive TPO-Ab.[7] Although most patients progress slowly to overt hypothyroidism, rapid progression over weeks to months has been reported.[195] Factors that may predispose to rapid progression include elderly age, high levels of TPO-Ab, intercurrent systemic infection or inflammation, iodinated contrast agents, and medications such as amiodarone and lithium.

The decision to treat with levothyroxine must also take into account the expense and inconvenience of a daily medication, which is not acceptable to some patients, and the possibility that overdosage with levothyroxine may exacerbate osteoporosis or cause cardiac arrhythmias. Ultimately, the decision to treat must depend on a careful consideration of the individual clinical situation and patient preference.[9] If a therapeutic trial is performed, the TSH concentration should be monitored carefully and should not be reduced below normal. If no therapy is given, patients should be monitored at intervals of 6 to 12 months, both clinically and by measurements of serum TSH.

Metabolic Insufficiency

Nonspecific symptoms of true hypothyroidism include mild lassitude, fatigue, slight anemia, constipation, apathy, cold intolerance, menstrual irregularities, loss of hair, and weight gain (see Fig. 13-5). Some patients with such complaints who have normal laboratory results for thyroid function have been considered candidates for levothyroxine therapy. The response to thyroid hormone therapy is sometimes gratifying, at least initially, but symptomatic improvement usually disappears after a time unless the dose is increased. Eventually, even larger doses fail to alleviate the symptoms, confirming that they do not arise from a deficiency of thyroid hormone.

Therefore, thyroid hormone therapy should be avoided in patients for whom there is no biochemical documentation of impaired thyroid function. Furthermore, even in patients with subclinical hypothyroidism, symptoms may be out of proportion to abnormalities in the fT_4 concentration. It is unwise to raise a patient's expectations that such symptoms will be relieved by correction of mild biochemical abnormalities.

Thyroid Function Testing in Patients Receiving Replacement Therapy for Unclear Reasons

Physicians are frequently confronted with patients who are receiving levothyroxine in whom the basis for the diagnosis cannot be established. It is often difficult to obtain previous clinical findings or laboratory data to determine whether thyroid hormone replacement is indicated. If serum TSH is in the normal range and primary hypothyroidism is suspected, a simple method of assessing the need for levothyroxine therapy is to switch levothyroxine to an every-other-day dosage or to reduce the daily dose by 50% and reevaluate TSH and fT_4 after 4 weeks. If there has been no significant increase in TSH concentration and fT_4 remains constant during that period, residual thyroid function is present, although it may still not be completely normal. To definitively answer this question, levothyroxine can then be withdrawn and blood tests repeated 4 to 8 weeks later.

If the initial TSH level is suppressed, indicating overreplacement, the levothyroxine dose should be reduced until TSH becomes detectable before this trial is instituted. If central hypothyroidism is suspected, the fT_4 must be monitored during these procedures.

Emergent Surgery in the Hypothyroid Patient

The perioperative course of patients with untreated hypothyroidism has been evaluated in several studies. In general, such patients were not recognized to be hypothyroid or did not require surgery despite the presence of significant hypothyroidism. Complications were uncommon. Perioperative hypotension, ileus, and central nervous system disturbances were more common in hypothyroid patients, and patients with major infections had fewer episodes of fever than did euthyroid control subjects.[196] Other complications were delayed recovery from anesthesia and abnormal hemostasis, possibly owing to an acquired form of von Willebrand's disease.[27]

From these studies, one may conclude that emergent surgery should not be postponed in hypothyroid patients but that such patients should be rigorously monitored for evidence of carbon dioxide retention, bleeding, infection, and hyponatremia. These findings are also relevant to the treatment of symptomatic coronary artery disease in hypothyroid individuals. Considering the lack of significant increase in perioperative complications, the option of surgery for remediable coronary artery lesions is open to hypothyroid individuals without the risk of a myocardial infarction in association with restitution of the euthyroid state (see later discussion).[197]

HEART DISEASE AND THYROID HORMONE THERAPY

Coexisting Coronary Artery Disease and Hypothyroidism

In many patients with coronary artery disease and primary hypothyroidism, cardiac function is improved in response to levothyroxine therapy because of a decrease in peripheral vascular resistance and improvement in myocardial function.[14,15] However, patients with preexisting angina pectoris should be evaluated for correctable lesions of the coronary arteries and treated appropriately before levothyroxine is administered.[197,198] Retrospective studies indicate that this approach is safer than the institution of replacement therapy before angiography and angioplasty or even coronary artery bypass grafting (CABG).[198,199]

In a few patients, lesions are not remediable or small-vessel disease is severe even after bypass grafting, so that complete replacement cannot be instituted. Such patients must receive optimal anti-anginal therapy combined with β-adrenergic receptor blockers in judicious quantities, and complete restitution of the euthyroid state may not be possible.

Thyroid Hormone for Compromised Cardiovascular Function

In addition to the issues raised in patients with combined hypothyroidism and coronary artery disease, there is interest in the potential therapeutic use of thyroid hormone in patients with cardiomyopathy and in those who have undergone CABG or other cardiac procedures.[14,15,199] As expected, T_3 levels are reduced in patients with advanced congestive heart failure, as with any illness. In one report, 23 patients with advanced heart failure (mean ejection fraction, 22%) were given up to 2.7 μg/kg of liothyronine over 6 hours and experienced increased cardiac output and decreased systemic vascular resistance but without an increase in heart or metabolic rate.[200] Similar effects were seen with a dose of liothyronine, 110 μg, administered over 6 hours after CABG.[199]

Liothyronine has also been given postoperatively for congenital heart disease; again, an improvement in cardiac output and a decrease in vascular resistance occurred without adverse side effects.[201] These results suggest that, in certain selected circumstances, liothyronine may be useful as adjunctive therapy in patients with congestive heart failure because of its effect of relaxing vascular smooth muscle.

Although most therapeutic trials of thyroid hormone treatment have used T_3, thyroid hormone analogues have also been used.[145] The most extensively studied one is 3,5-diiodothyropropionic acid (DITPA), an analogue that binds both TRα and TRβ with low affinity. A randomized study of DITPA in heart failure showed some improved cardiac performance, but the study was terminated due to significant metabolic side effects including weight loss.[202]

SCREENING FOR PRIMARY HYPOTHYROIDISM

The utility of screening for hypothyroidism has been addressed by a number of studies but remains controversial.[203] The conclusions depend, to a great extent, on assumptions regarding the effectiveness and economic value of identifying and treating patients with subclinical hypothyroidism.[8,204] One study concluded that the cost of TSH determinations performed every 5 years for women and men would be approximately $9000 per quality-adjusted life-year in women.[204] An evidenced-based medicine review of the literature by an expert panel concluded that there was insufficient evidence to support population-based screening.[8] Aggressive case finding, based on identification of risk factors such as family history, was advocated for pregnant women, women older than 60 years of age, and others at high risk. However, the fraction of patients with hypothyroidism missed when a case finding strategy is used is not known. A report from the U.S. Preventive Services Task Force also concluded that population screening for hypothyroidism in nonpregnant adults was not justified.[203] Large, randomized, prospective studies of levothyroxine treatment in patients with subclinical hypothyroidism to establish benefit have not yet been performed. Given the very high incidence of hypothyroidism in older women and the absence of robust clinical symptoms, an assessment of TSH levels at 5-year intervals in women older than 50 years of age seems justified until more extensive studies have been performed.

A second complex issue involves whether women planning pregnancy should be screened for hypothyroidism as a routine part of a prenatal visit. This question is raised because of the increasing association of adverse outcomes in pregnancy with even subclinical hypothyroidism, including impairment of mental development in infants of hypothyroid mothers, fetal loss, and preterm delivery.[49-51] The prevalence of overt hypothyroidism during pregnancy is approximately 2%,[205] and screening of all patients has been advocated by several professional organizations. Thyroid testing in high-risk patients (case finding), has been advocated, although a prospective study showed that approximately one third of pregnant women with underlying thyroid disease are missed by this testing approach.[207]

Maternal fT_4 concentrations in the lowest 10% of the normal range, even with normal TSH levels, have also been suggested as a risk factor for impaired neuropsychological development of the fetus.[206] It is not clear why this is a risk factor for impaired fetal neuropsychological development, because such patients are not hypothyroid.

A number of questions have been raised regarding the appropriate timing of testing, whether thyroid autoantibodies should be measured, the relative importance of TSH and fT_4, the influence of trimester on the normal ranges, and the appropriate threshold for intervention.[208] The association of maternal subclinical hypothyroidism and preterm delivery[46] is a much more proximal and defined end point to study, compared with intellectual performance in offspring. The morbidity and mortality from preterm delivery is significant for the newborn, and these findings are likely to allow for more focused intervention studies to determine the response to T_4 treatment.

For the moment, it appears that any patient with a family history of autoimmune thyroid disease who has symptoms suggesting hypothyroidism or thyroid enlargement should be tested for thyroid dysfunction before pregnancy or as soon after conception as is feasible. If it is possible, optimization of levothyroxine therapy for women known to have hypothyroidism before conception may be the most effective intervention to prevent hypothyroid-related complications of pregnancy. Although the data do not yet reach the threshold to mandate universal screening, the ease of testing, associated adverse outcomes, and demonstrated benefit of intervention make thyroid testing of all pregnant women a reasonable choice.

MYXEDEMA COMA

Myxedema coma is the ultimate stage of severe, long-standing hypothyroidism.[209,210] This state, which almost exclusively affects older patients, occurs most commonly during the winter months and is associated with a high mortality rate. It is usually accompanied by a subnormal temperature; values as low as 23° C have been recorded. The external manifestations of severe myxedema, bradycardia, and severe hypotension are invariably present. The characteristic delay in deep tendon reflexes may be lacking if the patient is areflexic. Seizures may accompany the comatose state. Although the pathogenesis of myxedema coma is not clear, factors that predispose to its development include exposure to cold, infection, trauma, and use of central nervous system depressants or anesthetics. Alveolar hypoventilation, leading to carbon dioxide retention and narcosis, and dilutional hyponatremia, resembling that seen with inappropriate secretion of arginine vasopressin (AVP), may also contribute to the clinical state.

From the foregoing, it appears that myxedema coma should be readily recognized from its clinical signs, but this is not the case. After a brain stem infarction, elderly patients with features suggestive of hypothyroidism may be both comatose and hypothermic. In addition, hypothermia of any cause (e.g., exposure to cold) may cause changes suggestive of myxedema, including delayed relaxation of deep tendon reflexes. The importance of the difficulty in diagnosing myxedema coma is that a delay in therapy worsens the prognosis. Consequently, a rapid serum T_4 measurement should be obtained on an emergency basis whenever possible. Otherwise, the diagnosis should be made on clinical grounds. After serum is sent for thyroid function tests, therapy should be initiated without awaiting the results of delayed confirmatory tests, because the mortality rate can be 20% or higher.

Treatment consists of administration of thyroid hormone and correction of the associated physiologic disturbances.[209-211] Because of the sluggish circulation and severe hypometabolism, absorption of therapeutic agents from the gut or from subcutaneous or intramuscular sites is unpredictable, and medications should be administered intravenously if possible. Administration of levothyroxine as a single intravenous dose of 500 to 800 μg serves to replete the peripheral hormone pool and may cause improvement within hours. Daily doses of intravenous levothyroxine, 100 μg, are given thereafter. Hydrocortisone (5 to 10 mg/hour) should also be given because of the possibility of relative adrenocortical insufficiency as the metabolic rate increases.

Alternatively, intravenous liothyronine may be given at a dose of 25 μg every 12 hours. Others have used a combination of 200 to 300 μg T_4 and 25 μg T_3 intravenously as a single dose, followed by 25 μg T_3 and 100 μg T_4 24 hours later and then 50 μg T_4 daily until the patient regains consciousness. *Hypotonic* fluids should not be given because of the danger of water intoxication owing to the reduced free water clearance of the hypothyroid patient. *Hypertonic* saline and glucose may be required to alleviate severe dilutional hyponatremia and the occasional hypoglycemia.

A critical element in therapy is support of respiratory function by means of assisted ventilation and controlled oxygen administration. Internal warming by gastric perfusion may be useful, but external warming should be avoided because it may lead to vascular collapse due to peripheral vasodilatation. Further heat loss can be prevented with blankets. An increase in temperature may be seen within 24 hours in response to levothyroxine. General measures applicable to the comatose patient should be undertaken, such as frequent turning, prevention of aspiration, and attention to fecal impaction and urinary retention.

Finally, the physician should assess the patient for the presence of coexisting disease, such as infection, cardiac disease, or cerebrovascular disease. In particular, the myxedematous patient may be afebrile despite the presence of a significant infection. As soon as the patient is able to take medication by mouth, treatment with oral levothyroxine should be instituted.

THYROIDITIS

Thyroiditis is a term indicating the presence of thyroid inflammation. It therefore comprises a large group of diverse inflammatory conditions: autoimmune or quasiautoimmune causes and viral or postviral conditions and infections, including those of bacterial and fungal origins; a chronic sclerosing form of thyroiditis, termed *Riedel's thyroiditis* (or struma); and miscellaneous causes of various types, including radiation-induced and granulomatous causes (e.g., sarcoidosis), as well as lithium-related thyroid disease.[212]

Not only are the causes of thyroiditis extremely varied, but their clinical presentations may also be diverse and are difficult to categorize in a simple fashion (Table 13-4). For example, autoimmune thyroiditis may manifest with hypothyroidism, but often patients remain euthyroid for long periods after the disease is initiated. On the other hand, if a euthyroid patient with Hashimoto's disease becomes pregnant, the postpartum period is often complicated by an acute form of hyperthyroidism caused by the transient exacerbation of thyroiditis, often followed by a period of hypothyroidism (see Chapter 12).

In nonpregnant patients, a similar syndrome, called *silent* or *painless thyroiditis,* is manifested primarily as thyrotoxicosis of sudden onset without localized pain and

TABLE 13-4

Causes of Thyroiditis

Autoimmune thyroiditis
Postpartum, silent, or painless thyroiditis (see Chapter 12)
Subacute (nonsuppurative) thyroiditis (see Chapter 12)
Acute infectious thyroiditis
Riedel's thyroiditis
Postirradiation (^{131}I or external-beam therapy) thyroiditis
Sarcoidosis

often without evidence of autoimmune disease. This condition may be viral in origin in some patients; however, the most classic presentation of viral thyroiditis is as *subacute, nonsuppurative thyroiditis,* also known as *de Quervain's thyroiditis, pseudotuberculous thyroiditis,* and *migratory* or *creeping thyroiditis*. Unlike typical autoimmune thyroiditis, this condition is characterized by extreme thyroid tenderness, with pain radiating to the oropharynx and ears, and must be differentiated from acute suppurative thyroiditis caused by bacterial or fungal infection.[213]

Inflammatory conditions of the thyroid present a dilemma because one must decide whether to discuss these entities as a group with the common denominator of inflammation or to categorize them according to their principal clinical effects, namely thyrotoxicosis or thyroid hormone deficiency. We have chosen the latter approach and have already discussed autoimmune thyroiditis, the major cause of thyroid gland failure (see Table 13-1). However, patients with acute autoimmune thyroiditis may also develop thyrotoxicosis (e.g., in postpartum silent thyroiditis, painless thyroiditis) (see Chapter 12). These patients must be differentiated from those with Graves' disease.

In addition, some patients with viral thyroiditis have thyrotoxicosis as a major manifestation, with varying degrees of neck discomfort ranging from none to full-blown subacute, nonsuppurative (granulomatous) thyroiditis. For that reason, this thyroiditis syndrome is also discussed in Chapter 12, even though the pain associated with the typical form of this condition makes the principal differential diagnosis lie between that and pyogenic thyroiditis. In that context, subacute thyroiditis is also mentioned later in this chapter.

ACUTE INFECTIOUS THYROIDITIS

Although the thyroid gland is remarkably resistant to infection, congenital abnormalities of the piriform sinus, underlying autoimmune disease, or immunocompromise of the host may lead to the development of an infectious disease of the thyroid gland.[213,214] The etiology can involve any bacterium, including *Staphylococcus, Pneumococcus, Salmonella,* or *Mycobacterium tuberculosis*.[213,215,216] In addition, infections with certain fungi, including *Coccidioides immitis, Candida, Aspergillus,* and *Histoplasma,* have been reported.[217]

The most common cause of repeated childhood pyogenic thyroiditis, particularly in the left lobe, is an internal fistula extending from the piriform sinus to the thyroid.[218,219] This sinus is the residual connection remaining along the path of migration of the ultimobranchial body from the fifth pharyngeal pouch to the thyroid gland. The predominance of thyroiditis of the left lobe is explained by the fact that the right ultimobranchial body is often atrophic, whereas this is not the case for the left side. Nonetheless, bacterial thyroiditis can develop in a patient with a completely normal thyroid gland. This is an extremely rare disease even as a complication of direct puncture of the thyroid gland (e.g., in fine-needle aspiration). In individuals with midline infections, persistence of the thyroglossal duct should be considered.

Incidence

Infectious thyroiditis is extremely rare, with no more than a few cases being seen in large tertiary care centers.

Clinical Manifestations

The clinical manifestations of infectious thyroiditis are dominated by local pain and tenderness in the affected lobe or in the entire gland. This is accompanied by painful swallowing and difficulty swallowing. Because of the tendency for referral of pain to the pharynx or ear, the patient may not recognize the tenderness in the anterior neck. Depending on the virulence of the organism and the presence of septicemia, symptoms such as fever and chills may also accompany the condition.

The major differential diagnosis lies between an infectious form of thyroiditis and subacute, nonsuppurative thyroiditis. It is instructive to compare the principal features of these two diseases to arrive at an accurate diagnosis (Table 13-5). By and large, patients with acute thyroiditis caused by a bacterium are much sicker than patients with subacute thyroiditis; they have more severe and localized tenderness and are less likely to have laboratory evidence of hyperthyroidism, which is present in approximately 60% of patients with subacute thyroiditis. Ultrasonographic examination often reveals the abscess in the thyroid gland or evidence of swelling, and needle aspiration may help pinpoint the responsible organism. A gallium scan will be positive as a result of the diffuseness of the inflammation. Particularly in children with thyroiditis of the left lobe, a barium swallow showing a fistula connecting the piriform sinus and the left lobe of the thyroid is diagnostic.[220,221]

Occasionally, pertechnetate scanning is useful in showing normal function in one lobe of the thyroid gland, which is much less common in subacute thyroiditis (which more often affects the entire gland). Needle aspiration should be used to drain the affected lobe, although occasionally surgical drainage is required. If a piriform sinus fistula can be demonstrated, it must be removed to prevent recurrence of the problem.

Antibiotics should be administered as appropriate for the offending organism. Fungal infections should be treated appropriately, especially because many of these patients are immunocompromised. Endemic organisms should be kept in mind as a cause, because both *Echinococcus* and *Trypanosomiasis* infections of the thyroid gland have been reported.

The prognosis is excellent—thyroid function is usually preserved, although post-thyroiditis thyroid function tests should be monitored to ascertain that thyroid failure has not occurred.

RIEDEL'S THYROIDITIS

Riedel's chronic sclerosing thyroiditis is rare and occurs primarily in middle-age women.[222,223] The etiologic mechanism is uncertain, although some cases appear to be a fibrotic form of Hashimoto's disease.[224,225] This condition is characterized by fibrosis of the thyroid gland and adjacent structures and may be associated with fibrosis elsewhere,

TABLE 13-5

Features That Are Useful in Differentiating between Acute Suppurative Thyroiditis and Subacute Thyroiditis

Characteristic	Acute Thyroiditis (% with Feature)	Subacute Thyroiditis (% with Feature)
History		
Preceding upper respiratory infection	88	17
Fever	100	54
Symptoms of thyrotoxicosis	Uncommon	47
Sore throat	90	36
Physical Examination of the Thyroid		
Painful thyroid swelling	100	77
Left side affected	85	Not specific
Migrating thyroid tenderness	Possible	27
Erythema of overlying skin	83	Not usually
Laboratory Findings		
Elevated white blood cell count	57	25-50
Elevated ESR (>30 mm/hr)	100	85
Abnormal thyroid hormone levels (elevated or depressed)	5-10	60
Alkaline phosphatase, transaminases increased	Rare	Common
Results of Needle Aspiration		
Purulent, bacteria or fungi present	~100	0
Lymphocytes, macrophages, some polyps, giant cells	0	~100
^{123}I uptake low	Uncommon	~100
Radiologic Findings		
Abnormal thyroid scan	92	—
Thyroid scan or ultrasound helpful in diagnosis	75	—
Gallium scan positive	~100	~100
Barium swallow showing fistula	Common	0
CT scan useful	Rarely	Not indicated
Clinical Course		
Clinical response to glucocorticoid treatment	Transient	100
Incision and drainage required	85	No
Recurrence following operative drainage	16	No
Piriform sinus fistula discovered	96	No

CT, computed tomography; ESR, erythrocyte sedimentation rate.

From DeGroot LJ, Larsen PR, Hennemann G. Acute and subacute thyroiditis. In: DeGroot LJ, Larsen PR, Hennemann G. The Thyroid and Its Diseases, 6th ed. New York: Churchill Livingstone; 1996:700.

especially in the retroperitoneal area.[223] The presence of eosinophils in specimens obtained by fine-needle aspiration has been demonstrated histologically, suggesting a unique autoimmune response to fibrous tissue.[226]

Symptoms develop insidiously and are related chiefly to compression of adjacent structures, including the trachea, esophagus, and recurrent laryngeal nerves. Systemic evidence of inflammation is uncommon. The thyroid gland is moderately enlarged, stony hard, and usually asymmetric. The consistency of the gland and the invasion of adjacent structures suggest carcinoma, but there is no enlargement of regional lymph nodes. Temperature, pulse, and leukocyte count are normal. Severe hypothyroidism is unusual but does occur, as does loss of parathyroid function. The RAIU may be normal or low. Elevated circulating thyroid autoantibodies are less common and are found in lower titers than in Hashimoto's disease.

Surgery may be required to preserve tracheal and esophageal function. If extensive involvement of perithyroid tissues is present, resection of the isthmus may relieve some symptoms. Treatment with thyroid hormone relieves the hypothyroidism but has no effect on the primary process, which may progress inexorably. Immunosuppressive treatment and even chemotherapy has been tried in individual cases. Glucocorticoids have been used for treatment, with sporadic improvement. The use of tamoxifen has also been successful in some patients.[227]

MISCELLANEOUS CAUSES

Only a few causes of generalized inflammation of the thyroid gland have been reported. These include inflammation arising after ^{131}I treatment for Graves' disease, a residual thyroid lobe in a patient with thyroid cancer of the contralateral lobe, and thyroiditis arising from external-beam therapy for conditions such as Hodgkin's or non-Hodgkin's lymphoma, breast carcinoma, or other lesions of the oropharynx. Anaplastic thyroid carcinoma has been reported in association with a diffuse thyroiditis and elevation of thyroid hormone levels. In general, only radioiodine-induced thyroiditis is associated with pain, and glucocorticoid treatment may be useful in symptomatic therapy.

REFERENCES

1. Roberts CG, Ladenson PW. Hypothyroidism. *Lancet.* 2004;363: 793-803.
2. Pearce EN, Farwell AP, Braverman LE. Thyroiditis. *N Engl J Med.* 2003;348:2646-2655.
3. Dayan CM, Panicker V. Novel insights into thyroid hormones from the study of common genetic variation. *Nat Rev Endocrinol.* 2009; 5:211-218.
4. Vanderpump MP, Tunbridge WM, French JM, et al. The incidence of thyroid disorders in the community: a twenty year follow-up of the Whickham Survey. *Clin Endocrinol (Oxf).* 1995;43:55-68.
5. Hollowell JG, Stehling NW, Flanders D, et al. Serum TSH, T4, and thyroid antibodies in the United States population (1988 to 1994): National Health and Nutrition Examination Survey (NHANES III). *J Clin Endocrinol Metab.* 2002;87:489-499.
6. Cooper DS. Subclinical hypothyroidism. *N Engl J Med.* 2001;345: 260-265.
7. Huber G, Staub J-J, Meier C, et al. Prospective study of the spontaneous course of subclinical hypothyroidism: prognostic value of thyrotropin, thyroid reserve, and thyroid antibodies. *J Clin Endocrinol Metab.* 2002;87:3221-3226.
8. Surks MI, Ortiz E, Daniels GH, et al. Subclinical thyroid disease: scientific review and guidelines for diagnosis and management. *JAMA.* 2004;291:228-238.
9. Col NF, Surks MI, Daniels GH. Subclinical thyroid disease: clinical applications. *JAMA.* 2004;291:239-243.
10. Kratzsch J, Pulzer F. Thyroid gland development and defects. *Best Pract Res Clin Endocrinol Metab.* 2008;22:57-75.
11. Smith TJ, Bahn RS, Gorman CA. Connective tissue, glycosaminoglycans, and diseases of the thyroid. *Endocr Rev.* 1989;10:366-391.
12. Safer JD, Crawford TM, Holick MF. Topical thyroid hormone accelerates wound healing in mice. *Endocrinology.* 2005;146:4425-4430.
13. Eisenbarth GS, Gottlieb PA. Autoimmune polyendocrine syndromes. *N Engl J Med.* 2004;50:2068-2079.
14. Klein I, Danzi S. Thyroid disease and the heart. *Circulation.* 2007; 116:1725-1735.
15. Kahaly GJ, Dillmann WH. Thyroid hormone action and the heart. *Endocr Rev.* 2005;26:704-728.
16. Kahaly GJ. Cardiovascular and atherogenic aspects of subclinical hypothyroidism. *Thyroid.* 2000;10:665-679.
17. Biondi B, Palmieri EA, Lombardi G, et al. Subclinical hypothyroidism and cardiac function. *Thyroid.* 2002;12:505-510.
18. Hardisty CA, Naik DR, Munro DS. Pericardial effusion in hypothyroidism. *Clin Endocrinol (Oxf).* 1980;13:349-354.
19. Keating FR, Parkin TW, Selby JB, et al. Treatment of heart disease associated with myxedema. *Prog Cardiovasc Dis.* 1961;3:364-381.
20. Hussein WI, Green R, Jacobsen DW, et al. Normalization of hyperhomocysteinemia with L-thyroxine in hypothyroidism. *Ann Intern Med.* 1999;131:348-351.
21. Ladenson PW, Sherman SI, Baughman KL, et al. Reversible alterations in myocardial gene expression in a young man with dilated cardiomyopathy and hypothyroidism. *Proc Natl Acad Sci U S A.* 1992;89: 5251-5255.
22. Biondi B, Cooper DS. Clinical significance of subclinical thyroid dysfunction. *Endocr Rev.* 2007;29:76-131.
23. Pearce EN, Wilson PW, Yang Q, et al. Thyroid function and lipid subparticle sizes in patients with short-term hypothyroidism and a population-based cohort. *J Clin Endocrinol Metab.* 2008;93:888-894.
24. Kvetny J, Heldgaard PE, Bladbjerg EM, et al. Subclinical hypothyroidism is associated with a low-grade inflammation, increased triglyceride levels and predicts cardiovascular disease in males below 50 years. *Clin Endocrinol (Oxf).* 2004;61:232-238.
25. Imaizumi M, Akahoshi M, Ichimaru S, et al. Risk for ischemic heart disease and all-cause mortality in subclinical hypothyroidism. *J Clin Endocrinol Metab.* 2004;89:3365-3370.
26. Cappola AR, Fried LP, Arnold AM, et al. Thyroid status, cardiovascular risk, and mortality in older adults. *JAMA.* 2006;295:1033-1041.
27. Tachman ML, Guthrie GP Jr. Hypothyroidism: diversity of presentation. *Endocr Rev.* 1984;5:456-465.
28. Checchi S, Montanaro A, Pasqui L, et al. L-Thyroxine requirement in patients with auotimmune hypothyroidism and parietal cell antibodies. *J Clin Endocrinol Metab.* 2008;93:465-469.
29. Elfstrom P, Montgomery SM, Kampe O, et al. Risk of thyroid disease in individuals with celiac disease. *J Clin Endocrinol Metab.* 2008; 93:3915-3921.
30. Malik R, Hodgson H. The relationship between the thyroid gland and the liver. *Q J Med.* 2002;95:559-569.
31. Volzke H, Robinson DM, John U. Association between thyroid function and gallstone disease. *World J Gastroenterol.* 2005;11:5530-5534.
32. Williams GR. Neurodevelopmental and neurophysiological actions of thyroid hormone. *J Neuroendocrinol.* 2008;20:784-794.
33. Bauer M, Goetz T, Glenn T, et al. The thyroid-brain interaction in thyroid disorders and mood disorders. *J Neuroendocrin.* 2008;20: 1101-1114.
34. Bauer M, Silverman DH, Schlagenhauf F. Brain glucose metabolism in hypothyroidism: a positron emission tomography study before and after thyroid hormone replacement. *J Clin Endocrinol Metab.* 2009;94:2922-2929.
35. Bland JH, Frymoyer JW. Rheumatic syndromes of myxedema. *N Engl J Med.* 1970;282:1171-1174.
36. Tan ZS, Vasan RS. Thyroid function and Alzheimer's disease. *J Alzheimers Dis.* 2009;16:503-507.
37. Kalmijn S, Mehta KM, Pols HA, et al. Subclinical hyperthyroidism and the risk of dementia: the Rotterdam study. *Clin Endocrinol (Oxf).* 2000;53:733-777.
38. Sampaolo S, Campos-Barros A, Mazziotti G, et al. Increased cerebrospinal fluid levels of 3,3′,5′-triiodothyronine in patients with Alzheimer's disease. *J Clin Endocrinol Metab.* 2005;90:198-202.
39. Schiess N, Pardo CA. Hashimoto's encephalopathy. *Ann N Y Acad Sci.* 2008;1142:254-265.
40. Murphy E, Williams GR. The thyroid and the skeleton. *Clin Endocrinol (Oxf).* 2004;61:285-298.
41. Rivkees SA, Bode HH, Crawford JD. Long-term growth in juvenile acquired hypothyroidism: the failure to achieve normal adult stature. *N Engl J Med.* 1988;31:599-602.
42. Iwasaki Y, Oiso Y, Yamauchi K, et al. Osmoregulation of plasma vasopressin in myxedema. *J Clin Endocrinol Metab.* 1990;70:534-539.
43. Squizzato A, Roumualdi E, Buller HR, et al. Thyroid dysfunction and effects on coagulation and fibrinolysis: a systematic review. *J Clin Endocrinol Metab.* 2007;92:2415-2420.
44. Lecky BRF, Williams TDM, Lightman SL, et al. Myxoedema presenting with chiasmal compression: resolution after thyroxine replacement. *Lancet.* 1987;1:1347-1350.
45. Kamilaris TC, DeBold CR, Pavlou SN, et al. Effect of altered thyroid hormone levels on hypothalamic-pituitary-adrenal function. *J Clin Endocrinol Metab.* 1987;65:994-999.
46. Barreto-Chaves ML, Carrillo-Sepulveda MA, Cameiro-Ramos MS, et al. The crosstalk between thyroid hormones and the renin-angiotensin system. *Vascul Pharmacol.* 2009;52:166-170.
47. Redmond GP. Thyroid dysfunction and women's reproductive health. *Thyroid.* 2004;14(suppl):S5-S15.
48. Yoshimura M, Hershman JM. Thyrotropic action of human chorionic gonadotropin. *Thyroid.* 1995;5:425-434.
49. Casey BM, Dashe JS, Wells CE, et al. Subclinical hypothyroidism and pregnancy outcomes. *Obstet Gynecol.* 2005;105:239-245.
50. Abalovich M, Amino N, Barbour LA, et al. Management of thyroid dysfunction during pregnancy and postpartum: and Endocrine Society Clinical Practice Guideline. *J Clin Endocrinol Metab.* 2007;92:S1-S47.
51. Negro R, Formoso G, Mangieri T, et al. Levothyroxine treatment in euthyroid pregnant women with autoimmune thyroid disease: effects on obstetrical complications. *J Clin Endocrinol Metab.* 2006;91: 2587-2591.
52. Krassas GE, Tziomalos K, Papdonpoulou F, et al. Erectile dysfunction in patients with hyper- and hypothyroidism: how common and should we treat? *J Clin Endocrinol Metab.* 2008;93:1815-1819.
53. Brenta G, Schnitman M, Gurfinkiel M, et al. Variations of sex hormone-binding globulin in thyroid dysfunction. *Thyroid.* 1999;9:273-277.
54. Silva JE, Bianco SDC. Thyroid-adrenergic interactions: physiological and clinical implications. *Thyroid.* 2008;18:157-165.
55. Haluzik M, Nedvidkova J, Bartak V, et al. Effects of hypo- and hyperthyroidism on noradrenergic activity and glycerol concentrations in human subcutaneous abdominal adipose tissue assessed with microdialysis. *J Clin Endocrinol Metab.* 2003;88:5605-5608.
56. Liu Y-Y, Brent GA. Thyroid hormone crosstalk with nuclear receptor signaling in metabolic regulation. *Trends Endocrinol Metab.* 2009; 21:166-173.
57. Crunkhorn S, Patti ME. Links between thyroid hormone action, oxidative metabolism, and diabetes risk? *Thyroid.* 2008;18:157-165.
58. Chidakel A, Mentuccia D, Celi FS. Peripheral metabolism of thyroid hormone and glucose homeostasis. *Thyroid.* 2005;15:899-903.
59. Canaris GJ, Manowitz NR, Mayor G, et al. The Colorado thyroid disease prevalence study. *Arch Intern Med.* 2000;160:526-534.
60. Vettor R. The metabolic actions of thyroid hormone and leptin: a mandatory interplay or not? *Diabetologia.* 2005;48:621-623.
61. Iglesias P, Alvarez Fidalgo P, Codoceo R, et al. Serum concentrations of adipocytokines in patients with hyperthyroidism and hypothyroidism before and after control of thyroid function. *Clin Endocrinol (Oxf).* 2003;59:621-629.
62. Zulewski H, Müller B, Exer P, et al. Estimation of tissue hypothyroidism by a new clinical score: evaluation of patients with various grades of hypothyroidism and controls. *J Clin Endocrinol Metab.* 1997;82: 771-776.
63. Rapa A, Monzani A, Moia S, et al. Subclinical hypothyroidism in children and adolescents: a range of clinical, biochemical, and genetic factors involved. *J Clin Endocrinol Metab.* 2009;94:2414-2420.
64. Greben B, Zavacki AM, Ribich S, et al. Cellular and molecular basis of deiodinase-regulated thyroid hormone signaling. *Endocr Rev.* 2008;29: 898-938.

65. Yamada M, Mori M. Mechanisms related to the pathophysiology and management of central hypothyroidism. *Nat Rev Endocrinol.* 2008; 4:683-694.
66. Hollowell JG, Staehling NW, Hannon WH, et al. Iodine nutrition in the United States—trends and public health implications: iodine excretion data from National Health and Nutrition Examination Surveys I and III (1971-1974 and 1988-1994). *J Clin Endocrinol Metab.* 1998;83:3401-3408.
67. Caldwell KL, Jones R, Hoolowell JG. Urinary iodine concentration: United States National Health and Nutrition Examination Survey 2001-2002. *Thyroid.* 2005;15:692-699.
68. Mariotti S, Franceschi C, Cossarizza A, et al. The aging thyroid. *Endocr Rev.* 1995;16:686-715.
69. Su SY, Grodski S, Serpell JW. Hypothyroidism following hemithyroidectomy. *Ann Surg.* 2009;250:991-994.
70. Davies TF, Amino N. A new classification for human autoimmune thyroid disease. *Thyroid.* 1993;3:331-333.
71. Tomer Y, Davies TF. Searching for the autoimmune thyroid disease susceptibility genes: from gene mapping to gene function. *Endocr Rev.* 2003;23:694-717.
72. Jacobson EM, Huber A, Tomer Y. The HLA gene complex in thyroid autoimmunity: from epidemiology to etiology. *J Autoimmun.* 2008; 30:58-62.
73. Giordano C, Stassi G, De Maria R, et al. Potential involvement of Fas and its ligand in the pathogenesis of Hashimoto's thyroiditis. *Science.* 1997;275:960-963.
74. Stassi G, Di Liberto D, Todaro M, et al. Control of target cell survival in thyroid autoimmunity by T-helper cytokines via regulation of apoptotic proteins. *Nat Immunol.* 2000;1:483-488.
75. Phelps E, Wu P, Bretz J, et al. Thyroid cell apoptosis: a new understanding of thyroid autoimmunity. *Endocrinol Metab Clin North Am.* 2000; 29:375-388.
76. Doniach D, Botttazo GF, Russell RCG. Goitrous autoimmune thyroiditis. *Clin Endocrinol (Oxf).* 1979;8:63-80.
77. Martin A, Davies TF. T cells and human autoimmune thyroid disease: emerging data show lack of need to invoke suppressor T-cell problems. *Thyroid.* 1992;2:247-261.
78. Tomer Y. Hepatitis C and interferon induced thyroiditis. *J Autoimmun.* 2010;34:J322-J326.
79. Wang SH, Bretz JD, Phelps E, et al. A unique combination of inflammatory cytokines enhances apoptosis of thyroid follicular cells and transforms nondestructive to destructive thyroiditis in experimental autoimmune thyroiditis. *J Immunol.* 2002;168:2470-2474.
80. Davies TF, Latif R, Yin X. Inheriting autoimmune thyroid disease. *Endocr Pract.* 2009;15:63-66.
81. Tomer Y, Greenberg DA, Concepcion E, et al. Thyroglobulin is a thyroid specific gene for the familial autoimmune thyroid diseases. *J Clin Endocrinol Metab.* 2002;87:404-407.
82. Ando T, Davies TF. Clinical review 160. Postpartum autoimmune thyroid disease: the potential role of fetal microchimerism. *J Clin Endocrinol Metab.* 2003;88:2965-2971.
83. Stagnaro-Green A. Clinical review 152. Postpartum thyroiditis. *J Clin Endocrinol Metab.* 2002;87:4042-4047.
84. Zimmerman MB. Iodine deficiency. *Endocr Rev.* 2009;30:376-408.
85. Martino E, Bartalena L, Bogazzi F, et al. The effects of amiodarone on the thyroid. *Endocr Rev.* 2001;22:240-254.
86. Sundick RS, Herdegen DM, Brown TR, et al. The incorporation of dietary iodine into thyroglobulin increases its immunogenicity. *Endocrinology.* 1987;120:2078-2084.
87. Nagataki S, Shibata Y, Inoue S, et al. Thyroid diseases among atomic bomb survivors in Nagasaki. *JAMA.* 1994;272:364-370.
88. Vermiglio F, Castagna MG, Volnova E, et al. Post-Chernobyl increased prevalence of humoral thyroid autoimmunity in children and adolescents from a moderately iodine-deficient area in Russia. *Thyroid.* 1999;9:781-786.
89. Skla C, Whitton J, Mertens A, et al. Abnormalities of the thyroid in survivors of Hodgkin's disease: data from the childhood cancer survivor study. *J Clin Endocrinol Metab.* 2000;85:3227-3232.
90. Imaizumi M, Usa T, Tominaga T, et al. Radiation dose-response relationships for thyroid nodules and autoimmune thyroid diseases in Hiroshima and Nagasaki atomic bomb survivors 55-58 years after radiation exposure. *JAMA.* 2006;295:1011-1022.
91. Tomer Y, Davies TF. Infection, thyroid disease, and autoimmunity. *Endocr Rev.* 1993;14:107-120.
92. Carle A, Pedersen IB, Knudsen N, et al. Thyroid volume in hypothyroidism due to autoimmune disease follows a unimodal distribution: evidence against thyroid atrophy and autoimmune thyroiditis being distinct diseases. *J Clin Endocrinol Metab.* 2009;94:833-839.
93. Graff-Baker A, Sosa JA, Roman SA. Primary thyroid lymphoma: a review of recent developments in diagnosis and histology-driven treatment. *Curr Opin Oncol.* 2010;22:17-22.
94. Baker J, Fosso CK. Immunological aspects of cancers arising from thyroid follicular cells. *Endocr Rev.* 1993;14:729-746.
95. Boyages SC. Clinical review 49. Iodine deficiency disorders. *J Clin Endocrinol Metab.* 1993;77:587-591.
96. Bottcher Y, Eszlinger M, Tonjes A, et al. The genetics of euthyroid familial goiter. *Trends Endocrinol Metab.* 2005;16:314-319.
97. Glinoer D. The regulation of thyroid function in pregnancy: pathways of endocrine adaptation from physiology to pathology. *Endocr Rev.* 1997;18:404-433.
98. Pearce EN, Pino S, He X, et al. Sources of dietary iodine: bread, cows' milk, and infant formula in the Boston area. *J Clin Endocrinol Metab.* 2004;89:3421-3424.
99. Pearce EN, Bazrafshan HR, He X, et al. Dietary iodine in pregnant women from the Boston, Massachusetts area. *Thyroid.* 2004;14: 327-328.
100. Leung AM, Pearce EN, Braverman LE. Iodine content of prenatal multivitamins in the United States. *N Eng J Med.* 2009;360:939-940.
101. Wolff J. Physiology and pharmacology of iodized oil in goiter prophylaxis. *Medicine (Baltimore).* 2001;80:20-36.
102. Silva JE. Effects of iodine and iodine-containing compounds on thyroid function. *Med Clin North Am.* 1985;69:881-898.
103. Wolff J, Chaikoff IL. Plasma inorganic iodide as a homeostatic regulator of thyroid function. *J Biol Chem.* 1948;174:555.
104. Muller B, Zulewski H, Huber P, et al. Impaired action of thyroid hormone associated with smoking in women with hypothyroidism. *N Engl J Med.* 1995;333:964-969.
105. Pearce EN, Braverman LE. Environmental pollutants and the thyroid. *Best Prac Res Clin Endocr Metab.* 2009;23:801-813.
106. Miller MD, Crofton KM, Rice DC, et al. Thyroid-disrupting chemicals: interpreting upstream biomarkers of adverse outcomes. *Environ Health Perspect.* 2009;117:1033-1041.
107. Hershman JM. Perchlorate and thyroid function: what are the environmental issues? *Thyroid.* 2005;15:427-431.
108. Tellez Tellez R, Michaud Chacon P, Reyes Abarca C, et al. Long-term environmental exposure to perchlorate through drinking water and thyroid function during pregnancy and the neonatal period. *Thyroid.* 2005;15:963-974.
109. Dohan O, De la Vieja A, Paroder V, et al. The sodium/iodide symporter (NIS): characterization, regulation, and medical significance. *Endocr Rev.* 2003;24:48-77.
110. Bakker B, Bikker H, Vulsma T, et al. Two decades of screening for congenital hypothyroidism in The Netherlands: TPO gene mutations in total iodide organification defects (an update). *J Clin Endocrinol Metab.* 2000;85:3708-3712.
111. Kopp P. Pendred's syndrome and genetic defects in thyroid hormone synthesis. *Rev Endocr Metab Disord.* 2000;1:109-121.
112. Vono-Toniolo J, Rivolta CM, Targovnik HM, et al. Naturally occurring mutations in the thyroglobulin gene. *Thyroid.* 2005;15:1021-1033.
113. Moreno JC, Klootwijk W, Toor HV, et al. Mutations in the iodotyrosine deiodinase gene and hypothyroidism. *N Engl J Med.* 2008;358: 1811-1818.
114. Best TB, Munro RE, Burwell S, et al. Riedel's thyroiditis associated with Hashimoto's thyroiditis, hypoparathyoidism, and retroperitoneal fibrosis. *J Endocrinol Invest.* 1991;14:767-772.
115. Kimura H, Yamashita S, Ashizawa K, et al. Thyroid dysfunction in patients with amyloid goitre. *Clin Endocrinol (Oxf).* 1997;46:769-774.
116. Oerter KE, Kamp GA, Munson PJ, et al. Multiple hormone deficiencies in children with hemochromatosis. *J Clin Endocrinol Metab.* 1993;76:357-361.
117. Gordon MB, Klein I, Dekker A, et al. Thyroid disease in progressive systemic sclerosis: increased frequency of glandular fibrosis and hypothyroidism. *Ann Intern Med.* 1981;95:431-435.
118. Rees Smith B, McLachlan SM, Furmaniak J. Autoantibodies to the thyrotropin receptor. *Endocr Rev.* 1988;9:106-121.
119. Brent GA. Graves' disease. *N Engl J Med.* 2008;358:2594-2605.
120. Biebermann H, Schoneberg T, Krude H, et al. Mutations of the human thyrotropin receptor gene causing thyroid hypoplasia and persistent congenital hypothyroidism. *J Clin Endocrinol Metab.* 1997;82: 3471-3480.
121. Spiegel AM, Shenker A, Weinstein LS. Receptor-effector coupling by G proteins: implications for normal and abnormal signal transduction. *Endocr Rev.* 1992;13:536-565.
122. Xie J, Pannain S, Pohlenz J, et al. Resistance to thyrotropin (TSH) in three families is not associated with mutations in the TSH receptor or TSH. *J Clin Endocrinol Metab.* 1997;82:3933-3940.
123. Huang SA, Tu HM, Harney JW, et al. Severe hypothyroidism caused by type 3 iodothyronine deiodinase in infantile hemangiomas. *N Engl J Med.* 2000;343:185-189.
124. Huang SA. Physiology and pathophysiology of type 3 deiodinase in humans. *Thyroid.* 2005;15:875-881.
125. Dumitrescu AM, Lio X-H, Abdullah SY, et al. Mutations in SECISBP2 result in abnormal thyroid hormone metabolism. *Nat Genet.* 2005;37: 1247-1252.
126. Canani LH, Capp C, Dora JM, et al. Type 2 deiodinase Thr92Ala polymorphism is associated with decreased enzyme velocity and severe insulin resistance in type 2 diabetes mellitus patients. *J Clin Endocrinol Metab.* 2005;90:3472-3478.

127. Torino F, Corsello SM, Longo R, et al. Hypothyroidism related to tyrosine kinase inhibitors: an emerging toxic effect of targeted therapy. *Nat Rev Clin Oncol.* 2009;6:219-228.
128. Desai J, Yassa L, Marqusee E, et al. Hypothyroidism after sunitinib treatment for patients with gastrointestinal stromal tumors. *Ann Intern Med.* 2006;145:660-664.
129. Sherman SI. Advances in chemotherapy of differentiated epithelial and medullary thyroid cancer. *J Clin Endocrinol Metab.* 2009;94:1493-1499.
130. Haugen BR. Drugs that suppress TSH or cause central hypothyroidism. *Best Pract Res Clin Endocrinol Metab.* 2009;23:793-800.
131. Comi RJ, Gesundheit N, Murray L. Response of thyrotropin-secreting pituitary adenomas to a long-acting somatostatin analogue. *N Engl J Med.* 1987;317:12-17.
132. Radovick S, Nations M, Du Y, et al. A mutation in the POU-homeodomain of Pit-1 responsible for combined pituitary hormone deficiency. *Science.* 1992;257:1115-1118.
133. Collu R, Tang J, Castagne J, et al. A novel mechanism for isolated central hypothyroidism: inactivating mutations in the thyrotropin-releasing hormone receptor gene. *J Clin Endocrinol Metab.* 1997;82:1561-1565.
134. Hayashizaki Y, Hiraoka Y, Tatsumi K. Deoxyribonucleic acid analyses of five families with familial inherited thyroid stimulating hormone deficiency. *J Clin Endocrinol Metab.* 1990;71:792.
135. Medeiros-Neto G, Herodotou DT, Rajan S, et al. A circulating, biologically inactive thyrotropin caused by a mutation in the beta subunit gene. *J Clin Invest.* 1996;97:1250-1256.
136. Refetoff S, Dumitrescu AM. Syndromes of reduced sensitivity to thyroid hormone: genetic defects in hormone receptors, cell transporters and deiodination. *Best Pract Res Clin Endocrinol Metab.* 2007;21:277-305.
137. Oetting A, Yen PM. New insights into thyroid hormone action. *Best Pract Res Clin Endocrinol Metab.* 2007;21:193-208.
138. Weiss RE, Refetoff S. Effect of thyroid hormone on growth: lessons from the syndrome of resistance to thyroid hormone. *Endocrinol Metab Clin North Am.* 1996;25:719-730.
139. Hauser PH, Zametkin AJ, Martinez P, et al. Attention deficit-hyperactivity disorder in people with generalized resistance to thyroid hormone. *N Engl J Med.* 1993;328:997-1001.
140. Brucker-Davis F, Skarulis MC, Grace MB, et al. Genetic and clinical features of 42 kindreds with resistance to thyroid hormone. *Ann Intern Med.* 1995;123:572-583.
141. Brucker-Davis F, Oldfield EH, Skarulis MC, et al. Thyrotropin-secreting pituitary tumors: diagnostic criteria, thyroid hormone sensitivity, and treatment outcome in 25 patients followed at the National Institutes of Health. *J Clin Endocrinol Metab.* 1999;84:476-486.
142. Reutrakul S, Sadow PM, Pannain S, et al. Search for abnormalities of nuclear corepressors, coactivators, and a coregulator in families with resistance to thyroid hormone without mutations in thyroid hormone receptor beta or alpha genes. *J Clin Endocrinol Metab.* 2000;85:3609-3617.
143. Weiss RE, Refetoff S. Treatment of resistance to thyroid hormone-primum non nocere. *J Clin Endocrinol Metab.* 1999;84:401-404.
144. Ueda S, Takamatsu J, Fukata S, et al. Differences in response of thyrotropin to 3,5,3′-triiodothyronine and 3,5,3′-triiodothyroacetic acid in patients with resistance to thyroid hormone. *Thyroid.* 1996;6:563-570.
145. Baxter JD, Webb P. Thyroid hormone mimetics: potential applications in atherosclerosis, obesity and type 2 diabetes. *Nat Rev Drug Discov.* 2009;8:308-320.
146. Roti E, Minelli R, Gardini E, et al. The use and misuse of thyroid hormone. *Endocr Rev.* 1993;14:401-423.
147. Mandel SJ, Brent GA, Larsen PR. Levothyroxine therapy in patients with thyroid disease. *Ann Intern Med.* 1993;119:492-502.
148. Toft AD. Thyroxine therapy. *N Engl J Med.* 1994;331:174-180.
149. Bach-Huynh TG, Nayak B, Loh J, et al. Timing of levothyroxine administration affects serum thyrotropin concentration. *J Clin Endocrinol Metab.* 2009;94:3905-3912.
150. Hennessey JV. Levothyroxine a new drug? Since when? How could that be? *Thyroid.* 2003;13:279-282.
151. Burman KD, Hennessey J, McDermott M, et al. The FDA revises requirements for levothyroxine products. *Thyroid.* 2008;18:487-490.
152. Santini F, Pinchera A, Marsili A, et al. Lean body mass is a major determinant of levothyroxine dosage in the treatment of thyroid disease. *J Clin Endocrinol Metab.* 2005;90:124-127.
153. Olveira G, Almaraz MC, Soriguer F, et al. Altered bioavailability due to changes in the formulation of a commercial preparation of levothyroxine in patients with differentiated thyroid carcinoma. *Clin Endocrinol (Oxf).* 1997;46:707-711.
154. Abramowicz M [editor]. Generic levothyroxine. *The Medical Letter of Drugs and Therapeutics.* 2004;46(1192):77-78.
155. Rees-Jones RW, Larsen PR. Triiodothyronine and thyroxine content of desiccated thyroid tablets. *Metabolism.* 1977;26:1213-1218.
156. LeBoff MS, Kaplan MM, Silva JE, et al. Bioavailability of thyroid hormones from oral replacement preparations. *Metabolism.* 1982;31:900-905.
157. Blumberg KR, Mayer WJ, Parikh DK, et al. Liothyronine and levothyroxine in Armour thyroid. *J Pharm Sci.* 1993;76:346-347.
158. Hays MT. Localization of human thyroxine absorption. *Thyroid.* 1991;3:241-248.
159. Centanni M, Gargano L, Canettieri G, et al. Thyroxine in goiter, *Helicobacter pylori* infection, and chronic gastritis. *N Engl J Med.* 2006;354:1787-1795.
160. Escobar-Morreale HF, Obregon MJ, Escobar del Ray F, et al. Replacement therapy for hypothyroidism with thyroxine alone does not ensure euthyroidism in all tissues, as studied in thyroidectomized rats. *J Clin Invest.* 1995;96:2828-2838.
161. Jonklaas J, Davidson B, Bhagat S, et al. Triiodothyronine levels in athyreotic individuals during levothyroxine therapy. *JAMA.* 2008;299:769-777.
162. Bunevicius R, Kazanavicius G, Zalinkevicius R, et al. Effects of thyroxine as compared with thyroxine plus triiodothyronine in patients with hypothyroidism. *N Engl J Med.* 1999;340:424-429.
163. Grozinsky-Glasberg S, Fraser A, Nahshoni E, et al. Thyroxine-trriodothyronine combination therapy versus thyroxine monotherapy for clinical hypothyroidism: meta-analysis of randomized controlled trials. *J Clin Endocrinol Metab.* 2006;91:2592-2599.
164. al-Adsani H, Hoffer LJ, Silva JE. Resting energy expenditure is sensitive to small dose changes in patients on chronic thyroid hormone replacement. *J Clin Endocrinol Metab.* 1997;82:1118-1125.
165. Henneman G, Docter R, Visser TJ, et al. Thyroxine plus low-dose, slow-release triiodothyronine replacement in hypothyroidism: proof of principle. *Thyroid.* 2004;14:271-275.
166. Carr K, Mcleod DT, Parry G, et al. Fine adjustment of thyroxine replacement dosage: comparison of the thyrotrophin releasing hormone tests using a sensitive thyrotrophin assay with measurement of free thyroid hormones and clinical assessment. *Clin Endocrinol (Oxf).* 1988;28:325-333.
167. Slawik M, Klawitter B, Meiser E, et al. Thyroid hormone replacement for central hypothyroidism randomized controlled trial comparing two doses of thyroxine (T4) with a combination of T4 and triiodothyronine. *J Clin Endocrinol Metab.* 2007;92:4115-4122.
168. Van Dop C, Conte FA, Koch TK, et al. Pseudotumor cerebri associated with initiation of levothyroxine therapy for juvenile hypothyroidism. *N Engl J Med.* 1983;308:1076-1080.
169. LaFranchi SH, Austin J. How should we be treating children with congenital hypothyroidism? *J Pediatr Endocrinol Metab.* 2007;20:559-578.
170. Fisher DA, Schoen EJ, La Franchi S, et al. The hypothalamic-pituitary-thyroid negative feedback control axis in children with treated congenital hypothyroidism. *J Clin Endocrinol Metab.* 2000;85:2722-2727.
171. Surks MI, Goswami G, Daniels GH. The thyrotropin reference range should remain unchanged. *J Clin Endocrinol Metab.* 2005;90:5489-5496.
172. Surks MI, Hallowell JG. Age-specific distribution of serum thyrotropin and antithyroid antibodies in the US population: implications for the prevelence of subclinical hypothyroidism. *J Clin Endocrinol Metab.* 2007;92:4575-4582.
173. Atzmon G, Barzilai N, Hollowell JG, et al. Extreme longevity is associated with increased serum thyrotropin. *J Clin Endocrinol Metab.* 2009;94:1251-1254.
174. Arafah BM. Decreased levothyroxine requirement in women with hypothyroidism during androgen therapy for breast cancer. *Ann Intern Med.* 1994;121:247-251.
175. Mandel SJ, Larsen PR, Seely EW, et al. Increased need for thyroxine during pregnancy in women with primary hypothyroidism. *N Engl J Med.* 1990;323:91-96.
176. Alexander EK, Marqusee E, Lawrence J, et al. Timing and magnitude of increases in levothyroxine requirements during pregnancy in women with hypothyroidism. *N Engl J Med.* 2004;351:241-249.
177. Loh JA, Wartofsky L, Jonklaas J, et al. The magnitude of increased levothyroxine requirements in hypothyroid pregnancy women depends upon the etiology of the hypothyroidism. *Thyroid.* 2009;19:269-275.
178. Vulsma T, Gons MH, DeVijlder JMM. Maternal fetal transfer of thyroxine in congenital hypothyroidism due to a total organification defect of thyroid dysgenesis. *N Engl J Med.* 1989;321:13-16.
179. Singh N, Singh PN, Hershman JM. Effect of calcium carbonate on the absorption of levothyroxine. *JAMA.* 2000;283:2822-2825.
180. Campbell NRC, Hasinoff BB, Stalts H, et al. Ferrous sulfate reduces thyroxine efficacy in patients with hypothyroidism. *Ann Intern Med.* 1992;117:1010-1013.
181. Demke DM. Drug interaction between thyroxine and lovastatin. *N Engl J Med.* 1989;321:1341-1342.
182. McLean M, Kirkwood I, Epstein M, et al. Cation-exchange resin and inhibition of intestinal absorption of thyroxine. *Lancet.* 1993;341:1286.

183. Isley WL. Effect of rifampin therapy on thyroid function tests in a hypothyroid patient on replacement L-thyroxine. *Ann Intern Med.* 1987;107:517-518.
184. DeLuca F, Arrigo T, Pandullo E, et al. Changes in thyroid function tests induced by 2-month carbamazepine treatment in L-thyroxine-substituted hypothyroid children. *Eur J Pediatr.* 1986;145:77-79.
185. Faber J, Lumholtz IB, Kirkegaard C, et al. The effects of phenytoin on the extrathyroidal turnover of thyroxine, 3,5,3′-triiodothyronine, 3,3′,5′-triiodothyronine, and 3′,5′-diiodothyronine in man. *J Clin Endocrinol Metab.* 1985;61:1093-1099.
186. McCowen KC, Garber JR, Spark R. Elevated serum thyrotropin in thyroxine-treated patients with hypothyroidism given sertraline. *N Engl J Med.* 1997;337:1010-1011.
187. Arafah BM. Increased need for thyroxine in women with hypothyroidism during estrogen therapy. *N Engl J Med.* 2001;344:1743-1749.
188. Messina M, Redmond G. Effects of soy protein and soybean isoflavones on thyroid function in healthy adults and hypothyroid patients: a review of the relevant literature. *Thyroid.* 2006;16:249-258.
189. Figge J, Dluhy RG. Amiodarone-induced elevation of thyroid stimulating hormone in patients receiving levothyroxine for primary hypothyroidism. *Ann Intern Med.* 1990;113:553-555.
190. Jochum F, Terwolbeck K, Meinhold H, et al. Effects of a low selenium state in patients with phenylketonuria. *Acta Paediatr.* 1997;86:775-777.
191. Marcocci C, Golia F, Bruno-Bosoro G, et al. Carefully monitored levothyroxine suppressive therapy is not associated with bone loss in premenopausal women. *J Clin Endocrinol Metab.* 1994;78:818-823.
192. Saravanan P, Chau WF, Roberts N, et al. Psychological well-being in patients on "adequate" doses of L-thyroxine: results of a large, controlled community-based questionnaire study. *Clin Endocrinol (Oxf).* 2002;57:577-585.
193. Kaplan MM, Swartz SL, Larsen PR. Partial peripheral resistance to thyroid hormone. *Am J Med.* 1981;70:1115-1121.
194. Nystrom E, Caidahl K, Fager G, et al. A double-blind cross-over 12-month study of L-thyroxine treatment of women with "subclinical" hypothyroidism. *Clin Endocrinol (Oxf).* 1988;29:63-76.
195. Heymann R, Brent GA. Rapid progression from subclinical to symptomatic overt hypothyroidism. *Endocr Prac.* 2005;11:115-119.
196. Sherman SI, Ladenson PW. Complications of surgery in hypothyroid patients. *Am J Med.* 1991;90:367-370.
197. Hay ID, Duick DX, Vlietstra RE, et al. Thyroxine therapy in hypothyroid patients undergoing coronary revascularization: a retrospective analysis. *Ann Intern Med.* 1981;95:456-457.
198. Sherman SI, Ladenson PW. Percutaneous transluminal coronary angioplasty in hypothyroidism. *Am J Med.* 1991;90:367-370.
199. Klemperer JD, Klein I, Gomez M, et al. Thyroid hormone treatment after coronary artery bypass surgery. *N Engl J Med.* 1995;333:1522-1527.
200. Hamilton MA, Stevenson LW, Fonarow GC, et al. Safety and hemodynamic effects of intravenous triiodothyronine in advanced congestive heart failure. *Am J Cardiol.* 1998;81:443-447.
201. Chowdhury D, Parnell VA, Ojamaa K, et al. Usefulness of triiodothyronine (T3) treatment after surgery for complex congenital heart disease in infants and children. *Am J Cardiol.* 1999;84:1107-1109, A10.
202. GoldmanS,McCarrenM,MorkinE,etal.DITPA(3,5-Diiodothyropropionic acid) a thyroid hormone analog to treat heart failure: phase II trial veterans affairs cooperative study. *Circulation.* 2009;119:3093-3100.
203. Helfand M. Screening for subclinical thyroid dysfunction in nonpregnant adults: a summary of the evidence for the U.S. preventative services task force. *Ann Intern Med.* 2004;140:128-141.
204. Danese MD, Powe NR, Sawin CT, et al. Screening for mild thyroid failure at the periodic health examination: a decision and cost-effectiveness analysis. *JAMA.* 1996;276:285-292.
205. Klein RZ, Haddow JE, Faix JD, et al. Prevalence of thyroid deficiency in pregnant women. *Clin Endocrinol (Oxf).* 1991;35:41-46.
206. Pop VJ, Kuijpens JL, van Baar AL, et al. Low maternal free thyroxine concentrations during early pregnancy are associated with impaired psychomotor development in infancy. *Clin Endocrinol (Oxf).* 1999;50:149-155.
207. Vaidya B, Anthony S, Bilous M, et al. Detection of thyroid dysfunction in early pregnancy: universal screening or targeted high-risk case finding. *J Clin Endocrinol Metab.* 2007;92:203-207.
208. Brent GA. Diagnosing thyroid dysfunction in pregnant women: is case finding enough? *J Clin Endocrinol Metab.* 2007;92:39-41.
209. Fliers E, Wiersinga WM. Myxedema coma. *Rev Endocr Metab Discord.* 2003;4:137-141.
210. Reinhardt W, Mann K. Incidence, clinical picture, and treatment of hypothyroid coma: results of a survey. *Med Klin.* 1997;92:521-524.
211. Nicoloff JT, LoPresti JS. Myxedema coma: a form of decompensated hypothyroidism. *Endocrinol Metab Clin North Am.* 1993;22:279-290.
212. Miller KK, Daniels GH. Association between lithium use and thyrotoxicosis caused by silent thyroiditis. *Clin Endocrinol (Oxf).* 2001;55:501-508.
213. Szabo SM, Allen DB. Thyroiditis-differentiation of acute suppurative and subacute: case report and review of the literature. *Clin Pediatr.* 1989;28:171-174.
214. Singer PA. Thyroiditis: acute, subacute, and chronic. *Med Clin North Am.* 1991;75:61-77.
215. Das DK, Pant CS, Chachra KL, et al. Fine-needle aspiration cytology diagnosis of tuberculous thyroiditis: a report of eight cases. *Acta Cytol.* 1992;36:517-522.
216. Chiovato L, Canale G, Maccherini D, et al. *Salmonella brandenburg:* a novel cause of acute suppurative thyroiditis. *Acta Endocrinol (Copenh).* 1993;128:439-442.
217. Gandhi RT, Tollin SR, Seely EW. Diagnosis of *Candida* thyroiditis by fine-needle aspiration. *J Infect.* 1994;28:77-81.
218. Miyauchi A, Matsuzuka F, Kuma K, et al. Piriform sinus fistula: an underlying abnormality common in patients with acute suppurative thyroiditis. *World J Surg.* 1990;14:400-405.
219. Lucaya J, Berdon WE, Enriquez G, et al. Congenital pyriform sinus fistula: a cause of acute left-sided suppurative thyroiditis and neck abscess in children. *Pediatr Radiol.* 1990;21:27-29.
220. Bernard PJ, Som PM, Urken ML, et al. The CT findings of acute thyroiditis and acute suppurative thyroiditis. *Otolaryngol Head Neck Surg.* 1988;99:489-493.
221. Hatabu H, Kasagi K, Yamamoto K, et al. Acute suppurative thyroiditis associated with piriform sinus fistula: sonographic findings. *Am J Med.* 1990;155:845-847.
222. Bartholomew LG, Cain JC, Woolner LB, et al. Sclerosing cholangitis: its possible association with Riedel's struma and fibrous retroperitonitis—report of two cases. *N Engl J Med.* 1963;269:8-13.
223. Chopra D, Wool MS, Grossen A, et al. Riedel's struma associated with subacute thyroiditis, hypothyroidism, and hypoparathyroidism. *J Clin Endocrinol Metab.* 1978;46:869-871.
224. Zelmanovitz F, Zelmanovitz T, Beck M, et al. Riedel's thyroiditis associated with high titers of antimicrosomal and antithyroglobulin antibodies and hypothyroidism. *J Endocrinol Invest.* 1994;17:733-737.
225. Julie C, Vieillefond A, Desligneres S, et al. Hashimoto's thyroiditis associated with Riedel's thyroiditis and retroperitoneal fibrosis. *Pathol Res Pract.* 1997;193:573-577.
226. Heufelder AE, Goellner JR, Bahn RS, et al. Tissue eosinophilia and eosinophil degranulation in Riedel's invasive fibrous thyroiditis. *J Clin Endocrinol Metab.* 1996;81:977-984.
227. Jung YJ, Schaub CR, Rhodes R, et al. A case of Riedel's thyroiditis treated with tamoxifen: another successful outcome. *Endocr Pract.* 2004;10:483-486.

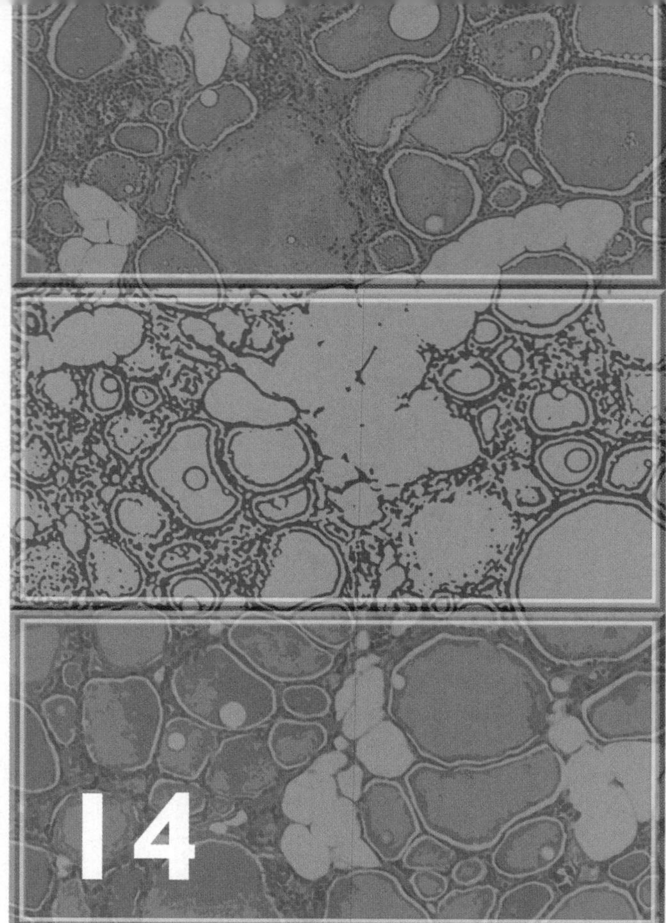

CHAPTER 14

Nontoxic Diffuse and Nodular Goiter and Thyroid Neoplasia

MARTIN-JEAN SCHLUMBERGER • SEBASTIANO FILETTI • IAN D. HAY

This chapter reviews the imaging techniques available for evaluating thyroid structural abnormalities; the units of measurement used in evaluation of the radiation dose and radioactivity are defined in Table 14-1.

Goiter resulting in thyrotoxicosis and other thyroid conditions arising from autoimmune thyroid disease are considered in Chapters 11 and 12.

This chapter then deals with the increasingly recognized problem of nodular thyroid disease. Thyroid neoplasia, both benign and malignant, is discussed authoritatively. We consider an appropriate histologic classification and staging of thyroid cancer and present a management program for the most common thyroid cancer types. This chapter is based on a consensus from the European Thyroid Association[1] and guidelines from the American Thyroid Association.[2,3]

EVALUATION OF STRUCTURAL ABNORMALITIES BY IMAGING TECHNIQUES

External Scintiscanning

Localization of functioning or nonfunctioning thyroid tissue in the area of the thyroid gland or elsewhere is made possible by techniques of external scintiscanning. The underlying principle is that isotopes selectively accumulated by thyroid tissue can be detected by a gamma camera and the data can be transformed into a visual display. Radioactivity in specific areas can be quantified.[4-7]

Several radioisotopes are employed in thyroid imaging. Technetium 99m (^{99m}Tc) pertechnetate is a monovalent anion that is actively concentrated by the thyroid gland

TABLE 14-1

Radiation Nomenclature: Traditional and International System (SI) Units*

Traditional Units	SI Units	Conversion Factors
Radiation Dose		
rad = radiation absorbed dose	Gy = gray 1 Gy = absorption of 1 joule/kg	1 Gy = 100 rad 1 rad = 0.01 Gy = 1 cGy
rem = roentgen-equivalent-man	Sv = sievert	1 Sv = 100 rem
Radioactivity (or Activity)		
Ci = curie	Bq = becquerel 1 Bq = 1 disintegration per second 1 GBq = 10^3 MBq = 10^6 kBq = 10^9 Bq	1 mCi = 37 MBq

*Prefixes: m (milli), c (centi), k (kilo), M (mega), G (giga).

but undergoes negligible organic binding and diffuses out of the gland as its concentration in the blood decreases. The short physical half-life of ^{99m}Tc (6 hours), its low fractional uptake, and its transient stay within the thyroid make the radiation delivered to the thyroid gland by a standard activity dose very low. Consequently, the intravenous administration of large activities (>37 MBq [1 mCi]) permits, about 30 minutes later, adequate imaging of the thyroid.

Two radioactive isotopes of iodine have been used in thyroid imaging. Iodine 131 (^{131}I) was commonly used in the past. However, ^{131}I is a beta emitter, its physical half-life is 8.1 days, and the energy of its main gamma ray is high and thus poorly adapted for its detection.[6] ^{123}I is, in many respects, ideal, but it is expensive. The energy of its main gamma ray is suitable for its detection by gamma cameras. Its short half-life (0.55 day) and absence of beta radiation result in a radiation dose to the thyroid that is about 1% of that delivered by a comparable activity of ^{131}I.[7]

The most important use of scintigraphic imaging of thyroid tissue is to define areas of increased or decreased function ("hot" or "cold" areas, respectively) relative to the function of the remainder of the gland. Almost all malignant nodules are hypofunctioning, but more than 80% of benign nodules are also nonfunctioning. Conversely, functioning nodules (hot nodules), particularly if the function of the surrounding tissue is decreased or absent, are rarely malignant.

Several nuclear medical tests (e.g., stimulation test after administration of exogenous thyroid-stimulating hormone [TSH], suppression test by administration of thyroid hormone) were used in the past to evaluate thyroid disorders but should no longer be used because sensitive TSH assays and scanning with a gamma camera permit the diagnosis of most hot nodules.

Scintiscanning with radioactive iodine can also be used to demonstrate that intrathoracic masses represent thyroid tissue and to detect ectopic thyroid tissue in the neck.

In patients with thyroid cancer, the total body scan is used to detect functioning metastases.[1,2] This scan is performed after the administration of larger activities of radioiodine, for diagnosis (1 to 5 mCi of ^{131}I or 1 to 5 mCi of ^{123}I) or for therapy (≥30 mCi of ^{131}I) and after intense stimulation with TSH. Superimposition of computed tomographic (CT) scans and gamma camera images greatly improves the sensitivity and specificity of the technique and the anatomic localization of any focus of uptake.[8,9]

Ultrasonography

Sonography is a noninvasive technique that is becoming an integral part of the clinical examination.[10] High-frequency sound waves are emitted by a transducer and reflected as they pass through the body, whereupon the returning echoes are received by the transducer, which also acts as a receiver. The amplitude of the reflections of the sound waves is influenced by differences in the acoustic impedance of the tissues encountered by the sound; for example, *fluid-filled* structures reflect few echoes and therefore have no or few internal echoes and well-defined margins; *solid* structures reflect varying amounts of sound and thus have varying degrees of internal echoes and less well-defined margins; and *calcified* structures reflect virtually all incoming sound and yield pronounced echoes with an acoustic "shadow" posteriorly.

Intrathyroidal nodules as small as 3 mm in diameter and cystic nodules as small as 2 mm can be readily detected. Color flow Doppler ultrasonography allows visualization of very small vessels, so that vascularity of thyroid nodules can be assessed.

The thyroid gland must be examined thoroughly in transverse and longitudinal planes. Imaging of patients with thyroid nodules and during follow-up of thyroid cancer should also include lymph node areas, classified as compartments, to identify enlarged cervical lymph nodes.[1,2,11-14]

The normal thyroid parenchyma has a characteristic homogeneous, medium-level echogenicity, with little identifiable internal architecture (Fig. 14-1). The surrounding muscles have the appearance of hypoechoic structures. The air-filled trachea in the midline gives a characteristic curvilinear reflecting surface with an associated reverberation artifact. The esophagus is usually hidden from sonographic visualization by the tracheal air shadow.

A diagrammatic representation of the neck showing the locations of any abnormal findings and their characteristics is a useful supplement to the routine film images recorded during an ultrasound examination. Such a cervical map with compartments[14] (Fig. 14-2) can help communicate the anatomic relationships of the pathology more clearly to the referring clinician and serves as a reference for the sonographer on follow-up examinations.

Neck ultrasonography is clinically useful at each step of thyroid evaluation (Table 14-2). It may confirm the presence of a thyroid nodule when the findings on physical examination are equivocal and may reveal the presence of other, nonpalpable nodules.

In patients with a thyroid nodule, gray-scale and color Doppler ultrasound are used to evaluate its sonographic features, including size, shape, echogenicity (hypoechoic or hyperechoic), and composition (cystic, solid, or mixed), and to determine the presence of coarse or fine calcifications, a halo and margins, and internal blood flow. It is used to examine the rest of the thyroid gland and lymph node areas. Elastography that assesses hardness as an indicator of malignancy in thyroid nodules has high specificity and sensitivity independent of nodule size, and this predictive value is maintained in follicular lesions, provided that the nodule is solid and devoid of coarse calcifications.[15] This promising technique requires additional validation with prospective studies.

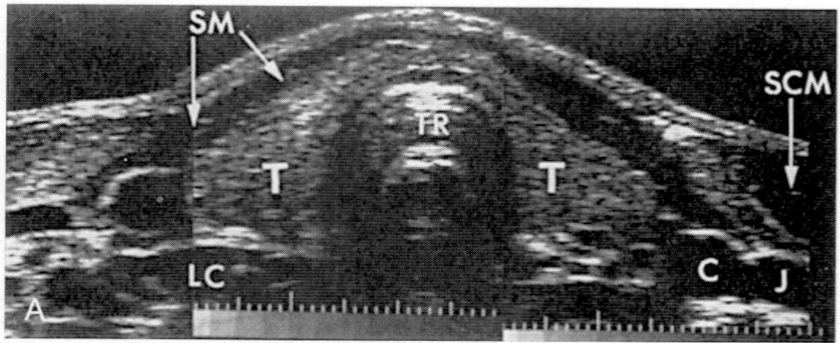

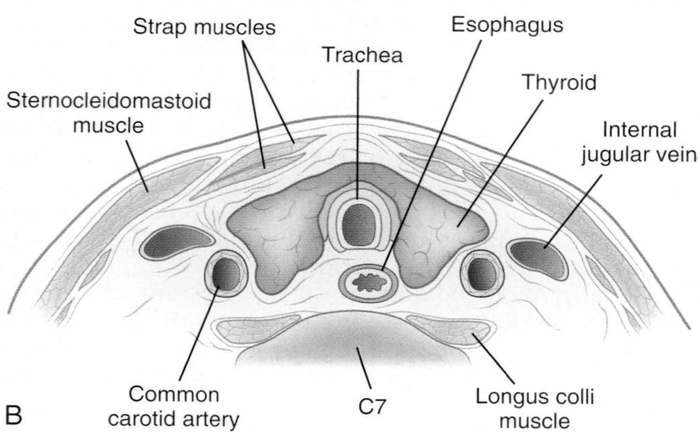

Figure 14-1 Transverse composite sonogram (**A**) and corresponding anatomic map (**B**) of the normal thyroid gland. C, common carotid artery; C7, seventh cervical vertebra; LC, longus colli muscle; SM, strap muscles; SCM, sternocleidomastoid muscle; T, thyroid; TR, trachea. (From Rifkin MD, Charboneau JW, Laing FC. Special course: ultrasound 1991. In: Reading CC [ed]. Syllabus: Thyroid, Parathyroid, and Cervical Lymph Nodes. Oak Brook, IL: Radiological Society of North America; 1991:363-377.)

In patients with known thyroid cancer, sonography can be useful in evaluating the extent of disease, both preoperatively and postoperatively. In those who present with cervical lymphadenopathy caused by papillary thyroid carcinoma (PTC) but have a gland that is palpably normal, sonography may be used preoperatively to detect an occult, primary intrathyroid focus. A preoperative sonogram should be obtained in all patients with PTC or medullary thyroid carcinoma (MTC), to identify the anatomic locations of any sonographically suspicious regional lymph nodes and thereby to permit planning of the extent of nodal dissection.[1-3,16] Occasionally, nonpalpable residual cancer that has been identified by preoperative ultrasonography and proved to be cytologically positive by ultrasound-guided fine-needle aspiration biopsy (FNAB) can be identified intraoperatively with the use of a hand-held ultrasound probe or by preoperative ultrasound-guided charcoal tattooing.[17]

After surgery for thyroid cancer, sonography is the preferred method for detecting residual, recurrent, or metastatic disease in the neck.[11-13] In patients who have undergone less than a near-total thyroidectomy, the sonographic appearance of the remaining thyroid tissue may be an important factor in the decision whether to recommend completion thyroidectomy. Also, it is more sensitive than neck palpation in detecting recurrent disease within the thyroid bed and metastatic disease in cervical lymph nodes.

Sonography may also be useful to guide FNAB of thyroid bed masses and lymph nodes.[2,10]

Computed Tomography

The CT appearance of the anatomic structures depends on the attenuation of the tissue examined. The thyroid gland, because of its high concentration of iodine, has higher attenuation than the surrounding soft tissues. Recent advances in spiral CT and in reconstruction algorithms have improved the performance of the method.[18,19]

CT scanning does not distinguish benign from malignant nodules and does not assess functional status; however, it can define the anatomic extent of large goiters with great clarity. CT scanning can provide useful information regarding the presence and extent of intrathoracic (substernal) goiters. The CT findings of an intrathoracic mass in continuity with the thyroid gland, with high attenuation on non—contrast-enhanced images and marked enhancement after injection of intravenous contrast material, suggests intrathoracic goiter. Radioiodine scanning can also be performed in this clinical setting, but false-negative results can occur if little or no functional tissue is present in the intrathoracic goiter. In aggressive pathologic processes such as anaplastic thyroid carcinoma, CT can define the extension of the tumor to the mediastinum and its relationships to surrounding structures and search for lung metastases.[18,19]

CT imaging is less sensitive than neck ultrasonography for the detection of lymph node metastases. Because of the necessity of infusing iodine-containing contrast agents for CT scanning of the neck and mediastinum, CT should be performed at least 4 weeks before any administration of radioiodine.

Magnetic Resonance Imaging

Because the hydrogen atoms of different tissues have different relaxation times (termed T1 and T2), a computer-assisted analysis of T1-weighted and T2-weighted signals may be used to differentiate thyroid gland from skeletal muscles, blood vessels, or regional lymph nodes. Normal thyroid tissue tends to be slightly more intense than muscles on a T1-weighted image, and tumors often appear more intense than normal thyroid tissue.

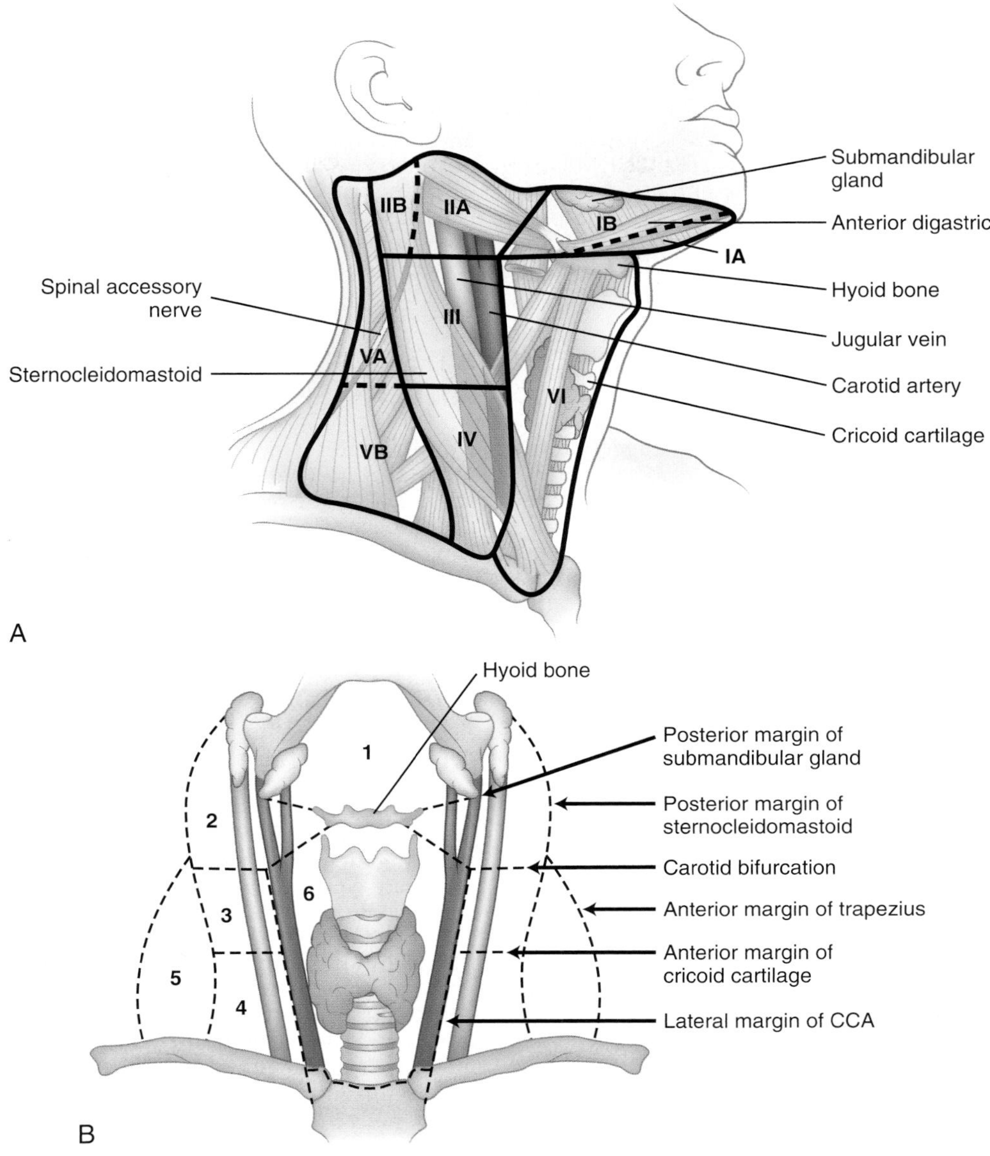

Figure 14-2 **A, Anatomic scheme of the neck with compartments.** (Reprinted with permission from Cooper DS, Doherty GM, Haugen BR, et al. Revised management guidelines for patients with thyroid nodules and differentiated thyroid cancer. *Thyroid,* 2009;19:1167-1214.) **B, Cervical map, derived from sonographic images, helps communicate anatomic relationships of pathology to clinicians and serves as a reference for follow-up examinations; standard colours are used to characterize any finding. CCA, common carotid artery.** (Reprinted with permission from J.W. Charboneau, Mayo Clinic.)

TABLE 14-2

Clinical Utility of Neck Ultrasound Examination

Map of the neck: thyroid and lymph node areas
Thyroid gland: size, volume, characteristics
Nodules: number and characteristics of each nodule—diameter, shape, echogenicity, composition, limits, presence of calcifications, vascularization
Lymph node areas
Follow-up: number and diameters of nodules
Guidance for fine-needle aspiration biopsy
Follow-up of thyroid cancer: thyroid bed and neck lymph node areas
Guidance for radiofrequency and ethanol ablation

Magnetic resonance imaging (MRI) does not distinguish benign from malignant nodules and does not assess functional status; however, it can define the anatomic extent of large goiters or aggressive tumors with the same clarity as CT scanning.

Recurrent neoplasms in the thyroid bed or regional lymph nodes can be detected with MRI; MRI is comparable in accuracy to CT. Recurrence is characterized by a mass with low to medium signal intensity on T1-weighted images and medium to high intensity on T2-weighted images. Conversely, scar tissue or fibrous tissue has low signal intensity on both T1- and T2-weighted images.[18,19] Tumor invasion of adjacent skeletal muscle has high signal intensity on T2-weighted images. Edema or inflammation in the muscle can cause a similar appearance and can be difficult to differentiate from recurrent tumor.

MRI is useful for assessment of the extent of bone involvement in cases of bone metastasis from follicular cell–derived carcinomas and MTC, which are poorly visualized on bone scintigraphy.[20,21] Contrast-enhanced MRI is more sensitive than three-phase contrast-enhanced CT for the detection of liver metastases from MTC, and spiral CT scanning is more sensitive than MRI for the detection of small lung metastases.[21]

Positron Emission Tomography

Positron emission tomography (PET) is both quantitative and tomographic. The radionuclide emits a positron that is converted into a pair of photons after a short path of a few millimeters in the tissue. The coincidence detection of the two photons, which travel on a line in opposite directions, permits localization of the site of the radionuclide decay.

The agent most widely used with PET is [^{18}F]-fluorodeoxyglucose (^{18}FDG). This agent is transported and phosphorylated as a glucose substitute but remains metabolically trapped inside tumor cells because of its inability to undergo glycolysis.

PET scanners permit in vivo images related to regional glucose metabolism, with high sensitivity and a spatial resolution of less than 5 mm. Superimposition of CT and PET images greatly improves the sensitivity and specificity of the technique and the anatomic localization of any focus of abnormal uptake. The uptake in any focus can be quantified; the most frequently used parameter is the standardized uptake value (SUV). The sensitivity of ^{18}FDG-PET scanning may be slightly improved with TSH stimulation.[22,23]

PET scanning should be performed only in selected patients with thyroid carcinoma. Low-risk patients are very unlikely to require ^{18}FDG-PET scanning as part of initial staging or follow-up. ^{18}FDG-PET scanning in thyroid cancer is used in the following circumstances[2,22]:

- To localize disease in thyroglobulin-positive (>10 ng/mL), radioiodine scan–negative patients; it is mostly useful for detection of lymph node metastases in the posterior neck and mediastinum or distant metastases
- For the initial staging and follow-up of patients with anaplastic, poorly differentiated, or Hürthle cell thyroid cancers, to identify sites of disease that may be missed with conventional imaging; in these cancers, FDG uptake is usually high
- In patients with known distant metastases in whom high FDG uptake in large metastases indicates a high risk for disease-specific mortality and poor response to radioiodine therapy[24]
- As a measurement of post-treatment response after local therapy (e.g., external-beam irradiation, surgical resection, radiofrequency ablation, embolization) or systemic therapy

Inflammatory lymph nodes, suture granulomas, and increased muscle activity are common causes of false-positive ^{18}FDG-PET findings. Also, asymmetric laryngeal uptake is frequently observed in patients with vocal cord paralysis. Therefore, cytologic or histologic confirmation is required before one can be certain that an ^{18}FDG-positive lesion represents metastatic disease.

High uptake has also been observed in several thyroid diseases such as thyroiditis, but PET cannot be used to differentiate benign from malignant thyroid nodules. The discovery of thyroid uptake on an FDG-PET scan performed for other reasons should lead to a complete workup, because a third of these nodules may prove to be malignant.[25,26]

In clinical research settings, PET scanning with ^{124}I has also been used for quantitation of uptake and for accurate dosimetry in distant metastases from thyroid cancer.[27] PET scanning with ^{18}F-labeled dihydroxyphenylalanine (DOPA) is used to visualize neoplastic foci of MTC,[28,29] because the FDG uptake is usually low in MTC patients, and FDG-PET is poorly informative.[21,30]

NONTOXIC GOITER: DIFFUSE AND NODULAR

Nontoxic goiter may be defined as any thyroid enlargement that is characterized by uniform or selective (i.e., restricted to one or more areas) growth of thyroid tissue, is not associated with overt hyperthyroidism or hypothyroidism, and does not result from inflammation or neoplasia. A thyroid nodule is defined as a discrete lesion, within the thyroid gland, caused by an abnormal, focal growth of thyroid cells.

Epidemiology

The prevalence of goiter, diffuse or nodular, varies widely depending on the iodine intake of the population living in a given area. Goiter may occur endemically (prevalence in children ≥5%), due mainly to iodine deficiency, or sporadically (prevalence <5%). In the general population, the Framingham survey indicated a 4.6% overall prevalence (6.4% in women and 1.5% in men), and the Wickham study reported a 3.2% prevalence (female-to-male ratio, 6.6 : 1).[31,32] However, variables such as regional variation in iodine intake, smoking habits, age and sex distribution, and especially the methodology used to determine thyroid volume (palpation versus sonography) may have biased many of these data. With sonography as the screening method, a goiter prevalence of up to 30% to 50% in an unselected adult population has been described. This prevalence is even higher in iodine-deficient areas and among older people.[31-35]

A prevalence of thyroid nodules of up to 50% has been described in autopsy series,[33] and greater than 60% in healthy adults screened with sonography.[34]

Etiology and Pathophysiology

Goiter has been traditionally regarded as the adaptive response of the thyroid follicular cell to any factor that impairs thyroid hormone synthesis. This classic concept no longer appears to encompass the many aspects of goiters. Indeed, goiter is characterized by a variety of clinical, functional, and morphologic presentations, and whether this heterogeneity represents different entities remains to be clarified. Also, iodine deficiency as the sole factor responsible for goiter appears to be an oversimplification. Not all inhabitants in an iodine-deficient region develop goiter. Moreover, endemic goiter has been observed in countries with no iodine deficiency, and even in some regions with iodine excess, and has not been observed in some regions with severe iodine deficiency. These findings suggest that other factors, both genetic and environmental, may play a role in the genesis of diffuse and nodular goiter, and some of these factors may act synergistically. Environmental factors include cigarette smoking, infections, drugs, and goitrogens.[35]

The role of genetic factors is suggested by several lines of evidence[36]: the clustering of goiters within families, the higher concordance rate for goiters in monozygotic compared with dizygotic twins, the female-to-male ratio (1:1 in endemic versus 7:1 to 9:1 in sporadic goiters), and the persistence of goiters in areas where a widespread iodine prophylaxis program has been properly implemented.

By studying families affected by goiter, researchers have been able to detect several gene abnormalities involving proteins related to thyroid hormone synthesis, such as mutations in genes encoding thyroglobulin (Tg), the sodium-iodide symporter (NIS), thyroid peroxidase (TPO), dual oxidase 2 (DUOX2), pendrin (Pendred syndrome, PDS), and the TSH receptor (TSHR). In addition, three loci for this disorder have been identified; they map to chromosomes 14q, Xp22, and 3q26, respectively.[37,38] Although an autosomal dominant inheritance has been demonstrated in several families, multiple genes may be involved in other families. This may explain why predisposing gene alterations remain unidentified in most patients with nontoxic goiter.

TSH has long been considered the major agent determining thyroid growth in response to any factor that impairs thyroid hormone synthesis. Indeed, in the rare clinical setting of a functioning TSH-secreting pituitary tumor, the increased blood TSH levels typically cause enlargement of the thyroid gland.[39] Similarly, goiter is also a typical feature of Graves' disease, in which a stimulatory growth effect on thyroid tissue is induced by TSHR-stimulating antibody through TSHR activation.[40] Moreover, thyroid enlargement may appear during the course of Graves' disease when increased TSH levels result from overtreatment with antithyroid drugs. In addition, toxic thyroid hyperplasia is usually present in non-autoimmune autosomal dominant hyperthyroidism, a disorder related to germline activating mutations of the TSHR gene.[41] This clinical condition further emphasizes the role of TSH-TSHR system activation in the genesis of thyroid hyperplasia.[36]

The serum TSH concentration is normal in most patients with nontoxic goiter.[35] Experimentally, it has been demonstrated in rats that iodine depletion enhances the promotion of thyroid growth despite normal levels of TSH.[42] Hence, any factor that impairs intrathyroidal iodine levels may lead to gradual development of goiter in response to normal concentrations of TSH.

Indeed, a complex network of both TSH-dependent and TSH-independent pathways directs thyroid follicular cell growth and function and plays a role in the goitrogenic process. In particular, a variety of growth factors, derived from the bloodstream or through autocrine or paracrine secretion, may serve to regulate thyroid cell proliferation and differentiation processes.[36]

Typically, early in the course of goiter formation, areas of microheterogeneity of structure and function are intermixed and include areas of functional autonomy and areas of focal hemorrhage. Analysis of hyperplastic nodules by rigid criteria have indicated that morphologically indistinguishable hyperplastic thyroid nodules may be either monoclonal or polyclonal. Monoclonal adenomas within hyperplastic thyroid glands may reflect a stage in progression along the hyperplasia-neoplasia spectrum; accumulation of multiple somatic mutations may subsequently confer a selective growth advantage to this single-cell clone.[43]

Histologically, nodules contain irregularly enlarged, involuted follicles distended with colloid or clusters of smaller follicles lined by taller epithelium and containing small colloid droplets. The nodules tend to be incompletely encapsulated; they are poorly demarcated from and merge with the internodular tissue, which also has an altered architecture. However, the nodules in some glands appear to be localized, with areas of apparently normal architecture elsewhere. Here, the distinction from a follicular adenoma may be difficult, and some pathologists apply terms such as *colloid* or *adenomatous* nodules to such lesions.

Natural History

Nontoxic goiter has a female preponderance. There appears to be no physiologic increase in thyroid volume during normal adolescence. Development of a goiter during adolescence, therefore, is a pathologic rather than a physiologic process.[44] However, as evidenced by sonographic measurement of thyroid volume in women living in an area of moderate iodine intake, normal pregnancy is goitrogenic, especially in women with preexisting thyroid disorders. The increased thyroid volume during pregnancy is associated with biochemical features of thyroid stimulation (i.e., an increased ratio of triiodothyronine [T_3] to thyroxine [T_4]) owing to slightly elevated serum TSH levels at delivery or a high concentration of human chorionic gonadotropin (hCG) during the first trimester.[45] Repeated pregnancies may play a role in the development of later thyroid disorders, and this relation might explain the higher prevalence of thyroid disorders in women.[46] The natural outcome of nontoxic nodular goiter was examined in an adult population with two main findings: (1) benign thyroid nodules are likely to grow (although slowly) over time, and (2) as a consequence, the concept that growing nodules are malignant whereas stable ones are benign should be discarded.[47]

Clinical Presentation

In an era when patients are advised on methods of self-examination to detect cancer at an early stage, the finding of a palpable abnormality in such a superficial location as the thyroid gland can be disconcerting. The affected patient is likely to seek medical evaluation. At the end of an appropriate investigation, the clinician can usually reassure the patient that the goiter or nodule is benign. Autonomous nodules, or autonomous functional areas in the context of a multinodular goiter, may result in increased thyroid hormone secretion and, subsequently, a subclinical or overt thyrotoxicosis. However, thyroid nodules are usually not associated with abnormal thyroid hormone secretion. Therefore, affected patients do not exhibit clinical symptoms or signs of thyroid dysfunction. The only clinical features of nontoxic goiter are those of thyroid enlargement. Almost 70% of patients with sporadic nontoxic goiter complain of neck discomfort; the remainder have cosmetic concerns or a fear of possible malignancy.[35]

Large goiters, which may displace or compress the trachea, esophagus, and neck vessels, can be associated with symptoms and signs including inspiratory stridor, dysphagia, and a choking sensation. These obstructive symptoms may be accentuated by the so-called Pemberton maneuver (see Chapter 11). Compression of the recurrent laryngeal nerve, with resulting hoarseness, suggests carcinoma rather than nontoxic goiter, but vocal cord paralysis can occasionally result from benign nodular goiters. Hemorrhage into a nodule or cyst produces acute, painful enlargement locally and may enhance or induce obstructive symptoms.[35]

Initial Investigation

Thyroid nodules are generally benign hyperplastic (or colloid) nodules or benign follicular adenomas, and only about 5% to 10% of nodules coming to medical attention are carcinomas. Differentiating true neoplasms from hyperplastic nodules and distinguishing between benign and malignant tumors are major challenges.

Moreover, with the widespread practice of medical checkups in healthy individuals and the increasing use of imaging technology, this problem is likely to become more common. High-resolution ultrasound studies suggest that the prevalence of nodular thyroid disease in healthy adults is greater than 60%.[34] However, during 2009 in the United States, only about 32,700 new cases of thyroid cancer were diagnosed.[48] Therefore, most of these so-called thyroid incidentalomas are obviously benign and do not progress to clinical tumors.[34]

In identifying the nodules that are likely to be malignant, a thorough history and a careful physical examination should be supplemented with laboratory testing, imaging procedures, and, most important, FNAB of the nodule in question. With this approach, it is possible to assess the likelihood of malignancy and to advise appropriate treatment for most patients.[35]

History and Physical Examination

Features of the history that favor benign disease include a family history of Hashimoto's thyroiditis, benign thyroid nodule, or goiter; symptoms of hypothyroidism or hyperthyroidism; and a sudden increase in size of the nodule with pain or tenderness, which suggests a cyst or localized subacute thyroiditis.[35] Features that suggest malignancy include young age (<20 years) or older age (>60 years); male gender; a history of external neck irradiation during childhood or adolescence; rapid growth; recent changes in speaking, breathing, or swallowing; and a family history of thyroid cancer or multiple endocrine neoplasia type 2 (MEN2).[35]

On physical examination, manifestations of thyroid malignancy should be sought, including firm consistency of the nodule, irregular shape, fixation to underlying or overlying tissues, vocal cord paralysis, and suspicious regional lymphadenopathy.[35]

Many studies have shown that a nodule size of less than 4 cm is not predictive of malignancy and that the incidence of cancer in incidentally identified or nonpalpable thyroid nodules is the same as in patients with palpable nodules. For nodules larger than 4 cm in diameter, the incidence of carcinoma may be higher.[49] However, given the excellent prognosis of micro-PTCs measuring less than 1 cm in diameter, most authors recommend investigation of only those nodules larger than 1 cm and nonpalpable nodules with clinical or sonographic suspicious findings.[2,10,34,50]

FDG-PET performed for nonthyroid disease detected incidental thyroid nodules in about 2% of patients. These nodules require an accurate assessment because of their increased rate of malignancy, up to 30%.[25,26] An evaluation of large groups of patients showed that the presence of multiple nodules does not decrease the likelihood of thyroid cancer. In patients with multiple nodules, the rate of malignancy per nodule decreases, but the decrease is approximately proportional to the number of nodules, so the overall rate per patient is the same as in patients with

TABLE 14-3

Clinical and Ultrasound Findings in Favor of Malignant Thyroid Nodules

Clinical Features	Ultrasound Findings
History	***Higher Suspicion***
Young age (<20 yr) or older age (>60 yr)	Hypoechoic lesions
Male gender	Irregular margins
Neck irradiation during childhood or adolescence	Presence of microcalcifications
Rapid growth	Absence of halo
Recent changes in speaking, breathing, or swallowing	Internal or central blood flow
Family history of thyroid malignancy or MEN2	
Physical Examination	***Low Suspicion***
Firm and irregular consistency of nodule	Echo-free (cystic) lesion
Fixation to underlying or overlying tissues	Spongiform lesion
Vocal cord paralysis	
Regional lymph adenopathy	

MEN2, multiple endocrine neoplasia type 2.

a solitary nodule. Also, thyroid cancers are often in the dominant nodule, but in approximately one third of cases, the cancer is in a nondominant nodule.[47]

In both prospective and retrospective studies, the sensitivity and specificity rates for detection of thyroid malignancy by history and physical examination (Table 14-3) were approximately 60% and 80%, respectively.[51,52] In these historical series, only about 20% of patients with later-confirmed malignancy had, when initially seen, neither suspicious features in the history nor evidence of potential malignancy on neck examination.

Laboratory Tests

As a first-line screening test, serum TSH may be measured with a highly sensitive immunometric assay and combined with a single measurement of free thyroid hormone concentrations.

A low or undetectable serum TSH, even if associated with normal free thyroid hormone levels, should suggest the possibility of toxic, autonomously functioning nodular areas in the goiter and should lead to thyroid scintigraphy. Such a finding should prompt further cardiac investigation, especially in elderly patients, whose risk of atrial fibrillation may be increased as much as threefold when serum TSH levels are less than 0.1 mU/L.[53] Patients with thyroid cancer rarely have abnormalities in serum TSH levels, but a higher serum TSH value, even if it is within the upper part of the reference range, is associated with increased risk of malignancy in a thyroid nodule.[54,55]

Measurement of serum anti-TPO antibody and anti-Tg antibody levels may be helpful in the diagnosis of chronic autoimmune thyroiditis, especially if serum TSH is elevated. Chronic thyroiditis has a typical hypoechoic appearance on sonography; the size and consistency of the thyroid gland may simulate either a solitary nodule or bilateral nodules; hypoechoic nodules should be submitted to FNAB, which will distinguish between foci of thyroiditis and nodules of epithelial origin.

Follicular cell–derived thyroid cancers (FCTCs), which include papillary, follicular, Hürthle cell, poorly differentiated, and anaplastic carcinomas, may release increased Tg into the bloodstream. Serum Tg levels in FCTCs and in a number of benign conditions overlap, so measurement of serum Tg levels is not useful in the initial workup of nodular thyroid disease. Some investigators routinely measure calcitonin levels in all patients with nodular thyroid disease to identify cases of MTC, because calcitonin is increased in almost all patients with clinical MTC.[56,57] However, because of the rarity of unsuspected MTC, there is a high frequency of false-positive results that may prompt a thyroidectomy despite a reassuring cytologic result; moreover, the clinical relevance of medullary microcarcinomas is unknown. Therefore, it is neither cost-effective nor necessary to measure calcitonin levels in patients with nodular thyroid disease in the absence of clinical suspicion of MTC or abnormal cytologic findings.[2,35] If the unstimulated serum calcitonin level is greater than 100 pg/mL, medullary cancer is likely to be present.[57]

The molecular abnormality in more than 95% of cases of familial MTC is a germline mutation of the *RET* proto-oncogene that is located on the long arm of chromosome 10.[58] Many investigators advocate *RET* mutation testing in all patients with MTC, including apparently sporadic cases, because 4% to 6% of such patients have germline mutations of the gene (see Chapter 41).[3] If a mutation is found, family members who are at risk are then tested to identify affected individuals. A negative result obviates the need for any further testing. Individuals who harbor such mutations should undergo prophylactic total thyroidectomy to prevent later development of the multicentric MTC that occurs in this disorder.[3]

Imaging in Nodular Goiter Evaluation

Today, when a nodular goiter is clinically present, ultrasonography represents by far the most useful thyroid imaging technique for providing helpful information for disease management and treatment. Ultrasonography should be used to assess both the morphology and the size of the goiter and may assist in screening and in follow-up of thyroid nodules.[1,2,10,35] Ultrasonography is capable of detecting even minute thyroid nodules. Of 1000 normal control subjects, 65% had detectable nodularity on high-resolution scanning.[34]

Attempts have been made to develop criteria for distinguishing benign and malignant nodules (see Table 14-3). Echo-free (cystic), spongiform, and homogeneously hyperechoic lesions are reputed to carry a low risk of malignancy.[10,35] Positive predictive criteria of malignancy include predominantly solid nodules and absence of cystic elements, hypoechoic nodules, presence of microcalcifications, irregular margins and absence of halo, and a taller rather than a wide shape measured in the transverse dimension.[59] Nodules that can be clearly identified as benign by sonography are uncommon. The color Doppler finding of predominantly internal or central blood flow appears to increase the risk that a nodule is malignant. However, like other sonographic features, color Doppler cannot be used to diagnose or exclude malignancy with a high degree of confidence.[10,35] Elastography is a promising technique that requires further evaluation to determine its usefulness in clinical practice.[15]

Recently, an equation was devised to predict the probability of malignancy in thyroid nodules, based on 12 ultrasound parameters. It was suggested that such a thyroid imaging reporting and data system could decide optimal strategies for managing thyroid nodules.[60]

Ultrasonography is useful in identifying hypoechoic solid nodules that should be submitted to FNAB, particularly in the presence of microcalcifications, and also in examining the rest of the thyroid gland and lymph node areas (Fig. 14-3).[2,10] It may also be used to direct the needle during FNAB—into the nodule in routine practice, or into solid portions in the case of partially cystic nodules—and in the setting of nonpalpable nodules, especially when the diameter of the nodule is 1 cm or more.[10] Cystic lesions may be treated by aspiration of the fluid and ethanol injection to avoid recurrence; this is optimally performed under ultrasonographic guidance.[61]

In patients with large goiters, CT or MRI is indicated to define the relationships with surrounding structures.

The traditional imaging procedure of the thyroid in past years has been scintigraphy using ^{131}I, ^{123}I, or ^{99m}Tc. Most thyroid carcinomas are inefficient in trapping and organifying iodine and appear on scans as areas of diminished isotope uptake, so-called cool or cold nodules. This feature reflects the early decrease of NIS expression during tumorigenesis.[62] However, most benign nodules also do not concentrate iodine and therefore are cold nodules. Furthermore, not all nodules with normal or slightly increased ^{99m}Tc uptake are benign, and some may appear cold on a thyroid scan with radioactive iodine.[4,5]

The only situation in which an iodine scan can exclude malignancy with reasonable certainty is in the case of a toxic adenoma, which is characterized by significantly increased uptake within the nodule (hot nodule) and markedly suppressed or absent uptake in the remainder of the gland. These lesions are suspected at clinical examination and are typically associated with a low or suppressed serum TSH level. They account for fewer than 10% of thyroid nodules and are almost invariably benign.[35] Thyroid scintigraphy should be used as a second-line technique to detect hyperfunctioning nodules in patients with low or undetectable serum TSH levels.

CT scanning and MRI in the initial diagnosis of thyroid malignancy do not provide higher-quality images of the thyroid and cervical nodes than those obtained by ultrasonography. CT examination of the lower central neck is preferable if tracheal or mediastinal invasion is suspected.[35]

Fine-Needle Aspiration Biopsy

FNAB of thyroid nodules has eclipsed all other techniques for diagnosis of thyroid cancer, with reported overall rates of sensitivity and specificity exceeding 90% in iodine-sufficient areas.[2,10,35,50,63,64] The technique is easy to perform and safe, only a handful of complications having been reported in the literature,[65] and causes little discomfort. However, care must be taken to obtain an adequate specimen; most authors recommend between three and six aspirations per nodule.[63,64] Routine use of ultrasound-guided biopsy even for clinically palpable solid nodules, combined with on-site cytologic examination, improves the accuracy of sampling and decreases the risk of inadequate sampling.[66-68] A satisfactory specimen contains at least five or six groups of 10 to 15 well-preserved cells. The cells are categorized by their cytologic appearances into *benign, indeterminate* or *suspicious*, and *malignant* groups (Table 14-4).

The diagnosis of PTC by FNAB on the basis of characteristic nuclear changes is particularly reliable and accurate, with sensitivity and specificity approaching 100%. For follicular neoplasms, however, the performance of FNAB is lower. If strict criteria for malignancy are used, sensitivity may be as low as 8%.[52] If any follicular neoplasm that is not clearly benign on cytologic examination is classified as cancerous, sensitivity rises to 90% or more, but with a considerable drop in specificity to less than 50% (i.e., a

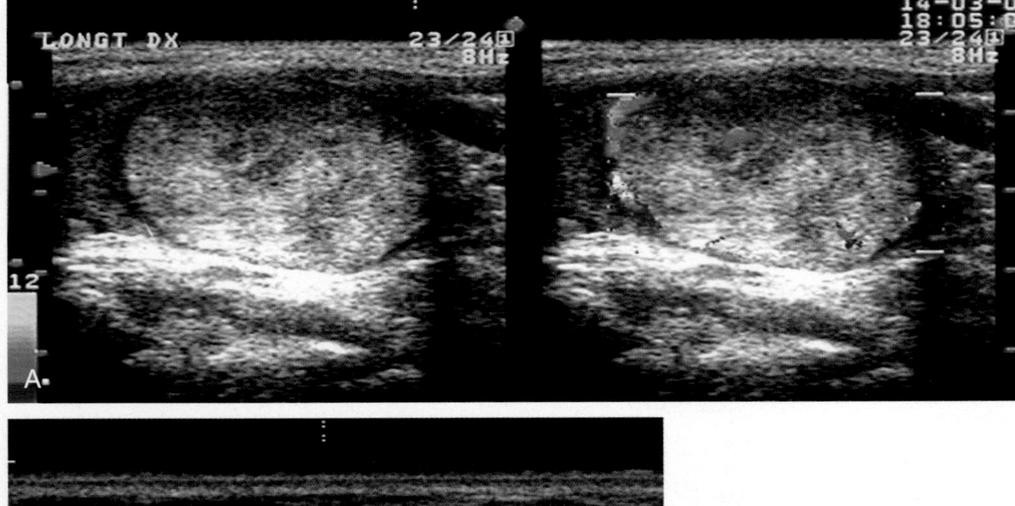

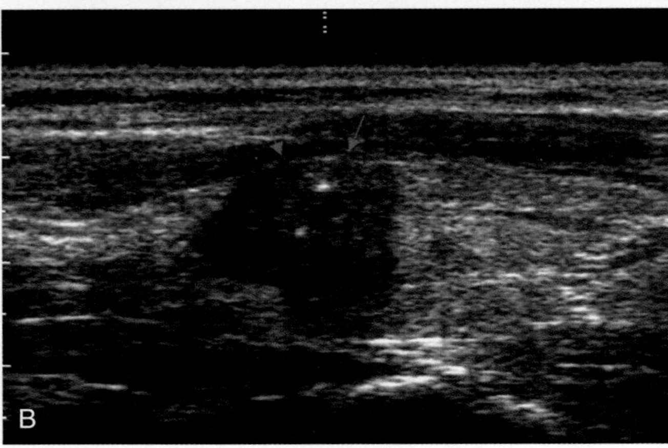

Figure 14-3 Conventional and color flow Doppler ultrasonography. **A,** Benign lesion. Sonogram shows well-defined, oval, hyperechoic nodule with perinodular and slight intranodular blood flow. **B,** Malignant lesion. Sonogram shows a nodule with inhomogeneous hypoechoic aspect, microcalcifications, irregular borders, and invasion of the thyroid capsule *(arrows)*.

TABLE 14-4

Probability of Malignancy at Histology Based on Fine-Needle Aspiration Biopsy Cytology (Summary of the Literature)

Cytology	Percentage of Cases, Mean (Range)	Probability of Malignancy (%)
Inadequate/nondiagnostic	16 (15-20)	10-20
Benign	70 (53-90)	1-2
Suspicious*	10 (5-23)	10-20
Malignant	4 (1-10)	>95

*The suspicious category includes follicular neoplasms (hyperplastic nodules, follicular adenomas, and follicular carcinomas) and some Hürthle cell tumors.

large number of false-positive results).[63] This seriously limits the usefulness of FNAB in iodine-deficient regions, where the incidence of follicular thyroid carcinoma (FTC) approaches that of PTC and where both follicular adenomas and hyperplastic adenomatous nodules are prevalent.[66]

The recent National Cancer Institute Thyroid Fine-Needle Aspiration State of the Science Conference proposed a more expanded classification for FNA cytology that adds two additional categories[69]:

1. Malignant (risk of malignancy, >95%)
2. Suspicious for malignancy (risk of malignancy, 50% to 75%)
3. Follicular or Hürthle cell neoplasm (risk of malignancy, 15% to 25%)
4. Follicular lesion of undetermined significance (risk of malignancy, 5% to 10%)
5. Benign lesions (risk of malignancy, <1%)

Attempts have been made to improve the accuracy of cytology and to decrease the percentage of indeterminate cases.[70] Results of FNAB should be combined with clinical and ultrasound characteristics. A PTC is usually solid or predominantly solid and hypoechoic, often with infiltrative irregular margins and increased nodular vascularity. Microcalcifications, if present, are highly specific for PTC but may be difficult to distinguish from colloid. The predictive value of ultrasonography is increased when several suspicious characteristics are present. Conversely, follicular cancer is more often isoechoic to hyperechoic and has a thick and irregular halo, but it does not have microcalcifications.[59,71]

Galectin 3 immunochemistry, alone or combined with TPO, may be a valuable adjunct to the standard cytologic techniques in cases of typical follicular lesions, either benign or malignant.[72] Prospective studies have confirmed the ability of genetic markers such as BRAF, RAS, and RET/PTC to improve preoperative diagnostic accuracy for patients with indeterminate cytology, but no medicoeconomic evaluation has been produced.[73] A combination of markers identified with microarray technology has also been advocated, but independent confirmation of their usefulness is required.[74-77]

The use of large-needle biopsy in addition to standard FNAB has improved diagnostic accuracy in difficult cases, but the technique is more exacting than FNAB alone and is associated with increased morbidity.[78] Particularly for cystic thyroid nodules, sampling from the margin of the nodule under ultrasonic guidance, rather than from the cystic fluid and debris in the center, increases accuracy.

In some centers FNAB is combined with preoperative FNAB with intraoperative frozen-section analysis. In the hands of experienced surgeon-pathologist teams, the rate of misdiagnosis with this approach is less than 5%, as evidenced by subsequent review of paraffin-embedded specimens. The approach avoids unnecessarily extensive surgery in patients with benign tumors, achieves resection of almost all malignant tumors, and rarely necessitates a second operation for completion thyroidectomy.[79] Such an approach is employed at the Mayo Clinic and at the Institut Gustave Roussy, where intraoperative frozen-section analysis is routine.

Apart from its limited utility in the evaluation of follicular neoplasms, the only other limitation of FNAB is with nondiagnostic specimens, which can account for as many as 20% of cases.[63,64] Although repeated aspiration increases both the accuracy and the rate of diagnostic aspirations, even repeated attempts sometimes fail. Ultrasound-guided FNAB can help overcome this problem in some patients.[67,68] The rate of cancer in surgically resected nodules with nondiagnostic FNAB results is 10% to 20%. Therefore, either close observation or surgical removal of the nodule is probably the best option. Some authorities recommend a trial of TSH suppression, which can sometimes shrink benign nodules. However, a significant proportion of benign nodules do not shrink, and some carcinomas do shrink; consequently, the diagnostic value of TSH suppression is doubtful. Figure 14-4 is an algorithm for the management of nodular thyroid disease in which FNAB is the first diagnostic test and subsequent management is based on cytologic results.

The most expeditious way to diagnose thyroid malignancy is to obtain a thorough history and physical examination, followed by ultrasonography, FNAB (preferably performed under ultrasound guidance), and evaluation of

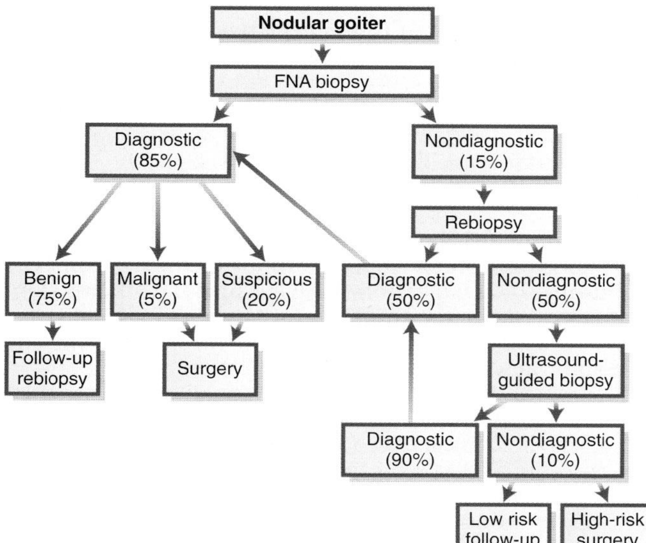

Figure 14-4 Management of nodular goiter based on fine-needle aspiration (FNA) biopsy as the first diagnostic test. Subsequent management is based on cytologic results. Percentages in parentheses indicate satisfactory or unsatisfactory biopsy results. (From Gharib H. Fine-needle aspiration biopsy of thyroid nodules: advantages, limitations, and effect. *Mayo Clin Proc.* 1994;69:44-49.)

the sample by an experienced cytologist. Imaging procedures in addition to ultrasonography and other tests may occasionally be helpful, but diagnostic thyroid scintiscanning, as traditionally practiced, is of little or no value and should be abandoned.[1,2,35]

In iodine-sufficient areas with a high relative prevalence of PTC, the combination of the history, physical examination, and FNAB is usually sufficient to confirm malignancy. Conversely, if the history and physical examination, ultrasonography, and FNAB do not suggest malignancy, the chances of missing a PTC are probably less than 1%.[63,64] In areas where the prevalence of follicular tumors is higher, more patients may require neck exploration because their FNAB is not conclusive.[66]

Surgery should also be considered for large tumors (>4 cm), especially in young subjects, to avoid repeated evaluations. In addition, because these tumors may be composed of various cell populations, results of FNAB are less reliable.[49]

Finally, micronodules smaller than 1 cm in diameter that are found incidentally during imaging do not need to be tested any further unless there are sonographic features suggestive of PTC or MTC. The usual advice is to repeat ultrasonography of such lesions after an interval of 6 to 12 months.[1,2,34]

MANAGEMENT OF BENIGN NONTOXIC DIFFUSE AND NODULAR GOITER

Patients with small, asymptomatic goiters may be monitored by clinical examination and evaluated periodically with ultrasound measurements. Goiter growth can be variable, and some patients have stable goiters for many years. For more than a century, thyroid "feeding" has been employed to reduce the size of nontoxic goiters. The 1953 report of Greer and Astwood, in which two thirds of patients' goiters regressed with thyroid therapy, led to widespread acceptance of suppressive therapy[80] despite some doubts about the value of such therapy.[81] An overview of studies performed from 1960 to 1992 suggested that 60% or more of sporadic nontoxic goiters respond to suppressive therapy.[81] In a prospective placebo-controlled, double-blind, randomized clinical trial, 58% of the T_4-treated group had a significant response at 9 months, as measured by ultrasonography, compared with 5% of the placebo-treated group.[82]

Nodular goiters appear to be less responsive than diffuse goiters. A 2002 meta-analysis failed to demonstrate a significant benefit of T_4 therapy, which was found to carry a relative risk of nodule shrinkage of only 1.9 (95% confidence interval, 0.95 to 3.81).[83] Statistical significance emerged from a multicenter randomized, double-blind, placebo-controlled trial: after 18 months of follow-up the nodule shrinkage was significantly greater in the group treated with levothyroxine than in the placebo group ($P = .01$); the proportion of responders was also significantly greater ($P = .04$).[84] It is likely that a subset of patients respond to T_4 suppressive therapy, particularly younger patients with small or recently diagnosed nodules.[83] However, thyroid nodules rapidly return to their pretreatment size after discontinuation of therapy,[35] so maintenance of size reduction may require continuous treatment.

A major concern in relation to long-term T_4 suppression therapy is the possibility of detrimental effects on the skeleton and heart. It has been reported that TSH suppression therapy is associated with variable degrees of bone loss, particularly in postmenopausal women.[85,86] However, other studies did not demonstrate significant change in bone mass after long-term T_4 therapy.[87] Furthermore, there is no evidence that treatment with the natural T_4 isomer, levothyroxine, is detrimental to the heart in young subjects when TSH is decreased to subnormal but still detectable values.[85,86]

Surgery for nontoxic goiter is physiologically unsound because it further restricts the ability of the thyroid to meet hormone requirements. Nevertheless, surgery may become necessary due to persistence of obstructive manifestations despite a trial of levothyroxine. Surgery should consist of a near-total or total thyroidectomy, but recurrence is seen in 10% to 20% of these patients within 10 years.[87] Surgical complications have been reported in 7% to 10% of cases and are more common with large goiters and with reoperation.[88] Prophylactic treatment with levothyroxine after goiter resection probably does not prevent goiter recurrence.[89]

Traditionally, the role of ^{131}I therapy for nontoxic goiter was to reduce the size of a massive goiter in elderly patients who were poor candidates for surgery or to treat goiter that had recurred after resection. Several studies demonstrated that primary treatment of nontoxic goiter with ^{131}I is followed by a reduction in thyroid volume.[90,91] In one study, thyroid volume (assessed by ultrasonography) was reduced by 40% after 1 year and 55% after 2 years with no further reduction thereafter, and 60% of the total reduction occurred within the first 3 months.[90] Considering its effectiveness in reducing the size of the thyroid gland, ^{131}I therapy has also been used for the treatment of nonautonomous thyroid nodules, and significant shrinkage, ranging from 31% to 60%, has been observed (Fig. 14-5).[92,93]

It was formerly argued that ^{131}I treatment of large goiters or goiters with substernal extension should be avoided because of the risks of acute swelling of the gland and consequent tracheal compression. However, ultrasonographic studies of thyroid volume after ^{131}I therapy have failed to demonstrate significant early volume increase. Moreover, decreased tracheal deviation and increased tracheal lumen size were demonstrated by MRI in patients who had compression from nontoxic goiter with substernal extension.[90]

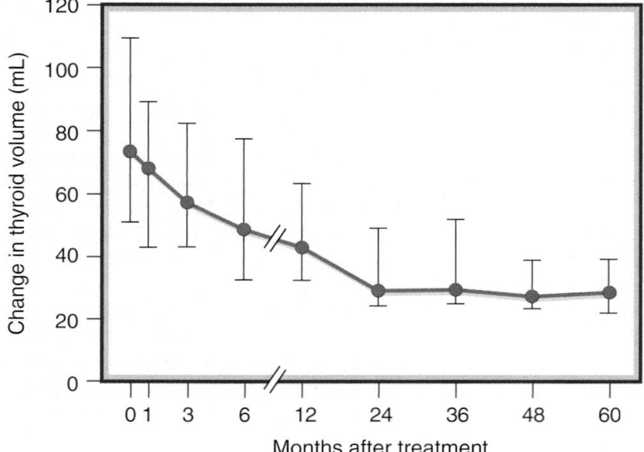

Figure 14-5 Median changes in thyroid volume after treatment with iodine 131 in 39 patients with nontoxic multinodular goiter who remained euthyroid after a single dose. Bars represent quartiles. (From Nygaard B, Hegedus L, Gervil M, et al. Radioiodine treatment of multinodular nontoxic goiter. *BMJ*, 1993;307:828-832.)

Therefore, it appears that ^{131}I treatment of nontoxic diffuse or multinodular goiter is effective and safe. Hypothyroidism has been reported in 20% to 40% of cases, and transient thyrotoxicosis and mild pain can occur.[90] Regular follow-up, preferably by a systematic annual recall scheme, is necessary. The activities used are in the range of those used for ^{131}I treatment of hyperthyroidism; the radiation doses are comparable, and long-term thyroid and nonthyroidal cancer risks after ^{131}I treatment for hyperthyroidism are reassuring.[94] Stimulation with low doses of recombinant human TSH (rhTSH), 0.01 to 0.03 mg, increases the thyroid ^{131}I uptake and may allow administration of a lower dosage of ^{131}I. However, such treatment also increases thyroid hormone production, and overproduction of thyroid hormones should be excluded before its use.[95] Long-term randomized studies comparing the effects, side effects, and costs and benefits of surgery and ^{131}I treatment need to be performed.

Percutaneous ethanol injection should be used only for recurrent symptomatic cystic nodules.[61] Laser therapy is still an experimental procedure and may be proposed, in experienced centers, for selected patients with symptomatic nodular goiters when surgery is not possible.[96]

MANAGEMENT OF MALIGNANT NODULAR GOITER

Thyroid tumors are the most common endocrine neoplasms. The management of a typical thyroid cancer is effective and usually consists of surgical resection followed by medical therapy and regular surveillance.[97-99] Some degree of consensus has been achieved with regard to the initial management of differentiated thyroid cancer, but important clinical and biologic questions remain unanswered. In the following discussion, we present a widely used scheme for classifying and staging tumors of the thyroid gland. We also review the features of the principal types of benign and malignant thyroid neoplasms and the controversies regarding the management of differentiated thyroid carcinoma, based on recent consensus statements and guidelines.[1-3]

Classification of Thyroid Tumors

Histologic Classification

Two monographs have had a major impact on the histologic classification of thyroid tumors. One is from the World Health Organization (WHO),[99] and the other is from the Armed Forces Institute of Pathology (AFIP).[100] The classification described in Table 14-5 is modified from the guidelines described by these organizations.

Lesions of follicular cell origin constitute more than 95% of the cases, and the remainder are largely made up of tumors exhibiting C-cell differentiation. Mixed medullary and follicular carcinomas, comprising cells with both C-cell and follicular differentiation, are rare and of uncertain histogenesis. Nonepithelial thyroid tumors mainly include malignant lymphomas, which may involve the thyroid gland as the only manifestation of the disease or as part of a systemic disease. True sarcomas and malignant hemangioendotheliomas are exceptional. Bloodborne metastases to the thyroid are not uncommon at autopsy in patients with widespread malignancy but rarely cause clinically detectable thyroid enlargement.

TABLE 14-5

Classification of Thyroid Neoplasms

Primary Epithelial Tumors
Tumors of Follicular Cells
Benign: Follicular Adenoma
Malignant: Carcinoma
Differentiated
Papillary
Follicular
Poorly differentiated
Undifferentiated (anaplastic)
Tumors of C Cells
Medullary carcinoma
Tumors of Follicular and C Cells
Mixed medullary-follicular carcinoma
Primary Nonepithelial Tumors
Malignant lymphomas
Sarcomas
Others
Secondary Tumors

TABLE 14-6

The Tumor-Node-Metastasis (TNM) Scoring System, 1992 and 2002 Versions

DEFINITION OF TNM	
1992 Version	**2002 Version**
Primary Tumor (T)	
T0—No evidence of primary tumor	T0—No evidence of primary tumor
T1—Tumor ≤1 cm limited to the thyroid	T1—Tumor ≤2 cm limited to the thyroid
T2—Tumor >1 and ≤4 cm limited to the thyroid	T2—Tumor >2 and ≤4 cm limited to the thyroid
T3—Tumor >4 cm limited to the thyroid	T3—Tumor >4 cm limited to the thyroid or any tumor with minimal extrathyroidal extension (e.g., to sternothyroid muscle, to parathyroid, to soft tissues)
T4—Tumor of any size extending beyond the thyroid capsule	T4a—Tumor of any size with extension beyond the thyroid capsule and invasion of any of the following: subcutaneous soft tissues, larynx, trachea, esophagus, recurrent laryngeal nerve
	T4b—Tumor invading prevertebral fascia or mediastinal vessels or encasing the carotid artery
Regional Lymph Nodes (N)	
N0—No regional lymph node metastasis	N0—No regional lymph node metastasis*
N1—Regional lymph node metastasis	N1—Regional lymph node metastasis
	N1a—Metastases in pretracheal and paratracheal lymph nodes, including prelaryngeal and Delphian lymph nodes
	N1b—Metastases in other unilateral, bilateral, or contralateral cervical or upper mediastinal lymph nodes
Distant Metastasis (M)	
M0—No distant metastasis	M0—No distant metastasis
M1—Distant metastasis	M1—Distant metastasis
TNM STAGING	
1992 Version	**2002 Version**
Age < 45 yr	
Stage I—Any T, any N, M0	Stage I—Any T, any N, M0
Stage II—Any T, any N, M1	Stage II—Any T, any N, M1
Stage III—None	Stage III—None
Stage IV—None	Stage IV—None
Age ≥ 45 yr	
Stage I—T1, N0, M0	Stage I—T1, N0, M0
Stage II—T2-T3, N0, M0	Stage II—T2, N0, M0
Stage III—T4, N0, M0 or any T, N1, M0	Stage III—T3, N0, M0 or any T1-3, N1a, M0
Stage IV—Any T, any N, M1	Stage IVA—T1-3, N1b, M0 or T4a, any N, M0
	Stage IVB—T4b, any N, M0
	Stage IVC—Any T, any N, M1

*To classify as N0, at least six lymph nodes should be examined at histology. Otherwise, the disease is classified as Nx.

From Beahrs OH, Henson DE, Hutter RVP, et al. *Manual for Staging of Cancer.* Philadelphia, PA: Lippincott, 1992; and American Joint Committee on Cancer. Thyroid. In: *AJCC Cancer Staging Handbook,* 6th ed. New York, NY: Springer; 2002:89-98.

Staging of Thyroid Carcinoma

In addition to the histologic classification of thyroid tumors developed by the WHO and AFIP groups, the International Union Against Cancer (UICC) and the American Joint Committee on Cancer (AJCC) have agreed on a staging system in thyroid cancer.[101,102] As stated by the AJCC, "the principal purpose served by international agreement on the classification of cancer cases by extent of disease was to provide a method of conveying clinical experience to others without ambiguity."

The AJCC based its system of classification on the older tumor-node-metastasis (TNM) system, which relies on assessing three components: the extent of the primary tumor (T), the absence or presence of regional lymph node metastases (N), and the absence or presence of distant metastases (M). The TNM system allows a reasonably precise description and recording of the anatomic extent of disease. The classification may be either *clinical* (cTNM), based on evidence (including biopsy) acquired before treatment, or *pathologic* (pTNM), by which intraoperative and surgical pathology data are available. Obviously, pTNM classification is preferable because a precise size can be assigned to the primary tumor, the histotype is identified, and extrathyroidal invasion is demonstrated unequivocally.

Typically, in the 1992 TNM classification,[101] the primary thyroid tumor status is defined according to the size of the primary lesion as T1 (greatest diameter ≤1 cm), T2 (>1 cm but ≤4 cm), T3 (>4 cm), or T4 with direct (extrathyroidal) extension or invasion through the thyroid capsule. A thyroid tumor with four degrees of T, two degrees of N, and two degrees of M can have 16 different TNM categories. For purposes of tabulation and analysis, these categories have been condensed into a convenient number of TNM stage-groupings (Table 14-6).

Whereas head and neck cancer is usually staged entirely on the basis of anatomic extent, in thyroid cancer staging both the histologic diagnosis and the age of the patient for

PTC and FTC are included because of their importance in predicting the behavior and prognosis of thyroid cancer. According to this staging scheme, all patients younger than 45 years of age with PTC or FTC are in stage I, unless they have distant metastases (DM), in which case they would be in stage II. In young patients and especially in children, the risk of recurrence is high and may be underestimated by the TNM staging system.[103] Older patients (≥45 years) with node-negative papillary or follicular microcarcinoma (T1 N0 M0) are in stage I. Tumors between 1.1 and 4.0 cm are classified as stage II, and those with either nodal spread (N1) or extrathyroidal invasion (T4) are stage III.

For MTC, the scheme is similar in that microcarcinoma is stage I and a node-positive tumor is stage III. There is no age distinction for MTC, although age is a significant independent prognostic indicator in most multivariate analyses,[104-106] and local (extrathyroidal) invasion is grouped within stage II. For patients with MTC and older patients with PTC or FTC, stage IV denotes the presence of distant metastases. Independent of age or tumor extent, all patients with undifferentiated (anaplastic) cancer are considered to be in stage IV.

The 2002 TNM classification is more complicated, and minimal or more extensive thyroid tumor extension may be difficult to define retrospectively.[102] At least six lymph nodes must be examined at histology to qualify for the definition of N0 status, and the prognostic difference between central lymph-node metastases and other regional metastases has yet to be validated. In fact, the risk of persistent or recurrent disease appears to be related to involvement of the central neck compartment and the numbers of involved lymph nodes and lymph nodes with capsular extension.[107] Currently, it is not possible to ascertain whether the modifications included in the 2002 TNM classification will significantly improve its prognostic value and have a clinical impact on therapeutic strategies. One risk is that some centers advocating lobectomy for tumors smaller than 1 cm (T1 in the 1992 classification) may extend this indication to the 2002-redefined T1 group (i.e., tumors up to 2 cm). This attitude, based on cause-specific mortality, may lead to undertreatment of some patients, exposing them to a higher risk of recurrence.

Follicular Adenoma

Follicular adenoma is a benign, encapsulated tumor with evidence of follicular cell differentiation.[99,100] It is the most common thyroid neoplasm and may be found in 4% to 20% of glands examined at autopsy.[108] The tumor has a well-defined fibrous capsule that is grossly and microscopically complete. There is a sharp demarcation and distinct structural difference from the surrounding parenchyma. These adenomas vary in size, but most have a diameter of 1 to 3 cm at the time of excision. Degenerative changes, such as necrosis, hemorrhage, edema, fibrosis, and calcification, are common features, particularly in larger tumors.

Follicular adenomas can be classified into subtypes according to the size or presence of follicles and degree of cellularity. Each adenoma tends to have a consistent architectural pattern. *Microfollicular, normofollicular,* and *macrofollicular* adenomas owe their names to the size of their follicles compared with follicles in the neighboring, nonneoplastic areas of the gland. *Trabecular adenomas* are cellular and consist of columns of cells arranged in compact cords. They show little follicle formation and rarely contain colloid. A variant, the *hyalinizing trabecular adenoma,* has unusually elongated cells and prominent hyaline changes in the extracellular space.[109] The histologic differences among these subtypes are striking but of no clinical importance. The only practical value of the classification is that the more cellular a follicular nodule is, the more one should search for evidence of malignancy in the form of invasion of blood vessels or of tumor capsule or both.[99,100]

Atypical adenomas are hypercellular or heterogeneous, or both, with gross and histologic appearances that suggest the possibility of malignancy but not invasion. They account for fewer than 3% of all follicular adenomas. Follow-up indicates that this lesion behaves in a benign fashion. The fact that the tumor does not recur or produce metastases after removal does not prove that it is actually benign; removal may have interrupted a natural history that would have culminated in invasion and metastases. This is why they are classified as tumors of "undefined malignancy."

The most important cytologic variant is the *oxyphilic* or *oncocytic (Hürthle cell) adenoma,* which is composed predominantly (at least 75%) or entirely of large cells with granular, eosinophilic cytoplasm.[110] Ultrastructurally, the cells are rich in mitochondria and may exhibit nuclear pleomorphism with distinct nucleoli. Although all such neoplasms are thought by some to be potentially malignant,[111] the biologic behavior and clinical course of oncocytic tumors correlate closely with the histology and the size of the initial lesion. The absence of invasion predicts a benign outcome,[110] but larger tumors may rarely be associated with later recurrence or metastasis, even in the absence of obvious microscopic evidence of invasion. Fortunately, such an occurrence is rare, and usually a diagnosis of benign Hürthle cell adenoma is reliable.[112,113]

Some normofollicular adenomas may contain pseudopapillary structures that can be confused with the papillae of PTC. These structures are probably an expression of localized hyperactivity and are most common in adenomas that show autonomous function.

In most hyperfunctioning follicular adenomas, activating point mutations have been identified in the TSHR or in the α-subunit of the stimulatory guanyl nucleotide protein ($G_s\alpha$) (Fig. 14-6).[41,114] Such mutations may trap the G protein in a state of constitutive activation, resulting in

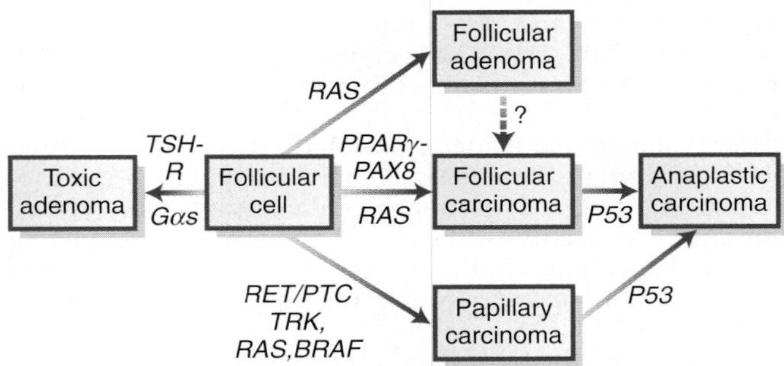

Figure 14-6 Genetic events in thyroid tumorigenesis. Activating point mutations of the *RAS* gene are found with a high frequency in follicular adenomas and follicular carcinomas and are considered to be an early event in follicular tumorigenesis. The PPARγ-PAX8 rearrangement is found only in follicular tumors. Rearrangements of transmembrane receptors with tyrosine kinase activity (*RET/PTC, TRK* genes) and activating point mutation of the *BRAF* gene are found only in PTCs. Inactivating point mutations of the *P53* gene are found only in poorly differentiated and anaplastic thyroid carcinomas. Activation of the cyclic adenosine monophosphate pathway, by point mutation of the thyrotropin receptor (TSH-R) or the α-subunit of the G protein genes, leads to the appearance of hyperfunctioning thyroid nodules. Gαs, stimulatory guanyl nucleotide protein; PPAR, peroxisome proliferator-activated receptor; PTC, papillary thyroid carcinoma.

enhanced cyclic adenosine monophosphate (cAMP) production and constitutive hyperstimulation of the cells. Genetic abnormalities found in hypofunctioning adenomas are detailed later.

Papillary Thyroid Carcinoma

PTC has been defined as "a malignant epithelial tumor showing evidence of follicular cell differentiation, and characterized by the formation of papillae and/or a set of distinctive nuclear changes."[99,100] The most common thyroid malignancy, PTC constitutes 50% to 90% of differentiated FCTCs worldwide.[98]

Papillary thyroid microcarcinoma (PTM) is defined by the WHO as a PTC 1.0 cm in diameter or smaller.[98-100,115-117] The incidence rate in the United States for clinically diagnosed PTM (approximately 1 per 100,000) is lower than that reported for tumors larger than 1 cm in diameter (approximately 5 per 100,000) and lower than the incidence of PTM in autopsy material from various continents (4% to 36%).[99,100] These findings suggest that more extensive screening is largely responsible for the apparently increasing incidence of thyroid carcinomas reported in recent years, which is largely due to increased detection of PTM.[118]

PTCs appear as firm, unencapsulated or partially encapsulated tumors. PTCs may be partly necrotic, and some are cystic. Typically, PTC shows a predominance of papillary structures, consisting of a fibrovascular core lined by a single layer of epithelial cells, but the papillae are usually admixed with neoplastic follicles having characteristic nuclear features.

The nuclei of PTC cells have a distinctive appearance that has a diagnostic significance comparable to that of the papillae. Indeed, the preoperative diagnosis of PTC can often be made on the basis of the characteristic nuclear changes seen in FNA material: Nuclei are larger than in normal follicular cells and overlap; they may be fissured like coffee beans; chromatin is hypodense (ground-glass nuclei); limits are irregular; and they frequently contain an inclusion corresponding to a cytoplasmic invagination.

Psammoma bodies are often present in the core of papillae or in the tumor stroma; they are microscopic structures made up of calcified layers.

Several subtypes exist and account for about 20% of all PTCs: The tumor is designated a *follicular variant* of PTC if the lining cells of the neoplastic follicles have the same nuclear features as seen in typical PTC and the follicular predominance over the papillae is complete.[99,100] The *diffuse sclerosing variant* is characterized by diffuse involvement of one or both thyroid lobes, widespread lymphatic permeation, prominent fibrosis, and lymphoid infiltration. The *tall cell variant* is characterized by well-formed papillae that are covered by cells twice as tall as they are wide. The *columnar cell variant* differs from other forms of PTC by the presence of prominent nuclear stratification of elongated cells. The tall cell and columnar cell variants are more aggressive, but controversy exists regarding outcome for the diffuse sclerosing variant.[98]

In children, tumor extension is usually substantial at diagnosis: tumors are large, unencapsulated, and invasive, with solid trabecular features. Extension beyond the thyroid capsule, lymph node metastases, and lung metastases are frequently observed.[103]

Molecular Pathogenesis

The thyroid follicular cell may give rise to benign or malignant tumors, and the malignancy can be of either papillary or follicular histotype. There is no evidence that human benign tumors ever undergo malignant transformation into classic PTC. Structural abnormalities of the chromosomes occur in about 50% of PTCs and frequently involve the long arm of chromosome 10.[114,119-122] The *RET* proto-oncogene is located on chromosome 10q11-12. It encodes a transmembrane receptor with a tyrosine kinase domain. Its ligands, such as the glial cell line–derived neutrophilic factor (GDNF), bind to the GDNF family receptor α-1 (GFRA1) and induce RET protein dimerization. *RET* (REarranged during Transfection) activation was first demonstrated in transfection experiments and subsequently was found only in PTC tumors. It was therefore called *RET/PTC*.

All activated forms of the *RET* proto-oncogene are the consequence of oncogenic rearrangements fusing the tyrosine kinase domain of the *RET* gene with the 5′ domain of other genes. The foreign gene is constitutively expressed, and its 5′ domain acts as a promoter, resulting in permanent expression of the *RET* gene. Furthermore, these genes have domains that induce *RET* activation by permanent dimerization. Because of this fusion, the chimeric protein is localized in the cytoplasm and not in the plasma cell membrane.

Three major classes of *RET/PTC* have been identified: *RET/PTC*$_1$ is formed by an intrachromosomal rearrangement fusing the *RET* tyrosine kinase domain to a gene designated *H4*, whose function is still unknown. *RET/PTC*$_2$ is formed by an interchromosomal rearrangement fusing the *RET* tyrosine kinase domain to a gene located on chromosome 17 that encodes the RIα regulatory subunit of protein kinase A. *RET/PTC*$_3$ is formed by an intrachromosomal rearrangement fusing the *RET* tyrosine kinase domain to a gene designated *ELE1*, whose function is still unknown. Several other variants of *RET/PTC* have been observed in post-Chernobyl thyroid tumors, including rearrangements formed by fusion of the tyrosine kinase domain of the RET gene at other breakpoint sites or with other partners.

The frequency of *RET/PTC* rearrangements occurring in adult PTC patients without prior childhood neck irradiation varies between 2.5% and 35%. In these tumors, the frequencies of *RET/PTC*$_1$ and *RET/PTC*$_3$ were similar and that of *RET/PTC*$_2$ was lower. The *RET/PTC* rearrangements were more frequently found (60% to 80% of cases) in cases of PTC occurring in children even in the absence of radiation exposure or in subjects of any age after radiation exposure during childhood (external irradiation or contamination after the Chernobyl nuclear accident).[114,122] *RET/PTC*$_3$ was more frequently found in aggressive tumors that occurred early after the accident and *RET/PTC*$_1$ in less aggressive tumors that occurred later. The finding of *RET/PTC* rearrangement in micro-PTCs suggests that it constitutes an early event in thyroid carcinogenesis. On the other hand, *RET/PTC*-positive tumors lack evidence of progression to poorly or undifferentiated tumor phenotypes.

An activating point mutation of the RAS genes is found in about 10% of PTCs, mostly in the follicular variant.[123] A single activating point mutation of the *BRAF* gene at codon 600 is found in 40% (range, 29% to 69%) of PTCs occurring in adults.[124] Its presence did not overlap with that of *RET/PTC*, and it was rarely found in PTCs occurring in children or after irradiation of the neck.[118,120] *BRAF* mutation is more frequently found in aggressive PTCs and in the tall cell variant, and it has not been found in other thyroid tumor types.[124] An intrachromosomal rearrangement of the *BRAF* gene with the *AKAP9* gene was found in PTCs occurring after the Chernobyl accident.[125]

Several additional oncogenes may occasionally be involved in PTC, including *NTRK1* (also named *TRKA*), which codes for a neural growth factor receptor with a tyrosine kinase domain and is activated by rearrangement in about 10% of PTCs. The receptor for hepatocyte growth factor is a transmembrane tyrosine kinase encoded by the *MET* oncogene; it is overexpressed in some patients with PTC, and low expression has been associated with the occurrence of distant metastases.

In conclusion, the mitogen-activated protein (MAP) kinase (RET/PTC, RAS, BRAF) pathway is activated in approximately 80% of sporadic or radiation-induced PTCs, and mutations affecting this pathway are considered to be initiating events of PTC and to mediate the mitogenic phenotype.[120] Other signal transduction pathways may also be activated, including the phosphatidyl inositol 3 (PI3) kinase pathway,[126] and activation by cross-talk among these pathways may exist.

A high incidence of PTC has been reported in patients with adenomatous polyposis coli; these cancers have a peculiar histologic appearance with solid areas and elongated cells. There is also a high incidence of follicular cell-derived tumors (mainly FTC) in Cowden's disease (the multiple hamartoma syndrome), suggesting that the predisposing genes may play a role in the occurrence of these tumors. The familial risk of thyroid cancer is higher than for other cancers, and 3% to 10% of cases of PTC are familial.[127] The behavior of familial thyroid cancers is similar to or slightly more aggressive than that of nonfamilial cases.[128] At least five loci of predisposition have been identified, but they do not explain all hereditary cases. The gene predisposing to familial thyroid tumors with cellular oxyphilia has been mapped to chromosome 19q13.2, but in a family with PTC and renal carcinoma a separate gene was mapped to chromosome 1p13.2.q22.[129] Recently, a genome-wide study in PTC identified an association with a single-nucleotide polymorphism (SNP) at chromosomal locus at 9q22, a region that contains the thyroid transcription factor gene, *FOXE1*[130]; the plausible implication of *FOXE1* in PTC was strengthened by a large gene candidate study.[131,132] A germline mutation in another thyroid transcription factor, TTF1, has also been reported in familial PTC.[132]

The expression of thyroid-specific genes has been studied at the messenger ribonucleic acid (mRNA) and protein levels in large series of human thyroid tumors. Expression of the NIS gene *(SLC5A5)* was profoundly decreased in benign and malignant thyroid hypofunctioning nodules; in malignant nodules, low expression of TPO, PDS, and Tg was also found.[62] These abnormalities clearly explain many of the metabolic defects typically observed in thyroid cancer tissues: a low iodine concentration, a low rate of iodine organification, a low hormonal synthesis, and a short intrathyroidal half-life of iodine. NIS expression is heterogeneous among tumor cells.[62] However, Tg is expressed in variable amounts in almost all FCTCs and can be shown by immunohistochemistry, which can prove useful in cases with atypical histology. Also, TSHRs are expressed in many FCTCs, and TSH may stimulate both their differentiation and growth.[62]

Multiple other abnormalities have been found in follicular cell–derived tumors, including overexpression of vascular endothelial growth factor (VEGF) and of VEGF receptors (VEGFRs), in line with the hypervascularization observed in these tumors.[133] VEGF, VEGFRs, and other angiogenic factors may be targets for experimental therapies.

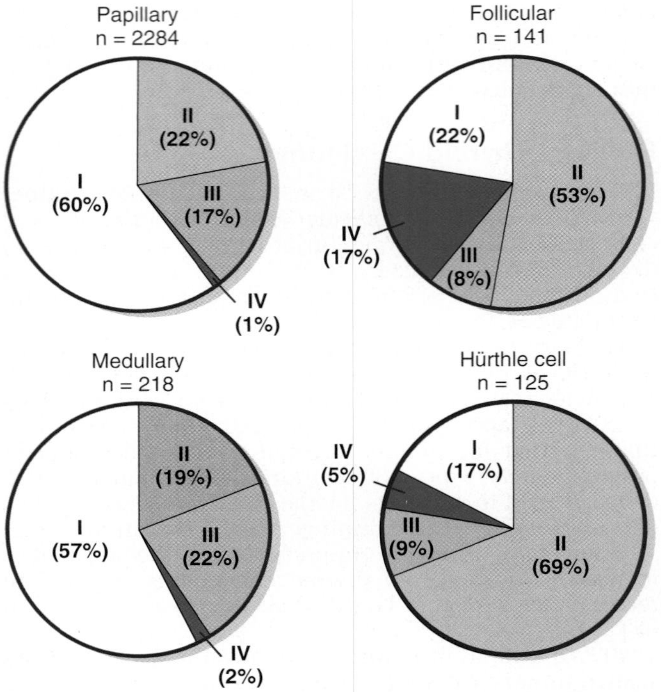

Papillary n = 2284: I (60%), II (22%), III (17%), IV (1%)
Follicular n = 141: I (22%), II (53%), III (8%), IV (17%)
Medullary n = 218: I (57%), II (19%), III (22%), IV (2%)
Hürthle cell n = 125: I (17%), II (69%), III (9%), IV (5%)

Figure 14-7 Distribution of pathologic tumor-node-metastasis (pTNM) stages I through IV in 2284 patients with papillary thyroid carcinoma (*upper left*), 218 patients with medullary thyroid cancer (*lower left*), 141 patients with follicular thyroid cancer (*upper right*), and 125 patients with Hürthle cell cancer (*lower right*) undergoing primary surgical treatment at the Mayo Clinic from 1940 to 1997.

Presenting Features

Although PTCs can occur at any age, most patients are between 30 and 50 years of age (mean age, 45 years). Women are affected more frequently then men (female predominance, 60% to 80%). Most primary tumors are 1 to 4 cm in size; they average about 2 to 3 cm in greatest diameter.[98,115] The increased incidence observed in recent years is mostly related to small PTCs.[118,134] PTC is frequently multifocal when it occurs in a single lobe, and it is bilateral in 20% to 80% of cases, depending on whether the thyroid was meticulously examined or not. Studies have suggested that contralateral PTC may have independent clonal origins, but this remains controversial.[135] Extrathyroidal invasion of adjacent soft tissues is present in about 15% of patients (range, 5% to 34%) at primary surgery, and about one third of PTC patients have clinically evident lymphadenopathy at presentation.[98,115] Between 35% and 50% of excised neck nodes have histologic evidence of involvement, and nodal involvement is present in up to 90% of patients 17 years of age or younger.[103,136] Only 1% to 7% of PTC patients have distant metastases at diagnosis.[98,115] Spread to superior mediastinal nodes is usually associated with extensive neck nodal involvement.

The TNM classification is a widely used system for tumor staging.[137] Most PTC patients present with stage I (60%) or stage II (22%) disease. Patients aged 45 years or older with either nodal metastases or extrathyroidal extension (stage III) account for fewer than 20% of cases.[98,115] As already noted, few PTC patients (1% to 7%) present with distant metastases and have stage IV disease. Figure 14-7 *(upper left)* illustrates the distribution of TNM stages in 2284 PTC cases seen at the Mayo Clinic, and Figure 14-8 demonstrates

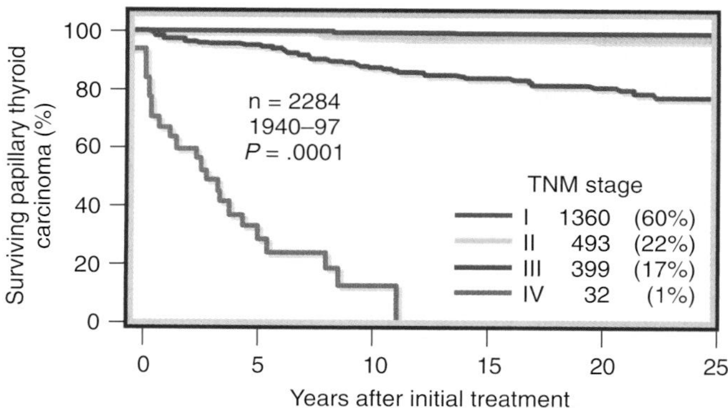

Figure 14-8 Cause-specific survival according to pathologic tumor-node-metastasis (pTNM) stage in a cohort of 2284 patients with papillary thyroid carcinoma treated at the Mayo Clinic from 1940 to 1997. The numbers in parentheses represent the percentage of patients in each pTNM stage grouping.

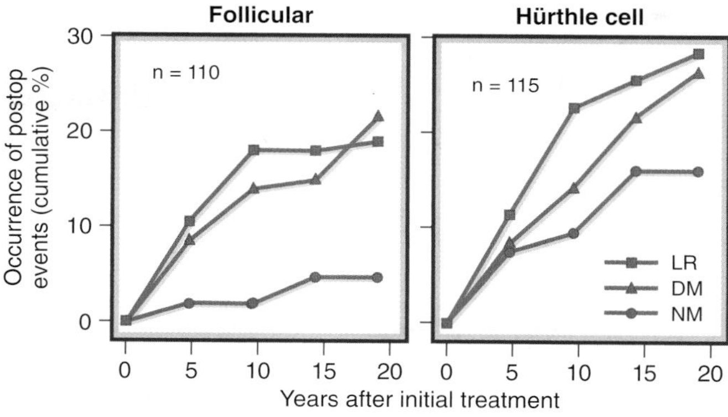

Figure 14-10 Development of neck nodal metastases (NM), local recurrences (LR), and distant metastases (DM) in the first 20 years after definitive surgery for follicular thyroid cancer (FTC) or Hürthle cell cancer (HCC) performed at the Mayo Clinic from 1940 to 1997. Based on 110 consecutive FTC patients and 115 HCC patients who had complete surgical resection and were without distant metastases on initial examination.

survival by TNM stage in this same cohort of PTC patients treated from 1940 to 1997. In these figures and also in the other figures in this chapter that illustrate outcome results from the Mayo Clinic 1940-1997 cohort of PTC patients, the pTNM stages are derived, in part, from the older (pre-2002) definition because of the challenges in defining from available records the N1a versus N1b status and the exact location of the extrathyroidal extension necessary to ascribe T4a or T4b status to the tumor extent at surgery.

Recurrence and Mortality

Three types of tumor recurrence may have been observed in patients with PTC: postoperative *nodal metastases* (NM), *local recurrence* (LR), and postoperative *distant metastases* (DM).

Local recurrence may be defined as "histologically confirmed tumor occurring in the resected thyroid bed, thyroid remnant, or other adjacent tissues of the neck (excluding lymph nodes)" after complete surgical removal of the primary tumor.[138] Metastases may be considered postoperative if discovered within 180 days for nodal metastases or 30 days for distant metastases.[98] Ideally, tumor recurrence should be considered only as it occurs in patients without initial distant metastases who had complete surgical resection of the primary tumors.

Figure 14-9 illustrates rates of PTC recurrence at local, nodal, and distant sites in 2150 patients with PTC treated at one institution from 1940 to 1997. After 20 years of follow-up, postoperative nodal metastases had been discovered in 9%, local recurrence in 5%, and distant metastases in 4%. Both local recurrence and distant metastases are less common in PTC than in FTC (Fig. 14-10). However, postoperative cases of nodal metastases were more frequent in PTC than in FTC.

Cause-specific mortality (CSM) rates for differentiated thyroid cancer are shown in Figure 14-11. CSM rates for PTC were 2% at 5 years, 4% at 10 years, and 5% at 20 years. Among those with lethal PTC, 20% of the deaths occurred during the first year after diagnosis, and 80% within 10 years. The 25-year cause-specific survival rate of 95% for PTC was significantly higher than the 79%, 71%, and 66% rates seen with MTC, Hürthle cell cancer (HCC), and FTC, respectively.

Outcome Prediction

Only a fraction (approximately 15%) of patients with PTC are likely to experience relapse of disease, and even fewer

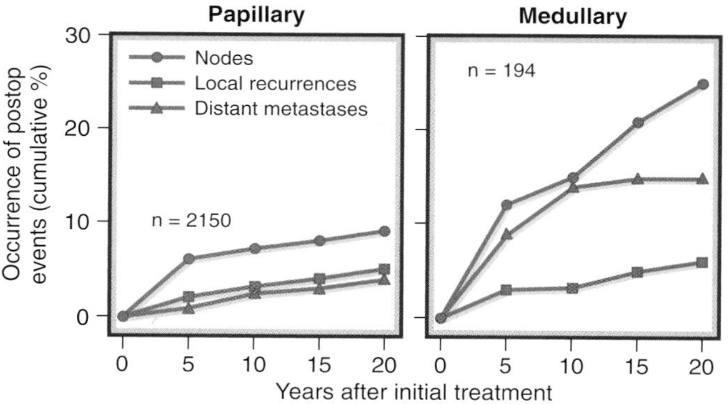

Figure 14-9 Development of neck nodal metastases, local recurrences, and distant metastases in the first 20 years after definitive surgery for papillary thyroid cancer (PTC) or medullary thyroid cancer (MTC) performed at the Mayo Clinic from 1940 to 1997. Based on 2150 consecutive PTC and 194 MTC patients who had complete surgical resection (i.e., no gross residual disease) and were without distant metastases on initial examination.

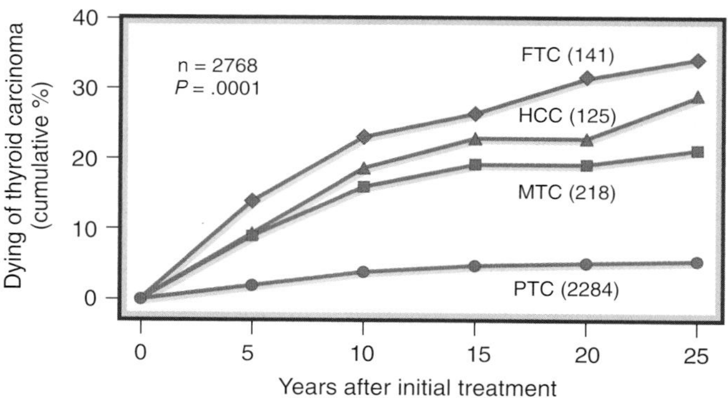

Figure 14-11 Cumulative cause-specific mortality rates for patients with differentiated thyroid carcinoma in the first 25 years after treatment with initial surgery performed at the Mayo Clinic from 1940 to 1997. Based on 2768 consecutively treated patients—2284 with papillary thyroid carcinoma (PTC), 141 with follicular thyroid cancer (FTC), 125 with Hürthle cell cancer (HCC), and 218 with medullary thyroid cancer (MTC).

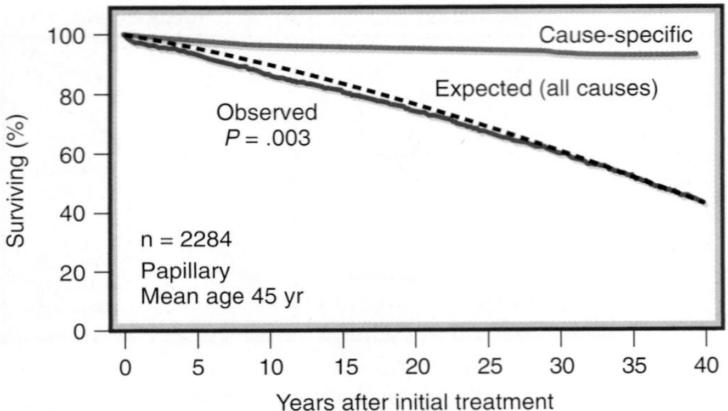

Figure 14-12 Observed survival to death from all causes and survival to death from thyroid cancer (cause-specific mortality) in 2284 consecutive patients with papillary thyroid carcinoma undergoing initial management at the Mayo Clinic from 1940 to 1997. Also plotted *(dashed line)* is the expected survival to death from all causes for patients of similar age and sex, based on appropriate Minnesotan life-tables.

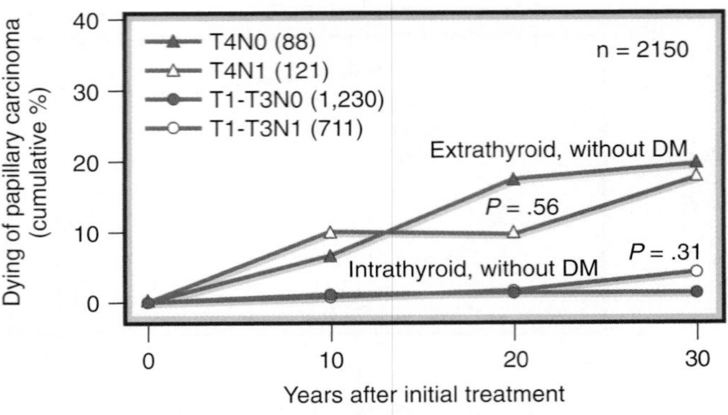

Figure 14-13 Lack of influence of nodal metastases at initial operation on cumulative mortality from papillary thyroid carcinoma in 1941 patients with pathologic T1 to T3 intrathyroidal tumors (i.e., completely confined to the thyroid gland) and 209 pathologic T4 patients with extrathyroidal (locally invasive) tumors, with (N1) or without (N0) nodal metastases. All patients had initial surgical treatment at the Mayo Clinic from 1940 to 1997. DM, distant metastases.

(approximately 5%) have a lethal outcome. Exceptional patients who have an aggressive course tend to experience relapse early (Fig. 14-12), and the rare fatalities usually occur within 5 to 10 years after diagnosis.[98,115] Multivariate analyses have been used to identify variables predictive of CSM.[115,139-145] Increasing age of the patient and the presence of extrathyroidal invasion were independent prognostic factors in all studies.

The presence of initial distant metastases and large size of the primary tumor are also significant variables in most studies,[115,139-141,144] and some groups[98,115,140,141,143] have reported that histopathologic grade (degree of differentiation) is an independent variable. The completeness of initial tumor resection (postoperative status) is also a predictor of mortality.[98,141,144] The presence of initial neck nodal metastases, although relevant to future nodal recurrence, does not influence CSM (Fig. 14-13).[98,115,144]

Several scoring systems based on these significant prognostic indicators have been devised. Each system allows one to assign the majority of PTC patients (≥80%) to a low-risk group, in which the CSM at 25 years is less than 2%, and the others (a small minority) to a high-risk group, in which almost all of the cancer-related deaths are observed. In general, these systems provide prediction of postoperative events comparable to that of the internationally accepted TNM staging system.[145]

One scoring index devised to assign PTC patients to prognostic risk groups[139] was named the AGES scheme, after the four independent variables: patient's *a*ge, tumor *g*rade, tumor *e*xtent (local invasion, distant metastases), and tumor *s*ize. With the use of such a scoring system, 86% of patients were placed in the minimal risk group (AGES score <4), and they experienced a 20-year CSM rate of only 1%.[98] By contrast, patients with AGES scores of 4 or higher (14% of the total) were considered to be at high risk and had a 20-year CSM of 36%.

Figure 14-14 compares the AGES scores with TNM staging and with two other schemes designed to stratify PTC patients as having either minimal risk or high risk of cancer-related death. Such a prognostic scoring system makes it possible to counsel patients and aids in the planning of individualized postoperative management programs in PTC.[139,144]

Although the AGES scheme had the potential for universal application, some academic centers could not include the differentiation (G) variable because their surgical pathologists did not recognize higher-grade PTC tumors.[145] Accordingly, a prognostic scoring system for predicting PTC mortality rates was devised with the use of candidate variables that included completeness of primary tumor resection but excluded histologic grade.[144] Cox model analysis and stepwise variable selection led to a final prognostic model, called MACIS, that included five variables: *m*etastasis, *a*ge, *c*ompleteness of resection, *i*nvasion, and *s*ize. The MACIS score is calculated as follows: 3.1 if the patient is 39 years of age or younger (or 0.08 × age if ≥40 years), plus 0.3 × tumor size in centimeters, plus 1 if the tumor was not completely resected, plus 1 if local invasion is present, plus 3 if distant metastases are present.

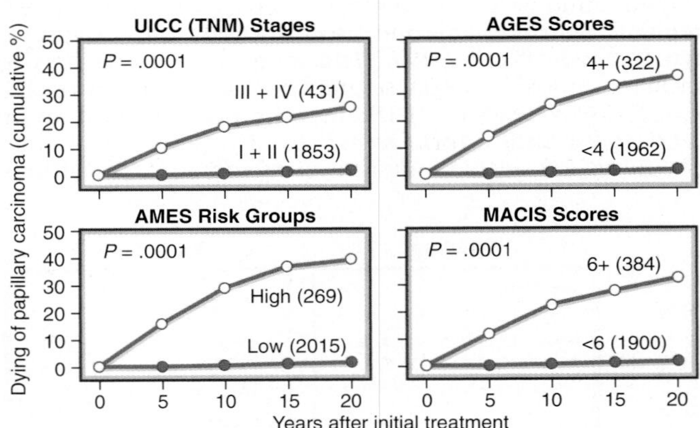

Figure 14-14 Cumulative mortality from papillary thyroid carcinoma in 2284 patients at either minimal risk or higher risk of cancer-related death as defined by International Union Against Cancer (UICC) pathologic tumor-node-metastasis (pTNM) stage *(upper left)*, AGES score *(upper right)*, AMES risk group *(lower left)*, and MACIS score *(lower right)*. The minimal risk group constituted 81% of the patients when defined by pTNM stage I or II, 86% as defined by an AGES score lower than 4, 88% as defined by the AMES low-risk criteria, and 83% when defined by an MACIS score lower than 6. The cause-specific mortality (CSM) rates at 20 years were 25% for those with TNM stage III or IV, 36% for an AGES score of 4 or higher, 39% for AMES high-risk status, and 32% for an MACIS score of 6 or higher. The ratios between the CSM rates for high-risk versus low-risk groups at 20 years were 19 for the pTNM system, 36 for AGES, 35 for AMES, and 40 for MACIS.

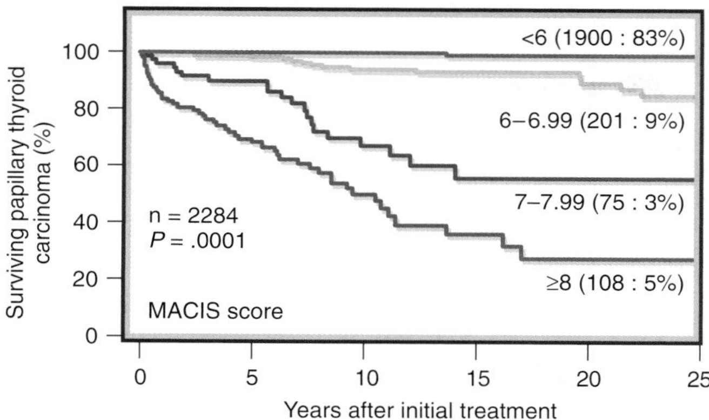

Figure 14-15 Cause-specific survival according to MACIS (*metastases, age*, completeness of resection, *invasion*, and *size*) score (<6, 6 to 6.99, 7 to 7.99, and ≥8) in a cohort of 2284 consecutive patients with papillary thyroid carcinoma (PTC) undergoing initial treatment at the Mayo Clinic from 1940 to 1997. The numbers and percentages of PTC patients in each of the four risk groups are shown in parentheses.

As illustrated by Figure 14-15, the MACIS scoring system permits identification of groups of patients with a broad range of risk of death from PTC. Twenty-year cause-specific survival rates for patients with MACIS scores lower than 6, between 6 and 6.99, between 7 and 7.99, and 8 or higher were 99%, 89%, 56%, and 27%, respectively ($P < .0001$). When cumulative mortality from all causes of death was considered, approximately 85% of PTC patients with AGES scores lower than 4 or MACIS scores lower than 6 had no excess mortality over rates predicted for control subjects.[139,144]

It should be emphasized that the five variables in the MACIS scoring system are easy to define after primary operation; consequently, the system can be applied in any clinical setting. The MACIS system can be used for counseling individual PTC patients and can help guide decision-making concerning the intensity of postoperative tumor surveillance and the appropriateness of adjunctive radioiodine therapy. Because the CIS variables (*c*ompleteness of resection, *i*nvasion, and *s*ize) require information obtained at surgery, the system probably should not be used to decide the extent of primary surgery.[146,147]

Follicular Thyroid Carcinoma

FTC is "a malignant epithelial tumor showing evidence of follicular cell differentiation but lacking the diagnostic features of papillary carcinoma."[99] Such a definition excludes the follicular variant of PTC, and it is also customary to exclude both the poorly differentiated carcinoma[148] and the rare mixed medullary and follicular carcinoma.[149] The correct classification of tumors with predominant oncocytic features (i.e., HCCs) is controversial.[110] The WHO committee has taken the stance that this tumor is an oxyphilic variant of FTC.[99] The AFIP monograph, by contrast, stated that "the tumors made up of this cell type have gross, microscopic, behavioral, cytogenetic (and conceivably etiopathogenic) features that set them apart from all others and justify discussing them in a separate section."[100]

Thus categorized, FTC is a relatively rare neoplasm whose identification requires invasion of the capsule, blood vessel, or adjacent thyroid. In epidemiologic surveys, FTC constituted 5% to 50% of differentiated thyroid cancers and tended to be more common in areas with iodine deficiency.[150] Owing to a combination of changing diagnostic criteria and an increase in the incidence of PTC associated with dietary iodine supplementation, the diagnosis of FTC has decreased in frequency; in one North American experience, minimally invasive nonoxyphilic FTCs made up fewer than 2% of thyroid malignancies.[151]

The microscopic appearance of FTC varies from well-formed follicles to a predominantly solid growth pattern.[99,100] Poorly formed follicles and atypical patterns (e.g., cribriform) may occur, and multiple architectural types may coexist. FTC is best divided into two categories on the basis of degree of invasiveness: minimally invasive (or encapsulated) and widely invasive. There is little overlap between these two types.

Minimally invasive FTC is an encapsulated tumor whose growth pattern resembles that of a trabecular or solid, microfollicular, or atypical adenoma. The diagnosis of malignancy depends on the demonstration of blood vessel or capsular invasion, or both. The criteria for invasion must therefore be strict.[99,100] Blood vessel invasion is almost never seen grossly. Microscopically, the vessels "should be of venous caliber, be located in or immediately outside of the capsule and contain one or more clusters of tumor cells attached to the wall and protruding into the lumen."[99] Interruption of the capsule must involve the full thickness to qualify as capsular invasion. Penetration of only the inner half or the presence of tumor cells embedded in the capsule does not qualify for the diagnosis of FTC. Foci of capsular invasion must be distinguished from the capsular rupture that can result from FNA. The acronym WHAFFT (*w*orrisome *h*istologic *a*lterations *f*ollowing *F*NA of the *t*hyroid) is applied to such changes.[152] The diagnosis of malignancy of these tumors can be difficult and may not be reproducible among pathologists. Immunohistochemistry with markers such as TPO, galectin 3, or HMBE1 may help for this purpose,[72] but these techniques did not reliably improve the accuracy of pathology in case of suspicious findings. Global gene expression studies with the microarray technology demonstrated different profiles between papillary carcinoma and follicular tumors,[74-76] but the reported distinction between follicular adenomas and minimally invasive follicular carcinoma with the expression study of a limited number of genes needs confirmation.[77]

In contrast, the rare *widely invasive* form of FTC can be distinguished easily from benign lesions. Although the tumor may be partially encapsulated, the margins are infiltrative even on gross examination, and vascular invasion is often extensive. The structural features are variable, but a follicular element is always present. If follicular differentiation is poor or absent, or in the presence of a trabecular, insular, or solid component, the tumor may be classified as a poorly differentiated carcinoma (see later discussion).[100,153]

Focal or extensive clear-cell changes can occur. A rare clear-cell variant of FTC has been described in which glycogen accumulation or dilatation of the granular endoplasmic reticulum is responsible for the clear cells.[154] If more than 75% of cells in an FTC exhibit Hürthle cell (or oncocytic) features, the tumor is classified as a Hürthle cell or oncocytic carcinoma[100,155] or as an oxyphilic variant FTC.[99]

Molecular Pathogenesis

There is still no accepted paradigm for the pathogenesis of FTC. A multistep adenoma-to-carcinoma pathogenesis, similar to that for colon cancer and other adenocarcinomas, is not universally accepted because pathologists do not recognize follicular carcinoma in situ and documentation of the evolution of adenoma to carcinoma is rare. Nevertheless, several facts about the pathogenesis of FTC are firmly established.[114,118,119,121,123] First, most follicular adenomas and all FTCs are probably of monoclonal origin. Second, oncogene activation, particularly by point mutation of the *RAS* oncogene, is common both in follicular adenomas (approximately 20%) and in FTCs (approximately 40%), supporting a role in early tumorigenesis.[123,156] The *RET* oncogene does not appear to be involved in follicular tumors.[114,118,119] Third, cytogenetic abnormalities and evidence of genetic loss are more common in FTC than in PTC and also occur in follicular adenomas.[119,121]

Of the cytogenetic abnormalities described in FTC, the most common are deletions, partial deletions, and deletion-rearrangements involving the short (p) arm of chromosome 3. Loss of heterozygosity (LOH) on chromosome 3p appears to be limited to FTC, because no evidence for 3p LOH has been found in follicular adenomas or in PTC. A translocation, t(2;3)(q13;p25), which results in fusion of the DNA binding domains of the thyroid transcription factor PAX8 to domains of the peroxisome proliferator-activated receptor (PPARγ1), was detected in 30% of FTCs (range, 11% to 63%) and in 10% of follicular adenomas but not in PTCs or multinodular hyperplasia.[157-159] The chimeric protein may retard the growth inhibition and follicular differentiation normally induced by PPARγ1.[158] The two main genetic alterations found in follicular carcinomas may act through distinct molecular pathways.[159]

Presenting Features

FTC tends to occur in older people, with the mean age in most studies being greater than 50 years, or about 10 years older than for typical PTC.[150] The average median age of patients with oxyphilic FTC (HCC) is about 60 years.[150,155] As in most thyroid malignancies, women outnumber men by more than 2 to 1. Most patients with FTC present with a painless thyroid nodule, with or without background thyroid nodularity, and they rarely (4% to 6%) have clinically evident lymphadenopathy at presentation.[150] Metastases to lymph nodes of the neck in FTC are so exceptional that "wherever they are observed, the alternative possibilities of follicular variant papillary carcinoma, oncocytic carcinoma, and poorly differentiated carcinoma should be considered."[100]

In most series in which tumor sizes were reported, the average tumor size in FTC (oxyphilic or nonoxyphilic) was larger than the average tumor size in PTC.[150,155] Direct extrathyroidal extension, by definition, does not occur with minimally invasive FTC but is common in the rare patients with invasive FTC. Between 5% and 20% of patients with FTC have distant metastases at presentation,[150] most commonly to lung or bone.[100,150] The bones most often involved are long bones (e.g., femur), flat bones (particularly pelvis, sternum, and skull), and vertebrae. If distant metastasis is the first manifestation of the disease, definitive proof of its thyroid origin should be obtained, usually by biopsy of a metastasis, before any thyroid surgery is performed. It is unusual for patients with FTC to have thyrotoxicosis caused by massive tumor burden.[160]

Most patients (53% to 69%) with FTC or HCC have pTNM stage II disease. Patients 45 years of age or older with nodal metastases or extrathyroidal extension (stage III) account for only 4% of FTCs and 9% of HCCs (see Fig. 14-7). About 5% of HCCs and 17% or more of nonoxyphilic FTCs have distant metastases at the time of diagnosis (stage IV).

Recurrence and Mortality

Nodal metastases are rare in typical FTC, and the nodal recurrence rate at 20 years after surgery is the lowest among

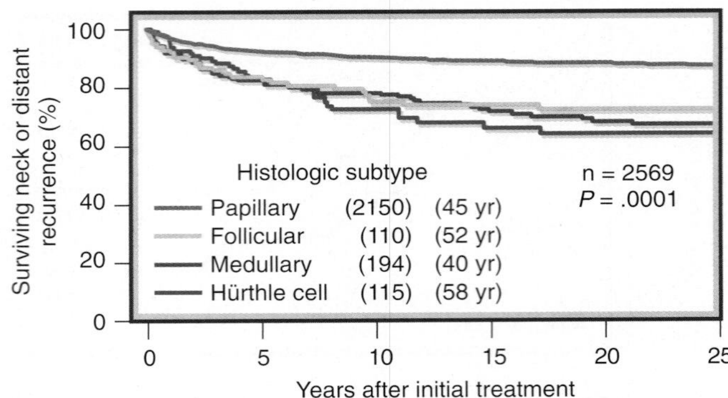

Figure 14-16 Postoperative recurrence (any site) during the first 20 years after definitive surgery for differentiated thyroid carcinoma performed at the Mayo Clinic from 1940 to 1997. Based on 2569 consecutive patients who had complete tumor resection and no distant metastases at presentation. The number of patients and the median age at diagnosis are shown in parentheses for each of the four histologic subtypes.

the differentiated thyroid carcinomas, approximately 2% (see Fig. 14-10). About 6% of patients with HCC have node involvement at presentation,[161] and within 25 years after primary surgery about 17% of HCC patients have nodal recurrence.[150] When recurrences at either neck or distant sites are taken into consideration, patients with HCC (Fig. 14-16) have the highest number of tumor recurrences after 10 to 20 years. As illustrated by Figure 14-10, local recurrences at 20 years are identified in 20% of FTCs and 30% of HCCs. Comparable distant metastases rates are 23% and 28%, respectively.

CSM rates vary with the presenting TNM stage in both FTC (Fig. 14-17) and HCC. The death rates tend to parallel the curves for development of distant metastases (see Fig. 14-10). In more than 5 decades of experience at the Mayo Clinic, the mortality rate for FTC has been found to exceeds that of HCC initially, but by 20 and 30 postoperative years there are no significant differences in cause-specific survival rates (80% and 70%, respectively) between FTC and HCC[150] (Fig. 14-18). Curves representing mortality from all causes differ in FTC and HCC. On average, patients with FTC are about 5 years younger, tend to die within the first 10 postoperative years, and have high all-cause mortality for 10 to 30 postoperative years (Fig. 14-19). Deaths related

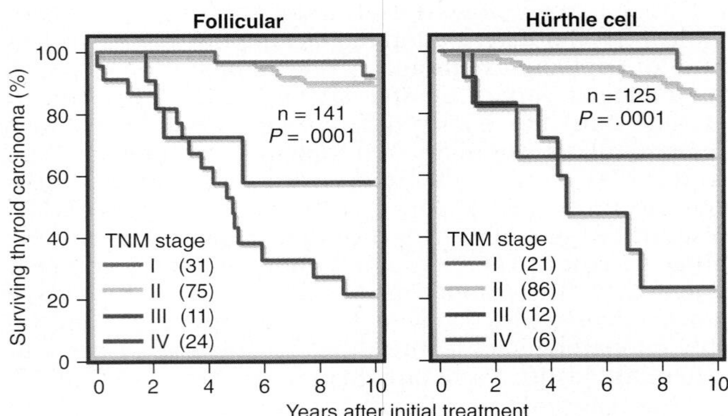

Figure 14-17 Cause-specific survival according to pathologic tumor-node-metastasis (pTNM) stage in a cohort of 141 patients with follicular thyroid carcinoma (*left panel*) and 125 patients with Hürthle cell carcinoma (*right panel*) treated at the Mayo Clinic from 1940 to 1997. Numbers in parentheses represent the number of patients in each pTNM stage grouping.

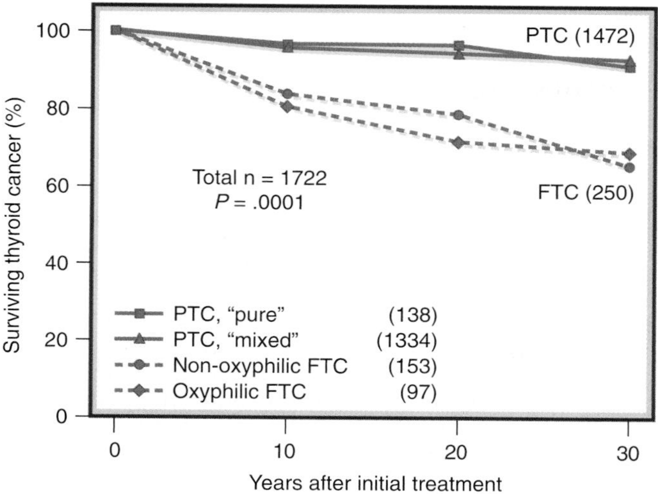

Figure 14-18 Comparison of cause-specific survival in 1472 patients with papillary thyroid carcinoma (PTC) and 250 patients with follicular thyroid carcinoma (FTC) treated at the Mayo Clinic from 1940 to 1990. Of the PTCs, 138 were "pure" papillary in histotype (no follicular elements); 97 of the FTC patients had predominantly oxyphilic tumors. There was a significant difference (P = .0001) between the cause-specific survival curves for PTC versus FTC. However, within each group, the survival curves are insignificantly different. (From Grebe SKG, Hay ID. Follicular thyroid cancer. *Endocrinol Metab Clin North Am.* 1995;24:761-801.)

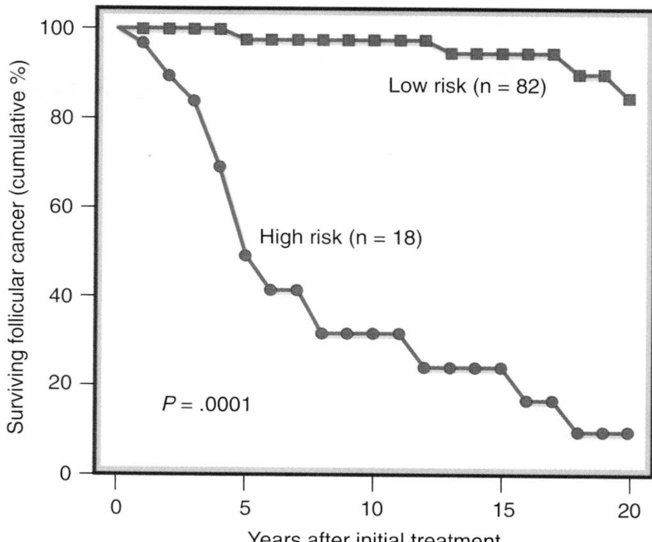

Figure 14-20 Cumulative cause-specific survival among 100 patients with nonoxyphilic follicular thyroid carcinoma treated at the Mayo Clinic from 1946 to 1970, plotted by high-risk and low-risk categories. High-risk patients were those for whom two or more of the following factors were present: age older than 50 years, marked vascular invasion, and metastatic disease at time of initial diagnosis. (From Brennan MD, Bergstralh EJ, van Heerden JA, et al. Follicular thyroid cancer treated at the Mayo Clinic, 1946 through 1970: initial manifestations, pathologic findings, therapy, and outcome. *Mayo Clin Proc.* 1991;66:11-22.)

to HCC occur gradually over the first 15 years; however, by 25 years, the average survivor of HCC is 84 years old, and by that time, almost 50% of the treated cohort would be predicted by the actuarial curve to have died from all causes.

Outcome Prediction

The risk factors that predict outcome in FTC are largely the same as in PTC[150,162-170]: distant metastases at presentation, increasing age of the patient, large tumor size, and the presence of local (extrathyroidal) invasion. To a lesser degree, increased mortality is associated with male gender and higher grade (less well-differentiated tumors). In addition, vascular invasiveness, lymphatic involvement at presentation, DNA aneuploidy, and oxyphilic histology are

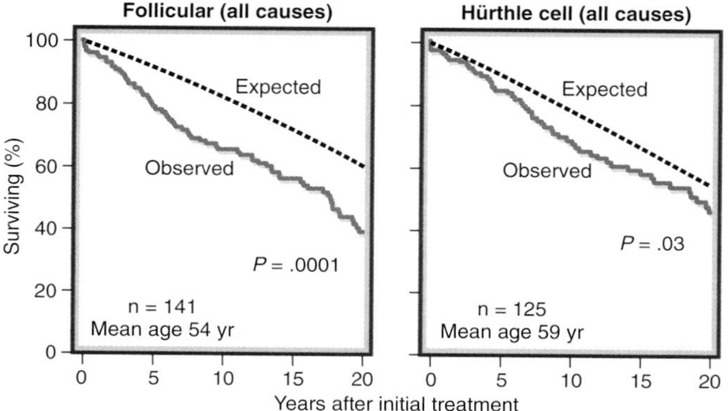

Figure 14-19 Survival to death from all causes in 141 consecutive patients with follicular thyroid carcinoma *(left)* and 125 patients with Hürthle cell cancer *(right)* undergoing initial management at the Mayo Clinic from 1940 to 1997. Also plotted is the expected survival (all causes) of persons of the same age and sex and with the same date of treatment but living under mortality conditions of the northwest central United States.

potential prognostic variables unique to FTC.[150] The importance of vascular invasion was underscored by a study showing that FTC patients with minimal capsular invasion and no evidence of vascular invasion had 0% CSM at 10-year follow-up.[162]

Prognostic scoring systems for FTC[150,163] allow stratification of patients into high-risk and low-risk categories. A multivariate analysis at the Mayo Clinic found that distant metastases at presentation, patient age greater than 50 years, and marked vascular invasion predict a poor outcome.[150] As illustrated by Figure 14-20, if two or more of these factors are present, the 5-year survival rate is only 47%, and 20-year survival is 8%. By contrast, if only one of these factors is present, 5-year survival is 99%, and 20-year survival is 86%.

Systems developed to predict outcome in either PTC or FTC have been applied to FTC patients. The pTNM and the AMES (*a*ge, *m*etastasis, *e*xtent, *s*ize) risk group categorization have proved to be useful in FTC.[164] From a multivariate analysis of 228 patients with FTC treated at the Memorial Sloan-Kettering Cancer Center, the following independent adverse prognostic factors were identified: age older than 45 years, Hürthle cell histotype, extrathyroidal extension, tumor size exceeding 4 cm, and the presence of distant metastases.[165] The prognostic importance in FTC of histologic grade was also confirmed,[165] and this factor was included in the assignment of low, intermediate, and high risk group categories (Fig. 14-21).

The AGES scheme, originally developed for PTC, has also been successfully applied to FTC.[166,167] Additionally, the MACIS classification has been demonstrated to be a more accurate predictor of survival in FTC than the TNM, AGES, and AMES prognostic schemes.[168] Therefore, scoring systems used in PTC may be cautiously applied to FTC as long as some of the unique features of this tumor, such as

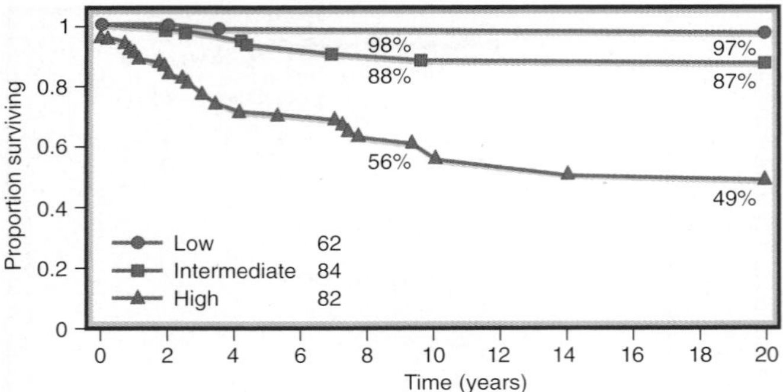

Figure 14-21 Survival differences in low-risk, intermediate-risk, and high-risk groups for 228 consecutive patients with follicular thyroid carcinoma who were seen and treated at the Memorial Sloan-Kettering Cancer Center during a period of 55 years from 1930 to 1985. The number of each patients in each group and the percentage of patients surviving at 10 and 20 years are shown. (From Shaha AR, Loree TR, Shah JP. Prognostic factors and risk group analyses in follicular carcinoma of the thyroid. *Surgery.* 1995;118: 1131-1138.)

vascular invasiveness and the remarkable significance of DNA aneuploidy in HCC, are kept in mind.[150]

Poorly Differentiated (Insular, Solid, or Trabecular) Carcinoma

Poorly differentiated thyroid carcinoma has been defined as "a tumor of follicular cell origin with morphological and biologic attributes intermediate between differentiated and anaplastic carcinomas of the thyroid."[100] New diagnostic criteria for poorly differentiated carcinoma have been proposed: (1) solid, trabecular, and insular pattern of growth; (2) absence of conventional nuclear features of papillary carcinomas; and (3) presence of at least convoluted nuclei, mitotic activity greater than 3 mitotic figures per 10 high-power fields, and tumor necrosis.[153] Similarly, in well differentiated cancer, necrosis, mitosis, and cellular atypia associated with vascular invasion are considered to be features of poor prognosis and of aggressiveness.[170] Most such tumors are larger than 5 cm in diameter at diagnosis, with extrathyroidal extension and blood vessel invasion. This type of tumor is viewed by the WHO committee[99] as a morphologic variant of FTC, but others view it as a poorly differentiated variant of either PTC or FTC.[100] *RET* rearrangement and *BRAF* mutation are infrequent in poorly differentiated carcinoma, NRAS mutation is found in 25% of tumors, and *TP53* mutation has been evidenced in a significant proportion of these tumors. Activation of the PI3 kinase pathway is frequent, as is overexpression of the vascular endothelial growth factor receptor.[126,171-173]

The mean age at diagnosis is about 55 years, and the female-to-male ratio is about 2 : 1.[100] Poorly differentiated carcinoma is aggressive and often lethal. Radioiodine uptake is rarely present, but FDG uptake on PET is frequently high. Production of Tg in blood may be lower than in differentiated carcinomas. Metastases are common in regional nodes and distant sites (lung, bone, brain). In one series, 56% of patients died from their tumor within 8 years of initial therapy.[148]

Undifferentiated (Anaplastic) Carcinoma

Anaplastic carcinoma constitutes about 1% to 2% of all thyroid carcinomas, usually occurs after the age of 60 years, and is slightly more common in women (female-to-male ratio, 1.3 : 1 to 1.5 : 1).[174-176] This carcinoma is highly malignant, is nonencapsulated, and extends widely. Evidence of invasion of adjacent structures, such as skin, muscles, nerves, blood vessels, larynx, and esophagus, is common. Distant metastases occur early in the course of the disease in lungs, liver, bones, and brain.

On histopathologic examination, the lesion is composed of atypical cells that exhibit numerous mitoses and form a variety of patterns. Spindle-shaped cells, multinucleated giant cells, and squamoid cells usually predominate. Areas of necrosis and polymorphonuclear infiltration are common, and the presence of PTC or FTC suggests that they may be the precursors of anaplastic carcinoma. Mutations of the *TP53* gene are present in many undifferentiated carcinomas but may not be found in the residual well-differentiated component, suggesting that these mutations occur after the development of the original tumor and may play a key role in tumor progression.[114,171]

The usual clinical complaint is that of a rapid, often painful enlargement of a mass that may have been present in the thyroid gland for many years. The tumor invades adjacent structures, causing hoarseness, inspiratory stridor, and difficulty in swallowing. On examination, the overlying skin is often warm and discolored. The mass is tender and often is fixed to adjacent structures. It is stony hard in consistency, but some areas may be soft or fluctuant. The regional lymph nodes are enlarged, and there may be evidence of distant metastases. Anaplastic carcinomas do not accumulate iodine and do not typically produce thyroglobulin; high FDG uptake is usually found on PET, and PET is the best tool for tumor staging and for control of treatment efficacy.[177]

Treatment should be initiated rapidly to avoid death from locally infiltrative disease and possible suffocation. Treatment consists of surgical resection of the tumor tissue present in the neck, if feasible, followed by a combination of external irradiation and chemotherapy.[175,176]

Medullary Thyroid Carcinoma

MTC accounts for fewer than 10% of thyroid malignancies (see Chapter 41). It arises from the parafollicular or C cells of the thyroid gland, and the tumor cells typically produce an early biochemical signal (hypersecretion of calcitonin). MTC readily invades the intraglandular lymphatics, spreading to other parts of the gland and to pericapsular and regional lymph nodes. It also regularly spreads through the bloodstream to the lungs, bones, and liver.[3,104-106,178]

MTC tumors are firm and usually nonencapsulated. On histopathologic examination, the tumor is composed of cells that vary in their morphologic features and arrangement. Round, polyhedral, and spindle-shaped cells form a variety of patterns, from solid and trabecular to endocrine or glandular-like structures. An amyloid stroma is commonly present.[99,100] Gross or microscopic foci of carcinoma may be present in other parts of the gland, and blood vessels may be invaded. In all cases, the diagnosis can be confirmed by positive immunostaining of tumor tissue for calcitonin and carcinoembryonic antigen (CEA).

MTC first appears either as a hard nodule or mass in the thyroid gland or as an enlargement of the regional lymph nodes. Occasionally, a metastatic lesion at a distant site is found first. The neck masses are frequently painful; they are sometimes bilateral and are often localized to the upper two thirds of each lobe of the gland, reflecting the anatomic location of the parafollicular cells.

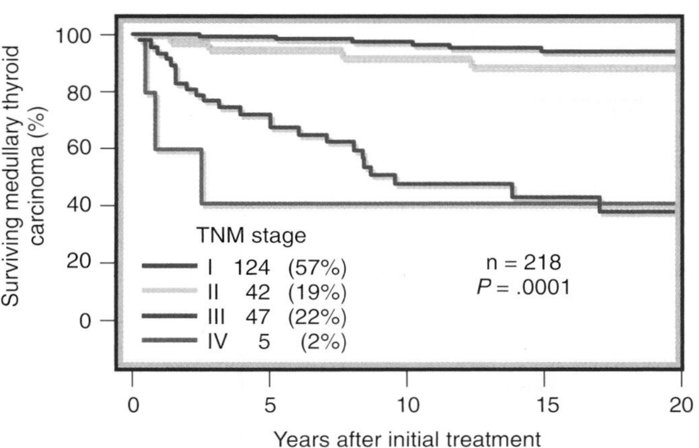

Figure 14-22 Cause-specific survival according to pathologic tumor-node-metastasis (pTNM) stage in a cohort of 218 patients with medullary thyroid carcinoma treated at the Mayo Clinic from 1940 to 1997. The number and percentage of patients in each pTNM stage group are shown.

The tumor occurs in both sporadic and hereditary forms, the latter making up about 20% of the total. The hereditary variety can be transmitted as a single entity (familial MTC), or it can arise as part of MEN2A or MEN2B syndrome. The hereditary form is typically bilateral and is usually preceded by a premalignant C-cell hyperplasia. Total thyroidectomy at this premalignant stage can cure the disease in more than 90% of cases.[3,56-58,178-180] *RET* proto-oncogene testing should be performed in all MTC patients. The finding of a germline mutation in this gene indicates a hereditary disease; the mutation should then be sought in all first-degree family members.

Early series of MTC mainly described sporadic cases, in which 80% of patients presented with TNM stage II or III disease. As more patients with familial MTC or MEN2A have been diagnosed, more patients have had curable (stage I) disease at presentation, and the survival rate has improved, a trend that should continue with widespread application of *RET* proto-oncogene testing.[178-180] Patients with MTC now have outcomes similar to or better than those of patients with nonpapillary FCTC (see Fig. 14-11). The cause-specific survival curves for 218 consecutive MTC cases treated from 1940 to 1997 at the Mayo Clinic, based on TNM stage, are presented in Figure 14-22.

Prognostic factors relevant to outcome in MTC include (1) age at diagnosis, (2) male gender, (3) initial extent of the disease (e.g., nodal metastases, distant metastases), (4) tumor size, (5) extrathyroidal invasion, (6) vascular invasion, (7) calcitonin immunoreactivity and amyloid staining in tumor tissue, (8) postoperative gross residual disease, and (9) postoperative plasma calcitonin levels.[104-106] In a multivariate analysis, only the age of the patient at initial treatment and the stage of the disease remained as significantly independent indicators of survival. This suggests that, in routine practice, clinicians attempting to predict outcome in MTC should take into account not only the presenting disease stage, as assessed by the pTNM system (see Fig. 14-22), but also the age of the patient at diagnosis.[104-106]

Cushing's syndrome may occur at an advanced stage of the disease, because of secretion of corticotropin by the tumor. Prostaglandins, serotonin, kinins, and vasoactive intestinal peptide may also be secreted and are variously responsible for flushing and for the attacks of watery diarrhea that about one third of patients experience, usually at an advanced stage of the disease.[104-106,178] In MEN2A, hyperparathyroidism occurs late and is usually due to parathyroid hyperplasia rather than adenoma. Pheochromocytomas invariably occur later than MTC; they are often bilateral and may be clinically silent, and patients at risk should be screened with measurements of urinary metanephrine excretion. In MEN2B, MTC and pheochromocytomas are associated with multiple mucosal neuromas *(bumpy lip syndrome)*, a marfanoid habitus, and typical facies, but such patients do not have hyperparathyroidism.[3,178]

Differentiation of sporadic MTC from other types of thyroid nodule on clinical grounds alone may be difficult. In patients with a family history of thyroid cancer associated with hypertension or hyperparathyroidism, the MEN2A syndrome should be suspected. FNAB has made it possible to diagnose MTC before surgery. In some patients, however, cytologic findings are misleading because the type of carcinoma is difficult to determine, and HCC may occasionally be confused with MTC.[99,100]

Positive immunocytochemical staining for calcitonin allows confirmation of the diagnosis. Basal plasma calcitonin levels are elevated in virtually all patients with clinical MTC.[56,57] Infusions of pentagastrin or calcium elicit secretion of calcitonin, and the response may be exaggerated in patients with MTC or the antecedent C-cell hyperplasia; the use of such infusions should be restricted to MTC patients with an undetectable or borderline plasma calcitonin level (see Chapter 41).

When the diagnosis of MTC is made based on calcitonin measurements or FNAB, patients should be evaluated for hyperparathyroidism and for pheochromocytoma. If these diagnoses are satisfactorily excluded, a total thyroidectomy with removal of regional nodes can safely be performed.[3,181,182] In patients with MEN syndrome, surgery should be performed for pheochromocytomas before the surgery for MTC is performed. First-degree relatives of patients with MEN or familial MTC should undergo DNA testing for presence of the mutant *RET* gene (see Chapter 41). Gene carriers should undergo prophylactic total thyroidectomy at an age that depends on the mutation: within the first year of life for those with MEN2B, and before 5 years of age for those with the 634 *RET* mutation (the most common type).[3,57,179,180] For carriers of other mutations, prophylactic total thyroidectomy may be delayed beyond age 5 years in the setting of a normal annual basal serum calcitonin level (and a normal stimulated level, if performed), normal findings on annual neck ultrasonography, a less aggressive MTC family history, and family preference. Surgery is indicated if none of these features is present.[3]

Primary Malignant Lymphoma

Primary thyroid lymphomas are rare tumors, accounting for 2.5% of all non-Hodgkin's lymphomas and fewer than 2% of all malignant thyroid tumors. The peak incidence is during the seventh decade of life, and the female-to-male ratio is 3:1.

Primary thyroid lymphoma almost always has a B-cell lineage.[183] Most thyroid malignant lymphomas are mucosa-associated lymphoid tissue (MALT) lymphomas that arise in a background of Hashimoto's thyroiditis. These small-cell lymphomas are characterized by a low grade of malignancy, a slow growth rate, and a tendency for recurrence at other MALT sites such as the gastrointestinal tract, respiratory tract, thymus, or salivary glands. At diagnosis, diffuse large-cell lymphomas account for about 70% to

80% of tumors, and a substantial proportion of clinical cases arise from the transformation of low-grade MALT lymphoma to high-grade B-cell lymphoma. Other histologies are rare.

Thyroid lymphomas almost invariably manifest as a rapidly enlarging, painless neck mass. One third of the patients have compressive symptoms. The mass is often fixed to surrounding tissues, and half of the patients have unilateral or bilateral cervical lymph node enlargement. Clinically evident distant disease is uncommon. About 20% of patients already have a long-standing goiter, and hypothyroidism is reported in up to 40% of cases. The palpated mass is solid and hypoechoic on ultrasonography, which often depicts a characteristic asymmetric, pseudocystic pattern. Most patients have serum anti-peroxidase and anti-thyroglobulin antibodies.

The diagnosis of lymphoma can often be established by FNA cytology, particularly the diffuse large B-cell type. Large-bore needle biopsy or open surgical biopsy may be needed for immunohistochemical staining to diagnose small-cell lymphomas and the frequently associated chronic autoimmune thyroiditis. Lymphocyte monoclonality for light-chain immunoglobulin may be necessary to confirm malignant lymphoma.

Accurate staging is critical for treatment planning. Staging includes a physical examination; complete blood count; serum lactate dehydrogenase; liver function tests; bone marrow biopsy; CT scan or MRI of the neck; CT scan of the thorax, abdomen, and pelvis; and appropriate biopsies at other sites where tumors are suspected. Involvement of Waldeyer's tonsillar ring and of the gastrointestinal tract has been associated with thyroid lymphomas, so upper gastrointestinal tract radiographs or endoscopy should be performed.

Treatment is guided by the histologic subtype, the extent of disease, and, in case of diffuse large B-cell lymphoma, by the age-adjusted international prognostic index.[184,185] Surgical debulking of thyroid lymphomas is neither feasible nor necessary. Small tumors are often treated initially as primary thyroid carcinomas with surgery, and additional radiotherapy may be necessary in case of indolent lymphoma.

For high-grade B-cell lymphoma, chemotherapy combined with rituximab (chimeric human-mouse anti-CD20 monoclonal antibody) has become the standard treatment.[186] The chemotherapy prescribed should be an anthracycline-based regimen. It usually consists of 4 to 6 cycles of the CHOP regimen (cyclophosphamide, 750 mg/m^2 on day 1; doxorubicin, 50 mg/m^2 on day 1; vincristine, 1.4 mg/m^2 on day 1; and prednisone, 40 mg/m^2 per day on days 1 through 5) every 3 weeks. For localized aggressive lymphoma, the combination of chemotherapy and radiotherapy used before the era of rituximab was found to reduce distant recurrence compared with radiotherapy alone. Radiation monotherapy should be used only for elderly patients who cannot receive medical treatment, because one third of the patients will experience recurrence at distant sites, usually within the first year after treatment.

For MALT lymphomas, if the disease is found to be localized after accurate staging, total thyroidectomy (predicted overall survival and disease-free survival, 100% at 5 years) or involved-field radiation therapy alone (2 Gy per fraction for 5 days/week up to a total dose of 30 to 40 Gy; 5-year overall survival rate, 90%) may be adequate.[187] For disseminated MALT lymphoma, chemotherapy alone (with single agent such as chlorambucil) or chemotherapy combined with local radiation therapy may be proposed.

SURGICAL TREATMENT OF THYROID CARCINOMA

Factors that influence the optimal extent of surgery include the histologic diagnosis, the size of the original lesion, the presence of lymph node and distant metastases, the patient's age, and the risk group category.[1-3] Obviously, the surgeon must be appropriately skilled in thyroid surgery, and the goal of surgery should be to remove all of the malignant neoplastic tissue that is present in the neck. A preoperative ultrasound examination of the thyroid gland and of neck lymph node areas should be routinely performed, and detected lesions should be adequately resected.[1-3]

In the case of PTC and FTC, a near-total thyroidectomy (i.e., leaving no more than 1 g of thyroid tissue) or a total thyroidectomy is recommended for all patients.[1,2,97,98,137-139,188] Total thyroidectomy reduces the recurrence rate, compared with more limited surgery, because many PTCs are both multifocal and bilateral. Removal of most, if not all, of the thyroid gland facilitates postoperative remnant ablation with ^{131}I.

For extremely low-risk patients (i.e., those with unifocal intrathyroidal PTM), a lobectomy may be an appropriate primary surgical procedure.[1,2,116,117] A completion thyroidectomy should be offered to those patients who have undergone a unilateral lobectomy for a supposedly benign tumor that proves to be a cancer and for whom a total thyroidectomy would have been recommended had the diagnosis been available before the initial surgery. This includes all patients with thyroid cancer except those with small (<1 cm), unifocal, intrathyroidal, node-negative, low-risk tumors.[2]

Surgical treatment of lymph nodes is based on the preoperative workup, including neck ultrasound examination. In the presence of clinically involved lymph nodes, a therapeutic lymph node dissection is routinely performed.[2,16] This includes dissection of the central compartment VI (paratracheal and tracheoesophageal areas) and may also include dissection of the ipsilateral supraclavicular area and the lower third of the jugulocarotid chain (compartments III and IV, respectively).[2,16,189] A modified ipsilateral neck dissection is performed if palpable lymph node metastases are present in the jugulocarotid chain or if a preoperative ultrasound examination demonstrates biopsy-proven lateral neck nodal disease; in such cases, a compartment VI dissection is also performed. Dissection is preferable to lymph node picking. In patients with PTC, in the absence of any evidence of lymph node involvement, a prophylactic central neck dissection is controversial and may be performed either routinely or only for advanced primary tumors (T3 or T4).[2,16,190,191]

Although this type of lymph node dissection has not been shown to improve the recurrence and survival rates,[107,161,162,191] several arguments support its routine use in patients with PTCs. Histologic evidence of lymph node metastases is present in up to two thirds of PTC patients, of whom more than 80% have involvement of the central compartment, and metastases are difficult to detect by palpation in lymph nodes located behind the vessels or in the paratracheal groove; moreover, preoperative neck ultrasound detects only half of the involved lymph nodes.[193] Knowledge of the initial lymph node status is a requisite for TNM classification, is useful for the indication of postsurgical radioiodine treatment,[189] and helps in the interpretation of any cervical abnormality identified during postoperative follow-up.[1,2] The major drawback of lymph node dissection is that it may increase the morbidity rate, and for this reason it should be performed by a skilled surgeon.

In the case of FTC, lymph node metastases are less frequent, and a lymph node dissection should be performed if involved lymph nodes are detected.

MTC is treated by total thyroidectomy, with a dissection of the central compartment of the neck and the lower two thirds of the jugulocarotid chains. A modified neck dissection is performed either routinely or for MTC affecting the lateral neck nodes.[180-182]

Ideally, patients with anaplastic carcinoma should be treated with near-total thyroidectomy and lymph node dissection, but lesions are frequently too extensive for any procedure but palliative surgery.[174-176] In these cases, surgery may be performed later in those patients with tumor regression after a combination of chemotherapy and external radiotherapy.

In recommending surgery, the endocrinologist should discuss potential operative complications with the patient. Unilateral lobectomy almost never causes permanent hypocalcemia but can cause temporary vocal cord paralysis in as many as 3% of patients. Total thyroidectomy causes temporary hypocalcemia in 7% to 10% of patients and permanent hypocalcemia in 0.5% to 1%; permanent vocal cord paralysis occurs in fewer than 1% and may benefit from specific treatments.[194] The risk of hypoparathyroidism should be reduced by identification of the parathyroid glands, possibly with the use of methylene blue staining and certainly, if viability is in doubt, by autotransplantion of the parathyroid glands at the time of initial neck exploration. The experience of the surgeon is important in regard to the finer technical points of thyroidectomy, including preservation of the external branch of the recurrent laryngeal nerve, which is important in the fine regulation of voice pitch.

A history of irradiation in childhood increases the risk of both benign and malignant thyroid nodules in later life.[195] The risk increases with younger age at exposure and with larger radiation dose. Several issues are relevant for the thyroidologist. With respect to the extent of surgery, a total thyroidectomy should be performed in all patients who have a thyroid carcinoma[195,196] and also in those with benign lesions.

Indeed, one must weigh the relative risk of complications associated with a more extensive surgical procedure against the possibility of recurrence of thyroid nodules in the residual thyroid tissue. In one irradiated population, both benign and malignant nodules recurred after subtotal thyroidectomy. The overall risk of recurrence in this study was approximately 20% and was lower in those who had more thyroid tissue removed than in those who underwent less extensive procedures. In those patients after surgery, suppression of TSH by thyroid hormone led to a reduction in recurrence from 35% to approximately 8%, but TSH suppression had no influence on the occurrence of malignant nodules.[195] Therefore, the recommendations for patients with thyroid nodules after neck exposure to radiation during childhood must take into account the estimated risk of developing a thyroid nodule and the experience of the operating surgeon. All irradiated patients who have had thyroid nodules removed should receive TSH-suppressive doses of levothyroxine regardless of the extent of surgery. The appearance of new thyroid nodules is, however, fairly common, and patients should be monitored indefinitely for this possibility.

It is not clear whether the experience just described should be extrapolated to prescribe routine TSH suppression therapy for all irradiated patients, even if nodularity is not present, because its beneficial effects have not been quantified and the risks of long-term TSH suppression in women, especially in regard to osteoporosis, have not been clearly defined and may be significant. At present, this approach cannot be recommended for all irradiated patients but can be recommended for patients who are at high risk for development of a thyroid nodule.[195]

POSTOPERATIVE MANAGEMENT

In view of the uncertainties reviewed in the previous section and the different needs of individual patients, postoperative treatment of thyroid carcinoma cannot always accord with a rigid algorithm.[1,2] One must consider the extent of disease at surgery, the histotype and differentiation of the tumor, the age of the patient, and the risk group category.

Iodine 131 Therapy

^{131}I is an effective agent for delivering high radiation doses to the thyroid tissue with low spillover to other portions of the body. The radiation dose to the thyroid tissue is related to the tissue concentration, the ratio between total tissue uptake and volume of functional tissue, and the effective half-life of ^{131}I in the tissue.[62,197] Thyroid tissue is able to concentrate iodine only after TSH stimulation, but even after optimal TSH stimulation, iodine uptake in neoplastic tissue is always lower than in normal thyroid tissue and may not be detectable in about one third of cases.[62]

^{131}I therapy is given postoperatively for three reasons.[1,2] First, it destroys normal thyroid remnants (this is termed *ablation*), thereby increasing the sensitivity of subsequent ^{131}I total-body scanning and the specificity of measurements of serum Tg for the detection of persistent or recurrent disease.[198] Second, it may destroy occult or known microscopic carcinomas, thereby potentially decreasing the long-term recurrence rate. Finally, it makes it possible to perform a postablative ^{131}I total-body scan, a sensitive tool for detecting persistent carcinoma.

It cannot be emphasized too strongly that postoperative ^{131}I therapy should be used *selectively* and that not all patients with a diagnosis of FCTC benefit from routine postoperative radioiodine ablative therapy.[1,2,91] In very-low-risk patients, the long-term prognosis after surgery alone is so favorable that ^{131}I ablation is not recommended.[1,2,199,200] However, patients who are at high risk of recurrence (Table 14-7) are routinely treated with ^{131}I because such therapy can potentially decrease both the recurrence rate and the death rate. Young children are also usually candidates for postoperative radioiodine therapy because they may have extensive neck lymph node involvement and frequently harbor pulmonary metastases that are not detectable with standard radiography or even with CT imaging of the chest.[103,136] In other patient groups, there is currently no evidence that ^{131}I therapy improves the long-term outcome; radioiodine is administered postoperatively if surgery was or could have been incomplete.

Postoperatively, no levothyroxine treatment is given for 4 to 6 weeks, but liothyronine can be substituted for at least 3 to 4 weeks and then discontinued for 2 weeks before radioiodine studies. At that time, the serum TSH level should be greater than an empirically determined level of 25 to 30 mU/L; an undetectable serum Tg level indicates a very low risk of finding persistent disease or of subsequent recurrence.[201] Intramuscular injections of rhTSH (0.9 mg/day for 2 consecutive days, with ^{131}I administered 1 day

TABLE 14-7

Indications for Iodine 131 Treatment in Patients with Papillary, Follicular, or Hürthle Cell Thyroid Carcinoma after Initial Definitive Near-Total Thyroidectomy

No Indication
Adult patients at very low risk for cause-specific mortality or relapse: complete surgical resection, favorable histology, and limited extent of disease (e.g., PTC patients with MACIS scores <6; patients with tumor size <1 cm, N0, and M0).
Definite Indications
Distant metastasis at diagnosis Incomplete tumor resection Complete tumor resection but high risk for mortality or recurrence (e.g., PTC patients with MACIS scores ≥6 and pTNM stage II/III FTC or HCC)
Probable Indications
Incomplete surgery (less than near-total thyroidectomy, no lymph node dissection) PTC or FTC in a child <16 yr of age If PTC, tall cell or columnar cell variant and diffuse sclerosing variant If FTC, widely invasive or poorly differentiated tumor Bulky nodal metastases

FTC, follicular thyroid carcinoma; HCC, Hürthle cell carcinoma; MACIS, scoring system based on metastasis, age, completeness of resection, invasion, and size; PTC, papillary thyroid carcinoma; pTNM, pathologic tumor-node-metastasis classification.

after the second injection) given on levothyroxine treatment may achieve an effective stimulation of radioiodine uptake by normal thyroid remnant, with ablation rates similar to those obtained with withdrawal[202]; its use prevents hypothyroidism because levothyroxine is initiated soon after surgery and is not discontinued, maintains quality of life, leads to a lower radiation exposure to the body, and permits earlier discharge from the hospital.[202-205] In addition, short-term recurrence rates have been found to be similar in patients prepared with thyroid hormone withdrawal versus rhTSH, even in patients with initial lymph node involvement.[206,207] rhTSH is approved for remnant ablation in the United States, Europe, and many other countries around the world.

In case of incomplete thyroidectomy, neck uptake may be measured with a tracer activity of ^{131}I or ^{123}I; the activity used should be small enough to avoid stunning (i.e., a decrease of thyroid uptake with the subsequent high activity of radioiodine).[208,209] High uptake (>10%) and high risk of persistent disease should lead to completion surgery. ^{131}I therapy can be administered to other patients, with no pretherapy total-body scan because of its low impact on the decision to ablate and because of concerns about ^{131}I-induced stunning, usually with 24-hour uptakes considerably less than 10%.[210] A total-body scan is performed 3 to 7 days after the radioiodine treatment and is highly informative in patients with a low uptake (<1%) in the thyroid bed. Additional metastatic foci have been reported in 10% to 26% of patients scanned after high-dose radioiodine treatment, compared with the diagnostic scan.[211] Single-photon emission computed tomography (SPECT)/CT fusion imaging with ^{131}I may provide superior lesion localization after remnant ablation.[8,9]

Levothyroxine therapy is then initiated or continued. Total ablation (defined as no visible uptake) may be verified by an ^{131}I total-body scan 6 to 12 months later, typically with 2 to 5 mCi (74 to 185 MBq). However, such control ^{131}I total-body scanning is not more routinely performed when postablation scan has been informative, because it does not afford any further information,[212,213] and total ablation is currently defined by an undetectable serum Tg level after rhTSH stimulation and normal findings on neck ultrasonography.[1,2]

Total ablation can be achieved after administration of either 100 mCi (3700 MBq) or 30 mCi (1100 MBq) in more than 80% of patients who had at least a near-total thyroidectomy, after preparation with either withdrawal or rhTSH.[214,215] After less extensive surgery, ablation is achieved in only two thirds of patients with 30 mCi (1100 MBq). Therefore, a near-total thyroidectomy should be performed in all patients who are to be treated with ^{131}I. Also, in high-risk patients, a high activity (100mCi or more) should be administered with the aims of ablating normal thyroid remnants and irradiating residual neoplastic tissue. Total ablation requires that a dose of at least 300 Gy (30,000 rad) be delivered to thyroid remnants. A dosimetric study can allow a more precise estimate of the ^{131}I activity to be administered and avoids the administration of excessive activities, particularly in elderly patients.[197,216]

^{131}I ablation therapy does not play a regular role in the management of anaplastic thyroid cancer, MTC, or thyroid lymphoma.

External Radiotherapy

External radiotherapy to the neck and mediastinum is indicated only for older patients (>45 years) with extensive PTC in whom complete surgical excision is impossible and in whom the tumor tissue does not take up ^{131}I. Retrospective studies have shown that, in these selected patients, external radiotherapy decreases the risk of neck recurrence.[217,218] The target volume encompasses the thyroid bed, bilateral neck lymph node areas, and the upper part of the mediastinum. Typically, 50 Gy (5000 rad) is delivered in 25 fractions over 5 weeks, with a boost of 5-10 Gy on any residual macroscopic focus.

In patients with MTC, this protocol may be applied after incomplete resection of the tumor. After apparently complete surgery, if plasma calcitonin remains detectable in the absence of distant metastases, it may decrease the risk of neck recurrence by a factor of 2 to 4.[104,178]

In patients with anaplastic thyroid carcinoma, if the extent of disease is limited and surgery is feasible, accelerated external radiotherapy in combination with chemotherapy permits local control of the disease in two thirds of patients and long-term survival in about 20%.[175,176]

Levothyroxine Treatment

The growth of thyroid tumor cells is controlled by TSH, and inhibition of TSH secretion with levothyroxine is thought to improve the recurrence and survival rates.[219] Therefore, levothyroxine should be given to all patients with FCTC, whatever the extent of thyroid surgery and other treatment. The initial effective dose is about 2 μg/kg body weight in adults; children require a higher dose and elderly patients a lower dose. The adequacy of therapy is monitored by measuring serum TSH 3 months after it is begun, the initial goal being a serum TSH concentration of less than 0.1 mU/L for high-risk thyroid cancer patients; maintenance of the TSH at or slightly below the lower limit of normal (0.1 to 0.5 mU/L) is appropriate for low-risk patients, including those who have not undergone remnant ablation.[1,2,219]

In patients with anaplastic thyroid carcinoma, MTC, or thyroid lymphoma, a replacement dose of levothyroxine is given, with the aim of obtaining a serum TSH level in the normal range.

FOLLOW-UP

In patients with PTC or FTC, the goals of follow-up after initial therapy are to maintain adequate levothyroxine therapy and to detect persistent or recurrent thyroid carcinoma. Most recurrences occur during the first years of follow-up, but some occur late. Therefore, follow-up is necessary throughout the patient's life.

Early Detection of Recurrent Disease

Clinical and Ultrasonographic Examinations

Palpation of the thyroid bed and lymph node areas is routinely performed at all follow-up visits for patients with thyroid cancer. Ultrasonography is more sensitive and may detect lymph nodes as small as 2 to 3 mm in diameter.[11-13] Metastatic lymph nodes should be differentiated from frequent benign lymph node hyperplasia, and false-positive findings can have deleterious consequences. If lymph nodes are small, thin, or oval; are located in the posterior neck chains; and, especially, decrease in size after an interval of 3 months, they are considered benign. By contrast, malignant lymph nodes are much more likely to occur in compartments III, IV, and VI. The feature with the highest sensitivity for malignancy is absence of a hilus (100%), but this has a low specificity of only 29%; the most specific criteria are short axis (>5 mm), hyperechogenicity, presence of hyperechoic punctuations and of a cystic component, and peripheral hypervascularization.[193] These characteristics can be difficult to recognize in patients with small lymph nodes, so they should be monitored at short intervals.

With the use of an assay that has a functional sensitivity of 1 ng/mL, serum Tg is undetectable in more than 20% of patients receiving levothyroxine treatment who have isolated lymph node metastases detected by palpation or by ^{131}I total-body scanning, and probably in a higher proportion of patients with lymph node metastases detected only by neck ultrasonography.[97,198] Therefore, undetectable values do not exclude metastatic lymph node disease. Ultrasonographically, suspicious lymph nodes larger than 5 to 8 mm in the smallest diameter should be biopsied for cytology with thyroglobulin measurement in the needle washout fluid.[220] The reverse transcriptase–polymerase chain reaction (RT-PCR) technique to amplify Tg mRNA in the fluid aspirate appears to be even more sensitive but is not yet being used by commercial laboratories.[221]

Radiography

Bone and chest radiographs are no longer routinely obtained for patients with undetectable serum Tg concentrations. The reason is that virtually all patients with abnormal radiographs have readily detectable serum Tg concentrations.

Serum Thyroglobulin Determinations

Tg is a glycoprotein that is produced only by normal or neoplastic thyroid follicular cells. Methods used for serum Tg determination and serum interferences are detailed in Chapter 11.[222] Tg should not be detectable in patients who have had total thyroid ablation, which improves both the sensitivity and the specificity for detection of persistent or recurrent disease.[198] Serum Tg antibodies may induce falsely negative results and should be *quantitatively* assessed with every measurement of serum Tg.[1,2,222] Serum Tg antibodies in patients who are in complete remission after total thyroid ablation decline gradually to low or undetectable levels, with a median time of 3 years.[223] Their persistence or reappearance during follow-up should be considered suspicious for persistent or recurrent disease.

There is a close relationship between tumor burden and the Tg level, both during levothyroxine therapy and after TSH stimulation.[222,224] This explains why serum Tg may be undetectable in patients who have isolated lymph node metastases in the neck or small lung metastases not visible on x-ray films. The production of Tg by both normal and neoplastic thyroid tissue is in part TSH dependent. High serum TSH concentrations can be achieved by withdrawing levothyroxine for 4 to 6 weeks. However, the resulting hypothyroidism is poorly tolerated by some patients. This effect can be attenuated by substituting the more rapidly metabolized liothyronine for levothyroxine for 3 to 4 weeks and withdrawing it for 2 weeks, or simply by reducing the dose of levothyroxine by 50%. The serum TSH concentration should be above an empirically determined value (25 to 30 mU/L) in patients treated in this way; if it is not, withdrawal should be prolonged until it is. Intramuscular injections of rhTSH (0.9 mg for 2 consecutive days) are an alternative because levothyroxine treatment need not be discontinued and side effects are minimal. After rhTSH stimulation, the peak of serum Tg is usually obtained 3 days after the second injection.[205,225] Although the increase in serum Tg is frequently less important after rhTSH than after withdrawal, the diagnostic efficiency of rhTSH for stimulating Tg production in the serum is comparable to that of levothyroxine withdrawal in most patients.[198,225]

If serum Tg is detectable during levothyroxine treatment, it will increase after TSH stimulation obtained by treatment discontinuation or injections of rhTSH. If the serum Tg is undetectable during levothyroxine treatment in a blood test performed 3 months after initial treatment, it will increase in 14% to 20% of patients after TSH stimulation at 9 to 12 months.[198,212,213] At that time, the serum Tg concentration is an excellent prognostic indicator.

Most patients with undetectable serum Tg concentrations who are not receiving levothyroxine therapy will remain free of relapse after more than 15 years of follow-up, and fewer than 1% will have a neck lymph node recurrence detected by sonography.[198,212,213] Persistent or recurrent disease is found in one third of the patients with detectable serum Tg concentrations and is twice as frequently located in neck lymph nodes than at distant sites; in these patients, serum Tg levels increase with time or remain elevated. In the other patients, serum Tg levels obtained after TSH stimulation at blood tests performed months or years later will decrease to low or undetectable levels, even in the absence of any further treatment, these patients can also be considered cured.[198,226] Persistent thyroid cells may produce Tg for several months after ^{131}I treatment, disappearing during subsequent months. These data demonstrate that the trend in serum Tg level is probably much more relevant than the actual serum Tg level by itself.

Modern Tg assays with a functional sensitivity of 0.1 ng/mL have an improved sensitivity for the detection of persistent disease during levothyroxine treatment, but at the expense of a decreased specificity; when using modern sensitive assays, the benefits of routine rhTSH stimulation in low-risk patients with undetectable serum Tg on levothyroxine treatment appear not to be significant.[227-229]

TABLE 14-8

Nonthyroidal Conditions Associated with ^{131}I Accumulation

Contamination
Skin, hair, clothes
Physiologic Accumulations
Salivary glands (mouth, esophagus), nose Stomach, colon (in hypothyroidism) Bladder Breast in young women Diffuse hepatic uptake (^{131}I-labeled iodoproteins)
Inflammatory Processes
Lung or bronchial, cutaneous, dental, sinusoidal
Other Conditions
Nonthyroidal neoplasms: salivary glands, stomach, lung, meningioma Struma ovarii Cysts: renal, pleuropericardial, hepatic, salivary, mammary, testicular hydrocele Thymus: normal or hyperplastic Ectasia of the common carotid artery with stasis Esophagus: dilatation, hiatal hernia Pericardial effusion, cardiac insufficiency

Iodine 131 Total-Body Scan

The results of a ^{131}I total-body scan depend on the ability of neoplastic thyroid tissue to take up ^{131}I in the presence of high serum TSH concentrations, which are achieved by withdrawal of levothyroxine or intramuscular injections of rhTSH (0.9 mg for 2 consecutive days, with radioiodine administration on the day following the second injection).[205]

If ^{131}I scanning is planned, patients should be instructed to avoid iodine-containing medications and iodine-rich foods, and urinary iodine should be measured in doubtful cases. Pregnancy must be excluded in women of childbearing age. For routine diagnostic scans, 2 to 5 mCi (74 to 185 MBq) of ^{131}I is given; higher activities may reduce the uptake of a subsequent therapeutic dose of ^{131}I.[208,209] The scan is done, and uptake, if any, is measured 48 to 72 hours after the administration of radioiodine, preferably with the use of a double-head gamma camera equipped with thick crystals and high-energy collimators. False-positive results are rare and usually are easily recognized (Table 14-8).

Total-Body Scans after Iodine 131 Therapy

Assuming equivalent fractional uptake after administration of either a diagnostic or a therapeutic dose of ^{131}I, uptake that is too low to be detected with 2 to 5 mCi (74 to 185 MBq) may be detectable after administration of 100 mCi (3700 MBq). Therefore, a total-body scan should be routinely performed 3 to 7 days after a high-activity of radioiodine (Fig. 14-23). This is also the rationale for administering a large activity of ^{131}I in patients with persistently elevated or increasing Tg levels (>10 ng/mL in the absence of levothyroxine treatment) even if the diagnostic scan is negative.[211]

Other Tests

Other tests should be performed only in selected cases and may include spiral CT or MRI of the neck and chest, bone scintigraphy, MRI of bones, and ^{18}FDG-PET scanning. FDG-PET scanning is performed both for diagnosis of remote neoplastic foci and for prognostic assessment. The sensitivity of FDG-PET may be improved by TSH stimulation, obtained after levothyroxine withdrawal or injections of rhTSH.[22-23] The FDG-PET scan is particularly useful for discovery of mediastinal lymph nodes, and it complements neck ultrasonography for detection of posterior neck lymph node metastases (Fig. 14-24). A spiral CT scan is more sensitive for discovery of small lung metastases. FDG uptake in metastases as quantified by SUV is closely related to clinical prognostic parameters: responses to radioiodine treatment are observed in metastases with radioiodine uptake and with no FDG uptake. Metastases with high SUV values are likely to progress rapidly and will not respond to therapy with radioiodine even when radioiodine uptake is present.[24]

Follow-Up Strategy

If the total-body scan performed after administration of ^{131}I to destroy the thyroid remnants is informative (when uptake in normal thyroid remnants is low, <1%) and does not show any uptake outside the thyroid bed, physical examination is performed and serum TSH and Tg levels are measured during levothyroxine treatment 3 months later (Fig. 14-25). In most centers, a neck ultrasonographic examination is performed and the serum Tg level is measured after thyroid hormone withdrawal or rhTSH

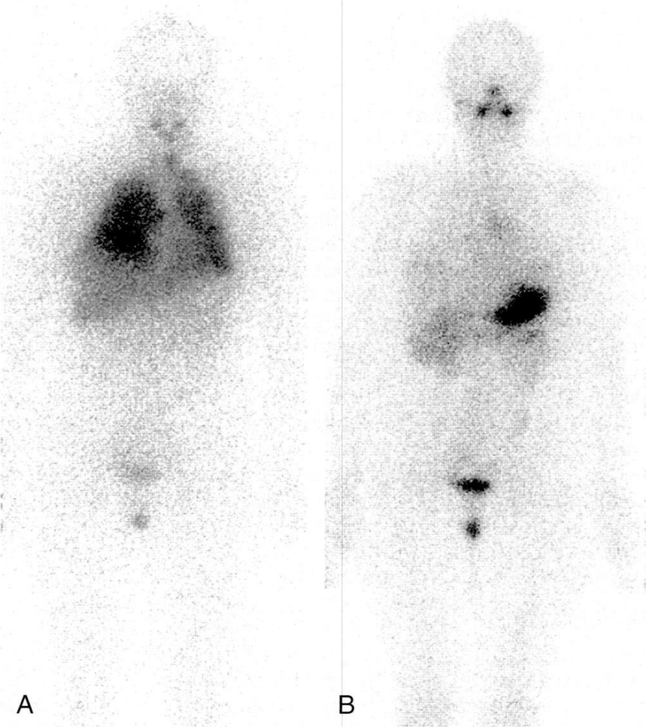

Figure 14-23 Total-body scans in an asymptomatic, 34-year-old patient who underwent surgery for a papillary thyroid carcinoma. The results of chest radiography were normal. **A,** This total-body scan was performed 4 days after postoperative administration of 100 mCi (3700 MBq) of radioactive iodine (^{131}I). Note the presence of diffuse uptake in the lungs and uptake in thyroid remnants and in the left supraclavicular lymph nodes. **B,** A total-body scan performed 6 months later, after the administration of a second treatment with 100 mCi of radioactive iodine, demonstrated the disappearance of all foci of uptake. The thyroglobulin level became undetectable during levothyroxine therapy, and 6 years later the patient is still considered to be in complete remission.

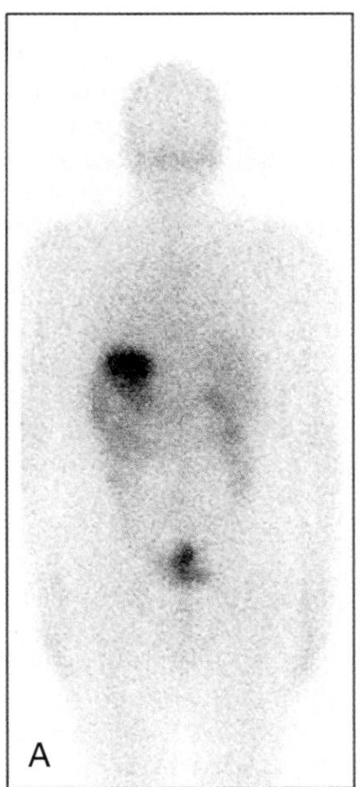

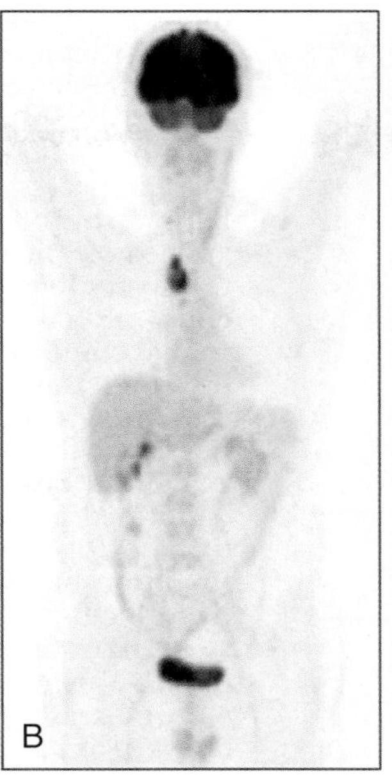

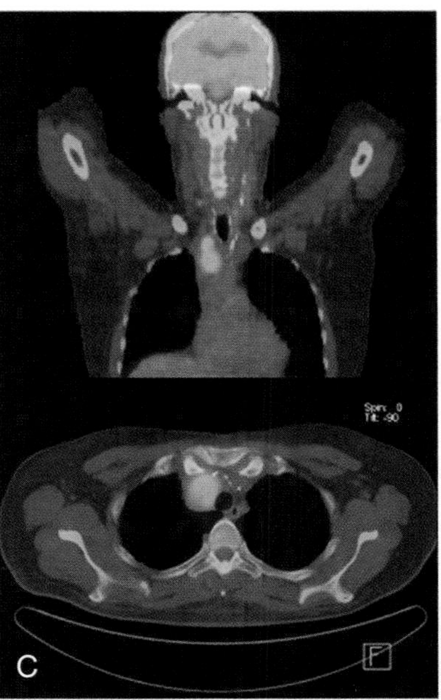

Figure 14-24 This patient was being monitored for a papillary thyroid carcinoma treated by total thyroidectomy and postoperative radioiodine. The serum thyroglobulin level was 45 ng/mL during levothyroxine suppressive treatment. **A,** A total-body scan was performed 3 days after administration of 100 mCi (3.7 GBq). There is no visible uptake in the neck and thorax. Notice the accumulation of radioiodine in the stomach, colon, and bladder. **B,** Positron emission tomography scan using [^{18}F]-fluorodeoxyglucose (^{18}FDG) with maximal intensity projection demonstrates significant uptake in the upper mediastinum. **C,** In fusion images of ^{18}FDG-PET and CT scans, axial and coronal slices localized the FDG uptake in the right paratracheal mediastinum, corresponding to a lymph node metastasis that was subsequently excised. Serum thyroglobulin became undetectable during thyroid hormone treatment.

stimulation 6 to 12 months later.[1,2] A diagnostic ^{131}I total-body scan is no longer routinely performed in low-risk patients with undetectable serum Tg, because almost all patients with ^{131}I uptake in their metastases also have detectable serum Tg levels. Visible uptake in the thyroid bed that is too low to be quantified should not be considered evidence of disease in the absence of any other abnormality. Ablation is currently established by an undetectable serum Tg level after TSH stimulation. Neck ultrasonography can identify lymph node metastases that are too small to produce detectable serum Tg levels and may be not seen on ^{131}I total-body scans (Table 14-9).[11-13]

Patients who have undetectable serum Tg after TSH stimulation and normal findings on neck ultrasonography are considered cured, the risk of long-term recurrence being less than 1%.[212,213] The dose of levothyroxine is decreased to maintain a serum TSH concentration within the normal range of 0.5 to 2.5 mU/L. In high-risk patients, higher doses of levothyroxine are given, the goal being a serum TSH concentration between 0.1 and 0.5 mU/L.[219,230] Clinical and biochemical evaluations with serum TSH and Tg determinations on levothyroxine treatment are performed annually; neck ultrasonography is performed in case of doubt and in high-risk patients, but any other testing is unnecessary as long as the patient's serum Tg concentration is undetectable and the patient does not produce an interfering anti-Tg autoantibody. There is no indication to obtain another rhTSH-stimulated Tg.[231] The use of sensitive assays for serum Tg determination should be permitted to avoid routine rhTSH stimulation in low-risk patients with undetectable serum Tg during levothyroxine treatment; rhTSH stimulation should still be performed in those low-risk patients with detectable serum Tg on levothyroxine treatment and in high-risk patients.[228] Such assays permit early diagnosis of persistent or recurrent disease and should be used in clinical practice during short- and long-term follow-up.[227-229] Tests performed at 9 to 12 months after initial treatment permit a reassessment of the initial prognostication; patients with no abnormal findings are considered to be at low risk and should be reassured, whereas those with any abnormal finding should be followed up more extensively.

Suspicious abnormalities discovered at neck ultrasonography should be submitted to FNAB, even if the serum Tg level remains undetectable after TSH stimulation. Lymph

TABLE 14-9

Sensitivity (%) of Various Methods and Combinations of Methods for Detection of Lymph Node Metastases*

	STUDY (N1/TOTAL NO. OF PATIENTS)		
Method	**Pacini[12] (27/340)**	**Frasoldati[11] (51/494)**	**Torlontano[13] (38/456)**
Tg/TSH	85 (rhTSH)	57 (WD)	82 (WD)
^{131}I TBS	21	45	34
Neck ultrasonography	70	94	100
Tg/TSH + ultrasonography	96	99.5	100

*Tg measurement and TBS were performed after either withdrawal (WD) or stimulation with rhTSH.

N1, number of patients in whom lymph node metastasis was detected; TBS, total-body scan; Tg, thyroglobulin; rhTSH, recombinant human thyrotropin (thyroid-stimulating hormone).

From Schlumberger M, Berg G, Cohen O, et al. Follow-up of low-risk patients with differentiated thyroid carcinoma: a European perspective. *Eur J Endocrinol.* 2004;50:105-112.

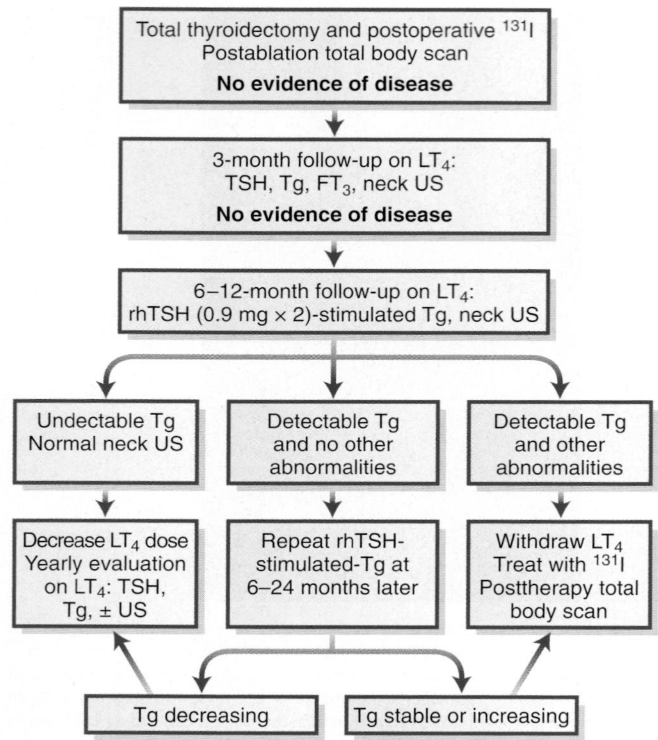

Figure 14-25 Follow-up of patients with papillary thyroid cancer (PTC) or follicular thyroid cancer (FTC) after near-total thyroidectomy and ablation with iodine 131, based on serum thyroglobulin (Tg) measurements and neck ultrasonography (US). Tg levels are considered undetectable if they are below the detection limit of the assay; the institutional threshold should be determined by each institution for each assay used for serum Tg determination. LT_4, levothyroxine; rhTSH, recombinant human thyroid-stimulating hormone; TBS, total-body scan; TSH, thyrotropin (thyroid-stimulating hormone). (From Pacini F, Schlumberger M, Dralle H, et al. European consensus for the management of patients with differentiated thyroid cancer of the follicular epithelium. *Eur J Endocrinol.* 2006;154:787-803.)

node metastases are indeed treated, but currently there is no evidence that treatment at a very early stage (i.e., <5 mm in diameter) improves the outcome, compared with treatment at a stage when they measure 5 to 10 mm in diameter.

At 9 to 12 months after initial treatment, serum Tg becomes detectable after TSH stimulation in 14% to 20% of patients. The discovery of any other abnormality will dictate specific treatments. Otherwise, suppressive levothyroxine treatment is maintained and another rhTSH stimulation test is performed months or years later, depending on the serum Tg level and the clinical context. Serum Tg decreases or becomes undetectable in the absence of any further treatment in two thirds of patients, who then will be considered cured. Serum Tg increases in the remaining third of patients, who should then be submitted to an extensive workup, which may include ultrasound of the neck, spiral CT of the lungs, bone scintigraphy, FDG-PET/CT scanning, and administration of a large activity of ^{131}I with a total-body scan 3 to 5 days later. Clinical recurrence will likely be found in time in most of this third of patients treated for PTC or FTC.[226]

In very low-risk PTC patients who have had a near-total or total thyroidectomy but were not given ^{131}I postoperatively, the intensity of the follow-up strategy depends largely on the serum Tg level and on the results of neck ultrasonography. If the Tg level is not detectable during levothyroxine treatment and a neck ultrasound study is negative, ^{131}I total-body scanning may be avoided. However, if the Tg is readily detectable despite adequate TSH suppression and increases with time, an ablative ^{131}I treatment may be necessary, with a post-treatment scan some days later.[211] The follow-up protocol previously described is then applied on the basis of serum Tg determinations.

In very low-risk PTC patients who have initially undergone only a unilateral lobectomy for PTM, yearly follow-up should consist of a careful neck examination and serum Tg determination during levothyroxine treatment. With time, ultrasonography is likely to show focal nodular abnormalities in the remaining lobe in most patients with detectable Tg concentrations. Usually, biopsies of these lesions can be performed under sonographic guidance, and most prove to be cytologically benign. However, if recurrent PTC is found on biopsy, a completion thyroidectomy should be performed.

In MTC patients, the tumor marker for follow-up is the plasma calcitonin level. In about 90% of young patients whose disease was treated at a preclinical stage on the basis of a *RET* oncogene mutation, the postoperative basal calcitonin level returns to normal and peak calcitonin levels, if measured after stimulation with pentagastrin or calcium, are absent.[179,180] About 5% of these patients have subsequent biologic recurrence of the disease.[106]

In adults with sporadic MTC, who most often present with TNM stage III (node-positive) disease, postoperative basal calcitonin levels are rarely normal.[232-234] In general, basal calcitonin levels correlate with MTC tumor mass, but many MTC patients who have undergone surgery with a curative intent still have postoperative elevations in calcitonin levels without clinical or imaging evidence of persistent disease. In these patients, the disease may be located in the neck if the basal calcitonin level is lower than 150 pg/mL; the risk of distant spread increases with higher calcitonin levels. The localization of neoplastic foci can be difficult and may require morphologic examinations, including neck and liver ultrasonography, CT scans of the neck and chest, or MRI of bones and liver[20,21]; if the results are negative, a venous sampling catheterization with calcitonin measurements may be indicated.[233,234] PET scanning with FDG is poorly sensitive,[21,30] and ^{18}F-DOPA PET seems more promising for localizing neoplastic MTC foci.[28,29] Reinterventions based on the results of selective venous sampling catheterization allow the removal of neoplastic foci in most patients but are not likely to improve the cure rate by more than 5% to 30%.[233-235] Such a situation may exist for several postoperative years, and slowly rising calcitonin levels may not necessarily imply a prognosis worse than that indicated by the presenting stage of disease.[232]

A second major tumor marker for MTC is CEA. In general, serum CEA levels are higher in patients with more malignant MTC, whereas the plasma calcitonin levels are higher in those with better differentiated tumors. The doubling times of calcitonin and CEA levels appear to be highly significant prognostic indicators for survival.[236,237]

Papillary and Follicular Thyroid Carcinoma

Locoregional Recurrences

Locoregional recurrences occur in 5% to 20% of patients with PTC or FTC. More than one third of reoperations for persistent or recurrent disease are related to inadequate initial thyroid surgery.[238] Small metastases may be treated with radioiodine, but their persistence after two or three treatments should lead to surgery.[239] A recurrence that is palpable or easily visualized with ultrasonography or CT scanning should be excised.[239,240] Compartmental dissection of previously unexplored compartments with clinically significant persistent or recurrent disease while sparing vital structures is performed, because microscopic lymph node metastases are commonly more extensive than would appear from imaging studies alone. Conversely, compartmental surgical dissections may not be feasible in compartments that have been previously explored due to extensive scarring, and only a more limited or targeted lymph node resection may be possible.

Total excision may be facilitated by total-body scanning 3 to 5 days after administration of 100 mCi (3700 MBq) of ^{131}I because it may identify additional tissue that should be excised. In some centers, surgery is performed 1 day later, typically with the use of an intraoperative probe. The completeness of resection is verified 1 to 2 days after surgery by another total-body scan, and in one series complete resection was achieved in 92% of cases.[240] In the absence of detectable uptake, other methods may be used to facilitate the excision of small neoplastic foci located in scar tissue or in sites that are difficult to redissect, such as intraoperative ultrasonography or preoperative ultrasound-guided charcoal tattooing.[17] External radiotherapy is indicated in FCTC patients with soft tissue recurrences that cannot be completely excised and do not take up ^{131}I.

Some patients with PTC who were not eligible for further surgery or ^{131}I therapy have been treated for regional nodal recurrence with ultrasound-guided radiofrequency ablation or percutaneous ethanol injections.[241-243] For tumors that invade the upper aerodigestive tract, patient outcome is related to complete resection of all gross disease, with techniques ranging from shaving tumor off the trachea or esophagus for superficial invasion, with preservation of function, to more aggressive techniques for direct intraluminal invasion, including tracheal resection and anastomosis or laryngopharyngoesophagectomy.[244] Surgery is usually combined with ^{131}I or external-beam irradiation, or both.

Distant Metastases

In a large group of patients with differentiated carcinoma (PTC, FTC, or HCC), only 9% developed distant metastases.[245] Mortality rates at 5 and 10 years after the diagnosis of metastasis were 65% and 75% for all patients with distant metastases, and almost 80% of the deaths were due to thyroid cancer.[245-247] Therefore, the development of distant metastases in FCTC portends an ominous prognosis. Lung metastases are more frequent in young patients with PTC, and the lung is almost the only site of distant spread in children. Bone metastases are more common in older patients and in those with FTC. Other less common sites are the brain, liver, and skin.[245-247]

Clinical symptoms of lung involvement are uncommon; in contrast, pain, swelling, or fracture occurs in more than 80% of patients with bone metastases. The pattern of lung involvement may vary and ranges from macronodular to diffuse infiltrates. The latter, when not detected by chest radiography, are usually diagnosed by ^{131}I total-body scanning and may be confirmed by spiral CT; enlarged mediastinal lymph nodes are often present in patients with PTC, especially children. Bone metastases are osteolytic and are often difficult to visualize on radiography or bone scintigraphy; bone involvement is better visualized by MRI. FDG-PET scanning is useful in these patients for determining the extent of disease and for prognostic assessment.[2,22] Almost all patients with distant metastases have high serum Tg concentrations unless the lung metastases are not visible on radiographs, and two thirds of such patients have ^{131}I uptake in their sites of metastasis.[246]

Palliative surgery is required for bone metastases if there are neurologic or orthopedic complications or a high risk of such complications. Radiofrequency ablation and cement injection may be effective alternatives. Surgery may also be performed with a curative intent in patients who have only one or a few bone metastases.[248]

Patients with distant metastases that take up ^{131}I are treated with 100 to 200 mCi (3700 to 7400 MBq) every 4 to 6 months during the first 2 years and then at longer intervals. Between ^{131}I treatments, suppressive doses of levothyroxine are given. In one study, the radiation dose to the tumor tissue and the outcome of ^{131}I therapy were correlated.[197] A radiation dose higher than 80 Gy (8000 rads) should be delivered to obtain cure; with radiation doses lower than 35 Gy (3500 rads), there is little chance for success. This is the rationale for using higher activities of radioiodine, either as a standard approach or based on individual dosimetry, and for using lithium salts in these patients, because their use may increase ^{131}I retention in tumor foci; however, there are no demonstrated benefits for any of these techniques.[249]

In patients with functioning metastases, PET scanning with ^{124}I showed that uptake in a given patient can vary among the metastases and also within a given metastasis.[27] Uptake may also be heterogeneous at the cellular level.[27,62] This heterogeneity in the dose distribution in neoplastic foci may explain the ineffectiveness of ^{131}I treatment despite significant uptake on total-body scanning. For treatment to be effective in this clinical setting, appropriate levels of TSH stimulation and absence of iodine contamination are essential. Prolonged withdrawal usually induces higher uptake in neoplastic foci than rhTSH does, and withdrawal should be the preferred method of TSH stimulation before radioiodine treatment in patients with metastatic disease.[250] Therapy mediated by rhTSH may be indicated in selected patients with underlying comorbidities that make iatrogenic hypothyroidism a potential risk, in patients with pituitary disease who are unable to raise their serum TSH, and in patients for whom a delay in therapy might be deleterious.[205] Such patients should be given the same or higher activity than would have been given had they been prepared with hypothyroidism or a dosimetrically determined activity. Lower doses, such as 1 mCi (37 MBq) per kilogram of body weight, are given to children. There is no limit to the cumulative activity of ^{131}I that can be given to patients with distant metastases, although the risk of leukemia and of solid cancers rises significantly with a cumulative activity greater than 500 mCi (18,500 MBq); moreover, further ^{131}I therapy may rarely provide significant benefit above this activity level.[246]

External radiotherapy is given to bone metastases visible on radiographs, even in the presence of iodine uptake.[246] Alternatively, embolization, radiofrequency ablation, or cement injection may be considered. Chemotherapy is poorly effective and should be given only to patients with radioresistant and progressing metastases.[251] Retinoic acid analogues that increased iodine uptake and decreased the growth rate of neoplastic tissue in several in vitro models were found to be poorly effective in clinical settings.[252,253] Kinase inhibitors that target tumor cells (MAP kinase pathway and eventually other targets) and endothelial cells (VEGFRs) and are anti-angiogenic are significantly more effective than cytotoxic chemotherapy agents and should be used as first-line treatment, preferably in the frame of a controlled trial.[254-259]

Disappearance of imaging abnormalities has been obtained overall in about 45% of patients with distant metastases showing avidity for ^{131}I, and responses are even more frequent in patients with radiosensitive disease, younger patients, those with small pulmonary metastases, and those who had a well-differentiated cancer and who have no FDG uptake on PET scanning; complete responses may be obtained several years after initiation of therapy.[245-247] When response was judged to have been complete after ^{131}I therapy, subsequent relapse rarely occurred even though serum Tg levels were persistently detectable in some patients.[246]

Overall survival after the discovery of distant metastasis is more favorable in young patients who have well-differentiated tumors that take up ^{131}I and whose metastases are small when discovered. When the tumor mass is considered, the location of the distant metastasis (lungs or bone) has no independent prognostic influence.[246] The poor prognosis of patients with bone metastases is linked to the large size of their lesions.[246-248] Large distant metastases with high FDG uptake on PET scanning almost never respond to ^{131}I therapy, confirming the clinical prognostic classification.[22,24] The prognostic importance of the small size of the metastases at their discovery has led to the administration of 100 mCi (3700 MBq) of ^{131}I activity to patients who have elevated serum Tg concentrations that increase with time in the absence of obvious disease.[211] Some believe that there is no conclusive evidence that ^{131}I treatment of these asymptomatic patients meaningfully prolongs life. Others have reported a 33% complete remission rate in treated patients who had a positive total-body scan after ^{131}I therapy.

Complications of Treatment with Iodine 131

Acute side effects (nausea, sialadenitis, loss of taste) after treatment with ^{131}I are common but are typically mild and resolve rapidly. Radiation thyroiditis is usually trivial, but if the thyroid remnant is large, the patient may have enough pain to warrant corticosteroid therapy for a few days. Tumors in certain locations, such as the brain, spinal cord, and paratracheal region, may swell in response to TSH stimulation or after ^{131}I therapy, causing compressive symptoms. Xerostomia and obstruction of lacrimal ducts occurs in 5% to 10% of patients treated with ^{131}I.[260,261] Radiation fibrosis may develop in patients with diffuse lung metastases and can eventually prove fatal if high activities (>150 mCi [5550 MBq]) are administered at short intervals (<3 months).[245-247]

Particular attention must be paid to avoiding administration of ^{131}I to pregnant women. After ^{131}I treatment, spermatogenesis may be transiently depressed,[262] and women may have transient ovarian failure. Genetic damage induced by exposure to ^{131}I before conception has been a major subject of concern, but no anomalies have been reported to date. Therefore, it is recommended that conception be postponed for 6 months after treatment with ^{131}I.[263] There is no evidence that pregnancy affects tumor growth in women receiving adequate levothyroxine therapy. In case of pregnancy in a patient treated with replacement levothyroxine, the dose of levothyroxine is increased by 30% as soon as the pregnancy is confirmed, and the serum TSH level is measured every month during the first half of pregnancy.[264] In a patient treated with a suppressive dose of levothyroxine, the serum TSH level is measured every month, and the daily dose of levothyroxine is increased when serum TSH is found increased.

Mild pancytopenia may occur after repeated ^{131}I therapy, especially in patients who have bone metastases also being treated with external radiotherapy. The overall relative risk of leukemia and of solid tumors was found to be increased in patients treated with a high cumulative dose of ^{131}I (>500 mCi [18,500 MBq]) and in association with external radiotherapy.[265]

Medullary Thyroid Carcinoma

For patients with locoregional recurrence of MTC, a complete diagnostic workup should be obtained, principally to exclude distant metastases. Surgery is performed, if feasible, and is typically followed by external radiotherapy.[2,178]

Distant metastases are usually multifocal in each involved organ and frequently involve multiple organs, including liver, lungs, and bones. They may progress slowly and may be compatible with decades of survival. Systemic chemotherapy is poorly efficient and may be indicated only in cases of rapid tumor progression.[266] Symptomatic treatments are given, in particular against diarrhea. Chemoembolization of liver metastases with adriamycin was reported to provide a high response rate for both symptoms and tumor mass.[267] Kinase inhibitors directed against tumor cells (RET and other kinases) and endothelial cells (VEGFRs) provide a significantly higher response rate than cytotoxic chemotherapy and should be proposed to MTC patients who have progressive disease as first-line treatment.[268,269]

REFERENCES

1. Pacini F, Schlumberger M, Dralle H, et al. European consensus for the management of patients with differentiated thyroid cancer of the follicular epithelium. *Eur J Endocrinol*. 2006;154:787-803.
2. Cooper DS, Doherty GM, Haugen BR, et al. Revised management guidelines for patients with thyroid nodules and differentiated thyroid cancer. *Thyroid*. 2009;19:1167-1214.
3. Kloos RT, Eng C, Evans DB, et al. Medullary thyroid cancer: management guidelines of the American thyroid. *Thyroid*. 2009;19:565-612.
4. Price DC. Radioisotopic evaluation of the thyroid and the parathyroids. *Radiol Clin North Am*. 1993;31:991-1015.
5. Meller J, Becker W. The continuing importance of thyroid scintigraphy in the era of high-resolution ultrasound. *Eur J Nucl Med Mol Imaging*. 2002;29(suppl 2):S425-S438.
6. Robbins RJ, Schlumberger MJ. The evolving role of ^{131}I for the treatment of differentiated thyroid carcinoma. *J Nucl Med*. 2005;46:28S-37S.
7. Loevinger R, Budinger TF, Watson EE. *MIRD Primer for Absorbed Dose Calculations*. New York, NY: Society of Nuclear Medicine; 1988.
8. Wong KK, Zarzhevsky N, Cahill JM, et al. 2008 Incremental value of diagnostic ^{131}I SPECT/CT fusion imaging in the evaluation of differentiated thyroid carcinoma. *AJR Am J Roentgenol*. 2008;191:1785-1794.
9. Aide N, Heutte N, Rame JP, et al. Clinical relevance of single-photon emission computed tomography/computed tomography of the neck and thorax in postablation (131)I scintigraphy for thyroid cancer. *J Clin Endocrinol Metab*. 2009;94:2075-2084.
10. Frates MC, Benson CB, Charboneau JW, et al. Management of thyroid nodules detected at US: Society of Radiologists in Ultrasound consensus conference statement. *Radiology*. 2005;237:794-800.
11. Frasoldati A, Pesenti M, Gallo M, et al. Diagnosis of neck recurrences in patients with differentiated thyroid carcinoma. *Cancer*. 2003;97:90-96.
12. Pacini F, Molinaro E, Castagna MG, et al. Recombinant human thyrotropin-stimulated serum thyroglobulin combined with neck ultrasonography has the highest sensitivity in monitoring differentiated thyroid carcinoma. *J Clin Endocrinol Metab*. 2003;88:3668-3673.
13. Torlontano M, Attard M, Crocetti U, et al. Follow-up of low risk patients with papillary thyroid cancer: role of neck ultrasonography in detecting lymph node metastases. *J Clin Endocrinol Metab*. 2004;89:3402-3407.
14. Robbins KT, Shaha AR, Medina JE, et al. Committee for Neck Dissection Classification, American Head and Neck Society 2008 Consensus statement on the classification and terminology of neck dissection. *Arch Otolaryngol Head Neck Surg*. 2008;134:536-538.
15. Rago T, Vitti P. Role of thyroid ultrasound in the diagnostic evaluation of thyroid nodules. *Best Pract Res Clin Endocrinol Metab*. 2008;22:913-928.

16. Stulak JM, Grant CS, Farley DR, et al. Value of preoperative ultrasonography in the surgical management of initial and reoperative thyroid cancer. *Arch Surg*. 2005;141:489-496.
17. Hartl DM, Chami L, Ghuzlan AA, et al. Charcoal suspension tattoo localization for differentiated thyroid cancer recurrence. *Ann Surg Oncol*. 2009;16:2602-2608.
18. Phan TT, Jager PL, van Tol KM, et al. Thyroid cancer imaging. *Cancer Treat Res*. 2004;122:317-343.
19. Alberico RA, Husain SH, Sirotkin I. Imaging in head and neck oncology. *Surg Oncol Clin North Am*. 2004;13:13-35.
20. Mirallie E, Vuillez JP, Bardet S, et al. High frequency of bone/bone marrow involvement in advanced medullary thyroid cancer. *J Clin Endocrinol Metab*. 2005;90:779-788.
21. Giraudet AL, Vanel D, Leboulleux S, et al. Imaging medullary thyroid carcinoma with persistent elevated calcitonin levels. *J Clin Endocrinol Metab*. 2007;92:4185-4190.
22. Leboulleux S, Schroeder PR, Schlumberger M, et al. The role of PET in follow-up of patients treated for differentiated epithelial thyroid cancers. *Nat Clin Pract Endocrinol Metab*. 2007;3:112-121.
23. Leboulleux S, Schroeder PR, Busaidy NL, et al. 2009 Assessment of the incremental value of recombinant TSH stimulation before FDG PET/CT imaging to localize residual differentiated thyroid cancer. *J Clin Endocrinol Metab*. 2009;94:1310-1316.
24. Robbins RJ, Wan QW, Grewal RK, et al. Real-time prognosis for metastatic thyroid carcinoma based on 2-[^{18}F] fluoro-2-deoxy-D-Glucose positron emission tomography. *J Clin Endocrinol Metab*. 2006;91:498-505.
25. Van den Bruel A, Maes A, De Potter T, et al. Clinical relevance of thyroid fluorodeoxyglucose-whole body positron emission tomography incidentaloma. *J Clin Endocrinol Metab*. 2002;87:1517-1520.
26. Kim JM, Ryu JS, Kim TY, et al. 18F-Fluorodeoxyglucose positron emission tomography does not predict malignancy in thyroid nodules cytologically diagnosed as follicular neoplasm. *J Clin Endocrinol Metab*. 2007;92:1630-1634.
27. Sgouros G, Kolbert KS, Sheikh A, et al. Patient specific dosimetry for ^{131}I thyroid cancer therapy using ^{124}I PET and 3-dimensional-internal dosimetry (3D-ID) software. *J Nucl Med*. 2004;45:1366-1372.
28. Gourgiotis L, Sarlis NJ, Reynolds JC, et al. Localization of medullary thyroid carcinoma metastasis in a multiple endocrine neoplasia type 2A patient by 6-(F-18)-fluorodopamine positron emission tomography. *J Clin Endocrinol Metab*. 2003;88:637-641.
29. Koopmans KP, de Groot JW, Plukker JT, et al. 18F-Dihydroxyphenylalanine PET in patients with biochemical evidence of medullary thyroid cancer: relation to tumor differentiation. *J Nucl Med*. 2008;49:524-531.
30. Ong SC, Schoder H, Patel SG, et al. Diagnostic accuracy of 18F-FDG PET in restaging patients with medullary thyroid carcinoma and elevated calcitonin levels. *J Nucl Med*. 2007;48:501-507.
31. Vander JB, Gaston EA, Dawber TR. The significance of nontoxic thyroid nodules: final report of a 15-year study of the incidence of thyroid malignancy. *Ann Intern Med*. 1968;69:537-540.
32. Tunbridge WM, Evered DC, Hall R, et al. The spectrum of thyroid disease in a community: the Whickham survey. *Clin Endocrinol (Oxf)*. 1977;7:481-493.
33. Mortensen JD, Woolner LB, Bennett WA. Gross and microscopic findings in clinically normal thyroid glands. *J Clin Endocrinol Metab*. 1955;15:1270-1280.
34. Tan GH, Gharib H. Thyroid incidentalomas: management approaches to nonpalpable nodules discovered incidentally on thyroid imaging. *Ann Intern Med*. 1997;126:226-231.
35. Hegedus L, Bonnema SJ, Bennedbaek FN. Management of simple nodular goiter: current status and future perspectives. *Endocr Rev*. 2003;24:102-132.
36. Krohn K, Fuhrer D, Bayer Y, et al. Molecular pathogenesis of euthyroid and toxic multinodular goiter. *Endocr Rev*. 2005;26:504-524.
37. Bignell GR, Canzian F, Shayeghi M, et al. Familial nontoxic multinodular thyroid goiter locus maps to chromosome 14q but does not account for familial nonmedullary thyroid cancer. *Am J Hum Genet*. 1997;61:1123-1130.
38. Capon F, Tacconelli A, Giardina E, et al. Mapping a dominant form of multinodular goiter to chromosome Xp22. *Am J Hum Genet*. 2000;67:1004-1007.
39. Abs R, Stevenaert A, Beckers A. Autonomously functioning thyroid nodules in a patient with a thyrotropin-secreting pituitary adenoma: possible cause-effect relationship. *Eur J Endocrinol*. 1994;131:355-358.
40. Salvi M, Fukazawa H, Bernard N, et al. Role of autoantibodies in the pathogenesis and association of endocrine autoimmune disorders. *Endocr Rev*. 1988;9:450-466.
41. Van Sande J, Parma J, Tonacchera M, et al. Genetic basis of endocrine disease: somatic and germline mutations of the TSH receptor gene in thyroid diseases. *J Clin Endocrinol Metab* 1995:80, 2577-2585.
42. Bray GA. Increased sensitivity of the thyroid in iodine-depleted rats to the goitrogenic effects of thyrotropin. *J Clin Invest*. 1968;47:1640-1647.
43. Apel RL, Ezzat S, Bapat BV, et al. Clonality of thyroid nodules in sporadic goiter. *Diagn Mol Pathol*. 1995;4:113-121.
44. Foley TP. Goiter in adolescents. *Endocrinol Metab Clin North Am*. 1993;22:593-606.
45. Glinoer D. The regulation of thyroid function during normal pregnancy: importance of the iodine nutrition status. *Best Pract Res Clin Endocrinol Metab*. 2004;18:133-152.
46. Hennemann G. Goiter and pregnancy: a new insight into an old problem [comment]. *Thyroid*. 1992;2:71-72.
47. Alexander EK, Hurwitz S, Heering JP, et al. Natural history of benign solid and cystic thyroid nodules. *Ann Intern Med*. 2003;138:315-318.
48. Jemal A, Siegel R, Ward E, et al. Cancer statistics, 2009. *CA Cancer J Clin*. 2009;59:225-249.
49. McCoy KL, Jabbour N, Ogilvie JB, et al. The incidence of cancer and rate of false-negative cytology in thyroid nodules greater than or equal to 4 cm in size. *Surgery*. 2007;142:837-844.
50. Papini E, Guglielmi R, Bianchini A, et al. Risk of malignancy in nonpalpable thyroid nodules: predictive value of ultrasound and color-Doppler features. *J Clin Endocrinol Metab*. 2002;87:1941-1946.
51. Blum M, Rothschild M. Improved nonoperative diagnosis of the solitary "cold" thyroid nodule: surgical selection based on risk factors and three months of suppression. *JAMA*. 1980;243:242-245.
52. Okamoto T, Yamashita T, Harasawa A, et al. Test performances of three diagnostic procedures in evaluating thyroid nodules: physical examination, ultrasonography and fine needle aspiration cytology. *Endocr J*. 1994;41:243-247.
53. Biondi B, Palmieri EA, Filetti S, et al. Mortality in elderly patients with subclinical hyperthyroidism. *Lancet*. 2002;359:799-800.
54. Boelaert K, Horacek J, Holder RL, et al. 2006 Serum thyrotropin concentration as a novel predictor of malignancy in thyroid nodules investigated by fine-needle aspiration. *J Clin Endocrinol Metab*. 2006;91:4295-4301.
55. Haymart MR, Repplinger DJ, Leverson GE, et al. Higher serum thyroid stimulating hormone level in thyroid nodule patients is associated with greater risks of differentiated thyroid cancer and advanced tumor stage. *J Clin Endocrinol Metab*. 2008;93:809-814.
56. Elisei R, Bottici V, Luchetti F, et al. Impact of routine measurement of serum calcitonin on the diagnosis and outcome of medullary thyroid cancer: experience in 10,864 patients with nodular thyroid disorders. *J Clin Endocrinol Metab*. 2004;89:163-168.
57. Costante G, Durante C, Francis Z, et al. Clinical interest of calcitonin determination in C cell disease. *Nat Clin Pract Endocrinol Metab*. 2009;5:35-44.
58. Marx SJ. Molecular genetics of multiple endocrine neoplasia types 1 and 2. *Nat Rev Cancer*. 2005;5:367-375.
59. Reading CC, Charboneau JW, Hay ID, et al. Sonography of thyroid nodules: a "classic pattern" diagnostic approach. *Ultrasound Q*. 2005;21:157-165.
60. Park JY, Lee HJ, Jang HW, et al. A proposal for a thyroid imaging reporting and data system for ultrasound features of thyroid carcinoma. *Thyroid*. 2009;19:1257-1264.
61. Zingrillo M, Torlontano M, Chiarella R, et al. Percutaneous ethanol injection may be a definitive treatment for symptomatic thyroid cystic nodules not treatable by surgery: five-year follow-up study. *Thyroid*. 1999;9:763-767.
62. Schlumberger M, Lacroix L, Russo D, et al. Defects in iodide metabolism in thyroid cancer and implications for the follow-up and treatment of patients. *Nat Clin Pract Endocrinol Metab*. 2007;3:260-269.
63. Hamburger JI. Diagnosis of thyroid nodules by fine needle biopsy: use and abuse. *J Clin Endocrinol Metab*. 1994;79:335-339.
64. Gharib H. Changing concepts in the diagnosis and management of thyroid nodules. *Endocrinol Metab Clin North Am*. 1997;26:777-800.
65. Hales MS, Hsu FS. Needle tract implantation of papillary carcinoma of the thyroid following aspiration biopsy. *Acta Cytol*. 1990;34:801-804.
66. Mikosch P, Gallowitsch HJ, Kresnik E, et al. Value of ultrasound-guided fine-needle aspiration biopsy of thyroid nodules in an endemic goitre area. *Eur J Nucl Med*. 2000;27:62-69.
67. Baloch ZW, Tam D, Langer J, et al. Ultrasound-guided fine-needle aspiration biopsy of the thyroid: role of on-site assessment and multiple cytologic preparations. *Diagn Cytopathol*. 2000;23:425-429.
68. Danese D, Sciacchitano S, Farsetti A, et al. Diagnostic accuracy of conventional versus sonography-guided fine-needle aspiration biopsy of thyroid nodules. *Thyroid*. 1998;8:15-21.
69. Baloch ZW, LiVolsi VA, Asa SL, et al. Diagnostic terminology and morphologic criteria for cytologic diagnosis of thyroid lesions: a synopsis of the National Cancer Institute Thyroid Fine-Needle Aspiration State of the Science Conference. *Diagn Cytopathol*. 2008;36:425-437.
70. Alexander EK. Approach to the patient with a cytologically indeterminate thyroid nodule. *J Clin Endocrinol Metab*. 2008;93:4175-4182.
71. Moon WJ, Jung SL, Lee JH, et al. Benign and malignant thyroid nodules: US differentiation-multicenter retrospective study. *Radiology*. 2008;247:762-770.
72. Bartolazzi A, Orlandi F, Saggiorato E, et al. Galectin-3-expression analysis in the surgical selection of follicular thyroid nodules with

indeterminate fine-needle aspiration cytology: a prospective multicentre study. *Lancet Oncol*. 2008;9:543-549.
73. Nikiforov YE, Nikiforov YE, Steward DL, et al. Molecular testing for mutations in improving the fine-needle aspiration diagnosis of thyroid nodules. *J Clin Endocrinol Metab*. 2009;94:2092-2098.
74. Chevillard S, Ugolin N, Vielh P, et al. Gene expression profiling of differentiated thyroid neoplasms: diagnostic and clinical implications. *Clin Cancer Res*. 2004;10:6586-6597.
75. Cerutti JM, Delcelo R, Amadei MJ, et al. A preoperative diagnostic test that distinguishes benign from malignant thyroid carcinoma based on gene expression. *J Clin Invest*. 2004;113:1234-1242.
76. Barden CB, Shister KW, Zhu B, et al. Classification of follicular thyroid tumors by molecular signature: results of gene profiling. *Clin Cancer Res*. 2003;9:1792-1800.
77. Weber F, Shen L, Aldred MA, et al. Genetic classification of benign and malignant thyroid follicular neoplasia based on a three-gene combination. *J Clin Endocrinol Metab*. 2005;90:2512-2521.
78. Carpi A, Nicolini A. The role of large-needle aspiration biopsy in the preoperative selection of palpable thyroid nodules: a summary of principal data. *Biomed Pharmacother*. 2000;54:350-353.
79. Furlan JC, Bedard YC, Rosen IB. Role of fine-needle aspiration biopsy and frozen section in the management of papillary thyroid carcinoma subtypes. *World J Surg*. 2004;28:880-885.
80. Greer MA, Astwood EB. Treatment of simple goiter with thyroid. *J Clin Endocrinol*. 1953;13:1312-1331.
81. Ross DS. Thyroid hormone suppressive therapy of sporadic nontoxic goiter. *Thyroid*. 1992;2:263-269.
82. Berghout A, Wiersinga WM, Drexhage HA, et al. Comparison of placebo with L-thyroxine alone or with carbimazole for treatment of sporadic nontoxic goitre. *Lancet*. 1990;336:193-197.
83. Castro MR, Caraballo PJ, Morris JC. Effectiveness of thyroid hormone suppressive therapy in benign solitary thyroid nodules: a meta-analysis. *J Clin Endocrinol Metab*. 2002;87:4154-4159.
84. Wemeau JL, Caron P, Schvartz C, et al. Effects of thyroid-stimulating hormone suppression with levothyroxine in reducing the volume of solitary thyroid nodules and improving extranodular nonpalpable changes: a randomized, double-blind, placebo-controlled trial by the French Thyroid Research Group. *J Clin Endocrinol Metab*. 2002;87:4928-4934.
85. Surks MI, Ortiz E, Daniels GH, et al. Subclinical thyroid disease: scientific review and guidelines for diagnosis and management. *JAMA*. 2004;291:228-238.
86. Biondi B, Palmieri EA, Klain M, et al. Subclinical hyperthyroidism: clinical features and treatment options. *Eur J Endocrinol*. 2005;152:1-9.
87. Berghout A, Wiersinga WM, Drexhage HA, et al. The long-term outcome of thyroidectomy for sporadic nontoxic goitre. *Clin Endocrinol (Oxf)*. 1989;31:193-199.
88. Agerback H, Pilegaard HK, Watt-Boolsen S, et al. Complications of 2,028 operations for benign thyroid disease. *Ugeskr Laeger*. 1988;150:533-536.
89. Bistrup C, Nielsen JD, Gregersen G, et al. Preventive effect of levothyroxine in patients operated for nontoxic goitre: a randomized trial of one hundred patients with nine years follow-up. *Clin Endocrinol (Oxf)*. 1994;40:323-327.
90. Bonnema SJ, Nielsen VE, Hegedus L. Long-term effects of radioiodine on thyroid function, size and patient satisfaction in non-toxic diffuse goitre. *Eur J Endocrinol* 2004:150:439-445.
91. Wesche MFT, Tiel-V Buul MCC, Lips P, et al. A randomized trial comparing levothyroxine with radioactive iodine in the treatment of sporadic nontoxic goiter. *J Clin Endocrinol Metab*. 2001;86:998-1005.
92. Manders JMB, Corstens FHM. Radioiodine therapy of euthyroid multinodular goiters. *Eur J Nucl Med Mol Imaging*. 2002;29(suppl 2):S466-S470.
93. Nygaard B, Faber J, Hegedus L. Acute changes in thyroid volume and function following ^{131}I therapy of multinodular goiter. *Clin Endocrinol (Oxf)*. 1994;41:715-718.
94. Holm LE, Hall P, Wiklund K, et al. Cancer risk after iodine-131 therapy for hyperthyroidism. *J Natl Cancer Inst*. 1991;83:1072-1077.
95. Huysmans DA, Nieuwlaat WA, Erdtsieck RJ, et al. Administration of a single low dose of recombinant human thyrotropin significantly enhances thyroid radioiodide uptake in nontoxic nodular goiter. *J Clin Endocrinol Metab*. 2000;85:3592-3596.
96. Papini E, Guglielmi R, Bizzarri G, et al. Ultrasound-guided laser thermal ablation for treatment of benign thyroid nodules. *Endocr Pract*. 2004;10:276-283.
97. Schlumberger MJ. Papillary and follicular thyroid carcinoma. *N Engl J Med*. 1998;338:297-306.
98. Hay ID. Papillary thyroid carcinoma. *Endocrinol Metab Clin North Am*. 1990;19:545-576.
99. Hedinger C, Williams ED, Sobin LH. *Histological Typing of Thyroid Tumours*. 2nd ed. Originally published by the World Health Organization as no 11 in the International Histological Classification of Tumours series. New York, NY: Springer-Verlag; 1988:1-20.
100. Rosai J, Carganio ML, Delellis RA. *Tumors of the Thyroid Gland*. Washington, DC: Armed Force Institute of Pathology; 1992.
101. Beahrs OH, Henson DE, Hutter RVP, et al. *Manual for Staging of Cancer*. Philadelphia, PA: Lippincott; 1992.
102. American Joint Committee on Cancer. Thyroid. In: Greene FL, Page DL, Fleming ID, et al, eds. *AJCC Cancer Staging Handbook*. 6th ed. New York, NY: Springer; 2002:89-98.
103. Schlumberger M, de Vathaire F, Travagli JP, et al. Differentiated thyroid carcinoma in childhood: long term follow-up of 72 patients. *J Clin Endocrinol Metab*. 1987;65:1088-1094.
104. Brierley J, Tsang R, Simpson WJ, et al. Medullary thyroid cancer: analyses of survival and prognostic factors and the role of radiation therapy in local control. *Thyroid*. 1996;6:305-310.
105. Kebebew E, Ituarte PH, Siperstein AE, et al. Medullary thyroid carcinoma: clinical characteristics, treatment, prognostic factors, and a comparison of staging systems. *Cancer*. 2000;88:1139-1148.
106. Modigliani E, Cohen R, Campos JM, et al. Prognostic factors for survival and for biochemical cure in medullary thyroid carcinoma: results in 899 patients. The GETC Study Group. Groupe d'étude des tumeurs à calcitonine. *Clin Endocrinol (Oxf)*. 1998;48:265-273.
107. Leboulleux S, Rubino C, Baudin E, et al. Prognostic factors for persistent or recurrent disease of papillary thyroid carcinoma with neck lymph node metastases and/or tumor extension beyond the thyroid capsule at initial diagnosis. *J Clin Endocrinol Metab*. 2005;90:5723-5729.
108. Bisi H, Fernandes VS, Asato de Camargo RY, et al. The prevalence of unsuspected thyroid pathology in 300 sequential autopsies, with special reference to the incidental carcinoma. *Cancer*. 1989;64:1888-1893.
109. Carney JA, Ryan J, Goellner JR. Hyalinizing trabecular adenoma of the thyroid gland. *Am J Surg Pathol*. 1987;11:583-592.
110. Carcangiu ML, Bianchi S, Savino D, et al. Follicular Hürthle cell neoplasms of the thyroid gland: a study of 153 cases. *Cancer*. 1991;68:1944-1953.
111. Gundry SR, Burney RE, Thompson NW, et al. Total thyroidectomy for Hürthle cell neoplasm of the thyroid. *Arch Surg*. 1983;118:529-532.
112. Grant CS, Barr D, Goellner JR, et al. Benign Hürthle cell tumors of the thyroid: a diagnosis to be trusted? *World J Surg*. 1988;12:488-494.
113. Chen H, Nicol TL, Zeiger MA, et al. Hürthle cell neoplasms of the thyroid: are there factors predictive of malignancy? *J Nucl Med*. 1998;34:1626-1631.
114. Kondo T, Ezzat S, Asa SL. Pathogenetic mechanisms in thyroid follicular-cell neoplasia. *Nat Rev Cancer*. 2006;6:292-303.
115. Hay ID, Thompson GB, Grant CS, et al. Papillary thyroid carcinoma managed at the Mayo Clinic during six decades (1940-1999): temporal trends in initial therapy and long-term outcome in 2444 consecutively treated patients. *World J Surg*. 2002;26:879-885.
116. Hay ID, Hutchinson ME, Gonzalez-Losada T, et al. Papillary thyroid microcarcinoma: a study of 900 cases observed in a 60-year period. *Surgery*. 2008;144:980-988.
117. Baudin E, Travagli J, Ropers J, et al. Microcarcinoma of the thyroid gland: the Gustave Roussy Institute experience. *Cancer*. 1998;83:553-559.
118. Davies L, Welch HG. Increasing incidence of thyroid cancer in the United States, 1973-2002. *JAMA*. 2006;295:2164-2167.
119. Pierotti MA, Bongarzone I, Borrello MG, et al. Cytogenetics and molecular genetics of carcinomas arising from thyroid epithelial follicular cells. *Genes Chromosom Cancer*. 1996;16:1-14.
120. Fagin JA. Challenging dogma in thyroid cancer molecular genetics: Role of RET/PTC and BRAF in tumor initiation. *J Clin Endocrinol Metab* 2004,89:4264-4266.
121. Herrmann MA, Hay ID, Bartlet DH, et al. Cytogenetic and molecular genetic studies of follicular and papillary thyroid cancers. *J Clin Invest*. 1991;88:1596-1603.
122. Williams ED. Cancer after nuclear fallout: lessons from the Chernobyl accident. *Nat Rev* 2002;2:543-549.
123. Vasko V, Ferrand M, Di Cristofaro J, et al. Specific pattern of RAS oncogene mutations in follicular thyroid tumors. *J Clin Endocrinol Metab*. 2003;88:2745-2752.
124. Xing M. BRAF mutation in papillary thyroid cancer: pathogenic role, molecular bases, and clinical implications. *Endocr Rev*. 2007;28:742-762.
125. Ciampi R, Knauf JA, Kerler R, et al. Oncogenic AKAP9-BRAF fusion is a novel mechanism of MAPK pathway activation in thyroid cancer. *J Clin Invest*. 2005;115:20-23.
126. Saji M, Ringel MD. The PI3K-Akt-mTOR pathway in initiation and progression of thyroid tumors. *Mol Cell Endocrinol*. 2009;321:20-28.
127. Goldgar DE, Easton DF, Cannon-Albright LA, Skolnick MH. Systematic population-based assessment of cancer risk in first-degree relatives of cancer probands. *J Natl Cancer Inst*. 1994;86:1600-1608.
128. Sturgeon C, Clark OH. Familial nonmedullary thyroid cancer. *Thyroid*. 2005;15:588-593.
129. Vriens MR, Suh I, Moses W, et al. Clinical features and genetic predisposition to hereditary nonmedullary thyroid cancer. *Thyoid*. 2009;19:1343-1349.

130. Gudmundsson J, Sulem P, Gudbjartsson DF, et al. Common variants on 9q22.33 and 14q13.3 predispose to thyroid cancer in European populations. *Nat Genet.* 2009;41:460-464.
131. Landa I, Ruiz-Llorente S, Montero-Conde C, et al. The variant rs1867277 in FOXE1 gene confers thyroid cancer susceptibility through the recruitment of USF1/USF2 transcription factors. *PLoS Genet.* 2009;5:e1000637.
132. Ngan ESW, Lang BHH, Liu T, et al. A germline mutation (A339V) in thyroid transcription factor-1 (TITF-1/NKX2.1) in patients with multinodular goiter and papillary thyroid carcinoma. *J Natl Cancer Inst.* 2009;101:162-175.
133. Mitchell JC, Parangi S. Angiogenesis in benign and malignant thyroid disease. *Thyroid.* 2005;15:494-510.
134. Colonna M, Grosclaude P, Remontet L, et al. Incidence of thyroid cancer in adults recorded by French Cancer registries (1978-1997). *Eur J Cancer.* 2002;38:1762-1768.
135. Shattuck TM, Westra WH, Ladenson PW, et al. Independent clonal origins of distinct tumor foci in multifocal thyroid carcinoma. *N Engl J Med.* 2005;352:2406-2412.
136. Zimmerman D, Hay ID, Gough IR, et al. Papillary thyroid carcinoma in children and adults: long-term follow-up of 1,039 patients conservatively treated at one institution during three decades. *Surgery.* 1988;104:1157-1166.
137. Kukkonen ST, Haapiainen RK, Fransila KO, et al. Papillary thyroid carcinoma: the new, age-related TNM classification system in a retrospective analysis of 199 patients. *World J Surg.* 1990;14:837-842.
138. Grant CS, Hay ID, Gough IR, et al. Local recurrence in papillary thyroid carcinoma: is extent of surgical resection important? *Surgery.* 1988;104:954-962.
139. Hay ID, Grant CS, Taylor WF, et al. Ipsilateral lobectomy versus bilateral lobar resection in papillary thyroid carcinoma: a retrospective analysis of surgical outcome using a novel prognostic scoring system. *Surgery.* 1987;102:1088-1095.
140. Tsang RW, Brierley JD, Simpson WJ, et al. The effects of surgery, radioiodine, and external radiation therapy on the clinical outcome of patients with differentiated thyroid carcinoma. *Cancer.* 1998;82:375-388.
141. DeGroot LJ, Kaplan EL, McCormick M, et al. Natural history, treatment and course of papillary thyroid carcinoma. *J Clin Endocrinol Metab.* 1990;71:414-424.
142. Shah JP, Loree TR, Dharker D, et al. Prognostic factors in differentiated carcinoma of the thyroid gland. *Am J Surg.* 1992;164:658-661.
143. Akslen LA, Livolsi VA. Prognostic significance of histologic grading compared with subclassification of papillary thyroid carcinoma. *Cancer.* 2000;88:1902-1908.
144. Hay ID, Bergstralh EJ, Goellner JR, et al. Predicting outcome in papillary thyroid carcinoma: development of a reliable prognostic scoring system in a cohort of 1,779 patients surgically treated at one institution during 1940 through 1989. *Surgery.* 1993;114:1050-1058.
145. Brierley JD, Panzarella T, Tsang RW, et al. A comparison of different staging systems predictability of patient outcome: thyroid carcinoma as an example. *Cancer.* 1997;79:2414-2423.
146. Hay ID. Management of patients with low-risk papillary thyroid carcinoma. *Endocr Pract.* 2007;13:521-533.
147. Pace-Asciak PZ, Payne RJ, Eski SJ, et al. Cost savings of patients with a MACIS score lower than 6 when radioactive iodine is not given. *Arch Otolaryngol Head Neck Surg.* 2007;133:870-873.
148. Carcangiu MC, Zempi G, Rosai J. Poorly differentiated ("insular") thyroid carcinoma: a reinterpretation of Langhans "wuchernde Struma." *Am J Surg Pathol.* 1984;8:655-668.
149. Sobrinho-Simoes M. Mixed medullary and follicular carcinoma of the thyroid. *Histopathology.* 1993;23:187-189.
150. Grebe SKG, Hay ID. Follicular thyroid cancer. *Endocrinol Metab Clin North Am.* 1996;24:761-801.
151. Livolsi VA, Asa SL. The demise of follicular carcinoma of the thyroid gland. *Thyroid.* 1994;4:233-236.
152. Livolsi VA, Merino MJ. Worrisome histologic alterations following fine-needle aspiration of the thyroid. *Pathol Annu.* 1994;29:99-120.
153. Volante M, Collini P, Nikiforov YE, et al. Poorly differentiated thyroid carcinoma: the Turin proposal for the use of uniform diagnostic criteria and an algorithmic diagnostic approach. *Am J Surg Pathol.* 2007;31:1256-1264.
154. Ishimaru Y, Fukuda S, Kurano R, et al. Follicular thyroid carcinoma with clear cell change showing unusual ultrastructural features. *Am J Surg Pathol.* 1988;12:240-246.
155. Watson RG, Brennan MD, Goellner JR, et al. Invasive Hürthle cell carcinoma of the thyroid: natural history and management. *Mayo Clin Proc.* 1984;59:851-855.
156. Challeton C, Bounacer A, Du Villard JA, et al. Pattern of ras and gsp oncogene mutations in radiation-associated human thyroid tumors. *Oncogene.* 1995;11:601-603.
157. Kroll TG, Sarraf P, Pecciarini L, et al. *PAX8-PPARγ1* fusion oncogene in human thyroid carcinoma. *Science.* 2000;289:1357-1360.
158. Powell GJ, Wang X, Allard BL, et al. The PAX8/PPAR gamma fusion oncoprotein transforms immortalized human thyrocytes through a mechanism probably involving wild-type PPAR gamma inhibition. *Oncogene.* 2004;23:3634-3641.
159. Nikiforova MN, Lynch RA, Biddinger PW, et al. RAS point mutations and PAX8-PPAR gamma rearrangement in thyroid tumors: evidence for distinct molecular pathways in thyroid follicular carcinoma. *J Clin Endocrinol Metab.* 2003;88:2318-2326.
160. Paul SJ, Sisson JC. Thyrotoxicosis caused by thyroid cancer. *Endocrinol Metab Clin North Am.* 1990;19:593-612.
161. Grebe SKG, Hay ID. Thyroid cancer nodal metastases: biologic significance and therapeutic considerations. *Surg Oncol Clin North Am.* 1996;5:43-63.
162. van Heerden JA, Hay ID, Goellner JR, et al. Follicular thyroid carcinoma with capsular invasion alone: a non-threatening malignancy. *Surgery.* 1992;112:1130-1136.
163. Mueller-Gaertner HW, Brzac HT, Rehpenning W. Prognostic indices for tumor relapse and tumor mortality in follicular thyroid carcinoma. *Cancer.* 1991;67:1903-1908.
164. Cady R, Rossi R. An expanded view of risk-group definition in differentiated thyroid carcinoma. *Surgery.* 1985;98:1171-1176.
165. Shaha AR, Loree TR, Shah JP. Prognostic factors and risk group analysis in follicular carcinoma of the thyroid. *Surgery.* 1995;118:1131-1138.
166. Emerick GT, Duh QY, Siperstein AE, et al. Diagnosis, treatment, and outcome of follicular thyroid carcinoma. *Cancer.* 1993;72:3287-3294.
167. Davis NL, Bugis SD, McGregor GI, et al. An evaluation of prognostic scoring systems in patients with follicular thyroid cancer. *Am J Surg.* 1995;170:476-480.
168. Asari R, Koperek O, Scheuba C, et al. Follicular thyroid carcinoma in an iodine-replete endemic goiter region: a prospectively collected, retrospectively analyzed clinical trial. *Ann Surg.* 2009;249:1023-1031.
169. LiVolsi VA, Baloch ZW. Predicting prognosis in thyroid carcinoma: can histology do it? *Am J Surg Pathol.* 2002;26:1064-1065.
170. d'Avanzo A, Ituarte P, Treseler P, et al. Prognostic scoring systems in patients with follicular thyroid cancer: a comparison of different staging systems in predicting the patient outcome. *Thyroid.* 2004;14:453-458.
171. Fagin JA, Matsuo K, Karmakar A, et al. High prevalence of mutations of the p53 gene in poorly differentiated human thyroid carcinomas. *J Clin Invest.* 1993;91:179-184.
172. Elliott DD, Sherman SI, Busaidy NL, et al. Growth factor receptors expression in anaplastic thyroid carcinoma: potential markers for therapeutic stratification. *Hum Pathol.* 2008;39:15-20.
173. Ricarte-Filho JC, Ryder M, Chitale DA, et al. Mutational profile of advanced primary and metastatic radioactive iodine-refractory thyroid cancers reveals distinct pathogenetic roles for BRAF, PIK3CA, and AKT1. *Cancer Res.* 2009;69:4885-4893.
174. McIver B, Hay ID, Giuffrida DF, et al. Anaplastic thyroid carcinoma: a 50-year experience at a single institution. *Surgery.* 2001;130:1028-1034.
175. Crevoisier R, Baudin E, Bachelot A, et al. Combined treatment of anaplastic thyroid carcinoma with surgery, chemotherapy, and hyperfractionated accelerated external radiotherapy. *Int J Radiation Oncology Biol Phys.* 2004;60:1137-1143.
176. Kebebew E, Greenspan FS, Clark OH, et al. Anaplastic thyroid carcinoma: treatment outcome and prognostic factors. *Cancer.* 2005;103:1330-1335.
177. Bogsrud TV, Karantanis D, Nathan MA, et al. 18F-FDG PET in the management of patients with anaplastic thyroid carcinoma. *Thyroid.* 2008;18:713-719.
178. Leboulleux S, Baudin E, Travagli JP, et al. Medullary thyroid carcinoma. *Clin Endocrinol (Oxf).* 2004;61:299-310.
179. Machens A, Niccoli-Sire P, Hoegel J, et al. Early malignant progression of hereditary medullary thyroid cancer. *N Engl J Med.* 2003;349:1517-1525.
180. Skinner MA, Moley JA, Dilley WG, et al. Prophylactic thyroidectomy in multiple endocrine neoplasia type 2A. *N Engl J Med.* 2005;353:1105-1113.
181. Moley JF, DeBenedetti MK. Patterns of nodal metastases in palpable medullary thyroid carcinoma: recommendations for extent of node dissection. *Ann Surg.* 1999;6:880-888.
182. Scollo C, Baudin E, Travagli JP, et al. Rationale for central and bilateral lymph node dissection in sporadic and hereditary medullary thyroid cancer. *J Clin Endocrinol Metab.* 2003;88:2070-2075.
183. Thieblemont C, Mayer A, Dumontet C, et al. Primary thyroid lymphoma is a heterogeneous disease. *J Clin Endocrinol Metab.* 2002;87:105-111.
184. Harris NL, Jaffe ES, Stein H, et al. A revised European-American classification of lymphoid neoplasms: a proposal from the International Lymphoma Study Group. *Blood.* 1994;84:1361-1392.
185. Shipp M, for The International Non-Hodgkin's Lymphoma Prognostic Factors Project. A predictive model for aggressive non-Hodgkin's lymphoma. *N Engl J Med.* 1993;329:987-994.
186. Coiffier B, Lepage E, Briere J, et al. CHOP chemotherapy plus rituximab compared with CHOP alone in elderly patients with diffuse large-B-cell lymphoma. *N Eng J Med.* 2002;346:235-242.

187. Tsang RW, Gosodarowicz MK, Pintilie M, et al. Localized mucosa-associated lymphoid tissue lymphoma treated with radiation therapy has excellent clinical outcome. *J Clin Oncol*. 2003;21:4157-4164.
188. Bilimoria KY, Bentrem DJ, Ko CY, et al. Extent of surgery affects survival for papillary thyroid cancer. *Ann Surg*. 2007;246:375-384.
189. Bonnet S, Hartl D, Leboulleux S, et al. 2009 Prophylactic lymph node dissection for papillary thyroid cancer less than 2 cm: implications for radioiodine treatment. *J Clin Endocrinol Metab*. 2009;94:1162-1167.
190. White MC, Gauger PG, Doherty GM. Central lymph node dissection in papillary thyroid carcinoma. *World J Surg*. 2007;31:895-904.
191. Mazzaferri EL, Doherty GM, Steward DL. The pros and cons of prophylactic central compartment lymph node dissection for papillary thyroid carcinoma. *Thyroid*. 2009;19:683-689.
192. Hay ID, Bergstralh EJ, Grant CS, et al. Impact of primary surgery on outcome in 300 patients with pathologic tumor-node-metastasis stage III papillary thyroid carcinoma treated at one institution from 1940 through 1989. *Surgery*. 1999;126:1173-1181.
193. Leboulleux S, Girard E, Rose M, et al. Ultrasound criteria of malignancy for cervical lymph nodes in patients followed up for differentiated thyroid cancer. *J Clin Endocrinol Metab*. 2007;92:3590-3594.
194. Hartl DM, Travagli JP, Leboulleux S, et al. Current concepts in the management of unilateral recurrent laryngeal nerve paralysis after thyroid surgery. *J Clin Endocrinol Metab*. 2005;90:3084-3088.
195. Schneider AB, Sarne DH. Long-term risks for thyroid cancer and other neoplasm after exposure to radiation. *Nat Clin Pract Endocrinol Metab*. 2005;1:82-91.
196. Rubino C, Cailleux AF, Abbas M, et al. Characteristics of follicular cell-derived thyroid carcinomas occurring after external radiation exposure: results of a case control study nested in a cohort. *Thyroid*. 2002;12:299-304.
197. Maxon HR, Thomas SR, Hertzberg VS, et al. Relation between effective radiation dose and outcome of radioiodine therapy for thyroid cancer. *N Engl J Med*. 1983;309:937-941.
198. Eustatia-Rutten CFA, Smit JWA, Romijn JA, et al. Diagnostic value of serum thyroglobulin measurements in the follow-up of differentiated thyroid carcinoma: a structured meta-analysis. *Clin Endocrinol (Oxf)*. 2004;61:61-74.
199. Hay ID. Selective use of radioiodine in the postoperative management of patients with papillary and follicular thyroid carcinoma. *J Surg Oncol*. 2006;94:692-700.
200. Hay ID, McDougall IR, Sisson JC. Perspective: the case against radioiodine remnant ablation in patients with well-differentiated thyroid carcinoma. *J Nucl Med* 2008:49:1395-1397.
201. Toubeau M, Touzery C, Arveux P, et al. Predictive value for disease progression of serum thyroglobulin levels measured in the postoperative period and after (131I) ablation therapy in patients with differentiated thyroid cancer. *J Nucl Med*. 2004;45:988-994.
202. Pacini F, Ladenson PW, Schlumberger M, et al. Radioiodine ablation of thyroid remnants after preparation with recombinant human thyrotropin in differentiated thyroid carcinoma: results of an international, randomized, controlled study. *J Clin Endocrinol Metab*, 2006 91:926-932.
203. Hänscheid H, Lassmann M, Luster M, et al. Iodine biokinetics and dosimetry in radioiodine therapy of thyroid cancer: procedures and results of a prospective international controlled study of ablation after rhTSH or hormone withdrawal. *J Nucl Med*. 2006;47:648-654.
204. Rémy H, Borget I, Leboulleux S, et al. Iodine 131 effective half-life and dosimetry in thyroid cancer patients. *J Nucl Med*. 2008;49:1445-1450.
205. Schlumberger M, Ricard M, De Pouvourville G, et al. How the availability of recombinant human TSH has changed the management of patients who have thyroid cancer. *Nat Clin Pract Endocrinol Metab*. 2007;3:641-650.
206. Tuttle RM, Brokhin M, Omry G, et al. RJ Recombinant human TSH-assisted radioactive iodine remnant ablation achieves short-term clinical recurrence rates similar to those of traditional thyroid hormone withdrawal. *J Nucl Med*. 2008;49:764-770.
207. Elisei R, Schlumberger M, Driedger A, et al. Follow-up of low-risk differentiated thyroid cancer patients who underwent radioiodine ablation of postsurgical thyroid remnants after either recombinant human thyrotropin or thyroid hormone withdrawal. *J Clin Endocrinol Metab*. 2009;94:4171-4179.
208. Lassman M, Luster M, Hanscheid H, et al. The impact of I-131 diagnostic activities on the biokinetics of thyroid remnants. *J Nucl Med*. 2004;45:619-625.
209. Nordén MM, Larsson F, Tedelind S, et al. Down-regulation of the sodium/iodide symporter explains 131I-induced thyroid stunning. *Cancer Res*. 2007;67:7512-7517.
210. Schlumberger M, Pacini F. The low utility of pretherapy scans in thyroid cancer patients. *Thyroid*. 2009;19:815-816.
211. Schlumberger M, Mancusi F, Baudin E, et al. ^{131}I therapy for elevated thyroglobulin levels. *Thyroid*. 1997;7:273-276.
212. Cailleux AF, Baudin E, Travagli JP, et al. Is diagnostic iodine-131 scanning useful after total thyroid ablation for differentiated thyroid cancer? *J Clin Endocrinol Metab*. 2000;85:175-178.
213. Pacini F, Capezzone M, Elisei R, et al. Diagnostic 131-iodine whole-body scan may be avoided in thyroid cancer patients who have undetectable stimulated serum Tg levels after initial treatment. *J Clin Endocrinol Metab*. 2002;87:1499-1501.
214. Bal CS, Kumar A, Pant GS. Radioiodine dose for remnant ablation in differentiated thyroid carcinoma: a randomized clinical trial in 509 patients. *J Clin Endocrinol Metab*. 2004;89:1666-1673.
215. Hackshaw A, Harmer C, Mallick U, et al. ^{131}I Activity for remnant ablation in patients with differentiated thyroid cancer: a systematic review. *J Clin Endocrinol Metab*. 2007;92:28-38.
216. Tuttle RM, Leboeuf R, Robbins RJ, et al. Empiric radioactive iodine dosing regimens frequently exceed maximum tolerated activity levels in elderly patients with thyroid cancer. *J Nucl Med*. 2006;47: 1587-1591.
217. Farahati J, Reiners C, Stuschke M, et al. Differentiated thyroid cancer: impact of adjuvant external radiotherapy in patients with perithyroidal tumor infiltration (stage pT4). *Cancer*. 1996;77:172-180.
218. Lee N, Tuttle M. The role of external beam radiotherapy in the treatment of papillary thyroid cancer. *Endocr Relat Cancer*. 2006;13: 971-977.
219. Biondi B, Filetti S, Schlumberger M. Thyroid-hormone therapy and thyroid cancer: a reassessment. *Nat Clin Pract Endocrinol Metab*. 2005;1:32-40.
220. Pacini F, Fugazzola L, Lippi F, et al. Detection of thyroglobulin in fine needle aspirates of nonthyroidal neck masses: a clue to the diagnosis of metastatic differentiated thyroid cancer. *J Clin Endocrinol Metab*. 1992;74:1401-1404.
221. Arturi F, Russo D, Giuffrida D, et al. Early diagnosis by genetic analysis of differentiated thyroid cancer metastases in small lymph nodes. *J Clin Endocrinol Metab*. 1997;82:1638-1641.
222. Demers LM, Spencer CA. *Laboratory Support for the Diagnosis and Monitoring of Thyroid Disease*. NACB Laboratory Medicine Practice Guidelines. Washington, DC: American Association for Clinical Chemistry; 2003. Available at http://www.nacb.org/lmpg/thyroid/LMPH.stm (accessed August 2010).
223. Chiovato L, Latrofa F, Braverman LE, et al. Disappearance of humoral thyroid autoimmunity after complete removal of thyroid antigens. *Ann Intern Med*. 2003;139:346-351.
224. Bachelot A, Cailleux AF, Klain M, et al. Relationship between tumor burden and serum thyroglobulin level in patients with papillary and follicular thyroid carcinoma. *Thyroid*. 2002;12:707-711.
225. Haugen BR, Pacini F, Reiners C, et al. A comparison of recombinant human thyrotropin and thyroid hormone withdrawal for the detection of thyroid remnant or cancer. *J Clin Endocrinol Metab*. 1999;84: 3877-3885.
226. Baudin E, Docao C, Cailleux AF, et al. Positive predictive value of serum thyroglobulin levels, measured during the first year of follow-up following thyroid hormone withdrawal, in thyroid cancer patients. *J Clin Endocrinol Metab*. 2003;88:1107-1111.
227. Smallridge RC, Meek SE, Morgan MA, et al. Monitoring thyroglobulin in a sensitive immunoassay has comparable sensitivity to recombinant human TSH-stimulated thyroglobulin in follow-up of thyroid cancer patients. *J Clin Endocrinol Metab*. 2007;92:82-87.
228. Schlumberger M, Hitzel A, Toubert ME, et al. Comparison of seven serum thyroglobulin assays in the follow-up of papillary and follicular thyroid cancer patients. *J Clin Endocrinol Metab*. 2007;92:2487-2495.
229. Snozek CL, Chambers EP, Reading CC, et al. Serum thyroglobulin, high-resolution ultrasound, and lymph node thyroglobulin in diagnosis of differentiated thyroid carcinoma nodal metastases. *J Clin Endocrinol Metab*. 2007;92:4278-4281.
230. Jonklaas J, Sarlis NJ, Litofsky D, et al. Outcomes of patients with differentiated thyroid carcinoma following initial therapy. *Thyroid*. 2006;16:1229-1242.
231. Castagna MG, Brilli L, Pilli T, et al. Limited value of repeat recombinant thyrotropin (rhTSH)-stimulated thyroglobulin testing in differentiated thyroid carcinoma patients with previous negative rhTSH-stimulated thyroglobulin and undetectable basal serum thyroglobulin levels. *J Clin Endocrinol Metab*. 2008;93:76-81.
232. van Heerden JA, Grant CS, Gharib H, et al. Long-term course of patients with persistent hypercalcitoninemia after apparent curative primary surgery for medullary thyroid carcinoma. *Ann Surg*. 1990;212:395-400.
233. Pellegriti G, Leboulleux S, Baudin E, et al. Long-term outcome of medullary thyroid carcinoma in patients with normal postoperative medical imaging. *Br J Cancer*. 2003;88:1537-1542.
234. Kebebew E, Kikuchi S, Duh QY, et al. Long-term results of reoperation and localizing studies in patients with persistent or recurrent medullary thyroid cancer. *Arch Surg*. 2000;135:895-901.
235. Fialkowski E, Debenedetti M, Moley J. Long-term outcome of reoperations for medullary thyroid carcinoma. *World J Surg*. 2008;32: 754-765.
236. Barbet J, Campion L, Kraeber-Bodéré F, et al. Prognostic impact of serum calcitonin and carcinoembryonic antigen doubling-times in patients with medullary thyroid carcinoma. *J Clin Endocrinol Metab*. 2005;90:6077-6084.

237. Giraudet AL, Al Ghulzan A, Aupérin A, et al. Progression of medullary thyroid carcinoma: assessment with calcitonin and CEA doubling times. *Eur J Endocrinol*. 2008;158:239-246.
238. Kouvaraki MA, Lee JE, Shapiro SE, et al. Preventable reoperations for persistent and recurrent papillary thyroid carcinoma. *Surgery*. 2004;136:1183-1191.
239. Pacini F, Cetani F, Miccoli P, et al. Outcome of 309 patients with metastatic differentiated thyroid carcinoma treated with radioiodine. *World J Surg*. 1994;18:600-604.
240. Travagli JP, Cailleux AF, Ricard M, et al. Combination of radioiodine (^{131}I) and probe-guided surgery for persistent or recurrent thyroid carcinoma. *J Clin Endocrinol Metab*. 1998;83:2675-2680.
241. Dupuy DE, Monchik JM, Decrea C, et al. Radiofrequency ablation of regional recurrence from well-differentiated thyroid malignancy. *Surgery*. 2001;130:971-977.
242. Hay ID, Reading CC, Charboneau JW. Long-term efficacy of ultrasound-guided percutaneous ethanol ablation of recurrent neck nodal metastases in pTNM stage I papillary thyroid carcinoma. *Thyroid*. 2005;15:S2-S3.
243. Kim BM, Kim MJ, Kim EK, et al. Controlling recurrent papillary thyroid carcinoma in the neck by ultrasonographically-guided percutaneous ethanol injection. *Eur Radiol*. 2008;18:835-842.
244. Gaissert HA, Honings J, Grillo HC, et al. Segmental laryngotracheal and tracheal resection for invasive thyroid carcinoma. *Ann Thorac Surg*. 2007;83:1952-1959.
245. Ruegemer JJ, Hay ID, Bergstralh EJ, et al. Distant metastases in differentiated thyroid carcinoma: a multivariate analysis of prognostic variables. *J Clin Endocrinol Metab*. 1988;63:960-967.
246. Durante C, Haddy N, Baudin E, et al. Long term outcome of 444 patients with distant metastases from papillary and follicular thyroid carcinoma: benefits and limits of radioiodine therapy. *J Clin Endocrinol Metab*. 2006;92:450-455.
247. Casara D, Rubello D, Saladini G, et al. Different features of pulmonary metastases in differentiated thyroid cancer: natural history and multivariate statistical analysis of prognostic variables. *J Nucl Med*. 1993;34:1626-1631.
248. Bernier MO, Leenhardt L, Hoang C, et al. Survival and therapeutic modalities in patients with bone metastases of differentiated thyroid carcinomas. *J Clin Endocrinol Metab*. 2001;86:1568-1573.
249. Koong S, Reynolds J, Movius E, et al. Lithium as a potential adjuvant to 131I therapy of metastatic, well-differentiated thyroid carcinoma. *J Clin Endocrinol Metab*. 1999;84:912-916.
250. Potzi C, Moameni A, Karanikas G, et al. Comparison of iodine uptake in tumour and nontumour tissue under thyroid hormone deprivation and with recombinant human thyrotropin in thyroid cancer patients. *Clin Endocrinol (Oxf)*. 2006;65:519-523.
251. Shimaoka K, Schoenfeld DA, DeWys WD, et al. A randomized trial of doxorubicin versus doxorubicin plus cisplatin in patients with advanced thyroid carcinoma. *Cancer*. 1985;56:2155-2160.
252. Kebebew E, Peng M, Reiff E, et al. A phase II trial of rosiglitazone in patients with thyroglobulin-positive and radioiodine-negative differentiated thyroid cancer. *Surgery*. 2006;140:960-966; discussion 966-967.
253. Gruning T, Tiepolt C, Zophel K, et al. Retinoic acid for redifferentiation of thyroid cancer: does it hold its promise? *Eur J Endocrinol*. 2003;148:395-402.
254. Baudin E, Schlumberger M. New therapeutic approaches for metastatic thyroid carcinoma. *Lancet Oncol*. 2007;8:148-156.
255. Schlumberger M, Sherman SI. Clinical trials for progressive differentiated thyroid cancer: patient selection, study design, and recent advances. *Thyroid*. 2009;19:1393-1400.
256. Sherman SI, Wirth LJ, Droz JP, et al. Motesanib diphosphate in progressive, differentiated thyroid cancer. *N Engl J Med*. 2008;359:31-42.
257. Gupta-Abramson V, Troxel AB, Nellore A, et al. Phase II trial of sorafenib in advanced thyroid cancer. *J Clin Oncol*. 2008;26:4714-4719.
258. Kloos RT, Ringel MD, Knopp MV, et al. Phase II trial of sorafenib in metastatic thyroid cancer. *J Clin Oncol*. 2009;27:1675-1684.
259. Cohen EEW, Rosen LS, Vokes EE, et al. Axitinib is an active treatment for all histologic subtypes of advanced thyroid cancer: results from a phase II study. *J Clin Oncol*. 2008;26:4708-4713.
260. Kloos RT, Duvuuri V, Jhiang SM, et al. Nasolacrimal drainage system obstruction from radioactive iodine therapy for thyroid carcinoma. *J Clin Endocrinol Metab*. 2002;87:5817-5820.
261. Mandel SJ, Mandel L. Radioactive iodine and the salivary glands. *Thyroid*. 2003;13:265-271.
262. Pacini F, Gasperi M, Fugazzola L, et al. Testicular function in patients with differentiated thyroid carcinoma treated with radioiodine. *J Nucl Med*. 1994;35:1418-1422.
263. Garsi JP, Schlumberger M, Rubino C, et al. Therapeutic administration of ^{131}I for differentiated thyroid cancer, radiation dose to ovaries and outcome of pregnancies. *J Nucl Med*. 2008;49:845-852.
264. Alexander EK, Marqusee E, Lawrence J, et al. Timing and magnitude of increase in levothyroxine requirements during pregnancy in women with hypothyroidism. *N Engl J Med*. 2004;351:241-249.
265. Rubino C, De Vathaire F, Dottorini ME, et al. Second primary malignancies in thyroid cancer patients. *Br J Cancer*. 2003;89:1638-1644.
266. Nocera M, Baudin E, Pellegriti G, et al. Treatment of advanced medullary thyroid cancer with an alternating combination of doxorubicin-streptozocin and 5 FU-dacarbazine. Groupe d'Étude des Tumeurs a Calcitonine (GETC). *Br J Cancer*. 2000;83:715-718.
267. Fromigué J, De Baere T, Baudin E, et al. Chemoembolization for liver metastases from medullary thyroid carcinoma. *J Clin Endocrinol Metab*. 2006;91:2496-2499.
268. Schlumberger M, Carlomagno F, Baudin E, et al. New therapeutic approaches for medullary thyroid carcinoma. *Nat Clin Pract Endocrinol Metab*. 2008;4:22-32.
269. Wells S, Gosnell J, Gagel R, et al. Vandetanib for the treatment of patients with locally advanced or metastatic hereditary medullary thyroid cancer. *J Clin Oncol*. 2009;28:767-772.

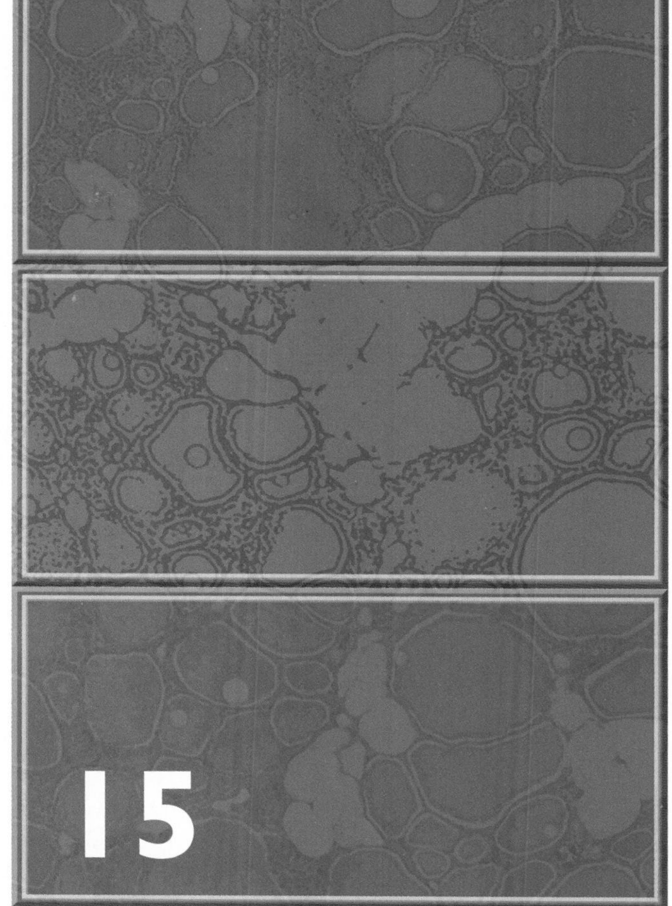

CHAPTER 15

The Adrenal Cortex

PAUL M. STEWART • NILS P. KRONE

THE ADRENAL CORTEX—HISTORICAL MILESTONES

The anatomy of the adrenal glands was described almost 450 years ago by Bartholomeo Eustacius,[1] and the zonation of the gland and its distinction from the medulla was elucidated shortly thereafter. However, a functional role for the adrenal glands was not accurately defined until the pioneering work of Thomas Addison, who described the clinical and autopsy findings in 11 cases of "Addison's disease" in his classic monograph in 1855.[2] Just a year later, Brown-Séquard demonstrated that the adrenal glands were "organs essential for life" by performing adrenalectomies in dogs, cats, and guinea pigs.[3] In 1896, William Osler first administered adrenal extract to a patient with Addison's disease, a feat that was repeated by others in animal and human studies over the next 40 years. Between 1937 and 1955, the adrenocorticosteroid hormones were isolated, and their structures were defined and synthesized.[4] Notable breakthroughs included the discovery of cortisone and clinical evaluation of its anti-inflammatory effect in patients with rheumatoid arthritis[5] and the isolation of aldosterone.[6]

The control of adrenocortical function by a pituitary factor was demonstrated in the 1920s, and this led to the isolation of sheep adrenocorticotropic hormone (ACTH) by Li, Evans, and Simpson in 1943.[7] Such a concept was supported through clinical studies, notably by Harvey Cushing in 1932, who associated his original clinical observations of 1912 (a "polyglandular syndrome" caused by pituitary basophilism) with adrenal hyperactivity.[8] The neural control of pituitary ACTH secretion by corticotropin-releasing factor (later renamed corticotropin-releasing hormone, or CRH) was defined by Harris and other workers in the 1940s, but CRH was not characterized and synthesized until 1981 in the laboratory of Wylie Vale.[9] Jerome Conn described primary aldosteronism in 1955,[10] and the control of adrenal aldosterone secretion by angiotensin II was confirmed shortly afterward. Advances in radioimmunoassay, and particularly molecular biology, have facilitated an exponential increase in the understanding of adrenal physiology and pathophysiology (Table 15-1).

ANATOMY AND DEVELOPMENT

The cells forming the adrenal cortex originate from the intermediate mesoderm. These cells derive from the urogenital ridge and have a common embryologic origin with the gonad and the kidney. Early differentiation of the adrenogonadal primordium from the urogenital ridge requires signaling cascades and transcription factors GLI3, SALL1, FOXD2, WT1, PBX1, WNT4, and the regulator of

TABLE 15-1

History of the Adrenal Cortex: Important Milestones

Year	Event
1563	Eustachius describes the adrenals (published by Lancisi in 1714).
1849	Thomas Addison, while searching for the cause of pernicious anemia, "stumbles" on a bronzed appearance associated with the adrenal glands—"melasma suprarenale."
1855	Thomas Addison describes the clinical features and autopsy findings in 11 cases of diseases of the suprarenal capsules, at least 6 of which were tuberculous in origin.
1856	In adrenalectomy experiments, Brown-Séquard demonstrates that the adrenal glands are essential for life.
1896	William Osler gives an oral glycerin extract derived from pig adrenals and demonstrates clinical benefit in patients with Addison's disease.
1905	Bulloch and Sequeria describe patients with congenital adrenal hyperplasia.
1929	Liquid extracts of cortical tissue are used to keep adrenalectomized cats alive indefinitely (Swingle and Pfiffner); subsequently, this extract was used successfully to treat a patient with Addison's disease (Rowntree and Greene).
1932	Harvey Cushing associates the "polyglandular syndrome" of pituitary basophilism, which he first described in 1912, with hyperactivity of the pituitary-adrenal glands.
1936	The concept of stress and its effect on pituitary-adrenal function are described by Seyle.
1937-1952	Isolation and structural characterization of adrenocortical hormones are reported by Kendall and Reichstein.
1943	Li and colleagues isolate pure adrenocorticotropic hormone from sheep pituitary.
1950	Hench, Kendall, and Reichstein share Nobel Prize in Medicine for describing the anti-inflammatory effects of cortisone in patients with rheumatoid arthritis.
1953	Isolation and analysis of the structure of aldosterone are reported by Simpson and Tait.
1956	Conn describes primary aldosteronism.
1981	Characterization and synthesis of corticotropin-releasing hormone are reported by Vale.
1980-present	The "molecular era": cloning and functional characterization of steroid receptors, steroidogenic enzymes, and adrenal transcription factors are reported, and the molecular basis for human adrenal diseases is defined.

telomerase activity, ACD (Fig. 15-1). The adrenogonadal primordium can be seen as the medial part of the urogenital ridge at 4 weeks. Separation of the adrenogonadal primordium and formation of the adrenal primordium seem to depend on the actions of transcription factors SF1, DAX1, WNT4, and CITED2. The adrenocortical primordium develops at approximately 8 weeks of gestation and can be differentiated into two distinct layers, the inner fetal zone (FZ) and the outer definitive zone (DZ). At approximately 9 weeks, the adrenal blastema encapsulates and the adrenal medulla develops when neural crest cells migrate into the adrenal gland.[11] During the second trimester, the FZ enlarges, becomes larger than the fetal kidney, and secretes abundant amounts of dehydroepiandrosterone (DHEA) and dehydroepiandrosterone sulfate (DHEAS). Concentrations of these hormones abruptly decline postnatally, in parallel with the postnatal involution of the FZ. The neocortex develops over the subsequent years into the adult adrenal gland.

In fetal life and up to 12 months of age, two distinct zones are evident, an inner, prominent FZ and an outer DZ that differentiates into the adult adrenal gland. After birth, the FZ regresses and the DZ, which contains an inner zona fasciculata (ZF) and an outer zona glomerulosa (ZG), proliferates.[12,13] The innermost zone, the zona reticularis (ZR), is evident after 2 years of life. The differentiation of the adrenal cortex into distinct zones has important functional consequences and is thought to depend on the temporal expression of transcription factors including Pref-1/ZOG, inner zone antigen, and steroidogenic factor 1 (SF1).[14,15] In preadrenachal children focal reticular zone islets can be found, but the ZG and ZF are clearly differentiated.[16] The occurrence of these ZR islets is consistent with the observation that DHEA and DHEAS concentrations gradually begin to rise from about 3 years of age.[17] At adrenache, the inner zone (ZR) thickens, corresponding with increased production of DHEA and DHEAS. Concurrently, changes in zone-specific enzyme expression patterns, such as decreased

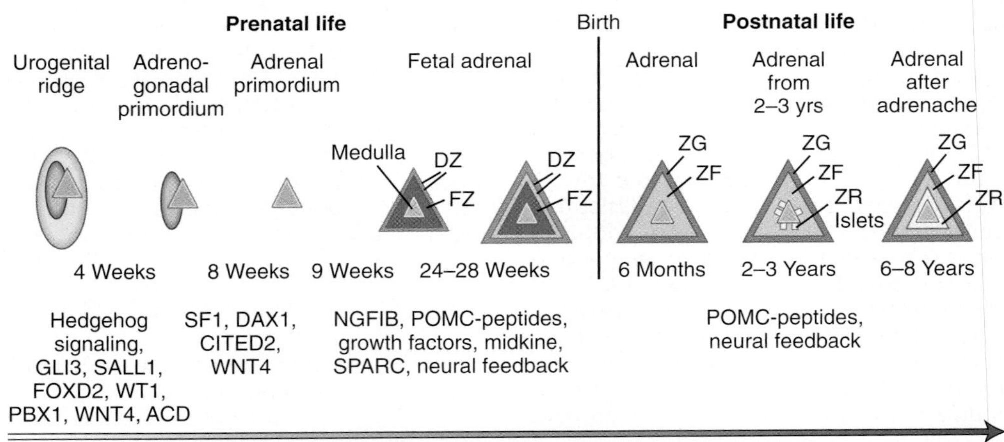

Figure 15-1 Schematic diagram of the development of the human adrenal cortex during prenatal and postnatal life. Transcription factors that are active at each stage (see text for details). DZ, definitive zone; FZ, fetal zone; POMC, pro-opiomelanocortin; SPARC, secreted protein, acidic, cysteine-rich (osteonectin); ZG, zona glomerulosa; ZF, zona fasciculata; ZR, zona reticularis.

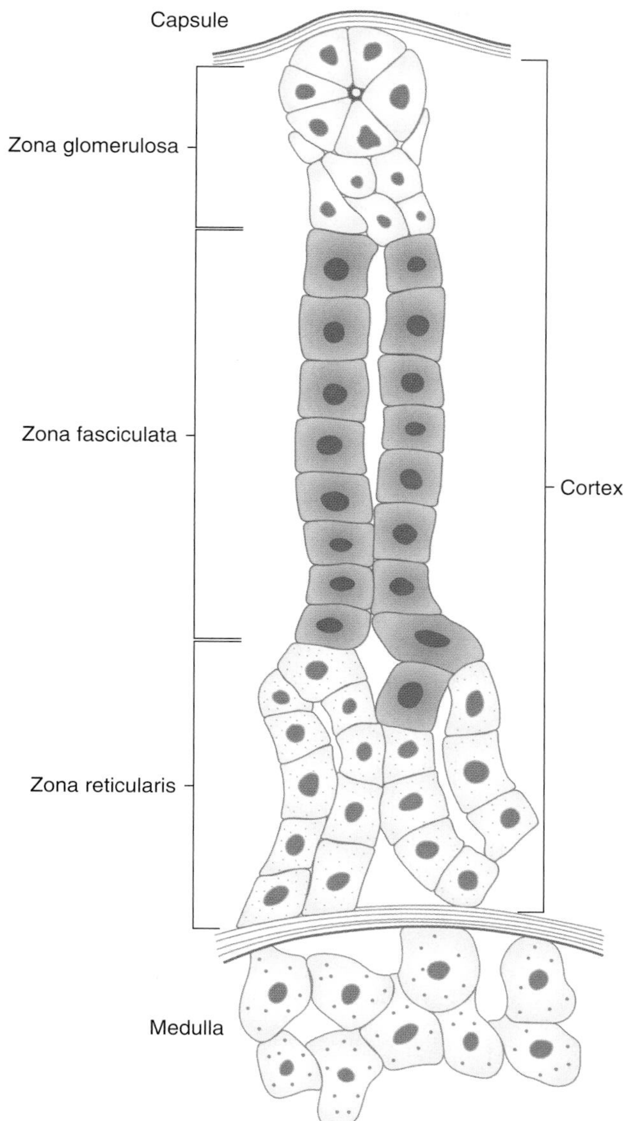

Figure 15-2 Schematic diagram of the structure of the human adrenal cortex, depicting the outer zona glomerulosa and inner zona fasciculata and zona reticularis.

3β-hydroxysteroid dehydrogenase type 2 (HSD3B2) and increased cytochrome b_5 and sulfotransferase (SULT2A1) in the ZR, lead to increased flux toward DHEA. Clinically, adrenarche becomes apparent at 6 to 8 years of age. Adrenal androgen production peaks in the third decade and then declines at a variable rate. Mineralocorticoids and glucocorticoids show a less age-specific variation.

The adult gland is a pyramidal structure, approximately 4 g in weight, 2 cm wide, 5 cm long, and 1 cm thick, that lies immediately above the kidney on its posteromedial surface. Beneath the capsule, the ZG comprises approximately 15% of the cortex (depending on sodium intake) (Fig. 15-2). Cells are clustered in spherical nests and are small, with smaller nuclei in comparison with cells in other zones. The ZF comprises 75% of the cortex; cells are large and lipid-laden and form radial cords within the fibrovascular radial network. The innermost ZR is sharply demarcated from both the ZF and the adrenal medulla. Cells there are irregular with little lipid content. The maintenance of normal adrenal size appears to involve a progenitor cell population lying between the ZG and ZF; cell migration and differentiation occur within the fasciculata and senescence occurs within the ZR, but the factors regulating this important aspect of adrenal regeneration are unknown. ACTH administration results in glomerulosa cells' adopting a fasciculata phenotype, and, in turn, the innermost fasciculata cells adopt a reticularis phenotype that is reversible on withdrawal of ACTH.

The vasculature of the adrenal cortex is complex. Arterial supply is conveyed by up to 12 small arteries from the aorta and the inferior phrenic, renal, and intercostal arteries. These branch to form a subcapsular arteriolar plexus from which radial capillaries penetrate deeper into the cortex. In the ZR, a dense sinusoidal plexus is created, which empties into a central vein. The right adrenal vein is short, draining directly into the inferior vena cava, whereas the longer left adrenal vein usually drains into the left renal vein.

ADRENAL STEROIDS AND STEROIDOGENESIS

Three main types of hormone are produced by the adrenal cortex—glucocorticoids (cortisol, corticosterone), mineralocorticoids (aldosterone, deoxycorticosterone), and sex steroids (mainly androgens). All steroid hormones are derived from the cyclopentanoperhydrophenanthrene structure, that is, three cyclohexane rings and a single cyclopentane ring (Fig. 15-3). Steroid nomenclature is defined in two ways: by trivial names (e.g., cortisol, aldosterone) or by the chemical structure as defined by the International Union of Pure and Applied Chemistry (IUPAC).[18] The IUPAC classification is inappropriate for clinical use but does provide an invaluable insight into steroid structure. The basic structure, trivial name, and IUPAC name of some common steroids are given in Figure 15-3 and Table 15-2. Estrogens have 18 carbon atoms (C18

TABLE 15-2

IUPAC and Trivial Names of Natural and Synthetic Steroids

Trivial Name	IUPAC Name
Aldosterone	4-Pregnen-11β,21-diol-3,18,20-trione
Androstenedione	4-Androsten-3,17-dione
Cortisol	4-Pregnen-11β,17α,21-triol-3,20-dione
Cortisone	4-Pregnen-17α,21-diol-3,11,20-trione
Dehydroepiandrosterone	5-Androsten-3β-ol-17-one
Deoxycorticosterone	4-Pregnen-21-ol-3,20-dione
Dexamethasone	1,4-Pregnadien-9α-fluoro-16α-methyl-11β,17α,21-triol-3,20-dione
Dihydrotestosterone	5α-Androstan-17β-ol-3-one
Estradiol	1,3,5(10)-Estratrien-3,17β-diol
Fludrocortisone	4-Pregnen-9α-fluoro-11β,17α,21-triol-3,20-dione
17-Hydroxyprogesterone	4-Pregnen-17α-ol-3,20-dione
Methylprednisolone	1,4-Pregnadien-6α-methyl-11β,17α,21-triol-3,20-dione
Prednisolone	1,4-Pregnadien-11β,17α,21-triol-3,20-dione
Prednisone	1,4-Pregnadien-17α,21-diol-3,11,20-trione
Pregnenolone	5-Pregnen-3β-ol-20-one
Progesterone	4-Pregnen-3,20-dione
Testosterone	4-Androsten-17β-ol-3-one
Triamcinolone	1,4-Pregnadien-9α-fluoro-11β,16α,17α,21-tetrol-3,20-dione

IUPAC, International Union of Pure and Applied Chemistry.

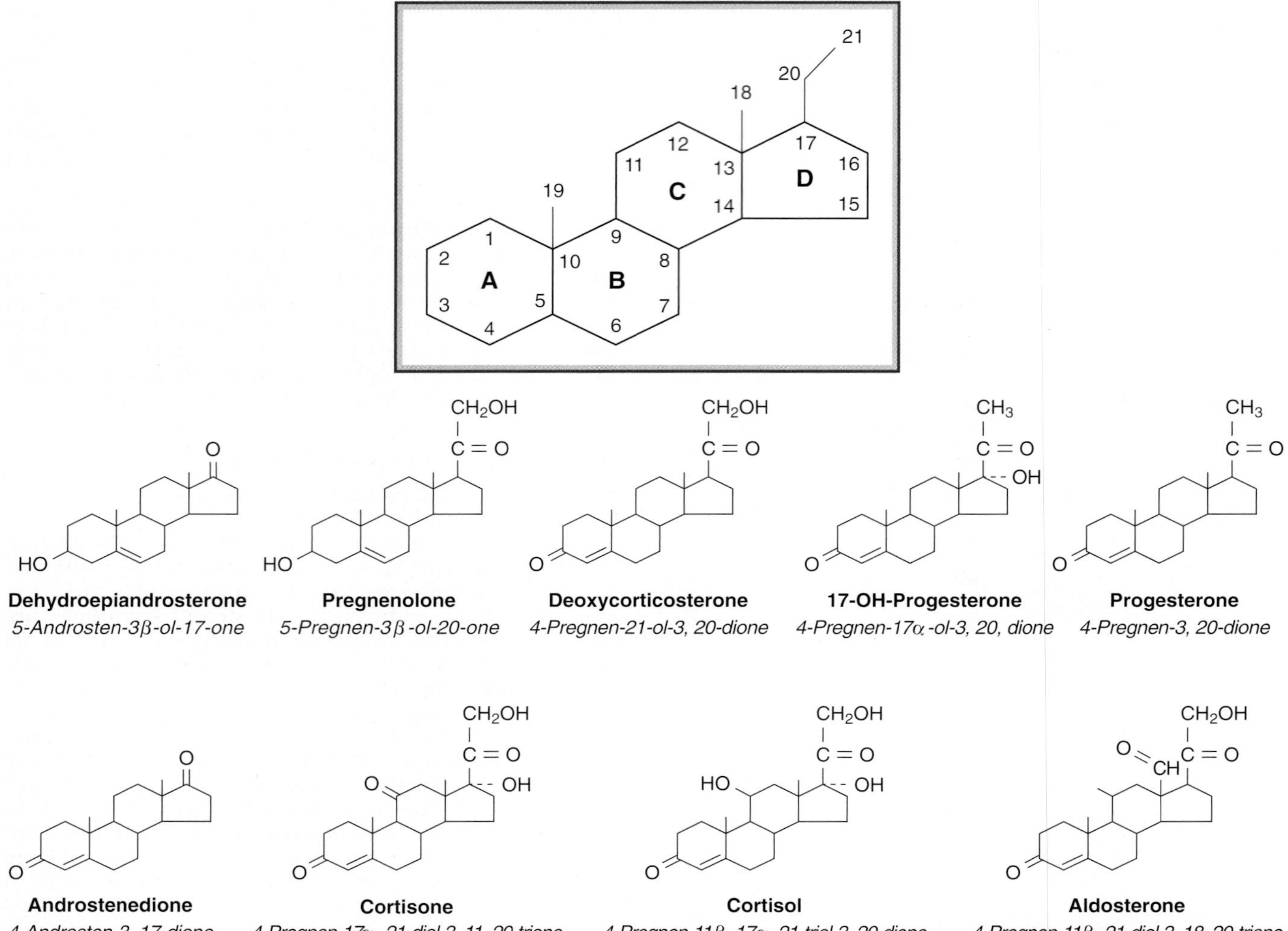

Figure 15-3 The cyclopentanoperhydrophenanthrene structure of corticosteroid hormones, highlighting the structure of some endogenous steroid hormones together with their nomenclature.

steroids) and androgens have 19 carbon atoms (C19), whereas glucocorticoids and progestogens are C21-steroid derivatives.

Cholesterol is the precursor for adrenal steroidogenesis. It is provided principally from the circulation, in the form of low-density lipoprotein (LDL) cholesterol.[19] Uptake is by specific cell-surface LDL receptors present on adrenal tissue[20]; LDL is then internalized via receptor-mediated endocytosis,[21] the resulting vesicles fuse with lysozymes, and free cholesterol is produced after hydrolysis. However, it is clear that this cannot be the sole source of adrenal cholesterol, because patients with abetalipoproteinemia who have undetectable circulating LDL and patients with defective LDL receptors in the setting of familial hypercholesterolemia still have normal basal adrenal steroidogenesis. Cholesterol can be generated de novo within the adrenal cortex from acetyl coenzyme A (CoA). In addition, there is evidence that the adrenal can utilize high-density lipoprotein (HDL) cholesterol after uptake through the putative HDL receptor, SR-B1.[22]

The biochemical pathways involved in adrenal steroidogenesis are shown in Figure 15-4. The initial hormone-dependent, rate-limiting step is the transport of intracellular cholesterol from the outer to inner mitochondrial membrane for conversion to pregnenolone by cytochrome P450 side-chain cleavage enzyme (P450scc). Naturally occurring human mutations have confirmed the importance of a 30-kd protein, steroidogenic acute regulatory protein (StAR), in mediating this effect. StAR is induced by an increase in intracellular cyclic adenosine monophosphate (cAMP) after binding of ACTH to its cognate receptor, providing the first important rate-limiting step in adrenal steroidogenesis.[23] Other transporters, including the peripheral benzodiazepine-like receptor, may be involved.[24]

Steroidogenesis involves the concerted action of several enzymes, including a series of cytochrome P450 enzymes, all of which have been cloned and characterized (Table 15-3). Cytochrome P450 enzymes are classified into two types according to their subcellular localization and their specific electron shuttle system. Mitochondrial (type I) cytochrome P450 enzymes such as CYP11A1 (P450scc), 11β-hydroxylase (CYP11B1, or P450c11b1), and aldosterone synthase (CYP11B2, or P450aldo) rely on electron-transfer facilitated by adrenodoxin and adrenodoxin reductase.[25,26] Micrososomal (type II) cytochrome P450 enzymes localized to the endoplasmic reticulum include the steroidogenic enzymes 17α-hydroxylase (CYP17A1, or P450c17), 21-hydroxylase (CYP21A2, or P450c21), and P450 aromatase (CYP19A1, or P450aro). The functions of

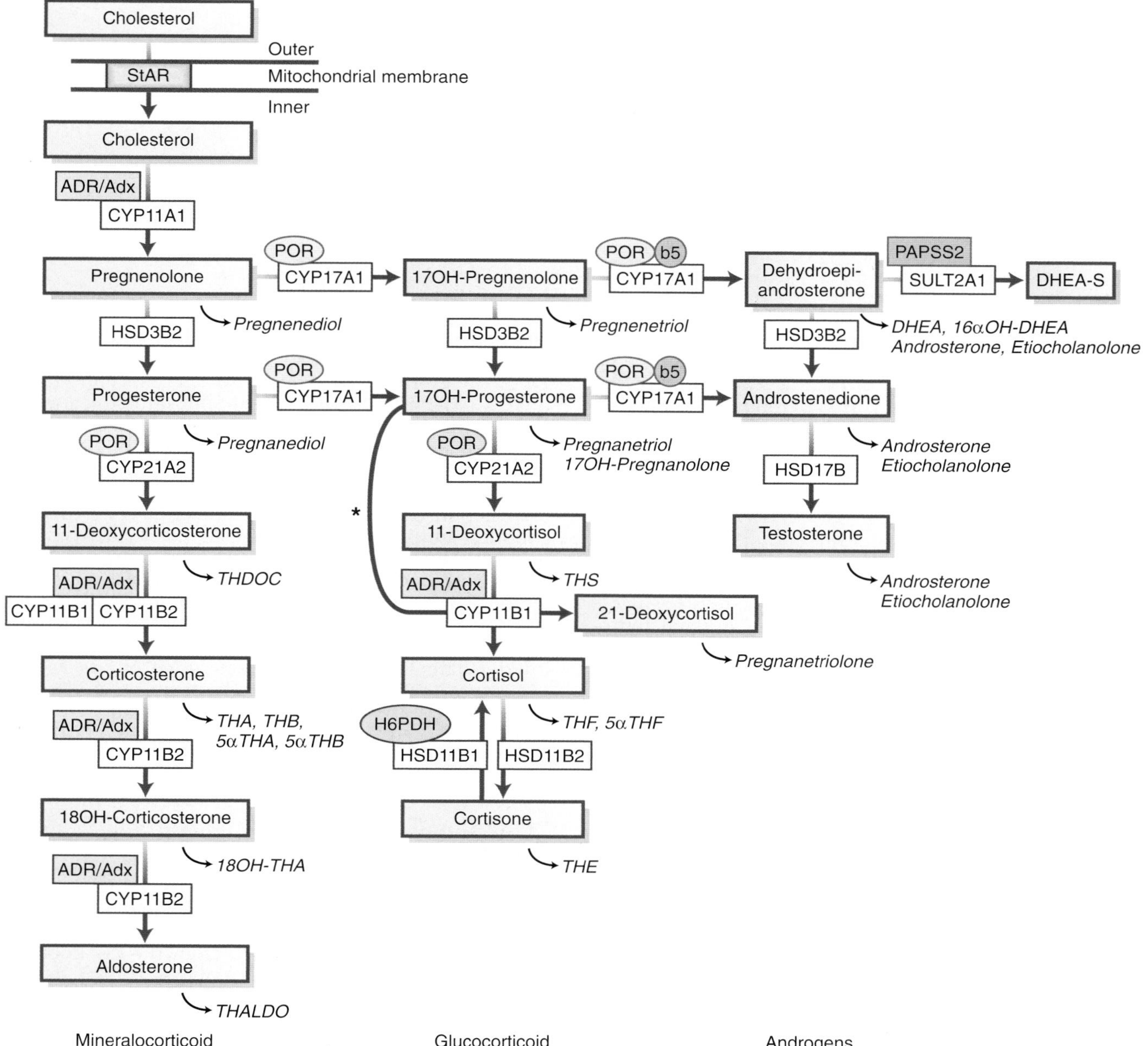

Figure 15-4 Adrenal steroidogenesis. After the steroidogenic acute regulatory (StAR) protein-mediated uptake of cholesterol into mitochondria within adrenocortical cells, aldosterone, cortisol, and adrenal androgens are synthesized through the coordinated action of a series of steroidogenic enzymes in a zone-specific fashion. The mitochondrial cytochrome P450 (CYP) type I enzymes (CYP11A1, CYP11B1, CYP11B2) requiring electron transfer via adrenodoxin reductase (ADR) and adrenodoxin (Adx) are marked with a box labeled *ADR/Adx*. The microsomal CYP type II enzymes (CYP17A1, CYP21A2) receive electrons from P450 oxidoreductase (circle labeled *POR*). The 17,20-lyase reaction catalyzed by CYP17A1 requires, in addition to POR, cytochrome b_5, indicated by a circle labeled b_5. Urinary steroid hormone metabolites are given in italics below the plasma hormones. The asterisk (*) indicates 11-hydroxylation of 17OH-progesterone to 21-deoxycortisol in cases of 21-hydroxylase deficiency. The adrenal conversion of androstenedione to testosterone is catalyzed by the aldo-keto reductase AKR1C3 (HSD17B5). CYP11A1, P450 side-chain cleavage enzyme; CYP11B1, 11β-hydroxylase; CYP11B2, aldosterone synthase; CYP17A1, 17α-hydroxylase; CYP21A2, 21-hydroxylase; DHEA, dehydroepiandrosterone; DHEA-S, dehydroepiandrosterone sulphate; H6PDH, hexose-6-phosphate dehydrogenase; HSD11B1, 11β-hydroxysteroid dehydrogenase 1; HSD11B2, 11β-hydroxysteroid dehydrogenase 2; HSD17B, 17β-hydroxysteroid dehydrogenase; HSD3B2, 3β-hydroxysteroid dehydrogenase type 2; 17OH-progesterone, 17α-hydroxyprogesterone; PAPSS2, 3′-phosphoadenosine 5′-phosphosulfate synthase 2; SULT2A1, sulfotransferase 2A1; THA, tetrahydro-11-dehydrocorticosterone; THB, tetrahydro-corticosterone; THALDO, tetrahydro-aldosterone; THDOC, tetrahydro-11-deoxycorticosterone; THF, tetrahydro-cortisol; THS, tetrahydro-11-deoxycortisol.

cytochrome P450 type II enzymes crucially depend on P450 oxidoreductase (POR), which provides electrons required for monooxygenase reaction catalyzed by the P450 enzyme.[26,27] This category also includes hepatic P450 enzymes involved in drug metabolism and enzymes involved in sterol and bile acid synthesis.[26,27] In addition, the 17,20-lyase activity of P450 CYP17A1 is dependent on a flavoprotein cytochrome b_5, which functions as an allosteric facilitator of CYP17A1, and POR interaction (Fig. 15-5; see Fig. 15-4).[28]

Mutations in the genes encoding these enzymes result in human disease, so some understanding of the underlying

TABLE 15-3

Nomenclature for Adrenal Steroidogenic Enzymes and Their Genes

Enzyme Name	Enzyme Family	Gene	Chromosome
P450 Cholesterol side-chain cleavage (SCC) (desmolase)	Cytochrome P450 type I	*CYP11A1*	15q23-q24
3β-Hydroxysteroid dehydrogenase (3β-HSD) (type II isozyme)	Short-chain alcohol dehydrogenase reductase superfamily	*HSD3B2*	1p13.1
17α-Hydroxylase/17,20 lyase	Cytochrome P450 type II	*CYP17A1*	10q24.3
21-Hydroxylase	Cytochrome P450 type II	*CYP21A2*	6p21.3
11β-Hydroxylase	Cytochrome P450 type I	*CYP11B1*	8q24.3
Aldosterone synthase	Cytochrome P450 type I	*CYP11B2*	8q24.3

pathways and steroid precursors is required.[29] After uptake of cholesterol to the mitochondrion, cholesterol is cleaved by the P450scc enzyme to form pregnenolone.[30] In the cytoplasm, pregnenolone is converted to progesterone by the type II isozyme 3β-HSD through a reaction involving dehydrogenation of the 3-hydroxyl group and isomerization of the double bond at C5.[31] Progesterone is hydroxylated to 17-hydroxyprogesterone (17-OHP) through the 17α-hydroxylase activity of CYP17A1. 17α-Hydroxylation is an essential prerequisite for glucocorticoid synthesis, and the ZG does not express 17α-hydroxylase. CYP17A1 also possesses 17,20-lyase activity, which results in production of the C19 adrenal androgens, dehydroepiandrosterone and androstenedione.[32] In humans, however, 17-OHP is not an efficient substrate for CYP17A1, and there is negligible conversion of 17-OHP to androstenedione. Adrenal androstenedione secretion is dependent on the conversion of dehydroepiandrosterone to androstenedione by 3β-HSD. This enzyme also converts 17-hydroxypregnenolone to 17-OHP, but the preferred substrate is pregnenolone. The human adrenal gland is capable of synthesis of small but significant amounts of testosterone, which increases in clinical conditions associated with androgen excess. This conversion is facilitated by the enzyme 17β-HSD type 5 (HSD17B5), also called aldoketoreductase 1C3 (AKR1C3).[33] 21-Hydroxylation of either progesterone (in the ZG) or 17-OHP (in the ZF) is carried out by the product of the *CYP21A2* gene, 21-hydroxylase, to yield deoxycorticosterone (DOC) or 11-deoxycortisol, respectively.[34] The final step in cortisol biosynthesis takes place in the mitochondria and involves the conversion of 11-deoxycortisol to cortisol by the enzyme CYP11B1 (11β-hydroxylase).[35] In the ZG, 11β-hydroxylase may also convert DOC to corticosterone. The enzyme CYP11B2 (aldosterone synthase) may also carry out this reaction, and in addition, it is required for conversion of corticosterone to aldosterone via the intermediate 18-OH corticosterone; CYP11B1 lacks these two enzymatic activities.[36,37] Therefore, CYP11B2 can carry out 11β-hydroxylation, 18-hydroxylation, and 18-methyloxidation to yield the characteristic C11-18 hemiacetyl structure of aldosterone.

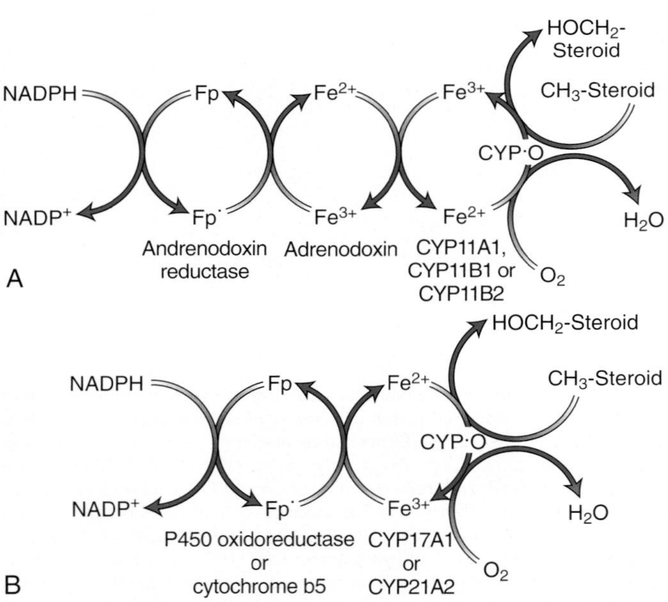

Figure 15-5 A, Electron shuttle system for the mitochondrial enzymes, CYP11A1, CYP11B1, and CYP11B2. Adrenodoxin reductase receives electrons from reduced nicotinamide adenine dinucleotide phosphate (NADPH) and reduces adrenodoxin, which transfers reducing equivalents to the cytochrome P450 (CYP) enzyme. The enzyme then transfers electrons, by way of oxygen, to the steroid. Fp, Flavoprotein; Fp′, reduced form of flavoprotein; $NADP^+$, nicotinamide adenine dinucleotide phosphate. **B,** Electron shuttle system for the microsomal enzymes, CYP17A1 and CYP21A2. P450 oxidoreductase, a flavoprotein, accepts electrons from NADPH and transfers them to the NADPH-P450 enzyme. The enzyme then transfers electrons, by way of oxygen, to the steroid. A second reducing equivalent may be supplied to CYP17A1 by NADPH-P450 oxidoreductase or cytochrome b_5.

Regulation of Adrenal Steroidogenesis: "Functional Zonation" of the Adrenal Cortex

Glucocorticoids are secreted in relatively high amounts (cortisol, 10 to 20 mg/day) from the ZF under the control of ACTH; mineralocorticoids are secreted in low amounts (aldosterone, 100 to 150 μg/day) from the ZG under the principal control of angiotensin II. As a class, adrenal androgens (DHEA, DHEAS, androstenedione) are the most abundant steroids secreted from the adult adrenal gland (>20 mg/day). In each case, secretion is facilitated through the expression of steroidogenic enzymes in a specific "zonal" manner. The ZG cannot synthesize cortisol because it does not express 17α-hydroxylase. In contrast, aldosterone secretion is confined to the outer ZG because of the restricted expression of CYP11B2. Although CYP11B1 and CYP11B2 share 95% homology, the 5′ promoter sequences differ, permitting regulation of the final steps in glucocorticoid and mineralocorticoid biosynthesis by ACTH and angiotensin II, respectively. In the ZR, high levels of cytochrome b_5 confer 17,20-lyase activity on CYP17A1 and androgen production. DHEA is sulfated in the ZR by the DHEA sulfotransferase (SULT2A1) to form DHEAS. This sulfonation reaction facilitated by SULT2A1 relies on the donor 3′-phosphoadenosine 5′-phosphosulfate (PAPS) to transfer a sulfonate group to an acceptor molecule. PAPS is synthesized by PAPS synthase, of which two isoenzymes exist (PAPSS1 and PAPSS2).[38]

In the fetal adrenal, steroidogenesis occurs primarily within the inner FZ. The FZ is a characteristic feature of higher primates, but the biologic role of fetal androgen production remains unclear. Because of a relative lack of 3β-HSD and high SULT2A1 activity, the principal steroidogenic products are DHEA and DHEAS, which are then aromatized by placental trophoblast to estrogens. Therefore, the majority of maternal estrogen across pregnancy is, indirectly, fetally derived.[39]

Classic endocrine feedback loops are in place to control the secretion of both hormones. Cortisol inhibits the secretion of CRH from the hypothalamus and ACTH from the pituitary, and aldosterone-induced sodium retention inhibits renal renin secretion.

Glucocorticoid Secretion: The Hypothalamus-Pituitary-Adrenal Axis

Pro-opiomelanocortin and ACTH

ACTH is the principal hormone stimulating adrenal glucocorticoid biosynthesis and secretion. ACTH has 39 amino acids but is synthesized within the anterior pituitary as part of a much larger, 241-amino-acid precursor called pro-opiomelanocortin (POMC). A transcription factor, TPIT, appears to be essential for differentiation of POMC-expressing cells within the anterior pituitary.[40] POMC is cleaved in a tissue-specific fashion to yield smaller peptide hormones. In the anterior pituitary, this results in the secretion of β-lipoprotein (β-LPH) and pro-ACTH, the latter being further cleaved to an amino-terminal peptide, joining peptide, and ACTH itself (Fig. 15-6).[41,42] Postsecretion cleavage of the precursor to γ-melanocyte stimulating hormone (pro-γ-MSH) by a serine protease (AsP) expressed in the outer adrenal cortex is thought to mediate the trophic action of "ACTH" on the adrenal cortex.[43] The first 24 amino acids of ACTH are common to all species, and a synthetic ACTH(1-24), Synacthen, is available commercially for clinical testing of the hypothalamic-pituitary-adrenal (HPA) axis and assessing adrenal glucocorticoid reserve. The hormones α-, β-, and γ-MSH are also cleaved products from POMC, but the increased pigmentation characteristic of Addison's disease is thought to arise directly from increased ACTH concentrations binding to the melanocortin-1 receptor (MC1R) rather than from α-MSH secretion.[44]

POMC is also transcribed in many extrapituitary tissues, notably brain, liver, kidney, gonad, and placenta.[41,45,46] In these normal tissues, POMC messenger RNA (mRNA) is usually shorter than the pituitary 1200-base-pair species due to lack of exons 1 and 2 and the 5′ region of exon 3.[47] As a result, it is probable that this POMC-like peptide is neither secreted nor active. However, in ectopic ACTH syndrome, additional POMC mRNA species are described that are longer than the normal pituitary POMC species (typically 1450 base pairs) due to the use of alternative promoters in the 5′ region of the gene.[48,49] This may in part explain the resistance of POMC secretion to glucocorticoid feedback in these tumors. Others factors, including interaction with tissue-specific transcription factors[50] and POMC methylation,[51] may explain the ectopic expression of ACTH in some malignant tissues. The cleavage of POMC is also tissue specific,[52] and it is possible, at least in some cases of ectopic ACTH syndrome, that circulating ACTH precursors (notably pro-ACTH) may cross-react in current ACTH radioimmunoassays.[53,54] The biologic activity of POMC itself on adrenal function is thought to be negligible.

POMC expression and processing within neurons in the hypothalamus, specifically the generation of α-MSH that interacts with melanocortin-4 receptors (MC4R), appears to be of crucial importance in appetite control and energy homeostasis (see later discussion).[55]

Corticotropin-Releasing Hormone and Arginine Vasopressin

POMC secretion is tightly controlled by numerous factors, notably CRH and arginine vasopressin (AVP) (Fig. 15-7).[56,57] Additional control is provided through an endogenous circadian rhythm and by stress and feedback inhibition by

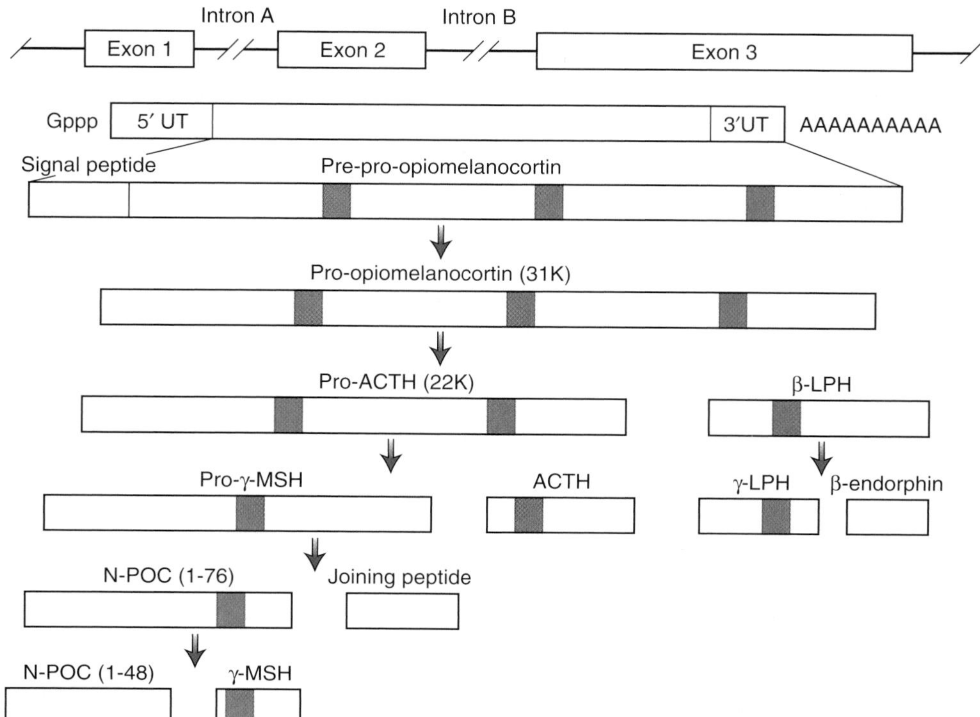

Figure 15-6 Synthesis and cleavage of pro-opiomelanocortin (POMC) within the human anterior pituitary gland. Prohormone convertase enzymes sequentially cleave POMC to adrenocorticotropic hormone (ACTH). *Shaded areas* represent melanocyte-stimulating hormone (MSH) structural units. β-LPH, β-lipoprotein; γ-LPH, γ-lipoprotein; N-POC, amino-terminal pro-opiomelanocortin.

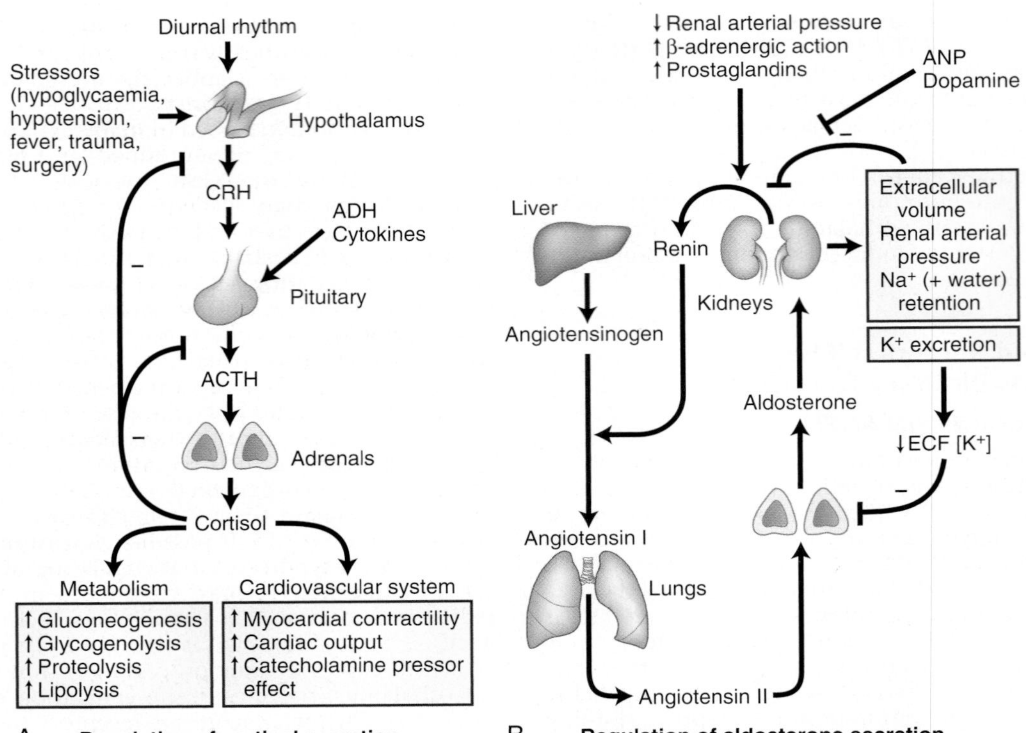

Figure 15-7 Normal negative feedback regulation of cortisol and aldosterone secretion. **A,** Hypothalamic-pituitary-adrenal axis. Adrenocorticotropic hormone (ACTH) is secreted from the anterior pituitary under the influence of two principal secretagogues, corticotropin-releasing hormone (CRH) and arginine vasopressin; other factors, including cytokines, also play a role. CRH secretion is regulated by an inbuilt circadian rhythm and by additional stressors operating through the hypothalamus. Secretion of CRH and ACTH is inhibited by cortisol, highlighting the importance of negative feedback control. **B,** Renin-angiotensin-aldosterone system (RAAS). Renin is secreted from the juxtaglomerular cells in the kidney dependent on renal arterial blood pressure. Renin converts angiotensinogen to angiotensin I, which is converted in the lungs by angiotensin converting enzyme (ACE) into angiotensin II. Angiotensin stimulates adrenal aldosterone synthesis. Extracellular fraction (ECF) of potassium has an important direct inhibitory influence on aldosterone secretion. ACE, Angiotensin converting enzyme; ACTH, adrenocorticotropic hormone; ADH, antidiuretic hormone; ANP, atrial natriuretic peptide; CRH, corticotropin-releasing hormone.

cortisol itself. CRH is a 41-amino-acid peptide that is synthesized in neurons within the paraventricular nucleus of the hypothalamus.[9,58,59] Human and rat CRH are identical, but ovine CRH differs by 7 amino acids[60,61]; ovine CRH is slightly more potent than human CRH in stimulating ACTH secretion but has a longer half-life and is therefore used diagnostically.

CRH is secreted into the hypophyseal portal blood, where it binds to specific type I CRH receptors on anterior pituitary corticotrophs[62] to stimulate POMC gene transcription through a process that includes activation of adenylate cyclase. It is unclear whether hypothalamic CRH contributes in any way to circulating levels; CRH is also synthesized in other tissues, and it is likely that circulating CRH reflects synthesis from testis, gastrointestinal tract, adrenal medulla, and particularly the placenta,[63] where the increased secretion across pregnancy results in a threefold increase in circulating CRH levels.[64] In the circulation, CRH is bound to CRH-binding protein (CRH-BP); levels of CRH-BP also increase during pregnancy so that cortisol secretion is not markedly elevated.[65]

CRH is the principal stimulus for ACTH secretion,[66] but AVP is able to potentiate CRH-mediated secretion.[67] In this case, AVP acts through the V1B receptor to activate protein kinase C. The peak response of ACTH to CRH does not differ across the day, but it is affected by endogenous function of the HPA axis in that responsiveness is reduced in subjects treated with corticosteroids but increased in subjects with Cushing's disease. Other reported ACTH secretagogues, including angiotensin II, cholecystokinin, atrial natriuretic factor, and vasoactive peptides, probably act to modulate the CRH control of ACTH secretion.[68]

The Stress Response and Immune-Endocrine Axis. The proinflammatory cytokines, notably interleukin 1 (IL-1), IL-6, and tumor necrosis factor-α also increase ACTH secretion, either directly or by augmenting the effect of CRH.[69,70] Leukemia inhibitory factor (LIF), a cytokine of the IL-6 family, is a further activator of the HPA axis.[71] This explains the response of the HPA axis to an inflammatory stimulus and is an important immune-endocrine interaction (see Chapter 7). Physical stresses increase ACTH and cortisol secretion, again through central actions mediated via CRH and AVP. Cortisol secretion rises in response to fever, surgery,[72] burn injury,[73] hypoglycemia,[74] hypotension, and exercise.[75] In all of these cases, this increased secretion can be viewed as a normal counterregulatory response to the insult. Acute psychological stress raises cortisol levels,[76] but secretion rates appear to be normal in patients with chronic anxiety states and underlying psychotic illness. However, depression is associated with high circulating cortisol concentrations, and this is an important consideration in the differential diagnosis of Cushing's syndrome (see later discussion).

Circadian Rhythm. ACTH is secreted in a pulsatile fashion with a circadian rhythm; levels are highest on wakening and decline throughout the day, reaching nadir values in the evening (Fig. 15-8).[77] The average ACTH pulse frequency is higher in normal adult men compared with women (18 versus 10 pulses/24 hours, respectively). The circadian ACTH rhythm appears to be mediated

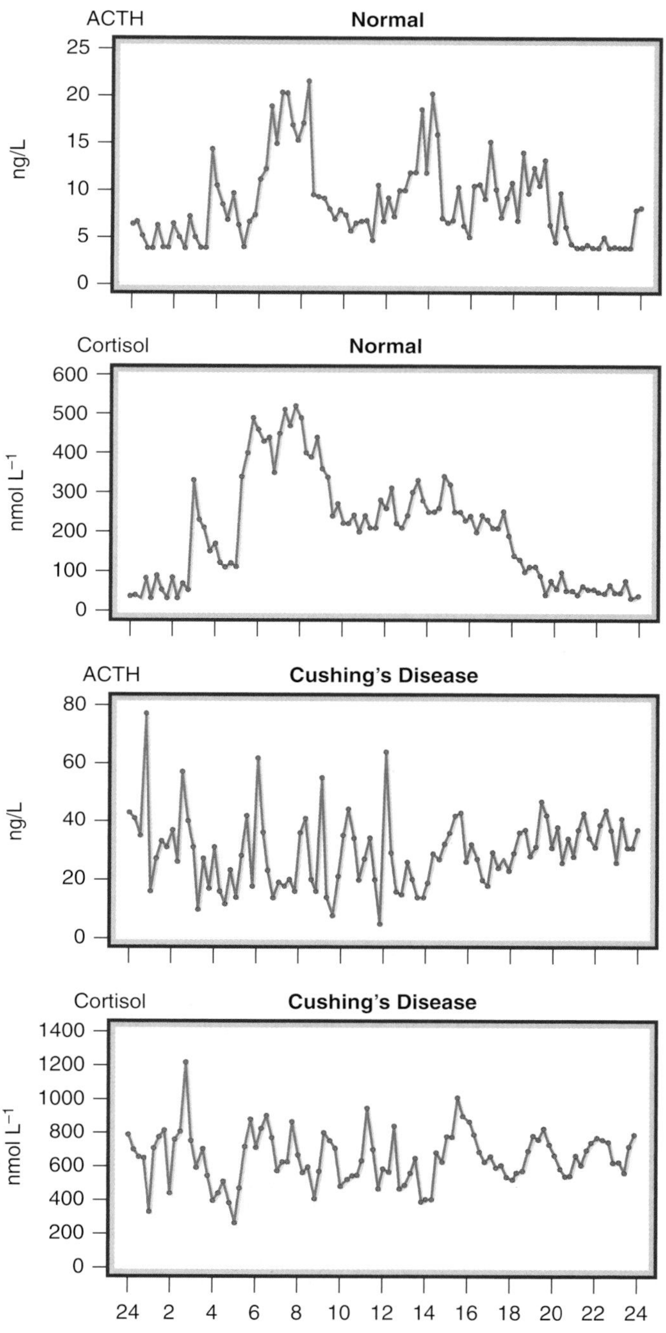

Figure 15-8 Circadian and pulsatile secretion of adrenocorticotropic hormone (ACTH) and cortisol in a normal subject *(top two panels)* and in a patient with Cushing's disease. In a normal subject, secretion of ACTH and cortisol is highest in early morning and falls to a nadir at midnight. ACTH pulse frequency and pulse amplitude are increased in Cushing's disease, and circadian rhythmic secretion is lost.

principally by an increased ACTH pulse amplitude occurring between 5 and 9 a.m. but also by a reduction in ACTH pulse frequency occurring between 6 p.m. and midnight.[78,79] Food ingestion is a further stimulus to ACTH secretion.

Circadian rhythm is dependent on both day-night[80] and sleep-wake[81] patterns and is disrupted by alternating day-night shift work and by long-distance travel across time zones.[82] It can take up to 2 weeks for the circadian rhythm to reset to an altered day-night cycle.

Negative Feedback. An important aspect of CRH and ACTH secretion is the negative feedback control exerted by glucocorticoids themselves. Glucocorticoids inhibit POMC gene transcription in the anterior pituitary[56] and CRH and AVP mRNA synthesis and secretion in the hypothalamus.[83,84] Annexin 1 (previously called lipocortin 1) may also play a critical role in effecting the negative feedback of glucocorticoids on ACTH and CRH release.[85] The negative feedback effect depends on the dose, potency, half-life, and duration of administration of the glucocorticoid and has important physiologic and diagnostic consequences. Suppression of the HPA axis by pharmacologic corticosteroids may persist for many months after cessation of therapy, and adrenocortical insufficiency should be anticipated. Diagnostically, the feedback mechanism explains ACTH hypersecretion in Addison's disease, as well as undetectable ACTH levels in patients with a cortisol-secreting adrenal adenoma. Feedback inhibition is principally mediated via the glucocorticoid receptor (GR); patients with glucocorticoid resistance resulting from mutations in the GR[86] and mice lacking the GR gene[87] have ACTH and cortisol hypersecretion due to perceived lack of negative feedback.

The ACTH Receptor and ACTH Effects on the Adrenal

ACTH binds to a G protein–coupled, melanocortin-2 receptor (MC2R),[88] of which there are approximately 3500 on each adrenocortical cell. Melanocortin-2 receptor accessory protein (MRAP) is required for correct localization and signaling of MC2R.[89] Current data suggest that MRAP might promote three different activities: as a chaperone assisting correct folding of MC2R in the endoplasmic reticulum, as an accessory protein essential for trafficking of MC2R to the plasma membrane, and as a coreceptor enabling MC2R to bind or to signal ACTH response.[90] Downstream signal transduction is mediated principally through the stimulation of adenylate cyclase and intracellular cAMP,[91] although both extracellular and intracellular Ca^{2+} play a role.[92] Other factors synergize with or inhibit the effects of ACTH on the adrenal cortex, including angiotensin II, activin, inhibin, and cytokines (tumor necrosis factor-α and leptin).[93] Cell-to-cell communication via gap junctions is also important in mediating the effects of ACTH.[94]

ACTH produces both immediate and chronic effects on the adrenal gland; the end result is the stimulation of adrenal steroidogenesis and growth. Acutely, steroidogenesis is stimulated through a StAR-mediated increase in cholesterol delivery to the CYP11A1 enzyme in the inner mitochondrial membrane.[23] Chronically (within 24 to 26 hours of exposure), ACTH acts to increase the synthesis of all steroidogenic CYP enzymes (CYP11A1, CYP17A1, CYP21A2, CYP11B1) in addition to adrenodoxin,[95,96] the effects of which are mediated at the transcriptional level. ACTH increases synthesis of the LDL and HDL receptors and possibly also synthesis of 3-hydroxy-3-methylglutaryl (HMG)-CoA reductase, the rate-limiting step in cholesterol biosynthesis. ACTH increases adrenal weight by inducing both hyperplasia and hypertrophy. Adrenal atrophy is a feature of ACTH deficiency.

Mineralocorticoid Secretion: The Renin-Angiotensin-Aldosterone Axis

Aldosterone is secreted from the ZG under the control of three principal secretagogues: angiotensin II, potassium, and, to a lesser extent, ACTH (Fig. 15-7). Other factors, notably somatostatin, heparin, atrial natriuretic factor, and dopamine, can directly inhibit aldosterone synthesis. The secretion of aldosterone and its intermediary 18-hydroxylated metabolites is restricted to the ZG because of the zone-specific expression of CYP11B2 (aldosterone synthase).[97] Corticosterone and DOC, synthesized in both the ZF and ZG, can act as mineralocorticoids, which becomes significant in some clinical diseases, notably some forms of congenital adrenal hyperplasia (CAH) and adrenal tumors. Similarly, it is now established that cortisol can act as a mineralocorticoid in the setting of impaired metabolism of cortisol to cortisone by the enzyme 11β-hydroxysteroid dehydrogenase type 2 (HSD11B2); this is important in patients with hypertension, ectopic ACTH syndrome, or renal disease. The renin-angiotensin system is described in detail in Chapter 16.

Angiotensin II and potassium stimulate aldosterone secretion principally by increasing the transcription of *CYP11B2* through common intracellular signaling pathways. cAMP response elements in the 5′ region of the *CYP11B2* gene are activated after an increase in intracellular Ca^{2+} and activation of calmodulin kinases. The potassium effect is mediated through membrane depolarization and opening of calcium channels, and the angiotensin II effect after binding of angiotensin II to the surface AT_1 receptor and activation of phospholipase C.[97]

The effect of ACTH on aldosterone secretion is modest and differs in the acute and chronic situation (see Chapter 16). An acute bolus of ACTH will increase aldosterone secretion, principally by stimulating the early pathways of adrenal steroidogenesis (see earlier discussion), but circulating levels increase by no more than 10% to 20% above baseline values. ACTH has no effect on *CYP11B2* gene transcription or enzyme activity. Chronic continual ACTH stimulation has either no effect or an inhibitory effect on aldosterone production, possibly because of receptor downregulation or suppression of angiotensin II–stimulated secretion because of a mineralocorticoid effect of cortisol, DOC, or corticosterone. Dopamine and atrial natriuretic peptide inhibit aldosterone secretion, as does heparin.

These separate lines of control—through the HPA axis for glucocorticoid biosynthesis and via the renin-angiotensin system for mineralocorticoid synthesis—have important clinical consequences. Patients with primary adrenal failure invariably have both cortisol and aldosterone deficiency, whereas patients with ACTH deficiency due to pituitary disease have glucocorticoid deficiency but normal aldosterone concentrations because the renin-angiotensin system is intact.

Adrenal Androgen Secretion

Adrenal androgens represent an important component (>50%) of circulating androgens in premenopausal women.[98] In men, this contribution is much smaller because of the testicular production of androgens, but adrenal androgen excess even in men may be of clinical significance, notably in patients with CAH, which results in a suppression of the hypothalamic-pituitary-gonadal axis. The adult adrenal secretes approximately 4 mg/day of DHEA, 7 to 15 mg/day of DHEAS, 1.5 mg of androstenedione, and 0.05 mg/day of testosterone.

DHEA is a crucial precursor of human sex steroid biosynthesis and exerts androgenic or estrogenic activity after conversion by the activities of the 3β-HSD superfamily (β-HSD isozymes and aromatase); these enzymes are expressed in peripheral target tissues, a fact that is of clinical importance in many diseases.[99] Some studies have postulated direct effects of DHEA acting as a classic hormone in peripheral tissues. Specific plasma membrane receptors have been identified but await full characterization.[100] Conventionally, desulfated DHEA is thought to be converted downstream to a biologically active hormone. Serum DHEAS was previously thought to represent a circulating storage pool for DHEA regeneration, but it was later suggested that conversion of DHEAS to DHEA by steroid sulfatase plays a minor role in adult physiology and that the equilibrium between serum DHEA and DHEAS is mainly regulated by SULT2A1 activity. This implies that serum DHEAS may not always appropriately reflect the active DHEA pool, particularly if SULT2A1 activity is impaired, as in the inflammatory stress response.[101]

TABLE 15-4

Dissociation of Adrenal Androgen and Glucocorticoid Secretion: Evidence for an Adrenal-Stimulating Hormone

Dexamethasone studies: Complete cortisol suppression with chronic high-dose dexamethasone; DHEA falls by only 20% (greater sensitivity of DHEA to acute low-dose dexamethasone administration).
Adrenarche: Clinically significant rise in circulating DHEA at 6 to 8 years of age; cortisol production unaltered.
Aging: Reduction in DHEA production; no change in cortisol.
Anorexia nervosa and illness: Fall in DHEA, no change (or increase) in cortisol.

DHEA, dehydroepiandrosterone.

DHEAS stimulates androgen secretion; DHEA (but not DHAS because of its increased plasma half-life) and androstenedione demonstrate a circadian rhythm similar to that of cortisol.[102] However, there are many discrepancies between adrenal androgen and glucocorticoid secretion, leading to the suggestion of an additional cortical androgen-stimulating hormone (CASH). Many putative CASHs have been proposed, including POMC derivatives such as joining peptide, prolactin, and insulin-like growth factor type 1 (IGF1), but conclusive proof is lacking. Efficient adrenal steroidogenesis toward androgen synthesis is crucially dependent on the relative activities of 3β-HSD and 17α-hydroxylase and, in particular, on the 17,20-lyase activity of 17α-hydroxylase. Factors that determine whether the 17-hydroxylated substrates, 17-OH pregnenolone and 17-OHP, will undergo 21-hydroxylation to form glucocorticoid or side-chain cleavage by 17α-hydroxylase to form DHEA and androstenedione are unresolved and seem likely to be important in defining the activity of any putative CASH (Table 15-4).

CORTICOSTEROID HORMONE ACTION

Receptors and Gene Transcription

Both cortisol and aldosterone exert their effects after uptake of free hormone from the circulation and binding to intracellular receptors; these are termed, respectively, the *glucocorticoid receptor* (GR, encoded by *NR3C1*) and the *mineralocorticoid receptor* (MR, encoded by *NR3C2*).[103-105] These are members of the thyroid/steroid hormone receptor superfamily of transcription factors; they consist of a carboxy-terminal ligand-binding domain, a central DNA-binding domain that interacts with specific DNA sequences on target genes, and an N-terminal hypervariable region. Although only single genes encode the GR and MR, splice

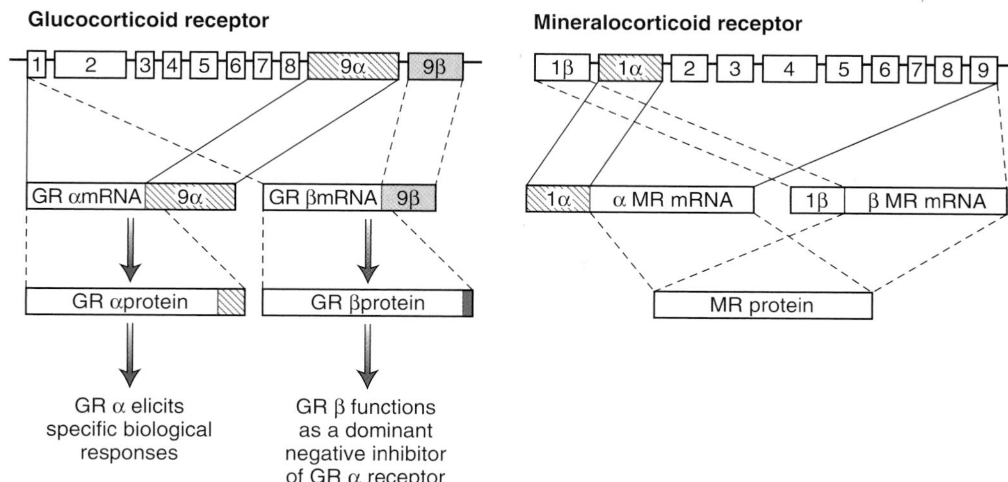

Figure 15-9 Schematic structure of the human genes encoding the glucocorticoid receptor (GR) and mineralocorticoid receptor (MR). In both cases, splice variants have been described. In the case of the GR, there is evidence that the GRβ isoform can act as a dominant negative inhibitor of GRα action. mRNA, messenger ribonucleic acid.

variants have been described in both receptor types; this, together with tissue-specific post-translational modification (phosphorylation, sumoylation, and ubiquitination) is thought to account for many of the diverse actions of corticosteroids (Fig. 15-9).[106,107]

Glucocorticoid hormone action has been studied in more depth than mineralocorticoid action. The binding of steroid to the GRα in the cytosol results in activation of the steroid-receptor complex through a process that involves the dissociation of heat shock proteins (HSP90 and HSP70).[108] Following translocation to the nucleus, gene transcription is stimulated or repressed after binding of the dimerized GR-ligand complex to a specific DNA sequence in the promoter regions of target genes.[109] This sequence, known as the glucocorticoid-response element (GRE), is invariably a palindromic CGTACAnnnTGTACT sequence that binds with high affinity to two loops of DNA within the DNA-binding domain of the GR (zinc fingers). This stabilizes the RNA polymerase II complex, facilitating gene transcription. The GRα variant may act as a dominant negative regulator of GRβ transactivation.[106]

Naturally occurring mutations in the GR (as seen in patients with glucocorticoid resistance) and GR mutants generated in vitro have highlighted critical regions of the receptor that are responsible for binding and transactivation,[110] but numerous others factors are required (e.g., coactivators, corepressors[111]), and this may make responses tissue specific. This is a rapidly evolving field and beyond the scope of this chapter. However, the interaction between GR and two particular transcription factors are important in mediating the anti-inflammatory effects of glucocorticoids and explain the effect of glucocorticoids on genes that do not contain obvious GREs in their promoter regions.[112] Activator protein 1 (AP1) comprises Fos and Jun subunits and is a proinflammatory transcription factor induced by a series of cytokines and phorbol ester. The GR-ligand complex can bind to c-Jun and prevent interaction with the AP1 site, thereby mediating the so-called transrepressive effects of glucocorticoids.[113] Similarly, functional antagonism exists between the GR and nuclear factor-κB (NF-κB), a ubiquitously expressed transcription factor that activates a series of genes involved in lymphocyte development, inflammatory response, host defense, and apoptosis (Fig. 15-10).[114] In keeping with the diverse array of actions of cortisol, many hundreds of glucocorticoid-responsive genes have been identified. Some glucocorticoid-induced genes and repressed genes are listed in Table 15-5.

In contrast to the diverse actions of glucocorticoids, mineralocorticoids have a more restricted role, principally stimulation of epithelial sodium transport in the distal nephron, distal colon, and salivary glands.[115] This action is mediated through induction of the apical sodium channel (comprising three subunits—α, β, and γ)[116] and the α_1 and β_1 subunits of the basolateral sodium-potassium adenosine triphosphatase pump (Na^+,K^+-ATPase)[117] through transcriptional regulation of serum- and glucocorticoid-induced kinase (SGK).[118] Aldosterone binds to the MR, principally in the cytosol (although there is evidence for expression of the unliganded MR in the nucleus), and the hormone-receptor complex is then translocated to the nucleus (Fig. 15-11).

The MR and GR share considerable homology—57% in the steroid-binding domain and 94% in the DNA-binding domain. It is perhaps not surprising, therefore, that there is promiscuity of ligand binding, with aldosterone (and the synthetic mineralocorticoid, fludrocortisone) binding to the GR and cortisol binding to the MR. For the MR, this is particularly impressive: in vitro, the MR has the same inherent affinity for aldosterone, corticosterone, or cortisol.[104] Specificity on the MR is conferred through the "prereceptor" metabolism of cortisol via the enzyme HSD11B2, which inactivates cortisol and corticosterone to inactive 11-keto metabolites, enabling aldosterone to bind to the MR.[119,120] Mineralocorticoid hormone action was extended beyond this classic action in sodium-transporting epithelia with the demonstration that aldosterone can induce cardiac fibrosis and inflammatory changes in renal vasculature. The underlying signaling pathways remain to be fully clarified, but the effects are reversible with MR antagonists.[121]

Finally, for both glucocorticoids and mineralocorticoids, there is accumulating evidence for so-called nongenomic effects involving hormone response obviating the genomic GR or MR. A series of responses have been reported to occur within seconds or minutes after exposure to corticosteroids and are thought to be mediated by as yet uncharacterized membrane-coupled receptors.[122,123]

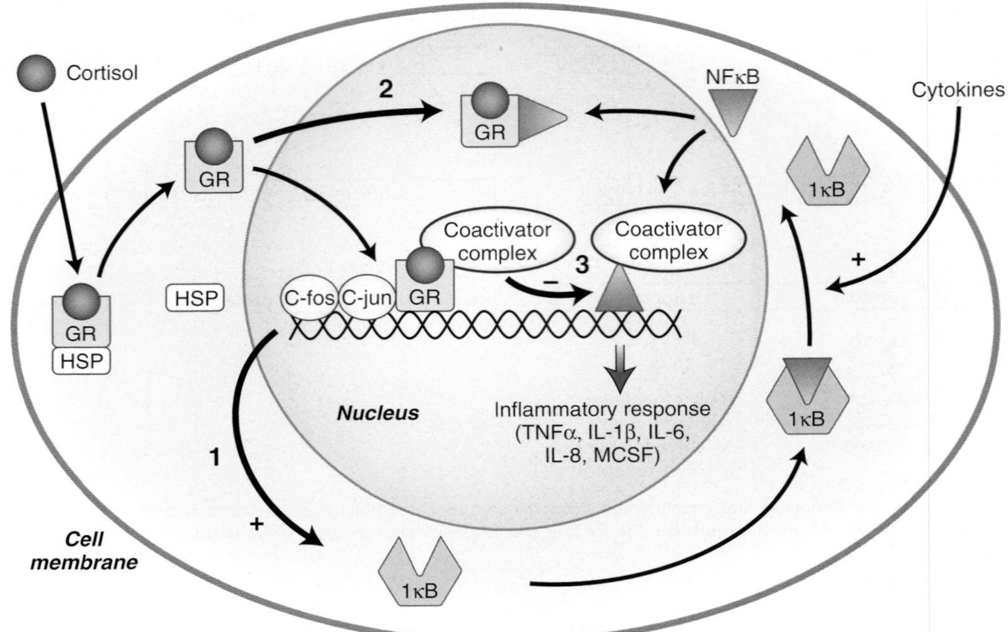

Figure 15-10 The anti-inflammatory action of glucocorticoids. Cortisol binds to the cytoplasmic glucocorticoid receptor (GR). Conformational changes in the receptor-ligand complex result in dissociation from heat shock proteins (HSP70 and HSP90) and migration to the nucleus. Binding occurs to specific DNA motifs—glucocorticoid response elements—in association with the activator protein 1 (AP1) comprising C-fos and C-jun. Glucocorticoids mediate their anti-inflammatory effects through several mechanisms: (1) the inhibitory protein IκB, which binds and inactivates nuclear factor-κB (NFκB), is induced; (2) the GR-cortisol complex is able to bind NFκB and thereby prevent initiation of an inflammatory process; (3) GR and NFκB compete for the limited availability of coactivators, which include cyclic adenosine monophosphate response element–binding protein (CREB) and steroid receptor coactivator-1. IL, interleukin; MCSF, macrophage colong stimulating factor; TNFα, tumor necrosis factor-α.

Cortisol-Binding Globulin and Corticosteroid Hormone Metabolism

More than 90% of circulating cortisol is bound, predominantly to the α_2-globulin, cortisol-binding globulin (CBG).[124] This 383-amino-acid protein is synthesized in the liver and binds cortisol with high affinity. Affinity for synthetic corticosteroids is negligible except for prednisolone, which has an affinity for CBG approximately half that of cortisol. Circulating CBG concentrations are approximately 700 nmol/L. Levels are increased by estrogens and in some patients with chronic active hepatitis; they are reduced by glucocorticoids and in patients with cirrhosis, nephrosis, and hyperthyroidism. The estrogen effect can be marked, with levels increasing twofold to threefold across pregnancy, a fact that should be taken into account when measuring plasma "total" cortisol in pregnancy and in women taking estrogens.

Inherited abnormalities in CBG synthesis are much rarer than those described for thyroxine-binding globulin but include cases of elevated CBG, partial or complete deficiency of CBG, and CBG variants with reduced affinity for cortisol.[125,126] In each case, alterations in CBG concentrations change the total circulating cortisol concentrations accordingly, but free cortisol concentrations are normal. Only this free circulating fraction is available for transport into tissues for biologic activity. The excretion of free cortisol through the kidneys is termed *urinary free cortisol* and represents only 1% of the total cortisol secretion.

The circulating half-life of cortisol varies between 70 and 120 minutes. The major steps in cortisol metabolism are depicted in Figure 15-12[127] and can be summarized as follows:

- Interconversion of the 11-hydroxyl group (cortisol, Kendall's compound F) to the 11-oxo group (cortisone, compound E) through activity of the 11β-HSD system (EC 1.1.1.146).[128,129] The metabolism of cortisol and that of cortisone then follow similar pathways.
- Reduction of the C4-5 double bond to form dihydrocortisol or dihydrocortisone, followed by hydroxylation of the 3-oxo group to form tetrahydrocortisol (THF) or tetrahydrocortisone (THE). The reduction of the C4-5 double can be carried out by either 5β-reductase or 5α-reductase, yielding, respectively, 5β-THF (THF) and 5α-THF (allo-THF). In normal subjects, the ratio of THF to allo-THF is 2:1. THF, allo-THF, and THE are rapidly conjugated with glucuronic acid and excreted in the urine.
- Further reduction of the 20-oxo group by either 20α- or 20β-HSD to yield α- and β-cortols and cortolones from cortisol and cortisone, respectively. Reduction of the C20 position may also occur without A-ring reduction, giving rise to 20α- and 20β-hydroxycortisol.
- Hydroxylation at C6 to form 6β-hydroxycortisol.
- Cleavage of THF and THE to the C19 steroids, 11-hydroxy- or 11-oxo- androsterone or etiocholanolone.
- Oxidation of the C21 position or cortols and cortolones to form the extremely polar metabolites, cortolic and cortolonic acids.

Approximately 50% of secreted cortisol appears in the urine as THF, allo-THF, and THE; 25% as cortols/cortolones; 10% as C19 steroids; and 10% as cortolic/cortolonic acids. The remaining metabolites are free unconjugated steroids (cortisol, cortisone, and their 6β-, and 20α/20β-metabolites).

The principal site of cortisol metabolism has been considered to be the liver, but many of the enzymes listed have been described in mammalian kidney, notably the interconversion of cortisol to cortisone by HSD11B2.

TABLE 15-5

Some of the Genes Regulated by Glucocorticoids or Glucocorticoid Receptors

Site of Action	Induced Genes	Repressed Genes
Immune system	IκB (nuclear factor-κB inhibitor)	Interleukins
	Haptoglobin	Tumor necrosis factor-α (TNF-α)
	T-cell receptor (TCR)-ζ	Interferon-γ
	p21, p27, and p57	E-selectin
	Lipocortin	Intercellular adhesion molecule-1
		Cyclooxygenase 2
		Inducible nitric oxide synthase (iNOS)
Metabolic	PPAR-γ	Tryptophan hydroxylase
	Tyrosine aminotransferase	Metalloprotease
	Glutamine synthase	
	Glycogen synthase	
	Glucose-6-phosphatase	
	PEPCK	
	Leptin	
	γ-Fibrinogen	
	Cholesterol 7α-hydroxylase	
	C/EBP/β	
Bone	Androgen receptor	Osteocalcin
	Calcitonin receptor	Collagenase
	Alkaline phosphatase	
	IGFBP6	
Channels and transporters	ENaC-α, -β, and -γ	
	SGK	
	Aquaporin 1	
Endocrine	Basic fibroblast growth factor (bFGF)	Glucocorticoid receptor
	Vasoactive intestinal peptide	Prolactin
	Endothelin	POMC/CRH
	Retinoid X receptor	PTHrP
	GHRH receptor	Vasopressin
	Natriuretic peptide receptors	
Growth and development	Surfactant proteins A, B, and C	Fibronectin
		α-Fetoprotein
		Nerve growth factor
		Erythropoietin
		G1 cyclins
		Cyclin-dependent kinases

CRH, corticotropin-releasing hormone; C/EBP/β, CAAT-enhancer binding protein-β; ENaC, epithelial sodium channel; GHRH, growth hormone–releasing hormone; IGFBP6, insulin-like growth factor–binding protein 6; PEPCK, phosphoenolpyruvate carboxykinase; POMC, pro-opiomelanocortin; PPAR, peroxisome proliferator-activated receptor; PTHrP, parathyroid hormone-related protein; SGK, serum- and glucocorticoid-induced kinase.
Modified from McKay LI, Cidlowski JA. Molecular control of immune/inflammatory responses: interactions between nuclear factor-κB and steroid receptor-signalling pathways. *Endocr Rev.* 1999;20:435-459.

Quantitatively, this is the most important pathway. Furthermore, the bioactivity of glucocorticoids is in part related to the hydroxyl group at C11; because cortisone with a C11-oxo group is an inactive steroid, expression of 11β-HSD in peripheral tissues plays a crucial role in regulating corticosteroid hormone action. Two distinct 11β-HSD isozymes have been reported—a type 1, reduced nicotinamide adenine dinucleotide phosphate (NADPH)-dependent oxo-reductase expressed principally in the liver, which confers bioactivity on orally administered cortisone by converting it to cortisol,[129] and a type 2, nicotinamide adenine dinucleotide (NAD)-dependent dehydrogenase. It is the HSD11B2, coexpressed with the MR in the kidney, colon, and salivary gland, that inactivates cortisol to cortisone and permits aldosterone to bind to the MR in vivo. If this enzyme-protective mechanism is impaired, cortisol is able to act as a mineralocorticoid; this explains some forms of endocrine hypertension (apparent mineralocorticoid excess, licorice ingestion) and the mineralocorticoid excess state that characterizes the ectopic ACTH syndrome.[128,130]

Hyperthyroidism results in increased cortisol metabolism and clearance, and hypothyroidism produces the converse, principally because of an effect of thyroid hormone on hepatic HSD11B1 and 5α/5β-reductases.[129] IGF1 increases cortisol clearance by inhibiting hepatic HSD11B1 (conversion of cortisone to cortisol).[131] 6β-Hydroxylation is normally a minor pathway, but cortisol itself induces 6β-hydroxylase so that 6β-hydroxycortisol excretion is markedly increased in patients with Cushing's syndrome.[132] Some drugs, notably rifampicin and phenytoin, increase cortisol clearance through this pathway.[133] Patients with renal disease have impaired cortisol clearance because of reduced conversion of renal cortisol to cortisone.[134] These observations have clinical implications for patients with thyroid disease, acromegaly, or renal disease and for patients taking cortisol replacement therapy. Adrenal crisis has been reported in steroid-replaced addisonian patients given rifampicin,[135] and hydrocortisone replacement therapy may need to be increased in treated patients who develop hyperthyroidism or reduced in patients with untreated growth-hormone deficiency.

Aldosterone is also metabolized in the liver and kidneys. In the liver, it undergoes tetrahydro reduction and is excreted in the urine as a 3-glucuronide tetrahydroaldosterone derivative. However, glucuronide conjugation at the

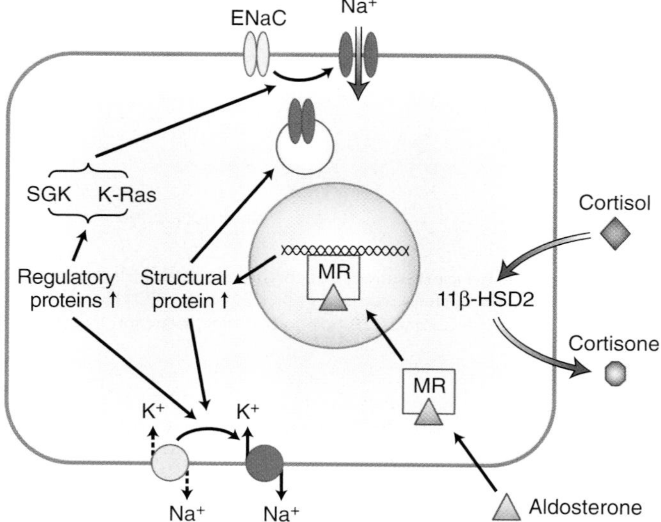

Figure 15-11 Mineralocorticoid hormone action. An epithelial cell in the distal nephron or distal colon is depicted. The much higher concentrations of cortisol are inactivated by the type 2 isozyme of 11β-hydroxysteroid dehydrogenase (11β-HSD2) to cortisone, permitting the endogenous ligand, aldosterone, to bind to the mineralocorticoid receptor (MR). Relatively few mineralocorticoid target genes have been identified, but they include serum- and glucocorticoid-induced kinase (SGK), subunits of the epithelial sodium channel (ENaC), and basolateral Na^+,K^+–adenosine triphosphatase.

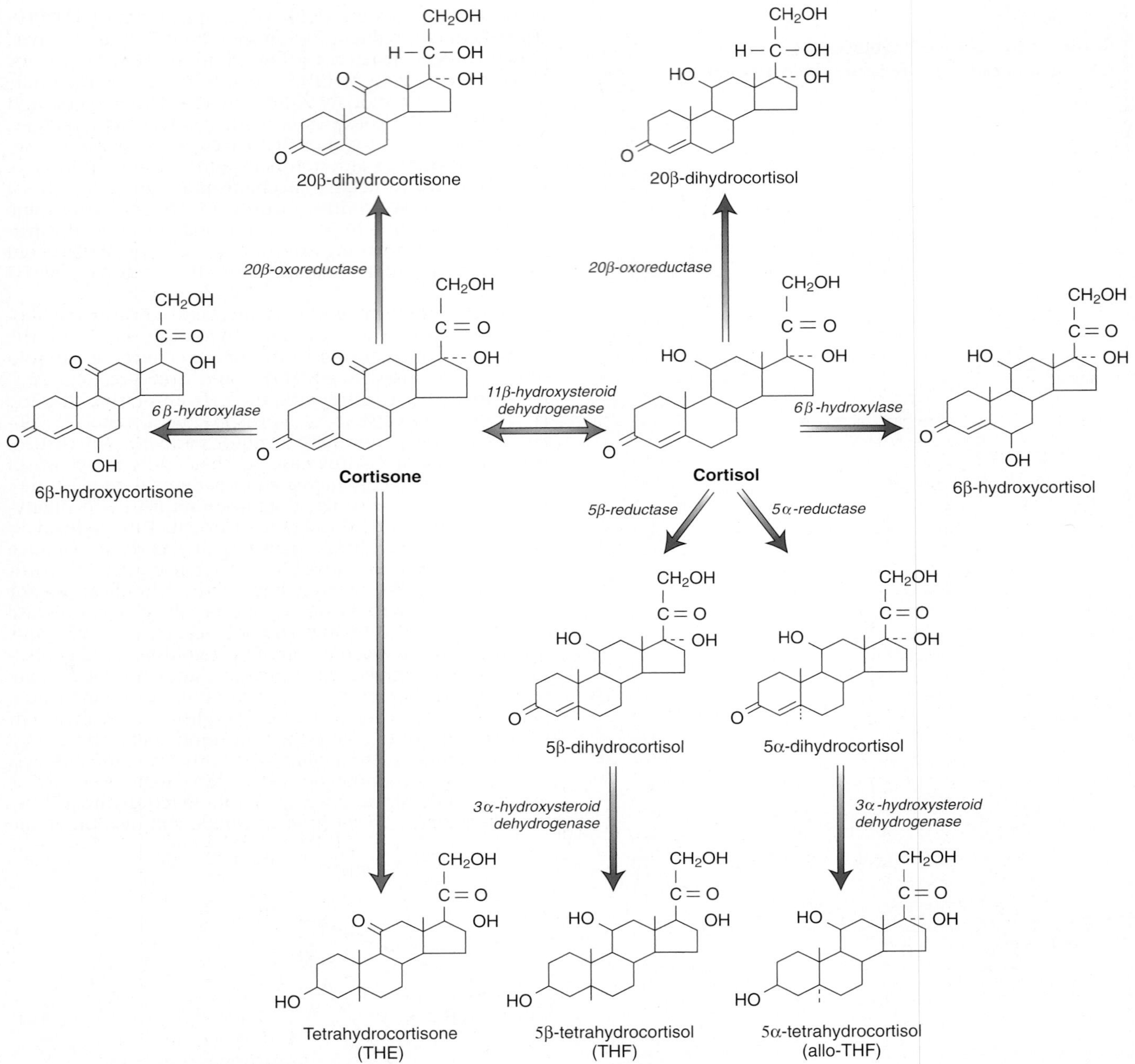

Figure 15-12 The principal pathways of cortisol metabolism. Interconversion of hormonally active cortisol to inactive cortisone is catalyzed by two isozymes of 11β-hydroxysteroid dehydrogenase (11β-HSD), with HSD11B1 principally converting cortisone to cortisol and HSD11B2 doing the reverse. Cortisol can be hydroxylated at the C6 and C20 positions. A ring reduction is undertaken by 5α-reductase or 5β-reductase and 3α-HSD.

18 position occurs directly in the kidney, as does 3α and 5α/5β metabolism of the free steroid.[136] Because of the aldehyde group at the C18 position, aldosterone is not metabolized by HSD11B2.[137] Hepatic aldosterone clearance is reduced in patients with cirrhosis, ascites, or severe congestive heart failure.

Effects of Glucocorticoids

The principal sites of action of glucocorticoids and some of the consequences of glucocorticoid excess are shown in Figure 15-13.

Carbohydrate, Protein, and Lipid Metabolism

Glucocorticoids increase blood glucose concentrations through their action on glycogen, protein, and lipid metabolism. In the liver, cortisol stimulates glycogen deposition by increasing glycogen synthase and inhibiting the glycogen-mobilizing enzyme, glycogen phosphorylase.[138] Hepatic glucose output increases through the activation of key enzymes involved in gluconeogenesis, principally glucose-6-phosphatase and phosphoenolpyruvate kinase (PEPCK).[139,140] In peripheral tissues (e.g., muscle, fat), cortisol inhibits glucose uptake and utilization.[141] In adipose

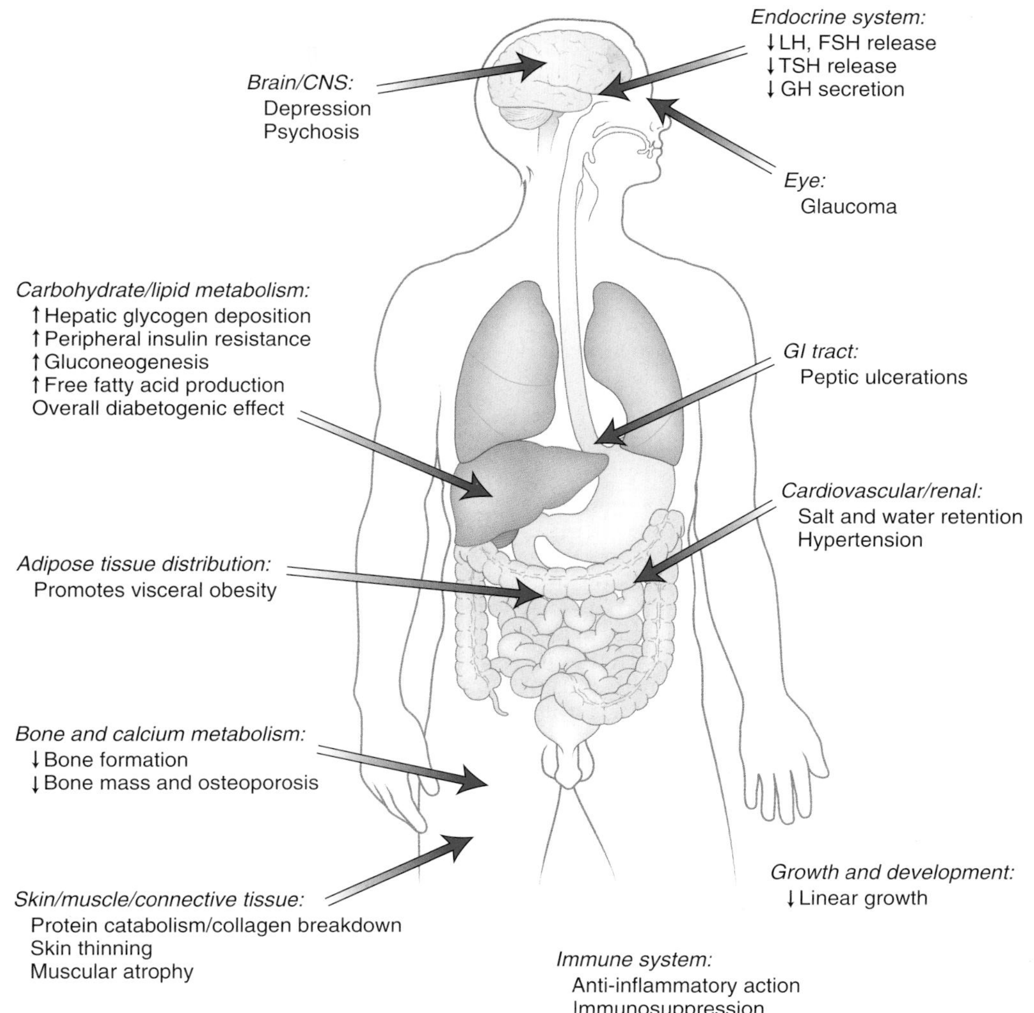

Figure 15-13 The principal sites of action of glucocorticoids in humans, highlighting some of the consequences of glucocorticoid excess. CNS, central nervous system; GI, gastrointestinal; FSH, follicle-stimulating hormone; GH, growth hormone; LH, luteinizing hormone; TSH, thyroid-stimulating hormone.

tissue, lipolysis is activated, resulting in the release of free fatty acids into the circulation. An increase in total circulating cholesterol and triglycerides is observed, but HDL-cholesterol levels fall. Glucocorticoids also have a permissive effect on other hormones, including catecholamines and glucagon. The result is insulin resistance and an increase in blood glucose concentrations, at the expense of protein and lipid catabolism.

Glucocorticoids stimulate adipocyte differentiation, promoting adipogenesis through the transcriptional activation of key differentiation genes, including lipoprotein lipase, glycerol-3-phosphate dehydrogenase, and leptin.[142] Long-term, the effects of glucocorticoid excess on adipose tissue is more complex, at least in humans, in whom the deposition of visceral or central adipose tissue is stimulated,[143] providing a useful discriminatory sign for the diagnosis of Cushing's syndrome. The predilection for visceral obesity may relate to the increased expression of the GR[144] and HSD11B1 in omental compared with subcutaneous adipose tissue.[145]

Skin, Muscle, and Connective Tissue

In addition to inducing insulin resistance in muscle tissue, glucocorticoids also cause catabolic changes in muscle, skin, and connective tissue. In the skin and connective tissue, glucocorticoids inhibit epidermal cell division and DNA synthesis and reduce synthesis and production of collagen.[146] In muscle, glucocorticoids cause atrophy (but not necrosis), which seems to be specific for type II (phasic) muscle fibers. Muscle protein synthesis is reduced.

Bone and Calcium Metabolism

Glucocorticoids inhibit osteoblast function, which is thought to account for the osteopenia and osteoporosis that characterize glucocorticoid excess.[147] Up to 1% of Western populations are taking long-term glucocorticoid therapy,[148] and glucocorticoid-induced osteoporosis is becoming a prevalent health concern, affecting 50% of patients treated with corticosteroids for longer than 12 months. However, the complication perhaps most feared by physicians is osteonecrosis. Osteonecrosis (also termed *avascular necrosis*) produces rapid and focal deterioration of bone quality and primarily affects the femoral head, leading to pain and ultimately to collapse of the bone, often necessitating hip replacement. It can affect individuals of any age and may occur with relatively low doses of glucocorticoids (e.g., during corticosteroid replacement therapy for adrenal failure).[149] Importantly, defects may not be detectable on conventional x-ray films but are readily seen on magnetic resonance imaging (MRI). Glucocorticoid-induced osteocyte apoptosis has been implicated in the pathogenesis of the condition,[150] and the lack of a direct role for an interrupted blood supply suggests that the term *osteonecrosis* is preferable to *avascular femoral necrosis*. However, there is still no explanation for individual susceptibility.

Glucocorticoids also induce negative calcium balance by inhibiting intestinal calcium absorption and increasing renal calcium excretion. As a consequence, parathyroid secretion is usually increased. In children, glucocorticoids suppress growth, but the increases in body mass index are thought to offset a deleterious effect on bone mineral density.[151]

Salt and Water Homeostasis and Blood Pressure Control

Glucocorticoids increase blood pressure by a variety of mechanisms involving actions on the kidney and vasculature.[152] In vascular smooth muscle, they increase sensitivity to pressor agents such as catecholamines and angiotensin II while reducing nitric oxide–mediated endothelial dilatation. Angiotensinogen synthesis is increased by glucocorticoids.[153] In the kidney, depending on the activity of HSD11B2, cortisol can act on the distal nephron to cause sodium retention and potassium loss (mediated via the MR).[130] Elsewhere across the nephron, glucocorticoids increase the glomerular filtration rate, proximal tubular epithelial sodium transport, and free water clearance.[154] This last effect involves antagonism of the action of vasopressin and explains the dilutional hyponatremia seen in patients with glucocorticoid deficiency.[155]

Anti-Inflammatory Actions and the Immune System

Glucocorticoids suppress immunologic responses, and this has been the stimulus to develop a series of highly potent pharmacologic glucocorticoids to treat a variety of autoimmune and inflammatory conditions. The inhibitory effects are mediated at many levels. In the peripheral blood, glucocorticoids reduce lymphocyte counts acutely (T lymphocytes > B lymphocytes) by redistributing lymphocytes from the intravascular compartment to the spleen, lymph nodes, and bone marrow. Conversely, neutrophil counts increase after glucocorticoid administration. Eosinophil counts rapidly fall, an effect that was historically used as a bioassay for glucocorticoids. The immunologic actions of glucocorticoids involve direct actions on both T and B lymphocytes, including inhibition of immunoglobulin synthesis and stimulation of lymphocyte apoptosis. Inhibition of cytokine production from lymphocytes is mediated through inhibition of the action of NF-κB. NF-κB plays a crucial and generalized role in inducing cytokine gene transcription; glucocorticoids can bind directly to NF-κB to prevent nuclear translocation, and they induce NF-κB inhibitor, which sequesters NF-κB in the cytoplasm, thereby inactivating its effect.[114]

Additional anti-inflammatory effects involve the inhibition of monocyte differentiation into macrophages and macrophage phagocytosis and cytotoxic activity. Glucocorticoids reduce the local inflammatory response by preventing the actions of histamine and plasminogen activators. Prostaglandin synthesis is impaired through the induction of lipocortins, which inhibit phospholipase A2 activity.[156]

Central Nervous System and Mood

Clinical observations of patients with glucocorticoid excess and deficiency reveal that the brain is an important target tissue for glucocorticoids, with depression, euphoria, psychosis, apathy, and lethargy being important manifestations. Both GRs and MRs are expressed in discrete regions of the rodent brain, including hippocampus, hypothalamus, cerebellum, and cortex.[157] Glucocorticoids cause neuronal death, notably in the hippocampus[158]; this may underlie the interest in glucocorticoids in relation to cognitive function, memory, and neurodegenerative diseases such as Alzheimer's.[159] Local blockade of cortisol generation by HSD11B1 has been shown to improve cognitive function.[160] DHEA has been shown to have neuroprotective effects in the hippocampus region.[161] CYP7B, an enzyme that metabolizes DHEA to its 7α-hydroxylated metabolite, is highly expressed in brain, but expression was decreased in dentate neurons in the hippocampus.[162]

Eye

In the eye, glucocorticoids act to raise intraocular pressure through an increase in aqueous humor production and deposition of matrix within the trabecular meshwork, which inhibits aqueous drainage. Steroid-induced glaucoma appears to have a genetic predisposition, but the underlying mechanisms are unknown.[163]

Gut

Long-term but not acute administration of glucocorticoids increases the risk of developing peptic ulcer disease.[164] Pancreatitis with fat necrosis is reported in patients with glucocorticoid excess. The GR is expressed throughout the gastrointestinal tract, and the MR in the distal colon; they mediate the corticosteroid control of epithelial ion transport.

Growth and Development

Although glucocorticoids stimulate transcription of the gene encoding growth hormone (GH) in vitro, glucocorticoids in excess inhibit linear skeletal growth,[151,165] probably as a result of catabolic effects on connective tissue, muscle, and bone and through inhibition of the effects of IGF1. The results of experiments on mice lacking the GR gene[87] have emphasized the role of glucocorticoids in normal fetal development. In particular, glucocorticoids stimulate lung maturation through the synthesis of surfactant proteins (SP-A, SP-B, and SP-C),[166] and mice lacking the GR die shortly after birth due to hypoxia from lung atelectasis. Glucocorticoids also stimulate the enzyme phenylethanolamine *N*-methyltransferase (PNMT), which converts noradrenaline to adrenaline in adrenal medulla and chromaffin tissue. Mice lacking the GR do not develop an adrenal medulla.[87]

Endocrine Effects

Glucocorticoids suppress the thyroid axis, probably through a direct action on the secretion of thyroid-stimulating hormone (TSH). In addition, they inhibit 5′ deiodinase activity that mediates the conversion of thyroxine to active triiodothyronine.

Glucocorticoids also act centrally to inhibit gonadotropin-releasing hormone (GnRH) pulsatility and release of luteinizing hormone (LH) and follicle-stimulating hormone (FSH).

TABLE 15-6

Therapeutic Use of Corticosteroids

Endocrine: Replacement therapy (Addison's disease, pituitary disease, congenital adrenal hyperplasia), Graves' ophthalmopathy
Skin: Dermatitis, pemphigus
Hematology: Leukemia, lymphoma, hemolytic anemia, idiopathic thrombocytopenic purpura
Gastrointestinal: Inflammatory bowel disease (ulcerative colitis, Crohn's disease)
Liver: Chronic active hepatitis, transplantation, organ rejection
Renal: Nephrotic syndrome, vasculitides, transplantation, rejection
Central nervous system: Cerebral edema, raised intracranial pressure
Respiratory: Angioedema, anaphylaxis, asthma, sarcoidosis, tuberculosis, obstructive airway disease
Rheumatology: Systemic lupus erythematosus, polyarteritis, temporal arteritis, rheumatoid arthritis
Muscle: Polymyalgia rheumatica, myasthenia gravis

Therapeutic Corticosteroids

Since the dramatic anti-inflammatory effect of cortisone was first demonstrated in the 1950s, a series of synthetic corticosteroids have been developed for therapeutic purposes. These are used to treat a diverse variety of human diseases, principally relying on their anti-inflammatory and immunologic actions (Table 15-6). The main corticosteroids used in clinical practice, together with their relative glucocorticoid and mineralocorticoid potencies, are listed in Table 15-7.

The structures of common synthetic steroids are depicted in Fig. 15-14. The biologic activity of a corticosteroid depends on a 4-3-keto, 11β-hydroxy, 17α,21-trihydroxyl configuration.[167] Conversion of the C11 hydroxyl group to a C11 keto group (i.e., cortisol to cortisone) inactivates the steroid. The addition of a 1,2 unsaturated bond to cortisol results in prednisolone, which is four times more potent than cortisol in classic glucocorticoid bioassays such as hepatic glycogen deposition, suppression of eosinophils, and anti-inflammatory actions. Prednisone, widely prescribed in the United States, is the cortisone-equivalent of prednisolone and relies on conversion by HSD11B1 in the liver for bioactivity.[168] Potency is further increased by the addition of a 6α-methyl group to prednisolone (methylprednisolone).

Fludrocortisone is a synthetic mineralocorticoid having 125-fold greater potency than cortisol in stimulating sodium reabsorption. This is achieved through the addition of a 9α-fluoro group to cortisol. Fludrocortisone also has glucocorticoid potency (12-fold greater than cortisol). The addition of a 16α-methyl group and 1,2, saturated bond to fludrocortisone results in dexamethasone, a highly potent glucocorticoid (25-fold greater than cortisol) that has negligible mineralocorticoid activity.[167,169]

TABLE 15-7

Relative Biologic Potencies of Synthetic Steroids in Bioassay Systems

Steroid	Anti-Inflammatory Action	Hypothalamic-Pituitary-Adrenal Suppression	Salt Retention
Cortisol	1	1	1
Prednisone	3	4	0.75
Prednisolone	3	4	0.75
Methylprednisolone	6.2	4	0.5
Fludrocortisone	12	12	125
Δ^1 Fludrocortisone	14	—	225
Triamcinolone	5	4	0
Dexamethasone	26	17	0

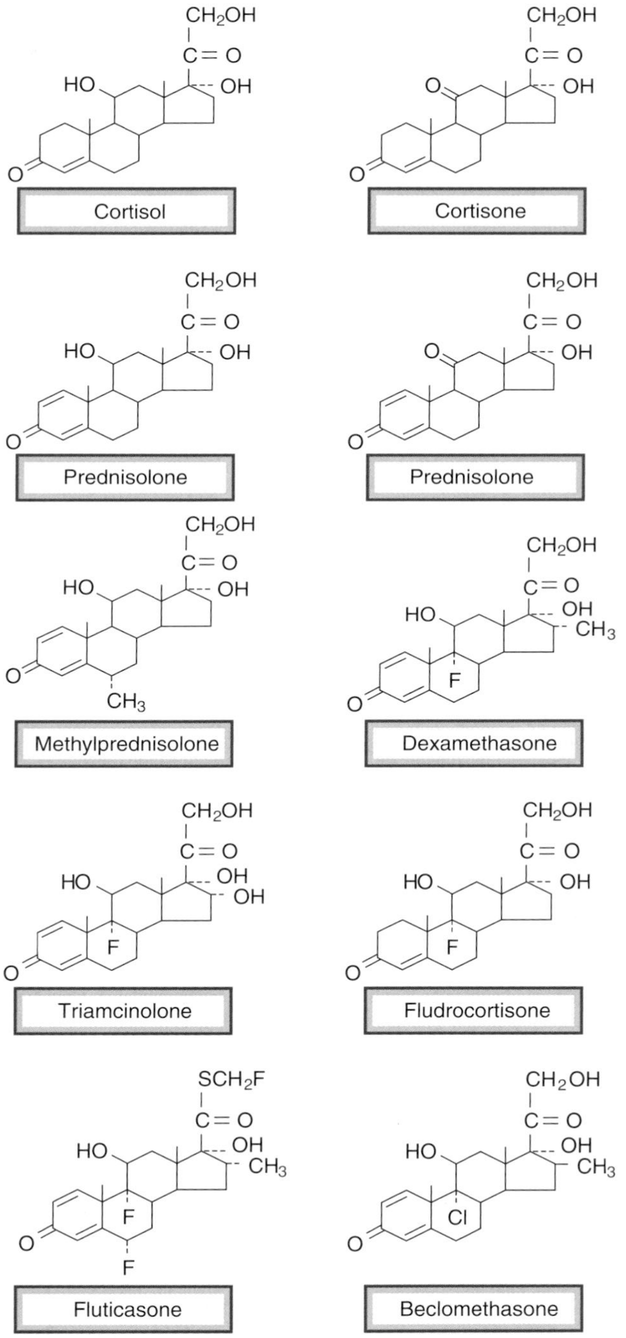

Cortisol
Cortisone
Prednisolone
Prednisolone
Methylprednisolone
Dexamethasone
Triamcinolone
Fludrocortisone
Fluticasone
Beclomethasone

Figure 15-14 Structures of the natural glucocorticoid cortisol, some of the more commonly prescribed synthetic glucocorticoids, and the mineralocorticoid fludrocortisone. Triamcinolone is identical to dexamethasone except that a 16α-hydroxyl group is substituted for the 16α-methyl group. Betamethasone, another widely used glucocorticoid, has a 16β-methyl group. Beclomethasone is derived from betamethasone by replacement of the 9α-fluoro group with a chloro group. Fluticasone is identical to dexamethasone except that an additional 6α-fluoro group has been added, and the hydroxymethyl group at position 21 has been exchanged by an S-fluoromethyl group.

Administration

Widely used synthetic glucocorticoids in respiratory and nasal aerosol sprays are betamethasone, beclomethasone, and fluticasone. Betamethasone has the same structure as dexamethasone but with a 16β-methyl group. Beclomethasone has the same structure as betamethasone apart from the replacement of the 9α-fluoro group with a 9α-chloro group. Fluticasone has the same structure as dexamethasone with an additional 6α-fluoro group and an 5-fluoromethyl group replacing the hydroxymethyl group.

Corticosteroids are given orally, parenterally, and by numerous topical routes (e.g., eyes, skin, nose, inhalation, rectal suppositories).[169] Unlike hydrocortisone, which has a high affinity for CBG, most synthetic steroids have low affinity for this binding protein and circulate as free steroid (approximately 30%) or bound to albumin (approximately 70%). Circulating half-lives vary depending on individual variability and underlying disease, particularly renal and hepatic impairment. Cortisone acetate should not be used parenterally because it requires metabolism by the liver to active cortisol.

It is beyond the scope of this chapter to describe which steroid should be given and by which route for the non-endocrine conditions listed in Table 15-6. Acute and long-term corticosteroid therapy in patients with hypoadrenalism or CAH is discussed in later sections.

Long-Term Therapy

In addition to the undoubted benefit that corticosteroids provide, there is an increasing incidence of overuse, particularly in patients with respiratory or rheumatologic disease, to such an extent that up to 1% of the population is now prescribed long-term corticosteroid therapy.[148] Because of their established euphoric effect, corticosteroids often make patients feel better but without any objective improvements in underlying disease parameters. In view of the long-term harm of chronic glucocorticoid excess,[170] decisions regarding treatment should be evidence based and subject to constant review based on efficacy and side effects. The endocrinologic consequences of chronic glucocorticoid excess, notably suppression of the HPA axis, are an important aspect of modern clinical practice. Endocrinologists need to be aware of the effects of long-term therapy and of steroid withdrawal. Selective glucocorticoid receptor agonists (SEGRAs) are being developed with the aim of dissociating the transrepressive, anti-inflammatory actions of glucocorticoids from the transactivating effects that, by and large, mediate deleterious side effects.[171]

The negative feedback control of the HPA axis by endogenous cortisol has been discussed. Synthetic corticosteroids similarly suppress the function of the HPA axis through a process that depends on the dose and duration of treatment. Consequently, the sudden cessation of corticosteroid therapy can result in adrenal failure.[169] This may also occur after treatment with high doses of the synthetic progestogen, medroxyprogesterone acetate, which possesses glucocorticoid agonist activity.[172] Among patients taking any steroid dose for less than 3 weeks' duration, clinically significant suppression of the HPA axis is rarely a problem, and patients can withdraw from steroids suddenly with no ill effect. The possible exception is the patient who receives frequent short courses of corticosteroid therapy (e.g., with recurrent episodes of severe asthma). Suppression of the HPA axis is inevitable in patients taking the equivalent of 15 mg/day or more of prednisolone for a long period[173]; with lower long-term doses (prednisolone 5 to 15 mg/day or equivalent), suppression of the HPA axis is variable. Defects in the response of the HPA axis to insulin-induced hypoglycemia or exogenous ACTH have been reported in patients taking doses as low as 5 mg/day of prednisolone,[174] but clinically significant suppression at these low doses is debatable. Alternate-day therapy has been associated with less suppression of the HPA axis. Inhaled steroids, particularly very potent synthetic corticosteroids such as the widely used beclomethasone and fluticasone preparations, can also cause HPA axis suppression.[175,176]

All patients receiving long-term therapy with corticosteroids should be treated in a similar fashion to patients with chronic ACTH deficiency; they should carry steroid cards and be offered steroid alert bracelets or necklaces. In the event of an intercurrent stress (e.g., infection, surgery), supplemental steroid cover should be given. If the patient is unable to take drugs orally, parenteral therapy is required.

Recovery from suppression may take 6 to 9 months. CRH secretion returns to normal, and within a few weeks the ACTH level begins to increase, rising above normal values until adrenal steroidogenesis recovers. In the interim, and without replacement therapy, patients may experience symptoms of glucocorticoid deficiency, including anorexia, nausea, weight loss, arthralgia, lethargy, skin desquamation, and postural dizziness (see the later discussions of adrenal insufficiency).[177]

To avoid symptoms of glucocorticoid deficiency, steroids should be cautiously withdrawn over a period of months.[178] Assuming that the underlying disease permits steroid reduction, doses should be reduced from pharmacologic levels to physiologic levels (equivalent to 7.5 mg/day prednisolone) over a few weeks. Thereafter, doses should be reduced by 1 mg/day of prednisolone every 2 to 4 weeks depending on patient well-being. An alternative approach is to switch the patient to hydrocortisone 20 mg/day and reduce the daily dose by 2.5 mg/day every week to a level of 10 mg/day. Corticosteroids should not be taken at night, because this results in greater suppression of early-morning ACTH secretion. After 2 to 3 months on reduced doses, endogenous function of the HPA axis can be assessed by a corticotropin (ACTH-Synacthen) stimulation test or an insulin-induced hypoglycemia test. A "pass" response to these tests indicates adequate function of the HPA axis, and corticosteroid therapy can be safely withdrawn. In those patients who are taking physiologic doses of prednisolone (less than 5 to 7.5 mg/day) or equivalent corticosteroid, a Synacthen stimulation test (SST) given 12 to 24 hours after omitted steroid therapy will provide an immediate answer as to whether sudden or gradual withdrawal of steroid therapy is indicated (Table 15-8).[176]

Iatrogenic-induced Cushing's syndrome occurs in patients who take suppressive doses of corticosteroids for longer than 3 weeks.[178] The rapidity of onset of clinical features depends on the administered dose but can occur within 1 month of therapy.

Adrenocortical Diseases

Adrenocortical diseases are relatively rare. Their importance lies in their high morbidity and mortality if untreated, coupled with the relative ease of diagnosis and the availability of effective therapy. The diseases are most readily classified on the basis of hormone excess or deficiency (Table 15-9).

TABLE 15-8

Suggested Plan for Steroid Replacement in Patients Withdrawing from Chronic Corticosteroid Therapy

Pred Dose (mg/day)	DURATION OF GLUCOCORTICOID TREATMENT			
	≤3 wk*	>3 wk		
≥7.5	Can stop	↓ rapidly (e.g., 2.5 mg q3-4d) THEN		
5-7.5	Can stop	↓ 1 mg q2-4 wk THEN	OR	Convert 5 mg pred to 20 mg HC, then ↓ 2.5 mg/wk to 10 mg/day THEN
<5	Can stop	↓ 1 mg q2-4 wk		After 2-3 mo at HC 10 mg/day, administer SST/ITT: Pass → Withdraw Fail → Continue

*Beware of frequent steroid courses (e.g., in asthma).
HC, hydrocortisone; ITT, insulin tolerance test; pred, prednisolone; SST, short Synacthen test.

Glucocorticoid Excess

Cushing's Syndrome

In 1912, Harvey Cushing first described a 23-year-old female with obesity, hirsutism, and amenorrhea, and 20 years later he postulated that this "polyglandular syndrome" was due to a primary pituitary abnormality causing adrenal hyperplasia.[8] Adrenal tumors were shown to cause the syndrome in some cases,[179] but ectopic ACTH production was not characterized until much later, in 1962.[180] The term *Cushing's syndrome* is used to describe all causes, whereas *Cushing's disease* is reserved for cases of pituitary-dependent Cushing's syndrome.

Cushing's syndrome comprises the symptoms and signs associated with prolonged exposure to inappropriately elevated levels of free plasma glucocorticoids. The use of the term *glucocorticoid* in the definition covers excess from both endogenous (cortisol) and exogenous (e.g., prednisolone, dexamethasone) sources. Iatrogenic Cushing's syndrome is common,[169,178] occurring to some degree in most patients taking long-term corticosteroid therapy. Endogenous causes of Cushing's syndrome are rare and result in loss of the normal feedback mechanism of the HPA axis and the normal circadian rhythm of cortisol secretion.

The incidence of pituitary-dependent Cushing's syndrome is estimated to be 5 to 10 cases per million population per year. The incidence of ectopic ACTH syndrome parallels that of bronchogenic carcinoma, and although 0.5% of lung cancer patients have ectopic ACTH syndrome, rapid progression of the underlying disease often precludes an early diagnosis. Cushing's disease and adrenal adenomas are four times more common in women, whereas ectopic ACTH syndrome is more common in men.

TABLE 15-9

Adrenocortical Diseases

Glucocorticoid Excess
Cushing's syndrome
Pseudo-Cushing's syndromes
Glucocorticoid Resistance
Glucocorticoid Deficiency
Primary hypoadrenalism
Secondary hypoadrenalism
Post-chronic corticosteroid replacement therapy
Congenital Adrenal Hyperplasia
Deficiencies of 21-hydroxylase, 3β-HSD, 17α-hydroxylase, 11β-hydroxylase, P450 oxidoreductase, P450 side chain cleavage, and StAR
Mineralocorticoid Excess
Mineralocorticoid Deficiency
Defects in aldosterone synthesis
Defects in aldosterone action
Hyporeninemic hypoaldosteronism
Adrenal Incidentalomas, Adenomas, and Carcinomas

HSD, hydroxysteroid dehydrogenase; StAR, steroidogenic acute regulatory (protein).

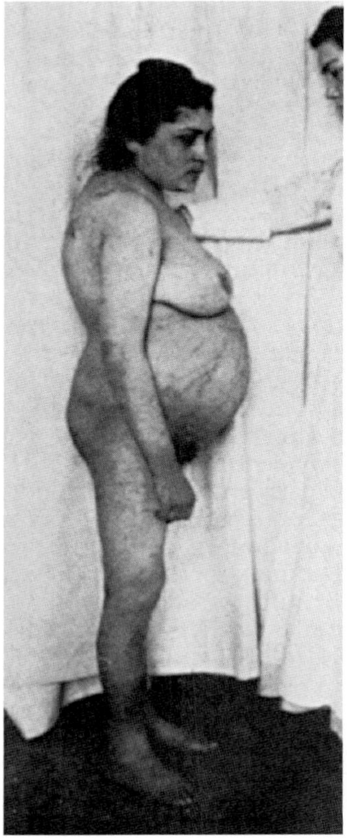

Clinical Features of Cushing's Syndrome

The classic features of Cushing's syndrome—centripetal obesity, moon face, hirsutism, and plethora—have been well known since Cushing's initial descriptions in 1912 and 1932 (Figs. 15-15, 15-16, and 15-17). However, this gross clinical picture is not always present, and a high index of suspicion is required in many cases. Once the

Figure 15-15 Minnie G., Cushing's index patient, at age 23 years. (From Cushing H. The basophil adenomas of the pituitary body and their clinical manifestations [pituitary basophilism]. *Bull Johns Hopkins Hosp.* 1932; 50:137-195.)

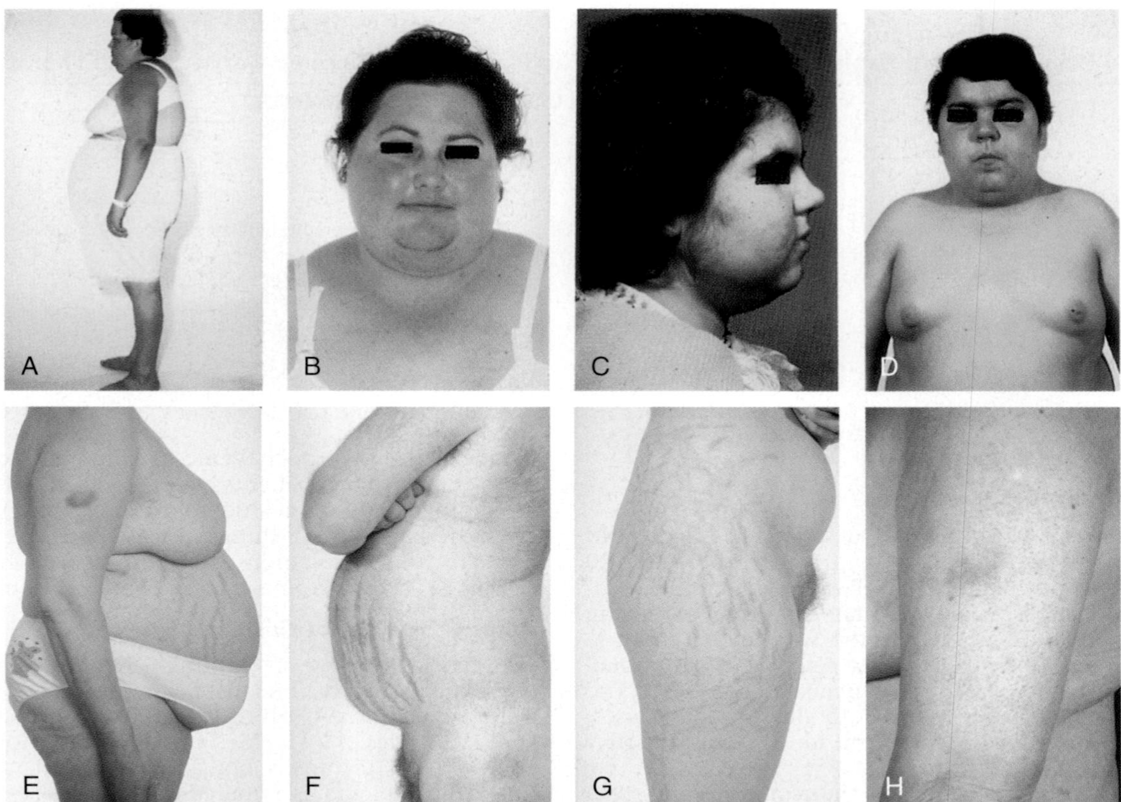

Figure 15-16 Clinical features of Cushing's syndrome. **A,** Centripetal and some generalized obesity and dorsal kyphosis in a 30-year-old woman with Cushing's disease. **B,** Same patient as in **A,** showing moon facies, plethora, hirsutism, and enlarged supraclavicular fat pads. **C,** Facial rounding, hirsutism, and acne in a 14-year-old girl with Cushing's disease. **D,** Central and generalized obesity and moon facies in a 14-year-old boy with Cushing's disease. **E** and **F,** Typical centripetal obesity with livid abdominal striae seen in a 41-year-old woman **(E)** and a 40-year-old man **(F)** with Cushing's syndrome. **G,** Striae in a 24-year-old patient with congenital adrenal hyperplasia treated with excessive doses of dexamethasone as replacement therapy. **H,** Typical bruising and thin skin of a patient with Cushing's syndrome. In this case, the bruising occurred without obvious injury.

normal physiologic effects of glucocorticoids are appreciated (see Fig. 15-13), the clinical features of glucocorticoid excess are easier to define. These are summarized in Table 15-10 together with the most discriminatory features that will assist in distinguishing Cushing's syndrome from simple obesity.[181,182]

Obesity. Weight gain and obesity are the most common signs of Cushing's syndrome. At least in adults, this weight gain is invariably centripetal in nature.[143,183] In fact, generalized obesity is more common in the general population than it is in patients with Cushing's syndrome. One exception is in pediatric patients, in whom glucocorticoid excess may result in generalized obesity. In addition to centripetal obesity, patients develop fat depots over the thoracocervical spine (buffalo hump), in the supraclavicular region, and over the cheeks and temporal regions, giving rise to the rounded, moon-like facies. The epidural space, another site of abnormal fat deposition, may lead to neurologic deficits.

Reproductive Organs. Gonadal dysfunction is common, with menstrual irregularity in females and loss of libido in both sexes. Hirsutism is frequently found in female patients, as is acne. The most common form of hirsutism is vellus hypertrichosis on the face; this should be distinguished from the darker, terminal differentiated hirsutism that may occur because of ACTH-mediated adrenal androgen excess. Hypogonadotropic hypogonadism occurs because of a direct inhibitory effect of cortisol on GnRH pulsatility and LH/FSH secretion, and it is reversible on correction of the hypercortisolism.[184,185]

Psychiatric Features. Psychiatric abnormalities occur in approximately 50% of patients with Cushing's syndrome, regardless of cause.[186,187] Agitated depression and lethargy are among the most common problems, but paranoia and overt psychosis are also well recognized. Memory and cognitive function may also be affected, and increased irritability may be an early feature. Insomnia is common, and both rapid eye movement and delta-wave sleep patterns are reduced.[188] Lowering of plasma cortisol by medical or surgical therapy usually results in a rapid improvement in the psychiatric state. Overall quality of life is significantly reduced in patients with Cushing's syndrome, particularly affecting physical health and functioning. Quality-of-life scores improve after treatment but do not return to normal.[189]

Bone. In childhood, the most common presentation is with poor linear growth and weight gain[149]; as discussed earlier, glucocorticoids have profound effects on growth and development.[165] Many patients with longstanding Cushing's syndrome have lost height because of osteoporotic vertebral collapse. This can be assessed by measuring the patient's sitting height or comparing the height with arm span; in normal subjects, height and arm span should be equal. Pathologic fractures, occurring spontaneously or

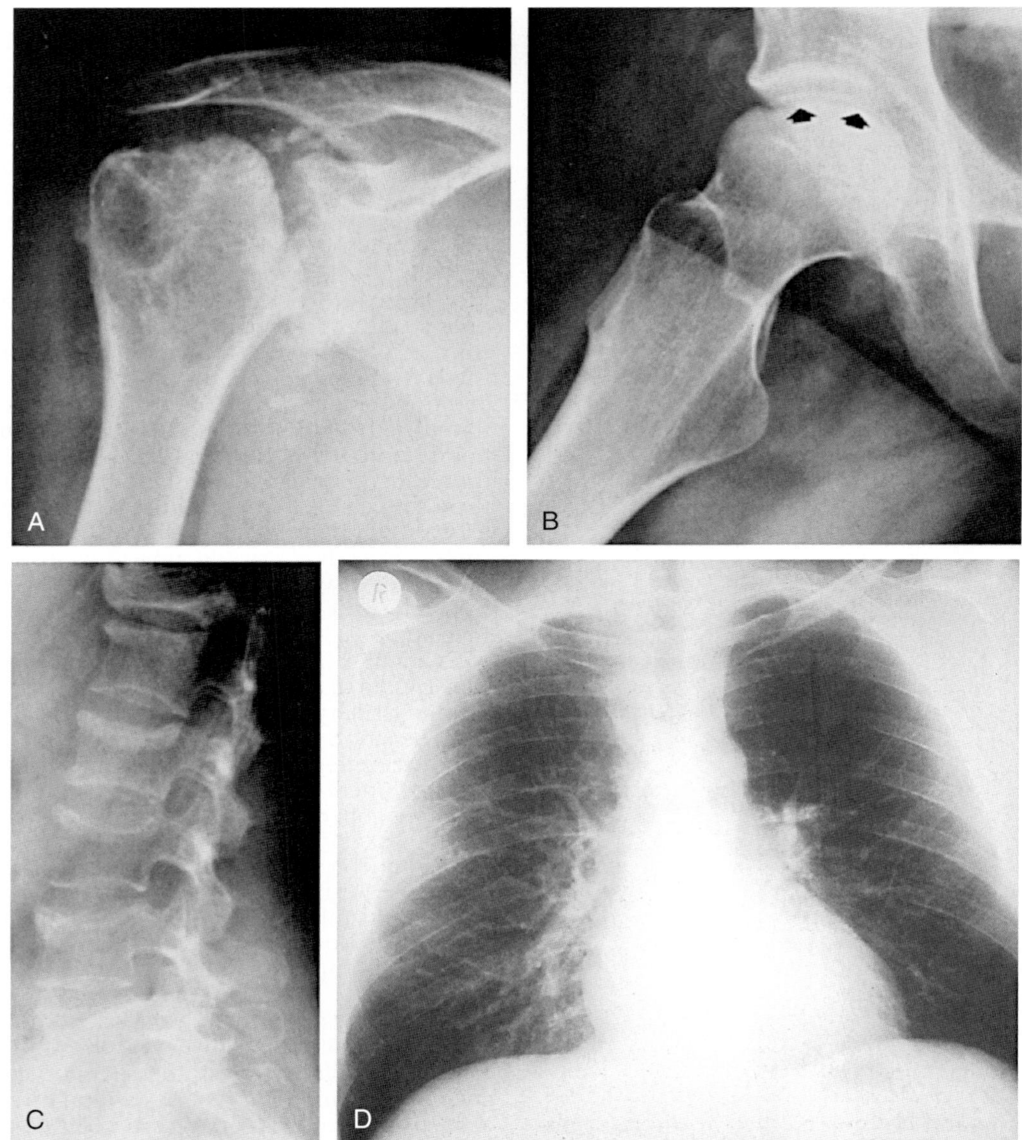

Figure 15-17 Bone abnormalities in Cushing's disease. **A,** Aseptic necrosis of the right humeral head in a 43-year-old woman with Cushing's disease of about 8 months' duration. **B,** Aseptic necrosis of the right femoral head in a 24-year-old woman with Cushing's disease of about 4½ years' duration. The *arrows* indicate the crescent subchondral radiolucency, best seen in this lateral view. **C,** Diffuse osteoporosis, vertebral collapse, and subchondral sclerosis in the same patient as in **A. D,** Rib fracture in a 38-year-old man with Cushing's disease. (**A** through **C**, from Phillips KA, Nance EP Jr, Rodriguez RM, et al. Avascular necrosis of bone: a manifestation of Cushing's disease. *South Med J.* 1986;79:825-829.)

after minor trauma, are not uncommon. Rib fractures, in contrast to those of the vertebrae, are often painless. The radiographic appearance is typical, with exuberant callus formation at the site of the healing fracture. In addition, osteonecrosis of the femoral and humeral heads is a recognized feature of endogenous Cushing's syndrome (see Fig. 15-17). Hypercalciuria may lead to renal calculi, but hypercalcemia is not a feature.

Skin. Hypercortisolism results in thinning of the skin and separation and exposure of the subcutaneous vascular tissue. On examination, wrinkling of the skin on the dorsum of the hand may be seen, resulting in a "cigarette paper" appearance (Liddle's sign). Minimal trauma may result in bruising, which frequently resembles the appearance of senile purpura. The plethoric appearance of the patient with Cushing's syndrome is secondary to the thinning of the skin[190] combined with loss of facial subcutaneous fat and is not caused by true polycythemia. Acne and papular lesions may occur over the face, chest, and back.

The typical, almost pathognomic, red-purple livid striae greater than 1 cm in width are most frequently found on the abdomen but may also be present on the upper thighs, breasts, and arms. They are very common in younger patients and less so in those older than 50 years of age. They must be differentiated from the paler, less pigmented striae that occur as a result of pregnancy (striae gravidarum) or in association with rapid weight loss.

Skin pigmentation is rare in Cushing's disease but common in the ectopic ACTH syndrome. It arises because of overstimulation of melanocyte receptors by POMC-derived peptides.

TABLE 15-10

Prevalence of Symptoms and Signs in Cushing's Syndrome and Discriminant Index Compared with Prevalence of Features in Patients with Simple Obesity

Findings	% of Patients	Discriminant Index
Symptoms		
Weight gain	91	
Menstrual irregularity	84	1.6
Hirsutism	81	2.8
Psychiatric dysfunction	62	
Backache	43	
Muscle weakness	29	8.0
Fractures	19	
Loss of scalp hair	13	
Signs		
Obesity	97	
Truncal	46	1.6
Generalized	55	0.8
Plethora	94	3.0
Moon facies	88	
Hypertension	74	4.4
Bruising	62	10.3
Red-purple striae	56	2.5
Muscle weakness	56	
Ankle edema	50	
Pigmentation	4	
Other Findings		
Hypertension	74	
Diabetes	50	
Overt	13	
Impaired glucose tolerance test	37	
Osteoporosis	50	
Renal calculi	15	

Data from Ross EJ, Linch DC. Cushing's syndrome-killing disease: discriminatory value of signs and symptoms aiding early diagnosis. *Lancet*. 1982;2:646-649.

Muscle. Myopathy and bruising are two of the most discriminatory features of the syndrome.[181] The myopathy of Cushing's syndrome involves the proximal muscles of the lower limbs and the shoulder girdle.[191] Complaints of weakness, such as inability to climb stairs or get up from a deep chair, are relatively uncommon, but testing for proximal myopathy by asking the patient to rise from a crouching position often reveals the problem.

Cardiovascular. Hypertension is another prominent feature, occurring in up to 75% of cases. Even though epidemiologic data show a strong association between blood pressure and obesity, hypertension is much more common in patients with Cushing's syndrome than in those with simple obesity.[152] This, together with the established metabolic consequences of the disease (diabetes, hyperlipidemia), is thought to explain the increased cardiovascular mortality in untreated cases.[192-194] Cardiovascular events are also more common in patients with presumed iatrogenic Cushing's syndrome resulting from prescribed corticosteroids.[170] In addition, thromboembolic events may be more common in Cushing's patients.

Infections. Infections are more common in patients with Cushing's syndrome.[195,196] In many instances, infections are asymptomatic and occur because the normal inflammatory response is suppressed. Reactivation of tuberculosis has been reported[197] and has even been the presenting feature in some cases. Fungal infections of the skin (notably tinea versicolor) and nails may occur, as may opportunistic fungal infections. Bowel perforation is more common in patients with extreme hypercortisolism, and the hypercortisolism may mask the usual symptoms and signs of the condition. Wound infections are more common and contribute to poor wound healing.

Metabolic and Endocrine Features. Glucose intolerance occurs, and overt diabetes mellitus is present in up to one third of patients in some series. Hepatic lipoprotein synthesis is stimulated, and increases in circulating cholesterol and triglycerides may be found.[198] Hypokalemic alkalosis is found in 10% to 15% of patients with Cushing's disease but in more than 95% of patients with ectopic ACTH syndrome. Several factors may contribute to this mineralocorticoid excess state, including corticosterone and DOC excess, but the principal culprit is thought to be cortisol itself. Depending on the prevailing cortisol production rate, cortisol swamps HSD11B2 in the kidney and acts as a mineralocorticoid. Hypokalemic alkalosis is more common in ectopic ACTH syndrome because cortisol production rates are higher than in patients with Cushing's disease.[130] This can be diagnosed by documenting an increase in the ratio of urinary cortisol to cortisone metabolites. In addition, hepatic 5α-reductase activity is inhibited, resulting in a greater excretion of 5α-cortisol metabolites.[199]

The functions of the pituitary-thyroid axis and the pituitary-gonadal axis are suppressed in patients with Cushing's syndrome because of a direct effect of cortisol on TSH and gonadotropin secretion.[200,201] Cortisol causes a reversible form of hypogonadotropic hypogonadism but also directly inhibits Leydig cell function. Growth hormone secretion is reduced, possibly mediated through an increase in somatostatinergic tone.

Eye. Ocular effects include raised intraocular pressure[202] and exophthalmos[203] (in up to one third of patients in Cushing's original series), the latter occurring because of increased retroorbital fat deposition. Cataracts, a well-recognized complication of corticosteroid therapy, seem to be uncommon,[204] except as a complication of diabetes. In our experience, chemosis is a sensitive and underreported feature of Cushing's syndrome.

CLASSIFICATION AND PATHOPHYSIOLOGY OF CUSHING'S SYNDROME

Cushing's syndrome is most readily classified into ACTH-dependent and ACTH-independent causes (Table 15-11).

ACTH-Dependent Causes

Cushing's Disease

When iatrogenic causes are excluded, the most common cause of Cushing's syndrome is Cushing's disease, accounting for approximately 70% of cases. The adrenal glands in these patients show bilateral adrenocortical hyperplasia with widening of the ZF and ZR.[182]

Cushing himself raised the question as to whether this disease was a primary pituitary condition or secondary to an abnormality in the hypothalamus, and there has been

TABLE 15-11

Classification of Causes of Cushing's Syndrome

ACTH-Dependent Causes
Cushing's disease (pituitary-dependent)
Ectopic ACTH syndrome
Ectopic CRH syndrome
Macronodular adrenal hyperplasia
Iatrogenic (treatment with 1-24 ACTH)
ACTH-Independent Causes
Adrenal adenoma and carcinoma
Primary pigmented nodular adrenal hyperplasia and Carney's syndrome.
McCune-Albright syndrome
Aberrant receptor expression (gastric inhibitory polypeptide, interleukin-1β)
Iatrogenic (e.g., pharmacologic doses of prednisolone, dexamethasone)
Pseudo-Cushing's Syndromes
Alcoholism
Depression
Obesity

ACTH, adrenocorticotrophic hormone; CRH, corticotropin-releasing hormone.

an ongoing debate on this issue ever since.[205] The hypothalamic theory states that ACTH-secreting adenomas arise because of dysfunctional regulation of corticotrophs through chronic stimulation by CRH (or AVP). Other studies provide data to support a primary pituitary defect as the cause of the condition (Table 15-12).

The hypothalamus may have an initiating role, but the overwhelming evidence is that, at presentation, the condition is pituitary dependent. In 85% to 90% of cases, the disease is caused by a pituitary adenoma of monoclonal origin[206,207]; basophil hyperplasia alone is found in 9% to 33% of pathologic series.[205] The majority of tumors are small microadenomas (<1 cm), but larger macroadenomas occur in up to 10% of cases and usually signify a more invasive tumor.[208] Selective surgical removal of a microadenoma results in cure with a very low recurrence rate. However, it is possible, particularly in cases with no identifiable pituitary adenoma, that Cushing's disease is heterogeneous with different subtypes.

A key biochemical hallmark of the disease is a relative resistance of ACTH secretion to normal glucocorticoid feedback inhibition.[209] ACTH-secreting pituitary adenomas function at a higher than normal set point for cortisol feedback. The predominant finding in Cushing's disease is an increase in ACTH pulse amplitude with loss of normal circadian rhythm, but ACTH pulse frequency is also increased in some cases (see Fig. 15-8).[210]

TABLE 15-12

Etiology of Cushing's Disease: Hypothalamic Theory Versus Pituitary Theory

Hypothalamic Theory	Pituitary Theory
Neuroendocrine abnormalities[282,283]	Lack of "cure" after pituitary stalk section
Loss of circadian rhythm, sleep disturbance, other "hypothalamic defects" (TSH, LH/FSH secretion)	Circulating and CSF CRH levels are suppressed.[284]
	Reversal of "hypothalamic defects" on correction of hypercortisolism
Efficacy of centrally acting drugs[285,286] (bromocriptine, cyproheptadine, sodium valproate)	High surgical cure rate (recurrences resulting from regrowth of inadequately resected tumor rather than "real" recurrence)[287,289]
Recurrences after pituitary surgery	Secondary hypoadrenalism after successful pituitary surgery (may be prolonged and associated with reduced ACTH expression in surrounding adjacent normal corticotrophs)[290]
Ectopic CRH-secreting tumors cause Cushing's disease,[281] but pathology shows basophil hyperplasia, not adenomas.	
	Pituitary ACTH-secreting adenoma in almost 90% of cases are monoclonal in origin.[291,292]

ACTH, adrenocorticotropic hormone; CRH, corticotropin-releasing hormone; CSF, cerebrospinal fluid; FSH, follicle-stimulating hormone; LH, luteinizing hormone; TSH, thyroid-stimulating hormone.

Ectopic ACTH Syndrome

In 15% of cases, Cushing's syndrome is associated with nonpituitary tumors secreting ACTH—the ectopic ACTH syndrome.[211-215] On clinical grounds, these can be divided into two entities: cases occurring in the setting of highly malignant tumors such as small-cell carcinoma of bronchus (Table 15-13) and more indolent cases occurring in patients with underlying neuroendocrine tumors such as bronchial carcinoids. In the former group, the clinical presentation more commonly resembles Addison's disease than Cushing's syndrome. Circulating ACTH concentrations and cortisol secretion rates can be extremely high. As a result, duration of symptoms from onset to presentation is short (<3 months); patients are commonly pigmented, and the metabolic manifestations of glucocorticoid excess are often rapid and progressive. Weight loss, myopathy, and glucose intolerance are prominent symptoms and signs. The association of these features with hypokalemic alkalosis and peripheral edema should alert the clinician to the diagnosis.

Depending on local referral practice, approximately 20% of cases of ectopic ACTH syndrome are explained by indolent tumors, such as benign bronchial carcinoids, that produce ACTH.[215,216] In these cases, symptoms and signs are commonly present for 18 months before clinical presentation. Such patients present with the typical features of Cushing's syndrome and may be biochemically similar to patients with Cushing's disease. Therefore, once a diagnosis of Cushing's syndrome is established, the principal diagnostic dilemma is in the distinction of pituitary-dependent Cushing's disease from these indolent causes of ectopic ACTH syndrome.[212,214]

POMC is expressed in some normal extrapituitary tissues and in many tumors (lung, testis) regardless of the presence of Cushing's syndrome, raising the appropriateness of the

TABLE 15-13

Tumors Associated with the Ectopic Adrenocorticotropic Hormone Syndrome

Tumor Type	Approximate Incidence (%)
Small-cell lung carcinoma	50
Non–small-cell lung carcinoma	5
Pancreatic tumors (including carcinoids)	10
Thymic tumors (including carcinoids)	5
Lung carcinoids	10
Other carcinoids	2
Medullary carcinoma of thyroid	5
Pheochromocytoma and related tumors	3
Rare carcinomas of prostate, breast, ovary, gallbladder, colon	10

designation "ectopic" ACTH syndrome.[217] Tumors most commonly associated with ectopic ACTH syndrome arise from neuroendocrine tissues, the cells of which possess the ability to uptake and decarboxylate amine precursors (APUD cells). However, only 0.5% to 1% of tumors in small-cell lung cancer are associated with ectopic ACTH syndrome, and the explanation for the development of ectopic ACTH secretion remains unclear. POMC mRNA transcripts are usually shorter in tumors not associated with ectopic ACTH syndrome, whereas those with the syndrome express larger POMC mRNA species as well as the "pituitary-size" transcript. In addition to aberrant transcriptional regulation of the POMC gene, interaction with tissue-specific transcription factors or methylation status of the POMC gene may be involved. Once secreted, POMC is cleaved in the pituitary by specific serine endoproteases to produce ACTH precursors; in ectopic ACTH syndrome, aberrant peripheral processing of POMC may lead to increased concentrations of circulating ACTH precursors (pro-ACTH, N-POC) (see Fig. 15-6). In contrast to ACTH secretion from pituitary adenomas, ectopic POMC/ACTH production is not responsive to normal glucocorticoid feedback[217] because of the defective GR or GR-signaling mechanism.[218] However, this sensitivity to glucocorticoid feedback is far from clearcut, which is one reason why the differential diagnosis of ACTH-dependent Cushing's syndrome can be challenging.[212]

Ectopic Corticotropin-Releasing Hormone Syndrome

Ectopic production of CRH is a very rare cause of pituitary-dependent Cushing's. A number of cases have now been described in which a tumor (usually bronchial carcinoid, medullary thyroid, or prostate carcinoma) has been shown to secrete CRH alone or in combination with ACTH.[215,219-221] Where available, pituitary histology has revealed corticotroph hyperplasia but not adenoma formation. Biochemically, these patients, like those with ectopic ACTH syndrome, lose the normal negative glucocorticoid feedback mechanism—50% have resistance to high-dose dexamethasone therapy. Ectopic CRH production may explain the suppression of cortisol secretion after high-dose dexamethasone that is observed in some patients with the "ectopic" ACTH syndrome.

Macronodular Adrenal Hyperplasia

In 10% to 40% of patients with Cushing's disease, there is bilateral adrenocortical hyperplasia associated with one or more nodules, which may be up to several centimeters in diameter.[222-225] Patients tend to be older and to have had symptoms for a longer time, but they otherwise present with the classic clinical features of Cushing's syndrome. Pathologically, the nodules are lobulated and can be markedly enlarged, but internodular hyperplasia is invariably found. Macronodular adrenal hyperplasia (MAH) is thought to result from long-standing adrenal ACTH stimulation, which leads to autonomous adrenal adenoma formation. Therefore, as the adrenals in a patient with Cushing's disease become more hyperplastic, they secrete more cortisol for a given ACTH level, which ultimately can lead to autosuppression. Individual clinical cases support this hypothesis, and MAH should be regarded as an ACTH-dependent form of Cushing's syndrome, even though ACTH levels may be relatively low and dexamethasone suppressibility less marked than in other cases of Cushing's disease.[226] The adenomas can be a trap for the unwary because they may be mistaken for primary adrenal tumors.

ACTH-Independent Causes

Cortisol-Secreting Adrenal Adenoma and Carcinoma

Excluding iatrogenic cases, adrenal adenomas are responsible for about 10% to 15% of Cushing's syndrome cases, and carcinomas for less than 5%. By contrast, 65% of cases of Cushing's syndrome in children have an adrenal etiology (15% adenomas, 50% carcinomas).[224-226] Onset of clinical features is gradual in patients with adenomas, but it is often rapid in adrenal carcinoma. In addition to the features of hypercortisolism, patients may complain of loin or abdominal pain, and a tumor may be palpable. The tumor may secrete other steroids, such as androgens or mineralocorticoids. Therefore, in females, there may be features of virilization, with hirsutism, clitoromegaly, breast atrophy, deepening of the voice, temporal recession, and severe acne. In "pure" cortisol-secreting adenomas, hirsutism is uncommon. Subclinical Cushing's syndrome has been reported in up to 10% of patients with adrenal "incidentalomas" (see later discussion).

Primary Pigmented Nodular Adrenal Hyperplasia and Carney's Syndrome

About 100 cases of ACTH-independent Cushing's syndrome have been reported in association with bilateral, small, pigmented adrenal nodules. Pathologically, these nodules are usually 2 to 4 mm in diameter (although they can be larger) and black or brown on cut section. Adjacent adrenal tissue is atrophic, distinguishing this primary pigmented nodular adrenal hyperplasia (PPNAD) from MAH. Presentation is with typical features of Cushing's syndrome in persons younger than 30 years of age and, in 50% of cases, in persons younger than 15 years of age.[227] Cases of PPNAD have been reported without Cushing's syndrome. Bilateral adrenalectomy is curative.

A familial autosomal dominant variant, called *Carney's complex* (Table 15-14), comprises mesenchymal tumors (especially atrial myxomas), spotty skin pigmentation, peripheral nerve tumors, and various other tumors including breast lesions, testicular tumors, and GH-secreting pituitary tumors.[228] Mutations of the gene encoding the protein kinase A (PKA) regulatory subunit type IA (*PRKAR1A*) lead

TABLE 15-14

Clinical Features of the Carney Complex

Feature	Prevalence (%)
Skin lesions	80
Pigmented lesions	
Blue nevi	
Cutaneous myxomas	
Cardiac myxomas	72
Pigmented nodular adrenal hyperplasia	45
Breast lesions	
Bilateral fibroadenomas	45 (females only)
Testicular tumors	56 (males only)
Pituitary lesions, usually growth hormone-secreting	10
Neural lesions (gastric schwannomas)	<5
Miscellaneous	
Thyroid cancers	Rare
Acoustic neuromas	Rare
Hepatomas	Rare

to abnormal PKA signaling and explain the phenotype in some cases.[229] Other cases have been mapped to chromosome 2p16, but the underlying genetic mutation is unknown.

McCune-Albright Syndrome

In McCune-Albright syndrome, fibrous dysplasia and cutaneous pigmentation may be associated with pituitary, thyroid, adrenal, and gonadal hyperfunction. The most common manifestation is with sexual precocity and GH excess, but Cushing's syndrome has been reported.[230] The underlying abnormality is a somatic mutation in the α-subunit of the stimulatory G protein, which is linked to adenyl cyclase. The mutation results in constitutive activation of the G protein, mimicking constant ACTH stimulation at the level of the adrenal. ACTH levels are suppressed, and adrenal adenomas may occur.

Macronodular Hyperplasia and Aberrant Receptor Expression

Although MAH commonly occurs in patients with ACTH-dependent Cushing's syndrome, truly ACTH-independent macronodular hyperplasia (AIMAH) is also recognized as a distinct entity.[231] The nodules are nonpigmented and greater than 5 mm in diameter; occasionally, the adrenals are massively enlarged. Most cases are explained on the basis of aberrant receptor expression within the adrenal cortex.[232] Food-induced hypercortisolism due to enhanced adrenal responsiveness to gastric inhibitory polypeptide (GIP) was the first cause of AIMAH described, due to expression of GIP receptors within the adrenal cortex, but aberrant expression of the vasopressin V_1, β-adrenergic, LH, serotonin, and angiotensin (AT_1) receptors have also been linked to AIMAH. Protocols have been suggested for the further investigation of AIMAH.[232]

Iatrogenic Cushing's Syndrome

The basis for iatrogenic Cushing's syndrome was discussed earlier. Development of the features of Cushing's syndrome depends on the dose, duration, and potency of the corticosteroids used in clinical practice. ACTH is rarely prescribed, but it will also result in cushingoid features if administered long-term. Some features, such as an increase in intraocular pressure, cataracts, benign intracranial hypertension, aseptic necrosis of the femoral head, osteoporosis, and pancreatitis, are more common in iatrogenic than endogenous Cushing's syndrome, whereas other features, notably hypertension, hirsutism, and oligomenorrhea/amenorrhea, are less prevalent.

Special Features of Cushing's Syndrome

Cyclic Cushing's Syndrome

Of particular clinical interest has been a group of patients with cyclic Cushing's syndrome, characterized by periods of excess cortisol production interspersed with intervals of normal cortisol production (Fig. 15-18). Some of these patients demonstrate a paradoxical rise in plasma ACTH and cortisol when treated with dexamethasone, and occasionally a patient is benefited by dopamine agonist (bromocriptine) or serotonin antagonist (cyproheptadine) therapy. Most patients have been thought to have pituitary-dependent disease, and in many of these patients, basophil adenomas have been removed, with long-term cure in some cases. However, cortisol secretion may show some evidence of cyclicity in patients with an ectopic source of ACTH.[233,234]

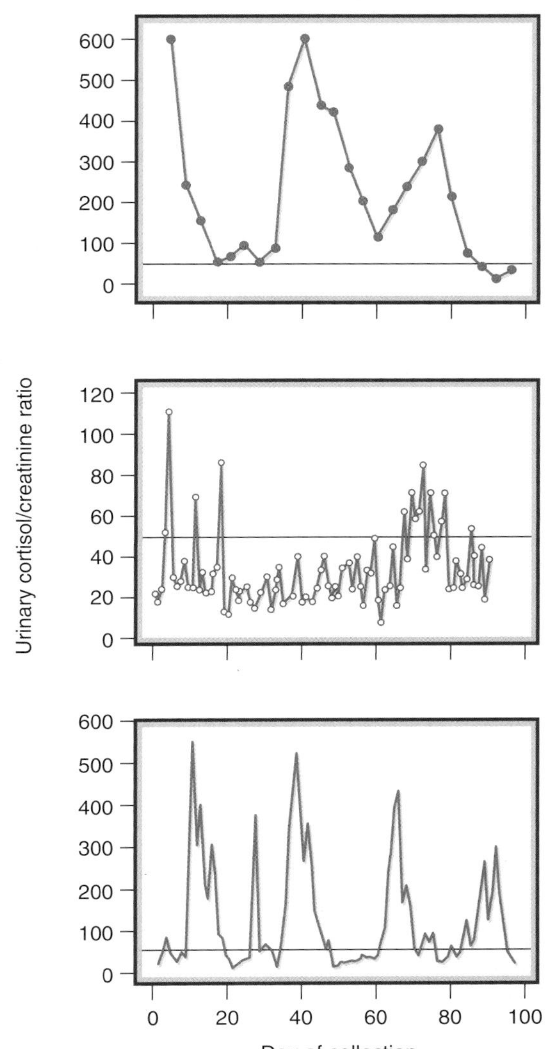

Figure 15-18 Patterns of cortisol secretion in three patients with cyclic Cushing's syndrome. In each case, the ratio of early-morning urinary cortisol (in nanomoles per liter) to creatinine (in millimoles per liter) are plotted against time. Variable periodicity in cortisol hypersecretion is shown. (From Atkinson AB, McCance DR, Kennedy L, et al. Cyclical Cushing's syndrome first diagnosed after pituitary surgery: a trap for the unwary. *Clin Endocrinol.* 1992;36:297-299.)

Children

Cushing's syndrome can occur at any age, but the causes differ across age groups (Fig. 15-19). In children, adrenal causes account for 65% of all cases, and in addition to the previously mentioned features, growth arrest is almost invariable.[235] The dissociation between height and weight is obvious, with the height most commonly below the mean, whereas the body mass index (BMI) is almost always above the mean. If the height and weight are increasing along the same percentile line, then the diagnosis of Cushing's syndrome is highly unlikely. Obesity in childhood Cushing's tends to be generalized. Most patients have a delayed bone age that is negatively correlated with height standard deviation score (SDS), duration of symptoms, and age at diagnosis. The observed growth failure often precedes other manifestations such as weight gain, pubertal arrest, fatigue, depression, hypertension, and acne. Pubertal development can be advanced in patients with virilizing

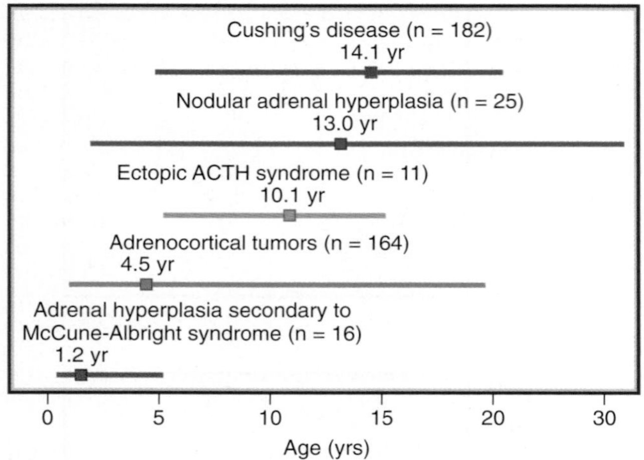

Figure 15-19 Etiology and age-dependency of pediatric Cushing's syndrome. (From Storr HL, Chan LF, Grossman AB, et al. Paediatric Cushing's syndrome: epidemiology, investigation and therapeutic advances. *Trends Endocrinol Metab.* 2007;18:167-174.)

tumors causing precocious pseudopuberty. However, in patients with true puberty, glucocorticoid-mediated suppression of gonadotropins may occur.[236]

Glucocorticoid excess influences not only the hypothalamic-pituitary-gonadal axis but also the GH-IGF1 axis, leading to both reduction of spontaneous GH secretion and pharmacologic GH response. Furthermore, direct effects of glucocorticoids on epiphyseal chrondocytes, probably together with disturbance of microvascularization of the growth plate, result in a negative effect on growth. Poor catch-up has been reported in children after cure of Cushing's disease, and evidence exists for GH inhibition by hypercortisolemia for 1 to 2 years after cure of Cushing's disease. GH secretion should be assessed 3 months after treatment. If GH deficiency is demonstrated, GH in a replacement dose of 25 μg/kg per day should be given. Catch-up growth is observed in most patients and target adult height is achieved. However, many patients remain obese.

Pregnancy

Pregnancy is rare in women with Cushing's syndrome because of associated amenorrhea due to androgen excess or hypercortisolism. However, pregnancy has been reported in approximately 100 such women, 50% of whom had adrenal adenomas.[237] A few cases of true pregnancy-induced Cushing's syndrome have been described, with regression after delivery.[238] In these cases, the etiology is unknown. Establishing a diagnosis and a cause can be difficult. Clinically, striae, hypertension, and gestational diabetes are common features in normal pregnancies, yet hypertension and diabetes are also the most common signs of Cushing's syndrome in a pregnant woman (70% and 30%, of all cases, respectively). Furthermore, biochemically normal pregnancy is associated with a threefold increase in plasma cortisol due to increased production of cortisol and cortisol-binding globulin. Urinary free cortisol also rises, and dexamethasone does not suppress plasma cortisol to the same degree as the nonpregnant state. Left untreated, the condition is associated with high maternal and fetal morbidity and mortality. Any adrenal or pituitary adenomas should be excised. Metyrapone, which is not teratogenic, has been effective in many cases in controlling the hypercortisolism.

Pseudo-Cushing's Syndromes

A pseudo-Cushing's state can be defined as the presence of some or all of the clinical features of Cushing's syndrome together with some evidence for hypercortisolism. Resolution of the underlying cause results in disappearance of the cushingoid state. Several causes are described.

Alcohol

In the original description of alcohol-related pseudo-Cushing's syndrome, urinary and plasma cortisol levels were elevated and failed to suppress with dexamethasone. Plasma ACTH has been found to be normal or suppressed. The condition is rare but should be suspected in a patient with an ongoing history of heavy alcohol intake and biochemical or clinical evidence of chronic liver disease.[239] The pathogenesis of this condition remains unknown, but a two-hit hypothesis has been put forward. Chronic liver disease of any cause is associated with impaired cortisol metabolism, but in alcoholic patients there is an increased cortisol secretion rate, rather than concomitant suppression in the face of impaired metabolism.[240] In some studies, alcohol has directly stimulated cortisol secretion; alternatively, AVP levels are elevated in patients with decompensated liver disease and may stimulate the HPA axis. With abstinence from alcohol, the biochemical abnormalities rapidly revert to normal.

Depression

Although the cause is unknown, it is recognized that patients with depression may exhibit the hormonal abnormalities of patients with Cushing's syndrome.[241] These abnormalities are reversible on correction of the psychiatric condition. Conversely, patients with Cushing's syndrome are frequently depressed, and a careful clinical and endocrinologic assessment is required.

Obesity

Although one of the most common referrals to a clinical endocrinologist is for exclusion of an underlying endocrine cause in a patient with obesity, the diagnosis of Cushing's syndrome in such patients should not cause difficulties. Patients with obesity have mildly increased cortisol secretion rates, and the data suggest that this is due to activation of the HPA axis.[242,243] However, circulating cortisol concentrations are invariably normal, and urinary free cortisol concentrations are either normal or only slightly elevated. The stimulus for the increased secretion of cortisol appears to be increased peripheral metabolism and clearance of cortisol—principally, reduced hepatic conversion of cortisone to cortisol by HSD11B1 and increased conversion of cortisol to 5α-reduced derivatives.[243]

Investigation of Patients with Suspected Cushing's Syndrome

There are two stages in the investigation of suspected Cushing's syndrome: (1) Does this patient have Cushing's syndrome? and (2) If the answer is "Yes," what is the cause? Unfortunately, many investigators fail to make this distinction and ill-advisedly use tests that are relevant to the second question in trying to answer the first question. In particular, it is essential that radiologic investigations not be undertaken until Cushing's syndrome has been confirmed biochemically. The major tests are listed in Table 15-15.[182,241,244,245]

TABLE 15-15

Tests Used in the Diagnosis and Differential Diagnosis of Cushing's Syndrome

Diagnosis—Does the Patient Have Cushing's Syndrome?
Circadian rhythm of plasma cortisol
Urinary free cortisol excretion*
Low-dose dexamethasone suppression test*
Differential Diagnosis—What Is the Cause of the Cushing's Syndrome?
Plasma ACTH
Plasma potassium, bicarbonate
High-dose dexamethasone suppression test
Metyrapone test
Corticotropin-releasing hormone
Inferior petrosal sinus sampling
CT, MRI scanning of pituitary, adrenals
Scintigraphy
Tumor markers

*Valuable outpatient screening tests (see text).
ACTH, Adrenocorticotropic hormone; CT, computed tomography; MRI, magnetic resonance imaging.

Question 1: "Does This Patient Have Cushing's Syndrome?"

Circadian Rhythm of Plasma Cortisol. In normal subjects, plasma cortisol levels are at their highest early in the morning and reach a nadir (<50 nmol/L [<2 μg/dL] in a nonstressed subject) at about midnight.[246] This circadian rhythm is lost in patients with Cushing's syndrome; in the majority, the 9 a.m. plasma cortisol is normal but nocturnal levels are raised. Random morning plasma cortisol levels are therefore of little value in making the diagnosis, whereas a midnight cortisol level greater than 200 nmol/L (>7.5 μg/dL) indicates Cushing's syndrome. However, various factors such as stress of venipuncture, intercurrent illness, and admission to hospital may lead to false-positive results. Ideally, patients should be hospitalized for 24 to 48 hours before the midnight cortisol level is measured, but some centers have reported discriminant results for midnight levels measured in outpatients.

Very few laboratories have developed methods for the measurement of free serum cortisol.[247] Because more than 90% of serum cortisol is protein bound, the results of the conventional assay are affected by drugs and by conditions that alter CBG levels. Estrogen therapy or pregnancy may elevate CBG and total serum cortisol. Loss of circadian rhythm is a sensitive diagnostic test, but for the reasons stated it is not a widely used screening test.

Salivary Cortisol. CBG is absent from saliva, and the use of salivary cortisol measurements offers a sensible alternative in that it does not require hospitalization. The diagnostic accuracy of a single midnight salivary cortisol level has been established in several studies: a cortisol value greater than 2.0 ng/mL (5.5 nmol/L) has a 100% sensitivity and a 96% specificity for diagnosis of Cushing's syndrome.[244,248,249]

Urinary Free Cortisol Excretion. For many years, the diagnosis of Cushing's syndrome was based on the measurement of urinary metabolites of cortisol (24-hour urinary 17-hydroxycorticosteroid or 17-oxogenic steroid excretion, depending on the method used). However, the sensitivity and specificity of these methods is poor, and most centers have replaced these assays with the more sensitive measurement of urinary free cortisol. This is an integrated measure of plasma free cortisol: as cortisol secretion increases, the binding capacity of CBG is exceeded, resulting in a disproportionate rise in urinary free cortisol. Normal values are less than 220 to 330 nmol/24 hours (80 to 120 μg/24 hours), depending on the assay used. Patients should make two or three complete consecutive collections to account for patient error in collecting samples and for episodic cortisol secretion, notably from adrenal adenomas. Simultaneous creatinine excretion (which differs by no more than 10% from day to day) may be used to ensure adequacy of collection. Urinary free cortisol is a useful screening test, although it is accepted that the value can be normal in up to 8% to 15% of patients with Cushing's syndrome.[244,245,250] Conversely, moderately elevated results should always be verified by further testing before a diagnosis of Cushing's syndrome is made.

Measurement of the cortisol-to-creatinine ratio in the first urine specimen passed on waking obviates the need for a timed collection and has been used as a screening test, particularly when cyclic Cushing's syndrome is suspected.[251] Urine aliquots may be sent to the local endocrinology laboratory, with cortisol-to-creatinine ratios greater than 25 nmol/mmol on repeated measurement being indicative of hypercortisolism.

Low-Dose Overnight Dexamethasone Suppression Tests. In normal subjects, the administration of a supraphysiologic dose of glucocorticoid results in suppression of ACTH and cortisol secretion. In Cushing's syndrome of whatever cause, there is a failure of this suppression when low doses of the synthetic glucocorticoid dexamethasone are given.[209]

The overnight test is a useful outpatient screening test.[241,244,252] Various doses of dexamethasone have been used, but usually 1 mg of dexamethasone is given at midnight. A normal response is a plasma cortisol level of less than 140 nmol/L (<5 μg/dL) between 8 and 9 a.m. the following morning. A dose of 1.5 or 2 mg gives a 30% false-positive rate, but after a dose of 1 mg this rate is only 12.5%, with a false-negative rate of less than 2%. In addition, sensitivity can be improved by reducing the plasma cortisol cut-off value: a postdexamethasone cortisol value of less than 50 nmol/L (<2 μg/dL) effectively excludes Cushing's syndrome. Therefore, the outpatient overnight test has high sensitivity (95%) but low specificity, and further investigation is often required.[253,254]

In the 48-hour low-dose dexamethasone test, plasma cortisol is measured at 9 a.m. on day 0 and again 48 hours later, after administration of dexamethasone 0.5 mg every 6 hours for 48 hours. Using a postdexamethasone plasma cortisol concentration of less than 50 nmol/L (<2 μg/dL) as the cutoff point, this test is reported to have a 97% to 100% true-positive rate and a false-positive rate of less than 1%.[241,253] Sensitivity is higher if plasma rather than urinary cortisol is measured.

Certain drugs (e.g., phenytoin, rifampicin) may increase the metabolic clearance rate of dexamethasone, leading to false-positive results. Simultaneous measurement of plasma dexamethasone may be useful in such cases and will also detect whether patients failed to take the drug.[254]

Pseudo-Cushing's or True Cushing's Syndrome? In patients with depression, urinary free cortisol concentrations may be elevated and may overlap with those seen in patients with true Cushing's syndrome. Compared with patients with Cushing's disease, depressed patients have greater suppressibility after dexamethasone and reduced response to CRH, but neither of these tests is diagnostic.[241,255] However, use of a CRH test after the standard 2-day low-dose dexamethasone suppression test has been reported to separate true from pseudo-Cushing's syndrome. In normal subjects and in patients with endogenous depression, insulin-induced hypoglycemia results in a rise in ACTH and cortisol levels, a response that usually is not seen in patients with Cushing's syndrome. Finally, loperamide lowers cortisol values in patients with pseudo-Cushing's but not in those with true Cushing's syndrome.[241]

Clinical Guidelines. The Endocrine Society, in collaboration with the European Society for Endocrinology, has issued evidence-based guidelines for the diagnosis of Cushing's syndrome.[256] Recommendations are to proceed initially with one of four highly sensitive screening tests: urinary free cortisol, late-night salivary cortisol, long overnight dexamethasone, or the 2-mg/48-hour dexamethasone screening test. Abnormality detected by of any of these tests in a patient with clinically suspected Cushing's syndrome should be confirmed with one of the additional tests; if both test results are abnormal, patients should then undergo testing for the cause of the Cushing's syndrome (Fig. 15-20).

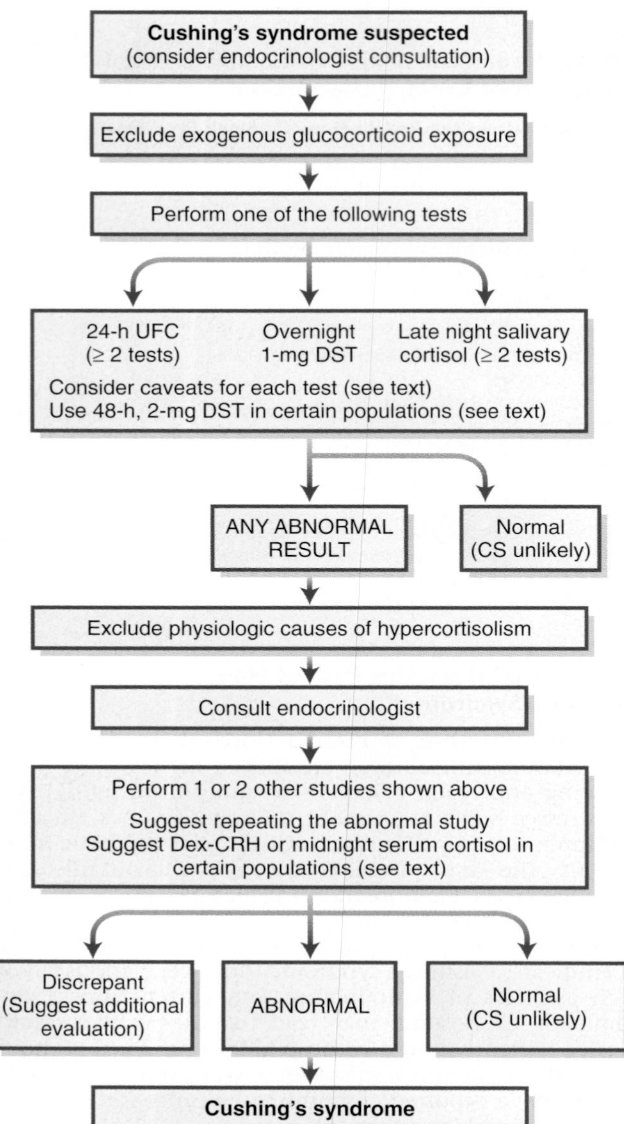

Figure 15-20 Algorithm for testing patients with suspected Cushing's syndrome (CS) according to the 2008 Endocrine Society clinical practice guideline. All statements are recommendations except for those prefaced by the word "Suggest." Diagnostic criteria that point to Cushing's syndrome are a urinary free cortisol (UFC) value greater than the normal range for the assay, a serum cortisol level greater than 1.8 μg/dL (>50 nmol/L) after administration of 1 mg dexamethasone (1-mg DST), and a late-night salivary cortisol concentration greater than 145 ng/dL (>4 nmol/L). CRH, corticotropin-releasing hormone; Dex, dexamethasone; DST, dexamethasone suppression test. (From Nieman LK, Biller BM, Findling JW, et al. The diagnosis of Cushing's syndrome: an Endocrine Society Clinical Practice Guideline. *J Clin Endocrinol Metab.* 2008;93:1526-1540.)

Question 2: "What Is the Cause of Cushing's Syndrome in This Patient?"

Having confirmed Cushing's syndrome clinically and biochemically, the clinician's the next step is to determine the cause (Fig. 15-21).

Morning Plasma ACTH. Ideally, ACTH should be measured with the use of a modern, two-site immunoradiometric assay. Such a test differentiates ACTH-dependent from ACTH-independent causes. In Cushing's disease, 50% of patients have a 9 a.m. ACTH level within the normal reference range (2 to 11 pmol/L [9 to 52 pg/mL]); in the remainder, it is modestly elevated. ACTH levels in the ectopic ACTH syndrome are high (usually >20 pmol/L [>90 pg/mL]); nevertheless, overlap values are seen in Cushing's disease in 30% of cases.[257] Therefore, this test cannot be used to differentiate the two conditions (Fig. 15-22). The most discriminatory time of day to measure ACTH is between 11 p.m. and 1 a.m., when ACTH/cortisol secretion is at a nadir; in our practice, ACTH is usually measured alongside cortisol in circadian rhythm studies. A midnight ACTH result greater than 5 pmol/L (>22 pg/mL) in a patient with biochemical hypercortisolism confirms that the underlying disease is ACTH dependent. The measurement of ACTH precursors (pro-ACTH, POMC) is not routinely available but may be more useful in detecting an ectopic source of ACTH; more data are required regarding "occult" tumors as a cause of the syndrome.

In patients with adrenal tumors, plasma ACTH is invariably undetectable (<1 pmol/L). This can also occur with degradation of ACTH; as a result, nonhemolyzed blood samples should be placed in ice and immediately separated.

The presence of plasma ACTH levels that are low-normal or intermittently detectable, which may occur in MAH, is problematic. The danger is that in some patients the asymmetry of the nodular hyperplasia may lead to a diagnosis of adrenal adenoma, the plasma ACTH is ignored, and an inappropriate adrenalectomy is performed. Conversely, in some patients with this syndrome, an autonomous adrenal tumor develops and unilateral adrenalectomy is required despite the detectable ACTH.

Plasma Potassium. Hypokalemic alkalosis is present in more than 95% of patients with the ectopic ACTH syndrome but in fewer than 10% of those with Cushing's disease. The etiology of this mineralocorticoid excess state is now established. Patients with the ectopic syndrome usually have higher rates of cortisol secretion. Cortisol saturates the renal-protective HSD11B2 enzyme, resulting in cortisol-induced mineralocorticoid hypertension (see

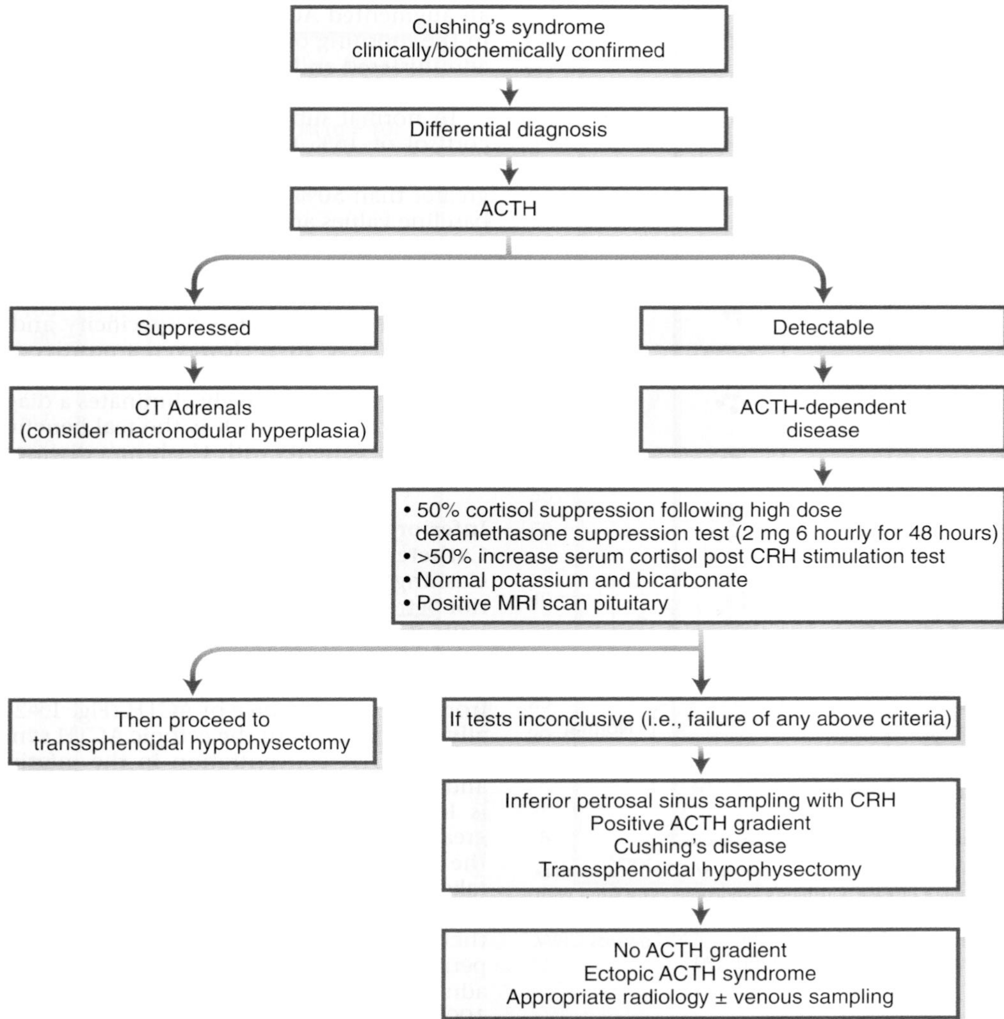

Figure 15-21 The tests to uncover the cause of Cushing's syndrome are debatable and differ in any given center depending on many factors, including familiarity and turnaround time of hormone assays and local expertise in techniques such as inferior petrosal sinus sampling. Depicted here is an algorithm in use within many endocrine units based on the reported sensitivity and specificity of each endocrine test. ACTH, adrenocorticotropin; CT, computed tomography; MRI. magnetic resonance imaging.

Chapter 16).[130] In addition, these patients have higher levels of the ACTH-dependent mineralocorticoid, DOC.

High-Dose Dexamethasone Suppression Test. The rationale for the high-dose dexamethasone suppression test is that in Cushing's disease the negative feedback control of ACTH is reset to a higher level than normal. Therefore, cortisol levels do not suppress with low-dose dexamethasone but do so after high doses. The original test introduced by Liddle was based on giving 2 mg dexamethasone every 6 hours for 48 hours and demonstrating a fall of greater than 50% in urinary 17-hydroxycorticosteroids.[209] In the modern test, the plasma or urinary free cortisol (or both) is measured at 0 and +48 hours, and a greater than 50% suppression of plasma cortisol from the basal value has been used to define a positive response. In all cases, the response is graded and is dependent on the original cortisol secretion rate: greater suppression is often observed in patients with lower basal cortisol values. About 90% of patients with Cushing's disease have a positive 48-hour test, compared with 10% of those with the ectopic ACTH syndrome. The robustness of the test can be improved by altering the cortisol cutoff value; the test has 100% specificity for diagnosing pituitary disease if more than 90% suppression in urinary free cortisol is used. Less commonly, 8 mg dexamethasone is given orally at 11 p.m., with plasma cortisol measured at 8 a.m. on the same day (basal sample) and at 8 a.m. on the following morning.[258] A further variation on this test is the timed (5- to 7-hour) infusion of dexamethasone (1 mg/hour).[259]

Up to 50% of patients with ectopic ACTH syndrome due to indolent bronchial carcinoid tumors exhibit some suppression after high-dose dexamethasone. Conversely, some patients with Cushing's disease, usually those with large, invasive ACTH-secreting pituitary macroadenomas, show no suppression after high-dose dexamethasone.[260]

Metyrapone Test. Metyrapone blocks the conversion of 11-deoxycortisol to cortisol, and DOC to corticosterone, by inhibiting 11β-hydroxylase (see Fig. 15-4). This lowers the plasma cortisol concentration and, via negative feedback control, increases plasma ACTH. This in turn stimulates increased secretion of adrenal steroids proximal to the block. Metyrapone is given in doses of 750 mg every 4

in diameter and should be considered for patients with ACTH-dependent Cushing's syndrome in whom pituitary disease has been excluded.[271]

Treatment of Cushing's Syndrome

Adrenal Causes

Unilateral adrenal adenomas should be removed by adrenalectomy; the cure rate is 100%.[272] With the increasing experience of laparoscopic adrenalectomy in most tertiary centers, this has now become the surgical treatment of choice for unilateral tumors, offering reduced surgical morbidity and postoperative hospital stay compared with traditional open approaches.[273] After the operation, it may take many months or even years for the contralateral suppressed adrenal to recover. It is wise, therefore, to give slightly suboptimal replacement therapy: dexamethasone 0.5 mg in the morning, with intermittent measurement of the morning plasma cortisol concentration before dexamethasone is taken. If the morning plasma cortisol is higher than 180 nmol/L (6.5 μg/dL), dexamethasone can be stopped. A subsequent insulin tolerance test may then demonstrate whether the response to stress is normal. In the interim, all patients should carry a steroid alert card and increase their dose of replacement therapy in the event of an intercurrent illness.

Adrenal carcinomas have had a very poor prognosis, and most patients have died within 2 years of diagnosis.[274] It is usual practice to try to remove the primary tumor, even though metastases may be present, so as to enhance the response to the adrenolytic agent *o,p′*-DDD[275] (mitotane). Radiotherapy to the tumor bed and to some metastases, such as those in the spine, may be of limited value. However, in recent years significant progress has been made by implementing collaborative multicenter studies. Phase III trials of mitotane therapy achieving therapeutic plasma mitotane levels have shown significant benefit[276]; drug combinations include etoposide, doxorubicine, and cisplatin plus mitotane or streptozotocin plus mitotane. Several targeted therapies, including IGF1 inhibitors, sunitinib, and sorafenib, may be of value in cases of "mitotane failure." The 10-year survival rate for patients with T1 N0 M0 disease is about 80% but is significantly impaired with increased tumor mass, positive lymph nodes, and distant metastases, reaching less than 20% for patients with T1-4 N0-1 M1.[277]

Pituitary-Dependent Cushing's Syndrome

The treatment of Cushing's disease has been significantly enhanced with transsphenoidal surgery conducted by an experienced surgeon.[278] Before the capability of selective removal of a pituitary microadenoma was developed, the treatment of choice was bilateral adrenalectomy. This had an appreciable mortality even in the best centers (up to 4%) and significant morbidity. The major risk was the subsequent development of Nelson's syndrome (postadrenalectomy hyperpigmentation with a locally aggressive pituitary tumor) (Fig. 15-29), which was attributed to loss of any negative feedback after adrenalectomy.[279] In an attempt to avoid this complication, pituitary irradiation was often carried out at the time of bilateral adrenalectomy.[280] In addition, these patients required lifelong replacement therapy with hydrocortisone and fludrocortisone. Currently, bilateral adrenalectomy is rarely indicated for patients with Cushing's disease but may be performed if pituitary surgery has failed or the condition has recurred.

The surgical outcome for transsphenoidal hypophysectomy varies from center to center and with surgical expertise.[281] Because of the hazards of untreated Cushing's disease and the potential complications of surgery, the endocrinologist should refer cases only to a recognized surgical specialist at a center in which outcome data have been established. In optimal centers, cure rates are 80% to 90% for microadenomas and 50% for macroadenomas.[282] Rates for postoperative hypopituitarism and permanent diabetes insipidus depend on how aggressive the surgeon was in removing pituitary tissue. The ideal outcome is a cured patient with intact pituitary function, but this may not be possible for a patient with Cushing's disease in whom a pituitary adenoma was not identified preoperatively or during the operation itself.

At the time of surgery, patients should be treated with corticosteroids, like other patient with potential or confirmed deficit of the HPA axis. In centers that lack facilities for frequent monitoring of cortisol levels, postoperative hydrocortisone cover is advised; this can be reduced to maintenance replacement doses usually within 3 to 7 days. On day 5 postoperatively, a 9 a.m. plasma cortisol level should be measured with the patient having omitted hydrocortisone for 24 hours. After selective removal of a microadenoma, the surrounding corticotrophs are usually suppressed (Fig. 15-30). As a result, plasma cortisol levels are less than 30 nmol/L (<1 μg/dL) postoperatively, and ongoing glucocorticoid replacement therapy is required. When the dexamethasone regimen described earlier (after removal of an adrenal adenoma) is used, the HPA axis usually (but not invariably) exhibits gradual recovery (Fig. 15-31). A nonsuppressed plasma cortisol postoperatively suggests that the patient is not "cured," even though cortisol secretion may have fallen to normal or subnormal values.[283,284] The recurrence rate in patients with an established "cure" after pituitary surgery is 2%, but this value is higher in children (up to 40%).[285,286] A detailed assessment of residual pituitary function is required in each case, and close follow-up of such individuals is warranted.

In the past, pituitary irradiation was often used in the treatment of Cushing's disease. However, because of the improvements in pituitary surgery, far fewer patients are so treated. In children, pituitary irradiation appears to be more effective.[287] Radiotherapy is not recommended as a primary treatment but is reserved for patients not responding to pituitary microsurgery, those who have undergone bilateral adrenalectomy, and patients with established Nelson's syndrome.

The management of recurrent Cushing's disease involves a consideration of repeat surgery, gamma knife radiosurgery, and medical therapies.[278,288]

Ectopic ACTH Syndrome

Treatment of the ectopic ACTH syndrome depends on the cause. If the tumor can be found and has not spread, then its removal can lead to cure (e.g., bronchial carcinoid, thymoma). However, the prognosis for small-cell lung cancer associated with the ectopic ACTH syndrome is poor. The cortisol excess and associated hypokalemic alkalosis and diabetes mellitus can be ameliorated by medical therapy. Treatment of the small-cell tumor itself will also, at least initially, produce improvement. Sometimes, if the ectopic source of ACTH cannot be found, it may be necessary to perform bilateral adrenalectomy and then monitor the patient carefully (sometimes for several years) before the primary tumor becomes apparent.

Medical Treatment of Cushing's Syndrome

Several drugs have been used in the treatment of Cushing's syndrome.[278] Metyrapone inhibits 11β-hydroxylase and

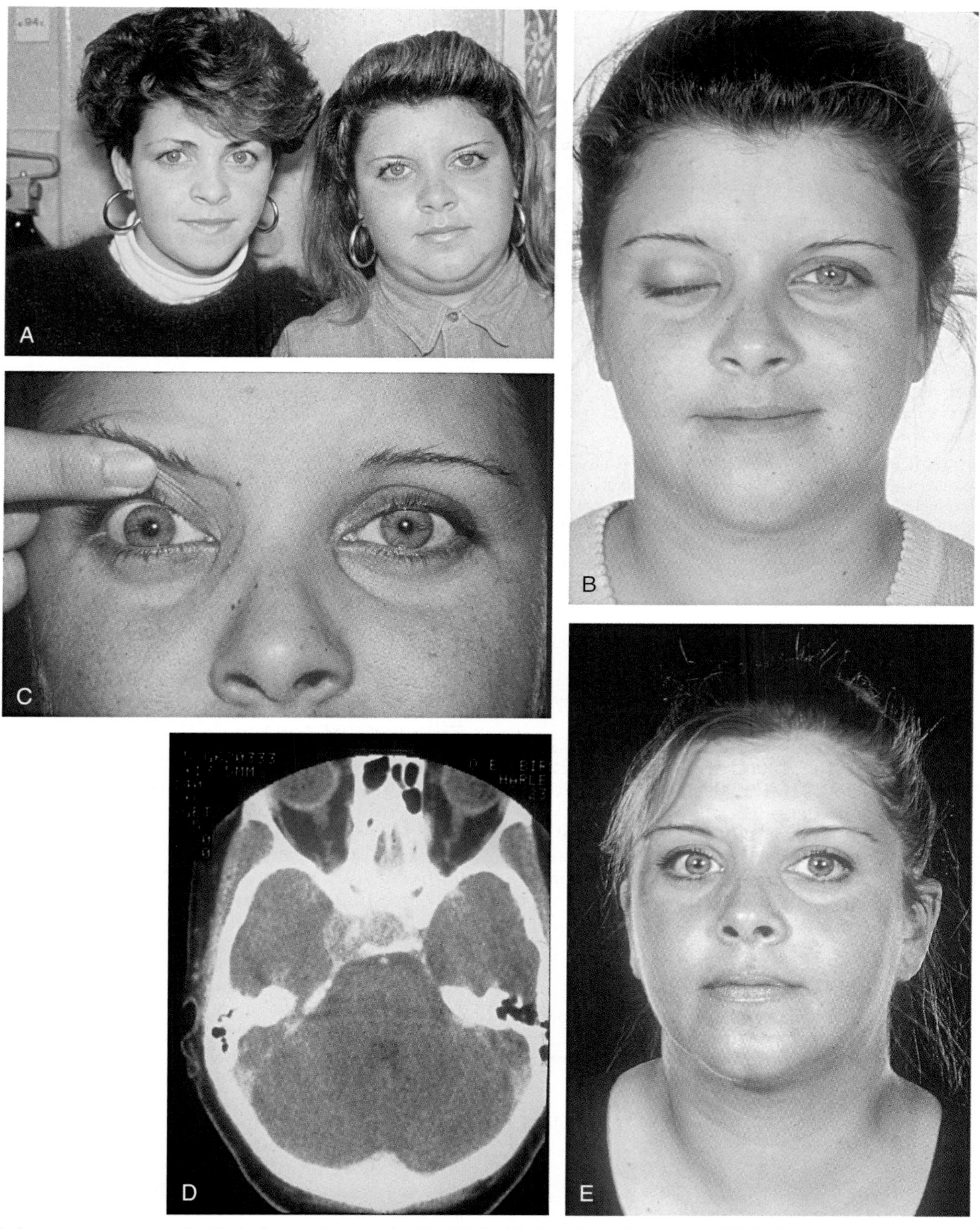

Figure 15-29 A young woman with Cushing's disease, photographed initially beside her identical twin sister **(A)**. In this case, treatment with bilateral adrenalectomy was undertaken. Several years later, the patient presented with Nelson's syndrome and a right third cranial nerve palsy (**B** and **C**) related to cavernous sinus infiltration from a locally invasive corticotropinoma **(D)**. Hypophysectomy and radiotherapy were performed with reversal of the third nerve palsy **(E)**. Note the advancing skin pigmentation of Nelson's syndrome.

has been the most commonly given agent, often with a goal of lowering cortisol concentrations before definitive therapy or while awaiting benefit from pituitary irradiation. The daily dose must be determined by measurements of plasma or urinary free cortisol. The aim should be to achieve a mean plasma cortisol concentration of about 300 nmol/L (11 µg/dL) during the day or a normal urinary free cortisol level. The drug is usually given in doses ranging from 250 mg twice daily to 1.5 g every 6 hours. Nausea is a side effect that can be helped (if it is not caused by adrenal insufficiency) by giving the drug with milk.[289]

Aminoglutethimide is a more toxic drug; high dose blocks earlier enzymes in the steroidogenic pathway and therefore affect the secretion of steroids other than cortisol. In doses of 1.5 to 3 g daily (starting with 250 mg every 8 hours), it commonly produces nausea, marked lethargy,

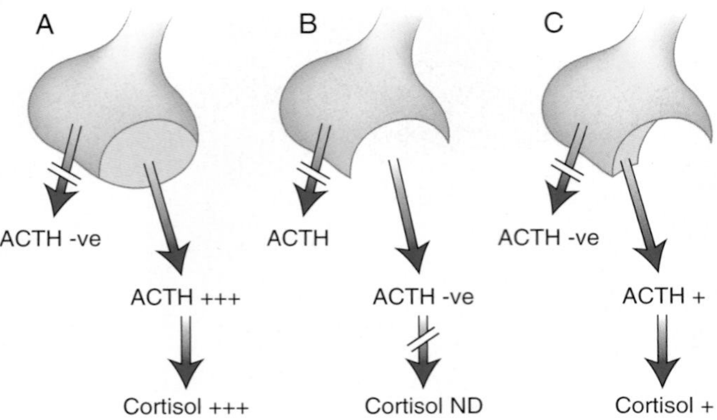

Figure 15-30 Selective removal of a microadenoma and its effect on the hypothalamic-pituitary-adrenal axis. **A,** Pretreatment. **B,** Total removal of adenoma. **C,** Incomplete excision. Because the surrounding normal pituitary corticotrophs are suppressed in a patient with an adrenocorticotropic hormone (ACTH)-secreting pituitary adenoma, successful removal of the tumor results in ACTH, and hence adrenocortical, deficiency, with an undetectable (<50 nmol/L [2 μg/dL]) plasma cortisol level. A postoperative plasma cortisol level higher than 50 nmol/L (2 μg/dL) implies that the patient is not cured. (Courtesy of Professor Peter Trainer.)

and a high incidence of skin rash.[290] It is commonly prescribed as combination therapy with metyrapone.

Trilostane, a 3β-HSD inhibitor, is ineffective in Cushing's disease, because the block in steroidogenesis is overcome by the rise in ACTH. However, it can be effective in patients with adrenal adenomas.[291]

Ketoconazole is an imidazole that has been widely used as an antifungal agent but causes abnormal liver function tests in about 15% of patients. Ketoconazole blocks a variety of steroidogenic cytochrome P450–dependent enzymes and thus lowers plasma cortisol levels. For effective control of Cushing's syndrome, 400 to 800 mg daily has been required.[292]

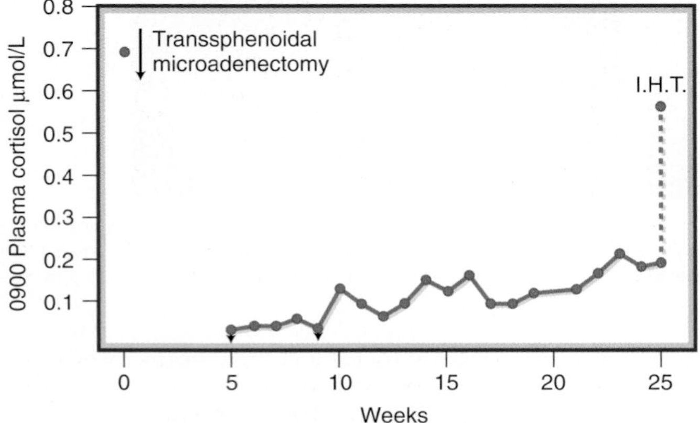

Figure 15-31 Gradual recovery of function of the hypothalamic-pituitary-adrenal axis in a patient after removal of a pituitary adrenocorticotropic hormone-secreting microadenoma. Morning (9 a.m.) plasma cortisol levels were measured. The insulin hypoglycemia test (I.H.T.) eventually demonstrated the return of a normal stress response.

Following the demonstration of the expression of the PPAR-γ receptor in ACTH-secreting pituitary tissue, a novel therapy for Cushing's disease was devised: the thiazolidinedione, rosiglitazone.[293] Doses up to 8 mg/day are required to suppress cortisol secretion, and the drug seems to have lasting benefit in approximately 20% of cases studied.[294] Further studies are required.

Mitotane (*o,p′*-DDD) is an adrenolytic drug that is taken up by both normal and malignant adrenal tissue, causing adrenal atrophy and necrosis.[275] Because of its toxicity, it has been used mainly in the management of adrenal carcinoma. Doses of up to 5 g/day are required to control glucocorticoid excess, although evidence that the drug causes tumor shrinkage or improves long-term survival is lacking. This agent also produces mineralocorticoid deficiency, and concomitant glucocorticoid and mineralocorticoid replacement therapy may be required. Side effects are common and include fatigue, skin rashes, neurotoxicity, and gastrointestinal disturbance.

Somatostatin analogues such as octreotide and lanreotide are generally ineffective in Cushing's disease. However, promising results have been reported with a novel somatostatin analogue, pasireotide, which demonstrates high-affinity binding to somatostatin receptor subtypes 1, 2, 3, and 5.[295] A fall in cortisol secretion was reported in 75% of Cushing's disease patients treated for 15 days with pasireotide, 600 μg given subcutaneously twice daily, but normalization of urinary free cortisol was achieved in fewer than 20% of these patients.

Prognosis of Cushing's Syndrome

Studies carried out before the introduction of effective therapy revealed that 50% of patients with untreated Cushing's syndrome died within 5 years, principally from vascular disease.[192] Even with modern management, an increased prevalence of cardiovascular risk factors persists for many years after an apparent "cure."[193,194] Paradoxically, on correction of the hypercortisolism, patients often feel worse. Skin desquamation, steroid-withdrawal arthropathy, profound lethargy, and mood changes may occur and can take several weeks or months to resolve.[296] In our experience, these features, together with postural hypotension, are particularly severe in "cured" patients who are also rendered vasopressin deficient. They can usually be ameliorated by a transient increase in glucocorticoid replacement therapy. Patients are invariably GH deficient, and GH replacement therapy may produce clinical benefit.

Features of Cushing's syndrome disappear over a period of 2 to 12 months after treatment. Hypertension and diabetes mellitus improve, but, as with other secondary causes, they may not resolve completely. The osteopenia of Cushing's syndrome improves rapidly during the first 2 years after treatment but resolves more slowly thereafter.[297] Vertebral fractures and osteonecrosis are irreversible, and permanent deformity results. Visceral obesity and myopathy are both reversible features. Reproductive and sexual function return to normal within 6 months, provided that anterior pituitary function was not compromised. Long-term health-related quality of life in adults significantly improves after treatment, but quality-of-life scores do not return to normal levels.[189] Similar observations have been made in pediatric patients, in whom significant improvement was noted before and after treatment but residual impairment of health-related quality of life persisted 1 year after cure.[298]

Glucocorticoid Resistance

A small number of patients have been described as having increased cortisol secretion but without the stigmata of Cushing's syndrome.[86,299] These patients are resistant to suppression of cortisol with low-dose dexamethasone but respond to high doses. ACTH levels are elevated and lead to increased adrenal production of androgens and DOC. Therefore, these patients may present with the features of androgen or mineralocorticoid excess, or both. Treatment with a dose of dexamethasone (usually >3 mg/day) adequate to suppress ACTH results in a fall in adrenal androgens and often returns plasma potassium and blood pressure to normal levels. Many of these patients have been found to have point mutations in the steroid-binding domain of the GR, with consequent reduction of glucocorticoid-binding affinity, but this is not invariable. A useful clinical discriminatory test to differentiate this condition from Cushing's syndrome is to measure bone mineral density: it is preserved in patients with glucocorticoid resistance or even increased in females because of the androgen excess. In addition, the circadian rhythm for ACTH and cortisol is preserved in patients with glucocorticoid resistance.

GLUCOCORTICOID DEFICIENCY

Primary and Secondary Hypoadrenalism

Primary hypoadrenalism refers to glucocorticoid deficiency occurring in the setting of adrenal disease, whereas secondary hypoadrenalism arises because of deficiency of ACTH (Table 15-16). A major distinction between these two is that mineralocorticoid deficiency invariably accompanies primary hypoadrenalism, but this does not occur in secondary hypoadrenalism: only ACTH is deficient, and the renin-angiotensin-aldosterone (RAA) axis is intact. A further important cause of adrenal insufficiency in which there may be dissociation of glucocorticoid and mineralocorticoid secretion is CAH.

Primary Hypoadrenalism

Addison's Disease

Thomas Addison described the condition now known as primary hypoadrenalism in his classic monograph published in 1855.[2] Addison's disease is a rare condition with an estimated incidence in the developed world of 0.8 cases per 100,000 and a prevalence of 4 to 11 cases per 100,000 population. Nevertheless, it is associated with significant morbidity and mortality, but once the diagnosis is made it can be easily treated.[300,301] Causes of Addison's disease are listed in Table 15-16.

TABLE 15-16

Etiology of Adrenocortical Insufficiency (Excluding Congenital Adrenal Hyperplasia)

Primary Causes: Addison's Disease
Autoimmune
Sporadic
Autoimmune polyendocrine syndrome type I (Addison's disease, chronic mucocutaneous candidiasis, hypoparathyroidism, dental enamel hypoplasia, alopecia, primary gonadal failure—see Chapter 42)
Autoimmune polyendocrine syndrome type II (Schmidt's syndrome) (Addison's disease, primary hypothyroidism, primary hypogonadism, insulin-dependent diabetes, pernicious anemia, vitiligo—Chapter 42)
Infections
Tuberculosis
Fungal infections
Cytomegalovirus
HIV
Metastatic tumor
Infiltrations
Amyloid
Hemochromatosis
Intra-adrenal hemorrhage (Waterhouse-Friderichsen syndrome) after meningococcal septicemia
Adrenoleukodystrophies
Congenital adrenal hypoplasia
DAX1 *(NR0B1)* mutations
SF1 mutations
ACTH resistance syndromes
MC2R gene mutations
MRAP gene mutations
AAAS (ALADIN) gene mutations (triple-A syndrome)
Bilateral adrenalectomy
Secondary Causes
Exogenous glucocorticoid therapy
Hypopituitarism
Selective removal of ACTH-secreting pituitary adenoma
Pituitary tumors and pituitary surgery, craniopharyngiomas
Pituitary apoplexy
Granulomatous disease (tuberculosis, sarcoid, eosinophilic granuloma)
Secondary tumor deposits (breast, bronchus)
Postpartum pituitary infarction (Sheehan's syndrome)
Pituitary irradiation (effect usually delayed for several years)
Isolated ACTH deficiency
Idiopathic
Lymphocytic hypophysitis
TPIT *(TBX19)* gene mutations
PCSK1 gene mutation (POMC processing defect)
POMC gene mutations
Multiple pituitary hormone deficiencies
HESX1 gene mutations
LHX4 gene mutations
SOX3 gene mutations
PROP1 gene mutations

ACTH, Adrenocorticotropic hormone; HIV, human immunodeficiency virus; POMC, pro-opiomelanocortin.

Autoimmune Adrenalitis. In the Western world, autoimmune adrenalitis accounts for more than 70% of all cases of primary hypoadrenalism.[302] Pathologically, the adrenal glands are atrophic with loss of most of the cortical cells, but the medulla is usually intact. In 75% of cases, adrenal autoantibodies can be detected.[303] Fifty percent of patients with this form of Addison's disease have an associated autoimmune disease (Table 15-17), thyroid disease being the most common. Conversely, only 1% to 2% of patients with more common autoimmune diseases such as insulin-dependent diabetes mellitus or thyrotoxicosis have antiadrenal autoantibodies and develop adrenal disease, although the figure is higher in patients with autoimmune hypoparathyroidism (16%). These autoimmune polyglandular syndromes (APS) have been classified into two distinct variants.[303] APS type I, or autoimmune polyendocrinopathy-candidiasis-ectodermal dysplasia (APECED), is a rare autosomal recessive condition comprising Addison's disease, chronic mucocutaneous candidiasis, and hypoparathyroidism. The more common APS type II, comprises Addison's disease, autoimmune thyroid disease, diabetes mellitus, and hypogonadism. Here, autoantibodies to 21-hydroxylase are usually present and are predictive for the development of adrenal destruction.[303] Polyglandular autoimmune syndromes are discussed in greater detail in Chapter 42.

TABLE 15-17

Incidence of Other Endocrine and Autoimmune Diseases in Patients with Autoimmune Adrenal Insufficiency

Disease	Incidence (%)
Thyroid disease	
Hypothyroidism	8
Nontoxic goiter	7
Thyrotoxicosis	7
Gonadal failure	
Ovarian	20
Testicular	2
Insulin-dependent diabetes mellitus	11
Hypoparathyroidism	10
Pernicious anemia	5
None	53

Infections. Worldwide, infectious diseases are the most common cause of primary adrenal insufficiency. These diseases include tuberculosis, fungal infections (histoplasmosis, cryptococcosis), and cytomegalovirus. Adrenal failure may also occur in the acquired immunodeficiency syndrome (AIDS).[304]

Tuberculous Addison's disease results from hematogenous spread of the infection from elsewhere in the body; extra-adrenal disease is usually evident. The adrenals are initially enlarged, with extensive epithelioid granulomas and caseation, and both the cortex and the medulla are affected. Fibrosis ensues, and the adrenals become normal or smaller in size, with calcification evident in 50% of cases.

The adrenals are frequently involved in patients with AIDS[304,305]; adrenalitis may occur after infection with cytomegalovirus or atypical mycobacteria, and Kaposi's sarcoma may result in adrenal replacement. Onset is often insidious, but if tested, more than 10% of patients with AIDS will demonstrate a subnormal cortisol response to a short Synacthen test. Adrenal insufficiency may be precipitated through the concomitant administration of appropriate anti-infectives such as ketoconazole (which inhibits cortisol synthesis) or rifampicin (which increases cortisol metabolism). Rarely, patients with AIDS and features of adrenal insufficiency are found to have elevated circulating ACTH and cortisol concentrations that fail to suppress normally after low-dose dexamethasone administration. This is thought to reflect an "acquired" form of glucocorticoid resistance resulting from reduced GR affinity, but the underlying cause remains unknown.[306]

Acquired Primary Adrenal Insufficiency

With the exception of tuberculosis and autoimmune adrenal failure, other causes of Addison's disease are rare (see Table 15-16). Adrenal metastases (most commonly from primary tumors in the lung or breast) are often found at postmortem examinations, but they uncommonly cause adrenal insufficiency,[307] perhaps because more than 90% of the adrenal cortex must be compromised before symptoms and signs become apparent. Necrosis of the adrenals due to intra-adrenal hemorrhage should be considered in any severely sick patient, particularly a patient with underlying infection, trauma, or coagulopathy.[308] Intra-adrenal bleeding may be found in patients with severe septicemia of any cause, particularly in children, in whom a common cause is infection with *Pseudomonas aeruginosa*. When caused by meningococci, the association with adrenal insufficiency is known as the Waterhouse-Friederichsen syndrome. Adrenal replacement may also occur with amyloidosis and hemochromatosis.

Inherited Primary Adrenal Insufficiency

Adrenal hypoplasia congenita (*AHC*) is an X-linked disorder comprising congenital adrenal insufficiency and combined primary and central hypogonadotropic hypogonadism. The condition is caused by mutations in the *DAX1* (*NROB1*) gene, a member of a nuclear receptor family that is expressed in the adrenal cortex, gonads, and hypothalamus.[309,310] Depending on the molecular defect, the clinical presentation can be highly variable. Severe cases often manifest with mineralocorticoid deficiency and gradually develop glucocorticoid deficiency. Hypogonadism is combined with primary testicular abnormalities and low gonadotropin levels. However, the so-called minipuberty of infancy can be normal.[311,312] Patients presenting with late-onset adrenal failure have also been described.[313]

Mutations in another transcription factor, steroidogenic factor-1 (SF1), may also result in adrenal insufficiency due to lack of development of a functional adrenal cortex. The transcriptional regulation of many P450 steroidogenic enzymes is dependent on SF1.[15] When it was first described, SF1 mutation was associated with complete sex reversal causing 46,XY disorder of sex development (DSD).[314] However, novel clinical phenotypes in SF1-deficient patients are now emerging; they range from isolated adrenal failure[315] to isolated gonadal failure[316] and ovarian insufficiency.[317] AHC may also occur in association with glycerol kinase deficiency and muscular dystrophy caused by gene deletion, including the *DAX1* gene.[318]

Adrenoleukodystrophy has a prevalence rate of 1:20,000 and is a cause of adrenal insufficiency in association with demyelination within the nervous system; demyelination results from a failure of β-oxidation of fatty acids within peroxisomes due to reduced activity of very-long-chain acyl-CoA synthetase.[319] Increased accumulation of very-long-chain fatty acids (VLCFA) occurs in many tissues, and serum assays can be used diagnostically. Only males have the fully expressed condition, and carrier females are usually normal. Several forms are recognized: a childhood cerebral form (30% to 40% of cases), adult adrenomyeloneuropathy (40%), and Addison's disease (7%). The childhood-onset form manifests at 5 to 10 years of age with progression eventually to a blind, mute, and severely spastic tetraplegic state. Adrenal insufficiency is usually present but does not appear to correlate with the neurologic deficit. Nevertheless, this is the most common form of adrenal insufficiency in a child younger than 7 years of age.[320] Adrenomyeloneuropathy, by contrast, manifests later in life with the gradual development of spastic paresis and peripheral neuropathy. Both the childhood and the adult condition result from mutations in the *ABCD1* gene on chromosome Xq28, which encodes for an ABC peroxisomal membrane protein involved in the import of VLCFA into the peroxisome.[321] So far, more than 400 mutations have been reported in the *ABCD1* gene with no relationship between genotype and phenotype.[322,323] Treatment options are few. Monounsaturated fatty acids, which block the synthesis of the saturated VLCFA, have been used; a combination of erucic acid and oleic acid (Lorenzo's oil) has led to normal levels of VLCFA. Treatment does not alter the rate of neurologic deterioration but may prevent new neurologic damage in asymptomatic cases.[323] Bone marrow transplantation is a further possibility.

Familial glucocorticoid deficiency (FGD), or inherited unresponsiveness to ACTH, is a rare autosomal recessive cause of hypoadrenalism that usually manifests in childhood.

Most patients present with neonatal hypoglycemia or later in life with increasing pigmentation, and they often have enhanced growth velocity. Primary adrenal failure in a child with normal activity of the RAA system is highly suggestive of FGD. The diagnosis can be confirmed by demonstrating low cortisol in combination with increased ACTH concentrations and normal plasma renin and aldosterone measurements.[90] The type 1 variant accounts for approximately 25% of all cases and is explained by inactivating mutations in the ACTH-binding receptor, MC2R.[324-326] The FGD type 2 variant caused by mutations in *MRAP* gene, which is thought to mediate intracellular trafficking of the *MC2R*, has been reported in some families.[89] However, 50% of patients with FGD do not have mutations in either *MC2R* or *MRAP*; other loci are being defined.

A variant called the *triple A syndrome* or *Allgrove's* syndrome refers to the triad of adrenal insufficiency due to ACTH resistance, achalasia, and alacrima. It is caused by mutations in the *AAAS* gene, which encodes ALADIN, a tryptophan/aspartate WD-repeat–containing protein of the nuclear pore complex.[327,328] The exact function of ALADIN is unknown, but its interaction with other proteins of the nuclear pore complex suggest that it is part of a structural scaffold.

Several syndromic disorders are associated with adrenal insufficiency for which the underlying molecular genetic defect remains to be elucidated.[11]

Secondary Hypoadrenalism (ACTH deficiency)

Acquired Secondary Adrenal Insufficiency

Acquired secondary adrenal insufficiency is a common clinical problem and is most often caused by a sudden cessation of exogenous glucocorticoid therapy. Such therapy suppresses the HPA axis with consequent adrenal atrophy, which may last for months after the glucocorticoid treatment is stopped. Adrenal atrophy and subsequent deficiency should be anticipated in any subject who has taken more than the equivalent of 30 mg hydrocortisone per day orally (>7.5 mg/day prednisolone or >0.75 mg/day dexamethasone) for longer than 3 weeks. In addition to the magnitude of the dose of glucocorticoid, the timing of administration may affect the degree of adrenal suppression. If prednisolone is given as 5 mg at night and 2.5 mg in the morning, there will be more marked suppression of the HPA axis compared with 2.5 mg at night and 5 mg in the morning, because the larger evening dose blocks the early-morning surge of ACTH.

Secondary hypoadrenalism may also occur after failure to give adequate glucocorticoid replacement therapy for intercurrent stress in a patient who has been on long-term glucocorticoid therapy.

Inherited Secondary Adrenal Insufficiency

Other causes of secondary adrenal insufficiency (see Table 15-16) reflect inadequate ACTH production from the anterior pituitary gland. In many of these conditions, other pituitary hormones are also deficient, so that the patient presents with partial or complete hypopituitarism. The clinical features of hypopituitarism make this a relatively easy diagnosis to make. Isolated ACTH deficiency is rare, and the diagnosis is difficult to make. It may occur in patients with lymphocytic hypophysitis. Mutations in the *TBX19*, the product of which (TPIT) regulates POMC expression, have been reported in a few cases of isolated ACTH deficiency occurring in neonatal life.[329] A rare but fascinating cause relates to a defect in the normal post-translational processing of POMC to ACTH by the prohormone convertase enzymes (PC1 and PC2).[330] Such patients may have more generalized defects in peptide processing (e.g., cleavage of proinsulin to insulin) giving rise to diabetes mellitus.

Some patients have mutations in the *POMC* gene that interrupt the synthesis of ACTH and causes ACTH deficiency. Elucidation of the phenotype of these patients has uncovered a novel role for POMC peptides in regulating appetite and hair color: in addition to adrenal insufficiency, *POMC* mutations result in severe obesity and red hair pigmentation.[331] A central role for α-MSH in regulating food intake via the hypothalamic MC4R has been established,[55] and in recombinant mice lacking the POMC gene, the obese phenotype can be reversed by giving an α-MSH agonist peripherally.[332]

Other rare inborn causes of secondary insufficiency are the result of mutations in genes involved in pituitary development, such as *HESX1*,[333] *LHX4*,[334] *SOX3*,[335] and *PROP1*.[336] These defects result in congenital hypopituitarism with multiple pituitary hormone deficiencies: ACTH deficiency may not be present at the time of diagnosis, it but develops progressively over time.

Secondary hypoadrenalism is also observed in patients with Cushing's disease after successful and selective removal of the ACTH-secreting pituitary adenoma. The function of adjacent "normal" pituitary corticotrophs is suppressed and may remain so for many months after curative surgery.[283-285]

Hypoadrenalism during Critical Illness

Hypoadrenalism may also complicate critical illness, even in individuals with a previously intact HPA axis.[337] This has been termed *functional adrenal insufficiency* to reflect the notion that hypoadrenalism is transient and is not caused by a structural lesion. Functional adrenal insufficiency has been difficult to define biochemically and is of uncertain etiology. Inability to mount an adequate and appropriate cortisol response to overwhelming stress or sepsis is frequently encountered in intensive care units and substantially increases the risk of death during acute illness.[338] This has stimulated attempts to define functional adrenal insufficiency quantitatively and to treat it with supplemental corticosteroids. Although this diagnosis remains highly contentious, if a suboptimal cortisol response is suspected, the current recommendations suggest (1) treatment with hydrocortisone, 200 mg/day in four divided doses or, preferably, 10 mg/hour as a continuous infusion, for patients with septic shock and (2) treatment with methylprednisolone, 1 mg/kg per day, for patients with severe early acute respiratory distress syndrome. Glucocorticoid treatment should be tapered off rather than stopped abruptly. Treatment of critical illness–related adrenal insufficiency with dexamethasone is not recommended.[339]

Clinical Features of Adrenal Insufficiency

Patients with primary adrenal failure usually have both glucocorticoid and mineralocorticoid deficiency. In contrast, those with secondary adrenal insufficiency have an intact RAA system. This accounts for differences in salt and water balance in the two groups of patients, which in turn result in different clinical presentations. The most obvious feature that differentiates primary from secondary hypoadrenalism is skin pigmentation (Table 15-18), which is almost always present in cases of primary adrenal insufficiency (unless of short duration) and absent in secondary insufficiency. The pigmentation is seen in sun-exposed

TABLE 15-18

Clinical Features of Primary Adrenal Insufficiency

Feature	Frequency (%)
Symptoms	
Weakness, tiredness, fatigue	100
Anorexia	100
Gastrointestinal symptoms	92
Nausea	86
Vomiting	75
Constipation	33
Abdominal pain	31
Diarrhea	16
Salt craving	16
Postural dizziness	12
Muscle or joint pains	13
Signs	
Weight loss	100
Hyperpigmentation	94
Hypotension (<110 mm Hg systolic)	88-94
Vitiligo	10-20
Auricular calcification	5
Laboratory Findings	
Electrolyte disturbances	92
Hyponatremia	88
Hyperkalemia	64
Hypercalcemia	6
Azotemia	55
Anemia	40
Eosinophilia	17

areas, recent rather than old scars, axillae, nipples, palmar creases, pressure points, and mucous membranes (buccal, vaginal, vulval, anal). The cause of the pigmentation has long been debated but is thought to reflect increased stimulation of the MC1R by ACTH itself. In autoimmune Addison's disease, there may be associated vitiligo (Fig. 15-32).

The clinical features relate to the rate of onset and the severity of adrenal deficiency.[300] In many cases, the disease has an insidious onset and a diagnosis is made only when the patient presents with an acute crisis during an intercurrent illness. Acute adrenal insufficiency, termed an adrenal crisis or Addisonian crisis, is a medical emergency manifesting as hypotension and acute circulatory failure (Table 15-19). Anorexia may be an early feature; it progresses to nausea, vomiting, diarrhea, and, sometimes, abdominal pain. Fever may be present, and hypoglycemia may occur.

TABLE 15-19

Clinical and Laboratory Features of an Adrenal Crisis

- Dehydration, hypotension, or shock out of proportion to severity of current illness
- Nausea and vomiting with a history of weight loss and anorexia
- Abdominal pain, so-called acute abdomen
- Unexplained hypoglycemia
- Unexplained fever
- Hyponatremia, hyperkalemia, azotemia, hypercalcemia, or eosinophilia
- Hyperpigmentation or vitiligo
- Other autoimmune endocrine deficiencies, such as hypothyroidism or gonadal failure

Patients presenting acutely with adrenal hemorrhage have hypotension; abdominal, flank, or lower chest pain; anorexia; and vomiting. The condition is difficult to diagnose, but evidence of occult hemorrhage (rapidly falling hemoglobin), progressive hyperkalemia, and shock should alert the clinician to the diagnosis.

Alternatively, the patient may present with vague features of chronic adrenal insufficiency—weakness, tiredness, weight loss, nausea, intermittent vomiting, abdominal pain, diarrhea or constipation, general malaise, muscle cramps, arthralgia, and symptoms suggestive of postural hypotension (see Table 15-18). Salt craving may be a feature, and a low-grade fever may be present. Supine blood pressure is usually normal, but almost invariably there is a fall in blood pressure on standing. Adrenal androgen secretion is lost; this is clinically more apparent in women, who may complain of loss of axillary and pubic hair and frequently have dry and itchy skin. Psychiatric symptoms may occur in long-standing cases and include memory impairment, depression, and psychosis. Formal quality-of-life measures indicate significant impairment in patients with primary or secondary adrenal insufficiency.[340] Tiredness is often profound, and patients may be inappropriately diagnosed with chronic fatigue syndrome or anorexia nervosa.

In secondary adrenal insufficiency due to hypopituitarism, the presentation may relate to deficiency of hormones other than ACTH, notably LH/FSH (infertility, oligorrhea/amenorrhea, poor libido) and TSH (weight gain, cold intolerance). Fasting hypoglycemia occurs because of loss of the gluconeogenic effects of cortisol. It is rare in adults unless there is concomitant alcohol abuse or additional GH deficiency. However, hypoglycemia is a common presenting feature of ACTH/adrenal insufficiency in childhood.[341] In addition, patients with ACTH deficiency present with malaise, weight loss, and other features of chronic adrenal insufficiency. Rarely, the presentation is more acute in patients with pituitary apoplexy.

Investigation of Hypoadrenalism

Routine Biochemical Profile

Among patients with established primary adrenal insufficiency, hyponatremia is present in about 90% and hyperkalemia in 65%. The blood urea concentration is usually elevated. Hyperkalemia occurs because of aldosterone deficiency, so it is usually absent in patients with secondary adrenal failure. Hyponatremia may be depletional in an Addisonian crisis, but in addition vasopressin levels are elevated, resulting in increased free water retention.[342] Therefore, in secondary adrenal insufficiency, there may be a dilutional hyponatremia with normal or low blood urea.

Reversible abnormalities in liver transaminases frequently occur. Hypercalcemia occurs in 6% of all cases[343] and may be particularly marked in patients with coexisting thyrotoxicosis. Free thyroxine concentrations are usually low or normal, but TSH values are frequently moderately elevated.[344] This is a direct effect of glucocorticoid deficiency and reverses with replacement therapy. Persistent elevation of TSH in association with positive thyroid autoantibodies suggests concomitant autoimmune thyroid disease.

Mineralocorticoid Status

In primary hypoadrenalism, mineralocorticoid deficiency usually occurs, manifested by elevated plasma renin activity and either low or low-normal plasma aldosterone. The investigation of ZG activity is frequently neglected in

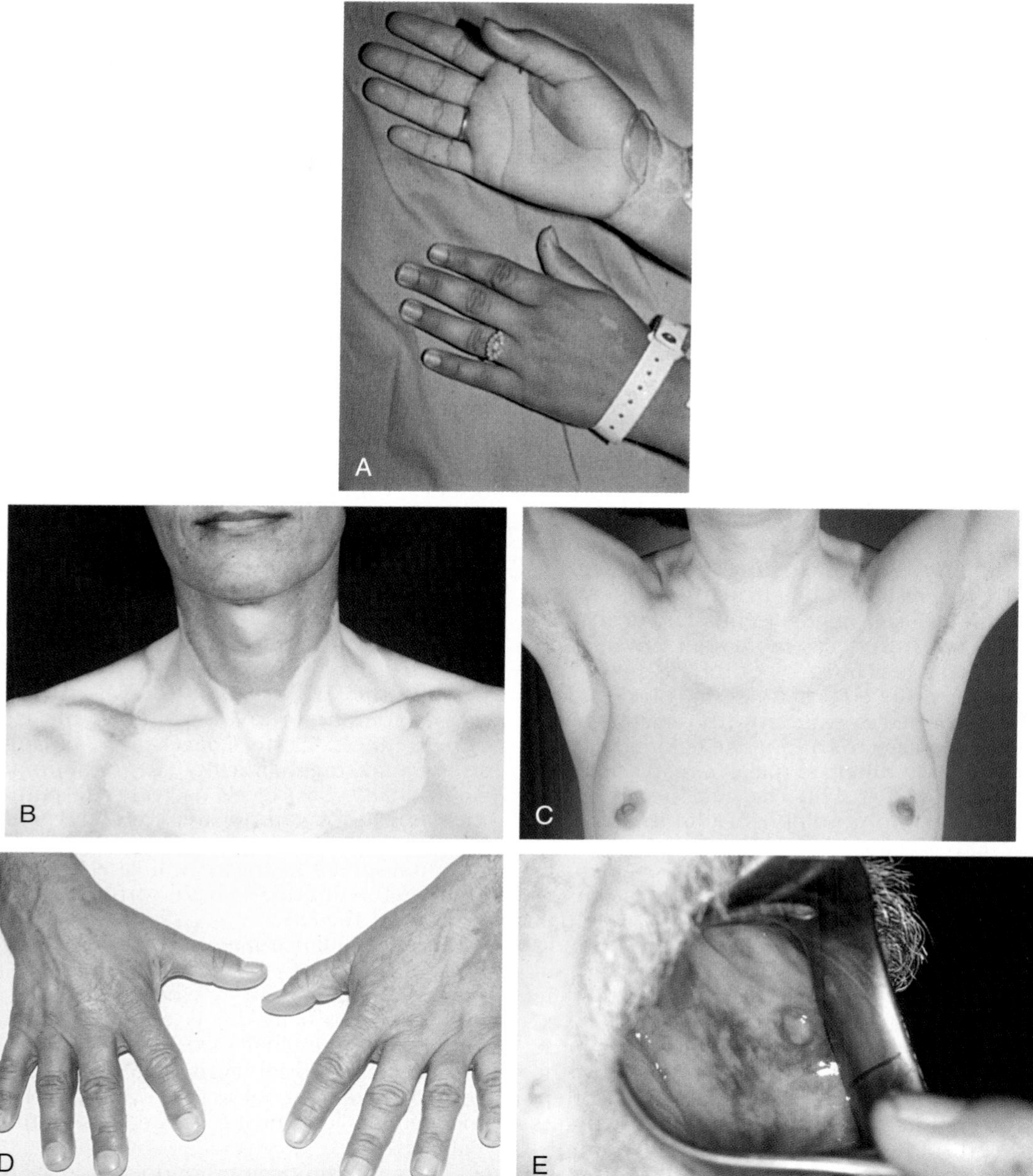

Figure 15-32 Pigmentation in Addison's disease. **A,** Hands of an 18-year-old woman with autoimmune polyendocrine syndrome and Addison's disease. Pigmentation in a patient with Addison's disease before (**B**) and after (**C**) treatment with hydrocortisone and fludrocortisone. Notice the additional presence of vitiligo. **D,** Similar changes in a 60-year-old man with tuberculous Addison's disease before (*left*) and after (*right*) corticosteroid therapy. **E,** Buccal pigmentation in the same patient as in **D**. (**B** and **C** courtesy of Professor C.R.W. Edwards.)

Addison's disease, compared with assessment of ZF function. In secondary adrenal insufficiency, the RAA system is intact.

Assessing Adequacy of Function of the HPA Axis

Clinical suspicion of the diagnosis should be confirmed with definitive diagnostic tests. Basal plasma cortisol and urinary free cortisol levels are often in the low-normal range and cannot be used to exclude the diagnosis. However, a basal cortisol value greater than 400 nmol/L (14.5 μg/dL) invariably indicates an intact HPA axis.[345] In practice, rather than wait for results of insensitive basal tests, all patients with suspected adrenal insufficiency should have an ACTH stimulation test; in patients with an Addisonian crisis, however, treatment should be instigated immediately and stimulation tests conducted at a later stage.

The ACTH stimulation test or SST involves intramuscular or intravenous administration of 250 μg tetracosactin, a synthetic ACTH(1-24) comprising the first 24 amino acids of normally secreted ACTH(1-39).[346] Plasma cortisol levels are measured at 0 and 30 minutes after ACTH administration, and a normal response is defined by a peak plasma cortisol level greater than 550 nmol/L (>20 μg/dL).[347] This value equates to the 5th percentile response in normal subjects but is very much assay-dependent, with different cortisol radioimmunoassays giving different results. Incremental responses (i.e., the difference between peak and basal values) are of no value in defining a "pass" response, with the possible exception of diagnosing relative adrenal insufficiency in patients with critical illness. Response is unaffected by the time of day of the test, and the test can be performed in patients who have commenced corticosteroid replacement therapy, so long as this therapy is of short duration and does not include hydrocortisone (which would cross-react in the cortisol assay). A prolonged ACTH stimulation test involving the administration of depot or intravenous infusions of tetracosactin for 24 to 48 hours differentiates primary from secondary hypoadrenalism. In normal subjects, the plasma cortisol level at 4 hours is greater than 1000 nmol/L (36 μg/dL); beyond that time, there is no further increase. Patients with secondary hypoadrenalism show a delayed response and usually have a much higher value at 24 and 48 hours than at 4 hours. In patients with primary hypoadrenalism, there is no response at either time. However, the test is rarely required if plasma ACTH has been appropriately measured at baseline. In primary adrenal insufficiency, the ACTH level is disproportionately elevated in comparison to plasma cortisol.[348]

Whereas there is agreement on the investigation of suspected primary adrenal failure, the diagnosis of secondary hypoadrenalism, notably in patients with existing hypothalamic/pituitary disease, is contentious. Based on correlations with the response of circulating cortisol to surgery, the insulin-induced hypoglycemia test or insulin tolerance test (ITT) was introduced more than 40 years ago as a laboratory test to assess integrity of the HPA axis, and it should be considered the gold standard in this regard.[349] It should not be performed in patients with ischemic heart disease (always check an electrocardiogram before the test), epilepsy, or severe hypopituitarism (i.e., 9 a.m. plasma cortisol <180 nmol/L [<6.5 μg/dL]). The test involves the intravenous administration of soluble insulin in a dose of 0.1 to 0.15 U/kg body weight, with measurement of plasma cortisol at 0, 30, 45, 60, 90, and 120 minutes. Adequate hypoglycemia (blood glucose <2.2 mmol/L with signs of neuroglycopenia—sweating and tachycardia) is essential. In normal subjects, the peak plasma cortisol concentration exceeds 500 nmol/L (18 μg/dL). However, the cortisol response to hypoglycemia can be reliably predicted by the SST—a safer, cheaper, and quicker test.[346,350]

The SST relies on the principle that the cortisol response to an exogenous bolus of ACTH is determined by the endogenous ACTH trophic drive to the adrenal cortex; impaired ACTH secretion from the anterior pituitary results in an impaired cortisol response after Synacthen administration. However, the ACTH test should not be used to diagnose secondary hypoadrenalism in patients with a recent pituitary insult (e.g., surgery, apoplexy). Total hypophysectomy results in a failed cortisol response to ITT immediately thereafter, but it takes 2 to 3 weeks for the adrenal cortex to readjust to the reduced level of ACTH secretion; in the interim, a false-positive cortisol response is seen. The SST should also be avoided in patients with a primary diagnosis of Cushing's disease, in whom an exaggerated cortisol response to ACTH may persist.

In clinical practice, if the ACTH test is normal, insulin hypoglycemia testing is not necessary in most cases unless there is also a need to document endogenous GH reserve in a patient with pituitary disease. In our practice, an ITT is performed in a patient with suspected hypopituitarism if there is a subnormal response to ACTH. Some patients have an inadequate response to ACTH but then respond normally to hypoglycemia[350]; they do not require corticosteroid replacement therapy. This approach is open to debate, and even taking into account the caveats listed, false-positive results have been reported for the SST.[351] Although these are rare (<2%), the possibility should be noted, particularly in patients with ongoing symptoms and signs indicative of hypoadrenalism.

A low-dose SST giving only 1 μg ACTH has been proposed as a screen for adequacy of function of the HPA axis, with the suggestion that it may be more sensitive than the conventional 250-μg test.[352-354] Other researchers dispute this suggestion,[355,356] and further validation of this test is required to support such a concept.

Two other tests have been advocated to assess adequacy of function of the HPA axis, but their use in modern clinical practice should be restricted to difficult diagnostic cases. In the overnight metyrapone test, 30 mg/kg (maximum, 3 g) metyrapone is given at midnight, and plasma cortisol and 11-deoxycortisol are measured at 8 a.m. the following morning. In patients with an intact axis, ACTH levels rise after the blockade of cortisol synthesis by metyrapone, and a normal result is signified by a peak 11-deoxycortisol value greater than 7 μg/dL.[357] The CRH stimulation test has been used to diagnose adrenal insufficiency; unlike the metyrapone test, it differentiates primary from secondary causes. Patients with primary adrenal failure have high ACTH levels that rise further after CRH stimulation. Patients with secondary adrenal failure have low ACTH levels that fail to respond to CRH. Patients with hypothalamic disease show a steady rise in ACTH levels after CRH administration.[358]

Testing the HPA Axis during Critical Illness. Many factors complicate investigation of the HPA axis during critical illness. Cortisol levels vary broadly with disease severity, making it difficult to define appropriate responses. Additionally, CBG levels decrease substantially, leading to increases in the ratio of free to bound serum cortisol; for this reason, tests that assess the whole axis (e.g., ITT) are not appropriate in the critical care setting. Investigations are therefore limited to basal cortisol levels or values measured after the SST.

Recent guidance has indicated that a random cortisol value of less than 400 nmol/L (<15 μg/dL) suggests corticosteroid insufficiency, whereas a level greater than 900 nmol/L (>33 μg/dL) is unlikely to occur in patients with compromised HPA axis function. For individuals with intermediate cortisol levels, an SST should be performed; a cortisol increment of less than 250 nmol/L (<9 μg/dL) is an independent prognostic marker for death in critically ill patients.[338]

An initial multicenter randomized trial of patients with septic shock showed that those with an increment less than 250 nmol/L across an SST had a significant improvement in mortality when given replacement corticosteroids.[359] However, in a more recent study hydrocortisone treatment hastened reversal of shock but did not improve overall survival in patients with septic shock.[360] The SST was not useful in predicting benefit from glucocorticoids. It is possible that differences in results between these two trials were due to differences in patient selection (e.g., severity of sepsis) and the speed of administration of glucocorticoids.

In light of this uncertainty, recent recommendations continue to suggest hydrocortisone treatment for septic shock and methylprednisolone for patients with severe early acute respiratory distress syndrome, particularly those with poor response to fluid resuscitation and vasopressor agents.[339] The role of glucocorticoids in the management of critically ill patients with other conditions requires further research.

Other Tests. Radioimmunoassays to detect autoantibodies such as those against the 21-hydroxylase antigen are now

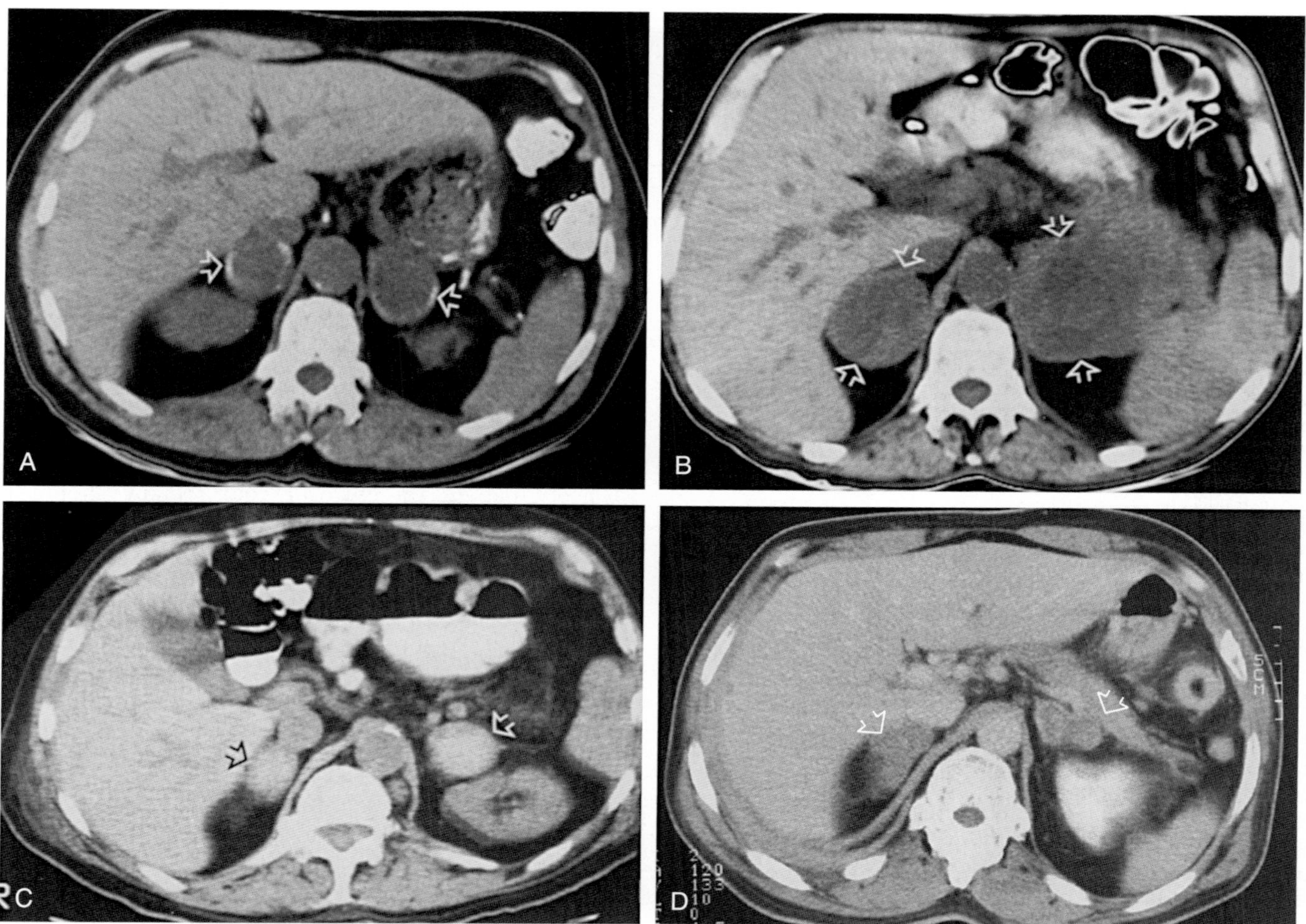

Figure 15-33 Computed tomographic (CT) scans of patients with primary adrenal insufficiency. The affected adrenal glands are indicated by arrows. **A,** CT scan of a 59-year-old man with histoplasmosis. Notice the subcapsular calcium in both glands. **B,** CT scan of a 59-year-old man with metastatic melanoma. **C,** CT scan of an 80-year-old man with bilateral adrenal hemorrhage resulting from anticoagulation for pulmonary emboli. **D,** Bilateral adrenal tuberculomas in a 79-year-old man with tuberculosis affecting the urogenital tract. (**A** and **B** courtesy of Dr. William D. Salmon, Jr.; **C,** courtesy of Dr. Craig R. Sussman.)

available and should be analyzed in patients with primary adrenal failure. In autoimmune Addison's disease, it is also important to look for evidence of other organ-specific autoimmune disease. A CT scan may reveal enlarged or calcified adrenals, suggesting an infective, hemorrhagic, or malignant diagnosis (Fig. 15-33). Chest radiography, tuberculin testing, and early-morning urine samples cultured for *Mycobacterium tuberculosis* should be performed if tuberculosis is suspected. CT-guided adrenal biopsy may reveal an underlying diagnosis in patients with suspected malignant deposits in the adrenal. Adrenoleukodystrophy can be diagnosed by measuring circulating levels of VLCFA. Finally, appropriate investigations, including pituitary MRI scans and an assessment of anterior function, are required for patients with suspected secondary hypoadrenalism who are not taking corticosteroid therapy.

Treatment of Acute Adrenal Insufficiency

Acute adrenal insufficiency is a life-threatening emergency, and treatment should not be delayed while waiting for definitive proof of diagnosis (Table 15-20). However, in addition to measurement of plasma electrolytes and blood glucose, appropriate samples for ACTH and cortisol should be taken before corticosteroid therapy is given. If the patient is not critically ill, an acute ACTH stimulation test can be performed.

In adults, intravenous hydrocortisone should be given in a dose of 100 mg every 6 to 8 hours. If this is not possible, then the intramuscular route should be used. In the patient with shock, 1 L of normal saline should be given intravenously over the first hour. Because of possible hypoglycemia, it is normal to give 5% dextrose in saline. Subsequent saline and dextrose therapy will depend on biochemical monitoring and the patient's condition. Clinical improvement, especially in the blood pressure, should be seen within 4 to 6 hours if the diagnosis is correct. It is important to recognize and treat any associated condition (e.g., infection) that may have precipitated the acute adrenal crisis.

After the first 24 hours, the dose of hydrocortisone can be reduced, usually to 50 mg intramuscularly every 6 hours and then to oral hydrocortisone, 40 mg in the morning and 20 mg at 6 p.m.. This can then be rapidly reduced to a more standard replacement dose of 20 mg on wakening and 10 mg at 6 p.m..

Long-Term Replacement Therapy

The aim of long-term therapy is to give replacement doses of hydrocortisone to mimic the normal cortisol secretion

TABLE 15-20

Treatment of Acute Adrenal Insufficiency (Adrenal Crisis) in Adults

Emergency Measures

1. Establish intravenous access with a large-gauge needle.
2. Draw blood for "stat" serum electrolytes and glucose and routine measurement of plasma cortisol and ACTH. Do not wait for laboratory results.
3. Infuse 2-3 L of 154 mmol/L NaCl (0.9% saline) solution, or 50 g/L (5%) dextrose in 154 mmol/L NaCl (0.9% saline) solution, as quickly as possible. Monitor for signs of fluid overload by measuring central or peripheral venous pressure and listening for pulmonary rales. Reduce infusion rate if indicated.
4. Inject intravenous hydrocortisone (100 mg immediately and every 6 hr)
5. Use supportive measures as needed.

Subacute Measures After Stabilization of the Patient

1. Continue intravenous 154 mmol/L NaCl (0.9% saline) solution at a slower rate for next 24-48 hr.
2. Search for and treat possible infectious precipitating causes of the adrenal crisis.
3. Perform a short ACTH stimulation test to confirm the diagnosis of adrenal insufficiency (if patient does not have known adrenal insufficiency).
4. Determine the type of adrenal insufficiency and its cause, if not already known.
5. Taper glucocorticoids to maintenance dosage over 1-3 days, if precipitating or complicating illness permits.
6. Begin mineralocorticoid replacement with fludrocortisones (0.1 mg by mouth daily) when saline infusion is stopped.

ACTH, adrenocorticotropic hormone.

rate (Table 15-21). In the past, this rate was thought to be approximately 25 to 30 mg/day, but stable isotope studies have indicated lower normal cortisol production rates of 8 to 15 mg/day.[361] Most patients can cope with less than 30 mg/day (usually 15 to 25 mg/day in divided doses). Doses are usually given on wakening, with a smaller dose at 6 p.m., but some patients feel better with three-times-a-day dosing. In cases of primary adrenal failure, cortisol day curves with simultaneous ACTH measurements are advocated to provide some insight into the adequacy of replacement therapy.[362] There are no good objective tests in secondary adrenal failure. Decisions regarding doses of replacement therapy are largely based on crude yet important end points such as weight, well-being, and blood pressure.[363] Bone mineral density is moderately reduced in a dose-dependent manner in patients treated with more than 25 mg/day of hydrocortisone,[364] highlighting the need to strive for minimally effective but safe doses.[365,366] Possibly because of the known action of IGF1 to increase cortisol clearance,[131] it is our experience that glucocorticoid requirements are slightly lower in hypopituitary, GH-deficient subjects than in patients with primary adrenal insufficiency.

In primary adrenal failure, mineralocorticoid replacement is usually also required in the form of fludrocortisone (or 9α-fluorinated hydrocortisone), 0.05 to 0.2 mg/day. The mineralocorticoid activity of this is about 125 times that of hydrocortisone. After the acute phase has passed, the adequacy of mineralocorticoid replacement should be assessed by measuring electrolytes, supine and erect blood pressures, and plasma renin activity.[367] Too little fludrocortisone may cause postural hypotension with elevated plasma renin activity, whereas too much causes the converse. Mineralocorticoid replacement therapy is all too frequently neglected in patients with adrenal failure.

Patients on glucocorticoid replacement therapy should be advised to double their daily dose in the event of intercurrent febrile illness, accident, or mental stress such as an important examination. If the patient is vomiting and cannot take medication by mouth, parenteral hydrocortisone must be given urgently. For minor surgery, 50 to 100 mg hydrocortisone hemisuccinate is given with the premedication. For major operations, this pretreatment is followed by the same regimen as for acute adrenal insufficiency (see Table 15-21). Pregnancy proceeds normally in patients taking replacement therapy, but daily doses of hydrocortisone are usually increased modestly (5 to 10 mg/day) in the last trimester. Progesterone is a mineralocorticoid antagonist, and the rising levels across pregnancy may necessitate an increased dose of fludrocortisone. During labor, patients should be well hydrated with a saline drip and should receive hydrocortisone 50 mg intramuscularly every 6 hours until delivery. Thereafter, doses can be rapidly tapered to prepregnancy levels.

Every patient on glucocorticoid therapy should be advised to register for a medical alert bracelet or necklace

TABLE 15-21

Treatment of Chronic Primary Adrenal Insufficiency in Adults

Maintenance Therapy

Glucocorticoid Replacement

- Hydrocortisone 15-20 mg on awakening and 5-10 mg in early afternoon
- Monitor clinical symptoms and morning plasma ACTH

Mineralocorticoid Replacement

- Fludrocortisone 0.1 (0.05-0.2) mg orally
- Liberal salt intake
- Monitor lying and standing blood pressure and pulse, edema, serum potassium, and plasma renin activity
- Educate patient about the disease, how to manage minor illnesses and major stresses, and how to inject steroid intramuscularly
- Obtain MedicAlert bracelet/necklace, Emergency Medical Information Card

Treatment of Minor Febrile Illness or Stress

- Increase glucocorticoid dose twofold to threefold for the few days of illness; do not change mineralocorticoid dose
- Contact physician if illness worsens or persists for more than 3 days or if vomiting develops
- No extra supplementation is needed for most uncomplicated, outpatient dental procedures with local anesthesia. General anesthesia or intravenous sedation should not be used in the office.

Emergency Treatment of Severe Stress or Trauma

- Inject contents of prefilled dexamethasone (4-mg) syringe intramuscularly
- Get to physician as quickly as possible

Steroid Coverage for Illness or Surgery in Hospital

- For moderate illness, give hydrocortisone 50 mg bid PO or IV. Taper rapidly to maintenance dose as patient recovers.
- For severe illness, give hydrocortisone 100 mg IV q8h. Taper to maintenance level by decreasing by half every day. Adjust dose according to course of illness.
- For minor procedures under local anesthesia and most radiologic studies, no extra supplementation is needed.
- For moderately stressful procedures such as barium enema, endoscopy, or arteriography, give a single 100-mg IV dose of hydrocortisone just before the procedure.
- For major surgery, give hydrocortisone 100 mg IV just before induction of anesthesia and continue q8h for first 24 hr. Taper dose rapidly, decreasing by half per day, to maintenance level.

ACTH, adrenocorticotropic hormone.

and to carry a "steroid card." Patients should receive regular education regarding the requirements of stress-related glucocorticoid dose adjustment, which should involve the patient's partner and family as well. Parental preparations of hydrocortisone for self-administration may be required for patients living far from hospitals and those planning vacations.

For patients with both primary and secondary adrenal failure, beneficial effects of adrenal androgen replacement therapy with 25 to 50 mg/day of DHEA have been reported. To date, reported benefit is principally confined to female patients and includes improvement in sexual function and well-being.[368] However, patients with adrenal insufficiency on current steroid replacement regimens have significantly impaired health-related subjective health status irrespective of the origin of disease or concomitant disease.[340]

CONGENITAL ADRENAL HYPERPLASIA

CAH comprises a group of autosomal recessive disorders caused by deficient adrenal corticosteroid biosynthesis.[369,370] It results from defects in one of the steroidogenic enzymes involved in cortisol biosynthesis or in the electron-providing factor, P450 oxidoreductase (POR). Congenital lipoid adrenal hyperplasia, caused by StAR deficiency affecting mitochondrial cholesterol uptake, is a subform of this disease complex with the unique feature of lipid accumulation leading to cell destruction. In each case, there is reduced negative feedback inhibition of cortisol and, depending on the steroidogenic pathway involved, alteration in adrenal mineralocorticoid and androgen secretion (Table 15-22).

Aldosterone synthase deficiency does not affect glucocorticoid biosynthesis and does not lead to adrenal hyperplasia, but it has been historically grouped into this disease complex. All forms of CAH together represent a disease continuum, ranging from severe forms caused by complete loss-of-function defects to milder forms in which the defective proteins have partial residual activity.

21-Hydroxylase Deficiency

Between 90% and 95% of cases of CAH are caused by 21-hydroxylase deficiency.[369] In Western societies, the incidence varies from 1 in 10,000 to 1 in 15,000 live births, but in isolated communities the incidence may be much higher (e.g., 1:300 in Alaskan Inuit populations). Nonclassic CAH is more common, with an incidence of about 1 in 500 to 1000 live births. The condition arises because of defective conversion of 17α-OHP to 11-deoxycortisol. Reduced cortisol biosynthesis results in reduced negative feedback drive and increased ACTH secretion; as a consequence, adrenal androgens are produced in excess (Fig. 15-34). Seventy-five percent of patients have clinically manifest mineralocorticoid deficiency because of failure to convert sufficient progesterone to DOC in the ZG.

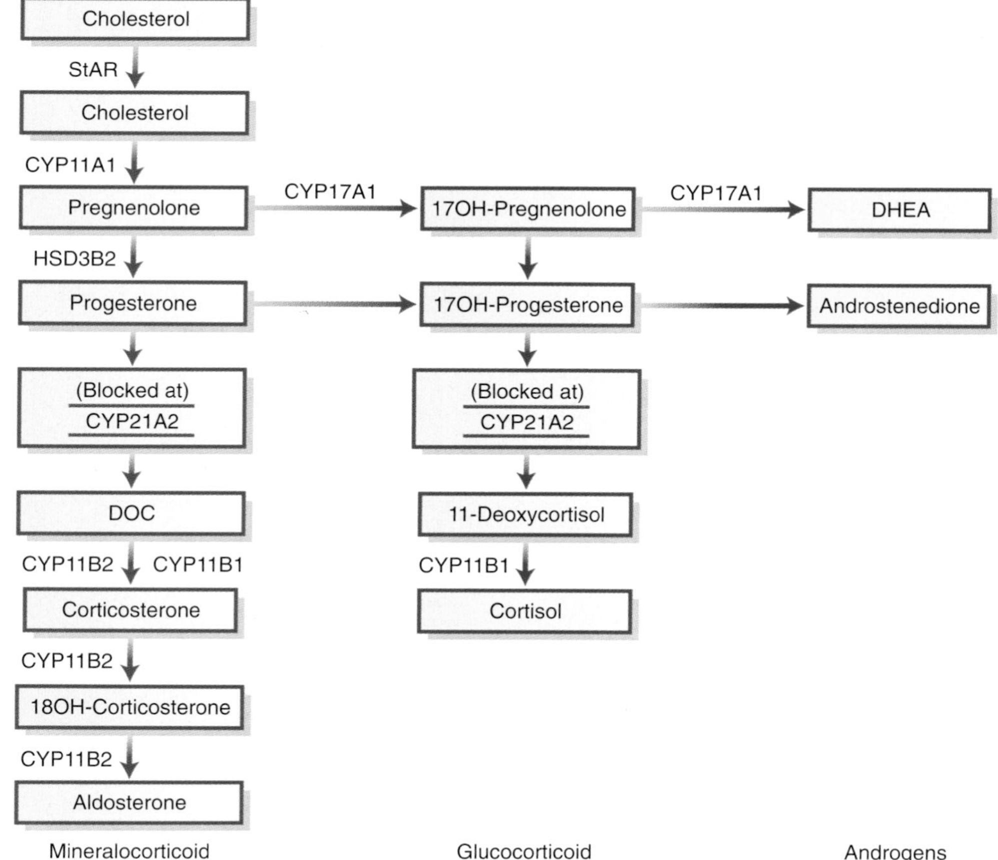

Figure 15-34 Congenital adrenal hyperplasia related to 21-hydroxylase deficiency. The normal synthesis of cortisol is impaired, and adrenocorticotropic hormone (ACTH) levels increase because of loss of normal negative feedback inhibition, resulting in an increase in adrenal steroid precursors proximal to the block. The results are cortisol deficiency, variable mineralocorticoid deficiency, and excessive secretion of adrenal androgens. CYP, cytochrome P450; DHEA, dehydroepiandrosterone; DOC, deoxycorticosterone; HSD, hydroxysteroid dehydrogenase; StAR, steroidogenic acute regulatory protein.

TABLE 15-22

Congenital Adrenal Hyperplasia: Features for Each Enzyme Defect

Deficiency	21-Hydroxylase	11β-Hydroxylase	17α-Hydroxylase	3β-HSD Type 2	P450 Oxidoreductase	Lipoid Adrenal Hyperplasia	P450 Side Chain Cleavage	Aldosterone Synthase	Apparent Cortisone Reductase
OMIM No.	+201910	#202010	#202110	+201810	#201750	*600617	+118485	*124080	*138090
Gene/Protein	CYP21A2	CYP11B1	CYP17A1	HSD3B2	POR	StAR	CYP11A1	CYP11B2	H6PDH
Alias	P450c21	P450c11	P450c17	3β-HSD	CPR, CYPOR		P450scc	P450aldo	
Incidence	*Classic:* 1:10,000 to 15,000 *Nonclassic:* 1:500 to 1:1,000	1:100,000 to 1; 200,000	Rare	Rare	Unknown	Rare	Rare	Rare	Rare
DSD	*Classic:* 46,XX *Nonclassic:* No	46,XX	46,XY	46,XY*	46,XX + 46,XY†	46,XY	46,XY	No	No
Primary affected organ	Adrenal	Adrenal	Adrenal, gonads	Adrenal, gonads	Adrenal, gonads, liver, all CYP type 2–expressing tissues	Adrenal, gonads	Adrenal, gonads	Adrenal	Liver, adrenal, all H6PDH/HSD11B1–expressing tissues
Glucocorticoids	*Classic:* Reduced *Nonclassic:* Normal	Reduced	Reduced	Reduced	Reduced to normal, impaired stress response	Reduced	Reduced	Normal	Normal, but reduced tissue levels due to increased cortisol clearance
Mineralocorticoids	*Classic:* Reduced in SW *Nonclassic:* Normal	Increased, mainly precursors	Increased	Reduced often	Reduced to increased	Reduced	Reduced	Reduced	Normal
Sex hormones	Increased	Increased	Reduced	Reduced in males, increased in females‡	Reduced	Reduced	Reduced	Normal	Increased
Increased marker metabolites in plasma	17-OHP, 21-DOF	DOC, S	Pregnenolone, progesterone, DOC, S	17-OH Pregnenolone, DHEA	Pregnenolone, progesterone, 17-OHP			DOC, B, 18-OHB	
Increased marker metabolites in urine	Pregnanetriol, 17-OH pregnanolone, pregnanetriolone	THDOC, THS	THDOC, THB, pregnenediol, pregnanediol	Pregnantriol	Pregnenediol, pregnanediol, pregnanetriol, 17-OH pregnanolone				
PRA	*Classic:* Increased *Nonclassic:* Normal to mildly increased	Reduced	Reduced	Increased		Increased	Increased	Increased	Normal
Hypertension	No	Yes	Yes	No	No or mild	No	No	No	No
Plasma sodium	*Classic:* Reduced in SW *Nonclassic:* Normal	Increased	Increased	Reduced in SW	Normal	Reduced	Reduced	Reduced	Normal
Plasma potassium	*Classic:* Increased in SW *Nonclassic:* Normal	Reduced	Reduced	Increased in SW	Normal	Increased	Increased	Increased	Normal
Urinary salt loss	*Classic:* Yes *Nonclassic:* No	No	No	Yes	No	Yes	Yes	Yes	No
Skeletal malformation	No	No	No	No	Yes§	No	No	No	No

*Masculinization of the external genitalia in females at birth is rare and usually mild; signs of increased androgens usually manifest later.

†DSD is observed in both sexes, and normal sex-specific sexual development is also reported.

‡Steroid hormone conversion by HSD3B1 in peripheral tissues.

§In most cases published thus far; however, absence of skeletal malformations does not rule out POR deficiency.

B, corticosterone; CYP, cytochrome P450; DHEA, dehydroepiandrosterone; DOC, 11-deoxycorticosterone; 21-DOF, 21-deoxycortisol; DSD, disorder of sex development; H6PDH, hexose-6-phosphate dehydrogenase; HSD, hydroxysteroid dehydrogenase; OMIM, Online Mendelian Inheritance in Man; 18-OHB, 18-hydroxycorticosterone; 17-OHP, 17-hydroxyprogesterone; POR, P450 oxidoreductase; PRA, plasma renin activity; S, 11-deoxycortisol; StAR, steroidogenic acute regulatory protein; SW, salt wasting; THB, tetrahydro-corticosterone; THS, tetrahydro-11-deoxycortisol; THDOC, tetrahydro-11-deoxycorticosterone.

TABLE 15-23

Forms of 21-Hydroxylase Deficiency

Phenotype	Classic Salt Wasting	Simple Virilizing	Nonclassic
Age at diagnosis	Newborn to 6 mo	*Female:* Newborn to 2 yr *Male:* 2-4 yr	Child to adult
Genitalia	*Female:* Ambiguous *Male:* Normal	*Female:* Ambiguous *Male:* Normal	*Female:* Virilized *Male:* Normal
Incidence	1:20,000	1:60,000	1:1000
Hormones			
Aldosterone	Reduced	Normal	Normal
Renin	Increased	Normal or increased	Normal
Cortisol	Reduced	Reduced	Normal
17-OHP	>5000 ng/dL	2500-5000 ng/dL	500-2500 ng/dL (ACTH stimulation)
Testosterone	Increased	Increased	Variable, increased
Growth	−2 to −3 SD	−1 to −2 SD	Probably normal
21-Hydroxylase activity (% of wild type)	0	1-5	20-50
Typical *CYP21A2* mutations	Deletions, conversions, nt656g G110Δ8nt, R356W I236N, V237E, M239K, Q318X	I172N Intron 2 splice site (nt656g)	V281L P30L

ACTH, adrenocorticotropic hormone; 17-OHP, 17-hydroxyprogesterone; SD, standard deviation.

Clinically, several distinct variants of 21-hydroxylase deficiency have been recognized (Table 15-23).

Simple Virilizing Form

In the simple virilizing form of 21-hydroxylase deficiency, the enhanced ACTH drive to adrenal androgen secretion in utero leads to virilization of an affected female fetus. Depending on the severity, clitoral enlargement, labial fusion, and development of a urogenital sinus may occur, leading to sexual ambiguity at birth and even inappropriate sex assignment. Males are phenotypically normal at birth and are at risk of not being diagnosed; this explains the skewed female-to-male ratio of simple virilizing CAH diagnosed in the preneonatal screening era. Such patients may present in early childhood with signs of precocious pseudopuberty such as sexual precocity, pubic hair development, or growth acceleration due to premature androgen excess. If left untreated, this stimulates premature epiphyseal closure and final adult height is invariably diminished.[371,372]

Salt-Wasting Form

Seventy-five percent of patients of both sexes who have the salt-wasting form of 21-hydroxylase deficiency also have concomitant, clinically manifested aldosterone deficiency. In addition to the described features, neonates commonly present after the first 2 weeks of life with a salt-wasting crisis and hypotension. The clinical signs and symptoms of salt wasting include poor feeding, vomiting, failure to thrive, lethargy, and sepsis-like symptoms. These features may alert the clinician to the diagnosis in a male baby, but the diagnosis is still delayed in many cases, and the condition carries a significant neonatal mortality rate.

Nonclassic or Late-Onset 21-Hydroxylase Deficiency

Patients with nonclassic 21-hydroxylase deficiency present in childhood or early adulthood with premature pubarche or with a phenotype that may masquerade as polycystic ovary syndrome (PCOS).[369,373,374] Indeed, nonclassic CAH is a recognized secondary cause of PCOS and appears to be more common than the classic variant. Recent evidence suggests that at least 30% of adult patients have an impaired cortisol response to ACTH(1-24)[375] and may be prone to stress-induced adrenal insufficiency. Routine assessment of adrenal glucocorticoid reserve is indicated. In some series from tertiary referral centers, nonclassic 21-hydroxylase deficiency accounts for up to 12% of all "PCOS" patients, but more realistic prevalence rates are probably 1% to 3%.[376] Females present with hirsutism, primary or secondary amenorrhea, or anovulatory infertility.[373] Androgenic alopecia and acne may be other presenting features.

Heterozygote 21-Hydroxylase Deficiency

Salt-wasting, simple virilizing, and late-onset 21-hydroxylase deficiency are all caused by homozygous or compound heterozygote mutations in the human 21-hydroxylase gene (*CYP21A2*). In the carrier or heterozygote state, only one allele is mutated. The clinical significance of the heterozygote state is uncertain; it does not appear to disadvantage reproductive capability but may cause signs of hyperandrogenism in adult women.[369]

Molecular Genetics

21-Hydroxylase deficiency is inherited as an autosomal recessive trait, and the higher incidence of the condition in some ethnic communities almost certainly relates to consanguinity. The *CYP21A2* gene and its highly homologous pseudogene (*CYP21A1P*) are located on the short arm of chromosome 6 (6p21.3). Because of the genomic localization within the human leukocyte antigen (HLA) locus, a region with a high frequency of genomic recombinations, most of the mutations causing 21-hydroxylase deficiency are generated by gene conversion events. Complete gene deletions or conversions of the *CYP21A2* gene, eight pseudogene-derived point mutations, and an 8-base-pair deletion are found in more than 95% of cases. Other rare pseudogene-independent *CYP21A2*-inactivating mutations have been reported in single families or small populations. Approximately 65% to 75% of CAH patients are compound heterozygous for the disease-causing mutations.[377]

The genotype-phenotype correlation in CAH due to 21-hydroxylase deficiency is well established. The clinical phenotype correlates with the less severely mutated allele and, consequently, with the residual 21-hydroxylase activity (Fig. 15-35).[378,379] This correlation appears to be high, although divergence between genotype and phenotype has been observed.[380] The 21-hydroxylase activity measured by in vitro analysis provides a possibility for estimating disease severity, although some phenotypic variability (e.g., salt wasting, age at onset) seems likely to depend on other

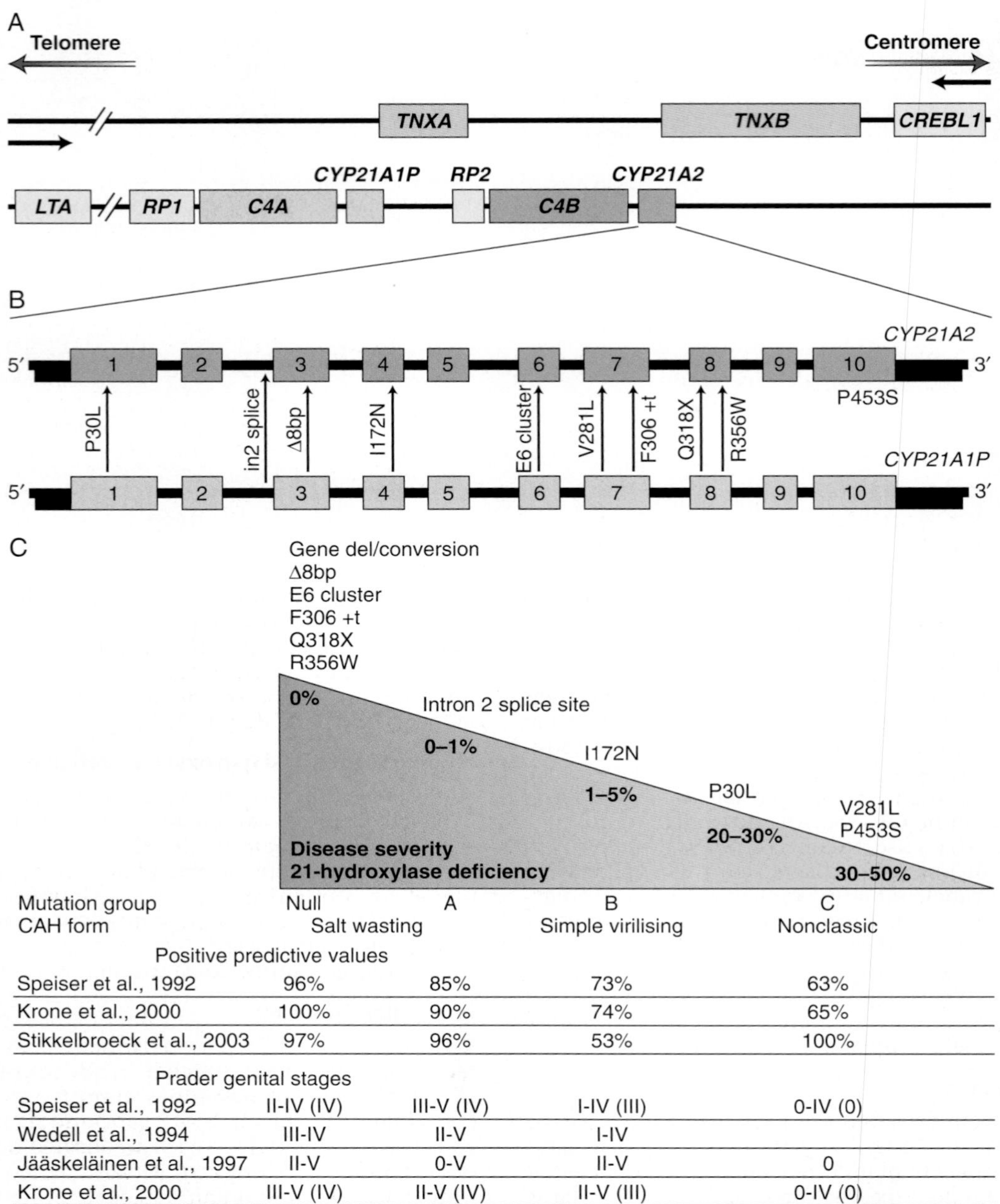

Positive predictive values	Null	A	B	C
Speiser et al., 1992	96%	85%	73%	63%
Krone et al., 2000	100%	90%	74%	65%
Stikkelbroeck et al., 2003	97%	96%	53%	100%

Prader genital stages	Null	A	B	C
Speiser et al., 1992	II-IV (IV)	III-V (IV)	I-IV (III)	0-IV (0)
Wedell et al., 1994	III-IV	II-V	I-IV	
Jääskeläinen et al., 1997	II-V	0-V	II-V	0
Krone et al., 2000	III-V (IV)	II-V (IV)	II-V (III)	0-IV (0)

Figure 15-35 Genetics of 21-hydroxylase deficiency. **A,** Genomic organization of the functional *CYP21A2* gene and its nonfunctional *CYP21A1P* pseudogene. **B,** Nine out of 10 common mutations are transferred by microconversions from the *CYP21A1P* pseudogene into the *CYP21A2* gene. **C,** Genotype-phenotype correlation in 21-hydroxylase deficiency is well established. Based on the in vitro enzyme activity, the *CYP21A2* gene-inactivating mutations can be categorized into four major mutation groups. Although variation has been reported for the milder mutations, the overall correlation is high regarding expression of the adrenal phenotype. Considerable variability exists for the correlation with genital virilization. CAH, congenital adrenal hyperplasia; NC, nonclassic congenital adrenal hyperplasia; SW, salt wasting; SV, simple virilizing.

interacting genes and maturation processes rather than *CYP21A2* itself. One such factor might be the length of the CAG repeats in the androgen receptor modulating androgen action.[381] Potential variations in the degree of recovery from glucocorticoid and mineralocorticoid deficiency during later life might be explained by significant 21-hydroxylase activity of the cytochrome P450 enzymes CYP2C19 and CYP3A4.[382]

Diagnostic Criteria

A diagnosis of 21-hydroxylase deficiency should be considered in any newborn infant with genital ambiguity and salt wasting, hypotension, or hypoglycemia. Hyponatremia and hypokalemia with raised plasma renin activity are found in salt-wasters. In later life, adrenal androgen excess (DHEAS, androstenedione) is found in patients presenting with sexual precocity or a PCOS-like phenotype. Randomly timed measurements of the plasma 17-OHP concentration are significantly increased in classic 21-hydroxylase deficiency. Commonly, 17-OHP concentrations in patients with salt-wasting CAH are higher than in non–salt-losing patients.

In nonclassic CAH, an SST is required to establish normal adrenal glucocorticoid reserve. Clinically useful

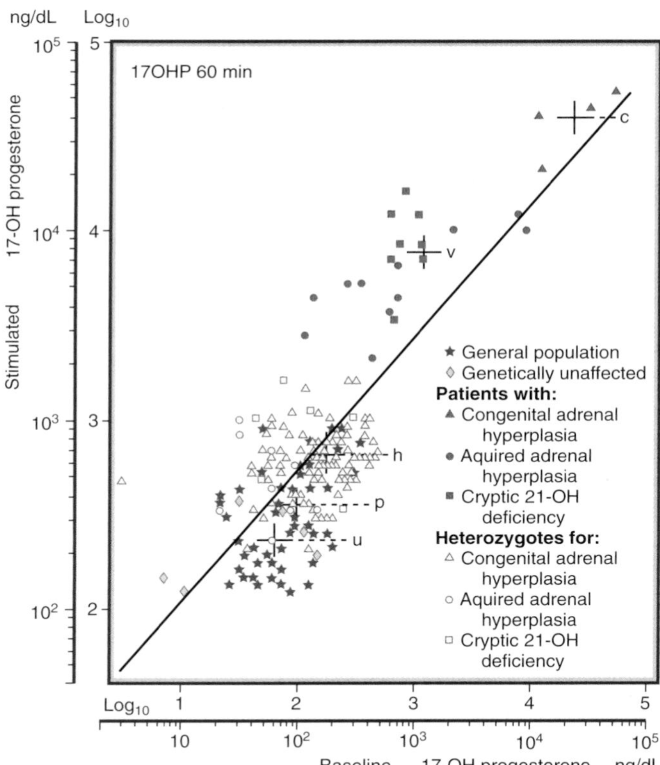

Figure 15-36 Basal and stimulated plasma 17α-hydroxyprogesterone (17-OHP) concentrations in patients with 21-hydroxylase (21-OH, CYP21A2) deficiency. To convert values to nmol/L, multiply by 0.0303. The mean for each group is indicated by a large cross and an adjacent letter: *c*, patients with classic CYP21A2 deficiency; *v*, patients with nonclassic (acquired and cryptic) CYP21A2 deficiency; *h*, heterozygotes for all forms of CYP21A2 deficiency; *p*, general population; *u*, known unaffected persons (e.g., siblings of patients with CYP21A2 deficiency who carry neither affected parental haplotype as determined by human leukocyte antigen typing). (From White PC, New MI, Dupont B. Congenital adrenal hyperplasia: part 1. *N Engl J Med.* 1987;316:1519-1524.)

nomograms have been developed that compare circulating concentrations of 17-OHP before and 60 minutes after exogenous ACTH administration to investigate borderline cases and to differentiate between nonclassic CAH and heterozygous carriers (Fig. 15-36).[383] This separates patients with classic and nonclassic 21-hydroxylase deficiency from heterozygote carriers and normal subjects, but there is some overlap between values seen in heterozygotes and in normal subjects. 17-OHP is measured basally and then 60 minutes after administration of 250 μg Synacthen. Stimulated values are invariably grossly elevated (>35 nmol/L [>11 μg/L]) in patients with classic and nonclassic forms of the disorder. Heterozygote patients usually have stimulated values between 10 and 30 nmol/L (330 to 1000 ng/dL) (see Fig. 15-36). Stimulation tests are not always required to make a diagnosis; for example, a basal 17-OHP concentration of less than 5 nmol/L (<150 ng/dL) in the follicular phase of the menstrual cycle effectively excludes late-onset 21-hydroxylase deficiency.[373] *CYP21A2* genotyping to confirm the clinical and biochemical diagnosis is a useful adjunct to hormonal measurements. Androgen excess in 21-hydroxylase deficiency is readily suppressed after glucocorticoid administration.

Prenatal diagnosis of 21-hydroxylase deficiency has been advocated, because treatment of an affected female may prevent masculinization in utero.[384] 17-OHP can be assayed in amniotic fluid, but the most robust approach is the rapid genotyping of fetal cells obtained by chorionic villous sampling in early gestation. In patients with known 21-hydroxylase deficiency (male or female) seeking fertility, determination of 17-OHP levels across an SST in the partner before conception will uncover nonclassic or heterozygote cases and provide the endocrinologist/geneticist with some assignment of risk before pregnancy.

Treatment

The objectives for treatment of 21-hydroxylase deficiency differ with age, but at all ages treatment and overall patient management can be fraught with difficulties.

In childhood, the overall goal is to replace glucocorticoid and mineralocorticoid, thereby preventing further salt-wasting crises, but also to normalize adrenal androgen secretion so that normal growth and skeletal maturation can proceed. Accurate replacement is essential; in excess, glucocorticoids will suppress growth, whereas inadequate replacement will result initially in accelerated linear growth and ultimately in short stature due to premature epiphyseal closure.[369] Response is best monitored through growth velocity and bone age, with biochemical markers from blood (17-OHP, androstenedione, testosterone), urine, and saliva (17-OHP, androstenedione, testosterone) being useful adjuncts. In difficult cases, a day curve study, as described for patients with primary adrenal failure but measuring the ACTH and 17-OHP response before and after corticosteroid replacement, may confirm overreplacement or underreplacement. The optimal glucocorticoid dose fails to suppress 17-OHP and its metabolites and maintains sex hormone concentrations in the middle of the age- and sex-specific normal range. Ideally, the biochemical investigations will indicate the need for dose adjustments before physical changes, growth, and skeletal maturation indicate inadequate or excessive glucocorticoid treatment.[385]

Corrective surgery (e.g., clitoral reduction, vaginoplasty) is frequently required during childhood. The method of choice should be a one-stage complete repair using the newest techniques of vaginoplasty, clitoral, and labial surgery.[385]

In late childhood and adolescence, appropriate replacement therapy is equally important. Overtreatment may result in obesity and delayed menarche/puberty with sexual infantilism, whereas underreplacement will result in sexual precocity. Compliance with regular medication is often an issue through adolescence.

Although much has been written about adequate control in childhood, adults with CAH often provide an ongoing dilemma for the endocrinologist. The follow-up of such patients should involve multidisciplinary clinics, initially with transition adolescence clinics to facilitate transfer from pediatric to adult care. Problems in adulthood relate to fertility concerns, hirsutism, and menstrual irregularity in women; obesity, metabolic consequences, probable increased cardiovascular risk, and impact of short stature; sexual dysfunction; and psychological problems.[369,386,387] Counseling is often required in addition to endocrine support. Males may develop enlargement of the testes due to so-called testicular adrenal rest tumors—that is, ectopic adrenal tissue, which may regress after glucocorticoid suppression. These patients need adequate endocrine therapy rather than urologic referral with ensuing risk of removal of testis mistaken for a tumor.[388]

In the absence of any evidence-based data, there are no prescriptive steroid regimens to treat patients with CAH at any age, and, as a result, many individualized regimens are used in clinical practice. Hydrocortisone is recommended for replacement therapy from the newborn period to adolescence.[385] Usual starting doses of hydrocortisone in childhood are 10 to 15 mg/m^2 per day in three divided doses per day, with up to 25 mg/m^2 in infancy only seldom required. These doses are higher than those employed for replacement of adrenal insufficiency because treatment also aims at normalization of ACTH-driven adrenal androgen excess. The optimal timing for providing the highest dose of hydrocortisone remains an ongoing matter of debate, with no data supporting either "circadian" replacement (giving the highest dose in the morning) or "reverse-phase" therapy (giving the largest dose of hydrocortisone at night). Long-acting steroids such as prednisone, prednisolone, and dexamethasone are more effective in this regard but should not be given before the end of puberty, to avoid oversuppression and reduction in linear growth.

Fludrocortisone is required for patients with salt wasting (although this may spontaneously improve with age). Fludrocortisone doses during the first year of life are commonly 150 μg/m^2 per day. Sodium needs to be supplemented, as milk feeds provide only maintenance sodium requirements. Adequate mineralocorticoid replacement usually leads to hydrocortisone dose reduction. The relative dose in relation to body surface decreases throughout life. Fludrocortisone doses of 100 μg/m^2 per day after the first 2 years of life are commonly sufficient. This requirement drops further with adolescence and adulthood to a daily dose of 100 to 200 μg (50 to 100 μg/m^2 per day). Mineralocorticoid substitution is monitored by measurements of plasma renin activity (low or suppressed levels indicating overtreatment) and blood pressure.[389]

Adrenomedullary dysplasia has been reported in the CAH adrenal, probably because of relative glucocorticoid deficiency, which results in epinephrine deficiency.[390] Benefits of epinephrine replacement on the metabolic response to exercise have been reported in children,[391] but further studies are required before routine catecholamine replacement therapy can be advocated. In clinical practice, sufficient supplementation of glucose during exercise and illness should be guaranteed, to prevent hypoglycemic episodes. Bilateral adrenalectomy is effective but should be regarded as a last resort[392]; in addition, the requirement for lifelong corticosteroid replacement therapy, patients could also develop feedback ACTH-secreting pituitary tumors.[393] This procedure bears also a number of risks, including surgical and anesthetic complications, and the patient is left completely adrenal insufficient.

Prenatal dexamethasone treatment is effective to avoid virilization of the external genitalia in the female fetus. Unlike hydrocortisone, which is inactivated by placental 11β-HSD, maternally administered dexamethasone can cross the placenta to suppress the fetal HPA axis. One approach is to advocate use of dexamethasone therapy as soon as pregnancy is confirmed in high-risk cases and to continue this therapy until the diagnosis is excluded in the female fetus. If the fetus is affected, only those of female sex require dexamethasone therapy across gestation. Therapy must be instigated at 6 to 7 weeks' gestation to be effective. The suggested dexamethasone dose is 20 to 25 μg/kg in three divided doses per day (total maximum dose, 1.5 mg/day).[369] However, because only one in eight pregnancies treated in this way will result in an affected female fetus, the use of steroid therapy in this setting has been questioned.[394] The fetal sex can be determined as early as week 6 of gestation with the use of novel molecular diagnostic methods that analyze free fetal DNA from maternal blood using real-time polymerase chain reaction. In this way, the number of unnecessarily treated cases can be reduced to three out of eight. Dexamethasone can lead to maternal Cushingoid effects in pregnancy[395] and may in turn have long-term, deleterious effects on the fetus, including metabolic and psycho-intellectual consequences. Prenatal treatment is controversial and has to be regarded as experimental; patients treated should be included in ongoing multicenter studies.[396]

In adult women with hyperandrogenism and untreated nonclassic CAH, there is no evidence that final height is affected. In this setting, glucocorticoid suppression in isolation rarely controls hirsutism, and additional antiandrogen therapy is often required (e.g., cyproterone acetate, spironolactone, flutamide together with an oral estrogen contraceptive pill). However, ovulation induction rates with gonadotropin therapy are improved after suppression of nocturnal ACTH levels with 0.25 to 0.5 mg dexamethasone. Hypogonadotropic hypogonadism in male patients is a consequence of increased aromatization of adrenal androgens, in particular androstenedione to estrone resulting in suppression of pituitary LH and FSH secretion. The condition is reversible after optimization of glucocorticoid therapy. However, overreplacement in men or women may also lead to hypogonadotropic hypogonadism due to glucocorticoid-mediated suppression of GnRH secretion.

Long-Term Complications and Comorbidities

Outcome assessed by final height is not optimal in many patients treated for 21-hydroxylase deficiency. In a meta-analysis including 18 studies published between 1977 and 2001, the mean adult height of patients with classic CAH was 10 cm (−1.4 SDS) below the population mean and −1.2 SDS calculated for target height. The pubertal growth spurt occurs earlier and is less pronounced than normal. An often overlooked problem is glucocorticoid overtreatment during the first 2 years of life; overtreatment suppresses the infant growth spurt, which is characterized by the highest postnatal growth velocity. Therefore, the lowest optimal dose of glucocorticoid replacement should be established as early in life as possible.

Increased fat mass and obesity are common among children and adolescents with CAH.[397-399] Glucocorticoid dose, chronologic age, advanced bone age maturation, and parental obesity all contribute to elevated BMI SDS.[398]

Increased fat mass and higher insulin levels have been described in women older than 30 years of age with CAH. However, clear evidence of cardiovascular risk factors had not been shown. Women with CAH do have a significantly higher rate of gestational diabetes, a possible forerunner for the development of type 2 diabetes,[400] and women with nonclassic CAH[401] and young adult CAH patients[402] have reduced insulin sensitivity. Increased intima media thickness as a marker of atherosclerosis has been detected.[402]

Daytime systolic blood pressure in children and adolescents with CAH is elevated, and the physiologic nocturnal dip in blood pressure is absent.[403] Elevated systolic blood pressure correlates with the degree of overweight and obesity.[404] There are no long-term outcome data on adults.

11β-Hydroxylase Deficiency

11β-Hydroxylase deficiency accounts for 7% of all cases of CAH, with an incidence of 1:100,000 live births.[405] The condition arises because of mutations in the 11β-hydroxylase *(CYP11B1)* gene that result in loss of enzyme activity and a block in the conversion of 11-deoxycortisol to cortisol. The *CYP11B1* gene is located on chromosome 8q24.3, approximately 40 kilobases from the highly homologous

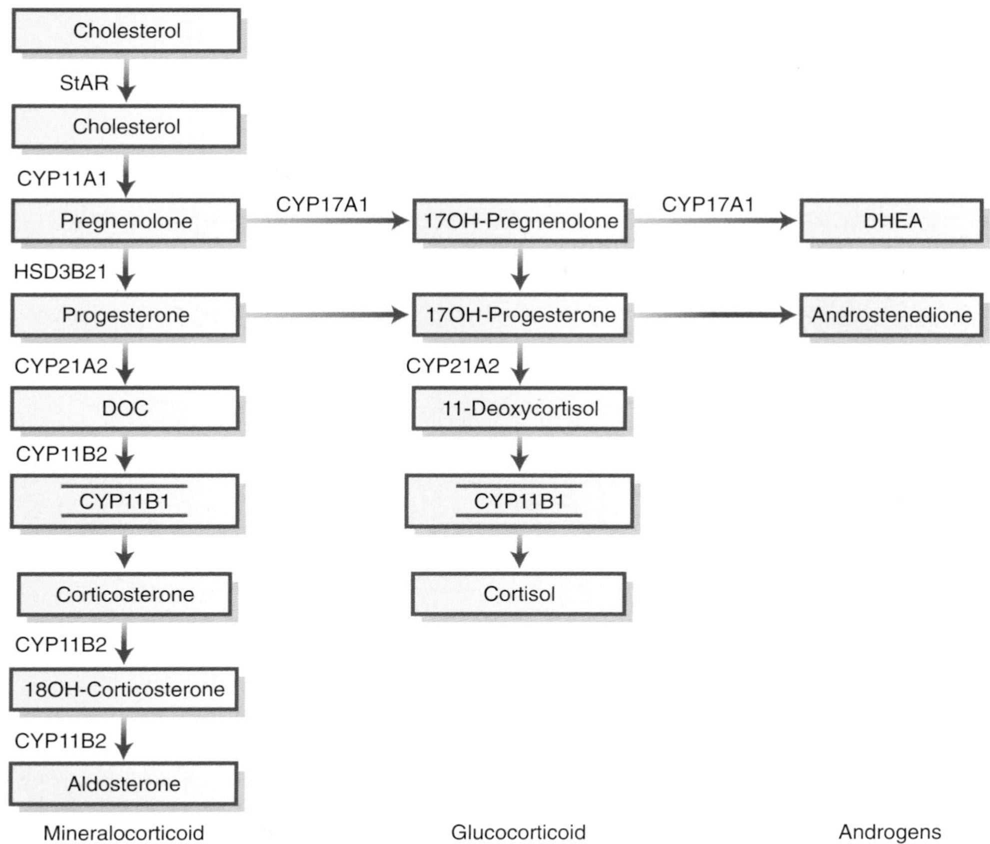

Figure 15-37 Congenital adrenal hyperplasia related to 11β-hydroxylase deficiency. The normal synthesis of cortisol is impaired, and adrenocorticotropic hormone (ACTH) levels increase because of the loss of normal negative feedback inhibition, which results in an increase in adrenal steroid precursors proximal to the block. The results are cortisol deficiency, mineralocorticoid excess related to excessive deoxycorticosterone (DOC) secretion, and excessive secretion of adrenal androgens. CYP, cytochrome P450; DHEA, dehydroepiandrosterone; DOC, deoxycorticosterone; HSD, hydroxysteroid dehydrogenase; StAR, steroidogenic acute regulatory protein.

aldosterone synthase gene (*CYP11B2*).[405] *CYP11B1*-inactivating mutations have been shown to be distributed over the entire coding region consisting of nine exons. Although mutation clusters are reported in exons 2, 6, 7, and 8,[377,405] real hot spots, as seen in 21-hydroxylase deficiency, do not exist. Most of the reported mutations lead to absent or almost absent 11β-hydroxylase enzyme activity, with only some cases of mild or nonclassic 11-hydroxylase deficiency reported.[406,407]

Loss of negative cortisol feedback and enhanced ACTH-mediated adrenal androgen excess occur in 11β-hydroxylase deficiency (Fig. 15-37). Clinical features therefore are very similar to those reported in the simple virilizing form of CAH (46,XX DSD including virilization of the external genitalia and sexual ambiguity); and again, milder cases can manifest later in childhood or even young adulthood. The principal difference from 21-hydroxylase deficiency is hypertension, which is thought to be secondary to the mineralocorticoid effect of DOC excess. However, there is a poor correlation between DOC secretion and the presence of hypertension, and unexplained salt wasting has been reported in few patients during early life. On this clinical background, the diagnosis can be made by measuring a plasma ACTH–stimulated 11-deoxycortisol value, which will be higher than three times the 95th percentile for an age-matched normal group. Basal concentrations of 17-OHP are commonly increased but may be normal even during the first weeks of life.[408]

Although established heterozygotes may not demonstrate an increase in 11-deoxycortisol above normal values after Synacthen stimulation[409] (unlike the 17-OHP response observed in heterozygote patients with 21-hydroxylase deficiency), exaggerated ACTH-stimulated responses have been observed in patients with hirsutism[410] and in patients with essential hypertension,[411] suggesting partial defects in 11β-hydroxylase activity.

Treatment is with replacement glucocorticoid therapy; with suppression of DOC secretion, the plasma renin activity, which is suppressed at baseline, increases into the normal range. In general, higher glucocorticoid doses are needed to suppress hyperandrogenism compared with the situation in 21-hydroxylase deficiency, and add-on antihypertensive therapy may be necessary in some cases. Antihypertensive treatment should be commenced at an early stage to avoid excessive glucocorticoid exposure.

17α-Hydroxylase Deficiency

Approximately 150 cases of 17α-hydroxylase deficiency have been reported.[412-414] Mutations within the *CYP17A1* gene result in failure to synthesize cortisol (17α-hydroxylase activity), adrenal androgens (17,20-lyase activity), and gonadal steroids (Fig. 15-38). Therefore, in contrast to 21- and 11β-hydroxylase deficiencies, 17α-hydroxylase deficiency results in adrenal and gonadal insufficiency and causes 46,XY DSD. A single enzyme is expressed in

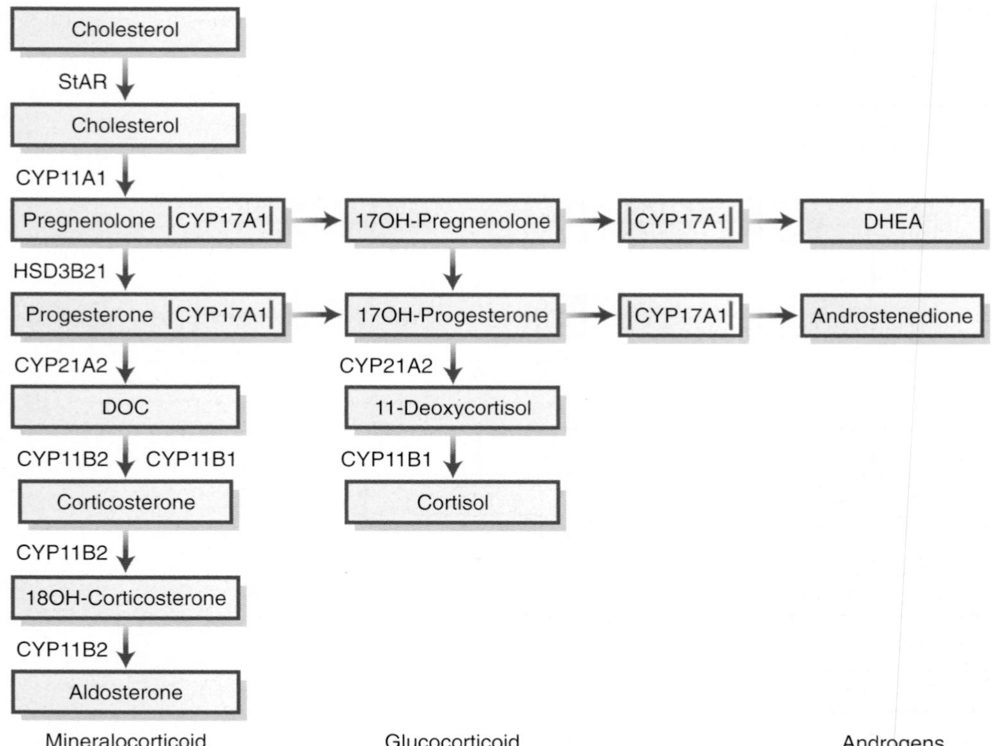

Figure 15-38 Congenital adrenal hyperplasia related to 17α-hydroxylase deficiency. The normal synthesis of cortisol is impaired, and adrenocorticotropic hormone (ACTH) levels increase because of loss of normal negative feedback inhibition resulting in an increase in adrenal steroid precursors proximal to the block. The result is cortisol deficiency and mineralocorticoid excess usually related to deoxycorticosterone (DOC) excess. Because gonadal 17α-hydroxylase activity is also absent, sex steroid secretion in addition to adrenal androgen secretion is severely impaired, resulting in hypogonadism. CYP, cytochrome P450; DHEA, dehydroepiandrosterone; DOC, deoxycorticosterone; HSD, hydroxysteroid dehydrogenase; StAR, steroidogenic acute regulatory protein.

the adrenal and the gonads and possesses both 17α-hydroxylation and 17,20-lyase activities, but rare patients with isolated deficiency in the hydroxylation of 17-OHP or 17,20-lyase deficiency have been reported.[413] Loss of negative feedback results in increased secretion of steroids proximal to the block, and mineralocorticoid synthesis is enhanced. Corticosterone has weaker glucocorticoid activity than cortisol, but corticosterone excess generally prevents adrenal crises. Accumulation of corticosterone and DOC results in severe hypokalemic hypertension. Sex steroid deficiency caused by loss of 17,20-lyase activity results in 46,XY DSD; this manifests as undervirilization in male newborns and primary amenorrhea in 46,XX individuals. There is lack of pubertal development due to hypergonadotropic hypogonadism in both sexes.[414]

The 17α-hydroxylase enzyme is a microsomal cytochrome P450 type II enzyme that requires electron transfer from NADPH via POR for catalytic activity.[26] For efficient catalysis of the 17,20-lyase reaction, the CYP17A1-POR complex requires additional allosteric interaction with cytochrome b_5.[415,416] The *CYP17A1* gene consists of eight exons and is located on chromosome 10q24.3. A variety of different mutations have been described, without evidence of a hot spot.[377,417] Relative hydroxylase/lyase activities of CYP17A1 mutants have been shown to vary in in vitro functional assays, but correlations with clinical phenotype are lacking. Patients with clinically "pure" 17,20-lyase deficiency have CYP17A1 mutations that selectively compromise 17,20-lyase activity.[415,418,419] Mutations underlying isolated 17,20-lyase deficiency are located within the area of the CYP17A1 molecule that is thought to interact with the cofactor cytochrome b_5, thereby disrupting the electron transfer from POR to CYP17A1, specifically for the conversion of 17-hydroxypregnenolone to DHEA.[415,418]

The diagnosis is usually made at the time of puberty when patients present with hypertension, hypokalemia, and hypergonadotropic hypogonadism, the last occurring because of lack of CYP17A1 expression within the gonad and impaired gonadal steroidogenesis. As a result, LH and FSH levels are elevated. Female patients (XX) have primary amenorrhea with absent sexual characteristics, whereas 46,XY individuals present with 46,XY DSD with female external genitalia but absent uterus and fallopian tubes. The intra-abdominal testes should be removed, and such patients are usually reared as females.

Glucocorticoid replacement reverses the DOC-induced suppression of the renin-angiotensin system and lowers blood pressure. Additional sex steroid replacement is required from puberty onward.

P450 Oxidoreductase Deficiency: Apparent Combined 17α-Hydroxylase and 21-Hydroxylase Deficiencies

Patients have been described with biochemical evidence of apparent combined 17α-hydroxylase and 21-hydroxylase deficiencies.[420] Urinary gas chromatography/mass spectrometry analysis reveals a typical pattern comprising increased pregnenolone and progesterone metabolites, slightly increased corticosterone metabolites, increased pregnanetriolone excretion, and low androgen metabolites (see Fig. 15-4). Mothers pregnant with an affected child present with low serum estriol and a characteristic urinary steroid profile, allowing for prenatal biochemical diagnosis.[421,422] The analysis of serum steroids only may lead to misdiagnosis.[423] Cortisol baseline secretion may be normal, but most, if not all, patients show an insufficient cortisol response to ACTH stimulation and therefore require glucocorticoid replacement. Impaired 17,20-lyase activity results in deficient androgen synthesis, and affected boys are often born undervirilized. Most of the affected girls are born with virilized genitalia. Therefore, patients can present with 46,XY or 46,XX DSD or with appropriate development of the external genitalia in both sexes. After birth, virilization does not progress, and circulating androgen concentrations are typically low. Some mothers develop signs of virilization during midpregnancy with an affected child; this commonly resolves soon after birth, further indicating intrauterine androgen excess.[421] In addition to these features of CAH, affected children may also present with bone malformations, including midface hypoplasia, craniosynostosis, and radiohumeral synostosis, in some cases resembling the Antley-Bixler congenital malformation syndrome.[424,425] The bone phenotype in affected patients with POR deficiency is most likely caused by an impairment of sterol biosynthesis, specifically of POR-dependent 14α-lanosterol demethylase (CYP51A1).

The paradox of fetal virilization but sex hormone deficiency in postnatal life might be mediated by a newly discovered "backdoor" pathway of androgen synthesis in fetal life that relies on neither androstenedione nor testosterone as an intermediate.[425-427] Pubertal development in POR deficiency appears to be dominated by the consequences of sex steroid deficiency,[427] and most patients require sex hormone substitution. The overall incidence of POR deficiency has not been established. However, a relatively large number of patients with POR deficiency were reported within a short period after the initial description of the molecular cause of the disease.[427,428]

The *POR* gene is located on chromosome 7q11.2 and consists of 15 translated exons spanning 32.9 kilobytes and encoding a protein of 680 amino acids. A variety of *POR*-inactivating mutations have been reported, including missense, frameshift, and splice site mutations. A287P is the most common mutation in Caucasians, whereas R457H is the most frequent founder mutation in the Japanese population. All patients carry *POR* mutations that are either partially inactivating or, in case of major loss-of-function mutations, manifest only in the compound heterozygous state. Homozygous mutations with total loss of function are most likely not viable—a view supported by the nonviability of complete *POR* gene deletion in the murine model.[429]

3β-Hydroxysteroid Dehydrogenase Deficiency

In this rare form of CAH, the secretion of all classes of adrenal and ovarian steroids is impaired due to mutations within the *HSD3B2* gene encoding 3β-HSD type 2.[430,431] There are two isoforms of 3β-HSD, encoded by *HSD3B1* and *HSD3B2*, respectively. The *HSD3B2* gene is located on chromosome Ip13·1 and consists of four exons. HSD3B2 is expressed mainly in the adrenal and the gonad, whereas HSD3B1 is expressed in the placenta and almost ubiquitously in peripheral target tissues.[27,431] The enzyme

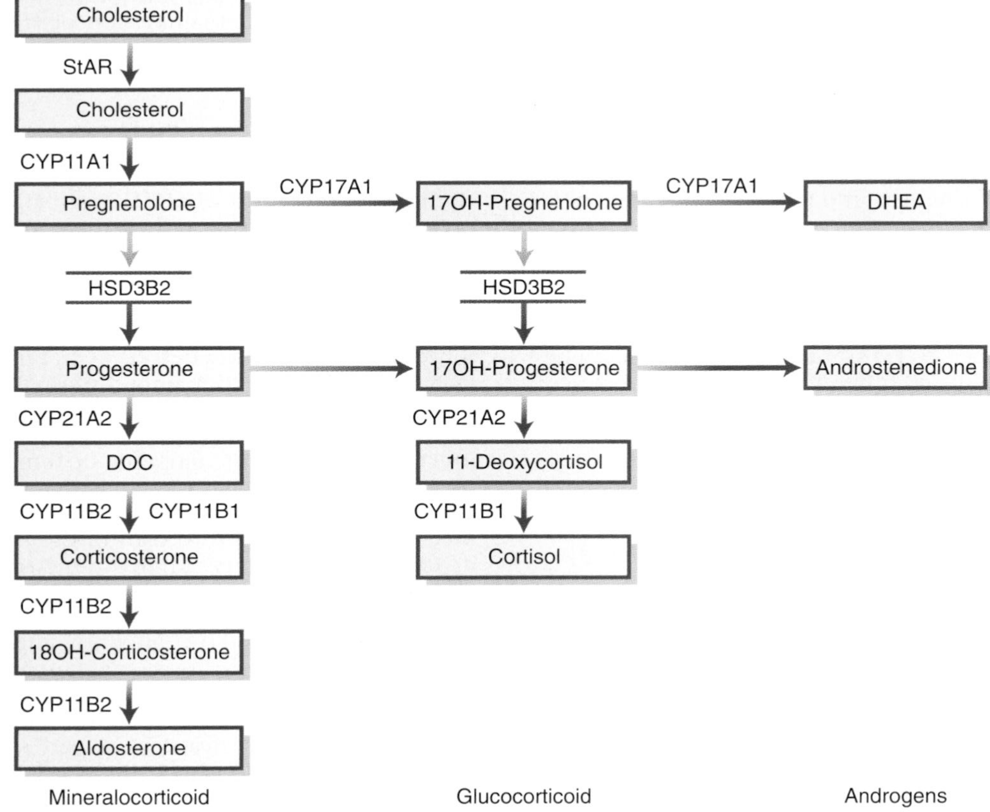

Figure 15-39 Congenital adrenal hyperplasia related to 3β-hydroxysteroid dehydrogenase (3β-HSD) type 2 deficiency resulting in cortisol deficiency and variable mineralocorticoid deficiency. Gonadal 3β-HSD type 2 activity is also absent, resulting in 46, XY DSD and hypogonadism or primary amenorrhea in females. Virilization in females can occur due to 3β-hydroxysteroid dehydrogenase type I activity. DOC, deoxycorticosterone; DHEA, dehydroepiandrosterone; DSD, disorder of sex development; StAR, steroidogenic acute regulatory protein.

HSD3B2 catalyzes three key reactions in adrenal steroidogenesis: the conversion of the Δ5-steroids pregnenolone, 17-hydroxypregnenolone, and DHEA to the Δ4-steroids progesterone, 17-OHP, and androstenedione, respectively. 3β-HSDII deficiency affects all three steroid hormone pathways (i.e., mineralocorticoids, glucocorticoids, and sex steroids).

The clinical spectrum shows a wide variety of disease expression. Patients usually present in early infancy with adrenal insufficiency. Loss of mineralocorticoid secretion results in salt wasting, although this is absent in 30% to 40% of cases (Fig. 15-39). As with 21-hydroxylase deficiency, absence of salt wasting may delay the presentation into childhood or puberty, ranging from a severe salt-wasting form with or without ambiguous genitalia in affected male neonates to isolated premature pubarche in infants and children of both sexes and a late-onset variant manifesting with hirsutism and menstrual irregularities. In general, the functional and biochemical data are in close agreement with the expressed phenotype in patients with the non–salt-wasting form of HSD3B2 deficiency. However, some variability exists, and identical mutations have been found in the *HSD3B2* gene in both salt-wasters and non–salt-wasters.[430,431] The correlation between the impairment in male sexual differentiation and salt wasting is poor. The spectrum of genital development is variable in both sexes. In males, because the HSD3B2 enzyme is also expressed within the gonad, 46,XY DSD may occur resulting in female external genitalia. However, most patients present with hypospadias, and even normal male genitalia may be found. In females, genital development can be normal, but usually there is evidence of mild virilization, presumably because of enhanced adrenal DHEA secretion, which is converted peripherally to testosterone. A late-onset form has been described in patients with premature pubarche[432] and a PCOS-like phenotype (i.e., hirsutism, oligorrhea/amenorrhea).[433]

Because activity of the HSD3B1 enzyme, present peripheral tissues, is intact, levels of circulating Δ4 steroids (progesterone, 17-OHP, androstenedione) may be normal (or even increased). However, a diagnosis is established by demonstration of an increased ratio of Δ5 steroids (pregnenolone, 17-hydroxypregnenolone, DHEA) to Δ4 steroids in plasma or urine. Hormonal criteria have been refined for the diagnosis of HSD3B2 deficiency based on genotyping of the *HSD3B2* gene. The 17-hydroxypregnenolone concentrations and the ratios of 17-hydroxypregnenolone to cortisol at baseline and after ACTH stimulation are of the highest discriminatory value in differentiating between patients affected by HSD3B2 deficiency and those with milder biochemical abnormalities, who are commonly negative for *HSD3B2* mutations.[434,435] Treatment is with replacement glucocorticoids, fludrocortisone (if indicated), and sex steroids from puberty onward.

StAR Deficiency: Congenital Lipoid Adrenal Hyperplasia

Mutations in the gene encoding StAR results in a failure of transport of cholesterol from the outer to the inner mitochondrial membrane in steroidogenic tissues. StAR-independent cholesterol transport occurs only at a low rate. As a result, there is deficiency of all adrenal and gonadal steroid hormones.[23,436] The adrenal glands are often massively enlarged and full of lipid; before the characterization of StAR, the condition was termed *congenital lipoid adrenal hyperplasia*.[436] StAR deficiency severely but incompletely abolishes pregnenolone synthesis. Cholesterol esters accumulate under the increased tone of ACTH stimulation. Consequently, the lipid accumulation worsens the dysfunction and leads to adrenal cell destruction. Presentation is with acute adrenal insufficiency in the neonatal period, and males exhibit 46,XY DSD due to absent gonadal steroids.

The most severe form of this disorder manifests with 46,XY DSD and combined adrenal insufficiency. Salt wasting typically develops in the neonatal period or after a few weeks of life, but later onset may also occur. Females can show spontaneous pubertal development. A milder form of StAR deficiency has also been described in normally virilized 46,XY individuals who present with adrenal failure during early childhood.[437] Treatment consists of glucocorticoid and mineralocorticoid replacement and substitution of sex hormones in later life.

P450 Side-Chain Cleavage Deficiency

Deficiency of P450scc (CYP11A1) enzyme is a rare inborn error of steroidogenesis, with only seven cases reported. It was previously thought that such mutations would not be viable, because the maintenance of human pregnancy relies on placentally produced progesterone. The production is facilitated by the fetal part of the placenta from the second trimester onward. P450scc deficiency manifests clinically and biochemically with similar signs and symptoms as StAR deficiency, but patients do not have enlarged adrenals.[438-440] Depending on the impairment of CYP11A1 function, a spectrum of clinical presentation ranges from 46,XY DSD with severe adrenal insufficiency in the newborn period to hypospadias and cryptorchidism and later manifestation of adrenal insufficiency during childhood.[441] Concentrations of all steroid hormones are decreased, in keeping with impaired conversion of cholesterol to pregnenolone. Treatment with glucocorticoid, mineralocorticoid, and sex steroid replacement is required.

Cortisone Reductase Deficiency

In cortisone reductase deficiency, adrenal glands become "hyperplastic" because of ACTH stimulation due to a defect in cortisol metabolism rather than an inherent defect within the gland itself.[129,442,443] Patients with this condition have a defect in the conversion of cortisone to cortisol, suggesting inhibition of 11-oxo-reductase activity and, by implication, inhibition of HSD11B1 (see Fig. 15-12). Cortisol clearance is increased and, as a consequence, ACTH secretion is elevated to maintain normal circulating cortisol concentrations but at the expense of adrenal androgen excess. Female patients present with hirsutism, menstrual irregularity, androgenic alopecia, or some combination of these features. Males may present with premature pubarche. Dexamethasone treatment to suppress ACTH has been used with some success to control the hyperandrogenism in these cases. Urinary tetrahydrometabolites of cortisol and cortisone show almost exclusively THE with little or no detectable THF or allo-THF; the ratio THF+allo-THF:THE is less than 0.05 (reference range, 0.8 to 1.3). The molecular bases for cortisone reductase deficiency are inactivating mutations in hexose-6-phosphate dehydrogenase (H6PDH).[443] H6PDH, located in the endoplasmic reticulum, catalyzes the conversion of glucose-6-phosphate to glucose-6-phosphogluconate, thereby generating NADPH, which is crucial in conveying oxo-reductase activity on HSD11B1.

Patients with PCOS share many of the same clinical characteristics as those with cortisone reductase deficiency. Whereas there is evidence to support increased cortisol

TABLE 15-24

Causes of Mineralocorticoid Deficiency

Addison's disease
Adrenal hypoplasia
Congenital adrenal hyperplasia (21-hydroxylase and 3β-hydroxysteroid dehydrogenase deficiencies)
Pseudohypoaldosteronism types I and II
Hyporeninemic hypoaldosteronism
Aldosterone biosynthetic defects
Drug induced

secretion rates in PCOS, perhaps indicating a defect in the conversion of cortisone to cortisol, a consensus with respect to THF+allo-THF:THE ratios is still lacking.[444] Association studies using single nucleotide polymorphic markers in the HSD11B1 and H6PDH genes have largely been negative.

Mineralocorticoid Deficiency

The mineralocorticoid deficiency syndromes are listed in Table 15-24. They can be divided into congenital and acquired syndromes. Mineralocorticoid deficiency may occur in some forms of CAH and with other causes of adrenal insufficiency (e.g., Addison's disease, CAH).

Primary Defects in Aldosterone Biosynthesis: Aldosterone Synthase Deficiency

Before the characterization of the *CYP11B2* gene, two diseases were recognized, *corticosterone methyl oxidase type I (CMO I) deficiency* and *corticosterone methyl oxidase type II (CMO II) deficiency*.[445] Subsequently, both variants were shown to be secondary to mutations in aldosterone synthase (CYP11B2), and they are now termed *aldosterone synthase deficiency, types I and II*.[446] Aldosterone synthase catalyzes the three terminal steps of aldosterone biosynthesis, 11β-hydroxylation of DOC to corticosterone, 18-hydroxylation to 18-hydroxycorticosterone, and 18-oxidation to aldosterone. Patients with type I aldosterone synthase deficiency have low to normal levels of 18-hydroxycorticosterone but undetectable levels of aldosterone (or urinary tetrahydroaldosterone), whereas patients with the type II variant have high levels of 18-hydroxycorticosterone and only subnormal or even normal levels of aldosterone. This suggests blockade of only the terminal 18-oxidation step, with some residual aldosterone synthase activity remaining. The explanation for the variable biochemical phenotype is unknown, particularly now that the same mutation in aldosterone synthase has been uncovered in both variants. It is possible that the phenotypic variation may reflect polymorphic variants in the residual and normal product of the *CYP11B1* gene, 11β-hydroxylase.

Both variants are rare and are inherited as autosomal recessive traits.[446] Patients usually present in neonatal life with a salt-wasting crisis involving severe dehydration, vomiting, and failure to grow and thrive. Hyperkalemia, metabolic acidosis, dehydration, and hyponatremia are found. The plasma renin activity is elevated, and plasma aldosterone levels are low. Plasma 18-hydroxycorticosterone levels, the ratio of plasma 18-hydroxycorticosterone to aldosterone, and the levels of their urinary metabolites are used to differentiate the type I and II variants. In most infants, the disorders become less severe as the child ages; indeed, in older children, adolescents, and adults, the abnormal steroid pattern described may be present and may persist throughout life without clinical manifestations.

Patients with CYP11B2 deficiency typically respond well to 9α-fludrocortisone (starting dose, 150 μg/m^2 per day in neonates and infants) and may also benefit from salt supplementation. Patients with failure to grow and thrive usually show a good catch-up growth. Electrolytes often tend to normalize spontaneously between 3 to 4 years of age. However, untreated patients are at significant risk for being growth retarded, although spontaneous normalization of growth can occur. Adults are usually asymptomatic but are more susceptible to salt loss. Rarely, presentation is in adulthood.[447] Mineralocorticoid treatment in later life has to be established on an individual basis.

Postadrenalectomy Hypoaldosteronism

In a patient with a unilateral aldosteronoma (Conn's syndrome), the contralateral ZG is frequently suppressed. Without reversal of the chronic volume expansion preoperatively, patients may develop severe hyperkalemia and hypotension lasting several days to several weeks after adrenalectomy. This effect may be exacerbated by the use of spironolactone preoperatively. Spironolactone has a long half-life and should be discontinued 2 to 3 days before surgery to minimize the risk of postoperative mineralocorticoid deficiency.

Defects in Aldosterone Action: Pseudohypoaldosteronism

Pseudohypoaldosteronism (PHA) is a rare, inherited salt-wasting disorder that was first described by Cheek and Perry in 1958 as a defective renal tubular response to mineralocorticoid in infancy. Patients present in the neonatal period with dehydration, hyponatremia, hypokalemia, metabolic acidosis, and failure to thrive despite normal glomerular filtration and normal renal and adrenal function.[448] Renin levels and plasma aldosterone are grossly elevated. When patients fail to respond to mineralocorticoid therapy, PHA is suspected as the underlying disorder.

PHA type I can be divided into two distinct disorders based on unique physiologic and genetic characteristics: the renal form of PHA, which is inherited as an autosomal dominant trait, and a generalized autosomal recessive form of PHA. The autosomal dominant form is usually less severe; the patient's condition often improves spontaneously within the first several years of life, allowing discontinuation of therapy. By contrast, the autosomal recessive form produces a multiorgan disorder, with mineralocorticoid resistance seen in the kidney, sweat, and salivary glands and the colonic mucosa. The condition does not spontaneously improve with age and is generally more severe than the autosomal dominant form.

The underlying basis for the autosomal dominant form of PHA is explained on the basis of inactivating mutations in the mineralocorticoid receptor (hMR, NR3C2).[448,449] By contrast, inactivating mutations in the α-subunit and, to a lesser extent, in the β- and γ-subunits of the epithelial sodium channel (ENaC) account for the generalized autosomal recessive form of mineralocorticoid resistance.[450,451] (In effect, this represents the opposite of Liddle's syndrome—see Chapter 16.) Generalized loss of ENaC activity leads to renal salt wasting (as seen in the renal form) in addition to recurrent respiratory infections and neonatal respiratory distress, cholelithiasis, and polyhydramnios.

PHA type I is resistant to mineralocorticoid therapy, so standard treatment involves supplementation with salt (2 to 8 g/day) in the form of sodium chloride and sodium bicarbonate as well as cation exchange resins. This usually corrects the patient's biochemical imbalance. However, if a patient shows signs of severe hyperkalemia, peritoneal dialysis may be necessary. Hypercalciuria has been reported in some cases of PHA-I. The recommended course of treatment for these patients usually involves indomethacin or hydrochlorothiazide. Indomethacin is thought to act by causing a reduction in the glomerular filtration rate or an inhibition of the effect of prostaglandin E_2 on renal tubules. Indomethacin has been shown to reduce polyuria, sodium loss, and hypercalciuria. Hydrochlorothiazide has been used to diminish hyperkalemia and reduce hypercalciuria in patients with PHA-I.

In patients with the autosomal dominant or renal form of PHA-I, the signs and symptoms of PHA decrease with age; nevertheless, these patients usually require salt supplementation for the first 2 to 3 years of life. In patients with the autosomal recessive or multiorgan type of PHA-I, resistance to therapy with sodium chloride or drugs that decrease serum potassium concentrations often occurs and may even lead to death in infancy from hyperkalemia. PHA-I patients with multiorgan involvement often require very high amounts of salt in their diet (up to 45 g NaCl per day). Carbenoxolone, a derivative of glycyrrhetinic acid in licorice, has been used with moderate success in helping to reduce the high levels of dietary salt needed by renal PHA-I patients. Carbenoxolone acts by inhibiting HSD11B2 activity and allows unmetabolized cortisol to bind to and activate MRs in a manner similar to that of aldosterone.[452] It was found to be ineffective in patients with multiorgan PHA-I.

Two other variants of PHA have been described—types II and III. Type II PHA, or Gordon's syndrome, is in retrospect a misnomer. Patients with Gordon's syndrome share some of the features of patients with PHA-I, notably hyperkalemia and metabolic acidosis, but they exhibit salt retention with mild hypertension and suppressed plasma renin activity rather than salt wasting. The condition is explained by mutations in a serine threonine kinase family (WNK1 and WNK4) that result in increased expression of these proteins with activation of the thiazide-sensitive sodium-chloride cotransporter in the cortical and medullary collecting ducts.[453] The condition represents the exact opposite of Gitelman's syndrome but is not a true form of PHA.

Type III PHA is an acquired and usually transient form of mineralocorticoid resistance seen in patients with underlying renal pathologies including obstruction and infection and in patients with excessive loss of salt through the gut or skin. Reduced glomerular filtration rate is a hallmark of the condition. The cause is unknown, although increased transforming growth factor-β–mediated aldosterone resistance has been suggested to be an underlying factor.

Hyporeninemic Hypoaldosteronism

Angiotensin II is a key stimulus to aldosterone secretion, and damage or blockade of the renin-angiotensin system may result in mineralocorticoid deficiency. Various renal diseases have been associated with damage to the juxtaglomerular apparatus and subsequent renin deficiency. These include systemic lupus erythematosus, myeloma, amyloid, AIDS, and damage related to use of nonsteroidal anti-inflammatory drugs, but the most common (>75% of cases) is diabetic nephropathy.[454,455]

The usual picture is that of an elderly patient with hyperkalemia, acidosis, and mild to moderate impairment of renal function. Plasma renin activity and aldosterone levels are low and fail to respond to sodium depletion, erect posture, or furosemide administration. In contrast to adrenal insufficiency, patients have normal or elevated blood pressure and no postural hypotension. Muscle weakness and cardiac arrhythmias may also occur. Other factors may contribute to the hyperkalemia, including the use of potassium-sparing diuretics, potassium supplementation, insulin deficiency, and use of β-adrenoceptor blocking drugs or prostaglandin synthetase inhibitors, which inhibit renin release.

Treatment of primary renin deficiency is with fludrocortisone in the first instance together with dietary potassium restriction. However, these patients are not salt depleted and may become hypertensive with fludrocortisone. In such a scenario, the addition of a loop-acting diuretic such as furosemide is appropriate. This will increase acid excretion and improve the metabolic acidosis.

ADRENAL ADENOMAS, INCIDENTALOMAS, AND CARCINOMAS

Adenomas

Cortisol-secreting adrenal adenomas were discussed earlier, and aldosterone-secreting adenomas (Conn's syndrome) are discussed in Chapter 16.

Pure virilizing benign adrenal adenomas are rare, with approximately 50 cases reported in the literature. Most cases occur in women; in males, the disorder is restricted to childhood, where presentation is with sexual precocity and accelerated bone age. Such tumors have to be considered in the differential diagnosis of CAH in patients presenting during childhood. In females, most patients present before the menopause with marked hirsutism, deepening of the voice, and amenorrhea. Clitoromegaly is found in 80% of cases. Testosterone is usually strikingly elevated, but gonadotropin levels may not be suppressed. By definition, urinary free cortisol is normal. Tumors vary in size and should be treated surgically. Postoperatively, clinical features invariably improve, and normal menses return.[456]

Incidentalomas

Autopsy series had defined the prevalence of adrenal adenomas greater than 1 cm in diameter to be between 1.5% and 7% before the advent of high-resolution imaging procedures such as CT and MRI; since that time, incidentally discovered adrenal masses have become a common clinical problem. An adrenal mass is uncovered in up to 4% of patients imaged for nonadrenal pathology.[457] Incidentalomas are uncommon in patients younger than 30 years of age but increase in frequency with age; they occur equally in males and females. Clinically, two issues arise: whether the lesion is functional (i.e., secreting hormones) and whether it is malignant. In more than 85% of cases, these lesions are nonfunctioning, benign adenomas. Occasionally they represent myelolipomas, hamartomas, or granulomatous infiltrations of the adrenal and result in a characteristic CT/MRI appearance (Fig. 15-40). Functioning tumors (pheochromocytomas and those secreting cortisol, aldosterone, or sex steroids) and carcinomas comprise the remainder. In addition, it is established that some incidentalomas cause abnormal hormone secretion without obvious clinical manifestations of a hormone excess state. The best example is so-called subclinical Cushing's syndrome, which occurs in up to 20% of all cases.[457,458] This

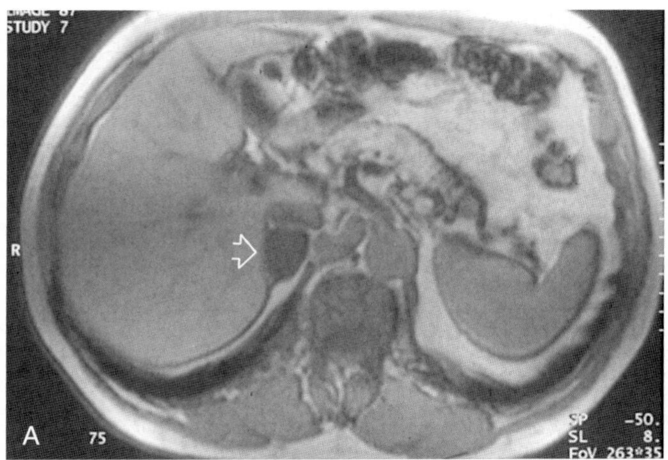
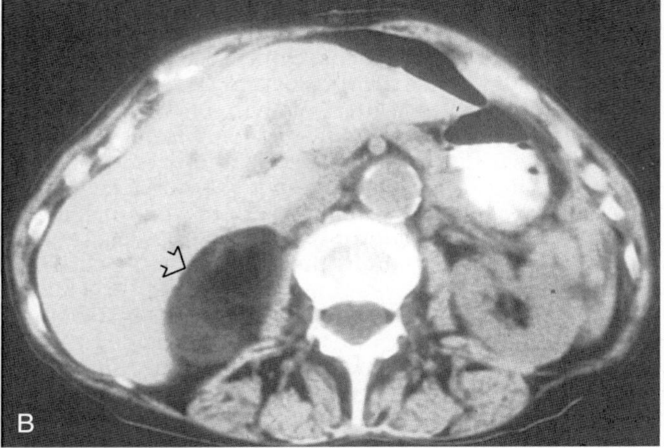

Figure 15-40 **A,** Adrenal incidentaloma discovered in a woman undergoing investigation for abdominal pain. **B,** Incidentally discovered right adrenal myelolipoma.

may explain why incidentalomas appear to be more common among patients with obesity and diabetes mellitus.[459]

As a result, all patients with incidentally discovered adrenal masses should undergo appropriate endocrine screening tests. This should comprise 24-hour urinary catecholamine collection or measurement of plasma metanephrines, 24-hour urinary free cortisol (or a midnight salivary cortisol level), and overnight dexamethasone suppression tests. Because of the reported poor sensitivity of serum potassium measurements in detecting primary aldosteronism, circulating levels of plasma renin activity and aldosterone are required in hypertensive patients. DHEAS should be measured as a marker of adrenal androgen secretion. Low levels may occur in patients with suppressed ACTH concentrations due to autonomous cortisol secretion from the adenoma.[460] Some studies have also documented high levels of 17-OHP after ACTH stimulation tests, suggesting partial defects in 21-hydroxylase in some tumors.

The possibility of malignancy should be considered in each case. In patients with a known extra-adrenal primary, the incidence of malignancy is obviously much higher; for example up to 20% of patients with lung cancer have adrenal metastases on CT scanning. In those with no evidence of malignancy, adrenal carcinoma is rare; in one study, only 26 of 630 incidentalomas were found to be adrenal carcinomas.[457] Many studies contain a positive bias, and true risk of malignancy may be much lower.[461] In true incidentalomas, size appears to be predictive of malignancy: fewer than 2% of incidentalomas smaller than 4 cm but 25% of those larger than 6 cm in diameter are malignant (Fig. 15-41).[462] Smooth, homogeneous adenomas on an enhanced adrenal scan with a Hounsfield unit score (a marker of radiodensity) less than 10 HU are invariably benign; malignancy is suspected in irregular, inhomogeneous adenomas with a score greater than 20 HU. On this background, adrenalectomy is indicated for functional tumors and for tumors larger than 4 cm in diameter. Repeat CT scanning in patients with smaller tumors can be used to guide management, but development of functional autonomy is very rare, and patients may be discharged if tumors are static. Laparoscopic adrenalectomy is the treatment of choice, offering shorter hospital stays and reduced operative complications (e.g., blood loss, morbidity) compared with open adrenalectomy. The possible exception is the patient with highly suggestive adrenal carcinoma, because breach of the tumor capsule is associated with a poorer outcome. Adequate preparation and close endocrine supervision perioperatively and postoperatively is required for functional tumors.

Carcinomas

Primary adrenal carcinoma is very rare, with an annual incidence of 1 per 1 million population. Women are more commonly affected than men, with a ratio of 2.5:1. The

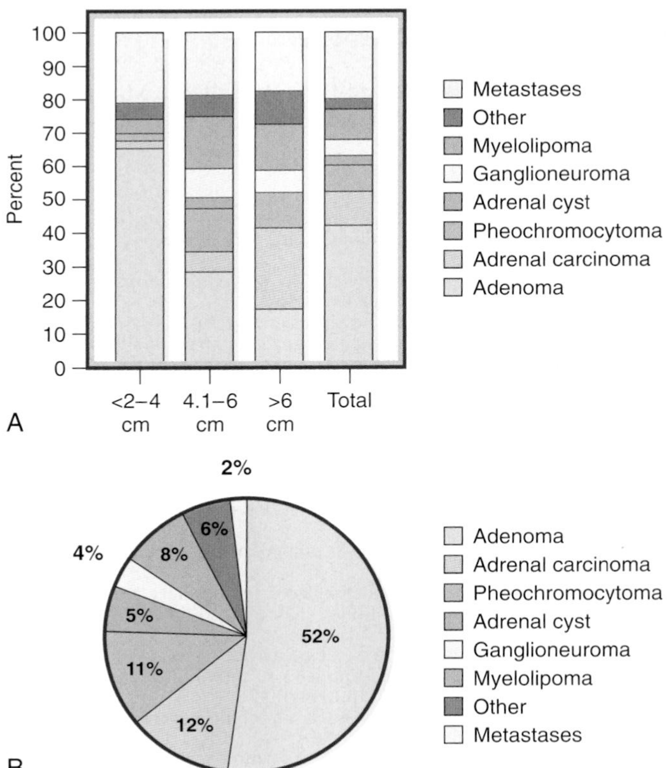

Figure 15-41 Distribution of diagnosis of adrenal incidentalomas. **A,** Data from eight studies with histologically determined diagnoses (n = 103) relating to tumor size. **B,** Distribution of 380 incidental adrenal masses by histologic diagnosis. (From Mansmann G, Lau L, Balk E, et al. The clinically inapparent adrenal mass: update in diagnosis and management. *Endocr Rev.* 2004;25:309-340.)

mean age at onset is between 40 and 50 years, although men tend to be older at presentation. Eighty percent of tumors are functional, most commonly secreting glucocorticoids alone (45%), glucocorticoids and androgens (45%), or androgens alone (10%). Fewer than 1% of all tumors secrete aldosterone. Patients present with features of the hormone excess state (glucocorticoid, androgen, or both) but abdominal pain, weight loss, anorexia, and fever occur in 25% of cases. An abdominal mass may be palpable. Current treatment choices for what is often an aggressive tumor are poor. Surgery offers the only chance of cure for patients with local disease, but metastatic spread is evident in 75% of cases at presentation. Radiotherapy is ineffective, as are most chemotherapeutic regimens. Mitotane in high doses offers benefit in reducing tumor growth,[276] and in controlling hormonal hypersecretion in 75% of cases.[275] Overall, the prognosis is poor, with 5-year survival rates of less than 20%. Newer chemotherapies are being evaluated.[277]

Etiology of Adrenal Tumors

The underlying basis for adrenal tumorigenesis is unknown. Clonal analysis suggests progression from a normal to an adenomatous to a carcinomatous lesion, but the molecular pathways involved remain obscure. Several factors have been associated with malignant transformation, including the genes encoding p53, p57 cyclin-dependent kinase, menin, IGF2, MC2R, and inhibin-α.[463] Mice lacking the inhibin-α gene develop adrenal tumors through a process that is also gonadotropin dependent.[464]

ACKNOWLEDGMENTS

Acknowledgment is given to Prof. W. Arlt, Dr. M.S. Cooper, Dr. J.W. Tomlinson, and Dr. W. Young for assistance with parts of this chapter.

REFERENCES

1. Eustachius B. Tabulae Anatomicae. In: Lancisius B, ed. Amsterdam: 1774.
2. Addison T. *On the Constitutional and Local Effects of Disease of the Supra-Renal Capsules*. London: Highley; 1866.
3. Brown-Sequard CE. Recherches experimentales sur la physiologie et la pathologie des capsules surrenales. *Arch Gen Med*. 1856;5:385-401.
4. Medvei VC. *A History of Clinical Endocrinology*. Pearl River, NY: Parthenon; 1993.
5. Hench PS, Kendall EC, et al. The effect of a hormone of the adrenal cortex (17-hydroxy-11-dehydrocorticosterone; compound E) and of pituitary adrenocorticotropic hormone on rheumatoid arthritis. *Mayo Clin Proc*. 1949;24:181-197.
6. Simpson SA, Tait JF. Recent progress in methods of isolation, chemistry, and physiology of aldosterone. *Recent Prog Horm Res*. 1955; 11:183-210.
7. Li CH, Evans HM, Simpson ME. Adrenocorticotrophic hormone. *J Biol Chem*. 1943;149:413-424.
8. Cushing H. The basophil adenomas of the pituitary body and their clinical manifestations (pituitary basophilism). *Bull Johns Hopkins Hosp*. 1932;50:137-195.
9. Vale W, Spiess J, Rivier C, et al. Characterization of a 41-residue ovine hypothalamic peptide that stimulates secretion of corticotropin and β-endorphin. *Science*. 1981;213:1394-1397.
10. Conn JW. Primary aldosteronism, a new clinical syndrome. *J Lab Clin Med*. 1955;45:3-17.
11. Else T, Hammer GD. Genetic analysis of adrenal absence: agenesis and aplasia. *Trends Endocrinol Metab*. 2005;16:458.
12. Mesiano S, Jaffe RB. Developmental and functional biology of the primate fetal adrenal cortex. *Endocr Rev*. 1997;18:378-403.
13. Jaffe RB, Mesiano S, Smith R, et al. The regulation and role of fetal adrenal development in human pregnancy. *Endocr Res*. 1998; 24:919-926.
14. Okamoto M, Takemori H. Differentiation and zonation of the adrenal cortex. *Curr Opin Endocrinol Diab*. 2000;7:122-127.
15. Luo X, Ikeda Y, Parker KL. A cell-specific nuclear receptor is essential for adrenal and gonadal development and sexual differentiation. *Cell*. 1994;77:481-490.
16. Havelock JC, Auchus RJ, Rainey WE. The rise in adrenal androgen biosynthesis: adrenarche. *Semin Reprod Med*. 2004;22:337-347.
17. Remer T, Boye KR, Hartmann MF, et al. Urinary markers of adrenarche: reference values in healthy subjects, aged 3-18 years. *J Clin Endocrinol Metab*. 2005;90:2015-2021.
18. IUPAC Commission on the Nomenclature of Organic Chemistry (CNOC) and IUPAC-IUB Commission on Biochemical Nomenclature (CBN). Definitive rules for the nomenclature of steroids. *Pure Appl Chem*. 1972;31:285-322.
19. Gwynne JT, Strauss JF 3rd. The role of lipoproteins in steroidogenesis and cholesterol metabolism in steroidogenic glands. *Endocr Rev*. 1982;3:299-329.
20. Faust JR, Goldstein JL, Brown MS. Receptor-mediated uptake of low density lipoprotein and utilization of its cholesterol for steroid synthesis in cultured mouse adrenal cells. *J Biol Chem*. 1977; 252:4861-4871.
21. Goldstein JL, Anderson RG, Brown MS. Coated pits, coated vesicles, and receptor-mediated endocytosis. *Nature*. 1979;279:679-685.
22. Landschulz KT, Pathak RK, Rigotti A, et al. Regulation of scavenger receptor, class B, type I, a high density lipoprotein receptor, in liver and steroidogenic tissues of the rat. *J Clin Invest*. 1996;98:984-995.
23. Stocco DM, Clark BJ. Regulation of the acute production of steroids in steroidogenic cells. *Endocr Rev*. 1996;17:221-244.
24. Amri H, Li H, Culty M, et al. The peripheral-type benzodiazepine receptor and adrenal steroidogenesis. *Curr Opin Endocrinol Diabetes*. 1999;6:179-184.
25. Bernhardt R. The role of adrenodoxin in adrenal steroidogenesis. *Curr Opin Endocrinol Diab*. 2000;7:109-115.
26. Miller WL. Minireview: Regulation of steroidogenesis by electron transfer. *Endocrinology*. 2005;146:2544-2550.
27. Payne AH, Hales DB. Overview of steroidogenic enzymes in the pathway from cholesterol to active steroid hormones. *Endocr Rev*. 2004;25:947-970.
28. Onoda M, Hall PF. Cytochrome b5 stimulates purified testicular microsomal cytochrome P-450 (C21 side-chain cleavage). *Biochem Biophys Res Commun*. 1982;108:454-460.
29. Miller WL. Molecular biology of steroid hormone synthesis. *Endocr Rev*. 1988;9:295-318.
30. John ME, John MC, Ashley P, et al. Identification and characterization of cDNA clones specific for cholesterol side-chain cleavage cytochrome P-450. *Proc Natl Acad Sci U S A*. 1984;81:5628-5632.
31. Lorence MC, Murry BA, Trant JM, et al. Human 3 β-hydroxysteroid dehydrogenase/delta 5-4 isomerase from placenta: expression in non-steroidogenic cells of a protein that catalyzes the dehydrogenation/isomerization of C21 and C19 steroids. *Endocrinology*. 1990; 126:2493-2498.
32. Bradshaw KD, Waterman MR, Couch RT, et al. Characterization of complementary deoxyribonucleic acid for human adrenocortical 17 alpha-hydroxylase: a probe for analysis of 17 alpha-hydroxylase deficiency. *Mol Endocrinol*. 1987;1:348-354.
33. Nakamura Y, Hornsby PJ, Casson P, et al. Type 5 17β-hydroxysteroid dehydrogenase (AKR1C3) contributes to testosterone production in the adrenal reticularis. *J Clin Endocrinol Metab*. 2009;94:2192-2198.
34. White PC, New MI, Dupont B. Cloning and expression of cDNA encoding a bovine adrenal cytochrome P-450 specific for steroid 21-hydroxylation. *Proc Natl Acad Sci U S A*. 1984;81:1986-1990.
35. Chua SC, Szabo P, Vitek A, et al. Cloning of cDNA encoding steroid 11 β-hydroxylase (P450c11). *Proc Natl Acad Sci U S A*. 1987;84: 7193-7197.
36. Mornet E, Dupont J, Vitek A, et al. Characterization of two genes encoding human steroid 11 β-hydroxylase (P-450(11) β). *J Biol Chem*. 1989;264:20961-20967.
37. Curnow KM, Tusie-Luna MT, Pascoe L, et al. The product of the CYP11B2 gene is required for aldosterone biosynthesis in the human adrenal cortex. *Mol Endocrinol*. 1991;5:1513-1522.
38. Strott CA. Sulfonation and molecular action. *Endocr Rev*. 2002; 23:703-732.
39. Siiteri PK, MacDonald PC. The utilization of dehydroisoandrosterone sulphate for estrogen synthesis during human pregnancy. *Steroids*. 1963;2:713-730.
40. Lamolet B, Pulichino AM, Lamonerie T, et al. A pituitary cell-restricted T box factor, Tpit, activates POMC transcription in cooperation with Pitx homeoproteins. *Cell*. 2001;104:849-859.
41. Smith AI, Funder JW. Proopiomelanocortin processing in the pituitary, central nervous system, and peripheral tissues. *Endocr Rev*. 1988; 9:159-179.
42. Donald RA. ACTH and related peptides. *Clin Endocrinol (Oxf)*. 1980;12:491-524.
43. Bicknell AB, Lomthaisong K, Woods RJ, et al. Characterization of a serine protease that cleaves pro-gamma-melanotropin at the adrenal to stimulate growth. *Cell*. 2001;105:903-912.

44. Suzuki I, Cone RD, Im S, et al. Binding of melanotropic hormones to the melanocortin receptor MC1R on human melanocytes stimulates proliferation and melanogenesis. *Endocrinology.* 1996;137:1627-1633.
45. DeBold CR, Nicholson WE, Orth DN. Immunoreactive proopiomelanocortin (POMC) peptides and POMC-like messenger ribonucleic acid are present in many rat nonpituitary tissues. *Endocrinology.* 1988;122:2648-2657.
46. de Keyzer Y, Lenne F, Massias JF, et al. Pituitary-like proopiomelanocortin transcripts in human Leydig cell tumors. *J Clin Invest.* 1990;86:871-877.
47. Clark AJ, Lavender PM, Coates P, et al. In vitro and in vivo analysis of the processing and fate of the peptide products of the short proopiomelanocortin mRNA. *Mol Endocrinol.* 1990;4:1737-1743.
48. de Keyzer Y, Bertagna X, Luton JP, et al. Variable modes of proopiomelanocortin gene transcription in human tumors. *Mol Endocrinol.* 1989;3:215-223.
49. Clark AJ, Lavender PM, Besser GM, et al. Pro-opiomelanocortin mRNA size heterogeneity in ACTH-dependent Cushing's syndrome. *J Mol Endocrinol.* 1989;2:3-9.
50. Picon A, Bertagna X, de Keyzer Y. Analysis of the human proopiomelanocortin gene promoter in a small cell lung carcinoma cell line reveals an unusual role for E2F transcription factors. *Oncogene.* 1999; 18:2627-2633.
51. Newell-Price J, King P, Clark AJ. The CpG island promoter of the human proopiomelanocortin gene is methylated in nonexpressing normal tissue and tumors and represses expression. *Mol Endocrinol.* 2001;15:338-348.
52. Zhou A, Bloomquist BT, Mains RE. The prohormone convertases PC1 and PC2 mediate distinct endoproteolytic cleavages in a strict temporal order during proopiomelanocortin biosynthetic processing. *J Biol Chem.* 1993;268:1763-1769.
53. Stewart PM, Gibson S, Crosby SR, et al. ACTH precursors characterize the ectopic ACTH syndrome. *Clin Endocrinol (Oxf).* 1994;40:199-204.
54. Oliver RL, Davis JR, White A. Characterisation of ACTH related peptides in ectopic Cushing's syndrome. *Pituitary.* 2003;6:119-126.
55. Coll AP, Farooqi IS, Challis BG, et al. Proopiomelanocortin and energy balance: insights from human and murine genetics. *J Clin Endocrinol Metab.* 2004;89:2557-2562.
56. Lundblad JR, Roberts JL. Regulation of proopiomelanocortin gene expression in pituitary. *Endocr Rev.* 1988;9:135-158.
57. Orth DN. Corticotropin-releasing hormone in humans. *Endocr Rev.* 1992;13:164-191.
58. Taylor AL, Fishman LM. Corticotropin-releasing hormone. *N Engl J Med.* 1988;319:213-222.
59. Antoni FA. Hypothalamic control of adrenocorticotropin secretion: advances since the discovery of 41-residue corticotropin-releasing factor. *Endocr Rev.* 1986;7:351-378.
60. Shibahara S, Morimoto Y, Furutani Y, et al. Isolation and sequence analysis of the human corticotropin-releasing factor precursor gene. *EMBO J.* 1983;2:775-779.
61. Furutani Y, Morimoto Y, Shibahara S, et al. Cloning and sequence analysis of cDNA for ovine corticotropin-releasing factor precursor. *Nature.* 1983;301:537-540.
62. Chen R, Lewis KA, Perrin MH, et al. Expression cloning of a human corticotropin-releasing-factor receptor. *Proc Natl Acad Sci U S A.* 1993;90:8967-8971.
63. Sasaki A, Sato S, Murakami O, et al. Immunoreactive corticotropin-releasing hormone present in human plasma may be derived from both hypothalamic and extrahypothalamic sources. *J Clin Endocrinol Metab.* 1987;65:176-182.
64. Campbell EA, Linton EA, Wolfe CD, et al. Plasma corticotropin-releasing hormone concentrations during pregnancy and parturition. *J Clin Endocrinol Metab.* 1987;64:1054-1059.
65. Linton EA, Wolfe CD, Behan DP, et al. A specific carrier substance for human corticotrophin releasing factor in late gestational maternal plasma which could mask the ACTH-releasing activity. *Clin Endocrinol (Oxf).* 1988;28:315-324.
66. Rivier C, Rivier J, Vale W. Inhibition of adrenocorticotropic hormone secretion in the rat by immunoneutralization of corticotropin-releasing factor. *Science.* 1982;218:377-379.
67. Hauger RL, Aguilera G. Regulation of pituitary corticotropin releasing hormone (CRH) receptors by CRH: interaction with vasopressin. *Endocrinology.* 1993;133:1708-1714.
68. Watanabe T, Oki Y, Orth DN. Kinetic actions and interactions of arginine vasopressin, angiotensin-II, and oxytocin on adrenocorticotropin secretion by rat anterior pituitary cells in the microperifusion system. *Endocrinology.* 1989;125:1921-1931.
69. Bateman A, Singh A, Kral T, et al. The immune-hypothalamic-pituitary-adrenal axis. *Endocr Rev.* 1989;10:92-112.
70. Chrousos GP. The hypothalamic-pituitary-adrenal axis and immune-mediated inflammation. *N Engl J Med.* 1995;332:1351-1362.
71. Ray DW, Ren SG, Melmed S. Leukemia inhibitory factor (LIF) stimulates proopiomelanocortin (POMC) expression in a corticotroph cell line: role of STAT pathway. *J Clin Invest.* 1996;97:1852-1859.
72. Udelsman R, Norton JA, Jelenich SE, et al. Responses of the hypothalamic-pituitary-adrenal and renin-angiotensin axes and the sympathetic system during controlled surgical and anesthetic stress. *J Clin Endocrinol Metab.* 1987;64:986-994.
73. Vaughan GM, Becker RA, Allen JP, et al. Cortisol and corticotrophin in burned patients. *J Trauma.* 1982;22:263-273.
74. Fish HR, Chernow B, O'Brian JT. Endocrine and neurophysiologic responses of the pituitary to insulin-induced hypoglycemia: a review. *Metabolism.* 1986;35:763-780.
75. Luger A, Deuster PA, Kyle SB, et al. Acute hypothalamic-pituitary-adrenal responses to the stress of treadmill exercise: physiologic adaptations to physical training. *N Engl J Med.* 1987;316:1309-1315.
76. Aguilera G. Regulation of pituitary ACTH secretion during chronic stress. *Front Neuroendocrinol.* 1994;15:321-350.
77. Weitzman ED, Fukushima D, Nogeire C, et al. Twenty-four hour pattern of the episodic secretion of cortisol in normal subjects. *J Clin Endocrinol Metab.* 1971;33:14-22.
78. Veldhuis JD, Iranmanesh A, Johnson ML, et al. Amplitude, but not frequency, modulation of adrenocorticotropin secretory bursts gives rise to the nyctohemeral rhythm of the corticotropic axis in man. *J Clin Endocrinol Metab.* 1990;71:452-463.
79. Horrocks PM, Jones AF, Ratcliffe WA, et al. Patterns of ACTH and cortisol pulsatility over twenty-four hours in normal males and females. *Clin Endocrinol (Oxf).* 1990;32:127-134.
80. Boivin DB, Duffy JF, Kronauer RE, et al. Dose-response relationships for resetting of human circadian clock by light. *Nature.* 1996; 379:540-542.
81. Czeisler CA, Dumont M, Duffy JF, et al. Association of sleep-wake habits in older people with changes in output of circadian pacemaker. *Lancet.* 1992;340:933-936.
82. Desir D, Van Cauter E, Fang VS, et al. Effects of "jet lag" on hormonal patterns: I. Procedures, variations in total plasma proteins, and disruption of adrenocorticotropin-cortisol periodicity. *J Clin Endocrinol Metab.* 1981;52:628-641.
83. Davis LG, Arentzen R, Reid JM, et al. Glucocorticoid sensitivity of vasopressin mRNA levels in the paraventricular nucleus of the rat. *Proc Natl Acad Sci U S A.* 1986;83:1145-1149.
84. Keller-Wood ME, Dallman MF. Corticosteroid inhibition of ACTH secretion. *Endocr Rev.* 1984;5:1-24.
85. Buckingham JC, John CD, Solito E, et al. Annexin 1, glucocorticoids, and the neuroendocrine-immune interface. *Ann N Y Acad Sci.* 2006;1088:396-409.
86. Lamberts SW, Koper JW, Biemond P, et al. Cortisol receptor resistance: the variability of its clinical presentation and response to treatment. *J Clin Endocrinol Metab.* 1992;74:313-321.
87. Cole TJ, Blendy JA, Monaghan AP, et al. Targeted disruption of the glucocorticoid receptor gene blocks adrenergic chromaffin cell development and severely retards lung maturation. *Genes Dev.* 1995; 9:1608-1621.
88. Mountjoy KG, Robbins LS, Mortrud MT, et al. The cloning of a family of genes that encode the melanocortin receptors. *Science.* 1992;257: 1248-1251.
89. Metherell LA, Chapple JP, Cooray S, et al. Mutations in MRAP, encoding a new interacting partner of the ACTH receptor, cause familial glucocorticoid deficiency type 2. *Nat Genet.* 2005;37:166-170.
90. Clark AJ, Chan LF, Chung TT, et al. The genetics of familial glucocorticoid deficiency. *Best Pract Res Clin Endocrinol Metab.* 2009;23: 159-165.
91. Cooke BA. Signal transduction involving cyclic AMP-dependent and cyclic AMP-independent mechanisms in the control of steroidogenesis. *Mol Cell Endocrinol.* 1999;151:25-35.
92. Enyeart JJ, Mlinar B, Enyeart JA. T-type Ca2+ channels are required for adrenocorticotropin-stimulated cortisol production by bovine adrenal zona fasciculata cells. *Mol Endocrinol.* 1993;7:1031-1040.
93. Ehrhart-Bornstein M, Hinson JP, Bornstein SR, et al. Intraadrenal interactions in the regulation of adrenocortical steroidogenesis. *Endocr Rev.* 1998;19:101-143.
94. Munari-Silem Y, Lebrethon MC, Morand I, et al. Gap junction-mediated cell-to-cell communication in bovine and human adrenal cells. A process whereby cells increase their responsiveness to physiological corticotropin concentrations. *J Clin Invest.* 1995;95:1429-1439.
95. Simpson ER, Waterman MR. Regulation of the synthesis of steroidogenic enzymes in adrenal cortical cells by ACTH. *Annu Rev Physiol.* 1988;50:427-440.
96. Waterman MR, Bischof LJ. Cytochromes P450 12: diversity of ACTH (cAMP)-dependent transcription of bovine steroid hydroxylase genes. *FASEB J.* 1997;11:419-427.
97. Rainey WE. Adrenal zonation: clues from 11β-hydroxylase and aldosterone synthase. *Mol Cell Endocrinol.* 1999;151:151-160.
98. Longcope C. Adrenal and gonadal androgen secretion in normal females. *Clin Endocrinol Metab.* 1986;15:213-228.
99. Labrie F, Belanger A, Simard J, et al. DHEA and peripheral androgen and estrogen formation: intracinology. *Ann N Y Acad Sci.* 1995;774:16-28.

100. Liu D, Dillon JS. Dehydroepiandrosterone activates endothelial cell nitric-oxide synthase by a specific plasma membrane receptor coupled to Galpha(i2,3). *J Biol Chem*. 2002;277:21379-21388.
101. Hammer F, Subtil S, Lux P, et al. No evidence for hepatic conversion of dehydroepiandrosterone (DHEA) sulfate to DHEA: in vivo and in vitro studies. *J Clin Endocrinol Metab*. 2005;90:3600-3605.
102. McKenna TJ, Fearon U, Clarke D, et al. A critical review of the origin and control of adrenal androgens. *Baillieres Clin Obstet Gynaecol*. 1997;11:229-248.
103. Weinberger C, Hollenberg SM, Rosenfeld MG, et al. Domain structure of human glucocorticoid receptor and its relationship to the v-erb-A oncogene product. *Nature*. 1985;318:670-672.
104. Arriza JL, Weinberger C, Cerelli G, et al. Cloning of human mineralocorticoid receptor complementary DNA: structural and functional kinship with the glucocorticoid receptor. *Science*. 1987;237:268-275.
105. Gustafsson JA, Carlstedt-Duke J, Poellinger L, et al. Biochemistry, molecular biology, and physiology of the glucocorticoid receptor. *Endocr Rev*. 1987;8:185-234.
106. Zhou J, Cidlowski JA. The human glucocorticoid receptor: one gene, multiple proteins and diverse responses. *Steroids*. 2005;70:407-417.
107. Pascual-Le Tallec L, Lombes M. The mineralocorticoid receptor: a journey exploring its diversity and specificity of action. *Mol Endocrinol*. 2005;19:2211-2221.
108. Pratt WB. The role of heat shock proteins in regulating the function, folding, and trafficking of the glucocorticoid receptor. *J Biol Chem*. 1993;268:21455-21458.
109. Beato M, Sanchez-Pacheco A. Interaction of steroid hormone receptors with the transcription initiation complex. *Endocr Rev*. 1996;17:587-609.
110. Bamberger CM, Schulte HM, Chrousos GP. Molecular determinants of glucocorticoid receptor function and tissue sensitivity to glucocorticoids. *Endocr Rev*. 1996;17:245-261.
111. McKenna NJ, Lanz RB, O'Malley BW. Nuclear receptor coregulators: cellular and molecular biology. *Endocr Rev*. 1999;20:321-344.
112. Rhen T, Cidlowski JA. Antiinflammatory action of glucocorticoids: new mechanisms for old drugs. *N Engl J Med*. 2005;353:1711-1723.
113. Schule R, Rangarajan P, Kliewer S, et al. Functional antagonism between oncoprotein c-Jun and the glucocorticoid receptor. *Cell*. 1990;62:1217-1226.
114. McKay LI, Cidlowski JA. Molecular control of immune/inflammatory responses: interactions between nuclear factor-kappa B and steroid receptor-signaling pathways. *Endocr Rev*. 1999;20:435-459.
115. Funder JW. Aldosterone action. *Annu Rev Physiol*. 1993;55:115-130.
116. Rossier BC, Alpern RJ. Cell and molecular biology of epithelial transport. *Curr Opin Nephrol Hypertens*. 1999;8:579-580.
117. Verrey F, Kraehenbuhl JP, Rossier BC. Aldosterone induces a rapid increase in the rate of Na,K-ATPase gene transcription in cultured kidney cells. *Mol Endocrinol*. 1989;3:1369-1376.
118. Chen SY, Bhargava A, Mastroberardino L, et al. Epithelial sodium channel regulated by aldosterone-induced protein sgk. *Proc Natl Acad Sci U S A*. 1999;96:2514-2519.
119. Edwards CR, Stewart PM, Burt D, et al. Localisation of 11 β-hydroxysteroid dehydrogenase: tissue specific protector of the mineralocorticoid receptor. *Lancet*. 1988;2:986-989.
120. Funder JW, Pearce PT, Smith R, et al. Mineralocorticoid action: target tissue specificity is enzyme, not receptor, mediated. *Science*. 1988;242:583-585.
121. Funder JW. New biology of aldosterone, and experimental studies on the selective aldosterone blocker eplerenone. *Am Heart J*. 2002;144:S8-11.
122. Iwasaki Y, Aoki Y, Katahira M, et al. Non-genomic mechanisms of glucocorticoid inhibition of adrenocorticotropin secretion: possible involvement of GTP-binding protein. *Biochem Biophys Res Commun*. 1997;235:295-299.
123. Funder JW. The nongenomic actions of aldosterone. *Endocr Rev*. 2005;26:313-321.
124. Hammond GL. Molecular properties of corticosteroid binding globulin and the sex-steroid binding proteins. *Endocr Rev*. 1990;11:65-79.
125. Roitman A, Bruchis S, Bauman B, et al. Total deficiency of corticosteroid-binding globulin. *Clin Endocrinol (Oxf)*. 1984;21:541-548.
126. Smith CL, Power SG, Hammond GL. A Leu-His substitution at residue 93 in human corticosteroid binding globulin results in reduced affinity for cortisol. *J Steroid Biochem Mol Biol*. 1992;42:671-676.
127. Fukushima DK, Bradlow HL, Hellman L, et al. Metabolic transformation of hydrocortisone-4-C14 in normal men. *J Biol Chem*. 1960;235:2246-2252.
128. White PC, Mune T, Agarwal AK. 11 β-hydroxysteroid dehydrogenase and the syndrome of apparent mineralocorticoid excess. *Endocr Rev*. 1997;18:135-156.
129. Tomlinson JW, Walker EA, Bujalska IJ, et al. 11β-hydroxysteroid dehydrogenase type 1: a tissue-specific regulator of glucocorticoid response. *Endocr Rev*. 2004;25:831-866.
130. Quinkler M, Stewart PM. Hypertension and the cortisol-cortisone shuttle. *J Clin Endocrinol Metab*. 2003;88:2384-2392.
131. Moore JS, Monson JP, Kaltsas G, et al. Modulation of 11β-hydroxysteroid dehydrogenase isozymes by growth hormone and insulin-like growth factor: in vivo and in vitro studies. *J Clin Endocrinol Metab*. 1999;84:4172-4177.
132. Voccia E, Saenger P, Peterson RE, et al. 6 β-hydroxycortisol excretion in hypercortisolemic states. *J Clin Endocrinol Metab*. 1979;48:467-471.
133. Yamada S, Iwai K. Induction of hepatic cortisol-6-hydroxylase by rifampicin (Letter). *Lancet*. 1976;2:366-367.
134. Whitworth JA, Stewart PM, Burt D, et al. The kidney is the major site of cortisone production in man. *Clin Endocrinol (Oxf)*. 1989;31:355-361.
135. Kyriazopoulou V, Parparousi O, Vagenakis AG. Rifampicin-induced adrenal crisis in addisonian patients receiving corticosteroid replacement therapy. *J Clin Endocrinol Metab*. 1984;59:1204-1206.
136. Morris DJ, Brem AS. Metabolic derivatives of aldosterone. *Am J Physiol*. 1987;252:F365-F373.
137. Edwards C, Hayman A. Enzyme protection of the mineralocorticoid receptor: evidence in favour of the hemi-acetal structure of aldosterone. In: Bonvalet JP, Farman N, Lombès M, et al, eds. *Aldosterone Fundamental Aspects*. London: Colloque INSERM/John Libbey Eurotext; 1991:67-76.
138. Stalmans W, Laloux M. Glucocorticoids and hepatic glycogen metabolism. In: Baxter JD, Rousseau GG, eds. *Glucocorticoid Hormone Action*. New York, NY: Springer-Verlag; 1979:518-533.
139. Watts LM, Manchem VP, Leedom TA, et al. Reduction of hepatic and adipose tissue glucocorticoid receptor expression with antisense oligonucleotides improves hyperglycemia and hyperlipidemia in diabetic rodents without causing systemic glucocorticoid antagonism. *Diabetes*. 2005;54:1846-1853.
140. Chakravarty K, Cassuto H, Reshef L, et al. Factors that control the tissue-specific transcription of the gene for phosphoenolpyruvate carboxykinase-C. *Crit Rev Biochem Mol Biol*. 2005;40:129-154.
141. Olefsky JM. Effect of dexamethasone on insulin binding, glucose transport, and glucose oxidation of isolated rat adipocytes. *J Clin Invest*. 1975;56:1499-1508.
142. Hauner H, Entenmann G, Wabitsch M, et al. Promoting effect of glucocorticoids on the differentiation of human adipocyte precursor cells cultured in a chemically defined medium. *J Clin Invest*. 1989;84:1663-1670.
143. Rebuffe-Scrive M, Krotkiewski M, Elfverson J, et al. Muscle and adipose tissue morphology and metabolism in Cushing's syndrome. *J Clin Endocrinol Metab*. 1988;67:1122-1128.
144. Bronnegard M, Arner P, Hellstrom L, et al. Glucocorticoid receptor messenger ribonucleic acid in different regions of human adipose tissue. *Endocrinology*. 1990;127:1689-1696.
145. Bujalska IJ, Kumar S, Stewart PM. Does central obesity reflect "Cushing's disease of the omentum"? *Lancet*. 1997;349:1210-1213.
146. Leibovich SJ, Ross R. The role of the macrophage in wound repair: a study with hydrocortisone and antimacrophage serum. *Am J Pathol*. 1975;78:71-100.
147. Canalis E. Mechanisms of glucocorticoid action in bone: implications to glucocorticoid-induced osteoporosis. Clinical Review 83. *J Clin Endocrinol Metab*. 1996;81:3441-3447.
148. van Staa TP, Leufkens HG, Abenhaim L, et al. Use of oral corticosteroids in the United Kingdom. *Q J Med*. 2000;93:105-111.
149. Williams PL, Corbett M. Avascular necrosis of bone complicating corticosteroid replacement therapy. *Ann Rheum Dis*. 1983;42:276-279.
150. Weinstein RS, Nicholas RW, Manolagas SC. Apoptosis of osteocytes in glucocorticoid-induced osteonecrosis of the hip. *J Clin Endocrinol Metab*. 2000;85:2907-2912.
151. Leonard MB, Feldman HI, Shults J, et al. Long-term, high-dose glucocorticoids and bone mineral content in childhood glucocorticoid-sensitive nephrotic syndrome. *N Engl J Med*. 2004;351:868-875.
152. Fraser R, Davies DL, Connell JM. Hormones and hypertension. *Clin Endocrinol (Oxf)*. 1989;31:701-746.
153. Saruta T, Suzuki H, Handa M, et al. Multiple factors contribute to the pathogenesis of hypertension in Cushing's syndrome. *J Clin Endocrinol Metab*. 1986;62:275-279.
154. Marver D. Evidence of corticosteroid action along the nephron. *Am J Physiol*. 1984;246:F111-F123.
155. Raff H. Glucocorticoid inhibition of neurohypophysial vasopressin secretion. *Am J Physiol*. 1987;252:R635-R644.
156. Peers SH, Flower RJ. The role of lipocortin in corticosteroid actions. *Am Rev Respir Dis*. 1990;141:S18-S21.
157. McEwen BS, De Kloet ER, Rostene W. Adrenal steroid receptors and actions in the nervous system. *Physiol Rev*. 1986;66:1121-1188.
158. Sapolsky RM, Krey LC, McEwen BS. Prolonged glucocorticoid exposure reduces hippocampal neuron number: implications for aging. *J Neurosci*. 1985;5:1222-1227.
159. Lupien SJ, de Leon M, de Santi S, et al. Cortisol levels during human aging predict hippocampal atrophy and memory deficits. *Nat Neurosci*. 1998;1:69-73.
160. Sandeep TC, Yau JL, MacLullich AM, et al. 11β-hydroxysteroid dehydrogenase inhibition improves cognitive function in healthy

elderly men and type 2 diabetics. *Proc Natl Acad Sci U S A*. 2004;101: 6734-6739.
161. Hajszan T, MacLusky NJ, Leranth C. Dehydroepiandrosterone increases hippocampal spine synapse density in ovariectomized female rats. *Endocrinology*. 2004;145:1042-1045.
162. Yau JL, Rasmuson S, Andrew R, et al. Dehydroepiandrosterone 7-hydroxylase CYP7B: predominant expression in primate hippocampus and reduced expression in Alzheimer's disease. *Neuroscience*. 2003;121:307-314.
163. Clark AF. Steroids, ocular hypertension, and glaucoma. *J Glaucoma*. 1995;4:354-369.
164. Messer J, Reitman D, Sacks HS, et al. Association of adrenocorticosteroid therapy and peptic-ulcer disease. *N Engl J Med*. 1983;309: 21-24.
165. Strickland AL, Underwood LE, Voina SJ, et al. Growth retardation in Cushing's syndrome. *Am J Dis Child*. 1972;123:207-213.
166. Ballard PL, Ertsey R, Gonzales LW, et al. Transcriptional regulation of human pulmonary surfactant proteins SP-B and SP-C by glucocorticoids. *Am J Respir Cell Mol Biol*. 1996;14:599-607.
167. Dluhy RG, Newmark SR, Lauler DP, et al. Pharmacology and chemistry of adrenal glucocorticoids. In: Azarnoff DL, ed. *Steroid Therapy*. Philadelphia, PA: Saunders; 1975:1-14.
168. Meikle AW, Weed JA, Tyler FH. Kinetics and interconversion of prednisolone and prednisone studied with new radioimmunoassays. *J Clin Endocrinol Metab*. 1975;41:717-721.
169. Axelrod L. Glucocorticoid therapy. *Medicine (Baltimore)*. 1976;55: 39-65.
170. Wei L, MacDonald TM, Walker BR. Taking glucocorticoids by prescription is associated with subsequent cardiovascular disease. *Ann Intern Med*. 2004;141:764-770.
171. Schacke H, Schottelius A, Docke WD, et al. Dissociation of transactivation from transrepression by a selective glucocorticoid receptor agonist leads to separation of therapeutic effects from side effects. *Proc Natl Acad Sci U S A*. 2004;101:227-232.
172. Loprinzi CL, Jensen MD, Jiang NS, et al. Effect of megestrol acetate on the human pituitary-adrenal axis. *Mayo Clin Proc*. 1992;67:1160-1162.
173. Christy NP. Corticosteroid withdrawal. In: Bardin CW, ed. *Current Therapy in Endocrinology and Metabolism*, 3rd ed. New York, NY: BC Decker; 1988:113-120.
174. Kane KF, Emery P, Sheppard MC, et al. Assessing the hypothalamo-pituitary-adrenal axis in patients on long-term glucocorticoid therapy: the short synacthen versus the insulin tolerance test. *QJM*. 1995;88: 263-267.
175. Casale TB, Nelson HS, Stricker WE, et al. Suppression of hypothalamic-pituitary-adrenal axis activity with inhaled flunisolide and fluticasone propionate in adult asthma patients. *Ann Allergy Asthma Immunol*. 2001;87:379-385.
176. Holme J, Tomlinson JW, Stockley RA, et al. Adrenal suppression in bronchiectasis and the impact of inhaled corticosteroids. *Eur Respir J*. 2008;32:1047-1052.
177. Dixon RB, Christy NP. On the various forms of corticosteroid withdrawal syndrome. *Am J Med*. 1980;68:224-230.
178. Hopkins RL, Leinung MC. Exogenous Cushing's syndrome and glucocorticoid withdrawal. *Endocrinol Metab Clin North Am*. 2005;34:371-384, ix.
179. Walters W, Wilder RM, Kepler EJ. The suprarenal cortical syndrome with presentation of ten cases. *Ann Surg*. 1934;100:670-688.
180. Meador CK, Liddle GW, Island DP, et al. Cause of Cushing's syndrome in patients with tumors arising from "nonendocrine" tissue. *J Clin Endocrinol Metab*. 1962;22:693-703.
181. Ross EJ, Linch DC. Cushing's syndrome—killing disease: discriminatory value of signs and symptoms aiding early diagnosis. *Lancet*. 1982;2:646-649.
182. Newell-Price J, Bertagna X, Grossman AB, et al. Cushing's syndrome. *Lancet*. 2006;367:1605-1617.
183. Wajchenberg BL, Bosco A, Marone MM, et al. Estimation of body fat and lean tissue distribution by dual energy X-ray absorptiometry and abdominal body fat evaluation by computed tomography in Cushing's disease. *J Clin Endocrinol Metab*. 1995;80:2791-2794.
184. Luton JP, Thieblot P, Valcke JC, et al. Reversible gonadotropin deficiency in male Cushing's disease. *J Clin Endocrinol Metab*. 1977;45:488-495.
185. Lado-Abeal J, Rodriguez-Arnao J, Newell-Price JD, et al. Menstrual abnormalities in women with Cushing's disease are correlated with hypercortisolemia rather than raised circulating androgen levels. *J Clin Endocrinol Metab*. 1998;83:3083-3088.
186. Jeffcoate WJ, Silverstone JT, Edwards CR, et al. Psychiatric manifestations of Cushing's syndrome: response to lowering of plasma cortisol. *Q J Med*. 1979;48:465-472.
187. Dorn LD, Burgess ES, Dubbert B, et al. Psychopathology in patients with endogenous Cushing's syndrome: "atypical" or melancholic features. *Clin Endocrinol (Oxf)*. 1995;43:433-442.
188. Friess E, Wiedemann K, Steiger A, et al. The hypothalamic-pituitary-adrenocortical system and sleep in man. *Adv Neuroimmunol*. 1995;5:111-125.
189. Lindsay JR, Nansel T, Baid S, et al. Long-term impaired quality of life in Cushing's syndrome despite initial improvement after surgical remission. *J Clin Endocrinol Metab*. 2006;91:447-453.
190. Ferguson JK, Donald RA, Weston TS, et al. Skin thickness in patients with acromegaly and Cushing's syndrome and response to treatment. *Clin Endocrinol (Oxf)*. 1983;18:347-353.
191. Pleasure DE, Walsh GO, Engel WK. Atrophy of skeletal muscle in patients with Cushing's syndrome. *Arch Neurol*. 1970;22:118-125.
192. Plotz CM, Knowlton AI, Ragan C. The natural history of Cushing's syndrome. *Am J Med*. 1952;13:597-614.
193. Etxabe J, Vazquez JA. Morbidity and mortality in Cushing's disease: an epidemiological approach. *Clin Endocrinol (Oxf)*. 1994;40:479-484.
194. Colao A, Pivonello R, Spiezia S, et al. Persistence of increased cardiovascular risk in patients with Cushing's disease after five years of successful cure. *J Clin Endocrinol Metab*. 1999;84:2664-2672.
195. Dale DC, Petersdorf RG. Corticosteroids and infectious diseases. *Med Clin North Am*. 1973;57:1277-1287.
196. Graham BS, Tucker WS Jr. Opportunistic infections in endogenous Cushing's syndrome. *Ann Intern Med*. 1984;101:334-338.
197. Hill AT, Stewart PM, Hughes EA, et al. Cushing's disease and tuberculosis. *Respir Med*. 1998;92:604-606.
198. Taskinen MR, Nikkila EA, Pelkonen R, et al. Plasma lipoproteins, lipolytic enzymes, and very low density lipoprotein triglyceride turnover in Cushing's syndrome. *J Clin Endocrinol Metab*. 1983;57:619-626.
199. Stewart PM, Walker BR, Holder G, et al. 11 β-hydroxysteroid dehydrogenase activity in Cushing's syndrome: explaining the mineralocorticoid excess state of the ectopic adrenocorticotropin syndrome. *J Clin Endocrinol Metab*. 1995;80:3617-3620.
200. Benker G, Raida M, Olbricht T, et al. TSH secretion in Cushing's syndrome: relation to glucocorticoid excess, diabetes, goitre, and the "sick euthyroid syndrome." *Clin Endocrinol (Oxf)*. 1990;33:777-786.
201. Saketos M, Sharma N, Santoro NF. Suppression of the hypothalamic-pituitary-ovarian axis in normal women by glucocorticoids. *Biol Reprod*. 1993;49:1270-1276.
202. Sayegh F, Weigelin E. Intraocular pressure in Cushing's syndrome. *Ophthalmic Res*. 1975;7:390-394.
203. Kelly W. Exophthalmos in Cushing's syndrome. *Clin Endocrinol (Oxf)*. 1996;45:167-170.
204. Bouzas EA, Mastorakos G, Friedman TC, et al. Posterior subcapsular cataract in endogenous Cushing syndrome: an uncommon manifestation. *Invest Ophthalmol Vis Sci*. 1993;34:3497-3500.
205. Biller BM. Pathogenesis of pituitary Cushing's syndrome: pituitary versus hypothalamic. *Endocrinol Metab Clin North Am*. 1994; 23:547-554.
206. Gicquel C, Le Bouc Y, Luton JP, et al. Monoclonality of corticotroph macroadenomas in Cushing's disease. *J Clin Endocrinol Metab*. 1992;75:472-475.
207. Biller BM, Alexander JM, Zervas NT, et al. Clonal origins of adrenocorticotropin-secreting pituitary tissue in Cushing's disease. *J Clin Endocrinol Metab*. 1992;75:1303-1309.
208. Woo YS, Isidori AM, Wat WZ, et al. Clinical and biochemical characteristics of adrenocorticotropin-secreting macroadenomas. *J Clin Endocrinol Metab*. 2005;90:4963-4969.
209. Liddle GW. Tests of pituitary-adrenal suppressibility in the diagnosis of Cushing's syndrome. *J Clin Endocrinol Metab*. 1960;20:1539-1560.
210. Stewart PM, Penn R, Gibson R, et al. Hypothalamic abnormalities in patients with pituitary-dependent Cushing's syndrome. *Clin Endocrinol (Oxf)*. 1992;36:453-458.
211. Jex RK, van Heerden JA, Carpenter PC, et al. Ectopic ACTH syndrome: diagnostic and therapeutic aspects. *Am J Surg*. 1985;149:276-282.
212. Howlett TA, Drury PL, Perry L, et al. Diagnosis and management of ACTH-dependent Cushing's syndrome: comparison of the features in ectopic and pituitary ACTH production. *Clin Endocrinol (Oxf)*. 1986;24:699-713.
213. Findling JW, Tyrrell JB. Occult ectopic secretion of corticotropin. *Arch Intern Med*. 1986;146:929-933.
214. Ilias I, Torpy DJ, Pacak K, et al. Cushing's syndrome due to ectopic corticotropin secretion: twenty years' experience at the National Institutes of Health. *J Clin Endocrinol Metab*. 2005;90:4955-4962.
215. Wajchenberg BL, Mendonca B, Liberman B, et al. Ectopic ACTH syndrome. *J Steroid Biochem Mol Biol*. 1995;53:139-151.
216. Limper AH, Carpenter PC, Scheithauer B, et al. The Cushing syndrome induced by bronchial carcinoid tumors. *Ann Intern Med*. 1992; 117:209-214.
217. Odell WD. Ectopic ACTH secretion: a misnomer. *Endocrinol Metab Clin North Am*. 1991;20:371-379.
218. Ray DW, Littlewood AC, Clark AJ, et al. Human small cell lung cancer cell lines expressing the proopiomelanocortin gene have aberrant glucocorticoid receptor function. *J Clin Invest*. 1994;93:1625-1630.
219. Carey RM, Varma SK, Drake CR Jr, et al. Ectopic secretion of corticotropin-releasing factor as a cause of Cushing's syndrome: a clinical, morphologic, and biochemical study. *N Engl J Med*. 1984;311:13-20.
220. Muller OA, von Werder K. Ectopic production of ACTH and corticotropin-releasing hormone (CRH). *J Steroid Biochem Mol Biol*. 1992;43:403-408.

221. Preeyasombat C, Sirikulchayanonta V, Mahachokelertwattana P, et al. Cushing's syndrome caused by Ewing's sarcoma secreting corticotropin releasing factor-like peptide. *Am J Dis Child.* 1992;146:1103-1105.
222. Aron DC, Findling JW, Fitzgerald PA, et al. Pituitary ACTH dependency of nodular adrenal hyperplasia in Cushing's syndrome: report of two cases and review of the literature. *Am J Med.* 1981;71:302-306.
223. Doppman JL, Nieman LK, Travis WD, et al. CT and MR imaging of massive macronodular adrenocortical disease: a rare cause of autonomous primary adrenal hypercortisolism. *J Comput Assist Tomogr.* 1991;15:773-779.
224. Samuels MH, Loriaux DL. Cushing's syndrome and the nodular adrenal gland. *Endocrinol Metab Clin North Am.* 1994;23:555-569.
225. Sturrock ND, Morgan L, Jeffcoate WJ. Autonomous nodular hyperplasia of the adrenal cortex: tertiary hypercortisolism? *Clin Endocrinol (Oxf).* 1995;43:753-758.
226. Hermus AR, Pieters GF, Smals AG, et al. Transition from pituitary-dependent to adrenal-dependent Cushing's syndrome. *N Engl J Med.* 1988;318:966-970.
227. Young WF Jr, Carney JA, Musa BU, et al. Familial Cushing's syndrome due to primary pigmented nodular adrenocortical disease: reinvestigation 50 years later. *N Engl J Med.* 1989;321:1659-1664.
228. Stratakis CA, Kirschner LS, Carney JA. Clinical and molecular features of the Carney complex: diagnostic criteria and recommendations for patient evaluation. *J Clin Endocrinol Metab.* 2001;86:4041-4046.
229. Kirschner LS, Carney JA, Pack SD, et al. Mutations of the gene encoding the protein kinase A type I-alpha regulatory subunit in patients with the Carney complex. *Nat Genet.* 2000;26:89-92.
230. Kirk JM, Brain CE, Carson DJ, et al. Cushing's syndrome caused by nodular adrenal hyperplasia in children with McCune-Albright syndrome. *J Pediatr.* 1999;134:789-792.
231. Malchoff CD, MacGillivray D, Malchoff DM. Adrenocorticotropic hormone-independent adrenal hyperplasia. *Endocrinologist.* 1996; 6:79-85.
232. Christopoulos S, Bourdeau I, Lacroix A. Aberrant expression of hormone receptors in adrenal Cushing's syndrome. *Pituitary.* 2004;7:225-235.
233. Atkinson AB, Kennedy AL, Carson DJ, et al. Five cases of cyclical Cushing's syndrome. *Br Med J (Clin Res Ed).* 1985;291:1453-1457.
234. Mantero F, Scaroni CM, Albiger NM. Cyclic Cushing's syndrome: an overview. *Pituitary.* 2004;7:203-207.
235. Leinung MC, Zimmerman D. Cushing's disease in children. *Endocrinol Metab Clin North Am.* 1994;23:629-639.
236. Storr HL, Chan LF, Grossman AB, et al. Paediatric Cushing's syndrome: epidemiology, investigation and therapeutic advances. *Trends Endocrinol Metab.* 2007;18:167-174.
237. Lindsay JR, Jonklaas J, Oldfield EH, et al. Cushing's syndrome during pregnancy: personal experience and review of the literature. *J Clin Endocrinol Metab.* 2005;90:3077-3083.
238. Wallace C, Toth EL, Lewanczuk RZ, et al. Pregnancy-induced Cushing's syndrome in multiple pregnancies. *J Clin Endocrinol Metab.* 1996;81:15-21.
239. Kirkman S, Nelson DH. Alcohol-induced pseudo-Cushing's disease: a study of prevalence with review of the literature. *Metabolism.* 1988;37:390-394.
240. Stewart PM, Burra P, Shackleton CH, et al. 11 β-hydroxysteroid dehydrogenase deficiency and glucocorticoid status in patients with alcoholic and non-alcoholic chronic liver disease. *J Clin Endocrinol Metab.* 1993;76:748-751.
241. Newell-Price J, Trainer P, Besser M, et al. The diagnosis and differential diagnosis of Cushing's syndrome and pseudo-Cushing's states. *Endocr Rev.* 1998;19:647-672.
242. Glass AR, Burman KD, Dahms WT, et al. Endocrine function in human obesity. *Metabolism.* 1981;30:89-104.
243. Stewart PM, Boulton A, Kumar S, et al. Cortisol metabolism in human obesity: impaired cortisone → cortisol conversion in subjects with central adiposity. *J Clin Endocrinol Metab.* 1999;84:1022-1027.
244. Arnaldi G, Angeli A, Atkinson AB, et al. Diagnosis and complications of Cushing's syndrome: a consensus statement. *J Clin Endocrinol Metab.* 2003;88:5593-5602.
245. Findling JW, Raff H. Screening and diagnosis of Cushing's syndrome. *Endocrinol Metab Clin North Am.* 2005;34:385-402, ix-x.
246. Newell-Price J, Trainer P, Perry L, et al. A single sleeping midnight cortisol has 100% sensitivity for the diagnosis of Cushing's syndrome. *Clin Endocrinol (Oxf).* 1995;43:545-550.
247. Hamrahian AH, Oseni TS, Arafah BM. Measurements of serum free cortisol in critically ill patients. *N Engl J Med.* 2004;350:1629-1638.
248. Raff H, Raff JL, Findling JW. Late-night salivary cortisol as a screening test for Cushing's syndrome. *J Clin Endocrinol Metab.* 1998; 83:2681-2686.
249. Yaneva M, Mosnier-Pudar H, Dugue MA, et al. Midnight salivary cortisol for the initial diagnosis of Cushing's syndrome of various causes. *J Clin Endocrinol Metab.* 2004;89:3345-3351.
250. Invitti C, Pecori Giraldi F, de Martin M, et al. Diagnosis and management of Cushing's syndrome: results of an Italian multicentre study. Study Group of the Italian Society of Endocrinology on the Pathophysiology of the Hypothalamic-Pituitary-Adrenal Axis. *J Clin Endocrinol Metab.* 1999;84:440-448.
251. Corcuff JB, Tabarin A, Rashedi M, et al. Overnight urinary free cortisol determination: a screening test for the diagnosis of Cushing's syndrome. *Clin Endocrinol (Oxf).* 1998;48:503-508.
252. Cronin C, Igoe D, Duffy MJ, et al. The overnight dexamethasone test is a worthwhile screening procedure. *Clin Endocrinol (Oxf).* 1990; 33:27-33.
253. Isidori AM, Kaltsas GA, Mohammed S, et al. Discriminatory value of the low-dose dexamethasone suppression test in establishing the diagnosis and differential diagnosis of Cushing's syndrome. *J Clin Endocrinol Metab.* 2003;88:5299-5306.
254. Meikle AW. Dexamethasone suppression tests: usefulness of simultaneous measurement of plasma cortisol and dexamethasone. *Clin Endocrinol (Oxf).* 1982;16:401-408.
255. Yanovski JA, Cutler GB, Jr., Chrousos GP, et al. Corticotropin-releasing hormone stimulation following low-dose dexamethasone administration. A new test to distinguish Cushing's syndrome from pseudo-Cushing's states. *JAMA.* 1993;269:2232-2238.
256. Nieman LK, Biller BM, Findling JW, et al. The diagnosis of Cushing's syndrome: an Endocrine Society Clinical Practice Guideline. *J Clin Endocrinol Metab.* 2008;93:1526-1540.
257. Findling JW. Clinical application of a new immunoradiometric assay for ACTH *Endocrinologist.* 1992;2:360-365.
258. Tyrrell JB, Findling JW, Aron DC, et al. An overnight high-dose dexamethasone suppression test for rapid differential diagnosis of Cushing's syndrome. *Ann Intern Med.* 1986;104:180-186.
259. Biemond P, de Jong FH, Lamberts SW. Continuous dexamethasone infusion for seven hours in patients with the Cushing syndrome: a superior differential diagnostic test. *Ann Intern Med.* 1990; 112:738-742.
260. Findling JW, Doppman JL. Biochemical and radiologic diagnosis of Cushing's syndrome. *Endocrinol Metab Clin North Am.* 1994;23: 511-537.
261. Avgerinos PC, Yanovski JA, Oldfield EH, et al. The metyrapone and dexamethasone suppression tests for the differential diagnosis of the adrenocorticotropin-dependent Cushing syndrome: a comparison. *Ann Intern Med.* 1994;121:318-327.
262. Trainer PJ, Faria M, Newell-Price J, et al. A comparison of the effects of human and ovine corticotropin-releasing hormone on the pituitary-adrenal axis. *J Clin Endocrinol Metab.* 1995;80:412-417.
263. Chrousos GP, Schulte HM, Oldfield EH, et al. The corticotropin-releasing factor stimulation test: an aid in the evaluation of patients with Cushing's syndrome. *N Engl J Med.* 1984;310:622-626.
264. Nieman LK, Oldfield EH, Wesley R, et al. A simplified morning ovine corticotropin-releasing hormone stimulation test for the differential diagnosis of adrenocorticotropin-dependent Cushing's syndrome. *J Clin Endocrinol Metab.* 1993;77:1308-1312.
265. Lindsay JR, Nieman LK. Differential diagnosis and imaging in Cushing's syndrome. *Endocrinol Metab Clin North Am.* 2005;34:403-421,x.
266. Oldfield EH, Doppman JL, Nieman LK, et al. Petrosal sinus sampling with and without corticotropin-releasing hormone for the differential diagnosis of Cushing's syndrome. *N Engl J Med.* 1991;325:897-905.
267. Kaltsas GA, Giannulis MG, Newell-Price JD, et al. A critical analysis of the value of simultaneous inferior petrosal sinus sampling in Cushing's disease and the occult ectopic adrenocorticotropin syndrome. *J Clin Endocrinol Metab.* 1999;84:487-492.
268. Hall WA, Luciano MG, Doppman JL, et al. Pituitary magnetic resonance imaging in normal human volunteers: occult adenomas in the general population. *Ann Intern Med.* 1994;120:817-820.
269. Korobkin M, Francis IR. Adrenal imaging. *Semin Ultrasound CT MRI.* 1995;16:317-330.
270. Miles JM, Wahner HW, Carpenter PC, et al. Adrenal scintiscanning with NP-59, a new radioiodinated cholesterol agent. *Mayo Clin Proc.* 1979;54:321-327.
271. de Herder WW, Krenning EP, Malchoff CD, et al. Somatostatin receptor scintigraphy: its value in tumor localization in patients with Cushing's syndrome caused by ectopic corticotropin or corticotropin-releasing hormone secretion. *Am J Med.* 1994;96:305-312.
272. Valimaki M, Pelkonen R, Porkka L, et al. Long-term results of adrenal surgery in patients with Cushing's syndrome due to adrenocortical adenoma. *Clin Endocrinol (Oxf).* 1984;20:229-236.
273. Young WF Jr, Thompson GB. Laparoscopic adrenalectomy for patients who have Cushing's syndrome. *Endocrinol Metab Clin North Am.* 2005;34:489-499, xi.
274. Kasperlik-Zaluska AA, Migdalska BM, Zgliczynski S, et al. Adrenocortical carcinoma: a clinical study and treatment results of 52 patients. *Cancer.* 1995;75:2587-2591.
275. Allolio B, Hahner S, Weismann D, et al. Management of adrenocortical carcinoma. *Clin Endocrinol (Oxf).* 2004;60:273-287.
276. Terzolo M, Angeli A, Fassnacht M, et al. Adjuvant mitotane treatment for adrenocortical carcinoma. *N Engl J Med.* 2007;356:2372-2380.
277. Fassnacht M, Allolio B. Clinical management of adrenocortical carcinoma. *Best Pract Res Clin Endocrinol Metab.* 2009;23:273-289.

278. Biller BM, Grossman AB, Stewart PM, et al. Treatment of adrenocorticotropin-dependent Cushing's syndrome: a consensus statement. *J Clin Endocrinol Metab.* 2008;93:2454-2462.
279. Assie G, Bahurel H, Coste J, et al. Corticotroph tumor progression after adrenalectomy in Cushing's disease: a reappraisal of Nelson's syndrome. *J Clin Endocrinol Metab.* 2007;92:172-179.
280. Jenkins PJ, Trainer PJ, Plowman PN, et al. The long-term outcome after adrenalectomy and prophylactic pituitary radiotherapy in adrenocorticotropin-dependent Cushing's syndrome. *J Clin Endocrinol Metab.* 1995;80:165-171.
281. Burch W. A survey of results with transsphenoidal surgery in Cushing's disease. *N Engl J Med.* 1983;308:103-104.
282. Utz AL, Swearingen B, Biller BM. Pituitary surgery and postoperative management in Cushing's disease. *Endocrinol Metab Clin North Am.* 2005;34:459-478, xi.
283. Trainer PJ, Lawrie HS, Verhelst J, et al. Transsphenoidal resection in Cushing's disease: undetectable serum cortisol as the definition of successful treatment. *Clin Endocrinol (Oxf).* 1993;38:73-78.
284. McCance DR, Besser M, Atkinson AB. Assessment of cure after transsphenoidal surgery for Cushing's disease. *Clin Endocrinol (Oxf).* 1996;44:1-6.
285. Leinung MC, Kane LA, Scheithauer BW, et al. Long term follow-up of transsphenoidal surgery for the treatment of Cushing's disease in childhood. *J Clin Endocrinol Metab.* 1995;80:2475-2479.
286. Joshi SM, Hewitt RJ, Storr HL, et al. Cushing's disease in children and adolescents: 20 years of experience in a single neurosurgical center. *Neurosurgery.* 2005;57:281-285; discussion 281-285.
287. Storr HL, Plowman PN, Carroll PV, et al. Clinical and endocrine responses to pituitary radiotherapy in pediatric Cushing's disease: an effective second-line treatment. *J Clin Endocrinol Metab.* 2003; 88:34-37.
288. Aghi MK. Management of recurrent and refractory Cushing disease. *Nat Clin Pract Endocrinol Metab.* 2008;4:560-568.
289. Verhelst JA, Trainer PJ, Howlett TA, et al. Short and long-term responses to metyrapone in the medical management of 91 patients with Cushing's syndrome. *Clin Endocrinol (Oxf).* 1991;35:169-178.
290. Child DF, Burke CW, Burley DM, et al. Drug controlled of Cushing's syndrome; combined aminoglutethimide and metyrapone therapy. *Acta Endocrinol (Copenh).* 1976;82:330-341.
291. Semple CG, Beastall GH, Gray CE, et al. Trilostane in the management of Cushing's syndrome. *Acta Endocrinol (Copenh).* 1983;102: 107-110.
292. McCance DR, Hadden DR, Kennedy L, et al. Clinical experience with ketoconazole as a therapy for patients with Cushing's syndrome. *Clin Endocrinol (Oxf).* 1987;27:593-599.
293. Heaney AP, Fernando M, Yong WH, et al. Functional PPAR-gamma receptor is a novel therapeutic target for ACTH-secreting pituitary adenomas. *Nat Med.* 2002;8:1281-1287.
294. Ambrosi B, Dall'Asta C, Cannavo S, et al. Effects of chronic administration of PPAR-gamma ligand rosiglitazone in Cushing's disease. *Eur J Endocrinol.* 2004;151:173-178.
295. Boscaro M, Ludlam WH, Atkinson B, et al. Treatment of pituitary-dependent Cushing's disease with the multireceptor ligand somatostatin analog pasireotide (SOM230): a multicenter, phase II trial. *J Clin Endocrinol Metab.* 2009;94:115-122.
296. Bhattacharyya A, Kaushal K, Tymms DJ, et al. Steroid withdrawal syndrome after successful treatment of Cushing's syndrome: a reminder. *Eur J Endocrinol.* 2005;153:207-210.
297. Hermus AR, Smals AG, Swinkels LM, et al. Bone mineral density and bone turnover before and after surgical cure of Cushing's syndrome. *J Clin Endocrinol Metab.* 1995;80:2859-2865.
298. Keil MF, Merke DP, Gandhi R, et al. Quality of life in children and adolescents 1 year after cure of Cushing syndrome: a prospective study. *Clin Endocrinol (Oxf).* 2009;71:326-333.
299. Charmandari E, Kino T, Souvatzoglou E, et al. Natural glucocorticoid receptor mutants causing generalized glucocorticoid resistance: molecular genotype, genetic transmission, and clinical phenotype. *J Clin Endocrinol Metab.* 2004;89:1939-1949.
300. Oelkers W. Adrenal insufficiency. *N Engl J Med.* 1996;335:1206-1212.
301. Arlt W, Allolio B. Adrenal insufficiency. *Lancet.* 2003;361:1881-1893.
302. Carey RM. The changing clinical spectrum of adrenal insufficiency. *Ann Intern Med.* 1997;127:1103-1105.
303. Betterle C, Dal Pra C, Mantero F, et al. Autoimmune adrenal insufficiency and autoimmune polyendocrine syndromes: autoantibodies, autoantigens, and their applicability in diagnosis and disease prediction. *Endocr Rev.* 2002;23:327-364.
304. Piedrola G, Casado JL, Lopez E, et al. Clinical features of adrenal insufficiency in patients with acquired immunodeficiency syndrome. *Clin Endocrinol (Oxf).* 1996;45:97-101.
305. Freda PU, Bilezikian JP. The hypothalamus-pituitary-adrenal axis in HIV disease. *AIDS Read.* 1999;9:43-50.
306. Norbiato G, Galli M, Righini V, et al. The syndrome of acquired glucocorticoid resistance in HIV infection. *Baillieres Clin Endocrinol Metab.* 1994;8:777-787.
307. Seidenwurm DJ, Elmer EB, Kaplan LM, et al. Metastases to the adrenal glands and the development of Addison's disease. *Cancer.* 1984;54: 552-557.
308. Xarli VP, Steele AA, Davis PJ, et al. Adrenal hemorrhage in the adult. *Medicine (Baltimore).* 1978;57:211-221.
309. Lalli E, Sassone-Corsi P. DAX-1 and the adrenal cortex. *Curr Opin Endocrinol Metab.* 1999;6:185-190.
310. Tabarin A, Achermann JC, Recan D, et al. A novel mutation in DAX1 causes delayed-onset adrenal insufficiency and incomplete hypogonadotropic hypogonadism. *J Clin Invest.* 2000;105:321-328.
311. Takahashi T, Shoji Y, Shoji Y, et al. Active hypothalamic-pituitary-gonadal axis in an infant with X-linked adrenal hypoplasia congenita. *J Pediatr.* 1997;130:485-488.
312. Kaiserman KB, Nakamoto JM, Geffner ME, et al. Minipuberty of infancy and adolescent pubertal function in adrenal hypoplasia congenita. *J Pediatr.* 1998;133:300-302.
313. Ozisik G, Mantovani G, Achermann JC, et al. An alternate translation initiation site circumvents an amino-terminal DAX1 nonsense mutation leading to a mild form of X-linked adrenal hypoplasia congenita. *J Clin Endocrinol Metab.* 2003;88:417-423.
314. Achermann JC, Ito M, Ito M, et al. A mutation in the gene encoding steroidogenic factor-1 causes XY sex reversal and adrenal failure in humans. *Nat Genet.* 1999;22:125-126.
315. Biason-Lauber A, Schoenle EJ. Apparently normal ovarian differentiation in a prepubertal girl with transcriptionally inactive steroidogenic factor 1 (NR5A1/SF-1) and adrenocortical insufficiency. *Am J Hum Genet.* 2000;67:1563-1568.
316. Lin L, Philibert P, Ferraz-de-Souza B, et al. Heterozygous missense mutations in steroidogenic factor 1 (SF1/Ad4BP, NR5A1) are associated with 46,XY disorders of sex development with normal adrenal function. *J Clin Endocrinol Metab.* 2007;92:991-999.
317. Lourenco D, Brauner R, Lin L, et al. Mutations in NR5A1 associated with ovarian insufficiency. *N Engl J Med.* 2009;360:1200-1210.
318. Scheuerle A, Greenberg F, McCabe ER. Dysmorphic features in patients with complex glycerol kinase deficiency. *J Pediatr.* 1995;126:764-767.
319. Moser HW, Moser AE, Singh I, et al. Adrenoleukodystrophy—survey of 303 cases: biochemistry, diagnosis, and therapy. *Ann Neurol.* 1984;16:628-641.
320. Laureti S, Casucci G, Santeusanio F, et al. X-linked adrenoleukodystrophy is a frequent cause of idiopathic Addison's disease in young adult male patients. *J Clin Endocrinol Metab.* 1996;81:470-474.
321. Mosser J, Douar AM, Sarde CO, et al. Putative X-linked adrenoleukodystrophy gene shares unexpected homology with ABC transporters. *Nature.* 1993;361:726-730.
322. Kemp S, Pujol A, Waterham HR, et al. ABCD1 mutations and the X-linked adrenoleukodystrophy mutation database: role in diagnosis and clinical correlations. *Hum Mutat.* 2001;18:499-515.
323. Moser HW, Raymond GV, Lu SE, et al. Follow-up of 89 asymptomatic patients with adrenoleukodystrophy treated with Lorenzo's oil. *Arch Neurol.* 2005;62:1073-1080.
324. Clark AJ, McLoughlin L, Grossman A. Familial glucocorticoid deficiency associated with point mutation in the adrenocorticotropin receptor. *Lancet.* 1993;341:461-462.
325. Tsigos C, Arai K, Hung W, et al. Hereditary isolated glucocorticoid deficiency is associated with abnormalities of the adrenocorticotropin receptor gene. *J Clin Invest.* 1993;92:2458-2461.
326. Huebner A, Elias LL, Clark AJ. ACTH resistance syndromes. *J Pediatr Endocrinol Metab.* 1999;12(Suppl 1):277-293.
327. Tullio-Pelet A, Salomon R, Hadj-Rabia S, et al. Mutant WD-repeat protein in triple-A syndrome. *Nat Genet.* 2000;26:332-335.
328. Handschug K, Sperling S, Yoon SJ, et al. Triple A syndrome is caused by mutations in AAAS, a new WD-repeat protein gene. *Hum Mol Genet.* 2001;10:283-290.
329. Pulichino AM, Vallette-Kasic S, Couture C, et al. Human and mouse TPIT gene mutations cause early onset pituitary ACTH deficiency. *Genes Dev.* 2003;17:711-716.
330. O'Rahilly S, Gray H, Humphreys PJ, et al. Brief report: impaired processing of prohormones associated with abnormalities of glucose homeostasis and adrenal function. *N Engl J Med.* 1995;333:1386-1390.
331. Krude H, Biebermann H, Luck W, et al. Severe early-onset obesity, adrenal insufficiency and red hair pigmentation caused by POMC mutations in humans. *Nat Genet.* 1998;19:155-157.
332. Yaswen L, Diehl N, Brennan MB, et al. Obesity in the mouse model of pro-opiomelanocortin deficiency responds to peripheral melanocortin. *Nat Med.* 1999;5:1066-1070.
333. Dattani MT, Martinez-Barbera JP, Thomas PQ, et al. Mutations in the homeobox gene HESX1/Hesx1 associated with septo-optic dysplasia in human and mouse. *Nat Genet.* 1998;19:125-133.
334. Machinis K, Pantel J, Netchine I, et al. Syndromic short stature in patients with a germline mutation in the LIM homeobox LHX4. *Am J Hum Genet.* 2001;69:961-968.
335. Lagerstrom-Fermer M, Sundvall M, Johnsen E, et al. X-linked recessive panhypopituitarism associated with a regional duplication in Xq25-q26. *Am J Hum Genet.* 1997;60:910-916.

336. Wu W, Cogan JD, Pfaffle RW, et al. Mutations in PROP1 cause familial combined pituitary hormone deficiency. *Nat Genet.* 1998;18: 147-149.
337. Cooper MS, Stewart PM. Corticosteroid insufficiency in acutely ill patients. *N Engl J Med.* 2003;348:727-734.
338. Annane D, Sebille V, Troche G, et al. A 3-level prognostic classification in septic shock based on cortisol levels and cortisol response to corticotropin. *JAMA.* 2000;283:1038-1045.
339. Marik PE, Pastores SM, Annane D, et al. Recommendations for the diagnosis and management of corticosteroid insufficiency in critically ill adult patients: consensus statements from an international task force by the American College of Critical Care Medicine. *Crit Care Med.* 2008;36:1937-1949.
340. Hahner S, Loeffler M, Fassnacht M, et al. Impaired subjective health status in 256 patients with adrenal insufficiency on standard therapy based on cross-sectional analysis. *J Clin Endocrinol Metab.* 2007;92: 3912-3922.
341. Artavia-Loria E, Chaussain JL, Bougneres PF, et al. Frequency of hypoglycemia in children with adrenal insufficiency. *Acta Endocrinol Suppl (Copenh).* 1986;279:275-278.
342. Laczi F, Janaky T, Ivanyi T, et al. Osmoregulation of arginine-8-vasopressin secretion in primary hypothyroidism and in Addison's disease. *Acta Endocrinol (Copenh).* 1987;114:389-395.
343. Muls E, Bouillon R, Boelaert J, et al. Etiology of hypercalcemia in a patient with Addison's disease. *Calcif Tissue Int.* 1982;34:523-526.
344. Topliss DJ, White EL, Stockigt JR. Significance of thyrotropin excess in untreated primary adrenal insufficiency. *J Clin Endocrinol Metab.* 1980;50:52-56.
345. Hagg E, Asplund K, Lithner F. Value of basal plasma cortisol assays in the assessment of pituitary-adrenal insufficiency. *Clin Endocrinol (Oxf).* 1987;26:221-226.
346. Lindholm J, Kehlet H. Re-evaluation of the clinical value of the 30 min ACTH test in assessing the hypothalamic-pituitary-adrenocortical function. *Clin Endocrinol (Oxf).* 1987;26:53-59.
347. Clark PM, Neylon I, Raggatt PR, et al. Defining the normal cortisol response to the short Synacthen test: implications for the investigation of hypothalamic-pituitary disorders. *Clin Endocrinol (Oxf).* 1998;49: 287-292.
348. Oelkers W, Diederich S, Bahr V. Diagnosis and therapy surveillance in Addison's disease: rapid adrenocorticotropin (ACTH) test and measurement of plasma ACTH, renin activity, and aldosterone. *J Clin Endocrinol Metab.* 1992;75:259-264.
349. Erturk E, Jaffe CA, Barkan AL. Evaluation of the integrity of the hypothalamic-pituitary-adrenal axis by insulin hypoglycemia test. *J Clin Endocrinol Metab.* 1998;83:2350-2354.
350. Stewart PM, Corrie J, Seckl JR, et al. A rational approach for assessing the hypothalamo-pituitary-adrenal axis. *Lancet.* 1988;1:1208-1210.
351. Streeten DH, Anderson GH Jr, Bonaventura MM. The potential for serious consequences from misinterpreting normal responses to the rapid adrenocorticotropin test. *J Clin Endocrinol Metab.* 1996;81: 285-290.
352. Oelkers W. Dose-response aspects in the clinical assessment of the hypothalamo-pituitary-adrenal axis, and the low-dose adrenocorticotropin test. *Eur J Endocrinol.* 1996;135:27-33.
353. Abdu TA, Elhadd TA, Neary R, et al. Comparison of the low dose short synacthen test (1 microg), the conventional dose short synacthen test (250 microg), and the insulin tolerance test for assessment of the hypothalamo-pituitary-adrenal axis in patients with pituitary disease. *J Clin Endocrinol Metab.* 1999;84:838-843.
354. Kazlauskaite R, Evans AT, Villabona CV, et al. Corticotropin tests for hypothalamic-pituitary-adrenal insufficiency: a metaanalysis. *J Clin Endocrinol Metab.* 2008;93:4245-4253.
355. Suliman AM, Smith TP, Labib M, et al. The low-dose ACTH test does not provide a useful assessment of the hypothalamic-pituitary-adrenal axis in secondary adrenal insufficiency. *Clin Endocrinol (Oxf).* 2002;56:533-539.
356. Stewart PM, Clark PM. The low-dose corticotropin-stimulation test revisited: the less, the better? *Nat Clin Pract Endocrinol Metab.* 2009;5:68-69.
357. Fiad TM, Kirby JM, Cunningham SK, et al. The overnight single-dose metyrapone test is a simple and reliable index of the hypothalamic-pituitary-adrenal axis. *Clin Endocrinol (Oxf).* 1994;40:603-609.
358. Schlaghecke R, Kornely E, Santen RT, et al. The effect of long-term glucocorticoid therapy on pituitary-adrenal responses to exogenous corticotropin-releasing hormone. *N Engl J Med.* 1992;326:226-230.
359. Annane D, Sebille V, Charpentier C, et al. Effect of treatment with low doses of hydrocortisone and fludrocortisone on mortality in patients with septic shock. *JAMA.* 2002;288:862-871.
360. Sprung CL, Annane D, Keh D, et al. Hydrocortisone therapy for patients with septic shock. *N Engl J Med.* 2008;358:111-124.
361. Esteban NV, Loughlin T, Yergey AL, et al. Daily cortisol production rate in man determined by stable isotope dilution/mass spectrometry. *J Clin Endocrinol Metab.* 1991;72:39-45.
362. Feek CM, Ratcliffe JG, Seth J, et al. Patterns of plasma cortisol and ACTH concentrations in patients with Addison's disease treated with conventional corticosteroid replacement. *Clin Endocrinol (Oxf).* 1981;14:451-458.
363. Arlt W, Rosenthal C, Hahner S, et al. Quality of glucocorticoid replacement in adrenal insufficiency: clinical assessment vs. timed serum cortisol measurements. *Clin Endocrinol (Oxf).* 2006;64: 384-389.
364. Lovas K, Gjesdal CG, Christensen M, et al. Glucocorticoid replacement therapy and pharmacogenetics in Addison's disease: effects on bone. *Eur J Endocrinol.* 2009;160:993-1002.
365. Peacey SR, Guo CY, Robinson AM, et al. Glucocorticoid replacement therapy: are patients over treated and does it matter? *Clin Endocrinol (Oxf).* 1997;46:255-261.
366. Howlett TA. An assessment of optimal hydrocortisone replacement therapy. *Clin Endocrinol (Oxf).* 1997;46:263-268.
367. Fiad TM, Conway JD, Cunningham SK, et al. The role of plasma renin activity in evaluating the adequacy of mineralocorticoid replacement in primary adrenal insufficiency. *Clin Endocrinol (Oxf).* 1996;45: 529-534.
368. Arlt W, Callies F, van Vlijmen JC, et al. Dehydroepiandrosterone replacement in women with adrenal insufficiency. *N Engl J Med.* 1999;341:1013-1020.
369. White PC, Speiser PW. Congenital adrenal hyperplasia due to 21-hydroxylase deficiency. *Endocr Rev.* 2000;21:245-291.
370. Merke DP, Bornstein SR. Congenital adrenal hyperplasia. *Lancet.* 2005;365:2125-2136.
371. Eugster EA, Dimeglio LA, Wright JC, et al. Height outcome in congenital adrenal hyperplasia caused by 21-hydroxylase deficiency: a meta-analysis. *J Pediatr.* 2001;138:26-32.
372. Cabrera MS, Vogiatzi MG, New MI. Long term outcome in adult males with classic congenital adrenal hyperplasia. *J Clin Endocrinol Metab.* 2001;86:3070-3078.
373. Azziz R, Dewailly D, Owerbach D. Nonclassic adrenal hyperplasia: current concepts. Clinical Review 56. *J Clin Endocrinol Metab.* 1994;78:810-815.
374. New MI. Extensive clinical experience: nonclassical 21-hydroxylase deficiency. *J Clin Endocrinol Metab.* 2006;91:4205-4214.
375. Bidet M, Bellanne-Chantelot C, Galand-Portier M-B, et al. Clinical and molecular characterization of a cohort of 161 unrelated women with nonclassical congenital adrenal hyperplasia due to 21-hydroxylase deficiency and 330 family members. *J Clin Endocrinol Metab.* 2009;94:1570-1578.
376. Azziz R, Sanchez LA, Knochenhauer ES, et al. Androgen excess in women: experience with over 1000 consecutive patients. *J Clin Endocrinol Metab.* 2004;89:453-462.
377. Krone N, Arlt W. Genetics of congenital adrenal hyperplasia. *Best Pract Res Clin Endocrinol Metab.* 2009;23:181-192.
378. Speiser PW, Dupont J, Zhu D, et al. Disease expression and molecular genotype in congenital adrenal hyperplasia due to 21-hydroxylase deficiency. *J Clin Invest.* 1992;90:584-595.
379. Krone N, Braun A, Roscher AA, et al. Predicting phenotype in steroid 21-hydroxylase deficiency? Comprehensive genotyping in 155 unrelated, well defined patients from southern Germany. *J Clin Endocrinol Metab.* 2000;85:1059-1065.
380. Wilson RC, Mercado AB, Cheng KC, et al. Steroid 21-hydroxylase deficiency: genotype may not predict phenotype. *J Clin Endocrinol Metab.* 1995;80:2322-2329.
381. Rocha RO, Billerbeck AE, Pinto EM, et al. The degree of external genitalia virilization in girls with 21-hydroxylase deficiency appears to be influenced by the CAG repeats in the androgen receptor gene. *Clin Endocrinol (Oxf).* 2008;68:226-232.
382. Gomes LG, Huang N, Agrawal V, et al. Extraadrenal 21-hydroxylation by CYP2C19 and CYP3A4: effect on 21-hydroxylase deficiency. *J Clin Endocrinol Metab.* 2009;94:89-95.
383. New MI, Lorenzen F, Lerner AJ, et al. Genotyping steroid 21-hydroxylase deficiency: hormonal reference data. *J Clin Endocrinol Metab.* 1983;57:320-326.
384. Forest MG, Betuel H, David M. Prenatal treatment in congenital adrenal hyperplasia due to 21-hydroxylase deficiency: up-date 88 of the French multicentric study. *Endocr Res.* 1989;15:277-301.
385. Joint LWPES/ESPE CAH Working Group. Consensus statement on 21-hydroxylase deficiency from the Lawson Wilkins Pediatric Endocrine Society and the European Society for Paediatric Endocrinology. *J Clin Endocrinol Metab.* 2002;87:4048-4053.
386. Meyer-Bahlburg HF. What causes low rates of child-bearing in congenital adrenal hyperplasia? *J Clin Endocrinol Metab.* 1999;84: 1844-1847.
387. Morgan JF, Murphy H, Lacey JH, et al. Long term psychological outcome for women with congenital adrenal hyperplasia: cross sectional survey. *BMJ.* 2005;330:340-341; discussion 341.
388. Claahsen-van der Grinten HL, Otten BJ, Stikkelbroeck MM, et al. Testicular adrenal rest tumours in congenital adrenal hyperplasia. *Best Pract Res Clin Endocrinol Metab.* 2009;23:209-220.
389. Hindmarsh PC. Management of the child with congenital adrenal hyperplasia. *Best Pract Res Clin Endocrinol Metab.* 2009;23: 193-208.

390. Merke DP, Chrousos GP, Eisenhofer G, et al. Adrenomedullary dysplasia and hypofunction in patients with classic 21-hydroxylase deficiency. *N Engl J Med.* 2000;343:1362-1368.
391. Weise M, Mehlinger SL, Drinkard B, et al. Patients with classic congenital adrenal hyperplasia have decreased epinephrine reserve and defective glucose elevation in response to high-intensity exercise. *J Clin Endocrinol Metab.* 2004;89:591-597.
392. Van Wyk JJ, Ritzen EM. The role of bilateral adrenalectomy in the treatment of congenital adrenal hyperplasia. *J Clin Endocrinol Metab.* 2003;88:2993-2998.
393. Charmandari E, Chrousos GP, Merke DP. Adrenocorticotropin hypersecretion and pituitary microadenoma following bilateral adrenalectomy in a patient with classic 21-hydroxylase deficiency. *J Pediatr Endocrinol Metab.* 2005;18:97-101.
394. Seckl JR, Miller WL. How safe is long-term prenatal glucocorticoid treatment? *Jama.* 1997;277:1077-1079.
395. Pang S, Clark AT, Freeman LC, et al. Maternal side effects of prenatal dexamethasone therapy for fetal congenital adrenal hyperplasia. *J Clin Endocrinol Metab.* 1992;75:249-253.
396. Lajic S, Nordenstrom A, Hirvikoski T. Long-term outcome of prenatal treatment of congenital adrenal hyperplasia. *Endocr Dev.* 2008;13:82-98.
397. Cornean RE, Hindmarsh PC, Brook CG. Obesity in 21-hydroxylase deficient patients. *Arch Dis Child.* 1998;78:261-263.
398. Volkl TM, Simm D, Beier C, et al. Obesity among children and adolescents with classic congenital adrenal hyperplasia due to 21-hydroxylase deficiency. *Pediatrics.* 2006;117:e98-e105.
399. Stikkelbroeck NM, Oyen WJ, van der Wilt GJ, et al. Normal bone mineral density and lean body mass, but increased fat mass, in young adult patients with congenital adrenal hyperplasia. *J Clin Endocrinol Metab.* 2003;88:1036-1042.
400. Falhammar H, Filipsson H, Holmdahl G, et al. Metabolic profile and body composition in adult women with congenital adrenal hyperplasia due to 21-hydroxylase deficiency. *J Clin Endocrinol Metab.* 2007;92:110-116.
401. Speiser PW, Serrat J, New MI, et al. Insulin insensitivity in adrenal hyperplasia due to nonclassical steroid 21-hydroxylase deficiency. *J Clin Endocrinol Metab.* 1992;75:1421-1424.
402. Sartorato P, Zulian E, Benedini S, et al. Cardiovascular risk factors and ultrasound evaluation of intima-media thickness at common carotids, carotid bulbs, and femoral and abdominal aorta arteries in patients with classic congenital adrenal hyperplasia due to 21-hydroxylase deficiency. *J Clin Endocrinol Metab.* 2007;92:1015-1018.
403. Roche EF, Charmandari E, Dattani MT, et al. Blood pressure in children and adolescents with congenital adrenal hyperplasia (21-hydroxylase deficiency): a preliminary report. *Clin Endocrinol.* 2003;58:589-596.
404. Volkl TMK, Simm D, Dotsch J, et al. Altered 24-hour blood pressure profiles in children and adolescents with classical congenital adrenal hyperplasia due to 21-hydroxylase deficiency. *J Clin Endocrinol Metab.* 2006;91:4888-4895.
405. White PC, Curnow KM, Pascoe L. Disorders of steroid 11 β-hydroxylase isozymes. *Endocr Rev.* 1994;15:421-438.
406. Joehrer K, Geley S, Strasser-Wozak EM, et al. CYP11B1 mutations causing non-classic adrenal hyperplasia due to 11 β-hydroxylase deficiency. *Hum Mol Genet.* 1997;6:1829-1834.
407. Peters CJ, Nugent T, Perry LA, et al. Cosegregation of a novel homozygous CYP11B1 mutation with the phenotype of non-classical congenital adrenal hyperplasia in a consanguineous family. *Horm Res.* 2007;67:189-193.
408. Peter M, Janzen N, Sander S, et al. A case of 11β-hydroxylase deficiency detected in a newborn screening program by second-tier LC-MS/MS. *Horm Res.* 2008;69:253-256.
409. Pang S, Levine LS, Lorenzen F, et al. Hormonal studies in obligate heterozygotes and siblings of patients with 11 β-hydroxylase deficiency congenital adrenal hyperplasia. *J Clin Endocrinol Metab.* 1980;50:586-589.
410. Gabrilove JL, Sharma DC, Dorfman RI. Adrenocortical 11-β-hydroxylase deficiency and virilism first manifest in the adult women. *N Engl J Med.* 1965;272:1189-1194.
411. de Simone G, Tommaselli AP, Rossi R, et al. Partial deficiency of adrenal 11-hydroxylase: a possible cause of primary hypertension. *Hypertension.* 1985;7:204-210.
412. Biglieri EG. 17 Alpha-hydroxylase deficiency: 1963-1966. *J Clin Endocrinol Metab.* 1997;82:48-50.
413. Zachmann M, Werder EA, Prader A. Two types of male pseudohermaphroditism due to 17, 20-desmolase deficiency. *J Clin Endocrinol Metab.* 1982;55:487-490.
414. Auchus RJ. The genetics, pathophysiology, and management of human deficiencies of P450c17. *Endocrinol Metab Clin North Am.* 2001;30:101-119, vii.
415. Geller DH, Auchus RJ, Miller WL. P450c17 mutations R347H and R358Q selectively disrupt 17,20-lyase activity by disrupting interactions with P450 oxidoreductase and cytochrome b5. *Mol Endocrinol.* 1999;13:167-175.
416. Auchus RJ, Lee TC, Miller WL. Cytochrome b5 augments the 17,20-lyase activity of human P450c17 without direct electron transfer. *J Biol Chem.* 1998;273:3158-3165.
417. Yanase T, Simpson ER, Waterman MR. 17 Alpha-hydroxylase/17,20-lyase deficiency: from clinical investigation to molecular definition. *Endocr Rev.* 1991;12:91-108.
418. Geller DH, Auchus RJ, Mendonca BB, et al. The genetic and functional basis of isolated 17,20/lyase deficiency. *Nat Genet.* 1997;17:201-205.
419. Sherbet DP, Tiosano D, Kwist KM, et al. CYP17 mutation E305G causes isolated 17,20-lyase deficiency by selectively altering substrate binding. *J Biol Chem.* 2003;278:48563-48569.
420. Peterson RE, Imperato-McGinley J, Gautier T, et al. Male pseudohermaphroditism due to multiple defects in steroid-biosynthetic microsomal mixed-function oxidases: a new variant of congenital adrenal hyperplasia. *N Engl J Med.* 1985;313:1182-1191.
421. Shackleton C, Marcos J, Arlt W, et al. Prenatal diagnosis of P450 oxidoreductase deficiency (ORD): a disorder causing low pregnancy estriol, maternal and fetal virilization, and the Antley-Bixler syndrome phenotype. *Am J Med Genet.* 2004;129A:105-112.
422. Cragun DL, Trumpy SK, Shackleton CH, et al. Undetectable maternal serum uE3 and postnatal abnormal sterol and steroid metabolism in Antley-Bixler syndrome. *Am J Med Genet.* 2004;129A:1-7.
423. Fukami M, Hasegawa T, Horikawa R, et al. Cytochrome P450 oxidoreductase deficiency in three patients initially regarded as having 21-hydroxylase deficiency and/or aromatase deficiency: diagnostic value of urine steroid hormone analysis. *Pediatr Res.* 2006;59:276-280.
424. Fluck CE, Tajima T, Pandey AV, et al. Mutant P450 oxidoreductase causes disordered steroidogenesis with and without Antley-Bixler syndrome. *Nat Genet.* 2004;36:228-230.
425. Arlt W, Walker EA, Draper N, et al. Congenital adrenal hyperplasia caused by mutant P450 oxidoreductase and human androgen synthesis: analytical study. *Lancet.* 2004;363:2128-2135.
426. Homma K, Hasegawa T, Nagai T, et al. Urine steroid hormone profile analysis in cytochrome P450 oxidoreductase deficiency: implication for the backdoor pathway to dihydrotestosterone. *J Clin Endocrinol Metab.* 2006;91:2643-2649.
427. Fukami M, Nishimura G, Homma K, et al. Cytochrome P450 oxidoreductase deficiency: identification and characterization of biallelic mutations and genotype-phenotype correlations in 35 Japanese patients. *J Clin Endocrinol Metab.* 2009;94:1723-1731.
428. Huang N, Pandey AV, Agrawal V, et al. Diversity and function of mutations in p450 oxidoreductase in patients with Antley-Bixler syndrome and disordered steroidogenesis. *Am J Hum Genet.* 2005;76:729-749.
429. Otto DM, Henderson CJ, Carrie D, et al. Identification of novel roles of the cytochrome p450 system in early embryogenesis: effects on vasculogenesis and retinoic acid homeostasis. *Mol Cell Biol.* 2003;23:6103-6116.
430. Rheaume E, Simard J, Morel Y, et al. Congenital adrenal hyperplasia due to point mutations in the type II 3 β-hydroxysteroid dehydrogenase gene. *Nat Genet.* 1992;1:239-245.
431. Simard J, Ricketts M-L, Gingras S, et al. Molecular biology of the 3β-hydroxysteroid dehydrogenase/δ5-δ4 isomerase gene family. *Endocr Rev.* 2005;26:525-582.
432. Marui S, Castro M, Latronico AC, et al. Mutations in the type II 3β-hydroxysteroid dehydrogenase (HSD3B2) gene can cause premature pubarche in girls. *Clin Endocrinol (Oxf).* 2000;52:67-75.
433. Pang SY, Lerner AJ, Stoner E, et al. Late-onset adrenal steroid 3 β-hydroxysteroid dehydrogenase deficiency: I. A cause of hirsutism in pubertal and postpubertal women. *J Clin Endocrinol Metab.* 1985;60:428-439.
434. Lutfallah C, Wang W, Mason JI, et al. Newly proposed hormonal criteria via genotypic proof for type II 3β-hydroxysteroid dehydrogenase deficiency. *J Clin Endocrinol Metab.* 2002;87:2611-2622.
435. Mermejo LM, Elias LLK, Marui S, et al. Refining hormonal diagnosis of type II 3β-hydroxysteroid dehydrogenase deficiency in patients with premature pubarche and hirsutism based on HSD3B2 genotyping. *J Clin Endocrinol Metab.* 2005;90:1287-1293.
436. Bose HS, Sugawara T, Strauss JF 3rd, et al. The pathophysiology and genetics of congenital lipoid adrenal hyperplasia. International Congenital Lipoid Adrenal Hyperplasia Consortium. *N Engl J Med.* 1996;335:1870-1878.
437. Baker BY, Lin L, Kim CJ, et al. Nonclassic congenital lipoid adrenal hyperplasia: a new disorder of the steroidogenic acute regulatory protein with very late presentation and normal male genitalia. *J Clin Endocrinol Metab.* 2006;91:4781-4785.
438. Tajima T, Fujieda K, Kouda N, et al. Heterozygous mutation in the cholesterol side chain cleavage enzyme (p450scc) gene in a patient with 46,XY sex reversal and adrenal insufficiency. *J Clin Endocrinol Metab.* 2001;86:3820-3825.
439. Hiort O, Holterhus PM, Werner R, et al. Heterozygous mutation in the cholesterol side chain cleavage enzyme (p450scc) gene in a patient with 46,XY sex. *J Clin Endocrinol Metab.* 2005;90:538-541.

440. Kim CJ, Lin L, Huang N, et al. Severe combined adrenal and gonadal deficiency caused by novel mutations in the cholesterol side chain cleavage enzyme, P450scc. *J Clin Endocrinol Metab*. 2008;93:696-702.
441. Rubtsov P, Karmanov M, Sverdlova P, et al. A novel homozygous mutation in CYP11A1 gene is associated with late-onset adrenal insufficiency and hypospadias in a 46,XY patient. *J Clin Endocrinol Metab*. 2009;94:936-939.
442. Jamieson A, Wallace AM, Andrew R, et al. Apparent cortisone reductase deficiency: a functional defect in 11β-hydroxysteroid dehydrogenase type 1. *J Clin Endocrinol Metab*. 1999;84:3570-3574.
443. Lavery GG, Walker EA, Tiganescu A, et al. Steroid biomarkers and genetic studies reveal inactivating mutations in hexose-6-phosphate dehydrogenase in patients with cortisone reductase deficiency. *J Clin Endocrinol Metab*. 2008;93:3827-3832.
444. Vassiliadi DA, Barber TM, Hughes BA, et al. Increased 5 alpha-reductase activity and adrenocortical drive in women with polycystic ovary syndrome. *J Clin Endocrinol Metab*. 2009;94:3558-3566.
445. Veldhuis JD, Melby JC. Isolated aldosterone deficiency in man: acquired and inborn errors in the biosynthesis or action of aldosterone. *Endocr Rev*. 1981;2:495-517.
446. White PC. Aldosterone synthase deficiency and related disorders. *Mol Cell Endocrinol*. 2004;217:81-87.
447. Kayes-Wandover KM, Schindler RE, Taylor HC, et al. Type 1 aldosterone synthase deficiency presenting in a middle-aged man. *J Clin Endocrinol Metab*. 2001;86:1008-1012.
448. Zennaro MC, Lombes M. Mineralocorticoid resistance. *Trends Endocrinol Metab*. 2004;15:264-270.
449. Geller DS, Rodriguez-Soriano J, Vallo Boado A, et al. Mutations in the mineralocorticoid receptor gene cause autosomal dominant pseudohypoaldosteronism type I. *Nat Genet*. 1998;19:279-281.
450. Chang SS, Grunder S, Hanukoglu A, et al. Mutations in subunits of the epithelial sodium channel cause salt wasting with hyperkalaemic acidosis, pseudohypoaldosteronism type 1. *Nat Genet*. 1996;12:248-253.
451. Strautnieks SS, Thompson RJ, Gardiner RM, et al. A novel splice-site mutation in the gamma subunit of the epithelial sodium channel gene in three pseudohypoaldosteronism type 1 families. *Nat Genet*. 1996;13:248-250.
452. Hanukoglu A, Joy O, Steinitz M, et al. Pseudohypoaldosteronism due to renal and multisystem resistance to mineralocorticoids respond differently to carbenoxolone. *J Steroid Biochem Mol Biol*. 1997; 60:105-112.
453. Wilson FH, Disse-Nicodeme S, Choate KA, et al. Human hypertension caused by mutations in WNK kinases. *Science*. 2001;293:1107-1112.
454. DeFronzo RA. Hyperkalemia and hyporeninemic hypoaldosteronism. *Kidney Int*. 1980;17:118-134.
455. Sunderlin FS Jr, Anderson GH Jr, Streeten DH, et al. The renin-angiotensin-aldosterone system in diabetic patients with hyperkalemia. *Diabetes*. 1981;30:335-340.
456. Gabrilove JL, Seman AT, Sabet R, et al. Virilizing adrenal adenoma with studies on the steroid content of the adrenal venous effluent and a review of the literature. *Endocr Rev*. 1981;2:462-470.
457. Kloos RT, Gross MD, Francis IR, et al. Incidentally discovered adrenal masses. *Endocr Rev*. 1995;16:460-484.
458. Terzolo M, Bovio S, Reimondo G, et al. Subclinical Cushing's syndrome in adrenal incidentalomas. *Endocrinol Metab Clin North Am*. 2005;34:423-439, x.
459. Catargi B, Rigalleau V, Poussin A, et al. Occult Cushing's syndrome in type-2 diabetes. *J Clin Endocrinol Metab*. 2003;88:5808-5813.
460. Flecchia D, Mazza E, Carlini M, et al. Reduced serum levels of dehydroepiandrosterone sulphate in adrenal incidentalomas: a marker of adrenocortical tumour. *Clin Endocrinol (Oxf)*. 1995;42: 129-134.
461. Cawood TJ, Hunt PJ, O'Shea D, et al. Recommended evaluation of adrenal incidentalomas is costly, has high false-positive rates and confers a risk of fatal cancer that is similar to the risk of the adrenal lesion becoming malignant: time for a rethink? *Eur J Endocrinol*. 2009;161:513-527.
462. Mansmann G, Lau J, Balk E, et al. The clinically inapparent adrenal mass: update in diagnosis and management. *Endocr Rev*. 2004; 25:309-340.
463. Gicquel C, Le Bouc Y, Luton JP, et al. Pathogenesis and treatment of adrenocortical carcinoma. *Curr Opin Endocrinol Diab*. 1998;5: 189-196.
464. Matzuk MM, Finegold MJ, Mather JP, et al. Development of cancer cachexia-like syndrome and adrenal tumors in inhibin-deficient mice. *Proc Natl Acad Sci U S A*. 1994;91:8817-8821.

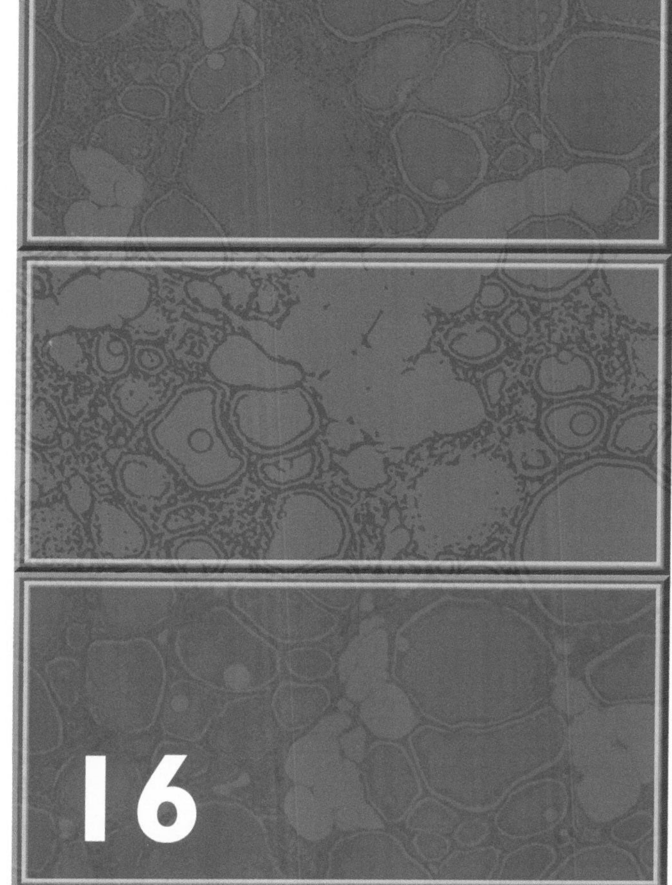

CHAPTER 16

Endocrine Hypertension

WILLIAM F. YOUNG, JR.

An estimated 85 million people in the United States are hypertensive.[1] In most, hypertension is *essential* or *idiopathic*, but a subgroup of approximately 15% have *secondary* hypertension. The secondary causes of hypertension can be divided into renal causes, such as renal parenchymal or renovascular disease, and endocrine causes. There are at least 14 endocrine disorders for which hypertension may be the initial clinical presentation (Table 16-1). An accurate diagnosis of endocrine hypertension provides the clinician with a unique treatment opportunity: to render a surgical cure or to achieve a dramatic response with pharmacologic therapy. The diagnostic and therapeutic approaches to endocrine hypertension—ranging from the classic adrenal causes of hypertension (e.g., pheochromocytoma, primary aldosteronism) to pituitary-dependent hypertension (e.g., Cushing's syndrome, acromegaly)—are reviewed in this chapter.

ADRENAL MEDULLA AND CATECHOLAMINES

The adrenal medulla occupies the central portion of the adrenal gland and accounts for 10% of total adrenal gland volume. There is no clear demarcation between the adrenal cortex and adrenal medulla. The adrenal glands derive blood supply from the superior, middle, and inferior branches of the inferior phrenic artery, from the renal arteries, and directly from the aorta. The adrenal arteries branch and form a plexus under the capsule. This plexus supplies the cortex. Some of the plexus arteries penetrate the cortex and supply the medulla, as do capillaries draining the cortical cells, forming the corticomedullary portal system. The right adrenal vein is short and drains directly into the inferior vena cava. The left adrenal vein merges with the inferior phrenic vein, and this larger vein (the common phrenic vein) drains into the left renal vein.

Adrenomedullary cells are called *chromaffin cells* (stain brown with chromium salts) or *pheochromocytes*. Cytoplasmic granules turn dark when stained with chromic acid because of the oxidation of epinephrine and norepinephrine to melanin. Chromaffin cells differentiate in the center of the adrenal gland in response to cortisol; some chromaffin cells also migrate to form paraganglia, collections of chromaffin cells located on both sides of the aorta. The largest cluster of chromaffin cells outside the adrenal medulla is located near the level of the inferior mesenteric artery and is referred to as the *organ of Zuckerkandl*; it is quite prominent in the fetus and is a major source of catecholamines during the first year of life. The preganglionic sympathetic neurons receive synaptic input from neurons within the pons, medulla, and hypothalamus, providing

TABLE 16-1

Endocrine Causes of Hypertension
Adrenal-Dependent Causes
Pheochromocytoma
Primary aldosteronism
Hyperdeoxycorticosteronism
Congenital adrenal hyperplasia
11β-Hydroxylase deficiency
17α-Hydroxylase deficiency
Deoxycorticosterone-producing tumor
Primary cortisol resistance
Cushing's syndrome
AME/11β-HSD Deficiency
Genetic
Type 1 AME
Acquired
Licorice or carbenoxolone ingestion (type 1 AME)
Cushing's syndrome (type 2 AME)
Thyroid-Dependent Causes
Hypothyroidism
Hyperthyroidism
Parathyroid-Dependent Causes
Hyperparathyroidism
Pituitary-Dependent Causes
Acromegaly
Cushing's syndrome

AME, apparent mineralocorticoid excess; HSD, hydroxysteroid dehydrogenase.

regulation of sympathetic activity by the brain. Axons from the lower thoracic and lumbar preganglionic neurons, via splanchnic nerves, directly innervate the cells of the adrenal medulla.

The term *catecholamine* refers to substances that contain catechol (ortho-dihydroxybenzene) and a side chain with an amino group—the catechol nucleus (Fig. 16-1).[2] Epinephrine is synthesized and stored in the adrenal medulla and released into the systemic circulation. Norepinephrine is synthesized and stored not only in the adrenal medulla but also in the peripheral sympathetic nerves. Dopamine, the precursor of norepinephrine, is found in the adrenal medulla and peripheral sympathetic nerves and acts primarily as a neurotransmitter in the central nervous system.

Catecholamines affect many cardiovascular and metabolic processes. They increase the heart rate, blood pressure, myocardial contractility, and cardiac conduction velocity. Specific receptors mediate the biologic actions of catecholamines. The dentification of three types of adrenergic receptors (α, β, and dopaminergic receptors), and their subtypes (α_1, α_2, β_1, β_2, β_3, D_1, and D_2) have led to understanding of the physiologic responses to endogenous and exogenous administration of catecholamines.[3] The α_1 subtype is a postsynaptic receptor that mediates vascular and smooth muscle contraction; stimulation causes vasoconstriction and increases blood pressure. The α_2 receptors are located on presynaptic sympathetic nerve endings; when activated, they inhibit release of norepinephrine. Stimulation causes suppression of central sympathetic outflow and decreased blood pressure.

There are three major β-receptor subtypes. The β_1 receptor mediates cardiac effects and is more responsive to isoproterenol than to epinephrine or norepinephrine. Stimulation causes positive inotropic and chronotropic effects on the heart, increased renin secretion in the kidney, and lipolysis in adipocytes. The β_2 receptor mediates bronchial, vascular, and uterine smooth muscle relaxation. Stimulation causes bronchodilation, vasodilatation in skeletal muscle, glycogenolysis, and increased release of norepinephrine from sympathetic nerve terminals. The β_3 receptor regulates energy expenditure and lipolysis.

D_1 receptors are localized to the cerebral, renal, mesenteric, and coronary vasculatures; stimulation causes vasodilation in these vascular beds. D_2 receptors are presynaptic; they are localized to sympathetic nerve endings, sympathetic ganglia, and brain. Stimulation of D_2 receptors in these locations inhibits the release of norepinephrine, inhibits ganglionic transmission, and inhibits prolactin release, respectively.

Most cells in the body have adrenergic receptors. The pharmacologic development of selective α- and β-adrenergic agonists and antagonists has advanced pharmacotherapy for various clinical disorders. For example, β_1 antagonists (e.g., atenolol, metoprolol) are now considered standard therapies for angina pectoris, hypertension, and cardiac arrhythmias.[4] Administration of β_2 agonists (e.g., terbutaline, albuterol) cause bronchial smooth muscle relaxation; these agents are commonly prescribed in inhaled formulations for the treatment of asthma.[5]

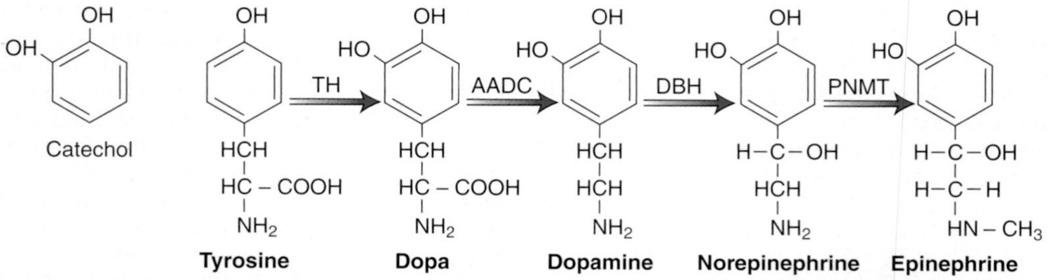

Figure 16-1 Biosynthetic pathway for catecholamines. The term *catecholamine* comes from the catechol (ortho-dihydroxybenzene) structure and a side chain with an amino group—the catechol nucleus(shown on left). Tyrosine is converted to 3,4-dihydroxyphenylalanine (dopa) by tyrosine hydroxylase (TH); this rate-limiting step provides the clinician with the option to treat pheochromocytoma with a TH inhibitor, α-methyl-paratyrosine (metyrosine). Aromatic L-amino acid decarboxylase (AADC) converts dopa to dopamine. Dopamine is hydroxylated to norepinephrine by dopamine β-hydroxylase (DBH). Norepinephrine is converted to epinephrine by phenylethanolamine *N*-methyltransferase (PNMT). Cortisol serves as a cofactor for PNMT, which explains why epinephrine-secreting neoplasms are almost exclusively localized to the adrenal medulla. (Modified and redrawn from Dluhy RG, Lawrence JE, Williams GH. Endocrine hypertension. In: Larsen PR, Kronenberg HM, Melmed S, et al., eds. *Williams Textbook of Endocrinology*. 10th ed. Philadelphia, PA: Saunders, 2003:555.)

Catecholamine Synthesis

Catecholamines are synthesized from tyrosine by a process of hydroxylation and decarboxylation (see Fig. 16-1). Tyrosine is derived from ingested food or synthesized from phenylalanine in the liver, and it enters neurons and chromaffin cells by active transport. Tyrosine is converted to 3,4-dihydroxyphenylalanine (dopa) by tyrosine hydroxylase, the rate-limiting step in catecholamine synthesis. Increased intracellular levels of catechols downregulate the activity of tyrosine hydroxylase; as catecholamines are released from secretory granules in response to a stimulus, cytoplasmic catecholamines are depleted and the feedback inhibition of tyrosine hydroxylase is released. Transcription of tyrosine hydroxylase is stimulated by glucocorticoids, cyclic adenosine monophosphate (cAMP)–dependent protein kinases, calcium/phospholipid-dependent protein kinase, and calcium/calmodulin-dependent protein kinase. α-Methyl-paratyrosine (metyrosine) is a tyrosine hydroxylase inhibitor that may be used therapeutically in patients with catecholamine-secreting neoplasms to decrease tumoral synthesis of catecholamines.

Aromatic L-amino acid decarboxylase catalyzes the decarboxylation of dopa to dopamine (see Fig. 16-1). Dopamine is actively transported into granulated vesicles to be hydroxylated to norepinephrine by the copper-containing enzyme dopamine β-hydroxylase. Ascorbic acid is a cofactor and hydrogen donor. The enzyme is structurally similar to tyrosine hydroxylase and may share similar transcriptional regulatory elements, and both are stimulated by glucocorticoids and cAMP-dependent kinases. These reactions occur in the synaptic vesicle of adrenergic neurons in the central nervous system, the peripheral nervous system, and the chromaffin cells of the adrenal medulla. The major constituents of the granulated vesicle are dopamine β-hydroxylase, ascorbic acid, chromogranin A, and adenosine triphosphate (ATP).

In the adrenal medulla, norepinephrine is released from the granule into the cytoplasm, where the cytosolic enzyme phenylethanolamine *N*-methyltransferase (PNMT) converts it to epinephrine (see Fig. 16-1). Epinephrine is then transported back into another storage vesicle. The *N*-methylation reaction by PNMT involves *S*-adenosylmethionine as the methyl donor as well as oxygen and magnesium. PNMT expression is regulated by the presence of glucocorticoids, which are in high concentration in the adrenal medulla through the corticomedullary portal system. Therefore, catecholamine-secreting tumors that secrete primarily epinephrine are localized to the adrenal medulla. In normal adrenal medullary tissue, approximately 80% of the catecholamines released are epinephrine.

Catecholamine Storage and Secretion

Catecholamines are found in the adrenal medulla and in sympathetically innervated organs. Catecholamines are stored in electron-dense granules that also contain ATP, neuropeptides (e.g., adrenomedullin, corticotropin [ACTH], vasoactive intestinal polypeptide), calcium, magnesium, and chromogranins. Uptake into the storage vesicles is facilitated by active transport by vesicular monoamine transporters (VMAT).[6] The VMAT ATP-driven pump maintains a steep electrical gradient. For every monoamine transported, ATP is hydrolyzed and two hydrogen ions are transported from the vesicle into the cytosol. Iodine 123 (^{123}I) and ^{131}I-labeled metaiodobenzylguanidine (MIBG) are imported by VMAT into the storage vesicles in the adrenal medulla, which makes ^{123}I-MIBG useful for imaging localization of catecholamine-secreting tumors and ^{131}I-MIBG potentially useful in treating malignant catecholamine-secreting tumors.[7,8] Catecholamine uptake, as well as that of MIBG, is inhibited by reserpine.[9] The catecholamine stores are dynamic, with constant leakage and reuptake.[10]

Stressful stimuli (e.g., myocardial infarction, anesthesia, hypoglycemia) trigger adrenal medullary catecholamine secretion. Acetylcholine from preganglionic sympathetic fibers stimulates nicotinic cholinergic receptors and causes depolarization of adrenomedullary chromaffin cells. Depolarization leads to activation of voltage-gated calcium channels, which results in exocytosis of secretory vesicle contents. A calcium-sensing receptor appears to be involved in the process of exocytosis. During exocytosis, all the granular contents are released into the extracellular space. Norepinephrine modulates its own release by activating the α_2-receptors on the presynaptic membrane. Stimulation of the presynaptic α_2-receptors inhibits norepinephrine release (the mechanism of action of some antihypertensive medications such as clonidine and guanfacine). Catecholamines are among the shortest-lived signaling molecules in plasma; the initial biologic half-life of circulating catecholamines is between 10 to 100 seconds. Approximately one half of the catecholamines circulate in plasma in loose association with albumin. Therefore, plasma concentrations of catecholamines fluctuate widely.

Catecholamine Metabolism and Inactivation

Catecholamines are removed from the circulation either by reuptake in sympathetic nerve terminals or by metabolism through two enzyme pathways (Fig. 16-2), followed by sulfate conjugation and renal excretion. Most of the metabolism of catecholamines occurs in the same cell in which they are synthesized.[10] Almost 90% of catecholamines released at sympathetic synapses are taken up locally by the nerve endings, termed *uptake-1*. Uptake-1 can be blocked by cocaine, tricyclic antidepressants, and phenothiazines. Extraneuronal tissues also take up catecholamines, and this is termed *uptake-2*. Most of these catecholamines are metabolized by catechol-*O*-methyltransferase (COMT).

Although COMT is found primarily outside neural tissue, *O*-methylation in the adrenal medulla is the predominant source of metanephrine (COMT converts epinephrine to metanephrine) and a major source of normetanephrine (COMT converts norepinephrine to normetanephrine) through methylation of the 3-hydroxy group.[10] *S*-Adenosylmethionine is used as the methyl donor, and calcium is required for this enzymatic step. Metanephrine and normetanephrine are oxidized by monoamine oxidase (MAO) to vanillylmandelic acid (VMA) by oxidative deamination. MAO may also oxidize epinephrine and norepinephrine to 3,4-dihydroxymandelic acid, which is then converted by COMT to VMA. MAO is located on the outer membrane of mitochondria. In the storage vesicle, norepinephrine is protected from metabolism by MAO. MAO and COMT metabolize dopamine to homovanillic acid (see Fig. 16-2).

PHEOCHROMOCYTOMA AND PARAGANGLIOMA

Catecholamine-secreting tumors that arise from chromaffin cells of the adrenal medulla and the sympathetic ganglia

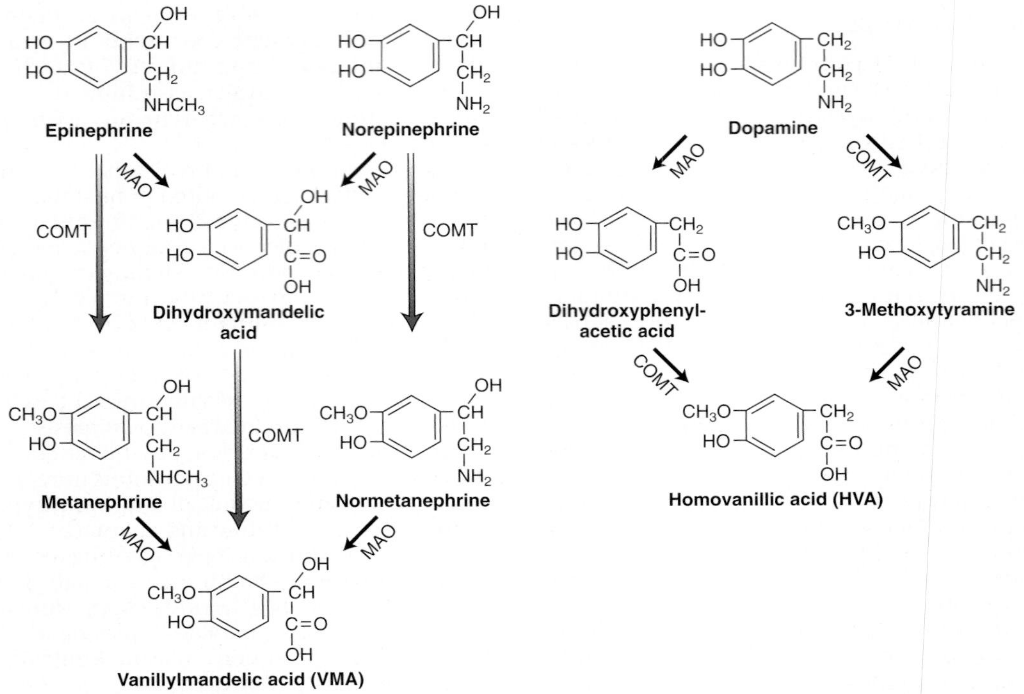

Figure 16-2 Catecholamine metabolism. Metabolism of catecholamines occurs through two enzymatic pathways. Catechol-*O*-methyltransferase (COMT) converts epinephrine to metanephrine and converts norepinephrine to normetanephrine through meta-*O*-methylation. Metanephrine and normetanephrine are oxidized by monoamine oxidase (MAO) to vanillylmandelic acid (VMA) by oxidative deamination. MAO also may oxidize epinephrine and norepinephrine to dihydroxymandelic acid, which is then converted by COMT to VMA. Dopamine is also metabolized by MAO and COMT to the final metabolite, homovanillic acid (HVA). (Modified and redrawn from Dluhy RG, Lawrene JE, Williams GH. Endocrine hypertension. In Larsen PR, Kronenberg HM, Melmed S, et al, eds. *Williams Textbook of Endocrinology*, 10th ed. Philadelphia, PA: Saunders, 2003:556.)

are referred to as *pheochromocytomas* and *catecholamine-secreting paragangliomas*, respectively.[11] Because the tumors have similar clinical presentations and are treated with similar approaches, many clinicians use the term *pheochromocytoma* to refer to both adrenal pheochromocytomas and extra-adrenal catecholamine-secreting paragangliomas. However, the distinction between pheochromocytoma and paraganglioma is an important one because of implications for associated neoplasms, risk for malignancy, and genetic testing. Catecholamine-secreting tumors are rare, with an annual incidence of 2 to 8 cases per 1 million people.[12] Based on screening studies for secondary causes of hypertension in outpatients, the prevalence of pheochromocytoma has been estimated at 0.1% to 0.6%.[13-15] Nevertheless, it is important to suspect, confirm, localize, and resect these tumors, because (1) the associated hypertension is curable with surgical removal of the tumor, (2) a risk of lethal paroxysm exists, (3) at least 10% of the tumors are malignant, and (4) between 10% and 20% of these tumors are familial, and their detection in the proband may result in early diagnosis in other family members.

History

The association between adrenal medullary tumors and symptoms was first recognized by Fränkel in 1886.[16] He described Fraulein Minna Roll, age 18, who had intermittent attacks of palpitation, anxiety, vertigo, headache, chest pain, cold sweats, and vomiting. She had a hard, noncompressible pulse and retinitis. Despite champagne therapy and injections of ether, she died. At autopsy, bilateral adrenal tumors were initially thought to be angiosarcomas, but later a positive chromaffin reaction confirmed pheochromocytoma. A subsequent study[17] published in 2007 documented the presence of a germline *RET* protooncogene mutation in four living relatives of Fraulein Roll—proving that the original patient and her family had multiple endocrine neoplasia type 2 (MEN2).

The term *pheochromocytoma*, proposed by Pick in 1912,[18] comes from the Greek words *phaios* ("dusky"), *chroma* ("color"), and *cytoma* ("tumor")—words that describe the dark staining reaction that is caused by the oxidation of intracellular catecholamines when they are exposed to dichromate salts. In 1926, César Roux in Lausanne, Switzerland, and Charles Mayo in Rochester, Minnesota, successfully surgically removed abdominal catecholamine-secreting tumors.[19] In 1929, it was discovered that a pheochromocytoma contained an excess amount of a pressor agent.[20] Subsequently, epinephrine (in 1936) and norepinephrine (in 1949) were isolated from pheochromocytoma tissue.[20] In 1950, it was found that patients with pheochromocytoma excreted increased amounts of epinephrine, norepinephrine, and dopamine in the urine.[21]

Clinical Presentation

Catecholamine-secreting tumors occur with equal frequency in men and women, primarily in the third, fourth, and fifth decades. These tumors are rare in children, and when discovered, they may be multifocal and associated with a hereditary syndrome. The symptoms, listed in Table 16-2, are caused by the pharmacologic effects of excess concentrations of circulating catecholamines.[22] The associated hypertension may be sustained or paroxysmal, and patients whose pheochromocytoma is diagnosed in the

TABLE 16-2

Signs and Symptoms Associated with Catecholamine-Secreting Tumors

Signs and Symptoms
Spell-Related Signs and Symptoms
Anxiety and fear of impending death
Diaphoresis
Dyspnea
Epigastric and chest pain
Headache
Hypertension
Nausea and vomiting
Pallor
Palpitation (forceful heartbeat)
Tremor
Chronic Signs and Symptoms
Anxiety and fear of impending death
Cold hands and feet
Congestive heart failure—dilated or hypertrophic cardiomyopathy
Constipation
Diaphoresis
Dyspnea
Ectopic hormone secretion–dependent symptoms (e.g., CRH/ACTH, GHRH, PTHrP, VIP)
Epigastric and chest pain
Fatigue
Fever
General increase in sweating
Grade II to IV hypertensive retinopathy
Headache
Hyperglycemia
Hypertension
Nausea and vomiting
Orthostatic hypotension
Painless hematuria (associated with urinary bladder paraganglioma)
Pallor
Palpitation (forceful heartbeat)
Tremor
Weight loss
Not Typical of Pheochromocytoma
Flushing

ACTH, adrenocorticotropic hormone; CRH, corticotropin-releasing hormone; GHRH, growth hormone–releasing hormone; PTHrP, parathyroid hormone–related peptide; VIP, vasoactive intestinal polypeptide.

(Adapted from Young WF Jr. Pheochromocytoma, 1926-1993. *Trends Endocrinol Metab.* 1993;4:122-127.)

presymptomatic stage may have normal blood pressure. The lability in blood pressure can be attributed to episodic release of catecholamines, chronic volume depletion, and impaired sympathetic reflexes. In addition to volume depletion, altered sympathetic vascular regulation may have a role in orthostasis, which is frequently observed in patients with pheochromocytoma.[23] Symptoms of orthostatic hypotension (e.g., lightheadedness, presyncope, syncope) may dominate the presentation, especially in patients with epinephrine- or dopamine-predominant tumors.[24,25]

Episodic symptoms may occur in spells, or paroxysms, that can be extremely variable in presentation but typically include forceful heartbeat, pallor, tremor, headache, and diaphoresis. The spell may start with a sensation of a "rush" in the chest and a sense of shortness of breath, followed by a forceful heart beat and a throbbing headache. Peripheral vasoconstriction associated with a spell results in cool or cold hands and feet and facial pallor. Increased sense of body heat and sweating are common symptoms that occur toward the end of the spell. Spells may be either spontaneous or precipitated by postural change, anxiety, medications (e.g., β-adrenergic antagonists, metoclopramide, anesthetic agents), exercise, or maneuvers that increase intra-abdominal pressure (e.g., change in position, lifting, defecation, exercise, colonoscopy, pregnancy, trauma). Although the types of spells experienced across the patient population are highly variable, spells tend to be stereotypical for each patient. Spells may occur multiple times daily or as infrequently as once monthly. The typical duration of a pheochromocytoma spell is 15 to 20 minutes, but it may be much shorter or last several hours. However, the clinician must recognize that most patients with spells do not have a pheochromocytoma[26] (Table 16-3).

Additional clinical signs of pheochromocytoma include hypertensive retinopathy, orthostatic hypotension, angina, nausea, constipation (megacolon may be the presenting

TABLE 16-3

Differential Diagnosis of Pheochromocytoma-Type Spells

Causes
Endocrine Causes
Carbohydrate intolerance
Hyperadrenergic spells
Hypoglycemia
Pancreatic tumors (e.g., insulinoma)
Pheochromocytoma
Primary hypogonadism (menopausal syndrome)
Thyrotoxicosis
Cardiovascular Causes
Angina
Cardiovascular deconditioning
Labile essential hypertension
Orthostatic hypotension
Paroxysmal cardiac arrhythmia
Pulmonary edema
Renovascular disease
Syncope (e.g., vasovagal reaction)
Psychological Causes
Factitious (e.g., drugs, Valsalva)
Hyperventilation
Severe anxiety and panic disorders
Somatization disorder
Pharmacologic Causes
Chlorpropamide-alcohol flush
Combination of a monoamine oxidase inhibitor and a decongestant
Illegal drug ingestion (cocaine, phencyclidine, lysergic acid diethylamide)
Sympathomimetic drug ingestion
Vancomycin ("red man syndrome")
Withdrawal of adrenergic-inhibitor
Neurologic Causes
Autonomic neuropathy
Cerebrovascular insufficiency
Diencephalic epilepsy (autonomic seizures)
Migraine headache
Postural orthostatic tachycardia syndrome
Stroke
Other Causes
Carcinoid syndrome
Mast cell disease
Recurrent idiopathic anaphylaxis
Unexplained flushing spells

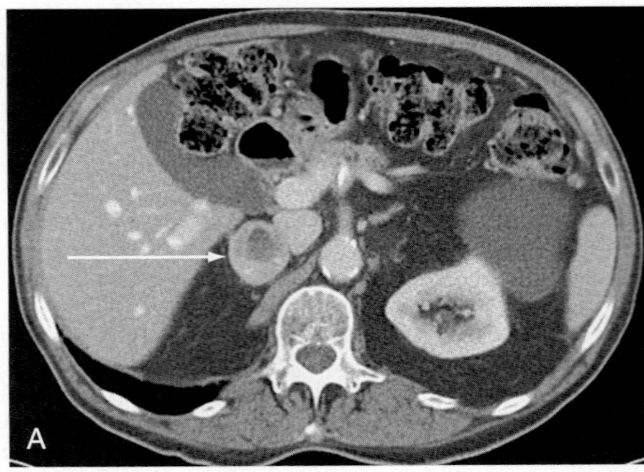

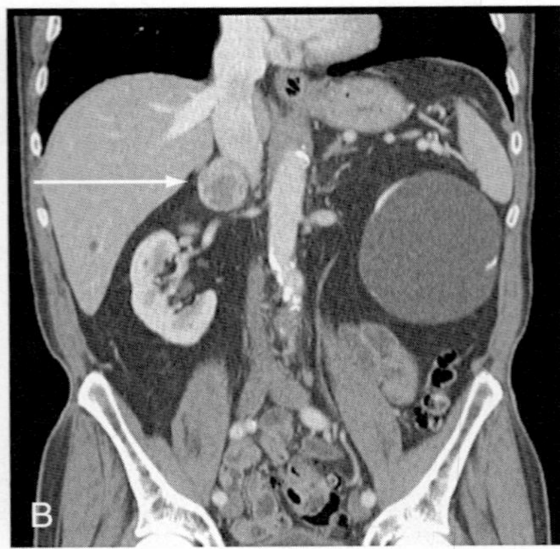

Figure 16-3 A computed tomographic (CT) scan of the abdomen with intravenous contrast in a 71-year-old man with an incidentally discovered right adrenal mass. The concentrations of plasma fractionated free metanephrines were abnormal: metanephrine, 0.34 nmol/L (normal, <0.5) and normetanephrine, 8.59 nmol/L (normal, <0.9). The 24-hour urine studies were abnormal: norepinephrine, 455 μg (normal, <170); epinephrine, 7.2 μg (normal, <35); dopamine, 160 μg (normal, <700); metanephrine, 173 μg (normal, <400); and normetanephrine, 3147 μg (normal, <900). **A,** The axial CT image shows a typical 3.8-cm heterogeneously enhancing right adrenal mass just lateral to the inferior vena cava and consistent with pheochromocytoma *(arrow)*. **B,** Coronal view shows the location *(arrow)* of the mass superior to the right kidney and inferior and medial to the liver. After α- and β-adrenergic blockade, a 2.5 × 1.5 × 1.5-cm, 20-g pheochromocytoma was removed laparoscopically.

symptom), hyperglycemia, diabetes mellitus, hypercalcemia, Raynaud's phenomenon, livedo reticularis, erythrocytosis, and mass effects from the tumor. Although hypercalcemia may be a sign of MEN2, it is usually isolated and resolves with resection of the catecholamine-secreting tumor. Calcitonin secretion is in part a catecholamine-dependent process; serum calcitonin concentrations are frequently mildly elevated in patients with pheochromocytoma, usually unrelated to MEN2. Fasting hyperglycemia and diabetes mellitus are caused in part by the α-adrenergic inhibition of insulin release. Painless hematuria and paroxysmal attacks induced by micturition and defication are associated with urinary bladder paragangliomas.

Some of the cosecreted hormones that may dominate the clinical presentation include ACTH (Cushing's syndrome), parathyroid hormone-related peptide (hypercalcemia), vasopressin (syndrome of inappropriate antidiuretic hormone secretion), vasoactive intestinal peptide (watery diarrhea), and growth hormone–releasing hormone (acromegaly).[27-29] Cardiomyopathy and congestive heart failure are the symptomatic presentations caused by pheochromocytoma that are most frequently unrecognized by clinicians.[30] The cardiomyopathy, whether dilated or hypertrophic, may be totally reversible with tumor resection. Myocarditis and myocardial infarction with normal coronary arteries seen on angiography are cardiac-based presentations that may not be recognized as pheochromocytoma.[31] The myocarditis is characterized by infiltration of inflammatory cells and focal contraction-band necrosis. Many physical examination findings can be associated with genetic syndromes that predispose to pheochromocytoma; these findings include retinal angiomas, iris hamartomas, marfanoid body habitus, café au lait spots, axillary freckling, subcutaneous neurofibromas, and mucosal neuromas on the eyelids and tongue. Some patients with pheochromocytoma are asymptomatic despite high circulating levels of catecholamines; this most likely reflects adrenergic receptor desensitization related to chronic stimulation.

A "rule of 10" has been quoted for describing the characteristics of catecholamine-secreting tumors: 10% are extra-adrenal, 10% occur in children, 10% are multiple or bilateral, 10% recur after surgical removal, 10% are malignant, 10% are familial, and 10% of benign sporadic adrenal pheochromocytomas are found as adrenal incidentalomas.[20] None of these figures is precisely 10%, however. For example, studies have suggested that up to 20% of catecholamine-secreting tumors are familial.[32] Also, in one study, 19 (58%) of 33 patients with adrenal pheochromocytoma had their adrenal tumors discovered incidentally on imaging performed for other reasons.[33] Because of the increased use of computed tomography (CT) and magnetic resonance imaging (MRI) and familial testing, pheochromocytoma is diagnosed in many patients before any symptoms develop. Although typically these incidentally discovered tumors in asymptomatic patients are small (<3 cm), they may be up to 10 cm in largest lesional diameter.

At the time of detection, pheochromocytomas have an average diameter of 4.5 cm[34] (Fig. 16-3). Paragangliomas are found where there is chromaffin tissue: along the para-aortic sympathetic chain, within the organ of Zuckerkandl (at the origin of the inferior mesenteric artery), in the wall of the urinary bladder, and along the sympathetic chain in the neck or mediastinum.[35] During early postnatal life, the extra-adrenal sympathetic paraganglionic tissues are prominent; later they degenerate, leaving residual foci associated with the vagus nerves, carotid vessels, aortic arch, pulmonary vessels, and mesenteric arteries. Odd locations for paragangliomas include the neck, intra-atrial cardiac septum, spermatic cord, vagina, scrotum, and sacrococcygeal region. Paragangliomas in the head and neck region (e.g., carotid body tumors, glomus tumors, chemodectomas) usually arise from parasympathetic tissue and typically do not hypersecrete catecholamines and metanephrines. Paragangliomas in the mediastinum, abdomen, and pelvis usually arise from sympathetic chromaffin tissue and usually do hypersecrete catecholamines and metanephrines.

Genetic and Syndromic Forms of Pheochromocytoma and Paraganglioma

Approximately 15% to 20% of patients with catecholamine-secreting tumors have germline mutations (inherited

TABLE 16-4

Autosomal Dominant Syndromes Associated with Pheochromocytoma and Paraganglioma

Syndrome	Gene	Gene Locus	Protein Product	Protein Function	Gene Mechanism	Typical Tumor Location
SDHD (familial paraganglioma type 1)*	*SDHD*	11q23	SDH D subunit	ATP production	Tumor suppressor	Skull base and neck; occasionally adrenal medulla, mediastinum, abdomen, pelvis
Familial paraganglioma type 2*	*SDHAF2*	11q13.1	Flavination cofactor	ATP production	Tumor suppressor	Skull base and neck; occasionally abdomen and pelvis
SDHC (familial paraganglioma type 3)	*SDHC*	1q21	SDH C subunit	ATP production	Tumor suppressor	Skull base and neck
SDHB (familial paraganglioma type 4)	*SDHB*	1p36.1-35	SDH B subunit	ATP production	Tumor suppressor	Abdomen, pelvis and medistinum; rarely adrenal medulla, skull base, and neck
MEN1	*MEN1*	11q13	Menin	Transcription regulation	Tumor suppressor	Adrenal medulla
MEN2A and MEN2B	*RET*	10q11.2	RET	Tyrosine kinase receptor	Protooncogene	Adrenal medulla, bilaterally
Neurofibromatosis type 1	*NF1*	17q11.2	Neurofibromin	GTP hydrolysis	Tumor suppressor	Adrenal-periadrenal
von Hippel-Lindau disease	*VHL*	3p25-26	VHL	Transcription elongation suppression	Tumor suppressor	Adrenal medulla, bilaterally; occasionally paraganglioma
Familial pheochromocytoma	*FP/TMEM127*	2q11	Transmembrane protein	Regulation of the mTORC1 signaling complex	Tumo suppressor	Adrenal medulla

*Associated with maternal imprinting.

ATP, adenosine triphosphate; GTP, guanosine triphosphate; MEN, multiple endocrine neoplasia; SDH, succinate dehydrogenase.

mutations present in all cells of the body) in genes associated with genetic disease[36,37] (Table 16-4). Hereditary catecholamine-secreting tumors typically manifest at a younger age than sporadic neoplasms do.[32] Sporadic pheochromocytoma typically is diagnosed on the basis of symptoms or as an incidental discovery on CT or MRI, whereas syndromic pheochromocytoma is frequently diagnosed earlier in the course of disease as a result of biochemical surveillance or genetic testing.[38]

Multiple Endocrine Neoplasia Type 2A

MEN2A (Sipple's syndrome) is an autosomal dominant disorder with age-related penetrance.[39] MEN2A is characterized by medullary thyroid cancer (MTC) in all patients, pheochromocytoma in 50% (usually bilateral and frequently asynchronous), primary hyperparathyroidism in 20%, and cutaneous lichen amyloidosis in 5%. Cutaneous lichen amyloidosis is a pruritic, papular, scaly, and pigmented skin lesion that is typically located in the interscapular region or on the extensor surfaces of the extremities.

MTC is usually detected before the pheochromocytoma is diagnosed. The prevalence of MEN2A is approximately 1 in 35,000 people. Numerous activating mutations throughout the *RET* proto-oncogene have been documented in persons with MEN2A. *RET*, located on chromosome 10q11.2, encodes a transmembrane receptor tyrosine kinase that is involved in the regulation of cell proliferation and apoptosis. Most mutations in MEN2A kindreds (>90%) involve one of six cysteine residues in the cysteine-rich region of the RET protein's extracellular domain encoded in *RET* exons 10 (codons 609, 611, 618, and 620) or 11 (codons 630 or 634). Eighty-five percent of individuals with MEN2A have a mutation in codon 634, particularly p.Cys634Arg (c.1900C>T).

Multiple Endocrine Neoplasia Type 2B

MEN2B is also an autosomal dominant disorder with age-related penetrance, and it represents approximately 5% of all MEN2 cases.[39] MEN2B is characterized by MTC in all patients, pheochromocytoma in 50%, mucocutaneous neuromas (typically involving the tongue, lips, and eyelids) in most patients, skeletal deformities (e.g., kyphoscoliosis, lordosis), joint laxity, myelinated corneal nerves, and intestinal ganglioneuromas (Hirschsprung's disease). Hirschsprung's disease is characterized by the absence of autonomic ganglion cells within the distal colon parasympathetic plexus, which results in chronic obstruction and megacolon.

MEN2B-associated tumors are caused by mutations in the RET protein's intracellular domain. A single methionine-to-threonine missense mutation in exon 16 (p.Met918Thr; c.2753T>C) is responsible for more than 95% of MEN2B cases. Another mutation, alanine to phenylalanine at codon 883 in exon 15, has been found in 4% of MEN2B kindreds.

Multiple Endocrine Neoplasia Type 2 Genetic Testing

More than 95% of patients with MEN2A and more than 98% of those with MEN2B have an identifiable mutation in the *RET* proto-oncogene. Genetic testing for mutations in the *RET* proto-oncogene is commercially available and should be considered for patients with bilateral pheochromocytoma, a family history of pheochromocytoma, or co-phenotype disorders. In a family with MEN2, a family member with a clinical diagnosis of MEN2 should be tested first. If a *RET* mutation is found, all family members of unknown status should be offered genotyping. Genetic counseling consultation should be considered before genetic testing is performed. In families with known MEN2, genetic testing shortly after birth facilitates prompt surgical management of the thyroid gland. Genetic testing shortly after birth is especially important in families with MEN2B, because the thyroid gland should be removed in the first 6 months of life (see Chapter 41 for further discussion of MEN2).

Multiple Endocrine Neoplasia Type 1

MEN1 is an autosomal dominant disorder characterized by pituitary adenomas, primary hyperparathyroidism, pancreatic islet cells tumors, adrenal adenomas, carcinoid tumors, collagenomas, angiofibromas, lipomas, and, very rarely, adrenal pheochromocytoma.[40,41] Pheochromocytoma has been documented in only a few patients with MEN1.[42,43] The prevalence of MEN1 is approximately 1 in 30,000 individuals.[40,41] MEN1 is caused by inactivating mutations in the tumor suppressor gene *MEN1,* which is located on chromosome 11q13. Genetic testing for mutations in *MEN1* is commercially available and should be considered only for patients with adrenal pheochromocytoma and MEN1 co-phenotype disorders.

von Hippel-Lindau Disease

Von Hippel-Lindau (VHL) syndrome is an autosomal dominant disorder that may manifest with a variety of benign and malignant neoplasms: pheochromocytoma (frequently bilateral), paraganglioma (mediastinal, abdominal, pelvic), hemangioblastoma (involving the cerebellum, spinal cord, or brainstem), retinal angioma, clear cell renal cell carcinoma, pancreatic neuroendocrine tumors, endolymphatic sac tumors of the middle ear, serous cystadenomas of the pancreas, and papillary cystadenomas of the epididymis and broad ligament. Patients with VHL syndrome may be divided into two groups: type 1 and type 2. Patients from kindreds with type 1 syndrome do not develop pheochromocytoma, whereas those from kindreds with type 2 syndrome are at high risk for developing pheochromocytoma. In addition, kindreds with type 2 VHL syndrome are subdivided into type 2A (low risk for renal cell carcinoma), type 2B (high risk for renal cell carcinoma), and type 2C (pheochromocytomas only).

The prevalence of VHL syndrome is approximately 1 in 35,000 people. The *VHL* tumor suppressor gene, located on chromosome 3p25-26, encodes a protein that regulates hypoxia-induced proteins.[44] More than 300 germline *VHL* mutations have been identified that lead to loss of function of the VHL protein. Almost 100% of patients with VHL syndrome have an identifiable gene mutation. Genotype-phenotype correlations have been documented for this disorder, and specific mutations are associated with particular patterns of tumor formation.[45,46] In up to 98% of cases, pheochromocytoma is associated with missense mutations (rather than truncating or null mutations) in the *VHL* gene. Genetic testing for VHL syndrome is commercially available and should be considered for patients with bilateral pheochromocytoma, a family history of pheochromocytoma, diagnosis of pheochromocytoma at a young age (≤30 years), or co-phenotype disorders.

Pheochromocytomas occurring in patients with MEN2 produce predominantly epinephrine and metanephrine, whereas those occurring in patients with VHL syndrome produce predominately norepinephrine and normetanephrine. These biochemical phenotypes result from mutation-specific differential gene expression. PNMT is overexpressed in MEN2-associated tumors (epinephrine and metanephrine profile) and underexpressed in VHL-associated tumors (norepinephrine and normetanephrine profile).[47] In addition, pheochromocytomas occurring in patients with MEN2 have increased tyrosine hydroxylase activity compared with those occurring in patients with VHL; this difference accounts for higher levels of catecholamines and metabolites in patients with MEN2.

Neurofibromatosis Type 1

Neurofibromatosis type 1 (NF1) is an autosomal dominant disorder characterized by neurofibromas, multiple café-au-lait spots, axillary and inguinal freckling, iris hamartomas (Lisch nodules), bony abnormalities, central nervous system gliomas, pheochromocytoma and paraganglioma, macrocephaly, and cognitive deficits. The expression of these features is variable. Approximately 2% of patients with NF1 develop catecholamine-secreting tumors.[48] In these patients, the catecholamine-secreting tumor is usually a solitary, benign adrenal pheochromocytoma, occasionally bilateral adrenal pheochromocytomas, and rarely an abdominal periadrenal paraganglioma. The prevalence of NF1 is approximately 1 in 3000 people. The *NF1* tumor suppressor gene, located on chromosome 17q11.2, encodes neurofibromin, a guanosine triphosphatase–activating protein that inhibits RAS activity. Inactivating *NF1* mutations cause the disorder. More than 95% of *NF1* mutations can be identified with a multistep testing protocol. However, unless a patient with pheochromocytoma presents with additional clinical characteristics consistent with an NF1 diagnosis, genetic testing of the *NF1* gene is not recommended.

Familial Paraganglioma

Familial paraganglioma is an autosomal dominant disorder characterized by paragangliomas that are located most often in the skull base and neck but also in the mediastinum, abdomen, pelvis, and urinary bladder. The occurrence of catecholamine hypersecretion in a patient with familial paraganglioma depends on tumor location; approximately 5% of skull base and neck paragangliomas and more than 50% of abdominal paragangliomas produce hormones.[35] The mean age at diagnosis is 30 to 35 years and can vary greatly within a family (mean difference among individuals ± standard deviation [SD], 14.3 ± 9.6 years; range, 0 to 37 years).[49] The prevalence of familial paraganglioma is unknown. Most cases of familial paraganglioma are caused by mutations in the succinate dehydrogenase (SDH; succinate:ubiquinone oxidoreductase) subunit genes (*SDHB, SDHC, SDHD, SHDA, and SDHAF2*), which make up portions of mitochondrial complex II.[50,51] Mitochondrial complex II is a tumor suppressor gene that is involved in the electron transport chain and the tricarboxylic acid (TCA) cycle.

Inactivating germline mutations in *SDHD,* located on chromosome 11q23, have been identified in multigenerational families with skull base and neck parasympathetic paragangliomas that are usually nonfunctional.[52] However, catecholamine-secreting paragangliomas may occur when mutations are located in the 5′ portion of *SDHD.*[53] Adrenal pheochromocytomas may also be found in patients with *SDHD* mutations.[54] Before the gene was characterized, affected families were said to have paraganglioma syndrome type 1. In patients with *SDHD* mutations, penetrance depends on the mutation's parent of origin. The disease is not manifested when the mutation is inherited from the mother but is highly penetrant when inherited from the father.[52,54] This phenomenon is known as *maternal imprinting.*

Missense mutations in *SDHC,* located on chromosome 1q21, have been reported in families with skull base and neck parasympathetic paragangliomas that are usually nonfunctional.[55] Before the gene was characterized, affected families were said to have paraganglioma syndrome type

3. Genetic testing for *SDHC* should be considered for families with skull base and neck paragangliomas that are negative for mutations in *SDHD*.

The gene associated with paraganglioma syndrome type 2, called SDH complex assembly factor 2 *(SDHAF2),* has recently been identified.[56] Multiple cofactors are required for normal activity of the SDH complex, including flavin-adenine dinucleotide (FAD) in Sdh1. FAD is covalently attached to Sdh1, and deletion of *SDHAF2* causes a complete loss of FAD cofactor attachment (flavination) of Sdh1. Germline loss-of-function mutations in the *SDHAF2* gene, located on chromosome 11q13.1, segregated with disease in a family with hereditary paraganglioma. Like families with mutations in *SDHD,* those with paraganglioma syndrome type 2 also exhibit maternal imprinting. This syndrome is associated with parasympathetic paragangliomas that typically occur in the skull base and neck.

Inactivating mutations in the tumor suppressor gene *SDHB,* located on chromosome 1p35-36, are associated with paragangliomas in the abdomen, pelvis, and mediastinum. Adrenal pheochromocytomas may also be found in patients with *SDHB* mutations.[54] Before the gene was characterized, affected families were said to have paraganglioma syndrome type 4. In families with *SDHB* mutations, imprinting has not been observed. Patients with *SDHB* mutations are at increased risk for malignant paraganglioma.[54,57,58] In a population-based study, patients with *SDHB* mutations also appeared to be at increased risk for renal cell carcinoma and papillary thyroid cancer,[54] but a referral center–based study did not find this apparent association.[59]

Genetic testing for *SDHB, SDHD,* and *SDHC* is available commercially and, because of the high prevalence among patients with paraganglioma, stepwise testing should be considered for all affected individuals (see later discussion). In addition, large germline deletions of *SDHB* and *SDHD* have been identified in families with paraganglioma[60]; thus, deletion detection testing should be performed if mutations are not found with gene sequencing.

Other Neurocutaneous Syndromes

Additional neurocutaneous syndromes associated with catecholamine-secreting tumors include ataxia-telangiectasia, tuberous sclerosis, and Sturge-Weber syndrome. The Carney triad (gastrointestinal stomal tumor, pulmonary chondroma, and catecholamine-secreting paraganglioma) is another syndrome associated with catecholamine-secreting tumors.[61] This syndrome is a rare, usually sporadic disorder of unknown etiology that primarily affects young women. The gastric stromal tumors are frequently multicentric and associated with early liver metastases. Nevertheless, most affected patients have a very indolent course. The pulmonary chondromas are benign and, if asymptomatic, require no specific therapy. The paragangliomas secrete catecholamines and should be resected when discovered. Additional features of the Carney triad include esophageal leiomyomas and adrenal cortical adenomas. The esophageal leiomyomas, found incidentally at the time of esophagogastroduodenoscopy, are benign and usually asymptomatic. The adrenal cortical adenomas may be nonfunctioning or secrete cortisol autonomously.

Genetic Testing

As previously outlined, genetic testing should be considered if a patient has one or more of the following: (1) paraganglioma, (2) bilateral adrenal pheochromocytoma, (3) unilateral adrenal pheochromocytoma and a family history of pheochromocytoma/paraganglioma, (4) unilateral adrenal pheochromocytoma with onset at a young age (<30 years), or (5) other clinical findings suggestive of one of the previously discussed syndromic disorders. An asymptomatic person at risk for disease on the basis of family history of pheochromocytoma/paraganglioma should have genetic testing only if an affected family member has a known mutation. Genetic testing can be complex, and testing of one family member has implications for related individuals. Genetic counseling is recommended to help families understand the implications of genetic test results, to coordinate testing of at-risk individuals, and to help families work through the psychosocial issues that may arise before, during, or after the testing process.

The clinician may obtain a list of clinically approved molecular genetic diagnostic laboratories at www.genetests.org (accessed December 2010). Given the considerable cost of genetic testing, use of a stepwise approach based on each patient's clinical scenario is prudent. Some examples follow:

- If a patient has a catecholamine-secreting abdominal, pelvic, or mediastinal paraganglioma, tests for mutations in the following genes should be ordered sequentially: *SDHB, SDHD, VHL, SDHC.* If a mutation is identified at any point in the testing algorithm, no further testing should be performed.
- If a patient presents with bilateral adrenal pheochromocytoma but without a history of MTC or goiter, tests for mutations in the following genes should be ordered sequentially: *VHL, RET.* If a *VHL* mutation is identified, genetic testing of the *RET* proto-oncogene should not be ordered. The biochemical phenotype—adrenergic (MEN2) or noradrenergic (VHL)—can also be used to guide genetic testing.
- If a patient who is 30 years of age or younger presents with apparent sporadic unilateral adrenal pheochromocytoma, tests for mutations in the following genes should be considered sequentially: *VHL, RET, SDHB, SDHD, SDHC,* and when clinically available, FP/TMEM127. If a mutation is identified at any point in the testing algorithm, no further testing should be performed.
- If a patient has a skull-base or neck paraganglioma, tests for mutations in the following genes should be ordered sequentially: *SDHD, SDHC, SDHAF2* (if clinically available)*, SDHB.* If the kindred shows a typical maternal imprinting inheritance pattern, then *SDHD* and *SDHAF2* should be ordered. If a mutation is identified at any point in the testing algorithm, no further testing should be performed.

Evaluation and Monitoring of Carriers of Succinate Dehydrogenase Mutations

If an SDH mutation is identified in a relative of a proband, biochemical and imaging studies are indicated. Prospective studies to guide the clinician in the frequency and type of testing are lacking. Biochemical testing for fractionated metanephrines in plasma or in a 24-hour urine collection should be performed annually in all carriers of SDH mutation. Because paragangliomas may be nonfunctioning or may be detected before catecholamine-secretory autonomy is evident, imaging studies are advised. For example, *SDHB* and at-risk *SDHD* (e.g., paternally inherited) mutation carriers should have CT or MRI of the chest, abdomen, and pelvis every 2 to 3 years; ^{123}I-MIBG scintigraphy should be performed every 5 years. *SDHC* and at-risk *SDHAF2* (e.g., paternally inherited) mutation carriers should have skull-base and neck imaging with ultrasound or MRI every 2 to

TABLE 16-5

Medications That May Increase Measured Levels of Fractionated Catecholamines and Metanephrines

Tricyclic antidepressants (including cyclobenzaprine)
Levodopa
Drugs containing adrenergic receptor agonists (e.g., decongestants)
Amphetamines
Buspirone and antipsychotic agents
Prochlorperazine
Reserpine
Withdrawal from clonidine and other drugs (e.g., illicit drugs)
Illicit drugs (e.g., cocaine, heroin)
Ethanol

3 years; ^{123}I-MIBG scintigraphy should be performed every 5 years; CT or MRI of the abdomen and pelvis every 5 years.

Diagnostic Investigation

Differential Diagnosis

Numerous disorders can cause signs and symptoms that may prompt the clinician to test for pheochromocytoma (see Table 16-3). The disorders span much of medicine and include endocrine disorders (e.g., primary hypogonadism), cardiovascular disorders (e.g., idiopathic orthostatic hypotension), psychologic disorders (e.g., panic disorder), pharmacologic causes (e.g., withdrawal from an adrenergic inhibitor), neurologic disorders (e.g., postural orthostatic tachycardia syndrome), and miscellaneous disorders (e.g., mast cell disease). Indeed, most patients tested for pheochromocytoma do not have it. In addition, levels of fractionated catecholamines and metanephrines may be elevated in several clinical scenarios, including withdrawal from medications or drugs (e.g., clonidine, alcohol), any acute illness (e.g., subarachnoid hemorrhage, migraine headache, preeclampsia), and administration of many drugs and medications (e.g., tricyclic antidepressants, levodopa, buspirone, antipyschiotic agents, cocaine, phencyclidine, amphetamines, ephedrine, pseudoephedrine, phenylpropanolamine, isoproterenol) (Table 16-5).

Case Detection

Pheochromocytoma should be suspected in patients who have one or more of the following:

- Hyperadrenergic spells (e.g., self-limited episodes of nonexertional palpitations, diaphoresis, headache, tremor, or pallor)
- Resistant hypertension
- A familial syndrome that predisposes to catecholamine-secreting tumors (e.g., MEN2, NF1, VHL)
- A family history of pheochromocytoma
- An incidentally discovered adrenal mass
- Hypertension and diabetes
- Pressor response during anesthesia, surgery, or angiography
- Onset of hypertension at a young age (<20 years)
- Idiopathic dilated cardiomyopathy
- A history of gastrointestinal stromal tumor or pulmonary chondromas (Carney triad)

Measurement of Fractionated Metanephrines and Catecholamines in Urine and Blood. The diagnosis must be confirmed biochemically by the presence of increased concentrations of fractionated catecholamines and fractionated metanephrines in urine or plasma (Fig. 16-4).[22] The metabolism of catecholamines is primarily intratumoral, with formation of metanephrine from epinephrine and normetanephrine from norepinephrine.[10] Most laboratories now measure fractionated catecholamines (dopamine, norepinephrine, and epinephrine) and fractionated metanephrines (metanephrine and normetanephrine) by high-performance liquid chromatography with electrochemical detection or tandem mass spectrometry.[62] These techniques have overcome the problems with fluorometric analysis, which include false-positive results caused by α-methyldopa, labetalol, sotalol, and imaging contrast agents.

At Mayo Clinic, the most reliable case-detection strategy is measurement of fractionated metanephrines and catecholamines in a 24-hour urine collection (sensitivity, 98%; specificity, 98%).[63,64] If clinical suspicion is high, then plasma fractionated metanephrines, which are products of intrapheochromocytoma catecholamine metabolism, should also be measured.[65] Some groups have advocated that plasma fractionated metanephrines should be a first-line test for pheochromocytoma[65,66]; the predictive value of a negative test is extremely high, and a normal result excludes pheochromocytoma except in patients with early preclinical disease and those with strictly dopamine-secreting neoplasms.[64] A plasma test is also attractive because of its simplicity. Although measurement of plasma fractionated metanephrines has a sensitivity of 96% to 100%,[64,65] the specificity is poor at 85% to 89%,[64,65,67] and the specificity falls to 77% in patients older than 60 years of age.[64] It has been estimated that 97% of patients with hypertension seen in a tertiary care clinic who have plasma fractionated metanephrine measurements above the reference range will not have a pheochromocytoma[67] and this results in excessive health care expenditures because of subsequent imaging and potentially inappropriate surgery.[68] Therefore, plasma fractionated metanephrines lack the necessary specificity to be recommended as a first-line test, and this measurement should be reserved for cases in which the index of suspicion is high (see Fig. 16-4).

The index of suspicion for pheochromocytoma should be high in the following scenarios: resistant hypertension; spells with associated pallor; a family history of pheochromocytoma; a genetic syndrome that predisposes to pheochromocytoma (e.g., MEN2); a past history of resected pheochromocytoma and present history of recurrent hypertension or spells; and an incidentally discovered adrenal mass that has imaging characteristics consistent with pheochromocytoma (Table 16-6). In addition, measurement of plasma fractionated metanephrines is a good first-line test for children, because obtaining a complete 24-hour urine collection is difficult in pediatric patients. Measurement of urinary dopamine or plasma methoxytyramine can be very useful in detecting the rare tumor with selective dopamine hypersecretion, because plasma metanephrine fractions are not direct metabolites of dopamine and may be normal in the setting of a dopamine-secreting tumor.[25,64]

The 24-hour urine collection for fractionated metanephrines and catecholamines should include measurement of urinary creatinine to verify an adequate collection. The normal ranges for plasma metanephrine and normetanephrine may be affected by the method used to obtain the blood sample. For example, use of an indwelling cannula for 20 minutes after an overnight fast before the blood draw has resulted in lower diagnostic cutoff points (metanephrine, <0.3 nmol/L; normetanephrine, <0.66 nmol/L)[69] to exclude pheochromocytoma compared

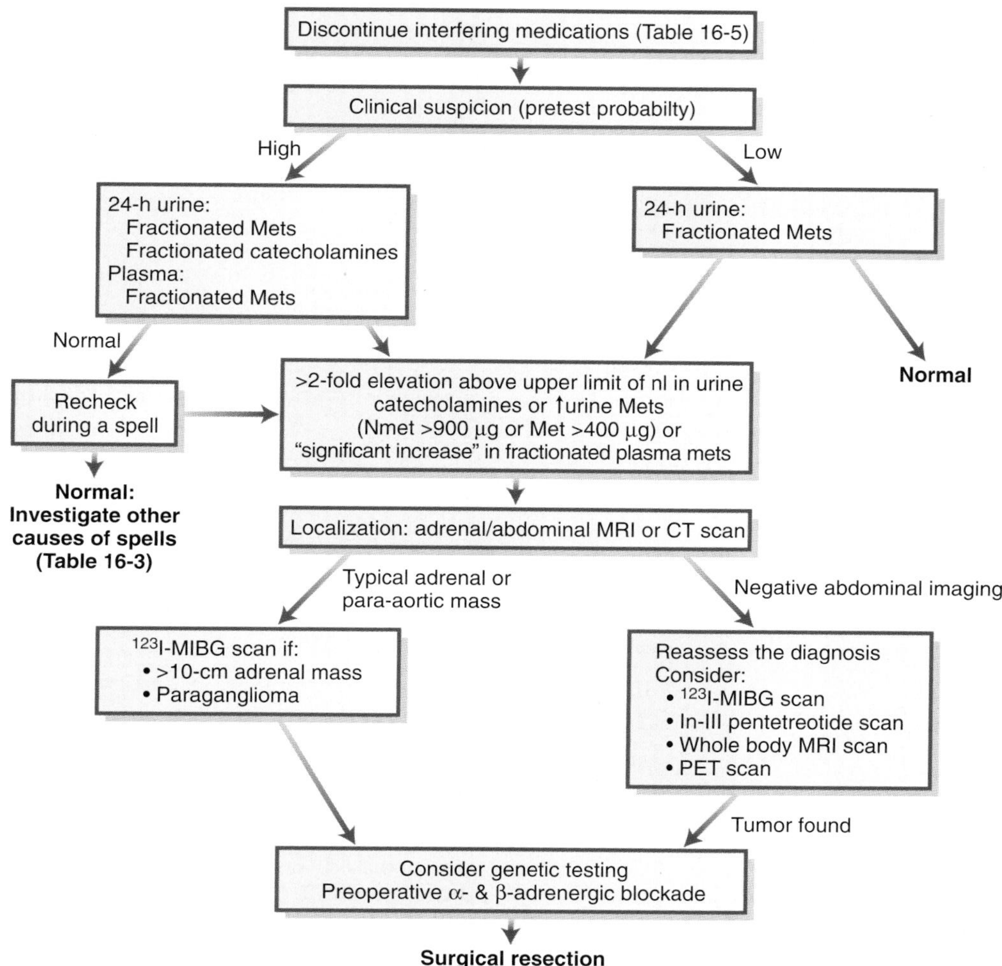

Figure 16-4 Evaluation and treatment of catecholamine-secreting tumors. Clinical suspicion is triggered by paroxysmal symptoms (especially hypertension); hypertension that is intermittent, unusually labile, or resistant to treatment; a family history of pheochromocytoma or associated conditions; or an incidentally discovered adrenal mass (see text for details). CT, computed tomography; In-111, indium 111; ^{123}I-MIBG, iodine 123–labeled metaiodobenzylguanidine; Mets, metanephrines; MRI, magnetic resonance imaging; nl, normal; Nmet, normetanephrine; PET, positron emission tomography. (Modified from Young WF Jr. Pheochromocytoma, 1926-1993. *Trends Endocrinol Metab.* 1993;4:122, with permission.)

with venipuncture in a seated ambulant nonfasting patient (metanephrine, <0.5 nmol/L; normetanephrine, <0.9 nmol/L).[64] The diagnostic cutoffs for most 24-hour urinary fractionated metanephrines assays are based on normal ranges derived from normotensive volunteer reference groups, and this can result in excessive false-positive test results. For example, in normotensive laboratory volunteers, the 95th percentiles are 428 μg for normetanephrine and 200 μg for metanephrine, whereas the corresponding values in individuals who are being tested for pheochromocytoma as part of routine clinical practice but who do not have the neoplasm are, respectively, 71% and 51% higher than those of the normal volunteers.[70]

Although it is preferred that patients not receive any medication during the diagnostic evaluation, treatment with most medications may be continued. Tricyclic antidepressants are the drugs that interfere most frequently with the interpretation of 24-hour urinary catecholamines and metabolites. To effectively screen for catecholamine-secreting tumors, treatment with tricyclic antidepressants and other psychoactive agents listed in Table 16-5 should be tapered and discontinued at least 2 weeks before any hormonal assessments. There are clinical situations for which it is contraindicated to discontinue certain medications (e.g., antipsychotics), and if case-detection testing is positive, then CT or MRI would be needed to exclude a catecholamine-secreting tumor. Furthermore, catecholamine secretion may be appropriately increased in situations of physical stress or illness (e.g., stroke, myocardial infarction, congestive heart failure, obstructive sleep apnea). Therefore, the clinical circumstances under which catecholamines and metanephrines are measured must be assessed in each case.

Other Tests That Have Been Used to Assess for Pheochromocytoma. Because of poor overall accuracy in testing for pheochromocytoma, measurement of plasma catecholamines no longer has a role.[69] Chromogranin A is stored and released from dense-core secretory granules of neuroendocrine cells and is increased in 80% of patients with pheochromocytoma.[71] Chromogranin A is not specific for pheochromocytoma, and elevations may be seen with other neuroendocrine tumors. Plasma neuropeptide Y levels are increased in 87% of patients with pheochromocytoma,[72] but they also lack the accuracy of 24-hour urinary fractionated metanephrines and catecholamines. The

TABLE 16-6

Typical Imaging Phenotypes of Adrenal Masses

Tumor Type	Size (cm)	Shape	Texture	Laterality	Contrast Enhancement	CT*	MRI†	Necrosis, Hemorrhage, or Calcifications	Growth
Cortical adenoma	≤3	Round to oval with smooth margins	Homogeneous	Usually unilateral	Limited	<10 HU; >50% washout	Isointense	Rare	Slow
Cortical carcinoma	>4	Irregular with unclear margins	Inhomogeneous	Usually unilateral	Marked	>10 HU; <50% washout	Hyperintense	Common	Rapid
Pheochromocytoma	>3	Round to oval with smooth margins	Inhomogeneous with areas of cystic degeneration	Usually solitary and unilateral	Marked	>10 HU; <50% washout	Hyperintense	Common	1 cm/yr
Metastasis	Variable	Oval to irregular with unclear margins	Inhomogeneous	Often bilateral	Marked	>10 HU; <50% washout	Hyperintense	Common	Variable

CT, computed tomography; HU, Hounsfield unit; MRI, magnetic resonance imaging.
*Precontrast radiodensity (HU) and percentage of contrast medium washout at 10 min.
†Relative intensity compared with liver on T2-weighted images.

24-hour urinary VMA excretion has poor diagnostic sensitivity and specificity compared with fractionated 24-hour urinary metanephrines.

Clonidine Suppression Test. The high false-positive rate for plasma catecholamines and fractionated metanephrines triggered the development of a confirmatory test, the clonidine suppression test. This test is intended to distinguish between pheochromocytoma and false-positive increases in plasma fractionated catecholamines and metanephrines. Clonidine is a centrally acting α_2-adrenergic receptor agonist that normally suppresses the release of catecholamines from neurons but does not affect the catecholamine secretion from a pheochromocytoma. Clonidine (0.3 mg) is administered orally, and plasma fractionated catecholamines or metanephrines are measured before and 3 hours after the dose.[73] In patients with essential hypertension, plasma catecholamine concentrations decrease (norepinephrine + epinephrine <500 pg/mL or >50% decrease in norepinephrine), as do plasma normetanephrine concentrations (into the normal range or >40% decrease). However, these concentrations remain increased in patients with pheochromocytoma.[73,74]

Provocative Testing and Suppression Testing. Because of advances in the methodology for measuring catecholamines and metanephrines, phentolamine, glucagon, histamine, metoclopramide, and tyramine tests are rarely needed. From 1975 to 1994 at Mayo Clinic, we performed histamine and glucagon stimulation testing in 542 patients in whom pheochromocytoma was highly suspected despite normal 24-hour urinary excretion of total metanephrines or catecholamines; not one patient had a positive stimulation test in this setting.[75]

Renal Failure. Measurements of urinary catecholamines and metabolites may be invalid if the patient has advanced renal insufficiency.[76] Serum chromogranin A levels have poor diagnostic specificity in these patients.[77] In patients without pheochromocytoma who are receiving hemodialysis, plasma norepinephrine and dopamine concentrations are increased, respectively, threefold and twofold above the upper limit of normal.[78,79] However, standard normal ranges can be used for interpreting plasma epinephrine concentrations.[80] Therefore, when patients with renal failure have plasma norepinephrine concentrations more than threefold above the upper normal limit or epinephrine concentrations greater than the upper normal limit, pheochromocytoma should be suspected. The findings of one study suggested that plasma concentrations of fractionated metanephrines are increased approximately twofold in patients with renal failure and may be useful in the biochemical evaluation of patients with marked renal insufficiency or renal failure.[81] However, the results of an earlier study suggested that concentrations of plasma fractionated metanephrines could not distinguish between 10 patients with pheochromocytoma and 11 patients with end-stage renal disease who required long-term hemodialysis.[82]

Factitious Pheochromocytoma. As with other similar disorders, factitious pheochromocytoma can be very difficult to confirm.[83] The patient usually has a medical background. The patient may "spike" the 24-hour urine container, or the catecholamines may be administered systemically.[84]

Localization

Localization studies should not be initiated until biochemical studies have confirmed the diagnosis of a catecholamine-secreting tumor (see Fig. 16-4). CT or MRI of the adrenal glands and abdomen should be the first localization test (sensitivity, >95%; specificity, >65%).[85-88] Approximately 85% of these tumors are found in the adrenal glands, and 95% are found in the abdomen and pelvis. The most common locations of catecholamine-secreting paragangliomas include superior abdominal para-aortic region, 46%;

inferior abdominal para-aortic region, 29%; urinary bladder, 10%; mediastinum, 10%; head and neck, 3%; and pelvis, 2%.[35]

Imaging Phenotype. The term *imaging phenotype* refers to the characteristics of the mass on CT or MRI (see Table 16-6). The lipid-rich nature of cortical adenomas is helpful in distinguishing these benign neoplasms from pheochromocytoma. On CT scans, the density of the image (with darker tissues being less dense) is attributed to x-ray attenuation. At the extremes of the CT density spectrum are air (black) and bone (white). The Hounsfield scale is a semiquantitative method of measuring x-ray attenuation. Typical Hounsfield unit (HU) values are −20 to −150 HU for adipose tissue and 20 to 50 HU for kidney. If an adrenal mass is less than 0 HU on unenhanced CT, it is almost certainly a benign adenoma.[89,90] Adrenal adenomas show a much earlier washout of contrast enhancement than do nonadenomas.[91] For example, Korobkin and colleagues[91] found that the mean percentage washout for adenomas was 51% at 5 minutes and 70% at 15 minutes, compared with 8% and 20%, respectively, for nonadenomas.

Although CT is still the primary adrenal imaging modality, MRI has advantages in certain clinical situations.[88] Several different MRI techniques have been used to characterize adrenal masses. Conventional spin-echo MRI was the first and is still the most frequently used technique. Early in the history of abdominal MRI, it became clear that with low- or midfield-strength magnets, T1- and T2-weighted imaging could be used to differentiate pheochromocytoma and malignancies from benign adenomas. On gadolinium-diethylenetriaminepenta-acetic acid (DPTA)-enhanced MRI, pheochromocytomas and malignant lesions show rapid and marked enhancement and a slower washout pattern, whereas adenomas demonstrate mild enhancement and a rapid washout of contrast.[92] Similar findings are made with CT.

Chemical shift MRI is a form of lipid-sensitive imaging. Chemical shift MRI is based on the principle that the hydrogen protons in water and lipid molecules resonate at different frequencies. Benign cortical adenomas contain approximately equal amounts of lipid and water, whereas the lipid content of pheochromocytomas is usually low. When the protons of water and lipid are aligned, they are said to be in phase, and when opposite each other, they are out of phase. When fat and water are in phase on MRI, the signal intensity is maximized; when they are out of phase, the signal intensity is reduced. This in-phase and out-of-phase process is the chemical shift technique. Benign adrenal cortical adenomas lose signal on out-of-phase images but appear relatively bright on in-phase images.[92] A modification of the chemical shift MRI technique uses gradient echo pulse sequences to produce a similar effect.

Imaging characteristics consistent with a benign cortical adenoma include round and homogeneous density, smooth contour with sharp margination, diameter usually less than 3 cm, unilateral location, low unenhanced CT attenuation values (<10 HU) with rapid contrast medium washout at 10 minutes after administration of contrast medium,[91,93] isointensity with liver on both T1- and T2-weighted MRI sequences, and chemical shift evidence of lipid on MRI (see Table 16-6). The imaging phenotype consistent with pheochromocytoma includes enhancement with intravenous contrast medium on CT (see Fig. 16-3), high signal intensity on T2-weighted MRI (Fig. 16-5), cystic and hemorrhagic changes, and variable size; also, the tumor may be bilateral. Although it has been suggested that patients with apparent simple adrenal cysts do not require hormonal evaluation, pheochromocytoma can mimic an adrenal cyst.

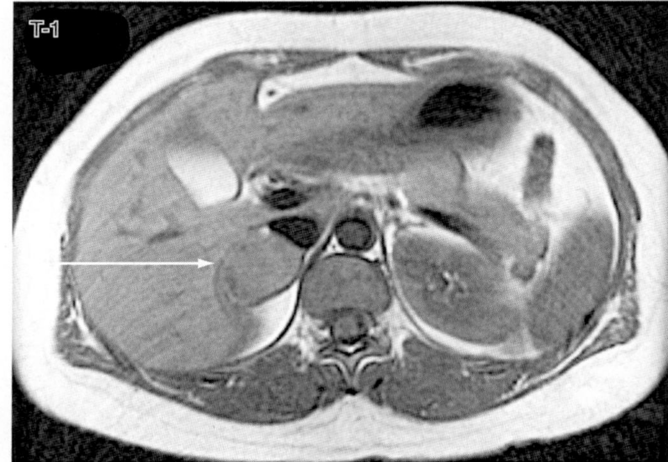

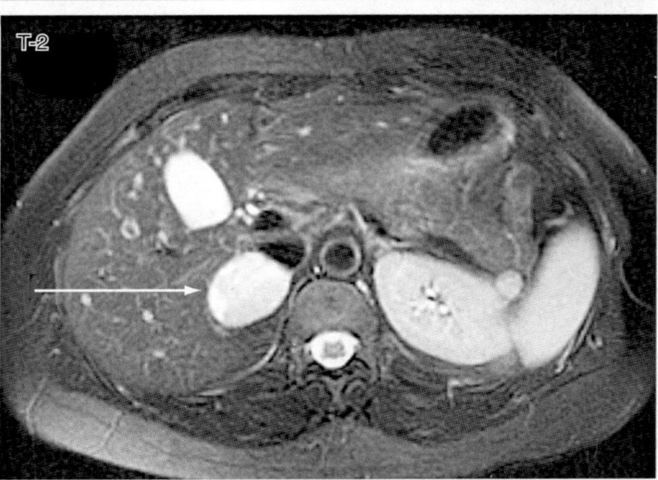

Figure 16-5 Magnetic resonance images of the abdomen of a 34-year-old woman with a recent onset of palpitations and hypertension. She presented with acute left ventricular failure after a single dose of a β-adrenergic blocker. The 24-hour urine test for total metanephrines and catecholamines showed the following: total metanephrines, 3800 μg (normal, <1000); norepinephrine, 37 μg (normal, <170); epinephrine, 7.7 μg (normal, <35); and dopamine, 147 μg (normal, <700). The images show a 3.3 × 3.5 × 4.5-cm, slightly heterogeneous, right adrenal mass consistent with pheochromocytoma *(arrows)* that has increased signal intensity on T2-weighted images *(lower panel)*. After α-adrenergic blockade and restoration of normal left ventricular function, the patient had a laparoscopic adrenalectomy to remove a 5 × 4 × 3 cm, 33-g pheochromocytoma. Postoperatively, the 24-hour urinary excretion of total metanephrines normalized.

^{123}I-MIBG Scintigraphy. If the results of abdominal imaging are negative, scintigraphic localization with ^{123}I-MIBG is indicated (Fig. 16-6). This radiopharmaceutical agent accumulates preferentially in catecholamine-producing tumors; however, this procedure is not as sensitive as was initially hoped (sensitivity, 80%; specificity, 99%).[86-88] ^{123}I-MIBG is superior to ^{131}I-MIBG because the photon energy allows single-photon emission computed tomographic (SPECT) images. Thyroid uptake of ^{123}I should be blocked with the administration of an iodide preparation (e.g., Lugol's solution). In a study of 282 patients with catecholamine-secreting tumors that were surgically confirmed, the overall sensitivity was 89% for CT, 98% for MRI, and 81% for ^{131}I-MIBG.[87] If a typical (<10 cm) unilateral

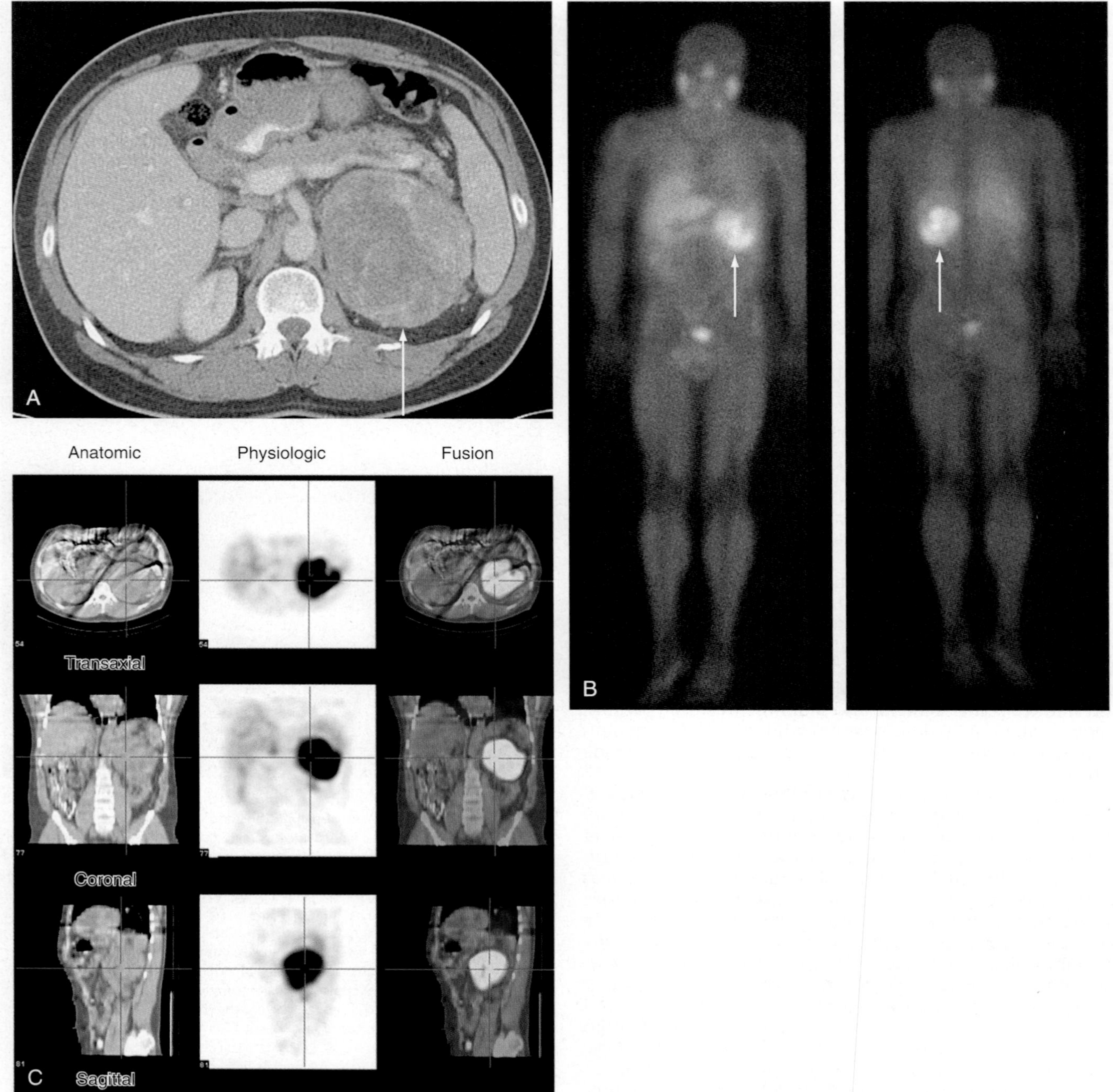

Figure 16-6 Computed tomography (CT) and ^{123}I-metaiodobenzylguanidine (^{123}I-MIBG) imaging from a 44-year-old man. He presented with a 9-year history of hypertension and recent onset of head throbbing, chest pressure, and abdominal pain. The 24-hour urine studies were abnormal: norepinephrine, 900 μg (normal, <170); epinephrine, 28 μg (normal, <35); dopamine, 468 μg (normal, <700); and total metanephrines, 17,958 μg (normal, <1000). **A,** Axial CT image with contrast shows a large, partially vascular and partially necrotic left adrenal tumor *(arrow)*. **B,** ^{123}I-MIBG whole-body scan shows a large focus of increased radiotracer uptake in the left upper abdomen *(arrow)* that corresponds to the mass seen on the CT image; no other abnormal uptake is seen. **C,** ^{123}I-MIBG and single-photon emission computed tomography (SPECT) fusion CT images correlate with the images seen on CT (anatomic) with those seen on ^{123}I-MIBG (physiologic) in the axial, coronal, and sagittal planes. After α- and β-adrenergic blockade, a 13.5 × 12 × 9-cm, 680-g pheochromocytoma was removed.

adrenal pheochromocytoma is found on CT or MRI, ^{123}I-MIBG scintigraphy is superfluous and the results may even confuse the clinician.[94,95] On the other hand, if the adrenal pheochromocytoma is more than 10 cm in diameter or if a paraganglioma is identified on CT or MRI, then ^{123}I-MIBG scintigraphy is indicated, because the patient has increased risk of malignant disease and additional paragangliomas. It is important for the clinician to recognize the medications that may interfere with ^{123}I-MIBG uptake (e.g., tricyclic antidepressants, labetalol, calcium channel blockers) and have the patient discontinue them before imaging is performed (Table 16-7).[96]

TABLE 16-7

Drugs That May Interfere with Metaiodobenzylguanidine (MIBG) Uptake

Uptake-1 Inhibition*
Antiemetics (e.g., prochlorperazine) Antipsychotics (e.g., chlorpromazine, haloperidol) Cocaine Labetalol Phenylpropanolamine Tricyclic antidepressants (e.g., amitriptyline, amoxapine, desipramine, doxepin, imipramine, nortriptyline)
Depletion of Storage Vesicle Contents†
Amphetamines (e.g., dextroamphetamine, fenfluramine, phentermine) Dopamine Labetalol Reserpine Sympathomimetics (e.g., ephedrine, phenylephrine, pseudoephedrine, salbutamol, terbutaline)
Inhibition of Vesicular Monoamine Transporters†
Reserpine
Unknown Mechanism*
Calcium channel blockers (e.g., diltiazem, nicardipine, nifedipine, nimodipine, verapamil)

*Should be stopped at least 48 hr before MIBG administration.
†Should be stopped at least 72 hr before MIBG administration.

Other Localizing Procedures. Localizing procedures that also can be used, but are rarely required, include computer-assisted imaging of the chest, neck, and skull base. Other localizing studies, such as somatostatin receptor imaging with ^{111}In-DTPA-pentetreotide, may also be considered. Although somatostatin receptors are usually expressed in pheochromocytomas and paragangliomas,[97] the sensitivity of somatostatin receptor imaging with ^{111}In-DTPA-pentetreotide is low. Although positron emission tomography (PET) scanning with ^{18}F-fluorodeoxyglucose (FDG) or ^{11}C-hydroxyephedrine or 6-[^{18}F]fluorodopamine can identify paragangliomas,[86,88] these expensive techniques probably should be reserved for identifying sites of metastatic disease in patients with negative ^{123}I-MIBG scintigraphic results. Selective venous sampling for catecholamines is usually misleading and should be avoided.

Treatment

The treatment of choice for pheochromocytoma is complete surgical resection. Surgical survival rates are 98% to 100% and are highly dependent on the skill of the endocrinologist, endocrine surgeon, and anesthesiologist team.[34,98] The most common adverse event after surgery is sustained hypertension. Careful preoperative pharmacologic preparation is crucial for successful treatment.[99] Most catecholamine-secreting tumors are benign and can be totally excised. Tumor excision usually cures hypertension.

Preoperative Management

Some form of preoperative pharmacologic preparation is indicated for all patients with catecholamine-secreting neoplasms. However, no randomized, controlled trials have compared the different approaches. Combined α- and β-adrenergic blockade is one approach to control blood pressure and prevent intraoperative hypertensive crises.[22] α-Adrenergic blockade should be started 7 to 10 days preoperatively to normalize blood pressure and expand the contracted blood volume. A longer duration of preoperative α-adrenergic blockade is indicated for patients with recent myocardial infarction, catecholamine cardiomyopathy, or catecholamine-induced vasculitis. Blood pressure should be monitored with the patient in the seated and standing positions twice daily. Target blood pressure is less than 120/80 mm Hg (seated), with systolic blood pressure greater than 90 mm Hg (standing); both targets should be modified on the basis of the patient's age and comorbid disease. On the second or third day of α-adrenergic blockade, patients are encouraged to start a diet high in sodium content (≥5000 mg/day) because of the catecholamine-induced volume contraction and the orthostasis associated with α-adrenergic blockade. This degree of volume expansion may be contraindicated in patients with congestive heart failure or renal insufficiency. After adequate α-adrenergic blockade has been achieved, β-adrenergic blockade is initiated, typically 2 to 3 days preoperatively.

α-Adrenergic Blockade. Phenoxybenzamine is the preferred drug for preoperative preparation to control blood pressure and arrhythmia. It is an irreversible, long-acting, nonspecific α-adrenergic blocking agent. The initial dosage is 10 mg once or twice daily, and the dose is increased by 10 to 20 mg in divided doses every 2 to 3 days as needed to control blood pressure and spells (Table 16-8). The final dosage of phenoxybenzamine is typically between 20 and 100 mg daily. The patient should be warned about the orthostasis, nasal congestion, and marked fatigue that occur in almost all patients. With their more favorable side effect profiles, selective α_1-adrenergic blocking agents (e.g., prazosin, terazosin, doxazosin) are preferable to phenoxybenzamine when long-term pharmacologic treatment is indicated (e.g., for metastatic pheochromocytoma). However, treatment with these agents is not routinely used preoperatively because of incomplete α-adrenergic blockade.

β-Adrenergic Blockade. The β-adrenergic antagonist should be administered only after α-adrenergic blockade is effective because with β-adrenergic blockade alone, hypertension may be more severe due to the unopposed α-adrenergic stimulation. Preoperative β-adrenergic blockade is indicated to control the tachycardia associated with both the high concentrations of circulating catecholamines and the α-adrenergic blockade. The clinician should exercise caution if the patient is asthmatic or has congestive heart failure. Chronic catecholamine excess can produce a myocardiopathy[30] that may become evident with the initiation of β-adrenergic blockade, resulting in acute pulmonary edema. Therefore, when the β-adrenergic blocker is administered, it should be used cautiously and at a low dose. For example, a patient is usually given 10 mg of propranolol every 6 hours to start. On the second day of treatment, the β-adrenergic blockade (assuming the patient tolerates the drug) is converted to a single long-acting dose. The dose is then increased as necessary to control the tachycardia (goal heart rate is 60-80 beats per minute).

Catecholamine Synthesis Inhibitor. Metyrosine should be used with caution and only after other agents have been ineffective or in patients in whom tumor manipulation or destruction (e.g., radiofrequency ablation of metastatic sites) will be marked. Although some centers advocate that this agent should be used routinely preoperatively, most reserve it primarily for patients who cannot be treated with

TABLE 16-8

Orally Administered Drugs Used to Treat Pheochromocytoma

Drug	Initial Dosage, mg/day* (Maximum)	Side Effects
α-Adrenergic Blocking Agents		
Phenoxybenzamine	10† (100)†	Postural hypotension, tachycardia, miosis, nasal congestion, diarrhea, inhibition of ejaculation, fatigue
Prazosin	1 (20)‡	First-dose effect, dizziness, drowsiness, headache, fatigue, palpitations, nausea
Terazosin	1 (20)†	First-dose effect, asthenia, blurred vision, dizziness, nasal congestion, nausea, peripheral edema, palpitations, somnolence
Doxazosin	1 (20)	First-dose effect, orthostasis, peripheral edema, fatigue, somnolence
Combined α- and β-Adrenergic Blocking Agent		
Labetalol	200† (1200)†	Dizziness, fatigue, nausea, nasal congestion, impotence
Calcium Channel Blocker		
Nicardipine sustained-release	30† (120)†	Edema, dizziness, headache, flushing, nausea, dyspepsia
Catecholamine Synthesis Inhibitor		
α-Methyl-ρ-L tyrosine (metyrosine)	1000‡ (4000)‡	Sedation, diarrhea, anxiety, nightmares, crystalluria, galactorrhea, extrapyramidal symptoms

*Given once daily unless otherwise indicated.
†Given in two doses daily.
‡Given in three or four doses daily.

the typical combined α- and β-adrenergic blockade protocol for cardiopulmonary reasons. Metyrosine inhibits catecholamine synthesis by blocking the enzyme tyrosine hydroxylase.[100] The side effects of metyrosine can be disabling; with long-term therapy, they include sedation, depression, diarrhea, anxiety, nightmares, crystalluria and urolithiasis, galactorrhea, and extrapyramidal signs. Metyrosine may be added to α- and β-adrenergic blockade if the resection will be difficult (e.g., malignant paraganglioma) or if destructive therapy is planned (e.g., radiofrequency ablation of hepatic metastases). Our typical protocol with short-term preprocedure preparation is to start with metyrosine 250 mg every 6 hours on day 1, 500 mg every 6 hours on day 2, 750 mg every 6 hours on day 3, and 1000 mg every 6 hours on the day before the procedure, with the last dose (1000 mg) given on the morning of the procedure. With this short-course therapy, the main side effect is hypersomnolence.

Calcium Channel Blockers. Calcium channel blockers, which block norepinephrine-mediated calcium transport into vascular smooth muscle, have been used successfully at several medical centers to preoperatively prepare patients with pheochromocytoma.[101-103] Nicardipine is the most commonly used calcium channel blocker in this setting; the starting dose is 30 mg twice daily of the sustained-release preparation (see Table 16-8). It is given orally to control blood pressure preoperatively and is given as an intravenous infusion intraoperatively (Table 16-9). Although there is less collective experience with calcium channel blockers than with α- and β-adrenergic blockers, when calcium channel blockers are used as the primary mode of antihypertensive therapy, they may be just as effective.[101,102] Clearly, the exclusive use of calcium channel blockers for the perioperative management of patients with catecholamine-secreting tumors does not prevent all hemodynamic changes; however, its use has been associated with low morbidity and mortality.[102] The main role for this class of drugs may be either to supplement the combined α- and β-adrenergic blockade protocol when blood pressure control is inadequate or to replace the adrenergic blockade protocol in patients with intolerable side effects.

Acute Hypertensive Crises

Acute hypertensive crises may occur before or during an operation, and they should be treated with intravenously administered sodium nitroprusside, phentolamine, or nicardipine (see Table 16-9). Sodium nitroprusside is an ideal

TABLE 16-9

Intravenously Administered Drugs Used to Treat Pheochromocytoma

Agent	Dosage Range
For Hypertension	
Phentolamine	Administer a 1-mg IV test dose, then 2- to 5-mg IV boluses as needed or continuous infusion.
Nitroprusside	IV infusion rates of 2 μg/kg of body weight per minute are suggested as safe. Rates >4 μg/kg per minute may lead to cyanide toxicity within 3 hr. Doses >10 μg/kg per minute are rarely required, and the maximal dose should not exceed 800 μg/min.
Nicardipine	Initiate therapy at 5.0 mg/hr; the IV infusion rate may be increased by 2.5 mg/hr q15 min up to a maximum of 15.0 mg/hr.
For Cardiac Arrhythmia	
Lidocaine	Initiate therapy with an IV bolus of 1-1.5 mg/kg (75-100 mg); additional boluses of 0.5-0.75 mg/kg (25-50 mg) can be given q5-10 min if needed up to a maximum of 3 mg/kg. Loading is followed by maintenance IV infusion of 2-4 mg/min (30-50 μg/kg per minute) adjusted for effect and settings of altered metabolism (e.g., heart failure, liver congestion) and as guided by blood level monitoring.
Esmolol	An initial IV loading dose of 0.5 mg/kg is infused over 1 min, followed by a maintenance infusion of 0.05 mg/kg per minute for the next 4 min. Depending on the desired ventricular response, the maintenance infusion may then be continued at 0.05 mg/kg per minute or increased stepwise (e.g., by 0.1 mg/kg per minute increments to a maximum of 0.2 mg/kg per minute), with each step being maintained for ≥4 min.

vasodilator for intraoperative management of hypertensive episodes because of its rapid onset of action and short duration of effect. It is administered as an intravenous infusion at 0.5 to 5.0 μg/kg of body weight per minute and adjusted every few minutes for target blood pressure response; to keep the steady-state thiocyanate concentration below 1 mmol/L, the rate of a prolonged infusion should be no more than 3 μg/kg per minute. Phentolamine is a short-acting, nonselective α-adrenergic blocker that is available in lyophilized form in 5-mg vials. An initial test dose of 1 mg is administered and is followed, if necessary, by repeat 5-mg boluses or continuous infusion. The response to phentolamine is maximal 2 to 3 minutes after a bolus injection and lasts 10 to 15 minutes. Nicardipine can be started at an infusion rate of 5 mg/hour and titrated for blood pressure control (the infusion rate may be increased by 2.5 mg/hour every 15 minutes up to a maximum of 15.0 mg/hour) (see Table 16-9).

Anesthesia and Surgery

Surgical resection of a catecholamine-secreting tumor is a high-risk surgical procedure, and an experienced surgeon-anesthesiologist team is required. The last oral doses of α- and β-adrenergic blockers can be administered early in the morning on the day of the operation. Fentanyl, ketamine, and morphine should be avoided, because they potentially can stimulate catecholamine release from a pheochromocytoma.[103] Also, parasympathetic nervous system blockade with atropine should be avoided because of the associated tachycardia. Anesthesia may be induced with intravenous injection of propofol, etomidate, or barbiturates in combination with synthetic opioids.[103] Most anesthetic gases can be used, but halothane and desflurane should be avoided. Cardiovascular and hemodynamic variables must be monitored closely. Continuous measurement of intra-arterial pressure and heart rhythm is required. If the patient has congestive heart failure or decreased cardiac reserve, monitoring of pulmonary capillary wedge pressure is indicated. The preoperative and perioperative treatment approach outlined here is the same for adults and children.[104,105]

In the past, an anterior midline abdominal surgical approach was typically used for resecting adrenal pheochromocytoma. However, the laparoscopic approach to the adrenal gland is currently the procedure of choice for patients with solitary intra-adrenal pheochromocytomas smaller than 8 cm in diameter.[106] In a series of 39 patients with pheochromocytoma who had laparoscopic adrenalectomy, the mean hospitalization was 1.7 days,[107] as opposed to the typical 5 to 7 days for open laparotomy. If the pheochromocytoma is in the adrenal gland, the entire gland should be removed. Laparoscopic adrenalectomy for pheochromocytoma should be converted to open adrenalectomy in cases of difficult dissection, invasion, adhesions, or surgeon inexperience.[108] If the tumor is malignant, as much of the tumor should be removed as possible. If a bilateral adrenalectomy is planned preoperatively, the patient should receive glucocorticoid stress coverage while awaiting transfer to the operating room. In addition, glucocorticoid coverage should be initiated in the operating room if unexpected bilateral adrenalectomy is necessary. Cortical-sparing bilateral adrenalectomies have been used to treat patients with VHL disease.

An anterior midline abdominal surgical approach is indicated for abdominal paragangliomas. The midline abdomen should be inspected carefully. Paragangliomas of the neck, chest, and urinary bladder require specialized approaches. "Unresectable" cardiac pheochromocytomas may require cardiac transplantation.

Hypotension may occur during and after surgical resection of the pheochromocytoma, and it should be treated with fluids and colloids and then intravenous pressor agents if necessary. Postoperative hypotension occurs less frequently in patients who have had adequate preoperative α-adrenergic blockade and volume expansion. If both adrenal glands were manipulated during surgery, adrenocortical insufficiency should be considered as a potential cause of postoperative hypotension. Because hypoglycemia can occur in the immediate postoperative period, blood glucose levels should be monitored, and fluid given intravenously should contain 5% dextrose. Blood pressure is usually normal by the time of hospital discharge. Some patients remain hypertensive for up to 4 to 8 weeks postoperatively. Long-standing, persistent hypertension does occur and may be related to accidental ligation of a polar renal artery, resetting of baroreceptors, hemodynamic changes, structural changes of the blood vessels, altered sensitivity of the vessels to pressor substances, functional or structural renal changes, or coincident primary hypertension.

Long-Term Postoperative Follow-Up

Approximately 1 to 2 weeks after surgery, fractionated catecholamines and metanephrines should be measured by collection of a 24-hour urine specimen. If the levels are normal, the resection of the pheochromocytoma should be considered complete. The survival rate after removal of a benign pheochromocytoma is almost equal to that of age- and sex-matched normal controls. Increased levels of catecholamines and metanephrines detected postoperatively are consistent with residual tumor (i.e., a second primary lesion or occult metastases). If bilateral adrenalectomy was performed, lifelong glucocorticoid and mineralocorticoid replacement therapy is prescribed. The 24-hour urinary excretion of fractionated catecholamines and metanephrines or plasma fractionated metanephrines should be checked annually for life. Annual biochemical testing assesses for metastatic disease, tumor recurrence in the adrenal bed, and delayed appearance of multiple primary tumors. Recurrence rates are highest for patients with familial disease, right-sided adrenal pheochromocytoma, or paraganglioma.[109] Follow-up CT or MRI is not needed unless metanephrine or catecholamine levels become elevated or the original tumor was associated with minimal catecholamine excess.

Genetic testing should be considered for patients with one or more of the following: a family history of pheochromocytoma; paraganglioma; and any sign that suggests a genetic cause, such as retinal angiomas, axillary freckling, café au lait spots, cerebellar tumor, MTC, or hyperparathyroidism. In addition, all first-degree relatives of a patient with pheochromocytoma or paraganglioma should have biochemical testing (e.g., 24-hour urine for fractionated metanephrines and catecholamines). If mutation testing in a patient is positive, first-degree relatives (the patient's parents, siblings, and children) should be offered genetic testing.

Malignant Pheochromocytoma and Paraganglioma

Distinguishing between benign and malignant catecholamine-secreting tumors is difficult on the basis of clinical, biochemical, or histopathologic characteristics. Malignancy is rare in patients with MEN2 or VHL syndrome, but it is common in those with familial paraganglioma caused by mutations in *SDHB*. Patients with *SDHB* mutations are more likely to develop malignant disease and nonparaganglioma neoplasms (e.g., renal cell carcinoma).[54,57,58] Although the 5-year survival rate for patients with malignant pheochromocytoma is less than 50%, the prognosis is variable: approximately 50% of patients have an indolent form of the disease, with a life expectancy of more than 20 years, and the other half have rapidly progressive disease, with death occurring within 1 to 3 years after diagnosis. The clinician should first assess the pace of the malignant disease and then target the level of therapy to the aggressiveness of tumor behavior. A multimodality, multidisciplinary, individualized approach is indicated to control catecholamine-dependent symptoms, local mass effect symptoms from the tumor, and overall tumor burden. Long-term pharmacologic therapy for the patient with metastatic pheochromocytoma is similar to that outlined for preoperative preparation in a patient with a catecholamine-secreting tumor.

Metastatic sites include local tissue invasion, liver, bone, lung, omemtum, and lymph nodes. Metastatic lesions should be resected, if possible, to decrease tumor burden. Skeletal metastatic lesions that are painful or threaten structural function can be treated with external radiotherapy or cryoablation or approached surgically. Thrombotic therapy for large, unresectable liver metastases and radiofrequency ablation for small liver metastases are options to be considered. In selected cases, long-acting octreotide has been beneficial. Because of the risk of massive catecholamine release, ablative therapy should be performed with great caution and only at centers with experience with these techniques; in addition to α- and β-adrenergic blockade, these patients are usually treated with metyrosine before the procedure. External radiotherapy can also be used to treat unresectable soft tissue lesions.

Local tumor irradiation with therapeutic doses of ^{131}I-MIBG has produced partial and temporary responses in approximately one third of patients.[7,8,110] If the tumor is considered aggressive and the patient's quality of life is affected, combination chemotherapy may be considered. In a nonrandomized, single-arm trial, the efficacy of chemotherapy with a combination CVD protocol (cyclophosphamide, 750 mg/m^2 body surface area on day 1; vincristine, 1.4 mg/m^2 on day 1; and dacarbazine 600 mg/m^2 on days 1 and 2; repeated every 21 days) was studied in 14 patients with malignant pheochromocytoma.[111,112] This protocol produced a complete and partial response rate of 57% (median duration, 21 months; range, 7 to >34). Complete and partial biochemical responses were seen in 79% of patients (median duration, >22 months; range, 6 to >35 months). All responding patients had objective improvement in performance status and blood pressure. CVD chemotherapy can be continued until the patient develops new lesions or there is a significant (e.g., >25%) increase in size of known tumor sites. Because CVD chemotherapy may induce massive catecholamine release, it is important that the patient be optimally α- and β-blocked, just as for surgery. In addition, the first cycle of CVD should be completed in the hospital and with close medical observation. Management of malignant pheochromocytoma can be frustrating because curative options are limited. Recent preliminary studies suggest that tyrosine kinase inhibitors (e.g., sunitinib) may have a role in the treatment of metastatic pheochromocytoma.[113]

Pheochromocytoma in Pregnancy

Pheochromocytoma in pregnancy can cause the death of both the fetus and the mother. The approach to the biochemical diagnosis is the same as for the nonpregnant patient. MRI (without gadolinium enhancement) is the preferred imaging modality, and ^{123}I-MIBG is contraindicated. The treatment of hypertensive crises is the same as for nonpregnant patients except that use of nitroprusside should be avoided. Although the most appropriate management is debated,[114] adrenal pheochromocytomas should be removed promptly if diagnosed during the first or second trimester of pregnancy. The preoperative preparation is the same as for a nonpregnant patient. If the pregnancy is already in the third trimester, a single operation is recommended, to perform a cesarean section and remove the adrenal pheochromocytoma at the same time. Spontaneous labor and delivery should be avoided. The management of catecholamine-secreting paragangliomas in pregnancy may require modification of these guidelines depending on tumor location.

RENIN-ANGIOTENSIN-ALDOSTERONE SYSTEM

The components of the renin-angiotensin-aldosterone (RAA) system are shown in Figure 16-7.[115] Aldosterone is secreted from the zona glomerulosa under the control of three primary factors: angiotensin II, potassium, and ACTH. The secretion of aldosterone is restricted to the zona glomerulosa because of zone-specific expression of aldosterone synthase (CYP11B2) (see Chapter 15). Dopamine, atrial natriuretic peptide, and heparin inhibit aldosterone secretion.

Renin and Angiotensin

Renin is an enzyme that is produced primarily in the juxtaglomerular apparatus of the kidney; it is stored in granules and released in response to specific secretagogues. The

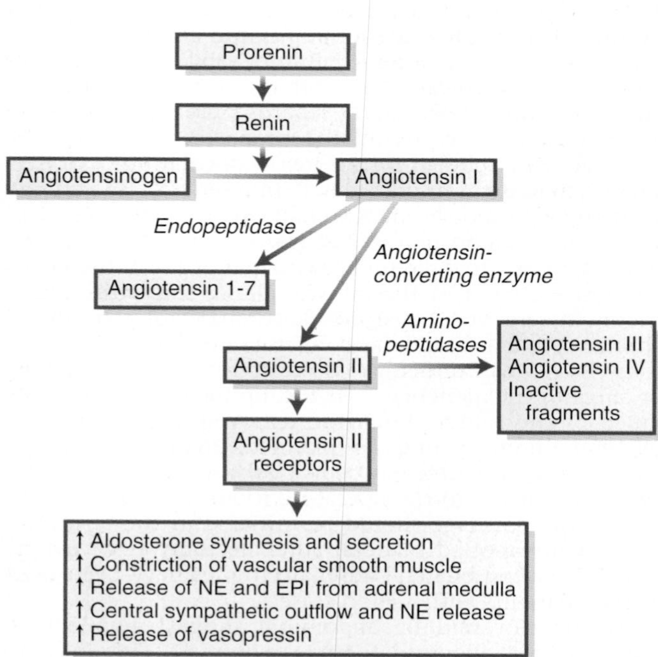

Figure 16-7 Components of the renin-angiotensin system. EPI, epinephrine; NE, norepinephrine. (Adapted and redrawn from Williams GH, Chao J, Chao L. Kidney hormones. In: Conn PM, Melmed S, eds. *Endocrinology: Basic and Clinical Principles*. Totowa, NJ, Humana Press, 1997:393-404.)

protein consists of 340 amino acids, of which the first 43 are a prosegment that is cleaved to produce the active enzyme. The release of renin into the circulation is the rate-limiting step in the RAA system. Renal renin release is controlled by four factors:

1. The macula densa, a specialized group of convoluted distal tubular cells that function as chemoreceptors for monitoring the sodium and chloride loads present in the distal tubule
2. Juxtaglomerular cells acting as pressure transducers that sense stretch of the afferent arteriolar wall and thus renal perfusion pressure
3. The sympathetic nervous system, which modifies the release of renin, particularly in response to upright posture
4. Humoral factors, including potassium, angiotensin II, and atrial natriuretic peptides

Renin release is maximized in conditions of low renal perfusion pressure or low tubular sodium content (e.g., renal artery stenosis, hemorrhage, dehydration). Renin release is suppressed by elevated perfusion pressure at the kidney (e.g., hypertension) and a high-sodium diet. Renin release is increased directly by hypokalemia and decreased by hyperkalemia.

Angiotensinogen, an α_2-globulin synthesized in the liver, is the only known substrate for renin and is broken down into the angiotensin peptides. The protein consists of 485 amino acids, 33 of which constitute a presegment that is cleaved after secretion. The action of renin on angiotensinogen produces angiotensin I. Angiotensin I comprises the first 10-amino-acid sequence after the presegment and does not appear to have biologic activity. Angiotensin II, the main biologically active angiotensin, is created by cleavage of the two carboxyl-terminal peptides of angiotensin I by angiotensin-converting enzyme (ACE) (see Fig. 16-7). ACE is localized to cell membranes in the lung and intracellular granules in certain tissues that produce angiotensin II. Amino peptidase A can remove the amino-terminal aspartic acid to produce the heptapeptide, angiotensin III. Angiotensin II and angiotensin III have equivalent efficacy in promoting aldosterone secretion and modifying renal blood flow. The half-life in the circulation of angiotensin II is short (<60 seconds). Elements of the RAA system are present in the adrenals, kidneys, heart, and brain. For example, the adrenal glomerulosa cells contain the proteins needed to produce and secrete angiotensin II. Other tissues contain one or more components of the system but require other cells or circulating components, or both, to generate angiotensin II.

Angiotensin II functions through the angiotensin receptor to maintain normal extracellular volume and blood pressure by (1) increasing aldosterone secretion from the zona glomerulosa via increased transcription of CYP11B2; (2) constricting vascular smooth muscle, thereby increasing blood pressure and reducing renal blood flow; (3) releasing norepinephrine and epinephrine from the adrenal medulla; (4) enhancing the activity of the sympathetic nervous system by increasing central sympathetic outflow, thereby increasing norepinephrine discharge from sympathetic nerve terminals; and (5) promoting the release of vasopressin.

Aldosterone

Approximately 50% to 70% of aldosterone circulates bound to albumin or weakly bound to corticosteroid-binding globulin; 30% to 50% of total plasma aldosterone is free. The half-life is relatively short at 15 to 20 minutes. In the liver, aldosterone is rapidly inactivated to tetrahydroaldosterone. The classic functions of aldosterone are regulation of extracellular volume and control of potassium homeostasis. These effects are mediated by the binding of free aldosterone to the mineralocorticoid receptor in the cytosol of epithelial cells, principally in the kidney.

Mineralocorticoid receptors have tissue-specific expression. For example, the tissues with the highest concentrations of these receptors are the distal nephron, colon, and hippocampus. Lower levels of mineralocorticoid receptors are found in the rest of the gastrointestinal tract and heart. Transport to the nucleus and binding to specific binding domains on targeted genes leads to their increased expression. Aldosterone-regulated kinase appears to be a key intermediary, and its increased expression leads to modification of the apical sodium channel, resulting in increased sodium ion transport across the cell membrane (see Chapter 15). The increased luminal negativity augments tubular secretion of potassium by the tubular cells and of hydrogen ion by the interstitial cells.

Glucocorticoids and mineralocorticoids bind equally to the mineralocorticoid receptor. Specificity of action is provided in many tissues by the presence of a glucocorticoid-inactivating enzyme, 11β-hydroxysteroid dehydrogenase, which prevents glucocorticoids from interacting with the receptor (see Chapter 15). Mineralocorticoid "escape" refers to the counterregulatory mechanisms that are manifested after 3 to 5 days of excessive mineralocorticoid administration. Several mechanisms contribute to this escape, including renal hemodynamic factors and increased levels of atrial natriuretic peptide.

In addition to the classic genomic actions mediated by aldosterone binding to cytosolic receptors, mineralocorticoids have acute, nongenomic actions resulting from activation of an unidentified cell surface receptor. This action involves a G protein signaling pathway and probably a modification of the sodium-hydrogen exchange activity. This effect has been demonstrated in both epithelial and nonepithelial cells.[116]

Aldosterone has additional, nonclassic effects primarily on nonepithelial cells.[117] These actions, although probably genomic and therefore mediated by activation of the cytosolic mineralocorticoid receptor, do not include modification of sodium-potassium balance. Aldosterone-mediated actions include the expression of several collagen genes; genes controlling tissue growth factors (e.g., transforming growth factor-β, plasminogen activator inhibitor type 1); and genes mediating inflammation.[118] The resultant actions lead to microangiopathy, necrosis (acutely), and fibrosis in various tissues such as the heart, the vasculature, and the kidney.[117] Increased levels of aldosterone are not necessary to cause this damage; an imbalance between the volume or sodium balance state and the level of aldosterone appears to be the critical factor.[117]

The action of angiotensin II on aldosterone involves a negative feedback loop that also includes extracellular fluid volume (Fig. 16-8).[119] The major function of this feedback loop is to modify sodium homeostasis and, secondarily, to regulate blood pressure. Sodium restriction activates the RAA axis. The effects of angiotensin II on both the adrenal cortex and the renal vasculature promote renal sodium conservation. On the other hand, with suppression of renin release and suppression of the level of circulating angiotensin, aldosterone secretion is reduced and renal blood flow is increased, promoting sodium loss. The RAA loop is very sensitive to dietary sodium intake. Sodium excess enhances the responsiveness of the renal and

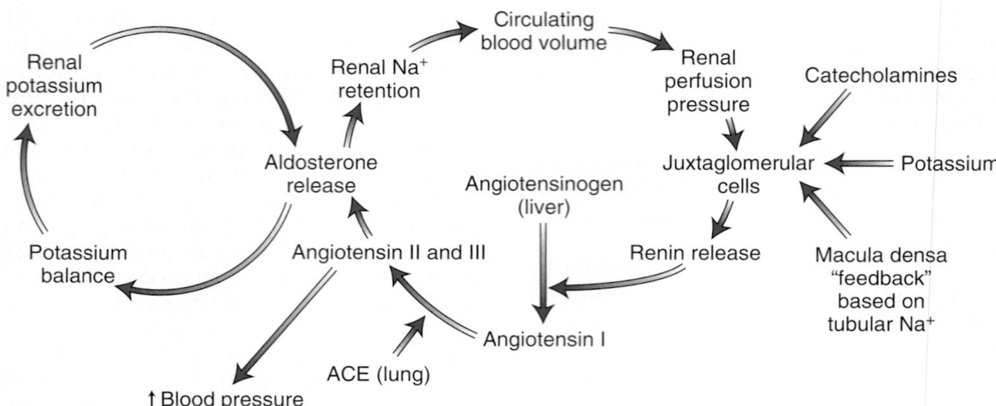

Figure 16-8 Renin-angiotensin-aldosterone and potassium-aldosterone negative feedback loops. Aldosterone production is determined by input from each loop. ACE, angiotensin-converting enzyme; BP, blood pressure; Na^+, sodium. (Adapted and redrawn from Williams GH, Dluhy RG. Diseases of the adrenal cortex. In: Braunwald E, Fauci AD, Kasper D, et al., eds. *Harrison's Principles of Internal Medicine*, 15th ed. New York, NY: McGraw-Hill, 2001:2087.)

peripheral vasculature and reduces the adrenal responsiveness to angiotensin II. Sodium restriction has the opposite effect. Therefore, sodium intake modifies target tissue responsiveness to angiotensin II, a fine-tuning mechanism that appears to be critical to maintaining normal sodium homeostasis without a chronic effect on blood pressure.

Excess aldosterone secretion causes hypertension through two main mechanisms: mineralocorticoid-induced expansion of plasma and extracellular fluid volume and increased total peripheral vascular resistance.

PRIMARY ALDOSTERONISM

Hypertension, suppressed plasma renin activity (PRA), and increased aldosterone excretion characterize the syndrome of primary aldosteronism, first described in 1955.[120] Aldosterone-producing adenoma (APA) and bilateral idiopathic hyperaldosteronism (IHA) are the most common subtypes of primary aldosteronism (Table 16-10). A much less common form, unilateral hyperplasia or primary adrenal hyperplasia (PAH), is caused by micronodular or macronodular hyperplasia of the zona glomerulosa of predominantly one adrenal gland. Familial hyperaldosteronism (FH) is also rare, and two types have been described. FH type I, or glucocorticoid-remediable aldosteronism (GRA), is autosomal dominant in inheritance and is associated with variable degrees of hyperaldosteronism, high levels of hybrid steroids (e.g., 18-hydroxycortisol, 18-oxocortisol), and suppression with exogenous glucocorticoids.[121] FH type II refers to the familial occurrence of APA or IHA or both.[122]

History

In his presidential address at the annual meeting of the Central Society for Clinical Research, Chicago, Illinois, October, 29, 1954, Dr. Jerome W. Conn stated[120]: "I have prepared no comprehensive review of my personal philosophy of clinical investigation. Instead, I plan to make a scientific report to you about a clinical syndrome, the investigation of which has been most exciting to me since I initiated it in April of this year." Conn, a Professor of Medicine at the University of Michigan, had been active in government-funded research on the mechanisms of human acclimatization to humid heat. He established that the body's acclimatization response was to rapidly diminish renal salt and water loss and to abruptly curtail the salt content of body sweat and saliva. He suggested that these responses were the result of increased adrenocortical

TABLE 16-10

Adrenocortical Causes of Hypertension
Low Renin and High Aldosterone
Primary Aldosteronism
Aldosterone-producing adenoma (APA)—35% of cases
Bilateral idiopathic hyperplasia (IHA)—60% of cases
Primary (unilateral) adrenal hyperplasia—2% of cases
Aldosterone-producing adrenocortical carcinoma—<1% of cases
Familial hyperaldosteronism (FH)
Glucocorticoid-remediable aldosteronism (FH type I)—<1% of cases
FH type II (APA or IHA)—<2% of cases
Ectopic aldosterone-producing adenoma or carcinoma—<0.1% of cases
Low Renin and Low Aldosterone
Hyperdeoxycorticosteronism
Congenital adrenal hyperplasia
11β-Hydroxylase deficiency
17α-Hydroxylase deficiency
Deoxycorticosterone-producing tumor
Primary cortisol resistance
Apparent mineralocorticoid excess (AME)/11β-HSD deficiency
Genetic
Type 1 AME
Acquired
Licorice or carbenoxolone ingestion (type 1 AME)
Cushing's syndrome (type 2 AME)
Cushing's Syndrome
Exogenous glucocorticoid administration—most common cause
Endogenous
ACTH-dependent—85% of cases
Pituitary
Ectopic
ACTH-independent—15% of cases
Unilateral adrenal disease (adenoma or carcinoma)
Bilateral adrenal disease
Massive macronodular hyperplasia (rare)
Primary pigmented nodular adrenal disease (rare)

ACTH, corticotropin; HSD, hydroxysteroid dehydrogenase.

function with elaboration of salt-retaining steroids. He also showed that intramuscular administration of deoxycorticosterone acetate (DOCA) produced similar changes in the electrolyte composition of urine, sweat, and saliva.

In April 1954, Professor Conn was asked to see M.W., a 34-year-old woman with a 7-year history of muscle spasms, temporary paralysis, tetany, and weakness and a 4-year history of hypertension. She was found to have a blood pressure of 176/104 mm Hg, severe hypokalemia (1.6 to 2.5 mEq/L), mild hypernatremia (146 to 151 mEq/L), and alkalosis (serum pH, 7.62). Because there were no signs or symptoms of glucocorticoid or androgen excess, Conn suspected, based on his past research, that M.W.'s clinical presentation could result from excess secretion of the adrenal salt-retaining corticoid. Conn studied M.W. in the Metabolism Research Unit for 227 days. Streeten's bioassay technique developed to measure sodium retention in adrenalectomized rats after intraperitoneal injection of human urine was used, and M.W. averaged 1333 µg DOCA equivalent per day, compared with normotensive controls at 61.4 µg/day. In his presidential address, Conn stated: "It is believed that these studies delineate a new clinical syndrome which is designated temporarily as primary aldosteronism." (Note: the word "temporarily" was used because aldosterone was yet to be measured in any human bodily fluid.)[120]

Conn planned for a bilateral adrenalectomy for his patient on December 10, 1954. In 1995, Gittler and Fajans described the surgical scene[123]: "To the immense delight of Conn and those in the operating room, the surgeon, Dr. William Baum, encountered a right 13-g adrenal tumor which was removed while leaving the contralateral gland intact. The patient's postoperative studies showed an almost total reversal of the preoperative metabolic and clinical abnormalities. Conn had achieved irrefutable proof of the validity of his investigative conclusions and established for the first time the relationship among adrenal aldosterone-producing tumors, hypertension, and hypokalemia. A new era had arrived in the study of hypertension and adrenal mineralocorticoids."

By 1964, Conn had collected 145 cases,[124] and he suggested that up to 20% of patients with essential hypertension might have primary aldosteronism.[125] This suggestion was downplayed by most as a gross overestimate.[126,127] Later, Conn decreased his predicted prevalence of primary aldosteronism to 10% of hypertensives,[128] a prediction that was substantiated nearly 40 years later.

Prevalence

In the past, clinicians would not consider the diagnosis of primary aldosteronism unless the patient presented with spontaneous hypokalemia, and then the diagnostic evaluation would require discontinuation of antihypertensive medications for at least 2 weeks. This diagnostic approach resulted in predicted prevalence rates of less than 0.5% of hypertensive patients.[126,127,129-133] However, it is now recognized that most patients with primary aldosteronism are not hypokalemic[134,135] and that screening can be completed while the patient is taking antihypertensive drugs with a simple blood test that yields the ratio of plasma aldosterone concentration (PAC) to PRA.[136-139] Use of the PAC/PRA ratio as a case-detection test, followed by aldosterone suppression for confirmatory testing, has resulted in much higher prevalence estimates for primary aldosteronism—5% to 10% of all patients with hypertension.[139-145]

Clinical Presentation

The diagnosis of primary aldosteronism is usually made in patients who are in the third to sixth decade of life. Few symptoms are specific to the syndrome. Patients with marked hypokalemia may have muscle weakness and cramping, headaches, palpitations, polydipsia, polyuria, nocturia, or a combination of these. Periodic paralysis is a very rare presentation in Caucasians, but it is not an infrequent presentation in patients of Asian decent.[146] For example, in a series of 50 patients with APA reported from Hong Kong, 21 (42%) presented with periodic paralysis.[146] Another rare presentation is tetany associated with the decrease in ionized calcium with marked hypokalemic alkalosis. The polyuria and nocturia are a result of hypokalemia-induced renal concentrating defect, and the presentation is frequently mistaken for prostatism in men. There are no specific physical findings. Edema is not a common finding because of the phenomenon of mineralocorticoid escape, described earlier. The degree of hypertension is typically moderate to severe and may be resistant to usual pharmacologic treatments.[134,147] In the first 262 cases of primary aldosteronism diagnosed at Mayo Clinic (1957-1986), the highest blood pressure was 260/155 mm Hg; the mean (± SD) was 184/112 ± 28/16 mm Hg.[147] Patients with APA tend to have higher blood pressures than those with IHA.[148] Hypokalemia is frequently absent, so all patients with hypertension are candidates for this disorder. In other patients, the hypokalemia becomes evident only with the addition of a potassium-wasting diuretic (e.g., hydrochlorothiazide, furosemide). Deep-seated renal cysts are found in up to 60% of patients with chronic hypokalemia.[149] Because of a reset osmostat, the serum sodium concentration tends to be high-normal or slightly above the upper limit of normal. This clinical clue is very useful in the initial assessment for potential primary aldosteronism.

Several studies have shown that patients with primary aldosteronism are at higher risk than other patients with hypertension for target-organ damage of the heart and kidney.[150,151] When matched for age, blood pressure, and duration of hypertension, patients with primary aldosteronism have greater left ventricular mass measurements than patients with other types of hypertension (e.g., pheochromocytoma, Cushing's syndrome, essential hypertension).[152] In patients with APA, the left ventricular wall thickness and mass were markedly decreased 1 year after adrenalectomy.[153] A case-control study of 124 patients with primary aldosteronism and 465 patients with essential hypertension (matched for age, sex, and systolic and diastolic blood pressure) found that patients presenting with either APA or IHA had a significantly higher rate of cardiovascular events (e.g., stroke, atrial fibrillation, myocardial infarction) than the matched patients with essential hypertension.[151] A negative effect of circulating aldosterone on cardiac function was found in young nonhypertensive subjects with GRA who had increased left ventricular wall thickness and reduced diastolic function compared with age- and sex-matched controls.[150]

Diagnosis

The diagnostic approach to primary aldosteronism can be considered in three phases: case-detection tests, confirmatory tests, and subtype evaluation tests.

Case-Detection Tests

Spontaneous hypokalemia is uncommon in patients with uncomplicated hypertension; when present, it strongly

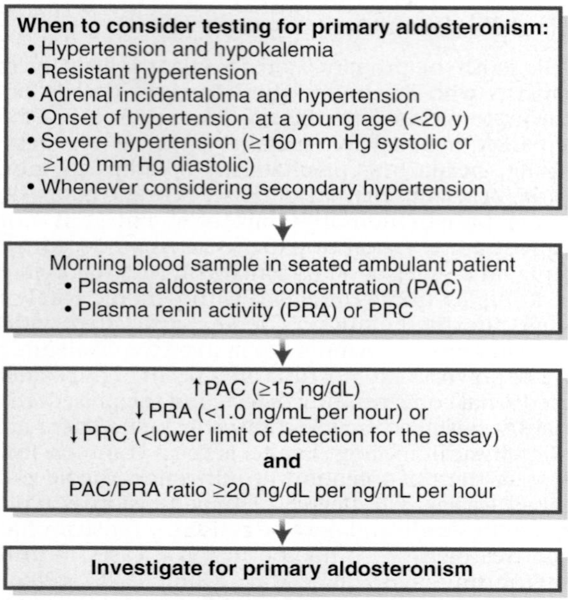

When to consider testing for primary aldosteronism:
- Hypertension and hypokalemia
- Resistant hypertension
- Adrenal incidentaloma and hypertension
- Onset of hypertension at a young age (<20 y)
- Severe hypertension (≥160 mm Hg systolic or ≥100 mm Hg diastolic)
- Whenever considering secondary hypertension

↓

Morning blood sample in seated ambulant patient
- Plasma aldosterone concentration (PAC)
- Plasma renin activity (PRA) or PRC

↓

↑PAC (≥15 ng/dL)
↓PRA (<1.0 ng/mL per hour) or
↓PRC (<lower limit of detection for the assay)
and
PAC/PRA ratio ≥20 ng/dL per ng/mL per hour

↓

Investigate for primary aldosteronism

Figure 16-9 Algorithm provides guidance on when to consider testing for primary aldosteronism and use of the ratio of plasma aldosterone concentration (PAC) to plasma renin activity (PRA) as a case-detection tool. PRC, plasma renin concentration.

suggests associated mineralocorticoid excess. However, several studies have shown that most patients with primary aldosteronism have baseline serum levels of potassium in the normal range.[134,139,154-156] Therefore, hypokalemia should not be the criterion used to trigger case detection testing for primary aldosteronism. Patients with hypertension and hypokalemia (regardless of presumed cause), treatment-resistant hypertension (poor control on three antihypertensive drugs), severe hypertension (≥160 mm Hg systolic or ≥100 mm Hg diastolic), hypertension and an incidental adrenal mass, or onset of hypertension at a young age should undergo screening for primary aldosteronism (Fig. 16-9).[134,135] In addition, patients should be screened for primary aldosteronism whenever a secondary hypertension evaluation is being considered, such as when a patient lacks a family history of hypertension or is being tested for renovascular disease or pheochromocytoma.

In patients with suspected primary aldosteronism, screening can be accomplished (see Fig. 16-9) by paired measurements of PAC and PRA in a random morning ambulatory blood sample (preferably obtained between 8 and 10 a.m.). This test may be performed while the patient is taking antihypertensive medications (with some exceptions, discussed later) and without posture stimulation.[134,135,138,139,157,158] Hypokalemia reduces the secretion of aldosterone, and it is optimal to restore the serum level of potassium to normal before performing diagnostic studies. Mineralocorticoid receptor antagonists (e.g., spironolactone, eplerenone) are the only medications that absolutely interfere with interpretation of the ratio and must be discontinued at least 6 weeks before testing. ACE inhibitors and angiotensin receptor blockers (ARBs) have the potential to falsely elevate the PRA. Therefore, the finding of a detectable PRA level or a low PAC/PRA ratio in a patient taking one of these drugs does not exclude the diagnosis of primary aldosteronism. However, an undetectably low PRA level in a patient taking an ACE inhibitor or ARB makes primary aldosteronism likely, and the PRA is suppressed (<1.0 ng/mL per hour) in almost all patients with primary aldosteronism.

The PAC/PRA ratio, first proposed as a case-detection test for primary aldosteronism in 1981,[137] is based on the concept of paired hormone measurements. The PAC is measured in nanograms per deciliter, and the PRA in nanograms per milliliter per hour. In a hypertensive hypokalemic patient, secondary hyperaldosteronism should be considered if both PRA and PAC are increased and the PAC/PRA ratio is less than 10 (e.g., renovascular disease). An alternative source of mineralocorticoid receptor agonism should be considered if both PRA and PAC are suppressed (e.g., hypercortisolism). Primary aldosteronism should be suspected if the PRA is suppressed (<1.0 ng/mL per hour) and the PAC is increased. At least 14 prospective studies have been published on the use of the PAC/PRA ratio in detecting primary aldosteronism.[159] Although there is some uncertainty about test characteristics and lack of standardization (see later discussion), the PAC/PRA ratio is widely accepted as the case-detection test of choice for primary aldosteronism.

It is important to understand that the lower limit of detection varies among different PRA assays and can have a dramatic effect on the PAC/PRA ratio. As an example, if the lower limit of detection for PRA is 0.6 ng/mL per hour and the PAC is 16 ng/dL, then the PAC/PRA ratio with an "undetectable" PRA would be 27; however, if the lower limit of detection for PRA is 0.1 ng/mL per hour, the same PAC level would yield a PAC/PRA ratio of 160. Thus, the cutoff for a "high" PAC/PRA ratio is laboratory dependent and, more specifically, PRA assay dependent. In a retrospective study, the combination of a PAC/PRA ratio greater than 30 and a PAC level greater than 20 ng/dL had a sensitivity of 90% and a specificity of 91% for APA.[160] At Mayo Clinic, the combination of a PAC/PRA ratio of 20 or higher, and a PAC level of at least 15 ng/dL is found in more than 90% of patients with surgically confirmed APA. In patients without primary aldosteronism, most of the variation occurs within the normal range.[161] A high PAC/PRA ratio is a positive screening test result, a finding that warrants further testing.[134,135]

It is critical for the clinician to recognize that the PAC/PRA ratio is only a case-detection tool, and all positive results should be followed by a confirmatory aldosterone suppression test to verify autonomous aldosterone production before treatment is initiated.[134,135] In a systematic review of 16 studies with 3136 participants, the PAC/PRA cutoff levels used varied between 7.2 and 100.[159] The sensitivity for APA varied between 64% and 100%, and the specificity between 87% and 100%. However, the description of the reference standard and the attribution of diagnosis at the end of the studies were incomplete, and there was a lack of standardization concerning the origin of the study cohort, ongoing antihypertensive medications, use of high-salt versus low-salt diet, and circumstances during blood sampling. The authors concluded that none of the studies provided any valid estimates of test characteristics (sensitivity, specificity, and likelihood ratio at various cutoff levels).[159] In a study of 118 subjects with essential hypertension, neither antihypertensive medications nor acute variation of dietary sodium affected the accuracy of the PAC/PRA ratio adversely; the sensitivities on and off therapy were 73% and 87%, respectively, and the specificities were 74% and 75%, respectively.[139] In a study of African American and Caucasian subjects with resistant hypertension, the PAC/PRA ratio was elevated (>20) in 45 of 58 subjects with primary aldosteronism and in 35 of 207 patients without primary aldosteronism (sensitivity, 78%;

specificity, 83%).[158] Furosemide and upright posture do not improve the post-test probability for APA more than the use of the baseline PAC/PRA ratio.[162]

The measurement of PRA is time-consuming, shows high interlaboratory variability, and requires special preanalytic prerequisites. To overcome these disadvantages, a monoclonal antibody against active renin is being used by several reference laboratories to measure the plasma renin concentration (PRC) instead of PRA. However, few studies have compared the different methods of testing for primary aldosteronism, and these studies lack confirmatory testing.[163,164] In one study with 76 normotensive volunteers and 28 patients with confirmed primary aldosteronism, the PAC/PRC ratio performed as well as the PAC/PRA ratio in differentiating the two groups.[165] Before a recommendation to replace PRA with PRC in testing for primary aldosteronism can be made, more studies with larger cohorts are needed. Until then, it is reasonable to consider a positive PAC/PRC test if the PAC is greater than 15 ng/dL and the PRC is lower below the lower limit of detection for the assay (see Fig. 16-9).

Confirmatory Tests

An increased PAC/PRA ratio is not diagnostic by itself, and primary aldosteronism must be confirmed by demonstration of inappropriate aldosterone secretion. The list of drugs and hormones capable of affecting the RAA axis is extensive, and a "medication-contaminated" evaluation is frequently unavoidable in patients with severe hypertension. Calcium channel blockers and α_1-adrenergic receptor blockers do not affect the diagnostic accuracy in most cases.[135] It is impossible to interpret data obtained from patients receiving treatment with mineralocorticoid receptor antagonists (e.g., spironolactone, eplerenone) when the PRA is not suppressed. Therefore, treatment with a mineralocorticoid receptor antagonist should not be initiated until the evaluation has been completed and the final decisions about treatment have been made. If primary aldosteronism is suspected in a patient receiving treatment with spironolactone or eplerenone, the treatment should be discontinued for at least 6 weeks before further diagnostic testing is undertaken. Aldosterone suppression testing can be performed with orally administered sodium chloride and measurement of urinary aldosterone or with intravenous sodium chloride loading and measurement of PAC.

Oral Sodium Loading Test. After hypertension and hypokalemia have been controlled, patients should receive a high-sodium diet (supplemented with sodium chloride tablets if needed) for 3 days, with a goal sodium intake of 5000 mg (equivalent to 218 mEq of sodium or 12.8 g sodium chloride).[147] The risk of increasing dietary sodium in patients with severe hypertension must be assessed in each case.[166] Because the high-salt diet can increase kaliuresis and hypokalemia, vigorous replacement of potassium chloride may be needed, and the serum level of potassium should be monitored daily. On the third day of the high-sodium diet, a 24-hour urine specimen is collected for measurement of aldosterone, sodium, and creatinine. To document adequate sodium repletion, the 24-hour urinary sodium excretion should exceed 200 mEq. Urinary aldosterone excretion of more than 12 µg/24 hours in this setting is consistent with autonomous aldosterone secretion.[167] The sensitivity and specificity of the oral sodium loading test are 96% and 93%, respectively.[168]

Intravenous Saline Infusion Test. The intravenous saline infusion test has also been used widely for the diagnosis of primary aldosteronism.[135,169-171] Normal subjects show suppression of PAC after volume expansion with isotonic saline; subjects with primary aldosteronism do not show this suppression. The test is done after an overnight fast. Two liters of 0.9% sodium chloride solution is infused intravenously with an infusion pump over 4 hours with the patient recumbent. Blood pressure and heart rate are monitored during the infusion. At the completion of the infusion, blood is drawn for measurement of PAC. PAC levels in normal subjects decrease to less than 5 ng/dL, whereas most patients with primary aldosteronism do not suppress to less than 10 ng/dL. Post-infusion PAC values between 5 and 10 ng/dL are indeterminate and may be seen in patients with IHA.[131,169,170,172]

Fludrocortisone Suppression Test. In the fludrocortisone suppression test, fludrocortisone acetate is administered for 4 days (0.1 mg every 6 hours) in combination with sodium chloride tablets (2 g three times daily with food). Blood pressure and serum potassium levels must be monitored daily. In the setting of low PRA, failure to suppress the upright 10 a.m. PAC to less than 6 ng/dL on day 4 is diagnostic of primary aldosteronism.[173] Increased QT dispersion and deterioration of left ventricular function have been reported during fludrocortisone suppression tests.[166] Most centers no longer use this test.

Subtype Studies

After case-detection and confirmatory testing, the third management issue guides the therapeutic approach by distinguishing APA and PAH from IHA and GRA. Unilateral adrenalectomy in patients with APA or PAH results in normalization of hypokalemia in all cases; hypertension is improved in all cases and is cured in 30% to 60%.[174-176] In IHA and GRA, unilateral or bilateral adrenalectomy seldom corrects the hypertension.[147] IHA and GRA should be treated medically. APA is found in approximately 35% of cases and bilateral IHA in approximately 60% (see Table 16-10). APAs are usually hypodense nodules (<2 cm in diameter) on CT and are golden yellow in color when resected. IHA adrenal glands may be normal on CT or may show nodular changes. Aldosterone-producing adrenal carcinomas are almost always larger than 4 cm in diameter and have an inhomogeneous phenotype on CT (see Table 16-6).

Computed Tomography of the Adrenal. Primary aldosteronism subtype evaluation may require one or more tests, the first of which is imaging of the adrenal glands with CT (Fig. 16-10). If a solitary unilateral hypodense (HU < 10) macroadenoma (>1 cm) and normal contralateral adrenal morphology are found on CT in a young patient (<40 years) with severe primary aldosteronism, unilateral adrenalectomy is a reasonable therapeutic option (see Fig. 16-10). However, in many cases, CT shows normal-appearing adrenals, minimal unilateral adrenal limb thickening, unilateral microadenomas (≤1 cm), or bilateral macroadenomas (Fig. 16-11). In these cases, additional testing is required to determine the source of excess aldosterone secretion.

Small APAs may be labeled incorrectly as IHA on the basis of CT findings of bilateral nodularity or normal-appearing adrenals. Also, apparent adrenal microadenomas may actually represent areas of hyperplasia, and unilateral adrenalectomy would be inappropriate. In addition, nonfunctioning unilateral adrenal macroadenomas are not uncommon, especially in older patients (>40 years).[177] Unilateral PAH may be visible on CT, or the PAH adrenal may appear normal on CT. In general, patients with APAs have more severe hypertension, more frequent hypokalemia,

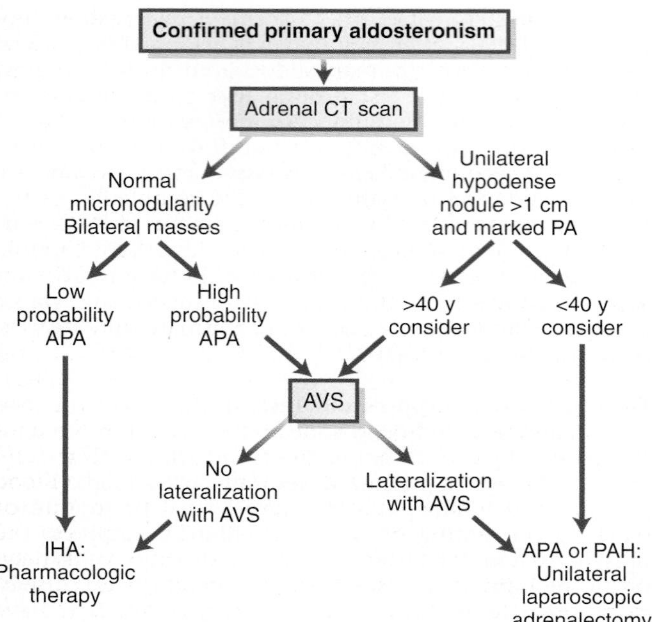

Figure 16-10 Subtype evaluation of primary aldosteronism. For patients who want to pursue a surgical treatment for their hypertension, adrenal venous sampling is frequently a key diagnostic step (see text for details). APA, aldosterone-producing adenoma; AVS, adrenal venous sampling; CT, computed tomography; IHA, idiopathic hyperaldosteronism; PA, primary aldosteronism; PAH, primary adrenal hyperplasia. (Modified from Young WF Jr, Hogan MJ: Renin-independent hypermineralocorticoidism. *Trends Endocrinol Metab.* 1994;5:97-106.)

and higher levels of plasma aldosterone (>25 ng/dL) and urinary aldosterone (>30 μg/24 hours), and are younger (<50 years), compared with those who have IHA.[147,148] Patients fitting these descriptors are considered to have a "high probability of APA" regardless of the CT findings (see Fig. 16-10), and 41% of patients with a "high probability of APA" and a normal adrenal CT scan prove to have unilateral aldosterone hypersecretion.[178]

Adrenal CT is not accurate in distinguishing between APA and IHA.[178,179] In one study of 203 patients with primary aldosteronism who were evaluated with both CT and adrenal venous sampling, CT was accurate in only 53% of patients[178]; based on the CT findings, 42 patients (22%) would have been incorrectly excluded as candidates for adrenalectomy, and 48 (25%) might have had unnecessary or inappropriate surgery.[178] In a systematic review of 38 studies involving 950 patients with primary aldosteronism, adrenal CT/MRI results did not agree with the findings from adrenal venous sampling in 359 patients (38%)[179]; based on CT/MRI, 19% of the 950 patients would have undergone noncurative surgery, and 19% would have been offered medical therapy instead of curative adrenalectomy.[179] Therefore, adrenal venous sampling is essential to direct appropriate therapy in patients with primary aldosteronism who have a high probability of APA and are seeking a potential surgical cure.

Adrenal Venous Sampling. Adrenal venous sampling is the criterion standard test to distinguish between unilateral and bilateral disease in patients with primary aldosteronism.[178,179] Adrenal venous sampling is an intricate procedure because the right adrenal vein is small and may be difficult to locate and cannulate; the success rate depends on the proficiency of the angiographer. A review of 47 reports found that the success rate for cannulation of the right adrenal vein in 384 patients was 74%.[147] With experience and focusing the expertise to one or two radiologists at a referral center, the AVS success rate can be as high as 96%.[178,180,181]

The five keys to a successful adrenal venous sampling program are: (1) appropriate patient selection, (2) careful patient preparation, (3) focused technical expertise, (4) defined protocol, and (5) accurate data interpretation.[182] A center-specific, written protocol is mandatory. The protocol should be developed by an interested group of endocrinologists, hypertension specialists, internists, radiologists, and laboratory personnel. Safeguards should be in place to prevent mislabeling of the blood tubes in the radiology suite and to prevent sample mixup in the laboratory.

At Mayo Clinic, we use continuous cosyntropin infusion during AVS (50 μg/hour starting 30 minutes before sampling and continuing throughout the procedure) for the following reasons: (1) to minimize stress-induced fluctuations in aldosterone secretion during nonsimultaneous AVS; (2) to maximize the gradient in cortisol from adrenal vein to inferior vena cava (IVC) and thus confirm successful sampling of the adrenal veins; and (3) to maximize the secretion of aldosterone from an APA.[171,178,181,182] The

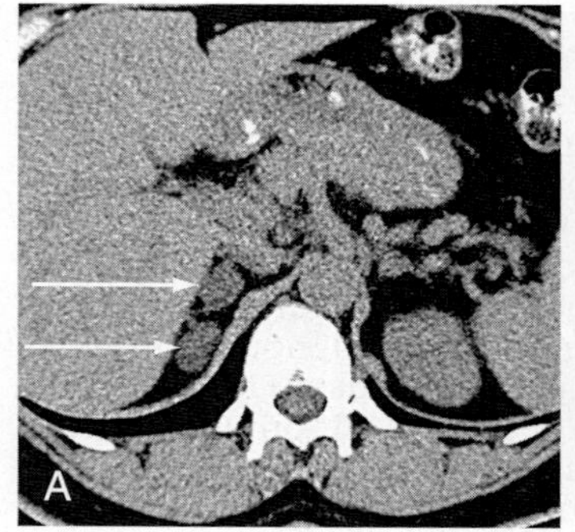

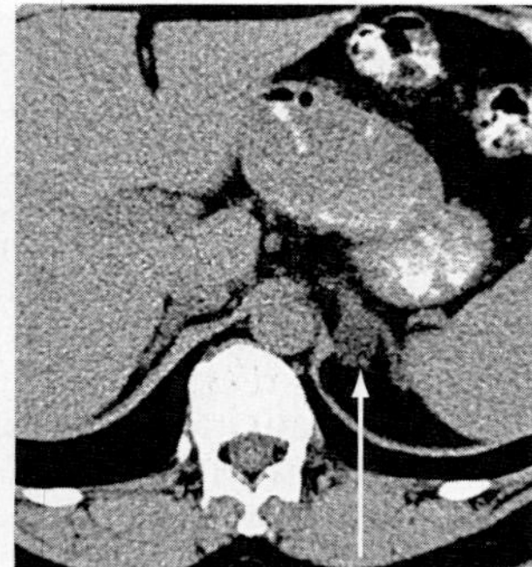

Results of bilateral adrenal venous sampling

Vein	Aldosterone (A), ng/dL	Cortisol (C), μg/dL	A/C ratio	Aldosterone ratio*
R adrenal vein	29,338	668	43.9	62.7
L adrenal vein	363	540	0.7	
Inferior vena cava	259	31	8.4	

*R adrenal vein A/C ratio divided by L adrenal vein A/C ratio.

B

Figure 16-11 A 43-year-old woman had a 2-year history of hypertension and hypokalemia. The screening test for primary aldosteronism was positive, with a plasma aldosterone concentration (PAC) of 37 ng/dL and low plasma renin activity (PRA) at less than 0.6 ng/mL per hour (PAC/PRA ratio >61). The confirmatory test for primary aldosteronism was also positive, with the 24-hour urinary excretion of aldosterone measured at 53 μg on a high-sodium diet (urinary sodium, 196 mEq/24 hours). **A,** Adrenal CT shows a 12-mm, low-density mass *(arrow, right panel)* in the medial limb of the left adrenal and two low-density, 10-mm nodules *(arrows, left panel)* within the right adrenal gland. **B,** Adrenal venous sampling lateralized aldosterone secretion to the right, and two cortical adenomas (1.8 × 1.2 × 0.8 cm and 2.5 × 1.5 × 1.2 cm) were found at laparoscopic right adrenalectomy. The postoperative plasma aldosterone concentration was less than 1.0 ng/dL. Hypokalemia was cured and blood pressure was normal without the aid of antihypertensive medications.

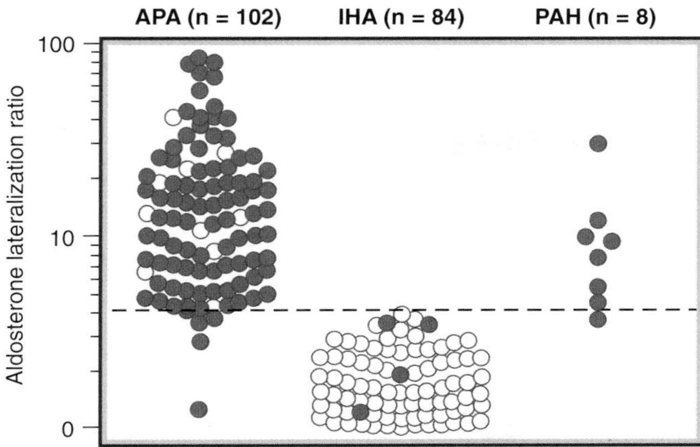

Figure 16-12 Adrenal vein aldosterone lateralization ratios for patients with unilateral aldosterone-producing adenomas (APA), bilateral idiopathic hyperplasia (IHA), and unilateral primary adrenal hyperplasia (PAH). Shaded symbols indicate that the diagnosis was confirmed surgically. The sensitivity and specificity of a cortisol-corrected plasma aldosterone concentration lateralization ratio greater than 4.0 for unilateral disease are 95.2% and 100%, respectively. (Reproduced with permission from Young WF Jr, Stanson AW, Thompson GB, et al. Role for adrenal venous sampling in primary aldosteronism. *Surgery.* 2004;136:1227-1235.)

adrenal veins are catheterized through the percutaneous femoral vein approach, and the position of the catheter tip is verified by gentle injection of a small amount of nonionic contrast medium and radiographic documentation. Blood is obtained from both adrenal veins and from the IVC below the renal veins and assayed for aldosterone and cortisol concentrations. To be sure that there is no cross-contamination, the "IVC" sample should be obtained from the external iliac vein. The venous sample from the left side typically is obtained from the common phrenic vein immediately adjacent to the entrance of the adrenal vein. The cortisol concentrations from the adrenal veins and IVC are used to confirm successful catheterization; the adrenal vein/IVC cortisol ratio is typically greater than 10:1.

Dividing the right and left adrenal vein PAC values by their respective cortisol concentrations corrects for the dilutional effect of the inferior phenic vein flow into the left adrenal vein; these are termed *cortisol-corrected ratios* (Fig. 16-12). In patients with APA, the mean cortisol-corrected aldosterone ratio (i.e., the ratio of PAC/cortisol from the APA side to that from the normal side) is 18:1.[178] A cutoff point of 4:1 for this ratio is used to indicate unilateral aldosterone excess (see Fig. 16-12).[178] In patients with IHA, the mean cortisol-corrected aldosterone ratio is 1.8:1 (high side to low side), and a ratio of less than 3.0:1 suggests bilateral aldosterone hypersecretion (see Fig. 16-12).[178] Therefore, most patients with a unilateral source of aldosterone have cortisol-corrected aldosterone lateralization ratios greater than 4.0, and ratios greater than 3.0 but less than 4.0 represent a zone of overlap. Ratios no higher than 3.0 are consistent with bilateral aldosterone secretion. The test characteristics of adrenal vein sampling for detection of unilateral aldosterone hypersecretion (APA or PAH) are 95% sensitivity and 100% specificity.[178] At centers with experience with adrenal vein sampling, the complication rate is 2.5% or less.[178,180] Complications can include symptomatic groin hematoma, adrenal hemorrhage, and dissection of an adrenal vein.

Some centers and clinical practice guidelines recommend that adrenal venous sampling should be performed in all patients who have the diagnosis of primary aldosteronism.[135,179] The use of adrenal venous sampling should be based on patient preference, patient age, clinical comorbidities, and the clinical probability of finding an APA.[134] A more practical approach is the selective use of adrenal venous sampling outlined in Figure 16-10.

Glucocorticoid-Remediable Aldosteronism: Familial Hyperaldosteronism Type I. GRA (FH type I) is inherited in an autosomal dominant fashion and is responsible for fewer than 1% of cases of primary aldosteronism (see Table 16-10).[121] GRA is characterized by early-onset hypertension that is usually severe and refractory to conventional antihypertensive therapies, aldosterone excess, suppressed PRA, and excess production of 18-hydroxycortisol and 18-oxycortisol. GRA is caused by a chimeric gene duplication that results from unequal crossover between the promoter sequence of the *CYP11B1* gene (which encodes 11β-hydroxylase) and the coding sequence of *CYP11B2* (which encodes aldosterone synthase).[121] This chimeric gene contains the 3′ corticotropin-responsive portion of the promoter from the 11β-hydroxylase gene fused to the 5′ coding sequence of the aldosterone synthase gene. The result is ectopic expression of aldosterone synthase activity in the cortisol-producing zona fasciculata. Mineralocorticoid production is regulated by corticotropin instead of by the normal secretagogue, angiotensin II. Therefore, aldosterone secretion can be suppressed by glucocorticoid therapy. In the absence of glucocorticoid therapy, this mutation results in overproduction of aldosterone and the hybrid steroids 18-hydroxycortisol and 18-oxycortisol, which can be measured in the urine to make the diagnosis.

Genetic testing is a sensitive and specific means of diagnosing GRA and obviates the need to measure the urinary levels of 18-oxycortisol and 18-hydroxycortisol or to perform dexamethasone suppression testing. Genetic testing for GRA should be considered for patients with primary aldosteronism who have a family history of primary aldosteronism, onset of primary aldosteronism at a young age (<20 years), or a family history of strokes at a young age.[182]

Familial Hyperaldosteronism Type II. FH type II is autosomal dominant and may be monogenic.[122] The hyperaldosteronism in FH type II does not suppress with dexamethasone, and GRA mutation testing is negative. FH type II is more common than FH type I, but it still accounts for fewer than 2% of all patients with primary aldosteronism. The molecular basis for FH type II is unclear, although a recent linkage analysis study showed an association with chromosomal region 7p22.[122]

Historical Perspectives. One of the first methods used to differentiate unilateral from bilateral adrenal disease in patients with primary aldosteronism was adrenal venous sampling.[183] However, other diagnostic methods were sought because of the suboptimal catheter technology in the 1960s and 1970s and the difficulty in successfully sampling from both adrenal veins. [^{131}I]-19-iodocholesterol scintigraphy[184] was first used in the early 1970s, and an improved agent, [^{131}I]-6β-iodomethyl-19-norcholesterol (NP-59), was introduced in 1977.[185] The sensitivity of this test depended heavily on the size of the adenoma.[186,187] In addition to its poor sensitivity, NP-59 is no longer available for use in the United States.

The posture stimulation test, also developed in the 1970s, was based on the finding that PAC in patients with APA shows diurnal variation and is relatively unaffected by changes in angiotensin II levels, whereas IHA is characterized by enhanced sensitivity to a small change in angiotensin II that occurs with standing.[188] In a review of 16 published reports, the accuracy of the posture stimulation test was found to be 85% in 246 patients with surgically verified APA.[147] However, it became clear that some APAs are sensitive to angiotensin II and some patients with IHA have diurnal variation in aldosterone secretion. Also, although the posture stimulation test may have predicted which patient had APA, it did not assist in localization.

18-Hydroxycorticosterone (18-OHB) is considered to be either the immediate precursor of aldosterone or a separate end product formed after 18-hydroxylation of corticosterone. Patients with APA typically have recumbent plasma 18-OHB levels greater than 100 ng/dL at 8 a.m., whereas patients with IHA usually have levels less than 100 ng/dL.[189] 18-OHB has actually proved to be a surrogate for PAC, which also tends to be higher in patients with APA than in those with IHA. However, the accuracy of supine morning 18-OHB and PAC levels in distinguishing between patients with APA and those with IHA is less than 80%.[147]

Principles of Treatment

The treatment goal is to prevent the morbidity and mortality associated with hypertension, hypokalemia, and cardiovascular damage.[190] Knowing the cause of the primary aldosteronism helps to determine the appropriate treatment. Normalization of blood pressure should not be the only goal. In addition to the kidney and colon, mineralocorticoid receptors are present in the heart, brain, and blood vessels. Excessive secretion of aldosterone is associated with increased risk of cardiovascular disease and morbidity. Therefore, normalization of circulating aldosterone or mineralocorticoid receptor blockade should be part of the management plan for all patients with primary aldosteronism.[154] However, clinicians must understand that most patients with long-standing primary aldosteronism have some degree of renal insufficiency that is masked by the glomerular hyperfiltration associated with aldosterone excess.[190,191] The true degree of renal insufficiency may become evident only after effective pharmacologic or surgical therapy.[190,191]

Surgical Treatment of Aldosterone-Producing Adenoma and Unilateral Hyperplasia

Unilateral laparoscopic adrenalectomy is an excellent treatment option for patients with APA or unilateral hyperplasia.[106] Although blood pressure control improves in almost 100% of patients postoperatively, average long-term cure rates of hypertension after unilateral adrenalectomy for APA range from 30% to 60%.[174,176] Persistent hypertension after adrenalectomy is correlated directly with having more than one first-degree relative with hypertension, use of more than two antihypertensive agents preoperatively, older age, increased serum creatinine level, and duration of hypertension and is most likely caused by coexistent primary hypertension.[174,176]

Laparoscopic adrenalectomy is the preferred surgical approach and is associated with shorter hospital stays and less long-term morbidity than the open approach.[192,193] Because APAs are small and may be multiple, the entire adrenal gland should be removed.[194] To decrease the surgical risk, hypokalemia should be corrected with potassium supplements or a mineralocorticoid receptor antagonist, or both, preoperatively. These medications should be discontinued postoperatively. PAC should be measured 1 to 2 days after the operation to confirm a biochemical cure. Serum potassium levels should be monitored weekly for 4 weeks after surgery, and a generous sodium diet should be followed to avoid the hyperkalemia of hypoaldosteronism that may occur because of the chronic suppression of the RAA axis. Clinically significant hyperkalemia develops after surgery in approximately 5% of APA patients, and short-term fludrocortisone supplementation may be required. Typically, the hypertension that was associated with aldosterone excess resolves in 1 to 3 months after the surgery. It has been found that adrenalectomy for APA is significantly less expensive than long-term medical therapy.[195]

Pharmacologic Treatment

IHA and GRA should be treated medically. In addition, APA may be treated medically if the medical treatment includes mineralocorticoid receptor blockade.[196] A sodium-restricted diet (<100 mEq of sodium per day), maintenance of ideal body weight, tobacco avoidance, and regular aerobic exercise contribute significantly to the success of pharmacologic treatment. No placebo-controlled, randomized trials have evaluated the relative efficacy of drugs in the treatment of primary aldosteronism.[197]

Spironolactone has been the drug of choice to treat primary aldosteronism for more than 4 decades.[198] It is available as 25-, 50-, and 100-mg tablets. The dosage is 12.5 to 25 mg per day initially and can be increased to 400 mg/day if necessary to achieve a high-normal serum potassium concentration without the aid of oral potassium chloride supplementation. Hypokalemia responds promptly, but hypertension can take as long as 4 to 8 weeks to be corrected. After several months of therapy, the dosage of spironolactone often can be decreased to as little as 25 to 50 mg/day; dosage titration is based on a goal serum potassium level in the high-normal range. Serum potassium and creatinine should be monitored frequently during the first 4 to 6 weeks of therapy (especially in patients with renal insufficiency or diabetes mellitus). Spironolactone increases the half-life of digoxin, and the digoxin dosage may need to be adjusted when treatment with spironolactone is started. Concomitant therapy with salicylates should be avoided because they interfere with the tubular secretion of an active metabolite and decrease the effectiveness of spironolactone. However, spironolactone is not selective for the mineralocorticoid receptor. For example, antagonism at the testosterone receptor may result in painful gynecomastia, erectile dysfunction, and decreased libido in men, and agonist activity at the progesterone receptor results in menstrual irregularity in women.[199]

Eplerenone is a steroid-based antimineralocorticoid that acts as a competitive and selective mineralocorticoid receptor antagonist and was approved by the U.S. Food and Drug Administration (FDA) for the treatment of uncomplicated essential hypertension in 2003.[198] The 9,11-epoxide group in eplerenone results in a marked reduction of the molecule's progestational and antiandrogenic actions; compared with spironolactone, eplerenone has 0.1% of the binding affinity to androgen receptors and less than 1% of the binding affinity to progesterone receptors. Treatment trials comparing the efficacy of eplerenone versus spironolactone for the treatment of primary aldosteronism have not been published. Presumably, eplerenone will be the superior drug if it is shown to be as effective as spironolactone for the treatment of mineralocorticoid-dependent hypertension, because it lacks the limiting antiandrogen side effects of spironolactone. Eplerenone is available as 25- and 50-mg tablets. For primary aldosteronism, it is reasonable to start with a dose of 25 mg twice daily (twice daily because of the shorter half-life of eplerenone compared with spironolactone) and titrated upward; the target is a high-normal serum potassium concentration without the aid of potassium supplements. The maximum dose approved by the FDA for hypertension is 100 mg/day. Potency studies with eplerenone show 25% to 50% less milligram-per-milligram potency compared with spironolactone. As with spironolactone, it is important to monitor blood pressure, serum potassium, and serum creatinine levels closely. Side effects include dizziness, headache, fatigue, diarrhea, hypertriglyceridemia, and elevated liver enzymes.

Patients with IHA frequently require a second antihypertensive agent to achieve good blood pressure control. Hypervolemia is a major reason for resistance to drug therapy, and low doses of a thiazide (e.g., 12.5 to 50 mg of hydrochlorothiazide daily) or a related sulfonamide diuretic are effective in combination with the mineralocorticoid receptor antagonist. Because these agents often lead to further hypokalemia, serum potassium levels should be monitored.

Before treatment is initiated, the diagnosis of GRA should be confirmed with genetic testing. In the GRA patient, chronic treatment with physiologic doses of a glucocorticoid normalizes blood pressure and corrects hypokalemia. The clinician should be cautious about iatrogenic Cushing's syndrome with excessive doses of glucocorticoids, especially when dexamethasone is used in children. Shorter-acting agents such as prednisone or hydrocortisone should be prescribed, using the smallest effective dose in relation to body surface area (e.g., hydrocortisone, 10 to 12 mg/m^2 per day). Target blood pressure in children should be guided by age-specific blood pressure percentiles.[200] Children should be monitored by pediatricians with expertise in glucocorticoid therapy, with careful attention paid to preventing retardation of linear growth due to overtreatment. Treatment with mineralocorticoid receptor antagonists in these patients may be just as effective as glucocorticoids and avoids the potential disruption of the hypothalamic-pituitary-adrenal axis and risk of iatrogenic side effects. In addition, glucocorticoid therapy or mineralocorticoid receptor blockade may even have a role in normotensive GRA patients.[150]

OTHER FORMS OF MINERALOCORTICOID EXCESS OR EFFECT

The medical disorders associated with excess mineralocorticoid effect from 11-deoxycorticosterone (DOC) and cortisol are listed in Table 16-10. These diagnoses should be considered if PAC and PRA are low in a patient with hypertension and hypokalemia.

Hyperdeoxycorticosteronism

Congenital Adrenal Hyperplasia

Congenital adrenal hyperplasia (CAH) is caused by enzymatic defects in adrenal steroidogenesis that result in deficient secretion of cortisol (see Chapter 15).[201] The lack of inhibitory feedback by cortisol on the hypothalamus and pituitary produces an ACTH-driven buildup of cortisol precursors proximal to the enzymatic deficiency. A deficiency of 11β-hydroxylase (CYP11B) or 17α-hydroxylase (CYP17) causes hypertension and hypokalemia because of hypersecretion of the mineralocorticoid DOC. The mineralocorticoid effect of increased circulating levels of DOC also decreases PRA and aldosterone secretion. These defects are autosomal recessive in inheritance and typically are diagnosed in childhood. However, partial enzymatic defects have been shown to cause hypertension in adults.

11β-Hydroxylase Deficiency. Approximately 5% of all cases of CAH are caused by 11β-hydroxylase deficiency; the prevalence in Caucasians is 1 in 100,000.[201] More than 40 mutations have been described in *CYP11B1*, the gene encoding 11β-hydroxylase.[202] There is an increased prevalence among Sephardic Jews from Morocco, suggestive of a founder effect. The impaired conversion of DOC to corticosterone results in high levels of DOC and 11-deoxycortisol; the substrate mass effect results in increased levels of adrenal androgens. Girls present in infancy or childhood with hypertension, hypokalemia, acne, hirsutism, and virilization, and boys present with pseudoprecocious puberty. Approximately two thirds of patients have mild to moderate hypertension. Markedly increased levels of DOC, 11-deoxycortisol, and adrenal androgens confirm the diagnosis. Glucocorticoid replacement normalizes the steroid abnormalities and hypertension.

17α-Hydroxylase Deficiency. 17α-Hydroxylase deficiency is a rare cause of CAH. 17α-Hydroxylase is essential for the synthesis of cortisol and gonadal hormones, and deficiency results in decreased production of cortisol and sex hormones. Genetic 46,XY males present with either pseudohermaphroditism or as phenotypic females, and 46,XX females present with primary amenorrhea. Therefore, a person with this form of CAH may not come to medical attention until puberty. The biochemical findings include low concentrations of plasma adrenal androgens, 17α-hydroxyprogesterone, aldosterone, and cortisol. The plasma concentrations of DOC, corticosterone, and 18-OHB are increased and PRA is suppressed. Although it is still rare, there is an increased prevalence of 17α-hydroxylase deficiency among Dutch Mennonites. As with 11β-hydroxylase deficiency, glucocorticoid replacement normalizes the steroid abnormalities and the hypertension.

Deoxycorticosterone-Producing Tumor

DOC-producing adrenal tumors are usually large and malignant.[203] Some of them secrete androgens and estrogens in addition to DOC, which may cause virilization in women or feminization in men. A high level of plasma DOC or urinary tetrahydrodeoxycorticosterone and a large adrenal tumor seen on CT confirm the diagnosis. Aldosterone secretion in these patients is typically suppressed. Optimal treatment is complete surgical resection.

Primary Cortisol Resistance

Increased cortisol secretion and plasma cortisol concentrations without evidence of Cushing's syndrome are found in patients with primary cortisol resistance (or glucocorticoid resistance), a rare familial syndrome.[204] The syndrome is characterized by hypokalemic alkalosis, hypertension, increased plasma concentrations of DOC, and increased adrenal androgen secretion. The hypertension and hypokalemia probably result from the combined effects of excess DOC and increased cortisol access to the mineralocorticoid receptor, resulting in high rates of cortisol production that overwhelm 11β-hydroxysteroid dehydrogenase type 2 (HSD11B2) activity (see discussion in next section). Primary cortisol resistance is caused by defects in the glucocorticoid receptor and the steroid-receptor complex. The treatment for the mineralocorticoid-dependent hypertension is blockade of the mineralocorticoid receptor with a mineralocorticoid receptor antagonist or suppression of ACTH secretion with dexamethasone.

Apparent Mineralocorticoid Excess Syndrome

Apparent mineralocorticoid excess is the result of impaired activity of the microsomal enzyme HSD11B2, which normally inactivates cortisol in the kidney by converting it to cortisone. Cortisol can be a potent mineralocorticoid, and because of the enzyme deficiency, high levels of cortisol accumulate in the kidney.[205] HSD11B2 normally excludes physiologic glucocorticoids from the nonselective mineralocorticoid receptor by converting them to the inactive 11-keto compound, cortisone. The characteristic abnormal urinary cortisol-cortisone metabolite profile seen in apparent mineralocorticoid excess reflects decreased HSD11B2 activity; the ratio of cortisol to cortisone is increased 10-fold above the normal value.[205]

Decreased HSD11B2 activity may be hereditary, or it may be secondary to pharmacologic inhibition of enzyme activity by glycyrrhizic acid, the active principle of licorice root (*Glycyrrhiza glabra*) and some chewing tobaccos. The congenital forms are rare autosomal recessive disorders; fewer than 50 patients have been identified worldwide. Children present with low birth weight, failure to thrive, hypertension, polyuria and polydipsia, and poor growth.[202] The clinical phenotype of patients with apparent mineralocorticoid excess includes hypertension, hypokalemia, metabolic alkalosis, low PRA, low PAC, and normal plasma cortisol levels. The diagnosis is confirmed by demonstration of an abnormal ratio of cortisol to cortisone in a 24-hour urine collection. Treatment includes blockade of the mineralocorticoid receptor with a mineralocorticoid receptor antagonist or suppression of endogenous cortisol secretion with dexamethasone.

The mineralocorticoid excess state caused by ectopic ACTH secretion, commonly seen in patients with Cushing's syndrome, is related to the high rates of cortisol production that overwhelm HSD11B2 activity. DOC levels may also be increased in severe ACTH-dependent Cushing's syndrome and contribute to the hypertension and hypokalemia in this disorder.

Liddle's Syndrome: Abnormal Renal Tubular Ionic Transport

In 1963, Liddle described an autosomal dominant renal disorder that appeared to be primary aldosteronism with hypertension, hypokalemia, and inappropriate kaliuresis.[206] However, PAC and PRA were very low in patients with Liddle's syndrome, so the disorder was termed *pseudoaldosteronism*. Liddle's syndrome is caused by mutations in the β or γ subunit of the amiloride-sensitive epithelial sodium channel.[202] This results in enhanced activity of the epithelial sodium channel, increased sodium reabsorption, potassium wasting, hypertension, and hypokalemia. Clinical genetic testing is available (see www.genetests.org). As would be predicted, amiloride and triamterene are very effective agents to treat the hypertension and hypokalemia of pseudoaldosteronism. However, spironolactone is ineffective in these patients. Liddle's syndrome can easily be distinguished from apparent mineralocorticoid excess based on the good clinical response to amiloride and triamterene, lack of efficacy of spironolactone and dexamethasone, and normal 24-hour urine cortisone/cortisol ratio.

Hypertension Exacerbated by Pregnancy

Hypertension exacerbated by pregnancy is a rare autosomal dominant disorder found in women who have early-onset hypertension with suppressed levels of aldosterone and renin. During pregnancy, both the hypertension and the hypokalemia are severely exacerbated. These patients have an activating mutation in the gene encoding the mineralocorticoid receptor that allows progesterone and other mineralocorticoid antagonists to become agonists.[207]

OTHER ENDOCRINE DISORDERS ASSOCIATED WITH HYPERTENSION

Cushing's Syndrome

Hypertension occurs in 75% to 80% of patients with Cushing's syndrome (see Chapter 15).[208,209] The mechanisms of hypertension include increased production of DOC, enhanced pressor sensitivity to endogenous vasoconstrictors (e.g., epinephrine, angiotensin II), increased cardiac output, activation of the RAA system by increased hepatic production of angiotensinogen, and cortisol inactivation overload with stimulation of the mineralocorticoid receptor. The source of excess glucocorticoids may be exogenous (iatrogenic) or endogenous. Mineralocorticoid production is usually normal in endogenous Cushing's syndrome; aldosterone and renin levels are usually normal, and DOC levels are normal or mildly increased. In adrenal carcinomas, DOC and aldosterone may be elevated.

The case-detection studies for endogenous cortisol excess include a midnight salivary cortisol measurement, the 1-mg overnight dexamethasone suppression test, and measurement of free cortisol in a 24-hour urine collection. Further studies to confirm Cushing's syndrome and to determine the cause of the cortisol excess state are outlined in Chapter 15.

The hypertension associated with Cushing's syndrome should be treated until a surgical cure is obtained. Mineralocorticoid receptor antagonists, at dosages used to treat primary aldosteronism, are effective in reversing the hypokalemia. Second-step agents (e.g., thiazide diuretics) may be added for optimal control of blood pressure. The hypertension associated with the hypercortisolism usually resolves over several weeks after a surgical cure, and antihypertensive agents may be tapered and withdrawn.

Thyroid Dysfunction

Hyperthyroidism

When excessive amounts of circulating thyroid hormones interact with thyroid hormone receptors on peripheral tissues, both metabolic activity and sensitivity to circulating catecholamines increase. Thyrotoxic patients usually have tachycardia, high cardiac output, increased stroke volume, decreased peripheral vascular resistance, and increased systolic blood pressure.[210] The initial management in patients with hypertension and hyperthyroidism includes use of a β-adrenergic blocker to treat hypertension, tachycardia, and tremor. The definitive treatment of hyperthyroidism is cause-specific (see Chapter 12).

Hypothyroidism

The frequency of hypertension (usually diastolic) is increased threefold in hypothyroid patients and may account for as many as 1% of cases of diastolic hypertension in the general population.[211] The mechanisms for the elevation in blood pressure include increased systemic vascular resistance and extracellular volume expansion. Treatment of thyroid hormone deficiency decreases blood pressure in most patients with hypertension and normalizes blood pressure in one third of them. Synthetic levothyroxine is the treatment of choice for hypothyroidism (see Chapter 13).

Primary Hyperparathyroidism

Hypercalcemia is associated with an increased frequency of hypertension. The most common cause of hypercalcemia is primary hyperparathyroidism. The frequency of hypertension in patients with primary hyperparathyroidism varies from 10% to 60%.[212] Most patients with primary hyperparathyroidism are asymptomatic, and the focus of the presentation may be the side effects of chronic hypercalcemia: polyuria and polydipsia, constipation, osteoporosis, renal lithiasis, peptic ulcer disease, and hypertension (see Chapter 28). The mechanisms of hypertension are unclear because there is no direct correlation with the elevated parathyroid hormone or calcium levels. The hypertension associated with hyperparathyroidism can also occur as a complication of hypercalcemia-induced renal impairment or when this disorder is part of MEN2 (pheochromocytoma). The treatment of hyperparathyroidism is surgical; hypertension may or may not remit after successful parathyroidectomy.[213]

Acromegaly

Chronic growth hormone excess from a growth hormone–producing pituitary tumor results in the clinical syndrome of acromegaly. The effects of chronic excess of growth hormone include acral and soft tissue overgrowth, progressive dental malocclusion, degenerative arthritis related to chondral and synovial tissue overgrowth within joints, low-pitched sonorous voice, excessive sweating and oily skin, perineural hypertrophy leading to nerve entrapment (e.g., carpal tunnel syndrome), cardiac dysfunction, and hypertension (see Chapter 9). Hypertension occurs in 20% to 40% of the patients and is associated with sodium retention and extracellular volume expansion.[214] Pituitary surgery is the treatment of choice; if necessary, it is supplemented with medical therapy or irradiation or both. The hypertension of acromegaly is treated most effectively by curing the excess of growth hormone. If a surgical cure is not possible, the hypertension usually responds well to diuretic therapy.

REFERENCES

1. Hajjar I, Kotchen TA. Trends in prevalence, awareness, treatment, and control of hypertension in the United States, 1988-2000. *JAMA*. 2003; 290:199-206.
2. Dluhy RG, Lawrence JE, Williams GH. Endocrine hypertension. In: Larsen PR, Kronenberg HM, Melmed S, et al. eds. *Williams Textbook of Endocrinology*, 10th ed. Philadelphia, PA: Saunders; 2003:555.
3. Milligan G, Svoboda P, Brown CM. Why are there so many adrenoceptor subtypes? *Biochem Pharmacol*. 1994;48:1059-1071.
4. Chobanian AV, Bakris GL, Black HR, et al. The seventh report of the Joint National Committee on Prevention, Detection, Evaluation, and Treatment of High Blood Pressure: the JNC 7 report. *JAMA*. 2003; 289:2560-2572.
5. Hospenthal MA, Peters JI. Long-acting beta(2)-agonists in the management of asthma exacerbations. *Curr Opin Pulm Med*. 2005;11:69-73.
6. Flatmark T, Almas B, Ziegler MG. Catecholamine metabolism: an update on key biosynthetic enzymes and vesicular monoamine transporters. *Ann N Y Acad Sci*. 2002;971:69-75.
7. Gonias S, Goldsby R, Matthay KK, et al. Phase II study of high-dose [131I]metaiodobenzylguanidine therapy for patients with metastatic pheochromocytoma and paraganglioma. *J Clin Oncol*. 2009;27: 4162-4168.
8. Rose B, Matthay KK, Price D, et al. High-dose 131I-metaiodobenzylguanidine therapy for 12 patients with malignant pheochromocytoma. *Cancer*. 2003;98:239-248.
9. Erickson JD, Eiden LE, Hoffman BJ. Expression cloning of a reserpine-sensitive vesicular monoamine transporter. *Proc Natl Acad Sci U S A*. 1992;89:10993-10997.
10. Eisenhofer G, Kopin IJ, Goldstein DS. Catecholamine metabolism: a contemporary view with implications for physiology and medicine. *Pharmacol Rev*. 2004;56:331-349.
11. Lloyd RV, Tischer AS, Kimura N, et al. Adrenal tumors: introduction. In: DeLellis RA, Lloyd RV, Heitz PU, et al. eds. *World Health Organization Classification of Tumours: Pathology and Genetics of Tumours of Endocrine Organs*. Lyon, France: IARC Press; 2004:136-138.
12. Stenstrom G, Svardsudd K. Phaechromocytoma in Sweden, 1958-1981: an analysis of the National Cancer Registry data. *Acta Med Scand*. 1986;220:225-232.
13. Sinclair AM, Isles CG, Brown I, et al. Secondary hypertension in a blood pressure clinic. *Arch Intern Med*. 1987;147:1289-1293.
14. Anderson GH Jr, Blakeman N, Streeten DH. The effect of age on prevalence of secondary forms of hypertension in 4429 consecutively referred patients. *J Hypertens*. 1994;12:609-615.
15. Omura M, Saito J, Yamaguchi K, et al. Prospective study on the prevalence of secondary hypertension among hypertensive patients visiting a general outpatient clinic in Japan. *Hypertens Res*. 2004;27:193-202.
16. Fränkel F. [Classics in oncology: A case of bilateral completely latent adrenal tumor and concurrent nephritis with changes in the circulatory system and retinitis—Felix Fränkel, 1886]. *CA Cancer J Clin*. 1984;34:93-106.
17. Neumann HPH, Vortmeyer A, Schmidt D, et al. Evidence of MEN-2 in the original description of classic pheochromocytoma. *N Engl J Med*. 2007;357:1311-1315.
18. Pick L. Das Ganglioma embryonale sympathicum (sympathoma embryonale), eine typische bösartige geschwuestform des sympathischen nervensystems. *Berl Klin Wochenschr*. 1912;49:16-22.
19. Welbourn RB. Early surgical history of phaeochromocytoma. *Br J Surg*. 1987;74:594-596.
20. Manger WM, Gifford RW. Background and importance and diagnosis. In: Manger WM, Gifford RW, eds. *Clinical and Experimental Pheochromocytoma*, 2nd ed. Cambridge, MA: Blackwell Science; 1996:1-7, 205-332.
21. Engel A, von Euler US. Diagnostic value of increased urinary output of noradrenaline and adrenaline in pheochromocytoma. *Lancet*. 1950;2:387.
22. Young WF Jr. Pheochromocytoma, 1926-1993. *Trends Endocrinol Metab*. 1993;4:122-127.
23. Munakata M, Aihara A, Imai Y, et al. Altered sympathetic and vagal modulations of the cardiovascular system in patients with pheochromocytoma: their relations to orthostatic hypotension. *Am J Hypertens*. 1999;12:572-580.
24. Dubois LA, Gray DK. Dopamine-secreting pheochromocytomas: in search of a syndrome. *World J Surg*. 2005;29:909-913.
25. Eisenhofer G, Goldstein DS, Sullivan P, et al. Biochemical and clinical manifestations of dopamine-producing paragangliomas: utility of plasma methoxytyramine. *J Clin Endocrinol Metab*. 2005;90:2068-2075.
26. Young WF Jr, Maddox DE. Spells: in search of a cause. *Mayo Clin Proc*. 1995;70:757-765.
27. O'Brien TO, Young WF Jr, Davila DG, et al. Cushing's syndrome associated with ectopic production of corticotrophin-releasing hormone, corticotrophin, and vasopressin by a phaeochromocytoma. *Clin Endocrinol (Oxf)*. 1992;37:460-467.
28. Onozawa M, Fukuhara T, Minoguchi M, et al. Hypokalemic rhabdomyolysis due to WDHA syndrome caused by VIP-producing composite pheochromocytoma: a case in neurofibromatosis type 1. *Jpn J Clin Oncol*. 2005;35:559-563.
29. Mune T, Katakami H, Kato Y, et al. Production and secretion of parathyroid hormone-related protein in pheochromocytoma: participation of an alpha-adrenergic mechanism. *J Clin Endocrinol Metab*. 1993;76:757-762.
30. Schifferdecker B, Kodali D, Hausner E, et al. Adrenergic shock: an overlooked clinical entity? *Cardiol Rev*. 2005;13:69-72.
31. Liao WB, Liu CF, Chiang CW, et al. Cardiovascular manifestations of pheochromocytoma. *Am J Emerg Med*. 2000;18:622-625.
32. Neumann HP, Bausch B, McWhinney SR, et al. Germ-line mutations in nonsyndromic pheochromocytoma. *N Engl J Med*. 2002;346: 1459-1466.
33. Motta-Ramirez GA, Remer EM, Herts BR, et al. Comparison of CT findings in symptomatic and incidentally discovered pheochromocytomas. *AJR Am J Roentgenol*. 2005;185:684-688.

145. Hamlet SM, Tunny TJ, Woodland E, et al. Is aldosterone/renin ratio useful to screen a hypertensive population for primary aldosteronism? *Clin Exp Pharmacol Physiol.* 1985;12:249-252.
146. Ma JT, Wang C, Lam KS, et al. Fifty cases of primary hyperaldosteronism in Hong Kong Chinese with a high frequency of periodic paralysis: evaluation of techniques for tumour localisation. *Q J Med.* 1986; 61:1021-1037.
147. Young WF Jr, Klee GG. Primary aldosteronism: diagnostic evaluation. *Endocrinol Metab Clin North Am.* 1988;17:367-395.
148. Blumenfeld JD, Sealey JE, Schlussel Y, et al. Diagnosis and treatment of primary hyperaldosteronism. *Ann Intern Med.* 1994;121:877-885.
149. Torres VE, Young WF Jr, Offord KP, et al. Association of hypokalemia, hypoaldosteronism, and renal cysts. *N Engl J Med.* 1990;322:345-351.
150. Stowasser M, Sharman J, Leano R, et al. Evidence for abnormal left ventricular structure and function in normotensive individuals with familial hyperaldosteronism type I. *J Clin Endocrinol Metab.* 2005;90:5070-5076.
151. Milliez P, Girerd X, Plouin PF, et al. Evidence for an increased rate of cardiovascular events in patients with primary aldosteronism. *J Am Coll Cardiol.* 2005;45:1243-1248.
152. Tanabe A, Naruse M, Naruse K, et al. Left ventricular hypertrophy is more prominent in patients with primary aldosteronism than in patients with other types of secondary hypertension. *Hypertens Res.* 1997;20:85-90.
153. Rossi GP, Sacchetto A, Visentin P, et al. Changes in left ventricular anatomy and function in hypertension and primary aldosteronism. *Hypertension.* 1996;27:1039-1045.
154. Young WF Jr. Minireview: primary aldosteronism—changing concepts in diagnosis and treatment. *Endocrinology.* 2003;144:2208-2213.
155. Williams JS, Williams GH, Raji A, et al. Prevalence of primary hyperaldosteronism in mild to moderate hypertension without hypokalaemia. *J Hum Hypertens.* 2006;20:129-136.
156. Calhoun DA, Nishizaka MK, Zaman MA, et al. Hyperaldosteronism among black and white subjects with resistant hypertension. *Hypertension.* 2002;40:892-896.
157. Mulatero P, Rabbia F, Milan A, et al. Drug effects on aldosterone/plasma renin activity ratio in primary aldosteronism. *Hypertension.* 2002;40: 897-902.
158. Nishizaka MK, Pratt-Ubunama M, Zaman MA, et al. Validity of plasma aldosterone-to-renin activity ratio in African American and white subjects with resistant hypertension. *Am J Hypertens.* 2005;18:805-812.
159. Montori VM, Young WF Jr. Use of plasma aldosterone concentration-to-plasma renin activity ratio as a screening test for primary aldosteronism: a systematic review of the literature. *Endocrinol Metab Clin North Am.* 2002;31:619-632.
160. Weinberger MH, Fineberg NS. The diagnosis of primary aldosteronism and separation of two major subtypes. *Arch Intern Med.* 1993; 153:2125-2129.
161. Young WF Jr. Primary aldosteronism: diagnosis. In: Mansoor GA, ed. *Secondary Hypertension: Clinical Presentation, Diagnosis, and Treatment.* Totowa, NJ: Humana Press; 2004:119-137.
162. Hirohara D, Nomura K, Okamoto T, et al. Performance of the basal aldosterone to renin ratio and of the renin stimulation test by furosemide and upright posture in screening for aldosterone-producing adenoma in low renin hypertensives. *J Clin Endocrinol Metab.* 2001;86:4292-4298.
163. Ferrari P, Shaw SG, Nicod J, et al. Active renin versus plasma renin activity to define aldosterone-to-renin ratio for primary aldosteronism. *J Hypertens.* 2004;22:377-381.
164. Olivieri O, Ciacciarelli A, Signorelli D, et al. Aldosterone to renin ratio in a primary care setting: the Bussolengo study. *J Clin Endocrinol Metab.* 2004;89:4221-4226.
165. Perschel FH, Schemer R, Seiler L, et al. Rapid screening test for primary hyperaldosteronism: ratio of plasma aldosterone to renin concentration determined by fully automated chemiluminescence immunoassays. *Clin Chem.* 2004;50:1650-1655.
166. Lim PO, Farquharson CA, Shiels P, et al. Adverse cardiac effects of salt with fludrocortisone in hypertension. *Hypertension.* 2001;37:856-861.
167. Young WF Jr, Hogan MJ, Klee GG, et al. Primary aldosteronism: diagnosis and treatment. *Mayo Clinic Proc.* 1990;65:96-110.
168. Bravo EL, Tarazi RC, Dustan HP, et al. The changing clinical spectrum of primary aldosteronism. *Am J Med.* 1983;74:641-651.
169. Kem DC, Weinberger MH, Mayes DM, et al. Saline suppression of plasma aldosterone in hypertension. *Arch Intern Med.* 1971;128: 380-386.
170. Holland OB, Brown H, Kuhnert L, et al. Further evaluation of saline infusion for the diagnosis of primary aldosteronism. *Hypertension.* 1984;6:717-723.
171. Weinberger MH, Grim CE, Hollifield JW, et al. Primary aldosteronism: diagnosis, localization, and treatment. *Ann Intern Med.* 1979;90: 386-395.
172. Arteaga E, Klein R, Biglieri EG. Use of the saline infusion test to diagnose the cause of primary aldosteronism. *Am J Med.* 1985;79: 722-728.
173. Stowasser M, Gordon RD. Primary aldosteronism: careful investigation is essential and rewarding. *Mol Cell Endocrinol.* 2004;217:33-39.
174. Sawka AM, Young WF, Thompson GB, et al. Primary aldosteronism: factors associated with normalization of blood pressure after surgery. *Ann Intern Med.* 2001;135:258-261.
175. Meyer A, Brabant G, Behrend M. Long-term follow-up after adrenalectomy for primary aldosteronism. *World J Surg.* 2005;29:155-159.
176. Celen O, O'Brien MJ, Melby JC, et al. Factors influencing outcome of surgery for primary aldosteronism. *Arch Surg.* 1996;131:646-650.
177. Kloos RT, Gross MD, Francis IR, et al. Incidentally discovered adrenal masses. *Endocr Rev.* 1995;16:460-484.
178. Young WF, Stanson AW, Thompson GB, et al. Role for adrenal venous sampling in primary aldosteronism. *Surgery.* 2004;136:1227-1235.
179. Kempers, MJ, Lenders, JW, van Outheusden, L, et al. Systematic review: diagnostic procedures to differentiate unilateral from bilateral adrenal abnormality in primary aldosteronism. *Ann Intern Med.* 2009;151: 329.
180. Daunt N. Adrenal vein sampling: how to make it quick, easy, and successful. *Radiographics.* 2005;25(suppl 1):S143-S158.
181. Doppman JL, Gill JR Jr. Hyperaldosteronism: sampling the adrenal veins. *Radiology.* 1996;198:309-312.
182. Young WF, Stanson AW. *What are the keys to successful adrenal venous sampling (AVS) in patients with primary aldosteronism? Clin Endocrinol (Oxf).* 2009;70:14-17.
183. Melby JC, Spark RF, Dale SL, et al. Diagnosis and localization of aldosterone-producing adenomas by adrenal-vein catheterization. *N Engl J Med.* 1967;277:1050-1056.
184. Conn JW, Morita R, Cohen EL, et al. Primary aldosteronism: photoscanning of tumors after administration of 131 I-19-iodocholesterol. *Arch Intern Med.* 1972;129:417-425.
185. Sarkar SD, Cohen EL, Beierwaltes WH, et al. A new and superior adrenal imaging agent, 131I-6beta-iodomethyl-19-nor-cholesterol (NP-59): evaluation in humans. *J Clin Endocrinol Metab.* 1977;45: 353-362.
186. Hogan MJ, McRae J, Schambelan M, et al. Location of aldosterone-producing adenomas with 131I-19-iodocholesterol. *N Engl J Med.* 1976;294:410-414.
187. Nomura K, Kusakabe K, Maki M, et al. Iodomethylnorcholesterol uptake in an aldosteronoma shown by dexamethasone-suppression scintigraphy: relationship to adenoma size and functional activity. *J Clin Endocrinol Metab.* 1990;71:825-830.
188. Ganguly A, Dowdy AJ, Luetscher JA, et al. Anomalous postural response of plasma aldosterone concentration in patients with aldosterone-producing adrenal adenoma. *J Clin Endocrinol Metab.* 1973;36: 401-404.
189. Biglieri EG, Schambelan M. The significance of elevated levels of plasma 18-hydroxycorticosterone in patients with primary aldosteronism. *J Clin Endocrinol Metab.* 1979;49:87-91.
190. Sechi LA, Di Fabio A, Bazzocchi M, et al. Intrarenal hemodynamics in primary aldosteronism before and after treatment. *J Clin Endocrinol Metab.* 2009;94:1191-1197.
191. Reincke M, Rump LC, Quinkler M, et al. Risk factors associated with a low glomerular filtration rate in primary aldosteronism. *J Clin Endocrinol Metab.* 2009;94:869-875.
192. Rossi H, Kim A, Prinz RA. Primary hyperaldosteronism in the era of laparoscopic adrenalectomy. *Am Surg.* 2002;68:253-256, discussion 256-257.
193. Gonzalez R, Smith CD, McClusky DA 3rd, et al. Laparoscopic approach reduces likelihood of perioperative complications in patients undergoing adrenalectomy. *Am Surg.* 2004;70:668-674.
194. Ishidoya S, Ito A, Sakai K, et al. Laparoscopic partial versus total adrenalectomy for aldosterone producing adenoma. *J Urol.* 2005; 174:40-43.
195. Sywak M, Pasieka JL. Long-term follow-up and cost benefit of adrenalectomy in patients with primary hyperaldosteronism. *Br J Surg.* 2002;89:1587-1593.
196. Ghose RP, Hall PM, Bravo EL. Medical management of aldosterone-producing adenomas. *Ann Intern Med.* 1999;131:105-108.
197. Lim PO, Young WF, MacDonald TM. A review of the medical treatment of primary aldosteronism. *J Hypertens.* 2001;19:353-361.
198. Sica DA. Pharmacokinetics and pharmacodynamics of mineralocorticoid blocking agents and their effects on potassium homeostasis. *Heart Fail Rev.* 2005;10:23-29.
199. Jeunemaitre X, Chatellier G, Kreft-Jais C, et al. Efficacy and tolerance of spironolactone in essential hypertension. *Am J Cardiol.* 1987;60: 820-825.
200. Morgenstern BZ. Hypertension in pediatric patients: current issues. *Mayo Clin Proc.* 1994;69:1089-1097.
201. Merke DP, Bornstein SR. Congenital adrenal hyperplasia. *Lancet.* 2005;365:2125-2136.
202. New MI, Geller DS, Fallo F, et al. Monogenic low renin hypertension. *Trends Endocrinol Metab.* 2005;16:92-97.
203. Mussig K, Wehrmann M, Horger M, et al. Adrenocortical carcinoma producing 11-deoxycorticosterone: a rare cause of mineralocorticoid hypertension. *J Endocrinol Invest.* 2005;28:61-65.

204. Kino T, Vottero A, Charmandari E, et al. Familial/sporadic glucocorticoid resistance syndrome and hypertension. *Ann N Y Acad Sci*. 2002;970:101-111.
205. Stewart PM, Corrie JE, Shackleton CH. Syndrome of apparent mineralocorticoid excess: a defect in the cortisol-cortisone shuttle. *J Clin Invest*. 1988;82:340-349.
206. Liddle GW, Blesdoe T, Coppage WS Jr. A familial renal disorder simulating primary aldosteronism but with negligible aldosterone secretion. *Trans Assoc Am Physicians*. 1963;76:199-213.
207. Geller DS, Farhi A, Pinkerton N, et al. Activating mineralocorticoid receptor mutation in hypertension exacerbated by pregnancy. *Science*. 2000;289:119-123.
208. Sacerdote A, Weiss K, Tran T, et al. Hypertension in patients with Cushing's disease: pathophysiology, diagnosis, and management. *Curr Hypertens Rep*. 2005;7:212-218.
209. Baid S, Nieman LK. Glucocorticoid excess and hypertension. *Curr Hypertens Rep*. 2004;6:493-499.
210. Danzi S, Klein I. Thyroid hormone and blood pressure regulation. *Curr Hypertens Rep*. 2003;5:513-520.
211. Streeten DH, Anderson GH Jr, Howland T, et al. Effects of thyroid function on blood pressure: recognition of hypothyroid hypertension. *Hypertension*. 1988;11:78-83.
212. Richards AM, Espiner EA, Nicholls MG, et al. Hormone, calcium and blood pressure relationships in primary hyperparathyroidism. *J Hypertens*. 1988;6:747-752.
213. Sancho JJ, Rouco J, Riera-Vida R, et al. Long-term effects of parathyroidectomy for primary hyperparathyroidism on arterial hypertension. *World J Surg*. 1992;16:732-736.
214. Terzolo M, Matrella C, Boccuzzi A, et al. Twenty-four hour profile of blood pressure in patients with acromegaly. Correlation with demographic, clinical and hormonal features. *J Endocrinol Invest*. 1999;22:48-54.

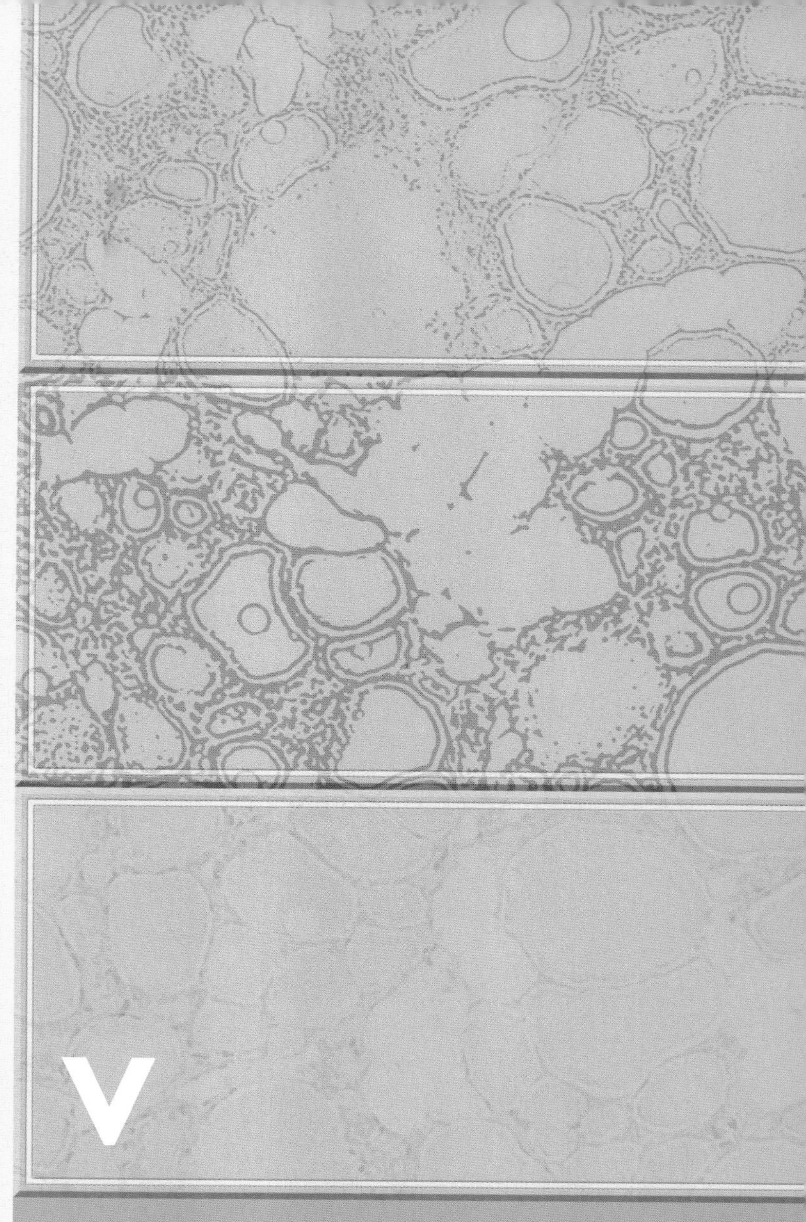

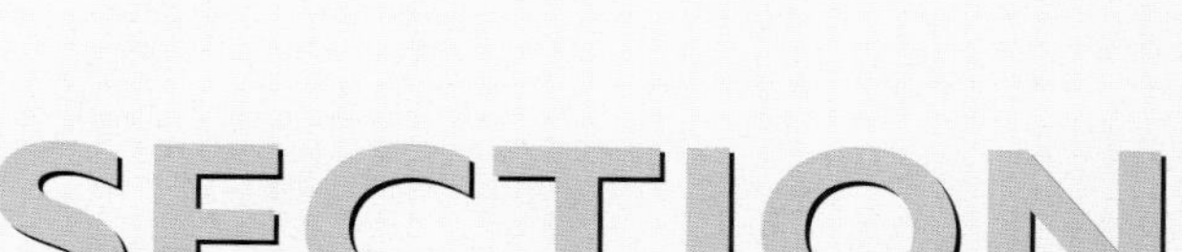

SECTION V

Reproduction

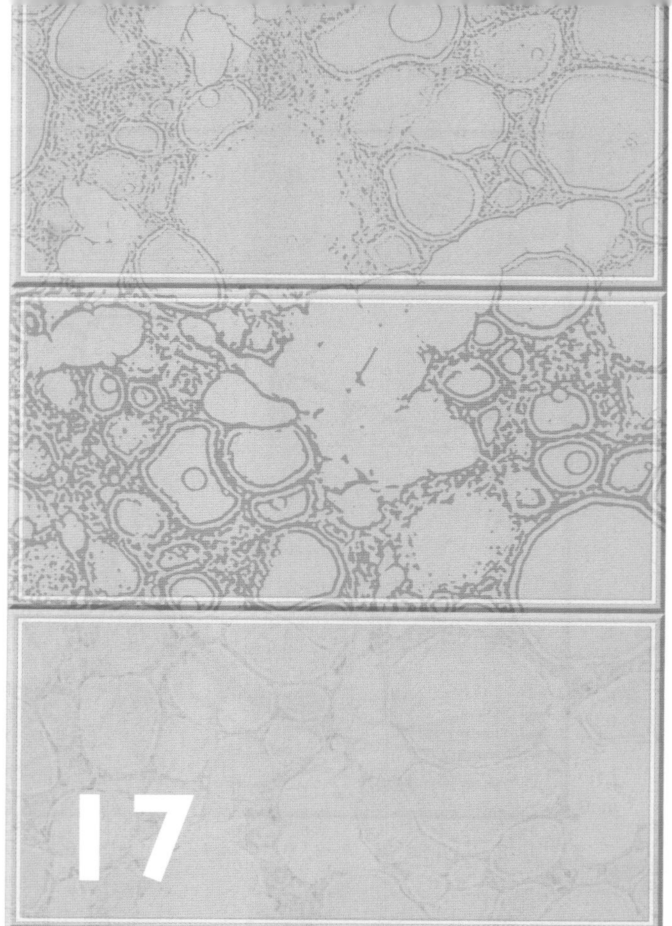

CHAPTER 17

Physiology and Pathology of the Female Reproductive Axis

SERDAR E. BULUN

REPRODUCTIVE PHYSIOLOGY

Tightly coordinated functions of the hypothalamus, pituitary, ovaries, and endometrium give rise to cyclic, predictable menses that indicate regular ovulation. Regular ovulation requires normal functioning of other endocrine glands, such as the thyroid and adrenals, and patients with hypothyroidism, hyperthyroidism, Cushing's syndrome, or glucocorticoid resistance may present with anovulation. Clinicians need a thorough knowledge of the functions and interactions of the hypothalamus, pituitary, ovaries, and uterus with other systems to correctly diagnose reproductive disorders and design treatment strategies.

A prominent reproductive function of the hypothalamus is pulsatile secretion of gonadotropin-releasing hormone (GnRH). Negative feedback effects of several factors, including ovarian steroids, regulate hypothalamic GnRH secretion into the portal vessels. Dopamine, norepinephrine, serotonin, and opioids produced in the brain may mediate the regulation of GnRH secretion by ovarian hormones or other stimuli. In response to GnRH, the anterior pituitary cells secrete follicle-stimulating hormone (FSH) and luteinizing hormone (LH). Steroids (e.g., estradiol, progesterone) and peptides (e.g., inhibin) of ovarian origin and activin and follistatin of pituitary origin modify secretion of FSH and LH. LH stimulates androstenedione production in theca cells of the ovary; FSH regulates estradiol and inhibin B production in the granulosa cells and follicular growth. Release of an egg from the mature follicle depends on a sudden rise in LH levels in midcycle. After ovulation, the follicle transforms into a corpus luteum that secretes estradiol and progesterone under the control of FSH and LH. LH also stimulates granulosa-lutein cells of the corpus luteum to secrete inhibin A (Fig. 17-1A).

The endocrine effects of FSH, LH, estradiol, progesterone, inhibin A, and inhibin B have been deduced from changes in their serum levels throughout the menstrual cycle (see Fig. 17-1A). The postulated endocrine effects were then demonstrated in cell-based and in vivo studies (see Fig. 17-1B). Activin and follistatin are produced in the ovary and the pituitary. They appear to act on FSH in the pituitary by autocrine or paracrine but not endocrine pathways. Activin stimulates FSH production, whereas follistatin suppresses this action of activin.

Endometrium, the mucosal lining of the uterine cavity, has extremely high concentrations of nuclear receptors for estrogen and progesterone and is extremely sensitive to

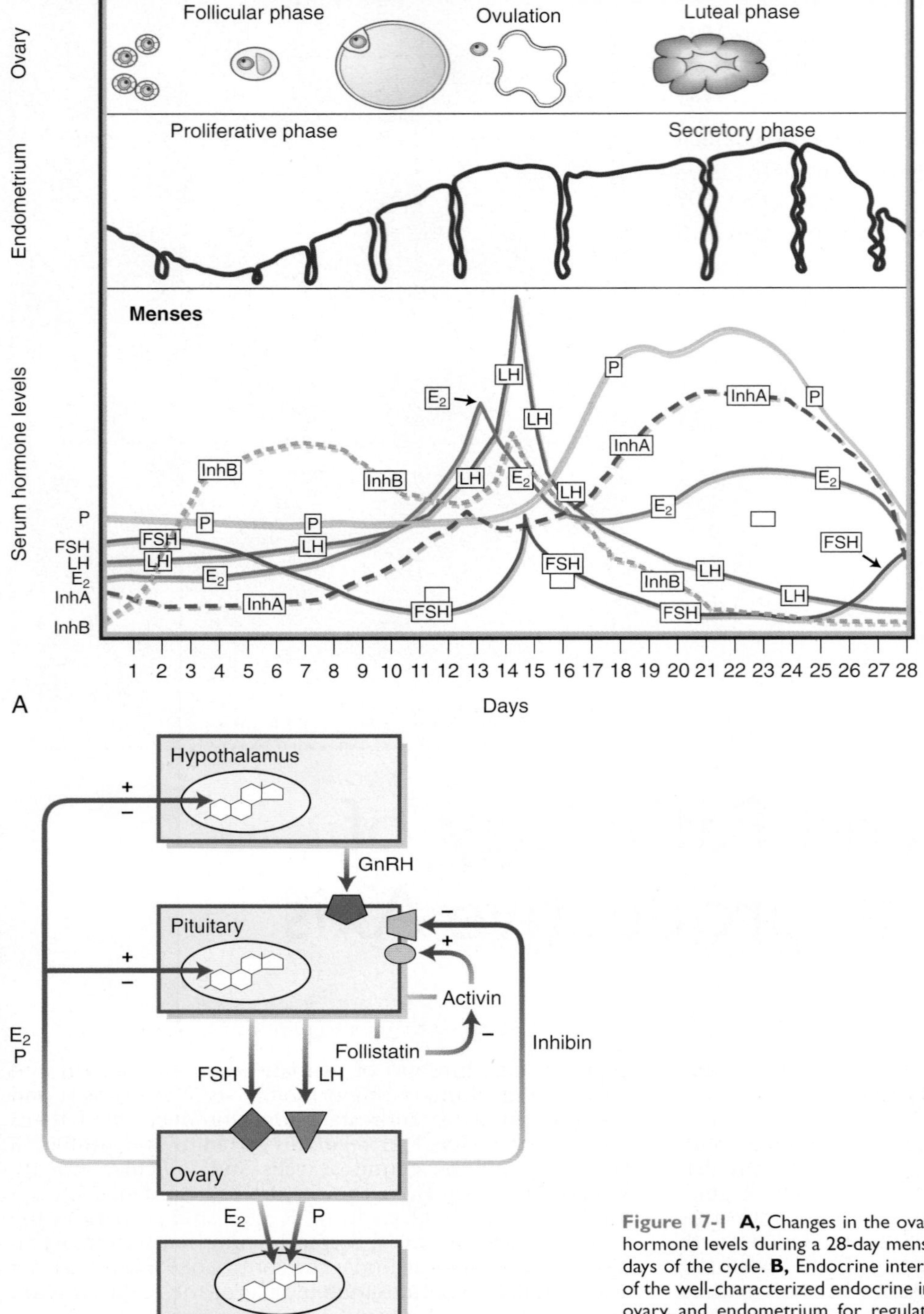

Figure 17-1 **A,** Changes in the ovarian follicle, endometrial thickness, and serum hormone levels during a 28-day menstrual cycle. Menses occur during the first few days of the cycle. **B,** Endocrine interactions in the female reproductive axis. Some of the well-characterized endocrine interactions among the hypothalamus, pituitary, ovary, and endometrium for regulation of the menstrual cycle are depicted. E_2, estradiol; FSH, follicle-stimulating hormone; GnRH, gonadotropin-releasing hormone; Inh, inhibin; LH, luteinizing hormone; P, progesterone.

these hormones. The biologically active estrogen, estradiol, induces the growth of endometrium; progesterone limits this estrogenic effect and enhances differentiation. Sloughing off the functional portion (functionalis) of the endometrium follows withdrawal of estrogen or progesterone. The remaining basal layer (basalis) is capable of full regeneration in response to estrogen.

Ovaries remain quiescent until puberty because the hypothalamus is immature in prepubertal children, and FSH and LH do not stimulate the ovaries. The entire reproductive function and most of the endocrine function of the ovaries cease after menopause because ovaries have lost all oocytes and surrounding steroidogenic cells by this time. These prepubertal and postmenopausal states, characterized by the absence of ovarian function, are associated with the lack of menses.

In summary, the female reproductive function from puberty to menopause can be viewed as an extremely delicate ticking clock. The normal function of this apparatus depends on coordinated actions of the hypothalamus, pituitary, ovaries, and endometrium. The result is regular menses every 24 to 35 days. Any disorder of these tissues or disorders of other systems that affect these reproductive units secondarily may result in anovulation and consequent irregular uterine bleeding.

REPRODUCTIVE FUNCTIONS OF THE HYPOTHALAMUS

Gonadotropin-Releasing Hormone

GnRH and its analogs are used for the treatment of hormone-dependent disorders and assisted reproductive technologies such as in vitro fertilization (IVF).[1] In a number of vertebrates, three GnRHs and three cognate receptors with distinct distributions and functions have been identified. In humans, the hypothalamic GnRH is primarily encoded by the GnRH type I (GnRH-I) gene (*GNRH1*) and regulates gonadotropin secretion through the pituitary GnRH type I receptor, which functions as a G protein–coupled receptor. Binding of GnRH-I to its type I receptor leads primarily to activation of G_q. A second form of GnRH, called GnRH-II is conserved in all higher vertebrates, including humans, and is present in extrahypothalamic brain and many reproductive tissues. Its cognate receptor has been cloned from various vertebrate species, including primates. The human gene homolog of this receptor has a frameshift and stop codon, and it appears that GnRH-II signaling occurs through the type I GnRH receptor. There is considerable plasticity in the use of different GnRHs, receptors, and signaling pathways for diverse functions.[1] For practical purposes, GnRH-I is referred to as GnRH in this chapter.

GnRH is a 10-amino-acid peptide that is synthesized primarily in specialized neuronal bodies of the arcuate nucleus of the medial basal hypothalamus.[2] Axons from GnRH neurons project to the median eminence and terminate in the capillaries that drain into the portal vessels.

The portal vein is a low-flow transport system that descends along the pituitary stalk and connects the hypothalamus to the anterior pituitary. The direction of the blood flow in this hypophyseal portal circulation is from the hypothalamus to the pituitary. GnRH originating in the neurons of the arcuate nucleus is secreted at the median eminence into the portal circulation, which delivers this hormone to the anterior pituitary (Fig. 17-2).

The mature decapeptide GnRH is derived from the posttranslational processing of a large precursor molecule, pre-pro-GnRH (see Fig. 17-2).[3] This precursor peptide is the product of a gene located in the short arm of chromosome 8.[4] The pre-pro-GnRH consists of 92 amino acids and contains four parts (from amino-terminal to carboxyl-terminal): a 23-amino-acid signal domain, the GnRH decapeptide, a 3-amino-acid proteolytic processing site, and a 56-amino-acid domain called GnRH-associated peptide.[5,6] The cleavage products of this precursor, GnRH and gonadotropin-releasing hormone–associated peptide (GAP), are transported to the nerve terminals and secreted into the portal circulation (see Fig. 17-2).[3,7,8] A physiologic role for GAP has not been established.[7]

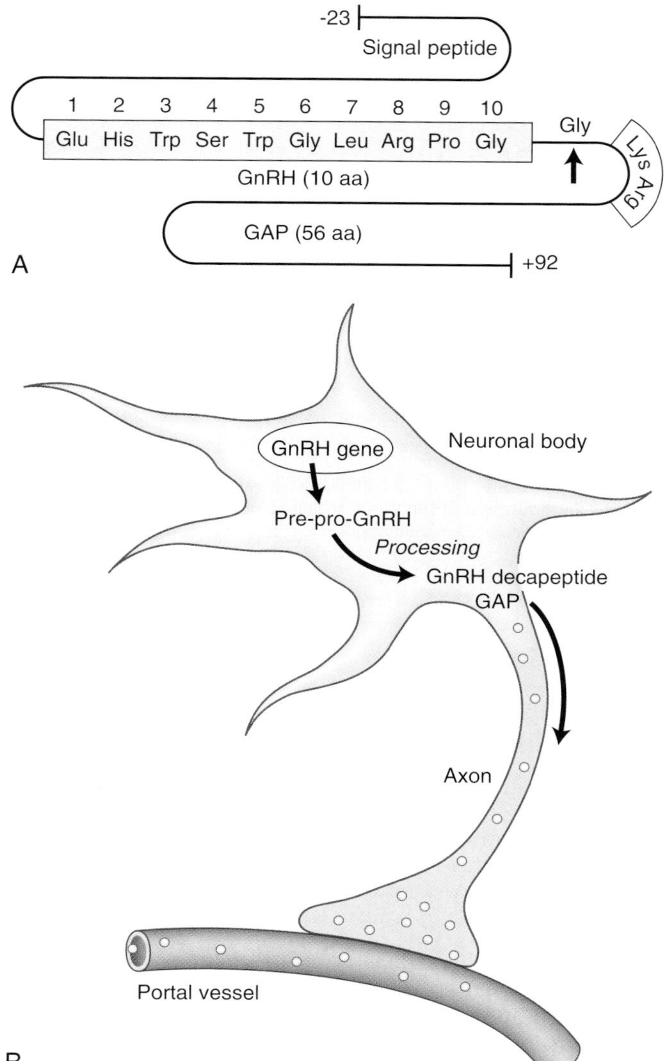

Figure 17-2 Gonadotropin-releasing hormone (GnRH) production. **A,** The GnRH gene encodes a precursor protein, pre-pro-GnRH, in the neuronal body. GnRH is released from this protein by proteolytic processing, which gives rise to GnRH and GnRH-associated protein (GAP) within the neuronal body. Both GnRH and GAP are transported in an axon to the nerve terminal and secreted into the portal circulation. **B,** Pre-pro-GnRH is a 92-amino-acid (aa) protein. The biologically active decapeptide (amino acids 1 through 10) is sandwiched between the 23-amino-acid signal peptide and the Gly-Lys-Arg sequence. The *arrow* indicates the site of proteolytic processing. The C-terminal 56-amino-acid peptide is cleaved to produce GAP. LHRH, luteinizing hormone–releasing hormone (gonadotropin-releasing hormone I). (From Yen SSC. Endocrine regulation of the reproductive system. In: Yen SSC, Jaffe RB, Barbieri RL, eds. *Reproductive Endocrinology,* 4th ed. Philadelphia, PA: Saunders; 1999:44.)

In humans, GnRH neurons are located primarily in the arcuate nucleus of the medial basal hypothalamus and the preoptic area of the anterior hypothalamus. The population of GnRH-producing neurons is relatively limited and is in the range of 1000 to 2000. The neurons that produce GnRH originate from the olfactory area during embryogenesis. GnRH and olfactory neurons migrate together along cranial nerves connecting the nose and forebrain to the hypothalamus during embryologic development, and disruption of this process causes idiopathic hypogonadotropic

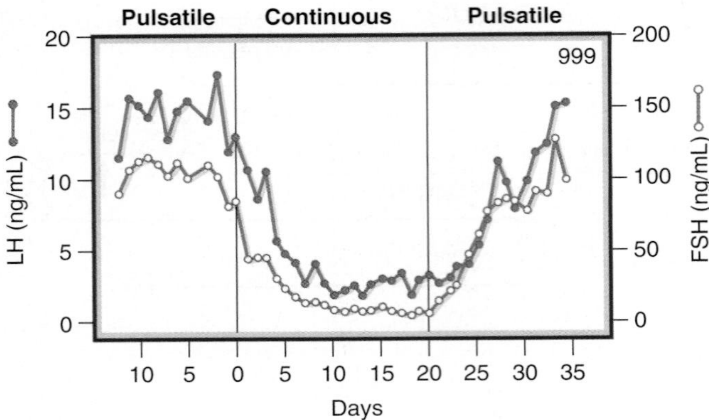

Figure 17-3 Effect of pulsatile or continuous administration of gonadotropin-releasing hormone (GnRH) to ovariectomized monkeys previously rendered GnRH deficient by placement of a lesion in the hypothalamus. Release of luteinizing hormone (LH) and follicle-stimulating hormone (FSH) was restored by hourly GnRH infusion, inhibited during a continuous infusion, and again restored after reinstitution of pulsatile GnRH administration. (Adapted from Belchetz PE, Plant TM, Nakai Y, et al. Hypophysial responses to continuous and intermittent delivery of hypothalamic gonadotropin releasing hormone. *Science*. 1978;202:631-633. Copyright © 1978, by American Association for the Advancement of Science.)

hypogonadism with anosmia, or Kallmann's syndrome. Individuals with Kallmann's syndrome usually have irreversible pubertal delay and subsequent infertility due to deficient GnRH and pituitary gonadotropins. The neuronal proteins anosmin 1 (encoded by the *KAL1* gene) and fibroblast growth factor receptor type 1 (encoded by the *FGFR1* gene) affect olfactory and GnRH neuron migration. Mutations in these genes cause Kallmann's syndrome. Data suggest that mutations of the genes for nasal embryonic luteinizing hormone–releasing hormone factor (*NELF*) and chromodomain helicase DNA-binding protein 7 (*CHD7*) may cause Kallmann's syndrome, but this correlation is not as conclusively established as it is for *KAL1* and *FGFR1*. Kallmann's syndrome associated with reproductive and olfactory dysfunction illustrates the important embryologic event of GnRH and olfactory neuron migration.[9]

Knobil and coworkers demonstrated in a pioneering series of experiments that normal gonadotropin secretion requires pulsatile GnRH discharge within a critical frequency and amplitude.[10] The periodicity and amplitude of the pulsatile rhythm of GnRH and gonadotropin secretion are crucial in regulating gonadal activities and therefore the entire reproductive axis (Fig. 17-3). The self-priming effect of GnRH in upregulating its receptors on pituitary gonadotropin-producing cells manifests only at the physiologic periodicity of 60 to 90 minutes.[11,12] Slower frequency causes anovulation and amenorrhea because of inadequate stimulation. Higher frequency or constant exposure to GnRH also gives rise to anovulation by downregulating expression of the GnRH receptor, thereby abolishing gonadotropin responses.

The activation of gene expression for gonadotropin subunits, including the common α-subunit and specific β-subunits for LH and FSH, dimerization of αβ subunits, and glycosylation appear to be governed by intermittency of GnRH inputs to pituitary gonadotrophs.[13] In humans, measurement of LH pulses is commonly used as an indication of GnRH pulsatile secretion.[14] The LH pulse frequency is approximately 90 minutes during the early follicular phase, 60 to 70 minutes during the late follicular phase, 100 minutes during the early luteal phase, and 200 minutes during the late luteal phase.[15] This variation is responsible for changes in FSH and LH levels and ovarian steroid release during these phases of the menstrual cycle. The relationship of gonadotropin secretion to GnRH pulse pattern has been studied in hypophysectomized animals receiving exogenous GnRH and in numerous in vitro systems. More rapid pulse frequencies favor LH secretion, whereas slower pulse frequencies favor FSH. It appears that variations in GnRH pulse frequency markedly influence both the absolute levels and the ratio of LH and FSH release.

Regulation of Gonadotropin-Releasing Hormone Secretion

Cyclic, predictable menses require the pulsatile release of GnRH within a critical range of frequencies. Pulsatile, rhythmic activity is an intrinsic property of GnRH neurons, and various hormones and neurotransmitters modulate this rhythm (Fig. 17-4).

The variations in GnRH pulse frequency are achieved, in part, by gonadal steroid feedback. Estradiol increases GnRH pulse frequency, and elevated progesterone levels decrease GnRH pulsatility.[13] Increased progesterone levels may decrease GnRH pulse frequency and thereby lead to preferential biosynthesis and secretion of FSH, as observed in the late luteal phase.[13]

GnRH pulsatility is also modulated by the actions of locally released neurotransmitters. Norepinephrine stimulates GnRH release, whereas dopamine exerts an inhibitory effect (see Fig. 17-4).[16] β-Endorphin and other opioids may suppress the hypothalamic release of GnRH.[17,18] The gonadal steroids modify endogenous opioid activity, and

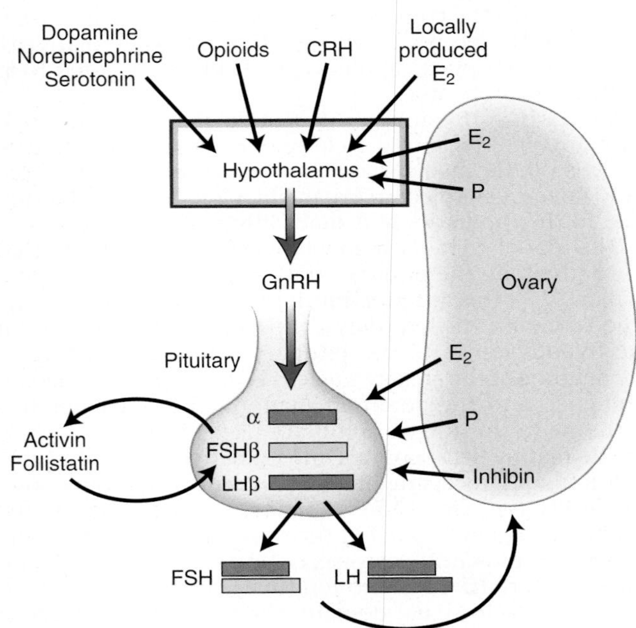

Figure 17-4 Regulation of gonadotropin-releasing hormone (GnRH), luteinizing hormone (LH), and follicle-stimulating hormone (FSH) secretion. Locally synthesized and systemic hormones regulate the pulsatile secretion of GnRH from the hypothalamus into the portal circulation. GnRH and a number of steroid and peptide hormones regulate the synthesis of α and β gonadotropin subunits and the formation and secretion of FSH and LH. CRH, corticotropin-releasing hormone; E_2, estradiol; P, progesterone.

the negative feedback of steroids on gonadotropins appears to be mediated in part by endogenous opioids.[19] It has been proposed that sex steroids enhance the activity of endogenous opioids that exert an inhibitory effect on GnRH secretion.[20] The negative effect of opioids on GnRH secretion is clinically explicable because the reduced GnRH secretion associated with hypothalamic amenorrhea may be mediated by an increase in endogenous opioid inhibitory tone.[21]

Estrogen signaling to GnRH neurons appears to be critical for suppressing FSH and LH and for coordinating the preovulatory surge release of LH. The precise roles of estrogen receptors α and β (ERα and ERβ, respectively) within the GnRH neurons or estradiol-sensitive afferent neurons in these negative and positive feedback effects of estrogen are not well understood.[22] Results of stimulation of FSH release after treatment of a premenopausal woman with an aromatase inhibitor and of in vitro studies suggest that estrogen locally produced by hypothalamic neurons may regulate gonadotropin secretion.[23,24]

Binding of the peptide kisspeptin to its G protein–coupled receptor KISS1R (previously known as GPR54), which is expressed in GnRH neurons, stimulates GnRH release in the hypothalamus.[25,26] Kisspeptin neurons contact GnRH neurons and act at the cell body and the nerve terminals. Kisspeptin can act directly on GnRH neurons or indirectly through synaptic input from other neurons to inhibit inwardly rectifying potassium channels and activate nonspecific cation channels, producing long-lasting depolarization and an increased action potential firing rate.[27] Mutations or targeted knockout of KISS1R produces isolated hypogonadotropic hypogonadism in humans and mice, indicating that signaling through this receptor is essential for sexual development and function.[25,26] Moreover, kisspeptin- and KISS1R-expressing neurons may be critical targets for the negative and positive feedback actions of estrogen and progestrone.[28]

Gonadotropin-Releasing Hormone Analogs

The half-life of GnRH is short (2 to 4 minutes) because it is degraded rapidly by peptidases in the hypothalamus and pituitary gland.[29] These peptidases cleave the bonds between amino acids 5 and 6, 6 and 7, and 9 and 10. Analogs of GnRH with different properties have been synthesized by alteration of amino acids at these positions. Many agonistic and antagonistic GnRH analogs with various biologic effects have been produced.

Peptide Gonadotropin-Releasing Hormone Agonists

Several GnRH agonist peptides are generated by substitution of amino acids at the 6 or 10 position (Fig. 17-5). The increased biologic activity of agonistic peptides has been attributed to their high binding affinity to GnRH receptors and their reduced susceptibility to enzymatic degradation. An amino acid substitution at position 6 gives rise to metabolic stability, whereas replacement of the C-terminal glycinamide residue by an ethylamide group increases strikingly the affinity for the receptors.[29-31] Peptide GnRH agonists are administered subcutaneously, intranasally, or intramuscularly. An initial agonistic action (i.e., flare effect) is associated with an increase in the circulating levels of LH and FSH.

The most prominent agonistic response is observed during the early follicular phase, when the combined effects of GnRH agonist and elevated levels of estradiol create a large reserve pool of gonadotropins.[32] Desensitization and downregulation of the pituitary produce hypogonadotropic hypogonadism. Administration of a long-acting

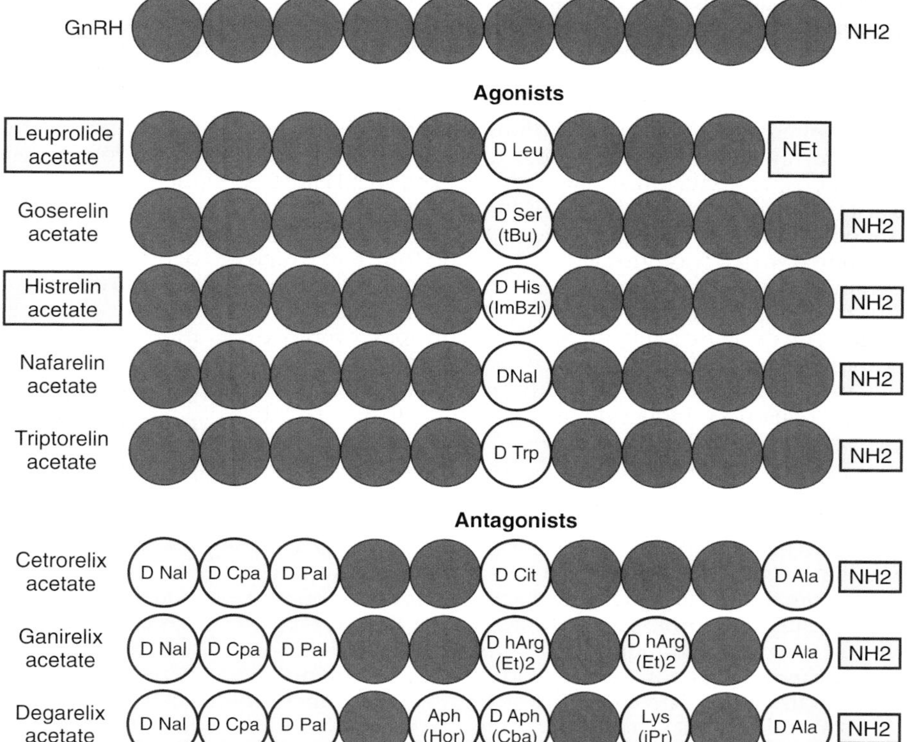

Figure 17-5 Gonadotropin-releasing hormone (GnRH) agonist and antagonist analogs in clinical practice. *Purple circles* indicate amino acids in the wild-type GnRH decapeptide, and *white circles* are labeled with the changes made to the analogs. (Modified from Millar RP, Lu Z, Pawson AJ, et al. Gonadotropin-releasing hormone receptors. *Endocr Rev.* 2004;25:235-275. Copyright © 2004 by the Endocrine Society.)

depot formulation of a GnRH agonist gives rise to downregulation of the gonadotropin-gonadal axis within 1 to 3 weeks. The initial downregulation effect is caused by desensitization, whereas the sustained response results from loss of receptors and the uncoupling of the receptor from its effector system. GnRH agonists may cause ovarian quiescence by the secretion of biologically inactive gonadotropins.

The U.S. Food and Drug Administration (FDA) has approved the use of these agonists for the treatment of GnRH-dependent precocious puberty, endometriosis, and prostate cancer. Another indication is preoperative hematologic improvement of patients with anemia caused by uterine leiomyomas. Off-label indications for GnRH agonists include downregulation of the pituitary during ovulation induction, induction of endometrial atrophy before endometrial ablation surgery, and prevention of menstrual bleeding in patients with coagulation defects. GnRH agonists have also been used to suppress ovarian steroidogenesis in hirsute patients.[33]

The most prominent side effects of long-term use of depot GnRH agonist formulations are caused by estrogen deficiency. Depot GnRH agonists induce a menopause-like state characterized by hot flashes, vaginal dryness, bone resorption, and osteopenia. Osteopenia is reversible in young women if treatment is maintained for no more than 6 months.[34,35] The risk/benefit ratio must be considered carefully before GnRH agonist treatment is extended for longer periods. Add-back regimens employing low-dose estrogens or progestins, or both, administered along with GnRH agonists have provided a means to overcome these side effects and to extend the length of agonist therapy.[36]

Peptide Gonadotropin-Releasing Hormone Antagonists

Inhibition of a premature LH rise by GnRH agonists requires at least 7 days, because it is accompanied by an initial stimulation of GnRH receptors before gonadotroph desensitization is achieved. In contrast, GnRH antagonists compete directly with endogenous GnRH for receptor binding and therefore rapidly inhibit secretion of gonadotropin and steroid hormones (see Fig. 17-5). This property conveys a potential advantage over GnRH agonists in the management of ovarian stimulation. However, because of the constant need to block endogenous GnRH, much higher doses of antagonists are required. The GnRH antagonists incorporate a number of amino acid substitutions in the N-terminal domain (involved in receptor activation) combined with a D-amino acid substitution for Gly6, which enhances the βII-type bend necessary for receptor binding.[1] GnRH antagonists have the advantage of inducing an immediate decrease in circulating gonadotropin levels with rapid reversal.[37-40] GnRH antagonists are alternative drugs to GnRH agonists for the prevention of a natural LH surge during ovulation induction by injectable FSH.[41] Use of GnRH antagonists has become popular in ovulation induction protocols for IVF (see Fig. 17-5).[41]

Nonpeptide Gonadotropin-Releasing Hormone Antagonists

Small molecular compound collections have been screened in mammalian cells that ectopically expressed human GnRH type I receptor. These studies led to the identification of synthetic compounds that bind to the GnRH type I receptor and block it. Several companies have manufactured orally administered GnRH antagonists intended for various indications, including endometriosis. None of these medications has yet reached the market.[1]

REPRODUCTIVE FUNCTIONS OF THE ANTERIOR PITUITARY

Gonadotrophs

Gonadotrophs are specialized cell types of the anterior pituitary that synthesize and secrete LH and FSH. These cells constitute 7% to 15% of the total number of anterior pituitary cells and are detected in this location from early fetal life.[42] Most gonadotrophs are capable of synthesizing both LH and FSH.[42,43] LH and FSH are each composed of two distinct, noncovalently associated protein subunits called α and β (see Fig. 17-4). In the gonadotroph, the subunit genes are transcribed into messenger ribonucleic acids (mRNAs), which are translated into the subunit precursors. Gonadotrophs contain cell surface GnRH type I receptors that mediate the action of GnRH. These receptors belong to the seven-transmembrane domain and G protein–coupled receptor family.

Gonadotropin-Releasing Hormone Receptor

In humans, hypothalamic GnRH regulates gonadotropin secretion through the pituitary GnRH type I receptor by activation of $G_{q/11}$.[44] Although the predominant coupling of the type I GnRH receptor in the gonadotroph is through $G_{q/11}$ stimulation, signal transduction can occur through other G proteins and potentially by G protein–independent means.[1,44] A number of downstream cascades are activated by GnRH. These include protein kinase C (PKC)-, Ca^{2+}-, and tyrosine kinase–dependent pathways.[1] In mouse pituitary gonadotrophs, the GnRH receptor activates several mitogen-activated protein (MAP) kinase cascades, including the ERK1/2, the JUN N-terminal kinase (JNK), the p38 MAP kinase, and the big MAP kinase (BMK1/ERK5).[1] The cross-talk between these pathways remains to be clarified.

Activation of G protein–coupled receptors is typically followed by their desensitization and internalization, and these processes involve rapid agonist-induced receptor phosphorylation by second messenger–dependent protein kinases and G protein–coupled receptor kinases. Because the serine and threonine residues that are phosphorylated by G protein–coupled receptor kinases are often located in the C-terminal tail, which is uniquely absent in the mammalian GnRH receptor, several studies have revealed that the tailless GnRH receptor neither undergoes rapid homologous desensitization nor exhibits agonist-induced receptor phosphorylation. The receptor internalizes slowly by means of clathrin-coated vesicles, and this process occurs independently of β-arrestin and dynamin.[1]

Luteinizing Hormone and Follicle-Stimulating Hormone

Each gonadotropin is a heterodimer. LH and FSH are made of two peptide subunits called α and β, which are associated with noncovalent bonds. The α-subunits of human LH, FSH, thyroid-stimulating hormone (TSH), and human chorionic gonadotropin (hCG) have an identical polypeptide structure. In contrast, the β-subunit of each hormone has a unique amino acid sequence and confers the specific activity of the αβ-heterodimer. Each subunit is rich in cysteine and contains multiple disulfide linkages. Each subunit also contains multiple carbohydrate moieties that play important roles in the biologic activity and metabolism of these hormones. The common α-subunit contains 92

TABLE 17-1

Properties of Gonadotropins

Gonadotropins	Location of β-Subunit Gene	Size of β-Subunit (No. of Amino Acids)	Half-Life in Serum
FSH	Chromosome 11p13	117	3-4 hr
LH	Chromosome 19q13.3	121	20 min
hCG	Chromosome 19q13.3	145	24 hr

FSH, follicle-stimulating hormone; hCG, human chorionic gonadotropin; LH, luteinizing hormone.

amino acids. The β-subunits of human FSH, LH, and hCG contain 117, 121, and 145 amino acids, respectively (Table 17-1).[45-48] On binding of GnRH to its receptor, the biosynthesis of the gonadotropins proceeds by transcription of the subunit genes, translation of the subunit mRNAs, post-translational modifications of the precursor subunits and subunit folding and combination, mature hormone packaging, and hormone secretion (see Fig. 17-4).

The human α-subunit gene is located on the short arm of chromosome 6. The encoded precursor polypeptide contains a 24-amino-acid leader sequence that is cleaved post-translationally to produce the mature 92-amino-acid α-subunit.

The human LH and hCG β-subunit genes are located on chromosome 19q13.3, which contains a cluster of seven β-subunit–like genes.[46] Five of these sequences are noncoding pseudogenes arranged in groups of tandem and inverted pairs. Only LH and hCG β-subunit genes give rise to two distinct and functional mRNA species. The LH β-subunit mRNA encodes a 145-amino-acid precursor protein that is later cleaved to produce a 24-amino-acid leader peptide and an 121-amino-acid, biologically active, mature peptide. The hCG β-subunit mRNA also encodes a 145-amino-acid protein. This protein, however, is not processed post-translationally and functions as the biologically active hCG β-subunit. The amino acid sequences of the human LH and hCG β–subunits are 82% homologous. These two β-subunits confer identical biologic activities when associated with the α-subunit.[46-48]

A single gene located on the short arm of chromosome 11 encodes the FSH β-subunit, which is 117 amino acids long.[49] Complementary DNA encoding human FSH-β, LH-β, or hCG-β in combination with the complementary DNA of the α-subunit is expressed in mammalian cells in culture. These cells can synthesize these proteins, modify them after translation, glycosylate and combine the subunits, and secrete them as intact FSH, LH, or hCG.[50] Recombinant gonadotropins produced through recombinant technology in mammalian cells are used clinically to stimulate gonadal function.[51]

Regulation of Circulating Levels of Follicle-Stimulating Hormone and Luteinizing Hormone

The molecular mechanisms responsible for formation and combination of the α- and β-subunits of FSH and LH are not completely understood. Production rates of α- and β-subunits are regulated in part by negative feedback by estrogen, which regulates the pulsatile release of GnRH from the hypothalamus.[50,52] The pituitary contains more α-subunit than β-subunit mRNA, and readily detectable levels of free α-subunit are present in serum. The free β-subunit is present at relatively low levels in the pituitary and is rarely found in serum or urine. The specific β-subunit may be the rate-limiting factor in the synthesis of these glycoprotein hormones.

Inhibin, activin, and follistatin were first identified as gonadal hormones that exerted selective effects on FSH secretion. Although the primary source of inhibin remains the ovary, activin and follistatin are produced in extragonadal tissues and can exert effects on FSH through an autocrine-paracrine mechanism. Inhibin B is secreted by ovarian granulosa cells during the follicular phase (under the control of FSH) and inhibin A by the corpus luteum in the luteal phase (under the control of LH). Inhibins act synergistically with estradiol to inhibit FSH secretion. Activin can directly stimulate FSH biosynthesis and release from the gonadotroph cells of the pituitary gland.[53] Follistatin can negatively regulate these effects by binding activin and preventing it from interacting with the activin receptor at the cell membrane.[54]

Serum levels of gonadotropins are proportional to their secretion rates and serum half-lives, which are regulated by the number of carbohydrate residues. The higher the content of carbohydrate residues, especially the sialic acid residues, the lower the rate of metabolism and the higher the serum half-life.[55] The sialic acid content of gonadotropic hormones and other glycoproteins has a marked effect on their rate of clearance and influences their apparent molecular size. The higher content of sialic acid in FSH compared with LH is responsible for slower clearance of FSH from the circulation; LH has the most rapid clearance rate. The hCG is highly sialylated and has the longest half-life (see Table 17-1).

OVARY

The ovary is essential for periodic release of oocytes and production of the steroid hormones, estradiol and progesterone. These activities are integrated into the cyclic repetitive process of follicular maturation, ovulation, and formation and regression of the corpus luteum. The ovary fulfills two major objectives: generation of a fertilizable ovum and preparation of the endometrium for implantation through the sequential secretion of estradiol and progesterone.[51] The ovarian follicle comprising the egg and surrounding granulosa and theca cells constitutes the fundamental functional unit of the ovary.

Adult human ovaries are oval bodies with a length of 2 to 5 cm, a width of 1.5 to 3 cm, and a thickness of 0.5 to 1.5 cm. The combined weight of normal ovaries during the reproductive years is 10 to 20 g (average, 14 g). The ovaries lie near the posterior and lateral pelvic wall and are attached to the posterior surface of the broad ligament by the peritoneal fold, called the *mesovarium*. Blood vessels, nerves, and lymphatic vessels traverse the mesovarium and enter the ovary at the hilum.[56]

The ovary consists of three structurally distinct regions: an outer cortex containing the surface germinal epithelium and the follicles; a central medulla consisting of stroma; and a hilum around the area of attachment of the ovary to the mesovarium. The functional anatomy of the adult ovary is illustrated in Figure 17-6. The hilum is the point of attachment of the ovary to the mesovarium. It contains nerves, blood vessels, and hilus cells, which have the

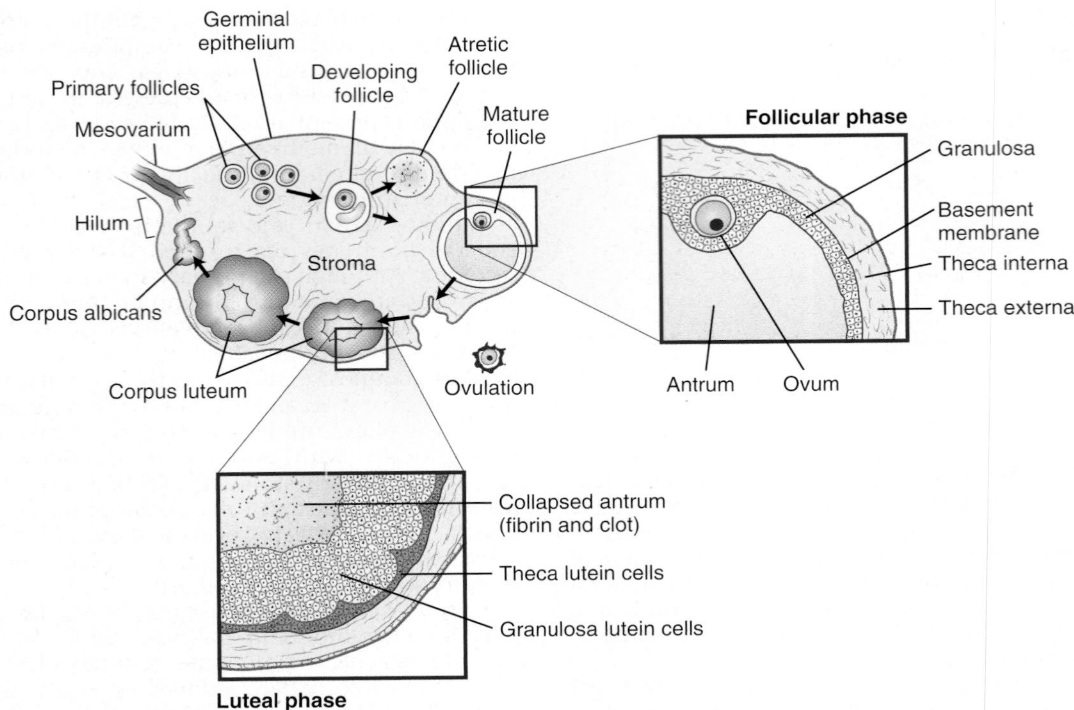

Figure 17-6 **Functional anatomy and changes in the adult ovary during an ovarian cycle.** (From Carr BR, Wilson JD. Disorders of the ovary and female reproductive tract. In: Braunwald E, Isselbacher KJ, Petersdorf RG, et al, eds. *Harrison's Principles of Internal Medicine,* 11th ed. New York, NY: McGraw-Hill; 1987:1818-1837.)

potential to become active in steroidogenesis or to form androgen-secreting tumors. These cells are similar to the testosterone-producing Leydig cells of the testes. The outermost portion of the cortex, called the *tunica albuginea,* is covered by a single layer of surface cuboidal epithelium called the *germinal epithelium.* The oocytes, enclosed in complexes called *follicles,* are in the inner part of the cortex, embedded in stromal tissue. One dominant follicle is recruited for ovulation during each cycle. The preovulatory follicle transforms into a corpus luteum after ovulation. In the absence of pregnancy, the corpus luteum regresses to become the corpus albicans. The stromal tissue is composed of connective tissue and interstitial cells, which are derived from mesenchymal cells and are presumed to have the ability to respond to LH or hCG with the production of androstenedione. The central medullary area of the ovary is derived largely from mesonephric cells.

Genetic Determinants of Ovarian Differentiation and Folliculogenesis

Nascent components of the human ovary develop long before a distinct ovary-like organ can be discerned. The female germ cells are created during embryogenesis when the precursors of primordial germ cells differentiate from somatic lineages of the embryo and take a unique route from the base of the yolk sac along the hindgut to reach the genital ridge. This starts the differentiation of female gonads (ovaries) at the genital ridge. The originally undifferentiated gonad differentiates along a female pathway, and the newly formed oocytes proliferate and subsequently enter meiosis.[51]

Ovarian differentiation and folliculogenesis depend on coordinated expression and interaction of a multitude of genes.[57] Targeted gene disruption or insertion in mice has made it possible to inquire about the function of specific genes in ovarian differentiation and folliculogenesis. Figure 17-7 summarizes the biologic roles of some of these genes.[57] Genetically altered mice represent a first step in attempts to understand in vivo the various gene interactions that result in a functional ovary. Ovarian pathologic conditions in transgenic mice closely resemble disorders observed in mutant human homologs, as exemplified in cases involving the FSH β-subunit and FSH receptor. Many mouse models of ovarian pathologic conditions are available. They can be divided into mice that have prenatal ovarian insufficiency with disordered gonad formation and diminished number of germ cells or absent germ cells and mice that have postnatal ovarian insufficiency as a result of defects at various stages of folliculogenesis (see Fig. 17-7).[57] These models should lead to the identification of genetic and molecular mechanisms responsible for the development and function of the human ovary.

In humans, certain gene defects give rise to specific defects in folliculogenesis. This was demonstrated by the discovery of a heterozygous mutation in the bone morphogenetic protein 15 gene *(BMP15)* that caused ovarian dysgenesis. BMP15 is an oocyte-specific growth and differentiation factor that stimulates folliculogenesis and granulosa cell growth. In vitro, mutant BMP15 reduced granulosa cell growth and antagonized the stimulatory activity of wild-type protein on granulosa cell proliferation. In vivo, this mutation was associated with familial ovarian dysgenesis, indicating that the action of BMP15 is required for progression of human folliculogenesis.[58] A comprehensive discussion of genes responsible for ovarian development, folliculogenesis, and ovulation is provided in an excellent review article by Edson and colleagues.[51]

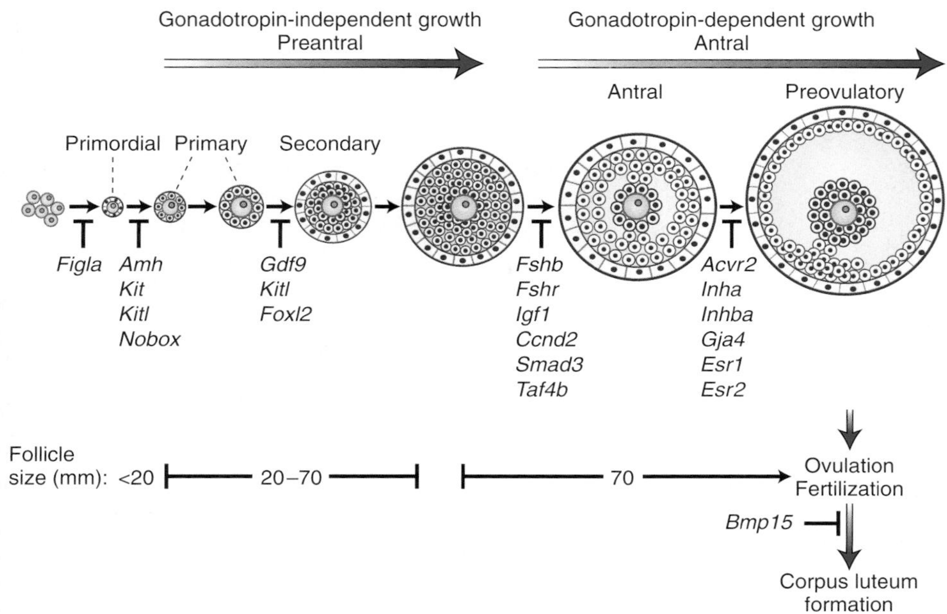

Figure 17-7 Developmental stages at which certain murine genes affect oogenesis. Data from transgenic mice with disruption of various genes have delineated critical roles of several genes during various phases of the follicular development. Preantral follicular growth is thought to be gonadotropin independent, whereas antrum formation and follicular maturation require the action of follicle-stimulating hormone (FSH). Acvr2, activin type II receptor; Amh, anti-Müllerian hormone; Bmp15, bone morphogenetic protein-15; Ccnd2, cyclin d2; Esr1, estrogen receptor-α; Esr2, estrogen receptor-β; Figla, factor in the germline-α; Foxl2, forkhead box L2; Fshb, FSH β-subunit; Fshr, FSH receptor; GDF-9, growth differentiation factor 9; Gja4, gap junction protein connexin 37; Igf1, insulin-like growth factor I; Inha, inhibin α-subunit; Inhba, activin β_A-subunit; Kit, kit receptor; Kitl, kit-ligand; Nobox, newborn oogenesis homeobox gene; Smad3, Sma mothers against decapentaplegic-3; Taf4b, TATA-box-binding protein-associated factor-4b. (Modified from Simpson JL, Rajkovic A. Ovarian differentiation and gonadal failure. *Am J Med Genet.* 1999;89:186-2000; and Choi Y, Rajkovic A. Genetics of mammalian folliculogenesis. *Cell Mol Life Sci.* 2006;63:579-590.)

Oocytes

The fertilization of an oocyte by a spermatozoon gives rise to a zygote that starts to divide rapidly. An eight-cell embryo is formed usually on the third day after fertilization. Up to that point, all embryonic cells are morphologically identical, truly totipotential, and capable of starting a new individual or any lineage. The formation of a 16-cell morula marks the beginning of the process of differentiation, with cells being allocated to the inside or outside of the embryo. At the next stage, the blastocyst, three lineages are defined: trophectoderm, which is the precursor of placenta; epiblast, which gives rise to the somatic cells of the embryo; and primitive endoderm, which eventually forms the yolk sac. After the embryo implants, a group of cells within the epiblast form the precursors of the primordial germ cells, the first cells of the future ovary to be defined.[51] The extraembryonic trophectoderm and primitive endoderm, which surround the epiblast cells of the postimplantation egg cylinder, are the sources of signals that instruct this small number of epiblast cells to become primordial germ cells; the rest of the cells commence differentiation into somatic tissues. The first primordial germ cell precursors express a key protein named PRDM1 (PRDI-BF1-RIZ domain containing 1, formerly called BLIMP1); these precursor cells represent the first cells of the mammalian embryo with committed cell fates.[51]

The primordial germ cells first become recognizable as a cluster of cells that stain intensely for alkaline phosphatase activity; these epiblast cells are observed at the base of the yolk sac before formation of the allantois.[51] Studies have confirmed that these cells are the only primordial germ cells, because their ablation results in embryos without germ cells, whereas transplantation of these cells leads to their proliferation followed by migration to the genital ridge.[51]

With the use of alkaline phosphatase as a marker, migration of these primordial germ cells from the yolk sac–epiblast junction to the indifferent gonad can be tracked; eventually, the ovary forms and permits the primordial germ cells to differentiate into oocytes. The oocytes enter meiosis and subsequently arrest. Entry into meiosis marks the developmental stage at which any progenitor cells that are capable of differentiating to oocytes disappear. The meiotically arrested oocytes eventually become surrounded by pre-granulosa cells and form individual primordial follicles, the resting pool of oocytes that have the potential to be recruited into the growing follicle pool during the postpubertal stage to be fertilized and to contribute to the next generation. These phenomena have been primarily observed in mice and are thought to be applicable to humans.[51]

Primordial germ cells of epiblast origin migrate to cross a remarkably long distance from the base of the yolk sac to the genital ridge in the fetus by ameboid movements with the aid of pseudopodia.[59] This long route of migration along the dorsal mesentery of the hindgut is interrupted only by the required lateral crossing of the celomic angle at the level of the genital ridge (Fig. 17-8). The exact trigger that initiates primordial germ cell migration and the chemoattractants that are required for directional movement toward the genital ridge are slowly beginning to be understood. The trigger may be expression of a key receptor on the primordial germ cell and expression of the secreted chemoattractants from the genital ridge. For example, suppression of transforming growth factor-β (TGF-β) signaling

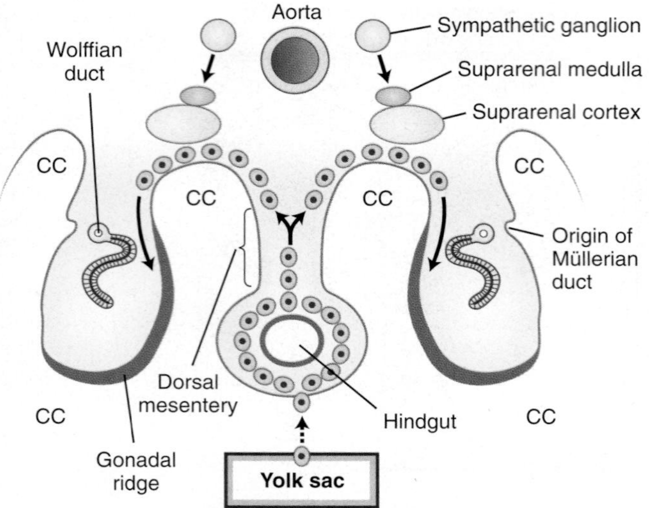

Figure 17-8 Transverse section of the caudal region of a 5-week embryo shows the location of gonadal ridges, the primordium of the adrenal glands, and the migration path of primordial germ cells. From the third week on, germ cells of epiblast origin located at the base of the yolk sac cross the dorsal mesentery of the hindgut and migrate to the gonadal ridges. By the end of the fifth week, rapid division of primordial germ cells, gonadal epithelium, and mesenchyme starts the early gonad that differentiates subsequently into the ovary in a 46,XX fetus. CC, celomic cavity. (Modified from Moore K. *The Developing Human.* Philadelphia, PA: WB Saunders; 1983.)

leads to enhanced migration due to reduction in the levels of TGF-β–induced collagen type 1 in the extracellular matrix.[60] An extracellular matrix gradient along the path of migration is important, and if too much matrix is laid down, germ cells show reduced migration. The KIT ligand (KITLG) may function as an effective chemoattractant for the primordial germ cells. The phosphatidylinositol 3 kinase (PI3K)/AKT and SRC kinase pathways are involved downstream of KIT in the primordial germ cell.[61]

Germ cells appear to be unable to persist outside the genital ridge, which may be viewed as the only region competent to sustain gonadal development. By the same token, germ cells play an indispensable role in the induction of gonadal development. No functional gonad can form in the absence of germ cells.

On arrival at the genital ridge by the fifth week of gestation, the premeiotic germ cells are referred to as *oogonia*.[62] During the subsequent 2 weeks of intrauterine life (weeks 5 to 7 of gestation, or the *indifferent stage*), the primordial gonadal structure constitutes no more than a bulge on the medial aspect of the urogenital ridge (see Fig. 17-8). This protuberance is created by proliferation of surface (celomic) germinal epithelium, by growth of the underlying mesenchyme, and by oogonial multiplication. The oogonia total 10,000 by about 6 to 7 weeks of intrauterine life. Because meiosis and oogonial atresia are not occurring, the actual number of germ cells is dictated by mitotic division at this time.

During the indifferent phase, the gonadal cortex and medulla are first delineated. However, short of cytogenetic evidence, the precise sexual identity of the gonadal ridge cannot be ascertained at this point. Nevertheless, the absence of testicular development beyond 7 weeks' gestation is considered presumptive evidence of formation of the ovary. Additional clues to the sexual identity of the gonad can be derived from the detection of oogonial meiosis at about 8 weeks' gestation, because no comparable process is observed in the testis until puberty. The sexual identity of the gonadal ridge is histologically clear by 16 weeks' gestation, when the first primordial follicles can be visualized.

By about 8 weeks of intrauterine life, persistent mitosis increases the total number of oogonia to 600,000 (Fig. 17-9). From this point on, the oogonial endowment is subject to three simultaneous processes: mitosis, meiosis, and oogonial atresia. Stated differently, the onset of oogonial meiosis and oogonial atresia is superimposed on oogonial mitosis. As a result of the combined impact of these processes, the number of germ cells peaks at 6 to 7 × 10^6 by 20 weeks' gestation (see Fig. 17-9). At this time, two thirds of the total germ cells are intrameiotic primary oocytes; the remaining third can still be viewed as oogonial. The midgestational peak and the postpeak decline are accounted for in part by the progressively decreasing rate of oogonial mitosis, a process destined to end entirely by about the seventh month of intrauterine life. Equally relevant is the increasing rate of oogonial atresia, which peaks at 5 months' gestation. During this period, regulation of the ovarian developmental process is complex and probably involves a diverse group of genes (see Fig. 17-7).[63,64]

From midgestation onward, relentless and irreversible attrition progressively diminishes the germ cell endowment of the gonad. About 50 years later, it is exhausted. For the most part, this is accomplished through follicular atresia rather than oogonial atresia, begins at about month

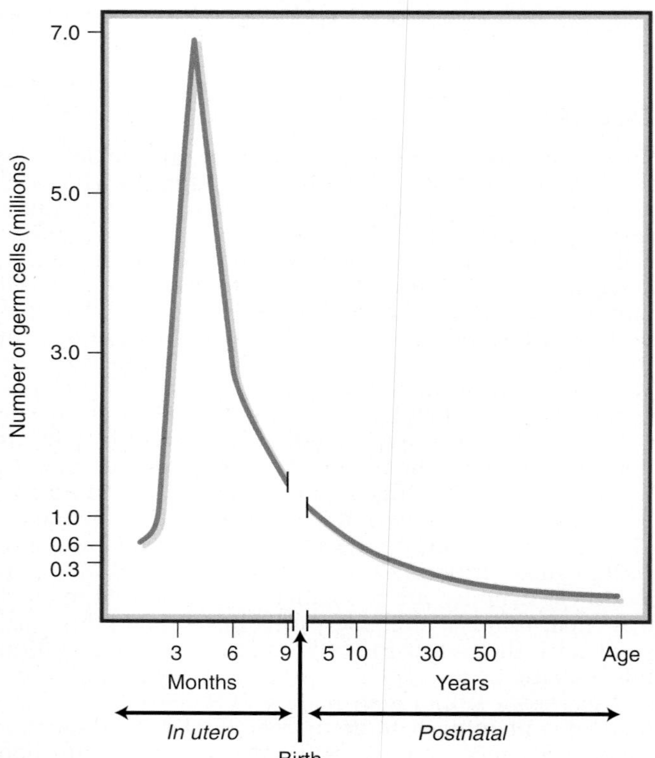

Figure 17-9 Age-dependent changes in germ cell number in the human ovary. The highest number of oocytes is found in the ovaries of a human fetus at midgestation. This number decreases sharply during the third trimester. After birth, the progressive decline in the number of ovarian follicles containing oocytes continues until complete depletion at menopause. (From Baker TG. A quantitative and cytological study of germ cells in the human ovaries. *Proc R Soc Biol Sci.* 1963;158:417-433.)

6 of gestation, and continues throughout life (see Fig. 17-9). In contrast, oogonial atresia is destined to end at 7 months of intrauterine life as follicular atresia sets in. Follicular atresia has a profound effect on germ cell endowment, because only 1 to 2 × 10^6 germ cells are present at birth (see Fig. 17-9).[65] Remarkably, this dramatic depletion of the germ cell mass occurs during a period as short as 20 weeks. No similar rate of depletion occurs earlier or subsequently. Consequently, newborn girls enter life still far from realizing their reproductive potential but having lost as much as 80% of their germ cell endowment. The germ cell mass decreases further to approximately 300,000 by the onset of puberty. Of these follicles, only 400 to 500 (<1% of the total) are recruited for ovulation in the course of a reproductive life span.

Between weeks 8 and 13 of fetal life, some of the oogonia depart from the mitotic cycle to enter the prophase of the first meiotic division. This change marks the conversion of these cells to primary oocytes well before actual follicle formation. Meiosis (beginning at about 8 weeks' gestation) provides temporary protection from oogonial atresia, allowing the germ cells to invest themselves with granulosa cells and to form primordial follicles. Oogonia that persist beyond the seventh month of gestation and have not entered meiosis are subject to oogonial atresia; consequently, no oogonia are usually present at birth.

Once formed, the primary oocyte persists in prophase of the first meiotic division until the time of ovulation, when meiosis is resumed and the first polar body is formed and extruded (Fig. 17-10). Although the exact cellular

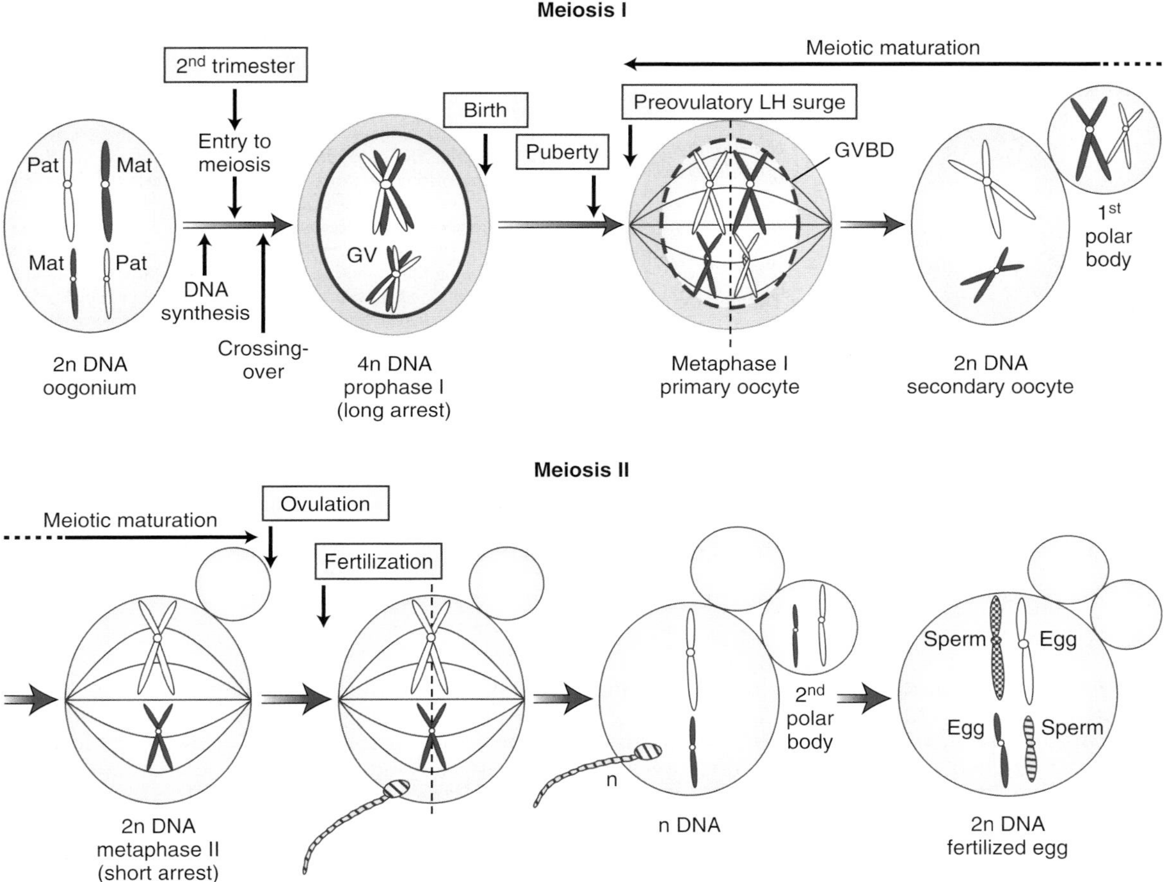

Figure 17-10 Meiotic cell division. During meiosis, the chromosomes that were inherited from the parents of the individual and stored in gonads are processed to prepare their genetic material for transmission to the offspring. Meiosis occurs exclusively in germ cells and serves two critical purposes: generation of germ cells genetically distinct from the somatic cells and generation of a mature egg (or sperm) with a reduction in the number of chromosomes from 46 to 23. Genetic recombination through crossover of genes between homologous chromosomes and random assortment of (grand-) maternal and (grand-) paternal chromosomes into daughter cells during the first meiotic division are responsible for the first function of meiosis, maintenance of genetic diversity. The second function is provided by a reduction in the number of chromosomes so that each daughter cell, or ovum, receives randomly one chromosome from each of the 23 pairs. During fertilization, the fusion of ovum and sperm, each of which contributes 23 chromosomes, produces a genetically novel individual with 46 chromosomes. The chromosome marked as *white* in the oogonium (*upper left corner*) originates from the father of the female fetus, whereas the *blue* chromosome comes from the mother of the fetus. The random exchange of genes (alleles) between homologous chromosomes (crossover) takes place before the meiotic arrest in the prophase I stage before birth. After birth, the oocytes of this child remain in meiotic arrest until puberty. In the developing oocyte in the graafian follicle, meiosis I is resumed immediately after the preovulatory luteinizing hormone (LH) surge during each ovulatory cycle. Meiotic maturation is defined as the period from the breakdown of the oocyte's nucleus (germinal vesicle [GV]) until the oocyte reaches metaphase II (i.e., transition from oocyte to egg). A second and short meiotic arrest occurs at metaphase II until the oocyte is fertilized by a sperm. DNA, deoxyribonucleic acid; GVBD, germinal vesicle breakdown; mat, maternal; n, amount of DNA material in the haploid number (23) of chromosomes; pat, paternal.

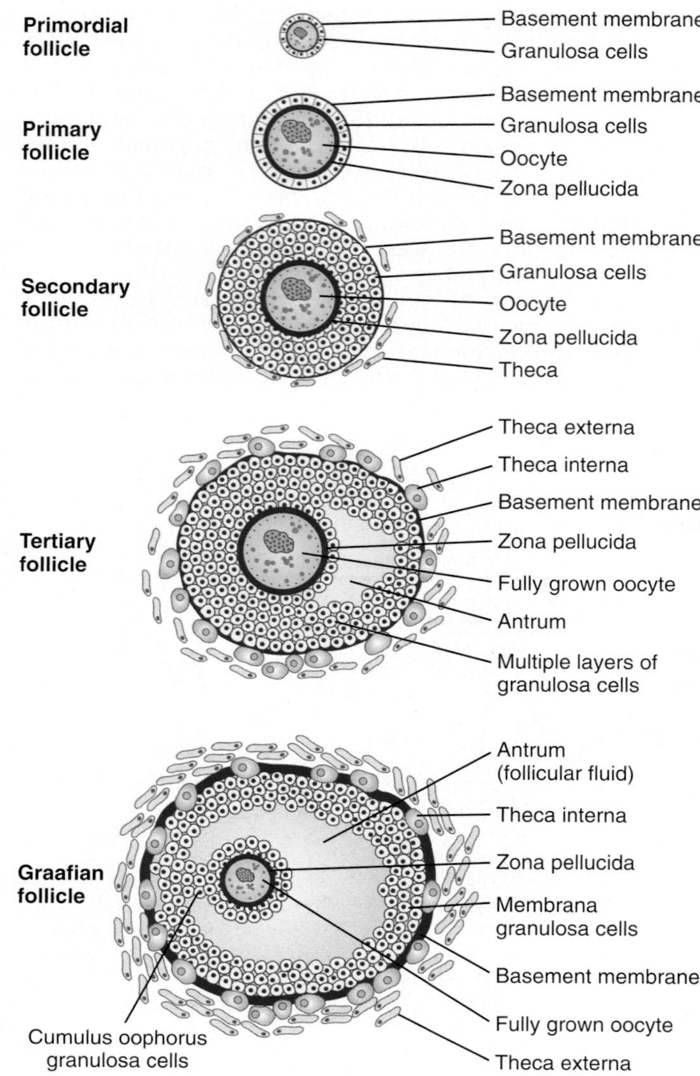

Figure 17-11 Developmental stages of the ovarian follicle. The primordial follicle is composed of a single layer of granulosa cells and a single immature oocyte arrested in the diplotene stage of the first meiotic division. The primordial follicle is separated from the surrounding stroma by a thin basal lamina (i.e., basement membrane). The oocyte and granulosa cells do not have a direct blood supply. The first sign of follicular recruitment is cuboidal differentiation in the spindle-shaped cells inside the basal lamina, which thereafter undergo successive mitotic divisions to form a multilayered granulosa cell zone. The oocyte enlarges and secretes a glycoprotein-containing mucoid substance called the *zona pellucida*, which surrounds the oocyte and separates the granulosa cells from the oocyte. This structure is a primary follicle. The secondary follicle is formed by further proliferation of granulosa cells and by the final phase of oocyte growth, in which the oocyte reaches 120 μm in diameter, coincident with proliferation of layers of cells immediately outside the basal lamina to constitute the theca. The portion of the theca adjacent to the basal lamina is called the *theca interna*. Theca cells that merge with the surrounding stroma are designated the *theca externa*. The secondary follicle acquires an independent blood supply consisting of one or more arterioles that terminate in a capillary bed at the basal lamina. Capillaries do not penetrate the basement membrane, and the granulosa and oocyte remain avascular. The tertiary follicle is characterized by further hypertrophy of the theca and the appearance of a fluid-filled space among the granulosa cells, called the *antrum*. The fluid in the antrum consists of a plasma transudate and secretory products of granulosa cells, some of which (estrogens) are found there in strikingly higher concentrations than in peripheral blood. The follicle rapidly increases in size under the influence of gonadotropins to form the mature or graafian follicle. In the graafian follicle, the granulosa and oocyte remain encased by the basal lamina and are devoid of direct vascularization. The antral fluid increases in volume, and the oocyte, surrounded by an accumulation of granulosa cells (i.e., *cumulus oophorus*), occupies a polar, eccentric position within the follicle. The mature graafian follicle is then ready to release the ovum by the process of ovulation. (Adapted from Erickson GF, Magoffin DA, Dyer CA. The ovarian androgen producing cells: a review of structure-function relations. *Endocr Rev.* 1985;6:371-379. Copyright © 1985 by The Endocrine Society.)

mechanisms responsible for this meiotic arrest remain uncertain, it is presumed that a granulosa cell–derived meiosis inhibitor is in play. This hypothesis is based on the observation that denuded (granulosa-free) oocytes are capable of spontaneously completing meiotic maturation in vitro.

The primary oocyte is converted into a secondary oocyte by completion of the first meiotic metaphase and formation of the first polar body, which occurs before ovulation but after the LH surge. At ovulation, the secondary oocyte and the surrounding granulosa cells (cumulus oophorus) are extruded and enter the fallopian tube. If sperm penetration occurs, the secondary oocyte undergoes a second meiotic division, after which the second polar body is eliminated (see Fig. 17-10).

Granulosa Cell Layer

In the developing ovaries of a human female fetus, oocytes initially exist as germ cell clusters before an ovarian follicle is formed. During the second half of in utero life, these germ cell clusters break down, and the surviving oocytes become individually surrounded with squamous pregranulosa cells to give rise to primordial follicles. The transition from primordial to primary follicle is marked histologically by a morphologic change in granulosa cells from squamous to cuboidal. By the secondary stage, there are at least two layers of cuboidal granulosa cells and an additional layer of somatic cells, the theca, which forms outside the basement membrane of the follicle (Fig. 17-11).[51] At puberty, FSH secreted by the pituitary promotes further granulosa cell proliferation and survival.

A basement lamina separates the oocyte and granulosa cells from the surrounding stromal cells.[66] The granulosa cells do not have direct access to the circulation before ovulation (Fig. 17-12).

The avascular nature of the granulosa cell compartment necessitates contact between neighboring cells. The granulosa cells are interconnected by extensive intercellular gap junctions, which result in their coupling to yield an expanded, integrated, and functional syncytium (Fig. 17-13).[67,68] Gap junctions are composed of proteins called *connexins*. Connexin-37 and other connexins have been demonstrated in gap junctions in follicles. Gap junction

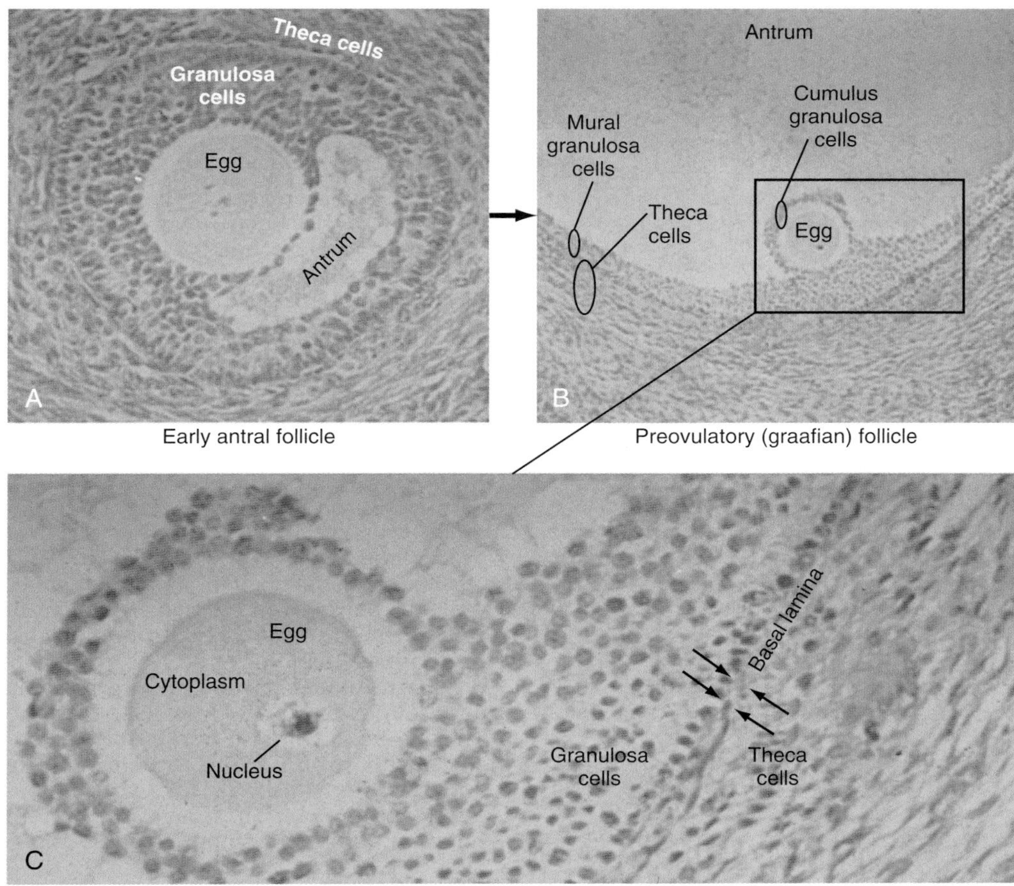

Figure 17-12 Histology of gonadotropin-dependent ovarian follicle development. **A,** Development of an antrum marks gonadotropin dependency. Multiple layers of granulosa and theca cells are present. **B,** The follicle destined to ovulate distinguishes itself from the rest of the cohort through accumulation of large quantities of antral fluid. The granulosa cells, which accumulate around the oocyte, are called *cumulus granulosa cells* and primarily function to support egg development. The mural granulosa cells in the periphery primarily serve as steroidogenic cells. **C,** A membrane called the *basal lamina (arrows)*, which has been formed at the primary stage, separates the granulosa cells from the theca component of the follicle.

protein connexin 37 (GJA4)-deficient mice lack graafian follicles, fail to ovulate, and develop inappropriate corpora lutea.[69] These specialized cell junctions may be important in metabolic exchange and in the transport of small molecules between neighboring granulosa cells. Moreover, the granulosa cells extend cytoplasmic processes that penetrate the zona pellucida to form gap junctions with the plasma membrane of the oocyte (see Fig. 17-13). In the GJA4-deficient mice, oocyte development is arrested before meiotic competence.[69] Gap junctions represent a crucial communication system that is needed for the tight control exerted by the cumulus granulosa cells on the resumption of meiosis by the enclosed primary oocyte.

Several gene products regulate the transition from primordial to primary follicle, which is marked by a change in the morphology of granulosa cells from squamous to cuboidal, followed by an increase in granulosa cell layers in the secondary follicle.[51] These genes are expressed in the oocyte or granulosa cells, emphasizing the active role of the oocyte in granulosa cell differentiation. Newborn oogenesis homeobox (NOBOX), spermatogenesis and oogenesis helix-loop-helix 1 (SOHLH1), and SOHLH2 are critical transcription factors during the transition from primordial to primary follicles.[51] Interactions between KITLG expressed in granulosa cells and the KIT tyrosine kinase receptor expressed in oocytes also appear to be critical in early folliculogenesis. The KITLG/KIT pathway induces the PI3K/AKT pathway, leading to phosphorylation and inactivation of forkhead box O3 (FOXO3), an inhibitor of primordial follicle activation.[51] These genetic studies supported a critical role of the PI3K/AKT/FOXO3 pathway in early follicle development and granulosa cell differentiation. Whereas FOXO3 is the key oocyte factor critical for suppressing primordial follicle activation, another forkhead domain transcription factor, forkhead box L2 (FOXL2), is crucial in the transition from squamous to cuboidal granulosa cells.[51]

Anti-müllerian hormone (AMH) produced by the granulosa cells of growing follicles appears to inhibit the growth of primordial follicles, and in its absence, there is a faster depletion of growing follicles, although it is unknown whether this is a direct or indirect effect of AMH. Clinically, serum AMH may be a useful biomarker of ovarian reserve. In women and mice, serum AMH declines with increasing age. Although it is difficult to establish a direct link between serum AMH and the primordial follicle pool in humans, antral follicle number is positively correlated with AMH levels.[51] More detailed information has been reviewed by Edson and colleagues.[51]

The granulosa cells in the fully developed graafian follicle shortly before ovulation are stratified in a manner that allows the distinction of a number of populations of

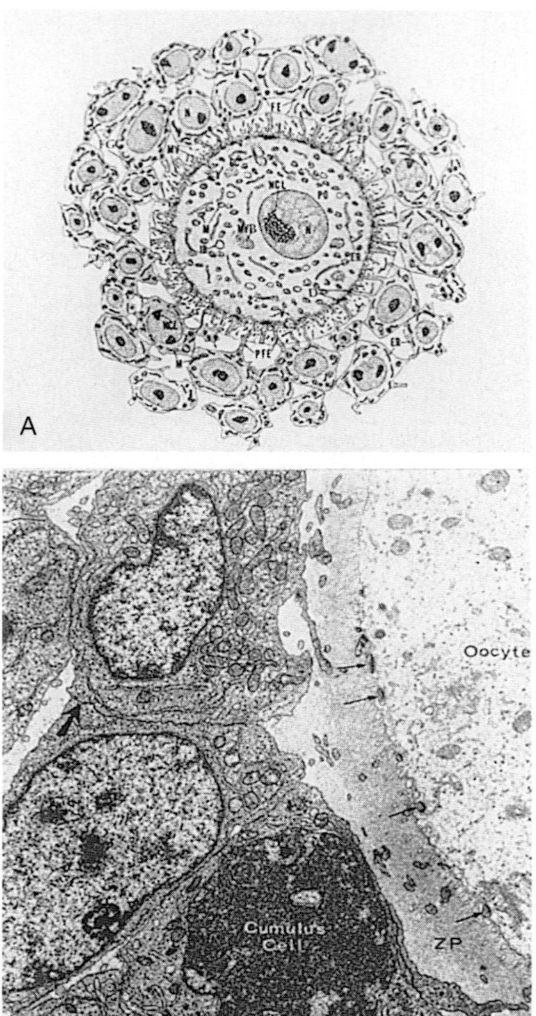

Figure 17-13 Structural relationship between the cumulus granulosa cell and the oocyte. **A,** Microvilli of an oocyte interdigitate with cytoplasmic extensions of granulosa cells, penetrating the zona pellucida. **B,** Notice the penetration of the zona pellucida by cytoplasmic processes of the granulosa cells. Small gap junctions *(thin arrows)* are observed between processes of the granulosa cell and the oocyte membrane. The *thick arrow* indicates a gap junction between granulosa cells. (From Erickson GF. An analysis of follicle development and ovum maturation. *Semin Reprod Endocrinol.* 1986;4:233, with permission of Thieme Medical Publishers, New York.)

cells.[70,71] Distinct populations of granulosa cells exhibit specific, specialized functions.[72-74] Mural granulosa cells within the outermost layer adjacent to the basement layer contain high levels of gonadotropin hormone receptors and steroidogenic enzymes and account for most of the steroidogenesis in the follicle.[70,71] The *cumulus oophorus* contains the egg and a surrounding mass of granulosa cells that have cell-cell interactions with the egg and seem to have critical roles in oocyte development (see Figs. 17-12 and 17-13).[72-74]

Mural and cumulus granulosa cells also exhibit distinct patterns of gene expression. For example, the tumor suppressor BRCA1 is highly expressed in ovarian granulosa cells of developing follicles.[75] However, in large antral or preovulatory follicles, BRCA1 expression significantly decreases in mural granulosa cells and becomes restricted to cumulus granulosa cells; these cells, unlike the mural ones, do not contain abundant aromatase, so this development gives rise to an intriguing inverse correlation of BRACA1 with aromatase mRNA and protein levels.[75] Stimulation of an FSH-dependent signaling pathway greatly induces aromatase but suppresses BRCA1 expression in granulosa cells. Moreover, BRCA1 binds to the aromatase promoter and inhibits its activity.[76] Therefore, BRCA1 may exert its tumor suppressor activity, in part, by limiting excessive estrogen formation in the ovary. A summary of ovarian follicle development is presented in Figure 17-11.

Theca Cell Layer

After the follicle achieves two layers of granulosa cells, another morphologically distinct layer of somatic cells, the theca, differentiates from ovarian stroma (see Figs. 17-11, 17-12, and 17-13).[51] The cells making up the theca-interstitial compartment are heterogeneous in nature.[77] Cells of the theca interna layer, which forms just outside the basement membrane surrounding the granulosa cells, show typical steroidogenic features, including mitochondria with tubular cristae, smooth endoplasmic reticulum, and abundant lipid vesicles (see Figs. 17-11 and 17-12). Theca interna cells are responsible for producing the C19 steroids that diffuse into the neighboring granulosa cells and serve as substrates for estrogen production. Theca externa is the outermost layer of the follicle and is composed of fibroblasts, smooth muscle–like cells, and macrophages (see Figs. 17-11 and 17-12). The theca externa is thought to have an important function during ovulation. Cells that contribute to the theca differentiate from mesenchymal precursor cells present in the ovarian stroma, adjacent to developing follicles. Like preantral folliculogenesis, theca formation is gonadotropin independent. Thecal precursor cells lack LH receptors, and the theca layer still forms in the ovaries of FSH-deficient mice.[51] After a discernible theca interna layer has developed, theca cell C19 steroid production is regulated primarily by LH.

The differentiated state of theca interna cells is marked by expression of a number of steroidogenic genes, including those of the LH receptor (*LHCGR*); steroidogenic acute regulatory protein (*STAR*); side-chain cleavage enzyme (*CYP11A1*); 3β-hydroxysteroid dehydrogenase-$\Delta^{5,4}$ isomerase type 2 (*HSD3B2*); and 17-hydroxylase/17,20-lyase (*CYP17A1*) in the human. Granulosa cells of the developing follicles appear to secrete factors that regulate theca cell differentiation. Candidate factors that may contribute to theca cell differentiation include insulin-like growth factor (IGF), KITLG, and growth differentiation factor 9 (GDF9). IGF1 induces expression of LHCGR, CYP11A1, and HSD3B type 1 (counterpart of human HDS3B type 2), whereas KITLG stimulates StAR protein and CYP17A1 expression in rat theca cells. In mice lacking the *GDF9* gene, a theca layer fails to form in the ovary. Whether GDF9 regulates theca cell recruitment or differentiation directly or indirectly through regulation of preantral granulosa cell development is unknown.

Follicles

The follicle represents the key functional unit in the ovary with respect to germ cell development and steroid production. The follicles are embedded in loose connective tissue of the ovarian cortex and can be subdivided into two functional types: nongrowing (primordial) and growing. Between 90% and 95% of follicles are nongrowing throughout reproductive life. Recruitment of a primordial follicle initiates dramatic changes in growth, structure, and function. The growing follicles are divided into four stages: primary, secondary, tertiary, and graafian (see Figs. 17-7 and 17-11). The first three stages of growth can occur in the absence of the pituitary and therefore appear to be controlled by intraovarian mechanisms (see Figs. 17-7 and 17-11). The follicle destined to ovulate is recruited during the first few days of the current cycle.[78]

The early growth of follicles occurs over several menstrual cycles, but the ovulatory follicle is one of a cohort recruited at the time of transition from the previous cycle's luteal phase to the current cycle's follicular phase.[79,80] The total time to achieve preovulatory status is approximately 85 days.[79,80] Most of this developmental period is FSH independent. Eventually, this cohort of follicles reaches a stage at which, unless recruited by FSH, the next step is atresia. A cohort of follicles measuring 2 to 5 mm in diameter is continuously available for a response to FSH. The late luteal increase in FSH is the critical feature in rescuing this cohort of follicles from atresia; it allows a dominant follicle to emerge and pursue a path to ovulation. The increase in the FSH level must be maintained for a critical period (see Fig. 17-1).[81]

Recruited primordial follicles either develop into dominant, mature graafian follicles destined to ovulate or degenerate as a result of atresia.[82] The average time for development of a selected follicle to the point of ovulation is 10 to 14 days. If a follicle is not recruited, it goes through a process called *atresia,* during which the oocyte and granulosa cells within the basal lamina die and are replaced by fibrous tissue. The theca cells outside the basal lamina do not seem to die but are thought to dedifferentiate and return to the pool of cells consisting of ovarian interstitial or stromal cells.[56] The process of atresia is thought to result from lack of the hormones or growth factors that are formed by the mature dominant follicle through intrinsic intraovarian mechanisms. There is general agreement that atresia of follicles occurs through apoptosis.[83] Apoptosis is an active and regulated process that is triggered by a cascade of caspase proteases that lead to characteristic fragmentation of DNA and eventual cell death.

Ovulation

There is a dramatic rise in circulating estradiol level as midcycle approaches. This is followed by a striking LH surge and, to a lesser extent, an FSH surge, which trigger the dominant follicle to ovulate. During each menstrual cycle, usually one follicle ovulates and gives rise to a corpus luteum. In women, LH or its surrogate hCG is essential to stimulate rupture of the mature follicle. It has been proposed that increased local prostaglandin biosynthesis in the follicle mediates the ovulatory effect of LH.[84,85]

Ovulation consists of rapid follicular enlargement followed by protrusion of the follicle from the surface of the ovarian cortex. This is followed by the rupture of the follicle and extrusion of an egg-cumulus complex into the peritoneal cavity (Fig. 17-14). Follicular rupture or ovulation occurs predictably 34 to 36 hours after the start of the LH surge. Elevation of a conical *stigma* on the surface of the protruding follicle precedes rupture (see Fig. 17-14). Rupture of this stigma is accompanied by a gentle rather than explosive expulsion of the ovum and antral fluid. A number of transcriptional regulators downstream of the LH receptor are required for ovulation. After the LH surge, progesterone receptor (PR) levels rapidly increase in the mural granulosa cells of the preovulatory follicle.[51] LH- or PR-dependent production of proteases acting locally on protein substrates in the basal lamina may play an important role in stigma formation and follicular rupture.[86,87] In particular, levels of plasminogen activator increase in the follicle before rupture.[88] Plasminogen activator–mediated conversion of plasminogen to plasmin may contribute to the proteolytic digestion of the follicular wall, which is a prerequisite for follicular rupture. Gene knockout studies in mice suggest that other factors important for ovulation or follicular rupture include endothelin 2, peroxisome proliferator-activated receptor-γ (PPARγ), CCAAT/enhancer-binding protein-β, liver receptor homolog 1, steroidogenic factor 1, and nuclear receptor interacting protein 1.[51]

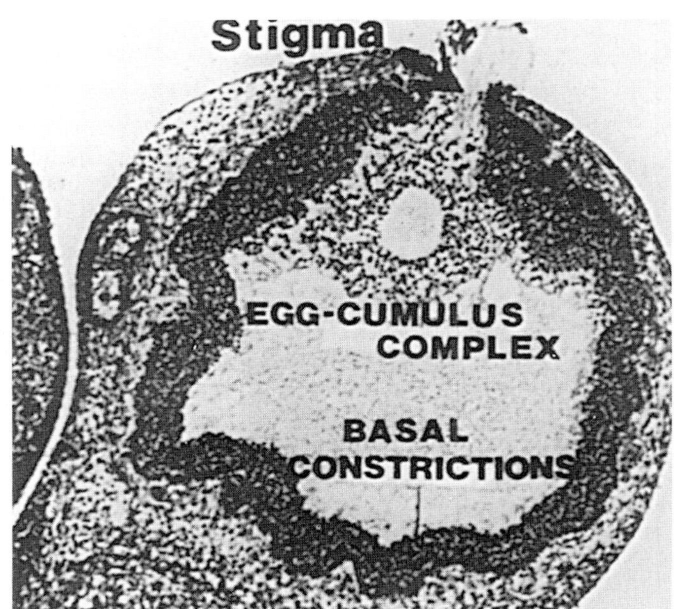

Figure 17-14 **Ovulation of the cumulus-oocyte complex through the stigma.** (From Erickson GF. An analysis of follicle development and ovum maturation. *Semin Reprod Endocrinol.* 1986; 4:233, Thieme Medical Publishers, New York, with permission.)

Corpus Luteum

After ovulation, the dominant follicle reorganizes to become the corpus luteum (Fig. 17-15). After rupture of the follicle, capillaries and fibroblasts from the surrounding stroma proliferate and penetrate the basal lamina (see Fig. 17-11). This rapid vascularization of the corpus luteum may be guided by angiogenic factors, some of which are detected in the follicular fluid.[89] Vascular endothelial growth factor has been isolated from corpora lutea and has been postulated, along with basic fibroblast growth factor, to be a potential angiogenic agent in corpora lutea.[90] Concurrently, the granulosa and theca cells undergo morphologic changes collectively referred to as *luteinization.* The granulosa cells become granulosa-lutein cells (large cells), and the theca cells are transformed into theca-lutein cells (small cells) (see Fig. 17-15).[91] The so-called K cells, scattered throughout the corpus luteum, are believed to be macrophages.

The corpus luteum is the endocrine gland that serves as the major source of sex steroid hormones secreted by the ovary during the postovulatory phase of the cycle. The human corpus luteum secretes as much as 40 mg of

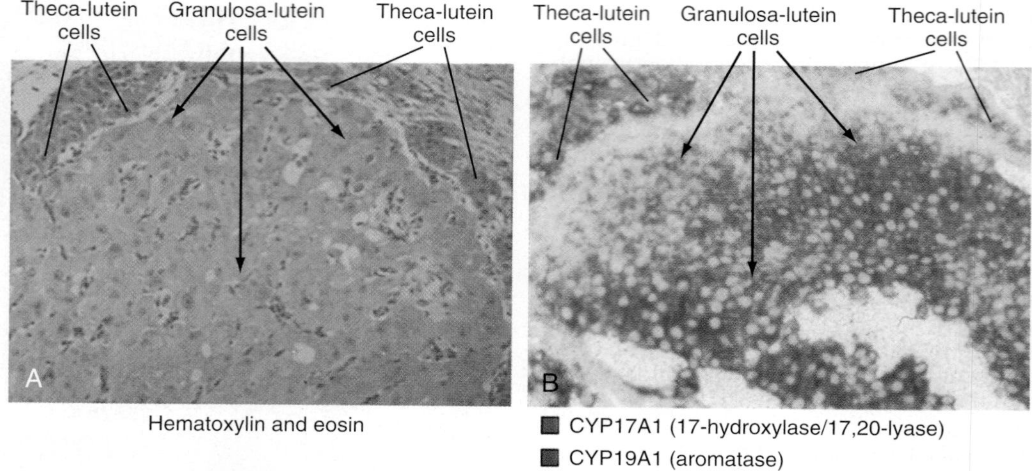

Figure 17-15 Corpus luteum. **A,** Hematoxylin and eosin stain shows the large granulosa-lutein cells occupying the center and smaller theca-lutein cells in the periphery. **B,** Immunoreactive aromatase, a product of the *CYP19A1* gene *(brown stain)*, is the hallmark of granulosa-lutein cells, whereas immunoreactive 17-hyroxylase/17,20-lyase, a product of the *CYP17A1* gene *(purple stain)*, is selectively localized to theca-lutein cells. (Courtesy of Dr. Hironobu Sasansendai, Japan.)

progesterone per day during the midluteal phase of the ovarian cycle.[92] In view of the small size of the corpus luteum, it is the most active steroidogenic tissue in humans. An important aspect of corpus luteum formation is the penetration of the follicle basement membrane by blood vessels, which provides the granulosa-lutein cells with low-density lipoprotein (LDL)-cholesterol.[89] LDL-cholesterol serves as the substrate for corpus luteum progesterone production.

A key regulator of steroidogenesis in the corpus luteum is LH. In humans, the LH receptor is maintained throughout the functional life span of the corpus luteum and not downregulated during the maternal recognition of pregnancy.[93] The rate-limiting step in LH-mediated progesterone formation in luteinized granulosa cells is the entry of cholesterol into the mitochondria, which is regulated by the StAR protein.[94] The availability of LDL-cholesterol and the StAR-mediated mitochondrial entry of cholesterol into the mitochondria seem to be the two critical factors that account for the production of large amounts of progesterone in the corpus luteum.

The functional life span of the corpus luteum is normally 14 ± 2 days, after which it spontaneously regresses. Unless pregnancy occurs, the corpus luteum is replaced by an avascular scar referred to as the *corpus albicans*.

Factors that may regulate luteal life span include hormones such as hCG, maintenance of luteal vascularization, and immune cells.[95] There is little doubt about the central role of LH in the maintenance of corpus luteum function. Withdrawal of LH support in a variety of experimental circumstances has almost invariably resulted in luteal regression.[95] In pregnancy, however, the LH surrogate hCG, secreted by the gestational trophoblast, maintains the ability of the corpus luteum to elaborate progesterone; this stimulus helps to maintain the early gestation until the luteoplacental shift.[96] The corpus luteum doubles in size (compared with the prepregnancy size) during the first 6 weeks of gestation (see Fig. 17-15). This increase results from proliferation of connective tissues and blood vessels, along with hypertrophy of the luteinized granulosa and theca cells. This early hypertrophy is followed by regression. The corpus luteum at term is only one half of its size during the menstrual cycle.

Hormones such as estrogens and prostaglandins have been suggested to be important factors in the promotion of luteal demise.[97,98] Immune factors may influence luteal life span because corpus luteal regression is associated with a progressive infiltration of lymphocytes and macrophages.[95]

Apoptosis is a critical end-point mechanism by which human corpora lutea are deleted. Corpora lutea during the early luteal phase of the menstrual cycle and the corpora lutea of early pregnancy show no evidence of apoptotic DNA fragmentation.[99] DNA fragmentation is detected in midluteal and late luteal corpora.[99] LH or hCG inhibits apoptosis in the corpus luteum. In the absence of these trophic factors, apoptosis ensues. The remaining corpus luteum, the corpus albicans, is composed of dense connective tissue.

Ovarian Follicle-Stimulating Hormone and Luteinizing Hormone Receptors

The FSH receptor is expressed exclusively by granulosa cells. The LH or hCG receptor (LHCGR) is expressed primarily by the theca-interstitial cells of all follicles and by granulosa cells of large preovulatory follicles.

Granulosa cells in primary or secondary follicles that are in the early developmental stages before antrum formation primarily bind FSH but not LH. In these preantral follicles, the binding of LH or hCG is confined to theca-interstitial cells.[100] Granulosa cells in more mature tertiary follicles with an antrum appear capable of binding both LH and FSH. The FSH receptors are found in granulosa cells from follicles of all sizes, but LH receptors are found only in granulosa cells of large preovulatory follicles.[101-103] These observations are consistent with the concept that the acquisition of LH receptors on granulosa cells is under the influence of FSH.[104,105]

The receptors for the glycoprotein hormones have related structures (Fig. 17-16). The receptors belong to the large family of G protein–coupled receptors, whose members all have a transmembrane domain that consists of seven membrane-traversing α-helices connected by three extracellular and three intracellular loops (see Fig. 17-16). The glycoprotein hormone receptors form a separate subgroup within this large family by virtue of their large extracellular hormone-binding domain at the N-terminus. FSH binds to the FSH receptor, and LH and hCG bind to the same LH receptor. The LH and FSH

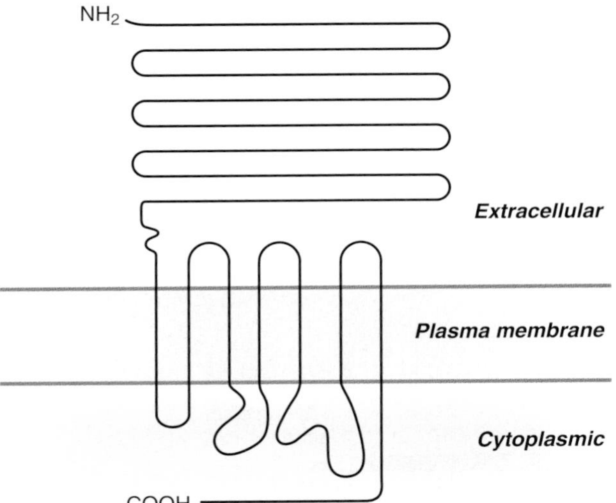

Figure 17-16 Gonadotropin receptor. The seven-transmembrane domain, G protein–coupled receptors for luteinizing hormone and follicle-stimulating hormone that are located in the membranes of ovarian granulosa and theca cells typically have large extracellular domains. (From Bulun SE, Simpson ER, Mendelson CR. The molecular basis of hormone action. In: Carr BR, Blackwell RE, eds. *Textbook of Reproductive Medicine*, 2nd ed. Stamford, CN: Appleton & Lange; 1998:137-156.)

receptor genes are located on chromosome 2 in the p21 region.[49] The relation of the glycoprotein hormone receptors to the other G protein–coupled receptors is indicated by their sequence homology in the C-terminal half of the receptor. This domain, encoded by a single, last exon, contains the seven-transmembrane segments and the G protein–coupling domain. The unusually large extracellular domain of the glycoprotein hormone receptors is encoded by the first 9 or 10 exons (Fig. 17-17).

Role of Follicle-Stimulating Hormone in Ovarian Function. FSH is the main promoter of follicular maturation. Given that FSH receptors have been exclusively localized to granulosa cells, it is presumed that FSH action in the ovary involves the granulosa cells. The ability of FSH to orchestrate follicular growth and differentiation depends on its ability to exert multiple actions concurrently.

Phenotypes of women with mutations that disrupt the function of the FSH β-subunit gene are in good agreement and demonstrate that FSH is necessary for normal follicular development, ovulation, and fertility.[49] Pubertal development is hampered in the absence of sufficient numbers of later-stage follicles with the granulosa cells needed for adequate estrogen production. Treatment of affected patients with exogenous FSH has resulted in follicular maturation, ovulation, and normal pregnancy.[49] The presenting phenotype of FSH β-subunit deficiency is practically identical to that caused by inactivating mutations of the FSH receptor.[49]

Women with FSH receptor mutations are clinically similar to patients with gonadal dysgenesis; they have absent or poorly developed secondary sexual characteristics and high serum levels of FSH and LH. The notable difference is the presence of ovarian follicles in women with mutated FSH receptors, consistent with the FSH independence of primordial follicle recruitment and early follicular growth and development. Total absence of any follicles, including those in the primordial stage, occurs in people in whom the FSH receptor mutation cannot be demonstrated.[49] The ovarian phenotype of FSH receptor deficiency is distinct from the common form of gonadal dysgenesis (Turner's syndrome), which is characterized by streak gonads and an absence of growing follicles.[49]

In vivo rodent studies suggest that FSH is capable of increasing the number of its own receptors in the granulosa cell. Whereas estradiol by itself may be without effect on the distribution, number, or affinity of granulosa cell FSH receptors, estrogens synergize with FSH to enhance the overall number of granulosa cell FSH receptors.[106] Changes in the production of estradiol by preantral follicles can increase their response to FSH through regulation of granulosa cell surface FSH receptors. This interaction between FSH and estradiol in follicular development has been well established in rodents. It appears that ERα and ERβ mediate the estrogenic effect on ovarian development and follicular maturation in mice.[107] However, it is not clear whether a similar relationship exists in the human ovary. ERα is not detected in the human ovary in significant quantities. Nevertheless, the demonstration of ERβ in the human ovary suggests an interaction between FSH and estrogen in the regulation of normal follicle development and ovulation in women.[108]

One of the major actions of FSH is induction of granulosa cell aromatase activity.[109,110] Little or no estrogen can be produced by FSH-unprimed granulosa cells even if they are supplied with aromatizable androgen precursors. Treatment with FSH enhances the aromatization capability of granulosa cells, an effect related to enhancement of the granulosa cell aromatase content.[111,112]

Treatment with FSH has also been shown to induce LH receptors in granulosa cells. The ability of FSH to induce LH receptors is augmented by the concomitant presence of estrogens.[113] Progestins, androgens, and LH itself may also induce LH receptors. After induction, the granulosa cell LH receptor requires the continued presence of FSH for its maintenance.

Circumstantial evidence, deduced from studies of women with disrupting mutations of the genes that encode FSH and LH receptors and aromatase (CYP19A1), indicates that FSH action, but not estrogen or LH action, is essential for follicular growth in humans.[49,114] Follicular growth and development up to the antral stage was observed in women with deficient LH action or estrogen biosynthesis, although these individuals were anovulatory.[49,114] Women with mutations of the FSH β-subunit or FSH receptor have only primordial follicles in their ovaries.[49] These data indicate that estrogen or LH is not critical for follicular development at least until the tertiary stage (see Figs. 17-11 and 17-12). However, FSH by itself is not sufficient to achieve normal follicular development and ovulation.

Role of Luteinizing Hormone in Ovarian Function. LH is essential for ovulation (follicular rupture) and the sustenance of corpus luteum function; in addition, it plays other important roles in follicular function. First, LH probably plays a major role in the promotion of theca-interstitial cell androgen production. Second, LH may well synergize with FSH in the more advanced phases of follicular development. Third, small and sustained increments in the circulating levels of LH are necessary and sufficient to cause small antral follicles to grow and develop to the preovulatory stage.[115,116]

It is presumed that LH acts on the theca-interstitial cells of small follicles, where it promotes the biosynthesis of C19 steroids.[117] The consequent increase in estrogen production is presumed to contribute to the growth and development of the follicles. Treatment with small doses of LH

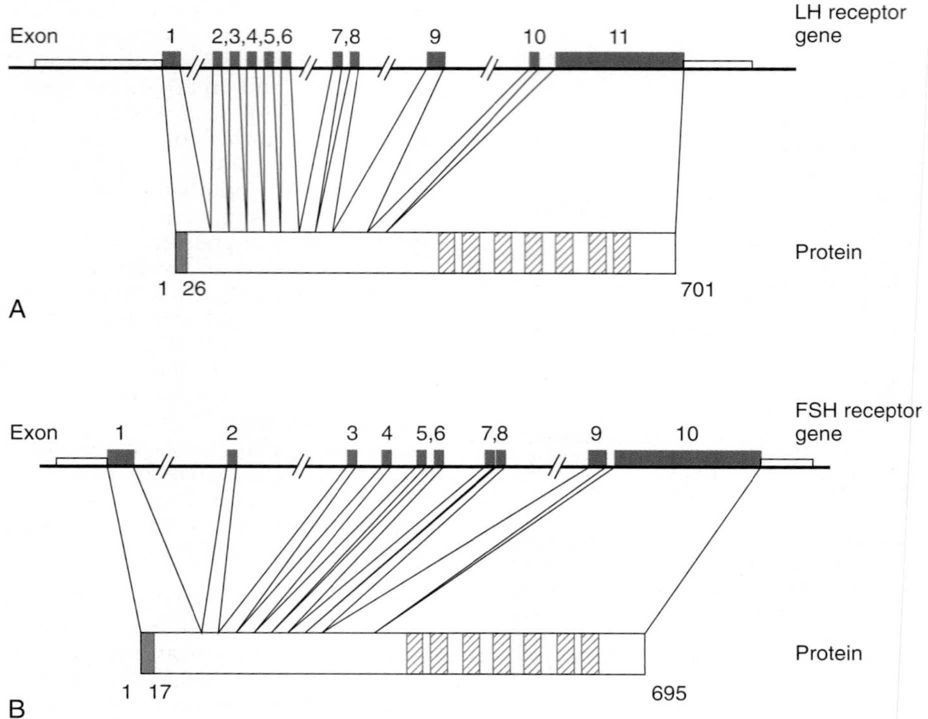

Figure 17-17 Human gonadotropin receptor genes. **A** and **B,** The structure of the genes is depicted at the top of the drawings. The *open bars* indicate sections of the exons that encode untranslated regions of the messenger ribonucleic acid; the *closed bars* indicate the sequences that encode the protein. Both genes are at least 80 kb long. The relation between the intron-exon structure of the gene and the domains on the protein is indicated by the *lines* connecting the gene to the protein. The *horizontally hatched* part of the protein indicates the signal peptide, and the *cross-hatched bars* signify the seven segments of the transmembrane domain. The numbers below the protein indicate the start and end of the signal peptide and the length of the total protein product, including the signal peptide. The receptor genes are similar in structure, with the exception of an additional exon in the luteinizing hormone (LH) receptor gene. Exon I encodes the signal peptide and a small part of the extracellular domain; the next eight or nine exons encode the rest of the extracellular domain, including the leucine-rich repeat motifs. In both receptor genes, the final exon is the largest and contains the information for the transmembrane signal transduction domain. FSH, follicle-stimulating hormone. (From Themmen APN, Huhtaniemi IT. Mutations of gonadotropins and gonadotropin receptors: elucidating the physiology and pathophysiology of pituitary-gonadal function. *Endocr Rev.* 2000;21:4551-583. Copyright © 2000 by The Endocrine Society.)

also presumably results in an increase in LH receptor content and in induction of the key steroidogenic proteins such as StAR, CYP11A1, HSD3B2, and CYP17A1.

The role of LH action in human ovarian physiology was exemplified by the phenotype of a woman with a disrupting mutation of the LH receptor gene.[49] She presented with amenorrhea, normally developed secondary sexual characteristics, increased circulating FSH and LH levels, and low levels of estradiol and progesterone that were unresponsive to hCG treatment.[49] The ovary contained follicles that developed up to antral stage with a well-developed theca layer but no preovulatory follicles or corpora lutea. These observations collectively support the view that LH is essential for ovulation and sufficient estrogen production, whereas follicular development is initially autonomous but at later stages depends on intact FSH action.

Ovarian Steroidogenesis

The steroid hormone contents of the ovarian vein effluents and peripheral venous blood were compared to distinguish steroids secreted by the ovary from those secreted by the adrenal or produced by peripheral conversion of precursors.[118] These studies revealed that the ovaries secrete pregnenolone, progesterone, 17α-hydroxyprogesterone, dehydroepiandrosterone (DHEA), androstenedione, testosterone, estrone, and estradiol.[119] Although such measurements provide insights into the steroidogenic pathways under study, they do not identify the specific ovarian cells involved. Studies using microdissected preovulatory follicles identified estrone and estradiol as the major steroid products (Fig. 17-18). Progesterone and 17α-hydroxyprogesterone proved to be the major products of the corpus luteum (see Fig. 17-18).

The general steroidogenic pathway for the production of estrogens and androgens is depicted in Figure 17-18. The biologically active ovarian steroids are estradiol and progesterone. The major C19 steroid product of the ovary, androstenedione, is not biologically active. However, it acts as a dual precursor and contributes to circulating levels of estrone and testosterone through conversion in extraglandular tissues such as adipose tissue and skin (discussed later).[120-122] It is likely that estrogenically weak estrone is further converted to the potent estrogen estradiol and androgenically weak testosterone is converted to the potent androgen dihydrotestosterone (DHT) locally in target tissues such as brain, breast, prostate, and genital skin and subsequently exert potent biologic effects.[122] This notion is supported by the presence in many human tissues of multiple proteins with overlapping enzymatic activities that catalyze these conversions (e.g., reductive 17β-HSD and 5α-reductase).[123]

The preovulatory follicle secretes estradiol during the first half of the menstrual cycle, and the corpus luteum secretes estradiol and progesterone during the second half of the cycle. The production of these two biologically

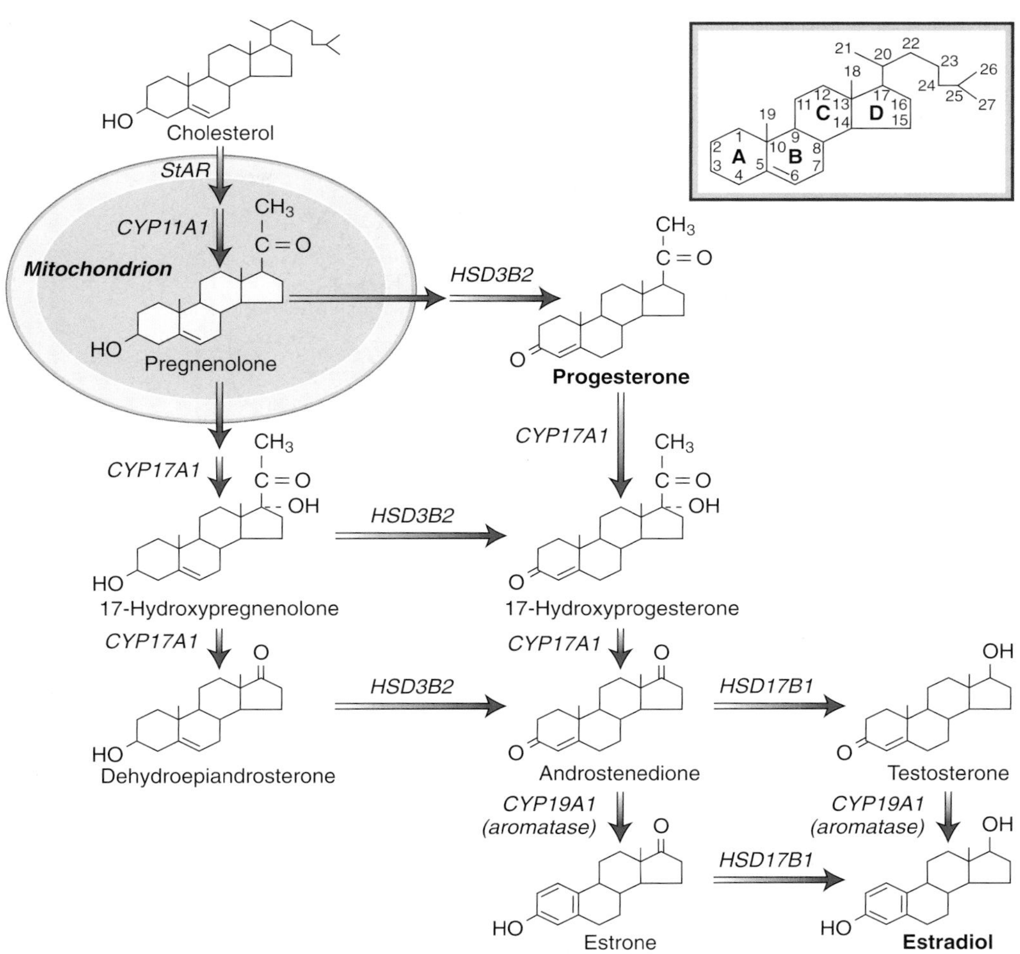

Figure 17-18 Steroidogenic pathway in the human ovary. The biologically active steroids progesterone and estradiol are produced primarily in the ovary of a woman of reproductive age. Estradiol production requires the activity of six steroidogenic proteins, including StAR, and six enzymatic steps. 17-Hydroxylase/17,20-lyase, the product of the *CYP17A1* gene, catalyzes two enzymatic reactions. The four rings of the cholesterol molecule and its derivative steroids are identified by the first four letters in the alphabet, and the carbons are numbered in the sequence shown in the *insert*. CYP17A1, 17-hydroxylase/17,20-lyase; CYP19A1, aromatase; HSD17B1, 17β-hydroxysteroid dehydrogenase type 1; HSD3B2, 3β-hydroxysteroid dehydrogenase-$\Delta^{5,4}$ isomerase type 2; StAR, steroidogenic acute regulatory protein.

active steroids is orchestrated in the follicle and corpus luteum in a cell-specific manner that is under the control of LH and FSH.

Steroids formed by the ovary and other steroid-producing organs are derived from cholesterol (see Fig. 17-18). Several sources of cholesterol can provide the ovary with substrate for steroidogenesis, including plasma lipoprotein cholesterol, cholesterol synthesized de novo within the ovary, and cholesterol from intracellular stores of cholesterol esters within lipid droplets. In the human ovary, LDL-cholesterol is an important source of cholesterol used for steroidogenesis.[92] LH stimulates the activity of adenylate cyclase, increasing production of cyclic adenosine monophosphate (cAMP), which serves as a second messenger to increase LDL receptor mRNA, binding and uptake of LDL-cholesterol, and the formation of cholesterol esters.[91,92] LDL-derived cholesterol is particularly essential for normal levels of progesterone production in the granulosa-lutein cells of the corpus luteum.[92]

Steroidogenic Genes and Their Functions in the Ovary

The first and rate-limiting step in the synthesis of all ovarian steroid hormones is the movement of cholesterol into the mitochondrion, which is regulated by the StAR protein encoded by the *STAR* gene (see Fig. 17-18).[124] This movement is followed by conversion of cholesterol to pregnenolone, which is catalyzed by the mitochondrial side-chain cleavage enzyme complex consisting of CYP11A1, adrenodoxin, and flavoprotein. LH induces steroidogenesis by increasing intracellular cAMP, which increases the conversion of cholesterol to pregnenolone in two distinct ways: acute regulation, which occurs over minutes through phosphorylation of preexisting StAR and rapid synthesis of new StAR, and chronic stimulation, which occurs within hours to days through the induction of CYP11A1 expression and consequent increased steroidogenesis (Fig. 17-19). StAR increases the flow of cholesterol to mitochondria, regulating substrate availability to CYP11A1 on the inner mitochondrial membrane.[124] In the absence of StAR, only 14% of the maximal StAR-induced level of steroidogenesis persists as StAR-independent steroidogenesis.[124]

StAR expression in the preovulatory graafian follicle is limited primarily to the theca cells (see Fig. 17-19).[125] The most important product of the theca cell during the follicular phase is the estrogen precursor androstenedione, and its production is thought to be controlled primarily by StAR. The biologically active steroid product of the ovary

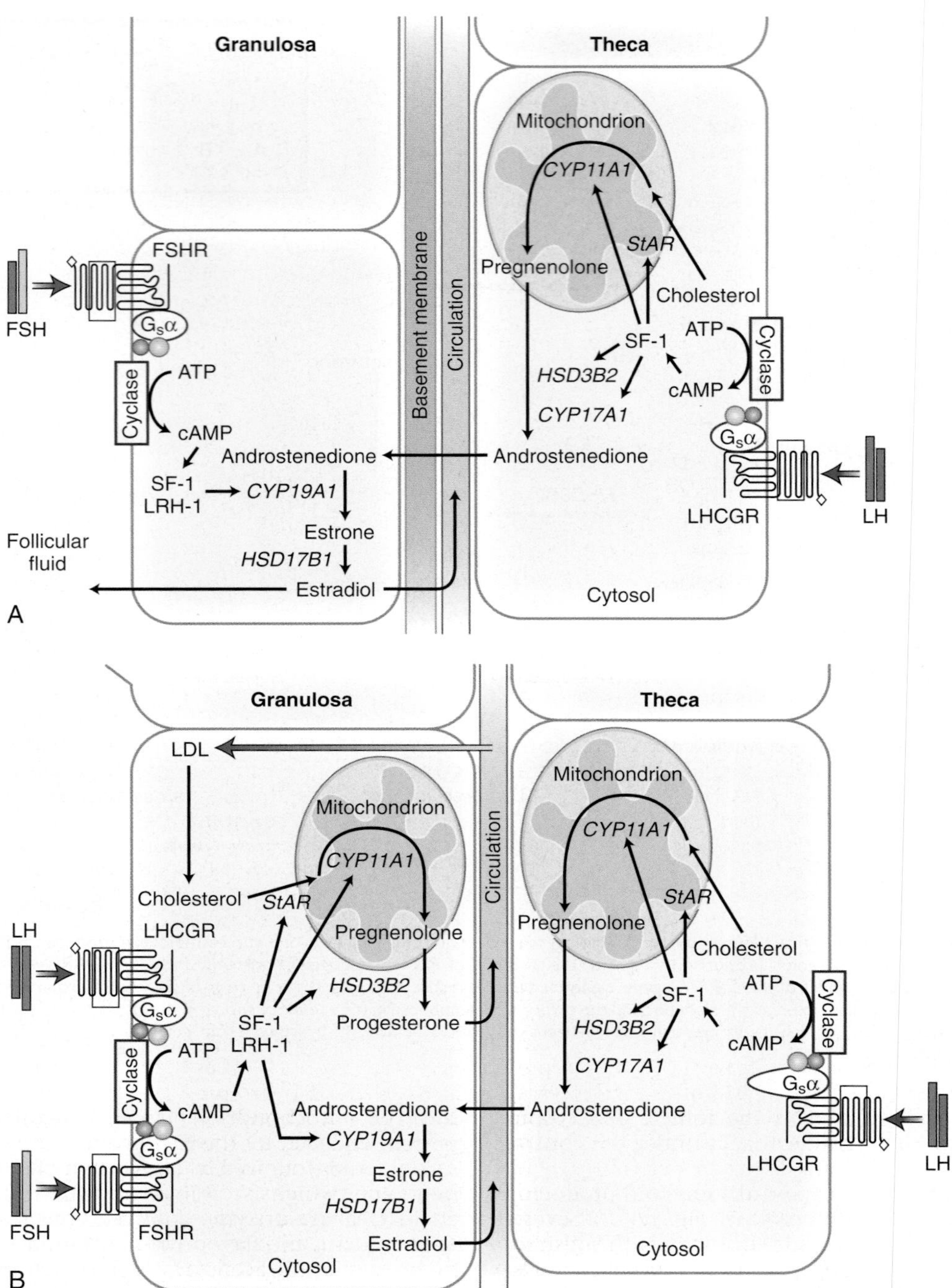

Figure 17-19 Two-cell hypothesis for ovarian steroidogenesis. **A,** The preovulatory follicle produces estradiol through a paracrine interaction between theca and granulosa cells. In response to stimulation with a gonadotropin, steroidogenic factor 1 (SF-1, a member of the nuclear receptor family) acts as a master switch to initiate transcription of a series of steroidogenic genes in theca cells. In follicular granulosa cells, another nuclear receptor, liver homolog receptor 1 (LRH-1), seems to primarily mediate the downstream effects of follicle-stimulating hormone (FSH) in the rodent ovary.[133,134] In humans, the roles of SF-1 and LRH-1 in steroidogenesis in preovulatory granulosa cells are not well understood. Because granulosa cells do not have a direct connection to the circulation, CYP19A1 (aromatase) in granulosa cells depends for substrate on androstenedione that diffuses from theca cells. Two critical steps in estradiol formation are the entry of cholesterol into mitochondria facilitated by steroidogenic acute regulatory protein (STAR) in theca cells and the conversion of androstenedione to estrone catalyzed by CYP19A1 in granulosa cells. **B,** In the corpus luteum, granulosa-lutein cells are heavily vascularized, a condition that is critical for entry of abundant quantities of cholesterol into this cell type through primarily low-density lipoprotein (LDL)-cholesterol receptors and for secretion of large amounts of progesterone into the circulation. The entry of cholesterol into mitochondria (mediated by STAR) is probably the most critical steroidogenic step for progesterone formation in granulosa-lutein cells. Androstenedione produced in theca-lutein cells serves as a substrate for estrone, which is further converted to estradiol in granulosa-lutein cells. Human data suggest that LRH-1 may mediate at least a portion of gonadotropin-dependent steroidogenesis in the corpus luteum.[136] Gonadotropins, SF-1, and possibly LRH-1 play key roles for important steroidogenic steps in the ovary. ATP, adenosine triphosphate; cAMP, cyclic adenosine monophosphate; FSHR, FSH receptor; HSD, hydroxysteroid dehydrogenase; LHCGR, LH receptor.

during the follicular phase is estradiol, which arises from the granulosa cells located adjacent to theca cells. The rate-limiting step for granulosa cell estradiol production is regulated by the FSH-dependent activity of the aromatase enzyme in a cyclic fashion.[110] During the luteal phase, cells of the corpus luteum, including granulosa-lutein cells, also show intense StAR immunoreactivity with a patchy distribution.[94,125] The delivery of cholesterol to the mitochondrial side-chain cleavage enzyme system in the corpus luteum is the rate-limiting step for progesterone biosynthesis and is regulated by StAR.[94] Estradiol production seems to be regulated primarily by StAR and CYP19A1, whereas progesterone biosynthesis may be primarily under the control of StAR.

The ovarian granulosa, theca, and corpus luteum cells possess StAR plus five distinct proteins with specific enzyme activities for steroid hormone formation. These steroidogenic enzymes are CYP11A1 (side-chain cleavage of P450), HSD3B2 (3β-hydroxysteroid dehydrogenase-$\Delta^{5,4}$ isomerase type 2), CYP17A1 (17-hydroxylase/17,20-lyase), CYP19A1 (aromatase P450), and HSD17B1 (17β-hydroxysteroid dehydrogenase type 1).[126] These enzymes are responsible for the conversion of cholesterol to the two major biologically active products: estradiol and progesterone.[127]

Steroidogenesis that depends on LH and FSH in theca and granulosa cells is mediated by common signaling molecules, including cAMP and the specific transcription factors steroidogenic factor 1 (SF1), product of the *NR5AI* gene, and liver receptor homolog 1 (LRH1), product of the *NR5A2* gene, which belong to the nuclear receptor family (see Fig. 17-19).[128,129] SF1 and LRH1 regulate the expression of genes that encode StAR, CYP11A1, HSD3B2, CYP17A1, and CYP19A1 (see Fig. 17-19). SF1 and possibly LRH1 can be regarded as downstream master switches that orchestrate ovarian steroidogenesis.[129]

All steroid hormones are derived from cholesterol. C27 cholesterol is coverted to the 18-, 19-, and 21-carbon steroid hormones that are secreted by the ovary.

C21 Steroids. The principal progestogens are C21 steroids and include pregnenolone, progesterone, and 17-hydroxyprogesterone (see Fig. 17-18). Pregnenolone is of primary importance in the ovary because of its key position as a precursor of all steroid hormones. Progesterone, the principal secretory product of the corpus luteum, is responsible for the progestational effects (i.e., cell differentiation and induction of secretory activity in the endometrium of the estrogen-primed uterus). Progesterone is essential for implantation of the fertilized ovum and maintenance of pregnancy. It also induces decidualization of the endometrium, inhibits uterine contractions, increases the viscosity of cervical mucus, promotes lateral (alveolar) development of the breast glands, and increases basal body temperature. However, 17-hydroxyprogesterone, also secreted by the corpus luteum, is thought to have little or no biologic activity.

C19 Steroids. The ovary secretes a variety of C19 steroids, including DHEA, androstenedione, and testosterone (see Fig. 17-18). They are produced by the theca cells and, possibly, to a lesser degree by the ovarian stroma. The major C19 steroid is androstenedione, part of which is secreted directly into plasma, with the remainder converted to estrogen by the granulosa cells. DHEA and androstenedione do not appear to have major androgenic actions. In the ovary and in peripheral tissues, DHEA is converted to androstenedione, which can be converted to estrone or testosterone. Testosterone is converted locally to DHT at target tissues for full androgenic action.

C18 Steroids. The naturally occurring estrogens are C18 steroids characterized by the presence of an aromatic A ring, a phenolic hydroxyl group at C3, and a hydroxyl group (estradiol) or a ketone group (estrone) at C17. Aromatase is the key enzyme for estrogen production in the ovary (see Fig. 17-18). The protein aromatase P450, encoded by the *CYP19A1* gene, confers the specific activity of the aromatase enzyme complex. CYP191A1 production in the ovarian granulosa cell is regulated primarily by FSH.[126] The principal and most potent estrogen secreted by the ovary is estradiol. Although estrone is also secreted by the ovary, another important source of estrone is extraglandular conversion of androstenedione in peripheral tissues.[130] Estriol (16-hydroxyestradiol) is the most abundant estrogen in urine and is produced by metabolism of estrone and estradiol in extraovarian tissues. All C18 steroids, including estrone, estradiol, and estriol, are commonly referred to as estrogens. However, estrone and estriol are only weakly estrogenic and must be converted to estradiol to show full estrogenic action. At least seven enzymes with overlapping activities are capable of converting estrone to estradiol in the ovary and extraovarian tissues.[131]

Catechol estrogens are formed by hydroxylation of estrogens at the C2 or C4 position. The physiologic role of catechol estrogen, if any, is unclear. Low body weight and hyperthyroidism are associated with increased formation of catechol estrogens.[132] Estrone sulfate, formed by peripheral conversion of estradiol and estrone, is the most abundant estrogen in blood, but it is not physiologically active. Estrone sulfate is presumed to serve as a reservoir for estrone formation in a number of tissues, including those that are targets of estrogen. Estradiol regulates gonadotropin secretion, development of the secondary sexual characteristics of women, uterine growth, thickening of the vaginal mucosa, thinning of the cervical mucus, linear growth of the ductal system of the breast, growth spurt, epiphyseal closure, and bone mineralization.

Two-Cell Theory for Ovarian Steroidogenesis

The classic two-cell theory is supported by molecular findings. Ovarian steroidogenesis in the preovulatory follicle takes place through LH receptors on theca cells and FSH (possibly also LH) receptors on granulosa cells (see Fig. 17-19). cAMP production and increased SF1 binding to multiple steroidogenic promoters mediate LH action in theca cells. The StAR protein is the primary regulator of production of androstenedione, which subsequently diffuses into granulosa cells to serve as the estrogen precursor. In the preovulatory follicle, cholesterol in theca cells arises from circulating lipoproteins and de novo biosynthesis. FSH is responsible for follicular growth and estrogen formation. FSH induces cAMP formation, activation of protein kinase A and certain mitogen-activated protein kinases, and increased binding activity of LRH1 or SF1 to the *CYP191A1* promoter in preovulatory granulosa cells to form estradiol primarily through aromatization of androstenedione (see Fig. 17-19). The relative roles of SF1 and LRH1 in estrogen formation in human ovarian granulosa cells are not well understood.[133-135]

In the corpus luteum, large deposits of cholesterol (which provides the yellow color) arise primarily from circulating lipoproteins to support the production of extremely high quantities of progesterone. Other key anatomic events in formation of the corpus luteum are the disruption of the basement membrane between the granulosa and theca cells and strikingly increased vascularization of granulosa–lutein cells (see Fig. 17-15). Theca-lutein cells possess LH receptors and produce androstenedione. Cyclic

AMP, SF1, and StAR induced by LH remain as the key regulators for biosynthesis of androstenedione, which serves as the estrogen precursor in neighboring granulosa-lutein cells (see Fig. 17-19).

The granulosa-lutein cell of the corpus luteum is anatomically and functionally different from its counterpart in the preovulatory follicle in several ways. First, these cells are luteinized and heavily vascularized and contain large quantities of cholesterol. Second, granulosa-lutein cells contain high levels of LH receptors in addition to FSH receptors. Third, they produce large quantities of progesterone that is regulated primarily by LH and StAR. Granulosa-lutein cells also aromatize androstenedione of thecal origin and eventually give rise to estradiol formation through FSH action and CYP19A1. The known mediators of LH and FSH in human granulosa-lutein cells are cAMP and increased LRH1 levels.[136] The relative roles of LRH1 and SF1 for progesterone and estradiol production in granulosa-lutein cells are not clear. Specific functions of the two gonadotropins (i.e., differentiation, growth, and progesterone formation versus estradiol formation) are probably determined by as yet unidentified modifying factors (see Fig. 17-19).

Peptide Hormones Produced by the Ovary

The ovary produces a large number of peptides that can act in an intracrine, autocrine, paracrine, or endocrine fashion. They include numerous growth factors (e.g., insulin-like growth factors [IGFs]) and cytokines (e.g., interleukin-1β). IGFs cross-talk with the FSH-dependent signaling cascade to augment the effects of FSH in granulosa cells.

These peptides, including inhibin, activin, and follistatin, are produced in ovarian granulosa cells under the control of FSH and LH (Fig. 17-20). Production of inhibin and activin is not limited to the ovary; a number of other tissues, including adrenal, pituitary, and placenta, synthesize these peptides. Two isoforms of inhibin have been isolated: inhibin A and inhibin B. They contain an identical α-subunit but distinct β-subunits (β_A and β_B), encoded by separate genes. The heterodimers of inhibin, $\alpha\beta_A$ and $\alpha\beta_B$, are called inhibin A and inhibin B, respectively (see Fig. 17-20). Although inhibin is produced by a number of tissues in the body, most of it is derived from the gonads. In the ovary, the source of inhibin is granulosa cells. The main role of inhibin is to suppress FSH production in the pituitary.

Although both inhibin isoforms seem to have similar biologic properties, their synthesis is regulated differently during the follicular and luteal phases (see Fig. 17-1A). Under the influence of FSH, inhibin B is secreted mainly during the early follicular phase, with levels decreasing in midfollicular phase and becoming undetectable after the LH surge.[135] LH-induced inhibin A levels are low during the first half of the follicular phase but increase gradually during midfollicular phase and peak during the luteal phase. All three subunits are detected in small antral follicles by immunohistochemistry and in situ hybridization.[137,138] The α- and β_A-subunits are found in the dominant follicle and in the corpus luteum. All three subunits are expressed in response to gonadotropins or factors that increase intracellular cAMP.[139]

Activin is structurally related to inhibin but exerts opposite actions. Activin contains two subunits that are identical to the β-subunits of inhibins A and B. The three activin isoforms are activin A ($\beta_A\beta_A$), activin B ($\beta_B\beta_B$), and activin AB ($\beta_A\beta_B$). In the pituitary, activin stimulates the release of FSH. In the ovarian follicle, activin enhances FSH action (see Fig. 17-20). As in the case of inhibin, activins are also produced in ovarian granulosa cells and pituitary gonadotrophs. Unlike inhibin, locally synthesized activin in the pituitary, rather than the ovarian-derived activin, is responsible for regulating FSH (see Fig. 17-4).

Follistatin is a single-unit peptide that is produced in several human tissues, including the pituitary and ovary (see Fig. 17-20). It binds and neutralizes the biologic

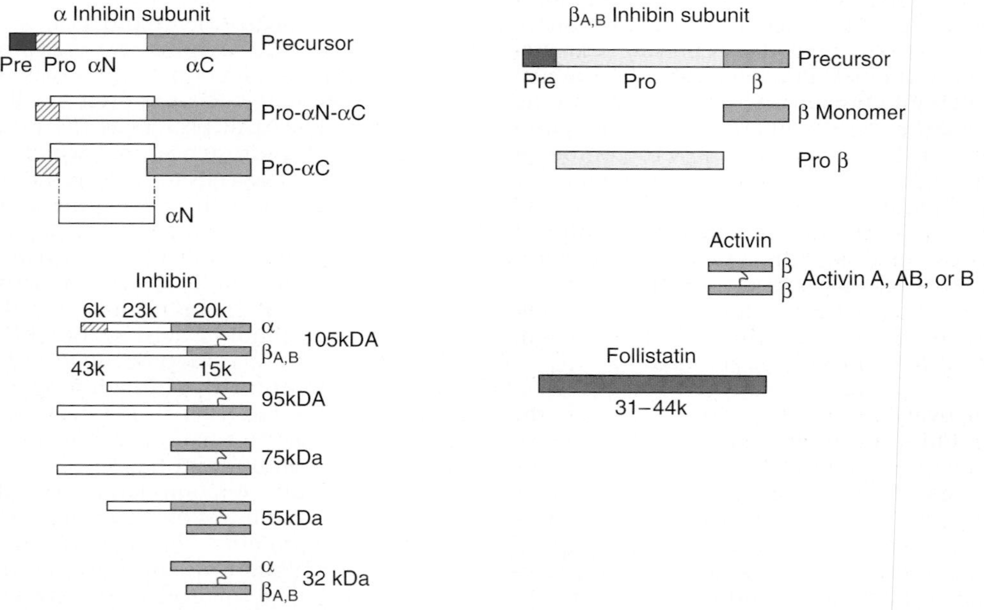

Figure 17-20 Structures of inhibin subunit precursors and processed forms in serum, the activins and the follistatins. The precise contribution of each molecular-weight form of inhibin to the biologic activity in serum is not known, but it has been established that the 55-kd and 32-kd forms are biologically active. (Modified from Burger H. Inhibin, activin and neoplasia. In: Yen SC, Jaffe RB, Barbieri RL, eds. *Reproductive Endocrinology,* 4th ed. Philadelphia, PA: Saunders; 1999:669-675.)

functions of activin. It appears that local follistatin levels in tissues modulate the effects of activin. This explains the inhibitory effect of follistatin on pituitary FSH secretion (see Fig. 17-4).

Overview of the Hormonal Changes during the Ovarian Cycle

FSH secretion is suppressed by negative feedback of the ovarian hormones estradiol, inhibin, and progesterone during the early and midluteal phase. The sharp decline of these hormones on regression of the corpus luteum during the late luteal phase abolishes this negative feedback (see Fig. 17-1A). This permits increased secretion of FSH just before and during menses. This initial increase in FSH is essential for follicle recruitment and growth and steroidogenesis. With continued growth of the follicle, autocrine and paracrine factors produced within the follicle maintain follicular sensitivity to FSH. Continuing and combined action of FSH and activin leads to the appearance of LH receptors on the granulosa cells, a prerequisite for ovulation and luteinization.

Ovulation is triggered by the rapid rise in circulating levels of estradiol. A positive feedback response at the level of the anterior pituitary and possibly at the hypothalamus results in the midcycle surge of LH that is necessary for expulsion of the egg and formation of the corpus luteum (see Fig. 17-1A). A rise in the progesterone level follows ovulation, along with a second rise in the estradiol level, producing the 14-day-long luteal phase characterized by low FSH and LH levels. Demise of the corpus luteum concomitant with a fall in hormone (progesterone, estradiol, and inhibin A) levels allows FSH to increase again toward the end of the luteal phase, initiating a new cycle. If pregnancy is established by implantation of a blastocyst, the structural integrity and function (i.e., progesterone and estradiol production) of the corpus luteum are maintained by hCG secreted from the trophoblast. The hCG acts as a surrogate for LH on the corpus luteum.

In addition to FSH and LH, local factors (e.g., activin, inhibin) regulate follicular development and steroidogenesis. In the early follicular phase, activin produced by granulosa cells in immature follicles enhances the action of FSH on aromatase activity and FSH and LH receptor formation while simultaneously suppressing C19-steroid formation in theca cells. In the late follicular phase, increased production of inhibin by the granulosa cells and decreased activin levels promote the synthesis of C19 steroids in the theca layer in response to LH and local growth factors and cytokines; this provides larger amounts of the precursor androstenedione for production of estrone and ultimately of estradiol in the granulosa cells.[140]

LH-mediated androstenedione production in theca cells and FSH-mediated estradiol production in granulosa cells are potentiated by IGFs.[141] The major endogenous IGF produced in the human ovarian follicle is IGF2 (rather than IGF1), which is produced by granulosa and theca cells. The actions of IGF1 and IGF2 are mediated by IGF receptor type 1 in both cells. IGF receptor type 1 is structurally similar to the insulin receptor. It appears that gonadotropin-related IGF action in the ovary is regulated primarily by IGF2 and IGF receptor type 1.[141]

In summary, ovulation is under the control of substances functioning as classic hormones (i.e., FSH, LH, estradiol, and inhibin), which transmit messages between the ovary and the hypothalamic-pituitary axis and of paracrine and autocrine factors such as IGF2, inhibin, and activin, which coordinate sequential activities within the follicle destined to ovulate. The negative feedback relationship between corpus luteum products (i.e., estradiol, progesterone, and inhibin) and FSH results in the critical initial rise in FSH immediately before and during menses, and the positive feedback relationship between estradiol and LH is responsible for the ovulatory stimulus (see Fig. 17-1). Within the ovary, IGF2, inhibin, and activin modify follicular responses necessary for growth and function. These endocrine, paracrine, and autocrine factors undoubtedly represent only a portion of the complete picture. The causes of anovulation are diverse and may be related to defects in cell surface receptors, intracellular elements of signal transduction, or cell-cell interactions.[142,143]

Extraovarian Steroidogenesis

Estradiol formation takes place in several tissues in the woman of reproductive age, including the ovary, peripheral tissues such as subcutaneous fat and skin, and physiologic and pathologic target sites such as the hypothalamus, breast cancer cells, and the cells of endometriosis (Fig. 17-21).[122] The latter two sources of estrogen are particularly critical in anovulatory premenopausal and postmenopausal women. Although only small quantities of estrogen are produced by an individual adipocyte or skin fibroblast in a continuous fashion, these cell types contribute to circulating estradiol levels because of their relative

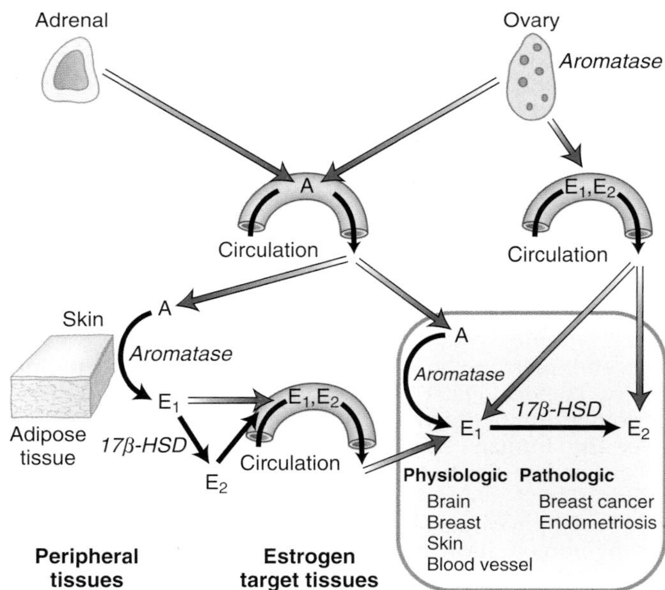

Figure 17-21 Estrogen biosynthesis in women. The biologically active estrogen, estradiol (E_2), is produced in at least three major sites: (1) by direct secretion from the ovary in reproductive-age women; (2) by conversion of circulating androstenedione (A), originating from the adrenal or ovary or both, to estrone (E_1) in peripheral tissues; and (3) by conversion of A to E_1 in estrogen target tissues. In the latter two instances, estrogenically weak estrone (E_1) is converted to E_2 within the same tissue. The expression of genes that encode the enzymes aromatase and reductive 17β-hydroxysteroid dehydrogenases (17β-HSD) is critical for E_2 formation at these sites. Reductive 17β-HSD activity in peripheral tissues may be conferred by protein products of several genes with overlapping functions. HSD17B1 is a distinct reductive 17β-HSD enzyme that is encoded by a specific gene expressed primarily in the ovary. Aromatase is encoded by a single gene (*CYP19A1*). E_2 formation by peripheral and local conversion is particularly important in postmenopausal women and in those with estrogen-dependent diseases such as breast cancer, endometriosis, or endometrial cancer.

abundance.[122] This effect is more pronounced in obese women because of increased mass of the adipose tissue and skin.[120]

Aromatase (CYP19A1) in adipocytes and skin fibroblasts is responsible for peripheral aromatization of androstenedione that arises from the ovary and the adrenal in premenopausal women and primarily from the adrenal in postmenopausal women (see Fig. 17-21).[122] However, the product of this reaction, estrone, is only weakly estrogenic. Estrone is further converted to estrone sulfate, which serves as a reservoir for estrone in blood and other tissues. Estrone (arising from androstenedione and estrone sulfate) is further converted to the biologically active estradiol in target tissues such as the endometrium and breast by a number of enzymatic proteins with overlapping reductive 17β-HSD activity (see Fig. 17-21).[131,144,145] It is likely that local CYP19A1 expression in hypothalamus is critical for the regulation of gonadotropin secretion.[146] Estrogen-dependent pathologic tissues such as those in breast cancer and endometriosis contain extremely high levels of CYP19A1 that enhances tissue growth by increasing local estradiol concentrations (see Fig. 17-21).[122] Circulating androstenedione is the major substrate for aromatase activity in these physiologic and pathologic target tissues.[144,147]

Significant quantities of circulating androstenedione can also be converted to testosterone in peripheral tissues (discussed later). This is probably accomplished by the presence of multiple 17β-HSDs with overlapping reductive activities in peripheral tissues.[131] Androgenic action of testosterone is strikingly amplified by its conversion to DHT in peripheral and target tissues (e.g., skin, prostate). At least two distinct proteins encoded by two separate genes, 5α-reductase type 1 and type 2, catalyze the conversion of testosterone to DHT in liver, prostate, and skin.[123] Local production of DHT in genital skin fibroblasts is critical for normal masculinization of external genitalia of male fetuses in utero.[123] DHT formation in the skin is an important cause of hirsutism.[148]

ENDOMETRIUM

The endometrium is the mucosal lining of the uterine cavity. The decidua is the highly modified and specialized endometrium of pregnancy. From an evolutionary perspective, the human endometrium is highly developed to accommodate the hemochorioendothelial type of placentation, which requires the presence of spiral arteries (Fig. 17-22). Trophoblasts of the blastocyst invade spiral arteries during implantation and placentation in the establishment of uteroplacental vessels.

Spiral arteries of the human endometrium confer another unique process, *menstruation*. Menstruation is shedding of endometrial tissue with hemorrhage that depends on sex steroid hormone–directed changes in blood flow in the spiral arteries. Spiral arteries are essential for menstruation; only humans and a few other primates that have endometrial spiral arteries experience menstruation. With nonfertile but ovulatory ovarian cycles, menstruation affects desquamation of the endometrium. New endometrial growth and development must be initiated with each ovarian cycle, so endometrial maturation corresponds with the next opportunity for pregnancy. There seems to be a narrow window of endometrial receptivity to blastocyst implantation, comprising the period between days 20 and 24 during a 28-day menstrual cycle.[149]

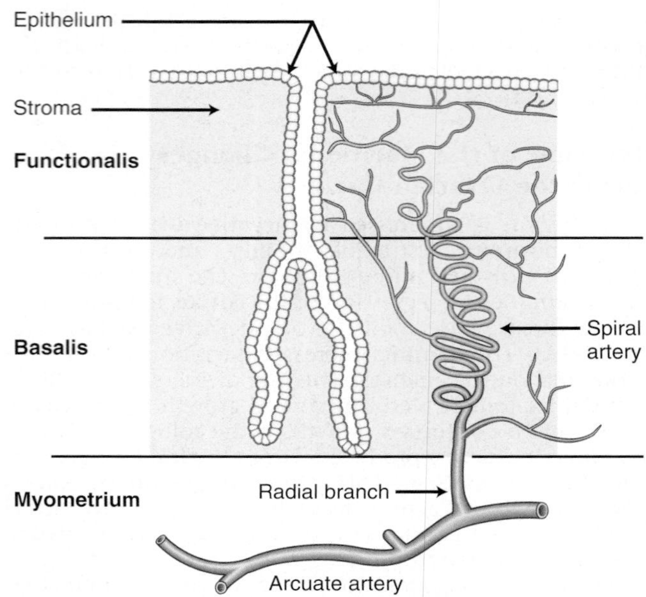

Figure 17-22 Functional anatomy of the endometrium. Endometrium is a multilayered mucosa specialized for implantation and support of pregnancy. A single, continuous layer of epithelial cells lines the surface of the stroma and penetrates the stroma with deep invaginations almost all the way down to the myometrium-endometrium junction. The entire thickness of the endometrium is penetrated by the spiral arteries and their capillaries. Spiral arteries originate from the radial branches of arcuate arteries, which arise from uterine arteries. The superficial layer (functionalis) is shed during menstruation, whereas the permanent bottom layer (basalis) gives rise to the regeneration of endometrium after each menstruation. The striking changes in the spiral arteries (i.e., coiling, stasis, and vasodilatation followed by intense vasoconstriction) are consistently observed before the onset of every menstruation episode. (Courtesy of Dr. Kristof Chwalisz, North Chicago, Illinois.)

Functional Anatomy of the Endometrium

The endometrium can be divided morphologically into an upper two-thirds *functionalis* layer and a lower one-third *basalis* layer (see Fig. 17-22). The purpose of the functionalis layer is to prepare for the implantation of the blastocyst; it is the site of proliferation, secretion, and degeneration. The purpose of the basalis layer is to provide the regenerative endometrium after menstrual loss of the functionalis.[150] Major histologic components of the endometrium include stromal cells, which constitute the skeleton of the tissue; a single layer of epithelial cells, which lines the lumen of the endometrial cavity and invaginations of the stroma; blood vessels; and resident immune cells. The epithelial cells that line the rather deep invaginations of the stroma are also referred to as *glandular cells*. However, these deep crypts represent extensions of the intracavitary lumen and are not true glands. These invaginations lined by epithelial cells extend from the surface of the functionalis layer (i.e., luminal epithelium) deep into the basalis level (i.e., glandular epithelium). After the functionalis layer is shed at the time of menstruation, the basalis, which contains epithelial and stromal cells, can give rise to a new functionalis layer for the upcoming cycle (Fig. 17-23).

The cellular components of the functionalis layer undergo a striking progression during the menstrual cycle, whereas the basalis shows only modest alterations. The sequence of endometrial changes associated with an ovulatory cycle has been carefully studied by Noyes and colleagues in humans and by Markee[151,152] and Bartelmez[153] in subhuman primates.

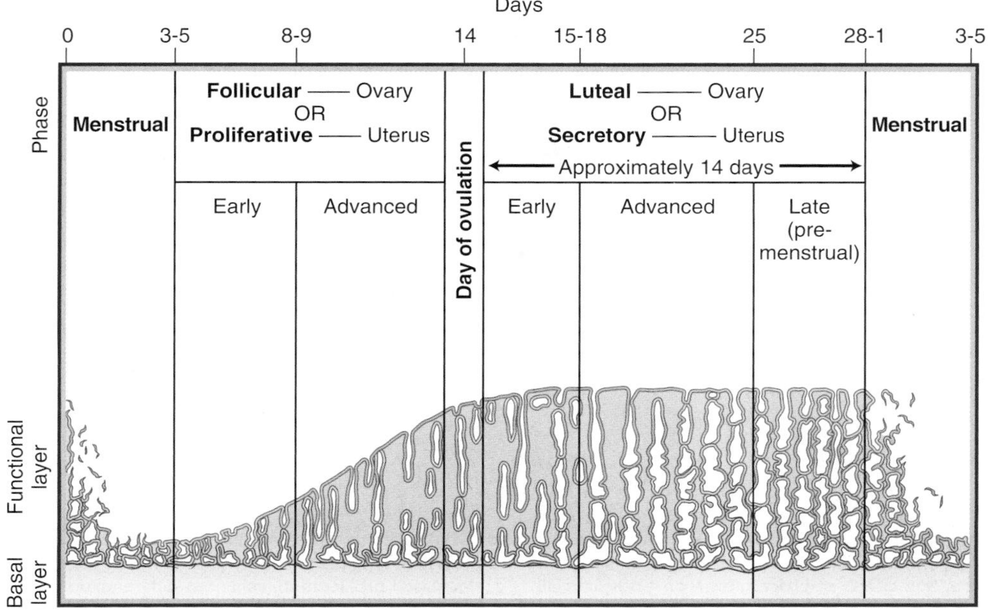

Figure 17-23 Cyclic changes in thickness and morphology of endometrium and the relation of these changes to those of the ovarian cycle. (From Cunningham FG, MacDonald PC, Gant NF, et al. The endometrium and decidua: menstruation and pregnancy. In: Cunningham FG, ed. *Williams Obstetrics*, 19th ed. Stamford, CN: Appleton & Lange, 1993:81-109.)

Hormone-Induced Morphologic Changes of the Endometrium

The cyclic changes in endometrial histology are faithfully reproduced during each ovulatory ovarian cycle. These sex steroid hormone–induced modifications can be summarized in several steps. First, during the preovulatory, or follicular, phase of the cycle, estradiol is secreted (principally by a single dominant follicle of one ovary) in increasing quantities until just before ovulation. Second, during the postovulatory, or luteal, phase of the cycle, progesterone is secreted by the corpus luteum in increasing amounts (up to 40 to 50 mg/day) until the midluteal phase. Third, beginning about 7 to 8 days after ovulation, the rates of progesterone and estradiol secretion by the corpus luteum begin to decline and then diminish progressively before menstruation (see Fig. 17-1).

In response to these cyclic changes in the rates of ovarian sex steroid hormone secretion, there are five main stages of the corresponding endometrial cycle: (1) menstrual-postmenstrual *reepithelialization*; (2) *endometrial proliferation* in response to stimulation by estradiol; (3) abundant *epithelial secretion*, occurring in response to the combined action of estradiol and progesterone; (4) *premenstrual ischemia*, the result of endometrial tissue volume involution, which causes stasis of blood in the spiral arteries; and (5) *menstruation*, which is preceded and accompanied by severe vasoconstriction of the endometrial spiral arteries and collapse and desquamation of all but the deepest layer of the endometrium. In the final analysis, menstruation is the consequence of the withdrawal of factors that maintain endometrial growth and differentiation (see Fig. 17-23).

Commonly, the initiation of menstruation is attributed to progesterone withdrawal. This concept was developed because the administration of estrogen to postmenopausal women and treatment with and then withdrawal of a progestin causes menstruation, even with continued estrogen treatment. Moreover, progesterone facilitates decidualization of the endometrium and the maintenance of pregnancy, whereas progesterone withdrawal favors the initiation of menstruation, lactation, and parturition. There are probably many additional coordinated and interactive processes other than progesterone withdrawal that are operative and essential for the success of each of these events.

The preovulatory (follicular or proliferative) phase and the postovulatory (luteal or secretory) phase of the ovarian-endometrial cycles are customarily divided into early and late stages (see Fig. 17-23). The normal secretory phase of the endometrial (menstrual) cycle can be subdivided almost daily by histologic criteria, from shortly after ovulation until the onset of menstruation. Noyes and other investigators have provided an extremely detailed description of the histologic features of the secretory phase endometrium, which permit accurate dating during the luteal phase.[154] Some gynecologists use histologic dating of endometrial biopsies obtained during the luteal phase to evaluate ovulation, progesterone production, or the degree of biologic response of the endometrium to progesterone. Normal endometrial development is assumed when the histologic and chronologic endometrial dating agree within 2 days. If they differ by more than 2 days, the endometrium is considered to be out of phase. Out-of-phase endometrial tissue may be a cause of implantation failure, producing infertility. However, the sensitivity and specificity of the dating of endometrial biopsy specimens for evaluation of infertility are unknown. It is important to understand this and other limitations of the test with respect to its routine clinical use as a basis for infertility treatments. For example, one important disadvantage of this test is interobserver variation in histologic interpretation of biopsies.

Effects of Ovarian Steroids on Endometrium

Estradiol or synthetic estrogens such as ethinyl estradiol cause a striking thickening of endometrial tissue. Stromal

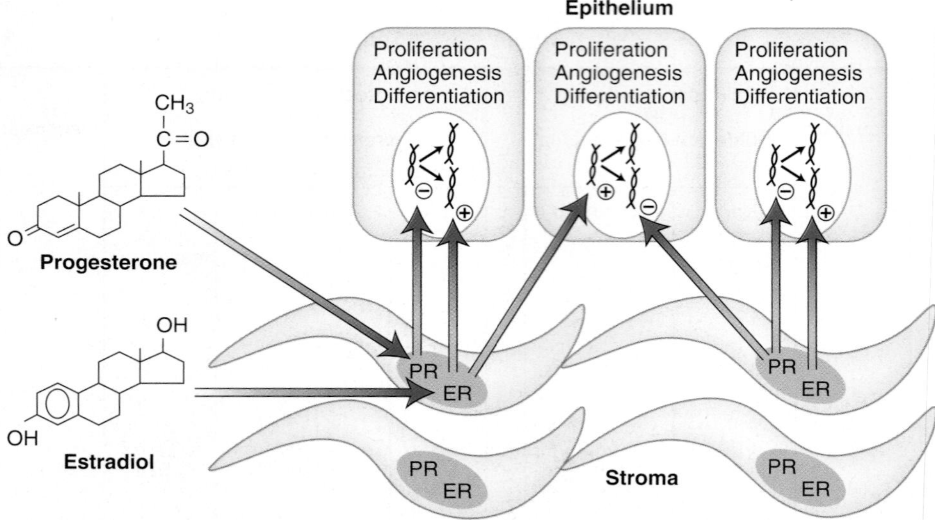

Figure 17-24 Critical epithelial effects of estrogen (i.e., deoxyribonucleic acid [DNA] synthesis, proliferation, and gene expression) are mediated primarily by estrogen receptor-α (ER) in stromal cells in a paracrine manner in the endometrium. This was demonstrated in mice.[156] It was also shown in mice and humans that the antiestrogenic effects of progesterone on epithelial cells (e.g., decreased proliferation, enhanced differentiation) are mediated primarily by progesterone receptors (PRs) in stromal cells.[157]

and epithelial cells of the endometrium proliferate rapidly under the influence of estradiol. Estradiol greatly increases mitotic activity and DNA synthesis in both cell types (Fig. 17-24). While promoting growth, estradiol also renders endometrial tissue responsive to progesterone by inducing the expression of progesterone receptors (PRs) in this tissue; progesterone action depends on previous or concurrent estrogen exposure of the endometrium.[155]

In contrast to the proliferative effects of estrogen, progesterone action primarily enables differentiation of the endometrium. For example, progesterone can inhibit and even reverse the proliferative action of estrogen on the functionalis layer (see Fig. 17-24). Moreover, progesterone action prepares the endometrium for implantation of the embryo through differentiation of epithelial and stromal cells. Progesterone induces the production and secretion of a glycogen-rich substance from the epithelial cells. Progesterone also causes an increase in stromal cell cytoplasm, a process called *pseudodecidualization*. The term *decidualization* is reserved for stroma differentiated under the combined influence of progesterone and hCG of placental origin during pregnancy.

Estrogen Action

Estradiol, the biologically potent, naturally occurring estrogen that is secreted by the granulosa cells of the dominant ovarian follicle, promotes responses of the endometrium through mechanisms similar to those used by other steroid hormones. Estradiol enters cells from blood by simple diffusion, but in estrogen-responsive cells, binding to the ER sequesters estradiol. ERs are proteins with a high affinity for estradiol and other biologically active estrogens (i.e., synthetic estrogens). Although ERα and ERβ are present in the endometrium, ERα seems to be the primary mediator of the estrogenic action in that tissue.[158,159] After transformational changes, the estradiol-receptor complex is a transcriptional factor that becomes associated with chromatin.[160] Estradiol-ERα complexes bind thousands of DNA sites across the entire genome and regulate the transcription of hundreds of genes at one time.[160,161] Contrary to a previous notion, most ERα binding sites are outside classically defined basal promoters, interact with the transcriptional start sites through DNA bending, and do not contain classically defined estrogen response elements.[160,161] This interaction brings about ER-specific initiation of gene transcription, which promotes the synthesis of specific mRNAs and, thereafter, specific proteins.[162] Among the many proteins synthesized in most estrogen-responsive cells are additional ERs and PRs. Estradiol acts in the endometrium and in other estrogen-responsive tissues to promote the perpetuation of estrogen action and the responsiveness of that tissue to progesterone.

The endometrial epithelial cells are estrogen responsive but probably do not replicate as a result of direct action of estradiol on them. Replication of human endometrial epithelial cells in culture is not increased appreciably, if at all, when estrogen is added to the medium. Estrogen acts on mouse uterine stromal cells to promote the synthesis of growth factors that act on epithelial cells (see Fig. 17-24).[156] These growth factors operate in a paracrine manner to cause increased DNA synthesis and replication in the adjacent epithelial cells. This type of paracrine arrangement may be a common mechanism that mediates estrogen action in hormone-responsive tissues.

Progesterone Action

Progesterone enters cells by diffusion, and in responsive tissues, it becomes associated with PRs that have a high affinity for progesterone. Two PR isoforms, PR-A and PR-B, are present in the human endometrium.[163] Because PR-B but not PR-A levels in the endometrium are tightly regulated during the human menstrual cycle, PR-B is presumed to play a more important biologic role.[163] The cellular content of PRs typically depends on previous estrogen action.

The progesterone-PR complex also promotes gene transcription, but the response to progesterone is strikingly different from that evoked by the estradiol-ER complex. Similar to ERα, PR binding sites are also widely distributed across the genome, lie frequently outside of basal promoters, and do not involve classically defined progesterone response elements.[164] Interaction of PR binding sites with basal promoters possibly requires DNA coiling.[164]

Progesterone actions include a decrease in the expression of ERs.[165] This is one means by which progesterone (and synthetic progestins) attenuates estrogen action. Progesterone also acts to increase the rate of enzymatic inactivation of estradiol to estrone through an increase in the activity of an oxidative-type 17β-HSD enzyme. Progesterone-dependent transcription of the *HSD17B2* gene is responsible for this enzyme activity.[166] Progesterone also acts to increase sulfation of estrogens (i.e., by estrogen sulfotransferase), another means of estrogen inactivation.[167] Progesterone acts as an antiestrogen in at least three ways: by reducing ER expression, by decreasing the tissue levels of estradiol through conversion to estrone, and by enhancing estrogen inactivation through sulfation. As in the case of estrogen action in the uterus, tissue recombination experiments using uteri of PR knockout and normal mice have demonstrated that many effects of progesterone on epithelial cells are also mediated in a paracrine fashion by PRs in stromal cells but not by those in epithelial cells (see Fig. 17-24).[157] Progesterone-dependent HSD17B2 enzyme induction and consequent estradiol inactivation are mediated primarily by stromal PRs in human endometrium.[168]

The most striking consequence of progesterone action is the differentiation of the endometrium. The histologic correlates of differentiation—stromal predecidualization and epithelial secretion—parallel increased levels of circulating progesterone during the luteal phase. The PR content of human endometrial tissue peaks during the late proliferative phase, just before ovulation, and declines sharply before circulating progesterone levels increase during the luteal phase.[163] This dyssynchrony between endometrial PR expression and circulating progesterone is not well understood. Molecular correlates of progesterone action with respect to differentiation include increased production of lactoferrin and glycodelin in epithelial cells and of prolactin and IGF-binding protein 1 in stromal cells of the endometrium.

The Receptive Phase of the Endometrium for Implantation

Unless the ovum is fertilized within 24 hours after ovulation, it does not survive. Fertilization takes place in the ampullary, the distal one third of the oviduct. Over the next 2 days, the fertilized ovum remains unattached within the tubal lumen; tubal fluids and residual attached cumulus granulosa cells sustain nutrition and energy for early cellular cleavage. After this stage, the embryo (which consists of a solid ball of cells called the morula) leaves the oviduct and enters the uterine cavity. By this time, endometrial secretions under the influence of luteal progesterone have filled the cavity and bathe the embryo in nutrients. This is the first of many neatly synchronized events that mark the conceptus-endometrial relationship. By 6 days after ovulation, the embryo (now a blastocyst) is ready to attach and implant. It finds an endometrial lining of sufficient depth, vascularity, and nutritional richness to sustain the important events of early placentation that are to follow. Just below the epithelial lining, a rich capillary plexus has been formed and is available for creation of the trophoblast-maternal blood interface. Later, the surrounding superficial portion of the functionalis zone, now occupying more and more of the endometrial cavity, provides a sturdy splint to retain endometrial architecture despite the invasive inroads of the burgeoning trophoblast.

Progesterone is essential for the maintenance of pregnancy. The blastocyst depends on progesterone produced by the corpus luteum at this time. The hCG secreted by the trophoblast prevents regression of the corpus luteum by acting as a surrogate LH. It maintains a continuous supply of progesterone to maintain the pregnancy until the placental tissue starts to produce sufficient quantities of progesterone (6 to 7 weeks after fertilization).

Studies in experimental and domestic animals have demonstrated that there must be synchronous development of the embryo and endometrium for normal implantation and development to occur. In laboratory animals, there is a discrete window for implantation, which in some species lasts only a matter of hours.

The receptive phase of the endometrium is the temporal window of endometrial maturation during which the trophectoderm of the blastocyst can attach to the endometrial epithelial cells and proceed to invade the endometrial stroma. In the study of human endometrial receptivity, a key question is the determination of the temporal window of implantation. Only factors expressed during this temporal window can be considered markers or functional mediators of the receptive state.

The window of uterine receptivity can be inferred from what has been learned from transfer of embryos to uteri of women primed with exogenous estrogen and progesterone preparations (Fig. 17-25). There is a distinct window for embryo transfer leading to implantation, which spans endometrial cycle days 16 to 20. Presumably, the actual window of implantation follows this window of transfer, because embryos need to develop further, from the four-cell to eight-cell stage to the blastocyst stage, before initiation of attachment and frank invasion can occur.

Based on serial measurements of serum hCG as a marker of initial embryonic-maternal interaction, the window of implantation in humans is estimated to be between days 20 and 24 of the cycle.[169] This relatively wide window agrees with the earlier morphologic data developed by Adams and colleagues.[170]

Mechanism of Menstruation

In the absence of pregnancy, failure of the appearance of hCG despite otherwise appropriate tissue reactions leads to the vasomotor changes associated with estrogen-progesterone withdrawal and menstrual desquamation. A program of endometrial remodeling is initiated; alterations in the extracellular matrix and infiltration of leukocytes lead to hypoxia-reperfusion injury and sloughing of the functionalis, followed by activation of hemostatic and regenerative processes. The main histologic features of the premenstrual phase are degradation of the stromal reticular network, stromal infiltration by polymorphonuclear and mononuclear leukocytes, and secretory exhaustion of the endometrial glands, whose epithelial cells now have basal nuclei. The endometrium shrinks preceding menstruation in part as a result of diminished secretory activity and the catabolism of extracellular matrix.

The most prominent and final effect of progesterone and estrogen withdrawal is menstruation. The classic studies of Markee suggested that an ischemic phase caused by vasoconstriction of the arterioles and coiled arteries precedes the onset of menstrual bleeding by 4 to 24 hours.[151] Bleeding occurs after the arterioles and arteries relax, leading to hypoxia-reperfusion injury. The superficial endometrial layers are distended by the formation of hematomas, and fissures develop, leading to the detachment of tissue fragments. Lysis and fragmentation of cells

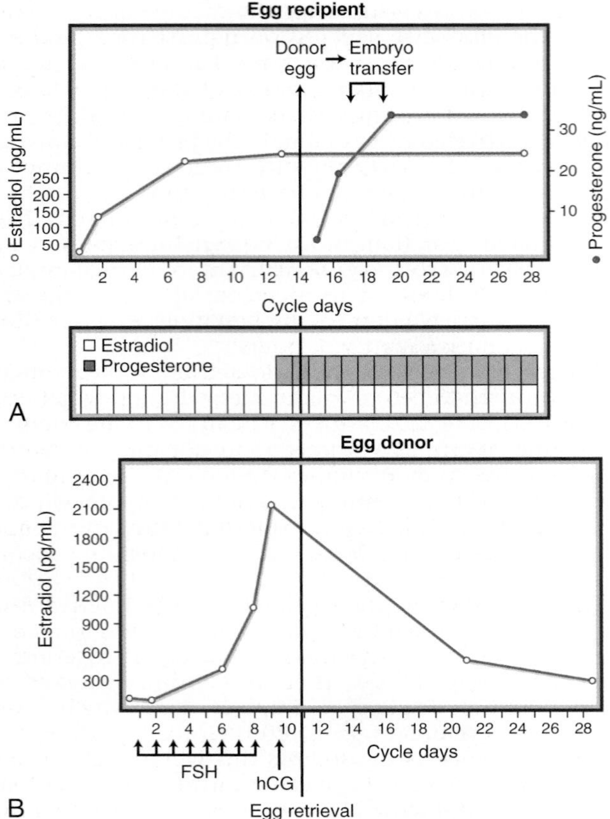

Figure 17-25 Donation of oocytes by a woman undergoing egg retrieval to a woman with ovarian insufficiency treated with exogenous estrogen and progesterone. The window of implantation in both women is synchronized by different but comparable hormonal treatments **A,** Woman with ovarian insufficiency is initially treated with oral micronized estradiol during days 1 through 14 of the cycle. Exogenous intramuscular progesterone is added to the estradiol treatment on days 15 through 28 and continued if pregnancy is diagnosed. Several donor eggs are fertilized with sperm from the recipient's husband, and one or two embryos are transferred to the uterus on day 16 to 19, depending on the stage of embryo development. These embryos are expected to implant between days 20 and 24. **B,** The egg donor is simultaneously treated with human recombinant follicle-stimulating hormone (FSH) with or without menopausal gonadotropin until cycle day 8 to 12, when human chorionic gonadotropin (hCG) is given to induce ovulation, and oocytes are harvested 32 to 36 hours later. One or two fertilized eggs are transferred to the uterus of the recipient. Progesterone supplement to the recipient is started before the embryo transfer. Serum levels of estradiol (E_2) or progesterone (P_4) in both women are shown. To convert estradiol values to picomoles per liter, multiply by 3.671. To convert progesterone values to nanomoles per liter, multiply by 3.180.

and apoptosis are evident. The menstrual efflux is composed of shed fragments of endometrium mixed with blood and liquefied by the fibrinolytic activity of the cellular debris (see Fig. 17-23). Clots of various sizes may be present if blood flow is excessive.

Control of Endometrial Function with the Use of Exogenous Hormones

The fertility potential of a woman is primarily determined by the biologic quality of her oocytes, reflected in part by the capacity of the fertilized ovum to divide at an optimal rate and contain a normal chromosomal complement. This biologic quality declines sharply after the age of 35 years. However, the biologic potential of the endometrium for successful implantation remains intact even at advanced ages.[171] Oocyte donation from a fertile woman and fertilization of the donor eggs in vitro with the recipient's male partner's sperm, followed by embryo transfer into the uterine cavity of the recipient woman with nonfunctioning ovaries (e.g., premature ovarian insufficiency), have been used successfully as a therapeutic strategy to treat infertility (see Fig. 17-25).[171,172] This clinical application has provided unique opportunities to examine the hormonal therapy for endometrial maturation. Several hormone replacement protocols have been proposed, and many pregnancies have resulted from donor oocytes in women with ovarian insufficiency (see Fig. 17-25). The success of these procedures (i.e., pregnancy rate) has averaged about 50% per embryo transfer.

The degree of endometrial differentiation in response to exogenous hormones has been evaluated by histologic analysis of endometrial biopsy specimens. The epithelial elements exhibit delayed maturation early during progesterone administration on days 20 to 22, but they catch up by day 26. Despite this apparent dyssynchrony, the pregnancy rate in these patients with donor oocytes is higher than in conventional IVF.[172]

The follicular phase is mimicked by administration of oral micronized estradiol in daily doses of up to 8 mg for about 10 days. Serum estradiol in these subjects during the replacement follicular phase reaches sufficiently high levels to stimulate endometrial growth. This is followed by up to 8 mg/day of oral estradiol combined with daily intramuscular progesterone (50 mg) to promote the secretory transformation. Intramuscular injection of 50 mg/day of progesterone in oil generates serum levels of progesterone usually greater than 20 ng/mL. The length of exposure to progesterone, but not the absolute plasma progesterone concentration achieved after adequate priming of the endometrium with estrogen, is a key factor for the development of uterine receptivity. The exogenous administration of only estradiol and progesterone is sufficient to prepare the endometrium for implantation in the absence of ovarian function. This observation further underscores the essential roles of these steroids in uterine physiology.

APPROACH TO THE WOMAN WITH REPRODUCTIVE DYSFUNCTION

Reproductive dysfunction in an adult woman is most often manifested by disruption of cyclic, predictable menses. Efficient diagnosis of the underlying disorder requires a thorough understanding of female reproductive physiology and pathology and an accurate history and physical examination. Without a critical analysis of clinical findings based on thorough knowledge of normal and abnormal reproductive function, the application of predetermined algorithms of laboratory testing causes unnecessary use of hormone measurements or imaging studies and delays diagnosis.

History

An essential tool for the evaluation of a woman with a reproductive disorder is a carefully recorded history. The history should be obtained from the patient with the aim of assessing the biologic effects of each of the various hormones. Recording the details of pubertal development as a reference for the onset of particular symptoms provides critical clues to the cause of certain reproductive disorders. For example, anovulation manifested by irregular uterine bleeding associated with the polycystic ovary syndrome (PCOS) most often begins during the pubertal years. The onset of gradually progressing hirsutism at about the time of puberty suggests nonclassic adrenal hyperplasia or PCOS. In these cases, measurement of serum 17-hydroxyprogesterone may help to differentiate nonclassic adrenal hyperplasia from PCOS. The appearance of hirsutism before puberty or several years after normal pubertal development should alert the clinician to the possibility of ovarian or adrenal neoplasms. Sudden onset of hirsutism at any age or the presence of virilization should prompt the physician to rule out steroid-secreting ovarian or adrenal tumors. Most women with symptomatic endometriosis suffer from severe episodes of painful menses (i.e., dysmenorrhea) that start during pubertal years.

Evaluation of female reproductive function depends on a detailed history of the menses. For example, PCOS is unlikely without a long-standing history of irregular periods since the menarche. A history of a period of cyclic, predictable menses before the onset of menstrual irregularities should draw attention to hypothalamic or other causes of anovulation. The current frequency, regularity, length, and quantity of uterine bleeding should be carefully recorded for several reasons. First, this information reflects tightly regulated interactions of several tissues, including the hypothalamus, pituitary, ovaries, and endometrium. Second, regular, predictable menses imply ovulation. Third, defining the type of menstrual irregularity may help with diagnosis of the underlying cause. For example, prolonged amenorrhea in a thin and estrogen-deficient woman suggests anovulation of hypothalamic origin. Infrequent periods of varying duration and with a varying amount of blood loss in a well-estrogenized, overweight woman suggest a primary ovarian dysfunction such as PCOS. Anovulation in a thin but well-estrogenized woman may also be caused by PCOS. Regular but heavy and prolonged menses with intermittent spotting may result from uterine anatomic disorders such as adenomyosis or leiomyomas. Fourth, neoplastic disorders of the endometrium, including endometrial polyps, hyperplasia, or malignancies, may be manifested by any pattern of irregular bleeding. The combination of vaginal ultrasonography and endometrial biopsy is extremely sensitive for the diagnosis of endometrial neoplasia.[173]

Disruption of cyclic and predictable menses is a common and alarming symptom that initially brings the patient to the clinician. After a careful evaluation of the menstrual symptoms, the clinician should identify other obvious symptoms of the endocrine disorder underlying the irregular periods. Pregnancy is the most common cause of amenorrhea (and other menstrual irregularities) in a woman of reproductive age. In a woman presenting with amenorrhea or any other menstrual irregularity, normal pregnancy, ectopic pregnancy, or gestational trophoblastic disease must be excluded at the onset. Careful evaluation of past reproductive history and the patient's sexual activity and contraceptive practices can provide useful indications of the likelihood of pregnancy. The reproductive history may suggest the possibility of Sheehan's syndrome of postpartum pituitary necrosis if menses did not resume after a delivery complicated by significant hemorrhage.[174] In such instances, evidence of adrenal and thyroid insufficiency should be sought. A classic symptom of Sheehan's syndrome is the absence of postpartum lactation, which is related to prolactin deficiency.

Amenorrhea is traditionally categorized as primary (no history of menstruation) or secondary (cessation of menses after a variable time). The diverse causes of primary amenorrhea are discussed extensively in Chapters 23 and 25. Although the distinction between primary and secondary amenorrhea may be useful for identifying the mechanism of disease and the differential diagnosis, the clinician should be aware that a disorder can initially manifest with either primary or secondary amenorrhea. For example, most women with gonadal dysgenesis have primary amenorrhea, but some patients have residual follicles and ovulate, and in these women with partial gonadal dysgenesis, some menstruation and rare pregnancies may occur before the cessation of ovarian function.[175,176] Patients with PCOS usually have secondary amenorrhea but occasionally have primary amenorrhea. Rarely, pregnancy may manifest as primary amenorrhea.

After pregnancy is ruled out, secondary amenorrhea is most often caused by chronic anovulation, which can be broadly categorized as hypothalamic dysfunction, galactorrhea-associated anovulation, ovarian insufficiency, androgen excess, or chronic illness or primary uterine disease (e.g., intrauterine adhesion formation after a postpartum curettage). Establishing any association of secondary amenorrhea with life events is extremely useful. Strenuous exercise is often associated with amenorrhea. Weight loss often precedes or accompanies secondary amenorrhea and has been suggested as evidence of hypothalamic dysfunction. An unusual dietary history may suggest bulimia or anorexia nervosa. A history of dilatation and curettage, postpartum endometritis, or disseminated tuberculosis with absent to scant menses suggests the possibility of intrauterine adhesion.[177] The presence of any signs or symptoms of estrogen deficiency, including painful intercourse, atrophic vagina, emotional lability, and vasomotor instability, suggests anovulation of a central nature with low concentrations of circulating gonadotropins (i.e., hypogonadotropic hypogonadism) or ovarian insufficiency with elevated gonadotropins (i.e., hypergonadotropic hypogonadism).

Galactorrhea in the absence of a recent history of pregnancy suggests a host of diagnostic possibilities and is frequently a manifestation of excessive prolactin secretion, although it may result from increased sensitivity of breast tissue to the hormones necessary for milk production. This history frequently reveals drug ingestion as the cause. Various drugs, including several psychotropic agents, antihypertensive agents, and oral contraceptives, have been implicated. Primary hypothyroidism may be associated with precocious puberty with galactorrhea in the child and with amenorrhea or galactorrhea, or both, in the adult woman. A history of excessive nipple manipulation or chest wall disease should be elicited because it may be the cause of galactorrhea. Prolactinomas, the prolactin-secreting adenomas of the pituitary, are a common cause of galactorrhea related to abnormally high serum levels of prolactin.

Physical Examination

The quantity and distribution of excessive hair growth should be considered in light of the familial history. Hypertrichosis—excessive growth of hair on the extremities, the head, and the back—must be distinguished from true hirsutism, which is the development of facial hair, chest hair, and a male escutcheon with or without signs of virilization in response to increased production of or sensitivity to biologically active androgens. Some degree of hypertrichosis is not uncommon in women of Mediterranean descent, whereas the occurrence of any facial hirsutism in the relatively hairless Asian woman may require thorough investigation. Hirsutism is best documented and quantified with the help of photographs. Virilization is characterized as thickening of the voice, severe cystic acne, hair loss, increased muscle mass, and clitoromegaly and implies a more severe degree of androgen excess than that found with hirsutism. The syndrome of complete androgen insensitivity is characterized by sparse to absent pubic and axillary hair due to resistance to androgen.

A careful inspection of the breasts is essential for a thorough physical examination. Classification of the stage of breast development according to the method of Marshall and Tanner[178] is a convenient and valuable adjunct. The physician should assess whether the breasts appear to have decreased in size recently (e.g., severe androgen excess), whether the areolae are well formed and pigmented (as they are in pregnancy), and whether a discharge (e.g., galactorrhea) can be expressed.

A woman with PCOS who has never ovulated or taken a progestin-containing medication may have Tanner stage 4 breast development related to adequate estrogen production, whereas the progression to Tanner stage 5 requires exposure to progesterone through ovulation or ingestion of a progestin (e.g., administration of oral contraceptives). Chapter 25 discusses Tanner staging of breast development.

The vulva, vagina, and cervix also represent sensitive indicators of gonadal steroid action. Because sensitivity of the genital skin and mucosa to androgen decreases with time from the early stages of fetal development to adulthood, the extent of any virilization can be helpful in suggesting the timing of androgen exposure. The most profound androgenic effects, such as posterior labial fusion with or without formation of a penile urethra, usually are observed in 46,XX fetuses exposed to androgens during the first 10 weeks of pregnancy. Similar findings have been described in patients with virilizing congenital adrenal hyperplasia, true hermaphroditism, and drug-induced virilization. Significant postnatal clitoromegaly, on the other hand, requires marked hormonal stimulation and, in the absence of significant exogenous steroids, strongly implicates an androgen-secreting tumor. The size of the glans clitoris can be quantitated by determining the clitoral index, which is the product of the sagittal and transverse diameters of the glans. Ninety-five percent of normal women have a clitoral index less than 35 mm^2.

The vagina and uterine cervix are the most sensitive indicators of estrogen action. Under the influence of estrogen, the vaginal mucosa progresses during sexual maturation from a tissue with a shiny, bright red appearance with sparse, thin secretions to a tissue with a dull, gray-pink, rugated surface with copious, thick secretions. Well-estrogenized vaginal mucosa with stretchable cervical mucus (i.e., *spinnbarkeit*) may indicate the proliferative phase of the menstrual cycle in an ovulatory woman or extraovarian estrogen formation in an anovulatory woman with PCOS. The biologic activity of estrogen can also be quantified by vaginal cytology.

To summarize, irregular uterine bleeding is a common symptom that brings the woman with reproductive dysfunction to the physician's office. Various disorders of the hypothalamus, pituitary, ovaries, or uterus or other issues that affect reproductive function may be responsible for this alarming symptom. After pregnancy is ruled out, a detailed history and results of the physical examination should be carefully recorded. In particular, the physician should pay attention to the salient features in the history and the biologic indicators of hormone action at target tissues during the physical examination. An analysis of these findings most often leads to a tentative diagnosis, which should be confirmed by laboratory testing.

DISORDERS OF THE FEMALE REPRODUCTIVE SYSTEM

Chronic Anovulation

Chronic anovulation is one of the most common gynecologic problems encountered by the practitioner. Patients may present with secondary amenorrhea, infrequent uterine bleeding (i.e., oligomenorrhea), or irregular episodes of excessive uterine bleeding. Infertility is an obvious consequence of chronic anovulation. Pregnancy or any cause related to end-organ insufficiency (e.g., intrauterine adhesions, müllerian agenesis), amenorrhea associated with genital ambiguity at birth (e.g., male or female pseudohermaphroditism, true hermaphroditism), or sexual infantilism due to gonadal dysgenesis should initially be ruled out.

For practical purposes, most of the etiologic factors giving rise to chronic anovulation in a woman of reproductive age fall into five broad categories: hypothalamic anovulation, hyperprolactinemia, androgen excess, premature ovarian insufficiency, and chronic illness (e.g., hepatic or renal insufficiency, acquired immunodeficiency syndrome [AIDS]). Salient features of the history and physical examination help to place a woman with anovulation in one or more of these categories.

One group of anovulatory patients is estrogen deficient. Common disorders in this group include hypothalamic anovulation, galactorrhea-hyperprolactinemia (e.g., hypothyroidism, prolactinoma, nonfunctioning pituitary tumor), and premature ovarian insufficiency in a woman of reproductive age. These patients are usually amenorrheic. All patients present with signs of estrogen deficiency (e.g., vaginal atrophy). Patients with hypothalamic anovulation or galactorrhea-hyperprolactinemia usually do not complain of hot flashes, whereas women with premature ovarian insufficiency present with vasomotor symptoms. One serious consequence of estrogen deficiency is bone loss giving rise to osteopenia and osteoporosis. If possible, the underlying cause should be corrected. Hormone therapy should be provided if ovulation cannot be restored.

Women with androgen excess constitute the second major group of anovulatory patients. A serious consequence of anovulation in this group is the greater risk for carcinoma of the endometrium because of unopposed action of estrogen formed continuously in extraovarian tissues. The most common disorder of the ovary associated with androgen excess and anovulation is PCOS. Insulin resistance plays a significant role in this condition and, along with hyperandrogenism, increases the risk of developing cardiovascular disease (CVD) or diabetes mellitus or both.[142] The clinician must recognize the long-term impact of PCOS and undertake therapeutic management of these anovulatory patients to avoid unwanted consequences. The clinician should also develop a plan with the patient to address long-term complications of unopposed estrogen formation associated with PCOS (e.g., endometrial neoplasia). Oral contraceptives or periodic progestin supplementation may be provided to prevent endometrial hyperplasia and cancer.

Many mechanisms may be responsible for anovulation in chronic illness. Effective treatment of the primary illness may restore normal menses. Alternatively, anovulatory bleeding may be managed with the use of exogenous hormones in these chronically ill patients (discussed later).

Measurements of FSH and prolactin help to categorize anovulatory patients. An undetectable or low-normal FSH level is consistent with hypothalamic amenorrhea, PCOS, or hyperprolactinemia, whereas high FSH levels suggest ovarian insufficiency. High prolactin levels may indicate a pituitary prolactinoma or hypothyroidism. The following sections describe specific disorders that cause chronic anovulation in women of reproductive age.

Hypothalamic Anovulation

Anovulation of hypothalamic origin usually manifests as amenorrhea. The terms *hypothalamic anovulation* and *hypothalamic amenorrhea* are used interchangeably in this chapter. A reduction in GnRH pulse frequency from the characteristic 60 to 120 minutes to intervals longer than 180 minutes leads to lower levels of LH and FSH secretion by the pituitary gland.[13,15] This functional gonadotropin deficiency fails to provide adequate stimulation to the ovarian follicles, and the normal sequence of follicular growth, maturation, follicular selection, and ovulation becomes attenuated. Downstream ovarian estradiol production remains low, and endometrial growth is reduced or arrested, resulting in a prolonged interval of amenorrhea. The transition from normal menstrual cyclicity to anovulation and amenorrhea can take place gradually and may be characterized by inadequate luteal phases, irregular menstrual bleeding, and amenorrhea. Patients with hypothalamic amenorrhea do not complain of hot flashes, even though circulating levels of estradiol are within the menopausal range. This suggests a significant role for GnRH or gonadotropins in the cause of hot flashes.

Any disorder of the central nervous system that interferes with normal GnRH pulse frequency can cause anovulation. Some of these disorders may be defined genetic or anatomic evidence such as isolated gonadotropin deficiency (with or without anosmia), infection, suprasellar tumors (e.g., pituitary adenomas, craniopharyngioma), and head trauma.[10] These genetic and anatomic disorders affect the function of the hypothalamus, and some of them may be ruled out by the medical history, physical examination, and imaging of the head (Table 17-2).

The most commonly observed form of hypothalamic anovulation is not associated with a demonstrable neuroanatomic finding.[180] This common form is called *functional hypothalamic amenorrhea* because it is presumed to involve aberrant but reversible regulation of otherwise normal neuroendocrine pathways. Changes in lifestyle may result in the return of normal ovulatory cycles. Functional hypothalamic amenorrhea may be associated with excessive exercise, abrupt weight loss, and emotional distress. It is hypothesized that these stress factors cause anovulation by affecting brain function and the GnRH pulse generator. Other causes of hypothalamic anovulation demonstrable by neuroanatomic or genetic evidence are uncommon (see Table 17-2).

Functional Hypothalamic Amenorrhea

Anovulation resulting from stress-associated changes is viewed as a functional disorder in which no anatomic or organic abnormalities of the hypothalamic-pituitary-ovarian axis can be identified. This condition typically manifests as amenorrhea of 6 months' duration and has also been called *functional hypothalamic amenorrhea*. The overall prevalence of functional hypothalamic amenorrhea among all amenorrhea disorders ranges from 15% to 48%.[180]

TABLE 17-2

Classification of Anovulation Caused by Disorders of the Hypothalamic-Pituitary Unit

Functional Hypothalamic Anovulation (Amenorrhea)
Stress (psychogenic or physical)
Dieting
Vigorous exercise
Chronic illness (e.g., chronic liver or renal insufficiency, AIDS)
Psychiatric-Medical Emergencies
Anorexia nervosa
Medications
Antipsychotics (e.g., olanzapine, risperidone, amisulpride, clozapine)[179]
Opiates
Hypothyroidism
Anatomically or Genetically Defined Pathologies of the Hypothalamic-Pituitary Unit
Pituitary tumors
Prolactinoma
Clinically nonfunctioning adenoma
GH-secreting adenoma (acromegaly)
ACTH-secreting adenoma (Cushing's disease)
Other pituitary tumors (e.g., metastasis, meningioma)
Pituitary stalk section
Hemorrhagic pituitary destruction, including pituitary apoplexy and Sheehan's syndrome
Pituitary aneurysm
Infiltrative disease of the pituitary (e.g., lymphocytic hypophysitis, sarcoidosis, histiocytosis X, tuberculosis)
Empty sella syndrome
Tumors that affect hypothalamic function (e.g., metastasis, craniopharyngioma)
Infiltrative granulomatous disease of the hypothalamus (e.g., sarcoidosis, histiocytosis X, tuberculosis)
Head trauma
Irradiation to the head
CNS infection
Isolated gonadotropin deficiency (including Kallmann's syndrome)
Other

ACTH, adrenocorticotropic hormone; AIDS, acquired immunodeficiency syndrome; CNS, central nervous system; GH, growth hormone.

Anovulation of hypothalamic origin is characterized by estrogen deficiency and low levels of gonadotropins. No genetic or anatomic disorders are identified in most patients. The concept of functional hypothalamic anovulation (i.e., amenorrhea) was first postulated in the 1940s as the failure of the hypothalamic-pituitary pathways to release LH from the anterior pituitary.[181] Since then, many clinical studies have confirmed this idea.[14] Accumulated data suggest that the common underlying defect is an alteration in the pulsatile secretion of GnRH. In patients with this disorder, diverse etiologic factors such as malnutrition or caloric restriction, depression, psychogenic stress, excessive energy expenditure related to exercise, or combinations of these disorders precede the onset of functional hypothalamic anovulation. Heightened awareness of diet or exercise and unrealistic expectations with respect to body image have most likely contributed to the epidemic of this anovulatory disorder.

Diagnosis of Functional Hypothalamic Amenorrhea

Patients with functional hypothalamic amenorrhea most commonly present with secondary amenorrhea characterized by absence of menstrual cycles for longer than 6 months without evidence of an organic disorder. The diagnosis of hypothalamic amenorrhea is one of exclusion. There are many neuroanatomic or genetic disorders that can mimic functional hypothalamic anovulation (see Table 17-2), and a careful and complete evaluation is essential to make this diagnosis.

Women with functional hypothalamic amenorrhea usually present with a history of regular menses for some time after menarche. This period of normal ovulatory function (determined by history) is interrupted by anovulation that usually manifests as secondary amenorrhea. Women with functional hypothalamic anovulation may occasionally present with primary amenorrhea.

Women with functional hypothalamic amenorrhea typically have a normal body weight or are thin. They are driven and involved in high-stress occupations. The occupation of the patient (e.g., ballerina, competitive athlete) may be an important clue. A detailed interview may reveal a variety of emotional crises or stressful events (e.g., divorce, death of a friend) preceding the onset of amenorrhea. During the interview, additional environmental and interpersonal factors may become evident, such as academic pressure, social maladjustment, or psychosexual problems. When evaluating the patient, the physician should take note of the current diet regimen, the use of any sedatives or hypnotics, and the nature and extent of the patient's exercise habits. Despite a careful interview, a history of stress, excessive physical exercise, or an eating disorder may not be readily revealed by some women with functional hypothalamic anovulation. These women usually do not complain of hot flashes, in contrast to women with ovarian insufficiency.

The physician should exclude a possible hyperprolactinemic cause (e.g., prolactinoma, hypothyroidism) and evidence of androgen excess (e.g., PCOS) during the physical examination. These women usually have normal secondary sexual characteristics. The pelvic examination usually shows a thinning vaginal mucosa accompanied by scant to absent cervical mucus with a normal to small uterus, which are all evidence of estrogen deficiency. Signs of a well-estrogenized vagina and cervix observed during the physical examination make the diagnosis of hypothalamic amenorrhea unlikely.

Laboratory tests are obtained to exclude other causes of anovulation and secondary amenorrhea. LH and FSH levels should be measured. Gonadotropin levels are usually lower than the normal values ordinarily found in the early follicular phase. TSH and prolactin levels are obtained to rule out hypothyroidism and hyperprolactinemia. The progestin challenge test (medroxyprogesterone acetate [MPA] at 5 mg/day for 10 days) elicits either a small spotting episode or an absence of withdrawal uterine bleeding in most patients. The administration of combined estrogen (2 mg/day of oral micronized estradiol) with progestin (5 mg/day of MPA for 10 days) will result in endometrial growth followed by vaginal bleeding because the uterine compartment remains functionally normal.

These results confirm that there is a scant or absent estrogenic effect on the endometrium, because circulating estradiol levels are typically in the low or early follicular phase range. Measurement of the serum estradiol level is not necessary. Because a suprasellar or large pituitary tumor is in the differential diagnosis, magnetic resonance imaging (MRI) of the head is necessary to rule out these possibilities. Imaging of the head is especially important if amenorrhea develops suddenly or is associated with a neurologic sign, both of which make the presence of a tumor more likely.

Pathophysiology of Functional Hypothalamic Anovulation

A critical defect in hypothalamic amenorrhea is the reduction in GnRH release from the medial basal hypothalamus, which leads to a reduction in GnRH pulse frequency. In humans, it is challenging and sometimes impossible to directly examine GnRH pulse frequency. LH pulse frequency is used as a surrogate measure to evaluate GnRH secretion because each GnRH pulse is accompanied by a concomitant LH pulse. It is possible to determine the temporal secretion of LH using frequent sampling of the peripheral blood at 10- to 15-minute intervals. Most clinical studies that focus on defining the GnRH pulse frequency use rapid, frequent blood sampling to measure the LH pulse frequency.[180]

A key observation in functional hypothalamic anovulation is the absence of increased gonadotropin secretion despite the lack of inhibitory factors of ovarian origin, such as estradiol and inhibin. The secretory pattern of LH is abnormal. A mechanistic factor in women with this type of anovulation is a slowdown in the frequency of pulsatile GnRH secretion.[14,182,183]

There is considerable variability in the amplitude and frequency of the pulsatile LH secretion in women with functional hypothalamic amenorrhea. When the LH secretory patterns are compared with that of the follicular phase of the menstrual cycle, a characteristic abnormality in LH pulse frequency and amplitude is seen, and occasionally, regression to a pronounced variability similar to what is seen in the prepubertal pattern is observed.[14,182,183] In severe cases, the frequency and amplitude of LH pulses are markedly reduced. These LH patterns also suggest that GnRH pulsatile secretion is not altered to the same degree in every patient. During the recovery phase of hypothalamic amenorrhea, reversal to a pattern of LH secretion seen early in puberty often occurs, and it is characterized by a sleep-associated increase in LH amplitude.[180]

The response of the pituitary gland to GnRH with respect to production and release of gonadotropins is not impaired in functional hypothalamic anovulation. Intravenous pulsatile GnRH administration can restore normal levels of LH and FSH.[184,185]

Norepinephrine, dopamine, and serotonin produced in the brain have been shown to modulate GnRH or LH release in animal studies. Patients receiving medication that alters these neurotransmitters (e.g., sedatives, antidepressants, stimulants, antipsychotics) have presented with abnormalities in their menstrual cycles. These responses to medications provide circumstantial evidence that disruptions of neural pathways can alter GnRH release in humans. From these observations, it appears that activation of the noradrenergic neurons principally stimulates release of GnRH, whereas dopaminergic and serotoninergic neurons can stimulate or inhibit GnRH-LH secretion.[186]

Another group of substances that have inhibitory influences on GnRH secretion are endogenous opioid peptides.[187,188] Blockade of endogenous opiate receptors by the administration of naloxone, an opiate antagonist, to women with this disorder causes an increase in the frequency and amplitude of pulsatile LH release.[189] Gonadotropin secretion resumes if the activity of the opiate receptor is blocked by long-term naloxone use in these anovulatory patients, and ovulatory function may be regained in some cases.[190] These studies suggest that there is an overall increase in endogenous opiate activity, which can reduce pulsatile GnRH secretion in functional hypothalamic amenorrhea.

The hypothalamic-pituitary-adrenal axis is hyperactive in many women with functional hypothalamic amenorrhea, with increased secretion of corticotropin-releasing hormone (CRH), adrenocorticotropic hormone (ACTH), and cortisol. Studies have demonstrated an increase in pulsatile ACTH secretion, increased adrenal sensitivity to ACTH, and increased cortisol secretion with a normal diurnal rhythm.[180] Reproductive function may be disrupted by chronic exposure to stress.[181] Activation of the pituitary-adrenocortical system is a common response in patients with chronic stress.[191] In functional hypothalamic amenorrhea, stressors such as exercise or emotional distress can chronically activate the hypothalamic-pituitary-adrenal axis.

The association between emotional or physical stress and disruption of the reproductive function of the hypothalamus is complex and involves several mechanisms. Daytime cortisol levels are markedly elevated, and the pituitary response to CRH is blunted.[185,192] In an animal model, CRH seems to be an important factor in the inhibition of GnRH pulsatility.[193,194] This inhibitory effect can be prevented by coadministration of a CRH antagonist or reversed by the opiate antagonist naloxone, suggesting that cross-talk occurs between the action of CRH and activation of the opioidergic system. Moreover, ACTH administration blocks the pituitary response to GnRH at the pituitary level.[195,196] Another stress hormone, oxytocin, can inhibit hypothalamic GnRH secretion.[188] In summary, overproduction of CRH and other stress-related hormones in the brain and activation of the pituitary-adrenocortical system by chronic stress seem to play causative roles in the inhibition of gonadotropin secretion in functional hypothalamic anovulation.

Leptin administration to correct the relative leptin deficiency in women with hypothalamic amenorrhea improves reproductive, thyroid, and growth hormone axes and markers of bone formation. This suggests that leptin, a peripheral signal reflecting the adequacy of energy stores, is required for normal reproductive and neuroendocrine function.[197]

The roles of energy balance–regulating peptides such as leptin and ghrelin were investigated in the mechanism of hypothalamic amenorrhea.[180] Leptin is a cytokine produced by the adipocytes and is considered to be an appetite-supressor peptide. Leptin is secreted in a pulsatile manner with a diurnal rhythm. A decrease in total circulating leptin with loss of the normal diurnal rhythm was reported in women with hypothalamic amenorrhea.[197] This relative hypoleptinemia is a common characteristic of several energy-deficient conditions and is associated with slowing of the LH pulse frequency.[197] Leptin administration to correct the relative leptin deficiency in women with hypothalamic amenorrhea was shown to improve reproductive, thyroid, and growth hormone axes and markers of bone formation, suggesting that leptin, a peripheral signal reflecting the adequacy of energy stores, is required for normal reproductive and neuroendocrine function.[197] In contrast to leptin, ghrelin is an appetite-inducing peptide secreted from the stomach. During the fasting state, ghrelin serves as the hunger signal from the periphery to the hypothalamic arcuate nucleus, a region that is known to control food intake. Ghrelin levels are reported to be elevated in women with hypothalamic amenorrhea.[198]

Hypothalamic Anovulation and Exercise

Regular vigorous exercise can lead to menstrual disturbances, a delay in menarche, luteal phase dysfunction, and secondary amenorrhea. Thirty percent of adolescent ballet dancers have problems with the progression of puberty. The mean age at menarche is delayed until the age of 15 years. Advancement of pubertal stages seems to coincide with times of prolonged rest or after recovery from an injury.[199-204] The intensity, length, and type of the sport determine the severity of the disease. Activities associated with an increased frequency of reproductive dysfunction are those that favor a lower body weight and include middle-distance and long-distance running, competitive swimming, gymnastics, and ballet dancing.

Competitive athletes show endocrine abnormalities in the central nervous system consistent with those in other forms of functional hypothalamic anovulation. Abnormalities include elevations of central CRH and β-endorphin levels.

The management of exercise-related anovulation depends on the patient's choices and expectations. Side effects such as osteoporosis and delay of puberty must be discussed thoroughly with the patient.[205] Decrease in exercise level and behavioral modification may be sufficient for the return of ovulatory function. Hormone therapy should be provided if sufficient results are not achieved. A low-dose oral contraceptive is a suitable option for women younger than 35 years of age.

Hypothalamic Anovulation Associated with Eating Disorders

Two common eating disorders associated with hypothalamic dysfunction are anorexia nervosa and bulimia. Patients with anorexia nervosa have extreme weight loss (>25% of original body weight) and a distorted body image accompanied by a striking fear of obesity. Bulimia is a related disorder characterized by alternating episodes of binge eating followed by periods of food restriction, self-induced vomiting, or excessive use of laxatives or diuretics. About 90% to 95% of these patients are women. The incidence of classic anorexia nervosa is about 1 case per 100,000 people in the general population.[206] Among female high school and college students, bulimia is fairly common. The incidence of anorexia nervosa peaks twice during the teen years, at ages 13 and 17. Bulimia usually begins at a later age, between 17 and 25 years. Anorexia nervosa has an extremely high mortality rate of 9% and is a true medical emergency. Death may result from cardiac arrhythmia, which may be precipitated by diminished heart muscle mass and associated electrolyte abnormalities.[207] These patients are also at increased risk for suicide.[208]

Gonadotropin secretion in anorexic women exhibits a prepubertal pattern that is similar to that observed in other forms of hypothalamic anovulation. Transitional patterns of LH secretion are seen with moderate degrees of weight recovery, and there is a normal or supranormal response to GnRH. Anovulation can persist in up to 50% of anorexic patients, even after normal weight is achieved. Anorexic and bulimic patients exhibit hyperactivation of the hypothalamus-pituitary system. Although the diurnal variation is maintained, persistent hypersecretion of cortisol occurs throughout the day.[209] Cushingoid features are not present, in part because of mild hypercortisolemia and a reduction of peripheral glucocorticoid receptors. Levels of CRH and β-endorphin are increased in the central nervous system.[210,211]

In anorexia nervosa, basal metabolism is decreased because peripheral conversion of thyroxine (T_4) to biologically potent triiodothyronine (T_3) is decreased. Instead, T_4 is converted to reverse T_3, an inactive isoform. This alteration is also observed in severely ill patients and during starvation.[212] Anorexics have partial diabetes insipidus and are unable to concentrate urine appropriately because of the impaired secretion of vasopressin.[213]

Anorexia nervosa and bulimia are extremely difficult to treat. The most accepted approaches include individual psychotherapy, group therapy, and behavior modification. Patients with eating disorders should have psychiatric consultation and follow-up. This helps with the diagnosis and treatment. For patients who weigh less than 75% of their ideal body weight, immediate hospitalization and aggressive treatment are recommended. Complications of anorexia nervosa include osteoporosis, estrogen deficiency, and generalized effects of malnutrition.[202] Hormone therapy in the form of a low-dose oral contraceptive should be provided until ovulatory function is achieved.

Treatment and Management of Functional Hypothalamic Anovulation

Treatment of chronic anovulation resulting from central nervous system–hypothalamic disorders should be directed at reversal of the primary cause (e.g., stress management, reduction of exercise, correction of weight loss). The importance of successful treatment of this disease state is underscored because these women are prone to the development of osteoporosis. For a considerable number of patients, spontaneous recovery of menstrual function takes place after a modification of lifestyle, psychological guidance, or accommodation to environmental stress. The initial treatment should be directed to a change in lifestyle and tailored to the individual patient. For individuals who remain amenorrheic, periodic assessment of reproductive status (every 4 to 6 months) is prudent.

Modification of the stress response through cognitive-behavioral therapy is a logical approach to lowering the endogenous stress levels in women with hypothalamic amenorrhea. This approach was explored in 16 subjects with hypothalamic amenorrhea randomized to cognitive-behavioral therapy or observation for a 20-week period.[214] The therapy design focused on attitudes and habits concerning eating, exercise, body image, problem-solving skills, and stress reduction. The results were encouraging. About 88% of those who underwent cognitive-behavioral therapy had evidence of ovulation, compared with only 25% of those who were observed.[214] These results suggest that endogenous stress is a major factor in the development and maintenance of hypothalamic amenorrhea and that modification of this stress response can restore normal menses.

If anovulation persists for longer than 6 months or if reversal of the primary cause is not practical (e.g., professional athletes, ballerinas), a major concern is the long-term effect of hypoestrogenism, especially on bone metabolism. In addition to estrogen deficiency, IGF1 deficiency, hypercortisolism, and nutritional factors may contribute to bone loss in this disorder.[215] However, epidemiologic data on the risk of fractures and the benefits of hormone therapy are scant.[205,215] On the basis of studies of reproductive-age women who were ovariectomized or underwent treatment with GnRH agonist for endometriosis, bone density is expected to decrease significantly, even within the first 6 months of amenorrhea. Because these patients are often reluctant to take medications, serial bone density studies of the lumbar spine and femur may be necessary to convince them of the necessity to begin estrogen replacement therapy. If the patient is not at risk for thromboembolism and does not smoke cigarettes, a low-dose combination oral contraceptive is a reasonable replacement option. Alternatively, a combination of conjugated estrogens (0.625 mg) and MPA (2.5 mg) daily may be administered to provide estrogenic support. The progestin (MPA) is added solely to prevent endometrial hyperplasia.

If the patient desires ovulation to achieve pregnancy, the most physiologic approach is ovulation induction with pulsatile GnRH. This is the best physiologic means of induction because the cause of the anovulatory state is decreased endogenous GnRH secretion. Pulsatile intravenous GnRH (5 µg every 90 minutes) was shown to be effective.[216] Monitoring of serum estradiol levels or follicular development can be minimized because the ovarian follicular response and gonadotropin output mimic the natural menstrual cycle. In these patients, continuation of pulsatile GnRH or hCG (1500 units administered intramuscularly every 3 days for a total of four doses) can support the function of the corpus luteum. Intravenous GnRH treatment results in ovulation rates of approximately 90%, pregnancy rates of up to 30%, and hyperstimulation rates of less than 1% per treatment cycle. Because the intravenous GnRH pump is not a practical choice for many women, an alternative strategy is the use of subcutaneous recombinant FSH for the development of one to three follicles and the induction of ovulation with intramuscular hCG followed by luteal support using intramuscular hCG or progesterone in oil.

The long-term prognosis for women with hypothalamic anovulation is encouraging. A group of investigators followed 93 women affected by functional hypothalamic amenorrhea for an average of 8.1 years.[217] At the end of the follow-up, 70.7% patients had recovered. Factors that predicted recovery included lowered mean cortisol levels, higher androstenedione levels, and an increase in body mass index. In recovered women, the body mass index increased or remained stable, whereas in nonrecovered women, it decreased or remained stable. At the end of the follow-up, 74.3% of patients treated with hormone therapy therapy and 80% of those with no therapy recovered, but only 41.7% of those taking oral contraceptive pills recovered.[217]

Chronic Anovulation Associated with Pituitary Disorders

The most common pituitary-related causes of anovulation are associated with hyperprolactinemia caused by prolactinomas or other functional or anatomic disorders of the pituitary. These disorders are frequently associated with dysregulation of gonadotropin secretion. Hyperprolactinemia and other pituitary disorders and their relation to reproduction are discussed in Chapter 9.

Chronic Anovulation Associated with Androgen Excess

The most common ovary-related disorder of chronic anovulation is PCOS. Irregular periods or amenorrhea and androgen excess are the most commonly observed features of PCOS. Other causes of ovary-related anovulation include steroid-secreting ovarian tumors and premature ovarian insufficiency. Androgen excess arising from extraovarian sources (e.g., adrenal disorders) is also associated with anovulation.

Approach to the Patient with Androgen Excess

Two natural androgens are testosterone, which is transported to target tissue by the circulation, and DHT, which is produced primarily by target tissues. Increased levels of these androgens can lead to hirsutism, which is excessive

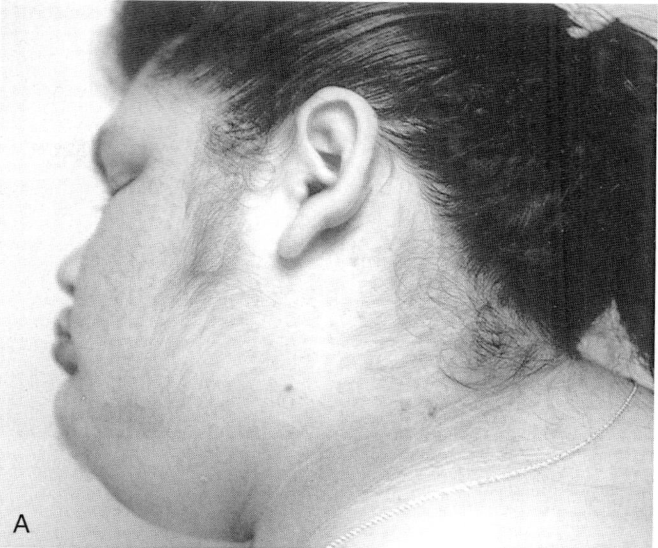

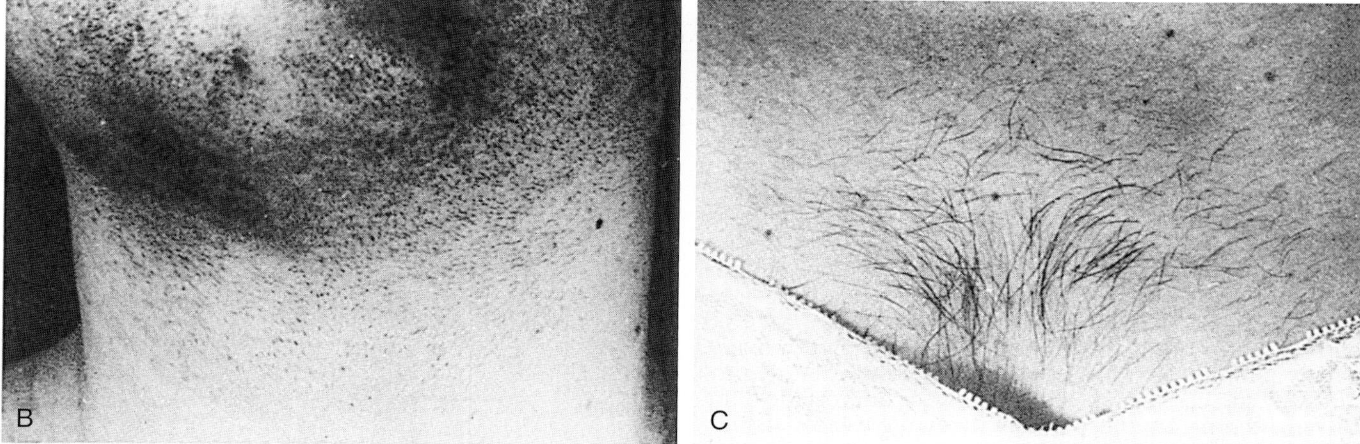

Figure 17-26 Hirsutism. **A,** Mild facial hirsutism. **B,** Severe facial hirsutism (chin), which requires regular shaving. **C,** Severe hirsutism on chest. (**B** and **C,** From Dunaif A, Hoffman AR, Scully RE, et al. The clinical, biochemical and ovarian morphologic features in women with acanthosis nigricans and masculinization. *Obstet Gynecol.* 1985;66:545-552.)

androgenic hair growth, or to virilization, a more severe form of androgen excess. Hirsutism is defined as the presence of terminal (coarse) hair in locations at which hair is not commonly found in women, including facial hair on the cheek, above the upper lip, and on the chin (Fig. 17-26A and B). The presence of midline chest hair is also significant (see Fig. 17-26 C). A male escutcheon, hair on the inner aspects of the thighs, and midline lower back hair entering the intergluteal area are hair growth patterns compatible with androgen excess. A moderate amount of hair on the forearms and lower legs by itself may not be abnormal, although it may be viewed by the patient as undesirable and may be mistaken for hirsutism. Numerous scoring systems are available for quantifying hirsutism. One of the most detailed scales was proposed by Ferriman and Gallwey.[218] A practical and clinically useful means of quantifying hirsutism is recording the hair growth in detail using simple drawings and photographs. In particular, photographs are invaluable for documenting hirsutism accurately.

Compared with hirsutism, virilization is a more severe form of androgen excess and implies significantly higher rates of testosterone production. Its manifestations include temporal balding, deepening of voice, decreased breast size, increased muscle mass, loss of female body contours, and clitoral enlargement (Fig. 17-27). Even if testosterone levels are moderately increased (<1.5 ng/mL), temporal balding and clitoromegaly may be observed after a long period (>1 year) in the presence of persistent androgen excess. A marked increase in androgen secretion, such as may occur from production by neoplasms, leads to a more full-blown picture of virilization in less than a few months.

Measurements of an enlarged clitoris may be used for the quantification of virilization. A clitoral length greater than 10 mm is considered abnormal (see Fig. 17-27). Clitoral length is quite variable, however. An increase in clitoral diameter is a much more sensitive indicator of androgen action. Normal values for clitoral diameter are less than 7 mm at the base of the glans (see Fig. 17-27). The most accurate definition of clitoromegaly involves use of the clitoral index (the product of the sagittal and transverse diameters of the glans clitoris). A clitoral index greater than 35 mm^2 is abnormal and correlates statistically with androgen excess.[219]

Origins of Androgens

Among the natural C19 steroids, DHT is a biologically potent androgen that is capable of acting through

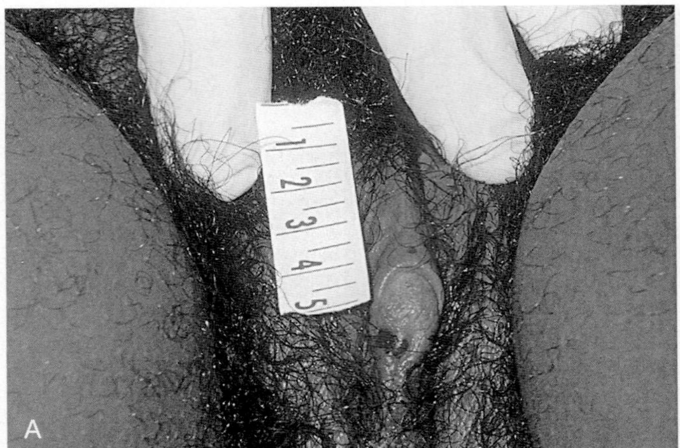

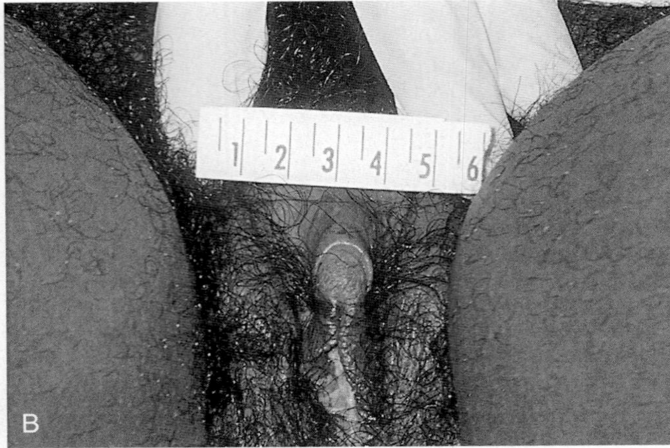

Figure 17-27 Severe clitoromegaly resulting from a testosterone-secreting ovarian tumor. **A,** The entire length of the clitoris is approximately 4 cm (normal, <1 cm). **B,** The transverse diameter of the clitoris measures 1.5 cm (normal, <0.7 cm).

androgen receptors on target cells. Testosterone is also thought to be a biologically active androgen, even though the direct androgenic effects of testosterone have not been clearly demonstrated in vivo. Almost all testosterone target tissues contain 5α-reductase activity, which converts testosterone to DHT, or aromatase activity, which produces estradiol in an intracrine fashion. It is not clear whether testosterone has any direct biologic effects independent of DHT or estradiol produced locally. There is no convincing evidence that the other C19 steroids, including androstenedione, DHEA, and dehydroepiandrosterone sulfate (DHEAS), are biologically active.

Testosterone in reproductive-age women is produced by two major mechanisms: direct secretion by the ovary, which accounts for roughly one third of testosterone production, and conversion of the precursor androstenedione to testosterone in the peripheral (extragonadal) tissues, which accounts for two thirds of testosterone production (Fig. 17-28).[220] These peripheral tissues include the skin and adipose tissue. Androstenedione, the direct precursor of testosterone, is produced in the ovary and the adrenal. The C19 steroids DHEAS and DHEA of adrenal origin and DHEA of ovarian origin indirectly contribute to testosterone formation by first being converted to androstenedione, which is subsequently converted to testosterone (see Fig. 17-28).

DHEA, DHEAS, and androstenedione are biologically inert steroids that serve as precursors for testosterone or estrone production. Up to 20 mg of DHEAS is produced daily, compared with only 3 mg of androstenedione and 8 mg of DHEA per day. These C19 steroids of adrenal origin (DHEAS and DHEA) exert their effects after conversion to testosterone (see Fig. 17-28). Only androstenedione can be converted directly to testosterone. The conversion rate of circulating androstenedione to testosterone in extragonadal tissues is about 5% in both men and women.

Testosterone binds nuclear androgen receptors but is converted to a more potent steroid, DHT, to exert full androgenic effects on certain target tissues such as hair follicles and external genitalia.[123,148] For example, intense androgen action in sex skin fibroblasts requires receptor occupancy by DHT. This conversion is catalyzed by the enzyme 5α-reductase and takes place in the liver and within androgen target cells such as sex skin fibroblasts (i.e., intracrine effect). The protein products of two genes (5α-reductase type 1 and type 2) exhibit this enzymatic activity.[123] DHT is necessary for hair growth and virilization of external genitalia, whereas a direct role of testosterone in these processes is questionable.

Androgen action in target tissues is determined at least in part by the level of local 5α-reductase activity and the androgen receptor content (see Fig. 17-28). Androgen receptors mediate androgenic action in critical target

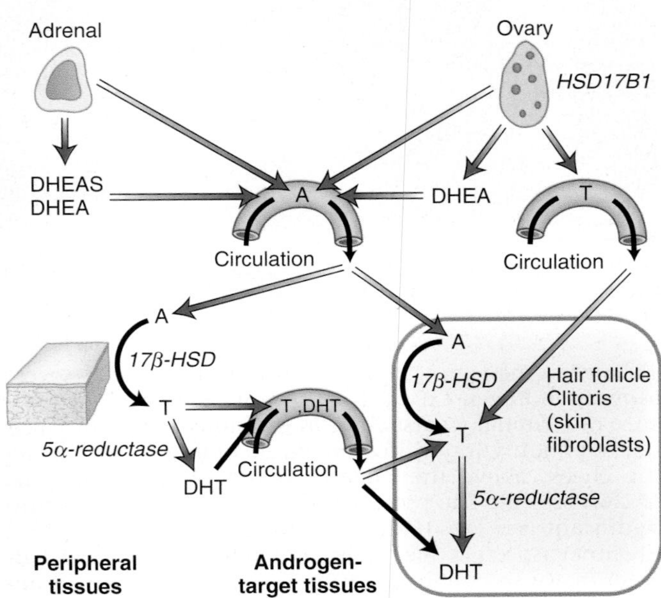

Figure 17-28 Androgen biosynthesis in women. Depending on the menstrual cycle phase or postmenopausal status, 20% to 30% of testosterone (T) is secreted by the ovary. The rest is accounted for by the conversion of circulating androstenedione (A) to T in various peripheral tissues. Both the adrenal and the ovary contribute to circulating A directly or indirectly, depending on the cycle phase or postmenopausal status and chronologic age. T may also be formed locally in androgen target tissues. T is converted to the biologically potent androgen dihydrotestosterone (DHT) within the target tissues and cells. For example, local conversion of T to DHT by 5α-reductase activity, which is conferred by products of at least two genes, in sex skin fibroblasts and hair follicles plays a key role in clitoral enlargement and hirsutism. The enzyme activity of 17β-HSD in peripheral tissues may be conferred by protein products of several genes with overlapping functions; HSD17B1, a distinct reductive 17β-HSD enzyme, is encoded by a specific gene expressed primarily in the ovary. DHEAS, dehydroepiandrosterone sulfate; 17β-HSD, reductive 17β-hydroxysteroid dehydrogenase.

tissues.[148,221] Local enzymes at target tissues other than 5α-reductase (e.g., aromatase, oxidative 17β-HSD) also regulate androgen action by metabolizing testosterone to the androgenically inactive androstenedione or to estradiol, a potent estrogen. There appears to be a balance between potent androgen action when DHT is formed and reduction of androgenicity when inactive C19 steroids or estradiol is formed from testosterone in target tissues and other extragonadal tissues. In particular, the metabolism of testosterone to DHT versus androstenedione or estradiol in these tissues is relevant for androgen-dependent disorders (e.g., hirsutism, virilization) and estrogen-dependent disorders such as malignancies of breast and endometrium (see Figs. 17-21 and 17-28).

Laboratory Evaluation of Androgen Action

Testosterone circulates in three forms: that which is bound to sex hormone–binding globulin (SHBG), the portion not bound to SHBG but loosely associated with albumin, and the fraction not bound by SHBG or albumin (i.e., free or dialyzable testosterone). The blood testosterone that is available to diffuse into target tissues includes the free and albumin-bound fractions and is referred to as bioavailable or non–SHBG-bound testosterone. The remainder is tightly bound to the protein SHBG.

SHBG is one of the primary regulators that determine the amounts of circulating bound and bioavailable testosterone available to act on target tissues. Conditions that decrease SHBG binding (e.g., androgen excess, obesity, acromegaly, hypothyroidism, liver disease) also increase bioavailable testosterone, augmenting the effect of testosterone. SHBG also regulates the circulating amounts of bioavailable estradiol by binding a significant fraction of circulating estradiol. Conditions that decrease SHBG levels give rise to increased bioavailable (non–SHBG-bound) estradiol.

The measurement of non–SHBG-bound (bioavailable) forms of testosterone has been advocated for states of androgen excess to detect more accurately subtle forms of hirsutism. Although the diagnostic yield of this measurement is superior to that of total serum testosterone, the correlation between total and non–SHBG-bound testosterone is excellent, so that bioavailable testosterone can usually be predicted from the total testosterone level.[222] The purpose of measuring serum testosterone is to establish the presence of circulating androgen excess and to detect extremely high values that may originate from an androgen-secreting neoplasm.

The normal serum levels of androgens, especially free testosterone determined by radioimmunoassay (RIA), vary from laboratory to laboratory. A group of investigators compared serum free testosterone levels measured by equilibrium dialysis with those measured by direct RIA and with those calculated from the free androgen index (100 × testosterone/SHBG), a simple index that correlates with the free testosterone level.[223] Calculated values for free testosterone using the free androgen index correlated well with those obtained from equilibrium dialysis. In contrast, the direct RIA method had unacceptably high systematic bias and random variability and did not correlate as well with equilibrium dialysis values. Moreover, the lower limit of detection was higher for the direct RIA than for equilibrium dialysis or calculated free testosterone.[223] The clinician should be aware of the limitations of RIAs performed without rigorous quality control.

Measuring the levels of all C19 steroids is not clinically necessary for most patients presenting with androgen excess. The most useful initial test is a serum total testosterone level. An abnormal level in the presence of hirsutism or virilization may be associated with PCOS, hyperthecosis, nonclassic adrenal hyperplasia, or an androgen-secreting neoplasm. Most androgen-secreting tumors are of ovarian origin. The likelihood of a neoplasm correlates roughly with increasing testosterone levels. The following tests may be added on the basis of the clinical presentation: serum 17-hydroxyprogesterone (i.e., nonclassic adrenal hyperplasia), serum prolactin and TSH (i.e., mild androgen excess associated with hyperprolactinemia), serum FSH and LH (i.e., elevated LH/FSH ratio in PCOS), serum DHEAS (i.e., adrenal tumors), and imaging of ovaries and adrenals (i.e., PCOS and steroid-secreting tumors).

Causes of Androgen Excess

Several disorders give rise to androgen excess. They include unusual causes such as iatrogenic or drug-induced androgen excess, congenital genital ambiguity (e.g., excessive in utero androgen formation in female pseudohermaphroditism), and conditions unique to pregnancy (e.g., luteoma of pregnancy, hyperreactio luteinalis). These uncommon causes and relatively more prevalent disorders associated with androgen excess are listed in Table 17-3. The term *extraovarian steroid formation* is used synonymously with *extraglandular, extragonadal*, or *peripheral steroid formation* in this text.

Overall, the prevalence of androgen-excess disorders was found to be as follows: 72.1% for PCOS (anovulatory patients, 56.6%; mildly affected ovulatory patients, 15.5%); 15.8% for idiopathic hyperandrogenism; 7.6% for idiopathic hirsutism; 4.3% for 21-hydroxylase-deficient nonclassic adrenal hyperplasia; and 0.2% for androgen-secreting tumors.[224]

In most hyperandrogenic disorders, androgen originates from more than one source (see Fig. 17-28). For example, testosterone secretion is somewhat increased from the ovary in PCOS, but the bulk of testosterone comes from extraovarian conversion of significantly elevated circulating androstenedione of ovarian origin to testosterone. Patients with PCOS also show increased adrenal output of

TABLE 17-3

Causes of Androgen Excess in Women of Reproductive Age

Ovarian
Polycystic ovary syndrome (PCOS) Hyperthecosis (a severe PCOS variant) Ovarian tumor (e.g., Sertoli-Leydig cell tumor)
Adrenal
Nonclassic adrenal hyperplasia Cushing's syndrome Glucocorticoid resistance Adrenal tumor (e.g., adenoma, carcinoma)
Specific Conditions of Pregnancy
Luteoma of pregnancy Hyperreactio luteinalis Aromatase deficiency in fetus
Other
Hyperprolactinemia, hypothyroidism Medications (danazol, testosterone, anabolizing agents) Idiopathic hirsutism (normal serum testosterone in an ovulatory woman) Idiopathic hyperandrogenism (patients who do not fall into any of the other categories listed)

DHEAS, which (after peripheral conversion to DHEA that is further converted to androstenedione) contributes indirectly to extraovarian testosterone formation.

If androgen excess is associated with primary amenorrhea, abnormal in utero sexual differentiation should be strongly suspected. These disorders are discussed in Chapter 23. Before embarking on a major workup for hirsutism or virilization, the physician is well advised to rule out exogenous androgen use. It is best to ask the patient to list all prescriptions and over-the-counter medications that she takes on her own, including injections. This is usually more rewarding than asking the patient whether she takes any androgens. Medications that can cause hirsutism or virilization are related to testosterone and include anabolic steroids and similar compounds.

The most common identifiable cause of androgen excess is PCOS, which is discussed elsewhere in this chapter. In this section, we first define some of the other disorders associated with hirsutism or virilization. This is followed by a simplified treatment strategy that may be applied to most hirsute patients within the categories of PCOS, nonclassic adrenal hyperplasia, and idiopathic hirsutism.

Idiopathic Hirsutism

Hirsutism is defined subjectively as the presence in a woman of terminal hair growth in a male-distribution pattern that affects quality of life sufficiently to prompt her to seek medical advice. Hirsutism should be distinguished from hypertrichosis, in which the excessive hair growth is not restricted to androgen-dependent areas and comprises vellus or lanugo-type hair. Hypertricosis is considered to be a phenotype not associated with male pattern hair growth and is unlikely to be modified by the known treatments of hirsutism.

Idiopathic (constitutional) hirsutism is characterized by excessive hair growth in the absence of excessive circulating androgen levels in ovulatory women, and it occurs more frequently in certain ethnic populations, particularly in women of Mediterranean ancestry.[148] It is defined as hirsutism in conjunction with regular menstrual cycles and normal levels of serum testosterone. Idiopathic hirsutism is not associated with any signs of virilization. Its cause is not understood completely. It has been proposed that women with idiopathic hirsutism have significantly increased cutaneous 5α-reductase activity,[225] but this association has not been confirmed. It is also unclear whether either of the 5α-reductase isoenzymes (type 1 or 2) is predominant in the development of idiopathic hirsutism.[148]

Idiopathic hirsutism is diagnosed in women who have hirsutism,[148] normal ovulatory function, and normal total or free testosterone levels. More than 80% of all women with cyclic predictable menses are ovulatory. Ovulatory function may be verified by a luteal phase day 7 progesterone level, which should be at least 5 ng/mL. Luteal phase day 7 corresponds to cycle day 17 for 24-day intervals, cycle day 21 for 28-day intervals, and cycle day 28 for 35-day intervals. The presence of oligo-ovulation or anovulation in hirsute women after exclusion of related disorders (e.g., hypothyroidism, hyperprolactinemia, nonclassic adrenal hyperplasia) is consistent with the diagnosis of PCOS.[148] Thyroid dysfunction and hyperprolactinemia should be excluded by the measurements of TSH and prolactin. The follicular-phase basal 17-hydroxyprogesterone level should be measured to exclude 21-hydroxylase–deficient, nonclassic adrenal hyperplasia. The use of exogenous androgens should also be excluded. In summary, the diagnosis of idiopathic hirsutism is one of exclusion in which ovulatory dysfunction, elevated circulating testosterone levels, and other causes of androgen excess are ruled out.

Androgen-Secreting Tumors of the Ovary and Adrenal

Most androgen-secreting tumors arise from the ovary. These ovarian tumors secrete large quantities of testosterone or its precursor, androstenedione. They include Sertoli-Leydig cell tumors, hilus cell tumors, lipoid cell tumors, and infrequently, granulosa-theca tumors. Steroidogenically inert ovarian neoplasms such as epithelial cystadenomas or cystadenocarcinomas may produce factors that stimulate steroidogenesis in adjacent non-neoplastic ovarian stroma and induce production of sufficient amounts of androgen precursors such as androstenedione to give rise to clinically detectable androgen excess. Approximately 5% of androstenedione is converted to testosterone in extraovarian tissues, ultimately producing androgen excess (see Fig. 17-28).

Sertoli-Leydig cell tumors, which account for fewer than 1% of all solid ovarian tumors, tend to occur during the second to fourth decades of life, whereas hilus cell tumors occur more frequently in postmenopausal women. By the time the signs and symptoms of androgen excess cause the patient to seek medical assistance, Sertoli-Leydig cell tumors are usually so large that they are readily palpable on pelvic examination, whereas hilus cell tumors are still small. In women with either type of tumor, the serum testosterone level is markedly elevated. Granulosa-theca tumors primarily produce estradiol but may occasionally produce testosterone.

Rapidly progressing symptoms of androgen excess suggest the presence of an androgen-producing tumor unless proved otherwise. This rapid progression is typical of both ovarian and adrenal androgen-producing tumors. Progression is usually associated with defeminizing signs, such as loss of female body contour and decreased breast size. As the tumor continues to grow, more and more testosterone is produced, resulting in rapidly worsening hirsutism and progressive virilization. Elevated serum testosterone levels are characteristically associated with ovarian tumors. This change may be mediated by production and secretion of testosterone directly by the tumor or by secretion of large quantities of androstenedione that are converted to testosterone in extragonadal tissues. The testosterone levels produced by certain ovarian tumors (e.g., Sertoli-Leydig cell tumors) may be suppressed by GnRH agonists,[226] so use of a GnRH agonist cannot be relied on to differentiate a neoplasm from another functional state.

In interpreting testosterone levels, the clinician should be familiar with the normal ranges of the clinical laboratory used. A value of three times the upper-normal range (or >2 ng/mL) suggests a neoplasm, particularly if the clinical history supports this diagnosis. Lower serum testosterone levels occasionally may be associated with virilizing ovarian tumors. If an androgen-secreting tumor is suspected, measurement of androstenedione is clinically useful. A severely elevated level of androstenedione is consistent with an ovarian or adrenal tumor. When an elevated level of testosterone is found and confirmed by clinical history, meticulously performed transvaginal ultrasonography should be able to detect the ovarian tumor. Transvaginal ultrasonography is the most sensitive method for the detection of an ovarian tumor.

In contrast to testosterone-secreting tumors of the ovary, testosterone-secreting tumors of the adrenal are rare. The cells of some testosterone-producing adrenal tumors may resemble ovarian hilus cells, which are analogous to Leydig cells. These tumor cells produce testosterone and may be stimulated by LH or hCG. In patients with testosterone-producing adrenal adenomas, testosterone secretion usually decreases after LH suppression and increases after hCG stimulation. Testosterone-secreting adrenal carcinomas also have been reported.[227]

Virilizing adrenal tumors commonly secrete large quantities of DHEAS, DHEA, and androstenedione, and testosterone is usually produced by extraovarian conversion of these precursors. Levels of serum DHEAS are highly elevated in most patients with virilizing adrenal tumors.[228] If DHEAS levels exceed 8 μg/mL, adrenal imaging by computed tomography (CT) or MRI should be ordered. Occasionally, such high levels of DHEAS are associated with a functional abnormality such as congenital adrenal hyperplasia caused by an enzymatic defect or an unexplained hyperfunctional adrenal state that is commonly associated with PCOS. These circumstances may explain a negative CT or MRI result, which warrants further investigation.

Levels of a variety of adrenal steroids, including corticosteroids, may be elevated in various combinations in the presence of an adrenal tumor. It is not possible to describe a particular pattern of hormones that defines an adrenal tumor.[228] Very high levels of serum DHEAS (>8 μg/mL) suggest an adrenal tumor. Testosterone-secreting adrenal tumors are rare. Virilizing ovarian tumors are encountered much more frequently than those of adrenal origin. If the presentation is compatible with an androgen-secreting tumor and the ovaries are normal by transvaginal ultrasonography, the adrenals should be evaluated next by imaging.

Testosterone levels three times the upper-normal range (i.e., >2 ng/mL) and DHEAS levels higher than 8 μg/mL have been used traditionally as guidelines to investigate further whether neoplasms of the ovary or adrenal are the sources of androgen excess. These numbers are provided only as guidelines, not as rules, and there are exceptions. First, because tumors secrete androgens episodically, more than one measurement may be required to detect a significantly elevated level.[229] Second, other precursor steroids are often elevated as well (particularly androstenedione), and their measurement should be considered. Third, some tumors may give rise to milder elevations of DHEAS and testosterone levels. Even mild elevations in a postmenopausal woman are highly suspicious for an androgen-secreting tumor. By the same token, greatly elevated serum testosterone levels may be observed in women with severe ovarian hyperthecosis (a severe variant of PCOS) in the absence of a tumor.

Virilization of recent onset and short duration warrants immediate investigation, even if testosterone and DHEAS levels are mildly elevated. With improvements in scanning techniques—vaginal ultrasonography for the ovary; abdominal ultrasonography, CT, and MRI for the adrenal—the diagnosis of even a small ovarian or adrenal tumor may be made. If no neoplasm can be localized, imaging of the ovary or adrenal after intravenous administration of radiolabeled iodomethylnorcholesterol (NP-59), which detects active steroid-producing tumors, has proved useful.[230] These diagnostic studies should be pursued aggressively before surgical exploration of a suspected tumor.

The clinician should question whether an ovarian or adrenal tumor detected by imaging is the actual source of androgen excess before resorting to its surgical resection. Occasionally, a hemorrhagic corpus luteum cyst of the ovary may mimic an androgen-secreting tumor, or a woman with androgen excess may have an adrenal "incidentaloma," which does not secrete androgen. Intraoperative selective ovarian or adrenal vein catheterization may be considered as a last resort to demonstrate significant steroid gradients before surgical exploration of an adrenal or ovary for a small tumor is undertaken, especially if the clinical picture is not certain.[231]

Non-Neoplastic Adrenal Disorders and Androgen Excess

Adrenal disorders such as classic congenital adrenal hyperplasia, Cushing's syndrome, and glucocorticoid resistance give rise to androgen excess related to overproduction of testosterone precursors from the adrenal. These disorders are discussed elsewhere in this text. In this chapter, we discuss nonclassic adrenal hyperplasia.

The diagnosis and prevalence of nonclassic adrenal hyperplasia continues to be debated, although the disorder clearly exists. Other terms that have been used to describe this syndrome include late-onset, adult-onset, attenuated, incomplete, and cryptic adrenal hyperplasia. This form of adrenal hyperplasia is caused by a partial deficiency in 21-hydroxylase activity. Although deficiencies in 11β-hydroxylase and 3β-HSD may result in the disorder, defects in 21-hydroxylase account for more than 90% of cases.[232]

The clinical presentation is almost identical to that of patients with PCOS. The prevalence of this disorder varies according to ethnic background, and the prevalence reported by different investigators has varied widely. The characteristic presentation consists of anovulatory uterine bleeding and progressive hirsutism of pubertal onset. These individuals are born with normal genitalia, do not exhibit salt wasting, and are symptom free until puberty. Patients of northern European ancestry have a low frequency of this disorder, whereas Ashkenazi Jews, Hispanics, and patients of central European ancestry have a much higher prevalence.[233] High-risk ethnic groups should be screened.

Screening may first be carried out by obtaining an 8:00 a.m. serum level of 17-hydroxyprogesterone in an anovulatory patient on any day. Although most women with nonclassic adrenal hyperplasia are anovulatory, some women with this disorder present with regular periods and hirsutism of pubertal onset or with only unexplained infertility.[232] If nonclassic adrenal hyperplasia is suspected in an ovulatory patient on the basis of clinical presentation, an 8:00 a.m. serum level of 17-hydroxyprogesterone should be obtained during the follicular phase, because 17-hydroxyprogesterone levels are higher in the luteal phase than in the proliferative phase in affected or disease-free ovulatory women.[232] A level of less than 2 ng/mL effectively rules out this diagnosis.[232]

The diagnosis of nonclassic adrenal hyperplasia can be made if the basal 17-hydroxyprogesterone level is higher than 8 ng/mL. No further testing is required in these cases. Values between 2 and 8 ng/mL are considered increased but not diagnostic of nonclassic adrenal hyperplasia. For example, disease-free women and patients with PCOS may also have basal levels of 17-hydroxyprogesterone in this indeterminate range.[232] In these circumstances, an ACTH stimulation test should be used to distinguish nonclassic adrenal hyperplasia from PCOS.[232] A rise of the 17-hydroxyprogesterone level to at least 10 ng/mL 60 minutes after intravenous injection of ACTH has been considered diagnostic of nonclassic adrenal hyperplasia.[234] A higher basal level of 17-hydroxprogesterone within the 2 to 8 ng/mL range is associated with a higher likelihood of nonclassic adrenal hyperplasia. For example, an 8:00 a.m.

17-hydroxyprogesterone level higher than 4 ng/mL had a sensitivity of 90% for the diagnosis of nonclassic adrenal hyperplasia.[232]

In a patient with androgen excess who belongs to an ethnic group in which there is a high prevalence of nonclassic adrenal hyperplasia, a baseline level of 17-hydroxyprogesterone should be measured at 8:00 a.m. A screening baseline level of 17-hydroxyprogesterone should be obtained for patients with premature pubarche, those with androgen excess of early pubertal onset, women with progressive hirsutism or virilization, and patients with strong family histories of severe androgen excess.

Laboratory Testing to Aid the Differential Diagnosis of Androgen Excess

Algorithms exist for the differential diagnosis of anovulation associated with hirsutism or virilization or both. Salient clinical features are of paramount importance to guide laboratory testing. The most important features are the onset and severity of the signs and the rapidity with which they progress. Rapidly progressing severe androgen excess implies an androgen-secreting tumor until proved otherwise. The possibility of a tumor is further underscored in a postmenopausal woman or in a reproductive-age woman with a recent history of cyclic, predictable periods. Ovarian hyperthecosis, a severe variant of PCOS, also gives rise to severe androgen excess that may progress rapidly, especially at the time of expected puberty. Androgen excess emerging at the time of puberty may be indicative of PCOS or nonclassic adrenal hyperplasia.

The most useful initial test to evaluate androgen excess is the serum level of total testosterone (Table 17-4). Testosterone levels in most normal ovulatory women are lower than 0.6 ng/mL, although the value may vary from laboratory to laboratory. Women with idiopathic hirsutism have cyclic menses and normal testosterone levels. No further testing for androgen excess is required in this group.

If the testosterone level is elevated in an anovulatory woman, serum levels of TSH and prolactin should be obtained to rule out anovulation associated with hyperprolactinemia. Ultrasonography of the ovaries also can help to identify an ovarian tumor or polycystic ovaries. If the ethnic background of the patient (i.e., Ashkenazi Jews, Hispanics, and those of central European ancestry), onset of hirsutism (i.e., puberty), or family history suggests nonclassic adrenal hyperplasia, a baseline serum level of 17-hydroxyprogesterone should be obtained at 8:00 a.m. Rare causes of androgen excess include an adrenal tumor, Cushing's syndrome, and glucocorticoid resistance. A serum level of DHEAS and adrenal imaging are required to assess the presence or absence of an adrenal tumor. CT, MRI, or abdominal ultrasonography may be used to assess the adrenals, depending on the expertise of the local radiology laboratory. A screening test for Cushing's syndrome and glucocorticoid resistance may be performed to explore rare adrenal causes of androgen excess (see Chapter 15).[235]

Most women with chronic anovulation and mild to moderate hirsutism of pubertal onset fall into the category of PCOS. These women have high normal or elevated testosterone levels and no other laboratory abnormalities. After other diagnoses are ruled out by laboratory testing or on clinical grounds, a diagnosis of PCOS can be made.

TABLE 17-4

Laboratory Tests for the Differential Diagnosis of Androgen Excess

Initial Testing
Total testosterone
Prolactin
Thyroid-stimulating hormone
Further Testing Based on Clinical Presentation*
17-Hydroxyprogesterone (8:00 a.m.)
17-Hydroxyprogesterone 60 min after intravenous ACTH
Cortisol (8:00 a.m.) after 1 mg dexamethasone at midnight
DHEAS
Androstenedione
Imaging of ovaries (transvaginal ultrasonography)
Imaging of adrenals (abdominal ultrasonography, CT, MRI)
Nuclear imaging after intravenous administration of radiolabeled cholesterol

*See text.
ACTH, adrenocorticotropic hormone; CT, computed tomography; DHEAS, dehydroepiandrosterone sulfate; MRI, magnetic resonance imaging.

Treatment of Hirsutism

Therapy for androgen excess should be directed toward its specific cause and suppression of abnormal androgen secretion. Specific treatments for hirsutism and virilization are indicated for ovarian and adrenal tumors, hyperthecosis, Cushing's syndrome, and adrenal hyperplasia. Neoplasms warrant surgical intervention and are not discussed in greater detail here. Suppression with a GnRH analogue may be tried initially for ovarian hyperthecosis. However, bilateral oophorectomy is ultimately necessary to control androgen excess arising from hyperthecosis in most patients (see later discussion). Patients with adrenal disease are treated specifically. For Cushing's syndrome, treatment correlates with the source of hypercortisolism. For nonclassic adrenal hyperplasia, glucocorticoid replacement should be implemented, as it is for adrenal insufficiency. When treating androgen excess associated with nonclassic adrenal hyperplasia, an antiandrogen (e.g., spironolactone) in combination with an oral contraceptive or a glucocorticoid may be used. The doses of glucocorticoids needed to suppress the adrenal can often cause symptoms and signs of glucocorticoid excess during long-term treatment. A combination oral contraceptive plus spironolactone is favored to treat androgen excess if the patient responds to this treatment with decreased hirsutism. More details of glucocorticoid therapy may be found in Chapter 15.

The general treatment of androgen excess is directed toward the prevention of abnormal hair growth and virilization. For practical purposes, the same approach is used for androgen excess associated with idiopathic hirsutism, PCOS, and nonclassic adrenal hyperplasia. The existing hair follicles and manifestations of virilization (e.g., thickening of voice, clitoromegaly, temporal balding) remain even after elimination of excessive androgen production. Terminal hair should be removed by mechanical methods (e.g., electrolysis) at least 3 months after androgen suppression is achieved. Patients with clitoromegaly may be referred to a urologist for clitoral reduction surgery after the source of virilization has been effectively eliminated. Several medications are available for the treatment of androgen excess and hirsutism.

Oral Contraceptives. Oral contraceptives reduce circulating testosterone and androgen precursors by suppression of LH and stimulation of SHBG levels, thereby reducing hirsutism in hyperandrogenic patients.[148] Oral contraceptives decrease circulating androgen in patients with PCOS and synergize with the effects of antiandrogens. Oral contraceptives may further improve the results of antiandrogen therapy in patients with idiopathic hirsutism or nonclassic adrenal hyperplasia. It is advisable to use an oral contraceptive containing 30 or 35 μg of ethinyl estradiol to achieve effective suppression of LH.[148] A meta-analysis showed that treatment with oral contraceptives for 6 months reduced Ferriman-Gallwey scores of hirsutism by an average of 27%.[236]

Spironolactone. The most common androgen blocker used for the treatment of hirsutism in the United States is spironolactone, an aldosterone antagonist structurally related to progestins. Spironolactone is effective for abnormal hair growth associated with PCOS or idiopathic hirsutism. Treatment with spironolactone for 6 months reduces Ferriman-Gallwey scores of hirsutism by an average of 38.4%.

Because spironolactone acts through mechanisms different from those of oral contraceptives, overall effectiveness is improved by combining these two medications in patients with hirsutism, including those with PCOS, idiopathic hirsutism, or nonclassic adrenal hyperplasia. Apart from inhibiting steroidogenesis and acting as an androgen antagonist, spironolactone has a significant effect in inhibiting 5α-reductase activity.[148,237] Basic experimental and several clinical studies have confirmed the efficacy of spironolactone for hyperandrogenism and suggest that the principal effect is related to its ability to block peripheral androgen production and action.[148]

Doses of spironolactone used in clinical studies have varied from 50 to 400 mg daily. Although doses of 100 mg/day usually are effective for the treatment of hirsutism, higher doses (200 to 300 mg/day) may be preferable in extremely hirsute or markedly obese women.[148,237] The initial recommended dosage is 100 mg/day, gradually increasing it by increments of 25 mg/day every 3 months up to 200 mg/day on the basis of the response. This approach may be helpful to minimize side effects such as gastritis, dry skin, and anovulation. In patients with normal renal function, hyperkalemia is almost never seen. Hypotension is rare except in older women. Monitoring for electrolytes and blood pressure is imperative within the first 2 weeks at each dose level. Adjustments in dose should be made only after 3 to 6 months, as with other antiandrogens, to account for the slow changes in the hair cycle.

Patients usually notice an initial transient diuretic effect. Some women with normal cycles complain of menstrual irregularity with spironolactone; this is remedied by a downward dose adjustment or the addition of an oral contraceptive. The mechanism for abnormal bleeding is unclear. In women with oligomenorrhea, such as those with PCOS, resumption of normal menses may occur. This change may be caused in part by an alteration in levels of circulating androgens; LH levels have only occasionally been reported to decrease.[238] Another important consideration is the potential in utero feminizing effect of this antiandrogen on the genitalia of a 46,XY fetus. Effective contraception should always be provided in women taking spironolactone.

Cyproterone Acetate. Cyproterone acetate is a 17-hydroxyprogesterone acetate derivative with strong progestagenic properties. Cyproterone acetate acts as an antiandrogen by competing with DHT and testosterone for binding to the androgen receptor. There is also some evidence that cyproterone acetate and ethinyl estradiol in combination can inhibit 5α-reductase activity in skin.[239] Cyproterone acetate is not available in the United States but has been used in other countries. The drug usually is administered daily in doses of 50 to 100 mg on days 5 through 15 of the treatment cycle. Because of its slow metabolism, it is administered early in the treatment cycle; when ethinyl estradiol is added, it is usually administered in 50-μg doses on days 5 through 26. This regimen is needed for menstrual control and is usually referred to as the *reverse sequential regimen*. Cyproterone acetate in doses of 50 to 100 mg/day, combined with ethinyl estradiol at 30 to 35 μg/day, is as effective as the combination of spironolactone (100 mg/day) and an oral contraceptive in the treatment of hirsutism.[148] In smaller doses (2 mg), cyproterone acetate has been administered as an oral contraceptive in daily combination with 50 or 35 μg of ethinyl estradiol. This regimen is primarily suited for individuals with a milder form of hyperandrogenism.[148]

Finasteride. Finasteride inhibits 5α-reductase activity and has been used primarily for the treatment of prostatic hyperplasia. It can also be used in the treatment of hirsutism.[240,241] At a dose of 5 mg/day, a significant improvement of hirsutism is observed after 6 months of therapy, without significant side effects. In hirsute women, the decline in circulating DHT levels is small and cannot be used to monitor therapy. Although this treatment regimen increases testosterone levels, SHBG levels remain unaffected.[240] A meta-analysis showed that finasteride treatment for 6 months reduced Ferriman-Gallwey scores of hirsutism by an average of 20.3%.[236]

Finasteride primarily inhibits 5α-reductase type 2. Because hirsutism results from the combined effects of type 1 and type 2, this agent is only partially effective. Although prolonged experience with finasteride is lacking, one of the potential advantages of this agent is its benign side effect profile. One study showed efficacy with 1 year of hirsutism treatment.[242] It was also reported that finasteride is less effective than spironolactone with respect to the reduction of hirsutism in women.[148] Nevertheless, finasteride at a dose of 5 mg/day for prolonged periods represents a useful option because of its benign side effect profile and good tolerance by patients. Like spironolactone, finasteride may cause congenital genital ambiguity in a 46,XY fetus, and effective contraception should be provided during its use.

Flutamide. Flutamide is a potent antiandrogen used in the treatment of prostate cancer. It has been shown to be effective in the treatment of hirsutism.[243,244] The mean Ferriman-Gallwey score is reduced by 41.3%.[236] Nevertheless, occasional severe hepatotoxicity makes this drug unsuitable for the indication of hirsutism.[245]

Metformin and Thiazolidinediones. Most studies conducted during the past decade have suggested that treatment with metformin (1500 to 2700 mg/day) for 6 months significantly reduces hirsutism as assessed by the Ferriman-Gallwey scoring system.[236] Most studies showed modest reductions in hirsutism scores (average, 19.1%).[236] In obese adolescent women with PCOS, metformin in combination with lifestyle modification (i.e., diet with a 500 kcal/day deficit and exercise 30 min/day) and oral contraceptives reduced the total testosterone level and waist circumference.[246] The thiazolidinediones (4 mg/day of rosiglitazone or 30 mg/day of pioglitazone), reduced Ferriman-Gallwey scores significantly.[236] These studies suggested that insulin-sensitizing agents may be used in the treatment of hirsutism, especially for women who do not wish to use other oral agents.

Lifestyle Modification. In obese adolescent women with PCOS, lifestyle modification (i.e., diet with a 500 kcal/day deficit and exercise 30 min/day) alone resulted in a 59% reduction in the testosterone/SHBG ratio, with a 122% increase in SHBG.[246] A moderate diet and exercise program should be recommended as part of hirsutism management, particularly for obese women.

Comprehensive Treatment Strategy for Hirsutism. The medications described in the previous paragraphs may be effective when administered as individual treatments. Patients with the most common form of hirsutism (i.e., PCOS) are often initially treated with a combination of two agents, one that suppresses the ovary (e.g., an oral contraceptive) and another that suppresses the extraovarian (peripheral) action of androgens (e.g., spironolactone). An oral contraceptive containing 30 to 35 μg of ethinyl estradiol combined with spironolactone (100 mg/day) is the initial treatment of choice. Even in women with idiopathic hirsutism, the addition of an oral contraceptive to the antiandrogen spironolactone can improve efficacy and prevent abnormal bleeding. For women with only minor complaints of hirsutism, the use of an oral contraceptive alone may be an appropriate first approach. Moderate lifestyle modification (i.e., diet with a 500 kcal/day deficit and 30 min/day of exercise) should be a part of hirsutism management in obese patients.

Because the growth phase of body hairs lasts 3 to 6 months, a response should not be expected before 6 months after onset of treatment. Objective means should be used to assess changes in hair growth. Scoring systems and evaluation of anagen hair shafts are difficult; taking photographs is the simplest and most objective tool. Patients are often unaware that change is taking place unless there is some objective measurement. Pictures of the face and selected midline body areas before and during therapy are especially useful for the encouragement of the patient and compliance with the treatment.

Suppression of androgen production and action inhibits only new hair growth. Existing coarse hair should be removed mechanically. Plucking, waxing, and shaving are ineffective for hair removal and cause irritation, folliculitis, and ingrown hairs. Electrolysis is still the method of choice. Laser epilation is relatively new and needs further evaluation.[148]

Most patients with PCOS and idiopathic hirsutism respond to this strategy within 1 year. Patients should be encouraged to continue treatment for at least 2 years. Then, depending on the wishes and clinical responses of patients, therapy can be stopped and the patient reevaluated. Many patients require continuous treatment for suppression of hirsutism.

Polycystic Ovary Syndrome

PCOS is the most common form of chronic anovulation associated with androgen excess; it occurs in perhaps 5% to 10% of reproductive-age women.[142] The diagnosis of PCOS is made by excluding other hyperandrogenic disorders (e.g., nonclassic adrenal hyperplasia, androgen-secreting tumors, hyperprolactinemia) in women with chronic anovulation and androgen excess.

During the reproductive years, PCOS is associated with important reproductive morbidity, including infertility, irregular uterine bleeding, and increased pregnancy loss. The endometrium of the patient with PCOS must be evaluated by biopsy, because long-term unopposed estrogen stimulation leaves these patients at increased risk for endometrial cancer. PCOS is also associated with increased metabolic and cardiovascular risk factors.[247] These risks are linked to insulin resistance and are compounded by the common occurrence of obesity, although insulin resistance also occurs in nonobese women with PCOS.[142]

PCOS is considered to be a heterogeneous disorder with multifactorial causes. PCOS risk is significantly increased with a positive family history of chronic anovulation and androgen excess, and this complex disorder may be inherited in a polygenic fashion.[248,249]

Historical Perspective

In their pioneering studies, Stein and Leventhal described an association between the presence of bilateral polycystic ovaries and signs of amenorrhea, oligomenorrhea, hirsutism, and obesity (Fig. 17-29).[250] At the time, these signs were strictly adhered to in the diagnosis of what was then known as *Stein-Leventhal syndrome*. These investigators also reported the results of bilateral wedge resection of the ovaries, in which at least half of each ovary was removed as a therapy for PCOS. Most of their patients resumed menses and achieved pregnancy after ovarian wedge resection. They postulated that removal of the thickened capsule of the ovary would restore normal ovulation by allowing the follicles to reach the surface of the ovary. The exact mechanism responsible for the therapeutic effect of removal or destruction of part of the ovarian tissue is still not well understood.

On the basis of Stein and Leventhal's work, a primary ovarian defect was inferred, and the disorder was commonly referred to as *polycystic ovarian disease*. Subsequent clinical, morphologic, hormonal, and metabolic studies uncovered multiple underlying pathologies, and the term *polycystic ovary syndrome* was introduced to reflect the heterogeneity of this disorder.

One of the most significant discoveries regarding the pathophysiology of PCOS was the demonstration of a unique form of insulin resistance and associated hyperinsulinemia.[142] Burghen and coworkers first reported this finding in 1980.[251] The presence of insulin resistance in PCOS has since been confirmed by a number of groups worldwide.[142]

Diagnosis of Polycystic Ovary Syndrome and Laboratory Testing

One of the most prominent features of PCOS is the history of ovulatory dysfunction (i.e., amenorrhea, oligomenorrhea, or other forms of irregular uterine bleeding) of pubertal onset. A clear history of cyclic predictable menses of menarchal onset makes the diagnosis of PCOS unlikely. Acquired insulin resistance associated with significant weight gain or an unknown cause may induce the clinical picture of PCOS in a woman with a history of previously normal ovulatory function. Hirsutism may develop prepubertally or during adolescence, or it may be absent until the third decade of life. Seborrhea, acne, and alopecia are other common clinical signs of androgen excess. In extreme cases of ovarian hyperthecosis (a severe variant of PCOS), clitoromegaly may be observed. Nonetheless, rapid progression of androgenic symptoms and virilization are rare in PCOS. Some women may never have signs of androgen excess because of hereditary differences in target tissue sensitivity to androgens.[148] Infertility related to the anovulation may be the only presenting symptom.

During the physical examination, it is essential to search for and document signs of androgen excess (hirsutism, virilization, or both), insulin resistance (acanthosis nigricans, Fig. 17-30), and the presence of unopposed estrogen action (well-rugated vagina and stretchable, clear cervical mucus) to support the diagnosis of PCOS. None of these signs is specific for PCOS, and each may be associated with any of the conditions listed in the differential diagnosis of PCOS (Table 17-5).

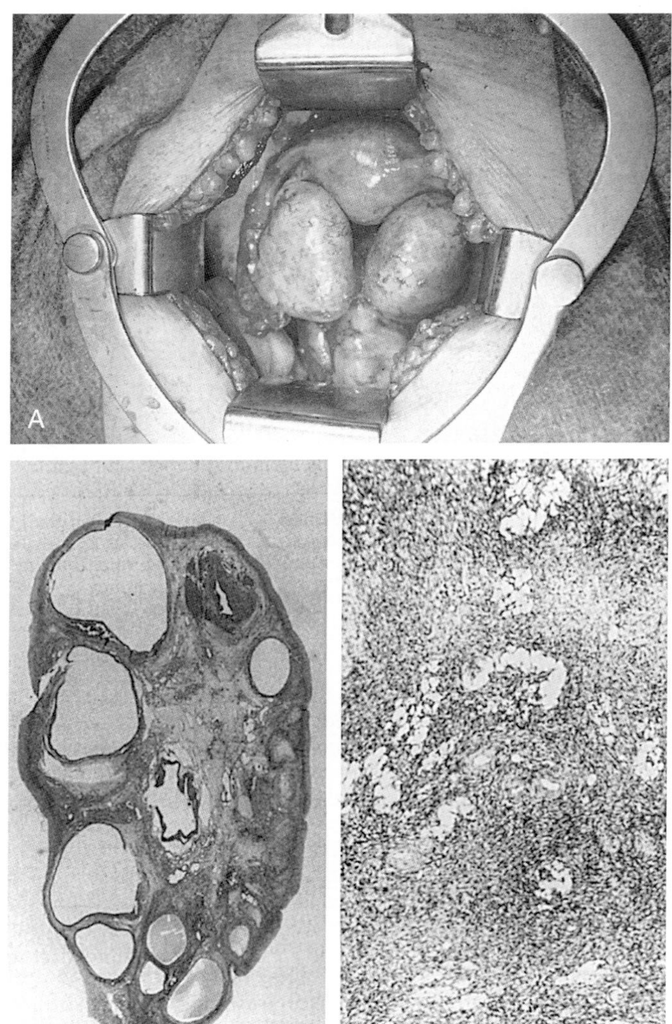

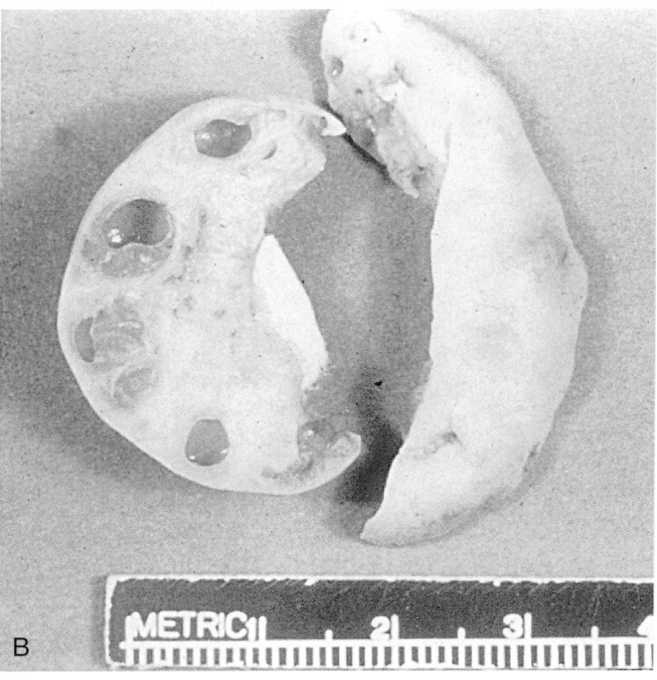

Figure 17-29 Polycystic ovaries. **A,** Operative findings of classic enlarged polycystic ovaries. The uterus is located adjacent to the two enlarged ovaries. **B,** Sectioned polycystic ovary with numerous follicles. **C,** Histologic section of a polycystic ovary with multiple subcapsular follicular cysts and stromal hypertrophy at low power *(left)*. At higher power (×100), islands of luteinized theca cells are visible in the stroma *(right)*. This morphologic change is called *stromal hyperthecosis*, and it appears to correlate directly with circulating insulin levels. (**C,** From Dunaif A. Insulin resistance and the polycystic ovary syndrome: mechanism and implications for pathogenesis. *Endocr Rev.* 1997;18:774-800. Copyright © 1997 by The Endocrine Society.)

PCOS was previously defined according to the proceedings of an expert conference sponsored by the National Institutes of Health (NIH) in 1990, which described the disorder as including hyperandrogenism or hyperandrogenemia (or both), oligo-ovulation, and exclusion of known disorders of androgen excess and anovulation.[252,253] Another expert conference held in Rotterdam in 2003 defined PCOS, after the exclusion of related disorders, by the presence of two of the following three features: oligo-ovulation or anovulation, clinical or biochemical signs of hyperandrogenism (or both), and polycystic ovaries (Fig. 17-31).[254] In essence, the Rotterdam 2003 criteria expanded the NIH 1990 definition by creating two new phenotypes: ovulatory women with polycystic ovaries plus hyperandrogenism and oligo-anovulatory women with polycystic ovaries but without hyperandrogenism. The clinical usefulness of including these new groups with respect to increased risk of infertility, insulin resistance, and long-term metabolic complications is not clear at this time.[255] More recently, the Androgen Excess Society published a broad consensus statement that included discussions of the merits and disadvantages of the NIH and Rotterdam criteria and suggested a practical definition that integrates both sets of diagnostic criteria (Table 17-6).[255]

TABLE 17-5

Differential Diagnosis of Polycystic Ovary Syndrome

Differential Diagnosis of Polycystic Ovary Syndrome
Idiopathic hirsutism
Hyperprolactinemia, hypothyroidism
Nonclassic adrenal hyperplasia
Ovarian tumors
Adrenal tumors
Cushing's syndrome
Glucocorticoid resistance
Other rare causes of androgen excess

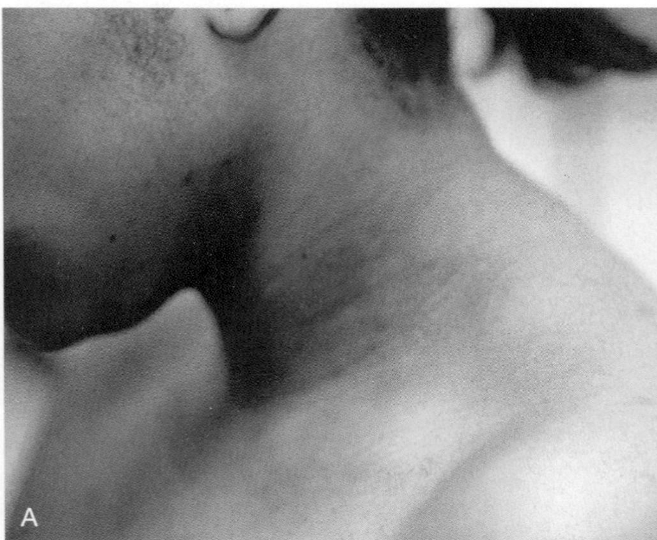

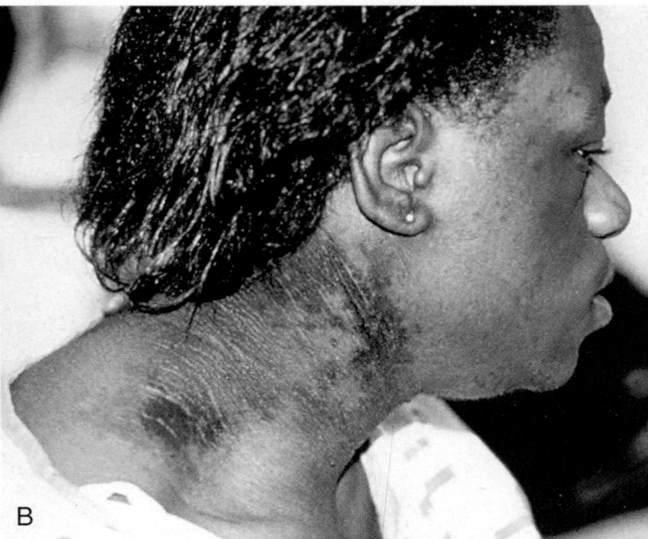

Figure 17-30 Acanthosis nigricans. **A,** Moderate acanthosis nigricans (i.e., darkening and thickening of skin) at the lateral lower fold of the neck. Notice facial hirsutism (sideburns) in the same patient. **B,** Severe acanthosis nigricans in another patient with severe insulin resistance. (**B,** Courtesy of Dr. R. Ann Word, Dallas, Texas.)

The exclusion of hyperprolactinemia, hypothyroidism, nonclassic adrenal hyperplasia, and tumors requires a careful history, physical examination, and laboratory testing, as detailed previously (see Table 17-4). Cushing's syndrome and glucocorticoid resistance may give rise to androgen excess and anovulation after a period of normal ovulatory function in teens. An 8:00 a.m. cortisol level after dexamethasone (1 mg) administration at midnight is a useful screening test for both conditions. Cushing's syndrome may be recognized by its typical signs, whereas 8:00 a.m. and 4:00 p.m. cortisol levels are essential to confirm the diagnosis of glucocorticoid resistance.[256] Glucocorticoid resistance is characterized by preserved diurnal rhythm despite significantly elevated cortisol, ACTH, and adrenal C19 steroid levels and absence of cushingoid symptoms and signs.[256]

Elevated total testosterone is the most direct evidence for androgen excess. Various levels of testosterone are found in women with PCOS. Rarely, serum testosterone levels higher than 2 ng/mL may be encountered in association with the most severe form of PCOS, ovarian hyperthecosis. Overall, it is much more common to observe

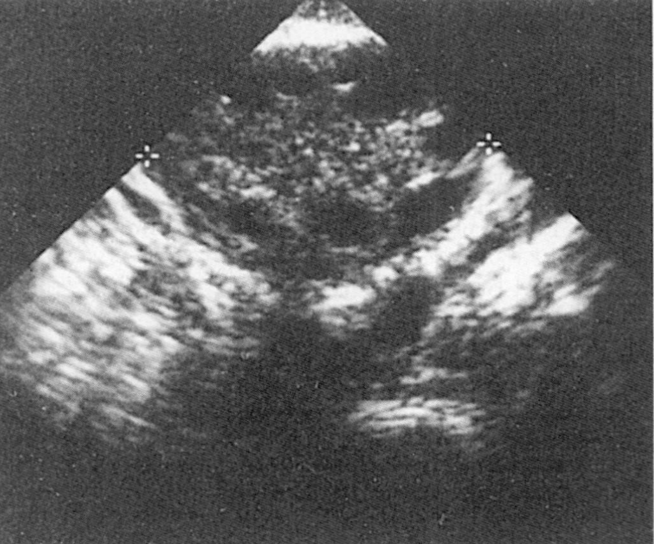

Figure 17-31 Transvaginal ultrasound image of a polycystic ovary. Notice the multiple, midsized follicles in the periphery and the increased solid area in the middle. (From Franks S. Medical progress: polycystic ovary syndrome. *N Engl J Med.* 1995;333:853-861.)

TABLE 17-6

Criteria for the Definition of PCOS

NIH Statement (1990)[253]
To include all of the following: 1. Hyperandrogenism and/or hyperandrogenemia 2. Oligo-ovulation 3. Exclusion of related disorders*
ESHRE/ASRM Statement (Rotterdam, 2003)[254]
To include two of the following, in addition to exclusion of related disorders*: 1. Oligo-ovulation or anovulation (e.g., amenorrhea, irregular uterine bleeding) 2. Clinical and/or biochemical signs of hyperandrogenism (e.g., hirsutism, elevated serum total or free testosterone) 3. Polycystic ovaries (by ultrasonography)
AES Suggested Criteria for the Diagnosis of PCOS (2006)[255]
To include all of the following: 1. Hyperandrogenism: hirsutism and/or hyperandrogenemia 2. Ovarian dysfunction: oligo-anovulation and/or polycystic ovaries 3. Exclusion of other androgen excess or related disorders*

*Including but not limited to 21-hydroxylase-deficient nonclassic adrenal hyperplasia, thyroid dysfunction, hyperprolactinemia, neoplastic androgen secretion, drug-induced androgen excess, the syndromes of severe insulin resistance, Cushing's syndrome, and glucocorticoid resistance.

NIH, National Institutes of Health; ESHRE, European Society for Human Reproduction and Embryology; ASRM, American Society for Reproductive Medicine; AES, Androgen Excess Society.

high-normal levels or borderline elevations of testosterone in women with PCOS.

Prolactin and TSH concentrations should be measured routinely to rule out mild androgen excess and anovulation that may be associated with hyperprolactinemia. If basal LH levels are used as a marker for PCOS, a significant number of patients will slip through the cracks because they do not manifest elevated LH levels or increased LH/FSH ratios. The NIH-sponsored consensus conference on diagnostic criteria for PCOS in 1990 recommended that LH and the LH/FSH ratio are not required for the diagnosis of PCOS.[253,257] The heterogeneity of LH values in PCOS may be caused by the pulsatile nature of LH secretion and negative effects of obesity on LH levels. An elevated LH/FSH ratio supports the diagnosis of PCOS and may be useful in differentiating mild cases of nonobese PCOS without prominent androgen excess from hypothalamic anovulation. However, failure to exhibit an elevated LH level is of no diagnostic value. By definition, nonclassic adrenal hyperplasia does not manifest as congenital virilization of external genitalia. Hyperandrogenic symptoms most commonly appear peripubertally or postpubertally. The clinical evaluation and laboratory-based diagnosis of nonclassic adrenal hyperplasia was discussed earlier. Chapters 15 describes the ACTH stimulation test. A screening test for Cushing's syndrome or glucocorticoid resistance should be performed as clinically indicated (see Chapter 15).

Serum DHEAS levels may be increased (up to 8 μg/mL) in about 50% of anovulatory women with PCOS. DHEAS originates almost exclusively from the adrenal.[258] The cause of adrenal hyperactivity in PCOS is unknown. Obtaining a DHEAS level routinely in a patient with PCOS is not recommended because it does not change the diagnosis or management. If an adrenal tumor is suspected, a DHEAS level should be obtained. DHEAS levels higher than 8 μg/mL may be associated with steroidogenically active adrenal tumors, and imaging is then indicated.

The Rotterdam 2003 criteria include the use of ultrasound as a diagnostic tool. The use of ultrasonography in the diagnosis of PCOS must be tempered by an awareness of the broad spectrum of women with ultrasonographic findings characteristic of polycystic ovaries. The typical polycystic-appearing ovary emerges in a nonspecific fashion when a state of anovulation persists for any length of time (see Fig. 17-31). About 75% of a cross-section of all anovulatory women will have polycystic-appearing ovaries as determined by ultrasonography.[259] There are numerous causes of anovulation, and there are numerous reasons for polycystic ovaries. A similar clinical picture and ovarian condition can reflect any of the dysfunctional states discussed previously. The polycystic-appearing ovary is the result of a functional derangement but not a specific central or local defect.

Biochemical evidence of insulin resistance or glucose intolerance is not necessary for the diagnosis of PCOS. Nonetheless, glucose intolerance should be investigated. Plasma glucose levels should be measured after a 75-g glucose load as a screen for glucose intolerance.

Women with PCOS commonly present with irregular uterine bleeding in the form of infrequent periods (i.e., oligomenorrhea) or amenorrhea. It is not necessary to document anovulation by ultrasonography, progesterone levels, or otherwise, especially if menstrual cycles are irregular with periods of amenorrhea. To confirm the diagnosis of chronic anovulation and unopposed estrogen exposure, most clinicians perform a progestin challenge test after a negative urine pregnancy test. Because endometrium is exposed to estradiol chronically in PCOS, these women respond to a challenge with a progestin (e.g., 5 mg/day of MPA given orally for 10 days) by uterine bleeding within a few days after the last pill of progestin. Reasons for lack of uterine bleeding after a progestin challenge include pregnancy, insufficient prior estrogen exposure of the endometrium, or an anatomic defect. If uterine bleeding does not follow progestin challenge, pregnancy should be ruled out again, along with other causes of chronic anovulation, as described in this chapter. An anatomic defect such as intrauterine adhesions may be ruled out with a hysterosalpingogram or hysteroscopy.

During the initial workup, an endometrial biopsy specimen should be obtained with the use of a plastic minisuction cannula (e.g., Pipelle) in the physician's office. If chronic anovulation persists, endometrial biopsies should be repeated periodically. Pregnancy should be ruled out by a urine or serum pregnancy test before each biopsy. Response to oral contraceptives or periodic progestin treatment with predictable withdrawal bleeding episodes is reassuring, and patients with predictable bleeding patterns do not need endometrial sampling during these treatments. In untreated patients, the risk of endometrial hyperplasia and malignancy is significantly increased even in young women with PCOS because of unopposed estrogen exposure.

Gonadotropin Production in Polycystic Ovary Syndrome

Women with PCOS have higher mean concentrations of LH but low or low-normal levels of FSH compared with levels found in normal women in the early follicular phase.[260] The elevated LH levels partly reflect increased sensitivity of the pituitary to GnRH stimulation, manifested by increases in LH pulse frequency and LH pulse amplitude.[261-263] An increased level of LH bioactivity accompanies high levels of LH in women with PCOS.[262]

The elevated LH levels in PCOS are presumed to be primarily caused by accelerated GnRH-LH pulsatile activity.[263] Central opioid tone appears to be suppressed because the pattern of LH secretion does not change in response to naloxone.[264] The enhanced pulsatile secretion of GnRH has been attributed to a reduction in hypothalamic opioid inhibition caused by the chronic absence of progesterone.[183] An increase in amplitude and frequency of LH secretion also correlates with steady-state levels of circulating estrogen.

In obese women with PCOS, LH levels may not be increased. The increase in LH pulse frequency is characteristic of the anovulatory state regardless of body fat content.[265] LH pulse amplitude, however, is comparatively normal in overweight women with PCOS, whereas it is increased in nonobese women with PCOS.[266] The overall LH reduction in obese women with PCOS may result from factors other than changes in LH pulse amplitude.[267] A low LH value does not rule out the diagnosis of PCOS, whereas a high LH/FSH ratio supports this diagnosis in an anovulatory woman.

Insulin has been implicated as a potential regulator of LH secretion in PCOS. Insulin enhances the transcription of the LH-β gene (*LHB*).[268,269] This laboratory observation was supported by an in vivo human study showing that insulin infusion suppresses pituitary response to GnRH in normal women and in women with PCOS.[270] These studies support the concept that insulin resistance or hyperinsulinemia may be responsible for abnormal gonadotropin release.

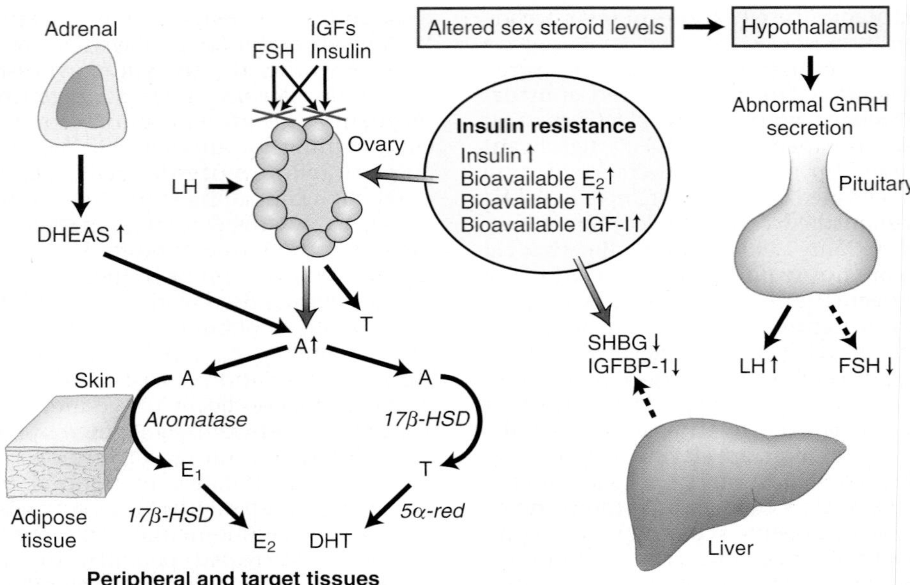

Figure 17-32 Pathologic mechanisms in polycystic ovary syndrome (PCOS). A deficient in vivo response of the ovarian follicle to physiologic quantities of follicle-stimulating hormone (FSH), possibly because of an impaired interaction between signaling pathways associated with FSH and insulin-like growth factors (IGFs) or insulin, may be an important defect responsible for anovulation in PCOS. Insulin resistance associated with increased circulating and tissue levels of insulin and bioavailable estradiol (E_2), testosterone (T), and IGF1 gives rise to abnormal hormone production in a number of tissues. Oversecretion of luteinizing hormone (LH) and decreased output of FSH by the pituitary, decreased production of sex hormone–binding globulin (SHBG) and IGF-binding protein 1 (IGFBP-1) in the liver, increased adrenal secretion of dehydroepiandrosterone sulfate (DHEAS), and increased ovarian secretion of androstenedione (A) all contribute to the feed-forward cycle that maintains anovulation and androgen excess in PCOS. Excessive amounts of E_2 and T arise primarily from the conversion of A in peripheral and target tissues. T is converted to the potent steroids estradiol or DHT (dihydrotestosterone). Reductive 17β-hydroxysteroid dehydrogenase (17β-HSD) enzyme activity may be conferred by protein products of several genes with overlapping functions; 5α-reductase (5α-red) is encoded by at least two genes, and aromatase is encoded by a single gene. GnRH, gonadotropin-releasing hormone.

Steroid Production in Polycystic Ovary Syndrome

Ovulatory cycles are characterized by cyclic fluctuating hormone levels that regulate ovulation and menses (see Fig. 17-1A). Anovulation in women with PCOS is associated with steady-state levels of gonadotropins and ovarian steroids. In patients with persistent anovulation, the average daily production of estrogen and androgens is increased and depends on LH stimulation (Fig. 17-32).[271] This is reflected in higher circulating levels of testosterone, androstenedione, DHEA, DHEAS, 17-hydroxyprogesterone, and estrone.[272] Testosterone, androstenedione, and DHEA are secreted directly by the ovary, whereas DHEAS, which is elevated in about 50% of anovulatory women with PCOS, is almost exclusively an adrenal contribution.[258] Circulating levels of androstenedione, secreted by polycystic ovaries, are particularly high.

Estrone arises primarily from peripheral aromatization of androstenedione and in part from ovarian secretion (Fig. 17-33).[272] Estrone is not a potent estrogen but can be viewed as a precursor that must be converted to estradiol to exert full estrogenic action. The presence of a number of reductive 17β-HSD isoenzymes with overlapping activities that catalyze the conversion of estrone to estradiol in peripheral (extraovarian) tissues is in part responsible for maintaining estradiol production in women with PCOS.[131,272] Increased androstenedione leads to a detectable increase in circulating levels of estradiol in women with PCOS compared with the levels measured during the first few days of an ovulatory cycle. This occurs through aromatase and 17β-HSD activities in extraovarian tissues such

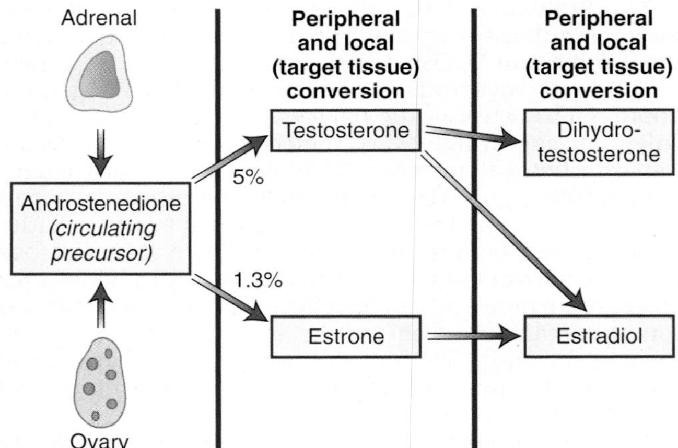

Figure 17-33 Extraovarian conversion of androstenedione to androgen and estrogen. Androstenedione of adrenal or ovarian origin, or both, acts as a dual precursor for androgen and estrogen. Approximately 5% of circulating androstenedione is converted to circulating testosterone, and approximately 1.3% of circulating androstenedione is converted to circulating estrone in peripheral tissues. Testosterone and estrone are further converted to biologically potent steroids, dihydrotestosterone and estradiol, in peripheral and target tissues. Biologically active amounts of estradiol in serum are measured in picograms per milliliter (pg/mL, or pmol/L), whereas biologically active levels of testosterone in serum are measured in nanograms per milliliter (ng/mL, or nmol/L). The 1.3% conversion of normal quantities of androstenedione to estrone may have a critical biologic impact in settings such as postmenopausal endometrial or breast cancer. Significant androgen excess is observed in conditions with abnormally increased androstenedione formation (e.g., polycystic ovary syndrome).

as skin and subcutaneous adipose tissue. Local conversion of estrone to estradiol is an important physiologic process for certain estrogen target tissues, such as disease-free breast and genital skin. Local conversion also can promote the growth of pathologic estrogen-dependent tissues, such as breast cancer and endometriosis (see Fig. 17-33).[122,131,273-275]

Androstenedione of ovarian origin is the most strikingly elevated steroid in PCOS. Androstenedione is not biologically active but serves as a dual precursor for androgen (i.e., testosterone that is further converted to the biologically far stronger androgen DHT) and estrogen (i.e., estrone that is further converted to biologically active estradiol in target tissues).[120] Estradiol is an extremely potent steroid. Biologically effective circulating levels of estradiol are measured in units of picograms per milliliter (pg/mL) or picomoles per liter (pmol/L); biologically effective levels of testosterone are measured in units of nanograms per milliliter (ng/mL) or nanomoles per liter (nmol/L) and circulate at 10 to 100 times the physiologic levels of estradiol. Even small rates of conversion of androstenedione to estrone may have a significant biologic impact, whereas markedly elevated production of androstenedione is required to produce significant amounts of testosterone and manifestations of androgen excess (see Fig. 17-33). Because elevated production of androstenedione does occur in PCOS, extraovarian production of testosterone is biologically significant in this disease. In postmenopausal women, who have much lower levels of androstenedione, extraovarian production of testosterone is less important. Relatively small quantities of estrone (and estradiol) produced primarily by peripheral aromatization of androstenedione have a biologic impact in men and postmenopausal women.[120]

Production of Sex Hormone–Binding Globulin in Polycystic Ovary Syndrome

SHBG binds testosterone and estradiol and decreases the biologic activities of these critical steroids. In PCOS, the net production of androgen and estrogen is increased. Amplified estrogenic and androgenic effects in PCOS also are caused by a decreased SHBG concentration, giving rise to increased free or biologically active quantities of estradiol and testosterone (see Fig. 17-32). The levels of SHBG are controlled by a balance of hormonal influences on its synthesis in the liver. Testosterone and insulin inhibit, whereas estrogen and T_4 stimulate SHBG formation.[276] In anovulatory women with PCOS, circulating levels of SHBG are reduced by approximately 50%; this may be a hepatic response to increased circulating levels of testosterone and insulin (see Fig. 17-32).[276] Circulating free estradiol and testosterone levels are increased because of the significant decrease in SHBG in patients with PCOS.

Three mechanisms contribute to the increased quantities of biologically available estradiol in PCOS: increased production of estradiol from estrone in peripheral (extraovarian) tissues, which gives rise to increased levels of circulating estradiol; increased, biologically available circulating estradiol levels due to decreased SHBG concentrations; and local conversion of estrone to estradiol at target tissues.[274] The local conversion mechanism is likely to be physiologically significant in estrogen targets such as the breast that proliferate in response to estrogen and in the central nervous system, which produces GnRH and gonadotropins under feedback regulation by estrogen (see Fig. 17-32).

In addition to giving rise to increased biologically available estradiol, decreased serum levels of SHBG cause elevations in biologically available free testosterone levels. Testosterone decreases serum SHBG levels, giving rise to a vicious feedback circle favoring low SHBG and high bioavailable testosterone levels (see Fig. 17-32). Insulin directly decreases serum SHBG concentrations in women with PCOS independent of any action of sex steroids.[276] Insulin increases free testosterone levels in PCOS by two mechanisms: increasing ovarian secretion of testosterone precursors (e.g., androstenedione) and suppressing SHBG.[276]

Follicular Fate in Polycystic Ovary Syndrome

Under the influence of relatively low but constant levels of FSH, follicular growth is continuously stimulated, although not to the point of full maturation and ovulation.[277] Despite the fact that full growth potential is not realized, the follicular life span may be extended by several months in the form of multiple follicular cysts. Most of these follicles in polycystic ovaries are 2 to 10 mm in diameter, and some can be as large as 15 mm. Hyperplastic theca cells, often luteinized in response to the high LH levels, surround these follicles (see Fig. 17-29). The accumulation of follicles arrested at various stages of development allows increased and relatively constant production of steroids in response to steady-state levels of gonadotropins.

These follicles are subject to atresia and are replaced by new follicles of similar limited growth potential. Steady-state turnover of stromal cells contributes to the stromal compartment of the ovary, and it is sustained by tissue derived from follicular atresia. A degenerating granulosa compartment, leaving the theca cells to contribute to the stromal compartment of the ovary, accompanies atresia (see Fig. 17-29). This functioning stromal tissue secretes significant amounts of androstenedione under the influence of increased LH. Androstenedione, by the mechanisms discussed previously, leads to increases in free testosterone and free estradiol levels and decreases in SHBG concentrations (see Fig. 17-32). From the point of view of steroidogenesis and steroid action, PCOS is the result of a complex vicious circle that includes a number of positive and negative feedback mechanisms.

Figure 17-32 summarizes the postulated mechanisms underlying PCOS. Because FSH and insulin or IGFs can synergize, it was postulated that this synergy does not occur in the presence of insulin resistance and might lead to relative resistance of the ovarian follicle to FSH. However, in vitro studies do not support this view. Cultured granulosa cells obtained from the small follicles of polycystic ovaries produce negligible amounts of estradiol but show a dramatic increase in estrogen production when FSH or IGF1 is added to the culture medium. When FSH and IGF1 were added together in vitro, they synergized to increase estrogen biosynthesis in granulosa cells from polycystic ovaries.[278]

Induction of ovulation in PCOS is achieved by increasing FSH levels that are hypothesized to overcome this postulated in vivo block to FSH at the granulosa cell level. Two popular treatments, oral clomiphene citrate and injectable recombinant FSH, can provide increased levels of endogenous or exogenous FSH that may lead to ovulation at various doses. Some PCOS patients require large doses of clomiphene citrate or FSH to achieve ovulation. Paradoxically, the polycystic ovary may overreact to pharmacologic levels of FSH by recruiting a large number of developing follicles at once; this occasionally gives rise to the ovarian hyperstimulation syndrome (discussed later).[279] The therapeutic window between ovarian nonresponsiveness and hyperreactivity is usually narrow. There are significant gaps of knowledge that do not permit reconciliation of clinical postulates with in vitro and in vivo findings related to the pathophysiology of PCOS.

Ovarian Hyperthecosis

Ovarian hyperthecosis is a severe variant of PCOS. The term refers to significantly increased stromal tissue with luteinized theca-like cells scattered throughout large sheets of fibroblast-like cells. The clinical and histologic findings represent an exaggerated version of PCOS.[280] This diagnosis can be made on clinical grounds; an ovarian biopsy is not necessary except to rule out an ovarian tumor.

Increased androgen production leads to the clinical picture of more intense androgenization. The higher testosterone levels may also lower LH levels by blocking estrogen action at the hypothalamic-pituitary level.[267] Hyperthecosis seems to be an exaggerated version of the same process that gives rise to chronic anovulation in PCOS. The severity of hyperthecosis correlates with the degree of insulin resistance.[267] Because insulin and IGF1 stimulate proliferation of thecal interstitial cells, hyperinsulinemia may be an important pathophysiologic factor in the cause of hyperthecosis.

It is not uncommon to encounter markedly high levels of testosterone, even above 2 ng/mL, in patients with ovarian hyperthecosis. Virilization is common. These patients usually do not ovulate in response to clomiphene or recombinant FSH. It is usually difficult to suppress testosterone production, even using a GnRH agonist. Bilateral oophorectomy should be a last resort, but it may be necessary to control testosterone production in some of these patients.

Genetics of Polycystic Ovary Syndrome

The strong trend of PCOS to aggregate in families suggests an underlying genetic basis.[281,282] Some key clinical features of PCOS are genetically transmitted. In particular, there is familial aggregation of hyperandrogenemia (with or without oligomenorrhea) in PCOS kindreds, suggesting that it is a genetic trait.[249] Another study showed that hyperinsulinism may be a familial characteristic in daughters of women with PCOS.[283]

The PCOS phenotype is a consequence of genes and environment. For example, obesity associated with unhealthy lifestyle choices aggravates the PCOS phenotype in genetically susceptible women. The lack of a clearcut phenotype adds further challenge to genetic studies of PCOS. Several genomic loci have been proposed to account for the PCOS phenotype. These include *CYP11A1*, the insulin gene, and the follistatin gene; however, no convincing evidence regarding any of these loci has been published.[284] Although independent studies identified a dinucleotide repeat marker near the insulin receptor gene that maps to chromosome 19p13.2, the particular PCOS gene in this locus has not been isolated.[285]

Insulin Resistance and Polycystic Ovary Syndrome

Insulin resistance is a major factor in the pathogenesis of non–insulin-dependent diabetes mellitus (NIDDM). The term *insulin resistance* can be defined as impaired whole-body insulin-mediated glucose disposal, as determined with the use of techniques such as the hyperinsulinemic glucose clamp technique.[142] Insulin resistance is defined clinically as the inability of a known quantity of exogenous or endogenous insulin to increase glucose uptake and use in an affected individual as much as it does in a normal person. Insulin resistance is frequently observed in lean and obese women with PCOS. More severe degrees of insulin resistance or impaired glucose tolerance are more common in obese women with PCOS.[142]

The association between a disorder of carbohydrate metabolism and androgen excess was first described in 1921 by Archard and Thiers and was called the "diabetes of bearded women." Since then, the association between PCOS and insulin resistance or impaired glucose tolerance has been well recognized.[142] This clinical association of insulin resistance and anovulatory hyperandrogenism is commonly found throughout the world and among different ethnic groups.[286] Androgen excess and insulin resistance are often associated with acanthosis nigricans. Acanthosis nigricans is a gray-brown, velvety discoloration and increased thickness of the skin, usually seen at the neck, groin, and axillae and under the breasts; it is a marker for insulin resistance (see Fig. 17-30). Hyperkeratosis and papillomatosis are the histologic characteristics of acanthosis nigricans. Acanthosis nigricans in hyperandrogenic women depends on the presence and severity of hyperinsulinemia and insulin resistance.[287] The mechanism responsible for the development of acanthosis nigricans is uncertain. This abnormal growth response of the skin may be mediated through receptors for various growth factors, including those for insulin and IGF1. Acanthosis nigricans is not specific for insulin resistance because it can be observed in the absence of insulin resistance or androgen excess.

Insulin resistance is characterized by an impaired glucose response to a specific amount of insulin. In many of these patients, normal glucose levels are maintained at the expense of increased circulating insulin to overcome the underlying defect. More severe forms of insulin resistance in PCOS range from impaired glucose tolerance to frank NIDDM. Resistance to insulin-stimulated glucose uptake is a relatively common phenomenon in the general population and is sometimes referred to as *syndrome X* or *dysmetabolic syndrome*. The fundamental abnormality leading to the manifestations that make up the metabolic syndrome is resistance to insulin-mediated glucose uptake in muscle and increased lipolysis, which produces elevated levels of circulating free fatty acids.[288] These individuals also have dyslipidemia, hypertension, and increased risk of developing CVD. Not surprisingly, the incidences of dyslipidemia and cardiovascular risk are increased significantly in women with PCOS.[289,290] The incidence of hypertension increases significantly after menopause in women with a history of PCOS.[142] There is a significant clinical and pathologic overlap between the metabolic syndrome and PCOS.[291]

The clinical presentation of patients with insulin resistance depends on the ability of the pancreas to compensate for the target tissue resistance to insulin. During the first stages of this condition, compensation is effective, and the only metabolic abnormality is hyperinsulinemia. In many patients, the beta cells of the pancreas eventually fail to meet the challenge, and declining insulin levels lead to impaired glucose tolerance and eventually to frank diabetes mellitus. Beta cell dysfunction is demonstrable in women with PCOS before the onset of glucose intolerance.[292]

Studies of well-characterized causes of hyperinsulinemia and androgen excess have illuminated various mechanisms of insulin resistance. Factors such as a decrease in insulin binding related to autoantibodies to insulin receptors, postreceptor defects, and a decrease in insulin receptor sites in target tissues are all involved in insulin resistance.[293] These rare syndromes are found in an extremely small portion of women with anovulation, androgen excess, and insulin resistance, leaving most PCOS patients without any demonstrable abnormalities in the number or quality of receptors or in antibody formation. The exact nature of insulin resistance in most women with PCOS is not well understood.

To understand the molecular defect underlying insulin resistance in PCOS, Dunaif and coworkers studied the differences between skin fibroblasts from women with and without PCOS with respect to insulin-dependent signal transduction.[142] The fibroblasts of women with PCOS showed no change in insulin binding or receptor affinity, but a postreceptor defect was observed in one half of the women with PCOS.[142] This defect is characterized by increased basal insulin receptor serine phosphorylation and a decreased in insulin-dependent tyrosine phosphorylation of the insulin receptor.[142] At about the same time, Miller and coworkers evaluated whether post-translational modification of the product of the *CYP17A1* gene alters the ratio of its hydroxylase to lyase activity; they found that serine phosphorylation of CYP17A1 dramatically increases the enzyme's 17,20-lyase but not its 17α-hydroxylase activity. These observations led the investigators to hypothesize that a dominantly inherited kinase (or kinases) phosphorylates serine residues at the insulin receptor-β and CYP17A1 product, leading to insulin resistance and increased androgen production, respectively. The cause of this abnormal phosphorylation pattern and consequences for insulin action and androgen production are important topics for further study.[294]

Within the context of a unified hypothesis, insulin resistance seems to be a critical defect that explains most of the endocrine abnormalities observed in PCOS (see Fig. 17-32). Insulin resistance is associated with abnormal responses of the ovarian follicle to FSH, which lead to anovulation and androgen secretion. This results in noncyclic formation of estrogen from androgens in peripheral tissues. Estradiol together with elevated androgen and insulin levels gives rise to abnormal gonadotropin secretion. This creates an anovulatory state favoring continuous formation of LH, steroid precursors, androgen, and estrogen (see Fig. 17-32).

Role of Obesity in Insulin Resistance and Anovulation. Increased waist-to-hip ratio compounded by significantly increased body mass index is called *android obesity* because this type of adipose tissue distribution is observed more commonly in men. Overweight women with anovulatory androgen excess commonly have this particular body fat distribution.[295] Android obesity is the result of fat deposition in the abdominal wall and in visceral mesenteric locations. This fat is more sensitive to catecholamines, less sensitive to insulin, and more active metabolically. Android obesity is associated with insulin resistance, glucose intolerance, diabetes mellitus, and an increase in androgen production rate and results in decreased levels of SHBG and increased levels of free testosterone and estradiol.[295] Android obesity is associated significantly with cardiovascular risk factors, including hypertension and dyslipidemia, and it has been tied to a notable increase in the risk of poor-prognosis breast cancer.[296,297] However, no direct association has been reported between PCOS and breast cancer risk.[298]

Although the combination of insulin resistance and androgen excess is often observed in obese women overall, women with android-type obesity appear to be at a significantly higher risk for insulin resistance and androgen excess. However, insulin resistance and androgen excess are not confined to obese anovulatory women but also occur in nonobese anovulatory women.[265] Although obesity by itself causes insulin resistance, the combination of insulin resistance and androgen excess is a specific feature of PCOS. Not surprisingly, the combination of obesity and PCOS is associated with more severe degrees of insulin resistance than those found in nonobese women with PCOS.[265,299] Android-type obesity, in contrast to general obesity, is a more specific risk factor for PCOS.

Diagnosis of Insulin Resistance. In everyday clinical practice, the criteria for diagnosing insulin resistance in an individual patient have not been standardized and present extremely complex issues. One fourth of the normal population has fasting and glucose-stimulated insulin levels that overlap with those of insulin-resistant individuals because of the great variability of insulin sensitivity in normal subjects.[142] Clinically available measures of insulin action, such as fasting or glucose-stimulated insulin levels, do not correlate well with more detailed measurements of insulin sensitivity in research settings.

In view of these constraints, it is reasonable to consider all women with PCOS at risk for insulin resistance and the associated abnormalities of the metabolic syndrome—dyslipidemia, hypertension, and CVD.[291] A lipid profile should be obtained in all cases of PCOS. Especially for obese women with PCOS, fasting glucose levels and glucose levels 2 hours after a 75-g glucose load should be obtained as a screen for glucose intolerance. The clinician should encourage the patient to take every possible measure (e.g., weight reduction, exercise) to reduce insulin resistance.

Use of Antidiabetic Drugs to Treat Anovulation and Androgen Excess. A logical approach to the management of PCOS includes using medications that improve insulin sensitivity in target tissues, achieving reductions in insulin secretion, and stabilizing glucose tolerance. The antidiabetic medication metformin (a biguanide) and the thiazolidinediones pioglitazone and rosiglitazone have been used to reduce insulin resistance. Although metformin appears to influence ovarian steroidogenesis directly, this effect does not appear to be primarily responsible for the attenuation of ovarian androgen production in women with PCOS. Rather, metformin inhibits the output of hepatic glucose, necessitating a lower insulin concentration and thereby probably reducing androgen production by theca cells.[300]

Metformin at a dose of 500 mg three times daily reduced hyperinsulinemia, basal and stimulated levels of LH, and free testosterone concentrations in overweight women with PCOS.[301,302] Some anovulatory women ovulated and achieved pregnancy; however, clomiphene is superior to metformin in achieving live births in infertile women with PCOS.[303-305] Among published studies of metformin use in women with PCOS, subject characteristics and control measures for effects of weight change, dose of metformin, and outcome vary widely. A meta-analysis of 13 studies in which metformin was administered to 543 participants reported that patients taking metformin had an odds ratio for ovulation of 3.88 (95% confidence interval [CI], 2.25 to 6.69) compared with placebo and an odds ratio for ovulation of 4.41 (95% CI, 2.37 to 8.22) for metformin plus clomiphene compared with clomiphene alone.[306] Although the addition of metformin to clomiphene seems to increase the ovulation rate, it does not result in a higher rate of live births.[304] Metformin also improved fasting insulin levels, blood pressure, and levels of LDL-cholesterol. These effects were judged to be independent of any changes in weight that were associated with metformin, but controversy persists about whether the beneficial effects of metformin are entirely independent of the weight loss that is typically seen early in the course of therapy.[305,306]

The thiazolidinediones are pharmacologic ligands for the nuclear receptor peroxisome proliferator-activated receptor-γ (PPARγ). They improve the action of insulin in the liver, skeletal muscle, and adipose tissue and have only a modest effect on hepatic glucose output. As with metformin, the thiazolidinediones are reported to affect ovarian steroid synthesis directly, although most evidence indicates that the reduction in insulin levels is responsible for decreased concentrations of circulating androgen.[300]

Women with PCOS who took troglitazone had consistent improvements in insulin resistance, pancreatic beta cell function, hyperandrogenemia, and glucose tolerance.[307,308] In a double-blind, randomized, placebo-controlled study, ovulation was significantly greater for women with PCOS who received troglitazone than for those who received placebo; free testosterone levels decreased, and levels of SHBG increased in a dose-dependent fashion.[309] Although troglitazone is no longer available because of its hepatotoxicity, subsequent studies using rosiglitazone and pioglitazone had similar results.[310-312] Because of concern about the use of thiazolidinediones in pregnancy and recent evidence linking these drugs to serious side effects such as heart failure and stroke, they have been less readily adopted for routine treatment of PCOS. The success of the strategy of reversing insulin resistance as a way to correct the critical abnormalities in PCOS argues for this defect as central to the pathogenesis of the disorder.

Management of Long-Term Deleterious Effects of Polycystic Ovary Syndrome

The long-term consequences of PCOS include irregular uterine bleeding, anovulatory infertility, androgen excess, chronically elevated levels of free estrogen associated with an increased risk of endometrial cancer, and insulin resistance associated with an increased risk of CVD and diabetes mellitus. Treatment must aid in achieving a healthy lifestyle and normal body weight, protect the endometrium from the effects of unopposed estrogen, and reduce testosterone levels.

Any woman with PCOS should be counseled to maintain a healthy lifestyle. In obese PCOS women, permanent lifestyle modification should be emphasized as the primary preventive measure to minimize short-term and long-term deleterious effects. Simple measures such as decreasing daily food intake by 500 kcal and introducing any type of moderate exercise for 30 minutes daily for 6 months can decrease hyperandrogenemia and diastolic blood pressure.[246] Because insulin resistance contributes to the abnormal lipid profile and increased cardiovascular risk in women with PCOS, weight loss is a high priority for patients who are overweight.[313] Insulin resistance and androgen excess can be reduced with a weight reduction of at least 5%.[314,315] Significant weight loss has also resulted in ovulation and pregnancy in a number of patients with PCOS.[316] Nutritional counseling and an emphasis on lifestyle changes are essential components of the long-term management of PCOS.

If the patient does not wish to become pregnant, medical therapy is directed toward the interruption of the effect of unopposed estrogen on the endometrium. Nonfluctuating levels of unopposed estradiol in the absence of progesterone cause irregular uterine bleeding, amenorrhea, and infertility and increase the risk of endometrial cancer. Anovulatory women with PCOS may have endometrial cancer even in their early 20s.[317] Endometrial biopsy should be performed periodically in untreated women with PCOS regardless of age. Pregnancy should be ruled out before each endometrial biopsy. The uterine bleeding pattern should not influence the decision to perform an endometrial biopsy. The presence of amenorrhea does not rule out endometrial hyperplasia. The critical factor that determines the risk of endometrial neoplasia is the duration of anovulation and exposure to unopposed estradiol. Long-term treatment with a progestin or oral contraceptive significantly decreases the risk of endometrial cancer.

One of the simplest and most effective ways to administer a progestin in the long term is to use an oral contraceptive. Oral contraceptives provide two additional benefits: reduction of androgen excess and contraception. Oral contraceptive pills reduce circulating androgen levels through suppression of circulating LH and stimulation of SHBG levels, and they have been shown to reduce hirsutism in hyperandrogenic patients.[148] Oral contraceptive treatment for anovulation and hyperinsulinemia in women with androgen excess does not increase cardiovascular risk.[318-320]

For the patient who does not complain of hirsutism but is anovulatory and has irregular bleeding, treatment with a single progestin may be attempted as an alternative to oral contraceptive use. Progestin therapy is directed toward interruption of the chronic exposure of endometrium to unopposed effects of estrogen. MPA may be administered intermittently (e.g., 5 mg daily for the first 10 days of every month) to ensure withdrawal bleeding and prevent endometrial hyperplasia. This treatment does not decrease androgen excess, nor does it provide contraception. Because newer oral contraceptives (with an ethinyl estradiol content of 30 μg or less and a new progestin) suppress androgen excess of ovarian origin, provide contraception, protect the endometrium, and do not increase insulin resistance, a low-dose oral contraceptive is the treatment of choice for nonsmokers with PCOS. An oral contraceptive together with the antiandrogen spirolactone (100 mg/day) is the recommended starting treatment for a hirsute woman with PCOS. The dose of spironolactone can be increased in increments to suppress hair growth, as described earlier.

Treatment with an oral contraceptive, with or without spironolactone, may not be effective in androgen suppression in severe cases of PCOS. In patients resistant to oral contraceptives, suppression of the ovary with a GnRH agonist may be required. Because glucocorticoids increase insulin resistance, they should be used with caution in patients with hyperinsulinemia. Spironolactone does not affect insulin sensitivity in anovulatory women and can be used safely without causing adverse effects on carbohydrate or lipid metabolism.[321]

The clinician must counsel women with PCOS regarding their increased risk of future diabetes mellitus. The age at onset of NIDDM is significantly earlier in these women than in the general population.[247] Women with PCOS are more likely to experience gestational diabetes.[322] Long-term follow-up studies have shown a significantly increased risk for frank diabetes mellitus in anovulatory patients with PCOS.[142] It is therefore important to monitor glucose tolerance with periodic measurements of glucose levels after fasting and after a 75-g glucose load. The place of insulin sensitizers, such as metformin and thiazolidinediones, in the long-term treatment of PCOS remains to be determined by data from future large clinical trials.[305,307,308,323]

The physician should alert the patient with PCOS that up to one half of first-degree relatives and sisters may be affected by PCOS or at least by androgen excess in the presence of regular menses.[249] These individuals may be at higher than average risk for CVD and may benefit from preventive measures that reduce this risk.

Ovulation Induction in Polycystic Ovary Syndrome

Clomiphene Citrate. Patient with PCOS who desire pregnancy are candidates for the medical induction of ovulation. When pregnancy is achieved, patients with PCOS appear to have an increased risk of spontaneous miscarriage.[324] This increased risk may be related to elevated levels of LH that may produce an adverse environment for the oocyte and the endometrium. LH levels should be suppressed with oral contraceptives before ovulation is induced. Suppression can be achieved in most patients with PCOS by the use of an oral contraceptive for 4 to 6 weeks before ovulation induction with clomiphene citrate or recombinant FSH.

To induce ovulation in women with PCOS, FSH levels are increased by administration of clomiphene citrate or by injection of recombinant FSH. Presumably, pharmacologic levels of FSH overcome the ovarian defect that is responsible for anovulation in PCOS.

Clomiphene citrate is a nonsteroidal, ovulation-inducing ER ligand with mixed agonistic-antagonistic properties.[325] Acting as an antiestrogen, clomiphene citrate is thought to displace endogenous estrogen from hypothalamic ERs, thereby removing the negative feedback effect exerted by endogenous estrogens. The resultant change in pulsatile GnRH release is thought to normalize the release of pituitary FSH and LH, which is followed by follicular recruitment and selection, assertion of dominance, and ovulation.[325]

Clomiphene citrate treatment can be started at any time in an amenorrheic and anovulatory patient provided that a pregnancy test is performed beforehand (Fig. 17-34). Alternatively, uterine bleeding may be induced after a 10-day treatment with a combination oral contraceptive or MPA (5 mg/day). On cycle day 2 or 3 (day 1 is the first day of uterine bleeding), a baseline ultrasound study is performed to rule out any ovarian follicular cyst of more than 25-mm average diameter. If one or more large cysts are seen, ovulation induction should be delayed until after gonadotropin suppression by continuous oral contraception treatment for 4 to 6 weeks to eliminate these cysts or decrease their size. Clomiphene citrate is started at 50 mg/day orally on day 3 of the cycle and continued for 5 days. Ultrasonography is performed on cycle day 13 or 14 to ensure follicular development (i.e., at least one new follicle measuring at least 16 mm in diameter). The patient should be encouraged to have intercourse every other day during the 10-day period following the last clomiphene citrate dose. Alternatively, measurement of urinary LH to detect an LH surge can be used to time intercourse. Intercourse is recommended on the day of a positive urinary LH peak and on the next day. Intercourse is recommended within 24 to 36 hours after an hCG injection.

If follicular development does not occur after the first course of therapy with clomiphene citrate at 50 mg/day, a second course of 100 mg daily for 5 days may be started. Lack of response at doses of 150 to 200 mg daily for 5 days should be an indication for a change of treatment. Most patients destined to conceive do so with the starting dose of clomiphene citrate (50 mg/day for 5 days). Most clomiphene citrate–initiated conceptions occur within the first 6 ovulatory cycles.[325] The incidence rate for multiple gestation in clomiphene citrate–induced pregnancies is 6% (4% for twins and 2% for triplets).[304] Failure to achieve pregnancy after 3 clomiphene cycles despite sonographic evidence of follicular development should prompt the clinician to perform a comprehensive infertility workup, including a semen analysis and evaluation of the uterine cavity and tubal patency.

Metformin. Head-to-head randomized trials showed that clomiphene alone is clearly superior to metformin only with respect to achieving ovulation and live births in women with PCOS.[304] However, the ovulatory response to clomiphene was increased in obese women with PCOS by decreasing insulin secretion with the addition of metformin.[307,308,323] A later randomized study showed that the higher rate of ovulation in the users of clomiphene plus metformin seemed to be offset by a higher rate of pregnancy losses, producing similar live birth rates in clomiphene-only and clomiphene plus metformin groups.[304] The benefit of the addition of metformin to clomiphene in obese clomiphene-nonresponders with PCOS needs to be assessed further.

Aromatase Inhibitors. Aromatase inhibitors reduce hypothalamic-pituitary estrogen feedback that leads to increased GnRH secretion, concomitant elevations in LH and FSH, and increased ovarian follicular development in premenopausal women.[114,326] The gonadotropin-stimulating aromatase inhibitors letrozole and anastrozole have been used off-label in the treatment of patients with ovulatory dysfunction, such as PCOS, and for increasing the number of ovarian follicles recruited for ovulation in women who are already ovulatory.[326-328] Oral administration of letrozole (2.5 or 5 mg/day) or anastrozole (1 mg/day) on days 3 to

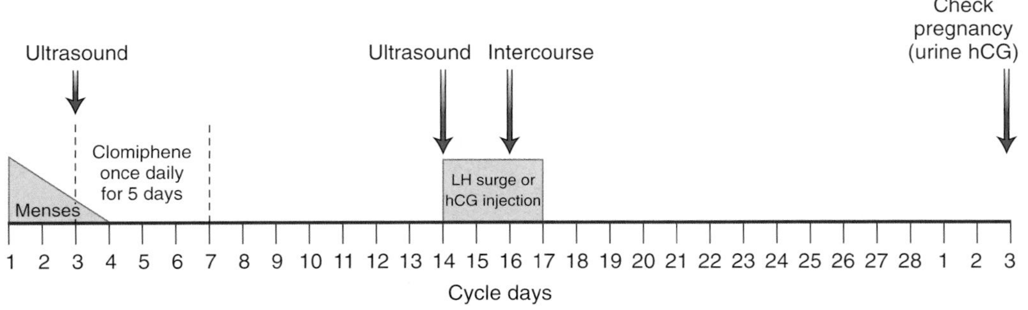

Figure 17-34 Monitoring of clomiphene citrate-initiated ovulation. On cycle day 2 or 3, a baseline ultrasound examination is performed to rule out any large ovarian follicular cyst. Clomiphene citrate is started on day 3 of the cycle and continued for 5 days. Ultrasonography is performed on cycle day 13 or 14 to ensure follicular development. The patient should be encouraged to have intercourse every other day during the 10-day period after the last clomiphene citrate dose. Urinary human chorionic gonadotropin (hCG) levels are checked to determine whether pregnancy has occurred.

7 after uterine bleeding is effective for ovulation induction in women with anovulatory infertility.[328-330] Clomiphene resistance in women with PCOS has been particularly studied as a potential indication for aromatase inhibitors; no difference between anastrozole (1 mg/day) and letrozole (2.5 mg/day) was demonstrated.[328] A head-to-head randomized study did not show any advantage to the use of letrozole (5 mg/daily) over clomiphene citrate (100 mg daily) as first-line treatment for induction of ovulation in women with PCOS.[329] Another randomized study, however, demonstrated that letrozole (2.5 mg/day) and metformin (1500 mg/day) plus clomiphene (150 mg/day) were equally effective for inducing ovulation and achieving pregnancy in patients with clomiphene-resistant PCOS.[330] A retrospective study did not show any difference in the overall rates of major and minor congenital malformations among newborns from mothers who conceived after letrozole or clomiphene treatment.[332] Although worldwide experience with aromatase inhibitors for ovulation induction is increasing, definitive studies in the form of randomized, controlled trials comparing live birth rates and safety associated with clomiphene citrate and an aromatase inhibitor are lacking.[331]

Low-Dose Gonadotropin Therapy. For women who do not ovulate in response to clomiphene citrate, FSH injections are started on day 3 of spontaneous or progestin-induced uterine bleeding. Recombinant FSH is administered subcutaneously starting with a daily dose of 75 IU for up to 10 days, if necessary, and using small incremental dose increases (12.5 to 37.5 IU) from then on at 3- to 7-day intervals until serum estradiol concentrations begin to increase. The dose is then maintained until follicular rupture, which is induced by subcutaneous injection of recombinant hCG (250 µg). Follicular growth is monitored by transvaginal ultrasonography and blood estradiol levels, which serve as biochemical markers for the granulosa cell mass in the growing follicle.[333] This regimen induces development of a single follicle in most cycles and has succeeded in reducing the rate of multiple pregnancies to as low as 6% in some series.[279] The low-dose regimen also practically eliminated the complication of severe ovarian hyperstimulation syndrome (OHSS).[279] Conception rates are comparable to those achieved with conventional therapy. The miscarriage rate remains somewhat higher than that after spontaneous conceptions (20% to 25%).

Conventional-dose gonadotropin therapy (starting FSH dose, 150 IU daily) should not be used as first-line treatment in patients with PCOS because it causes two important complications: an alarming number of multiple pregnancies (14% to 50% of treatment cycles) and a significantly increased risk of severe ovarian hyperstimulation syndrome (1.3% to 9.4% of treatment cycles). Three important complications of gonadotropin therapy in PCOS patients are significantly increased rates of multiple pregnancies, severe ovarian hyperstimulation syndrome, and spontaneous miscarriage.[334]

OHSS is a more common complication of conventional-dose gonadotropin treatment. Milder forms are relatively common and are characterized by weight gain, abdominal discomfort, and enlarged ovaries. Home bedrest and oral intake of fluids are sufficient to manage this form. Severe OHSS occurs in 0.1% to 0.2% of stimulation attempts and is accompanied by severe ascites, pleural effusion, electrolyte imbalance, and hypovolemia with oliguria. The most dreaded complication is deep venous thrombosis and embolism. Its cause is poorly understood. Large number of follicles, peak estradiol levels greater than 2000 pg/mL, and pregnancy are associated with a higher likelihood of OHSS. Prevention includes withholding of hCG injections and intrauterine insemination. Treatment of severe OHSS includes hospitalization, maintenance of fluid and electrolyte balance, prophylaxis of thromboembolism by heparin, and drainage of severe ascites or pleural effusions. Frequently, supportive measures are sufficient to manage this self-limited condition.

Premature Ovarian Insufficiency

Premature ovarian insufficiency, which is defined as early depletion of ovarian follicles (before the age of 40 years), is a state of hypergonadotropic hypogonadism. These patients go through a normal puberty and a variable period of cyclic menses followed by oligomenorrhea or amenorrhea accompanied by hot flashes and urogenital atrophy. Premature ovarian insufficiency should always be included in the differential diagnosis of chronic anovulation. History and physical examination may reveal menstrual irregularity or secondary amenorrhea accompanied by symptoms and signs of estrogen deficiency, such as hot flashes and urogenital atrophy. Elevated FSH levels greater than the 95% CIs of the midcycle gonadotropin peak of the normal menstrual cycle (>40 IU/L) on at least two occasions confirm the diagnosis.[335]

On average, menopause occurs at the age of 50 years, with 1% of women continuing to menstruate beyond the age of 60 years and another 1% whose menopause occurs before 40 years. Premature menopause or ovarian insufficiency has been arbitrarily defined as the cessation of menses before 40 years of age.[336]

The cause or genetic basis of premature ovarian insufficiency is not well understood. Two genetic syndromes associated with premature ovarian insufficiency are gonadal dysgenesis with primarily mosaic X-chromosome defects and *FMR1* gene premutation, a variant of fragile X syndrome.[337] Syndromes resulting from single-gene mutations (e.g., blepharophimosis-ptosis-epicanthus inversus syndrome [*FOXL2* mutation], galactosemia [*GALT* mutation]) may be associated with premature ovarian insufficiency.[337] Despite these observations, the cause of premature ovarian insufficiency remains unknown in most cases.

The underlying ovarian defect may manifest at various ages, depending on the number of functional follicles left in the ovaries. The different symptoms may be regarded as phases in the process of perimenopausal change, regardless of the actual age of the patient. If loss of follicles occurs rapidly before puberty, primary amenorrhea and lack of secondary sexual development ensue. The degree to which the adult phenotype develops and the age at which secondary amenorrhea actually occurs depend on whether follicle loss took place during or after puberty. In cases of primary amenorrhea associated with sexual infantilism, the ovarian remnants exist as streaks, and transvaginal ultrasonography usually cannot detect any ovaries. Many gene defects (e.g., *FSHR, CYP17A1, CYP19A1*) involve ovarian failure at the expected time of puberty, and the phenotypes manifest with primary amenorrhea and lack of secondary sexual development (see Chapter 25).[337]

Premature ovarian insufficiency can result from an autoimmune process, and it is frequently associated with autoimmune polyendocrine syndromes.[338] Other causes of premature insufficiency can be related to the sudden destruction of follicles by chemotherapy, irradiation, or infections such as mumps oophoritis. The effect of irradiation depends on the patient's age and the x-ray dose.[339] Steroid levels begin to fall and gonadotropins rise within

2 weeks after irradiation of the ovaries. Young women exposed to radiation are less likely to have permanent ovarian insufficiency because of the higher number of oocytes present at younger ages. When the radiation field excludes the pelvis or the ovaries are transposed out of the pelvis by laparoscopic surgery before irradiation, there is no risk of premature ovarian insufficiency.[340] Most chemotherapeutic agents used for eradication of malignancies are toxic to the ovaries and cause ovarian insufficiency.[341] Resumption of menses and pregnancy have been reported after radiotherapy or chemotherapy,[342] but premature ovarian insufficiency may occur years after these therapies.[316]

Diagnosis and Management of Premature Ovarian Insufficiency

Premature ovarian insufficiency should be suspected in a woman younger than 40 years of age who presents with amenorrhea, oligomenorrhea, or another form of menstrual irregularity. Menopausal serum FSH levels (40 IU/L) on at least two occasions are sufficient for the diagnosis of premature ovarian insufficiency. These young women can be diagnosed with ovarian insufficiency and infertility if gonadotropin levels are repeatedly elevated.

Case reports of pregnancies in affected women occurring during hormone replacement therapy have been published.[343,344] In particular, young women with premature ovarian insufficiency may experience intermittent periods of ovarian function, with antral follicles present at ovarian ultrasonography and ovulation described in cases that followed up with regular endocrine assessments. A randomized trial of hormone therapy in this setting showed that folliculogenesis occurred often but was less frequently followed by ovulation and even less frequently by pregnancy (up to 14%); conventional-dose estrogen therapy did not improve the rate of folliculogenesis, ovulation, or pregnancy.[335] Later pilot studies or case reports suggested that lowering FSH levels to less than 15 IU/L by use of high-dose estrogen or a GnRH antagonist in young women with premature ovarian insufficiency may trigger ovulation or permit ovulation induction and pregnancy in a small number of patients.[345,346]

The clinician should inform patients diagnosed with premature ovarian insufficiency that there is a small but significant likelihood of spontaneous pregnancy or pregnancy after ovulation induction in the future. Women who desire pregnancy are still best served by assisted reproductive technology employing donor oocytes, because the probability of pregnancy with an autologous egg is low. Use of donor oocytes followed by IVF with the partner's sperm and intrauterine embryo transfer after synchronization of the recipient patient's endometrium with the donor's cycle using exogenous estrogen and progesterone is offered to the patient who wishes to carry a pregnancy in her uterus (see Fig. 17-25). This approach offers an excellent chance of pregnancy (>50% per donor oocyte IVF cycle).

Patients with premature ovarian insufficiency have an increased incidence of an abnormal complement of chromosomes.[347] The risk of having an abnormal karyotype increases with decreasing age at onset of the ovarian insufficiency. A chromosomal analysis is recommended for some of these patients because of the increased risk of a gonadal tumor associated with the presence of a Y chromosome.[348] The arbitrarily chosen age group for chromosomal analysis includes women 30 years of age or younger because it is rare to encounter a gonadal tumor in patients with premature ovarian insufficiency after the age of 30 years.[349]

Mosaicism that includes a Y chromosome has been associated with a high incidence of gonadal tumors.[348] These malignant tumors arise from germ cells and include gonadoblastomas, dysgerminomas, yolk sac tumors, and choriocarcinoma. Secondary virilization in patients with karyotypic abnormalities and premature ovarian insufficiency significantly increases the risk of a dysontogenetic gonadal tumor. The precise risk of a tumor in various subsets of these patients is not well known because a significant number of women carrying a Y chromosome do not have symptoms of virilization. The frequency of Y chromosomal material determined by polymerase chain reaction is high in those with Turner's syndrome (12.2%), but the occurrence of a gonadal tumor among these Y-positive patients seems to be as low as 7% to 10%.[350]

Fragile X–associated disorders are caused by a CGG trinucleotide repeat expansion in the promoter region of the *FMR1* gene. Expansion of the CGG trinucleotide repeats to more than 200 copies induces methylation of the *FMR1* gene, with an outcome of transcriptional silencing.[351] This so-called full mutation was linked to mental retardation or autism. Individuals who carried the premutation (defined as >55 but <200 CGG repeats) have increased FMR1 mRNA levels with decreased levels of fragile X mental retardation protein (FMRP). Convincing evidence relates the *FMR1* premutation to altered ovarian function and loss of fertility.[352] The natural history of the altered ovarian function in women who carry the *FMR1* premutation is still not well understood. Women with premature ovarian failure are at increased risk for an *FMR1* premutation and should be informed of the availability of fragile X testing.

Premature ovarian insufficiency usually occurs as an isolated autoimmune disorder. Rarely, it may be associated with hypothyroidism, diabetes mellitus, hypoadrenalism, hypoparathyroidism, or systemic lupus erythematosus.[353] It can be part of an autoimmune polyendocrine syndrome.[338] Thyroid insufficiency, adrenal insufficiency, and diabetes mellitus are the endocrine disorders most frequently associated with premature ovarian insufficiency.[354] Periodic endocrine testing for glucose intolerance, adrenal or parathyroid function, and autoimmune disease (e.g., systemic lupus erythematosus) should be considered based on the clinical presentation (Table 17-7).

Treatment of premature ovarian insufficiency should be directed toward its specific cause. In most cases, however, it is not possible to identify a specific cause if there are no karyotypic anomalies. Besides infertility, long-term ovarian steroid deficiency has far-reaching health implications. Early menopause has been associated with increased cardiovascular mortality and stroke, bone fracture, and colorectal cancer risks.[337] Despite reduced risks for development of breast cancer, overall quality of life and life expectancy decline with early menopause.[337] Hormone therapy, using combined estrogen and progestin or a low-dose oral

TABLE 17-7

Laboratory Evaluation of Premature Ovarian Insufficiency

Follicle-stimulating hormone (to establish the diagnosis of premature ovarian insufficiency)
Karyotype (<30 yr of age or sexual infantilism)
Testing for *FMR1* gene premutation carrier state
Thyroid-stimulating hormone (hypothyroidism)

FMR1, fragile-X mental retardation 1.

contraceptive, is the cornerstone of the management for these women. The added value of androgen replacement remains uncertain.[337]

DIAGNOSIS AND MANAGEMENT OF ANOVULATORY UTERINE BLEEDING

Acyclic production of estrogen during anovulatory cycles gives rise to irregular shedding of the endometrium. These bleeding manifestations of anovulatory cycles in the absence of uterine pathology or systemic illness are commonly referred to as *dysfunctional uterine bleeding*. Anovulatory uterine bleeding, which is the most common cause of chronic menstrual irregularities, is a diagnosis of exclusion. Pregnancy, uterine leiomyomas, endometrial polyps, and adenomyosis should be ruled out as anatomic causes of irregular uterine bleeding. Malignancies of the vagina, cervix, endometrium, myometrium, fallopian tubes, and ovaries should also be ruled out before a diagnosis of anovulatory uterine bleeding is made. Coagulation abnormalities should be excluded.

Anovulatory uterine bleeding can be managed without surgical intervention by either restoring ovulation or mimicking the ovulatory hormonal profile by providing exogenous steroids. The rationale for use of exogenous steroids is based on the knowledge of predictable responses of the endometrium to estrogen and progesterone. Physiologic responses of the endometrium to natural ovarian steroids have been uncovered by observation of the gross and microscopic changes occurring in the endometrium during thousands of normal ovulatory cycles in humans and other primates.[151,153,355] The pharmacologic application of exogenous estrogens and progestins in women with anovulatory bleeding aims to correct the production of local tissue factors that mediate physiologic steroid action and reverse the excessive and prolonged flow typical of anovulatory cycles.

Clinical management of irregular uterine bleeding with exogenous hormones is a time-honored method, and it has diagnostic value. Failure to control vaginal bleeding with hormonal therapy, despite appropriate application and use, makes the diagnosis of anovulatory uterine bleeding considerably less likely. In such cases, attention is directed to an anatomic pathologic entity within the reproductive axis as the cause of abnormal bleeding.

Heavy but regular menstrual bleeding (i.e., hypermenorrhea) can be encountered in ovulatory women. It may have an anatomic cause, such as a leiomyoma impinging on the endometrial cavity or the diffuse and pathologic presence of benign endometrial glands in the myometrium (i.e., adenomyosis). In the absence of a specific pathologic cause, it is presumed that hypermenorrhea reflects subtle disturbances in the endometrial tissue mechanism. In essentially all cases, evaluation and treatment are identical to the approach detailed in this section.

Characteristics of Normal Menses

Normal menstruation takes place about 14 days after each ovulation episode as a consequence of postovulatory estrogen-progesterone withdrawal. The quantity and duration of bleeding are quite reproducible. This predictability leads many women to expect a certain characteristic flow pattern. Any slight deviations, such as plus or minus 1 day in duration or minor deviation from expected tampon use, are causes for major concern in the patient. Most women of reproductive age can predict the timing of their flows so accurately that even minor variability may require reassurance by the clinician. Although variability of menstrual cycles is a common feature during the teenage years and perimenopausal transition, the characteristics of menstrual bleeding do not undergo appreciable change between ages 20 and 40.[356]

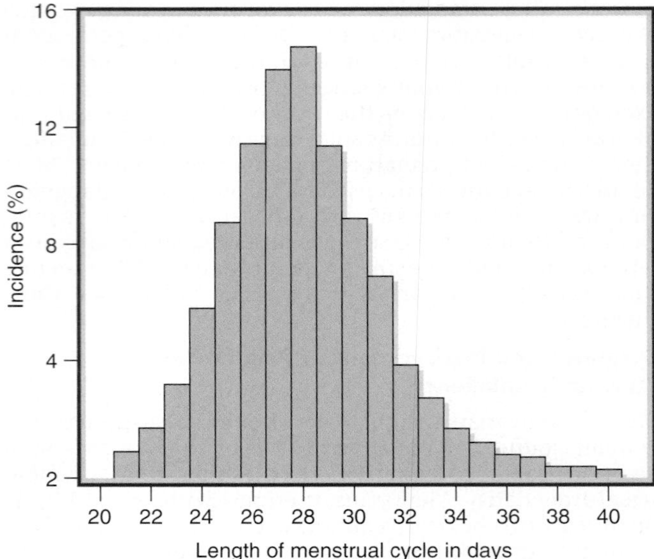

Figure 17-35 Variation of the duration of the menstrual cycle in women with regular cycles. (From Cunningham FG, MacDonald PC, Gant NF, et al. The endometrium and decidua: menstruation and pregnancy. In: Cunningham FG, ed. *Williams Obstetrics*, 19th ed. Stamford, CN: Appleton & Lange, 1993:81-109.)

For ovulatory women, the changes in the length of the menstrual cycle over the period of reproductive age are predictable. Between menarche and age 20, the cycle length for most ovulatory women is relatively longer. Between 20 and 40 years, there is increased regularity as cycles shorten. In the 40s, cycles begin to lengthen again. The highest incidence of anovulatory cycles occurs before age 20 and after age 40.[357] In these age groups, the average length of a cycle is between 25 and 28 days. Among ovulatory women, the frequency of a cycle of less than 21 days or more than 35 days is rare (<2%).[358] Overall, most women have cycles that last 24 to 35 days (Fig. 17-35).[356] Between ages 40 and 50, menstrual cycle length increases and anovulation becomes more prevalent.[359]

The average postovulatory bleeding lasts from 4 to 6 days. The normal volume of menstrual blood loss is 30 mL. More than 80 mL is considered abnormal. Most of the blood loss occurs during the first 3 days of a period, so excessive flow may exist without prolongation of flow.[360,361]

During an ovulatory cycle, the duration from ovulation to menses is relatively constant and averages 14 days (see Fig. 17-1A). Greater variability in the length of the proliferative phase, however, produces a distribution in the duration of the menstrual cycle. Menstrual bleeding more often than every 24 days or less often than every 35 days requires evaluation.[356,359] Flow that lasts 7 or more days also requires evaluation. A flow that totals more than 80 mL per month usually leads to anemia and should be treated.[362] In clinical practice, however, it is difficult to quantify menstrual flow because evaluation and treatment are based solely on the patient's perceptions regarding the duration, amount, and timing of her menstrual bleeding. Despite this difficulty in quantifying menstrual blood loss, the clinician should evaluate the cause of excessive uterine bleeding. Anemia should be ruled out by a complete blood cell count.[363] A low hemoglobin value accompanied by microcytic and hypochromic red blood cells suggests excessive blood loss during menses. These patients should be provided with iron supplementation. The likely presence of coagulation defects, uterine leiomyomas, or adenomyosis underlying prolonged menses should be evaluated in anemic patients through a meticulous history and physical examination followed by relevant laboratory tests.

Terminology Describing Abnormal Uterine Bleeding

Oligomenorrhea is defined as intervals between episodes of uterine bleeding longer than 35 days, and the term *polymenorrhea* is used to describe intervals shorter than 24 days. *Hypermenorrhea* refers to regular intervals (24 to 35 days) but excessive flow or duration of bleeding, or both. *Hypomenorrhea* refers to diminution of the flow or shortening of the duration of regular menses, or both.

Uterine Bleeding in Response to Steroid Hormones

Estrogen Withdrawal Bleeding

Uterine bleeding follows acute cessation of estrogen support to the endometrium. This type of uterine bleeding can occur after bilateral oophorectomy, irradiation of mature follicles, or administration of estrogen to a castrate followed by discontinuation of therapy. Similarly, the bleeding that occurs after castration can be delayed by concomitant estrogen therapy. Flow occurs on discontinuation of exogenous estrogen. Estrogen withdrawal by itself (in the absence of progesterone) almost invariably causes uterine bleeding.

Estrogen Breakthrough Bleeding

Chronic exposure to various quantities of estrogen stimulates the growth of endometrium continuously in the absence of progesterone, as in the case of excessive extragonadal estrogen production in PCOS. After a certain point, the amount of estrogen produced in extraovarian tissue remains insufficient to maintain structural support for the endometrium. This gives rise to unpredictable episodes of shedding of the surface endometrium. Relatively low doses of estrogen yield intermittent spotting that may be prolonged, but the quantity is light. High levels of estrogen and sustained availability lead to prolonged periods of amenorrhea followed by acute, often profuse episodes of bleeding with excessive loss of blood.

Progesterone Withdrawal Bleeding

Typical progesterone withdrawal bleeding occurs after ovulation in the absence of pregnancy. Removal of the corpus luteum also leads to endometrial desquamation. Pharmacologically, a similar event can be achieved by administration and then discontinuation of progesterone or a synthetic progestin. Progesterone withdrawal bleeding occurs only if the endometrium is initially primed by endogenous or exogenous estrogen. If estrogen therapy is continued as progesterone is withdrawn, the progesterone withdrawal bleeding still occurs. Only if estrogen levels are increased markedly is progesterone withdrawal bleeding delayed.[364] Progesterone withdrawal bleeding is quite predictable in the presence of previous or concomitant estrogen exposure.

Progestin Breakthrough Bleeding

The pharmacologic phenomenon of breakthrough bleeding occurs in the setting of an unfavorably high ratio of progestin to estrogen. In the absence of sufficient estrogen, continuous progestin therapy leads to intermittent bleeding of variable duration, similar to the low-dose estrogen breakthrough bleeding described previously. This type of bleeding is associated with combination oral contraceptives that contain low-dose estrogen and the long-acting, progestin-only contraceptive methods such as Norplant and Depo-Provera.[365] Progestin breakthrough bleeding is highly unpredictable and is characterized by extensive variability among women.

Causes of Irregular Uterine Bleeding

Pregnancy and its complications represent one of the most common causes of irregular uterine bleeding (Table 17-8). Pregnancy should be ruled out by a urine test in any woman of reproductive age who presents with irregular bleeding (Table 17-9).

Anovulatory uterine bleeding arising from responses of the endometrium to inappropriate production of ovarian steroids has also been called *dysfunctional uterine bleeding* because treatments that restore ovulatory function potentially reverse the irregular bleeding pattern. Common examples of anovulatory bleeding include those associated with exercise-related anovulation, hyperprolactinemia, hypothyroidism, or PCOS.[366] In these cases, restoration of ovulatory menses by correction of the underlying disorder or use of exogenous hormones can achieve predictable uterine bleeding. Various pathologic entities of the genital tract (i.e., ovaries, uterus, vagina, or vulva) or coagulation abnormalities can cause deviation from normal menses (see Table 17-8).

Anovulatory uterine bleeding is a diagnosis of exclusion for several reasons. Vulvar, vaginal, or uterine malignancies or an estrogen- or androgen-secreting ovarian tumor may cause abnormal uterine bleeding (see Table 17-8). Pregnancy and pregnancy-related problems such as ectopic pregnancy or spontaneous miscarriage are extremely common causes of abnormal uterine bleeding. The most common cause of disruption of a normal menstrual pattern is pregnancy or a complication of pregnancy. Another common cause of irregular uterine bleeding is observed in oral contraceptive users in the form of progestin breakthrough bleeding. Progestin breakthrough bleeding during postmenopausal hormone therapy is also common. Patients may be unknowingly using other hormonal medications with an impact on the endometrium. For example, the use of ginseng, an herbal root, has been associated with estrogenic activity and abnormal bleeding.[367] Although uterine bleeding is a common benign side effect of various long-term hormone treatments, the clinician should always be convinced first that no other pathology is present. Anatomically demonstrable pathologies of the menstrual outflow tract include endometrial hyperplasia and cancer, endometrial polyps, uterine leiomyomas, adenomyosis, and endometritis. Irregular, serious bleeding may be associated with chronic illness, such as renal insufficiency, liver insufficiency, or AIDS. Careful examination may discover genital injury or a foreign object (see Table 17-8).

At puberty, the most common cause of irregular uterine bleeding is anovulation. Approximately 20% of adolescents with excessive irregular uterine bleeding have a coagulation defect.[368,369] Among all women of reproductive age with hypermenorrhea, the prevalence of a coagulation

TABLE 17-8

Causes of Irregular Uterine Bleeding
Complications of Pregnancy
Threatened miscarriage
Incomplete miscarriage
Ectopic pregnancy
Anovulation
Physiologic
Uncomplicated pregnancy (amenorrhea)
Pubertal (postmenarchal) anovulation
Anovulation immediately before menopause
Medications (e.g., oral contraceptives, GnRH agonists, danazol)
Hypothalamic (frequently presents as amenorrhea)
Functional (e.g., diet, exercise, stress)
Anatomic (e.g., tumor, granulomatous disease, infection)
Medications
Other
Hyperprolactinemia, other pituitary disorders
Prolactinoma
Other pituitary tumors, granulomatous disease
Hypothyroidism
Medications
Other
Androgen excess
PCOS, hyperthecosis
Ovarian tumor (e.g., Sertoli-Leydig cell tumor)
Nonclassic adrenal hyperplasia
Cushing's syndrome
Glucocorticoid resistance
Adrenal tumor (e.g., adenoma, carcinoma)
Medications (e.g., testosterone, danazol)
Other
Premature ovarian insufficiency (frequently presents as amenorrhea)
Chronic illness
Liver insufficiency
Renal insufficiency
AIDS
Other
Anatomic Defects Affecting the Uterus
Uterine leiomyomas
Endometrial polyps
Adenomyosis (usually manifests as hypermenorrhea)
Intrauterine adhesions (usually manifests as amenorrhea)
Endometritis
Endometrial hyperplasia, cancer
Chronic estrogen exposure (e.g., PCOS, medication, liver insufficiency)
Estrogen-secreting ovarian tumor (e.g., granulosa cell tumor)
Advanced cervical cancer
Other
Coagulation Defects (Usually Manifest as Hypermenorrhea)
Von Willebrand's disease
Factor XI deficiency
Other
Extrauterine Genital Bleeding (May Mimic Uterine Bleeding)
Vaginitis
Genital trauma
Foreign body
Vaginal neoplasia
Vulvar neoplasia
Other

AIDS, acquired immunodeficiency syndrome; GnRH, gonadotropin-releasing hormone; PCOS, polycystic ovary syndrome.

TABLE 17-9

Diagnostic Tests to Evaluate Irregular Uterine Bleeding
Commonly Used Tests
Urine hCG test
Serum hCG level (incomplete miscarriage, ectopic pregnancy)
Transvaginal pelvic ultrasonography (intrauterine or ectopic pregnancy, uterine leiomyoma, endometrial polyp or neoplasia, ovarian tumor)
Serum FSH, LH (anovulation; ovarian insufficiency)
Serum prolactin, TSH (anovulation; hyperprolactinemia)
Complete blood count, PT, PTT (evaluation for anemia, coagulation defect)
Liver and renal functions, HIV (anovulation; chronic disease)
Endometrial biopsy (endometrial disease; polyp, neoplasia, endometritis)
Less Commonly Used Tests
Evaluation for PCOS, ovarian or adrenal tumor, nonclassic adrenal hyperplasia, Cushing's syndrome, and glucocorticoid resistance (androgen excess)
Head CT or MRI scan (hypothalamic anovulation, hyperprolactinemia)
Pelvic MRI scan (adenomyosis, uterine leiomyoma)
Hysterosonography with intrauterine saline installation (endometrial polyp, uterine leiomyoma)
Hysteroscopy (endometrial polyp, uterine leiomyoma)
Dilatation and curettage (endometrial disease not diagnosed by ultrasonography or biopsy)

CT, computed tomography; FSH, follicle-stimulating hormone; hCG, human chorionic gonadotropin; HIV, human immunodeficiency virus; LH, luteinizing hormone; MRI, magnetic resonance imaging; PCOS, polycystic ovary syndrome; PT, prothrombin time; PTT, partial thromboplastin time; TSH, thyroid-stimulating hormone.

disorder is 17%; von Willebrand's disease is the most common defect, and factor XI deficiency is the second common diagnosis. Bleeding because of a coagulation defect usually consists of a heavy flow with regular, cyclic menses (i.e., hypermenorrhea), and the same pattern can be seen in patients being treated with anticoagulants.[370] Bleeding disorders are usually associated with hypermenorrhea since menarche and a history of bleeding with surgery or trauma. Hypermenorrhea may be the only sign of an inherited bleeding disorder.[371]

Early pregnancy or its complications should always be ruled out first by a sensitive urine hCG measurement in any reproductive-age woman presenting with irregular bleeding. Threatened or incomplete miscarriage and ectopic pregnancy are common causes of irregular uterine bleeding. Other tests should be ordered on the basis of the initial clinical evaluation, including tests to evaluate anovulatory disorders of various causes (see Table 17-9). In patients with a history of prolonged heavy menses (i.e., hypermenorrhea) of pubertal origin, coagulation studies (e.g., prothrombin time, partial thromboplastin time, bleeding time) and a complete blood cell count should be obtained.

Pelvic ultrasonography through a vaginal probe is an extremely useful test for the evaluation of normal or abnormal pregnancy, uterine leiomyomas, endometrial neoplasia, and ovarian tumors (see Table 17-9). Other imaging studies may be used judiciously to rule out pathologies of the hypothalamus, pituitary, and adrenal (discussed earlier). Pelvic MRI is used to rule out adenomyosis, a uterine disorder characterized by the abnormal presence of diffuse endometrial tissue in the myometrial layer. Advanced adenomyosis is associated with diffuse enlargement of the uterus, hypermenorrhea, and anemia.

Endometrial histology should be determined by an endometrial biopsy performed in the physician's office in patients at risk for endometrial hyperplasia or cancer (e.g., PCOS, liver insufficiency, obesity, diabetes mellitus, hormone therapy). A benign endometrial polyp or a uterine leiomyoma protruding into the uterine cavity can be diagnosed by hysterosonography using intrauterine saline installation or by hysteroscopy. Hysterosonography and hysteroscopy are not appropriate tests to evaluate endometrial hyperplasia or cancer because these procedures may cause dissemination of malignant cells. If malignancy is suspected, it should be ruled out by an office endometrial biopsy (see Table 17-9). Occasionally, an office endometrial biopsy cannot be performed or is not diagnostic of endometrial neoplasia. In these rare instances, endometrial curettage under anesthesia is performed for a reliable tissue diagnosis.

A careful history and physical examination eliminate the need for most of these diagnostic tests. Before ordering a certain diagnostic study, it is useful to consider whether a particular test result would alter the ultimate clinical management.

Management of Anovulatory Uterine Bleeding

The terms *dysfunctional uterine bleeding* and *anovulatory bleeding* are used interchangeably and denote inappropriate stimulation of the endometrium during dysfunctional states of the reproductive system. If ovulatory function can be restored, anovulatory bleeding usually gives way to predictable cyclic periods. Because restoration of ovulatory function may not be possible or practical in many of these women, exogenous estrogen and progestin are administered for several purposes. The indications for hormonal treatment of uterine bleeding include the need to stop acute uterine bleeding, to maintain predictable bleeding episodes, or to prevent endometrial hyperplasia. Hormonal treatments are used to stop anovulatory uterine bleeding and to induce predictable bleeding episodes.

Anovulatory uterine bleeding is a diagnosis of exclusion. Various anatomically demonstrable pathologies of the genital tract (see Table 17-8) should be ruled out before administration of estrogen, progestin, or GnRH analogues.

Oral Contraceptives

Use of combination oral contraceptives in an acute or chronic fashion is the most common treatment for irregular uterine bleeding. The estrogen component of the combination pill stabilizes the endometrial tissue and stops shedding within hours; it decreases ovarian secretion of sex steroids by suppression of gonadotropins within several days. The progestin component of the pill directly affects endometrial tissue to decrease shedding over days and potentiates ovarian suppression induced by estrogen. The progestin (in the presence of estrogen) induces differentiation of the endometrial tissue into a stable form called *pseudodecidua*. Typically, a monophasic oral contraceptive preparation that contains 30 or 35 μg of ethinyl estradiol is preferred. Triphasic oral contraceptives and those with less than 30 μg of ethinyl estradiol are not suitable for the treatment of excessive anovulatory uterine bleeding. A combination oral contraceptive in high doses (2 or 3 pills per day) can be used for short intervals (i.e., weeks) to treat an acute episode of excessive uterine bleeding. A usual dose of 1 pill per day may be administered for years to manage chronic anovulatory bleeding associated with PCOS or hyperprolactinemia.

Oral Contraceptives and Acute Excessive Uterine Bleeding Associated with Anemia. Unopposed estrogen exposure in women with anovulatory uterine bleeding is commonly associated with chronic endometrial buildup and heavy bleeding episodes. Therapy is administered as 1 combination oral contraceptive pill twice daily for 1 week. In obese women, the oral contraceptive may be given three times daily. This therapy is maintained despite cessation of flow within 2 days. If flow does not abate, other diagnostic possibilities (e.g., polyps, incomplete abortion, neoplasia) should be reevaluated. In case of anovulatory bleeding, the flow does diminish rapidly within 2 days after the beginning of high-dose oral contraceptive treatment (i.e., 1 pill two or three times daily). Specific causes of anovulation and possible coagulation disorders should be evaluated during the next few days. The physician also should consider whether blood replacement or initiation of iron therapy is necessary. The high-dose estrogen-progestin combination has produced the structural rigidity intrinsic to the compact pseudodecidual reaction. Continued random breakdown of formerly fragile tissue is avoided, and blood loss stopped. However, a large quantity of tissue remains to react to estrogen-progestin withdrawal. The patient must be warned to anticipate a heavy flow with severe cramping a few days after stopping this therapy. The patient should also be warned of possible nausea that may be caused by high-dose oral contraceptive treatment.

At the end of a week of high-dose oral contraceptive treatment, the pill is stopped temporarily. A heavy flow usually starts within a few days. On the third day of this withdrawal bleeding, a regular dose of combination oral contraceptive medication (1 pill/day) is started. This is repeated for several 3-week treatments interrupted by 1-week withdrawal intervals. A decrease in volume with each successive cycle is expected. Oral contraceptives reduce menstrual flow by more than one half in most women.[372]

Early application of the estrogen-progestin combination limits growth and allows orderly regression of excessive endometrial height to normal levels. Because oral contraceptives do not treat the underlying cause of anovulation but provide symptomatic relief by directly affecting the endometrium, cessation of oral contraceptives results in the return of erratic uterine bleeding. Regardless of the requirement for contraception, use of oral contraceptives represents the best choice for hormonal management of heavy anovulatory bleeding and should be offered as long-term management.

Oral Contraceptives and Chronic Irregular Uterine Bleeding. PCOS is a common form of anovulation associated with chronic steady-state levels of unopposed estrogen that may give rise to endometrial hyperplasia and cancer (discussed earlier). Hypothalamic anovulation and hyperprolactinemia are associated with low estrogen levels that are insufficient to prevent bone loss. A combination oral contraceptive is a suitable long-term treatment for both forms of chronic anovulation.

Oral contraceptives represent the most suitable long-term symptomatic management option for any kind of anovulatory uterine bleeding, including oligomenorrhea. Before the administration of an oral contraceptive, pregnancy should be ruled out. One pill per day is ordinarily administered for 3-week periods interrupted by 1-week hormone-free intervals. Withdrawal bleeding is expected during the hormone-free interval. The progestin component serves to prevent endometrial hyperplasia associated with steady-state unopposed estrogen exposure in PCOS. In cases of anovulation associated with hypoestrogenism (e.g., hypothalamic anovulation, hyperprolactinemia), the estrogen component of the pill provides sufficient replacement to prevent bone loss. The risk of thromboembolism, stroke, or myocardial infarction associated with long-term administration is extremely low in current nonsmokers and in the absence of a history of thromboembolism. Provided that the oral contraceptive controls the abnormal uterine bleeding effectively, a chronically anovulatory woman can continue this regimen until menopause.

Synthetic Progestins

Synthetic progestins enhance endometrial differentiation and antagonize the proliferative effects of estrogen on the endometrium (see Fig. 17-24).[165,373] The effects of progestins or natural progesterone include limitation of estrogen-induced endometrial growth and prevention of endometrial hyperplasia. The absence of naturally synthesized progesterone in anovulatory states is the rationale for administering a progestin.

The most common indication for long-term cyclic progestin administration is to prevent endometrial malignancy in a patient with PCOS and unopposed chronic estrogen exposure of the endometrium. A combination oral contraceptive is the treatment of choice in these cases. If the patient cannot use an oral contraceptive for some reason (e.g., history of thromboembolism), a progestin may be administered in a cyclic fashion to prevent endometrial hyperplasia. Before the administration of a progestin (or oral contraceptive), pregnancy should be ruled out. In the treatment of oligomenorrhea associated with PCOS, orderly, limited withdrawal bleeding can be accomplished by administration of a progestin such as MPA (5 mg/day) for at least 10 days every 2 months. Alternatively, norethindrone acetate at 5 mg/day or megestrol acetate at 20 mg/day may be administered for 10 days every 2 months. Absence of withdrawal bleeding requires further workup.

In the treatment of excessive uterine bleeding (i.e., hypermenorrhea or polymenorrhea), these progestins at higher daily doses (20 mg/day of MPA, 10 mg/day of norethindrone acetate, or 40 mg/day of megestrol acetate) are prescribed for 2 weeks to induce predecidual stromal changes in the endometrium. A heavy progestin withdrawal flow usually follows within 3 days after the last dose is administered. Thereafter, repeated progestin treatment (5 mg/day of MPA, 5 mg/day of norethindrone acetate, or 20 mg/day of megestrol acetate) is offered cyclically for at least the first 10 days of every other month to ensure therapeutic effect. Failure of progestin to correct irregular bleeding requires diagnostic reevaluation such as endometrial biopsy. Predictable withdrawal bleeding within several days after each cycle of progestin administration suggests the absence of endometrial malignancy.

High-Dose Estrogen for Acute Excessive Uterine Bleeding

An oral contraceptive given two or three times daily is the treatment of choice to stop heavy anovulatory bleeding. A high-dose oral contraceptive regimen should be offered to women with heavy uterine bleeding with or without asymptomatic anemia after anatomically demonstrable pathology of the genital tract has been ruled out (see Table 17-8). A patient with acute and severe anovulatory bleeding accompanied by symptomatic anemia represents a medical emergency. These patients should be hospitalized immediately and offered a blood transfusion. After genital tract pathology has been ruled out by history, physical examination, and pelvic ultrasonography, intravenously administered high-dose estrogen is the treatment of choice to stop life-threatening bleeding. A well-established regimen is to administer 25 mg of conjugated estrogen intravenously every 4 hours until bleeding markedly slows down or for at least 24 hours.[374] Estrogen most likely acts on the capillaries to induce clotting.[375] Before intravenous estrogen treatment is discontinued, an oral contraceptive pill is started three times daily. Oral contraceptive treatment is then continued as described previously.

Because high-dose estrogen is a risk factor for thromboembolism, taking two or three oral contraceptive pills per day for a week or large doses of intravenous conjugated estrogens for 24 hours should be regarded as presenting a significant risk. However, no data are available to evaluate any risk associated with this type of acute use of hormonal therapy for such short intervals. The physician and patient should make a decision regarding high-dose hormone therapy after considering its risks and benefits. Alternative treatment options may be offered to patients with significant risk factors. Exposure to high doses of estrogen should be avoided in women with a past episode of idiopathic venous thromboembolism or a strong family history. High-dose hormone treatment should also be avoided in women with severe chronic illness such as liver insufficiency or renal insufficiency. One alternative for these patients is dilatation and curettage, followed by treatment with an oral contraceptive (one pill per day) until the uterine bleeding is under control.

Gonadotropin-Releasing Hormone Analogues for Excessive Anovulatory Uterine Bleeding

A GnRH analogue may be given to women with excessive anovulatory bleeding or hypermenorrhea related to severe chronic illness such as liver insufficiency or coagulation disorders. Monthly depot injections of GnRH agonists are not effective for acute excessive uterine bleeding and may increase uterine bleeding for the first 2 weeks. GnRH antagonists downregulate FSH and LH without a delay and achieve amenorrhea more rapidly. The GnRH agonist leuprolide acetate depot (3.75 mg/month intramuscularly) may be administered for 6 months or longer to control uterine bleeding due to chronic illness. GnRH antagonists can probably be used to halt acute or chronic anovulatory bleeding; however, insufficient published data are available to provide dose recommendations. Long-term side effects of GnRH analogues, including osteoporosis, make this an undesirable choice for long-term therapy. If long-term treatment with GnRH analogues is chosen, norethindrone acetate (2.5 mg daily) should be added back. This add-back regimen is usually sufficient to prevent osteoporosis and does not ordinarily worsen the uterine bleeding.

HORMONE-DEPENDENT BENIGN GYNECOLOGIC DISORDERS

Endometriosis

Endometriosis is defined as the presence of endometrium-like tissue in ectopic sites outside the uterine cavity, primarily on pelvic peritoneum and ovaries, and it is associated with chronic pelvic pain, pain during intercourse, and infertility.[376] It is an estrogen-dependent inflammatory disease that affects 5% to 10% of U.S. women of reproductive age.[376] This classic presentation may represent a common phenotype resulting from diverse anatomic or biochemical aberrations of uterine function. As cellular and molecular mechanisms in endometriosis are uncovered, this condition is coming to be viewed as a systemic and chronic complex disease such as diabetes mellitus or asthma.[377] Endometriosis may be inherited in a polygenic manner, because its incidence is increased by up to sevenfold in relatives of women with endometriosis.[378]

Pathology

There are three clinically distinct forms of endometriosis: endometriotic implants on the surface of pelvic peritoneum and ovaries (i.e., peritoneal endometriosis), ovarian cysts lined by endometrioid mucosa (i.e., endometriomas), and a complex, solid mass composed of endometriotic tissue blended with adipose and fibromuscular tissue and residing between rectum and vagina (i.e., rectovaginal nodule). These three types of lesions may be variant phenotypes of the same pathologic process, or they may be caused by different mechanisms.[379,380] Their common histology is the presence of endometrial stromal or epithelial cells, chronic bleeding, and inflammatory changes. These lesions may occur singly or in combination and are associated with significantly increased risk of infertility and chronic pelvic pain.[379,380] The inflammatory process in endometriosis may stimulate nerve endings in the pelvis to cause pain, impair the function of the uterine tubes, decrease receptivity of the endometrium, and impair development of the oocyte and embryo. Endometriosis may also cause infertility by physically blocking the tubes.

Clinical evidence points to a deleterious effect of uninterrupted ovulatory cycles on the development and persistence of endometriosis.[377] First, symptoms of endometriosis usually appear after menarche and vanish after menopause. Occasionally, a rectovaginal nodule remains symptomatic in a postmenopausal woman, suggesting that its persistence is independent of ovarian estrogen. Second, multiparity is associated with a decreased risk of endometriosis. Third, disruption of ovulation by GnRH analogues, oral contraceptives, or progestins reduces pelvic disease and associated pain. In line with these observations, basic and clinical research findings indicate major roles of the ovarian steroids estrogen and progesterone in the pathology of endometriosis. In humans and primate models, estrogen stimulates the growth of endometriotic tissue, whereas aromatase inhibitors that block estrogen formation and antiprogestins are therapeutic.[377] Levels of nuclear receptors for estrogen and progesterone in endometriotic tissue are strikingly different from those in normal endometrium.[377] Fourth, biologically significant quantities of progesterone and estrogen are produced locally by an abnormally active steroidogenic cascade that includes aromatase.[377]

Mechanism

A number of hypotheses have been proposed regarding the histologic origin of endometriosis. Sampson suggested that fragments of menstrual endometrium pass retrograde through the tubes and then implant and persist on peritoneal surfaces.[381] This mechanism has been demonstrated in primate models and observed naturally in human disease, and it is supported by the observation that spontaneous endometriosis occurs exclusively in species that menstruate. Alternatively, the celomic-metaplasia hypothesis describes the genesis of endometriotic lesions within the peritoneal cavity by differentiation of mesothelial cells into endometrium-like tissue. A third hypothesis argues that menstrual tissue from the endometrial cavity reaches other body sites through veins or lymphatic vessels.[377] Finally, it has been proposed that circulating blood cells originating from bone marrow differentiate into endometriotic tissue at various body sites.[382] Sampson's implantation hypothesis offers a plausible mechanism for most endometriotic lesions but does not explain why only some women develop endometriosis. Although most women of reproductive age have reflux menstruation into the peritoneal cavity, endometriosis is encountered in only 5% to 10% of this population.

Two possible mechanisms may explain the successful implantation of refluxed endometrium to the peritoneal surface. First, the eutopic endometrium of women with endometriosis exhibits multiple subtle but significant molecular abnormalities, including activation of oncogenic pathways or biosynthetic cascades favoring increased production of estrogen, cytokines, prostaglandins, and metalloproteinases.[377] When this biologically distinct tissue attaches to mesothelial cells, the magnitude of these abnormalities is amplified drastically to enhance implant survival.[377] A second mechanism suggests that a defective immune system fails to clear implants off the peritoneal surface.[377] It is possible that both mechanisms may contribute to the same phenotype.

Clear molecular distinctions, such as overproduction of estrogen, prostaglandins, and cytokines, are observed between endometriotic tissue and endometrium (Fig. 17-36).[377] More subtle forms of these abnormalities are also observed in endometrium from an patient with endometriosis compared with endometrium from a disease-free woman. Inflammation is a hallmark of endometriotic tissue that overproduces prostaglandins, metalloproteinases, cytokines, and chemokines.[377] Increased levels of acute inflammatory cytokines such as interleukin-1β (IL-1β), IL-6, and tumor necrosis factor (TNF) likely enhance adhesion of shed endometrial tissue fragments on peritoneal surfaces, and proteolytic membrane metalloproteinases may further promote their implantation.[377] Monocyte chemoattractant protein 1, IL-8, and RANTES (i.e., *r*egulated on *a*ctivation, *n*ormal *T* cell *e*xpressed and *s*ecreted) attract the granulocytes, natural killer cells, and macrophages typically observed in endometriosis.[383] Autoregulatory positive feedback loops ensure further accumulation of these immune cells, cytokines, and chemokines in established lesions.

Basic biologic functions such as inflammation, immune response, angiogenesis, and apoptosis are altered in favor of survival and replenishment of endometriotic tissue.[377] These functions depend in part on estrogen or progesterone action. Excessive formation of estrogen and prostaglandin and development of progesterone resistance have emerged as clinically useful concepts, because targeting of aromatase in the estrogen biosynthetic pathway, cyclooxygenase 2 (COX2) in the prostaglandin pathway, or the progesterone receptor (PR) significantly reduces laparoscopically visible endometriosis or pelvic pain (see Fig. 17-36).[377] These three critical mechanisms have been linked by specific epigenetic (hypomethylation) defects that cause overexpression of the nuclear receptors SF1 and ERβ.[377]

Diagnosis

Reliable diagnosis of peritoneal endometriosis can be made only by direct visualization of these lesions by laparoscopy or laparotomy. Ovarian endometriotic cysts filled with a thick, bloody fluid (i.e., endometriomas) can be diagnosed accurately by vaginal ultrasonography.

Treatment

Treatment of infertility caused by endometriosis consists of surgical removal with or without assisted reproductive

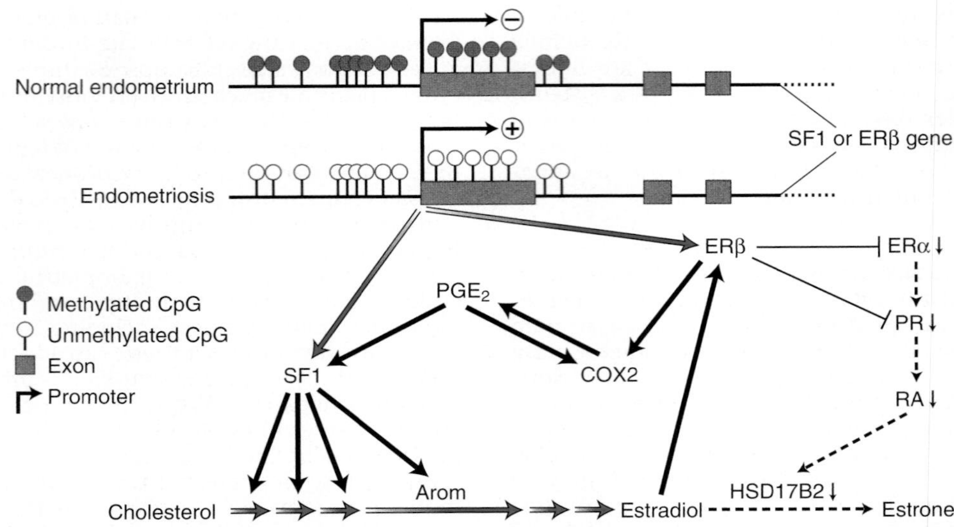

Figure 17-36 Molecular mechanisms in endometriosis. Two nuclear receptors, steroidogenic factor 1 (SF1) and estrogen receptor-β (ERβ), play significant roles in the pathology of endometriosis. In normal endometrial stromal cells, cytosine-phosphate-guanine (CpG) islands located at the SF1 and ERβ promoters are robustly methylated and silenced. A lack of promoter methylation is associated with promoter activation and the presence of extraordinarily large quantities of these nuclear receptors in endometriotic stromal cells. Prostaglandin E_2 (PGE_2) induces multiple steroidogenic genes, including aromatase (arom), and formation of estradiol from cholesterol. SF1 mediates this steroidogenic action of PGE_2. ERβ suppresses ERα and progesterone receptors (PRs). This results in defective retinoic acid (RA) production and action, leading to 17β-hydroxysteroid dehydrogenase 2 (HSD17B2) deficiency and failure to metabolize estradiol. ERβ also induces cyclooxygenase 2 (COX2) and formation of PGE_2. Estradiol and PGE_2 are produced in large quantities and enhance cell survival and inflammation in endometriotic tissue.

technology, whereas pain is usually treated with a combination of medical suppression of ovulation and surgery. Peritoneal implants are resected or vaporized by electric current or laser. Ovarian endometriomas and rectovaginal endometriotic nodules may be effectively removed only by full dissection. Epidemiologic and laboratory data suggest a link between ovarian endometriosis and distinct types of ovarian cancer.[377]

Although current hormonal therapy for infertility associated with endometriosis is not of proven value, it is somewhat successful for pelvic pain associated with endometriosis.[384] However, the duration of relief provided by medical treatment is relatively short.[385] Various agents used are comparable in terms of efficacy. Most of the current medical treatments were designed to suppress ovulation (e.g., GnRH agonists, oral contraceptives, danazol, progestins). A possible alternative mechanism of action of the androgenic steroid danazol or a progestin is a direct antiproliferative effect on endometriotic tissue.

Many patients and physicians do not favor danazol because of its anabolic and androgenic side effects of weight gain and muscle cramps and occasional irreversible virilization (e.g., clitoromegaly, voice changes).[386] Up to 50% of patients with endometriosis fail to complete 6 months of treatment with danazol.[387] The rest of the hormonal agents—oral contraceptives, progestins, and GnRH agonists—show comparable efficacy for control of endometriosis-associated pain.[388-390] A 6-month course using any one of these agents results in a significant reduction of pain in more than 50% of patients.[388-390] Induction of pain relief with a continuously administered oral contraceptive or progestin takes longer than with a GnRH agonist.

There is a high incidence of persistence of the disease after all of these medical therapies.[391] Six months after completion of a 6-month course of treatment with a progestin, oral contraceptive, or GnRH agonist, moderate to severe pain symptoms recurred in 50% of initial responders.[389] The recurrence rate of pain in the rest of the patients was approximately 5% to 20% per year during a 5-year follow-up.[391] A 6-month course of GnRH agonist treatment is currently the most popular regimen. The most serious side effect of GnRH agonist treatment for endometriosis is bone loss related to estrogen deficiency, and oral estrogen-progestin preparations or bisphosphonates are usually added back to minimize bone loss.[36]

We are still far from the cure of endometriosis, and current treatments are not satisfactory for effective control of pain. The radical treatment is removal of both ovaries, and even this was not found to be effective in a number of cases of postmenopausal endometriosis.[389] New alternative strategies are needed to offer women with endometriosis a reasonable chance to live without suffering from chronic pelvic pain for decades.

There are two important caveats about GnRH agonist treatment. First, large quantities of estrogen can be produced locally within the endometriotic cells. This represents an intracrine mechanism of estrogen action, in contrast to ovarian secretion, which is an endocrine means of supplying this steroid to target tissues (see Fig. 17-21).[275,389] Second, estradiol produced in peripheral tissue sites (e.g., adipose tissue, skin fibroblasts) may give rise to pathologically significant circulating levels of estradiol in a subset of women.[275] GnRH agonists do not inhibit peripheral estrogen formation or local estrogen production within the estrogen-responsive lesion. Moreover, endometriosis is resistant to selective effects of progesterone and progestins.[377]

Aromatase inhibitors and selective progesterone response modulators are candidate therapeutic agents for endometriosis. Aromatase expression and local estrogen biosynthesis in endometriotic implants prompted pilot studies to target aromatase in endometriosis using its third-generation inhibitors. Among these inhibitors, anastrozole and letrozole were used successfully to treat endometriosis in postmenopausal and premenopausal women.[387,392-395] These studies suggested the following:

1. Aromatase inhibitors effectively treat pelvic pain associated with endometriosis, which is resistant to existing therapeutic modalities.
2. An aromatase inhibitor is the medical treatment of choice for persistent postmenopausal endometriosis.
3. Use of aromatase inhibitors in premenopausal women with endometriosis requires ovarian suppression by the addition of a GnRH analogue, progestin, or combination oral contraceptive.
4. Pilot data showed that side effect profiles were quite favorable and did not include bone loss in regimens that combined an aromatase inhibitor with an oral contraceptive or a progestin.[393,395]

Aromatase inhibitors represent one of the most promising new treatments for pain associated with endometriosis.

Uterine Leiomyomas

Uterine leiomyomas (fibroids) originate from the myometrium and are the most common solid tumor of the pelvis.[396] Leiomyomas are responsible for more than 200,000 hysterectomies per year in the United States. They are almost invariably benign and represent clonal expansion of individual myometrial cells. Leiomyomas can cause a variety of symptoms, including irregular and excessive uterine bleeding, pressure sensation in the lower abdomen, pain during intercourse, pelvic pain, recurrent pregnancy loss, infertility, and compression of adjacent pelvic organs, or they may be totally asymptomatic. Uterine fibroids are reported to occur in 20% to 40% of reproductive-age women with symptoms.[397] Leiomyomas are more common in African American women and have a polygenic inheritance pattern. Diagnosis can be made by abdominal and transvaginal ultrasonography. Transvaginal ultrasonography is a sensitive method for determining the size, number, and location of uterine leiomyomas.

Uterine leiomyomas appear during the reproductive years and regress after menopause, indicating their ovarian steroid–dependent growth potential, although the role of steroids or other growth factors in the initiation and growth of these tumors is not well understood. The neoplastic transformation of myometrium to leiomyoma probably involves somatic mutations of normal myometrium and the complex interactions of sex steroids and growth factors.[398] Traditionally, estrogen has been considered the major promoter of myoma growth. Later biochemical, histologic, and clinical data suggest an important role for progesterone in the growth of uterine leiomyomas. Progesterone and progestins, acting through the PR, enhance proliferative activity in leiomyomas.[164,399,400]

The therapeutic choices depend on the goals of therapy, with hysterectomy most often used for definitive treatment and myomectomy used when preservation of child-bearing capability is desired. Intracavitary and submucous leiomyomas can be removed by hysteroscopic resection. Laparoscopic myomectomy is technically possible but involves an increased risk of uterine rupture during pregnancy. The overall recurrence rate after myomectomy varies widely, from 10% to 50%. Other FDA-approved treatment options include selective uterine artery embolization and extracorporeal ablation of uterine fibroids with MRI-guided, high-intensity, focused ultrasound.[397]

Although GnRH agonist–induced hypogonadism can reduce the overall volume of the uterus containing leiomyomas and tumor vascularity, the severe side effects and prompt recurrences make GnRH agonists useful only for short-term goals such as reducing anemia related to uterine bleeding or decreasing tumor vascularity before hysteroscopic resection. Trials have consistently demonstrated that treatment with an antiprogestin such as mifepristone reduces fibroid size.[397] This observation underscores the role of progesterone in the cause of uterine fibroids and opens a new area of therapeutic investigation.

MANAGEMENT OF MENOPAUSE

Consequences of Menopause

Perimenopause

Menopause is the permanent cessation of menses as a result of the irreversible loss of a number of ovarian functions, including ovulation and estrogen production. Perimenopause is a critical period of life during which striking endocrinologic, somatic, and psychological alterations occur in the transition to menopause. Perimenopause encompasses the change from ovulatory cycles to cessation of menses and is marked by irregularity of menstrual bleeding.

The most sensitive clinical indication of perimenopause is the progressively increasing occurrence of menstrual irregularities. The menstrual cycle for most ovulatory women lasts 24 to 35 days, and approximately 20% of all reproductive-age women experience irregular cycles.[356] When women are in their 40s, anovulation becomes more prevalent and the menstrual cycle length increases beginning several years before menopause.[359] The median age at the onset of perimenopause is 47.5 years.[401] Regardless of the age at onset, menopause (i.e., cessation of menses) is consistently preceded by a period of prolonged cycle intervals.[402] Elevated circulating levels of FSH mark this menstrual cycle change before menopause and are accompanied by decreased inhibin levels, normal levels of LH, and slightly elevated levels of estradiol.[403] These changes in serum hormone levels reflect a decreasing ovarian follicular reserve and can be detected most reliably on day 2 or 3 of the menstrual cycle.

Serum estradiol levels do not begin to decline until less than a year before menopause. The average circulating estradiol levels in perimenopausal women are estimated to be somewhat higher than those in younger women because of an increased follicular response to elevated FSH levels.[404] The decline in inhibin production by the follicle, which allows a rise in FSH levels, in the later reproductive years reflects diminishing follicular reserve and competence. Ovarian follicular output of inhibin begins to decrease after 30 years of age, and this decline becomes much more pronounced after age 40. These hormonal changes parallel a sharp decline in fecundity, which starts at age 35.

Perimenopause is a transitional period during which postmenopausal levels of FSH can be observed despite continued menses; LH levels remain in the normal range. Pregnancy is still possible in the perimenopausal woman, because occasional ovulation and functional corpus luteum formation can occur. Until complete cessation of menses is observed or FSH levels higher than 40 IU/L are measured on two separate occasions, some form of contraception should be recommended to prevent unwanted pregnancy.

Perimenopause represents an optimal period in which to evaluate the general health of the mature woman and introduce measures to prepare her for the striking physiologic changes that come with menopause. The patient and her clinician should attempt to achieve several important aims during perimenopause. The long-term goal is to maintain an optimal quality of physical and social life. Another immediate objective is the detection of any major chronic disorders that occur with aging. The clinician should counsel the perimenopausal woman about the symptoms and long-term consequences of menopause. The benefits and risks of hormone therapy should be discussed thoroughly at this time.

Menopause

The median age at menopause is approximately 51 years.[405] The age at menopause is probably determined in part by genetic factors, because mothers and daughters tend to experience menopause at the same age.[406-408] Environmental factors may modify the age at menopause. For example, current smoking is associated with an earlier menopause, whereas alcohol consumption delays menopause.[405] Oral contraceptive use does not affect the age at which menopause begins.

The symptoms frequently seen and related to decreased estrogen production in menopause include irregular frequency of menses followed by amenorrhea, vasomotor instability manifested as hot flashes and sweats, urogenital atrophy giving rise to pain during intercourse and a variety of urinary symptoms, and consequences of osteoporosis and CVD. The combination and extent of these symptoms vary widely for each patient. Some patients experience multiple severe symptoms that may be disabling, whereas others have no symptoms or only mild discomfort associated with perimenopause.

Biosynthesis of Estrogen and Other Steroids in the Postmenopausal Woman

No follicular units can be detected histologically in the ovaries after menopause.[409] In reproductive-age women, the granulosa cell of the ovulatory follicle is the major source of inhibin and estradiol. In the absence of these factors that inhibit gonadotropin secretion, FSH and LH levels increase sharply after menopause. These levels peak a few years after menopause and decrease gradually and slightly thereafter.[410] The postmenopausal serum level of either gonadotropin may be more than 100 IU/L. FSH levels are usually higher than LH levels because LH is cleared from the blood much more quickly and possibly because the low levels of inhibin in menopause selectively lead to increased FSH secretion. Nevertheless, increased LH is a major factor that maintains significant quantities of androstenedione and testosterone secretion from the ovary, although the total production rates of both steroids decline after menopause.

The primary steroid products of the postmenopausal ovary are androstenedione and testosterone.[411] The average premenopausal rate of production of androstenedione of 3 mg/day is decreased by one half to approximately 1.5 mg/day.[411] The decrease primarily results from a substantial reduction in the ovarian contribution to the circulating androstenedione pool. Adrenal secretion accounts for most of the androstenedione production in the postmenopausal woman, with only a small amount secreted from the ovary.[412] DHEA and DHEAS originate almost exclusively from the adrenal and decline steadily with advancing age independent of menopause. The serum levels of DHEA and DHEAS after menopause are about one fourth of those in young adult women.[413]

Testosterone production is decreased by approximately one third after menopause.[411] Total testosterone production can be approximated by the sum of ovarian secretion and peripheral formation from androstenedione (see Fig. 17-28). In the premenopausal woman, significant amounts of testosterone are produced by conversion of androstenedione in extraovarian tissues. Because ovarian androstenedione secretion is substantially decreased after menopause, the decrease in postmenopausal testosterone production is accounted for in large measure by a decrease in the relative contribution of extraovarian sources.[411] With the disappearance of follicles and decreased estrogen, the elevated gonadotropins drive the remaining stromal tissue in the ovary to maintain testosterone secretion at levels observed during the premenopausal years. The contribution of the postmenopausal ovary to the total testosterone production is increased in the presence of seemingly unaltered ovarian secretion.

The most dramatic endocrine alteration of perimenopause involves the decline in the circulating level and production rate of estradiol. The average menopausal level of circulating estradiol is less than 20 pg/mL. The estradiol and estrone levels in postmenopausal women are usually slightly less than those in adult men. Circulating estradiol in postmenopausal women (and men) is derived from the peripheral conversion of androstenedione to estrone, which is converted peripherally to estradiol (see Fig. 17-21).[414] The mean circulating level of estrone in postmenopausal women (37 pg/mL) is higher than that of estradiol. The average postmenopausal production rate of estrone is approximately 42 μg per 24 hours. After menopause, almost all estrone and estradiol is derived from the peripheral aromatization of androstenedione. There is a drastic change in the androgen-to-estrogen ratio because of the sharp decrease in estradiol level and the only slightly reduced testosterone. The frequent onset of mild hirsutism after menopause reflects this striking shift in the hormone ratio. During the postmenopausal years, DHEAS and DHEA levels continue to decline steadily with advancing age, whereas serum androstenedione, testosterone, estrone, and estradiol levels do not change significantly.[410]

The aromatization of androstenedione to estrone in extraovarian tissues correlates positively with weight and advancing age (see Figs. 17-21 and 17-33).[121] Body weight correlates positively with the circulating levels of estrone and estradiol. Because aromatase enzyme activity is present in significant quantities in adipose tissue, increased aromatization of androstenedione in overweight individuals may reflect the increased bulk of tissue containing the enzyme.[120] There is a twofold to fourfold increase in the specific activity of aromatase per cell with advancing age.[122] An increased overall number of adipose fibroblasts with aromatase activity and a decrease in the levels of SHBG increase the free estradiol level and contribute to the increased risk of endometrial cancer in obese women.[122] The production rate and circulating levels of estradiol after menopause are insufficient to provide support for urogenital tissues and bone. Osteoporosis and urogenital atrophy are some of the most dramatic and unwanted consequences of estradiol deficiency during menopause.

Estrogen is produced locally in pathologic tissues such as breast cancer through the aromatase and reductive 17β-HSD enzymes (Fig. 17-37).[122,415] In postmenopausal women, androstenedione of adrenal origin is the most important substrate for aromatase in tumor tissue.[122,415] Estrone is produced primarily by aromatase that resides in undifferentiated adipose fibroblasts surrounding malignant epithelial cells (see Fig. 17-37).[122,415] Estrone then

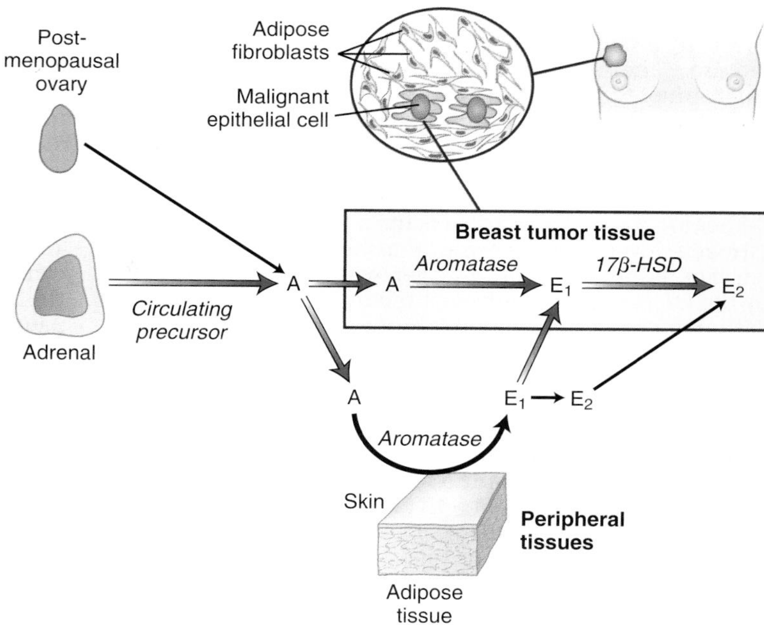

Figure 17-37 Tissue sources of estrogen in postmenopausal breast cancer. The important pathologic roles of extraovarian (peripheral) and local estrogen biosynthesis are shown for an estrogen-dependent disease in postmenopausal women. The estrogen precursor androstenedione (A) originates primarily from the adrenal in the postmenopausal woman. Aromatase expression and enzyme activity in extraovarian tissues such as fat increase with advancing age. The aromatase activity in skin and subcutaneous adipose fibroblasts gives rise to formation of systemically available estrone (E_1) and, to a smaller extent, estradiol (E_2). The conversion of circulating A to E_1 in undifferentiated breast adipose fibroblasts compacted around malignant epithelial cells and subsequent conversion of E_1 to E_2 in malignant epithelial cells provide high tissue concentrations of E_2 for tumor growth. The clinical relevance of these findings is exemplified by the successful use of aromatase inhibitors to treat breast cancer in postmenopausal women. 17β-HSD, reductive-type 17β-hydroxysteroid dehydrogenase.

diffuses into malignant epithelial cells that contain reductive 17β-HSD activity and is converted to biologically active estradiol (see Fig. 17-37).[144] Paracrine interactions in breast tumor tissue produce estradiol in malignant epithelial cells that enhances proliferation. The clinical relevance of these findings was exemplified by the successful use of aromatase inhibitors as first-line and second-line endocrine treatments for postmenopausal breast cancer.[416,417]

Management of Postmenopausal Uterine Bleeding

Perimenopausal or postmenopausal bleeding can be caused by hormone administration or excessive extraovarian estrogen formation. Irregular uterine bleeding is commonly observed during the perimenopausal transition as anovulatory cycles alternate with ovulatory cycles. Uterine bleeding after menopause is less common if the patient is not receiving hormone therapy treatment. Obese women are more likely to experience postmenopausal bleeding because of increased peripheral aromatization of adrenal androstenedione. Patients receiving a continuous combination regimen of hormone therapy may experience unpredictable uterine bleeding. The major objective in these circumstances is to rule out endometrial malignancy. This can be best achieved by tissue diagnosis through an office endometrial biopsy using a plastic cannula. Transvaginal ultrasonographic measurement of endometrial thickness may be used in postmenopausal women to avoid unnecessary biopsies.[173] A biopsy is required if an endometrial thickness of 5 mm or greater is observed.

Before employing ultrasonography and endometrial biopsy to explore the cause of bleeding that is assumed to arise from the intrauterine cavity, the clinician should rule out diseases of the vulva, vagina, and cervix. Careful inspection of these organs along with a normal cervical Pap smear within the past year is sufficient to rule out the vulva, vagina, and cervix as potential sources of bleeding. Postmenopausal uterine bleeding is the most common initial event that alerts the patient and her physician to the possibility of endometrial cancer. The causes of postmenopausal uterine bleeding are benign most of the time. Endometrial malignancy is encountered in patients with bleeding in only about 1% to 2% of postmenopausal endometrial biopsies.[418] Approximately three fourths of these biopsies reveal no pathology or an atrophic endometrium. Other histologic findings include hyperplasia (15%) and endometrial polyps (3%). Persistent unexplained uterine bleeding requires repeated evaluation, biopsy, hysteroscopy, or dilatation and curettage.

Unpredictable irregular uterine bleeding is observed in approximately 20% of postmenopausal women receiving a long-term (>1 year) continuous estrogen-progestin combination. This should also be evaluated appropriately with ultrasonography or biopsy, or both.[173]

Hot Flashes

The most frequent and striking symptom during perimenopause is the hot flash. It typically occurs during the transition from perimenopause to postmenopause. The flash is also a major symptom of postmenopause, and it can occur up to 5 years after menopause.[419] More than four fifths of postmenopausal women experience hot flashes within 3 months after the cessation of ovarian function, whether natural or surgical in origin. Of these women, more than three fourths have hot flashes for more than 1 year, and approximately one half have them for up to 5 years.[419] Hot flashes lessen in frequency and intensity with advancing age, unlike other sequelae of menopause, which progress with time.

A hot flash is a subjective sensation of intense warmth of the upper body, which typically lasts for approximately 4 minutes but may range in duration from 30 seconds to 5 minutes. It can follow a prodrome of palpitations or headache and is frequently accompanied by weakness, faintness, or vertigo. The episode usually ends in profuse sweating and a cold sensation. Hot flashes may occur rarely or recur every few minutes. At night, hot flashes are more frequent and can be severe enough to awaken a woman from sleep. They are also more intense during times of stress. In a cool environment, hot flashes are fewer, less intense, and shorter in duration than in a warm environment.[420]

The hot flash results from a sudden reduction of estrogen levels rather than from hypoestrogenism itself. Regardless of the cause of menopause—natural, surgical, or estrogen withdrawal caused by a GnRH agonist—hot flashes are associated with an acute and significant drop in estrogen level. The consistent association between the onset of flashes and acute estrogen withdrawal is supported by the effectiveness of estrogen therapy and the absence of flashes in prolonged hypoestrogenic states, such as gonadal dysgenesis or hypothalamic amenorrhea. Hypogonadal women experience hot flashes only after estrogen is administered and withdrawn.[421]

Not all hot flashes are caused by menopause. Sudden episodes of sweating and flashes may be caused by catecholamine- or histamine-secreting tumors (e.g., pheochromocytoma, carcinoid), hyperthyroidism, or chronic infection (e.g., tuberculosis). The hot flash may also be psychosomatic in origin. In these circumstances, the clinician should obtain a serum FSH level to confirm perimenopause or menopause before initiating hormone therapy. The relation of obesity to hot flashes has been debated. Early work was suggestive that body fat protected against vasomotor symptoms due to the aromatization of androgens to estrogens in fat tissue.[422] Recent evidence, however, indicates that higher body mass index, and body fat in particular, is associated with greater vasomotor symptom reporting, primarily hot flashes.[423] These findings are consistent with a thermoregulatory model of vasomotor symptoms in which body fat acts as an insulator, rendering vasomotor symptoms, a putative heat dissipation event, more likely.[423]

Urogenital Atrophy

The urogenital sinus gives rise to development of the lower vagina, vulva, and urethra during embryonic development, and these tissues are estrogen dependent. The decrease in estrogen at menopause causes the vaginal walls to become pale because of diminished vascularity and to thin down to only three or four cell layers. The vaginal epithelial cells in postmenopausal women contain less glycogen; before menopause glycogen is metabolized by lactobacilli to create an acidic pH, thereby protecting the vagina from bacterial overgrowth. Loss of this protective mechanism leaves the thin, friable tissue vulnerable to infection and ulceration. The vagina also loses its rugae and becomes shorter and inelastic. Postmenopausal women may complain of symptoms caused by vaginal dryness, such as pain during intercourse, vaginal discharge, burning, itching, or bleeding. Genitourinary atrophy leads to a variety of symptoms that affect the ease and quality of living.

Urethritis with dysuria, stress urinary incontinence, urinary frequency, and dyspareunia are further results of mucosal thinning of the urethra and bladder. Intravaginal estrogen treatment can effectively alleviate recurrent urinary tract infections and vaginal symptoms in the postmenopausal patient.[424]

Postmenopausal Osteoporosis

Osteoporosis is a disease characterized by low bone mass and microarchitectural deterioration of bone tissue, leading to enhanced bone fragility and a consequent increase in fracture risk. The most frequent sites of fracture are the vertebral bodies, distal radius, and femoral neck. Osteoporosis has become a global health issue. It is at epidemic proportions in the United States, affecting more than 20 million people.[425] Most osteoporotic patients are postmenopausal women.

Osteoporosis in postmenopausal women is a function of advancing age and estrogen deficiency. Seventy-five percent or more of the bone loss in women during the first 15 years after menopause is attributed to estrogen deficiency rather than to aging.[426,427] For the first 20 years after the cessation of ovarian estrogen secretion, postmenopausal osteoporosis accounts for a 50% reduction in trabecular bone and 30% loss of cortical bone.[426,427] Vertebral bone is especially vulnerable because the trabecular portion of the vertebral bodies is metabolically very active and decreases dramatically in amount in response to estrogen deficiency. Vertebral bone mass is already significantly decreased in perimenopausal and early postmenopausal women who have rising FSH and decreasing estrogen levels, whereas bone loss from the radius is not detected until at least 1 year after menopause.[427]

The risk of fracture depends on two factors: the peak bone mass achieved at maturity (at approximately age 30) and the subsequent rate of bone loss. An accelerated rate of bone loss after menopause strongly predicts an increased risk of fracture. The unfavorable effects of low premenopausal bone mass and accelerated loss of bone after menopause are additive, and these individuals are at the highest risk for fracture. An increased rate of average bone loss during menopause is an indicator of lower endogenous estrogen levels, possibly because postmenopausal bone loss is considerably slower in women with increased adipose tissue mass and consequent increased peripheral estrogen formation.[273]

Numerous studies show that hormone therapy started at perimenopause prevents postmenopausal bone loss.[428] Hormone therapy started at any age in a postmenopausal woman has potential beneficial effects by at least preventing additional bone loss. However, the incidence of fractures or rate of height loss was not reduced during a 4-year follow-up of women starting hormone therapy at a mean age of 66.7 (±6.7) years. The Women's Health Initiative (WHI) trial results revealed a decreased number of vertebral and hip fractures in the group of postmenopausal women receiving estrogen plus progestin or estrogen only; this important evidence was the first from randomized trials suggesting that estrogen prevents fractures.[122]

POSTMENOPAUSAL HORMONE THERAPY

Postmenopausal women who have undergone a hysterectomy should receive hormone therapy with estrogen only (HT-E). A progestin is added to estrogen (HT-EP) in the postmenopausal woman with a uterus to prevent endometrial hyperplasia or cancer. HT-EP is much more commonly prescribed than is HT-E, because most postmenopausal women do not undergo hysterectomy. The risks and benefits of these two regimens are distinct, and we refer to each separately in this section.

Until late 1990s, the most common practice was to treat all women disturbed by the symptoms of hormone deprivation (e.g., hot flashes) with estrogen and to use long-term hormonal prophylaxis against osteoporosis. The assumption that HT was cardioprotective played an important role in encouraging postmenopausal women to stay on this regimen indefinitely.[431] Estrogens and progestins used for postmenopausal HT were among the most commonly prescribed medications in the United States. A national survey suggested that there was a significant upward trend for the use of any form of HT from the 1970s until the 1990s. Many women started HT at menopause or later and remained on it. At one point, 46% of women who had experienced a natural menopause and 71% of women who had undergone bilateral oophorectomy reported having used postmenopausal HT.[432] The average duration of use in the United States in 1992 was 6.6 years, but only 20% of users had maintained treatment for at least 5 years.

This trend changed drastically in the early 2000s, after publication of the principal results of two large randomized trials, the Heart and Estrogen/Progestin Replacement Study (HERS) in 1998 and the WHI trial in 2002.[433-435] WHI results constituted the direct cause of discontinuation of HT in approximately 30% of postmenopausal women.[435] A discussion of HERS and WHI trials and how they changed HT practices is warranted. Debate continues regarding the applicability of the WHI and HERS results to all or various subsets of postmenopausal women.[431] Although the use of HT has dramatically decreased, these influential studies raised a number of important issues that require further studies to address.[431,436]

The WHI trial was a tremendously important contribution to understanding menopausal therapy. Most earlier cohort, retrospective, and prospective observational studies had demonstrated significant (40% to 60%) reductions in coronary heart disease (CHD) in postmenopausal women taking HT-E or HT-EP. These studies also showed reductions in all-cause mortality and osteoporotic fractures. However, there were modest increases in the risk of breast cancer, on the order of 20% to 30% (attributable as a risk of approximately 1 case per 1000 person-years).[433-435] These earlier studies also demonstrated a reduced incidence of Alzheimer's-type dementia in women who had used HT-EP compared with women who had not.[437] Given the inherent biases that confound observational studies, randomized clinical trials were needed to establish whether HT protects against CVD or dementias.[431,437]

The HERS and other secondary prevention studies demonstrated no benefit for women with known CVD initiating HT 8 to 23 years beyond menopause.[433-435] In the WHI hormone trials, women with no prior history of clinical CVD who started HT-EP (i.e., combined conjugated equine estrogens [CEEs] and MPA) an average of 12 years after menopause increased their CHD risk slightly and nonsignificantly, whereas HT-E (i.e., CEEs given without MPA) did not increase CHD risk but failed to significantly reduce it.[437] There were modest increases in thromboembolic disease and stroke in both trials and a borderline statistically significant increase in breast cancer only in the HT-EP arm of the WHI. Cognitive evaluation of older women (>65 years) in the WHI cohort demonstrated increases in incidence of new dementia and no difference in overall rates of cognitive decline.[437] Surprisingly, both HT preparations were associated with adverse effects on urinary incontinence.[437]

It was concluded that the overall risk/benefit ratio for HT was unfavorable. Results from the WHI study indicated that the combination of CEE (0.625 mg/day) and MPA (2.5 mg/day) should not be initiated or continued for the primary prevention of CHD in postmenopausal women. The substantial risks for CVD and breast cancer must be weighed against the beneficial effect on fracture risk when selecting from the available agents to prevent osteoporosis.

Historical Perspective of Scientific Studies Regarding Hormone Therapy

In the 1950s, a growing number of physicians and their patients believed that replacement of the estrogen lost at menopause would prevent many of the manifestations of aging, including CHD, osteoporotic fractures, and a decline in cognitive and sexual function. This led to widespread use of HT-E after menopause. Other evidence in support of the CHD benefit were also consistent. Observational studies showed less heart disease among women taking estrogen, pathophysiologic mechanisms provided biologic plausibility, and clinical trials revealed improvements in blood lipid levels and other surrogate measures.[431,437,438]

The most commonly used form of HT-E was CEEs. In the 1980s, it was recognized that postmenopausal HT-E treatment was causing endometrial cancer. Although uncommon and usually curable, this cancer can be prevented by antagonizing the estrogen with a progestin, and several HT-EP combinations were explored in the search for one that preserved the benefits of estrogen. In the 1990s, after it was demonstrated that lipid effects remained largely favorable when CEEs were combined with MPA, this particular estrogen plus progestin regimen became the most widely used form of HT in the United States for postmenopausal women with a uterus.[438]

In the late 1980s and 1990s, it became apparent that HT-EP increased the breast cancer incidence.[439] This increase was significant but minimal. In view of HT's perceived cardiovascular benefits and bone-protective effects, many women and their clinicians still considered the overall benefit largely to exceed the risk.[438]

In 1998, the HERS study, the first major randomized trial of HT, unexpectedly found an increase in CHD events during the first year and no overall cardiovascular benefit with longer follow-up when HT-EP was compared with placebo in 2763 women with prior coronary disease.[440] This trial also found that HT-EP caused venous thromboembolism. In 2002, the WHI HT-EP trial was interrupted prematurely because of a perceived net harm.[429] Among 16,608 healthy postmenopausal women with a uterus, HT-EP caused an increased risk of coronary events, stroke, venous thromboembolism, breast cancer, and pulmonary embolism. A global index formulated by the investigators found these harmful outcomes to outweigh the decreased risk of hip fracture and colon cancer (Table 17-10). A subsequent report showing a significant twofold increase in dementia among WHI women older than 65 years accentuated these concerns.[441] Results from the HERS and WHI led the FDA to require a warning of harm and to recommend that estrogen preparations not be used to prevent CHD and not be considered first-line therapy for prevention of osteoporosis. In view of these WHI study findings, a number of professional societies changed their guidelines to recommend that HT not be used for prevention of disease and that its use for treatment of symptoms should be at the lowest dose and for the shortest time possible.[431]

Women and their clinicians anxiously awaited the results of the WHI HT-E trial in 10,739 healthy women with hysterectomy who were randomly assigned to receive CEEs only or placebo.[430] As in the HERS and WHI HT-EP trials, HT-E did not reduce the risk of CHD, although early CHD harm, which may be a consequence of progestin, appeared to be less pronounced.[430]

TABLE 17-10

Results of the Women's Health Initiative Randomized Controlled Trial of Postmenopausal Hormone Therapy with Estrogen Alone (E-alone) or Estrogen Plus Progestin (E+P)*

		E+P			E-alone		
Factor	**Hypothesized Effect**	**HR**	**95% CI**	**AR**	**HR**	**95% CI**	**AR**
Coronary heart disease	↓	1.24	1.00-1.54	+6	0.95	0.79-1.15	−3
Stroke	↔ ↓	1.31	1.02-1.68	+8	1.37	1.09-1.73	+12
Pulmonary embolism	↑	2.13	1.45-3.11	+10	1.37	0.90-2.07	+4
Venous thromboembolism	↑	2.06	1.57-2.70	+18	1.32	0.99-1.75	+8
Breast cancer	↑	1.24	1.02-1.50	+8	0.80	0.62-1.04	−6
Colorectal cancer	↓	0.56	0.38-0.81	−7	1.08	0.75-1.55	+1
Endometrial cancer		0.81	0.48-1.36	−1	NA		
Hip fracture	↓	0.67	0.47-0.96	−5	0.65	0.45-0.94	−7
Total fractures	↓	0.76	0.69-0.83	−47	0.71	0.64-0.80	−53
Total mortality	↓	0.98[‡]	0.82-1.18	−1	1.04[‡]	0.91-1.12	+3
Global index[†]		1.15[‡]	1.03-1.28	+19	1.01[‡]	1.09-1.12	+2
Diabetes		0.79	0.67-0.93		0.88	0.77-1.01	
Gallbladder disease	↑	1.59	1.28-1.97		1.67	1.35-2.06	
Stress incontinence		1.87	1.61-2.18		2.15	1.77-2.62	
Urge incontinence		1.15	0.99-1.34		1.32	1.10-1.58	
Peripheral artery disease		0.89	0.63-1.25		1.32	0.99-1.77	
Probable dementia	↓	2.05	1.21-3.48		1.49	0.83-2.66	

*Hazard ratio (HR), 95% confidence interval (CI), and attributable risk (AR) per 10,000 person-years are shown for various clinical outcomes. HR estimates are based on proportional hazards analysis stratified by age (5-year categories) and randomization in the dietary modification trial.

†Global index is defined for each woman as the time to the earliest diagnosis of coronary heart disease, stroke, pulmonary embolism, breast cancer, colorectal cancer, endometrial cancer (for E+P), hip fracture, or death from other causes.

‡Based on an average follow-up of 5.2 and 8.6 years for E+P and E-alone, respectively. All other values are based on an average of 5.6 (E+P) and 7.1 (E-alone) years of follow-up.

From Prentice RL, Anderson GL. The Women's Health Initiative: lessons learned. *Annu Rev Public Health* 2008;29:131-150.

Resolution of the Discrepancies between Observational and Randomized Studies

The WHI program included a randomized, controlled trial and a large observational study.[437] Results from the observational component of the WHI were in agreement with the many observational studies performed earlier in the 1990s.[437] A confusing debate followed the conflicting conclusions from the observational studies and randomized trials on the effect of HT on CHD and breast cancer. HT appeared to be protective against CHD in observational studies, but randomized trials showed an increase in CHD during the first years of use.[437] Moreover, HT-EP use was associated with a lesser risk of breast cancer in the randomized WHI trial than in observational studies.[437] HT-E was associated with a smaller breast cancer risk than HT-EP in observational studies, but it carried no risk in the randomized WHI trial.[437] This led investigators to reanalyze data from randomized trials and observational studies with a different perspective.

With respect to CHD risk, the results of observational studies and randomized trials were well aligned, primarily by analyzing the data according to time since initiation of HT.[442] This analysis was naturally performed in randomized trials, because HT was started at randomization. In the WHI and HERS studies, HT-EP did increase CHD risk, which later vanished. In observational studies, in which current users were contrasted with never-users at the time of enrollment, most current users were already past the window of increased CHD risk and were in a phase of diminished risk. For example, when cohort data from the observational part of the WHI were reanalyzed according to time since start of therapy, the same pattern emerged as in the randomized trials: an initial increase in risk followed by a decrease.[437] The misleading conclusions drawn from the observational studies were not necessarily because of poor-quality data; the problem was that the initial analysis of these data did not take into account that HT might produce different effects over a period of time.[437] The reanalysis of the Nurses Health Study on HT-EP and CHD confirmed this conclusion by finding the same pattern of an initial increase in risk, whereas the original analysis had suggested overall protection.[442]

The discrepancy between the conclusions from randomized trials and those from observational studies with respect to breast cancer risk was explicable by a similar "timing hypothesis." Women in the randomized trials had on average been in menopause longer, whereas in the observational study, the women had started HT closer to menopause.[437,442] The findings of observational and randomized studies fell in line after the randomized trial data were reanalyzed and adjusted for the interval between menopause and treatment.[437] This reanalysis showed a clear increase in risk for HT-EP and a slight increase for HT-E. In this case, the observational studies had indicated a true risk for the women closer to menopause. In the randomized trial, that risk was diluted because fewer women close to menopause were included. In clinical practice, this risk is important because HT is usually started close to menopause. The discrepancies were not caused by differences in study design but instead reflected a lack of appreciation for the timing of initiation of treatment relative to menopause.[437,442] These reanalyses confirmed that the CHD and stroke risks are significant and slightly higher in older women, whereas the actual breast cancer risk is higher in women closer to menopause.[437]

Risks and Contraindications of Hormone Therapy

Coronary Heart Disease

Data suggest that initiation of HT many years after menopause is associated with excess CHD risk, whereas HT given for a limited period soon after menopause is not. HT-EP or HT-E does not prevent CHD as was previously proposed. To the contrary, there may be a small but significant increase in the rate of CHD among women taking HT-EP.[429,440] Women with preexisting CHD and healthy women are at risk. HT-E, on the other hand, does not increase the risk for CHD in healthy women.[430]

Stroke

Another outcome that was consistent across the three trials is the increased risk of stroke among women assigned to HT-E or HT-EP. Increased stroke risk may be attributable to the estrogen component of the hormone regimen, because it is the only statistically significant adverse effect of HT-E.[429,430,440]

Pulmonary Embolism

A pattern of increased pulmonary embolism was observed in all randomized studies, although the risk was attenuated and was not statistically significant in the WHI HT-E trial.[429,430,440]

Breast Cancer

Findings of the WHI HT-E trial were markedly different from those of the HERS and WHI HT-EP trials with respect to breast cancer risk. The WHI HT-E trial indicated a trend, albeit statistically not significant, toward a lower breast cancer risk, in contrast to an observational literature that mostly reports a moderate increase in risk with estrogen-alone preparations. However, after control for prior use of postmenopausal hormone therapy and additional control for time from menopause to first use of postmenopausal hormone therapy, the hazard ratios agreed closely between the observational and randomized trial data.[443] Nonetheless, the higher risk for breast cancer observed in the HT-EP trials probably represents a harmful additional effect of MPA, the progestin used in these studies. The increased breast cancer risk was statistically significant in the WHI HT-EP trial, which demonstrated an attributable risk of 6 cases per 10,000 person-years.[437] This was matched by a trend of the same magnitude in the HERS study and was supported by evidence from large observational studies suggesting that the addition of MPA or another progestin to estrogen may significantly increase the risk for breast cancer (see Table 17-10).

Ovarian Cancer

A retrospective 1979-1998 cohort study of 44,241 postmenopausal women revealed that HT-E, particularly when taken for 10 or more years, significantly increases risk of ovarian cancer. The relative risks for 10 to 19 years and for 20 or more years were 1.8 (95% CI, 1.1 to 3.0) and 3.2 (95% CI, 1.7 to 5.7), respectively (*P* value for trend, <.001). This study did not show an increased risk among women who used short-term HT-EP, but the investigators suggested that the risk associated with longer-term HT-EP use warrants further investigation.[444] The WHI HT-EP study found a trend for increased ovarian cancer risk that was not significant.[430]

Lung Cancer

One report suggested that HT-EP significantly increases the number of deaths from non–small-cell lung cancer in postmenopausal women.[445] However, the observed trend toward increased lung cancer incidence was not statistically significant.[445]

Dementia

In postmenopausal women 65 years of age or older, HT-EP significantly increased risk and resulted in an additional 23 cases of probable dementia per 10,000 women per year.[446] Alzheimer's disease was the most common classification of dementia. A similar trend was observed for HT-E but did not reach statistical significance.[446] When the data were pooled, HT significantly increased probable dementia risk.[446]

Hyperlipidemia

Hyperlipidemia is a rare side effect observed in patients with severe familial hypertriglyceridemia. An oral estrogen regimen can hasten development of severe hypertriglyceridemia or pancreatitis in women with severely elevated triglyceride levels.[447] Estrogen replacement is relatively contraindicated in women with substantially increased triglyceride levels.

Gallbladder Disease

Both WHI trials (HT-E and HT-EP) showed greater risk for any gallbladder disease or surgery with estrogen.[448] Both trials indicated a higher risk for cholecystitis and for cholelithiasis. Women on either HT regimen were more likely to undergo cholecystectomy.[429,430] These data suggest an increase in risk of biliary tract disease among postmenopausal women using estrogen therapy. The morbidity and cost associated with these outcomes may need to be considered in decisions regarding the use of estrogen therapy. Preexisting gallbladder disease is a relative contraindication for estrogen replacement.

Benefits of Hormone Therapy

Hot Flashes

HT-E or HT-EP reliably treats hot flashes in most women. Currently, hot flashes constitute the most common indication for a short course of HT (<5 years).

Fractures

HT-EP or HT-E significantly decreased the incidence of hip, vertebral, and other osteoporotic fractures. In this case, the results of observational studies of estrogen and fracture risk and of trials using a surrogate end point (i.e., bone mineral density) agree with the results of clinical trials of fracture prevention.

Colon Cancer

Colon cancer was significantly less common with HT-EP in the WHI study but not with HT-E, for reasons that are not clear.[429,430] It is possible that progestin is the protective hormone in this case.

Negative Women's Health Initiative Results Relevant to Previously Postulated Benefits

In the WHI study, HT-EP resulted in no significant effects on general health, vitality, mental health, depressive symptoms, or sexual satisfaction.[449] Contrary to expectations, HT-EP and HT-E increased symptoms of urinary incontinence.[437] HT-EP was associated with a statistically significant but small benefit in terms of sleep disturbance, physical functioning, and bodily pain after 1 year.[449] At 3 years, however, there were no significant benefits in any quality-of-life outcomes.[449] The group that received HT-E in the WHI trial also did not have a meaningful improvement in health-related quality of life after 1 or 3 years.[450]

HT-EP did not improve cognitive improvement, as was previously anticipated.[441] The group receiving HT-E showed a trend for worsened mild cognitive impairment, although this was not significant.[441] Among postmenopausal women 65 years old or older, HT-EP did not improve cognitive function when compared with placebo, whereas HT-E had an adverse effect on cognition, which was greater among women with lower cognitive function at initiation of treatment.[451,452]

Interpretation of the WHI and HERS Results in a Broader Perspective

The mean age of participants in all three randomized trials was in the mid-60s, raising the concern that these results may not apply to treatment begun early in menopause.[429,430,440] In this regard, the WHI HT-E trial found that the subgroup of women in the youngest age group (50 to 59 years) appeared to respond to estrogen more favorably than older women for many of the outcomes, including the global index. However, differences in hazard ratios among subgroups were statistically significant for only 1 of 23 tests and could well have occurred by chance.[430]

Even if hazard ratios are similar in women of all ages, the absolute risks differ substantially. The absolute risk for many diseases approximately doubles with each decade of age. Women in their 50s have about one half of the risk of women in their 60s and one fourth of the risk of women in their 70s. This means that any effect of hormone therapy on these diseases will be less marked in younger than in older women. The possibility of more favorable findings in 50- to 59-year-old women and the low absolute risk of adverse outcomes at this age suggest that use of HT-E to treat menopausal symptoms for a limited duration early in menopause is reasonable.

The WHI trials suggested that HT-E has advantages over HT-EP for treatment in postmenopausal women. It has only one or two adverse outcomes (i.e., increased strokes and probably pulmonary emboli) rather than four (i.e., increased strokes, CHD, pulmonary emboli, and breast cancer), and both regimens have an important benefit (i.e., decreased fractures). However, this risk/benefit assessment does not take into account the dementia findings, and even in their absence, HT-E produced no improvement in the overall global index. HT-E in women with a uterus increases the risk of uterine cancer and rates of uterine bleeding, biopsy, and hysterectomy. As more deliberate and exhaustive analyses of this trial become available, they will likely contribute to new practice guidelines.

There is considerable debate regarding the type of estrogen and mode of administration. Estradiol may have advantages over CEEs, and transdermal administration, by avoiding high levels in the portal circulation and delivery to the liver, may have advantages over oral delivery.[453] Trials employing transdermal estradiol are being conducted.[454]

Post-WHI Recommendations for Hormone Therapy

Decision making for women interested in HT involves balancing the potential benefits of hormone therapy against the potential risks.[455] HT is effective for treatment of hot flashes, and for this indication, HT-E seems to be associated with less risk than HT-EP. However, HT-E does have adverse effects, and it is prudent to keep the dose low and the duration of treatment short. A progestin should be added only to prevent endometrial cancer. Women without a uterus should receive HT-E.

Many clinicians and epidemiologists agree that short-term estrogen therapy using the lowest effective estrogen dose is a reasonable option for recently menopausal women who have moderate to severe symptoms and no previous history or elevated risk of CHD, stroke, breast cancer, or venous thromboembolism. HT usually lasts for 2 to 3 years but rarely more than 5 years, because menopausal symptoms diminish after several years, whereas the risk of breast cancer increases with longer duration of HT.

A small group of women may need long-term therapy for severe, persistent symptoms after stopping HT. These few women may be encouraged to first try nonhormonal options such as gabapentin; estrogen treatment should be resumed only if these alternatives are not helpful. For isolated symptoms of genitourinary atrophy, low-dose vaginal estrogens with minimal systemic absorption and endometrial effects are highly beneficial.[455]

In the absence of evidence for an overall net benefit of postmenopausal treatment with HT-E and with the evidence that HT-EP is harmful, neither therapy should be used for preventing CHD or improving mental function.

Target Groups for Hormone Therapy

In women with gonadal dysgenesis and surgical menopause, the duration of estrogen deprivation is prolonged. Estrogen replacement is recommended for these patients for reduction of hot flashes and for long-term prophylaxis against osteoporosis and target organ atrophy. A low-dose contraceptive may be offered to nonsmoking women until the age of 45 years. After that point, doses of estrogen equivalent to 0.625 mg of conjugated estrogens may be more appropriate because of a sharp age-related increase in risk for thromboembolic events. The physician should recommend a continuous estrogen-progestin combination to those women with a uterus and an estrogen-only regimen to women without a uterus.

During perimenopause, hot flashes can be suppressed with an estrogen-progestin combination. Because bone loss related to estrogen deprivation also begins during this period, a benefit for women who take HT to prevent hot flashes is that bone loss will not start for the few years of therapy.[456] In perimenopausal women, unexplained uterine bleeding should be evaluated with an endometrial biopsy before the start of hormone therapy.

Estrogen Preparations and Beneficial Dose of Estrogen

Oral Estrogens: Combined Conjugated Equine Estrogens

The amount of estrogen that is effective for hot flashes varies. For this purpose, it is reasonable to start with CEEs at 0.3 mg/day (or micronized estradiol at 0.5 mg/day) and gradually increase this dose to CEEs at 0.625 mg/day (equivalent to micronized estradiol at 1 mg/day) and 1.25 mg/day (equivalent to micronized estradiol at 2 mg/day). If hot flashes in a postmenopausal woman are not alleviated by 1.25 mg/day of CEEs or an equivalent transdermal estradiol dose, it is unlikely that higher doses will be effective. In this case, alternative diagnoses (e.g., tuberculosis, depression, thyroid disease) should be ruled out.

Low-dose estrogen (0.3 mg/day of CEEs or 0.5 mg/day of micronized estradiol) maintain blood estradiol levels between 17 to 32 pg/mL (average, 22 pg/mL) and may be sufficient for preserving bone density and for alleviating menopausal symptoms in early postmenopausal women.[457] The effect of estrogen on arterial thrombosis is probably dose related.[457] For example, oral contraceptives with higher doses of estrogen are more likely to be associated with increased risks of myocardial infarction and stroke, especially in smokers. When choosing a dose for HT, it is imperative to achieve and maintain the lowest beneficial levels of circulating estradiol and to avoid higher levels, to minimize the risk of thrombosis.

The addition of a progestin, either cyclically or continuously, to concomitant estrogen replacement reduces the risk of estrogen-induced endometrial hyperplasia or carcinoma but poses additional problems.[458] These include regular withdrawal bleeding in up to 90% of women treated with cyclic therapy and irregular spotting in 20% of women treated with continuous estrogen plus progestin. Progestins appear to reduce the beneficial effects of estrogen on high-density lipoprotein (HDL)- and LDL-cholesterol and to increase the risks of pulmonary embolism, CHD, and breast cancer.[429,430,440]

A time-honored sequential regimen involves oral administration of 0.625 mg of CEEs or the equivalent dose of a variety of available products on days 1 through 25 of each month (Fig. 17-38). A daily dose of 5 mg of MPA is added on days 12 through 25 or on days 16 through 25. Withdrawal bleeding is expected on or after day 26 of each month. Another common cyclic regimen involves continuous oral administration of 0.625 mg of conjugated estrogens or the equivalent daily dose (see Fig. 17-38). A daily dose of 5 mg of MPA is added for the first 10 to 14 days of every month. One-year randomized trial data indicate that the 5-mg dose protects the endometrium as well as the 10-mg dose does.[459] Progestin withdrawal bleeding occurs in 90% of women with a sequential or cyclic regimen.[460,461] These regimens can also cause adverse symptoms related to the relatively high daily doses of progestin, including breast tenderness, bloating, fluid retention, and depression. The lowest possible dose of a progestin is recommended.

The continuous combined method of treatment has the potential benefit of reduced bleeding and amenorrhea, but it is occasionally complicated by breakthrough bleeding (see Fig. 17-38).[460,461] In this regimen, a combination of 0.625 mg of conjugated estrogens and 2.5 mg of MPA is given orally every day. The continuous combination regimen is simple and convenient, and it is associated with an incidence of amenorrhea in 80% of patients after at least 6 months of use. The other 20% of patients continue to experience some degree of unpredictable spotting. Overall compliance is much better in users of the continuous combination regimen. Moreover, the lower daily dose of MPA is associated with a lower incidence of breast tenderness with this regimen. Other estrogen-progestin combinations are also available for similar continuous use.

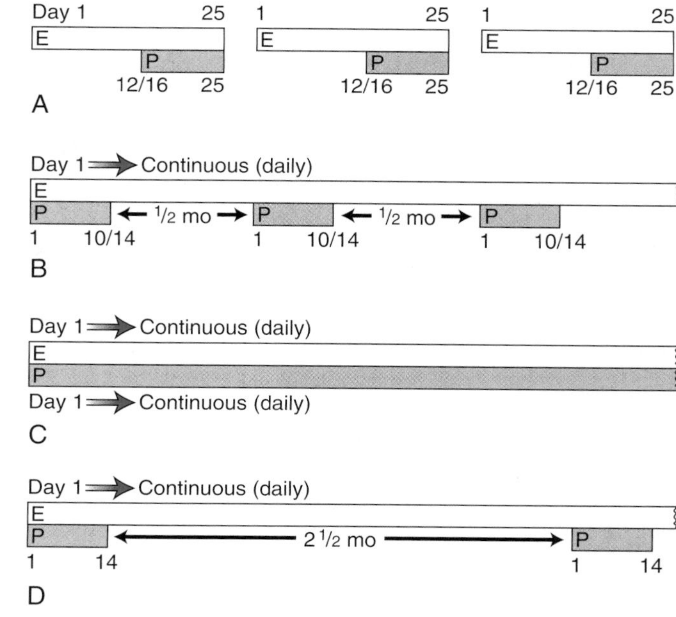

Figure 17-38 Regimens of hormone therapy. Estrogen (E) is replaced in a postmenopausal woman to prevent osteoporosis, urogenital atrophy, and hot flashes. In the postmenopausal woman with a uterus, a progestin (P) should be added to estrogen to prevent endometrial hyperplasia and cancer. E and P can be administered in several ways. **A** and **B,** Postmenopausal women receiving hormone therapy have predictable withdrawal bleeding episodes after each P course. **C,** E and P are administered together. After a year of continuous combination therapy, the rate of unpredictable breakthrough spotting is 20%. **D,** This relatively new regimen was introduced to minimize the harmful effects of a progestin. Its long-term safety for endometrial hyperplasia or cancer risk is unknown. Predictable bleeding after each P course every 3 months is presumed to be reassuring.

Cyclic progestin has also been used at less frequent intervals, such as every 3 to 6 months. When added to standard-dosage estrogen, 10 mg of MPA every 3 months for 14 days produced a 1.5% rate of hyperplasia (a rate low enough to be interpreted as endometrial protection), and long-term use of MPA at 6-month intervals was associated with a low rate of endometrial cancer. However, clinicians have not determined the optimal progestin dosage and schedule to use with low-dosage estrogen. Low-dosage estrogen use can reasonably be assumed to require less progestin for protection of the endometrium.

Most postmenopausal women can switch their HT regimen from standard-dosage HT to low-dosage estrogen opposed by MPA at 3-month intervals or start HT at this low dose.[457] Although its long-term safety has not been proved with respect to endometrial hyperplasia, the following regimen appears to be a reasonable compromise for treating hot flashes and preventing osteoporosis while minimizing the harmful effects of progestins and high-dose estrogen[457]: 0.3 mg/day of CEEs or 0.025 mg of transdermal estradiol is administered continuously. Every 3 months, a 14-day course of 5 mg of MPA is added (see Fig. 17-38 D). Endometrial biopsy is not required in the presence of withdrawal bleeding after each periodic progestin intake and in the absence of irregular bleeding. This regimen may be continued for up to 5 years. After discontinuation of HT, the postmenopausal woman can be switched to a bisphosphonate or a selective estrogen receptor modulator (SERM) for bone protection.

Transdermal Estrogen

Transdermal estrogen preparations appear to be as effective as oral estrogens for treating hot flashes and maintaining bone mineral density, but they have different metabolic profiles. Oral estrogens are easier to administer and seem to have favorable effects on lipoprotein profiles. However, oral estrogens are associated with several disadvantages, including unfavorable changes in serum levels of triglycerides, C-reactive protein, fibrinogen, factor VII, and plasminogen activator inhibitor type 1.[455] A meta-analysis of clinical trials suggested a higher risk of venous thromboembolic events among oral HT users compared with transdermal estrogen users.[455] Clinical trial data that address the effect of transdermal estrogen on CHD and stroke risk are limited.[455]

A daily dose of 0.05 mg of transdermal estradiol is equivalent to 0.625 mg of oral CEEs or 1 mg of oral micronized estradiol. A lower-dose transdermal preparation includes 0.025 mg of estradiol (equivalent to 0.3 mg of oral CEEs). An ultra-low-dose transdermal estradiol preparation (0.014 mg) is also available. In women with symptoms not responding to smaller doses, high-dose transdermal estradiol at 0.1 mg/day (equivalent to CEEs at 1.25 mg/day) may be used. For the average menopausal woman with hot flashes, it is reasonable to start with a daily dose of 0.025 mg. This should be accompanied by a progestin in a woman with a uterus.

Management of Breakthrough Bleeding during Postmenopausal Hormone Therapy

Approximately 90% of women receiving estrogen plus cyclic administration of a progestin have monthly progestin withdrawal bleeding in a predictable fashion. Continuous combined estrogen-progestin therapy causes breakthrough bleeding in approximately 40% of women during the first 6 months, with the remaining 60% being amenorrheic. The pattern of vaginal bleeding in women taking the continuous combined regimen is unpredictable and causes anxiety in most patients, but the incidence of breakthrough bleeding decreases to 20% after 1 year of treatment.[460-462] Nevertheless, breakthrough bleeding remains the most important reason for discontinuance of this therapy. Most patients find it unacceptable and prefer to switch to a cyclic progestin regimen or to discontinue hormone therapy altogether. There is no effective pharmacologic method to manage the breakthrough bleeding associated with continuous combined estrogen-progestin regimens. The physician can only reassure the patient that the bleeding is likely to subside within 1 year from the start of HT. If breakthrough bleeding continues beyond 1 year, the regimen should be changed to daily estrogen plus cyclic progestin.

HT can be started in the amenorrheic postmenopausal patient at any time. Perimenopausal women with oligomenorrhea, hot flashes, or other associated symptoms can also be treated with HT. In the oligomenorrheic patient, a hormone therapy regimen may be initiated on day 3 of one of the infrequent menses. If the candidate for hormone therapy does not have irregular uterine bleeding, it is not essential to perform endometrial biopsies routinely before beginning treatment. Studies indicate that asymptomatic postmenopausal women rarely have endometrial abnormalities.[462-464] Pretreatment biopsies using a thin plastic biopsy cannula in the office may be limited to patients who are at higher risk for endometrial hyperplasia (e.g., unpredictable uterine bleeding, history of PCOS or chronic anovulation, obesity, liver disease, diabetes mellitus).

Giving a woman a combined estrogen-progestin regimen does not preclude the development of endometrial cancer.[465] Therefore it is necessary to rule out endometrial malignancy in women receiving HT who are experiencing irregular uterine bleeding. The important task is to differentiate breakthrough bleeding from bleeding induced by hyperplasia or cancer. Because breakthrough bleeding is extremely common, many biopsies must be performed to detect a rare case of endometrial abnormality during HT. To decrease the number of endometrial biopsies, a screening method using transvaginal ultrasonography has been introduced.[173] The thickness of the postmenopausal endometrium as measured by transvaginal ultrasonography in postmenopausal women correlates with the presence or absence of pathology.[173] Patients receiving a cyclic or daily combination hormone therapy regimen who have an endometrial thickness of less than 5 mm can be managed conservatively.[466-468] An endometrial thickness equal to or greater than 5 mm requires biopsy. Based on this algorithm, it is estimated that 50% to 75% of bleeding patients receiving HT and evaluated by ultrasonography require biopsy.[173]

Management of Menopausal Symptoms in Breast Cancer Survivors

Vasomotor symptoms constitute a major problem for survivors of breast cancer. Approximately 65% of women become symptomatic with hot flashes (mostly severe) after treatment for breast cancer.[469] Hot flashes are encountered more frequently among tamoxifen users and women treated with chemotherapy. Up to 90% of premenopausal women who receive chemotherapy and tamoxifen have vasomotor symptoms.[469]

Breast cancer survivors often seek relief from hot flashes. HT is typically withheld from women with breast cancer because of concerns that estrogen may stimulate recurrence. One randomized study showed that after extended follow-up, there was a statistically significant increased risk of a new breast cancer event in survivors who took HT.[470] In this randomized, non–placebo-controlled study, 442 women assigned to receive HT-EP/HT-E or best symptomatic management without hormones were followed for a median of 4 years. Thirty-nine of the 221 women in the HT arm and 17 of the 221 women in the control arm had a new breast cancer diagnosed (hazard risk, 2.4; 95% CI, 1.3 to 4.2). Cumulative breast cancer incidences at 5 years were 22.2% in the HT arm and 8.0% in the control arm. No difference in mortality from breast cancer was found.[470]

Because of higher breast cancer recurrence associated with HT, many breast cancer survivors have sought nonhormonal alternatives,[469] including other pharmaceutical agents, herbal or dietary remedies, and mind-body or behavioral therapies. Mind-body or behavioral treatments for hot flashes are particularly attractive to survivors of breast cancer because they do not have the side effects caused by pharmaceutical agents, but it is not yet known whether they are effective.[469]

Several nonhormonal pharmaceutical agents have been used off-label for women who cannot take or elect not to take HT. Among the non-HT treatments, selective serotonin reuptake inhibitors (SSRIs), serotonin-norepinephrine reuptake inhibitors (SNRIs), clonidine, and gabapentin were found to be more effective than placebo.[455] Although all of these nonsteroidal medications could reduce the number of hot flashes per day, their beneficial effects were far less than what has been observed with estrogen, and these drugs are all associated with significant side effects that can limit their use in some women. Extracts of black cohosh or red clover were found to be ineffective, and the results for soy isoflavone extracts were mixed.[455] The beneficial doses for hot flashes include paroxetine (an SSRI) at 10 to 20 mg/day, paroxetine controlled release at 12.5 to 25 mg/day, venlafaxine (an SNRI) at 75 mg/day, desvenlafaxine (an SNRI) at 100 mg/day, and gabapentin at 900 mg/day. Gabapentin should be started with a smaller dose given at bedtime, and the dose should be gradually increased. Paroxetine reduces the metabolism of tamoxifen to its most active metabolite, endoxifen, and should be avoided in women with breast cancer who are receiving tamoxifen.[455]

Tibolone, a synthetic steroid with estrogenic, androgenic, and progestagenic properties, is approved in 90 countries for treatment of menopausal symptoms and in 45 countries for prevention of osteoporosis. Tibolone preserves bone mineral density, reduces hot flashes, and may increase libido and vaginal lubrication in postmenopausal women.[471] A randomized study showed that tibolone reduced the risks of fracture and breast cancer and possibly colon cancer but increased the risk of stroke in older women with osteoporosis.[471] Tibolone is not available in the United States.

For long-term prophylaxis against osteoporosis in breast cancer survivors, tamoxifen, raloxifene, or a bisphosphonate are viable options. However, tamoxifen and raloxifene intensify hot flashes.

Selective Estrogen Receptor Modulators and Bisphosphonates as Alternatives to Hormone Therapy

SERMs are compounds that act like estrogen in some target tissues but antagonize estrogenic effects in others (see Chapter 30).[472] One of the first SERMs was tamoxifen, for which estrogen-like agonist activity on bone was observed to occur simultaneously with estrogen antagonist activity on the breast.[472] Tamoxifen had been approved initially for treatment and prevention of breast cancer. An unwanted effect of tamoxifen is its estrogen-like action on the endometrium. Second-generation compounds have since been developed, most notably raloxifene, which has estrogen-like actions on bone, lipids, and the coagulation system; estrogen antagonist effects on the breast; and no detectable action in the endometrium.[473] In 2007, the FDA approved raloxifene for reducing the risk of invasive breast cancer in postmenopausal women with osteoporosis and in postmenopausal women who are at high risk for invasive breast cancer. Raloxifene is most often used to prevent and treat osteoporosis in postmenopausal women.

In placebo-controlled trials, raloxifene reduced vertebral fractures, whereas tamoxifen reduced nonvertebral fractures.[473] Tamoxifen and raloxifene had similar effects on fractures at multiple sites in a randomized, head-to-head trial.[473] Tamoxifen or raloxifene reduced risk for invasive breast cancer compared with placebo by approximately 7 to 10 cases per 1000 women per year.[473] Tamoxifen and raloxifene reduced ER-positive breast cancer but not ER-negative breast cancer, noninvasive breast cancer, or mortality.[473] Tamoxifen and raloxifene increase thromboembolic events by 4 to 7 cases per 1000 women per year; raloxifene causes fewer events than tamoxifen. Tamoxifen increases risk for endometrial cancer compared with placebo by 4 cases per 1000 women per year and causes cataracts.[473] Raloxifene use is not associated with endometrial cancer or cataract risk.[473] The most common side effects for tamoxifen are hot flashes and other vasomotor symptoms and vaginal discharge, itching, or dryness. For raloxifene, vasomotor symptoms and leg cramps are most common. In a head-to-head trial, raloxifene users reported more musculoskeletal problems, dyspareunia, and weight gain, whereas tamoxifen users had more gynecologic problems, vasomotor symptoms, and bladder control symptoms.[473] Tamoxifen and raloxifene may be used to reduce the incidence of vertebral fractures and invasive breast cancer in postmenopausal women. The major drawbacks include hot flashes and increased thromboembolic events for both drugs and endometrial cancer for tamoxifen. Data are lacking on optimal doses, duration, timing, long-term effects, and effects in nonwhite women.

The major treatment goal in postmenopausal osteoporosis is to prevent fractures by maintaining or increasing bone mineral density and reducing excessive bone turnover.[474] Bisphosphonates suppress resorption by inhibiting the attachment of osteoclasts to bone matrix and enhancing programmed cell death in osteoclasts. They have increased bone mineral density and reduced the risk for osteoporotic fractures in numerous clinical trials.[474] The FDA has approved four bisphosphonates for treatment or prevention of osteoporosis. Oral alendronate and oral risedronate were approved in 1995 and 2000, respectively. In 2003, oral ibandronate was approved, followed by intravenous ibandronate in 2006. Intravenous zoledronic acid was approved in 2007. A 5-mg dose of zoledronic acid is infused over 15 minutes once each year. Alendronate is given as a once-weekly 35- or 70-mg tablet or a once-daily 5- or 10-mg tablet; risedronate is given as a once-daily 5-mg tablet, a once-weekly 35-mg tablet, or a once-monthly 150-mg tablet, and ibandronate is given as a once-monthly 150-mg tablet or as 3 mg intravenously every 3 months.[475]

Compared with placebo controls, all four approved bisphosphonates reduce the relative risk of new vertebral fractures by on average 50% in women with postmenopausal osteoporosis.[475,476] Alendronate, risedronate, and zoledronic acid reduce the relative risk of new nonvertebral and hip fractures.[474] Clinical trial extensions of up to 10 years with alendronate and 7 years with risedronate have shown that efficacy is maintained during long-term treatment.[474] Moreover, discontinuation of long-term (≥5 years) alendronate therapy results in minimal bone loss over the ensuing 3 to 5 years.[477] As in the case of SERMs, definitive data are lacking on optimal doses, duration, timing, long-term effects, and effects in nonwhite women. Once-yearly zoledronic acid infusions appear to be an attractive choice because of better compliance and lack of esophagitis, a side effect associated with oral bisphosphonates.

Osteonecrosis of the jaw is a rare but serious side effect of bisphosphonate therapies. Bisphosphonate users who plan to undergo tooth extraction should discuss this side effect to their dental surgeons, because tooth extraction may predispose them to osteonecrosis of the jaw.[478] The addition of zoledronic acid to adjuvant endocrine therapy reduced disease recurrence in all body sites and improved disease-free survival in premenopausal patients with estrogen-responsive early breast cancer.[479] Further studies are required to explore the potential of bisphosphonates in preventing breast cancer in postmenopausal women with no previous history of breast cancer.

A number of case reports and a recent retrospective study suggested that the risk of esophageal cancer increased with oral bisphosphonate use over about a 5-year period. In western countries, the incidence of esophageal cancer in patients over the age of 60 is estimated to increase from 1 to 2 per 1000 population with 5 years' use of an oral bisphosphonate.[480,481] Another retrospective study, however, did not find such a link.[482] Until more accurate data are available, health-care providers should avoid prescribing oral bisphosphonates to patients with Barrett esophagus, a known risk factor for esophageal cancer.[480]

REFERENCES

1. Cheng CK, Leung PC. Molecular biology of gonadotropin-releasing hormone (GnRH)-I, GnRH-II, and their receptors in humans. *Endocr Rev*. 2005;26:283-306.
2. Seeburg PH, Adelman JP. Characterization of cDNA for precursor of human luteinizing hormone releasing hormone. *Nature*. 1984;311:666-668.
3. Seeburg PH, Mason AJ, Stewart TA, et al. The mammalian GnRH gene and its pivotal role in reproduction. *Recent Prog Horm Res*. 1987;43:69-98.
4. Hayflick JS, Adelman JP, Seeburg PH. The complete nucleotide sequence of the human gonadotropin-releasing hormone gene. *Nucleic Acids Res*. 1989;17:6403-6404.
5. Chavali GB, Nagpal S, Majumdar SS, et al. Helix-loop-helix motif in GnRH-associated peptide is critical for negative regulation of prolactin secretion. *J Mol Biol*. 1997 Oct 10;272(5):731-740.
6. Nikolics K, Mason AJ, Szonyi E, et al. A prolactin-inhibiting factor within the precursor for human gonadotropin-releasing hormone. *Nature*. 1985;316:511-517.
7. Ackland JF, Nikolics K, Seeburg PH, et al. Molecular forms of gonadotropin-releasing hormone associated peptide (GAP): changes within the rat hypothalamus and release from hypothalamic cells in vitro. *Neuroendocrinology*. 1988;48:376-386.
8. Ronnekleiv OK, Naylor BR, Bond CT, et al. Combined immunohistochemistry for gonadotropin-releasing hormone (GnRH) and pro-GnRH, and in situ hybridization for GnRH messenger ribonucleic acid in rat brain. *Mol Endocrinol*. 1989;3:363-371.
9. Kim HG, Bhagavath B, Layman LC. Clinical manifestations of impaired GnRH neuron development and function. *Neurosignals*. 2008;16:165-182.
10. Knobil E. The neuroendocrine control of the menstrual cycle. *Recent Prog Horm Res*. 1980;36:53-88.
11. Van Vugt DA, Diefenbach WD, Alston E, et al. Gonadotropin-releasing hormone pulses in third ventricular cerebrospinal fluid of ovariectomized rhesus monkeys: correlation with luteinizing hormone pulses. *Endocrinology*. 1985;117:1550-1558.
12. Gross KM, Matsumoto AM, Southworth MB, et al. Evidence for decreased luteinizing hormone-releasing hormone pulse frequency in men with selective elevations of follicle-stimulating hormone. *J Clin Endocrinol Metab*. 1985;60:197-202.
13. Haisenleder DJ, Dalkin AC, Ortolano GA, et al. A pulsatile gonadotropin-releasing hormone stimulus is required to increase transcription of the gonadotropin subunit genes: evidence for differential regulation of transcription by pulse frequency in vivo. *Endocrinology*. 1991;128:509-517.
14. Reame NE, Sauder SE, Case GD, et al. Pulsatile gonadotropin secretion in women with hypothalamic amenorrhea: evidence that reduced frequency of gonadotropin-releasing hormone secretion is the mechanism of persistent anovulation. *J Clin Endocrinol Metab*. 1985;61:851-858.
15. Filicori M, Santoro N, Merriam GR, et al. Characterization of the physiological pattern of episodic gonadotropin secretion throughout the human menstrual cycle. *J Clin Endocrinol Metab*. 1986;62:1136-1144.
16. Herbison AE. Noradrenergic regulation of cyclic GnRH secretion. *Rev Reprod*. 1997;2:1-6.
17. Gindoff PR, Ferin M. Endogenous opioid peptides modulate the effect of corticotropin-releasing factor on gonadotropin release in the primate. *Endocrinology*. 1987;121:837-842.
18. Rabinovici J, Rothman P, Monroe SE, et al. Endocrine effects and pharmacokinetic characteristics of a potent new gonadotropin-releasing hormone antagonist (Ganirelix) with minimal histamine-releasing properties: studies in postmenopausal women. *J Clin Endocrinol Metab*. 1992;75:1220-1225.
19. Shoupe D, Montz FJ, Lobo RA. The effects of estrogen and progestin on endogenous opioid activity in oophorectomized women. *J Clin Endocrinol Metab*. 1985;60:178-183.
20. Goodman RL, Parfitt DB, Evans NP, et al. Endogenous opioid peptides control the amplitude and shape of gonadotropin-releasing hormone pulses in the ewe. *Endocrinology*. 1995;136:2412-2420.
21. Wildt L, Leyendecker G, Sir-Petermann T, et al. Treatment with naltrexone in hypothalamic ovarian failure: induction of ovulation and pregnancy. *Hum Reprod*. 1993;8:350-358.
22. Petersen SL, Ottem EN, Carpenter CD. Direct and indirect regulation of gonadotropin-releasing hormone neurons by estradiol. *Biol Reprod*. 2003;69:1771-1778.
23. Yilmaz MB, Wolfe A, Cheng YH, et al. Aromatase promoter I.f is regulated by estrogen receptor alpha (ESR1) in mouse hypothalamic neuronal cell lines. *Biol Reprod*. 2009;81:956-965.
24. Casper RF. Aromatase inhibitors in ovarian stimulation. *J Steroid Biochem Mol Biol*. 2007;106:71-75.
25. Seminara SB, Messager S, Chatzidaki EE, et al. The GPR54 gene as a regulator of puberty. *N Engl J Med*. 2003;349:1614-1627.
26. de Roux N, Genin E, Carel JC, et al. Hypogonadotropic hypogonadism due to loss of function of the KiSS1-derived peptide receptor GPR54. *Proc Natl Acad Sci U S A*. 2003;100:10972-10976.
27. Colledge WH. Kisspeptins and GnRH neuronal signalling. *Trends Endocrinol Metab*. 2009;20:115-121.
28. Popa SM, Clifton DK, Steiner RA. The role of kisspeptins and GPR54 in the neuroendocrine regulation of reproduction. *Annu Rev Physiol*. 2008;70:213-238.
29. Handelsman DJ, Swerdloff RS. Pharmacokinetics of gonadotropin-releasing hormone and its analogs. *Endocr Rev*. 1986;7:95-105.
30. Galbiati M, Zanisi M, Messi E, et al. Transforming growth factor-beta and astrocytic conditioned medium influence luteinizing hormone-releasing hormone gene expression in the hypothalamic cell line GT1. *Endocrinology*. 1996;137:5605-5609.
31. Karten MJ, Rivier JE. Gonadotropin-releasing hormone analog design: structure-function studies toward the development of agonists and antagonists—rationale and perspective. *Endocr Rev*. 1986;7:44-66.
32. Lemay A, Maheux R, Faure N, et al. Reversible hypogonadism induced by a luteinizing hormone-releasing hormone (LH-RH) agonist (Buserelin) as a new therapeutic approach for endometriosis. *Fertil Steril*. 1984;41:863-871.
33. Carr BR, Breslau NA, Givens C, et al. Oral contraceptive pills, gonadotropin-releasing hormone agonists, or use in combination for treatment of hirsutism: a clinical research center study. *J Clin Endocrinol Metab*. 1995;80:1169-1178.
34. Cann CE, Martin MC, Genant HK, et al. Decreased spinal mineral content in amenorrheic women. *JAMA*. 1984;251:626-629.
35. Matta WH, Shaw RW, Hesp R, et al. Reversible trabecular bone density loss following induced hypo-oestrogenism with the GnRH analogue buserelin in premenopausal women. *Clin Endocrinol (Oxf)*. 1988;29:45-51.
36. Surrey ES. Add-back therapy and gonadotropin-releasing hormone agonists in the treatment of patients with endometriosis: can a consensus be reached? Add-Back Consensus Working Group. *Fertil Steril*. 1999;71:420-424.
37. Pavlou SN, Debold CR, Island DP, et al. Single subcutaneous doses of a luteinizing hormone-releasing hormone antagonist suppress serum gonadotropin and testosterone levels in normal men. *J Clin Endocrinol Metab*. 1986;63:303-308.
38. Pavlou SN, Wakefield G, Schlechter NL, et al. Mode of suppression of pituitary and gonadal function after acute or prolonged administration of a luteinizing hormone-releasing hormone antagonist in normal men. *J Clin Endocrinol Metab*. 1989;68:446-454.
39. Edelstein MC, Gordon K, Williams RF, et al. Single dose long-term suppression of testosterone secretion by a gonadotropin-releasing hormone antagonist (Antide) in male monkeys. *Contraception*. 1990;42:209-214.
40. Behre HM, Kliesch S, Puhse G, et al. High loading and low maintenance doses of a gonadotropin-releasing hormone antagonist effectively suppress serum luteinizing hormone, follicle-stimulating hormone, and testosterone in normal men. *J Clin Endocrinol Metab*. 1997;82:1403-1408.
41. Gonzalez-Barcena D, Alvarez RB, Ochoa EP, et al. Treatment of uterine leiomyomas with luteinizing hormone-releasing hormone antagonist Cetrorelix. *Hum Reprod*. 1997;12:2028-2035.
42. Childs GV, Hyde C, Naor Z, et al. Heterogeneous luteinizing hormone and follicle-stimulating hormone storage patterns in subtypes of gonadotropes separated by centrifugal elutriation. *Endocrinology*. 1983;113:2120-2128.
43. Childs GV. Functional ultrastructure of gonadotropes: a review. *Curr Top Neuroendocrinol*. 1986;7:49-97.
44. Millar RP, Lu ZL, Pawson AJ, et al. Gonadotropin-releasing hormone receptors. *Endocr Rev*. 2004;25:235-275.
45. Gharib SD, Wierman ME, Shupnik MA, et al. Molecular biology of the pituitary gonadotropins. *Endocr Rev*. 1990;11:177-199.
46. Talmadge K, Vamvakopoulos NC, Fiddes JC. Evolution of the genes for the beta subunits of human chorionic gonadotropin and luteinizing hormone. *Nature*. 1984;307:37-40.
47. Jameson JL, Becker CB, Lindell CM, et al. Human follicle-stimulating hormone beta-subunit gene encodes multiple messenger ribonucleic acids. *Mol Endocrinol*. 1988;2:806-815.

48. Jameson L, Chin WW, Hollenberg AN, et al. The gene encoding the beta-subunit of rat luteinizing hormone: analysis of gene structure and evolution of nucleotide sequence. *J Biol Chem.* 1984;259:15474-15480.
49. Themmen APN, Huhtaniemi IT. Mutations of gonadotropins and gonadotropin receptors: elucidating the physiology and pathophysiology of pituitary-gonadal function. *Endocr Rev.* 2000;21:551-583.
50. Shupnik MA. Gonadotropin gene modulation by steroids and gonadotropin-releasing hormone. *Biol Reprod.* 1996;54:279-286.
51. Edson MA, Nagaraja AK, Matzuk MM. The mammalian ovary from genesis to revelation. *Endocr Rev.* 2009;30:624-712.
52. Abbud RA, Ameduri RK, Rao JS, et al. Chronic hypersecretion of luteinizing hormone in transgenic mice selectively alters responsiveness of the alpha-subunit gene to gonadotropin-releasing hormone and estrogens. *Mol Endocrinol.* 1999;13:1449-1459.
53. Thackray VG, Mellon PL, Coss D. Hormones in synergy: regulation of the pituitary gonadotropin genes. *Mol Cell Endocrinol.* 2009;314:192-203.
54. Bernard DJ, Fortin J, Wang Y, Lamba P. Mechanisms of FSH synthesis: what we know, what we don't, and why you should care. *Fertil Steril.* 2010 May 15;93(8):2465-2485.
55. de Leeuw R, Mulders J, Voortman G, et al. Structure-function relationship of recombinant follicle stimulating hormone (Puregon). *Mol Hum Reprod.* 1996;2:361-369.
56. Mossman KD. *Comparative Morphology of the Mammalian Ovary.* Madison, WI: University of Wisconsin Press; 1973.
57. Simpson JL, Rajkovic A. Ovarian differentiation and gonadal failure. *Am J Med Genet.* 1999;89:186-200.
58. Di Pasquale E, Beck-Peccoz P, Persani L. Hypergonadotropic ovarian failure associated with an inherited mutation of human bone morphogenetic protein-15 (BMP15) gene. *Am J Hum Genet.* 2004;75:106-111.
59. Witschi E. Migration of the germ cells of human embryos from the yolk sac to the primitive gonadal folds. *Contrib Embryol.* 1948;32:67.
60. Chuva S, van den Driesche S, Carvalho S, et al. Altered primordial germ cell migration in the absence of transforming growth factor β signaling via ALK5. *Devel Biol.* 2005;284:194-203.
61. Farini D, La Sala G, Tedesco M, et al. Chemoattractant action and molecular signaling pathways of Kit ligand on mouse primordial germ cells. *Devel Biol.* 2007;306:572-583.
62. Baker TG, Franchi LL. The fine structure of oogonia and oocytes in human ovaries. *J Cell Sci.* 1967;2:213-224.
63. Shifren JL, Osathanondh R, Yeh J. Human fetal ovaries and uteri: developmental expression of genes encoding the insulin, insulin-like growth factor I, and insulin-like growth factor II receptors. *Fertil Steril.* 1993;59:1036-1040.
64. Bennett RA, Osathanondh R, Yeh J. Immunohistochemical localization of transforming growth factor-alpha, epidermal growth factor (EGF), and EGF receptor in the human fetal ovary. *J Clin Endocrinol Metab.* 1996;81:3073-3076.
65. Himelstein-Braw R, Byskov AG, Peters H, et al. Follicular atresia in the infant human ovary. *J Reprod Fertil.* 1976;46:55-59.
66. Oktem O, Oktay K. The ovary: anatomy and function throughout human life. *Ann N Y Acad Sci.* 2008;1127:1-9.
67. Albertini DF, Anderson E. The appearance and structure of intercellular connections during the ontogeny of the rabbit ovarian follicle with particular reference to gap junctions. *J Cell Biol.* 1974;63:234-250.
68. Amsterdam A, Knecht M, Catt KJ. Hormonal regulation of cytodifferentiation and intercellular communication in cultured granulosa cells. *Proc Natl Acad Sci U S A.* 1981;78:3000-3004.
69. Simon AM, Goodenough DA, Li E, et al. Female infertility in mice lacking connexin 37. *Nature.* 1997;385:525-529.
70. Zoller LC, Weisz J. Identification of cytochrome P-450, and its distribution in the membrana granulosa of the preovulatory follicle, using quantitative cytochemistry. *Endocrinology.* 1978;103:310-313.
71. Zoller LC, Weisz J. A quantitative cytochemical study of glucose-6-phosphate dehydrogenase and delta 5-3 beta-hydroxysteroid dehydrogenase activity in the membrana granulosa of the ovulable type of follicle of the rat. *Histochemistry.* 1979;62:125-135.
72. Hillensjo T, LeMaire WJ. Gonadotropin releasing hormone agonists stimulate meiotic maturation of follicle-enclosed rat oocytes in vitro. *Nature.* 1980;287:145-146.
73. Lawrence TS, Dekel N, Beers WH. Binding of human chorionic gonadotropin by rat cumuli oophori and granulosa cells: a comparative study. *Endocrinology.* 1980;106:1114-1118.
74. Magnusson C, Billig H, Eneroth P, et al. Comparison between the progestin secretion responsiveness to gonadotrophins of rat cumulus and mural granulosa cells in vitro. *Acta Endocrinol (Copenh).* 1982;101:611-616.
75. Hu Y, Ghosh S, Amleh A, et al. Modulation of aromatase expression by BRCA1: a possible link to tissue-specific tumor suppression. *Oncogene.* 2005;24:8343-8348.
76. Lu M, Chen D, Lin Z, et al. BRCA1 negatively regulates the cancer-associated aromatase promoters I.3 and II in breast adipose fibroblasts and malignant epithelial cells. *J Clin Endocrinol Metab.* 2006;91:4514-4519.
77. Erickson GF, Magoffin DA, Dyer CA, et al. The ovarian androgen producing cells: a review of structure/function relationships. *Endocr Rev.* 1985;6:371-399.
78. Mais V, Kazer RR, Cetel NS, et al. The dependency of folliculogenesis and corpus luteum function on pulsatile gonadotropin secretion in cycling women using a gonadotropin-releasing hormone antagonist as a probe. *J Clin Endocrinol Metab.* 1986;62:1250-1255.
79. Gougeon A. Regulation of ovarian follicular development in primates: facts and hypotheses. *Endocr Rev.* 1996;17:121-155.
80. Gougeon A. Dynamics of follicular growth in the human: a model from preliminary results. *Hum Reprod.* 1986;1:81-87.
81. Schipper I, Hop WC, Fauser BC. The follicle-stimulating hormone (FSH) threshold/window concept examined by different interventions with exogenous FSH during the follicular phase of the normal menstrual cycle: duration, rather than magnitude, of FSH increase affects follicle development. *J Clin Endocrinol Metab.* 1998;83:1292-1298.
82. Peters H, McNatty KP. *The Ovary: A Correlation of Structure and Function in Mammals.* Berkeley, CA: University of California Press; 1980:12-34.
83. Tilly JL, Kowalski KI, Johnson AL, et al. Involvement of apoptosis in ovarian follicular atresia and postovulatory regression. *Endocrinology.* 1991;129:2799-2801.
84. Bauminger A, Lindner HR. Periovulatory changes in ovarian prostaglandin formation and their hormonal control in the rat. *Prostaglandins.* 1975;9:737-751.
85. Tsafriri A, Lindner HR, Zor U, et al. Physiological role of prostaglandins in the induction of ovulation. *Prostaglandins.* 1972;2:1-10.
86. Espey LL. Ovarian proteolytic enzymes and ovulation. *Biol Reprod.* 1974;10:216-235.
87. Bjersing L, Cajander S. Ovulation and the mechanism of follicle rupture: IV. Ultrastructure of membrana granulosa of rabbit graafian follicles prior to induced ovulation. *Cell Tissue Res.* 1974;153:1-14.
88. Beers WH, Strickland S, Reich E. Ovarian plasminogen activator: relationship to ovulation and hormonal regulation. *Cell.* 1975;6:387-394.
89. Frederick JL, Shimanuki T, diZerega GS. Initiation of angiogenesis by human follicular fluid. *Science.* 1984;224:389-390.
90. Kamat BR, Brown LF, Manseau EJ, et al. Expression of vascular permeability factor/vascular endothelial growth factor by human granulosa and theca lutein cells: role in corpus luteum development. *Am J Pathol.* 1995;146:157-165.
91. Ohara A, Mori T, Taii S, et al. Functional differentiation in steroidogenesis of two types of luteal cells isolated from mature human corpora lutea of menstrual cycle. *J Clin Endocrinol Metab.* 1987;65:1192-1200.
92. Carr BR, MacDonald PC, Simpson ER. The role of lipoproteins in the regulation of progesterone secretion by the human corpus luteum. *Fertil Steril.* 1982;38:303-311.
93. Duncan WC, McNeilly AS, Fraser HM, et al. Luteinizing hormone receptor in the human corpus luteum: lack of down-regulation during maternal recognition of pregnancy. *Hum Reprod.* 1996;11:2291-2297.
94. Strauss JF 3rd, Christenson LK, Devoto L, et al. Providing progesterone for pregnancy: control of cholesterol flux to the side-chain cleavage system. *J Reprod Fertil Suppl.* 2000;55:3-12.
95. Bukovsky A, Caudle MR, Keenan JA, et al. Is irregular regression of corpora lutea in climacteric women caused by age-induced alterations in the "tissue control system"? *Am J Reprod Immunol.* 1996;36:327-341.
96. Casper RF, Yen SS. Induction of luteolysis in the human with a long-acting analog of luteinizing hormone-releasing factor. *Science.* 1979;205:408-410.
97. Schoonmaker JN, Victery W, Karsch FJ. A receptive period for estradiol-induced luteolysis in the rhesus monkey. *Endocrinology.* 1981;108:1874-1877.
98. O'Grady J, Kohorn EI, Glass RH, et al. Inhibition of progesterone synthesis in vitro by prostaglandin F2a. *J Reprod Fertil.* 1972;30:153-156.
99. Shikone T, Yamoto M, Kokawa K, et al. Apoptosis of human corpora lutea during cyclic luteal regression and early pregnancy. *J Clin Endocrinol Metab.* 1996;81:2376-2380.
100. Bortolussi M, Marini G, Dal Lago A. Autoradiographic study of the distribution of LH(HCG) receptors in the ovary of untreated and gonadotrophin-primed immature rats. *Cell Tissue Res.* 1977;183:329-342.
101. Nimrod A, Erickson GF, Ryan KJ. A specific FSH receptor in rat granulosa cells: properties of binding in vitro. *Endocrinology.* 1976;98:56-64.
102. Nimrod A, Bedrak E, Lamprecht SA. Appearance of LH-receptors and LH-stimulable cyclic AMP accumulation in granulosa cells during follicular maturation in the rat ovary. *Biochem Biophys Res Commun.* 1977;78:977-984.
103. Jaaskelainen K, Markkanen S, Rajaniemi H. Internalization of receptor-bound human chorionic gonadotrophin in preovulatory rat granulosa cells in vivo. *Acta Endocrinol (Copenh).* 1983;103:406-412.

104. Uilenbroek JT, Richards JS. Ovarian follicular development during the rat estrous cycle: gonadotropin receptors and follicular responsiveness. *Biol Reprod.* 1979;20:1159-1165.
105. Zeleznik AJ, Midgley AR Jr, Reichert LE Jr. Granulosa cell maturation in the rat: increased binding of human chorionic gonadotropin following treatment with follicle-stimulating hormone in vivo. *Endocrinology.* 1974;95:818-825.
106. Richards JS, Ireland JJ, Rao MC, et al. Ovarian follicular development in the rat: hormone receptor regulation by estradiol, follicle stimulating hormone and luteinizing hormone. *Endocrinology.* 1976;99: 1562-1570.
107. Couse JF, Korach KS. Estrogen receptor null mice: what have we learned and where will they lead us? *Endocr Rev.* 1999;20:358-417.
108. Brandenberger AW, Tee MK, Jaffe RB. Estrogen receptor alpha (ER-alpha) and beta (ER-beta) mRNAs in normal ovary, ovarian serous cystadenocarcinoma and ovarian cancer cell lines: down-regulation of ER-beta in neoplastic tissues. *J Clin Endocrinol Metab.* 1998;83:1025-1028.
109. Dorrington JH, Moon YS, Armstrong DT. Estradiol-17beta biosynthesis in cultured granulosa cells from hypophysectomized immature rats: stimulation by follicle-stimulating hormone. *Endocrinology.* 1975; 97:1328-1331.
110. Simpson ER, Mahendroo MS, Means GD, et al. Aromatase cytochrome P450, the enzyme responsible for estrogen biosynthesis. *Endocr Rev.* 1994;15:342-355.
111. Moon YS, Dorrington JH, Armstrong DT. Stimulatory action of follicle-stimulating hormone on estradiol-17 beta secretion by hypophysectomized rat ovaries in organ culture. *Endocrinology.* 1975;97:244-247.
112. Armstrong DT, Papkoff H. Stimulation of aromatization of exogenous and endogenous androgens in ovaries of hypophysectomized rats in vivo by follicle-stimulating hormone. *Endocrinology.* 1976;99: 1144-1151.
113. Rani CS, Salhanick AR, Armstrong DT. Follicle-stimulating hormone induction of luteinizing hormone receptor in cultured rat granulosa cells: an examination of the need for steroids in the induction process. *Endocrinology.* 1981;108:1379-1385.
114. Bulun S. Aromatase deficiency and estrogen resistance: from molecular genetics to clinic. *Semin Reprod Med.* 2000;18:31-39.
115. Richards JS, Jonassen JA, Kersey K. Evidence that changes in tonic luteinizing hormone secretion determine the growth of preovulatory follicles in the rat. *Endocrinology.* 1980;107:641-648.
116. Richards JS, Bogovich K. Effects of human chorionic gonadotropin and progesterone on follicular development in the immature rat. *Endocrinology.* 1982;111:1429-1438.
117. Bogovich K, Richards JS. Androgen biosynthesis in developing ovarian follicles: evidence that luteinizing hormone regulates thecal 17 alpha-hydroxylase and C17-20-lyase activities. *Endocrinology.* 1982;111: 1201-1208.
118. Barlow JJ, Emerson K Jr, Saxena BN. Estradiol production after ovariectomy for carcinoma of the breast. *N Engl J Med.* 1969;280:633-637.
119. Baird DT, Fraser IS. Concentration of oestrone and oestradiol in follicular fluid and ovarian venous blood of women. *Clin Endocrinol (Oxf).* 1975;4:259-266.
120. Hemsell DL, Grodin JM, Brenner PF, et al. Plasma precursors of estrogen: II. Correlation of the extent of conversion of plasma androstenedione to estrone with age. *J Clin Endocrinol Metab.* 1974;38:476-479.
121. Bulun SE, Simpson ER. Competitive reverse transcription-polymerase chain reaction analysis indicates that levels of aromatase cytochrome P450 transcripts in adipose tissue of buttocks, thighs, and abdomen of women increase with advancing age. *J Clin Endocrinol Metab.* 1994;78:428-432.
122. Bulun SE, Zeitoun K, Sasano H, et al. Aromatase in aging women. *Semin Reprod Endocrinol.* 1999;17:349-358.
123. Mahendroo MS, Russell DW. Male and female isoenzymes of steroid 5alpha-reductase. *Rev Reprod.* 1999;4:179-183.
124. Miller WL, Strauss JF 3rd. Molecular pathology and mechanism of action of the steroidogenic acute regulatory protein, StAR. *J Steroid Biochem Mol Biol.* 1999;69:131-141.
125. Pollack SE, Furth EE, Kallen CB, et al. Localization of the steroidogenic acute regulatory protein in human tissues. *J Clin Endocrinol Metab.* 1997;82:4243-4251.
126. Simpson ER, Mahendroo MS, Means GD, et al. Aromatase cytochrome P450, the enzyme responsible for estrogen biosynthesis. *Endocr Rev.* 1994;15:342-355.
127. Ying SY. Inhibins, activins, and follistatins: gonadal proteins modulating the secretion of follicle-stimulating hormone. *Endocr Rev.* 1988;9:267-293.
128. Leers-Sucheta S, Morohashi K, Mason JI, et al. Synergistic activation of the human type II 3beta-hydroxysteroid dehydrogenase/delta5-delta4 isomerase promoter by the transcription factor steroidogenic factor-1/adrenal 4-binding protein and phorbol ester. *J Biol Chem.* 1997;272:7960-7967.
129. Hanley NA, Ikeda Y, Luo X, et al. Steroidogenic factor 1 (SF-1) is essential for ovarian development and function. *Mol Cell Endocrinol.* 2000;163:27-32.
130. Siiteri PK, MacDonald PC. Role of extraglandular estrogen in human endocrinology. In: Greep RO, Astwood EB, eds. Handbook of Physiology, vol 2. Washington, DC: American Physiological Society; 1973:619-629.
131. Peltoketo H, Luu-The V, Simard J, et al. 17β-Hydroxysteroid dehydrogenase (HSD)/17-ketosteroid reductase (KSR) family: nomenclature and main characteristics of the 17HSD/KSR enzymes. *J Mol Endocrinol.* 1999;23:1-11.
132. Merriam GR, Pfeiffer DG, Loriaux DL, et al. Catechol estrogens and the control of gonadotropin and prolactin secretion in man. *J Steroid Biochem.* 1983;19:619-625.
133. Hinshelwood MM, Repa JJ, Shelton JM, et al. Expression of LRH-1 and SF-1 in the mouse ovary: localization in different cell types correlates with differing function. *Mol Cell Endocrinol.* 2003;207:39-45.
134. Falender AE, Lanz R, Malenfant D, et al. Differential expression of steroidogenic factor-1 and FTF/LRH-1 in the rodent ovary. *Endocrinology.* 2003;144:3598-3610.
135. Weck J, Mayo KE. Switching of NR5A proteins associated with the inhibin α-subunit gene promoter following activation of the gene in granulosa cells. *Mol Endocrinol.* 2006;20:1090-1103.
136. Peng N, Kim JW, Rainey WE, et al. The role of the orphan nuclear receptor, liver receptor homologue-1, in the regulation of human corpus luteum 3beta-hydroxysteroid dehydrogenase type II. *J Clin Endocrinol Metab.* 2003;88:6020-6028.
137. Jaatinen TA, Penttila TL, Kaipia A, et al. Expression of inhibin alpha, beta A and beta B messenger ribonucleic acids in the normal human ovary and in polycystic ovarian syndrome. *J Endocrinol.* 1994;143: 127-137.
138. Roberts VJ, Barth S, el-Roeiy A, et al. Expression of inhibin/activin subunits and follistatin messenger ribonucleic acids and proteins in ovarian follicles and the corpus luteum during the human menstrual cycle. *J Clin Endocrinol Metab.* 1993;77:1402-1410.
139. Eramaa M, Tuuri T, Hilden K, et al. Regulation of inhibin alpha- and beta A-subunit messenger ribonucleic acid levels by chorionic gonadotropin and recombinant follicle-stimulating hormone in cultured human granulosa-luteal cells. *J Clin Endocrinol Metab.* 1994;79:1670-1677.
140. Groome NP, Illingworth PJ, O'Brien M, et al. Measurement of dimeric inhibin B throughout the human menstrual cycle. *J Clin Endocrinol Metab.* 1996;81:1401-1405.
141. Adashi EY. The IGF family and folliculogenesis. *J Reprod Immunol.* 1998;39:13-19.
142. Dunaif A. Insulin resistance and the polycystic ovary syndrome: mechanism and implications for pathogenesis. *Endocr Rev.* 1997;18: 774-800.
143. Franks S, Stark J, Hardy K. Follicle dynamics and anovulation in polycystic ovary syndrome. *Hum Reprod Update.* 2008 Jul-Aug;14(4): 367-378.
144. Sasano H, Frost A, Saitoh R, et al. Aromatase and 17beta-hydroxysteroid dehydrogenase type 1 in human breast carcinoma. *J Clin Endocrinol Metab.* 1996;81:4042-4046.
145. Zeitoun KM, Takayama K, Sasano H, et al. Deficient 17beta-hydroxysteroid dehydrogenase type 2 expression in endometriosis: failure to metabolize estradiol-17alpha. *J Clin Endocrinol Metab.* 1998;83:4474-4480.
146. Konkle AT, McCarthy MM. Developmental time course of estradiol, testosterone, and dihydrotestosterone levels in discrete regions of male and female rat brain. *Endocrinology.* 2011 Jan;152(1):223-235.
147. Bulun SE, Noble LS, Takayama K, et al. Endocrine disorders associated with inappropriately high aromatase expression. *J Steroid Biochem Mol Biol.* 1997;61:133-139.
148. Azziz R, Carmina E, Sawaya ME. Idiopathic hirsutism. *Endocr Rev.* 2000;21:347-362.
149. Psychoyos A. Uterine receptivity for nidation. *Ann N Y Acad Sci.* 1986;476:36-42.
150. Wynn RM. Histology and ultrastructure of the human endometrium. In: Wynn RM, ed. *Biology of the Uterus*. New York, NY: Plenum Press; 1977:341-376.
151. Markee JE. Menstruation in intraocular endometrial transplants in the rhesus monkey. *Contr Embryol Carneg Instn.* 1940;28:219-308.
152. Markee J. Morphological basis for menstrual bleeding: relation of regression to the initiation of bleeding. *Bull N Y Acad Med.* 1948;24:253-268.
153. Bartelmez G. The phases of the menstrual cycle and their interpretation in terms of the pregnancy cycle. *Am J Obstet Gynecol.* 1957;74;931-955.
154. Noyes RW, Hertig AT, Rock J. Dating the endometrial biopsy. *Fertil Steril.* 1950;1:3-25.
155. Eckert R, Katzenellenbogen B. Human endometrial cells in primary tissue culture: modulation of the progesterone receptor level by natural and synthetic estrogens in vitro. *J Clin Endocrinol Metab.* 1981;52:699-708.
156. Cooke PS, Buchanan DL, Young P, Setiawan T, et al. Stromal estrogen receptors mediate mitogenic effects of estradiol on uterine epithelium. *Proc Natl Acad Sci U S A.* 1997;94:6535-6540.
157. Kurita T, Young P, Brody JR, et al. Stromal progesterone receptors mediate the inhibitory effects of progesterone on estrogen-induced

uterine epithelial cell deoxyribonucleic acid synthesis. *Endocrinology*. 1998;139:4708-4713.
158. Matsuzaki S, Fukaya T, Suzuki T, et al. Oestrogen receptor alpha and beta mRNA expression in human endometrium throughout the menstrual cycle. *Mol Hum Reprod*. 1999:5559-5564.
159. Cooke P, Buchanan D, Lubahn D, et al. Mechanism of estrogen action: lessons from the estrogen receptor-alpha knockout mouse. *Biol Reprod*. 1998;59:470-475.
160. Carroll JS, Liu XS, Brodsky AS, et al. Chromosome-wide mapping of estrogen receptor binding reveals long-range regulation requiring the forkhead protein FoxA1. *Cell*. 2005;122:33-43.
161. Lin Z, Reierstad S, Huang CC, et al. Novel estrogen receptor-α binding sites and estradiol target genes identified by chromatin immunoprecipitation cloning in breast cancer. *Cancer Res*. 2007;67:5017-5024.
162. Katzenellenbogen B. Estrogen receptors: bioactivities and interactions with cell signaling pathways. *Biol Reprod*. 1996;54:287-293.
163. Attia GR, Zeitoun K, Edwards D, et al. Progesterone receptor isoform A but not B is expressed in endometriosis. *J Clin Endocrinol Metab*. 2000;85:2897-2902.
164. Yin P, Lin Z, Reierstad S, et al. Krüppel-like transcription factor 11 integrates progesterone receptor signaling and proliferation in uterine leiomyoma cells. *Cancer Res*. 2010;70:1722-1730.
165. Tseng L, Gurpide E. Effects of progestins on estradiol receptor levels in human endometrium. *J Clin Endocrinol Metab*. 1975;41:402-404.
166. Casey ML, MacDonald PC, Andersson S. 17b-Hydroxysteroid dehydrogenase type 2: chromosomal assignment and progestin regulation of gene expression in human endometrium. *J Clin Invest*. 1994;94: 2135-2141.
167. Tseng L, Liu HC. Stimulation of acylsulfotransferase activity by progestin in human endometrium in vitro. *J Clin Endocrinol Metab*. 1981;53:418-421.
168. Yang S, Fang Z, Gurates B, et al. Stromal progesterone receptors mediate induction of 17beta-hydroxysteroid dehydrogenase type 2 expression in human endometrial epithelium: a paracrine mechanism for inactivation of estradiol. *Mol Endocrinol*. 2001;15:2093-2105.
169. Bergh PA, Navot D. The impact of embryonic development and endometrial maturity on the timing of implantation. *Fertil Steril*. 1992;58:537-542.
170. Adams EC, Hertig AT, Rock J. A description of 34 human ova within the first 17 days of development. *Am J Anat*. 1956;98:435-493.
171. Sauer MV, Paulson RJ, Lobo RA. Reversing the natural decline in human fertility: an extended clinical trial of oocyte donation to women of advanced reproductive age. *JAMA*. 1992;268:1275-1279.
172. Rosenwaks Z. Donor eggs: their application in modern reproductive technologies. *Fertil Steril*. 1987;47:895-909.
173. Langer RD, Pierce JJ, O'Hanlan KA, et al. Transvaginal ultrasonography compared with endometrial biopsy for the detection of endometrial disease. Postmenopausal Estrogen/Progestin Interventions Trial. *N Engl J Med*. 1997;337:1792-1798.
174. Sheehan HL. The recognition of chronic hypopituitarism resulting from postpartum pituitary necrosis. *Am J Obstet Gynecol*. 1971;111:852-854.
175. Simpson JL, Christakos AC, Horwith M, et al. Gonadal dysgenesis in individuals with apparently normal chromosomal complements: tabulation of cases and compilation of genetic data. *Birth Defects Orig Artic Ser*. 1971;7:215-228.
176. Hague WM, Adams J, Reeders ST, et al. 45 X Turner's syndrome in association with polycystic ovaries (case report). *Br J Obstet Gynaecol*. 1989;96:613-618.
177. Asherman JG. Amenorrhea traumataica (atretica). *J Obstet Gynecol Br Emp*. 1948;55:23-30.
178. Marshall W, Tanner JM. Variations in patterns of pubertal changes in girls. *Arch Dis Child*. 1969;44:291-303.
179. Novick D, Haro JM, Perrin E, et al. Tolerability of outpatient antipsychotic treatment: 36-month results from the European Schizophrenia Outpatient Health Outcomes (SOHO) study. *Eur Neuropsychopharmacol*. 2009;19:542-550.
180. Liu JH, Bill AH. Stress-associated or functional hypothalamic amenorrhea in the adolescent. *Ann N Y Acad Sci*. 2008;1135:179-184.
181. Klinefelter HJ, Albright F, Griswold GC. Experience with a quantitative test for normal or decreased amounts of follicle-stimulating hormone in urine in endocrinological diagnosis. *J Clin Endocrinol Metab*. 1943;3:529-544.
182. Khoury SA, Reame NE, Kelch RP, et al. Diurnal patterns of pulsatile luteinizing hormone secretion in hypothalamic amenorrhea: reproducibility and responses to opiate blockade and an alpha 2-adrenergic agonist. *J Clin Endocrinol Metab*. 1987;64:755-762.
183. Berga SL, Mortola JF, Girton L, et al. Neuroendocrine aberrations in women with functional hypothalamic amenorrhea. *J Clin Endocrinol Metab*. 1989;68:301-308.
184. Yen SS, Rebar R, VandenBerg G, Judd H. Hypothalamic amenorrhea and hypogonadotropinism: responses to synthetic LRF. *J Clin Endocrinol Metab*. 1973;36:811-816.
185. Loucks AB, Mortola JF, Girton L, et al. Alterations in the hypothalamic-pituitary-ovarian and the hypothalamic-pituitary-adrenal axes in athletic women. *J Clin Endocrinol Metab*. 1989;68:402-411.
186. Kalra SP. Catecholamine involvement in preovulatory LH release: reassessment of the role of epinephrine. *Neuroendocrinology*. 1985;40: 139-144.
187. Ropert JF, Quigley ME, Yen SS. Endogenous opiates modulate pulsatile luteinizing hormone release in humans. *J Clin Endocrinol Metab*. 1981;52:583-585.
188. Gambacciani M, Yen SS, Rasmussen DD. GnRH release from the mediobasal hypothalamus: in vitro inhibition by corticotropin-releasing factor. *Neuroendocrinology*. 1986;43:533-536.
189. Quigley ME, Yen SS. Evidence for increased dopaminergic inhibition of secretion of thyroid-stimulating hormone in hyperprolactinemic patients with pituitary microadenoma. *Am J Obstet Gynecol*. 1980;137:653-655.
190. Genazzani AD, Petraglia F, Gastaldi M, et al. Naltrexone treatment restores menstrual cycles in patients with weight loss-related amenorrhea. *Fertil Steril*. 1995;64:951-956.
191. Selye H. The stress syndrome. *Nature*. 1936;138:32.
192. Suh BY, Liu JH, Berga SL, et al. Hypercortisolism in patients with functional hypothalamic-amenorrhea. *J Clin Endocrinol Metab*. 1988;66:733-739.
193. Xiao E, Luckhaus J, Niemann W, et al. Acute inhibition of gonadotropin secretion by corticotropin-releasing hormone in the primate: are the adrenal glands involved? *Endocrinology*. 1989;124:1632-1637.
194. Rivier C, Vale W. Influence of corticotropin-releasing factor on reproductive functions in the rat. *Endocrinology*. 1984;114:914-921.
195. Matteri RL, Moberg GP, Watson JG. Adrenocorticotropin-induced changes in ovine pituitary gonadotropin secretion in vitro. *Endocrinology*. 1986;118:2091-2096.
196. Kamel F, Kubajak CL. Modulation of gonadotropin secretion by corticosterone: interaction with gonadal steroids and mechanism of action. *Endocrinology*. 1987;121:561-568.
197. Welt CK, Chan JL, Bullen J, et al. Recombinant human leptin in women with hypothalamic amenorrhea. *N Engl J Med*. 2004;351: 987-997.
198. Schneider LF, Monaco SE, Warren MP. Elevated ghrelin level in women of normal weight with amenorrhea is related to disordered eating. *Fertil Steril*. 2008;90:121-128.
199. Baranowska B, Rozbicka G, Jeske W, et al. The role of endogenous opiates in the mechanism of inhibited luteinizing hormone (LH) secretion in women with anorexia nervosa: the effect of naloxone on LH, follicle-stimulating hormone, prolactin, and beta-endorphin secretion. *J Clin Endocrinol Metab*. 1984;59:412-416.
200. Atkinson RL. Naloxone decreases food intake in obese humans. *J Clin Endocrinol Metab*. 1982;55:196-198.
201. Morley JE, Levine AS. Stress-induced eating is mediated through endogenous opiates. *Science*. 1980;209:1259-1261.
202. Rigotti NA, Neer RM, Skates SJ, et al. The clinical course of osteoporosis in anorexia nervosa: a longitudinal study of cortical bone mass. *JAMA*. 1991;265:1133-1138.
203. Frisch RE, Wyshak G, Vincent L. Delayed menarche and amenorrhea in ballet dancers. *N Engl J Med*. 1980;303:17-19.
204. Frisch RE, Gotz-Welbergen AV, McArthur JW, et al. Delayed menarche and amenorrhea of college athletes in relation to age of onset of training. *JAMA*. 1981;246:1559-1563.
205. Drinkwater BL, Nilson K, Chesnut CH 3rd, et al. Bone mineral content of amenorrheic and eumenorrheic athletes. *N Engl J Med*. 1984;311:277-281.
206. Willi J, Grossmann S. Epidemiology of anorexia nervosa in a defined region of Switzerland. *Am J Psychiatry*. 1983;140:564-567.
207. Schwartz DM, Thompson MG. Do anorectics get well? Current research and future needs. *Am J Psychiatry*. 1981;138:319-323.
208. Swift WJ. The long-term outcome of early onset anorexia nervosa: a critical review. *J Am Acad Child Psychiatry*. 1982;21:38-46.
209. Boyar RM, Hellman LD, Roffwarg H, et al. Cortisol secretion and metabolism in anorexia nervosa. *N Engl J Med*. 1977;296:190-193.
210. Gold PW, Gwirtsman H, Avgerinos PC, et al. Abnormal hypothalamic-pituitary-adrenal function in anorexia nervosa: pathophysiologic mechanisms in underweight and weight-corrected patients. *N Engl J Med*. 1986;314:1335-1342.
211. Kaye WH, Gwirtsman HE, George DT, et al. Elevated cerebrospinal fluid levels of immunoreactive corticotropin-releasing hormone in anorexia nervosa: relation to state of nutrition, adrenal function, and intensity of depression. *J Clin Endocrinol Metab*. 1987;64:203-208.
212. Moshang T Jr, Utinger RD. Low triiodothyronine euthyroidism in anorexia nervosa. In: Vigersky RS, ed. *Anorexia Nervosa*. New York, NY: Raven Press; 1977:263-270.
213. Gold PW, Kaye W, Robertson G, et al. Abnormalities in plasma and cerebrospinal-fluid arginine vasopressin in patients with anorexia nervosa. *N Engl J Med*. 1983;308:1117-1123.
214. Berga SL, Loucks TL. Use of cognitive behavior therapy for functional hypothalamic amenorrhea. *Ann N Y Acad Sci*. 2006;1092: 114-129.
215. Soyka LA, Grinspoon S, Levitsky LL, et al. The effects of anorexia nervosa on bone metabolism in female adolescents. *J Clin Endocrinol Metab*. 1999;84:4489-4496.

216. Liu JH, Yen SS. The use of gonadotropin-releasing hormone for the induction of ovulation. *Clin Obstet Gynecol.* 1984;27:975-982.
217. Falsetti L, Gambera A, Barbetti L, et al. Long-term follow-up of functional hypothalamic amenorrhea and prognostic factors. *J Clin Endocrinol Metab.* 2002;87:500-505.
218. Ferriman D, Gallwey JD. Clinical assessment of body hair growth in women. *J Clin Endocrinol Metab.* 1961;21:1440-1447.
219. Tagatz GE, Kopher RA, Nagel TC, et al. The clitoral index: a bioassay of androgenic stimulation. *Obstet Gynecol.* 1979;54:562-564.
220. Bardin CW, Lipsett MB. Testosterone and androstenedione blood production rates in normal women and women with idiopathic hirsutism or polycystic ovaries. *J Clin Invest.* 1967;46:891-902.
221. Mowszowicz I, Melanitou E, Doukani A, et al. Androgen binding capacity and 5 alpha-reductase activity in pubic skin fibroblasts from hirsute patients. *J Clin Endocrinol Metab.* 1983;56:1209-1213.
222. Schwartz U, Moltz L, Brotherton J, et al. The diagnostic value of plasma free testosterone in non-tumorous and tumorous hyperandrogenism. *Fertil Steril.* 1983;40:66-72.
223. Miller KK, Rosner W, Lee H, et al. Measurement of free testosterone in normal women and women with androgen deficiency: comparison of methods. *J Clin Endocrinol Metab.* 2004;89:525-533.
224. Carmine E, Rosato F, Janni A, et al. Extensive clinical experience: relative prevalence of different androgen excess disorders in 950 women referred because of clinical hyperandrogenism. *J Clin Endocrinol Metab.* 2006;91:2-6.
225. Paulson RJ, Serafini PC, Catalino JA, et al. Measurements of 3 alpha,17 beta-androstanediol glucuronide in serum and urine and the correlation with skin 5 alpha-reductase activity. *Fertil Steril.* 1986;46:222-226.
226. Kennedy L, Traub AI, Atkinson AB, et al. Short term administration of gonadotropin-releasing hormone analog to a patient with a testosterone-secreting ovarian tumor. *J Clin Endocrinol Metab.* 1987;64:1320-1322.
227. Bavdekar SB, Kasla RR, Parmar RC, et al. Selective testosterone secreting adrenocortical carcinoma in an infant. *Indian J Pediatr.* 2001;68:95-97.
228. Derksen J, Nagesser SK, Meinders AE, et al. Identification of virilizing adrenal tumors in hirsute women. *N Engl J Med.* 1994;331:968-973.
229. Friedman CI, Schmidt GE, Kim MH, et al. Serum testosterone concentrations in the evaluation of androgen-producing tumors. *Am J Obstet Gynecol.* 1985;153:44-49.
230. Taylor L, Ayers JW, Gross MD, et al. Diagnostic considerations in virilization: iodomethyl-norcholesterol scanning in the localization of androgen secreting tumors. *Fertil Steril.* 1986;46:1005-1010.
231. Bricaire C, Raynaud A, Benotmane A, et al. Selective venous catheterization in the evaluation of hyperandrogenism. *J Endocrinol Invest.* 1991;14:949-956.
232. Azziz R, Hincapie LA, Knochenhauer ES, et al. Screening for 21-hydroxylase-deficient nonclassic adrenal hyperplasia among hyperandrogenic women: a prospective study. *Fertil Steril.* 1999;72:915-925.
233. Speiser PW, Dupont B, Rubinstein P, et al. High frequency of nonclassical steroid 21-hydroxylase deficiency. *Am J Hum Genet.* 1985;37:650-667.
234. New MI, Lorenzen F, Lerner AJ, et al. Genotyping steroid 21-hydroxylase deficiency: hormonal reference data. *J Clin Endocrinol Metab.* 1983;57:320-326.
235. Stratakis CA, Karl M, Schulte HM, et al. Glucocorticosteroid resistance in humans: elucidation of the molecular mechanisms and implications for pathophysiology. *Ann N Y Acad Sci.* 1994;746:362-374; discussion 374-376.
236. Koulouri O, Conway GS. A systematic review of commonly used medical treatments for hirsutism in women. *Clin Endocrinol (Oxf).* 2008;68:800-805.
237. Lobo RA, Shoupe D, Serafini P, et al. The effects of two doses of spironolactone on serum androgens and anagen hair in hirsute women. *Fertil Steril.* 1985;43:200-205.
238. Evron S, Shapiro G, Diamant YZ. Induction of ovulation with spironolactone (Aldactone) in anovulatory oligomenorrheic and hyperandrogenic women. *Fertil Steril.* 1981;36:468-471.
239. Mowszowicz I, Wright F, Vincens M, et al. Androgen metabolism in hirsute patients treated with cyproterone acetate. *J Steroid Biochem.* 1984;20:757-761.
240. Rittmaster RS. Finasteride. *N Engl J Med.* 1994;330:120-125.
241. Wong IL, Morris RS, Chang L, et al. A prospective randomized trial comparing finasteride to spironolactone in the treatment of hirsute women. *J Clin Endocrinol Metab.* 1995;80:233-238.
242. Castello R, Tosi F, Perrone F, et al. Outcome of long-term treatment with the 5 alpha-reductase inhibitor finasteride in idiopathic hirsutism: clinical and hormonal effects during a 1-year course of therapy and 1-year follow-up. *Fertil Steril.* 1996;66:734-740.
243. Diamanti-Kandarakis E, Mitrakou A, Raptis S, et al. The effect of a pure antiandrogen receptor blocker, flutamide, on the lipid profile in the polycystic ovary syndrome. *J Clin Endocrinol Metab.* 1998;83:2699-2705.
244. Moghetti P, Castello R, Negri C, et al. Flutamide in the treatment of hirsutism: long-term clinical effects, endocrine changes, and androgen receptor behavior. *Fertil Steril.* 1995;64:511-517.
245. Wysowski DK, Freiman JP, Tourtelot JB, et al. Fatal and nonfatal hepatotoxicity associated with flutamide. *Ann Intern Med.* 1993;118:860-864.
246. Hoeger K, Davidson K, Kochman L, et al. The impact of metformin, oral contraceptives, and lifestyle modification on polycystic ovary syndrome in obese adolescent women in two randomized, placebo-controlled clinical trials. *J Clin Endocrinol Metab.* 2008;93:4299-4306.
247. Legro RS, Kunselman AR, Dodson WC, et al. Prevalence and predictors of risk for type 2 diabetes mellitus and impaired glucose tolerance in polycystic ovary syndrome: a prospective, controlled study in 254 affected women. *J Clin Endocrinol Metab.* 1999;84:165-169.
248. Urbanek M, Legro RS, Driscoll DA, et al. Thirty-seven candidate genes for polycystic ovary syndrome: strongest evidence for linkage is with follistatin. *Proc Natl Acad Sci U S A.* 1999;96:8573-8578.
249. Legro RS, Driscoll D, Strauss JF 3rd, et al. Evidence for a genetic basis for hyperandrogenemia in polycystic ovary syndrome. *Proc Natl Acad Sci U S A.* 1998;95:14956-14960.
250. Stein I, Leventhal M. Amenorrhea associated with bilateral polycystic ovaries. *Am J Obstet Gynecol.* 1935;29:181-191.
251. Burghen GA, Givens JR, Kitabchi AE. Correlation of hyperandrogenism with hyperinsulinism in polycystic ovarian disease. *J Clin Endocrinol Metab.* 1980;50:113-116.
252. Tamura M, Deb S, Sebastian S, et al. Estrogen up-regulates cyclooxygenase-2 via estrogen receptor in human uterine microvascular endothelial cells. *Fertil Steril.* 2004;81:1351-1356.
253. Zawadzki JK, Dunaif A. Diagnostic criteria for polycystic ovary syndrome: towards a rational approach. In: Dunaif A, Givens JR, Haseltine FP, et al, eds. *Polycystic Ovary Syndrome.* 1992:377-384.
254. Rotterdam ESHRE/ASRM-Sponsored PCOS Consensus Workshop Group. Revised 2003 consensus on diagnostic criteria and long-term health risks related to polycystic ovary syndrome. *Fertil Steril.* 2004;81:19-25.
255. Azziz R. Controversy in clinical endocrinology: diagnosis of polycystic ovarian syndrome—the Rotterdam criteria are premature. *J Clin Endocrinol Metab.* 2006;91:781-785.
256. Stratakis CA, Karl M, Schulte HM, et al. Glucocorticosteroid resistance in humans: elucidation of the molecular mechanisms and implications for pathophysiology. *Ann N Y Acad Sci.* 1994;746:362-374.
257. Dunaif A. Insulin resistance in polycystic ovarian syndrome. *Ann N Y Acad Sci.* 1993;687:60-64.
258. Hoffman D, Klove K, Lobo R. The prevalence and significance of elevated dehydroepiandrosterone sulfate levels in anovulatory women. *Fertil Steril.* 1980;42:853-861.
259. Franks S. Polycystic ovary syndrome. *N Engl J Med.* 1995;333:853-861.
260. Kletzky OA, Davajan V, Nakamura RM, et al. Clinical categorization of patients with secondary amenorrhea using progesterone-induced uterine bleeding and measurement of serum gonadotropin levels. *Am J Obstet Gynecol.* 1975;121:695-703.
261. Venturoli S, Porcu E, Fabbri R, et al. Episodic pulsatile secretion of FSH, LH, prolactin, oestradiol, oestrone, and LH circadian variations in polycystic ovary syndrome. *Clin Endocrinol (Oxf).* 1988;28:93-107.
262. Imse V, Holzapfel G, Hinney B, et al. Comparison of luteinizing hormone pulsatility in the serum of women suffering from polycystic ovarian disease using a bioassay and five different immunoassays. *J Clin Endocrinol Metab.* 1992;74:1053-1061.
263. Hayes FJ, Taylor AE, Martin KA, et al. Use of a gonadotropin-releasing hormone antagonist as a physiologic probe in polycystic ovary syndrome: assessment of neuroendocrine and androgen dynamics. *J Clin Endocrinol Metab.* 1998;83:2343-2349.
264. Barnes RB, Lobo RA. Central opioid activity in polycystic ovary syndrome with and without dopaminergic modulation. *J Clin Endocrinol Metab.* 1985;61:779-782.
265. Morales AJ, Laughlin GA, Butzow T, et al. Insulin, somatotropic, and luteinizing hormone axes in lean and obese women with polycystic ovary syndrome: common and distinct features. *J Clin Endocrinol Metab.* 1996;81:2854-2864.
266. Taylor AE, McCourt B, Martin KA, et al. Determinants of abnormal gonadotropin secretion in clinically defined women with polycystic ovary syndrome. *J Clin Endocrinol Metab.* 1997;82:2248-2256.
267. Nagamani M, Van Dinh T, Kelver ME. Hyperinsulinemia in hyperthecosis of the ovaries. *Am J Obstet Gynecol.* 1986;154:384-389.
268. Dorn C, Mouillet JF, Yan X, et al. Insulin enhances the transcription of luteinizing hormone-beta gene. *Am J Obstet Gynecol.* 2004;191:132-137.
269. Adashi EY, Hsueh AJ, Yen SS. Insulin enhancement of luteinizing hormone and follicle-stimulating hormone release by cultured pituitary cells. *Endocrinology.* 1981;108:1441-1449.

270. Lawson M, Jain S, Sun S, et al. Evidence for insulin suppression of baseline luteinizing hormone in women with polycystic ovarian syndrome and normal women. *J Clin Endocrinol Metab*. 2008;93:2089-2096.
271. Chang RJ. Ovarian steroid secretion in polycystic ovarian disease. *Semin Reprod Endocrinol*. 1984;2:244.
272. Wajchenberg BL, Achando SS, Mathor MM, et al. The source(s) of estrogen production in hirsute women with polycystic ovarian disease as determined by simultaneous adrenal and ovarian venous catheterization. *Fertil Steril*. 1988;49:56-61.
273. Chen D, Reierstad S, Lu M, Lin Z, Ishikawa H, Bulun SE. Regulation of breast cancer–associated aromatase promoters. *Cancer Lett*. 2009;273:15-27.
274. Reed MJ, Singh A, Ghilchik MW, et al. Regulation of estradiol 17beta-hydroxysteroid dehydrogenase in breast tissues: the role of growth factors. *J Steroid Biochem Mol Biol*. 1991;39:791-798.
275. Bulun SE, Lin Z, Imir G, et al. Regulation of aromatase expression in estrogen-responsive breast and uterine disease: from bench to treatment. *Pharmacol Rev*. 2005;57:359-383.
276. Nestler JE. Obesity, insulin, sex steroids and ovulation. *Int J Obes Relat Metab Disord*. 2000;24(suppl 2):S71-S73.
277. Fauser BC. Observations in favor of normal early follicle development and disturbed dominant follicle selection in polycystic ovary syndrome. *Gynecol Endocrinol*. 1994;8:75-82.
278. Mason HD, Margara R, Winston RM, et al. Insulin-like growth factor-I (IGF-I) inhibits production of IGF-binding protein-1 while stimulating estradiol secretion in granulosa cells from normal and polycystic human ovaries. *J Clin Endocrinol Metab*. 1993;76:1275-1279.
279. Homburg R, Howles CM. Low-dose FSH therapy for anovulatory infertility associated with polycystic ovary syndrome: rationale, results, reflections and refinements. *Hum Reprod Update*. 1999;5:493-499.
280. Judd HL, Scully RE, Herbst AL, et al. Familial hyperthecosis: comparison of endocrinologic and histologic findings with polycystic ovarian disease. *Am J Obstet Gynecol*. 1973;117:976-982.
281. Cooper HE, Spellacy WN, Prem KA, et al. Hereditary factors in the Stein-Leventhal syndrome. *Am J Obstet Gynecol*. 1968;100:371-387.
282. Ferriman D, Purdie AW. The inheritance of polycystic ovarian disease and a possible relationship to premature balding. *Clin Endocrinol (Oxf)*. 1979;11:291-300.
283. Kent S, Gnatuk C, Kunselman A, et al. Hyperandrogenism and hyperinsulinism in children of women with polycystic ovary syndrome: a controlled study. *J Clin Endocrinol Metab*. 2008;93:1662-1669.
284. Diamanti-Kandarakis E, Kandarakis H, Legro RS. The role of genes and environment in the etiology of PCOS. *Endocrine*. 2006;30:19-26.
285. Urbanek M. The genetics of the polycystic ovary syndrome. *Nat Clin Pract Endocrinol Metab*. 2007;3:103-111.
286. Osei K, Schuster DP. Ethnic differences in secretion, sensitivity, and hepatic extraction of insulin in black and white Americans. *Diabet Med*. 1994;11:755-762.
287. Dunaif A, Green G, Phelps RG, et al. Acanthosis nigricans, insulin action, and hyperandrogenism: clinical, histological, and biochemical findings. *J Clin Endocrinol Metab*. 1991;73:590-595.
288. Reaven GM, Lithell H, Landsberg L. Hypertension and associated metabolic abnormalities: the role of insulin resistance and the sympathoadrenal system. *N Engl J Med*. 1996;334:374-381.
289. Mather KJ, Kwan F, Corenblum B. Hyperinsulinemia in polycystic ovary syndrome correlates with increased cardiovascular risk independent of obesity. *Fertil Steril*. 2000;73:150-156.
290. Talbott E, Guzick D, Clerici A, et al. Coronary heart disease risk factors in women with polycystic ovary syndrome. *Arterioscler Thromb Vasc Biol*. 1995;15:821-826.
291. Ehrmann DA, Liljenquist DR, Kasza K, et al. Prevalence and predictors of the metabolic syndrome in women with polycystic ovary syndrome. *J Clin Endocrinol Metab*. 2006;91:48-53.
292. Dunaif A, Finegood DT. Beta-cell dysfunction independent of obesity and glucose intolerance in the polycystic ovary syndrome. *J Clin Endocrinol Metab*. 1996;81:942-947.
293. Reddy SS, Kahn CR. Epidermal growth factor receptor defects in leprechaunism: a multiple growth factor-resistant syndrome. *J Clin Invest*. 1989;84:1569-1576.
294. Bremer AA, Miller WL. The serine phosphorylation hypothesis of polycystic ovary sybdrome: a unifying mechanism for hyperandrogenemia and insulin resistance. *Fertil Steril*. 2008;89:1039-1048.
295. Kirschner MA, Samojlik E, Drejka M, et al. Androgen-estrogen metabolism in women with upper body versus lower body obesity. *J Clin Endocrinol Metab*. 1990;70:473-479.
296. Schapira DV, Kumar NB, Lyman GH, et al. Abdominal obesity and breast cancer risk. *Ann Intern Med*. 1990;112:182-186.
297. Kumar NB, Cantor A, Allen K, et al. Android obesity at diagnosis and breast carcinoma survival: evaluation of the effects of anthropometric variables at diagnosis, including body composition and body fat distribution and weight gain during life span, and survival from breast carcinoma. *Cancer*. 2000;88:2751-2757.
298. Anderson KE, Sellers TA, Chen PL, et al. Association of Stein-Leventhal syndrome with the incidence of postmenopausal breast carcinoma in a large prospective study of women in Iowa. *Cancer*. 1997;79:494-499.
299. Campbell PJ, Gerich JE. Impact of obesity on insulin action in volunteers with normal glucose tolerance: demonstration of a threshold for the adverse effect of obesity. *J Clin Endocrinol Metab*. 1990;70:1114-1118.
300. Ehrmann DA. Polycystic ovary syndrome. *N Engl J Med*. 2005;352:1223-1236.
301. Velazquez EM, Mendoza S, Hamer T, et al. Metformin therapy in polycystic ovary syndrome reduces hyperinsulinemia, insulin resistance, hyperandrogenemia, and systolic blood pressure, while facilitating normal menses and pregnancy. *Metabolism*. 1994;43:647-654.
302. Nestler JE, Jakubowicz DJ. Decreases in ovarian cytochrome P450c17 alpha activity and serum free testosterone after reduction of insulin secretion in polycystic ovary syndrome. *N Engl J Med*. 1996;335:617-623.
303. Velazquez E, Acosta A, Mendoza SG. Menstrual cyclicity after metformin therapy in polycystic ovary syndrome. *Obstet Gynecol*. 1997;90:392-395.
304. Legro RS, Barnhart HX, Schlaff WD, et al. Clomiphene, metformin, or both for infertility in the polycystic ovary syndrome. *N Engl J Med*. 2007;356:551-566.
305. Palomba S, Falbo A, Zullo F, et al. Evidence-based and potential benefits of metformin in the polycystic ovary syndrome: a comprehensive review. *Endocr Rev*. 2009;30:1-50.
306. Tang T, Lord JM, Norman RJ, et al. Insulin-sensitising drugs (metformin, rosiglitazone, pioglitazone, D-chiro-inositol) for women with polycystic ovary syndrome, oligo amenorrhea, and subfertility. *Cochrane Database Syst*. Rev 2010(1):CD003053.
307. Dunaif A, Scott D, Finegood D, et al. The insulin-sensitizing agent troglitazone improves metabolic and reproductive abnormalities in the polycystic ovary syndrome. *J Clin Endocrinol Metab*. 1996;81:3299-3306.
308. Ehrmann DA, Schneider DJ, Sobel BE, et al. Troglitazone improves defects in insulin action, insulin secretion, ovarian steroidogenesis, and fibrinolysis in women with polycystic ovary syndrome. *J Clin Endocrinol Metab*. 1997;82:2108-2116.
309. Azziz R, Ehrmann D, Legro RS, et al. Troglitazone improves ovulation and hirsutism in the polycystic ovary syndrome: a multicenter, double blind, placebo-controlled trial. *J Clin Endocrinol Metab*. 2001;86:1626-1632.
310. Ghazeeri G, Kutteh WH, Bryer-Ash M, et al. Effect of rosiglitazone on spontaneous and clomiphene citrate-induced ovulation in women with polycystic ovary syndrome. *Fertil Steril*. 2003;79:562-566.
311. Belli SH, Graffigna MN, Oneto A, et al. Effect of rosiglitazone on insulin resistance, growth factors, and reproductive disturbances in women with polycystic ovary syndrome. *Fertil Steril*. 2004;81:624-629.
312. Romualdi D, Guido M, Ciampelli M, et al. Selective effects of pioglitazone on insulin and androgen abnormalities in normo- and hyperinsulinaemic obese patients with polycystic ovary syndrome. *Hum Reprod*. 2003;18:1210-1218.
313. Wild RA, Alaupovic P, Parker IJ. Lipid and apolipoprotein abnormalities in hirsute women: I. The association with insulin resistance. *Am J Obstet Gynecol*. 1992;166:1191-1196; discussion 1196-1197.
314. Kiddy DS, Hamilton-Fairley D, Bush A, et al. Improvement in endocrine and ovarian function during dietary treatment of obese women with polycystic ovary syndrome. *Clin Endocrinol (Oxf)*. 1992;36:105-111.
315. Guzick DS, Wing R, Smith D, et al. Endocrine consequences of weight loss in obese, hyperandrogenic, anovulatory women. *Fertil Steril*. 1994;61:598-604.
316. Clark AM, Ledger W, Galletly C, et al. Weight loss results in significant improvement in pregnancy and ovulation rates in anovulatory obese women. *Hum Reprod*. 1995;10:2705-2712.
317. Gitsch G, Hanzal E, Jensen D, et al. Endometrial cancer in premenopausal women 45 years and younger. *Obstet Gynecol*. 1995;85:504-508.
318. Kjos SL, Peters RK, Xiang A, et al. Contraception and the risk of type 2 diabetes mellitus in Latina women with prior gestational diabetes mellitus. *JAMA*. 1998;280:533-538.
319. Garg SK, Chase HP, Marshall G, et al. Oral contraceptives and renal and retinal complications in young women with insulin-dependent diabetes mellitus. *JAMA*. 1994;271:1099-1102.
320. Petersen KR, Skouby SO, Sidelmann J, et al. Effects of contraceptive steroids on cardiovascular risk factors in women with insulin-dependent diabetes mellitus. *Am J Obstet Gynecol*. 1994;171:400-405.
321. Diamanti-Kandarakis E, Mitrakou A, Hennes MM, et al. Insulin sensitivity and antiandrogenic therapy in women with polycystic ovary syndrome. *Metabolism*. 1995;44:525-531.
322. Lanzone A, Fulghesu AM, Cucinelli F, et al. Preconceptional and gestational evaluation of insulin secretion in patients with polycystic ovary syndrome. *Hum Reprod*. 1996;11:2382-2386.

323. Nestler JE, Jakubowicz DJ, Evans WS, et al. Effects of metformin on spontaneous and clomiphene-induced ovulation in the polycystic ovary syndrome. *N Engl J Med*. 1998;338:1876-1880.
324. Regan L, Owen EJ, Jacobs HS. Hypersecretion of luteinising hormone, infertility, and miscarriage. *Lancet*. 1990;336:1141-1144.
325. Adashi EY. Clomiphene citrate-initiated ovulation: a clinical update. *Semin Reprod Endocrinol*. 1986;4:225-276.
326. Mitwally MF, Casper RF. Use of an aromatase inhibitor for induction of ovulation in patients with an inadequate response to clomiphene citrate. *Fertil Steril*. 2001;75:305-309.
327. Al-Omari WR, Sulaiman WR, Al-Hadithi N. Comparison of two aromatase inhibitors in women with clomiphene-resistant polycystic ovary syndrome. *Int J Gynaecol Obstet*. 2004;85:289-291.
328. Badawy A, Mosbah A, Shady M. Anastrozole or letrozole for ovulation induction in clomiphene-resistant women with polycystic ovarian syndrome: a prospective randomized trial. *Fertil Steril*. 2008;89:1209-1212.
329. Badawy A, Abdel Aal I, Abulatta M. Clomiphene citrate or anastrozole for ovulation induction in women with polycystic ovary syndrome? A prospective controlled trial. *Fertil Steril*. 2009;92:860-863.
330. Abu Hasim H, Shokeir T, Badawy A. Letrozole versus combined metformin and clomiphene citrate for ovulation induction in clomiphene-resistant women with polycystic ovary syndrome: a randomized controlled trial. *Fertil Sterol*. 2010;94:1405-1409.
331. Casper RF, Mitwally MF. Aromatase inhibitors for ovulation induction (review). *J Clin Endocrinol Metab*. 2006;91:760-771.
332. Tulandi T, Martin J, Al-Fadhli R, et al. Congenital malformations among 911 newborns conceived after infertility treatment with letrozole or clomiphene citrate. *Fertil Steril*. 2006;86:1761-1765.
333. Marci R, Senn A, Dessole S, et al. A low-dose stimulation protocol using highly purified follicle-stimulating hormone can lead to high pregnancy rates in in vitro fertilization patients with polycystic ovaries who are at risk of a high ovarian response to gonadotropins. *Fertil Steril*. 2001;75:1131-1135.
334. Hamilton-Fairley D, Franks S. Common problems in induction of ovulation. *Baillieres Clin Obstet Gynaecol*. 1990;4:609-625.
335. Taylor AE, Adams JM, Mulder JE, et al. A randomized, controlled trial of estradiol replacement therapy in women with hypergonadotropic amenorrhea. *J Clin Endocrinol Metab*. 1996;81:3615-3621.
336. Conway GS. Premature ovarian failure. *Br Med Bull*. 2000;56:643-649.
337. Broekmans FJ, Soules MR, Fauser BC. Ovarian aging: mechanisms and clinical consequences. *Endocr Rev*. 2009;30:465-493.
338. Myhre AG, Halonen M, Eskelin P, et al. Autoimmune polyendocrine syndrome type 1 (APS I) in Norway. *Clin Endocrinol (Oxf)*. 2001;54:211-217.
339. Wallace WH, Shalet SM, Crowne EC, et al. Ovarian failure following abdominal irradiation in childhood: natural history and prognosis. *Clin Oncol (R Coll Radiol)*. 1989;1:75-79.
340. Morice P, Thiam-Ba R, Castaigne D, et al. Fertility results after ovarian transposition for pelvic malignancies treated by external irradiation or brachytherapy. *Hum Reprod*. 1998;13:660-663.
341. Bines J, Oleske DM, Cobleigh MA. Ovarian function in premenopausal women treated with adjuvant chemotherapy for breast cancer. *J Clin Oncol*. 1996;14:1718-1729.
342. Byrne J, Mulvihill JJ, Myers MH, et al. Effects of treatment on fertility in long-term survivors of childhood or adolescent cancer. *N Engl J Med*. 1987;317:1315-1321.
343. Rebar RW, Connolly HV. Clinical features of young women with hypergonadotropic amenorrhea. *Fertil Steril*. 1990;53:804-810.
344. Nelson LM, Anasti JN, Kimzey LM, et al. Development of luteinized graafian follicles in patients with karyotypically normal spontaneous premature ovarian failure. *J Clin Endocrinol Metab*. 1994;79:1470-1475.
345. Check JH, Katsoff B. Ovulation induction and pregnancy in a woman with premature menopause following gonadotropin suppression with the gonadotropin releasing hormone antagonist, cetrorelix: a case report. *Clin Exp Obstet Gynecol*. 2008;35:10-12.
346. Tartagni M, Cicinelli E, De Pergola G, et al. Effects of pretreatment with estrogens on ovarian stimulation with gonadotropins in women with premature ovarian failure: a randomized, placebo-controlled trial. *Fertil Steril*. 2007;87:858-861.
347. Dewald G, Spurbeck JL. Sex chromosome anomalies associated with premature gonadal failure. *Semin Reprod Endocrinol*. 1983;1:79-92.
348. Giltay JC, Ausems MG, van Seumeren I, et al. Short stature as the only presenting feature in a patient with an isodicentric (Y)(q11.23) and gonadoblastoma: a clinical and molecular cytogenetic study. *Eur J Pediatr*. 2001;160:154-158.
349. Manuel M, Katayama PK, Jones HW Jr. The age of occurrence of gonadal tumors in intersex patients with a Y chromosome. *Am J Obstet Gynecol*. 1976;124:293-300.
350. Gravholt CH, Fedder J, Naeraa RW, et al. Occurrence of gonadoblastoma in females with Turner syndrome and Y chromosome material: a population study. *J Clin Endocrinol Metab*. 2000;85:3199-3202.
351. Peprah E, He W, Allen E, et al. Examination of FMR1 transcript and protein levels among 74 premutation carriers. *J Hum Genet*. 2010;55:66-68.
352. Wittenberger MD, Hagerman RJ, Sherman SL, et al. The FMR1 premutation and reproduction. *Fertil Steril*. 2007;87:456-465.
353. Nelson L. Autoimmune ovarian failure: comparing the mouse model and the human disease. *J Soc Gynecol Investig*. 2001;8(1 suppl):S55-S57.
354. Wheatcroft NJ, Salt C, Milford-Ward A, et al. Identification of ovarian antibodies by immunofluorescence, enzyme-linked immunosorbent assay or immunoblotting in premature ovarian failure. *Hum Reprod*. 1997;12:2617-2622.
355. Ramathal CY, Bagchi IC, Taylor RN, Bagchi MK. Endometrial decidualization: of mice and men. *Semin Reprod Med*. 2010;28:17-26.
356. Belsey EM, Pinol AP. Menstrual bleeding patterns in untreated women. Task Force on Long-Acting Systemic Agents for Fertility Regulation. *Contraception*. 1997;55:57-65.
357. Chiazze L Jr, Brayer FT, Macisco JJ Jr, et al. The length and variability of the human menstrual cycle. *JAMA*. 1968;203:377-380.
358. Munster K, Schmidt L, Helm P. Length and variation in the menstrual cycle: a cross-sectional study from a Danish county. *Br J Obstet Gynaecol*. 1992;99:422-429.
359. Treloar AE, Boynton RE, Behn BG, et al. Variation of the human menstrual cycle through reproductive life. *Int J Fertil*. 1967;12:77-126.
360. Rybo G. Menstrual blood loss in relation to parity and menstrual pattern. *Acta Obstet Gynecol Scand*. 1966;45(suppl 7):25-45.
361. Haynes PJ, Hodgson H, Anderson AB, et al. Measurement of menstrual blood loss in patients complaining of menorrhagia. *Br J Obstet Gynaecol*. 1977;84:763-768.
362. Higham JM, O'Brien PM, Shaw RW. Assessment of menstrual blood loss using a pictorial chart. *Br J Obstet Gynaecol*. 1990;97:734-739.
363. Fraser IS, McCarron G, Markham R. A preliminary study of factors influencing perception of menstrual blood loss volume. *Am J Obstet Gynecol*. 1984;149:788-793.
364. de Ziegler D, Bergeron C, Cornel C, et al. Effects of luteal estradiol on the secretory transformation of human endometrium and plasma gonadotropins. *J Clin Endocrinol Metab*. 1992;74:322-331.
365. Belsey EM. Vaginal bleeding patterns among women using one natural and eight hormonal methods of contraception. *Contraception*. 1988;38:181-206.
366. Wilansky DL, Greisman B. Early hypothyroidism in patients with menorrhagia. *Am J Obstet Gynecol*. 1989;160:673-677.
367. Hopkins MP, Androff L, Benninghoff AS. Ginseng face cream and unexplained vaginal bleeding. *Am J Obstet Gynecol*. 1988;159:1121-1122.
368. Claessens EA, Cowell CA. Acute adolescent menorrhagia. *Am J Obstet Gynecol*. 1981;139:277-280.
369. Smith YR, Quint EH, Hertzberg RB. Menorrhagia in adolescents requiring hospitalization. *J Pediatr Adolesc Gynecol*. 1998;11:13-15.
370. van Eijkeren MA, Christiaens GC, Haspels AA, et al. Measured menstrual blood loss in women with a bleeding disorder or using oral anticoagulant therapy. *Am J Obstet Gynecol*. 1990;162:1261-1263.
371. Edlund M, Blomback M, von Schoultz B, Andersson O. On the value of menorrhagia as a predictor for coagulation disorders. *Am J Hematol*. 1996;53:234-238.
372. Nilsson L, Rybo G. Treatment of menorrhagia. *Am J Obstet Gynecol*. 1971;110:713-720.
373. Kirkland JL, Murthy L, Stancel GM. Progesterone inhibits the estrogen-induced expression of c-fos messenger ribonucleic acid in the uterus. *Endocrinology*. 1992;130:3223-3230.
374. DeVore GR, Owens O, Kase N. Use of intravenous Premarin in the treatment of dysfunctional uterine bleeding: a double-blind randomized control study. *Obstet Gynecol*. 1982;59:285-291.
375. Livio M, Mannucci PM, Vigano G, et al. Conjugated estrogens for the management of bleeding associated with renal failure. *N Engl J Med*. 1986;315:731-735.
376. Giudice LC, Kao LC. Endometriosis. *Lancet*. 2004;364:1789-1799.
377. Bulun SE. Endometriosis. *N Engl J Med*. 2009;360:268-279.
378. Simpson JL, Elias S, Malinak LR, et al. Heritable aspects of endometriosis: I. Genetic studies. *Am J Obstet Gynecol*. 1980;137:327-331.
379. Garry R. The endometriosis syndromes: a clinical classification in the presence of aetiological confusion and therapeutic anarchy. *Hum Reprod*. 2004;19:760-768.
380. Brosens I. Endometriosis rediscovered? *Hum Reprod*. 2004;19:1679-1680; author reply 1680-1681.
381. Sampson JA. Peritoneal endometriosis due to the menstrual dissemination of endometrial tissue into the peritoneal cavity. *Am J Obstet Gynecol*. 1927;14:422-469.
382. Sasson IE, Taylor HS. Stem cells and the pathogenesis of endometriosis. *Ann N Y Acad Sci*. 2008;1127:106-115.
383. Hornung D, Ryan IP, Chao VA, et al. Immunolocalization and regulation of the chemokine RANTES in human endometrial and endometriosis tissues. *J Clin Endocrinol Metab*. 1997;82:1621-1628.
384. Olive D, Schwartz LB. Endometriosis. *N Eng J Med*. 1993;328:1759-1769.

385. Waller KG, Shaw RW. Gonadotropin-releasing hormone analogues for the treatment of endometriosis: long-term follow-up. *Fertil Steril.* 1993;59:511-515.
386. Shaw RW. An open randomized comparative study of the effect of goserelin depot and danazol in the treatment of endometriosis. Zoladex Endometriosis Study Team. *Fertil Steril.* 1992;58:265-272.
387. A decision tree for the use of estrogen replacement therapy or hormone replacement therapy in postmenopausal women: consensus opinion of the North American Menopause Society. *Menopause.* 2000;7:76-86.
388. Vercellini P, Cortesi I, Crosignani P. Progestins for symptomatic endometriosis: a critical analysis of the evidence. *Fertil Steril.* 1997;68: 393-401.
389. Takayama K, Zeitoun K, Gunby RT, et al. Treatment of severe postmenopausal endometriosis with an aromatase inhibitor. *Fertil Steril.* 1998;69:709-713.
390. Vercellini P, Trespidi L, Colombo A. A gonadotropin-releasing hormone agonist versus a low-dose oral contraceptive for pelvic pain associated with endometriosis. *Fertil Steril.* 1993;60:75-79.
391. Waller KG, Shaw RW. Gonadotropin-releasing hormone analogues for the treatment of endometriosis: long-term follow-up. *Fertil Steril.* 1993;59:511-515.
392. Amsterdam L, Gentry W, Rubin S, Jobanputra S, Bulun SE. Treatment of endometriosis-related pelvic pain with a combination of an aromatase inhibitor (anastrozole) plus a combination oral contraceptive: a novel approach. *Proceedings of the 85th Annual Endocrine Society Meeting.* 2003;1:360.
393. Ailawadi R, Jobanputra S, Kataria M, et al. Treatment of endometriosis and chronic pelvic pain with letrozole and norethindrone acetate: a pilot study. *Fertil Steril.* 2004;81:290-296.
394. Soysal S, Soysal M, Ozer S, et al. The effects of post-surgical administration of goserelin plus anastrozole compared to goserelin alone in patients with severe endometriosis: a prospective randomized trial. *Hum Reprod.* 2004;19:160-167.
395. Attar E, Bulun SE. Aromatase inhibitors: the next generation of therapeutics for endometriosis? *Fertil Steril.* 2006;85:1307-1318.
396. Stewart EA. Uterine fibroids. *Lancet.* 2001;357:293-298.
397. Tropeano G, Amoroso S, Scambia G. Non-surgical management of uterine fibroids. *Hum Reprod Update.* 2008;14:259-274.
398. Maruo T, Matsuo H, Samoto T, et al. Effects of progesterone on uterine leiomyoma growth and apoptosis. *Steroids.* 2000;65:585-592.
399. Yin P, Lin Z, Cheng YH, et al. Progesterone receptor regulates Bcl-2 gene expression through direct binding to its promoter region in uterine leiomyoma cells. *J Clin Endocrinol Metab.* 2007;92:4459-4466.
400. Ishikawa H, Ishi K, Sema VA, et al. Progesterone is essential for maintenance and growth of uterine leiomyoma. *Endocrinology.* 2010;151: 2433-2442.
401. McKinlay SM, Brambilla DJ, Posner JG. The normal menopause transition. *Maturitas.* 1992;14:103-115.
402. den Tonkelaar I, te Velde ER, Looman CW. Menstrual cycle length preceding menopause in relation to age at menopause. *Maturitas.* 1998;29:115-123.
403. Buckler HM, Evans CA, Mamtora H, et al. Gonadotropin, steroid, and inhibin levels in women with incipient ovarian failure during anovulatory and ovulatory rebound cycles. *J Clin Endocrinol Metab.* 1991;72:116-124.
404. Santoro N, Brown JR, Adel T, et al. Characterization of reproductive hormonal dynamics in the perimenopause. *J Clin Endocrinol Metab.* 1996;81:1495-1501.
405. McKinlay SM, Bifano NL, McKinlay JB. Smoking and age at menopause in women. *Ann Intern Med.* 1985;103:350-356.
406. Torgerson DJ, Avenell A, Russell IT, et al. Factors associated with onset of menopause in women aged 45-49. *Maturitas.* 1994;19:83-92.
407. Torgerson DJ, Thomas RE, Campbell MK, et al. Alcohol consumption and age of maternal menopause are associated with menopause onset. *Maturitas.* 1997;26:21-25.
408. Cramer DW, Xu H, Harlow BL. Family history as a predictor of early menopause. *Fertil Steril.* 1995;64:740-745.
409. Gosden RG. Follicular status at the menopause. *Hum Reprod.* 1987;2:617-621.
410. Jiroutek MR, Chen MH, Johnston CC, et al. Changes in reproductive hormones and sex hormone-binding globulin in a group of postmenopausal women measured over 10 years. *Menopause.* 1998;5:90-94.
411. Adashi EY. The climacteric ovary as a functional gonadotropin-driven androgen-producing gland. *Fertil Steril.* 1994;62:20-27.
412. Grodin JM, Siiteri PK, MacDonald PC. Source of estrogen production in postmenopausal women. *J Clin Endocrinol Metab.* 1973;36:207-214.
413. Labrie F, Belanger A, Cusan L, et al. Marked decline in serum concentrations of adrenal C19 sex steroid precursors and conjugated androgen metabolites during aging. *J Clin Endocrinol Metab.* 1997;82: 2396-2402.
414. Judd HL, Shamonki IM, Frumar AM, et al. Origin of serum estradiol in postmenopausal women. *Obstet Gynecol.* 1982;59:680-686.
415. Bulun SE, Noble LS, Takayama K, et al. Endocrine disorders associated with inappropriately high aromatase expression. *J Steroid Biochem Mol Biol.* 1997;61:133-139.
416. Bonneterre J, Buzdar A, Nabholtz JM, et al. Anastrozole is superior to tamoxifen as first-line therapy in hormone receptor positive advanced breast carcinoma. *Cancer.* 2001;92:2247-2258.
417. BIG 1-98 Collaborative Group, Mouridsen H, Giobbie–Hurder A, Goldhirsch A, et al. Letrozole therapy alone or in sequence with tamoxifen in women with breast cancer. *N Engl J Med.* 2009 Aug 20;361(8): 766-776.
418. Feldman S, Shapter A, Welch WR, et al. Two-year follow-up of 263 patients with post/perimenopausal vaginal bleeding and negative initial biopsy. *Gynecol Oncol.* 1994;55:56-59.
419. Oldenhave A, Jaszmann LJ, Haspels AA, et al. Impact of climacteric on well-being: a survey based on 5213 women 39 to 60 years old. *Am J Obstet Gynecol.* 1993;168:772-780.
420. Kronenberg F, Barnard R. Modulation of menopausal hot flasheds by ambient temperature. *J Therm Biol.* 1992;17:43-49.
421. Yen SS. The biology of menopause. *J Reprod Med.* 1977;18:287-296.
422. Erlik Y, Meldrum DR, Judd HL. Estrogen levels in postmenopausal women with hot flashes. *Obstet Gynecol.* 1982;59:403-407.
423. Thurston RC, Sowers MR, Sternfeld B, et al. Gains in body fat and vasomotor symptom reporting over the menopausal transition: the study of women's health across the nation. *Am J Epidemiol.* 2009; 170:766-774.
424. Raz R, Stamm WE. A controlled trial of intravaginal estriol in postmenopausal women with recurrent urinary tract infections. *N Engl J Med.* 1993;329:753-756.
425. Dempster DW, Lindsay R. Pathogenesis of osteoporosis. *Lancet.* 1993;341:797-801.
426. Richelson LS, Wahner HW, Melton LJ 3rd, et al. Relative contributions of aging and estrogen deficiency to postmenopausal bone loss. *N Engl J Med.* 1984;311:1273-1275.
427. Nilas L, Christiansen C. Bone mass and its relationship to age and the menopause. *J Clin Endocrinol Metab.* 1987;65:697-702.
428. Christiansen C. Hormone replacement therapy and osteoporosis. *Maturitas.* 1996;23(suppl):S71-S76.
429. Rossouw JE, Anderson GL, Prentice RL, et al. Risks and benefits of estrogen plus progestin in healthy postmenopausal women: principal results from the Women's Health Initiative randomized controlled trial. *JAMA.* 2002;288:321-333.
430. Anderson GL, Limacher M, Assaf AR, et al. Effects of conjugated equine estrogen in postmenopausal women with hysterectomy: the Women's Health Initiative randomized controlled trial. *JAMA.* 2004;291: 1701-1712.
431. American College of Obstetrics and Gynecology. ACOG Committee Opinion No. 420, November 2008: hormone therapy and heart disease. *Obstet Gynecol.* 2008;112:1189-1192.
432. Brett KM, Madans JH. Use of postmenopausal hormone replacement therapy: estimates from a nationally representative cohort study. *Am J Epidemiol.* 1997;145:536-545.
433. Ness J, Aronow WS, Newkirk E, et al. Use of hormone replacement therapy by postmenopausal women after publication of the Women's Health Initiative Trial. *J Gerontol A Biol Sci Med Sci.* 2005;60:460-462.
434. Hoffmann M, Hammar M, Kjellgren KI, et al. Changes in women's attitudes towards and use of hormone therapy after HERS and WHI. *Maturitas.* 2005;52:11-17.
435. Thunell L, Milsom I, Schmidt J, et al. Scientific evidence changes prescribing practice: a comparison of the management of the climacteric and use of hormone replacement therapy among Swedish gynaecologists in 1996 and 2003. *BJOG.* 2006;113:15-20.
436. Miller VM, Black DM, Brinton EA, et al. Using basic science to design a clinical trial: baseline characteristics of women enrolled in the kronos early estrogen prevention study (KEEPS). *J Cardiovasc Transl Res.* 2009;2:228-239.
437. Prentice RL, Anderson GL. The women's health initiative: lessons learned. *Annu Rev Public Health.* 2008;29:131-150.
438. Nicholson WK, Brown AF, Gathe J, et al. Hormone replacement therapy for African American women: missed opportunities for effective intervention. *Menopause.* 1999;6:147-155.
439. Bergkvist L, Adami HO, Persson I, et al. The risk of breast cancer after estrogen and estrogen-progestin replacement. *N Engl J Med.* 1989;321: 293-297.
440. Hulley S, Grady D, Bush T, et al. Randomized trial of estrogen plus progestin for secondary prevention of coronary heart disease in postmenopausal women. Heart and Estrogen/progestin Replacement Study (HERS) Research Group. *JAMA.* 1998;280:605-613.
441. Shumaker SA, Legault C, Rapp SR, et al. Estrogen plus progestin and the incidence of dementia and mild cognitive impairment in postmenopausal women: the Women's Health Initiative Memory Study—a randomized controlled trial. *JAMA.* 2003;289:2651-2662.
442. Vandenbroucke JP. The HRT controversy: observational studies and RCTs fall in line. *Lancet.* 2009;373:1233-1235.
443. Prentice RL, Chlebowski RT, Stefanick ML, et al. Estrogen plus progestin therapy and breast cancer in recently postmenopausal women. *Am J Epidemiol.* 2008;167:1207-1216.
444. Lacey JV Jr, Mink PJ, Lubin JH, et al. Menopausal hormone replacement therapy and risk of ovarian cancer. *JAMA.* 2002;288:334-341.

445. Chlebowski RT, Schwartz AG, Wakelee H, et al. Oestrogen plus progestin and lung cancer in postmenopausal women (Women's Health Initiative trial): a post-hoc analysis of a randomised controlled trial. *Lancet*. 2009;374:1243-1251.
446. Shumaker SA, Legault C, Kuller L, et al. Conjugated equine estrogens and incidence of probable dementia and mild cognitive impairment in postmenopausal women: Women's Health Initiative Memory Study. *JAMA*. 2004;291:2947-2958.
447. Glueck CJ, Lang J, Hamer T, et al. Severe hypertriglyceridemia and pancreatitis when estrogen replacement therapy is given to hypertriglyceridemic women. *J Lab Clin Med*. 1994;123:59-64.
448. Cirillo DJ, Wallace RB, Rodabough RJ, et al. Effect of estrogen therapy on gallbladder disease. *JAMA*. 2005;293:330-339.
449. Hays J, Ockene JK, Brunner RL, et al. Effects of estrogen plus progestin on health-related quality of life. *N Engl J Med*. 2003;348:1839-1854.
450. Brunner RL, Gass M, Aragaki A, et al. Effects of conjugated equine estrogen on health-related quality of life in postmenopausal women with hysterectomy: results from the Women's Health Initiative Randomized Clinical Trial. *Arch Intern Med*. 2005;165:1976-1986.
451. Rapp SR, Espeland MA, Shumaker SA, et al. Effect of estrogen plus progestin on global cognitive function in postmenopausal women: the Women's Health Initiative Memory Study—a randomized controlled trial. *JAMA*. 2003;289:2663-2672.
452. Espeland MA, Rapp SR, Shumaker SA, et al. Conjugated equine estrogens and global cognitive function in postmenopausal women: Women's Health Initiative Memory Study. *JAMA*. 2004;291: 2959-2968.
453. Reed SD, Newton KM, Lacroix AZ. Indications for hormone therapy: the post-Women's Health Initiative era. *Endocrinol Metab Clin North Am*. 2004;33:691-715.
454. Harman SM, Naftolin F, Brinton E, et al. Is the estrogen controversy over? Deconstructing the Women's Health Initiative Study: a critical evaluation of the evidence. *Ann N Y Acad Sci*. 2005;1052:43-56.
455. Martin KA, Manson JE. Approach to the patient with menopausal symptoms. *J Clin Endocrinol Metab*. 2008;93:4567-4575.
456. Riis BJ, Hansen MA, Jensen AM, et al. Low bone mass and fast rate of bone loss at menopause: equal risk factors for future fracture—a 15-year follow-up study. *Bone*. 1996;19:9-12.
457. Ettinger B, Pressman A, Van Gessel A. Low-dosage esterified estrogens opposed by progestin at 6-month intervals. *Obstet Gynecol*. 2001; 98:205-211.
458. Lindheim SR, Presser SC, Ditkoff EC, et al. A possible bimodal effect of estrogen on insulin sensitivity in postmenopausal women and the attenuating effect of added progestin. *Fertil Steril*. 1993;60:664-667.
459. Woodruff JD, Pickar JH. Incidence of endometrial hyperplasia in postmenopausal women taking conjugated estrogens (Premarin) with medroxyprogesterone acetate or conjugated estrogens alone. The Menopause Study Group. *Am J Obstet Gynecol*. 1994;170:1213-1223.
460. Archer DF, Pickar JH, Bottiglioni F. Bleeding patterns in postmenopausal women taking continuous combined or sequential regimens of conjugated estrogens with medroxyprogesterone acetate. Menopause Study Group. *Obstet Gynecol*. 1994;83:686-692.
461. The Postmenopausal Estrogen/Progestin Interventions (PEPI) trial. Effects of estrogen or estrogen/progestin regimens in heart disease risk factors in postmenopausal women. *JAMA*. 1995;273:199-208.
462. Nand SL, Webster MA, Baber R, et al. Bleeding pattern and endometrial changes during continuous combined hormone replacement therapy. The Ogen/Provera Study Group. *Obstet Gynecol*. 1998;91:678-684.
463. Archer DF, McIntyre-Seltman K, Wilborn WW Jr, et al. Endometrial morphology in asymptomatic postmenopausal women. *Am J Obstet Gynecol*. 1991;165:317-320; discussion 320-322.
464. Korhonen MO, Symons JP, Hyde BM, et al. Histologic classification and pathologic findings for endometrial biopsy specimens obtained from 2964 perimenopausal and postmenopausal women undergoing screening for continuous hormones as replacement therapy (CHART 2 Study). *Am J Obstet Gynecol*. 1997;176:377-380.
465. McGonigle KF, Karlan BY, Barbuto DA, et al. Development of endometrial cancer in women on estrogen and progestin hormone replacement therapy. *Gynecol Oncol*. 1994;55:126-132.
466. Karlsson B, Granberg S, Wikland M, et al. Transvaginal ultrasonography of the endometrium in women with postmenopausal bleeding: a Nordic multicenter study. *Am J Obstet Gynecol*. 1995;172:1488-1494.
467. Bakos O, Smith P, Heimer G. Transvaginal ultrasonography for identifying endometrial pathology in postmenopausal women. *Maturitas*. 1994;20:181-189.
468. Granberg S, Ylostalo P, Wikland M, et al. Endometrial sonographic and histologic findings in women with and without hormonal replacement therapy suffering from postmenopausal bleeding. *Maturitas*. 1997;27:35-40.
469. Avis NE. Breast cancer survivors and hot flashes: the search for nonhormonal treatments. *J Clin Oncol*. 2008;26:5008-5010.
470. Holmberg L, Iversen OE, Rudenstam CM, et al. Increased risk of recurrence after hormone replacement therapy in breast cancer survivors. *J Natl Cancer Inst*. 2008;100:475-482.
471. Cummings SR, Ettinger B, Delmas PD, et al. The effects of tibolone in older postmenopausal women. *N Engl J Med*. 2008;359:697-708.
472. Jordan VC, O'Malley BW. Selective estrogen-receptor modulators and antihormonal resistance in breast cancer. *J Clin Oncol*. 2007;25: 5815-5824.
473. Nelson HD, Fu R, Griffin JC, et al. Systematic review: comparative effectiveness of medications to reduce risk for primary breast cancer. *Ann Intern Med*. 2009;151:703-715, W-226-35.
474. Bilezikian JP. Efficacy of bisphosphonates in reducing fracture risk in postmenopausal osteoporosis. *Am J Med*. 2009;122:S14-S21.
475. Jansen JP, Bergman GJ, Huels J, et al. Prevention of vertebral fractures in osteoporosis: mixed treatment comparison of bisphosphonate therapies. *Curr Med Res Opin*. 2009;25:1861-1868.
476. Bianchi G, Sambrook P. Oral nitrogen-containing bisphosphonates: a systematic review of randomized clinical trials and vertebral fractures. *Curr Med Res Opin*. 2008;24:2669-2677.
477. Bonnick S, Saag KG, Kiel DP, et al. Comparison of weekly treatment of postmenopausal osteoporosis with alendronate versus risedronate over two years. *J Clin Endocrinol Metab*. 2006;91:2631-2637.
478. Lodi G, Sardella A, Salis A, et al. Tooth extraction in patients taking intravenous bisphosphonates: a preventive protocol and case series. *J Oral Maxillofac Surg*. 2010;68:107-110.
479. Gnant M, Mlineritsch B, Schippinger W, et al. Endocrine therapy plus zoledronic acid in premenopausal breast cancer. *N Engl J Med*. 2009; 360:679-691.
480. Wysowski DK. Reports of esophageal cancer with oral bisphosphonate use. *N Engl J Med*. 2009 Jan 1;360(1):89-90.
481. Green J, Czanner G, Reeves G, et al. Oral bisphosphonates and risk of cancer of oesophagus, stomach, and colorectum: case-control analysis within a UK primary care cohort. *BMJ*. 2010 Sep 1;341:c4444.
482. Cardwell CR, Abnet CC, Cantwell MM, Murray LJ. Exposure to oral bisphosphonates and risk of esophageal cancer. *JAMA*. 2010 Aug 11;304(6):657-663.

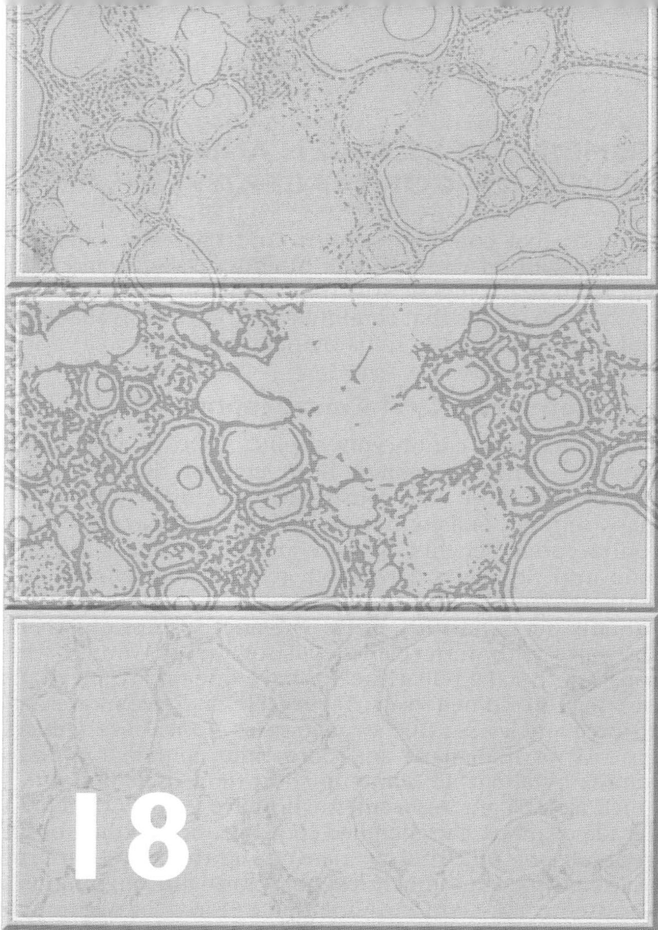

CHAPTER 18

Hormonal Contraception

MARTHA HICKEY • ANDREW M. KAUNITZ

Prevention of unplanned pregnancy continues to challenge clinicians and consumers in developed and developing countries. In the United States and other developed countries, the birth rate continues to fall according to the U.S. National Center for Health Statistics. On average, women devote more than 3 decades of their lives to avoiding unintended pregnancy. In developing countries, childbirth and unsafe abortion are important causes of maternal mortality and morbidity.

Contraceptive advice and provision should start before the commencement of sexual activity and continue through the reproductive years. The United States has one of the highest teenage pregnancy rates in the developed world.[1] Teenaged parenting commonly has adverse consequences for the adolescent, her children, and her family.[2] Programs to prevent unplanned pregnancy by promoting abstinence have largely been ineffective. Nonhormonal contraceptives, such as male condoms, may offer benefits in terms of protection against sexually transmitted infection (STI), but they are highly user dependent and do not reliably prevent unplanned pregnancy in many populations. Female hormonal contraception is the most effective and acceptable reversible contraceptive option; male hormonal contraception has not achieved this goal. Despite the wide variety of female hormonal contraceptive methods and other methods available, about one half of all pregnancies in developed countries are unplanned. In the United States, almost 3.2 million unintended pregnancies occur annually.[3] Figures are not available for most developing countries, but it is likely that the proportion of pregnancies that are unintended is much higher.

The ideal contraceptive would be safe, highly effective, discreet, cheap, long acting, easily reversible, and under the patient's control. It would not need to be activated at or around the time of intercourse and would not disrupt vaginal bleeding patterns. The ideal contraceptive would also protect against STI. Because an ideal contraceptive does not exist, the challenge for clinicians is to tailor the available methods to the medical, personal, and social needs of the consumer and her partner as they evolve throughout her reproductive life span. The clinician must also learn to recognize and address barriers to the safe and effective implementation of the selected methods. Hormonal contraceptives are most effectively used by consumers who are well informed about the advantages and likely side effects of the method and who have actively participated in selecting the method. Expert contraceptive advice and provision can significantly reduce maternal mortality and can improve the social and educational status of women worldwide.

COMBINED ESTROGEN AND PROGESTIN CONTRACEPTIVES

Methods that combine estrogen and progestin offer the advantage of relatively regular bleeding patterns and high efficacy if used consistently. Increasing flexibility in delivery systems means that combined methods are available in oral, transdermal, and transvaginal preparations.

The Combined Oral Contraceptive Pill

Combined oral contraceptive pills (COCPs) offer safe, reversible, and convenient birth control that is highly effective for those who consistently take pills correctly. In many settings, oral contraception provides important noncontraceptive benefits. By individualizing counseling and follow-up strategies based on relevant behavioral and medical considerations, physicians can maximize their patients' success with COCPs. The effectiveness of COCPs correlates with correct and consistent use. Women who consistently take pills correctly have one or two pregnancies per 100 women-years. Teenagers may have more than 15 pregnancies per 100 women-years. COCP use reduces the risk of malignant and borderline epithelial ovarian tumors by about 40% among short-term users and by as much as 80% among women who have used COCPs for a decade or more. Unscheduled spotting and bleeding occur in about one fourth of women during the first 3 months of use but become much less common with ongoing use. Counseling patients to anticipate early breakthrough bleeding and reassuring those who experience this side effect may improve continuation rates.

Women who are bothered by hormone withdrawal symptoms or who may benefit from less frequent withdrawal bleeding may benefit from the newer formulations of oral contraceptives that shorten or eliminate the hormone-free interval. Perimenopausal women benefit from the regularity of menses, relief from vasomotor symptoms, and positive impact on bone mineral density (BMD) offered by combination oral contraception. Women with diabetes, controlled hypertension, lupus, or obesity may be candidates for a trial of low-dose oral contraception provided they are younger than 35 years, nonsmokers, and otherwise show no evidence of vascular damage.

COCPs have been available for more than 50 years and have gradually been refined to improve safety, efficacy, and acceptability. COCPs are used by more than 10 million U.S. women, making them the most widely used hormonal contraceptive method. Current methods contain estrogen, usually as ethinyl estradiol at doses of 20 to 50 μg/day and with a range of progestins. COCPs offer women safe, convenient, effective, and reversible fertility regulation. Use of COCPs also confers important noncontraceptive health benefits that should be discussed during counseling. This section describes COCPs available in the United States, focusing on education, counseling, and management measures to maximize contraceptive efficacy.

Composition and Formulations

Over time, the dose of estrogen and progestin in COCPs has gradually decreased, and the type of progestin has changed. Currently, the highest-dose formulations marketed in the United States contain 50 μg of estrogen, and most COCPs prescribed contain 35 μg or less. All modern COCPs formulated with 35 μg of estrogen or less use the potent estrogen ethinyl estradiol. Older COCP preparations contain one of five progestins: norethindrone, norethindrone acetate, ethynodiol diacetate, norgestrel, or levonorgestrel. Newer formulations contain the less-androgenic progestins, norgestimate, desogestrel, and drospirenone.

Many COCP formulations are marketed in the United States (Table 18-1). These products are not different in terms of safety or efficacy if used correctly.[4] COCPs were originally formulated to mimic the normal menstrual cycle by providing 21 days of combined estrogen and progestin, followed by a 7-day pill-free week when withdrawal bleeding occurred. Modern COCPs mainly continue to follow this regimen and contain active pills for 21 to 24 days, although there is no evidence that a hormone-free interval provides any health benefits. Hormone-withdrawal symptoms, including pelvic pain and mood symptoms, may occur during the pill-free week.[5] COCP regimens differ in whether the dose of ethinyl estradiol and progestin is the same throughout the 21 days of use or the doses vary. Monophasic preparations have a constant dose of estrogen and progestin in each of the 21 or 24 active hormone tables in each cycle pack. Phasic preparations alter the dose of the progestin and, in some formulations, the estrogen component among the active tablets in each pack. COCPs typically come in 28-day packages designed to be simple to use. Pills are still taken during the hormone-free interval, but they do not contain sex steroids.

The hormone-free interval can be modified or eliminated. This may improve contraceptive success; reduce hormone-withdrawal symptoms; improve treatment of problems such as dysmenorrhea, pelvic pain, and anemia; and be more convenient for some women.[6] Newer oral contraception pills offer extended-cycle regimens of 91 pills, with inert tablets or tablets containing 10 μg of ethinyl estradiol in place of the conventional hormone-free interval.

Mechanism of Action, Efficacy, Administration, and Effect on Pregnancy

Administration of COCPs prevents ovulation by inhibiting gonadotropin secretion through the effect of estrogen and progestin on the pituitary and hypothalamus. The progestin component of the pill primarily suppresses luteinizing hormone secretion, whereas the estrogenic component suppresses follicle-stimulating hormone. Both steroids in COCPs contribute to the suppression of ovulation. Because the contraceptive efficacy of COCPs relies on daily use, failure rates are largely attributable to poor adherence. Pregnancies range from less than 1 per 100 women-years (Pearl index) with excellent adherence to more than 15 pregnancies per 100 women-years with low adherence. Typical first-year combination oral contraception failure rates are estimated at 8 per 100 women.[7]

Traditionally, COCPs have been started on the first day of menses, but the pills can be safely started at any time if pregnancy has been excluded (quick start method).[8] This approach may reduce unplanned pregnancies occurring while women are waiting to start the pills. If the COCPs are inadvertently taken during pregnancy, they do not appear to increase the rate of miscarriage or adversely affect the developing fetus.[9]

Because daily use is critical to ensure contraceptive efficacy, some women prefer to link pill taking with a daily ritual (e.g., tooth brushing). Clear instructions for managing missed pills are an essential component of COCP counseling. If a woman misses 1 or 2 tablets, she should take 1 pill as soon as possible. She should then continue to take 1 tablet twice daily until each of the missed tablets have

TABLE 18-1

Oral Contraceptive Formulations Available in the United States

	Name	Estrogen	Progestin	Progestin Dose (mg)
EE, 50 μg monophasic	Ovcon 50*	EE	Norethindrone	1.0
	Ortho-Novum 1/50*	Mestranol	Norethindrone	1.0
	Norinyl 1 + 50*	Mestranol	Norethindrone	1.0
EE, 35 μg monophasic	Femcon Fe†	EE	Norethindrone	0.4
	Modicon*	EE	Norethindrone	0.5
	Brevicon*	EE	Norethindrone	0.5
	Ovcon 35*	EE	Norethindrone	0.4
	Ortho-Cyclen*	EE	Norgestimate	0.25
	Demulen 1/35*	EE	Ethynodiol diacetate	1.0
	Ortho-Novum 1/35*	EE	Norethindrone	1.0
	Norinyl 1 + 35*	EE	Norethindrone	1.0
EE, 35 μg biphasic	Ortho-Novum 10/11*	EE	Norethindrone	0.5/1.0
EE, 35 μg triphasic	Ortho-Novum 7/7/7*	EE	Norethindrone	0.5/0.75/1.0
	Ortho Tri-Cyclen*‡	EE	Norgestimate	0.18/0.215/0.25
	Tri-Norinyl*	EE	Norethindrone	0.5/1.0/0.5
	Estrostep*‡	EE (20/30/35)	Norethindrone acetate	1.0
EE, 30 μg monophasic	Loestrin 1.5/30*	EE	Norethindrone acetate	1.5
	Ortho-Cept*	EE	Desogestrel	0.15
	Desogen*	EE	Desogestrel	0.15
	Lo-Ovral*	EE	Norgestrel	0.3
	Nordette*	EE	Levonorgestrel	0.15
	Levlen*	EE	Levonorgestrel	0.15
	Yasmin*	EE	Drosperinone	3.0
EE, 30 μg triphasic	Triphasil*	EE (30/40/30)	Levonorgestrel	0.05/0.075/0.125
	Tri-Levlen*	EE (30/40/30)	Levonorgestrel	0.05/0.075/0.125
Extended cycle (84 active tablets)	Seasonale*	EE	Levonorgestrel	0.150
Extended cycle (84 estrogen/progestin tablets, 7 tablets 10 μg EE)	Seasonique	EE	Levonorgestrel	0.150
EE, 25 μg	Cyclessa*	EE	Desogestrel	0.10/0.125/0.150
	Ortho Tri-Cyclen Lo	EE	Norgestimate	0.18/0.215/0.25
EE, 20 μg monophasic	Loestrin 1/20*	EE	Norethindrone acetate	1.0
	Levlite*	EE	Levonorgestrel	0.1
	Alesse*	EE	Levonorgestrel	0.1
21 Hormonally active tablets (2 inert tablets, 5 tablets 10 μg EE)	Mircette*	EE	Desogestrel	0.15
24 Hormonally active tablets	Yaz‡§	EE	Drosperinone	3.0
	Loestrin 24Fe	EE	Norethindrone acetate	1.0
Extended cycle (84 estrogen/progestin tablets, 7 tablets 10 μg EE)	LoSeasonique	EE	Levonorgestrel	0.1
28 Hormonally active tablets	Lybrel	EE	Levonorgestrel	0.09
Progestin-only	Micronor*		Norethindrone	0.35

EE, ethinyl estradiol.
*Generic versions available.
†Chewable tablets.
‡Indicated for the treatment of acne in women desiring to use oral contraception.
§Indicated for the treatment of premenstrual dysphoric disorder in women desiring to use oral contraception.

been taken. If she has missed more than two consecutive tablets, she should use an additional form of contraception (e.g., condoms) until the current pack of pills is finished and she experiences expected withdrawal bleeding. COCPs are not suitable for women who consistently miss pills, because this undermines contraceptive efficacy. In these cases, a method that does not require daily adherence (e.g., contraceptive rings; patches; an injectable, intrauterine, or implantable method) should be considered.

After discontinuation of COCPs, most women rapidly recommence ovulation. Some women may ovulate if the hormone-free interval is extended beyond 7 days. In some women, ovulation may be delayed for several months after discontinuing oral contraception.[10]

Noncontraceptive Health Benefits

For some users, COCPs offer substantial noncontraceptive health benefits. These advantages include reducing in dysmenorrhea and symptoms of premenstrual syndrome, creating predictable withdrawal bleeding in women with dysfunctional uterine bleeding, reducing the daily intensity and duration of menstrual flow, improving anemia, and markedly reducing the risk of ovarian and endometrial cancer. Educating COCP candidates and users regarding these noncontraceptive benefits can assist the patient in making a choice and can increase oral contraception adherence and continuation.

Benign breast diseases, including fibroadenoma and cystic changes, occur less commonly in COCP users.

Functional cysts are not reliably suppressed by modern COCP formulations containing 35 μg of estradiol or less. COCP use reduces the incidence of pelvic inflammatory disease (PID)[11] and ectopic pregnancy,[12] two common and potentially life-threatening conditions. In perimenopausal women, COCPs can maintain BMD, improve reduced BMD, and possibly reduce the risk of postmenopausal fracture. Skeletal health benefits associated with COCP use may also apply to women who have been hypoestrogenic and those with hypothalamic amenorrhea.[13]

Reducing the risk of epithelial ovarian and endometrial cancer is perhaps the most important noncontraceptive benefit of COCP use. Although the incidence is low, epithelial ovarian cancer is the most common cause of death from gynecologic malignancy in the United States. The reduction in borderline and invasive ovarian cancer risk with COCP use is consistently about 40% among short-term users and as much as 80% among women who have taken COCPs for more than 10 years; risk reduction persists for more than 15 years after discontinuation of oral contraception.[14] A woman in her late 30s or 40s taking COCPs reduces her risk of ovarian cancer during the peak presentation of this disease (i.e., 50 to 60 years). Worldwide, an estimated 100,000 deaths from epithelial ovarian cancer have been prevented since COCPs first became available in the 1960s; current COCP use is estimated to prevent an additional 30,000 such deaths each year.[15] Epidemiologic data suggest that COCP use reduces the risk of ovarian cancer for those at increased risk for this disease.[16]

Endometrial adenocarcinoma is the most common gynecologic cancer in U.S. women. The risk of endometrial adenocarcinoma is reduced by 50% with COCP use, and the protection persists for at least 20 years after oral contraception discontinuation.[17] COCP use may also decrease the risk of colorectal cancer.[18]

All COCP formulations appear to treat acne. Selected COCP formulations are approved by the U.S. Food and Drug Administration (FDA) for the treatment of acne (i.e., ethinyl estradiol/triphasic norgestimate, estrophasic norethindrone acetate, and ethinyl estradiol/drospirenone)[19] and for premenstrual dysphoric disorder (24/4 20-μg ethinyl estradiol/3-mg drospirenone).[20]

Side Effects

Although COCPs are well tolerated by most users, some experience side effects that may affect quality of life, contraceptive continuation, and patient satisfaction. Counseling about side effects is an important aspect of contraceptive care and may improve patient tolerance when they occur.

Nausea and breast tenderness affect about 10% to 15% of COCP users, particularly during the initial months of use, and they tend to resolve with long-term use.[21] Contrary to popular perception, randomized, placebo-controlled trials have not shown that the pills cause weight gain.

Unscheduled vaginal bleeding is common, affecting about 25% of COCP users during the initial 3 months of use, but the incidence declines with ongoing COCP use. Unscheduled bleeding is more common with lower-dose (20 μg) than standard-dose (30 or 35 μg) ethinyl estradiol preparations.[21] Because irregular bleeding may be a manifestation of pathology such as cervical or endometrial infection, polyps, or neoplasia, persistent or new-onset bleeding should be investigated. There are no FDA-approved treatments for unscheduled bleeding associated with hormonal contraception. Amenorrhea may occur with long-term COCP use, and it is variably tolerated by patients. It may be more acceptable with counseling that provides appropriate reassurance. Urine pregnancy tests should be made readily available to women who experience absence of withdrawal bleeding or who for other reasons suspect they could be pregnant during use of any method of hormonal contraception.

Headaches affect up to 10% of COCP users and do not require neurologic evaluation unless migraines with focal neurologic symptoms are reported. A history of migraine plus aura is a contraindication for use of COCPs.[22] For women 35 years old or older, combination estrogen-progestin contraceptives should be avoided by all with migraines.[23] Similarly, any COCP users who experience increased frequency or intensity of any type of migraine headache should discontinue estrogen-containing contraceptives. If migraine headaches occur only during withdrawal bleeding, elimination of the hormone-free interval may be therapeutic.

Health Risks

Extensive studies in large populations have established the risks and benefits of COCPs for most women. Results indicate that for most women, use of COCPs represents a safe contraceptive choice. However, clinicians should be aware of circumstances in which the COCP may pose health risks. The World Health Organization (WHO) has developed guidelines to help clinicians determine the safety of COCP and other contraceptive methods.[24] The safety of COCP is considered in four categories:

1. Conditions with no restriction on the use of the contraceptive method
2. Conditions in which the advantages of the method usually outweigh the theoretical or proven risks
3. Conditions in which the theoretical or proven risks usually outweigh the advantages; examples include gallbladder disease, less than 21 days after delivery, lactation up to 6 months after delivery, and taking medications that may interfere with COCP efficacy
4. Conditions that present an unacceptable health risk if the contraceptive method is used; examples include a personal history of deep venous thrombosis or pulmonary embolism, cardiovascular accident, known thrombophilia tendency, and migraine headaches with aura or other neurologic signs.

Thromboembolic Disease. The established increased risk of venous thromboembolism (VTE) is related to the estrogenic component. Low-dose preparations carry a lower risk, but the incidence of VTE is still increased.[25] COCPs containing less than 50 mg of ethinyl estradiol are associated with a fourfold increased risk of VTE. No differences in VTE risk between 35- and 20-μg preparations have been established. Cigarette smoking further increases the risk of for arterial and venous thrombotic events.[26,27] In otherwise healthy women taking COCPs, the absolute risk of VTE remains small at 1 to 1.5 cases per 10,000 women-years compared with nonpregnant nonusers (0.4 per 10,000 women-years). The VTE risk for COCP use is significantly lower than that for pregnancy (6 per 10,000 women-years).[25] The pill is contraindicated for those at increased risk for VTE: these high-risk women include those with a personal history of VTE, women immediately after delivery, those with known inherited thrombophilic conditions, and obese women 35 years old or older. Routine screening of women for familial thrombophilic markers is not recommended before initiating COCP use.[28] However, women with known thrombophilic conditions should be encouraged to use progestin-only and intrauterine contraceptives.

Myocardial Infarction and Thrombotic and Hemorrhagic Stroke. The relationship between COCP use and cardiovascular disease is complex. Retrospective studies in humans and animal data suggest that COCP use does not increase the risk of atherosclerosis.[29] Myocardial infarction occurs rarely in COCP users, and these users are almost exclusively smokers; in these women, the infarctions usually are linked to thrombotic rather than atherosclerotic causes.[29] Because cigarette smoking and COCP may act synergistically to increase the risk of myocardial infarction, COCPs are contraindicated in smokers older than 35 years. Among other women with risk factors for myocardial infarction or stroke, including hypertension, diabetes, and migraine headache, COCPs should be avoided by those older than 35 years.

Breast Cancer. The association between use of menopausal estrogen-progestin therapy and breast cancer has led many to assume that COCP use is associated with an increased risk of breast cancer. However, findings from a large, long-term cohort study in Britain and large case-control studies in the United States found that regardless of duration of use, neither current nor prior use of COCP is associated with an increased risk of invasive or in situ breast cancer or death from breast cancer.[23] Although many women at elevated risk for breast cancer due to affected family members are concerned that use of COCP is unsafe, a large, Canadian, prospective study of women with a family history of breast cancer found that neither current nor prior use of COCP was associated with an elevated risk of breast cancer.[30] Studies of women with known *BRCA* gene mutations have yielded mixed results with respect to the impact of COCP use on breast cancer risk.[31]

Cervical Cancer. Pooled data from 24 studies including more than 16,000 women with cervical cancer and 35,000 without cervical cancer found that for current COCP users, the risk of invasive cervical cancer increased with increasing duration of use (relative risk for ≥5 years' use versus never use =1.90; 95% confidence interval [CI], 1.69 to 2.13). The risk declined after use ceased, and after 10 or more years, it returned to the risk level of never users. A similar pattern of risk was seen for invasive and in situ cancer and for women who tested positive for high-risk human papillomavirus (HPV) strains. Ten years' use of oral contraceptives from about age 20 to 30 years is estimated to increase the cumulative incidence of invasive cervical cancer by age 50 from 7.3 to 8.3 cases per 1000 women in less developed countries and from 3.8 to 4.5 cases per 1000 women in more developed countries.[32] Regular cytologic screening according to national protocols is advised for all sexually active women, regardless of contraceptive use. A history of cervical intraepithelial neoplasia or genital HPV infection is not a contraindication for COCP use.

Use of Combined Oral Contraceptive Pills after Abortion, after Delivery, or during Lactation

COCPs may be initiated immediately after induced or spontaneous termination of a first- or second-trimester pregnancy but not immediately after term delivery because the risk of VTE is elevated during the puerperium. Because COCPs may reduce milk production, some experts do not think they represent an optimal contraceptive choice in lactating women.[33] However, ovulation may occur as early as 3 weeks after delivery, and this consideration may be foremost for some COCP users. The use of COCP at 4 weeks after delivery is within the range approved by the FDA and other medical authorities. The use of progestin-only contraceptives in postpartum and lactating women is addressed later in this chapter.

Use of Concomitant Medications with Combined Oral Contraceptive Pills

Anticonvulsants and antibiotics that induce hepatic enzymes may reduce the contraceptive efficacy of COCPs. In these cases, high-dose progestin-only methods such as depot medroxyprogesterone acetate (DMPA) or intrauterine contraceptives may be preferable.[34]

Contraceptive Vaginal Ring and Contraceptive Patch

The transdermal and transvaginal routes are safe and acceptable alternatives to COCPs to deliver combined estrogen-progestin contraception. The contraceptive patch (Ortho Evra) and the contraceptive vaginal ring (NuvaRing) offer women combination estrogen-progestin contraception without taking pills daily. The ring is inserted in the vagina for 3 weeks and then withdrawn for 1 week, during which withdrawal bleeding is anticipated.

In consistent users, the contraceptive failure rates with the patch and ring are similar to or somewhat lower than with oral contraceptives. In the absence of adequate evidence to determine how the risks and noncontraceptive benefits of the patch and the ring compare with the COCP, they are usually considered to be equivalent. The incidence of unscheduled (breakthrough) bleeding and spotting may be somewhat lower with the ring than with COCPs.[35]

Transdermal Contraceptive Patch

The only contraceptive patch available in the United States is Ortho Evra. It is a 4.5-cm, tan square that releases 20 μg of ethinyl estradiol daily along with norelgestromin, the biologically active metabolite of the progestin norgestimate (Fig. 18-1). A new patch is applied each week on the same day for 3 weeks, followed by a patch-free week, during which withdrawal bleeding is anticipated. Sweating associated with vigorous exercise, swimming, and use of a hot

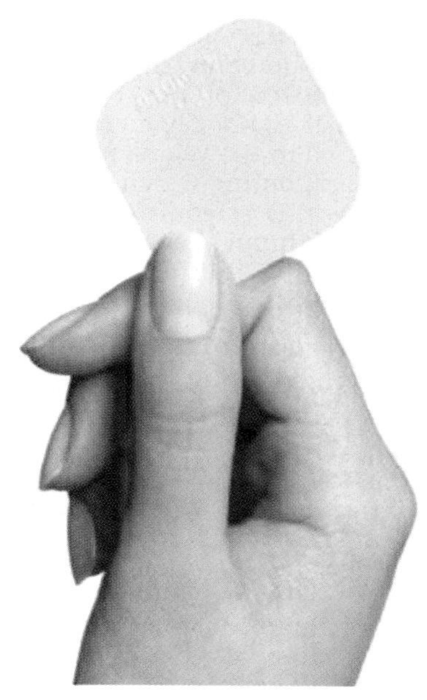

Figure 18-1 The contraceptive patch, Ortho Evra.

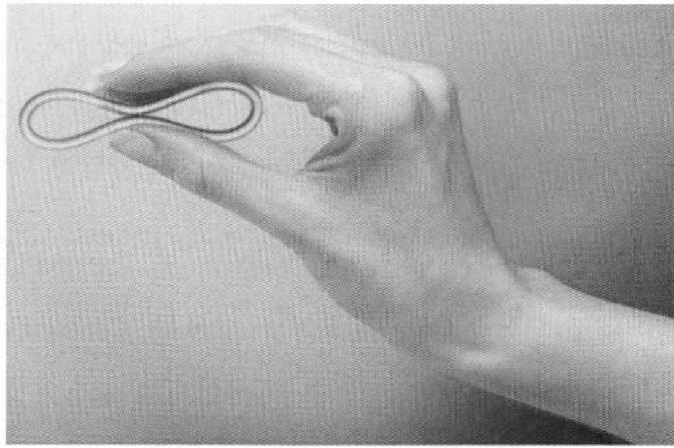

Figure 18-2 The contraceptive vaginal ring.

tub or sauna do not result in patch detachment or clinically relevant changes in serum hormonal contraceptive levels.[36]

Unscheduled bleeding in patch users is similar to that seen with COCPs.[37] Compared with COCP users, patch users may be more likely to report breast discomfort, dysmenorrhea, nausea, and vomiting. Mild local skin reactions are common.[37] The patch is easy to use for many women, but for those at high risk for unintended pregnancy, the patch may be associated with a higher failure rate than COCPs.[38]

Contraceptive Vaginal Ring

The vaginal mucosa offers excellent absorption of sex steroids. The only contraceptive vaginal ring available in the United States is the NuvaRing, a flexible plastic ring that is 4 mm thick and has an outside diameter of 54 mm. The ring releases 15 μg daily of ethinyl estradiol along with etonogestrel, the biologically active metabolite of the progestin desogestrel (Fig. 18-2). The ring does not require individual fitting; as long as it remains in the vagina, appropriate absorption of steroids occurs. Expulsion is uncommon. Women's interest in using a contraceptive vaginal ring varies; some women are highly motivated and comfortable with this method. Some users keep the ring in place during sexual relations; in this setting, male discomfort is not common. Other users prefer to remove the ring before intercourse, and removal for 3 hours or less does not impair efficacy.[39] Back-up contraception is required for 7 days if the ring is removed for longer than 3 hours.

Like the traditional COCP regimen, the contraceptive vaginal ring is inserted in the vagina for 3 weeks and then withdrawn for 1 week, during which withdrawal bleeding is anticipated. A new ring is required every 4 weeks. Rates of unscheduled (breakthrough) bleeding and spotting are lower with the ring than with COCPs.[35]

Contraceptive Mechanism of Action, Initiation, and Efficacy of the Patch and Ring

The contraceptive patch and vaginal ring act by suppression of ovulation.[40] The patch and ring are immediately effective if commenced on day 1 of menstruation, but starting at any other time requires 7 days of backup contraception, such as condoms.

The contraceptive efficacy of the patch and the vaginal ring is high when used correctly.[40,41] Typical annual user failure rates are thought to be similar to those for the COCP at about 8%.[7] Contraceptive efficacy may be reduced in patch users weighing more than 90 kg.[42] Contraindications to the patch and the vaginal ring are the same as for COCPs.

Estrogen Levels with the Patch, Oral Contraceptives, and the Ring: Risk of Venous Thromboembolism

The contraceptive patch generates higher circulating levels of ethinyl estradiol than the COCP and vaginal ring generate.[43] It is uncertain whether use of the patch is associated with a higher risk of VTE than use of the COCP.[44]

PROGESTIN-ONLY CONTRACEPTIVE METHODS

Progestin-only contraception is an option for women for whom an estrogen-containing contraceptive is contraindicated or causes additional health concerns. Progestin-only contraceptives offer many advantages over estrogen-containing methods. They can be used immediately after delivery and in women considered at risk for VTE. They are formulated in long-acting preparations that provide a high level of contraceptive efficacy and acceptability. The main disadvantage of the progestin-only contraceptives is changes in vaginal bleeding patterns. This is common in progestin-only oral contraceptives users and represents the most frequent cause for contraceptive discontinuation. Types of progestin-only contraceptives include the following:

- Oral progestin-only contraception (minipills)
- Progestin implants (Implanon)
- Intrauterine contraception (Mirena)
- Injectable contraception (DMPA Depo-provera)

Oral Progestin-Only Contraception

Only one progestin-only oral contraceptive formulation is marketed in the United States: norethindrone in 0.35-mg tablets (e.g., Micronor, Nor-QD, generics). The progestin dose is substantially lower than the dose in any combination oral contraceptive. It is dispensed in packs of 28 active pills, which are taken continuously (i.e., no pill-free or nonhormonal pill week) (see Table 18-2).

Mechanism of Action

The mechanism of action of progestin-only oral contraceptives varies among patients and may include suppression of ovulation, thickening cervical mucus, and inducing

TABLE 18-2

Summary and Recommendations for Progestin-Only Oral Contraceptive Use

1. Progestin-only contraception is an option for women in whom an estrogen-containing contraceptive is either contraindicated or causes additional health concerns.
2. Ovulation is not consistently suppressed; the main contraceptive actions of progestin-only oral contraception are effects on cervical mucus and the endometrium.
3. The typical user failure rate with progestin-only oral contraception is estimated to be >8%. Women choosing progestin-only oral contraception are often subfertile as a result of breast-feeding or older reproductive age, so the failure rate in these populations may be lower than in more fertile populations.
4. It is essential that the pill be taken at the same time each day to maximize contraceptive efficacy.
5. Menstrual irregularities are common in users of progestin-only oral contraception and represent the most frequent cause for contraceptive discontinuation.

endometrial atrophy. Unlike the mechanism of COCPs, ovulation is not consistently suppressed with progestin-only contraceptives, and the progestin effects on cervical mucus and the endometrium are critical factors in preventing conception. Within hours of administration, progestin-only oral contraceptives reduce the volume of cervical mucus and increase its viscosity, which prevents sperm from passing through the cervical canal and endometrial cavity. However, these changes persist for only 20 hours.[45]

Efficacy

The efficacy of progestin-only oral contraceptives is not well established. National survey data used to estimate contraceptive failure rates with typical use have failed to distinguish between COCPs (the larger group) and progestin-only oral contraceptives. It is thought that the typical first-year failure rates with progestin-only oral contraceptives are higher than those seen with COCPs (8%).[46] Another confounding factor is that the women using progestin-only oral contraceptives may have reduced fertility as a result of breast-feeding or older reproductive age. The failure rate of progestin-only oral contraceptives in these populations is lower than it would be in more fertile populations. For women of normal fertility (e.g., women who are not breast-feeding), some experts recommend off-label use of 2 progestin-only tablets daily, with the assumption that this strategy enhances contraceptive efficacy. However, published reports have not assessed this approach, and there are no data regarding contraceptive efficacy of progestin-only oral contraceptives in obese, fertile women (discussed later).

Starting the Progestin-Only Pill

Progestin-only oral contraceptives can be initiated on the first day of menses, but a backup contraceptive should be used during the first week. Some clinicians initiate progestin-only oral contraceptives at any time in the cycle, as long as the clinician is reasonably certain that the patient is not pregnant. With this strategy, backup contraception should be used for the first 7 days of use. Because of the short duration of action and the short half-life of progestin-only oral contraceptives, the pill must be taken at the same time each day to maximize contraceptive efficacy. A backup contraceptive (e.g., condoms) should be used for at least 2 days if the progestin-only oral contraceptive is taken more than 3 hours late or forgotten on any day. The patient should also resume taking daily progestin-only oral contraceptives as soon as possible.

Side Effects of the Progestin-Only Oral Contraceptives

Follicular Cysts. Sonographic studies have shown that follicular cysts are more common among progestin-only oral contraceptive users than among other women, but they may come and go over time.[47] No intervention is required in asymptomatic women, other than reassurance and sonographic follow-up. If a follow-up sonogram in 6 to 8 weeks demonstrates resolution or decrease in size of follicular cysts, no further evaluation is required. Progestin-only oral contraceptive users who have persistent concerns about ovarian follicular changes should be offered another method of contraception.

Side effects with the progestin-only pill other than changes in bleeding patterns are relatively uncommon. Androgenic progestins may exacerbate acne. Weight gain has not been objectively documented, and headaches are uncommon.

TABLE 18-3

Conditions in Which Progestin-Only Contraception May Be Preferable to Estrogen-Containing Methods*

Migraine headaches, especially those with aura
Cigarette smoking or obesity in women >35 years
History of thromboembolic disease
Hypertension with vascular disease or age >35 years
Systemic lupus erythematosus with vascular disease, nephritis, or antiphospholipid antibodies
Less than 3 weeks postpartum
Hypertriglyceridemia
Coronary artery disease
Congestive heart failure
Cerebrovascular disease

*In women with the conditions listed, use of progestin-only contraceptives may be safer than combination oral, transdermal, or vaginal ring contraceptives.

From ACOG Committee on Practice Bulletins–Gynecology. ACOG practice bulletin no. 73: Use of hormonal contraception in women with coexisting medical conditions. *Obstet Gynecol.* 2006;107:1453-1472.

Contraindications to Progestin-Only Contraceptives. Progestin-only contraceptives may be appropriate for many women with contraindications to contraceptive doses of estrogen, including women age 35 or older who are obese, who smoke, who have hypertension, or who have diabetes. Progestin-only contraceptives are also appropriate for women with a prior medical history of VTE (Table 18-3). Unfortunately, package labeling for some progestin-only contraceptives does not reflect this distinction. For example, package labeling for DMPA inappropriately lists a history of VTE as a contraindication.[28]

Use of Progestin-Only Contraceptives When Estrogen Is Contraindicated. Use of progestin-only oral contraceptives, injectables, and implants may be appropriate when contraceptive doses of estrogen are contraindicated. COCP use (like pregnancy) confers an increased risk of morbidity and mortality in women older than 35 years who smoke, are obese, or have hypertension; women with coronary artery disease; women at increased risk for thromboembolism; and women with active systemic lupus erythematosus. Progestin-only methods should be considered safe and effective contraceptive choices for these women (see Table 18-3).

Effect of Carbohydrate Metabolism. Most studies have reported that progestin-only oral contraceptives have little impact on carbohydrate metabolism.[48] However, one study conducted in Latina women observed that lactating women with a history of gestational diabetes who used progestin-only oral contraceptives after delivery had an almost tripled risk of diabetes compared with those who used low-dose COCPs.[49] Clinicians should monitor glucose tolerance in high-risk lactating women using progestin-only oral contraceptives.

Ectopic Pregnancy Risk. Progestin-only oral contraceptives lower the overall risk of ectopic pregnancy and intrauterine pregnancy. A history of ectopic pregnancy does not contraindicate progestin-only oral contraceptive use. However, if pregnancy occurs, the likelihood that the pregnancy is ectopic is higher in progestin-only oral contraceptive users than in nonusers of contraceptives (5% versus 2%).[50]

Effect on Bone Mineral Density. The only study assessing skeletal health in progestin-only oral contraceptive users was conducted in breast-feeding women. Progestin-only oral contraceptives protected against small, reversible losses in BMD occurring during lactation.[51]

Effect on Cancer Risk. Progestins usually suppress endometrial growth.[47] However, few epidemiologic data address the effect of progestin-only oral contraceptives on endometrial cancer risk or on any cancer risk.

Effect on Sexually Transmitted Infections. Use of progestin-only oral contraceptives has not been shown to protect users from acquiring STIs.

Use After Abortion or Delivery. Progestin-only oral contraceptives may be initiated immediately after abortion or delivery. They should be initiated within 2 weeks to ensure effectiveness.

Progestin-Only Oral Contraceptives during Lactation. The progestin-only oral contraceptive does not interfere with the quality or quantity of breast milk.[52] Very little progestin is passed from nursing mothers into their breast milk, and no adverse impact on infant growth has been observed. Package labeling advises delaying administration in lactating women until 6 weeks after delivery. Based on the absence of data suggesting harm to the infant or mother and the contraceptive benefits of early initiation, some experts recommend initiation of progestin-only pills or DMPA before hospital discharge and no later than the third postpartum week, regardless of lactation status.[53]

Abnormal Bleeding. Unscheduled bleeding, spotting, and amenorrhea are common menstrual patterns during progestin-only oral contraceptive use, and users should be counseled accordingly. Interpreting signs and symptoms of pregnancy, whether intrauterine or extrauterine, can be challenging. Pregnancy testing is appropriate for progestin-only oral contraceptive users experiencing nausea, breast tenderness, a change in menstrual pattern, or lower abdominal pain (see Table 18-2).

TABLE 18-4

Timing of Depot Medroxyprogesterone Acetate (DMPA) Injections

Method	Depot Medroxyprogesterone Acetate
First Injection	
Spontaneous menstrual cycle	Within 5 days of menses onset
Spontaneous or elective first-trimester abortion	Within 7 days
Term delivery	Within 3 wk after delivery if not lactating; within 6 wk if lactating
Switching from combined oral contraceptive pills	While on active pills or within 7 days after taking the pill pack's last active tablet
Switching from combination contraceptive patch (Ortho Evra)	While on weekly patch or within 7 days after patch removal
Switching from combination contraceptive vaginal ring (NuvaRing)	While ring is in place or within 7 days after ring removal
Switching from levonorgestrel IUD (Mirena)	First injection should occur before IUD removal and within 5 yr after IUD insertion; if patient is menstruating, a condom should be used as backup if the first injection is not given within 5 days of menses onset
Switching from Copper T 380A IUD	First injection should occur before IUD removal and within 10 yr after IUD insertion; backup contraception such as condoms should be used if the first injection is not given within 5 days of menses onset
Subsequent Injections	
Injection interval	Every 12 wk (3 mo); earlier reinjections are acceptable
Grace period	Two weeks; after 1 wk manufacturer recommends pregnancy testing before repeat injection

IUD, intrauterine device.
From Kaunitz AM. Current concepts regarding use of DMPA. *J Reprod Med.* 2002;47:785-789.

Depot Medroxyprogesterone Acetate for Contraception

DMPA is an injectable, progestin-only contraceptive that provides highly effective, private, and reversible contraception. It avoids the need for user action daily or near the time of sexual intercourse and the need for partner cooperation (Table 18-4).

Formulations and Pharmacology

DMPA is available in two formulations: 150 mg/1 mL for intramuscular injection and 104 mg/0.65 mL for subcutaneous injection. The newer subcutaneous injection may be less painful and is available in a prefilled syringe, offering the potential for self-administration. The injections can be given every 3 months because low solubility of the microcrystals at the injection site allows pharmacologically active drug levels to persist for several months. Intramuscular DMPA is available as a generic formulation, which is less costly than subcutaneous DMPA. Otherwise, the benefits and risks are similar for intramuscular and subcutaneous administration.[54]

DMPA primarily acts by inhibiting follicular maturation and ovulation through inhibition of gonadotropin secretion. Unlike other progestin-only contraceptives, mean estradiol levels may be lower than normal for cycling premenopausal women. Although the endometrium becomes atrophic, vasomotor symptoms are uncommon. Because of its progestin effect, it also causes changes in cervical mucus and tubal motility that are hostile to sperm migration.[55]

For the 150-mg intramuscular injection, failure rates in clinical trials have ranged from 0.0 to 0.7 per 100 woman-years. The typical-user failure rate is 7 failures per 100 woman-years, reflecting the fact that some users do not return for their injections as scheduled.[46] Because progestin levels are high, efficacy has not been reduced by high body weight or use of concurrent medications. For the 104-mg subcutaneous injection, no contraceptive failures were reported in phase III clinical trials.[56] As this formulation is relatively new, and typical-user failure rates are not available, but they are expected to be similar to those for the intramuscular preparation.

Administration of Depot Medroxyprogesterone Acetate

Starting Injections. The ideal time to initiate DMPA is within 5 days of the onset of menses. This approach ensures that the patient is not pregnant at the time of injection and prevents ovulation during the first month of use, so that backup contraception is unnecessary. Most women have pharmacologically active drug levels and a poor cervical mucus score within 24 hours after injection.[55] The "same-day," "quick-start," or "Depo-now" approach when a pregnancy test result is negative facilitates DMPA initiation for many users, and it may prevent some pregnancies.[57] However, there is a small possibility of undiagnosed pregnancy despite a negative pregnancy test result. Back-up contraception should be used for 3 days because ovulation may occur within 24 hours of the initial injection. DMPA given during pregnancy does not appear to be teratogenic.[58]

Repeat Injections. Repeat injections of DMPA should be given every 3 months. After a 150-mg injection, ovulation does not occur for at least 14 weeks. A 2-week grace period is appropriate for women receiving injections every 3 months. In women more than 1 to 2 weeks late for an injection, a urine pregnancy test should be performed before administering further DMPA. Timing of DMPA injections is summarized in Table 18-4.[55]

Side Effects of Depot Medroxyprogesterone Acetate

Candid counseling regarding the side effects of DMPA and the need for timed injections should be provided. Women who are well informed when they choose this method of contraception are more likely to become satisfied users with high continuation rates.[55] Common side effects of DMPA (>5% of long-term users) include menstrual irregularities (i.e., bleeding or amenorrhea), weight changes, headache, abdominal pain or discomfort, nervousness, dizziness, and asthenia.[55]

Menstrual Changes. Menstrual changes occur in almost all women using DMPA and are the most frequent cause for discontinuation of these and all other progestin-only contraceptives.[59] Proactive patient education before initiation of DMPA and supportive follow-up can improve tolerance of menstrual changes. During the first months of use, episodes of unpredictable bleeding and spotting lasting 7 days or longer are common. Bleeding decreases with use, and at 1 year, 50% of women experience amenorrhea; this rate increases to 75% with long-term use.[60] Similar bleeding patterns are reported with the subcutaneous preparation.[61] Some women may view amenorrhea (along with a reduction or elimination of menstrual cramps) as one of the advantages of using this method.

There are no established methods for predicting, preventing, or treating unscheduled bleeding in DMPA users. In new DMPA users, 50 mg of mifepristone (not marketed in the United States for this indication) taken every 2 weeks decreases the incidence of unscheduled bleeding.[62] Some studies have shown that estrogen supplements (e.g., 1.25 mg of oral conjugated estrogen, 1 to 2 mg of oral micronized estradiol or 0.1-mg estradiol patches) may terminate a bleeding episode.[59] However, a systematic review concluded that there is a lack of high-quality data to support routine clinical use of any interventions to treat persistent unscheduled bleeding with progestin-only contraceptives.[63]

Weight Changes. The impact of DMPA on weight has been controversial. Level 1 data has failed to show that DMPA causes weight gain.[55,64] Weight gain with the use of DMPA may be associated with user subgroups at particular risk for obesity, including adolescents and ethnic minorities.[65]

Other Side Effects. Observational studies have not reported any consistent effects of DMPA on mood. Some evidence indicates that progestins may cause or exacerbate depressive symptoms in certain subpopulations of women, including those with a history of premenstrual syndrome or mood disorders.[55]

Risks and Benefits of Depot Medroxyprogesterone Acetate

DMPA has been used to manage a variety of gynecologic and nongynecologic disorders. The tendency of DMPA to cause amenorrhea makes it a particularly appropriate contraceptive choice for women with menorrhagia, dysmenorrhea, or iron-deficiency anemia. DMPA is a useful means of suppressing menstrual bleeding and managing menstrual hygiene in individuals with special needs (e.g., cognitive impairment, military personnel). Use of DMPA has been associated with hematologic improvement (i.e., fewer painful crises) in women with sickle cell disease.[66]

DMPA users have a decreased risk of PID, although rates of *Chlamydia* infection are increased.[67] The increased risk of *Chlamydia* infection may indicate that women who choose DMPA contraception engage in higher-risk sexual behavior than women choosing other methods. The decreased risk of PID may reflect progestational changes in the cervical mucus and endometrium, along with reduced menstrual flow. Progestins inhibit endometriotic tissue growth by directly causing initial decidualization and eventual atrophy and by inhibiting pituitary gonadotropin secretion and ovarian estrogen production. Randomized trials have shown that DMPA is more effective than oral contraceptives and danazol and as effective as leuprolide injections for treatment of pain associated with endometriosis.[68] In the United States, subcutaneous DMPA is approved for the treatment of pain associated with endometriosis.

The efficacy of DMPA does not appear to be attenuated by the use of enzyme-inducing anticonvulsants,[34] and DMPA may have intrinsic anticonvulsant properties. For these reasons, DMPA may be a good contraceptive for many women with seizure disorders.

Effect on Cancer Risk. Large case-control studies conducted by the WHO have shown that use of DMPA is associated with an 80% reduced risk of endometrial cancer and does not affect the incidence of ovarian, cervical, or liver cancer. Multicountry data from the WHO and data from the United States, South Africa, and New Zealand provide reassurance that use of DMPA is not associated with an increased risk of breast cancer.[69,70]

Effect on Cardiovascular Risk. DMPA has an adverse effect on circulating lipids but does not increase production of coagulation factors and has no adverse effect on blood pressure. No adverse clinical effects on cardiovascular disease have been observed.[55] Based on these findings, the American College of Obstetricians and Gynecologists (ACOG) stated that DMPA and other progestin-only contraceptives might be appropriate contraceptive options for women with a history of VTE and those in whom use of combination estrogen-progestin contraceptive is contraindicated.[28] This recommendation is different from package labeling for DMPA (written in the 1960s), which indicates that a prior history of VTE is a contraindication to DMPA use. In women with multiple risk factors for cardiovascular disease (e.g., smoking, older age, hypertension, diabetes), the WHO classifies DMPA as category 3, indicating that the risks of use may exceed the benefits. The basis for this caution is uncertain.

Effect on Skeletal Health. DMPA's impact on BMD has generated much controversy. In suppressing gonadotropin production and ovulation,[71] DMPA also suppresses ovarian production of estradiol.[72] The resulting hypoestrogenemia causes a decline in BMD.[73] Compared with nonusers, BMD at the hip and spine of DMPA users decreases by 0.5% to 3.5% after 1 year and by 5.7% to 7.5% after 2 years of use.[74] The rate of loss is greatest during the first 1 to 2 years of use.[75,76] The intramuscular and subcutaneous formulations of DMPA have similar effects on BMD.[54] Although it is well established that DMPA leads to BMD declines in current users, the long-term impact of injectable contraception on skeletal health, if any, is uncertain. Particular concern surrounds the long-term skeletal health impact in two groups of women[77]: young women, who have not yet reached their peak bone mass, and older reproductive-age women, who are experiencing accelerated declines in BMD as they approach menopause.

Published data do not suggest that DMPA use reduces peak bone mass or increases the risk of postmenopausal osteoporotic fractures.[78] One prospective and one retrospective study in high-risk groups, however, suggested an increased risk of fracture in DMPA users.[79,80] A Danish case-control study also suggested that DMPA is associated with an increased fracture risk.[81] However, use of DMPA is rare in Danish women, and this study did not assess baseline risk factors such as smoking or body mass index (BMI). It is difficult to draw clinical inferences from this study's findings. To our knowledge, no prospective study has assessed the impact of DMPA contraceptive use on subsequent fracture risk in postmenopausal women.

Notwithstanding the lack of a known increase in fracture risk, the FDA added a black box warning to DMPA package labeling in 2004: "Women who use DMPA may lose significant bone mineral density. Bone loss is greater with increasing duration of use and may not be completely reversible. It is unknown if use of DMPA during adolescence or early adulthood, a critical period of bone accretion, will reduce peak bone mass and increase the risk for osteoporotic fracture in later life. DMPA should be used as a long-term birth control method (e.g., longer than 2 years) only if other birth control methods are inadequate." The addition of this warning to DMPA's package labeling appears to have led some physicians to limit the duration of DMPA use and to order BMD assessment in women using DMPA.[82]

The clinical impact of decreased BMD in current DMPA users is uncertain. Studies involving premenopausal women and adolescents treated with DMPA for up to 5 years indicate that the decline in BMD associated with injectable contraception is largely reversed after discontinuation.[64,83-87] Overall, DMPA-associated declines in bone density at the spine appear to reverse more rapidly than BMD declines occurring at the hip. Recovery of BMD deficits associated with DMPA use appears to occur more rapidly after use by adolescents than after use in adult women.[85]

To summarize, current use of DMPA is associated with BMD declines, but a significant increase in risk of fractures in DMPA users has not been demonstrated.[88] Professional organizations, including the ACOG,[28,74] the Society for Adolescent Medicine,[74,89] the WHO,[90] and the Society of Obstetricians and Gynaecologists of Canada,[91] state that the advantages of DMPA use as a contraceptive outweigh the theoretical concerns regarding skeletal harm. Skeletal health concerns should not restrict initiation or continuation of DMPA in reproductive age women, including teens and women older than 35 years. Published evidence does not support limiting the duration of DMPA therapy. The effect of DMPA on BMD is similar to that with pregnancy (decrease in BMD of 2% to 8%) or lactation (decrease in BMD of 3% to 5%).[74] Use of DMPA is not an indication for BMD testing before, during, or as follow-up of administration.[28,78] Likewise, antiresorptive agents, including bisphosphonates, are not appropriate to prevent bone loss in women using injectable contraception.[78]

As with all reproductive-age patients, clinicians should encourage DMPA users to consume adequate amounts of calcium and vitamin D. Clinical judgment is called for when helping women with risk factors for osteoporosis make sound choices regarding DMPA and alternative contraceptives.

Effect on Sexually Transmitted Infections. Use of DMPA does not protect users from acquiring STIs. Whether it increases the risk of acquiring these infections is less clear. Results of primate studies suggest that DMPA may lead to thinning of vaginal mucosa, facilitating penetration of the HIV virus. However, human studies have failed to show any impact of DMPA or other hormonal contraceptives on HIV transmission.[92] In HIV-infected women, DMPA does not appear to increase the rates of STI acquisition.[93]

DMPA use may be associated with an increased incidence of endocervical chlamydial and gonococcal infection.[94] However, women who chose to use DMPA may be more likely to have STIs at baseline, which may bias study results.

Effect on Return of Fertility. Although DMPA does not permanently impact endocrine function, return of fertility may be delayed. Within 10 months of the last injection, 50% of women who discontinue DMPA to become pregnant will conceive. However, in some women, fertility is not reestablished until up to 18 months after the last injection.[55] The persistence of ovulation suppression after DMPA discontinuation is not related to the duration of use, but it is related to weight. Before initiating DMPA contraception, clinicians should counsel candidates about the possible prolonged duration of action. Women who may want to become pregnant within the next 1 or 2 years should choose an alternative contraceptive.

DMPA may be initiated immediately after abortion or delivery. It should be initiated by 2 weeks after delivery to ensure effectiveness.[55]

Progestin-only contraceptives appear to be safe to use during lactation. However, high-quality studies are lacking.[33]

Use When Estrogen Is Contraindicated. DMPA appears to be safe for many women with contraindications to estrogen-containing contraceptives (e.g., migraine with aura; women older than 35 years who smoke, are obese, or have hypertension; cardiovascular disease; or lupus) (Table 18-5).

Potential Drug Interactions. The contraceptive efficacy of DMPA in women taking hepatic enzyme inducers has not been explicitly studied; however, physicians with substantial experience prescribing DMPA (150 mg every 3 months) for women taking anticonvulsants have not reported contraceptive failure among such patients.[34]

TABLE 18-5

Summary and Recommendations for Depot Medroxyprogesterone Acetate (DMPA) Use

1. DMPA is an excellent method of contraception for women who desire a long-term, reversible contraceptive method.
2. DMPA primarily acts by inhibiting follicular maturation and ovulation through inhibition of gonadotropin secretion; it also affects cervical mucus.
3. DMPA is available in two formulations: 150 mg/1 mL for IM injection and 104 mg/0.65 mL for SC injection.
4. The ideal time to initiate DMPA is within 5 days of the onset of menses, so as to ensure absence of pregnancy. The dose is repeated every 3 months, with a 2-week grace period.
5. Although DMPA does not permanently affect endocrine function, return of fertility may be delayed.
6. Thorough, candid counseling about side effects is important. Women who are well-informed when they choose this method of contraception are much more likely to become highly satisfied users with high continuation rates.
7. Menstrual changes occur in all women using DMPA and are the most frequent cause for discontinuation.
8. Because DMPA induces amenorrhea, it can be used for managing a variety of gynecologic and nongynecologic disorders, such as menorrhagia, dysmenorrhea, and iron deficiency anemia.
9. There is no high-quality evidence that use of DMPA increases the risk of developing cancer, cardiovascular disease, or sexually transmitted infection. DMPA use significantly reduces the risk of developing endometrial cancer.
10. There is an association between current DMPA use and decreased bone mineral density; losses in bone mineral density are temporary, reverse after discontinuation of DMPA, and have not been linked to postmenopausal osteoporosis or fractures.

Cost Issues. In addition to enhancing quality of life by allowing couples to choose whether and when they wish to bear children, effective contraception saves health care costs. Male and female sterilization and long-acting reversible methods (e.g., intrauterine devices, subdermal implant) constitute the most cost-effective contraceptive options, followed by other hormonal methods (e.g., oral contraceptives). DMPA is more cost-effective than oral contraception. Barrier and behavioral methods (i.e., male condom and withdrawal, respectively) are least cost-effective compared with other contraceptive options. Nevertheless, when compared with no method, they still prevent a large number of unintended pregnancies, leading to important cost savings.[95]

Intrauterine Progestins for Contraception

The levonorgestrel-containing intrauterine system (LNG-IUS) is an effective, safe, and convenient form of long-term, reversible contraception. Intrauterine contraception use in the United States fell dramatically after early studies reported an association between intrauterine contraception use and later tubal infertility. Modern intrauterine contraception is highly effective and safe to use in selected populations. The addition of progestin to the intrauterine device (IUD) increases contraceptive efficacy and offers the added benefit of markedly reducing uterine blood loss. The LNG-IUS provides other therapeutic benefits, including treatment of heavy menstrual bleeding (i.e., menorrhagia) and endometriosis and suppression of endometrial growth.

IUDs are highly effective, require little patient effort, and are cost-effective. Hormone-containing devices have many potential noncontraceptive benefits and can address the medical and contraceptive needs of an individual patient.

Contraceptive Uses

Mirena (Bayer, Wayne, NJ) is the only progestin-containing IUD approved in the United States. It is a T-shaped device with a reservoir containing 52 mg of levonorgestrel. It delivers 20 mg of levonorgestrel per day and maintains its contraceptive efficacy for at least 5 years. The maximum plasma levels are reached within a few hours, and they plateau between 100 and 200 pg/mL, levels that are lower than those with implants or oral contraceptives. Data from large international studies confirm extremely low pregnancy rates, ranging between 0.1 per 100 and 0.3 per 100 women-years.[96] Despite endometrial suppression, fertility resumes rapidly after contraceptive removal.[97]

The mechanism of action of the contraceptive effects of LNG-IUS is not well defined. Most LNG-IUS users continue to ovulate, even when there is amenorrhea.[98] The principal mechanism of contraceptive action cervical mucus changes and appears to be profound endometrial suppression. The latter may contribute to the reduction in uterine bleeding seen with this device.[98]

Abnormal Bleeding, Expulsion, and Uterine Perforation

As with DMPA and other progestin-only contraceptives, unpredictable uterine bleeding is the most common reason for discontinuation of the LNG-IUS.[59] Unscheduled bleeding is most common during the early months of LNG-IUS use and tends to resolve with time. By 12 months, up to 50% of women have amenorrhea or infrequent bleeding.[99] Addressing patient preferences and assessing acceptance of menstrual disturbances are integral to efforts aimed at reducing early discontinuation rates. Adequate and specific counseling about likely changes in bleeding patterns before placement is essential to increase patient acceptability.

Expulsion, the most common cause of IUD failure, occurs in about 5% of users. Those at increased risk for expulsion include nulliparous women, women with severe dysmenorrhea, those with uterine cavity abnormalities, and women with insertions immediately after delivery or abortion.[100] The WHO recommends immediate insertion after first (category 1) and second (category 2) trimester abortions. Postpartum insertion is recommended after a 4-week interval, with more immediate insertion recommended only if the clinician decides that the risks outweigh the benefits. Because expulsion usually occurs within the first few months, women are encouraged to follow up with their care provider within 12 weeks of insertion.

Uterine perforation is an uncommon but potentially serious complication of LNG-IUS placement. Perforation rates are up to 2.6 cases per 1000 women and may be increased for lactating women.[101]

Upper Genital Tract Infection

Widespread concerns regarding a strong causative association between intrauterine contraception and pelvic infection appear to have been largely unsubstantiated. After early reports, subsequent studies have not confirmed this association.

A clinical history (including sexual history) should be taken as part of the routine assessment for intrauterine contraception to identify women at high risk for STIs; testing before insertion should be performed selectively, not routinely. Prophylactic antibiotics are not recommended. PID among users of intrauterine contraception is most strongly related to the insertion process and to the background risk of STIs. Conditions that represent an unacceptable health risk if an IUD is inserted are current PID, current purulent cervicitis, and chlamydial or gonorrheal infection.[102] If a woman develops PID with an LNG-IUS in place, Centers for Disease Control and Prevention (CDC) guidelines for treatment (available at http://www.cdc.gov/std/treatment/2006/updated-regimens.htm [accessed August 2010]) should be followed, and if the patient responds to therapy, the IUD can remain in place.

Infertility

The issues regarding intrauterine contraception and subsequent infertility have been the source of controversy for years. Current best evidence does not support a causative relationship. In light of the available data, the ACOG and the WHO include nulliparous women as IUC candidates (category 2).[103]

Metabolic and Systemic Effects

Low but detectable circulating levels of androgenic progestins in LNG-IUS users has raised concerns that glucose control, lipid profile, and blood pressure may be negatively affected. However, these concerns have not been substantiated in high-quality clinical trials.[98] The data suggest that the LNG-IUS is safe to use in patients with diabetes, hypertension, or hyperlipidemia.[104] Progestins are not thought to increase the risk of thromboembolic disease, but no studies have specifically examined the comparative risk of thromboembolism among LNG-IUS users.

Noncontraceptive Uses of the Levonorgestrel-Containing Intrauterine System

Heavy Menstrual Bleeding. The LNG-IUS is a well-established and highly effective treatment intervention for heavy menstrual bleeding. In comparative studies, it offers efficacy equal to or greater than other uterine-conserving treatments (e.g., balloon ablation, transcervical endometrial resection, medical management), is an acceptable alternative to hysterectomy for many women,[105] and offers comparable improvement in health-related quality of life for menstrual disorders. However, more patients in the LNG-IUS group reported systemic side effects, irregular bleeding, and breast tenderness than those in the oral progestin or endometrial ablation group.

Although up to 43% of women using the LNG-IUS to treat abnormal uterine bleeding will eventually undergo hysterectomy, the system still offers lower direct and indirect health costs at 5 years ($2817 per participant) than the hysterectomy group ($4660 per participant).[105]

Symptomatic Fibroids and Uterine Adenomyosis. Preliminary data suggest that the LNG-IUS is also an effective treatment for heavy menstrual bleeding associated with uterine fibroids. Submucous fibroids may be more likely to cause heavy bleeding and are more likely to lead to LNG-IUS expulsion because they distort the uterine cavity.[106] Additional trials are needed to define the role of the LNG-IUS in the treatment of symptomatic fibroids.

Uterine adenomyosis also is a common, benign cause of heavy menstrual bleeding; dysmenorrhea is commonly associated with this condition. Published reports suggest that the LNG-IUS reduces bleeding and pain in women with this condition.[107]

Endometriosis. Results of small, prospective studies using the LNG-IUS as a treatment for pelvic pain and dysmenorrhea associated with endometriosis are encouraging. The system may offer effective symptom relief, at least in the short term. However, these studies are limited by small sample sizes and vary significantly with regard to enrollment criteria and by stage and location of disease. A short-term, randomized trial found that the LNG-IUS was as effective as a gonadotropin-releasing hormone agonist in reducing pain in women with endometriosis. One advantage of the LNG-IUS in this setting is the absence of hypoestrogenic effects associated with the use of gonadotropin-releasing hormone agonists.[108] Follow-up of these women for 3 years showed no further improvement in pelvic pain after 12 months of use.[109] Additional studies are needed to confirm the original findings and to determine how to best integrate its use into current clinical protocols. As expected, all studies also reported increased menstrual disturbances in the LNG-IUS groups.

Uterine Protection with Estrogen Replacement Therapy. Good-quality evidence supports the long-term use of LNG-IUS for endometrial suppression during estrogen replacement therapy.[110] However, the intrauterine levonorgestrel is relatively large and may be difficult to insert into a postmenopausal woman in an outpatient setting and is likely to cause irregular bleeding. Availability of a smaller progestin-releasing IUD would facilitate use in menopausal women. Acceptability studies are needed, and more studies are necessary to determine the lowest effective dose of LNG required to attain effective endometrial suppression.

Uterine Protection with Tamoxifen Use. Tamoxifen is commonly used as adjuvant endocrine therapy in the treatment of estrogen receptor–positive breast cancer in premenopausal women and in selected postmenopausal women. In postmenopausal women, tamoxifen appears to increase the risk of endometrial polyps, hyperplasia, and cancer. A systematic review of the LNG-IUS in the prevention of endometrial pathology in tamoxifen users concluded that Mirena reduced the risk of endometrial polyps in tamoxifen users, but no data demonstrate that it reduces the risk of endometrial hyperplasia or cancer. Mirena users had a higher incidence of unscheduled bleeding, which may increase the need for diagnostic intervention in this high-risk group.[111]

Treatment for Endometrial Hyperplasia or Carcinoma. Small, prospective studies have show that the LNG-IUS is an effective and safe alternative in the treatment of perimenopausal and postmenopausal women with (simple) endometrial hyperplasia without atypia.[112] When there is atypia, the device may be less effective. The best treatment for early endometrial cancer is hysterectomy. Progestins are sometimes used as palliative or adjuvant therapy. No randomized, controlled trials have examined the role of LNG-IUS in the treatment of atypical endometrial hyperplasia or carcinoma. Small studies of selected patients suggest that intrauterine progestin in surgical high-risk candidates with endometrial cancer may be an alternative management option.[113] Larger studies are needed to better determine the value of LNG-IUS in this context.

Expanding the Use of Intrauterine Devices

There is growing consensus that it is time to broaden our use of IUDs, including the LNG-IUS. One of the greatest challenges will be to effectively counsel patients seeking contraceptives to best meet their needs and to prepare them for possible side effects. Among the demonstrated and potential noncontraceptive uses of LNG-IUS, research supports the use of this device to reduce heavy menstrual bleeding and protect the endometrium in women during use of menopausal estrogen therapy. Other uses, such as for endometriosis, adenomyosis, or endometrial hyperplasia or carcinoma, are less clear. As with all progestin-only contraceptives, bleeding changes represent the most common reason for user dissatisfaction and premature discontinuation.

Contraceptive Implants

Contraceptive implants provide long-acting, highly effective, convenient, and reversible contraception. All subdermal implants for clinical use in humans use progestins. These methods offer an excellent contraceptive option for women who have contraindications to combined hormonal methods and an option for any woman who desires long-term protection against pregnancy that is rapidly reversible. The only subdermal implant available to women in the United States is Implanon (Schering-Plough, Kenilworth, NJ) (Fig. 18-3).

Implanon contains etonogestrel as a single-rod subdermal implant. It has been available in the United States since 2006 but has been extensively used internationally for many years. Implanon is approved for 3 years of use, provides excellent efficacy throughout its use, and is easy to insert and remove. Implanon can be used during lactation, may improve dysmenorrhea, and does not significantly affect BMD, lipids, or liver enzymes.[114,115] Like other progestin-only contraceptives, Implanon commonly causes irregular vaginal bleeding.

Description and Pharmacology

The Implanon rod releases the gonane progestin etonogestrel, formerly known as 3-ketodeosogestrel, the biologically active metabolite of desogestrel. Etonogestrel is the same progestin used in the contraceptive vaginal ring. The implant is 4 cm long and 2 mm in diameter, and it has a core made from a nonbiodegradable solid composed of ethylene vinyl acetate impregnated with 68 mg of etonogestrel (see Fig. 18-3). The ethylene vinyl acetate copolymer of Implanon allows controlled release of hormone over 3 years of use.[115] Each implant is provided in a disposable sterile inserter for subdermal application. Maximum serum concentrations of etonogestrel are usually seen by day 4 after implant insertion. Etonogestrel levels decrease slightly by 1 year and further by 3 years but remain above the threshold needed to suppress ovulation.[116] After removal, serum levels are undetectable by 1 week in most users, who resume ovulation within 6 weeks of implant removal.

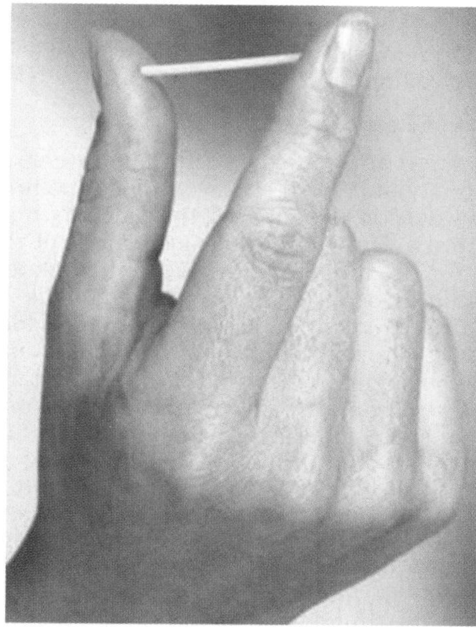

Figure 18-3 Implanon.

Despite effective suppression of ovulation, estradiol levels only fall into the early follicular level range, and Implanon does not cause hypoestrogenism. An initial decrease in the estradiol level is followed by a gradual rise to normal levels.[115]

Mechanism of Action and Efficacy

The contraceptive action of Implanon is primarily effective inhibition of ovulation, although some thickening of cervical mucus may also occur.[117]

Implanon provides highly effective contraception. In an integrated analysis of 11 international clinical trials that included more than 900 healthy women between 18 and 40 years old, no pregnancies were reported while the etonogestrel implants were in place. Six pregnancies occurred during the first 14 days after etonogestrel implant removal. Including these six pregnancies, the cumulative Pearl index (number of pregnancies per 100 women-years) was 0.38 (year 1 and 2 Pearl indices were 0.27 and 0.30, respectively).[117] After the Implanon has been removed, normal ovulation and fertility rapidly return.

Reported pregnancies among Implanon users primarily been due unrecognized pregnancies at the time of insertion and those caused by clinician failure when inserting the device. Postmarketing data from Australia show a failure rate of 1.07 per 1000 insertions.[118] For the total number of confirmed pregnancies, 21% of cases had insufficient data to detect the reason for failure, and the remaining 19% of pregnancies were caused by method failure. However, even when these method failures are accounted for, Implanon continues to have one of the highest efficacies of any method available.

There are reports of Implanon failure in women using anticonvulsants, particularly carbamazepine,[34] and contraceptive implants are not recommended in women taking anticonvulsants or other medications that induce hepatic enzymes. Although no reports suggest higher etonogestrel implant failure rates in overweight and obese women, insufficient data address implant efficacy in these subgroups of women.

Safety and Side Effect Profile

Bleeding Patterns. Implanon users commonly experience irregular and unpredictable bleeding patterns, similar to the experience of users of other continuous progestin-only contraceptives. Combined data from 11 clinical trials showed that the most common bleeding patterns with Implanon were amenorrhea (22.2%), infrequent bleeding (33.6%), frequent bleeding (6.7%), and frequent or prolonged bleeding, or both (17.7%). The number of bleeding days usually was not increased, but the pattern was unpredictable. Of clinical relevance is that bleeding patterns experienced during the initial 3 months predicted future patterns for most women. The group of women with favorable bleeding patterns during the first 3 months tended to continue with this pattern throughout the first 2 years of use, whereas the group with unfavorable initial patterns had at least a 50% chance that the pattern would improve. Only 11.3% of patients discontinued use because of bleeding irregularities, mainly because of prolonged flow and frequent irregular bleeding. Most women (77%) who had baseline dysmenorrhea experienced complete resolution of symptoms. Effective preinsertion counseling on the possible changes in bleeding patterns may improve continuation rates.[119]

Despite extensive clinical trials of agents to improve bleeding patterns with long-acting progestin-only contraceptives, there are no reliable ways of predicting or improving bleeding patterns. COCPs containing high-dose estrogen (50 μg of ethinyl estradiol/250 μg LNG for 20 days) can effectively stop a bleeding episode, but they may cause nausea.[120] Lower-dose COCPs may shorten bleeding episodes but do not decrease their frequency.[63] Data from a large, randomized, controlled trial enrolling Implanon users with frequent or prolonged bleeding have shown that mifepristone in combination with ethinyl estradiol or doxycycline was significantly more effective in stopping an episode of bleeding compared with doxycycline, alone or in combination with ethinyl estradiol, or with placebo. However, there was no improvement in subsequent bleeding patterns.[121] Mifepristone is not readily available in the United States for the treatment of abnormal bleeding. Treatment options for problematic bleeding in progestin contraceptive users are limited, and there are no studies supporting a long-term beneficial effect of any therapeutic regimen.

Acne. Some studies have shown an improvement in acne in Implanon users, but others have found deterioration. The opposing nature of these data and the lack of control groups make it difficult to provide patients with a clear expectation regarding the incidence or severity of acne while using the etonogestrel implant. Patients should be counseled that there is no apparent trend with regard to acne incidence or improvement while using the etonogestrel implant.[117]

Bone Mineral Density. Implanon does not reduce mean circulating estradiol levels. Consistent with that observation, limited data from clinical trials does not show an adverse effect of Implanon on BMD.[115]

Dysmenorrhea. Studies of Implanon and dysmenorrhea show a consistent pattern of symptom improvement.[115] Effective suppression of ovulation means that Implanon may also be an effective treatment for patients with cyclic exacerbation of symptoms who wish to avoid estrogen.

Weight Changes. Several studies have observed a small (<1 kg) weight increase in Implanon users.[117] However, only 3% to 7% of women chose to remove Implanon because of weight changes.

Ovarian Cysts. Similar to the effect seen in women using progestin-only pills, ovarian cysts occur in up to 15% of Implanon users. They may take up to 2 months to resolve but usually are not symptomatic. Most cysts regress spontaneously and do not need additional treatment.[117]

Breast-Feeding. Implanon does not appear to change the content of breast milk and does not influence infant growth up to 3 years. Limited data show that Implanon is safe for use during lactation.[115]

Effect on Lipid Profile. Lipid measurements reveal an overall decrease in serum total cholesterol, high-density lipoprotein (HDL) cholesterol, and low-density lipoprotein (LDL) cholesterol. Some studies have also shown a decrease in triglyceride levels. Minor reductions in the HDL/LDL ratio have been observed, although not into ranges thought to be clinically significant. Implanon use should not significantly increase the risk of cardiovascular disease.[122] In those with known abnormal cholesterol or lipid profiles, these levels should be followed during Implanon use.

Effect on Liver Function. Mixed results on liver function tests have been observed for implant users. Some studies have shown mild changes, including an increase in mean total and unconjugated bilirubin and aspartate transaminase levels.[123] Others have shown no effect.[116] Although results are mixed, clinicians should be aware that there may be mild changes in liver function test results during etonogestrel implant use. These changes may not be clinically significant in healthy women, but they may have clinical relevance in women with preexisting liver disease.

Before recommending Implanon, providers should review the indications and contraindications for its use. Contraindications to etonogestrel implant use listed on the package insert include known or suspected pregnancy, active venous thromboembolic disease, active liver disease, undiagnosed genital tract bleeding, known or suspected breast cancer, progesterone-dependent tumors, and allergy to any of the implant's components.[117] Although the package insert lists VTE disease as a contraindication to etonogestrel implant use, there is no evidence to support this restriction. Because of concerns regarding an increased risk of contraceptive failure, women chronically using hepatic enzyme–inducing medications are not proper candidates for this type of contraception.

When explaining the etonogestrel implant, the physician needs to address any concerns and fears a woman may have about this method of contraception. In particular, women may have concerns about implant removal, although removal problems with single-rod devices such as Implanon are uncommon. Side effects (particularly irregular bleeding) should be discussed in advance, because an unexpected side effect may cause women to request early removal of the implant. All women should be reminded about safe sexual practices, because the implant does not provide protection against STIs. Patients who are good candidates for this form of contraception are those who desire long-term reversible birth control, have no contraindications to etonogestrel implant use, accept implant insertion and removal, and are ready to accept a change in menstrual bleeding patterns.

Insertion and Removal

Proper insertion and removal techniques are essential for clinical efficacy and for the prevention of complications. Timing of insertion depends on the patient's prior use of contraception and the clinician's evaluation of the appropriateness for the individual. In the United States, Implanon has been made available only to clinicians who have completed insertion and removal training provided by the manufacturer. Proper training of clinicians appears to reduce the incidence of complications at insertion and removal. Complications of Implanon insertion are rare (<2%) but may include local pain, infection, and bleeding.[124] There is no indication for routine follow-up.

Implanon is licensed for 3 years of use and should then be removed. Prolonged use beyond 3 years has not been associated with any specific nonpregnancy complications. Before removal, the clinician needs to palpate the implant. Under sterile conditions, a 2- to 3-mm incision is made vertically over the implant. The rod is then removed using the pop-out technique described elsewhere for Norplant

System removal.[125] If inserted correctly, removal is usually simple and should take less than 5 minutes.[116] The most common reason for difficulty is implants that were placed too deeply. If the clinician cannot palpate the implant, imaging techniques may be necessary before proceeding.

Future Use of Implanon

Implanon provides women with an additional highly effective, non–user-dependent, reversible contraceptive option. The primary advantages of the etonogestrel implant over other types of contraception are the convenience and high level of contraception associated with implant use and, for women with contraindications to contraceptive use of estrogen, the absence of estrogen. The trade-off for women is the erratic bleeding that occurs throughout implant use.

Emergency Contraception

Emergency contraception is defined as a drug or device used to prevent pregnancy after unprotected sexual intercourse (including sexual assault) or after a recognized contraceptive failure. In the United States, 1.5 mg of levonorgestrel, packaged as Plan B, and the Copper T 380A IUD are the most common emergency contraceptives available to women and are effective up to 5 days after unprotected sexual intercourse. In August 2006, Plan B was approved for over-the-counter sale to women 18 years old or older in the United States. It is not known whether the increased availability of emergency contraception will decrease unintended pregnancy and induced abortion rates. Such reductions unfortunately have not been observed in countries where over-the-counter emergency contraception has been available for longer periods.

Unintended pregnancies, those that are mistimed or undesired at the time of conception, are common in the United States. Of the 6.4 million pregnancies recorded in 2001, approximately one half were unintended. Of these 3.1 million unintended pregnancies, 42% resulted in induced abortions. Among women with unintended pregnancies, 48% were using contraceptives during the month of conception, although not always correctly.[126] Emergency contraception is intended as a backup method for occasional use, rather than a regular method of contraception. Although emergency contraception is sometimes called postcoital contraception or the morning-after pill, these labels are confusing, because they imply that emergency contraception can be taken only the morning after unprotected sexual intercourse. Emergency contraception can reduce the risk of unintended pregnancy up to 5 days after unprotected sex. Emergency contraception should be available to all women at risk for unplanned pregnancy, including adolescents and victims of sexual assault.

Emergency contraception has the potential to reduce unintended pregnancy rates, thereby reducing the number of induced abortions. Providing education about how to use and access emergency contraception is an integral part of women's health care.

Emergency Contraception Regimens

The oral emergency contraception regimen most commonly used in the United States consists of 1.5 mg of the progestin levonorgestrel. Makers of this product, packaged and marketed as Plan B (Barr Pharmaceuticals Inc., Pomona, NY) instruct women to take the first 0.75-mg levonorgestrel tablet as soon as possible after unprotected intercourse and to take the second 0.75-mg tablet 12 hours after the first dose. The FDA approved Plan B for use as an emergency contraceptive in 1999. Previous regimens combined progestin and estrogen, often called the Yuzpe regimen.[127] This combined regimen has been superseded by the levonorgestrel-only preparation because it is more effective and causes fewer side effects.[128]

Oral emergency contraception is maximally effective within 72 hours of unprotected intercourse but may have some effect up to 120 hours later.[129] However, given the reduced efficacy of oral hormonal emergency contraception with delayed use, women should also be informed about the copper-bearing IUD as an alternative if appropriate.[126]

Emergency contraception with the antiprogestin mifepristone (25 to 50 mg) is superior to other hormonal regimens. Low doses of mifepristone (<25 mg) may be more effective than 0.75 mg of levonorgestrel (two doses).[128] In the United States, mifepristone is not used for emergency contraception because of its high cost and because it is not manufactured or marketed in an appropriate dose. Other progesterone receptor modulators for emergency contraception are undergoing clinical trials.

Mechanism of Action

The mode of action of hormonal emergency contraception is multifactorial and not completely understood. Because sperm are viable in the female reproductive tract for up to 5 days but eggs can be fertilized only within 1 day of ovulation, the mechanism of action most likely depends on when levonorgestrel-only emergency contraception is given in relation to the time of intercourse and time of ovulation. No evidence supports the theory that hormonal emergency contraception interferes with postfertilization events, and most evidence suggests that it prevents pregnancy by preventing conception. Because levonorgestrel-only emergency contraception does not interrupt an established pregnancy, defined as beginning with implantation, hormonal emergency contraception is not considered an abortifacient.[130]

Efficacy

The probability of pregnancy after a single act of unprotected intercourse varies (3% to 8%) according to the day of the menstrual cycle and the couple's fertility status.[131] Calculating the efficacy of emergency contraception is complex because it is impossible to know how many pregnancies would otherwise have occurred. It is known, however, that the use of levonorgestrel-only emergency contraception is more effective than no treatment at all after a single episode of unprotected intercourse.[132] Plan B labeling cites an average preventive action of 89%. If 100 women had unprotected intercourse once during the second or third week of the cycle and were not treated with emergency contraception, about 8 would become pregnant, but after treatment with emergency contraception, typically only 1 woman would become pregnant. A meta-analysis concluded that 1.5 mg of levonorgestrel (Plan B) was superior to the Yuzpe regimen, with a combined relative risk of pregnancy of 0.51 (95% CI, 0.31 to 0.83) compared with Yuzpe.[2] Taking a total of 1.5 mg of levonorgestrel in a single dose is as effective as the 0.75-mg split dose and more user-friendly.[128]

The timing of oral emergency contraception influences its effectiveness significantly. Waiting 12 hours to initiate treatment after unprotected intercourse increases the odds of pregnancy by almost 50%, and its efficacy decreases linearly with time. Oral emergency contraception should be taken as soon as possible after unprotected intercourse or contraceptive failure.

Indications

Emergency contraception is indicated for any woman at risk for unintended pregnancy from an identified episode of contraceptive failure or unprotected intercourse. However, surveys have found that the level of knowledge and use of emergency contraception in the United States by women and their health care providers is low. Relatively few women presenting for termination of pregnancy or antenatal care were aware of emergency contraception.[126]

No clinical examination or pregnancy testing is required before using oral hormonal emergency contraception. There are no medical contraindications to the use of oral emergency contraception regimens because of their short duration of use. Plan B's labeling lists three contraindications: pregnancy, hypersensitivity to any component of the product, and undiagnosed abnormal genital bleeding. Pregnancy is a relative contraindication because emergency contraception is ineffective if a pregnancy is already established. On the basis of studies of the teratogenic risk of combined oral contraceptives, however, there is no increased risk to the fetus if oral emergency contraception is taken while pregnant. Despite information in the package labeling, there is no medical rationale to justify denying women with undiagnosed genital bleeding access to emergency contraception.[126]

WHO recommendations[133] state that women with previous ectopic pregnancy, cardiovascular disease, migraines, or liver disease and women who are breast-feeding can use emergency contraception. There may be reduced efficacy of oral emergency contraception in women with severe malabsorption syndromes and those taking liver enzyme–inducing drugs. There is no evidence that hormonal emergency contraception increases the risk of VTE disease. There have been case reports of levonorgestrel-only emergency contraception interfering with warfarin anticoagulant action. Women taking liver enzyme–inducing medications (including but not limited to rifampin, carbamazepine, phenytoin, phenobarbital, and St. John's wort) or warfarin should seek clinical advice regarding emergency contraception use. However, there is no need to delay emergency contraception use in these women, for whom an unintended pregnancy may carry additional health risks.

Side Effects

The FDA has determined that Plan B is safe enough to be available as an over-the-counter preparation only for women at least 18 years old. Women 17 years old or younger must obtain Plan B with a prescription or without a prescription in states with direct pharmacy access. Not all pharmacies stock Plan B or participate in this program, but lists of participating pharmacies are available (http://www.ec-help.org/PharmacyLocations.asp or http://www.not-2-late.com [accessed August 2010]).

There have been no deaths or serious complications directly linked to emergency contraception. The most common short-term side effects include nausea, vomiting, and irregular bleeding, which affect up to 20% of users. Other minor adverse effects reported by women in clinical trials included dizziness, fatigue, breast tenderness, headache, and abdominal pain.[128] The levonorgestrel-only regimen results in less nausea and vomiting than the Yuzpe regimen. If vomiting occurs within 1 to 2 hours of taking Plan B, most experts recommend that the dose be repeated.

Irregular bleeding caused by hormonal emergency contraception typically resolves by the next menstrual cycle. There is a low incidence of intermenstrual spotting after using hormonal emergency contraception, ranging from 3% to 37% in trials. After hormonal emergency contraception is taken, menses usually occurs within 1 week before or after the expected time. If the delay in the onset of menses is greater than 1 week or if the expected menses is lighter than usual, a pregnancy test should be performed. Because hormonal emergency contraception can postpone ovulation, making a woman vulnerable to pregnancy later in the cycle, women should be counseled to begin a regular method of contraception *immediately* after using emergency contraception. A woman should also be advised to seek medical attention for continued irregular bleeding or abdominal pain, because these symptoms may be a sign of a spontaneous abortion or ectopic pregnancy.

Research has shown that although increased access to emergency contraception improves use, it does not seem to reduce the rates of unintended pregnancy or abortion.[134] Although access is an important factor, how women use emergency contraception may be a stronger determinant of its ultimate effect. Studies show that even when women have emergency contraception at home, they often fail to use it after unprotected sexual intercourse. The most common reason for this is a lack of recognition of the risk of pregnancy or neglect of the perceived risk.

Future of Emergency Contraception

Emergency contraception reduces the chance of pregnancy when used correctly up to 5 days after an identified episode of contraceptive failure or unprotected sexual intercourse. The most common regimens used in the United States are levonorgestrel-only emergency contraception (Plan B) and the Copper T 380A IUD (ParaGard). In the United States, given limitations in access, advance prescriptions for Plan B are still recommended for women 18 years old or older despite its over-the-counter status. Although increasing knowledge of and access to emergency contraception is a public health priority, the use of regular, ongoing contraception must be emphasized. The worldwide experience has not shown that improved access to emergency contraception has a population-level effect of reduced unintended pregnancies. This is consistent with the hypothesis that only a small proportion of women with access to emergency contraception actually take the pills to prevent pregnancy. Along with increased access, better educating women about how to use emergency contraception and encouraging its use are required to produce a demonstrable population-level effect.

ANTIPROGESTINS AND SELECTIVE PROGESTERONE RECEPTOR MODULATORS

Use for Contraception

Although not available for contraception in the United States, mifepristone and other progestin antagonists have contraceptive potential, acting by several mechanisms. At low doses, they inhibit ovulation by blocking the luteinizing hormone surge. Low doses also retard endometrial development by virtue of their antiproliferative action. As a consequence, the endometrium cannot support implantation. Higher doses can block follicular maturation and induce follicular atresia. When administered in the late luteal phase, progestin antagonists induce endometrial bleeding, preventing implantation.[135]

Long-Term Contraceptive Potential

Daily doses of 2 to 10 mg of mifepristone suppress follicular development, block the luteinizing hormone surge, and delay ovulation. A multicenter, double-blind, randomized, controlled trial comparing mifepristone with the progestin-only pill showed that mifepristone (5 mg) was as effective as the progestin-only pill for contraception and had higher rates of amenorrhea. Almost one half of the mifepristone users had cystic glandular dilatation of the endometrium, but none showed hyperplasia or atypia.[136]

The lowest daily dose of mifepristone capable of inhibiting ovulation is 2 mg daily. Lower doses interfere with endometrial maturation but do not suppress ovulation.[135] Mifepristone (200 mg) in the early luteal phase can prevent embryo implantation.[137] Combined with prostaglandin, mifepristone in the late luteal phase is an effective menses regulator.[137]

Management of Irregular Bleeding Induced by Progestin-Only Contraception

Unscheduled bleeding is one of the main drawbacks of progestin-only contraception. Mifepristone and other progestin antagonists may be effective treatments for abnormal bleeding with these methods. Mifepristone (150 mg monthly) reduced unscheduled bleeding in users of the progestin-only pill containing desogetrel.[138] Mifepristone (50 mg monthly) reduced the duration of bleeding in Norplant users.[139] In new users of DMPA, 50 mg of mifepristone over 2 weeks reduced unscheduled bleeding,[62] and low-dose mifepristone in combination with ethinyl estradiol or doxycycline was effective in stopping bleeding in Implanon users.[121] The action of mifepristone in improving bleeding patterns is not fully understood but is likely to be endometrial rather than permitting ovulation in these contraceptive users.[139]

Emergency Contraception

In addition to providing more effective emergency contraception than other hormonal regimens, mifepristone has the distinct advantage of being effective up to 120 hours after unprotected intercourse, whereas other methods are maximally effective up to 72 hours.[128] However, a disadvantage is that more women using mifepristone have a delay in the expected onset of their next menstrual period compared with other methods. This is a drawback because the onset of menses reassures the woman that emergency contraception has been successful. Despite the proven effectiveness of mifepristone as an emergency contraceptive agent, China is the only country to have licensed and approved mifepristone for this indication.[135]

CLINICAL CHALLENGES IN CONTRACEPTIVE CARE

Hormonal Contraception for Adolescents

The United States has the highest rate of teenage pregnancy and birth in the Western industrialized world.[140] Approximately 80% of these pregnancies are unplanned, of which about 30% end in termination, 57% in live births, and 14% in miscarriage. Teenage pregnancy and parenting are precursors of poor medical, educational, and psychosocial outcomes for mother and child. Children of teenage mothers are at greater risk for preterm birth, low birth weight, neonatal death, and later behavioral problems and poor academic performance. Teenage parenting contributes to the intergenerational transmission of poverty.[2]

Considerations for clinicians advising adolescents about contraception should include the potentially high fertility rates in these young women, their high rates of unprotected intercourse, increased risk of STIs, and low compliance with contraceptive methods that require daily use.[140] Because rates of COCPs discontinuation and unintended pregnancy are so high among adolescents, long-acting methods, including DMPA injection, contraceptive implants, and IUDs, should be made available to teens.[141,142] The clinician should also be aware of the legal conditions surrounding prescribing contraception to minors (http://www.guttmacher.org; click on *adolescents* and *state policies in brief* [accessed August 2010]).

All adolescents should receive health guidance annually regarding responsible health behaviors, including abstinence, latex condoms to prevent STIs, and appropriate methods of birth control, along with instructions on ways to use them effectively.[140] Adolescents should also be counseled in a nonjudgmental manner about the need to use condoms during anal and oral intercourse. Barriers to effective contraception use by adolescents include lack of forward planning, lack of confidential care, fear of disapproval by parents and doctors, absence of adolescent-friendly services, language and cultural barriers, fear of pelvic examination, and cost. Misconceptions about contraception, including effects on weight gain, future fertility, acne, and risk of cancer, may also prevent adolescents from using effective contraception and should be addressed in counseling. No matter how effective the method and how easy it is to use, detailed counseling is required for adolescents. Practitioners should recommend the new quadrivalent human papillomavirus (HPV) vaccine to sexually active adolescent girls.

Oral Contraceptive Pills in Adolescents

Although COCPs are potentially safe and effective methods for adolescents, many young women are not effectively educated about correct use and potential unwanted effects. They may use oral contraception inconsistently, which will lead to very high pregnancy rates.[140] During counseling it is important to provide clear verbal and written instructions about starting COCP use, ways to ensure daily compliance, and what to do if one or more pills is missed.

Initiating or continuing hormonal contraception does not require pelvic examination, cervical cytology, or sexually transmitted disease screening in adolescents or older reproductive-age women. A history excluding contraindications, blood pressure measurement, and a negative urinary pregnancy test result are sufficient before initiating hormonal contraception. Before beginning COCPs, education about appropriate use, missed pills, and adverse effects is appropriate. Screening for STIs or Pap smears (should be started 3 years after the onset of sexual activity or when 21 years old) should be considered regardless of contraceptive use.[140] The use of condoms should be encouraged in conjunction with the COCPs to prevent STIs.

Initial follow-up should be at 6 to 8 weeks after commencing the COCPs to monitor correct use and adverse events and should be done thereafter at 6 to 12 months. Education and ongoing counseling are essential to ensure correct usage. Many adolescents are concerned that the COCPs will cause weight gain or acne, and these issues should be directly addressed. A newly available chewable pill (Femcon Fe) has a mint flavor and may be more acceptable to young women who find it difficult to swallow pills. Unscheduled bleeding may be less acceptable to adolescents compared with adult women. Clinicians must consider the possibility that unscheduled bleeding represents cervicovaginal infection in this high-risk population and investigate and treat it accordingly. Few data specifically address the use of transdermal or vaginal ring contraception in adolescents.

Injectable Contraceptives in Adolescents

Discontinuation rates for DMPA in adolescents are extremely high, with 33% not receiving a second injection at 3 months. Three fourths of adolescents initiating DMPA have discontinued it by 12 months.[140] However, because DMPA suppresses ovulation for an extended period of time, prior use of DMPA protects many adolescents from unintended pregnancy despite inconsistent use. Weight gain is the most commonly cited reason for adolescents to discontinue DMPA, and it may be more common in African American adolescents.[143] Although loss of bone density has been a concern in adolescents using DMPA, the position statement of the Society for Adolescent Medicine is that DMPA is an extremely effective contraceptive and that clinical concerns about loss of BMD must be placed within the context of likely bone recovery on discontinuation, low risk of fractures, and benefits of preventing unintended pregnancy among adolescents.[89]

Contraception in Women with Underlying Medical Conditions

Because pregnancy in women with underlying medical conditions is associated with higher risks of maternal and perinatal morbidity and mortality, achieving effective contraception is particularly important in this setting. Although numerous studies have addressed the safety and effectiveness of hormonal contraceptive use in healthy women, data unfortunately are far less complete for women with underlying medical problems or other special circumstances. Using the best available scientific evidence, this chapter provides information to help clinicians and women with coexisting medical conditions make sound decisions regarding the selection and appropriateness of various hormonal contraceptives, including the levonorgestrel IUD.

Decisions regarding contraception for women with coexisting medical problems may be complicated. In some cases, medications taken for certain chronic conditions may alter the effectiveness of hormonal contraception, and pregnancy in these cases may pose substantial risks to the mother and her fetus. Differences in content and delivery methods of hormonal contraceptives may affect patients with certain conditions differently. Because transdermal and vaginal ring contraception is relatively new, few data address its use in women with medical concerns. In the absence of more extensive data, contraindications to the use of estrogen-progestin COCPs should also be considered as contraindications to the use of transdermal and vaginal ring contraception. Practitioners should recognize that the use of other nonhormonal forms of contraception, such as the copper IUD, remains a safe, effective choice for many women with medical conditions.

Package labeling approved by the FDA for progestin-only contraceptives is occasionally the same as that for combined estrogen-progestin methods without supporting evidence, further complicating decisions for women with coexisting medical conditions. For instance, labeling for norethindrone progestin-only oral contraceptives no longer lists a history of thromboembolism as a contraindication. Such a history, however, remains listed as a contraindication in package labeling for DMPA injections and the contraceptive implant.

Hormonal Contraception in Women Older Than 35 Years

Use of estrogen-progestin oral contraceptives, patches, and vaginal rings should be considered safe in healthy, lean, nonsmoking women older than 35 years (Table 18-6).[23] Large U.S. population-based case-control studies have found no increased risk of myocardial infarction or stroke among healthy, nonsmoking women older than 35 years who use oral contraceptives formulated with less than 50 μg of estrogen.[28] Perimenopausal women may benefit from the positive effect on BMD offered by COCPs.[13]

Use of COCPs may reduce vasomotor symptoms in perimenopausal women.[144] The reduced risk of endometrial and ovarian cancers associated with COCP use is of particular importance to older women of reproductive age. Age, COCP use, and obesity each represent independent risk factors for thrombosis. Because VTE risk has been observed

TABLE 18-6

World Health Organization (WHO) and American College of Obstetrics and Gynecology (ACOG) Guidelines Regarding Use of Combination Estrogen-Progestin Contraceptives (Oral Contraception, Ring, Patch) in Women 35 Years of Age and Older

Variable	ACOG Guidelines	WHO Guidelines
Obesity	Progestin-only or intrauterine contraception* may be safer	Benefit usually outweighs risks†
Smoker	Progestin-only or intrauterine contraception* should be used	Risk unacceptable
Hypertension	Progestin-only or intrauterine contraception* should be used	Risk unacceptable
Diabetes	Progestin-only or intrauterine contraception* should be used	Risk unacceptable
Migraine	Progestin-only or intrauterine contraception* should be used	Risk unacceptable
None of the above risk factors	Healthy nonsmoking women doing well on a combination contraceptive can continue their method until age 50-55 yr, after weighing the risks and benefits	For women ≥40 yr, the risk of cardiovascular disease increases with age and may also increase with use of combined hormonal contraceptives. In the absence of other adverse clinical conditions, combined hormonal contraceptives may be used until menopause.

*Includes progestin-only oral contraception, depot medroxyprogesterone acetate (DMPA), contraceptive implants, copper intrauterine devices (IUDs), and progestin-releasing IUDs.

†Obesity in women age 35 and older not specifically addressed.

to rise sharply after age 39 for COCP users, these pills should be used with caution by women older than 35 years who are obese.

Discontinuation of Combined Oral Contraceptive Pills at Menopause

As increasing numbers of women in their late 40s and early 50s use combination contraceptives, the question of when women no longer need contraception will arise more frequently. Assessment of follicle-stimulating hormone levels to determine when hormonal contraceptive users have become menopausal and no longer need contraception is expensive, and results may be misleading. Until a well-validated tool to confirm menopause is available, an alternative approach is for healthy, nonsmoking women doing well on a combination contraceptive to discontinue her method between the ages of 50 and 55 years.[23]

Hormonal Contraception in Cigarette Smokers

In women who use COCPs, smoking and hypertension represent synergistic risk factors for myocardial infarction and stroke. Some studies conducted outside the United States have found an increased risk of myocardial infarction and stroke with COCPs use. The prevalence of smoking and untreated hypertension was high among participants in these studies.[28,145] Current guidelines indicate that, as with all medication, contraceptive hormones should be selected and initiated by weighing risks and benefits for the individual patient. For women 35 years old or older who have cardiovascular risk factors, including obesity, hypertension, smoking, diabetes, or migraines, progestin-only and intrauterine contraceptives are preferable to combination estrogen-progestin contraceptives (i.e., COCPs, transdermal patch, and vaginal ring).[23,28]

Existing data are mixed with regard to possible protection from COCPs for atherosclerosis and cardiovascular events; longer-term cardiovascular follow-up of menopausal women with regard to prior COCP use, including subgroup information regarding adequacy of ovulatory cycling, the presence of hyperandrogenic conditions, and the presence of prothrombotic genetic disorders, is needed to address this important issue.[146]

Hormonal Contraception and Chronic Hypertension

Even low-dose COCPs may increase blood pressure. The ACOG guidelines advise that women younger than 35 years with well-controlled hypertension are candidates for a trial of low-dose COCPs provided they are otherwise healthy with no evidence of end-organ vascular disease and do not smoke.[28] Blood pressure should be closely monitored in these women. If blood pressure remains well controlled with careful monitoring several months after contraceptive initiation, use can be continued. Progestin-only methods may be a safer option for hypertensive women. Prospective studies of progestin-only pills and DMPA have not shown any increase in baseline blood pressure.[29]

In healthy women of reproductive age, the incidence of myocardial infarction or stroke with the use of low-dose COCPs is extremely low. Although the relative risk of these events is increased in women with hypertension, the absolute risk remains low. Because of the increased risk of myocardial infarction and stroke associated with hypertension alone and the likelihood of additional risks associated with use of estrogen-progestin contraceptives, the decision to use combination hormonal contraceptives in these patients should be weighed against the adverse pregnancy outcomes associated with hypertension. The noncontraceptive benefits of COCPs also should be taken into account. The ACOG recommends that use of progestin-only contraceptives such as DMPA, progestin-only oral contraceptives, or the levonorgestrel-containing IUD are preferable to estrogen-progestin contraceptives in women 35 years old or older who have hypertension.[23,28]

Hormonal Contraception in Women with Lipid Disorders

The term *dyslipidemia* includes disorders of lipoprotein metabolism that lead to atherosclerosis. These abnormalities arise from genetic and secondary factors and are caused by excessive entry of lipoproteins into the bloodstream or an impairment in their removal, or both.

The estrogen component of COCPs enhances removal of LDL cholesterol and increases levels of HDL cholesterol. Oral estrogen also increases triglyceride levels; however, in the setting of concomitantly increased HDL and decreased LDL levels, the moderate triglyceride elevations caused by oral estrogen use do not appear to increase the risk of atherogenesis.[146] The progestin component of COCPs antagonizes these estrogen-induced lipid changes, which increases LDL levels and decreases HDL and triglyceride levels. Among women taking COCPs with an identical dose of estrogen, the choice and dose of the progestin component may affect net lipid changes. COCPs formulated with more androgenic progestins raise HDL and triglyceride levels less than formulations with less androgenic progestins.[147] Use of the transdermal contraceptive patch increases HDL and triglyceride levels and lowers LDL levels, similar to the lipid changes observed in women using COCPs formulated with more androgenic progestins. As with COCPs, use of the contraceptive vaginal ring increases triglyceride levels. In contrast to COCPs, use of DMPA lowers HDL levels, raises LDL levels, and does not raise triglyceride levels.[29] The LNG-IUS has not been shown to affect circulating lipid or triglyceride levels.[148]

Lipids are surrogate measures, however, and the effect of contraceptives on lipids may not necessarily correlate with effects on cardiovascular disease or mortality. It is not known whether the differential lipid effects of distinct hormonal contraceptive formulations or means of administration have any clinical significance in women with normal baseline lipid levels or those with lipid disorders. Because the absolute risk of cardiovascular events is low, most women with controlled dyslipidemia can use COCPs formulated with 35 μg estrogen or less. Fasting serum lipid levels should be monitored as frequently as each month after initiating COCPs in dyslipidemic women. Less frequent monitoring is appropriate after stabilization of lipid parameters has been observed. In women with uncontrolled LDL cholesterol levels greater than 160 mg/dL or with multiple additional risk factors for cardiovascular disease (including smoking, diabetes, obesity, hypertension, family history of premature coronary artery disease, HDL level <35 mg/dL, or triglyceride level >250 mg/dL), use of alternative contraceptives should be considered.[133] Use of progestin-only contraceptives does not increase triglyceride levels. The use of DMPA and other progestin-only contraceptives is appropriate in women with hypertriglyceridemia, who may be at increased risk for pancreatitis if they used COCPs.[28]

Hormonal Contraception in Women with Diabetes

COCPs do not appear to impair carbohydrate metabolism or affect vascular disease in diabetic women. A systematic review concluded that hormonal contraceptives have limited effect on carbohydrate metabolism in women without diabetes. However, studies are limited and do not inform the management of diabetic women who are overweight.[149]

Although the existing data support the use of combination hormonal contraceptives by women with diabetes, use should be limited to nonsmoking, otherwise healthy women with diabetes who are younger than 35 years and show no evidence of hypertension, nephropathy, retinopathy, or other vascular disease.[28] A clinical trial found that metabolic control was similar in women with uncomplicated diabetes randomized to a copper IUD or the LNG-IUS.[150] The levonorgestrel-containing IUD is an appropriate option for women with diabetes.

In the general population, hormonal contraceptives do not appear to increase the risk of developing diabetes.[29] However, limited data from populations at increased risk for diabetes (i.e., Hispanic and Navajo women) suggest that progestin-only contraceptives may increase the risk of diabetes.[28]

Hormonal Contraception for Women with Migraine Headaches

Headaches are common in women of reproductive age. Most of these headaches are tension headaches, not migraines. Some women with migraines experience improvement in their symptoms with the use of hormonal contraceptives, and some women's symptoms worsen. Because the presence of true migraine headaches affects the decision to use estrogen-containing contraception, careful consideration of the diagnosis is important.[28]

Most migraines occur without aura. Nausea, vomiting, photophobia, phonophobia, visual blurring, generalized visual spots, or flashing occurring before or during a migraine headache do not constitute aura. Typical auras last 5 to 60 minutes before headache and are visual. Several reversible visual symptoms indicate the presence of aura: flickering, uncolored zigzag line progressing laterally to the periphery of one visual field; laterally spreading, scintillating scotoma (i.e., area of lost or depressed vision within a visual field, surrounded by an area of normal or less depressed vision or loss of vision) (http://64.227.208.149/NS_BASH/BASH_guideline31Aug05.pdf).

The risk of stroke is increased in women who have migraine with aura. Although cerebrovascular events occur rarely among women with migraines who use COCPs, the impact of a stroke is so devastating that clinicians should consider the use of progestin-only, intrauterine, or barrier contraceptives in this setting. Estrogen-containing contraceptives are contraindicated in women migraine sufferers with aura and should be discontinued in patients suffering from migraine without aura if aura symptoms appear.[22] Current COCP formulations usually are well tolerated by patients with migraine without aura. The latest International Classification of Headache Disorders identifies at least two entities related to the use of COCPs: exogenous hormone-induced headache and estrogen-withdrawal headache (http://ihs-classification.org/en/ [accessed August 2010]). Other risk factors (e.g., tobacco use, hypertension, hyperlipidemia, obesity, diabetes) must be carefully considered when prescribing estrogen-containing contraceptives for patients with migraine without aura. For women older than 35 years with migraines, combination estrogen-progestin contraceptives should be avoided in favor of progestin-only and intrauterine methods.[23,28]

Hormonal Contraception in Women with Fibrocystic Breast Changes, Fibroadenoma, or a Family History of Breast Cancer

Women with benign breast disease with epithelial hyperplasia with or without atypia or with a family history of breast cancer are at increased risk for breast cancer.[151] Large cohort studies have consistently shown that COCPs appear to decrease the risk of benign breast disease.[152] A history of benign breast disease should not be regarded as a contraindication to COCP use.

Neither current nor prior use of COCPs appears to elevate the risk of breast cancer in women with a family history of this common malignancy.[30] Studies among women with known *BRCA* gene mutations have yielded mixed results with respect to impact on breast cancer risk.[153] *BRCA1* and *BRCA2* mutations are associated with a 45% and 25% lifetime risk, respectively, for epithelial ovarian cancer.[154] Use of COCPs reduces the subsequent risk of ovarian cancer in high-risk and low-risk women and offers important potential benefits for women with *BRCA1* or *BRCA2* mutations, particularly those who have not completed their families or have not yet undergone risk-reducing bilateral salpingo-oophorectomy.[28]

Hormonal Contraception in Women with Uterine Leiomyomata

Uterine fibroids are common, affecting up to 50% of women of reproductive age.[155] Fibroids tend to be larger and clinically manifest at an earlier age in black women compared with white women in the United States.[156] Uterine fibroids may be asymptomatic, but they are also associated with heavy menstrual bleeding. Use of COCPs may be effective in reducing menstrual blood loss in women with heavy menstrual bleeding who do not have uterine fibroids, but the evidence to support this is not strong.[157] There is insufficient information to conclude how hormonal contraceptives affect symptoms, including heavy menstrual bleeding, in women with uterine fibroids. COCPs do not appear to induce the growth of uterine fibroids.[158]

There is limited information about the role of other hormonal contraceptives in the development, growth, and management of uterine fibroids. Small studies suggest that DMPA may reduce abnormal bleeding in symptomatic women with uterine fibroids, and the levonorgestrel-releasing IUD may also reduce heavy menstrual bleeding associated with uterine fibroids. However, the presence of fibroids may increase the risk of expulsion of the levonorgestrel-containing IUD.[106]

Hormonal Contraception in Postpartum and Lactating Women

Postpartum women remain in a hypercoagulable state for weeks after childbirth. Product labeling for COCPs advises deferring use until 4 weeks after delivery in non–breast-feeding women. Because progestin-only oral contraceptives and DMPA do not contain estrogen, these methods may be safely initiated immediately by postpartum women.[28] There is no established effect of COCPs on the quality or quantity of breast milk.

Traditionally, COCPs have not been recommended as the first choice for breast-feeding mothers because of concerns that the estrogenic component can reduce the volume of milk production and the caloric and mineral content of breast milk in lactating women.[33] However, use of COCPs by well-nourished breast-feeding women does not appear to result in problems with infant development. A systematic review of randomized, controlled trials concluded that existing data is of poor quality and insufficient to establish an effect of hormonal contraception on lactation.[159] Use of combination hormonal contraceptives can be considered after milk flow is well established. Evidence from limited studies suggests that progestin-only contraception does not interfere with lactation or infant development and does not increase the risk of thromboembolic disease.[159] It appears reasonable to initiate progestin-only contraception, including DMPA, progestin-only pills, and implants, immediately after delivery, regardless of whether mothers are nursing their infants.[53]

Hormonal Contraception in Women Taking Anticonvulsants

Effective contraception is a critical component of the management of the female patient with epilepsy because of the increased risk of seizures in pregnancy and the multitude of interactions between antiepileptic drugs (AEDs) and hormonal contraception. Steroid hormones and many of the AEDs are substrates for the cytochrome P450 enzyme system, in particular, the CYP3A4 isoenzyme. Concomitant use of hormonal contraceptives and AEDs may pose a risk of unexpected pregnancy, seizures, and drug-related adverse effects.[34] The risk of COCP failure is slightly increased in the presence of CYP3A4 enzyme-inducing AEDs. Several AEDs induce the production of sex hormone–binding globulin (SHBG) to which the progestins are tightly bound, resulting in lower concentrations of free progestin that may also lead to COCP failure. There is no increase in the risk of COCP failure in women taking non–enzyme-inducing AEDs. Oral contraceptives significantly increase the metabolism of lamotrigine, posing a risk of seizures when hormonal agents are initiated and of toxicity during pill-free weeks. There is no evidence that COCPs increase seizures in women with epilepsy.[34] Although higher-dose COCPs are one contraceptive option for women on enzyme-inducing AEDs, a variety of other options are available. Injectable contraception (DMPA) appears effective with concomitant AED use, and a potential advantage of using DMPA in women with seizure disorders is DMPA's intrinsic anticonvulsant effect.[55]

Contraceptive failures are reported in women taking AEDs and using the etonogestrel implant system (Implanon). Small, observational studies suggest that the levonorgestrel intrauterine system continues to be highly effective in women taking anticonvulsants.[160]

Hormonal Contraception in Women Taking Antibiotics

Although there have been many anecdotal reports of COCP failure in women taking concomitant antibiotics, pharmacokinetic evidence of lower serum steroid levels exists only for rifampin. Women taking rifampin should not rely on oral, transdermal, vaginal ring, or implantable contraception alone for protection. Approximately 20% of pregnant women visiting family planning or abortion clinics reported concomitant COCP and antibiotic use. It is possible that individual differences in pharmacokinetic responses to antibiotics underlie these reported contraceptive failures.[161] In contrast to rifampin, use of ampicillin, doxycycline, fluconazole, metronidazole, miconazole, quinalones, and tetracycline have not lowered steroid levels in women using COCPs.[28]

Hormonal Contraception in HIV-Positive Women

More than 15 million women, many of reproductive age, are infected with human immunodeficiency virus (HIV). Heterosexual intercourse is increasingly linked to HIV transmission. The role of hormonal contraception in HIV-positive women has been controversial. Studies in female sex workers suggest that some hormonal contraceptives may increase the risk of HIV acquisition, but the effect is not seen in women at low risk for HIV infection. Hormonal contraception does not interfere with antiviral drug effectiveness or disease progression in women taking antiretrovirals. However, in those not receiving antiretroviral medication, COCP use has been associated with accelerated disease progression.[162] Pharmacokinetic studies have shown changes in circulating sex steroid levels in women taking antiretrovirals, but the clinical implications of these observations are unclear. All the available hormonal contraceptive methods can be used by women at risk for HIV infection and by HIV-infected women, but further studies are needed to investigate the safety and efficiency of hormonal contraception in women living with HIV infection or acquired immunodeficiency syndrome (AIDS).

The LNG-IUS appears to be safe in HIV-positive women taking antiretroviral therapy; available evidence suggests that use does not increase a women's risk of overall complications or infection-related complications. The device may also be useful in the treatment of heavy menstrual bleeding in HIV-positive women.[163]

Hormonal Contraception in Women with a History of Thromboembolism

Women with a documented history of unexplained VTE or VTE associated with pregnancy or exogenous estrogen use should not use estrogen-containing hormonal contraceptives unless they are taking anticoagulants. A COCP candidate who experienced a single episode of VTE years earlier associated with a nonrecurring risk factor (e.g., VTE occurring after immobilization after a motor vehicle accident) may not currently be at increased risk for VTE. The decision to initiate estrogen-containing contraceptives in these candidates can be individualized.[28]

Limited data have assessed the risk of VTE associated with use of progestin-only contraceptives. A large WHO study did not find an increased VTE risk with use of progestin-only contraceptions.[164] A systematic review suggested increased VTE risk with use of progestin-only contraceptives, but it might reflect that higher-risk women were more likely to be prescribed progestin-only methods.[165]

Hormonal Contraception in Women Awaiting Surgery

VTE with pulmonary embolism remains a major cause of fatalities associated with surgical (including gynecologic) procedures. Findings of a large, British, prospective, cohort study suggested that the risk of postoperative VTE was approximately twice as high ($P > .05$) in COCP users as in nonusers.[166] The procoagulant changes of COCPs take 6 weeks or longer to resolve after discontinuation.[167]

The benefits associated with stopping combination contraceptives 1 month or more before major surgery should be balanced against the risks of an unintended pregnancy. If oral contraceptives are continued before major surgical procedures, heparin prophylaxis should be considered. Use of COCPs at the time of arthroscopic surgery has increased VTE risk.[168] Because of the low perioperative risk of VTE, it is not considered necessary to discontinue combination contraceptives before laparoscopic tubal sterilization or other brief surgical procedures not known to be associated with an elevated VTE risk.

Hormonal Contraception in Women with Hypercoagulable States

Women with familial thrombophilic syndromes, including factor V Leiden mutation, prothrombin G2010 A mutation, and protein C, protein S, or antithrombin deficiency have an elevated risk for VTE during COCP use and pregnancy and can develop VTE earlier during use than lower-risk users.[169] Women with factor V Leiden mutation have an increased risk of VTE of about eightfold compared with women without the mutation, and the risk is more than 30 times higher for carriers who used COCPs compared with nonusers who are not carriers of the mutation.[170] Approximately 5% of women of reproductive age are thought to carry the factor V Leiden mutation, but many of them will never experience a thrombotic event. In light of this, screening for factor V Leiden mutations or other thrombophilias is not considered to be cost-effective in the U.S. population considering estrogen-containing contraception in the absence of a clear family or personal history of thrombosis.[170] However, women with known familial thrombophilic conditions should be encouraged to use progestin-only and intrauterine contraception.

Hormonal Contraception in Women Taking Anticoagulation Therapy

The long-term risks of warfarin for reproductive-age women include heavy or prolonged menstrual bleeding and rarely include hemoperitoneum after rupture of ovarian cysts. Warfarin is a teratogen. Because COCPs can reduce menstrual blood loss and do not appear to increase the risk of recurrent thrombosis in well-anticoagulated women,[171] some authorities recommend their use in these patients. However, no large studies address the safety of estrogen-containing contraceptives in women taking oral anticoagulation, and many experts recommend the use of progestin-only or intrauterine contraception in this setting. Because use of the copper IUD increases menstrual flow, use of the LNG-IUS is more appropriate in this situation.[172] Since intramuscular injection of DMPA consistently suppresses ovulation and anecdotal experience has not revealed injection site problems such as hematoma in anticoagulated women, DMPA represents another potential contraceptive choice in this patient population.

Hormonal Contraception in Obese Women

The proportion of Americans who are obese (BMI ≥ 30) has risen to 30% (http://www.cdc.gov/nchs/ [accessed August 2010]). Concerns about obesity and contraception include possible complications such as VTE or reduced efficacy (particularly with low-dose methods) and the increased risk of pregnancy associated with obesity. The prospect of effective contraception with weight loss may also provide a window of opportunity for obese women to achieve a normal BMI, increase their chances of successful pregnancy, and reduce pregnancy complications. There is some evidence that obese sexually active women (and diabetic women) may be less likely to use contraception than normal-weight women.[173] Because pregnancy confers increased risks to mother and child in these pregnancies, the clinician must ensure that safe and effective contraception is provided when pregnancy is not planned.

The efficacy of COCPs, contraceptive rings, and transdermal patches primarily reflects the suppression of ovulation that results from the dose of progestin. Time to reach steady-state levels of levonorgestrel after ingestion appears to be twice as long among obese women compared with women of normal weight; the interval until hypothalamic-pituitary-ovarian activity is suppressed may be lengthened, placing obese women at higher risk for ovulation.[174]

The true rate of contraceptive failure in overweight and obese women is unknown, because past clinical trials of efficacy routinely excluded women who weighed more than 90 kg. The failure rate among obese COCP users is estimated to be between 60% and 120% greater than among those with a normal BMI.[174] Despite this observation, COCPs are more effective than barrier methods in obese women.

In clinical trials of the transdermal patch, women in the highest weight decile (≥90 kg) had a substantially higher contraceptive failure rate.[42] The incrementally higher rates in this setting with oral and transdermal methods should not exclude their use in overweight women motivated to use these methods in preference to less effective methods.

Obese women who are concerned about the possibility of decreased efficacy of the COCPs can consider using an IUD or implant as highly effective alternatives, especially because many obese women have hypertension and other risk factors for vascular disease that may be exacerbated by exogenous estrogen. There is relatively little high-quality information regarding the efficacy of DMPA in obese women, but in overweight women, higher pregnancy rates have not been observed with use of the 150-mg intramuscular or 106-mg subcutaneous formulations of DMPA.[56] Although DMPA does not appear to increase BMI in all women, adolescents who are already obese may gain more weight when using DMPA compared with other methods.[175]

The health risks associated with use of estrogen-containing contraceptives may be increased in obese women. Exogenous estrogen and obesity are independent risk factors for VTE. Case-control studies suggest that higher BMI values (>25) may increase the risk of VTE by up to 10-fold in COCP users.[176] Because age also represents an independent risk factor for VTE, the ACOG recommends use of progestin-only and intrauterine contraceptives in obese women older than 35 years.[28] In helping overweight women make sound contraceptive choices, practitioners should incorporate these observations in discussions with patients. Because obese women have an elevated risk for dysfunctional uterine bleeding and endometrial neoplasia, use of the LNG-IUS may represent a particularly sound choice.

Hormonal Contraception in Women with Systemic Lupus Erythematosus

Although effective contraception is important for women with lupus, concerns about increasing disease activity and thrombosis have resulted in clinicians rarely prescribing combination estrogen-progestin oral contraceptives to women with this disease. However, level 1 data indicate that COCPs are safe in women with systemic lupus erythematosus (SLE) if they have stable, mild disease; are seronegative for antiphospholipid antibodies; and have no history of thrombosis.[177] Among those with the antiphospholipid syndrome, there may be a high incidence of thrombosis in COCP users, suggesting that estrogen-containing contraceptives should be avoided.[178]

Providing effective contraception for women with SLE is extremely important. Pregnancy carries marked maternal and fetal risks, and almost one fourth of women with SLE who conceive choose to terminate their pregnancies.[179] Although there are limited data regarding the safety of IUDs in women with SLE, they provide highly effective birth control and may represent a sensible option for these patients.[180]

Hormonal Contraception in Women with Sickle Cell Disease

Similar to pregnancy in SLE patients, pregnancy in women with sickle cell disease increases maternal and fetal morbidity and mortality. The safety of hormonal contraceptives in women with homozygous sickle cell (SS) disease has been controversial. Only one small, randomized, controlled trial has addressed this issue. Twenty-five patients were randomized to three monthly DMPA or intramuscular saline placebo injections in a crossover design. DMPA users were less likely to experience painful sickle episodes (odds ration = 0.23; 95% CI, 0.05 to 1.02).[181] No randomized studies have addressed estrogen-containing products. These limited data suggest that DMPA is a safe contraceptive option for women with sickle cell disease. In addition to providing effective contraception, DMPA may reduce sickle pain crises.[66]

No well-controlled study has assessed whether VTE risk in oral contraception users with sickle cell disease is higher than in other combination oral contraception users. However, a small, U.S., case-control study found that COCP use was associated with a nonsignificantly elevated risk of VTE.[182] Cross-sectional studies of women with sickle cell disease have observed no differences in markers for platelet activation, thrombin generation, fibrinolysis, or red cell deformability between users of combination oral contraception methods, progestin-only methods, and nonusers of hormonal contraception.[183] On the basis of these observations, studies of pregnant women with sickle cell disease, and small, observational studies of women with sickle cell disease who use COCPs and on theoretical considerations, the ACOG concludes that pregnancy carries a greater risk than estrogen-containing contraceptive use.[28]

Hormonal Contraception in Depression

Depression and mood disorders are extremely common in women of reproductive age. The issues to consider are the impact of hormonal contraceptives on mood and the potential impact of treatments for depression on contraceptive efficacy.

Data on the use of hormonal contraceptives in women with depression are limited but usually show no effect. Women with depressive disorders do not appear to suffer worsening of symptoms with use of hormonal methods of contraception. However, depression is one of the most commonly stated reasons for discontinuation of COCPs.[184] Unfortunately, few data help clinicians advise women with a history of anxiety or depression regarding appropriate contraceptive choices.

Prescription antidepressants do not affect the efficacy of hormonal contraceptives.[28] Data from randomized, controlled trials of fluoxetine have failed to confirm any effect of COCPs on the response to fluoxetine.[185] However, the herbal remedy St. John's wort, a hepatic enzyme inducer, increased progestin and estrogen metabolism, breakthrough bleeding, and the likelihood of ovulation in women using COCPs.[186] The relationship between DMPA use and depression has been controversial, and studies have failed to identify a causal relationship between the two.[55]

CHOOSING A CONTRACEPTIVE METHOD

Given the number of contraceptive options available to women, it is important that providers concentrate their efforts on helping women chose the best contraceptive method and focus on counseling that helps improve continuation. The best birth control method is one that provides the safest and most effective contraceptive for a woman and is the method she chooses to use and has access to. This approach places a strong value on medical considerations but also includes consideration of a woman's lifestyle, preferences, and level of prevention desired. Long-acting contraceptives (i.e., IUD and implant) offer women the advantages of high contraceptive efficacy and high rates of continuation. When discussing contraception, physicians should present all suitable options to their patients, including long-acting methods.

When helping women make sound contraceptive decisions, clinicians should consider the patient's age, lifestyle, and other relevant circumstances, including the recognition that contraceptive needs are likely to change during different phases of reproductive life and that the risks and benefits may alter according to age and background health factors. For those considering pregnancy in the future, contraceptive reversibility and time to return of fertility should be discussed. Affordability must be considered, because it may affect continuation rates and therefore affect efficacy.

All contraceptives have potential side effects. Discussion of these effects and other areas of patient preparation may increase acceptability. The clinician should provide information about adverse events that are individualized and provided in the context of how they compare with the effects of an unplanned pregnancy. Information about contraceptive failure and access to emergency contraception should be offered. For those at risk for sexually transmitted diseases, hormonal contraception cannot provide reliable protection. The physician should encourage consistent condom use and minimizing the number of partners, regardless of contraceptive choice. No method of contraception is perfect. Each woman must consider the advantages and disadvantages of each method in making her decision. The most effective method is likely to be the one that she can use successfully.

REFERENCES

1. Manlove J, Ikramullah E, Mincieli L, et al. Trends in sexual experience, contraceptive use, and teenage childbearing: 1992-2002. *J Adolesc Health*. 2009;44:413-423.
2. Skinner SR, Hickey M. Current priorities for adolescent sexual and reproductive health in Australia. *Med J Aust*. 2003;179:158-161.
3. Sarkar NN. Barriers to emergency contraception (EC): does promoting EC increase risk for contracting sexually transmitted infections, HIV/AIDS? *Int J Clin Pract*. 2008;62:1769-1775.
4. Dinger JC, Heinemann LA, Kühl-Habich D. The safety of a drospirenone-containing oral contraceptive: final results from the European Active

Surveillance Study on oral contraceptives based on 142,475 women-years of observation. *Contraception*. 2007;75:344-354.
5. Coffee AL, Kuehl TJ, Willis S, et al. Oral contraceptives and premenstrual symptoms: comparison of a 21/7 and extended regimen. *Am J Obstet Gynecol*. 2006;195:1311-1319.
6. Archer DF. Menstrual-cycle-related symptoms: a review of the rationale for continuous use of oral contraceptives. *Contraception*. 2006; 74:359-366.
7. Trussell J. Understanding contraceptive failure. *Best Pract Res Clin Obstet Gynaecol*. 2009;23:199-209.
8. Westhoff C, Heartwell S, Edwards S, et al. Initiation of oral contraceptives using a quick start compared with a conventional start: a randomized controlled trial. *Obstet Gynecol*. 2007;109:1270-1276.
9. Bracken M. Oral contraception and congenital malformations in offspring: a review and meta-analysis of the prospective studies. *Obstet Gynecol*. 1990;76:552-557.
10. Hassan MA, Killick SR. Is previous use of hormonal contraception associated with a detrimental effect on subsequent fecundity? *Hum Reprod*. 2004;19:344-351.
11. Panser LA, Phipps WR. Type of oral contraceptive in relation to acute, initial episodes of pelvic inflammatory disease. *Contraception*. 1991;43:91-99.
12. Franks AL, Beral V, Cates W Jr, et al. Contraception and ectopic pregnancy risk. *Am J Obstet Gynecol*. 1990;163:1120-1123.
13. Martins SL, Curtis KM, Glasier AF. Combined hormonal contraception and bone health: a systematic review. *Contraception*. 2006; 73:445-469.
14. Tworoger SS, Fairfield KM, Colditz GA, et al. Association of oral contraceptive use, other contraceptive methods, and infertility with ovarian cancer risk. *Am J Epidemiol*. 2007;166:894-901.
15. Collaborative Group on Epidemiological Studies of Ovarian Cancer, Beral V, Doll R, et al. Ovarian cancer and oral contraceptives: collaborative reanalysis of data from 45 epidemiological studies including 23,257 women with ovarian cancer and 87,303 controls. *Lancet*. 2008;371:303-314.
16. Antoniou AC, Rookus M, Andrieu N, et al. Reproductive and hormonal factors, and ovarian cancer risk for BRCA1 and BRCA2 mutation carriers: results from the International BRCA1/2 Carrier Cohort Study. *Cancer Epidemiol Biomarkers Prev*. 2009;18:601-610.
17. Jick SS, Walker AM, Jick H. Oral contraceptives and endometrial cancer. *Obstet Gynecol*. 1993;82:931-935.
18. Fernandez E, La Vecchia C, Balducci A, et al. Oral contraceptives and colorectal cancer risk: a meta-analysis. *Br J Cancer*. 2001;84: 722-727.
19. George R, Clarke S, Thiboutot D. Hormonal therapy for acne. *Semin Cutan Med Surg*. 2008;27:188-196.
20. Lopez LM, Kaptein A, Helmerhorst FM. Oral contraceptives containing drospirenone for premenstrual syndrome. Cochrane Database Syst Rev 2009;(2):CD006586.
21. Gallo MF, Nanda K, Grimes DA, et al. 20 microg versus >20 microg estrogen combined oral contraceptives for contraception. Cochrane Database Syst Rev 2008;(4):CD003989.
22. Allais G, Gabellari IC, De Lorenzo C, et al. Oral contraceptives in migraine. *Expert Rev Neurother*. 2009;9:381-393.
23. Kaunitz AM. Hormonal contraception for the older reproductive age woman. *N Engl J Med*. 2008;358:1262-1270.
24. Stang A, Schwingl P, Rivera R. New contraceptive eligibility checklists for provision of combined oral contraceptives and depot-medroxyprogesterone acetate in community-based programmes. *Bull World Health Organ*. 2000;78:1015-1023.
25. Martínez F, Avecilla A. Combined hormonal contraception and venous thromboembolism. *Eur J Contracept Reprod Health Care*. 2007; 12:97-106.
26. Severinsen MT, Kristensen SR, Johnsen SP, et al. Smoking and venous thromboembolism: a Danish follow-up study. *J Thromb Haemost*. 2009;8:1297-1303.
27. Lowe GD. Common risk factors for both arterial and venous thrombosis. *Br J Haematol*. 2008;140:488-495.
28. ACOG Committee on Practice Bulletins–Gynecology. ACOG practice bulletin no. 73: Use of hormonal contraception in women with coexisting medical conditions. *Obstet Gynecol*. 2006;107:1453-1472.
29. ESHRE Capri Workshop Group. Hormones and cardiovascular health in women. *Hum Reprod Update*. 2006;12:483-497.
30. Silvera SA, Miller AB, Rohan TE. Oral contraceptive use and risk of breast cancer among women with a family history of breast cancer: a prospective cohort study. *Cancer Causes Control*. 2005;16:1059-1063.
31. Bermejo-Pérez MJ, Márquez-Calderón S, Llanos-Méndez A. Effectiveness of preventive interventions in BRCA1/2 gene mutation carriers: a systematic review. *Int J Cancer*. 2007;121:225-231.
32. International Collaboration of Epidemiological Studies of Cervical Cancer, Appleby P, Beral V, et al. Cervical cancer and hormonal contraceptives: collaborative reanalysis of individual data for 16,573 women with cervical cancer and 35,509 women without cervical cancer from 24 epidemiological studies: I. *Lancet*. 2007;370: 1609-1621.
33. Truitt ST, Fraser AB, Grimes DA, et al. Hormonal contraception during lactation: systematic review of randomized controlled trials. *Contraception*. 2003;68:233-238.
34. Dutton C, Foldvary-Schaefer N. Contraception in women with epilepsy: pharmacokinetic interactions, contraceptive options, and management. *Int Rev Neurobiol*. 2008;83:113-134.
35. Bjarnadóttir RI, Tuppurainen M, Killick SR. Comparison of cycle control with a combined vaginal ring and oral levonorgestrel/ethinyl estradiol. *Am J Obstet Gynecol*. 2002;186:389-395.
36. Abrams LS, Skee DM, Wong FA, et al. Pharmacokinetics of norelgestromin and ethinyl estradiol from two consecutive contraceptive patches. *J Clin Pharmacol*. 2001;41:1232-1237.
37. Lopez LM, Grimes DA, Gallo MF, et al. Skin patch and vaginal ring versus combined oral contraceptives for contraception. Cochrane Database Syst Rev 2010;(1):CD003552.
38. Thurman AR, Hammond N, Brown HE, et al. Preventing repeat teen pregnancy: postpartum depot medroxyprogesterone acetate, oral contraceptive pills, or the patch? *J Pediatr Adolesc Gynecol*. 2007;20:61-65.
39. Shimoni N, Westhoff C. Review of the vaginal contraceptive ring (NuvaRing). *J Fam Plann Reprod Health Care*. 2008;34:247-250.
40. Mulders TM, Dieben TO. Use of the novel combined contraceptive vaginal ring NuvaRing for ovulation inhibition. *Fertil Steril*. 2001;75:865-870.
41. Roumen FJME, Apter D, Mulders TMS, et al. Efficacy, tolerability and acceptability of a novel contraceptive vaginal ring releasing etonogestrel and ethinyl estradiol. *Hum Reprod*. 2001;16:469-475.
42. Zieman M, Guillebaud J, Weisberg E, et al. Contraceptive efficacy and cycle control with Ortho Evra/Evra transdermal system: the analysis of pooled data. *Fertil Steril*. 2002;77:S13-S18.
43. van den Heuvel MW, van Bragt AJ, Alnabawy AK, et al. Comparison of ethinylestradiol pharmacokinetics in three hormonal contraceptive formulations: the vaginal ring, the transdermal patch and an oral contraceptive. *Contraception*. 2005;72:168-174.
44. Jick S, Kaye JA, Li L, Jick H. Further results on the risk of nonfatal venous thromboembolism in users of the contraceptive transdermal patch compared to users of oral contraceptives containing norgestimate and 35 microg of ethinyl estradiol. *Contraception*. 2007;76:4-7.
45. Erkkola R, Landgren BM. Role of progestins in contraception. *Acta Obstet Gynecol Scand*. 2005;84:207-216.
46. Trussell J. Contraceptive failure in the United States. *Contraception*. 2004;70:89.
47. ESHRE Capri Workshop Group. Ovarian and endometrial function during hormonal contraception. *Hum Reprod*. 2001;16:1527-1535.
48. Godsland IF, Crook D, Simpson R, et al. The effects of different formulations of oral contraceptive agents on lipid and carbohydrate metabolism. *N Engl J Med*. 1990;323:1375-1381.
49. Kjos SL, Peters RK, Xiang A, et al. Contraception and the risk of type 2 diabetes in Latino women with prior gestational diabetes. *JAMA*. 1998;280:533-538.
50. Furlong L. Ectopic pregnancy risk when contraception fails: a review. *J Reprod Med*. 2002;47:881-885.
51. Caird LE, Reid-Thomas V, Hannan WJ, et al. Oral progestogen-only contraception may protect against loss of bone mass in breast-feeding women. *Clin Endocrinol (Oxf)*. 1994;41:739-745.
52. Halderman LD, Nelson AL. Impact of early postpartum administration of progestin-only hormonal contraceptives compared with nonhormonal contraceptives on short-term breast-feeding patterns. *Am J Obstet Gynecol*. 2002;186:1250-1256; discussion 1256-1258.
53. Rodriguez MI, Kaunitz AM. An evidence-based approach to postpartum use of depot medroxyprogesterone acetate in breastfeeding women. *Contraception*. 2009;80:4-6.
54. Kaunitz AM, Darney PD, Ross D, et al. Subcutaneous DMPA vs. intramuscular DMPA: a 2-year randomized study of contraceptive efficacy and bone mineral density. *Contraception*. 2009;80:7-17.
55. Kaunitz AM. Current concepts regarding use of DMPA. *J Reprod Med*. 2002;47:785-789.
56. Jain J, Jakimiuk AJ, Bode FR, et al. Contraceptive efficacy and safety of DMPA-SC. *Contraception*. 2004;70:269-275.
57. Lopez LM, Newmann SJ, Grimes DA, et al. Immediate start of hormonal contraceptives for contraception. Cochrane Database Syst Rev 2008;(2):CD006260.
58. Borgatta L, Murthy A, Chuang C, et al. Pregnancies diagnosed during Depo-Provera use. *Contraception*. 2002;66:169-172.
59. d'Arcangues C. Management of vaginal bleeding irregularities induced by progestin-only contraceptives. *Hum Reprod*. 2000;15:24-29.
60. Belsey EM. Menstrual bleeding patterns in untreated women and with long-acting methods of contraception. Task Force on Long-Acting Systemic Agents for Fertility Regulation. *Adv Contracept*. 1991;7:257-270.
61. Arias RD, Jain JK, Brucker C, et al. Changes in bleeding patterns with depot medroxyprogesterone acetate subcutaneous injection 104 mg. *Contraception*. 2006;74:234-238.
62. Jain JK, Nicosia AF, Nucatola DL, et al. Mifepristone for the prevention of breakthrough bleeding in new starters of depo-medroxyprogesterone acetate. *Steroids*. 2003;68:1115-1119.

63. Abdel-Aleem H, d'Arcangues C, Vogelsong KM, et al. Treatment of vaginal bleeding irregularities induced by progestin only contraceptives. Cochrane Database Syst Rev 2007;(4):CD003449.
64. Crosignani PG, Luciano A, Ray A, et al. Subcutaneous depot medroxyprogesterone acetate versus leuprolide acetate in the treatment of endometriosis-associated pain. *Hum Reprod.* 2006;21:248-256.
65. Mangan SA, Larsen PG, Hudson S. Overweight teens at increased risk for weight gain while using depot medroxyprogesterone acetate. *J Pediatr Adolesc Gynecol.* 2002;15:79-82.
66. Manchikanti A, Grimes DA, Lopez LM, et al. Steroid hormones for contraception in women with sickle cell disease. Cochrane Database Syst Rev 2007;(2):CD006261.
67. Baeten JM, Nyange PM, Richardson BA, et al. Hormonal contraception and risk of sexually transmitted disease acquisition: results from a prospective study. *Am J Obstet Gynecol.* 2001;185:380-385.
68. Practice Committee of American Society for Reproductive Medicine. Treatment of pelvic pain associated with endometriosis. *Fertil Steril.* 2008;90:S260-S269.
69. Kaunitz AM. Depot medroxyprogesterone acetate contraception and the risk of breast and gynecologic cancer. *J Reprod Med.* 1996; 41:419-427.
70. Skegg DC, Noonan EA, Paul C, et al. Depot medroxyprogesterone acetate and breast cancer: a pooled analysis of the World Health Organization and New Zealand studies. *JAMA.* 1995;273:799-804.
71. Mishell DJ. Pharmacokinetics of depot medroxyprogesterone acetate contraception. *J Reprod Med.* 1996;41:381-390.
72. Clark MK, Sowers M, Levy BT, et al. Magnitude and variability of sequential estradiol and progesterone concentrations in women using depot medroxyprogesterone acetate for contraception. *Fertil Steril.* 2001;75:871-877.
73. Gbolade BA. Depo-Provera and bone density. *J Fam Plann Reprod Health Care.* 2002;28:7-11.
74. American College of Obstetricians and Gynecologists Committee on Gynecologic Practice. ACOG Committee Opinion No. 415: Depot medroxyprogesterone acetate and bone effects. *Obstet Gynecol.* 2008;112:727-730.
75. Clark MK, Sowers MFR, Nichols S, et al. Bone mineral density changes over two years in first-time users of depot medroxyprogesterone acetate. *Fertil Steril.* 2004;82:1580-1586.
76. Scholes D, LaCroix AZ, Ichikawa LE. Injectable hormone contraception and bone density: results from a prospective study. *Epidemiology.* 2002;13:581-587.
77. Westhoff C. Depot-medroxyprogesterone acetate injection (Depo-Provera): a highly effective contraceptive option with proven long-term safety. *Contraception.* 2003;68:75-87.
78. Kaunitz AM, Arias R, McClung M. Bone density recovery after depot medroxyprogesterone acetate injectable contraception use. *Contraception.* 2008;77:67-76.
79. Lappe JM, Stegman MR, Recker RR. The impact of lifestyle factors on stress fractures in female Army recruits. *Osteoporos Int.* 2001;12: 35-42.
80. Watson KC, Lentz MJ, Cain KC. Associations between fracture incidence and use of depot medroxyprogesterone acetate and anti-epileptic drugs in women with developmental disabilities. *Womens Health Issues.* 2006;16:346-352.
81. Vestergaard P, Rejnmark L, Mosekilde L. The effects of depot medroxyprogesterone acetate and intrauterine device use on fracture risk in Danish women. *Contraception.* 2008;78:459-464.
82. Paschall S, Kaunitz AM. Depo-Provera and skeletal health: a survey of Florida obstetrics and gynecologist physicians. *Contraception.* 2008;78: 370-376.
83. Kaunitz AM, Miller P, Rice VM, et al. Bone mineral density in women aged 25-35 years receiving depot medroxyprogesterone acetate: recovery following discontinuation. *Contraception.* 2006;74:90-99.
84. Clark MK, Sowers MFR, Nichols S, et al. Bone mineral density loss and recovery during 48 months in first-time users of depot medroxyprogesterone acetate. *Fertil Steril.* 2006;86:1466-1474.
85. Scholes D, Lacroix AZ, Ichikawa LE, et al. Change in bone mineral density among adolescent women using and discontinuing depot medroxyprogesterone acetate contraception: change in bone mineral density among adolescent women using and discontinuing depot medroxyprogesterone acetate contraception. *Arch Pediatr Adolesc Med.* 2005;158:139-144.
86. Orr-Walker BJ, Evans MC, Ames RW, et al. The effect of past use of the injectable contraceptive depot medroxyprogesterone acetate on bone mineral density in normal post-menopausal women. *Clin Endocrinol (Oxf).* 1998;49:615-618.
87. Petitti DB, Piaggio G, Mehta S, et al. Steroid hormone contraception and bone mineral density: a cross-sectional study in an international population. The WHO Study of Hormonal Contraception and Bone Health. *Obstet Gynecol.* 2000;95:736-744.
88. Curtis KM, Martins SL. Progestogen-only contraception and bone mineral density: a systematic review. *Contraception.* 2006;73:470-487.
89. Cromer BA, Scholes D, Berenson A, et al. Depot medroxyprogesterone acetate and bone mineral density in adolescents—the Black Box Warning: a Position Paper of the Society for Adolescent Medicine. *J Adolesc Health.* 2006;39:296-301.
90. World Health Organization. *WHO Statement on Hormonal Contraception and Bone Health.* Geneva, Switzerland: 2005:1-2.
91. Black A. Canadian contraception consensus—update on depot medroxyprogesterone acetate (DMPA). *J Obstet Gynaecol Can.* 2006;28:305-313.
92. Myer L, Denny L, Wright TC, et al. Prospective study of hormonal contraception and women's risk of HIV infection in South Africa. *Int J Epidemiol.* 2007;36:166-174.
93. Overton ET, Shacham E, Singhatiraj E, et al. Incidence of sexually transmitted infections among HIV-infected women using depot medroxyprogesterone acetate contraception. *Contraception.* 2008; 78:125-130.
94. Morrison CS, Turner AN, Jones LB. Highly effective contraception and acquisition of HIV and other sexually transmitted infections. *Best Pract Res Clin Obstet Gynaecol.* 2009;23:263-284.
95. Mavranezouli I. Health economics of contraception. *Best Pract Res Clin Obstet Gynaecol.* 2009;23:187-198.
96. Jensen JT. Contraceptive and therapeutic effects of the levonorgestrel intrauterine system: an overview. *Obstet Gynecol Surv.* 2005; 60:604-612.
97. Andersson K, Batar I, Rybo G. Return to fertility after removal of a levonorgestrel-releasing intrauterine device and Nova-T. *Contraception.* 1992;46:575-584.
98. Lähteenmäki P, Rauramo I, Backman T. The levonorgestrel intrauterine system in contraception. *Steroids.* 2000;65:693-697.
99. French R, Sorhaindo AM, Van Vliet H, et al. Progstogen-releasing intrauterine systems versus other forms of reversible contraceptives for contraception. Cochrane Database Syst Rev 2004;3:CD001776.
100. ESHRE Capri Workshop Group. Intrauterine devices and intrauterine systems. *Hum Reprod Update.* 2008;14:197-208.
101. Van Houdenhoven K, van Kaam KJ, van Grootheest AC, et al. Uterine perforation in women using a levonorgestrel-releasing intrauterine system. *Contraception.* 2006;73:257-260.
102. Martínez F, López-Arregui E. Infection risk and intrauterine devices. *Acta Obstet Gynecol Scand.* 2009;88:246-250.
103. ACOG Committee on Practice Bulletins–Gynecology. ACOG practice bulletin: Clinical management guidelines for obstetrician-gynecologists. Number 59, January 2005: Intrauterine device. *Obstet Gynecol.* 2005;105: 223-232.
104. Practice Committee of American Society for Reproductive Medicine. Hormonal contraception: recent advances and controversies. *Fertil Steril.* 2008;90(5 suppl):S103-S113.
105. Lethaby AE, Cooke I, Rees M. Progesterone or progestogen-releasing intrauterine systems for heavy menstrual bleeding. Cochrane Database Syst Rev 2005;(4):CD002126.
106. Kaunitz AM. Progestin-releasing intrauterine systems and leiomyoma. *Contraception.* 2007;75:S130-S133.
107. Sheng J, Zhang WY, Zhang JP, et al. The LNG-IUS study on adenomyosis: a 3-year follow-up study on the efficacy and side effects of the use of levonorgestrel intrauterine system for the treatment of dysmenorrhea associated with adenomyosis. *Contraception.* 2009;79:189-193.
108. Petta CA, Ferriani RA, Abrao MS, et al. Randomized clinical trial of a levonorgestrel-releasing intrauterine system and a depot GnRH analogue for the treatment of chronic pelvic pain in women with endometriosis. *Hum Reprod.* 2005;20:1993-1998.
109. Petta CA, Ferriani RA, Abrão MS, et al. A 3-year follow-up of women with endometriosis and pelvic pain users of the levonorgestrel-releasing intrauterine system. *Eur J Obstet Gynecol Reprod Biol.* 2009;143:128-129.
110. Wildemeersch D, Pylyser K, De Wever N, et al. Endometrial safety after 5 years of continuous combined transdermal estrogen and intrauterine levonorgestrel delivery for postmenopausal hormone substitution. *Maturitas.* 2007;57:205-209.
111. Chin J, Konje J, Hickey M. Levonorgestrel intrauterine system for endometrial protection in women with breast cancer on adjuvant tamoxifen. Cochrane Database Syst Rev 2009;(4):CD007245.
112. Haimovich S, Checa MA, Mancebo G, et al. Treatment of endometrial hyperplasia without atypia in peri- and postmenopausal women with a levonorgestrel intrauterine device. *Menopause.* 2008;15: 1002-1004.
113. Montz FJ, Bristow RE, Bovicelli A, et al. Intrauterine progesterone treatment of early endometrial cancer. *Am J Obstet Gynecol.* 2002;186: 651-657.
114. Díaz S. Contraceptive implants and lactation. *Contraception.* 2002;65: 39-46.
115. Hohmann H, Creinin MD. The contraceptive implant. *Clin Obstet Gynecol.* 2007;50:907-917.
116. Funk S, Miller MM, Mishell DR Jr, et al. The Implanon US Study Group. Safety and efficacy of Implanon, a single-rod implantable contraceptive containing etonogestrel. *Contraception.* 2005;71:319-326.
117. Darney P, Patel A, Rosen K, et al. Safety and efficacy of a single-rod etonogestrel implant (Implanon): results from 11 international clinical trials. *Fertil Steril.* 2009;91:1646-1653.

118. Weisberg E, Fraser I. Australian women's experience with Implanon. *Aust Fam Physician*. 2005;34:694-696.
119. Mansour D, Korver T, Marintcheva-Petrova M, et al. The effects of Implanon on menstrual bleeding patterns. *Eur J Contracept Reprod Health Care*. 2008;13:13-28.
120. Diaz S, Croxatto HB, Pavez M, et al. Clinical assessment of treatments for prolonged bleeding in users of Norplant implants. *Contraception*. 1990;42:97-109.
121. Weisberg E, Hickey M, Palmer D, et al. A randomized controlled trial of treatment options for troublesome uterine bleeding in Implanon users. *Hum Reprod*. 2009;24:1852-1861.
122. Merki-Feld GS, Imthurn B, Seifert B. Effects of the progestagen-only contraceptive implant Implanon on cardiovascular risk factors. *Clin Endocrinol (Oxf)*. 2008;68:355-360.
123. Biswas A, Biswas S, Viegas OA. Effect of etonogestrel subdermal contraceptive implant (Implanon) on liver function tests: a randomized comparative study with Norplant implants. *Contraception*. 2004;70: 379-382.
124. Croxatto HB. Progestin implants. *Steroids*. 2000;65:681-685.
125. Pymar HC, Creinin MD, Schwartz JL. "Pop-out" method of levonorgestrel implant removal. *Contraception*. 1999;59:383-387.
126. Allen RH, Goldberg AB. Emergency contraception: a clinical review. *Clin Obstet Gynecol*. 2007;50:927-936.
127. Yuzpe AA. Postcoital contraception. *Int J Gynaecol Obstet*. 1978; 16:497-501.
128. Cheng L, Gülmezoglu AM, Oel CJ, et al. Interventions for emergency contraception. Cochrane Database Syst Rev 2008;(2):CD001324.
129. Rodrigues I, Grou F, Joly J. Effectiveness of emergency contraceptive pills between 72 and 120 hours after unprotected sexual intercourse. *Am J Obstet Gynecol*. 2001;184:531-537.
130. Davidoff F, Trussell J. Plan B and the politics of doubt. *JAMA*. 2006;296:1775-1778.
131. Wilcox AJ, Dunson DB, Weinberg CR, et al. Likelihood of conception with a single act of intercourse: providing benchmark rates for assessment of post-coital contraceptives. *Contraception*. 2001;63: 211-215.
132. Raymond E, Taylor D, Trussell J, et al. Minimum effectiveness of the levonorgestrel regimen of emergency contraception. *Contraception*. 2004;69:79-81.
133. World Health Organization. *Medical Eligibility Criteria for Contraceptive Use*, 3rd ed. Geneva: WHO; 2004. (4th ed. in press 2009).
134. Raymond EG, Trussell J, Polis CB. Population effect of increased access to emergency contraceptive pills: a systematic review. *Obstet Gynecol*. 2007;109:181-188.
135. Chabbert-Buffet N, Meduri G, Bouchard P, et al. Selective progesterone receptor modulators and progesterone antagonists: mechanisms of action and clinical applications. *Hum Reprod Update*. 2005;11: 293-307.
136. Lakha F, Ho PC, Van der Spuy ZM, et al. A novel estrogen-free oral contraceptive pill for women: multicentre, double-blind, randomized controlled trial of mifepristone and progestogen-only pill (levonorgestrel). *Hum Reprod*. 2007;22:2428-2436.
137. von Hertzen H, Van Look PF. Antiprogestins for contraception? *Semin Reprod Med*. 2005;23:92-100.
138. Gemzell-Danielsson K, van Heusden AM, Killick SR, et al. Improving cycle control in progestogen-only contraceptive pill users by intermittent treatment with a new anti-progestogen. *Hum Reprod*. 2002;17:2588-2593.
139. Cheng L, Zhu H, Wang A, et al. Once a month administration of mifepristone improves bleeding patterns in women using subdermal contraceptive implants releasing levonorgestrel. *Hum Reprod*. 2000;15: 1969-1972.
140. Gupta N, Corrado S, Goldstein M. Hormonal contraception for the adolescent. *Pediatr Rev*. 2008;29:386-396.
141. Tolaymat LL, Kaunitz AM. Long-acting contraceptives in adolescents. *Curr Opin Obstet Gynecol*. 2007;19:453-460.
142. American College of Obstetricians and Gynecologists. ACOG Committee Opinion 392: Intrauterine device and adolescents. *Obstet Gynecol*. 2007;210:1493-1495.
143. Berenson AB, Rahman M. Changes in weight, total fat, percent body fat, and central-to-peripheral fat ratio associated with injectable and oral contraceptive use. *Am J Obstet Gynecol*. 2009;200:329.e1-329.e8.
144. Casper RF, Dodin S, Reid RL. The effect of 20 μg ethinyl estradiol/1 mg norethindrone acetate (Minestrin™), a low-dose oral contraceptive, on vaginal bleeding patterns, hot flashes, and quality of life in symptomatic perimenopausal women. *Menopause*. 1997;4:139-147.
145. Tanis BC, van den Bosch MA, Kemmeren JM, et al. Oral contraceptives and the risk of myocardial infarction. *N Engl J Med*. 2001;345:1787-1793.
146. Shufelt CL, Bairey Merz CN. Contraceptive hormone use and cardiovascular disease. *J Am Coll Cardiol*. 2009;53:221-231.
147. van Rooijen M, von Schoultz B, Silveira A, et al. Different effects of oral contraceptives containing levonorgestrel or desogestrel on plasma lipoproteins and coagulation factor VII. *Am J Obstet Gynecol*. 2002;186:44-48.
148. Ng YW, Liang S, Singh K. Effects of Mirena (levonorgestrel-releasing intrauterine system) and Ortho Gynae T380 intrauterine copper device on lipid metabolism: a randomized comparative study. *Contraception*. 2009;79:24-28.
149. Lopez LM, Grimes DA, Schulz KF. Steroidal contraceptives: effect on carbohydrate metabolism in women without diabetes mellitus. Cochrane Database Syst Rev 2009;(4):CD00613.
150. Rogovskaya S, Rivera R, Grimes DA, et al. Effect of a levonorgestrel intrauterine system on women with type 1 diabetes: a randomized trial. *Obstet Gynecol*. 2005;105:811-815.
151. Hartmann LC, Sellers TA, Frost MH, et al. Benign breast disease and the risk of breast cancer. *N Engl J Med*. 2005;353:229-237.
152. Vessey M, Yeates D. Oral contraceptives and benign breast disease: an update of findings in a large cohort study. *Contraception*. 2007;76: 418-424.
153. Milne RL, Knight JA, John EM, et al. Oral contraceptive use and risk of early-onset breast cancer in carriers and non-carriers of BRCA 1 and BRCA 2 mutations. *Cancer Epidemiol Biomarkers Prev*. 2005;14: 350-356.
154. Antoniou A, Pharoah PD, Narod S, et al. Average risks of breast and ovarian cancer associated with BRCA1 or BRCA2 mutations detected in case series unselected for family history: a combined analysis of 22 studies. *Am J Hum Genet*. 2003;72:1117-1130.
155. Parker WH. Etiology, symptomatology, and diagnosis of uterine myomas. *Fertil Steril*. 2007;87:725-736.
156. Day Baird D, Dunson DB, Hill MC, et al. High cumulative incidence of uterine leiomyoma in black and white women: ultrasound evidence. *Am J Obstet Gynecol*. 2003;188:100-107.
157. Farquhar C, Brown J. Oral contraceptive pill for heavy menstrual bleeding. Cochrane Database Syst Rev 2009;(4):CD000154.
158. Parazzini F, Negri E, LaVecchia C, et al. Oral contraceptive use and risk of uterine fibroids. *Obstet Gynecol*. 1992;79:430-433.
159. Truitt ST, Fraser AB, Grimes DA, et al. Hormonal contraception during lactation: systematic review of randomized controlled trials. *Contraception*. 2003;68:233-228.
160. Bounds W, Guillebaud J. Observational series on women using the contraceptive Mirena concurrently with anti-epileptic and other enzyme-inducing drugs. *Fam Plann Reprod Health Care*. 2002;28: 78-80.
161. Dickinson BD, Altman RD, Nielsen NH, et al. Drug interactions between oral contraceptives and antibiotics. *Obstet Gynecol*. 2001;98: 853-860.
162. Heikinheimo O, Lähteenmäki P. Contraception and HIV infection in women. *Hum Reprod Update*. 2009;15:165-176.
163. Lehtovirta P, Paavonen J, Heikinheimo O. Experience with the levonorgestrel-releasing intrauterine system among HIV-infected women. *Contraception*. 2007;75:37-39.
164. [No authors listed]. Cardiovascular disease and use of oral and injectable progestogen-only contraceptives and combined injectable contraceptives: results of an international, multicenter, case-control study. World Health Organization Collaborative Study of Cardiovascular Disease and Steroid Hormone Contraception. *Contraception*. 1998;57: 315-324.
165. Bergendal A, Odlind V, Persson I, et al. Limited knowledge on progestogen-only contraception and risk of venous thromboembolism. *Acta Obstet Gynecol Scand*. 2009;88:261-266.
166. Vessey M, Mant D, Smith A, et al. Oral contraceptives and venous thromboembolism: findings in a large prospective study. *Br Med J*. 1986;292:526.
167. Robinson GE, Burren T, Mackie IJ, et al. Changes in haemostasis after stopping the combined contraceptive pill: implications for major surgery. *BMJ*. 1991;302;269-271.
168. Black C, Kaye JA, Jick H. Clinical risk factors for venous thromboembolus in users of the combined oral contraceptive pill. *Br J Clin Pharmacol*. 2002;53:637-640.
169. Bloemenkamp KW, Rosendaal FR, Helmerhorst FM, et al. Higher risk of venous thrombosis during early use of oral contraceptives in women with inherited clotting defects. *Arch Intern Med*. 2000;160:49-52.
170. Vandenbroucke JP, Rosing J, Bloemenkamp KW, et al. Oral contraceptives and the risk of venous thrombosis. *N Engl J Med*. 2001;344: 1527-1535.
171. Comp PC. Thrombophilic mechanisms of OCs. *Int J Fertil Womens Med*. 1997;suppl 1:170-176.
172. Kadir RA, Chi C. Levonorgestrel intrauterine system: bleeding disorders and anticoagulant therapy. *Contraception*. 2007;75:S123-S129.
173. Vahratian A, Barber JS, Lawrence JM, et al. Family-planning practices among women with diabetes and overweight and obese women in the 2002 National Survey for Family Growth. *Diabetes Care*. 2009;32:1026-1031.
174. Trussell J, Schwarz EB, Guthrie K. Obesity and oral contraceptive pill failure. *Contraception*. 2009;79:334-338.
175. Bonny AE, Ziegler J, Harvey R, et al. Weight gain in obese and nonobese adolescent girls initiating depot medroxyprogesterone, oral contraceptive pills, or no hormonal contraceptive method. *Arch Pediatr Adolesc Med*. 2006;160:40-45.

176. Abdollahi M, Cushman M, Rosendaal F. Obesity: risk of venous thrombosis and the interaction with coagulation factor levels and oral contraceptive use. *Thromb Haemost.* 2003;89:493-498.
177. Petri M, Buyon JP. Oral contraceptives in systemic lupus erythematosus: the case for (and against). *Lupus.* 2008;17:708-710.
178. Lakasing L, Khamashta M. Contraceptive practices in women with systemic lupus erythematosus and/or antiphospholipid syndrome: what advice should we be giving? *J Fam Plann Reprod Health Care.* 2001;27:7-12.
179. Bermas BL. Oral contraceptives in systemic lupus erythematosus: a tough pill to swallow? *N Engl J Med.* 2005;353:2602-2604.
180. Sánchez-Guerrero J, Uribe AG, Jiménez-Santana L, et al. A trial of contraceptive methods in women with systemic lupus erythematosus. *N Engl J Med.* 2005;353:2539-2549.
181. De Ceulaer K, Gruber C, Hayes R, et al. Medroxyprogesterone acetate and homozygous sickle-cell disease. *Lancet.* 1982;2:229-231.
182. Austin H, Lally C, Benson JM, et al. Hormonal contraception, sickle cell trait, and risk for venous thromboembolism among African American women. *Am J Obstet Gynecol.* 2009;200:620.e1-620.e3.
183. Yoong WC, Tuck SM, Pasi KJ, et al. Markers of platelet activation, thrombin generation and fibrinolysis in women with sickle cell disease: effects of differing forms of hormonal contraception. *Eur J Haematol.* 2003;70:310-314.
184. Kulkarni J. Depression as a side effect of the contraceptive pill. *Expert Opin Drug Saf.* 2007;6:371-374.
185. Koke SC, Brown EB, Miner CM. Safety and efficacy of fluoxetine in patients who receive oral contraceptive therapy. *Am J Obstet Gynecol.* 2002;187:551-555.
186. Murphy PA, Kern SE, Stanczyk FZ, et al. Interaction of St. John's wort with oral contraceptives: effects on the pharmacokinetics of norethindrone and ethinyl estradiol, ovarian activity and breakthrough bleeding. *Contraception.* 2005;71:402-408.

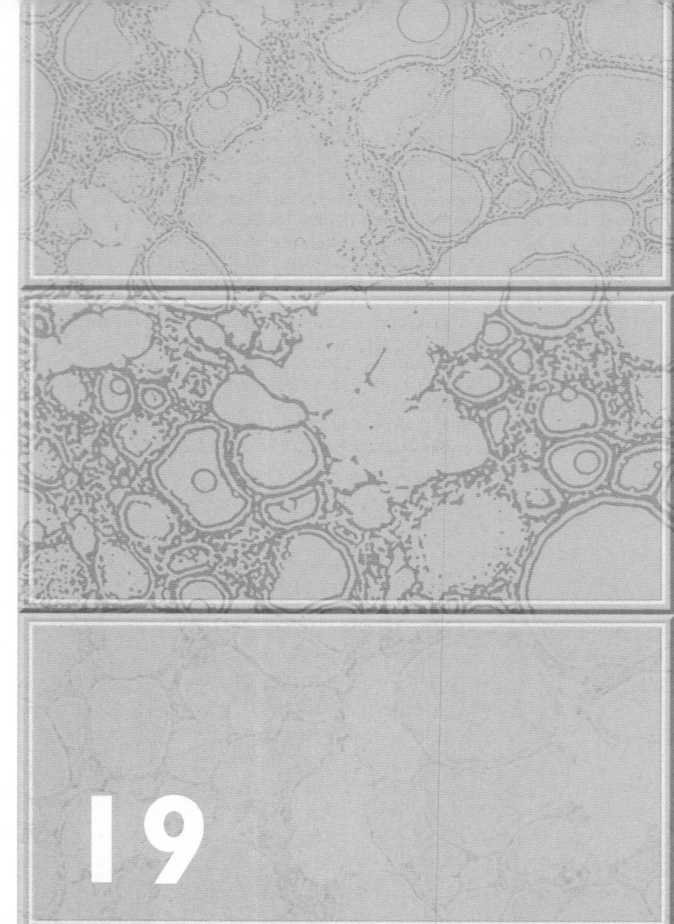

Testicular Disorders

ALVIN M. MATSUMOTO • WILLIAM J. BREMNER

The testes have critical physiologic roles during different stages of development. During early fetal life, production of testosterone and anti-müllerian hormone (AMH) by the fetal testis is required for the differentiation and development of normal male internal and external genitalia. During puberty, activation of the hypothalamic-pituitary-testicular axis and testosterone production by the testis are necessary for the induction of secondary (adult) male sexual characteristics, stimulation of sexual function, and initiation of sperm production. In adults, testis production of testosterone and sperm is required for the maintenance of adult male characteristics (virilization), sexual function, spermatogenesis, and fertility potential. Therefore, disorders of the testis may result in abnormalities in sexual development and function, body habitus and function, and fertility that have profound effects on health and well-being.

Disorders of the testis are common. Klinefelter's syndrome, the most common human sex chromosome abnormality and the primary testicular disorder causing testosterone deficiency and impaired spermatogenesis, affects approximately 1 in 500 to 600 men.[1,2] Isolated disorders of sperm production are the main causes of male infertility, which affects approximately 5% to 6% of otherwise healthy men in the reproductive age group.[3] Testicular disorders resulting in testosterone deficiency may contribute to complaints of reduced libido (sexual interest and desire), erectile dysfunction, gynecomastia (benign breast enlargement), and reduced bone mass (osteoporosis), all of which are common in men, particularly as they age. Finally, disordered hypothalamic-pituitary-testicular function is commonly associated with chronic systemic illnesses, wasting syndromes, morbid obesity, chronic use of certain medications (e.g., opiates, glucocorticoids), and aging. These conditions often result in testosterone deficiency that, if severe and prolonged, may contribute to clinical manifestations and morbidity.[4,5]

The treatment of testicular disorders usually results in significant clinical improvements in function and quality of life. In prepubertal boys and adults with severe testosterone deficiency, testosterone therapy results in dramatic transformations in body composition and function.[6] In men with infertility and impaired spermatogenesis due to gonadotropin deficiency, gonadotropin or gonadotropin-releasing hormone (GnRH) therapy may stimulate sperm and testosterone production and effectively restore fertility. Finally, advances in assisted reproductive technology (ART) have permitted previously infertile men with testicular disorders to have children. For example, although men with Klinefelter's syndrome and azoospermia (no spermatozoa in their ejaculate) were once thought to have untreatable infertility, testicular sperm extraction using microsurgical techniques combined with intracytoplasmic sperm injection (ICSI) may permit some of these men to father children.[7]

FUNCTIONAL ANATOMY AND HISTOLOGY

The Testis

Adult testes are paired, ovoid organs that hang from the inguinal canal by the *spermatic cord* (which is composed of a neurovascular pedicle, vas deferens, and cremasteric muscle); they are located outside the abdominal cavity within the scrotum. The left testis hangs lower in the scrotum than the right in about 60% of men, and the right testis hangs lower in approximately 30% of men. Each testis has a volume of 15 to 30 mL and measures 3.5 to 5.5 cm in length by 2.0 to 3.0 cm in width.[8,9]

The testis comprises two structurally and functionally distinct compartments: the *seminiferous tubule compartment*, which is composed of Sertoli cells and developing germ cells at various stages of spermatogenesis and accounts for 80% to 90% of the volume of the testis, and the *interstitial compartment*, which is composed of Leydig cells that secrete testosterone, the main male sex steroid hormone, as well as peritubular myoid cells, fibroblasts, neurovascular cells, and macrophages (Fig. 19-1).[10] Because germ cells constitute most of the testis volume, small testes are usually an indication of significantly impaired spermatogenesis.

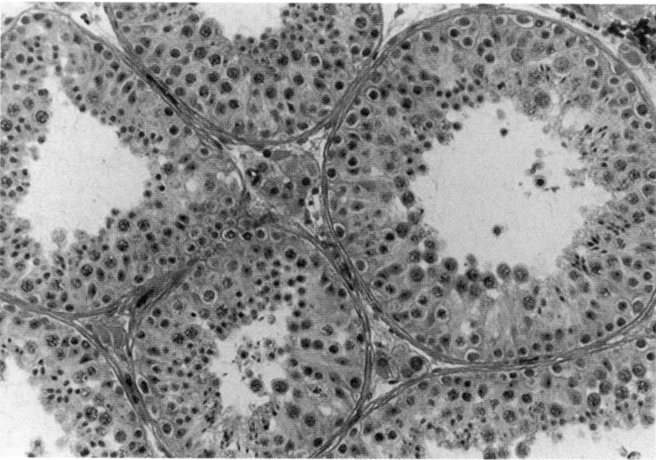

Figure 19-1 Light photomicrograph of the seminiferous tubule and interstitial compartments of the human testes. The seminiferous tubule compartment makes up the majority of the testis and is composed of developing germ cells enveloped by Sertoli cells. Spermatogonia line the basal lamina of the seminiferous tubules, spermatocytes at various stages of development are present in the middle layers of the tubules, and spermatids at various steps of maturation are present in the luminal aspect of the seminiferous tubules. Within each tubule, there are germ cells at different stages of spermatogenesis. In the interstitial compartment, there are prominent clusters of Leydig cells nestled between seminiferous tubules, peritubular myoid cells within the basal lamina of the tubules, and scattered blood vessels and macrophages. (From Matsumoto AM. Spermatogenesis. In: Adashi EY, Rock JA, Rosenwaks Z, eds. *Reproductive Endocrinology, Surgery, and Technology.* Philadelphia, PA: Lippincott-Raven; 1996:359-384.)

The testis is surrounded by a fibrous capsule, the *tunica albuginea*. Fibrous septa that emanate from the tunica albuginea separate the parenchyma of the testis into lobules. The arterial blood supply of the testes is derived primarily from the testicular (internal spermatic) arteries that arise from the abdominal aorta and descend through the inguinal canal in the spermatic cord. Collateral blood supply is provided by the cremasteric and deferential arteries. This collateral supply permits survival of the testis after a testicular artery ligation associated with surgical fixation of a high undescended testis into the scrotum (orchiopexy). However, twisting of the spermatic cord, known as *testicular torsion,* results in strangulation of the blood supply to the testis and causes testicular necrosis and infarction after 6 to 8 hours, making this condition a surgical emergency.[11] A testis that has a *bell-clapper deformity* (i.e., is not attached to the scrotal wall) is more susceptible to testicular torsion. Lymphatic drainage from the testes follows the testicular arteries to periaortic lymph nodes; this is a common route for metastasis of testicular cancer.

A network of veins that comprise the pampiniform plexus provides venous drainage from the testes. The pampiniform plexus coalesces into the testicular (internal spermatic) vein. The right testicular vein drains into the inferior vena cava, and the left testicular vein empties at a right angle into the left renal vein. One-way valves in testicular veins prevent backflow of blood into the scrotum. Abnormal enlargement of the venous plexus draining a testicle, known as a *varicocele,* occurs if valves are defective or absent or if there is extrinsic venous compression impeding normal venous drainage.[12] Increased pressures associated with the backflow of blood and altered temperature regulation may contribute to testicular dysfunction associated with a varicocele. Ninety-eight percent of varicoceles occur in the left scrotum, possibly because of absent or defective valves in the left testicular vein. The presence of a prominent unilateral right-sided varicocele or new-onset varicocele on either side should prompt evaluation for venous obstruction by an abdominal or pelvic malignancy (e.g., renal cell carcinoma) or lymphadenopathy; a chronic right-sided varicocele may also indicate *situs inversus.* Rarely, an anatomic anomaly of the superior mesenteric artery that compresses the left renal vein causes a left-sided varicocele; this is known as the *nutcracker syndrome.*

Because the testes are located outside the abdominal cavity, they are exposed to temperatures approximately 2° C lower than core body temperature. The position of the testes within the scrotum and the testicular temperature are regulated by the cremasteric muscle. The cremasteric muscle contracts when warming is needed, resulting in shortening of the spermatic cord and drawing of the testis toward the abdomen; when cooling is needed, it relaxes, resulting in lowering of the testis into scrotum. Also, the pampiniform venous plexus provides a concurrent heat exchange mechanism to cool the testis by surrounding the testicular artery with cooler venous blood. A testis temperature slightly lower than core body temperature is important for normal spermatogenesis. Exposure of the testes to higher temperatures, such as with failure of the testes to descend normally into the scrotum (*cryptorchidism*) or excessive external heat exposure due to frequent hot tub use, impairs spermatogenesis.

Seminiferous Tubule

Seminiferous tubules contain epithelium consisting of Sertoli cells that envelop and support germ cells undergoing progressive differentiation and development into mature spermatozoa. Once released into the lumen, mature spermatozoa are transported within seminiferous tubules, which measure up to 70 cm in length and are tightly coiled within lobules of the testis, to the rete testis, the efferent ducts, the epididymis, and, finally, the vas deferens for ultimate ejaculation. The seminiferous tubules are surrounded by a basal lamina composed of extracellular matrix that serves to separate them from the interstitial compartment, provides structural integrity to the tubules, and regulates the function of cells in contact with it. Histologic examination of a testis biopsy specimen in cross-section reveals many different seminiferous tubules surrounded by basal lamina and clusters of Leydig cells in the interstitial compartment between each tubule (see Fig. 19-1).[10]

Sertoli cells extend from the basal lamina to the lumen of tubules, and adjacent Sertoli cells envelop and provide a structural scaffold for germ cells as they differentiate within the tubule (Fig. 19-2).[8] Undifferentiated spermatogenic stem cells, called *spermatogonia*, lie along the basal lamina at the periphery of tubules, interspersed between Sertoli cells. Adjacent Sertoli cells surround spermatogonia and form specialized junctional complexes or tight junctions that divide the seminiferous tubule into the *basal compartment,* in which spermatogonia reside, and the *adluminal compartment,* which is occupied by differentiating germ cells. Sertoli cell tight junctions impede the passage of large molecules, steroids, and ions into the seminiferous tubule and constitute the cytologic basis of the *blood-testis barrier*, analogous to the blood-brain barrier. In the adluminal compartment, *spermatocytes* derived from spermatogonia in the basal compartment undergo meiosis to form *spermatids* that progressively mature (*spermiogenesis*), with the more mature germ cells occupying positions closer to the lumen, until mature spermatozoa are released into the lumen of the tubule (*spermiation*).

Because of the blood-testis barrier, only Sertoli cells and spermatogonia are directly accessible to endocrine and paracrine regulation from the circulation and cells of the interstitial compartment. Sertoli cells need to synthesize and secrete a number of products, some of which are present in circulation but not accessible to developing germ cells in the adluminal compartment, in order to nurture and regulate spermatogenesis. Sertoli cells contain receptors for follicle-stimulating hormone (FSH) and androgens, and they mediate the regulation of spermatogenesis by circulating FSH and testosterone produced locally by Leydig cells in response to stimulation from circulating luteinizing hormone (LH). Sertoli cells also produce the glycoprotein hormones—AMH, which causes regression of müllerian ducts and prevents the development of female accessory sex organs in the male fetus, and inhibin B, which participates in negative feedback suppression of FSH—and extracellular matrix components.

Spermatogenesis

In male humans, the process of spermatogenesis supports a production rate of approximately 120 million mature spermatozoa per day by the human testis (approximately

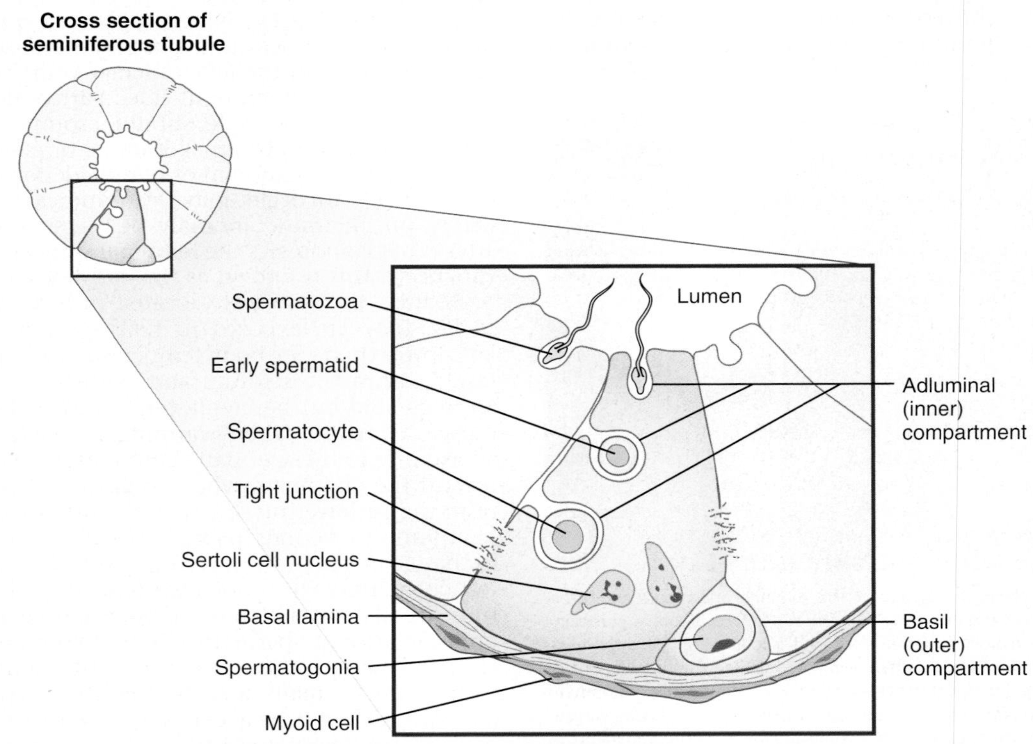

Figure 19-2 Schematic diagram of the cells in the seminiferous tubule (*top*). The seminiferous tubule consists of Sertoli cells that surround developing germ cells (*middle*). Sertoli cells extend from the basal lamina to the lumen. Tight junctions between adjoining Sertoli cells separate the seminiferous tubule into basal and adluminal compartments and are the anatomic basis for the blood-testis barrier (*bottom*). The basal compartment, which contains spermatogonia lining the basal lamina and peritubular myoid cells, is exposed to the interstitial compartment, which contains Leydig cells and blood vessels that deliver endocrine regulators of testis function (e.g., gonadotropins). The adluminal compartment contains developing spermatocytes, spermatids, and mature spermatozoa that are released into the lumen of the seminiferous tubule. (From Matsumoto AM. The testis. In: Felig P, Frohman LA, eds. *Endocrinology and Metabolism,* 4th ed. New York, NY: McGraw-Hill; 2001:635-705.)

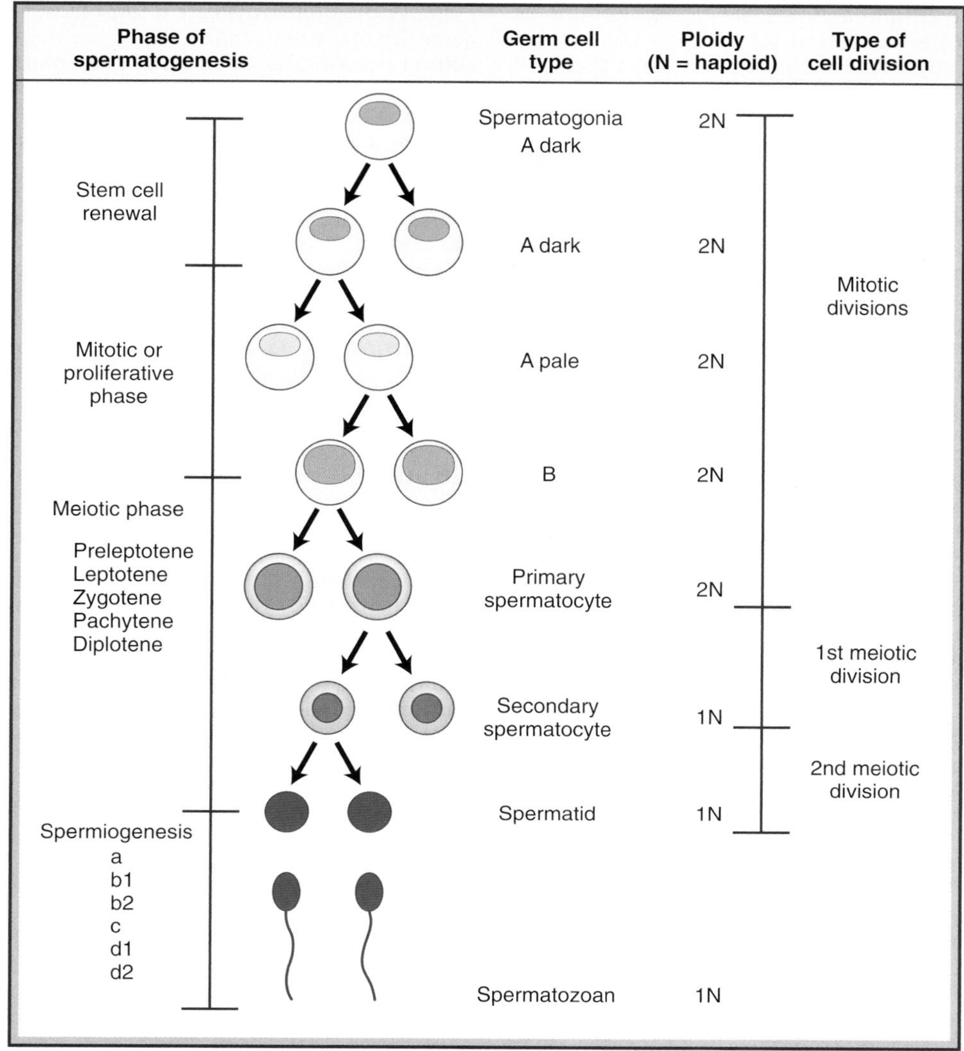

Figure 19-3 Schematic diagram of human spermatogenesis. Spermatogonial stem cells undergo self-renewal by mitotic division. At the initiation of spermatogenesis, some spermatogonia undergo differentiation into primary spermatocytes, which contain a diploid number of chromosomes (2N = 46 chromosomes). The primary spermatocytes then undergo two successive meiotic divisions to form spermatids, which contain a haploid number of chromosomes (1N = 23 chromosomes). Spermatids undergo spermiogenesis to form mature spermatozoa, which also contain a haploid number of chromosomes. (From Matsumoto AM. Spermatogenesis. In: Adashi EY, Rock JA, Rosenwaks Z, eds. *Reproductive Endocrinology, Surgery, and Technology.* Philadelphia, PA: Lippincott-Raven; 1996:359-384.)

1000 per heartbeat!).[13] Spermatogenesis, the process by which stem cells (spermatogonia) differentiate into mature spermatozoa, proceeds in three functionally distinct phases: (1) the *mitotic or proliferative phase,* during which the majority of spermatogonia undergo mitosis to renew the stem cell pool and a minority become committed to further differentiation to produce spermatocytes; (2) the *meiotic phase,* during which spermatocytes undergo successive meiotic divisions to produce haploid germ cells (spermatids); and (3) *spermiogenesis,* during which immature, round spermatids differentiate into mature spermatozoa (Fig. 19-3).[10,14]

Proliferative Phase

Based on chromatin staining and pattern, spermatogonia may be classified as A dark (A_d), A pale (A_p), or B spermatogonia. Because of their relatively low mitotic rate, A_d spermatogonia are thought to be the spermatogonial stem cells. A_d spermatogonia are relatively resistant to external insults (e.g., ionizing radiation), and in response to such insults, they undergo mitotic proliferation. However, severe or complete depletion of A_d spermatogonia, such as occurs with high-dose x-irradiation or vascular compromise, results in irreversible impairment or loss of sperm production.

A small number of A_d spermatogonia undergo mitotic divisions to form A_p and then B spermatogonia. In humans, the rate of formation of B spermatogonia is low, so that only a small number of B spermatogonia are available to enter meiosis and undergo further differentiation.[15] This limits the efficiency of spermatogenesis in humans. B spermatogonia are the most sensitive germ cells to the effects of ionizing radiation, and their numbers are reduced after irradiation of the testes.[16]

B spermatogonia that become committed to further differentiation undergo mitotic division to form *preleptotene* or *resting* spermatocytes, which enter a prolonged meiotic phase of 24 days. Spermatogonia do not completely separate after mitosis *(incomplete cytokinesis)*. Groups of spermatogonia remain connected via cytoplasmic bridges, forming a syncytium, and undergo meiosis and spermiogenesis in synchrony.

Meiotic Phase

Preleptotene primary spermatocytes contain a diploid complement of chromosomes (46 chromosomes or 2N, where N is the number of haploid chromosomes), and they are the last germ cells to undergo DNA synthesis. Preleptotene spermatocytes undergo an initial round of meiotic division (*meiosis I*), lasting longer than 2 weeks, to form secondary spermatocytes that contain a haploid complement of chromosomes (1N). Secondary spermatocytes, which are present for only about 8 hours, undergo a second meiotic division (*meiosis II*) to form haploid spermatids.

Improper segregation of chromosomes (*meiotic nondisjunction*) resulting in an abnormal number of chromosomes (*aneuploidy*) occurs in 0.7% of live births and 50% of first-trimester abortuses.[17,18] Klinefelter's syndrome, a common cause of primary hypogonadism, occurs in about 1 in 500 live births and is associated classically with a 47, XXY karyotype caused by paternal meiotic nondisjunction in 50% of cases.[19] Down syndrome (trisomy 21) occurs in approximately 1 in 700 live births and is caused by paternal meiotic nondisjunction in 5% to 20% of cases.[20]

Spermiogenesis

The final phase of spermatogenesis is the maturation of spermatids from round to elongated spermatids and then to mature spermatozoa; this process, known as spermiogenesis, is followed by release of spermatozoa into the lumen of seminiferous tubules (spermiation). The major changes that occur during spermiogenesis include formation of the sperm head with condensation of chromosomes (DNA and nucleoproteins) and formation of the *acrosomal cap,* which contains proteolytic enzymes needed for sperm penetration of the ovum; formation of the sperm tail or *flagellum* (pointing into the lumen), which permits motility; phagocytic removal of excess spermatid cytoplasm (known as the *residual body*) by Sertoli cells; and release of mature spermatozoa into the lumen. Progressive maturation of spermatids is accompanied by progressive movement of more mature spermatids toward the lumen of the seminiferous tubule. Spermiogenesis is directed by the Sertoli cells that sustain and support developing spermatids and by the major endocrine regulators of Sertoli cells, FSH and testosterone.

Germ Cell Loss

Compared to most other species, the efficiency of spermatogenesis in humans is relatively poor, and the germ cell degeneration and loss that occurs predominantly during mitosis and meiosis is a major contributor to the low efficiency of sperm production.[21] Significant degrees of germ cell degeneration occurring during meiosis account for a decrease of approximately 40% in the ratio of the number of spermatids to preleptotene spermatocytes. This ratio is reduced further as men age, resulting in a reduction of daily sperm production in elderly men. It is hypothesized that germ cell degeneration prevents abnormal germ cells from further development, thereby serving an important quality control function.

Organization of Spermatogenesis

Histologic examination of a human testis in cross-section reveals that germ cells at particular phases of development cluster in six cellular associations, referred to as *stages,* which together constitute a complete *cycle* of spermatogenesis. In most mammals, stages are organized sequentially along the longitudinal axis of the tubules, so that all of the germ cells present in a cross-section of a tubule are in the same stage of spermatogenesis.[22,23] In contrast, three or more different stages of a cycle may variably be present in a cross-section of human testis. Although some have proposed a helical pattern of stages along the tubule to explain this seemingly chaotic arrangement, this has not been confirmed by others.

In humans, the duration of spermatogenesis from A_p spermatogonia to release of mature spermatozoa is 74 ± 4 days.[24] The epididymal transit time of spermatozoa is approximately 12 to 21 days.[25] Therefore, external insults to the testis (e.g., ionizing radiation) or induction of gonadotropin deficiency (e.g., by male contraceptive regimens) that affects early germ cell development and reduces spermatogenesis may not be reflected in reduced sperm counts in the ejaculate until months later.

Sperm Transport and Fertilization

Mature spermatozoa released into the lumen of the seminiferous tubule are transported to the rete testis, to the efferent ducts of the testis, and then to the caput epididymis primarily by peristaltic contractions and intratubular fluid flow. In the epididymis, sperm undergo functional modifications that result in the capacity for sustained forward motility. After ejaculation from the vas deferens and penis into the female reproductive tract, human sperm undergo *capacitation* in the uterus; the resulting biochemical alterations in the acrosomal cap increase the fluidity and hyperactivated motility induced by uterine secretory products so that the spermatozoa acquire the capacity to fertilize an ovum.[26,27] After capacitation, as the spermatozoon meets an ovum in the ampulla of the fallopian tube, the sperm binds to the egg and releases hyaluronidase to penetrate the zona pellucida that surrounds the ovum, a process known as the *acrosome reaction.* Fertilization then occurs as the plasma membranes of sperm and ovum fuse.

Spermatozoa

Morphologically, most ejaculated human spermatozoa are composed of an oval-shaped head that contains condensed chromatin and nucleoproteins; an acrosomal cap that covers approximately the anterior two thirds of the head; a short neck that contains centrioles important for attachment of the tail and cleavage of the zygote after fertilization; a middle piece that consists of axial filaments surrounded by a spiral of mitochondria containing oxidative enzymes that provide energy for motility; and a long tail or flagellum that permits normal progressive forward motility of the spermatozoa (Fig. 19-4).[10] The flagellum consists of a microtubule-based cytoskeleton, the *axoneme,* which has a characteristic structure composed of two central microtubules surrounded by nine microtubule doublets (9 × 2 + 2 pattern) that serves as a scaffold for motor protein complexes (i.e., *dynein arms*).[28]

In humans, the normal sperm concentration in the ejaculate is greater than 15 million/mL, with 4% or more having normal morphology by strict criteria (≥30% by previous criteria) and 40% or more having total motility, according to the most recent World Health Organization criteria.[29,30] Men with infertility may exhibit abnormal morphology of the sperm head (tapered, amorphous, or double-headed forms) or of the tail (coiled forms) and reduced or absent motility. Alterations in the structural or

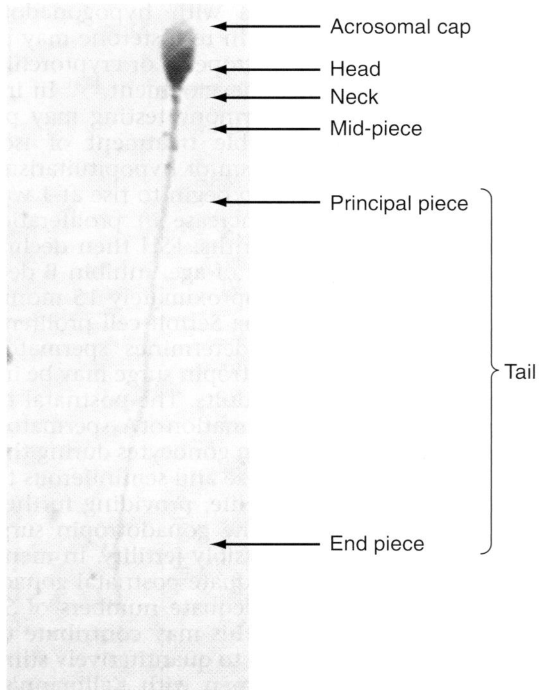

Figure 19-4 Light photomicrograph of an ejaculated mature human spermatozoon, composed of a head, neck, mid-piece, and tail (principal piece and end piece). (From Matsumoto AM. Spermatogenesis. In: Adashi EY, Rock JA, Rosenwaks Z, eds. *Reproductive Endocrinology, Surgery, and Technology.* Philadelphia, PA: Lippincott-Raven; 1996:359-384.)

functional components of the axoneme (e.g., absence of dynein arms) result in altered motility, and deficiency of dynein adenosine triphosphatase (ATPase) results in primary ciliary dyskinesia or immotile cilia syndrome.[31]

Interstitium

The interstitial compartment of the testis contains clusters of Leydig cells, the primary sex steroid-producing cells of the testis, which comprise only about 5% of testis volume (see Fig. 19-1).[23,32] Leydig cells produce testosterone, which acts as a paracrine regulator within the seminiferous tubules of the testis on Sertoli cells in close proximity to stimulate spermatogenesis. Testosterone is secreted into adjacent testicular capillaries and then into the general circulation to act as an endocrine signal on androgen target organs throughout the body. Leydig cells also produce *insulin-like factor 3* (*INSL3*), a peptide hormone in the relaxin-insulin family, which plays an important role in the first phase of testicular descent from the abdomen into the scrotum during development.[33] INSL3 also may be an important autocrine regulator of Leydig cells and a paracrine regulator of germ cells directly.[34]

Peritubular myoid cells, which surround the seminiferous tubules, are contractile, smooth, muscle-like cells that serve to facilitate forward transport of spermatozoa and testicular fluid within the tubular lumen, provide structural integrity to the tubule, secrete extracellular matrix components and putative regulatory factors such as growth factors, and are involved in retinol metabolism.[23,35] These cells contain androgen receptors (ARs) and are thought to mediate some of the paracrine effects of testosterone on Sertoli cells within the seminiferous tubules, although their precise role in human testicular physiology remains unclear.

The interstitial compartment also contains macrophages that may regulate Leydig cell steroidogenesis by secretion of cytokines and may play a role in phagocytosis of degenerating cells and necrotic debris. The interstitium contains arterioles and a rich network of capillaries that permit secretion of testosterone and other products into the circulation and delivery of the main endocrine regulators of testis function, the gonadotropins LH and FSH.

TESTIS DEVELOPMENT

Fetal Development

During embryogenesis, the Y chromosome directs the development of the testis from an undifferentiated anlage that has the potential to develop into either a testis or an ovary.[36] The *SRY (sex-determining region of the Y chromosome) gene,* located on the pseudoautosomal region of the Y chromosome, encodes a transcription factor that increases the expression of SRY-box 9 *(SOX9),* which in turn drives the formation of Sertoli cells and testis differentiation. *SRY* gene expression is activated by a number of factors, including steroidogenic factor 1 (SF1) and the binding protein GATA4.[37] *SRY*-independent *SOX9* expression may also be driven by SF1. *SOX9* directs the expression of other genes that are essential in testis differentiation, such as fibroblast growth factor 9 (*FGF9*) and *AMH,* and in repression of ovarian differentiation, such as *WNT4* and *DAX1* (now designated *NR0B1*). In the absence of SRY or SRY action, SOX9 is repressed by a number of factors, including *β-catenin,* and development of the follicular cells and ovaries follows.

Primordial germ cells originate in the yolk sac and migrate to the genital ridges. Together with celomic epithelial and mesenchymal cells that eventually differentiate, respectively, into Sertoli cells and interstitial cells (Leydig and peritubular myoid cells), they form the *genital blastema* by 6 weeks of gestation. Primordial germ cells that fail to migrate normally explain the location of extragonadal germ cell cancers in men. Under the influence of gene products activated by SRY, primordial germ cells become surrounded by primitive Sertoli cells to form seminiferous or sex cords that eventually develop into seminiferous tubules.

Leydig cells begin to form at 8 weeks of gestation. Then, under the influence of maternal human chorionic gonadotropin (hCG) initially and later LH and FSH from the fetal pituitary gland, immature Leydig cells, Sertoli cells, and germ cells undergo differentiation, proliferation, and organization. Testosterone production from fetal Leydig cells increases progressively and induces development of the epididymis, vas deferens, and seminal vesicles from wolffian or mesonephric ducts. Conversion of testosterone to 5α-dihydrotestosterone (5α-DHT) in the urogenital tract leads to the formation of the prostate from the urogenital sinus, the penis from the genital tubercles and folds, and the scrotum from the urogenital swelling.[38] In the absence of testosterone production or action, female internal and external genitalia develop. AMH secretion from the fetal Sertoli cells causes regression of the müllerian or paramesonephric ducts and prevents the formation of a uterus and fallopian tubes.

Male phenotypic development is complete by about 15 weeks of gestation, after which the proliferation of Sertoli grows, the scrotum develops, libido and erections are stimulated, and the gender role may change from female to male. Cryptorchidism is common but not invariable and is associated with oligozoospermia or azoospermia. Testes may descend at the time of puberty. Normal sperm counts may occur in individuals with descended testes, and fertility has been reported in men with SRD5A2 deficiency. However, in adults, the prostate remains underdeveloped and is not palpable, facial and body hair are diminished, sebum is not produced, and male-pattern baldness does not occur, supporting the importance of normal SRD5A2 activity and DHT for hair growth, sebaceous function, and prostate development. Serum DHT concentrations are low, testosterone levels are normal to slightly elevated, and gonadotropin concentrations are modestly elevated.

Within the prostate gland, conversion of testosterone to DHT produces concentrations of DHT that are approximately 10-fold higher than those in serum, serving to amplify androgen activity in the prostate. Intraprostatic androgen concentrations may contribute to prostate pathology, such as BPH or prostate cancer.[117]

Inhibitors of SRD5A2 (finasteride) or of both SRD5A1 and SRD5A2 (dutasteride) are used to treat lower urinary tract symptoms, improve urinary flow, and prevent complications related to BPH, as well as to treat male-pattern baldness and androgenic alopecia.[118] Treatment with finasteride or dutasteride reduces, respectively, the prevalence or the incidence of prostate cancer found on biopsy but is possibly associated with a greater number of cancers with high Gleason grade.[119,120] An important aspect of the effect of androgens on the prostate is that intraprostatic androgen concentrations are not reflected in serum levels, underscoring the importance of local paracrine and autocrine actions of androgens in the physiology and pathology of the prostate and probably other androgen target tissues.

Catabolism of Testosterone. The primary site of catabolism of circulating testosterone and 5α-DHT is the liver.[121] Testosterone and 5α-DHT are taken up in the liver, and testosterone is converted to an inactive metabolite, 5β-DHT, by the enzyme 5β-reductase. Both 5α- and 5β-DHT then undergo 3α-reduction by the enzyme 3α-HSD to form 3α,5α-androstanediol (also called 3α-diol) and 3α,5β-androstanediol, respectively; this is followed by 17β-reduction by the enzyme 17β-HSD to form androsterone and etiocholanolone as catabolic products. In peripheral tissues such as skin, 5α-DHT may also be converted to 3α-diol, which is further metabolized in the liver.

In the liver, testosterone, DHT, 3α-androstanediols, androsterone, and etiocholanolone undergo glucuronidation and, to a lesser degree, sulfation to form more hydrophilic conjugates that are released into circulation and excreted in urine and bile. Metabolic inactivation of testosterone primarily involves its conversion to metabolites such as testosterone (about 50%), androsterone (20%), and etiolocholanolone (20%) glucuronides (as well as sulfates) and lesser conversion to 3α-diol glucuronides. Because 3α-diol comes mostly from skin, blood and urine measurements of 3α-diol glucuronide (3α-diol G) has been used as a marker of peripheral androgen action.[121] In men with 5α-reductase deficiency, 3α-diol G concentrations are reduced. The amount of body hair and acne correlates with 3α-diol G levels.

Epitestosterone (17α-hydroxy-4-androsten-3-one) is a biologically inactive 17α-hydroxy epimer of testosterone (17β-hydroxy-4-androsten-3-one) that is produced by the testes in response to LH.[122] The production rate of epitestosterone is about 3% that of testosterone, but its clearance rate is 33% that of testosterone, and there is no interconversion of epitestosterone and testosterone. Similar to testosterone, epitestosterone is conjugated in the liver, primarily to glucuronides and sulfates, and excreted in the urine. Because epitestosterone conjugates are rapidly cleared in the urine, excretion rates of testosterone and epitestosterone are similar, and the ratio of urinary testosterone to epitestosterone (T/E ratio) is approximately 1 : 1.

Measurements of the T/E ratio and other metabolites in urine by sensitive gas chromatography/mass spectrometry methods are used to detect androgenic anabolic steroid doping by competitive athletes.[122] Administration of androgenic anabolic steroids suppresses the production and clearance of epitestosterone relative to testosterone, resulting in an elevated T/E ratio in urine. The World and United States Anti-Doping Agencies have set a threshold T/E ratio of greater than 4 : 1 as suspicious for anabolic steroid doping.

Testosterone is glucuronidated primarily by the enzyme uridine diphosphate glucuronyl transferase 2B17 (UGT2B17), whereas epitestosterone is glucuronidated mostly by another UGT isoform, UGT2B7. Although testosterone may be glucuronidated by other UGT isoforms (e.g., UGT2B15), individuals with an inactivating genetic polymorphism of UGT2B17 (common in Asian populations) have reduced testosterone glucuronidation and clearance, resulting in lower T/E ratios that do not reach threshold levels with androgen administration.[121,123,124] Realization that there were populations with naturally low T/E led to a reduction in the T/E ratio cutoff from the previous threshold for suspicion of doping of (>6 : 1) to the present one (>4 : 1). Also, there are individuals with a naturally high T/E ratios, perhaps because of other genetic polymorphisms or environmental factors such as excessive alcohol consumption that may increase T/E ratio transiently.[125] In the absence of environmental perturbations, the T/E ratio in a single individual is remarkably stable over time, and longitudinal measurements of urinary T/E ratio may be used to detect illicit androgen use. Coadministration of epitestosterone with testosterone has been used by athletes to avoid detection.

If a urinary T/E ratio is suspicious for doping, exogenous androgen use is confirmed by gas chromatography combustion isotope ratio mass spectrometry (GC/C/IRMS), which can detect small differences in the ratio of carbon 13 to carbon 12 ($^{13}C/^{12}C$) isotopes of testosterone or its metabolites.[122] Because synthetic androgens are synthesized from plant sources (yams or soy), their $^{13}C/^{12}C$ ratio is lower than that of endogenously produced testosterone and other steroids that reflect an animal source or dietary ingestion of both animal and plant products. However, $^{13}C/^{12}C$ IRMS will not detect doping by administration of hCG or LH-like activity to stimulate endogenous testosterone production or administration of androgens derived from animal sources that have a $^{13}C/^{12}C$ ratio similar to that of endogenous testosterone.

Mechanisms of Androgen Action

In androgen target tissues, testosterone and DHT in circulation diffuse through the plasma membrane and bind to intracellular ARs.[126] Binding of androgen to the AR induces a conformational change in the AR that causes dissociation of heat shock proteins bound to AR, permitting translocation into the nucleus, induction of phosphorylation and homodimerization, and interaction with DNA, specifically on AREs located in regulatory sites of target genes. The AR dimer actively recruits tissue-specific coregulators

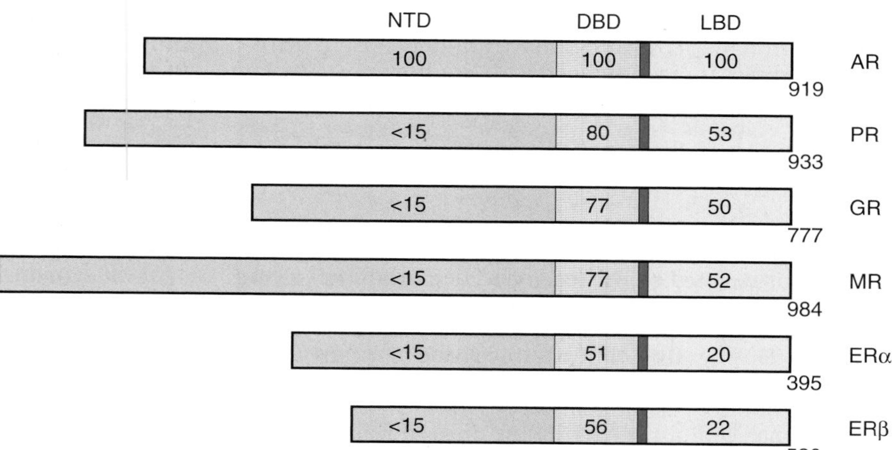

Figure 19-12 Schematic diagram of the structure of the human androgen receptor (AR) gene and homology to other steroid hormone receptors: progesterone receptor (PR), glucocorticoid receptor (GR), mineralocorticoid receptor (MR), estrogen receptor-α (ERα), and estrogen receptor-β (ERβ). The AR is a 919-amino-acid protein that is composed of three functional domains: a ligand-binding domain (LBD), a DNA-binding domain (DBD), and an N-terminal transactivation domain (NTD). The DBD shares the greatest degree of homology (>51% versus AR) and the NTD the least degree of homology (<15% versus AR) among steroid hormone receptors. (From Li J, Al-Azzawi F. Mechanism of androgen receptor action. *Maturitas.* 2009;63:142-148.)

(coactivators and corepressors) to form the transcriptional apparatus necessary to control androgen-regulated gene transcription and subsequent protein synthesis.

The *AR* gene is located on the long arm of the X chromosome (Xq11-12). *AR* is organized into functional domains (Fig. 19-12)[126]: (1) an *N-terminal domain* (NTD) comprising two transactivation domains (AF1 and AF5) that mediate the majority of *AR* transcriptional activity and coregulator interaction and two trinucleotide repeat segments (CAG and GGN, encoding polyglutamine and polyglycine tracts, respectively) of varying number that modify *AR* transactivation; (2) a *DNA-binding domain* (DBD) comprising two finger motifs, the first mediating DNA recognition and binding and the second stabilizing DNA interaction and mediating dimerization of *AR*; (3) a small *hinge region* (H); and (4) a *ligand-binding domain* (LBD) that mediates high-affinity binding of androgen to the AR and also contains another transactivation domain (AF2).

AR is a member of the nuclear receptor superfamily that includes other steroid hormone receptors. It shares approximately 80% sequence homology in the DBD, and 50% in the LBD, with its most closely related steroid receptors, the progesterone receptor (PR), the glucocorticoid receptor (GR), and the mineralocorticoid receptor (MR).[126] This may explain why, for example, some progestins (e.g., medroxyprogesterone acetate) have AR agonist activity, others (e.g., cyproterone acetate) have AR antagonist activity, and a mineralocorticoid antagonist, spironolactone, has AR antagonist activity. Compared with the binding of testosterone, DHT binds to AR with higher affinity, greater stability, and a slower rate of dissociation, conferring greater androgen activity to DHT, the most potent endogenous androgen in humans.

Inactivating mutations of the *AR* may cause qualitative or quantitative abnormalities of receptor function, resulting in variably impaired androgen action.[127] *AR* mutations manifest phenotypic variability, ranging from that of a male who is phenotypically female with normal female external genitalia and breast development (*complete testicular feminization*), which occurs in individuals with complete androgen insensitivity or resistance, to that of an otherwise normal male with incomplete hypospadias, mild undervirilization, or infertility.

In a normal population, the number of trinucleotide CAG repeats in the first exon of the *AR* gene varies from 11 to 35. In general, the number of CAG repeats appears to correlate inversely with AR function and action, both in vitro and in vivo, in transgenic mice and humans. *Kennedy's disease,* or *X-linked spinal and bulbar muscular atrophy* (*SBMA*), is a rare adult-onset neurodegenerative disease of motor neurons that results in progressive muscle weakness; it is associated with a markedly expanded number of CAG repeats, varying from 40 to 62, which does not overlap with the normal population.[128] Neurodegeneration in this disorder is thought to be caused by toxicity from intracellular aggregation of the AR and associated cofactors that is worsened by androgen binding to the mutant AR and translocation into the nucleus.

Most men with Kennedy's disease also manifest clinical findings of partial androgen resistance, including gynecomastia, reduced libido, erectile dysfunction, decreased facial hair, testicular atrophy, and oligozoospermia or azoospermia in association with high testosterone and high or normal gonadotropin levels.[129] The severity of the latter biochemical indices of androgen insensitivity is directly related to CAG repeat length. Although it is not found consistently, some studies have reported an association between CAG repeat number and manifestations of androgen action in normal men.[130] In these studies, a low number of CAG repeats within the normal range was associated with higher androgenicity (e.g., earlier onset of prostate cancer, male pattern baldness, lower HDL-cholesterol), and a high number of repeats within the normal range was associated with lower androgenicity (e.g., gynecomastia, impaired spermatogenesis, lower bone density, depressive symptoms). CAG repeat number also seems to be associated with the clinical manifestations of men with androgen deficiency due to Klinefelter's disease and their response to testosterone treatment, the latter suggesting a possible pharmacogenetic influence of this AR polymorphism.

Studies in vitro and in experimental animals suggest that some actions of androgens may occur within seconds to minutes, too rapidly to be caused by classic genomic effects of androgens acting through the AR on gene transcription and subsequent protein synthesis, which usually take hours to produce effects.[131] Rapid, nongenomic effects of androgens may be mediated by cell surface interactions and receptors and by the activation of conventional signal transduction mechanisms, including activation of PKA and PKC, which increase intracellular calcium and MAPK pathways. Binding of androgen to intracellular AR may also activate coregulators that do not require gene transcription to signal, such as the tyrosine kinase, steroid receptor coactivator (SRC). Nongenomic actions of androgens have been described in testis (Sertoli cells), brain, muscle, cardiovascular tissues, prostate, and immune cells. In humans, the rapid vasodilatory effect of testosterone on myocardial ischemia in patients with coronary artery disease is attributed to a direct nongenomic effect of androgens on vascular cells.

Androgen Effects at Various Stages of Sexual Development

Levels of testosterone and its actions differ at various stages of sexual development (Fig. 19-13).[132] During *fetal life*, testosterone is secreted by the fetal testis beginning at 7 weeks of gestation.[36] Testosterone secretion is primarily under the control of hCG, initially, and then LH secreted by the fetal pituitary. During this time, testosterone concentrations increase to almost adult male levels, and testosterone and its conversion to DHT are critical for normal male internal and external genital differentiation (e.g., development of primary sexual characteristics). Testosterone concentrations remain elevated through most of the second trimester, after which they decline.

Shortly after birth, during *neonatal life*, LH secretion increases and stimulates a second rise in testosterone levels, almost to adolescent concentrations, between 3 to 6 months of age; this is followed by a fall to low prepubertal levels.[133] The neonatal surge in testosterone levels may have a role in development of normal phallus size and completion of testicular descent. The neonatal increase in testosterone and FSH levels at this time also stimulates Sertoli cell proliferation and spermatogonial development, which may play a role in determining spermatogenic capacity.

During *puberty*, testosterone concentrations increase to adult male levels in response to activation of hypothalamic GnRH secretion and its stimulation of pituitary gonadotropin secretion.[43,134] The progressive increase in testosterone and its active metabolites, estradiol and DHT, is responsible for the development of secondary sexual characteristics (*virilization* or *masculinization*) and other changes. Pubertal changes induced by testosterone may be categorized as those related to body, brain, and sexual function. *Body function changes* include the following:

- Growth and development of the penis and scrotum and the appearance of rugal folds and pigmentation in scrotal skin
- Enlargement of the prostate and seminal vesicles and production of accessory sexual gland secretion and seminal fluid
- Androgen-dependent hair growth and development of a male hair distribution—facial (moustache and beard), external auditory canal, chest, axillary, pubic and lower abdomen (male escutcheon), perianal, inner thigh, and leg and arm hair growth and frontal scalp hair recession
- Increase in sebum production
- Stimulation of IGF1 production together with that of growth hormone (GH)
- Long bone growth and eventually closure of long bone epiphyses resulting in cessation of growth
- Increase in BMD and stimulation of peak bone mass
- Increase in skeletal muscle mass and strength, especially in shoulder and pectoral muscles
- Decrease and redistribution of body fat
- Enlargement of the larynx and thickening of vocal cords, resulting in a lower-pitched voice
- Stimulation of erythropoiesis resulting in an increase in hematocrit, primarily by direct bone marrow induction of erythroid differentiation and stimulation of erythropoietin secretion
- Suppression of HDL-cholesterol.

Brain function changes include stimulation of libido (sexual interest, desire, and motivation); increase in motivation, initiative, and social aggressiveness; and increase in aspects of cognitive function (e.g., visuospatial abilities). *Sexual function changes* include initiation of spermatogenesis and acquisition of fertility potential and increase in spontaneous erections.

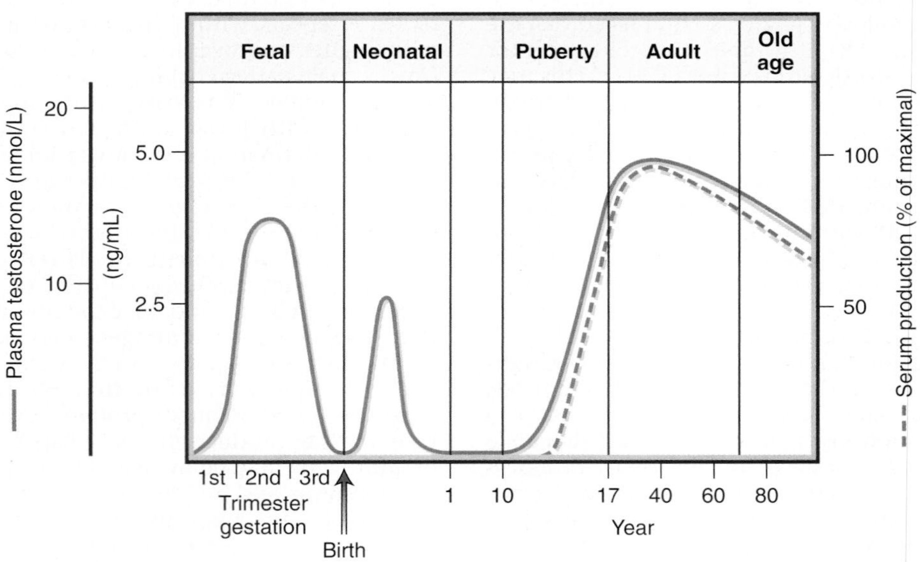

Figure 19-13 Schematic diagram of changes in serum testosterone concentration and sperm production during different phases of life. During fetal life, testosterone levels increase almost to adult male levels, peaking during the first trimester and remaining elevated throughout the second trimester, after which they decline. During neonatal life, testosterone increases almost to adolescent levels at 3 to 6 months of age, then declines to prepubertal levels. During puberty, testosterone concentrations and sperm production increase to adult male levels over several years. With aging, there is a variable, gradual, and progressive decline in serum testosterone levels and sperm production, beginning at age 40 years. (From Griffin JE, Wilson JD. The testis. In: Bondy PK, Rosenberg LE, eds. *Metabolic Control and Disease*, 8th ed. Philadelphia, PA: WB Saunders; 1980:1535-7158.)

In *adult life*, normal adult male levels of testosterone serve to maintain many of the changes induced during puberty. This includes maintenance of body function changes such as normal amounts of androgen-dependent hair and male hair distribution, sebum production, BMD, muscle mass and strength, hematocrit in the male range (higher than the female range), and HDL-cholesterol in the male range (lower than the female range); brain function changes such as libido, motivation, initiative, social aggressiveness, energy and vitality, mood, and possibly some aspects of cognitive function; and sexual function changes such as sperm production and fertility potential and spontaneous erections. Some of the masculinizing changes induced by testosterone during puberty are permanent. Once they are developed, testosterone is not necessary for maintenance of penis size, scrotal development, linear growth, laryngeal size, vocal cord thickness, or voice pitch.[110]

With *aging*, there is a gradual and progressive decline in serum testosterone concentrations associated with reductions in muscle mass and strength, BMD, libido, energy and vitality, mood, aspects of cognitive function, sperm production and fertility, and erections.[135]

MALE HYPOGONADISM

The two major functions of the testis are to produce sufficient amounts of testosterone and of sperm to support the development and maintenance of male sexual function, body function, and fertility. *Male hypogonadism* is a clinical syndrome that results from a failure of the testes to produce adequate amounts of testosterone; this is almost always associated with impaired sperm production (*androgen deficiency and impairment of sperm production*) or with an *isolated impairment of sperm production or function* with normal testosterone production. Hypogonadism is the most common disorder of testis function encountered in clinical practice.

Because testis function is controlled by the hypothalamus and the pituitary, male hypogonadism may be caused by a primary disorder of the testis (*primary hypogonadism*); it may be secondary to a disorder of the pituitary or hypothalamus (*secondary hypogonadism*); or, in some instances, there may be defects at both levels (*combined primary and secondary hypogonadism*).

Identifying men with secondary hypogonadism has important clinical implications that may affect management.[110] For example, secondary hypogonadism can be caused by a pituitary adenoma that may be associated with clinical manifestations related to tumor mass (e.g., headaches, visual field defects); to deficiency or excessive secretion of other anterior pituitary hormones; or to diabetes insipidus resulting from hypothalamic antidiuretic hormone deficiency. Such patients require management of the primary disorder in addition to testosterone replacement therapy. Secondary hypogonadism may be reversible with treatment of the underlying condition (e.g., nutritional deficiency) or discontinuation of an offending medication (e.g., glucocorticoids, opiates), or it may be associated with a chronic systemic illness that is not curable, such as chronic kidney disease (CKD). Impaired spermatogenesis and infertility caused by gonadotropin deficiency in men with secondary hypogonadism may be treated with gonadotropin or GnRH therapy, and sperm production and fertility may be restored. In contrast, infertility caused by primary testicular disease is usually not treatable with hormone therapy and requires other fertility options, such as the use of donor sperm, ART (e.g., ICSI), or adoption.

Clinical Manifestations

Because testosterone has different roles during sexual life, the manifestations of androgen deficiency differ depending on the stage of sexual development.[8,110]

Androgen Deficiency and Impairment in Sperm Production

Fetal Androgen Deficiency. During fetal development, testosterone and its conversion to DHT have vital roles in directing male internal and external genital differentiation and development. Fetal androgen deficiency (e.g., from congenital defects in testosterone biosynthesis enzymes) or androgen resistance (e.g., from AR mutations or 5α-reductase deficiency) manifests at birth with varying degrees of ambiguous genitalia and DSDs (i.e., male pseudohermaphroditism) (Table 19-1).[36,62] Depending on the severity of androgen deficiency or resistance, the phenotype of individuals with these disorders may range from that of a normal female to that of an otherwise normal male with microphallus, pseudovaginal perineoscrotal hypospadias, bifid scrotum, and cryptorchidism of varying severity. These disorders are described in greater detail in Chapter 23.

Prepubertal Androgen Deficiency. The increase in testosterone levels that occurs at the time of puberty is responsible for development of secondary sexual characteristics; an increase in muscle mass and reduction and redistribution of body fat; long bone growth and eventually closure of epiphyses resulting in cessation of growth; stimulation of sexual interest (libido), erections, and sexual activity; and initiation of spermatogenesis and seminal fluid production.[136] Prepubertal androgen deficiency causes *eunuchoidism* (Fig. 19-14; see Table 19-1),[136] which is characterized most notably by infantile genitalia with a small penis and a poorly developed scrotum that lacks rugal folds and pigmentation. The testes are small, usually less than 2 cm in length and from 2 mL to less than 4 mL in volume. Hair is thin and fine, and there is a lack of androgen-dependent hair growth (i.e., absence of a male hair pattern in all body areas) and no temporal hair recession. The pubic hair pattern is more typical of females, with the shape of an inverted triangle in the pubic area (female escutcheon) rather in a diamond shape with hair extending from the pubic area to the umbilicus (male escutcheon), and there is little hair extending to the thighs. Acne does not develop because sebum production is not stimulated by androgens.

Eunuchoidism is typified by a distinctive body habitus, characterized by poor muscle mass development (especially in the shoulders and chest), prepubertal fat distribution (predominantly in the face, chest, and hips), and excessively long arms and legs relative to height. Arm span exceeds height, and the distance from the crown of the head to the symphysis pubis exceeds that from the symphysis to the floor, both differences being greater than 5 cm. The voice is high-pitched in the absence of androgen-dependent laryngeal enlargement and vocal cord thickening. Relatively long arms and legs result from a failure of long bone epiphyses to close; epiphyseal closure is mediated normally by increased estradiol derived from aromatization of the increased testosterone produced at the time of puberty.

TABLE 19-1

Clinical Manifestations of Androgen Deficiency

Symptoms	Signs
FETAL ANDROGEN DEFICIENCY	
Ambiguous genitalia	Ambiguous genitalia (47,XY DSD)
	Normal female genitalia
	Microphallus (resembling clitoromegaly)
	Pseudovaginal perineoscrotal hypospadias
	Bifid scrotum
	Cryptorchidism
PREPUBERTAL ANDROGEN DEFICIENCY	
Symptoms	**Signs**
Delayed puberty	Eunuchoidism
Lack of sexual interest or desire (libido)	Infantile genitalia
Reduced nighttime or morning spontaneous erections	Small testes
Breast enlargement and tenderness	Lack of male hair pattern growth, no acne
Reduced motivation and initiative	Disproportionately long arms and legs relative to height
Diminished strength and physical performance	Pubertal fat distribution
No ejaculate or ejaculation (spermarche)	Poorly developed muscle mass
Inability to father children (infertility)	High-pitched voice
	Reduced peak bone mass, osteopenia or osteoporosis
	Gynecomastia
	Small prostate gland
	Aspermia, severe oligozoospermia or azoospermia
ADULT ANDROGEN DEFICIENCY	
Symptoms	**Signs**
Incomplete sexual development	Eunuchoidism
Lack of sexual interest or desire (libido)	Small or shrinking testes
Reduced nighttime or morning spontaneous erections	Loss of male hair (axillary and pubic hair)
Breast enlargement and tenderness	Gynecomastia
Inability to father children (infertility)	Aspermia or azoospermia or severe oligozoospermia
Height loss, history of minimal-trauma fracture	Low bone mineral density (osteopenia or osteoporosis)
Hot flushes, sweats	Height loss, minimal-trauma or vertebral compression fracture
Reduced shaving frequency	Unexplained reduction in prostate size or PSA
Less Specific Symptoms	**Less Specific Signs**
Decreased energy, vitality	Mild normocytic, normochromic anemia (normal female range)
Decreased motivation, self-confidence	Depressed mood, mild depression or dysthymia
Feeling sad or blue, irritability	Reduced muscle bulk and strength
Weakness, decreased physical or work performance	Increased body fat or body mass index
Poor concentration and memory	Fine facial skin wrinkling (lateral to orbits and mouth)
Increased sleepiness	

DSD, disorders of sex development; PSA, prostate-specific antigen.

Prepubertal androgen deficiency may not be recognized or diagnosed until adulthood. Compromise in peak bone mass accrual due to androgen deficiency may manifest as low BMD for age, and prolonged severe androgen deficiency increases the risk of osteoporosis and fractures as these men become older. Despite the absence of pubertal development, these individuals may develop gynecomastia (benign breast enlargement) that is caused by androgen deficiency rather than by the relatively high ratio of estradiol to testosterone levels associated with pubertal gynecomastia. Motivation and initiative are reduced and, together with poor muscle mass and strength, may contribute to poor physical performance (e.g., in athletics or the military). These men have reduced sexual interest or desire (libido) and have spontaneous erections at night or on awakening in the morning. Hematocrit remains in the female range due to inadequate androgen stimulation of erythropoiesis. The prostate and seminal vesicles remain small without androgen stimulation, and seminal fluid production is absent, resulting in aspermia (lack of ejaculate) and failure to undergo spermarche (first ejaculation). Seminal fluid may be present in men with partial prepubertal androgen deficiency or in those treated with androgens. However, these men usually have severe oligozoospermia or azoospermia, and most are infertile.

Adult Androgen Deficiency. Some individuals with prepubertal androgen deficiency who are not diagnosed or are inadequately treated as boys present as adults with features of eunuchoidism and other manifestations of prepubertal androgen deficiency (see Table 19-1). Their condition is usually clinically obvious because of inadequate sexual development for chronologic age.

In adults, testosterone is needed to maintain sexual function, some secondary sexual characteristics, muscle and bone mass, and sperm production. Clinical manifestations of androgen deficiency are nonspecific and may be modified by the severity and duration of androgen deficiency, the presence of comorbid illnesses, previous testosterone treatment, or variations in target-organ sensitivity to androgens. Therefore, the clinical diagnosis of androgen deficiency acquired as an adult can be challenging, particularly in older men.[110]

Some clinical symptoms and signs are suggestive of androgen deficiency. Adults most commonly present with *sexual dysfunction* (diminished libido as manifested by reduced sexual interest or desire, reduced spontaneous and sexually evoked erections, and erectile dysfunction); *gynecomastia* (benign breast enlargement that may be accompanied by tenderness); and *infertility* (inability to father children despite unprotected intercourse) associated with oligozoospermia or azoospermia and small or shrinking testes with severe impairment in spermatogenesis. Secondary sexual characteristics do not regress to a prepubertal state; however, with long-standing, severe androgen deficiency, there may be loss of androgen-dependent hair, such as reduced facial hair associated with reduced shaving frequency and loss of axillary and pubic hair (Fig. 19-15). Men with rapid and profound decreases in testosterone levels (e.g., from GnRH treatment of prostate cancer) may have hot flushes and sweats due to vasomotor instability, similar to those experienced by menopausal women. Because testosterone and its active metabolite, estradiol, have an important role in the maintenance of bone mass, men with chronic androgen deficiency may present with osteopenia or osteoporosis on BMD measurement (e.g., by dual energy x-ray absorptiometry [DEXA] scan) or with a minimum-trauma bone or vertebral compression fracture that may be

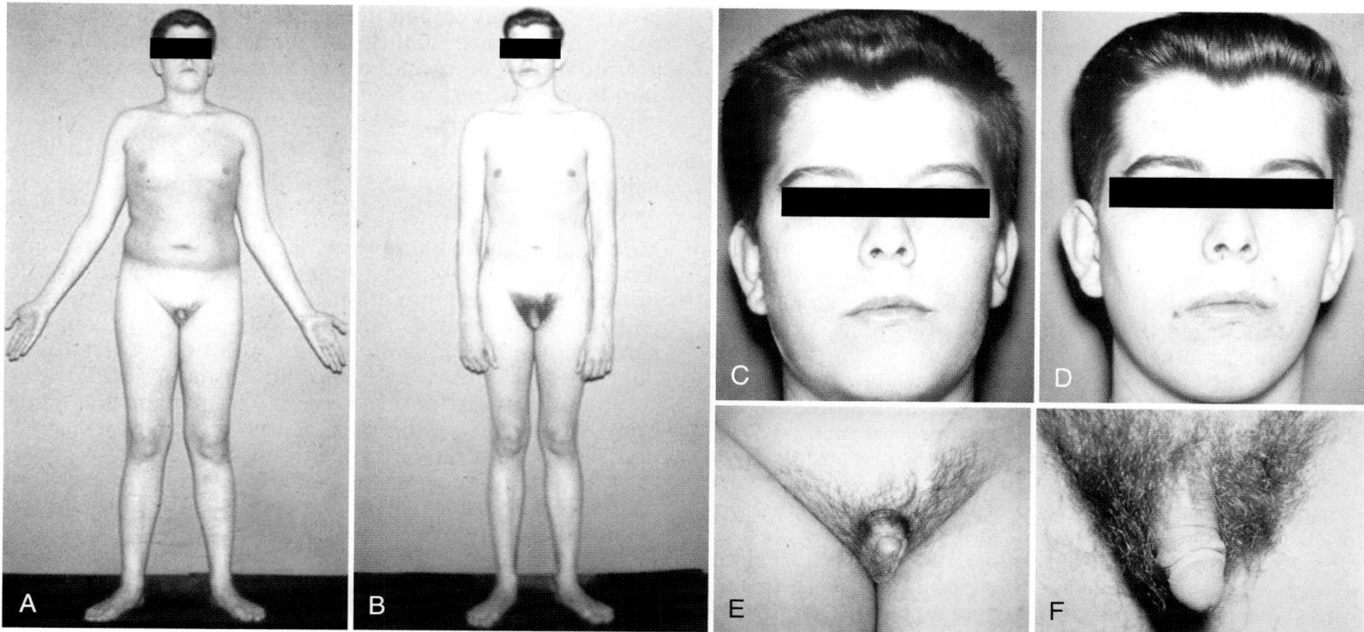

Figure 19-14 A 19-year-old patient with prepubertal androgen deficiency caused by congenital anorchia before (**A, C,** and **E**) and after (**B, D,** and **F**) 5 years of testosterone treatment, which ended when he was 19 years old. Before testosterone treatment, the patient had features of eunuchoidism, characterized by infantile genitalia (small penis and poorly developed scrotum); lack of chest, pubic, and facial hair; long arms and legs relative to height; and poorly developed muscle mass in the upper body with accumulation of fat in the face, chest, and hips. After testosterone treatment, there was an increase in penis size; an increase in chest, pubic, and facial hair with scalp recession and development of acne; an increase in muscle mass, particularly in the upper body; and loss of fat in the face, chest, and hips. (From Matsumoto AM. The testis. In: Felig P, Frohman LA, eds. *Endocrinology and Metabolism,* 4th ed. New York, NY: McGraw-Hill; 2001:635-705.)

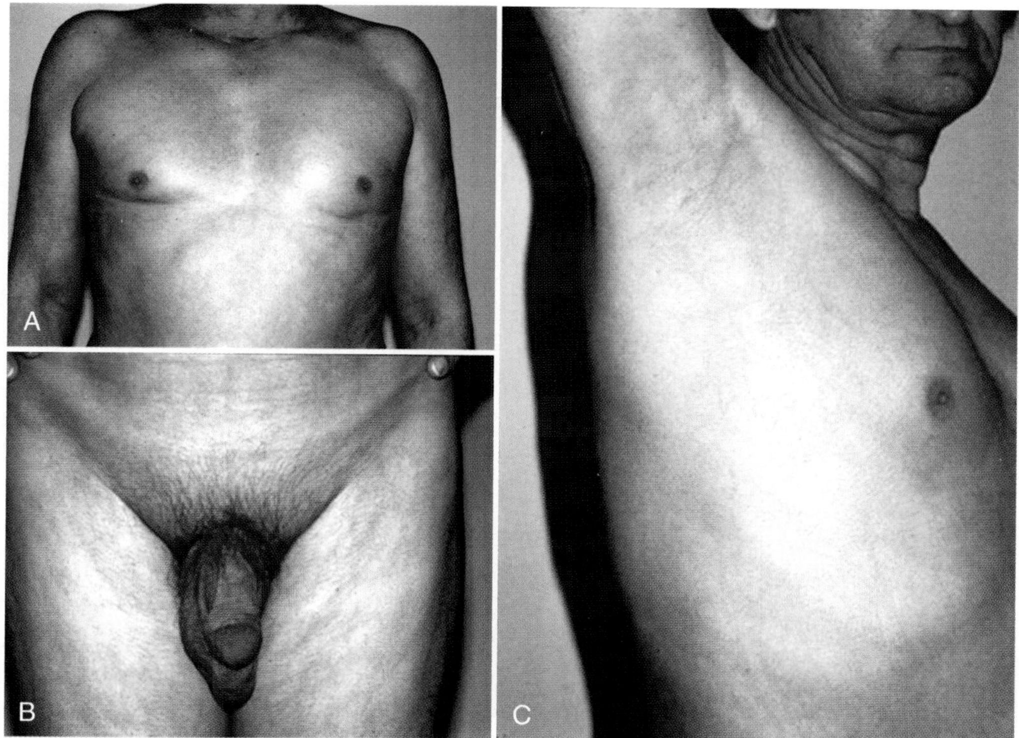

Figure 19-15 A 54-year-old man with adult androgen deficiency caused by hypopituitarism who presented with sexual dysfunction (reduced libido and erectile dysfunction); loss of chest, axillary, and pubic hair (**A, B,** and **C**); and gynecomastia (**A**). His penis and testes were normal in size (**B**). He had normal facial hair (**C**), but his shaving frequency was less.

associated with height loss. An unexplained reduction in prostate size or in the level of prostate-specific antigen (PSA) is uncommon but may occur as a result of acquired androgen deficiency.

Other symptoms and signs are much less specific for androgen deficiency but may occur, commonly in conjunction with clinical manifestations described previously that are more suggestive of androgen deficiency. Men with low testosterone concentrations often complain of diminished energy and *joie de vivre* (vitality), poor motivation and social aggressiveness, depressed mood and irritability that may be diagnosed as subsyndromal depression (mild depression or dysthymia), increased sleepiness, or poor concentration and memory. Men with severe androgen deficiency may have a mild hypoproliferative normocytic, normochromic anemia within the female range in the absence of androgen stimulation of erythropoiesis. With long-standing deficiency, reduced muscle bulk and strength associated with weakness and reduced physical and work performance occur. The latter symptoms may occur in conjunction with an increase in body fat, but androgen deficiency is not a cause of clinically obvious obesity per se. Skin changes and reduced sebum production with severe, long-standing androgen deficiency may be associated with fine facial wrinkling that is particularly noticeable on the lateral corners of the orbits (lateral canthus) and mouth. Testis size may be small, especially with severe impairment of spermatogenesis, but in most men with acquired adult androgen deficiency, testis size is normal to slightly reduced.

Because clinical manifestations are nonspecific, older men may have a number of medical conditions or comorbidities and medications that contribute to symptoms and signs that are consistent with androgen deficiency, presenting a particular diagnostic challenge (Fig. 19-16). Symptoms and signs of comorbid illnesses may mask, mimic, or contribute to clinical manifestations of androgen deficiency in older men. Elderly men may present with muscle loss and mobility impairment, fragility fracture or osteoporosis, and reduced vitality and depressed mood. On close examination, however, older men with severe, long-standing androgen deficiency usually manifest objective evidence of androgen deficiency.

Isolated Impairment of Sperm Production or Function

Most men with male infertility have hypogonadism manifested by an isolated impairment of sperm production with normal androgen production. These men present as adults with infertility and demonstrate oligozoospermia or azoospermia, sperm with abnormal morphology (*teratospermia*) or reduced or absent motility (*asthenospermia*), or a combination of abnormalities on seminal fluid analysis. They do not have manifestations of androgen deficiency, and serum testosterone concentrations are normal. Testes may be small (if spermatogenesis is severely impaired) or normal-sized. Testes may not be palpable if cryptorchidism or anorchia is present.

History and Physical Examination

Clinical evaluation of male hypogonadism involves a careful history and physical examination directed at determining whether there are symptoms and signs of androgen deficiency or isolated impairment of sperm production and at identifying potential common etiologies of hypogonadism.[8] Because adults with androgen deficiency present commonly with sexual dysfunction, gynecomastia, and infertility, the differential diagnosis of these conditions and causes other than hypogonadism of these presenting complaints should be considered. Laboratory evaluation of serum testosterone, gonadotropins, and seminal fluid (in men who are concerned with infertility) are performed to confirm the diagnosis of hypogonadism and to determine

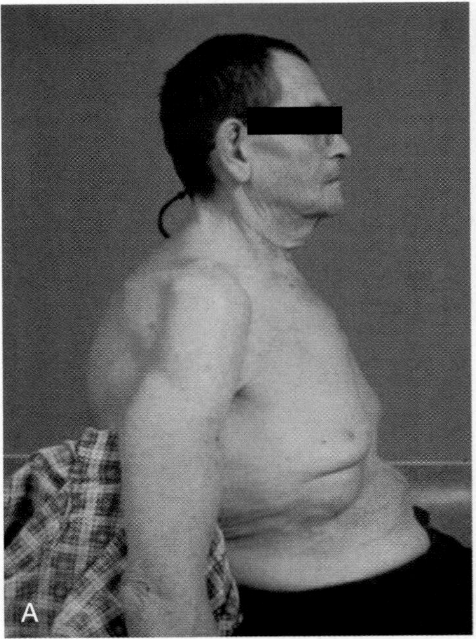

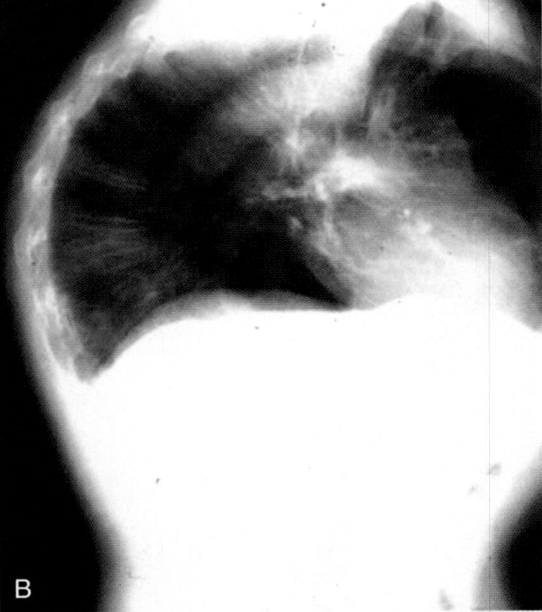

Figure 19-16 A 70-year-old man with severe androgen deficiency caused by Kallmann's syndrome (hypogonadotropic hypogonadism and anosmia) who presented to a geriatric evaluation and management unit with functional and mobility disability caused by upper (**A**) and lower muscle wasting and severe back pain from multiple vertebral compression fractures (**B**) due to osteoporosis. He was noted to have gynecomastia and absence of chest, axillary, and pubic hair.

whether there is predominantly primary or secondary hypogonadism.

The history should include inquiry regarding symptoms of androgen deficiency. These may be grouped as relating to several areas:

1. *Development*: genital abnormalities and the potential need for surgical correction (e.g., hypospadias, microphallus, cryptorchidism); delayed sexual development or growth and need for hormone therapy; family history of delayed puberty or reproductive disorders; psychological impact of delayed puberty or growth; difficulty in school or learning disability; inability or reduced ability to smell
2. *Sexual function*: poor erections; reduced spontaneous, nighttime, or morning erections; inability to perform sexually; decreased sexual activity; inability to father children despite unprotected sexual relations (>1 year); small or shrinking testes
3. *Brain function*: poor general well-being; reduced sexual desire, interest, and motivation (libido); poor energy and vitality and excessive fatigue; poor motivation and initiative, passivity, low self-confidence, and low self-esteem; depressed mood and irritability; difficulty sleeping; hot flushes and sweats; poor concentration and memory
4. *Body function*: decreased muscle bulk and strength; reduced physical activity or performance; breast enlargement or tenderness, especially if recent in onset; height loss, history of low-trauma or vertebral compression fractures, osteopenia, or osteoporosis; body hair loss (chest, axillary, or pubic); reduced beard growth and shaving frequency.

The initial history may also include inquiry concerning the potential etiology of hypogonadism. With *primary hypogonadism,* there may be a history of mumps involving the testes; testicular trauma, irradiation, or surgery; medication use (spironolactone, ketoconazole, cytotoxic agents); or chronic liver or kidney failure. With *secondary hypogonadism,* headaches; visual complaints or reduced peripheral vision; history of pituitary disease; chronic lung disease or chronic heart failure (CHF); wasting conditions (e.g., AIDS, cancer); nutritional deficiencies; recent acute illness; morbid obesity; or use of certain medications (e.g., opiates, CNS-active drugs, glucocorticoids, anabolic steroids, megestrol acetate, medroxyprogesterone acetate, nutritional supplements) may be noted.

The patient should be questioned regarding conditions that are relative or absolute contraindications to testosterone treatment, including a history of severe BPH and lower urinary tract symptoms as measured by the American Urological Association (AUA) symptom score or International Prostate Symptom Score (IPSS); history of prostate or breast cancer; history or symptoms of untreated obstructive sleep apnea syndrome (daytime sleepiness, snoring with sleep disruption, witnessed apnea episodes); history of severe congestive heart failure; and polycythemia or hyperviscosity.

In patients with suspected prepubertal androgen deficiency, total arm span, height, and the distances from the crown of the head to the symphysis pubis and from the symphysis pubis to the floor should be measured (see Fig. 19-14). Eunuchoidal body proportions are characterized by an arm span that is at least 5 cm greater than height and a crown-to-symphysis distance that is at least 5 cm greater than the symphysis-to-floor distance; such proportions are indicative of prepubertal androgen deficiency. Men with Klinefelter's syndrome may have disproportionately long legs relative to arms and a greater ratio of lower- to upper-body segment measurements but a relatively normal ratio of arm span to height. Eunuchoidism is also characterized by infantile genitalia (micropenis or small penis, unrugated and nonpigmented scrotum); small testes or, rarely, absence of the testes; cryptorchidism; sparse or absent facial, axillary, chest, extremity, and pubic hair; poorly developed upper body musculature; fat predominance in the face, chest, and hips; and gynecomastia. Patients with Kallmann's syndrome may have anosmia or hyposmia that may be tested with an odor identification and threshold test using readily identifiable, common household odorants (e.g., alcohol swab, peppermint, cinnamon, cocoa, coffee, cigarette, orange, soap) or more formally, such as with the University of Pennsylvania scratch and sniff test.

The physical findings of androgen deficiency acquired in adulthood are usually more subtle than those of prepubertal androgen deficiency (see Fig. 19-15). In patients with severe, long-standing adult androgen deficiency, there may be loss of androgen-dependent facial, axillary, chest, extremity, and pubic hair; however, there are ethnic variations in body hair in androgen-dependent areas (e.g., less in Asians and Hispanics). The skin may be dry, and there may be fine wrinkling lateral to orbits or mouth in patients with severe, long-standing androgen deficiency. Patients should be carefully examined for the presence of palpable breast tissue or gynecomastia; presence, size, and consistency of the testes; and palpable abnormalities in the scrotum, such as varicocele, epididymal enlargement, or tenderness or absence of the vas deferens. A digital rectal examination (DRE) should be performed to primarily determine whether there are palpable abnormalities, such as a prostate nodule or induration, and also to assess the size of the prostate. Careful examination for kyphosis and measurement of height are useful for detecting significant height loss (>5 cm) associated with osteoporotic vertebral compression fractures that may be asymptomatic.

Proper technique is needed to examine the male breast. The thumb and index finger are used to grasp and gently pinch the periareolar area of the breast and to palpate glandular breast tissue, which is rubbery in consistency and firmer than the surrounding adipose tissue (Fig. 19-17). With this technique, gynecomastia can usually be distinguished from excessive breast adipose tissue, called *pseudogynecomastia*, which is often associated with generalized obesity. Gynecomastia is usually bilateral and relatively symmetric, but occasionally it is asymmetric and more prominent on one side. If present, asymmetric gynecomastia may suggest breast carcinoma, which is usually rock-hard and irregular and may be associated with skin dimpling (*peau d'orange*), nipple retraction or discharge, and axillary lymphadenopathy. The diameter of palpable breast tissue is used as an objective measure of gynecomastia. Gynecomastia of recent onset is usually tender on palpation, and men usually complain of nipple irritation associated with rubbing against clothing.

Examination of the testes and scrotum may be performed with the patient either lying on his back or standing, but the latter position is preferred because it relaxes the scrotum, making some abnormalities (e.g., varicocele) more easily detected. In patients with retractile testes positioned high in the scrotum, it may be possible to palpate the testes only after placing the scrotum in warm water, after a warm bath, or by having the patient assume a squatting position. The testes may be very difficult to examine and palpate in morbidly obese men who have excessive folds of fat overlying the scrotum, in the presence of a large hydrocele, if the testis is tender (e.g., with

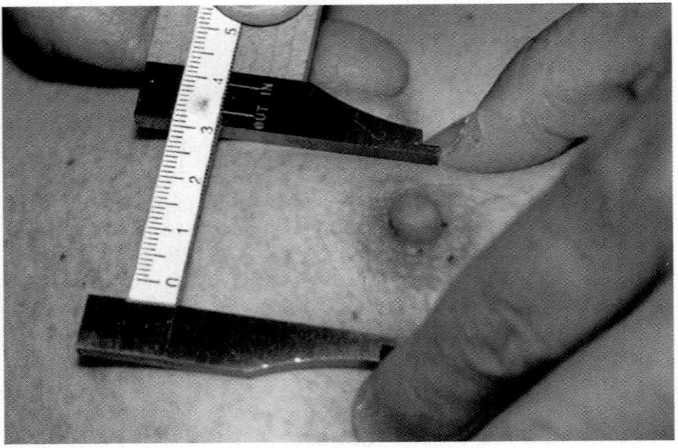

Figure 19-17 The proper method of examining the male breast is to use the thumb and index finger to grasp the periareolar area of the breast and to gently pinch the thumb and index finger together on either side of the breast toward the nipple. Glandular breast tissue feels like a rubbery disc of tissue that extends concentrically from under the nipple and subareolar area and is firmer than the surrounding adipose tissue. The size of gynecomastia is estimated by measurement of the diameter of palpable breast tissue. (From Matsumoto AM. The testis. In: Felig P, Frohman LA, eds. *Endocrinology and Metabolism*, 4th ed. New York, NY: McGraw-Hill; 2001:635-705.)

epididymo-orchitis or testicular torsion), or occasionally in some men who are sensitive to palpation for unclear reasons. In these instances, testicular ultrasound may be required to confirm the presence of the testis, estimate its size, and detect abnormalities.

Although ultrasonographic size estimates are more accurate, testis size can be estimated by measuring length and width with a ruler or calipers or by comparing testis volume with that of ellipsoid models of known volume (Prader orchidometer) (Fig. 19-18). Normal testis size varies with age and ethnicity. Normal prepubertal testis size is approximately 1.6 to 2.9 cm in length and 1.0 to 1.8 cm in width, or 1 to 4 mL in volume. Testis size greater than 4 mL suggests the onset of puberty. In adults, normal testes usually measure 3.5 to 5.5 cm in length and 2.0 to 3.0 cm in width, or 15 to 30 mL in volume.[9,137] In addition to size, testes should be palpated for consistency or firmness and for presence of a mass representing a benign or malignant testicular tumor. The testicular examination in men with Klinefelter's syndrome is notable for very small (usually <3 mL), firm testes.

Differential Diagnosis

Because sexual dysfunction, gynecomastia, and infertility are often presenting complaints in adults with androgen deficiency, it is important to consider the differential diagnosis and to be familiar with other common causes of these manifestations when evaluating men who present with these complaints.

Sexual Dysfunction

Normal sexual function requires successive, coordinated physiologic events—libido, erection, ejaculation, orgasm, and detumescence—that occur in a defined sequence and require normal psychological, CNS, peripheral nerve, vascular, and genital function.[138]

Sexual dysfunction may involve specific disorders of libido or sexual desire, erectile dysfunction, ejaculatory disorders, orgasmic dysfunction, or failure of detumescence. These may occur in isolation, but specific disorders of sexual function commonly occur together because these processes are interrelated and because a specific etiology (e.g., androgen deficiency) can affect more than one of the physiologic processes that mediate normal sexual function. Male sexual dysfunction is detailed in Chapter 20. Men with androgen deficiency often present with sexual dysfunction, and it is important to consider the differential diagnosis of this complaint in the evaluation.

Androgen deficiency often results in reduced libido or sexual desire (hypoactive sexual desire disorder), loss or reduction of spontaneous evening and morning or sexually stimulated erections (erectile dysfunction), and, if severe, reduced or absent ejaculation. In many men with androgen deficiency, erectile response to intense erotic stimuli (and, occasionally, spontaneous erections) may be preserved, suggesting that the androgen requirement for sexual function is variable.[139] However, persistent erectile dysfunction may cause performance anxiety, and, together with hypoactive sexual desire and depressed mood associated with androgen deficiency, this may contribute to the eventual loss of erotically stimulated erections and, secondarily, to orgasmic dysfunction. Androgen deficiency may also affect nitric oxide production and maximal smooth muscle relaxation and vasodilatation within the penis, reducing the ability to produce an erection that is sufficient to satisfactorily complete sexual intercourse and further contributing to the severity of erectile dysfunction.[140,141]

Clinically, men with androgen deficiency most commonly present with hypoactive sexual desire disorder and erectile dysfunction. Severely androgen-deficient men may

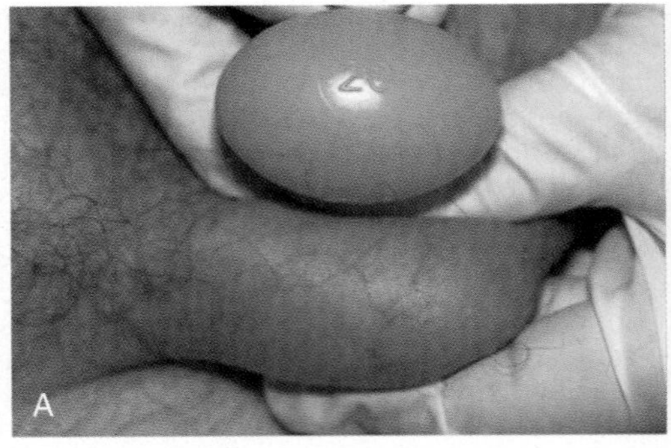

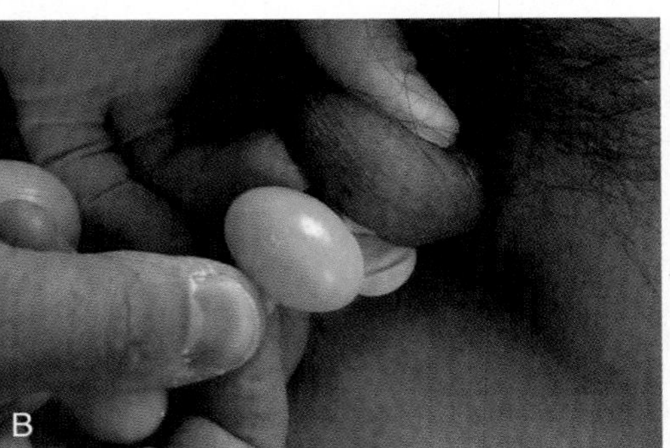

Figure 19-18 The assessment of testis size using a Prader orchidometer in a normal man (**A**), who has a right testis size of 20 mL, and in a man with Kallmann's syndrome (**B**), who has a right testis size of 5 mL. Care must be taken not to include the head of the epididymis when estimating testis size. (From Matsumoto AM. The testis. In: Felig P, Frohman LA, eds. *Endocrinology and Metabolism*, 4th ed. New York, NY: McGraw-Hill; 2001:635-705.)

present with reduced ejaculation, but these individuals usually also complain of hypoactive sexual desire disorder and erectile dysfunction.

Hypoactive Sexual Desire Disorder and Erectile Dysfunction. Libido, the desire or drive for sexual activity, is generated by external visual, auditory, and tactile stimuli as well as internal psychic stimuli acting on cortical and subcortical brain regions such as the limbic system (amygdala, hippocampus, anterior thalamic nuclei, and prefrontal cortex) and the temporal lobe. Stimuli from these areas are relayed to the medial preoptic area, which serves to integrate central inputs and sends impulses to the paraventricular nuclei; these, in turn, send projections to the thoracolumbar and sacral spinal cord centers that regulate penile erection. This neural pathway explains why brain disorders that cause hypoactive sexual desire disorder are usually accompanied by varying degrees of erectile dysfunction (see later discussion).[138] In particular, there is a loss of the spontaneous evening and morning erections that are associated with brain activation of sexual neural pathways during rapid-eye-movement (REM) sleep and dreaming. Clinically, libido may be influenced by previous or recent sexual activity and by experiences, psychosocial background, overall state of general health, androgen sufficiency, and brain function.

The neurotransmitter systems that regulate the physiology of normal libido are not known precisely. However, there is evidence that central dopamine neurotransmission may be important in mediating CNS regulation of sexual desire and erections. In humans, treatment with dopamine receptor agonists (e.g., bromocriptine, pergolide) may stimulate spontaneous erections, and in 20% to 30% of men with Parkinson's disease, levodopa therapy is associated with stimulation of libido and spontaneous erections. The use of pharmacologic agents with dopamine receptor antagonist activity is frequently associated with reduced libido and erectile dysfunction. However, these agents also affect a number of other neurotransmitter systems. Dopamine antagonism (e.g., by neurolytic agents) results in elevated prolactin levels that suppress endogenous gonadotropin and testosterone secretion and may contribute to reduced libido and erectile dysfunction.

Hypoactive sexual desire disorder is defined as persistent or recurrent deficiency or absence of desire for sexual activity resulting in marked personal distress or interpersonal difficulty or both.[138,142] It is estimated to affect more than 15% of men. The causes of hypoactive sexual desire disorder are primarily disorders that affect normal brain function and are usually associated with erectile dysfunction, in particular loss of spontaneous evening or morning erections (Table 19-2). *Erectile dysfunction* is defined as the inability to achieve or maintain penile erection that is adequate for completion of satisfactory sexual intercourse or activity.[143] Erectile dysfunction is a common condition that increases with aging. It is estimated to affect fewer than 10% of men younger than 40 years of age but approximately 50% of men between 40 and 70 years of age, with 35% of men in the latter age group having moderate or complete erectile dysfunction.

Hypoactive Sexual Desire Disorder and Erectile Dysfunction Due to Brain Disorders. *Psychogenic disorders* commonly cause hypoactive sexual desire and erectile dysfunction; these disorders include stress or preoccupation associated with life circumstances or situations, illness, marital discord, or underlying maternal transference or gender identity issues; performance anxiety associated with fear of failure or preoccupation with the adequacy of erections during sexual intercourse; major depression or dysthymia (moderate or complete erectile dysfunction occurs in 60% to 90% of men with moderate to severe depression); and major psychiatric illness such as psychotic or personality disorders.[138,142,143]

TABLE 19-2

Causes of Hypoactive Sexual Desire Disorder and Erectile Dysfunction

Cause	Examples
BRAIN DISORDERS	
Psychogenic disorders	Stress or preoccupation, performance anxiety, depression, major psychiatric illness
Chronic systemic illness	Heart, respiratory, kidney, or liver failure; cancer
CNS-active drugs	Alcohol; antihypertensive, narcotic, sedative-hypnotic, anticonvulsant, antidepressant, antipsychotic medications
Structural brain disease	Temporal lobe or limbic system disorders, Parkinson's or other neurodegenerative brain disease, vascular brain disorders
Androgen deficiency	Primary and secondary hypogonadism
Other endocrine disorders	Hyperprolactinemia, Cushing's syndrome, hyperthyroidism, hypothyroidism
SPINAL CORD AND PERIPHERAL DISORDERS	
Spinal cord disorders	Trauma, vascular compromise, spinal stenosis, epidural abscess, tumor, transverse myelitis, multiple sclerosis, other spinal cord lesions
Peripheral nerve disorders	Diabetes mellitus; pelvic, prostate, or retroperitoneal surgery or damage; other causes of peripheral neuropathy
PNS-active drugs	Anticholinergic, antihistamine, antidepressant, sympathomimetic, α-adrenergic agonist, β-adrenergic antagonist medications
Peripheral vascular disease	Aorto-iliac atherosclerosis, diabetes mellitus, trauma, surgery, vasculitis, venous incompetence (venous leakage), smoking
Antihypertensive drugs	Diuretics, α- and β-adrenergic antagonists, ACE inhibitors, calcium channel antagonists
Penile abnormalities	Peyronie's disease, chordee, micropenis, trauma, priapism, phimosis

ACE, angiotensin-converting enzyme; CNS, central nervous system; PNS, peripheral nervous system.

Chronic systemic illness (chronic heart, respiratory, kidney, or liver failure or cancer) and poor general health are usually associated with reduced libido and spontaneous erections.[138,142,143] A number of *CNS-active medications* may cause hypoactive sexual desire disorder and erectile dysfunction, including alcohol, centrally acting antihypertensive medications, narcotics, sedative-hypnotic drugs, anticonvulsants, antidepressants, and antipsychotic medications. In addition to their direct effects on brain neurotransmitter function, both chronic illness and CNS-active medications may also be associated with androgen deficiency. *Structural brain disease*, such as infiltrative or destructive lesions of the temporal lobe or limbic system, Parkinson's or other neurodegenerative brain disease, or vascular brain disorders such as stroke or vasculitis, may reduce libido and spontaneous erections.

Androgen deficiency is commonly associated with reduction or loss of libido and spontaneous erections.[144,145] Sexual dysfunction is usually a prominent presenting complaint in young, severely androgen-deficient men and in older men who are treated with medical therapies (e.g., GnRH agonist treatment) or surgical castration for advanced prostate cancer. In contrast, older men with less severe androgen deficiency may have sexual dysfunction that is also related to underlying chronic systemic illness or use of certain medications.[146] Comorbid conditions contribute to the nonspecificity of presenting complaints of androgen deficiency (e.g., sexual dysfunction) as men age. Testosterone treatment of severe androgen deficiency in young men usually improves sexual desire, interest, and thoughts; attentiveness to erotic stimuli; and the frequency, duration, and rigidity of spontaneous evening and morning erections.[145,147]

Other endocrine disorders can cause hypoactive sexual desire disorder and erectile dysfunction; examples include hyperprolactinemia, Cushing's syndrome (glucocorticoid excess), hyperthyroidism, and hypothyroidism. In addition to their direct effects on brain function, hyperprolactinemia and glucocorticoid excess also suppress GnRH and gonadotropin secretion and induce androgen deficiency that contributes to sexual dysfunction. Anecdotally, some men with androgen deficiency due to severe hyperprolactinemia who are treated with testosterone treatment alone do not fully recover sexual function and may require additional therapy with dopamine receptor agonists, but this has not been demonstrated conclusively. Dopamine receptor agonists lower elevated prolactin levels and may also have direct affects in the brain to activate neuronal systems involved in stimulating libido and erections.

Erectile Dysfunction Due to Spinal Cord or Peripheral Disorders. External and internal erotic stimuli from the brain are relayed via descending neural pathways in the lateral spinal columns to stimulate the parasympathetic sacral (S2-4) spinal erection center, resulting in *psychogenic erections*. Efferent parasympathetic nervous system stimulation from the sacral center travels via the nervi erigentes (pelvic splanchnic nerve) and the pelvic plexus and enters the penis via the cavernosal nerve. This stimulation causes relaxation of the smooth muscles that form sponge-like interconnected trabecular spaces within the corpora cavernosa of the penis and vasodilation of the cavernosal arterioles and vascular sinusoids. As a result, blood flow and pressure into the trabecular spaces within the corpora increase several-fold and causes engorgement of the penis (tumescence). Expansion of the trabecular spaces against the thick fibrous sheath (tunica albuginea) surrounding the corpora compresses subtunical venules and impedes venous outflow, resulting in sustained penile tumescence (i.e., an erection).[138,143]

Afferent somatic (via the pudendal nerve) and parasympathetic impulses in response to sensory stimulation of the penis with sexual intercourse or masturbation also act to stimulate erections via a reflex arc through the sacral spinal erection center, resulting in *reflexogenic erections*. Pudendal nerve stimulation also triggers the reflex contraction of the ischiocavernosus and bulbocavernosus muscles, resulting in vascular compression at the base of the penis, further increasing cavernosal blood pressure and maximal penile rigidity, leading to the plateau phase of erection.

The primary neurotransmitter that mediates penile smooth muscle relaxation and erection is nitric oxide (NO). In response to parasympathetic cholinergic (acetylcholine-mediated) stimulation, NO is synthesized from its precursor, L-arginine, by the enzyme nitric oxide synthase (NOS) and is released by corporal sinusoidal endothelial cells and postganglionic noncholinergic, nonadrenergic nerve terminals. NO then enters adjacent smooth muscle cells, where it activates guanylate cyclase and increases intracellular cyclic guanosine monophosphate (cGMP). cGMP activates cGMP-dependent protein kinase, which phosphorylates a number of proteins, including myosin light chains and ion channels that ultimately decrease intracellular calcium concentrations, causing smooth muscle relaxation, increase in penile blood flow, and erection. cGMP is hydrolyzed and inactivated by the enzyme, phosphodiesterase type 5 (PDE5). In addition to cGMP, other neurotransmitters induce cavernosal smooth muscle relaxation, including prostaglandin E_1 (PGE_1), which activates adenylate cyclase and increases cAMP and cAMP-dependent protein kinase.

Knowledge of the neurotransmitter systems that control erections has been used to design pharmacologic treatments for erectile dysfunction (detailed in Chapter 20).[143,148,149] The most commonly used treatments are oral PDE5 inhibitors, such as sildenafil, vardenafil, and tadalafil, which act to inhibit the breakdown of cGMP, resulting in more sustained smooth muscle relaxation and improved penile erection after erotic stimulation. Injection of intracavernosal PGE_1 or insertion of intraurethral PGE_1 pellets acts to increase cavernosal cAMP concentrations and induce smooth muscle relaxation and penile erection even in the absence of sexual stimulation. Intracavernosal injections of papaverine, a nonspecific phosphodiesterase inhibitor (which inhibits the breakdown of both cGMP and cAMP), combined with phentolamine, an α_1- and α_2-adrenergic receptor antagonist vasodilator (bi-mix), or the two combined together with PGE_1 (tri-mix), are also used to induce smooth muscle relaxation and erection.

Studies in experimental animals and in vitro have found that androgen deficiency impairs penile nerve, trabecular smooth muscle, vascular endothelial, and tunica albuginea structure and function; reduces both endothelial and neuronal NOS synthesis and activity; and causes accumulation of adipocytes in the subtunical region of the corpora cavernosa.[141] These changes are reversed with androgen administration, suggesting a direct penile effect of androgens in addition to their central role in maintaining penile erections. In humans, ARs are expressed in the corpora cavernosa tissue. However, there is no conclusive evidence to support the notion that androgen treatment has a direct effect in the penis to enhance the response to PDE5 inhibitor therapy in androgen-deficient men with erectile dysfunction. In practice, symptomatic men with androgen deficiency and sexual dysfunction are usually treated with testosterone replacement; if erectile dysfunction does not improve, they are given additional therapy for erectile dysfunction (e.g., a PDE5 inhibitor).

In addition to the brain disorders that cause hypoactive sexual desire disorder and erectile dysfunction, spinal cord and peripheral disorders (e.g., peripheral nervous system disorders, peripheral vascular disease, medications that affect peripheral nerve and vascular function, penile abnormalities) may also cause erectile dysfunction that is usually not associated with hypoactive sexual desire (see Table 19-2). However, long-standing, severe erectile dysfunction may cause performance anxiety or depression, which may secondarily reduce libido. Furthermore, peripheral disorders that cause erectile dysfunction may also affect brain function and alter sexual interest and drive, contributing to erectile dysfunction. Tricyclic antidepressants may affect both peripheral and CNS function.

Spinal cord disorders, such as spinal cord injury due to trauma, vascular compromise, spinal stenosis, epidural abscess, tumor, transverse myelitis, multiple sclerosis, or other spinal cord lesions, usually cause erectile dysfunction. In general, the severity of erectile dysfunction associated with spinal cord injury and the response to treatment vary with the cord level involved, the severity of the lesion (i.e., complete versus incomplete), and the time since the injury. *Peripheral nerve disorders*, particularly those that affect the autonomic nervous system, may disrupt the normal regulation of penile erectile tissue and cause erectile dysfunction. For example, erectile dysfunction may be caused by diabetes mellitus or other causes of peripheral neuropathy (e.g., amyloidosis, vasculitis, heavy metal toxicity, renal failure, multiple system atrophy, acute intermittent porphyria) or by pelvic, prostate, or retroperitoneal surgery or damage (e.g., abdominoperineal resection of the rectum, pelvic lymph node dissection, prostatectomy, aorto-iliac bypass, lumbar sympathectomy). Peripheral nervous system medications, including anticholinergic agents, antihistamines, antidepressants, sympathomimetic medications, α-adrenergic agonists, and β-adrenergic antagonists, often impair erectile function by affecting peripheral nervous system regulation of erectile tissue of the penis, and many also cause erectile dysfunction by altering neurotransmitter function in the CNS.

The blood supply of the penis is derived from the internal iliac (hypogastric) artery, a branch of the common iliac artery that bifurcates from the aorta.[138] The internal iliac artery gives rise to the internal pudendal artery, which branches into the dorsal penile, bulbourethral, and cavernosal arteries. The cavernosal arteries run through the middle of the corpora cavernosa and give off corkscrew-shaped branches, the helicine arteries, that open directly into the lacunar spaces. Smooth muscle relaxation of lacunar spaces increases blood flow into the corpora cavernosa, resulting in penile tumescence. Blood from the lacunar spaces or cavernosal sinusoids collects in the subtunical plexus and is delivered via emissary veins to the deep dorsal vein, which ultimately drains into the internal and common internal iliac veins and then into the inferior vena cava. With filling of the lunar spaces of the corpora cavernosa and penile tumescence against the fibrous tunica albuginea, venous outflow from the subtunical venous plexus is impeded, and sustained tumescence or erection ensues. Disorders of arterial inflow or venous output may cause erectile dysfunction.

Peripheral vascular disease due to aorto-iliac atherosclerosis is probably the most common cause of erectile dysfunction in aging men.[138,143] These men usually have absent or severely diminished femoral artery pulses, and some present clinically with Leriche syndrome (absent femoral pulses, buttock or leg claudication, and erectile dysfunction). Other men with iliac atherosclerosis may be able to achieve an erection, but with penetration and use of the hip muscles for thrusting during sexual intercourse, blood is diverted from the penis to the hips, resulting in premature detumescence and loss of erection; this is known as the *pelvic steal syndrome*. Atherosclerotic large- and small-vessel disease may contribute to erectile dysfunction in men with diabetes mellitus, hypertension, CKD, smoking, and other atherosclerotic risk factors. Erectile dysfunction occurs in about 50% of men with diabetes mellitus. Smoking, specifically nicotine, also causes direct vasoconstriction of the corpora cavernosum and erectile dysfunction. Other conditions that compromise aorto-iliac circulation, such as pelvic trauma, irradiation, and vasculitis, are less common causes of erectile dysfunction. Chronic pressure on the pudendal artery from bicycle riding, especially with some bicycle seats, may cause penile ischemia and erectile dysfunction; in addition, pressure on the pudendal nerve may cause penile numbness and contribute to sexual dysfunction. *Penile venous incompetence* (venous leakage) may cause premature loss of erections and inability to maintain erections sufficient to complete intercourse.

Many *antihypertensive medications*, including diuretics, α- and β-adrenergic antagonists, angiotensin-converting enzyme inhibitors, and calcium channel antagonists, have been implicated as causes of erectile dysfunction. *Penile abnormalities*, such as Peyronie's disease or chordee (fibrosis or scarring of the tunica albuginea resulting in bending of the penis), micropenis or microphallus, penile trauma, phimosis (inability to retract the foreskin over the penis), and priapism (painful extended erections) may also cause erectile dysfunction.

Evaluation of Erectile Dysfunction. The etiology of erectile dysfunction is usually strongly suspected on the basis of a careful medical, psychiatric, and medication history and physical examination.[138,143] Erectile dysfunction of psychogenic origin usually occurs abruptly, is transient, is intermittent or associated with a stressful situation, or occurs with only some partners but not with others or not with masturbation. Spontaneous evening and morning erections are usually maintained in psychogenic erectile dysfunction but lost with organic causes. Spontaneous erections may be detected by formal measurements of nocturnal penile tumescence (NPT) in a sleep laboratory or by breakage of wires of different tensile strength in a snap gauge (RigiScan), but these assessments are not routinely performed in practice and usually are not necessary.

Patients with nonpsychogenic brain disorders, spinal cord or peripheral nervous system disorders, vascular disorders, or penile abnormalities that cause organic erectile dysfunction usually exhibit clinical manifestations of the underlying disorder, and offending drugs that impair erectile function are revealed with a careful review of medications. Androgen deficiency is a cause of reduced libido and erectile dysfunction and occurs in 15% to 20% of men who complain of sexual dysfunction in a general medical clinic.[150] Therefore, evaluation of men who present with sexual dysfunction should include inquiry regarding other symptoms of androgen deficiency, examination for signs such as small testis size and gynecomastia, and confirmation of androgen deficiency by measurement of serum testosterone levels (see later discussion).

Peripheral pulses, in particular the presence of femoral pulses, should be tested to assess for peripheral vascular disease. Diagnosis of penile vascular insufficiency may be suspected by Doppler ultrasound measurement of the ratio of penile to brachial systolic blood pressure (penile/brachial index). A penile/brachial index greater than 0.75 is normal, whereas an index of less than 0.60 is suggestive of vascular erectile dysfunction. If there is a clinical suspicion of spinal cord disease, perineal and penile sensation should be assessed. A cremasteric reflex (stroking of the inner thigh associated with contraction of the ipsilateral cremasteric muscle and pulling up of the scrotum and testis) and a bulbocavernosus reflex (squeezing of the glans penis associated with contraction of the anal sphincter) should be elicited to assess spinal cord levels L1-2 and S2-4, respectively. Finally, the penis should be examined for abnormalities, such as penile plaques, angulation, or tight, unretractable foreskin.

Ejaculatory Disorders and Orgasmic Dysfunction. After the plateau phase of erection is achieved, sympathetic nervous system stimulation from the thoracolumbar (T10-L2) spinal erection center travels via the hypogastric nerve and pelvic plexus, enters the penis via the cavernosal nerve, and causes α-adrenergic receptor–mediated contraction of the cauda epididymis, vas deferens, accessory sex glands (the bulbourethral or Cowper's glands and the urethral glands or glands of Littre), prostate, seminal vesicles, and ejaculatory ducts to move sperm and semen to the posterior urethra (*emission*). It also stimulates closure of the internal urethral sphincter to prevent retrograde ejaculation of sperm into the bladder.[138] After emission, continued sensory stimulation of the penis with sexual intercourse or masturbation stimulates reflex rhythmic contractions of the ischiocavernosus and bulbocavernosus muscles, resulting in expulsion of semen from the urethra (*ejaculation*).[138]

Like erection, ejaculation is under considerable control by higher brain centers, with both voluntary and involuntary regulation.[138] *Premature ejaculation* is ejaculation that occurs before or shortly after vaginal penetration during sexual intercourse and is followed by a rapid loss of erection.[151] The etiology of premature ejaculation is usually a psychological disturbance such as performance anxiety; it is rarely the result of an organic cause. There is evidence that serotoninergic neurotransmission inhibits sexual function and ejaculation. Selective serotonin reuptake inhibitors retard ejaculation, an effect that is used therapeutically to treat premature ejaculation.[152] Other men with psychological disorders such as excessive anxiety may have *retarded ejaculation* (inability to ejaculate), either in isolation or in combination with impaired libido and erections. The ejaculate is composed of spermatozoa (10%) and seminal fluid (90%), the latter derived mostly from the seminal vesicles (65%) and the prostate gland (30%). Because secretions from these accessory sex glands are androgen dependent, severe androgen deficiency may result in *absent or reduced ejaculation*. Absent or reduced ejaculation may also be caused by urethral abnormalities. Autonomic neuropathy, such as that caused by diabetes mellitus, sympatholytic drugs, thoracolumbar sympathectomy, extensive retroperitoneal or pelvic surgery, or bladder neck surgery, may be associated with absent or reduced ejaculation by causing *retrograde ejaculation* into the bladder.

Orgasm, the pleasurable sensation associated with ejaculation, usually occurs simultaneously with ejaculation and is mediated by CNS activation via ascending pathways from the spinal cord erection centers to regions of the temporal lobe and limbic system.[138] Because of impaired libido and erectile dysfunction, men with androgen deficiency may also fail to achieve an orgasm. Isolated absence of orgasm in the presence of normal libido, erections, and ejaculation is relatively rare and is almost always caused by a psychological disorder.

Disorders of Detumescence. After ejaculation, the thoracolumbar sympathetic outflow acts via α-adrenergic receptor stimulation to cause contraction of trabecular smooth muscle, which results in collapse of lacunar spaces, vasoconstriction of arterioles of the corpora cavernosa (reducing blood flow into the penis), and decompression of subtunical venules, leading to an increase in venous outflow and a flaccid penis (*detumescence*).[138] Premature detumescence may contribute to erectile dysfunction, such as that caused by penile venous incompetence. Intracorporal injection of an α-adrenergic receptor antagonist, phentolamine, together with papaverine and PGE_1, causes sustained lacunar smooth muscle relaxation, arteriole vasodilatation, and penile tumescence and is used to treat erectile dysfunction caused by premature detumescence.

Priapism is failure of detumescence with persistence of erection lasting for longer than 4 hours that is unrelated to sexual stimulation and is usually painful.[138] An erection that persists for more than 4 hours is an emergency and may be complicated by ischemia, thrombosis, and vascular damage that contribute further to erectile dysfunction; if ischemia is severe, it can cause gangrene and eventual loss of the penis. Priapism may be idiopathic, or it may be caused by medications (e.g., intracavernosal injection therapy for erectile dysfunction, phenothiazines, trazodone, cocaine); by hematologic disorders such as sickle cell disease or chronic myelogenous leukemia; by neurologic disorders such as spinal cord injury; or by infiltrative diseases such as amyloidosis. The initial treatment is administration of the α-adrenergic receptor agonist, pseudoephedrine; if this is unsuccessful, aspiration of blood from the corpora cavernosa is performed with local anesthesia.

Gynecomastia

Gynecomastia is benign enlargement of the male breast caused by proliferation of glandular breast tissue.[153-155] On inspection, it is difficult to distinguish gynecomastia from increased adipose tissue deposition within the breast in the absence of glandular proliferation (pseudogynecomastia), which is commonly present in obese men and boys. Detection of glandular breast tissue requires a careful and properly performed physical examination (see earlier discussion), feeling for a firm, rubbery, finely lobular, freely mobile disc of tissue that extends concentrically from under the nipple and areola. Initially, gynecomastia of relatively recent and rapid onset may be painful and associated with tenderness. With time, glandular tissue is replaced by fibrous tissue and tenderness resolves, although palpable tissue remains. In contrast, pseudogynecomastia is soft, nondiscrete, and irregularly lobular, similar to subcutaneous fat in the abdomen.

Gynecomastia is usually present bilaterally but may be asymmetric in size and symptoms. If palpable breast tissue is present unilaterally, the major concern is male breast cancer. Breast cancer is usually rock-hard and indurated, eccentrically located from the nipple and areola, and fixed to underlying tissue; it may be associated with skin dimpling with retraction of hair follicles (*peau d'orange*), nipple retraction, nipple bleeding or discharge, or axillary lymphadenopathy.[156] Other chest wall tumors may cause unilateral breast enlargement, including lipomas, sebaceous or dermoid cysts, hematomas, fat necrosis, lymphangiomas, neurofibromas, and lymphomas.

The primary hormones that regulate breast tissue development are estrogens, which stimulate the growth and differentiation of breast epithelium to form ducts (ductal hyperplasia), and progesterone, which controls acinar development and the formation of glandular buds (glandular formation).[155] Growth hormone, IGF1, insulin, thyroid hormone, and cortisol play permissive roles in breast development. Androgens inhibit the growth and differentiation of breast tissue. Prolactin stimulates differentiated breast acinar cells to produce milk, but high progesterone levels inhibit lactogenesis. Therefore, milk production requires a reduction in high progesterone levels in the presence of high prolactin levels, as occurs in the first few days after delivery. Milk production (galactorrhea) is rarely seen in men with hyperprolactinemia and gynecomastia, because progesterone levels are not usually high enough for breast acinar development to occur, and they do not decline in the presence of high prolactin levels to stimulate lactogenesis.

Gynecomastia develops in clinical situations in which the levels or activity of estrogens is relatively high in comparison with androgens (i.e., high estrogen-to-androgen ratio). This hormonal milieu may result from high estrogen or low androgen concentrations or activity. Androgen deficiency, because it decreases the inhibitory influence of androgens on breast development, is a major cause of gynecomastia. However, the differential diagnosis of other causes of gynecomastia should be considered in patients who present with breast enlargement with or without tenderness.

Causes of Gynecomastia. *Physiologic gynecomastia* occurs normally in neonatal and pubertal boys. Transient gynecomastia (neonatal gynecomastia) occurs in 60% to 90% of neonatal boys as a result of exposure in utero to high concentrations of maternal estrogens; it resolves within several weeks after delivery (Table 19-3).[153-155] At the time of puberty, breast enlargement greater than 0.5 cm in diameter, which is often tender, initially occurs in 60% to 70% of boys by 14 years of age and then regresses within 1 to 2 years. This pubertal gynecomastia is thought to be caused by a transient rise in serum concentrations of estrogen relative to testosterone during puberty.

Pathologic gynecomastia may result from excessive estrogen levels or action or from androgen deficiency or resistance in isolation. In some conditions, both estrogen excess and androgen deficiency contribute to proliferation of glandular breast tissue.[153-155] For example, in most conditions that cause gynecomastia as a result of excessive estrogen exposure, high circulating estrogen concentrations inhibit endogenous gonadotropin and testosterone secretion and cause secondary hypogonadism, which also contributes to the growth of breast tissue. Also, some disorders of the testes that cause androgen deficiency (i.e., primary hypogonadism), such as Klinefelter's syndrome, result in high circulating LH levels that stimulate aromatase activity in Leydig cells, leading to higher levels of estradiol relative to testosterone and contributing to the pathogenesis of gynecomastia.

Estrogen excess disorders that cause gynecomastia include exposure to exogenous estrogens (e.g., diethylstilbestrol treatment of prostate cancer, contact with an estrogen-containing cream or cosmetic, accidental occupational exposure to estrogens, ingestion of estrogen-containing nutritional supplements or excessive amounts of phytoestrogens) and exposure to estrogen receptor (ER) agonists such as marijuana smoke (unidentified phenolic components but not active cannabinoids[157]) or digitoxin. Ingestion of normal dietary amounts of phytoestrogens (e.g., soybean isoflavones) does not usually cause gynecomastia.[158] Uncommonly, administration of testosterone or other aromatizable androgens, usually to prepubertal boys or men with long-standing, severe androgen deficiency, induces or worsens gynecomastia by initially causing relatively higher estradiol than testosterone levels.

Increased peripheral aromatase activity with increased conversion of androgens to estrogens in excessive amounts of adipose tissue is thought to cause mild to moderate gynecomastia in men with obesity.[153-155] Also, increased aromatization of androgens to estrogens with increasing amounts of adipose tissue (including that within the breast) probably contributes substantially to the increased prevalence of gynecomastia with aging, which occurs in up to 65% of men 50 to 80 years of age.[153-155] Familial gynecomastia, an autosomal dominant or X-linked genetic disorder caused by constitutive activation of the *CYP19A1* (aromatase) gene that results in increased peripheral conversion of androgen to estrogen, is a very rare cause of gynecomastia that manifests as prepubertal gynecomastia persisting into adulthood.

Estrogen-secreting tumors of the adrenal gland or testis are uncommon causes of gynecomastia. Feminizing adrenal tumors are usually malignant and large, manifesting with a palpable abdominal mass. In contrast, estrogen-secreting Leydig or Sertoli tumors are usually small and benign. Feminizing Sertoli tumors (in particular, the large-cell calcifying variety) may occur in isolation or in association with autosomal dominant disorders such as Peutz-Jeghers syndrome (multiple intestinal polyps and mucocutaneous

TABLE 19-3

Causes of Gynecomastia

Cause	Examples
PHYSIOLOGIC CAUSES	
Maternal estrogen exposure	Neonatal gynecomastia
Transient increase in estrogen to androgen concentrations	Pubertal gynecomastia
ESTROGEN EXCESS	
Estrogens or estrogen receptor agonists	Estrogens, marijuana smoke, digitoxin, testosterone or other aromatizable androgens
Increased peripheral aromatase activity	Obesity, aging, familial
Estrogen-secreting tumors	Adrenal carcinoma, Leydig or Sertoli cell tumor
hCG-secreting tumors	Germ cell, lung, hepatic carcinoma
hCG treatment	
ANDROGEN DEFICIENCY OR RESISTANCE	
Androgen deficiency	Primary of secondary hypogonadism
Hyperprolactinemia causing androgen deficiency	
Androgen resistance disorders	Congenital and acquired androgen resistance
Drugs that interfere with androgen action	Spironolactone, androgen receptor antagonists, marijuana, 5α-reductase inhibitors, histamine 2 receptor antagonists
SYSTEMIC DISORDERS	
Organ failure	Hepatic cirrhosis, chronic kidney disease
Endocrine disorders	Hyperthyroidism, acromegaly, growth hormone treatment, Cushing's syndrome
Nutritional disorders	Refeeding, recovery from chronic illness (hemodialysis, insulin, isoniazid, antituberculous medications, HAART)
IDIOPATHIC CAUSES	
Drugs Adult-onset idiopathic gynecomastia	HAART, calcium channel antagonists, amiodarone, antidepressants (SSRIs, tricyclic antidepressants), alcohol, amphetamines, penicillamine, sulindac, phenytoin, omeprazole, theophylline
Persistent prepubertal macromastia	

HAART, highly active antiretroviral therapy; hCG, human chorionic gonadotropin; SSRIs, selective serotonin reuptake inhibitors.

pigmented macules) or the Carney complex (cardiac or cutaneous myxomas, pigmented skin lesions, and endocrinopathy, including functioning endocrine tumors of the adrenal and testis). *hCG-secreting tumors* (e.g., germ cell, lung, gastric, renal cell, or hepatic carcinomas in adults; hepatoblastomas in boys) or *hCG treatment* of gonadotropin deficiency increases aromatase activity in Leydig cells and stimulates excessive secretion of estradiol relative to testosterone, causing relative rapid onset of symptomatic gynecomastia.

Disorders and drugs that cause *androgen deficiency*, such as conditions that cause either primary or secondary hypogonadism (including medications such as cytotoxic agents) or androgen resistance, are major causes of gynecomastia.[153-155] Although prolactin acts on the breast to facilitate milk production in developed glandular tissue, the major mechanism by which hyperprolactinemia causes gynecomastia is inhibition of endogenous gonadotropin and testosterone production (inducing androgen deficiency), which acts indirectly to stimulate breast development by reducing the inhibitory influence of androgens on the breast. Hyperprolactinemia is a main reason that a number of CNS-active medications, such as antipsychotics, antidepressants, and sedatives, are associated with gynecomastia. Drugs that interfere with androgen action, such as spironolactone (in contrast to eplerenone, a selective aldosterone receptor antagonist that does not cause gynecomastia), AR antagonists (e.g., flutamide, bicalutamide, nilutamide), marijuana, and histamine 2 (H_2) receptor antagonists, may cause gynecomastia.

Androgen deficiency contributes to the pathogenesis of gynecomastia in *systemic disorders* such as major organ failure—and, in particular, in hepatic cirrhosis and CKD, which are commonly associated with combined primary and secondary hypogonadism—and in *endocrine disorders* such as acromegaly and Cushing's syndrome, which may be associated with secondary hypogonadism.[153-155] In hepatic cirrhosis, there is reduced catabolism of Δ^4-androstenedione, resulting in increased peripheral conversion of Δ^4-androstenedione to estrone and increased circulating estrogen levels. Also, in both hepatic cirrhosis and hyperthyroidism, increased serum concentrations of SHBG, which binds testosterone with greater affinity than estradiol, result in relatively higher free estradiol compared with free testosterone levels and thereby contribute to stimulation of breast tissue and development of gynecomastia. LH levels are often elevated in men with hyperthyroidism, which stimulates relatively more estradiol than testosterone secretion by Leydig cells of the testes. Excessive GH with acromegaly or GH treatment and excessive cortisol with Cushing's syndrome directly stimulate breast tissue growth in addition to causing secondary hypogonadism, both of which contribute to the pathogenesis of gynecomastia.

Gynecomastia often accompanies *nutritional disorders*, in particular during nutritional repletion after a period of starvation and weight loss (refeeding gynecomastia) and analogously during recovery from chronic illness.[153-155] In both starvation and severe chronic illness that is commonly associated with anorexia and weight loss, central GnRH production and concomitant gonadotropin and testosterone secretion are markedly suppressed. With refeeding or restitution of appetite and weight gain, there is activation of the hypothalamic-pituitary-testicular axis and restoration of gonadal function, similar to what occurs during puberty but more rapid (a "second puberty"), resulting in transiently higher levels of estrogen relative to androgen and inducing gynecomastia. Refeeding gynecomastia was described initially in World War II prisoners who developed painful gynecomastia after liberation and nutritional repletion. Analogously, refeeding-like gynecomastia may occur in stage 5 CKD with the initiation of hemodialysis, in type 1 diabetes mellitus (T1DM) with insulin therapy, in tuberculosis with antituberculosis medications, and in human immunodeficiency virus (HIV) infection or AIDS with highly active antiretroviral treatment (HAART). As mentioned, these chronic systemic disorders also cause androgen deficiency that may contribute to the pathogenesis of gynecomastia. HAART also may cause lipohypertrophy and fat accumulation in the breast (pseudogynecomastia), and efavirenz has estrogenic activity.

The mechanisms of gynecomastia associated with a number of *drugs* are not entirely clear, and these cases are usually classified as idiopathic. Such drugs include HAART, calcium channel blockers (e.g., nifedipine, verapamil), amiodarone, antidepressants (selective serotonin reuptake inhibitors, tricyclic antidepressants), alcohol, amphetamines, penicillamine, sulindac, phenytoin, omeprazole (much less commonly than H_2-receptor antagonists), and theophylline.[153-155,159]

In a number of cases of adult-onset gynecomastia, the etiology remains idiopathic. Most of these cases are probably caused by increased aromatization of androgens to estrogens associated with increased peripheral adiposity, enhanced breast production of estrogens, enhanced sensitivity to estrogens, or some combination of these factors. Rarely, boys may develop severe pubertal gynecomastia (female size breast development, Tanner stage III through V) that persists to adulthood (persistent pubertal macromastia). This disorder is not associated with specific hormonal or receptor abnormalities and remains idiopathic.

Evaluation. Most gynecomastia is asymptomatic and of mild degree but can be appreciated on a properly performed, careful physical examination (as described earlier). Mild, asymptomatic gynecomastia found incidentally on examination and in isolation does not warrant evaluation. However, breast enlargement that is recent and rapid in onset, large (>5 cm in obese men, >2 cm in lean men), symptomatic (i.e., associated with breast pain, tenderness, or galactorrhea), asymmetric, or suspicious for malignancy (eccentrically located, rock-hard, fixed to overlying or underlying tissues, or associated with bloody nipple discharge or lymphadenopathy) should trigger further evaluation.

A careful history, including medication history, and physical examination usually identify potential predisposing conditions or medications causing gynecomastia that in older men may be mulifactorial.[153-155] Clinical evaluation should focus on evidence of androgen deficiency; assessment of prescription and over-the-counter medications, substance abuse, herbal or nutritional supplement intake, cosmetic use, and usual dietary intake; symptoms and signs of systemic illness (e.g., hepatic or renal disease), malignancy, or endocrine disorders (e.g., thyroid, GH, cortisol excess); and history of recent recovery from malnutrition, severe weight loss, or chronic illness. At a minimum, the initial laboratory evaluation comprises serum testosterone, LH, FSH, TSH, and renal and liver function tests. Evaluation also usually includes measurements of estradiol, prolactin, and β-hCG, although elevations of these hormones usually affect testosterone and gonadotropin concentrations. Breast enlargement suspicious for malignancy should be evaluated by mammography and biopsy.

Treatment. Pubertal gynecomastia usually regresses spontaneously without treatment in 1 to 2 years and by age 17 in about 90% of cases. In adults, spontaneous regression of symptoms (breast pain and tenderness, nipple sensitivity) associated with inflammatory glandular proliferation usually occurs within 6 months, after which progressive stromal fibrosis causes more or less permanent palpable breast tissue and only partial regression of gynecomastia by 1 year.

Initial treatment of gynecomastia is directed at correction of the underlying cause of breast enlargement or discontinuation or replacement of a potentially offending medication.[160] Testosterone replacement therapy in androgen-deficient men may result in partial regression of gynecomastia, especially if breast enlargement is of recent onset. Prophylactic low-dose breast irradiation (10 to 15 Gy over 1 to 3 days) may be used before androgen deprivation therapy in men with prostate cancer to prevent the development of gynecomastia; this is more common in surgical orchidectomy and in AR antagonist monotherapy rather than combined therapy with a GnRH agonist or antagonist. ER antagonists (tamoxifen, 10 to 20 mg daily, or raloxifene, 60 mg daily) are effective in treating pubertal and adult gynecomastia and preventing gynecomastia induced by androgen deprivation therapy. For unclear reasons, aromatase inhibitors (e.g., anastrazole) are not effective. Although tamoxifen is not approved for treatment of gynecomastia, it has been shown to be effective in the treatment of idiopathic gynecomastia, resulting in partial regression in approximately 80% and complete regression in about 60% of cases. A gel formulation of DHT, a nonaromatizable androgen, is used to treat gynecomastia in some countries outside the United States.

Gynecomastia of recent onset, during the initial phase of ductal proliferation, periductal inflammation and edema, and subareolar fat accumulation, is usually responsive to medical therapy (e.g., androgen replacement in hypogonadal men, ER antagonist therapy). With longstanding gynecomastia (>1 year), there is progressive stromal fibrosis of the breast that is not responsive to medical treatment. In these cases, surgical reduction mammoplasty (i.e., removal of breast tissue [subcutaneous mastectomy] with or without periareolar adipose tissue [liposuction]) is necessary, especially if breast enlargement is severe, painful, socially embarrassing, or disfiguring.

Infertility

Infertility is defined as the inability of a sexually active couple to achieve conception despite 1 year of unprotected intercourse. The probability of conception in a sexually active couple is approximately 85% by 1 year. Approximately 15% of couples in the reproductive age group are infertile, and a male factor contributes to the cause (either in isolation or in combination with a female factor) in about half of the cases. Therefore, male infertility is a common condition, affecting approximately 7% of men.[161]

Causes of Male Infertility. In about 80% to 90% of infertile men, infertility is caused by primary or secondary hypogonadism, manifested mostly by an isolated impairment of sperm production or function, much less commonly by androgen deficiency and impaired spermatogenesis, and rarely by androgen resistance (Table 19-4).[162,163] The evaluation and specific causes of hypogonadism are discussed in detail in subsequent sections. Most men with isolated impairment in sperm production have a primary disorder of the testes that is idiopathic in 60% to 70% of cases (if one includes both idiopathic oligozoospermia or azoospermia and varicocele, although their relationship to the pathogenesis of infertility is unclear). If isolated impairment of spermatogenesis is severe in men with primary hypogonadism, serum FSH levels may be selectively elevated as a result of reduced negative feedback by inhibin B from Sertoli cells of the testis. In men with less severely impaired spermatogenesis, serum gonadotropin levels are normal, but this is still classified with disorders of primary hypogonadism because gonadotropin treatment has not been demonstrated to improve fertility.

Disorders of spermatogenesis caused by primary hypogonadism may be associated with chromosomal or genetic disorders. There is an 8- to 10-fold increase in the prevalence of chromosomal abnormalities among infertile men with impaired spermatogenesis—specifically, sex chromosomal aneuploidy (e.g., Klinefelter's syndrome) or robertsonian translocations of two nonhomologous chromosomes, most commonly involving chromosomes 13 and 14 or chromosomes 14 and 21.[164] The long arm of the Y chromosome (Yq), specifically the azoospermia factor *(AZF)* region (Yq11), contains a number of genes that encode for proteins that have important roles in spermatogenesis. This region contains highly homologous palindromic DNA repeat sequences that are susceptible to

TABLE 19-4
Causes of Male Infertility

Cause	Examples
HYPOGONADISM	
Isolated impairment of sperm production or function	
Androgen deficiency and impaired sperm production	
Androgen resistance	
DISORDERS OF SPERM TRANSPORT	
Genital tract obstruction	Congenital bilateral absence of the vas deferens, cystic fibrosis, other congenital defects, vasectomy, postinfectious fibrosis, Young syndrome
Accessory gland dysfunction	Androgen deficiency or resistance, infection or inflammation, anti-sperm antibodies (immunologic)
Sympathetic nervous system dysfunction	Autonomic neuropathy, sympatholytic drugs, sympathectomy, retroperitoneal or abdominopelvic surgery, spinal cord injury or disease, vasovasostomy
EJACULATORY DYSFUNCTION	
Premature or retarded ejaculation	
Retrograde ejaculation	Prostatectomy, bladder neck surgery, autonomic neuropathy, SNS dysfunction
Reduced ejaculation	Androgen deficiency or resistance, SNS dysfunction, ureteral abnormalities
COITAL DISORDERS	
Erectile dysfunction	
Defects in coital technique	Infrequent intercourse, excessive intercourse or masturbation, poor timing in relation to ovulation, premature withdrawal of penis

SNS, sympathetic nervous system.

rearrangement and deletions. Small deletions in the *AZF* region *(Y chromosome microdeletions)* are the most common genetic cause of impaired sperm production and male infertility; they are found in 5% to 10% of men with azoospermia or severe oligozoospermia (sperm concentration <5 million/mL).[164] Y chromosome microdeletions have been identified in three regions: in the *AZFa* region, microdeletions are uncommon but are usually associated with azoospermia and Sertoli cell–only histology; in the *AZFb* region, they are usually associated with severe oligozoospermia and germ cell arrest at the pachytene primary spermatocyte stage; and in the *AZFc* region, where the majority of Y chromosome microdeletions reside, they are usually associated with germ cell arrest at the spermatid stage or hypospermatogenesis with some mature spermatids present. Occasionally, microdeletions in the *AZFb* and *AZFc* regions are associated with azoospermia and Sertoli cell–only histology. Genes encoding a number of candidate proteins for male infertility include *DDX3Y* (DEAD box Y, an ATP-dependent RNA helicase), *RBMY* (RNA-binding motif Y-linked, an RNA-binding protein), and *DAZ* (deleted in azoospermia, another RNA-binding protein) in the *AZFa, AZFb,* and *AZFc* regions, respectively.[164,165]

Approximately 15% to 20% of male infertility is caused by *disorders of sperm transport* from the testes to the urethra, most commonly by genital tract obstruction. *Congenital bilateral absence of the vas deferens* (CBAVD) is present in 1% to 2% of men with infertility.[164,166,167] Seventy-five percent of men with CBAVD are heterozygous for the cystic fibrosis transmembrane conductance regulator gene *(CFTR),* which encodes for an epithelial chloride channel, or carry compound heterozygous mutations of *CTFR*. They do not have obvious clinical manifestations of cystic fibrosis, although some manifest abnormalities on sweat chloride testing and sinopulmonary infections. Conversely, almost all men with cystic fibrosis have CBAVD. CBAVD is also commonly associated with absence of the seminal vesicles, ejaculatory ducts, and epididymides due to fetal atrophy of these wolffian duct derivatives; in 10% of cases, there is also renal agenesis or hypoplasia.

Other causes of genital tract obstruction include other congenital defects of the epididymides and vas deferens (e.g., epididymal cysts associated with prenatal diethylstilbestrol exposure); vasectomy (surgical ligation of the vas deferens); postinfectious fibrosis (e.g., associated with gonorrhea, *Chlamydia* infection, other sexually transmitted diseases; tuberculosis; leprosy); and Young syndrome, a rare, congenital primary ciliary dyskinesia syndrome characterized by bronchiectasis, recurrent sinopulmonary infections, and obstructive azoospermia caused by thickened, inspissated mucous secretions obstructing the epididymides.

Although a causal link to infertility has not been clearly established, other genital tract abnormalities may contribute to impaired sperm transport and the pathogenesis of infertility in some men. *Accessory gland dysfunction,* such as reduced seminal vesicle and prostate secretions associated with disorders that cause severe androgen deficiency or resistance, may contribute to reduced fertility, although the main effects of these disorders are to impair spermatogenesis and cause sexual dysfunction. *Infection or inflammation* of the epididymides, seminal vesicles, or prostate gland may affect fertility directly by impairing sperm maturation or function or secondarily by causing scarring of the genital tract or induction of *anti-sperm antibodies* in semen (resulting in sperm agglutination and impaired sperm function).[168,169] *Sympathetic nervous system dysfunction* (e.g., associated with autonomic neuropathy, sympatholytic drugs, sympathectomy, retroperitoneal or abdominopelvic surgery, spinal cord injury or disease, vasovasostomy) may contribute to impaired sperm transport and male infertility.

Ejaculatory dysfunction may cause or contribute to male infertility by preventing normal or efficient deposition of sperm into the vagina and female genital tract. Premature or retarded ejaculation may contribute to infertility if ejaculation occurs during arousal or foreplay before vaginal penetration or after withdrawal from the vagina. Retrograde ejaculation of semen into the bladder rather than the urethra occurs with neuromuscular failure of normal bladder sphincter contraction during ejaculation. Retrograde ejaculation may be associated with prostatectomy or bladder neck surgery (e.g., transurethral resection of the prostate [TURP]), autonomic neuropathy (e.g., complicating diabetes mellitus), or sympathetic nervous system dysfunction, and in particular with sympatholytic drugs (e.g., α-adrenergic receptor antagonists such as prazosin or terazosin), retroperitoneal or abdominopelvic surgery (e.g., retroperitoneal lymph node dissection), and spinal cord injury or disease. Reduced ejaculation caused by androgen deficiency or resistance, sympathetic nervous system dysfunction, or urethral abnormalities may contribute to reduced sperm delivery to the female genital tract.

Erectile dysfunction may contribute to male infertility by causing unsuccessful completion of intercourse. Coital disorders are uncommon causes of male infertility, but they are potentially correctable with proper education. Infrequent sexual intercourse, excessive intercourse with other partners or masturbation, intercourse during menses rather than just before or around the time of ovulation, and premature withdrawal of the penis during intercourse may contribute to reduced fertility.

Evaluation. Because a coexisting female factor contributes to infertility in 30% of cases, it is important for the female partner to undergo evaluation for ovulation (menstrual periods, androgenization) and for cervical disorders (postcoital testing) and uterine and tubal disorders (hysterosalpingogram, pelvic ultrasound). In men, the history and physical examination are usually able to identify the potential etiology of male infertility.[162-164]

In addition to an assessment of general health and medical comorbidities, the initial clinical evaluation should focus on the following:

- Symptoms and signs of androgen deficiency or resistance (as detailed elsewhere in this chapter)
- Scrotal examination for presence of a varicocele, presence and size of the testes, and presence or absence of firm, fibrous cords of the vas deferens
- Family history or evidence of cystic fibrosis
- Previous vasectomy or vasovasostomy
- History or manifestations of genitourinary infections
- Medications, particularly ones that cause androgen deficiency or resistance and sympatholytic agents
- Ejaculatory problems, in particular absent or reduced ejaculate
- Autonomic neuropathy (e.g., complicating diabetes mellitus)
- Retroperitoneal or abdominopelvic surgery
- Spinal cord injury or disease
- Erectile dysfunction
- Coital practices and techniques.

The initial laboratory evaluation of male infertility should begin with at least two or three seminal fluid analyses performed over a period of a few months (see later discussion) to assess semen volume, sperm count and concentration, and sperm motility and morphology, with the aim of identifying men who have impaired sperm production or function, the major cause of male infertility. The presence of leukocytes in semen (>10^6/mL, termed *leukospermia* or *pyospermia*) may suggest a genitourinary inflammation or infection, but routine cultures are not usually helpful in guiding treatment. Agglutination of spermatozoa in semen (i.e., sticking of motile sperm to each other) suggests the presence of *anti-sperm antibodies,* which can be measured in semen and in serum and may indicate an immunologic cause of male infertility.

Seminal fluid fructose is derived mostly from the seminal vesicles (60%) and to a lesser extent from the prostate gland (30%). Absent or low seminal fluid fructose and low semen volume suggest either congenital absence of the vas deferens and seminal vesicles or obstruction of the ejaculatory ducts. Dilated seminal vesicles may be detected on transrectal ultrasonography to confirm the presence of ejaculatory duct obstruction. In men who have little or no ejaculate, a postejaculatory urine specimen should be collected and examined for the presence of sperm, indicating retrograde ejaculation.

If there are clinical manifestations of androgen deficiency, serum testosterone levels should be measured on at least two occasions to confirm androgen deficiency, and measurements of LH and FSH should be performed to determine whether the patient has primary or secondary hypogonadism (see later discussion). Identification of infertile men with secondary hypogonadism potentially has important therapeutic implications. In men with impaired sperm production due to gonadotropin deficiency, spermatogenesis may be stimulated and fertility restored with the use of gonadotropin or GnRH therapy. Secondary hypogonadism is one of few treatable causes of male infertility. Elevated levels of testosterone, LH, and FSH suggest androgen resistance.

Measurements of FSH levels specifically as a marker of Sertoli cell and seminiferous tubule function are useful in identifying men with severe defects in spermatogenesis and impairment of seminiferous tubule and Sertoli cell function; such patients often demonstrate selective elevation in serum FSH concentrations with normal or high-normal LH levels due to loss of negative feedback inhibition of pituitary FSH secretion by inhibin B.[170] However, men with less severe seminiferous tubule dysfunction and impairment of spermatogenesis and those with azoospermia due to genital tract obstruction (obstructive azoospermia) have normal serum FSH levels.

Genetic disorders make up a small but significant proportion of the causes of male infertility. Because ART, and specifically ICSI, which involves direct injection of spermatozoa into the cytoplasm of an ovum (discussed later), is commonly used to treat male infertility, the potential exists for transmission of genetic defects to offspring. Therefore, genetic testing and counseling should be undertaken for men who are considering ICSI, particularly for those with severe oligozoospermia or azoospermia.[162-164]

Men in whom bilateral congenital absence of the vas or genital tract obstruction is suspected (i.e., those with low semen volume, low fructose level, and nonpalpable vas deferens in the scrotum) and those who have unexplained obstructive azoospermia should undergo genetic testing for *CFTR* mutations and genetic counseling before ICSI. In men with severe oligozoospermia (sperm concentration <5 million/mL) or azoospermia, testing for Y chromosome microdeletions in the *AZF* region should routinely be performed. There is a high prevalence of sex chromosome and autosomal chromosome defects, often in the absence of other phenotypic abnormalities, in men with moderately impaired spermatogenesis and infertility. Therefore, karyotyping is recommended before ICSI for infertile men with impaired sperm production, and in particular for those with a sperm concentration of less than 10 million/mL.

In azoospermic men with normal semen volume, a normal fructose level, and a normal FSH level in whom it is unclear whether azoospermia is caused by germ cell failure, genital tract obstruction, or both, surgical exploration of the scrotum and testis biopsy are needed. Biopsy is also used to harvest sperm for ICSI, even in men with known severe impairment in spermatogenesis, such as those with Klinefelter's syndrome.[162,163,171]

Specialized tests of in vitro sperm function, such as detailed examination of sperm motility using computer-assisted semen analysis (CASA), cervical mucus penetration tests, acrosome reaction, and human zona pellucida binding tests, may be useful in some men who are considering intrauterine insemination or in vitro fertilization. However, these tests should be performed only in highly specialized laboratories that have demonstrated excellent quality control. Even in such laboratories, there is a high rate of clinical false-positive and false-negative results, limiting the clinical utility of these tests.

Treatment. In men with infertility caused by primary hypogonadism (whether due to androgen deficiency and impairment of sperm production or to isolated impairment of sperm production or function), defects in sperm production are not treatable, although spontaneous recovery of spermatogenesis may occur at variable times after discontinuation of cytotoxic drugs or ionizing radiation. Because intratesticular testosterone concentrations are normally approximately 100-fold higher than serum levels, exogenous testosterone treatment of men with androgen deficiency cannot deliver sufficient amounts of testosterone to support sperm production in the testis.

In men with secondary hypogonadism, on the other hand, sperm production can be stimulated with gonadotropin or GnRH treatment, or spermatogenesis may recover sufficiently to restore fertility after discontinuation of drugs that suppress gonadotropins, such as androgenic anabolic steroids, progestins, glucocorticoids, and drugs causing hyperprolactinemia.

Most men with a varicocele and infertility have abnormal seminal fluid. However, varicocele repair has not be been demonstrated to be effective in restoring fertility to these men. Therefore, unless a varicocele is very large or symptomatic, surgical repair is not recommended.[12] Although the efficacy of treatment is unclear, infertile men with leukospermia or sperm agglutination are usually treated empirically with a 14-day course of antibiotics, such as doxycycline, trimethoprim-sulfamethoxazole, or a fluoroquinolone. Although high-dose prednisone (40 to 60 mg for several months) has been shown to be effective in treating infertile men with anti-sperm antibodies, the risks of high-dose glucocorticoid treatment are substantial, and this therapy cannot be recommended given the safer alternative of ICSI.

Although ICSI is costly, it is used increasingly to treat male infertility, and it dramatically improves the prognosis for men with impaired sperm production regardless of the cause.[172] Spermatozoa that are ejaculated or obtained by testicular biopsy *(testicular sperm extraction [TESE])* or from the epididymis (*microsurgical epididymal sperm aspiration [MESA]*) are used for ICSI and other ARTs. With ICSI, fertilization rates of about 60% and pregnancy rates of approximately 20% are achieved, irrespective of the etiology of male infertility or source of spermatozoa. ICSI after TESE using microsurgical testis biopsy or fine-needle aspiration to retrieve sperm has been successful in restoring fertility to men with primary hypogonadism who had severe impairments in spermatogenesis and azoospermia that were previously thought to be untreatable (e.g., Klinefelter's syndrome, prolonged azoospermia after chemotherapy).[173] Because of the potential for chromosomal abnormalities and transmission of Y chromosome microdeletions and *CFTR* mutations that cause infertility in male offspring, genetic testing and counseling should be conducted if ICSI is being considered (see earlier discussion).[164]

Obstruction of the epididymides or the ejaculatory ducts can be corrected surgically, such as with end-to-end anastomosis of the epididymides or transurethral resection of the ejaculatory ducts. More commonly, MESA is used to obtain spermatozoa that can be incubated with ova in vitro (*in vitro fertilization [IVF]*) or directly injected into an ovum (ICSI), and this is more successful in restoring fertility than surgical options. In contrast, microsurgical reanastomosis of the vas (vasovasostomy) to reverse vasectomy is less costly and more successful in restoring fertility than MESA followed by IVF or ICSI. Return of sperm in the ejaculate occurs in approximately 90% of men who undergo vasectomy reversal, but restoration of fertility occurs in only about 50%, probably because of stenosis or blockage of the previous vasovasostomy, epididymal blockage, or the development of anti-sperm antibodies in response to the vasectomy.[174]

In men with retrograde ejaculation, collection of spermatozoa in alkalinized postejaculation urine, followed by extensive washing and *intrauterine insemination* (*IUI*) or ICSI, has been used successfully to treat infertility. With proper education, coital disorders that contribute to infertility may be corrected. Also, the timing of intercourse may be optimized to occur a few days before ovulation (the period of highest probability for conception) based on basal body temperature measurements or, more accurately, on commercially available rapid urinary LH kits to estimate the timing of ovulation in the female partner.

If the treatment options described previously are not available or affordable to infertile couples who desire children, artificial insemination with donor sperm or adoption may be considered.

Diagnosis of Male Hypogonadism

Clinical Manifestations of Androgen Deficiency

The diagnosis of male hypogonadism requires clinical manifestations consistent with androgen deficiency and unequivocally low serum testosterone levels. In community-dwelling middle-aged to older men, the crude prevalence of symptomatic androgen deficiency is 2% to 9%, depending on the constellation of symptoms and signs and the biochemical definition of androgen deficiency used.[175-177] This prevalence increases with age and is much higher in a primary care setting.[178] In community populations, the prevalence of low testosterone levels alone, without consideration of symptoms and signs of androgen deficiency, is much higher than that of clinical androgen deficiency. This underscores the importance of making a diagnosis of hypogonadism only in men who have clinical manifestations and consistently low testosterone levels. Both the clinical and the biochemical diagnosis of androgen deficiency can be challenging, especially in older adults.

Although the manifestations of fetal androgen deficiency or resistance (ambiguous genitalia and DSDs) and those of prepubertal androgen deficiency (eunuchoidism) are usually clinically obvious, the clinical diagnosis of androgen deficiency in adults is more difficult. As described previously, the symptoms and signs of androgen deficiency are nonspecific and have a broad differential diagnosis. Moreover, clinical manifestations may be modified by a number of factors, such as the severity and duration of androgen deficiency, age, comorbid illnesses, medications, previous testosterone treatment, and individual variations in androgen sensitivity, all of which contribute to variability in clinical presentation that may confound the diagnosis.[110]

The degree and duration of androgen deficiency have impressive effects on clinical manifestations. The severe and relatively rapid suppression of testosterone levels in men with prostate cancer treated with a GnRH agonist or orchidectomy results in prominent clinical manifestations with notable reductions in erectile function, libido, energy, and mood; hot flushes and sleep disturbances; infertility; decreases in muscle mass and strength, BMD (associated with an increase in fracture risk), and body hair; gynecomastia; increases in body fat; anemia; and possibly increases in the risks for diabetes mellitus and for cardiovascular events.[179,180] In contrast, men with mild androgen deficiency may have few or no referable manifestations; such patients have "subclinical" androgen deficiency that may or may not be associated with clinically significant outcomes. The latter situation is analogous to that observed in other endocrine disorders such as subclinical hypothyroidism or asymptomatic primary hyperparathyroidism.

Aging is associated with alterations in body functions, such as declines in sexual function, muscle mass and strength, and BMD, that result in clinical manifestations similar to those of androgen deficiency.[135] These alterations associated with aging may also be caused in part by age-related androgen deficiency. To add to the clinical complexity in older men, age-associated comorbid illnesses and medications used to treat these illnesses may modify the symptoms and signs of androgen deficiency, and in many instances, they may also contribute to the etiology of androgen deficiency. Therefore, it is understandable why the diagnosis of clinical androgen deficiency is challenging in older men, and particularly in frail elderly men who have multiple comorbidities and are taking numerous medications.

Previous testosterone treatment that has been discontinued may affect the clinical manifestations of androgen deficiency, depending on the duration of therapy and the time since discontinuation. It is also likely that clinical manifestations of androgen deficiency are affected by individual variations in androgen action on specific target organs. Alterations in androgen sensitivity may result from individual or tissue-specific differences in the activity of the AR or the ER and associated coregulators or from differences in active metabolism or inactivation of testosterone.

In men with clinical manifestations suggestive of androgen deficiency, the diagnosis of hypogonadism is confirmed biochemically by measurement of consistently low serum testosterone concentrations (Fig. 19-19).[110]

Testosterone Measurements

As with the clinical manifestations, the biochemical confirmation of androgen deficiency presents its own difficulties. Testosterone levels exhibit both biologic and assay variability. Total testosterone concentrations are affected

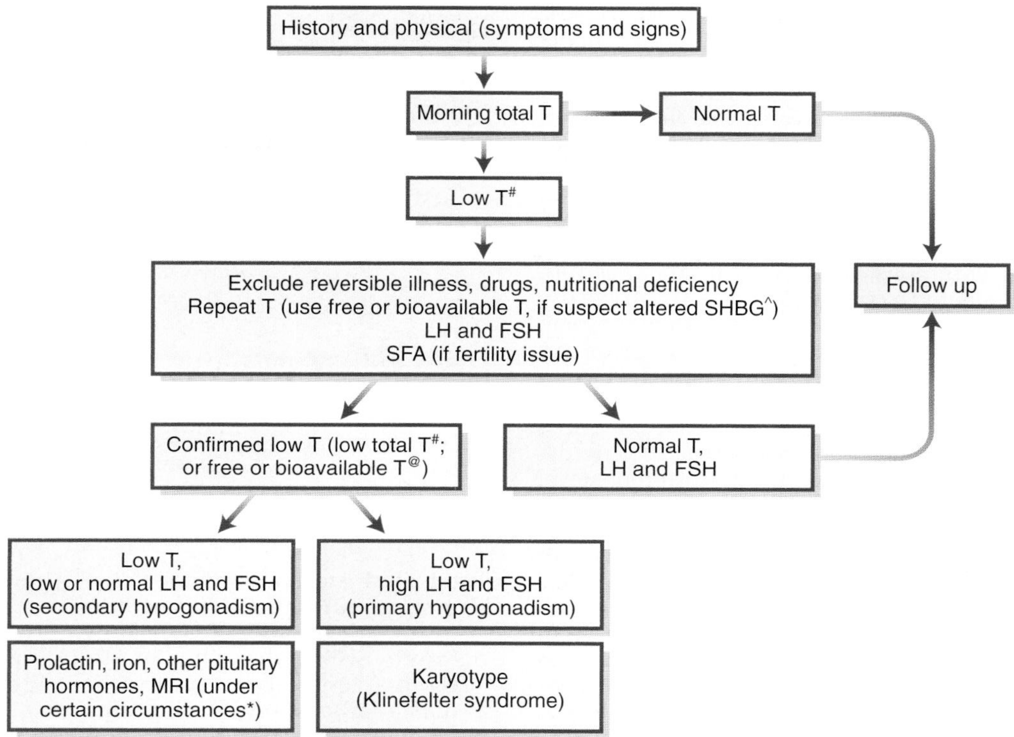

Figure 19-19 Algorithm for the diagnosis and evaluation of suspected androgen deficiency. In men with clinical manifestations (symptoms and signs) consistent with androgen deficiency, a morning serum total testosterone (T) measurement should be obtained. #The normal range for total T in healthy young men varies in different laboratories, but the lower limit of normal for most reliable assays is 280 to 300 ng/dL (9.8 to 10.4 nmol/L). If the initial total T concentration is low, the measurement should be repeated to confirm the presence of biochemical androgen deficiency. Reversible illnesses, drugs, or nutritional deficiencies that can transiently lower T levels should be ruled out before making a diagnosis of male hypogonadism. ^If a condition is present that could cause an alteration in the level of sex hormone–binding globulin (SHBG), an accurate measurement of free or bioavailable T (instead of total T) should be obtained to confirm the presence of biochemical androgen deficiency. @The normal range for accurate measurements of free testosterone (free T by equilibrium dialysis and calculated free T) in healthy young men varies in different laboratories but is usually 5 to 6 ng/dL (0.17 to 0.31 nmol/L). Levels of luteinizing hormone (LH) and follicle-stimulating hormone (FSH) should be obtained with T to determine whether androgen deficiency is caused by secondary hypogonadism (low T with low or normal LH and FSH) or by primary hypogonadism (low T with high LH and FSH). *In men with secondary hypogonadism, assessment of serum prolactin, serum iron, and other pituitary hormones, with or without magnetic resonance imaging (MRI), should be considered for further evaluation. In men with primary hypogonadism and consistent clinical features (e.g., very small testes), a karyotype should be considered to confirm the diagnosis of Klinefelter's syndrome. SFA, seminal fluid analysis. (From Bhasin S, Cunningham GR, Hayes FJ, et al. Testosterone therapy in men with androgen deficiency syndromes: an Endocrine Society clinical practice guideline. *J Clin Endocrinol Metab.* 2010;95:2536-2559.)

by alterations in SHBG, and testosterone levels may be suppressed transiently with illness, certain medications, and some nutritional deficiencies.[110] Therefore, the biochemical diagnosis of androgen deficiency requires demonstration of consistently and unequivocally low serum testosterone levels on at least two occasions and preferably measured in the morning. In men who have conditions that alter SHBG, accurate and reliable free or bioavailable testosterone measurements are needed to confirm the diagnosis of hypogonadism. Finally, the diagnosis of hypogonadism should not be made during acute or subacute illness.

The threshold level of circulating total or free testosterone below which symptoms and signs of androgen deficiency occur and for which testosterone treatment will improve clinical manifestations is not known. However, the concept of a single threshold testosterone level is probably not valid, nor is it clinically useful, because thresholds vary with the specific symptom and the androgen target organ or tissue. In general, symptoms and signs of androgen deficiency are more likely to occur with a total testosterone level that is below the lower limit of the normal range for young healthy men (approximately 280 to 300 ng/dL or 2.8 to 3.0 ng/mL [9.7 to 10.4 nmol/L], when using an accurate and reliable assay). The likelihood and severity of clinical manifestations of androgen deficiency increases with a greater decline in testosterone level below normal.

Variability in Testosterone Levels. Because serum testosterone levels exhibit both biologic and assay variability, a single measurement is not a reliable indicator of an individual's average concentration. Serum testosterone levels exhibit both ultradian and circadian variation, providing physiologic sources of biologic variability. Ultradian fluctuations in serum testosterone levels, characterized by peaks of incremental amplitude that average approximately 240 ng/dL (40% fractional amplitude) with a 95-minute duration,[45] have been reported in a small number of young men; more chaotic peaks with lower amplitude have been reported in older men.[181] As described previously, the circadian variation in serum testosterone peaks at about 8 a.m. and has a maximum excursion averaging 140 ng/dL.[64] The circadian variation in testosterone is blunted but still present in older men, with a maximum excursion averaging 60 ng/dL. In young men, serum testosterone levels are 20% to 25% lower at 4 p.m. than at 8 a.m. (i.e., over the course of usual clinic hours).[182] This difference decreases with age: in 70-year-old men, testosterone levels are 10% lower at 4 p.m. than at 8 a.m. Most importantly, many young and old men who have testosterone concentrations that are below normal in the afternoon have consistently normal levels in the morning. Given these findings and the fact that normal ranges of testosterone concentration are usually based on morning blood samples, testosterone measurements to confirm the diagnosis of hypogonadism should preferably be performed in the morning.

There is also substantial day-to-day variation in serum testosterone concentrations, underscoring the need to repeat the measurement to confirm low levels, particularly if the first result was only moderately below normal. Among men with serum testosterone levels of less than 300 ng/dL on an initial test, 30% were found to have a normal level on repeat testing.[183] Among community-dwelling middle-aged to older men who had an initial serum testosterone concentration of less than 250 ng/dL, 20% were found to have an average testosterone level higher than 300 ng/dL (i.e., within the normal range) when six samples were drawn over the subsequent 6 months.[184] However, none of the subjects who had an initial average serum testosterone concentration of less than 250 ng/dL on two separate samples obtained 1 to 3 days apart had an average level higher than 300 ng/dL in six samples drawn over the next 6 months. These findings support the need to measure testosterone on at least two occasions to confirm the diagnosis of androgen deficiency.

Total Testosterone Assays. Total testosterone assays are performed in most local laboratories and are readily available to clinicians. Therefore, total testosterone is recommended as the initial measurement for the assessment of androgen deficiency. In local clinical laboratories, total testosterone is usually measured by automated platform-based immunoassays. However, there is substantial variability in results from different assays, mostly because the accreditation of laboratories has been based on the reproducibility of results in comparison to other laboratories using the same method or kit, rather than on the accuracy of results. For example, when identical quality control samples were assayed by different methods or kits, the reported measured values ranged from 160 to 508 ng/dL. Moreover, the lower limit of the normal range in some assays was as low as 132 to 210 ng/dL (clearly in the hypogonadal range for most conventional assays).[185] In contrast, the lower limit of the normal range based on conventional radioimmunoassays is approximately 280 to 300 ng/dL.

Most commercial laboratories now measure testosterone by liquid chromatography tandem mass spectrometry methods that have the potential to be more accurate than immunoassays. To address the problems in the quality control of testosterone assays, the U.S. Centers for Disease Control and Prevention (CDC) has initiated a program to standardize and harmonize testosterone assays using accuracy-based quality control standards.[186]

The prevalence of low testosterone concentrations is high in a number of clinical conditions, namely presence of a pituitary or sellar mass; irradiation; disease; use of certain medications, such as opiates or high-dose glucocorticoids; HIV disease with weight loss; late-stage CKD, especially with hemodialysis; moderate to severe chronic lung disease; infertility; BMD levels that reveal osteoporosis or low-trauma fracture; and type 2 diabetes mellitus (T2DM). If clinical manifestations consistent with androgen deficiency are present in men with these conditions, testosterone measurements should be performed.[110]

TABLE 19-5

Conditions Associated with Alterations in SHBG Concentrations

Decreased SHBG Concentrations	Increased SHBG Concentrations
Moderate obesity, type 2 diabetes mellitus	Aging
Nephrotic syndrome	Hepatic cirrhosis and hepatitis
Glucocorticoids, progestins, and androgens	Estrogens
Hypothyroidism	Hyperthyroidism
Acromegaly	Anticonvulsants
Familial SHBG deficiency	HIV disease

HIV, human immunodeficiency virus; SHBG, sex hormone–binding globulin.
(From Bhasin S, Cunningham GR, Hayes FJ et al. Testosterone therapy in men with androgen deficiency syndromes; an Endocrine Society clinical practice guideline. *J Clin Endocrinol Metab*. 2010;95:2536-2559.)

Total Testosterone Affected by Alterations in Sex Hormone–Binding Globulin. Because a substantial proportion (30% to 40%) of circulating testosterone is bound tightly to SHBG, alterations in SHBG concentration may affect total testosterone levels without altering free or bioavailable testosterone. Conditions that suppress SHBG levels (even within the broad normal range) lower total testosterone (sometimes to below the normal range) without affecting circulating free or bioavailable testosterone levels (Table 19-5).[110] Common conditions that lower SHBG concentrations include moderate obesity, often associated with T2DM; protein-losing states, such as nephrotic syndrome; administration of glucocorticoids, progestins, or androgens; hypothyroidism; acromegaly; and familial SHBG deficiency. SHBG concentrations are increased with increasing age; hepatic cirrhosis and inflammation (hepatitis of any cause); estrogens; hyperthyroidism; anticonvulsants; and HIV disease.

If conditions that affect SHBG concentration are present in a patient or if total testosterone concentrations are close to the lower limit of the normal range, serum free or bioavailable testosterone measurements should be obtained to confirm androgen deficiency. Unfortunately, accurate and reliable assays for free or bioavailable testosterone are not performed routinely in most local clinical laboratories. Although direct free testosterone assays using automated platform-based analog immunoassay methods are available, these assays are inaccurate and are affected by alterations in SHBG, so they offer no advantage over total testosterone measurements and are not recommended.[187-189]

The gold standard method for measurement of free testosterone levels is equilibrium dialysis or centrifugal ultrafiltration. Free testosterone concentrations may be calculated accurately from measurements of total testosterone, SHBG, and albumin using affinity constants for binding of testosterone to its binding proteins and published formulas. Calculated free testosterone values are comparable to those measured by equilibrium dialysis.[188] However, calculated values depend on the specific testosterone and SHBG assays employed and the formula used to estimate free testosterone.[190] Bioavailable testosterone is measured by ammonium sulfate precipitation of SHBG-bound testosterone and measurement of free and albumin-bound testosterone in the supernatant. Bioavailable testosterone levels may also be calculated from measurements of total testosterone, SHBG, and albumin. These accurate and reliable measurements of free and bioavailable testosterone are available in commercial laboratories and should be used to confirm androgen deficiency in men who have conditions that affect SHBG and in those with total testosterone levels near the lower limit of the normal range.

Transient Suppression of Testosterone. In evaluating men for a diagnosis of male hypogonadism, it is important to recognize that serum testosterone levels may be suppressed transiently during acute (particularly critical) and subacute illness and recovery; with the short-term use of certain medications, such as opiates, high-dose glucocorticoids, and CNS-active medications or recreational drugs that affect gonadotropin and testosterone production; and during transient malnutrition, such as that associated with illness, eating disorders, or excessive or prolonged strenuous exercise. In such situations, measurement of serum testosterone should be delayed until the patient is completely recovered from the illness, the offending drugs are discontinued, the malnutrition is corrected, or the excessive exercise is stopped.[110]

Case-Finding in Androgen Deficiency

In the absence of evidence for long-term clinical benefits greater than risks for testosterone treatment of androgen deficiency, screening for androgen deficiency in the general population or in all elderly men is not indicated. Existing case-finding instruments lack sufficient specificity and sensitivity to be clinically useful. In certain clinical conditions, there is a high prevalence of low testosterone concentrations, and measurement of serum testosterone should be performed. These conditions include hypothalamic-pituitary mass, disease, surgery, or radiation therapy; medications that suppress testosterone production (e.g., opiates, glucocorticoids); HIV-associated weight loss and other wasting syndromes; and osteoporosis or minimal-trauma fragility fracture, especially in young men. In patients with a chronic disease in which low testosterone is common (e.g., T2DM, CKD, chronic obstructive pulmonary disease [COPD]), serum testosterone should be measured if symptoms or signs indicative of androgen deficiency (e.g., sexual dysfunction, weakness) are present.[110]

Seminal Fluid Analysis

If infertility is a main complaint, whether or not androgen deficiency is also present, seminal fluid analysis should be performed to determine the presence and degree of impairment of sperm production. Seminal fluid analyses are performed on ejaculated semen samples obtained by masturbation after a standardized period (usually 48 hours) of abstinence from ejaculation. Semen collection after withdrawal of the penis from the partner just before ejaculation during sexual intercourse (coitus interruptus) is usually incomplete and is not recommended, but it may be an option if masturbation is not possible or is not permitted for personal or religious reasons. Seminal fluid analyses should be performed in a specialized laboratory that employs standardized procedures, such as those outlined by the World Health Organization (WHO), and is certified and qualified to carry out these procedures.[29]

According to recently revised WHO criteria based on approximately 1800 to 1900 men from 14 countries whose partners became pregnant in 12 months or less (Table 19-6), the lower limit of normal sperm concentration is 15 million/mL; semen volume is 1.5 mL; total sperm count is 39 million per ejaculate; total sperm motility (both progressive and nonprogressive) is 40% and progressive sperm motility is 32%; and sperm morphology (percentage of normal forms) using strict criteria to eliminate spermatozoa with even mild abnormalities is 4%.[29] Values below these lower limits may be classified as falling into the subfertile range, and such values are found in independent (unscreened) populations. In another study, the subfertile ranges were defined as follows: sperm concentration, less than 13.5 million/mL; motility, less than 32%; and strict morphology, less than 9%. The respective fertile ranges were higher than 48 million/mL for sperm concentration, 63% for motility, and 12% for strict morphology. Values between these ranges indicated indeterminate fertility.[191]

TABLE 19-6
Normal Seminal Fluid Analysis

Parameter	Normal Value
Sperm concentration	≥15 million/mL
Semen volume	≥1.5 mL
Sperm count	≥39 million per ejaculate
Sperm motility	≥40% (progressive sperm motility >32%)
Sperm morphology	≥4% normal forms (by strict criteria excluding sperm with mild abnormalities)

From *WHO Laboratory Manual for the Examination and Processing of Human Semen*, 5th ed. Geneva, Switzerland: World Health Organization, 2010.

Sperm counts and concentrations exhibit extreme variability (Fig. 19-20)[8] for a number of reasons, including variations in sexual activity and abstinence, completeness of collection, recent illness (especially febrile illness) that may suppress spermatogenesis, and lifestyle factors such as frequent hot tub use. Therefore, at least two or three seminal fluid analyses, separated by at least 2 weeks, should be performed to assess sperm production adequately. Also, to assess motility, freshly collected semen (within 1 hour of ejaculation) should be used, necessitating collection at or near the laboratory in which the analysis is to be performed.

Gonadotropin Measurements

Androgen Deficiency and Impaired Sperm Production. The diagnosis of hypogonadism is confirmed in men with symptoms and signs consistent with androgen deficiency if low testosterone levels are found on at least two occasions in the absence of acute illness, medication use, or nutritional deficiency that could transiently lower testosterone, provided that an accurate assay of low free or bioavailable testosterone is performed for men who have conditions that alter SHBG or a total testosterone level near the lower limit of normal. Measurements of serum gonadotropins, LH, and FSH should be obtained to distinguish primary from secondary hypogonadism (see Fig. 19-19).[110]

Men with primary hypogonadism caused by a disorder of the testis have low serum testosterone in association with elevated LH and FSH levels as a result of reduced negative feedback suppression of gonadotropin secretion by testosterone and inhibin B (Fig. 19-21).[8] In contrast, men with secondary hypogonadism caused by a disorder of the pituitary or the hypothalamus (or both) have low testosterone in association with low gonadotropin levels or inappropriately normal LH and FSH given the presence of the low testosterone level (Fig. 19-22).[8] In most local clinical laboratories, LH and FSH are measured by newer-generation, nonradioactive immunoassays that have sufficient sensitivity to distinguish between normal and low concentrations.

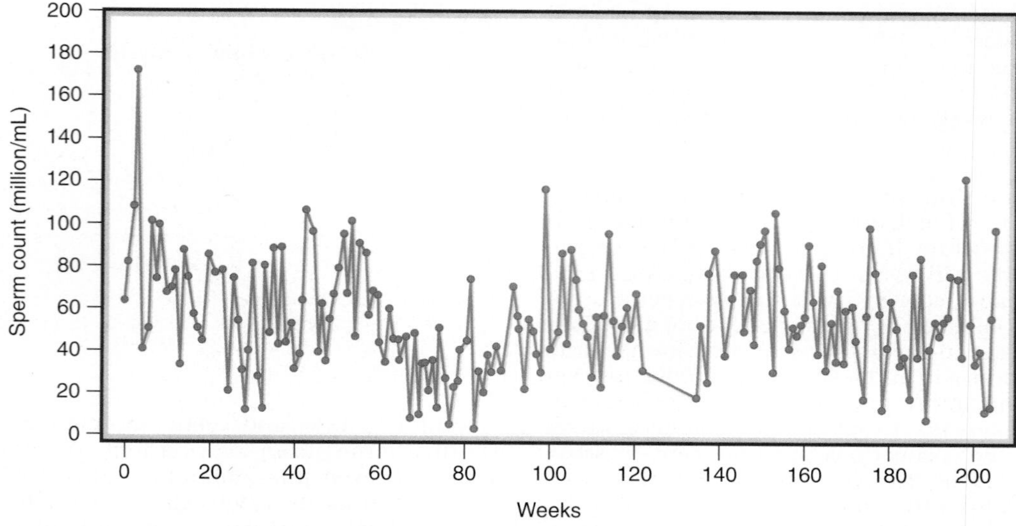

Figure 19-20 Normal variation in sperm concentration (millions of spermatozoa per milliliter of ejaculate) in a healthy young man: results of frequent sampling over a period of 210 weeks. At several times during this period, sperm concentrations dropped below the normal range (15 million/mL). (From Matsumoto AM. The testis. In: Felig P, Frohman LA, eds. *Endocrinology and Metabolism*, 4th ed. New York, NY: McGraw-Hill; 2001:635-705.)

Aging, some systemic illnesses (e.g., hemochromatosis), and certain medications (e.g., glucocorticoids) may cause defects in both the testes and the hypothalamus or pituitary, resulting in combined primary and secondary hypogonadism. In most cases, a hormonal pattern consistent with either primary or secondary hypogonadism predominates. For example, men with hemochromatosis have defects in both the pituitary and the testis due to iron overload, but they usually have low testosterone and gonadotropin levels, consistent mostly with secondary hypogonadism. Men with late-stage CKD have both testis and hypothalamic-pituitary dysfunction but usually have

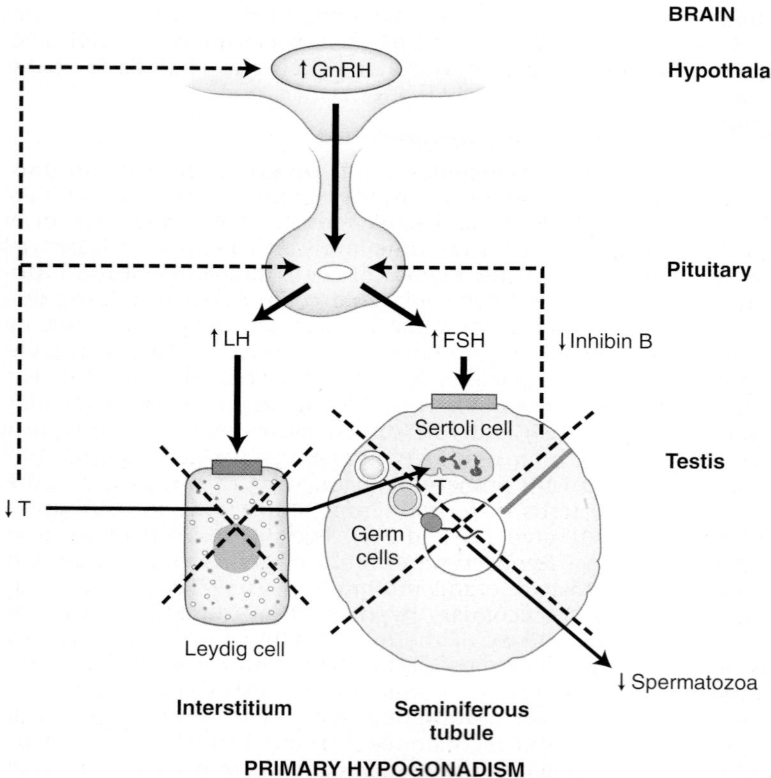

Figure 19-21 Schematic diagram of alterations in the hypothalamic-pituitary-testicular axis with primary hypogonadism due to testicular disease, which results in both androgen deficiency and impairment of sperm production and elevated luteinizing hormone (LH) and follicle-stimulating hormone (FSH) levels (hypergonadotropic hypogonadism) due to loss of negative feedback regulation of gonadotropins. GnRH, gonadotropin-releasing hormone; T, testosterone. (From Matsumoto AM. The testis. In: Felig P, Frohman LA, eds. *Endocrinology and Metabolism*, 4th ed. New York, NY: McGraw-Hill; 2001:635-705.)

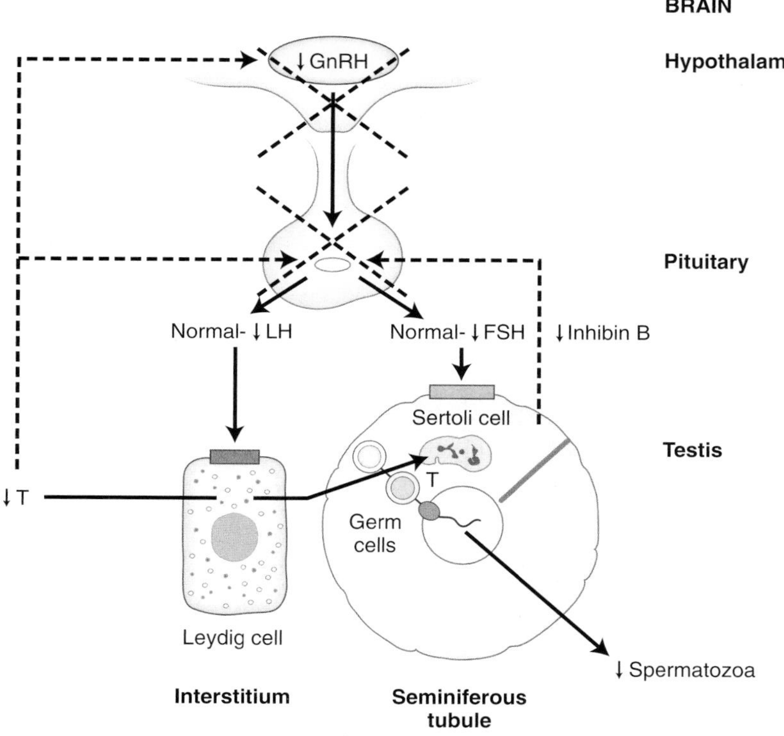

Figure 19-22 Schematic diagram of alterations in the hypothalamic-pituitary-testicular axis with secondary hypogonadism due to hypothalamic and/or pituitary disease, which results in both androgen deficiency and impairment of sperm production and inappropriately normal or low luteinizing hormone (LH) and follicle-stimulating hormone (FSH) levels (hypogonadotropic hypogonadism). GnRH, gonadotropin-releasing hormone; T, testosterone. (From Matsumoto AM. The testis. In: Felig P, Frohman LA, eds. *Endocrinology and Metabolism,* 4th ed. New York, NY: McGraw-Hill; 2001:635-705.)

low testosterone and elevated LH and FSH concentrations, the latter mostly due to reduced clearance of gonadotropins by the kidney. Some men have more than one disorder influencing the gonadal axis, one affecting the testis and another affecting the hypothalamus or pituitary. This may result in a hormonal pattern that is predominantly consistent with either primary or secondary hypogonadism or in a combined pattern (e.g., very low testosterone levels with only slightly elevated or high-normal gonadotropin levels that are lower than expected given the presence of very low testosterone concentrations).

Distinguishing primary from secondary hypogonadism helps to define the specific etiology of hypogonadism and has important clinical and therapeutic implications.[8] Secondary hypogonadism may be caused by a destructive process in the pituitary or hypothalamus, such as a pituitary adenoma. A large pituitary adenoma (macroadenoma) may cause space-occupying tumor mass effects such as headaches, visual field defects, hydrocephalus, or cerebrospinal fluid rhinorrhea, or it may result in impaired or excessive secretion of some anterior pituitary hormones, leading to clinical manifestations and therapeutic implications beyond the treatment of androgen deficiency alone. Secondary hypogonadism may be caused by disorders that are transient, such as an acute illness, certain medications (e.g., opiates, glucocorticoids), or malnutrition associated with illness. In such cases, androgen deficiency may resolve with treatment of and recovery from the illness or malnutrition or discontinuation of the offending medication. Finally, in men with secondary hypogonadism who have gonadotropin deficiency but otherwise normal testes, gonadotropin or GnRH treatment may be used to stimulate spermatogenesis and androgen production and to restore fertility in men who wish to father children. In contrast, infertility in men with primary hypogonadism is not treatable with hormone therapy.

Isolated Impairment of Sperm Production or Function. Most men with isolated impairment of sperm production have low sperm counts or abnormalities in sperm motility or morphology (or both) but no clinical manifestations of androgen deficiency and normal levels of testosterone and gonadotropins. Most men with isolated impairment of sperm production or function are classified as having primary hypogonadism with an isolated defect in the seminiferous tubule compartment of the testes (Table 19-7); in such cases, there is no response to gonadotropin treatment, as there is in secondary hypogonadism. Men with severe seminiferous tubule failure and azoospermia or severe oligozoospermia may demonstrate a selective elevation in FSH levels as a result in reduced negative feedback from inhibin B with normal LH levels (Fig. 19-23).[8] Occasionally, isolated impairment in sperm production is caused by gonadotropin deficiency (i.e., secondary hypogonadism) (Table 19-8); this may occur in men who are taking high doses of testosterone and in those who have androgen-secreting tumors, congenital adrenal hyperplasia, or, rarely, isolated FSH deficiency.

Men with nonfunctioning or gonadotropin-secreting pituitary tumors often have secondary hypogonadism with clinical manifestations of androgen deficiency and low testosterone levels.[53] Many of these men secrete excessive amounts of intact FSH and biologically inactive free α-,

TABLE 19-7

Causes of Primary Hypogonadism

Common Causes	Uncommon Causes
ANDROGEN DEFICIENCY AND IMPAIRMENT OF SPERM PRODUCTION	
Congenital or Developmental Disorders	
Klinefelter's syndrome (XXY) and variants	Myotonic dystrophy Uncorrected cryptorchidism Noonan syndrome Bilateral congenital anorchia Polyglandular autoimmune syndrome Testosterone biosynthetic enzyme defects CAH (testicular adrenal rest tumors) Complex genetic syndromes Down syndrome LH receptor mutation
Acquired Disorders	
Bilateral surgical castration or trauma Drugs (spironolactone, ketoconazole, alcohol, chemotherapy agents) Ionizing radiation	Orchitis
Systemic Disorders	
Chronic liver disease (hepatic cirrhosis)* Chronic kidney disease* Aging*	Malignancy (lymphoma, testicular cancer) Sickle cell disease* Spinal cord injury Vasculitis (polyarteritis) Infiltrative disease (amyloidosis, leukemia)
ISOLATED IMPAIRMENT OF SPERM PRDUCTION OR FUNCTION	
Congenital or Developmental Disorders	
Cryptorchidism Varicocele Y chromosome microdeletions	Myotonic dystrophy Sertoli cell–only syndrome Primary ciliary dyskinesia Down syndrome FSH receptor mutation
Acquired Disorders	
Orchitis Ionizing radiation Chemotherapy agents Thermal trauma	Environmental toxins
Systemic Disorders	
Acute febrile illness Malignancy (testicular cancer, Hodgkin's disease)* Idiopathic azoospermia or oligozoospermia	Spinal cord injury

*Combined primary and secondary hypogonadism.
CAH, congenital adrenal hyperplasia; FSH, follicle-stimulating hormone; LH, luteinizing hormone.

TABLE 19-8

Causes of Secondary Hypogonadism

Common Causes	Uncommon Causes
ANDROGEN DEFICIENCY AND IMPAIRMENT OF SPERM PRODUCTION	
Congenital or Developmental Disorders	
Constitutional delayed puberty Hemochromatosis	IHH and variants IHH Kallmann's syndrome Congenital adrenal hypoplasia Isolated LH deficiency, LHβ mutations Complex genetic syndromes
Acquired Disorders	
Hyperprolactinemia Opiates Androgenic anabolic steroids, progestins, estrogen excess GnRH agonist or antagonist	Hypopituitarism Pituitary or hypothalamic tumor Surgical hypophysectomy, pituitary or cranial irradiation Vascular compromise, traumatic brain injury Granulomatous or infiltrative disease Infection Pituitary stalk disease Lymphocytic hypophysitis
Systemic Disorders	
Glucocorticoid excess (Cushing's syndrome)* Chronic organ failure* Chronic liver disease (hepatic cirrhosis), chronic kidney disease, chronic lung disease, chronic heart failure Chronic systemic illness* Diabetes mellitus Malignancy Rheumatic disease (rheumatoid arthritis) HIV disease Starvation,* malnutrition,* eating disorders, endurance exercise Morbid obesity, obstructive sleep apnea Acute and critical illness Aging*	Chronic systemic illness* Spinal cord injury Transfusion-related iron overload (β-thalassemia) Sickle cell disease Cystic fibrosis
ISOLATED IMPAIRMENT OF SPERM PRODUCTION OR FUNCTION	
Congenital or Developmental Disorders	
	Congenital adrenal hyperplasia (21-hydroxylase deficiency, 11β- hydroxylase deficiency) Isolated FSH deficiency, FSHβ mutations
Acquired Disorders	
Testosterone, androgenic anabolic steroids Malignancy (Hodgkin's disease, testicular cancer)*	Androgen- or hCG-secreting tumors Hyperprolactinemia

*Combined primary and secondary hypogonadism.
FSH, follicle-stimulating hormone; GnRH, gonadotropin-releasing hormone; hCG, human chorionic gonadotropin; HIV, human immunodeficiency virus; IHH, idiopathic hypogonadotropic hypogonadism; LH, luteinizing hormone.

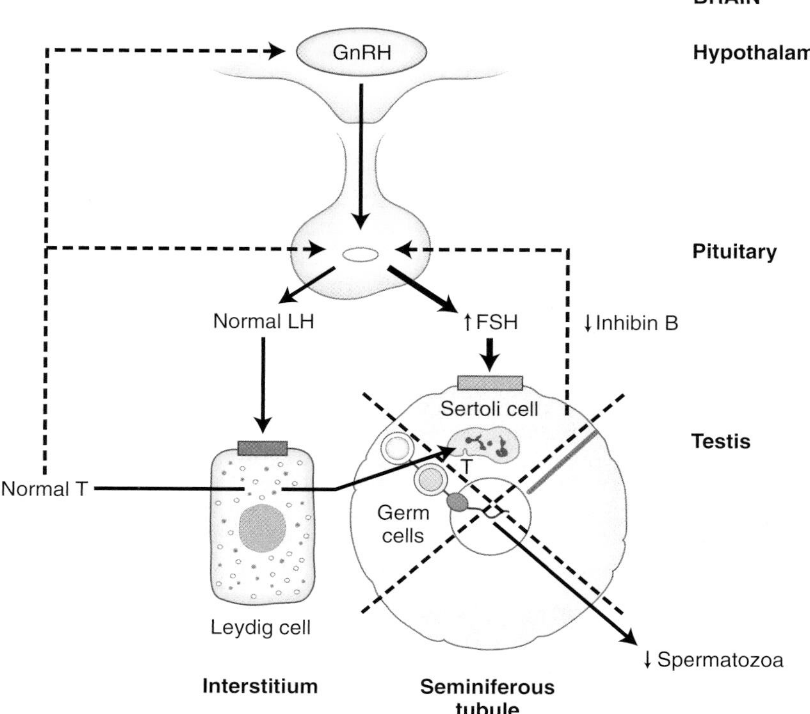

Figure 19-23 Schematic diagram of alterations in the hypothalamic-pituitary-testicular axis with primary hypogonadism due to an isolated seminiferous tubule defect, which results in isolated impairment of sperm production and/or function and elevation of follicle-stimulating hormone (FSH) levels with normal luteinizing hormone (LH) levels. With less severe seminiferous tubule defects, both FSH and LH levels are normal. GnRH, gonadotropin-releasing hormone; T, testosterone. (From Matsumoto AM. The testis. In: Felig P, Frohman LA, eds. *Endocrinology and Metabolism,* 4th ed. New York, NY: McGraw-Hill; 2001:635-705.)

FSHβ-, and LHβ-subunits but rarely intact LH. Therefore, a gonadotropin-secreting pituitary tumor should be suspected in a man who has clinical manifestations of androgen deficiency, low testosterone, and elevated FSH but normal or low LH (or, rarely, elevated LH but normal FSH), which is an atypical gonadotropin pattern for men with androgen deficiency.

Rarely, disorders of androgen action or androgen resistance manifest in adults (Table 19-9). These men usually present with clinical manifestations similar to those of men with mild androgen deficiency, usually with an almost normal male phenotype and frequently with varying degrees of hypospadias, cryptorchidism, scrotal abnormalities, or impairment in sperm production. Usually, both serum testosterone and gonadotropin levels are elevated (Fig. 19-24).[8]

TABLE 19-9

Causes of Androgen Resistance

Common Causes	Uncommon Causes
Congenital or Developmental Disorders	
	Kennedy disease (spinal and bulbar muscular atrophy) Partial androgen insensitivity syndrome (AR mutations) 5α-reductase type 2 deficiency Complete androgen insensitivity syndrome (female phenotype)
Acquired Disorders	
AR antagonists (bicalutamide, nilutamide) Drugs (spironolactone, cyproterone acetate, marijuana, histamine 2 receptor antagonists)	Celiac disease

AR, androgen receptor.

Further Evaluation

Testosterone measurements and assessment of sperm production, combined with measurement of gonadotropin levels, allow classification of the causes of male hypogonadism into primary or secondary hypogonadism and subclassification of the latter into disorders causing androgen deficiency and impairment in sperm production and those causing isolated impairment of sperm production or function (see Tables 19-7 and 19-8).

Once hypogonadism has been classified, further evaluation includes a history (including medication review), physical examination, and laboratory testing to identify a specific etiology. For example, in men with primary hypogonadism and suggestive clinical manifestations such as very small testes and gynecomastia, low or low-normal testosterone, azoospermia, and markedly elevated gonadotropins, a karyotype may be obtained to confirm the diagnosis of Klinefelter's syndrome.

In men with secondary hypogonadism, further evaluation may include measurements of serum prolactin (in almost all cases) to exclude hyperprolactinemia; iron saturation to screen for hereditary hemochromatosis, especially in men with other manifestations of iron overload (e.g., liver failure, diabetes, CHF) and in young men with unexplained selective gonadotropin deficiency; further testing to exclude excessive secretion or deficiency of anterior pituitary hormones; and magnetic resonance imaging

(MRI) of the sella turcica to exclude a pituitary or hypothalamic tumor or infiltrative disease. Computed tomography of the sella turcica usually detects a pituitary macroadenoma but is less sensitive than sella MRI in detecting smaller tumors and infiltrative disease.[110]

It is not cost-effective to perform sella MRI in all men with secondary hypogonadism. This modality should be reserved for men with severe androgen deficiency (e.g., serum testosterone <150 ng/dL) due to secondary hypogonadism, particularly with distinctly low gonadotropin levels[192,193]; discordant LH and FSH levels associated with androgen deficiency; hyperprolactinemia (especially with prolactin levels >100 to 200 ng/mL); clinical and biochemical evidence of excessive secretion of other pituitary hormones (e.g., free α-subunit secretion, Cushing's syndrome, acromegaly), panhypopituitarism, or diabetes insipidus; and tumor mass effects, such as severe headache, visual field defects, or visual impairment.

In men who have severe androgen deficiency caused by primary or secondary hypogonadism or who have sustained a low-trauma or fragility fracture, DEXA scanning to assess BMD should be performed to exclude osteopenia or osteoporosis.[110]

Causes of Primary Hypogonadism

Androgen Deficiency and Impairment in Sperm Production

Congenital or Developmental Disorders

Klinefelter's Syndrome. Classically, Klinefelter's syndrome is characterized by very small, firm testes; azoospermia and infertility; varying degrees of androgen deficiency and eunuchoidism; and uniformly elevated gonadotropin levels.[194-196] It is the most common sex chromosome abnormality and the most common cause of primary hypogonadism resulting in androgen deficiency and impaired sperm production. It occurs prenatally and neonatally in 1 of every 500 to 700 males, and the prevalence in adults is 1 in 2500.[1,2] Because the syndrome does not cause premature mortality in boys, the low adult prevalence indicates that Klinefelter's syndrome is often overlooked and underdiagnosed in men. This is surprising, given the almost uniform finding of extremely small testes and other phenotypic abnormalities in these men. The risk of having a child with Klinefelter's syndrome increases with both maternal and paternal age.

The fundamental chromosomal abnormality in Klinefelter's syndrome is the presence of one or more extra X chromosomes due to maternal meiotic nondisjunction (mostly in meiosis I) in approximately 50% of the cases or paternal meiotic nondisjunction in the remaining cases.[194-196] The principal karyotype in 90% of men with Klinefelter's syndrome is 47,XXY. Most of the remaining 10% have mosaic Klinefelter's syndrome (47,XXY/46,XY), in which there is a 47,XXY karyotype in some tissues and a normal 46,XY karyotype in other tissues. Mosaicism occurs as a result of postfertilization mitotic nondisjunction. Men with mosaic Klinefelter's syndrome usually demonstrate a variable and less severe phenotype that depends on the specific tissues in which an extra X chromosome is present. Some men with mosaicism have a normal karyotype in the testis with intact spermatogenesis and fertility. Rarely, men with Klinefelter's syndrome have more than one extra X chromosome (e.g., 48,XXXY, 49,XXXXY). Men with these variants manifest a more severe phenotype than is seen in classic Klinefelter's syndrome.

Infants with Klinefelter's syndrome may manifest micropenis, hypospadias, cryptorchidism, or developmental delay.[197] During childhood, boys with the syndrome commonly have small testes and reduced penile length relative

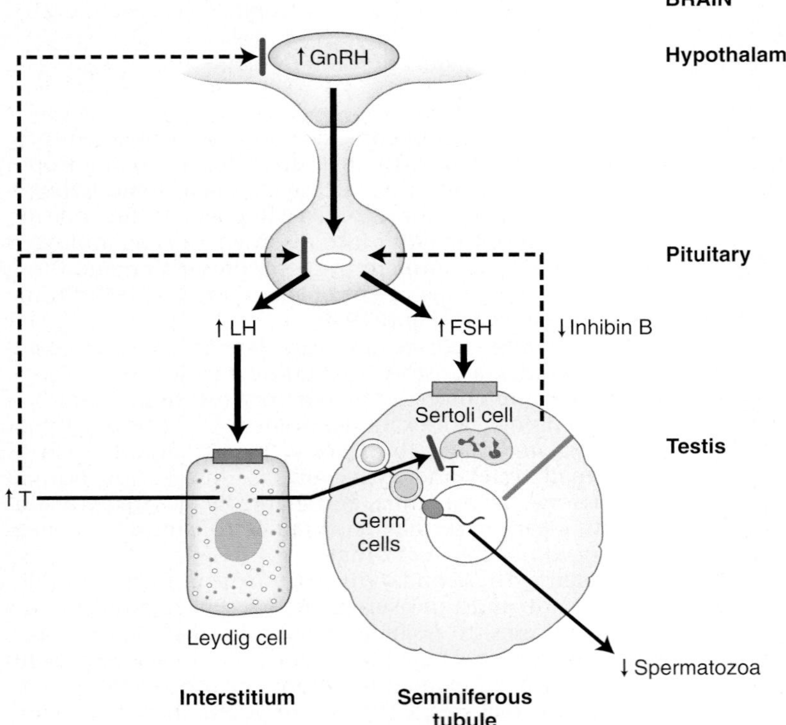

Figure 19-24 Schematic diagram of alterations in the hypothalamic-pituitary-testicular axis with androgen resistance due to impaired androgen action (e.g., androgen receptor mutation), which results in high testosterone (T) levels but reduced androgen action. This leads to manifestations of androgen deficiency, impaired sperm production, and elevated luteinizing hormone (LH) and follicle-stimulating hormone (FSH) levels due to impaired androgen-mediated negative feedback regulation of gonadotropins. GnRH, gonadotropin-releasing hormone. (From Matsumoto AM. The testis. In: Felig P, Frohman LA, eds. *Endocrinology and Metabolism*, 4th ed. New York, NY: McGraw-Hill; 2001:635-705.)

to age-matched normal individuals and may manifest relatively tall stature, clinodactyly, hypertelorism, gynecomastia, elbow dysplasia, high-arched palate, hypotonia, language delay or learning and reading disabilities requiring therapy, and behavioral problems. However, these manifestations may be mild and are often missed. Fewer than 10% of boys with Klinefelter's syndrome (usually those with the most severe phenotype) are diagnosed before puberty. At puberty, the testes fail to increase in size and become firm due to a progressive loss of germ cells and seminiferous tubule hyalinization and fibrosis; Sertoli cell products, inhibin B, and AMH decline to very low or undetectable levels; testosterone levels increase but to less than normal levels in some boys, resulting in varying degrees of eunuchoidism and gynecomastia; and FSH levels are disproportionately elevated relative to LH levels.

In adults, the most prominent and consistent clinical feature of Klinefelter's syndrome is very small testes, <4 mL (<2.5 cm) in length; this feature is easily detected on examination and should alert the clinician to possibility of Klinefelter's syndrome (Fig. 19-25).[9,198] Men with this syndrome may present with a complaint of infertility and subsequently be found to have azoospermia and very small testes.[199] Other manifestations include varying degrees of androgen deficiency, eunuchoidism, and gynecomastia (Fig. 19-26).[196] In contrast to the classic long arms and legs of eunuchoidism seen in patients with prepubertal androgen deficiency, Klinefelter's syndrome results in a disproportionate increase in lower- compared with upper-extremity long bone growth. Gynecomastia occurs in 50% to 80% of men with the syndrome and may be quite prominent and embarrassing. Learning and developmental disabilities occur in about 70% of men with Klinefelter's syndrome. Character and personality disorders and behavioral problems occur commonly, possibly in part because of the psychosocial consequences of androgen deficiency. Men with Klinefelter's syndrome have intelligence quotient (IQ) scores that are reduced by 10 to 15 points but not into the intellectual disability range. Taurodontism, characterized by enlarged molar teeth resulting from enlargement and extension of the pulp chamber, is present in 40% of men with Klinefelter's syndrome.

As described previously, the *AR* gene is located on the X chromosome, and the length of the highly polymorphic CAG repeat in exon 1 of the *AR* gene is inversely related to AR activity. In Klinefelter's syndrome, the X chromosome carrying the *AR* gene with a short CAG repeat length (i.e., greater AR activity) undergoes inactivation preferentially.[130] Klinefelter's syndrome patients with short CAG repeat lengths were found to have more stable relationships, higher educational levels, and greater responses to testosterone treatment. In contrast, men with long CAG repeat length (i.e., reduced AR activity) had longer arms and legs, smaller testes, a greater degree of gynecomastia, and lower BMD. Therefore, skewed inactivation of the X chromosome resulting in preferential activity of the long CAG repeat may contribute to phenotypic severity and variability of Klinefelter's syndrome.

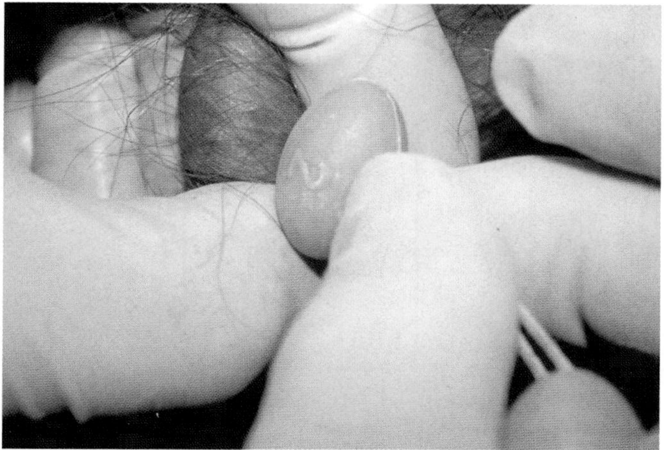

Figure 19-25 Testis size in a man with classic 47,XXY Klinefelter's syndrome is characteristically very small (e.g., 2 mL).

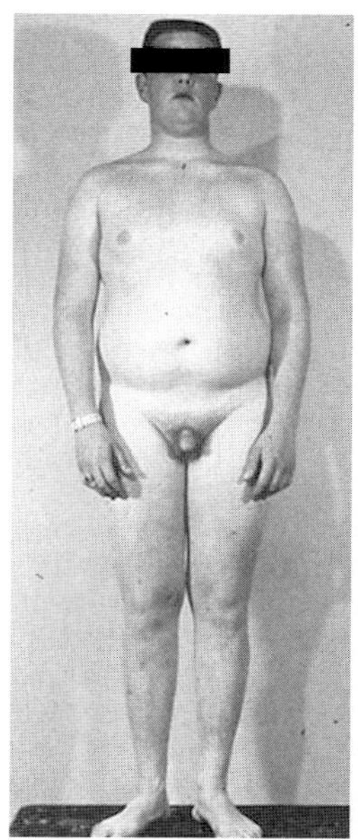

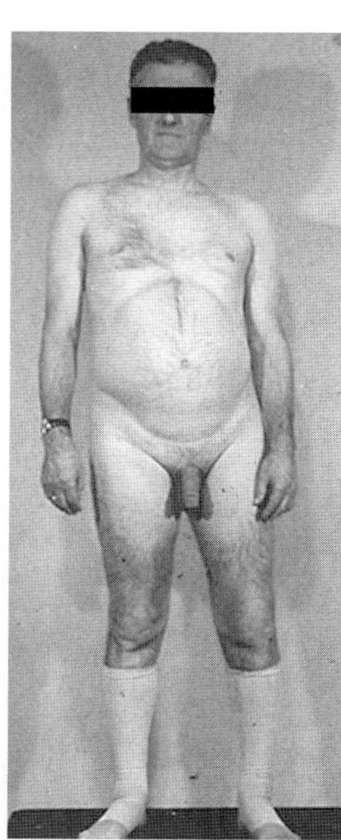

Figure 19-26 Variability in the degree of androgen deficiency manifested in men with Klinefelter's syndrome. The man on the left, who has classic 47,XXY Klinefelter's syndrome, demonstrates prepubertal androgen deficiency with eunuchoidal body proportions, small penis, sparse chest and pubic hair, poor muscle development, prepubertal fat distribution, and very small testes (2 mL bilaterally). The man on the right, who has mosaic 47,XXY/46,XY Klinefelter's syndrome, demonstrates normal body proportions, penis size, and body hair but small testis size (8 mL bilaterally). (From Smyth CM, Bremner WJ. Klinefelter syndrome. *Arch Intern Med.* 1998;158:1309-1314.)

Most men with mosaic Klinefelter's syndrome exhibit less severe clinical manifestations than those with the classic syndrome. Men with more than two extra X chromosomes have more severe manifestations and a higher incidence of intellectual disability and somatic abnormalities such as hypospadias, cryptorchidism, and radioulnar synostosis. Very rarely, some phenotypic males with a 46,XX karyotype exhibit typical clinical manifestations of Klinefelter's syndrome except that they have shorter stature and a greater incidence of cryptorchidism, gynecomastia, and androgen deficiency.[200] In most of these cases, there has been a translocation of an SRY-containing segment of the Y chromosome onto an X chromosome.

In addition to infertility, variable androgen deficiency, and gynecomastia, patients with Klinefelter's syndrome have an approximately 20-fold increased risk in breast cancer compared with normal men (although the absolute lifetime risk of <1% is low); such patients account for approximately 4% of all cases of male breast cancer.[201] Klinefelter's syndrome is also associated with increased risk for mitral valve prolapse; lower-extremity varicose veins, venous stasis ulcers, deep vein thrombosis, and pulmonary embolism; autoimmune diseases such as systemic lupus erythematosus, rheumatoid arthritis, and Sjögren's syndrome; other cancers such as extragonadal germ cell cancer and non-Hodgkin's lymphoma; T2DM and the metabolic syndrome; and psychiatric illnesses such as depression and schizophrenia. There is a minimal reduction in life expectancy of approximately 2 years in men with Klinefelter's syndrome, associated with excess deaths due to a variety of common causes.[202,203]

Azoospermia is present in more than 95% of men with classic Klinefelter's syndrome, and infertility in more than 99%. Serum total testosterone levels are usually low but may fall in the low-normal to mid-normal range in 40% to 50% of cases (Fig. 19-27).[195,196] Relative to normal men, men with Klinefelter's syndrome have elevated serum estradiol levels, which probably contributes to the development of gynecomastia, and increased SHBG concentrations. Increased SHBG levels provide a partial explanation for normal total testosterone levels in the presence of low concentrations of free testosterone. Serum FSH levels are almost always elevated; serum LH levels are usually elevated but may fall into the high-normal range in some men (see Fig. 19-27).[195,196]

A *Barr body analysis* may be used as a rapid and reliable screening test for Klinefelter's syndrome. In a normal female with two X chromosomes, one X chromosome is inactivated and may be detected as sex chromatin (Barr body) on staining of the nucleus in epithelial cells obtained from a scraping of the buccal mucosa (buccal smear). In a normal 46,XY male, the single X chromosome is not inactivated, and no Barr body is present. In contrast, X inactivation occurs in a 47,XXY man with Klinefelter's syndrome, resulting in a detectable Barr body. Men with variant syndromes characterized by more than two extra X chromosomes may exhibit more than one Barr body per nucleus; the number of Barr bodies is one less than the number of extra X chromosomes. Although Barr body analysis may be helpful in screening for Klinefelter's syndrome, it is subject to false-negative and false-positive results and is no longer performed commonly.

The diagnosis of Klinefelter's syndrome is confirmed by *karyotype analysis,* which is usually performed on cultured peripheral blood lymphocytes. Occasionally, karyotype analysis is performed on cultured skin fibroblasts and testis tissue if mosaicism is suspected. If a fetus is diagnosed on prenatal testing with 47,XY Klinefelter's syndrome, genetic counseling should be provided. Despite a reasonably good prognosis, 75% of couples choose termination of a fetus with a prenatal diagnosis of Klinefelter's syndrome.

Treatment of Klinefelter's syndrome is directed at correction of androgen deficiency. Infants with micropenis may benefit from topical testosterone treatment. For boys with Klinefelter's syndrome, early intervention with speech and reading therapy is important if speech delay and dyslexia are present. At puberty, testosterone treatment may be needed for adequate development of secondary sexual characteristics; peak bone mass and BMD; muscle mass and strength; and energy, motivation, mood, and behavior. Adults with Klinefelter's syndrome who have clinical manifestations of androgen deficiency and consistently low levels of serum total or free testosterone (or both) should receive testosterone replacement therapy. Also, men who have symptoms and signs of androgen deficiency but normal total and free testosterone levels should be offered a trial of testosterone treatment.

Although azoospermia and infertility are irreversible, TESE permits identification of the relatively few seminiferous tubules that contain active spermatogenesis and harvesting of sperm from the small testes of men with Klinefelter's syndrome for use in ICSI; this approach results in live birth rates of approximately 45% in specialized centers.[7] Because there is an increased risk of sex chromosome and autosomal aneuploidy, genetic counseling and prenatal or preimplantation testing should be provided to couples who undergo ICSI.

Prominent gynecomastia does not resolve with testosterone treatment and requires reduction mammoplasty.

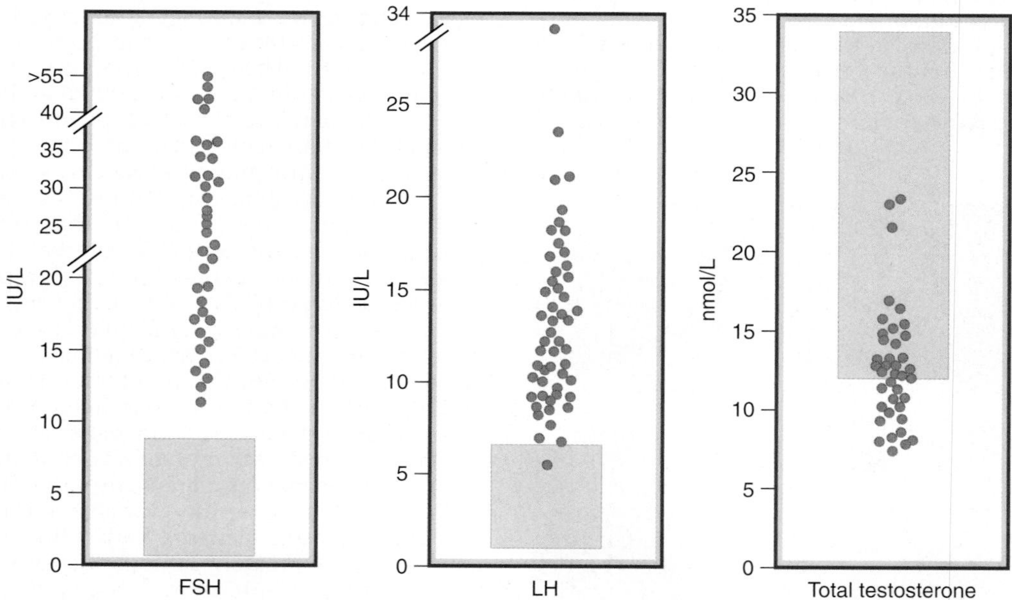

Figure 19-27 Serum levels of follicle-stimulating hormone (FSH, *left*), luteinizing hormone (LH, *middle*) and total testosterone (T, *right*) in men with Klinefelter's syndrome *(dots)* compared with normal men (normal range depicted by *shaded boxes*). A substantial proportion of men with Klinefelter's syndrome have total testosterone levels within the normal range, but almost all have elevated LH and FSH levels. (From Smyth CM, Bremner WJ. Klinefelter syndrome. *Arch Intern Med.* 1998;158:1309-1314.)

Psychological counseling for patients and spouses and participation in support groups may be extremely helpful for men with Klinefelter's syndrome.

Myotonic Dystrophy. Myotonic dystrophy is an autosomal dominant, multisystem disorder that is characterized by progressive muscle weakness and wasting (particularly in the lower legs, hands, neck, and face) and results in physical disability; myotonia (involuntary sustained contraction of muscles); cataracts; cardiac conduction defects; respiratory insufficiency; dysphagia; testicular atrophy, impaired spermatogenesis, infertility, and androgen deficiency; premature frontal balding; and intellectual disability.[204] Features of the disease usually develop in young adults but can occur at any age, and their severity varies widely among affected individuals. There are two types of myotonic dystrophy, caused by expansion of CTG trinucleotide repeats in two different genes. Myotonic dystrophy type 1 has more severe clinical features and is caused by CTG repeat expansion in the dystrophia myotonica protein kinase gene *(DMPK)*; it accounts for 98% of cases. Myotonic dystrophy type 2 is less severe and is caused by CTG repeat expansion in the CCHC-type zinc finger, nucleic acid–binding protein gene *(CNBP)*.

Primary hypogonadism occurs in approximately 80% of young to middle-aged men with myotonic dystrophy.[205,206] Most of these men have isolated impairment of sperm production or function with testicular atrophy, oligozoospermia or azoospermia, moderate to severe testicular damage on testis biopsy, infertility, and disproportionately elevated FSH compared with LH levels. Approximately 20% to 40% of men with myotonic dystrophy have variable degrees of androgen deficiency with low testosterone levels and elevated LH and FSH; testosterone replacement therapy is appropriate for these men. High-dose testosterone therapy has been demonstrated to improve muscle mass but did not affect muscle strength.[207] Infertility is irreversible, and patients who desire children need to pursue ART or other options; genetic counseling and preimplantation or prenatal testing should be provided, given the autosomal dominant nature of the disease.

Cryptorchidism. Cryptorchidism is the failure of one or both testes to descend normally from within the abdomen through the inguinal canal into the scrotum. It is the most common congenital disorder of the male genital tract in children, affecting 2% to 4% of full-term male births.[208,209] It is more common in premature, low-birth-weight, and small-for-gestational-age infants. Spontaneous descent of the testis occurs during the first year in most infants (probably induced by the neonatal surge of gonadotropins and testosterone), so the prevalence of cryptorchidism in boys and adults is lower, approximately 0.3% to 1.0%. Because a patent processus vaginalis is usually also present, inguinal hernia is found in conjunction with cryptorchidism in 50% to 80% of cases. Both unilateral and bilateral cryptorchidism are associated with impaired sperm production and infertility and an increased risk of testicular cancer.

In contrast to cryptorchidism, *ectopic testes* are located outside the normal path of testicular descent.[210] Ectopic testes may be located anywhere in the perineum or in the femoral or superficial inguinal regions. It is also important to distinguish cryptorchidism from *retractile testes* (pseudocryptorchidism). Retractile testes are located in the scrotum but withdraw into the inguinal canal or abdomen with minimal stimulation due to a hyperactive cremasteric reflex; they are not usually associated with impaired sperm production, infertility, or increased risk of testicular cancer. However, impaired spermatogenesis and fertility have been reported in men with bilateral retractile testes located high in the inguinal canal or, sometimes, in the abdomen.

Bilateral cryptorchidism may be associated with a number of disorders causing primary hypogonadism (including Klinefelter's syndrome variants and Noonan syndrome), secondary hypogonadism (including IHH, Kallmann's syndrome, and complex genetic disorders associated with multiple congenital anomalies or defects, such as Prader-Labhart-Willi syndrome or Laurence-Moon-Biedl syndrome), and androgen resistance syndromes (e.g., Reifenstein syndrome).[211] Cryptorchidism may also be caused by mutations of the Leydig cell product, INSL3, which controls growth of the gubernaculum, or of its receptor (RXFP2) in up to 5% of cases.

Unilateral or bilateral cryptorchidism that is not related to known causes of hypogonadism or androgen resistance usually results in primary hypogonadism, causing isolated impairment of sperm production associated with low sperm counts, normal testosterone concentrations, a selective elevation in FSH levels, and, occasionally, high LH levels as well.[208,209] Rarely, cryptorchidism causes Leydig cell failure and androgen deficiency (e.g., in adults with uncorrected bilateral cryptorchidism), producing low serum testosterone with high LH and FSH levels.[212,213] Azoospermia occurs in 50% to 60% and oligozoospermia in 75% to 100% of men with bilateral cryptorchidism; among men with unilateral cryptorchidism, these figures are, respectively, 15% to 20% and 20% to 40%. This suggests that the function of both testes is compromised in unilateral cryptorchidism. An underlying developmental or environmental disorder affecting both testes (*testicular dysgenesis*) may contribute to impaired spermatogenesis in these individuals.[208,209] The formation of A_d spermatogonia from neonatal gonocytes is inhibited in undescended testes. Uncommonly, normal testicular descent is impeded by an anatomic abnormality such as a large external inguinal hernia. In this instance, both testes function normally, and correction of the anatomic abnormality with orchiopexy before puberty usually preserves spermatogenesis and fertility.

The risk of testicular cancer in an undescended testis is 2.5- to 8-fold greater than in a scrotal testis, and the risk remains higher even after the testis is surgically relocated into the scrotum, supporting the notion that cryptorchidism is a manifestation of a underlying testicular disorder (i.e., testicular dysgenesis).[208-211] Even though the incidence of testicular cancer is only 1 or 2 per 100,000 males, the lifetime risk of malignancy in a cryptorchid testis is substantial. The prevalence of testicular carcinoma in situ, which is thought to precede testicular cancer, is about 3% in the cryptorchid testis. Testicular cancer usually occurs in men 20 to 40 years of age.

A careful physical examination should be performed to assess the location of testes within the scrotum or inguinal canal; the presence of an inguinal hernia, hydrocele, or other scrotal mass; the cremasteric reflex induced by stroking of the upper medial thigh; and penile size and the position of the urethral meatus. The examination should be performed with the patient standing, squatting, or supine with legs abducted. Scrotal examination may be difficult in a morbidly obese man with a large abdominal panniculus. Techniques that may be helpful in the detection of retractile testes include examination during a Valsalva maneuver, with pressure applied to the lower abdomen, or after scrotal warming or a hot bath to facilitate testicular descent. Also, elicitation of the cremasteric reflex may cause a localized puckering of the scrotal skin if a retractile testis is present in the scrotum. Often, a low undescended testis may be confirmed by pushing with one hand on the lower abdomen, with firm strokes from the anterior superior iliac spine through the groin and to the pubis, toward and into the scrotum, and then grasping the testis with the other hand. After the testis has been held in the scrotum until the cremasteric muscle fatigues, it is released. If the testis then retracts, it is considered a retractile testis; a low cryptorchid testis returns to its undescended position after release. Absence of a palpable testis in the scrotum after repeated examinations may be a result of cryptorchidism, an extremely atrophic testis, or anorchia (absent testis). Up to 50% of men with a unilateral, nonpalpable testis in the scrotum have a severely atrophic or absent testis rather than cryptorchidism; in these instances, the contralateral testis may be relatively large (by about 2 mL). High-resolution ultrasonography or MRI may help to localize testes that are not palpable.

Treatment for persistent cryptorchidism should be started before puberty, when greater germ cell degeneration occurs.[208,209] The exact timing of treatment is controversial, but recent recommendations suggest that treatment should be instituted between 6 to 12 months or up to 24 months of age. Hormonal treatment with hCG or GnRH in prepubertal boys is effective in stimulating descent of a cryptorchid testis in approximately 10% to 20% of cases. A trial of hormonal therapy may be attempted in the hope of avoiding surgery. If hormonal treatment is unsuccessful or not attempted, an orchiopexy (surgical relocation and fixation of the testis into the scrotum with ligation of the hernia sac at the external or internal inguinal ring) should be performed to allow examination of the testes (e.g., as in monitoring for malignancy) and preservation of remaining testis function. Despite orchiopexy, spermatogenesis remains impaired and fertility rates are reduced, particularly with bilateral cryptorchidism (65% paternity rate after orchiopexy). If orchiopexy is performed before puberty, the risk of testicular cancer is reduced but is still increased twofold to threefold. In patients with a history of unilateral cryptorchidism, the risk of malignancy in the contralateral testis is also increased, by about 70%. Because the risk of malignancy is two to six times higher in men who underwent orchiopexy after puberty and the fertility potential is poor, some clinicians recommend orchidectomy for men with cryptorchidism discovered after puberty. The majority of testis cancers found in persistently cryptorchid testes are seminomas, whereas those in cryptorchid testes after orchiopexy are mostly non-seminoma testicular cancers.

Noonan Syndrome. Noonan syndrome is an autosomal dominant or occasional sporadic genetic disorder that is characterized by short stature; unusual facial features (hypertelorism, downward-slanting eyes, ptosis, strabismus, low-set ears with thickened helices, high nasal bridge, micrognathia and triangular-shaped face, high-arched palate, low hairline, dental malocclusion); short, webbed neck; shield-like chest, pectus excavatum or carinatum, scoliosis, cubitus valgus, and joint laxity; intellectual disability; cardiac disease (pulmonic stenosis, hypertrophic cardiomyopathy); hepatosplenomegaly; lymphedema; and cryptorchidism.[214,215]

Because a number of these clinical features resemble those of females with Turner syndrome, Noonan syndrome was previously called male Turner syndrome. However, the karyotype in these men is normal. Noonan syndrome affects approximately 1 in 1000 to 2500 live births and is caused by mutations in genes in the Ras-MAPK signaling pathway.[214,215] Approximately 50% of men with Noonan syndrome have mutations in the *PTPN11* (the protein tyrosine phosphatase nonreceptor type 11) gene, and the remainder have mutations in the *SOS1* (son of sevenless homolog 1), *RAF1*, or *KRAS* genes.

Men with Noonan syndrome may demonstrate primary hypogonadism characterized by androgen deficiency and impaired sperm production with elevated gonadotropin levels; they usually present with delayed puberty.[216] Cryptorchidism is present in more than 50% of men with the syndrome and contributes to the etiology of hypogonadism.

Bilateral Congenital Anorchia. Congenital anorchia (also known as functional prepubertal castrate or vanishing testis syndrome) is a rare condition in which one or both testes are absent in a phenotypically and genotypically normal male.[217,218] Normal fetal testes function is needed for normal male internal and external genital differentiation and development during early gestation. The presence of otherwise normal male internal and external genitalia without müllerian duct–derived structures or descent of the spermatic cord structures (e.g., vas deferens, blood vessels) into the scrotum implies that normally functioning testes must have been present during the first 16 weeks of gestation and subsequently lost during fetal or neonatal life. The prevalence of bilateral congenital anorchia is 1 in 20,000, and that of unilateral congenital anorchia is 1 in 5000 males. The etiology is not known but is probably heterogeneous. It is hypothesized that congenital anorchia may be caused by spermatic vascular compromise due to torsion or trauma during or after testicular descent.

Infants with bilateral anorchia present with micropenis in almost 50% of cases, supporting a prenatal origin of the disorder.[217,218] Males with congenital anorchia usually present with prepubertal primary hypogonadism with delayed puberty and eunuchoidism (see Fig. 19-14), very low testosterone levels in the castrate range, and elevated gonadotropin levels. On examination, palpable testes are absent but blind-ending spermatic cords and epididymides are usually present. Normal testosterone and gonadotropin concentrations in pubertal or adult patients with absent testes exclude the diagnosis of congenital anorchia and should raise the possibility of bilateral cryptorchidism, which carries an increased risk for testicular malignancy.

An hCG stimulation test may be performed to distinguish congenital anorchia from bilateral cryptorchidism. In patients with congenital anorchia, serum testosterone concentrations do not increase in response to prolonged hCG administration (e.g., 1000 to 2000 IU three times weekly for 2 weeks), whereas most patients with bilateral cryptorchidism respond to hCG. However, lack of testosterone response to hCG administration for 6 weeks has been reported in men with bilateral cryptorchidism.[219] Serum AMH concentrations are usually undetectable in patients with congenital anorchia.[220] Measurements of AMH levels are more sensitive than those of testosterone concentrations but equally specific. If clinical examination and endocrine biochemical tests do not distinguish bilateral anorchia from cryptorchidism, imaging studies (e.g., MRI) and laparoscopy or surgical abdominal exploration may be necessary to confirm the diagnosis.

Treatment of bilateral congenital anorchia consists of testosterone replacement to stimulate penile length in patients with micropenis and to induce and maintain sexual development in boys with delayed puberty and eunuchoidism. Implantation of testicular prostheses in the scrotum may be of psychological and cosmetic value.

Autoimmune Polyglandular Syndrome. Autoimmune polyglandular syndromes are characterized by a clustering of organ-specific autoimmune disorders that involve a number of endocrine and nonendocrine tissues and are associated with circulating autoantibodies to components of these tissues. Autoimmune polyglandular syndrome type 1, also called autoimmune polyendocrinopathy-candidiasis-ectodermal dystrophy (APECED), is a rare autosomal recessive disorder that is caused by a mutation in the autoimmune regulator *(AIRE)* gene.[221] Its main features are mucocutaneous candidiasis, hypoparathyroidism, primary adrenal insufficiency, and the presence of autoimmune disorders including primary hypogonadism. The prevalence of primary hypogonadism is much more common in females than in males. In females, hypogonadism is manifested as premature ovarian failure and is present in 35% to 70% of cases, whereas in males, it is present in 8% to 28% of cases and is manifested by either androgen deficiency and impairment in sperm production or isolated impairment in sperm production (azoospermia) with elevated gonadotropin levels.

Autoimmune polyglandular syndrome type 2 is a common polygenic disorder associated with the genes for human leukocyte antigens (HLA) DR3 and DR4.[222] It is characterized by autoimmune primary adrenal insufficiency, thyroid disease (Hashimoto's or Graves' disease), and T1DM in addition to other autoimmune disorders including primary hypogonadism (again, more common in females than in males). In autoimmune polyglandular syndrome type 2, primary hypogonadism is associated with circulating steroid-producing cell autoantibodies (SCA) and with specific autoantibodies to CYP11A1 and 17α-hydroxylase.

Defects in Testosterone Biosynthetic Enzymes. Males with uncommon defects in 17,20-lyase/17α-hydroxylase, 17β-HSD/17-ketoreductase, or 3β-HSD, resulting from mutations in the *CYP17, HSD17B3,* and *HSD3B3* genes, respectively, usually present at birth as phenotypic females with partial virilization or with ambiguous genitalia. However, patients with incomplete defects in these enzymes may present as phenotypic males with hypospadias, gynecomastia, and primary hypogonadism with androgen deficiency manifested by delayed puberty.

Because 17,20-lyase and 17α-hydroxylase activities reside in the same enzyme, mutations in *CYP17* usually cause deficiencies in both activities, leading to elevated levels of progesterone, corticosterone, and deoxycorticosterone (DOC).[223] Rarely, males exhibiting isolated 17,20-lyase deficiency with elevated 17-hydroxyprogesterone levels have been reported.[224] Patients with 17α-hydroxylase deficiency may have hypertension and hypokalemia due to excessive production of the aldosterone precursor DOC, which has potent mineralocorticoid activity, but this is relatively uncommon in males compared with females. Patients with this deficiency usually do not manifest adrenal insufficiency because of increased production of the cortisol precursor, corticosterone, which has glucocorticoid activity. Males with either 17,20-lyase/17α-hydroxylase deficiency or isolated 17,20-lyase deficiency have primary hypogonadism with low testosterone and elevated LH and FSH levels; they require testosterone treatment at the time of puberty.

Patients with 17β-HSD/17-ketoreductase deficiency may have ambiguous genitalia and be raised as females, but at puberty, their testosterone levels increase sufficiently to induce virilization, resulting in gender reassignment (similar to individuals with androgen resistance due to 5α-reductase deficiency).[225] Serum testosterone levels are low to normal, but androstenedione and gonadotropin levels are increased.

Incomplete deficiency of 3β-HSD is a rare disorder that may manifest in adolescents with mild ambiguous genitalia, delayed virilization, gynecomastia, low testosterone levels, and elevated LH and FSH levels.[226] Levels of pregnenolone, 17-hydroxypregnenolone, and DHEA are elevated. Spontaneous virilization and puberty due to direct effects of high levels of the weak androgen DHEA or conversion of DHEA to testosterone (or both) has been reported. A eugonadal male with partial 3β-HSD deficiency who presented with gynecomastia has also been reported.[227]

Congenital Adrenal Hyperplasia. Adolescent and adult male patients with congenital adrenal hyperplasia due to 21-hydroxylase deficiency may develop *testicular adrenal rest tumors* that resemble Leydig cell tumors but do not contain intracytoplasmic Reinke crystalloids, which are commonly found (approximately 40%) on histologic analysis in the latter.[228-230] Testicular adrenal rest tumors may be large and easily palpable, or they may be detectable only on testicular ultrasonography. These tumors are thought to originate embryologically from aberrant adrenal tissue, and they are responsive to adrenocorticotropic hormone (ACTH). They regress with adequate glucocorticoid therapy for congenital adrenal hyperplasia and suppression of ACTH, and they grow with inadequate glucocorticoid treatment.

21-Hydroxylase deficiency is an autosomal recessive condition caused by a mutation in the *CYP21* gene. It is the most common enzymatic defect causing congenital adrenal hyperplasia. 21-Hydroxylase deficiency produces an accumulation of steroid substrates (17-hydroxyprogesterone and progesterone) that results in excessive production of adrenal androgens (androstenedione and DHEA), which are subsequently converted to testosterone. In addition, 21-hydroxylase deficiency causes reduced production of cortisol and aldosterone, resulting in deficiency of glucocorticoid and mineralocorticoid, respectively, and increased ACTH secretion (due to reduced cortisol negative feedback). Elevated ACTH secretion stimulates adrenal gland growth, resulting in adrenal hyperplasia. Glucocorticoid treatment suppresses ACTH secretion, reduces excessive adrenal androgen production, treats clinical adrenal insufficiency, and prevents excessive adrenal hyperplasia.

Excessive adrenal androgen production due to untreated or inadequate glucocorticoid therapy for 21-hydroxylase deficiency suppresses gonadotropin secretion by sex steroid negative feedback regulation and causes secondary hypogonadism. Because androgen levels are maintained by excessive adrenal production, men with 21-hydroxlase deficiency may not have clinical androgen deficiency. However, they usually have isolated impairment of sperm production due to gonadotropin deficiency. Adequate glucocorticoid therapy reduces excessive adrenal androgen production and usually restores gonadotropin secretion and normalizes testis function. Adequate and early glucocorticoid treatment also causes regression of adrenal rest tumors, which otherwise may affect testicular function directly or cause mechanical obstruction of seminiferous tubules.[228-230]

If testicular adrenal rest tumors are present, inadequate glucocorticoid treatment stimulates their growth, often resulting in very large tumors that can cause irreversible testicular damage.[228-230] In this circumstance, although adequate glucocorticoid therapy reduces tumor size, the patient will manifest primary hypogonadism with androgen deficiency due to loss of Leydig cells and impaired sperm production due to loss of seminiferous tubules. On adequate glucocorticoid treatment, tumors may regress completely, but testis size usually remains small, serum testosterone levels and sperm counts low, and gonadotropin levels elevated.

Complex Genetic Syndromes. Primary hypogonadism resulting in androgen deficiency and impaired sperm production or in isolated impairment in sperm production or function may occur as a manifestation of complex genetic syndromes, usually in association with a number of congenital anomalies or defects and distinct morphologic developmental manifestations.[231] Examples include the Alström, ataxia telangiectasia, H-, Marinesco-Sjögren, Robinow, Rothmund-Thomson, Sohval-Soffer, Weinstein, Werner, and Wolfram syndromes.[232-241] Primary hypogonadism may also occur in some patients with Prader-Labhart-Willi syndrome (associated with cryptorchidism), Laurence-Moon-Bardet-Biedl syndrome, and Alström syndrome, disorders that are more commonly associated with secondary hypogonadism.[242-244]

Down Syndrome. Down syndrome, or trisomy 21, is a chromosomal disorder in which all or part of an extra chromosome 21 is present.[245] It affects 1 of every 700 to 800 infants and is the most common cause of intellectual disability in children. Down syndrome is characterized by moderate to severe intellectual disability, spontaneous warm and cheerful personality, short stature, characteristic mongoloid facial features (most notably round facies with microgenia, upward-slanting and almond-shaped eyes resulting from bilateral epicanthal folds, macroglossia, and flat nasal bridge), congenital heart defects, hypothyroidism, and defects affecting most other body systems. Males with Down syndrome usually manifest primary hypogonadism, most commonly characterized by isolated impairment in sperm production with normal or selective elevation of FSH levels. Histologically, they may manifest hypospermatogenesis (moderate to severe reduction in all germ cell types), maturation arrest, or Sertoli cell–only syndrome with loss of all germ cells. Less commonly, they demonstrate mild to moderate androgen deficiency with low or low-normal testosterone and elevated LH and FSH levels.

Luteinizing Hormone Receptor Mutations. Inactivating mutations of the LH receptor in males usually cause Leydig cell aplasia or hypoplasia. These patients present with DSDs involving a female phenotype without breast development at puberty (Leydig cell aplasia) or genital ambiguity (hypoplasia) and cryptorchidism.[58] Rarely, partially inactivating LH receptor mutations lead to presentation of a male with micropenis, hypospadias, delayed sexual development, undervirilization, low testosterone, impaired sperm production, and high LH levels, consistent with primary hypogonadism. However, they usually have normal FSH levels. An individual with an LH receptor mutation was reported to exhibit normal levels of testosterone and spermatogenesis after hCG stimulation, suggesting that hCG action via the LH receptor may be dissociated from that of LH.[246]

Acquired Disorders

Bilateral Surgical Castration and Trauma. Bilateral surgical castration causes a rapid and profound decline in testosterone levels within hours, resulting in severe clinical manifestations of androgen deficiency, including hot flushes. Severe blunt trauma to the testes and associated vascular compromise may result in testicular atrophy and loss of testes function, including androgen deficiency and impaired spermatogenesis or isolated impairment in sperm production or function.

Drugs and Ionizing Radiation. Certain drugs that affect androgen production may cause androgen deficiency. The antifungal agent, ketoconazole, inhibits 17,20-lyase and 17α-hydroxylase activity at high doses (>400 mg daily) and has been used, in conjunction with other agents, to lower both adrenal and testicular androgen production in the treatment of prostate cancer.[247,248] Spironolactone, a nonspecific aldosterone antagonist, acts mainly as a competitive AR antagonist and inhibits androgen action.[249] However, it also inhibits 17,20-lyase and 17α-hydroxylase activity and testosterone biosynthesis at high doses. Excessive intake of alcohol inhibits testosterone production, but it may also suppress gonadotropins; it may be associated with nutritional deficiency or chronic liver disease, which may contribute to androgen deficiency and impairment in sperm production.[250,251]

In general, because spermatogenesis involves active cell replication, the germ cell compartment is much more sensitive to external or environmental influences (e.g., chemotherapy agents, ionizing radiation) than are Leydig cells. Exposure to such agents often results in primary hypogonadism characterized by an isolated impairment in sperm production or function and elevated gonadotropins. However, severe testis damage induced by these agents may cause Leydig cell dysfunction or damage, resulting in both androgen deficiency and impairment of sperm production.

Combination chemotherapy regimens that include alkylating agents (e.g., cyclophosphamide, ifosfamide, procarbazine, busulfan, chlorambucil), such as those used for the treatment of Hodgkin's and non-Hodgkin's lymphoma and leukemia, are particularly toxic to the testes and may result in androgen deficiency in up to 20% of patients.[16,252-254] High-dose chemotherapy and total body irradiation before bone marrow transplantation may also cause androgen deficiency in a substantial proportion of men. In contrast, men with testicular cancer who undergo combination chemotherapy that includes platinum drugs (together with unilateral orchidectomy and, often, radiation therapy) have a relatively low prevalence of usually mild androgen deficiency with slightly low to low-normal testosterone levels and elevated LH levels.[255]

Exposure of testes to ionizing irradiation commonly suppresses spermatogenesis in a dose-dependent manner, and doses greater than 600 to 800 cGy may compromise Leydig cell function and reduce testosterone production.[252,253]

Orchitis. Viral infection of the testes may result in testicular atrophy, impaired sperm production, and, in severe cases, androgen deficiency. *Mumps orchitis* was common before the introduction of the measles/mumps/rubella (MMR) vaccine in 1968, after which rates of mumps infection decreased profoundly.[256,257] Because of worldwide shortage of the MMR vaccine approximately 15 years ago, there has been a resurgence of mumps infection and orchitis in adolescents and young adults. Prepubertal mumps orchitis is very uncommon and is not associated with subsequent testicular dysfunction. Orchitis is the most common complication of mumps infection in pubertal boys and adults; it usually causes permanent seminiferous tubule damage, impaired spermatogenesis, and, in severe cases, Leydig cell failure and androgen deficiency.

Mumps infection usually manifests with headache, fever, and malaise followed by unilateral or bilateral parotid swelling due to parotiditis.[256,257] Testis pain and swelling due to orchitis occurs in about 10 days or up to 6 weeks after the onset of parotiditis and may be subclinical in up to 50% of cases. Epididymitis accompanies orchitis in 85% of cases. Mumps orchitis is usually unilateral but may be bilateral in 15% of cases in adolescents and in 30% of cases in young adults. Even if orchitis is clinically unilateral, degenerative changes may occur in the apparently unaffected testis. Germ cell sloughing occurs as a result of acute infection, inflammation, and ischemia resulting from pressure induced by swelling of the testes within the tunica albuginea. The acute phase is followed by seminiferous tubule fibrosis and then testicular atrophy (30% to 50% of cases) for the next several months, resulting impaired spermatogenesis in 25% to 40% of cases. In severe cases, prednisone may be used to reduce inflammation and swelling associated with mumps orchitis, but it does not prevent testis damage.

HIV infection usually causes gonadotropin suppression and secondary hypogonadism. However in 20% to 30% of cases, HIV infection causes primary hypogonadism characterized by low testosterone and elevated gonadotropin levels. The etiology of primary hypogonadism is orchitis that is caused by HIV infection of the testis or occurs secondary to opportunistic infection (e.g., by cytomegalovirus [CMV], *Mycobacterium avium intracellulare, Toxoplasma gondii*) associated with the patient's immunocompromised state.[258,259]

Other causes of infectious orchitis usually associated with epididymitis include echovirus, arbovirus, or lymphocytic choriomeningitis infection; gonorrhea or *Chlamydia* infection in young adults and urinary pathogens such as *Escherichia coli* in older men; leprosy and tuberculosis; brucellosis, glanders, and syphilis; and parasitic infections such as filariasis and bilharziasis.[258,260]

Systemic Disorders. Low serum testosterone levels associated with symptoms and signs consistent with androgen deficiency are commonly associated with chronic diseases affecting the liver, kidney, heart, and lungs.[4,5] The underlying cause of both clinical and biochemical hypogonadism in these conditions is complex and multifactorial. The illness itself, associated complications, nutritional compromise, and medications used to treat the illness may contribute to or confound the clinical manifestations of androgen deficiency and also may suppress gonadotropin and testosterone production, thereby playing an etiologic role. Chronic systemic diseases usually have effects both on testis and hypothalamic-pituitary function and cause combined primary and secondary hypogonadism. Clinically, however, measurements of gonadotropin levels usually suggest predominantly primary hypogonadism (i.e., elevated gonadotropins) or secondary hypogonadism (i.e., normal or low gonadotropins). The benefits and risks of testosterone therapy in patients with these systemic disorders have not been evaluated in long-term randomized, controlled outcome studies.

Chronic Liver Disease. In men with chronic liver disease of any etiology (and particularly in those with hepatic cirrhosis or liver failure), sexual dysfunction, gynecomastia, and testicular atrophy resulting in impaired androgen and sperm production occur commonly, affecting 50% to 75% of these patients.[4,5,261-263] Total testosterone levels may be low but are often normal or high-normal, because SHBG levels are increased substantially with cirrhosis and chronic active hepatitis. Therefore, measurements of free or bioavailable testosterone using accurate assay methods should be used to assess androgen deficiency. Free and bioavailable testosterone levels are usually low, and LH levels are usually elevated or in the high-normal range in patients with mild to moderate hepatic cirrhosis (Child-Pugh class A or B).

Estrogen (estrone and estradiol) levels are usually high due to increased production (e.g., induced by alcohol excess) and reduced clearance of adrenal androgens (e.g., androstenedione), which provide increased substrates for aromatization of androgens to estrogens. High estrogen levels contribute to the development of gynecomastia (high estrogen-to-androgen ratio), palmar erythema and spider angiomata, and increased prolactin levels. Treatment of ascites and edema with spironolactone may further lower testosterone levels and block androgen action, contributing to gynecomastia and other manifestations of androgen deficiency. High LH levels may be suppressed by high estrogen and prolactin levels and by the malnutrition that occur commonly in men with hepatic cirrhosis and liver failure. Oligozoospermia or azoospermia associated with abnormalities in sperm motility and morphology occurs in approximately 30% to 50% of men with chronic liver disease.

Testosterone treatment of androgen deficiency is usually well tolerated but occasionally may worsen gynecomastia and rarely may increase edema and ascites by causing fluid retention. Because immunosuppressive medications such as prednisone and cyclosporine are used to prevent rejection, liver transplantation only partially reverses hypogonadism associated with chronic liver disease.[261,262]

Chronic Kidney Disease. Late-stage CKD commonly causes combined primary and secondary hypogonadism, resulting in androgen deficiency and impairment in sperm production in 50% to 60% of these patients.[4,5,264] Serum testosterone levels are low, and LH and FSH levels are high, in large part because of markedly reduced renal clearance of gonadotropins as well as increased secretion resulting from reduced negative feedback. SHBG levels are usually not affected by CKD unless nephrotic syndrome is present, in which case levels of SHBG and, consequently, total testosterone may be low. In the latter situation, free or bioavailable testosterone measurements should be performed to assess androgen deficiency. Sperm production is impaired, and sperm motility and the percentage of sperm with normal morphology are reduced. The Leydig cell response to hCG administration is reduced, consistent with primary testicular dysfunction. The frequency and amplitude of pulsatile LH secretion are altered, suggesting an alteration in hypothalamic-pituitary function as well. Hyperprolactinemia that suppresses gonadotropins and zinc deficiency that affects testicular function may contribute to testicular dysfunction in men with CKD.

Hemodialysis and peritoneal dialysis do not improve testosterone or sperm production.[264,265] Successful renal transplantation usually brings testosterone and sperm production to almost normal levels, although immunosuppression by rapamycin inhibitors (e.g., sirolimus) may impair testis function slightly.[264,266,267]

Aging. After age 40 years, there is a gradual and progressive decline in total testosterone levels (by approximately 1% per year), such that an increasing proportion of older men have low serum testosterone concentrations in the hypogonadal range.[268-270] Because SHBG levels increase with age, free and bioavailable testosterone concentrations decline even more rapidly (2% to 3% per year). Daily sperm production, sperm motility, percentage of sperm with normal morphology, Sertoli cell number, and inhibin B levels also decline with aging.[135] Leydig cell number and testosterone production in response to stimulation by hCG and pulsatile LH are reduced, consistent with primary testicular dysfunction.[135] In older men, circadian variation in testosterone concentration is present but blunted.[64] Furthermore, pulsatile LH secretion is more irregular and disorderly and LH pulse amplitude is reduced in older compared with young men. Pulsatile GnRH administration normalizes pulsatile LH but not testosterone secretion, consistent with an impairment of hypothalamic GnRH secretion occurring in combination with a primary defect in testosterone production by the testis.[271,272]

Serum LH and FSH levels increase (by about 1% to 2% per year) with aging but do not usually rise above the normal range until very old age (>70 years).[268-270,273] Therefore, the most common hormonal profile associated with aging observed in middle-aged to older men is low testosterone with normal LH and FSH levels, consistent with "secondary hypogonadism." As men get older, gonadotropins continue to rise. A hormonal pattern of low testosterone and elevated LH and FSH levels, consistent with "primary hypogonadism," is more prevalent in elderly men, particularly after 70 years of age.

As men age, they may develop chronic organ failure or systemic illnesses, take an increasing number of medications, and develop nutritional deficiency or wasting syndromes that are associated with low testosterone concentrations.[274] It is likely that these comorbid conditions contribute to low testosterone and clinical hypogonadism associated with aging in men. Conversely, the age-related decline in testosterone levels may contribute to the susceptibility or severity of clinical hypogonadism observed in these conditions.

In community-dwelling middle-aged to older men, the prevalence of low testosterone increased from 12% among men in their 50s to 48% among men older than 80 years of age.[269] The prevalence of clinical androgen deficiency (i.e., symptoms and signs consistent with androgen deficiency and low testosterone levels) was 6% to 9% and increased with age, reaching 18% to 23% among men in their 70s.[175,176] When more stringent criteria for the diagnosis of androgen deficiency associated with aging were used (i.e., three sexual symptoms and a low testosterone level defined as late-onset hypogonadism), the prevalence was 2% and also increased with age, reaching 5% among men in their 70s.[177]

In addition to the decline in testosterone levels, aging is associated with alterations in body function that could be related to androgen deficiency.[135] These include a decline in muscle mass and strength associated with reduced physical function and performance; decreased BMD and increased risk of osteoporosis and fractures; increased body fat; reduction in sexual function and activity, including reduced libido and erectile dysfunction; decline in vitality, energy, mood, and cognitive function; and alterations in sleep quality. Similar changes occur in younger hypogonadal men and improve with testosterone treatment, raising the possibility that the decline in testosterone levels that occurs with aging may contribute to these age-associated changes in body function.

Relatively small, short-term (up to 3 years) studies of testosterone treatment in heterogeneous groups of older men with low or low-normal testosterone levels without regard to the presence of symptoms or signs of androgen deficiency have produced conflicting results. Most have found beneficial effects of testosterone treatment on body composition, with increasing lean or muscle mass and decreasing fat mass, but less consistent effects on muscle strength and performance, BMD, sexual function, vitality, and cognitive function. The only adverse effect found in these studies was excessive erythrocytosis in some men. More recent studies of testosterone treatment in frail older men with low testosterone levels found beneficial effects on muscle strength and physical performance,[275,276] but there was an increase in cardiovascular events in one small study.[275] Larger, long-term, randomized trials are needed to determine the balance of clinical benefits and risks (particularly as related to prostate cancer and cardiovascular disease) of testosterone treatment in elderly men. Until results from these outcome studies are available, testosterone treatment should be considered only for older men who have clinically significant manifestations of androgen deficiency and unequivocally low serum testosterone levels, and only after a careful discussion of the uncertainty concerning the long-term benefits and risks of treatment.[110,277]

Other Systemic Disorders. Primary hypogonadism with low testosterone levels or elevated LH levels (or both) occurs in up to 20% of men with *malignancy* such as advanced Hodgkin's disease or testicular cancer before gonadotoxic chemotherapy and radiation therapy.[278-280] Impairment of sperm production is found more frequently, in about 30% to 50% of men with Hodgkin's disease or testicular cancer before therapy. The mechanism of gonadal dysfunction before treatment is not clear.

Sickle cell disease is an autosomal recessive disorder caused by a point mutation in the β-globulin chain. It results in an abnormal hemoglobin (hemoglobin S) that polymerizes, leading to sickle-shaped, rigid, and fragile red blood cells. The disease is characterized by recurrent episodes of painful, vaso-occlusive events in a variety of organs due to thrombosis, ischemia and infarction, and hemolysis. Sickle cell disease is a common disorder, affecting approximately 1 in 700 African American infants. Sickle cell disease may cause primary hypogonadism characterized by low to low-normal testosterone concentrations, clinical manifestations consistent with androgen deficiency, testicular atrophy and impaired spermatogenesis, and elevated gonadotropin levels, possibly due to repeated testicular vaso-occlusive events and infarction.[281-283] Hydroxyurea therapy and possibly zinc deficiency may contribute to impaired spermatogenesis. Men with sickle cell disease may experience priapism due to penile vaso-occlusion, and this may be precipitated by restoration of libido with testosterone treatment of hypogonadism.

Within the first few months to 1 year after a *spinal cord injury*, testosterone levels and sperm production are suppressed and gonadotropins are usually normal. However, in some men, LH or FSH levels or both may be elevated in the presence of low to low-normal testosterone, consistent with primary hypogonadism.[284] Chronically after a spinal cord injury, serum testosterone remains low and gonadotropins are usually suppressed or normal, consistent with secondary hypogonadism.[285,286] The latter condition may be caused by hyperprolactinemia associated with medications, nutritional deficiency, obstructive sleep apnea, or debilitation from chronic spinal cord injury. Testis biopsy revealed impaired spermatogenesis in approximately 40% of men with spinal cord injury, but mature sperm that could be used for TESE and ICSI were present in almost 90%.[287]

Vasculitis (e.g., periarteritis nodosa, Wegener's granulomatosis, Henoch-Schönlein purpura, Behçet's disease) or *infiltrative disease* (e.g., systemic amyloidosis) involving both testes may cause testicular damage and may necessitate orchidectomy, resulting in both androgen deficiency and impaired sperm production.[288,289]

Isolated Impairment of Sperm Production or Function

Congenital or Developmental Disorders. As described previously, cryptorchidism, myotonic dystrophy, and Down syndrome most commonly manifest with primary hypogonadism characterized by isolated impairment in sperm production without androgen deficiency and selectively elevated FSH levels. In men with less severely impaired spermatogenesis, serum gonadotropin levels are normal, but it is most appropriate to classify these men as having primary hypogonadism with isolated impairment in sperm production, because gonadotropin treatment has not been demonstrated to improve fertility.

Varicocele. Varicocele is a dilatation of the pampiniform venous plexus surrounding the spermatic cord in the scrotum. It is caused by retrograde blood flow into the internal spermatic vein, which is usually caused by defective or absent valves in spermatic veins or, rarely, by obstruction of normal venous drainage by extrinsic or intrinsic venous compression (e.g., from a tumor). It usually occurs on the left side, and most cases are asymptomatic. A varicocele is present in 10% to 15% of men in the general population and more frequently in infertile men (up to 30% to 40%).[12,290,291]

The relationship of varicocele to impaired sperm production and infertility is unclear.[12,290,291] Approximately 50% of men who have a varicocele demonstrate normal semen analyses, and many are fertile. Men with a large varicocele and infertility usually exhibit low sperm counts with reduced motility and increased numbers of sperm with abnormal morphology (e.g., tapered or amorphous sperm heads), but these abnormalities are not specific for varicocele. Testis size and serum levels of testosterone, LH, and FSH are usually normal. Varicocele is painful in 2% to 10% of men with infertility. Testis biopsy in men with a varicocele and abnormal semen parameters reveals a spectrum of histopathologic findings, including hypospermatogenesis, maturation arrest, and Sertoli cell–only histology.

It is unclear whether varicocele ligation improves fertility in men who present with infertility. Controlled trials to investigate the efficacy of varicocele ligation have not demonstrated improved fertility. However, these trials were generally small, heterogeneous, and of poor quality. A small number of controlled trials of infertile men with palpable varicocele and at least one abnormal semen parameter have suggested improvement in the spontaneous pregnancy rate with varicocele ligation. Some organizations have recommended surgical ligation for infertile men who have a large, palpable varicocele with an abnormal seminal fluid analysis.[12,290,291]

Y Chromosome Microdeletion. Yq chromosome microdeletions are the most common genetic cause of impaired sperm production and male infertility. They are found in 5% to 10% of men with severe oligozoospermia and in 10% to 15% of men with azoospermia.[164] As mentioned earlier, microdeletions have been identified in three regions of the long arm of the Y chromosome (Fig. 19-28).[164,165]

Microdeletions in the *AZFa* region, which contains the *DDX3Y* and *USP9Y* (ubiquitin specific peptidase 9, Y-linked) genes, are usually associated with azoospermia and Sertoli cell–only histology. Microdeletions in the *AZFb* region, which contains multiple copies of the *RBMY* and *PRY* (PTPM13-like, Y-linked) genes, are usually associated with severe oligozoospermia and germ cell arrest at the pachytene primary spermatocyte stage and occasionally with hypospermatogenesis. Microdeletions in the *AZFc* region, which contains the *DAZ* (deleted in azoospermia) gene and is where the majority of Y chromosome microdeletions reside, are usually associated with germ cell arrest at the spermatid stage or with hypospermatogenesis with some mature spermatids present. *AZFc* microdeletions are found in approximately 12% of men with nonobstructive azoospermia and 6% of men with severe oligozoospermia. Microdeletions in both the *AZFb* and the *AZFc* region are usually associated with azoospermia and Sertoli cell–only histology.

Yq microdeletion analysis should be considered for couples who are contemplating ICSI, because these microdeletions have been shown to be transmitted to male offspring with the ICSI procedure.[164] If ICSI is performed in men with Y chromosome microdeletions, genetic counseling and preimplantation or prenatal testing should be considered.

Sertoli Cell–Only Syndrome (Germ Cell Aplasia). Sertoli cell–only syndrome, or germ cell aplasia, is an uncommon histologic diagnosis in which the seminiferous tubules are completely devoid of germ cells and are lined only with Sertoli cells with little to no fibrosis or hyalinization.[292] Men with this disorder present with infertility, normal androgenization, moderately small testes (10 to 20 mL in volume), azoospermia, normal testosterone and LH levels,

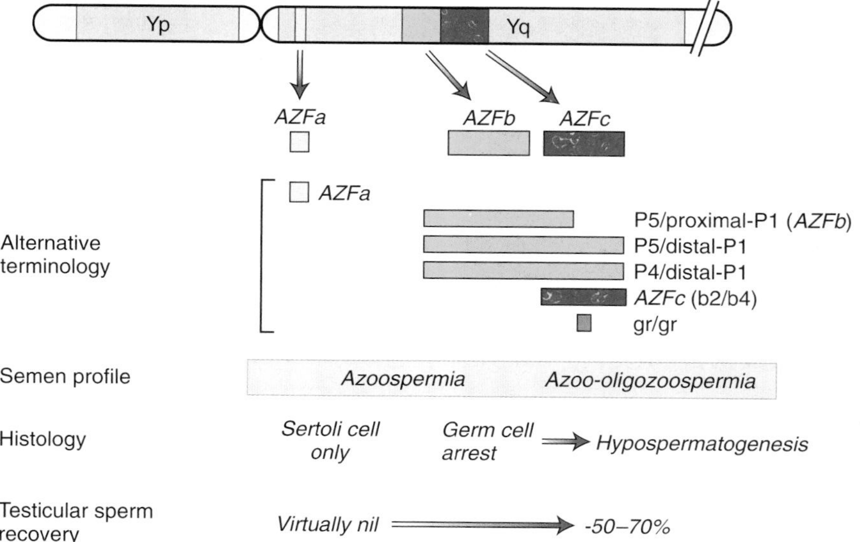

Figure 19-28 Schematic diagram of the short (Yp) and long (Yq) arms of the human Y chromosome. Deletions in regions of Yq, specifically in azoospermia factor (AZF) regions, are associated with severe defects in sperm production. Microdeletions in the AZFa region are usually associated with azoospermia and Sertoli cell–only histology. Microdeletions most commonly affect the AZFc region and may be associated with severe oligozoospermia or azoospermia. However, even if oligozoospermia or azoospermia is present, sperm for use in intracytoplasmic sperm injection (ICSI) are recoverable from half of the patients by testicular sperm extraction (TESE) at biopsy. (From McLachlan RI, O'Bryan MK. Clinical Review: state of the art for genetic testing of infertile men. *J Clin Endocrinol Metab.* 2010;95:1013-1024.)

and selectively elevated FSH levels (indicating severe seminiferous tubule dysfunction).[293] Occasionally, LH levels are slightly high and the testosterone response to hCG stimulation is reduced, suggesting mild Leydig cell dysfunction.

The cause of Sertoli cell–only syndrome is not known, but it is thought to result from congenital absence of germ cells due to a failure of gonocyte migration. In some families, however, germ cells were present before puberty but were subsequently lost during or after puberty. As described previously, a Sertoli cell–only histology may be associated with microdeletions in the long arm of the Y chromosome in the *AZF* regions.[294] Severe germ cell damage and loss occurring with Klinefelter's syndrome, mumps orchitis, cryptorchidism, ionizing radiation, or alkylating agents may result in seminiferous tubules lined only with Sertoli cells. However, in these cases of acquired Sertoli cell–only syndrome, there is usually extensive seminiferous tubule sclerosis or hyalinization, and the testes are usually smaller. Infertility is irreversible in congenital Sertoli cell–only syndrome, but it may be reversible with time in some cases of acquired Sertoli cell–only syndrome.

Primary Ciliary Dyskinesia (Immotile Cilia Syndrome). Primary ciliary dyskinesia, or immotile cilia syndrome, is a rare, heterogeneous, autosomal recessive genetic disorder of cilia. It is characterized primarily by recurrent respiratory infections (sinusitis and bronchitis) that lead to the development of bronchiectasis, caused by impaired mucociliary clearance due to dyskinesia of respiratory tract cilia, and to infertility caused by asthenozoospermia (nonmotile or poorly motile sperm) due to impaired sperm tail movement.[295] In half of the cases, primary ciliary dyskinesia is associated with situs inversus and is known as Kartagener's syndrome. Some men exhibit abnormalities of sperm motility in the absence of respiratory tract involvement.

Patients with primary ciliary dyskinesia and impaired sperm motility demonstrate ultrastructural abnormalities of the axoneme, the microtubule cytoskeleton of the sperm flagellum, especially in the dynein arms (motor protein complexes). Almost all men with primary ciliary dyskinesia have mutations of the genes encoding the dynein axonemal heavy chain 5 *(DNAH5)*, dynein intermediate chain 1 *(DNAI1)*, or dynein axonemal heavy chain 11 *(DNAH11)*. These men present with infertility and an isolated impairment in sperm motility with normal sperm counts and morphology and normal testosterone and gonadotropin levels.

Follicle-Stimulating Hormone Receptor Mutations. Rare inactivating FSH receptor mutations have been described in males.[58,86] In contrast to females with FSH receptor mutations, who have primary amenorrhea and infertility, men have a more variable presentation. Some demonstrate severe oligozoospermia, whereas others have moderate oligozoospermia or normal sperm concentrations with abnormal sperm morphology and some have normal fertility. Serum testosterone levels are normal, FSH levels are elevated, and LH levels are slightly high to normal. It is possible that normal testosterone production within the testes contributes to the persistence of spermatogenesis and fertility in the absence of FSH action.

Acquired Disorders. Because seminiferous tubule function is more susceptible to damage than Leydig cell function, most men with primary hypogonadism due to chemotherapy agents, ionizing radiation, or orchitis caused by mumps or other infections manifest isolated impairment of sperm production without androgen deficiency.

Alkylating agents (e.g., cyclophosphamide, ifosfamide, procarbazine, busulfan, chlorambucil) used in combination chemotherapy regimens to treat lymphoma and leukemia almost uniformly cause azoospermia that recovers after 5 years in up to two thirds of men.[254,296,297] High-dose chemotherapy and total body irradiation before bone marrow transplantation commonly causes irreversible germ cell damage associated with azoospermia or severe oligozoospermia and elevated FSH levels. Sperm production is suppressed initially in men with testicular cancer who undergo combination chemotherapy that includes platinum drugs, unilateral orchidectomy, and often radiation therapy.[255] However, sperm production recovers in 80% of men by 5 years. Before chemotherapy begins, cryopreservation of sperm for subsequent use in IUI, IVF, or ICSI should be offered to men who desire future fertility.

Approaches aimed at suppressing gonadotropins with GnRH agonists or exogenous testosterone administration have not been effective in preventing germ cell damage by chemotherapy. Methotrexate and sulfasalazine may cause oligozoospermia and low sperm motility and contribute to infertility.[298] The processes of human spermatogenesis, and particularly the spermatogonia, are very sensitive to the effects of exposure to ionizing radiation.[16,252-254] X-radiation doses as low as 15 cGy may suppress sperm production temporarily. The time required to recover spermatogenesis after x-irradiation is dose dependent. Recovery of sperm counts to baseline takes 9 to18 months after exposure to 100 cGy or less and up to 5 years after 400 to 600 cGy. Although Leydig cell function is more resistant to ionizing radiation, x-irradiation of greater than 800 cGy may cause Leydig cell damage and androgen deficiency. As with chemotherapy, sperm banking before radiation therapy for later use in ART offers hope for subsequent fertility.

Prolonged and repeated *thermal trauma* (e.g., with excessive hot tub use) to the testes may suppress sperm production, usually transiently.[299,300]

A number of chemical agents used in industry and laboratories have been implicated as direct toxins to the testes. Examples of *environmental toxins* include carbon disulfide, a solvent used in rayon production; dibromochloropropane, an insecticide; lead; deuterium oxide; ethyl glycol; cadmium; fluoroacetamide; nitrofurans; dinitropyroles; diamines; and α-chlorohydrin. Furthermore, it is postulated that environmental or xenobiotic agents such as phthalates act as anti-androgens or estrogens to alter reproductive function; these agents have been termed *endocrine disruptors*.[301] Such environmental agents have been implicated in causing the increased incidence of testicular dysgenesis syndrome (i.e., hypospadias, cryptorchidism, declining sperm counts, and testicular cancer).[302]

Systemic Disorders. An acute febrile illness may cause a temporary suppression of spermatogenesis.[302] In men with spinal cord injury resulting in tetraplegia or paraplegia, impaired sperm production may be caused in part by increased scrotal temperature due to loss of lumbar sympathetic innervations.[284-287] Men with malignancy, in particular Hodgkin's lymphoma or testicular cancer, may have impaired spermatogenesis with azoospermia or oligozoospermia in 30% to 80% of cases before treatment.[278-280]

In the majority of men who present with infertility and an isolated impairment of sperm production, an etiology cannot be identified. Idiopathic oligozoospermia or azoospermia occurs in 60% to 80% of cases (including men with varicocele).[161-163] If isolated impairment of spermatogenesis is severe in men with primary hypogonadism, serum FSH levels may be selectively elevated. As mentioned earlier, men with less severely impaired spermatogenesis and normal serum gonadotropin levels are still classified as having a disorder of primary hypogonadism, because gonadotropin treatment has not been demonstrated to improve fertility in such cases.

Causes of Secondary Hypogonadism

Androgen Deficiency and Impairment in Sperm Production

Congenital or Developmental Disorders

Constitutional Delay of Growth and Puberty. It is important to consider *constitutional delay of growth and puberty (CDGP)* in the differential diagnosis of secondary hypogonadism because it is a transient cause of secondary hypogonadism and is the most common cause of pubertal delay usually associated with growth delay and short stature in boys.[136,303,304]

The initial endocrine event that precedes the phenotypic changes of puberty is activation of the CNS mechanisms that regulate GnRH production, which results in pulsatile LH followed by testosterone secretion, initially at night (see Fig. 19-5) and then throughout the day.[42] Under the influence of increasing testosterone concentrations, secondary sexual characteristics appear at between 9 and 13 years of age.

The first physical sign of pubertal development is an increase of testis size to greater than 4 mL in volume (or >2.5 cm in length) and thinning of the scrotum, which is followed by development of rugal folds and increased pigmentation.[136,303,304] Subsequently, penile length increases and pubic hair develops over the next 1 to 2 years, followed by long bone growth (with peak height velocity occurring approximately 3 years later) and development of other secondary sexual characteristics, such as laryngeal enlargement and deepening of the voice. In boys, peak bone mass usually is not reached until the third decade. There is considerable variability in the onset and progression of puberty and the degree of virilization, and this is attributable in large part to an individual's genetic and ethnic background.

Delayed puberty is suspected if there is no evidence of sexual maturation and testis size is less than 4 mL at 14 years of age.[136,303,304] Boys with delayed puberty often experience considerable psychosocial distress due to the lack of sexual and physical development that results in their being considered younger than their peer group and having difficulty competing in athletics. In addition to the lack of sexual development, both boys and their parents are usually also concerned about the boy's failure to undergo a growth spurt and short stature.

CDGP, or transient secondary hypogonadism, is the cause of delayed puberty in approximately 65% of cases.[136,303,304] Permanent secondary hypogonadism (e.g., due to IHH, pituitary or hypothalamic tumors, infiltrative diseases), which initially may be clinically indistinguishable from CDGP, is the cause of delayed puberty in fewer than 10% of cases. Other causes of delayed sexual development and growth, which are usually clinically apparent on presentation, include functional secondary hypogonadism (e.g., due to chronic systemic illness, hypothyroidism, medications) in about 20% and primary hypogonadism (e.g., due to Klinefelter's syndrome, mumps, chemotherapy, radiation therapy) or androgen resistance in approximately 5% of cases.

CDGP is a physiologic variant of normal puberty that is characterized by a slowing of the growth rate and of the timing and tempo of pubertal development.[136,303,304] Because there is an increased prevalence of CDGP in families with GnRH deficiency (IHH), CDGP could represent a mild variant of IHH.[305] No genes or genetic polymorphisms have been identified that determine the variations in the timing of normal puberty. However, a family history of delayed puberty or being a "late bloomer" is found in 80% of boys with CDGP.

Clinically, a boy with this condition typically has a height age (i.e., the age that corresponds to the boy's height at the 50th percentile) and a degree of sexual development (usually prepubertal or early pubertal) that are concordant with his bone age, but all of these measures are similarly delayed with respect to chronologic age; in other words, growth, sexual development, and bone age are retarded.[136,303,304] Height velocity usually proceeds at a prepubertal rate or slightly more slowly, relative to peers of the same chronologic age whose height velocity has accelerated at 12 to 13 years of age.

In the absence of anosmia, hyposmia, or other morphologic abnormalities, CDGP cannot be distinguished clinically or biochemically from permanent IHH (see later discussion). If spontaneous puberty does not develop by 18 years of age in a normosmic patient, the diagnosis is usually IHH rather than CDGP. However, spontaneous reversal of hypogonadism has been reported in some men with normosmic IHH.[306]

Eventually, boys with CDGP undergo normal growth and sexual development, but several years after their peers.[136,303,304] Normal height is usually attained, but target midparental height may not be achieved. Also, acquisition of peak bone mass may be compromised in some men. Boys with CDGP may experience severe emotional distress and social exclusion or isolation as a result of immature sexual development and short stature. Therefore, after exclusion of organic causes of delayed puberty, testosterone treatment is usually initiated in boys with CDGP at age 14, or sometimes sooner, to induce sexual maturation and growth that is more consistent with that of their peers. Testosterone is usually started at a low dose and gradually increased over several years; it is stopped intermittently to assess whether spontaneous puberty occurs (see later discussion).

Hereditary Hemochromatosis. Hereditary hemochromatosis is a common autosomal recessive disorder that is characterized by inappropriately high gastrointestinal iron absorption resulting in excessive iron storage in a number of tissues, most prominently liver, pancreas, heart, joints, skin, testes, and pituitary gland.[307,308] In most cases, hereditary hemochromatosis is caused by mutations in the hemochromatosis gene *(HFE)*, most commonly homozygous C282Y/C282Y mutations (70% to 85%) or compound heterozygote C282Y/H63D mutations (5% to 10%), or rarely by other mutations in iron-regulating genes such as transferring receptor 2 *(TFR2)*, hepcidin antimicrobial peptide *(HAMP)*, hemojuvelin *(HJV)*, and solute carrier family 40 A1 *(SLC40A1)*. Homozygous C282Y mutations occur in approximately 1 of every 200 to 400 Caucasians of Northern European descent.

Regardless of the specific mutation causing hereditary hemochromatosis, iron overload results from insufficient hepatic production of hepcidin, a peptide hormone that degrades the iron-exporter protein, ferroportin; this causes unregulated iron absorption in the duodenum and iron overload in tissues.[307,308] Initially, iron overload causes an increase in transferrin iron saturation, followed by an increase in ferritin concentrations in most men with hemochromatosis. Therefore, the biochemical penetrance is high. Evaluation for hemochromatosis should be considered if iron saturation is greater than 45% in men. In the absence of inflammation or cancer, a serum ferritin level higher than 1000 μg/L is associated with greater risk of hepatic cirrhosis in patients with hemochromatosis, and a liver biopsy or MRI for hepatic iron content should be considered.

In contrast to biochemical abnormalities consistent with iron overload, the clinical penetrance of hereditary hemochromatosis is quite low (0.5% to 2.0%), and manifestations of iron overload (hepatic cirrhosis or carcinoma, diabetes mellitus, heart failure or arrhythmias, arthralgias or arthritis, bronzing of skin, hypogonadism) are far less common.[307,308] This may be related to the importance of secondary insults to end organs (e.g., alcoholic liver damage) that contribute to clinical manifestations or to earlier diagnosis with increased awareness and screening. Clinical manifestations, when present, usually appear at between 40 and 60 years of age.

Men with hereditary hemochromatosis almost always manifest secondary hypogonadism resulting in androgen deficiency and impairment in sperm production due to iron overload in the pituitary gland that causes selective gonadotropin deficiency.[309] Serum testosterone levels and sperm counts are low, LH and FSH levels are usually low, and gonadotropin response to GnRH stimulation is absent or markedly attenuated. In the presence of hepatic cirrhosis caused by hemochromatosis, SHBG levels may be elevated; as a result, serum testosterone levels may be normal in the presence of low free testosterone levels. Therefore, accurate and reliable measurements of free testosterone are needed to confirm biochemical androgen deficiency in men with hepatic cirrhosis due to hemochromatosis. Iron deposition in the pituitary may be detected by MRI. Iron overload also occurs in the testes and may occasionally cause a modest reduction in testosterone response to gonadotropin stimulation, resulting in combined primary and secondary hypogonadism. However, in most cases, gonadotropin treatment is able to stimulate normal testicular function, including spermatogenesis and fertility.

After diabetes, secondary hypogonadism is the most common endocrinopathy associated with hereditary hemochromatosis.[307-309] It usually occurs in men with hepatic cirrhosis and ferritin levels higher than 1500 μg/L (i.e., later in the course of iron overload). Because serum SHBG concentrations may be elevated in hepatic cirrhosis, accurate measurements of free rather than total testosterone should be performed to evaluate androgen status in men with hemochromatosis. The prevalence of hypogonadism in iron overload has declined from between 10% and 100% in older reports to approximately 6% more recently, associated with earlier diagnosis and less severe iron overload. Hypogonadism may be reversed with therapeutic phlebotomy, usually early in the course of iron overload.

Idiopathic Hypogonadotropic Hypogonadism. IHH, also referred to as hypogonadotropic eunuchoidism or congenital hypogonadotropic hypogonadism, is an uncommon, clinically heterogeneous group of disorders characterized by isolated gonadotropin deficiency of varying degree with otherwise normal pituitary function.[310] Males with IHH fail to undergo normal puberty, resulting in incomplete sexual maturation or eunuchoidism, androgen deficiency with very low testosterone (usually in the prepubertal range), low to low-normal LH and FSH levels, and impaired sperm production. Gonadotropin deficiency is caused by a defect in normal GnRH production or action, as evidenced by absent or abnormal patterns of pulsatile LH secretion (see Fig. 19-7)[47] and the ability of exogenous pulsatile GnRH treatment to restore normal gonadotropin secretion and testis function. Infants with IHH may have micropenis or cryptorchidism. Rarely, a man with normal virilization develops IHH as an adult.[311]

In approximately 60% of cases, IHH is associated with anosmia or hyposmia and is known as Kallmann's syndrome.[312] Developmental failure of olfactory bulbs (detectable on brain MRI) is responsible for the anosmia or hyposmia. The remaining 40% of men have normosmic IHH. In addition, some men with IHH exhibit other developmental defects, including synkinesia (mirror movements); unilateral renal agenesis; cleft lip/palate or high-arched palate; sensorineural hearing loss; digital skeletal abnormalities such as syndactyly or brachydactyly (fourth metacarpal); dental agenesis; eye movement abnormalities or color blindness (deuteranopia); and agenesis of the corpus callosum.

The prevalence of Kallmann's syndrome is approximately 1 in 8000 to 10,000 men, and there is a marked male predominance (male-to-female ratio, 4:1 to 5:1).[312] X-linked recessive, autosomal dominant, and autosomal recessive modes of inheritance are observed, but many cases are sporadic. Family members of a man with Kallmann's syndrome may have variable clinical expressions, such as normosmic IHH, isolated anosmia, or CDGP.[50,313] In approximately 30% to 40% of cases, Kallmann's syndrome is caused by a known mutation of genes that play important roles in the migration of GnRH neurons from the olfactory placode to the hypothalamus and in normal development of the olfactory bulbs during fetal development. These include mutations of *KAL1* (10% to 20%), *FGFR1/KAL2* (10%), *PROK2* (5%), and *PROKR2* (5%).[50,313]

The *KAL1* gene is located on the X chromosome and encodes an extracellular adhesion glycoprotein known as anosmin 1.[50,313] Mutation or deletion of *KAL1* results in failure of the normal migration of GnRH neurons from the olfactory placode to the hypothalamus, resulting in severe GnRH deficiency; it is the main cause of X-linked recessive Kallmann's syndrome (type 1). The phenotype of Kallmann's syndrome caused by *KAL1* mutations is more severe and less variable than that of other known genetic defects. Synkinesia is present in 80% and unilateral renal agenesis in 30% of cases. The *FGFR1* gene encodes for a fibroblast growth factor receptor that also plays an important role in the migration of GnRH neurons during development.[50,313] Mutations in this gene cause a spectrum of phenotypes, from severe autosomal dominant Kallmann's syndrome (type 2) and normosmic IHH to CDGP associated with cleft lip/palate (in 30% of cases), dental agenesis, and skeletal abnormalities such as brachydactyly and syndactyly. *PROK2* and *PROKR2* encode for a peptide and its G protein–coupled receptor that play important roles in normal GnRH neuronal migration and olfactory bulb development.[50,313] The clinical phenotypes in men with *PROK2* or *PROKR2* mutations are quite variable, ranging from severe Kallmann's syndrome (type 4 or type 3, respectively) to normosmic IHH.

In approximately 30% of cases, normosmic IHH is caused by mutations in genes involved in hypothalamic-pituitary function (particularly during puberty). These include mutations in *GNRHR,* the GnRH receptor (10% to 20%); *KISS1R,* which encodes the receptor for kisspeptin 1/metastin, an important GnRH stimulatory neuropeptide particularly at the time of puberty (2% to 5%); *TAC3,* which encodes neurokinin B, another important GnRH stimulatory neuropeptide, and the gene for its receptor, TAC3R; *FGFR1/KAL2* (2% to 5%); *PROK2*; the genes for leptin *(LEP)* and its receptor *(LEPR)*, which are associated with massive obesity; and, rarely, the GnRH gene, *GNRH1*.[50,313]

Hypogonadotropic hypogonadism is a component of complex genetic syndromes associated with specific dysmorphic features or combined hormonal defects. For example, the *CHARGE syndrome*, characterized by *c*oloboma of the eye or CNS anomalies, *h*eart anomalies, nasal choanal *a*tresia, growth *r*etardation, *g*enital defect (hypogonadism), and *e*ar anomalies (deafness, dysmorphic ears, and hypoplasia of the semicircular canals), may be associated with Kallmann's syndrome or normosmic IHH.[314,315] In approximately 60% of cases, CHARGE syndrome is caused by a mutation in the chromodomain helicase DNA binding protein 7 (*CHD7*) gene, which encodes for a chromatin remodeling protein. *CDH7* mutations have been found in approximately 3% to 4% of men with Kallmann's syndrome or normosmic IHH, and it is hypothesized that IHH may be a mild variant of the CHARGE syndrome.

X-linked congenital adrenal hypoplasia, characterized by adrenal insufficiency due to adrenal hypoplasia and normosmic IHH, is caused by a mutation in the dose-sensitive sex reversal–adrenal hypoplasia (DSS-AHC) critical region on the X chromosome protein 1 (*DAX1*) gene, now known as *NR0B1* (nuclear receptor subfamily 0, group B, member 1), which encodes for an orphan nuclear receptor. Mutations of the SF-1 gene *(NR5A1)*, which encodes another orphan nuclear receptor; the prohormone convertase 1 *(PC1)* gene, which encodes an enzyme involved in post-translational processing of pituitary prohormones and neuropeptides; and genes for a number of pituitary transcription factors such as *HESX1* (septo-optic dysplasia or deMorsier syndrome), *LHX3, LHX4, POUF1,* and *PROP1* cause deficiencies in multiple anterior pituitary and other hormones in addition to gonadotropin deficiency. Mutations in the latter transcription factors may also be associated with specific dysmorphic features. Unlike men with IHH, those with multiple hormone defects usually fail to normalize gonadotropin and testicular function in response to chronic pulsatile GnRH administration.[50,313]

In the absence of anosmia, hyposmia, or features of Kallmann's syndrome (e.g., synkinesia), it is not possible to confidently distinguish an individual who has normosmic IHH not associated with a complex genetic syndrome from one who has CDGP.[136,303,304] In both conditions, there may be a family history of delayed puberty, IHH, or Kallmann's syndrome; a history of cryptorchidism; clinical manifestations of delayed sexual maturation or eunuchoidism; and low serum testosterone and low to low-normal gonadotropin levels. In contrast to boys with IHH, who have normal height for their chronologic age, those with CDGP usually manifest some growth delay and short stature. Boys with IHH may have a history of micropenis and usually demonstrate pubertal delay after 19 years of age, although some individuals undergo spontaneous puberty after 20 years of age or reversal of IHH in adulthood.[306] Currently, there is no diagnostic test that completely and reliably distinguishes isolated normosmic IHH from CDGP.

As discussed previously, after organic causes of delayed puberty (e.g., craniopharyngioma) have been excluded, testosterone therapy is usually initiated in boys with delayed puberty at about 14 years of age to induce sexual maturation and growth.[136,303,304] Testosterone is usually discontinued intermittently to assess whether spontaneous puberty occurs, as determined by an increase in testis size. Boys with IHH usually require continued testosterone treatment to achieve and maintain sexual maturation, whereas those with CDGP do not require further treatment after spontaneous secretion of gonadotropin and testosterone commences. Sustained reversal occurs after discontinuation of therapy in about 10% of men with Kallmann's syndrome or normosmic IHH who present initially with absent or partial sexual maturation.[306] Therefore, it is reasonable to discontinue treatment briefly to assess the reversibility of hypogonadotropic hypogonadism.

If fertility is desired, testosterone therapy is stopped and treatment with gonadotropin or, in some specialized centers, pulsatile GnRH is instituted to stimulate sperm production. Previous treatment with testosterone, which might be expected to suppress endogenous gonadotropin further, does not alter the subsequent response of spermatogenesis to gonadotropin therapy.[316,317] Gonadotropin or GnRH therapy is much more likely to stimulate spermatogenesis if there is some evidence of sexual maturation and larger testes at baseline and no history of cryptorchidism or another primary testicular disorder.[318] Even in the absence of clinical evidence of hypothalamic-pituitary-testicular disorder, some men with IHH do not have an adequate gonadotropin or testicular response to chronic pulsatile GnRH therapy, suggesting underlying pituitary or testicular defects.[319]

Men with IHH have varying degrees of gonadotropin deficiency, as evidenced by a persistent but abnormal pattern of pulsatile LH secretion (see Fig. 19-7).[47] In some men with IHH, FSH secretion predominates relative to LH secretion, resulting in some germ cell maturation and spermatogenesis and a rare variant form of IHH known as *isolated LH deficiency* or the "fertile eunuch syndrome."[320-322] This syndrome is characterized by prepubertal androgen deficiency or eunuchoidism caused by LH deficiency but pubertal or almost adult-sized testes in which advanced-stage spermatogenesis is present due to relatively preserved FSH secretion. However, spermatogenesis usually is not completely normal in these men, and they are not fertile, as the name of the syndrome might imply. Because there is only relative gonadotropin deficiency and some spermatogenesis is present, treatment with LH-like activity (hCG) stimulates Leydig cell testosterone production and ameliorates androgen deficiency, stimulating spermatogenesis sufficient for induction of fertility. Men with *isolated FSH deficiency* in the absence of an FSHβ mutation have been reported, but the degree and nature of the defect in pulsatile gonadotropin secretion has not been well documented.[323-325]

Men with inactivating *LHβ mutations* usually demonstrate a lack of pubertal development, impaired spermatogenesis or azoospermia, and infertility.[59,326,327] Recently, however, a man with an LHβ mutation resulting in a partially active LH molecule (as indicated by expression of steroidogenic enzymes in a few mature Leydig cells and low intratesticular testosterone levels) was reported to have complete and quantitatively normal spermatogenesis.[80] Complete spermatogenesis was achieved in the presence of very low LH and intratesticular testosterone concentrations and high serum FSH levels in this man. Men with inactivating *FSHβ mutations* have been found generally to have azoospermia with undetectable FSH, low or low-normal testosterone, and high LH levels.[82-85]

Complex Genetic Syndromes. Secondary hypogonadism may be present in a number of complex genetic syndromes, such as Prader-Labhart-Willi, Laurence-Moon-Bardet-Biedl, Alström, Bjornstad, Börjeson-Forssman-Lehmann, Bosma, Chudley, Costello, Gordon-Holmes, Johnson-McMillin, Juberg-Marsidi, LEOPARD (multiple lentigines), Martsof, Moebius-Poland, Roifman, Rud, and

Woodhouse-Sakati syndromes.[231,244,328-343] Most of these syndromes are diagnosed by pediatricians and pediatric endocrinologists based on the clustering of specific dysmorphic features and congenital anomalies that are characteristic of the syndrome.[231] Secondary hypogonadism in these disorders usually causes prepubertal androgen deficiency. Many but not all of these syndromes are associated with CNS abnormalities or intellectual disability. Obesity may contribute to the etiology of hypogonadism and may alert clinicians to the potential presence of a complex genetic syndrome. Some, such as the Prader-Labhart-Willi, Laurence-Moon-Bardet-Biedl, and Alström syndromes, have been reported to be associated with primary as well as secondary hypogonadism.[242-244]

Acquired Disorders

Hyperprolactinemia. Hyperprolactinemia is a common cause of secondary hypogonadism. These patients have low testosterone concentrations and low to low-normal gonadotropin levels and present with sexual dysfunction (reduced libido and erectile dysfunction), infertility, and gynecomastia.[344] Because the male breast usually is not exposed to a relatively high estrogen and progestin milieu such as that associated with induction of ductal hyperplasia and glandular formation, high prolactin levels rarely result in galactorrhea. Hyperprolactinemia causes gonadotropin deficiency primarily by suppressing pulsatile hypothalamic GnRH secretion, as evidenced by reduced spontaneous LH pulse frequency and amplitude and restoration of normal LH pulsatility and testosterone levels with dopamine agonist treatment or pulsatile GnRH administration.[345]

Common causes of hyperprolactinemia resulting in clinical secondary hypogonadism are a prolactin-secreting adenoma, pituitary stalk disease (e.g., stalk compression from a non–prolactin-secreting adenoma, traumatic stalk section); hypothalamic disease (e.g., hypothalamic tumors, granulomatous disease); and medications.[344]

In contrast to women, men with prolactin-secreting adenomas usually present with large macroadenomas because of a lack of symptoms, delay in seeking medical care for symptoms such as sexual dysfunction, or possibly a gender-specific difference in the biologic behavior of the tumor.[346,347] In approximately 10% of cases, there is excessive cosecretion of both prolactin and GH. In men with prolactin-secreting macroadenomas, serum prolactin levels are usually higher than 250 ng/mL, and they can be higher than 1000 ng/mL with tumors larger than 2 cm in diameter. If a patient with a very large pituitary macroadenoma is found to have only modestly elevated prolactin levels, this may be a false-negative result caused by saturation of both the capture and the detection antibodies used in two-site sandwich immunoassays.[348] This phenomenon is known as the prozone or "hook" effect and necessitates dilution of serum samples.

Diseases affecting the pituitary stalk and hypothalamic diseases may cause hyperprolactinemia because of disruption of the hypothalamic hypophyseal portal tract and transport of dopamine from the hypothalamus to the pituitary in the former condition or loss of hypothalamic dopamine-containing neurons in the latter. Suprasellar extension of a large, non–prolactin-secreting pituitary macroadenoma that compresses the pituitary stalk usually causes hyperprolactinemia with serum prolactin levels in the 20 to 250 ng/mL range, although higher levels are occasionally seen.[344]

Medications that cause hyperprolactinemia (prolactin concentration usually <100 ng/mL) interfere with hypothalamic dopamine production or action or affect the regulation of dopamine secretion by CNS neurotransmitters (e.g., serotonin).[349,350] The medications that most commonly cause hyperprolactinemia are dopamine D_2 receptor antagonists, such as typical antipsychotic drugs (phenothiazines, thioxanthenes, and butyrophenones), some atypical antipsychotic agents (e.g., risperidone, molindone) and gastrointestinal pro-motility agents (e.g., metoclopramide, domperidone). In contrast, newer atypical antipsychotic medications such as clozapine, olanzapine, quetiapine, ziprasidone, and aripiprazole much less commonly increase prolactin. Other medications that less commonly cause hyperprolactinemia include some tricyclic antidepressants (e.g., clomipramine), monoamine oxidase inhibitors (e.g., pargyline; clorgiline, which is rarely used), and antihypertensive agents (verapamil; α-methyldopa and reserpine, which are rarely used). Selective serotonin and serotonin/norepinephrine reuptake inhibitors in general have minimal to no effect on prolactin levels.

Serum prolactin levels may be elevated in patients with CKD, in proportion to the degree of renal failure, because of both increased secretion and decreased clearance, and this may contribute to the hypogonadism associated with chronic renal failure. The mild hyperprolactinemia associated with primary hypothyroidism does not usually suppress gonadotropin secretion significantly or cause clinical secondary hypogonadism in men. However, if primary hypothyroidism is severe and long-standing, it may cause slight enlargement of the pituitary gland, which may be confused with a pituitary adenoma.

Treatment is aimed initially at the underlying cause of hyperprolactinemia. In men with prolactin-secreting macroadenomas, treatment is initiated with a dopamine agonist medication such as bromocriptine or carbergoline.[344,346,351] Dopamine agonist therapy usually results in a reduction of serum prolactin, decreased tumor size, and improvement in visual field defects. Treatment with these agents may also improve sexual dysfunction, normalize testosterone levels, and improve semen quality. In men who remain persistently hypogonadal despite adequate dopamine agonist treatment, testosterone therapy may be initiated to treat manifestations of androgen deficiency. Testosterone is aromatized to estradiol, which may act directly on lactotrophs in the pituitary and may increase prolactin levels and tumor growth and cause resistance to dopamine agonist therapy.[352] Therefore, careful monitoring is required during testosterone replacement therapy.

In some men who do not respond to dopamine agonist treatment alone, gonadotropin or pulsatile GnRH therapy may be necessary to stimulate spermatogenesis sufficient to induce fertility. Surgery or radiation therapy may be needed for tumors that are resistant to dopamine agonists, and urgent surgery may be needed for pituitary apoplexy or rapidly progressive tumor mass effects such as visual loss. Medications that cause hyperprolactinemia may be stopped or switched to ones that do not elevate prolactin. For antipsychotic and antidepressant medications, such changes should be made in consultation with the patient's psychiatrist.[349] If discontinuing or switching drugs is not an option, testosterone treatment may be needed to treat androgen deficiency. Addition of a dopamine agonist while administration of an offending antipsychotic medication is continued should be done with extreme caution, because there is a risk of exacerbating psychosis.

Opiates. Use of opiates or opioid medications, particularly potent, long-acting narcotic analgesics such as methadone (>60 mg daily); controlled-release or intrathecal morphine sulfate or the transdermal fentanyl patch; and drugs of abuse such as heroin (diacetylmorphine) or time-released oxycodone (OxyContin) profoundly suppress gonadotropin secretion, resulting in severe androgen deficiency.[353-355]

Prolonged use of opiates causes symptomatic androgen deficiency, resulting in sexual dysfunction and long-term consequences such as loss of BMD and increased risk of osteoporosis; this is a common cause of secondary hypogonadism associated with androgen deficiency and impairment in sperm production. As such, testosterone treatment should be considered in cases of severe secondary hypogonadism due to chronic use of opiates. However, short-term use of opiates or use of short-acting opiates (e.g., postoperatively) may cause only a transient suppression of gonadotropins and testosterone that does not require treatment.

Administration of opiate antagonists such as naloxone or naltrexone results in an increase in LH pulse frequency in normal men, suggesting that endogenous opiate neuronal systems within the hypothalamus exert a negative regulation on pulsatile GnRH secretion.[356] Therefore, exogenous administration of opiates most likely causes gonadotropin secretion by suppressing hypothalamic GnRH secretion. The action of exogenous opiates on GnRH secretion is probably mediated by μ-opioid receptors. In this regard, the pure μ-opioid receptor agonist, methadone, more severely suppresses gonadotropins and testosterone than does buprenorphine, which is a partial μ-receptor, δ-receptor, and opioid receptor–like 1 (ORL1)/nociceptin receptor agonist and κ-opioid receptor antagonist.[355] Both methadone and buprenorphine are used clinically for detoxification and maintenance treatment of opioid addiction.

In men taking chronic high-dose, long-acting opiates, serum testosterone, LH, and FSH are usually severely suppressed, and sperm production is impaired.[357] The most prominent abnormality demonstrated on seminal fluid analysis in men taking methadone is reduced sperm motility (asthenospermia), but abnormalities in sperm morphology (teratospermia) and oligozoospermia are also seen. Functional δ-, κ-, and μ-opioid receptors have been reported to be present on human spermatozoa.[358] Therefore, exogenous opiates may have a direct effect by slowing sperm motility, independent of their effects on the hypothalamic-pituitary-testicular axis.

Sex Steroids. Administration of sex steroids, androgens, progestins, or estrogens suppresses gonadotropin secretion by negative feedback mechanisms at the hypothalamus or the pituitary gland or both; chronic administration may cause secondary hypogonadism, resulting in androgen deficiency and impaired sperm production.

Synthetic androgens (androgenic anabolic steroids) and testosterone are being used increasingly by boys and men to increase muscle bulk and strength and enhance athletic performance or physical appearance. For these purposes, these androgens are used in extremely high doses in a variety of combinations and patterns for prolonged periods. The prevalence of anabolic steroid abuse ranges from approximately 1% to 6% in various populations including high school and college students, young recreational athletes, and competitive athletes.[122,359,360]

During chronic administration of high-dose androgenic anabolic steroids, serum levels of testosterone, LH, and FSH are very low and sperm counts are usually suppressed to severe oligozoospermia or azoospermia.[122,359,360] Unless testosterone is being administered, serum testosterone concentrations are low, because synthetic anabolic steroids do not cross-react in testosterone assays. Although serum testosterone levels are low, abused anabolic steroids are themselves androgens, so individuals taking these agents usually do not complain of androgen deficiency symptoms.

After discontinuation of even prolonged anabolic steroid use, recovery of the hypothalamic-pituitary-testicular axis usually occurs within weeks to months. However, for unclear reasons, some men experience a protracted period of symptomatic hypogonadism that may last for several months to several years.[122,359,360] It usually is not possible to know whether these men had underlying hypogonadism before taking anabolic steroids; therefore, if secondary hypogonadism is severe, an appropriate workup including sellar imaging is usually needed. Prolonged secondary hypogonadism after androgenic anabolic steroid use often causes sexual dysfunction and depressed mood. Severe symptoms may lead to continued use of these agents and anabolic steroid dependence. Treatment with testosterone to relieve symptoms of androgen deficiency or with gonadotropins (hCG) to stimulate sperm production and induce fertility may be needed. Off-label treatment with clomiphene citrate has also been reported to stimulate gonadotropin and testosterone secretion in these men.[361]

Chronic administration of high doses of progestins such as megestrol acetate or depo-medroxyprogesterone acetate or estrogens such as diethylstilbestrol also suppresses gonadotropins and testicular function, resulting in secondary hypogonadism. Megestrol acetate is used to stimulate appetite in wasting conditions such as cancer and HIV disease. At the doses used for this purpose, it causes severe symptomatic androgen deficiency and suppression of sperm production.[362] Weight gain induced by megestrol acetate is mostly fat rather than lean mass, in part because of the androgen deficiency that it causes.[363] Most importantly, megestrol acetate may cause symptomatic and potentially life-threatening secondary adrenal insufficiency.[362] Both megestrol and depo-medroxyprogesterone acetate have been used to induce medical castration in patients with prostate cancer.[364] Medroxyprogesterone acetate has also been used to reduce libido in psychiatric conditions manifested by deviant sexual behavior (paraphilia), and it is used in combination with testosterone (to prevent androgen deficiency) for suppression of spermatogenesis in male contraceptive development trials.[104,365] Administration of estrogens (e.g., diethylstilbestrol for prostate cancer), exposure to estrogen-containing substances, or excessive estradiol production by estrogen-secreting tumors (e.g., Sertoli cell tumors) suppresses gonadotropin and testosterone production and causes secondary hypogonadism, usually with prominent gynecomastia.[366-368]

Gonadotropin-Releasing Hormone Analogues. GnRH analogues, both agonists and antagonists, severely suppress endogenous gonadotropin and testosterone production (i.e., medical castration); they are used to treat androgen-dependent pathologic states such as locally advanced or metastatic prostate cancer and central precocious puberty.[180,369] Administration of GnRH agonists (e.g., leuprolide, goserelin) produces an initial stimulation of gonadotropin and testosterone secretion (known as a "flare"), which is followed in 1 to 2 weeks by GnRH receptor downregulation and marked suppression of gonadotropins and testosterone to castrate levels.[180] The initial surge in testosterone levels has been associated with clinical flares in metastatic prostate cancer, and there have been reports of increased bladder outlet obstruction, bone pain, pathologic fracture, spinal cord compression, and death. However, these complications are very uncommon, and it is not clear that they are directly related to the initial increase in testosterone concentrations. To prevent the potential complications associated with the testosterone flare, AR antagonists (e.g., bicalutamide) are usually coadministered with a GnRH agonist for men with metastatic prostate cancer.[370] In contrast to agonists, GnRH antagonists (e.g., degarelix) cause an immediate suppression of gonadotropin and testosterone secretion without a flare.[369]

Continuous administration of GnRH agonists in men with locally advanced or metastatic prostate cancer induces castrate or near-castrate testosterone levels and causes symptoms of severe androgen deficiency, including sexual dysfunction with reduced libido and reduced spontaneous erections; diminished energy and motivation; depressed mood and irritability; hot flushes and sleep disturbance; decreased memory and concentration; reduced in muscle mass and strength; increased fat mass and insulin resistance; decreased BMD resulting in osteopenia or osteoporosis; gynecomastia and loss of male hair pattern; and decreased hemoglobin and hematocrit, resulting in significant decline in quality of life.[179,180] As a result, increasingly, GnRH agonist therapy is administered intermittently in the treatment of advanced prostate cancer. However, in a substantial number of men who stop GnRH agonist therapy, testicular function remains suppressed and testosterone levels persist within the castrate or hypogonadal range for prolonged periods (up to 1 to 3 years).[371,372] Risk factors for prolonged testicular suppression are longer duration of GnRH agonist therapy, older age (>70 years), and possibly low testosterone levels before treatment.

Large population studies have found that prolonged GnRH agonist therapy increases the risk of diabetes mellitus, coronary heart disease, myocardial infarction, sudden cardiac death, stroke, and fractures. Consequently, the U.S. Food and Drug Administration has recommended that the risk factors for these diseases should be assessed and the benefits and risks of GnRH agonist therapy weighed before it is used and that monitoring for these conditions should be continued during treatment.[180,369,373,374]

Hypopituitarism. A destructive or infiltrative lesion of the pituitary gland or hypothalamus commonly causes impaired pituitary hormone production (hypopituitarism) and gonadotropin deficiency resulting in androgen deficiency and impairment in sperm production. The prevalence of hypopituitarism has been estimated to be approximately 1 in 2200.[375,376]

Hypopituitarism is most commonly caused by *pituitary adenomas* and their treatment (hypophysectomy or radiation therapy) or by *hypothalamic or parasellar tumors* such as craniopharyngioma, meningioma, optic glioma or astrocytoma, metastatic carcinoma (from breast, lung, colon, or prostate), pinealoma, germinoma, cordoma, and ependymoma; together, these tumors account for approximately 90% of cases.[375,376]

Other conditions of the pituitary or hypothalamus (or both) that cause hypopituitarism include cranial radiation therapy (intracranial tumors, acute lymphoblastic leukemia prophylaxis, nasopharyngeal carcinoma, total body irradiation); vascular compromise (traumatic brain injury, infarction or pituitary apoplexy, subarachnoid hemorrhage, ischemic stroke, vascular malformation); granulomatous or infiltrative disease (sarcoidosis, histiocytosis X, Wegener's granulomatosis, hemochromatosis, transfusion-induced iron overload); infection (tuberculosis, fungal infections such as aspergillosis or coccidiomycosis, basilar meningitis, encephalitis, syphilis, Whipple's disease); pituitary stalk disease (traumatic injury such as basilar skull fracture or surgical pituitary stalk section, granulomatous disease, lymphocytic infundibuloneurohypophysitis, infection, tumor); and lymphocytic hypophysitis (in particular, lymphocytic infundibuloneurohypophysitis, which is more common in men, rather than lymphocytic adenohypophysitis, which is more common in women).[375,376] These conditions are discussed in detail in Chapter 9.

Destructive or infiltrative lesions of the pituitary gland (e.g., nonfunctioning pituitary adenoma) usually result in a gradual, progressive loss of anterior pituitary function. In these instances, GH and gonadotropin (FSH and LH) deficiency (i.e., secondary hypogonadism) usually occur initially, followed by deficiencies of TSH (secondary hypothyroidism) and, eventually, ACTH (secondary adrenal insufficiency), resulting in *panhypopituitarism*.[375,376] However, there are many exceptions to this order of loss, depending on the specific location of the pituitary lesion and the nature of the underlying disease process. For example, lymphocytic hypophysitis usually causes ACTH and TSH deficiency without impairment of gonadotropin production, and ACTH deficiency is more common than TSH deficiency after radiation therapy involving the hypothalamic-pituitary axis. Anterior pituitary hormone loss is even less predictable in disease processes involving the hypothalamus, in part because of the more disperse anatomic arrangement in the hypothalamus of nuclei that produce releasing factors for pituitary hormones. Acute destructive processes such as pituitary apoplexy usually cause panhypopituitarism.

Diseases of the hypothalamus or high in the pituitary stalk may be associated with *diabetes insipidus*, which is caused by destruction or retrograde degeneration of neurons producing arginine vasopressin (AVP) in the supraoptic or the paraventricular nuclei, respectively.[375-377] Processes involving only the pituitary gland do not cause diabetes insipidus.

Hypothalamic and pituitary stalk diseases may cause hyperprolactinemia due to loss of dopamine-containing neurons or interruption of the hypothalamic hypophyseal portal tract and transport of dopamine from the hypothalamus to the pituitary. Pituitary microadenomas or macroadenomas may produce prolactin, and suprasellar extension of nonsecretory pituitary macroadenomas or those secreting other hormones (e.g., GH) may cause hyperprolactinemia by interrupting the hypothalamic-hypophyseal portal system.

Prepubertal boys who have hypopituitarism resulting in gonadotropin deficiency present with delayed puberty and eunuchoidism, and men present with adult androgen deficiency and complaints of reduced libido and erectile dysfunction. However, in patients with secondary hypogonadism, clinicians must be alert to the possibility and clinical manifestations of *deficiencies of other pituitary hormones* (ACTH, TSH, GH, and AVP); *excessive pituitary hormone production* by pituitary adenomas and resulting clinical syndromes, such as excessive prolactin production resulting hyperprolactinemia, ACTH resulting in Cushing's syndrome, GH resulting in acromegaly, gonadotropin and free α- and β-subunits (which usually do not result in a hormone excess syndrome but rarely cause precocious puberty), or, rarely, TSH resulting in hyperthyroidism; and *tumor mass effects* such as headache, visual disturbance, and visual field defects (typically bilateral superior quadrantanopsia or bitemporal hemianopsia, but a unilateral effect and a variety of visual field defects may be present) and, uncommonly, cerebrospinal fluid rhinorrhea, cranial nerve palsies, temporal lobe epilepsy, and personality changes.[375,376] It is important to have a high index of suspicion for the presence of secondary adrenal insufficiency in patients with hypothalamic or pituitary disease, because it is a life-threatening and treatable condition that manifests with nonspecific symptoms and signs. In boys with hypopituitarism who present with a clinical picture of CDGP, GH deficiency may occur in conjunction with gonadotropin deficiency and may contribute to short stature and growth delay.

Usually in men with secondary hypogonadism due to hypopituitarism, the serum testosterone level and sperm count are very low, and LH and FSH levels are distinctly low or, less commonly, in the low-normal to slightly low range. The gonadotropin response to acute or chronic GnRH stimulation is not a clinically useful differential diagnostic test because it does not reliably distinguish between pituitary and hypothalamic disease causing gonadotropin deficiency in hypopituitarism. If hypopituitarism is suspected on the basis of the initial clinical and laboratory evaluation, further evaluation should include hypothalamic-pituitary imaging, preferably an MRI with gadolinium contrast enhancement, which can better define the presence and extent of hypothalamic and pituitary disease compared with a computed tomographic scan (although the latter is able to detect pituitary macroadenoma and microcalcifications found frequently in craniopharyngioma); formal visual field examination; and investigation of anterior pituitary hormone deficiency or excess.[375,376]

Treatment is aimed at the underlying etiology of the hypopituitarism and treatment of pituitary hormone deficiency, including treatment of androgen deficiency secondary to gonadotropin deficiency with testosterone replacement therapy.[375,376] With transsphenoidal surgical treatment of pituitary adenomas, pituitary function is improved in approximately 50% of cases. Dopamine agonist treatment of prolactin-secreting pituitary adenomas improves pituitary function in 60% to 75% of cases. If fertility is desired, testosterone treatment is stopped and gonadotropin therapy is initiated, initially with hCG. In men with acquired gonadotropin deficiency without coexisting testicular disease, hCG treatment alone may stimulate spermatogenesis to levels sufficient to restore fertility.[79]

Systemic Disorders

Glucocorticoid Excess (Cushing's Syndrome). Excessive levels of either exogenous or endogenous glucocorticoids (the latter due to pituitary Cushing's disease or adrenal adenoma) is a common acquired cause of secondary hypogonadism resulting in symptomatic prepubertal or adult androgen deficiency and impaired sperm production.[378-381] In contrast to those patients with adrenal adenoma, some men with glucocorticoid excess due to adrenal carcinoma secrete excessive amounts of androgens (and mineralocorticoids) and do not demonstrate hypogonadism.

Glucocorticoids act primarily to suppress gonadotropins via inhibition of hypothalamic GnRH secretion, but they may also have direct suppressive effects on testis function and therefore produce combined primary and secondary hypogonadism. However, high-dose immunosuppressive glucocorticoid therapy is most commonly associated with a hormone pattern characterized by low testosterone and low-normal gonadotropin levels, consistent with secondary hypogonadism. Occasionally in men receiving glucocorticoid treatment, gonadotropins are high-normal or slightly elevated, suggesting primary hypogonadism.

Although it occurs most commonly with high-dose glucocorticoid treatment, doses as low as 7.5 mg of prednisone may cause hypogonadism, particularly in older men. Because high doses of glucocorticoids may suppress SHBG concentrations, it is important to confirm the biochemical diagnosis of hypogonadism using an accurate measurement of free testosterone (i.e., calculated free testosterone or free testosterone by equilibrium dialysis). In preliminary studies of men receiving chronic glucocorticoid therapy, testosterone treatment was found to improve muscle mass, BMD, and quality of life.[382]

Chronic Organ Failure. Chronic organ failure, such as in hepatic cirrhosis, CKD, chronic lung disease, or CHF, is a common cause of symptomatic secondary hypogonadism.[4,5] As discussed previously, chronic systemic illness commonly affects the hypothalamic-pituitary-testicular axis at multiple levels and usually causes combined primary and secondary hypogonadism, but many disorders are associated with a hormone pattern characterized by low serum testosterone and low to low-normal gonadotropin levels, indicative of secondary hypogonadism.

The etiology of clinical and biochemical hypogonadism in these cases is multifactorial and encompasses both the chronic disease itself and its associated conditions of malnutrition, wasting, a pro-inflammatory state (with elevated cytokines such as IL-1 and tumor necrosis factor-α [TNF-α]), medication use (e.g., alcohol, opiates, glucocorticoids), chronic stress, and other comorbid illnesses. These associated factors play a large role in suppressing gonadotropin levels and contribute to the hormonal pattern of secondary hypogonadism associated with chronic organ failure. The degree to which these factors contribute to the clinical and biochemical manifestations of hypogonadism varies considerably among individuals. Furthermore, biochemical confirmation of low testosterone in patients with chronic organ failure or systemic illness may be confounded by alterations in SHBG. Therefore, accurate and reliable measurements of free testosterone are needed to establish biochemical androgen deficiency in the presence of chronic systemic illness.

Hepatic cirrhosis from any etiology (e.g., alcoholic or nonalcoholic liver disease) is commonly associated with a hormone pattern that is consistent with primary hypogonadism (i.e., low free testosterone, high LH, and normal to high-normal FSH levels) in mild to moderate disease (Child-Pugh class A or B) and with secondary hypogonadism (i.e., low free testosterone and low-normal LH and FSH levels) in severe to end-stage liver disease (Child-Pugh class C).[262,263] SHBG concentrations increase progressively with the severity of cirrhosis, resulting in normal or high serum total testosterone levels despite low free testosterone concentrations and clinical manifestations of androgen deficiency. Sperm production is commonly impaired and sperm motility is reduced in men with hepatic cirrhosis.

In alcoholic cirrhosis, serum estrone and estradiol levels are relatively high due to increased production of adrenal androgens (e.g., androstenedione) induced by alcohol and its metabolite, acetaldehyde; reduced clearance of these by the liver; and subsequent aromatization of androstenedione to estrone and its conversion to estradiol.[4,5] Relative hyperestrogenism is responsible for a number of the clinical manifestations commonly observed in men with alcoholic compared with nonalcoholic cirrhosis, including gynecomastia, palmar erythema, plethora, spider angiomata, and loss of male body hair (reduced axillary and pubic hair and a female escutcheon). Men with severe alcoholic cirrhosis usually have atrophic testes due to direct toxic effects of alcohol.

In men with severe hepatic cirrhosis, pulsatile GnRH secretion and the pituitary response to GnRH are diminished, contributing to secondary hypogonadal failure.[383] Spironolactone, which is used to treat edema and ascites associated with portal hypertension, is an AR antagonist and an androgen biosynthesis inhibitor. Its use may contribute to symptoms of androgen deficiency, gynecomastia, and hypogonadism. Protein-calorie malnutrition, complications of cirrhosis such as infection, and continued alcohol abuse contribute to the clinical manifestations and etiology of low testosterone in these chronically ill men. Successful liver transplantation improves but does not normalize gonadal function, probably because of chronic immunosuppressive treatment with glucocorticoids and other agents.[262]

As described in a previous section, *CKD* is commonly associated with a hormone pattern of low serum testosterone and elevated gonadotropin concentrations resulting from reduced renal clearance, consistent with primary hypogonadism.[4,5,264,265,267] However, the amplitude of pulsatile LH secretion is reduced, suggesting impaired hypothalamic-pituitary function in men with CKD.[384] Gonadotropin secretion may also be suppressed by coexisting uremia, hyperprolactinemia, malnutrition, a pro-inflammatory state, comorbid conditions (e.g., diabetes), and obesity, and some men demonstrate a hormone pattern that is more consistent with secondary hypogonadism (i.e., with low testosterone and normal to high-normal gonadotropin levels). Successful renal transplantation usually normalizes levels of testosterone and gonadotropins and sperm production.[264,265]

Men with *chronic lung disease*, especially COPD, commonly have low serum testosterone levels.[385,386] The prevalence of biochemical hypogonadism depends on the population studied and varies from 12% in a community-based population to 38% in male veterans, the latter being a population with high comorbidity. In the population of veterans, approximately 75% of men with COPD with low serum testosterone have low or low-normal gonadotropin levels, consistent with secondary hypogonadism, and the remainder have elevated gonadotropins, indicative of primary hypogonadism.[386] Coexisting factors that contribute to the clinical symptoms and biochemical diagnosis of hypogonadism in men with severe COPD include muscle wasting, inactivity, and deconditioning; malnutrition and cachexia; chronic stress and inflammation; medications (e.g., glucocorticoids); and hypoxia. Hypoxia suppresses gonadotropin and testosterone secretion independent of glucocorticoid therapy in men with COPD or idiopathic pulmonary fibrosis.[385-387] Preliminary studies have demonstrated an increase in lean mass with testosterone treatment in men with COPD and low testosterone levels but inconsistent improvements in muscle strength, including respiratory muscle function, and no effects on endurance or quality of life.

CHF is associated with biochemical androgen deficiency in approximately 25% to 30% of cases.[388-390] Men with CHF who have low serum testosterone usually have normal to low-normal gonadotropin levels, suggesting secondary hypogonadism. However, it is unclear whether men with CHF and low testosterone differ from those with normal testosterone in regard to symptoms and signs or response to testosterone therapy.[389] In limited initial clinical trials in men with CHF, testosterone treatment improved exercise tolerance, muscle strength, and oxygen capacity in men with either low or normal testosterone levels, suggesting a pharmacologic effect of testosterone independent of the presence of androgen deficiency.

Chronic Systemic Illness. A number of chronic systemic illnesses, such as diabetes mellitus, malignancy, rheumatic disease, and HIV disease, may also cause secondary hypogonadism characterized by low serum testosterone concentrations and low or low-normal gonadotropin levels.[4,5] As in men with chronic organ failure, the etiology of clinical and biochemical hypogonadism is multifactorial due to the chronic illness itself and associated obesity (e.g., with diabetes mellitus) or malnutrition (e.g., with malignancy), wasting, pro-inflammatory state, medication use (e.g., opiates, glucocorticoids), chronic stress, or other comorbid illnesses. These factors suppress gonadotropin levels and contribute variably to the clinical and biochemical androgen deficiency seen in individuals with systemic illness. Because systemic illnesses and associated comorbidities and medications may alter SHBG concentrations, measurements of free testosterone are needed to confirm biochemical androgen deficiency.

Low serum free testosterone and low or low-normal gonadotropin levels, consistent with secondary hypogonadism, occur in 30% to 50% of men with *T2DM*.[391,392] Low testosterone levels are associated with nonspecific clinical manifestations that may be caused by androgen deficiency, such as erectile dysfunction. Insulin resistance and moderate obesity are commonly associated with T2DM. In patients with T2DM and moderate obesity, low total testosterone levels may result from reduced SHBG concentrations caused by insulin resistance and action on the liver. Therefore, it is important to confirm biochemical androgen deficiency in these men by using calculated free testosterone values or measurements of free testosterone by equilibrium dialysis.

Secondary hypogonadism and clinical manifestations of androgen deficiency may also be caused by comorbidities and complications associated with diabetes, such as obesity, atherosclerotic vascular disease, the pro-inflammatory state of diabetes, diabetic neuropathy, and CKD. Therefore, testosterone treatment should be considered only in those diabetic men with symptomatic androgen deficiency that has been confirmed by accurate free testosterone measurements. If symptoms do not improve with an adequate trial of testosterone therapy (e.g., 6 months), discontinuation of treatment should be considered, particularly in men who had borderline or slightly low testosterone levels before therapy.

Men with poorly controlled T1DM may have reduced serum testosterone and gonadotropin levels and reduced LH pulse amplitude and frequency, which are not present in those with well controlled disease.[393]

Men with *malignancy* commonly have secondary hypogonadism characterized by low serum testosterone concentrations and low or low-normal gonadotropin levels.[394-396] As mentioned previously, some men with malignancy present with low testosterone and elevated gonadotropin concentrations, consistent with primary hypogonadism. Malnutrition, wasting (cancer cachexia), systemic inflammation, medication use (e.g., opiate pain medications, glucocorticoids), chronic stress, and concomitant comorbid illnesses contribute to clinical and biochemical hypogonadism in men with cancer. Because SHBG may be reduced as a result of these associated conditions, free testosterone measurements are needed to confirm androgen deficiency.

Primary or secondary hypogonadism may be present before systemic chemotherapy or radiation therapy as well as after treatment. A low free testosterone concentration with normal or elevated gonadotropin levels was found in 40% to 60% of men with advanced malignancy (i.e., metastatic cancer) presenting with malnutrition and men with various stages of Hodgkin's disease before chemotherapy.[279,280] Low levels of free testosterone and bioavailable testosterone were present, respectively, in approximately 78% and 66% of men with a variety of cancers, excluding those with androgen-dependent cancer (prostate, breast) or testicular cancer, most of whom received chemotherapy or radiation therapy or both.[394,396] Low testosterone was associated with reduced quality of life and sexual function.[395]

Men with *rheumatic diseases*, in particular the systemic autoimmune disorder rheumatoid arthritis, may manifest symptoms of sexual dysfunction (reduced libido and erectile dysfunction) and low serum free or bioavailable testosterone and gonadotropin levels in approximately 30% of cases.[397] Secondary hypogonadism in rheumatoid arthritis may be due in part to systemic inflammation (with elevated cytokines such as IL-1 and TNF-α), complications such as rheumatoid lung, and treatment with glucocorticoids, but it may also occur early in the course of rheumatoid arthritis in the absence of complications and before glucocorticoid therapy.[398] In men with long-standing rheumatoid arthritis, low free testosterone levels do not normalize after marked suppression of inflammation induced by anti-TNF therapy.[399] Testosterone treatment may improve symptoms of androgen deficiency, but it does not reduce disease activity.[400]

Men with systemic lupus erythematosus also may demonstrate low free testosterone concentrations in conjunction with normal or low-normal gonadotropin levels, indicative of secondary hypogonadism, or elevated gonadotropins, consistent with primary hypogonadism.[401-403] Factors that contribute to gonadotropin suppression and secondary hypogonadism include chronic systemic illness and inflammation, major organ involvement or organ failure (heart, lung, brain, kidney), and glucocorticoid therapy. Factors that contribute to primary testicular dysfunction include systemic and local inflammation or vasculitis, organ failure, and treatment with cytotoxic agents such as cyclophosphamide.

It is also possible that the hypogonadism contributes to the immunologic pathophysiology of rheumatic disorders.[404,405] Autoimmune diseases, and in particular autoimmune rheumatic diseases (e.g., Sjögren syndrome, systemic lupus erythematosus, rheumatoid arthritis), thyroid disease (Hashimoto's disease, Graves' disease), and autoimmune neurologic diseases (e.g., myasthenia gravis, multiple sclerosis), occur more commonly in women than in men. Sex steroid hormones, primarily estrogens and androgens, modulate immune function by direct actions on immune cell function and may play a role in sex differences in autoimmunity and in the pathophysiology of autoimmune disorders.

Men with *HIV disease* commonly have hypogonadism characterized by symptomatic androgen deficiency and impaired sperm production with low free testosterone levels due to combined primary and secondary hypogonadism.[406,407] Hypogonadism occurred in up to 50% of men with HIV wasting before the advent of HAART. Although androgen deficiency is less common since the advent of HAART, it occurs in approximately 20% of HIV-infected men. In 75% to 90% of cases, low free testosterone is associated with low or low-normal gonadotropin levels, consistent with secondary hypogonadism.[408,409] In the remaining 10% to 25% of cases, gonadotropin concentrations are elevated, indicating primary hypogonadism.

As in other chronic systemic illnesses, the etiology of hypogonadism in men with HIV disease is multifactorial.[4,5] In addition to HIV infection itself, gonadotropin suppression and secondary hypogonadism may be caused by malnutrition, wasting, and cachexia; opportunistic infections resulting in hypothalamic-pituitary function (e.g., CMV, *T. gondii*); systemic inflammation (with elevated levels of cytokines such as IL-1 and TNF-α); medications (e.g., opiates, glucocorticoids, megestrol acetate); ongoing substance abuse (e.g., alcohol); and acute and chronic illnesses. Conditions that may play a role in causing primary hypogonadism include opportunistic infections affecting the testes (CMV, *M. avium intracellulare*, *T. gondii*), malignancies involving the testes (Kaposi's sarcoma, lymphoma), systemic inflammation, and medications (chemotherapy for secondary neoplasms, ketoconazole).[406,407]

Protein-calorie malnutrition may suppress SHBG concentrations, and advancing HIV infection is associated with increased SHBG levels. Therefore, accurate measurements of free testosterone levels should be used to evaluate men with HIV disease for androgen deficiency.[408,409] Sperm production associated with abnormalities in sperm motility and morphology and testicular atrophy may be present. It is important to recognize that HIV may be present in semen even when it is undetectable in plasma.[407]

In small clinical trials, treatment with testosterone and androgenic anabolic steroid has been demonstrated to improve libido and sexual function; increase muscle mass and strength and BMD; decrease fat mass; improve mood, well-being, and quality of life; and increase hematocrit in HIV-infected men with low serum testosterone levels.[110]

Men with chronic *spinal cord injury* at any level resulting in tetraplegia or paraplegia may have secondary hypogonadism with low serum testosterone and low or normal gonadotropin levels.[285,286] In men with lower spinal cord injury causing paraplegia, there may be a transient suppression of testosterone levels within 4 months after the injury that resolves in most cases.[410] Gonadotropin suppression is caused in part by a number of conditions associated with spinal cord injury, such as acute and chronic trauma and stress associated with the injury and attendant complications; obstructive sleep apnea; obesity or nutritional compromise; hyperprolactinemia (usually associated with medications); and medication use (e.g., glucocorticoids, opiates, CNS-active drugs). The benefits and risks of testosterone treatment in patients with spinal cord injury are not clear.

Thalassemia major, or β-thalassemia, is an autosomal recessive disorder characterized by absent or severely deficient synthesis of β-globulin chains of hemoglobin resulting in severe anemia that requires lifelong blood transfusions. It is common in the Mediterranean region, in India, and in Southeast Asia. Chronic blood transfusions in patients with β-thalassemia cause *transfusion-related iron overload* in tissues and produce clinical manifestations similar to those that occur in patients with hereditary hemochromatosis. Transfusion-related iron overload may also occur in patients with sickle cell anemia, refractory aplastic anemia, or myelodysplastic syndrome.

Iron deposition in the testes and pituitary gland usually causes combined primary and secondary hypogonadism.[411,412] However, males with transfusion-related iron overload usually exhibit a hormonal pattern indicative of secondary hypogonadism, with low serum free testosterone and low to low-normal gonadotropin concentrations in most cases. Hypogonadism due to transfusion-related iron overload may manifest with prepubertal or adult androgen deficiency and impaired sperm production; affected boys usually have short stature and growth delay.[413] Treatment requires iron chelation therapy with agents such as deferoxamine, deferasirox, or deferiprone. In men with long-standing β-thalassemia, chelation therapy does not reverse hypogonadism.[414]

Sickle cell disease may be associated with low serum testosterone and low to low-normal gonadotropin levels, indicative of secondary hypogonadism.[415-417] Gonadotropin suppression may be caused by transfusion-induced iron overload (although much less commonly than in men with β-thalassemia[418]); hypothalamic-pituitary microinfarctions; medications (e.g., opiates for chronic pain); systemic inflammation; nutritional deficiencies; and chronic systemic illness and stress secondary to repeated painful vaso-occlusive events. As discussed earlier, men with sickle cell disease may present with primary hypogonadism due to testicular microinfarctions caused by vaso-occlusive events or iron overload affecting the testes. Priapism, which may occur with vaso-occlusive events, has been reported in patients receiving testosterone therapy.[419]

Uncommonly, boys or men with *cystic fibrosis* have low serum testosterone and low to low-normal gonadotropin concentrations, a hormonal pattern consistent with secondary hypogonadism.[420] Chronic systemic illness and inflammation, malnutrition, and glucocorticoid use may contribute to gonadotropin suppression.

Nutritional Disorders or Endurance Exercise. Starvation, malnutrition, and eating disorders (anorexia nervosa) suppress gonadotropin and testosterone secretion, resulting in symptomatic secondary hypogonadism with androgen deficiency (usually manifested by reduced libido, sexual activity, and performance) and impaired sperm production; these effects are reversed with restoration of food/calorie intake and weight gain. Fasting for periods of 3 to 5 days suppresses gonadotropin and testosterone secretion and decreases LH pulse amplitude and frequency.[421-423] These changes are reversed completely by pulsatile GnRH administration or low-dose recombinant methionyl human leptin replacement, suggesting that short-term starvation suppresses leptin production, which in turn suppresses the hypothalamic GnRH pulse generator.[424,425] Severe protein-calorie malnutrition, often associated with other nutritional deficiencies, may cause severe suppression of testosterone and elevation of gonadotropin levels, indicative of primary hypogonadism.[422,426]

Chronic *endurance exercise* results in low serum testosterone, low to low-normal gonadotropin concentrations, and impaired sperm production and motility, consistent with secondary hypogonadism.[427,428] High-intensity endurance training, such as occurs in the military and with overtraining in athletes, is associated with relative calorie deprivation and intense stress and causes more severe suppression of gonadotropin and testosterone levels than is seen with chronic lower-intensity endurance exercise.[421,429] Suppression of the hypothalamic-pituitary-testicular axis resolves with cessation of training and increased calorie intake. Other than reduced spermatogenesis, the clinical consequences of androgen deficiency induced by endurance exercise are not clear.[430] In contrast to chronic endurance exercise, short-term endurance or resistance exercise in some men results in an acute and transient increase in testosterone levels that is modified by the intensity of exercise and prior training and is possibly related to hemoconcentration, reduced metabolic clearance, or increases in serum LH levels.[431]

Mild to moderate obesity results in reduced SHBG and total testosterone levels. Free testosterone is usually normal but may be reduced in association with low or low-normal gonadotropin levels in some men, particularly in those with comorbid conditions such as T2DM or obstructive sleep apnea.[432-434] In men with *morbid obesity,* particularly those with a body mass index (BMI) greater than 40 kg/m^2 or massive obesity (BMI >45 kg/m^2), serum free testosterone is low, gonadotropin levels are low or low-normal, and LH pulse amplitude (but not frequency) is reduced, indicative of secondary hypogonadism.[435] Morbidly and massively obese men often complain of reduced libido and sexual dysfunction, but these symptoms are confounded by obesity and comorbidities associated with morbid obesity, such as depression, diabetes, and obstructive sleep apnea. Bariatric surgery and rapid weight loss induced by a very low-calorie diet increase serum testosterone and gonadotropin concentrations.

Morbid obesity may be complicated by *obstructive sleep apnea* syndrome. Men with untreated or inadequately treated obstructive sleep apnea have low gonadotropin and testosterone concentrations independent of obesity and age.[433,436] Adequate treatment with continuous positive airway pressure (CPAP) may improve symptoms attributed to androgen deficiency and reverse biochemical secondary hypogonadism in some men, particularly those with massive obesity and comorbid conditions that cause hypogonadism independent of sleep apnea. Whereas obstructive sleep apnea may induce androgen deficiency, treatment of hypogonadism with relatively high doses of testosterone (e.g., doses associated with the use of parenteral testosterone esters) may induce or worsen obstructive sleep apnea in men with predisposing conditions such as obesity and in older men.[433,437,438]

Acute and Critical Illness. Acute and critical illnesses, including medical and surgical illnesses requiring hospital or intensive care unit admission (e.g., myocardial infarction, respiratory illness, sepsis, burns, surgery, polytrauma, stroke, traumatic brain injury, liver disease), suppress gonadotropin and testosterone secretion as a result of combined primary and secondary testicular dysfunction.[439,440] However, the predominant hormone pattern during acute or critical illness is low serum testosterone with low or low-normal gonadotropin levels, suggesting secondary hypogonadism. Spontaneous LH pulse amplitude is reduced, but pulse frequency is maintained, and pulsatile GnRH administration only partially corrects secondary hypogonadism, underscoring the presence of concomitant pituitary and testicular defects.[441] For unclear reasons, aromatization of testosterone to estradiol and serum levels of estradiol may be elevated, sometimes markedly, in patients with acute or critical illness despite low testosterone levels.[442] Estradiol levels are associated with mortality in critically ill and injured patients.[443]

The severity and duration of testosterone suppression are related to the severity of the acute or critical illness, the presence of underlying chronic systemic illnesses, and the medications used (e.g., glucocorticoids, opiates).[439,440] Recovery of testosterone and gonadotropin levels may take several weeks to months, depending on the severity and duration of the acute illness, duration of subacute recovery and rehabilitation, complications including malnutrition, medications, and underlying chronic systemic illnesses or organ failure. In the presence of underlying chronic disease or organ failure, hypogonadism may persist long after recovery from the acute illness. Evaluation for underlying hypogonadism should not be performed during acute or subacute illness. It should be delayed for several months, until recovery to the individual's baseline or near-baseline clinical condition has occurred.

Aging. As discussed earlier, aging is associated with a gradual and progressive decline in total and free testosterone levels; as a result, an increasing proportion of older men have low serum testosterone concentrations in the hypogonadal range.[268-270] The prevalence of clinical androgen deficiency is 6% to 9% and increases with age, reaching 18% to 23% among men in their 70s.[175,176] Serum gonadotropin levels increase with aging but do not usually rise above the normal range until very old age, usually beyond

70 years of age.[270] Therefore, the most common hormonal profile observed clinically in middle-aged to older men is low testosterone with normal LH and FSH levels, indicative of secondary hypogonadism. Pulsatile LH secretion is abnormal and is characterized by disorderly LH pulses of reduced amplitude; it is normalized by exogenous pulsatile GnRH administration, suggesting a defect in hypothalamic GnRH secretion.[272]

The presence of chronic systemic illness or organ failure, medications, or malnutrition or wasting syndromes may contribute to suppression of gonadotropin and testosterone production. Conversely, the age-related decline in testosterone may contribute to the susceptibility and severity of clinical hypogonadism that occurs in these conditions.[274]

Relatively small, short-term studies of testosterone treatment in heterogenous populations of older men have produced conflicting results, with most finding beneficial effects of testosterone treatment on body composition (increasing lean mass and decreasing fat mass) but less consistent effects on muscle strength and performance, BMD, sexual function, vitality, and cognitive function. Larger, long-term, randomized trials are needed to determine the balance of clinical benefits and risks (particularly, prostate cancer and cardiovascular risks) associated with testosterone treatment in elderly men. For now, testosterone treatment should be considered on an individual basis only for older men who have clinically significant symptoms and signs of androgen deficiency and unequivocally low serum testosterone levels and only after a careful discussion of the uncertainty regarding the benefits and risks of treatment.[110]

Isolated Impairment of Sperm Production or Function

Congenital or Developmental Disorders

Congenital Adrenal Hyperplasia. If untreated or inadequately treated with glucocorticoids, congenital adrenal hyperplasia caused by deficiency of 21-hydroxlase or 11β-hydroxylase results in excessive secretion of adrenal androgens (androstenedione and DHEA) that are converted to testosterone. Elevated circulating androgen concentrations suppress gonadotropin secretion by negative feedback regulation, which in turn decreases endogenous testosterone secretion and sperm production, resulting in secondary hypogonadism. Excessive androgen production prevents androgen deficiency, so secondary hypogonadism is manifested by isolated impairment of sperm production and function.[444]

Adequate glucocorticoid therapy reduces excessive adrenal androgen production and usually restores gonadotropin secretion and normalizes testis function, including spermatogenesis. However, despite adequate treatment, some men with congenital adrenal hyperplasia continue to manifest impaired sperm production and function, most commonly as a result of long-standing inadequate glucocorticoid treatment and irreversible testicular damage caused by large adrenal rest tumors or excessive glucocorticoid treatment. As discussed previously, excessive glucocorticoid treatment of congenital adrenal insufficiency also suppresses gonadotropin secretion and results in androgen deficiency and impairment in sperm production.

Isolated Follicle-Stimulating Hormone Deficiency and FSHB Mutations. Rare cases of men with isolated FSH deficiency in the absence of *FSHB* gene mutations have been reported; these patients had isolated impairment in sperm production characterized by azoospermia or severe oligozoospermia, and hypospermatogenesis or maturation arrest was found in the few who underwent testis biopsy.[323-325] These men had normal virilization, normal levels of testosterone and LH, low to undetectable serum FSH levels with poor or no response to GnRH administration, normal LH, and normal inhibin B and activin A levels when tested. In one man, administration of recombinant human FSH (rhFSH) alone resulted in a robust increase in sperm counts and induced fertility on two occasions.

Men with inactivating mutations of *FSHB* have been found generally to have azoospermia with undetectable FSH, low or low-normal testosterone, and high LH levels.[82-85] In one man, rhFSH administration was demonstrated to increase testosterone levels, suggesting that FSH-stimulated Sertoli cells may enhance LH-induced Leydig cell production of testosterone via a paracrine mechanism.[445]

Acquired Disorders

Androgen Administration or Excess. Exogenous testosterone administration (in normal men or in men with partial hypogonadism)[446] or stimulation of endogenous testosterone production by hCG administration[447] or ectopic hCG-secreting tumors (e.g., testis cancer, lung cancer)[448] suppresses pituitary gonadotropin secretion by negative feedback regulation; this in turn suppresses spermatogenesis by the testes in the presence of normal or high testosterone levels (i.e., secondary hypogonadism with isolated impairment of sperm production).[449,450] Use of some androgenic anabolic steroids (e.g., nandrolone) may also produce low gonadotropin levels and isolated reduction in spermatogenesis while providing sufficient androgen activity to avoid clinical androgen deficiency.

Discontinuation of androgen or hCG administration results in restoration of normal gonadotropin secretion and recovery of normal sperm production and testosterone production by the testis. Long-term anabolic steroid abuse in athletes has been reported to be associated with testicular atrophy and severe oligozoospermia or azoospermia that persists for several months to years after discontinuation of the performance-enhancing agents. Suppressed sperm production induced by anabolic steroids may respond to treatment with hCG or with clomiphene citrate (off-label use).[361,451] Administration of testosterone in combination with progestins in normal men has been the main strategy used to suppress sperm production in recent male contraceptive development trials.[90]

Malignancy. Malignancies that occur commonly in men of reproductive age (e.g., testicular cancer, Hodgkin's disease) manifest with impaired sperm production and function before chemotherapy or radiation therapy in 30% to 80% of cases.[278-280] Among men with cancer who provided semen samples for cryopreservation before treatment, approximately 64% had abnormal semen parameters and 12% had no viable sperm.[452]

In population studies, testicular cancer is associated with infertility. This association may reflect abnormal testicular development, termed *testicular dysgenesis syndrome*, caused by exposure to environmental gonadotoxins or endocrine disruptors (e.g., estrogens) or by an underlying genetic predisposition.[278,453] Testicular dysgenesis syndrome is also associated with cryptorchidism and hypospadias, and the former is associated with an increased risk of testicular cancer and abnormal spermatogenesis. Ectopic hCG secretion and possibly increased scrotal temperature associated with cancer within the testis may also contribute to impaired spermatogenesis in men with testicular cancer.[453] Hodgkin's disease and other lymphomas and leukemias may be associated with fever, weight loss, and systemic inflammation.[453] These cancers may also involve the testis. All of these factors may play a role in impairing sperm production. Men with these cancers who have systemic disease, symptoms, or inflammation may present with low-normal testosterone, suppressed gonadotropin levels, and abnormal semen analysis, consistent with secondary hypogonadism causing isolated impairment of sperm production or function.

Hyperprolactinemia. As discussed previously, men with severe hyperprolactinemia (e.g., prolactin levels >200 ng/mL) develop secondary hypogonadism causing androgen deficiency and impaired sperm production. Mild hyperprolactinemia may be associated with isolated impairment of sperm production.[454] In most of these cases, gonadotropin and testosterone levels are normal and spermatogenesis is not improved with dopamine agonist treatment.[455] Therefore, hyperprolactinemia does not contribute to impairment in sperm production and probably is not clinically significant in most cases. In most instances, abnormal sperm production and function are caused by a primary testicular disorder, such as idiopathic oligozoospermia or azoospermia. Rarely, some men with moderate hyperprolactinemia (e.g., prolactin levels 100 to 200 ng/mL) have low-normal testosterone and gonadotropin levels and isolated impairment of sperm production that responds to dopamine agonist treatment.[454]

Androgen Resistance Syndromes

Congenital Disorders

Congenital androgen resistance and insensitivity syndromes are usually caused by defects in androgen action due to mutations in the *AR* gene or in the steroid 5α-reductase type 2 gene, *SRD5A2*.[116,127,456,457] Males with severe defects in androgen action present at birth either as phenotypic females, as occurs with *complete androgen insensitivity syndrome* (CAIS, previously known as testicular feminization syndrome), or as males with ambiguous genitalia and *46,XY DSDs* (previously termed male pseudohermaphroditism).[457] Individuals with *partial androgen insensitivity syndrome (PAIS)* present with varying degrees of prepubertal or adult androgen deficiency and mildly to severely disordered male sexual development.

Males with CAIS usually present as females with normal breast development, primary amenorrhea, and absence of body hair.[457] Severe androgen insensitivity results in absence of male facial, axillary, and pubic hair; normal-appearing female external genitalia and distal two thirds of the vagina; and poorly developed or absent male internal genitalia (prostate, epididymides, seminal vesicles, and vasa deferentia) as a result of fetal androgen insensitivity. In adults with CAIS, female breast development is present due to conversion of normal to high concentrations of testosterone (which are secreted by the testes at puberty) to estradiol, which stimulates breast development. Because testes that are intra-abdominal or inguinal in location secrete AMH during fetal development, female internal genitalia (proximal vagina, uterus, and fallopian tubes) are absent.

There is considerable variation in the presentation of individuals with PAIS.[457] Some of these males present at birth with ambiguous genitalia, whereas others present at puberty or in adulthood with mild genital abnormalities or relatively normal genital development. Clinical manifestations of androgen deficiency and disordered male sexual development range from severe undervirilization to near-normal virilization with infertility. In men with PAIS, manifestations that are indicative of disordered sexual development, such as microphallus, hypospadias, scrotal abnormalities (e.g., bifid scrotum), cryptorchidism, and gynecomastia, are common. Gynecomastia is present in almost all of these individuals.

As a result of the variability in clinical manifestations, PAIS encompasses a number of disorders previously referred to as Reifenstein, Lubs, Rosewater, and Gilbert-Dreyfus syndromes. For example, Reifenstein syndrome is characterized by hypospadias, gynecomastia, undervirilization, a small prostate gland, cryptorchidism, and impaired spermatogenesis. However, even in the same family, different members may have different clinical manifestations. Some family members may not have hypospadias, and others may be normally virilized. Given this degree of variability in manifestations, the older eponyms are not clinically useful.[457]

Some men with PAIS have no evidence of disordered male sexual development and present with isolated impairment of sperm (idiopathic oligozoospermia or azoospermia), occasionally in association with gynecomastia, high to high-normal testosterone levels, and elevated LH levels. This disorder is referred to as *minimal AIS*.[127,456]

In both CAIS and PAIS, serum testosterone levels are high or high-normal and LH concentrations are elevated, but FSH levels are usually normal. Most men with CAIS or PAIS have autosomal recessive mutations of the *AR* gene on the X chromosome that alter its primary sequence and structure (almost always resulting in CAIS) or its function, resulting in impaired androgen binding to AR, AR binding to DNA, or AR transactivation.[127,456] In men with androgen insensitivity syndromes, the correlation of *AR* genotype and clinical phenotype is relatively poor. In some men with PAIS or minimal AIS, no mutations in *AR* are identifiable and are possibly due to high CAG repeat length in the *AR* gene, mutations of *SRD5A2*, or mutations of coactivators or corepressors that regulate AR function.

An increase in the number of trinucleotide CAG repeats in the first exon of the *AR* gene results in expansion of the polyglutamine tract in the NTD of the AR.[130] The CAG repeat length is inversely correlated with AR function and action. Pathologic increase to more than 40 to 62 CAG repeats (normal range, 11 to 35) causes Kennedy's disease (SBMA), a rare neurodegenerative disease that is thought to be caused by neurotoxicity from intracellular aggregation of the abnormal AR and associated coregulator proteins (see earlier discussion).[128,129] Men with Kennedy's disease have clinical manifestations of partial androgen resistance, including gynecomastia, sexual dysfunction, oligozoospermia or azoospermia, and infertility, associated with high testosterone and high or normal gonadotropin levels. Higher CAG repeat numbers within the normal range have been reported to be associated with decreased virilization, impaired spermatogenesis and infertility, and gynecomastia in some studies but not in others.[130]

5α-Reductase deficiency, caused by an autosomal recessive mutation in *SRD5A2*, is a rare cause of PAIS.[116] Affected individuals typically present with markedly ambiguous genitalia, usually characterized by a clitoris-like phallus, a severely bifid scrotum, an apparent vaginal opening with perineal and scrotal hypospadias (termed *pseudovaginal perineoscrotal hypospadias*), an atrophic prostate, and testes located in the inguinal canal or scrotum or sometimes intra-abdominally (cryptorchidism). In contrast to men with androgen insensitivity syndromes, wolffian duct differentiation is unaffected, and patients with 5α-reductase deficiency have normal epididymides, seminal vesicles, ejaculatory ducts, and vasa deferentia. AMH secretion by the fetal testes causes regression of müllerian duct structures, so no female internal genitalia develop.

Because ambiguous genitalia resemble female more than male external genitalia, individuals with 5α-reductase deficiency are usually raised as females.[116] However, with the marked increase in testosterone production by the testes at puberty, partial virilization occurs (i.e., penile growth, rugation and pigmentation of the scrotum, increased muscle mass and height, deepening of the voice, increase in libido, and spontaneous erections), and some of these individuals take on a male gender role at puberty, depending on complex psychosocial factors and cultural background. Sebum production is normal in these men. Because normal androgen action in the skin and prostate requires conversion of testosterone to DHT by 5α-reductase, men with 5α-reductase deficiency do not develop a male body hair pattern, and the prostate gland remains nonpalpable. Prostate cancer and BPH have not been reported in these men.

Men with 5α-reductase deficiency have high-normal to high serum testosterone, elevated LH, and normal to elevated FSH levels. Serum DHT levels are low. Spermatogenesis is impaired (oligozoospermia or azoospermia) as a result of cryptorchidism, but normal sperm production has been reported in some men with descended testes.

Individuals with CAIS are usually raised as females and undergo orchidectomy (particularly if cryptorchidism is present) and treatment with estrogen replacement.[457] In men with PAIS or 5α-reductase deficiency, virilization has been induced with high-dose testosterone treatment, which increases serum testosterone concentrations to above the normal range and normalizes DHT levels.[457]

Acquired Disorders

AR antagonists (flutamide, bicalutamide or nilutamide) induce androgen resistance and are used to treat androgen-dependent prostate cancer.[458] Drugs such as spironolactone, cyproterone acetate, marijuana, and H_2 receptor antagonists (specifically cimetidine) have AR antagonist activity.[459-463]

Men with *celiac disease* or gluten-sensitive enteropathy may experience manifestations of androgen deficiency, including reduced virilization, sexual dysfunction, impaired sperm production and function, and infertility. They may also demonstrate high to high-normal levels of serum total and free testosterone and high LH levels, indicative of androgen resistance.[464-466] Manifestations of androgen deficiency and biochemical androgen resistance may improve with dietary gluten restriction and improvement in small bowel atrophy in some men.[466] Malnutrition, nutritional deficiencies, chronic systemic illness, and hyperprolactinemia may occur in men with celiac disease and may contribute to their clinical manifestations. Serum DHT concentrations may be low despite high testosterone levels in men with celiac disease, suggesting that partial 5α-reductase deficiency may also be present and may play a role in androgen resistance. The main source of circulating DHT is from conversion of testosterone to DHT by 5α-reductase type 1 in skin.[465] However, 5α-reductase is also present in the gut, so it is possible that loss of enzyme activity in the small bowel with active celiac sprue contributes to low DHT levels.

Treatment of Androgen Deficiency

Treatment of Reversible Causes

As detailed earlier, it is important before starting testosterone treatment of androgen deficiency to consider whether a low serum testosterone level might represent transient suppression caused by a critical, acute, or subacute illness or recovery from an acute illness; short-term use of certain medications; transient malnutrition (e.g., associated with illness); or excessive and chronic strenuous endurance exercise. In these clinical situations, serum testosterone measurements and therapy should be delayed until the patient has recovered completely from illness, offending drugs have been discontinued, malnutrition has been corrected, or excessive exercise has been stopped.[110]

Testosterone Replacement Therapy

Therapeutic Goals and Management. The overall goal of testosterone replacement therapy is to correct or improve the clinical manifestations of androgen deficiency in men with primary or secondary hypogonadism. Because specific manifestations vary with the stage of sexual development, the specific goals of testosterone treatment vary depending on whether the patient is a prepubertal boy or an adult.[6,110]

In boys with prepubertal androgen deficiency and delayed puberty, the goals of testosterone treatment are the following[136,303,304]:

- To induce and maintain secondary sexual characteristics, including growth of the penis and scrotum, and a male body hair pattern
- To increase muscle mass and strength
- To stimulate BMD, acquisition of peak bone mass, and long bone growth without compromising adult height by inducing premature closure of epiphyses
- To stimulate libido and spontaneous erections
- To improve energy, mood, and motivation
- To induce laryngeal enlargement and deepening of the voice
- To increase red blood cell production into the normal adult male range

Testosterone treatment also stimulates the growth of accessory sex glands (seminal vesicles and prostate), resulting in seminal fluid production and an increase in ejaculate volume, but it does not stimulate sperm production to a degree sufficient for induction of fertility. The most common cause of delayed puberty is not a pathologic condition but rather CDGP. Testosterone therapy in boys who present with delayed puberty is usually of low dosage to avoid premature epiphyseal closure and compromise of adult height, and it is given intermittently until spontaneous puberty occurs (see later discussion). If spontaneous puberty does not occur, the testosterone dose is increased gradually to adult levels.[136,303,304]

The goals of testosterone therapy in adults with hypogonadism are the following[6,110]:

- To improve sexual function and activity by restoring libido and improving erectile function
- To increase muscle mass and strength, potentially improving physical function and performance
- To increase BMD, potentially reducing the risk of fractures
- To improve energy, vitality, mood, and motivation
- To increase hematocrit into the normal adult male range
- To restore male hair growth

Recent-onset gynecomastia that is usually symptomatic may respond to testosterone treatment, but severe or long-standing gynecomastia requires surgical excision. Spermatogenesis requires relatively high intratesticular concentrations of testosterone that cannot be achieved by exogenous androgen administration. Therefore, testosterone replacement therapy does not stimulate sperm production or testis size, nor does it restore fertility. Treatment of infertility in hypogonadal men is usually possible only in those men with secondary hypogonadism and gonadotropin deficiency; gonadotropin or GnRH therapy is used.[467]

The normal adult range of serum testosterone levels is broad and is usually based on results in healthy young men using blood samples drawn in the morning. In young men with androgen deficiency, testosterone replacement therapy produces beneficial clinical effects as serum testosterone concentrations are increased into this normal range. Serum testosterone levels decline gradually and progressively with age, but the physiologic significance of this age-related decline is unclear. Initial studies in older men with low serum testosterone levels demonstrated some clinical beneficial effects with testosterone treatment that increased testosterone levels into the normal young adult range. Therefore, the goal of testosterone treatment of hypogonadism is to restore serum testosterone concentrations to within the normal adult range, irrespective of age.[110]

The dose-response effects of testosterone vary in different target organs and for different clinical outcomes.[468] For example, the action of testosterone on muscle mass demonstrates a continuous dose-response relationship. With testosterone administration, muscle mass increases when testosterone levels are increased from below normal to within the normal range, and it continues to increase as levels are raised from within to above the normal range. In contrast, the actions of testosterone on libido exhibit threshold dose-response characteristics: testosterone administration increases libido when serum testosterone concentrations are increased from low to low-normal levels but does not continue to stimulate libido further as serum testosterone is increased to normal or supraphysiologic levels.

In men with severe, long-standing androgen deficiency, testosterone replacement therapy induces profound alterations in sexuality, behavior, and physical appearance that may be upsetting to patients and their partners and may result in serious adjustment problems. To reduce the likelihood of problems, it is important to inform and counsel hypogonadal men and their partners regarding changes in body characteristics and behavior that are expected during testosterone replacement therapy. In some men with severe, long-standing hypogonadism, initiation of testosterone replacement with a low-dose regimen (e.g., testosterone enanthate or cypionate 100 mg every 2 weeks, testosterone patch 2.5 mg daily, testosterone gel 2.5 g daily) for several months, followed by an increase to full testosterone replacement, may produce a more gradual symptomatic transition from hypogonadism to eugonadism and may result in fewer adjustment difficulties.[523]

Because the metabolic clearance rate of testosterone is reduced in older men with hypogonadism, therapeutic testosterone levels may be achieved with lower doses of testosterone.[469] In some clinical situations, such as severe symptomatic BPH or the presence of a number of comorbid illnesses, full testosterone replacement may be ill advised. In these instances, low-dose testosterone supplementation (e.g., testosterone enanthate or cypionate 50 mg to 100 mg IM every 2 weeks, testosterone patch 2.5 mg daily, testosterone gel 2.5 g daily) may be more prudent than full testosterone replacement therapy. Low doses of testosterone may be sufficient to induce some beneficial effects while minimizing potential adverse stimulatory effects on prostate growth.

The potential effectiveness of low-dose testosterone supplementation is suggested by studies of short-acting testosterone formulations (testosterone undecanoate and cyclodextrin) that produced anabolic effects despite serum testosterone concentrations that were not sustained within the normal range.[470,471] An analogy may be made to the use of hydrocortisone for glucocorticoid replacement therapy, in which the duration of biologic action of hydrocortisone on tissues is not reflected by its serum concentrations. Short-term administration of low-dose testosterone enanthate (50 mg/week IM) was found to increase muscle strength and power in some young men in whom hypogonadism was induced by concomitant GnRH agonist treatment.[472]

Hypogonadism due to gonadotropin deficiency may be caused by hypothalamic-pituitary disease that requires specific management in addition to testosterone replacement. Therefore, careful evaluation to determine the cause of secondary hypogonadism should be performed before testosterone treatment is started. For example, pituitary or hypothalamic tumors may cause mass effects such as visual field defects, or they may be associated with deficiency or excessive secretion of other pituitary hormones. These tumors may require surgery or radiation therapy, additional hormonal replacement, medical therapy, or some combination of these treatments to reduce excessive pituitary hormone secretion. In some cases, treatment of the underlying cause of secondary hypogonadism corrects the androgen deficiency (e.g., stopping a medication that causes hyperprolactinemia or gonadotropin deficiency). In men with gonadotropin deficiency and normal testes who are interested in fathering children, gonadotropin therapy may be used instead of testosterone replacement to stimulate sperm production, restore fertility, and correct androgen deficiency. Similarly, men with secondary hypogonadism due to hypothalamic disease may be treated with pulsatile GnRH to stimulate testosterone and sperm production and restore fertility.

A comprehensive clinical approach is important for optimal management of hypogonadism. It is important to consider etiologies other than androgen deficiency that might contribute to clinical manifestations and to manage them appropriately. In hypogonadal men who complain primarily of sexual dysfunction, an underlying neurovascular disease or use of certain medications is usually the major cause of erectile dysfunction. In these men, testosterone treatment alone is insufficient to completely restore erections and permit satisfactory sexual intercourse. Additional treatment with a type 5 phosphodiesterase inhibitor (sildenafil, vardenafil, or tadalafil), intracavernosal or intraurethral PE_1 (alprostadil [Muse]), or a penile vacuum device may be needed for a satisfactory clinical outcome. In hypogonadal men who present with osteoporosis, it is critical to perform a thorough evaluation for other common causes of bone loss (e.g., vitamin D deficiency, alcohol abuse, smoking, medications, inactivity, primary hyperparathyroidism) and to treat them as well. It is also important to institute measures to prevent falls to reduce the risk of fractures.

Testosterone Formulations. Testosterone formulations that are used to treat male hypogonadism are summarized in Table 19-10.[6,110] In the United States, these include parenteral testosterone esters that are administered by IM injection, a transdermal testosterone patch and testosterone gels, and a transbuccal testosterone tablet.

Oral 17α-alkylated testosterone derivatives, such as methyltestosterone and fluoxymesterone, should not be used for testosterone replacement therapy.[6] It is difficult to achieve full androgen replacement with these oral formulations because they are weak androgens that have low bioavailability. They also have the potential for serious

TABLE 19-10

Treatment of Adult Male Hypogonadism

Formulation	Dosage	Advantages	Disadvantages
TREATMENT OF ANDROGEN DEFICIENCY			
Formulations Available in the United States			
Parenteral Testosterone Esters			
Testosterone enanthate or cypionate, IM injections	*Adults:* 150-200 mg IM every 2 wk or 75-100 mg IM every wk. *Prepubertal boys:* 50-100 mg monthly or 25-50 mg every 2 wk, increasing to 50-100 mg every 2 wk and then to adult replacement dosage over 2-4 yr OR until spontaneous pubertal development occurs	Extensive clinical use Inexpensive with self-injection Some dose flexibility	IM injections, discomfort Symptomatic fluctuation of T levels (supraphysiologic after injection to low-normal or low before next injection) Frequent IM injections to reduce fluctuations of T levels More erythrocytosis than with transdermal T
Transdermal Testosterone			
Testosterone patch (nonscrotal)	2.5 or 5 mg (one patch) or 7.5 mg or 10 mg (one 2.5-mg plus 5.0-mg patch or two 5-mg patches) applied daily over non-pressure areas	Low- to mid-normal physiologic T levels Mimics normal circadian variation when applied nightly No injections Less erythrocytosis than with parenteral T Rapid withdrawal of T replacement if adverse effects occur	Frequent skin irritation Low-normal T levels: Two patches may be needed Skin adhesion poor with excessive sweating Daily application More expensive than parenteral T
Testosterone gels (1%)	5-10 g of gel (delivering 5-10 mg of T) applied daily over shoulders or trunk Available in foil sachets of 2.5 or 5.0 g, tubes of 5 or 10 g, and metered-dose pumps delivering 1.25 g per pump depression	Low- to high-normal steady-state physiologic T levels No injections Little skin irritation Dose flexibility Rapid withdrawal of T replacement if adverse effects occur	Potential for contact transfer of T to women or children Daily application More expensive than parenteral T, especially with higher doses Moderately high DHT levels One formulation has a musk odor and another is associated with stickiness or skin dryness Slight skin irritation in some men
Transbuccal testosterone	30 mg tablet applied between cheek and gum bid	Mid-normal steady-state physiologic T levels No injections, patch or gel application, or their associated disadvantages Rapid withdrawal of T replacement if adverse effects occur	Twice-daily application Gum irritation or inflammation Altered or bitter taste High learning curve; requires careful instruction or poor acceptability occurs Tablets may be difficult to remove or may fall off prematurely No dose flexibility Moderately high DHT levels More expensive than parenteral T
Testosterone pellets	2-6 pellets (each 8-9 mm containing 75 mg of T) implanted SQ every 3-6 mo	Maintenance of normal T levels for a longer duration	Requires surgical incision Extrusion, bleeding, and infection can occur uncommonly Large number of pellets Not easily removed; fibrosis may occur Lack of ability for rapid withdrawal of T replacement if adverse effects occur Infrequent use
Testosterone Formulations Available Outside the United States			
Oral testosterone undecanoate	40-80 mg PO with meals bid to tid	Oral administration is convenient for many	Twice- or thrice-daily administration Variable T levels and clinical responses Requires administration with meal High DHT levels
Parenteral testosterone undecanoate	1000 mg IM initially and at 6 wk, then 1000 mg IM every 10-14 wk	Less frequent IM injections Maintenance of normal T levels for a longer duration No apparent fluctuations in T levels or symptoms	IM injections, discomfort Large-volume injection (4 mL) Self-injection not possible Rarely, cough immediately after injection Prolonged maintenance of T level after discontinuation for adverse effects
Testosterone-in-adhesive matrix patch	Two patches (delivering 4.8 mg of T per day) applied every 2 days	Low- to mid-normal physiologic T levels Duration 2 days No injections	Some skin irritation Two patches needed

Table continued on following page

TABLE 19-10

Treatment of Adult Male Hypogonadism (Continued)

Formulation	Dosage	Advantages	Disadvantages
Testosterone gel 2%	3-4 g (60-80 mg of T) applied to abdomen or both inner thighs daily	Low-normal to high-normal steady-state physiologic T levels No injections Little skin irritation Dose flexibility Rapid withdrawal of T replacement if adverse effects occur	Potential for contact transfer of T to women or children Daily application
TREATMENT TO INITIATE AND MAINTAIN SPERM PRODUCTION IN MEN WITH HYPOGONADOTROPIC HYPOGONADISM			
Initially to Stimulate Testosterone and Potentially Sperm Production			
Human chorionic gonadotropin (hCG)	500-2000 IU given SQ 2-3 times weekly to maintain serum T levels within the normal range for 6-12 mo	Effective in stimulating endogenous T production In men with acquired and some men with partial congenital hypogonadotropic hypogonadism, sperm production may be stimulated with hCG treatment alone SQ injections easier than IM injections (smaller needle, injection not as deep) Less fluctuation in T levels compared with IM T ester injections No injection, patch, or buccal tablet	Injections 2-3 times weekly Expensive Higher doses needed in men with concomitant primary testicular disease (e.g., cryptorchidism) Breast tenderness or gynecomastia secondary to high estradiol production by testes May require dilution Occasional burning sensation with injection Ineffective in primary hypogonadism
Added to hCG to Stimulate Sperm Production			
FSH Human menopausal gonadotropin (hMG), human FSH (hFSH), or recombinant human FSH (rhFSH)	After 6-12 mo of hCG treatment alone resulting in normal T levels, add FSH 75-300 IU is given SQ three times weekly for an additional 6-12 mo or longer	Effective in stimulating sperm production in men with hypogonadotropic hypogonadism	Injections 3 times weekly Extremely expensive, prohibitive cost for most Breast tenderness or gynecomastia secondary to high estradiol production by testes May require dilution Occasional burning sensation with injection In men with concomitant primary testicular disease (e.g., cryptorchidism), stimulation of spermatogenesis is not likely
To Stimulate Testosterone and Sperm Production			
Gonadotropin-releasing hormone (GnRH)	5-25 ng/kg SC every 2 hr by programmable infusion pump for 6-12 mo	Effective in stimulating both endogenous T and sperm production	GnRH not readily available Requires pump use and management, usually in a specialized center Expensive Infrequently used except at certain sites Rarely, local irritation, infection

DHT, dihydrotestosterone; FSH, follicle-stimulating hormone; IM, intramuscular; SQ, subcutaneous; T, testosterone.

hepatotoxicity.[360] 17α-Alkylated androgens most commonly cause cholestasis that is reversible with discontinuation. More concerning is the potential for these agents to cause peliosis hepatis (blood-filled cysts in the liver) or benign or malignant hepatic tumors. 17α-Alkylated androgens also lower HDL- and raise LDL-cholesterol, causing a pro-atherogenic lipid profile, and they are relatively expensive. Therefore, these oral androgens carry greater potential risks with few therapeutic benefits compared with other testosterone formulations, and they should not be used to treat male hypogonadism.

Parenteral Testosterone Esters. Relatively long-acting parenteral 17β-hydroxyl esters of testosterone, *testosterone enanthate* and *testosterone cypionate*, are administered by IM injection. These are effective, safe, and relatively practical and inexpensive preparations that have been used for testosterone replacement in hypogonadal men for decades. Transdermal testosterone gel formulations provide more physiologic testosterone levels and are now used more commonly than testosterone ester injections. However, testosterone esters are preferred over transdermal formulations by some hypogonadal men because they are the least expensive formulation available, require less frequent administration, and usually produce higher average serum testosterone concentrations. Given proper instruction, most hypogonadal men (or a family member) are able to self-administer IM testosterone ester injections. Otherwise, testosterone injections need to be administered in a clinic setting.

Esterification of testosterone at the 17β-hydroxyl group increases its hydrophobicity and solubility within an oil vehicle (sesame oil for testosterone enanthate, cottonseed oil for testosterone cypionate). After IM injection, testosterone esters are released slowly from the oil vehicle within muscle and hydrolyzed rapidly to testosterone, which is released into circulation, resulting in relatively high peak serum testosterone concentrations but an extended duration of release. Testosterone enanthate and testosterone cypionate have similar pharmacokinetic profiles, duration of action, and therapeutic efficacy, so they are considered clinically equivalent.[473,474]

In adults with hypogonadism, the usual starting dose of testosterone enanthate or cypionate is 150 mg to 200 mg IM every 2 weeks. After IM administration of 200 mg of testosterone enanthate, serum testosterone levels usually rise above the normal range for 1 to 3 days and then decline gradually over 2 weeks to the lower end of the normal range, or sometimes to below-normal levels, before the next injection (Fig. 19-29).[475,476] The extreme rise and fall of serum testosterone concentrations may cause fluctuations in energy, mood, and libido that are disturbing to some men. Shortening the dosing interval to every 10 days and reducing the dose to 150 mg (i.e.,150 mg IM every 10 days) may alleviate symptoms associated with nadir testosterone levels occurring before the next injection. Alternatively, some patients prefer changing the dose of testosterone enanthate or cypionate to 75 to 100 mg IM every week to reduce swings in testosterone concentrations and associated symptoms. Administration of testosterone enanthate at doses of 300 mg IM every 3 weeks or 400 mg IM every 4 weeks produces extremely wide fluctuations in serum testosterone concentrations with markedly supraphysiologic levels for several days after an injection and levels below normal 3 weeks after an injection (see Fig. 19-29).[475,476]

Because CDGP in which puberty eventually occurs spontaneously is clinically indistinguishable from delayed puberty caused by permanent hypogonadotropic hypogonadism (e.g., IHH),[136,303,304] testosterone treatment usually

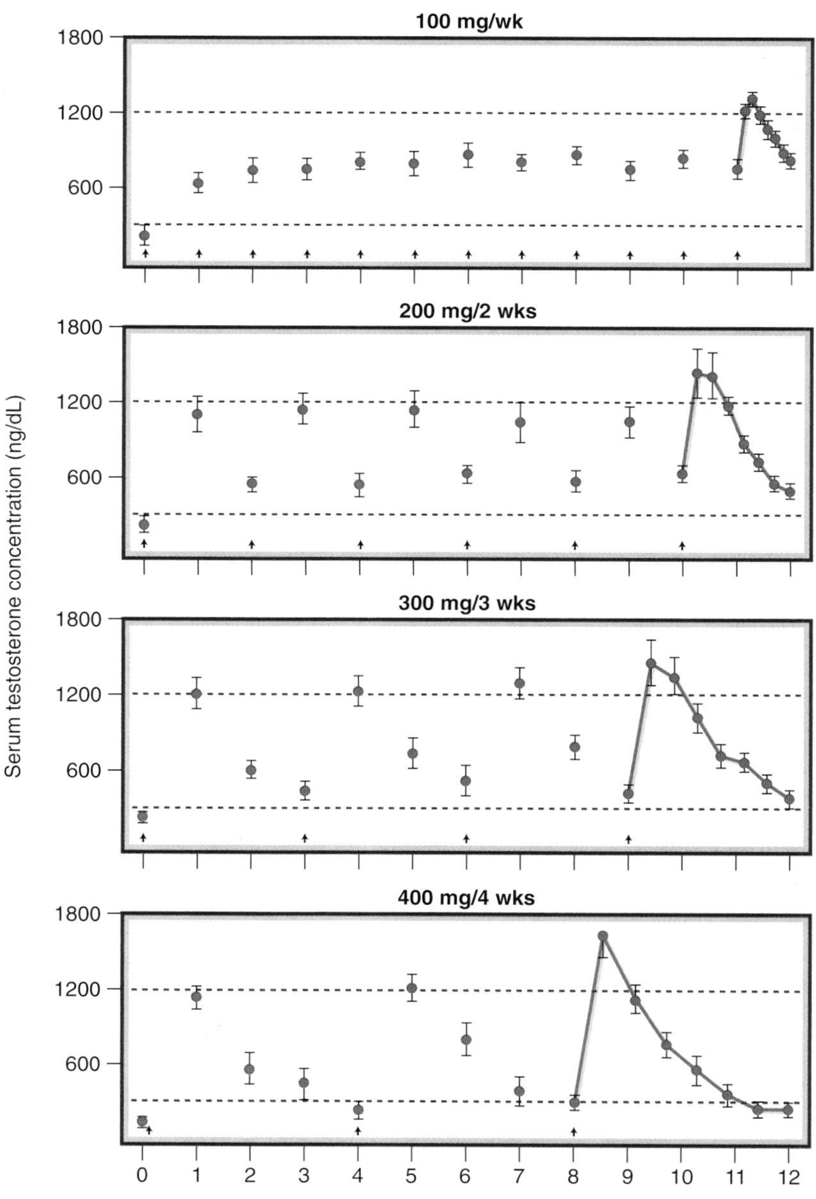

Figure 19-29 Serum total testosterone concentrations in men with primary hypogonadism treated with intramuscular injections of testosterone enanthate for 12 weeks at a dose of 100 mg weekly, 200 mg every 2 weeks, 300 mg every 3 weeks, or 400 mg every 4 weeks. Blood was sampled weekly until the last injection, after which it was sampled more frequently, demonstrating that the optimal dosage to maintain serum testosterone levels within the normal range *(dashed lines)* is every 200 mg every 2 weeks or 100 mg every week. (From Snyder PJ, Lawrence DA. Treatment of male hypogonadism with testosterone enanthate. *J Clin Endocrinol Metab.* 1980;51:1335-1339.)

is not initiated in boys with prepubertal androgen deficiency until they are about 14 years of age (with a bone age of at least 10.5 years). Testosterone therapy is administered intermittently to allow determination of spontaneous puberty, if it occurs. Occasionally, testosterone therapy is started at a younger age if delayed genital development and growth is causing severe psychological distress in affected boys and their families.

In boys with prepubertal androgen deficiency, treatment is initiated with a very low dose of testosterone enanthate or cypionate (e.g., 50 to 100 mg IM monthly or 25 to 50 mg every 2 weeks) to prevent premature closure of long bone epiphyses that would compromise adult height.[136,303,304] These low doses of testosterone are sufficient to induce some virilization and long bone growth without interfering with the spontaneous puberty that occurs eventually in boys with CDGP. Testosterone treatment is continued for 3 to 6 months and then stopped for 3 to 6 months to assess whether spontaneous pubertal onset occurs. If there is indication that spontaneous puberty is occurring (e.g., testes size is >8 mL), testosterone therapy is discontinued. If there is no evidence of spontaneous puberty, intermittent testosterone treatment is continued. The dose of testosterone enanthate or cypionate is increased gradually to 50 to 100 mg IM every 2 weeks and then to full adult replacement doses over the next several years to mimic the gradual increase in testosterone concentrations that occurs during puberty.

At present, transdermal testosterone formulations are not approved for use in boys with delayed puberty. However, because they circumvent the need for IM injections, low-dose transdermal testosterone patches and gels would provide very useful alternatives for the treatment of prepubertal androgen deficiency in boys, and they are currently being tested for this indication.

Transdermal Testosterone. Transdermal testosterone formulations available for testosterone replacement therapy for male hypogonadism include an adhesive testosterone patch and two 1% testosterone gels (see Table 19-10). Transdermal delivery of testosterone is used in hypogonadal men who prefer this method or are unable to tolerate or self-administer IM injections of testosterone ester. Testosterone gel is the most frequently used formulation for treatment of male hypogonadism in the United States.

In contrast to testosterone ester injections, which produce transient supraphysiologic testosterone levels, patch and gel formulations produce a more physiologic range of testosterone concentrations; use of the patch results in a normal circadian variation, and the gel formulations produce steady-state serum testosterone levels.

Testosterone stimulates red blood cell production, and testosterone replacement therapy may result in excessive erythrocytosis. In men with hypogonadism, excessive erythrocytosis occurs less commonly with testosterone patch therapy than with testosterone enanthate injections, suggesting that physiologic testosterone levels produced by transdermal testosterone therapy may be associated with fewer androgenic adverse effects.[477] Compared with testosterone ester injections, transdermal formulations have a short half-life in subcutaneous tissue and in the circulation; consequently, their discontinuation results in a rapid fall in serum testosterone concentrations and a shorter duration of action. Therefore, an advantage of transdermal testosterone is the ability to withdraw androgen replacement relatively rapidly if adverse effects such as excessive erythrocytosis develop or prostate cancer is detected.

Disadvantages of transdermal formulations include the requirement for daily application, greater expense compared with testosterone ester injections, skin irritation or rash with testosterone patches[478] (less common with testosterone gels), and the potential with gel formulations for transfer of testosterone to others through skin contact at the application site.

The first transdermal testosterone delivery system for treatment of male hypogonadism was a scrotal testosterone patch.[479] Treatment required daily application of two relatively large, nonadhesive patches to clean, dry, and preferably shaven scrotal skin and the use of brief-style underwear to hold them in place. These requirements were not acceptable to some hypogonadal men. Also, in some men with long-standing, severe prepubertal androgen deficiency, the scrotum was too small to accommodate even the smaller-sized testosterone patch. Because of poor adherence to scrotal skin, thin adhesive strips were added as an option to this patch. Some men using this testosterone patch experienced skin irritation and itching. The scrotal testosterone patch produced serum DHT levels in the upper-normal range or above the normal range as a result of high 5α-reductase activity within sexual skin of the scrotum. The nonscrotal testosterone patch and testosterone gels have supplanted the scrotal testosterone patch for testosterone replacement therapy, and it is no longer available in the United States.

A nonscrotal testosterone patch, *Androderm* (Watson, Corona, CA), is available for testosterone replacement therapy in male patients with hypogonadism.[480] This patch is composed of a central reservoir containing testosterone and permeation enhancers in an alcohol-based gel surrounded by an adhesive patch that is applied to the skin of the back, abdomen, upper arms, or thighs, avoiding areas over a bony prominence. When applied at night, the testosterone patch produces serum testosterone levels that peak in the morning, mimicking the circadian variation of endogenous testosterone concentrations in normal men. Androderm patches are available in two sizes, delivering either 2.5 mg (37 cm^2) or 5 mg (44 cm^2) of testosterone daily. Long-term use of the testosterone patch usually maintains serum testosterone levels within the mid- to low-normal range and improves the clinical manifestations of androgen deficiency. Usually, to achieve consistent mid- to high-normal testosterone concentrations, application of two patches is necessary—either one 2.5-mg patch plus one 5-mg patch or two 5-mg patches.[481]

The major limitation of Androderm is skin irritation or rash of varying severity; this side effect occurs in at least 30% to 60% of patients.[478] Mild to moderate erythema and irritation are almost always present, probably because of a skin reaction to the permeation-enhancing agent or adhesive. Uncommonly, severe contact dermatitis or burn-like skin reactions occur. Pretreatment of the skin under the reservoir of the patch with a topical corticosteroid such as triamcinolone acetonide 0.1% cream reduces the incidence and severity of skin irritation produced by testosterone patches.[482]

Two transdermal formulations containing testosterone in a 1% hydroalcoholic gel, AndroGel (Abbott, Abbott Park, Ill.) and Testim (Auxilium, Norristown, Penn.), are available for testosterone replacement therapy in hypogonadal men.[483] AndroGel was the first testosterone gel formulation to be marketed, and it has rapidly become the testosterone formulation most frequently used for treatment of male hypogonadism in the United States.

AndroGel is dispensed into the palm of the hand and applied daily in the morning to clean, dry skin over the shoulders and upper arms or the abdomen and flanks but not on the scrotum.[6] The alcohol-based gel dries rapidly after application, and testosterone is absorbed into the subcutaneous space, where it is released steadily over the remainder of the day, producing relatively steady-state testosterone levels. Residual testosterone remains on the surface of the skin of the hands and at the sites of application. Therefore, the hands should be washed with soap and water after application, the sites of gel application should be covered with clothing, and skin contact with these sites by others (especially women and children) should be avoided to prevent transfer of testosterone.[484] Residual testosterone on the skin at application sites may be washed off (e.g., by showering or bathing), but this should be avoided for the first 5 to 6 hours after application (or 1 to 2 hours if done infrequently) to maximize testosterone absorption.

Long-term use of AndroGel in hypogonadal men maintains steady-state physiologic serum testosterone concentrations and improves the clinical manifestations of androgen deficiency (Fig. 19-30).[183,485-487] AndroGel is available in foil sachets at two different doses: 2.5 g of gel containing 25 mg of testosterone or 5 g of gel containing 50 mg of testosterone. (Because only about 10% of the medication is absorbed, these sachets deliver, respectively, 2.5 mg or 5.0 mg of testosterone.) The starting dose of AndroGel is 5 g daily. Based on testosterone levels or clinical response approximately 2 weeks after initiation of therapy, the dose may be increased to 7.5 g (i.e., one 2.5 g packet plus one 5.0 g packet) or to 10.0 g (two 5.0 g packets) daily or decreased to 2.5 g daily. A metered-dose pump delivering increments of 1.25 g of AndroGel per pump depression is also available to provide greater flexibility in dose adjustment.

In contrast to testosterone patches, local skin irritation with testosterone gel formulations is relatively uncommon, occurring in fewer than 5% of men, and is probably related mostly to drying of the skin by the alcohol. Some men complain of stickiness of the skin after the alcohol-based gel dries. AndroGel produces serum DHT levels at the upper end or above the normal range as a result of 5α-reductase activity in the relatively large surface area of skin over

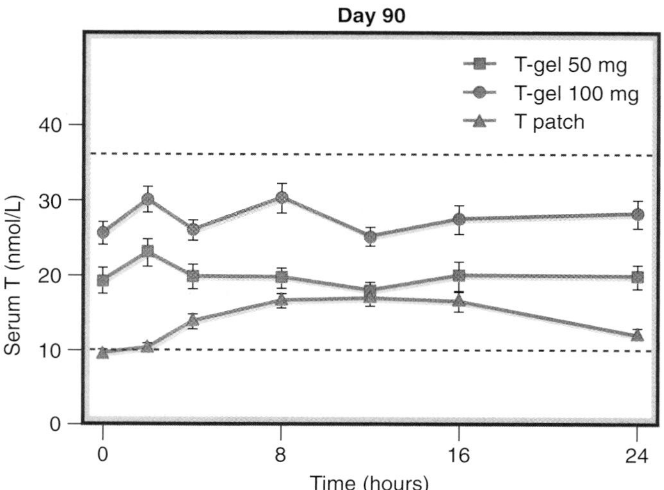

Figure 19-30 Serum total testosterone (T) levels after application of T-gel 50 mg (5 g of gel containing 50 mg of T and delivering approximately 5 mg of T) daily, or T-gel 100 mg (10 g of gel containing 100 mg of T and delivering approximately 10 mg of T) daily, or two T patches (delivering a total 5 mg of T) daily in hypogonadal men treated for 90 days. All three treatments achieved T levels within the low-normal, mid-normal, and upper-normal range *(dashed lines)* over the first 24 hours after application. (From Swerdloff RS, Wang C, Cunningham G, et al. Long-term pharmacokinetics of transdermal testosterone gel in hypogonadal men. *J Clin Endocrinol Metab.* 2000;85:4500-4510.)

which the gel is applied. A major limitation to the use of AndroGel for testosterone replacement therapy is its expense, particularly if more than one packet is needed daily for adequate testosterone replacement. The cost may be prohibitive for patients who do not have adequate third-party medication coverage.

Testim is the other 1% hydroalcoholic testosterone gel that is available for treatment of male hypogonadism.[488] It is applied daily in the morning to intact, clean, dry skin over the shoulders and arms but not over the abdomen or on scrotal skin. Like AndroGel, Testim produces steady-state testosterone levels over 24 hours and has the potential for contact transfer of residual testosterone on the skin surface at application sites. Similar precautions are recommended to prevent contact transfer, and washing off of residual testosterone on the skin surface should be avoided for at least 2 hours to maintain normal testosterone levels.

In short-term, placebo-controlled trials, Testim maintained steady-state physiologic serum testosterone levels in hypogonadal men and improved the clinical manifestations of androgen deficiency.[489] After the initial application of Testim, serum testosterone levels are approximately 30% higher than those achieved after application of AndroGel. However, no direct comparison of steady-state testosterone levels with long-term use of the two testosterone gels is available.[489]

Testim is packaged in two doses, a 5-g tube containing 50 mg of testosterone and a 10-g tube containing 100 mg of testosterone; these deliver approximately 5 mg and 10 mg of testosterone, respectively (i.e., 10% absorption). The starting dose of Testim is 5 g daily. Based on testosterone levels or clinical response approximately 2 weeks after initiation of therapy, the dose may be increased to 10 g daily. In contrast to AndroGel, Testim is not available in a dose of 2.5 g or in a metered-dose dispenser, limiting dose adjustments with this formulation.

Although AndroGel is odorless, Testim has a musk-like scent. Depending on the individual patient and his partners, this odor may be thought of as pleasant or objectionable. Testim contains a skin emollient and is less drying to the skin than AndroGel. However, both testosterone gels are tolerated well with very little skin irritation compared to the testosterone patch. Like AndroGel, Testim produces high-normal to slightly high serum DHT levels and is expensive.

Recently, two new transdermal formulations for the treatment of male hypogonadism were approved in the United States: *Fortesta* (Endo Pharmaceuticals, Chadds Ford, Penn.) is a 2% testosterone gel that is applied to the inner thighs at a dosage of 40-70 mg daily by a metered-dose pump that delivers 10 mg per pump depression. *Axiron* (Eli Lilly, Indianapolis, Ind.) is a 2% testosterone solution that is applied to axillary skin at a dosage of 30-120 mg daily by a metered-dose pump applicator that delivers 30 mg per pump depression.

Transbuccal Testosterone. A transbuccal testosterone tablet, *Striant* (Columbia Laboratories, Livingston, NJ), is available for testosterone replacement therapy in hypogonadal men (see Table 19-10).[490,491] This formulation is a small mucoadhesive tablet that contains 30 mg of testosterone in an oil-water emulsion carrier vehicle. The tablet contains polycarbophil, which, after application, remains attached to buccal mucosa until epithelial cells turn over (approximately 12 to 15 hours). The tablet is placed in the mouth between the inner cheek and gum, above the incisors, with the monoconvex side toward the gum and the flat side toward the cheek. After placement, the tablet softens and swells with hydration and becomes gelatinous and sticky, causing it to adhere to the gum. Testosterone is released at a controlled and sustained, constant rate from the tablet through the buccal mucosa into the systemic circulation, circumventing first-pass hepatic metabolism.

Striant tablets are placed on the buccal mucosa twice daily, with one tablet applied in the morning and removed after 12 hours and another applied in the evening on the opposite side.[490,491] Use of Striant requires careful instruction to orient the tablet with the rounded side against the gum and to hold it firmly in place with a finger over the lip for approximately 30 seconds. If the tablet falls off or is dislodged, a new tablet should be applied and left in place until the next regularly scheduled dose. Swallowing of the tablet is not harmful. The buccal tablet is removed by gently sliding it downward toward the incisor to avoid scratching the gum.

Application of a Striant tablet containing 30 mg of testosterone every 12 hours produces average steady-state testosterone levels in the mid-normal range throughout the day.[490,491] Although a formal study has not been conducted, unrestricted intake of food and beverage (including alcohol), tooth-brushing, mouth-washing, and gum-chewing did not appear to affect the absorption of testosterone in pharmacokinetic studies. Contact transfer of testosterone in saliva to others has not been reported to occur. Like the transdermal testosterone gels, Striant produces high-normal to high serum DHT concentrations, probably because of 5α-reductase activity in the buccal mucosa. In general, transbuccal testosterone tablets are tolerated well. Approximately 10% to 15% of men developed gum or mouth irritation or inflammation, and 5% experienced an altered or bitter taste in the mouth.[490]

Like the transdermal testosterone formulations, Striant is relatively expensive compared with testosterone ester injections. Initially, patients are aware and bothered by the tablet between their cheek and gum, resulting in premature discontinuation of the formulation. However, with continued use, the unusual sensation and awareness of the buccal tablet diminishes and it becomes less bothersome. Twice-daily application of Striant is required to sustain physiologic testosterone levels, and this makes compliance challenging. Informing patients that awareness of the buccal tablet diminishes over time and linking application of the transbuccal tablet to a routine daily activity such as morning and evening tooth-brushing may help to improve and maintain compliance.

Testosterone Pellets. Subcutaneous testosterone pellets are used infrequently in the United States but more commonly in Australia and some European countries for testosterone replacement therapy in men with hypogonadism.[492,493] In the United States, *Testopel Pellets* (Slate Pharmaceuticals, Durham, NC) are available for testosterone replacement (see Table 19-10). These are cylindrically shaped pellets, 3.2 mm diameter by 8 to 9 mm in length, that contain 75 mg of testosterone. Testopel Pellets are used at doses that range from 225 to 450 mg (i.e., three to six 75-mg pellets) and are implanted every 3 to 4 months.[492]

Pharmacokinetic profiles for testosterone pellets depend on the specific pellet formulation.[493,494] In European studies using a different formulation, subcutaneous implantation of three to six 200-mg pellets (for a total of 600 to 1200 mg of testosterone) produced the almost zero-order, sustained release of testosterone and maintained steady-state physiologic serum testosterone levels for 4 to 6 months in hypogonadal men.[494] Testosterone pellets are implanted subcutaneously with the use of a trocar that is introduced through a small skin incision. This minor surgical procedure is repeated two to three times yearly to maintain normal serum testosterone levels.

Although spontaneous extrusion of pellets and local bleeding or infection may occur occasionally, these are uncommon in experienced hands. If adverse effects develop after implantation, a major concern is that removal of the testosterone pellets will be difficult, if not impossible. Therefore, the use of testosterone pellets is inappropriate for testosterone replacement in older patients, who are predisposed to erythrocytosis and prostate disease during treatment, and is not an acceptable formulation for many physicians and patients.

Testosterone Formulations Available Outside the United States

Oral Testosterone Undecanoate. In many countries outside the United States, an oral 17β-hydroxyl ester of testosterone, testosterone undecanoate (Andriol Testocaps; Organon, Oss, Netherlands), is available to provide testosterone replacement therapy in hypogonadal men.[495,496] Testosterone undecanoate, which is formulated in a castor oil vehicle, is absorbed directly from the gastrointestinal tract into the lymphatic system and then into the systemic circulation, thereby avoiding first-pass hepatic accumulation and inactivation. Serum testosterone concentrations peak approximately 5 hours after administration of testosterone undecanoate and fall to pretreatment levels within 8 to 12 hours. For testosterone replacement therapy, it is administered at relatively high doses, 40 to 80 mg two to three times daily (total dose, 80 to 240 mg daily). The frequency of administration makes compliance difficult for many men. Absorption of testosterone undecanoate requires concomitant food ingestion, and serum testosterone levels and clinical responses are highly variable. Because of 5α-reductase activity in the gastrointestinal tract, serum DHT concentrations are often very high.

The use of castor oil and propylene glycol laurate instead of oleic acid, the vehicle used in the original formulation, permits storage at room temperature and extends the shelf-life of Andriol Testocaps for up to 3 years while maintaining pharmacokinetic and pharmacodynamic characteristics similar to those of the original formulation. Testosterone levels fall quickly after discontinuation of testosterone undecanoate. Therefore, it may be particularly useful for testosterone replacement therapy in older men with clinically significant prostate disease and comorbidities, in whom rapid withdrawal of androgen action is desirable if adverse effects develop, and in those for whom only low-dose testosterone supplementation is needed.

Injectable Testosterone Undecanoate. An injectable formulation of testosterone undecanoate in a castor oil vehicle (Nebido; Bayer Schering Pharma AG, Berlin, Germany) has been approved and is used in Europe and other countries for testosterone replacement therapy in hypogonadal men.[497-501] Testosterone undecanoate in castor oil is administered initially as a slow IM injection in the gluteus muscle at a dose of 1000 mg in 4 mL, followed by another injection of the same dose 6 weeks later and then every 10 to 14 weeks, to produce and maintain serum testosterone levels within the normal range in most hypogonadal men and to correct clinical manifestations of androgen deficiency. Because of the large volume of drug administered and the need for proper injection technique, self-administration is not possible. Coughing may occur in a small number of men immediately after injection of testosterone undecanoate. Although there is no direct evidence for the cause of coughing, it is hypothesized to be related to fat droplet microembolism emanating from the large volume of castor oil vehicle that is injected into the muscle with this formulation.

A different formulation of testosterone undecanoate in castor oil (Aveed, Endo Pharmaceuticals, Chadds Ford, PA) is awaiting approval in the United States. This formulation will be administered in a dose of 750 mg in 3 mL initially, followed by another, similar injection 4 weeks later and then every 10 weeks.[485]

Transdermal Testosterone Formulations. A *testosterone-in-adhesive matrix patch* (Testopatch, Pierre Fabre, Castres, France) is available in a number of countries in Europe for testosterone replacement therapy in patients with male hypogonadism.[502,503] This patch is composed of an adhesive matrix that contains testosterone (0.5 mg per cm^2) and excipients that comes in three sizes—30, 45, and 60 cm^2. Two 60-cm^2 patches (delivering approximately 4.8 mg of testosterone daily) are applied to the skin of the arms, trunk, or thighs every 2 days to maintain serum testosterone levels in the normal range in hypogonadal men. Skin irritation has been reported to occur in about 20% of patients using this patch.

A *testosterone gel 2%* formulation (Tostran or Tostrex, ProStrakan, Galashiels, UK) is available in some countries in Europe for testosterone replacement therapy.[504] One gram of gel contains 20 mg of testosterone in butylhydroxytoluene and propylene glycol, and it comes in a metered-dose canister that delivers 0.5 g of gel (10 mg of testosterone). The dose of testosterone gel is 3 to 4 g (60 to 80 mg of testosterone) applied to the skin of the abdomen or both inner thighs daily. Precautions must be taken to avoid contact transfer of testosterone to women and children.

Selective Androgen Receptor Modulators. There is considerable interest in the development of selective androgen receptor modulators (SARMs), nonsteroidal molecules that interact with AR and have differential effects on various androgen target organs.[505,506] The goal is to develop an orally active, nonsteroidal SARM that will maintain the beneficial anabolic and androgenic actions of testosterone on muscle, bone, sexual function, and mood but have reduced potential for adverse effects (e.g., on the prostate gland). These novel drugs are being developed primarily for use in muscle-wasting conditions such as age-related sarcopenia and cancer cachexia but not at present for treatment of male hypogonadism. The mechanisms by which SARMs act in a tissue-specific manner are unclear. It is possible that SARMs have less stimulatory effect on the prostate because they are not actively metabolized by 5α-reductase, or they may act by unique interactions with tissue-specific AR coactivator and corepressor molecules.

Nonsteroidal SARMs have been developed that have anabolic actions in muscle and bone but reduced stimulatory effects on the prostate gland in animals.[505,506] SARMs do not have intrinsic ER activity, and if they suppress endogenous gonadotropin, testosterone, and estradiol secretion, they will produce a state of relative estrogen deficiency. Therefore, studies evaluating the clinical benefits and risks of an SARM must consider potential adverse effects on target actions that are regulated by estradiol in men, such as effects on BMD, lipids (HDL-cholesterol), cardiovascular function, and brain function. The importance of estrogens on bone, for example, was underscored by a recent long-term study of the potent, nonaromatizable androgen, DHT gel, administered to older men. Compared with placebo, DHT gel stimulated lean body mass and reduced fat mass but suppressed BMD.[99]

Monitoring Clinical Response and Testosterone Levels. The clinical responses to testosterone replacement and serum testosterone levels are used to monitor the adequacy testosterone therapy in androgen-deficient men (Table 19-11).[110] Symptoms and signs of androgen deficiency should be assessed before the initiation of testosterone treatment, 3 to 6 months after starting testosterone, and then yearly. By 3 to 6 months, most hypogonadal men experience improvements in libido, sexual function and activity, energy, vitality, motivation, and mood.[507] Increases in body hair growth, muscle mass and strength, and BMD occur over the subsequent months to years of testosterone therapy.

Serum testosterone concentrations are monitored to determine the adequacy of therapy and to avoid overreplacement or underreplacement. This is particularly important in men treated with transdermal testosterone patches and gels, because the bioavailability of these formulations is highly variable among individuals. The goal of testosterone replacement therapy is to achieve serum testosterone levels in the mid-normal range.[110]

For testosterone ester injections, testosterone concentrations should be measured at 3 to 6 months of treatment, midway between two injections (e.g., 1 week after an injection if the injections are given every 2 weeks). Serum testosterone levels measured at the nadir of the injection interval (i.e., just before the next injection) may help to document an inadequate dosing interval. For the testosterone patch, testosterone levels should be measured after approximately 3 to 4 weeks of daily use, 8 to 10 hours after application of a patch on the previous evening. For testosterone gels, testosterone levels should be measured after about 2 weeks of daily use, at any time after application of the gel. For buccal testosterone, serum testosterone should be measured 4 to 6 weeks after initiation of therapy, at any time after application of the buccal tablet, preferably in the morning.

Risks and Adverse Effects

Contraindications and Precautions. Testosterone treatment is contraindicated in men with metastatic prostate cancer or breast cancer.[110] The primary concern is that testosterone administration could stimulate the growth of these androgen-dependent malignancies. Testosterone therapy is particularly risky in men with metastatic prostate cancer, in whom rapid growth of metastatic tumors may worsen bone pain or cause spinal cord compression. In fact, the mainstay of treatment for metastatic prostate cancer is androgen-deprivation therapy to reduce endogenous testosterone production and action; this is achieved by GnRH agonist and AR antagonist treatment or by surgical orchidectomy.[508] The effect of testosterone replacement in hypogonadal men with localized prostate cancer is not known. However, in the absence of evidence, testosterone treatment in men with clinical evidence of prostate cancer should be avoided.

The safety of testosterone therapy in hypogonadal men who have been surgically cured of organ-confined, low-grade prostate cancer and have had clinically undetectable disease and an undetectable PSA level for several years also is not clear. Because these men would not have been treated with androgen-deprivation therapy, testosterone replacement to restore eugonadal levels of testosterone seems reasonable. In these patients, a careful discussion of the potential benefits and risks of testosterone replacement should be undertaken, and therapy should be initiated only after informed consent and with careful monitoring by DRE and measurement of PSA levels.

Before testosterone replacement therapy is started in middle-aged and older men (>40 years) with androgen deficiency, a PSA measurement and a careful DRE to look

TABLE 19-11

Monitoring During Testosterone Treatment

Parameter	Timing	Further Management
	MEASURES OF EFFICACY	
Symptoms and signs of androgen deficiency	At baseline, after 3-6 mo, and then yearly For men at high risk for fracture, BMD before treatment; for men with osteoporosis or minimum-trauma fracture, BMD after 1-2 yr	Continue testosterone treatment in men with clinical improvement and no adverse effects Consider discontinuing testosterone treatment in men if no clinical improvement Institute appropriate treatment for men with osteoporosis, including calcium and vitamin D
Serum testosterone	*Testosterone ester injection:* after 3-6 mo, measured midway between injections or at end of dosing interval (if androgen deficiency symptoms are present at that time) *Testosterone patch:* after 3-4 wk, at 8-10 hr after application *Testosterone gel:* after 2 wk, at any time after application *Buccal testosterone:* after 4-6 wk, at any time after application (preferably in the morning) *Testosterone pellets:* at end of dosing interval *Oral testosterone undecanoate:* after 1 wk, at 3-5 hr after oral dose *Testosterone undecanoate injection:* at end of dosing interval	Adjust dose or dosing interval to achieve serum testosterone levels in mid-normal range
	ADVERSE EFFECTS	
Hematocrit	At baseline, after 3-6 mo, and then yearly	If hematocrit >54%, stop or reduce dosage of testosterone until hematocrit declines to normal and reinitiate testosterone at lower dosage Investigate for hypoxic condition such as obstructive sleep apnea, chronic lung disease
PSA level, DRE, and IPSS in men > 40 yr	At baseline, after 3-6 mo, and then according to accepted guidelines	Urologic evaluation if any of the following: PSA increase >1.4 ng/mL within any 12-mo period PSA velocity >0.4 ng/mL per year after 6 mo of testosterone treatment (only if 2 yr of PSA values are available) Palpable abnormality (nodule or induration) on DRE IPSS score >19
Obstructive sleep apnea (snoring, witnessed apnea, daytime somnolence, unexplained erythrocytosis, worsening hypertension or edema)	At baseline, after 3-6 mo, and then yearly	Evaluation for obstructive sleep apnea or adjustment of CPAP settings Evaluation of other causes of hypoxia
Formulation-specific adverse effects	At baseline, after 3-6 mo, and then yearly	
Testosterone ester injections	Discomfort, bleeding, or hematoma with IM injections Fluctuations in energy, mood, libido Allergy to oil vehicle (rare)	Reinstruct on self-injection site technique Consider shortening injection interval if nadir testosterone level low
Testosterone patch	Skin irritation Adhesion to skin	Coadministration of corticosteroid cream may reduce skin irritation
Testosterone gel	Contact transfer to others Skin dryness	Reinstruct on washing hands and covering application area after gel dries or showering 4-6 hr after application, avoiding prolonged skin-to-skin contact of application site with women and children
Buccal testosterone tablets	Gum irritation or inflammation Poor adhesion to gums Altered or bitter taste	Reinstruct on proper application and reassure to complete an adequate trial with correct technique
Subcutaneous testosterone pellets	Pellet extrusion Implantation-site infection, bleeding, fibrosis	Reimplant pellets Treat infection with appropriate drainage and antibiotics

BMD, bone mineral density; CPAP, continuous positive airway pressure; DRE, digital rectal examination; IM, intramuscular; IPSS, International Prostate Symptom Score; PSA, prostate-specific antigen.

for a suspicious prostate nodule or induration should be performed.[110] Hypogonadal men with an abnormal DRE or a consistently elevated PSA value (e.g., >4 ng/mL in Caucasian men, >3 ng/mL in African American men and men at high risk for prostate cancer) should have a urologic evaluation that may include a transrectal ultrasound study and biopsy of the prostate before starting testosterone. Older men, African American men, men with an abnormal DRE, and men with a history of a first-degree relative with prostate cancer have an increased risk of prostate cancer; men with a previous negative prostate biopsy and men who are taking a 5α-reductase inhibitor have a reduced risk. A prostate cancer risk calculator, based on data from placebo-treated men in the Prostate Cancer Prevention Trial, is available to assess the risk of clinical (biopsy-detectable) and high-grade (Gleason score ≥7) prostate cancer according to ethnicity, age, PSA level, family history of prostate cancer, normal or abnormal DRE, results of prior prostate biopsy, and use of a 5α-reductase inhibitor. This calculator is available at http://deb.uthscsa.edu/URORiskCalc/Pages/uroriskcalc.jsp (accessed January 2010).[509,510] Although it has not been validated for men with androgen deficiency, this prostate cancer risk calculator may be helpful in assessing the risk of clinical or high-grade prostate cancer that may be present in a hypogonadal man before testosterone replacement is instituted.

Although breast cancer in men is rare, some disorders that cause androgen deficiency, such as Klinefelter's syndrome, are associated with an increased risk of breast cancer.[201] Therefore, a careful breast examination for suspicious masses should be performed in hypogonadal men before starting testosterone treatment. The conversion of testosterone to estradiol may stimulate growth of ER-positive breast cancer.

Relative contraindications to testosterone replacement therapy include the following[110]:

- Untreated obstructive sleep apnea, because higher-dose testosterone treatment may rarely worsen sleep-disordered breathing and its complications
- Baseline hematocrit in the high-normal range (e.g., hematocrit >50 at or near sea level), because further stimulation of erythropoiesis induced by testosterone therapy may result in erythrocytosis and, potentially, hyperviscosity and vascular complications, particularly in elderly men with underlying vascular disease
- Severe edematous conditions (e.g., uncontrolled or poorly controlled congestive heart failure), because the fluid retention associated with testosterone therapy may worsen preexisting edema
- Severe LUTS due to BPH, such as in men with IPSS greater than 19

Potential Adverse Effects and Monitoring. Monitoring for potential adverse effects of testosterone therapy is sumarized in Table 19-11.

Hematocrit. Testosterone replacement stimulates erythropoiesis in hypogonadal men, increasing the hemoglobin concentration and hematocrit from the female range into the normal adult male range.[511] Occasionally, testosterone treatment causes excessive erythrocytosis (e.g., hematocrit >54%) that may require temporary discontinuation of therapy or lowering of the testosterone dose until the hematocrit declines to normal, reinitiation of testosterone at a lower dose, or sometimes therapeutic phlebotomy.[512] Excessive erythrocytosis occurs more commonly in older men and in those treated with parenteral testosterone esters rather than transdermal testosterone patches, probably related to the supraphysiologic testosterone levels that are present for a few days after administration and the higher average testosterone concentrations produced by IM testosterone.[477] A greater erythropoietic response to testosterone is associated with greater suppression of hepcidin, a liver-derived peptide that is the main regulator of iron bioavailability.[513]

Adverse effects of erythrocytosis induced by testosterone are poorly documented. However, there is concern that an excessive increase in red cell volume and blood viscosity could cause vascular complications such as thrombosis, especially older men with underlying atherosclerotic cardiovascular disease, resulting in stroke or myocardial infarction. Therefore, hematocrit should be measured before testosterone therapy is initiated, 3 to 6 months after starting treatment, and then yearly.[110] If erythrocytosis develops during testosterone replacement therapy, testosterone should be stopped and an evaluation should be performed to determine whether an underlying predisposing condition, such as hypoxia due to obstructive sleep apnea syndrome or chronic lung disease, is stimulating or contributing to erythrocytosis. Subsequently, testosterone may be restarted at a lower dosage.

Prostate. Prostate size is reduced in men with androgen deficiency, and testosterone replacement therapy increases prostate volume to that of age-matched eugonadal men.[514] Testosterone therapy does not cause excessive prostate enlargement, and there is no evidence that it worsens LUTS, reduces urinary flow rate, causes urinary retention, or increases the need for invasive intervention for BPH (e.g., TURP). However, long-term, controlled studies have not been performed to evaluate these outcomes in middle-aged to older hypogonadal men, who are most at risk for development of clinically significant, symptomatic BPH. Therefore, in hypogonadal men older than 40 years of age, LUTS should be monitored with the use of the IPSS or the AUA Symptom Index before testosterone treatment, at 3 to 6 months after starting treatment, and then in accordance with accepted guidelines.[110] Concomitant therapy for LUTS (e.g., α-adrenergic receptor antagonists, 5α-reductase inhibitors, surgical bladder outlet procedures) should be considered in hypogonadal men with bothersome severe LUTS that affects quality of life.

There is no evidence that testosterone treatment causes prostate cancer. In middle-aged to older men with androgen deficiency, there is concern that long-term testosterone therapy might stimulate previously unrecognized or clinically undetectable localized or metastatic prostate cancer or accelerate the growth of preexisting subclinical disease into clinically apparent prostate cancer. There is evidence that testosterone treatment stimulates the growth of metastatic prostate cancer, but its effect on progression of subclinical prostate cancer is not known. Small, short-term, controlled studies (up to 3 years in duration) have not found an increased incidence of prostate cancer in older men treated with testosterone.[512] Larger, longer-term, prospective, randomized, controlled trials are needed to determine whether testosterone therapy stimulates the growth and progression of subclinical prostate cancer into clinically evident and significant high-grade disease.

Along with reduced prostate size, serum PSA concentrations in androgen-deficient men are decreased, and testosterone replacement increases PSA to levels observed in age-matched eugonadal men.[514] Because testosterone replacement is a potentially disease-modifying intervention that may alter the natural history of prostate cancer, initial monitoring of PSA is prudent and should be performed to detect marked rises in PSA that might indicate stimulation of previously unrecognized prostate cancer growth.[110] PSA monitoring is distinct from PSA screening for prostate cancer, which is more controversial and has been demonstrated recently to have no effect or only modest effect on mortality in the general population of men.[515-517]

Therefore, in men older than 40 years of age, both PSA measurement and DRE should be performed before testosterone therapy is initiated, 3 to 6 months after starting treatment, and then in accordance with accepted guidelines. More intensive PSA monitoring should not be performed, because abnormal levels that would trigger a prostate biopsy are more likely to occur in older hypogonadal men on testosterone therapy, resulting in an increased likelihood of detecting localized prostate cancer, for which the management is unclear.[518] The diagnosis of subclinical or localized low-grade prostate cancer may not affect overall mortality, but the potential medical, surgical, psychological, and socioeconomic consequences and morbidity of this diagnosis may be considerable.

Hypogonadal men receiving testosterone therapy who demonstrate a verified increase in PSA greater than 1.4 ng/mL in any 12-month period during therapy; a PSA velocity of greater than 0.4 ng/mL per year using the value at 3 to 6 months as baseline (and only if 2 or more years of PSA values are available); an abnormal finding on DRE (nodule or induration); or an AUA Symptom Index or IPSS greater than 19 should undergo urologic evaluation.[110] Elevated PSA levels should be confirmed with a repeat measurement. If prostatitis or urinary tract infection that can markedly elevate PSA concentrations is suspected, PSA measurements should be repeated after appropriate antibiotic treatment.

Sleep Apnea. Testosterone treatment has been reported to induce or worsen obstructive sleep apnea, but the prevalence of clinically significant obstructive sleep apnea during testosterone replacement therapy is probably very low and may be dose related.[433,437,438] Short-term, high-dose testosterone treatment in older hypogonadal men significantly worsened obstructive sleep apnea, increased the duration of hypoxemia, and shortened total sleep time as assessed by polysomnography. In contrast, older men treated with a scrotal testosterone patch for 3 years did not demonstrate a significant worsening of sleep apnea as assessed by a portable device.[519] As discussed earlier, sleep apnea may conversely cause gonadotropin and testosterone suppression and secondary hypogonadism, probably because of the stress of oxygen desaturation and sleep disturbance.

Sleep apnea is associated with significant morbidity and mortality. Therefore, hypogonadal men, and especially those at increased risk (e.g., obese men), should be monitored for symptoms of obstructive sleep apnea syndrome (e.g., loud snoring, apnea witnessed by a bed partner, daytime somnolence, unexplained erythrocytosis, worsening or recent onset of hypertension or edema) before starting testosterone therapy, after 3 to 6 months, and then yearly.[110] If symptoms suggest sleep apnea, a formal sleep study (polysomnography) should be performed. If obstructive sleep apnea is confirmed, appropriate treatment (e.g., CPAP) should be instituted before testosterone treatment is started or continued.

Reduced Sperm Production and Fertility. In men who have androgen deficiency and persistence of some sperm production with either partial primary or secondary hypogonadism, testosterone treatment suppresses gonadotropin production by negative feedback regulation, which in turn suppresses spermatogenesis and may further impair fertility.[446] Suppression of sperm production is most important in men with secondary hypogonadism and normal testes who wish to father children. In these men, testosterone therapy should be discontinued and gonadotropin therapy should be started, initially with hCG alone and then, if necessary, with combined hCG and FSH treatment to stimulate spermatogenesis.[79] In the absence of coexisting testicular disease (e.g., cryptorchidism), prior testosterone therapy does not impair the subsequent induction of sperm production with gonadotropins.[316,317]

Acne and Oily Skin. Boys with prepubertal androgen deficiency who are receiving testosterone therapy to induce puberty and men with severe hypogonadism who are treated with full replacement doses of testosterone may develop acne and increased oiliness of the skin.[136,303] These conditions usually respond to local skin measures (e.g., benzoyl peroxide, retinoic acid) and antibiotics, reduction in testosterone dose, or both.

Gynecomastia. Occasionally, breast tenderness or gynecomastia develops or worsens during testosterone replacement therapy, particularly in boys who are receiving testosterone for induction of puberty, men with severe androgen deficiency who are treated with full replacement or high-dose testosterone, and hypogonadal men with predisposing conditions such as hepatic cirrhosis. Gynecomastia is commonly found in boys and men with androgen deficiency before the initiation of testosterone therapy. A careful breast examination should be performed before and again during testosterone replacement therapy to detect the presence or worsening of gynecomastia and the rare occurrence of breast cancer.

Lipids. In hypogonadal men, testosterone replacement results in no change or only a slight decrease in HDL-cholesterol and no change in total cholesterol or LDL-cholesterol levels.[512,520] The reduction in HDL-cholesterol is greater in men with more severe androgen deficiency and in those treated with supraphysiologic testosterone doses or with nonaromatizable, oral 17α-alkylated androgens.[360]

The clinical significance of HDL-cholesterol suppression induced by testosterone in terms of cardiovascular risk is not known. Understanding of the effects of testosterone therapy on major cardiovascular outcomes (e.g., myocardial infarction, stroke, cardiovascular mortality) will require larger, longer-term, randomized, controlled studies. Cardiovascular risk and lipid measurements should be evaluated as recommended by available practice guidelines; at present, more intensive monitoring in hypogonadal men receiving therapy is not justified.

Other Potential Adverse Effects. Frontal balding or androgenic alopecia may develop or worsen in genetically predisposed hypogonadal men during testosterone replacement therapy. Mild to moderate *weight gain* usually occurs during testosterone treatment, because of the anabolic actions of testosterone on muscle mass and associated fluid retention. Testosterone therapy usually does not cause clinically significant edema, except occasionally in hypogonadal men with underlying edematous states such as congestive heart failure or hepatic cirrhosis.

Stimulation of excessive libido and erections by testosterone is rare and usually occurs in boys or young men with severe, long-standing androgen deficiency who are treated with full replacement or high-dose testosterone therapy. These symptoms usually resolve spontaneously or with a reduction in testosterone dose. Contrary to popular opinion, testosterone treatment does not cause pathologic aggressiveness, anger, or rage.[521,522] Instead, testosterone replacement therapy increases social aggressiveness, motivation, and initiative and reduces irritability and anger.

Profound behavioral and physical changes induced by testosterone treatment in men with severe, long-standing androgen deficiency may be upsetting to both patients and their partners. Therefore, changes that are expected to occur with testosterone replacement should be discussed with patients and their partners before and during treatment. Oral 17α-alkylated androgens may cause cholestasis or potentially serious hepatotoxicity.[360] However, liver toxicity does not occur with testosterone replacement therapy, and routine monitoring of liver enzymes is not necessary in hypogonadal men.

Formulation-Specific Adverse Effects. Testosterone ester injections may cause local discomfort, bleeding, or hematoma at the site of IM injections.[110] Instruction on proper injection technique minimizes the likelihood of these adverse effects. Fluctuations in energy, mood, and libido associated with the peak and nadir swings of testosterone levels after testosterone ester injections may be disturbing to some hypogonadal men and may require reduction of the dose injected and shortening of the injection interval or switching to transdermal testosterone. Rarely, an allergy may occur to the sesame oil (enanthate) or cottonseed oil (cypionate) vehicle used.

Testosterone patches frequently cause local skin erythema, irritation, itching, and contact dermatitis and occasionally lead to more severe reactions.[110] Use of a topical corticosteroid cream under the reservoir of the patch may reduce skin irritation and reactions, but often men prefer to switch to another testosterone formulation. Testosterone patches may adhere poorly to skin, particularly with excessive perspiration.

In contrast to testosterone patches, *testosterone gels* cause little to no skin irritation. However, residual testosterone remains on the skin surface at the application sites, and there is a potential for transfer of testosterone to women and children who have prolonged intimate contact with these sites.[110] Precautions to avoid contact transfer of testosterone include washing the hands immediately after application of testosterone gel, covering the application site with clothing, washing off residual testosterone on skin by showering or bathing (4 to 6 hours after application), and avoiding prolonged skin-to-skin contact of the application site with women or children.

Buccal testosterone tablets may cause gum irritation or inflammation or an altered or bitter taste sensation, and they may adhere poorly to gums if not they are not properly applied.[110]

Subcutaneous testosterone pellets may uncommonly extrude spontaneously; rarely, there may be bleeding or infection at the site of implantation.[110]

Gonadotropin Therapy

Secondary hypogonadism manifests as prepubertal or adult androgen deficiency and impairment of sperm production due to gonadotropin deficiency. The primary goal of gonadotropin therapy in men with secondary hypogonadism is to initiate and maintain spermatogenesis in order to establish and restore fertility.[523] Because gonadotropin therapy is more complex (requiring multiple injections weekly) and more expensive than testosterone replacement therapy, symptomatic androgen deficiency is usually treated with the latter. In patients with partial gonadotropin deficiency, testosterone treatment may suppress remaining gonadotropin secretion by negative feedback regulation. When fertility is desired and stimulation of sperm production is needed in a man with secondary hypogonadism, testosterone is discontinued and gonadotropin therapy is initiated. Previous testosterone treatment does not compromise subsequent stimulation of spermatogenesis by gonadotropins.[316,317]

The gonadotropin preparations most commonly used to treat secondary hypogonadism are purified urinary gonadotropins. Human recombinant gonadotropin preparations are now available and have much higher purity than urinary preparations, but they are more expensive. Because urinary gonadotropins are highly effective in treating gonadotropin deficiency, they remain the most commonly used preparations for treatment of secondary hypogonadism.

hCG is used to provide LH-like activity because its half-life is longer than that of LH. In contrast to LH, which would require pulsatile administration approximately every 2 hours, hCG is administered two to three times per week. Purified urinary preparations of hCG (derived from urine of pregnant women) that contain LH-like activity are used almost exclusively in gonadotropin therapy. FSH activity is usually provided by purified urinary *human menopausal gonadotropin (hMG),* which is derived from urine of menopausal women and contains both FSH and LH; by highly purified urinary *human FSH*; or, rarely, by *recombinant human FSH (rhFSH).* FSH preparations are administered three times daily. hCG and FSH preparations may be administered either intramuscularly or subcutaneously.[524,525] Both are equally effective, but the latter is better tolerated and more easily self-administered.

In patients with prepubertal gonadotropin deficiency, initiation of sperm production requires treatment with both hCG and FSH (Fig. 19-31).[79] Gonadotropin therapy is initiated with administration of hCG alone at a dose of 500 to 2000 IU subcutaneously (SQ) two to three times weekly to stimulate sufficient endogenous testosterone production to increase and maintain circulating testosterone levels in the normal range and to correct manifestations of androgen deficiency.[6] The dose of hCG is increased until serum testosterone concentrations are within eugonadal range. Despite the more frequent injections, some men with secondary hypogonadism prefer hCG over testosterone treatment because costs are comparable (if purified urinary preparations are used), SQ injections using smaller needles are better tolerated, and testes size and spermatogenesis may increase slightly, particularly in patients with partial prepubertal gonadotropin deficiency.

Men with gonadotropin deficiency who also have primary testicular disease (e.g., cryptorchidism) or severe prepubertal isolated hypogonadotropic hypogonadism may require larger doses of hCG (e.g., up to 3000 to 5000 IU two to three times weekly, or occasionally much more). Men with secondary hypogonadism who have coexisting severe testicular damage may be completely unresponsive to hCG treatment (see Fig. 19-31). Because hCG stimulates Leydig cell aromatase activity within the testes, serum estradiol concentrations may increase disproportionately relative to testosterone levels, resulting in breast tenderness or gynecomastia more frequently than with testosterone replacement therapy. Some men may complain of burning at the site of SQ injections of hCG.

hCG stimulates Leydig cell testosterone production, resulting in relatively high intratesticular testosterone concentrations that cause Sertoli cells to mature and sperm production to be initiated to varying degrees. In a small proportion of patients with partial prepubertal deficiency and in almost all men with acquired postpubertal gonadotropin deficiency, treatment with hCG alone may stimulate sperm production (see Fig. 19-31).[79] Evidence for partial gonadotropin deficiency includes testes size larger than 4 mL, physical examination evidence of partial androgenization, low-normal gonadotropin concentrations, and low-normal levels of inhibin B.[526-530] Most patients with severe prepubertal gonadotropin deficiency require FSH treatment in addition to hCG to stimulate complete spermatogenesis and induce fertility.[530-533]

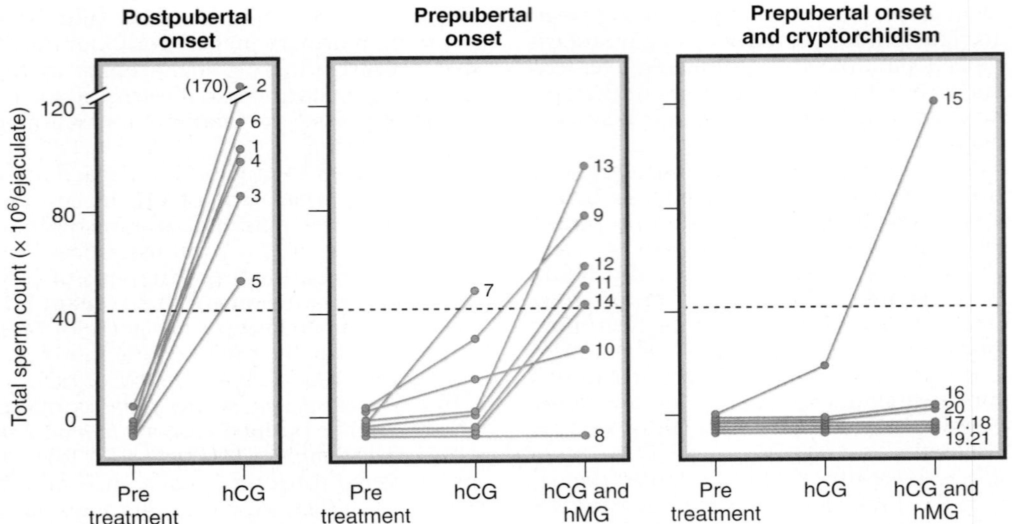

Figure 19-31 Total sperm count response to gonadotropin therapy with human chorionic gonadotropin (hCG) alone or in combination with human menopausal gonadotropin (hMG) in males with hypogonadotropic hypogonadism of postpubertal onset *(left)*, prepubertal onset without cryptorchidism *(middle)*, or prepubertal onset with cryptorchidism *(right)*. Sperm production was induced by hCG alone in all men with postpubertal hypogonadotropic hypogonadism and in some with prepubertal onset who did not have cryptorchidism. Both hCG and hMG treatment was required to increase sperm production above the lower limit of normal *(dashed line)* in patients with prepubertal hypogonadotropic hypogonadism who did not have cryptorchidism. With one exception, men with prepubertal hypogonadotropic hypogonadism who also had cryptorchidism failed to respond to hCG alone or to combined hCG and hMG therapy. (From Finkel DM, Phillips JL, Snyder PJ. Stimulation of spermatogenesis by gonadotropins in men with hypogonadotropic hypogonadism. *N Engl J Med.* 1985;313:651-655.)

If no sperm is present in the ejaculate after 6 to 12 months of treatment with hCG and serum testosterone concentrations in the eugonadal range, hMG or FSH at a dose of 75 IU three times weekly (increasing to 300 IU SQ three times weekly) is added, in combination with the same dose of hCG, for an additional 6 to 12 months or longer, until spermatogenesis is induced.

The induction of sperm production by gonadotropin therapy may take 12 to 24 months. Factors that limit the duration of gonadotropin treatment are impatience by patients or their partners and the expense of gonadotropins, in particular hMG or FSH preparations, which are very costly. Some couples may opt for alternative means to have children (e.g., adoption). In patients with prepubertal gonadotropin deficiency, sperm output is often low, possibly because of inadequate gonadotropin stimulation of Sertoli cell number and maturation during development.[534] Despite quantitatively low sperm production during gonadotropin therapy, fertility may be possible, sometimes at very low sperm counts (e.g., <1 million/mL).[526] Some patients who have very low sperm counts and remain infertile on gonadotropin treatment may elect to use ejaculated sperm for ICSI.

Once spermatogenesis has been initiated with combined hCG and FSH treatment in patients with prepubertal gonadotropin deficiency, sperm production may be maintained with hCG treatment alone.[467] In men with acquired postpubertal gonadotropin deficiency, reinitiation of spermatogenesis can usually be accomplished with hCG therapy alone.[79]

In men with secondary hypogonadism due to hypothalamic GnRH deficiency (e.g., IHH, Kallmann's syndrome), pulsatile GnRH therapy may be used to stimulate production of endogenous gonadotropins (both LH and FSH) and testosterone and to initiate and maintain sperm production sufficient for fertility.[319] GnRH is administered SQ with the use of a portable infusion pump that delivers small doses (pulses) of GnRH every few hours (e.g., GnRH 5 to 25 ng/kg SQ every 2 hours, increasing to higher doses if needed); this treatment mimics a near-normal physiologic stimulus to the pituitary gland. In men with IHH, pulsatile GnRH treatment is successful in stimulating gonadotropin, testosterone, and sperm production in approximately 75% of cases; in the other 25% of cases, men fail to respond due to concomitant pituitary or testicular defects.[319] The effectiveness of pulsatile GnRH replacement in stimulating sperm production is comparable to that of gonadotropin therapy. Practically, however, the use of pulsatile GnRH therapy is limited to specialized centers because GnRH is not readily available, the infusion pump requires additional expertise and management, and therapy is expensive.

REFERENCES

1. Bojesen A, Juul S, Gravholt CH. Prenatal and postnatal prevalence of Klinefelter syndrome: a national registry study. *J Clin Endocrinol Metab.* 2003;88:622-626.
2. Morris JK, Alberman E, Scott C, et al. Is the prevalence of Klinefelter syndrome increasing? *Eur J Hum Genet.* 2008;16:163-170.
3. Irvine DS. Epidemiology and aetiology of male infertility. *Hum Reprod.* 1998;13(suppl 1):33-44.
4. Kalyani RR, Gavini S, Dobs AS. Male hypogonadism in systemic disease. *Endocrinol Metab Clin North Am.* 2007;36:333-348.
5. Karagiannis A, Harsoulis F. Gonadal dysfunction in systemic diseases. *Eur J Endocrinol.* 2005;152:501-513.
6. Matsumoto AM. Androgen treatment of male hypogonadism. In: Kandeel FR, ed. *Male Sexual Function Pathophysiology and Treatment.* New York, NY: Informa Healthcare; 2007:433-452.
7. Ramasamy R, Ricci JA, Palermo GD, et al. Successful fertility treatment for Klinefelter's syndrome. *J Urol.* 2009;182:1108-1113.
8. Matsumoto AM. The testis. In: Felig P, Frohman LA, eds. *Endocrinology and Metabolism*, 4th ed. New York, NY: McGraw-Hill; 2001:635-705.
9. Lubs HA. Testicular size in Klinefelter's syndrome in men over fifty. *N Engl J Med.* 1962;267:326-331.
10. Matsumoto AM. Spermatogenesis. In: Adashi EY, Rock JA, Rosenwaks Z, eds. *Reproductive Endocrinology, Surgery, and Technology.* Philadelphia, PA: Lippincott-Raven; 1996:359-384.

11. Kapoor S. Testicular torsion: a race against time. *Int J Clin Pract.* 2008;62:821-827.
12. Zini A, Boman JM. Varicocele: red flag or red herring? *Semin Reprod Med.* 2009;27:171-178.
13. Amann RP, Howards SS. Daily spermatozoal production and epididymal spermatozoal reserves of the human male. *J Urol.* 1980;124:211-215.
14. Holstein AF, Schulze W, Davidoff M. Understanding spermatogenesis is a prerequisite for treatment. *Reprod Biol Endocrinol.* 2003;1:107.
15. Russell LD, Ettlin RA, Sinha Hikim AP, et al. Mammalian spermatogenesis. In: Russell LD, Ettlin RA, Sinha Hikim AP, et al., eds. *Histological and Histopathological Evaluaton of the Testis.* Clearwater, FL: Cache River Press; 1990:1-40.
16. Rowley MJ, Leach DR, Warner GA, et al. Effect of graded doses of ionizing radiation on the human testis. *Radiat Res.* 1974;59:665-678.
17. Hook EB. Maternal age, paternal age, and human chromosome abnormality: nature, magnitude, etiology, and mechanisms of effects. *Basic Life Sci.* 1985;36:117-132.
18. Hook EB, Cross PK, Schreinemachers DM. Chromosomal abnormality rates at amniocentesis and in live-born infants. *JAMA.* 1983;249:2034-2038.
19. Paduch DA, Fine RG, Bolyakov A, et al. New concepts in Klinefelter syndrome. *Curr Opin Urol.* 2008;18:621-627.
20. Petersen MB, Antonarakis SE, Hassold TJ, et al. Paternal nondisjunction in trisomy 21: excess of male patients. *Hum Mol Genet.* 1993;2:1691-1695.
21. Johnson L. Efficiency of spermatogenesis. *Microsc Res Tech.* 1995;32:385-422.
22. Clermont Y. The cycle of the seminiferous epithelium in man. *Am J Anat.* 1963;112:35-51.
23. Kerr JB. Functional cytology of the human testis. *Baillieres Clin Endocrinol Metab.* 1992;6:235-250.
24. Heller CG, Clermont Y. Spermatogenesis in man: an estimate of its duration. *Science.* 1963;140:184-186.
25. Rowley MJ, Teshima F, Heller CG. Duration of transit of spermatozoa through the human male ductular system. *Fertil Steril.* 1970;21:390-396.
26. Geraci E, Giudice G. Sperm activation and sperm-egg interaction. *J Submicrosc Cytol Pathol.* 2006;38:11-20.
27. Suarez SS. Control of hyperactivation in sperm. *Hum Reprod Update.* 2008;14:647-657.
28. Inaba K. Molecular basis of sperm flagellar axonemes: structural and evolutionary aspects. *Ann N Y Acad Sci.* 2007;1101:506-526.
29. Cooper TG, Noonan E, von Eckardstein S, et al. World Health Organization reference values for human semen characteristics. *Hum Reprod Update.* 2010;16:231-245.
30. Menkveld R. Clinical significance of the low normal sperm morphology value as proposed in the fifth edition of the WHO Laboratory Manual for the Examination and Processing of Human Semen. *Asian J Androl.* 2010;12:47-58.
31. Leigh MW, Pittman JE, Carson JL, et al. Clinical and genetic aspects of primary ciliary dyskinesia/Kartagener syndrome. *Genet Med.* 2009;11:473-487.
32. Haider SG. Cell biology of Leydig cells in the testis. *Int Rev Cytol.* 2004;233:181-241.
33. Hughes IA, Acerini CL. Factors controlling testis descent. *Eur J Endocrinol.* 2008;159(suppl 1):S75-S82.
34. Foresta C, Zuccarello D, Garolla A, et al. Role of hormones, genes, and environment in human cryptorchidism. *Endocr Rev.* 2008;29:560-580.
35. Maekawa M, Kamimura K, Nagano T. Peritubular myoid cells in the testis: their structure and function. *Arch Histol Cytol.* 1996;59:1-13.
36. Biason-Lauber A. Control of sex development. *Best Pract Res Clin Endocrinol Metab.* 2010;24:163-186.
37. Sekido R, Lovell-Badge R. Sex determination and SRY: down to a wink and a nudge? *Trends Genet.* 2009;25:19-29.
38. Tapanainen J, Kellokumpu-Lehtinen P, Pelliniemi L, et al. Age-related changes in endogenous steroids of human fetal testis during early and midpregnancy. *J Clin Endocrinol Metab.* 1981;52:98-102.
39. Quigley CA. The postnatal gonadotropin and sex steroid surge: insights from the androgen insensitivity syndrome (Editorial). *J Clin Endocrinol Metab.* 2002;87:24-28.
40. Grumbach MM. A window of opportunity: the diagnosis of gonadotropin deficiency in the male infant. *J Clin Endocrinol Metab.* 2005;90:3122-3127.
41. Main KM, Schmidt IM, Skakkebaek NE. A possible role for reproductive hormones in newborn boys: progressive hypogonadism without the postnatal testosterone peak. *J Clin Endocrinol Metab.* 2000;85:4905-4907.
42. Boyar RM, Rosenfeld RS, Kapen S, et al. Human puberty: simultaneous augmented secretion of luteinizing hormone and testosterone during sleep. *J Clin Invest.* 1974;54:609-618.
43. Patton GC, Viner R. Pubertal transitions in health. *Lancet.* 2007;369:1130-1139.
44. Nielsen CT, Skakkebaek NE, Richardson DW, et al. Onset of the release of spermatozoa (spermarche) in boys in relation to age, testicular growth, pubic hair, and height. *J Clin Endocrinol Metab.* 1986;62:532-535.
45. Veldhuis JD, King JC, Urban RJ, et al. Operating characteristics of the male hypothalamo-pituitary-gonadal axis: pulsatile release of testosterone and follicle-stimulating hormone and their temporal coupling with luteinizing hormone. *J Clin Endocrinol Metab.* 1987;65:929-941.
46. Whitcomb RW, O'Dea LS, Finkelstein JS, et al. Utility of free alpha-subunit as an alternative neuroendocrine marker of gonadotropin-releasing hormone (GnRH) stimulation of the gonadotroph in the human: evidence from normal and GnRH-deficient men. *J Clin Endocrinol Metab.* 1990;70:1654-1661.
47. Santoro N, Filicori M, Crowley WF Jr. Hypogonadotropic disorders in men and women: diagnosis and therapy with pulsatile gonadotropin-releasing hormone. *Endocr Rev.* 1986;7:11-23.
48. Matsumoto AM, Gross KM, Bremner WJ. The physiological significance of pulsatile LHRH secretion in man: gonadotrophin responses to physiological doses of pulsatile versus continuous LHRH administration. *Int J Androl.* 1991;14:23-32.
49. Wierman ME, Kiseljak-Vassiliades K, Tobet S. Gonadotropin-releasing hormone (GnRH) neuron migration: initiation, maintenance and cessation as critical steps to ensure normal reproductive function. *Front Neuroendocrinol.* 2010;32:43-52.
50. Brioude F, Bouligand J, Trabado S, et al. Non-syndromic congenital hypogonadotropic hypogonadism: clinical presentation and genotype-phenotype relationships. *Eur J Endocrinol.* 2010;162:835-851.
51. Bliss SP, Navratil AM, Xie J, et al. GnRH signaling, the gonadotrope and endocrine control of fertility. *Front Neuroendocrinol.* 2010;31:322-340.
52. Ulloa-Aguirre A, Maldonado A, Damian-Matsumura P, et al. Endocrine regulation of gonadotropin glycosylation. *Arch Med Res.* 2001;32:520-532.
53. Snyder PJ. Gonadotroph cell adenomas of the pituitary. *Endocr Rev.* 1985;6:552-563.
54. Tsatsoulis A, Shalet SM, Robertson WR. Changes in the qualitative and quantitative secretion of luteinizing hormone (LH) following orchidectomy in man. *Clin Endocrinol (Oxf).* 1988;29:189-194.
55. Yen SC, Llerena LA, Pearson OH, et al. Disappearance rates of endogenous follicle-stimulating hormone in serum following surgical hypophysectomy in man. *J Clin Endocrinol Metab.* 1970;30:325-329.
56. Ascoli M, Fanelli F, Segaloff DL. The lutropin/choriogonadotropin receptor: a 2002 perspective. *Endocr Rev.* 2002;23:141-174.
57. Miller WL. Molecular biology of steroid hormone synthesis. *Endocr Rev.* 1988;9:295-318.
58. Huhtaniemi I, Alevizaki M. Gonadotrophin resistance. *Best Pract Res Clin Endocrinol Metab.* 2006;20:561-576.
59. Valdes-Socin H, Salvi R, Daly AF, et al. Hypogonadism in a patient with a mutation in the luteinizing hormone beta-subunit gene. *N Engl J Med.* 2004;351:2619-2625.
60. Reiter EO, Norjavaara E. Testotoxicosis: current viewpoint. *Pediatr Endocrinol Rev.* 2005;3:77-86.
61. Bhasin S. Testicular disorders. In: Kronenberg HM, Melmed S, Polonsky KS, et al., ed. *Williams Textbook of Endocrinology.* 11th ed. Philadelphia, PA: Elsevier; 2008:645-698.
62. Mendonca BB, Costa EM, Belgorosky A, et al. 46,XY DSD due to impaired androgen production. *Best Pract Res Clin Endocrinol Metab.* 2010;24:243-262.
63. Hammond GL, Ruokonen A, Kontturi M, et al. The simultaneous radioimmunoassay of seven steroids in human spermatic and peripheral venous blood. *J Clin Endocrinol Metab.* 1977;45:16-24.
64. Bremner WJ, Vitiello MV, Prinz PN. Loss of circadian rhythmicity in blood testosterone levels with aging in normal men. *J Clin Endocrinol Metab.* 1983;56:1278-1281.
65. Nankin HR, Murono E, Lin T, et al. Morning and evening human Leydig cell responses to hCG. *Acta Endocrinol (Copenh).* 1980;95:560-565.
66. Ivell R, Anand-Ivell R. Biology of insulin-like factor 3 in human reproduction. *Hum Reprod Update.* 2009;15:463-476.
67. Bay K, Hartung S, Ivell R, et al. Insulin-like factor 3 serum levels in 135 normal men and 85 men with testicular disorders: relationship to the luteinizing hormone-testosterone axis. *J Clin Endocrinol Metab.* 2005;90:3410-3418.
68. Simoni M, Gromoll J, Nieschlag E. The follicle-stimulating hormone receptor: biochemistry, molecular biology, physiology, and pathophysiology. *Endocr Rev.* 1997;18:739-773.
69. Rannikko A, Penttila TL, Zhang FP, et al. Stage-specific expression of the FSH receptor gene in the prepubertal and adult rat seminiferous epithelium. *J Endocrinol.* 1996;151:29-35.
70. Bremner WJ, Millar MR, Sharpe RM, et al. Immunohistochemical localization of androgen receptors in the rat testis: evidence for stage-dependent expression and regulation by androgens. *Endocrinology.* 1994;135:1227-1234.
71. Jegou B. The Sertoli cell. *Baillieres Clin Endocrinol Metab.* 1992;6:273-311.

72. Petersen C, Soder O. The Sertoli cell: a hormonal target and "super" nurse for germ cells that determines testicular size. *Horm Res*. 2006;66: 153-161.
73. Avvakumov GV, Cherkasov A, Muller YA, et al. Structural analyses of sex hormone-binding globulin reveal novel ligands and function. *Mol Cell Endocrinol*. 2010;316:13-23.
74. Selva DM, Hammond GL. Human sex hormone-binding globulin is expressed in testicular germ cells and not in Sertoli cells. *Horm Metab Res*. 2006;38:230-235.
75. McLean DJ, Friel PJ, Pouchnik D, et al. Oligonucleotide microarray analysis of gene expression in follicle-stimulating hormone-treated rat Sertoli cells. *Mol Endocrinol*. 2002;16:2780-2792.
76. O'Shaughnessy PJ, Verhoeven G, De Gendt K, et al. Direct action through the Sertoli cells is essential for androgen stimulation of spermatogenesis. *Endocrinology*. 2010;151:2343-2348.
77. Welsh M, Saunders PT, Atanassova N, et al. Androgen action via testicular peritubular myoid cells is essential for male fertility. *FASEB J*. 2009;23:4218-4230.
78. Ruwanpura SM, McLachlan RI, Meachem SJ. Hormonal regulation of male germ cell development. *J Endocrinol*. 2010;205:117-131.
79. Finkel DM, Phillips JL, Snyder PJ. Stimulation of spermatogenesis by gonadotropins in men with hypogonadotropic hypogonadism. *N Engl J Med*. 1985;313:651-655.
80. Achard C, Courtillot C, Lahuna O, et al. Normal spermatogenesis in a man with mutant luteinizing hormone. *N Engl J Med*. 2009;361: 1856-1863.
81. Bruysters M, Christin-Maitre S, Verhoef-Post M, et al. A new LH receptor splice mutation responsible for male hypogonadism with subnormal sperm production in the propositus, and infertility with regular cycles in an affected sister. *Hum Reprod*. 2008;23:1917-1923.
82. Layman LC. Mutations in the follicle-stimulating hormone-beta (FSH beta) and FSH receptor genes in mice and humans. *Semin Reprod Med*. 2000;18:5-10.
83. Layman LC, Porto AL, Xie J, et al. FSH beta gene mutations in a female with partial breast development and a male sibling with normal puberty and azoospermia. *J Clin Endocrinol Metab*. 2002;87: 3702-3707.
84. Lindstedt G, Nystrom E, Matthews C, et al. Follitropin (FSH) deficiency in an infertile male due to FSHbeta gene mutation: a syndrome of normal puberty and virilization but underdeveloped testicles with azoospermia, low FSH but high lutropin and normal serum testosterone concentrations. *Clin Chem Lab Med*. 1998;36:663-665.
85. Phillip M, Arbelle JE, Segev Y, et al. Male hypogonadism due to a mutation in the gene for the beta-subunit of follicle-stimulating hormone. *N Engl J Med*. 1998;338:1729-1732.
86. Meduri G, Bachelot A, Cocca MP, et al. Molecular pathology of the FSH receptor: new insights into FSH physiology. *Mol Cell Endocrinol*. 2008;282:130-142.
87. Matsumoto AM, Bremner WJ. Endocrine control of human spermatogenesis. *J Steroid Biochem*. 1989;33:789-790.
88. Gromoll J, Simoni M, Nieschlag E. An activating mutation of the follicle-stimulating hormone receptor autonomously sustains spermatogenesis in a hypophysectomized man. *J Clin Endocrinol Metab*. 1996;81:1367-1370.
89. Matthiesson KL, McLachlan RI, O'Donnell L, et al. The relative roles of follicle-stimulating hormone and luteinizing hormone in maintaining spermatogonial maturation and spermiation in normal men. *J Clin Endocrinol Metab*. 2006;91:3962-3969.
90. Page ST, Kalhorn TF, Bremner WJ, et al. Intratesticular androgens and spermatogenesis during severe gonadotropin suppression induced by male hormonal contraceptive treatment. *J Androl*. 2007;28: 734-741.
91. Roth MY, Page ST, Lin K, et al. Dose-dependent increase in intratesticular testosterone by very low-dose human chorionic gonadotropin in normal men with experimental gonadotropin deficiency. *J Clin Endocrinol Metab*. 2010;95:3806-3813.
92. Drincic A, Arseven OK, Sosa E, et al. Men with acquired hypogonadotropic hypogonadism treated with testosterone may be fertile. *Pituitary*. 2003;6:5-10.
93. Matthiesson KL, Stanton PG, O'Donnell L, et al. Effects of testosterone and levonorgestrel combined with a 5alpha-reductase inhibitor or gonadotropin-releasing hormone antagonist on spermatogenesis and intratesticular steroid levels in normal men. *J Clin Endocrinol Metab*. 2005;90:5647-5655.
94. Pitteloud N, Dwyer AA, DeCruz S, et al. The relative role of gonadal sex steroids and gonadotropin-releasing hormone pulse frequency in the regulation of follicle-stimulating hormone secretion in men. *J Clin Endocrinol Metab*. 2008;93:2686-2692.
95. Pitteloud N, Dwyer AA, DeCruz S, et al. Inhibition of luteinizing hormone secretion by testosterone in men requires aromatization for its pituitary but not its hypothalamic effects: evidence from the tandem study of normal and gonadotropin-releasing hormone-deficient men. *J Clin Endocrinol Metab*. 2008;93:784-791.
96. Boepple PA, Hayes FJ, Dwyer AA, et al. Relative roles of inhibin B and sex steroids in the negative feedback regulation of follicle-stimulating hormone in men across the full spectrum of seminiferous epithelium function. *J Clin Endocrinol Metab*. 2008;93:1809-1814.
97. Canovatchel WJ, Volquez D, Huang S, et al. Luteinizing hormone pulsatility in subjects with 5-alpha-reductase deficiency and decreased dihydrotestosterone production. *J Clin Endocrinol Metab*. 1994;78: 916-921.
98. Iranmanesh A, Veldhuis JD. Combined inhibition of types I and II 5 alpha-reductase selectively augments the basal (nonpulsatile) mode of testosterone secretion in young men. *J Clin Endocrinol Metab*. 2005; 90:4232-4237.
99. Idan A, Griffiths KA, Harwood DT, et al. Long-term effects of dihydrotestosterone treatment on prostate growth in healthy, middle-aged men without prostate disease: a randomized, placebo-controlled trial. *Ann Intern Med*. 2010;153:621-632.
100. Oakley AE, Clifton DK, Steiner RA. Kisspeptin signaling in the brain. *Endocr Rev*. 2009;30:713-743.
101. Silveira LG, Tusset C, Latronico AC. Impact of mutations in kisspeptin and neurokinin B signaling pathways on human reproduction. *Brain Res*. 2010;1364:72-80.
102. de Kretser DM, Buzzard JJ, Okuma Y, et al. The role of activin, follistatin and inhibin in testicular physiology. *Mol Cell Endocrinol*. 2004;225:57-64.
103. Bilezikjian LM, Blount AL, Donaldson CJ, et al. Pituitary actions of ligands of the TGF-beta family: activins and inhibins. *Reproduction*. 2006;132:207-215.
104. Page ST, Amory JK, Bremner WJ. Advances in male contraception. *Endocr Rev*. 2008;29:465-493.
105. Dunn JF, Nisula BC, Rodbard D. Transport of steroid hormones: binding of 21 endogenous steroids to both testosterone-binding globulin and corticosteroid-binding globulin in human plasma. *J Clin Endocrinol Metab*. 1981;53:58-68.
106. Vermeulen A. Physiology of the testosterone-binding globulin in man. *Ann N Y Acad Sci*. 1988;538:103-111.
107. Mendel CM. The free hormone hypothesis: distinction from the free hormone transport hypothesis. *J Androl*. 1992;13:107-116.
108. Willnow TE, Nykjaer A. Cellular uptake of steroid carrier proteins: mechanisms and implications. *Mol Cell Endocrinol*. 2010;316:93-102.
109. Hammes A, Andreassen TK, Spoelgen R, et al. Role of endocytosis in cellular uptake of sex steroids. *Cell*. 2005;122:751-762.
110. Bhasin S, Cunningham GR, Hayes FJ, et al. Testosterone therapy in men with androgen deficiency syndromes: an Endocrine Society clinical practice guideline. *J Clin Endocrinol Metab*. 2010;95:2536-2559.
111. Horton R. Sex steroid production and secretion in the male. *Andrologia*. 1978;10:183-194.
112. Grumbach MM, Auchus RJ. Estrogen: consequences and implications of human mutations in synthesis and action. *J Clin Endocrinol Metab*. 1999;84:4677-4694.
113. Lombardi G, Zarrilli S, Colao A, et al. Estrogens and health in males. *Mol Cell Endocrinol*. 2001;178:51-55.
114. Zirilli L, Rochira V, Diazzi C, et al. Human models of aromatase deficiency. *J Steroid Biochem Mol Biol*. 2008;109:212-218.
115. Thigpen AE, Silver RI, Guileyardo JM, et al. Tissue distribution and ontogeny of steroid 5 alpha-reductase isozyme expression. *J Clin Invest*. 1993;92:903-910.
116. Imperato-McGinley J, Zhu YS. Androgens and male physiology the syndrome of 5alpha-reductase-2 deficiency. *Mol Cell Endocrinol*. 2002;198:51-59.
117. Randall VA. Role of 5 alpha-reductase in health and disease. *Baillieres Clin Endocrinol Metab*. 1994;8:405-431.
118. Aggarwal S, Thareja S, Verma A, et al. An overview on 5alpha-reductase inhibitors. *Steroids*. 2010;75:109-153.
119. Andriole GL, Bostwick DG, Brawley OW, et al. Effect of dutasteride on the risk of prostate cancer. *N Engl J Med*. 2010;362:1192-1202.
120. Thompson IM, Goodman PJ, Tangen CM, et al. The influence of finasteride on the development of prostate cancer. *N Engl J Med*. 2003;349:215-224.
121. Belanger A, Pelletier G, Labrie F, et al. Inactivation of androgens by UDP-glucuronosyltransferase enzymes in humans. *Trends Endocrinol Metab*. 2003;14:473-479.
122. Basaria S. Androgen abuse in athletes: detection and consequences. *J Clin Endocrinol Metab*. 2010;95:1533-1543.
123. Schulze JJ, Lorentzon M, Ohlsson C, et al. Genetic aspects of epitestosterone formation and androgen disposition: influence of polymorphisms in CYP17 and UGT2B enzymes. *Pharmacogenet Genomics*. 2008;18:477-485.
124. Swanson C, Mellstrom D, Lorentzon M, et al. The uridine diphosphate glucuronosyltransferase 2B15 D85Y and 2B17 deletion polymorphisms predict the glucuronidation pattern of androgens and fat mass in men. *J Clin Endocrinol Metab*. 2007;92:4878-4882.
125. van de Kerkhof DH, de Boer D, Thijssen JH, et al. Evaluation of testosterone/epitestosterone ratio influential factors as determined in doping analysis. *J Anal Toxicol*. 2000;24:102-115.
126. Li J, Al-Azzawi F. Mechanism of androgen receptor action. *Maturitas*. 2009;63:142-148.

127. Hughes IA, Deeb A. Androgen resistance. *Best Pract Res Clin Endocrinol Metab*. 2006;20:577-598.
128. Finsterer J. Bulbar and spinal muscular atrophy (Kennedy's disease): a review. *Eur J Neurol*. 2009;16:556-561.
129. Dejager S, Bry-Gauillard H, Bruckert E, et al. A comprehensive endocrine description of Kennedy's disease revealing androgen insensitivity linked to CAG repeat length. *J Clin Endocrinol Metab*. 2002;87:3893-3901.
130. Zitzmann M. The role of the CAG repeat androgen receptor polymorphism in andrology. *Front Horm Res*. 2009;37:52-61.
131. Rahman F, Christian HC. Non-classical actions of testosterone: an update. *Trends Endocrinol Metab*. 2007;18:371-378.
132. Griffin JE, Wilson JD. The testis. In: Bondy PK, Rosenberg LE, eds. *Metabolic Control and Disease*. 8th ed. Philadelphia, PA: WB Saunders; 1980:1535-1578.
133. Chemes HE. Infancy is not a quiescent period of testicular development. *Int J Androl*. 2001;24:2-7.
134. Marshall WA, Tanner JM. Variations in the pattern of pubertal changes in boys. *Arch Dis Child*. 1970;45:13-23.
135. Kaufman JM, Vermeulen A. The decline of androgen levels in elderly men and its clinical and therapeutic implications. *Endocr Rev*. 2005;26:833-876.
136. Richmond EJ, Rogol AD. Male pubertal development and the role of androgen therapy. *Nat Clin Pract Endocrinol Metab*. 2007;3:338-344.
137. Sherins RJ, Howards SS. Male infertility. In: Harrison JH, Gittes RF, Perlmutter AD, et al., eds. *Campbell's Urology*. 4th ed. Philadelphia, PA: WB Saunders; 1978:715-776.
138. Kandeel FR, Koussa VK, Swerdloff RS. Male sexual function and its disorders: physiology, pathophysiology, clinical investigation, and treatment. *Endocr Rev*. 2001;22:342-388.
139. Carani C, Granata AR, Bancroft J, et al. The effects of testosterone replacement on nocturnal penile tumescence and rigidity and erectile response to visual erotic stimuli in hypogonadal men. *Psychoneuroendocrinology*. 1995;20:743-753.
140. Corona G, Maggi M. The role of testosterone in erectile dysfunction. *Nat Rev Urol*. 2010;7:46-56.
141. Traish AM. Androgens play a pivotal role in maintaining penile tissue architecture and erection: a review. *J Androl*. 2009;30:363-369.
142. Meuleman EJ, van Lankveld JJ. Hypoactive sexual desire disorder: an underestimated condition in men. *BJU Int*. 2005;95:291-296.
143. McVary KT. Clinical practice: erectile dysfunction. *N Engl J Med*. 2007;357:2472-2481.
144. Buvat J, Maggi M, Gooren L, et al. Endocrine aspects of male sexual dysfunctions. *J Sex Med*. 2010;7:1627-1656.
145. Wylie K, Rees M, Hackett G, et al. Androgens, health and sexuality in women and men. *Maturitas*. 2010;67:275-289.
146. Wylie K, Kenney G. Sexual dysfunction and the ageing male. *Maturitas*. 2010;65:23-27.
147. Bolona ER, Uraga MV, Haddad RM, et al. Testosterone use in men with sexual dysfunction: a systematic review and meta-analysis of randomized placebo-controlled trials. *Mayo Clin Proc*. 2007;82:20-28.
148. Qaseem A, Snow V, Denberg TD, et al. Hormonal testing and pharmacologic treatment of erectile dysfunction: a clinical practice guideline from the American College of Physicians. *Ann Intern Med*. 2009;151:639-649.
149. Tsertsvadze A, Fink HA, Yazdi F, et al. Oral phosphodiesterase-5 inhibitors and hormonal treatments for erectile dysfunction: a systematic review and meta-analysis. *Ann Intern Med*. 2009;151:650-661.
150. Buvat J, Bou Jaoude G. Significance of hypogonadism in erectile dysfunction. *World J Urol*. 2006;24:657-667.
151. Rowland DL. Psychophysiology of ejaculatory function and dysfunction. *World J Urol*. 2005;23:82-88.
152. Linton KD, Wylie KR. Recent advances in the treatment of premature ejaculation. *Drug Des Devel Ther*. 2010;4:1-6.
153. Braunstein GD. Clinical practice: gynecomastia. *N Engl J Med*. 2007;357:1229-1237.
154. Johnson RE, Murad MH. Gynecomastia: pathophysiology, evaluation, and management. *Mayo Clin Proc*. 2009;84:1010-1015.
155. Narula HS, Carlson HE. Gynecomastia. *Endocrinol Metab Clin North Am*. 2007;36:497-519.
156. Gomez-Raposo C, Zambrana Tevar F, Sereno Moyano M, et al. Male breast cancer. *Cancer Treat Rev*. 2010;36:451-457.
157. Lee SY, Oh SM, Chung KH. Estrogenic effects of marijuana smoke condensate and cannabinoid compounds. *Toxicol Appl Pharmacol*. 2006;214:270-278.
158. Messina M. Soybean isoflavone exposure does not have feminizing effects on men: a critical examination of the clinical evidence. *Fertil Steril*. 2010;93:2095-2104.
159. Eckman A, Dobs A. Drug-induced gynecomastia. *Expert Opin Drug Saf*. 2008;7:691-702.
160. Gruntmanis U, Braunstein GD. Treatment of gynecomastia. *Curr Opin Investig Drugs*. 2001;2:643-649.
161. Gnoth C, Godehardt E, Frank-Herrmann P, et al. Definition and prevalence of subfertility and infertility. *Hum Reprod*. 2005;20:1144-1147.
162. Bhasin S. Approach to the infertile man. *J Clin Endocrinol Metab*. 2007;92:1995-2004.
163. Dohle GR, Colpi GM, Hargreave TB, et al. EAU guidelines on male infertility. *Eur Urol*. 2005;48:703-711.
164. McLachlan RI, O'Bryan MK. Clinical Review: state of the art for genetic testing of infertile men. *J Clin Endocrinol Metab*. 2010;95:1013-1024.
165. Vogt PH, Falcao CL, Hanstein R, et al. The AZF proteins. *Int J Androl*. 2008;31:383-394.
166. Radpour R, Gourabi H, Dizaj AV, et al. Genetic investigations of CFTR mutations in congenital absence of vas deferens, uterus, and vagina as a cause of infertility. *J Androl*. 2008;29:506-513.
167. Walsh TJ, Pera RR, Turek PJ. The genetics of male infertility. *Semin Reprod Med*. 2009;27:124-136.
168. Comhaire FH, Mahmoud AM, Depuydt CE, et al. Mechanisms and effects of male genital tract infection on sperm quality and fertilizing potential: the andrologist's viewpoint. *Hum Reprod Update*. 1999;5:393-398.
169. Pellati D, Mylonakis I, Bertoloni G, et al. Genital tract infections and infertility. *Eur J Obstet Gynecol Reprod Biol*. 2008;140:3-11.
170. Adamopoulos DA, Koukkou EG. "Value of FSH and inhibin-B measurements in the diagnosis of azoospermia": a clinician's overview. *Int J Androl*. 2010;33:e109-e113.
171. Jarow JP. Diagnostic approach to the infertile male patient. *Endocrinol Metab Clin North Am*. 2007;36:297-311.
172. Palermo GD, Neri QV, Takeuchi T, et al. ICSI: where we have been and where we are going. *Semin Reprod Med*. 2009;27:191-201.
173. Schlegel PN. Nonobstructive azoospermia: a revolutionary surgical approach and results. *Semin Reprod Med*. 2009;27:165-170.
174. Nagler HM, Jung H. Factors predicting successful microsurgical vasectomy reversal. *Urol Clin North Am*. 2009;36:383-390.
175. Araujo AB, Esche GR, Kupelian V, et al. Prevalence of symptomatic androgen deficiency in men. *J Clin Endocrinol Metab*. 2007;92:4241-4247.
176. Araujo AB, O'Donnell AB, Brambilla DJ, et al. Prevalence and incidence of androgen deficiency in middle-aged and older men: estimates from the Massachusetts Male Aging Study. *J Clin Endocrinol Metab*. 2004;89:5920-5926.
177. Wu FC, Tajar A, Beynon JM, et al. Identification of late-onset hypogonadism in middle-aged and elderly men. *N Engl J Med*. 2010;363:123-135.
178. Mulligan T, Frick MF, Zuraw QC, et al. Prevalence of hypogonadism in males aged at least 45 years: the HIM study. *Int J Clin Pract*. 2006;60:762-769.
179. Grossmann M, Zajac JD. Androgen deprivation therapy in men with prostate cancer: how should the side effects be monitored and treated? *Clin Endocrinol (Oxf)*. 2010, Nov 30 (Epub ahead of print).
180. Moreau JP, Delavault P, Blumberg J. Luteinizing hormone-releasing hormone agonists in the treatment of prostate cancer: a review of their discovery, development, and place in therapy. *Clin Ther*. 2006;28:1485-1508.
181. Pincus SM, Mulligan T, Iranmanesh A, et al. Older males secrete luteinizing hormone and testosterone more irregularly, and jointly more asynchronously, than younger males. *Proc Natl Acad Sci U S A*. 1996;93:14100-14105.
182. Brambilla DJ, Matsumoto AM, Araujo AB, et al. The effect of diurnal variation on clinical measurement of serum testosterone and other sex hormone levels in men. *J Clin Endocrinol Metab*. 2009;94:907-913.
183. Swerdloff RS, Wang C, Cunningham G, et al. Long-term pharmacokinetics of transdermal testosterone gel in hypogonadal men. *J Clin Endocrinol Metab*. 2000;85:4500-4510.
184. Brambilla DJ, O'Donnell AB, Matsumoto AM, et al. Intraindividual variation in levels of serum testosterone and other reproductive and adrenal hormones in men. *Clin Endocrinol (Oxf)*. 2007;67:853-862.
185. Wang C, Catlin DH, Demers LM, et al. Measurement of total serum testosterone in adult men: comparison of current laboratory methods versus liquid chromatography-tandem mass spectrometry. *J Clin Endocrinol Metab*. 2004;89:534-543.
186. Rosner W, Vesper H. Toward excellence in testosterone testing: a consensus statement. *J Clin Endocrinol Metab*. 2010;95:4542-4548.
187. Swerdloff RS, Wang C. Free testosterone measurement by the analog displacement direct assay: old concerns and new evidence. *Clin Chem*. 2008;54:458-460.
188. Vermeulen A, Verdonck L, Kaufman JM. A critical evaluation of simple methods for the estimation of free testosterone in serum. *J Clin Endocrinol Metab*. 1999;84:3666-3672.
189. Winters SJ, Kelley DE, Goodpaster B. The analog free testosterone assay: are the results in men clinically useful? *Clin Chem*. 1998;44:2178-2182.
190. Ly LP, Sartorius G, Hull L, et al. Accuracy of calculated free testosterone formulae in men. *Clin Endocrinol (Oxf)*. 2010;73:382-388.
191. Guzick DS, Overstreet JW, Factor-Litvak P, et al. Sperm morphology, motility, and concentration in fertile and infertile men. *N Engl J Med*. 2001;345:1388-1393.

192. Citron JT, Ettinger B, Rubinoff H, et al. Prevalence of hypothalamic-pituitary imaging abnormalities in impotent men with secondary hypogonadism. *J Urol*. 1996;155:529-533.
193. Dobs AS, El-Deiry S, Wand G, et al. Central hypogonadism: distinguishing idiopathic low testosterone from pituitary tumors. *Endocr Pract*. 1998;4:355-359.
194. Bojesen A, Gravholt CH. Klinefelter syndrome in clinical practice. *Nat Clin Pract Urol*. 2007;4:192-204.
195. Lanfranco F, Kamischke A, Zitzmann M, et al. Klinefelter's syndrome. *Lancet*. 2004;364:273-283.
196. Smyth CM, Bremner WJ. Klinefelter syndrome. *Arch Intern Med*. 1998;158:1309-1314.
197. Zeger MP, Zinn AR, Lahlou N, et al. Effect of ascertainment and genetic features on the phenotype of Klinefelter syndrome. *J Pediatr*. 2008;152:716-722.
198. Boisen E. Testicular size and shape of 47,XYY and 47,XXY men in a double-blind, double-matched population survey. *Am J Hum Genet*. 1979;31:697-703.
199. Okada H, Fujioka H, Tatsumi N, et al. Klinefelter's syndrome in the male infertility clinic. *Hum Reprod*. 1999;14:946-952.
200. Vorona E, Zitzmann M, Gromoll J, et al. Clinical, endocrinological, and epigenetic features of the 46,XX male syndrome, compared with 47,XXY Klinefelter patients. *J Clin Endocrinol Metab*. 2007;92:3458-3465.
201. Brinton LA, Carreon JD, Gierach GL, et al. Etiologic factors for male breast cancer in the U.S. Veterans Affairs medical care system database. *Breast Cancer Res Treat*. 2010;119:185-192.
202. Bojesen A, Juul S, Birkebaek N, et al. Increased mortality in Klinefelter syndrome. *J Clin Endocrinol Metab*. 2004;89:3830-3834.
203. Swerdlow AJ, Higgins CD, Schoemaker MJ, et al. Mortality in patients with Klinefelter syndrome in Britain: a cohort study. *J Clin Endocrinol Metab*. 2005;90:6516-6522.
204. Turner C, Hilton-Jones D. The myotonic dystrophies: diagnosis and management. *J Neurol Neurosurg Psychiatry*. 2010;81:358-367.
205. Al-Harbi TM, Bainbridge LJ, McQueen MJ, et al. Hypogonadism is common in men with myopathies. *J Clin Neuromuscul Dis*. 2008;9:397-401.
206. Vazquez JA, Pinies JA, Martul P, et al. Hypothalamic-pituitary-testicular function in 70 patients with myotonic dystrophy. *J Endocrinol Invest*. 1990;13:375-379.
207. Griggs RC, Pandya S, Florence JM, et al. Randomized controlled trial of testosterone in myotonic dystrophy. *Neurology*. 1989;39:219-222.
208. Ashley RA, Barthold JS, Kolon TF. Cryptorchidism: pathogenesis, diagnosis, treatment and prognosis. *Urol Clin North Am*. 2010;37:183-193.
209. Hutson JM, Balic A, Nation T, et al. Cryptorchidism. *Semin Pediatr Surg*. 2010;19:215-224.
210. Mathers MJ, Sperling H, Rubben H, et al. The undescended testis: diagnosis, treatment and long-term consequences. *Dtsch Arztebl Int*. 2009;106:527-532.
211. Virtanen HE, Bjerknes R, Cortes D, et al. Cryptorchidism: classification, prevalence and long-term consequences. *Acta Paediatr*. 2007;96:611-616.
212. Atkinson PM, Epstein MT, Rippon AE. Plasma gonadotropins and androgens in surgically treated cryptorchid patients. *J Pediatr Surg*. 1975;10:27-33.
213. Lee PA, Coughlin MT. Leydig cell function after cryptorchidism: evidence of the beneficial result of early surgery. *J Urol*. 2002;167:1824-1827.
214. Allanson JE. Noonan syndrome. *Am J Med Genet C Semin Med Genet*. 2007;145C:274-279.
215. Romano AA, Allanson JE, Dahlgren J, et al. Noonan syndrome: clinical features, diagnosis, and management guidelines. *Pediatrics*. 2010;126:746-759.
216. Kelnar CJ. Noonan syndrome: the hypothalamo-adrenal and hypothalamo-gonadal axes. *Horm Res*. 2009;72(suppl 2):24-30.
217. Aynsley-Green A, Zachmann M, Illig R, et al. Congenital bilateral anorchia in childhood: a clinical, endocrine and therapeutic evaluation of twenty-one cases. *Clin Endocrinol (Oxf)*. 1976;5:381-391.
218. Zenaty D, Dijoud F, Morel Y, et al. Bilateral anorchia in infancy: occurence of micropenis and the effect of testosterone treatment. *J Pediatr*. 2006;149:687-691.
219. McEachern R, Houle AM, Garel L, et al. Lost and found testes: the importance of the hCG stimulation test and other testicular markers to confirm a surgical declaration of anorchia. *Horm Res*. 2004;62:124-128.
220. Lee MM, Donahoe PK, Silverman BL, et al. Measurements of serum mullerian inhibiting substance in the evaluation of children with nonpalpable gonads. *N Engl J Med*. 1997;336:1480-1486.
221. Husebye ES, Perheentupa J, Rautemaa R, et al. Clinical manifestations and management of patients with autoimmune polyendocrine syndrome type I. *J Intern Med*. 2009;265:514-529.
222. Falorni A, Laureti S, Santeusanio F. Autoantibodies in autoimmune polyendocrine syndrome type II. *Endocrinol Metab Clin North Am*. 2002;31:369-389, vii.
223. Yanase T. 17 alpha-Hydroxylase/17,20-lyase defects. *J Steroid Biochem Mol Biol*. 1995;53:153-157.
224. Sherbet DP, Tiosano D, Kwist KM, et al. CYP17 mutation E305G causes isolated 17,20-lyase deficiency by selectively altering substrate binding. *J Biol Chem*. 2003;278:48563-48569.
225. Faienza MF, Giordani L, Delvecchio M, et al. Clinical, endocrine, and molecular findings in 17beta-hydroxysteroid dehydrogenase type 3 deficiency. *J Endocrinol Invest*. 2008;31:85-91.
226. Pang S. Congenital adrenal hyperplasia owing to 3 beta-hydroxysteroid dehydrogenase deficiency. *Endocrinol Metab Clin North Am*. 2001;30:81-99, vi-vii.
227. Cavanah SF, Dons RF. Partial 3 beta-hydroxysteroid dehydrogenase deficiency presenting as new-onset gynecomastia in a eugonadal adult male. *Metabolism*. 1993;42:65-68.
228. Cabrera MS, Vogiatzi MG, New MI. Long term outcome in adult males with classic congenital adrenal hyperplasia. *J Clin Endocrinol Metab*. 2001;86:3070-3078.
229. Claahsen-van der Grinten HL, Otten BJ, Stikkelbroeck MM, et al. Testicular adrenal rest tumours in congenital adrenal hyperplasia. *Best Pract Res Clin Endocrinol Metab*. 2009;23:209-220.
230. Stikkelbroeck NM, Otten BJ, Pasic A, et al. High prevalence of testicular adrenal rest tumors, impaired spermatogenesis, and Leydig cell failure in adolescent and adult males with congenital adrenal hyperplasia. *J Clin Endocrinol Metab*. 2001;86:5721-5728.
231. Rimoin DL, Conner JM, Pyeritz RE, et al. *Principles and Practice of Medical Genetics*. Philadelphia, PA: Elsevier Health Sciences; 2007.
232. Imura H, Nakao Y, Kuzuya H, et al. Clinical, endocrine and metabolic aspects of the Werner syndrome compared with those of normal aging. *Adv Exp Med Biol*. 1985;190:171-185.
233. Lee PA, Danish RK, Mazur T, et al. Micropenis: III. Primary hypogonadism, partial androgen insensitivity syndrome, and idiopathic disorders. *Johns Hopkins Med J*. 1980;147:175-181.
234. Marshall JD, Beck S, Maffei P, et al. Alström syndrome. *Eur J Hum Genet*. 2007;15:1193-1202.
235. Medlej R, Wasson J, Baz P, et al. Diabetes mellitus and optic atrophy: a study of Wolfram syndrome in the Lebanese population. *J Clin Endocrinol Metab*. 2004;89:1656-1661.
236. Molho-Pessach V, Agha Z, Aamar S, et al. The H syndrome: a genodermatosis characterized by indurated, hyperpigmented, and hypertrichotic skin with systemic manifestations. *J Am Acad Dermatol*. 2008;59:79-85.
237. Slavotinek A, Goldman J, Weisiger K, et al. Marinesco-Sjögren syndrome in a male with mild dysmorphism. *Am J Med Genet A*. 2005;133A:197-201.
238. Sohval AR, Soffer LJ. Congenital familial testicular deficiency. *Am J Med*. 1953;14:328-348.
239. Weinstein RL, Kliman B, Scully RE. Familial syndrome of primary testicular insufficiency with normal virilization, blindness, deafness and metabolic abnormalities. *N Engl J Med*. 1969;281:969-977.
240. Werder EA, Murset G, Illig R, et al. Hypogonadism and parathyroid adenoma in congenital poikiloderma (Rothmund-Thomson syndrome). *Clin Endocrinol (Oxf)*. 1975;4:75-82.
241. Zadik Z, Levin S, Prager-Lewin R, et al. Gonadal dysfunction in patients with ataxia telangiectasia. *Acta Paediatr Scand*. 1978;67:477-479.
242. Hirsch HJ, Eldar-Geva T, Benarroch F, et al. Primary testicular dysfunction is a major contributor to abnormal pubertal development in males with Prader-Willi syndrome. *J Clin Endocrinol Metab*. 2009;94:2262-2268.
243. Leroith D, Farkash Y, Bar-Ziev J, et al. Hypothalamic-pituitary function in the Bardet-Biedl syndrome. *Isr J Med Sci*. 1980;16:514-518.
244. Marshall JD, Paisey RB, Carey C, et al. Alström syndrome. In: Pagon RA, Bird TC, Dolan CR, et al., eds. *GeneReviews [Internet]*. 2003 [updated 2010 Jun 08].
245. Hawli Y, Nasrallah M, El-Hajj Fuleihan G. Endocrine and musculoskeletal abnormalities in patients with Down syndrome. *Nat Rev Endocrinol*. 2009;5:327-334.
246. Muller T, Gromoll J, Simoni M. Absence of exon 10 of the human luteinizing hormone (LH) receptor impairs LH, but not human chorionic gonadotropin action. *J Clin Endocrinol Metab*. 2003;88:2242-2249.
247. Feldman D. Ketoconazole and other imidazole derivatives as inhibitors of steroidogenesis. *Endocr Rev*. 1986;7:409-420.
248. Rajfer J, Sikka SC, Rivera F, et al. Mechanism of inhibition of human testicular steroidogenesis by oral ketoconazole. *J Clin Endocrinol Metab*. 1986;63:1193-1198.
249. Loriaux DL, Menard R, Taylor A, et al. Spironolactone and endocrine dysfunction. *Ann Intern Med*. 1976;85:630-636.
250. Adler RA. Clinical review 33: clinically important effects of alcohol on endocrine function. *J Clin Endocrinol Metab*. 1992;74:957-960.
251. Emanuele MA, Emanuele NV. Alcohol's effects on male reproduction. *Alcohol Health Res World*. 1998;22:195-201.
252. Clifton DK, Bremner WJ. The effect of testicular x-irradiation on spermatogenesis in man: a comparison with the mouse. *J Androl*. 1983;4:387-392.

253. Shalet SM, Tsatsoulis A, Whitehead E, et al. Vulnerability of the human Leydig cell to radiation damage is dependent upon age. *J Endocrinol.* 1989;120:161-165.
254. Steffens M, Beauloye V, Brichard B, et al. Endocrine and metabolic disorders in young adult survivors of childhood acute lymphoblastic leukaemia (ALL) or non-Hodgkin lymphoma (NHL). *Clin Endocrinol (Oxf).* 2008;69:819-827.
255. Travis LB, Beard C, Allan JM, et al. Testicular cancer survivorship: research strategies and recommendations. *J Natl Cancer Inst.* 2010;102:1114-1130.
256. Davis NF, McGuire BB, Mahon JA, et al. The increasing incidence of mumps orchitis: a comprehensive review. *BJU Int* 2010, Jan 11 (Epub ahead of print).
257. Ternavasio-de la Vega HG, Boronat M, Ojeda A, et al. Mumps orchitis in the post-vaccine era (1967-2009): a single-center series of 67 patients and review of clinical outcome and trends. *Medicine (Baltimore).* 2010;89:96-116.
258. Hagley M. Epididymo-orchitis and epididymitis: a review of causes and management of unusual forms. *Int J STD AIDS.* 2003;14:372-377; quiz 378.
259. Pudney J, Anderson D. Orchitis and human immunodeficiency virus type 1 infected cells in reproductive tissues from men with the acquired immune deficiency syndrome. *Am J Pathol.* 1991;139:149-160.
260. Trojian TH, Lishnak TS, Heiman D. Epididymitis and orchitis: an overview. *Am Fam Physician.* 2009;79:583-587.
261. Floreani A, Mega A, Tizian L, et al. Bone metabolism and gonad function in male patients undergoing liver transplantation: a two-year longitudinal study. *Osteoporos Int.* 2001;12:749-754.
262. Foresta C, Schipilliti M, Ciarleglio FA, et al. Male hypogonadism in cirrhosis and after liver transplantation. *J Endocrinol Invest.* 2008;31:470-478.
263. Zietz B, Lock G, Plach B, et al. Dysfunction of the hypothalamic-pituitary-glandular axes and relation to Child-Pugh classification in male patients with alcoholic and virus-related cirrhosis. *Eur J Gastroenterol Hepatol.* 2003;15:495-501.
264. Handelsman DJ, Liu PY. Androgen therapy in chronic renal failure. *Baillieres Clin Endocrinol Metab.* 1998;12:485-500.
265. Prem AR, Punekar SV, Kalpana M, et al. Male reproductive function in uraemia: efficacy of haemodialysis and renal transplantation. *Br J Urol.* 1996;78:635-638.
266. Huyghe E, Zairi A, Nohra J, et al. Gonadal impact of target of rapamycin inhibitors (sirolimus and everolimus) in male patients: an overview. *Transpl Int.* 2007;20:305-311.
267. Xu LG, Xu HM, Zhu XF, et al. Examination of the semen quality of patients with uraemia and renal transplant recipients in comparison with a control group. *Andrologia.* 2009;41:235-240.
268. Feldman HA, Longcope C, Derby CA, et al. Age trends in the level of serum testosterone and other hormones in middle-aged men: longitudinal results from the Massachusetts male aging study. *J Clin Endocrinol Metab.* 2002;87:589-598.
269. Harman SM, Metter EJ, Tobin JD, et al. Longitudinal effects of aging on serum total and free testosterone levels in healthy men. Baltimore Longitudinal Study of Aging. *J Clin Endocrinol Metab.* 2001;86:724-731.
270. Morley JE, Kaiser FE, Perry HM 3rd, et al. Longitudinal changes in testosterone, luteinizing hormone, and follicle-stimulating hormone in healthy older men. *Metabolism.* 1997;46:410-413.
271. Mulligan T, Iranmanesh A, Kerzner R, et al. Two-week pulsatile gonadotropin releasing hormone infusion unmasks dual (hypothalamic and Leydig cell) defects in the healthy aging male gonadotropic axis. *Eur J Endocrinol.* 1999;141:257-266.
272. Veldhuis JD, Keenan DM, Liu PY, et al. The aging male hypothalamic-pituitary-gonadal axis: pulsatility and feedback. *Mol Cell Endocrinol.* 2009;299:14-22.
273. Tajar A, Forti G, O'Neill TW, et al. Characteristics of secondary, primary, and compensated hypogonadism in aging men: evidence from the European Male Ageing Study. *J Clin Endocrinol Metab.* 2010;95:1810-1818.
274. Wu FC, Tajar A, Pye SR, et al. Hypothalamic-pituitary-testicular axis disruptions in older men are differentially linked to age and modifiable risk factors: the European Male Ageing Study. *J Clin Endocrinol Metab.* 2008;93:2737-2745.
275. Basaria S, Coviello AD, Travison TG, et al. Adverse events associated with testosterone administration. *N Engl J Med.* 2010;363:109-122.
276. Srinivas-Shankar U, Roberts SA, Connolly MJ, et al. Effects of testosterone on muscle strength, physical function, body composition, and quality of life in intermediate-frail and frail elderly men: a randomized, double-blind, placebo-controlled study. *J Clin Endocrinol Metab.* 2010;95:639-650.
277. Wang C, Nieschlag E, Swerdloff R, et al. Investigation, treatment, and monitoring of late-onset hypogonadism in males: ISA, ISSAM, EAU, EAA, and ASA recommendations. *J Androl.* 2009;30:1-9.
278. Petersen PM, Giwercman A, Skakkebaek NE, et al. Gonadal function in men with testicular cancer. *Semin Oncol.* 1998;25:224-233.
279. Vigersky RA, Chapman RM, Berenberg J, et al. Testicular dysfunction in untreated Hodgkin's disease. *Am J Med.* 1982;73:482-486.
280. Viviani S, Ragni G, Santoro A, et al. Testicular dysfunction in Hodgkin's disease before and after treatment. *Eur J Cancer.* 1991;27:1389-1392.
281. Abbasi AA, Prasad AS, Ortega J, et al. Gonadal function abnormalities in sickle cell anemia: studies in adult male patients. *Ann Intern Med.* 1976;85:601-605.
282. Brachet C, Heinrichs C, Tenoutasse S, et al. Children with sickle cell disease: growth and gonadal function after hematopoietic stem cell transplantation. *J Pediatr Hematol Oncol.* 2007;29:445-450.
283. Parshad O, Stevens MC, Preece MA, et al. The mechanism of low testosterone levels in homozygous sickle-cell disease. *West Indian Med J.* 1994;43:12-14.
284. Celik B, Sahin A, Caglar N, et al. Sex hormone levels and functional outcomes: a controlled study of patients with spinal cord injury compared with healthy subjects. *Am J Phys Med Rehabil.* 2007;86:784-790.
285. Kostovski E, Iversen PO, Birkeland K, et al. Decreased levels of testosterone and gonadotrophins in men with long-standing tetraplegia. *Spinal Cord.* 2008;46:559-564.
286. Naderi AR, Safarinejad MR. Endocrine profiles and semen quality in spinal cord injured men. *Clin Endocrinol (Oxf).* 2003;58:177-184.
287. Elliott SP, Orejuela F, Hirsch IH, et al. Testis biopsy findings in the spinal cord injured patient. *J Urol.* 2000;163:792-795.
288. Richter JG, Becker A, Specker C, et al. Hypogonadism in Wegener's granulomatosis. *Scand J Rheumatol.* 2008;37:365-369.
289. Scalvini T, Martini PR, Obici L, et al. Infertility and hypergonadotropic hypogonadism as first evidence of hereditary apolipoprotein A-I amyloidosis. *J Urol.* 2007;178:344-348.
290. Biyani CS, Cartledge J, Janetschek G. Varicocele. *Clin Evid (Online)* 2009 Jan 6.
291. Kim HH, Goldstein M. Adult varicocele. *Curr Opin Urol.* 2008;18:608-612.
292. Nistal M, Jimenez F, Paniagua R. Sertoli cell types in the Sertoli-cell-only syndrome: relationships between Sertoli cell morphology and aetiology. *Histopathology.* 1990;16:173-180.
293. Micic S, Ilic V, Micic M, et al. Endocrine profile of 45 patients with Sertoli cell only syndrome. *Andrologia.* 1983;15:228-232.
294. Kamp C, Huellen K, Fernandes S, et al. High deletion frequency of the complete AZFa sequence in men with Sertoli-cell-only syndrome. *Mol Hum Reprod.* 2001;7:987-994.
295. Storm van's Gravesande K, Omran H. Primary ciliary dyskinesia: clinical presentation, diagnosis and genetics. *Ann Med.* 2005;37:439-449.
296. Brydoy M, Fossa SD, Dahl O, et al. Gonadal dysfunction and fertility problems in cancer survivors. *Acta Oncol.* 2007;46:480-489.
297. Kiserud CE, Fossa A, Bjoro T, et al. Gonadal function in male patients after treatment for malignant lymphomas, with emphasis on chemotherapy. *Br J Cancer.* 2009;100:455-463.
298. Grunewald S, Paasch U, Glander HJ. Systemic dermatological treatment with relevance for male fertility. *J Dtsch Dermatol Ges.* 2007;5:15-21.
299. Jung A, Schuppe HC. Influence of genital heat stress on semen quality in humans. *Andrologia.* 2007;39:203-215.
300. Wang C, Cui YG, Wang XH, et al. transient scrotal hyperthermia and levonorgestrel enhance testosterone-induced spermatogenesis suppression in men through increased germ cell apoptosis. *J Clin Endocrinol Metab.* 2007;92:3292-3304.
301. Diamanti-Kandarakis E, Bourguignon JP, Giudice LC, et al. Endocrine-disrupting chemicals: an Endocrine Society scientific statement. *Endocr Rev.* 2009;30:293-342.
302. Yiee JH, Baskin LS. Environmental factors in genitourinary development. *J Urol.* 2010;184:34-41.
303. Ambler GR. Androgen therapy for delayed male puberty. *Curr Opin Endocrinol Diabetes Obes.* 2009;16:232-239.
304. Traggiai C, Stanhope R. Delayed puberty. *Best Pract Res Clin Endocrinol Metab.* 2002;16:139-151.
305. Waldstreicher J, Seminara SB, Jameson JL, et al. The genetic and clinical heterogeneity of gonadotropin-releasing hormone deficiency in the human. *J Clin Endocrinol Metab.* 1996;81:4388-4395.
306. Raivio T, Falardeau J, Dwyer A, et al. Reversal of idiopathic hypogonadotropic hypogonadism. *N Engl J Med.* 2007;357:863-873.
307. Clark P, Britton LJ, Powell LW. The diagnosis and management of hereditary haemochromatosis. *Clin Biochem Rev.* 2010;31:3-8.
308. Pietrangelo A. Hemochromatosis: an endocrine liver disease. *Hepatology.* 2007;46:1291-1301.
309. McDermott JH, Walsh CH. Hypogonadism in hereditary hemochromatosis. *J Clin Endocrinol Metab.* 2005;90:2451-2455.
310. Pallais JC, Au M, Pitteloud N, et al. Isolated gonadotropin-releasing hormone (GnRH) deficiency overview. In: Pagon RA, Bird TC, Dolan CR, et al., eds. *GeneReviews [Internet].* 2007 [updated 2010 Oct 14].
311. Dwyer AA, Hayes FJ, Plummer L, et al. The long-term clinical follow-up and natural history of men with adult-onset idiopathic hypogonadotropic hypogonadism. *J Clin Endocrinol Metab.* 2010;95:4235-4243.

312. Pallais JC, Au M, Pitteloud N, et al. Kallmann syndrome. In: Pagon RA, Bird TC, Dolan CR, et al., eds. *GeneReviews [Internet]*. 2007 [updated 2011 Jan 04].
313. Semple RK, Topaloglu AK. The recent genetics of hypogonadotrophic hypogonadism: novel insights and new questions. *Clin Endocrinol (Oxf)*. 2010;72:427-435.
314. Jongmans MC, van Ravenswaaij-Arts CM, Pitteloud N, et al. CHD7 mutations in patients initially diagnosed with Kallmann syndrome: the clinical overlap with CHARGE syndrome. *Clin Genet.* 2009;75:65-71.
315. Zentner GE, Layman WS, Martin DM, et al. Molecular and phenotypic aspects of CHD7 mutation in CHARGE syndrome. *Am J Med Genet A.* 2010;152A:674-686.
316. Burger HG, de Kretser DM, Hudson B, et al. Effects of preceding androgen therapy on testicular response to human pituitary gonadotropin in hypogonadotropic hypogonadism: a study of three patients. *Fertil Steril.* 1981;35:64-68.
317. Ley SB, Leonard JM. Male hypogonadotropic hypogonadism: factors influencing response to human chorionic gonadotropin and human menopausal gonadotropin, including prior exogenous androgens. *J Clin Endocrinol Metab.* 1985;61:746-752.
318. Pitteloud N, Hayes FJ, Dwyer A, et al. Predictors of outcome of long-term GnRH therapy in men with idiopathic hypogonadotropic hypogonadism. *J Clin Endocrinol Metab.* 2002;87:4128-4136.
319. Sykiotis GP, Hoang XH, Avbelj M, et al. Congenital idiopathic hypogonadotropic hypogonadism: evidence of defects in the hypothalamus, pituitary, and testes. *J Clin Endocrinol Metab.* 2010;95:3019-3027.
320. Pitteloud N, Boepple PA, DeCruz S, et al. The fertile eunuch variant of idiopathic hypogonadotropic hypogonadism: spontaneous reversal associated with a homozygous mutation in the gonadotropin-releasing hormone receptor. *J Clin Endocrinol Metab.* 2001;86: 2470-2475.
321. Shiraishi K, Naito K. Fertile eunuch syndrome with the mutations (Trp8Arg and Ile15Thr) in the beta subunit of luteinizing hormone. *Endocr J.* 2003;50:733-737.
322. Smals AG, Kloppenborg PW, van Haelst UJ, et al. Fertile eunuch syndrome versus classic hypogonadotrophic hypogonadism. *Acta Endocrinol (Copenh).* 1978;87:389-399.
323. Giltay JC, Deege M, Blankenstein RA, et al. Apparent primary follicle-stimulating hormone deficiency is a rare cause of treatable male infertility. *Fertil Steril.* 2004;81:693-696.
324. Mantovani G, Borgato S, Beck-Peccoz P, et al. Isolated follicle-stimulating hormone (FSH) deficiency in a young man with normal virilization who did not have mutations in the FSHbeta gene. *Fertil Steril.* 2003;79:434-436.
325. Murao K, Imachi H, Muraoka T, et al. Isolated follicle-stimulating hormone (FSH) deficiency without mutation of the FSHbeta gene and successful treatment with human menopausal gonadotropin. *Fertil Steril.* 2008;90:2012 e17-e39.
326. Bhagavath B, Layman LC. The genetics of hypogonadotropic hypogonadism. *Semin Reprod Med.* 2007;25:272-286.
327. Lofrano-Porto A, Barra GB, Giacomini LA, et al. Luteinizing hormone beta mutation and hypogonadism in men and women. *N Engl J Med.* 2007;357:897-904.
328. Carter MT, Picketts DJ, Hunter AG, et al. Further clinical delineation of the Borjeson-Forssman-Lehmann syndrome in patients with PHF6 mutations. *Am J Med Genet A.* 2009;149A:246-250.
329. Chudley AE, Lowry RB, Hoar DI. Mental retardation, distinct facial changes, short stature, obesity, and hypogonadism: a new X-linked mental retardation syndrome. *Am J Med Genet.* 1988;31:741-751.
330. Ehara H, Utsunomiya Y, Ieshima A, et al. Martsolf syndrome in Japanese siblings. *Am J Med Genet A.* 2007;143A:973-978.
331. Graham JM Jr, Lee J. Bosma arhinia microphthalmia syndrome. *Am J Med Genet A.* 2006;140:189-193.
332. Johnson VP, McMillin JM, Aceto T Jr, et al. A newly recognized neuroectodermal syndrome of familial alopecia, anosmia, deafness, and hypogonadism. *Am J Med Genet.* 1983;15:497-506.
333. Lopez de Lara D, Cruz-Rojo J, Sanchez del Pozo J, et al. Moebius-Poland syndrome and hypogonadotropic hypogonadism. *Eur J Pediatr.* 2008;167:353-354.
334. Miller JL, Goldstone AP, Couch JA, et al. Pituitary abnormalities in Prader-Willi syndrome and early onset morbid obesity. *Am J Med Genet A.* 2008;146A:570-577.
335. Robertson SP, Rodda C, Bankier A. Hypogonadotrophic hypogonadism in Roifman syndrome. *Clin Genet.* 2000;57:435-438.
336. Robin G, Jonard S, Vuillaume I, et al. [Hypogonadotropic hypogonadism discovered in a patient with cerebellar ataxia]. *Ann Endocrinol (Paris).* 2005;66:545-551.
337. Saugier-Veber P, Abadie V, Moncla A, et al. The Juberg-Marsidi syndrome maps to the proximal long arm of the X chromosome (Xq12-q21). *Am J Hum Genet.* 1993;52:1040-1045.
338. Selvaag E. Pili torti and sensorineural hearing loss: a follow-up of Bjornstad's original patients and a review of the literature. *Eur J Dermatol.* 2000;10:91-97.
339. Stoll C, Eyer D. A syndrome of congenital ichthyosis, hypogonadism, small stature, facial dysmorphism, scoliosis and myogenic dystrophy. *Ann Genet.* 1999;42:45-50.
340. Waters AM, Beales PL. Bardet-Biedl Syndrome. In: Pagon RA, Bird TC, Dolan CR, et al., eds. *GeneReviews [Internet]*. 2003 [updated 2010 Nov 18].
341. White SM, Graham JM Jr, Kerr B, et al. The adult phenotype in Costello syndrome. *Am J Med Genet A.* 2005;136:128-135.
342. Woodhouse NJ, Sakati NA. A syndrome of hypogonadism, alopecia, diabetes mellitus, mental retardation, deafness, and ECG abnormalities. *J Med Genet.* 1983;20:216-219.
343. Swanson SL, Santen RJ, Smith DW. Multiple lentigines syndrome: new findings of hypogonadotrophism, hyposmia, and unilateral renal agenesis. *J Pediatr.* 1971;78:1037-1039.
344. Chahal J, Schlechte J. Hyperprolactinemia. *Pituitary.* 2008;11: 141-146.
345. Bouchard P, Lagoguey M, Brailly S, et al. Gonadotropin-releasing hormone pulsatile administration restores luteinizing hormone pulsatility and normal testosterone levels in males with hyperprolactinemia. *J Clin Endocrinol Metab.* 1985;60:258-262.
346. Casanueva FF, Molitch ME, Schlechte JA, et al. Guidelines of the Pituitary Society for the diagnosis and management of prolactinomas. *Clin Endocrinol (Oxf).* 2006;65:265-273.
347. Klibanski A. Clinical practice: prolactinomas. *N Engl J Med.* 2010;362:1219-1226.
348. Frieze TW, Mong DP, Koops MK. "Hook effect" in prolactinomas: case report and review of literature. *Endocr Pract.* 2002;8:296-303.
349. Madhusoodanan S, Parida S, Jimenez C. Hyperprolactinemia associated with psychotropics: a review. *Hum Psychopharmacol.* 2010;25:281-297.
350. Molitch ME. Medication-induced hyperprolactinemia. *Mayo Clin Proc.* 2005;80:1050-1057.
351. Colao A, Di Sarno A, Guerra E, et al. Drug insight: cabergoline and bromocriptine in the treatment of hyperprolactinemia in men and women. *Nat Clin Pract Endocrinol Metab.* 2006;2:200-210.
352. Molitch ME. Pharmacologic resistance in prolactinoma patients. *Pituitary.* 2005;8:43-52.
353. Mendelson JH, Mendelson JE, Patch VD. Plasma testosterone levels in heroin addiction and during methadone maintenance. *J Pharmacol Exp Ther.* 1975;192:211-217.
354. Abs R, Verhelst J, Maeyaert J, et al. Endocrine consequences of long-term intrathecal administration of opioids. *J Clin Endocrinol Metab.* 2000;85:2215-2222.
355. Hallinan R, Byrne A, Agho K, et al. Hypogonadism in men receiving methadone and buprenorphine maintenance treatment. *Int J Androl.* 2009;32:131-139.
356. Veldhuis JD, Rogol AD, Samojlik E, et al. Role of endogenous opiates in the expression of negative feedback actions of androgen and estrogen on pulsatile properties of luteinizing hormone secretion in man. *J Clin Invest.* 1984;74:47-55.
357. Ragni G, De Lauretis L, Bestetti O, et al. Gonadal function in male heroin and methadone addicts. *Int J Androl.* 1988;11:93-100.
358. Agirregoitia E, Valdivia A, Carracedo A, et al. Expression and localization of delta-, kappa-, and mu-opioid receptors in human spermatozoa and implications for sperm motility. *J Clin Endocrinol Metab.* 2006;91:4969-4975.
359. Kanayama G, Brower KJ, Wood RI, et al. Anabolic-androgenic steroid dependence: an emerging disorder. *Addiction.* 2009;104:1966-1978.
360. van Amsterdam J, Opperhuizen A, Hartgens F. Adverse health effects of anabolic-androgenic steroids. *Regul Toxicol Pharmacol.* 2010;57: 117-123.
361. Tan RS, Vasudevan D. Use of clomiphene citrate to reverse premature andropause secondary to steroid abuse. *Fertil Steril.* 2003;79:203-205.
362. Dev R, Del Fabbro E, Bruera E. Association between megestrol acetate treatment and symptomatic adrenal insufficiency with hypogonadism in male patients with cancer. *Cancer.* 2007;110:1173-1177.
363. Oster MH, Enders SR, Samuels SJ, et al. Megestrol acetate in patients with AIDS and cachexia. *Ann Intern Med.* 1994;121:400-408.
364. Venner P. Megestrol acetate in the treatment of metastatic carcinoma of the prostate. *Oncology.* 1992;49(suppl 2):22-27.
365. Briken P, Kafka MP. Pharmacological treatments for paraphilic patients and sexual offenders. *Curr Opin Psychiatry.* 2007;20:609-613.
366. Aggarwal R, Weinberg V, Small EJ, et al. The mechanism of action of estrogen in castration-resistant prostate cancer: clues from hormone levels. *Clin Genitourin Cancer.* 2009;7:E71-E76.
367. Finkelstein JS, McCully WF, MacLaughlin DT, et al. The mortician's mystery: gynecomastia and reversible hypogonadotropic hypogonadism in an embalmer. *N Engl J Med.* 1988;318:961-965.
368. Mineur P, De Cooman S, Hustin J, et al. Feminizing testicular Leydig cell tumor: hormonal profile before and after unilateral orchidectomy. *J Clin Endocrinol Metab.* 1987;64:686-691.
369. Herbst KL. Gonadotropin-releasing hormone antagonists. *Curr Opin Pharmacol.* 2003;3:660-666.
370. Oh WK, Landrum MB, Lamont EB, et al. Does oral antiandrogen use before leuteinizing hormone-releasing hormone therapy in patients

with metastatic prostate cancer prevent clinical consequences of a testosterone flare? *Urology*. 2010;75:642-647.

371. Bong GW, Clarke HS Jr, Hancock WC, et al. Serum testosterone recovery after cessation of long-term luteinizing hormone-releasing hormone agonist in patients with prostate cancer. *Urology*. 2008;71:1177-1180.
372. Kaku H, Saika T, Tsushima T, et al. Time course of serum testosterone and luteinizing hormone levels after cessation of long-term luteinizing hormone-releasing hormone agonist treatment in patients with prostate cancer. *Prostate*. 2006;66:439-444.
373. Keating NL, O'Malley AJ, Freedland SJ, et al. Diabetes and cardiovascular disease during androgen deprivation therapy: observational study of veterans with prostate cancer. *J Natl Cancer Inst*. 2010;102:39-46.
374. Keating NL, O'Malley AJ, Smith MR. Diabetes and cardiovascular disease during androgen deprivation therapy for prostate cancer. *J Clin Oncol*. 2006;24:4448-4456.
375. Prabhakar VK, Shalet SM. Aetiology, diagnosis, and management of hypopituitarism in adult life. *Postgrad Med J*. 2006;82:259-266.
376. Schneider HJ, Aimaretti G, Kreitschmann-Andermahr I, et al. Hypopituitarism. *Lancet*. 2007;369:1461-1470.
377. Rupp D, Molitch M. Pituitary stalk lesions. *Curr Opin Endocrinol Diabetes Obes*. 2008;15:339-345.
378. Luton JP, Thieblot P, Valcke JC, et al. Reversible gonadotropin deficiency in male Cushing's disease. *J Clin Endocrinol Metab*. 1977;45:488-495.
379. MacAdams MR, White RH, Chipps BE. Reduction of serum testosterone levels during chronic glucocorticoid therapy. *Ann Intern Med*. 1986;104:648-651.
380. McKenna TJ, Lorber D, Lacroix A, et al. Testicular activity in Cushing's disease. *Acta Endocrinol (Copenh)*. 1979;91:501-510.
381. Reid IR, Ibbertson HK, France JT, et al. Plasma testosterone concentrations in asthmatic men treated with glucocorticoids. *Br Med J (Clin Res Ed)*. 1985;291:574.
382. Crawford BA, Liu PY, Kean MT, et al. Randomized placebo-controlled trial of androgen effects on muscle and bone in men requiring long-term systemic glucocorticoid treatment. *J Clin Endocrinol Metab*. 2003;88:3167-3176.
383. Bannister P, Handley T, Chapman C, et al. Hypogonadism in chronic liver disease: impaired release of luteinising hormone. *Br Med J (Clin Res Ed)*. 1986;293:1191-1193.
384. Veldhuis JD, Wilkowski MJ, Zwart AD, et al. Evidence for attenuation of hypothalamic gonadotropin-releasing hormone (GnRH) impulse strength with preservation of GnRH pulse frequency in men with chronic renal failure. *J Clin Endocrinol Metab*. 1993;76:648-654.
385. Svartberg J. Androgens and chronic obstructive pulmonary disease. *Curr Opin Endocrinol Diabetes Obes*. 2010;17:257-261.
386. Laghi F, Antonescu-Turcu A, Collins E, et al. Hypogonadism in men with chronic obstructive pulmonary disease: prevalence and quality of life. *Am J Respir Crit Care Med*. 2005;171:728-733.
387. Semple PD, Beastall GH, Brown TM, et al. Sex hormone suppression and sexual impotence in hypoxic pulmonary fibrosis. *Thorax*. 1984;39:46-51.
388. Iellamo F, Rosano G, Volterrani M. Testosterone deficiency and exercise intolerance in heart failure: treatment implications. *Curr Heart Fail Rep*. 2010;7:59-65.
389. Jankowska EA, Biel B, Majda J, et al. Anabolic deficiency in men with chronic heart failure: prevalence and detrimental impact on survival. *Circulation*. 2006;114:1829-1837.
390. Malkin CJ, Channer KS, Jones TH. Testosterone and heart failure. *Curr Opin Endocrinol Diabetes Obes*. 2010;17:262-268.
391. Dhindsa S, Miller MG, McWhirter CL, et al. Testosterone concentrations in diabetic and nondiabetic obese men. *Diabetes Care*. 2010;33:1186-1192.
392. Grossmann M, Gianatti EJ, Zajac JD. Testosterone and type 2 diabetes. *Curr Opin Endocrinol Diabetes Obes*. 2010;17:247-256.
393. Lopez-Alvarenga JC, Zarinan T, Olivares A, et al. Poorly controlled type I diabetes mellitus in young men selectively suppresses luteinizing hormone secretory burst mass. *J Clin Endocrinol Metab*. 2002;87:5507-5515.
394. Chlebowski RT, Heber D. Hypogonadism in male patients with metastatic cancer prior to chemotherapy. *Cancer Res*. 1982;42:2495-2498.
395. Fleishman SB, Khan H, Homel P, et al. Testosterone levels and quality of life in diverse male patients with cancers unrelated to androgens. *J Clin Oncol*. 2010;28:5054-5060.
396. Vigano A, Piccioni M, Trutschnigg B, et al. Male hypogonadism associated with advanced cancer: a systematic review. *Lancet Oncol*. 2010;11:679-684.
397. Tengstrand B, Carlstrom K, Hafstrom I. Bioavailable testosterone in men with rheumatoid arthritis–high frequency of hypogonadism. *Rheumatology (Oxford)*. 2002;41:285-289.
398. Tengstrand B, Carlstrom K, Hafstrom I. Gonadal hormones in men with rheumatoid arthritis: from onset through 2 years. *J Rheumatol*. 2009;36:887-892.
399. Straub RH, Harle P, Atzeni F, et al. Sex hormone concentrations in patients with rheumatoid arthritis are not normalized during 12 weeks of anti-tumor necrosis factor therapy. *J Rheumatol*. 2005;32:1253-1258.
400. Hall GM, Larbre JP, Spector TD, et al. A randomized trial of testosterone therapy in males with rheumatoid arthritis. *Br J Rheumatol*. 1996;35:568-573.
401. Koller MD, Templ E, Riedl M, et al. Pituitary function in patients with newly diagnosed untreated systemic lupus erythematosus. *Ann Rheum Dis*. 2004;63:1677-1680.
402. Mok CC, Lau CS. Profile of sex hormones in male patients with systemic lupus erythematosus. *Lupus*. 2000;9:252-257.
403. Vilarinho ST, Costallat LT. Evaluation of the hypothalamic-pituitary-gonadal axis in males with systemic lupus erythematosus. *J Rheumatol*. 1998;25:1097-1103.
404. Jimenez-Balderas FJ, Tapia-Serrano R, Fonseca ME, et al. High frequency of association of rheumatic/autoimmune diseases and untreated male hypogonadism with severe testicular dysfunction. *Arthritis Res*. 2001;3:362-367.
405. McCombe PA, Greer JM, Mackay IR. Sexual dimorphism in autoimmune disease. *Curr Mol Med*. 2009;9:1058-1079.
406. Crum NF, Furtek KJ, Olson PE, et al. A review of hypogonadism and erectile dysfunction among HIV-infected men during the pre- and post-HAART eras: diagnosis, pathogenesis, and management. *AIDS Patient Care STDs*. 2005;19:655-671.
407. Lo JC, Schambelan M. Reproductive function in human immunodeficiency virus infection. *J Clin Endocrinol Metab*. 2001;86:2338-2343.
408. Moreno-Perez O, Escoin C, Serna-Candel C, et al. The determination of total testosterone and free testosterone (RIA) are not applicable to the evaluation of gonadal function in HIV-infected males. *J Sex Med* 2010, Jul 7 (Epub ahead of print).
409. Wunder DM, Bersinger NA, Fux CA, et al. Hypogonadism in HIV-1-infected men is common and does not resolve during antiretroviral therapy. *Antivir Ther*. 2007;12:261-265.
410. Schopp LH, Clark M, Mazurek MO, et al. Testosterone levels among men with spinal cord injury admitted to inpatient rehabilitation. *Am J Phys Med Rehabil*. 2006;85:678-684; quiz 685-687.
411. Ghosh S, Bandyopadhyay SK, Bandyopadhyay R, et al. A study on endocrine dysfunction in thalassaemia. *J Indian Med Assoc*. 2008;106:655-656, 658-659.
412. Safarinejad MR. Evaluation of semen quality, endocrine profile and hypothalamus-pituitary-testis axis in male patients with homozygous beta-thalassemia major. *J Urol*. 2008;179:2327-2332.
413. Soliman AT, Nasr I, Thabet A, et al. Human chorionic gonadotropin therapy in adolescent boys with constitutional delayed puberty vs those with beta-thalassemia major. *Metabolism*. 2005;54:15-23.
414. Wang C, Tso SC, Todd D. Hypogonadotropic hypogonadism in severe beta-thalassemia: effect of chelation and pulsatile gonadotropin-releasing hormone therapy. *J Clin Endocrinol Metab*. 1989;68:511-516.
415. el-Hazmi MA, Bahakim HM, al-Fawaz I. Endocrine functions in sickle cell anaemia patients. *J Trop Pediatr*. 1992;38:307-313.
416. Landefeld CS, Schambelan M, Kaplan SL, Embury SH. Clomiphene-responsive hypogonadism in sickle cell anemia. *Ann Intern Med*. 1983;99:480-483.
417. Modebe O, Ezeh UO. Effect of age on testicular function in adult males with sickle cell anemia. *Fertil Steril*. 1995;63:907-912.
418. Fung EB, Harmatz PR, Lee PD, et al. Increased prevalence of iron-overload associated endocrinopathy in thalassaemia versus sickle-cell disease. *Br J Haematol*. 2006;135:574-582.
419. Slayton W, Kedar A, Schatz D. Testosterone induced priapism in two adolescents with sickle cell disease. *J Pediatr Endocrinol Metab*. 1995;8:199-203.
420. Leifke E, Friemert M, Heilmann M, et al. Sex steroids and body composition in men with cystic fibrosis. *Eur J Endocrinol*. 2003;148:551-557.
421. Friedl KE, Moore RJ, Hoyt RW, et al. Endocrine markers of semistarvation in healthy lean men in a multistressor environment. *J Appl Physiol*. 2000;88:1820-1830.
422. Lado-Abeal J, Prieto D, Lorenzo M, et al. Differences between men and women as regards the effects of protein-energy malnutrition on the hypothalamic-pituitary-gonadal axis. *Nutrition*. 1999;15:351-358.
423. Wabitsch M, Ballauff A, Holl R, et al. Serum leptin, gonadotropin, and testosterone concentrations in male patients with anorexia nervosa during weight gain. *J Clin Endocrinol Metab*. 2001;86:2982-2988.
424. Aloi JA, Bergendahl M, Iranmanesh A, et al. Pulsatile intravenous gonadotropin-releasing hormone administration averts fasting-induced hypogonadotropism and hypoandrogenemia in healthy, normal weight men. *J Clin Endocrinol Metab*. 1997;82:1543-1548.
425. Chan JL, Williams CJ, Raciti P, et al. Leptin does not mediate short-term fasting-induced changes in growth hormone pulsatility but increases IGF-I in leptin deficiency states. *J Clin Endocrinol Metab*. 2008;93:2819-2827.
426. Smith SR, Chhetri MK, Johanson J, et al. The pituitary-gonadal axis in men with protein-calorie malnutrition. *J Clin Endocrinol Metab*. 1975;41:60-69.

427. Hackney AC. Endurance exercise training and reproductive endocrine dysfunction in men: alterations in the hypothalamic-pituitary-testicular axis. *Curr Pharm Des.* 2001;7:261-273.
428. Hackney AC, Fahrner CL, Gulledge TP. Basal reproductive hormonal profiles are altered in endurance trained men. *J Sports Med Phys Fitness.* 1998;38:138-141.
429. Sewani-Rusike CR, Mudambo KS, Tendaupenyu G, et al. Effects of the Zimbabwe Defence Forces training programme on body composition and reproductive hormones in male army recruits. *Cent Afr J Med.* 2000;46:27-31.
430. Arce JC, De Souza MJ. Exercise and male factor infertility. *Sports Med.* 1993;15:146-169.
431. Tremblay MS, Copeland JL, Van Helder W. Effect of training status and exercise mode on endogenous steroid hormones in men. *J Appl Physiol.* 2004;96:531-539.
432. Allan CA, McLachlan RI. Androgens and obesity. *Curr Opin Endocrinol Diabetes Obes.* 2010;17:224-232.
433. Liu PY, Caterson ID, Grunstein RR, et al. Androgens, obesity, and sleep-disordered breathing in men. *Endocrinol Metab Clin North Am.* 2007;36:349-363.
434. Mah PM, Wittert GA. Obesity and testicular function. *Mol Cell Endocrinol.* 2010;316:180-186.
435. Vermeulen A, Kaufman JM, Deslypere JP, et al. Attenuated luteinizing hormone (LH) pulse amplitude but normal LH pulse frequency, and its relation to plasma androgens in hypogonadism of obese men. *J Clin Endocrinol Metab.* 1993;76:1140-1146.
436. Yee B, Liu P, Phillips C, et al. Neuroendocrine changes in sleep apnea. *Curr Opin Pulm Med.* 2004;10:475-481.
437. Matsumoto AM, Sandblom RE, Schoene RB, et al. Testosterone replacement in hypogonadal men: effects on obstructive sleep apnoea, respiratory drives, and sleep. *Clin Endocrinol (Oxf).* 1985;22:713-721.
438. Schneider BK, Pickett CK, Zwillich CW, et al. Influence of testosterone on breathing during sleep. *J Appl Physiol.* 1986;61:618-623.
439. Spratt DI, Cox P, Orav J, et al. Reproductive axis suppression in acute illness is related to disease severity. *J Clin Endocrinol Metab.* 1993;76:1548-1554.
440. Spratt DI, Kramer RS, Morton JR, et al. Characterization of a prospective human model for study of the reproductive hormone responses to major illness. *Am J Physiol Endocrinol Metab.* 2008;295:E63-E69.
441. van den Berghe G, Weekers F, Baxter RC, et al. Five-day pulsatile gonadotropin-releasing hormone administration unveils combined hypothalamic-pituitary-gonadal defects underlying profound hypoandrogenism in men with prolonged critical illness. *J Clin Endocrinol Metab.* 2001;86:3217-3226.
442. Spratt DI, Morton JR, Kramer RS, et al. Increases in serum estrogen levels during major illness are caused by increased peripheral aromatization. *Am J Physiol Endocrinol Metab.* 2006;291:E631-E638.
443. May AK, Dossett LA, Norris PR, et al. Estradiol is associated with mortality in critically ill trauma and surgical patients. *Crit Care Med.* 2008;36:62-68.
444. Reisch N, Flade L, Scherr M, et al. High prevalence of reduced fecundity in men with congenital adrenal hyperplasia. *J Clin Endocrinol Metab.* 2009;94:1665-1670.
445. Lofrano-Porto A, Casulari LA, Nascimento PP, et al. Effects of follicle-stimulating hormone and human chorionic gonadotropin on gonadal steroidogenesis in two siblings with a follicle-stimulating hormone beta subunit mutation. *Fertil Steril.* 2008;90:1169-1174.
446. Matsumoto AM. Effects of chronic testosterone administration in normal men: safety and efficacy of high dosage testosterone and parallel dose-dependent suppression of luteinizing hormone, follicle-stimulating hormone, and sperm production. *J Clin Endocrinol Metab.* 1990;70:282-287.
447. Matsumoto AM, Karpas AE, Bremner WJ. Chronic human chorionic gonadotropin administration in normal men: evidence that follicle-stimulating hormone is necessary for the maintenance of quantitatively normal spermatogenesis in man. *J Clin Endocrinol Metab.* 1986;62:1184-1192.
448. de Bruin D, de Jong IJ, Arts EG, et al. Semen quality in men with disseminated testicular cancer: relation with human chorionic gonadotropin beta-subunit and pituitary gonadal hormones. *Fertil Steril.* 2009;91:2481-2486.
449. Knuth UA, Behre H, Belkien L, et al. Clinical trial of 19-nortestosterone-hexoxyphenylpropionate (Anadur) for male fertility regulation. *Fertil Steril.* 1985;44:814-821.
450. Schurmeyer T, Knuth UA, Belkien L, et al. Reversible azoospermia induced by the anabolic steroid 19-nortestosterone. *Lancet.* 1984;1:417-420.
451. Turek PJ, Williams RH, Gilbaugh JH 3rd, et al. The reversibility of anabolic steroid-induced azoospermia. *J Urol.* 1995;153:1628-1630.
452. Hendry WF, Stedronska J, Jones CR, et al. Semen analysis in testicular cancer and Hodgkin's disease: pre- and post-treatment findings and implications for cryopreservation. *Br J Urol.* 1983;55:769-773.
453. Magelssen H, Brydoy M, Fossa SD. The effects of cancer and cancer treatments on male reproductive function. *Nat Clin Pract Urol.* 2006;3:312-322.
454. Micic S, Dotlic R, Ilic V, et al. Hormone profile in hyperprolactinemic infertile men. *Arch Androl.* 1985;15:123-128.
455. Vandekerckhove P, Lilford R, Vail A, et al. Bromocriptine for idiopathic oligo/asthenospermia. Cochrane Database Syst Rev. 2000;(2):CD000152.
456. Rajender S, Singh L, Thangaraj K. Phenotypic heterogeneity of mutations in androgen receptor gene. *Asian J Androl.* 2007;9:147-179.
457. Werner R, Grotsch H, Hiort O. 46,XY disorders of sex development: the undermasculinised male with disorders of androgen action. *Best Pract Res Clin Endocrinol Metab.* 2010;24:263-277.
458. Hirawat S, Budman DR, Kreis W. The androgen receptor: structure, mutations, and antiandrogens. *Cancer Invest.* 2003;21:400-417.
459. Barradell LB, Faulds D. Cyproterone: a review of its pharmacology and therapeutic efficacy in prostate cancer. *Drugs Aging.* 1994;5:59-80.
460. Doggrell SA, Brown L. The spironolactone renaissance. *Expert Opin Investig Drugs.* 2001;10:943-954.
461. Funder JW, Mercer JE. Cimetidine, a histamine H2 receptor antagonist, occupies androgen receptors. *J Clin Endocrinol Metab.* 1979;48:189-191.
462. Peden NR, Boyd EJ, Browning MC, et al. Effects of two histamine H2-receptor blocking drugs on basal levels of gonadotrophins, prolactin, testosterone and oestradiol-17 beta during treatment of duodenal ulcer in male patients. *Acta Endocrinol (Copenh).* 1981;96:564-568.
463. Purohit V, Ahluwahlia BS, Vigersky RA. Marihuana inhibits dihydrotestosterone binding to the androgen receptor. *Endocrinology.* 1980;107:848-850.
464. Farthing MJ, Edwards CR, Rees LH, et al. Male gonadal function in coeliac disease: 1. Sexual dysfunction, infertility, and semen quality. *Gut.* 1982;23:608-614.
465. Farthing MJ, Rees LH, Dawson AM. Male gonadal function in coeliac disease: III. Pituitary regulation. *Clin Endocrinol (Oxf).* 1983;19:661-671.
466. Green JR, Goble HL, Edwards CR, et al. Reversible insensitivity to androgens in men with untreated gluten enteropathy. *Lancet.* 1977;1:280-282.
467. Matsumoto AM, Bremner WJ. Endocrinology of the hypothalamic-pituitary-testicular axis with particular reference to the hormonal control of spermatogenesis. *Baillieres Clin Endocrinol Metab.* 1987;1:71-87.
468. Bhasin S, Woodhouse L, Casaburi R, et al. Testosterone dose-response relationships in healthy young men. *Am J Physiol Endocrinol Metab.* 2001;281:E1172-E1181.
469. Coviello AD, Lakshman K, Mazer NA, et al. Differences in the apparent metabolic clearance rate of testosterone in young and older men with gonadotropin suppression receiving graded doses of testosterone. *J Clin Endocrinol Metab.* 2006;91:4669-4675.
470. Gooren LJ, Bunck MC. Androgen replacement therapy: present and future. *Drugs.* 2004;64:1861-1891.
471. Wang C, Alexander G, Berman N, et al. Testosterone replacement therapy improves mood in hypogonadal men: a clinical research center study. *J Clin Endocrinol Metab.* 1996;81:3578-3583.
472. Bhasin S, Woodhouse L, Casaburi R, et al. Older men are as responsive as young men to the anabolic effects of graded doses of testosterone on the skeletal muscle. *J Clin Endocrinol Metab.* 2005;90:678-688.
473. Schulte-Beerbuhl M, Nieschlag E. Comparison of testosterone, dihydrotestosterone, luteinizing hormone, and follicle-stimulating hormone in serum after injection of testosterone enanthate of testosterone cypionate. *Fertil Steril.* 1980;33:201-203.
474. Schurmeyer T, Nieschlag E. Comparative pharmacokinetics of testosterone enanthate and testosterone cyclohexanecarboxylate as assessed by serum and salivary testosterone levels in normal men. *Int J Androl.* 1984;7:181-187.
475. Snyder PJ. Clinical use of androgens. *Annu Rev Med.* 1984;35:207-217.
476. Snyder PJ, Lawrence DA. Treatment of male hypogonadism with testosterone enanthate. *J Clin Endocrinol Metab.* 1980;51:1335-1339.
477. Dobs AS, Meikle AW, Arver S, et al. Pharmacokinetics, efficacy, and safety of a permeation-enhanced testosterone transdermal system in comparison with bi-weekly injections of testosterone enanthate for the treatment of hypogonadal men. *J Clin Endocrinol Metab.* 1999;84:3469-3478.
478. Jordan WP Jr, Atkinson LE, Lai C. Comparison of the skin irritation potential of two testosterone transdermal systems: an investigational system and a marketed product. *Clin Ther.* 1998;20:80-87.
479. Amory JK, Matsumoto AM. The therapeutic potential of testosterone patches. *Expert Opin Investig Drugs.* 1998;7:1977-1985.
480. Arver S, Dobs AS, Meikle AW, et al. Long-term efficacy and safety of a permeation-enhanced testosterone transdermal system in hypogonadal men. *Clin Endocrinol (Oxf).* 1997;47:727-737.
481. Singh AB, Norris K, Modi N, et al. Pharmacokinetics of a transdermal testosterone system in men with end stage renal disease receiving maintenance hemodialysis and healthy hypogonadal men. *J Clin Endocrinol Metab.* 2001;86:2437-2445.
482. Wilson DE, Kaidbey K, Boike SC, et al. Use of topical corticosteroid pretreatment to reduce the incidence and severity of skin reactions

associated with testosterone transdermal therapy. *Clin Ther.* 1998;20:299-306.
483. Lakshman KM, Basaria S. Safety and efficacy of testosterone gel in the treatment of male hypogonadism. *Clin Interv Aging.* 2009;4:397-412.
484. de Ronde W. Hyperandrogenism after transfer of topical testosterone gel: case report and review of published and unpublished studies. *Hum Reprod.* 2009;24:425-428.
485. Wang C, Harnett M, Dobs AS, et al. Pharmacokinetics and safety of long-acting testosterone undecanoate injections in hypogonadal men: an 84-week phase III clinical trial. *J Androl.* 2010;31:457-465.
486. Wang C, Swerdloff RS, Iranmanesh A, et al. Transdermal testosterone gel improves sexual function, mood, muscle strength, and body composition parameters in hypogonadal men. *J Clin Endocrinol Metab.* 2000;85:2839-2853.
487. Wang C, Swerdloff RS, Iranmanesh A, et al. Effects of transdermal testosterone gel on bone turnover markers and bone mineral density in hypogonadal men. *Clin Endocrinol (Oxf).* 2001;54:739-750.
488. Bouloux P. Testim 1% testosterone gel for the treatment of male hypogonadism. *Clin Ther.* 2005;27:286-298.
489. Steidle C, Schwartz S, Jacoby K, et al. AA2500 testosterone gel normalizes androgen levels in aging males with improvements in body composition and sexual function. *J Clin Endocrinol Metab.* 2003;88:2673-2681.
490. Korbonits M, Kipnes M, Grossman AB. Striant SR: a novel, effective and convenient testosterone therapy for male hypogonadism. *Int J Clin Pract.* 2004;58:1073-1080.
491. Wang C, Swerdloff R, Kipnes M, et al. New testosterone buccal system (Striant) delivers physiological testosterone levels: pharmacokinetics study in hypogonadal men. *J Clin Endocrinol Metab.* 2004;89:3821-3829.
492. Cavender RK, Fairall M. Subcutaneous testosterone pellet implant (Testopel) therapy for men with testosterone deficiency syndrome: a single-site retrospective safety analysis. *J Sex Med.* 2009;6:3177-3192.
493. Fennell C, Sartorius G, Ly LP, et al. Randomized cross-over clinical trial of injectable vs. implantable depot testosterone for maintenance of testosterone replacement therapy in androgen deficient men. *Clin Endocrinol (Oxf).* 2010;73:102-109.
494. Handelsman DJ, Conway AJ, Boylan LM. Pharmacokinetics and pharmacodynamics of testosterone pellets in man. *J Clin Endocrinol Metab.* 1990;71:216-222.
495. Gooren LJ. Advances in testosterone replacement therapy. *Front Horm Res.* 2009;37:32-51.
496. Kohn FM, Schill WB. A new oral testosterone undecanoate formulation. *World J Urol.* 2003;21:311-315.
497. Edelstein D, Basaria S. Testosterone undecanoate in the treatment of male hypogonadism. *Expert Opin Pharmacother.* 2010;11:2095-2106.
498. Gooren LJ. New long-acting androgens. *World J Urol.* 2003;21:306-310.
499. Harle L, Basaria S, Dobs AS. Nebido: a long-acting injectable testosterone for the treatment of male hypogonadism. *Expert Opin Pharmacother.* 2005;6:1751-1759.
500. Minnemann T, Schubert M, Hubler D, et al. A four-year efficacy and safety study of the long-acting parenteral testosterone undecanoate. *Aging Male.* 2007;10:155-158.
501. Yassin AA, Haffejee M. Testosterone depot injection in male hypogonadism: a critical appraisal. *Clin Interv Aging.* 2007;2:577-590.
502. Raynaud JP, Aumonier C, Gualano V, et al. Pharmacokinetic study of a new testosterone-in-adhesive matrix patch applied every 2 days to hypogonadal men. *J Steroid Biochem Mol Biol.* 2008;109:177-184.
503. Raynaud JP, Legros JJ, Rollet J, et al. Efficacy and safety of a new testosterone-in-adhesive matrix patch applied every 2 days for 1 year to hypogonadal men. *J Steroid Biochem Mol Biol.* 2008;109:168-176.
504. Winters SJ, Wang C. LH and non-SHBG testosterone and estradiol levels during testosterone replacement of hypogonadal men: further evidence that steroid negative feedback increases as men grow older. *J Androl.* 2010;31:281-287.
505. Bhasin S, Jasuja R. Selective androgen receptor modulators as function promoting therapies. *Curr Opin Clin Nutr Metab Care.* 2009;12:232-240.
506. Gao W, Dalton JT. Expanding the therapeutic use of androgens via selective androgen receptor modulators (SARMs). *Drug Discov Today.* 2007;12:241-248.
507. Snyder PJ, Peachey H, Berlin JA, et al. Effects of testosterone replacement in hypogonadal men. *J Clin Endocrinol Metab.* 2000;85:2670-2677.
508. Quon H, Loblaw DA. Androgen deprivation therapy for prostate cancer: review of indications in 2010. *Curr Oncol.* 2010;17(suppl 2):S38-S44.
509. Eyre SJ, Ankerst DP, Wei JT, et al. Validation in a multiple urology practice cohort of the Prostate Cancer Prevention Trial calculator for predicting prostate cancer detection. *J Urol.* 2009;182:2653-2658.
510. Parekh DJ, Ankerst DP, Higgins BA, et al. External validation of the Prostate Cancer Prevention Trial risk calculator in a screened population. *Urology.* 2006;68:1152-1155.
511. Coviello AD, Kaplan B, Lakshman KM, et al. Effects of graded doses of testosterone on erythropoiesis in healthy young and older men. *J Clin Endocrinol Metab.* 2008;93:914-919.
512. Fernandez-Balsells MM, Murad MH, Lane M, et al. Clinical review 1. Adverse effects of testosterone therapy in adult men: a systematic review and meta-analysis. *J Clin Endocrinol Metab.* 2010;95:2560-2575.
513. Bachman E, Feng R, Travison T, et al. Testosterone suppresses hepcidin in men: a potential mechanism for testosterone-induced erythrocytosis. *J Clin Endocrinol Metab.* 2010;95:4743-4747.
514. Behre HM, Bohmeyer J, Nieschlag E. Prostate volume in testosterone-treated and untreated hypogonadal men in comparison to age-matched normal controls. *Clin Endocrinol (Oxf).* 1994;40:341-349.
515. Andriole GL, Crawford ED, Grubb RL 3rd, et al. Mortality results from a randomized prostate-cancer screening trial. *N Engl J Med.* 2009;360:1310-1319.
516. Barry MJ. Screening for prostate cancer: the controversy that refuses to die. *N Engl J Med.* 2009;360:1351-1354.
517. Schroder FH, Hugosson J, Roobol MJ, et al. Screening and prostate-cancer mortality in a randomized European study. *N Engl J Med.* 2009;360:1320-1328.
518. Calof OM, Singh AB, Lee ML, et al. Adverse events associated with testosterone replacement in middle-aged and older men: a meta-analysis of randomized, placebo-controlled trials. *J Gerontol A Biol Sci Med Sci.* 2005;60:1451-1457.
519. Snyder PJ, Peachey H, Hannoush P, et al. Effect of testosterone treatment on bone mineral density in men over 65 years of age. *J Clin Endocrinol Metab.* 1999;84:1966-1972.
520. Whitsel EA, Boyko EJ, Matsumoto AM, et al. Intramuscular testosterone esters and plasma lipids in hypogonadal men: a meta-analysis. *Am J Med.* 2001;111:261-269.
521. O'Connor DB, Archer J, Wu FC. Effects of testosterone on mood, aggression, and sexual behavior in young men: a double-blind, placebo-controlled, cross-over study. *J Clin Endocrinol Metab.* 2004;89:2837-2845.
522. Wang C, Cunningham G, Dobs A, et al. Long-term testosterone gel (AndroGel) treatment maintains beneficial effects on sexual function and mood, lean and fat mass, and bone mineral density in hypogonadal men. *J Clin Endocrinol Metab.* 2004;89:2085-2098.
523. Matsumoto AM. Hormonal therapy of male hypogonadism. *Endocrinol Metab Clin North Am.* 1994;23:857-875.
524. Saal W, Glowania HJ, Hengst W, et al. Pharmacodynamics and pharmacokinetics after subcutaneous and intramuscular injection of human chorionic gonadotropin. *Fertil Steril.* 1991;56:225-229.
525. Saal W, Happ J, Cordes U, et al. Subcutaneous gonadotropin therapy in male patients with hypogonadotropic hypogonadism. *Fertil Steril.* 1991;56:319-324.
526. Burris AS, Clark RV, Vantman DJ, et al. A low sperm concentration does not preclude fertility in men with isolated hypogonadotropic hypogonadism after gonadotropin therapy. *Fertil Steril.* 1988;50:343-347.
527. Burris AS, Rodbard HW, Winters SJ, et al. Gonadotropin therapy in men with isolated hypogonadotropic hypogonadism: the response to human chorionic gonadotropin is predicted by initial testicular size. *J Clin Endocrinol Metab.* 1988;66:1144-1151.
528. McLachlan RI, Finkel DM, Bremner WJ, et al. Serum inhibin concentrations before and during gonadotropin treatment in men with hypogonadotropic hypogonadism: physiological and clinical implications. *J Clin Endocrinol Metab.* 1990;70:1414-1419.
529. Miyagawa Y, Tsujimura A, Matsumiya K, et al. Outcome of gonadotropin therapy for male hypogonadotropic hypogonadism at university affiliated male infertility centers: a 30-year retrospective study. *J Urol.* 2005;173:2072-2075.
530. Warne DW, Decosterd G, Okada H, et al. A combined analysis of data to identify predictive factors for spermatogenesis in men with hypogonadotropic hypogonadism treated with recombinant human follicle-stimulating hormone and human chorionic gonadotropin. *Fertil Steril.* 2009;92:594-604.
531. Bouloux PM, Nieschlag E, Burger HG, et al. Induction of spermatogenesis by recombinant follicle-stimulating hormone (puregon) in hypogonadotropic azoospermic men who failed to respond to human chorionic gonadotropin alone. *J Androl.* 2003;24:604-611.
532. Farhat R, Al-zidjali F, Alzahrani AS. Outcome of gonadotropin therapy for male infertility due to hypogonadotrophic hypogonadism. *Pituitary.* 2010;13:105-110.
533. Matsumoto AM, Snyder PJ, Bhasin S, et al. Stimulation of spermatogenesis with recombinant human follicle-stimulating hormone (follitropin alfa; GONAL-f): long-term treatment in azoospermic men with hypogonadotropic hypogonadism. *Fertil Steril.* 2009;92:979-990.
534. Johnson L, Thompson DL Jr, Varner DD. Role of Sertoli cell number and function on regulation of spermatogenesis. *Anim Reprod Sci.* 2008;105:23-51.

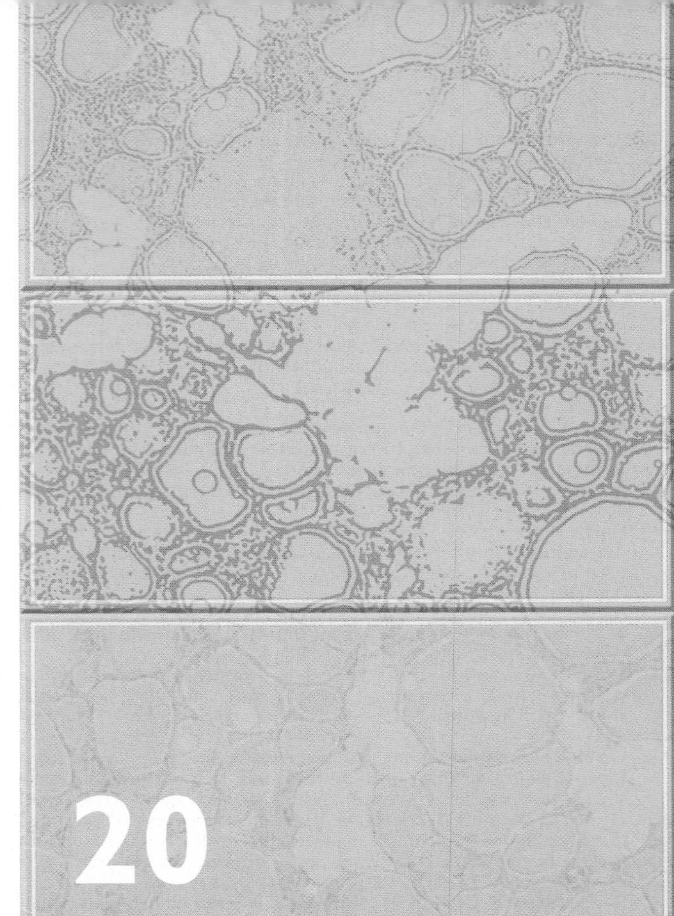

CHAPTER 20

Sexual Dysfunction in Men and Women

SHALENDER BHASIN • ROSEMARY BASSON

Endocrine disease and its treatment can frequently disturb sexual function in men and women.[1] In addition, many patients believe, often incorrectly, that their sexual dysfunction must be due to "hormonal imbalance" and seek management from endocrinologists.[2] Patients consider their sexual lives to be important, and, recognizing the importance of sexual function as a determinant of quality of life, the World Health Organization has declared sexual health a fundamental right of men and women.

Michael Kinsey's pioneering epidemiologic investigations provided the first evidence of the considerable variability in sexual practices of American men and women.[3] Excellent epidemiologic surveys using modern sampling techniques, such as the Massachusetts Male Aging Study (MMAS) led by John McKinlay[4] and the National Health and Social Life Survey (NHSLS) led by Laumann and Rosen,[5,6] revealed high prevalence rates of sexual dysfunction among community-dwelling, middle-aged and older men. Ongoing and distressing sexual dysfunction affects 10% of people, and prevalence rates are even higher among older men.[7,8] Temporary or nondistressing dysfunction is frequently reported by up to 40% of the population.

William Masters and Virginia E. Johnson[9] found that both men and women display predictable physiologic responses after sexual stimulation. Their landmark descriptions of the human sexual response cycle provided the basis for rational classification of human sexual disorders. Sigmund Freud ascribed sexual problems in adult men and women to earlier difficulties in maturation of childhood sexuality and development of parent-child relationships. Recent advances in understanding of the physiologic and biochemical mechanisms of penile erection and the development of mechanism-specific therapies for erectile dysfunction (ED) have largely supplanted Freud's psychoanalytic theories.

The 1980s and 1990s witnessed remarkable progress in understanding of the physicochemical mechanisms that lead to penile tumescence and rigidity. It was recognized that penile erections are the result of cavernosal smooth muscle relaxation and increased penile blood flow.[10-12] The appreciation of nitric oxide (NO) as a key vasodilator in the vascular smooth muscle was a pivotal discovery that was later recognized by the awarding of the Nobel Prize in Physiology or Medicine to Robert F. Furchgott, Louis J.

Ignarro, and Ferid Murad. The recognition that NO caused cavernosal smooth muscle relaxation by simulating guanylyl cyclase provided the foundation for the development of highly effective oral therapies for the treatment of ED.

Historically, the classification and nomenclature for sexual disorders were based on the *Diagnostic and Statistical Manual* (DSM), which is primarily a psychiatric nomenclature, reflecting the belief that sexual disorders in men and women are psychogenic in their origin.[13] In the 1990s, several expert groups updated the clinical definitions of sexual disorders in men.[14,15] The growing recognition that ED is commonly a manifestation of systemic disease and the availability of easy-to-use therapeutic options, including oral and intraurethral drugs, have duly placed sexual disorders in men within the purview of the endocrinologist and the primary care provider. In middle-aged and older men, but less so in women, sexual dysfunction is often related to comorbid medical conditions.[16-20] Sexual dysfunction can be a manifestation of serious underlying medical disease, such as a pituitary neoplasm, diabetes, or coronary artery disease.[20] ED may signal asymptomatic coronary artery disease.[19] In women, sexual dysfunction is more strongly linked to mental health.[16-18]

The clinical definitions of sexual dysfunction, especially in women, remain shrouded in debate. In women, there is poor correlation between a clinician's diagnosis of sexual dysfunction and a woman's perception of the problem.[21] For instance, in one study,[21] some 20% of middle-aged women were given a diagnosis of sexual dysfunction even though they reported no problem, whereas a similar number did not receive a diagnosis of sexual dysfunction but reported problematic sex. The definitions of sexual dysfunction are being revised by both the American Psychiatric Association's DSM5 committee and the International Classification of Diseases (ICD) committee and will be published in 2013. It is hoped that patients' and clinicians' perceptions of dysfunction will become more aligned.

This chapter describes the current conceptualization of sexual response in men and women, the underlying pathophysiologic mechanisms, the sexual sequelae of various endocrine disorders, and clinical assessment of sexual dysfunction and its management. Management strategies for sexual dysfunction stemming from hormonal and nonhormonal factors are outlined.

HUMAN SEXUAL RESPONSE CYCLE

Masters and Johnson[9] found that both men and women display predictable physiologic responses after sexual stimulation that can be categorized in four phases: the excitement phase, the plateau phase, the orgasmic phase, and the resolution phase (Fig. 20-1A). The traditional model of human sexual response stemming from the research of Masters, Johnson and Kaplan was that of a linear progression—from desire, to arousal, to a plateau of high arousal, followed by orgasm/ejaculation, and finally a phase of resolution. However, recent studies have revealed greater variability and flexibility and a more circular nature of human sexual response than was appreciated before (see Fig. 20-1B). In both men and women, the relationship between desire and arousal is variable and complex; women are often unable to separate the two.[22,23] The motivations and incentives for sex are multiple and varied. A wish to increase emotional intimacy between the partners is important for both men and women.[23-27] Sexual "desire," as in lust or drive, is only one of many reasons people engage in sex.[25] The new models reflect this complexity, including the multiple reasons to initiate or agree to sex, a variable order and overlap of the phases of desire and arousal, and the potential for gradually increasing arousal to allow more intense stimulation to be effective and desired (see Fig. 20-1B).[22]

Bancroft and Graham proposed dual control theories for sexual motivation in men and women.[28-31] Their dual control model envisions a balance between sexual activation and sexual inhibition in an individual's brain, with this balance determining whether sexual stimulation leads to arousal.[29,30] A questionnaire was used to characterize the specific factors associated with an individual's sexual excitation and sexual inhibition (due to the threat of performance failure, the threat of performance consequences, or both).[30] In women, factor analysis identified five factors related to excitation and three related to inhibition. The excitation factors included sexual arousability, partner characteristics, sexual power dynamics, smell, and setting. The inhibition factors were relationship importance (reflecting the need for sex to occur within a specific type of relationship), concerns about sexual function (the tendency of worries and distractions about sexual function to impair arousal), and arousal contingency (the potential for arousal to be inhibited by some contextual/situational factor).[30,31] This model explains certain basic neurophysiologic aspects of individual variability and is open to further refinement and validation.

PHYSIOLOGIC MECHANISMS OF HUMAN SEXUAL RESPONSE

Physiology of Desire and Arousal

Functional Brain Imaging of Sexual Arousal

Brain imaging studies indicate that many brain regions are involved in sexual response.[32,33] In healthy individuals, erotic images activate limbic and paralimbic regions that are thought to be important for sexual motivation and parietal areas (among others) that modulate the emotional and motor response.[32,33] Specific inhibitory regions deactivate these sexual responses.[32,33] Many additional brain areas also are activated, including those associated with visual processing, attention, motor and somatosensory function, emotion, and reward.

Men generally show greater responsiveness to visual sexually arousing stimuli than women do.[34,35] When men and women viewed couples interacting in nonsexual ways, men showed significantly greater activation in the amygdala than the women did, yet the women rated their arousal higher.[34,35] It is possible that amygdala activation is not related to sexual arousal per se. These researchers suggest that the amygdala may mediate the more important role of visual stimuli in male sexual behavior.[34,35] Men showed greater activation of the amygdala in response to those stimuli that generated higher subjective arousal. In contrast, women showed significantly greater amygdala activation in response to less arousing stimuli. When viewing sexually explicit couple images, the men showed greater activation in some brain areas, including the hypothalamus, than the women did. Moreover, in women, viewing the sexually explicit images did not lead to greater activation in these regions than viewing the neutral couple scenes. In other studies, during the sexual arousal phase of genital stimulation, women displayed more activation in

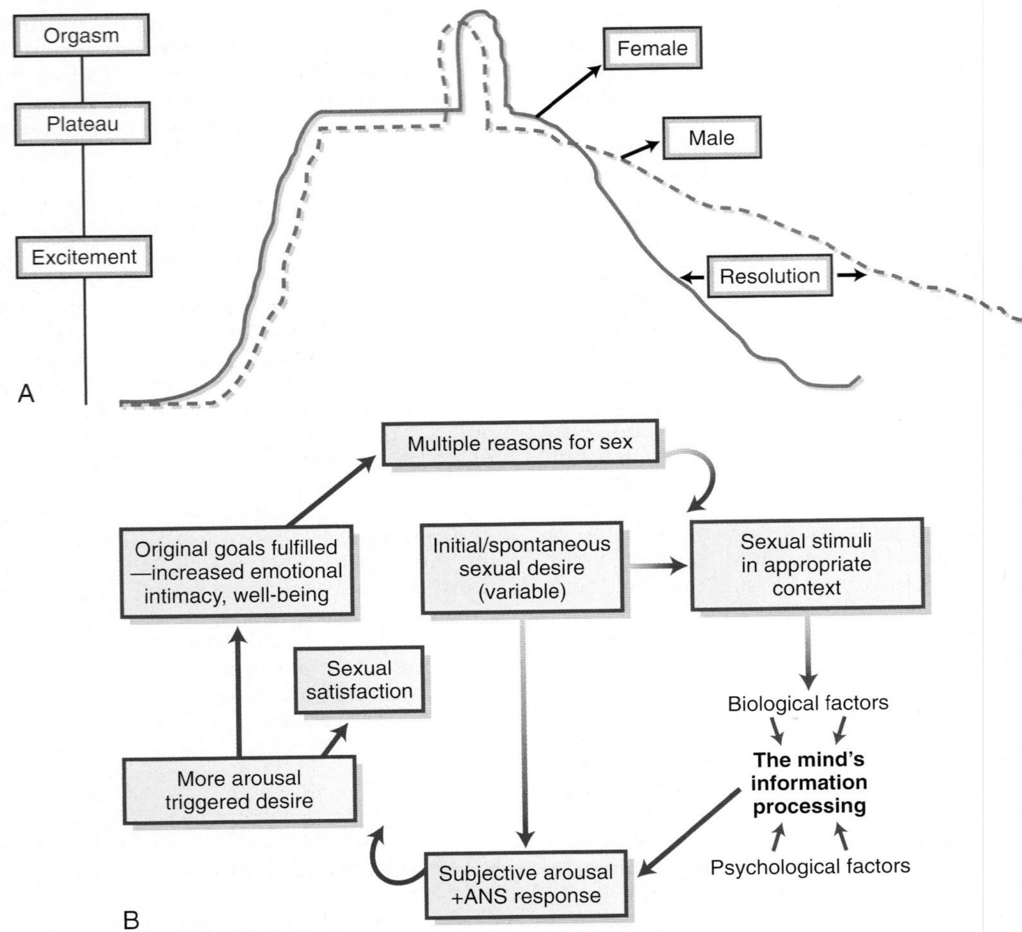

Figure 20-1 **A,** The four phases of the human sexual response cycle as postulated by Masters and Johnson.[9] Because the resolution phase is prolonged considerably in men, men can experience refractoriness to further stimulation for varying lengths of time before they can achieve another orgasm. As discussed in the text, understanding of the human sex response cycle has evolved substantially since the publication of this work. **B,** The circular human response cycle of overlapping phases. It is increasingly recognized that the human sexual response involves much more complexity, circularity, and flexibility than is reflected in Masters and Johnson's original model. "Desire" may or may not be present initially; it can be triggered during the experience. Arousal and desire overlap. Multiple psychological and biological factors influence the information processing of sexual stimuli. Underlying this processing may be the individual's unique tendency for excitation versus inhibition. ANS, autonomic nervous system.

the left frontoparietal areas, whereas men showed more activation in the right claustrum and ventral occipitotemporal cortex.[34,35]

The complexity of these systems was reflected in a study of surgically menopausal women who were sexually active but were receiving no hormonal therapy.[36] When these women viewed erotica during functional magnetic resonance imaging (MRI), they failed to display the brain activation observed in premenopausal women or in themselves when they were treated with testosterone and estrogen; yet, they reported sexual arousal from the erotic videos, both without and with hormonal supplementation.[36]

Neurotransmitters and Hormones Involved in Sexual Desire and Subjective Arousal

A variety of hormones and peptides are involved in the sexual response.[35-41] The interplay among androgens and neurotransmitters is complex: androgens influence neurotransmitter release, and neurotransmitters may modulate androgen receptor signaling.[35,38,41] The role of testosterone in desire and arousal is better documented in men than in women. In animal models, steroid hormones modulate sexual arousal by directing synthesis of the enzymes and the receptors for a number of neurotransmitters, including dopamine, noradrenalin, melanocortin, and oxytocin.[35-41] Systems that act within the hypothalamus and limbic regions of the brain are involved in the process of arousal, attention, and sexual behavior. It is thought that dopamine transmission in the medial preoptic area and the nucleus accumbens focuses the person's attention on sexual stimuli (the incentives or motivations for sexual activity).[35-41] It is postulated that the behavioral pattern stimulated by those systems and the subjective feelings that accompany them constitute the phenomenon commonly referred to as *sexual desire* or *arousal* when genital sensations triggered by these systems are subjectively felt. The main part of this neural pathway includes the medial preoptic area and its outputs to the ventral tegmental area. The latter contains dopamine cell bodies that project to various limbic and cortical regions, including the prefrontal cortex, the nucleus accumbens, the anterior cingulate cortex, and the amygdala.

Brain pathways for sexual inhibition include opioid, endocannabinoid, and serotonin neural transmissions feeding back to various levels of the excitatory pathways.[38-42] It is thought that the behavioral pattern stimulated by the inhibitory pathways includes both sexual reward and satiety refractoriness.[38-42]

Exogenous opiates are sexually inhibiting independent of their inhibitory effect on luteinizing hormone (LH), LH-releasing hormone, and testosterone. Endogenous opioids modulate the feedback effects of sex steroids on the hypothalamus and pituitary. β-Endorphin is synthesized in the anterior pituitary, the hypothalamus, and the nucleus of the solitary tract in the brain stem. The sexual inhibiting effects occur mainly through opioid action in the medial preoptic area and in the amygdala.[43] Low doses of opiates can have facilitatory effects, possibly through actions in the ventral tegmental area to activate the mesolimbic dopamine system. Exogenous opiates can induce an intense feeling of pleasure which has been likened to orgasm followed by a state of relaxation and calm.[44]

Melanocortins are derived from pro-opiomelanocortin and modulate sexual response through a specific receptor subtype, the melanocortin-4 receptor. Administration of melanocortin receptor agonists has been associated with an increase in spontaneous erection in healthy men and in men with ED and with increased desire, but not genital responses, in women.[45,46]

Oxytocin levels increase close to orgasm. This hormone is known to be involved in pair bonding in some animal species,[47] but its relevance in humans is not known.

The physiologic role of prolactin in the human sexual response remains unclear. Because a generalized reduction of dopamine activity in the hypothalamus results in increased prolactin secretion, it has been difficult to distinguish between the effects of raised prolactin itself and the possible effects of the reduced dopamine transmission.[48] High levels of prolactin are associated with impaired sexual function in men and women.[49,50]

The effects of the biologic factors are intertwined with those of the environmental and social factors. For instance, dopamine and progesterone, acting on their cognate receptors in the hypothalamus, can increase sexual behavior in oophorectomized, estrogenized female rats, and the presence of a male animal alongside the cage can cause an identical stimulation of the sexual behavior without the administration of either progesterone or dopamine.[51] In rodents, birds, and fish, complex neural networks enable the animal to assess the context of potential sexual activity and relate it to past experience and to expectation of reward.[52]

Genital Sexual Congestion and Arousal

Men and women differ substantially with respect to the correlation between genital congestion and subjective sexual arousal (excitement). Whereas subjective arousal is typically concordant with genital congestion in men, there is a poor correlation between subjective arousal and measures of genital congestion in women.[53,54] Also, in contrast to men's assessment of their erections, women's assessment of their degree of genital congestion is less accurate. It is thought that genital congestion in women is a prompt, automatic reflex that occurs within seconds of an erotic stimulus; it may not be deemed at all sexually arousing by the woman, or it may even be deemed emotionally negative.[55] Viewing primates engaging in sexual activity subjectively arouses neither young men nor young women. However, young women display marked genital congestion, as measured by vaginal photoplethysmography (VPP), whereas no genital response is recorded in the men.[53,54] Similarly, heterosexual women viewing lesbian women engaged in sexual activity report minimal subjective arousal but show a prompt vasocongestive response; in contrast, heterosexual men viewing male same-sex activity show little genital or subjective response.[54]

Physiologic Mechanisms of Penile Erection

Penile Anatomy and Blood Flow

The erectile tissue of the penis consists of two dorsally positioned corpora cavernosa and a ventrally placed corpus spongiosum.[10-12,56] The erectile tissue of both the corpora cavernosa and the corpus spongiosum is composed of numerous cavernous spaces separated by trabeculae.[10-12,56] These trabeculae are composed mainly of smooth muscle cells that are arranged in a syncytium. Endothelial cells cover the surfaces of the trabeculae.

The penile arterial blood supply is derived from pudendal arteries, which are branches of the internal iliac arteries (Fig. 20-2). The pudendal artery divides into cavernosal, dorsal penile, and bulbourethral arteries. The cavernosal arteries and their branches, the helicine arteries, provide blood flow to the corpora cavernosa.[10,11] Dilatation of the helicine arteries increases blood flow and pressure in the cavernosal sinuses.[10-12,56]

Penile Innervation

The neural input to the penis consists of sympathetic (T11 through L2), parasympathetic (S2 through S4), and somatic nerves (Table 20-1).[57] Sympathetic and parasympathetic fibers converge in the inferior hypogastric plexus, where the autonomic input to the penis is integrated and communicated to the penis through the cavernosal nerves. In humans, the inferior hypogastric ganglionic plexus is located retroperitoneally, near the rectum.[12,57]

Several brain regions, including the amygdala, the medial preoptic area, the paraventricular nucleus of the hypothalamus, and the periaqueductal gray matter, act coordinately to affect penile erections.[57] The medial preoptic area of the hypothalamus serves as the integration site

TABLE 20-1
Innervation of the Penis

Type of Fiber	Location of Neurons in Spinal Cord	Nerves Carrying the Fibers	General Function
Sympathetic	T10-L2	Prevertebral outflow through the hypogastric and cavernous nerves; paravertebral outflow through the parasympathetic ganglia and pudendal or pelvic and cavernous nerves	Generally antierectile; sympathetic innervation plays an important role in regulating seminal emission
Parasympathetic	S2-S4	Cavernosal and pelvic nerves	Proerectile
Somatic	S2-S4	Pudendal nerve	Penile sensation, contraction of the striated muscles during ejaculation

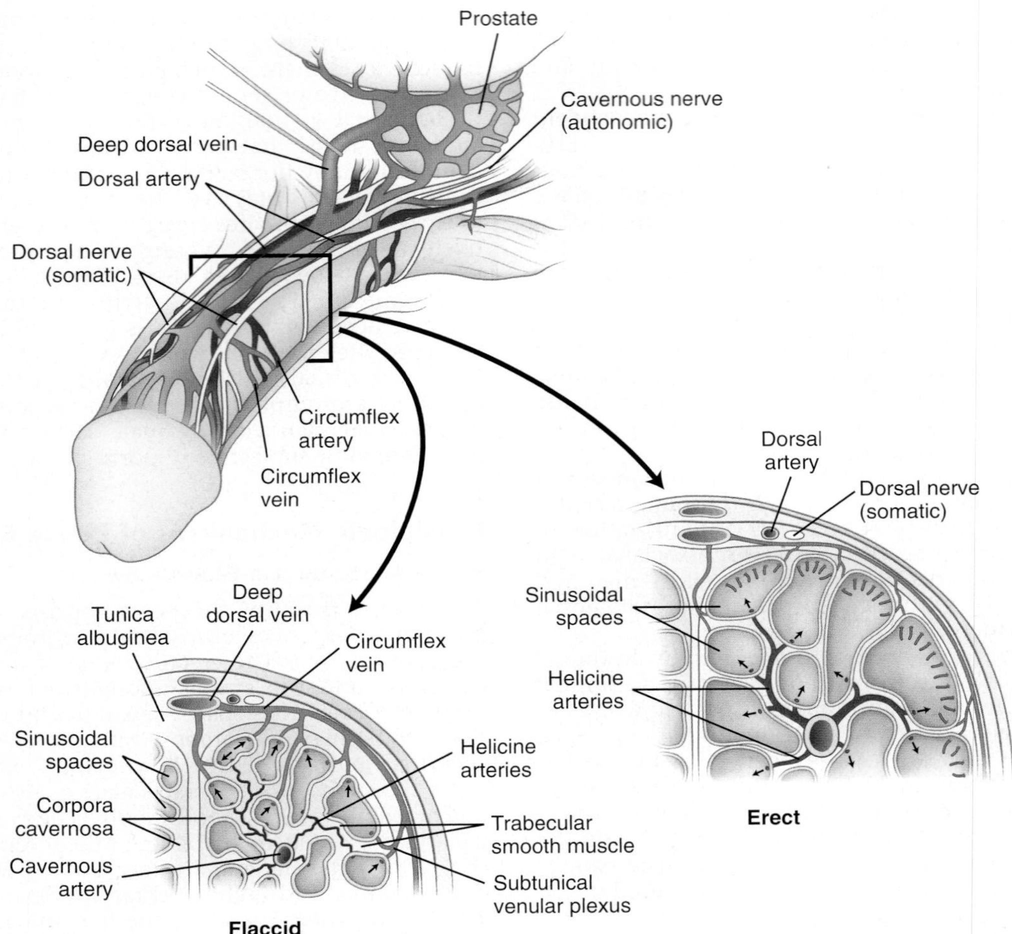

Figure 20-2 Anatomy and mechanism of penile erection. The corpora cavernosa are made up of trabecular spaces that are surrounded by cavernosal smooth muscle. Helicine arteries provide the arterial supply to the cavernosal spaces. The dorsal nerve provides the sensory innervation to the penis. During erection, relaxation of the trabecular smooth muscle and increased blood flow result in engorgement of the sinusoidal spaces in the corpora cavernosa. The expansion of the sinusoids compresses the venous return against the tunica albuginea, resulting in entrapment of blood. This imparts rigidity to the tumescent penis. (Adapted from Lue TF. Erectile dysfunction. *N Engl J Med.* 2000;342:1802-1813.)

for the central nervous system control of erections; it receives sensory input from the amygdala and sends impulses to the paraventricular nuclei of the hypothalamus and the periaqueductal gray matter. Neurons in paraventricular nuclei project onto the thoracolumbar and sacral nuclei associated with erections.

The parasympathetic input to the penis is proerectile, and sympathetic input is mainly inhibitory.[57] The stimuli from the perineum and lower urinary tract are carried to the penis through the sacral reflex arc.[57]

Hemodynamic Changes during Penile Erection

Penile erection results from a series of biochemical and hemodynamic events that are associated with activation of central nervous system sites involved in regulation of erections, relaxation of cavernosal smooth muscle, increased blood flow into cavernosal sinuses, and venous occlusion resulting in penile engorgement and rigidity.[10,56] Normal penile erection requires coordinated involvement of intact central and peripheral nervous systems, corpora cavernosa and spongiosa, and normal arterial blood supply and venous drainage.[10,56]

As cavernosal smooth muscle relaxes and the blood flow to the penis increases, the increased pooling of blood in the cavernosal spaces results in penile engorgement (see Fig 20-2).[10,56] The expanding corpora cavernosa compress the venules against the rigid tunica albuginea, restricting the venous outflow from the cavernosal spaces.[10,56] This facilitates entrapment of blood in the cavernosal sinuses, imparting rigidity to the erect penis.

Biochemical Regulation of Cavernosal Smooth Muscle Tone

The tone of the corporal smooth muscle cells determines the erectile state of the penis.[10-12,56] When the cavernosal smooth muscle cells are relaxed, the penis is engorged with blood and erect. When the cavernosal smooth muscle cells are contracted, there is predominance of sympathetic neural activity, and the penis is flaccid.[56]

The smooth muscle tone in the corpora cavernosa is maintained by the release of stored intracellular calcium (Ca^{2+}) into the cytoplasm and influx of calcium through membrane channels.[58-61] The transmembrane influx of calcium in the cavernosal smooth muscle cells is mediated mostly by L-type voltage-dependent calcium channels, although T-type calcium channels are also expressed in cavernosal smooth muscle cells.[58-61] An increase in

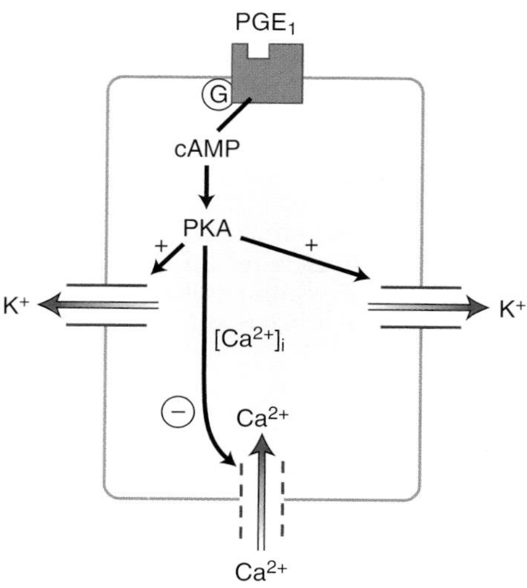

Figure 20-3 Regulation of cavernosal smooth muscle contractility by prostaglandin E_1 (PGE_1). Relaxation of the cavernosal smooth muscle is regulated by intracellular 3′,5′-cyclic adenosine monophosphate (cAMP) and cyclic guanosine monophosphate (cGMP). These intracellular second messengers, by activating specific protein kinases, cause sequestration of intracellular calcium (Ca^{2+}) and closure of Ca^{2+} channels and opening of potassium K^+ channels. This results in a net decrease in intracellular Ca^{2+}, leading to smooth muscle relaxation. PGE_1 by binding to PGE_1 receptors, increases the intracellular concentrations of cAMP, which activates protein kinase A (PKA). PKA promotes the sequestration of intracellular Ca^{2+}, inhibits Ca^{2+} influx, and stimulates K^+ channels. The net result is a decrease in intracytoplasmic Ca^{2+} and smooth muscle relaxation. PGE_1 stimulates cAMP generation. (Adapted from Bhasin S, Benson GS. Male sexual function. In: De Kretser D, ed. *Knobil and Neill's Physiology of Reproduction,* 3rd ed. Boston, MA: Academic Press; 1173-1194; and Lue TF. Erectile dysfunction. *N Engl J Med.* 2000;342:1802-1813.)

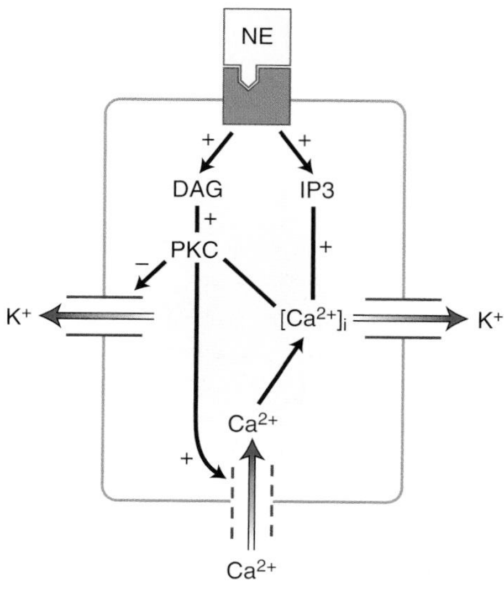

Figure 20-4 Regulation of cavernosal smooth muscle contractility by norepinephrine (NE). NE, which mediates adrenergic signals, binds to adrenergic receptors and stimulates diacyl glycerol (DAG) and inositol 1,4,5-triphosphate (IP3). DAG stimulates protein kinase C (PKC), which, along with IP3, causes an increase in intracytoplasmic calcium (Ca^{2+}) and inhibition of potassium (K^+) channels. Increased intracellular Ca^{2+} causes cavernosal smooth muscle contraction and loss of penile erection. (Adapted from Bhasin S, Benson GS. Male sexual function. In: De Kretser D, ed. *Knobil and Neill's Physiology of Reproduction,* 3rd ed. Boston, MA: Academic Press; 1173-1194; and Lue TF. Erectile dysfunction. *N Engl J Med.* 2000;342:1802-1813.)

intracellular calcium activates myosin light-chain kinase, resulting in phosphorylation of myosin light chain, actin-myosin interactions, and smooth muscle contraction.[61]

The transmembrane and intracellular calcium flux in the cavernosal smooth muscle cells is regulated by a number of cellular processes that involve potassium (K^+) flux through potassium channels, connexin43-derived gap junctions, and a number of cholinergic, adrenergic, and noradrenergic noncholinergic mediators (Figs. 20-3 through 20-6).[58-65] The nonadrenergic noncholinergic mediators include vasoactive intestinal peptide (VIP), calcitonin gene-related peptide (CGRP), and NO.[66]

Adrenergic pathways, acting through norepinephrine and α_1-adrenergic receptors, activate phospholipase C, which generates diacyl glycerol and inositol triphosphate.[61] Diacyl glycerol activates protein kinase C, which inhibits potassium channels and activates transmembrane calcium influx by activating L-type calcium channels (see Fig. 20-4).[19] Inositol triphosphate increases intracellular calcium by promoting the release of calcium from intracellular calcium stores.[20,21] The net increase in intracellular calcium promotes actin-myosin interactions, resulting in smooth muscle contraction and a flaccid penis.

Prostaglandin E_1 (PGE_1), binding to its cognate receptor, results in generation of cyclic adenosine monophosphate (cAMP), which activates protein kinase A. Activated protein kinase A stimulates potassium channels resulting in K^+ efflux from the cell (see Fig. 20-3). The protein kinase A–mediated processes also result in a net decrease in intracellular calcium, favoring smooth muscle cell relaxation.

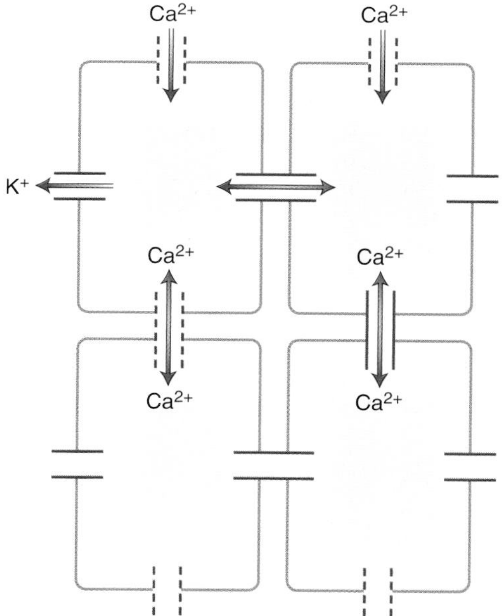

Figure 20-5 The interconnection of cavernosal smooth muscle cells in the penis. Connexin43-derived gap junctions connect adjacent corporal smooth muscle cells and allow flow of ions among interconnected smooth muscle cells. Therefore, alterations in action potential and potassium-channel activity in any myocyte affect the adjacent myocytes. Ca^{2+}, calcium ions; K^+, potassium ions. (Adapted from Melman A, Christ GJ. Integrative erectile biology: the effects of age and disease on gap junctions and ion channels and their potential value to the treatment of erectile dysfunction. *Urol Clin North Am.* 2001;28:217-230.)

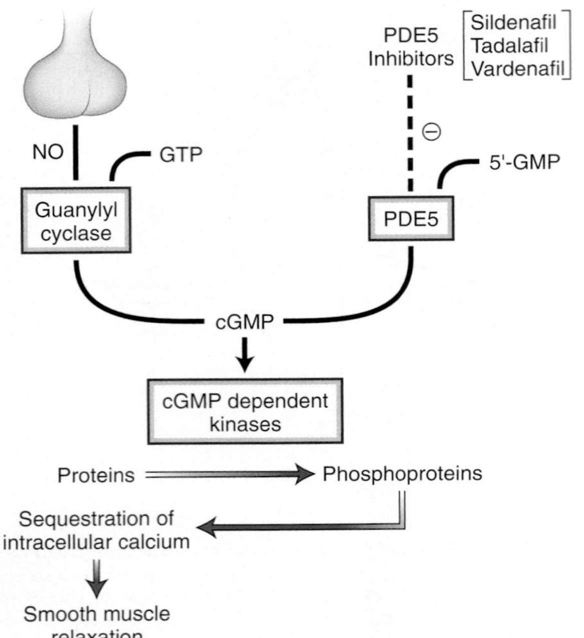

Figure 20-6 Regulation of cavernosal smooth muscle relaxation by nitric oxide (NO). Cyclic guanosine monophosphate (cGMP) regulates cavernosal smooth muscle relaxation by promoting sequestration of cytoplasmic calcium. NO is released from noradrenergic norcholinergic nerve endings and possibly from the endothelium. NO activates guanylyl cyclase, which generates cGMP from guanosine triphosphate (GTP), which in turn activates cGMP-dependent kinases, resulting in sequestration of intracellular calcium and smooth muscle relaxation. cGMP is degraded by cyclic nucleotide phosphodiesterases. Sildenafil, vardenafil, and tadalafil are selective inhibitors of phosphodiesterase isoform 5 (PDE5), which is present in cavernosal smooth muscles. (Adapted from Bhasin S, Benson GS. Male sexual function. In: De Kretser D, ed. *Knobil and Neill's Physiology of Reproduction*, 3rd ed. Boston, MA: Academic Press; 1173-1194; and Lue TF. Erectile dysfunction. *N Engl J Med.* 2000;342:1802-1813.)

Potassium Channels. At least three types of potassium channels—K_{ATP}, Kv, and the calcium-sensitive K^+ channels, referred to as BK_{Ca} or maxi-K channels—are expressed in the cavernosal smooth muscle cells.[58] Of these, the BK_{Ca} channels are the most important, because they account for 90% of K^+ efflux from the cavernosal smooth muscle cells. BK_{Ca} channel openers have been shown to relax cavernosal smooth muscle cells in vitro.[64] Strategies that increase BK_{Ca} channel expression in vivo improve erectile capacity in diabetic and older rodents[65] and are being explored as therapies for ED. A phase I human gene therapy trial has shown the feasibility of this approach.[67]

Connexin43 Gap Junctions. The smooth muscle cells in the corpora cavernosa are connected by connexin43 gap junctions that allow the ions and some signaling molecules such as inositol triphosphate to diffuse freely across smooth muscle cells.[58,68] The ionic changes induced by a stimulus in one smooth muscle cell are communicated rapidly across other smooth muscle cells, resulting in coordinated regulation of the entire corpora cavernosum.[58,68] Therefore, the corpora cavernosa can be viewed functionally as a syncytium of interconnected smooth muscle cells (see Fig. 20-5).[58,68]

Nitric Oxide. NO, derived from the nerve terminals innervating the corpora cavernosa, the endothelial lining of penile arteries, and the cavernosal sinuses, is an important biochemical regulator of cavernosal smooth muscle relaxation. NO also induces arterial dilatation.[69] The actions of NO on the cavernosal smooth muscle and the arterial blood flow are mediated through the activation of guanylyl cyclase, the production of cyclic guanosine monophosphate (cGMP), and activation of cGMP-dependent protein kinase (also called protein kinase G, or PKG) (see Fig. 20-6). cGMP causes smooth muscle relaxation by lowering intracellular calcium. There is some evidence that NO inhibits Rho kinase–induced cavernosal smooth muscle sensitivity to calcium.[70]

Cyclic Nucleotide Phosphodiesterases. Cyclic nucleotide phosphodiesterases (PDEs) hydrolyze cAMP and cGMP, thereby reducing their concentrations within the cavernosal smooth muscle. Of the 13 or more isoforms of PDEs that have been identified, isoforms 2, 3, 4, and 5 are expressed in the penis.[71-78] Only phosphodiesterase 5 (PDE5) is specific to the NO/cGMP pathway in the corpora cavernosa.[71-77] Hydrolysis of cGMP by this enzyme results in reversal of the smooth muscle relaxation and reversal of penile erection. Sildenafil, vardenafil, and tadalafil are potent and selective inhibitors of the activity of PDE5; they prevent breakdown of cGMP and thereby enhance penile erection.[73,76,77,79]

Regulation of Sensitivity to Intracellular Calcium by Rho A/Rho Kinase Signaling. Considerable attention has focused on the role of Rho kinase in modulating the sensitivity of cavernosal smooth muscle to intracellular calcium.[60] A growing body of evidence suggests that sensitization to intracellular calcium is regulated by the balance between phosphorylation of the regulatory light chain of myosin II by a myosin light-chain kinase and its dephosphorylation by a myosin light-chain phosphatase (Fig. 20-7).[60,80-85] Phosphorylation of the regulatory light chain of myosin II is necessary for activation of myosin II adenosine triphosphatases (ATPases) by actin, and its dephosphorylation prevents activation of myosin II

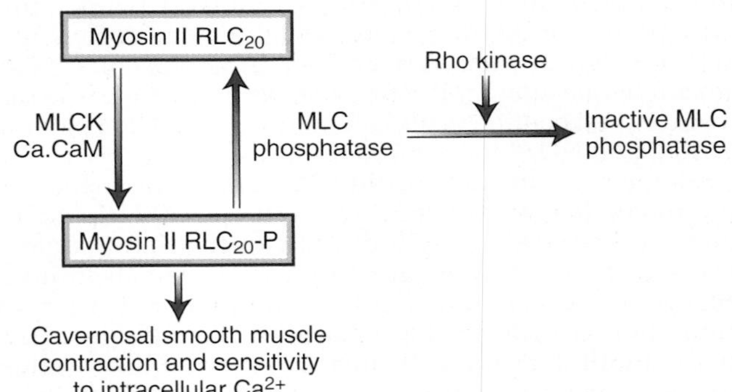

Figure 20-7 The role of Rho A/Rho kinase in regulation of cavernosal smooth muscle sensitivity to intracellular calcium (Ca^{2+}). Sensitivity to calcium and smooth muscle contractility is regulated by the Rho A/Rho kinase system. The balance between phosphorylation (P) of myosin regulatory light-chain (Myosin II RLC_{20}) kinase and its dephosphorylation by a myosin light-chain phosphatase is a major determinant of the smooth muscle sensitization to Ca^{2+}. By inhibiting the activity of MLC phosphatase, Rho kinase, the downstream effector of Rho A, can regulate smooth muscle responsiveness to calcium. Ca.CaM, calcium calmodulin. (Adapted from Somlyo AP, Somlyo AV. Ca^{2+} sensitivity of smooth muscle and nonmuscle myosin II: modulated by G proteins, kinases, and myosin phosphatase. *Physiol Rev.* 2003; 83:1325-1358.)

ATPases.[60,80-85] The ratio of kinase to phosphatase activities is an important determinant of the contractile sensitivity of the cavernosal smooth muscle cell to intracellular calcium.[60]

Rho A is a guanosine triphosphatase (GTPase) of approximately 20 kd that modulates Rho kinase activity, myosin light-chain phosphorylation, and calcium sensitivity in smooth muscle cells.[60] The Rho A–GDP complex is associated with a GDP dissociation inhibitor (RhoGDI) in its inactive state.[31] A number of intracellular signals can promote an exchange of GDP for GTP on Rho A through the mediation of guanine nucleotide exchange factors.[60] The Rho A–GTP interacts with its downstream effector, Rho kinase,[80,81] increasing the sensitivity of vascular smooth muscle to intracellular calcium by inhibiting the myosin light-chain phosphatases. Although the Rho A/Rho kinase expression is not significantly different between young and older rats, the activity of Rho kinase is higher in the older rats[84]; the age-related increase in Rho kinase activity has been proposed as one possible mechanism to explain the age-related decrease in erectile capacity.[84,85] Inhibition of Rho kinase activity in experimental animals increases cavernosal smooth muscle relaxation and improves intracavernosal pressures and penile erections.[85] Therefore, inhibitors of Rho A/Rho kinase signaling promise to provide attractive targets for the development of therapies for ED.[85]

Mechanisms of Ejaculation

The ejaculatory mechanisms consist of three processes: emission, ejection, and orgasm.[86-89] Although orgasm and seminal fluid ejection often occur contemporaneously, these two processes are regulated by separate mechanisms. *Emission,* the deposition of seminal fluid into the posterior urethra, is dependent on the integrity of the vasa deferentia, seminal vesicles, prostate gland, and bladder neck.[88,89] *Ejaculation* refers to the ejection of seminal fluid containing sperm and the secretions of seminal vesicles, prostate, and bulbourethral glands from the posterior urethra out through the urethral meatus; it is regulated primarily by central nervous system activation of the sympathetic nervous system.[88] This emission is ejaculated out of the urethra by contractions of the bulbospongiosus and levator ani muscles, closure of the bladder sphincter due to sympathetic activation, and synchronized opening of the external urinary sphincter.[88] The sensation associated with the rhythmic contractions of these pelvic floor muscles is referred to as the *orgasm.*

The stria terminalis, the posteromedial amygdala, the subparafascicular thalamus, the medial preoptic area of the hypothalamus, the periaqueductal gray matter in the midbrain region, and the paragigantocellular nucleus in the pons integrate seminal fluid emission and ejection during copulatory behavior.[89,90] The paragigantocellular nucleus, through serotoninergic pathways, inhibits the lumbosacral motor nuclei that are involved in ejaculation[89,90]; input from the medial preoptic area to the paragigantocellular nucleus causes loss of this inhibition, resulting in ejaculation.[90,91] An ejaculation generator in the spinal cord integrates the central and peripheral, sympathetic and parasympathetic signals to control ejaculation.[89-91] The parasympatheic fibers from the spinal ejaculation generator feed into the sacral parasympathetic nucleus and are carried from there through the pelvic nerve and the major parasympathetic ganglion into the seminal tract.[91] Sympathetic fibers are carried from the spinal ejaculation generator into the dorsal gray commissure and intermediolateral cell column and then through the lumbar sympathetic chain, pelvic nerve, superior hypogastric plexus, and major pelvic ganglion into the seminal tract.[90]

Neural pathways that use serotonin and dopamine as neurotransmitters play an important role in regulating ejaculation.[90] Administration of selective serotonin reuptake inhibitors (SSRIs) is being explored for the treatment of premature ejaculation.[92,93] At least 14 different serotonin receptor subtypes have been identified in different brain regions; the 5-HT1A somatodendritic receptors in the mesencephalic and medullary raphe nuclei reduce ejaculatory latency.[89,90] A better understanding of the neurochemical mechanisms that regulate ejaculation may provide mechanism-specific targets for treatment of ejaculatory disorders.

ROLE OF TESTOSTERONE IN REGULATING SEXUAL FUNCTION IN MEN

Testosterone regulates many domains of sexual function in men. Although androgen-deficient men can achieve penile erections in response to visual erotic stimuli, their overall sexual activity is decreased.[94] Spontaneous but not stimulus-bound erections are testosterone responsive (Table 20-2).[94] Testosterone promotes sexual thoughts and desire[94-101] and increases sexual arousal and attentiveness to erotic auditory and other stimuli.[95,96] Nocturnal erections, temporally related to peaks of nighttime testosterone secretion, are of lower amplitude and duration in androgen-deficient men, and testosterone therapy increases the frequency, fullness, and duration of nocturnal penile tumescence.[101,102] Maximum rigidity may require a threshold level of androgen activity.[103-107] Testosterone regulates nitric oxide synthase (NOS) in the cavernosal smooth muscle,[104,105] exerts trophic effects on cavernosal smooth muscle[106] and the ischiocavernosus and bulbospongiosus muscles, and is necessary for the veno-occlusive response.[103,104] Androgen-deficient men show delayed orgasm and low ejaculatory volume.

TABLE 20-2

Domains of Sexual Function Regulated by Testosterone: Effects of Testosterone Therapy in Androgen-Deficient Men*

Domains That Are Improved by Testosterone Therapy
Sexual desire
Spontaneous sexual thoughts
Attentiveness to erotic auditory stimuli
Frequency of nighttime and daytime erections
Duration, magnitude, and frequency of nocturnal penile erections
Overall sexual activity score
Volume of ejaculate
Domains That Are Not Improved or for Which There Is Insufficient or Inconclusive Evidence
Erectile response to visual erotic stimulus
Erectile function in men who have normal testosterone levels
Therapeutic response to selective phosphodiesterase inhibitors
Orgasms

*Testosterone administration in androgen-deficient men improves overall sexual activity scores through its effects on specific domains of sexuality.

Reproduced with permission from Bhasin S, Enzlin P, Coviello A, et al. Sexual dysfunction in men and women with endocrine disorders. *Lancet.* 2007;369: 597-611.

Testosterone therapy in androgen-deficient men improves overall sexual activity, sexual desire, spontaneous sexual thoughts, and attentiveness to erotic auditory stimuli; frequency of nighttime and daytime erections; duration, magnitude, and frequency of nocturnal penile erections; overall sexual activity scores; and the volume of ejaculate.[94,98,101,103,105,110] However, testosterone does not improve erectile response to visual erotic stimului,[94] or erectile function in men with ED who have normal testosterone levels, or orgasms.[107-110]

Brain imaging studies suggest that processing of sexual stimuli may be altered in androgen-deficient men, with decreased activation in those brain areas that typically are activated in eugonadal men and in androgen-deficient men after testosterone replacement in response to erotic stimuli.[98]

Acting on dopaminergic receptors in the medial preoptic area of the hypothalamus, testosterone elicits reward-seeking behavior in male mammals.[99] This may be the basis for testosterone's motivational effects on mammalian sexual behavior.[99] The roles of cytochrome P450 (CYP19) aromatase and steroid 5α-reductase systems in mediating androgen effects on sexual function remain unclear.[100] Studies suggest that 5α-reduction of testosterone is not necessary for mediation of testosterone's effects on desire, but investigations of men with mutations of the CYP19 aromatase gene suggest that aromatization to estradiol may be important in mediating testosterone's effects on sexual desire.[111,112]

There is some, albeit inconclusive, evidence to support the proposal that testosterone improves therapeutic response to selective PDE inhibitors.[113-115] Androgen deficiency and ED are two independently distributed disorders that coexist in 6% to 10% of middle-aged and older men.[116] Testosterone trials after failure of sildenafil therapy have been inconclusive.[113]

PHYSIOLOGY OF PHYSICAL SEXUAL AROUSAL IN WOMEN

A number of physical changes accompany subjective excitement or arousal in women, including genital swelling; increased vaginal lubrication; breast engorgement and nipple erection; increased skin sensitivity to sexual stimulation; changes in heart rate, blood pressure, muscle tone, breathing, and temperature; and mottling of the skin, a sexual flush of vasodilatation over the chest and face.[9] These changes result from the reflex action of the autonomic nervous system. Within seconds there is increased blood flow to the vagina: vasodilatation of the arterioles in the submucosal plexus increases transudation of interstitial fluid from the capillaries across the epithelium and into the vaginal lumen. Simultaneously, there is relaxation of smooth muscle cells around the clitoral sinusoids. MRI studies have confirmed the presence of extensive clitoral tissue far beyond the visible portion of the clitoris.[117] The clitoris comprises the head, the shaft, the rami that extend along the pubic arch, and the periurethral tissue in front of the anterior vaginal wall, as well as the bulbar tissue that surrounds the anterior distal vagina and is contiguous with the periurethral tissue. The vagina lengthens and dilates during arousal, elevating the uterus. The labia become swollen and darker red, and the lower third of the vagina swells. As the clitoris becomes more swollen, it elevates to lie nearer the symphysis pubis.

When increases in genital congestion in response to visual erotic stimuli were recorded using VPP, the correlation between genital congestion and subjective arousal was found to be highly variable.[53,118] This was true in sexually healthy women and in women reporting a lack of desire or arousal or sexual pain. Women reporting chronic lack of arousal showed prompt increases in vaginal congestion, comparable to those in control women, but reported no subjective sexual excitement in response to the erotic stimulation. Functional MRI studies showed that, unlike in men, activation of the areas organizing genital vasocongestion in women does not correlate with a woman's subjective excitement.[34]

The neurobiology of the genital vasocongestive response in women is incompletely understood but involves release of NO from the parasympathetic nerves, along with release of VIP.[119] Acetylcholine, which blocks noradrenergic vasoconstricting mechanisms and promotes NO release from the endothelium, is also released. There is communication between the NO-containing cavernous nerve to the clitoris and the distal portion of the somatic dorsal nerve of the clitoris from the pudendal nerve. Pelvic sympathetic nerves release primarily vasoconstrictive noradrenalin, adrenalin, and adenosine triphosphate (ATP), but some release acetylcholine, NO, and VIP. The provoked anxiety in the laboratory situation can increase the vasocongestive response of the genitalia to erotic stimulation in sexually healthy women.[120] The melanocortin-4 receptors and oxytocin also may be involved in clitoral and vaginal efferent pathways.

There is some evidence for a "cervical motor reflex," such that touch to the cervix reduces pressure in the upper portion of the vagina but increases pressure in the middle and lower portions.[121] Reduced uterine tone can occur in response to mechanical or electrical stimulation of the clitoris. Possibly, this reflex contributes to an increase in size and elevation of the uterus with sexual arousal.[121]

The clitoris is the most sexually sensitive area of the body. Immunohistologic studies have identified neurotransmitters thought to be associated with sensation (substance P and CGRP) that are concentrated immediately under the epithelium of the glans clitoris. The physiology of nongenital physical changes and their correlation with subjective excitement remain poorly understood.

PHYSIOLOGY OF ORGASM

Orgasm is a brain event, triggered typically by genital stimulation but also by sleep, stimulation of other parts of the body (including breast and nipple), fantasy, certain medications, and, in women with spinal cord injury, vibrostimulation of the cervix.

Orgasm is a subjective experience in both men and women, and it has been difficult to determine an objective marker. In healthy men, there is the associated ejaculation, and in both genders, there are involuntary (reflexive) muscular contractions of the striated perineal muscles. One objective and quantitative measure has been established that shows strong correspondence with the subjective experience of orgasm.[122,123] The researchers performed spectral analysis of rectal pressure data while volunteers imitated orgasm, tried to achieve orgasm and failed, or experienced orgasm. The most significant and important difference in spectral power between orgasm in both control tasks was found in the alpha band.[122] Outbursts of alpha fluctuations in rectal pressure occurred only during orgasm.[122]

Positron emission tomography studies during orgasm have shown largely similar brain activations and deactivations in both men and women: activations mainly in the anterior lobe of the cerebellar vermis and deep cerebellar nuclei and deactivations in the left ventromedial and orbitofrontal cortex.[34] The only major difference between the genders during orgasm itself was the activation in the periaqueductal gray matter in men.[34] The lateral orbitofrontal cortex is thought to be involved in urge suppression and behavioral release, whereas the medial parts encode hedonic experiences, becoming activated with increasing satiation and subjective pleasantness and deactivated with feelings of satiety. It is thought that the orgasm-related deactivation of the middle orbitofrontal cortex reflects satiety and not the hedonic experience of orgasm. The medial orbitofrontal cortex is part of the neuronal network that includes the amygdala, whose deactivation during orgasm is associated with a more carefree state of mind.[33]

The role of oxytocin in orgasm is unclear. Oxytocin levels increase at the time of orgasm.[124] Possibly, the increase in oxytocin modulates the experience of orgasm stemming from the action of the smooth muscles in the genitalia.[124] The periorgasmic release of oxytocin may contribute to the postorgasmic refractory period in men.[125]

DEFINITIONS OF SEXUAL DYSFUNCTION IN MEN

Both the DSM and the ICD definitions of sexual disorder are under revision, with new editions to be published in 2013. Changes are expected, especially in women, given the blurring of the phases of sexual response and the common comorbidity of dysfunction in various phases.[126-131]

Hypoactive Sexual Desire in Men

Hypoactive sexual desire disorder is persistent or recurrent deficiency (or absence) of sexual fantasies and desire for sexual activity that causes marked distress or interpersonal difficulty and that is not better explained by another disorder, direct physiologic effects of a substance (i.e., medication), or general medical condition.[132-134] A diagnosis of hypoactive sexual desire disorder is appropriate only if the person reports "distress or interpersonal difficulty" due to low sexual desire.[132-134] Low sexual desire is not necessarily pathologic; it may be an appropriate adaptation to relationship and health-related issues.[132-134]

Hypoactive sexual desire disorder in men, when it is generalized—that is, when self-stimulation (masturbation) is also absent—is a multifactorial disorder that can result from androgen deficiency, use of medications (e.g., SSRIs, antiandrogens, gonadotropin-releasing hormone [GnRH] analogs, antihypertensives, cancer chemotherapeutic agents, anticonvulsants), systemic illness, depression and other psychological problems, other causes of sexual dysfunction, or relationship and differentiation problems. Androgen deficiency is an important, treatable cause of hypoactive sexual desire disorder and should be excluded by measuring serum total testosterone levels.

True incidence and prevalence rates of hypoactive sexual desire disorder in the general population are unknown. In studies of referred patient populations, the prevalence rate has been estimated at 5% in men and 22% in women.[7,8,134] Prevalence rates increase with age.[134,135] Whether these figures include situational hypoactive sexual desire disorder (i.e., desire for partnered sex is absent but self-stimulation continues) is unclear. Hypoactive sexual desire disorder often coexists with other sexual disorders, such as ED, and may develop as a consequence of other preexisting sexual disorders.[134-136]

Appropriate evaluation and treatment of hypoactive sexual desire disorder is important, because evaluation may lead to the detection of treatable androgen deficiency. Also, hypoactive sexual desire in one partner can strain the relationship between sexual partners[136,137] and lead to ED. Low sexual desire may impede or reduce the effectiveness of treatments for other sexual dysfunctions.

Erectile Dysfunction

Erectile dysfunction, previously referred to as impotence, is the inability to attain or to maintain an erection sufficient for satisfactory sexual intercourse.[11,14-15] *Sexual dysfunction* is a more general term that also includes libidinal, orgasmic, and ejaculatory dysfunction, in addition to the inability to attain or maintain penile erection. The MMAS[4] and NHSLS[6,7] investigations revealed a surprisingly high prevalence of ED in men (see later discussion). ED significantly affects quality of life of both the affected individual and his partner. In one study, ED had a negative impact on the sexual life of female partners, specifically on their sexual satisfaction and sexual drive.[137]

Prevalence and Incidence Rates

The best data on the prevalence of ED in men have emerged from two cross-sectional studies that used population-based sampling techniques, the MMAS[4,138]; and the NHSLS.[6,7] The MMAS was a cross-sectional and longitudinal, community-based epidemiologic survey in which 1709 men, 40 to 70 years of age, residing in the greater Boston area, were surveyed between 1987 and 1989.[4,138] Of these, 847 men were resurveyed between 1995 and 1997.[138] This study revealed that 52% of men between the ages of 40 and 70 were affected by ED of some degree; 17.2% of surveyed men reported minimal ED, 25.2% moderate ED, and 9.6% complete ED.[4,138] The NHSLS was a national probability survey of English-speaking Americans, 18 to 59 years of age, living in the United States.[6,7] This survey also revealed a high prevalence of ED in men, and the prevalence increased with increasing age.[6,7]

These two landmark studies and data from several other studies are in agreement that ED is a common problem worldwide.[4,6,7,135,138-143] ED has been estimated to affect 20 to 30 million men in the United States alone and 150 to 200 million men worldwide. The prevalence of ED increases with age; it affects fewer than 10% of men before 45 years of age but is present in 75% of men older than 80 years of age.[4] Men with other medical problems, such as hypertension, diabetes, cardiovascular disease, or end-stage renal disease, have a significantly higher prevalence of ED than healthy men.[4]

There is a paucity of longitudinal data on the incidence rates of ED in men. In the MMAS, the crude incidence rate among white men in the Boston area was 25.9 cases per 1000 man-years overall[138]: 12.4 cases per 1000 in the group aged 40 to 49 years, 29.8 per 1000 among 50- to 59-year-olds, and 46.4 per 1000 in the 60- to 69-year-old group.[138] In another study, incidence rates were derived from a survey of men seen at a preventive medicine clinic.[8] This study found the incidence rates of ED to be less than 3 cases per 1000 man-years among men younger than 45 years of age and 52 cases per 1000 man-years among men aged 65 years or older. These studies suggest a worldwide incidence of ED of 152 million in 1995 and an annual incidence of 600,000 to 700,000 in the United States.[142]

Risk Factors for Erectile Dysfunction

The risk factors for ED include age, diabetes mellitus, hypertension, smoking, medication use, depression, dyslipidemia, and cardiovascular disease.[4,140,141] Advancing age is an important risk factor for ED in men[4,140,141]: less than 10% of men younger than 40 years and more than 50% of those older than 70 have ED. In both the MMAS and the NHSLS, the prevalence of ED increased with each decade of life.[4,6]

Among the chronic diseases associated with ED, diabetes mellitus is the most important risk factor. In the MMAS, the age-adjusted risk of complete ED was three times higher in men with a history of treated diabetes mellitus than in those without a history of diabetes mellitus.[4,138] Fifty percent of men with diabetes mellitus will experience ED sometime during the course of their illness. In the MMAS, treated heart disease, treated hypertension, and hyperlipidemia were associated with significantly increased risk of ED. Among men with treated heart disease and hypertension, the probability of ED was more than two times greater for smokers than for nonsmokers. Smoking also increases the risk of ED in men taking medications for cardiovascular diseases. Cardiovascular disorders, including hypertension, stroke, coronary artery disease, and peripheral vascular disease, are all associated with increased risk of ED. Physical activity is associated with reduced risk of ED.[140]

Several reviews have emphasized the relationship between prescription medications and the occurrence of ED. In the MMAS, use of antihypertensives, cardiac medications, or oral hypoglycemic drugs was associated with an increased risk of ED.[4] Thiazide diuretics and psychotropic medications used in the treatment of depression may be the drugs most commonly associated with ED, simply because of the high prevalence of their use. However, a variety of drugs, including almost all antihypertensives, digoxin, histamine-2 receptor antagonists, anticholinergics, cytotoxic agents, and androgen antagonists, have been implicated in the pathophysiology of ED.

Erectile Dysfunction as a Marker of Cardiovascular Disease

Cardiovascular disease and ED share common risk factors, including diabetes mellitus, obesity, hypertension, smoking, and dyslipidemia.[144-152] ED precedes the symptoms of coronary artery disease by 2 to 3 years and cardiovascular events such as myocardial infarction or stroke by 3 to 5 years.[144-146] ED in men is associated with increased risk of death, particularly mortality due to cardiovascular disease.[147] The presence of ED is a good predictor of subsequent coronary artery disease, especially in younger men, independent of traditional coronary risk factors; however, it does not enhance the predictive ability of models that include traditional risk factors, likely reflecting the common pathophysiologic mechanisms of ED and coronary artery disease.[147] Men reporting ED are 1.3 to 1.6 times more likely to experience a cardiovascular event within 10 years than men without ED.[145-148]

Lower Urinary Tract Symptoms and Erectile Dysfunction

Surveys have revealed an association between lower urinary tract symptoms (LUTS) and ED,[153-159] even after adjusting for age and other risk factors. The Cologne Male Study and the Multinational Study of the Aging Male revealed that the presence and severity of LUTS is an predictor of ED irrespective of age.[154] LUTS and age are stronger predictors of ED than all other risk factors, including diabetes, dyslipidemia, and hypertension. Because LUTS and ED are two common conditions in middle-aged and older men, it is possible that this association reflects the coexistence of two highly prevalent conditions. However, there is growing evidence that the two conditions may be mechanistically linked, because the biochemical mechanisms that regulate bladder detrusor and cavernosal smooth muscle function share many similarities.[159,160]

Potassium channels, especially the calcium-sensitive BK_{Ca} channels, Rho A/Rho kinase signaling, L-type calcium channels, and gap junctions are important mediators of both detrusor and cavernosal smooth muscle contractility and relaxation. Increased myocyte contractility that characterizes both bladder detrusor dysfunction and ED may be mechanistically related to increased Rho kinase activity, impairments of potassium channel function,[159-161] α-adrenergic receptor imbalance, and endothelial dysfunction. Additional proposed hypotheses include increased sympathetic activity and autonomic dysfunction and alterations in NO generation or PKG activity in the detrusor and cavernosal smooth muscles.[159-161] Some therapies for LUTS, such as some types of surgery and 5α-reductase inhibitors, may worsen sexual dysfunction. PDE5 inhibitors are being investigated for the treatment of LUTS.[161-164]

Ejaculatory Disorders

Ejaculatory disorders include premature ejaculation, delayed ejaculation, retrograde ejaculation, anejaculation/anorgasmia, and painful ejaculation.[86,89] Recent surveys have highlighted the high prevalence and clinical importance of ejaculatory disorders.[89,165,166] Although the availability of oral PDE5 inhibitors has increased awareness of ED, ejaculatory disorders are at least as prevalent and may be even more prevalent than ED.[165,166] *Premature ejaculation,* defined as ejaculation associated with lack of or poor ejaculatory control that causes distress in one or both partners, is the most prevalent sexual disorder in men 18 to 59 years of age.[86,89,165] *Delayed ejaculation* refers to inability to ejaculate in a reasonable period that interferes with sexual or emotional satisfaction and is associated with distress.

Retrograde ejaculation is the failure of the semen to be ejected out through the urethral meatus; instead, the semen is propelled backward into the urinary bladder. Retrograde ejaculation can be the result of autonomic neuropathy associated with diabetes mellitus; sympathectomy; therapy with adrenergic antagonists, some types of antihypertensives, antipsychotics, or antidepressants; bladder neck incompetence; or urethral obstruction. Retrograde ejaculation due to diabetes-associated autonomic neuropathy is the second most prevalent ejaculatory disorder. After transurethral resection of the prostate, the bladder neck closure mechanism may be damaged. Patients remain continent because of a second, more distal, continence mechanism that is present in the region of the membranous urethra; however, many patients who have undergone transurethral resection of the prostate experience retrograde ejaculation. Ejaculatory disorders can lead to infertility among men.

DEFINITIONS OF SEXUAL DISORDERS IN WOMEN

The Third International Consensus on Sexual Dysfunctions in Men and Women in 2009 endorsed the interim revisions to the current DSM (Fourth Edition, Text Revised)

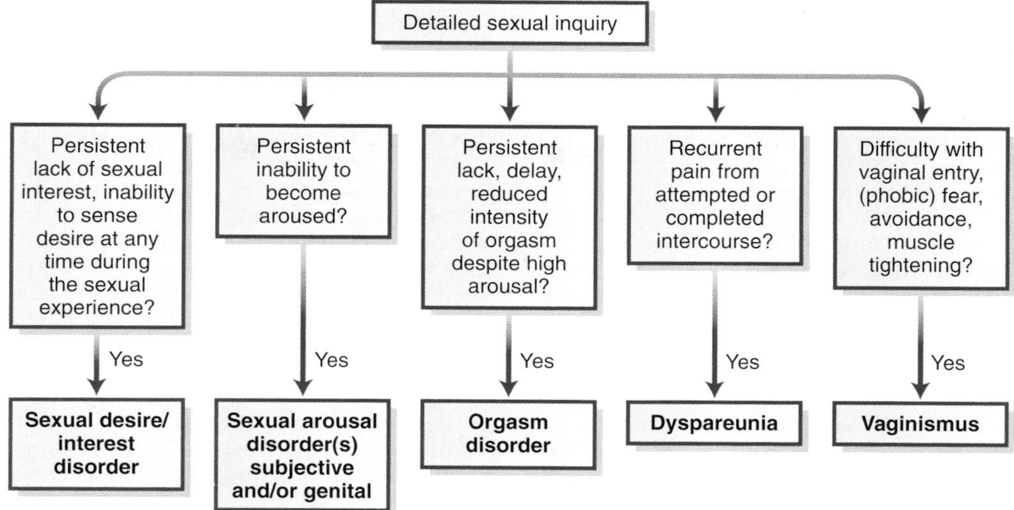

Figure 20-8 Currently recommended definitions for women's sexual dysfunction. Comorbidity is usual, especially sexual desire/interest disorder with one of the sexual arousal disorders. (From Basson R, Leiblum S, Brotto L, et al. Definitions of women's sexual dysfunctions reconsidered: advocating expansion and revision. *J Psychosom Obstet Gynaecol.* 2003;24:221-229.)

definitions of women's sexual dysfunction proposed in 2003.[167] Definitive changes (DSM5) are expected in 2013. The currently recommended definitions for women's sexual dysfunction are shown in Figure 20-8.

Sexual Desire/Interest Disorder

In sexual desire/interest disorder, feelings of sexual interest or desire are absent or diminished, sexual thoughts or fantasies are absent, and there is a lack of responsive desire. Motivations (here defined as reasons or incentives) for attempting to become sexually aroused are scarce or absent. The lack of interest is considered to be beyond the normative lessening with lifecycle and relationship duration.[167]

Apparently innate or "spontaneous" desire, present before sexual stimulation begins, is often present for women especially early in a relationship and sometimes is associated with the menstrual cycle. However, absence of sexual desire does not equate to dysfunction: typically, initial or spontaneous desire lessens with relationship duration.[168]

Prevalence is unclear given the lack of consistency of definition of hypoactive sexual desire in the different studies. Studies reporting low desire and distress have had reported prevalence rates of about 10%, not increasing with age.

Risk factors include negative feelings for the partner and mood disorders. Depression, either currently or in the past, and, in the absence of any diagnosed depression, more depressive and anxious thoughts and low self-esteem are found significantly more commonly than in control women.[169]

Arousal Disorders

Most women complaining of lack of arousal show physiologically healthy vasocongestive responses in the genitalia to erotic sexual stimulation, as measured by VPP, but do not experience subjective arousal; it is their lack of subjective arousal that is the key to their distress, rather than failure of genital congestion.[53] The subtypes of sexual arousal disorder include subjective sexual arousal disorder, genital sexual arousal disorder, and persistent genital arousal disorder.

Subjective Arousal Disorder

In subjective arousal disorder, feelings of sexual arousal (sexual excitement and sexual pleasure) from any type of sexual stimulation are absent or markedly diminished. Vaginal lubrication or other signs of physical response still occur.[167](See Fig. 20-10.)

Genital Sexual Arousal Disorder

In patients with complaints of impaired genital sexual arousal, the self-report may include minimal vulvar swelling or vaginal lubrication with any type of sexual stimulation and reduced sexual sensations from caressing of the genitalia. Subjective sexual excitement still occurs from nongenital sexual stimuli.[167]

A woman diagnosed with the genital subtype of arousal disorder indicates that she can still be subjectively aroused by, for instance, viewing an erotic film, pleasuring her partner, being kissed, or receiving breast stimulation. She complains of the marked loss of intensity of any genital response including orgasm. Awareness of throbbing, swelling, and lubrication is absent or markedly diminished.

It is the woman's self-report of absent or impaired genital congestion and lubrication that is the basis of the definition. There may or may not be demonstrable physical pathophysiology if such testing were available. Moreover, loss of sexual quality of sensations despite apparently adequate engorgement can occur and is little understood.

Interim publications referring to DSM5 revisions to definitions advocate that desire and arousal disorders be merged.[126,127] Increasing evidence that desire ahead of and at the outset of sexual engagement, although welcomed probably by both partners, is not mandatory for a woman's sexual enjoyment and satisfaction.[136,127] It is the inability to trigger desire and arousal during sexual engagement (as well as an absence of desire initially) that constitutes disorder. Therefore, merging of sexual and desire difficulties into one disorder appears logical.

Persistent Genital Arousal Disorder

In persistent genital arousal disorder, there is spontaneous, intrusive, and unwanted genital arousal (e.g., tingling, throbbing, pulsating) in the absence of sexual interest and desire. Any awareness of subjective arousal is typically, but not invariably, unpleasant. The arousal is unrelieved by one or more orgasms, and the feelings of arousal persist for hours or days.[167]

The disorder is poorly understood but is becoming a more frequently recognized syndrome. The definition is recommended to facilitate investigation of prevalence and etiology.

Women's Orgasmic Disorder

In women with orgasm disorder, despite self-reports of high sexual arousal or excitement, there is either lack of orgasm, markedly diminished intensity of orgasmic sensations, or marked delay of orgasm from any kind of stimulation.[167]

The prevalence is unclear, because many studies include women with low arousal who do not reach orgasm. Risk factors include anxiety about the partner's presence, fear of being vulnerable, fear of not being in control, and fear of intimacy. These factors often stem from childhood (nonsexual) experiences.

Dyspareunia

In dyspareunia, there is persistent or recurrent pain with attempted or complete vaginal entry or penile vaginal intercourse.[167] It is recommended that the experience of women who cannot tolerate full penile entry and the movements of intercourse because of pain be included in the definition of dyspareunia. Clearly, the outcome depends on the woman's pain tolerance and her partner's hesitancy or insistence.

Reported prevalence rates vary between 20% and 35%. The most common form of dyspareunia, provoked vestibulodynia (PVD), affects some 16% of (mostly young) women.[170] Risk factors for PVD include some personality traits—perfectionism, reward dependency, fear of negative evaluation—as well as harm avoidance, hypervigilance for pain, higher levels of trait anxiety, and shyness.[170] For a small subset, vaginal candidiasis appears to precipitate and maintain the condition.

Vaginismus

A woman with vaginismus has persistent or recurrent difficulties in allowing vaginal entry of a penis, a finger, and/or any object, despite her expressed will to do so. There is often (phobic) avoidance, involuntary pelvic muscle contraction, and anticipation or fear of pain or the experience of pain. Structural and other physical abnormalities must be ruled out or addressed.[167]

Prevalence rates are unclear. Risk factors include depression, anxiety, social phobia, somatization, and hostility. Some studies identify increased catastrophic thinking in women with vaginismus compared with women without dyspareunia or women with other forms of pain (e.g., PVD); moreover, women with vaginismus show higher disgust propensity.[170] Despite the theories, there is no scientific evidence that vaginismus is secondary to religious orthodoxy, negative sexual upbringing, or concerns about sexual orientation. There is typically extreme fear of vaginal entry, fear that harm will come from something the size of a penis entering the vagina, and fear of damage by vaginal delivery.

SEXUAL DYSFUNCTION IN THE CONTEXT OF ENDOCRINE DISEASE

This section focuses on sexual sequelae of endocrine disease and its treatment, but in any given person, nonendocrine factors may be more important. These include psychological, relational, contextual, cultural, and nonendocrine medical influences, especially depression, hypertension, neurologic disease, and LUTS.[21] For patients with chronic disease, the disease itself, its treatment, its psychological effects, and interpersonal, personal, and contextual issues affect sexual response.[21,171]

In healthy women, factors such as attitudes toward sex, feelings for the partner, past sexual experiences, duration of the relationship, and mental and emotional health have been shown to modulate desire and arousability more strongly than biologic factors.[16,171-174] Contrary to gender stereotypes, recent analysis of the 1035 sexually active adults who participated in the NHSLS in 1992 showed that men's physical sexual pleasure was more closely linked to relational factors than was the case for women.[26] Similarly, in a recent international study of midlife and older couples, men rated the importance of sex for closeness and intimacy to their partner more highly than did their female partners.[27] Qualitative research also suggests that men as well as women note that positive self-esteem and feeling attractive enhance desire and arousal.[24,30] Sexual context is also important for both men and women.[24,30,174]

Endocrine Disorders and Sexual Dysfunction in Men

Androgen Deficiency Syndromes

Androgen deficiency can occur because of primary testicular dysfunction or as a result of disorders affecting the hypothalamus or the pituitary.[107] Common causes of primary testicular dysfunction include Klinefelter's syndrome, uncorrected cryptorchidism, human immunodeficiency virus (HIV) disease, orchitis, trauma, torsion, and irradiation and cancer chemotherapy.[107] Before arriving at a diagnosis of idiopathic hypogonadotropic hypogonadism, systemic illness, excessive exercise, recreational drugs (especially marijuana, cocaine, and alcohol), central hypogonadism from pituitary or suprasellar tumors, hemochromatosis, hyperprolactinemia, and infiltrative disorders should be considered.[107] The testosterone levels required to maintain sexual function are close to the lower limit of the normal male range.[109,175-177] Therefore, some men with pituitary tumors may remain asymptomatic until their tumor has grown substantially and testosterone levels have declined to a level below this threshold.

Diabetes and Sexual Dysfunction in Men

Men with diabetes mellitus are at increased risk for ED, retrograde ejaculation, and low testosterone levels. Peyronie's disease is an important comorbid condition in older diabetic men with ED.[178-186] Men with diabetes have significantly lower scores for sexual desire, activity, arousal, and satisfaction,[179,180] in part due to the medical and psychological factors associated with diabetes, such as the variations in glycemic control, reduced energy, altered self-image, and interpersonal difficulties regarding dietary compliance, glucose monitoring, and medications. Diabetes also is associated with increased risk of low testosterone levels.[177,187-190] In population studies, sex hormone–binding globulin (SHBG) and total testosterone are more strongly associated with diabetes risk than free testosterone levels; these data suggest that the observed association of testosterone with diabetes risk may be related to factors such as insulin sensitivity and inflammation that regulate SHBG.[191]

The prevalence of ED in men with diabetes increases with age and has been as high as 75% in some studies. ED in men with type 2 diabetes, even without other risk factors for coronary artery disease, may signal silent cardiac ischemia.[192] Among men with diabetes, those with ED are more likely to be older smokers with longer duration of diabetes, poor metabolic control, untreated hypertension, and presence of neuropathy, microalbuminuria, macroalbuminuria, retinopathy, cardiovascular disease, diuretic treatment, low testosterone levels, and psychological vulnerability.[183-186] Increased physical activity and consumption of small amounts of alcohol have been found to be protective. The risk of ED generally increases with chronic elevation of glycosylated hemoglobin (HbA_{1c}).[183]

Endothelial and smooth muscle dysfunction, autonomic neuropathy, and psychological and interpersonal issues contribute to sexual dysfunction in men with diabetes.[193-195] Endothelial dysfunction is evident in penile blood vessels and in nongenital vascular beds.[194] Endothelial NOS (eNOS) is reduced, possibly due to overexpression of arginase or lack of reduced nicotinamide adenine dinucleotide phosphate (NADPH), an essential cofactor for NOS.[193-200] Additionally, accumulation of oxygen free radicals, including those from advanced glycosylation end products, quench NO and attenuate the action of potassium channels.[196] The low NADPH is also associated with increased diacylglycerol and protein kinase C and, consequently, increased smooth muscle contractility.[193,195] Increased activation of the RhoA/Rho kinase pathway may increase the sensitivity of cavernosal smooth muscle to calcium.[197] Autonomic neuropathy affecting the pelvic nerves may lead to ED as well as ejaculatory dysfunction.[198]

Retrograde ejaculation and partial ejaculatory incompetence affect up to one third of men with diabetes.[201] Autonomic nerve damage in diabetes may be associated with dysfunction of the internal sphincter so that all or a part of the seminal fluid is propelled into the bladder.[198] *Partial ejaculatory incompetence* refers to the condition in which ejaculatory emission remains intact but the expulsion phase is inhibited; consequently, the semen trickles out of the penis and the experience of orgasm is altered in quality. Both ejaculatory problems may be a cause of infertility.

Sexual Dysfunction Associated with Therapies for Benign Prostatic Hypertrophy

Benign prostatic hypertrophy is frequently associated with LUTS and sexual dysfunction.[154-157,202] Although treatment with some α_1-adrenergic receptor blockers can improve erectile function, others (e.g., tamsulosin) are associated with ejaculatory dysfunction.[203] Treatment of men with LUTS with 5α-reductase inhibitors has been associated with increased risk of ejaculatory disorder, ED, and decreased libido.[204,205]

Hyperprolactinemia and Sexual Dysfunction

Hyperprolactinemic men often present with decreased libido or ED; 75% of men with macroprolactinomas and 50% of men with microprolactinomas report reduced desire or ED, and almost all have subnormal nocturnal penile erections.[206-209] Hyperprolactinemia affects 1% to 5% of men presenting with ED[206-207]; a fraction of these men have prolactin-secreting pituitary adenomas.

Prolactin lowers testosterone levels through its inhibitory effects on GnRH secretion and on the pituitary response to GnRH. Most, but not all, men with sexual dysfunction and hyperprolactinemia have low testosterone levels.[208,209] Whether and how hyperprolactinemia directly affects erectile function through target organ effects is not well understood. Erectile function usually improves in hyperprolactinemic men after treatment with dopamine agonists.[210]

Sexual Dysfunction in Patients with Thyroid Disease

Hypothyroidism has been associated with increased risk of hypoactive sexual desire and ED.[211-215] The exact prevalence of sexual dysfunction in men with hypothyroidism is unknown. Free testosterone levels are lower in hypothyroid men than in controls and become normal after thyroxine replacement.[211-215] Serum LH and follicle-stimulating hormone (FSH) levels are typically not elevated in men with primary hypothyroidism.[211] Hyperprolactinemia is noted in a small fraction of hypothyroid men.[211]

Free testosterone levels are typically normal in men with hyperthyroidism, but SHBG and estradiol levels are elevated, resulting in a high ratio of estradiol to testosterone and gynecomastia in some hyperthyroid men.[211-213] Hyperthyroidism has been observed in a small fraction of men with ED.[79]

Sexual Dysfunction in Men with Metabolic Syndrome

Men with metabolic syndrome have a higher prevalence of ED than men without the metabolic syndrome.[216-219] The risk of ED is correlated with the number of identified components of metabolic syndrome.[216-219]

Endocrine Disorders and Sexual Dysfunction in Women

Diabetes in Women

That women with diabetes mellitus are more likely than age-matched controls to report sexual dissatisfaction is confirmed in most studies.[220-225] In contrast to men with diabetes and ED, in whom glycemic control and disease duration correlate with the incidence of ED, usually no such correlation has been observed in women with diabetes and sexual dysfunction. A review of sexual dysfunction in women with diabetes mellitus confirmed a consistent link with comorbid depression.[226]

Past studies often failed to differentiate between type 1 and type 2 diabetes, and many did not separate premenopausal and postmenopausal women with diabetes mellitus. The rates of decreased desire are generally similar in women with and without diabetes, but decreased arousal and reduced lubrication are more common in women with diabetes. However, in one study, younger women with diabetes had low desire but otherwise normal sexual responses, whereas all phases of sexual response, including sexual desire, were blunted in women older than 50 years of age, compared with controls.[225] A recent large study of women enrolled in the long-term Epidemiology of Diabetes, Interventions, and Complications (EDIC) study, albeit without a comparison group of control subjects, confirmed dysfunction in 35% of those women who were sexually active. Low desire was present in more than one half of the women; problems with orgasm, arousal, and lubrication in 40% to 50%; and pain in 21%.[227] In multivariate analysis, only depression and marital status predicted sexual dysfunction. Data on dyspareunia and orgasmic difficulties are conflicting.

In women, hyperandrogenism is associated with increased risk of diabetes due to increased insulin resistance and pancreatic beta cell dysfunction.[228-231] Lower SHBG levels are associated with type 2 diabetes in both genders.[187,191] In women with polycystic ovary syndrome, the length of the polyglutamine tract in exon 1 of the androgen receptor gene has been reported to modulate the association between increased testosterone and insulin resistance.[232] Estrogen therapy has been shown to decrease androgen levels and improve glucose control.[233,234] The protective effects of estrogen on pancreatic insulin secretion, insulin sensitivity, and genital tissue health in women need further investigation.

Diabetes has been associated with reduced clitoral blood flow and cavernosal smooth muscle content and decreased sensation in the clitoris, labia, and vagina as well as extragenital sites.[235,236] The peripheral vascular dysfunction and neuropathy in diabetes also potentially impair sexual response.

Metabolic Syndrome in Women

Metabolic syndrome has been shown to have a negative effect on women's sexuality, independent of associated diabetes and obesity.[237-239] This negative effect seems to be more prevalent in premenopausal rather than postmenopausal women.[237-239]

Polycystic Ovary Syndrome

Limited research has shown that women with polycystic ovary syndrome may be less sexually satisfied and may find themselves less attractive than controls.[240-242] The presumption is that these findings are related to obesity and androgen-related symptoms.[240,241] There is minimal information on treatment of androgen excess with antiandrogens: one small case study reported that desire increased in 6 women and decreased in 13 women treated with an antiandrogen.[243] Another study showed that the insulin sensitizer, metformin, improved psychosexual function in women with polycystic ovary syndrome.[244]

Congenital Adrenal Hyperplasia

Nonclassic forms of congenital adrenal hyperplasia may manifest with signs of hyperandrogenism in childhood or adulthood, depending on the severity of the 21-hydroxylase enzyme deficiency.[245] The presenting features of 21-hydroxylase enzyme deficiency may include menstrual disorders such as amenorrhea, anovulation, hirsutism, or oligomenorrhea with infertility.[245,246] Limited research suggests that sexual functioning of women with nonclassic 21-hydroxylase deficiency is not different from that of controls. However, women with classic congenital adrenal hyperplasia may show gender-atypical behavior[247]; in one study, male-typical role-playing in childhood correlated with reduced satisfaction with the female gender role and reduced heterosexual interest in adulthood.[248] Disturbed body image, repeated genital examinations, and genital surgery may also affect sexual function in women with congenital adrenal hyperplasia.[247] Clearly, caring for these women requires careful individualized treatment with appropriate therapy for signs and symptoms of androgen excess as well as psychosexual counseling.

Hyperprolactinemia in Women

Hyperprolactinemia is associated with increased risk of sexual dysfunction.[249-251] Women with hyperprolactinemia report lower overall satisfaction with sexual function and lower scores for sexual desire, arousal, lubrication, and orgasm domains than women with normal prolactin levels.[250] Prolactin inhibits GnRH pulses, attenuates gonadotropin response to GnRH, and is associated with reduced ovarian secretion of estrogen and androgen. Therefore, sexual dysfunction in women with hyperprolactinemia may be related to changes in sex hormones. Although menstrual disturbance or infertility is more commonly the presenting symptom of hyperprolactinemia, lower scores for sexual function and desire have also been found in women with hyperprolactinemia who have regular menses.[249-251] Normal menstruation, younger age, and small tumor size are more likely to be associated with normal sexual function than the actual level of prolactin or testosterone.[249-251] Sexual outcomes of treatment of hyperprolactinemic women with dopamine agonists have not been well studied.

Pituitary Disease in Women

There is limited research on sexual function in women who have deficiencies of various pituitary hormones. Most women with pituitary disease report menstrual irregularity or problems with sexual function, including decreased sexual desire and problems with lubrication or orgasm.[251] In one randomized trial of 51 women, testosterone therapy in women who were receiving estrogen therapy was associated with some benefit in sexual function and mood, compared with placebo, and a higher frequency of androgenic side effects than placebo.[252] The effects of dehydroepiandrosterone (DHEA) on sexual function and mood in women with hypopituitarism are poorly understood.[253]

Adrenal Insufficiency

In addition to the deficiency of cortisol and aldosterone, women with adrenal insufficiency also have low levels of testosterone and DHEA.[253-257] Adrenal insufficiency in women has been associated with low sexual desire, general lack of well-being, and poor quality of life. However, clinical trials of DHEA replacement in women with adrenal insufficiency have reported inconsistent results, possibly due, in part, to their small size.[253-257] An earlier small trial in women with primary or secondary adrenal insufficiency reported greater improvements in sexual interest and satisfaction and in mood for women receiving DHEA, compared with placebo[253]; however, two other studies did not find significant improvements in sexual function.[254,255]

Natural Menopause

A majority of women who discontinue postmenopausal estrogen supplementation develops signs of vulval vaginal atrophy, which is a risk factor for sexual dysfunction.[258] Among sexually active women, those with sexual dysfunction are 3.8 times more likely to have atrophy than those with normal sexual function.[258] However, epidemiologic studies have not shown an increase in the prevalence of dyspareunia with age.[259-261] Clearly, not all postmenopausal women develop sexual symptoms of estrogen deficiency. It is likely that multiple factors contribute to sexual symptoms, including variations in the intracrine production of estrogen from adrenal precursors, in the number and sensitivity of estrogen receptors, and in the degree of sexual arousal or excitement at the time of vulval stimulation and vaginal entry.[262-264]

Most studies report a decrease in sexual desire with advancing age[265] that is not easily explained by estrogen deficiency alone. Adaptive changes occur in the brain in response to the reductions in circulating levels of sex hormones associated with age and menopause.[266,267] Sex hormones may be produced locally within the brain: in women, steroidogenic enzymes and sex receptors in the brain are upregulated in response to decreased circulating levels of sex hormones.[266,267] Investigation of the question of biologic adaptation to reduced amounts of sex hormones is in its infancy.

Surgical Menopause

Surgical menopause is a state of both androgen and estrogen deficiency and has often been viewed as a risk factor for sexual dysfunction in women. However, studies have shown that most women undergoing bilateral salpingo-oophorectomy (BSO) for benign clinical indications do not develop sexual dysfunction.[268-270] Three prospective studies found that women choosing BSO plus hysterectomy for benign indications did not develop sexual dysfunction over the next 1 to 3 years.[268-270]

A large national survey of 2207 American women confirmed an increased prevalence of distress about low sexual desire in women with a relatively recent BSO. However, both older and younger women with a relatively recent BSO reported low sexual desire per se as often as age-matched subjects with intact ovaries. Moreover, despite their continued hormonal deficit, women older than 45 years who underwent oophorectomy before menopause had fewer complaints of low desire than women of similar age with intact ovaries.[265]

Aging-Associated Decline in Sex Hormone Precursors in Women

From the middle 30s to the early 60s, a woman's adrenal production of precursor hormones—DHEA, androstenedione, and DHEA sulfate (DHEAS)—declines by 70%.[262,263,271,273] However, the trajectories of decline in these precursor steroids vary among women.[261-263,271,274] The relationship of the age-related decline in these circulating precursors to sexual function remains poorly understood. On the population level, variation in circulating levels of sex steroids and their precursors[271-274] is related to variation in the activities of steroidogenic enzymes such as 3β-hydroxysteroid dehydrogenase (3β-HSD), 17β-HSD, 17,20-lyase, and aromatase and to variation in the plasma clearance of these hormones and precursors.[262-264] Total androgen production is measured by means of androgen metabolites, most notably androsterone glucuronide (ADT-G).[263] A recent study of 250 women carefully evaluated for sexual dysfunction found that ADT-G levels in the 124 control women were comparable to those in the 121 women with sexual dysfunction.[275]

Selective Estrogen Receptor Modulators

Selective estrogen receptor modulators (SERMs) are a class of ligands that bind estrogen receptor subtypes and induce a unique profile of tissue-specific gene expression. Accordingly, each SERM may also be associated with a unique set of clinical responses. Currently available SERMS do not ameliorate the genital sexual symptoms of estrogen lack. Sexual symptoms and hot flushes are more frequent in women receiving raloxifene than in those receiving tamoxifen.[276] Ospemifene is a novel SERM under trial for the treatment of vaginal atrophy in postmenopausal women.[277]

Oral Contraceptives

Combined oral contraceptives containing ethinyl estradiol increase SHBG and thus decrease available free testosterone. The decrease in sexual desire and subjective arousability in some women receiving oral contraceptives has been attributed to the decrease in free testosterone levels.[278,279] However, oral contraceptives exert multiple psychological and biologic actions, some of which may positively affect sexuality (e.g., by reducing anxiety about unwanted pregnancy and diminishing dysmenorrhea).[278,279]

Androgen Insensitivity Syndrome

Research on sexual function in 46,XY women with androgen insensitivity syndrome due to mutations in the androgen receptor is very limited. Women with complete androgen insensitivity syndrome have a female phenotype with full breast development but variable shallow vaginal development.[280] These women are often confronted with complex psychosocial issues related to the mismatch between their genetic sex and their gender role, the timing of diagnosis and timing of disclosure to the woman, and infertility. However, limited information from retrospective case series suggests that, despite androgen insensitivity, these women have normal sexual desire and function.[280]

ASSESSMENT OF SEXUAL DYSFUNCTION

Assessment of sexual function is an important part of the general assessment of patients with endocrine diseases. Open-ended, nonjudgmental questions such as, "Many men with diabetes notice changes in their erections or ejaculation—are you having any difficulties?" can facilitate further discussion of sexual problems. When sexual problems are identified, sensitive and respectful inquiry into their nature and the current and past sexual context is necessary. Evaluating both partners together as well as individually can often uncover problems that may not be apparent in individual interviews (see Table 20-4).

Evaluation of Men with Sexual Dysfunction

There are four important considerations in the evaluation of men with hypoactive sexual desire disorders. First, an important initial step in the evaluation is an interview of the couple to determine which dysfunctions are present, such as ED, problematic sexual desire, and difficulties with ejaculation or orgasm. Second, the clinician should ascertain whether the couple has a relationship problem. It should be established whether self-stimulation continues despite lack of desire for partnered sex. With the availability of Internet sites, sex alone, possibly on a frequent basis, may allow sexual expression in spite of relationship difficulties. Third, a general health evaluation is necessary to exclude systemic illness, depression, and medication use. Fourth, testosterone levels should be measured to exclude androgen deficiency, which is an important treatable cause of hypoactive sexual desire disorder.

The diagnostic workup of men with ED should start with an evaluation of general health (Tables 20-3 and 20-4). The presence of diabetes mellitus, coronary artery disease, peripheral vascular disease, hypertension, stroke, spinal cord or back injury, multiple sclerosis, depression, or dementia should be verified. Information about use of

TABLE 20-3

Diagnostic Evaluation of Erectile Dysfunction

History
Ascertain Psychosexual History The nature of sexual dysfunction: whether the primary problem is decreased desire, ED, premature or delayed ejaculation, or difficulty in achieving orgasms The strength of the marital relationship and marital discord Depression Stress Sexual performance anxiety Knowledge and beliefs about sexuality
Ascertain Risk Factors The presence of diabetes mellitus, hypertension, CAD, end-stage renal disease, or peripheral vascular disease History of spinal cord injury, stroke, or Alzheimer's disease Prostate or pelvic surgery Pelvic injury Medications such as antihypertensives, antidepressants, antipsychotics, antiandrogens, and inhibitors of androgen production The use of recreational drugs such as alcohol, cocaine, opiates, and tobacco
Ascertain Factors That Might Affect Choice of Therapy or the Patient's Response to Therapy Coexisting CAD and its symptoms and severity Exercise tolerance The use of nitrates or nitrate donors The use of α-adrenergic blockers The use of vasodilators for hypertension or congestive heart failure The use of foods (e.g., cranberry juice) or drugs (e.g., erythromycin, protease inhibitors, ketoconazole, itraconazole) that might affect the metabolism of PDE5 inhibitors
Physical Examination
Ascertain signs of androgen deficiency, such as loss of secondary sex characteristics, eunuchoidal proportions, small testicular volume, or breast enlargement Evaluate genital and perineal sensation to evaluate neurologic deficit due to spinal cord lesion, previous stroke, or peripheral neuropathy Measure blood pressure and postural change in blood pressure Evaluate femoral and pedal pulses and evidence of lower-extremity ischemia Conduct a penile examination to exclude Peyronie's disease and other penile deformities
Basic Laboratory Evaluation* for All Men with Erectile Dysfunction
Fasting blood glucose level Serum testosterone level

*Basic tests that should be performed in all men with ED.
CAD, coronary artery disease; ED, erectile dysfunction; PDE5, phosphodiesterase isoform 5.

recreational drugs such as alcohol, marijuana, cocaine, or tobacco; prescription medications, particularly antihypertensives, antiandrogens, antidepressants, and antipsychotic drugs; and nonprescription, over-the-counter supplements is important, because almost a quarter of all cases of ED can be attributed to medications. A detailed sexual history, including the nature of relationships, partner expectations, situational erectile failure, performance anxiety, and marital discord or dissatisfaction, needs to be elicited. It is important to distinguish between inability to achieve erection, changes in sexual desire, and failure to achieve orgasm and ejaculation, because the etiologic factors vary with the type of sexual disorder.

A directed physical examination should focus on secondary sex characteristics, the presence or absence of breast enlargement, testicular volume, evaluation of femoral and pedal pulses; neurologic examination to determine the presence of motor weakness, perineal sensation, anal sphincter tone, and bulbocavernosus reflex; and examination of the penis to evaluate any unusual curvature, palpable plaques, or superficial lesions.[276,277]

The laboratory tests in the evaluation of a man with ED usually include the measurements of hemoglobin, blood glucose, blood urea nitrogen, creatinine, plasma lipids, and testosterone levels.

The initial diagnostic work in most men presenting with ED consists of general health evaluation, evaluation of cardiovascular risk, and the measurements of hemoglobin, blood glucose, BUN and creatinine, plasma lipids, and measurement of serum testosterone levels. Further evaluation using more invasive diagnostic testing is limited to those men who do not respond to an empiric trial of oral PDE5 inhibitors; these patients should be referred to a specialist for detailed evaluation of sexual function.[278-281]

The diagnosis of androgen deficiency should be made only in men with consistent symptoms and signs and unequivocally low early-morning serum testosterone levels that are below the lower limit of the normal range for healthy young men (e.g., testosterone <300 ng/dL in some laboratories) on at least two occasions.[107] Initial evaluation is directed at excluding systemic illness, eating disorders, excessive exercise, and the use of medicines and recreational drugs that can suppress testosterone levels. Measurement of the morning total testosterone level by a reliable assay remains the best initial test. Measurements of free or bioavailable testosterone levels may be useful in men with suspected SHBG abnormalities due to aging, obesity, chronic illness, thyroid disease, or liver disease.

In men found to be androgen-deficient, measurement of LH levels helps distinguish between testicular (LH elevated) and hypothalamic-pituitary (LH low or inappropriately normal) defects. Men with hypogonadotropic hypogonadism may require measurement of serum prolactin, serum transferring, evaluation of other pituitary hormones, and pituitary MRI. The diagnostic yield of pituitary imaging to exclude pituitary tumors can be improved by selecting men with testosterone levels lower than 150 ng/dL, panhypopituitarism, persistent hyperprolactinemia, or symptoms of tumor mass.[282,283]

There is considerable debate about the usefulness and cost-effectiveness of hormonal evaluation and the extent to which androgen deficiency should be investigated in men presenting with ED. Between 8% and 10% of men with ED have low testosterone levels; the prevalence of androgen deficiency increases with advancing age.[284-287] The prevalence of low testosterone levels is not significantly different among men who present with ED and men in an age-matched population.[116] These data are consistent with the proposal that ED and androgen deficiency are two common but independently distributed disorders.[116] However, it is important to exclude androgen deficiency in this patient population. Androgen deficiency is a correctable cause of sexual dysfunction, and in some men, ED and low testosterone levels respond to testosterone replacement. Androgen deficiency can have additional deleterious effects on the individual's health; for instance, it may contribute to osteoporosis and loss of muscle mass and function.

In large studies,[116,282,283] only a small fraction of men with ED and low testosterone levels have been found to

TABLE 20-4

Assessment of Sexual Dysfunction

Assessment Questions	Comments
Questions Asked of Both Partners	
1. Sexual problems and reason for presenting at this time	Ask patients to describe sexual problems in their own words; clarify further with direct questions, giving options rather than leading questions, support and encouragement, acknowledgement of embarrassment, and reassurance that sexual problems are common
2. Duration, consistency, and priority if more than one problem is present	Are problems present in all situations? Which problem is most troubling?
Context of sexual problems	Emotional intimacy between partners, activity or behavior just before sexual activity, privacy, sexual communication, time of day and fatigue level, birth control (adequacy, type), risk of STDs, usefulness of sexual stimulation, sexual knowledge.
3. Rest of each partner's sexual response, other than the given problem area	Both currently and before the onset of the sexual problems
4. Reaction of each partner	How each has reacted emotionally, sexually, and behaviorally.
5. Previous help	Compliance with recommendations and effectiveness
Questions Asked of Each Partner When Seen Alone*	
1. Partner's own assessment of the situation	Sometimes it is easier to disclose symptom severity (e.g., total lack of desire) in the partner's absence
2. Sexual response with self-stimulation	Also inquire about sexual thoughts and fantasies
3. Past sexual experiences	Positive and negative aspects
4. Developmental history	Relationships to others in the home while growing up; losses, traumas, to whom (if anyone) was the patient close; was he or she shown physical affection, love, respect?
5. Past or current sexual, emotional, and physical abuse	Explain that abuse questions are routine and do not necessarily imply causation of the problems; it is helpful to ask whether the patient ever felt hurt or threatened in the relationship and, if so, whether he or she wishes to give more information
6. Physical health, especially conditions leading to debility and fatigue, difficulty with mobility (e.g., in caressing a partner, performing self-stimulation), and difficulties with self-image (e.g., from obesity, hypogonadism)	Specifically, ask about medications with known sexual side effects, including SSRIs, β-blockers, antiandrogens, GnRH agonists, oral contraceptives
7. Evaluation of mood	A significant correlation of sexual function and mood (including anxiety and depression) warrants routine screening for mood disorder using either a questionnaire, e.g., Beck Inventory or semi-structured series of questions.

*Items 3 through 5 of the single-patient interview may sometimes be omitted (e.g., for a recent problem after decades of healthy sexual function).
SSRIs, selective serotin reuptake inhibitors; GnRH, gonadotropin-releasing hormone; STDs, sexually transmitted diseases.
Adapted with permission from Basson R. Sexual dysfunction in women. *N Engl J Med.* 2006;354:1497-1506.

have space-occupying lesions of the hypothalamic-pituitary region. In one large survey, all of the hypothalamic-pituitary lesions were found in men with serum testosterone levels lower than 150 ng/dL.[282,283] Therefore, the cost-effectiveness of the diagnostic workup to rule out an underlying lesion of the hypothalamic-pituitary region can be increased by limiting the workup to men with serum testosterone levels lower than 150 ng/dL.[107]

If the history, physical examination, and laboratory tests do not identify medical problems needing further workup, then a cost-effective approach is to prescribe a trial of an oral PDE5 inhibitor, provided there are no contraindications (e.g., nitrate use).

Tests that evaluate the integrity of penile vasculature and blood flow[288,289] are not needed in most patients with ED; they are reserved for patients in whom the results of these tests would alter the management or prognosis. These tests should be performed only by those with considerable experience with their use. The penile brachial blood pressure index is a simple and specific, but not a sensitive, index of vascular insufficiency.[288] It is rarely used today in the evaluation of ED.

Intracavernosal injection of a vasoactive agent such as PGE_1 can be useful as a diagnostic as well as a potential therapeutic modality. This procedure can reveal whether there will be a response to this therapeutic modality, and it facilitates patient education about the procedure and its potential side effects. Failure to respond to intracavernosal injection can raise the suspicion of vascular insufficiency or a venous leak that might need further evaluation and treatment.

Most men with ED do not need duplex color sonography, cavernosography, or pelvic angiography.[11,277,289] Angiography could be useful in a young man with arterial insufficiency associated with pelvic trauma. Suspicion of congenital or traumatic venous leak in a young man presenting with ED would justify a cavernosography. In each instance, confirmation of the vascular lesion might lead to consideration of surgery. Duplex ultrasonography can provide a noninvasive evaluation of vascular function.[289]

Nocturnal penile tumescence testing is not needed for most patients being evaluated for ED; it is recommended only when there is high clinical suspicion of psychogenic ED or situational problems or to document poor penile rigidity preoperatively, or for medicolegal reasons. Although recording of nocturnal penile tumescence in a sleep laboratory on successive nights can help differentiate organic from psychogenic impotence, this test is expensive and labor intensive. For most cases, a careful history of nighttime or early-morning erections provides a reasonable correlation with nocturnal penile tumescence and RigiScan studies.[290]

The introduction of portable RigiScan devices in 1985 provided clinicians with a reliable means of continuously monitoring penile tumescence and rigidity at home.[290] It is a multicomponent device that the patient wears at bedtime for two or three nights. It has two wire gauge loops that are placed around the base and tip of the penis and record changes in penile circumference and rigidity. Data are stored and downloaded by means of a software program that allows for interpretation.

Evaluation of Women with Sexual Dysfunction

Physical examination, including pelvic and genital examination, is part of routine care (Table 20-5; see Table 20-4) and can be reassuring to the patient by confirming normal anatomy and tissue health. Unless dyspareunia is involved, it is not often that physical examination identifies the cause of sexual dysfunction. For some women with a history of coercive or abusive sexual experiences, such an examination can cause extreme anxiety. The reason for the examination and an explanation of what will and will not be done should be provided before the examination begins. In women with vaginismus, the vaginal examination should be delayed until psychological therapy renders it possible without undue discomfort to the patient.

Laboratory testing plays a small role in women's sexual evaluation. Estrogen activity is best evaluated by history and examination. The commercially available estradiol radioimmunoassays lack the sensitivity and precision required to measure the low concentrations present in the older woman; also, these assays do not measure estrone, the major estrogen in postmenopausal women. Serum levels of testosterone do not correlate with sexual function, and the available radioimmunoassays currently do not have the required sensitivity or accuracy at the low levels found in women. Liquid chromatography/mass spectrometry can provide accurate measurements of testosterone levels in women and is now available from several commercial laboratories. However, the levels of testosterone so measured were similar in women with and without sexual dysfunction in a recent study of 250 carefully evaluated women.[275]

The circulating testosterone levels may not reflect intracrine production or metabolism of androgens. Measurement of testosterone metabolites has been proposed as a marker of intracrine plus gonadal production of testosterone, but the circulating levels of these metabolites have been shown to be similar in women with and without sexual dysfunction.[275] Prolactin or thyrotropin should be measured if there are other symptoms that suggest abnormality.[1]

TABLE 20-5

Physical Examination for the Woman with Sexual Dysfunction: What to Look For

General Examination
Signs of systemic disease leading to low energy, low desire, low arousability, such as anemia, bradycardia, and slow relaxing reflexes of hypothyroidism
Signs of connective tissue disease, such as scleroderma or Sjögren's syndrome, that are associated with vaginal dryness
Disabilities that might preclude movements involved in caressing a partner, self-stimulation, or intercourse
Disfigurements or presence of stomas or catheters that may decrease sexual self-confidence leading to low desire, low arousability
External Genitalia
Sparsity of pubic hair suggesting low adrenal androgens
Vulval skin disorders, including lichen sclerosis, that may cause soreness with sexual stimulation
Cracks or fissures in the interlabial folds suggestive of chronic candidiasis
Labial abnormalities that may cause embarrassment or sexual hesitancy
Introitus
Vulval disease involving introitus, such as pallor, friability, loss of elasticity and moisture of vulval atrophy, lichen sclerosis, recurrent splitting of the posterior fourchette manifested as just visible white lines perpendicular to the fourchette edge
Abnormalities of the hymen, adhesions of the labia minora, swellings in the area of the major vestibular glands, allodynia (pain sensation from touch stimulus) of the crease between the outer hymenal edge and the inner edge of the labia minora—typical of provoked vestibulodynia
Presence of cystocele, rectocele, prolapse interfering with the woman's sexual self-image
Inability to tighten and relax perivaginal muscles often associated with hypertonicity of pelvic muscles and midvaginal dyspareunia; abnormal vaginal discharge associated with burning dyspareunia
Internal Examination
Pelvic muscle tone, presence of tenderness, "trigger points" on palpation of deep levator ani due to underlying hypertonicity
Full Bimanual Examination
Presence of nodules or tenderness in the cul-de-sac or vaginal fornix and along uterosacral ligaments, retroverted fixed uterus as causes of deep dyspareunia
Tenderness on palpation of posterior bladder wall from anterior vaginal wall suggestive of bladder pathology

Adapted with permission from Basson R. Sexual dysfunction in women. *N Engl J Med.* 2006;354:1497-1506.

MANAGEMENT OF SEXUAL DYSFUNCTION IN MEN

Treatment of Hypoactive Sexual Desire in Men

It is important to distinguish between a generalized condition, in which there is no desire for any sexual activity, and a situational disorder, in which the man still self-stimulates but has little desire to be sexually active with a partner. The latter situation reflects difficulties with intimacy rather than a sexual disorder. It is necessary to focus on the couple when the patient has an ongoing sexual relationship. Treating the sexual dysfunction in the male partner improves the female partner's sexual function and satisfaction. Comorbid depression should be treated and relationship difficulties addressed. The efficacy of cognitive and behavioral therapies has not been evaluated systematically in men with hypoactive sexual desire disorder.

Testosterone therapy should be considered in men with hypoactive sexual desire who have androgen deficiency, even though there are no randomized trials of testosterone in men with hypoactive sexual desire disorder. Much of the information about the effects of testosterone on sexual desire has emerged from open-label trials of testosterone in hypogonadal men, which recruited participants based on low testosterone levels.[291-294] Testosterone therapy in these trials was associated with significant improvements in overall sexual activity, sexual desire, attention to erotic cues, and duration and frequency of nocturnal penile erections.[94,97,101,102,109,110,291,294] Meta-analyses of randomized testosterone trials, mostly in middle-aged and older men, reported greater improvements in nocturnal erections, sexual thoughts and motivation, number of successful attempts at intercourse, scores of erectile function, and

TABLE 20-6

A Step-Wise Approach to Treatment of Erectile Dysfunction

1. All patients and their sexual partners can benefit from and should receive psychosexual counseling.
2. First-line therapies: oral selective phosphodiesterase inhibitors (sildenafil, vardenafil, or tadalafil)
3. Second-line therapies: external vacuum devices, intraurethral alprostadil, intracavernosal injection of alprostadil
4. Third-line therapies: penile prosthesis, vascular surgery

overall sexual satisfaction in men receiving testosterone compared with placebo.[107,110,295]

Treatment of Erectile Dysfunction

The current practice employs a step-wise approach that first applies minimally invasive therapies that are easy to use and have fewer adverse effects and progresses to more invasive therapies that may require injections or surgical intervention after the first-line choices have been exhausted (Table 20-6 and Fig. 20-9). The physician should discuss the risks, benefits, and alternatives of all therapies with the couple. The selection of the therapeutic modality should be based on the underlying etiology, patient preference, the nature and strength of the patient's relationship with his sexual partner, and the absence or presence of underlying cardiovascular disease and other comorbid conditions.[11,276,277] All patients with ED can benefit from psychosexual counseling.[11,276,277]

In the execution of good medical practice, treatment of all associated medical disorders should be optimized. In men with diabetes mellitus, efforts to optimize glycemic control should be instituted, although improving glycemic control may not improve sexual function. In men with hypertension, control of blood pressure should be optimized; if possible, the therapeutic regimen may be modified to remove antihypertensive drugs that impair sexual function. This strategy is not always feasible, because almost all antihypertensive agents have been associated with sexual dysfunction; the frequency of this adverse event is less with angiotensin converting enzyme inhibitors and angiotensin receptor blockers than with other agents.

First-Line Therapies

Psychosexual Counseling. As Rosen emphasized, the major goals of psychosexual therapy are to reduce performance anxiety, develop the patient's sexual skills and knowledge, modify negative sexual attitudes, and improve communication between partners.[296] Counseling can be of benefit in patients with psychogenic or organic causes of sexual dysfunction (Table 20-7).[296]

Masters and Johnson postulated that an individual's focus on sexual performance rather than erotic stimulation is a major factor in the pathophysiology of psychogenic ED[296,297]; they referred to this behavior as "spectatoring." Many experts recommend a "sensate focus" treatment approach in which the couple avoids intercourse and engages in nongenital, nondemanding, pleasure-seeking exercises to reduce performance anxiety.[296]

Involving the partner in the counseling process helps dispel misperceptions about the problem, decreases stress,

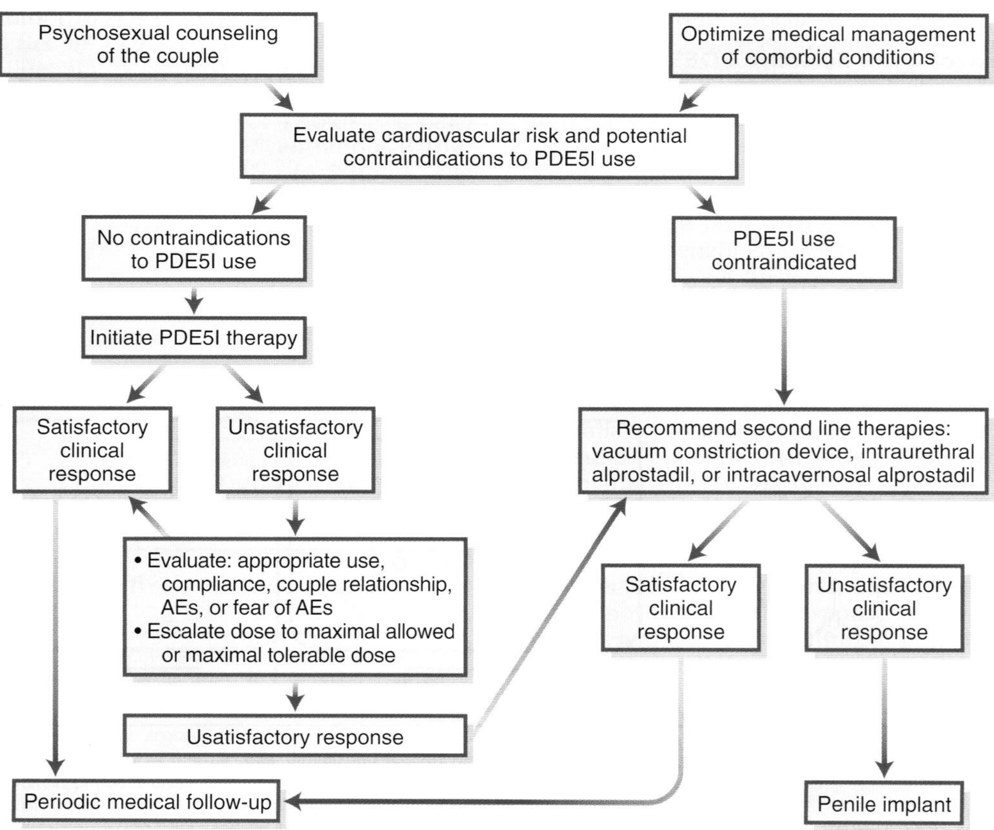

Figure 20-9 An algorithmic approach to the treatment of erectile dysfunction in men. AE, adverse effects; PDE5I, phosphodiesterase 5 inhibitor.

218. Demir O, Akgul K, Akar Z, et al. Association between severity of lower urinary tract symptoms, erectile dysfunction and metabolic syndrome. *Aging Male*. 2009;12:29-34.
219. Demir T, Demir O, Kefi A, et al. Prevalence of erectile dysfunction in patients with metabolic syndrome. *Int J Urol*. 2006;13:385-388.
220. Basson RJ, Rucker BM, Laird PG, et al. PG Sexuality of women with diabetes. *J Sex Reprod Med*. 2001;1:11-20.
221. Enzlin P, Mathieu C, Van den Bruel A, et al. Sexual dysfunction in women with type 1 diabetes: a controlled study. *Diabetes Care*. 2002;25:672-677.
222 Erol B, Tefekli A, Ozbey I, et al. Sexual dysfunction in type II diabetic females: a comparative study. *J Sex Marital Ther*. 2002;28(suppl 1):55-62.
223. Erol B, Tefekli A, Sanli O, et al. Does sexual dysfunction correlate with deterioration of somatic sensory system in diabetic women? *Int J Impot Res*. 2003;15:198-202.
224. Doruk EH, Akabay E, Çayan S, et al. Effect of diabetes mellitus on female sexual function and risk factors. *Arch Androl*. 2005;51: 1-6.
225. Abu Ali RM, Al Hajeri RM, Khader YS, et al. Sexual dysfunction in Jordanian diabetic women. *Diabetes Care*. 2008;31:1580-1581.
226. de Groot M, Anderson R, Freedland KE, et al. Association of depression and diabetes complications: a meta-analysis. *Psychosom Med*. 2001; 63:619-630.
227. Enzlin P, Rosen R, Wiegel M, et al. Sexual dysfunction in women with type-1 diabetes: long-term findings from the DCCT/EDIC study cohort. *Diabetes Care* 2009 32:780-783.
228. Dunaif A, Segal KR, Futterweit W, et al. Profound peripheral insulin resistance, independent of obesity, in polycystic ovary syndrome. *Diabetes*. 1989;38:1165-1174.
229. Diamond MP, Grainger D, Diamond MC, et al. Effects of methyltestosterone on insulin secretion and sensitivity in women. *J Clin Endocrinol Metab*. 1998;83:4420-4425.
230. Dunaif A, Finegood DT. Beta-cell dysfunction independent of obesity and glucose intolerance in the polycystic ovary syndrome. *J Clin Endocrinol Metab*. 1996;81:942-947.
231. Holte J, Bergh T, Berne C, et al. Enhanced early insulin response to glucose in relation to insulin resistance in women with polycystic ovary syndrome and normal glucose tolerance. *J Clin Endocrinol Metab*. 1994;78:1052-1058.
232. Möhlig M, Jürgens A, Spranger J, et al. The androgen receptor CAG repeat modifies the impact of testosterone on insulin resistance in women with polycystic ovary syndrome. *Eur J Endocrinol*. 2006;155: 127-130.
233. Alonso A, González-Pardo H, Garrido P, et al. Acute effects of 17beta-estradiol and genistein on insulin sensitivity and spatial memory in aged ovariectomized female rats. Age (Dordr). 2010 May 14 [Epub ahead of print].
234. Crespo CJ, Smit E, Snelling A, et al. Hormone replacement therapy and its relationship to lipid and glucose metabolism in diabetic and nondiabetic postmenopausal women: results from the Third National Health and Nutrition Examination Survey (NHANES III). *Diabetes Care*. 2002;25:1675-1680.
235. Park K, Ahn K, Chang JS, et al. Diabetes induced alteration of clitoral hemodynamics and structure in the rabbit. *J Urol*. 2002;168: 1269-1272.
236. Caruso S, Rugolo S, Mirabella D, et al. Changes in clitoral blood flow in premenopausal women affected by type 1 diabetes after single 100-mg administration of sildenafil. *Urology*. 2006;68:161-165.
237. Esposito K, Maiorino MI, Bellastella G, et al. Determinants of female sexual dysfunction in type 2 diabetes. *Int J Impot Res*. 2010;22: 179-184.
238. Ponholzer A, Temml C, Rauchenwald M, et al. Is the metabolic syndrome a risk factor for female sexual dysfunction in sexually active women? *Int J Impot Res*. 2008;20:100-104.
239. Esposito K, Ciotola M, Marfella R, et al. The metabolic syndrome: a cause of sexual dysfunction in women. *Int J Impot Res*. 2005;17: 224-226.
240. Janssen OE, Hahn S, Tan S, et al. Mood and sexual function in polycystic ovary syndrome. *Semin Reprod Med*. 2008;26:45-52.
241. Elsenbruch S, Hahn S, Kowalsky D, et al. Quality of life, psychosocial well-being, and sexual satisfaction in women with polycystic ovary syndrome. *J Clin Endocrinol Metab*. 2003;88:5801-5807.
242. Hahn S, Janssen OE, Tan S, et al. Clinical and psychological correlates of quality-of-life in polycystic ovary syndrome. *Eur J Endocrinol*. 2005;153:853-860.
243. Conaglen HM, Conaglen JV. Sexual desire in women presenting for antiandrogen therapy. *J Sex Marital Ther*. 2003;29:255-267.
244. Hahn S, Benson S, Elsenbruch S, et al. Metformin treatment of polycystic ovary syndrome improves health-related quality-of-life, emotional distress and sexuality. *Hum Reprod*. 2006;21:1925-1934.
245. Dewailly D, Vantyghem-Haudiquet MC, Sainsard C, et al. Clinical and biological phenotypes in late-onset 21-hydroxylase deficiency. *J Clin Endocrinol Metab*. 1986;63:418-423.
246. Lobo RA, Goebelsmann U. Adult manifestation of congenital adrenal hyperplasia due to incomplete 21-hydroxylase deficiency mimicking polycystic ovarian disease. *Am J Obstet Gynecol*. 1980;138:720-726.
247. Frisén L, Nordenström A, Falhammar H, et al. Gender role behavior, sexuality, and psychosocial adaptation in women with congenital adrenal hyperplasia due to CYP21A2 deficiency. *J Clin Endocrinol Metab*. 2009;94:3432-3439.
248. Hines M, Brook C, Conway GS. Androgen and psychosexual development: core gender identity, sexual orientation and recalled childhood gender role behavior in women and men with congenital adrenal hyperplasia (CAH). *J Sex Res*. 2004;41:75-81.
249. Wierman M, Nappi R, Avis N, et al. Endocrine aspects of women's sexual function. *J Sex Med*. 2010 Jan 5 [Epub ahead of print].
250. Kadioglu P, Yalin AS, Tiryakioglu O, et al. Sexual dysfunction in women with hyperprolactinemia: a pilot study report. *J Urol*. 2005;174: 1921-1925.
251. Hulter BM, Lundberg PO. Sexual function in women with hypothalamo-pituitary disorders. *Arch Sex Behav*. 1994;23:171-183.
252. Miller KK, Biller BM, Beauregard C, et al. Effects of testosterone replacement in androgen-deficient women with hypopituitarism: a randomized, double-blind, placebo-controlled study. *J Clin Endocrinol Metab*. 2006;91:1683-1690.
253. Arlt W, Callies F, van Vlijmen JC, et al. Dehydroepiandrosterone replacement in women with adrenal insufficiency. *N Engl J Med*. 1999;341:1013-1020.
254. Hunt PJ, Gurnell EM, Huppert FA, et al. Improvement in mood and fatigue after dehydroepiandrosterone replacement in Addison's disease in a randomized, double blind trial. *J Clin Endocrinol Metab*. 2000;85:4650-4656.
255. Gurnell EM, Hunt PJ, Curran SE, et al. Long-term DHEA replacement in primary adrenal insufficiency: a randomized, controlled trial. *J Clin Endocrinol Metab*. 2008;93:400-409.
256. Libè R, Barbetta L, Dall'Asta C, et al. Effects of dehydroepiandrosterone (DHEA) supplementation on hormonal, metabolic and behavioral status in patients with hypoadrenalism. *J Endocrinol Invest*. 2004;27: 736-741.
257. Binder G, Weber S, Ehrismann M, et al. South German Working Group for Pediatric Endocrinology. Effects of dehydroepiandrosterone therapy on pubic hair growth and psychological well-being in adolescent girls and young women with central adrenal insufficiency: a double-blind, randomized, placebo-controlled phase III trial. *J Clin Endocrinol Metab*. 2009;94:1182-1190.
258. Levine KB, Williams RE, Hartmann KE. Vulvovaginal atrophy is strongly associated with female sexual dysfunction among sexually active postmenopausal women. *Menopause*. 2008;15:661-666.
259. Lindau ST, Schumm LP, Laumann EO, et al. The study of sexuality and health among older adults in the United States. *N Engl J Med*. 2007;357:762-774.
260. Öberg K, Sjögern Fugl-Myer K. On Swedish women's distressing sexual dysfunctions: some concomitant conditions and life satisfaction. *J Sex Med*. 2005;2:169-180.
261. Valadares ALR, Pinto Neto AM, Osis MJD, et al. Dyspareunia: a population based study with Brazilian women between 40 and 65 years old. *Menopause*. 2006;13:P-98-P-1016.
262. Labrie F. Intracrinology. *Mol Cell Endocrinol*. 1991;78:C113-C118.
263. Labrie F, Bélanger A, Bélanger P, et al. Androgen glucuronides, instead of testosterone, as the new markers of androgenic activity in women. *J Steroid Biochem*. 2006;99:182-188.
264. Woods NF, Mitchell ES, Tao Y, et al. Polymorphisms in the estrogen synthesis and metabolism pathways and symptoms during the menopausal transition: observations from the Seattle Midlife Women's Health Study. *Menopause*. 2006;13:902-910.
265. West SL, D'Aloisio AA, Agans RP, et al. Prevalence of low sexual desire and hypoactive sexual desire disorder in a nationally representative sample of US women. *Arch Intern Med*. 2008;168:1441-1449.
266. Melcangi RC, Panzica GC. Neuroactive steroids: old players in a new game. *Neuroscience*. 2006;138:733-739.
267. Ishunina TA, Swaab DF. Alterations in the human brain in menopause. *Maturitas*. 2007;57:20-22.
268. Aziz A, Brannstrom M, Bergquist C, et al. Perimenopausal androgen decline after oophorectomy does not influence sexuality or psychological well-being. *Fertil Steril*. 2005;83:1021-1028.
269. Farquar CM, Harvey SA, Yu Y, et al. A prospective study of three years of outcomes after hysterectomy with and without oophorectomy. *Obstet Gynecol*. 2006;194:714-717.
270. Teplin V, Vittinghoff E, Lin F, et al. Oophorectomy in premenopausal women: health-related quality of life and sexual functioning. *Obstet Gynecol*. 2007;109:347-354.
271. Guay A, Munarriz R, Jacobson J, et al. Serum androgen levels in healthy premenopausal women with and without sexual dysfunction: part A. Serum androgen levels in women aged 20-49 years with no complaints of sexual dysfunction. *Int J Impot Res*. 2004;16:112-120.
272. Tannenbaum C, Barrett-Connor E, Laughlin GA, et al. A longitudinal study of dehydroepiandrosterone sulphate (DHEAS) change in older

men and women: the Rancho Bernardo Study. *Eur J Endocrinol.* 2004;151:717-725.
273. Berr C, Lafont S, Debuire B, et al. Relationships of dehydroepiandrosterone sulfate in the elderly with functional, psychological, and mental status, and short-term mortality: a French community-based study. *Proc Natl Acad Sci U S A.* 1996;93:13410-13415.
274. Cappola AR, O'Meara ES, Guo W, et al. Trajectories of dehydroepiandrosterone sulfate predict mortality in older adults: the Cardiovascular Health Study. *Gerontol A Biol Sci Med Sci.* 2009;64:1268-1274.
275. Basson R, Brotto LA, Petkau J, et al. Role of androgens in women's sexual dysfunction. *Menopause.* 2010;17:962-971.
276. Montague DK, Jarow JP, Broderick GA, et al. Erectile Dysfunction Guideline Update Panel. *J Urol.* 2005;174:230-239.
277. Lobo JR, Nehra A. Clinical evaluation of erectile dysfunction in the era of PDE-5 inhibitors. *Urol Clin North Am.* 2005;32:447-455.
278. Cappelleri JC, Rosen RC, Smith MD, et al. Diagnostic evaluation of the erectile function domain of the International Index of Erectile Function. *Urology.* 1999;54:346-351.
279. Lue TF, Giuliano F, Montorsi F, et al. Summary of recommendations on sexual dysfunctions in men. *J Sex Med.* 2004;1:6-23.
280. O'Leary MP, Fowler FJ, Lenderking WR, et al. A brief male sexual function inventory. *Urology.* 1995;46:697-706.
281. Rosen RC, Cappelleri JC, Smith MD, et al. Development and evaluation of an abridged, 5-item version of the International Index of Erectile Function (IIEF-5) as a diagnostic tool for erectile dysfunction. *Int J Impot Res.* 1999;11:319-326.
282. Buvat J, Lemaire A. Endocrine screening in 1,022 men with erectile dysfunction: clinical significance and cost-effective strategy [see comments]. *J Urol.* 1997;158:1764-1767.
283. Citron JT, Ettinger B, Rubinoff H, et al. Prevalence of hypothalamic-pituitary imaging abnormalities in impotent men with secondary hypogonadism. *J Urol.* 1996;155:529-533.
284. Wu FC, Tajar A, Pye SR, et al. European Male Aging Study Group. Hypothalamic-pituitary-testicular axis disruptions in older men are differentially linked to age and modifiable risk factors: the European Male Aging Study. *J Clin Endocrinol Metab.* 2008;93:2737-2745.
285. Wu FC, Tajar A, Beynon JM, et al. EMAS Group. Identification of late-onset hypogonadism in middle-aged and elderly men. *N Engl J Med.* 2010;363:123-135.
286. Harman SM, Metter EJ, Tobin JD, et al. Baltimore Longitudinal Study of Aging. Longitudinal effects of aging on serum total and free testosterone levels in healthy men. Baltimore Longitudinal Study of Aging. *Clin Endocrinol Metab.* 2001;86:724-731.
287. Orwoll E, Lambert LC, Marshall LM, et al. Testosterone and estradiol among older men. *J Clin Endocrinol Metab.* 2006;91:1336-1344.
288. Atchison M, Aitchison J, Carter R. Is the penile brachial index a reproducible and useful measurement? *Br J Urol.* 1990;66:202-204.
289. Mueller SC, Wallenberg-Pachaly H, Voges GE, et al. Comparison of selective internal iliac pharmaco-angiography, penile brachial index and duplex sonography with pulsed Doppler analysis for the evaluation of vasculogenic (arteriogenic) impotence. *J Urol.* 1990;143: 928-932.
290. Brock G. Tumescence monitoring devices: past and present. In: Hellstrom WJ, ed. *Handbook of Sexual Dysfunction.* San Francisco, CA: The American Society of Andrology; 1999:65-69.
291. Steidle C, Schwartz S, Jacoby K, et al. North American AA2500 T Gel Study Group. AA2500 testosterone gel normalizes androgen levels in aging males with improvements in body composition and sexual function. *J Clin Endocrinol Metab.* 2003;88:2673-2681.
292. Wang C, Swerdloff RS, Iranmanesh A, et al. Testosterone Gel Study Group. Transdermal testosterone gel improves sexual function, mood, muscle strength, and body composition parameters in hypogonadal men. *J Clin Endocrinol Metab.* 2000;85:2839-2853.
293. Wang C, Cunningham G, Dobs A, et al. Long-term testosterone gel (AndroGel) treatment maintains beneficial effects on sexual function and mood, lean and fat mass, and bone mineral density in hypogonadal men. *J Clin Endocrinol Metab.* 2004;89:2085-2098.
294. Arver S, Dobs AS, Meikle AW, et al. Improvement of sexual function in testosterone deficient men treated for 1 year with a permeation enhanced testosterone transdermal system. *J Urol.* 1996;155: 1604-1608.
295. Boloña ER, Uraga MV, Haddad RM, et al. Testosterone use in men with sexual dysfunction: a systematic review and meta-analysis of randomized placebo-controlled trials. *Mayo Clin Proc.* 2007;82:20-28.
296. Rosen RC. Psychogenic erectile dysfunction: classification and management. *Urol Clin North Am.* 2001;28:269-278.
297. Abrahamson DJ, Barlow DH, Beck JG, et al. The effects of attentional focus and partner responsiveness on sexual responding: replication and extension. *Arch Sex Behav.* 1985;14:361-371.
298. Melnik T, Soares BG, Nasselo AG. Psychosocial interventions for erectile dysfunction. Cochrane Database Syst Rev. 2007;(3):CD004825.
299. Melnik T, Soares BG, Nasello AG. The effectiveness of psychological interventions for the treatment of erectile dysfunction: systematic review and meta-analysis, including comparisons to sildenafil treatment, intracavernosal injection, and vacuum devices. *J Sex Med.* 2008;5:2562-2574.
300. Hatzimouratidis K, Amar E, Eardley I, et al. Guidelines on male sexual dysfunction: erectile dysfunction and premature ejaculation. *Eur Urol.* 2010;57:804-814.
301. Haning H, Niewohner U, Bischoff E. Phosphodiesterase type 5 (PDE5) inhibitors. *Prog Med Chem.* 2003;41:249-306.
302. Qaseem A, Snow V, Denberg TD, et al. Clinical Efficacy Assessment Subcommittee of the American College of Physicians. Hormonal testing and pharmacologic treatment of erectile dysfunction: a clinical practice guideline from the American College of Physicians. *Ann Intern Med.* 2009;151:639-649.
303. Bischoff E. Potency, selectivity, and consequences of nonselectivity of PDE inhibition. *Int J Impot Res.* 2004;16(suppl 1):S11-S14.
304. Jeremy JY, Ballard SA, Naylor AM, et al. Effects of sildenafil, a type-5 cGMP phosphodiesterase inhibitor, and papaverine on cyclic GMP and cyclic AMP levels in the rabbit corpus cavernosum in vitro. *Br J Urol.* 1997;79:958-963.
305. Stief CG, Uckert S, Becker AJ, et al. The effect of the specific phosphodiesterase (PDE) inhibitors on human and rabbit cavernous tissue in vitro and in vivo. *J Urol.* 1998;159:1390-1393.
306. Reference deleted in proofs.
307. Saenz de Tejada I, Angulo J, Cuevas P, et al. The phosphodiesterase inhibitory selectivity and the in vitro and in vivo potency of the new PDE5 inhibitor vardenafil. *Int J Impot Res.* 2001;13:282-290.
308. Yu G, Mason H, Wu X, et al. Substituted pyrazolopyridopyridazines as orally bioavailable potent and selective PDE5 inhibitors: potential agents for treatment of erectile dysfunction. *J Med Chem.* 2003; 46:457-460.
309. Seftel AD. Phosphodiesterase type 5 inhibitor differentiation based on selectivity, pharmacokinetic, and efficacy profiles. *Clin Cardiol.* 2004; 27:I14-I19.
310. Rajagopalan P, Mazzu A, Xia C, et al. Effect of high-fat breakfast and moderate-fat evening meal on the pharmacokinetics of vardenafil, an oral phosphodiesterase-5 inhibitor for the treatment of erectile dysfunction. *J Clin Pharmacol.* 2003;43:260-267.
311. Nichols DJ, Muirhead GJ, Harness JA. Pharmacokinetics of sildenafil after single oral doses in healthy male subjects: absolute bioavailability, food effects and dose proportionality. *Br J Clin Pharmacol.* 2002;53(suppl 1):5S-12S.
312. Rendell MS, Rajfer J, Wicker PA, et al. Sildenafil for treatment of erectile dysfunction in men with diabetes: a randomized controlled trial. Sildenafil Diabetes Study Group [see comments]. *JAMA.* 1999;281:421-426.
313. Blanker MH, Thomas S, Bohnen AM. Systematic review of Viagra RCTs. *Br J Gen Pract.* 2002;52:329.
314. Burls A, Gold L, Clark W. Systematic review of randomised controlled trials of sildenafil (Viagra) in the treatment of male erectile dysfunction. *Br J Gen Pract.* 2001;51:1004-1012.
315. Fink HA, Mac Donald R, Rutks IR, et al. Sildenafil for male erectile dysfunction: a systematic review and meta-analysis. *Arch Intern Med.* 2002;162:1349-1360.
316. Markou S, Perimenis P, Gyftopoulos K, et al. Vardenafil (Levitra) for erectile dysfunction: a systematic review and meta-analysis of clinical trial reports. *Int J Impot Res.* 2004;16:470-478.
317. Montorsi F, McCullough A. Efficacy of sildenafil citrate in men with erectile dysfunction following radical prostatectomy: a systematic review of clinical data. *J Sex Med.* 2005;2:658-667.
318. Moore RA, Derry S, McQuay HJ. Indirect comparison of interventions using published randomised trials: systematic review of PDE-5 inhibitors for erectile dysfunction. *BMC Urol.* 2005;5:18.
319. Jarow JP, Burnett AL, Geringer AM. Clinical efficacy of sildenafil citrate based on etiology and response to prior treatment [see comments]. *J Urol.* 1999;162:722-725.
320. Vardi M, Nini A. Phosphodiesterase inhibitors for erectile dysfunction in patients with diabetes mellitus. Cochrane Database Syst Rev. 2007;(1):CD002187.
321. Donatucci C, Eardley I, Buvat J, et al. Vardenafil improves erectile function in men with erectile dysfunction irrespective of disease severity and disease classification. *J Sex Med.* 2004;1:301-309.
322. Hatzichristou D, Montorsi F, Buvat J, et al. The efficacy and safety of flexible-dose vardenafil (Levitra) in a broad population of European men. *Eur Urol.* 2004;45:634-641; discussion 641.
323. Hellstrom WJ, Gittelman M, Karlin G, et al. Vardenafil for treatment of men with erectile dysfunction: efficacy and safety in a randomized, double-blind, placebo-controlled trial. *J Androl.* 2002;23:763-771.
324. Nehra A, Grantmyre J, Nadel A, et al. Vardenafil improved patient satisfaction with erectile hardness, orgasmic function and sexual experience in men with erectile dysfunction following nerve sparing radical prostatectomy. *J Urol.* 2005;173:2067-2071.
325. Rosen R, Shabsigh R, Berber M, et al. Efficacy and tolerability of vardenafil in men with mild depression and erectile dysfunction: the depression-related improvement with vardenafil for erectile response study. *Am J Psychiatry.* 2006;163:79-87.

326. Brock GB, McMahon CG, Chen KK, et al. Efficacy and safety of tadalafil for the treatment of erectile dysfunction: results of integrated analyses. *J Urol*. 2002;168:1332-1336.
327. Carson C, Shabsigh R, Segal S, et al. Efficacy, safety, and treatment satisfaction of tadalafil versus placebo in patients with erectile dysfunction evaluated at tertiary-care academic centers. *Urology*. 2005;65: 353-359.
328. Padma-Nathan H, McMurray JG, Pullman WE, et al. On-demand IC351 (Cialis) enhances erectile function in patients with erectile dysfunction. *Int J Impot Res*. 2001;13:2-9.
329. Porst H, Padma-Nathan H, Giuliano F, et al. Efficacy of tadalafil for the treatment of erectile dysfunction at 24 and 36 hours after dosing: a randomized controlled trial. *Urology*. 2003;62:121-125; discussion 125-126.
330. Saenz de Tejada I, Anglin G, Knight JR, et al. Effects of tadalafil on erectile dysfunction in men with diabetes. *Diabetes Care*. 2002;25: 2159-2164.
331. Morales A, Gingell C, Collins M, et al. Clinical safety of oral sildenafil citrate (Viagra) in the treatment of erectile dysfunction. *Int J Impot Res*. 1998;10:69-73.
332. Coelho OR. Tolerability and safety profile of sildenafil citrate (Viagra) in Latin American patient populations. *Int J Impot Res*. 2002;14(suppl 2):S54-S59.
333. Giuliano F, Jackson G, Montorsi F, et al. Safety of sildenafil citrate: review of 67 double-blind placebo-controlled trials and the postmarketing safety database. *Int J Clin Pract*. 2010;64:240-255.
334. Aversa A, Mazzilli F, Rossi T, et al. Effects of sildenafil (Viagra) administration on seminal parameters and post-ejaculatory refractory time in normal males. *Hum Reprod*. 2000;15:131-134.
335. Hellstrom WJG, Gittelman M, Jarow J, et al. An evaluation of semen characteristics in men 45 years of age after daily dosing with tadalafil 20 mg: results of a multicenter, randomized, double-blind, placebo-controlled, 9-month study. *Eur Urol*. 2008;53:1058-1065.
336. Hatzichristou DG. Phosphodiesterase 5 inhibitors and nonarteritic anterior ischemic optic neuropathy (NAION): coincidence or causality. *J Sex Med*. 2004;2:751-758.
337. Buono L, Foroozan R, Sergott RC, et al. Nonarteritic anterior ischemic optic neuropathy. *Curr Opin Ophthamol*. 2002;13:357-361.
338. Snodgrass AJ, Campbell HM, Mace DL, et al. Sudden sensorineural hearing loss associated with vardenafil. *Pharmacotherapy*. 2010;30: 112.
339. McGwin G Jr. Phosphodiesterase type 5 inhibitor use and hearing impairment. *Arch Otolaryngol Head Neck Surg*. 2010;136:488-492.
340. Feenstra J, Drie-Pierik RJ, Lacle CF, et al. Acute myocardial infarction associated with sildenafil [letter] [see comments]. *Lancet*. 1998;352: 957-958.
341. Zusman RM, Morales A, Glasser DB, et al. Overall cardiovascular profile of sildenafil citrate. *Am J Cardiol*. 1999;83:35C-44C.
342. Herrmann HC, Chang G, Klugherz BD, et al. Hemodynamic effects of sildenafil in men with severe coronary artery disease. *N Engl J Med*. 2000;342:1622-1626.
343. Thadani U, Smith W, Nash S, et al. The effect of vardenafil, a potent and highly selective phosphodiesterase-5 inhibitor for the treatment of erectile dysfunction, on the cardiovascular response to exercise in patients with coronary artery disease. *J Am Coll Cardiol*. 2002;40: 2006-2012.
344. Jackson G. Hemodynamic and exercise effects of phosphodiesterase 5 inhibitors. *Am J Cardiol*. 2005;96:32M-36M.
345. Cheitlin MD, Hutter AM Jr, Brindis RG, et al. Use of sildenafil (Viagra) in patients with cardiovascular disease. Technology and Practice Executive Committee [published erratum appears in *Circulation*. 1999;7; 100:2389] [see comments]. *Circulation*. 1999;99:168-177.
346. Muller JE, Mittleman A, Maclure M, et al. Triggering myocardial infarction by sexual activity: low absolute risk and prevention by regular physical exertion. Determinants of Myocardial Infarction Onset Study Investigators [see comments]. *JAMA*. 1996;275:1405-1409.
347. Conti CR, Pepine CJ, Sweeney M. Efficacy and safety of sildenafil citrate in the treatment of erectile dysfunction in patients with ischemic heart disease. *Am J Cardiol*. 1999;83:29C-34C.
348. Carson CC 3rd. Cardiac safety in clinical trials of phosphodiesterase 5 inhibitors. *Am J Cardiol*. 2005;96:37M-41M.
349. Kloner RA. Novel phosphodiesterase type 5 inhibitors: assessing hemodynamic effects and safety parameters. *Clin Cardiol*. 2004;27:I20-I25.
350. Highleyman L. Protease inhibitors and sildenafil (Viagra) should not be combined. *Beta*. 1999;12:3.
351. Bailey DG, Dresser GK. Interactions between grapefruit juice and cardiovascular drugs. *Am J Cardiovasc Drugs*. 2004;4:281-297.
352. Carson CC. Combination of phosphodiesterase-5 inhibitors and alpha-blockers in patients with benign prostatic hyperplasia: treatments of lower urinary tract symptoms, erectile dysfunction, or both? *BJU Int*. 2006;97(suppl 2):39-43; discussion 44-45.
353. Liguori G, Trombetta C, De Giorgi G, et al. Efficacy and safety of combined oral therapy with tadalafil and alfuzosin: an integrated approach to the management of patients with lower urinary tract symptoms and erectile dysfunction. Preliminary report. *J Sex Med*. 2009;6:544-545.
354. Kaplan SA, Gonzalez RR, Te AE. Combination of alfuzosin and sildenafil is superior to monotherapy in treating lower urinary tract symptoms and erectile dysfunction. *Eur Urol*. 2007;51:1717-1723.
355. McCullough AR, Barada JH, Fawzy A, et al. Achieving treatment optimization with sildenafil citrate (Viagra) in patients with erectile dysfunction. *Urology*. 2002;60:28-38.
356. McMahon C. Comparison of efficacy, safety, and tolerability of on-demand tadalafil and daily dosed tadalafil for the treatment of erectile dysfunction. *J Sex Med*. 2005;2:415-425; discussion 425-417.
357. Porst H, Rajfer J, Casabé A, et al. Long-term safety and efficacy of tadalafil 5 mg dosed once daily in men with erectile dysfunction. *J Sex Med*. 2008;5:2160-2169.
358. Hellstrom WJG, Gittelman M, Jarow J, et al. An evaluation of semen characteristics in men 45 years of age after daily dosing with tadalafil 20 mg: results of a multicenter, randomized, double-blinds, placebo-controlled, 9-month study. *Eur Urol*. 2008;53:1058-1065.
359. Lau DHW, Kommu S, Mumtaz FH, et al. The management of phosphodiesterase inhibitor failure. *Curr Vasc Pharmacol*. 2006;4:89-93.
360. Martinez JM. Prognostic factors for response to sildenafil in patients with erectile dysfunction. *Eur Urol*. 2001;40:641-646.
361. Wespes E, Rammal A, Garbar C. Sildenafil no-responders: hemodynamic and morphometric studies. *Eur Urol*. 2005;48:136-139.
362. McGarvey MR. Tough choices: the cost-effectiveness of sildenafil [editorial; comment]. *Ann Intern Med*. 2000;132:994-995.
363. Smith KJ, Roberts MS. The cost-effectiveness of sildenafil [see comments]. *Ann Intern Med*. 2000;132:933-937.
364. Tan HL. Economic cost of male erectile dysfunction using a decision analytic model: for a hypothetical managed-care plan of 100,000 members. *Pharmacoeconomics*. 2000;17:77-107.
365. Sun P, Seftel A, Swindle R, et al. The costs of caring for erectile dysfunction in a managed care setting: evidence from a large national claims database. *J Urol*. 2005;174:1948-1952.
366. Plumb JM, Guest JF. Annual cost of erectile dysfunction to UK Society. *Pharmacoeconomics*. 1999;16:699-709.
367. Vrijhof HJ, Delaere KP. Vacuum constriction devices in erectile dysfunction: acceptance and effectiveness in patients with impotence of organic or mixed aetiology. *Br J Urol*. 1994;74:102-105.
368. Cookson MS, Nadig PW. Long-term results with vacuum constriction device. *J Urol*. 1993;149:290-294.
369. Lewis JH, Sidi AA, Reddy PK. A way to help your patients who use vacuum devices. *Contemp Urol*. 1993;3:15-21.
370. Engelhardt PF, Plas E, Hubner WA, et al. Comparison of intraurethral liposomal and intracavernosal prostaglandin-E1 in the management of erectile dysfunction. *Br J Urol*. 1998;81:441-444.
371. Kim ED, McVary KT. Topical prostaglandin-E1 for the treatment of erectile dysfunction [see comments]. *J Urol*. 1995;153:1828-1830.
372. Peterson CA, Bennett AH, Hellstrom WJ, et al. Erectile response to transurethral alprostadil, prazosin and alprostadil-prazosin combinations. *J Urol*. 1998;159:1523-1527.
373. Fulgham PF, Cochran JS, Denman JL, et al. Disappointing initial results with transurethral alprostadil for erectile dysfunction in a urology practice setting. *J Urol*. 1998;160:2041-2046.
374. Linet OI, Ogrinc FG. Efficacy and safety of intracavernosal alprostadil in men with erectile dysfunction. The Alprostadil Study Group. *N Engl J Med*. 1996;334:873-877.
375. El-Sakka AI. Intracavernosal prostaglandin E1 self vs office injection therapy in patients with erectile dysfunction. *Int J Impot Res*. 2006;18:180-185.
376. Heaton JP, Lording D, Liu SN, et al. Intracavernosal alprostadil is effective for the treatment of erectile dysfunction in diabetic men. *Int J Impot Res*. 2001;13:317-321.
377. Tsai YS, Lin JS, Lin YM. Safety and efficacy of alprostadil sterile powder (S. Po., CAVERJECT) in diabetic patients with erectile dysfunction. *Eur Urol*. 2000;38:177-183.
378. Shabsigh R, Padma-Nathan H, Gittleman M, et al. Intracavernous alprostadil alfadex is more efficacious, better tolerated, and preferred over intraurethral alprostadil plus optional actis: a comparative, randomized, crossover, multicenter study. *Urology*. 2000;55:109-113.
379. Chew KK. Intracavernosal injection therapy: does it still have a role in erectile dysfunction? *Aust Fam Physician*. 2001;30:43-46.
380. The European Alprostadil Study Group. The long-term safety of alprostadil (prostaglandin-E1) in patients with erectile dysfunction. *Br J Urol*. 1998;82:538-543.
381. Dinsmore WW, Gingell C, Hackett G, et al. Treating men with predominantly nonpsychogenic erectile dysfunction with intracavernosal vasoactive intestinal polypeptide and phentolamine mesylate in a novel auto-injector system: a multicentre double-blind placebo-controlled study. *BJU Int*. 1999;83:274-279.
382. Mulhall JP, Daller M, Traish AM, et al. Intracavernosal forskolin: role in management of vasculogenic impotence resistant to standard 3-agent pharmacotherapy. *J Urol*. 1997;158:1752-1758; discussion 1758-1759.

383. Usta MF, Bivalacqua TJ, Sanabria J, et al. Patient and partner satisfaction and long-term results after surgical treatment for Peyronie's disease. *Urology*. 2003;62:105-109.
384. Hellstrom WJ, Usta MF. Surgical approaches for advanced Peyronie's disease patients. *Int J Impot Res*. 2003;15(suppl 5):S121-S124.
385. Carson CC, Mulcahy JJ, Govier FE. Efficacy, safety and patient satisfaction outcomes of the AMS 700CX inflatable penile prosthesis: results of a long-term multicenter study. AMS 700CX Study Group. *J Urol*. 2000;164:376-380.
386. Wilson SK, Cleves MA, Delk JR 2nd. Comparison of mechanical reliability of original and enhanced Mentor Alpha I penile prosthesis. *J Urol*. 1999;162:715-718.
387. Mills TM, Lewis RW, Stopper VS. Androgenic maintenance of inflow and veno-occlusion during erection in the rat. *Biol Reprod*. 1998; 59:1413-1418.
388. Fink HA, MacDonald R, Rutks IR, et al. Trazodone for erectile dysfunction: a systematic review and meta-analysis. *BJU Int*. 2003;92: 441-446.
389. Lebret T, Herve JM, Gorny P, et al. Efficacy and safety of a novel combination of L-arginine glutamate and yohimbine hydrochloride: a new oral therapy for erectile dysfunction. *Eur Urol*. 2002;41:608-613; discussion 613.
390. Fleshner N, Harvey M, Adomat H, et al. Evidence for pharmacological contamination of herbal erectile function products with type 5 phosphodiesterase inhibitors [abstract]. *J Urol*. 2004;171:314.
391. Hong B, Ji YH, Hong JH, et al. A double-blind crossover study evaluating the efficacy of Korean red ginseng in patients with erectile dysfunction: a preliminary report. *J Urol*. 2002;168:2070-2073.
392. Jang DJ, Lee MS, Shin BC, et al. Red ginseng for treating erectile dysfunction: a systematic review. *Br J Clin Pharmacol*. 2008;66:444-450.
393. Harraz A, Shindel AW, Lue TF. Emerging gene and stem cell therapies for the treatment of erectile dysfunction. Nat *Rev Urol*. 2010; 7:143-152.
394. Strong TD, Gebska MA, Burnett AL, et al. Endothelium-specific gene and stem cell-based therapy for erectile dysfunction. *Asian J Androl*. 2008;10:14-22.
395. Deng W, Bivalacqua TJ, Hellstrom WJ, et al. Gene and stem cell therapy for erectile dysfunction. *Int J Impot Res*. 2005;17(suppl 1):S57-S63.
396. Garban H, Marquez D, Magee T, et al. Cloning of rat and human inducible penile nitric oxide synthase: application for gene therapy of erectile dysfunction. *Biol Reprod*. 1997;56:954-963.
397. Christ GJ, Rehman J, Day N, et al. Intracorporal injection of hSlo cDNA in rats produces physiologically relevant alterations in penile function. *Am J Physiol*. 1998;275:H600-H608.
398. Bivalacqua TJ, Champion HC, Mehta YS, et al. Adenoviral gene transfer of endothelial nitric oxide synthase (eNOS) to the penis improves age-related erectile dysfunction in the rat. *Int J Impot Res*. 2000;12(suppl 3):S8-S17.
399. Champion HC, Bivalacqua TJ, Hyman AL, et al. Gene transfer of endothelial nitric oxide synthase to the penis augments erectile responses in the aged rat. *Proc Natl Acad Sci U S A*. 1999;96:11648-11652.
400. Burchardt M, Burchardt T, Anastasiadis AG, et al. Application of angiogenic factors for therapy of erectile dysfunction: protein and DNA transfer of VEGF 165 into the rat penis. *Urology*. 2005;66:665-670.
401. Rogers RS, Graziottin TM, Lin CS, et al. Intracavernosal vascular endothelial growth factor (VEGF) injection and adeno-associated virus-mediated VEGF gene therapy prevent and reverse venogenic erectile dysfunction in rats. *Int J Impot Res*. 2003;15:26-37.
402. Deng W, Bivalacqua TJ, Chattergoon NN, et al. Adenoviral gene transfer of eNOS: high-level expression in ex vivo expanded marrow stromal cells. *Am J Physiol Cell Physiol*. 2003;285:C1322-C1329.
403. Gholami SS, Rogers R, Chang J, et al. The effect of vascular endothelial growth factor and adeno-associated virus mediated brain derived neurotrophic factor on neurogenic and vasculogenic erectile dysfunction induced by hyperlipidemia. *J Urol*. 2003;169:1577-1581.
404. Melman A, Bar-Chama N, McCullough A, et al. Plasmid-based gene transfer for treatment of erectile dysfunction and overactive bladder: results of a phase I trial. *Isr Med Assoc J*. 2007;9:143-146.
405. Melman A, Bar-Chama N, McCullough A, et al. hMaxi-K gene transfer in males with erectile dysfunction: results of the first human trial. *Hum Gene Ther*. 2006;17:1165-1176.
406. Morishita R, Aoki M, Hashiya N, et al. Safety evaluation of clinical gene therapy using hepatocyte growth factor to treat peripheral arterial disease. *Hypertension*. 2004;44:203-209.
407. Kim HJ, Jang SY, Park JI, et al. Vascular endothelial growth factor-induced angiogenic gene therapy in patients with peripheral artery disease. *Exp Mol Med*. 2004;36:336-344.
408. Kusumanto YH, van Weel V, Mulder NH, et al. Treatment with intramuscular vascular endothelial growth factor gene compared with placebo for patients with diabetes mellitus and critical limb ischemia: a double-blind randomized trial. *Hum Gene Ther*. 2006;17:683-691.
409. Alexander JH, Ferguson TB Jr, Joseph DM, The PRoject of Ex-vivo Vein graft Engineering via Transfection IV (PREVENT IV) trial: study rationale, design, and baseline patient characteristics. *Am Heart J*. 2005;150:643-649.
410. Gaffney MM, Hynes SO, Barry F, et al. Cardiovascular gene therapy: current status and therapeutic potential. *Br J Pharmacol*. 2007;152: 175-188.
411. Powell RJ, Simons M, Mendelsohn FO, et al. Results of a double-blind, placebo-controlled study to assess the safety of intramuscular injection of hepatocyte growth factor plasmid to improve limb perfusion in patients with critical limb ischemia. *Circulation*. 2008;118:58-65.
412. Shigematsu H, Yasuda K, Iwai T, et al. Randomized, double-blind, placebo-controlled clinical trial of hepatocyte growth factor plasmid for critical limb ischemia. *Gene Ther*. 2010;17:1152-1161.
413. Garcia MM, Fandel TM, Lin G, et al. Treatment of erectile dysfunction in the obese type 2 diabetic ZDF rat with adipose tissue-derived stem cells. *J Sex Med*. 2010;7(1 Pt 1):89-98.
414. Bivalacqua TJ, Deng W, Kendirci M, et al. Mesenchymal stem cells alone or ex vivo gene modified with endothelial nitric oxide synthase reverse age-associated erectile dysfunction. *Am J Physiol Heart Circ Physiol*. 2007;292:H1278-H1290.
415. Abdel Aziz MT, El-Haggar S, Mostafa T, et al. Effect of mesenchymal stem cell penile transplantation on erectile signaling of aged rats. *Andrologia*. 2010;42:187-192.
416. Tomasi PA, Fanciulli G, Delitala G. Successful treatment of retrograde ejaculation with the alpha1-adrenergic agonist methoxamine: case study. *Int J Impot Res*. 2005;17:297-299.
417. Ochsenkühn R, Kamischke A, Nieschlag E. Imipramine for successful treatment of retrograde ejaculation caused by retroperitoneal surgery. *Int J Androl*. 1999;22:173-177.
418. Safarinejad MR. Midodrine for the treatment of organic anejaculation but not spinal cord injury: a prospective randomized placebo-controlled double-blind clinical study. *Int J Impot Res*. 2009;21: 213-220.
419. Kamischke A, Nieschlag E. Treatment of retrograde ejaculation and anejaculation. *Hum Reprod Update*. 1999;5:448-474.
420. Shifren JL, Davis SR, Moreau M, et al. Testosterone patch for the treatment of hypoactive sexual desire disorder in naturally menopausal women: results from the INTIMATE NM1 Study. *Menopause*. 2006;13:770-779.
421. Buster JE, Kingsberg SA, Aguirre O, et al. Testosterone patch for low sexual desire in surgically menopausal women: a randomized trial. *Obstet Gynecol*. 2005;105:944-952.
422. Simon J, Braunstein G, Nachtigall L, et al. Testosterone patch increases sexual activity and desire in surgically menopausal women with hypoactive sexual desire disorder. *J Clin Endocrinol Metab*. 2005;90:5226-5233.
423. Davis SR, van der Mooren MJ, van Lunsen RHW, et al. Efficacy and safety of a testosterone patch for the treatment of hypoactive sexual desire disorder in surgically menopausal women. A randomized, placebo controlled trial. *Menopause*. 2006;13:387-396.
424. Braunstein G, Sundwall DA, Katz M, et al. Safety and efficacy of a testosterone patch for the treatment of hypoactive sexual disorder in surgically menopausal women: a randomized, placebo-controlled trial. *Arch Intern Med*. 2005;165:1582-1589.
425. Arlt W. Androgen therapy in women. *Eur J Endocrinol*. 2006;154: 1-11.
426. Davis S, Moreau M, Kroll R, et al. Testosterone for low libido in postmenopausal women not taking estrogen. *N Eng J Med*. 2008; 359:2005-2017.
427. Panay N, Al-Azzawi F, Bouchard C, et al. Testosterone treatment of HSDD in naturally menopausal women: the ADORE study. *Climacteric*. 2010;13:121-131.
428. Baron DL, Wender DB, Sloan JA, et al. Randomized controlled trial to evaluate transdermal testosterone in female cancer survivors with decreased libido: North Central Cancer Treatment Group Protocol N02C3. *J Nat Cancer Inst*. 2007;99:672-679.
429. Davis S, Papalia MA, Norman RJ, et al. Safety and efficacy of a testosterone metered-dose transdermal spray for treatment of decreased sexual satisfaction in premenopausal women: a placebo-controlled randomized, dose ranging study. *Ann Intern Med*. 2008;148:569-577.
430. Basson R. Testosterone supplementation to improve women's sexual satisfaction: complexities and unknowns [editorial]. *Ann Intern Med*. 2008;148:620-621.
431. Padero MC, Bhasin S, Friedman TC. Androgen supplementation in older women: too much hype, not enough data. *J Am Geriatr Soc*. 2002;50:1131-1140.
432. Schover LR. Androgen therapy for loss of desire in women: is the benefit worth the breast cancer risk? *Fertil Steril*. 2008;90:129-140.
433. Braunstein GD. Management of female sexual dysfunction in postmenopausal women by testosterone administration: safety issues and controversies. *J Sex Med*. 2007;4(4 Pt 1):859-866.
434. Wild RA. Endogenous androgens and cardiovascular risk. *Menopause*. 2007;14:609-610.
435. Wierman ME, Basson R, Davis SR, et al. Androgen therapy in women: an Endocrine Society Clinical practice guideline. *J Clin Enocrinol Metab*. 2006;91:3697-3710.

436. Van der Nadem F, Bloemers J, Yassem WE, et al. The influence of testosterone combined with a PDE5-inhibitor on cognitive, effective, and physiological sexual functioning in women suffering from sexual dysfunction. *J Sex Med*. 2009;6:777-790.
437. Labrie F, Archer D, Bouchard C, et al. Effect of Intravaginal Prasterone (DHEA) on libido and sexual dysfunction in postmenopausal women. *Menopause*. 2009;16:923-931.
438. Chollet JA, Carter G, Meyn LA, et al. Efficacy and safety of vaginal estrogen and progesterone in post-menopausal women with atrophic vaginitis. *Menopause*. 2009;16:978-993.
439. Bachman GA, Schaefers M, Uddin A, et al. Microdose transdermal estrogen therapy for relief of vulvovaginal symptoms in post-menopausal women. *Menopause*. 2009;16:877-882.
440. Hays J, Ockene JK, Brunner RL, et al. Effects of estrogen plus progestin on health-related quality of life. *N Engl J Med*. 2003;348:1839-1854.
441. Trudel G, Marchand A, Ravart M, et al. The effect of a cognitive-behavioral group treatment program on hypoactive sexual desire in women. *Sex Rel Ther*. 2001;16:145-164.
442. Brotto LA, Basson R, Luria M. A mindfulness-based group psychoeducational intervention targeting sexual arousal disorder in women. *J Sex Med*. 2008;5:1646-1659.
443. Sarwer DB, Durlak JA. A field trial of the effectiveness of behavioral treatment for sexual dysfunctions. *J Sex Marital Ther*. 1997;23:87-97.
444. Basson R, McKinnes R, Smith MD, et al. Efficacy and safety of sildenafil citrate in women with sexual dysfunction associated with female sexual arousal. *Gend Based Med*. 2002;11:367-377.
445. Heiman JR, LoPiccolo J. *Becoming Orgasmic: A Sexual and Personal Growth Program for Women*. New York, NY: Fireside; 1988.
446. Jankovich R, Miller PR. Response of women with primary orgasmic dysfunction to audiovisual education. *J Sex Marital Ther*. 1978;4:16-19.
447. Brotto LA, Heiman JR, Goff B, et al. A psychoeducational intervention for sexual dysfunction in women with gynecologic cancer. *Arch Sex Behav*. 2008;37:317-329.
448. Segraves RT, Clayton A, Croft H, et al. Bupropion sustained release for the treatment of hypoactive sexual desire disorder in premenopausal women. *J Clin Psychopharmacol*. 2004;24:339-342.
449. Nijland EA, Weijmar Schultz WC, Nathorst-Boos J, et al. Tibolone and transdermal E2/NETA for the treatment of female sexual dysfunction in naturally menopausal women: results of a randomized active-controlled trial. *J Sex Med*. 2008;5:646-656.
450. Meston CM, Worcel M. The effects of yohimbine plus l-arginine glutamate on sexual arousal in postmenopausal women with sexual arousal disorder. *Arch Sex Behav*. 2002;31:323-332.
451. Meston CM, Heiman JR. Ephedrine-activated physiological sexual arousal in women. *Arch Gen Psychiatry*. 1998;55:652-656.
452. Caruso S, Rugolo S, Agnello C, et al: Sildenafi l improves sexual functioning in premenopausal women with type 1 diabetes who are affected by sexual arousal disorder: a double-blind, crossover, placebo-controlled pilot study. *Fertil Steril*. 2006;85:1496-1501.
453. Dasgupta R, Wiseman OJ, Kanabar G, et al: Efficacy of sildenafil in the treatment of female sexual dysfunction due to multiple sclerosis. *J Urol*. 2004;171:1189-1193.
454. Ito TY, Trant AS, Polan ML. A double-blind placebo-controlled study of Argin Max, a nutritional supplement for enhancement of female sexual function. *J Sex Marital Ther*. 2001;27:541-549.
455. Heiman JR, Meston CM. Empirically validated treatment for sexual dysfunction. *Ann Rev Sex Res*. 1997;8:148-194.
456. Nurnberg HG, Hensley PL, Heiman JR, et al. Sildenafil treatment of women with antidepressant-associated sexual dysfunction: a randomized controlled trial. *JAMA*. 2008;300:395-404.
457. Bachmann G, Rosen R, Pinn V, et al. Vulvodynia: a state-of-the-art consensus on definitions, diagnosis and management. *J Reprod Med*. 2006;51:447-456.
458. Petersen CD, Giraldi A, Lundvall L, et al. Botulinum toxin type A: a novel treatment for provoked vestibulodynia? Results from a placebo controlled randomized double blinded study. *J Sex Med*. 2009;6: 2523-2537.
458a. Anderson RU, Wise D, Sawyer T, Chan C. Integration of myofascial trigger point release and paradoxical relaxational training treatment of chronic pelvic pain in men. *J Urol*. 2005;174:155-160.
459. McGuire H, Hawton K. Interventions for vaginismus. Cochrane Database Syst Rev. 2003;(1):CD001760.
460. van Lankveld JJ, ter Kuile MM, de Groot HE, et al. Cognitive-behavioral therapy for women with lifelong vaginismus: a randomized waiting-list controlled trial of efficacy. *J Consult Clin Psychol*. 2006;74:168-178.
461. Magee TR, Ferrini MG, Davila HH, et al. Protein inhibitor of nitric oxide synthase (NOS) and the N-methyl-D-aspartate receptor are expressed in the rat and mouse penile nerves and colocalize with penile neuronal NOS. *Biol Reprod*. 2003 Feb;68(2):478-488.
462. Bivalacqua TJ, Kendirci M, Champion HC, et al. Dysregulation of cGMP-dependent protein kinase 1 (PKG-1) impairs erectile function in diabetic rats: influence of in vivo gene therapy of PKG1alpha. *BJU Int*. 2007 Jun;99(6):1488-1494.
463. Burchardt M, Burchardt T, Anastasiadis AG, et al. Application of angiogenic factors for therapy of erectile dysfunction: protein and DNA transfer of VEGF 165 into the rat penis. *Urology*. 2005 Sep;66(3): 665-670.
464. Dall'Era JE, Meacham RB, Mills JN, et al. Vascular endothelial growth factor (VEGF) gene therapy using a nonviral gene delivery system improves erectile function in a diabetic rat model. *Int J Impot Res*. 2008 May-Jun;20(3):307-314.
465. Jin HR, Kim WJ, Song JS, et al. Intracavernous delivery of synthetic angiopoietin-1 protein as a novel therapeutic strategy for erectile dysfunction in the type II diabetic db/db mouse. *J Sex Med*. 2010 Nov; 7(11):3635-3646.
466. Ryu JK, Cho CH, Shin HY, et al. Combined angiopoietin-1 and vascular endothelial growth factor gene transfer restores cavernous angiogenesis and erectile function in a rat model of hypercholesterolemia. *Mol Ther*. 2006 Apr;13(4):705-715.
467. Bakircioglu ME, Lin CS, Fan P, et al. The effect of adeno-associated virus mediated brain derived neurotrophic factor in an animal model of neurogenic impotence. *J Urol*. 2001 Jun;165(6 Pt 1):2103-2109.
468. Bennett NE, Kim JH, Wolfe DP, et al. Improvement in erectile dysfunction after neurotrophic factor gene therapy in diabetic rats. *J Urol*. 2005 May;173(5):1820-1824.
469. Kato R, Wolfe D, Coyle CH, et al. Herpes simplex virus vector-mediated delivery of neurturin rescues erectile dysfunction of cavernous nerve injury. *Gene Ther*. 2009 Jan;16(1):26-33.
470. Shen ZJ, Wang H, Lu YL, et al. Gene transfer of vasoactive intestinal polypeptide into the penis improves erectile response in the diabetic rat. *BJU Int*. 2005 Apr;95(6):890-894.
471. Bivalacqua TJ, Usta MF, Kendirci M, et al. Superoxide anion production in the rat penis impairs erectile function in diabetes: influence of in vivo extracellular superoxide dismutase gene therapy. *J Sex Med*. 2005 Mar;2(2):187-197.
472. Pu XY, Hu LQ, Wang HP, et al. Improvement in erectile dysfunction after insulin-like growth factor-1 gene therapy in diabetic rats. *Asian J Androl*. 2007 Jan;9(1):83-91.

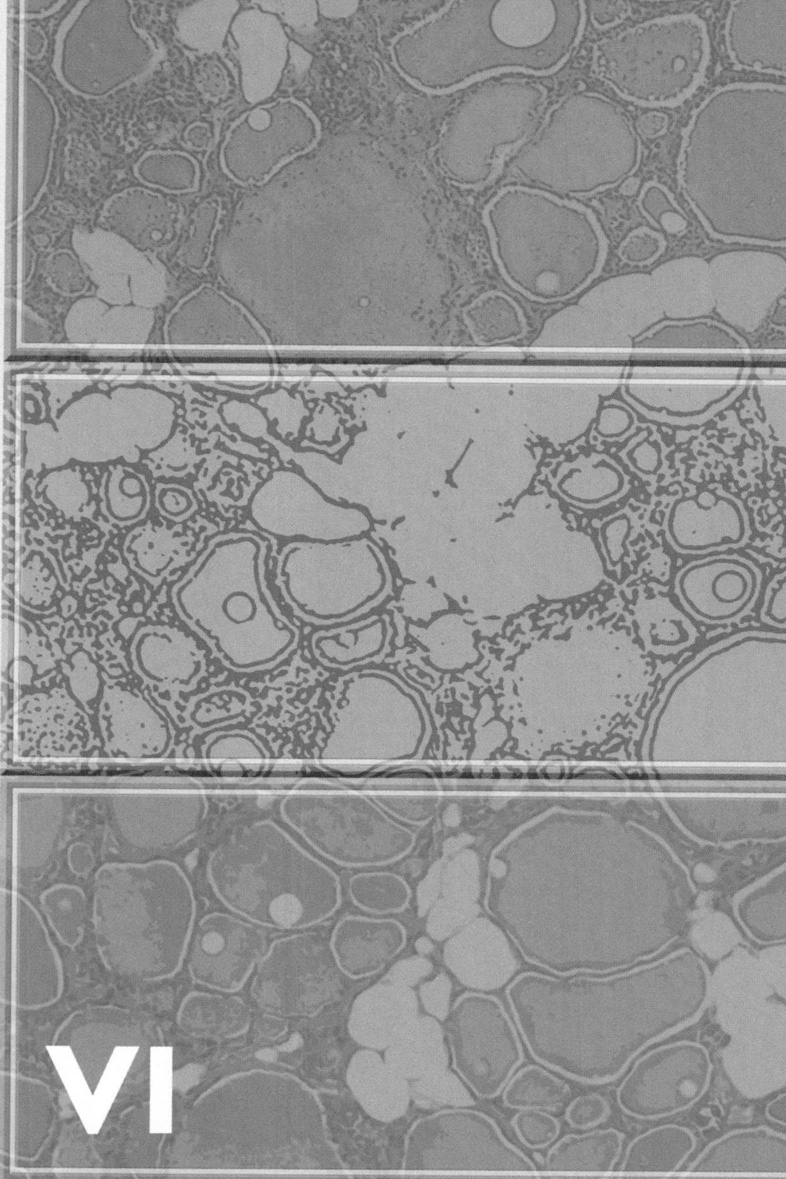

SECTION VI

Endocrinology and the Life Span

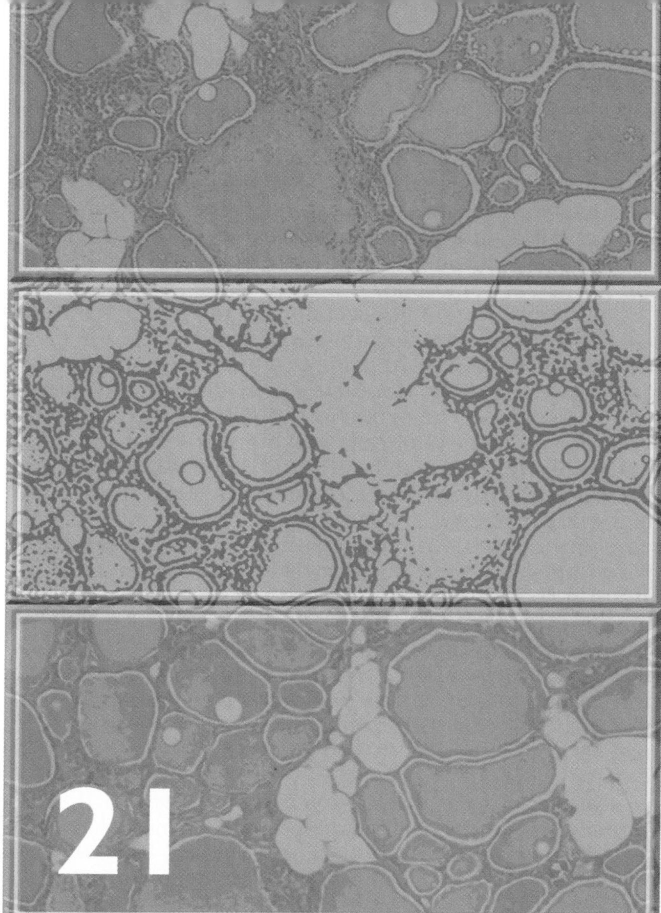

CHAPTER 21

Endocrine Changes in Pregnancy

GLENN D. BRAUNSTEIN

PLACENTAL DEVELOPMENT

Normal placentation requires a coordinated series of events, beginning with fertilization. The fertilization rate after unprotected regular intercourse during a single menstrual cycle is 25% to 30%. However, in approximately one third of conceptions, there is either failure of implantation or clinical or subclinical spontaneous abortion.[1]

For the first 5 days, preimplantation development takes place within the fallopian tube. During this period, the zygote undergoes cleavage division, and at least through the eight-cell stage, the blastomeres remain totipotential. In the 16-cell stage, differentiation of the innermost cells into the *inner cell mass* and the surrounding cells into the *trophectoderm* occurs. The inner cell mass develops into the fetus, and the trophectoderm gives rise to the placenta and membranes. On approximately day 5 or 6 after fertilization, the blastocyst enters the uterus, but implantation does not occur for another 1 to 2 days. Implantation occurs after the zona pellucida disappears from around the embryo.[2]

Implantation is a complex process that involves apposition of the microvilli on the trophectoderm cells with the pinocytes (i.e., fused microvilli) on the endometrial cells, followed by removal of fluid between the cells through pinocytosis by the endometrial cells, a process stimulated by progesterone.[3] Progesterone synthesis by the corpus luteum is stimulated and sustained during this time and for the first 6 to 7 weeks of pregnancy by secretion of human chorionic gonadotropin (hCG) by the trophoblast cells. The hCG is first detected in the maternal serum 6 to 9 days after conception.[4] Attachment of the embryo is enhanced through the expression of a variety of adhesion molecules, including mucins, integrins, and trophinin, a trophoblast-specific cell membrane adhesion protein; cytokines; growth factors; and a variety of transcription factors encoded by homeobox genes.[3,5,6]

After the trophoblast attaches to the endometrium during the window of implantation 6 to 10 days after ovulation, the embryo invades the endometrium through a complex process involving matrix metalloproteinases and differentiation of the trophectoderm into *cytotrophoblasts* or *syncytiotrophoblasts*. The syncytiotrophoblasts are multinucleated cells formed by the fusion of cytotrophoblasts. The cytotrophoblasts form a column of cells that invade the endometrium, form anchoring villi, and enter the maternal vasculature, eventually replacing the endothelial layer of the endometrial and myometrial spiral arterioles with a layer of cytotrophoblasts (i.e., vascular trophoblasts).[5] This process converts the high-resistance, low-capacity uterine vessels into low-resistance, high-volume vessels, which are essential for growth of the placenta and fetus.[7] At the site of implantation, the endometrial cells undergo decidualization, enlarging and increasing their metabolic activity with enhanced production of tissue inhibitors or metalloproteinase, extracellular matrix proteins, cytokines, and growth factors that modulate the extent of trophoblast invasion and influence trophoblast function.[3,4,8]

The trophoblast cells secrete several angiogenic proteins, including vascular endothelial growth factor, platelet-derived growth factor (PDGF), and basic fibroblast growth factor (bFGF), which stimulate blood vessel development within the villi.[5] The syncytiotrophoblasts form an outer layer of cells in the chorionic villi between the cytotrophoblast cells and the maternal blood space on the exterior surface. Only three tissues separate the fetal blood from maternal blood: the endothelium of the fetal vessels in the villi, connective tissue, and the trophoblasts; this form of placentation is referred to as *hemochorial*. Therefore, in addition to hCG secretion, which is responsible for maintaining early pregnancy; progesterone secretion, which is required for continuation of pregnancy after the luteal-placental shift; and the synthesis and secretion of other hormones and growth factors (Table 21-1), the syncytiotrophoblasts provide the major site for transportation of oxygen and nutrients to and removal of waste from the fetus.

Substances are transferred across the placenta through transcellular pathways that include carrier-mediated transport (e.g., immunoglobulin G through the Fcγ receptor) and simple extracellular diffusion. The degree of transplacental passage of a hormone from the mother to the fetus through diffusion depends on the rate of placental blood flow, the maternal concentration of hormone that is free or readily dissociable from binding proteins, and the molecular mass, lipid solubility, charge, and degree of placental metabolic degradation of the hormone. Maternal-to-fetal transfer occurs for hormones smaller than 700 d, but the placenta is not permeable to hormones larger than 1200 d.[9]

The trophoblast anchors the placenta and fetus to the uterus and helps protect the fetus, which contains paternal antigens, from rejection by the maternal immune system. This immunologic protection may be mediated by high concentrations of progesterone at the trophoblast-maternal interface and the expression by the trophoblasts of a histocompatibility complex antigen, human leukocyte antigen G (HLA-G), which exhibits reduced polymorphism compared with other major HLA antigens.[10] The mass of the trophoblast increases logarithmically during the first trimester, followed by a more gradual increase throughout the remainder of pregnancy. Trophoblastic mass closely correlates with maternal serum concentrations of human placental lactogen (hPL) and pregnancy-specific β_1-glycoprotein throughout pregnancy and with hCG during the first trimester but not during the subsequent trimesters.[11]

MATERNAL ADAPTATIONS TO PREGNANCY

Myriad physiologic changes take place beginning shortly after implantation. During early pregnancy, these effects are hormonally mediated. In the second and third trimesters, the uteroplacental vascular system and mechanical factors associated with the enlarging gravid uterus combine with the hormonal milieu to alter the function of every system.

TABLE 21-1

Hormones, Peptides, and Growth Factors Produced by the Placenta

Hormones, Peptides, and Growth Factors
Hypothalamic Analogues and Neuropeptides
Anandamide (endocannabinoid)
Corticotropin-releasing hormone
Dopamine
Met-enkephalin
Ghrelin
Gonadotropin-releasing hormone
Growth hormone–releasing hormone
Melatonin
Neuropeptide Y
Oxytocin
Somatostatin
Substance P
Thyrotropin-releasing hormone
Urocortin
Vasoactive intestinal peptide
Pituitary Analogues
α-Melanocyte-stimulating hormone
β-Endorphin
Chorionic corticotropin
Chorionic gonadotropin
Placental lactogen
Placental variant growth hormone
Steroid Hormones
Estrogens
Progesterone
Growth Factors and Other Hormones
Activins
Adrenomedullin
Angiotensinogen
Basic fibroblast growth factor
Calcitonin
Colony-stimulating factor
Endothelin 1
Epidermal growth factor
Erythropoietin
Follistatin
Hepatocyte growth factor
Inhibins
Insulin-like growth factor type 1
Insulin-like growth factor type 2
Interleukins
Leptin
Leukemia inhibitory factor
Metastin
Nerve growth factor
Oncomodulin
Osteopontin
Parathyroid hormone–related protein
Platelet-derived growth factor
Pro-early placental insulin-like peptide
Renin
Transforming growth factor-α and -β
Tumor necrosis factor-α
Vascular endothelial growth factor
Other
Corticotropin-releasing hormone–binding protein
Insulin-like growth factor–binding protein
Nitric oxide
Prostate-specific antigen

General Adaptations

Weight gain averages 12.5 kg, of which the fetus accounts for about 3.4 kg, the placenta for 0.65 kg, amniotic fluid for 0.8 kg, uterus for 1 kg, breasts for 0.4 kg, blood for 1.5 kg, extravascular fluid for 1.5 kg, and maternal fat stores for approximately 3.3 kg.[12] The volume of the uterine cavity increases from about 10 mL to an average of 5 L at term, and blood flow through the uteroplacental circulation reaches 450 to 650 mL/minute.[12]

To maintain appropriate perfusion of the mother and the fetal-placental unit, blood volume increases throughout pregnancy and is 40% to 45% higher at term than in the nonpregnant state. The plasma volume increases by about 45% to 50% as a result of aldosterone-stimulated sodium and water retention. The red cell mass increases approximately 20% because of increased production resulting from a twofold to threefold increase in erythropoietin secretion. The net effect is a decrease in the hematocrit by about 15% at term.[12]

The renal blood flow and glomerular filtration rate (GFR) increase rapidly and peak during the second trimester, and a 50% increase in creatinine clearance results in a reduction in the serum creatinine level. Atrial natriuretic peptide (ANP) levels increase during pregnancy and may in part be responsible for increased renal blood flow, GFR, 24-hour urine volume, and natriuresis.[13] An alteration in the osmotic thresholds for the release of vasopressin and activation of the hypothalamic thirst centers, possibly caused by an extragonadal effect of hCG, lead to an approximately 4% reduction in serum osmolality (approximately 10 mOsm/kg).[14]

Several hemodynamic changes are induced by the low-resistance, high-capacity uteroplacental vessels, which in many respects act like an arteriovenous malformation; the increased blood volume; and the large quantities of estrogens, progesterone, prostaglandins, and angiotensin present during pregnancy. Changes include an increase in the heart rate by 10 to 15 beats/minute, a 30% to 50% increase in cardiac output resulting from increased stroke volume in early pregnancy and heart rate during the third trimester, a reduction in diastolic blood pressure of 10 to 15 mm Hg with little or no change in systolic pressure, and an approximately 20% reduction in peripheral vascular resistance.[12]

The pulmonary vascular resistance is reduced by about one third. Pregnancy also is associated with increases in pulmonary tidal volume by about 30%, which results in a respiratory alkalosis that is compensated by increased bicarbonate excretion by the kidneys; in minute ventilatory volume by 30% to 40%; and in minute oxygen uptake. There are no changes in respiratory rate, maximum breathing capacity, or forced or timed vital capacity. However, there is an approximately 40% reduction in the expiratory reserve because of the elevation of the diaphragm by the enlarged uterus.[12]

Gastrointestinal tract function is altered during pregnancy. Gastric emptying time is unchanged until labor, when it becomes prolonged. Reduced lower esophageal sphincter tone and displacement of the abdominal contents by the pregnant uterus result in a marked increase in gastroesophageal reflux disease. Motility of the intestine is also reduced, contributing to the constipation that is common during pregnancy. Decreased motility of the gallbladder leads to an increased gallbladder volume and reduced emptying of bile after meals, producing a more lithogenic bile and increasing cholelithiasis during pregnancy.[12]

Maternal Endocrine Alterations

Pituitary Gland

The anterior pituitary gland enlarges by an average of 36% during pregnancy, primarily because of a 10-fold increase in lactotroph size and number. This enlargement increases the height and convexity of the pituitary that is observed on magnetic resonance imaging. Numbers of somatotrophs and gonadotrophs are reduced, and there are no changes in corticotrophs or thyrotrophs.[15] The size of the posterior pituitary gland diminishes during pregnancy.[16]

The marked increase in estrogen levels during pregnancy enhances prolactin synthesis and secretion, and maternal prolactin serum levels increase in parallel with the enlargement of the lactotrophs. At term, the mean serum prolactin concentration is 207 ng/mL (range, 35 to 600 ng/mL), in contrast to a mean of 10 ng/mL in nonpregnant, premenopausal women. Prolactin also is present in the amniotic fluid and appears to be primarily of decidual origin because the decidua actively synthesizes prolactin. Amniotic fluid prolactin levels are 10 to 100 times higher than in the maternal circulation in early pregnancy, and maternal bromocriptine ingestion does not reduce the amniotic fluid prolactin levels but does reduce the maternal and fetal serum concentrations.[17] Prolactin levels return to the baseline of nonpregnancy approximately 7 days after delivery in the absence of breast-feeding. With breast-feeding, the basal prolactin levels remain elevated for several months but gradually decrease; however, with suckling, there is a brisk rise in prolactin levels within 30 minutes.[15]

Growth hormone (GH) levels in maternal serum remain unchanged throughout pregnancy, although the source of immunoreactive GH during gestation does change. Relaxin, secreted by the corpus luteum of pregnancy, and estrogens stimulate GH secretion during early pregnancy.[18] Pituitary GH is known as GH1 or hGH-N; its messenger ribonucleic acid (mRNA) and GH1 secretion decrease after the 25th week of pregnancy, and beginning in the fourth month of gestation, the placental syncytiotrophoblast secretes a variant of GH (called GH2 or hGH-V) in a nonpulsatile pattern.[19,20] In concert with the different sources of GH during the first and second halves of pregnancy, the GH response to provocative stimuli differs in each half. Insulin hypoglycemia or arginine infusion results in an enhanced GH response during the first half of gestation, and during the second half, the response is decreased compared with the response in nonpregnant women.[15]

Maternal serum concentrations of insulin-like growth factor type 1 (IGF1) are elevated during the second half of pregnancy, probably through the combined effect of the placental GH variant and hPL, which is evolutionarily related to GH and prolactin. HPL has somatotropic biologic activity, and its serum concentration increases throughout pregnancy, paralleling that of IGF1.[19-22] It is likely that the suppression of GH1 synthesis and secretion is caused by the high IGF1 concentrations, which in late pregnancy are five times higher than those in nonpregnant women.[20]

Although the placenta synthesizes and secretes biologically active gonadotropin-releasing hormone (GnRH), pituitary gonadotropin production decreases throughout pregnancy, as indicated by a marked reduction in gonadotropin immunoreactivity in the gonadotrophs beginning at 10 weeks' gestation and by a reduction in serum levels of luteinizing hormone (LH) and follicle-stimulating hormone (FSH).[15] Suppression is probably mediated through the elevated blood levels of ovarian and placental

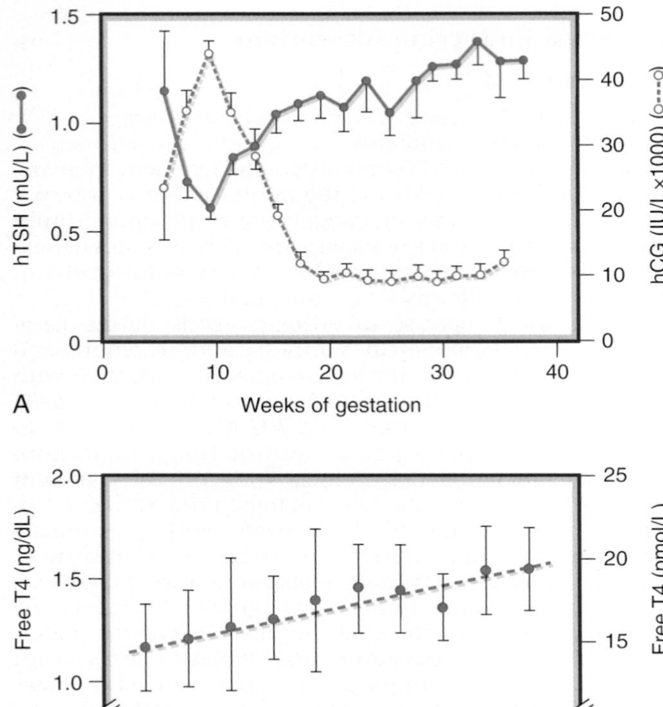

Figure 21-1 **A,** Concentrations of serum thyrotropin (hTSH, *filled circles*) and human chorionic gonadotropin (hCG, *open circles*) throughout pregnancy. Between 8 and 14 weeks of gestation, there is a significant negative correlation between the individual hTSH and hCG levels ($P < .001$). Each point represents the mean (± standard error). **B,** Linear regression of maternal serum free thyroxine (T_4) and hCG concentrations during the first half of gestation ($P < .001$). (From Glinoer D, de Nayer P, Bourdoux P, et al. Regulation of maternal thyroid during pregnancy. *J Clin Endocrinol Metab.* 1990;71:276.)

sex steroid hormones and by placental production of inhibin. Suppression is incomplete because administration of exogenous GnRH leads to release of gonadotropins, although the response is blunted compared with that of nonpregnant women and does not return to normal until a month after birth.[15]

The mean concentrations of human thyroid-stimulating hormone (thyrotropin or hTSH) during the first trimester are significantly lower than in the second and third trimesters or in the nonpregnant state.[23] Much of this early decrease may be accounted for by the intrinsic thyrotropic activity of hCG. The maximal biologic thyrotropic activity in maternal serum corresponds to the peak concentration of hCG at 10 to 12 weeks after the last menstrual period, when there is a reciprocal relationship between the rising hCG levels and falling hTSH concentrations (Fig. 21-1).[23,24] The only time during pregnancy when the free thyroxine concentration in the maternal serum is elevated corresponds to the time of peak hCG and lowest hTSH, suggesting that the depressed hTSH is the result of feedback suppression by thyroxine. Despite the lower mean hTSH during early pregnancy, the hTSH response to exogenous thyrotropin-releasing hormone (TRH) is normal.[15]

Maternal adrenocorticotropic hormone (ACTH, or corticotropin) levels rise during pregnancy, increasing fourfold over concentrations in the nonpregnant state between 7 and 10 weeks' gestation. There is a further gradual rise to weeks 33 to 37, when a mean fivefold increase over prepregnancy values is found, followed by a 50% drop just before parturition and a marked 15-fold increase during the stress of delivery.[25] The ACTH concentration returns to the prepregnancy level within 24 hours of delivery. The pituitary gland and placenta are sources of circulating ACTH during pregnancy, and exogenous corticotropin-releasing hormone (CRH) stimulates the release of ACTH from both tissues in a dose-dependent manner.[25] Biologically active CRH is synthesized and secreted by the placenta and, to a lesser extent, by the decidual and fetal membranes, but unlike the inhibitory effect on pituitary CRH, glucocorticoids stimulate the expression of placental CRH.[25]

There appears to be a disconnect between CRH and ACTH during pregnancy. Although biologically active CRH would be expected to stimulate ACTH production, the qualitative patterns of CRH production, which shows an exponential rise during the sixth month of gestation, and ACTH secretion, which demonstrates a more gradual rise during pregnancy, are quite different. The lack of a significant correlation between maternal plasma CRH and ACTH during pregnancy suggests that factors such as the elevated levels of free cortisol in the maternal serum may modulate the response to CRH. The circadian rhythm and the ability to respond to stress are maintained throughout pregnancy; however, the ACTH response to exogenous CRH during the third trimester is blunted, whereas the responsiveness to vasopressin is maintained, suggesting that the elevation of CRH in the maternal serum downregulates the responsiveness to CRH.[25]

Arginine vasopressin (AVP) concentrations in the maternal serum are similar to those in nonpregnant women.[26] During pregnancy, however, there is increased synthesis of AVP, which is offset by the increased metabolic clearance of the hormone through destruction by a trophoblast-derived cysteine aminopeptidase (i.e., vasopressinase), whose levels rise throughout pregnancy in parallel with the increase in trophoblastic mass.[26,27] The osmolar set point for thirst is reduced, and the release of AVP is related to the 10 mOsm/kg average decrease in plasma osmolality during pregnancy, possibly reflecting an extragonadotropic effect of hCG.[14] Taking into account the reduced set point, the AVP response to dehydration and water loading is normal.

Oxytocin levels progressively increase in the maternal blood and parallel the increase in maternal serum levels of estradiol and progesterone.[28] The levels increase further with cervical dilation and vaginal distention during labor and delivery, stimulating contraction of the uterine smooth muscles and enhancing fetal ejection.[28] Uterine oxytocin receptors also increase throughout pregnancy, resulting in a 100-fold increase in oxytocin binding at term in the myometrium.[29]

Thyroid Gland

The thyroid gland enlarges by an average of 18% during pregnancy.[23] Enlargement is associated with an increase in the size of the follicles with increased amounts of colloid and enhanced blood volume. This enlargement may be a response to the thyrotropic effect of hCG and asialo-hCG, which may account for some of the increase in serum thyroglobulin concentrations observed during pregnancy. Enhanced iodine I 131 uptake by the maternal thyroid gland reflects the combined effects of hCG stimulation and reduction of the blood levels of iodide by increased renal iodide clearance.[23]

Rising estrogen concentrations during pregnancy induce increased hepatic synthesis of thyroxine-binding globulin (TBG) and enhanced sialylation of TBG, which decreases its metabolic clearance rate.[24] The results are a twofold increase in TBG and increased total thyroxine (T_4) and triiodothyronine (T_3) levels in maternal serum throughout pregnancy,[23] whereas for most of the gestation, the free T_4 and free T_3 concentrations remain normal. There are no significant changes in the levels of thyroxine-binding prealbumin, but albumin levels are decreased because of the increase in vascular volume.

Parathyroid Glands

During pregnancy, approximately 30 g of calcium is transferred from the maternal compartment to the fetus, with most of the transfer occurring during the last trimester. Maternal total serum calcium levels decrease during pregnancy, with a nadir at 28 to 32 weeks related to the decrease in albumin levels that accompanies the increase in vascular volume. However, the albumin-adjusted total calcium and the ionized calcium concentrations rise slightly above the level in the nonpregnant state.[30] The urinary calcium excretion rate increases in parallel with the increased GFR, and intestinal calcium absorption undergoes a twofold increase.[30]

Although some studies have suggested that parathyroid hormone (PTH) levels increase during pregnancy, measurements of intact PTH levels by two-site immunometric assays indicate that they are within the normal, nonpregnancy range throughout pregnancy.[30] In contrast, the circulating concentrations of PTH-related protein (PTHrP) increase throughout pregnancy.[30] Many normal tissues produce this protein, and the source of the elevated levels during pregnancy is unclear, although the two most likely sites are the mammary tissue and the placenta. PTHrP is probably involved in placental calcium transport. Serum calcitonin levels increase during pregnancy, which may reflect the combined contribution of the thyroid C cells, the breast, and the placenta.[30]

The serum levels of 25-hydroxyvitamin D are unchanged during pregnancy, but the estrogen-induced rise in vitamin D–binding globulin results in a twofold increase in 1,25-dihydroxyvitamin D concentrations in maternal serum.[30] The biologically active free fraction of 1,25-dihydroxyvitamin D_3 (calcitriol) also increases, which may reflect both increased maternal renal 1α-hydroxylase activity, stimulated in part by pregnancy-induced increased calcitonin secretion, and the synthesis and secretion of calcitriol by the placenta.[30] This increase in the active metabolite of vitamin D may be responsible in part for the enhanced intestinal calcium absorption.

Pancreas

Hyperplasia and hypertrophy of the beta cells in the islets of Langerhans are probably the result of stimulation by estrogen and progesterone.[31] During early pregnancy, the glucose requirements of the fetus lead to enhanced transport of glucose across the placenta by facilitated diffusion, and maternal fasting hypoglycemia may occur. Although basal insulin levels may be normal, there is hypersecretion of insulin in response to a meal. Because studies have shown no change or an increase in insulin clearance during pregnancy, this increase represents an increase in synthesis and secretion.[32] The results are enhanced glycogen storage and decreased hepatic glucose production.

As pregnancy progresses, the levels of hPL rise, as do the levels of glucocorticoids, progesterone, free fatty acids, and tumor necrosis factor-α, leading to the insulin resistance found during the last half of pregnancy.[32] In late pregnancy, glucose ingestion produces higher and more sustained levels of glucose and insulin and a greater degree of glucagon suppression than in the nonpregnant state.

Adrenal Glands

As a result of the hyperestrogenemia of pregnancy, hepatic production of cortisol-binding globulin is increased. Amplified production results in a doubling of the maternal serum levels of cortisol-binding globulin, which decreases metabolic clearance of cortisol and produces a threefold rise in total plasma cortisol by week 26, when the levels reach a plateau until they rise at the onset of labor.[25,33] The rate of cortisol production is increased, and the plasma free cortisol concentrations are also increased. Cortisol production is enhanced by an increase in the maternal plasma ACTH concentration and hyperresponsiveness of the adrenal cortex to ACTH stimulation during pregnancy.[25] Cortisol secretion follows that of ACTH, and the diurnal rhythm is maintained during pregnancy.[33] Despite the elevated free cortisol levels, pregnant women do not develop the stigma of glucocorticoid excess, possibly because of the antiglucocorticoid activities of the elevated concentrations of progesterone.

Plasma renin substrate levels are increased as a consequence of the effects of estrogen on the liver. Renin levels are also increased, and increased renin activity produces higher levels of angiotensin II, which lead to an 8- to 10-fold increase in aldosterone production and serum aldosterone levels.[25] The aldosterone levels peak in midpregnancy and are maintained until delivery.

Despite their baseline elevations, the various components of the renin-angiotensin-aldosterone system demonstrate normal responses to positional changes, sodium restriction, and sodium loading. Elevated aldosterone levels do not result in increased serum sodium concentrations, decreased serum potassium levels, or increased blood pressure; this may reflect the high concentrations of progesterone, which can displace aldosterone from its renal receptors. Another mineralocorticoid, 11-deoxycorticosterone, shows a 6- to 10-fold increase in concentration at term.[25] Elevated levels of this hormone are caused by estrogen-induced extraglandular 21-hydroxylation of progesterone produced by the placenta.[34]

Levels of androstenedione and testosterone, whether they are of adrenal or ovarian origin, are elevated because of the estrogen-induced increase in hepatic synthesis of sex hormone–binding globulin. However, the free androgen levels remain normal or low. Adrenal production rates of dehydroepiandrosterone (DHEA) and dehydroepiandrosterone sulfate (DHEAS) are increased twofold, but the maternal serum concentration of DHEAS is reduced to one third to one half of the nonpregnancy levels because of enhanced 16-hydroxylation and placental use of 16-hydroxydehydroepiandrosterone sulfate in estrogen formation.[34]

Adrenal medullary function remains normal throughout pregnancy. The 24-hour urine catecholamine and plasma epinephrine and norepinephrine levels are similar to concentrations in the nonpregnant state.[35,36]

PLACENTAL HORMONE PRODUCTION

Steroid Hormones

Placental steroidogenesis takes place in the syncytiotrophoblast, and synthesis and secretion of estrogens and progesterone increase throughout pregnancy in concert with the increase in the trophoblast mass (Fig. 21-2).[11] The placenta does not express steroidogenic factor 1 (SF1), a transcription factor that is an important regulator of genes involved in adrenal and gonadal steroid hormone synthesis.[37] The trophoblast has reduced levels of, or lacks, several enzymes that are important for the de novo production of estrogens and progesterone and therefore depends on precursors of maternal and fetal origin. This dependence underlies the concept of the *maternal-fetal-placental unit*.[38] These interactions are outlined in Figure 21-3.[39,40]

Progesterone

Although the trophoblast can synthesize cholesterol from acetate, the amount of an essential enzyme needed for cholesterol synthesis, hydroxymethylglutaryl-coenzyme A reductase, in placental microsomes is low because of the inhibitory effects of the high intracellular concentrations of cholesterol that result from progesterone inhibition of cholesterol esterification.[41] Steroid synthesis by the placenta depends on the delivery of low-density lipoprotein (LDL) and very-low-density lipoprotein (VLDL) from the maternal circulation. The syncytiotrophoblast contains receptors for LDL, VLDL, and high-density lipoprotein (HDL). Receptor-mediated uptake of LDL cholesterol is stimulated by estrogens, as is the activity of the cholesterol side-chain cleavage/desmolase enzyme (CYP11A1), which converts cholesterol to pregnenolone.[38,42] The placenta lacks the steroidogenic acute regulatory (STAR) protein, which mediates the transport of cholesterol from the outer to inner mitochondrial membrane, the site where CYP11A1 acts, so another mitochondrial transport mechanism must be present in the placenta. Altered placental steroid production is not seen in pregnancies with STAR mutations that result in congenital lipoid hyperplasia affecting the adrenals and gonads.[43]

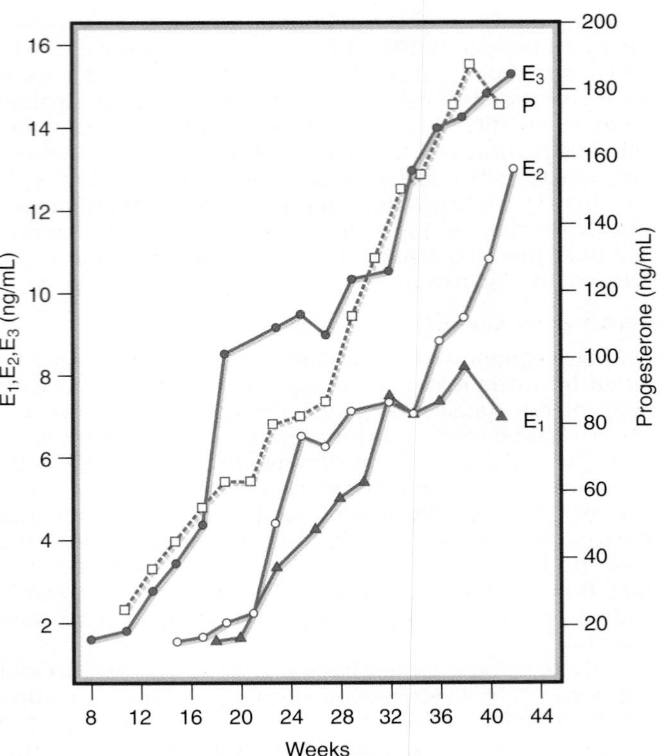

Figure 21-2 Mean plasma concentrations of estrone (E_1), estradiol (E_2), estriol (E_3), and progesterone (P) during pregnancy. (Data from Tulchinsky D, Hobel CJ, Yeager E, et al. Plasma estrone, estradiol, estriol, progesterone, and 17-hydroxyprogesterone in human pregnancy: I. Normal pregnancy. *Am J Obstet Gynecol.* 1972;112:1095; and Levitz M, Young BK. Estrogens and pregnancy. *Vitam Horm.* 1977;35:109.)

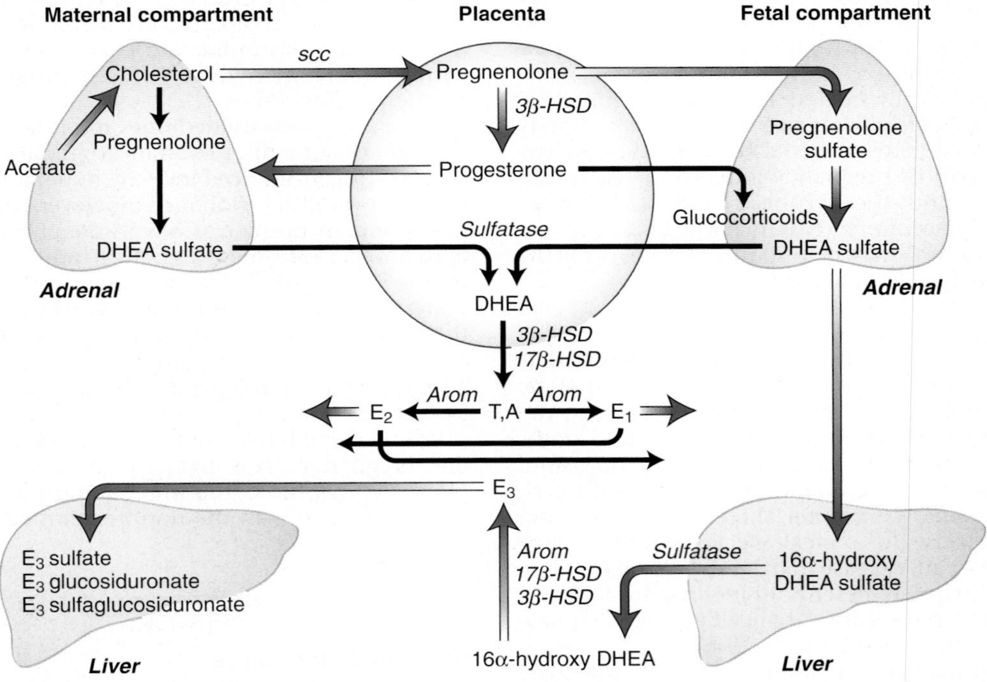

Figure 21-3 Steroidogenesis in the maternal-fetal-placental unit. A, androstenedione; Arom, aromatase-enzyme complex; DHEA, dehydroepiandrosterone; E_1, estrone; E_2, estradiol; E_3, estriol; HSD, hydroxysteroid dehydrogenase; SCC, cholesterol side-chain cleavage enzyme; T, testosterone.

Progesterone is synthesized in the trophoblast from pregnenolone by a placental isoform of 3β-hydroxysteroid dehydrogenase 1 (3β-HSD1).[42] Approximately 90% of the progesterone synthesized is secreted into the maternal compartment, and at term, the mean maternal serum concentration is about 150 ng/mL. The fetal adrenals lack 3β-HSD activity and therefore are not essential for progesterone production.[42] Progesterone production continues after fetal death.[44]

Progesterone appears to have multiple functions during pregnancy, the most important of which is preparation of the uterus for implantation and maintenance of the pregnancy.[38] The corpus luteum is the primary source of progesterone during the first 6 to 8 weeks of pregnancy, after which ovarian progesterone production declines and placental synthesis and secretion become the major source of the hormone (i.e., luteal-placental shift).[44]

Luteectomy, or removal of the ovary containing the corpus luteum, within the first 35 days after conception leads to abortion, but the pregnancy usually continues if these procedures are performed 46 or more days after conception. This indicates that placental progesterone production is sufficient to maintain the pregnancy even before the luteal-placental shift.[44] Administration of the progesterone receptor antagonist mifepristone during the first 49 days after conception results in abortion, demonstrating that progesterone is essential for the maintenance of early pregnancy.[45]

Progesterone is an important substrate for fetal adrenal glucocorticoid and mineralocorticoid synthesis and for maintenance of myometrial quiescence, possibly through inhibition of prostaglandin formation.[38,42] A possible role for the high concentrations of progesterone at the trophoblast-decidua junction is suppression of cell-mediated rejection of the fetus, which expresses paternal antigens, by maternal T lymphocytes.[38]

Estrogens

Because the trophoblast lacks 17α-hydroxylase and 17,20-lyase (CYP17) activities, it cannot directly convert progesterone to estrogen. Pregnenolone produced in the placenta enters the fetal compartment, where it is taken up by the fetal zone of the adrenal cortex, which also synthesizes pregnenolone from fetal LDL cholesterol. Pregnenolone is conjugated with sulfate by fetal steroid sulfotransferase in the fetal liver and adrenals to form pregnenolone sulfate; this is converted in the fetal adrenals to 17α-hydroxypregnenolone sulfate and then to DHEAS by 17α-hydroxylase and 17,20-lyase (CYP17) activities.[46]

DHEAS enters the fetal circulation and undergoes hydroxylation in the fetal liver to form 16α-hydroxy-DHEAS, which is converted to 16α-DHEA in the placenta through the action of placental sulfatase. Further metabolism in the trophoblast by 3β-HSD1, 17β-hydroxysteroid dehydrogenase (17β-HSD), and aromatase (CYP19) leads to the generation of estriol, which is quantitatively the major estrogen in the maternal circulation during pregnancy. The maternal liver actively conjugates estriol with glucosiduronate and sulfate, which are excreted into the urine. Because approximately 90% of the estriol in maternal serum and urine is derived from fetal precursors, these estriol levels serve as an index of fetal well-being.[46]

DHEAS from the fetus and mother is taken up by the placenta and converted to estradiol by the actions of sulfatase, 3β-HSD1, 17β-HSD, and aromatase or converted to estrone by sulfatase, 3β-HSD1, and aromatase. An estrogen unique to pregnancy, estetrol, is generated by 15α-hydroxylation of 16α-DHEAS in the fetal adrenal and enzymatically converted by placental sulfatase, 3β-HSD1, 17β-HSD, and aromatase.[47] During pregnancy, estrogens have several actions[38]:

- They enhance receptor-mediated uptake of LDL cholesterol, which is important for normal placental steroid production.
- They increase uteroplacental blood flow.
- They increase endometrial prostaglandin synthesis.
- They increase uterine sensitivity to progesterone in late pregnancy.
- They prepare the breasts for lactation.

However, estrogen action does not appear to be essential in maintaining pregnancy, because a fetus with deletion of the gene encoding placental sulfatase cannot remove the sulfate moiety from 16α-hydroxy-DHEAS and therefore has maternal estrogen levels approaching only about 10% of normal.[48] Similarly, pregnancies complicated by fetal aromatase deficiency may continue to term, suggesting that the high concentrations of estrogens found in normal pregnancy are not necessary.[49]

Protein Hormones

Human Chorionic Gonadotropin

Chemistry. The glycoprotein hCG is composed of two dissimilar subunits, α and β, which are noncovalently linked through hydrophobic bonding. This molecule shares structural homology with the other glycoprotein hormones: hLH, hFSH, and hTSH. These hormones have α-subunits that contain the same sequence of 92 amino acids and differ only in their carbohydrate composition; the β-subunits differ in amino acid and carbohydrate structures and are responsible for the biologic and immunologic specificity of the heterodimeric (intact) hormones. The 22,200-d β-subunit of hCG is composed of 145 amino acids. Approximately 80% of the first 115 amino acids are homologous to those in the β-subunit of hLH. The hCG molecule has an additional 24 amino acids on its carboxy-terminal end that enhance its biologic activity.

Both subunits of hCG contain two oligosaccharide chains attached to asparagine residues through *N*-glycosidic linkages, and the β-subunit contains an additional four *O*-serine-linked oligosaccharide units in the C-terminal peptide. The carbohydrate composition of hCG contains microheterogeneity that affects hormone clearance and biologic activity. The tertiary structure of hCG is determined by the carbohydrate composition and multiple disulfide bonds within each subunit. The α-subunit contains five disulfide bonds, and the β-subunit has six. In each of the subunits, three of the disulfide bonds form a cystine knot, similar to that found in PDGF-β and transforming growth factor-β (TGF-β).[50-52]

Biosynthesis. The single α-subunit gene, located on chromosome 6, is actively expressed in the cytotrophoblast and syncytiotrophoblast. In contrast, the β-subunit is encoded by a cluster of six genes located on chromosome 19 in proximity to the hLH-β gene *(LHB)*. Three of the hCG-β genes are actively transcribed during pregnancy, primarily in the syncytiotrophoblast, which has the ability to synthesize and secrete free subunits and intact hCG. After synthesis of the protein core, each subunit is glycosylated, undergoes further post-translational modification through trimming of the carbohydrate, and then combines to form intact hCG.[50-52]

Secretion of hCG differs from that of many of the other placental proteins, whose secretory patterns parallel that

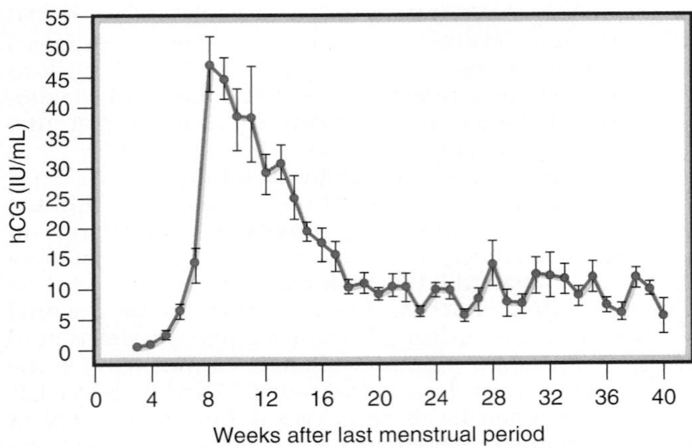

Figure 21-4 Mean (± standard error) levels of maternal serum human chorionic gonadotropin (hCG) throughout normal pregnancy. (From Braunstein GD, Rasor J, Danzer H, et al. Serum human chorionic gonadotropin levels throughout normal pregnancy. *Am J Obstet Gynecol.* 1976;126:678.)

of the trophoblastic mass. HCG is first detected in maternal serum 6 to 9 days after conception.[4] The levels rise in a logarithmic fashion, peaking 8 to 10 weeks after the last menstrual period, followed by a decline to a nadir at 18 weeks, with subsequent levels remaining constant until delivery (Fig. 21-4).[53] A hyperglycosylated form of hCG produced by the cytotrophoblasts is the major form of hCG during the first 2 to 3 weeks after implantation; afterward, the normally glycosylated form produced by the syncytiotrophoblast predominates throughout the rest of pregnancy.[51,52] The placenta also secretes free subunits. During the first 13 weeks of pregnancy, relatively more β-subunit is synthesized than α-subunit, and throughout the remainder of pregnancy, the opposite occurs.[53] A hyperglycosylated form of the α-subunit (called "big α") is unable to combine with the free β-subunit and is secreted into the maternal serum.

The physiologic factors that regulate hCG secretion in vivo are unknown. Much of the data concerning factors that stimulate or inhibit hCG synthesis and secretion have been derived from in vitro studies and are difficult to extrapolate to the in vivo situation. There is strong circumstantial evidence that GnRH, synthesized in the cytotrophoblast and the syncytiotrophoblast, may be an important factor in hCG secretion. This peptide is identical to hypothalamic GnRH and stimulates placental hCG production in vitro and in vivo, whereas GnRH antagonists decrease basal hCG secretion.[50,54,55]

Immunohistochemical staining for GnRH in placental tissue is highest at 8 weeks' gestation and lower afterward,[56] roughly paralleling the pattern of hCG production, as do the circulating levels of GnRH measured in maternal serum.[57] The placenta contains GnRH receptors.[58] Placental GnRH release is stimulated by cyclic adenosine monophosphate (cAMP), prostaglandin E_2, prostaglandin F_2, epinephrine, epidermal growth factor, insulin, and vasoactive intestinal peptide (VIP), factors that also increase hCG secretion in vitro.[50,54,59]

Two other peptides synthesized by the cytotrophoblast, activin and inhibin, modulate GnRH and hCG secretion; activin increases both, and inhibin inhibits the action of GnRH on the syncytiotrophoblast.[54] Increases in hCG production have been found after trophoblast exposure to FGF, calcium, glucocorticoids, phorbol esters, and leptin.[54,60] Decreased production occurs with TGF-β, follistatin, and progesterone.[54] The decidua may influence hCG production through paracrine mechanisms.[8] Decidual interleukin-1 stimulates hCG secretion in cultured trophoblasts,[61] whereas decidual prolactin and an 8- to 10-kd decidual protein inhibit hCG production.[62]

HCG may regulate its own production to some extent. The hCG receptors are present on the surface of trophoblastic cells, and the addition of hCG to placental cells in culture stimulates cAMP production and promotes proliferation and differentiation of the cytotrophoblasts into syncytiotrophoblasts.[50] Both hCG mRNA and hCG production are stimulated by analogues of cAMP or agents that activate adenylate cyclase, probably through a protein kinase.[50,60] The net effect of an increase in syncytiotrophoblast mass and cAMP levels is enhancement of hCG secretion.

The placenta is not the only site of hCG synthesis. Immunoreactive hCG has been found by immunocytochemistry or by immunoassay of extracts of a wide variety of normal tissues, including spermatozoa, testes, endometrium, kidney, liver, colon, gastric tissue, lung, spleen, heart, fibroblast, brain, and pituitary gland,[63] and the hormone is synthesized in some fetal tissues.[50] The pituitary appears to be the major source of hCG or an hCG-like material present in nonpregnant individuals. Immunoactive and bioactive hCG has been partially purified from pituitary glands; the material is secreted in vitro by fetal pituitary cells and has been shown by immunocytochemistry to be present in gonadotroph-type cells that do not contain hLH or human FSH.[63,64]

Immunoreactive hCG has been measured in sera from normal, nonpregnant individuals, with the highest concentrations found in postmenopausal women.[51,65] In postmenopausal women, this material is secreted in a pulsatile fashion in parallel with hLH pulses, and during the normal menstrual cycle, the immunoreactive hCG shows a midcycle peak concomitant with the hLH peak.[65] In men and postmenopausal women, GnRH stimulates secretion of the hormone, whereas its secretion is inhibited by oral contraceptives in women and by a GnRH agonist in agonadal men.[51,65]

Gestational and nongestational trophoblastic tumors secrete hCG and its free subunits. The syncytiotrophoblastic cells of nongestational trophoblastic neoplasms secrete hCG, as do the trophoblastic giant cells of seminomas.[66] In many instances, the tumors produce incomplete forms of hCG or its subunits, and differences in carbohydrate content from the hCG variants in pregnancy have been especially apparent. A wide variety of nontrophoblastic tumors also secrete hCG, although the predominant moiety appears to be the free β-subunit of hCG.[51,66]

Metabolism. After it is secreted, hCG exhibits biexponential clearance from the circulation, with a fast half-life ($T_{1/2}$) of 6 hours and a slow $T_{1/2}$ of approximately 36 hours. In contrast, the free β-subunit has a fast $T_{1/2}$ of 41 minutes and a slow $T_{1/2}$ of 4 hours, and the free α-subunit has a 13-minute fast $T_{1/2}$ and a 76-minute slow $T_{1/2}$.[67] Approximately 22% of the intact hormone appears in the urine unchanged; the rest undergoes metabolic degradation (Fig. 21-5). One of the early steps is proteolytic cleavage ("nicking") of the β-subunit at Val44-Leu45 and Gly47-Val48. Human leukocyte elastase, present in macrophages and leukocytes, appears to be responsible for some of the nicking of the β-subunit.[67]

Nicked hCG is unstable and dissociates into free α-subunit and nicked free β-subunit. The latter is further metabolized, primarily in the kidney, to produce the β-core

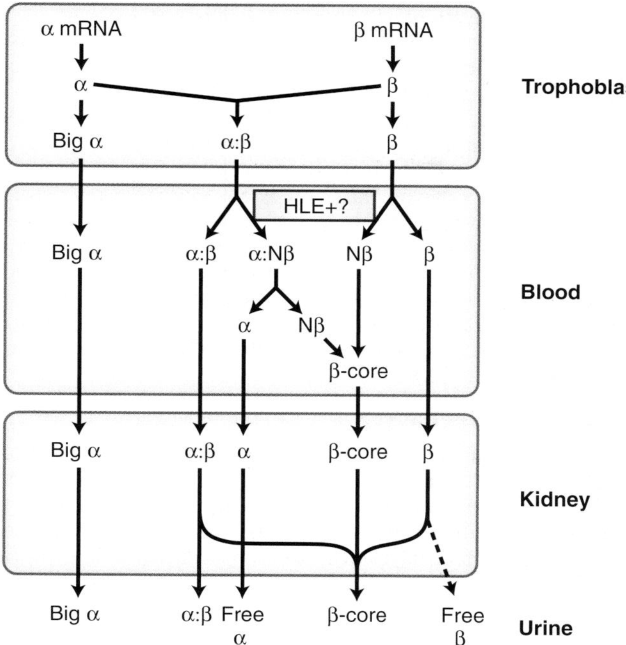

Figure 21-5 Proposed pathways for metabolism of human chorionic gonadotropin (hCG). α:β, intact hCG; α:Nβ, hCG with nicked β-subunit; Big α: hyperglycosylated form of the α-subunit; HLE, human leukocyte elastase; Nβ, free nicked β-subunit; CTP fragment, carboxy-terminal fragment; mRNA, messenger RNA. (From Braunstein GD. Physiologic functions of human chorionic gonadotropin during pregnancy. In: Mochizuki M, Hussa R, eds. *Placental Protein Hormones*. Amsterdam: Elsevier Science, 1988:33.)

fragment, which is composed of the β-subunit amino acids 6 to 40 disulfide-bridged to amino acids 55 to 92, trimmed of a portion of carbohydrate. The β-core fragment has a molecular mass of 10,479 d.[67] This fragment is the major form of immunoreactive hCG in the urine in pregnancy. In normal pregnancy, the urine also contains variable quantities of the big α, free α-subunit, free β-subunit, nicked hCG, nicked free β-subunit, C-terminal fragments of the β-subunit, and fragments of the α-subunit.[67]

Physiologic Functions. The physiologic functions of hCG occur after interaction of the hormone with the hLH-hCG receptor. The receptor gene *(LHCGR)* is located on chromosome 2 and encodes a G protein–coupled receptor with seven hydrophobic transmembrane domains and a large extracellular amino-terminus that binds to hCG and hLH. The receptor is part of superfamily of receptors, including those for hFSH, hTSH, AVP, VIP, PTH, and receptors for a variety of biogenic amines and neurotransmitters.[50] The hCG-receptor interaction results in increased cAMP production and, in some tissues, increased activation of the phosphatidylinositol pathway.[44]

Because of the close structural homology of the hLH-hCG receptor with the other glycoprotein hormone receptors, hCG may interact with the hTSH and hFSH receptors and may therefore have weak intrinsic hTSH and hFSH biologic activity. The hTSH-like activity of hCG clinically manifests during normal pregnancy by the reciprocal decrease in maternal hTSH at the time of the hCG peak between 8 and 12 weeks after the last menstrual period. It is especially important in patients with hydatidiform moles and other forms of trophoblastic disease, in which hCG levels may exceed 100,000 IU/L and result in clinical thyrotoxicosis (see Fig. 21-1).[23,24]

One of the major functions of hCG during pregnancy is the "rescue" of the corpus luteum during the conception cycle.[44] During a menstrual cycle without conception, progesterone concentrations in the serum increase for the first 6 to 7 days of the luteal phase, followed by a 3- to 4-day plateau and then a decrease that results in shedding of the endometrial lining. After conception and implantation, the corpus luteum continues to secrete progesterone and 17-hydroxyprogesterone for another 4 to 6 weeks. The maternal serum progesterone and 17-hydroxyprogesterone concentrations then decrease, indicating a marked diminution in corpus luteum function.[68] The fall in 17-hydroxyprogesterone concentrations continues, but the drop in progesterone levels is only transient. This marks the transition from dependence on ovarian progesterone production to placental progesterone secretion (i.e., luteal-placental shift). Luteectomy during the first 50 days after the last menstrual period is associated with a decline in progesterone levels and expulsion of the products of conception. After a therapeutic abortion, progesterone levels drop rapidly.

The fetal-placental unit is responsible for the signal to maintain the corpus luteum. Several data support the idea that hCG is that physiologic signal,[44] including

- The presence of hLH-hCG receptors on the corpus luteum
- The early production of hCG by the implanting trophoblast
- The dose-dependent increases in cAMP, progesterone, and estradiol from luteal cells cultured in vitro after exposure to hCG
- The parallel rise of progesterone and hCG in early pregnancy
- The enhanced progesterone secretion and prolongation of the menstrual cycle in nonpregnant women given exogenous hCG during their luteal phase

The inability of hCG to prolong the life of the corpus luteum of pregnancy beyond the sixth to eighth week of pregnancy results from homologous desensitization of the adenylate cyclase system and the inhibitory effects of the high estrogen levels on progesterone synthesis through inhibition of 3β-hydroxysteroid dehydrogenase and $\Delta^{5\text{-}4}$-isomerase in the corpus luteum.

Another physiologic role for hCG is in the differentiation of fetal male genitalia through stimulation of the hLH-hCG receptors on the fetal testicular Leydig cells during the period when differentiation of wolffian duct structures and development of the external genitalia occur. The maximum testosterone production per unit weight of the testes coincides with the maximum binding of ^{125}I-labeled hCG to the fetal testicular receptors at 10 to 12 weeks of development, and fetal Leydig cells produce cAMP and testosterone in vitro after exposure to hCG. The hCG concentrations in fetal serum parallel the fetal testicular testosterone levels at a time when the amount of fetal pituitary hLH is not sufficient to stimulate the testosterone production.[69]

During normal pregnancy, hCG has several other possible actions. In vitro, hCG stimulates the differentiation of cytotrophoblast to syncytiotrophoblast and therefore may play an important paracrine role in regulating syncytiotrophoblast mass and production of trophoblast hormones.[62,70] Additional data supporting this autoregulatory effect of hCG include the in vitro stimulation of placental synthesis of cAMP, activation of glycogen phosphorylase, and incorporation of radiolabeled galactose and leucine into placental proteins on exposure to hCG.[69] HCG stimulates the secretion of vascular endothelial growth factor (VEGF) from the cytotrophoblast, which may be important for placental angiogenesis.[50] Vasodilation of myometrial blood vessels mediated by hCG binding to vascular hCG receptors may enhance uterine blood flow in early pregnancy.[50] The fetal zone of the adrenal releases DHEAS in response to hCG exposure in vitro; hCG may have adrenocorticotropic activities in concert with fetal pituitary ACTH and placental ACTH.[69]

It has been suggested that hCG plays a role in the immunosuppression that occurs during pregnancy. Many early studies on this topic were hampered by the use of impure preparations of hCG or the presence of preservatives such as phenol that can alter the end points of the test systems used to define immunosuppression. The immunosuppressive effects may be caused by gonadal steroid secretion in response to the hCG in the in vivo models used in some of the studies.[71] Relaxin secretion from the corpus luteum is stimulated by hCG in vivo and in vitro.[50]

The decreased osmotic threshold for thirst and AVP release during pregnancy is clearly related to hCG.[26] It may be a direct effect of hCG or an indirect effect through stimulation of gonadal steroids or interaction with hLH-hCG receptors in vascular smooth muscle.

Gestational Trophoblastic Disease. Gestational trophoblastic disease (GTD) includes complete and partial hydatidiform moles, choriocarcinoma, and placental-site trophoblastic tumor.[72] Complete molar pregnancy is the most common variety, occurring in 1 to 2 of 1000 pregnancies. Patients classically present in the second trimester with vaginal bleeding, a uterus that is larger than expected for the duration of pregnancy, anemia, and excessive vomiting, although with the increased use of ultrasound examination early in pregnancy, the diagnosis is often made in the first trimester before the classic signs and symptoms develop.[73] Pathologically, trophoblast hyperplasia, marked edema of the chorionic villi, and absence of fetal tissues are observed. In contrast, partial moles demonstrate focal trophoblast hyperplasia and villous swelling, and they often have fetal tissues with congenital malformations. Approximately 20% of patients with complete moles develop persistent trophoblastic disease, whereas only 2% to 4% of patients develop persistent disease after partial molar pregnancy. Persistent trophoblastic disease also can occur after a normal term pregnancy and in pregnancies that end in spontaneous or induced abortion.

Choriocarcinoma is the most aggressive malignant form of persistent trophoblastic disease and may involve complications from local uterine disease, such as bleeding and rupture of the uterus, or from the effects of metastases, especially those involving the liver, lungs, and brain. The least common form of GTD is placental-site trophoblastic tumor, which is derived from the intermediate trophoblast and is often associated with vaginal bleeding and amenorrhea.[72]

All of these neoplasms secrete hCG and free β-subunit, and they often secrete additional forms of these molecules. With the exception of placental-site trophoblastic tumor, which secretes relatively low amounts of hCG, the serum and urine concentrations of hCG roughly parallel the tumor burden and provide prognostic information. The hCG measurements in concert with clinical and radiologic findings, especially vaginal ultrasonographic findings, are useful for making the diagnosis of GTD. Rarely, false-positive, low-level hCG results may be found in some women who have heterophilic antibodies and other interfering substances in their sera. This may lead to a misdiagnosis of GTD. Because these substances are not excreted in the urine, a urine pregnancy test result will be negative in the presence of such "phantom hCG."[72,73]

Hydatidiform moles are initially treated with uterine dilation and evacuation with or without adjunctive single-agent chemotherapy with methotrexate or actinomycin D. Approximately 90% of patients with low-risk, persistent trophoblastic disease are cured by single-agent chemotherapy; 75% of patients with high-risk, metastatic disease are cured by multiagent chemotherapy, including etoposide, methotrexate, actinomycin D, cyclophosphamide, and vincristine. Serial hCG measurements are invaluable for monitoring because they accurately reflect the effect of therapy on the tumor.[51,72,73]

Human Placental Lactogen

Also called chorionic somatomammotropin, hPL is a single-chain, nonglycosylated polypeptide composed of 191 amino acid residues and two disulfide bridges, with a molecular mass of 21,600 d.[19,74] It is closely related chemically and biologically to both GH (85% amino acid homology) and prolactin (13% amino acid homology). The GH-hPL gene cluster is located on the long arm of chromosome 17 and consists of five genes—one coding for the pituitary GH1, one for the placental GH2, and three for placental hPL: chorionic somatomammotropin hormone 1 or hPL-A *(CSH1)*, chorionic somatomammotropin hormone 2 or hPL-B *(CSH2)*, and chorionic somatomammotropin hormone-like 1 or hPL-L *(CSHL1)*, of which only *CSH1* and *CSH2* are transcribed).[20,74]

HPL is synthesized and secreted by the syncytiotrophoblast and is detected in maternal serum between 20 and 40 days of gestation.[19] The maternal serum levels rise rapidly and peak at 34 weeks, followed by a plateau (Fig. 21-6).[75] The serum concentrations and placental hPL mRNA concentrations are closely correlated with placental weight and syncytiotrophoblastic mass.[74-76] The maternal serum concentrations at term average between 6 and 7 μg/mL; at that time, on the basis of the 9- to 15-minute $T_{1/2}$ of disappearance from the circulation, the placental production rate of hPL is in excess of 1 g/day. The fetal serum levels are 1/50 to 1/100 of the maternal levels.[74]

The physiologic in vivo regulation of hPL synthesis and secretion, other than the constitutive production related to placental mass, is unknown. Several studies have examined the possible role of nutrients in hPL secretion in pregnant women. Neither acute hyperglycemia nor hypoglycemia appeared to alter the hPL concentrations, although prolonged glucose infusions decreased and prolonged fasting increased the concentrations.[19,54,74,77] Arginine infusions, dexamethasone administration, and changes in plasma free fatty acid levels did not affect the maternal hPL concentrations.[78,79] Glucose, estrogens, glucocorticoids, prostaglandins, epinephrine, oxytocin, TRH, GnRH, and L-dopa have been examined in in vitro systems and found to be without consistent effects.[80-83]

Angiotensin II, IGF1, phospholipase A_2, arachidonic acid, and epidermal growth factor stimulated hPL release in vitro.[54,84] Epidermal growth factor probably enhances production through promotion of cytotrophoblast-to-syncytiotrophoblast differentiation.[84] Apolipoprotein AI also stimulated hPL synthesis and release through cAMP-dependent and arachidonic acid–dependent pathways.[19,85,86] Because changes in the maternal plasma apolipoprotein AI concentrations parallel those of hPL during pregnancy, it is likely that this apoprotein, alone and as part of circulating HDL, is important in the secretion of hPL.[86]

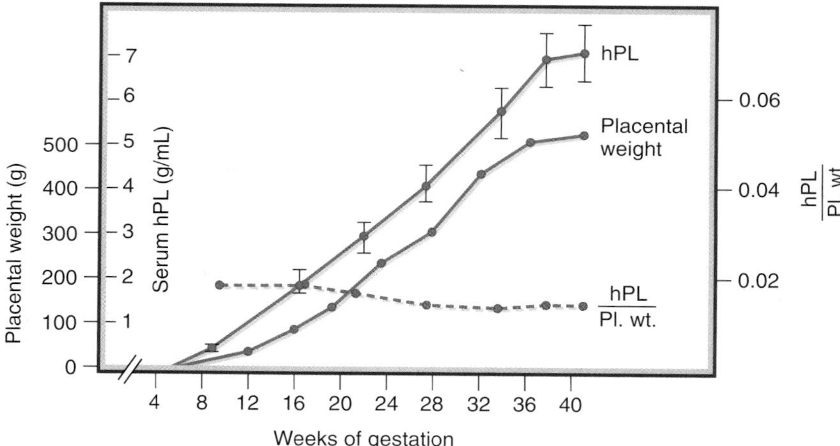

Figure 21-6 Placental weight (Pl. wt.), maternal serum concentrations of human placental lactogen (hPL), and the ratio of hPL to Pl. wt. during pregnancy. (From Selenkow HA, Saxena BN, Dana CL. Measurement and pathophysiologic significance of human placental lactogen. In: Pecile A, Finzi C, eds. *The Feto-Placental Unit.* Amsterdam: Excerpta Medica, 1969:340.)

Several biologic activities of hPL are qualitatively similar to those of GH and prolactin, and hPL can bind to both GH and prolactin receptors.[87] In various bioassay systems, hPL had weak somatotropic and lactogenic effects.[87,88] It appears to be a major regulator of IGF1 production, and during pregnancy, hPL concentrations correlate with those of IGF1.[19,88] HPL also affects the metabolism of maternal nutrients. It stimulates pancreatic islet insulin secretion directly and after carbohydrate administration,[87,88] and it is a diabetogenic factor during pregnancy through its promotion of insulin resistance. It enhances lipolysis, leading to a rise in free fatty acid levels, which may in part be responsible for insulin resistance.[87]

The various biologic activities of hPL suggest that the role of hPL during pregnancy is to provide the fetus with a constant supply of glucose and amino acids.[87] The hPL-stimulated lipolysis allows the mother to use free fatty acids for energy during fasting, allowing glucose, amino acids, and ketone bodies to cross the placenta for use by the fetus. In addition, hPL promotes amino acid uptake by muscle and stimulates protein production, IGF1 production, and glycogen synthesis in the fetus.[88,89]

Despite the proposed importance of hPL in maternal and fetal metabolic homeostasis during pregnancy, its absence does not appear to impair pregnancy. Deficient or absent hPL production related to gene defects has been described in several women who experienced normal pregnancies and delivered normal infants.[90]

Placental Growth Hormone

GH2 is synthesized and secreted by the syncytiotrophoblast.[19,20] Alternate splicing of the *GH2* gene results in two nonglycosylated isoforms with molecular masses of 22 and 26 kd.[20,74] The 22-kd variant may be glycosylated and circulate as a 26-kd protein.[79] GH2 is detected in the maternal plasma from 10 weeks' gestation and peaks during the third trimester (Fig. 21-7).[19,20,91]

GH2 has somatotropic activity and stimulates IGF1 production, and the increased IGF1 concentrations may be responsible for the suppression of maternal pituitary hGH secretion (see Fig. 21-7).[20,91] GH2 also may modulate trophoblast invasion.[92] Unlike GH1, GH2 is not secreted in a pulsatile fashion, nor is it released from the trophoblast by growth hormone–releasing hormone (GHRH); however, it is inhibited by glucose. At term, 85% of the GH biologic activity in maternal serum may be attributed to GH2, 12% to hPL, and only 3% to GH1.[93] Within 48 hours after delivery, GH1 secretion by the pituitary returns to normal.

Human Chorionic Corticotropin

The syncytiotrophoblast synthesizes an ACTH-like peptide, human chorionic corticotropin (hCC), and several

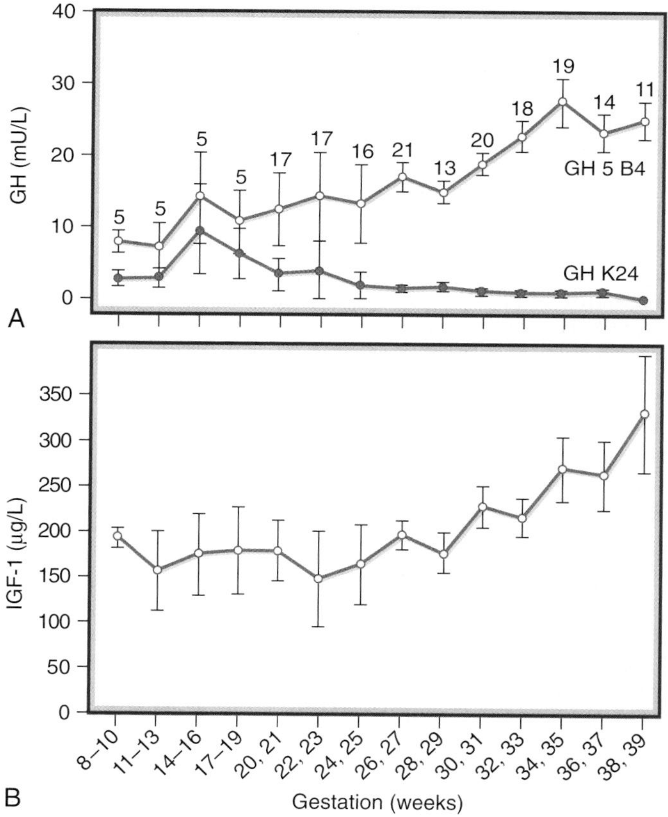

Figure 21-7 Mean (± standard error) of plasma human growth hormone (GH) **(A)** and insulin-like growth factor type I (IGF1) **(B)** levels throughout pregnancy. The number of individual assays of growth hormone (GH) and IGF1 at each gestational stage is indicated in **A** at the top of vertical bars. GH 5 B4 indicates placental GH (GH2); GH K24 indicates pituitary GH (GH1). (From Mirlesse V, Frankenne F, Alsat E, et al. Placental growth hormone levels in normal pregnancy and in pregnancies with intrauterine growth retardation. *Pediatr Res.* 1993;34:39.)

pro-opiomelanocortin-derived peptides, including β-lipotropin, β-endorphin, and α-melanocyte–stimulating hormone.[25] The maternal serum concentrations of ACTH increase as pregnancy progresses, and the elevation of free cortisol levels during pregnancy may be related in part to placental hCC and pituitary ACTH production.[25]

The hCC secretion is stimulated by CRH, which is probably the most important factor regulating the local production of the peptide through paracrine or autocrine mechanisms, or both, because it is also produced by the cytotrophoblast and the syncytiotrophoblast. Unlike the situation with the pituitary, glucocorticoids and oxytocin stimulate hCC release from placental cultures.[25] The resistance of maternal plasma ACTH concentrations to suppression after glucocorticoid administration may reflect the placental hCC contribution to the total pool of circulating immunoreactive ACTH.[25]

Hypothalamic Peptides

Gonadotropin-Releasing Hormone. The cytotrophoblast and the syncytiotrophoblast synthesize and secrete GnRH, which has the same chemical structure and biologic activity as hypothalamic GnRH.[54,56] Although the GnRH mRNA levels in the placenta are similar throughout gestation, the highest concentrations of the peptide in the placenta and serum are found during the first trimester and correlate with the mass of the cytotrophoblast and peak hCG concentrations.[56,94]

In vitro, GnRH production by placental explants or purified trophoblasts is stimulated by prostaglandins, epinephrine, activin, insulin, epidermal growth factor, VIP, estradiol, and estriol, and secretion is reduced by inhibin, progesterone, and κ-opiate and μ-opiate agonists.[95,96] The syncytiotrophoblast contains low-affinity GnRH receptors, whose concentrations parallel the hCG secretory pattern.[58]

Because GnRH stimulates hCG secretion by placental explants and purified trophoblast cells in vitro, with the response of early to midtrimester placentas being greater than that of term trophoblast, it is reasonable to conclude that GnRH is an important autocrine or paracrine regulator of hCG secretion.[95] The hCG-stimulatory effect of GnRH can be blocked by administration of a GnRH antagonist.[55] Because GnRH stimulates metalloproteinases in cytotrophoblasts, the peptide may be important during implantation.[97]

Corticotropin-Releasing Hormone. The cytotrophoblast and the syncytiotrophoblast synthesize and secrete a 41-amino-acid peptide that is identical to hypothalamic CRH.[25,98] CRH mRNA is first detected in the trophoblast at 7 weeks' gestation. The levels remain low during the first 30 weeks of pregnancy but rise 20-fold during the final 5 weeks, a pattern that parallels the rise of CRH content in the placenta and concentrations in maternal plasma.[98] In maternal plasma, CRH circulates bound to a 37-kd protein that is synthesized by the placenta, liver, and brain and that reduces the biologic activity of the CRH.[25,98]

In vitro, placental CRF production is stimulated by prostaglandins (E_2 and $F_{2\alpha}$), norepinephrine, acetylcholine, oxytocin, neuropeptide Y, AVP, angiotensin II, and interleukin-1. Glucocorticoids increase CRH mRNA and peptide, whereas in the hypothalamus, suppression is found. CRH secretion is reduced by progesterone and nitric oxide donors. The placenta contains CRH binding sites, and the addition of CRH to cultured placental cells results in a dose-dependent increase in hCC, β-endorphin, and α-melanocyte-stimulating hormone secretion.[25,54,98] It is likely that CRH has an autocrine or paracrine effect in the placenta.

Whether CRH has a physiologic effect on the maternal pituitary secretion of ACTH is unclear; the circulating CRH may be biologically inactive because of the binding protein. However, just before parturition, the binding protein concentration decreases by approximately 50%, and the CRH levels rise.[25,98] At this time, CRH stimulates the synthesis and release of prostaglandins from the decidua, amnion, and chorion, which enhances cervical ripening.[99] The myometrium contains CRH receptors, and CRH may increase myometrial contractility.[98] In this way, CRH may have a role in initiating and promoting parturition. CRH may also stimulate the fetal pituitary production of ACTH, which may lead to increased fetal adrenal DHEA production and ultimately to estriol synthesis by the fetal-placental unit.[98] In addition to CRH, the syncytiotrophoblast and fetal membranes secrete urocortin-1, which in vitro stimulates placental ACTH, prostaglandin E_2, and activin secretion through the CRH receptor.[100]

Other Peptides. A peptide with properties of TRH that is not identical to hypothalamic TRH has been identified in the placenta.[101,102] It can stimulate the release of hTSH in vitro and in vivo.[103,104] It has unknown physiologic significance because there is no convincing evidence that a chorionic thyrotropin exists, and hCG appears to be the major trophoblastic thyrotropin-like substance.

Immunoreactive somatostatin has been identified in the cytotrophoblast in first-trimester placentas.[105,106] The levels decrease as pregnancy advances.[105] This pattern has led to the speculation that somatostatin inhibits hPL production and that the loss of inhibition allows the placenta to secrete increasing quantities of hPL.[105] The finding of somatostatin receptors in the placenta adds some indirect support to this hypothesis.[106] However, somatostatin does not inhibit hPL (or GH2) production by placental cells exposed to the peptide in vitro.[106]

A substance with GHRH-like activity has been found in the placenta.[107] However, because exposure of placental cells to hypothalamic GHRH does not result in stimulation of hPL or GH2 secretion, it is unlikely that human placental GHRH is physiologically important. Ghrelin also is produced by the placenta, with the highest maternal serum levels found during midgestation, which corresponds to the highest ghrelin mRNA levels.[108]

Several other neuropeptides have been found in the placenta, usually through immunohistochemical techniques. They include methionine enkephalin,[54,109] leucine enkephalin,[110] dynorphin,[109,110] neuropeptide Y,[54,111] and oxytocin.[54,112] The physiologic functions of these placental peptides are unknown. It has been suggested that dynorphin may have a role in the paracrine regulation of hPL release through its binding to placental κ-opiate receptors.[109,110] Neuropeptide Y and oxytocin stimulate the secretion of CRH from placental cells in culture.[59]

Growth Factors

Several growth factors, growth factor–binding proteins, and growth factor receptors have been identified in the placenta. They include IGF1, IGF2, relaxin, epidermal growth factor, PDGF, nerve growth factor, FGF, TGF-β, inhibin, activin, and folliculostatin.[54,59] As reviewed earlier, a number of these factors have been implicated in the autocrine or paracrine regulation of placental hormone synthesis and release and in placental angiogenesis, and they may have important actions in fetal development. In addition to the placenta, the human endometrium is a rich source of growth factors, cytokines, and vasoactive neuropeptides that are important for uteroplacental function.[8]

REFERENCES

1. Wilcox AJ, Weinberg CR, O'Connor JF, et al. Incidence of early loss of pregnancy. *N Engl J Med.* 1988;319:189.
2. Staun-Ram E, Shalev E. Human trophoblast function during the implantation process. *Reprod Biol Endocrinol.* 2005;3:56.
3. Achache H, Revel A. Endometrial receptivity markers, the journey to successful embryo implantation. *Human Reprod Update.* 2006;12: 731.
4. Braunstein GD, Grodin JM, Vaitukaitis J, et al. Secretory rates of human chorionic gonadotropin by normal trophoblast. *Am J Obstet Gynecol.* 1973;115:447.
5. Ferretti C, Bruni L, Dangles-Marie V, et al. Molecular circuits shared by placental and cancer cells, and their implications in the proliferative, invasive and migratory capacities of trophoblasts. *Human Reprod Update.* 2007;13:121.
6. Fukuda MN, Sugihara K, Nakayama J. Trophinin: what embryo implantation teaches us about human cancer. *Cancer Biol Therapy.* 2008;7:1165.
7. Murphy VE, Smith R, Giles WB, et al. Endocrine regulation of human fetal growth: the role of the mother, placenta, and fetus. *Endocr Review* 2006:27:141.
8. Hannan NJ, Salamonsen LA. Role of cytokines in the endometrium and in embryo implantation. *Curr Opin Obstet Gynecol.* 2007;19: 266.
9. Fisher DA. Fetal and neonatal endocrinology. In: DeGroot LJ, Jameson JL, de Kretser D, et al, eds. *Endocrinology.* 5th ed. Philadelphia: Elsevier Saunders; 2006:3369.
10. Moffett A, Loke C. Immunology of placentation in eutherian mammals. *Nat Rev Immunol.* 2006;6:584.
11. Braunstein GD, Rasor JL, Engvall E, et al. Interrelationships of human chorionic gonadotropin, human placental lactogen, and pregnancy-specific beta 1-glycoprotein throughout normal human gestation. *Am J Obstet Gynecol.* 1980;138:1205.
12. Cunningham EG, Leveno KJ, Bloom SL, et al, eds. *Maternal physiology.* In Williams Obstetrics, New York: McGraw-Hill; 2005:121.
13. Castro LC, Hobel CJ, Gornbein J. Plasma levels of atrial natriuretic peptide in normal and hypertensive pregnancies: a meta-analysis. *Am J Obstet Gynecol.* 1994;171:1642.
14. Lindheimer MD, Davison JM. Osmoregulation, the secretion of arginine vasopressin and its metabolism during pregnancy. *Eur J Endocrinol.* 1995;132:133.
15. Foyouzi N, Frisbaek Y, Norwitz ER. Pituitary gland and pregnancy. *Obstet Gynecol Clin North Am.* 2004;31:873.
16. Elster AD, Sanders TG, Vines FS, et al. Size and shape of the pituitary gland during pregnancy and post partum: measurement with MR imaging. *Radiology.* 1991;181:531.
17. Lehtovirta P, Ranta T. Effect of short-term bromocriptine treatment on amniotic fluid prolactin concentration in the first half of pregnancy. *Acta Endocrinol.* 1981;97:559.
18. Emmi AM, Skurnick J, Goldsmith LT, et al. Ovarian control of pituitary hormone secretion in early human pregnancy. *J Clin Endocrinol Metab.* 1991;72:1359.
19. Handwerger S, Brar A. Placental lactogen, placental growth hormone, and decidual prolactin. *Semin Reprod Endocrinol.* 1992;10:106.
20. Fuglsang J, Ovesen P. Aspects of placental growth hormone physiology. *Growth Horm IGF Res.* 2006;16:67.
21. Walker WH, Fitzpatrick SL, Barrera-Saldana HA, et al. The human placental lactogen genes: structure, function, evolution and transcriptional regulation. *Endocr Rev.* 1991;12:316.
22. Zimkeller W. Current topic: the role of growth hormone and insulin-like growth factors for placental growth and development. *Placenta.* 2000;21:451.
23. Glinoer D. The regulation of thyroid function in pregnancy: pathways of endocrine adaptation from physiology to pathology. *Endocr Rev.* 1997;18:404.
24. Glinoer D, de Nayer P, Bourdoux P, et al. Regulation of maternal thyroid during pregnancy. *J Clin Endocrinol Metab.* 1990;71:276.
25. Lindsay JR, Nieman LK. The hypothalamic-pituitary-adrenal axis in pregnancy: challenges in disease detection and treatment. *Endocr Rev.* 2005;26:775.
26. Davison JM, Shiells EA, Philips PR, et al. Serial evaluation of vasopressin release and thirst in human pregnancy: role of human chorionic gonadotrophin in the osmoregulatory changes of gestation. *J Clin Invest.* 1988;81:798.
27. Davison JM, Sheills EA, Barron WM, et al. Changes in the metabolic clearance of vasopressin and in plasma vasopressinase throughout human pregnancy. *J Clin Invest.* 1989;83:1313.
28. Leake RD, Weitzman RE, Glatz TH, et al. Plasma oxytocin concentrations in men, nonpregnant women, and pregnant women before and during spontaneous labor. *J Clin Endocrinol Metab.* 1981;53:730.
29. Zeeman GG, Khan-Dawood FS, Dawood MY. Oxytocin and its receptor in pregnancy and parturition: current concepts and clinical implications. *Obstet Gynecol.* 1997;89:873.
30. Kovacs CS, Fuleihan G-H. Calcium and bone disorders during pregnancy and lactation. *Endocrinol Metab Clin North Am.* 2006;35:21.
31. Costrini NV, Kalkhoff RK. Relative effects of pregnancy, estradiol, and progesterone on plasma insulin and pancreatic islet insulin secretion. *J Clin Invest.* 1971;50:992.
32. Lain KY, Catalano PM. Metabolic changes in pregnancy. *Clin Obstet Gynecol.* 2007;4:938.
33. Carr BR, Parker CR Jr, Madden JD, et al. Maternal plasma adrenocorticotropin and cortisol relationships throughout human pregnancy. *Am J Obstet Gynecol.* 1981;139:416.
34. Rainey WE, Rehman KS, Carr BR. Fetal and maternal adrenals in human pregnancy. *Obstet Gynecol Clin North Am.* 2004;31:817.
35. Zuspan FP. Urinary excretion of epinephrine and norepinephrine during pregnancy. *J Clin Endocrinol Metab.* 1970;30:357.
36. Tunbridge RD, Donnai P. Plasma noradrenaline in normal pregnancy and in hypertension of late pregnancy. *Br J Obstet Gynaecol.* 1981; 88:105.
37. Ramayya MS, Zhou J, Kino T, et al. Steroidogenic factor 1 messenger ribonucleic acid expression in steroidogenic and nonsteroidogenic human tissues: Northern blot and in situ hybridization studies. *J Clin Endocrinol Metab.* 1997;82:1799.
38. Pepe GJ, Albrecht ED. Actions of placental and fetal adrenal steroid hormones in primate pregnancy. *Endocr Rev.* 1995;16:608.
39. Tulchinsky D, Hobel CJ, Yeager E, et al. Plasma estrone, estradiol, estriol, progesterone, and 17-hydroxyprogesterone in human pregnancy: I. Normal pregnancy. *Am J Obstet Gynecol.* 1972;112:1095.
40. Levitz M, Young BK. Estrogens in pregnancy. *Vitam Horm.* 1977;35:109.
41. Simpson ER, Burkhart MF. Regulation of cholesterol metabolism by human choriocarcinoma cells in culture: effect of lipoproteins and progesterone on cholesteryl ester synthesis. *Arch Biochem Biophys.* 1980;200:86.
42. Kallen CB. Steroid hormone synthesis in pregnancy. *Obstet Gynecol Clin North Am.* 2004;31:795.
43. Bose HS, Sugawara T, Strauss JF III, et al. The pathophysiology and genetics of congenital lipoid adrenal hyperplasia. International Congenital Lipoid Adrenal Hyperplasia Consortium. *N Engl J Med.* 1996; 335:1870.
44. Braunstein GD. Evidence favoring human chorionic gonadotropin as the physiological "rescuer" of the corpus luteum during early pregnancy. *Early Pregnancy.* 1996;2:183.
45. Spitz IM, Bardin CW. Drug therapy: mifepristone (RU486)—a modulator of progestin and glucocorticoid action. *N Engl J Med.* 1993;329: 404.
46. Miller WL. Steroid hormone biosynthesis and actions in the materno-feto-placental unit. *Clin Perinatol.* 1998;25:799.
47. Heikkila J, Luukkainen T. Urinary excretion of estriol and 15 alpha-hydroxyestriol in complicated pregnancies. *Am J Obstet Gynecol.* 1971;110:509.
48. Ryan KJ. Placental synthesis of steroid hormones. In: Tulchinsky D, Ryan KJ, eds. *Maternal-Fetal Endocrinology.* Philadelphia, PA: WB Saunders; 1980:3.
49. Shozu M, Akasofu K, Harada T, et al. A new cause of female pseudohermaphroditism: placental aromatase deficiency. *J Clin Endocrinol Metab.* 1991;72:560.
50. Keay SD, Vatish M, Karteris E, et al. The role of hCG in reproductive medicine. *Br J Obstet Gynaecol.* 2004;111:1218.
51. Stenman U-H, Tiitinen A, Alfthan H, et al. The classification, functions and clinical use of different isoforms of HCG. *Human Reprod Update.* 2006;12:769.
52. Braunstein GD, Rasor J, Danzer H, et al. Serum human chorionic gonadotropin levels throughout normal pregnancy. *Am J Obstet Gynecol.* 1976;126:678.
53. Cole LA. New discoveries on the biology and detection of human chorionic gonadotropin. *Reprod Biol Endocrinol.* 2009;7:8.
54. Sullivan MHF. Endocrine cell lines from the placenta. *Mol Cell Endocrinol.* 2004;228:103.
55. Siler-Khodr TM, Khodr GS, Vickery BH, et al. Inhibition of hCG, alpha hCG and progesterone release from human placental tissue in vitro by a GnRH antagonist. *Life Sci.* 1983;32:2741.
56. Miyake A, Sakumoto T, Aono T, et al. Changes in luteinizing hormone-releasing hormone in human placenta throughout pregnancy. *Obstet Gynecol.* 1982;60:444.
57. Siler-Khodr TM, Khodr GS, Valenzuela G. Immunoreactive gonadotropin-releasing hormone level in maternal circulation throughout pregnancy. *Am J Obstet Gynecol.* 1984;150:376.
58. Currie AJ, Fraser HM, Sharpe RM. Human placental receptors for luteinizing hormone releasing hormone. *Biochem Biophys Res Commun.* 1981;99:332.
59. Petraglia F, Santuz M, Florio P, et al. Paracrine regulation of human placenta: control of hormonogenesis. *J Reprod Immunol.* 1998;39:221.
60. Maymó JL, Pérez A, Sánchez-Margalet V, et al. Up-regulation of placental leptin lay human chorionic gonadotropin. *Endocrinology.* 2009 Jan;150(1):304-313.
61. Masuhiro K, Matsuzaki N, Nishino E, et al. Trophoblast-derived interleukin-1 (IL-1) stimulates the release of human chorionic gonadotropin by activating IL-6 and IL-6-receptor system in first trimester human trophoblasts. *J Clin Endocrinol Metab.* 1991;72:594.

62. Ren SG, Braunstein GD. Decidua produces a protein that inhibits choriogonadotrophin release from human trophoblasts. *J Clin Invest.* 1991;87:326.
63. Braunstein GD, Kamdar V, Rasor J, et al. Widespread distribution of a chorionic gonadotropin-like substance in normal human tissues. *J Clin Endocrinol Metab.* 1979;49:917.
64. Odell WD, Griffin J, Bashey HM, et al. Secretion of chorionic gonadotropin by cultured human pituitary cells. *J Clin Endocrinol Metab.* 1990;71:1318.
65. Odell WD, Griffin J. Pulsatile secretion of human chorionic gonadotropin in normal adults. *N Engl J Med.* 1987;317:1688.
66. Braunstein GD. Placental proteins as tumor markers. In: Herberman RB, Mercer DW, eds. *Immunodiagnosis of Cancer.* New York: Marcel Dekker; 1991:673.
67. Braunstein GD. Beta core fragment: structure, production, metabolism, and clinical utility. In: Lustbader JW, Puett D, Ruddon RW, eds. *Glycoprotein Hormones.* New York: Springer-Verlag; 1994:293.
68. Yoshimi T, Strott CA, Marshall JR, et al. Corpus luteum function in early pregnancy. *J Clin Endocrinol Metab.* 1969;29:225.
69. Braunstein GD. Physiologic functions of human chorionic gonadotropin during pregnancy. In: Mochizuki M, Hussa R, eds. *Placental Protein Hormones.* Amsterdam: Elsevier Science; 1988:33.
70. North RA, Whitehead R, Larkins RG. Stimulation by human chorionic gonadotropin of prostaglandin synthesis by early human placental tissue. *J Clin Endocrinol Metab.* 1991;73:60.
71. Nisula B, Bartocci A. Choriogonadotropin and immunity: a reevaluation. *Ann Endocrinol.* 1984;45:315.
72. Soper JT, Mutch DG, Schink JC. Diagnosis and treatment of gestational trophoblastic disease. ACOG Practice Bulletin No. 53. *Gynecol Oncol.* 2004;93:575.
73. Berkowitz RS, Goldstein DP. Molar pregnancy. *N Engl J Med.* 2009; 360:1639.
74. Barrera-Saldana HA. Growth hormone and placental lactogen: biology, medicine and biotechnology. *Gene.* 1998;211:11.
75. Selenkow HA, Saxena BN, Dana CL. Measurement and pathophysiologic significance of human placental lactogen. In: Pecile A, Finzi C, eds. *The Feto-Placental Unit.* Amsterdam: Excerpta Medica; 1969:340.
76. Hoshina M, Boothby M, Boime I. Cytological localization of chorionic gonadotropin alpha and placental lactogen mRNAs during development of the human placenta. *J Cell Biol.* 1982;93:190.
77. Gaspard U, Sandront H, Luyckx A. Glucose-insulin interaction and the modulation of human placental lactogen (HPL) secretion during pregnancy. *J Obstet Gynaecol Br Commonw.* 1974;81:201.
78. Morris HH, Vinik AI, Mulvihal M. Effects of acute alterations in maternal free fatty acid concentration on human chorionic somatomammotropin secretion. *Am J Obstet Gynecol.* 1974;119:224.
79. Ylikorkala O, Kauppila A. Effect of dexamethasone on serum levels of human placental lactogen during the last trimester of pregnancy. *J Obstet Gynaecol Br Commonw.* 1974;81:368.
80. Niven PA, Buhi WC, Spellacy WN. The effect of intravenous oestrogen injections on plasma human placental lactogen levels. *J Obstet Gynaecol Br Commonw.* 1974;81:466.
81. Belleville F, Lasbennes A, Nabet P, et al. Study of compounds capable of intervening in the in vitro regulation of the secretion of chorionic somatomammotropin by placenta in culture. *C R Seances Soc Biol Fil.* 1974;168:1057.
82. Handwerger S, Barrett J, Tyrey L, et al. Differential effect of cyclic adenosine monophosphate on the secretion of human placental lactogen and human chorionic gonadotropin. *J Clin Endocrinol Metab.* 1973;36:1268.
83. Hershman JM, Kojima A, Friesen HG. Effect of thyrotropin-releasing hormone on human pituitary thyrotropin, prolactin, placental lactogen, and chorionic thyrotropin. *J Clin Endocrinol Metab.* 1973;36:497.
84. Wilson EA, Jawad MJ, Vernon MW. Effect of epidermal growth factor on hormone secretion by term placenta in organ culture. *Am J Obstet Gynecol.* 1984;149:579.
85. Handwerger S, Quarfordt S, Barrett J, et al. Apolipoproteins AI, AII, and CI stimulate placental lactogen release from human placental tissue: a novel action of high density lipoprotein apolipoproteins. *J Clin Invest.* 1987;79:625.
86. Desoye G, Schweditsch MO, Pfeiffer KP, et al. Correlation of hormones with lipid and lipoprotein levels during normal pregnancy and postpartum. *J Clin Endocrinol Metab.* 1987;64:704.
87. Eberhardt NL, Jiang SW, Shepard AR, et al. Hormonal and cell-specific regulation of the human growth hormone and chorionic somatomammotropin genes. *Prog Nucleic Acid Res Mol Biol.* 1996;54:127.
88. Handwerger S, Freemark M. The roles of placental growth hormone and placental lactogen in the regulation of human fetal growth and development. *J Pediatr Endocrinol Metab.* 2000;13:343.
89. Sorenson RL, Brelje TC. Adaptation of islets of Langerhans to pregnancy: beta-cell growth, enhanced insulin secretion and the role of lactogenic hormones. *Horm Metab Res.* 1997;29:301.
90. Sideri M, De Virgiliis G, Guidobono F, et al. Immunologically undetectable human placental lactogen in a normal pregnancy. *Br J Obstet Gynaecol.* 1983;90:771.
91. Mirlesse V, Frankenne F, Alsat E, et al. Placental growth hormone levels in normal pregnancy and in pregnancies with intrauterine growth retardation. *Pediatr Res.* 1993;34:39.
92. Lacroix M-C, Guibourdenche J, Fournier T, et al. Stimulation of human trophoblast invasion by placental growth hormone. *Endocrinology.* 2005;146:2434.
93. Petraglia F, Florio P, Nappi C, et al. Peptide signaling in human placenta and membranes: autocrine, paracrine, and endocrine mechanisms. *Endocr Rev.* 1996;17:156.
94. Kelly AC, Rodgers A, Dong KW, et al. Gonadotropin-releasing hormone and chorionic gonadotropin gene expression in human placental development. *DNA Cell Biol.* 1991;10:411.
95. Petraglia F, Lim AT, Vale W. Adenosine 3′,5′-monophosphate, prostaglandins, and epinephrine stimulate the secretion of immunoreactive gonadotropin-releasing hormone from cultured human placental cells. *J Clin Endocrinol Metab.* 1987;65:1020.
96. Petraglia F, Vaughan J, Vale W. Steroid hormones modulate the release of immunoreactive gonadotropin-releasing hormone from cultured human placental cells. *J Clin Endocrinol Metab.* 1990;70:1173.
97. Chou CS, Zhu H, MacCalman CD, et al. Regulatory effects of gonadotropin-releasing hormone (GnRH) I and GnRH II on the levels of matrix metalloproteinase (MMP)-2, MMP-9, and tissue inhibitor of metalloproteinase-1 in primary cultures of human extravillous cytotrophoblasts. *J Clin Endocrinol Metab.* 2003;88:4781.
98. Fadalti M, Pezzani I, Cobellis L, et al. Placental corticotrophin-releasing factor: an update. *Ann N Y Acad Sci.* 2000;900:89.
99. Jones SA, Challis JR. Local stimulation of prostaglandin production by corticotropin-releasing hormone in human fetal membranes and placenta. *Biochem Biophys Res Commun.* 1989;159:192.
100. Florio P, Vale W, Petraglia F. Urocortins in human reproduction. *Peptides.* 2004;25:1751.
101. Youngblood WW, Humm J, Lipton MA, et al. Thyrotropin-releasing hormone-like bioactivity in placenta: evidence for the existence of substances other than Pyroglu-His-Pro-NH2 (TRH) capable of stimulating pituitary thyrotropin release. *Endocrinology.* 1980;106:541.
102. Bajoria R, Babawale M. Ontogeny of endogenous secretion of immunoreactive-thyrotropin releasing hormone by the human placenta. *J Clin Endocrinol Metab.* 1998;83:4148.
103. Gibbons JM Jr, Mitnick M, Chieffo V. In vitro biosynthesis of TSH- and LH-releasing factors by the human placenta. *Am J Obstet Gynecol.* 1975;121:127.
104. Shambaugh G III, Kubek M, Wilber JF. Thyrotropin-releasing hormone activity in the human placenta. *J Clin Endocrinol Metab.* 1979;48:483.
105. Watkins WB, Yen SS. Somatostatin in cytotrophoblast of the immature human placenta: localization by immunoperoxidase cytochemistry. *J Clin Endocrinol Metab.* 1980;50:969.
106. Caron P, Buscail L, Beckers A, et al. Expression of somatostatin receptor SST4 in human placenta and absence of octreotide effect on human placental growth hormone concentration during pregnancy. *J Clin Endocrinol Metab.* 1997;82:3771.
107. Berry SA, Srivastava CH, Rubin LR, et al. Growth hormone-releasing hormone-like messenger ribonucleic acid and immunoreactive peptide are present in human testis and placenta. *J Clin Endocrinol Metab.* 1992;75:281.
108. Fuglsang J. Ghrelin in pregnancy and lactation. *Vitam Horm.* 2008;77:259.
109. Ahmed MS, Cemerikie B, Agbas A. Properties and functions of human placental opioid system. *Life Sci.* 1992;50:83.
110. Lemaire S, Valette A, Chouinard L. Purification and identification of multiple forms of dynorphin in human placenta. *Neuropeptides.* 1983;3:181.
111. Petraglia F, Calza L, Giardino L, et al. Identification of immunoreactive neuropeptide-gamma in human placenta: localization, secretion, and binding sites. *Endocrinology.* 1989;124:2016.
112. Fields PA, Eldridge RK, Fuchs AR, et al. Human placental and bovine corpora luteal oxytocin. *Endocrinology.* 1983;112:1544.

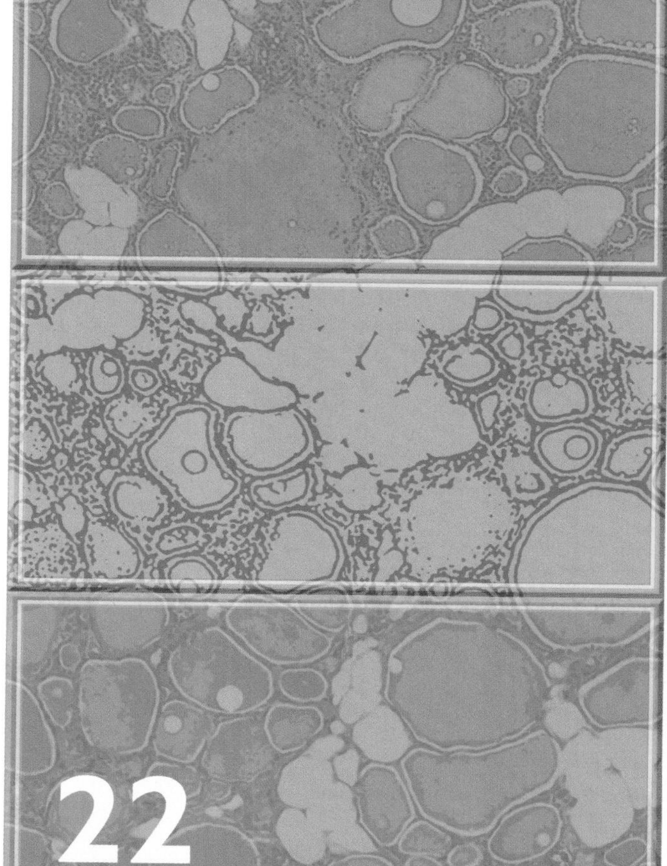

CHAPTER 22

Endocrinology of Fetal Development

MEHUL T. DATTANI • PETER C. HINDMARSH • DELBERT A. FISHER

The unfolding of our understanding of mammalian pregnancy and fetal development represents one of the dramatic chapters of scientific progress during the past half-century. Successful pregnancy involves complex genetic, cellular, and hormonal interactions facilitating implantation, placentation, embryonic and fetal development, parturition, and fetal adaptation to extrauterine life. An array of signaling molecules, transcription factors, and epigenetic events program embryogenesis and fetal development in concert with autocrine, paracrine, and endocrine networks of hormones and growth factors that provide the cellular communication coordinating maternal-placental-fetal interactions and fetal maturation. Unique features of the placental-fetal endocrine environment include a growing spectrum of placental hormones and growth factors and a variety of fetal endocrine adaptations to the intrauterine environment (Table 22-1).[1] The fetal adrenal cortex, the para-aortic chromaffin system including the paired organs of Zuckerkandl, and the intermediate lobe of the pituitary are prominent among these. Vasotocin, the parent neurohypophyseal hormone in submammalian species, is expressed transiently during fetal life, and calcitonin, a largely vestigial hormone in adult mammals, plays a significant role in fetal calcium and bone metabolism.

In addition, the active adrenal glucocorticoid, cortisol, and the thyroid hormones are largely inactive during much of fetal life because of the production of inactive analogues. Hormones and growth factors that play prominent roles in the fetus include catecholamines, parathyroid hormone–related protein (PTHrP), anti-müllerian hormone (AMH), insulin-like growth factor 2 (IGF2), transforming growth factor-β (TGF-β), and the neuroregulins. In the perinatal period, cortisol serves to modulate the functional adaptations that are required for extrauterine survival. In addition, hormonal programming during the fetal-perinatal period conditions the adult functional characteristics of selected endocrine systems. This chapter reviews the current status of our understanding of the maternal-placental-fetal endocrine and growth factor milieu, maturation of the fetal endocrine systems, and adaptations of the fetal endocrine systems to extrauterine life.

TABLE 22-1

Features of the Fetal Endocrine Environment

Placental Hormone Production
Estrogens Progesterone Neuropeptides Growth factors
Neutralization of Hormone Actions
Growth hormone Cortisol Thyroxine Catecholamines
Unique Fetal Endocrine Systems
Fetal adrenal cortex Para-aortic chromaffin system Intermediate lobe of the pituitary
Prominent Fetal Hormones or Metabolites
Vasotocin Calcitonin Cortisone Reverse triiodothyronine (rT_3) Sulfated iodothyronines Ectopic neuropeptides
Fetal Endocrine System Adaptations
Adrenal-placental interactions Testicular control of male phenotypic differentiation Developmentally regulated growth factor control of fetal growth Neuropeptides and fetal water metabolism Parathyroid glands and placental calcium transport Catecholamine and vasopressin responses to hypoxia Cortisol programming for extrauterine exposure Catecholamine and cortisol control of extrauterine adaptation Perinatal hormonal programming

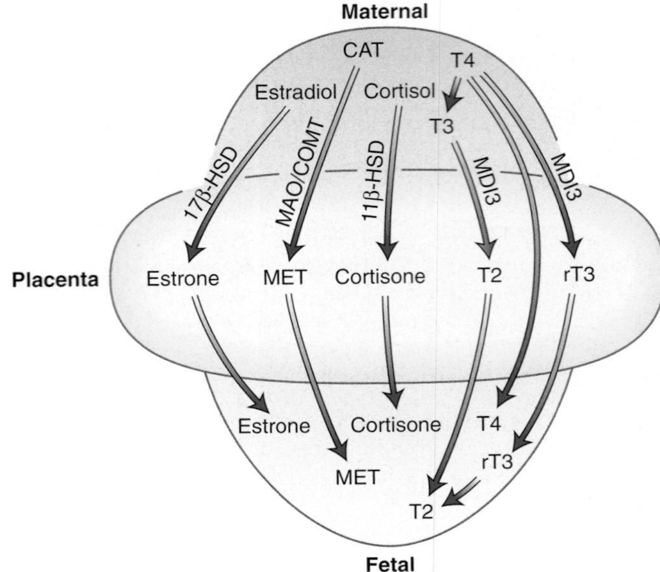

Figure 22-1 Placental neutralization of biologic activity of hormones during maternal-fetal transfer. The neutralizing enzymes, 17β-hydroxysteroid dehydrogenase (17β-HSD) and 11β-HSD, are shown. See text for details. CAT, catecholamines; COMT, catechol *O*-methyltransferase; MAO, monoamine oxidase; MDI3, type 3 iodothyronine monodeiodinase; MET, metanephrines; rT_3, 3,3′5′ (reverse) triiodothyronine; T_2, diiodothyronine; T_3, 3,5,3′ triiodothyronine; T_4, thyroxine.

PLACENTAL HORMONE TRANSFER

The fetal endocrine milieu is largely independent of maternal hormones because the placenta is impermeable to most peptide hormones. Hormones larger than 0.7 to 1.2 kd have little or no access to the fetal compartment.[2] The exception is immunoglobulin G, which is actively transported from mother to fetus during the latter half of gestation.[3] Steroid and thyroid hormones and catecholamines do cross the placenta, but several of these are metabolized en route, including cortisol, estradiol, thyroxine, triiodothyronine, and catecholamines.[4-8]

In particular, the placental cells contain an active 11β-hydroxysteroid dehydrogenase (11β-HSD) that catalyzes the conversion of most of the maternal cortisol to inactive cortisone.[5,6] This is important considering the steep gradient between the maternal cortisol concentration and that of the fetus—almost a 10-fold difference. This enzymatic inactivation can be bypassed with dexamethasone, leading to fetal exposure to glucocorticoid, which, in rodent models, has adverse effects on blood pressure, blood glucose, and memory.[9,10] This altered metabolism is used by physicians to promote glucocorticoid maturation of the fetal lung in cases of preterm delivery and in the management of fetuses affected by a virilizing form of congenital adrenal hyperplasia. Single doses appear to be safe for mother and child,[11] but the safety of more chronic exposure is not established.

Placental 17β-HSD is considered to prevent passage of excessive estrogens to the fetus by catalyzing inactivation of estradiol to estrone.[7] Placental tissue also contains an iodothyronine inner ring monodeiodinase, which deiodinates most of the thyroxine (T_4) to inactive reverse triiodothyronine (rT_3) and converts active 3,5,3′-triiodothyronine (T_3) to inactive diiodothyronine.[8,12] Nonetheless, there is some transplacental passage of T_4 to the fetus in early pregnancy, and this may be of importance, because observational studies have suggested altered intellectual function, albeit mild, in infants born to mothers with mild untreated hypothyroidism.[13,14]

Catecholamine-degrading enzymes in placental tissue include monoamine oxidase and catechol *O*-methyltransferase, 3,9 and both metanephrine and dihydroxymandelic acid metabolites of catecholamines are present in placental homogenates (Fig. 22-1).[15]

ECTOPIC FETAL HORMONE PRODUCTION

Kidney, liver, and testes from 16- to 20-week-old human fetuses produce immunoreactive and bioactive human chorionic gonadotropin (hCG) in vitro.[16,17] Kidney tissue produces almost half as much hCG per milligram of protein as placenta; liver activity is lower. Adrenocorticotropic hormone (ACTH)-like immunoreactivity is present in relatively high concentrations in neonatal rat pancreas and kidney.[18] This material is presumably derived from a pro-opiomelanocortin (POMC) parent molecule. Hypothalamic neuropeptides are present in a variety of adult tissues, particularly in the pancreas and gut.[19-23] In the fetus, hypothalamic neuropeptides are also present in the gut and tissues derived from it. High concentrations of thyrotropin-releasing hormone (TRH) and somatostatin immunoreactivity have been reported in neonatal rat pancreas and gastrointestinal tract tissues, whereas hypothalamic concentrations of these immunoreactive substances are low.[24,25] These neuropeptides have immunoreactive and chromatographic properties similar to those of the synthetic hypothalamic peptides.

Encephalectomy does not alter the circulating TRH levels in the neonatal rat, whereas significant reductions are produced by pancreatectomy. In the sheep fetus, thyroid hormones modulate pancreatic and gut TRH concentrations, pointing to thyroid hormone control of extrahypothalamic *TRH* gene transcription or translation in the fetus.[26] TRH and somatostatin also are present in the human neonatal pancreas and in blood of the human newborn, with both hormones derived mostly from extrahypothalamic sources.[27-30] The presence of TRH at high concentrations in fetal ovine blood and the modulation of fetal pancreatic, placental, and blood TRH levels by thyroid hormones suggest a role for extrahypothalamic TRH in the control of fetal pituitary thyrotropin secretion before the near-term maturation of hypothalamic TRH.[26] The role of extraneural somatostatin in the fetus is undefined.

FETAL ENDOCRINE SYSTEMS

Anterior Pituitary and Target Organs

The anterior and intermediate lobes of the pituitary gland are derived from oral ectoderm, whereas the posterior pituitary is derived from neural ectoderm.[31,32] The human fetal forebrain is identifiable by 3 weeks of gestation, the diencephalon and telencephalon by 5 weeks. Rathke's pouch, the buccal precursor of the anterior pituitary gland, separates from the primitive pharyngeal stomodeum by 5 weeks of gestation.[31,33,34] The neural components of the transducer system (hypothalamus, pituitary stalk, and posterior pituitary) are largely developed by 7 weeks of gestation, and the bony floor of the sella turcica is also present by that time, separating the adenohypophysis from the primitive gut. Capillaries develop within the proliferating anterior pituitary mesenchymal tissue around Rathke's pouch and the diencephalon by 8 weeks of gestation, and intact hypothalamic-pituitary portal vessels are present by 12 to 17 weeks. Maturation of the pituitary portal vascular system continues, and the system becomes functionally intact during the period of histologic differentiation of the hypothalamus and development of the portal vascular extension into hypothalamic tissue; this maturation process extends to 30 to 35 weeks of gestation.

The hypothalamic cell condensations, which represent the hypothalamic nuclei, and the interconnecting fiber tracts are demonstrable histologically by 15 to 18 weeks of gestation.[26,33] Hypothalamic cells and diencephalic fiber tracts for the hypothalamic neuropeptides somatostatin, corticotropin-releasing hormone (CRH), growth hormone–releasing hormone (GHRH), and gonadotropin-releasing hormone (GnRH) are also visible by that time. Concentrations of dopamine, TRH, GnRH, and somatostatin are significant in hypothalamic tissue by 10 to 14 weeks of gestation. Specialized anterior pituitary cell types, including lactotropes, somatotropes, corticotropes, thyrotropes, and gonadotropes, can be recognized in the anterior pituitary between 7 and 16 weeks of gestation. Anterior pituitary hormones—including growth hormone (GH), prolactin (PRL), thyroid-stimulating hormone (TSH), luteinizing hormone (LH), follicle-stimulating hormone (FSH), and ACTH—are detectable by radioimmunoassay between 10 and 17 weeks of gestation. Therefore, the anatomy and biosynthetic mechanisms that make up the hypothalamic-pituitary neuroendocrine transducer appear to be functional by 12 to 17 weeks of gestation in humans.

Development of the pituitary gland has been extensively studied in the mouse. Although little is known about pituitary development in humans, it would appear to mirror that seen in the rodent, because pituitary development is similar in all vertebrates. The development of the anterior pituitary occurs in four distinct stages of differentiation leading to the formation of a complicated secretory organ containing five different cell types secreting six different hormones:

Stage 1. Formation of the pituitary placode from oral ectoderm. Cell types of the pituitary gland are derived from the most anterior midline portion of the embryo in a region contiguous with the anterior neural ridge. The anterior neural ridge is displaced ventrally to form the oral epithelium, which gives rise to the roof of the oral cavity. Onset of pituitary organogenesis coincides with a thickening (pituitary placode) in the roof of the oral ectoderm at embryonic day (E) 8.5 in the mouse, corresponding to 4 to 6 weeks' gestation in humans.

Stage 2. Formation of rudimentary Rathke's pouch. Invagination of the oral ectoderm forms a rudimentary pouch, and evagination of the ventral diencephalon forms the posterior pituitary. The pituitary placode makes contact with the floor of the ventral diencephalon. Apposition between the rudimentary Rathke's pouch and neural ectoderm of the diencephalon is critical to normal development and is maintained throughout early pituitary organogenesis.

Stage 3. Formation of definitive Rathke's pouch. The rudimentary Rathke's pouch deepens and folds on itself until it closes, forming a definitive pouch. The infundibulum or pituitary stalk is formed by evagination of the posterior part of the presumptive diencephalon.

Stage 4. Formation of the adult pituitary gland. The definitive pouch is completely detached from the oral cavity. Spatial and temporal differentiation of various cell types within the pituitary gland results in the development of individual hormone secreting cells in a sequential order.

Complex genetic interactions dictate normal pituitary development. A cascade of signaling molecules and transcription factors plays a crucial role in organ commitment, cell proliferation, cell patterning, and terminal differentiation, and the final product is a culmination of this coordinated process (Fig. 22-2). Initially, cells within the primordium of the pituitary gland are competent to differentiate into all cell types. After expression of the earliest markers of pituitary gland development, such as homeobox gene expressed in embryonic stem cells (*Hesx1*), further signaling pathways are established from within the gland and ventral diencephalon that direct these cells toward terminal differentiation into mature hormone-secreting cell types. Signaling molecules and transcription factors are expressed sequentially at critical periods of pituitary development, and expression of many of these factors is attenuated subsequently (Fig. 22-3). Genes that are expressed early are implicated in organ commitment but are also implicated in repression and activation of downstream target genes that have specific roles in directing the cells toward a particular fate.

Spontaneous or artificially induced mutations in the mouse have led to significant insights into human pituitary disease, and identification of mutations associated

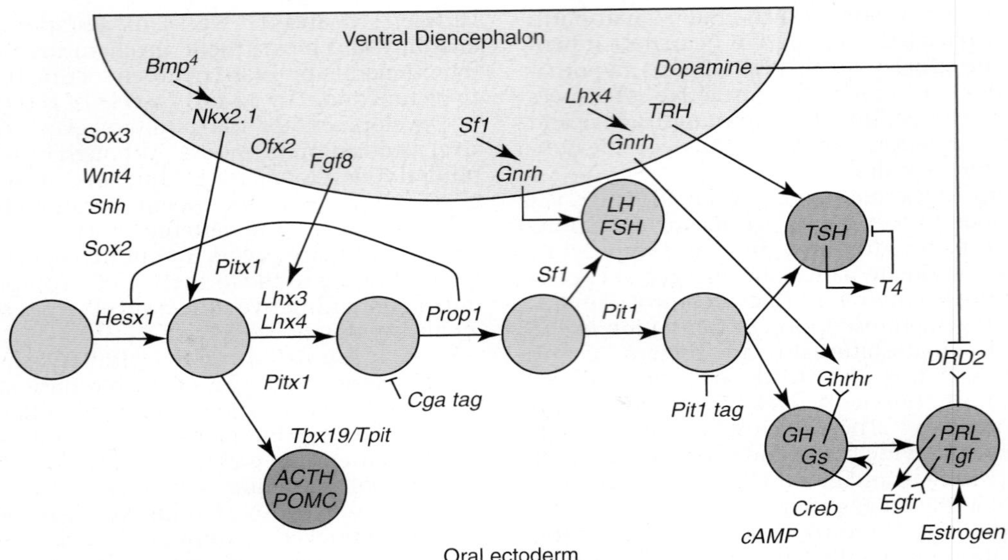

Figure 22-2 Schematic representation of the developmental cascade of genes implicated in human pituitary development with particular reference to pituitary cell differentiation.

with human pituitary disease have, in turn, been invaluable in defining the genetic cascade responsible for the development of this embryologic tissue. Mutations involved specifically in human hypothalamopituitary disease are listed in Table 22-2 and are briefly discussed here.

Extrinsic molecules within the ventral diencephalon and surrounding structures, such as bone morphogenetic proteins 2 and 4 (*Bmp2, Bmp4*), fibroblast growth factor 8 (*Fgf8*), sonic hedgehog (*Shh*), wingless (*Wnt4*), thyroid transcription factor 1 (*Ttf1*; also called *Nkx2-1*), and molecules involved in Notch signaling play critical roles in early organogenesis.[31,34,35] Recent studies in the mouse have shown that a close interaction between oral ectoderm and neural ectoderm is critical for initial development of the pituitary gland. Rathke's pouch develops in a two-step process that requires at least two sequential inductive signals from the diencephalon. First, induction and formation of the rudimentary pouch is dependent upon *Bmp4*, and second, *Fgf8* activates two key regulatory genes, LIM

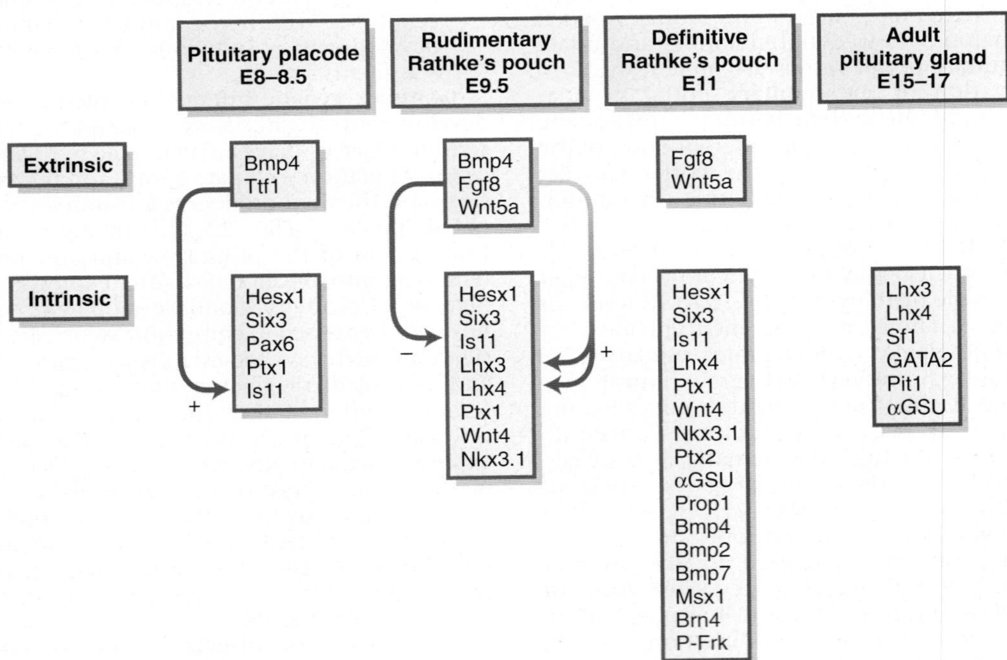

Figure 22-3 Transcription factors and signaling molecules involved in anterior pituitary development.

TABLE 22-2

Comparison of Murine and Human Phenotypes in Pituitary Development

Gene	Protein	Murine Loss-of-Function Phenotype	Human Phenotype	Inheritance (Murine and Human)
HESX1	HESX1	Anophthalmia or microphthalmia, agenesis of corpus callosum, absence of septum pellucidum, pituitary dysgenesis or aplasia	Variable: SOD, CPHD, IGHD with EPP Anterior pituitary hypoplastic or absent Posterior pituitary ectopic or eutopic Frequency of mutations: <1%	Dominant or recessive in humans, recessive in mouse
OTX2	OTX2	Lack of forebrain and midbrain, olfactory placode, optic placodes	Anophthalmia, APH, ectopic posterior pituitary, absent infundibulum Frequency of mutations: 2-3% of anophthalmia/microphthalmia cases	Heterozygous: haploinsufficiency/dominant negative
SOX2	SOX2	Homozygous null mutants: embryonic lethal Heterozygous mice and further dose reduction: poor growth, reduced fertility, CNS abnormalities, anophthalmia; pituitary hypoplasia with reduction in all cell types	Hypogonadotropic hypogonadism; APH, abnormal hippocampi, bilateral anophthalmia/microphthalmia, abnormal corpus callosum, learning difficulties, esophageal atresia, sensorineural hearing loss, hypothalamic hamartoma Frequency of mutations: 8/235	De novo haploinsufficiency in humans, heterozygous mutation associated with haploinsufficiency in mouse
SOX3	SOX3	Poor growth, weakness, craniofacial abnormalities, ACC, hypothalamic and infundibular abnormalities	IGHD and mental retardation, hypopituitarism; APH, infundibular hypoplasia, EPP, midline abnormalities Frequency of mutations: 6% (duplications), 1.5% (mutations)	X-linked recessive in both mice and humans
GLI2	GLI2	N/A	Holoprosencephaly, hypopituitarism, craniofacial abnormalities, polydactyly, single nares, single central incisor, partial ACC Frequency of mutations: 1.5%	Haploinsufficiency in humans
LHX3	LHX3	Hypoplasia of Rathke's pouch	GH, TSH, gonadotropin deficiency with pituitary hypoplasia ACTH insufficiency variable Short, rigid cervical spine Variable sensorineural hearing loss. Frequency of mutations: 1.3%	Recessive in both
LHX4	LHX4	Mild hypoplasia of anterior pituitary	GH, TSH, cortisol deficiency, persistent craniopharyngeal canal and abnormal cerebellar tonsils; APH, ectopic/eutopic posterior pituitary, absent infundibulum Frequency of mutations: 1.2%	Recessive in mouse, dominant in humans
PROP1	PROP1	Hypoplasia of anterior pituitary with reduced somatotropes, lactotropes, thyrotropes, corticotropes, and gonadotropes	GH, TSH, PRL, and gonadotropin deficiency Evolving ACTH deficiency Enlarged pituitary with later involution Frequency of mutations: 1.1% sporadic cases, 29.5% familial cases	Recessive in both
POU1F1	POU1F1 (PIT1)	Anterior pituitary hypoplasia with reduced somatotropes, lactotropes, and thyrotropes	Variable anterior pituitary hypoplasia with GH, TSH, and PRL deficiencies Frequency of mutations: 3.8% sporadic cases, 18% familial cases	Recessive in mouse, dominant/recessive in humans

ACC, agenesis of corpus callosum; ACTH, adrenocorticotropic hormone; APH, anterior pituitary hypoplasia; CNS, central nervous system; CPHD, combined pituitary hormone deficiencies; EPP, ectopic posterior pituitary; GH, growth hormone; IGHD, isolated growth hormone deficiency; N/A, not applicable; PRL, prolactin; SOD, septo-optic dysplasia; TSH, thyroid-stimulating hormone.

homeobox 3 (*Lhx3*) and LIM homeobox 4 (*Lhx4*), that are essential for subsequent development of the rudimentary pouch into a definitive pouch.

Bmp4 and *Fgf8* are present only in the diencephalon and not in Rathke's pouch. Murine mutations within the Ttf1/Nkx2-1 (also called thyroid-specific enhancer binding protein), which is expressed only in the presumptive ventral diencephalon, can cause severe defects in the development of the diencephalon and the anterior pituitary gland. Conditional deletion of *Rbp-J*, which encodes the major mediator of the Notch pathway, leads to conversion of the late (pituitary-specific transcription factor 1 [*Pit1*]) lineage into the early (corticotroph) lineage. Notch signaling is required for maintaining expression of *Prop1* (prophet of Pit1), which is required for generation of the *Pit1* lineage. Attenuation of Notch signaling is necessary for terminal differentiation in *Pit1* cells and for maturation and proliferation of the GH-producing somatotroph.[35] There have been no reported mutations of these early morphogenetic signals in humans.

Mutations of the sonic hedgehog (SHH) signaling pathway (SHH, TGIF, ZIC2, PTCH1, GLI2) and the transcription factor SIX3 have been identified in patients with holoprosencephaly, with and without hypothalamo-pituitary defects.[36-38] Mutations in *HESX1* have been identified in patients with septo-optic dysplasia (SOD; a combination of pituitary, eye, and midline forebrain defects), combined pituitary hormone deficiencies (CPHD), and isolated growth hormone deficiency (IGHD).[31,39] Mutations in *SOX2* and *OTX2* have recently been described in association with severe eye defects, hypogonadotropic hypogonadism, and variable hypopituitarism.[40-44] Mutations and genomic duplications in *SOX3* have been identified in patients with hypopituitarism with and without learning defects.[45]

Mutations in the gene encoding the LIM homeodomain transcription factor LHX3 have been identified in patients with hypopituitarism, neck abnormalities, and sensorineural deafness, whereas mutations in *LHX4* have been identified in patients with hypopituitarism and cerebellar abnormalities.[46-48] Mutations in genes expressed later in pituitary development, such as *PROP1* and *POU1F1* (previously known as *PIT1*), are associated with more specific pituitary phenotypes (variable GH, TSH, ACTH, PRL, and gonadotropin deficiencies and often a large anterior pituitary that later involutes with *PROP1* mutations; GH, TSH, and PRL deficiencies with *POU1F1* mutations), in keeping with a role for these genes in cellular proliferation and differentiation and hormone secretion.[31,49-51] Mutations in the T-box transcription factor *TBX19/TPIT* have been described in patients with early-onset isolated ACTH deficiency.[52] No genetic etiology has been identified in most cases of congenital hypopituitarism to date, suggesting a role for other, unidentified genes or environmental factors.

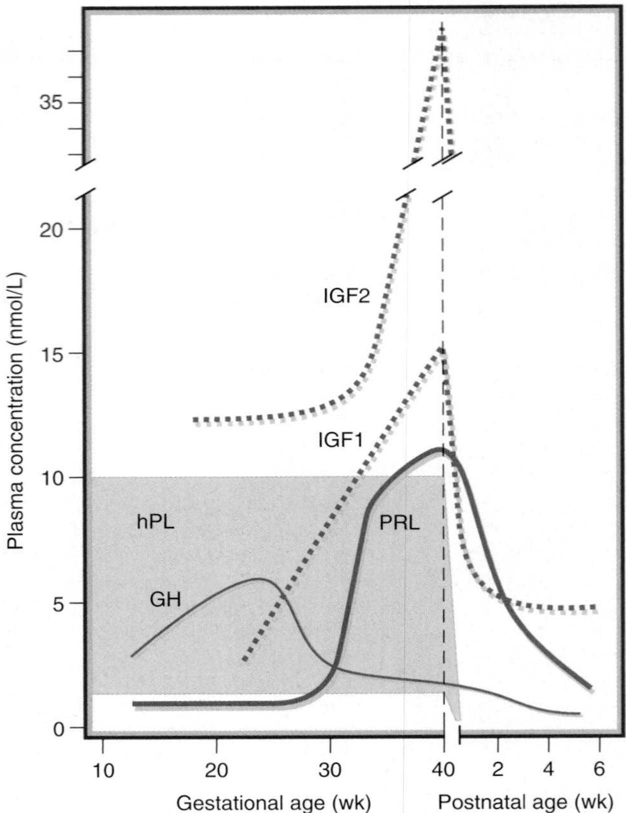

Figure 22-4 Patterns of change of fetal plasma human placental lactogen (hPL), growth hormone (GH), prolactin (PRL), insulin-like growth factor I (IGF1), and insulin-like growth factor 2 (IGF2) during gestation and in the neonatal period. The shaded area indicates the range of fetal plasma hPL concentrations. (Data from references 323-325.)

Growth Hormone and Prolactin

The human fetal pituitary gland can synthesize and secrete GH by 8 to 10 weeks of gestation.[2,33] Pituitary GH content increases from about 1 nmol (20 ng) at 10 weeks to 45 nmol (1000 ng) at 16 weeks of gestation. Fetal plasma GH concentrations in cord blood samples are in the range of 1 to 4 nmol/L during the first trimester and increase to a mean peak of approximately 6 nmol/L at midgestation. Plasma GH concentrations fall progressively during the second half of gestation, to a mean value of 1.5 nmol/L at term.[33] Pituitary GH messenger RNA (mRNA) and GH content generally parallel the increase in plasma GH concentration between 16 and 24 weeks of gestation.[53] This pattern of ontogenesis of plasma GH reflects a progressive maturation of hypothalamic-pituitary and forebrain function. The responses of plasma GH to somatostatin and GHRH and to insulin and arginine are mature at term in human infants.[33,54]

The high plasma GH concentrations at midgestation after development of the pituitary portal vascular system may reflect unrestrained secretion.[33] Studies of 9- to 16-week-old human fetal pituitary cells in culture showed a predominant response to GHRH and a limited effect of somatostatin, suggesting that the inhibitory action of somatostatin develops later in gestation.[55] This interpretation was substantiated by in vivo studies in the sheep fetus, which showed a failure of somatostatin to inhibit GHRH-stimulated GH release early in the third trimester and maturation of the inhibitory effect of somatostatin near term.[33] The predominant GHRH enhancement and limited somatostatin inhibition of GH secretion at midgestation presumably relate to a limited capacity for inhibition of GH release by somatomedin feedback. In addition, there may be unrestrained GH secretion at the pituitary cell level, or immaturity of limbic and forebrain inhibitory circuitry that modulates hypothalamic function, or both.[33] Whatever the mechanisms, control of GH secretion matures progressively during the last half of gestation and the early weeks of postnatal life, so that mature responses to sleep, glucose, and L-dopa are present by 3 months of age.

The ontogenesis of fetal plasma PRL differs significantly from that of GH; concentrations are low until 25 to 30 weeks of gestation and increase to a mean peak value of approximately 11 nmol/L at term (Fig. 22-4).[33] Pituitary PRL content increases progressively from 12 to 15 weeks, and in vitro fetal pituitary cells from midgestation fetuses show limited autonomous PRL secretion, although PRL release increases in response to TRH and decreases in response to dopamine. Brain and hypothalamic control of PRL matures late in gestation and during the first months of extrauterine life.[33,54] Estrogen stimulates PRL synthesis and release by pituitary cells, and the marked increase in fetal plasma PRL concentration in the last trimester parallels the increase in fetal plasma estrogen levels, although lagging by several weeks.[33,54] Anencephalic fetuses have plasma PRL concentrations in the normal or low-normal range. These data support a role for estrogen in stimulating fetal PRL release. The fetal sheep exhibits a similar pattern of fetal plasma PRL levels, indicating that maturation and integration of brain and hypothalamic mechanisms modulating PRL release develop late in gestation and in the postnatal period, accounting for the delayed postnatal fall in plasma PRL level in the neonate of this species.[33]

There is a general tendency toward hypersecretion of fetal pituitary hormones during the last half of gestation, and pituitary hormones found at high levels in cord blood from aborted human fetuses and premature human infants include GH, TSH, ACTH, β-endorphin, β-lipotropin, LH, and FSH.[33,54] Development of hypothalamic-pituitary control is complex, involving maturational events in the cortex and midbrain, the hypothalamus and hypothalamic-pituitary portal vascular system, peripheral endocrine systems, and the placenta itself, including hormone, growth factor, and neuropeptide production. The fetal pituitary hyperfunction appears to be related more to relatively delayed maturation of the central nervous system (CNS) and hypothalamic control with unrestrained secretion of stimulating hypothalamic hormones than to the action of placental neuropeptides.[33]

Postnatally, GH acts through receptors in liver and other tissues to stimulate production of IGF1 and, to a lesser degree, IGF2. Prenatally, GH receptor mRNA levels and receptor binding are low in fetal liver, although receptor mRNA is present in other fetal tissues.[33] The growth of anencephalic fetuses is almost normal, suggesting that factors other than GH stimulate fetal IGF production. Nutritional factors are known to play a role.[56,57]

PRL receptors are present in most fetal tissues during the first trimester of gestation, and it is likely that lactogenic hormones have a significant role in organ and tissue development early in gestation.[56,58] The coordinated increase in fetal adipose tissue and the adipose tissue PRL receptors PRLR1 and PRLR2 suggests that PRL may play a role in growth and maturation of fetal adipose tissue later in gestation.[59] PRL may also play a role in fetal skeletal maturation.[59] Ovine placental lactogen stimulates glycogen synthesis in fetal ovine liver, and HPL stimulates amino acid transport, DNA synthesis, and IGF1 production in human fetal fibroblasts and muscle cells. GH and PRL have little activity in these tissues (see "Fetal Growth").[58]

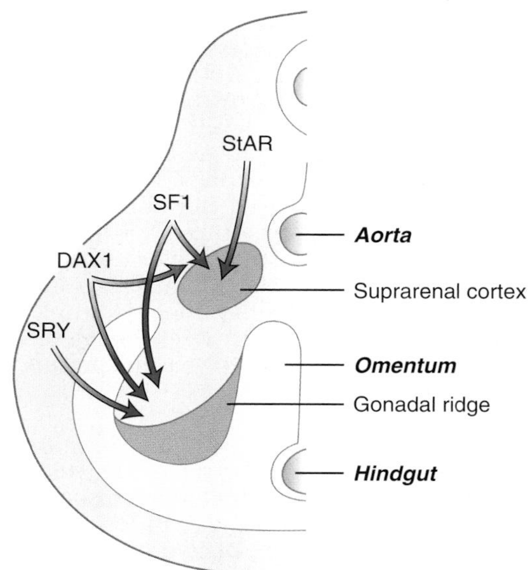

Figure 22-5 Hemi-cross-section of a 5-week human embryo showing the locations of the adrenal primordia (suprarenal cortices) and gonadal ridges. The homeobox genes programming adrenal and gonadal embryogenesis are indicated. Steroidogenic factor 1 (SF1) is involved in testicular and ovarian development. *SRY* is the single critical regulator of testicular embryogenesis. Inactivation of the *DAX1* gene leads to adrenal hypoplasia. The steroidogenic acute regulatory protein (StAR) is the rate-limiting factor for adrenal steroidogenesis. See text for details.

Adrenal System

Embriology

The primordia of the adrenal glands can be recognized just cephalad of the bilaterally developing mesonephros by 3 to 4 weeks of gestation.[60,61] The adrenal cortex is derived from a thickening of the intermediate mesoderm at 4 to 5 weeks of gestation in humans, in contrast to the adrenal medulla, which derives from the ectoderm. This region, known as the *gonadal ridge*, contains adrenogonadal progenitor cells that give rise to the steroidogenic cells of the adrenal gland and the gonad. The gonadal cells migrate caudally. Cells destined to become adrenal tissue migrate retroperitoneally to the upper pole of the mesonephros. They are then infiltrated at 7 to 8 weeks of gestation by sympathetic cells derived from the neural crest that will form the adrenal medulla. Encapsulation of the adrenal gland occurs after 8 weeks of gestation and results in the formation of a distinct organ just above the developing kidney.

The fetal adrenal is composed of three functional zones: an outer definitive zone capable of producing both glucocorticoids and mineralocorticoids, a transitional zone with enzymes for cortisol production, and a much larger inner fetal zone capable of producing significant amounts of C19 androgens such as dehydroepiandrosterone (DHEA) and dehydroepiandrosterone sulphate (DHEAS), which are then converted to estrogens by the placenta. The large eosinophilic cells of the fetal zone are well differentiated by 9 to 12 weeks of gestation and are capable of active steroidogenesis. The fetal adrenal glands grow rapidly and progressively in mass and form 0.4% of body weight at term; the combined glandular weight is approximately 8 g at term, when the fetal zone makes up about 80% of the mass of the gland with a relative size 10- to 20-fold that of the adult adrenal.[16,60,61] The fetal zone is identified only in higher primates. The adrenal gland undergoes rapid involution postnatally, largely due to regression of the fetal zone, which is absent by 6 months of age in most cases.

Genetic Regulation of Adrenal Development

Fetal adrenal cortical development is under the control of several genes and growth factors. Much of our understanding of adrenal development derives from studies of transgenic mice and of patients with various forms of adrenal hypoplasia. The earliest stages of adrenal development may be regulated by a number of transcription factors (e.g., SALL1, FOXD2, PBX1, WT1, SF1 [NR5A1], DAX1 [NROB1]), coregulators (e.g., CITED2), signaling molecules (e.g., Hedgehog/GLI3, WNT3/WNT4/WNT11, midkine), matrix proteins (e.g., SPARC), and regulators of telomerase activity (e.g., ACD). Of these molecules, the genes encoding the orphan nuclear receptors SF1 (steroidogenic factor 1) and DAX1 (dosage-sensitive sex reversal, adrenal hypoplasia congenita, X-chromosome factor)[62-64] appear to be critical for early development (Fig. 22-5). These genes show coordinated expression in adrenal cortex, testis, ovary, hypothalamus, and pituitary tissues.

SF1 gene knockout mice manifest adrenal and gonadal agenesis, gonadotropin deficiency, and absence of the hypothalamic ventromedial nucleus.[63] Inactivating *DAX1* gene mutations are associated with adrenal hypoplasia and gonadotropin deficiency.[63] Several other transcription factors including *WT1, LIM1,* and *PBX1* are involved earlier in the complex genetic cascade programming adrenal gland organogenesis from the celomic epithelium and urogenital ridge.[63,64] The steroidogenic acute regulatory protein *(StAR)* is a rate-limiting factor in adrenal steroidogenesis. *StAR* knockout mice manifest glucocorticoid and mineralocorticoid deficiency and female genitalia in XY animals.[65] In humans, inactivating *StAR* mutations cause adrenal hypoplasia and adrenal hormone insufficiency, and 46XY males with normal male genitalia have been described in association with *StAR* mutations.[65,66]

Later adrenal gland development and growth is mediated by a variety of growth factors. Proliferation of the fetal and definitive zones is stimulated by basic fibroblast growth factor (bFGF) and epidermal growth factor (EGF), and the fetal adrenal expresses high levels of IGF2 mRNA and protein, which are responsive to ACTH.[16] Moreover, IGF2 augments ACTH-stimulated expression of steroidogenic enzymes and stimulates steroid hormone production in fetal adrenal cortical cells, suggesting a role in adrenal regulation during fetal and postnatal life.[16] The pattern of enzyme maturation in the fetal adrenal suggests that cortisol production by the definitive zone does not occur de novo from cholesterol until 30 weeks of gestation, but some production using progesterone as the precursor probably occurs earlier.[16]

Adrenal Steroidogenetics

The fetal adrenal expresses the same five steroidogenic apoenzymes as the adult gland. One microsomal enzyme has 17-hydroxylase/17-20-lyase (CYP17A1 or P450c17) activities, and another has 21-hydroxylase (CYP21A2 or P450c21) activity. Two mitochondrial cytochrome P450 enzymes provide cholesterol side-chain cleavage (CYP11A1 or P450scc) and C11/C18 hydroxylation of the parent steroid structure (CYP11B1/CYP11B2 or P450c11/aldosterone synthase). A fifth enzyme, expressed by the smooth endoplasmic reticulum, exhibits both 3β-HSD and Δ^4, Δ^5-isomerase activities.[60,61] Quantitative differences in the relative activities of these enzymes are found between cells derived from the fetal versus the definitive zones, and these differences are largely due to regulated steroidogenic gene transcription.[60]

The fetal zone has relatively high steroid sulfotransferase activity, and because of the low 3β-HSD and high sulfotransferase activities, the major steroid products of the fetal adrenal are DHEA, DHEAS, pregnenolone sulfate, several $\Delta^5$3β-hydroxysteroids, and limited amounts of $\Delta^5$3-ketosteroids, including cortisol and aldosterone.[60,61] The definitive zone contributes only a small fraction of total fetal adrenal steroid output. Glucocorticoids are synthesized in the first trimester due to transient expression of type 2 3β-hydroxysteroid dehydrogenase (HSD3B2), which is maximal between 8 and 9 months of gestation.[67] The hypothalamic-pituitary-adrenal axis is sensitive to glucocorticoid-mediated feedback at this time; 46XX fetuses with steroidogenic defects (e.g., in CYP21 or CYP11) lack cortisol and have an elevated ACTH drive that results in excess production of fetal androgens at a time when the genital and scrotal folds are sensitive to androgen exposure, resulting in virilization of female genitalia.[67]

Cholesterol, the major substrate for fetal adrenal steroidogenesis, is derived from circulating low-density lipoprotein (LDL) and from de novo adrenal synthesis. LDL-cholesterol, largely of fetal liver and testicular origin, contributes 70% of the total. The fetal zone contains more LDL binding sites and manifests a greater rate of de novo cholesterol synthesis than does the definitive zone, in keeping with its greater steroidogenic activity. Both ACTH and angiotensin II receptors (AT_1 and AT_2) are present on fetal adrenal cells early in gestation. ACTH stimulates steroid production by activating StAR and increasing delivery of substrate cholesterol to P450scc; angiotensin II inhibits 3β-HSD activity and promotes DHEA production in the fetal zone.[60] Both fetal adrenal cortisol and placental estradiol regulate hepatic synthesis of cholesterol in the fetus.

The major stimulus to fetal adrenal function is fetal pituitary ACTH.[16,60,68] Although placental hCG may support early adrenal growth, the involution of the adrenal gland that occurs after 15 weeks in the anencephalic fetus suggests a crucial role for pituitary-derived factors. CRH protein has been demonstrated in fetal baboon pituitary, adrenal, liver, kidney, and lung tissues during the last third of gestation. The levels are highest in the pituitary (300 to 500 pg/mg protein); levels in adrenal and lung average 20 to 30 pg/mg protein, and those in liver and kidney tissues average 5 to 10 pg/mg protein.[69] *CRH* gene knockout in mice leads to neonatal death due to pulmonary hypoplasia, suggesting that CRH-stimulated glucocorticoid production is essential for adrenergic chromaffin and normal lung development.[70] Circulating CRH levels are elevated in the fetus, largely from extrahypothalamic and placental sources.[16,69,71] Maternal levels of CRH are elevated during the last trimester of gestation and reach values of 0.5 to 1 nmol/L at term; normal values in nonpregnant women are lower than 0.01 nmol/L.[72] This placental CRH is bioactive, and levels correlate with maternal cortisol concentrations, suggesting that this circulating placental CRH plays a role in stimulating maternal corticotropin release. Fetal plasma CRH levels at term are approximately 0.03 nmol/L; relative to the presumably high level in pituitary portal blood, plasma CRH probably has little role in modulating fetal corticotropin release. Midgestation fetal plasma corticotropin concentrations average about 55 pmol/L (250 pg/mL), levels that maximally stimulate fetal adrenal steroidogenesis, and concentrations are higher throughout gestation than in postnatal life, although they fall near term (Fig. 22-6).[16,60] Arginine vasopressin (AVP) and catecholamines also are significant stimuli for fetal ACTH secretion.[73]

The paradox of human fetal adrenal function is that steroidogenesis is programmed largely to production of inactive products.[60] The gland is maximally stimulated to

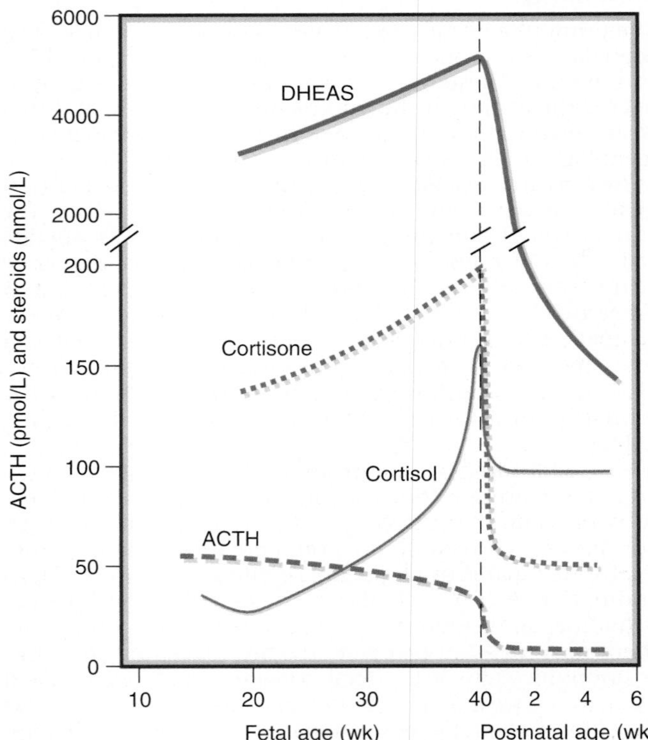

Figure 22-6 Patterns of change of fetal plasma adrenocorticotropic hormone (ACTH), cortisol, cortisone, and dehydroepiandrosterone sulfate (DHEAS) during gestation and in the neonatal period. The trend of average values is shown for each hormone in nanomoles per liter. Notice the broken scale for DHEAS. (Data from references 60, 326-328.)

maintain fetal cortisol levels and ACTH feedback homeostasis but is programmed by the steroidogenic enzyme expression pattern (e.g., relative 3β-HSD deficiency) to produce inactive DHEA and pregnenolone and their sulfate conjugates. Much of the DHEA is converted to 16-hydroxy-DHEAS by the fetal adrenal and fetal liver. As already discussed, this programming is designed to provide DHEA substrate for placental estrone and estradiol production: 16-hydroxy-DHEA undergoes metabolism to estriol in the placenta. Fetal DHEAS production and maternal estriol concentrations increase progressively to term; DHEAS production approximates to 200 mg/day near term.[16] In the anencephalic fetus, placental estrogen production is reduced to about 10% of normal.[16,60] In pregnant baboons with placental estrogen production suppressed by administration of an aromatase inhibitor, the volume of the fetal zone of the fetal adrenal increased markedly.[74] This effect was reversed by administration of inhibitor plus estrogen, suggesting that estrogen selectively suppresses fetal zone growth and development during the second half of primate pregnancy. It is proposed that this represents a feedback system to regulate secretion of fetal adrenal DHEA, thereby maintaining normal fetal-placental function and development.[74] Near term, the fetal cortisol production rate in blood, per unit body weight, is similar to that in the adult.[60] About two thirds of fetal cortisol is derived from the fetal adrenal glands, and one third is derived from placental transfer.[60] The metabolic clearance of cortisol in the fetus is rapid; 80% is oxidized in fetal tissues or placenta to cortisone or further metabolites.[60]

The corticotropin feedback control system matures progressively during the second half of gestation and the early neonatal period. Dexamethasone can suppress the human fetal pituitary-adrenal axis at term but not at 18 to 20 weeks of gestation.[60] In the fetal sheep, hypothalamic and pituitary glucocorticoid receptors are present at midgestation, and corticotropin suppressibility can be demonstrated by the midpoint of the third trimester of gestation.[75] The number of glucocorticoid receptors in the sheep fetal hypothalamus increases at term, at the time of increasing glucocorticoid levels, suggesting that some process in the fetus allows the normal autoregulation of glucocorticoid receptors to be overridden at term.[76]

Adrenal hormone receptors, including glucocorticoid receptors (GRs) and mineralocorticoid receptors (MRs), are members of the nuclear receptor superfamily of steroid hormone, thyroid hormone, vitamin D, and retinoid receptors.[77] GRs are present in most body tissues by the second trimester and play an important role in fetal development. Mice lacking GR function manifest enlarged and disorganized adrenal cortices, adrenal medullary atrophy, lung hypoplasia, and defective gluconeogenesis.[72,77] They appear normal at birth but are not viable.

GRs are present at birth and are probably present at midgestation in most tissues, including placenta, lung, brain, liver, and gut.[60,76,78] Fetal cortisol is converted to cortisone through 11HSDB2 in fetal tissues, and levels of circulating cortisone in the fetus at midgestation are fourfold to fivefold higher than cortisol concentrations (see Fig. 22-6). Cortisone is a relatively inactive glucocorticoid, and this metabolism protects the anabolic milieu of the fetus, because cortisol can retard both placental and fetal growth.[79] As term approaches, selected fetal tissues including liver and lung express 11HSDB1, a reductase that promotes local conversion of cortisone to cortisol.[60] Cortisol serves as an important stimulus to prepare the fetus for extrauterine survival. An increase in fetal cortisol concentration occurs during the last 10 weeks of gestation and is the result of increased cortisol secretion and decreased conversion to cortisone.[60] This increase in fetal cortisol production has an important role in the maturation of several fetal systems or functions that are critical to extrauterine survival (see "Transition to Extrauterine Life").[60,80]

The human fetal adrenal gland is capable of aldosterone secretion near term with the development of the zona glomerulosa, and fetal plasma aldosterone concentrations in infants who are born by cesarean section are threefold to fourfold higher than maternal levels.[60,81] Vaginal delivery and maternal salt restriction increase concentrations in both mother and infant. The increased aldosterone levels in the fetus are a result of increased fetal adrenal secretion and persist during the first year of extrauterine life.[81] However, there is a poor correlation between plasma renin activity (PRA) and aldosterone concentrations in cord blood.[82] Aldosterone secretion is low in the midgestation human fetal adrenal and is unresponsive to the secretagogues that are known to modulate aldosterone production in the adult. In sheep, fetal aldosterone becomes responsive to PRA and angiotensin II in the neonatal period.[83] In this species, in which late fetal aldosterone levels are also high compared with adult levels, furosemide stimulates PRA but not aldosterone during the third trimester; the aldosterone response to furosemide (and PRA) is delayed until the neonatal period.[83,84] This situation also appears to be the case in the human fetus and neonate.

MRs are present in fetal tissues from 12 to 16 weeks of gestation.[85] MR immunoreactivity is detectable in fetal kidney, skin, hair follicles, trachea and bronchioles, esophagus, stomach, small intestine, colon, and pancreatic exocrine ducts. The role of MRs in these fetal tissues remains unclear. MR knockout mice appear normal at birth but demonstrate defects in mineralocorticoid and renin-angiotensin system functions in the postnatal period.[86]

Angiotensin II levels in the sheep fetus are similar to maternal values, and blockade of fetal production with angiotensin-converting enzyme inhibitors decreases the fetal glomerular filtration rate.[84] Both subtypes of angiotensin receptors, AT_1 and AT_2, are detectable in various tissues early in fetal development.[87] AT_1 receptor mRNA expression in the fetal sheep kidney is low early in gestation, increases in the latter third of pregnancy, and decreases postnatally. AT_2 mRNA levels are high at midgestation and decrease during the third trimester.[87] These changes are believed to reflect growth factor–mediated changes in cells that contain AT in various tissues. Hormonal factors modulate fetal renal AT gene expression in sheep: angiotensin II suppresses both AT_1 and AT_2, and cortisol increases AT_1 gene expression in kidney and lungs.[87,88]

The role of the fetal renin-angiotensin system is not clear; rather than modulating renal sodium excretion through aldosterone, it may maintain renal excretion of salt and water into amniotic fluid to prevent oligohydramnios.[84] This renal effect is presumably mediated by modulation of arterial pressure. The mechanism for the high aldosterone concentrations in the fetal and neonatal periods remains unclear. Atrial natriuretic peptide (ANP), a cardiac hormone, is known to inhibit aldosterone secretion. Because plasma atrial natriuretic factor concentrations (ANP, BNP, and CNP) are high in the fetus, the increased PRA and aldosterone levels are not caused by relative atrial natriuretic factor deficiency.[89]

Aldosterone affects renal sodium excretion in the fetal sheep and in premature infants.[60,83] Manifestations of mineralocorticoid deficiency in the newborn term infant can occur as a result of aldosterone deficiency or competition for binding to renal MRs by other steroids such as

17-hydroxyprogesterone.[60] Relatively reduced glomerular filtration in the newborn limits sodium loss initially, but by 1 week of age, aldosterone deficiency produces the characteristic manifestations of hyponatremia, hyperkalemia, and volume depletion.

Defects of Adrenal Steroidogenesis

Adrenal insufficiency may occur secondary to ACTH deficiency, or it may be primary, resulting from adrenal failure. The mature ACTH peptide is cleaved from the larger precursor molecule, POMC, together with other small peptides such as β-endorphin and α- and β-melanocyte-stimulating hormone (MSH). Defects in ACTH synthesis, processing, or release can lead to secondary adrenal hypoplasia resulting in neonatal hypoglycemia, prolonged jaundice, or collapse. Given that mineralocorticoid secretion is largely independent of ACTH secretion, it is preserved, and salt loss is therefore unusual. Nevertheless, mineralocorticoid deficiency can be an issue in some patients with ACTH insensitivity. Low serum concentrations of ACTH, absence of hyperpigmentation, and the presence of associated features such as pale skin, red hair, diarrhea, and obesity (*POMC/PC1* mutations) are important diagnostic clues.

The presence of multiple pituitary hormone deficiencies (e.g., GH, ACTH, TSH, gonadotropins, vasopressin, and PRL) may point to a diagnosis of multiple pituitary hormone deficiency (MPHD), often in association with structural abnormalities of the pituitary gland, eye abnormalities, and forebrain abnormalities (SOD). Signs such as those of congenital hypothyroidism, hypoglycemia, congenital hypogonadotropic hypogonadism (micropenis, undescended testes), and severe postnatal growth failure may be suggestive of the diagnosis. A number of single-gene defects have now been associated with this disorder (e.g., mutations in *HESX1, SOX3, LHX3, LHX4, PROP1*).[31] Occasionally, ACTH insufficiency may not be present at the time of diagnosis but may develop progressively with time.

Recessive mutations in the T-box factor *TPIT* (*TBX19*) have been identified in patients with severe, early-onset isolated ACTH deficiency with profound hypoglycemia, prolonged jaundice, and sudden neonatal death.[52] TPIT is required for the specification, maturation, and maintenance of both precorticotrope and premelanotrope populations and for the suppression of gonadotrope fate. It is also required to activate the expression of POMC in conjunction with the transcription factor PTX1. Murine transgenesis resulted in ACTH and glucocorticoid deficiencies, adrenal hypoplasia, and pigmentation defects in mice deleted for TPIT.[52]

ACTH resistance can occur in a number of well-defined entities, such as defects in the ACTH receptor (melanocortin 2 receptor [*MC2R*], familial glucocorticoid deficiency [FGD] type 1), in MC2R accessory protein (*MRAP*, FGD type 2), or as part of the triple-A syndrome (alacrimia, achalasia, addisonism; also known as Allgrove syndrome, caused by defects in ALADIN/AAAS). These disorders are characterized by isolated glucocorticoid deficiency, hyperpigmentation, and markedly elevated concentrations of ACTH.[90,91] Nevertheless, approximately 15% of individuals with triple-A syndrome have evidence of mineralocorticoid insufficiency, those with the most severe loss of function manifesting hyponatremia on presentation.

Primary adrenal failure may be caused by congenital adrenal hypoplasia (or adrenal hypoplasia congenital [AHC]).[92] This results in severe salt-losing primary adrenal failure in early infancy or childhood, although milder, delayed onset forms of the condition exist. The most common form of the condition is X-linked. Patients have mutations in the nuclear receptor DAX1 (*NROB1*), and, in addition to adrenal failure, the males also suffer from hypogonadotropic hypogonadism. Rarely, patients present with isolated mineralocorticoid deficiency with normal cortisol levels; however, glucocorticoid deficiency usually develops later. The exact role of DAX1 in adrenal development remains unknown, although data suggest that it probably acts as a repressor of SF1 transcription. It may also act to regulate adrenal progenitor cell development and maturation, because loss of function is associated with aberrant cellular differentiation.[93]

Heterozygous and homozygous mutations in SF1 have been associated with adrenal failure in 46XY phenotypic females, as well as in at least one 46XX girl, although the latter phenotype is rare.[92] Recently, mutations in SF1 have been associated with gonadal dysgenesis in 46XY individuals, in the absence of adrenal involvement.[94] Additionally, SF1 mutations have recently also been associated with primary ovarian failure.[95]

Various forms of congenital adrenal hyperplasia may be associated with variable adrenal failure (e.g., mutations in CYP11A1, StAR, HSD3B2I, CYP17, CYP21, CYP11B1) with varying degrees of genital ambiguity. The enzyme P450c11 (aldosterone synthase), which is found in the zona glomerulosa, has 11β-hydroxylase, 18-hydroxylase, and 18-methyl-oxidase activities and catalyses all the reactions needed to convert 11-deoxycorticosterone (DOC) to aldosterone. Mutations in the gene encoding the enzyme are associated with isolated mineralocorticoid deficiency. Functional mineralocorticoid deficiency with severe salt loss resulting in hyponatremia and hyperkalemia may also arise as a result of mutations in the mineralocorticoid receptor or in the gene encoding the epithelial sodium channel, ENaC.

Thyroid System

Embriology

The thyroid gland is a derivative of the primitive buccopharyngeal cavity and develops from contributions of two anlagen: a midline thickening of the pharyngeal floor (median anlage) that acts as the precursor of the T_4-producing follicular cells and paired caudal extensions of the fourth pharyngobranchial pouches (lateral anlagen) that give rise to the parafollicular calcitonin-secreting cells (C cells).[96,97] These structures are discernible by 16 to 17 days of gestation, and by 24 days the median anlage develops a thin, flask-like diverticulum extending from the floor of the buccal cavity, at a point that is later known as the foramen cecum on the developing tongue, to the fourth branchial arch. At 24 to 32 days, this median anlage has already become a bilobed structure, and by 50 days of gestation, the median and lateral anlagen have fused and the buccal stalk has ruptured.

During this period, the thyroid gland, which initially consists of a round cluster of cells, migrates caudally from the pharyngeal floor, through the anterior midline of the neck, to its definitive location in the anterior neck; during this time, the cells multiply. Data suggest that localization of growing thyroid tissue along the anteroposterior axis is linked to the development of the ventral aorta in the zebrafish; in other words, vessels provide guidance cues in zebrafish thyroid morphogenesis.[98] In mouse thyroid development, the midline primordium bifurcates and two lobes relocalize cranially along the bilateral pair of carotid arteries. In sonic hedgehog–deficient mice, thyroid tissue always develops along the ectopically and asymmetrically positioned carotid arteries, suggesting that in mice, as in zebrafish, codeveloping arteries define the presence of the thyroid.[98]

Additionally, Fagman and colleagues[99] implicated Tbx1 in the development of the thyroid gland, although it cannot be detected in the thyroid primordium at any embryonic stage. In Tbx1$^{-/-}$ mice, the downward translocation of Titf1/Nkx2.1-expressing thyroid progenitor cells is much delayed. In late mutant embryos, the thyroid fails to form symmetric lobes but persists as a single mass that is approximately one quarter of the normal size. The hypoplastic gland mostly attains a unilateral position resembling thyroid hemiagenesis. The data suggest that failure of the thyroid primordium to reestablish contact with the aortic sac is a major factor in the prevention of normal growth of the midline anlage along the third pharyngeal arch arteries. This interaction may be facilitated by *Tbx1*-expressing mesenchyme filling the gap between the pharyngeal endoderm and the detached thyroid primordium.[99] Conditional ablation of *Fgf8* in *Tbx1*-expressing cells caused an early thyroid phenotype similar to that of *Tbx1* mutant mice. In addition, expression of an *Fgf8* complementary DNA in the *Tbx1* domain rescued the early size defect of the thyroid primordium in *Tbx1* mutants. These data suggest that a Tbx1-Fgf8 pathway in the pharyngeal mesoderm is a key regulator of mammalian thyroid development.[99]

At 51 days, the gland exhibits its definitive external form, with an isthmus connecting the two lateral lobes, and it reaches its final position below the thyroid cartilage by the 7th week of embryonic life. At the same time, connection of the median anlage with the ultimobranchial body, developed from the endoderm of the fourth pharyngeal pouch, occurs, resulting in incorporation of the C cells into the thyroid. During its descent, the developing thyroid gland retains an attachment to the pharynx by a narrow epithelial stalk known as the thyroglossal duct.[100] By 37 days, this structure that connects the median thyroid anlage with the point of origin of its migration on the floor of the pharynx has usually disappeared,[101] and normally the only remnant of the thyroglossal duct is the foramen cecum itself. An ectopic thyroid and persistent thyroglossal duct or cyst may occur as a consequence of abnormalities of thyroid descent.

Usually, the terminal differentiation of thyroid follicular cells—as evidenced by expression of the genes encoding the TSH receptor (*TSHR*), the sodium-iodide symporter (*NIS*), thyroglobulin (*Tg*), and thyroperoxidase (*TPO*) and the formation of follicles—occurs in the normal embryo only after migration is complete.[102] Gene expression studies performed on thyroid tissues derived from human embryos and fetuses showed that *TITF1*, *FOXE1*, *PAX8*, TSHR, and *DUOX2* were stably expressed from the 7th to the 33rd gestational weeks.[103-106] Genes encoding Tg, TPO, and pendrin were expressed as early as 7 weeks' gestational age. NIS expression appeared last and showed the highest fit by the broken line regression model of all genes. Immunohistochemical studies detected TITF1, TSHR, and Tg in unpolarized thyrocytes before follicle formation. T_4 and NIS labeling were found in developing follicles from the 11th gestational week onward. These studies suggest a key role for NIS in the onset of human thyroid function.[103]

By 70 days of gestation, colloid is visible histologically and thyroglobulin synthesis and iodide accumulation can be demonstrated within the gland. During the final follicular phase of development, colloid spaces increase in size, and there is progressive cell growth and accumulation of thyroid hormones. Terminal differentiation of the human thyroid is characterized by the onset of follicle formation and thyroid hormone synthesis at 11 weeks' gestation. At

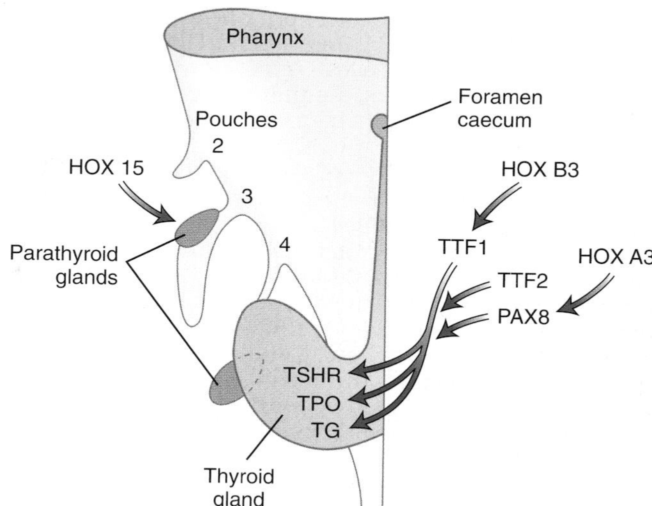

Figure 22-7 Illustration of the homeobox genes that program development of the thyroid and parathyroid glands. *HEX* is involved early in the integrated cascade that programs thyroid gland embryogenesis. *HOXB3* and *HOXA3* may be responsible for activation of thyroid transcription factors TTF1 and TTF2, respectively, during early embryogenesis. *PAX8* is essential in the cascade. These factors are also involved in thyroid follicular cell function, promoting thyroglobulin (TG), thyroid peroxidase (TPO), and thyroid-stimulating hormone receptor (TSHR) gene transcription. *HOX15* gene knockout in mice causes parathyroid gland aplasia. See text for details.

12 weeks of gestation, the fetal thyroid gland weighs about 80 mg, and at term it weighs 1 to 1.5 g. The parathyroid glands develop between 5 and 12 weeks of gestation from the third and fourth pharyngeal pouches.

At least five developmental genes are involved in thyroid and parathyroid gland embryogenesis. These include the genes for thyroid transcription factors *HEX* (*Hex* in the mouse), *TTF1* (*Titf1/Nkx2.1*), *FOXE1* (*Titf2/Foxe1*), *NKX2-5*, and *PAX8* (Fig. 22-7).[97,104-107] *Hex* gene knockout in mice is associated with thyroid agenesis or severe hypoplasia. *Ttf2* knockout results in thyroid dysgenesis and cleft palate. *Ttf1* knockout leads to pulmonary hypoplasia and thyroid agenesis. Inactivating *Pax8* mutations lead to thyroid hypoplasia and renal anomalies. *Ttf1* knockout is also associated with parafollicular C-cell aplasia. The *HOX* genes appear to be important in the expression of *Ttf1* and *Pax8*. *HOX15* gene disruption in mice results in parathyroid gland aplasia.[108] *TTF1/NKX2.1* and *PAX8* also play a role in the survival of thyroid cell precursors and regulation of thyroid-specific gene expression, whereas *FOXE1/TTF2* is critical for cellular migration.

TTF1, TTF2, PAX8, NKX2-5, and *TSHR* gene mutations account for fewer than 10% of patients with familial thyroid dysgenesis and congenital hypothyroidism; no mutations have been identified in *HEX* as yet.[106] Most cases of congenital hypothyroidism occur sporadically, and the pathogenesis in these cases remains unclear. It is known that signaling molecules such as those in the FGF pathway and the SHH pathway are also implicated in murine thyroid development.[108] In late organogenesis, the *SHH* gene appears to have an important role in the symmetric bilobation of the thyroid; it also suppresses the ectopic expression of thyroid follicular cells. It is not inconceivable that mutations in these genes may be identified in patients with congenital hypothyroidism.[98]

In the rat, at fetal day 15, despite early evidence of *Tg*, *TPO,* and *TSHR* gene expression, the thyroid gland is difficult to distinguish from the surrounding structures, and iodine organification, thyroid hormoneogenesis, and evidence of a follicular structure are absent. These data suggest that TTF1/NKX2-1 and PAX8 are necessary but not sufficient for the expression of the fully differentiated thyroid phenotype. Expression of the *TSHR* gene is significantly upregulated on fetal day 17, and this is accompanied by significant growth and rapid development in terms of structure and function. The expression of *Tg* and *TPO* is increased and thyroid follicles are seen with thyroid hormoneogenesis, suggesting that the TSHR has an important role to play in these events. Murine mutation of the *TSHR* gene is associated with the *hyt/hyt* phenotype in mice, which exhibits severe hypothyroidism and a hypoplastic but normally located thyroid gland with a poorly developed follicular structure. In humans, a similar phenotype is observed in babies of mothers with potent TSHR-blocking antibodies and in babies with severe loss-of-function mutations in *TSHR*.

Embryogenesis is largely complete by 10 to 12 weeks' gestation, equivalent to fetal day 15 to 17 in the rat, and thyroid follicle precursors are first seen at this stage. Tg is also detected in follicular spaces, and evidence of iodine uptake and organification is obtained at this stage. Pituitary and plasma thyrotropin (TSH) concentrations begin to increase during the second trimester in the human fetus, at about the time that pituitary portal vascular continuity develops (Fig. 22-8).[103,109] Plasma thyrotropin levels increase progressively during the last half of gestation. Plasma concentrations of T_4-binding globulin and total T_4 increase progressively, from low levels at 16 to 18 weeks of gestation to maximal levels at 35 to 40 weeks. Free T_4 levels also increase as a consequence of the increase in T_4 production. The increases in plasma TSH and T_4 levels during the third trimester reflect a progressive maturation of hypothalamic pituitary control and of thyroid gland responsiveness to TSH. Pituitary TSH secretion is responsive to hypothyroxinemia and to TRH early in the third trimester.[106] Hypothyroxinemia results in an elevated fetal serum TSH concentration, whereas hyperthyroidism due to maternal Graves' disease is associated with a suppressed fetal TSH concentration. Premature infants born at 26 to 28 weeks of gestation respond to exogenous TRH with an increase in plasma TSH concentration comparable to that in adults.[110] However, their TSH response to extrauterine exposure is reduced, indicating hypothalamic immaturity.

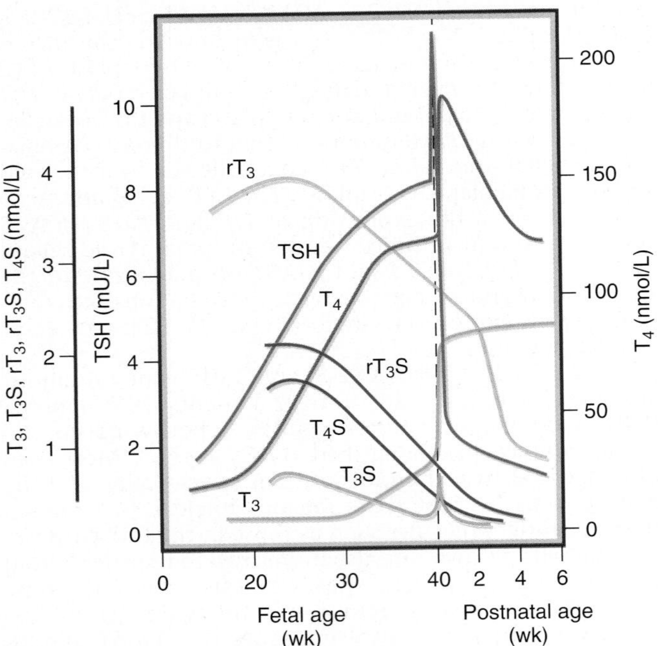

Figure 22-8 Patterns of change of fetal plasma thyroid-stimulating hormone (TSH), thyroxine (T_4), triiodothyronine (T_3), reverse T_3 (rT_3), and iodothyronine sulfates (T_4S, rT_3S, and T_3S) during gestation and in the neonatal period. The patterns for T_4S and rT_3S are based on limited 30-week data. (Data from references 109, 329, 330.)

Thyroid Hormonogenesis

Hypothalamic-pituitary-thyroid control matures during an interval corresponding to the late third trimester and early neonatal period of human development.[109,111] The period of parallel increases in fetal TSH and free T_4 levels during the latter half of gestation is followed by the sequential TSH and free T_4 surges in the early neonatal period and a final slow equilibration of the TSH/free T_4 ratio to adult values during infancy and childhood.[111-113] This maturation includes coordinated maturation of hypothalamic TRH secretion, pituitary TRH sensitivity, thyrotropin negative-feedback control, and thyroid follicular cell responsiveness to TSH. Fetal serum TRH levels are higher than in maternal blood, and this is the consequence of extrahypothalamic (placenta and pancreas) TRH production and decreased TRH degradation in fetal serum. Functionally, the fetus progresses from a state of both primary (thyroidal) and tertiary (hypothalamic) hypothyroidism at midgestation, through a state of mild tertiary hypothyroidism during the final weeks in utero, to a fully mature hypothalamic-pituitary-thyroid axis by 2 months after birth. The neonatal free T_4 increments also are reduced (compared with term infants) in premature infants born at 31 to 34 weeks, attenuated at 28 to 30 weeks, and absent in 23- to 27-week infants.[113]

The adult thyroid follicular cell can modify iodine transport or uptake with changes in dietary iodine intake, independent of variations in serum thyrotropin levels.[114,115] Before 36 to 40 weeks of gestation, the thyroid gland lacks this autoregulatory mechanism and is susceptible to iodine-induced inhibition of thyroid hormone synthesis.[110,115] The fetal thyroid follicular cell, when exposed to high circulating levels of iodide, is unable to reduce iodide trapping and prevent the high intracellular iodide concentrations that produce the blockade of hormone synthesis referred to as the *Wolff-Chaikoff effect*. Failure of the immature thyroid to exhibit autoregulation is probably due to failure of downregulation of thyroid cell membrane NIS units, which may be related to the absence or reduced iodination of an 8- to 10-kd protein in the thyroid follicular cell.[114,115] In addition to maturation of autoregulation, thyroidal responsiveness to thyrotropin increases during the last trimester.[97]

The metabolism of thyroid hormones occurs through a progressive series of monodeiodinations.[109,116] Three deiodinase enzymes act to remove an iodine atom from the outer (phenolic) ring or the inner (tyrosyl) ring of the tetraiodothyronine (T_4) molecule, thus, respectively, activating or inactivating the hormone. The deiodinases are encoded by separate genes and share sequence homology. Most of the circulating, biologically active T_3 in adults is derived by outer-ring monodeiodination of T_4 in liver and other nonthyroidal tissues; biologically inactive rT_3 derives from inner-ring deiodination of T_4 in peripheral tissues. The type I enzyme (D1), an outer-ring monodeiodinase, is a high-Michaelis-constant (K_m) enzyme inhibited by propylthiouracil and stimulated by thyroid hormone. It

TABLE 22-3

Deiodinase Expression in Human and Rodent Tissues

Tissue	D1	D2	D3
Brain	X	X	X
Pituitary	X	X	
Thyroid	X	X*	
Liver	X		X†
Kidney	X		
Ovary	X		X
Ear		X*	
Heart		X*	
Muscle		X†	
Skin		X	X
Testes		X	X
Uterus		X	X
Brown fat		X	

*Expressed in human only.
†Expressed only in fetus.
Modified from St. Germain DL, Hernandez A, Schneider MJ, et al. Insights into the role of deiodinases from studies of genetically modified animals. *Thyroid*. 2005;15:905-916.

deiodinates T_4 to T_3 and rT_3 to T2. D1 also has inner-ring deiodinase activity, converting T_3 to T_2. Activity of D1 is low throughout gestation. The type 2 outer-ring monodeiodinase (D2) is a low-K_m enzyme that is insensitive to propylthiouracil and inhibited by thyroid hormone. It deiodinates T_4 to T_3 and rT_3 to T_2, and it is highly expressed in brain and pituitary. Type 3 monodeiodinase (D3) inactivates T_4 and T_3 via inner-ring deiodination of T_4 to rT_3 and of T_3 to T_2; it is highly expressed in fetal tissues and placenta. D1 is largely responsible for production of T_3 that escapes from the cells, especially liver and kidney, into the circulation, whereas D2 is responsible for production of local tissue T_3. Inactive rT_3 also diffuses out of most tissues to appear in plasma.

The distribution of the deiodinases has been characterized in rodent and human tissues (Table 22-3).[116] D2 is detectable by midgestation and plays an important role in supplying T_3 to developing brain tissue, regulating thermogenesis in brown adipose tissue in the neonatal period, and regulating pituitary TSH secretion. D3 activity is present in placenta, liver, and perhaps fetal skin, accounting for the higher levels of rT_3 in the fetus and limiting the metabolic effects of thyroid hormones during much of fetal life. There is little conversion of T_4 to circulating T_3 via D1 deiodination until midgestation in the human fetus; plasma T_3 levels are low (<0.2 nmol/L or <15 ng/dL) until 30 weeks of gestation, after which the mean value increases to 0.7 nmol/L (50 ng/dL) at term (Fig. 22-7).[117] On the other hand, fetal brain T_3 concentrations are 60% to 80% of those in the adult by fetal age 20 to 26 weeks due to D2 activity. In the presence of fetal hypothyroidism, D2 increases while D3 decreases in an effort to maintain near-normal brain T_3 concentrations. Sulfation is active in fetal tissues, and the predominant thyroid hormone metabolites in the fetus are iodothyronine sulfates.[109,118,119]

High levels of phenolsulfotransferases (SULT) have been characterized in fetal liver, lung, and brain by midgestation. SULT activities decrease rapidly in the neonatal period.[119] In the last third of gestation in fetal sheep, the mean plasma production rates for T_4 and metabolites (in micrograms per kilogram of body weight per day) are as follows: T_4, 40; T_4 sulfate (T_4S), 10; rT_3, 5; rT_3S, 12; T_3, 2; and T_3S, 2. All metabolites are biologically inactive except T_3 and perhaps T_3S, so that 90% of the T_4 metabolites in the fetus are biologically inactive.[118] The sulfated metabolites accumulate in fetal serum as a result of the low D1 activity in fetal tissues and because the sulfated iodothyronines are not substrates for D3.[114,118] The production rate of T_3 increases progressively between 30 weeks of gestation and term because of maturation of D1 activity in the liver and other tissues and because of decreasing D3 activity in placenta.[97,120] In the fetal sheep, hepatic D1 activity increases progressively during the last trimester.[121]

It has long been assumed that thyroid hormones passively diffuse into cells. However, several classes of cell membrane iodothyronine transporters have been described, questioning this hypothesis.[122-124] These transporters belong to different families of organic anion, amino acid, and monocarboxylate solute carriers, including the organic anion transporting polypeptide (OATP) family and the solute carrier family 21 (SLC21).[122-124] The significance of these transporters is not yet clear, but mutation of the human monocarboxylate transporter 8 (MCT8), a member of the SLC21 family shown to be a specific thyroid hormone transporter present in developing brain, leads to a syndrome of combined thyroid dysfunction and psychomotor retardation.[123,124] *Mct8* expression in neonatal mice has been localized to neurons in the olfactory bulb, cerebral cortex, hippocampus, and amygdala. Presumably, all thyroid hormone-sensitive cell populations express iodothyronine membrane transporters. A cell surface T_4 receptor has been characterized as an $\alpha_V\beta_3$ integrin that serves as the initiation site for T_4-induced activation of the mitogen-activated protein kinase (MAPK) pathway for angiogenesis and perhaps actin polymerization and neuronal migration.[125] The ontogenesis and significance of these cell surface receptors and membrane transporters in fetal development remain to be further defined.

Thyroid Hormone Action

Classic thyroid hormone actions are mediated via functional thyroid hormone nuclear receptors, members of the steroid/retinoid/vitamin D family of nuclear transcription factors. Two genes code for the receptors: *THRA* on chromosome 17 encodes TRα, and *THRB* on chromosome 3 encodes TRβ.[126] These genes code for four classic receptor isoforms (TRα1, TRα2, TRβ1, and TRβ2), three of which bind thyroid hormones (T_3/T_4 affinity, 10:1) and bind to DNA to effect gene transcription. The TRα2 isoform does not bind thyroid hormone but binds to DNA and can inhibit binding of other TRs. The TRs exist as monomers, homodimers, and heterodimers with other nuclear receptor family members such as retinoid X (RXR). Other TR transcripts, including TRΔα1 and TRΔα2, have been characterized. These do not bind DNA or T_3 but can inhibit TR and retinoid receptor activities.[127]

The TRs are expressed developmentally and differentially in various fetal and adult tissues. TRα proteins are present in most tissues. TRβ1 is expressed in liver, kidney, and lung and in developing brain, cochlea, and pituitary. TRβ2 expression is restricted largely to the pituitary gland, retina, and cochlea.[97,126] The receptors function redundantly, as indicated by knockout studies in mice, but predominant effects of one or another TR have been characterized (Table 22-4). Knockout of both the TRα and TRβ genes in mice is not lethal but results in elevated TSH levels, deafness, bradycardia, and decreased postnatal growth with delayed bone maturation.[97,126,127] Lethality occurs because of improper intestinal development associated with persistent TRΔα isoforms in TRα or combined

TABLE 22-4

Predominant Thyroid Hormone Receptor Subtype Functions in Developing Mice

Brain	Thermogenesis
TRα1, TRβ1	TRα1, TRβ1, TRβ2
Pituitary TSH secretion	Inner ear
	TRα1, TRβ2
	TRβ2, TRα1
Pituitary GH secretion	Retina
	TRβ2
	TRα1
Bone maturation	Intestine
TRα1	TRα1
Liver	Heart
TRβ1	TRα1

Modified from Yen P. Genomic and nongenomic actions of thyroid hormones. In Braverman LE, Utiger RD, eds. *The Thyroid*, 9th ed. Philadelphia, PA: Lippincott Williams and Wilkins, 2005:135-150; and Flamant F, Samarut J. Thyroid hormone receptors: lessons from knockout and knockin mutant mice. *Trends Endocrinol Metab.* 2005;14:85-90.

TRα and TRβ knockout mice.[127] In the fetal rat brain, TRα1 mRNA and receptor binding are detectable by 12 to 14 days of gestation (term is 21 days), increasing to maximal levels at birth. The TRβ1 isoform is detected at birth and increases approximately 40-fold in the early postnatal period.[97,128] In human fetal brain, TRα1 and TRβ1 isoforms and receptor binding are present by 8 to 10 weeks of gestation; TRα1 transcripts and receptor occupancy increase 8- to 10-fold by 16 to 18 weeks.[97,129,130] Liver, heart, and lung receptor binding can be identified by 13 to 18 weeks.[97,130,131]

Ontogeny of Thyroid Hormone Secretion

The role of maternal thyroid hormone during fetal development remains controversial. The high placental concentration of D3 inactivates most of the thyroid hormone presented from the maternal circulation. The iodide released in this manner is used for fetal thyroid hormone synthesis. Despite the limited maternal-fetal placental transfer of T_4 and the predominant production of inactive thyroid hormone metabolites in the human fetus, significant levels of free T_4 are present in fetal fluids, from placental transfer early in gestation and from fetal thyroid production during later gestation.[97,128] Early in gestation, placental transfer is the only source of T_4 in fetal fluids and is essential for normal fetal neurodevelopment. T_4 is detectable in human celomic fluid at levels of 0.5 to 2 nmol/L between 6 and 11 weeks of gestation, before the onset of fetal thyroid function.[132] Low concentrations of T_4 are detectable in the fetal brain at about 10 weeks of gestation. Significant placental transfer continues to term, when serum T_4 levels in the athyroid fetus range from 30 to 70 nmol/L (2.3 to 5.4 μg/dL).[133] Isotopic equilibrium studies with pregnant rats at term suggest that 15% to 20% of the T_4 in fetal tissues is of maternal origin.[134] As indicated, thyroid hormones cross the placenta early in gestation, supplying the low levels of free T_4 that are essential for brain development between 12 and 20 weeks, before the onset of fetal thyroid hormone production.[128] Most thyroid hormone in the fetal compartment is inactivated to sulfated and deiodinated analogues until the perinatal period.[109,118,119] This neutralization of active circulating thyroid hormone maintains the low T_3 metabolic state, facilitating fetal growth and programmed tissue maturation.

Thyroid hormone–programmed development of selective fetal tissues requires the interaction of local tissue D1, D2, thyroid receptors, receptor coactivators, and thyroid-responsive genes. In most responsive tissues, the timing of maturation events is controlled by the state of the thyroid receptors acting as a molecular switch.[127,135] In the absence of T_3, the unliganded receptor (aporeceptor) recruits corepressors, repressing gene transcription. Non–T_3-binding receptors also can repress transcription by inhibiting receptor DNA binding. Local tissue maturation events are initiated by the coincident availability of T_3, liganded T_3 receptor, T_3-mediated receptor exchange of co-repressor with coactivators for creation of an active holoreceptor, and activation of responsive gene transcription.

These programming events have been investigated in studies of transgenic mice, including brain, liver, heart, intestine, and bone tissues, thermogenesis, and spleen erythropoiesis.[135-141] The timing of these events in the mouse range from early midbrain neuronal development at gestational day 15; through perinatal activation of hepatic enzymes, cardiac ion channels, and spleen erythropoiesis; to postnatal brain, intestinal, and bone maturation and thermogenesis. Parturition occurs at a gestational age equivalent to human midgestation. In hypothyroid mice, repressive effects of aporeceptors have been shown to delay tissue maturation in brain, bone, intestine, spleen, and heart.[138] The increase in circulating T_3 levels associated with parturition in mice and humans normally triggers development of tissue functions essential to postnatal metabolism and homeostasis (e.g., hepatic, intestinal, and cardiac functions and brown fat thermogenesis). Thyroid hormone–stimulated maturation of vision and hearing appear to be triggered by the local expression of D2, mediating local T_3 production, postnatally in the mouse and probably toward the end of the second midtrimester in the human fetus.[116]

In humans, T_3-mediated maturation of fetal tissues, including liver, heart, brown adipose tissue, and bone, allows them to become thyroid hormone–responsive during late gestation and in the perinatal period. Paracrine actions of thyroid hormone are critical for normal fetal development—for example, in the cochlea, where D2 is expressed in connective tissue immediately adjacent to the sensory epithelium and spiral ganglion, where thyroid hormone receptors are located. This implies that D2-containing cells in the connective tissue take up T_4 from the circulation, convert it to T_3, and then release D3 to adjacent responsive cells. Similarly, in the brain, D2 is expressed predominantly in glial cells, whereas TRs are expressed in adjacent neurons and oligodendrocytes. In other areas of the brain, such as the pituitary gland, hippocampus, and caudate nucleus, there is coexpression of D2 and TRs. On the other hand, D3 is coexpressed with TRs in neurons, thereby protecting sensitive tissues from the effects of excess thyroid hormone.

The actions of thyroid hormones and their developmental regulation in the brain are complex. Functionally, thyroid hormones are critical for the establishment of neural circuits during a critical window of brain development. They provide inductive cues for the differentiation and maturation of a number of processes such as neurogenesis and neural cell migration (occurring between 5 and 24 weeks of gestation), neuronal differentiation, dendritic and axonal growth, synaptogenesis, gliogenesis (late fetal period to 6 months postpartum), myelination (second trimester to 24 months postpartum), and neurotransmitter enzyme synthesis. TRs are found in highest concentration in developing neurons and in multiple areas of the fetal brain, including the cerebrum, the cerebellum, and the auditory and visual cortex. The hormones bind to receptors and stimulate a number of genes such as myelin, neurotropins and their receptors, cytoskeletal components, transcription factors, extracellular matrix proteins and adhesion molecules, intracellular signaling molecules, and mitochondrial and cerebellar genes.

Thyroid hormone is also important for normal bone growth. T_3 regulates endochondral ossification and controls chondrocyte differentiation in the growth plate both in vivo and in vitro. TRs are expressed on osteoblasts and growth plate chondrocytes, and T_3 target genes have been identified in bone. T_3 stimulates skull suture closure in vivo.

In the perinatal period, thyroid hormone stimulates the transcription of thermogenin (also known as uncoupling protein 1 [UCP1]), a protein that uncouples nucleotide phosphorylation and the storage of energy as adenosine triphosphate ATP, actions that are important for nonshivering thermogenesis by brown adipose tissue.

Congenital Hypothyroidism

Classic signs of congenital hypothyroidism (jaundice, lethargy, feeding difficulties, macroglossia, myxedema, hypothermia, growth retardation, and progressive developmental delay and IQ deterioration) accrue during the early weeks and months of extrauterine life as maternal T_4 becomes unavailable and the non-CNS tissues become responsive to thyroid hormone.[97,109] Rarely, hypothyroidism is associated with respiratory distress in the neonatal period. Maternal hypothyroxinemia has been associated with attention deficit-hyperactivity disorder and with 5 to 10 points of IQ deficit in the offspring of such pregnancies.[14,97,128] The period of brain dependency for thyroid hormone extends postnatally to 2 to 3 years of age, but the early weeks and months of life are most critical. Untreated thyroid agenesis is associated with a loss of 5 to 7 IQ points monthly during the first months of postnatal life, and over 6 to 8 months this can amount to a 30- to 40-point IQ deficit.[128] Most countries, therefore, have a rigorous screening program to ensure early diagnosis and treatment.

In congenital hypothyroidism, there is an increased net flux of maternal thyroid hormone to the fetus, resulting in cord T_4 concentrations that are 25% to 50% of normal. There is increasing evidence of maternal-fetal T_4 transfer in the first half of pregnancy, when fetal thyroid hormone levels are low.[142] The transplacental passage of thyroid hormone, in conjunction with adjustments in brain deiodinase activity, has a critical role in minimizing the adverse effects of fetal hypothyroidism and helps explain the normal or near-normal outcome of hypothyroid fetuses (provided that prompt and adequate treatment of hypothyroidism ensues postnatally) as well as the relatively normal clinical appearance of the majority of babies with congenital hypothyroidism at birth. On the other hand, in the presence of both maternal and fetal hypothyroidism—such as that observed in the presence of potent TSH receptor–blocking antibodies, maternal and fetal POU1F1 deficiency, and severe iodine deficiency—there is severe neurocognitive impairment despite early and adequate commencement of thyroid replacement. Importantly, the presence of maternal hypothyroxinemia or inadequately controlled hypothyroidism is also associated with significant neurocognitive deficit in the offspring that is not reversible by early postnatal therapy.[13,14]

Pituitary-Gonadal Axis

The mammalian gonad originates from the intermediate mesoderm from which the bipotential genital ridge differentiates. The gonad is derived from two tissue anlagen: the primordial germ cells of the yolk sac wall and the somatic, stromal cells that migrate from the primitive mesonephros.[143,144] By 4 to 5 weeks of gestation, the germ cells have begun their migration from the yolk sac, and the gonadal ridge has appeared as a derivative of the mesonephros. The germ cells are incorporated into the developing gonadal ridge during the 6th week, when the primitive gonad is composed of a surface epithelium, primitive gonadal cords continuous with the epithelium, and a dense cellular mass referred to as the *gonadal blastema*, which includes the steroidogenic cell precursors.[143]

Until the appearance of testicular cords made up of Sertoli cells at 6 weeks, the fetal testis and ovary are indistinguishable. Embryogenesis of the gonads is programmed by genes encoding the male sexual determinant SRY as well as SF1, SOX9, and DAX1.[145,146] SRY is a critical regulator of male gonadal differentiation. Three other genes—WT1, SOX9, and SF1—are expressed in the bipotential gonadal ridge during its differentiation from the intermediate mesoderm and are critical for normal male sexual differentiation. WT1, the Wilms' tumor suppressor gene located at 11p13, is expressed in both the primitive kidney and the genital ridge. Its expression is related to the transition from mesenchyme to epithelium. WT1 is a transcription factor that contains four zinc fingers and binds to an ERG1 consensus binding sequence. SRY is activated by certain WT1 isoforms in vitro.

SF1 is required for testicular and ovarian development and mediates müllerian-inhibiting hormone (AMH) gene expression and gonadotropin production. SF1 and DAX1 are orphan receptors of the steroid/thyroid hormone family of nuclear receptors and appear to interact as heterodimers coordinately involved in the regulation of target genes in the adrenal glands and in hypothalamic gonadotrope cells and the ventromedial hypothalamic nucleus.[145,146] SF1 also regulates the expression of the cytochrome P450 enzymes. Recent data suggest that SRY binds to multiple elements within a SOX9 gonad-specific enhancer in mice and that it does so along with SF1. SF1 and SRY cooperatively upregulate SOX9; then, together with SF1, SOX9 also binds to the enhancer to help maintain its own expression after that of SRY has declined.[147]

A current view of the pathways for genes programming gonadal differentiation is shown in Figure 22-9. The full menu of downstream gene targets remains to be defined, but the net result is the highly organized pattern of gonadal development and phenotypic sexual differentiation. Fetal pituitary gonadotropins are not required for gonadal development or sexual differentiation; LH or FSH receptor knockout mice are born phenotypically normal.[148]

Human mutations in several of the genes programming gonadal differentiation have been described.[144] Loss-of-function mutations of *SRY* or *SOX9* produce XY sex reversal, whereas gain-of-function mutations or duplications produce XX sex reversal. Mutations in *SOX9* are associated with camptomelic dysplasia and 46XY sex reversal. *SF1* mutations have been associated with 46XY sex reversal with gonadal dysgenesis, with or without adrenal failure. More recently, the phenotypic spectrum of *SF1* mutations has widened to encompass gonadal dysgenesis, premature ovarian failure, and the vanishing testis syndrome.[94,95,149] Mutations may be heterozygous or recessive, the latter likely to be associated with a more severe loss of function. *WT1* mutations produce several syndromes associated with abnormal testicular embryogenesis (WAGR syndrome [Wilms' tumor, aniridia, genitourinary anomalies, and mental retardation], Denys-Drash syndrome, and Frasier syndrome) and renal abnormalities such as Wilms' tumor or glomerulosclerosis. *WNT4* gain-of-function mutations

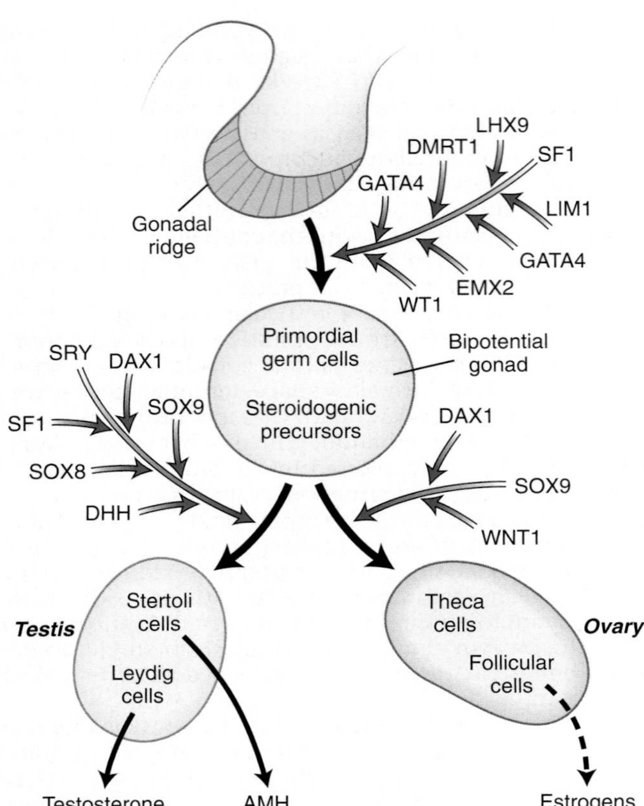

Figure 22-9 Summary of the molecular and cellular events of gonadal differentiation. AMH, antimüllerian hormone or müllerian inhibiting substance; DHH, desert hedgehog. See text for details. (Molecular cascades developed from Harley VR, Clarkson MJ, Argentaro A. The molecular action and regulation of the testis-determining factors, SRY (sex determining region of the Y chromosome) and SOX9 (SRY-related high-mobility group [HMG] Box 9). *Endocr Rev.* 2003;24:466-487; and Park SY, Jameson JL. Minireview: transcriptional regulation of gonadal development and differentiation. *Endocrinology.* 2005;146:1035-1042.)

result in XX sex reversal, whereas *Dax1* duplication is associated with XY sex reversal.[144]

In the presence of SRY, male gonadal differentiation begins at 7 weeks of gestation with organization of the gonadal blastema into interstitium and germ cell–containing testicular cords. The primitive cords lose their connections with the epithelium, primitive Sertoli cells and spermatogonia become visible within the cords, and the epithelium differentiates to form the tunica albuginea.[150] Leydig cells derived from the undifferentiated interstitium are visible by the end of the 8th week of gestation and are capable of androgen synthesis at that time. By 14 weeks of gestation, these cells make up as much as 50% of the cell mass, but as the tubules develop, they account for a smaller percentage of the tissue. The fetal testes grow from approximately 20 mg at 14 weeks of gestation to 800 mg at birth; at 5 to 6 months they descend into the inguinal canal in association with the epididymis and the ductus deferens.[150] The gonad, adrenal, and kidney all initially develop in close proximity, and as the testes descend, they may carry rests of adrenocortical cells with them. These adrenal rests may become hyperplastic with resulting testicular enlargement if subjected to prolonged ACTH stimulation (e.g., in patients with poorly controlled congenital adrenal hyperplasia). In the mouse, testicular descent is regulated by Insl3, which is a member of the insulin-like family and is secreted by Leydig cells.[151] Targeted disruption of the *Insl3* gene is associated with maldevelopment of the gubernaculum and bilateral cryptorchidism.[151] *Insl3* is also secreted by theca cells of the postnatal ovary, and females homozygous for *Insl3* mutations are subfertile with deregulation of the estrous cycle.

In human females, differentiation of ovaries begins during the 7th week of gestation, in the absence of *SRY*. The gonadal blastema differentiates into interstitium and medullary cords containing the primitive germ cells, referred to as *oogonia*. The cords degenerate, and cortical layers of surface epithelium, containing individual small oogonia, appear. By 11 to 12 weeks of gestation, clusters of dividing oogonia are surrounded by cord cells within the cortex; the medulla at this time consists largely of connective tissue.[152] At 12 weeks of gestation, primitive granulosa cells begin to replicate and many of the large oogonia in the deepest layers of the cortex enter their first meiotic division. Primordial follicles are first observed at about 18 weeks of gestation, and the number increases rapidly thereafter.[153] However, the number of oocytes progressively declines, from a peak of 3 to 6 million at 5 months' gestation to approximately 2 million at term.[16,153] Germ cell proliferation and apoptosis are ongoing simultaneously. Proliferating oocytes cluster, but the clusters break down with the development of follicles because only those oocytes enfolded by developing granulosa cells (as primordial follicles) survive.[16,153] By 5 months of gestation and during the 7th month, stroma-derived thecal cells develop around the primordial follicles as they mature to primary follicles. This process continues after birth, again progressing toward the superficial layers. Each fetal ovary weighs about 15 mg at 14 weeks of gestation and 300 to 350 mg at birth.[152] The number of surviving primary follicles at birth correlates with the duration of subsequent postpubertal ovulation. Interstitial cells with characteristics of steroid-producing cells are present after 12 weeks, and during the third trimester theca cells with steroidogenic capacity surround the developing follicles.[16] Significant aromatase activity also is present, but few if any steroids are produced by the ovary during development.[16,152]

The specific genetic mechanisms dictating ovarian development are largely unknown, but recently, mutations in *RSPO1* have been reported in association with 46XX sex reversal.[155,156] RSPO1 belongs to the R-spondin family of proteins that is implicated in Wnt/β-catenin signaling, and the gene encoding the protein may be ovary-determining.

In the male, the development of Leydig cells leads to an increase in fetal testosterone production between gestational weeks 10 and 20 (Fig. 22-10).[150] In vitro studies in the rat have shown that hCG binding to fetal testis cells does not downregulate LH receptors. If this is true in vivo in the human, continuous exposure of the Leydig cell to hCG would not desensitize the fetal testis and would allow the maintenance of augmented testosterone production during development. Fetal LH may contribute to fetal Leydig cell function, but quantitatively hCG is the predominant gonadotropin. Testosterone itself, acting through the androgen receptor, stimulates differentiation of the primitive mesonephric ducts into bilateral ductus deferens, epididymides, seminal vesicles, and ejaculatory ducts. Androgen receptors appear in the mesenchyme of urogenital structures at 8 weeks of gestation, followed by appearance of the receptors in the epithelium during development at 9 to 12 weeks.[154] There was no difference in receptor expression in male and female fetuses. Dihydrotestosterone stimulates male differentiation of the urogenital sinus

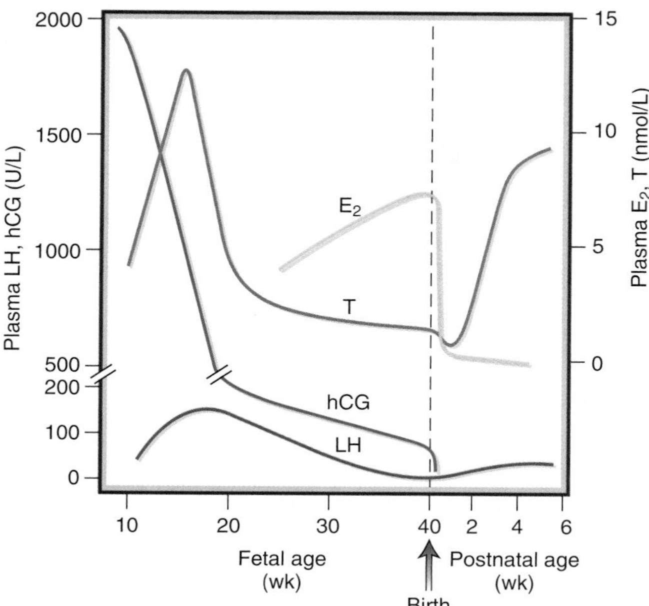

Figure 22-10 Patterns of change of plasma concentrations of human chorionic gonadotropin (hCG), luteinizing hormone (LH), testosterone (T), and estradiol (E_2) in a male fetus during gestation and in the neonatal period. (Data from references 277, 331-334.)

and external genitalia, including differentiation of the prostate, growth of the genital tubercle to form a phallus, and fusion of the urogenital folds to form the penile urethra. Dihydrotestosterone is formed from testosterone by the 5α-reductase enzyme within the urogenital sinus and urogenital tubercle, and it acts through the same androgen receptor that mediates the action of testosterone in the wolffian ducts. Mutations in the gene encoding the enzyme 5α-reductase are associated with variable disorders of sex development with 46XY phenotypes.

The fetal testis also produces AMH, which causes dedifferentiation of the müllerian duct system in the male fetus.[157,158] AMH is a glycoprotein with a monomer molecular size of approximately 72 kd and multimer sizes ranging from 145 to 235 kd. It is produced by testicular Sertoli cells and reaches the müllerian ducts largely by diffusion; duct regression in vitro requires a 24- to 36-hour exposure to AMH. AMH is synthesized early in gestation, with production peaking at the time of müllerian duct regression; biosynthesis continues throughout gestation and decreases after birth. *AMH* gene expression is activated by the *SRY* and *SF1* genes.[157] AMH also has autocrine and paracrine effects on testicular steroidogenic function during fetal life.[158] Male phenotypic differentiation is mediated by testicular testosterone and AMH and occurs between 8 and 14 weeks of gestation. In the female fetus, the müllerian duct system differentiates in the absence of AMH, the mesonephric ducts fail to develop in the absence of testosterone, and the undifferentiated urogenital sinus and external genitalia mature into female structures. Mutation of the AMH gene results in a persistent müllerian duct syndrome in the XY fetus.[157]

Estrogen effects are mediated by cognate receptors, members of the large family of steroid and thyroid hormone, vitamin D, and retinoid receptors.[159,160] Two receptors, ERα and ERβ, have been identified, with 96% and 58% homology in the DNA-binding and ligand-binding domains, respectively. ERα is encoded by *ESR1* on chromosome 6 and ERβ by *ESR2* on chromosome 14. Expression profiles of mRNAs of both receptors have been characterized in the 16- to 23-week human fetus. One or both receptor mRNAs are present in most tissues. The ERβ message is predominant, particularly in testis, ovary, spleen, thymus, adrenal, brain, kidney, and skin. The ERα message is prominent in the uterus, with relatively low levels in most other tissues.[159,160] The significance of ERs in fetal development is unclear. Knockout of the *ERα* gene in mice does not impair fetal development of any tissue, but adult females are infertile, with hypoplastic uteri and polycystic ovaries, and adult males manifest decreased fertility.[160] ERβ knockout mice develop normally, and female adults are fertile with normal sexual behavior; adult males reproduce normally but have prostate and bladder hyperplasia.[159] It is known that estrogens regulate DHEA production in the baboon and human fetal adrenal.[159] Knockout of both *ERα* and *ERβ* genes also has little impact on fetal development, but after birth the uterus, fallopian tubes, vagina, and cervix in females are hypoplastic and unresponsive to estrogen.[160]

Both androgens and estrogens are involved in the structural development of the rat brain.[161] Gonadal hormones also control gonadotropin production in the brain that results in cyclic ovarian function and normal function of the testes.[162,163] Testosterone administration to neonatal female rats produces permanent inhibition of cyclic hypothalamic control through local aromatization to estradiol and ER binding. In primates and humans, estrogens seem to be more effective in this regard. However, there is no evidence for permanent programming in the primate, and there appear to be no major tissue biochemical differences between the sexes in utero to account for sexual dimorphic behavioral or gonadotropic programming.[163] Therefore, the mechanisms for these effects are not yet clear in the primate and human fetus.

Intermediate Lobe of the Pituitary

The intermediate lobe of the pituitary gland is prominent in both the human and the sheep fetus. Intermediate lobe cells begin to disappear near term and are virtually absent in the adult human pituitary, although the intermediate lobe in the adult of some lower species is anatomically and functionally distinct.[164] The major secretory products of the intermediate lobe are α-MSH and β-endorphin, both derived from cleavage of the POMC molecule.[165] Cleavage of POMC in the anterior lobe results predominantly in corticotropin and β-lipotropin formation. In rhesus monkeys and humans, the fetal pituitary contains high concentrations of compounds resembling α-MSH and corticotropin-like intermediate lobe peptide (CLIP).[166] In the human fetus, α-MSH levels decrease with increasing fetal age.[167] The circulating levels of β-endorphin and β-lipotropin are high in the fetal lamb, and the ratio of β-endorphin to β-lipotropin increases during hypoxic stimulation of the anterior pituitary.[167] Because hypoxia provokes corticotropin release and β-lipotropin production from the anterior pituitary, these data have been interpreted to suggest that basal β-endorphin levels in the fetus originate in the intermediate lobe. α-MSH and CLIP may play a role in fetal adrenal activation, and α-MSH may play a role in fetal growth.[168,169] However, these effects are probably minor. The processing of pituitary POMC in the human fetus by the end of the second trimester is similar to that in the adult, but the role of these intermediate lobe peptides in the fetus remains obscure.[170]

Posterior Pituitary

The fetal neurohypophysis is well developed by 10 to 12 weeks of gestation and contains both AVP (also called *antidiuretic hormone*) and oxytocin (OT).[171,172] In addition, arginine vasotocin (AVT), the parent neurohypophyseal hormone in submammalian vertebrates, is present in the fetal pituitary and pineal glands and in adult pineal glands from several mammalian species, including humans.[173] AVT is present in the pituitary during fetal life and disappears in the neonatal period. In adult mammals, instillation of AVT into cerebrospinal fluid inhibits gonadotropin and corticotropin release, stimulates PRL release by the anterior pituitary, and induces sleep; however, the physiologic importance of these effects remains unclear. The role of AVT in the fetal pineal gland is unknown.

In the fetal sheep, the baseline fetal plasma AVP concentrations are similar to maternal levels after midgestation. During the last trimester of gestation, fetal hypothalamic and pituitary responsiveness to both volume and osmolar stimuli for AVP secretion are well developed, and AVP exerts antidiuretic effects on the fetal kidney.[171,172] Baseline plasma levels of AVT in fetal sheep during the last trimester approximate values for AVP and OT.[173] Presumably this AVT is derived from the posterior pituitary, but the stimuli for AVT secretion in the fetus are not defined. The neurohypophyseal peptides are synthesized as large precursor molecules (neurophysins) and processed to bioactive amidated peptides.[174] Enzymatic processing involves progressive cleavage of carboxyl terminal–extended peptides, sequentially producing (for OT) OT-glycine-lysine-arginine (OTGKR), OTGK, OTG, and OT. Similar progressive processing yields AVPG and AVP from the AVP neurophysin. Enzymatic processing of neurophysins matures progressively in the fetus so that early in gestation fetal plasma contains relatively large concentrations of the extended peptides. For OT, the ratio of OT-extended peptides to OT in fetal sheep serum is approximately 35 : 1 early in gestation and 3 : 1 late in gestation.[174]

In the fetus, AVP appears to function as a stress-responsive hormone. Perhaps the major potential stress for the fetus is hypoxia, and the response of AVP to hypoxia is increased compared with the maternal response and with fetal AVP responses to osmolar stimuli.[172,175-177] Plasma AVP concentrations in human cord blood are elevated in association with intrauterine bradycardia and meconium passage.[176] The vasopressor action of AVP may be important in the maintenance of fetal circulatory homeostasis during hemorrhage and hypoxia; AVP has a limited effect on fetoplacental blood flow.[171,177] Fetal hypoxia is also a major stimulus for catecholamine release. There is little information on interactions between AVP and catecholamines during fetal hypoxia, but both fetal hypoxia and AVP stimulate anterior pituitary function.[177] A role for AVP as a corticotropin-releasing hormone is established in the adult, and the ovine fetal pituitary responds separately and synergistically to AVP and CRH early in the third trimester.[178] The role of AVP in controlling fetal corticotropin release seems to decrease with gestational age. It is not known whether AVT functions as a corticotropin-releasing hormone in the fetus.

OT receptors have been demonstrated in human fetal membranes at term, and AVP receptors have been found in renal medullary membranes of newborn sheep.[179-181] Both AVP and AVT evoke antidiuretic actions in the sheep fetus during the last third of gestation, and both hormones act to conserve water for the fetus by inhibiting fluid loss into amniotic fluid through the lungs and kidneys.[171,172] Aquaporin-1, -2, and -3 water channel receptors are present in the human fetal and newborn kidney, and the ability of the newborn infant to regulate free water clearance in response to volume and osmolar stimuli has been demonstrated.[182,183] Whether AVT exerts its effects through AVP receptors or separate fetal AVT receptors is not clear. Maximal concentrating capacity by the fetal kidney is limited to about 600 mmol/L. This limitation is not related to inadequate AVP stimulation but rather to inherent immaturity of the renal tubules.

Lack of AVP is associated with diabetes insipidus and with a failure to retain water in the body leading to polyuria and polydipsia. Although most cases of diabetes insipidus are from acquired causes such as pituitary germinoma, craniopharyngioma, or Langerhans' cell histiocytosis, the condition may rarely be due to mutations in the AVP-neurophysin gene. Mutations in *WFS1* are associated with autosomal recessive Wolfram syndrome that includes diabetes insipidus, diabetes mellitus, optic atrophy, and sensorineural hearing loss.[184]

Fetal Autonomic Nervous System

The primordia of the sympathetic trunk ganglia are visible in the human fetus by 6 to 7 weeks of gestation. The preaortic sympathetic primordia at that time are composed of primitive sympathetic neurons and chromaffin cells, which condense into chains of cell masses along the abdominal aorta. By 10 to 12 weeks of gestation, the paired adrenal masses are well developed. In addition, numerous extramedullary paraganglia (derived from preaortic condensations of sympathetic neurons and chromaffin cells) are scattered throughout the abdominal and pelvic sympathetic plexuses.[185] Each of these extramedullary paraganglia may reach a maximal diameter of 2 to 3 mm by 28 to 30 weeks of gestation. The largest of the paraganglia, the organs of Zuckerkandl near the origin of the inferior mesenteric arteries, enlarge to 10 to 15 mm in length at term. After birth, the paraganglia gradually atrophy and disappear by 2 to 3 years of age. With increasing gestational age, there is progressive growth of the adrenal medullae, increasing catecholamine content of the adrenal medullae, and progressive maturation of medullary functional capacity. Histologically, the adrenal medullae are somewhat immature at birth, but by 1 year they resemble the adult glands.

Both chromaffin and sympathetic nerve cells are derived from common neuroectodermal stem cells. In mice, the sympathoadrenal progenitor cells first aggregate at the dorsal aorta, where they migrate in a dorsolateral direction to form sympathetic ganglia or ventrally to colonize the adrenal glands.[186] In the adrenal glands, they differentiate into neuroendocrine cells, expressing tyrosine hydroxylase and dopamine β-hydroxylase in response to a series of transcription factors including PHOX2B, MASH1, PHOX2A, and dHAND.[186] The *PHOX2B* gene is pivotal in development of most relays of the autonomic nervous system; mutation of this gene has been associated with the congenital hypoventilation syndrome, with Hirschsprung's disease, and with a predisposition to neuroblastoma.[187] Sympathetic nervous system development is nerve growth factor (NGF) dependent, and injections of NGF antiserum into neonatal rats led to degeneration of immature chromaffin cells, sympathetic cells, and pheochromoblasts.[188] Whether NGF and other growth factors are involved in the transient life span and function of the paraganglia in the human fetus and neonate is not clear. The role of placental NGF in maturation of the fetal autonomic nervous system is also unclear.

Catecholamines are present in the para-aortic chromaffin tissue by 10 to 15 weeks of gestation, and concentrations increase until term. The predominant catecholamine is norepinephrine (NE), presumably because of low activity of phenylethanolamine *N*-methyltransferase (PNMT) in para-aortic chromaffin tissue. This enzyme, which catalyzes the methylation of NE to epinephrine, appears to be activated by the high levels of cortisol that diffuse into the adrenal medulla from the adrenal cortex; in contrast, cortisol levels in extramedullary chromaffin tissue are low.[185,189,190] In fetal mammals, the chromaffin cells of the adrenal medulla can respond directly to asphyxia, long before splanchnic innervation develops, by secreting NE; the noninnervated para-aortic tissue responds similarly. In the fetal sheep, a similar developmental transition occurs between days 120 and 135 of the 150-day gestation.[185,189,190] The CNS responds to stimuli that evoke sympathetic nervous system responses before the adrenomedullary splanchnic innervation, but the adrenal medulla is relatively unresponsive to such stimuli. The transition is heralded by an adrenomedullary response to hypoglycemia mediated by the CNS.[189] This response is present in developing sheep, monkeys, and human fetuses during the third trimester of gestation.[191-193] Central and adrenal enkephalins are also involved in fetal autonomic nervous system function, and pretreatment with naloxone potentiates and methadone inhibits the catecholamine response to hypoxia.[185,190]

Basal plasma epinephrine, NE, and dopamine levels during the last third of gestation in sheep decrease as term approaches.[193,194] The metabolic clearance rate of epinephrine increases with gestational age, whereas the production rate remains unchanged, indicating that the decrease in basal catecholamine levels that occurs with fetal age is due to maturation of clearance mechanisms.[194] The fetal sheep responds to maternal exercise or hypoxia with increased catecholamine levels.[195] The human neonate responds to parturition with an increase in plasma epinephrine and NE concentrations, and these responses are augmented by hypoxia and acidosis.[195-197] In the newborn infant, catecholamine secretion also increases after cold exposure and hypoglycemia.[189,192]

Catecholamines are critical for fetal cardiovascular function and fetal survival. Gene knockout studies in mice, targeting either tyrosine hydroxylase or dopamine β-hydroxylase, produced fetal catecholamine deficiency and midgestation fetal death in 90% of the mutant embryos.[196,197] In addition, fetal catecholamines are the major stress hormones in the fetus.[189-192] The fetal adrenal and the para-aortic chromaffin masses discharge large amounts of catecholamines directly into the circulation in response to fetal hypoxia.[189] Moreover, the defense against fetal hypoxia involves catecholamine actions mediated through cardiac α-receptors that are unique to immature animals. α-Adrenergic receptors predominate in immature cardiac tissue and gradually decline in number as β-adrenergic receptors increase with maturation. Chromaffin tissue in the fetus is also innervated by opiate receptors and contains relatively large amounts of opiate peptides that appear to be cosecreted with the catecholamines.[189] The extent to which these peptides or pituitary endorphins are involved in modulating fetal catecholamine secretion remains unclear.

Parathyroid Hormone/Calcitonin System

Parathyroid gland development from the third and fourth pharyngeal pouches proceeds in synchrony with thyroid embryogenesis.[96,97] The third pouches encounter the migrating thyroid anlage, and the parathyroid anlagen are carried caudally with the thyroid gland, finally coming to rest at the lower poles of the thyroid lobes as the inferior parathyroid glands. The fourth pouches encounter the thyroid anlage later and come to rest at the upper poles of the thyroid lobes as the superior parathyroid glands. The individual parathyroid glands increase in diameter from less than 0.1 mm at 14 weeks of gestation to 1 to 2 mm at birth. The fifth pouches contribute paired ultimobranchial bodies that are incorporated into the developing thyroid gland as the parafollicular or C cells that secrete calcitonin. Both endocrine systems are functional during the second and third trimesters (see Fig. 22-8). Disruption of the *HOX15* gene in mice results in parathyroid gland aplasia, indicating that this gene functions as part of the gene cascade programming normal thyroid-parathyroid gland development. Additional genes involved in parathyroid gland embryogenesis include *SOX3, GCM2, GATA3, CRKL*, and *TBX1*.[198-200] *CRKL* and *TBX1* mutations have been associated with the DiGeorge syndrome and *GATA3* mutation with a DiGeorge-like syndrome; *GCM2* mutation leads to isolated hypoparathyroidism.[198] *SOX3* mutations are generally associated with variable hypopituitarism, but studies have implicated the gene in parathyroid development.[200]

Studies in fetal sheep and monkeys and measurements in human preterm and term infants indicate that high concentrations of fetal calcium (averaging 2.75 to 3 mmol/L in the last trimester) are maintained by active placental transport from maternal blood.[201,202] The transport of calcium occurs across the syncytiotrophoblast, which contains a calcium-binding protein that buffers intracellular calcium ions as they are transported across the syncytial cell to the basement membrane. An ATP-dependent calcium pump transports the calcium across the cell membrane to the fetal circulation.[202] The placental calcium pump is stimulated by a midmolecule portion of PTHrP secreted by the fetal parathyroid gland and by the placenta, where it may exert a paracrine effect.[202-204] The placenta is impermeable to parathyroid hormone (PTH), PTHrP, and calcitonin, but 25-hydroxyvitamin D and 1,25-dihydroxyvitamin D (calcitriol) are transported across the placenta, and free vitamin D levels in fetal blood are similar to or higher than maternal values.[201,202]

Thyroparathyroidectomy in the fetal sheep causes a rapid decrease in fetal plasma calcium concentration and a loss of the placental calcium gradient.[201] In mice, knockout of the gene for PTHrP abolished the maternal-fetal calcium gradient and reduced placental transport of calcium.[202,205] Placental calcium transport in these models was restored by the midmolecule fragment of PTHrP (amino acids 67 to 86) but not by PTH or the PTHrP(1-34) fragment, both of which activate the PTH/PTHrP receptor.[204,205] Therefore, a second, as yet unidentified PTHrP receptor recognizing the PTHrP(38-94) ligand appears to be involved in placental calcium pump activation.[202]

Other factors are also involved in maintenance of fetal serum calcium levels, because knockout of the mouse gene for PTH-PTHrP also results in hypocalcemia in the presence of normal or increased placental calcium transport.[201,203] PTH and PTHrP, through the PTH/PTHrP receptor, presumably modulate fetal skeletal calcium flux, calcium excretion through the fetal kidney, and perhaps reabsorption of calcium from amniotic fluid. PTHrP has a major role in fetal bone development and metabolism as well as fetal calcium homeostasis. PTHrP knockout mice display increased ossification of the basal portion of the skull, long bones, vertebral bodies, and pelvic bones and mineralization of the normally cartilaginous portions of the ribs and sternum; as a result of the cartilaginous mineralization, the animals die of asphyxiation in the early neonatal period.[202,204,205]

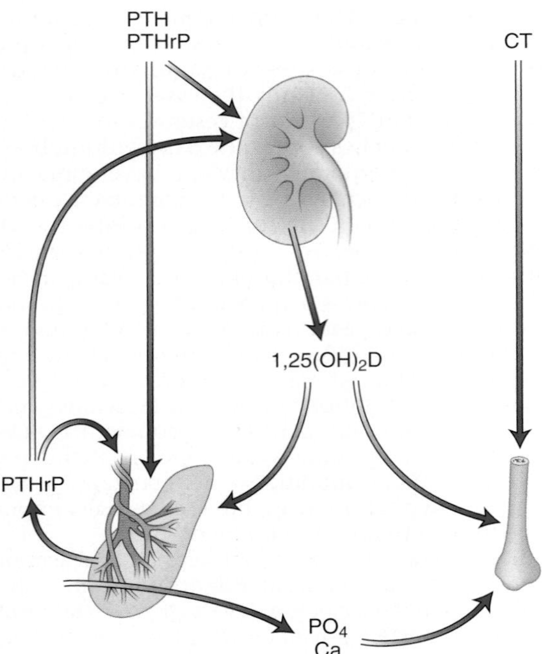

Figure 22-11 Proposed actions of parathyroid hormone (PTH), PTH-related protein (PTHrP), and calcitonin (CT) in the fetus. PTHrP and perhaps PTH from the parathyroid glands and PTHrP from the placenta act on the placenta to promote calcium (Ca) and phosphate (PO_4) transport from the maternal to the fetal circulation to maintain the relative fetal hypercalcemia and the high rate of fetal bone formation during the last half of gestation. PTHrP also acts on the kidney to promote 1-hydroxylation of 25-hydroxycholecalciferol to $1,25(OH)_2D$ (1,25-dihydroxyvitamin D, calcitriol), which augments placental calcium transport and promotes fetal bone growth. High fetal CT levels tend to promote bone accretion. See text for details.

Fetal nephrectomy also reduces fetal calcium concentrations, and the hypocalcemia can be prevented by administration of $1,25(OH)_2D$ (calcitriol).[201] Moreover, infusion into the sheep fetus of antibody to $1,25(OH)_2D$ reduced the placental calcium gradient.[201] Therefore, fetal PTHrP and PTH appear to stimulate fetal renal $1,25(OH)_2D$ production, which acts to enhance maternal-fetal transport of calcium by the placenta. The fetal kidney can synthesize $1,25(OH)_2D$ via 1-hydroxylation of 25-hydroxycholecalciferol, and the placenta contains both $1,25(OH)_2D$ receptors and a vitamin D–dependent calcium-binding protein. In the sheep fetus, the endogenous production rate of $1,25(OH)_2D$ during the last third of gestation was six times greater than that in the mother.[206] The metabolic clearance of $1,25(OH)_2D$ was also higher in the fetus than in the mother.

The fetal parathyroid-placental axis promotes maternal-fetal transfer of bone mineral and accretion of fetal bone mineral. The high blood levels of calcitonin in the fetus, probably resulting from the chronic stimulation by fetal hypercalcemia, are thought to contribute to the fetal bone mineral accretion.[199,201] A prominent effect of calcitonin is to inhibit bone resorption, and the high fetal serum calcium concentrations coupled with high circulating calcitonin promote bone mineral anabolism.[199] Placental calcitonin production may contribute to the calcitonin in fetal plasma, but the persistence of high plasma levels in neonatal plasma argues for predominant fetal production. Also, $1,25(OH)_2D$ or $24,25(OH)_2D$ may play a role in fetal cartilage growth and bone mineral accretion.[206] These concepts are summarized in Figure 22-11.

Endocrine Pancreas: Insulin and Glucagon

Embryogenesis of the pancreas is mediated in the mouse by a series of homeobox genes and transcription factors that program pancreatic budding from the gut tube, development of branching ducts and undifferentiated epithelium, differentiation of exocrine and endocrine cell lineages that originate from endodermal tissue, and organization of the endocrine cells into islets of Langerhans. The process begins at day 8 of the 21-day gestation and extends 2 to 3 weeks after birth (Fig. 22-12).[207] Studies in mice have shown that knockout of the *Pdx1, HlxB9, Isl1,* or *Hes1* genes results in pancreatic agenesis or dysgenesis. In humans, mutations in PDX1 are associated with neonatal diabetes mellitus due to pancreatic agenesis. In mice, *NGN3* or *Beta2* knockout leads to complete absence of endocrine cells, whereas knockout of the lower pathway genes shown in Figure 22-13 impairs specific islet cell differentiation.[207] Members of the EGF family of growth factors, laminin, and perhaps other growth factors including the IGFs contribute to pancreatic growth and differentiation.[208,209]

The human fetal pancreas is identifiable by 4 weeks of gestation, and alpha and beta cells can be recognized by 8 to 9 weeks. Insulin, glucagon, somatostatin, and pancreatic polypeptide are measurable by 8 to 10 weeks of gestation.[210] Alpha cells are more numerous than beta cells in the early fetal pancreas and reach a relative peak at midgestation; beta cells continue to increase throughout the second half of gestation, so that, by term, the ratio of alpha to beta cells is approximately 1 : 1. The insulin content of

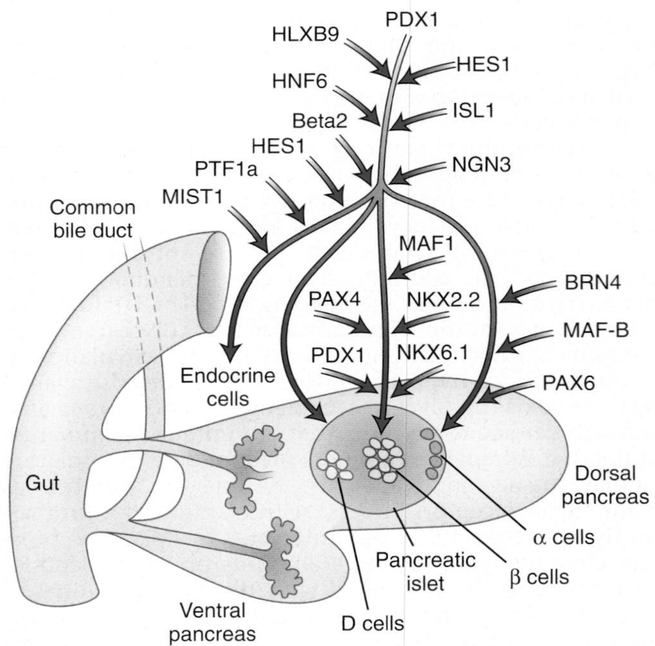

Figure 22-12 Expression of transcription factors during pancreatic embryogenesis. Knockout of *PDX1, HLXB9,* or *ISL1* is associated with early arrest of pancreatic development. *HLXB9* knockout leads to failure of the pancreatic dorsal bud to develop with decreased beta cell number in the remnant pancreas. *HES1* or neurogenin 3 *(NGN3)* disruption leads to aplasia or hypoplasia of the islets of Langerhans. Disruption of the downstream transcription factors impairs formation of the beta cells or alpha cells. *SOX9* and *HNF3B* (not shown) are required for early foregut formation and pancreas specification. (From Habener JF, Kemp DM, Thomas MJ. Mini review: transcriptional regulation in pancreatic development. *Endocrinology.* 2005;146: 1025-1034.)

the pancreas increases from less than 3.6 pmol/g (0.5 U/g) at 7 to 10 weeks to 30 pmol/g (4 U/g) at 16 to 25 weeks of gestation and 93 pmol/g (13 U/g) near term; the concentration in the adult pancreas is approximately 14 pmol/g (2 U/g).[211] Endocrine cells are dispersed throughout the exocrine tissues by 20 weeks, and the islets of Langerhans are clearly differentiated by 31 weeks.

Although the fetal beta cell is functional by 14 to 24 weeks of gestation, secretion of insulin into the bloodstream by the fetal pancreas is low. Insulin release from the fetal rat pancreas in vitro in response to glucose or pyruvate is minimal but can be stimulated by leucine, arginine, tolbutamide, or potassium chloride, indicating that parts of the secretory mechanism are functional in the fetus.[211-213] Insulin secretion in adult islets is mediated by two or more mechanisms, including stimulation of the adenylate cyclase system with production of cyclic adenosine monophosphate (cAMP) and inhibition of potassium efflux, which leads to depolarization of the cell membrane and opening of voltage-dependent calcium channels. The former mechanism, although suppressed in the fetal islets, can be augmented by theophylline, but calcium channel activation does not occur in fetal islets in response to initiators of insulin release that cause depolarization of adult islet cells.[213] Infusion of glucose or arginine to pregnant women before hysterotomy fails to provoke fetal insulin secretion at midgestation or near term, and plasma insulin concentrations in the late human fetus are relatively unresponsive to high glucose concentrations before the onset of labor.[211]

Similar observations have been made in the monkey: neither glucose nor arginine stimulated fetal insulin release near term, but glucagon evoked prompt insulin secretion.[211] Late in gestation in the ovine fetus, epinephrine inhibits insulin release through a receptor pathway.[211] In the anencephalic human fetus, the endocrine pancreas develops normally if maternal carbohydrate metabolism is not impaired; however, beta cell hypertrophy and hyperplasia do not occur in the anencephalic fetus nor in decapitated fetal rabbits exposed to chronic hyperglycemia. This lack of beta cell response to hyperglycemia may be the result of deficiency of GH or IGF1 or both, because GH

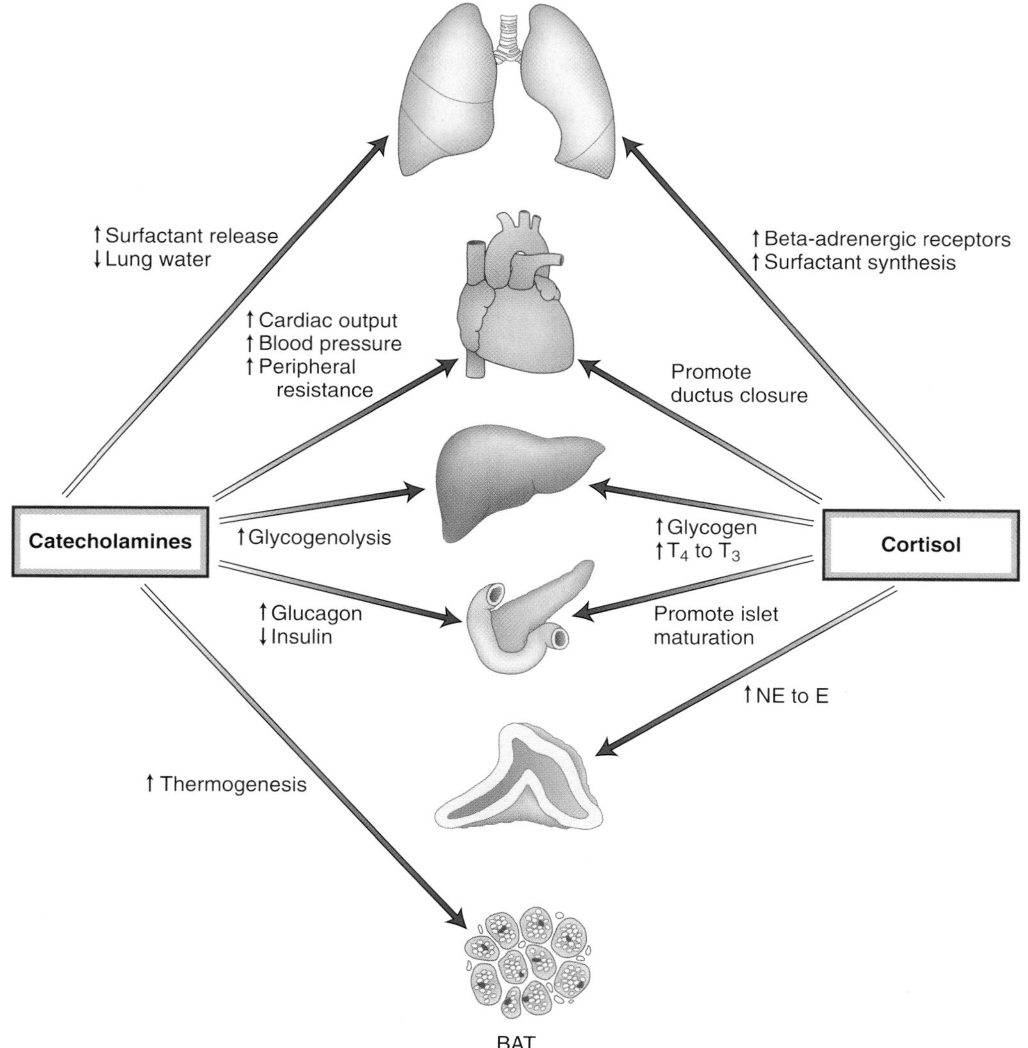

Figure 22-13 Actions of cortisol and catecholamines during fetal adaptation to the extrauterine environment. The prenatal cortisol surge acts to promote functional maturation of several organ systems. The neonatal catecholamine surge triggers or potentiates a number of the extrauterine cardiopulmonary and metabolic functional adaptations that are critical to extrauterine survival. See text for details. *BAT*, brown adipose tissue; *E*, epinephrine; *NE*, norepinephrine; T_3, triiodothyronine; T_4, thyroxine.

stimulates insulin gene expression and may play a permissive role in beta cell hyperplasia and hypertrophy.[209]

Pancreatic glucagon concentrations are relatively high in fetal plasma and increase progressively with fetal age.[211,212] The fetal pancreatic glucagon content at midgestation is approximately 6 μg/g, compared with an adult level of 2 μg/g. As is true for insulin, the capacity for glucagon secretion is blunted in the fetus. Hyperglycemia does not suppress fetal plasma glucagon concentrations in rats, monkeys, or sheep, and acute hypoglycemia does not evoke glucagon secretion in the rat fetus. Amino acids, which are important secretagogues for insulin and glucagon in the adult, probably have little role in modulating insulin and glucagon secretion in the preterm fetus. However, infusion of alanine into women at term increases both maternal and cord blood glucagon concentrations, indicating a fetal glucagon response to amino acids in the term fetus. Catecholamines also evoke glucagon release in the near-term ovine fetus.[211]

Therefore, the fetal pancreatic islet cells, although histologically mature and capable of hormone synthesis and hyperplasia, are relatively immature functionally at birth with regard to their capacity to secrete insulin and glucagon. The rapid maturation of responsiveness to glucose in the neonatal period in both premature and mature infants suggests that this blunted state may be a secondary result of the relatively stable fetal serum glucose concentrations maintained by placental transfer of maternal glucose rather than a primary, temporally fixed maturation process. Alternatively, the lack of any enteric signal to the pancreas from feeding via release of incretins may also account for this stability. The blunted capacity for insulin and glucagon secretion has been related to a deficient capacity of the fetal pancreatic islet cells to generate cAMP or to rapid destruction of cAMP by phosphodiesterase, or both.[211]

In rodents, a period of a rapid increase in beta cell mass at the time of birth and shortly thereafter has been observed, and this rapid change is attenuated by a period of apoptosis before adult mass is achieved. Beta cell mass is more difficult to determine from a developmental standpoint in humans. At birth in the human, there are some 200 to 300 $\times 10^6$ beta cells, which is approximately one third of the population present in adulthood. However, most of the actual mass change takes place in the newborn period and is associated with changes in beta cell size rather than number.[214] Thereafter, there is rapid further expansion in terms of cell numbers, but the waxing and waning of the beta cell mass, particularly with pregnancy, is poorly understood. How much beta cell mass is a determinant of duration to type 2 diabetes mellitus is unclear.

Insulin and glucagon are normally not necessary for substrate metabolism in the fetus.[212] Glucose is obtained by placental transfer through facilitated diffusion. The fetal respiratory quotient is approximately 1, which suggests that glucose is the primary energy substrate for the fetus. Other substrates, such as amino acids and lactate, may also be utilized in the human as in the sheep fetus. However, at least early in gestation, hepatic metabolism and substrate utilization appear to be independent of insulin and to be modulated in an autoregulatory fashion by glucose.[211] In addition, the constant supply of glucose normally precludes the necessity for endogenous gluconeogenesis, and gluconeogenic enzyme activities are low in the fetal liver.

Glycogen storage in the fetus is modulated by fetal glucocorticoids and probably by placental lactogen (hPL). Fetal insulin plays a role near term, when insulin also has the capacity to increase fetal glucose uptake and lipogenesis.[211,212] Insulin receptors are present on most fetal cells in higher numbers than on adult cells; moreover, hyperinsulinemia fails to downregulate fetal insulin receptors.[211] Fetal hepatic glucagon receptors, in contrast, are reduced in number, and fetal liver is relatively resistant to the glycemic effect of glucagon. These conditions tend to potentiate the fetal anabolic milieu during the period of rapid growth in the last trimester of gestation.

Poorly controlled maternal diabetes mellitus is associated with fetal macrosomia, an increased risk of spontaneous abortion, and fetal malformation. Maternal hyperglycemia also leads to hyperinsulinism and beta cell hyperplasia in the infant. Infants of diabetic mothers are prone to polycythemia, renal vein thrombosis, hypocalcemia, respiratory distress syndrome, jaundice, persistent fetal circulation, cardiomyopathy, congenital heart disease, and malformations of other organs.

NEUTRALIZATION OF HORMONE ACTIONS IN THE FETUS

After the period of embryogenesis, the fetal milieu is programmed to optimize body growth and organ development through an array of generalized and specialized growth factors (see "Fetal Growth"). These function in a stable metabolic environment with substrate supply maintained by the placenta. The endocrine and metabolic systems characterizing the extrauterine environment are programmed to maintain metabolic stability in a changing external environment with intermittent substrate provision. Hormonal systems in the fetus are programmed to maintain anabolism with minimal hormonal perturbation. Therefore, production of catabolic and thermogenic hormones is limited, and the effects of the hormones altering metabolic substrate supply and distribution pathways are muted (Table 22-5).

TABLE 22-5

Neutralization of Hormone Actions in the Fetus*

PRODUCTION OF INACTIVE METABOLITES	
Active Hormone	**Inactive Metabolites**
Cortisol	Cortisone
Thyroxine (T_4)	rT_3, T_4S, rT_3S
Triiodothyronine (T_3)	T_3S, T_2
DELAYED EXPRESSION OR NEUTRALIZATION OF RECEPTORS	
Active Hormone	**Receptor**
Growth hormone (GH)	GHR
Thyroid hormone	TRα, TRβ
Catecholamines	β-AR
Estrogens	ER
Glucagon	GR
LIMITED HORMONE SECRETION	
Active Hormone	**Secretory Cell**
Insulin	Islet cell beta
Glucagon	Islet cell alpha

*See text for details.

AR, adrenergic receptor; T_2, diiodothyronine; rT_3, reverse T_3; T_4S, T_4 sulfate.

Limitation of Hormone Secretion

The human fetal pancreas is functional during the second trimester, but secretion of insulin in response to glucose or pyruvate is minimal until the neonatal period.[211,212] Glucagon secretion is also blunted, although fetal blood glucagon levels are relatively high. Fetal islet hyperplasia and increased insulin secretion occur in response to chronic hyperglycemia (e.g., in the infant of a diabetic mother), and insulin release can be stimulated by acute fetal infusions of leucine, arginine, or tolbutamide.[211,213] Moreover, responsiveness of both insulin and glucagon secretion to glucose develops rapidly in the neonatal period.[211] It is not clear whether the limited fetal islet cell responsiveness results from the relatively stable fetal serum glucose levels or from a temporally fixed maturation process (see earlier discussion).

Production of Inactive Metabolites

Throughout the second half of gestation, cortisol is metabolized in fetal tissues to inactive cortisone through the activity of HSD11B2. The placenta is permeable to steroid hormones, including cortisol. During midgestation, placental HSD11B2 activity is low, and some cortisol is transferred to the fetus. Placental HSD11B2 activity increases during the second half of pregnancy under the control of placental estrogens, and enzyme activity near term is high.[16,215] Maternal-fetal cortisol transfer decreases progressively. In addition, although many adult tissues can convert cortisone to cortisol, conversion is limited during most of fetal life. Consequently, most of the cortisol that crosses the placenta or is produced by the fetus is inactivated to cortisone by the placenta or by fetal tissues.

Levels of cortisone in fetal plasma exceed those of cortisol by threefold to fourfold until after 30 weeks of gestation (see Fig. 22-6). Teleologically, this would help preserve the anabolic and growth-promoting milieu of the fetus and minimize premature maturational and parturitional effects of cortisol. After 30 weeks, the ratio of cortisol to cortisone in fetal tissues and plasma increases as a result of increased fetal secretion and decreased conversion of cortisol to cortisone within the placenta and fetal tissues.[215] Cortisol has an important maturational action on several fetal tissues near term (see later discussion).

Fetal thyroid hormone metabolism is characterized by conversion of active thyroid hormones to inactive rT_3 and inactive sulfated iodothyronines and by limited receptor and postreceptor responsiveness to thyroid hormone in selected tissues.[109,118] The placenta contains an iodothyronine inner-ring monodeiodinase that catalyzes conversion of maternal T_4 to rT_3. The fetal sheep liver and kidney, in contrast to the adult liver and kidney, manifest low levels of D1 outer-ring monodeiodinase activity, so conversion of T_4 to active T_3 is limited and large amounts of inactive iodothyronine sulfoconjugates accumulate.[109,120] As a consequence, plasma T_3 levels in the fetus remain low until the last few weeks of gestation (see Fig. 22-8). Selected fetal tissues (brain, brown adipose tissue) have active D2 outer-ring monodeiodinase activities that contribute to local tissue T_3 concentrations; local T_3 is important in development, particularly in the hypothyroid fetus.[109,216] Near term and in the neonatal period in the human fetus, the dramatic increase in plasma T_3 levels, and presumably in T_3 production, heralds the onset of thyroid hormone actions on growth and development and on metabolism (see Fig. 22-8).

Neutralization of Receptor Response

Selected ovine fetal tissues seem relatively unresponsive to thyroid hormones. Fetal ovine liver and kidney thermogenesis—as evidenced by oxygen consumption, sodium-potassium pump (Na^+,K^+-ATPase) activity, and mitochondrial α-glycerophosphate activity—is unresponsive to exogenous T_3 during the third trimester, and thyroid hormone responsiveness in a number of tissues (cardiac, hepatic, renal, and skin) develops only during the perinatal period.[217] β-Adrenergic receptor binding in heart and lung of the ovine fetus is unresponsive to T_3 late in the third trimester but increases in response to T_3 in the neonatal period.[97,217] In rodent species, in which development at birth is comparable to human fetal development at midgestation, pituitary GH concentrations become responsive to thyroid hormone only during the first weeks of extrauterine life.[218] Mouse submandibular gland EGF and NGF levels become responsive to thyroid hormone during the second week of life, as do urine and kidney EGF concentrations and hepatic EGF receptor levels.[219,220] Mouse skin EGF levels and EGF receptors are responsive during the first neonatal week.[221,222] Therefore, despite the presence of nuclear T_3 receptors in significant concentrations in developing rat and sheep fetuses, many thyroid hormone actions in these species are delayed.[223] The mechanism of this delayed thyroid hormone responsiveness is not clear; developmental programming of iodothyronine monodeiodinase expression and gene expression programming via unliganded TRs or TR-interacting corepressors probably all play a role.

The effect of the high circulating concentrations of GH in the fetus is also limited. Fetal somatic growth is only partially GH dependent; indeed, the GH-deficient fetus has little or no growth retardation.[58,,224] The paucity of fetal GH effects is due to delayed maturation of GH receptors or postreceptor mechanisms. In animals such as sheep, hepatic GH receptor binding appears only during the neonatal period.[58] Receptor deficiency may also be a factor in the limited PRL bioactivity in the fetus near term.[58]

There is less information on fetal hormone responsiveness in other systems. β-Adrenergic receptor binding in heart and lung of the sheep fetus is relatively low near term and increases in the neonatal period in response to thyroid hormones.[217] Premature lambs have an augmented plasma catecholamine surge at birth but have a relatively mild increase in plasma free fatty acid levels, which suggests reduced catecholamine responsiveness.[225] The high concentrations of progesterone and estrogens in fetal blood also seem to have limited effects in the fetus. Progesterone receptors are present in low concentration in fetal guinea pig kidney, lung, and uterus at midgestation and increase progressively until term.[226] ERs appear in neonatal rat uterus, oviduct, cervix, and vagina during the first 10 days of extrauterine life, and both ERα and ERβ mRNAs are present in human fetal tissues during the second trimester.[159,227] The human neonate often manifests mild breast enlargement at birth, and vaginal estrogenization may be evident in female infants at birth. Estrogen effects otherwise appear to be limited (see Table 22-5).

FETAL GROWTH

Insulin-Like Growth Factors

The IGFs are involved in regulation of uterine and placental growth during pregnancy. In early embryonic and fetal development, IGF1, EGF, and estrogens are mitogens for endometrial stromal cells, and the endometrial contents of IGF1 and IGF1 mRNA are high at implantation and during early embryogenesis in the sow.[228] Uterine IGF1 and IGF1 mRNA levels decrease progressively with advancing gestation.[228] Placental tissue also contains IGF1 and IGF2 mRNAs, significant concentrations of the respective proteins, and IGF1 receptors.[16] Autocrine and paracrine roles for the IGFs in uterine and placental tissues are postulated. IGF1 and insulin are produced by embryonic tissues during the prepancreatic stage of mouse development, and both factors stimulate growth of embryonic mouse cells.[229]

IGF2 is genomically imprinted and paternally expressed in the fetus and placenta. The mature IGF2 protein is generated from the biologically inactive pro-IGF2 peptide by the action of proprotein convertase 4. Recent studies have shown a role of IGF2 in determining placental nutrient supply and, hence, fetal growth.[230] In mutant mice lacking the imprinted placental-specific IGF2 transcript, growth of the placenta is altered from early gestation, but fetal growth is normal until late gestation, suggesting functional adaptation of the placenta to meet the fetal demands. It is believed that this adaptation may be mediated by the altered expression of placental transporters GLUT3 and Slc38a4.[231]

Studies of transgenic mice with null mutations of the genes encoding *IGF1, IGF2,* or the IGF1 receptor have defined the role of the somatomedins; the birth weight of the embryos lacking IGF1 or IGF2 was only 60% that of control mice. When both genes were inactive, birth weight was reduced another 30%, and mice lacking the IGF1 receptor had birth weights averaging 45% of control values.[56] IGF2-deficient mice also manifested intrauterine growth retardation in association with a small placenta. They had near-normal postnatal growth but delayed bone development.[56] IGF2-receptor knockout fetal mice are 30% overweight, suggesting a negative growth-modulating effect of this receptor.

The normal growth in fetuses with both IGF1 and IGF2 receptor knockout is caused by IGF1 signaling via the insulin receptor; combined IGF1, IGF2, and insulin receptor knockout results in severe intrauterine growth retardation and fetal death. Knockout of individual IGF binding proteins has little effect on fetal or placental growth.[56] In humans, mutations in *IGFI* or *IGFIR* are associated with intrauterine growth retardation,[232,233] suggesting that IGF1 signaling contributes significantly to fetal growth.

Hypomethylation of the 11p15 imprinted region has been associated with the phenotype of Silver-Russell syndrome.[234] This results in the relaxation of imprinting and biallelic expression of *H19* and downregulation of *IGF2*. Additionally, abnormal processing of IGF2 by proprotein convertase 4 in the placenta has been implicated in the etiology of fetal growth restriction.[235] Pregnant women carrying fetuses with intrauterine growth retardation (IUGR, low birth weight for gestational age) had higher levels of pro-IGF2 compared with controls. More recently, Murphy and colleagues reported severe intrauterine growth retardation and atypical diabetes mellitus secondary to insulin resistance in association with disruption of regulation of the *IGF2* gene.[236] On the other hand, overexpression of IGF2 as a result of loss of imprinting associated with uniparental paternal disomy, *CDKN1C* gene loss of function, alteration in the KvLQT1 differentially methylated region (DMR), or microdeletions in the human H19 DMR is associated with overgrowth in the form of Beckwith-Wiedemann syndrome.[237]

IGF-binding proteins (IGFBPs) are present as early as 5 weeks of gestation; prenatally as postnatally, the IGFs circulate in association with binding proteins.[56] High concentrations of circulating IGFBP1 are associated with fetal growth restriction in the mouse, as is overexpression of fetal IGFBP1 in the human.[238,239] Therefore, during fetal and postnatal life, plasma concentrations of IGFs are relatively high compared with tissue concentrations. In the fetus, IGF2 levels are five to six times higher than those of IGF1, in contrast to these concentrations in children and adults, and concentrations of both increase progressively throughout gestation.[240] Fetal concentrations of both peptides at term are 30% to 50% of the adult concentrations.

In most studies, cord blood IGF1 concentrations correlate with birth size.[56] Despite the fetal growth–enhancing effects of IGF2, blood concentrations are only weakly related to size at birth, largely because of the inhibiting effect of soluble IGF2 receptor (IGF2R)[241] but also because IGF2 appears to exert most of its growth effects in the earlier part of gestation. Soluble IGF2R is derived through proteolytic cleavage of the transmembrane region of the receptor in many tissues. IGF receptors have been identified as early as 5 weeks of gestation and are widespread in fetal tissues.[56] IGF1 stimulates glycogenesis in cultured fetal rat hepatocytes and induces formation of myotubes in cultured myoblasts. IGF2 is active in cultured muscle and neonatal rat astroglial cells. Insulin receptors are increased in fetal cells and are resistant to downregulation; no similar data are available for the IGF1 receptor.

As discussed earlier, the control of IGF production differs in fetal and postnatal life. GH receptors are relatively deficient, and receptors for hPL predominate in fetal tissues.[58,59] GH does play a minor role in the fetus, as reflected in the low IGF concentrations and slight reduction in birth weight and length in infants with GH resistance (Laron dwarfism) and growth hormone deficiency.[224] hPL stimulates IGF1 production and augments amino acid transport and DNA synthesis in human fetal fibroblasts and muscle cells.[58] IGF1 and IGF2 levels are reduced in fetuses of protein-starved pregnant rats, and the low IGF2 levels are reversed by hPL.[242] Thyroidectomy of the third-trimester sheep fetus impairs skeletal muscle growth in association with a decrease in muscle GH receptor mRNA and IGF1 mRNA without an effect on IGF2 levels.[243] This period is equivalent to the postnatal period in the human, and there is no evidence that thyroid hormones modulate GH receptor or IGF1 levels in the human fetus. Glucocorticoids can inhibit fetal growth, presumably by inhibiting IGF gene transcription.[243]

Nutrition is the major factor modulating IGF production in the fetus. IGF concentrations fall in suckling rats deprived of milk, and IGF1 and IGF2 concentrations are reduced in fetuses of protein-starved pregnant rats and placentally restricted sheep.[56,57] These data support the view that the IGFs are important in embryonic and fetal growth and that in the fetus they are regulated, at least in part, by hPL and by nutritional substrate derived transplacentally. The high concentrations of IGF2 in fetal rat serum, the high levels of IGF2 mRNA in fetal tissues, and the presence of a truncated form of IGF1 in human fetal brain tissue suggest unique developmental actions of these peptides.

Insulin

Insulin has been proposed to act as a fetal growth factor. Infants born to women with diabetes mellitus may have hyperinsulinemia associated with increased birth weight.[244] Most of this increased weight is accounted for by body fat; there is little increase in body length, but some organomegaly may occur. Infants with hyperinsulinemia caused by congenital hyperinsulinism or the Beckwith-Wiedemann syndrome may also have increased somatic growth in utero. Conversely, the human fetus with pancreatic agenesis is small and has decreased muscle bulk and little or no adipose tissue.[244]

Mice with insulin or insulin receptor gene mutations have a 10% decrease in birth weight and early neonatal death with hyperglycemia and ketonemia.[56] Insulin receptor mutations in humans lead to severe intrauterine growth retardation and limited postnatal weight gain.[56] In contrast to mice, the human fetus during the latter half of gestation has a significant increase in adipose mass, and adipose tissue is highly sensitive to insulin. In clinical conditions associated with fetal hyperinsulinemia, the human neonate is born large for gestation age, primarily due to increased lipogenesis mediated by insulin or IGF1 receptors.

Epidermal Growth Factor/Transforming Growth Factor System

The EGF/TGF-α system has been characterized in considerable detail.[245,246] EGF is a 6-kd peptide product of a large, 1207-amino-acid precursor molecule and acts through a 170-kd membrane receptor glycoprotein. This receptor, like the IGF receptor, has intrinsic tyrosine kinase activity, and tyrosine kinase–mediated autophosphorylation is a critical event in EGF signal transduction. TGF-α, which has 35% amino acid homology with murine EGF and 44% homology with human EGF, also acts through the EGF receptor system.[245,246] Several additional family members have been characterized, including amphiregulin, heparin-binding EGF, betacellulin, and neuregulins.[246] Three additional receptors are referred to as ErbB2, ErbB3, and ErbB4 in animals; the human receptors are called human EGF receptor 2 (HER2), HER3, and HER4.[246]

EGF, pre-pro-EGF mRNA, and EGF receptors are present in most tissues in the postnatal rodent, but mRNA levels are highest in salivary glands and kidneys. EGF and pre-pro-EGF mRNA levels are absent or low in the fetal mouse and remain low in mouse tissues during the early neonatal period.[247] Nonetheless, the EGF receptor knockout mouse exhibits epithelial immaturity and multiorgan failure with early death.[247] Tissue concentrations of both EGF and EGF mRNA increase in the mouse during the first 2 months of postnatal life; indeed, concentrations of EGF in the salivary glands increase several thousand-fold between 3 weeks and 3 months of age. Mouse urinary levels increase 200-fold and kidney concentrations increase 10-fold between 1 week and 2 months of age. EGF concentrations in mouse ocular tissues increase 100-fold during the first week of life.[245] Liver EGF concentrations increase more slowly, as do serum levels, and there is a high degree of correlation between serum and liver EGF levels in the developing mouse.[245] Therefore, the production of EGF in the rodent is accelerated during the early neonatal period, and it is during this time that most hormone-stimulated growth and development occur.

Fetal mouse and human tissues have high concentrations of TGF-α.[246,248,249] Immunoreactive TGF-α concentrations in mice are measurable at relatively high levels in lung, brain, liver, and kidney tissues in the fetal/neonatal rat, and the ontogenic pattern of TGF-α is tissue specific; most late fetal tissues studied contained TGF-α, and levels persisted or increased in most tissues through the period of growth and development.[248] In rodents and sheep, EGF provokes precocious eyelid opening and tooth eruption in neonatal animals; stimulates lung maturation; promotes palatal development in organ culture; stimulates gastrointestinal maturation; evokes secretion of pituitary hormones including GH, PRL, and corticotropin; and stimulates secretion of chorionic gonadotropin and placental lactogen by the placenta.[245,247] Both EGF and TGF-α compete for binding to the EGF receptor, and both factors accelerate eye opening and tooth eruption in the neonatal rodent, presumably through interaction with the same EGF receptor.[245]

Considerable evidence suggests a role for the EGF family of growth factors in mammalian CNS development.[259] EGF, TGF-α, neuregulins, and the EGF receptors are widely distributed in the nervous system.[245,250-253] EGF promotes proliferation of astroglial cells, acts as an astroglial differentiation factor, and enhances survival and outgrowth of selected neuronal cells.[250,251] Transgenic mice with a deficiency of neuregulin, ErbB2, ErbB3, or ErbB4 die in utero with cardiac anomalies and developmental anomalies of the hindbrain, midbrain, and ventral forebrain (see Table 22-5).[252,253]

EGF also plays an important role in rodent pregnancy. Maternal salivary gland and plasma EGF concentrations in the mouse increase fourfold to fivefold during pregnancy.[254] Removal of the salivary glands prevents the increase in plasma EGF; moreover, salivary gland removal reduces the number of mice completing term pregnancy (by 50%), decreases the percentage of live pups, and decreases the crown-rump length of fetuses delivered.[254] Administration of EGF antiserum to pregnant mice without salivary glands further increases the abortion rate, whereas administration of EGF improves pregnancy outcome.[254] Because maternal EGF is too large a molecule to traverse the placental barrier, an effect on maternal metabolism or on the placenta is likely.[254] The placenta is richly endowed with EGF receptors, and placental tissue binds and degrades EGF to constituent amino acids.[245] TGF-α is also produced by the maternal deciduus in rodents and stimulates proliferation of decidual tissue and decidual PRL production.

Nerve Growth Factor

NGF is a 13-kd protein that is present at high concentrations in mouse salivary gland and at low concentrations in many adult tissues.[246] It is also produced by human placental tissue. It is the original member of an expanding family of neurotropic growth factors that now includes brain-derived neurotropic factor, neurotropin 3, and two less well-characterized factors; these ligands act via two receptors, NGF and NGF2 (or Trk).[246,255] NGF binds to high-affinity plasma membrane receptors and is internalized and transported to subcellular organelles, including the nucleus, in neurons of the peripheral nervous system. It promotes neurite outgrowth and enhances tyrosine hydroxylase and dopamine β-hydroxylase activities in developing sympathetic neurons. NGF acts on undifferentiated sympathetic cell precursors to evoke both hyperplastic and hypertrophic effects and plays a permissive role in stimulating the development of immature autonomic neurons along either a sympathetic or a cholinergic pathway.[246,256]

The injection of NGF in neonatal mice causes a marked increase in the volume of the superior cervical ganglia and increases the nerve supply of body organs. Likewise, injection of NGF antiserum during early neonatal life results in a decrease in the size of the superior cervical ganglia, reduction in tyrosine hydroxylase activity, and permanent sympathectomy.[256] Maternal NGF autoantibodies in rats and rabbits impair autonomic nervous system development in utero.[257] This impairment affects sympathetic and dorsal root ganglia and autonomic innervation of peripheral organs. NGF is produced by neonatal mouse astroglial cells in tissue culture, is present in developing mouse brain tissue, and, together with brain-derived neurotropic factor and neurotropin 3, plays an important role in brain development.[254,255,258] Thyroid hormones and testosterone modulate postnatal NGF levels in the submandibular gland of the mouse. Thyroid hormones increase NGF, neurotropin 3, and brain-derived neurotropic factor mRNA levels in adult rat brain.[245,259]

Other Factors

Additional growth factors are involved in fetal growth and development, including hematopoietic growth factors, platelet-derived growth factors (PDGFs), fibroblast growth factors (FGFs), vascular endothelial growth factor (VEGF), and members of the TGF-β family.[56,246] Hematopoietic growth factors are also active in the fetus during development; erythropoietin in fetal sheep is produced by the liver rather than the kidney, and erythropoietin gene expression in fetal sheep is regulated by glucocorticoids.[260] A switch to kidney production occurs after parturition.[261] Postnatally, thyroid hormones, testosterone, and hypoxia modulate erythropoietin production. PDGF represents a family of homodimers and heterodimers of PDGFA and PDGFB chains derived from two gene loci.[262] Two PDGF receptors have been characterized, PDGFα and PDGFβ. The genes for PDGF and its receptors are expressed in many tissues. *PDGFA* gene inactivation in mice leads to defects in lung, skin, intestine, testes, and brain resulting in early postnatal death.[262] *PDGFB* gene inactivation leads to microvessel disruption and leakage with hemorrhage, edema, and intrauterine death.

The FGF family of heparin-binding growth factors now includes 17 members with diverse effects on development, angiogenesis, wound healing, and other biologic systems.[263,264] These effects are mediated by ligand-activated tyrosine protein kinase receptors (FGFRs) transcribed from four related genes. Several receptor isoforms are products of alternative RNA splicing.[56,246] Targeted disruptions of *FGF* and *FGFR* genes in mice have defined critical roles in development.[246,263] FGF3-deficient mice show tail and inner ear defects. Knockout of the *FGF4* gene is lethal, leading to early death. Knockout of the *FGFR1* gene also leads to early fetal death. *FGF10* knockout mice die at birth because of pulmonary agenesis. Deficiency of FGF4, FGF8, FGF9, FGF10, or FGF17 is associated with limb deformities. FGF8 deficiency leads to abnormal left-right axis patterning. In mice, *FGFR3* knockout results in chondrocyte hypertrophy and increased bone length.[246] In humans, a variety of gain-of-function *FGFR* mutations are associated with chondrodysplasias and craniosynostosis syndromes.[246] FGF, like EGF, stimulates the production of hCG from a choriocarcinoma cell line.[264] These observations and the fact that the placenta contains FGF, NGF, TGF-α, TGF-β, IGF1, and IGF2 suggest that the placenta plays an important role in modulating fetal growth.

TRANSITION TO EXTRAUTERINE LIFE

The transition to extrauterine life involves abrupt delivery from the protected intrauterine environment and succor by the placenta into the relatively hostile extrauterine environment. The neonate must initiate air breathing and defend against hypothermia, hypoglycemia, and hypocalcemia as the placental supply of energy and nutritional substrate is removed. Both the adrenal cortex and the autonomic nervous system, including the para-aortic chromaffin system, are essential for extrauterine adaptation. Longer-term transition requires adaptation to an environment of intermittent nutrient supply and transient substrate deficiency and requires maturation of the secretory control mechanisms for the PTH-calcitonin system and the endocrine pancreas.

Cortisol Surge

In most mammals, a cortisol surge occurs near term and is mediated by increased cortisol production by the fetal adrenal and a decreased rate of conversion of cortisol to cortisone. Pepe and Albrecht have proposed that the preterm fetal cortisol surge is due to the progressive stimulation by estrogens of placental HSD11B2 activity and the subsequent increase in placental conversion of cortisol to cortisone.[215] The resulting decrease in maternal-to-fetal cortisol transfer results in stimulation of fetal CRH and corticotropin secretion through the negative-feedback control loop. The concomitant estrogen-stimulated increase in HSD11B2 activity in fetal tissues potentiates the relative fetal cortisol deficiency and the CRH-corticotropin response.[215] Placental CRH may also potentiate fetal adrenal activation. Recent data suggest an increase in HSD11B1 expression and activity in placenta and intrauterine fetal membranes during late gestation, with a consequent increase in local cortisol production in preparation for parturition.[265]

The cortisol surge augments surfactant synthesis in lung tissue; increases lung liquid reabsorption; increases adrenomedullary PNMT activity, which in turn increases methylation of NE to epinephrine; increases hepatic iodothyronine outer-ring monodeiodinase activity and hence conversion of T_4 to T_3; decreases sensitivity of the ductus arteriosus to prostaglandins, facilitating ductus closure; induces maturation of several enzymes and transport processes of the small intestine; and stimulates maturation of hepatic enzymes (see Fig. 22-13).[80,266] In some cases, these events involve increased synthesis of specific proteins or enzymes. In other instances, such as the action on the ductus arteriosus, the mechanism remains obscure.

Secondary effects of cortisol also promote extrauterine adaptations. The increased T_3 levels stimulate β-adrenergic receptor binding, potentiate surfactant synthesis in lung tissue, and increase the sensitivity of brown adipose tissue to NE. The significance of prenatal cortisol is demonstrated by the effects of gene-targeted CRH or glucocorticoid receptor deficiency in mice; the progeny of homozygous CRH-deficient or glucocorticoid receptor–deficient animals die in the first 12 hours with lung dysplasia and surfactant deficiency.[267,268]

Catecholamine Surge

Parturition also evokes a dramatic catecholamine surge in the newborn, resulting in extraordinarily high levels of NE, epinephrine, and dopamine in cord blood.[185] As discussed earlier, plasma NE concentrations exceed epinephrine concentrations because of peripheral and adrenomedullary and para-aortic catecholamine release. Cord blood NE levels of 15 nmol/L (2500 pg/mL) and epinephrine concentrations of 2 nmol/L (370 pg/mL) are common after spontaneous delivery of term infants.[185] Concentrations of 25 nmol/L (4200 pg/mL) of NE and 35 nmol/L (640 pg/mL) of epinephrine are common in cord blood of premature infants. These changes evoke critical cardiovascular adaptations, including increased blood pressure and increased cardiac inotropic effects; increased glucagon secretion; decreased insulin secretion; increased thermogenesis in brown adipose tissue and increased plasma free fatty acid levels; and pulmonary adaptation, including mobilization of pulmonary fluid and increased surfactant release.[185,189,265]

Thermogenesis in Neonatal Brown Adipose Tissue

Brown adipose tissue is the major site of thermogenesis in the newborn and is especially prominent in the mammalian fetus. The largest accumulations of brown adipose tissue envelop the kidneys and adrenal glands, and smaller amounts surround the blood vessels of the mediastinum and neck.[269] The mass of brown adipose tissue peaks at the time of birth and gradually decreases during the early weeks of life. Surgical removal of this tissue leads to neonatal hypothermia. NE, through β-adrenergic receptors, stimulates thermogenesis by brown adipose tissue, and optimal responsiveness of this tissue to NE is dependent on thyroid hormone.[269,270] Brown adipose tissue is rich in mitochondria containing a unique 32-kd protein (thermogenin) that uncouples oxidation and phosphorylation of adenosine diphosphate, reduces ATP production, and consequently enhances thermogenesis.[269,271] Thermogenin is T_3 dependent, and brown adipose tissue contains a 5′-monoiodothyronine deiodinase that deiodinates T_4 locally to T_3.[269,271] Full maturation of catecholamine-stimulated cellular respiration in brown adipose tissue occurs before delivery in the ovine fetus and requires thyroid hormone.[269,272] Fetal thyroidectomy in this species leads to marked hypothermia, with low plasma free fatty acid levels and increased plasma epinephrine concentrations.[272] In vitro, basal brown adipose tissue thermogenesis and NE-stimulated and dibutyryl cAMP-stimulated thermogenesis are decreased by fetal thyroidectomy.

The rapid onset of thermogenesis in brown adipose tissue is essential for survival in newborn infants. Catecholamine release is the stimulus for brown adipose tissue thermogenesis in the early neonatal period, and responsiveness to catecholamines is markedly increased by cutting of the umbilical cord.[270] Fetal hypoxia and placental inhibitors, including prostaglandin E_2 and adenosine, appear to inhibit brown adipose tissue thermogenesis in utero.[270] Cord cutting, neonatal cooling, catecholamine stimulation, and augmented conversion of T_4 to T_3 in brown adipose tissue in the neonatal period are the essential features that mediate and condition newborn thermogenesis.

Calcium Homeostasis

The neonate must adjust rapidly from a high-calcium environment regulated by PTHrP and calcitonin to a low-calcium environment that requires regulation by PTH and vitamin D. With removal of the placenta in term infants, plasma total calcium concentration falls, reaching a nadir of approximately 2.3 mmol/L (9 mg/dL),[202] and the ionized calcium concentration reaches a low level of about 1.2 mmol/L (4.8 mg/dL) by 24 hours of life.[273] Plasma PTH levels are relatively low in the neonatal period and are minimally responsive to hypocalcemia during the first 2 to 3 days of life. Calcitonin concentrations are high in cord blood (approximately 2000 ng/L), increase further during the early neonatal period, and remain high for several days after birth.[202,274] The relatively obtunded PTH response and the high calcitonin levels lead to a 2- to 3-day period of transient neonatal hypocalcemia.[274,275] Inhibition of calcitonin secretion and stimulation of PTH secretion gradually result in increased serum calcium levels in the neonate. The disappearance of PTHrP in the neonatal lamb is approximately coincident with the time of restoration of calcium levels to the adult range.[202] The mechanism of transition from PTHrP to PTH secretion by the neonatal parathyroid glands is not clear.

Calcium homeostasis is also affected in the human newborn by the low level of glomerular filtration that persists for several days.[274,275] In addition, renal responsiveness to PTH is reduced in the first few days of life. These factors limit phosphate excretion and predispose the neonate to hyperphosphatemia, particularly if the diet includes high-phosphate milk such as unmodified cow's milk. Premature infants, compared with term infants, tend to have lower PTH and higher calcitonin levels and more immature kidney function; in these infants, neonatal hypocalcemia may be more marked and prolonged, and the incidence of symptomatic hypocalcemia is higher. Birth asphyxia also predisposes the neonate to hypocalcemia.[275] Infants born to mothers with hypercalcemia related to hyperparathyroidism have a high incidence of symptomatic hypocalcemia. These infants have a more marked suppression of parathyroid function and a longer period of transient hypoparathyroidism in the neonatal period. PTH secretion and calcium homeostasis usually return to normal in 1 to 2 weeks in full-term infants and within 2 to 3 weeks in the small premature infant.

Glucose Homeostasis

The abrupt withdrawal of the placental glucose supply leads to a prompt fall in plasma glucose in the term neonate.[211,212] The low glucose and high catecholamine levels stimulate glucagon secretion, and the plasma glucagon level peaks within 2 hours after birth.[211,212] Plasma insulin levels are low at birth and tend to fall further with hypoglycemia. The early glucagon response is short-lived; however, concentrations remain at about 100 ng/L for the first 12 to 24 hours, and the glucagon/insulin ratio is high enough to stabilize glucose levels in the range of 2.8 to 4 mmol/L (50 to 70 mg/dL) during this period. The early glucagon and catecholamine surges deplete hepatic glycogen stores, so the return of plasma glucose concentrations to normal after 12 to 18 hours requires maturation of hepatic gluconeogenesis under the stimulus of a high plasma glucagon/insulin ratio.[212] Glucagon secretion gradually increases during the early hours after birth, especially with protein feeding, which stimulates gut glucagon release and pancreatic glucagon secretion.[211,212] Premature infants have more severe and more prolonged hypoglycemia because of reduced glycogen stores and impaired hepatic gluconeogenesis. Infants born to diabetic mothers have more severe neonatal hypoglycemia because of relative hyperinsulinism. In the healthy term infant, glucose homeostasis is achieved within 5 to 7 days of life; in premature infants, 1 to 2 weeks may be required.

Other Hormonal Adaptations

Delivery of the placenta results in decreases in fetal blood concentrations of estrogens, progesterone, hCG, and hPL. The fall in estrogen concentrations presumably removes the major stimulus to fetal pituitary PRL release, and PRL concentrations decrease within several weeks. The relatively delayed fall may be due to lactotrope hyperplasia in the fetal pituitary or to delayed maturation of hypothalamic dopamine secretion. The gradual fall of GH concentrations during the early weeks of life is due to delayed maturation of hypothalamic-pituitary feedback control of GH release.[33] In the neonatal primate, there are concomitant decreases in plasma GH concentrations and GH responsiveness to exogenous GHRH.[276] The mechanisms remain unclear; changes in secretion or in pituitary sensitivity to GHRH or somatostatin, or both, may be involved. IGF1 and IGF2 levels fall to infantile values within a few days, presumably because of the removal of placental hPL and placental IGF production (see Fig. 22-4).

In male infants (see Fig. 22-10), after a transient fall in testosterone concentrations as the hCG stimulus abates, pituitary LH secretion rebounds modestly, and there is a secondary surge of plasma testosterone that persists at significant levels for several weeks.[33,277] This surge is mediated by hypothalamic GnRH; blockade of neonatal activation of the pituitary-testicular axis with a GnRH agonist in neonatal monkeys ablates the neonatal increments in LH and testosterone.[278] Such a blockade also results in subnormal increments in plasma LH and testosterone levels and subnormal testicular enlargement at puberty in these animals, suggesting that neonatal GnRH release with pituitary-testicular activation may be critical for normal sexual maturation of male primates.[278] In females, a transient, secondary surge in FSH may transiently elevate estrogen concentrations.

Delivery results in a reversal of the high fetal cortisone/cortisol ratio, and plasma cortisol concentrations are higher in the neonate despite relatively lower plasma corticotropin concentrations (see Fig. 22-6). Presumably, this increase is due to decreased inhibition of adrenal 3β-HSD by estrogen and perhaps to removal of a placental CRH action on fetal pituitary corticotropin release. Plasma DHEAS and DHEA levels fall as the fetal adrenal atrophies.

The increase in serum thyrotropin levels during the early minutes after birth is due to cooling of the neonate in the extrauterine environment.[97,109] In term infants, the thyrotropin surge peaks at 30 minutes at a concentration of about 70 mU/L (see Fig. 22-8). This peak evokes increased secretion of T_4 and T_3 by the thyroid gland. In addition, increased conversion of T_4 to T_3 by liver and other tissues maintains the T_3 concentration in the extrauterine range of 1.6 to 3.4 nmol/L (105 to 220 ng/dL). The re-equilibration of thyrotropin levels to the normal extrauterine range is probably a result of the readjustment of prevailing serum T_3 concentrations and maturation of feedback control of thyrotropin by thyroid hormones during the early weeks of life.[97,111] Production of rT_3 by fetal and neonatal tissues abates by 3 to 4 weeks of age, at which time serum rT_3 reaches adult levels.

PROGRAMMING OF DEVELOPING ENDOCRINE SYSTEMS

During the past several decades, the concept of the plasticity of fetal endocrine systems has evolved from experiments in several mammalian species indicating that hormonal programming occurs during a critical fetal or perinatal period of development. There is a growing list of examples. In the female rodent, transient neonatal androgen administration masculinizes the pattern of hypothalamic control of GnRH secretion and pituitary gonadotropin secretion, masculinizes adult behavior and adult sexual activity, permanently alters the pattern of GH secretion, increases longitudinal bone growth and body weight, and masculinizes the pattern of hepatic steroid metabolism.[279,280] Prenatal androgens program the timing of neuroendocrine puberty in sheep: the higher the dose of prenatal testosterone, the earlier the initiation of the pubertal LH rise.[281] Estrogen administration to pregnant rats during the last third of gestation produces cryptorchid male offspring and may permanently suppress spermatogenesis in adult males.[282] Transient levothyroxine administration to neonatal rodents leads to growth retardation, delayed puberty, decreased adult pituitary weight, decreased pituitary TRH concentrations, low serum thyrotropin levels, and decreased thyrotropin responsiveness to propylthiouracil challenge.[283,284] Administration of insulin or alloxan to neonatal rats produces permanent alteration of glucose tolerance.[285] A single dose of vasopressin to the neonatal rat permanently enhances the adult response to vasopressin.[286] Fetal exposure to high maternal glucocorticoid levels in the rat inhibits fetal growth and leads to subsequent hypertension in the offspring.[287] Moreover, it has been observed that the permanent programming can be transmitted to later generations, leading to the concept of epigenetic effects.[285,288]

The concept of fetal programming was extended with the observation of ecologic associations between fetal and early-life health indicators (e.g., birth size, infant mortality) and adult diseases. The concept, advanced in the 1980s, that adult diseases have fetal and perinatal genesis has been referred to as the *Barker hypothesis*.[289] There is now extensive documentation of the association of IUGR with an increased risk of later hypertension, insulin resistance, diabetes, and cardiovascular and coronary heart disease.[290-297] The programming involves epigenetic, neuroendocrine, hormonal receptor, and metabolic alterations involving the placenta and fetus.[298-306]

Epigenetic effects include genetic imprinting. Imprinted genes are a class of genes in placental mammals and marsupials whose expression depends on the parental origin.[298-304] Imprinting is controlled epigenetically (by such factors as nutrition) via DNA methylation and chromatin modifications. In mice, imprinted genes in the placenta regulate the supply of nutrients; in the fetus, they control nutrient metabolism.[298] In mice, approximately 60 imprinted genes have been identified, and for most the imprinting status is conserved in humans; many of these genes are involved in the control of fetal growth.[304] Paternally expressed imprinted genes tend to enhance and maternally expressed genes tend to suppress fetal growth. Knockout of paternally expressed genes for IGF2, PEG1, PEG2, and insulin result in IUGR, whereas knockout of the maternal genes *H19*, *IGF2R*, or overexpression of *IGF2* results in fetal overgrowth.[298] Other genetic alterations including modification of tandem repeats in the insulin gene have been described.[299]

Hormones in the fetus are derived from the placenta, from the mother, from fetal endocrine glands, and from circulating precursors in fetal or placental tissues. These extensive networks linking maternal-placental-fetal endocrine interactions, and the apparent plasticity of developing endocrine and metabolic systems, facilitate endocrine system programming. As discussed earlier, the programming may be relatively system limited.[279-287] Other examples include the observation many years ago that diethylstilbestrol administration to pregnant women increased the prevalence of vaginal adenocarcinoma in female offspring during the second and third decades of life.[295] More recently, it was shown that prenatal or neonatal diethylstilbestrol exposure in hamsters and mice perturbs normal uterine development by affecting the genetic pathways programming uterine differentiation and results in hyperplastic and neoplastic uterine lesions with increased levels of cJun, cFos, Myc, Bax, and Bcl-x.[307,308] Excessive androgen exposure during fetal life has been associated with later polycystic ovary syndrome.[295] Hormonal programming also is demonstrable in cell lines and in unicellular organisms, in which a single exposure to a hormone can produce persistent alteration of the hormonal response characteristics or of prohormone processing.[309,310] Undernutrition during pregnancy in the rat results in the development of obesity, hyperinsulinemia, and hyperleptinemia during adult life; this phenotype is potentiated when the offspring are fed a high-fat diet.[311] Neonatal leptin treatment normalized the programmed phenotype, indicating that metabolic programming may be reversible during the period of developmental plasticity.[311]

The effects of maternal undernutrition and fetal IUGR extend to several systems, and it is hypothesized that excessive maternal-fetal glucocorticoids play a significant programming role. Glucocorticoids have wide-ranging effects in the fetus, altering receptors, enzymes, ion channels, and transporters in a variety of cells and tissues in the late-gestation fetus, and can induce programming of other endocrine systems. Throughout gestation, they modify *GLUT* gene expression in placenta and fetus, influence IGF and glucocorticoid receptor gene expression in various tissues, affect expression of several transcription factors, and affect a wide variety of enzymes in placenta, liver, kidney, intestine, and lung.[301] Maternal undernutrition, stress, and placental dysfunction are associated with increased maternal and fetal glucocorticoid levels, which contribute importantly to IUGR and programmed alterations in adult endocrine systems and metabolism.[293,301,302]

MATERNAL AND FETAL MEDICINE

The foregoing review summarizes current understanding of the intrauterine endocrine milieu and highlights progress in this challenging frontier of medicine. This progress has set the stage for fetal endocrine disease diagnosis, therapy for fetal endocrine and metabolic disorders, management of disorders of fetal growth, and diagnosis and management of perinatal or neonatal endocrine dysfunction. In addition, understanding of developmental endocrinology is increasingly relevant to management strategies for premature infants and infants and children with fetal growth retardation and for understanding of the pathogenesis of adult endocrine and metabolic diseases.

We are now entering an era of direct access to and management of the intrauterine environment with provision of medical and surgical fetal therapy, entailing both potential advantages and risks.[312] With expansion of the application and scope of amniotic fluid fetal cell sampling, maternal plasma DNA analysis, and the advent of fetal visualization and intrauterine fetal blood sampling, direct access for fetal diagnosis is now possible.[313-316] Intrauterine diagnosis and treatment of fetal adrenal and thyroid disorders have become the standard of care.[317,318] Intravenous nutritional supplementation of fetal sheep can prevent some forms of growth retardation, and chronic fetal therapy through indwelling pumps is feasible in animal fetuses.[319] These approaches, coupled with increasing availability of synthetic hormones and growth factor agonists and antagonists, facilitate direct fetal endocrine therapy. In addition, intrauterine stem cell transplantation has been successful in the correction of congenital hematologic disease. The fetus in early gestation is a favorable recipient of cellular therapy, and fetal cell transplantation may be applicable to therapy for selected endocrine and metabolic disease.[320,321] Finally, there is a growing experience with fetal and neonatal gene therapy in animals.[322]

REFERENCES

1. Murphy VE, Smith R, Giles WB, et al. Endocrine regulation of human fetal growth: the role of the mother, placenta, and fetus. *Endocrine Rev.* 2006;27:141-169.
2. Fisher DA. Fetal and neonatal endocrinology. In: DeGroot LJ, Jameson JL, eds. *Endocrinology*. 5th ed. Philadelphia, PA: Elsevier Saunders; 2006:3369-3386.
3. Palfi M, Selbing A. Placental transport of maternal immunoglobulin G. *Am J Reprod Immunol.* 1998;39:24-26.
4. Sodha RJ, Proegler M, Schneider H. Transfer and metabolism of norepinephrine studied from maternal to fetal and fetal to maternal sides in the in vitro perfused human placental life. *Am J Obstet Gynecol.* 1984;148:474-481.
5. Benediktsson R, Calder A, Edwards CRW, et al. Placental 11β-hydroxysteroid dehydrogenase: a key regulator of fetal glucocorticoid exposure. *Clin Endocrinol (Oxf).* 1997;46:161-166.
6. Murphy BEP. Cortisol and cortisone in human fetal development. *J Steroid Biochem.* 1979;11:509-513.
7. Takeyama J, Sasano H, Suzuki T, et al. 17β-Hydroxysteroid dehydrogenase types 1 and 2 in human placenta: an immunohistochemical study with correlation to placental development. *J Clin Endocrinol Metab.* 1998;83:3710-3715.
8. Krysin E, Brzezinska-Slebodzinska E, Slebodzinski AB. Divergent deiodination of thyroid hormones in the separated parts of the fetal and maternal placenta in pigs. *J Endocrinol.* 1997;155:295-303.
9. Benediktsson R, Lindsay RD, Noble J, et al. Glucocorticoid exposure in utero: new model for adult hypertension. [Erratum in *Lancet.* 1993;341572.] *Lancet.* 1993;341:339-341.
10. Yau JL, Olsson T, Morris RG, et al. Glucocorticoids, hippocampal corticosteroid receptor gene expression and antidepressant treatment: relationship with spatial learning in young and aged rats. *Neuroscience.* 1995;66:571-581.
11. Roberts D, Dalziel SR. Antenatal corticosteroids for accelerating fetal lung maturation for women at risk of preterm birth. *Cochrane Database Syst Rev.* 2006;(3):CD004454.
12. Roti E, Gnudi A, Braverman LE. The placental transport, synthesis and metabolism of hormones and drugs which affect thyroid function. *Endocr Rev.* 1983;4:131-149.
13. Pop VJ, Brouwers EP, Vader HL, et al. Maternal hypothyroxinaemia during early pregnancy and subsequent child development: a 3-year follow-up study. *Clin Endocrinol (Oxf).* 2003;59:282-288.
14. Haddow JE, Palomaki GE, Allan WC, et al. Maternal thyroid deficiency during pregnancy and subsequent neuropsychological development of the child. *N Engl J Med.* 1999;341:549-555.
15. Iisalo E, Castren O. The enzymatic inactivation of noradrenaline in human placental tissue. *Ann Med Exp Biol Fenn.* 1967;45:253-257.
16. Mesiano S, Jaffe RB. Neuroendocrine-metabolic regulation of pregnancy. In: Strauss JF III, Barbieri RL, eds. *Reproductive Endocrinology*. 5th ed. Philadelphia, PA: WB Saunders; 2004:327-366.
17. Goldsmith PC, McGregor WG, Raymoure WJ, et al. Cellular localization of chorionic gonadotropin in human fetal liver and kidney. *J Clin Endocrinol Metab.* 1983;57:654-661.
18. Kapcala LP. Immunoassayable adrenocorticotropin in peripheral organs: concentrations during early development. *Life Sci.* 1985;37:2283-2290.
19. Martino E, Lernmark A, Seo H, et al. High concentration of thyrotropin releasing hormone in pancreatic islets. *Proc Natl Acad Sci U S A.* 1978;75:4265-4267.
20. Pekary AE, Meyer NV, Vaillant C, et al. Thyrotropin releasing hormone and a homologous peptide in the male rat reproductive system. *Biochem Biophys Res Commun.* 1980;95:993-1000.
21. Suda T, Tomori N, Tozawa F, et al. Distribution and characterization of immunoreactive corticotropin-releasing factor in human tissues. *J Clin Endocrinol Metab.* 1984;59:861-866.
22. Thompson RC, Seasholtz AF, Herbert E. Rat corticotropin releasing hormone gene: sequence and tissue specific expression. *Mol Endocrinol.* 1987;1:363-370.
23. Shibaski T, Kiyosawa Y, Masuda A, et al. Distribution of growth hormone releasing hormone-like immunoreactivity in human tissue extracts. *J Clin Endocrinol Metab.* 1984;59:263-268.
24. Wu P, Jackson IMD. Identification, characterization and localization of thyrotropin releasing hormone precursor peptides in perinatal rat pancreas. *Regul Pept.* 1988;22:347-360.

25. Koshimizu T. The development of pancreatic and gastrointestinal somatostatin-like immunoreactivity and its relationship to feeding in neonatal rats. *Endocrinology*. 1983;112:911-916.
26. Polk DH, Reviczky AL, Lam RW, et al. Thyrotropin releasing hormone in the ovine fetus: ontogeny and effect of thyroid hormone. *Am J Physiol*. 1991;23:E53-E58.
27. Rahier J, Wallon J, Henquin JC. Abundance of somatostatin cells in the human neonatal pancreas. *Diabetologia*. 1980;18:251-254.
28. Leduque P, Aratan-Spire S, Czernichow P, et al. Ontogenesis of thyrotropin-releasing hormone in the human fetal pancreas. *J Clin Invest*. 1986;78:1028-1034.
29. Saito H, Saito S, Sano T, et al. Fetal and maternal plasma levels of immunoreactive somatostatin at delivery: evidence for its increase in the umbilical artery and its arteriovenous gradient in the fetoplacental circulation. *J Clin Endocrinol Metab*. 1983;56:567-571.
30. Koshimizu T, Ohyama Y, Yokota Y, et al. Peripheral plasma concentrations of somatostatin-like immunoreactivity in newborns and infants. *J Clin Endocrinol Metab*. 1985;61:78-82.
31. Kelberman D, Rizzoti K, Lovell-Badge R, et al. Genetic Regulation of pituitary gland development in human and mouse. *Endocr Rev*. 2009;30:790-829.
32. Dasen JS, Rosenfeld MG. Signaling and transcriptional mechanisms in pituitary development. *Annu Rev Neurosci*. 2001;24:327-355.
33. Grumbach MM, Gluckman PD. The human fetal hypothalamus and pituitary gland: the maturation of neuroendocrine mechanisms controlling secretion of fetal pituitary growth hormone, prolactin, gonadotropins, adrenocorticotropin-related peptides, and thyrotropin. In: Tulchinsky D, Little AB, eds. *Maternal Fetal Endocrinology*. 2nd ed. Philadelphia, PA: WB Saunders; 1994:193-261.
34. Cohen LE, Radovik S. Molecular basis of combined pituitary hormone deficiencies. *Endocr Rev*. 2002;23:431-442.
35. Zhu X, Zhang J, Tollkuhn J, et al. Sustained Notch signaling in progenitors is required for sequential emergence of distinct cell lineages during organogenesis. *Genes Dev*. 2006;20:2739-2753.
36. Roessler E, Belloni E, Gaudenz K, et al. Mutations in the human Sonic Hedgehog gene cause holoprosencephaly. *Nat Genet*. 1996;14:357-360.
37. Brown SA, Warburton D, Brown LY, et al. Holoprosencephaly due to mutation in ZIC1, a homologue of *Drosophila* odd-paired. *Nat Genet*. 1998;20:180-183.
38. Roessler E, Muenke M. The molecular genetics of holoprosencephaly. *Am J Med Genet C Semin Med Genet*. 2010;154C(1):52-61.
39. Dattani MT, Martinez-Barbera JP, Thomas PQ, et al. Mutations in the homeobox gene HESX1/Hesx1 associated with septo-optic dysplasia in human and mouse. *Nat Genet*. 1998;19:125-133.
40. Kelberman D, Rizzoti K, Avilion A, et al. Mutations within Sox2/SOX2 are associated with abnormalities in the hypothalamo-pituitary-gonadal axis in mice and humans. *J Clin Invest*. 2006;116:2442-2455.
41. Kelberman D, de Castro SC, Huang S, et al. SOX2 plays a critical role in the pituitary, forebrain and eye during human embryonic development. *J Clin Endocrinol Metab*. 2008;93:1865-1873.
42. Tajima T, Ohtake A, Hoshino M, et al. OTX2 loss of function mutation causes anophthalmia and combined pituitary hormone deficiency with a small anterior and ectopic posterior pituitary. *J Clin Endocrinol Metab*. 2008;94:314-319.
43. Dateki S, Fukami M, Sato N, et al. OTX2 mutation in a patient with anophthalmia, short stature, and partial growth hormone deficiency: functional studies using the IRBP, HESX1, and POU1F1 promoters. *J Clin Endocrinol Metab*. 2008;93:3697-3702.
44. Diaczok D, Romero C, Zunich J, et al. A novel dominant negative mutation of OTX2 associated with combined pituitary hormone deficiency. *J Clin Endocrinol Metab*. 2008;93:4351-4359.
45. Woods KS, Cundall M, Turton J, et al. Over- and underdosage of SOX3 is associated with infundibular hypoplasia and hypopituitarism. *Am J Hum Genet*. 2005;76:833-849.
46. Netchine I, Sobrier ML, Krude H, et al. Mutations in LHX3 result in a new syndrome revealed by combined pituitary hormone deficiency. *Nat Genet*. 2000;25:182-186.
47. Rajab A, Kelberman D, de Castro SC, et al. Novel mutations in LHX3 are associated with hypopituitarism and sensorineural hearing loss. *Hum Mol Genet*. 2008;17:2150-2159.
48. Machinis K, Pantel J, Netchine I, et al. Syndromic short stature in patients with a germline mutation in the LIM homeobox LHX4. *Am J Hum Genet*. 2001;69:961-968.
49. Wu W, Cogan JD, Pfaffle RW, et al. Mutations in PROP1 cause familial combined pituitary hormone deficiency. *Nat Genet*. 1998;18:147-149.
50. Radovick S, Nations M, Du Y, et al. A mutation in the POU-homeodomain of Pit-1 responsible for combined pituitary hormone deficiency. *Science*. 1992;257:1115-1118.
51. Ohta K, Nobukuni Y, Mitsubuchi H, et al. Mutations in the Pit-1 gene in children with combined pituitary hormone deficiency. *Biochem Biophys Res Commun*. 1992;189:851-855.
52. Pulichino AM, Vallette-Kasic S, Couture C, et al. Human and mouse TPIT gene mutations cause early onset pituitary ACTH deficiency. *Genes Dev*. 2003;17:711-716.
53. Mulchahey JJ, DiBlasio AM, Martin MC, et al. Hormone production and peptide regulation of the human fetal pituitary gland. *Endocr Rev*. 1987;8:406-425.
54. Suganuma N, Seo H, Yamamoto N, et al. The ontogeny of growth hormone in the human fetal pituitary. *Am J Obstet Gynecol*. 1989;160:729-733.
55. Goodyear CG, Sellen JM, Fuks M, et al. Regulation of growth hormone secretion from human fetal pituitaries, interactions between growth hormone releasing factor and somatostatin. *Reprod Nutr Dev*. 1987;27:461-470.
56. DeLeon DD, Cohen P, Katz LEL. Growth factor regulation of fetal growth. In: Polin RA, Fox WW, Abman SH, eds. *Fetal and Neonatal Physiology*. 3rd ed. Philadelphia, PA: WB Saunders; 2004:1880-1890.
57. Kind KL, Owens JA, Robinson JS, et al. Effect of restriction of placental growth on expression of IGFs in fetal sheep: relationship to fetal growth, circulating IGFs and binding proteins. *J Endocrinol*. 1995;146:23-34.
58. Gluckman PD, Pinal CS. Growth hormone and prolactin. In: Polin RA, Fox WW, Abman SH, eds. *Fetal and Neonatal Physiology*. 3rd ed. Philadelphia, PA: WB Saunders; 2004:1891-1895.
59. Clement-Lacroix P, Ormandy C, Lepescheux L, et al. Osteoblasts are a new target for prolactin analysis of bone formation in prolactin receptor knockout mice. *Endocrinology*. 1999;140:3404-3410.
60. Winter JSD. Fetal and neonatal adrenocortical physiology. In: Polin RA, Fox WW, Abman SH, eds. *Fetal and Neonatal Physiology*. Philadelphia, PA: WB Saunders; 2004:1915-1925.
61. Geller DH, Miller WL. Molecular development of the adrenal gland. In: Pescovitz OH, Eugster EA, eds. *Pediatric Endocrinology*. Philadelphia, PA: Lippincott Williams & Wilkins; 2004:548-567.
62. Ikeda Y, Swain A, Weber TH, et al. Steroidogenic factor 1 and DAX-1 localize in multiple cell lineages: potential links in endocrine development. *Mol Endocrinol*. 1996;10:1261-1272.
63. Hammer GD, Parker KL, Schimmer BP. Minireview: transcriptional regulation of adrenocortical development. *Endocrinology*. 2005;146:1018-1024.
64. Fujieda K, Tajima T. Molecular basis of adrenal insufficiency. *Pediatric Res*. 2005;57:62R-69R.
65. Miller WL. Steroid hormone biosynthesis and actions in the materno-feto-placental unit. *Clin Perinatal*. 1998;25:799-817.
66. Baker BY, Lin L, Kim CJ, et al. Nonclassic congenital lipoid adrenal hyperplasia: a new disorder of the steroidogenic acute regulatory protein with very late presentation and normal male genitalia. *J Clin Endocrinol Metab*. 2006;91:4781-4785.
67. Goto M, Piper Hanley K, Marcos J, et al. In humans, early cortisol biosynthesis provides a mechanism to safeguard female sexual development. *J Clin Invest*. 2006;116:953-960.
68. Leavitt MG, Albrecht EO, Pepe GJ. Development of the baboon fetal adrenal gland: regulation of the ontogenesis of the definitive and transitional zones by adrenocorticotropin. *J Clin Endocrinol Metab*. 1999;84:3831-3835.
69. Dotzler DA, Digeronimo JJ, Yoder BA, et al. Distribution of corticotrophin releasing hormone in the fetus, newborn, juvenile and adult baboon. *Pediatr Res*. 2004;55:120-125.
70. Cole TJ, Blendy JA, Monaghan AD, et al. Targeted disruption of the glucocorticoid receptor gene blocks adrenergic chromaffin development and severely retards lung maturation. *Genes Dev*. 1995;9:1608-1625.
71. Thompson M, Smith R. The action of hypothalamic and placental corticotrophin releasing factor on the corticotrope. *Mol Cell Endocrinol*. 1989;62:1-12.
72. Goland RS, Wardlow SL, Blum M, et al. Biologically active corticotropin-releasing hormone in maternal and fetal plasma during pregnancy. *Am J Obstet Gynecol*. 1988;159:884-890.
73. Rivier C, Vale W. Neuroendocrine interactions between corticotrophin releasing factor and vasopressin on adrenocorticotropic hormone secretion in the rat. In: Schrier WW, ed. *Vasopressin*. New York, NY: Raven; 1985:181-188.
74. Albrecht ED, Aberdeen GW, Pepe GJ. Estrogen elicits cortical zone specific effects on development of the primate fetal adrenal gland. *Endocrinology*. 2005;146:1737-1744.
75. Rose JC, Turner CS, Ray DeW, et al. Evidence that cortisol inhibits basal adrenocorticotropin secretion in the sheep fetus by 0.70 gestation. *Endocrinology*. 1988;123:1307-1313.
76. Yang K, Jones SA, Challis JRG. Changes in glucocorticoid receptor number in the hypothalamus of the sheep fetus with gestational age and after adrenocorticotropin treatment. *Endocrinology*. 1990;126:11-17.
77. McKenna NT, Moore DD. Nuclear receptors: structure, function and cofactors. In: DeGroot LJ, Jameson JL, eds. *Endocrinology*. 5th ed. Philadelphia, PA: Elsevier Saunders; 2006:277-287.
78. Pavlik A, Buresova M. The neonatal cerebellum: the highest level of glucocorticoid receptors in the brain. *Dev Brain Res*. 1984;12:13-20.

79. Johnson JW, Mitzner W, Beck JC, et al. Long term effects of betamethasone in fetal development. *Am J Obstet Gynecol*. 1981;141:1053-1064.
80. Liggins GC. The role of cortisol in preparing the fetus for birth. *Reprod Fertil Dev*. 1994;6:141-150.
81. Beitins IZ, Graham GG, Kowarski A, et al. Adrenal function in normal infants and in marasmus and kwashiorkor: plasma aldosterone concentration and aldosterone secretion rate. *J Pediatr*. 1974;84:444-451.
82. Katz FH, Beck P, Makowski EL. The renin-aldosterone system in mother and fetus at term. *Am J Obstet Gynecol*. 1974;118:51-55.
83. Siegel SR, Fisher DA. Ontogeny of the renin-angiotensin-aldosterone system in the fetal and newborn lamb. *Pediatr Res*. 1980;14:99-102.
84. Lumbers ER. Functions of the renin-angiotensin system during development. *Clin Exp Pharmacol Physiol*. 1995;22:499-505.
85. Berger S, Bleich M, Schmid N, et al. Mineralocorticoid receptor knockout mice: pathophysiology of Na^+ metabolism. *Proc Natl Acad Sci U S A*. 1998;95:9424-9429.
86. Hirasawa G, Sasano H, Suzuki T, et al. 11β-Hydroxysteroid dehydrogenase type 2 and mineralocorticoid receptor in human fetal development. *J Clin Endocrinol Metab*. 1999;84:1453-1458.
87. Robillard JE, Page WV, Matthews MS, et al. Differential gene expression and regulation of renal angiotensin II receptor subtypes (AT1 and AT2) during fetal life in sheep. *Pediatr Res*. 1995;38:896-904.
88. Chen K, Carey LC, Liu J, et al. The effect of hypothalamo-pituitary disconnection on the renin-angiotensin system in the late gestation sheep. *Am J Physiol Regul Integr Comp Physiol*. 2005;288:R1279-R1287.
89. Walther T, Schultheiss HP, Tschope C, et al. Natriuretic peptide system in fetal heart and circulation. *J Hypertens*. 2002;20:785-791.
90. Clark AJ, Chan LF, Chung TT, et al. The genetics of familial glucocorticoid deficiency. *Best Pract Res Clin Endocrinol Metab*. 2009;23:159-165.
91. Cooray SN, Chan L, Metherell L, et al. Adrenocorticotropin resistance syndromes. *Endocr Devel*. 2008;13:99-116.
92. Ferraz-de-Souza B, Achermann JC. Disorders of adrenal development. *Endocr Devel*. 2008;13:19-32.
93. Kim AC, Barlaskar FM, Heaton JH, et al. In search of adrenocortical stem and progenitor cells. *Endocr Rev*. 2009;30:241-263.
94. Kohler B, Lin L, Ferraz-de-Souza B, et al. Five novel mutations in steroidogenic factor 1 (SF1/Ad4BP, NR5A1) are associated with 46XY disorders of sex development with normal adrenal function. *Human Mutation*. 2008;29:59-64.
95. Lourenco D, Brauner R, Lin L, et al. Mutations in NR5A1 associated with ovarian insufficiency. *N Engl J Med*. 2009;360:1200-1210.
96. Santisteban P. Development and anatomy of the hypothalamic-pituitary axis. In: Braverman LE, Utiger RD, eds. *The Thyroid*. 9th ed. Philadelphia, PA: JB Lippincott; 2005:8-25.
97. Brown RS, Huang SA, Fisher DA. The maturation of thyroid function in the perinatal period and during childhood. In: Braverman LE, Utiger RD, eds. *The Thyroid*. 9th ed. Philadelphia, PA: JB Lippincott; 2005:1013-1028.
98. Alt B, Elsalini OA, Schrumpf P, et al. Arteries define the position of the thyroid gland during its developmental relocalization. *Development*. 2006;133:3797-3804.
99. Fagman H, Liao J, Westerlund J, et al. The 22q11 deletion syndrome candidate gene Tbx1 determines thyroid size and positioning. *Hum Mol Genet*. 2007;16:276-285.
100. O'Rahilly R. The timing and sequence of events in the development of the human endocrine system during the embryonic period proper. *Anat Embryol (Berlin)*. 1983;166:439-451.
101. Sprinzl GM, Koebke J, Wimmers-Klick J, et al. Morphology of the human thyroglossal tract: a histologic and macroscopic study in infants and children. *Ann Otol Rhinol Laryngol*. 2000;109(12 Pt 1):1135-1139.
102. Macchia P. Recent advances in understanding the molecular basis of primary congenital hypothyroidism. *Mol Med Today*. 2000;6:36-42.
103. Szinnai G, Lacroix L, Carre A, et al. Sodium/iodide symporter (NIS) gene expression is the limiting step for the onset of thyroid function in the human fetus. *J Clin Endocrinol Metab*. 2007;92:70-76.
104. Parlato R, Rosica A, Rodriguez-Mallon A, et al. An integrated regulatory network controlling survival and migration in thyroid organogenesis. *Dev Biol*. 2004;276:464-475.
105. Trueba SS, Auge J, Mattei G, et al. PAX8, TITF1 and FOXE1 gene expression patterns during human development: new insights into human thyroid development and thyroid dysgenesis-associated malformations. *J Clin Endocrinol Metab*. 2005;90:455-462.
106. De Felice M, Di Lauro R. Thyroid development and its disorders: genetics and molecular mechanisms. *Endocr Rev*. 2004;25:722-746.
107. Dentice M, Cordeddu V, Rosica A, et al. Missense mutation in the transcription factor NKX2-5: a novel molecular event in the pathogenesis of thyroid dysgenesis. *J Clin Endocrinol Metab*. 2006;91:1428-1433.
108. Chisaka O, Capecchi MR. Regionally restricted developmental defects resulting from targeted disruption of the mouse homeobox gene hox-1.5. *Nature*. 1991;350:473-479.
109. Burrow GN, Fisher DA, Larsen PR. Maternal and fetal thyroid function. *N Engl J Med*. 1994;331:1072-1078.
110. Roti E. Regulation of thyroid stimulating hormone (TSH) secretion in the fetus and neonate. *J Endocrinol Invest*. 1988;11:145-158.
111. Fisher DA, Nelson JC, Carlton EI, et al. Maturation of human hypothalamic-pituitary-thyroid function and control. *Thyroid*. 2000;10:229-234.
112. Murphy N, Home R, vanToor H, et al. The hypothalamic-pituitary-thyroid axis in preterm infants: changes in the first 24 hours of postnatal life. *J Clin Endocrinol Metab*. 2004;89:2824-2831.
113. Williams FLR, Simpson J, Delahunty C, et al. Developmental trends in cord and postpartum serum thyroid hormones in preterm infants. *J Clin Endocr Metab*. 2004;89:5314-5320.
114. Eng PHK, Cardona GR, Fang SL, et al. Escape from the acute Wolff-Chaikoff effect is associated with a decrease in thyroid sodium/iodide symporter messenger ribonucleic acid and protein. *Endocrinology*. 1999;140:3404-3410.
115. Sherwin JR. Development of regulatory mechanisms in the thyroid: failure of iodide to suppress iodide transport activity. *Proc Soc Exp Biol Med*. 1982;169:458-462.
116. St. Germain DL, Hernandez A, Schneider MJ, et al. Insights into the role of deiodinases from studies of genetically modified animals. *Thyroid*. 2005;15:905-916.
117. Hume R, Simpson J, Delahunty C, et al. Human fetal and cord serum thyroid hormones: developmental trends and interrelationships. *J Clin Endocrinol Metab*. 2004;89:4097-4103.
118. Polk DH, Reviczky A, Wu SY, et al. Metabolism of sulfoconjugated thyroid hormone derivatives in developing sheep. *Am J Physiol*. 1994;266:E892-E896.
119. Kerry R, Hume R, Kaptein E, et al. Sulfation of thyroid hormone and dopamine during human development: ontogeny of phenol sulfotransferases and arylsulfatase in liver, lung, and brain. *J Clin Endocrinol Metab*. 2001;86:2734-2742.
120. Richard K, Hume R, Kaptein E, et al. Ontogeny of iodothyronine deiodinases in human liver. *J Clin Endocrinol Metab*. 1998;83:2868-2874.
121. Polk DH, Wu WY, Wright C, et al. Ontogeny of thyroid hormone effect on tissue 5′-monodeiodinase activity in fetal sheep. *Am J Physiol*. 1988;254:E337-E341.
122. Jansen J, Friesema ECH, Milici C, et al. Thyroid hormone transporters in health and disease. *Thyroid*. 2005;15:757-768.
123. Heuer H, Maier ML, Iden S, et al. The monocarboxylate transporter 8 linked to human psychomotor retardation is highly expressed in thyroid hormone-sensitive neuron populations. *Endocrinology*. 2005;146:1701-1706.
124. Dumitrescu AM, Liao XH, Best TB, et al. A novel syndrome combining thyroid and neurological abnormalities is associated with mutations in a monocarboxylate transporter gene. *Am J Hum Genet*. 2004;74:168-175.
125. Bergh JJ, Lin HY, Lansing L, et al. Integrin αVβ3 contains a cell surface receptor site for thyroid hormone that is linked to activation of mitogen-activated protein kinase and induction of angiogenesis. *Endocrinology*. 2005;146:2864-2871.
126. Yen P. Genomic and nongenomic actions of thyroid hormones. In: Braverman LE, Utiger RD, eds. *The Thyroid*. 9th ed. Philadelphia, PA: Lippincott Williams and Wilkins; 2005:135-150.
127. Flamant F, Samarut J: Thyroid hormone receptors: lessons from knockout and knockin mutant mice. *Trends Endocrinol Metab*. 2005;14:85-90.
128. Morreale de Escobar G, Obregon MJ, Escobar del Rey F. Role of thyroid hormone during early brain development. *Eur J Endocrinol*. 2004;151:U25-U37.
129. Kilby MD, Giltoes N, McCabe C, et al. Expression of thyroid receptor isoforms in the human fetal central nervous system and the effects of intrauterine growth retardation. *Clin Endocrinol (Oxf)*. 2000;53:469-477.
130. Iskaros J, Pickard M, Evans I, et al. Thyroid hormone receptor gene expression in first trimester human fetal brain. *J Clin Endocrinol Metab*. 2000;85:2620-2623.
131. Rajatapiti P, Kester MHA, de Krijger RR, et al. Expression of glucocorticoid, retinoid, and thyroid hormone receptors during human lung development. *J Clin Endocrinol Metab*. 2005;90:4309-4314.
132. Contempre B, Jauniaux E, Calvo R, et al. Detection of thyroid hormones in human embryonic cavities during the first trimester of pregnancy. *J Clin Endocrinol Metab*. 1993;77:1719-1722.
133. Vulsma T, Gons MH, de Vijlder JJ. Maternal-fetal transfer of thyroxine in congenital hypothyroidism due to a total organification defect or thyroid agenesis. *N Engl J Med*. 1989;321:13-16.
134. Morreale De Escobar G, Calvo R, Obregon MJ, et al. Contribution of maternal thyroxine to fetal thyroxine pools in normal rats near term. *Endocrinology*. 1990;126:2765-2767.
135. Sadow PM, Chassande O, Koo EK, et al. Regulation of expression of thyroid hormone receptor isoforms and coactivators in liver and heart by thyroid hormone. *Mol Cell Endocrinol*. 2003;203:65-75.
136. Quignodon L, Legrand C, Allioli N, et al. Thyroid hormone signaling is highly heterogeneous during pre- and postnatal brain development. *J Molec Endocrinol*. 2004;33:467-476.

137. Plateroti M, Gauthier K, Domon-Dell C, et al. Functional interference between thyroid hormone receptor α (TRα) and natural truncated TRΔα isoforms in the control of intestinal development. *Mol Cell Biol.* 2001;21:4761-4772.
138. Mai W, Janier MF, Allioli N, et al. Thyroid hormone receptor α is a molecular switch of cardiac function between fetal and postnatal life. *Proc Natl Acad Sci U S A.* 2004;101:10332-10337.
139. Harvey CB, O'Shea PJ, Scott AJ, et al. Molecular mechanisms of thyroid hormone effects on bone growth and function. *Mol Gen Metab.* 2002;75:17-30.
140. Marrit H, Schifman A, Stepanyan Z, et al. Temperature homeostasis in transgenic mice lacking thyroid receptor α gene products. *Endocrinology.* 2004;146:2872-2884.
141. Angelin-Duclos C, Domenget C, Kolbus A, et al. Thyroid hormone T3 acting through the thyroid hormone α receptor is necessary for implementation of erythropoiesis in the neonatal spleen environment in the mouse. *Development.* 2005;132:925-934.
142. Morreale de Escobar G, Obregon MJ, Escobar del Rey F. Is neuropsychological development related to maternal hypothyroidism or to maternal hypothyroxinemia? *J Clin Endocrinol Metab.* 2000;85: 3975-3987.
143. Erickson RP, Blecher SR. Genetics of sex determination and differentiation. In: Polin RA, Fox WW, Abman SH, eds. *Fetal and Neonatal Physiology.* 3rd ed. Philadelphia, PA: WB Saunders; 2004:1935-1941.
144. Lee MM. Molecular genetic control of sex differentiation. In: Pescovitz OH, Eugster EA, eds. *Pediatric Endocrinology.* Philadelphia, PA: Lippincott Williams & Wilkins; 2004:231-242.
145. Harley VR, Clarkson MJ, Argentaro A. The molecular action and regulation of the testis-determining factors, SRY (sex determining region of the Y chromosome) and SOX9 (SRY-related high-mobility group [HMG] Box 9). *Endocr Rev.* 2003;24:466-487.
146. Park SY, Jameson JL. Minireview: transcriptional regulation of gonadal development and differentiation. *Endocrinology.* 2005;146:1035-1042.
147. Sekido R, Lovell-Badge R. Sex determination involves synergistic action of SRY and SF1 on a specific Sox9 enhancer. *Nature.* 2008;453:930-934.
148. Zang FP, Poutanen M, Wilbertz J, et al. Normal prenatal but arrested postnatal sexual development of luteinizing hormone receptor knockout (LURKO) mice. *Mol Endocrinol.* 2001;15:172-183.
149. Philibert P, Zenaty D, Lin L, et al. Mutational analysis of steroidogenic factor 1 (*NR5a1*) in 24 boys with bilateral anorchia: a French collaborative study. *Hum Reprod.* 2007;22:3255-3261.
150. Aslan AR, Kogan BA, Gondos B. Testicular development. In: Polin RA, Fox WW, Abmans SH, eds. *Fetal and Neonatal Physiology.* 3rd ed. Philadelphia, PA: WB Saunders; 2004:1950-1955.
151. Nef S, Parada LF. Cryptorchidism in mice mutant for Insl3. *Nat Genet.* 1999;22:295-299.
152. Byskov AG, Westergaard LG. Differentiation of the ovary. In: Polin RA, Fox WW, Abman SH, eds. *Fetal and Neonatal Physiology.* 3rd ed. Philadelphila, PA: WB Saunders; 2004:1941-1949.
153. Fulton N, da Silva SJM, Bayne RAL, et al. Germ cell proliferation and apoptosis in the developing human ovary. *J Clin Endocrinol Metab.* 2005;90:4664-4670.
154. Sajjad Y, Quenby S, Nickson P, et al. Immunohistochemical localization of androgen receptors in the urogenital tracts of human embryos. *Reproduction.* 2004;128:331-339.
155. Tomaselli S, Megiorni F, De Bernardo C, et al. Syndromic true hermaphroditism due to an R-spondin 1 (RSPO1) homozygous mutation. *Hum Mutation.* 2008;29:220-226.
156. Parma P, Radi O, Vidal V, et al. R-spondin 1 is essential in sex determination, skin differentiation and malignancy. *Nat Genet* 2006, 38:1304-1309.
157. Josso N, Belville C, Dicard JY. Mutations in AMH and its receptors. *Endocrinology.* 2003;13:247-251.
158. Roviller Fabre V, Carmona S, Abou Merhi A, et al. Effect of anti-müllerian hormone on Sertoli and Leydig cell functions in fetal and immature rats. *Endocrinology.* 1998;139:1213-1220.
159. Brandenberger AW, Tee MK, Lee JY, et al. Tissue distribution of estrogen receptors alpha (ERα) and beta (ERβ) mRNA in the midgestation human fetus. *J Clin Endocrinol Metab.* 1997;82:3509-3512.
160. Couse JF, Korach KS. Estrogen receptor null mice: what have we learned and where will they lead us? *Endocrine Rev.* 1999;20:358-417.
161. Falgueras AG, Pinos H, Collado P, et al. The role of the androgen receptor in CNS masculinization. *Brain Res.* 2005;1035:13-23.
162. Naftolin F, Brawer JB. The effect of estrogens on hypothalamic structure and function. *Am J Obstet Gynecol.* 1978;132:758-765.
163. Sholl SA, Goy RW, Kim KL. 5α-Reductase, aromatase, and androgen receptor levels in the monkey brain during fetal development. *Endocrinology.* 1989;124:627-634.
164. Visser M, Swaab DF. Life span changes in the presence of alpha-melanocyte-stimulating-hormone-containing cells in the human pituitary. *J Dev Physiol.* 1979;1:161-178.
165. Perry RA, Mulvogue HM, McMillen IC, et al. Immunohistochemical localization of ACTH in the adult and fetal sheep pituitary. *J Dev Physiol.* 1985;7:397-404.
166. Silman RE, Holland T, Chard T, et al. The ACTH family tree of the rhesus monkey changes with development. *Nature.* 1978;276:526-528.
167. Charles MA, Suh H, Hjalt TA, et al. PITX genes are required for cell survival and Lhx3 activation. *Mol Endocrinol.* 2005;19:1893-1903.
168. Glickman JA, Carson GD, Challis JRG. Differential effects of synthetic adrenocorticotropin and melanocyte stimulating hormone on adrenal formation in human and sheep fetus. *Endocrinology.* 1979;104:34-39.
169. Swaab DF, Martin JT. Functions of alpha melanotropin and other opiomelanocortin peptides in labour, intrauterine growth and brain development. *Ciba Found Symp.* 1981;81:196-217.
170. Facchinetti F, Storchi AR, Petraglia F, et al. Ontogeny of pituitary β-endorphin and related peptides in the human embryo and fetus. *Am J Obstet Gynecol.* 1987;156:735-739.
171. Leake RD, Fisher DA. Ontogeny of vasopressin in man. In: Czernichow P, Robinson AG, eds. Diabetes Insipidus in Man: Frontiers in Hormone Research, vol 13. Basel: S Karger; 1985:42-51.
172. Leake RD. The fetal-maternal neurohypophysial system. In: Polin RA, Fox WW, eds. *Fetal and Neonatal Physiology.* 2nd ed. Philadelphia, PA: WB Saunders; 1998:2442-2446.
173. Ervin MG, Leake RD, Ross MG, et al. Arginine vasotocin in ovine maternal and fetal blood, fetal urine, and amniotic fluid. *J Clin Invest.* 1985;75:1696-1701.
174. Morris M, Castro M, Rose JC. Alterations in prohormone processing during early development in the fetal sheep. *Am J Physiol.* 1992; 263:R738-R740.
175. Zhao X, Nijland MJM, Ervin G, et al. Regulation of hypothalamic arginine vasopressin content in fetal sheep: effect of acute tonicity alterations and fetal maturation. *Am J Obstet Gynecol.* 1998;179: 899-905.
176. DeVane GW, Porter JC. An apparent stress-induced release of arginine vasopressin by human neonates. *J Clin Endocrinol Metab.* 1980; 51:1412-1416.
177. Matthews SG, Challis JRG. Regulation of CRH and AVP mRNA in the developing ovine hypothalamus: effects of stress and glucocorticoids. *Am J Physiol.* 1995;268:E1096-E1107.
178. Brooks AN, White A. Activation of pituitary adrenal function in fetal sheep by corticotrophin-releasing factor and arginine vasopressin. *J Endocrinol.* 1990;124:27-35.
179. Benedetto MT, DeCicco F, Rossiello F, et al. Oxytocin receptor in human fetal membranes at term and during labor. *J Steroid Biochem.* 1990;35:205-208.
180. Tribollet E, Charpak S, Schmidt A, et al. Appearance and transient expression of oxytocin receptors in fetal, infant and peripubertal rat brain studied by autoradiography and electrophysiology. *J Neurosci.* 1989;9:1764-1773.
181. Ervin MG, Miller SJ, Ramseyer LJ, et al. Renal arginine vasopressin receptors in newborn and adult sheep. *Clin Res.* 1990;38:170A.
182. Devuyst O, Burrow CR, Smithe BL, et al. Expression of aquaporins 1 and 2 during nephrogenesis and in autosomal dominant polycystic kidney disease. *Am J Physiol.* 1996;271:F169-F183.
183. Baum MA, Ruddy MK, Hosselet CA, et al. The perinatal expression of aquaporin-2 and aquaporin-3 in developing kidney. *Pediatr Res.* 1998;43:783-790.
184. Cryns K, Sivakumaran TA, Van den Ouweland JM, et al. Mutational spectrum of the WFS1 gene in Wolfram syndrome, nonsyndromic hearing impairment, diabetes mellitus and psychiatric disease. *Hum Mutation.* 2003;22:275-287.
185. Padbury JF. Functional maturation of the adrenal medulla and peripheral sympathetic nervous system. *Baillieres Clin Endocrinol Metab.* 1989;33:689-705.
186. Huber K, Karch N, Ernsberger U, et al. The role of PHOX2B in chromaffin cell development. *Dev Biol.* 2005;279:501-508.
187. Gaultier C, Trang H, Dauger S, et al. Pediatric disorders with autoimmune dysfunction: What role for PHOX2B? *Pediatr Res.* 2005;58:1-6.
188. Aloe L, Levi-Montalcini R. Nerve growth factor-induced transformation of immature chromaffin cells in vivo into sympathetic neurons: effect of antiserum to nerve growth factor. *Proc Natl Acad Sci U S A.* 1979;76:1246-1250.
189. Slotkin TA, Seidler FJ. Adrenomedullary catecholamine release in the fetus and newborn: secretory mechanisms and their role in stress and survival. *J Dev Physiol.* 1988;10:1-16.
190. Stonestreet BS, Piasecki GJ, Susa JB, et al. Effects of insulin infusion on catecholamine concentration in fetal sheep. *Am J Obstet Gynecol.* 1989;160:740-745.
191. Cohen WR, Piasecki GJ, Cohn HE, et al. Plasma catecholamines in the hypoxaemic fetal rhesus monkey. *J Dev Physiol.* 1987;9:507-515.
192. Pryds O, Christensen NJ, Friis-Hansen B. Increased cerebral blood flow and plasma epinephrine in hypoglycemic, preterm neonates. *Pediatrics.* 1990;85:172-176.
193. Palmer SM, Oakes GK, Lam RW, et al. Catecholamine physiology in the ovine fetus. I: Gestational age variation in basal plasma concentrations. *Am J Obstet Gynecol.* 1984;149:420-425.

194. Palmer SM, Oakes GK, Lam RW, et al. Catecholamine physiology in the ovine fetus. II: Metabolic clearance rate of epinephrine. *Am J Physiol*. 1984;246:E350-E355.
195. Palmer SM, Oakes GK, Champion JA, et al. Catecholamine physiology in the ovine fetus. III: Maternal and fetal response to acute maternal exercise. *Am J Obstet Gynecol*. 1984;149:426-434.
196. Zhou QY, Ouaife CJ, Palmiter RD. Targeted disruption of the tyrosine hydroxylase gene reveals that catecholamines are required for mouse fetal development. *Nature*. 1995;374:640-643.
197. Thomas SA, Matsumoto AM, Palmiter RD. Noradrenaline is essential for mouse fetal development. *Nature*. 1995;374:643-646.
198. Hochberg Ze'ev, Tiosano D. Disorders of mineral metabolism. In: Pescovitz OH, Eugster EA, eds. *Pediatric Endocrinology*. Philadelphia, PA: Lippincott Williams & Wilkins; 2004:614-640.
199. Miao D, He B, Karaplis C, et al. Parathyroid hormone is essential for normal fetal bone formation. *J Clin Invest*. 2002;109:1173-1182.
200. Bowl MR, Nesbit MA, Harding B, et al. An interstitial deletion/insertion involving chromosomes 2p25.3 and Xq27.1 near SOX3 causes X-linked recessive hypoparathyroidism. *J Clin Invest*. 2005;115: 2822-2831.
201. Prada JA. Calcium-regulating hormones. In: Polin RA, Fox WW, eds. *Fetal and Neonatal Physiology*. 2nd ed. Philadelphia, PA: WB Saunders; 1998:2287-2296.
202. Kovaks CS, Kronenberg HM: Maternal-fetal calcium and bone metabolism during pregnancy, puerperium and lactation. *Endocr Rev*. 1997;18:832-872.
203. Care AD, Abbas SK, Pickard DW, et al. Stimulation of ovine placental transport of calcium and magnesium by mid-molecule fragments of human parathyroid hormone-related protein. *J Exp Physiol*. 1990; 75:605-608.
204. Kovacs CS, Lanske B, Hunzelman JL, et al. Parathyroid hormone-related peptide (PTHrP) regulates fetal-placental calcium transport through a receptor distinct from the PTH/PTHrP receptor. *Proc Natl Acad Sci U S A*. 1996;93:15233-15238.
205. Karaplis AC, Luz A, Glowacki J, et al. Lethal skeletal dysplasia from targeted disruption of the parathyroid hormone-related protein gene. *Genes Dev*. 1994;8:277-289.
206. Ross R, Halbert K, Tsang RC. Determination of the production and metabolic clearance rates of 1,25-dihydroxyvitamin D_3 in the pregnant sheep and its chronically catheterized fetus by primed infusion technique. *Pediatr Res*. 1989;26:633-638.
207. Habener JF, Kemp DM, Thomas MJ. Mini review: transcriptional regulation in pancreatic development. *Endocrinology*. 2005;146:1025-1034.
208. Jiang FX, Harrison LC. Laminin-1 and epidermal growth factor family members co-stimulate fetal pancreas cell proliferation and colony formation. *Differentiation*. 2005;73:45-49.
209. Formby B, Ullrich A, Coussens L, et al. Growth hormone stimulates insulin gene expression in cultured human fetal pancreatic islets. *J Clin Endocrinol Metab*. 1988;66:1075-1079.
210. Edlund H. Pancreatic organogenesis: developmental mechanisms and implications for therapy. *Nat Rev Genet*. 2002;3:524-532.
211. Sperling MA. Carbohydrate metabolism: insulin and glucagons. In: Tulchinsky D, Little AB, eds. *Maternal-Fetal Endocrinology*. 2nd ed. Philadelphia, PA: WB Saunders; 1994:380-400.
212. Girard J. Control of fetal and neonatal glucose metabolism by pancreatic hormones. *Baillieres Clin Endocrinol Metab*. 1989;3:817-836.
213. Ammon HP, Glocker C, Waldner RG, et al. Insulin release from pancreatic islets of fetal rats mediated by leucine, b-BCH, tolbutamide, glibenclamide, arginine, potassium chloride, and theophylline does not require stimulation of Ca^{2+} net uptake. *Cell Calcium*. 1989;10: 441-450.
214. Meier JJ, Butler AE, Saisho Y, et al. Beta-cell replication is the primary mechanism subserving the postnatal expansion of beta-cell mass in humans. *Diabetes*. 2008;57:1584-1594.
215. Pepe GJ, Albrecht ED. Actions of placental and fetal adrenal steroid hormones in primate pregnancy. *Endocr Rev*. 1995;16:608-648.
216. Ruiz de Ona C, Obregon MJ, Escobar del Rey F, et al. Developmental changes in rat brain 5′-deiodinase and thyroid hormones during the fetal period: the effects of fetal hypothyroidism and maternal thyroid hormones. *Pediatr Res*. 1988;24:588-594.
217. Polk DH, Cheromcha D, Reviczky A, et al. Nuclear thyroid hormone receptors: ontogeny and thyroid hormone effects in sheep. *Am J Physiol*. 1989;256:E543-E549.
218. Coulombe P, Ruel J, Dussault JH. Effects of neonatal hypo- and hyperthyroidism on pituitary growth hormone content in the rat. *Endocrinology*. 1980;107:2027-2033.
219. Lakshmanan J, Perheentupa J, Macaso T, et al. Acquisition of urine, kidney and submandibular gland epidermal growth factor responsiveness to thyroxine administration in neonatal mice. *Acta Endocrinol*. 1985;109:511-516.
220. Alm J, Scott SM, Fisher DA. Epidermal growth factor receptor ontogeny in mice with congenital hypothyroidism. *J Dev Physiol*. 1986;8: 377-385.
221. Hoath SB, Lakshmanan J, Fisher DA. Thyroid hormone effects on skin and hepatic epidermal growth factor concentrations in neonatal and adult mice. *Biol Neonate*. 1984;45:49-52.
222. Hoath SB, Lakshmanan J, Fisher DA. Epidermal growth factor binding to neonatal mouse skin explants and membrane preparations: effect of triiodothyronine. *Pediatr Res*. 1985;19:277-280.
223. Perez Castillo A, Bernal J, Ferriero B, et al. The early ontogenesis of thyroid hormone receptor in the rat fetus. *Endocrinology*. 1985;117:2457-2461.
224. Mehta A, Hindmarsh PC, Stanhope RG, et al. The role of growth hormone in determining birth size and early postnatal growth, using congenital growth hormone deficiency (GHD) as a model. *Clin Endocrinol (Oxf)*. 2005;63:223-231.
225. Padbury JF, Lam RW, Newnham JP, et al. Neonatal adaptation: greater neurosympathetic system activity in preterm than full term sheep at birth. *Am J Physiol*. 1985;248:E443-E449.
226. Pasqualini JR, Sumida C, Gelly C, et al. Progesterone receptors in the fetal uterus and ovary of the guinea pig: evolution during fetal development and induction and stimulation in estradiol-primed animals. *J Steroid Biochem*. 1976;7:1031-1038.
227. Yamashita S, Newbold RR, McLachlan JA, et al. Developmental pattern of estrogen receptor expression in female mouse genital tracts. *Endocrinology*. 1989;125:2888-2896.
228. Simmen FA, Simmon RCM, Letcher LR, et al. IGFs in pregnancy: developmental expression in uterus and mammary gland and paracrine actions during embryonic and neonatal growth. In: LeRoith D, Raizada MK, eds. *Molecular and Cellular Biology of Insulin-Like Growth Factors and Their Receptors*. New York, NY: Plenum; 1989:195-208.
229. Spaventi R, Antica M, Pavelic K. Insulin and insulin-like growth factor I (IGF I) in early mouse embryogenesis. *Development*. 1990;108: 491-495.
230. Sibley CP, Coan PM, Ferguson-Smith AC, et al. Placental-specific insulin-like growth factor 2 (Igf2) regulates the diffusional exchange characteristics of the mouse placenta. *Proc Natl Acad Sci U S A*. 2004;101:8204-8208.
231. Constancia M, Angiolini E, Sandovici I, et al. Adaptation of nutrient supply to fetal demand in the mouse involves interaction between the Igf2 gene and placental transporter systems. *Proc Natl Acad Sci U S A*. 2005;102:19219-19224.
232. Woods KA, Camacho-Huebner C, Savage MO, et al. Intrauterine growth retardation and postnatal growth failure associated with deletion of the insulin-like growth factor 1 gene. *N Engl J Med*. 1996; 335:1383-1387.
233. Abuzzahab MJ, Schneider A, Goddard A, et al. IGF-1 receptor mutations resulting in intrauterine and postnatal growth retardation. *N Engl J Med*. 2003;349:2211-2222.
234. Gicquel C, Rossignol S, Cabrol S, et al. Epimutation of the telomeric imprinting center region on chromosome 11p15 in Silver-Russell syndrome. *Nat Genet*. 2005;37:1003-1007.
235. Qiu Q, Basak A, Mbikay M, et al. Role of pro-IGF-11 processing by proprotein convertase 4 in human placental development. *Proc Natl Acad Sci U S A*. 2005;102:11047-11052.
236. Murphy R, Baptista J, Holly J, et al. Severe intrauterine growth retardation and atypical diabetes associated with a translocation breakpoint disrupting regulation of the insulin-like growth factor 2 gene. *J Clin Endocrinol Metab*. 2008;93:4373-4380.
237. Sparago A, Cerrato F, Vernucci M, et al. Microdeletions in the human H19 DMR result in loss of IGF2 imprinting and Beckwith-Wiedemann syndrome. *Nat Genet*. 2004;36:958-960.
238. Watson CS, Bialek P, Arizo M, et al. Elevated circulating insulin-like growth factor-binding protein-1 is sufficient to cause fetal growth restriction. *Endocrinology*. 2006;147:1175-1186.
239. Ben Lagha N, Seurin D, Le Bouc Y, et al. Insulin-like growth factor-binding protein (IGFBP-1) involvement in intrauterine growth retardation: study on IGFBP-1 overexpressing transgenic mice. *Endocrinology*. 2006;147:4730-4737.
240. Forhead AJ, Li J, Gilmour RS, et al. Thyroid hormone and the mRNA of the GH receptor and IGFs in skeletal muscle of fetal sheep. *Am J Physiol Endocrinol Metab*. 2002;282:E80-E86.
241. Ong K, Kratzsch J, Kiess W, et al. Size at birth and cord blood levels of insulin, insulin-like growth factor (IGF-I), IGF-II, IGF binding protein-1 (IGFBP-1), IGFBP-3 and the soluble IGF-II/mannose-6-phosphate receptor in term human infants. *J Clin Endocrinol Metab*. 2000;85: 4266-4269.
242. Pilistine SJ, Moses AC, Munro HN. Placental lactogen administration reverses the effect of low protein diet on maternal and fetal somatomedin levels in the pregnant rat. *Proc Natl Acad Sci U S A*. 1984;81: 5853-5857.
243. Gohlke BC, Fahnenstich H, Dame C, et al. Longitudinal data for intrauterine levels of fetal IGF-I and IGF-II. *Horm Res*. 2004;61:200-204.
244. Accili D, Drago J, Lee EJ, et al. Early neonatal death in mice homozygous for a null allele of the insulin receptor gene. *Nat Genet*. 1996;12:106-109.
245. Fisher DA, Lakshmanan J. Metabolism and effects of EGF and related growth factors in mammals. *Endocr Rev*. 1990;11:418-442.

246. Rotwein P. Peptide growth factors other than insulin-like growth factors or cytokines. In: DeGroot LJ, Jameson JL, eds. *Endocrinology*. 5th ed. Philadelphia, PA: Elsevier Saunders; 2006:675-695.
247. Meittinen PJ, Berger JE, Menesses J, et al. Epithelial immaturity and multiorgan failure in mice lacking epidermal growth factor receptor. *Nature*. 1995;376:337-341.
248. Brown PI, Lam R, Lakshmanan J, et al. Transforming growth factor alpha in developing rats. *Am J Physiol*. 1990;259:E256-E260.
249. Hemmings R, Langlais J, Falcone T, et al. Human embryos produce transforming growth factor α activity and insulin-like growth factor II. *Fertil Steril*. 1992;58:101-104.
250. Mazzoni IE, Kenigsberg RL. Effects of epidermal growth factor in the mammalian central nervous system. *Drug Dev Res*. 1992;26:111-128.
251. Kitchens DL, Snyder EY, Gottlieb DI. FGF and EGF are mitogens for immortalized neural progenitors. *J Neurobiol*. 1990;21:356-375.
252. Santa-Olalla J, Covarrubias L. Epidermal growth factor, transforming growth factor-α, and fibroblast growth factor differentially influence neural precursor cells of mouse embryonic mesencephalon. *J Neurosci Res*. 1995;42:172-183.
253. Lee KF, Simon H, Chen C, et al. Requirement for neuregulin receptor erbB2 in neural and cardiac development. *Nature*. 1995;378:394-398.
254. Kamei Y, Tsutsumi O, Kuwabara Y, et al. Intrauterine growth retardation and fetal losses are caused by epidermal growth factor deficiency in mice. *Am J Physiol*. 1993;264:R597-R600.
255. Yan Q, Elliott J, Snider WD. Brain derived neurotrophic factor rescues spinal motor neurons from axotomy-induced cell death. *Nature*. 1992;360:753-755.
256. Gospodarowicz D. Epidermal and nerve growth factors in mammalian development. *Annu Rev Physiol*. 1981;43:251-263.
257. Padbury JF, Lam RW, Polk DH, et al. Autoimmune sympathectomy in fetal rabbits. *J Dev Physiol*. 1986;8:369-376.
258. Tarris RH, Weichsel ME Jr, Fisher DA. Synthesis and secretion of a nerve growth stimulating factor by neonatal mouse astrocyte cells in vitro. *Pediatr Res*. 1986;20:367-372.
259. Giordano T, Pan JB, Casuto D, et al. Thyroid hormone regulation of NGF, NT3 and BDNF RNA in the adult rat brain. *Mol Brain Res*. 1992;16:239-245.
260. Lim GB, Dodic M, Earnest L, et al. Regulation of erythropoietin gene expression in fetal sheep by glucocorticoids. *Endocrinology*. 1996;137:1658-1663.
261. Moritz KM, Lim GB, Wintour EM. Developmental regulation of erythropoietin and erythropoiesis. *Am J Physiol*. 1997;273:R1829-R1844.
262. Betsholtz C. Functions of platelet-derived growth factor and its receptors deduced from gene inactivation in mice. *J Clin Ligand Assay*. 2000;23:206-213.
263. Lewandoski M, Sun X, Martin GR. Fgf8 signalling from the AER is essential for normal limb development. *Nat Genet*. 2000;26:460-463.
264. Oberbauer AM, Linkhart TA, Mohan S, et al. Fibroblast growth factor enhances human chorionic gonadotropin synthesis independent of mitogenic stimulation in Jar choriocarcinoma cells. *Endocrinology*. 1988;123:2696-2700.
265. Alfaidy N, Li W, Macintosh T, et al. Late gestation increase in 11beta-hydroxysteroid dehydrogenase 1 expression in human fetal membranes: a novel intrauterine source of cortisol. *J Clin Endocrinol Metab*. 2003;88:5033-5038.
266. Wallace MJ, Hooper SB, Harding R. Effects of elevated fetal cortisol concentrations on the volume, secretion, and reabsorption of lung liquid. *Am J Physiol*. 1995;269:R881-R887.
267. Muglia L, Jacobson L, Dikkes P, et al. Corticotropin-releasing hormone deficiency reveals major fetal but not adult glucocorticoid need. *Nature*. 1995;373:427-432.
268. Cole TJ, Blendy JA, Monaghan P, et al. Targeted disruption of the glucocorticoid receptor gene blocks adrenergic chromaffin cell development and severely retards lung maturation. *Genes Dev*. 1995;9:1608-1621.
269. Polk DH. Thyroid hormone effects on neonatal thermogenesis. *Semin Perinatol*. 1988;12:151-156.
270. Gunn TR, Gluckman PD. Perinatal thermogenesis. *Early Hum Dev*. 1995;42:169-183.
271. Obregon MJ, Pitamber R, Jacobsson A, et al. Euthyroid status is essential for the perinatal increase in thermogenin mRNA in brown adipose tissue of rat pups. *Biochem Biophys Res Commun*. 1987;148:9-14.
272. Polk DH, Padbury JF, Callegari CC, et al. Effect of fetal thyroidectomy on newborn thermogenesis in lambs. *Pediatr Res*. 1987;21:453-457.
273. Longhead JL, Minouni F, Tsang RC. Serum ionized calcium concentrations in normal neonates. *Am J Dis Child*. 1988;142:516-518.
274. Venkataraman PS, Tsang RC, Chen IW, et al. Pathogenesis of early neonatal hypocalcemia: studies of serum calcitonin, gastrin and plasma glucagon. *J Pediatr*. 1987;110:599-603.
275. Mimoumi F, Tsang RC. Perinatal mineral metabolism. In: Tulchinsky D, Little AB, eds. *Maternal-Fetal Endocrinology*. 2nd ed. Philadelphia, PA: WB Saunders; 1994:402-417.
276. Wheeler MD, Styne DM. Longitudinal changes in growth hormone response to growth hormone-releasing hormone in neonatal rhesus monkeys. *Pediatr Res*. 1990;28:15-18.
277. Penny R, Parlow AF, Frasier SD. Testosterone and estradiol concentrations in paired maternal and cord sera and their correlation with the concentration of chorionic gonadotropin. *Pediatrics*. 1979;64:604-608.
278. Mann DR, Gould KG, Collins DC, et al. Blockade of neonatal activation of the pituitary-testicular axis: effect on peripubertal luteinizing hormone and testosterone secretion and on testicular development in male monkeys. *J Clin Endocrinol Metab*. 1989;68:600-607.
279. Dohler KD. The special case of hormonal imprinting: the neonatal influence on sex. *Experientia*. 1986;42:759-769.
280. Resko JA, Roselli CE. Prenatal hormones organize sex differences in the neuroendocrine reproductive system: observations on guinea pigs and nonhuman primates. *Cell Mol Neurobiol*. 1997;17:627-648.
281. Kosut SS, Wood RI, Herbosa-Encaracion C, et al. Prenatal androgens time neuroendocrine puberty in the sheep: effect of testosterone dose. *Endocrinology*. 1997;138:1072-1077.
282. Grocock CA, Charlton HM, Pike MC. Role of fetal pituitary in cryptorchidism induced by exogenous maternal oestrogen during pregnancy in mice. *J Reprod Fertil*. 1988;83:295-300.
283. Martin SM, Moberg GP. Effects of early neonatal thyroxine treatment on development of the thyroid and adrenal axes in rats. *Life Sci*. 1981;29:1683-1688.
284. Walker P, Courtin F. Transient neonatal hyperthyroidism results in hypothyroidism in the adult rat. *Endocrinology*. 1985;116:2246-2250.
285. Csaba G, Inczefi-Gonda A, Dobozy O. Hereditary transmission in the F_1 generation of hormonal imprinting (receptor memory) induced in rats by neonatal exposure to insulin. *Acta Physiol Hung*. 1984;63:93-99.
286. Csaba G, Ronai A, Laszlo V, et al. Amplification of hormone receptors by neonatal oxytocin and vasopressin treatment. *Horm Metab Res*. 1980;12:28-31.
287. Benediktsson R, Lindsay RD, Noble J, et al. Glucocorticoid exposure in utero: new model for adult hypertension. *Lancet*. 1993;341:339-341.
288. Drake AJ, Walker BR, Seckl JR. Intergenerational consequences of fetal programming by in utero exposure to glucocorticoids in rats. *Am J Physiol Regul Integr Comp Physiol*. 2005;288:R34-R38.
289. Lackland DR. Fetal and early life determinants of hypertension in adults: implications for study. *Hypertension*. 2004;44:811-812.
290. Barker DJP. Fetal programming of coronary heart disease. *Trends Endocrinol Metab*. 2002;13:364-368.
291. Barker DJP. The developmental origins of chronic adult disease. *Acta Paediatr Suppl*. 2004;336:26-33.
292. Ozanne SE, Hales CN. Early programming of glucose-insulin metabolism. *Trends Endocrinol Metab*. 2002;13:368-373.
293. Matthews SG. Early programming of the hypothalamo-pituitary-adrenal axis. *Trends Endocrinol Metab*. 2002;13:373-380.
294. Young BS. Programming of sympatho-adrenal function. *Trends Endocrinol Metab*. 2002;13:381-385.
295. Davies MJ, Norman RJ. Programming and reproductive function. *Trends Endocrinol Metab*. 2002;13:386-392.
296. Holt RIG. Fetal programming of the growth hormone–insulin-like growth factor axis. *Trends Endocrinol Metab*. 2002;13:392-402.
297. Dodic M, Moritz K, Koukoulas I, et al. Programmed hypertension: kidney, brain or both. *Trends Endocrinol Metab*. 2002;13:403-408.
298. Reik W, Constancia M, Fowdey A, et al. Regulation of supply and demand for maternal nutrients in mammals by imprinted genes. *J Physiol*. 2003;547:35-44.
299. Ibanez L, Ong K, Potau N, et al. Insulin gene variable number of tandem repeat genotype and the low birth weight, precocious pubarche, and hyperinsulinism sequence. *J Clin Endocrinol Metab*. 2001;86:5788-5793.
300. Ijzerman RG, Stehouwer CDA, de Geus EJ, et al. Low birth weight is associated with increased sympathetic activity: dependence on genetic factors. *Circulation*. 2003;108:566-571.
301. Fowden AL, Forhead AJ. Endocrine mechanisms of intrauterine programming. *Reproduction*. 2004;127:515-526.
302. Slone-Wilcoxon J, Redei EE. Maternal-fetal glucocorticoid milieu programs hypothalamic-pituitary-thyroid function of adult offspring. *Endocrinology*. 2004;145:4068-4072.
303. Lavcola L, Perrini S, Belsanti G, et al. Intrauterine growth restriction in humans is associated with abnormalities in placental insulin-like growth factor signaling. *Endocrinology*. 2005;146:1498-1505.
304. Waterland RA, Jirtle RL. Early nutrition, epigenetic changes at transposons and imprinted genes, and enhanced susceptibility to adult chronic diseases. *Nutrition*. 2004;20:63-68.
305. McMullen S, Langley-Evans SC. Maternal low-protein diet in rat pregnancy programs blood pressure through sex-specific mechanisms. *Am J Physiol Regul Integr Physiol*. 2005;288:R85-R90.
306. Bunt JC, Tataranni PA, Salbe AD. Intrauterine exposure to diabetes is a determinant of hemoglobin A(1)c and systolic blood pressure in Pima Indian children. *J Clin Endocrinol Metab*. 2005;90:3225-3229.

307. Zheng X, Hendry WJ III. Neonatal stilbestrol treatment alters the estrogen-related expression of both cell proliferation and apoptosis-related proto-oncogene (c-jun, dfos, cmyc, bax, bcl-2 and bcl-x) in the hamster uterus. *Cell Growth Diff.* 1997;8:425-434.
308. Huang WW, Yin Y, Bi Q, et al. Developmental diethylstilbestrol exposure alters genetic pathways of uterine cytodifferentiation. *Mol Endocrinol.* 2005;19:669-682.
309. Csaba G. Receptor ontogeny and hormonal imprinting. *Experientia.* 1986;42:750-759.
310. Sato SM, Mains MI, Adzick MS, et al. Plasticity in the adrenocorticotropin-related peptides produced by primary cultures of neonatal rat pituitary. *Endocrinology.* 1988;122:68-77.
311. Vickers MH, Gluckman PD, Coveny HH, et al. Neonatal leptin treatment reverses developmental programming. *Endocrinology.* 2005;146: 4211-4216.
312. Flake AW. Fetal therapy: medical and surgical approaches. In: Creasy RK, Resnik R, eds. *Maternal-Fetal Medicine.* 4th ed. Philadelphia, PA: WB Saunders; 1999:365-377.
313. Harman CR. Assessment of fetal health. In: Creasy RK, Resnik R, eds. *Maternal-Fetal Medicine.* 5th ed. Philadelphia, PA: WB Saunders; 2004:357-401.
314. Resnick R, Creasy RK. Intrauterine growth restriction. In: Creasy RK, Resnick R, eds. *Maternal Fetal Medicine.* 5th ed. Philadelphia, PA: WB Saunders; 2004:495-512.
315. Bianchi DW. Prenatal exclusion of recessively inherited disorders: should maternal plasma analysis precede invasive techniques. *Clin Chem.* 2002;48:689-690.
316. Manning FA. General principles and applications of ultrasonography. In: Creasy RK, Resnik R, eds. *Maternal-Fetal Medicine.* 5th ed. Philadelphia, PA: WB Saunders; 2004:315-355.
317. Fisher DA. Fetal thyroid function: diagnosis and management of fetal thyroid disorders. *Clin Obstet Gynecol.* 1997;40:16-31.
318. New MI, Carlton A, Obeid J, et al. Update: prenatal diagnosis for congenital adrenal hyperplasia in 595 pregnancies. *Endocrinologist.* 2003;13:233-239.
319. Charlton V, Johengen M. Fetal intravenous nutritional supplementation ameliorates the development of embolization-induced growth retardation in sheep. *Pediatr Res.* 1987;22:55-61.
320. Flake AW, Zanjani ED. In utero hematopoietic stem cell transplantation. *JAMA.* 1997;278:932-937.
321. Lin RY, Kubo A, Keller GM, et al. Committing embryonic stem cells to differentiate into thyrocyte-like cells in vitro. *Endocrinology.* 2003;144: 2644-2649.
322. Waddington SN, Kennea NL, Buckley SMK, et al. Fetal and neonatal gene therapy: benefits and pitfalls. *Gene Therapy.* 2004;11:592-597.
323. Bennett A, Wilson DM, Liu R, et al. Levels of insulin-like growth factors I and II in human cord blood. *J Clin Endocrinol Metab.* 1983;57: 609-612.
324. Kaplan SL, Grumbach MM, Aubert ML. The ontogenesis of pituitary hormones and hypothalamic factors in the human fetus: maturation of central nervous system regulation of anterior pituitary function. *Recent Prog Horm Res.* 1976;32:161-243.
325. Bala RM, Lopatka J, Leung A, et al. Serum immunoreactive somatomedin levels in normal adults, pregnant women at term, children at various ages, and children with constitutionally delayed growth. *J Clin Endocrinol Metab.* 1981;52:508-512.
326. Winters AJ, Oliver C, Colston C, et al. Plasma ATH levels in the human fetus and neonate as related to age and parturition. *J Clin Endocrinol Metab.* 1974;39:269-273.
327. Murphy BEP. Human fetal serum cortisol levels related to gestational age: evidence of a midgestational fall and a steep late gestational rise, independent of sex or mode of delivery. *Am J Obstet Gynecol.* 1982;144:276-282.
328. Beitins IZ, Bayard F, Ances FIG, et al. The metabolic clearance rate, blood production, interconversion and transplacental passage of cortisol and cortisone in pregnancy near term. *Pediatr Res.* 1973;7: 509-513.
329. Fisher DA, Klein AH. Thyroid development and disorders of thyroid function in the newborn. *N Engl J Med.* 1981;304:702-712.
330. Santini F, Chiovato L, Ghirri P, et al. Serum iodothyronines in the human fetus and the newborn: evidence for an important role of placenta in fetal thyroid hormone homeostasis. *J Clin Endocrinol Metab.* 1999;84:493-498.
331. Reyes FI, Boroditsky RS, Winter JS, et al. Studies on human sexual development: II. Fetal and maternal serum gonadotropin and sex steroid concentrations. *J Clin Endocrinol Metab.* 1974;38:612-617.
332. Kaplan SL, Grumbach MM, Aubert ML. The ontogenesis of pituitary hormones and hypothalamic factors in the human fetus: maturation of central nervous system regulation of anterior pituitary function. *Recent Prog Horm Res.* 1976;32:161-243.
333. Winter JS, Faiman C, Hobson WC, et al. Pituitary-gonadal relations in infancy: I. Patterns of serum gonadotropin concentrations from birth to four years of age in man and chimpanzee. *J Clin Endocrinol Metab.* 1975;40:545-551
334. Forest MG, Cathiard AM. Pattern of plasma testosterone and delta4-androstenedione in normal newborns; evidence for testicular activity at birth. *J Clin Endocrinol Metab.* 1975;41:977-980.

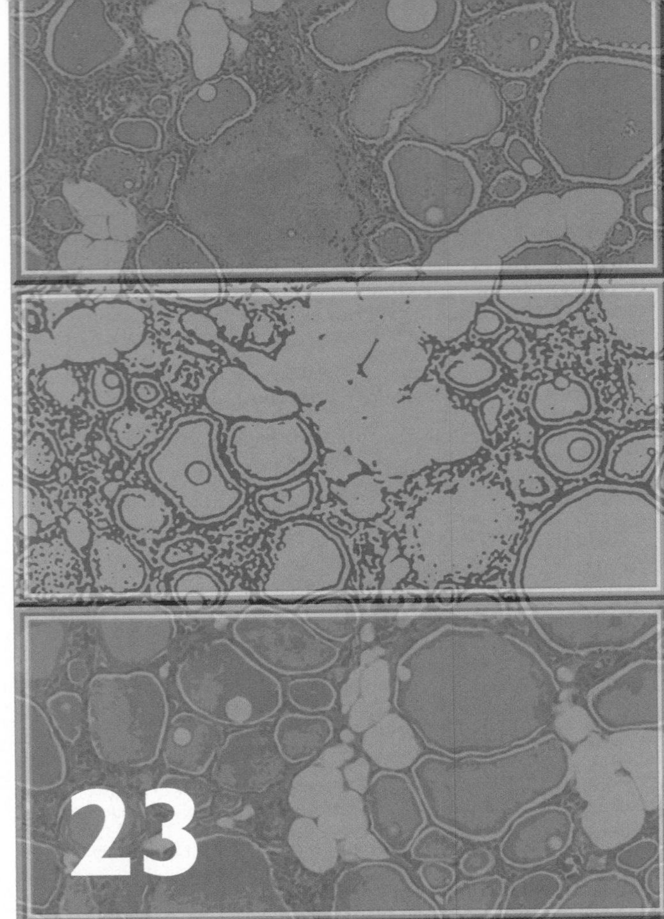

CHAPTER 23

Disorders of Sex Development

JOHN C. ACHERMANN • IEUAN A. HUGHES

Under most circumstances, the distinction between male and female is considered to be absolute, and sex assignment at birth is instantaneous. The sex assignment based on the birth phenotype is simultaneously accompanied by gender assignment and sex of rearing as male or female. When genital anomalies preclude initial sex assignment, the consensus is that assigning male or female sex remains the preferred option in most societies. Nevertheless, reaching a final decision may be delayed by the nature and complexity of the investigations and assessments required. Ambiguity of the external genitalia sufficient to prevent immediate sex assignment at birth is rare, but it is estimated that abnormalities of the external genitalia that need formal investigation occur in 1 of every 4000 births.[1]

Investigation and management of disorders of sex development in infants and young people require an understanding of the embryology of the urogenital system, the genes that control organ development, and the mechanism of normal hormone production and action. Previous editions of this textbook have held that tenet and emphasized the scientific advances that allow the many causes of abnormal genital development to be better characterized.[2] Many of the advances in identifying key genes involved in normal sex determination and sex differentiation have resulted from detailed clinicopathologic assessment of prismatic cases. However, causation remains unexplained for many forms of gonadal dysgenesis and for the male who has normal testis determination, androgen production, and action but abnormal external genital development. Application of techniques such as array comparative genome hybridization and high-throughput sequencing is providing information about the disorders that remain unexplained.

Clarity in terminology is essential to understand disorders of sex development and their management. The importance of this element of management was a key component of a statement known as the Chicago Consensus, published by a group of experts working in this field.[3] It was resolved that the term *intersex* should be abandoned in view of pejorative elements and be replaced by the generic term *disorders of sex development* (DSDs). Linked to this change was the recommendation to abandon nomenclature such as *male pseudohermaphroditism, female pseudohermaphroditism,* and *true hermaphroditism.* Already there is evidence that centers providing a service for DSDs are embracing these new developments, and the terminology is appearing in scientific literature.[4] The alternative nomenclature is shown in Table 23-1; its use for classification of the causes of DSDs is discussed later.

There has been a major change in how DSDs are managed, with families and the affected individual at an appropriate age being fully engaged in the decision-making

TABLE 23-1

Proposed Revised Nomenclature

Previous Terms	Proposed Terms
Intersex	Disorders of sex development (DSDs)
Male pseudohermaphrodite Undervirilization of an XY male Undermasculinization of an XY male	46,XY DSD
Female pseudohermaphrodite Overvirilization of an XX female Masculinization of an XX female	46,XX DSD
True hermaphrodite	Ovotesticular DSD
XX male or XX sex reversal	46,XX testicular DSD
XY sex reversal	46,XY complete gonadal dysgenesis

Reproduced with permission from Hughes IA, Houk C, Ahmed SF, et al. Consensus statement on management of intersex disorders. *Arch Dis Child.* 2006;91:554-562.

process that involves disclosure commensurate with changing cognitive and psychological development. The need to understand the embryology and genetic and hormonal control of typical sex development underpins the investigation and management of a DSD.

DEVELOPMENT OF REPRODUCTIVE SYSTEMS

Development of reproductive systems begins at 4 to 5 weeks' gestation in humans and may be considered complete with the development of secondary sexual characteristics and fertility (i.e., production of viable gametes) after puberty. Sex development is a dynamic process that requires the appropriate and timely interaction of a multitude of genes, proteins, signaling molecules, paracrine factors, and endocrine stimuli.[5-9] Marked differences in the basic mechanisms of sex determination, differentiation, and reproductive strategy have evolved in different species, with variability in sex chromosome complement, gonad development, and gametogenesis throughout the animal kingdom.[10,11] In this chapter, we focus on the basic mechanisms of reproductive development in humans. We also include important insights obtained from studies of normal and transgenic mice and discuss the relevance of these findings to individuals with DSDs.

The three basic processes of normal development are sex determination and sex differentiation, development of the hypothalamic-gonadotroph axis in the fetus, and function of the hypothalamic-pituitary-gonadal (HPG) axis in infancy and childhood. A more detailed explanation of pituitary development is provided in Chapter 22 and of normal and disordered puberty in Chapter 25.

Sex Determination and Sex Differentiation

Sex determination is the process whereby the bipotential gonad develops into a testis or an ovary. *Sex differentiation* requires the developing gonad to function appropriately to produce peptide hormones and steroids.

In the male, the process of sex differentiation involves regression of Müllerian structures (uterus, fallopian tubes, and the upper one third of the vagina), stabilization of Wolffian structures (seminal vesicles, vasa deferentia, and epididymides), androgenization of the external genitalia (penis and scrotum), and descent of the testes from their origin in the urogenital ridge to their final position in the scrotum (Fig. 23-1).

In the female, the ovary usually is steroidogenically quiescent until the time of puberty, when estrogen synthesis stimulates breast and uterine development and follicular development results in regular menstrual cycles. Defects in ovarian development usually first manifest in adolescence. Ovarian development and differentiation has been viewed in the past as a default process that occurs in the absence of the chromosomal, genetic, and endocrine signals deemed actively necessary to "make a male." Although male sex differentiation is undoubtedly a more active developmental process—as defined in the classic experiments of Alfred Jost[12]—studies of gene expression

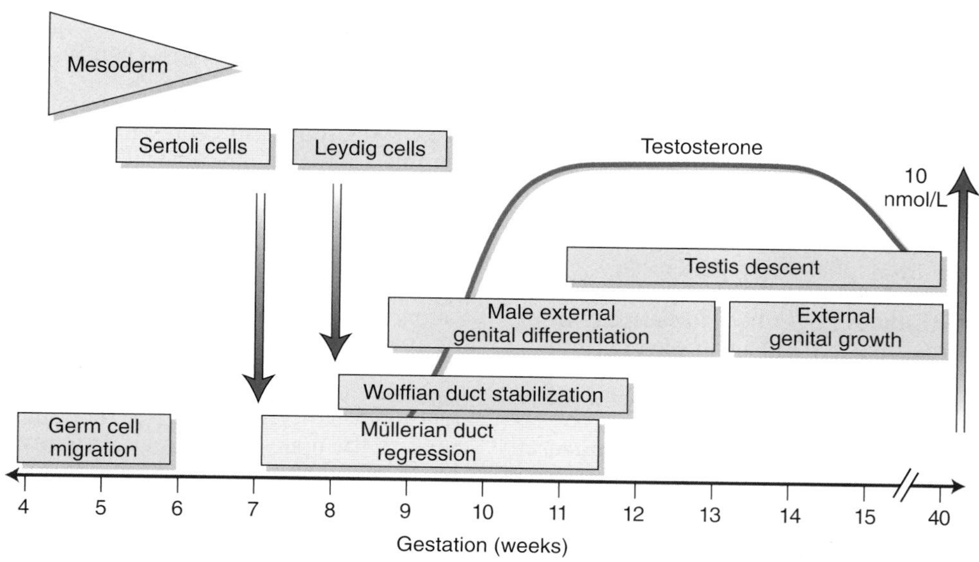

Figure 23-1 Events temporally related to sex differentiation in the male fetus. Mesoderm refers to the tissue source for Sertoli and Leydig cell formation. The continuous line depicts the rise in fetal serum testosterone, with a peak concentration of about 10 nmol/L (300 ng/dL).

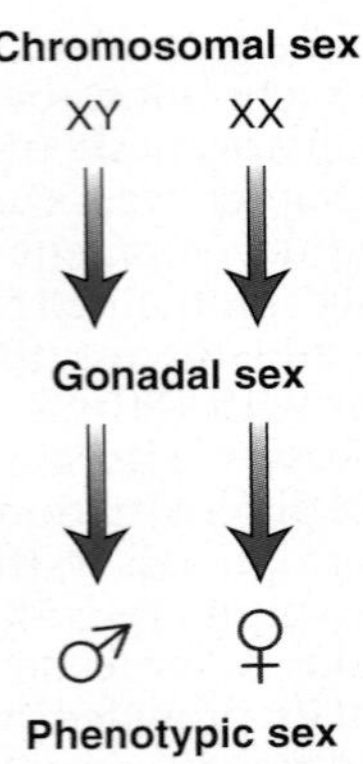

Figure 23-2 Division of sex development into three major components provides a useful framework for diagnosis and classification. Chromosomal sex refers to the karyotype (46,XX, 46,XY, or variants). Gonadal sex refers to the presence of a testis or ovary after the process of sex determination. Phenotypic (anatomic) sex refers to the appearance of the external genitalia and internal structures after the process of sex differentiation.

show that a specific complement of genes are implicated in ovarian development and integrity, some of which (e.g., *RSPO1*) may actively antagonize testis differentiation.[13-15] Even the concept of a fixed and quiescent population of ovarian germ cells at birth has been challenged by some.[16] Ovarian development probably involves many active processes rather than being simply a default mechanism.

Classically, sex determination and sex differentiation can be divided into three major components: chromosomal sex (i.e., presence of a Y or X chromosome), gonadal sex (i.e., presence of a testis or ovary), and phenotypic or anatomic sex (i.e., presence of male or female external and internal genitalia) (Fig. 23-2). None of these processes absolutely defines a person's "sex," and psychosexual development ("brain sex") may be an unpredictable outcome of several biologic factors, as well as environmental and social influences. The presence or absence of a Y chromosome or well-formed testes should not be the focus of how a physician views an individual with a DSD after a diagnosis or management plan has been established. Consideration of sex development in terms of chromosomal sex, gonadal sex, and phenotypic (or anatomic) sex can be a useful way of understanding the processes involved in reproductive development, and it can be a helpful construct for the investigation and diagnosis of patients with these conditions, especially because the (somatic) karyotype is usually readily available as one of the first and potentially guiding investigations. The chromosomal-gonadal-phenotypic model is described in this chapter.

Chromosomal Sex

Chromosomal sex describes the complement of sex chromosomes present in an individual (e.g., 46,XY; 46,XX). In humans, the usual complement of 46 chromosomes consists of 22 pairs of autosomes (identified numerically from 1 to 22 based on decreasing size) and a pair of sex chromosomes (XX or XY) (Fig. 23-3). Other species have different numbers of chromosomes, or they may have sexually dimorphic autosomes.[10,11]

In humans, chromosomal sex usually is determined at the time of fertilization, when two haploid gametes (ova and sperm, with 23 chromosomes each) fuse to generate a diploid zygote (46 chromosomes). Gametes are ultimately derived from germ cells, which initially replicate their chromosome complement and then undergo a series of two meiotic divisions, meiosis I (reduction division) and meiosis II, to produce haploid ova or sperm. Normal ova have a single X chromosome. Normal sperm contain a single Y chromosome or a single X chromosome, resulting, respectively, in a 46,XY or 46,XX zygote after fertilization.

Nondisjunction is the failure of either of a pair of sister chromatids to separate during anaphase (Fig. 23-4).[17,18] *Meiotic nondisjunction* during gametogenesis can result in ova or sperm with gain or loss of sex chromosomal material. Fertilization by such gametes can give rise to a zygote with an imbalance in sex chromosome number, called *sex chromosome aneuploidy*. For example, a zygote with a single X chromosome (i.e., 45,X) defines Turner syndrome, and the presence of an extra X causes Klinefelter syndrome (47,XXY) or triple-X syndrome (47,XXX).[18] Zygotes with no X chromosomal material (45,Y) are nonviable.

Mitotic nondisjunction can occur in the zygote, resulting in an imbalance in sex chromosome number in a proportion or subset of cells, and this is called *sex chromosome mosaicism* (e.g., 45,X/46,XY). In such cases, the two (or more) cell lines originate from a single zygote. This situation differs from *chimerism,* which is the existence of two or more cell lines with different genetic origins in one individual. Chimerism can occur through double fertilization (dispermy) of a binucleate ovum, fusion of two complete zygotes or morulae before implantation, or fertilization by separate sperm of an ovum and its polar body.

Chimerism is difficult to detect if the separate cell lines have the same sex chromosomes. However, if the different cell lines are of different sexes, a 46,XX/46,XY karyotype occurs. This form of true *sex chromosome chimerism* is rare in humans, but it is seen more frequently in cattle in a condition called *freemartinism,* which results from admixture of hematopoietic and primordial germ cells (PGCs) between biovular twins of opposite sex through anastomotic placental channels. A 46,XX/46,XY karyotype also can result from mosaicism. The consequences of some of these events in humans are discussed later (see "Sex Chromosome Disorders of Sex Development").

The Y Chromosome. Although the Y chromosome was initially thought to be "inert," detection of a 46,XY karyotype in males and a 47,XXY karyotype in men with Klinefelter syndrome provided evidence that the Y chromosome carries a gene (or genes) responsible for male sex determination. In fact, a single Y chromosome usually is sufficient to drive testis development, even in the presence of multiple copies of chromosome X.

The human Y chromosome is approximately 60 megabases (Mb) long and represents only 2% of the human genome DNA (Fig. 23-5).[19,20] The Y chromosome consists of the highly variable and largely genetically inactive heterochromatic region on the long arm, the remnants of a conserved male-specific region, and autosomal-derived regions that are estimated to have been added approximately 80 to 130 million years ago. It is thought that Y-chromosomal genes encode only 60 proteins and that the male-specific regions are undergoing rapid evolution, with marked differences even between humans and chimpanzees.[21] Although some of these genes have putative roles in growth, cognition, and tooth development, several genes in the male-specific region are involved in reproductive development and function. For example, a cluster of genes at Yq11.22 (e.g., the *AZFc* region) is essential for spermatogenesis, and genes within the gonadoblastoma locus (e.g., *TSPY*) increase the risk of malignancy when present in dysgenetic gonads. Deletions of other genetic loci, such as a 1.6-Mb deletion of the Y chromosome that

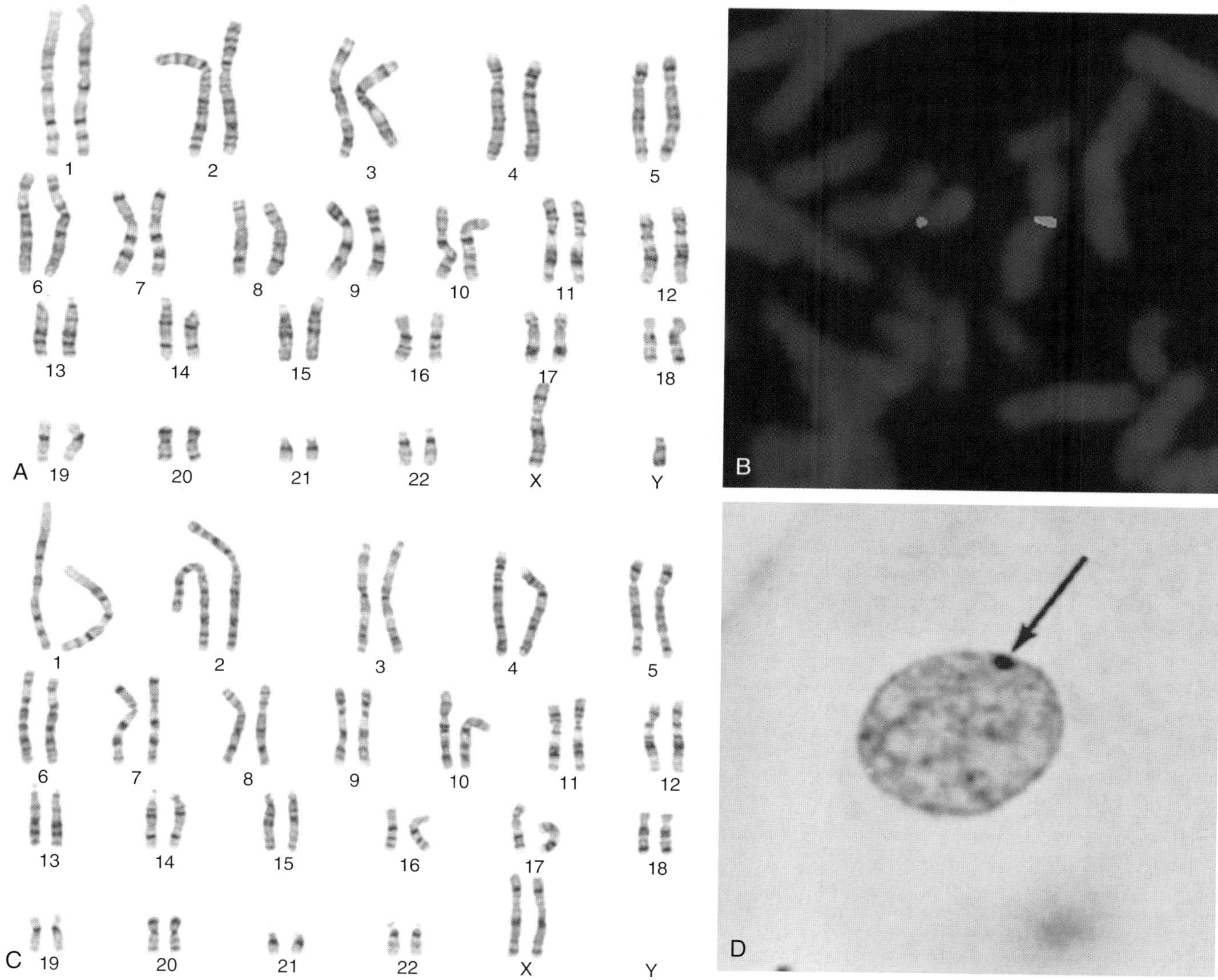

Figure 23-3 Cytogenetic and fluorescence in situ hybridization (FISH) studies. **A,** Male (46,XY) G-banded karyotype. **B,** FISH analysis of a male (46,XY) using fluorescent probes directed against SRY (spectrum red) and against the X centromere (spectrum green). **C,** Female (46,XX) G-banded karyotype. **D,** Photomicrograph shows the X chromatin body (Barr body, *arrow*) in the nucleus of buccal mucosa cells from a 46,XX female (thionine stain; original magnification, ×2000). (**A** through **C,** Courtesy of Lee Grimsley and Jonathan Waters, MD, North East London Regional Cytogenetics Laboratory, Great Ormond Street Hospital NHS Trust, London, UK.)

removes part of the *AZF*c region, known as the *gr/gr* deletion, result in susceptibility to germ cell tumors.[22-24]

The euchromatic (conserved) portion of the Y chromosome consists of a Y-specific segment and regions at the distal ends of the short and long arms, called the *pseudoautosomal regions* (PARs) (see Fig. 23-5).[19] These PARs are homologous to the distal ends of the short and long arms of the X chromosome and are the only regions involved in pairing and recombination during meiosis. This process is essential for proper distribution of recombined sex chromosomal material to daughter cells. PAR1 (distal short arm, Yp and Xp) contains at least 10 genes, including the homeobox gene *SHOX* (formerly called *PHOG*). SHOX haploinsufficiency contributes to the short stature associated with Turner syndrome, Xp– or Yp–deletions, and Léri-Weill syndrome (i.e., dyschondrosteosis). These regions are not subject to dosage compensation (i.e., gene inactivation). PAR2 (distal long arm) contains genes that mostly encode growth factors and signaling molecules.

The quest for a testis-determining factor on the Y chromosome began more than 50 years ago. The discovery by Eichwald and Silmser in 1955 of a male cell membrane–specific antigen that causes rejection of skin grafts by female mice led to pursuit of the H-Y antigen as a candidate testis-determining factor.[25] In 1987, Mardon and Page proposed that the sex-determining function of the Y chromosome is located within a 140-kb segment of the short arm, within the Y-specific euchromatic portion.[26] A zinc finger transcription factor, ZFY, was the initial candidate in this region. However, in 1989, Palmer and colleagues described several 46,XX *males* who harbored Y-to-X translocations of Y chromosomal material that was distal (telomeric) to the ZFY locus; this discovery finally refuted the role of ZFY as the putative testis-determining gene and focused attention

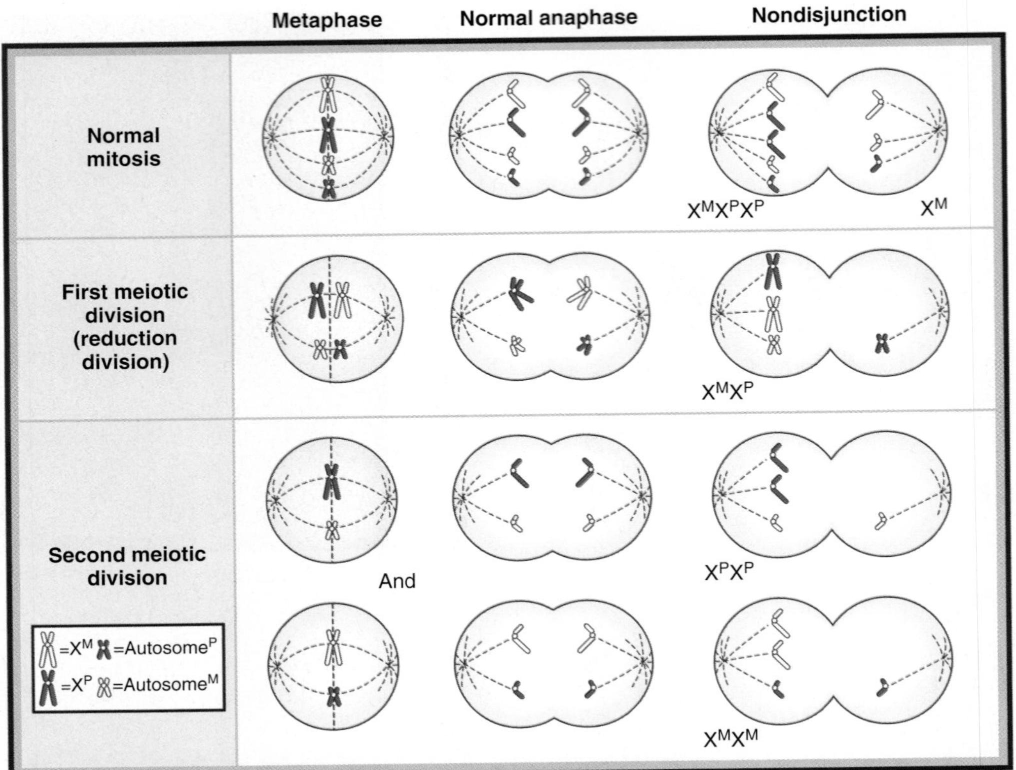

Figure 23-4 A female somatic cell is represented to show the types of cell division. At the metaphase plate are two X chromosomes and two homologous autosomes of group 21 to 22. Division occurs through the centromere, giving rise to two daughter cells of identical chromosomal composition. Replication of each arm into two chromatids takes place while the chromosomes are extended and before the next metaphase. The first meiotic division involves pairing of homologous chromosomes. The centromere does not divide in this cell division. Chance determines whether the maternal (X^M) or paternal (X^P) member of each pair goes to a specific daughter cell. During the complex prophase of first meiotic division (not shown), multiple chiasmata are formed between the chromosomes of each pair, facilitating exchanges of chromosomal segments (crossover) between them. During the second meiotic division, the centromere again divides, giving rise to daughter cells identical to the parent cell. This division more nearly resembles mitosis than the first meiotic division. Nondisjunction can take place in mitosis or in the first or second meiotic division.

on a 35-kb region of the Y chromosome close to the pseudoautosomal boundary.[27] This region contained a putative transcription factor subsequently called *sex-determining region Y (SRY)* that was expressed in appropriate tissues (see Fig. 23-5).

A series of elegant studies in mice and humans established *SRY* as the likely primary Y-chromosomal testis-determining gene.[28-30] The first definitive proof came with the generation of transgenic XX mice specifically expressing the *SRY* locus (14 kb); some of these mice had a male phenotype, developed testes (without spermatogenesis), and showed male sexual mating behavior (Fig. 23-6).[31] This work was supported by reports of deletions and loss-of-function mutations in *SRY* in humans with 46,XY complete gonadal dysgenesis (Swyer syndrome) (see later discussion).[29,32,33]

The X Chromosome. The X chromosome is a relatively large and gene-rich chromosome compared with the Y chromosome, and it consists of about 160 Mb of genomic DNA (see Fig. 23-5).[19,34,35] This DNA contains 5% of the haploid genome and more than 1000 expressed genes, of which about 800 encode proteins. Genes on the X chromosome play an important role in sex development in males and females at the level of the gonad and gametogenesis and also in hypothalamic-pituitary (gonadotroph) function (e.g., androgen receptor [AR], KAL1, DAX1 [NR0B1], MAMLD1, SOX3). More than 100 X-chromosome genes are expressed in the testis.[34] However, most X-linked genes are unrelated to sex development and have a diverse range of cellular functions.

The X chromosome contains PARs at the distal end of each arm, similar to the Y chromosome (see Fig. 23-5).[19] These regions and several genes in their boundaries do not undergo X inactivation; they function in an autosomal fashion with their homologs on the Y-chromosome PARs. A large number of genes on the X chromosome are located outside the PARs and do not have homologs on the Y chromosome. Because many of these genes are involved in a wide range of cellular processes unrelated to sex development or sex-specific function, a process must exist to maintain the balance in expressed copy number (i.e., gene dosage) of these genes in both males with a single X chromosome and females with two X chromosomes.

The first insight into a mechanism that could explain correction of this potential imbalance came after identification in 1949 of the X chromatin body (i.e., Barr body) in a proportion of cells in females (see Fig. 23-3). Subsequent studies showed that this X chromatin is derived from only one of the two X chromosomes in interphase nuclei of these somatic cells.[36] Grumbach and colleagues showed that the X chromosome giving rise to X chromatin completes DNA synthesis later than any other chromosome.[36] These findings led to the concept that only one X chromosome is genetically active during interphase, whereas the other X chromosome is heterochromatinized and relatively inactive. This change in activation state occurs in early gestation in humans (12 to 18 days, late blastocyte stage)

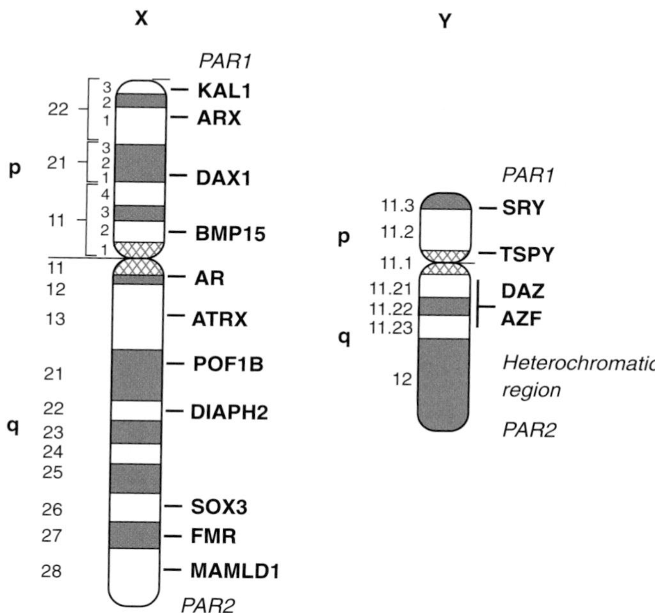

Figure 23-5 Schematic diagrams of the X chromosome *(left)* and Y chromosome *(right)* show key regions and genes involved in sex development and reproduction. AR, androgen receptor; ARX, aristaless-related homeobox, X-linked; ATRX, α-thalassemia, X-linked mental retardation; AZF, azoospermia factor; BMP15, bone morphogenetic protein 15; DAX1, dosage-sensitive sex reversal congenital adrenal hypoplasia critical region on the X chromosome type 1; DAZ, deleted in azoospermia; DIAP2, human homolog of the *Drosophila* diaphanous gene; FMR, fragile X, mental retardation; KAL1, Kallmann syndrome type 1; MAMLD1, mastermind-like domain containing 1 (CXorf6); p, short arm; PAR, pseudoautosomal region; POF1B, actin-binding protein, 34 kd; q, long arm; SOX3, SRY-related HMG box 3; SRY, sex-determining region Y; TSPY, testes-specific protein Y.

and is a multistep process leading to stable and epigenetic silencing of genes on all X chromosomes in excess of one (Lyon hypothesis).[37] However, female germ cells beyond the stage of oogonia are exempt from X inactivation, in keeping with the need for a second X chromosome for germ cell and ovarian development.

X inactivation involves a number of important steps, including chromosome counting, random selection of which X chromosome to inactivate (maternal or paternal), and silencing—the initiation, establishment, and maintenance of X inactivation. These complex molecular and cellular silencing processes involve DNA methylation, histone acetylation, and maintenance of inactivation by a noncoding RNA gene *XIST,* located in the X-inactivating center (Xq13), and its antisense transcript TSIX.[38,39] After inactivation has occurred, the inactive state of that particular X chromosome is transmitted to all descendants of that cell, so that normal females effectively function as genetic mosaics insofar as X-linked traits are concerned. If the initial population of cells is small, skewed X inactivation can occur as a chance event despite random inactivation. In these situations, heterozygous female carriers of an X-linked disorder may manifest symptoms of the condition. Profiles of X inactivation exhibit extensive variability.[40] Some studies have proposed that certain genes on the X chromosome in males and the active chromosome in females undergo a further process of upregulation so that the ratio of sex chromosome to autosome expression is maintained.[38,39,41] A subset of genes on the X chromosome may be imprinted.

It was hoped that studying families with ovarian failure or women with Turner syndrome who have chromosomal variations such as partial loss of X material would lead to identification of the loci for key genes involved in ovarian development and function.[42-44] Although several X-chromosomal loci and genes for premature ovarian failure (POF) or primary ovarian insufficiency (POI) have been identified, including those for POF1 (*FMR1* permutations on Xq26-q28), POF2A (*DIAPH2* on Xq22), POF2B (*POF1B* [an actin-binding protein] on Xq21), and POF4 (*BMP15* on Xp11.2), the gene for POF3 (*FOXL2*) is on 3q23, that for POF5 (*NOBOX*) is on 7q35, that for POF6 (*FIGLA*) is on 2p12, and that for steroidogenic factor 1 or SF1 (*NR5A1*) is on 9q33.[45-51] Certain variants of Turner syndrome are more likely to involve ovarian dysfunction (e.g., isochromosome for Xq), but it is likely that the accelerated oocyte atresia in Turner syndrome also reflects impaired meiosis and subsequent germ cell apoptosis caused by sex chromosome imbalance, rather than only the loss of certain genetic loci containing ovarian development genes.[42]

Gonadal Sex

Gonadal sex refers to the development of the gonadal tissue as testis or ovary. The principal embryologic and morphologic changes involved in gonad development are shown in Figure 23-7 and have been described in excellent reviews by Brennan and Capel[5] and by Wilhelm and colleagues.[7]

The Bipotential Gonad. The primitive gonad arises from a condensation of the medioventral region of the urogenital ridge at approximately 4 to 5 weeks after conception in humans (see Fig. 23-7). The primitive gonad separates from the adrenal primordium at about 5 weeks but remains bipotential ("indifferent") until about 42 days' post-conception. Testes and ovaries are morphologically indistinguishable from each other until approximately the 6th week of post-conception (13-mm stage).

Several important genes are expressed in the developing urogenital ridge in mice that facilitate formation of the bipotential gonad; they include *Emx2, Lim1, Lhx9, M33/CBX2, Pod1, Gata4/Fog2, Map3k4, Wt1,* and *Nr5a1/Sf1* (Fig. 23-8). Deletion of these genes causes gonadal dysgenesis in mice, but only some of them have been associated with human DSDs.

Emx2 is a mouse homolog of the *Drosophila* empty spiracles (*Ems*) homeobox gene involved in head morphogenesis. It is expressed early in the development of the urogenital system; *Emx2* null mice have absent kidneys, ureters, gonads, and genital tracts and have developmental abnormalities of the brain.[52] Although heterozygous mutations in *EMX2* have been found in patients with schizencephaly (without gonadal dysgenesis), mutations causing a gonadal phenotype in humans have not been reported.[53]

The homeobox gene *Lhx1* (also called *Lim1*) is expressed in the intermediate mesoderm and nephrogenic cords. Targeted deletion of this gene in mice results in a failure to develop kidneys, gonads, and anterior brain structures.[54] Human *LHX1* mutations have not been described, although the expected phenotype would be quite severe. The related homeobox gene *Lhx9* is also expressed in the brain, limb buds, and urogenital ridge, but deletion of this gene in mice leads to gonadal dysgenesis alone.[55] No human *LHX9* mutations have been identified, despite a study of 41 patients with 46,XY gonadal dysgenesis.[56]

Other genes implicated in early gonad development in mice are *M33/CBX2, Pod1, Gata4/Fog2,* and *Map3k4.*[57-59] *M33* is the mouse homolog of the *Drosophila* polycomb

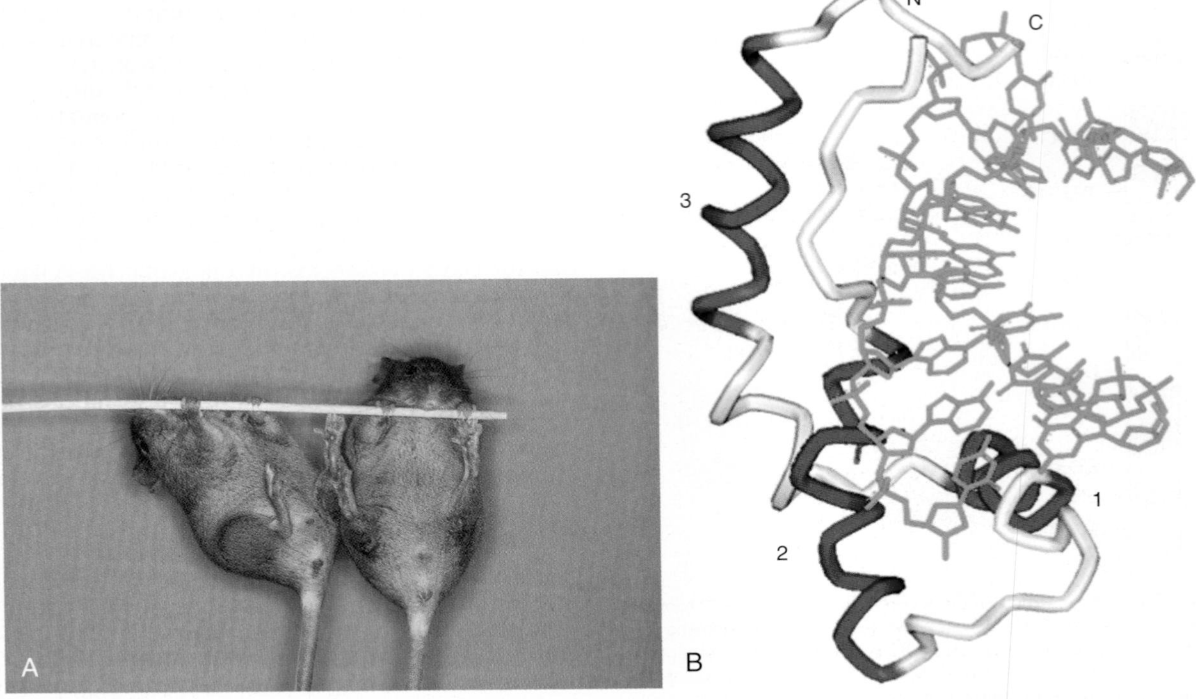

Figure 23-6 **A,** The XX*SRY*$^{+}$ mouse *(right)* has testis development and a male phenotype, providing convincing evidence that *SRY* is a testis-determining gene. A normal XY male littermate is shown for comparison *(left)*. **B,** Model of the structure of the SRY high-mobility group (HMG) box bound to DNA. The HMG domain contains three α-helices *(red)*, which adopt an L-shaped conformation. Binding of this region of SRY to the minor groove of DNA *(green)* causes it to bend and unwind. (**A,** Courtesy of Professor Robin Lovell-Badge, National Institute of Medical Research, London, UK; **B,** From Harley VR, Clarkson MJ, Argentaro A. The molecular action and regulation of the testis-determining factors, SRY [sex-determining region on the Y chromosome] and SOX9 [SRY-related high-mobility group {HMG} box 9]. *Endocr Rev.* 2003;24:466-487, with permission of The Endocrine Society, copyright 2003.)

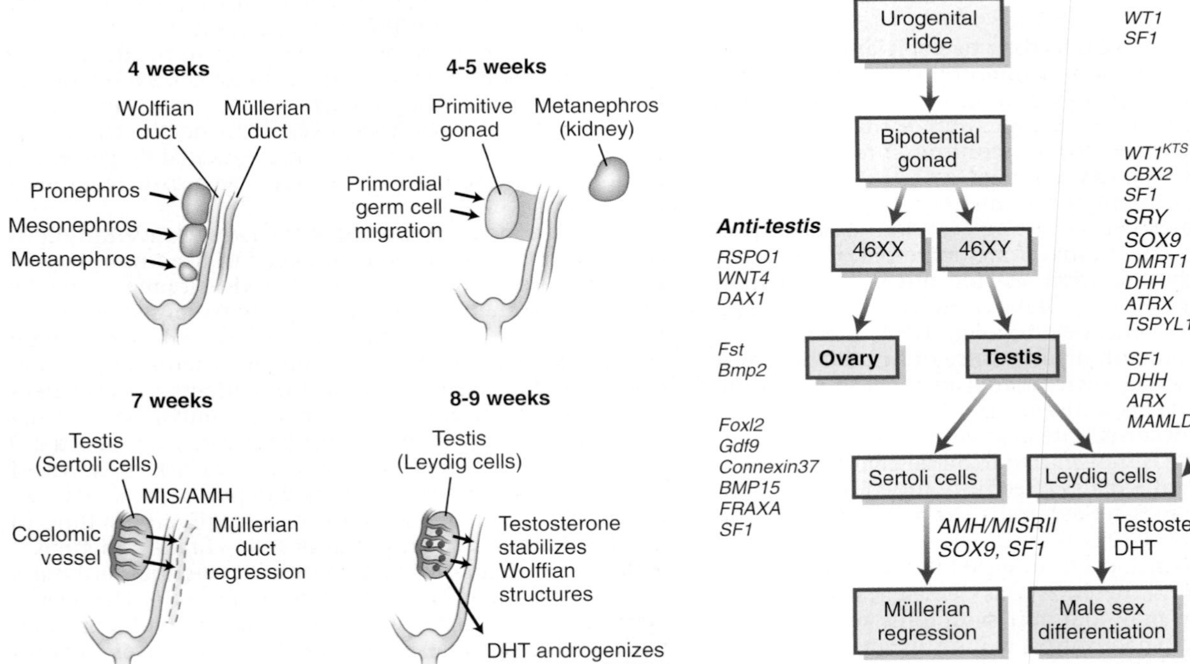

Figure 23-7 Schematic representation of the principal morphologic and functional events during early gonad or testis development in humans. DHT, dihydrotestosterone. (Modified from Achermann JC, Jameson JL. Testis determination. *Top Endocrinol.* 2003;22:10-14, with permission of Chapterhouse Codex.)

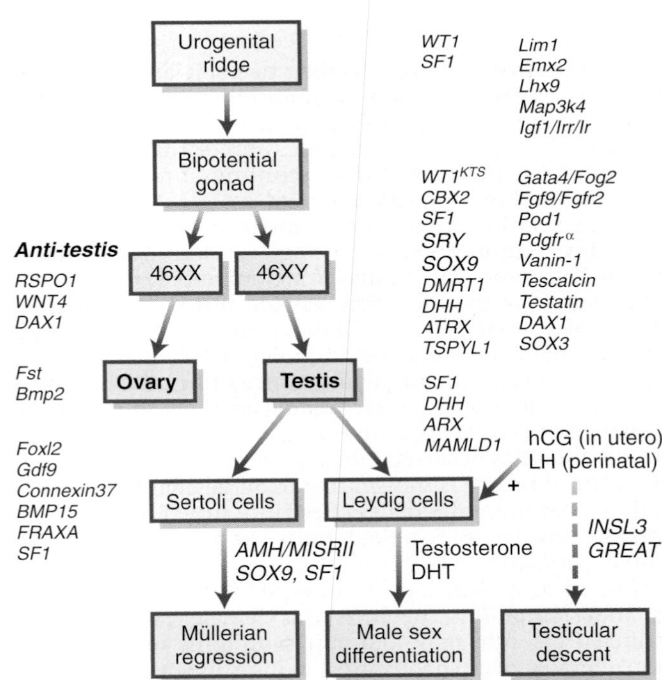

Figure 23-8 The flow chart provides an overview of the major events involved in sex determination and sex differentiation. Mutations or deletions in the genes reported to cause disorders of sex development in humans are shown in upper case. The genes and factors shown in lower-case letters have been proposed to play an important role in sex development, largely based on results from studies of mice.

gene, which may play a role in chromatin modification and gene silencing. Deletion of this gene in mice causes impaired 46,XY sex development through effects early in the sex development pathway, and disruption of the human homolog, *CBX2*, has been reported in a 46,XY child with a female phenotype and ovaries.[57,58] *Pod1* encodes a basic helix-loop-helix transcription factor that appears to be essential for gonad development in both sexes in mice.[59] *Gata4* (and its cofactor, *Fog2*) encodes a transcriptional regulator involved in early gonadal and cardiac development. Mice with deletions of these genes have cardiac defects and variable gonadal phenotypes.[60,61] Haploinsufficiency and point mutations in *GATA4* have been identified in patients with cardiac defects, and resulting human mutations associated with gonadal dysgenesis has been reported.[61a]

Signaling pathways may play a role in early gonad development. For example, deletions of multiple components of the insulin signaling pathway (i.e., insulin receptor, insulin-related receptor, and insulin-like growth factor 1 receptor) disrupt the early stages of testis development and downstream *SRY* expression in mice, whereas alterations in *Map3k4* (formerly called *Mekk4*) affect mitogen-activated protein kinase kinase kinase signaling, resulting in impaired gonadal growth, altered mesonephric cell migration, and reduced *SRY* and *SOX9* expression.[62,63] This work adds to the body of literature showing the importance of signaling factors in endocrine development. Other factors implicated in gonadal development in mice include the transcription regulators Cited2 and Pbx1.[64,65]

The role of transcription factors such as the product of the Wilms' tumor 1 gene (*WT1*) and SF1 in early gonad development has become better understood as murine models are characterized, and alterations in these genes have been found in patients with impaired gonad development (see "46,XY Disorders of Sex Development" and Fig. 23-8).

The *WT1* gene (11p13) encodes a four–zinc finger transcription factor expressed in the developing genital ridge, kidney, gonads, and mesothelium.[66,67] Homozygous deletion of the gene encoding Wt1 in mice prevents gonad and kidney development.[68] The WT1 protein is subject to complex post-translational modification and splicing processes, and it is thought that at least 24 WT1 isoforms exist.[69] The two most common variants are an isoform with alternative splicing of exon 5 and insertion of an additional 17 amino acids in the middle of the protein and an isoform that uses an alternative splice donor site for exon 9, resulting in the addition of three amino acids (lysine, threonine, and serine; called +KTS) between zinc finger 3 and 4. It is thought that +KTS and −KTS isoforms have different cellular functions and differential effects on gonad and renal development.[70] The ratio of +KTS to −KTS isoforms may be important in testis development, with the +KTS isoform having a cell-autonomous role in regulating SRY expression and influencing cellular proliferation and Sertoli cell differentiation.[71] WT1 also regulates expression of Sf1 and SOX9 in mice and may oppose β-catenin pathways. Although significant insight into the roles of different WT1 isoforms is being obtained from transgenic mice, the overall role of WT1 in cellular biology is complex and incompletely understood.

In humans, WT1 transcripts can be detected in the indifferent gonadal ridge when it first forms at 32 days after ovulation.[72] Deletions or mutations of WT1 cause well-defined syndromes in humans. Haploinsufficiency of WT1 due to deletion of the chromosomal locus containing *WT1* and *PAX6* (11p13) causes WAGR syndrome (Wilms' tumor, aniridia, genitourinary abnormalities, and mental retardation).[73] Dominant negative point mutations in *WT1* cause Denys-Drash syndrome (gonadal dysgenesis, genital ambiguity, nephropathy, and predisposition to Wilms' tumor),[74] whereas mutations in the exon 9 splice site of *WT1*, causing an altered ratio of +KTS to −KTS isoforms of WT1, result in Frasier syndrome (gonadal dysgenesis, late-onset nephropathy, and predisposition to gonadoblastoma) (see "46,XY Disorders of Sex Development" and Fig. 23-20).[75,76] Although these isoforms may play different roles in regulating various stages of renal and gonad development, it is likely that significant phenotypic overlap in the latter two conditions exists.[77]

Another key transcription factor expressed in the urogenital ridge is steroidogenic factor 1 (SF1, *NR5A1*).[78] SF1 is a member of the nuclear receptor superfamily that regulates the transcription of at least 30 genes known to be involved in gonadal development, adrenal development, steroidogenesis, and reproduction. In mice, complete deletion of the gene encoding SF1 results in apoptosis of the developing gonad and adrenal gland during early embryonic development.[79] Other features of these homozygous-deleted animals include persistent Müllerian structures and impaired androgenization in XY animals, hypogonadotropic hypogonadism, abnormalities of the ventromedial hypothalamus, altered stress responses, and late-onset obesity in adult animals rescued by adrenal transplantation.[80] Heterozygous animals have reduced gonadal size and impaired adrenal stress responses.[81]

SF1 is expressed during the early stages of urogenital ridge formation in humans (32 days after ovulation), where it is involved in maintaining gonadal integrity and permitting testicular differentiation.[72] Consistent with the mouse phenotype, heterozygous or homozygous loss-of-function mutations have been described in two patients with primary adrenal failure, severe 46,XY gonadal dysgenesis, and persistent Müllerian structures (see later discussion).[82,83] Haploinsufficiency of SF1 is emerging as a relatively frequent cause of 46,XY DSD.[78,84] Data for mice suggest that Sf1 plays a critical role in testis development and facilitates SRY regulation of *SOX9* expression.[85] Although SF1 was originally thought to play a less significant role in the ovary compared with the testis, studies in mice and humans show that SF1 is also an important regulator of ovarian integrity and function.[51,86,87]

In addition to the single-gene defects outlined previously, several chromosomal duplications or deletions have been associated with impaired gonad development in patients. Dosage-sensitive overexpression or underexpression of key factors in these regions may interfere with normal sex development. For example, duplication of a region of the X chromosome (Xp21, dosage-sensitive sex reversal) containing the gene encoding *DAX1* (*NROB1*) has been reported in several 46,XY patients with impaired testicular development or ovotestes.[88] These reports suggest that the orphan nuclear receptor DAX1 may act to antagonize testis development as an anti-testis gene. This concept was supported by studies in mice (*Mus poshiavinus*) in which overexpression of *DAX1* caused impaired male development in the presence of a weakened *SRY* locus.[89] However, targeted deletion of *Dax1* in a similar mouse strain also caused impaired testis development or ovotestis. Patients with X-linked adrenal hypoplasia congenita due to mutations in DAX1 have abnormal testis architecture and infertility, suggesting that critical doses of these factors have important roles; underactivity or overactivity could have deleterious effects at different stages of gonadal development.[90]

Impaired gonadal development has been described in a 46,XY individual with duplication of 1p35 that resulted in overexpression of the signaling molecules WNT4 and RSPO1, further supporting the concept that genes in certain loci have a role in opposing testis development.[91]

In addition to these regions of genomic duplication, many chromosomal rearrangements and deletions have been described in individuals with reproductive disorders. The most frequent ones associated with abnormalities of testis development (i.e., 9p24, 10q25-qter, Xq13, or 16p13.3-pter) are considered in later sections of this chapter.

Primordial Germ Cell Migration. PGCs are the embryonic precursors of gametes (spermatocytes or ova). Surprisingly, in all species, PGCs arise some distance from the developing gonad and undergo a process of migration during the early stages of embryogenesis.[92,93] In humans, PGCs arise from pluripotent epiblast cells and are initially located in the 24-day embryo in a region of the dorsal endoderm of the yolk sac, close to the allantoic evagination (see Fig. 23-7). After mitotic division, PGCs migrate into the primitive gonad (between 4 and 5 weeks' gestation) under the influence of signaling molecules, receptors, and extracellular matrix proteins such as KIT, the KIT ligand KITLG (formerly called Steel), β_1-integrin, E-cadherin, interferon-induced transmembrane protein 1 (IFITM1), and IFITM3.[94] Hindgut expansion may also regulate or facilitate this process. Gonadal colonization is mediated by CXCL12 (previously called SDF1) and its receptor CXCR4 and influenced by CXCR7.

In the first few months of gestation, PGCs undergo multiple cycles of mitotic division. In the testis, a self-renewing population of germ cells exists. These undifferentiated PGCs are maintained by factors such as POU5F1 (also called OCT4), but they commit to differentiation in response to the expression of specific signaling molecules and transcription factors. After several cycles of mitotic division, these cells enter mitotic arrest.[95] Subsequent testicular development can occur in the absence of this germ cell population.[96] Meiosis occurs only during the progress of spermatogenesis during puberty (see Chapter 19).

In the developing ovary, primordial ova (oogonia) undergo mitotic expansion in the first few months of gestation (5 to 24 weeks), followed by meiotic division (8 to 36 weeks) and a process of meiotic arrest (oocytes).[94,95] Although it was originally thought that entry into meiosis occurred autonomously, data suggest that retinoic acid signaling from the mesonephros stimulates this process.[97,98] Male germ cells may be protected from this signal by their location within the testis cord and by Sertoli cell expression of the cytochrome P450 isoenzyme 26B1 (CYP26B1), which breaks down retinoic acid. Meiotic arrest occurs in the first prophase, when the chromatids of homologous pairs have begun to separate but are fixed by chiasmata (diplotene stage), and it is maintained by G protein–coupled protein 3 (GPR3).[99] The presence of these PGCs and subsequent meiotic oocytes is critical for differentiation of prefollicular cells into follicular cells and for the maintenance of ovarian development (see Chapter 17).

More than 6 million oogonia and prophase oocytes exist in the developing ovary at about 16 weeks' gestation, and formation of oogonia from PGCs ceases by the 7th month. At that stage, some oocytes remain in undifferentiated nests, whereas others associate with somatic pregranulosa cells to form primitive or primordial follicles. However, approximately 80% of oogonia fail to form follicles and undergo apoptosis, so that only 1 million germ cells are present in the ovary at the time of birth. These "resting" primordial follicles can remain in that stage of development throughout the woman's reproductive life, and meiosis progresses only in response to ovulation of the graafian follicle (approximately 400 times in a woman's reproductive lifetime). It was once widely held that the population of germ cells present at birth represented a fixed pool that was gradually reduced with time through apoptosis and ovulation; however, this view has been challenged by reports of a potential self-renewing population of germline stem cells in the mouse ovary that are active into adult life.[16] Whether such mechanisms exist in primates remains a subject of debate.[94,100]

Testis Determination. Testis determination is an active process that begins at about 6 weeks' post-conception in humans and consists of several distinct genetic and morphologic events.[5,7] One of the first and most significant events in testis determination is a transient wave of SRY expression through the undifferentiated gonad. Data from several species indicate that SRY expression must reach a certain threshold within a definite time window for testis development to occur.[7,101,102] Initially, this occurs centrally, followed by expression in cells located at the cranial and caudal poles.

In humans, *SRY* is a single-exon gene (Yp11.3) that encodes a 204-amino-acid, high-mobility group (HMG)–box transcription factor.[28,101] Mutations and deletions in *SRY* tend to cluster within the region encoding the HMG box and have been reported in approximately 10% to 15% of patients with sporadic or familial 46,XY gonadal dysgenesis (see "46,XY Disorders of Sex Development" and Fig. 23-21).[29,32,101] As described earlier, translocation or transgenic expression of *SRY* is sufficient to induce testis development in XX patients and mice (see "The Y Chromosome" and Fig. 23-6).[31]

In humans, SRY is first detected in the XY gonad at approximately 42 days' post-conception, just before differentiation of the bipotential gonad into a testis.[103] Expression levels peak from approximately day 44, when testicular cords are first visible, but unlike in the mouse, SRY expression does not switch off completely in humans. Instead, low-level SRY expression is confined to Sertoli cells (day 52), where it persists into adulthood.

The HMG box of human SRY is a 79-amino-acid structure that has moderate homology with SRY in other species (approximately 70%) and with the HMG box of related SOX (SRY-like HMG box) proteins (60%) (see "46,XY Disorders of Sex Development" and Fig. 23-21).[101] The HMG box consists of three α-helices, which are able to adopt an L-shaped or boomerang-shaped configuration (see Fig. 23-6). The HMG box binds to variations on specific response elements (AACAAT/A) in the minor groove of DNA and induces a 40- to 85-degree structural bend in its target, depending on the sequence. The precise function of protein-directed DNA bending is not known, although this interaction results in minor groove expansion, DNA unwinding, and altered base stacking.[101,104-106] These effects likely alter DNA architecture in chromatin and may permit the interaction of other protein complexes with the DNA, resulting in activation or repression.

Other important domains in SRY are two nuclear localization signals that can interact with calmodulin and importin-β to regulate cellular localization[107]; several serine residues in the amino-terminus of SRY that can undergo phosphorylation and influence DNA binding[108]; and a carboxyl-terminal, 7-amino-acid motif that interacts with PDZ domains of SRY-interacting protein 1 (SIP1).[109] This interacting protein is thought to be important for SRY function in humans, because it can replace the function of the long C-terminal, glutamate-rich repeat domain (285 amino acids) of *SRY* found in mice. Human SRY lacks a classic transactivation domain; most human mutations in SRY interfere with DNA binding or nuclear localization.[101,105,110,111]

SRY expression is thought to switch the fate of the progenitor cells to that of pre-Sertoli cells; elegant studies of chimeric XX-XY gonads have shown that most Sertoli cells are XY derived.[112] These SRY-positive cells can signal to other cell lineages to induce male-specific differentiation.[5,113-116] The onset of SRY expression is followed by marked cellular proliferation and the migration of mesonephric cells into developing testis (Fig. 23-9).[5,117-119] These mesonephric cells are thought to differentiate into Leydig, endothelial, and peritubular myoid cells, depending on their interactions with somatic cells in the gonad. However, although SRY was shown convincingly to be the primary testis-determining gene more than 15 years ago, relatively little is known about the regulation of SRY expression.

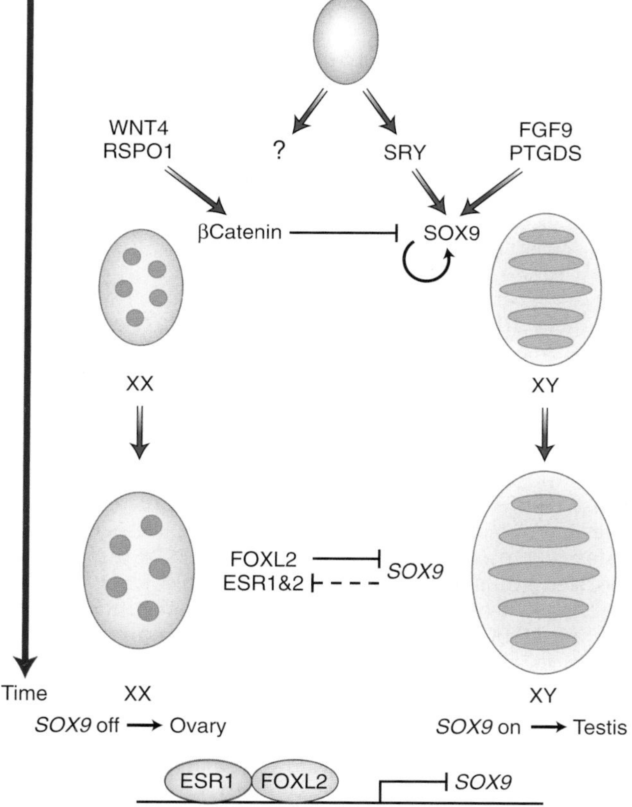

Figure 23-9 Model of *SOX9* regulation required for maintenance of gonadal phenotype in mammals. During initial phases of sex determination, SRY upregulates *SOX9* expression. *SOX9* expression in male gonads is activated and maintained by subsequent positive autoregulatory loops involving SOX9 itself, together with FGF9 and prostaglandin D_2 signaling. In contrast, β-catenin stabilization by WNT4 and RSPO1 signaling suppresses *SOX9* expression in female gonads. After birth, β-catenin activity declines. In adult female gonads, FOXL2 and estrogen receptors (ESR1 and 2) are required to actively repress *SOX9* expression to ensure ovarian somatic cell fate. The transcriptional repression of *SOX9* by FOXL2 and estrogen receptors is necessary throughout the lifetime of the female to prevent transdifferentiation of the somatic compartment of the ovary into a testis. PTGDS, prostaglandin D synthase. (From Uhlenhaut NH, Jakob S, Anlag K, et al. Somatic sex reprogramming of adult ovaries to testes by FOXL2 ablation. *Cell.* 2009;139:1130-1142, with permission of Cell Press, copyright 2009.)

Some studies have shown that SF1, WT1, and SP1 can all regulate SRY promoter activity in vitro, and signaling pathways may be important, but the exact mechanisms that activate SRY in vivo remain poorly understood.[120] The downstream targets of SRY are also unknown, although SOX9 is an obvious candidate. Recent evidence has demonstrated that SRY and SF1 can synergistically regulate SOX9 expression through a testis-specific enhancer region (TESCO).[85,113] It is unclear whether other direct SRY target genes exist or whether SRY also acts as a negative regulator of factors involved in testis repression, such as R-spondin 1 or β-catenin.[121]

SOX9 is an SRY-related HMG box factor comprising 3 exons (509 amino acids) that shows upregulation and nuclear localization in the developing male gonad shortly after the initial wave of SRY expression.[101,122-125] In humans, SOX9 becomes strongly localized to the developing sex cords at 44 to 52 days after ovulation and is expressed in Sertoli cells thereafter.[103] SOX9 is also expressed in the developing cartilage under the regulation of parathyroid hormone–related protein (PTHRP)/Indian hedgehog signaling pathways. Heterozygous mutations or deletions in SOX9 cause camptomelic dysplasia, a form of severe skeletal dysplasia associated with variable gonadal dysgenesis in approximately 75% of patients.[101,106,122,123] Mutations have been found in the HMG box of SOX9, in the C-terminal transactivation domain, and in a region that interacts with heat shock proteins (e.g., HSP70) (see "46,XY Disorders of Sex Development" and Fig. 23-21).[101,126]

Although SOX9 is a key target of SRY, an important body of evidence has emerged to show that SOX9 can be a testis-determining factor in its own right. In addition to the gonadal dysgenesis caused by loss-of-function mutations in SOX9, overexpression of SOX9 due to mosaic duplication of the locus containing *SOX9* (17q24.3-q25.1) has been reported in a 46,XX individual with ambiguous genitalia.[127] Transgenic expression of SOX9 in mice results in testis development in XX animals, and the XX *odsex* (*Ods*) mouse develops as a male due to disruption of a regulatory element 1 Mb upstream of *SOX9* that causes testis-specific overexpression of SOX9 during development.[128-130] Similar disruption of an upstream *cis*-regulatory region resulting in SOX9 overexpression has been proposed as a cause of 46,XX testicular DSD.[131] The regulatory region of the *SOX9* promoter is very large. Breakpoints have been reported up to 350 kb from the start of the *SOX9* gene in patients with camptomelic dysplasia and gonadal dysgenesis. In mice, *SOX9* may mediate its effects through direct interactions with other target genes (e.g., *FGF9, PTGDs, AMH*) and through the mutual degradation of β-catenin, thereby promoting testis development pathways rather than those opposing testis development (see Fig. 23-9).[113] Autoregulatory loops may also be important in maintaining SOX9 expression.

Around the time of SRY and SOX9 expression (and nuclear localization), the developing testis undergoes a series of distinct cellular and morphologic changes (Fig. 23-10). Understanding of these processes has resulted largely from studies in mice.[5] As outlined earlier, the first stage of testis development in mice involves a proliferation of Sf1-positive somatic cells that results in an increase in Sertoli cell precursors and Sertoli cell differentiation. This process is influenced by growth factors such as Fgf9 and the receptor Fgfr2.[132] These primitive Sertoli cells coalesce with peritubular myoid cells to form primary sex cords, which then condense to form primitive seminiferous cords (at about 7 weeks' post-conception in humans). Sex cord development is supported by a striking reorganization of the gonadal vasculature in the developing testis, but not

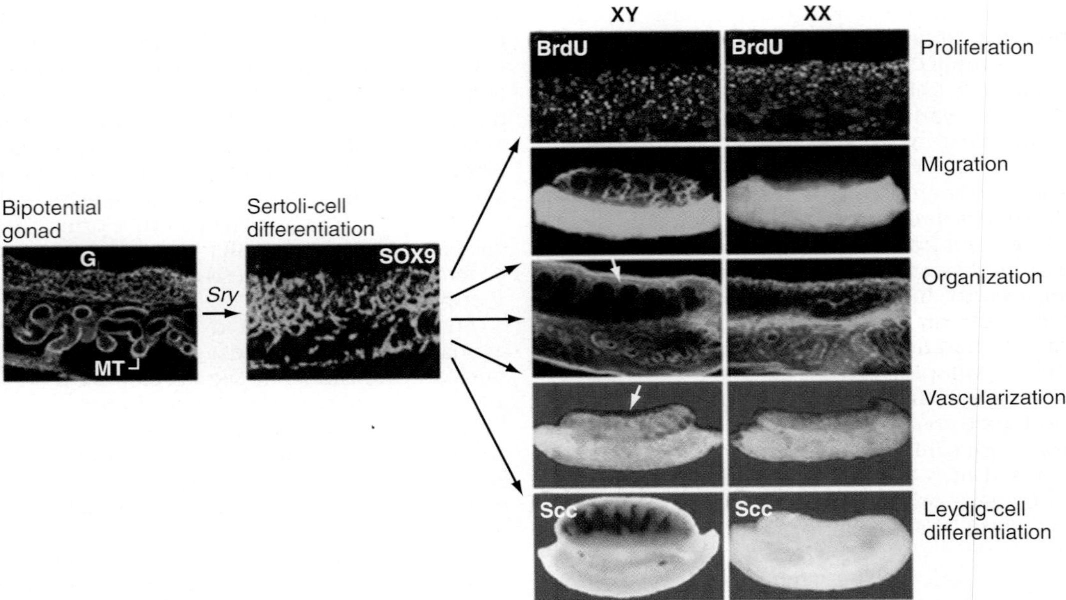

Figure 23-10 Key morphologic changes in the developing testis in mice. No morphologic differences between the XY and XX gonad are seen during the bipotential gonad stage at 10.5 to 11.5 days postcoitum (dpc) *(far left)*. In XY gonads, *SRY* expression is followed by expression and nuclear localization of SOX9 *(blue)* in pre-Sertoli cells *(middle)*, resulting in Sertoli cell differentiation by 11.5 dpc (vasculature and germ cells are labeled with platelet–endothelial cell adhesion molecule [PECAM] and appear *green*). Between 11.5 and 12.5 dpc, distinct changes occur in the XY gonad *(near right column)*, which are not seen in the XX gonad *(far right)*. These changes include proliferation of coelomic epithelial cells (measured by BrdU incorporation; *red, arrow*); migration of cells from the mesonephros (shown by recombinant culture of a wild-type gonad and a mesonephros in which the cells express *green* fluorescent protein); structural organization of testis cords (detected by laminin deposition, *green*); male-specific vascularization (by light microscopy with blood cells indicated by an *arrow*); and Leydig cell differentiation (detected by mRNA in situ hybridization for the steroidogenic enzyme P450scc). MT, basal lamina of mesonephric tubules; G, gonad. (From Brennan J, Capel B. One tissue, two fates: molecular genetic events that underlie testis versus ovary development. *Nat Rev Genet.* 2004;5:509-521, with permission of Macmillan Publishers Ltd.)

in the ovary (see Fig. 23-10).[5,133] These changes include the development of a discrete coelomic vessel, restriction of endothelial cells to the interstitial space between the sex cords, and increased branching of blood vessels. The development of these vascular systems is influenced by growth factor signaling systems, such as Pdgfra/Ptgds, and can be repressed by the Wnt4/β-catenin/follistatin systems.[134-136] These changes in vascular architecture play an important role in determining cellular patterning and organization in the developing testis, in supporting paracrine interactions, and in the export of androgens from the developing Leydig cells to the perineal and systemic circulation.

Although the expression of SRY plays a crucial role as a testis-determining factor, it is becoming clear that many other factors are necessary for early testis development (see Fig. 23-8). Some of these factors may be expressed exclusively within the developing testis, whereas others may play a facilitative role in supporting gonad development and are also expressed in other developing tissues (e.g., brain).

Desert hedgehog (DHH) is a member of the hedgehog signaling pathway that is expressed in mouse embryonic Sertoli cells and interstitium, and it plays a key role in the differentiation of peritubular myoid cells through its action on the Patched receptor.[137] The peritubular myoid cells are flat, smooth muscle–like cells that ensheath the testis cords and are necessary for cord development and structural integrity. Deletion of the *Dhh* gene in the mouse leads to impaired differentiation of peritubular myoid cells and Leydig cells and to impaired androgenization in males.[138,139] In humans, *DHH* mutations have been reported in patients with impaired testicular development, with or without minifascicular neuropathy.[140]

DMRT1 (double sex, Mab3–related transcription factor 1; 9p24.3) encodes a 373-amino-acid protein that is homologous to the sex-development *double sex* gene of *Drosophila* and the *Mab3* gene of *Caenorhabditis elegans*. DMRT1 shows a male-specific pattern expression in the developing genital ridge and is expressed in the developing Sertoli cells by 7 weeks' post-conception.[141,142] Deletion of *Dmrt1* in the mouse results in normal androgenization but regression of testes later in embryonic development.[143] No specific point mutations in *DMRT1* have been described in humans, but impaired gonadal development and 46,XY DSDs are well-established features of the 9p deletion syndrome. Disruption of *DMRT* is the most likely explanation for this condition.[144]

ARX (aristaless-related homeobox, X-linked gene) encodes a transcription factor that regulates neuronal migration, brain development, and Leydig cell development. Deletion of *Arx* in the mouse causes abnormal neuronal development and a block in Leydig cell differentiation.[145] Mutations in *ARX* in humans cause a condition known as X-linked lissencephaly and ambiguous genitalia (XLAG).[145] *MAMLD1* (mastermind-like domain–containing 1; previously called *CXORF6*) is a regulator of fetal Leydig cell function. Defects in *MAMLD1* have been reported in infants with severe hypospadias.[146] Signaling through Pdgf and the Pdgfra also has been shown to be important in fetal and adult Leydig cell differentiation after deletion of these genes in mice.[147]

Other genes proposed to play a role in early testis development have been identified from chromosome deletions or differential expression studies. For example, *Tescalcin* encodes a calcium-binding protein that is expressed in the early mouse fetal testes.[148] ATRX (Xq13.3; also known as

XH2 or *XNP*) is a transcription factor deleted in the α-thalassemia mental retardation syndrome.[149,150] The syndrome includes a range of genital phenotypes from partial gonadal dysgenesis to micropenis. The locus containing *SOX8* is deleted in the ATR-16 (α-thalassemia mental retardation) syndrome affecting the tip of chromosome 16p,[151] and terminal deletions of chromosome 10 (10q25-qter) are frequently associated with urogenital abnormalities and sometimes with complete gonadal dysgenesis.[152] More than 50 syndromic conditions or human chromosomal rearrangements have been associated with a range of urogenital phenotypes.[153] Furthermore, gene expression profiling in the embryonic mouse gonad is revealing a host of expressed and differentially expressed genes involved in testicular and ovarian development. Higher-resolution analysis of chromosomal changes using techniques such as array comparative genome hybridization is allowing the identification of much smaller chromosomal deletions, duplications, and rearrangements that may affect genes related to sex development.[154]

Ovary Development. For many years, ovary development was thought to be a constitutive (default) process, because an external female phenotype occurs in the absence of gonadal tissue and Müllerian structures persist in the absence of anti-Müllerian hormone (AMH; also known as Müllerian-inhibiting substance [MIS]). Although the presence of PGCs was known to be necessary to maintain ovarian integrity, evidence now shows that ovarian development is an active process that requires expression of a set of specific genes and factors necessary to actively prevent testis development.

Several genes, including *Dazl, Bmp8b, Smad5, Gja4* (previously known as *Cx37*), *Foxl2*, and the POF family of genes listed previously, have been implicated in ovarian and follicular development in mice.[9,45-51] Studies comparing gene expression profiles in the testes and ovaries of mice at critical stages of fetal development (e10.5 to e13.5) have shown that a specific subset of ovarian genes (e.g., follistatin, cyclin kinase inhibitors) are turned on soon after the onset of testis determination.[13,14] It is unclear whether any ovary-determining genes exist or whether these factors play a role in maintaining ovarian development in the absence of testis-determining gene expression. However, it seems likely that certain active processes are involved, because many of the genes and proteins (e.g., WNT4, RSPO1/β-catenin, FOXL2, estrogen receptors), as well as meiotic germ cells, may antagonize testis development or prevent development of a male-type cell lineage.[15,155-160] Data in mice suggest that these processes may be ongoing, even in the postnatal ovary (see Fig. 23-9).[160]

Phenotypic or Anatomic Sex

The developing gonad produces several steroid and peptide hormones that mediate sexual differentiation and result in the phenotypic sex seen at birth. Alfred Jost first showed the importance of fetal testicular androgens in this process in 1947.[12] In his classic experiments, Jost demonstrated that surgical removal of the gonads during embryonic development of the rabbit resulted in development of female reproductive characteristics, regardless of chromosomal sex of the embryo.

Male Sexual Differentiation

Sertoli Cells and Müllerian Regression. Sertoli cells play a key role in supporting germ cell survival, and they produce two important peptide hormones: AMH and inhibin B. AMH, a glycoprotein homodimer, is a member of the transforming growth factor-β (TGF-β) superfamily and is first secreted in humans from about 7 weeks' post-conception under the regulation of key transcription factors such as SOX9, SF1, WT1, and GATA4 (see Figs. 23-1 and 23-7).[161,162] AMH causes regression of Müllerian structures (e.g., fallopian tubes, uterus, upper two thirds of the vagina) by its paracrine action on the AMH type 2 receptor (AMHR2). This receptor forms a serine/threonine kinase heterodimeric receptor complex with ALK2 (ACVR1) to induce apoptosis through secondary paracrine signals, such as matrix metalloproteinase 2 (MMP2).[162]

Müllerian structures appear to be maximally sensitive to AMH between 9 and 12 weeks' gestation, a time when the developing testis is producing peak concentrations of AMH but before the onset of significant AMH production by the developing ovary. Consequently, boys with mutations in the *AMH* or *AMHR2* genes can present with persistent Müllerian duct syndrome (PMDS) and undescended testes but otherwise normal external genitalia. In contrast, severe forms of 46,XY gonadal dysgenesis can result in persistent Müllerian structures due to impaired Sertoli cell development and AMH release. In some cases, a hemiuterus is present if testicular development is more severely affected on that same side, but it is likely that androgenization of the external genitalia also is impaired. Defects confined to Leydig cell steroidogenesis in 46,XY DSD are not associated with persistent Müllerian structures, because Sertoli cell production of AMH is unaffected. In normal boys, a small Müllerian remnant sometimes persists as a testicular appendage. Inhibin B suppresses pituitary follicle-stimulating hormone (FSH) activity, but its local role during testis development is less clear. AMH and inhibin B may have important functions throughout life at multiple levels of the HPG axis.[163]

Fetal Leydig Cells and Steroidogenesis. Fetal Leydig cells develop within the interstitium of the developing testis and secrete androgens by 8 to 9 weeks' post-conception (see Fig. 23-1).[164] Luteinizing hormone/human chorionic gonadotropin (LH/hCG) receptors are present on the Leydig cells only from 10 to 12 weeks' post-conception, suggesting that the initial secretion of testosterone is independent of hCG and fetal LH. A massive expansion in fetal Leydig cells occurs between 14 and 18 weeks' gestation, resulting in marked increase in testosterone secretion at about 16 weeks.[165,166] Fetal Leydig cell steroidogenesis is stimulated by placental hCG during the first two trimesters of pregnancy, but the developing hypothalamic-gonadotroph system produces significant amounts of LH from about 20 weeks' gestation.[167]

The pathways of testicular steroidogenesis are shown in Figure 23-11. The role of individual enzymes is discussed in relation to individual steroidogenic defects later in this chapter and in several excellent reviews.[8,168] Cholesterol is taken up into Leydig cells by low-density lipoprotein or high-density lipoprotein receptors or is generated de novo by cholesterol synthesis pathways or from cholesterol ester. Stimulation of the LH/hCG receptor by the appropriate glycoprotein hormone increases the ability of steroidogenic acute regulatory protein (StAR) to facilitate movement of cholesterol from the outer to the inner mitochondrial membrane. The first and rate-limiting step in steroid hormone synthesis involves three distinct reactions: 20α-hydroxylation, 22-hydroxylation, and cleavage of the cholesterol side chain to generate pregnenolone and isocaproic acid. These steps are catalyzed by a single enzyme, P450scc (CYP11A1).

Pregnenolone is converted to progesterone by the microsomal enzyme 3β-hydroxysteroid dehydrogenase

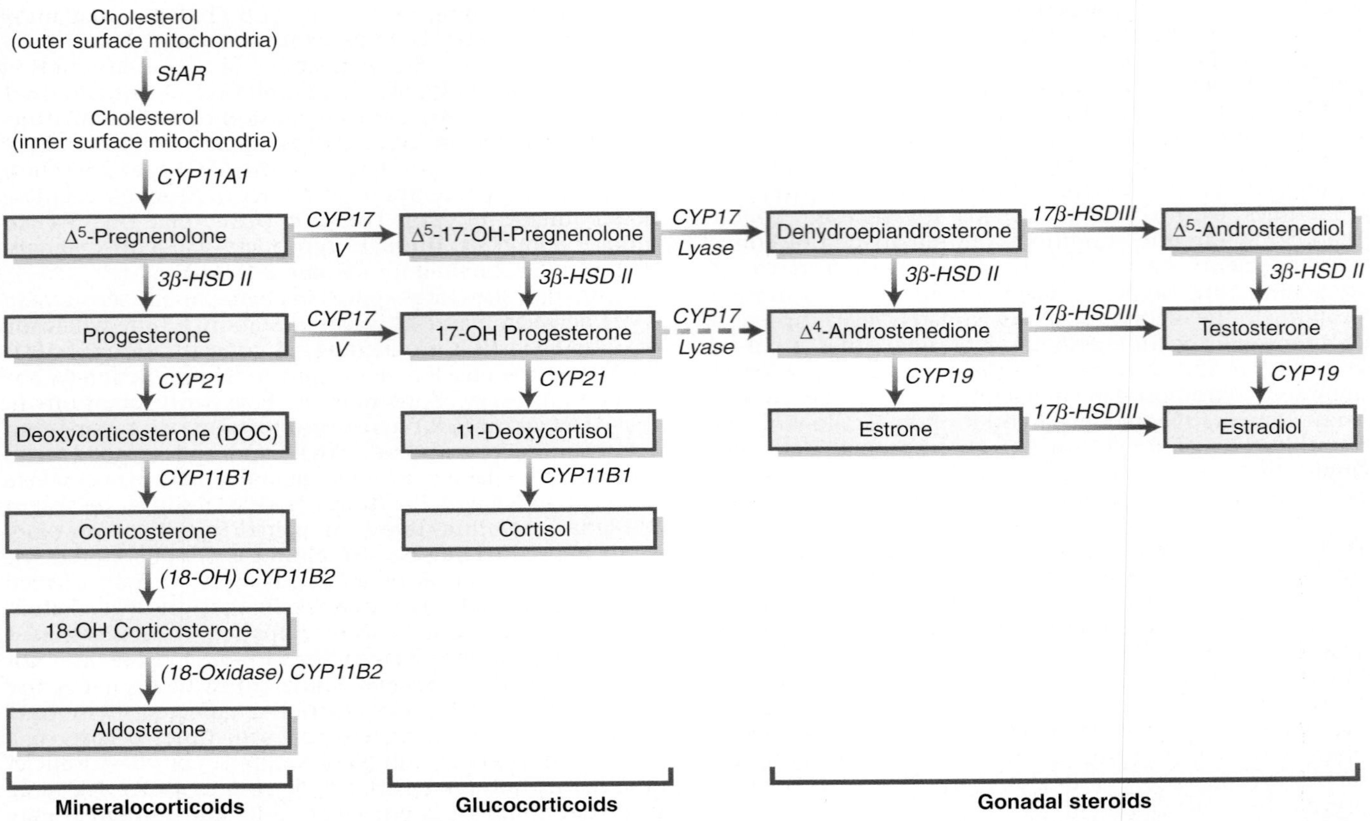

Cholesterol (outer surface mitochondria)
↓ StAR
Cholesterol (inner surface mitochondria)
↓ CYP11A1

Mineralocorticoids		Glucocorticoids		Gonadal steroids		
Δ^5-Pregnenolone	CYP17 V →	Δ^5-17-OH-Pregnenolone	CYP17 Lyase →	Dehydroepiandrosterone	17β-HSDIII →	Δ^5-Androstenediol
↓ 3β-HSD II		↓ 3β-HSD II		↓ 3β-HSD II		↓ 3β-HSD II
Progesterone	CYP17 V →	17-OH Progesterone	CYP17 Lyase - - →	Δ^4-Androstenedione	17β-HSDIII →	Testosterone
↓ CYP21		↓ CYP21		↓ CYP19		↓ CYP19
Deoxycorticosterone (DOC)		11-Deoxycortisol		Estrone	17β-HSDIII →	Estradiol
↓ CYP11B1		↓ CYP11B1				
Corticosterone		Cortisol				
↓ (18-OH) CYP11B2						
18-OH Corticosterone						
↓ (18-Oxidase) CYP11B2						
Aldosterone						

Figure 23-11 Schematic diagram shows the steroid biosynthetic pathways leading to androgen production in the testis. In humans, the main pathway to androgen production is through conversion of 17-hydroxypregnenolone to dehydroepiandrosterone (DHEA) rather than through conversion of 17-hydroxyprogesterone to androstenedione. Subsequent testosterone biosynthesis can occur through conversion of DHEA to androstenedione (by 3β-hydroxysteroid dehydrogenase type 2 [3β-HSD II]), followed by the actions of 17α-hydroxysteroid dehydrogenase type 3 (17β-HSD III) to generate testosterone, or through the intermediate metabolite androstenediol. During male sex development, testosterone undergoes local conversion to dihydrotestosterone (DHT) by 5α-reductase type 2 (not shown). The high-affinity action of dihydrotestosterone on the androgen receptor results in androgenization of the external genitalia. The pathways responsible for mineralocorticoid and glucocorticoid synthesis are present in the adrenal gland. Additional or alternative pathways to dihydrotestosterone production may exist in the fetal testis.

type 2 (HSD3B2), or it can undergo 17α-hydroxylation by P450c17 (CYP17) to yield 17-hydroxypregnenolone. CYP17 also has 17,20-lyase activity, which can cleave the C17,20 carbon bond of 17-hydroxypregnenolone to generate dehydroepiandrosterone (DHEA). This 17,20-lyase activity is favored by the presence of Δ^5-substrates, redox partners such as P450 oxidoreductase (POR) and cytochrome b_5, and serine phosphorylation. These reactions are facilitated by the relative abundance of these factors in Leydig cells in humans, and the main pathway to androgen production is through conversion of 17-hydroxypregnenolone to DHEA rather than through conversion of 17-hydroxyprogesterone (17-OHP) to androstenedione.[169] Subsequent testosterone production can occur through conversion of DHEA to androstenedione (by HSD3B2), followed by the actions of HSD17B3 to generate testosterone, or by the intermediate metabolite androstenediol (see Fig. 23-11). During male sex development, testosterone undergoes local conversion to dihydrotestosterone (DHT) by 5α-reductase type 2. DHT's high-affinity action on the androgen receptor results in androgenization of the external genitalia. Studies based on the phenotype of patients with POR deficiency and the fetal Tammar wallaby have proposed that an alternative pathway to DHT production may exist in the human fetal testis (see "P450 Oxidoreductase Deficiency").[170,171]

Local production of testosterone is thought to be necessary for stabilization of Wolffian structures such as the epididymides, vasa deferentia, and seminal vesicles, whereas the potent metabolite DHT induces androgenization of the external genitalia and urogenital sinus (Fig. 23-12). In the male, the urogenital sinus develops into the prostate and prostatic urethra, the genital tubercle develops into the glans penis, the urogenital (urethral) folds fuse to form the shaft of the penis, and the urogenital (labioscrotal) swellings form the scrotum (Figs. 23-13 and 23-14). The distinction between a clitoris and a penis at this stage is based primarily on size and whether the labia minora fuse to form a corpus spongiosum. The effects of androgenization on the genital tubercle between 8 and 10 weeks' post-conception were shown by Goto and colleagues (see Fig. 23-14).[172]

Testosterone and DHT mediate their effects through the androgen receptor (AR; Xq11-q12), which is a transcription factor (see "46,XY Disorders of Sex Development"). Surprisingly little is known about AR targets in the developing Wolffian structures (testosterone responsive) and in the key target tissues (DHT responsive). However, various degrees of impaired androgen action are seen in a range of syndromic conditions and may reflect defects in genes that mediate target-tissue responsiveness and genital tubercle growth (e.g., *HOXA10, HOXA13*).[7] Studies in mice have

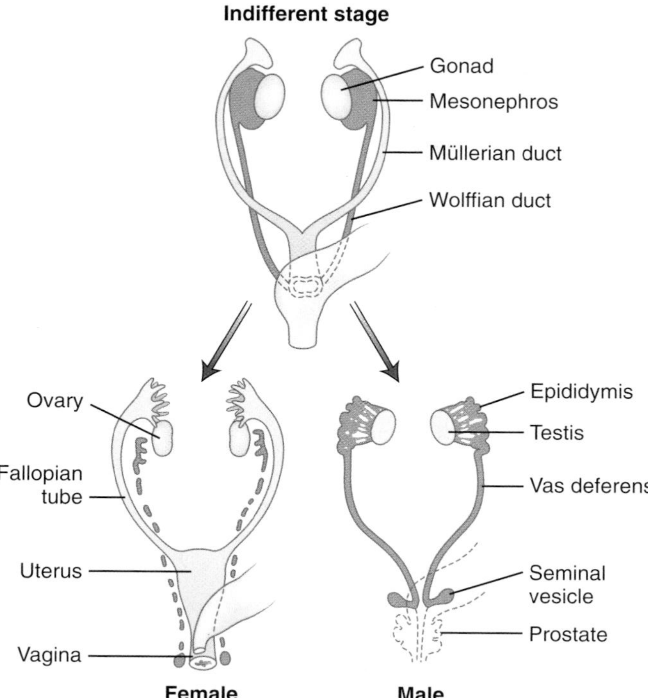

Figure 23-12 Embryonic differentiation of female and male genital ducts from Wolffian and Müllerian primordial tissue before descent of the testes into the scrotum. In females, Müllerian structures persist to form the fallopian tubes, uterus, and upper portion of the vagina. The lower portion of the vagina and urethra are derived from the urogenital sinus. In males, Wolffian structures develop into the epididymises, vasa deferentia, and seminal vesicles, whereas the prostate and prostatic urethra are derived from the urogenital sinus. In some cases, a small Müllerian remnant can persist in males as a testicular appendage.

revealed a number of factors that are necessary for development of the Wolffian ducts (e.g., Gdf7, Bmps4, Bmps7, Bmps8a, Bmps8b, Hoxa10, Hoxa11) and for growth of the genital tubercle (e.g., Fgfs, Shh, Wnts, Hoxa13, Hoxd13, Bmp/noggin, ephrin signaling).[7]

Testis Descent. Testicular descent is a two-stage process that starts at about 8 weeks' gestation and is usually complete by the middle of the third trimester.[173] The initial *transabdominal* stage of testicular descent (8 to 15 weeks) involves contraction and thickening of the gubernacular ligament and degeneration of the craniosuspensory ligament. This stage is mediated by the testis itself after secretion of factors such as insulin-like 3 (INSL3, a relaxin-like factor) and its G protein–coupled receptor, GREAT (also called LGR8 or RXFP2).[174] Other testicular factors are likely to be involved in testicular descent, because most dysgenetic testes are intra-abdominal. The subsequent *transinguinal* (or inguinoscrotal) phase of testicular descent (25 to 35 weeks) is primarily driven by androgens. The genitofemoral nerve and its neurotransmitter, calcitonin gene–related peptide (CGRP), have also been implicated in this process.

Subsequent Testicular Development. During the second and third trimesters, the testes show several distinct morphologic changes, including a reduction in fetal Leydig cell mass and elongation and coiling of seminiferous cords. There is no further significant development of germ cells during this time, and seminiferous cords do not canalize until later in childhood. Nevertheless, certain developmental insults can affect the testis at this stage. For example, vanishing (absent) testis syndrome is most likely a late fetal event, because boys with this condition have adequate androgenization and no Müllerian structures.

Female Sexual Differentiation. The processes of female sexual differentiation are less obvious than in the male and do not involve significant changes in the external genitalia. Müllerian structures persist to form the fallopian tubes, uterus, and upper portion of the vagina (see Fig. 23-12). Normal uterine development in mice occurs in the absence of the ovary, but it is not a passive process, because a host of factors are required for uterine development (e.g., Pax2, Lim1, Emx2, Wnt4/Lp, Hoxa13) and differentiation (e.g., Wnt7a, Hoxa10, Hoxa11, Hoxa13, progesterone and estrogen receptors).[175] The lack of local testosterone production leads to degeneration of Wolffian structures. The urogenital sinus develops into the urethra and lower portion of the vagina, the genital tubercle develops into the clitoris, the urogenital (urethral) folds form the labia minora, and the urogenital (labioscrotal) swellings form the labia majora (see Figs. 23-12 and 23-13).

In contrast to the testis, the developing ovary does not express FSH and LH/hCG receptors until after 16 weeks' gestation. At about 20 weeks' gestation, plasma concentrations of FSH reach a peak and the first primary follicles are formed.[167] By 25 weeks' gestation, the ovary has developed definitive morphologic characteristics. Folliculogenesis can proceed, and a few Graafian follicles have developed by the third trimester. However, the amount of estrogen secreted by the developing ovary is likely to be insignificant compared with placental estrogen synthesis, and the ovary is thought to remain generally quiescent until activation at the time of puberty. Abnormalities in several factors (e.g., connexin 37, GDF9, FSH receptors, estrogen receptor-α, progesterone receptor) can interfere with this early folliculogenesis.

Several conditions can affect female sexual development in utero. Exposure of the fetus to androgens results in androgenization of the external genitalia.[172] A uterus is present, but the local testosterone concentration typically is not sufficient to stabilize Wolffian structures because the androgens are usually adrenal in origin. Most frequently, androgenization of the 46,XX fetus results from disorders of adrenal steroidogenesis (e.g., 21-hydroxylase [CYP21] deficiency, 11β-hydroxylase deficiency, POR deficiency) or from mild androgenic effects after conversion of excess DHEA in HSD3B2 deficiency (discussed later). Rare causes of androgenization include aromatase deficiency, glucocorticoid resistance, ovotesticular DSD, and maternal virilizing tumors (e.g., luteoma of pregnancy). Exposure to certain chemical agents in pregnancy has been proposed as a cause of fetal androgenization. For other developmental abnormalities of the female genital tract (e.g., Mayer-Rokitansky-Küster-Hauser syndrome) see "46,XX Disorders of Sex Development."

Psychosexual Development

Psychosexual development is traditionally viewed as having several distinct components (Table 23-2). *Gender identity* refers to a person's self-representation or identification as male or female (with the caveat that some individuals may not identify exclusively with either). *Gender role* (sex-typical behaviors) describes the expression or portrayal of psychological characteristics that are sexually dimorphic within the general population, such as toy preferences and physical aggression. *Sexual orientation* refers to choice of sexual partner and erotic interest (e.g., heterosexual, bisexual, homosexual) and includes behavior, fantasies, and attractions.

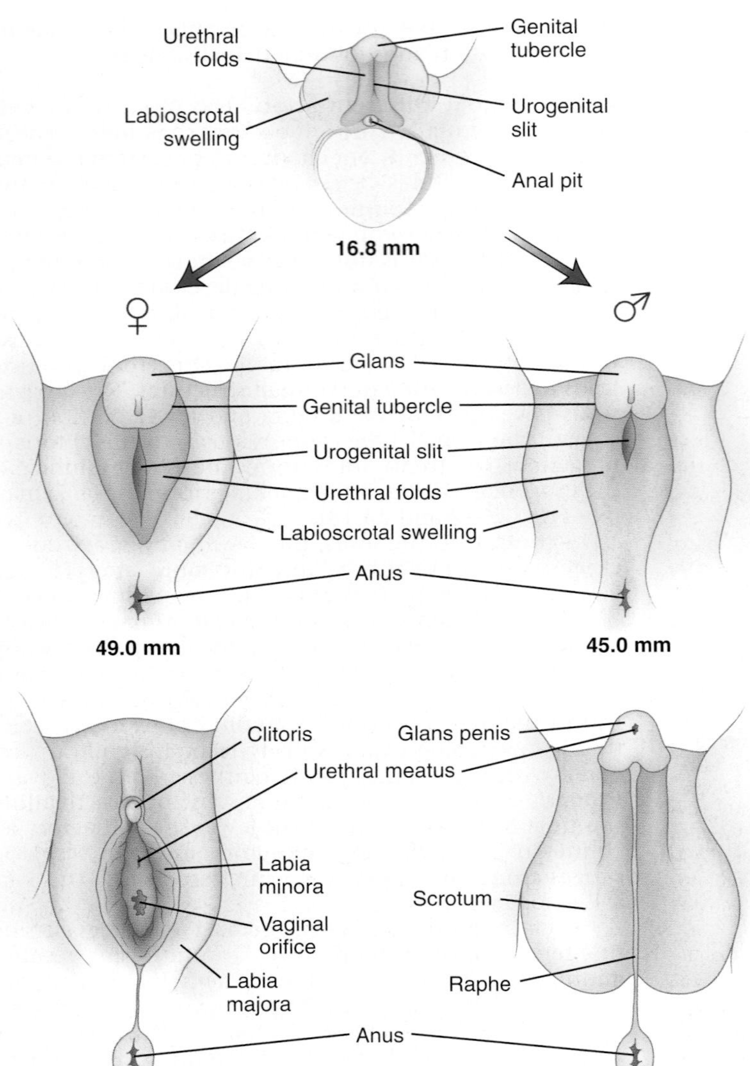

Figure 23-13 **Differentiation of male and female external genitalia.** (Adapted from Spaulding MH. The development of the external genitalia in the human embryo. *Contrib Embryol Carnegie Inst.* 1921;13:69-88.)

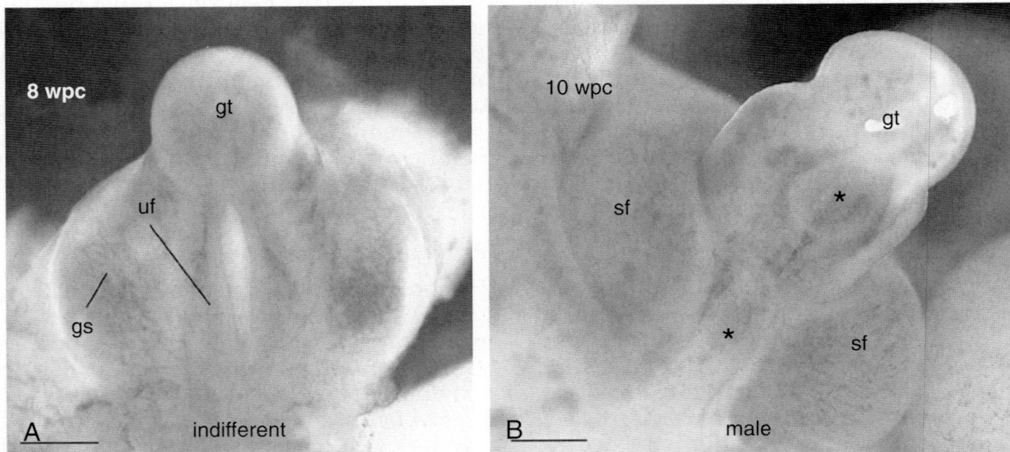

Figure 23-14 Differentiation of male external genitalia in humans between 8 and 10 weeks postconception (wpc). **A,** Undifferentiated human external genitalia at 8 wpc. **B,** Differentiation of scrotal folds and fusion of the urethral folds (*asterisks* indicate patent regions on either side) at 10 wpc. gs, genital swelling; gt, genital tubercle; sf, scrotal folds; uf, urethral folds. Scale bars: 500 μm. (From Goto M, Piper Hanley K, Marcos J, et al. In humans, early cortisol biosynthesis provides a mechanism to safeguard female sexual development. *J Clin Invest.* 2006;116:872-874, with permission of the American Society for Clinical Investigation, copyright 2006.)

TABLE 23-2

Terminology for Gender-Related Behavior

Gender identity	Identification of sex as male or female
Gender role	Expression of sexually dimorphic behavior
	Aggression
	Parenting rehearsal
	Peer and group interactions
	Labeling (e.g., "tomboy")
	Grooming behavior
Sexual orientation	Choice of sexual partner

The past 50 years have seen a number of opposing theories about the origins of psychosexual development and debate about the relative contributions of chromosomes, hormones, brain structure, and societal and family influences on the various components. Much of this work has focused on the study of rodents and nonhuman primate species. For example, Young and colleagues first showed in 1959 that exposure of guinea pigs to testosterone during pregnancy resulted in altered mating behavior of female offspring.[176] These effects may be most pronounced during a critical window of exposure and, in rodents, may depend in part on aromatization of the androgens to estrogens, receptor availability, and social environment.[177,178] More recently, interest has focused on the role of genes and chromosomes in sex behavior. For example, studies of differential gene expression patterns in the developing mouse brain have shown upregulation of different X and Y chromosomal genes in early embryonic life, even before the onset of significant androgen secretion by the developing testis in males.[179] Studies of mice in which SRY was deleted (XYSRY$^-$) or transgenically expressed (XXSRY) showed certain neuroanatomic differences between XY and XX mice independent of gonad development and endocrine status.[180] These findings suggest that factors related to chromosome complement have at least the potential to affect psychosexual development independent of sex hormone action, and a model integrating classic organizational and activational effects with sex chromosome effects may be more appropriate.[181]

Understanding the complex issues related to human psychosexual development is much more challenging, especially because gender identity is a component of psychosexual development that cannot readily be assessed in nonhuman species. For many years, it was thought that gender identity would be concordant with assigned sex, provided that the child was raised unambiguously and appropriate surgical "correction" and hormone therapies were instituted concordant with the gender chosen. This theory assumed psychosexual neutrality at birth, but it has been challenged by a refocusing on the potential importance of prenatal (e.g., endocrine) and innate (e.g., chromosomal) influences on psychosexual development. Direct data to assess such effects in humans are limited, but studies in women with complete androgen insensitivity syndrome (CAIS) argue against a strong behavioral role for Y chromosome genes alone in human psychosexual development, because the karyotype is 46,XY but psychosexual development is female.[182] However, the gender characteristics of individuals with a Y chromosome and a degree of androgen exposure or responsiveness (e.g., partial androgen insensitivity syndrome [PAIS], 5α-reductase deficiency) can vary, and long-term gender identity can be difficult to predict.[183]

Prenatal exposure to androgens can also influence certain aspects of psychosexual development in 46,XX individuals.[184,185] Girls with congenital adrenal hyperplasia (CAH) who harbor more severe mutations and have more marked genital androgenization are more likely to play more with boys' toys, with long-term effects evident into adulthood.[186] Prenatal androgen exposure can also be associated with other psychological characteristics, such as sexual orientation.[186,187] However, the association between high prenatal androgen exposure and gender identity is less marked, except perhaps in some cases of testicular DSD.[188] Although gender dissatisfaction (i.e., unhappiness with assigned sex) is more common in individuals with DSD, more than 90% of 46,XX individuals with CAH who are assigned female gender in infancy later identify as female.[189] The causes of gender dissatisfaction are poorly understood and are hard to predict from karyotype, prenatal androgen exposure, degree of genital virilization, or assigned gender.[190-192] Because gender identity, sex-typical behavior, and sexual orientation are separate components of psychosexual development, it is important to appreciate that homosexual orientation (relative to sex of rearing) or strong cross-sex interest in an individual with DSD is not necessarily an indication of incorrect gender assignment.[3]

Challenges in assessing gender identity in young children make it difficult to know when this is established, although it is thought to be between 18 and 36 months and possibly younger.[193] Many of the sexually dimorphic differences in brain structures reported at puberty or in adulthood are not seen in early childhood and are therefore not useful for guiding gender assignment.[194,195] Potential plasticity in psychosexual development may exist, as is evident from studies of some patients with conditions such as 5α-reductase deficiency who may change their gender role in adolescence. A better understanding of the processes of human psychosexual development and of the influences of different forms of DSD is needed to help make early gender assignment decisions and to guide psychological support in the future.

Development of the Hypothalamic-Gonadotroph Axis in the Fetus

Fetal hypothalamic-gonadotroph development occurs from 6 weeks' post-conception, in parallel with the processes of sex determination and sexual differentiation in humans. Pituitary gonadotropin release probably does not influence the gonad until about 20 weeks of gestation.[167] Detailed descriptions of the development of the neuroendocrine system and congenital disorders of the hypothalamic-pituitary axis are provided in other Chapters. However, development of the hypothalamic-gonadotroph axis has some unique features, and abnormalities in this process can cause congenital forms of hypogonadotropic hypogonadism (HH).

Development and Migration of Gonadotropin-Releasing Hormone–Synthesizing Neurons

Embryonic development of the hypothalamic gonadotropin-releasing hormone (GnRH) neurosecretory system is intimately related to development of the extracranial and intracranial olfactory apparatus, and in all species studied, the GnRH-synthesizing neurons originate extracranially before migrating to their final position in the fetal hypothalamus (Fig. 23-15).[196]

In humans, GnRH-synthesizing neurons first appear in the embryonic medial olfactory placode at about 6 weeks' post-conception and begin to migrate along axons of the terminal vomeronasal nerve complex on a neural cell

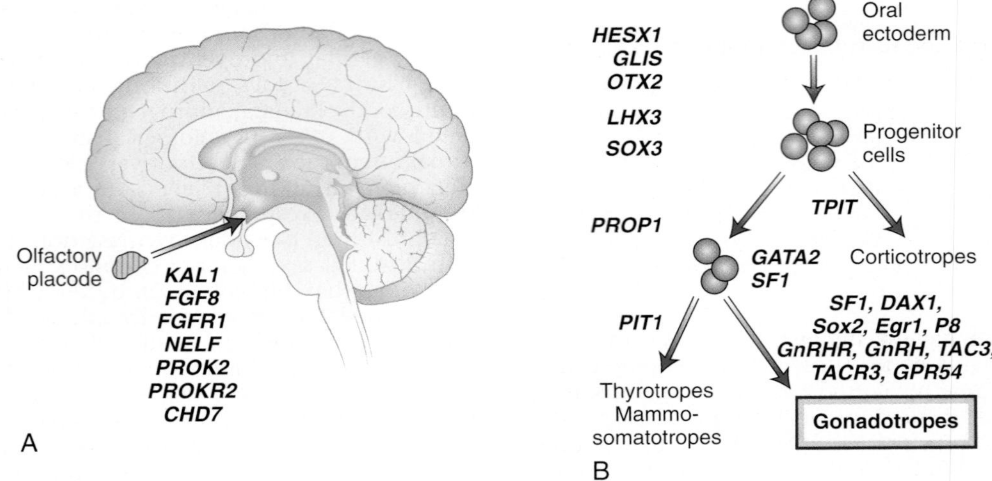

Figure 23-15 Development of the hypothalamic-gonadotroph axis in humans. **A,** Migration of gonadotropin-releasing hormone (GnRH) neurons from the olfactory placode to the fetal hypothalamus is facilitated by proteins such as anosmin 1 (now called KAL1), fibroblast growth factor 8 (FGF8), FGF receptor 1 (FGFR1), NELF, prokineticin 2 (PROK2), its receptor PROKR2, and CHD7. Defects in these factors have been reported in association with Kallmann syndrome (i.e., hypogonadotropic hypogonadism and anosmia), although in some cases, sense of smell can be normal. **B,** Differentiation of the anterior pituitary gland. The gradient of factors such as GATA2/SF1 and TPIT (TBX19) may provide a switch for gonadotroph differentiation. Variations in several transcription factors (e.g., HESX1, GLI2, LHX3, OTX2, SOX3, PROP1) are associated with multiple pituitary hormone deficiency in humans. Mutations affecting isolated gonadotroph factors have not been described, except as part of complex phenotypes associated with mutations in SF1, DAX1, and SOX2. Defects in GnRH, the GnRH receptor, and GPR54 have also been reported in individuals with congenital hypogonadotropic hypogonadism.

adhesion molecule (NCAM)–rich scaffold. At about 6.5 weeks', these migrating neurons pass through the primitive cribriform plate and penetrate the forebrain medial and caudal to the developing olfactory bulbs. GnRH neurons then migrate posteriorly in the submeningeal space by the interhemispheric fissure before proceeding laterally to reach their final position in the fetal mediobasal hypothalamus starting at about 14 weeks' gestation.[196] Fetal GnRH neuron migration is complete by approximately 19 weeks' gestation, by which stage pulsatile GnRH release is established.

Several cell adhesion molecules and signaling factors have been implicated in this migratory process, including anosmin 1/KAL1, FGFR1, NELF, and AXL/GAS6, and GnRH neurons express different transcription factors at different stages of maturation. Other neuroendocrine cells co-migrate with GnRH-synthesizing neurons. Some of these cells synthesize neurotransmitters and hormones such as neuropeptide Y, leptin, corticotropin-releasing factor (CRF), and glutamate; these factors may interact with GnRH neurons along the migratory path or in their final position in the hypothalamus. The association of GnRH neuronal migration with development of the olfactory system explains the association of some forms of HH with anosmia (i.e., lack of a sense of smell) in Kallmann syndrome. This condition can result from mutations in several X-linked and autosomal genes, which often represent ligand-and-receptor pairs (e.g., *KAL1, FGF8/FGFR1, PROK2/PROKR2, NELF, CHD7*). However, clinical features can vary within families (e.g., normosmic HH rather than anosmia), and inheritance patterns may be influenced by changes in more than one of these genes (i.e., digenic pattern). These features are discussed in more detail in other chapters.[197,198]

Gonadotropin-Releasing Hormone Synthesis and Action

GnRH-synthesizing neurons are located throughout the hypothalamus, with a concentration in the arcuate nucleus. GnRH is synthesized as a precursor polypeptide; this precursor undergoes cleavage and enzymatic processing to form a mature, 10-amino-acid hormone that is stored in secretory granules. GnRH is released from neuronal projections at the medial eminence into the portal blood system in a pulsatile manner to stimulate GnRH receptors on the anterior pituitary gonadotrophs. GnRH pulsatility is thought to be established in the second trimester and may be modulated at various stages of development by a G protein–coupled receptor (KISS1R, formerly called GPR54) and its ligand kisspeptin, as well as a host of other neuroendocrine factors and regulators (e.g., neurokinin B). Congenital HH has been reported in patients with defects in GnRH or the GnRH receptor, loss of function of KISS1R, and defects in the neurokinin B system (TAC3/TACR3).[197-198] In humans, HH can results from abnormalities in GnRH processing (e.g., prohormone convertase 1 [PCSK1]) and leptin/leptin receptor signaling.

Pituitary Gonadotroph Development and Function

During development, cells destined to form the anterior pituitary arise within the oral ectoderm and Rathke's pouch, and they undergo a process of differentiation into corticotrophs, thyrotrophs, mammosomatotrophs, and gonadotrophs (see Fig. 23-15). The mechanisms underlying these processes are discussed in Chapter 22. Developmental events that affect differentiation of early progenitor cells can cause congenital gonadotropin insufficiency as part of a multiple pituitary hormone deficiency. For example, mutations or variations in transcription factors such as HESX1, GLI2, OTX2, LHX3, SOX3, and PROP1 have been associated with HH, although in some conditions the onset of HH is often delayed until adolescence (e.g., with PROP1 variants).[199]

Differentiation of the gonadotropin cell line from other pituitary lineages may be controlled by gradient-dependent switches such as GATA2 and TBX19 (previously called TPIT). A limited number of factors that appear to affect gonadotroph function have been identified, including SF1

(*NRSA1*), DAX1 (NROβ1), and SOX2. Individuals with changes in SF1 may have partial deficits in gonadotropin synthesis, but the phenotype is more complex because it also involves gonadal dysgenesis. Mutations in DAX1 cause X-linked adrenal hypoplasia congenita. HH is an established part of this condition, but only about 10% of affected boys have evidence of congenital gonadotropin insufficiency, and the HPG axis is usually intact in early postnatal life.[200] SOX2 mutations can cause congenital HH with developmental delay and microphthalmia.[201]

Gonadotropins

Fetal pituitary gonadotropin synthesis and release begins at about 14 weeks' gestation and peaks at 20 to 22 weeks.[167] Synthesis of these hormones is regulated by hypothalamic GnRH, downstream signaling mechanisms such as pituitary adenylate cyclase–activating peptide (PACAP, now called ADCYAP1), and transcription factors such as SF1, DAX1, PITX1, early growth response 1 (EGR1), and the stress protein p8. The α-subunits of these hormones undergo post-translational modification and heterodimerize with a common α-subunit to form the mature glycoprotein hormones FSH and LH.

Gonadotropin hormones are influenced by inhibin, activin, and follistatin. Inhibin is a heterodimeric hormone comprising an α-subunit bound to one of two distinct β-subunits, β_A or β_B. Inhibin A and inhibin B are produced by the gonads (predominantly ovarian granulosa cells and testicular Sertoli cells, respectively) and placenta, and they suppress FSH. Activins stimulate FSH and consist of homodimers or heterodimers of inhibin β-subunits (i.e., activin A, activin B, or activin AB). Follistatin binds activin to attenuate its action and reduce FSH release. These hormones are likely to function at a local (paracrine) level in the pituitary, to have a systemic influence on gonadotropin release, and to signal through TGF-β/SMAD pathways.

Mutations in genes encoding the gonadotropin hormones LH and FSH have been described in a small number of patients with abnormalities of puberty or spermatogenesis, but severe congenital abnormalities associated with these conditions have not been described. Males with inactivating mutations of the LHβ subunit had descended testes and small penises but no evidence of hypospadias. These findings support the role of placental hCG signaling through the LH/hCG receptor as the primary mediator of fetal Leydig cell androgen production.

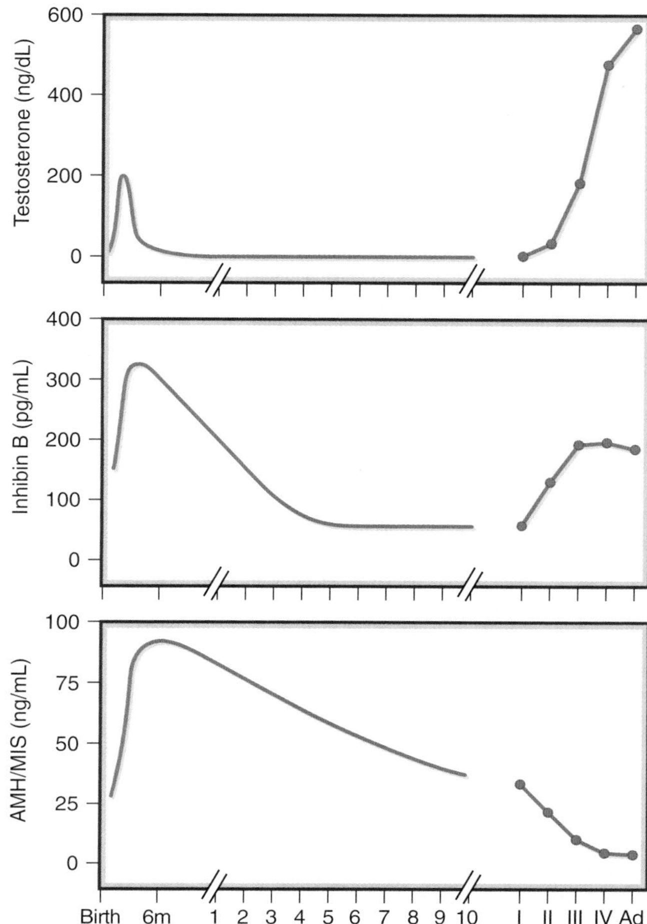

Figure 23-16 Typical postnatal changes are shown for testosterone, anti-Müllerian hormone (AMH/MIS), and inhibin B in normal males from birth to adulthood. Pubertal stages (I through IV) are indicated. Conversions: testosterone, ng/dL × 0.0347 for nmol/L; AMH/MIS, ng/mL × 7.14 for pmol/L; ranges may vary with the assay.

The Hypothalamic-Pituitary-Gonadal Axis in Infancy and Childhood

At birth, the infant is removed from the influence of maternal and placental hormones and undergoes a series of distinct endocrine changes.

Postnatal Endocrine Changes in Boys

In boys, low concentrations of testosterone can be detected by standard assays at birth, but these levels fall during the first few days of life. Thereafter, a reactivation of the HPG axis occurs, beginning at about 6 weeks of age, which results in peaks of testosterone nearing midpubertal levels between 2 and 3 months after birth (Fig. 23-16).[202,203] This peak of testosterone is associated with an acceleration in penile growth.[203] The HPG axis then becomes relatively quiescent by 4 to 6 months of age, until the onset of puberty in late childhood.

Inhibin B concentrations are high at birth and fall during the first 2 years of life before rising with the onset of puberty between 11 and 15 years of age (see Fig. 23-16).[204,205] In contrast, AMH concentrations remain high from birth through childhood and decline to low concentrations with the onset of puberty (see Fig. 23-16).[161,206] AMH and inhibin B can be useful markers of active testicular tissue in boys with cryptorchidism, anorchia, and 46,XY DSD. INSL3 assays may provide a useful additional marker of testicular integrity in the future.

Postnatal Endocrine Changes in Girls

The early postnatal endocrine events in girls are less well understood. Placental estrogen exposure can result in breast development before birth, and a small episode of menstrual bleeding can occur several days after birth from withdrawal of estrogen and progesterone. It is likely that girls also have a discrete activation of the HPG axis in infancy. However, detectable concentrations of estradiol (5 to 20 pg/mL [20 to 80 pmol/L]) and inhibin B (50 to 200 pg/mL) can be measured in the first few months of life, and surprisingly high concentrations of FSH with marked interindividual variability can be found during infancy and early childhood (median, 3.8 IU/L; range, 1.2 to 18.8 IU/L [2.5% to 97.5%] at 3 months of age in healthy, term girls).[207] Inhibin A has been proposed as a test of ovarian tissue in the newborn period in children with possible ovotesticular DSD, but this hormone is below the limits of detection in many normal, term newborn girls, and FSH stimulation may be needed to detect it.

DISORDERS OF SEX DEVELOPMENT

DSDs can have a wide range of presenting phenotypes depending on the underlying condition and its severity. Individuals with these conditions can present to many different health care professions, including neonatologists, geneticists, urologists, gynecologists, and internists. When an infant is born with ambiguous genitalia, the need for further investigation is usually clear. However, 46,XY individuals with complete 17α-hydroxylase/17,20-lyase deficiency may first present in early adolescence with hypertension and delayed puberty, or a young woman with CAIS (46,XY) may first present to a gynecologist with amenorrhea.

Significant progress in understanding of the molecular basis of gonad development has occurred during the past 20 years. Although several single-gene disorders causing gonadal dysgenesis in humans have been described and many more candidate genes are emerging from studies in mice, the percentage of patients with disorders of gonad development who can be diagnosed at the molecular level remains disappointingly low (15% to 20%). Defining the exact bases of different DSDs can have important implications for gender assignment, predicting response to treatment (e.g., androgen supplementation), assessing associated features (e.g., adrenal dysfunction) or the risk of tumorigenesis, and determining likely fertility options and long-term counseling for the individual and family. However, long-term outcome studies are often inadequate, and an evidence-based approach to management is not possible in many cases.

Nomenclature and Classification of Disorders of Sex Development

The proposal to change terminology by replacing *intersex* with the *DSD* acronym has led to a new classification for DSDs.[3,4] DSD has been defined as "congenital conditions in which development of chromosomal, gonadal, or anatomic sex is atypical."[3] This definition is wide ranging enough to cover conditions such as cloacal extrophy but sufficiently specific not to embrace, for example, disorders of puberty. The most common cause of ambiguous genitalia of the newborn, CAH, is classified as 46,XX DSD, and the next most common cause, PAIS, is classified as 46,XY DSD. Table 23-3 shows how such a classification system can be applied to DSDs. The list is not exhaustive but provides a framework for the following discussion of the more common causes of DSD, which classifies them as sex chromosome variations (sex chromosome DSD), disorders of

TABLE 23-3

Example of a DSD Classification

Sex Chromosome DSD	46,XY DSD	46,XX DSD
A: 47,XXY (Klinefelter syndrome and variants) B: 45,X (Turner syndrome and variants) C: 45,X/46,XY (mixed gonadal dysgenesis) D: 46,XX/46,XY (chimerism)	A: Disorders of gonadal (testis) development 1. Complete or partial gonadal dysgenesis (e.g., *SRY, SOX9, SF1, WT1, DHH*) 2. Ovotesticular DSD 3. Testis regression B: Disorders in androgen synthesis or action 1. Disorders of androgen synthesis Luteinizing hormone (LH) receptor mutations Smith-Lemli-Opitz syndrome StAR protein mutations Cholesterol side-chain cleavage (*CYP11A1*) 3β-Hydroxysteroid dehydrogenase 2 (*HSD3B2*) 17α-Hydroxylase/17,20-lyase (*CYP17*) P450 oxidoreductase (*POR*) Cytochrome b_5 (*CYB5A*) 17β-Hydroxysteroid dehydrogenase (*HSD17B3*) 5α-Reductase 2 (*SRD5A2*) 2. Disorders of androgen action Androgen insensitivity syndrome Drugs and environmental modulators C: Other 1. Syndromic associations of male genital development (e.g., cloacal anomalies, Robinow, Aarskog, hand-foot-genital, popliteal pterygium) 2. Persistent Müllerian duct syndrome 3. Vanishing testis syndrome 4. Isolated hypospadias (*MAMLD1*) 5. Congenital hypogonadotropic hypogonadism 6. Cryptorchidism (*INSL3, GREAT*) 7. Environmental influences	A: Disorders of gonadal (ovary) development 1. Gonadal dysgenesis 2. Ovotesticular DSD 3. Testicular DSD (e.g., *SRY*+, dup *SOX9, RSPO1, WNT4*) B: Andro of gen excess 1. Fetal 3β-Hydroxysteroid dehydrogenase 2 (*HSD3B2*) 21-Hydroxylase (*CYP21A2*) P450 oxidoreductase (*POR*) 11β-Hydroxylase (*CYP11B1*) Glucocorticoid receptor mutations 2. Fetoplacental Aromatase (*CYP19*) deficiency Oxidoreductase (*POR*) deficiency 3. Maternal Maternal virilizing tumors (e.g., luteomas) Androgenic drugs C: Other 1. Syndromic associations (e.g., cloacal anomalies) 2. Müllerian agenesis/hypoplasia (e.g., MURCS) 3. Uterine abnormalities (e.g., MODY5) 4. Vaginal atresias (e.g., McKusick-Kaufman) 5. Labial adhesions

CYP, cytochrome P450 isoenzyme; DSDs, disorders of sex development; MODY5, maturity-onset diabetes of the young type 5; MURCS, Müllerian, renal, and cervical spine syndrome; StAR, steroidogenic acute regulatory (protein).

testis development and androgenization (46,XY DSD), and disorders of ovary development and androgen excess (46,XX DSD) (see Fig. 23-2).

Sex Chromosome Disorders of Sex Development

Differences in the number of sex chromosomes (i.e., sex chromosome aneuploidy) can be considered *sex chromosome DSDs*. These conditions include Klinefelter syndrome (47,XXY and its variants), Turner syndrome (45,X and its variants), mixed gonadal dysgenesis (45,X/46,XY mosaicism and its variants), and true sex chromosome chimerism (46,XY/46,XX) (Table 23-4). A 45,Y cell line is nonviable.

Mixed gonadal dysgenesis and sex chromosome chimerism can manifest with ambiguous genitalia at birth, but such a presentation is unlikely in Klinefelter syndrome unless multiple X chromosomes are present or in Turner syndrome unless there is a Y fragment. In many cases of classic sex chromosome aneuploidy, the diagnosis is made in adolescence or adult life as a result of associated features, impaired pubertal development, or infertility. More detailed descriptions of the long-term management of some of these conditions are provided in the relevant chapters (e.g., Turner syndrome and Klinefelter syndrome in Chapter 25).

Klinefelter Syndrome and Its Variants

Klinefelter syndrome is the most common forms of sex chromosome aneuploidy, with a reported incidence of 1 in 500 to 1 in 1000 live births.[208,209] This incidence may be increasing.[210] The classic form of Klinefelter syndrome is associated with a 47,XXY karyotype and is caused by meiotic nondisjunction of the sex chromosomes during gametogenesis (Fig. 23-17; see Fig. 23-4).[209,210] This abnormality occurs during spermatogenesis in approximately 40% of patients and during oogenesis in approximately 60%. Mosaic forms of Klinefelter syndrome (46,XY/47,XXY) represent mitotic nondisjunction within the developing zygote and are thought to occur in approximately 10% of individuals with this condition (see Fig. 23-4). Other chromosomal variants associated with Klinefelter syndrome (e.g., 48,XXXY) have been reported.

The clinical features of Klinefelter syndrome and its variants are summarized in Table 23-4.[208,209] In the most severe situations, a young man may be diagnosed because of small testes, gynecomastia, poor androgenization at puberty, eunuchoid proportions, or infertility. Diagnosis before puberty is the exception. Other features, such as learning difficulties, language delay, and altered motor development, may occur.[211,212] However, it is likely that the clinical detection of Klinefelter syndrome based on postnatal karyotyping is biased toward detection of those individuals with a more severe phenotype. As few as 25% of men with Klinefelter syndrome may be diagnosed throughout their life span.[209]

The development of testes and a male phenotype in individuals with Klinefelter syndrome provides important evidence for the key role of the Y chromosome in testis determination and subsequent prenatal androgen production. However, micropenis and hypospadias may be presenting features in some cases (personal observation), and some studies report elevated early postnatal gonadotropin concentrations.[213]

A more predictable elevation in gonadotropin concentrations (e.g., FSH, LH) occurs in the preadolescent and periadolescent periods in patients with Klinefelter syndrome, after activation of the HPG axis.[214,215] By adolescence, plasma concentrations of FSH are increased in 90% of patients with Klinefelter syndrome, and plasma concentrations of LH are increased in 80%. Other serum markers of testicular function (e.g., prepubertal AMH, peripubertal inhibin B, midpubertal INSL3) are often below the normal ranges.[216,217] Although some androgenization usually occurs during puberty in classic Klinefelter syndrome, plasma testosterone is decreased in 50% to 75% of cases.[214] Testes usually remain small and firm; the median length and volume are 2.5 cm (4 mL), but most are smaller than 3.5 cm (12 mL). They typically appear inappropriately small for the degree of androgenization. The serum estradiol concentration is often elevated, which contributes to the gynecomastia observed during the adolescent period.

Testicular biopsy is not warranted clinically, because the diagnosis can usually be made on karyotyping from

TABLE 23-4

Clinical Features of Sex Chromosome DSDs

Condition	Karyotype	Gonad	Internal Genitalia	Features
Klinefelter syndrome	47,XXY and variants	Hyalinized testes	No uterus	Small testis, azoospermia, hypoandrogenemia; tall stature and increased leg length; increased incidence of learning difficulties, obesity, breast tumors, varicose veins, impaired glucose tolerance
Turner syndrome	45,X and variants	Streak gonad or immature ovary	Uterus	*Childhood:* Lymphedema, shield chest, web neck, low hairline; cardiac defects and coarctation of the aorta; renal and urinary abnormalities; short stature, cubitus valgus, hypoplastic nails, scoliosis; otitis media and hearing loss; ptosis and amblyopia; nevi; autoimmune thyroid disease; visuospatial learning difficulties *Adulthood:* Pubertal failure, primary amenorrhea; hypertension; aortic root dilatation and dissection; sensorineural hearing loss; increased risk of CVD, IBD, colon cancer, thyroid disease, glucose intolerance and diabetes mellitus, osteoporosis (note that some of these may be related to estrogen deficiency)
Mixed gonadal dysgenesis	45,X/46, XY and variants	Testis or dysgenetic gonad	Variable	Increased risk of gonadal tumors; short stature; some features of Turner syndrome may be present
Ovotesticular DSD	46,XX/46,XY chimerism	Testis, ovary, or ovotestis	Variable	Possible increased risk of gonadal tumors

CVD, cardiovascular disease; DSDs, disorders of sex development; IBD, inflammatory bowel disease.

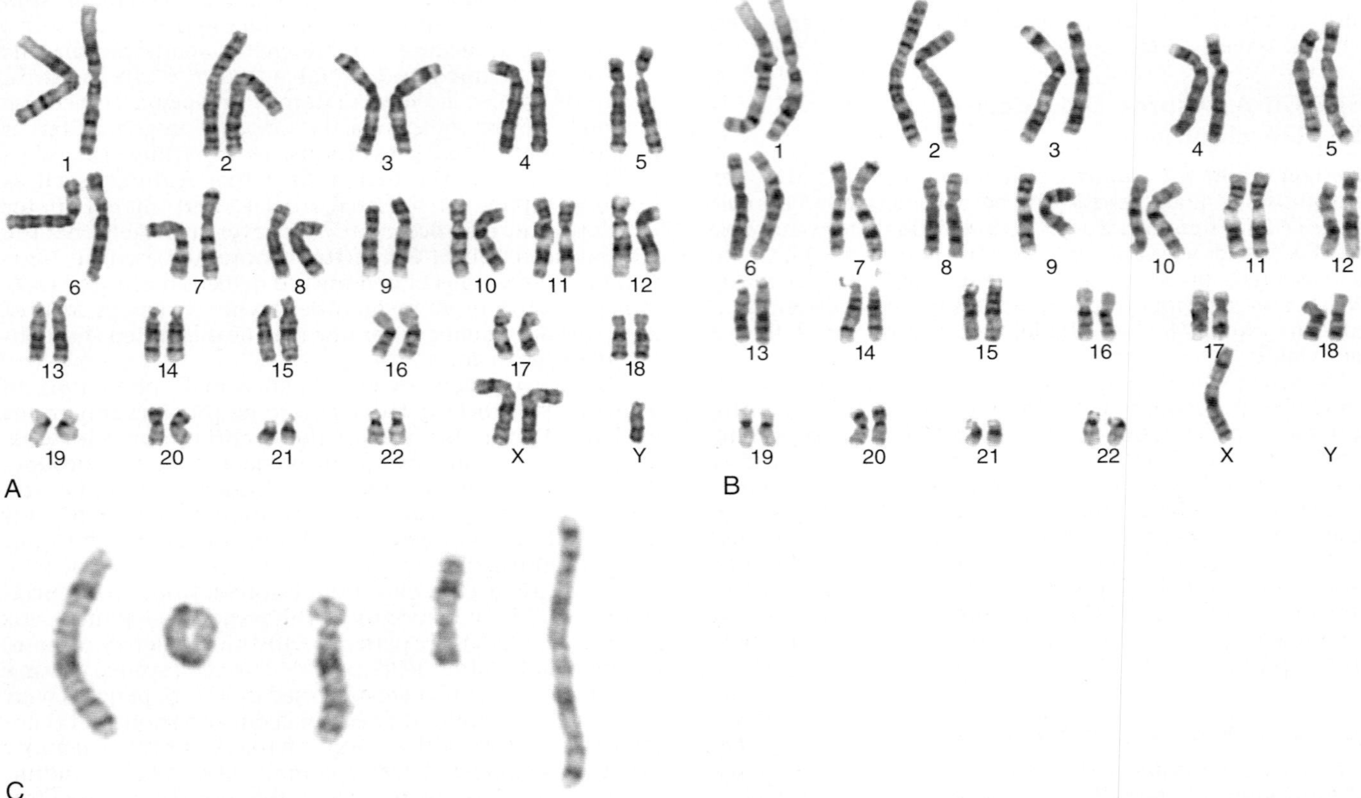

Figure 23-17 G-banded karyotypes of Klinefelter syndrome (47,XXY) **(A)** and Turner syndrome (45,X) **(B)**. **C,** Structural changes of the X chromosome seen in variants of Turner syndrome (*from left to right:* normal X; ring chromosome [r(X)(p22.3q22)]; short-arm deletion [del(X)(p21)]; long-arm deletion [del(X)(q21.31)]; isochromosome [I(X)(q10)]). (Images courtesy of Lee Grimsley and Jonathan Waters, MD, North East London Regional Cytogenetics Laboratory, Great Ormond Street Hospital NHS Trust, London, UK.)

peripheral blood cells. However, studies in which testicular histology has been obtained report germ cell depletion, progressive hyalinization of seminiferous tubules, and Leydig cell hyperplasia after chronic LH stimulation. A significant proportion of men with Klinefelter syndrome receive testosterone supplementation to fully induce puberty and to support sexual characteristics, libido, and bone mineralization into adult life. Management of Klinefelter syndrome in adolescence and adulthood is discussed in Chapters 23 and 25. Although some cases of spontaneous fertility have been reported for mosaic forms of Klinefelter syndrome (46,XY/47,XXY), the prospects for fertility in classic Klinefelter syndrome have been thought to be poor. However, testicular sperm extraction (TESE) combined with intracytoplasmic sperm injection (ISCI) has reportedly led to successful pregnancy for approximately 50% of men with classic Klinefelter syndrome (47,XXY) in specialist centers.[218,219] The potential risk of transmission of the sex chromosome aneuploidy must be considered, although it seems to be low. Benefits of this approach may decrease with age, suggesting that progressive deterioration in testicular function is a feature of Klinefelter syndrome.

Turner Syndrome and Its Variants

Turner syndrome is the second most frequent form of sex chromosome aneuploidy, with an incidence of approximately 1 case in 2500.[42] The classic form of Turner syndrome is associated with a 45,X karyotype, which occurs in approximately one half of individuals with this condition (see Fig. 23-17). Mosaic forms of Turner syndrome (45,X/46,XX) account for approximately one fourth of the patients, and the remainder have structural abnormalities of the X chromosome, such as long arm or short arm deletions, isochromosomes, or ring chromosomes (see Fig. 23-17).[42,220]

A 45,X chromosome constitution may be the consequence of nondisjunction or chromosome loss during gametogenesis in either parent that results in a sperm or ovum that lacks a sex chromosome (see Fig. 23-4). Although errors in mitosis in normal zygotes often lead to mosaicism, a purely 45,X constitution may arise at the first cleavage division from anaphase lag with loss of a sex chromosome or, less often, from mitotic nondisjunction with failure of the complementary 47,XXX or 47,XYY cell line to survive.[17] An estimated 2% of all zygotes have a 45,X karyotype, and approximately 7% of spontaneous abortuses have a 45,X karyotype, making this the most frequent chromosomal anomaly in humans.

The clinical features of Turner syndrome are highly variable and depend on the age of the child and time of diagnosis. For example, a prenatal diagnosis of Turner syndrome may be made incidentally after amniocentesis or chorionic villous sampling for another reason, such as advanced maternal age, or after the detection of increased nuchal translucency on fetal ultrasound scanning.[220,221] In early infancy, the diagnosis should be considered in females with lymphedema, nuchal folds, low hair line, or left-sided cardiac defects. Unexplained growth failure or somatic features (e.g., abnormal nails, shield chest, abnormal carrying angle, recurrent ear infections) may point to the diagnosis during childhood, and Turner syndrome should be considered in all girls with pubertal delay or pubertal failure. The clinical features of Turner syndrome are summarized in Table 23-4, and the diagnosis and management of this condition are discussed in Chapter 25. Timely and appropriate introduction of estrogens is necessary in adolescence to ensure adequate breast and uterine development, thereby optimizing the opportunity to carry a pregnancy by ovum donation in the future.[221,222] Women with Turner syndrome benefit from dedicated transition in adolescence and long-term follow-up with a focus on issues such as cardiovascular, bone, and reproductive health and hearing.[42,221-223]

Girls with classic Turner syndrome show ovarian dysgenesis, which highlights the importance of having two copies of the X chromosome for ovarian development and integrity. Studies of Turner syndrome embryos have shown normal germ cell migration and normal ovarian development until the third month of gestation.[224] Then, accelerated germ cell apoptosis and subsequent oocyte atresia occur, resulting in progressive degeneration of the ovary in the prenatal or postnatal period. With these gonadal changes, LH and FSH tend to rise in late childhood, after activation of the hypothalamic pulse generator. Nevertheless, sufficient estrogen synthesis for puberty to commence in adolescence occurs in approximately 25% of girls with Turner syndrome (10% of those with 45,X; 30% to 40% of those with 45,X/46,XX mosaicism), and menstruation occurs in about 2% of cases.[42,225] Gonadectomy is not usually required except when a Y fragment containing the *TSPY* locus is present; in such patients, the risk of gonadoblastoma is increased.[23,226] It is unclear whether any follicular tissue can be usefully cryopreserved for girls in whom spontaneous puberty has occurred, although oocyte cryopreservation has been used successfully in several women with Turner mosaicism.[227-229]

45,X/46,XY Mosaicism and Variants

A mosaic 45,X/46,XY karyotype, sometimes referred to as *mixed gonadal dysgenesis*, probably arises through anaphase lag during mitosis in the zygote, although Y chromosomal abnormalities are sometimes seen, and interchromosomal rearrangements with loss of structural abnormal Y material may be a common mechanism for variants of this condition. Although the classic form of this condition is associated with 45,X/46,XY mosaicism, 45,X/47,XYY or 45,X/46,XY/47,XYY mosaic karyotypes have also been reported.

The clinical phenotype associated with a 45,X/46,XY mosaicism is highly variable, and the true prevalence of this condition is unknown (see Table 23-4). Historically, individuals with the most severe forms of 45,X/46,XY mosaicism have been referred for further assessment, and most series of patients reported in the literature have probably reflected this bias.[230,231]

Reported genital phenotypes associated with 45,X/46,XY mosaicism range from female external genitalia or mild clitoromegaly through all stages of ambiguous genitalia to hypospadias or a normal penis.[230,231] Gonadal phenotypes range from streak gonads through dysgenetic testes to testes with normal histologic architecture. In rare cases, ovarian-like stroma and sparse primordial follicles may be present. The gonads may be positioned anywhere along the pathway of testicular descent, with streak gonads more likely to be intra-abdominal and well-formed testes more likely to be in the inguinoscrotal region. Müllerian structures may be present in the most severe cases because of impaired AMH production by Sertoli cells. Marked differences in gonadal development and histology can be seen between the right and the left sides or even within a single gonad (hence, the term *mixed gonadal dysgenesis*).[2] The presence of a hemiuterus and fallopian tube on the side of the most severely affected gonad in some cases provides important evidence for the paracrine actions of AMH on developing Müllerian structures.

Somatic features associated with a 45,X/46,XY karyotype are highly variable and do not always correlate well with the gonadal phenotype.[231] At the most severe end of the spectrum, clinical features reminiscent of Turner syndrome may be seen, such as short stature, nuchal folds, low-set hairline, and cardiac and renal abnormalities. Detailed evaluation and long-term follow-up of these patients may be warranted, as for Turner syndrome (see Chapter 25). In other cases, a reduction in predicted height may be the only somatic manifestation. It is unclear whether detailed, ongoing monitoring for features associated with Turner syndrome (e.g., thyroid function, hearing, cardiac anomalies) is required for this group of individuals, but a low threshold should be maintained if there are any concerns.

Gender assignment can be difficult in individuals with 45,X/46,XY, and several factors should be considered, including genital appearance and urogenital anatomy, risk of gonadal malignancy, fertility and reproductive options, potential need for hormone replacement, and probable gender identity, sex role behavior, and psychosexual functioning.

Most infants with female or minimally androgenized genitalia are raised as female, and the presence of a uterus or hemiuterus allows the potential for pregnancy by ovum donation in the future. Intra-abdominal streak and dysgenetic gonads are thought to pose a significant risk of malignancy and should be removed.[3,23,232,233] Estrogen replacement is required to induce breast and uterine development in adolescence, and the addition of progestins allows menstruation when a uterus is present. Growth-promoting agents have been used on an individual basis when short stature or Turner syndrome–like features are present, but no proper trials have been performed to assess this group of patients. Similarly, no long-term outcome data on gender identity or psychosexual functioning are available.

Infants with hypospadias and reasonable phallic development are usually raised as male. Testosterone can be given to promote phallic growth in infancy, and hypospadias repair is usually undertaken as a two-stage procedure. Attempts should be made to perform orchidopexy as a one- or two-stage procedure, because there may be a significant risk of malignancy in these gonads, and careful monitoring is necessary.[23] Gonads that cannot be placed within the scrotum are usually removed.[3,233] Gonads that can be secured within the scrotum need careful monitoring and biopsy in early adolescence to assess for carcinoma in situ.[23,233] Puberty should be carefully monitored to ensure adequate endogenous testosterone production, and in some cases, testosterone supplementation is needed. Loss of height potential is generally unpredictable but needs careful monitoring.

Assignment of gender and management of a 45,X/46,XY child with *highly ambiguous genitalia* can be a difficult situation for parents and physicians, and long-term outcome data for this group are not available. Limited data suggest that approximately 60% of infants with this phenotype are raised female, but they are infertile, have no uterus, require gonadectomy, and are likely to undergo urogenital surgery.[2] In contrast, those raised as male require multiple hypospadias operations, may have poor corporal tissue, are infertile if dysgenetic gonads are present that need to be removed, and may have a significantly reduced height potential. These situations highlight the need for a multidisciplinary approach to initial assessment and management and for long-term monitoring and support. Long-term outcome data from larger studies may provide better guidance on the management of this group of individuals in the future.

In addition to the most severe cases described earlier, a 45,X/46,XY mosaic karyotype can be associated with a male phenotype and apparently normal testis development. Initial cases of normal males with a 45,X/46,XY karyotype were described after screening of family members as potential bone marrow transplant donors,[2] but later studies of amniocentesis showed that 90% of fetuses diagnosed as 45,X/46,XY by amniocentesis and confirmed as having this karyotype have normal male genitalia and apparently normal testes postnatally.[234,235] Moreover, there seems to be limited correlation between the degree of mosaicism on peripheral blood sampling and gonadal or somatic phenotype. Follow-up data on this cohort are limited, HPG function has not been reported in detail, and fertility outcome and tumor risk are not known. Although a 45,X/46,XY karyotype is an uncommon finding in men presenting with testicular tumors or in the infertility clinic, more detailed long-term studies of the 45,X/46,XY male cohort are required to know whether extensive follow-up is necessary. It may seem prudent to monitor gonadal function in this cohort and to assess for evidence of testicular carcinoma in situ in adolescence, but evidence for the best approach is lacking.

Ovotesticular Disorders of Sex Development: 46,XX/46,XY Chimerism and Variants

The diagnosis of ovotesticular DSD (true hermaphroditism) requires the presence of ovarian tissue (containing follicles) and testicular tissue in the same or the opposite gonad (Fig. 23-18; see Table 23-4). Gonadal stroma arranged in whorls, similar to those found in the ovary but lacking oocytes, is not considered sufficient evidence to designate the rudimentary gonad as an ovary.[2]

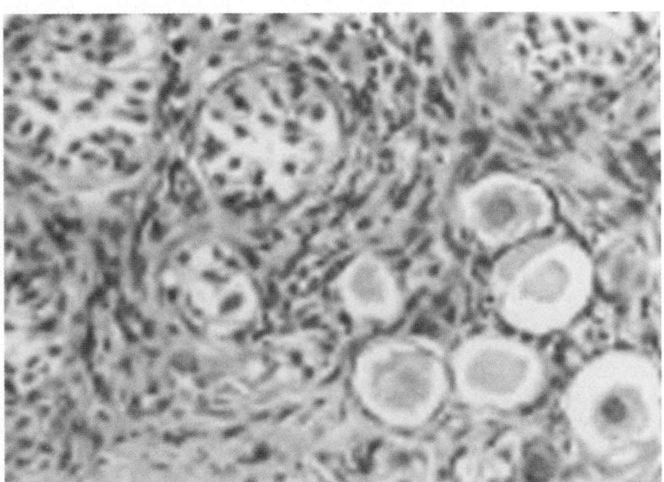

Figure 23-18 Ovotestis, showing immature seminiferous tubules lined with Sertoli cells and germ cells *(upper left)* and ovarian tissue with follicles *(lower right)* (Hematoxylin-eosin stain; original magnification, ×400). (Courtesy of Neil Sebire, MD, Great Ormond Street Hospital NHS Trust, London, UK.)

TABLE 23-5

Relative Frequency (%) of Different Karyotypes in Ovotesticular DSD (True Hermaphroditism)

Location	46,XX/46,XY	46,XX	46,XY
North America	21	72	7
Europe	41	52	7
Africa	—	97	—

Adapted from Krob G, Braun A, Kuhnle U. True hermaphroditism: geographical distribution, clinical findings, chromosomes and gonadal histology. *Eur J Pediatr.* 1994;153:2-10.

Ovotesticular DSD is an uncommon condition that has been reported in approximately 500 individuals worldwide. Although 46,XX/46,XY chimerism (sometimes caused by double fertilization or ovum fusion; see "Chromosomal Sex") does occur in a proportion of these patients, especially in North America and Europe, most individuals with 46,XX/46,XY chimerism do not have this condition (Table 23-5).[236] Rather, most patients with ovotesticular DSD, especially those in South and Western Africa, have a 46,XX karyotype.[236-238] The molecular basis of this disorder is not known, but familial cases have been reported, and autosomal recessive and sex-limited autosomal dominant transmission have been proposed. *RSPO1* mutations have been found occasionally, but *SRY* translocations are rare.[239,240] Ovotesticular DSD associated with a 46,XY karyotype is not prevalent and may represent cryptic gonadal mosaicism for a Y chromosome deletion or early sex-determining gene mutation. Ovotesticular DSD likely has several causes.

Patients with ovotesticular DSD may be subclassified according to the type and location of the gonads.[2] *Lateral* cases (20%) have a testis on one side and an ovary on the other. *Bilateral* cases (30%) have testicular and ovarian tissue present bilaterally, usually as ovotestes. *Unilateral* cases (50%) have an ovotestis present on one side and an ovary or testis on the other. The ovary (or ovotestis) is more frequently found on the left side of the body, whereas the testis (or ovotestis) is found more often on the right. An ovary is likely to be in its normal anatomic position, whereas a testis or ovotestis can be anywhere along the pathway of testicular descent and is often found in the right inguinal region.

Differentiation of the genital tract and development of secondary sex characteristics vary in ovotesticular DSD.[241] Most patients who present early have ambiguous genitalia or significant hypospadias. Cryptorchidism is common, but at least one gonad is palpable, usually in the labioscrotal fold or inguinal region, more often on the right, and often associated with an inguinal hernia. The differentiation of the genital ducts usually follows that of the gonad, and a hemiuterus or rudimentary uterus is often present on the side of the ovary or ovotestis.

Breast development at the time of puberty is common in ovotesticular DSD. Menses occurs in a significant proportion of cases, and ovulation and pregnancy have been reported in a number of patients with a 46,XX karyotype, especially when an ovary is present. However, progressive androgenization can occur in girls with significant testicular tissue, which can result in voice changes and clitoral enlargement during adolescence if left untreated. Individuals raised as male often present with hypospadias and undescended testes, although bilateral scrotal ovotestes have been reported. These individuals can experience significant estrogenization at the time of puberty and may have cyclic hematuria if a uterus is present. Spermatogenesis is rare, and interstitial fibrosis of the testis is common.

Although ovotesticular DSD is rare, the diagnosis should be considered in all patients with ambiguous genitalia, especially if there is more pronounced scrotalization or detection of a gonad on the right. A 46,XX/46,XY karyotype strongly supports the diagnosis, but the detection of a 46,XX or 46,XY karyotype does not exclude the diagnosis. Pelvic imaging with ultrasound or magnetic resonance imaging (MRI) is useful for visualizing internal genitalia. The presence of testicular tissue may be detected by measurement of basal testosterone, AMH, and inhibin B in the first months of life, and by measuring basal AMH and testosterone inverse of hCG stimulation thereafter. Ovarian tissue is more difficult to detect in early childhood, although estradiol, inhibin A, and follicular response to repeated injection of recombinant human FSH can provide useful information.[242] Examination under anesthesia and laparoscopy may provide the most detailed information about internal structures and allow a biopsy to confirm the diagnosis of ovotesticular DSD when other forms of DSD have been excluded.

The management of ovotesticular DSD depends on the age at diagnosis, genital development, internal structures, and reproductive capacity. Male or female assignment may be appropriate for the young infant in whom a strong gender identity has not been established. Individuals with a 46,XX karyotype and a uterus are likely to have functional ovarian tissue, and female assignment is likely to be appropriate. Potentially functional testicular tissue should be removed and monitored postoperatively by measuring serum AMH levels and by demonstrating a lack of testosterone response to hCG stimulation. The risk of malignant transformation in ovarian tissue of 46,XX patients is not known.

A male gender assignment may be more appropriate if there is reasonable phallic development and müllerian structures are absent or very poorly formed. Ovarian tissue is usually removed to prevent estrogenization at puberty, and remnant Müllerian structures can be removed by an experienced surgeon. The prevalence of gonadoblastoma or germinoma arising in the testicular tissue of patients with 46,XX ovotesticular DSD has been estimated at 3% to 4 %. Because the ovotesticular tissue is usually dysgenetic, removal of this testicular tissue has been advocated.[23] However, management of a histologically normal, scrotally positioned testis is more difficult, and careful monitoring and biopsy for carcinoma in situ in adolescence may be an appropriate strategy.

Gender identity is an important consideration in patients with ovotesticular DSD who first present in late childhood or adolescence due to androgenization in girls or estrogenization in boys. In most cases, gender identity is consistent with sex of rearing. After appropriate counseling, the discordant gonad and dysgenetic tissue should be removed to prevent further androgenization in girls and estrogenization in boys. Sex hormone supplementation may be required for complete pubertal development.

46,XY Disorders of Sex Development

The 46,XY DSDs can be categorized as disorders of testis development, disorders of androgen synthesis, disorders of androgen action, and other conditions affecting sex development (Table 23-6; see also Fig. 23-8).

Disorders of Testis Development

Disorders of testis development can have a spectrum of phenotypes and presentations. In the most extreme cases, *complete testicular dysgenesis* is associated with a complete lack of androgenization of the external genitalia and persistent Müllerian structures due to insufficient AMH production—a condition sometimes called Swyer syndrome. In contrast, *partial gonadal dysgenesis* may be associated with clitoromegaly or ambiguous genitalia. A uterus and vagina may or may not be present. A subset of less severe forms of male reproductive development, such as isolated hypospadias, testicular regression, micropenis, or male infertility, may represent milder variants of the more severe phenotypes.

Several single-gene disorders have been described in patients with various degrees of testicular dysgenesis. Table 23-6 summarizes these factors, and their role in development has already been discussed (see "Testis Determination"). Candidate genes for these disorders have been discovered based largely on mouse phenotypes and on cases of gonadal dysgenesis occurring as part of a more complex syndrome. In such cases, the presence of any associated features can help to direct genetic analysis appropriately. A genetic diagnosis is reached only in 20% to 30% of cases of 46,XY testicular dysgenesis at present.

Single-Gene Disorders

***Steroidogenic Factor 1:* NR5A1.** SF1 (encoded by *NR5A1*) is a member of the nuclear receptor superfamily that regulates the transcription of at least 30 genes involved in gonadal development, adrenal development, steroidogenesis, and reproduction.[78,243] Complete deletion of the gene encoding Sf1 in mice results in apoptosis of the developing gonad and adrenal gland during early embryonic development.[79] XY animals are phenotypically female and have persistent müllerian structures. Abnormalities of the ventromedial hypothalamus and variable HH are also described.

Based on the phenotypic findings in the mouse, SF1 mutations were first reported in two 46,XY individuals with female external genitalia, persistent Müllerian structures, and primary adrenal failure.[82,83] These changes resulted in impaired DNA binding. The first mutation was a de novo heterozygous Gly35Glu change in the P-box primary DNA-binding region of SF1, and the second was a recessively inherited homozygous Arg92Gln mutation in the A-box secondary DNA-binding region (Fig. 23-19).

An increasing number of heterozygous nonsense, frameshift, and missense mutations in *NR5A1* have been associated with 46,XY DSD (see Fig. 23-19).[78,84,244] These changes result in haploinsufficiency of SF1 and a spectrum of phenotypes, most commonly mild gonadal dysgenesis and significantly impaired androgenization but with normal adrenal function.[78,84,245] These variations usually arise de novo but may be inherited from the mother in a sex-limited dominant fashion (i.e., the mother carries the mutation but is unaffected).[84] In other cases, there is a family history of ovarian insufficiency.[51] Loss of SF1 function also is reported in some boys with severe hypospadias and undescended testes, bilateral anorchia, and a small penis, and in men with infertility.[246-247] Therefore, variable loss of SF1 activity is associated primarily with testicular dysfunction or variable ovarian dysfunction in humans. Adrenal function may need to be monitored over time.

***Chromobox Homolog 2:* CBX2.** Chromobox homolog 2 *(CBX2)* is a human homolog of the polycomb protein M33. Deletion of its gene causes XY sex reversal in mice. Loss-of-function mutations in *CBX2* were described in a 46,XY girl with a uterus and ovaries who was diagnosed by prenatal karyotyping.[248]

***Wilms' Tumor 1 Gene:* WT1.** *WT1* (11p13) is a four-zinc finger transcription factor expressed in the developing genital ridge, kidney, gonads, and mesothelium.[66-67]

TABLE 23-6

Overview of Important Genes Involved in DSDs

Gene	Protein	OMIM	Locus	Inheritance	Gonad	Müllerian Structures	External Genitalia	Associated Features/Variants
A. Causes of 46,XY DSD								
Disorders of Gonadal (Testicular) Development: Single-Gene Disorders								
WT1	TF	607102	11p13	AD	Dysgenetic testis	±	Female or ambiguous	Wilms' tumor, renal abnormalities, gonadal tumors (WAGR, Denys- Drash, and Frasier syndromes)
CBX2	Polycomb protein	602770	17q25	AR	Ovary (one case)	+	Female	
NR5A1 (SF1)	Nuclear receptor TF	184757	9q33	AD/AR	Dysgenetic testis (variable)	±	Female, ambiguous, or hypospadias	More severe phenotypes include primary adrenal failure; milder phenotypes have isolated partial gonadal dysgenesis or impaired androgenization or both
SRY	TF	480000	Yp11.3	Y	Dysgenetic testis or ovotestis	±	Female or ambiguous	
SOX9	TF	608160	17q24-q25	AD	Dysgenetic testis or ovotestis	±	Female or ambiguous	Camptomelic dysplasia (17q24 rearrangements have a milder phenotype than point mutations)
DHH	Signaling molecule	605423	12q13.1	AR	Dysgenetic testis, testis	–	Female	The severe phenotype of one patient included minifascicular neuropathy; other patients have isolated gonadal dysgenesis
ARX	TF	300382	Xp22.13	X	Dysgenetic testis (Leydig)	–	Ambiguous	X-linked lissencephaly, epilepsy, temperature instability
TSPYL1	? Chromatin remodeling	604714	6q22-23	AR	Dysgenetic testis	–	Female or ambiguous	Sudden infant death
MAMLD1 (CXORF6)	Unknown	300120	Xq28	X	Normal (Leydig cell dysfunction)	–	Hypospadias	
*Disorders of Gonadal (Testicular) Development: Chromosomal Changes Involving Key Candidate Genes**								
DMRT1	TF	602424	9p24.3	Monosomic deletion	Dysgenetic testis	±	Female or ambiguous	Mental retardation
ATRX	Helicase (? chromatin remodeling)	300032	Xq13.3	X	Dysgenetic testis	–	Female, ambiguous, or male	α-Thalassemia, mental retardation
NR0B1 (DAX1)	Nuclear receptor TF	300018	Xp21.3	dupXp21	Dysgenetic testis or ovary	±	Female or ambiguous	
WNT4	Signaling molecule	603490	1p35	dup1p35	Dysgenetic testis	+	Ambiguous	Mental retardation
Disorders in Hormone Synthesis or Action								
DHCR7	Enzyme	602858	11q12-q13	AR	Testis	–	Variable	Smith-Lemli-Opitz syndrome: coarse facies, second-third toe syndactyly, failure to thrive, developmental delay, cardiac and visceral abnormalities
LHCGR	G-protein receptor	152790	2p21	AR	Testis	–	Female, ambiguous, or micropenis	Leydig cell hypoplasia
STAR	Mitochondrial associated protein	600617	8p11.2	AR	Testis	–	Female, ambiguous, or micropenis	Lipoid CAH (primary adrenal failure), pubertal failure
CYP11A1	Enzyme	118485	15q23-q24	AR	Testis	–	Female or ambiguous	CAH (primary adrenal failure), pubertal failure
HSD3B2	Enzyme	201810	1p13.1	AR	Testis	–	Ambiguous	CAH, primary adrenal failure, ↑ Δ^5:Δ^4 ratio
CYP17A1	Enzyme	202110	10q24.3	AR	Testis	–	Female, ambiguous, or micropenis	CAH, hypertension due to DOC (except in isolated 17,20-lyase deficiency)

POR (P450 oxidoreductase)	CYP enzyme electron donor	124015	7q11.2	AR	Testis	–	Male or ambiguous	Mixed features of 21-hydroxylase deficiency, 17α-hydroxylase/17,20-lyase deficiency, and aromatase deficiency; sometimes associated with Antley-Bixler craniosynostosis
CYB5A	Cofactor	613218	18q23	AR	Testis	–	Ambiguous or hypospadiac	Methemoglobinemia
HSD17B3	Enzyme	605573	9q22	AR	Testis	–	Female or ambiguous	Partial androgenization at puberty, ↑ ratio of androstenedione to testosterone
SRD5A2	Enzyme	607306	2p23	AR	Testis	–	Ambiguous or micropenis	Partial androgenization at puberty, ↑ ratio of testosterone to DHT
Androgen receptor	Nuclear receptor TF	313700	Xq11-q12	X	Testis	–	Female, ambiguous, micropenis, or normal male	Phenotypic spectrum from complete AIS (female external genitalia) to partial AIS (ambiguous) to normal male genitalia/infertility
AMH	Signaling molecule	600957	19p13.3-p13.2	AR	Testis	+	Normal male	Persistent müllerian duct syndrome (PMDS)
AMH receptor	Serine/threonine kinase transmembrane receptor	600956	12q13	AR	Testis	+	Normal male	Male external genitalia, bilateral cryptorchidism
B. Causes of 46,XX DSD								
Disorders of Gonadal (Ovarian) Development								
SRY	TF	480000	Yp11.3	Translocation	Testis or ovotestis	–	Male or ambiguous	
SOX9	TF	608160	17q24	dup17q24	Not determined	–	Male or ambiguous	
RSPO1	Thrombospondin (Wnt signaling)	609595	1p34.3	AR	Testis or ovotestis	–	Male	Palmar-plantar hyperkeratosis, squamous cell carcinoma
WNT4	Wnt signaling	611812	1p35	AR	Testis or ovotestis	–	Male or ambiguous	SERKAL syndrome
Androgen Excess								
HSD3B2	Enzyme	201810	1p13	AR	Ovary	+	Clitoromegaly (mild)	CAH, primary adrenal failure, partial androgenization due to ↑ conversion of DHEA
CYP21A2	Enzyme	201910	6p21-p23	AR	Ovary	+	Ambiguous; rarely Prader V	CAH, phenotypic spectrum from severe salt-losing forms associated with adrenal failure to simple virilizing forms with compensated adrenal function, ↑ 17-OHP
CYP11B1	Enzyme	202010	8q21-q22	AR	Ovary	+	Ambiguous; rarely Prader V	CAH, hypertension due to ↑ 11-deoxycorticosterone
POR (P450 oxidoreductase)	CYP enzyme electron donor	124015	7q11.2	AR	Ovary	+	Normal or ambiguous	Mixed features of 21-hydroxylase deficiency, 17α-hydroxylase/17,20-lyase deficiency and aromatase deficiency; associated with Antley-Bixler craniosynostosis
CYP19	Enzyme	107910	15q21	AR	Ovary	+	Ambiguous	Maternal androgenization during pregnancy, absent breast development at puberty except in partial cases
Glucocorticoid receptor†	Nuclear receptor TF	138040	5q31	AR	Ovary	+	Normal or ambiguous	↑ ACTH, 17-OHP, cortisol, mineralocorticoids, and androgens; failure of dexamethasone suppression

*Chromosomal rearrangements likely to include key genes are included.

†Note: patient heterozygous for a mutation in CYP21.

–, absent; +, present; ACTH, adrenocorticotropin; AD, autosomal dominant (often de novo mutation); AIS, androgen insensitivity syndrome; AR, autosomal recessive; CAH, congenital adrenal hyperplasia; CYP, cytochrome P450 enzyme; DHEA, dehydroepiandrosterone; DHT, dihydrotestosterone; DOC, 11-deoxycorticosterone; DSDs, disorders of sex development; 17-OHP, 17-hydroxyprogesterone; LHCGR, the luteinizing hormone (LH) or human chorionic gonadotropin (hCG) receptor; OMIM, *Online Mendelian Inheritance in Man*; SERKAL, sex-reversal, kidney, adrenal and lung dysgenesis; TF, transcription factor; WAGR, Wilms' tumor, aniridia, genitourinary anomalies, and mental retardation.

Adapted from Achermann JC, Ozisik G, Meeks JJ, et al. Genetic causes of human reproductive disease. *J Clin Endocrinol Metab.* 2002;87:2447-2454, with permission.

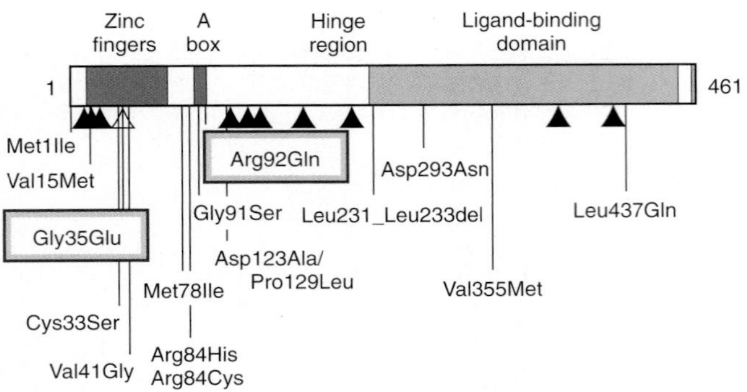

Figure 23-19 Schematic diagram of steroidogenic factor 1 (SF1) shows key domains and mutations associated with a gonadal phenotype. The Gly35Glu (heterozygous) and Arg92Gln (homozygous) changes *(boxes)* affect DNA-binding regions of the protein (P box and A box, respectively) and are associated with marked underandrogenization, dysgenetic gonads, Müllerian structures, and primary adrenal failure. Heterozygous frameshift and nonsense mutations *(triangles)*, as well as missense mutations, have been described in 46,XY individuals with milder phenotypes of disorders of sex development and in women with primary ovarian insufficiency. (From Lin L, Philibert P, Ferraz-de-Souza B, et al. Heterozygous missense mutations in steroidogenic factor-1 [SF1/Ad4BP, NR5A1] are associated with 46,XY disorders of sex development with normal adrenal function. *J Clin Endocrinol Metab.* 2007;92:991-999, with permission of The Endocrine Society, copyright 2007.)

Homozygous deletion of *WT1* in mice prevents development of the gonads and kidneys.[68] The WT1 protein has several different isoforms that have complex roles in sex development, as outlined previously and shown in Figure 23-20. The important role of WT1 in human testis development has been confirmed through the description of various WT1 mutations in patients with WAGR syndrome, Denys-Drash syndrome, and Frasier syndrome.

WAGR syndrome is caused by deletion of a region of chromosome 11p13.[249] The resultant phenotype is likely to be the consequence of haploinsufficiency of WT1, together with loss of developmental genes such as *PAX6,* which is involved in eye development.[73] Renal abnormalities include renal agenesis and horseshoe kidney. Genitourinary abnormalities are usually relatively mild and include hypospadias, cryptorchidism, and ureteral atresia.

Denys-Drash syndrome is characterized by gonadal dysgenesis, severe congenital or early-onset nephropathy (i.e., diffuse mesangial sclerosis), and predisposition to Wilms' tumor.[74] Most 46,XY patients with Denys-Drash syndrome present with genital ambiguity in the newborn period, although normal male or female phenotypes have been described. The presence or absence of Müllerian structures depends on the degree of Sertoli cell dysfunction. Denys-Drash syndrome usually results from heterozygous de novo point mutations in *WT1* that have a dominant negative effect on the function of the wild-type protein. These point mutations usually affect the DNA-binding region (zinc fingers) of WT1. The risk of early-onset end-stage renal failure is high, and Wilms' tumor usually develops in the first decade of life. Gonadoblastoma occurs in fewer than 10% of cases.

Frasier syndrome usually results from heterozygous mutations in the donor splice site of exon 9 of *WT1*.[75,76] These changes are predicted to result in an imbalance in the ratio of +KTS to −KTS isoforms of WT1. Frasier syndrome is characterized by streak gonads, a 46,XY female phenotype with Müllerian structures, and later-onset nephropathy (i.e., focal segmental glomerulosclerosis) that usually causes renal failure in the second decade of life. There is a high risk of gonadal tumors such as gonadoblastoma in patients with Frasier syndrome.[23] In practice, Denys-Drash syndrome and Frasier syndrome may represent a continuum of phenotypes rather than distinct conditions.[77] Milder variants of these conditions may also occur; for example, a man with hypospadias was found to have late-onset nephropathy due to a *WT1* mutation.[250] Taken together, these cases highlight the importance of considering this diagnosis in 46,XY DSD and of performing urinalysis for proteinuria in cases of 46,XY DSD.

Management of patients with *WT1* mutations includes monitoring and treatment of renal function and assessment for Wilms' tumor, as well as gonadectomy in individuals with Frasier syndrome and in patients with Denys-Drash syndrome who have a Y chromosome.[23] Meacham syndrome (i.e., DSD, cardiac defects, and diaphragmatic hernia) also may result from changes in *WT1*.[251]

***Sex-Determining Region of the Y Chromosome:* SRY.** The sequence of events leading to the identification of *SRY* as the primary testis-determining gene and the actions of SRY in testis development were described earlier. SRY is a 204-amino-acid, HMG box transcription factor that is encoded by a single exon on the Y chromosome (Yp11.3) (see Fig. 23-5).[28,29,101] The discovery of inactivating mutations in SRY in patients with 46,XY gonadal dysgenesis confirmed the key role played by this factor in testis determination in humans.[29,32,33,101]

Approximately 15% of individuals with the complete form of 46,XY gonadal dysgenesis have inactivating mutations in *SRY*.[101] Most of the mutations occur in the HMG box DNA-binding domain of the SRY protein (Fig. 23-21), a region that is involved in binding and bending of DNA.[101,104] Rare mutations in the 5′ and 3′ flanking regions

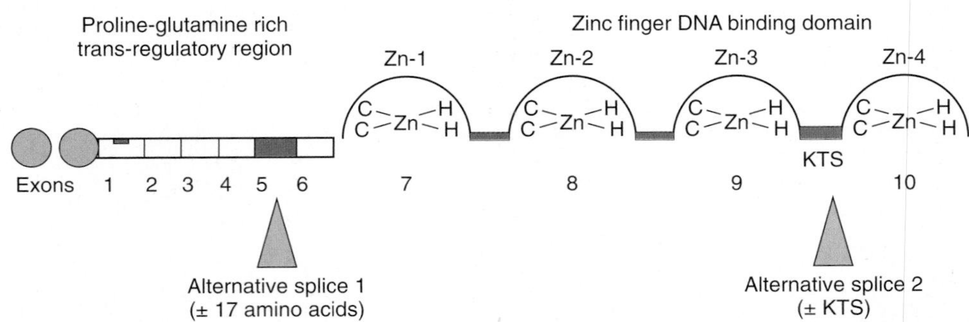

Figure 23-20 Schematic diagram shows the structure of WT1 and the changes associated with exon 5 and exon 9 (addition of lysine, threonine, and serine) in +KTS isoforms. Many point mutations associated with Denys-Drash syndrome are located within zinc fingers 2 and 3 (especially Arg394). Mutations affecting the exon 9 splice site are associated with Frasier syndrome. (Modified from Koziell A, Grundy R. Frasier and Denys-Drash syndromes: different disorders or part of a spectrum? *Arch Dis Child.* 1999;81:365-369, with permission of the BMJ Publishing Group, copyright 1999.)

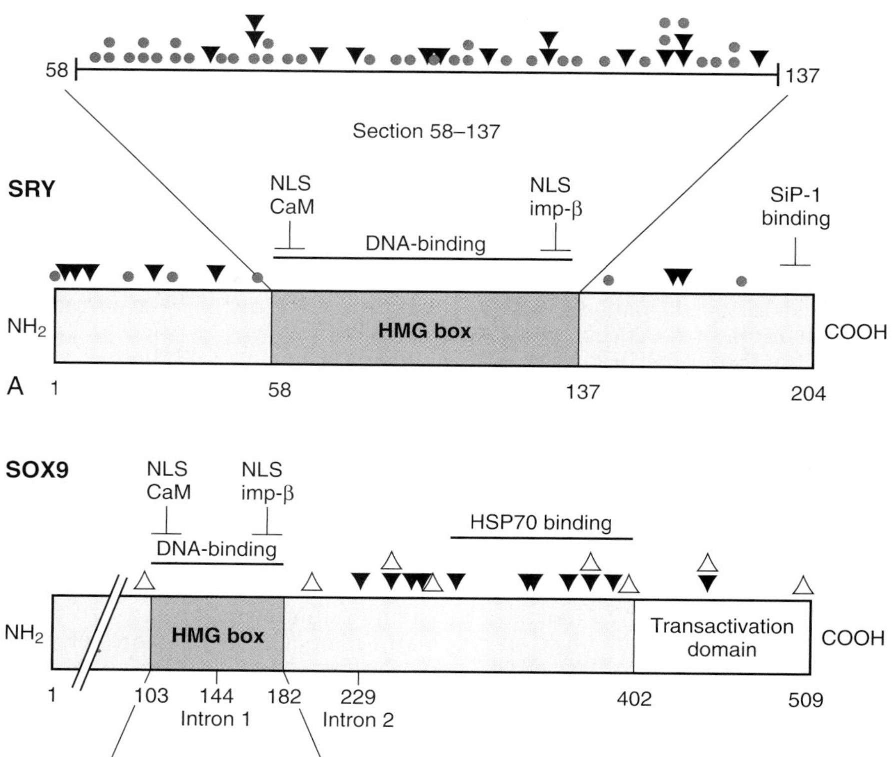

Figure 23-21 Structure of human SRY and SOX9 proteins and a selection of reported mutations. **A,** Diagram of SRY. The high-mobility group (HMG) box is an 80-amino-acid, DNA-binding domain with nuclear localization signals (NLSs) at either end, one of which binds calmodulin (CaM) and the other importin-β (imp-β). The last seven amino acids of SRY can bind to either of the PDZ domains found in SRY-interacting protein 1 (SIP1). The *solid circles* indicate missense mutations reported in the SRY protein that affect testicular development and cluster within the HMG box. Nonsense and frameshift mutations in SRY are indicated by *solid triangles*. **B,** Diagram of SOX9. SOX9 has an HMG box with two NLSs, similar to SRY. However, SOX9 is encoded by three exons, binds to heat shock protein 70 (HSP70), and has a *trans*-activation domain at the carboxyl-terminal end, unlike SRY. Selected mutations causing 46,XY DSD and camptomelic dysplasia are indicated by the *solid circles* (missense) and *solid triangles* (nonsense and frameshift). Mutations that cause only camptomelia or a bony phenotype in 46,XY males or affect 46,XX females are indicated by *open triangles*.

lead, respectively, to complete and partial gonadal dysgenesis.[252-255] The HMG box contains two nuclear localization signals that bind calmodulin and importin B.[101] Mutations in these nuclear localization signal domains in the HMG box of SRY result in failure to transport the SRY protein into the nucleus and consequent XY gonadal dysgenesis.[107]

***SRY Box 9:* SOX9.** Heterozygous mutations of the autosomal *SOX9* gene (17q24-q25) cause camptomelic dysplasia.[101,122,123] Features of this condition include bowed long bones, hypoplastic scapula, a deformed pelvis, 11 pairs of ribs, a small thoracic cage, cleft palate, macrocephaly, micrognathia, hypertelorism, and a variety of cardiac and renal defects. Death from respiratory distress often occurs in the neonatal period, but long-term survival has been reported.

SOX9 is emerging as an important testis-determining gene in its own right, and it may be one of the key regulators of testis determination downstream of *SRY* (see "Testis Determination").[85] Consistent with this hypothesis, three fourths of affected 46,XY patients have dysgenetic gonads, but a complete spectrum of genital phenotypes can be seen, from completely male to completely female appearance.[101] Histologic examination of the gonads from 46,XY patients with ambiguous or female external genitalia shows various degrees of testicular dysgenesis extending to streak gonads with primordial follicles or even ovaries.[256] Müllerian structures may or may not be present, depending on the degree of gonadal dysgenesis. Affected 46,XX females have normal external genitalia and apparently normal ovaries.

The locus for camptomelic dysplasia with 46,XY DSD was mapped to 17q24.3-q25.1 after studies of three patients with balanced, de novo reciprocal translocations and the proposal of *SOX9* as a candidate gene based on expression studies in the mouse.[124,125] Subsequently, missense, nonsense, frameshift, and splice junction mutations have been detected in *SOX9* in patients with camptomelic dysplasia with or without gonadal dysgenesis.[101] These mutations are usually heterozygous de novo changes. In one kindred, multiple siblings were affected due to germline mosaicism for a *SOX9* mutation in a parent.[256] The gonadal phenotype in this kindred varied in the two affected 46,XY siblings: one of them had dysgenetic gonads, and the other was reported to have normal ovaries.

The *SOX9* gene has three exons and two introns; it encodes a 509-residue protein that contains an HMG box with 71% homology to that of the SRY protein and a C-terminal, *trans*-activation domain (see Fig. 23-21). Unlike SRY, in which most mutations are located within the HMG box, SOX9 mutations are located throughout the protein, with little relation between functional domains and phenotype. Chromosomal translocations that disrupt regulatory elements upstream of the SOX9 promoter can be associated with a less severe phenotype or camptomelic dysplasia without gonadal abnormalities. Heterozygous changes that allow residual DNA binding and transactivation may also be associated with the acamptomelic variant and variable or absent DSD.

***Desert Hedgehog:* DHH.** The hedgehog signaling pathways play an important role in many aspects of neuronal, skeletal, and endocrine development. A homozygous mutation in the desert hedgehog gene (*DHH*) was reported in a patient with partial gonadal dysgenesis and minifascicular neuropathy.[140] Subsequently, a number of *DHH* changes were reported in patients with complete 46,XY gonadal dysgenesis but no apparent neurologic features.[257]

***Aristaless-Related Homeobox, X-Linked Gene:* ARX.** ARX is a transcription factor that plays a central role in neuronal migration, and the *Arx* knockout mouse has a profound myelination defect. *ARX* was considered a candidate gene for the X-linked lissencephaly ambiguous genitalia (XLAG) syndrome, and mutations in *ARX* have been described in several patients with this condition.[145] This unusual form of lissencephaly is associated with severe epilepsy and thermal instability. The genital abnormality most likely represents a defect in Leydig cell function. Additional *ARX* mutations have been described in patients with neurologic defects (e.g., infantile spasms) without significant DSDs.

***Testis-Specific Protein, Y-Linked–Like 1 Gene:* TSPYL1.** An association between 46,XY gonadal dysgenesis and sudden infant death syndrome was characterized in a large Amish kindred and named sudden infant death, dysgenetic testes (SIDDT).[258] An autosomal recessive gene responsible for this condition, *TSPYL1,* encodes a protein of unknown function that may be involved in chromatin remodeling. Additional variants of *TSPYL1* and 46,XY DSD have recently been described.[259]

***Mastermind-Like Domain-Containing 1:* MAMLD1.** *MAMLD1* (formerly called *CXORF6*) is a gene on the X chromosome that encodes a protein expressed in the developing testes. Hemizygous mutations in *MAMLD1* were originally described in cases of isolated severe hypospadias, although a range of severities has been described.[146,260] *MAMLD1* disruption results in a defect in fetal Leydig cell development and function.[261]

Chromosomal Rearrangements Associated with Gonadal Dysgenesis. Abnormalities of genital development are associated with a number of chromosomal deletions, duplications, and rearrangements.[153] The most frequently seen changes are deletions of 9p24-pter, 10q25-qter, and Xq13 and duplications of Xp21.

Deletions of 9p24-pter likely disrupt *DMRT1*, a gene with sex-specific homologs in *Drosophila (double sex* gene) and *Caenorhabditis elegans* (*Mab3*) that is expressed in early gonad development (see "Normal Sex Development").[141,143] No specific point mutations in *DMRT1* have been described in humans, but impaired gonadal development and 46,XY DSD are well-established features of the 9p-deletion syndrome, suggesting that haploinsufficiency of the *DMRT* locus may be a cause of testicular dysgenesis in humans.[142,144]

Terminal deletions of chromosome 10 (10q25-qter) are frequently associated with urogenital abnormalities and sometimes with complete gonadal dysgenesis.[152] The gene in this locus has not been identified.

Deletions of Xq13.3 and of the tip of chromosome 16p cause α-thalassemia mental retardation (ATR) syndromes that may have gonadal dysgenesis as part of the phenotype.[150,151] The Xq13.3 locus contains the transcription factor gene *ATRX* (also known as *XH2* or *XNP*), and the *SOX8* gene is located on 16p.[150,151]

Duplications of the Xp21.3 region that contains the *DAX1* gene can cause abnormal testis development in some cases.[88] The role of *DAX1* and the *WNT4* pathway (duplication 1p35) in opposing testis development was discussed previously (see "Development of Reproductive Systems").[89,91]

Syndromic Causes of 46,XY Disorders of Sex Development. In addition to the specific syndromes outlined earlier, various degrees of testicular dysgenesis and impaired genital development (e.g., hypospadias, cryptorchism, scrotal transposition) are seen in many discrete syndromes.[153] In some situations, a genetic basis has been identified, but in many cases the cause is unknown.

46,XY DSD is often associated with intrauterine growth restriction (IUGR). Monozygotic twins can show disparate genital development, with the growth-restricted twin having ambiguous genitalia and the larger twin appearing as a normal male. The mechanism of this association is unclear. However, more common genetic causes of 46,XY DSD (e.g., mutations of SRY, SF1, androgen receptor, and steroidogenic enzymes) are rarely found in this group of IUGR patients. In these conditions, the birth weight usually is normal for gestational age (personal observation).

Disorders of Androgen Synthesis

Defects anywhere along the pathway of androgen synthesis and target organ action can result in impaired androgenization and 46,XY DSD (i.e., male pseudohermaphroditism) (see Table 23-6 and Fig. 23-11).

Cholesterol Synthesis Defects: Smith-Lemli-Opitz Syndrome. Smith-Lemli-Opitz syndrome has a broad phenotypic spectrum but typically includes microcephaly, mental retardation, cardiac defects, ptosis, upturned nose, micrognathia, cleft palate, polydactyly, syndactyly of toes (especially the second and third toes), severe hypospadias, micropenis, and growth failure.[262] The abnormalities of the external genitalia in approximately 65% of 46,XY patients vary from micropenis and hypospadias to complete failure of androgenization, resulting in a female phenotype.

Smith-Lemli-Opitz syndrome is caused by a deficiency of 7-dehydrocholesterol reductase (3β-hydroxysterol Δ7-reductase [DHCR7]), the phylogenetically conserved sterol-sensing domain–containing enzyme required for the last step in the biosynthetic pathway from acetate to cholesterol. Cholesterol is necessary as a substrate for steroid synthesis, and intermediates of cholesterol synthesis may have important interactions with hedgehog signaling pathways.

The syndrome is diagnosed by finding elevated plasma levels of 7-dehydrocholesterol (7-DHC) and low levels of cholesterol. The *DHCR7* gene maps to 11q12-q13, and more than 70 mutations have been described.[262] Measurement of serum 7-DHC should be considered in all underandrogenized males with relevant phenotypic features, however mild. Testis development is apparently normal, and normal, elevated, or low concentrations of plasma testosterone have been described in affected male infants with intact HPG function. Compromised adrenal function can occur in rare cases.

Luteinizing Hormone Receptor Mutations. Mutations in the LH/hCG receptor cause impaired responsiveness to hCG and LH, resulting in Leydig cell agenesis or hypoplasia.[263] Phenotypically, the external genitalia vary from a female appearance to a male with a micropenis (Table 23-7). Müllerian derivatives are absent in all patients, and rudimentary Wolffian derivatives may be present, even in some patients with severely underandrogenized external genitalia. This finding may reflect some early hCG-independent mechanisms of testosterone synthesis between 8 and 10 weeks' gestation.[2] Small, undescended testes are usually found in the inguinal region in the most severe forms of this Leydig cell hypoplasia. Patients with milder

TABLE 23-7

Clinical Features of Leydig Cell Hypoplasia in 46,XY Individuals

Karyotype	46,XY
Inheritance	Autosomal recessive; mutations in *LHCGR* gene
Genitalia	Female, hypospadias, or micropenis
Wolffian duct derivatives	Hypoplastic
Müllerian duct derivatives	Absent
Gonads	Testes
Habitus	Underandrogenization with variable failure of sex hormone production at puberty
Hormone profile	Low T and DHT; elevated LH (and FSH); exaggerated LH response to LHRH stimulation; poor T and DHT response to hCG stimulation

DHT, dihydrotestosterone; FSH, follicle-stimulating hormone; hCG, human chorionic gonadotropin; LH, luteinizing hormone; LHCGR, the LH or hCG receptor; LHRH, luteinizing hormone–releasing hormone; T, testosterone.

phenotypes may have appropriately descended testes of relatively normal size because the Leydig cell population contributes only about 10% to testicular volume. On histologic examination, the testes lack distinct Leydig cells in prepubertal patients. Postpubertal patients have absent or decreased numbers of Leydig cells without Reinke's crystalloids, normal-appearing Sertoli cells, and discrete seminiferous tubules with spermatogenic arrest. This observation highlights the important role of intratesticular androgen in the final stages of sperm maturation.

The typical biochemical profile of patients with Leydig cell hypoplasia includes elevated basal and luteinizing hormone–releasing hormone (LHRH)–stimulated LH (and FSH) levels in early infancy or at puberty. In childhood, when the GnRH pulse generator is quiescent, basal LH levels may sometimes be detected above the normal range. Plasma levels of 17-OHP, androstenedione, and testosterone are low, with little or no response to prolonged hCG stimulation. Plasma LH falls after testosterone administration. Less marked biochemical changes can occur with milder forms of this condition.

More than 30 different homozygous or compound heterozygous mutations have been reported in the LH/hCG receptor gene (*LHCGR*) in individuals with various forms of this condition (Fig. 23-22).[264,265] The original reports of Kremer and colleagues[264] and Latronico and associates[265] described homozygous Ala593Pro and Arg554Stop mutations, respectively, in 46,XY phenotypic females with Leydig cell hypoplasia, hypergonadotropic hypogonadism, and no testosterone response to hCG stimulation. An affected 46,XX sister showed normal sexual maturation at puberty but had an elevated LH level and amenorrhea,

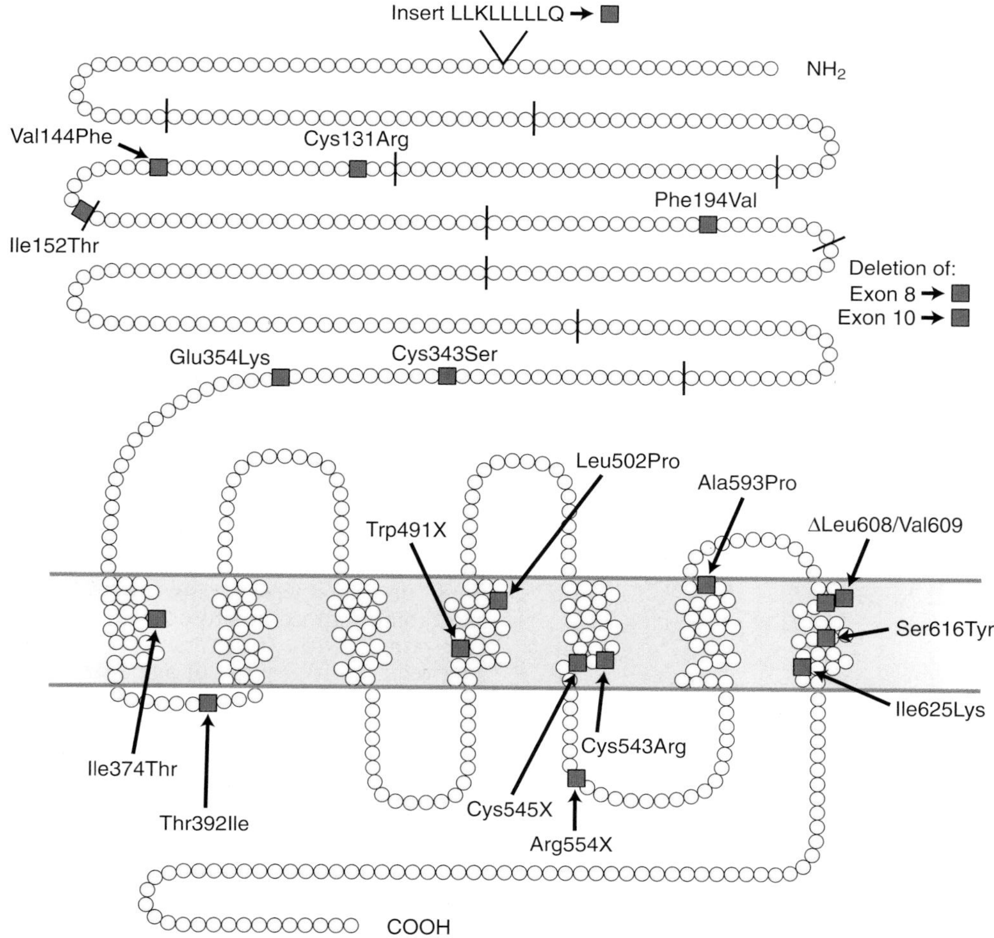

Figure 23-22 Diagram of the seven transmembrane domain of the luteinizing hormone/human chorionic gonadotropin (LH/hCG) receptor with selected inactivating mutations shown by *squares*. Most of these changes are associated with marked underandrogenization. However, the changes at residues 616 and 625 in the seventh transmembrane domain are associated with a milder phenotype of micropenis.

demonstrating that the LH receptor is not necessary for estrogen synthesis but is necessary for normal ovulation in females. These mutations impair hCG stimulation of intracellular cyclic adenosine monophosphate (cAMP) in in vitro studies through disturbances in hCG binding, intracellular signaling, or receptor stability and trafficking, depending on the nature of the change. Defects in a novel cryptic exon of the LH receptor (exon 6A) have also been described as a cause of 46,XY DSD.[266] Partial loss-of-function mutations in the LH/hCG receptor causing milder phenotypes such as micropenis have tended to localize within the seventh transmembrane domain (Ser616Tyr, Ile625Lys) (see Fig. 23-22).[265,267] Individuals with complete Leydig cell hypoplasia are usually raised as females and require estrogens at puberty. Gonadectomy is usually performed. If a male gender assignment is chosen, testosterone supplements may be given in early infancy and to support puberty. The risk of gonadal malignancy is unknown.[23]

Steroidogenic Acute Regulatory Protein Defects. Steroidogenic acute regulatory protein (StAR) is a 30-kd mitochondrial protein that is present in the adrenal gland and gonads. It plays a key role in facilitating the rapid movement of cholesterol from the outer to the inner mitochondrial membrane.[268,269] This process is necessary to allow de novo steroid biosynthesis in response to an increase in adrenocorticotropic hormone (ACTH) or angiotensin II in the adrenal gland or an LH pulse in the gonad. The exact mechanism by which StAR facilitates this movement is unclear, but it is likely that the protein remains on the mitochondrial surface in a molten globule structure.[269] Although a limited amount of cholesterol transfer is StAR independent (14%), this protein certainly plays a central role in the acute regulation of adrenal and gonadal steroidogenesis.

Consistent with these actions, patients with recessively inherited defects in StAR develop a severe form of primary adrenal failure called *lipoid congenital adrenal hyperplasia* (lipoid CAH).[270] Patients with this condition tend to present with severe glucocorticoid deficiency (e.g., hypoglycemia, hyperpigmentation) early in life and progressive mineralocorticoid insufficiency resulting in hyponatremia, hyperkalemia, dehydration, acidosis, and collapse (Table 23-8). Little or no C18, C19, and C21 steroids are detectable in plasma or urine, even after corticotropin or hCG stimulation. Females (46,XX) with lipoid CAH have normal genitalia and a uterus. In 46,XY individuals, mutations in *STAR* typically cause a marked deficiency in testosterone synthesis by fetal Leydig cells so that completely female genitalia are seen. Testes may be abdominal, inguinal, or labial. A blind vaginal pouch is present, and Müllerian structures have regressed. A karyotype should be performed in all apparent girls presenting with early-onset adrenal failure.

The typical finding in lipoid CAH is lipid accumulation within steroidogenic cells. In the steroid-deficient state, the tropic drive by ACTH, angiotensin II, and LH causes increased cholesterol uptake and synthesis by steroidogenic cells. Coupled with the inability of StAR to facilitate cholesterol movement into mitochondria, this leads to marked accumulation of cholesterol in cells and results in the appearance of enlarged, lipid-laden adrenal glands seen on MRI or computed tomography (CT). Eventually, cholesterol accumulation causes engorgement and results in disruption of the structural and functional integrity of the cell—the two-hit hypothesis (Fig. 23-23).[271] The StAR-knockout mouse has a comparable phenotype to patients with lipoid CAH, consistent with the two-hit hypothesis model.[272] StAR is not necessary for placental progesterone production, unlike P450scc (CYP11A1).

The two-hit hypothesis also explains why 46,XX girls with lipoid CAH show evidence of estrogenization and breast development at puberty but have progressive hypergonadotropic hypogonadism.[271,273] Follicular cells are relatively quiescent in utero and before puberty and are therefore undamaged. At the beginning of each cycle, they are recruited, and a small amount of estradiol can be produced as a result of StAR-independent mechanisms. This can occur until the follicular cells are engorged and rendered nonfunctional. Puberty can occur, but any cycles are anovulatory because progesterone synthesis in the latter half of the cycle is disturbed. Without treatment, polycystic ovaries and progressive ovarian failure usually ensue.

Although more than 20 different StAR mutations have been described in patients from around the world, lipoid CAH is especially prevalent in Japan and Korea, where it is the second most common steroidogenic disorder after CYP21 deficiency (Fig. 23-24).[271,274] Most Japanese patients and virtually all Korean patients harbor the Gln258Stop mutation, which is estimated to be carried by 1 in 300 Japanese people.[274] Other geographic clusters include the Leu260Pro mutation in patients of Swiss ancestry, Arg182His in Eastern Saudi Arabia, and Arg182Leu in Palestinians. Most of these mutations show complete loss of function. However, a nonclassic form of lipoid CAH has been described that is caused by point mutations in StAR, and retains approximately 20% function.[275] These patients presented with progressive glucocorticoid deficiency between 2 and 4 years of age; affected males had normal androgenization of the external genitalia. StAR mutations may also be associated with hypospadias and adrenal failure.[276]

Treatment of classic lipoid CAH includes glucocorticoid and mineralocorticoid replacement and salt supplementation in early life. Gonadectomy is usually performed in individuals with a 46,XY karyotype. Estrogen treatment is given to induce puberty and is administered to 46,XX females when gonadal failure occurs.

TABLE 23-8

Clinical Features of Lipoid CAH in 46,XY Individuals

Karyotype	46,XY
Inheritance	Autosomal recessive; mutations in *STAR* gene
Genitalia	Female; sometimes ambiguous, hypospadiac, or male
Wolffian duct derivatives	Hypoplastic or normal
Müllerian duct derivatives	Absent
Gonads	Testes
Habitus	Severe adrenal insufficiency in infancy with salt loss; failure of pubertal development; rare "nonclassic" cases associated with isolated glucocorticoid deficiency
Hormone profile	Usually deficiency of glucocorticoids, mineralocorticoids, and sex steroids except in rare "nonclassic" cases

CAH, congenital adrenal hyperplasia; STAR, steroidogenic acute regulatory protein.

P450 Side-Chain Cleavage Enzyme Deficiency. P450scc (CYP11A1) is the mitochondrial enzyme that converts cholesterol to pregnenolone by three distinct enzymatic

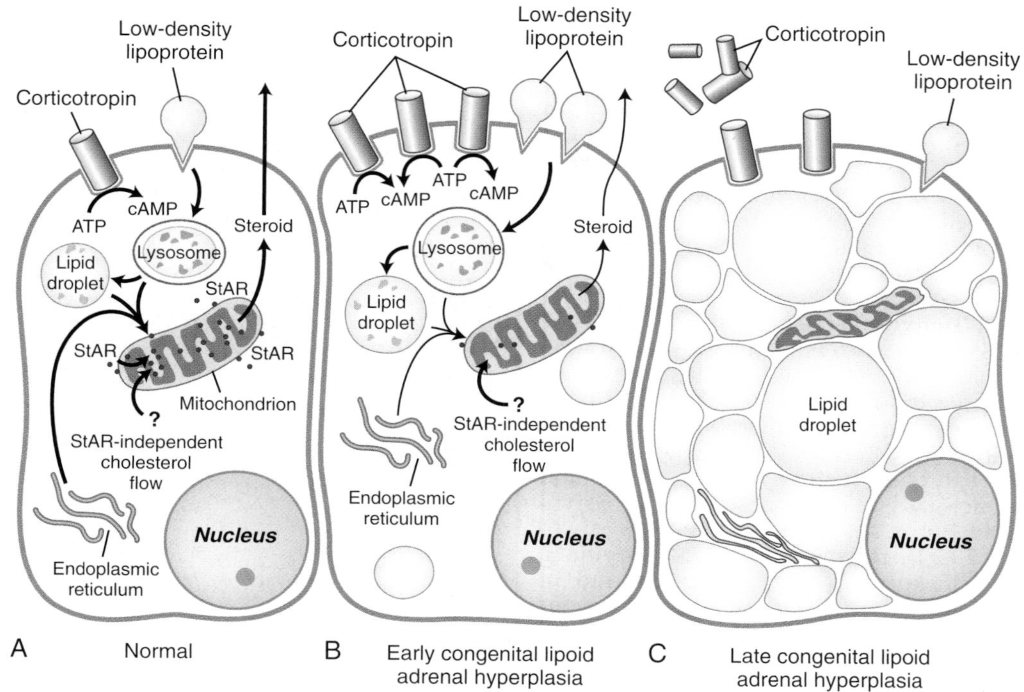

Figure 23-23 Model of the steroid-synthesizing cell (adrenal/gonadal) showing conversion of cholesterol to steroids. **A,** Cholesterol from low-density lipoprotein, from cholesterol esters stored in lipid droplets, and from endogenous synthesis in the endoplasmic reticulum is transported from the outer mitochondrial membrane to the inner membrane. This transport is facilitated by the steroidogenic acute regulatory protein (StAR) and by other, StAR-independent mechanisms. In the mitochondria, steroid synthesis begins with the conversion of cholesterol to Δ^5-pregnenolone by the enzyme CYP11A1 (P450scc). **B,** In patients with lipoid congenital adrenal hyperplasia, a mutation in the gene encoding StAR results in little or no activity of the mutant StAR, greatly reducing cholesterol transport into the mitochondria. Low levels of steroidogenesis by mechanisms independent of StAR can occur; however, increased secretion of corticotropin (or luteinizing hormone or follicle-stimulating hormone) results in cholesterol accumulation in the cells as lipid droplets. **C,** Continued stimulation and resultant accumulation of cholesterol causes engorgement of these cells, with mechanical and chemical perturbation of cell function. This results in primary adrenal insufficiency and impaired androgen biosynthesis by fetal Leydig cells. Females with lipoid congenital adrenal hyperplasia feminize at puberty and menstruate but have progressive hypergonadotropic hypogonadism. This may occur because the follicular cells are relatively quiescent in utero and before puberty and therefore are undamaged. At the beginning of each cycle, follicles are recruited, and a small amount of estradiol can be produced as a result of StAR-independent mechanisms. This can occur until the follicular cells are engorged and rendered nonfunctional. ATP, adenosine triphosphate; cAMP, cyclic adenosine monophosphate. (From Bose HS, Sujiwara T, Strauss JF III, et al. The pathophysiology and genetics of congenital lipoid adrenal hyperplasia. *N Engl J Med.* 1996;335:1870-1878, with permission of the Massachusetts Medical Society, copyright 1996.)

reactions: 20α-hydroxylation, 22-hydroxylation, and cleavage of the cholesterol side chain. P450scc is therefore responsible for the first and rate-limiting step in steroid synthesis, which is necessary for pregnenolone production by the placenta and for mineralocorticoid, glucocorticoid, and androgen production by the adrenal glands and gonads.

Although a natural model of lipoid CAH due to P450scc deficiency exists in the rabbit, it was thought that severe loss of P450scc activity in humans would be incompatible with survival. Placental progesterone production is necessary to support pregnancy (i.e., luteoplacental shift) after the second trimester in higher primates but not in rodents.

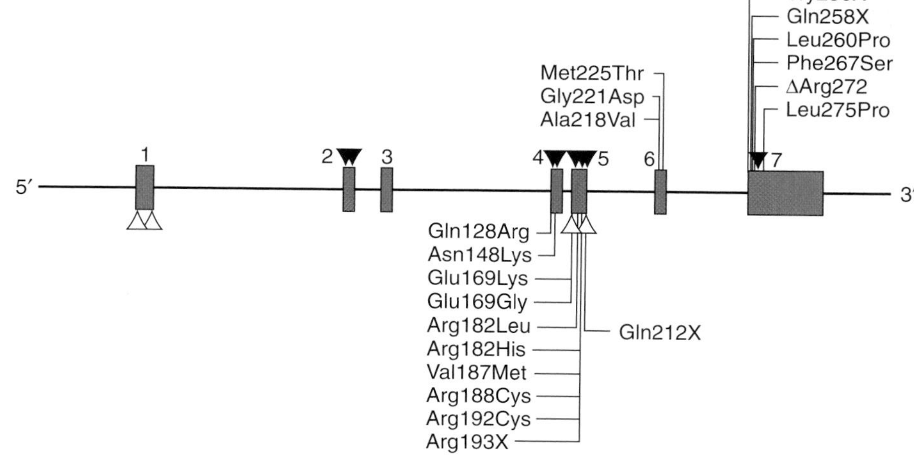

Figure 23-24 Diagram of selected mutations identified in the *STAR* gene associated with lipoid congenital adrenal hyperplasia. Numbered *solid boxes* depict the exons. The three-letter abbreviations for amino acids are used to indicate the position of missense mutations; X indicates a nonsense (stop) mutation; insertions and deletions resulting in frameshift mutations *(solid triangles)* and splice site mutations *(open triangles)* are shown. Although *STAR* mutations are common in Japan, Korea, and regions of the Middle East, an increasing number of sporadic changes in the steroidogenic acute regulatory (StAR) protein are being detected in other countries. Two missense mutations at residues 187 and 188 have been associated with a nonclassic late-onset phenotype of glucocorticoid insufficiency.

However, complete disruption of P450 activity due to a frameshift mutation in *CYP11A1* has been reported in a 46,XY infant with a female phenotype and severe early-onset, salt-losing adrenal failure.[277] A small number of other mutations in P450scc have also been described, usually in 46,XY phenotypic females with severe salt-losing adrenal failure (Table 23-9).[278] Partial loss of function defects in P450scc have been described in boys with hypospadias who developed adrenal failure in late childhood.[279] This condition is now well established as a cause of combined adrenal and gonadal failure.

3β-Hydroxysteroid Dehydrogenase/$\Delta^{4,5}$-Isomerase Type 2 Deficiency. 3β-HSD deficiency is a rare cause of CAH and is one of the steroidogenic deficiencies that affects both adrenal and gonadal steroid production. The autosomal recessive disorder is a consequence of mutations in *HSD3B2,* the gene encoding the 3β-HSD/$\Delta^{4,5}$-isomerase type 2 isozyme, which is expressed mainly in the adrenals and gonads. This enzyme catalyses a crucial step in the biosynthesis of all steroid hormones, the conversion of Δ^5- to Δ^4-steroids (see Fig. 23-11). The other 3β-HSD isoenzyme in humans, *HSD3B1,* is expressed in the placenta and in peripheral tissues such as the skin (mainly sebaceous glands), breast, and prostate; it is not associated with CAH. Type 1 and 2 isoenzymes are 93.5% homologous in protein structure, and their genes are located on chromosome lp13.1.[280] Human pregnancy is maintained by high levels of progesterone produced by placental HSD3B1 activity, and a homozygous type 1 gene defect would not be compatible with survival of an affected fetus.

Classic HSD3B2 deficiency is subdivided into salt-losing and non–salt-losing forms. Males with HSD3B2 deficiency have clinical features as summarized in Table 23-10. The external genitalia are usually ambiguous, with a small penis, severe hypospadias, partial labioscrotal fusion, a urogenital sinus, and a blind vaginal pouch.

Newborns with severe HSD3B2 deficiency develop adrenal insufficiency soon after birth. The 46,XY males with partial deficiency of HSD3B2 are not salt losers because they have mutant enzymes that retain 2% to 10% of HSD3B2 enzymatic activity, as assessed by transient expression of the mutant in intact cells.[281] Gynecomastia can occur at puberty in affected males and females. This is presumably the result of HSD3B1-mediated peripheral conversion of Δ^5-C19-steroids to Δ^4-C19-steroids and aromatization to estrogens.[282] Normal puberty and fertility have been reported in males with a null mutation in the *HSD3B2* gene.[283,284]

The straightforward biochemical profile of classic HSD3B2 deficiency is based on an elevated ratio of Δ^5- to Δ^4-steroids, determined in plasma or urine. The most specific analyte to confirm the diagnosis is 17-hydroxypregnenolone, which is present at levels greater than 100 nmol/L basally or after ACTH stimulation.[281] However, this steroid is measured only in specialist laboratories. The concentrations of Δ^4-steroids such as 17-OHP and androstenedione may also be elevated in HSD3B2 deficiency because of peripheral HSD3B1 activity. In a neonatal screening program, an elevated 17-OHP level in a salt-losing person with HSD3B2 deficiency may invoke a diagnosis of CYP21 deficiency.[285]

HSD3B2 is a four-exon gene that encodes 371 amino acids. About 36 mutations have been reported, and many affected individuals are compound heterozygotes (Fig. 23-25). The concordance between genotype and phenotype is close, so that the presence or absence of salt losing in HSD3B2 deficiency is quite predictable. Examples of mutants that retain no enzyme activity and cause severe salt losing include Gly15Asp, Leu108Trp, Glu142Lys, Pro186Leu, Leu205Pro, Pro222Gln, Tyr253Asn, and Thr259Arg. In contrast, mutations such as Ala10Val and Ala245Pro retain considerable enzyme activity and have been found in males with perineoscrotal hypospadias and no salt loss. A late-onset form of HSD3B2 deficiency usually manifests as premature pubarche and idiopathic hirsutism in females. Clearer biochemical markers consistent with mutation-proven HSD3B2 deficiency have been derived for this late-onset group.[286,287] These markers include ACTH-stimulated 17-hydroxypregnenolone and 17-hydroxypregnenolone-to-cortisol ratios that are 54 and 38 standard deviations above the control means, respectively. However, biochemical phenotyping is not possible for carrier detection in families with known *HSD3B2* mutations.[288] Targeting analysis of this gene in patients with idiopathic hypospadias yields, at best, only subtle changes in a few cases.[289]

17α-Hydroxylase/17,20-Lyase Deficiency. P450c17 (CYP17) is a microsomal enzyme with 17α-hydroxylase and

TABLE 23-9

Clinical Features of CYP11A1 Deficiency in 46,XY Individuals

Karyotype	46,XY
Inheritance	Autosomal recessive; mutations in *CYP11A1* gene
Genitalia	Female; rarely ambiguous or hypospadiac male
Wolffian duct derivatives	Hypoplastic or normal
Müllerian duct derivatives	Absent
Gonads	Testes (or absent)
Habitus	Severe adrenal insufficiency in infancy with salt loss ranging to milder adrenal insufficiency with onset in childhood; prematurity associated in one case
Hormone profile	Usually deficiency of glucocorticoids, mineralocorticoids, and sex steroids

CYP11A1, cytochrome P450 side-chain cleavage enzyme.

TABLE 23-10

Clinical Features of HSD3B2 Deficiency in 46,XY Individuals

Karyotype	46,XY
Inheritance	Autosomal recessive; mutations in *HSD3B2* gene
Genitalia	Ambiguous; hypospadiac male
Wolffian duct derivatives	Normal
Müllerian duct derivatives	Absent
Gonads	Testes
Habitus	Severe adrenal insufficiency in infancy; poor virilization at puberty with gynecomastia *Mild form:* no mineralocorticoid deficiency, premature adrenarche → mild virilization
Hormone profile	Increased concentrations of Δ^5 C_{21}- and C_{19}-steroids (e.g., 17-hydroxypregnenolone/cortisol ratio response to corticotropin, 17-hydroxypregnenolone, DHEA suppressible by dexamethasone)

DHEA, dehydroepiandrosterone; HSD3B2, 3β-hydroxysteroid dehydrogenase type 2.

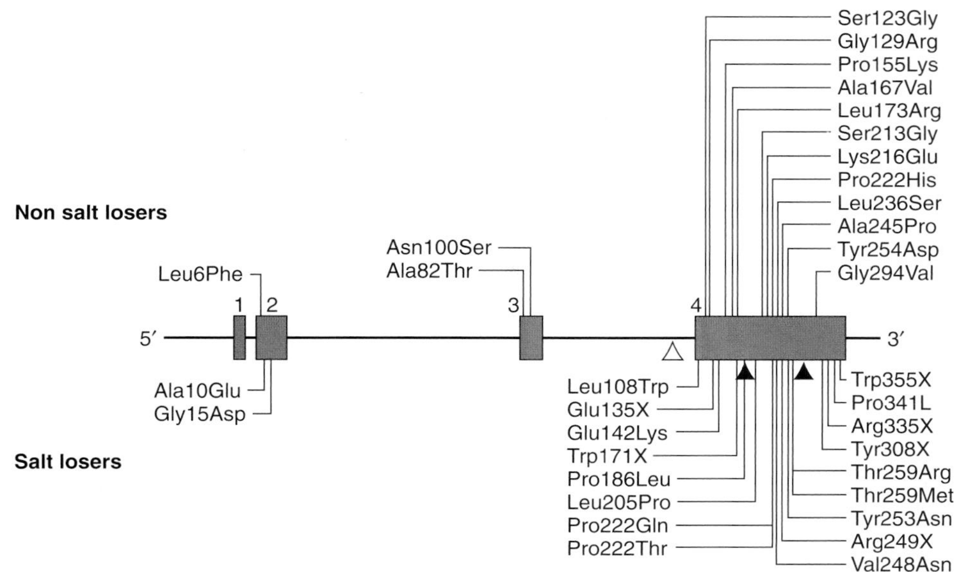

Figure 23-25 Diagram of the 3β-hydroxysteroid dehydrogenase type 2 gene *(HSD3B2)* shows the mutations that result in deficiency of the enzyme. The numbered *solid boxes* depict the exons. Mutations are subdivided according to their association with salt-losing and non–salt-losing states. The three-letter abbreviations for amino acids are used to indicate the position of missense mutations; X indicates a nonsense (stop) mutation; insertions and deletions resulting in frameshift mutations *(solid triangles)* and splice site mutations *(open triangles)* are shown.

17,20-lyase activity that is expressed in the adrenals and gonads but not in the placenta or in ovarian granulosa cells.[290-292] The 17α-hydroxylase action of P450c17 catalyzes the conversion of pregnenolone (Δ^5) to 17-hydroxypregnenolone and the conversion of progesterone (Δ^4) to 17-OHP (see Fig. 23-11). The 17,20-lyase action of P450c17 can covert 17-hydroxypregnenolone (Δ^5) to DHEA and 17-OHP (Δ^4) to androstenedione (see Fig. 23-11). P450c17 is bound to the smooth endoplasmic reticulum, where it accepts electrons from a specific flavoprotein, reduced nicotinamide adenine dinucleotide phosphate (NADPH)-POR. The 17,20-lyase activity of P450c17 is favored by the presence of Δ^5 substrates, redox partners such as POR and cytochrome b_5, and serine phosphorylation. Unlike in rodents, the Δ^5-17,20-lyase activity of human P450c17 is 50 times more efficient than its Δ^4-17,20-lyase activity; therefore very little androstenedione is formed directly from 17-OHP, and the principal pathway to androgen production is through DHEA.[169] P450c17 also has 16α-hydroxylase activity.

Defects in P450c17 action can result in two different forms of CAH. Most often, combined 17α-hydroxylase/17,20-lyase deficiency is seen, but rare cases of isolated 17,20-lyase deficiency have been reported (Tables 23-11 and 23-12).[292]

Combined 17α-hydroxylase/17,20-lyase deficiency is an uncommon form of CAH, although an increasing number of cases are being reported from many different countries.[293] A prevalence of approximately 1 case per 50,000 individuals is reported. The classic phenotype of complete combined 17α-hydroxylase/17,20-lyase deficiency is that of a phenotypic female (46,XX, or underandrogenized 46,XY) who presents with an absence of secondary sexual characteristics (i.e., hypergonadotropic hypogonadism) at puberty and is found to have low-renin hypertension and hypokalemic alkalosis (see Table 23-11).

The classic phenotype and underlying biochemistry can be explained by the enzyme deficiency (see Fig. 23-11).[262] A defect in 17α-hydroxylation in the adrenal cortex and gonads results in impaired synthesis of 17-OHP and 17-hydroxypregnenolone and therefore of cortisol, androgens, and estrogens. Decreased cortisol synthesis causes increased corticotropin secretion, which results in excessive secretion of 17-deoxysteroids by the adrenal cortex, including the mineralocorticoids 11-deoxycorticosterone (DOC), corticosterone, and 18-hydroxycorticosterone. Excess DOC secretion leads to hypertension, hypokalemic alkalosis, and suppression of the renin-angiotensin system. Diminished aldosterone synthesis and secretion are sometimes reported. Corticosterone is a weak glucocorticoid; the high plasma concentrations in this disorder prevent the signs and symptoms of cortisol deficiency (e.g., hypoglycemia) and modulate the secretion of corticotropin.

Affected 46,XX females have normal female internal and external genital tracts, but the ovaries cannot secrete

TABLE 23-11

Clinical Features of Combined CYP17 Deficiency in 46,XY Individuals

Karyotype	46,XY
Inheritance	Autosomal recessive; mutations in *CYP17* gene
Genitalia	Female, ambiguous, or hypospadiac male
Wolffian duct derivatives	Absent or hypoplastic
Müllerian duct derivatives	Absent
Gonads	Testes
Habitus	Absent or poor virilization at puberty, gynecomastia, hypertension
Hormone profile	Decreased T; increased LH and FSH; increased plasma deoxycorticosterone, corticosterone, and progesterone; decreased plasma renin activity
	Low renin hypertension with hypokalemic alkalosis

CYP17, 17α-hydroxylase/17,20-lyase; FSH, follicle-stimulating hormone; LH, luteinizing hormone; T, testosterone.

TABLE 23-12

Clinical Features of Isolated 17,20-Lyase Deficiency in 46,XY Individuals

Karyotype	46,XY
Inheritance	Autosomal recessive; mutations in *CYP17* gene, usually affecting key redox domains
Genitalia	Female, ambiguous, or hypospadiac male
Wolffian duct derivatives	Absent or hypoplastic
Müllerian duct derivatives	Absent
Gonads	Testes
Habitus	Absent or poor virilization at puberty; gynecomastia
Hormone profile	Decreased plasma T, DHEA, androstenedione, and estradiol; abnormal increase in plasma 17-hydroxyprogesterone and 17-hydroxypregnenolone; increased LH and FSH; increased ratio of C_{21}-deoxysteroids to C_{19}-steroids (DHEA, androstenedione) after hCG stimulation

CYP17, 17α-hydroxylase/17,20-lyase; DHEA, dehydroepiandrosterone; FSH, follicle-stimulating hormone; hCG, human chorionic gonadotropin; LH, luteinizing hormone; T, testosterone.

estrogens at puberty, resulting in absent breast development and hypogonadism with elevated plasma FSH and LH levels. The lack of adrenal and ovarian androgens can result in little or no growth of pubic and axillary hair. In affected 46,XX individuals, the ovaries have a high proportion of atretic follicles, and some ovaries contain an increased number of enlarged follicular cysts.

Affected 46,XY individuals with complete combined 17α-hydroxylase/17,20-lyase deficiency who are diagnosed in adolescence usually have female external genitalia and a blind vaginal pouch (see Table 23-11). Testes may be intra-abdominal, in the inguinal canal, or in the labioscrotal folds. Inguinal hernias are common, Müllerian structures are absent, and Wolffian derivatives are hypoplastic. Bone age is frequently delayed, and prolonged linear growth can lead to tall stature. Pubic and axillary hair is absent or sparse, and hypergonadotropic hypogonadism is associated with a failure to develop secondary sexual characteristics at puberty. Excessive secretion of DOC and corticosterone usually leads to low-renin hypertension and hypokalemic alkalosis, as in 46,XX girls with this condition.

Complete 17α-hydroxylase/17,20-lyase deficiency is associated with a variety of mutations in the *CYP17* gene that cause complete loss of function in assays of enzyme activity. These changes include a range of missense, frameshift, and nonsense mutations (Fig. 23-26). A common mutation is the 4-base-pair duplication in exon 8, which is shared by Mennonites and individuals in the Friesland region of the Netherlands and is attributed to a founder effect originating in Friesland. Other geographic clusters include an in-frame deletion of residues 487 to 489 in Southeast Asia and the Arg362Cys and Trp406Arg missense mutations found among Brazilians of Portuguese and Spanish ancestry, respectively.[292,294] However, many different changes occur in other populations and are located throughout the enzyme.[295]

Partial forms of combined 17α-hydroxylase/17,20-lyase deficiency have been described. This condition most frequently manifests in a 46,XY infant with ambiguous genitalia or severe hypospadias for whom the steroid profile is consistent with the diagnosis of P450c17 deficiency. Hypertension may or may not be present in partial forms of combined 17α-hydroxylase/17,20-lyase deficiency, and aldosterone secretion may be normal or even elevated. Corticosterone levels, which are usually 50- to 100-fold higher than normal, provide adequate glucocorticoid effects and prevent symptoms of cortisol deficiency. The development of male secondary sexual characteristics at puberty may be incomplete, and gynecomastia is often seen. This rare condition has been associated with a

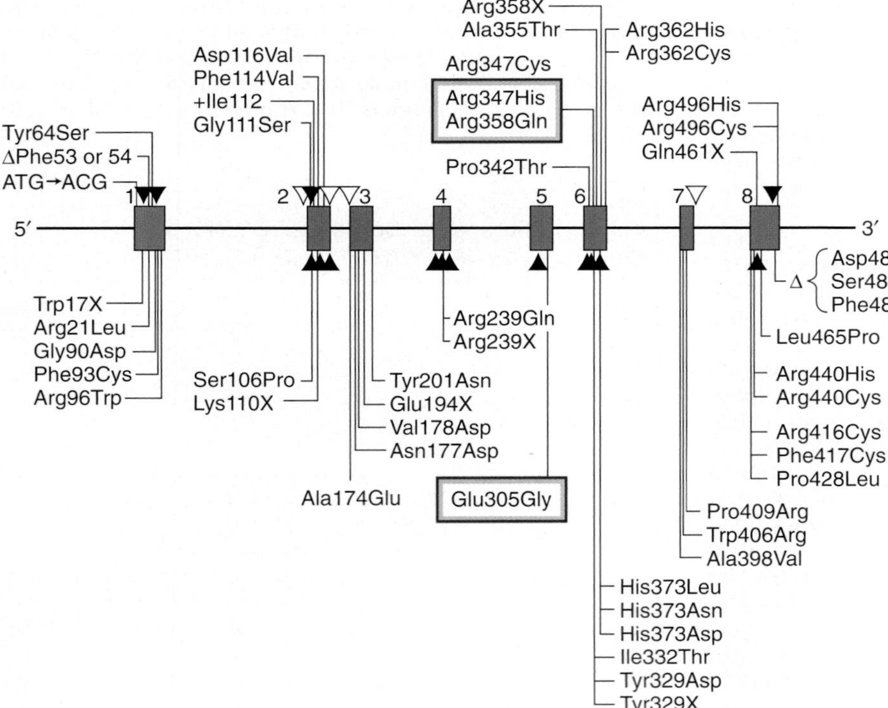

Figure 23-26 Diagram of selected mutations in the *CYP17* gene causing 17α-hydroxylase/17,20-lyase deficiency. The numbered *solid boxes* depict the exons. The three-letter abbreviations for amino acids are used to indicate the position of missense mutations; X indicates a nonsense (stop) mutation; insertions and deletions resulting in frameshift and splice site mutations are shown by *solid triangles* and *open triangles*, respectively. All of these mutations cause 17α-hydroxylase deficiency. Several missense mutations, such as those at codons 305, 347, and 358 *(boxes)*, have been associated with "isolated" 17,20-lyase deficiency.

phenylalanine deletion at codon 53 or 54[296]; in a patient compound heterozygous for a null mutation in P450c17, a Pro342Thr mutation, and 20% of normal 17α-hydroxylase activity[297]; and in a small number of additional cases in which some residual enzyme function was retained. Analysis of these patients suggests that 5% of normal activity in a 46,XX female is sufficient to allow estrogen production with normal secondary sexual characteristics and irregular menses, whereas more than 25% of normal activity appears to be necessary to achieve normal androgenization of the external genitalia of affected 46,XY males.

Isolated 17,20-lyase activity has been reported in a small number of patients.[298] These 46,XY individuals usually have genital ambiguity, normal secretion of glucocorticoids and mineralocorticoids, and marked reduction in sex steroid synthesis (see Table 23-12). The first two patients shown to have a molecular defect in P450c17 harbored homozygous point mutations in the enzyme (Arg347His, Arg358Gln) that specifically interfered with 17,20-lyase activity by changing the distribution of surface charges in the redox-partner binding site.[299] Other patients have been reported with similar mutations or with a point mutation (Glu305Gly) that specifically alters the conformation of the substrate binding site.[300]

The diagnosis of 17α-hydroxylase deficiency should be suspected in all cases of 46,XY DSD, and it is strongly supported by the discovery of hyporeninemic hypertension and hypokalemic alkalosis and by a lack of secondary sex characteristics at puberty. Plasma concentrations of corticotropin, DOC, corticosterone, and progesterone are high, and those of 17α-OHP, cortisol, and gonadal steroids are low. Replacement therapy with physiologic doses of glucocorticoids suppresses DOC and corticosterone secretion and normalizes serum potassium levels, blood pressure, and plasma renin and aldosterone levels. Gonadectomy is usually performed in 46,XY patients who have a female gender assignment. Appropriate gonadal steroid replacement therapy is indicated at puberty.

Cytochrome b_5 Deficiency. A splice site mutation in the 17,20-lyase redox partner cytochrome b_5 was first reported in a 46,XY child with ambiguous genitalia and methemoglobinemia, although extensive endocrinologic data were not reported.[301] However, a homozygous nonsense mutation in this gene (*CYB5A*) was recently described in a 46,XY child with severe hypospadias and a biochemical profile consistent with isolated 17,20-lyase deficiency.[302] Methemoglobin was elevated above the normal range in this case, but it did not result in clinical signs.

P450 Oxidoreductase Deficiency. POR is a membrane-bound flavoprotein that plays a central role in electron transfer from NADPH to P450 enzymes (Fig. 23-27).[303] POR is crucial in the 17,20-lyase reaction of P450c17, and it interacts with all 57 microsomal P450 enzymes, including P450c21 (21-hydroxylase) and P450c19 (aromatase), and with many others involved in hepatic drug metabolism.

A potential role for POR in human steroidogenesis emerged after the description of several patients with apparent combined deficiencies of CYP17 and CYP21.[304] Ambiguous genitalia and unusual patterns of combined steroidogenic defects have been described in a subset of patients with Antley-Bixler syndrome, a form of skeletal dysplasia that is characterized by craniosynostosis, brachycephaly, midface hypoplasia, proptosis, choanal stenosis, radioulnar or radiohumeral synostosis, bowed femora, and arachnodactyly.

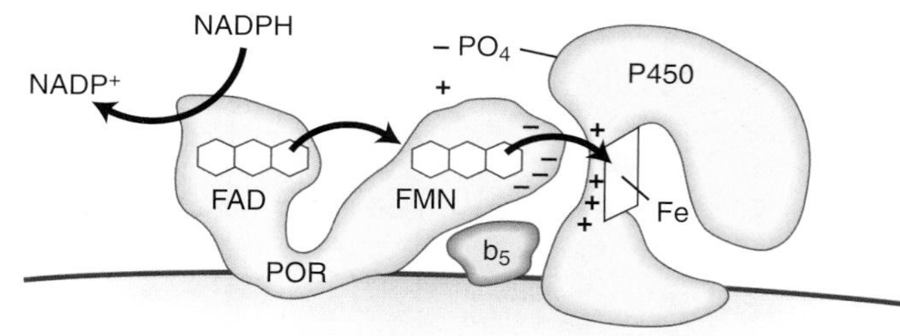

Figure 23-27 Role of P450 oxidoreductase (POR) in electron transfer to microsomal (type II) P450 enzymes. Reduced nicotinamide adenine dinucleotide phosphate (NADPH) interacts with POR, which is bound to the endoplasmic reticulum, and transfers a pair of electrons to the FAD moiety. This change in charge results in altered conformation, which allows the electrons to pass from the FAD to the FMN moiety. After further realignment, the FMN domain can interact with the redox partner binding site of the P450 enzyme (e.g., P450c17, P450c21, P450c19), permitting electron transfer to the active heme group of the enzyme, which results in substrate catalysis. The interaction of POR and the P450 enzymes is coordinated by negatively charged acidic residues on the surface of the FMN domain of POR and positively charged basic residues in the redox partner binding site of the P450 enzyme. In the case of human P450c17, this interaction is facilitated by the allosteric action of cytochrome b_5 and by serine phosphorylation of P450c17. (From Miller WL. Minireview: regulation of steroidogenesis by electron transfer. *Endocrinology.* 2005;146:2544-2550, with permission of The Endocrine Society, copyright 2005.)

The first recessively inherited human mutations in POR were described in 2004, and a significant number of changes have been described in patients with marked phenotypic variations (Table 23-13).[170,305,306] At the most severe end of the spectrum are Antley-Bixler syndrome with ambiguous genitalia and apparent combined CYP17 and CYP21 deficiency with no skeletal phenotype. Milder defects in POR have also been seen in women with a form of polycystic ovary syndrome and in men with mild gonadal insufficiency. A range of POR activity is associated with this spectrum of phenotypes, and skeletal features can be subtle. Two common mutations are emerging: Arg287Pro is the most prevalent mutation in patients of European ancestry, whereas the Arg457His mutation is common in Japan.[170,306-307] Activating mutations in fibroblast growth factor receptor 2 (FGFR2) have also been reported in

TABLE 23-13

Clinical Features of P450 Oxidoreductase Deficiency in 46,XY Individuals

Karyotype	46,XY
Inheritance	Autosomal recessive; mutations in *POR* gene
Genitalia	Ambiguous; hypospadias or male
Wolffian duct derivatives	Absent or hypoplastic
Müllerian duct derivatives	Absent
Gonads	Testes
Habitus	Variable androgenization at birth; variable virilization at puberty; glucocorticoid deficiency; no severe mineralocorticoid deficiency; features of Antley-Bixler syndrome (craniosynostosis, skeletal dysplasia) in some cases
Hormone profile	Evidence of combined CYPC17 and CYPC21 insufficiency; normal or low cortisol with poor response to ACTH stimulation; elevated 17-OHP; T low

ACTH, adrenocorticotropin; CYP, cytochrome P450 enzyme; 17-OHP, 17-hydroxyprogesterone; POR, P450 oxidoreductase; T, testosterone.

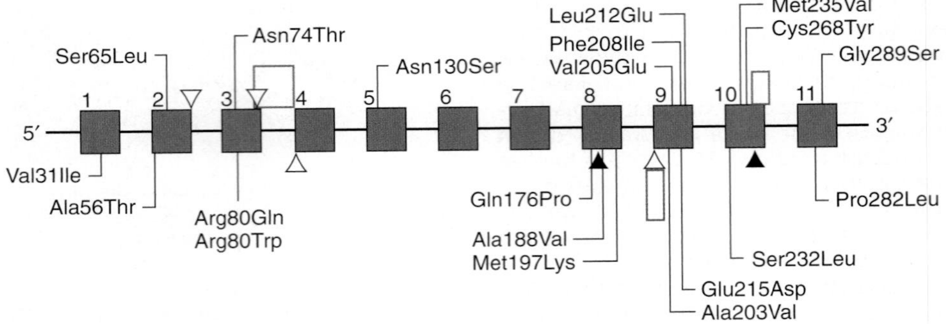

Figure 23-28 Diagram of the 17β-hydroxysteroid dehydrogenase type 3 gene *(HSD17B3)* shows the mutations that result in deficiency of the enzyme. The numbered *solid boxes* depict the exons. The three-letter abbreviations for amino acids are used to indicate the position of missense mutations; X indicates a nonsense (stop) mutation; insertions and deletions resulting in frameshift mutations *(solid triangles)* and splice site mutations *(open triangles)* are shown.

association with Antley-Bixler syndrome; these patients do not have ambiguous genitalia or steroidogenic defects.

Most patients with POR deficiency have normal electrolytes and mineralocorticoid function (see Table 23-13).[308] Cortisol insufficiency may be present, or if basal levels are adequate, the response to ACTH stimulation is reduced. The serum 17-OHP concentration is usually elevated, with a variable response to ACTH stimulation, and levels of sex steroids tend to be low, especially outside the early neonatal period. POR deficiency can be associated with ambiguous genitalia in both sexes (46,XY and 46,XX). Underandrogenization of 46,XY males can occur and may result from disturbed 17,20-lyase activity during fetal Leydig cell steroidogenesis. The partial androgenization of 46,XX infants is more prevalent and may be the result of a disturbance in aromatase activity, because POR is an electron donor for this enzyme and aromatase deficiency causes prenatal androgenization of the developing 46,XX fetus (see "Aromatase Deficiency"). Alternatively, a backdoor pathway of androgen biosynthesis has been described in certain species, such as the fetal Tammar wallaby.[170,171] In this model system, 17-OHP can be converted to DHT without the use of androstenedione or testosterone as an intermediate. Emerging data indicate that this pathway may also be functional during human development.

17β-Hydroxysteroid Dehydrogenase Type 3 Deficiency. The 17β-hydroxysteroid dehydrogenase type 3 (HSD17B3) reaction in the human is mediated by isozymes that catalyze the reduction of androstenedione, DHEA, and estrone to testosterone, Δ^5-androstenediol, and estradiol, respectively, as well as the reverse reaction (see Fig. 23-11).[309] The HSD17B3 enzyme uses NADPH as a cofactor. The *HSD17B3* gene contains 11 exons and is located on chromosome 9q22. The type 3 isoenzyme is expressed primarily in the testes, where it favors the conversion of the weak androgen substrate, androstenedione, to the more biologically active testosterone (see Fig. 23-11). The family of 17β-HSDs comprise at least 14 isoenzymes that have physiologic relevance to a range of human disorders such as breast and prostate cancer, endometriosis, and disturbances in fatty acid metabolism, as well as 46,XY DSDs.[310]

A deficiency of HSD17B3, which is also called 17-ketosteroid reductase, was first reported as one of the causes of 46,XY DSD by Saez and colleagues (Fig. 23-28).[310,311] Many cases have been reported, and the phenotype is well characterized (Table 23-14).[312-314] Most affected males have female external genitalia at birth, although a few infants present with ambiguous genitalia. The testes are usually located in the inguinal canal; the wolffian ducts are stabilized to form epididymides, vas deferens, seminal vesicles, and ejaculatory ducts; and there is a blind vaginal pouch. Affected infants are invariably assigned a female sex and may mistakenly be assumed to have CAIS. Profound virilization occurs at puberty in the form of deepening of the voice, hirsutism, muscle development, and clitoromegaly. This is often how the condition must be distinguished from other causes of virilization arising at puberty in children raised female.

The pubertal increase in testosterone is mostly from extraglandular conversion from androstenedione. We have speculated that this is mediated by genetic or environmental induction of enzyme activities of the aldoketoreductase family 1C (AKR1C), such as the 17β-HSD17B5 type 5 isoenzyme, also known as AKR1C3.[315,316] The androstenedione substrate is increased at puberty, and the testes have partial HSD17B3 activity in some cases. In a large cohort of patients from a consanguineous population in the Gaza Strip, the phallus was described as reaching lengths of 4 to 8 cm.[317] The *HSD17B3* mutation reported in this population (Arg80Gln) is associated with 15% to 20% retention of normal HSD17B3 activity (see Fig. 23-28). The development of gynecomastia at puberty occurs because of estrogens derived from the conversion of androstenedione by aromatase in extraglandular tissue and the action of the HSD17B1 or HSD17B2 isoenzymes.

TABLE 23-14
Clinical Features of HSD17B3 Deficiency in 46,XY Individuals

Karyotype	46,XY
Inheritance	Autosomal recessive; mutations in *HSD17B3* gene
Genitalia	Female → ambiguous; blind vaginal pouch
Wolffian duct derivatives	Present
Müllerian duct derivatives	Absent
Gonads	Testes (usually undescended)
Habitus	Virilization at puberty (phallus enlargement, deepening of voice, and development of facial and body hair); gynecomastia variable
Hormone profile	Increased plasma estrone and androstenedione; decreased ratio of plasma testosterone/androstenedione and estradiol after hCG stimulation test; increased plasma FSH and LH levels

FSH, follicle-stimulating hormone; hCG, human chorionic gonadotropin; HSD17B3, 17β-hydroxysteroid dehydrogenase 3; LH, luteinizing hormone.

The striking virilization at puberty, similar to that of patients with 5α-reductase type 2 deficiency, has resulted in gender role reassignment from female to male in some cases. Patients presenting as androgenized females at puberty usually undergo urgent gonadectomy, reduction clitoroplasty, and maintenance of female gender. In a series of women with diverse forms of DSD, there was evidence of significant psychological distress.[318] However, only two subjects with 17β-HSD deficiency were included in this pilot study. The typical biochemical profile in HSD17B3 deficiency is an elevated androstenedione level relative to testosterone (see Table 23-14). Expressed as a ratio of testosterone to androstenedione (after an hCG stimulation test before puberty), values less than 0.8 are typically found in these patients.[319] Testicular vein sampling at the time of gonadectomy shows a markedly increased androstenedione gradient relative to that of testosterone.

Only mutations in the *HSD17B3* gene that encodes the testis-specific enzyme are a cause of this form of 46,XY DSD. The range of mutations reported in patients with HSD17B3 deficiency is shown in Figure 23-28. Most are missense mutations, and some patients are compound heterozygotes. Expression studies of the mutant enzymes in heterologous cells usually show complete absence of activity in the conversion of androstenedione to testosterone compared with the normal enzyme. A study of women with polycystic ovary syndrome showed no association with polymorphisms in the *HSD17B3* gene.[320] Women homozygous or compound heterozygous for *HSD17B3* mutations are asymptomatic. The presence of Wolffian duct derivatives in the form of a normal vas deferens and epididymis in patients with homozygous mutations that result in complete absence of enzymatic activity is intriguing. A similar finding occurs in a significant number of patients with CAIS due to a missense mutation in the *AR* gene.[321] Androgens can diffuse directly into the adjacent Wolffian ducts to elicit a paracrine effect. Fetal androstenedione levels are expected to be increased. Although this is a weak androgen, a reporter gene assay indicated that it was almost as potent as testosterone and DHT when tested at concentrations greater than 10 nmol/L.[322]

Establishment of the diagnosis of HSD17B3 deficiency soon after birth, because of finding inguinal testes in a phenotypic female infant or because of ambiguity of the external genitalia, raises the question of sex assignment. Because of the experience of gender role change at puberty in affected families as reported in Gaza, it has been proposed that these patients be given male sex assignment at diagnosis.[323] In this study, 46,XY males with female external genitalia were treated early with testosterone, followed later by first-stage genitoplasty. Most achieved a reasonable cosmetic result and a penile length within the normal range. No more recent studies have reported on outcomes for infants assigned a male sex of rearing. Phenotypic variability within affected families can also influence gender assignment.[315] Gender role changes at puberty were reported in 39% to 64% of patients raised as girls in one study, but the numbers of subjects on which these figures were based were fewer than for 5α-reductase deficiency.[190]

Steroid 5α-Reductase Type 2 Deficiency. Steroid 5α-reductase type 2 deficiency is a defect in androgen biosynthesis. As with 17β-HSD deficiency, it is characterized by a 46,XY karyotype, normally differentiated testes, and male internal ducts but external genitalia that may be more ambiguous at birth. There is a striking degree of virilization at puberty in patients raised as female. Classic features of this enzyme deficiency are summarized in Table 23-15.

TABLE 23-15

Clinical Features of 5α-Reductase Type 2 Deficiency in 46,XY Individuals

Karyotype	46,XY
Inheritance	Autosomal recessive; mutations in *SRD5A2* gene
Genitalia	Usually ambiguous with small, hypospadiac phallus; blind vaginal pouch
Wolffian duct derivatives	Normal
Müllerian duct derivatives	Absent
Gonads	Normal testes
Habitus	Decreased facial and body hair; no temporal hair recession, prostate not palpable
Hormone profile	Decreased ratio of 5α/5β C21 and C19 steroids in urine; increased T/DHT ratio before and after hCG stimulation; modest increase in plasma LH; decreased conversion of T to DHT in vitro

DHT, dihydrotestosterone; hCG, human chorionic gonadotropin; LH, luteinizing hormone; SRD5A2, steroid-5α-reductase type 2; T, testosterone.

The description of a genetic isolate from villages in the southwestern part of the Dominican Republic and a subsequent review of the biochemical and molecular features underlines the importance of DHT in the development of the male phenotype.[324-327] At birth, there is a bifid scrotum, a urogenital sinus, a blind vaginal pouch, and a clitoris-like, hypospadiac phallus. Testes differentiate normally and are located in the inguinal canal or in the labioscrotal folds. No Müllerian structures are present. The Wolffian ducts are stabilized so that the epididymides, vasa deferentia, and seminal vesicles are well differentiated; the ejaculatory ducts usually terminate in the blind vaginal pouch. The prostate is hypoplastic.

Affected males virilize to various degrees at puberty. The voice deepens, muscle mass increases, the phallus lengthens to 4 to 8 cm, the bifid scrotum becomes rugated and pigmented, and the testes enlarge and descend into the labioscrotal folds. Postpubertal affected males do not have acne, temporal hair recession, or enlargement of the prostate, and they do not develop gynecomastia. There is normal libido with penile erections. Histologic examination of the testes shows Leydig cell hyperplasia and decreased spermatogenesis. This is caused by failure to transform spermatogonia into spermatocytes, rather than associated cryptorchidism.[328] Nevertheless, some members of the Dominican cohort had a normal sperm count. One man fathered a child after intrauterine insemination, and two affected brothers in a Swedish family were spontaneously fertile after hypospadias repair performed in childhood.[329,330] Gender role changes occur frequently in 5α-reductase deficiency, particularly where clusters of cases occur in geographic regions (e.g., Dominican Republic, New Guinea,[331] South Lebanon, Turkey). Overall, gender role is changed in 56% to 63% of cases.[190] Females (46, XX) homozygous for 5α-reductase deficiency undergo normal puberty but delayed menarche, and fertility is normal.[332]

The biochemical profile in 5α-reductase deficiency typically shows an elevated testosterone-to-DHT ratio, which needs to be determined after hCG stimulation when investigations are undertaken before puberty (see Table 23-15). A ratio exceeding 20:1 suggests the diagnosis. Serum LH and FSH levels may be normal or elevated after puberty. Analysis of a urinary steroid profile by gas chromatography and mass spectrometry is usually specific to demonstrate a diminished ratio of urinary 5α- to 5β-reduced C19 and C21 steroids.[333] The diagnosis can still be confirmed biochemically after gonadectomy because of persistent effects on 5α/5β-reduced C21 steroids. However, the results may not be sufficiently reliable in early infancy.

Early diagnosis of 5α-reductase type 2 deficiency is important because of its bearing on sex assignment. The natural history of this condition, with a tendency for change to a male gender role with virilization at puberty, indicates that male gender assignment must be an option when there is ambiguous or severely underandrogenized genitalia at birth.[334] This enzyme deficiency can masquerade as PAIS in newborns.[335] DHT, which may be applied topically as a cream, increases penile length and facilitates repair of the hypospadias.[336]

5α-reductase type 2 deficiency is transmitted as an autosomal recessive trait. Two microsomal 5α-reductase enzymes catalyze the NADPH-dependent conversion of testosterone to DHT. 5α-Reductase type 2 is a 254-amino-acid protein encoded by the *SRD5A2* gene on chromosome 2p23.[326] The type 2 isozyme is expressed predominantly in the primordia of the prostate and external genitalia but not in the Wolffian ducts until after their differentiation into the male internal genital ducts.[337] The type 1 isoenzyme is expressed in skin, including human genital skin fibroblasts. This isoenzyme may contribute to the virilization that occurs in 5α-reductase–deficient patients at puberty.[338]

The 5α-reductase type 2 deficiency is genetically heterogeneous, and the more than 50 mutations detected in the *SRD5A2* gene are distributed among all five exons (Fig. 23-29). Most are missense mutations, and a complete gene deletion is found in the New Guinea population. There is a predominance of mutations in exon 4, mostly localized between codons 197 and 230, where the effect is complete inactivation of the mutant enzyme. A stretch of 21 amino acids in this region probably functions as a transmembrane domain.[327] There is little correlation between the severity of the clinical phenotype and the nature of the mutation, although the highly prevalent proline-to-arginine mutation in the Mexican population is associated with severe undervirilization at birth and female sex assignment.[327] A significant number of cases are compound heterozygotes, and consanguinity is common. Male heterozygotes are normal.

Disorders of Androgen Action

The key role of androgens in male sex differentiation cannot be better illustrated than by the consequence of total lack of response to androgens in target tissues—a complete female phenotype in a 46,XY individual with normally formed testes producing age-appropriate testosterone levels. This is the paradigm of a hormone resistance syndrome. The pathophysiology of clinical syndromes associated with complete or partial resistance to androgens is related to the mechanism of normal androgen action.[339,340]

Male sex differentiation, the subsequent acquisition of secondary sex characteristics at puberty, and the onset of spermatogenesis are all mediated by androgens binding to a single intracellular AR ubiquitously expressed in target tissue. The AR is one of a quartet of nuclear receptors (i.e., glucocorticoid, mineralocorticoid, progesterone, and androgen) that are closely related within a large superfamily and activate gene transcription through hormone response elements. The single-copy eight exon gene encoding the AR is located on Xq11-q12; the AR is a protein of 919 amino acid residues. The major functional domains are an N-terminal transactivation domain (NTD) encoded by exon 1; a central, highly conserved DNA-binding domain (DBD) encoded by exons 2 and 3; a hinge region that connects the DBD to the ligand-binding domain; and a C-terminal ligand-binding domain (LBD) encoded by exons 4 through 8 (Fig. 23-30). The 70-amino-acid DBD is highly conserved among nuclear receptors and contains

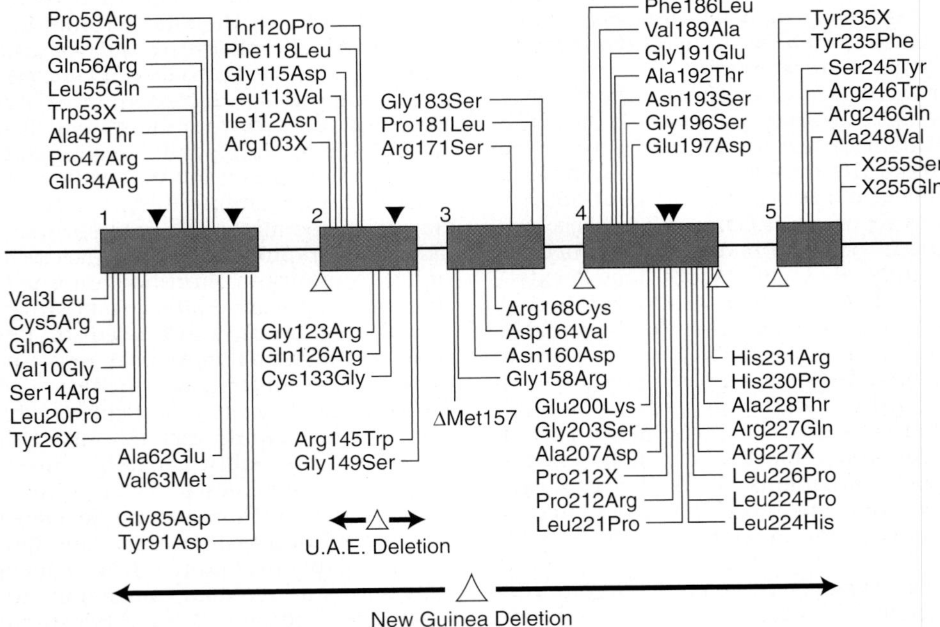

Figure 23-29 Diagram of the 5α-reductase type 2 gene *(SRD5A2)* shows the mutations that result in 5α-reductase deficiency. The numbered *solid boxes* depict the exons. The three-letter abbreviations for amino acids are used to indicate the position of missense mutations; X indicates a nonsense (stop) mutation; insertions and deletions resulting in frameshift and splice site mutations are shown by *solid triangles* and *open triangles*, respectively. Large deletions found in affected United Arab Emirates (UAE) and New Guinea populations are shown. (Adapted from Grumbach MM, Hughes IA, Conte FA. Disorders of sex differentiation. In Larsen PR, Kronenberg HM, Melmed S, et al., eds. *Williams Textbook of Endocrinology,* 10th ed. Philadelphia, PA: Saunders, 2003, with additional data provided courtesy of Dr. Julianne Imperato-McGinley, Department of Medicine, Weill Medical College of Cornell University, Ithaca, NY.)

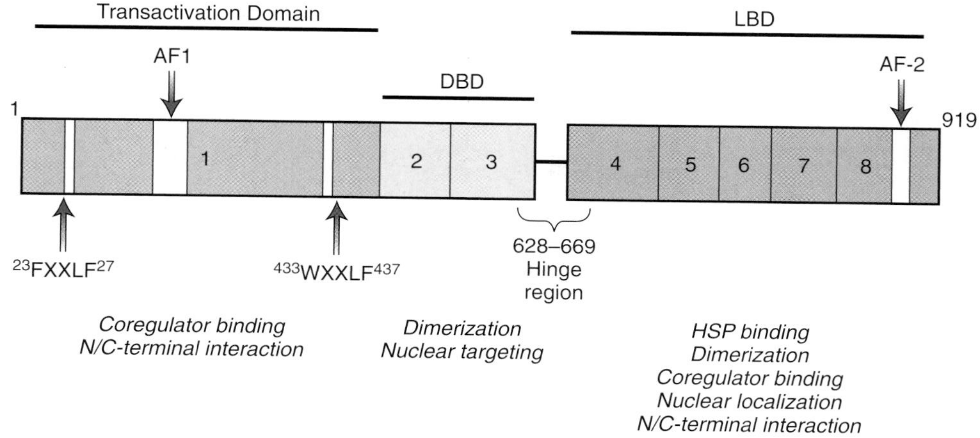

Figure 23-30 Schematic diagram of the androgen receptor (AR) shows the major functional domains and subsidiary functions. Single-amino-acid codes are used, and X represents any amino acid. Numbers outside the structure refer to amino acids (AR comprises 919 amino acid residues); numbers 1 through 8 inside the structure refer to AR exons. AF, activation function; DBD, DNA-binding domain; LBD, ligand-binding domain; HSP, heat shock protein.

cysteine residues that coordinate zinc atoms to form the zinc fingers characteristic of nuclear receptors and many other transcription factors. The first zinc finger contains a P box that enters the major grove of DNA to form specific base-pair contacts that are identical for all classic steroid receptors. The second zinc finger containing the D box is involved in protein-protein interactions and also stabilizes the unit for receptor dimerization. This requires recognition of selective androgen response elements.[341] The subsidiary functions operated by these domains are shown in Figure 23-30 and include dimerization, binding to coregulator proteins, interaction with HSPs, and transcriptional regulation.

The two subdomains most involved in activation of transcription are the motif activation function 1 (AF1) in the NTD and the motif activation function 2 (AF2) in the LBD. AF1 is ligand independent, whereas AF2 is ligand dependent and interacts with p160 steroid receptor coactivators such as NCOA1 (formerly called SRC1), NCOA2 (formerly SRC2 or TIF2), and NCOA3 (formerly SRC3).[342] For most nuclear receptors, there is a strong interaction between the AF2 subdomain and LXXLL motifs (in which L is leucine and X is any amino acid) in the coactivators. In the case of the AR, this interaction is weaker, and the AF2 subdomain interacts in an intramolecular manner with its cognate AF1 subdomain in the NTD. This N-terminal and C-terminal (N-C) interaction is a relatively unique feature of the AR and is mediated by interaction with the FXXLF motif (in which F is phenylalanine) in AF1 comprising amino acid residues 23 to 27. The N-C interaction stabilizes the AR and slows down the dissociation of the ligand from its receptor. Further modulation of AR function occurs posttranslationally by processes such as phosphorylation and sumoylation.

A unique feature of the AR is the homopolymeric stretches of amino acids within the NTD. A sequence of CAG repeats in exon 1 encodes for a stretch of glutamines that ranges from 11 to 31 repeats (mean, 21 repeats) in the general population. Another repeat ranges from 10 to 25 glycines (mean, 23 glycines) in the general population. In vitro studies show that the length of the CAG repeat is inversely proportional to the activity of the AR as a transcription factor.[343]

Figure 23-31 illustrates androgens interacting with the AR on entering target cells and subsequent activation of target genes. A single receptor binds all androgens; testosterone is converted to DHT, which is biologically more potent because it dissociates from the AR at a slower rate. The AR in the unliganded state is located in the cytoplasm complexed to HSPs such as HSP70 and HSP90 and complexed to co-chaperone proteins such as FKBP4 (also called FKBP52). Binding of ligand to its receptor initiates dissociation from these complexes to allow translocation of the AR into the nucleus, where it binds as a homodimer to inverted repeats of 5′-AGAACA-2′–like motifs with a three-nucleotide spacer (nnn). The action of the AR is further modulated by interaction with coregulatory proteins that function as coactivators or corepressors.[342] Many coactivators act in a generic fashion (e.g., SRC and CBP/p300-interacting transactivator [CITED] family of proteins), but others, RAN (formerly called ARA24), RNF 14 (formerly ARA54), TGFB1I1 (formerly ARA55), and NCOA4 (formerly ARA70) are relatively specific to the AR.

The crystal structure of the AR LBD bound to natural and synthetic androgens is shown in Figure 23-32. The three-dimensional structure of a nuclear receptor LBD comprises 12 α-helices associated with antiparallel β-sheets arranged in the form of a tripartite sandwich. A hydrophobic pocket is formed by helices 3, 4, 5, 7, 11, and 12, to which the ligand is bound on contact with its cognate receptor. Helix 12, the outermost α-helix, folds back on top of the ligand hydrophobic pocket like a lid closing on a box. This has been referred to as the *mousetrap effect;* the ligand is captured and retained by slowing the rate of ligand-receptor dissociation. This trapping effect by helix 12 also permits interaction between the LBD and AF2 subdomain and the LXXLL motif in associated coregulator proteins. Information about the structural and functional aspects of the AR has been gathered from analysis of AR mutations that lead to various degrees of androgen resistance, which are clinically manifested as syndromes of androgen insensitivity that are classified as complete, partial, and minimal according to severity of hormone resistance.[339]

Complete Androgen Insensitivity Syndrome. The phenotype of CAIS is that of a female (Table 23-16). Estimates of the prevalence of this X-linked recessive disorder range from 1 case in 20,400 to 1 in 99,000 genetic males.[344] The typical mode of presentation is that of an adolescent female who has breast development with a pubertal growth spurt but who has not had menarche. Pubic and axillary hair is

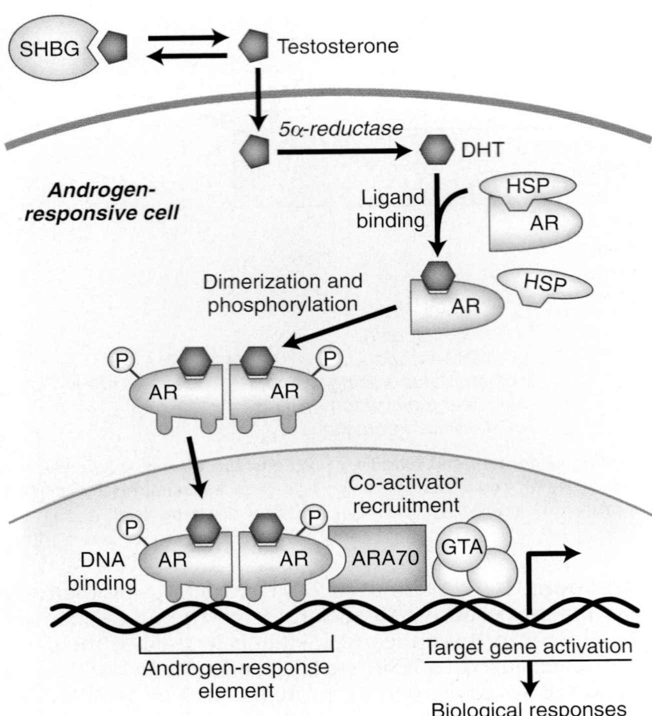

Figure 23-31 Androgen action in a target cell. Circulating testosterone bound predominantly to sex hormone–binding globulin (SHBG) enters the cell in free form, where it is converted to dihydrotestosterone (DHT), a more potent androgen. Both androgens bind to a single cytoplasmic androgen receptor (AR) complexed to heat shock proteins (HSPs) and other co-chaperones such as FKBP52. Androgen binding dissociates the AR from HSPs, and AR-bound androgen translocates to the nucleus, binding to DNA response elements as a homodimer. Coactivators such as NCOA4(ARA70) bind to the AR complex to mediate interaction with the general transcription apparatus (GTA). This results in transcription of androgen-responsive genes and pleiotropic biologic responses, including male sex differentiation, growth, muscle and bone development, spermatogenesis, and prostate growth. P, phosphorylation. (Adapted from Feldman BJ, Feldman D. The development of androgen-independent prostate cancer. *Nature Ref Cancer.* 2001;1:34-45, with permission of Nature Publishing Group, copyright 2001.)

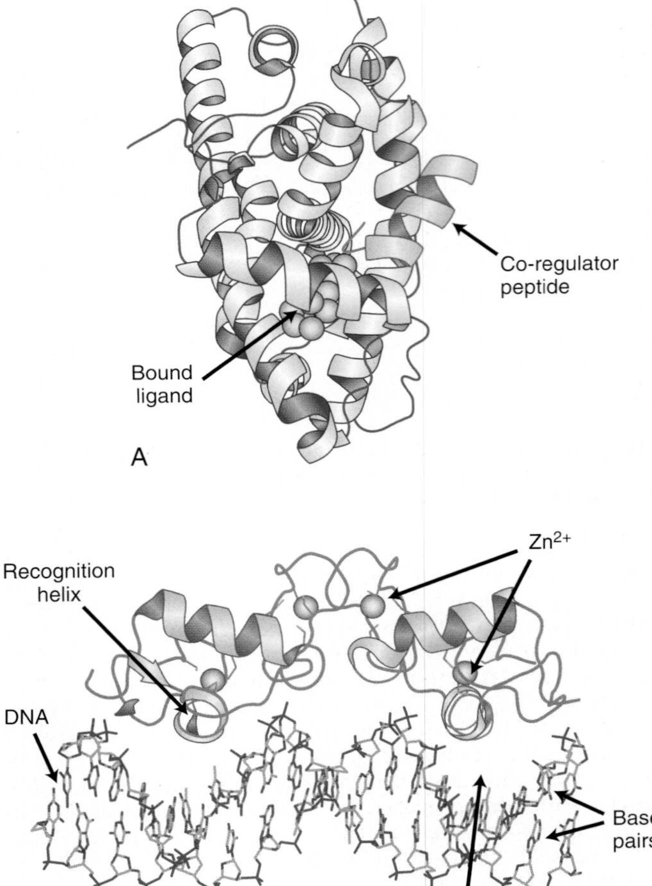

Figure 23-32 **A,** Schematic diagram of the androgen receptor (AR) shows the tripartite sandwich arrangement of the helices, the position of the bound ligand in the pocket, and a coregulator FXXLF peptide bound to the activation function 2 (AF2) region. **B,** The DNA-binding domain structure of the AR binds through its two zinc fingers to DNA response elements.

TABLE 23-16

Clinical Features of Complete Androgen Insensitivity Syndrome

Karyotype	46,XY
Inheritance	X-linked recessive; mutations in *AR* gene
Genitalia	Female with blind vaginal pouch
Wolffian duct derivatives	Often present, depending on mutation type
Müllerian duct derivatives	Absent or vestigial
Gonads	Testes
Habitus	Scant or absent pubic and axillary hair; breast development and female habitus at puberty; primary amenorrhea
Hormone and metabolic profile	Increased LH and testosterone levels; increased estradiol (for male reference range); FSH levels often normal or slightly increased; resistance to androgenic and metabolic effects of testosterone

AR, androgen receptor; FSH, follicle-stimulating hormone; LH, luteinizing hormone.

usually absent or scanty. The uterus is absent as a result of normal AMH action, although there may be Müllerian remnants. The Wolffian ducts are stabilized in many patients, with well-developed vas deferens and epididymis observed when gonadectomy is performed.[321] The main differential diagnosis at this age is XY complete gonadal dysgenesis (i.e., Swyer syndrome), which is distinguished by poor breast development, taller stature, decreased ratio of upper to lower body segments, and a different hormone profile.[345] CAIS may occur in early infancy with bilateral inguinal or labial swellings. 17β-HSD deficiency may also manifest in this manner. Bilateral inguinal hernias are rare in girls, and it has been estimated that 1% to 2% of such patients have CAIS.[346] A CAIS diagnosis should be considered in all girls with this type of hernia, and the presence of a Y chromosome should be checked by fluorescence in situ hybridization (FISH) or a full karyotype. If the hernial sac contains gonads, a biopsy should be performed in concert with the cytogenetic studies.[347] It is not unusual to obtain the history of an older female sibling who had an inguinal hernia repair in infancy, and when the karyotype is subsequently checked, the sibling is also found to have CAIS.

It is increasingly common for the sex of the infant to be determined before birth by analysis of the fetal karyotype because of maternal risk factors for congenital malformations. Fetal sexing is possible by three-dimensional ultrasound as early as the first trimester. Consequently, a mismatch between fetal sexing and birth phenotype may be the presentation.

Partial Androgen Insensitivity Syndrome. The terminology of PAIS implies some biologic response to androgens that results in incomplete masculinization (Table 23-17). The external genitalia may be ambiguous at birth, but the prototypic phenotype for PAIS is characterized by perineoscrotal hypospadias, micropenis, and a bifid scrotum. The testes may be undescended. The more severe form of PAIS, manifesting as isolated clitoromegaly, is only marginally different from CAIS. The milder end of the spectrum of PAIS includes isolated hypospadias; isolated micropenis does not appear to be a manifestation of PAIS.

The list of differential diagnoses within the 46,XY DSD category is lengthy for the PAIS phenotype. Causes include partial gonadal dysgenesis, a defect in androgen biosynthesis (e.g., LH receptor, SF1, 17β-HSD, and 5α-reductase deficiencies), mixed gonadal dysgenesis in association with 45,X/46,XY mosaicism, and ovotesticular DSD.

Minimal or Mild Androgen Insensitivity Syndrome. This category of androgen insensitivity syndrome (AIS) emerged after investigations for male factor infertility, which suggested a defect in androgen action in some cases.[348] Studies of males who have oligospermia and normal testosterone levels with increased LH concentrations show that a small percentage have a mutation in the *AR* gene. High doses of androgens may overcome the spermatogenic defect. Minimal or mild androgen insensitivity syndrome (MAIS) may manifest with gynecomastia in young adulthood, and there may be a history of minor hypospadias repair in childhood. Cancer of the breast is rare in males, but the risk is increased in those with MAIS or PAIS, with an association between longer glutamine repeats in the AR and male breast cancer.[349] Breast cancer has not been reported in women with CAIS.

Hormone Profiles in Androgen Insensitivity Syndromes. The typical hormone profile in a postpubertal patient with CAIS and intact gonads comprises a testosterone level within or above the adult male range, an inappropriately increased concentration of LH, and a normal or slightly elevated FSH level. The serum estradiol level also is increased because of direct contributions from the testis and peripheral aromatization. A similar gonadotrophin and sex steroid profile occurs in PAIS.[350] Concentrations of sex hormone–binding globulin (SHBG) are sexually dimorphic, with levels in patients with CAIS similar to those found in normal females. The SHBG response to a stanozolol, a nonaromatizable androgen, has been suggested as a biomarker of androgen responsiveness, but it is not sufficiently reliable for clinical use in PAIS.[351] The serum concentration of inhibin is normal, and the AMH concentration is even increased in CAIS, whereas these levels are low in gonadal dysgenesis.[352]

Male infants have an LH-induced surge in serum testosterone concentrations during the first few months of life, which manifests as some growth of the penis. Isolated case reports suggested that the surge does not occur in CAIS, and this was confirmed in a study of 10 infants with CAIS who proved to have an *AR* mutation.[353] Testosterone levels did increase after hCG stimulation in these patients. In contrast, infants with PAIS have a spontaneous neonatal testosterone surge.

Such observations provide some insight into the control mechanisms of HPG cyclicity.[354] Although a female infant with bilateral inguinal swellings and a 46,XY karyotype suggests a diagnosis of CAIS, measurement of baseline gonadotropins and sex steroids before and after hCG stimulation should be performed to exclude other causes.

TABLE 23-17

Clinical Features of Partial Androgen Insensitivity Syndrome

Karyotype	46, XY
Inheritance	X-linked recessive; mutations in *AR* gene
External genitalia	Ambiguous with blind vaginal pouch → undermasculinized → isolated hypospadias → normal male with infertility (mild AIS)
Wolffian duct derivatives	Often normal
Müllerian duct derivatives	Absent
Gonads	Testes (usually undescended)
Habitus	Decreased to normal axillary and pubic hair; beard growth, and body hair; gynecomastia common at puberty
Hormone and metabolic profile	Increased LH and testosterone concentrations; increased estradiol (for men); FSH levels may be normal or slightly increased
	Partial resistance to androgenic and metabolic effects of testosterone

AIS, androgen insensitivity syndrome; AR, androgen receptor; FSH, follicle-stimulating hormone; LH, luteinizing hormone.

Molecular Pathogenesis of Androgen Insensitivity Syndromes. Information about the various mutations that affect the AR and give rise to clinical disease is recorded on an International Mutation Database at McGill University (http://www.androgendb.mcgill.ca). A map that includes most of the reported mutations is shown in Figure 23-33. Most mutations are related to syndromes of androgen insensitivity, but somatic mutations identified in prostate carcinoma also are listed. The database comprises almost 1000 entries, encompassing more than 300 mutations that can cause AIS. There is no specific hot spot of mutations, but certain locations, such as exons 5 and 7, are affected more frequently. About two thirds of reported mutations are located in the LBD, approximately 20% in the DBD, and a few in the NTD encoded by the large first exon. The NTD has not been crystallized, but its distinct disordered molten-globular structure reflects a reduced spectrum of missense mutations found in the DBD and LBD.[340] Nonsense mutations are evenly distributed throughout the *AR* gene, and all result in a CAIS phenotype.

Figure 23-34 illustrates the range of mutations recorded on the Cambridge DSD Database for CAIS and PAIS. The most common functional AR defect is a mutation that disrupts the hydrophobic ligand-binding pocket in the LBD. Repositioning of helix 12 generates the AF2 coregulator interaction surface. Most LBD mutations causing CAIS cluster within amino acid residues 688 to 712, 739 to 784, and 827 to 870. The first two clusters cover most of the ligand-binding pocket. One example is a mutation in helix 5, which changes the polar arginine to glutamine at codon 752. This results in a CAIS phenotype that is also found in the spontaneous *Tfm* rat model of CAIS.[355]

The phenotype can vary according to different substitutions at the same codon. Phenylalanine at codon 754 in helix 5 has a side chain that points away from the ligand-binding pocket. Figure 23-35 illustrates that when

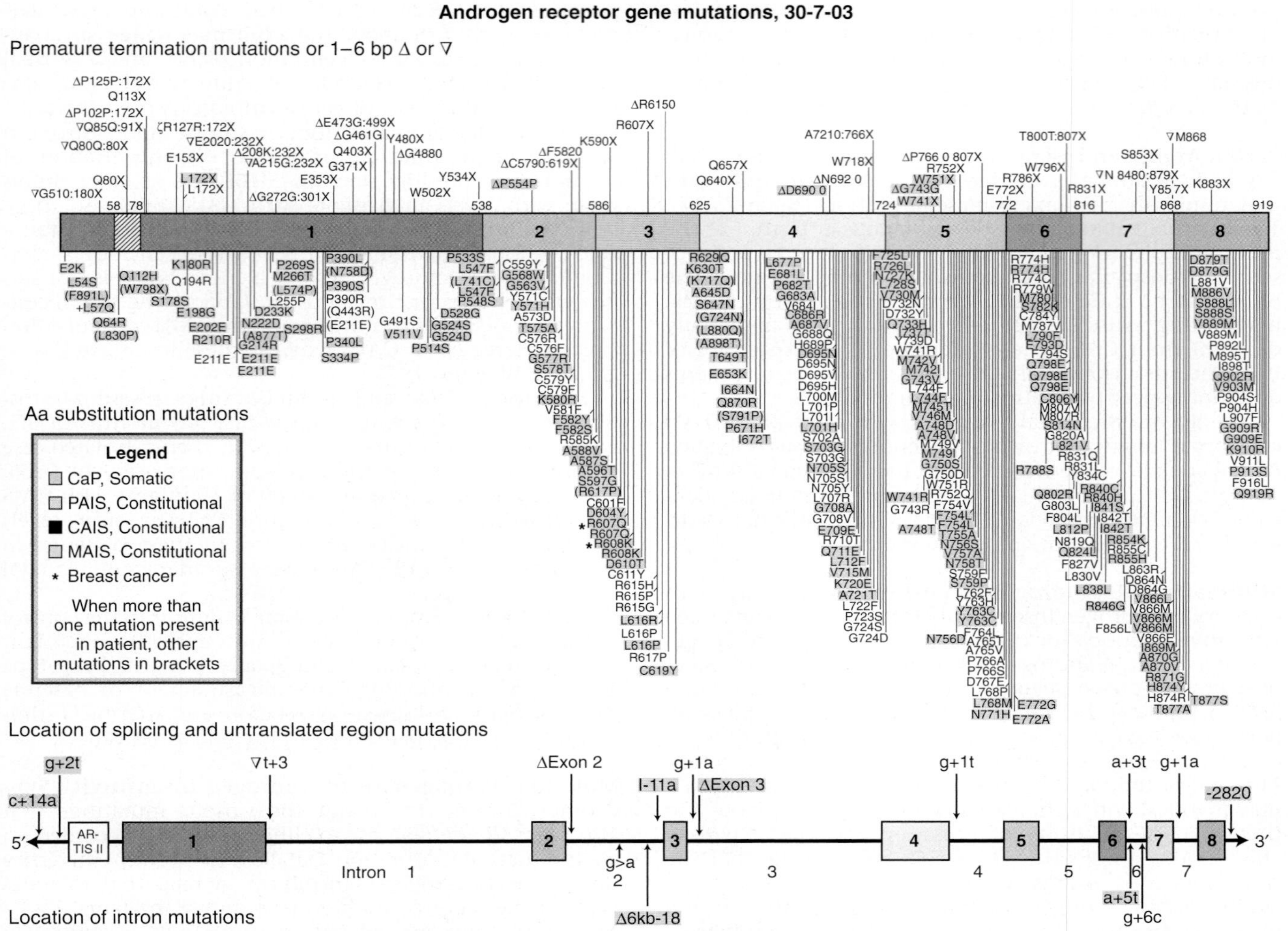

Androgen receptor gene mutations, 30-7-03

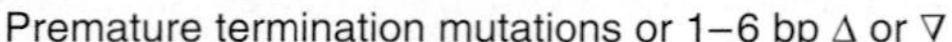

Figure 23-33 Overview of androgen receptor (AR) mutations that cause different forms of androgen insensitivity syndrome (AIS). CAIS, complete androgen insensitivity syndrome; MAIS, minimal or mild androgen insensitivity syndrome; PAIS, partial androgen insensitivity syndrome. (From the McGill Androgen Receptor Gene Mutation Database. Available at http://www.androgendb.mcgill.ca [accessed November 2010]).

phenylalanine is substituted for a valine, the mutant AR is transcriptionally inactive and causes CAIS.[356] In contrast, serine and leucine substitutions result in a PAIS phenotype, explained by some residual transcriptional activity as measured in vitro. It is possible to rescue androgen action in vitro by administering high doses of androgens, as shown in Figure 23-35 in the case of a asparagine substituted for glutamic acid at codon 690. Linking the DBD to the LBD is a flexible hinge region defined by residues 628 to 669. This region stabilizes receptor interaction with selective androgen response elements and signals nuclear localization. Deletion of the hinge region by site-directed mutagenesis results in enhanced gene transcription, suggesting that it has a role in repression. This may not be the case in human studies, based on reduced N-C interactions as the sole explanation for the phenotype in PAIS subjects with an arginine-to-tryptophan substitution at codon 629 in the hinge region.[357]

There can be considerable heterogeneity in the phenotypic expression of a particular mutation, sometimes even within families. A mutation at codon 703 in exon 4 of the LBD, which changes a serine to a glycine, is reported in four individuals listed in the McGill Database. One patient had a normal female phenotype consistent with CAIS. The other three all had ambiguous genitalia consistent with PAIS, but the degree of androgenization of the external genitalia was sufficiently variable that two were raised male and the other was raised female.[358] X-linked disorders are associated with a high rate of de novo mutations; the rate in AIS is about 30%. Such mutations arise as a single mutational event in a parental germ cell (the mother in the case of AIS) or as germ cell mosaicism in the maternal gonad. When the mutation arises at the postzygotic stage, the index case is a somatic mosaic. This gives rise to expression of mutant and wild-type ARs in different target tissues, including the external genitalia. Perhaps one third of de novo mutations in AIS arise at the postzygotic stage, which could explain some of the variable phenotype in PAIS, whereas no somatic mosaicism is found in CAIS.[359,360] Other modulatory factors include differences in 5α-reductase type 2 expression and reduced *AR* transcription and translation.[361,362]

Several in vitro assays are used to define mutant AR function. The techniques are particularly important to apply when a novel mutation associated with a PAIS phenotype is discovered and is located in the LBD. Measurement of androgen binding in genital skin fibroblasts derived from foreskin, scrotal, or labial skin obtained at surgery can provide information on AR number and binding affinity to ligand. Typically, binding is absent in CAIS, whereas the

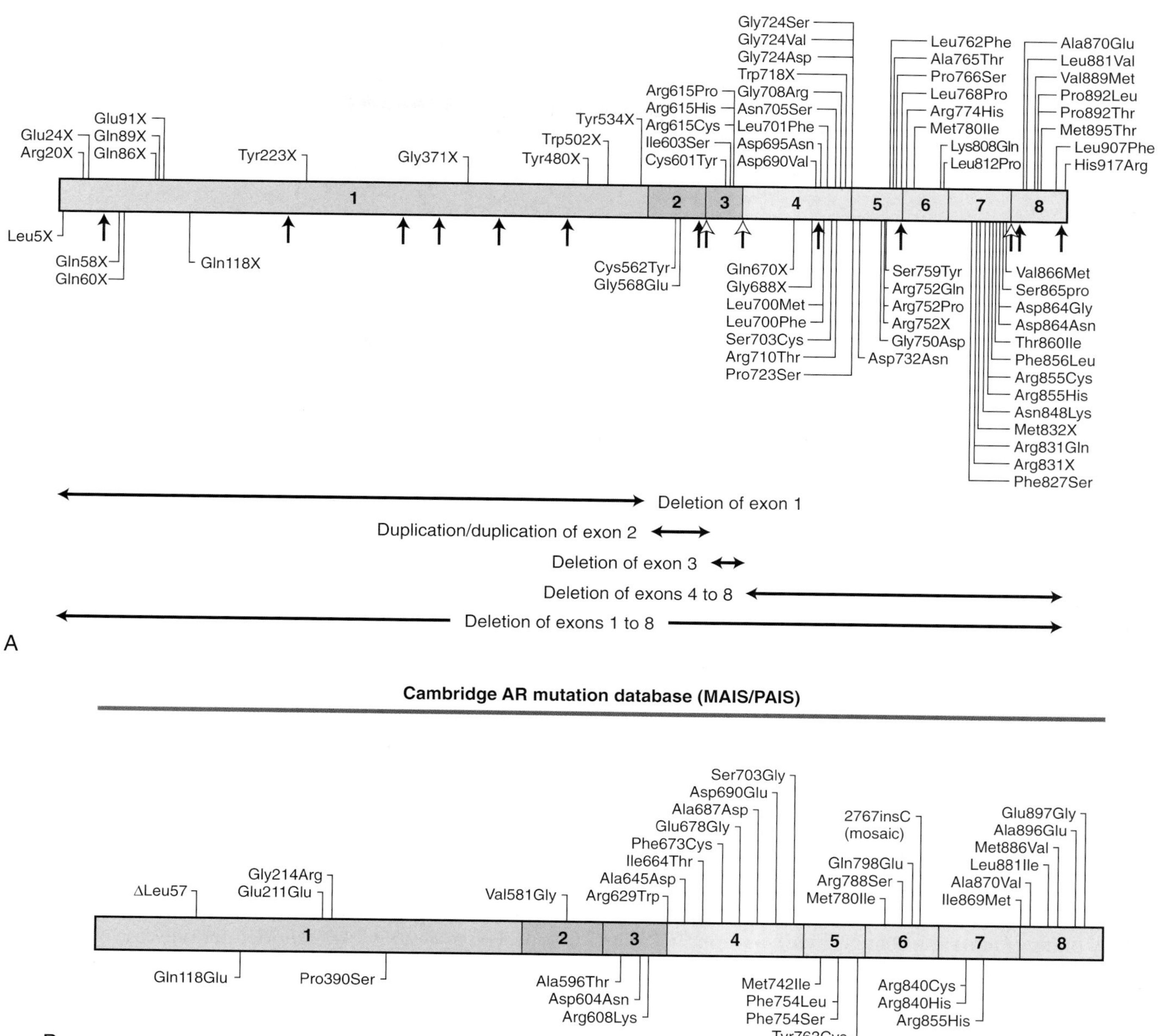

Figure 23-34 Androgen receptor (AR) mutations recorded in the Cambridge DSD Database. *Closed arrows* indicate deletions; *open arrows* indicate splice site mutations. **A,** Complete androgen insensitivity syndrome (CAIS). **B,** Partial androgen insensitivity syndrome (PAIS) or minimal or mild androgen insensitivity syndrome (MAIS). (Courtesy of Trevor Bunch, University of Cambridge, Cambridge, UK.)

kinetics of binding is altered in PAIS. Using this resource to analyze androgen-dependent gene expression, there is evidence that *AR* mutations induce lasting changes in genital skin fibroblast transcripts independent of biopsy site.[363] Similar data from genome-wide profiling can be obtained from transcriptomes of blood leukocytes in a range of disorders affecting genital development.[364]

The standard assay used to study the function of a mutant AR is a promoter-luciferase assay applied after transient transfection into a receptor-negative cell line such as Cos-1, Hela, CV-1, or the PC3 prostate cancer cell line. Figure 23-35 illustrates the application of such an assay for analysis of four AR missense mutations. The data provide an indication of potential mutant AR recovery over a range of androgen concentrations. This has particular relevance for subjects with PAIS who are raised male and may require large doses of androgens to induce puberty or to stimulate spermatogenesis. The mammalian two-hybrid assay is particularly useful for functional analysis of AR mutants in view of the unique requirement for intramolecular N-C terminal interaction in the AR. Several mutations located in the LBD do not affect ligand binding, and AR dysfunction is explained by disruption of the androgen-induced interaction between the N-terminal FXXLF motif and the

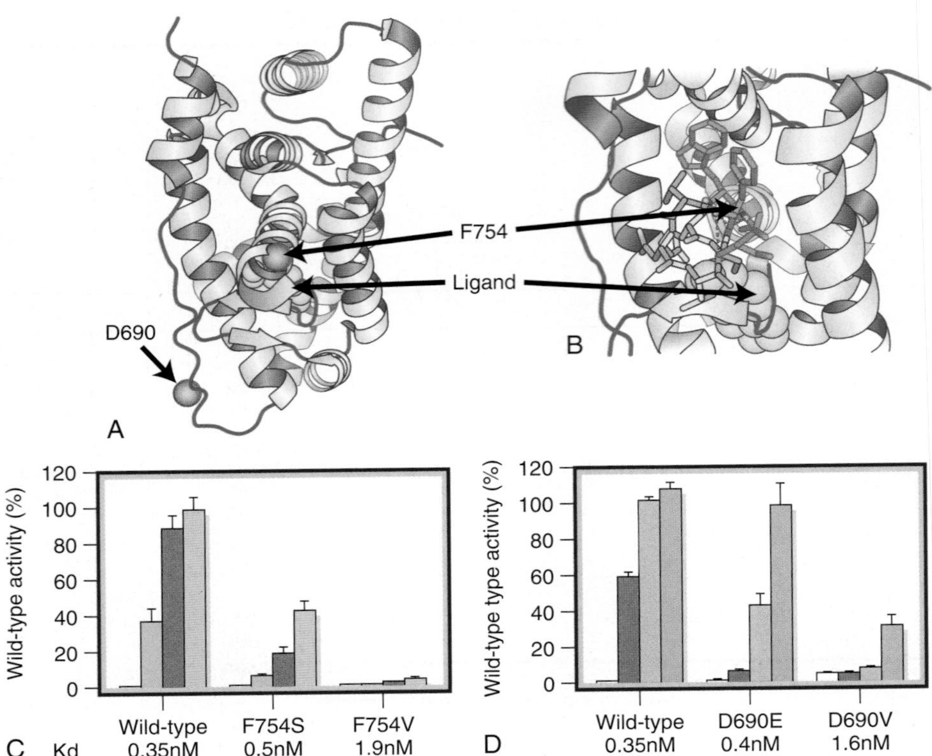

Figure 23-35 Schematic diagram of the androgen receptor (AR). **A,** Position of mutated residues Phe754 and Asp690 *(pink)*. **B,** Residue Phe754 forms hydrogen bonds with neighboring residues *(orange)* that help to stabilize helices 5, 6, and 7. **C** and **D,** Luciferase reporter assays demonstrate mutant trans-activation activity relative to wild-type AR. The *bars* represent the responses to increasing concentrations of dihydrotestosterone (1, 3.3, and 10 nmol/L). Kd values for binding affinity are shown.

AF2 subdomain in the C-terminus.[365,366] Other in vitro studies relevant to analysis of the AR include Western immunoblotting, ligand dissociation kinetics, oligonucleotide electrophoretic mobility shift assay, and use of the green fluorescent protein (GFP) technique to determine trafficking of the AR from the cytoplasm to the nucleus. Allied to functional studies in vitro, structure-guided modeling of the nuclear receptor can be used to predict the likely consequences of a mutant AR.[356,365] As sequencing the entire *AR* gene has become more straightforward, discovery of novel mutations has become common.[367,368] Nevertheless, it is necessary to undertake functional assays of the AR variant to determine its pathogenicity, particularly in cases of PAIS.

Androgen Insensitivity Syndromes without an Androgen Receptor Mutation. An *AR* gene mutation is identified in about 90% of subjects when the clinical and biochemical phenotype is consistent with CAIS. In contrast, the yield of mutations is less than 25% in PAIS, even when other causes of a similar phenotype have been excluded.[358] In a study of two AR-related coactivators, RAN (formerly called ARA24) and NCOA4 (formerly ARA70), no substantive variations were found in amino acid residues in a series of patients with PAIS who had a normal AR.[369,370] In studies relating to prostate cancer, NCOA3 (formerly SRC3) was identified as the preferred coactivator for the AR in the ligand-activated state.[371] The *NCOA3* gene contains a variable tract of CAG/CAA triplets that encode a polyglutamine repeat. The lengths of glutamine repeats were found to be shorter in PAIS subjects compared with controls.[372] Variation in the NCOA3 protein may modulate or destabilize receptor-coactivator interactions. Targeted disruption of Fkbp4 (also called Fkbp52), an AR co-chaperone, causes infertility and hypospadias in male mice.[373] However, no mutations were found in a cohort of boys with nonsyndromic hypospadias.[374] Hyperexpansion of the polyglutamine repeat in the N-terminus of the AR leads to toxic gain-of-function and Kennedy's disease or spinal and bulbar muscular atrophy (SBMA).[375] Affected males have testicular atrophy, decreased spermatogenesis, gynecomastia, and elevated androgen levels in keeping with androgen resistance. An abnormally expanded CAG repeat to 44 residues was reported for one case of hypospadias.[376] Variations in the length of the polyglutamine tract within the normal range have been found in a remarkable number of clinical scenarios, as summarized in Table 23-18. Even behavior in adolescent males and the physiologic response to hypoxic training in young men have been associated with the number of glutamine repeats.[377,378] When CAG (glutamine) and GGN (glycine) lengths are analyzed together in the context of a missense mutation in the *AR* gene causing AIS, the combined effects appear to modulate the phenotypic expression of a given AR mutant in different affected individuals.[379]

Management of Androgen Insensitivity Syndromes. Gender assignment and sex of rearing is uniformly female in CAIS. However, one case was reported of male gender identity that resulted in complete sex reassignment involving androgen treatment and phalloplasty.[380] An inactivating *AR* mutation was identified. Such an isolated case does not alter the premise that the sex of rearing is female in CAIS, but the observation raises the question of what role a functional AR plays in the development of male gender identity. Inguinal hernias need repair when patients present in

TABLE 23-18

Disease Associations with Variations in the Androgen Receptor Glutamine Repeat

Shortened (CAG)n	Increased (CAG)n
Prostate cancer	*Above normal range*
Ovarian hyperandrogenism	SBMA (Kennedy's disease)
Androgenetic alopecia	Hypospadias (one reported case)
Aspects of Klinefelter phenotype	*Within normal range*
Response to androgen treatment	Male infertility
Central obesity	Gynecomastia
Mental retardation	Hypospadias
Endometrial cancer	Aspects of Klinefelter phenotype
Coronary artery disease severity	Bone density
	Breast cancer

(CAG)n, number of CAG (glutamine) repeats; SBMA, spinal and bulbar muscular atrophy.

infancy, with an option at this stage to perform gonadectomy. There is no uniform practice concerning early versus late gonadectomy. There is merit in having spontaneous puberty from gonads in situ compared with induction of puberty with estrogen replacement. However, there is a small risk of a gonadal tumor if gonadectomy is delayed until adulthood. If early gonadectomy is undertaken, estrogen replacement should be started when the child is 10 to 11 years old with ethinyl estradiol (initially 2 μg (micrograms) daily and up to 20 to 30 μg daily by 14 to 15 years of age). Thereafter, adult estrogen replacement may continue orally with natural estrogens (1 mg daily) or changed to transdermal delivery (40 to 50 μg [micrograms]). Adjunctive replacement with progestins is seldom used because of the absence of a uterus, and depot estrogen is preferred by some women. Adults with CAIS report improved well-being with androgen replacement, particularly when it is introduced after gonadectomy. The mechanism of this androgenic effect is not understood. If gonads are left in situ, the onset of puberty occurs at the same age as in girls in their peer group.[381] Pubic hair occurs slightly later (median age, 14 years), and axillary hair usually is absent. Adult height of persons with CAIS is close to target male height and taller when gonadectomy is delayed.[345] Bone mineral density is decreased in CAIS compared with 5α-reductase deficiency, illustrating the direct role of androgens in bone mineralization. Adult bone mineral density in CAIS is similar whether gonadectomy occurs before or after puberty.

There is an increased risk of gonadal tumors in DSDs, particularly in the presence of a Y chromosome.[23,382,383] Seminoma, an invasive type II germ cell tumor, can develop in later adulthood in patients with AIS. This is preceded by an in situ neoplastic change called *intratubular germ cell neoplasia unclassified* (ITGNU). A more commonly recognized histologic term for this lesion is carcinoma in situ (CIS). The outcome of CIS is more likely to be a gonadoblastoma when the gonad is not well differentiated. The abundance of primordial germ cells in the tubules (i.e., ITGNU lesion) represents a delay in germ cell maturation into spermatogonia, and the arrested gonocyte underlies the cause of common germ cell cancer in young men.[384] In the context of testicular germ cell tumors in young men, the presence of testicular microlithiasis strongly predicts concurrence of germ cell tumor and ITGNU.[385] CIS cells originate from primordial germ cells (i.e., gonocytes) and express immunohistochemical markers such as placenta-like alkaline phosphatase (PLAP), KIT (the receptor for the stem cell factor KITLG), TAFP2C (formerly called AP2G), POU5F1 (formerly OCT 3/4), and NANOG.[386] Immunohistochemical detection of POU5F1 and KITLG represents particularly informative markers for CIS.[387]

The initiating events for neoplastic transformation from the CIS state are not known. Normal androgen production and action are required for germ cell maturation. Environmental chemicals acting as endocrine disruptors on the mother and developing fetus may disrupt germ cell maturation in a particular genetic background.[388] This theory aims to explain the increased incidence of testis tumors, which is often associated with abnormal spermatogenesis, undescended testes, and hypospadias. The prevalence of germ cell tumors among CAIS adults has been reported as 25% to 30%.[389] However, later estimates from larger numbers of affected individuals have been as low as 0.8% for CAIS and 5.5% for AIS overall.[23,390] Gonadectomy usually is performed in early adulthood, and some adults with CAIS decline gonadectomy.

Surgery in CAIS is confined to gonadectomy and perhaps to vaginoplasty procedures. Laparoscopic procedures are routine for removal of intra-abdominal testes. Those in the inguinal region can be removed during herniorrhaphy or by a laparoscopy-assisted transinguinal approach. The vagina in CAIS ends blindly and is shortened. The regular use of graded vaginal dilators during adolescence usually is successful.[391] The prepubertal girl with CAIS requires an examination under anesthesia at puberty to evaluate the vaginal anatomy.

The early management of PAIS centers on gender assignment and the subsequent plan and timing for surgery. The phenotypic heterogeneity seen in PAIS has been emphasized; most PAIS infants are raised male. Surgical procedures required include orchidopexy, chordee correction, and urethral reconstruction for the hypospadias. In some cases, several procedures implemented into adult life are required before full penile reconstruction is successful. Large doses of androgen may be required to promote phallic growth; the results of functional studies of any mutant AR that has been identified can be a useful predictor of the likely response. An approach involving high-content analysis of AR function at the cellular level by multiple assays has been proposed as a means to target androgen pharmacotherapy according to the type of AR mutation.[392] In practice, a course of androgen injections in early infancy is often used to assess androgen responsiveness. A monthly course of three 25-mg intramuscular injections of Sustanon (mixture of testosterone esters) is a common protocol. It is important to quantify the response, and an androgenization score, which takes account of penis size, testis position, and site of urethral orifice, is reliable and simple to apply.[393]

The risk of germ cell tumor of the testis is 15% or greater in patients with PAIS if the gonad is nonscrotal in position.[394] A patient with PAIS who is raised male should have careful monitoring of scrotal testes. It is recommended that a biopsy be performed at puberty. If CIS is diagnosed, there is debate about whether the contralateral testis should be biopsied. Unilateral CIS is treated by gonadectomy; bilateral CIS, which is rare, is managed with local low-dose radiotherapy, which effectively eradicates CIS.[395] Regular self-examination and testicular ultrasonography to screen for microliths is also recommended.[396]

The management of PAIS is complicated by the low incidence of proven *AR* mutations in cases that meet the phenotypic criteria consistent with incomplete resistance to androgens. In most reported series, which have included molecular analysis of the *AR* gene in a large number of cases, only about 25% of patients have a mutation in the coding region of the gene.[397,398] What causes the phenotype in most PAIS cases with a normal *AR* is not known, but there is a strong association between hypospadias and low birth weight linked to placental insufficiency, and the outcome of mutations in *NR5A1* may mimic PAIS in some cases.[84,399,400] Information on outcome in adult life for parameters such as physical health, sexual function, fertility, quality of life, and social participation is scanty for males with PAIS. Some were dissatisfied with their gender assignment and had major impairment in sexual function.[401-403]

Sex assignment in MAIS is male. Clinical presentation occurs in adolescence because of gynecomastia or for investigation of male factor infertility in adulthood. Reduction mammoplasty is required for the gynecomastia.

Counseling. AIS is an X-linked recessive condition; in 30% of cases, the mutation arises spontaneously. In cases with a PAIS phenotype, X linkage can be tested among family members by analysis of the CAG repeats. Even if a mutation has been identified, it is important to emphasize the phenotypic variability in the manifestation of a mutant receptor. An important component of counseling in AIS is disclosure of the diagnosis at an appropriate age and cognitive stage. Historically, the principles of beneficence (i.e., commitment by health care professionals to deliver care that provides the maximum benefit to the patient) and nonmaleficence (i.e., duty to avoid causing harm) were applied to AIS in the mistaken belief that nondisclosure of the diagnosis was the appropriate management.[404] Most clinicians now ensure that adults with AIS and the parents of affected children are fully informed about the condition and are apprised of the management options. Much of the enlightened change in practice has arisen from improved team networking with, and support from, advocacy groups.[405,406]

Other Conditions Affecting 46,XY Sex Development

Persistent Müllerian Duct Syndrome. AMH is a glycoprotein homodimer that is secreted by the Sertoli cells of the developing testes from approximately 7 weeks' post-conception. It acts through the AMH type 2 receptor (AMHR2) between 8 and 12 weeks' post-conception to cause regression of the Müllerian duct (see "Development of Reproductive Systems").[161,162]

AMH is encoded by a 2.75-kb gene containing five exons in the region of chromosome 19p13.3. The AMHR2 is a serine/threonine kinase with a single transmembrane domain that is encoded by an 11-exon gene on 12q13.[161] Exons 1 to 3 code for the signal sequence and the extracellular domain of the AMHR2, exon 4 codes for the transmembrane domain, and exons 5 through 11 code for the intracellular serine/threonine domain.

Persistent Müllerian duct syndrome (PMDS), also known as herniae uteri inguinale, is a condition in which 46,XY males have well-developed testes and normal male ducts and external genitalia but also have Müllerian duct derivatives. The diagnosis is often not made until a fallopian tube and uterus are encountered in patients undergoing inguinal hernia repair, orchiopexy, or abdominal surgery. Because of the trend for early surgical repair of an inguinal hernia or undescended testis, more cases are detected in infancy or early childhood. There are two anatomic forms. In the more prevalent form, a hernia contains a partially descended or scrotal testis, and the ipsilateral tube and uterus are in the hernia. In some instances, the contralateral testis and tube also are present in the hernial sac. The presence of transverse testicular ectopia should suggest PMDS. In the second form, the uterus, tubes, and testes are in the pelvis.

PMDS in normally differentiated males can result from failure of the testes to synthesize or secrete bioactive AMH or from a defect in the response of the duct to AMH because of an AMHR2 defect. Approximately one half of all genetically proven cases of PMDS result from defects in AMH, and half are caused by mutations in its receptor (Fig. 23-36).[407] *AMH* gene mutations are most commonly found in Mediterranean, Northern African, and Middle Eastern countries,[408] and most familial mutations are homozygous. In contrast, mutations in the gene encoding AMHR2 are more commonly found in France and Northern Europe and are often compound heterozygous mutations.[409] In an extensive study of 69 families with PMDS, 28 different mutations in the *AMH* gene were detected in 31 families (see Fig. 23-36).[407,408] Homozygous and compound heterozygous mutations were found in affected families, including splicing, missense, nonsense, and deletion mutations affecting the whole gene, but they mainly affected exon 1 and the 3[1] region of exon 5 (see Fig. 23-36). Deleterious mutations in *AMHR2* were detected in 27 families and included deletion, missense, and nonsense mutations (see Fig. 23-36). The most common mutation was a 27-bp deletion in exon 10.[410] No abnormality in *AMH* or *AMHR2* genes was detected in 11 families (16% of the total number). Measurement of serum AMH levels can provide a useful means for guiding genetic analysis; patients with PMDS caused by mutations of the *AMH* gene have low or undetectable levels of serum AMH, whereas AMH concentrations are often high normal or elevated in patients with mutations of *AMHR2*.

Treatment of PMDS includes an attempt to ensure fertility in males, which is a difficult issue because of the anatomic findings. Testicular differentiation and function are normal in these patients, but an increased prevalence of testicular degeneration has been described, which probably results from torsion of the testes. Anatomic abnormalities of the epididymis and the vas deferens are common. Infertility may result from late orchiopexy or from mechanical problems associated with entrapment of the vas deferens in the Müllerian derivatives. Early orchiopexy, proximal salpingectomy (leaving the epididymis attached to the fimbriae of the fallopian tube), dissection of the vas deferens from the lateral walls of the uterus, and a complete hysterectomy are recommended as a useful surgical approach. These structures can be left in place if there is risk of damage to the genital ducts. Men with high pelvic testes rarely have successful orchiopexy, and many of these individuals are androgen deficient.

Hypospadias. Hypospadias is incomplete fusion of the penile urethra defined by an arrest in development of the urethral spongiosum and ventral prepuce.[411] The normal embryologic correction of penile curvature is also interrupted. It is a common congenital anomaly, with an estimated birth prevalence of 3 to 4 cases per 1000 live births. Although it has been suggested that the rates of hypospadias have been increasing, this is not borne out in contemporaneous studies.[411-417] The cause is unknown in most cases, but it is assumed that there is an interplay of genetic and environmental factors.[418] Mutations in the *MAMLD1* gene on chromosome Xq28 cause hypospadias in a minority of cases.[146,419,420] Mutations in *HOXA13*, including expansion of polyalamine tracts, and in related fibroblast growth factors (FGFs) and bone morphogenetic proteins (BMPs) are found in the hand-foot-genital syndrome.[421-423] Hypospadias may also be a presenting

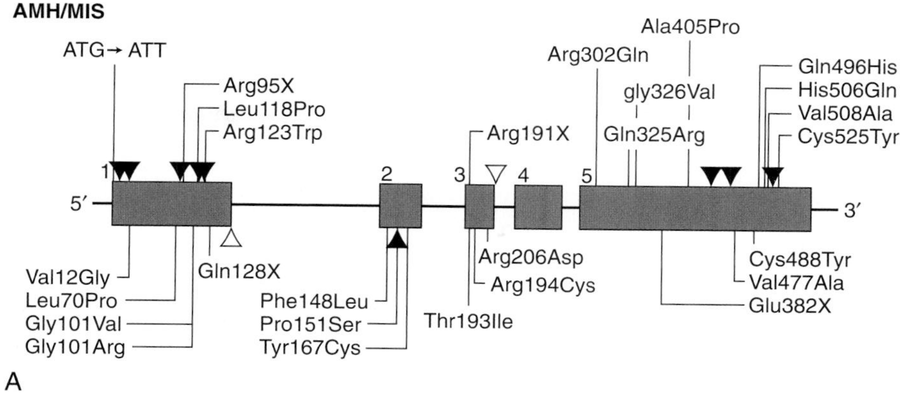

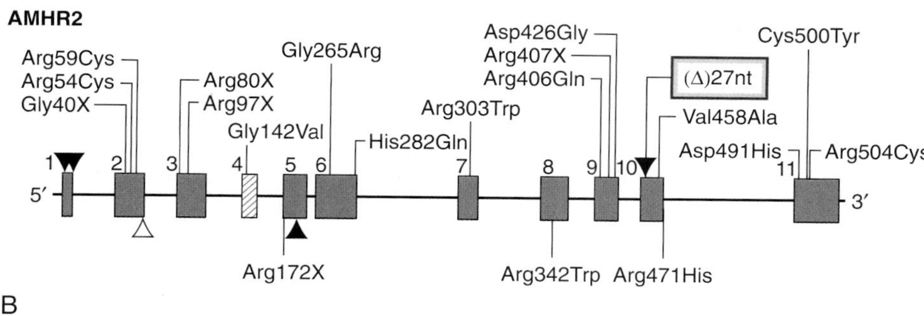

Figure 23-36 **A,** Diagram of the mutations in the anti-Müllerian hormone (AMH/MIS) gene that cause persistent Müllerian duct syndrome. The numbered *solid boxes* depict the exons. The three-letter abbreviations for amino acids are used to indicate the positions of missense mutations; X indicates a nonsense (stop) mutation; insertions and deletions resulting in frameshift and splice site mutations are shown by *solid triangles* and *open triangles*, respectively. **B,** Diagram of selected mutations in the gene for the AMH receptor type 2 *(AMHR2)*. The numbered *solid boxes* depict the exons. Exons 1 to 3 encode the extracellular domain of the receptor. Exon 4 *(diagonal lines)* encodes the transmembrane domain, and exons 5 through 11 encode the intracytoplasmic domain. Different forms of mutation are depicted, as in part A. The Δ27nt *(open box)* is a 27-nucleotide deletion, the most common *AMHR2* mutation causing the persistent Müllerian duct syndrome. (**A,** Redrawn from Imbeaud S, Carré Eusebe D, Rey R, et al. Molecular genetics of the persistent müllerian duct syndrome: a study of 19 families. *Hum Mol Genet.* 1994;3:125-131, with permission of Oxford University Press. **B,** Redrawn from Imbeaud S, Belville C, Messike-Zeitoun L, et al. A 27 base-pair deletion of the antimüllerian type II receptor gene is the most common cause of the persistent müllerian duct syndrome. *Hum Mol Genet.* 1996;5:1269-1277, with permission of Oxford University Press.)

feature of milder forms of disorders of testicular dysgenesis or steroidogenic defects (e.g., mutated NR5A1), especially if the penis is small or the testes undescended.[246] The prevalence of these conditions in isolated hypospadias is likely to be much lower. There is a familial clustering of cases in hypospadias, with a 7% incidence of one or more additional affected family members.[424]

Hypospadias is associated with increased maternal age, multiple births, maternal exposure to diethylstilbestrol in utero, paternal subfertility, maternal vegetarian diet, maternal smoking, assisted reproductive techniques, paternal exposure to pesticides, and fetal growth restriction.[425] The association with low birth weight is remarkably consistent across all studies of idiopathic hypospadias.[426,427]

Management is surgical. The urethral meatus is relocated to the glans, and the penis is straightened by correcting any chordee to give a normal, forward-directed urinary stream and the ability to have satisfactory sexual intercourse. Numerous techniques are described; repairs may require more than one stage, usually starting at 6 to 12 months of age. The true severity of the hypospadias may not be apparent until release of the chordee. Complications include fistula formation, meatal stenosis, urethral stricture, and residual chordee. Outcome data from large series are lacking, but there is evidence of satisfactory sexual function and cosmetic appearance after surgery.[428,429] Proximal hypospadias was associated with a lower maximum urinary flow outcome.

Anorchia and Cryptorchidism. The term *vanishing testis syndrome* was coined for the phenotype of bilateral anorchia in an otherwise normally developed male infant.[2] It recognizes the presence of normal testes in early gestation operating to induce Müllerian duct regression, stabilize Wolffian duct development, and differentiate male external genitalia. Any ambiguity of the external genitalia suggests a variant of the syndrome related to some form of XY gonadal dysgenesis. Bilateral anorchia with a normally differentiated but small phallus (micropenis) is also a recognized variant of the syndrome, and it may be represent a milder variant of testicular dysgenesis in some cases.[247] The cause of classic anorchia is unknown, but an interruption of the testis blood supply by a torsion or vascular occlusion event in utero has been proposed. Surgical exploration and histologic findings typically show testicular nubbins as remnants of gonads, which are associated with a vas deferens in most patients and with some epididymal tissue. The presence of hemosiderin-laden macrophages and dystrophic calcification is consistent with the vascular accident hypothesis in some cases.

The diagnosis of complete anorchia is based on a combination of biochemical tests, imaging studies, and surgical exploration. An undetectable serum AMH level is a reliable marker when evaluating infants with nonpalpable gonads. This, coupled with elevated serum levels of gonadotropins and no testosterone response to hCG stimulation, predicts the absence of testes. A low inhibin B level is also supportive, although levels normally fall during childhood (see Fig. 23-16). Imaging with CT or MRI may be useful before laparoscopy. Most centers undertake surgical exploration to remove testicular remnants even though usually no evidence of malignancy is found. The procedure can be deferred until the time of insertion of prostheses.

Testes that have not descended at birth (i.e., cryptorchidism) is the most common congenital abnormality in boys, affecting 2% to 4% of term infants.[173,430] There are geographic differences in prevalence, with the rate as high as 9% in Denmark and as low as 2.4% in Finland.[431] There is epidemiologic evidence of an increasing prevalence to 6% in populations studied in the United Kingdom.[432] Longitudinal studies demonstrated the expected decline in prevalence in early infancy to 2.4% but a subsequent rise to 7% by 2 years of age.

Ascending testis or acquired cryptorchidism is common and accounts for more than one half of cases of undescended testes seen in childhood.[433] The strong association with low birth weight is well recognized, as are disorders of the pituitary-gonadal axis such as HH and the AIS. These observations are consistent with the role of androgens in the inguinoscrotal phase of testis descent. The first phase of transabdominal migration is under the control of INSL3, which is produced by Leydig cells.[174] Mutations in *INSL3* and the gene for its receptor, *RXFP2,* are found in a very small proportion of boys with cryptorchidism.[434] Higher exposure to persistent endocrine-disrupting chemicals has been found in cryptorchid boys based on analyses of breast milk samples as a proxy for fetal exposure.[435]

Environmental Chemicals. The proposed increase in male reproductive tract disorders (testis cancer, abnormal spermatogenesis, cryptorchidism, and hypospadias) led to the concept that testicular dysgenesis syndrome (TDS) of fetal origin might be triggered by lifestyle factors and exposure to endocrine-disrupting chemicals operating during the fetal and perinatal periods.[436] The clearest evidence that certain chemicals such as herbicides, fungicides, bisphenol A, and phthalates can act as endocrine disruptors is derived from observations of wildlife and laboratory animal experiments. It remains uncertain whether there is a new and emerging public health problem.[437]

Not all components of the quartet of male reproductive disorders can be assigned to TDS, particularly for cases of isolated hypospadias and men with solely impaired sperm quality.[438] It has been questioned on epidemiologic grounds whether the TDS exists at all.[439] Direct evidence of toxic effects in humans has not been established. The anogenital distance in newborn rodents is a sensitive index after maternal exposure to androgens and antiandrogens. Data on this anthropometric measure are available from normal male infants studied longitudinally from birth to 2 years of age.[440] A preliminary study reported reduced anogenital distance in male infants related to prenatal phthalate exposure.[441] The U.S. Environmental Protection Agency (EPA) has recommended measurement of anogenital distance as one of the markers in reproductive toxicity studies in humans.[442]

The relevance of these epidemiologic and experimental findings to the assessment of an individual case of DSD remains uncertain.[443] Major programs of research such as the Cluster of Research into Endocrine Disruption in Europe (CREDO) supported by the European Commission and the endocrine-disrupting chemicals research program of the EPA are being conducted to determine the risks posed to human health by environmental chemicals. The maxim that exposure to chemicals should be reduced to as low a level as is reasonably practicable seems to be a sensible precautionary approach while further data are being gathered in humans.

46,XX Disorders of Sex Development

46,XX DSDs can be divided into disorders of ovary development, disorders of androgen synthesis, and other conditions affecting sex development (see Table 23-3).

Disorders of Ovary Development

Disorders of ovary development (i.e., ovarian dysgenesis or resistance) do not usually manifest until puberty, when a failure of estrogenization becomes apparent. In contrast, several well-defined but poorly understood disorders of gonadal development can result in a 46,XX individual with an ovary containing testicular tissue (i.e., 46,XX ovotesticular DSD) or even the development of a testis capable of producing enough androgen for a male phenotype and sufficient AMH to regress the uterus (i.e., 46,XX testicular DSD).

Ovarian Dysgenesis. Ovarian dysgenesis is most frequently seen in association with sex chromosome aneuploidy (e.g., Turner syndrome; 45,X and variants) when progressive ovarian apoptosis is evident. Ovarian resistance results from mutations in the FSH receptor and manifests at puberty.[207] Ovarian dysfunction can also occur with a wide range of multisystem syndromes, often involving DNA-repair mechanisms (e.g., Perrault, Maximilian, Quayle and Copeland, Pober, Malouf, Nijmegen, Cockayne, Rothmund-Thompson, Werner syndromes; ataxia telangiectasia).[153] Several nonmetabolic causes of POI or POF have been described,[43-51] including POF1, Xq26-q28, *FMR* premutations; POF2A, Xq22, *DIAPH2;* POF2B, Xq21, POF1B [actin-binding protein]*;* POF3, 3q22, *FOXL2;* POF4, Xp11.2, *BMP15*; POF5, 7q35, *NOBOX*; also 9q33, *NR5A1*), as well as mitochondrial disorders such as mutations in POLG.[444] Although these conditions usually manifest with POI and early menopause, more severe forms of some of these disorders can interfere with earlier aspects of ovarian development and function and can manifest with absent puberty.

46,XX Ovotesticular and 46,XX Testicular Disorders of Sex Development. In rare conditions, the developing ovary may contain an element of testicular tissue (i.e., 46,XX ovotesticular DSD) or may even develop as a functioning testis (i.e., 46,XX testicular DSD). In 46,XX ovotesticular DSD, the patient usually presents with ambiguous genitalia at birth and progressive virilization at puberty if the gonad is not removed. In contrast, 46,XX testicular DSD is usually associated with a normal male phenotype and absence of Müllerian structures. However, the testis is not capable of supporting spermatogenesis because crucial genes on the Y chromosome are absent.

A detailed review of the presentation, endocrinology, and management of 46,XX ovotesticular DSD was given earlier (see "Sex Chromosome Disorders of Sex Development") because many of the issues faced are similar to those with 46,XX/46,XY chimerism. However, a 46,XX karyotype is the most frequent finding in ovotesticular DSD, especially in patients from sub-Saharan Africa.[238]

Familial cases have been described, and it is likely that a genetic basis exists in some cases, although the exact cause is unknown. Translocation of a testis-determining gene (e.g., *SRY, SOX9*) has been found in rare cases.[131] Partial dysfunction of the ovarian-testis repressor gene *RSPO1* has been described.[239]

Patients with 46,XX testicular DSD often present first with male factor infertility. In some cases, a family history is present. Because different family members can have different phenotypes, it is possible that 46,XX testicular DSD represents the most severe end of the spectrum of ovarian transdifferentiation phenotypes. Up to 80% of 46,XX males harbor translocations of Y-chromosomal material containing SRY, the testis-determining factor.[27,101] This finding helped considerably in mapping the *SRY* gene in the first instance (see "Development of Reproductive Systems"), and in some situations, residual ovarian tissue (ovotestis) develops. Individuals with *SRY* translocations can be diagnosed by FISH analysis using a probe directed to that gene (see Fig. 23-3). A number of *SRY*-negative cases have been reported. Loss-of-function mutations in *RSPO1* (an ovarian gene encoding Respondin 1) have been reported in individuals with 46,XX testicular DSD with palmar-plantar hyperkeratosis and squamous cell carcinoma.[15] This factor, which mediates the WNT4 signaling pathway, was the first ovarian-specific repressor of testis development to be described. Loss of function of Respondin 1 in the developing gonad of 46,XX individuals results in testis development and an infertile male phenotype. It is likely that additional factors may act as repressors of SRY and testis determination. Severe disruption of WNT4 can result in 46,XX sex reversal as part of the SERKAL syndrome, which consists of female-to-male sex reversal and renal, adrenal, and lung dysgenesis.[445]

Disorders of Androgen Excess

The steroid biosynthetic disorders causing androgen excess and 46,XX DSD are summarized in Table 23-6. Although CYP21 deficiency is by far the most common form of this condition, alternative diagnoses should be considered because approaches to counseling and management may vary.

3β-Hydroxysteroid Dehydrogenase Type 2 Deficiency. 3β-HSD/$\Delta^{4,5}$-isomerase catalyzes the conversion of Δ^5-steroids to Δ^4-steroids and is required for the generation of mineralocorticoids, glucocorticoids, and more potent androgens (e.g., testosterone, DHT) by the adrenal glands and gonads (see Fig. 23-11). The actions of 3β-HSD and the consequences of deficiency of the type 2 enzyme (HSD3B2) were described earlier, because this deficiency results in adrenal insufficiency with variable defects in androgenization of the developing male fetus.

Defects in HSD3B2 also manifest in 46,XX females. Severe, recessively inherited defects in enzyme function can cause mild clitoral enlargement at birth in girls with glucocorticoid deficiency (with or without salt loss). This mild androgenization occurs not as a direct androgenic effect of the excess DHEA but as a result of its conversion and that of other Δ^5-3β-hydroxy-C19-steroids to testosterone by HSD3B1 in the placenta and in the peripheral tissues of the fetus. This conversion, coupled with the limited capacity of the placenta to aromatize androgens to estrogens early in gestation, can increase circulating levels of androgens in the female fetus and cause modest clitoromegaly in a minority of patients. Milder, nonclassic forms of HSD3B2 deficiency can cause premature pubarche in girls. Breast development can occur at puberty in affected females, presumably by peripheral conversions of Δ^5-C19 steroids to Δ^4-C19 steroids by HSD3B1 expressed principally in peripheral tissues and by the subsequent aromatization of androgens to estrogens. The presence of menses has been reported in treated females with this condition.

The diagnosis of HSD3B2 deficiency can be challenging in nonclassic forms of this condition.[288] The levels of Δ^5-steroids (e.g., 17-hydroxypregnenolone, DHEA, and its sulfate, DHEAS) usually are increased, and the ratio of Δ^5-steroids to Δ^4-steroids (e.g., the ratio of 17-OHP to cortisol) is markedly increased, especially after stimulation with intravenous ACTH. The urinary steroid profile can also be informative, because 17-ketosteroids and especially DHEAS and 16-hydroxy-DHEAS are elevated. Basal plasma concentrations of 17-OHP can be increased as a result of peripheral conversion of Δ^5-17-hydroxypregnenolone to 17-OHP by the type 1 enzyme. This finding may lead to confusion with alternative forms of CAH, such as CYP21 deficiency or POR deficiency. Mild forms of HSD3B2 deficiency may manifest in a fashion similar to that of virilizing adrenal tumors. Suppression of the increased plasma and urinary levels of C19 and C21 3β-hydroxysteroids by glucocorticoids distinguishes 3β-HSD deficiency in such cases. Treatment for 3β-HSD deficiency is glucocorticoid, mineralocorticoid, and salt supplementation, as appropriate, and estrogen replacement to induce puberty.

21-Hydroxylase Deficiency. In the context of DSD, CYP21 deficiency (see Fig. 23-11) is the most common cause of ambiguous genitalia of the newborn. It is primarily a disorder of adrenal steroidogenesis (see Chapter 15).

A female fetus with CYP21 deficiency can become androgenized to various degrees, as illustrated by the Prader classification (Fig. 23-37). The fact that CYP21 deficiency can androgenize a female sufficiently to result in a male phenotype at birth (with nonpalpable testes) is indicative of exposure to extremely high circulating concentrations of androgens. Serum concentrations of testosterone are invariably within the adult male range and sometimes higher in CAH caused by CYP21 deficiency. Androgenization can be prevented if dexamethasone is administered to the mother early enough in gestation, indicating an intact fetal pituitary-adrenal axis that is responsive to negative-feedback regulation. This model is based on studies of human fetal adrenal explants that synthesize cortisol, androstenedione, and testosterone under ACTH regulation, which is subject to negative feedback by glucocorticoids.[172] The route to increased adrenal production may be through the backdoor pathway to androgen synthesis.[170,171] Nevertheless, high fetal concentrations of 17-OHP, androstenedione, and testosterone are the hallmark of androgenization in CAH due to CYP21 deficiency. More than 75% of patients are also salt losers because of their inability to synthesize sufficient mineralocorticoids. The two forms are readily explained by the nature of the mutation, which affects the *CYP21* gene on chromosome 6p21.3. The concordance

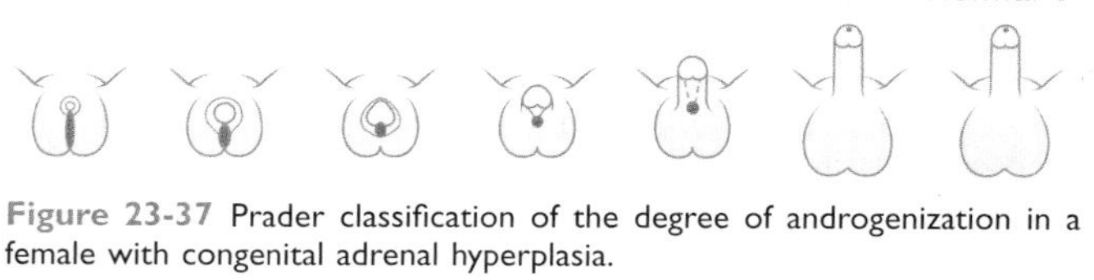

Figure 23-37 Prader classification of the degree of androgenization in a female with congenital adrenal hyperplasia.

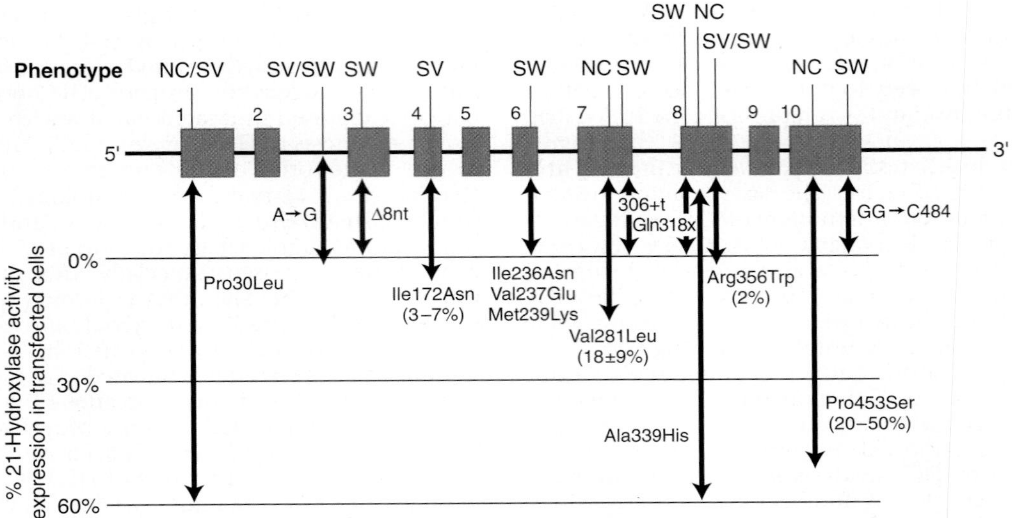

Figure 23-38 Diagram of the *CYP21* gene and locations of the mutations that cause more than 90% of cases of 21-hydroxylase deficiency. The numbered boxes depict the exons. The three-letter abbreviations for amino acids are used; X indicates a nonsense (stop) mutation. An adenine (A) to guanine (G) transition in intron 2 causes a common splice site mutation. Other mutations include an 8-nucleotide deletion (Δnt) in exon 3, a thymidine insertion at codon 306 (306+T), and a guanine (G) to cytosine (C) transition at codon 484. The activities of the mutant enzymes, expressed as a percentage of the wild type, are indicated on the vertical axis and in parentheses for some missense mutations. NC, nonclassic form; SV, simple virilizing; SW, salt wasting.

between genotype and phenotype for the single-gene disorder is remarkably precise (Fig. 23-38). In patients who are compound heterozygotes, the phenotype usually is concordant with the milder allele. More than 90% of cases result from *CYP21* deletion or one of nine mutations derived from the nonfunctional pseudogene *CYP21P* (see Fig. 23-38). About 5% of *CYP21* mutations arise spontaneously.[446] Worldwide, almost 100 non–pseudogene-derived mutations are reported for the *CYP21A2* allele.

The diagnosis of CYP21 deficiency in a newborn with ambiguous genitalia is readily confirmed by markedly elevated serum 17-OHP concentrations (>300 nmol/L) after the first 48 hours. Sick, preterm infants can have moderately increased steroid levels, so ACTH stimulation may be needed to resolve any diagnostic confusion. The affected male usually has no alerting clinical signs at birth and, if a salt loser, does not decompensate with hypokalemia, hyperkalemia, and weight loss until 1 to 2 weeks after birth. Newborn screening programs to measure blood spot 17-OHP concentrations soon after birth have been introduced in some countries.[447,448]

Of major relevance to DSD is the potential to prevent ambiguous genitalia of the newborn through prenatal treatment with dexamethasone.[449] Treatment is effective if dexamethasone is started by 6 to 7 weeks' gestation. However, in current practice, karyotype analysis and *CYP21* genotype analysis is not available until approximately 5 weeks later. Seven unaffected or male fetuses would need to be treated with dexamethasone during this initial period for every one affected female fetus who might benefit.

Several concerns have been raised about the potential effects of dexamethasone on the developing fetus. Although no apparent somatic abnormalities have been observed in fetuses treated with dexamethasone to term and monitored through infancy and early childhood, and cognitive and motor development based on questionnaires appeared not to be adversely affected by exposure to dexamethasone, direct examination of 26 children who had been exposed to dexamethasone from gestational age 6 to 7 weeks did show adverse effects on verbal working memory compared with controls.[450-453] All of these studies were observational, and a meta-analysis emphasized the paucity of good-quality, long-term follow-up data to inform a risk/benefit analysis.[454] This aspect should be considered when counseling families about prenatal treatment. Clinical practice guidelines have suggested that prenatal therapy should be undertaken using protocols approved by institutional review boards and at centers capable of collecting long-term outcome data as part of multicenter studies.[455] Analysis of free fetal DNA in maternal blood for fetal sex determination using real-time quantitative polymerase chain reaction (PCR) techniques appears to be reliable at a median gestational age of 9 weeks.[456] This would allow some reduction in unnecessary exposure to dexamethasone in male fetuses. It may be possible to reduce the dose of dexamethasone used later in gestation without altering efficacy,[172,455] but significantly more research and long-term follow-up data are needed.

P450 Oxidoreductase Deficiency. POR is a membrane-bound flavoprotein that plays a central role in electron transfer from NADPH to all microsomal P450 enzymes, including CYP17, CYP21, and CYP19 (aromatase) (see Fig. 23-27). Defects in POR can cause apparent combined CYP17 and CYP21 deficiency, with or without Antley-Bixler syndrome, a form of craniosynostosis. These conditions were described earlier (see "Disorders of Androgen Synthesis").[170,305-308] POR deficiency can be associated with ambiguous genitalia in both 46,XX and 46,XY infants. The androgenization of 46,XX fetuses may result from a defect in aromatase activity or occur through a proposed backdoor pathway of DHT production that does not involve androstenedione or testosterone as intermediates.[170,171] Children with this condition usually have cortisol deficiency, but mineralocorticoid function is relatively preserved.

11β-Hydroxylase Deficiency. 11β-Hydroxylase (CYP11B1) deficiency is a disorder of adrenal steroidogenesis. It can profoundly androgenize an affected female fetus and accounts for 5% to 8% of patients with CAH; there is a clustering of cases among Moroccan Jews. Apart from causing ambiguous genitalia in the newborn, 11β-hydroxylase deficiency manifests later with hypertension. Accumulation of 11-deoxycorticosterone leads to salt and fluid retention, and plasma renin is suppressed.

11β-Hydroxylase is encoded by the *CYP11B1* gene, which is located on chromosome 8q21-22 in tandem with *CYP11B2,* which encodes aldosterone synthase, the enzyme catalyzing the conversion of deoxycorticosterone to corticosterone and then to aldosterone.[457] Some *CYP11B1* mutations that cause 11β-hydroxylase deficiency are shown in Figure 23-38. Fifty-three mutations are listed in the Human Gene Mutation Database at the Institute of Medical Genetics at Cardiff University, and most are missense mutations. Arg448 appears to be a relative hot spot for mutations, with Arg448His possibly a founder mutation in the Moroccan Jewish population. A null mouse model of 11β-hydroxylase deficiency showed the expected phenotype of glucocorticoid deficiency, mineralocorticoid excess, hyperplastic adrenals, hypertension, and hypokalaemia.[458] However, affected female mice were not virilized because rodent adrenals do not synthesize androgens.

Familial Glucocorticoid Resistance. Glucocorticoid resistance is a rare disorder that is usually caused by sporadic heterozygous mutations in the glucocorticoid receptor α-isoform (GRα).[459] Partial end-organ insensitivity to glucocorticoid action coupled with impaired feedback mechanisms results in excess ACTH secretion and elevated circulating cortisol levels without the clinical features of Cushing's syndrome. In many cases, elevated levels of mineralocorticoids cause hypertension and hypokalemia, and elevated levels of adrenal androgens cause hirsutism and acne.

Most GRα mutations are heterozygous changes that cause a partial loss of function through altering ligand binding, nuclear localization, coactivator interactions, and target gene transcription, often with some degree of dominant negative activity. Complete loss of the GRα gene (*NR3C1*) is lethal in mice, and one case of complete glucocorticoid resistance has been described in a male infant with profound hypoglycemia and hypertension. One homozygous *NR3C1* mutation (Val571Ala) was reported in a Brazilian girl who had a large clitoris, posterior labioscrotal fusion, and a urogenital sinus at birth.[460] This mutation caused marked reduction in GRα function without complete loss of receptor activity. She also harbored a heterozygous mutation in *CYP21.* More severe GRα mutations may manifest as mild 46,XX DSD, although the phenotype might have been modified in this case by the coexistence of a heterozygous CYP21 change.

Aromatase Deficiency. Aromatase (CYP19A1), formerly called estrogen synthetase, is the only cytochrome P450 enzyme known to catalyze the conversion of androgens (C19 steroids) to estrogens (C18 steroids) in vertebrate species.[461] Aromatase is expressed in many tissues, including the placenta, ovary, brain, bone, vascular endothelium, breast, and adipose tissue, where it is regulated by a number of tissue-specific promoters to convert testosterone to estradiol and androstenedione to estrone (Fig. 23-39). Aromatase plays a crucial role in the local production of estrogens and in the synthesis of circulating estrogens from the ovary at the time of puberty.

Aromatase deficiency due to recessively inherited mutations in *CYP19* has been described in approximately 13 girls with 46,XX DSD (see Fig. 23-40). The clinical and biochemical features of this condition underscore the key role aromatase plays in the fetoplacental unit, and this condition is sometimes referred to as *placental aromatase deficiency.* Aromatase plays a critical role in protecting the fetus from excessive androgen exposure in utero (Fig. 23-41). In the absence of aromatase, estrogen cannot be synthesized by the placenta, and large quantities of placental testosterone and androstenedione are transferred to the fetal and maternal circulation, resulting in androgenization of the female fetus and virilization of the mother during pregnancy.[462]

Females (46,XX) with aromatase insufficiency are born with clitoromegaly, various degrees of posterior fusion, scrotalization of the labioscrotal folds, and, in some infants with a urogenital sinus, a single perineal orifice.[463-465] There is often a striking history of maternal virilization after the second trimester of pregnancy (e.g., acne, hair growth, voice changes) coupled with elevated maternal androgen levels, which usually resolve after the infant is born. As expected for a steroidogenic defect, affected girls (46,XX) have normal Müllerian structures. The histology of the ovaries in infancy is normal, but under increased FSH

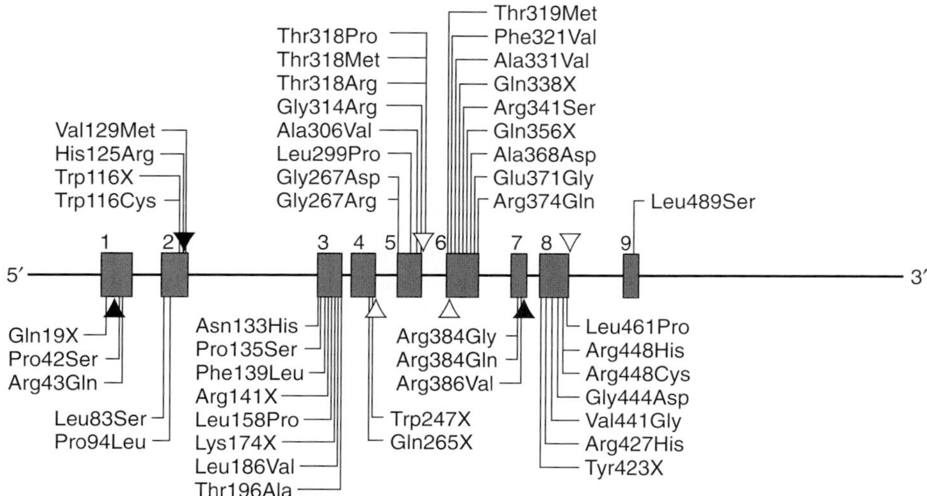

Figure 23-39 Diagram of the *CYP11B1* gene and locations of the mutations causing 11β-hydroxylase deficiency. The numbered solid boxes depict the exons. The three-letter abbreviations for amino acids are used; X indicates a nonsense (stop) mutation. A deletion of cytosine (C) at codon 32 and the addition of two nucleotides at codon 394 cause frameshift mutations; insertions and deletions resulting in a frameshift and splice site are shown by *solid triangles* and *open triangles*, respectively.

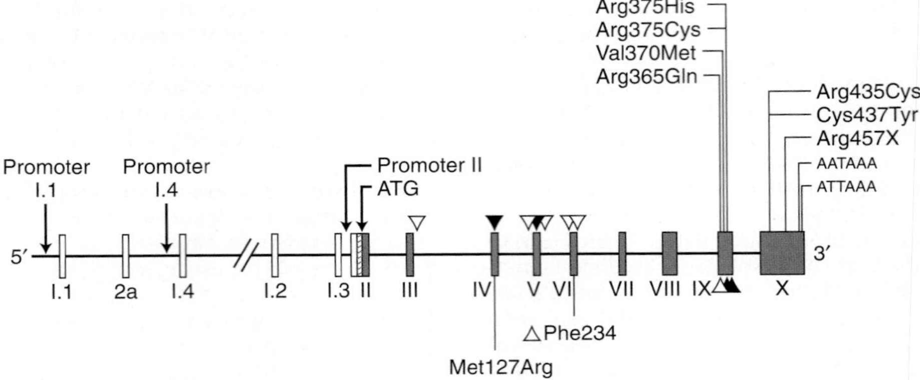

Figure 23-40 Diagram of the *CYP19* gene and selected mutations causing aromatase deficiency. The numbered *solid boxes* represent translated exons. The septum in the *open box* in exon II represents the 3′ acceptor splice junction for the untranslated exons. Multiple alternative promoters and the untranslated exons *(open boxes)* are indicated. The three-letter abbreviations for amino acids are used to indicate the positions of missense mutations; X indicates a nonsense (stop) mutation; insertions and deletions resulting in frameshift and splice site mutations are shown by *solid triangles* and *open triangles*, respectively. In addition to the mutations causing classic aromatase deficiency, a homozygous Arg435Cys mutation and deletion of a phenylalanine residue at position 234 are both associated with a partial aromatase insufficiency phenotype. (Modified from Morishima A, Grumbach MM, Simpson ER, et al. Aromatase deficiency in male and female siblings caused by a novel mutation and the physiological role of estrogens. *J Clin Endocrinol Metab.* 1995;80:3689-3698, with permission of The Endocrine Society, copyright 1995.)

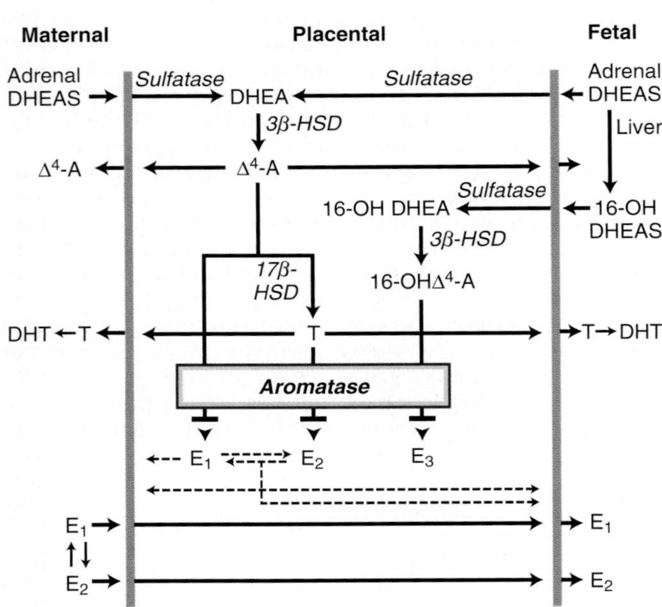

Figure 23-41 Aromatase plays a crucial role in protecting the fetus from excessive androgen exposure in utero. The placenta lacks CYP17 enzymatic activity and cannot convert C21 steroids such as progesterone to C19 steroids and thereafter to estrogens. During gestation, large quantities of dehydroepiandrosterone sulfate (DHEAS) are produced in the fetal and maternal adrenal glands. DHEAS is 16α-hydroxylated in the fetal adrenal and liver. The 16α-hydroxy-DHEAS from the fetus and DHEAS from the fetus and mother are transferred to the placental unit, where the sulfate moiety is cleaved by placental sulfatase. These steroids can then be converted to androstenedione (A) and 16α-hydroxyandrostenedione by 3β-hydroxysteroid dehydrogenase (HSD) type I/$\Delta^{4,5}$-isomerase; to testosterone and 16α-hydroxytestosterone by 17β-HSD; and to estrogens (mainly estriol from 16α-hydroxy-DHEA) by placental aromatase. Androstenedione and 16α-hydroxyandrostenedione may be aromatized directly to estrogens. DHT, dihydrotestosterone; E_1, estrone; E_2, estradiol; E_3, estriol; T, testosterone. (Modified and redrawn from Conte FA, Grumbach MM, Ito Y, et al. A syndrome of female pseudohermaphrodism, hypergonadotropic hypogonadism, and multicystic ovaries associated with missense mutations in the gene encoding aromatase ($P450_{arom}$). *J Clin Endocrinol Metab.* 1994;78:1287-1292, with permission of The Endocrine Society, copyright 1994.)

stimulation in the absence of ovarian aromatase, multiple, enlarged follicular cysts develop. At puberty, affected females have hypergonadotropic hypogonadism, typically fail to develop female secondary sexual characteristics, and exhibit progressive virilization. Plasma androstenedione and testosterone levels are elevated, and estrone and estradiol levels are low or not measurable. The ovaries enlarge and develop multiple cysts at puberty; in one affected female, polycystic ovaries were detected in infancy. The hypergonadotropism and the multiple ovarian cysts respond to estrogen replacement therapy, but in some cases, temporary treatment with an antiandrogen is necessary.[466]

In addition to a role in the reproductive axis, aromatase deficiency has implications for bone development, metabolism, and immune function, as determined by the long-term follow-up of the small numbers of women (46,XX) and men (46,XY) with aromatase deficiency and by studies of aromatase-knockout mice.[461] Males present only after puberty and have tall stature, delayed bone maturation and epiphyseal fusion, and osteopenia, suggesting that estrogens are essential for the prevention of osteoporosis in males and females and for normal skeletal maturation and proportions.[467] This phenotype is similar to that of a man with an inactivating estrogen receptor-α mutation.[468] Hyperinsulinemia and abnormal plasma lipids have also been reported in aromatase deficiency, which may in part reflect estrogen insufficiency but may also reflect specific actions of aromatase itself. The finding of apparently normal psychosexual development in the three aromatase-deficient adolescent or adult patients and in the man with an estrogen receptor defect suggests that estrogen does not play a critical role in sex differentiation of the human brain, as has been reported in nonprimate mammals.

Approximately 18 *CYP19A1* mutations have been described in males and females with aromatase deficiency (see Fig. 23-40). These changes are inherited in a recessive fashion and are present in a homozygous or compound heterozygous state. Functional assays of aromatase activity have shown severe loss of enzyme function (approximately 0.3%) in all cases associated with classic aromatase deficiency, other than approximately 1% activity for the Arg-435Cys change found in a compound heterozygte together with the null Cys437Tyr mutation.[464] Although this patient had a classic presentation at birth, maternal virilization during pregnancy was reportedly absent. A homozygous Arg435Cys change has been reported in a girl who presented with androgenized genitalia at birth but showed limited breast development during puberty.[469] Deletion of a single phenylalanine residue (Phe234del) causing partial loss of aromatase activity was described in an androgenized 46,XX individual who showed significant breast development (Tanner stage 4) during puberty.[469]

A spectrum of phenotypes may be seen with aromatase insufficiency in humans. This important diagnosis should be considered in all androgenized 46,XX infants when more common forms of CAH (e.g., CYP21 deficiency) have been excluded. A history of maternal virilization in pregnancy should always be sought, and increased levels of Δ^4-androstenedione, testosterone, and DHT and low levels of plasma estriol, urinary estriol, and amniotic fluid estrone, estradiol, and estriol may be detected.

Maternal Androgen Excess. Maternal sources of androgens that may virilize a female fetus may be endogenous from adrenal and ovarian tumors or exogenous from maternal ingestion of androgenic compounds. Danazol, a synthetic derivative of ethisterone with androgenic, antiestrogenic, and antiprogestogenic activities, is used in diverse conditions such as endometriosis, benign fibrocystic breast disease, and hereditary angioedema and in women with unexplained subfertility. It crosses the placenta and is contraindicated in pregnancy in view of reports that a female fetus may become androgenized.[470] Ovarian causes of virilization include primary malignancy, benign lesions such as luteoma and hyperreactio luteinalis, and polycystic ovary syndrome. Recurrence in subsequent pregnancies and maternal virilization can occur with luteomas.[471] As in fetal aromatase deficiency, a similar pattern of recurrent hyperandrogenization without evidence of placental aromatase deficiency has been reported.[472]

Other Conditions Affecting 46,XX Sex Development

Several syndromic associations can cause developmental genital abnormalities in 46,XX females, although these are less common than the syndromic associations resulting in underandrogenization in 46,XY males. Complex urogenital anomalies such as cloacal extrophy can affect both sexes and require major reconstructive surgery for bladder and bowel function and for the lower genital system.

Abnormalities in uterine development can result in bicornate uterus (i.e., Fryns syndrome), uterine hemiagenesis or hypoplasia, or uterine agenesis. These conditions can be associated with renal, cardiac, and cervical spinal abnormalities as part of Mayer-Rokitansky-Küster-Hauser (MRKH) syndrome or MURCS (Müllerian, renal, and cervical spine syndrome).[473] The cause of these conditions is unknown for most women, although some familial cases have been described, and a mutation in *WNT4* was reported in a patient with absent Müllerian structures (uterus and upper vagina), unilateral renal agenesis, and mild hyperandrogenemia.[474] Uterine abnormalities have also been associated with maturity-onset diabetes of the young type 5 (MODY5, *HNF1B*) and with vaginal abnormalities in patients with hand-foot-genital syndrome *(HOXA13)* and McKusick-Kaufman syndrome (*MKKS*, formerly called *BBS6*). Because a prominent clitoris can be associated with conditions such as Fraser syndrome or neurofibromatosis, careful evaluation is necessary before a hyperandrogenic cause is diagnosed.

Other common conditions that may be mistaken for a more serious underlying disorder include apparent clitoromegaly seen in premature or former premature babies or when little labial adipose tissue is present. Assessment by a surgeon or physician with experience of normal variability in clitoral size is important. Labial adhesions are a common finding in female newborns. They often resolve spontaneously, although estrogen cream can be used to accelerate the process. Transient menstrual bleeding during the first week of life can be seen frequently in female infants with the withdrawal of large amounts of estrogens and progesterones after birth. This finding can be alarming for parents, but it rapidly resolves, and no treatment is needed.

INVESTIGATION AND MANAGEMENT OF DISORDERS OF SEX DEVELOPMENT

The general principles of the approach to the management of DSD apply regardless of the underlying diagnosis. In the case of presentation in the newborn period, the prototypical example of DSD is ambiguous genitalia for which instantaneous sex assignment is not possible. Although final assignment will be delayed pending the results of investigations, the principle applies that all infants should be designated as male or female. DSD presentations in the newborn period may be less overtly ambiguous when there is less doubt about the sex, but there is significant undermasculinization of a male infant or masculinization of a female infant. An apparent male with nonpalpable testes (possible CAH) or an apparent female with inguinal hernias (possible CAIS or 17β-HSD deficiency) also should be investigated. A family history of DSD or a mismatch between prenatal genotype and the birth phenotype should prompt investigation. Problems in infants that merit investigation are listed in Table 23-19.

It is debatable whether deviation from the genital anatomy of the typical male or female, estimated to occur in 1.7% of live births, should be a guide for investigation. More realistic evidence suggests that some form of genital anomaly at birth may have a prevalence as high as 1 in 300,[475] whereas ambiguity of the external genitalia has a prevalence of approximately 1 in 5000 births.[476] Against such a background, it is useful to provide reference to normative data on measurements of the genitalia in infants (Table 23-20) and to methods to assess the degree of external virilization in CAH (Fig. 23-37) or as an external masculinization score[393] (Fig. 23-42). The latter system has the merit of providing a quantitative score for four

TABLE 23-19

Problems in Newborns That Merit Investigation for DSDs

Ambiguous genitalia
Apparent female genitalia
- Enlarged clitoris
- Posterior labial fusion
- Inguinal/labial mass

Apparent male genitalia
- Nonpalpable testes
- Isolated perineoscrotal hypospadias
- Severe hypospadias, undescended testes, micropenis

Family history of DSD, such as complete AIS
Discordance between genital appearance and prenatal karyotype

AIS, androgen insensitivity syndrome; DSD, disorders of sex development.

TABLE 23-20

Anthropometric Measurements of the External Genitalia (Mean ± SD)

Population	Age	Stretched Penile Length (cm) or Clitoral Length	Penile Width (cm) or Clitoral Width	Testicular Volume (mL) or Perineum Length
Males				
USA	30 wk GA	2.5 ± 0.4		
USA	Full term	3.5 ± 0.4	1.1 ± 0.1	0.52 (median)
Japan	Term to 14 yr	2.9 ± 0.4 to 8.3 ± 0.8		
Australia	24 to 36 wk GA	2.27 + (0.16 GA)		
Chinese	Term	3.1 ± 0.3	1.07 ± 0.09	
India	Term	3.6 ± 0.4	1.14 ± 0.07	
North America	Term	3.4 ± 0.3	1.13 ± 0.08	
Europe	10 yr	6.4 ± 0.4		0.95 to 1.20
Europe	Adult	13.3 ± 1.6		16.5 to 18.2
Females				
USA	Full term	4.0 ± 1.24 mm	3.32 ± 0.78 mm	
USA	Adult, nulliparous	15.4 ± 4.3 mm		
USA	Adult	19.1 ± 8.7 mm	5.5 ± 1.7 mm	31.3 ± 8.5 mm

GA, gestational age; SD, standard deviation.

Reproduced from Hughes IA, Houk C, Ahmed SF, Lee PA. Consensus statement on management of intersex disorders. *Arch Dis Child.* 2006;91:554-562, with permission. From Feldman KW, Smith DW. Fetal phallic growth and penile standards for newborn male infants. *J Pediatr.* 1975;86395-86398; Schonfield WA, Beebe GW. Normal growth and variation in the male genitalia from birth to maturity. *J Urol.* 1942;48759-48777; Fujieda K, Matsuura N. Growth and maturation in the male genitalia from birth to adolescence. II Change of penile length. *Acta Paediatr Japan.* 1987;29220-29223; Tuladhar R, Davis PG, Batch J. et al. Establishment of a normal range of penile length in preterm infants. *J Paediatr Child Health.* 1998;34471-34473; Cheng PK, Chanoine JP. Should the definition of micropenis vary according to ethnicity? *Horm Res.* 2001;55278-55281; Zachmann M, Prader A, Kind H P. et al. Testicular volume during adolescence: cross-sectional and longitudinal studies. *Helv Paediatr Acta.* 1974;2961-2972; Oberfield SE, Mondok A, Shahrivar F. et al. Clitoral size in full-term infants. *Am J Perinatol.* 1989;6453-6454; Verkauf BS, Von Thron J, O'Brien WF. Clitoral size in normal women. *Obstet Gynecol.* 1992;8041-8044; Lloyd J, Crouch NS, Minto CL. et al. Female genital appearance: "normality" unfolds. *BJOG.* 2005;112643-112646.

components of male genital development, and it can be applied objectively when assessing the response to androgen treatment. The score is also useful as a guide to decide which infants require further evaluation and investigation. The diagnostic yield in terms of finding chromosomal abnormalities in isolated mild hypospadias or isolated cryptorchidism ranges from 2% to 7%; the rate increases to 12.5% when both conditions are present.[477] A cause was identified for more than one third of severe cases when hypospadias was comprehensively investigated.[478]

Investigations

Before embarking on a process of investigation that may be complex and lengthy, an adequate history should be obtained and a thorough physical examination should be performed. The information obtained may add urgency to complete initial investigations and start treatment if a life-threatening condition affecting the adrenal is suspected. The history should cover facets such as family history of DSD, adrenal disorders, or infertility and details of the current pregnancy, such as the need for assisted reproductive technologies, maternal exposure to medications, maternal virilization during pregnancy, and birth weight.[479] The examination should take note of features suggesting particular DSD-related syndromes or indications of metabolic decompensation or hyperpigmentation. Specific examination of the external genitalia should assess the appearance and size of the phallus, the location of a urethral opening, the presence of a vaginal opening, the nature of the scrotum or labioscrotal folds, and the site of any palpable gonads. If possible, the phallic length along its dorsal surface should be documented (see Table 23-20). Often, the sex of the infant is not easily determined after the examination, and investigations are needed urgently.

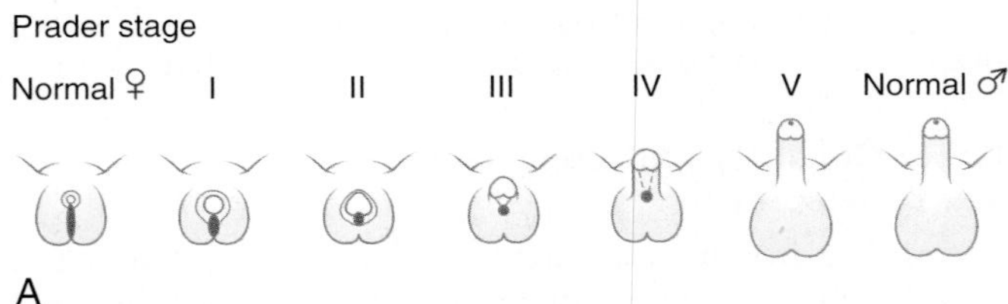

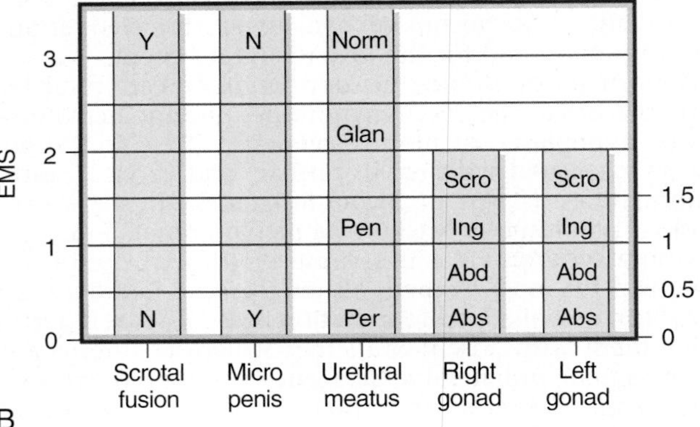

Figure 23-42 **A,** Prader staging for scoring the degree of androgenization of the external genitalia in a female infant with congenital adrenal hyperplasia. **B,** The external masculinization score (EMS) is used to assess degree of underandrogenization in an individual with 46,XY disorder of sex development. The score is based on the presence or absence of a micropenis and bifid scrotum, the location of the urethral meatus, and the position of the testes. (From Ahmed SF, Khwaja O, Hughes JA. The role of a clinical score in the assessment of ambiguous genatalia. *BJU Int.* 2000;85;120-124.)

TABLE 23-21

Investigations in a Newborn with Ambiguous Genitalia

Genetics	FISH* (X- and Y-specific probes)
	Karyotype*
	Save DNA with consent
Endocrine	17-hydroxyprogesterone,* 11-deoxycortisol, 17-hydroxypregnenolone
	Routine serum biochemistry*; urinalysis*
	Renin, ACTH
	Testosterone*, androstenedione, DHT
	Gonadotropins, AMH, inhibin B
	Urinary steroids by GC/MS
	Dynamic tests: ACTH stimulation
	hCG stimulation
	Save serum
Imaging	Abdominopelvic and renal ultrasound*
	CT, MRI
	Cystourethroscopy, sinogram
Surgical	Laparoscopy
	Gonadal biopsies

*Indicates first-line investigations for which results are available within days (see Table 23-19). For images of G-banded karyotypes and FISH analysis, see Fig. 23-3.

ACTH, adrenocorticotropic hormone; AMH, anti-Müllerian hormone; CT, computed tomography; DHT, dihydrotestosterone; FISH, fluorescent in situ hybridization; GC-MS, gas chromatography–mass spectrometry; hCG, human chorionic gonadotropin; MRI, magnetic resonance imaging.

Investigations should be targeted initially to answer specific questions that would be informative about sex assignment, even though a definitive diagnosis may not be achieved until another batch of tests are undertaken. A first-line set of investigations, as listed in Table 23-21, usually achieves the first target. Obtaining an indication of the sex chromosomes by FISH using X- and Y-specific probes within hours after birth has been a major advance in management. A definitive karyotype is necessary, but the result is often available within days. Concomitant endocrine tests include measurement of serum 17-OHP, testosterone, and AMH. The latter peptide is proving to be a highly reliable indicator of the presence of testicular tissue.[480] Urine should be collected and stored pending a later decision about analysis by specific gas chromatography and mass spectrometry. For the more uncommon forms of CAH, this test can provide the definitive diagnosis.[333] Imaging by pelvic ultrasound may be most informative when a cervix or uterus is clearly visualized in the context of a 46,XX karyotype and elevated serum 17-OHP concentration. In a term infant, the diagnosis is CAH, the most common cause of ambiguous genitalia of the newborn. Ultrasound imaging alone should not always be relied on to delineate the internal genital anatomy or to locate the site of gonads. MRI or laparoscopy may be a more definitive investigation to answer such questions. An ACTH stimulation test may be required to confirm a diagnosis of CAH in some cases and to verify adequate cortisol production in some rare forms of 46,XY DSD.

Second-line investigations usually are required when the karyotype is 46,XY or perhaps 45,X/46,XY. In this instance, the question is whether testes are present and, if so, whether they are capable of producing normal, age-related levels of androgens. The lynchpin of this assessment is the hCG stimulation test, for which several protocols have been employed. We are most familiar with the 3-day stimulation test comprising 1500 units daily, with samples for steroid analysis collected before the first injection and 24 hours after the last injection.[481] Measurement of testosterone is essential, but in addition, androstenedione and DHT are measured when an androgen biosynthetic defect is suspected. The stimulation test may be prolonged for another 2 weeks (using twice-weekly hCG injections) to determine whether the gonads are dysgenetic. The hCG stimulation test is often preceded by an acute LHRH stimulation test, which occasionally may be useful for suggesting primary gonadal dysgenesis (i.e., exaggerated peak LH and especially peak FSH levels) or some hypothalamic-pituitary dysfunction (i.e., absent LH and FSH responses). Analysis of DNA for specific gene mutations and androgen-binding assays using genital skin fibroblasts are investigations that may be required later. At this stage, an underlying diagnosis of DSD is often not established, particularly for phenotypes similar to PAIS (but with no *AR* mutation detected), partial gonadal dysgenesis, or a phenotype associated with an unknown dysmorphic syndrome. Laparoscopy and gonadal biopsy for histology and karyotyping may be needed in some cases to obtain a definitive diagnosis. In rare cases of possible 46,XX ovotesticular DSD manifesting at birth, measurement of estradiol and inhibin A levels after recombinant FSH stimulation may provide an assessment of ovarian tissue.[242]

Management

The pillars of management are effective communication with the family from the outset of having a newborn with a DSD, clear explanation of the steps to be taken to investigate their child, joint discussion about sex assignment, and description of the sequential road map for management through childhood, through puberty, and into young adulthood. The information provided and the manner with which it is delivered has a long-lasting effect on how parents perceive and understand their child's problem. Providing appropriate written information, adapted to local circumstances, is essential, and audiotaping consultations and providing edited transcripts can be valuable. Later, families find support from patient advocacy groups or benefit from being put in touch with another family affected by DSD.

Who should act as the key contact for affected families and be the conduit for communication among the multidisciplinary team? The team may include a pediatric endocrinologist, a pediatric surgeon/urologist, a clinical psychologist, a specialist in pediatric and adolescent gynecology, a clinical geneticist, a neonatologist, a social worker, and a medical ethicist. Not all of these professionals are routinely involved from the outset, but the mechanism must be in place for all to engage in management discussions as part of regular meetings of the multidisciplinary team. Each team member should be trained in the skills of communication relevant to the management of an infant with DSD. In reality, the trio of the pediatric endocrinologist, pediatric surgeon/urologist, and clinical psychologist take a major share of this responsibility and make themselves readily available. The family's primary care physician must be constantly informed of developments.

How a multidisciplinary team operates in practice in the management of DSD is exemplified by the 20 years of experience gleaned at the Great Ormond Street Hospital for Children in London and transitional care in the Adolescent Unit at the neighboring University College Hospital.[482] Although many DSD centers can report their own practice, the London model provides a comprehensive report of a holistic approach to the management of DSD from birth through adolescence. Each member of the multidisciplinary team understands his or her responsibilities and what is required for input, but success depends on well-organized, regular meetings of the multidisciplinary team. This provides an opportunity to review the results of investigations across a range of disciplines (e.g., biochemistry, imaging, genetics, histopathology), opinions on diagnosis and sex assignment, and the action plans in the immediate and longer term. The factual information should be presented in a formal manner (e.g., PowerPoint) and in the context of an up-to-date review of the relevant literature. An electronic record must be secured appropriately and medical confidentiality ensured. A gathering of the multidisciplinary team in this manner may provide an opportunity for an educational exercise to a wider audience, perhaps supplemented at the end of the meeting with formal talks stemming from a syllabus of DSD topics.

Management of DSD is an ongoing process in which the team meeting can review newly obtained information, including feedback on the outcome of consultations with each of the team professionals. Over a 2-year period, the multidisciplinary team in London reviewed more than 100 cases of DSD, with approximately two thirds categorized as 46,XY DSDs.[482] Within this category were disorders of gonadal development, disorders of androgen synthesis or action, and a significant number of syndromic disorders. As expected, various forms of CAH predominated within the 46,XX category, and there were a significant number of cases of isolated clitoromegaly of unknown cause. Mixed gonadal dysgenesis (45,X/46,XY mosaicism) predominated in the sex chromosome DSD category when classic Turner syndrome was excluded.

Outcomes

Several issues should be considered after the initial assessment, attempted diagnosis, and decisions about sex assignment are completed. Sex assignment is based on several factors, including the underlying diagnosis, likely gender identity, appearance of the genitalia and options for urologic and sexual function, the probable need for hormone replacement, potential for fertility, and tumor risk (Table 23-22). These factors should be considered within the context of the views of the family and social and cultural circumstances. Female sex assignment is assumed in 46,XX DSD due to CAH on early diagnosis and in 46,XY due to CAIS. However, such decisions are not as straightforward for mixed gonadal dysgenesis (45,X/46,XY mosaicism), ovotesticular DSD, partial gonadal dysgenesis, severe PAIS, or the androgen biosynthetic defects (i.e., 17β-HSD and 5α-reductase enzyme deficiencies).

Exposure to androgens in the prenatal and postnatal periods is considered to be a factor that leads to brain masculinization and increased male-typical behavior. The evidence that this may be the case is more persuasive for prenatal androgen exposure, based on studies of girls with CAH[483] and on play behavior in normal children.[484] In contrast, studies in infant rhesus macaques treated with a GnRH agonist after birth showed that expression of infant sex differences in behavior was not altered by manipulation of the postnatal surge in testosterone.[485] Boys with congenital anorchia and otherwise normal development of the external genitalia at birth showed no difference in male-typical sex behavior in young adulthood compared with controls.[486] Consequently, the relevance of the postnatal testosterone surge to brain masculinization is unsubstantiated. The sex difference in toy preferences in early childhood may relate more to socialization and cognitive gender development than to inborn factors.[487]

The surgical options are a function of sex assignment, and procedures are planned accordingly. The timing of surgery may be delayed, allowing the child to engage in discussions at the appropriate time. This is increasingly the practice adopted for female sex assignment for conditions such as CAH. In some cases, surgery may not be considered necessary. Outcome studies involving assessment of genital sensitivity and sexual function in women with CAH show clear impairment related to previous feminizing genital surgery.[488,489] Although surgical procedures have changed, these data have had a profound bearing on decisions taken during infancy and childhood for the surgical management of conditions such as CAH. It is generally accepted that clitoroplasty should be reserved only for the most

TABLE 23-22

Risk of Germ Cell Malignancy according to Diagnosis

Risk Group	Disorder	Malignancy Risk (%)	Recommended Action	No. Studies	No. Patients
High	GD* (+Y)† intra-abdominal	15-35	Gonadectomy‡	12	350
	Partial AIS nonscrotal	50	Gonadectomy‡	2	24
	Frasier syndrome	60	Gonadectomy‡	1	15
	Denys-Drash syndrome (+Y)	40	Gonadectomy‡	1	5
Intermediate	Turner syndrome (+Y)	12	Gonadectomy‡	11	43
	17β-HSD	28	Watchful waiting	2	7
	GD (+Y)† scrotal	Unknown	Biopsy§ and irradiation?	0	0
	Partial AIS scrotal gonad	Unknown	Biopsy§ and irradiation?	0	0
Low	Complete AIS	2	Biopsy§ and?	2	55
	Ovotesticular DSD	3	Testis tissue removal?	3	426
	Turner syndrome (−Y)	1	None	11	557
No (?)	5α-Reductase	0	Unresolved	1	3
	Leydig cell hypoplasia	0	Unresolved	1	2

*GD including disorders not further specified, 46XY, 45X/46XY, mixed, partial, and complete).
†GBY region positive, including the *TSPY* gene.
‡At time of diagnosis.
§At puberty, allowing investigation of at least 30 seminiferous tubules, preferentially diagnosis based on OCT3/4 immunohistochemistry.
AIS, androgen insensitivity syndrome; DSD, disorder of sex development; GD, gonadal dysgenesis; 17β-HSD, 17β-hydroxysteroid dehydrogenase.
Reproduced with permission from Hughes IA, Houk C, Ahmed SF, et al. Consensus statement on management of intersex disorders. *Arch Dis Child.* 2006;91:554-562.

severe degree of clitoromegaly, and vaginal surgery is deferred until after puberty. The long-term outcome of vaginal reconstruction procedures performed before puberty for a variety of conditions (e.g., CAH, AIS, mixed gonadal dysgenesis, persistent cloaca) suggests that complications may be reduced by undertaking the surgery later.[490] In adulthood, vaginal length in conditions such as CAIS and the MRKH syndrome can be normalized by dilator treatment alone.[391,491]

Subjects with DSD raised male require surgery to correct hypospadias and orchidopexy for testis maldescent.[492,493] Hypospadias repair usually is scheduled for between 6 and 24 months of age. More than one procedure is often required. It is the surgeon's responsibility to map out these procedures for the parents and to ensure that their expectations are realistic when questions are raised later about the role of phalloplasty in adulthood.[494] The topic of gonadectomy planned before puberty in 46,XY individuals raised female to prevent virilization and in others with DSD to avoid gonadal tumors was covered earlier. The irreversible nature of such a procedure has created uncertainty among professionals, particularly when the procedure is performed before the affected child can be engaged in discussions. This is another issue that requires the collective discussion of the multidisciplinary team and often includes input from an ethicist. The practice of cryopreserving excised gonads with unrealistic expectations for preservation of reproductive potential should be viewed cautiously, especially because current knowledge is based primarily on the gonadal effects of cancer therapies.[495-497]

Disclosure policies about sharing diagnostic information in relation to the karyotype, gonads, internal and external genital anatomy, and levels of circulating sex hormones are relevant across the spectrum of DSD presentations. It is germane whether the problem is congenital anorchia, undescended testes, micropenis, isolated hypospadias or ambiguous genitalia, or a phenotype completely at variance with the karyotype or gonadotype. The need for planned disclosure is most apparent for the girl who has had previous gonadectomy, has an XY karyotype, and is now in late childhood. Counseling in this setting should be undertaken only by a psychologist skilled in DSD management and should be provided in a stepwise manner. A more immediate need for professional input occurs in adolescence when, for example, investigations for primary amenorrhea reveal a diagnosis such as CAIS or complete gonadal dysgenesis. The historical practice of concealment is no longer acceptable.[404] It is encouraging that younger adults with DSD who participated in a survey of disclosure experiences reported more positively about appropriate information sharing, compared with participants of an older age.[498] Nevertheless, there remains considerable scope for improving communication and investing in more resources for psychosocial support.

Transitional Care and Adulthood

Various forms of transitional care have been reported for chronic endocrine-related disorders such as CAH, Turner syndrome, and growth hormone deficiency.[499-501] A model of transitional care is of paramount importance in DSD, as exemplified by the increasing role of gynecologists and adult endocrinologists in the management of female adolescents, urologists for young men, and, above all, clinical psychologists for many patients. Transition is an opportunity to take stock of the diagnosis, the appropriateness of hormone replacement therapy, and the need for further surgical interventions. The accuracy of the diagnosis may be questionable for many individuals, particularly females with an XY karyotype.[502] The hinterland between pediatric and adult practice may be the time when DSD comes to light, that is, in the adolescent girl with primary amenorrhea or with virilization and in the boy with gynecomastia (Table 23-23). An appropriately constituted multidisciplinary team is as important at this stage in the DSD management process as it is at birth and is vital for coordinating the long-term endocrine, gynecologic, urologic, and psychological issues related to DSD into adult life.[503]

TABLE 23-23

DSD Manifesting in Adolescence

Prepubertal Sex of Rearing	Karyotype	DSD
Female	46,XY	17β-HSD deficiency
		5α-reductase deficiency
		Partial AIS
		Complete AIS*
		Swyer syndrome (complete gonadal dysgenesis)*
		CYP17 deficiency*
Male	46,XX	Ovotesticular DSD (feminization from ovarian tissue, infertility)
		XX male
		Congenital adrenal hyperplasia (usually manifests earlier with precocious puberty)

*Presentation is with primary amenorrhea ± lack of puberty.
AIS, androgen insensitivity syndrome; CYP, cytochrome P450 enzyme; DSD, disorders of sex development; 17β-HSD, 17β-hydroxysteroid dehydrogenase.

Future Development

The Chicago Consensus has been the catalyst for a sea change in the approach to management of DSD. The change in nomenclature and the development of a new classification system has incited a quiet revolution in this branch of medicine.[504] DSD centers are incorporating the changes in their clinical practice and the new nomenclature is being used abundantly in the biomedical literature.[505] There is a consensus among professionals working in the field of DSD to make progress in tackling the challenges that the multidisciplinary team face in management. Disclosure strategy merits research that can draw on experiences in other areas of practice, such as adoption and studies of donor conception.[506] No single center is able to gather sufficient numbers of cases and experience in management to make strides in elucidating the genetic and endocrine mechanisms causing gonadal dysgenesis, PAIS-like phenotypes, or isolated hypospadias and in gathering more data to interpret age-related changes in steroid production and metabolism. National and international forms of collaboration are essential for progress.

ACKNOWLEDGMENTS

We recognize the major contributions made to this chapter by previous editors Melvin Grumbach, MD, and Felix Conte, MD. John C. Achermann holds a Wellcome Trust Senior Research Fellowship in Clinical Science (079666). Ieuan A. Hughes is supported by the NIHR Cambridge Biomedical Research Centre for his work on disorders of sexual development, and both authors acknowledge the support of the European Commission–funded EuroDSD Programme.

REFERENCES

1. Sax L. How common is intersex? A response to Anne Fausto-Sterling. *J Sex Res*. 2002;39:174-178.
2. Grumbach MM, Hughes IA, Conte FA. Disorders of sex differentiation. In: Larsen PR, Kronenberg HM, Melmed S, et al., eds. *Williams Textbook of Endocrinology*. 10th ed. Philadelphia, PA: WB Saunders; 2003: 842-1002.
3. Hughes IA, Houk C, Ahmed SF, et al. Consensus statement on management of intersex disorders. *Arch Dis Child*. 2006;91:554-563.
4. Pasterski V, Prentice P, Hughes IA. Consequences of the Chicago consensus on disorders of sex development (DSD): current practices in Europe. *Arch Dis Child*. 2010;95:618-623.
5. Brennan J, Capel B. One tissue, two fates: molecular genetic events that underlie testis versus ovary development. *Nat Rev Genet*. 2004;5:509-521.
6. DiNapoli L, Capel B. SRY and the standoff in sex determination. *Mol Endocrinol*. 2008;22:1-9.
7. Wilhelm D, Palmer S, Koopman P. Sex determination and gonadal development in mammals. *Physiol Rev*. 2007;87:1-28.
8. Scott HM, Mason JI, Sharpe RM. Steroidogenesis in the fetal testis and its susceptibility to disruption by exogenous compounds. *Endocr Rev*. 2009;30:883-925.
9. Edson MA, Nagaraja AK, Matsuk MM. The mammalian ovary from genesis to revelation. *Endocr Rev*. 2009;30:624-712.
10. Matsubara K, Tarui H, Toriba M, et al. Evidence for different origin of sex chromosomes in snakes, birds, and mammals and step-wise differentiation of snake chromosomes. *Proc Natl Acad Sci U S A*. 2006;103:18031-18032.
11. Marshall Graves JA. Weird animal genomes and the evolution of vertebrate sex and sex chromosomes. *Annu Rev Genet*. 2008;42:565-586.
12. Jost A. Recherches sur la differentiation sexualle de l'embryo de lapin. *Arch Anat Microsc Morph Exp*. 1947;36:271-315.
13. Nef S, Schaad O, Stallings NR, et al. Gene expression during sex determination reveals a robust female genetic program at the onset of ovarian development. *Dev Biol*. 2005;287:361-367.
14. Beverdam A, Koopman P. Expression profiling of purified mouse gonadal somatic cells during the critical time window of sex determination reveals novel candidate genes for human sexual dysgenesis syndromes. *Hum Mol Genet*. 2006;15:417-431.
15. Parma P, Radi O, Vidal V, et al. R-spondin1 is essential in sex determination, skin differentiation and malignancy. *Nat Genet*. 2006;38: 1304-1309.
16. Johnson J, Canning J, Kaneko T, et al. Germline stem cells and follicular renewal in the postnatal mammalian ovary. *Nature*. 2004;428: 145-150.
17. Hall H, Hunt P, Hassold T. The origin of human aneuploidy: where we have been, where we are going. *Hum Mol Genet*. 2007;16(Spec. no. 2):R203-R208.
18. Thomas NS, Hassold TJ. Aberrant recombination and the origin of Klinefelter syndrome. *Hum Reprod Update*. 2003;9:309-317.
19. Ross MT, Bentley DR, Tyler-Smith C. The sequences of the human sex chromosomes. *Curr Opin Genet Dev*. 2006;16:213-218.
20. Tilford CA, Kuroda-Kawaguchi T, Skaletsky H, et al. A physical map of the human Y chromosome. *Nature*. 2001;409:943-945.
21. Hughes JF, Skaletsky H, Pyntikova T, et al. Chimpanzee and human Y chromosomes are remarkably divergent in structure and gene content. *Nature*. 2010;463:536-539.
22. McElreavey K, Ravel C, Chantot-Bastaraud S, et al. Y chromosome variants and male reproductive function. *Int J Androl*. 2006;29: 298-303.
23. Cools M, Drop SL, Wolffenbuttel KP, et al. Germ cell tumors in the intersex gonad: old paths, new directions, moving frontiers. *Endocr Rev*. 2006;27:468-484.
24. Nathanson KL, Kanetsky PA, Hawes R, et al. The Y deletion gr/gr and susceptibility to testicular germ cell tumor. *Am J Hum Genet*. 2005;77:1034-1043.
25. Goldberg E. HY antigen and sex determination. *Philos Trans R Soc Lond B Biol Sci*. 1988;322:72-81.
26. Mardon G, Page DC. The sex determining region of the mouse Y chromosome encodes a protein with a highly acidic domain and 13 zinc fingers. *Cell*. 1989;56:765-770.
27. Palmer MS, Sinclair AH, Berta P, et al. Genetic evidence that ZFY is not the testis-determining factor. *Nature*. 1989;342:937-939.
28. Sinclair AH, Berta P, Palmer MS, et al. A gene from the human sex determining region encodes a protein with homology to a conserved DNA-binding motif. *Nature*. 1990;346:240-244.
29. Berta P, Hawkins RJ, Sinclair AH, et al. Genetic evidence equating SRY and the testis determining factor. *Nature*. 1990;348:448-450.
30. Koopman P, Munsterberg A, Capel B, et al. Expression of a candidate sex determining gene during mouse testis differentiation. *Nature*. 1990;348:450-452.
31. Koopman P, Gubbay J, Vivian N, et al. Male development of chromosomally female mice transgenic for SRY. *Nature*. 1991;351:117-121.
32. Jager RJ, Anvret M, Hall K, et al. A human XY female with a frame shift mutation in the candidate testis-determining gene SRY. *Nature*. 1990;348:452-454.
33. Goodfellow PN, Lovell-Badge R. SRY and sex determination in mammals. *Annu Rev Genet*. 1993;27:271-292.
34. Ross MT, Grafham DV, Coffey AJ, et al. The DNA sequence of the human X chromosome. *Nature*. 2005;434:325-337.
35. Harsha HC, Suresh S, Amanchy R, et al. A manually curated functional annotation of the human X chromosome. *Nat Genet*. 2005;37: 331-332.
36. Grumbach MM, Morishima A, Taylor JH. Human sex chromosome abnormalities in relation to DNA replication and heterochromatinization. *Proc Natl Acad Sci U S A*. 1963;49:581-589.
37. Lyon MF. The X inactivation centre and X chromosome imprinting. *Eur J Hum Genet*. 1994;2:255-261.
38. Heard E, Disteche CM. Dosage compensation in mammals: fine-tuning the expression of the X-chromosome. *Genes Dev*. 2006;20:1848-1867.
39. Payer B, Lee JT. X chromosome dosage compensation: how mammals keep the balance. *Annu Rev Genet*. 2008;42:733-772.
40. Carrel L, Willard HF. X-inactivation profile reveals extensive variability in X-linked gene expression in females. *Nature*. 2005;434:400-404.
41. Nguyen DK, Disteche CM. Dosage compensation of the active X chromosome in mammals. *Nat Genet*. 2006;38:47-53.
42. Elsheikh M, Dunger DB, Conway GS, et al. Turner's syndrome in adulthood. *Endocr Rev*. 2002;23:120-140.
43. Schlessinger D, Herrera L, Crisponi L, et al. Genes and translocations involved in POF. *Am J Med Genet*. 2002;222:328-333.
44. Bondy CA, Cheng C. Monosomy for the X chromosome. *Chromosome Res*. 2009;17:649-658.
45. Murray A, Webb J, Grimley S, et al. Studies of FRAXA and FRAXE in women with premature ovarian failure. *J Med Genet*. 1998;35: 637-640.
46. Sala C, Arrigo G, Torri G, et al. Eleven X chromosome breakpoints associated with premature ovarian failure (POF) map to a 15-Mb YAC contig spanning Xq21. *Genomics*. 1997;40:123-131.
47. Lacombe A, Lee H, Zahed L, et al. Disruption of POF1B binding to nonmuscle actin filaments is associated with premature ovarian failure. *Am J Hum Genet*. 2006;79:113-119.
48. Di Pasquale E, Beck-Peccoz P, Persani L. Hypergonadotropic ovarian failure associated with an inherited mutation of human bone morphogenetic protein-15 (BMP15) gene. *Am J Hum Genet*. 2004;75:106-111.
49. Moumné L, Batista F, Benayou BA, et al. The mutations and potential targets of the forkhead transcription factor FOXL2. *Mol Cell Endocrinol*. 2008;282:2-11.
50. Qin Y, Choi Y, Zhao H, et al. NOBOX homeobox mutation causes premature ovarian failure. *Am J Hum Genet*. 2007;81:576-581.
51. Lourenço D, Brauner R, Lin L, et al. Mutations in NR5A1 associated with ovarian insufficiency. *N Engl J Med*. 2009;360:1200-1210.
52. Miyamoto N, Yoshida M, Kuratani S, et al. Defects of urogenital development in mice lacking *Emx2*. *Development*. 1997;124:1653-1664.
53. Brunelli S, Faiella A, Capra V, et al. Germline mutation in the homeobox gene EMX2 in patients with severe schizencephaly. *Nat Genet*. 1996;12:94-96.
54. Shawlot W, Behringer RR. Requirement for Lim1 in head-organizer function. *Nature*. 1995;374:425-430.
55. Birk OS, Casiano DE, Wassif CA, et al. The LIM homeobox gene *Lhx9* is essential for mouse gonad formation. *Nature*. 2000;403:909-913.
56. Ottolenghi C, Moreira-Filho C, Mendonca BB, et al. Absence of mutations involving the LIM homeobox domain gene LHX9 in 46,XY gonadal agenesis and dysgenesis. *J Clin Endocrinol Metab*. 2001;86: 2465-2469.
57. Katoh-Fukui Y, Tsuchiya R, Shiroishi T, et al. Male-to-female sex reversal in M33 mutant mice. *Nature*. 1998;393:688-692.
58. Biason-Lauber A, Konrad D, Meyer M, et al. Ovaries and female phenotype in a girl with 46,XY karyotype and mutations in the CBX2 gene. *Am J Hum Genet*. 2009;84:658-663.
59. Cui S, Ross A, Stallings N, et al. Disrupted gonadogenesis and male-to-female sex reversal in Pod1 knockout mice. *Development*. 2004;131: 4095-5105.
60. Tevosian SG, Albrecht KH, Crispino JD, et al. Gonadal differentiation, sex determination and normal *SRY* expression in mice require direct interaction between transcription partners GATA4 and FOG2. *Development*. 2002;129:4627-4634.
61. Bouma GJ, Washburn LL, Albrecht KH, et al. Correct dosage of Fog2 and Gata4 transcription factors is critical for fetal testis development in mice. *Proc Natl Acad Sci U S A*. 2007;104:14994-14999.

61a. Lourenio D, Brauner R, Rybczynska N, et al. Loss-of-function mutation in *GATA4* causes anomalies of human testicular development. *Proc Natl Acad Sci USA*. 2011;102:1597-1602.

62. Nef S, Verma-Kurvari S, Merenmies J, et al. Testis determination requires insulin receptor family function in mice. *Nature*. 2003;426: 291-295.
63. Bogani D, .Siggers P, Brixey R, et al. Loss of mitogen-activated protein kinase kinase kinase 4 (MAP3K4) reveals a requirement for MAPK signalling in mouse sex determination. *PloS Biol*. 2009;7:e1000196.
64. Buaas FW, Val P, Swain A. The transcriptional co-factor CITED2 functions during sex determination and early gonad development. *Hum Mol Genet*. 2009;18:2989-3001.
65. Schnabel CA, Selleri L, Cleary ML. Pbx1 is essential for adrenal development and urogenital ridge differentiation. *Genesis*. 2003;37: 123-130.
66. Call KM, Glaser T, Ito CY, et al. Isolation and characterization of a zinc finger polypeptide gene at the human chromosome 11 Wilms tumor locus. *Cell*. 1990;60:509-520.
67. Pritchard-Jones K, Fleming S, Davidson D, et al. The candidate Wilms' tumor gene is involved in genitourinary development. *Nature*. 1990;346:194-197.
68. Kreidberg JA, Sariola H, Loring JM, et al. WT1 is required for early kidney development. *Cell*. 1993;74:679-691.
69. Hohenstein P, Hastie ND. The many facets of the Wilms' tumour gene, WT1. *Hum Mol Genet*. 2006;15:R196-R201.
70. Nachtigal MW, Hirokawa Y, Enyeart-VanHouten DL, et al. Wilms' tumor 1 and Dax-1 modulate the orphan nuclear receptor SF-1 in sex-specific gene expression. *Cell*. 1998;93:445-454.
71. Bradford ST, Wilhelm D, Bandiera R, et al. A cell-autonomous role for WT1 in regulating SRY in vivo. *Hum Mol Genet*. 2009;18:3429-3438.
72. Hanley NA, Ball SG, Clement-Jones M, et al. Expression of steroidogenic factor 1 and Wilms' tumour 1 during early human gonadal development and sex determination. *Mech Dev*. 1999;87:175-180.
73. Francke U, Holmes LB, Atkins L, et al. Aniridia–Wilms' tumor association: evidence for specific deletion of 11p13. *Cytogenetics Cell Genet*. 1979;24:185-192.
74. Pelletier J, Bruening W, Kashtan CE, et al. Germline mutations in the Wilms tumor suppressor gene are associated with abnormal urogenital development in Denys-Drash syndrome. *Cell*. 1991;67:437-447.
75. Barbaux X, Niandet P, Gubler M-C, et al. Donor splice-site mutations in WTI are responsible for Frasier syndrome. *Nat Genet*. 1997;17:467-470.
76. Klamt B, Koziell A, Poulat F, et al. Frasier syndrome is caused by defective alternative splicing of WT1 leading to an altered ratio of WT1 +/−KTS splice isoforms. *Hum Mol Genet*. 1998;7:709-714.
77. Koziell A, Charmandari E, Hindmarsh PC, et al. Frasier syndrome: part of the Denys Drash continuum or simply a WT1 gene associated disorder of intersex and nephropathy? *Clin Endocrinol*. 2000;52: 519-524.
78. Lin L, Achermann JC. Steroidogenic factor-1 (SF-1, NR5A1, Ad4BP) and disorders of testis development. *Sex Dev*. 2008;2:200-209.
79. Luo X, Ikeda Y, Parker KL. A cell-specific nuclear receptor is essential for adrenal and gonadal development and sexual differentiation. *Cell*. 1994;77:481-490.
80. Majdic G, Young M, Gomez-Sanches E, et al. Knockout mice lacking steroidogenic factor 1 are a novel genetic model of hypothalamic obesity. *Endocrinology*. 2002;143:607-614.
81. Park SY, Meeks JJ, Raverot G, et al. Nuclear receptors Sf1 and Dax1 function cooperatively to mediate somatic cell differentiation during testis development. *Development*. 2005;132:2415-2423.
82. Achermann JC, Ito M, Ito M, et al. A mutation in the gene encoding steroidogenic factor-1 causes XY sex reversal and adrenal failure in humans. *Nat Genet*. 1999;22:125-126.
83. Achermann JC, Ozisik G, Ito M, et al. Gonadal determination and adrenal development are regulated by the orphan nuclear receptor, steroidogenic factor-1 in a dose dependent manner. *J Clin Endocrinol Metab*. 2002;87:1829-1833.
84. Lin L, Pascal P, Ferraz-de-Souza B, et al. Heterozygous missense mutations in steroidogenic factor 1 (SF1/Ad4BP, NR5A1) are associated with 46,XY disorders of sex development with normal adrenal function. *J Clin Endocrinol Metab*. 2007;92:991-999.
85. Sekido R, Lovell-Badge R. Sex determination involves synergistic action of SRY and SF1 on a specific SOX9 enhancer. *Nature*. 2008; 453:930-934.
86. Biason-Lauber A, Schoenle EJ. Apparently normal ovarian differentiation in a prepubertal girl with transcriptionally inactive steroidogenic factor 1 (NR5A1/SF-1) and adrenocortical insufficiency. *Am J Hum Genet*. 2000;67:1563-1568.
87. Pelusi C, Ikeda Y, Zubair M, et al. Impaired follicle development and infertility in female mice lacking steroidogenic factor 1 in ovarian granulosa cells. *Biol Reprod*. 2008;79:1074-1083.
88. Bardoni B, Zanaria E, Guioli S, et al. A dosage sensitive locus at chromosome Xp21 is involved in male to female sex reversal. *Nat Genet*. 1994;7:497-501.
89. Swain A, Narvaez V, Burgoyne P, et al. Dax1 antagonizes SRY action in mammalian sex determination. *Nature*. 1998;391:761-767.
90. Meeks JJ, Weiss J, Jameson JL. Dax1 is required for testis determination. *Nat Genet*. 2003;34:32-33.
91. Jordan BK, Mohammed M, Ching ST, et al. Up-regulation of WNT-4 signaling and dosage-sensitive sex reversal in humans. *Am J Hum Genet*. 2001;68:1102-1109.
92. Molyneaux KA, Stallock J, Schaible K, et al. Time-lapse analysis of living mouse germ cell migration. *Dev Biol*. 2001;240:488-498.
93. Richardson BE, Lehmann R. Mechanisms guiding primordial germ cell migration: strategies from different organisms. *Nat Rev Mol Cell Biol*. 2010;11:37-49.
94. Oktem O, Oktay K. Current knowledge in the renewal capability of germ cells in the adult ovary. *Birth Defects Res C Embryo Today*. 2009;87:90-95.
95. McLaren A. Germ and somatic cell lineages in the developing gonad. *Mol Cell Endocrinol*. 2000;163:3-9.
96. Kurohmaru M, Kanai Y, Hayashi Y. A cytological and cytoskeletal comparison of Sertoli cells without germ cell and those with germ cells using the W/WV mutant mouse. *Tissue Cell*. 1992;24: 895-903.
97. Bowles J, Knight D, Smith C, et al. Retinoid signaling determines germ cell fate in mice. *Science*. 2006;312:596-600.
98. Koubova J, Menke DB, Zhou Q, et al. Retinoic acid regulates sex-specific timing of meiotic initiation in mice. *Proc Natl Acad Sci U S A*. 2006;103:2474-2479.
99. Mehlmann LM. Stops and starts in mammalian oocytes: recent advances in understanding the regulation of meiotic arrest and oocyte maturation. *Reproduction*. 2005;130:791-799.
100. Telfer EE, Gosden RG, Byskov AG, et al. On regenerating the ovary and generating controversy (Editorial). *Cell*. 2005;122:821-822.
101. Harley VR, Clarkson MJ, Argentaro A. The molecular action and regulation of the testis-determing factors, SRY (sex-determining region on the Y chromosome) and SOX9 (SRY-related high-mobility group [HMG] box 9). *Endocr Rev*. 2003;24:466-487.
102. Hiramatsu R, Matoa S, Kanai-Azuma M, et al. A critical time window of SRY action in gonadal sex determination in mice. *Development*. 2009;136:129-138.
103. Hanley NA, Hagan DM, Clement-Jones M, et al. SRY, SOX9, and DAX1 expression patterns during human sex determination and gonadal development. *Mech Dev*. 2000;91:403-407.
104. Harley VR, Jackson DI, Hextall PJ, et al. DNA binding activity of recombinant SRY from normal males and XY females. *Science*. 1992;255:453-456.
105. Werner MH, Huth JR, Gronenborn AM, et al. Molecular basis of human 46,XY sex reversal revealed from the three-dimensional solution structure of the human SRY DNA complex. *Cell*. 1995;81:705-714.
106. Sim H, Argentaro A, Harley VR. Boys, girls and shuttling of SRY and SOX9. *Trends Endocrinol Metab*. 2008;19:213-222.
107. Sim H, Rimmer K, Kelly S, et al. Defective calmodulin-mediated nuclear transport of the sex-determining region of the Y chromosome (SRY) in XY sex reversal. *Mol Endocrinol*. 2005;7:1884-1892.
108. Desclozeaux M, Poulat F, de Santa Barbara P, et al. Phosphorylation of an N-terminal motif enhances DNA-binding activity of the human SRY protein. *J Biol Chem*. 1998;273:7988-7995.
109. Poulat F, Barbara PS, Desclozeaux M, et al. The human testis determining factor SRY binds a nuclear factor containing PDZ protein interaction domains. *J Biol Chem*. 1997;272:7167-7172.
110. Jäger R, Harley V, Pfeiffer R, et al. A familial mutation in the testis-determining gene *SRY* shared by both sexes. *Hum Genet*. 1992;90: 350-355.
111. Li B, Zhang W, Chan G, et al. Human sex reversal due to impaired nuclear localization of SRY: a clinical correlation. *J Biol Chem*. 2001;276:46480-46484.
112. Burgoyne PS, Buehr M, Koopman P. Cell-autonomous action of the testis-determining gene: Sertoli cells are exclusively XY in XX-XY chimaeric mouse testes. *Development*. 1988;102:443-450.
113. Sekido R, Lovell-Badge R. Sex determination and SRY: down to a wink and a nudge? *Trends Genet*. 2009;25:19-29.
114. Albrecht KH, Eicher EM. Evidence that SRY is expressed in pre-Sertoli cells and Sertoli and granulosa cells have a common precursor. *Dev Biol*. 2001;240:92-107.
115. Wilhelm D, Martinson F, Bradford S, et al. Sertoli cell differentiation is induced both cell-autonomously and through prostaglandin signaling during mammalian sex determination. *Dev Biol*. 2005;287: 111-124.
116. Malki S, Nef S, Notarnicola C, et al. Prostaglandin D2 induces nuclear import of the sex-determining factor SOX9 via its cAMP-PKA phosphorylation. *EMBO J*. 2005;24:1798-1809.
117. Schmahl J, Eicher EM, Washburn LL, et al. SRY induces cell proliferation in the mouse gonad. *Development*. 2000;127:65-73.
118. Martineau J, Nordqvist K, Tilmann C, et al. Male-specific cell migration into the developing gonad. *Curr Biol*. 1997;7:958-968.
119. Capel B, Albrecht KH, Washburn LL, et al. Migration of mesonephric cells into the mammalian gonad depends on SRY. *Mech Dev*. 1999; 84:127-131.
120. Ross DG, Bowles J, Koopman P, et al. New insights into SRY regulation through identification of 5′ conserved sequences. *BMC Mol Biol*. 2008;8:85.

121. Bernard P, Sim H, Knower K, et al. Human SRY inhibits beta-catenin-mediated transcription. *Int J Biochem Cell Biol.* 2008;40:2889-2900.
122. Foster JW, Dominguez-Steglich MA, Guioli S, et al. Camptomelic dysplasia and autosomal sex reversal caused by mutations in an SRY-related gene. *Nature.* 1994;372:525-530.
123. Wagner T, Wirth J, Meyer J, et al. Autosomal sex reversal and camptomelic dysplasia are caused by mutations in and around the *SRY*-related gene *SOX9*. *Cell.* 1994;79:1111-1120.
124. Morais da Silva S, Hacker A, Harley V, et al. SOX 9 expression during gonadal development implies a conserved role for the gene in testis differentiation in mammals and birds. *Nat Genet.* 1996;14: 62-68.
125. Kent J, Wheatley SC, Andrews JE, et al. A male-specific role for SOX9 in vertebrate sex determination. *Development.* 1996;122:2813-2822.
126. Südbeck P, Schmitz ML, Baeuerle PA, et al. Sex reversal by loss of the C-terminal transactivation domain of human SOX9. *Nat Genet.* 1996;13:230-232.
127. Huang B, Wang S, Ning Y, et al. Autosomal XX sex reversal caused by duplication of SOX9. *Am J Med Genet.* 1999;87:349-353.
128. Vidal VP, Chaboissier MC, de Rooij DG, et al. SOX9 induces testis development in XX transgenic mice. *Nat Genet.* 2001;28:216-217.
129. Qin Y, Bishop CE. SOX9 is sufficient for functional testis development producing fertile male mice in the absence of SRY. *Hum Mol Genet.* 2005;14:1221-1229.
130. Bishop CE, Whitworth DJ, Qin Y, et al. A transgenic insertion upstream of SOX9 is associated with dominant XX sex reversal in the mouse. *Nat Genet.* 2000;26:490-494.
131. Refai O, Friedman A, Terry L, et al. De novo 12;17 translocation upstream of SOX9 resulting in 46,XX testicular disorder of sex development. *Am J Med Genet A.* 2010;152A:422-426.
132. Kim Y, Bingham N, Sekido R, et al. Fibroblast growth factor receptor 2 regulates proliferation and Sertoli cell differentiation during male sex determination. *Proc Natl Acad Sci U S A.* 2007;104:16558-16563.
133. Coveney D, Cool J, Oliver T, et al. Four-dimensional analysis of vascularization during primary development of an organ, the gonad. *Proc Natl Acad Sci U S A.* 2008;105:7212-7217.
134. Jeays-Ward K, Hoyle C, Brennan J, et al. Endothelial and steroidogenic cell migration are regulated by WNT4 in the developing mammalian gonad. *Development.* 2003;130:3663-3670.
135. Yao HH, Matsuk MM, Jorgez CJ, et al. Follistatin operates downstream of Wnt4 in mammalian ovary organogenesis. *Dev Dyn.* 2004;230: 210-215.
136. Kim Y, Kobayashi A, Sekido R, et al. Fgf9 and Wnt4 act as antagonistic signals to regulate mammalian sex determination. *PloS Biol.* 2006; 4:e187.
137. Clark AM, Garland KK, Russell LD. *Desert hedgehog* (*Dhh*) gene is required in the mouse testis for formation of adult-type Leydig cells and normal development of peritubular cells and seminiferous tubules. *Biol Reprod.* 2000;63:1825-1838.
138. Yao HH, Whoriskey W, Capel B. Desert Hedgehog/Patched 1 signaling specifies fetal Leydig cell fate in testis organogenesis. *Genes Dev.* 2002;16:1433-1440.
139. Park SY, Tong M, Jameson JL. Distinct roles for steroidogenic factor 1 and desert hedgehog pathways in fetal and adult Leydig cell development. *Endocrinology.* 2007;148:3704-3710.
140. Umehara F, Tate G, Itoh K, et al. A novel mutation of desert hedgehog in a patient with 46,XY partial gonadal dysgenesis accompanied by minifascicular neuropathy. *Am J Hum Genet.* 2000;67:1302-1305.
141. Moniot B, Berta P, Scherer G, et al. Male specific expression suggests role of DMRT1 in human sex determination. *Mech Dev.* 2000;91: 323-325.
142. Ottolenghi C, Veitia R, Quintana-Murci L, et al. The region on 9p associated with 46,XY sex reversal contains several transcripts expressed in the urogenital system and a novel double sex-related domain. *Genomics.* 2000;64:170-178.
143. Raymond CS, Murphy MW, O'Sullivan MG, et al. Dmrt1, a gene related to worm and fly sexual regulators, is required for mammalian testis differentiation. *Genes Dev.* 2000;14:2587-2595.
144. Barbaro M, Balsamo A, Anderlid BM, et al. Characterization of deletions at 9p affecting the candidate regions for sex reversal and deletion 9p syndrome by MLPA. *Eur J Hum Genet.* 2009;17:1439-1447.
145. Kitamura K, Yanazawa M, Sugiyama N, et al. Mutation of ARX causes abnormal development of forebrain and testes in mice and X-linked lissencephaly with abnormal genitalia in humans. *Nat Genet.* 2002;32:359-369.
146. Fukami M, Wada Y, Miyabayashi K, et al. CXorf6 is a causative gene for hypospadias. *Nat Genet.* 2006;38:1369-1371.
147. Brennan J, Tilmann C, Capel B. Pdgfr-α mediates testis cord organization and fetal Leydig cell development in the XY gonad. *Genes Dev.* 2003;17:800-810.
148. Perera EM, Martin H, Seeherunvong T, et al. Tescalcin, a novel gene encoding a putative EF-hand Ca(2)-binding protein, Col9a3, and renin are expressed in the mouse testis during the early stages of gonadal differentiation. *Endocrinology.* 2001;142:455-463.
149. Gibbons RJ, Higgs DR. Molecular-clinical spectrum of the ATR-X syndrome. *Am J Med Genet.* 2000;97:204-212.
150. Ion A, Telvi L, Chaussain JL, et al. A novel mutation in the putative DNA helicase XH2 is responsible for male to female sex reversal associated with an atypical form of ATRX syndrome. *Am J Hum Genet.* 1996;58:1185-1191.
151. Pfeifer D, Poulat F, Holinski-Feder E, et al. The SOX8 gene is located within 700 kb of the tip of chromosome 16p and is deleted in a patient with ATR-16 syndrome. *Genomics.* 2000;63:108-116.
152. Waggoner DJ, Chow CK, Dowton SB, et al. Partial monosomy of distal 10q: three new cases and a review. *Am J Med Genet.* 1999;86:1-5.
153. Pinsky L, Erickson RP, Schimke RN, eds. Genetic Disorders of Human Sexual Development. New York, NY: Oxford University Press; 1999.
154. Bashamboo A, Wieacker P, Ledig S, et al. New technologies for the identification of novel genetic markers of disorders of sex development (DSD). *Sex Dev.* 2010;4:213-224.
155. Yao HH, DiNapoli L, Capel B. Meiotic germ cells antagonize mesonephric cell migration and testis cord formation in mouse gonads. *Development.* 2003;130:5895-5902.
156. Vainio S, Heikkila M, Kispert A, et al. Female development in mammals is regulated by Wnt-4 signalling. *Nature.* 1999;397:405-409.
157. Chassot AA, Gregoire EP, Magliano M, et al. Genetics of ovarian differentiation: Rspo1, a major player. *Sex Dev.* 2008;2:219-227.
158. Liu CF, Bingham N, Parker K, et al. Sex specific roles of beta-catenin in mouse gonadal development. *Hum Mol Genet.* 2009;18:405-417.
159. Couse JF, Hewitt SC, Bunch DO, et al. Postnatal sex reversal of the ovaries in mice lacking estrogen receptors alpha and beta. *Science.* 1999;286:2328-2331.
160. Uhlenhaut NH, Jakob S, Anlag K, et al. Somatic sex reprogramming of adult ovaries to testes by FOXL2 ablation. *Cell.* 2009;139:1130-1142.
161. Teixeira J, Maheswaran S, Donahoe PK. Müllerian inhibiting substance: an instructive developmental hormone with diagnostic and possible therapeutic applications. *Endocr Rev.* 2001;22:657-674.
162. Josso N, Clemente N. Transduction pathway of anti-müllerian hormone, a sex-specific member of the TGF-beta family. *Trends Endocrinol Metab.* 2003;14:91-97.
163. Bedecarrats GY, O'Neill FH, Norwitz ER, et al. Regulation of gonadotropin gene expression by müllerian inhibiting substance. *Proc Natl Acad Sci U S A.* 2003;100:9348-9353.
164. Siiteri PK, Wilson JD. Testosterone formation and metabolism during male sexual differentiation in the human embryo. *J Clin Endocrinol Metab.* 1974;38:113-125.
165. Murray TJ, Fowler PA, Abramovich DR, et al. Human fetal testis: second trimester proliferative and steroidogenic capacities. *J Clin Endocrinol Metab.* 2000;85:4812-4817.
166. Tapanainen JS, Kellokumpu-Lehtinen P, Pelliniemi L, et al. Age-related changes in endogenous steroids of human fetal testis during early and midpregnancy. *J Clin Endocrinol Metab.* 1981;52:98-102.
167. Kaplan SL, Grumbach MM. Pituitary and placental gonadotrophins and sex steroids in the human and sub-human primate fetus. *Clin Endocrinol Metab.* 1978;7:487-511.
168. Payne AH, Hales DB. Overview of steroidogenic enzymes in the pathway from cholesterol to active steroid hormones. *Endocr Rev.* 2004;25:947-970.
169. Fluck CE, Miller WL, Auchus RJ. The 17,20-lyase activity of cytochrome p450c17 from human fetal testis favors the delta5 steroidogenic pathway. *J Clin Endocrinol Metab.* 2003;88:3762-3766.
170. Arlt W, Walker EA, Draper N, et al. Congenital adrenal hyperplasia caused by mutant P450 oxidoreductase and human androgen synthesis: analytical study. *Lancet.* 2004;363:2128-2135.
171. Auchus RJ. The backdoor pathway to dihydrotestosterone. *Trends Endocrinol Metab.* 2004;15:432-438.
172. Goto M, Piper Hanley K, Marcos J, et al. In humans, early cortisol biosynthesis provides a mechanism to safeguard female sexual development. *J Clin Invest.* 2006;116:953-960.
173. Hughes IA, Acerini CL. Factors controlling testis descent. *Eur J Endocrinol.* 2008;159(suppl 1):S75-S82.
174. Zimmermann S, Steig G, Emmen JM, et al. Targeted disruption of the Insl3 gene causes bilateral cryptorchidism. *Mol Endocrinol.* 1999;13: 681-691.
175. Kobayashi A, Behringer RR. Developmental genetics of the female reproductive tract in mammals. *Nat Rev Genet.* 2003;4:751-766.
176. Phoenix CH, Goy RW, Gerall AA, et al. Organizing action of prenatally administered testosterone proprionate on the tissues mediating mating behaviour in the female guinea pig. *Endocrinology.* 1959;65: 369-382.
177. Wallen K. Hormonal influences on sexually differentiated behavior in nonhuman primates. *Front Neuroendocrinol.* 2005;26:7-26.
178. Wallen K. Nature needs nurture: the interaction of hormonal and social influences on the development of behavioral sex differences in rhesus monkeys. *Horm Behav.* 1996;30:364-378.
179. Dewing P, Shi T, Horvath S, et al. Sexually dimorphic gene expression in mouse brain precedes gonadal differentiation. *Brain Res Mol Brain Res.* 2003;118:82-90.

180. Arnold AP, Chen X. What does the "four core genotypes" mouse model tell us about sex differences in the brain and other tissues? *Front Neuroendocrinol.* 2009;30:1-9.
181. Arnold AP. The organizational-activational hypothesis as the foundation for a unified theory of sexual differentiation in all mammalian tissues. *Horm Behav.* 2009;55:570-578.
182. Hines M, Ahmed F, Hughes IA. Psychological outcomes and gender-related development in complete androgen insensitivity syndrome. *Arch Sex Behav.* 2003;32:93-101.
183. Wisniewski AB, Mazur T. 46,XY DSD with female or ambiguous external genitalia at birth due to androgen insensitivity syndrome, 5α-reductase-2 deficiency, or 17β-hydroxysteroid dehydrogenase deficiency: a review of quality of life outcomes. *Int J Paediatr Endocrinol.* 2009:567430.
184. Cohen-Bendahan CCC, van de Beek C, Berenbaum SA. Prenatal sex hormone effects on child and adult sex-typed behavior: methods and findings. *Neurosci Biobehav Rev.* 2005;29:353-384.
185. Hines M. Early androgen influences on human neural and behavioural development. *Early Hum Dev.* 2008;84:805-807.
186. Frisén L, Nordenström A, Falhammar H, et al. Gender role behavior, sexuality, and psychosocial adaptation in women with congenital adrenal hyperplasia due to CYP21A2 deficiency. *J Clin Endocrinol Metab.* 2009;94:3432-3439.
187. Meyer-Bahlburg HF, Dolezal C, Baker SW, et al. Sexual orientation in women with classical or non-classical congenital adrenal hyperplasia as a function of degree of prenatal androgen excess. *Arch Sex Behav.* 2008;37:85-99.
188. Meyer-Bahlburg HF, Dolezal C, Baker SW, et al. Prenatal androgenization affects gender-related behavior but not gender identity in 5-12-year-old girls with congenital adrenal hyperplasia. *Arch Sex Behav.* 2004;33:97-104.
189. Dessens AB, Slijper FM, Drop SL. Gender dysphoria and gender change in chromosomal females with congenital adrenal hyperplasia. *Arch Sex Behav.* 2005;32:389-397.
190. Cohen-Kettenis PT. Gender change in 46,XY persons with 5-alpha-reductase-2 deficiency and 17-beta-hydroxysteroid dehydrogenase-3 deficiency. *Arch Sex Behav.* 2005;34:399-410.
191. Meyer-Bahlburg HF. Gender identity outcome in female-raised 46,XY persons with penile agenesis, cloacal exstrophy of the bladder, or penile ablation. *Arch Sex Behav.* 2005;34:423-438.
192. Zucker KJ. Intersexuality and gender identity differentiation. *Annu Rev Sex Res.* 1999;10:1-69.
193. Martin CL, Ruble DN, Szkrybalo J. Cognitive theories of early gender development. *Psychol Bull.* 2002;128:903-933.
194. Luders E, Narr K, Thompson PM, et al. Gender differences in cortical complexity. *Nat Neurosci.* 2004;7:799-800.
195. Ernst M, Maheu FS, Schroth E, et al. Amygdala function in adolescents with congenital adrenal hyperplasia: a model for the study of early steroid abnormalities. *Neuropsychologia.* 2007;45:2104-2113.
196. Schwarting GA, Wierman ME, Tobet SA. Gonadotropin-releasing hormone neuronal migration. *Semin Reprod Med.* 2007;25:305-312.
197. Semple RK, Kemal Topaloglu A. The recent genetics of hypogonadotropic hypogonadism: novel insights and new questions. *Clin Endocrinol.* 2010;72:427-435.
198. Bianco SD, Kaiser UB. The genetic and molecular basis of idiopathic hypogonadotropic hypogonadism. *Nat Rev Endocrinol.* 2009;5:569-576.
199. Kelberman D, Rizzoti K, Lovell-Badge R, et al. Genetic regulation of pituitary gland development in human and mouse. *Endocr Rev.* 2009;30:790-829.
200. Lin L, Gu WX, Ozisik G, et al. Analysis of DAX1 (NR0B1) and steroidogenic factor-1 (NR5A1) in children and adults with primary adrenal failure: ten years' experience. *J Clin Endocrinol Metab.* 2006;91:3048-3054.
201. Kelberman D, Rizzoti K, Avilion A, et al. Mutations within SOX2/SOX2 are associated with abnormalities in the hypothalamo-pituitary-gonadal axis in mice and humans. *J Clin Invest.* 2006;116:2442-2455.
202. Forest MG, Sizonenko PC, Cathiard AM, et al. Hypophyso-gonadal function in humans during the first year of life: 1. Evidence for testicular activity in early infancy. *J Clin Invest.* 1974;53:819-828.
203. Boas M, Boisen KA, Virtanen HE, et al. Postnatal penile length and growth rate correlate to serum testosterone levels: a longitudinal study of 1962 normal boys. *Eur J Endocrinol.* 2006;154:125-129.
204. Crofton PM, Illingworth PJ, Groome NP, et al. Changes in dimeric inhibin A and B during normal early puberty in boys and girls. *Clin Endocrinol.* 1997;46:109-114.
205. Kubini K, Zachmann M, Albers N, et al. Basal inhibin B and the testosterone response to human chorionic gonadotropin correlate in prepubertal boys. *J Clin Endocrinol Metab.* 2000;85:134-138.
206. Lee MM, Misra M, Donahoe PK, et al. MIS/AMH in the assessment of cryptorchidism and intersex conditions. *Mol Cell Endocrinol.* 2003;211:91-98.
207. Chellakooty M, Schmidt IM, Haavisto AM, et al. Inhibin A, inhibin B, follicle-stimulating hormone, luteinizing hormone, estradiol, and sex hormone-binding globulin levels in 473 healthy infant girls. *J Clin Endocrinol Metab.* 2003;88:3515-3520.
208. Lanfranco F, Kamischke A, Zitzmann M, et al. Klinefelter syndrome. *Lancet.* 2004;364:273-283.
209. Boiesen A, Gravholt CH. Klinefelter syndrome in clinical practice. *Nat Clin Pract Urol.* 2007;4:192-204.
210. Morris JK, Alberman E, Scott C, et al. Is the prevalence of Klinefelter syndrome increasing? *Eur J Hum Genet.* 2008;16:163-170.
211. Boada R, Janusz J, Hutaff-Lee C, et al. The cognitive phenotype in Klinefelter syndrome: a review of the literature including genetic and hormonal factors. *Dev Disabil Res Rev.* 2009;15:284-294.
212. Ross JL, Roeltgen DP, Stefanatos G, et al. Cognitive and motor development during childhood in boys with Klinefelter syndrome. *Am J Med Genet A.* 2008;146(A):708-719.
213. Salbenblatt JA, Bender BG, Puck MH, et al. Pituitary-gonadal function in Klinefelter syndrome before and during puberty. *Pediatr Res.* 1985;19:82-86.
214. Wikstrom AM, Dunkel L. Testicular function in Klinefelter syndrome. *Horm Res.* 2008;69:317-326.
215. Aksglaede L, Andersson AM, Jorgensen N, et al. Primary testicular failure in Klinefelter syndrome: the use of bivariate luteinizing hormone-testosterone reference charts. *Clin Endocrinol.* 2007;66:276-281.
216. Wikstrom AM, Hoei-Hansen CE, Dunkel L, et al. Immunoexpression of androgen receptor and nine markers of maturation in the testes of adolescent boys with Klinefelter syndrome: evidence for degeneration of germ cells at the onset of meiosis. *J Clin Endocrinol Metab.* 2007;92:714-719.
217. Wikstrom AM, Bay K, Hero M, et al. Serum insulin-like factor 3 levels during puberty in healthy boys and boys with Klinefelter syndrome. *J Clin Endocrinol Metab.* 2006;91:4705-4708.
218. Schiff JD, Palermo GD, Veeck LL, et al. Success of testicular sperm extraction and intracytoplasmic sperm injection in men with Klinefelter syndrome. *J Clin Endocrinol Metab.* 2005;90:6263-6267.
219. Fullerton G, Hamilton M, Maheshwari M. Should non-mosaic Klinefelter syndrome men be labeled as infertile in 2009? *Hum Reprod.* 2010;25:588-597.
220. Sybert VP, McCauley E. Turner's syndrome. *N Engl J Med.* 2004;351:1227-1238.
221. Bondy CA. Turner Syndrome Study Group. Care of girls and women with Turner syndrome: a guideline of the Turner Syndrome Study Group. *J Clin Endocrinol Metab.* 2007;92:10-25.
222. Davenport ML. Approach to the patient with Turner syndrome. *J Clin Endocrinol Metab.* 2010;95:1487-1495.
223. Devernay M, Ecosse E, Coste J, et al. Determinants of medical care for young women with Turner Syndrome. *J Clin Endocrinol Metab.* 2009;94:3408-3413.
224. Singh RF, Carr DH. The anatomy and histology of XO human embryos and fetuses. *Anat Rec.* 1966;155:369-384.
225. Pasquino AM, Passeri F, Pucarelli I, et al. Spontaneous pubertal development in Turner's syndrome. Italian Study Group for Turner's syndrome. *J Clin Endocrinol Metab.* 1997;82:1810-1813.
226. Gravholt CH, Fedder J, Naeraa RW, et al. Occurrence of gonadoblastoma in females with Turner syndrome and Y chromosome material: a population study. *J Clin Endocrinol Metab.* 2000;85:3199-3202.
227. Hreinsson JG, Otala M, Fridstrom M, et al. Follicles are found in the ovaries of adolescent girls with Turner's syndrome. *J Clin Endocrinol Metab.* 2002;87:3618-3623.
228. El-Shawarby SA, Sharif F, Conway G, et al. Oocyte cryopreservation after controlled ovarian hyperstimulation in mosaic Turner syndrome: another fertility preservation option in a dedicated UK clinic. *BJOG.* 2010;117:234-237.
229. Oktay K, Rodriguez-Wallberg KA, Sahin G. Fertility preservation by ovarian stimulation and oocyte cryopreservation in a 14-year-old adolescent with Turner syndrome mosaicism and impending ovarian failure. *Fert Steril.* 2010;94:753.e15-753.e19.
230. Knudtzon J, Aarskog D. 45,X/46,XY mosaicism: a clinical review and report of ten cases. *Eur J Pediatr.* 1987;146:266-271.
231. Telvi L, Lebbar A, Del Pino O, et al. 45,X/46,XY mosaicism: report of 27 cases. *Pediatrics.* 1999;104:304-308.
232. Müller J, Skakkebaek NE, Ritzen M, et al. Carcinoma in situ of the testis in children with 45,X/46,XY gonadal dysgenesis. *J Pediatr.* 1985;106:431-436.
233. Müller J, Ritzen EM, Ivarsson SA, et al. Management of males with 45,X/46,XY gonadal dysgenesis. *Horm Res.* 1999;52:11-14.
234. Hsu LY. Prenatal diagnosis of 45,X/46,XY mosaicism: a review and update. *Prenat Diagn.* 1989;9:31-48.
235. Chang HJ, Clark RD, Bachman H. The phenotype of 45,X/46,XY mosaicism: an analysis of 92 prenatally diagnosed cases. *Am J Hum Genet.* 1990;46:156-167.
236. Krob G, Braun A, Kuhnle U. True hermaphroditism: geographical distribution, clinical findings, chromosomes and gonadal histology. *Eur J Pediatr.* 1994;153:2-10.
237. Wiersma R, Ramdial PK. The gonads of 111 South African patients with ovotesticular disorder of sex differentiation. *J Pediatr Surg.* 2009;44:556-560.

238. Wiersma R. Management of the African child with true hermaphroditism. *J Pediatr Surg*. 2001;36:397-399.
239. Tomaselli S, Megiorni F, De Bernardo C, et al. Syndromic true hermaphroditism due to an R-spondin (RSPO1) homozygous mutation. *Hum Mutation*. 2008;29:220-226.
240. McElreavey K, Rappaport R, Vilain E, et al. A minority of 46,XX true hermaphrodites are positive for the Y DNA sequence including SRY. *Hum Genet*. 1992;90:121-125.
241. Damiani D, Fellous M, McElreavey K, et al. True hermaphroditism: clinical aspects and molecular studies in 16 cases. *Eur J Endocrinol*. 1997;136:201-204.
242. Steinmetz L, Rocha MN, Longui CA, et al. Inhibin A production after gonadotropin stimulus: a new method to detect ovarian tissue in ovotesticular disorder of sex development. *Horm Res*. 2009;71: 94-99.
243. Schimmer BP, White PC. Minireview: steroidogenic factor 1—its roles in differentiation, development, and disease. *Mol Endocrinol*. 2010;24:1322-1337.
244. Correa RV, Domenice S, Bingham NC, et al. A microdeletion in the ligand binding domain of human steroidogenic factor 1 causes XY sex reversal without adrenal insufficiency. *J Clin Endocrinol Metab*. 2004;89:1767-1772.
245. Kohler B, Lin L, Ferraz-de-Souza B, et al. Five novel mutations in steroidogenic factor 1 (SF1, NR5A1) in 46,XY patients with severe underandrogenization but without adrenal insufficiency. *Hum Mutat*. 2008; 29:59-64.
246. Kohler B, Lin L, Mazen I, et al. The spectrum of phenotypes associated with mutations in steroidogenic factor 1 (SF-1, NR5A1, Ad4BP) includes severe penoscrotal hypospadias in 46,XY males without adrenal insufficiency. *Eur J Endocrinol*. 2009; 161:237-242.
247. Philibert P, Zenaty D, Lin L, et al. Mutational analysis of steroidogenic factor 1 (NR5a1) in 24 boys with bilateral anorchia: a French collaborative study. *Hum Reprod*. 2007; 22:3255-3261.
248. Biason-Lauber A, Konrad D, Meyer M, et al. Ovaries and female phenotype in a girl with 46,XY karyotype and mutations in the CBX2 gene. *Am J Hum Genet*. 2009; 84:658-663.
249. Fischbach BV, Trout KL, Lewis J, et al. WAGR syndrome: a clinical review of 54 cases. *Pediatrics*. 2005;116:984-988.
250. Kohler B, Schumacher V, l'Allemand D, et al. Germline Wilms tumor suppressor gene (WT1) mutation leading to isolated genital malformation without Wilms tumor or nephropathy. *J Pediatr*. 2001;138: 421-424.
251. Suri M, Kelehan P, O'Neill D, et al. WT1 mutations in Meacham syndrome suggest a coelomic mesothelial origin of the cardiac and diaphragmatic malformations. *Am J Med Genet A*. 2007; 143A:2312-2320.
252. Brown S, Yu C, Lanzano P, et al. A de novo mutation (Gln2Stop) at the 5′ end of the SRY gene leads to sex reversal with partial ovarian function. *Am J Hum Genet*. 1998;62:189-192.
253. Hawkins JR, Taylor A, Goodfellow PN, et al. Evidence for increased prevalence of SRY mutations in XY females with complete rather than partial gonadal dysgenesis. *Am J Hum Genet*. 1992;51:979-984.
254. McElreavey K, Vilain E, Abbas N, et al. XY sex reversal associated with a deletion 5′ to the SRY "HMG box" in the testis-determining region. *Proc Natl Acad Sci U S A*. 1992;89:11016-11020.
255. Vilain E, McElreavey K, Jaubert F, et al. Familial case with sequence variant in the testis-determining region associated with two sex phenotypes. *Am J Hum Genet*. 1992;50:1008-1011.
256. Cameron FJ, Hageman RM, Cooke-Yarborough C, et al. A novel germ line mutation in SOX9 causes familial camptomelic dysplasia and sex reversal. *Hum Mol Genet*. 1996;5:1625-1630.
257. Canto P, Soderlund D, Reyes E, et al. Mutations in the desert hedgehog (DHH) gene in patients with 46,XY complete pure gonadal dysgenesis. *J Clin Endocrinol Metab*. 2004;89:4480-4483.
258. Puffenberger EG, Hu-Lince D, Parod JM, et al. Mapping of sudden infant death with dysgenesis of the testes syndrome (SIDDT) by a SNP genome scan and identification of TSPYL loss of function. *Proc Natl Acad Sci U S A*. 2004;101:11689-11694.
259. Vinci G, Brauner R, Tar A, et al. Mutations in the TSPYL1 gene associated with 46,XY disorder of sex development and male infertility. *Fertil Steril*. 2009;92:1347-1350.
260. Chen Y, Thai HT, Lundin J, et al. Mutational study of the MAMLD1-gene in hypospadias. *Eur J Med Genet*. 2010; 53:122-126.
261. Ogata T, Wada Y, Fukami M. MAMLD1 (CXorf6): a new gene for hypospadias. *Sex Dev*. 2008; 2:244-250.
262. Porter FD. Smith-Lemli-Opitz syndrome: pathogenesis, diagnosis and management. *Eur J Hum Genet*. 2008;16:535-541.
263. Berthezene F, Forest MG, Grimaud JA, et al. Leydig cell agenesis: a cause of male pseudohermaphroditism. *N Engl J Med*. 1976;295: 969-972.
264. Kremer H, Kraaij R, Toledo S, et al. Male pseudohermaphroditism due to a homozygous missense mutation of the luteinizing hormone receptor gene. *Nat Genet*. 1995;9:160-164.
265. Latronico AC, Anasti J, Arnhold IJP, et al. Brief report: testicular and ovarian resistance to luteinizing hormone caused by homozygous inactivating mutations of the luteinizing hormone receptor gene. *N Engl J Med*. 1996;334:507-512.
266. Kossack N, Simoni M, Richter-Unruh A, et al. Mutations in a novel, cryptic exon of the luteinizing hormone/chorionic gonadotropin receptor gene cause male pseudohermaphroditism. *PLoS Med*. 2008;5:e88.
267. Martens JWM, Verhoef-Post M, Abelin N, et al. A homozygous mutation in the luteinizing hormone receptor causes partial Leydig cell hypoplasia: correlation between receptor activity and phenotype. *Mol Endocrinol*. 1998;12:775-784.
268. Lin D, Sugawara T, Strauss JF III, et al. Role of steroidogenic acute regulatory protein in adrenal and gonadal steroidogenesis. *Science*. 1995;267:1828-1831.
269. Miller WL. StAR search: what we know about how the steroidogenic acute regulatory protein mediates mitochondrial cholesterol import. *Mol Endocrinol*. 2007;21:589-601.
270. Prader A, Gurtner HP. Das Syndrom des Pseudohermaphroditismus masculinus bei kongenitaler NebennierenrindenHyperplasie ohne Androgenuberproduktion (adrenaler Pseudohermaphrotidismus masculinus). *Helv Paediatr Acta*. 1955;10:397-412.
271. Bose HS, Sugawara T, Strauss JF III, et al. The pathophysiology and genetics of congenital lipoid adrenal hyperplasia. *N Engl J Med*. 1996;335:1870-1878.
272. Caron K, Soo S-C, Wetsel W, et al. Targeted disruption of the mouse gene encoding steroidogenic acute regulatory protein provides insights into congenital lipoid adrenal hyperplasia. *Proc Natl Acad Sci U S A*. 1997;94:11540-11545.
273. Bose HS, Pescouitz OH, Miller WL. Spontaneous feminization in a 46,XX female patient with adrenal hyperplasia due to a homozygous frame shift mutation in the steroidogenic reactive protein. *J Clin Endocrinol Metab*. 1997;82:1511-1515.
274. Nakae J, Tajima T, Sugawara T, et al. Analysis of the steroidogenic acute regulatory protein (StAR) gene in Japanese patients with congenital lipoid adrenal hyperplasia. *Hum Mol Genet*. 1997;6:571-576.
275. Baker BY, Lin L, Kim CJ, et al. Nonclassic congenital lipoid adrenal hyperplasia: a new disorder of the steroidogenic acute regulatory protein with very late presentation and normal male genitalia. *J Clin Endocrinol Metab*. 2006;91:4781-4785.
276. Sahakitrungruang T, Soccio RE, Lang-Muritano M, et al. Clinical, genetic, and functional characterization of four patients carrying partial loss-of-function mutations in the steroidogenic acute regulatory protein (StAR). *J Clin Endocrinol Metab*. 2010;95:3352-3359.
277. Hiort O, Holterhus PM, Werner R, et al. Homozygous disruption of P450 side-chain cleavage (CYP11A1) is associated with prematurity, complete 46,XY sex reversal, and severe adrenal failure. *J Clin Endocrinol Metab*. 2005;90:538-541.
278. Kim CJ, Lin L, Huang N, et al. Severe combined adrenal and gonadal deficiency caused by novel mutations in the cholesterol side chain cleavage enzyme, P450scc. *J Clin Endocrinol Metab*. 2008; 93:696-702.
279. Rubtsov P, Karmanov M, Sverdlova P, et al. A novel homozygous mutation in CYP11A1 gene is associated with late-onset adrenal insufficiency and hypospadias in a 46,XY patient. *J Clin Endocrinol Metab*. 2009;94:936-939.
280. Simard J, Ricketts M-L, Gingras S, et al. Molecular biology of the 3β-hydroxysteroid dehydrogenase/Δ^5-Δ^4 isomerase gene family. *Endocr Rev*. 2005;26:525-582.
281. Moisan AM, Ricketts ML, Tardy V, et al. New insight into the molecular basis of 3β-hydroxysteroid dehydrogenase deficiency: identification of eight mutations in the HSD3B2 gene eleven patients from seven new families and comparison of the functional properties of twenty-five mutant enzymes. *J Clin Endocrinol Metab*. 1999;84:4410-4425.
282. Alos N, Moisan AM, Ward L, et al. A novel A10E homozygous mutation in the HSD3B2 gene causing severe salt-wasting 3β-hydroxysteroid dehydrogenase deficiency in 46,XX and 46,XY French-Canadians: evaluation of gonadal function after puberty. *J Clin Endocrinol Metab*. 2000;85:1968-1974.
283. Parks GA, Bermudez JA, Anast CS, et al. Pubertal boy with the 3β-hydroxysteroid dehydrogenase defect. *J Clin Endocrinol Metab*. 1971;33:269-278.
284. Rheaume E, Simard J, Morel Y, et al. Congenital adrenal hyperplasia due to point mutations in the type II 3 beta-hydroxysteroid dehydrogenase gene. *Nat Genet*. 1992;1:239-245.
285. Johannsen TH, Mallet D, Dige-Petersen H, et al. Delayed diagnosis of congenital adrenal hyperplasia with salt wasting due to type II 3β-hydroxysteroid dehydrogenase deficiency. *J Clin Endocrinol Metab*. 2005;90:2076-2080.
286. Lutfallah C, Wang W, Mason JI, et al. Newly proposed hormonal criteria via genotypic proof for type II 3beta-hydroxysteroid dehydrogenase deficiency. *J Clin Endocrinol Metab*. 2002;87:2611-2622.
287. Mermejo LM, Elias LL, Marui S, et al. Refining hormonal diagnosis of type II 3 beta-hydroxysteroid dehydrogenase deficiency in patients with premature pubarche and hirsutism based on HSD3B2 genotyping. *J Clin Endocrinol Metab*. 2005;90:1287-1293.
288. Pang S, Carbunaru G, Haider A, et al. Carriers for type II 3beta-hydroxysteroid dehydrogenase (HSD3B2) deficiency can only be

identified by HSD3B2 genotype study and not by hormone test. *Clin Endocrinol*. 2003;58:323-331.
289. Codner E, Okuma C, Iniguez G, et al. Molecular study of the 3 beta-hydroxysteroid dehydrogenase gene type II in patients with hypospadias. *J Clin Endocrinol Metab*. 2004;89:957-964.
290. New MI. Male pseudohermaphrodism due to a 17-alpha-hydroxylase deficiency. *J Clin Invest*. 1970;49:1930-1941.
291. Winter JSD, Couch RM, Muller J, et al. Combined 17-hydroxylase and 17/20 desmolase deficiencies: evidence for synthesis of a defective cytochrome P450c17. *J Clin Endocrinol Metab*. 1989;68:309-316.
292. Auchus RJ. The genetics, pathophysiology, and management of human deficiencies of P450c17. *Endocrinol Metab Clin North Am*. 2001;30:101-119.
293. Miller WL. Steroid 17alpha-hydroxylase deficiency: not rare everywhere. *J Clin Endocrinol Metab*. 2004;89:40-42.
294. Costa-Santos M, Kater CE, Auchus RJ. Brazilian Congenital Adrenal Hyperplasia Multicenter Study Group. Two prevalent CYP17 mutations and genotype-phenotype correlations in 24 Brazilian patients with 17-hydroxylase deficiency. *J Clin Endocrinol Metab*. 2004;89:49-60.
295. Dhir V, Reisch N, Bleicken CM, et al. Steroid 17alpha-hydroxylase deficiency: functional characterization of four mutations (A174E, V178D, R440C, L465P) in the CYP17A1 gene. *J Clin Endocrinol Metab*. 2009;94:3058-3064.
296. Yanase T, Kagimoto M, Suzuki B, et al. Deletion of a phenylalanine in the N-terminal region of human cytochrome P-450(17α) results in combined 17α-hydroxylase/17,20-lyase deficiency. *J Biol Chem*. 1989;264:18076-18082.
297. Ahlgren R, Yanase T, Simpson ER, et al. Compound heterozygous mutations (Arg239stop, Pro342Thr) in the CYP17 (P450 17-alpha) gene lead to ambiguous external genitalia in a male with partial combined 17 alpha-hydroxylase/17,20 lyase deficiency. *J Clin Endocrinol Metab*. 1992;74:667-672.
298. Geller DH, Auchus RJ, Mendonca BB, et al. The genetic and functional basis of isolated 17,20 lyase deficiency. *Nat Genet*. 1997;17:201-205.
299. Geller DH, Auchus RJ, Miller WL. P450c17 mutations R347H and R358Q selectively disrupt 17,20-lyase activity by disrupting interactions with P450 oxidoreductase and cytochrome b5. *Mol Endocrinol*. 1999;13:167-175.
300. Sherbert DP, Tosiano D, Kwist KM, et al. CYP17 mutation E305G causes isolated 17,20-lyase deficiency by selectively altering substrate binding. *J Biol Chem*. 2003;278:48563-48569.
301. Giordano SJ, Kaftory A, Steggles AW. A splicing mutation in the cytochrome b_5 gene from a patient with congenital methemoglobinemia and pseudohermaphrodism. *Hum Genet*. 1994;93:568-570.
302. Kok RC, Timmerman MA, Wolffenbuttel KP, et al. Isolated 17,20-lyase deficiency due to the cytochrome b5 mutation W27X. *J Clin Endocrinol Metab*. 2010;95:994-999.
303. Miller WL. Minireview: regulation of steroidogenesis by electron transfer. *Endocrinology*. 2005;146:2544-2550.
304. Peterson RE, Imperato-McGinley J, Gautier T, et al. Male pseudohermaphroditism due to multiple defects in steroid-biosynthetic microsomal mixed-function oxidases: a new variant of congenital adrenal hyperplasia. *N Engl J Med*. 1985;313:1182-1191.
305. Fluck CE, Tajima T, Pandey AV, et al. Mutant P450 oxidoreductase causes disordered steroidogenesis with and without Antley-Bixler syndrome. *Nat Genet*. 2004;36:228-230.
306. Miller WL, Huang N, Agrawal V, et al. Genetic variation in human P450 oxidoreductase. *Mol Cell Endocrinol*. 2009; 300:180-184.
307. Fukami M, Nishimura G, Homma K, et al. Cytochrome P450 oxidoreductase deficiency: identification and characterization of biallelic mutations and genotype-phenotype correlations in 35 Japanese patients. *J Clin Endocrinol Metab*. 2009; 94:1723-1731.
308. Miller WL, Huang N, Pandey AV, et al. P450 oxidoreductase deficiency: a new disorder of steroidogenesis. *Ann N Y Acad Sci*. 2005;1061:100-108.
309. Labrie F, Luu-The V, Lin SX, et al. Role of 17 beta-hydroxysteroid dehydrogenases in sex steroid formation in peripheral intracrine tissues. *Trends Endocrinol Metab*. 2000;11:421-427.
310. Saez JM, de Perett E, Morera AM, et al. Familial male pseudohermaphroditism with gynaecomastia due to a testicular 17-ketosteroid reductase defect: I. In vivo studies. *J Clin Endocrinol Metab*. 1971;32:604-610.
311. Saez JM, Morera AM, de Peretti E, et al. Further in vivo studies in male pseudohermaphroditism with gynaecomastia due to a testicular 17-ketosteroid reductase defect (compared to a case of testicular feminization). *J Clin Endocrinol Metab*. 1972;34:598-600.
312. Andersson S, Geissler WM, Wu L, et al. Molecular genetics and pathophysiology of 17 beta-hydroxysteroid dehydrogenase 3 deficiency. *J Clin Endocrinol Metab*. 1996;81:130-136.
313. Boehmer AL, Brinkmann AO, Sandkuijl LA, et al. 17 Beta-hydroxysteroid dehydrogenase-3 deficiency: diagnosis, phenotypic variability, population genetics, and worldwide distribution of ancient and de novo mutations. *J Clin Endocrinol Metab*. 1999;84:4713-4721.
314. Twesten W, Holterhus P, Sippell WG, et al. Clinical, endocrine and molecular genetic findings in patients with 17beta-hydroxysteroid dehydrogenase deficiency. *Horm Res*. 2002;53:26-31.
315. Lee YS, Kirk JM, Stanhope RG, et al. Phenotypic variability in 17β-hydroxysteroid dehydrogenase-3 deficiency and diagnostic pitfalls. *Clin Endocrinol (Oxf)*. 2007;67:20-28.
316. Qiu W, Zhou M, Labrie F, et al. Crystal structures of the multispecific 17beta-hydroxysteroid dehydrogenase type 5: critical androgen regulation in human peripheral tissues. *Mol Endocrinol*. 2004;18:1798-1807.
317. Rösler A. Steroid 17 beta-hydroxysteroid dehydrogenase deficiency in man: an inherited form of male pseudohermaphroditism. *J Steroid Biochem Mol Biol*. 1992;43:989-1002.
318. Schützmann K, Brinkmann L, Schacht M, et al. Psychological distress, self-harming behavior, and suicidal tendencies in adults with disorders of sex development. *Arch Sex Behav*. 2009;38:16-33.
319. Faisal SF, Iqbal A, Hughes IA. The testosterone : androstenedione ratio in male undermasculinization. *Clin Endocrinol*. 2000;53:697-702.
320. Moghrabi N, Hughes IA, Dunaif A, et al. Deleterious missense mutations and silent polymorphism in the human 17beta-hydroxysteroid dehydrogenase 3 gene (HSD17B3). *J Clin Endocrinol Metab*. 1998:83;2855-2860.
321. Hannema SE, Scott IS, Hodapp J, et al. Residual activity of mutant androgen receptors explains wolffian duct development in the complete androgen insensitivity syndrome. *J Clin Endocrinol Metab*. 2004;89:5815-5822.
322. Khan N, Sharma KK, Andersson S, et al. Human 17beta-hydroxysteroid dehydrogenases types 1, 2 and 3 catalyse bi-directional equilibrium reactions, rather than unidirectional metabolism, in HEK-293 cells. *Arch Biochem Biophys*. 2004;429:50-59.
323. Gross DJ, Landau H, Kohn G, et al. Male pseudohermaphroditism due to 17 beta-hydroxysteroid dehydrogenase deficiency: gender assignment in early infancy. *Acta Endocrinol*. 1986;112:238-246.
324. Imperato-McGinley J, Guerrero L, Gautier T, et al. Steroid 5α-reductase deficiency in man: an inherited form of male pseudohermaphroditism. *Science*. 1974;186:1213-1215.
325. Andersson S, Berman DM, Jenkins EP, et al. Deletion of steroid 5-alpha-reductase 2 gene in male pseudohermaphroditism. *Nature*. 1991;354:159-161.
326. Wilson JD, Griffin JE, Russell DW. Steroid 5a-reductase 2 deficiency. *Endocr Rev*. 2003;14:577-593.
327. Vilchis F, Ramos L, Mendez JP, et al. Molecular analysis of the SRD5A2 in 46,XY subjects with incomplete virilization: the P212R substitution of the steroid 5 α-reductase-2 may constitute an ancestral founder mutation in Mexican patients. *J Androl*. 2009;31:358-364.
328. Cai LQ, Fratianni CM, Gautier T, et al. Dihydrotestosterone regulation of semen in male pseudohermaphrodites with 5 alpha-reductase-2 deficiency. *J Clin Endocrinol Metab*. 1994;79:409-414.
329. Katz MD, Kligman I, Cai L-Q, et al. Paternity by intrauterine insemination with sperm from a man with 5α-reductase-2 deficiency. *N Engl J Med*. 1997;336:994-997.
330. Nordenskjold A, Ivarsson SA. Molecular characterization of 5 alpha-reductase type 2 deficiency and fertility in a Swedish family. *J Clin Endocrinol Metab*. 1998;83:3236-3238.
331. Herdt GH, Davidson J. The Sambia "Turnim-Man": sociocultural and clinical aspects of gender formation in male pseudohermaphrodites with 5-alpha-reductase deficiency in Papua, New Guinea. *Arch Sex Behav*. 1988;17:33-56.
332. Katz MD, Cai LQ, Zhu YS, et al. The biochemical and phenotypic characterization of females homozygous for 5 alpha-reductase 2 deficiency. *J Clin Endocrinol Metab*. 1995;80:3160-3167.
333. Krone N, Hughes BA, Lavery GG, et al. Gas chromatography/mass spectrometry (GC/MS) remains a pre-eminent discovery tool in clinical steroid investigations even in the era of fast liquid chromatography tandem mass spectrometry (LC/MS/MS). *J Steroid Biochem Mol Biol*. 2010;121:496-504.
334. Forti G, Falchetti A, Santoro S, et al. Steroid 5 alpha-reductase 2 deficiency: virilization in early infancy may be due to partial function of mutant enzyme. *Clin Endocrinol*. 1996;44:477-482.
335. Maimoun L, Philibert P, Cammas B, et al. Undervirilization in XY newborns may hide a 5alpha-reductase deficiency: report of three new SRD5A2 gene mutations. *Int J Androl*. 2010;33:841-847.
336. Charmandari E, Dattani MT, Perry LA, et al. Kinetics and effect of percutaneous administration of dihydrotestosterone in children. *Horm Res*. 2001;56:177-181.
337. Levine AC, Wang JP, Ren M, et al. Immunohistochemical localization of steroid 5 alpha-reductase 2 in the human male fetal reproductive tract and adult prostate. *J Clin Endocrinol Metab*. 1996;81:384-389.
338. Thiele S, Hoppe U, Holterhus P-M, et al. Isoenzyme type 1 of 5alpha-reductase is abundantly transcribed in normal human genital skin fibroblasts and may play an important role in masculinisation of 5alpha-reductase type 2 deficient males. *Eur J Endocrinol*. 2005;152:875-880.
339. Quigley C, De Bellis A, Marschke KB, et al. Androgen receptor defects: historical, clinical, and molecular perspectives. *Endocr Rev*. 1995;16:271-321.

340. Claessens F, Denayer S, Van Tilborgh N, et al. Diverse roles of androgen receptor (AR) domains in AR-mediated signaling. *Nucl Recept Signal.* 2008;6:e008.
341. Denayer S, Helsen C, Thorrez L, et al. The rules of DNA recognition by the androgen receptor. *Mol Endocrinol.* 2010;24:898-913.
342. Lonard DM, Kumar R, O'Malley BW. Minireview: the SRC family of coactivators: an entrée to understanding a subset of polygenic diseases? *Mol Endocrinol.* 2010;24:279-285.
343. Tut TG, Ghadessy FJ, Trifiro MA, et al. Long polyglutamine tracts in the androgen receptor are associated with reduced trans-activation, impaired sperm production, and male infertility. *J Clin Endocrinol Metab.* 1997;82:3777-3782.
344. Boehmer AL, Brinkmann AO, Bruggenwirth H, et al. Genotype versus phenotype in families with androgen insensitivity syndrome. *J Clin Endocrinol Metab.* 2001;86:4151-4160.
345. Han TS, Goswami D, Trikudanathan S, et al. Comparison of bone mineral density and body proportions between women with complete androgen insensitivity syndrome and women with gonadal dysgenesis. *Eur J Endocrinol.* 2008;159:179-185.
346. Hurme T, Lahdes-Vasama T, Makela E, et al. Clinical findings in prepubertal girls with inguinal hernia with special reference to the diagnosis of androgen insensitivity syndrome. *Scand J Urol Nephrol.* 2009;43:42-46.
347. Deeb A, Hughes IA. Inguinal hernia in female infants: a cue to check the sex chromosomes? *BJU Int.* 2005;96:401-403.
348. Yong EL, Loy CJ, Sim KS. Androgen receptor gene and male infertility. *Hum Reprod Update.* 2003;9:1-7.
349. MacLean HE, Brown RW, Beilin J, et al. Increased frequency of long androgen receptor CAG repeats in male breast cancers. *Breast Cancer Res Treat.* 2004;88:239-246.
350. Ahmed SF, Cheng A, Hughes IA. Assessment of the gonadotropin-gonadal axis in androgen insensitivity syndrome. *Arch Dis Child.* 1999;80:324-329.
351. Werner R, Grötsch H, Hiort O. 46,XY disorder of sex development—the undermasculinised male with disorders of androgen action. *Best Pract Res Clin Endocrinol.* 2010;24:263-277.
352. Boukari K, Meduri G, Brailly-Tabard S, et al. Lack of androgen receptor expression in Sertoli cells accounts for the absence of anti-müllerian hormone repression during early human testis development. *J Clin Endocrinol Metab.* 2009;94:1818-1825.
353. Bouvattier C, Carel JC, Lecointre C, et al. Postnatal changes of T, LH, and FSH in 46,XY infants with mutations in the AR gene. *J Clin Endocrinol Metab.* 2002;87:29-32.
354. Quigley CA. The postnatal gonadotropin and sex steroid surge: insights from the androgen insensitivity syndrome (Editorial). *J Clin Endocrinol Metab.* 2002;87:24-28.
355. Yarbrough WG, Quarmby VE, Simental JA, et al. A single base mutation in the androgen receptor gene causes androgen insensivity in the testicular feminized rat. *J Biol Chem.* 1990;265:8893-8900.
356. Tadokoro R, Bunch T, Schwabe JW, et al. Comparison on the molecular consequences of different mutations at residue 754 and 690 of the androgen receptor (AR) and androgen insensitivity syndrome (AIS) phenotype. *Clin Endocrinol.* 2009;71:253-260.
357. Deeb, A, Jääskeläinen J, Dattani M, et al. A novel mutation in the human androgen receptor suggests a regulatory role for the hinge region in amino-terminal and carboxy-terminal interactions. *J Clin Endocrinol Metab.* 2008;93:3691-3696.
358. Deeb A, Mason C, Lee YS, et al. Correlation between genotype, phenotype and sex of rearing in 111 patients with partial androgen insensitivity syndrome. *Clin Endocrinol.* 2005;63:56-62.
359. Kohler B, Lumbroso S, Leger J, et al. Androgen insensitivity syndrome: somatic mosaicism of the androgen receptor in seven families and consequences for sex assignment and genetic counselling. *J Clin Endocrinol Metab.* 2005;90:106-111.
360. Cheikhelard A, Morel Y, Thibaud E, et al. Long-term follow up and comparison between genotype and phenotype in 29 cases of complete androgen insensitivity syndrome. *J Urol.* 2008;180:1496-1501.
361. Boehmer AL, Brinkmann AO, Nijman RM, et al. Phenotypic variation in a family with partial androgen insensitivity syndrome explained by differences in 5alpha dihydrotestosterone availability. *J Clin Endocrinol Metab.* 2001;86:1240-1246.
362. Holterhus PM, Werner R, Hoppe U, et al. Molecular features and clinical phenotypes in androgen insensitivity syndrome in the absence and presence of androgen receptor gene mutations. *J Mol Med.* 2005;83:1005-1113.
363. Holterhus PM, Deppe U, Werner R, et al. Intrinsic androgen-dependent gene expression patterns revealed by comparison of genital fibroblasts from normal males and individuals with complete and partial androgen insensitivity syndrome. *BMC Genomics.* 2007;8:376.
364. Holterhus PM, Bebermeier JH, Werner R, et al. Disorders of sex development expose transcriptional autonomy of genetic sex and androgen-programmed hormonal sex in human blood leukocytes. *BMC Genomics.* 2009;10:292.
365. Jääskeläinen J, Deeb A, Schwabe JW, et al. Human androgen receptor gene ligand-binding domain mutations leading to disrupted interaction between the N- and C-terminal domains. *J Mol Endocrinol.* 2006;36:361-368.
366. Elfferich P, Juniarto AZ, Dubbink HJ, et al. Functional analysis of novel androgen receptor mutations in a unique cohort of Indonesian patients with a disorder of sex development. *Sex Dev.* 2009;3:237-244.
367. Werner R, Grötsch H, Hiort O. 46,XY disorders of sex development—the undermasculinised male with disorders of androgen action. *Best Pract Res Clin Endocrinol Metab.* 2010;24:263-277.
368. Audi L, Fernandez-Cancio M, Carrascosa A, et al. Novel (60%) and recurrent (40%) androgen receptor gene mutations in a series of 59 patients with a 46,XY disorder of sex development. *J Clin Endocrinol Metab.* 2010;95:1876-1888.
369. Mongan NP, Lim HN, Hughes IA. Genetic evidence to exclude the androgen receptor-polyglutamine associated coactivator, ARA-24, as a cause of male undermasculinisation. *Eur J Endocrinol.* 2001;145:809-811.
370. Lim HN, Hawkins JR, Hughes IA. Genetic evidence to exclude the androgen receptor co-factor, ARA70 (NCOA4) as a candidate gene for the causation of undermasculinised genitalia. *Clin Genet.* 2001;59:284-286.
371. Zhou XE, Suino-Powell KM, Li J, et al. Identification of SRC3/A1B1 as a preferred coactivator for hormone-activated androgen receptor. *J Biol Chem.* 2010;285:9161-9171.
372. Mongan NP, Jääskeläinen J, Bhattacharyya S, et al. Steroid receptor coactivator-3 glutamine repeat polymorphism and the androgen insensitivity syndrome. *Eur J Endocrinol.* 2003;148:277-279.
373. Cheung-Flynn J, Prapapanich V, Cox MB, et al. Physiological role for the cochaperone FKBP52 in androgen receptor signalling. *Mol Endocrinol.* 2005;19:1654-1666.
374. Beleza-Meireles A, Barbaro M, Wedell A, et al. Studies of a co-chaperone of the androgen receptor, FKBP52, as candidate for hypospadias. *Reprod Biol Endocrinol.* 2007;5:8.
375. La Spada AR, Wilson EM, Lubahn DB, et al. Androgen receptor gene mutations in X-linked spinal and bulbar muscular atrophy. *Nature.* 1991;352:77-79.
376. Ogata T, Muroya K, Ishii T, et al. Undermasculinized genitalia in a boy with an abnormally expanded CAG repeat length in the androgen receptor gene. *Clin Endocrinol.* 2001;54:835-838.
377. Vermeersch H, T'sjoen G, Kaufman JM, et al. Testosterone, androgen receptor gene CAG repeat length, mood, and behaviour in adolescent males. *Eur J Endocrinol.* 2010;163:319-328.
378. Wang HY, Hu Y, Wang SH, et al. Association of androgen receptor CAG repeat polymorphism with VOmax response to hypoxic training in North China Han men. *Int J Androl.* 2010;33:794-799.
379. Werner R, Holterhus PM, Binder G, et al. The A645D mutation in the hinge region of the human androgen receptor (AR) gene modulates AR activity, depending on the context of the polymorphic glutamine and glycine repeats. *J Clin Endocrinol Metab.* 2006;91:3515-3520.
380. T'sjoen G, De Cuypere G, Monstrey S, et al. Male gender identity in complete androgen insensitivity syndrome. *Arch Sex Behav.* 2010; April 1 (Epub ahead of print).
381. Papadimitriou DT, Linglart A, Morel Y, et al. Puberty in subjects with complete androgen insensitivity syndrome. *Horm Res.* 2006;65:126-131.
382. Savage MO, Lowe DG. Gonadal neoplasia and abnormal sexual differentiation. *Clin Endocrinol.* 1990;32:519-533.
383. Looijenga LH, Hersmus R, de Leeuw BH, et al. Gonadal tumours and DSD. *Best Pract Res Clin Endocrinol Metab.* 2010;24:291-310.
384. Sonne SB, Almstrup K, Dalgaard M, et al. Analysis of gene expression profiles of microdissected cell populations indicates that testicular carcinoma in situ is an arrested gonocyte. *Cancer Res.* 2009;69:5241-5250.
385. Tan IB, Ang KK, Ching BC, et al. Testicular microlithiasis predicts concurrent testicular germ cell tumors and intratubular germ cell neoplasia of unclassified type in adults: a meta-analysis and systematic review. *Cancer.* 2010;116:4520-4532.
386. Almstrup K, Sonne SB, Hoei-Hansen CE, et al. From embryonic stem cells to testicular germ cell cancer: should we be concerned? *Int J Androl.* 2006;29:211-218.
387. Stoop H, Honecker F, van de Geijn GJ, et al. Stem cell factor as a novel diagnostic marker for early malignant germ cells. *J Pathol.* 2008;216:43-54.
388. Rajpert-de Meyts E, Hoei-Hansen CE. From gonocytes to testicular cancer: the role of impaired gonadal development. *Ann N Y Acad Sci.* 2007;1120:168-180.
389. Rutgers JL, Scully RE. The androgen insensitivity syndrome (testicular feminization): a clinicopathologic study of 43 cases. *Int J Gynecol Pathol.* 1991;10:126-144.
390. Hannema SE, Scott IS, Rajpert-De Meyts E, et al. Testicular development in the complete androgen insensitivity syndrome. *J Pathol.* 2006;208:518-527.
391. Ismail-Pratt IS, Bikoo M, Liao L-M, et al. Normalization of the vagina by dilator treatment alone in complete androgen insensitivity syndrome and Mayer-Rokitansky-Kuster-Hauser syndrome. *Hum Reprod.* 2007;22:2020-2024.

392. Szafran AT, Hartig S, Sun H, et al. Androgen receptor mutations associated with androgen insensitivity syndrome: a high content analysis approach leading to personalized medicine. *PLoS One*. 2009;4:e8179.
393. Ahmed SF, Khwaja O, Hughes IA. The role of a clinical score in the assessment of ambiguous genitalia. *BJU Int*. 2000;85:120-124.
394. Pleskacova J, Hersmus R, Oosterhuis JW, et al. Tumor risk in disorders of sex development. *Sex Dev*. 2010:4:259-269.
395. Hoei-Hansen CE, Rajpert-De Meyts E, Daugaard G, et al. Carcinoma in situ testis, the progenitor of testicular germ cell tumours: a clinical review. *Ann Oncol*. 2005;16:863-868.
396. Holm M, Hoei-Hansen CE, Rajpert-De Meyts E, et al. Increased risk of carcinoma in situ in patients with testicular germ cell cancer with ultrasonic microlithiasis in the contralateral testicle. *J Urol*. 2003;170:1163-1167.
397. Ahmed SF, Cheng A, Dovey L, et al. Phenotypic features, androgen receptor binding, and mutational analysis in 278 clinical cases reported as androgen insensitivity syndrome. *J Clin Endocrinol Metab*. 2000; 85:658-665.
398. Morel Y, Rey R, Teinturier C, et al. Aetiological diagnosis of male sex ambiguity: a collaborative study. *Eur J Pediatr*. 2002;161:49-59.
399. Hughes IA, Northstone K, Golding J, ALSPAC Study Team. Reduced birth weight in boys with hypospadias: an index of androgen dysfunction? *Arch Dis Child Fetal Neonatal Ed*. 2002;87:F150-F151.
400. Main KM, Jensen RB, Asklund C, et al. Low birth weight and male reproductive function. *Horm Res*. 2006;65:116-122.
401. Migeon CJ, Wisniewski AB, Gearhart JP, et al. Ambiguous genitalia with perineoscrotal hypospadias in 46,XY individuals: long-term medical, surgical, and psychosexual outcome. *Pediatrics*. 2002;110:e31.
402. Bouvattier C, Mignot B, Lefevre H, et al. Impaired sexual activity in male adults with partial androgen insensitivity. *J Clin Endocrinol Metab*. 2006;91:3310-3315.
403. Wisniewski AB, Migeon CJ, Meyer-Bahlburg HF, et al. Complete androgen insensitivity syndrome: long-term medical, surgical and psychosexual outcome. *J Clin Endocrinol Metab*. 2000;85:2664-2669.
404. Conn J, Gillam L, Conway GS. Revealing the diagnosis of androgen insensitivity syndrome in adulthood. *BMJ*. 2005;331:628-630.
405. Warne G. Support groups for CAH and AIS. *Endocrinologist*. 2003;13:175-178.
406. Garrett CC, Kirkman M. Being an XY female: an analysis of accounts from the website of the androgen insensitivity syndrome support group. *Health Care Women Int*. 2009;30:428-446.
407. Josso N, Belville C, de Clemente N, et al. AMH and AMH receptor defects in persistent müllerian duct syndrome. *Hum Reprod Update*. 2005;11:351-356.
408. Imbeaud S, Carre-Eusebe D, Rey R, et al. Molecular genetics of the persistent müllerian duct syndrome: a study of 19 families. *Hum Mol Genet*. 1994;13:25-131.
409. Imbeaud S, Faure E, Lamarre I, et al. Insensitivity to anti müllerian hormone due to a mutation in the human antimüllerian hormone receptor. *Nat Genet*. 1995;11:382-388.
410. Imbeaud S, Belville C, Messika-Zeitoun L, et al. A 27 base pair deletion of the antimüllerian type II receptor gene is the most common cause of the persistent müllerian duct syndrome. *Hum Mol Genet*. 1996;5:1269-1277.
411. Baskin LS, Ebbers MB. Hypospadias: anatomy, etiology, and technique. *J Pediatr Surg*. 2006;41:463-472.
412. Paulozzi LJ. International trends in rates of hypospadias and cryptorchidism. *Environ Health Perspect*. 1999;107:297-302.
413. Nelson CP, Park JM, Wan J, et al. The increasing incidence of congenital penile anomalies in the United States. *J Urol*. 2005;174: 1573-1576.
414. Ahmed SF, Dobbie R, Finlayson AR, et al. Prevalence of hypospadias and other genital anomalies among singleton births, 1988-1997, in Scotland. *Arch Dis Child Fetal Neonatal Ed*. 2004;89:F149-F151.
415. Abdullah N, Pearce M, Parker L, et al. Birth prevalence of cryptorchidism and hypospadias in northern England, 1993-2000. *Arch Dis Child*. 2007;92:576-579.
416. Fisch H, Lambert SM, Hensle TW, et al. Hypospadias rates in New York state are not increasing. *J Urol*. 2009;181:2291-2294.
417. Fisch H, Hyun G, Hensle TW. Rising hypospadias rates: disproving a myth. *J Pediatr Urol*. 2010;6:37-39.
418. Kalfa N, Philibert P, Sultan C. Is hypospadias a genetic, endocrine or environmental disease, or still an unexplained malformation? *Int J Androl*. 2009; 32:187-197.
419. Kalfa N, Liu B, Klein O, et al. Mutations of CXorf6 are associated with a range of severities of hypospadias. *Eur J Endocrinol*. 2008;159:453-458.
420. Chen Y, Thai HT, Lundin J, et al. Mutational study of the MAMLD1-gene in hypospadias. *Eur J Med Genet*. 2010; 53:122-126.
421. Goodman FR, Bacchelli C, Brady AF, et al. Novel *HOXA13* mutations and the phenotypic spectrum of hand-foot-genital syndrome. *Am J Hum Genet*. 2000;67:197-202.
422. Beleza-Meireles A, Lundberg F, Lagerstedt K, et al. FGFR2, FGF8, FGF10 and BMP7 as candidate genes for hypospadias. *Eur J Hum Genet*. 2007;15:405-410.
423. Utsch B, McCabe CD, Galbraith K, et al. Molecular characterization of HOXA13 polyalanine expansion proteins in hand-foot-genital syndrome. *Am J Med Genet A*. 2007; 143A:3161-3168.
424. Fredell L, Kockum I, Hansson E, et al. Heredity of hypospadias and the significance of low birth weight. *J Urol*. 2002;167:1423-1427.
425. Brouwers MM, Feitz WFJ, Roelofs LA, et al. Risk factors for hypospadias. *Eur J Pediatr*. 2007;166:671-678.
426. Fujimoto T, Suwa T, Kabe K, et al. Placental insufficiency in early gestation is associated with hypospadias. *J Pediatr Surg*. 2008;43:358-361.
427. Brouwers MM, van der Zanden LF, de Gier RP, et al. Hypospadias: risk factor patterns and different phenotypes. *BJU Int*. 2010;105:254-262.
428. Rynja SP, Wouters GA, Van Schaijk M, et al. Long-term follow up of hypospadias: functional and cosmetic results. *J Urol*. 2009;182: 1736-1743.
429. Aulagne MB, Harper L, de Napoli-Cocci S, et al. Long-term outcome of severe hypospadias. *J Pediatr Urol*. 2010;6:469-472.
430. Hutson JM, Balic A, Nation T, et al. Cryptorchidism. *Semin Pediatr Surg*. 2010;19:215-224.
431. Boisen KA, Kaleva M, Main KM, et al. Difference in prevalence of congenital cryptorchidism in infants between two Nordic countries. *Lancet*. 2004;363:1264-1269.
432. Acerini CL, Miles HL, Dunger DB,et al. The descriptive epidemiology of congenital and acquired cryptorchidism in a UK infant cohort. *Arch Dis Child*. 2009;94:868-872.
433. Wohlfahrt-Veje C, Boisen KA, Boas M, et al. Acquired cryptorchidism is frequent in infancy and childhood. *Int J Androl*. 2009;32: 423-428.
434. Ferlin A, Zuccarello D, Garolla A, et al. Mutations in *INSL3* and *RXFP2* genes in cryptorchid boys. *Ann N Y Acad Sci*. 2009;1160:213-214.
435. Krysiak-Baltyn K, Toppari J, Skakkebaek NE, et al. Country-specific chemical signatures of persistent environmental compounds in breast milk. *Int J Androl*. 2010;33:270-278.
436. Main KM, Skakkebaek NE, Virtanen HE, et al. Genital anomalies in boys andd the environment. *Best Pract Res Clin Endocrinol Metab*. 2010;24:279-289.
437. Acerini CL, Hughes IA. Endocrine disrupting chemicals: a new and emerging public health problem? *Arch Dis Child*. 2006;91:633-641.
438. Jorgensen N, Meyts ER, Main KM, et al. Testicular dysgenesis syndrome comprises some but not all cases of hypospadias and impaired spermatogenesis. *Int J Androl*. 2010;33:298-303.
439. Akre O, Richiardi L. Does a testicular dysgenesis syndrome exist? *Hum Reprod*. 2009;24:2053-2060.
440. Thankamony A, Ong KK, Dunger DB, et al. Anogenital distance from birth to 2 years: a population study. *Environ Health Perspect*. 2009;117:1786-1790.
441. Swan SH, Main KM, Liu F, et al. Decrease in anogenital distance among male infants with prenatal phthalate exposure. *Environ Health Perspect*. 2005;113:1056-1061.
442. Arbuckle TE, Hauser R, Swan SH, et al. Meeting report: measuring endocrine-sensitive endpoints within the first years of life. *Environ Health Perspect*. 2008;116:948-951.
443. Yiee JH, Baskin LS. Environmental factors in genitourinary development. *J Urol*. 2010; 184:34-41.
444. Pagnamenta AT, Taanman JW, Wilson CJ, et al. Dominant inheritance of premature ovarian failure associated with mutant mitochondrial DNA polymerase gamma. *Hum Reprod*. 2006;21:2467-2473.
445. Mandel H, Shemer R, Borochowitz ZU, et al. SERKAL syndrome: an autosomal-recessive disorder caused by a loss-of-function mutation in WNT4. *Am J Hum Genet*. 2008; 82:39-47.
446. Robins T, Bellanne-Chantelot C, Barbaro M, et al. Characterization of novel missense mutations in *CYP21* causing congenital adrenal hyperplasia. *J Mol Med*. 2007;85:243-251.
447. White PC. Medscape. Neonatal screening for congenital adrenal hyperplasia. *Nat Rev Endocrinol*. 2009;5:490-498.
448. Hughes IA. Prenatal treatment of congenital adrenal hyperplasia: do we have enough evidence? *Treat Endocrinol*. 2006;5:1-6.
449. Nimkarn S, New MI. Congenital adrenal hyperplasia due to 21-hydroxylase deficiency: a paradigm for prenatal diagnosis and treatment. *Ann N Y Acad Sci*. 2010;1192:5-11.
450. New MI, Carlson A, Obeid J, et al. Prenatal diagnosis for congenital adrenal hyperplasia in 532 pregnancies. *J Clin Endocrinol Metab*. 2001;86:5651-5657.
451. Lajic S, Nordenstrom A, Hirvikoski T. Long-term outcome of prenatal treatment of congenital adrenal hyperplasia. *Endocr Dev*. 2008;13: 82-98.
452. Meyer-Bahlburg HF, Dolezal C, Baker SW, et al. Cognitive and motor development of children with and without congenital adrenal hyperplasia after early-prenatal dexamethasone. *J Clin Endocrinol Metab*. 2004;89:610-614.
453. Hirvikoski T, Nordenström A, Lindholm T, et al. Cognitive functions in children at risk for congenital adrenal hyperplasia treated prenatally with dexamethasone. *J Clin Endocrinol Metab*. 2007;92:542-548.
454. Fernández-Balsells M, Muthusamy K, Smushkin G, et al. Prenatal dexamethasone use for the prevention of virilization in pregnancies at risk for classical congenital adrenal hyperplasia due to 21 hydroxylase

(CYP21A2) deficiency: a systematic review and meta-analyses. *Clin Endocrinol*. 2010; June 9 (Epub ahead of print).

455. Speiser PW, Azziz R, Baskin LS. Congenital adrenal hyperplasia due to 21-hydroxylase deficiency: an Endocrine Society clinical practice guideline. *J Clin Endocrinol Metab*. 2010;95:4133-4160.
456. Scheffer PG, van der Schoot CE, Page-Christiaens GC, et al. Reliability of fetal sex determination using maternal plasma. *Obstet Gynecol*. 2010;115:117-126.
457. Nimkarn S, New MI. Steroid 11beta-hydroxylase deficiency congenital adrenal hyperplasia. *Trends Endocrinol Metab*. 2008;19:96-99.
458. Mullins LJ, Peter A, Wrobel N, et al. Cyp11b1 null mouse, a model of congenital adrenal hyperplasia. *J Biol Chem*. 2009;284:3925-3934.
459. Charmandari E, Kino T, Ichijo T, et al. Generalized glucocorticoid resistance: clinical aspects, molecular mechanisms, and implications of a rare genetic disorder. *J Clin Endocrinol Metab*. 2008;93:1563-1572.
460. Mendonca BB, Leite MV, de Castro M, et al. Female pseudohermaphroditism caused by a novel homozygous missense mutation of the GR gene. *J Clin Endocrinol Metab*. 2002;87:1805-1809.
461. Santen RJ, Brodie H, Simpson ER, et al. History of aromatase: saga of an important biological mediator and therapeutic target. *Endocr Rev*. 2009;30:343-375.
462. Shozu M, Akasofu K, Harada T, et al. A new cause of female pseudohermaphroditism: placental aromatase deficiency. *J Clin Endocrinol Metab*. 1991;72:560-566.
463. Belgorosky A, Guercio G, Pepe C, et al. Genetic and clinical spectrum of aromatase deficiency in infancy, childhood and adolescence. *Horm Res*. 2009;72:321-330.
464. Ito Y, Fisher CR, Conte FA, et al. Molecular basis of aromatase deficiency in an adult female with sexual infantilism and polycystic ovaries. *Proc Natl Acad Sci U S A*. 1993;90:11673-11677.
465. Conte FA, Grumbach MM, Ito Y, et al. A syndrome of female pseudohermaphrodism, hypergonadotropic hypogonadism, and multicystic ovaries associated with missense mutations in the gene encoding aromatase (P450arom). *J Clin Endocrinol Metab*. 1994;78:1287-1292.
466. Mullis PE, Yoshimura N, Kuhlmann B, et al. Aromatase deficiency in a female who is compound heterozygote for two new point mutations in the P450arom gene: impact of estrogens on hypergonadotropic hypogonadism, multicystic ovaries, and bone densitometry in childhood. *J Clin Endocrinol Metab*. 1997;82:1739-1745.
467. Carani C, Qin K, Simoni M, et al. Effect of testosterone and estradiol in a man with aromatase deficiency. *N Engl J Med*. 1997;337:91-95.
468. Smith EP, Boyd J, Frank GR, et al. Estrogen resistance caused by a mutation in the estrogen receptor gene in a man. *N Engl J Med*. 1994;331:1056-1061.
469. Lin L, Ercan O, Raza J, et al. Variable phenotypes associated with aromatase (CYP19) insufficiency in humans. *J Clin Endocrinol Metab*. 2007;92:982-990.
470. Brunskill J. The effects of fetal exposure to Danazol. *Br J Obstet Gynaecol*. 1992;99:212-214.
471. VanSlooten AJ, Rechner SF, Dodds WG. Recurrent maternal virilization during pregnancy caused by benign androgen-producing ovarian lesions. *Am J Obstet Gynecol*. 1992;167:1342-1343.
472. Holt HB, Medbak S, Kirk D, et al. Recurrent severe hyperandrogenism during pregnancy: a case report. *J Clin Pathol*. 2005;58:439-442.
473. Oppelt P, Renner SP, Kellermann A, et al. Clinical aspects of Mayer-Rokitansky-Kuester-Hauser syndrome: recommendations for clinical diagnosis and staging. *Hum Reprod*. 2006;21:792-797.
474. Biason-Lauber A, Konrad D, Navratil F, et al. A WNT4 mutation associated with müllerian-duct regression and virilization in a 46,XX woman. *N Engl J Med*. 2004;351:792-798.
475. Ahmed SF, Rodie M. Investigation and initial management of ambiguous genitalia. *Best Pract Res Clin Endocrinol Metab*. 2010;24:197-218.
476. Thyen U, Lanz K, Holterhus PM, et al. Epidemiology and initial management of ambiguous genitalia at birth in Germany. *Horm Res*. 2006;66:195-203.
477. Moreno-Garcia M, Miranda EB. Chromosomal anomalies in cryptorchidism and hypospadias. *J Urol*. 2002;168:2170-2172.
478. Boehmer AI, Nijman RJ, Lammers BA, et al. Etiological studies of severe or familial hypospadias. *J Urol*. 2001;165:1246-1254.
479. Jensen TK, Sobotka T, Hansen MA, et al. Declining trends in conception rates in recent birth cohorts of native Danish women: a possible role of deteriorating male reproductive health. *Int J Androl*. 2008;31:81-92.
480. Ahmed SF, Keir L, McNeilly J, et al. The concordance between serum anti-müllerian hormone and testosterone concentrations depends on duration of hCG stimulation in boys undergoing investigation of gonadal function. *Clin Endocrinol*. 2010;72:814-819.
481. Ahmed SF, Cheng A, Hughes IA. Biochemical evaluation of the gonadotrophin-gonadal axis in androgen insensitivity syndrome. *Arch Dis Child*. 1999;80:324-329.
482. Brain CE, Creighton SM, Mushtaq I, et al. Holistic management of DSD. *Best Pract Res Clin Endocrinol Metab*. 2010;24: 335-354.
483. Hines M. *Brain Gender*. New York, NY: Oxford University Press; 2004.
484. Auyeung B, Baron-Cohen S, Ashwin E, et al. Fetal testosterone predicts sexually differentiated childhood behaviour in girls and in boys. *Psychol Sci*. 2009; 20:144-148.
485. Brown GR, Dixson AF. Investigation of the role of postnatal testosterone in the expression of sex differences in behaviour in infant rhesus macaques (*Macaca mulatta*). *Horm Behav*. 1999;35:186-194.
486. Poomthavorn P, Stargatt R, Zacharin M. Psychosexual and psychosocial functions of anorchid young adults. *J Clin Endocrinol Metab*. 2009;94:2502-2505.
487. Jadva V, Hines M, Golombok S. Infants' preferences for toys, colours, and shapes: sex differences and similarities. *Arch Sex Behav*. 2010; 39:1261-1273.
488. Crouch NS, Creighton SM. Long-term functional outcomes of female genital reconstruction in childhood. *BJU Int*. 2007;100:403-406.
489. Crouch NS, Liao LM, Woodhouse CR, et al. Sexual function and genital sensitivity following feminizing genitoplasty for congenital adrenal hyperplasia. *J Urol*. 2008;179:634-638.
490. Burgu B, Duffy PG, Cuckow P, et al. Long-term outcome of vaginal reconstruction: comparing techniques and timing. *J Paediatr Urol*. 2007;3:316-320.
491. Gargollo PC, Cannon GM, Diamond DA, et al. Should progressive perineal dilation be considered first line therapy for vaginal agenesis? *J Urol*. 2009;182:1882-1889.
492. Kraft KH, Shukla AR, Canning DA. Hypospadias. *Urol Clin North Am*. 2010;37:167-181.
493. Vidal I, Gorduza DB, Haraux E, et al. Surgical options in disorders of sex development (DSD) with ambiguous genitalia. *Best Pract Res Clin Endocrinol Metab*. 2010;24:311-314.
494. Columbo F, Casarico A. Penile enlargement. *Curr Opin Urol*. 2008;18: 583-588.
495. Paris MC, Schlatt S. Ovarian and testicular tissues xenografting: its potential for germline preservation of companion animals, non-domestic and endangered species. *Reprod Fertil Dev*. 2007;19:771-782.
496. Stukenborg JB, Schlatt S, Simoni M, et al. New horizons for in vitro spermatogenesis? An update on novel three-dimensional culture systems as tools for meiotic and post-meiotic differentiation of testicular germ cells. *Mol Hum Reprod*. 2009;15:521-529.
497. Rodriguez-Wallberg KA, Oktay K. Fertility preservation medicine: options for young adults and children with cancer. *J Pediatr Hematol Oncol*. 2010;32:390-396.
498. Liao LM, Green H, Creighton SM, et al. Service users' experiences of obtaining and giving information about disorders of sex development. *BJOG*. 2010;117:193-199.
499. Kirk J, Clayton P. Specialist services and transitional care in paediatric endocrinology in the UK and Ireland. *Clin Endocrinol*. 2006;65: 59-63.
500. Merke DP. Approach to the adult with congenital adrenal hyperplasia due to 21-hydroxylase deficiency. *J Clin Endocrinol Metab*. 2008;93: 653-660.
501. Conway GS. Adult care of pediatric conditions: lessons from Turner's syndrome. *J Clin Endocrinol Metab*. 2009;94:3185-3187.
502. Minto CL, Crouch NS, Conway GS, et al. XY females: revisiting the diagnosis. *BJOG*. 2005;112:1407-1410.
503. Berra M, Liao LM, Creighton SM, et al. Long-term health issues of women with XY karyotype. *Maturitas*. 2010;65:172-178.
504. Hughes IA. The quiet revolution. *Best Pract Res Clin Endocrinol Metab*. 2010;24:159-162.
505. Pasterski V, Prentice P, Hughes IA. Impact of the consensus statement and the new DSD classification system. *Best Prac Res Clin Endocrinol Metab*. 2010;24:187-195.
506. MacCallum F, Golombok S. Embryo donation families: mothers' decisions regarding disclosure of donor conception. *Hum Reprod*. 2007;22: 2888-2895.

Note added in proof: Mutations in *GATA4* and *MAP3K1* have been reported in 46,XY DSD (testicular dysgenesis) and upregulation of SOX3 has been described with 46,XX testicular DSD.

Pearlman A, Loke J, Le Caignec C, et al. Mutations in *MAP3K1* cause 46,XY disorders of sex development and implicate a common signal transduction pathway in human testis development. *Am J Hum Genet*. 2010;87:898-906.

Sutton E, Hughes, White S, et al. Identification of SOX3 in XX male sex reversal gene in mice and humans. *J Clin Invest*. 2011;121:318-341.

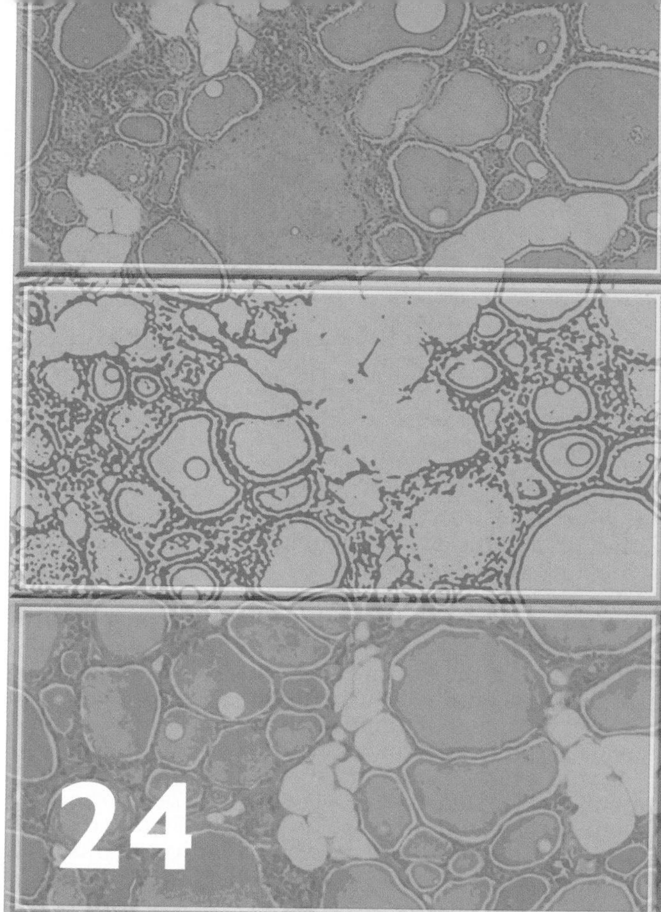

CHAPTER 24

Normal and Aberrant Growth

DAVID W. COOKE • SARA A. DIVALL • SALLY RADOVICK

NORMAL GROWTH

Overview

Growth is a fundamental, intrinsic aspect of childhood health. It is also a complex yet tightly regulated process. An individual's final height and the path taken to reach that end point are significantly determined by that person's genetic composition. But growth and final height can also be affected by external factors, including the quality and quantity of nutrition, and by psychosocial factors. This process is regulated by multiple hormones and growth factors interacting with an array of membrane receptors that activate seemingly redundant intracellular signaling cascades. And yet, as complex as this process is, 1 standard deviation (SD) of adult height represents about only 4% of the mean adult height.

Whether linear growth occurs as a continuous process or with periodic bursts of growth and arrest[1-4] has been hard to characterize definitively. There do appear to be seasonal variations of growth, with slower growth in autumn and winter and greater growth in spring and early summer.[5,6] Some normal children have a broad growth channel, with many showing diverse but characteristic growth tracks.[7] Nonetheless, even though the process of growth is multifactorial and complex, children usually grow in a remarkably predictable manner. Deviation from such a normal pattern of growth can be the first manifestation of a wide variety of disease processes, including endocrine and nonendocrine disorders and involving virtually any organ system of the body. Therefore, frequent and accurate assessment of growth is of primary importance in the care of children.

Measurement

Assessment of growth requires accurate and reproducible determinations of height. Supine length is routinely measured in children younger than 2 years of age, and erect height is assessed in older children. It can be useful to measure both length and height in children between 2 and 3 years of age, to allow comparisons to prior length measurements and to begin to record height measurement for ongoing comparisons. The inherent inaccuracies involved in measuring length in infants are often obscured by the rapid skeletal growth during this period. For measurement of supine length (Fig. 24-1), it is best to use a firm box with an inflexible board, against which the head lies, and a movable footboard, on which the feet are placed perpendicular to the plane of the supine length of the infant. Optimally, the child should be relaxed, the legs should be fully extended, and the head should be positioned in the

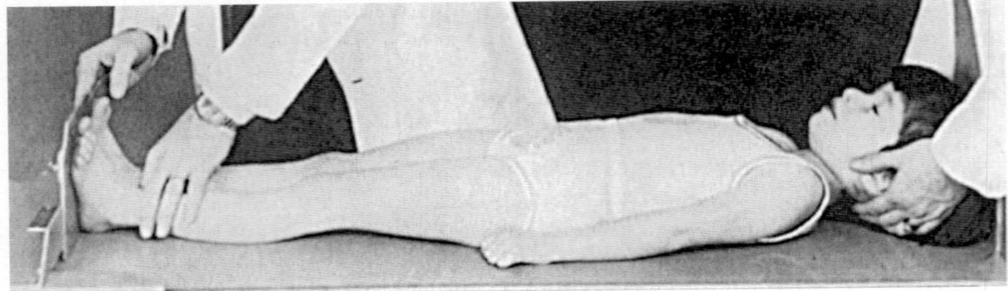

Figure 24-1 Technique for measuring recumbent length. (A device suitable for measurement of length of infants can be purchased from Raven Equipment Limited, Essex, United Kingdom.) (Photograph courtesy of Noel Cameron.)

Frankfurt plane, with the line connecting the outer canthus of the eyes and the external auditory meatus perpendicular to the long axis of the trunk.

When children are old enough (and physically capable) to stand erect, it is best to employ a wall-mounted Harpenden stadiometer similar to that designed by Tanner and Whitehouse for the British Harpenden Growth Study. The traditional measuring device of a flexible arm mounted to a weight balance is notoriously unreliable and does not provide accurate serial measurements.

As with length measurements in infants, positioning of the child in the stadiometer is critical (Fig. 24-2). The child should be fully erect, with the head in the Frankfurt plane; the back of the head, thoracic spine, buttocks, and heels should touch the vertical axis of the stadiometer, and the heels should be together. Every effort should be made to correct discrepancies related to lordosis or scoliosis. Ideally, serial measurements should be made at the same time of day, because standing height may undergo diurnal variation.

Height determinations should be performed by a trained individual rather than an inexperienced member of the staff. We recommend that lengths and heights be measured in triplicate, that variation should be no more than 0.3 cm, and that the mean height should be recorded. For determination of height velocity when several measurements are being made within a short period, the same individual should perform the determinations to eliminate interobserver variability. Even when every effort is made to obtain accurate height measurements, a minimum interval of 6 months is necessary for meaningful height velocity computation. Nine to 12 months' data are preferable so that errors of measurement are minimized and the seasonal variation in height velocity is assimilated into the data.

Growth Charts

Evaluation of a child's height must be done in the context of normal standards. Most American pediatric endocrine clinics use the cross-sectional data provided by the National Center for Health Statistics (NCHS), which were originally introduced in 1977. Revised and updated growth charts have been available on the Centers for Disease Control (CDC) web site since 2000 (www.cdc.gov/growthcharts; Figs. 24-3 through 24-8).[8] The data for these charts encompass measurements obtained in the United States between 1963 and 1995, and they include a broader representation of the U.S. population for all measures than was available in earlier charts.

These charts allow comparison of individual children with the 3rd, 10th, 25th, 50th, 75th, 90th, and 97th percentiles of normal American children. There are, however, two limitations of these charts when applied to the individual child. First, they do not satisfactorily define children below the 3rd or above the 97th percentiles—the very children in whom it is most critical to define the degree to which they deviate from the normal growth centiles. However, the NCHS data tables (also available on the CDC web site) can be used to compute standard deviation scores (SDS). For example, a short child below the 3rd percentile can be described more precisely as being

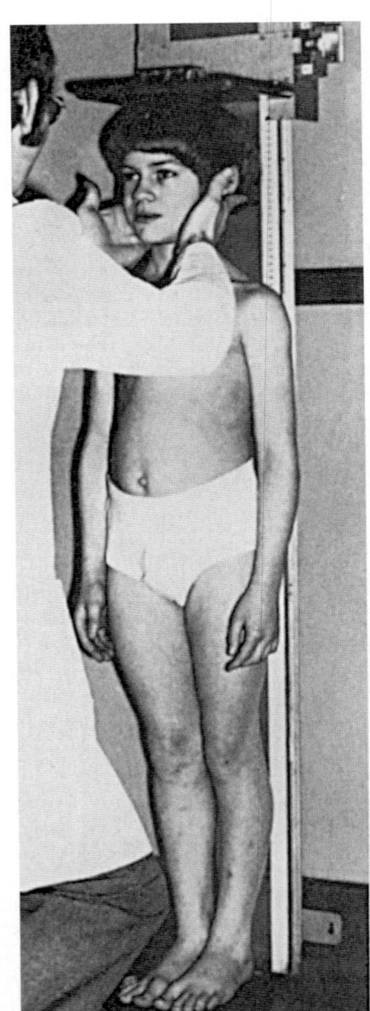

Figure 24-2 Technique for measuring erect height using the Harpenden stadiometer with direct digital display of height. (Devices of this type are available from Holtain Ltd, Wales, United Kingdom, and Seritex Inc, Carlstadt, NJ.)

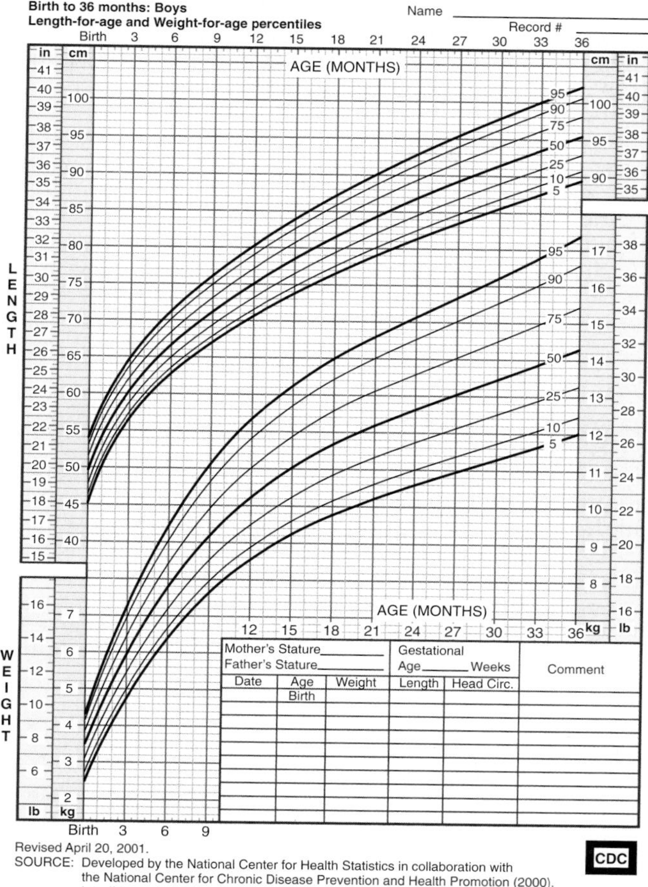

Figure 24-3 Length-for-age and weight-for-age percentiles for boys (birth to 36 months) developed by the National Center for Health Statistics in collaboration with the National Center for Chronic Disease Prevention and Health Promotion (2000). Available at http://www.cdc.gov/growthcharts (accessed October 2010).

approximately 4.2 SDS below the mean for age. A height SDS for age is calculated as follows: the SDS equals the child's height, minus the mean height for normal children of the child's age and gender, divided by the SD of the height for normal children of this age and gender. Second, cross-sectional data are of greater value during infancy and childhood than in adolescence, because differences in the timing of pubertal onset can considerably influence normal growth rates. To address this issue, Tanner and colleagues[9] developed longitudinal growth charts, in an effort to construct the curve shapes with centile widths obtained from a large cross-sectional survey, thus accounting for variability in the timing of puberty. Such charts are of particular value in assessing growth during adolescence and puberty and for plotting sequential growth data for any individual child.

The data from cross-sectional and longitudinal growth studies have been employed to develop *height velocity* standards (Figs. 24-9 and 24-10). It is important to emphasize that carefully documented height velocity data are invaluable in assessing a child with abnormalities of growth. There is considerable variability in normal height velocity of children at different ages; however, between the age of 2 years and the onset of puberty, children grow with remarkable fidelity relative to the normal growth curves. Any crossing of percentile curves on the height chart during this age period should be considered abnormal and warrants further evaluation.

Syndrome-specific growth curves have been developed for a number of clinical conditions associated with growth failure, such as Turner syndrome (TS),[10] achondroplasia,[11] and Down syndrome.[12] Such growth profiles are invaluable for tracking the growth of children with these clinical conditions. Deviation of growth from the appropriate disease-related growth curve suggests the possibility of a second underlying cause, such as acquired autoimmune hypothyroidism in children with Down syndrome or TS.

Body Proportions

Many abnormal growth states, including both short stature and excessive stature, are characterized by *disproportionate* growth. The following determinations should be made as part of the evaluation of short stature:

1. Occipitofrontal head circumference
2. Lower body segment: distance from top of pubic symphysis to the floor
3. Upper body segment: the difference between total height and lower body segment (it can also be measured as the sitting height, subtracting the height of the chair or stool)
4. Arm span

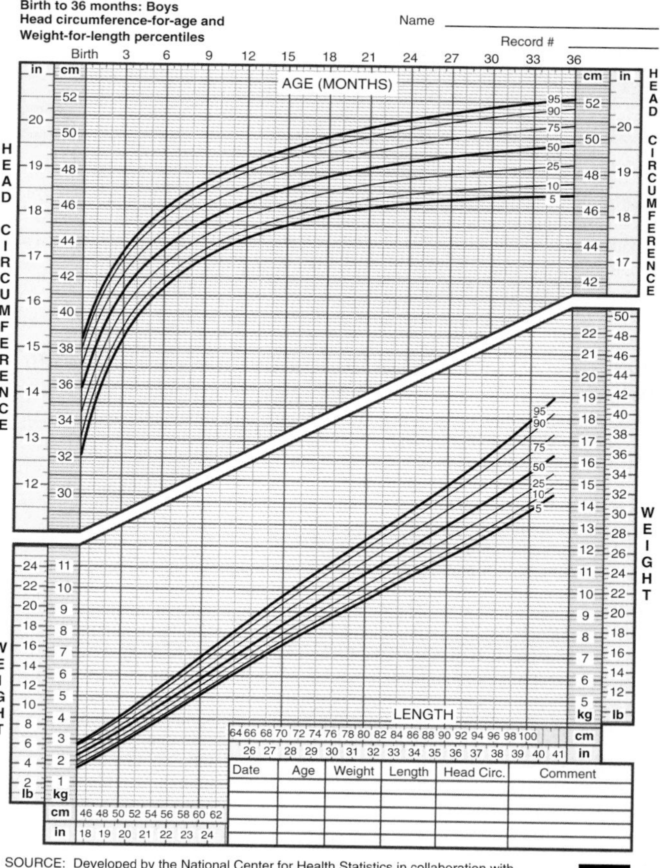

Figure 24-4 Head circumference-for-age and weight-for-length percentiles for boys (birth to 36 months) developed by the National Center for Health Statistics in collaboration with the National Center for Chronic Disease Prevention and Health Promotion (2000). Available at http://www.cdc.gov/growthcharts (accessed October 2010).

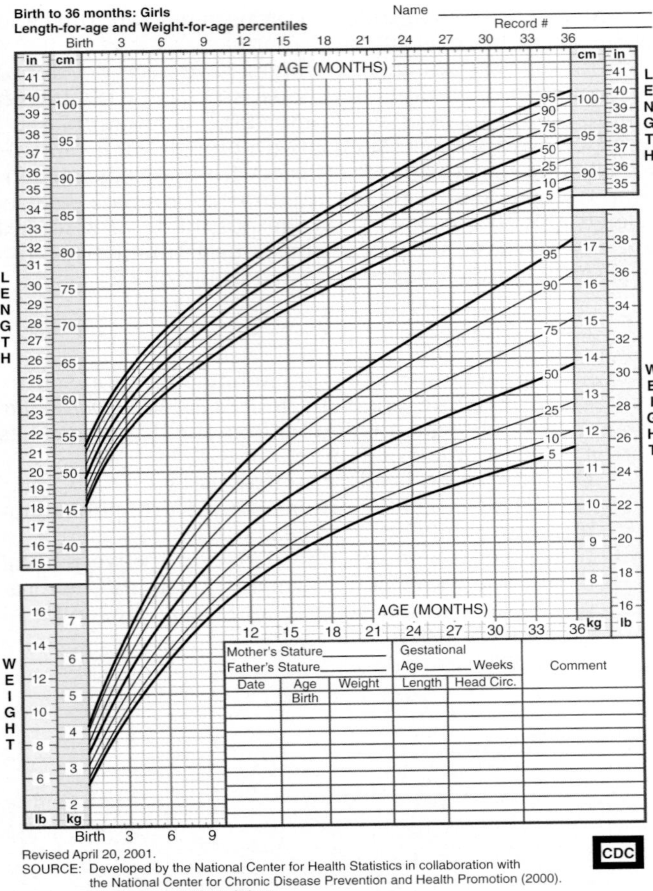

Figure 24-5 Length-for-age and weight-for-age percentiles for girls (birth to 36 months) developed by the National Center for Health Statistics in collaboration with the National Center for Chronic Disease Prevention and Health Promotion (2000). Available at http://www.cdc.gov/growthcharts (accessed October 2010).

Published standards exist for these body proportion measurements, which must be evaluated relative to the patient's age.[13] The ratio of upper segment to lower segment ranges from 1.7 in the neonate to slightly less than 1.0 in the adult (Fig. 24-11).

Parental Target Height

Genetic factors are important determinants of growth and height potential. Therefore, it is useful to assess a patient's stature relative to that of siblings and parents. Tanner and associates developed a growth chart that factored parents' heights into the evaluation of the heights of children ages 2 to 9 years.[14] One can also calculate a child's expected final height based on the parents' heights by calculating the midparental height. This is the average of the parents' heights, after accounting for the average difference in height between adult men and women (13 cm). In other words, a boy's midparental height equals the average of his parents' heights plus 6.5 cm, and a girl's midparental height equals the average of her parents' heights minus 6.5 cm.

Because of regression to the mean,[15,16] children of short parents are likely to be less short than their parents, and children of tall parents are likely to be less tall than their parents. Therefore, a child's genetic *target height range* centers on the point that represents 80% of the difference between the child's midparental height and the mean adult height for the child's gender.[15] For example, if a boy's father is 168 cm tall and his mother is 153 cm tall, his midparental height is 167 cm, which is 10 cm below the mean height of adult men (177 cm). Therefore, the boy's target height range centers on 169 cm, which is 8 cm below the mean adult height for men. In more than 95% of children, the adult height falls within 10 cm of the point thus calculated.[14,15] In children with extremely short stature (>–3 SD), the father's height may more strongly correlate with the patient's height, and the mother's height may more greatly influence birth length.[17]

Skeletal Maturation

The growth potential in the tubular bones can be assessed by evaluation of the progression of ossification within the epiphyses. The ossification centers of the skeleton appear and progress in a predictable sequence in normal children, and this skeletal maturation can be compared with normal age-related standards. This forms the basis of the *bone age* or *skeletal age*, a quantitative determination of net somatic maturation that serves as a mirror of the tempo of growth and maturation. The bone age also reflects the degree of growth plate senescence and therefore is a useful adjunct

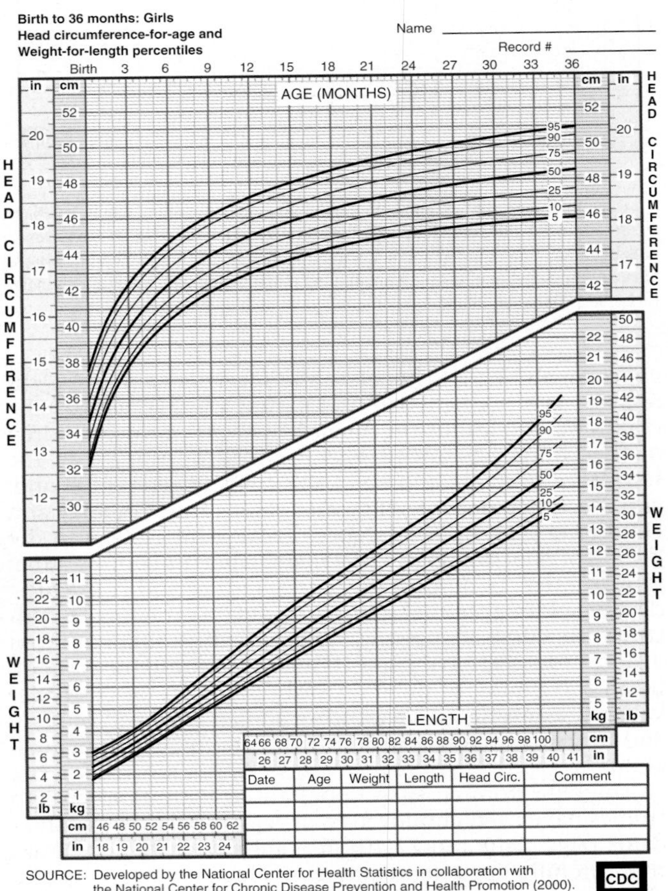

Figure 24-6 Head circumference-for-age and weight-for-length percentiles for girls (birth to 36 months) developed by the National Center for Health Statistics in collaboration with the National Center for Chronic Disease Prevention and Health Promotion (2000). Available at http://www.cdc.gov/growthcharts (accessed October 2010).

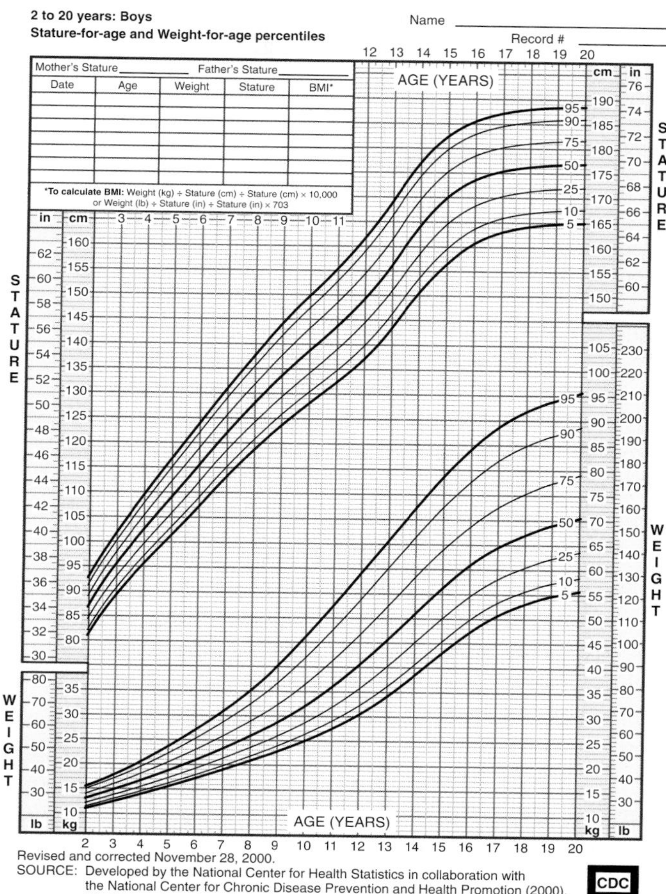

Figure 24-7 Stature-for-age and weight-for-age percentiles for boys (2 to 20 years) developed by the National Center for Health Statistics in collaboration with the National Center for Chronic Disease Prevention and Health Promotion (2000). Available at http://www.cdc.gov/growthcharts (accessed October 2010).

in estimating growth opportunity (i.e., the ultimate adult height), as discussed later in this chapter.

Not all of the factors that determine the normal pattern of skeletal maturation have been identified, but genetic factors and multiple hormones, including thyroxine, growth hormone (GH), and gonadal steroids, are involved.[18] Ultimately, growth cessation occurs after exhaustion of the proliferative capacity of the growth plate chondrocyte.[19] Estrogen plays an important role in this process: animal studies have indicated that estrogen accelerates growth plate senescence,[20] and studies in patients with mutations of the gene for the estrogen receptor[21] or for the aromatase enzyme[22-24] demonstrated that estrogen is primarily responsible for epiphyseal fusion.[25]

Phases of Normal Growth

Growth occurs at differing rates during intrauterine life, early and middle childhood, and adolescence, then ceases after fusion of long bone and vertebral epiphyseal growth plates. Karlberg and associates resolved the normal linear growth curve into three additive, partially superimpossible phases[26,27]: an "infancy" phase, starting in midgestation and then rapidly decelerating until about 3 to 4 years of age; a "childhood" phase, slowly decelerating during early adolescence; and a sigmoid-shaped "puberty" phase that comprises the adolescent growth spurt. Prenatal growth averages 1.2 to 1.5 cm per week but varies dramatically (Fig. 24-12); the midgestational length growth velocity of 2.5 cm per week falls to almost 0.5 cm per week immediately before birth. Growth velocity (see Figs. 24-2 and 24-3) averages about 15 cm per year during the first 2 years of life; it then slows to approximately 6 cm per year during middle childhood. During this time, a normal child's height, plotted on a growth curve, typically remain within a given growth channel; that is, it does not cross percentile lines on the growth curve.

Prepubertal growth is similar between boys and girls. The height difference between men and women, an average of 13 cm, is accounted for by two factors. First, boys grow for an average of 2 years longer than girls do, because girls have an earlier onset of puberty and, consequently, earlier cessation of growth. Therefore, prepubertal growth is greater for boys; they are 8 to 10 cm taller when their puberty starts, compared with girls' heights when their puberty starts.[15] Second, boys achieve a greater maximal pubertal growth velocity than girls do, giving them 3 to 5 cm greater pubertal growth. The time of onset of puberty varies in normal children, resulting in a normal variation in the timing of the pubertal growth spurt. However, in most normal children, the final height is not influenced by the chronologic age at onset of the pubertal growth spurt,

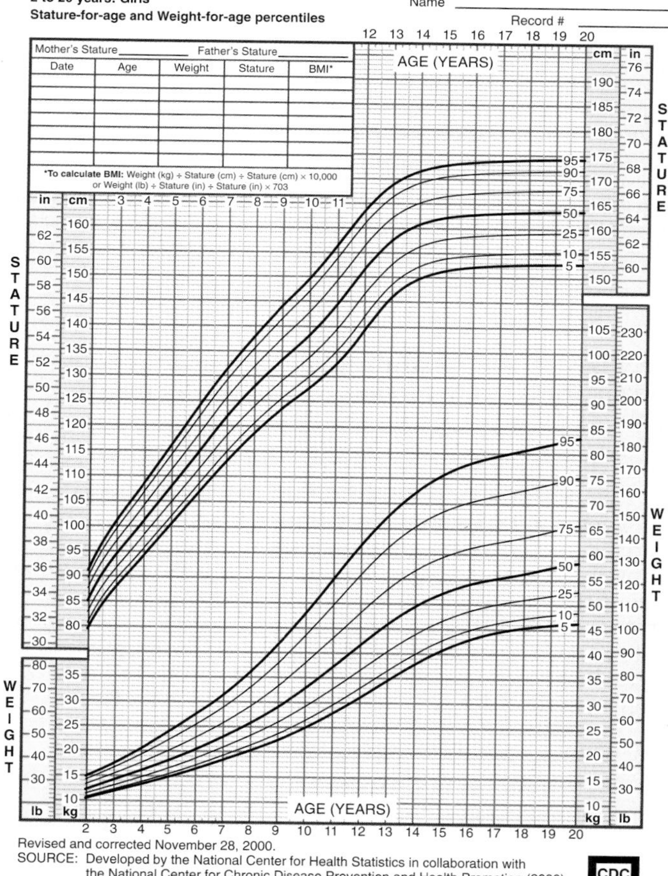

Figure 24-8 Stature-for-age and weight-for-age percentiles for girls (2 to 20 years) developed by the National Center for Health Statistics in collaboration with the National Center for Chronic Disease Prevention and Health Promotion (2000). Available at http://www.cdc.gov/growthcharts (accessed October 2010).

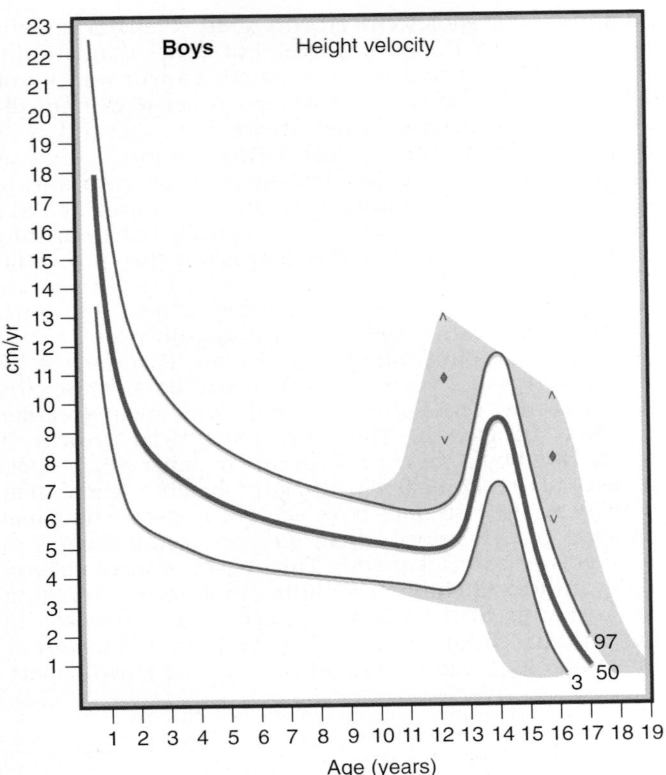

Figure 24-9 Height velocity chart for boys constructed from longitudinal observations of British children. The 97th, 50th, and 3rd percentile curves define the general pattern of growth during puberty. Shaded areas indicate velocities in those children with peak velocities occurring up to 2 standard deviations before or after the average age depicted by the percentile lines (*Up arrows*, *diamonds*, and *down arrows* mark, respectively, the 97th, 50th, and 3rd percentiles of peak velocity when the peak occurs at these early or late limits.) (Modified from charts prepared by Tanner JM and Whitehouse RH from data published in references 9, 1211, and 1899. Reproduced with permission of J.M. Tanner and Castlemead Publications, Ward's Publishing Services, Herts, United Kingdom.)

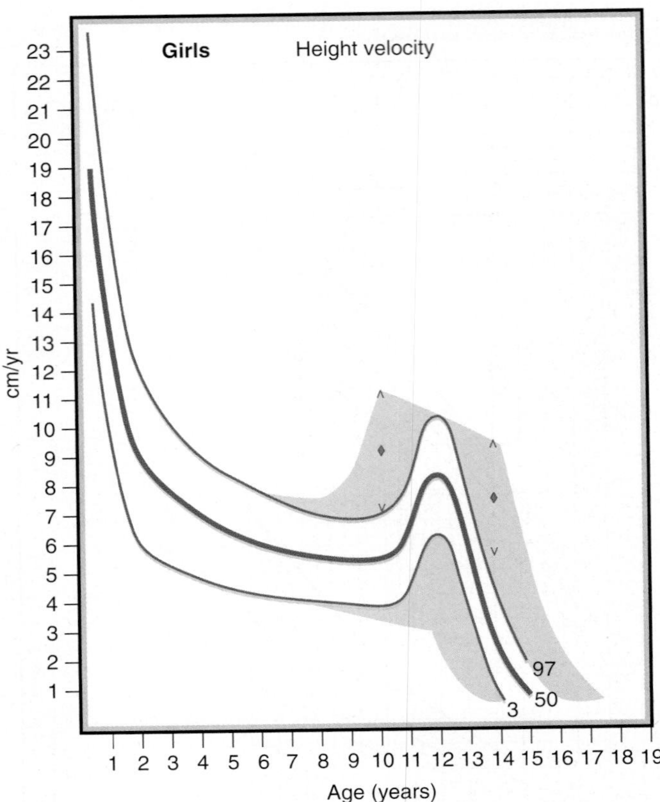

Figure 24-10 Height velocity chart for girls constructed from longitudinal observations of British children. The 97th, 50th, and 3rd percentile curves define the general pattern of growth during puberty. Shaded areas indicate velocities in those children with peak velocities occurring up to 2 standard deviations before or after the average age depicted by the percentile lines (*Up arrows*, *diamonds*, and *down arrows* mark, respectively, the 97th, 50th, and 3rd percentiles of peak velocity when the peak occurs at these early or late limits.) (Modified and reproduced with permission of J.M. Tanner and Castlemead Publications, Ward's Publishing Services, Herts, United Kingdom.)

because the additional time for prepubertal growth that occurs when puberty is late is balanced by the fact that pubertal growth is smaller the later it occurs (see Figs. 24-2 and 24-3). After puberty, chondrocyte proliferation in the growth plate slows and senescence occurs due to depletion of stem-like cells in the resting zone of the growth plate.[28,29]

There are two variants of normal growth whose characteristic patterns are such that children exhibiting these growth variants are often evaluated for a growth disorder. These two variants are crossing linear percentiles of infancy, and constitutional delay of growth and development (CDGD). In many cases, it is difficult to differentiate children with these normal growth variants from children with a growth disorder.

Crossing Linear Percentiles of Infancy

As in postnatal growth, genetic and environmental factors are important determinants of fetal growth and of the size of an infant (weight and length) at birth. However, there are significant differences between the factors affecting birth size and those affecting childhood growth and adult stature. There is much less correlation between length at birth and ultimate adult height than between length at birth and height in the later years of childhood.[30]

Parental stature affects birth length, as it does adult stature; this is an indicator of the genetic influence on

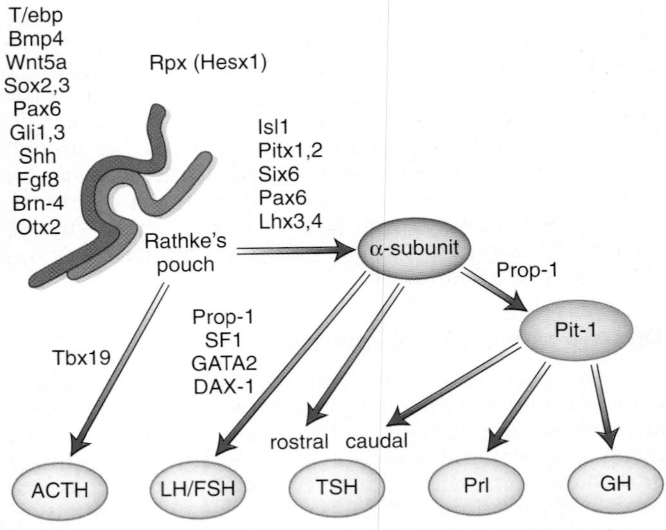

Figure 24-11 Ratio of upper to lower body segment from birth to 18 years of age. (From data in Wilkins L. *The Diagnosis and Treatment of Endocrine Disorders in Childhood and Adolescence*. Springfield, IL: Charles C Thomas; 1957.)

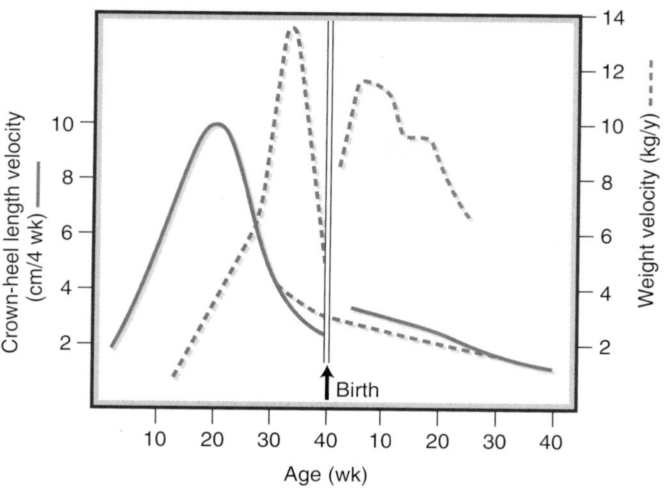

Figure 24-12 Rate of linear growth and weight gain in utero and during first 40 weeks after birth. Length velocity is expressed in centimeters per week. The solid line depicts the actual linear growth rate; the dashed line connecting the prenatal and postnatal length velocity lines depicts the theoretical curve for no uterine restriction late in gestation. The lighter dashed line depicts weight velocity. (From data in Tanner JM. *Fetus into Man.* Cambridge, MA: Harvard University Press; 1978.)

growth. Although maternal and paternal stature contribute equally to childhood growth and adult stature, the effect of maternal stature may predominate over that of paternal stature on length at birth.[31,32] However, some studies have found equal effects of maternal and paternal stature on birth size.[33] Maternal nutrition and health have significant effects on fetal growth. Maternal weight has a positive effect, and smoking during pregnancy has a negative effect. Maternal diabetes has a strong positive effect on fetal growth. It is possible for the prenatal determinants of growth to result, for example, in a child who will ultimately grow to below-average stature but is above average size at birth. For this reason, it is common for infants' lengths to cross percentiles on the growth curve. Indeed, it is more common for the growth of an infant to cross percentiles than to follow a single percentile from birth into childhood: approximately one third of infants have lengths that cross percentiles moving upward on the growth curves, and approximately one third have lengths that cross percentiles moving downward.[32,34] Most normal infants crossing percentiles do so in the first 6 to 12 months, although some normal infants cross percentiles after 1 year of age.

Infants who are small at birth can be divided into (1) those who are small only because of prematurity and are therefore of a size appropriate for gestational age (AGA) and (2) those who are small for gestational age (SGA). SGA is usually defined as a birth weight or length (or both) below the 3rd percentile (or, sometimes, below the 10th percentile) for gestational age.[35] Some infants born SGA represent the small percentage of individuals whose genetic potential leads to small size at birth, and they can be expected to remain small throughout childhood and adulthood. However, many infants are SGA due to intrauterine growth retardation (IUGR) and have a genetic potential that would not be expected to result in small adult stature. Most infants who are born small, either AGA or SGA, have catch-up growth and achieve lengths greater than the 3rd percentile within the first 2 years of life. However, up to 10% of SGA infants do not show such catch-up growth.[36,37] The pathologic aspects of IUGR and of SGA in infants who do not have catch-up growth are discussed later.

Constitutional Delay of Growth and Development

CDGD is a normal variant of growth.[38] It describes the growth pattern of children who will experience a later than average timing of puberty. Their birth size is normal, and their final height is within their genetic potential. However, during most of their childhood, they grow at a height percentile below that expected based on their genetic potential. Typically, these children have a low growth velocity during the first years of life, crossing downward on the length percentile growth curves, so that by 2 years of age their heights are at or slightly below the 5th percentile. After age 3 years, their growth rate is typically normal, so that their height growth usually remains parallel to the 5th percentile until adolescence, although the height SDS may gradually drift slightly lower during the middle childhood years in some cases.[38,39] Their height diverges even further from that of average children during the early teen years due to the declining prepubertal growth velocity of these children compared with the accelerating growth rate of average children with onset of puberty.

Ultimately, children with CDGD have a late growth spurt, consistent with their late puberty, and this brings their height into the normal adult range. Final height is often in the lower part of the parental target height range, and few patients exceed the parental target height,[40-42] although this finding is probably, at least in part, the result of a selection bias of the children examined for such studies. However, there is evidence that a delayed growth spurt may adversely affect growth of the spine, resulting in a decrease in the final ratio of the upper to the lower segment and perhaps contributing to a limited final height.[43] Studies have also reported that prepubertal boys with CDGD have decreased bone mineral density (BMD),[44] and this decreased BMD may persist into adulthood, although not all studies have confirmed this finding.[45]

Secular Changes in Height

There are surprisingly few data concerning the stature of modern humans before the measurement of military recruits became customary in the 18th century. Skeletal remains from the last ice age appear to indicate that adult stature 10,000 to 20,000 years ago was not substantially different from that of contemporary adults, although this record is obviously fragmentary.[46] It has been suggested that a reduction in stature was observed with the introduction of agriculture approximately 5000 years ago, with growth attenuation resulting from the combined effects of nutrient deficiency, population growth, and spread of infectious diseases.

Military recruits in the 18th and 19th centuries were clearly shorter than those of today, although it must be recognized that soldiers were commonly recruited from the lower socioeconomic classes, and poor health and nutrition would have contributed to both poor growth and late maturity.[47] Whereas men in the 20th century averaged 5 to 10 cm greater in height than those in the 18th century for whom we have records, much of this height gain has occurred over the last 100 years and probably reflects the dramatic improvement in overall nutrition and health seen in the Western world.

Therefore, secular changes in height appear to reflect fundamental alterations in the standard of living rather than major genomic differences among populations; future economic advances in developing countries can be predicted to lead to improvement in adult stature and a reduction in international differences in growth.

ENDOCRINE REGULATION OF GROWTH

The Hypothalamic-Pituitary Axis: Embryogenesis and Anatomy

The pituitary gland is central to the regulation of mammalian growth. The pituitary gland develops from oral ectoderm in response to inductive signals from the neuroepithelium of the ventral diencephalon and intrinsic signaling gradients determining expression patterns of pituitary-specific transcription factors in the developing anterior pituitary gland.[48] The primordium of the anterior pituitary, Rathke's pouch, forms as an upward invagination of a single-cell-thick layer of ectoderm that contacts the neuroectoderm of the primordium of the ventral hypothalamus at embryonic day 8.5 (E8.5) in the mouse embryo[49,50] and can be identified by the third week of pregnancy in humans.[51] The neurohypophysis (posterior pituitary) originates in the neural ectoderm of the floor of the forebrain, which also develops into the third ventricle. During anterior pituitary development, overlapping but regionally specific and temporally distinct patterns of homeobox transcription factor expression lead to the sequential appearance of the terminally differentiated cell types from E12.5 to birth.[50]

The initiation of anterior pituitary gland development depends on the competency of the oral ectoderm to respond to inducing factors from the neural epithelium of the ventral diencephalon.[52] The bone morphogenic protein 4 (BMP4) signal from the ventral diencephalon is the critical dorsal neuroepithelial signal required for organ commitment of the anterior pituitary gland. Wnt5a and fibroblast growth factor 8 (FGF8) are also expressed in the diencephalon in distinct overlapping patterns with BMP4. Subsequently, a BMP2 signal arises from the boundary of a region of oral ectoderm in which Sonic hedgehog (SHH) expression, initially expressed uniformly in the oral ectoderm, is selectively excluded from the developing Rathke's pouch. The ventral-dorsal BMP2 signal and the dorsal-ventral FGF8 signal appear to create opposing activity gradients that are suggested to dictate overlapping patterns of specific transcription factors underlying cell lineage specification. The various extensions of these transcription factors in their fields are theorized to combinatorially determine the specific cell types. The FGF8 gradient determines the dorsal cell phenotypes,[52,53] and dorsally expressed transcription factors include Nkx-3.1, Six3, Pax6,[54] and prophet of PIT1 (PROP1).[55] Temporally specific attenuation of the BMP2 signal is required for terminal differentiation of the ventral cell types, and ventrally expressed transcription factors include islet-1 (Isl1), Brn4, P-Frk, and GATA2.[52,55,56] PIT1 (encoded by the gene *POU1F1*) is required for somatotroph, lactotroph, and thyrotroph development,[57,58] whereas the orphan nuclear receptor steroidogenic factor 1 (SF1) is selectively expressed in the gonadotrophs.[59,60]

The ventral-dorsal gradient induces GATA2 in a corresponding gradient in presumptive gonadotrophs and thyrotrophs, and high levels of GATA2 in the most ventral aspect of the developing anterior pituitary directly or indirectly restrict expression of *POU1F1* out of the presumptive gonadotrophs. In the absence of PIT1, GATA2 expression appears sufficient to induce the entire set of transcription factors that are typical of the gonadotroph cell type, including SF-1, P-Frk, and Isl-1. Conversely, the absence of GATA2 dorsally is critical for differentiation of PIT1-positive cells to somatotroph/lactotroph fates. It is hypothesized that the level of GATA2 expression in the thyrotrophs is below the threshold required to inhibit activation of the *POU1F1* gene early enhancer, permitting the emergence of a PIT1+, GATA2+ cell that results in the thyrotroph fate.[56] Pax6 has a role in the sharp boundary of attenuation of the ventral signals that dictate thyrotroph and gonadotroph cell lineages. In the absence of Pax6, the ventral lineages, particularly thyrotrophs, become dorsally extended at the expense of somatotroph and lactotroph cell types,[54] and Pax6 mutant mice are GH and PRL deficient.[61]

The earliest marker of the anterior pituitary is expression of the glycoprotein α-subunit (αGSU), which appears at E11.5 in the mouse. These αGSU-positive cells also express the transcription factor Isl1 and mark a population of differentiating thyrotrophs that disappears after birth.[53,57,62,63] αGSU is expressed in mature thyrotrophs and gonadotrophs. At E12.5, corticotrophs start to differentiate and produce pro-opiomelanocortin (POMC).[53,63] Intensified cell proliferation within Rathke's pouch results in formation of a visible nascent anterior pituitary lobe on E12.5.[50] Definitive thyrotrophs are observed at 14.5 dpc, characterized by the expression of *Tshb* at E14.5 and followed by the expression of GH and prolactin (PRL) in somatotrophs and lactotrophs, respectively, at E15.5. The gonadotrophs are the last cell type to develop, at E16.5, marked by expression of luteinizing hormone (LH) and later by follicle-stimulating hormone (FSH). Eventually, the mature gland is populated by at least five highly differentiated cell types; ventrally to dorsally, they are the gonadotrophs, thyrotrophs, somatotrophs, lactotrophs, and corticotrophs.[52] Ultimately, some of these same transcription factors are also involved in the cell-specific expression and regulation of the gene products of these pituitary cell types, with corticotrophs producing adrenocorticotropin (ACTH), thyrotrophs producing thyrotropin (thyroid-stimulating hormone, TSH), gonadotrophs producing gonadotropins (LH and FSH), somatotrophs producing GH, and lactotrophs producing PRL. The developmental factors that play an in vivo role in pituitary gland development and differentiation are shown in Fig. 24-13.

In humans, GH-producing cells can be found in the anterior pituitary gland by 9 weeks of gestation,[64] and vascular connections between the anterior lobe of the pituitary and the hypothalamus develop at about the same time,[65,66] although hormone production can occur in the pituitary in the absence of connections with the hypothalamus. Somatotrophs can be demonstrated in the pituitary in anencephalic newborns.[67]

In the newborn, the pituitary weighs about 100 mg. In the adult, the mean weight is about 600 mg, with a range of 400 to 900 mg; the pituitary is slightly heavier in women than in men and increases during pregnancy.[68] The mean adult pituitary size is 13 × 9 × 6 mm.[69] The anterior pituitary normally constitutes 80% of the weight of the pituitary. The pituitary resides in the sella turcica, immediately above and partially surrounded by the sphenoid bone. The volume of the sella turcica is a good index of pituitary size and may be reduced in the child with pituitary hypoplasia. The optic chiasm is located superior to the pituitary gland, so suprasellar growth of a pituitary tumor may initially manifest with visual complaints or evidence of decreases in peripheral vision. Furthermore, development of the neurohypophysis and the pituitary are intimately related, leading to potential anatomic associations of central nervous system (CNS) abnormalities with pituitary hypoplasia. For example, septo-optic dysplasia is associated with several CNS anatomic abnormalities and pituitary hormone

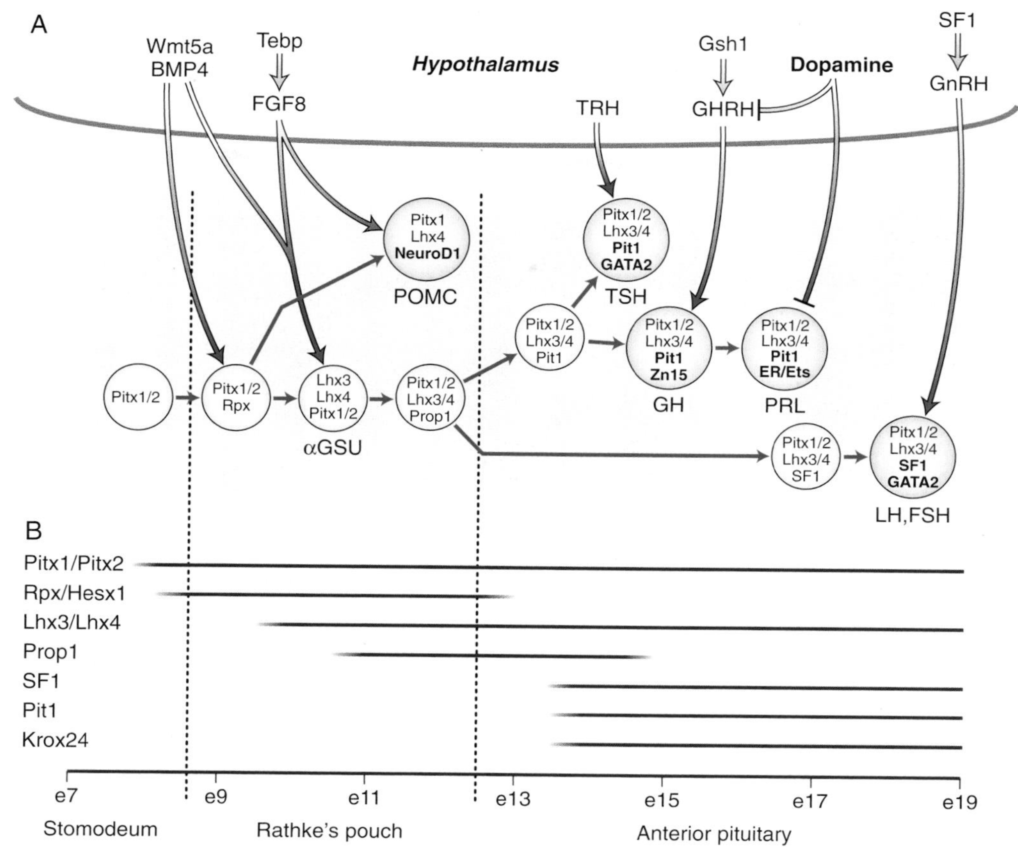

Figure 24-13 Development of pituitary cell lineages. **A,** Schematic representation of pituitary cell precursors shows the expression of prevalent transcription factors at each stage of development. Terminally differentiated cells are shown as larger and shaded circles together with the hormones produced (lineage-specific transcription factors are highlighted in bold in these cells). The interaction with transcription factors and signaling molecules in the hypothalamus is also depicted. Transcription factors are represented in lower case (except for SF1 and GATA2), whereas signaling molecules appear in upper case. **B,** The timing of appearance and disappearance of pituitary transcription factors during mouse embryogenesis. *BMP4,* bone morphogenic protein 4; *e,* embryonic day; *ER,* estrogen receptor; *FGF8,* fibroblast growth factor 8; *FSH,* follicle-stimulating hormone; *GHRH,* growth hormone–releasing hormone; *GnRH,* gonadotropin-releasing hormone; *αGSU,* glycoprotein α-subunit; *LH,* luteinizing hormone; *POMC,* pro-opiomelanocortin; *PRL,* prolactin; *SF1,* steroidogenic factor 1; *TRH,* thyrotropin-releasing hormone; *TSH,* thyroid-stimulating hormone; *Wmt5a,* wingless type MMTV integration site family, member 5A; *Hesx1,* homeobox expressed in ES1 cells (Rathke's pouch homeobox, Rpx). (Reprinted with permission from Lopez-Bermejo A, Buckway CK, Rosenfeld RG. Genetic defects of the growth hormone-insulin-like growth factor axis. *Trends Endocrinol.* 2000;11:43.)

deficiencies.[70] For this reason, children with congenital blindness or nystagmus should be monitored for hypopituitarism.

The anterior pituitary receives controlling signals from the hypothalamus through the portal circulatory system (Fig. 24-14).[65,66] The hypothalamus integrates signals from other brain regions and the environment, resulting in the release of factors that control pituitary hormone synthesis and secretion. Hypothalamic neurons that synthesize peptides terminate in the infundibulum, enter the primary plexus of the hypophyseal portal circulation, and are transported via the hypophyseal portal veins to the capillaries of the anterior pituitary. This portal system in the pituitary stalk provides a means of communication between the neurons of the hypothalamus and the anterior pituitary. Magnetic resonance imaging (MRI) of the pituitary stalk conveys important anatomic information in patients with hypopituitarism.

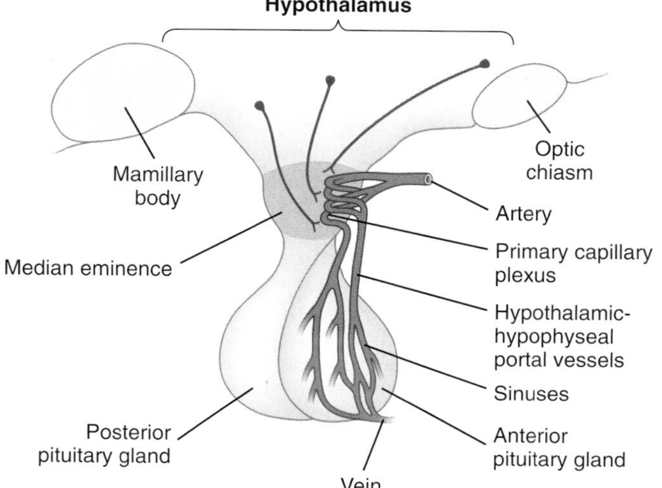

Figure 24-14 The main components of the hypothalamic-pituitary portal system. (From Guyton AC, Hall JC. *Human Physiology and Mechanisms of Disease,* 6th ed. Philadelphia, PA: WB Saunders; 1997:600, with permission.)

Growth Hormone

Human GH is produced as a single-chain, 191-amino-acid, 22-kd protein containing two intramolecular disulfide bonds (Fig. 24-15).[71] GH shares sequence homology with

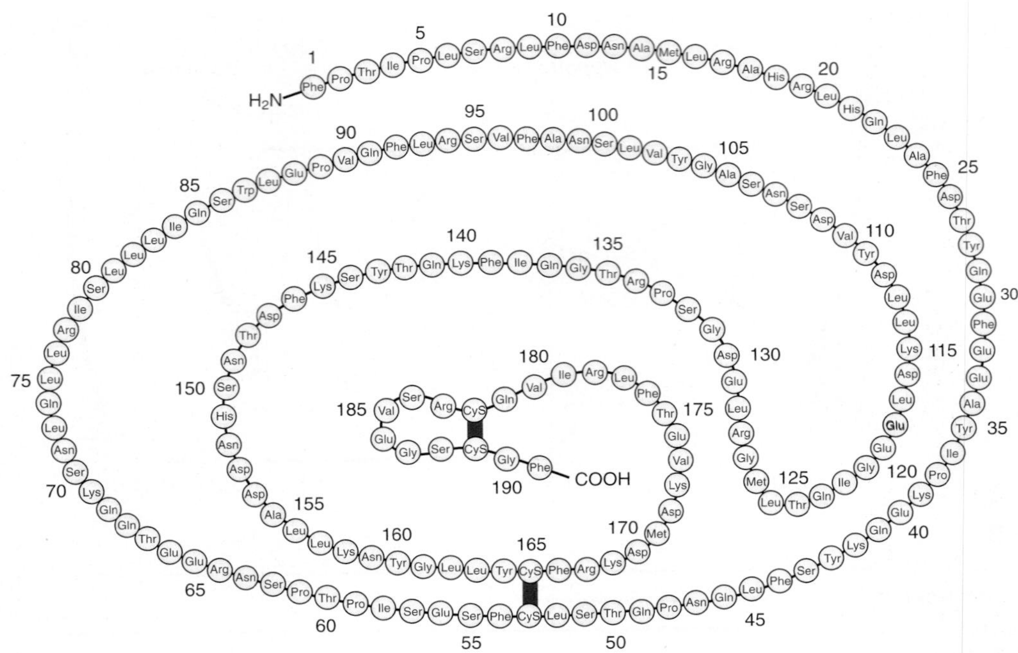

Figure 24-15 **Covalent structure of human growth hormone.** (From Chawla RK, Parks JS, Rudman D. Structural variants of human growth hormone: biochemical, genetic and clinical aspects. *Annu Rev Med.* 1983;34:519-547.)

PRL, chorionic somatomammotropin (CS, placental lactogen), and a 22-kd GH variant (GH-V) that is secreted only by the placenta and differs from pituitary GH by 13 amino acids.[72] The genes encoding these proteins most likely evolved from a common ancestral gene, despite being located on different chromosomes (chromosome 6 for PRL and chromosome 17 for GH).[73] The genes for GH, PRL, and placental lactogen share a common structural organization, with four introns separating five exons. The GH subfamily contains five members, with genes located on a 78-kilobase (kb) section of chromosome 17; the 5′ to 3′ order of the genes is GH, a CS pseudogene, CS-A, GH-V, and CS-B.[74] Normally, about 75% of GH produced by the pituitary is of the mature, 22-kd form. Alternative splicing of the second codon results in deletion of amino acids 32 through 46, yielding a 20-kd form that normally accounts for 5% to 10% of pituitary GH.[73] The remainder of pituitary GH includes desamidated and *N*-acetylated forms and various GH oligomers.

The pulsatile pattern characteristic of GH secretion reflects the interplay of two hypothalamic regulatory peptides, growth hormone–releasing hormone (GHRH) and somatostatin (also called somatotropin release–inhibiting factor, or SRIF), with modulation by other putative GH-releasing factors.[75] GHRH is secreted from nerve cells within the hypothalamus binds to receptors in the anterior pituitary to stimulate somatotroph cell proliferation, differentiation, and growth[76-78] and to stimulate the secretion and synthesis of GH.[79-84] Regulation of GH production by GHRH is mediated largely at the level of transcription and is enhanced by increases in intracellular cyclic adenosine monophosphate (cAMP) levels. The GHRH receptor is a member of the G protein–coupled receptor family B-III.[85,86] In a dwarf transgenic mouse model with diminished GHRH production, pituitary somatotroph proliferation is markedly decreased.[87,88] Transgenic mice that overexpress GHRH grow at a faster rate than control mice.[89]

Somatostatin appears to have its major effect on the timing and amplitude of pulsatile GH secretion and lesser effects on the regulation of GH synthesis. The pulsatile secretion of GH in vivo is believed to result from a simultaneous reduction in hypothalamic somatostatin release and increased GHRH release.[90] Conversely, a trough of GH secretion occurs when somatostatin is released in the face of diminished GHRH activity.

Regulation of the reciprocal secretion of GHRH and somatostatin is imperfectly understood. The hypothalamus integrates signals for stress, sleep, hemorrhage, fasting, hypoglycemia, and exercise through the secretion of multiple neurotransmitters and neuropeptides to regulate the release of these hypothalamic factors and ultimately to influence GH secretion. This physiologic phenomenon forms the basis for a number of GH-stimulatory tests employed in the evaluation of GH secretory capacity or reserve. GH secretion is also influenced by a variety of nonpeptide hormones, including androgens,[91,92] estrogens,[93] thyroxine,[94] and glucocorticoids.[95,96] The mechanisms by which these hormones regulate GH secretion may involve actions at the hypothalamus and the pituitary. For example, hypothyroidism and glucocorticoid excess may each blunt spontaneous and provocative GH secretion. Gonadal steroids appear to be responsible for the rise in GH secretion that characterizes puberty.

Synthetic hexapeptides capable of stimulating GH secretion are termed GH secretagogues.[97,98] These peptides stimulate GH release and enhance the GH response to GHRH, although they work at receptors distinct from those for GHRH, at hypothalamic and pituitary sites.[97,98] Kojima and colleagues[99] identified a natural ligand called *ghrelin*, a 28-amino-acid protein with the serine 3 residue *n*-octanoylated. It is produced mainly by the oxyntic cells of the stomach (and throughout the gastrointestinal tract[100]) and in the hypothalamus, heart, lung, and adipose tissue. Ghrelin has a potent, dose-related, GH-releasing effect[101] and potentiates the GHRH-dependent secretion of GH.[102] GH release results from the binding of ghrelin to the growth hormone secretagogue 1a receptor (GHSR-1a) on somatotrophs in the pituitary[101] and on GHRH-containing neurons in the hypothalamus.[103] Many studies have demonstrated that ghrelin has a wide range of effects, including immune function, cognition, gonadal axis regulation, bone metabolism, gastrointestinal motility, cell proliferation, and effects on the cardiovascular system.[104] However, it is difficult to separate the direct effects of ghrelin from those related to GH secretion. Although ghrelin has documented physiologic effects in vivo, Ghsr-1a knockout mice have a phenotype similar to that of wild-type animals, suggesting that ghrelin does not have a role in growth. However, compensatory mechanisms may provide an explanation for these findings.[105,106]

More recently, studies have documented a positive correlation between ghrelin and anthropometric parameters in the first months of life, which strengthens the hypothesis that ghrelin exerts an influence on growth.[107] Two reports of mutations in GHSR-1a in familial short stature provide evidence to the contrary.[108,109] Further studies indicate that the aging process may be associated with decreased expression of GHSRs in the hypothalamus[110] and with systemic concentration of ghrelin.[111] In addition to direct effects on linear growth, ghrelin has been shown to increase energy stores by stimulating appetite and affecting peripheral glucose and lipid metabolism.[112-114] These data suggest that ghrelin is an important stimulus for nutrient allocation for growth and metabolism and a central component of the GH regulatory system. Orally active ghrelin analogues have been considered as therapeutic agents in the treatment of GH deficiency (GHD), because they may provide a more physiologic approach to increasing the pulsatile release of endogenous GH compared with a single daily dose of recombinant human GH. However, there has been no definite evidence of the therapeutic efficacy of ghrelin analogues in the treatment of GH-deficiency states.

Pituitary adenylate cyclase–activating polypeptide (PACAP) is a hypothalamic peptide that has been shown to be effective in releasing GH from cultured pituitary cells. It belongs to a superfamily of hormones that includes glucagon, secretin, glucagon-like peptide 1 (GLP1), GLP2, GHRH, vasoactive intestinal polypeptide (VIP), peptide histidine methionine (PHM), and glucose-dependent insulinotropic polypeptide (GIP). Gene knockout of the specific PACAP receptor (PAC1R) resulted in 60% mortality in the PAC1R null mice in the first 4 weeks after birth, providing insight into the importance of PACAP even though other superfamily members may compensate some of its functions.[115] The surviving knockout mice showed reduced glucose-stimulated insulin release and glucose intolerance. This observation suggests that PACAP is important in carbohydrate metabolism, potentially through GH.

The synthesis and secretion of GH is also regulated by the insulin-like growth factor (IGF) peptides. Receptors specific for IGF1 and IGF2 have been identified in the hypothalamus and pituitary.[116,117] Inhibition of GH secretion by IGF1 or IGF2 or both has been demonstrated,[118] and spontaneous GH secretion is diminished in humans treated with synthetic IGF1.[119]

Growth Hormone Secretion in Humans

The episodic release of GH from the pituitary somatotrophs results in intermittent increases in serum levels of GH separated by periods of low or undetectable levels, during which time GH secretion is minimal.[120,121] The pulsatile nature of GH secretion has been demonstrated by frequent serum sampling coupled with the use of sensitive immunofluorometric or chemoluminescent assays of GH.[121] Under normal circumstances, serum GH levels are less than 0.04 mg/L between secretory bursts. It is impractical to assess GH secretion by random serum sampling. Extensive sampling studies at different ages in normal persons and in many abnormal conditions have defined GH pulses, basal secretion, and diurnal variability. Computer programs have been developed to indicate whether changes in GH levels in various life periods and under diverse clinical circumstances occur because of a change of secretory mass or pulse frequency, altered clearance, or a combination of these processes.[120-123] Deconvolution techniques allow accurate estimates of the quantity of GH secreted per burst, GH clearance kinetics, and pulse amplitudes and frequencies, as well as an overall calculation of endogenous GH production. Approximate entropy, a model-free measure, is applied to quantify the degree of orderliness of GH release patterns.[124,125] The impact of the specific nature of pulsatile GH secretion on its biologic actions is under study.[120,121] For example, it appears that better statural growth is associated with large swings of GH output of relatively uniform magnitude in an irregular sequence (high approximate entropy).[126,127]

GH-secreting cells have been identified by 9 to 12 weeks of gestation, and immunoreactive pituitary GH is present by 7 to 9 weeks of gestation.[128,129] Fetal pituicytes secrete GH in vitro by 5 weeks,[130] before the hypothalamic-portal vascular system is differentiated.[131] PIT1 mRNA and PIT1 protein are expressed by at least 6 weeks of gestation; their abundant presence early in gestation suggests an important role in cytodifferentiation and cell proliferation.[132] GH can be identified in fetal serum by the end of the first trimester, with peak levels of approximately 150 mg/L in midgestation.[128,129] Serum levels fall throughout the latter part of pregnancy and are lower in full-term than in premature infants, perhaps reflecting feedback by the higher serum levels of IGF peptides that characterize the later stages of gestation.[133,134]

Mean levels of GH decrease from values of 25 to 35 mg/L in the neonatal period to approximately 5 to 7 mg/L through childhood and early puberty.[129,135,136] Twenty-four hour GH secretion peaks during adolescence, undoubtedly contributing to the high serum levels of IGF1 that are characteristic of puberty. The increase in GH production during middle to late puberty is caused by enhanced pulse amplitude and increased mass of GH per secretory burst, rather than by a change in pulse frequency (Figs. 24-16 and 24-17).[120,124,135,136] Greater irregularity in GH secretion corresponds to greater linear growth.[137] In the face of stable levels of the growth hormone–binding protein (GHBP),[138,139] the enhanced pubertal GH production appears to be associated with higher levels of "free" GH (Fig. 24-18), potentially facilitating the delivery of IGF1 to target tissues. This enhanced activity of the GH-IGF axis contributes to the insulin resistance that occurs during puberty.[140] Production of GH and IGF begins to decline by late adolescence[122] and continues to fall throughout adult life. Normal young adult men experience 6 to 10 GH secretory bursts per 24 hours, a value similar to that observed in younger children and adolescents.[121,135] On the other hand, 24-hour GH production rates for normal men range from 0.25 to 0.52 mg/m^2 surface area,[96,141] about 20% to 30% of pubertal levels; this is largely due to decreased GH pulse amplitude with age.[135] Indeed, puberty may be considered, with some justification, a period of "physiologic acromegaly," whereas aging, with its decrease in GH secretion, has been termed "the somatopause."[93,142]

Physiologic states that affect GH secretion, in addition to maturation and aging, include sleep,[143] nutritional status,[144] fasting, exercise,[145] stress,[145] and gonadal steroids.[91] Maximal GH secretion occurs during the night,

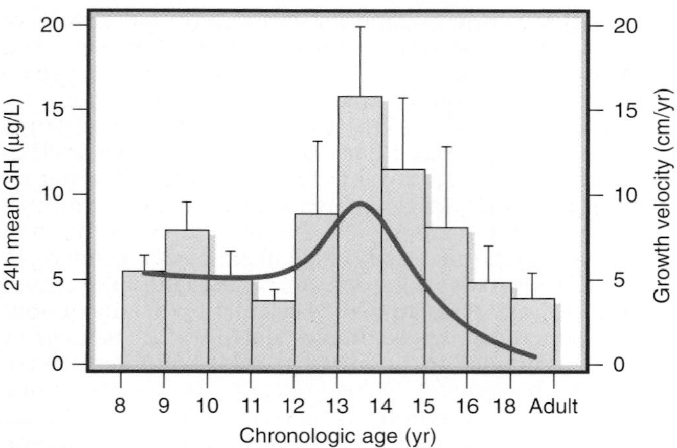

Figure 24-16 Relation between 24-hour mean growth hormone (GH) levels and age in boys and men. The bars represent the 24-hour mean and standard error (+SE) values of GH *(left axis)* obtained from 60 24-hour GH profiles of healthy boys and men subdivided according to chronologic age. An idealized growth velocity curve reproduced from the 50th percentile values for whole-year height velocity of North American boys[15] is superimposed. (From Martha PM Jr, Rogol AD, Veldhuis JD, et al. Alterations in the pulsatile properties of circulating growth hormone concentrations during puberty in boys. *J Clin Endocrinol Metab.* 1989;69:563-570.)

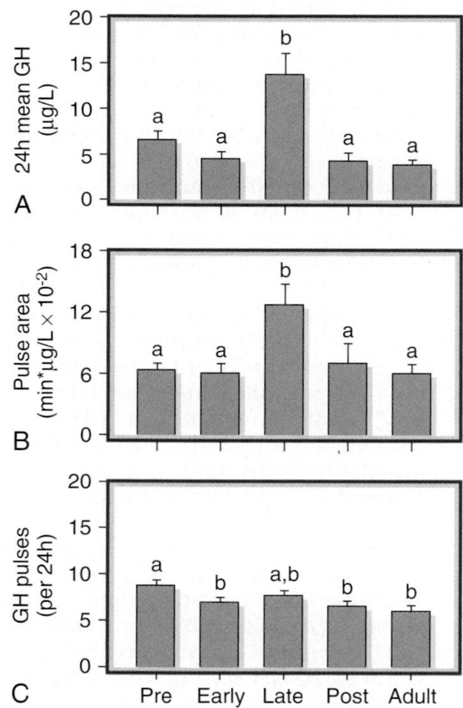

Figure 24-17 **A,** The 24-hour and standard error (+SE) levels of growth hormone (GH) for groups of normal boys at varied stages of pubertal maturation. **B,** The mean (+SE) area under the GH concentration-versus-time curve for individual GH pulses, as identified by the cluster pulse detection algorithm. **C,** The number of GH pulses (+SE), as detected by the cluster algorithm, in the 24-hour GH concentration profiles for boys in each of the pubertal study groups. Notice that the mean 24-hour GH concentration changes are largely mediated by changes in the amount of GH secreted per pulse, rather than the frequency of pulses. In each panel, bars bearing the same letter are statistically indistinguishable. (From Martha PM Jr, Rogol AD, Veldhuis JD, et al. Alterations in the pulsatile properties of circulating growth hormone concentrations during puberty in boys. *J Clin Endocrinol Metab.* 1989;69:563-570.)

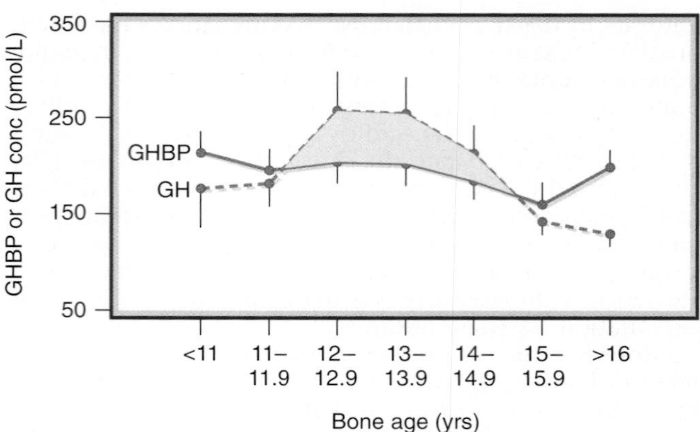

Figure 24-18 Levels of growth hormone (GH) and growth hormone–binding protein (GHBP) measured in normal pubertal boys throughout adolescence. The GHBP levels do not significantly change during puberty, but there is a significant increment of GH production and, therefore, of GH levels during this same time. These data suggest that there may be greater amounts of "free GH" during this period, leading to greater production of insulin-like growth factor 1. (Based on data from references 136 and 138.)

especially at the onset of the first slow-wave sleep period (stages III and IV). Rapid eye movement (REM) sleep, on the other hand, is associated with low GH secretion.[143,146] A circadian rhythm of somatostatin secretion, upon which is superimposed episodic bursts of GHRH release, may help explain the nocturnal augmentation of GH production.[147]

When testosterone was administered to boys with delayed puberty, spontaneous GH release was enhanced, but such a change was not duplicated by administration of nonaromatizable androgens, emphasizing the possible unique importance of estrogen in GH secretion.[122,148-150] The effects of testosterone on serum IGF1 levels may in part be independent of GH, because individuals with mutations of the GH receptor (GHR) still experience a modest rise in serum IGF1 during puberty.[151] With a combination of deconvolution analysis, approximate entropy, and cosine regression analysis, Veldhuis and associates[124,150] carefully evaluated intensive GH sampling data derived from measurements in sensitive GH assays in prepubertal and pubertal children of both genders. In addition to the amplified secretory burst mass caused by jointly increased GH pulse amplitude and duration, they found that sex steroids selectively affect facets of GH neurosecretory control: estrogen increases the basal GH secretion rate and the irregularity of GH release patterns, whereas testosterone stimulates greater GH secretory burst mass and greater IGF1 concentrations.

Obesity is characterized by lowered GH production, reflected by a diminished number of GH secretory bursts and shorter half-life duration.[144,152] Obesity in childhood and adolescence is characterized by decreased GH production with normal IGF and increased GHBP levels and often by increased linear growth.[152] The hyperinsulinism associated with obesity causes lowered levels of IGF-binding protein 1 (IGFBP1) and, perhaps, higher levels of "free" IGF1.[153] Endogenous GH secretion and levels achieved during provocative tests in obese subjects[154] approximated the diagnostic range of GHD. Fasting increased both the number and the amplitude of GH secretory bursts, presumably reflecting decreased somatostatin secretion and enhanced GHRH release, while lowering GHBP concentrations. Rapid changes in levels of IGFBPs in response to altered nutrition and changes in insulin levels may modify the effect of IGF1 on its negative feedback and effector sites.[121,152] Body mass also influences GH production in normal prepubertal and pubertal children and adults.[135,155,156]

The Growth Hormone Receptor and Growth Hormone Binding Protein

The gene for the human GHR is located on chromosome 5p13.1-p12, where it spans more than 87 kb.[157] The GHR gene (*GHR*) contains 10 exons: exon 1 contains the 5′ untranslated region, whereas exons 2 through 10 encode the three domains of the GHR—the extracellular ligand-binding domain, a single transmembrane domain, and a cytoplasmic domain for signal transduction.[158] The highest level of *GHR* expression is in the liver, followed by muscle, fat, kidney, and heart. Although ubiquitously expressed transcription factors have been found to bind the *GHR* promoter, little is known about how these transcription factors coordinate regulation of *GHR* expression. The receptor is 620 amino acids long, with a predicted molecular weight of 70 kd before glycosylation. It is a member of the class I hematopoietic cytokine family[159] and has sequence homology to PRL, erythropoietin, granulocyte-macrophage colony-stimulating factor, and interferon receptors as well as the interleukin 2 (IL2), IL3, IL4, IL6, and IL7 receptors.[158]

Two isoforms of the *GHR* have been found in humans—a full-length form and a form that has a deletion of exon 3 (*GHRd3*) with a loss of a 22-amino-acid segment of the extracellular domain of the receptor.[160] The *GHRd3* allele is present in approximately 33% of a general population.[160] Several studies have investigated the clinical significance of the *GHRd3* allele on growth and GH responsiveness in specific disease states.

GH must bind to a homodimer complex of GHR to activate its intracellular signaling pathways (Fig. 24-19). Whether dimerization of the GHR subunits occurs before or after GH binding is a matter of debate. It was initially thought that dimerization would occur only after GH binding; GH would bind to the first subunit, after which the GH-GHR complex would diffuse within the membrane

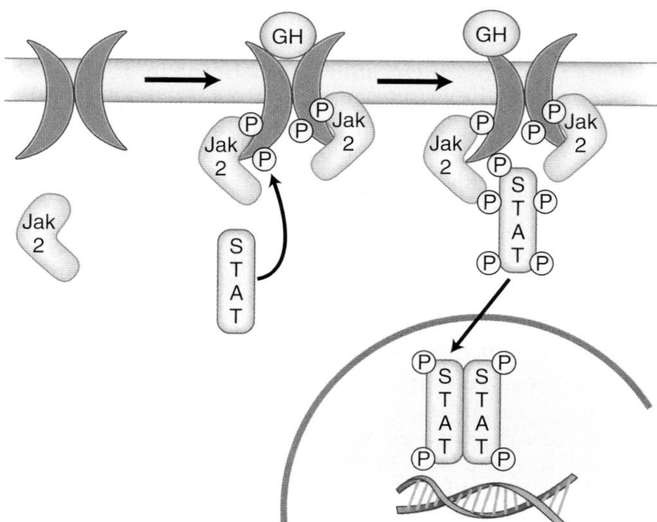

Figure 24-19 A model depicting intracellular signaling intermediates induced by binding of growth hormone (GH) with the GH receptor (GHR). Jak, Janus kinase; P, phosphorylation; STAT, signal transducer and activator of transcription. (From Le Roith DC, Bondy S, Yakar J-L, et al. The somatomedin hypothesis: 2001. *Endocrine Rev.* 2001;22:53-74.)

until contacted by a second subunit, leading to receptor activation.[161,162] However, it was shown in live cells that the subunits of the GHR are constitutively dimerized in an inactive (i.e., unbound) state.[163,164] The two subunits are joined by their transmembrane domains through leucine zipper interactions, with steric hindrance from extracellular domains preventing interactions between identical receptor partners. The GH binding sites on the extracellular domains of the two subunits are placed asymmetrically. Therefore, once GH binds to the constitutive dimer, it induces rotation of the two subunits of the dimer that is transmitted via the transmembrane domain to the intracellular domain, allowing downstream kinase activation by transphosphorylation.

After binding to its receptor, GH stimulates phosphorylation of JAK2 (Janus kinase 2), a tyrosine kinase associated with the GHR (see Fig. 24-19). On recruitment or activation, the JAK2 molecule causes phosphorylation of critical tyrosines on the intracellular portion of the GHR, a sort of transphosphorylation. The phosphorylated tyrosines on the GHR provide docking sites for critical intermediary STAT proteins (signal transducers and activators of transcription).[161,165] STAT proteins dock, via their SRC homology 2 (SH2) domain to phosphotyrosines on ligand-activated receptors, such as the GHR. After docking, phosphorylation occurs on single tyrosines at the carboxyl-terminus of the protein. Then STATs dissociate from the GHR, dimerize, translocate to the nucleus, and bind to DNA through their DNA-binding domain to regulate gene transcription. There are seven known mammalian STATs; of these, STAT5B appears to be most critically involved in mediating the growth-promoting actions of the GHR, as was indicated by several gene disruption studies in rodent models.[166-169] GH- and JAK2-dependent phosphorylation and activation have been demonstrated for many cytoplasmic signaling molecules which, after forming homodimers or heterodimers, translocate into the nucleus, bind DNA, and activate transcription.[170-172]

It has been shown that GHR signaling can also lead to activation of extracellular related kinase 1 (ERK1) and ERK2 to increase transcription.[173] How GHR activation leads to ERK1/2 activation is a matter of debate. A JAK2-independent but SRC-dependent phosphorylation has been modeled,[174,175] as has a JAK2-dependent but SRC-independent mechanism.[176] Experiments were conducted in different cell lines, so it is possible that the mechanisms of ERK1/2 activation by GHR are different in different cell lines. It is unclear what role these pathways play in the GH stimulation of growth.

Inhibition of GH signaling by several members of the GH-inducible suppressor of cytokine signaling (SOCS) family has been reported.[177] The importance of SOCS proteins in controlling growth is demonstrated by the finding of gigantism in Socs-2 knockout mice,[178] an effect that appears to require the presence of GH and activation of STAT5B.[179] Endotoxin and the proinflammatory cytokines IL1 and tumor necrosis factor-α (TNF-α) can induce SOCS proteins[180] and GH insensitivity. It has been proposed that IL1 and TNF-α are factors that play a role in the GH insensitivity of sepsis by inducing SOCS3.[181]

GHBP prolongs the half-life of GH, presumably by impairing glomerular filtration, and modulates its binding to the GHR. It binds GH with high specificity and affinity but with low capacity; only about 45% of circulating GH is bound.[139,182,183] GHBP is derived from proteolytic cleavage of the extracellular domain of the receptor.[184] GHBP levels reflect GHR levels and activity; that is, low levels are associated with states of GH insensitivity.[139] Levels of GHBP are low early in life, rise through childhood, and plateau during the pubertal years and adulthood.[138,185,186] Levels are constant for an individual once puberty is reached and correlate inversely with 24-hour GH production.[138] Impaired nutrition, diabetes mellitus, hypothyroidism, chronic liver disease, and inherited abnormalities of the GHR are associated with low levels of GHBP, whereas obesity, refeeding, early pregnancy, and estrogen treatment are associated with elevated levels of GHBP.[139] In general, GHBP levels reflect GHR levels and activity. Patients with GH insensitivity due to defects of the extracellular domain of the GHR have low GHBP levels, and GHBP levels therefore can be useful in identifying these individuals. Patients with GH insensitivity due to nonreceptor abnormalities, defects of the intracellular domain of the GHR, or inability of the receptor to dimerize may have normal levels of GHBP.[151,187-189]

GHR signaling affects the transcription of many genes immediately (<3 hours after stimulation) and other genes over a longer period of stimulation. After acute GH stimulation in GH-deficient rats, hepatic genes immediately induced by GH included signal transducers (STAT3, gp130, p38), DNA repair proteins, receptor proteases, and metabolic regulators such as Igf1, Igfbp3, and Mct1.[190] Studies using *Ghr*$^{-/-}$ mice or mice overexpressing *Gh* indicate that Ghr signaling is involved in regulation of expression of genes involved in carbohydrate, fat, and steroid metabolism.[168,191-193]

The development of mice that lack *Ghr* or downstream components of Ghr signaling has shed light on the role of GH in normal physiology. *Ghr*$^{-/-}$ mice exhibit normal size at birth but have attenuated postnatal growth, with body weight about half of normal and length about two-thirds of normal.[194] *Ghr*$^{-/-}$ mice also exhibit delayed pubertal maturation, longer life span, and increased insulin sensitivity compared with controls.

To determine which cytoplasmic regions of the GHR are involved in growth-promoting actions, mice with truncated *Ghr* were engineered via homologous recombination (so-called knock-in mice). One knock-in mouse had a mutation that resulted in removal of the C-terminal region of the receptor (mutant 569), including some recognized Stat5 and Socs2 recruitment sites; a second knock-in mouse had a mutation that resulted in truncation of the receptor downstream from the Jak2, mitogen-activated protein (MAP) kinase, and phosphatidylinositol 3 (PI3) kinase interaction sites, a region that included the majority of Stat5 recruitment sites (mutant 391).[168] Homozygous mutant 569 mice exhibited a body size 44% of that of wild-type mice on loss of 70% of Stat5 signaling and with IGF1 levels 80% lower than in the wild-type mouse. As expected, homozygous mutant 391 mice had more severe growth attenuation, with a body size 11% of that of wild-type mice on complete loss of Stat5 signaling. The fact that these mice had some growth implicates other signaling pathways, such as MAP kinase, in growth-promoting roles.

Mice with *Ghr* deleted only in the liver were produced and were found to have low IGF1 levels and high GH levels. These mice exhibited normal growth but had significantly lower bone density than controls. They also exhibited liver steatosis with insulin resistance and elevated serum free fatty acid levels.[195] This mouse model sheds light on the metabolic function of excessive GHR signaling independent of IGF1 signaling.

Deletion of *Jak2* in mice is embryonically lethal,[196] as is deletion of *Stat3*. Deletion of *Stat1* or *Stat5a* does not affect body size. However, deletion of *Stat5b* leads to decreased size in male but not female mice. The *Stat5a/b*$^{-/-}$ mouse is smaller than the *Stat5b*$^{-/-}$ mouse.[197] Deletion of *Socs2*,[178] but not of other *Socs* genes,[179] produced gigantism in mice, indicating the specific role of *Socs2* in the negative regulation of GHR action. The combined *Igf1* and *Ghr*$^{-/-}$ mouse had a more severe attenuation of postnatal growth than mice with knockout of either gene alone, indicating that GH and IGF1 promote growth by both common and independent functions.[198] The liver-specific IGF1 knockout mouse with extremely low serum IGF1 levels has normal linear growth, suggesting IGF-independent actions of GH or paracrine production and effects of IGF1, or both.[199]

Historically, the anabolic actions of GH were thought to be mediated entirely by the IGF peptides (the so-called somatomedin hypothesis).[200,201] Although a majority of GH actions are mediated by IGFs, the opposite effects of GH and IGFs on metabolism and in knockout mouse models suggest that there are IGF-independent actions of GH. Indeed, the "diabetogenic" actions of GH are contradictory to the glucose-lowering effects of IGFs. In vitro studies suggest potential IGF-independent action of GH in the following tissues:

1. Epiphysis—stimulation of epiphyseal growth
2. Bone—stimulation of osteoclast differentiation and activity, stimulation of osteoblast activity, and increase in bone mass through endochondral bone formation
3. Adipose tissue—acute insulin-like effects, followed by increased lipolysis, inhibition of lipoprotein lipase, stimulation of hormone-sensitive lipase, decreased glucose transport, and decreased lipogenesis[202-204]
4. Muscle—increased amino acid transport, increased nitrogen retention, increased lean tissue, and increased energy expenditure[205,206]

The concept of IGF-independent actions of GH is supported by results of in vivo studies in which IGF1 could not duplicate all of the effects of GH, such as nitrogen retention and insulin resistance.[207]

Insulin-Like Growth Factors

Historical Background

The IGFs (somatomedins) are a family of peptides that are, in part, GH dependent and mediate many of the anabolic and mitogenic actions of GH. They were originally identified in 1957 by their ability to stimulate [^{35}S]-sulfate incorporation into rat cartilage and were called *sulfation factors*.[200] In 1972, that term was replaced with *somatomedin*,[208] and purification of somatomedin from human serum yielded a basic peptide (somatomedin-C) and a neutral peptide (somatomedin-A).[209,210] In 1978, Rinderknecht and Humbel[211,212] isolated two active somatomedins from human plasma and, after demonstrating a striking structural resemblance to proinsulin, renamed them *insulin-like growth factors* (IGFs).

IGF Genes and Protein Structure

There are two IGFs circulating in humans, IGF1 and IGF2. IGF1 is a basic peptide of 70 amino acids, and IGF2 is a peptide of 67 amino acids. The two peptides share 45 of 73 possible amino acid positions and have 50% amino acid homology to insulin.[200,211,212] Like insulin, both IGFs have A and B chains connected by disulfide bonds. The connecting C-peptide region is 12 amino acids for IGF1 and 8 amino acids for IGF2, bearing no homology for the C-peptide region of proinsulin. The D-peptide region contains C-terminal extensions of 8 amino acids for IGF1 and 6 amino acids for IGF2. The E-peptide is a trailer peptide

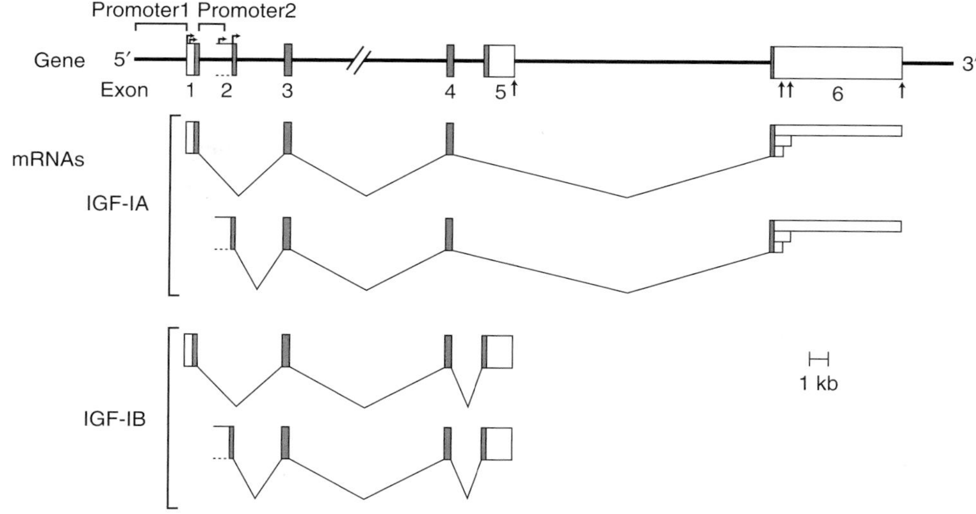

Figure 24-20 Structure and expression of the human insulin-like growth factor I (IGF-I) gene. The structure of the different human IGF-I messenger RNAs (mRNAs) is displayed below the map of the gene. Sites of pre-mRNA processing are indicated by the *thin lines*. Sites of differential polyadenylation are marked at the 3′ end of the gene by *vertical arrows* and in the mRNAs by *horizontal boxes* of varying length. (From Rotwein P. Structure, evolution, expression and regulation of insulin-like growth factors I and II. *Growth Factors.* 1991;5:3-18.)

that is cleaved in post-translational processing. The structural similarity explains the ability of both IGFs to bind to the insulin receptor and the ability of insulin to bind to the type I IGF receptor (encoded by *IGF1R*). On the other hand, structural differences probably explain the failure of insulin to bind with high affinity to the IGFBPs.

Insulin-Like Growth Factor I

Gene Regulation. The human IGF1 gene (*IGF1*) is located on the long arm of chromosome 12[213-215] and contains at least six exons (Fig. 24-20). Exons 1 and 2 encode alternative signal peptides, each containing several transcription start sites; that is, the multiple existing *IGF1* transcripts consist of either exon 1 or exon 2. Two different promoters regulated in a tissue-specific manner[216,217] control the use of exon 1 or 2. Exons 3 and 4 encode the remaining signal peptide, the remainder of the mature IGF1 molecule, and part of the trailer peptide (E peptide). Exons 5 and 6 encode alternatively used segments of the trailer peptide and 3′ untranslated sequences with multiple different polyadenylation sites. As a result, multiple mRNA species exist, allowing for tissue-specific, developmental, and hormonal regulation of *IGF1* gene expression.

GH appears to be the primary regulator of *Igf1* transcription, which begins as early as 30 minutes after intraperitoneal injection of GH into hypophysectomized rats.[218] Transcriptional activation by GH results in a 20-fold rise in *Igf1* mRNA, but there may be tissue-to-tissue variability in extent of GH-induced expression of *Igf1* mRNA.[219] Another influential factor is estrogen, which stimulates *Igf1* mRNA expression in the uterus but inhibits GH-stimulated *Igf1* transcription in the liver.[220] Estradiol administration to a $Ghr^{-/-}$ mouse can stimulate hepatic *Igf1* synthesis and growth.[221] The sex-steroid effects on *IGF1* transcription plays a role in the pubertal rise of IGF1 levels in humans (see later discussion).

The mechanisms involved in regulation of IGF gene expression include the existence of multiple promoters, heterogeneous transcription initiation within each of the promoters, alternative splicing of various exons, differential RNA polyadenylation, and variable mRNA stability. Translation of *IGF1* may also be under complex control. The transcription factor STAT5B is the most critical mediator of GH-induced activation of IGF1 transcription, as detailed earlier. Two adjacent STAT5B binding sites have been identified in the second intron of the rat *Igf1* gene, within a region previously identified as undergoing acute changes in chromatin structure after GH treatment.[169]

Once translated, IGF1 pre-propeptides require processing to form the mature IGF1 peptide (Fig. 24-21). After processing, all transcript isoforms result in an identical 70-amino-acid protein containing the A, B, C, and D domains. Pro-IGF1 also contains the E peptide. Proteases from the subtilisin-related proprotein convertase family (SPC) cleave pro-IGF1 at Arg71, located in the D portion of the peptide.[222] Several reports have demonstrated the secretion of pro-IGF1 from fibroblasts and other cells,[223,224] although the biologic significance of the pro-IGF1 peptide is unclear. It has been shown that the *IGF1* splice variant (see Fig. 24-20) that includes exon 5 increases in rabbit muscle subjected to stretch.[225] The ability to express this transcript diminishes with age.[226,227] This transcript, when injected into rabbit muscle, promoted increased muscle mass within 2 weeks.[228] However, viral delivery of this transcript to skeletal muscle did not cause a greater increase

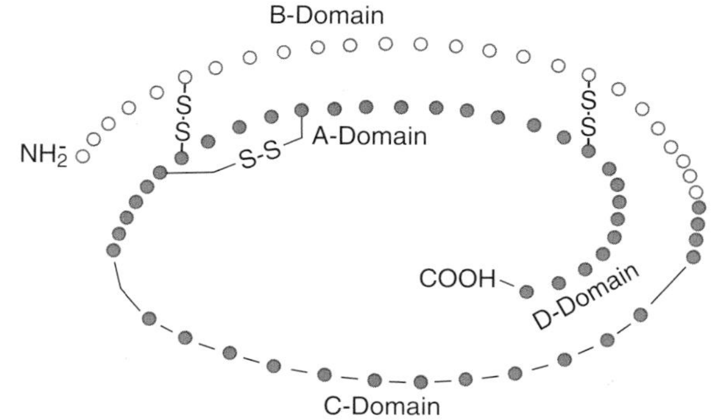

Figure 24-21 Structure of the insulin-like growth factor IGF-I peptide. (Reproduced from Yakar S, Wu Y, Setser J, et al. The role of circulating IGF-I. *Endocrine.* 2002;19:239-248.)

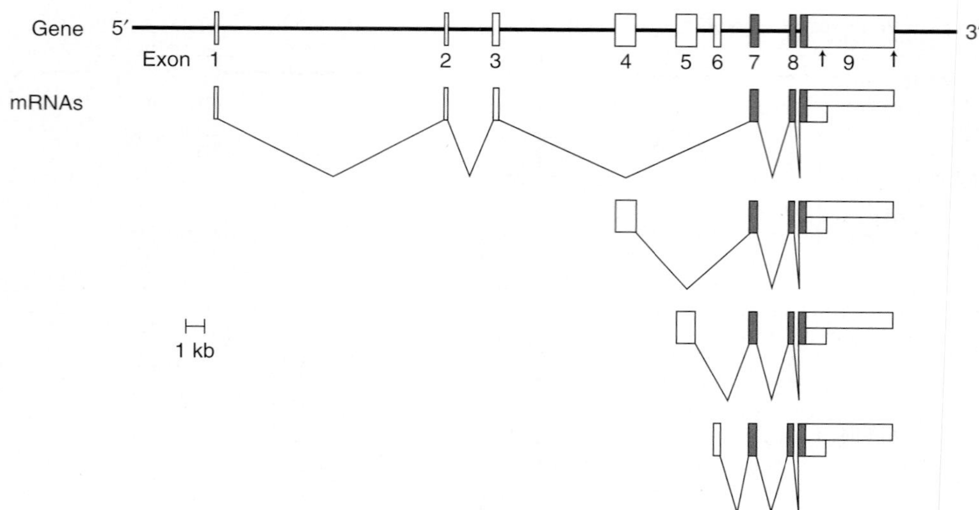

Figure 24-22 Structure and expression of the human insulin-like growth factor 2 (IGF2) gene. The structure of different human IGF2 messenger RNAs (mRNAs) is displayed below the map of the gene. The patterns of mRNA processing are indicated by the *thin lines*. Sites of differential polyadenylation are marked at the 3′ end of the gene by *vertical arrows* and in the mRNAs by horizontal boxes of varying length. (From Rotwein P. Structure, evolution, expression and regulation of insulin-like growth factors I and II. *Growth Factors.* 1991;5:3-18.)

in muscle mass over other IGF1 transcripts. It was postulated that muscle damage, caused by injection but not by viral delivery of the transcript, must occur for the transcript to have a differential effect on muscle mass.[229] These studies demonstrate potential roles of the various *IGF1* transcripts.

Serum Levels. In human fetal serum, IGF1 levels are relatively low and are positively correlated with gestational age.[230,231] There is a reported correlation between fetal cord serum IGF1 levels and birth weight,[230-232] but this relationship is controversial.[233] IGF1 levels in newborn serum are typically 30% to 50% of adult levels. Serum levels rise during childhood. During puberty, IGF1 levels rise to 2 to 3 times the adult range. Levels during adolescence correlate better with Tanner stage or bone age than with chronologic age.[234,235] The pubertal rise in gonadal steroids may stimulate IGF1 production indirectly by contributing to a rise in GH secretion and directly by augmenting liver synthesis and secretion of IGF1. Girls with gonadal dysgenesis show no adolescent increase in serum IGF1, providing evidence of the association of the pubertal rise in IGF1 with the production of gonadal steroids.[236-238] As further evidence, patients with GH insensitivity due to GHR mutations exhibit a modest rise in IGF1 during puberty despite a decline in GH levels. After 20 to 30 years of age, serum IGF1 levels gradually and progressively fall.[239,240] The age-associated decline in IGF1 levels has been implicated in the negative nitrogen balance, decrease in muscle mass, and osteoporosis of aging.[239]

Insulin-Like Growth Factor 2

Gene Regulation. The gene for IGF2 (*IGF2*) is located on the short arm of chromosome 11,[213-215] adjacent to the insulin gene, and contains 9 exons (Fig. 24-22). Exons 1 through 6 encode 5′ untranslated RNA, exon 7 encodes the signal peptide and most of the mature protein, and exon 8 encodes the C-terminal portion of the protein. As with *IGF1*, multiple mRNA species exist to allow for developmental and hormonal regulation of expression. *IGF2* mRNA expression is high in fetal life and has been detected as early as the blastocyst stage in mice.[241] Fetal tissues generally have high *IGF2* mRNA levels that decline postnatally.

IGF2 is imprinted—that is, only one allele is active, depending on parental origin. In the case of *IGF2*, only the paternally expressed allele is active. Most imprinted genes occur in clusters with reciprocally imprinted genes, and *IGF2* is no exception. The noncoding gene *H19* is downstream from *IGF2* and is oppositely imprinted, meaning that only the maternal allele is expressed and the paternal allele is inactive. The promoters of *IGF2* and *H19* share a set of enhancers that act on either gene. On the paternal allele, the *H19* promoter region is methylated and thus inactivated (so-called epigenetic regulation of expression).[242] The *IGF2* promoter does not contain regions that can be methylated. Instead, upstream from the *H19* and *IGF2* promoter region is a so-called differentially methylated region (DMR). When it is methylated, binding of CCCTC binding factor (CTCF) is prevented, allowing enhancers to act on the *IGF2* promoter to activate transcription.[243] On the maternal chromosome, the DMR region is not methylated, allowing CTCF to bind and preventing transcription (Fig. 24-23).[244]

The fact that *IGF2* is monoallelically expressed emphasizes the importance of gene dosage to normal physiology and development. Loss of imprinting of *IGF2* can lead to

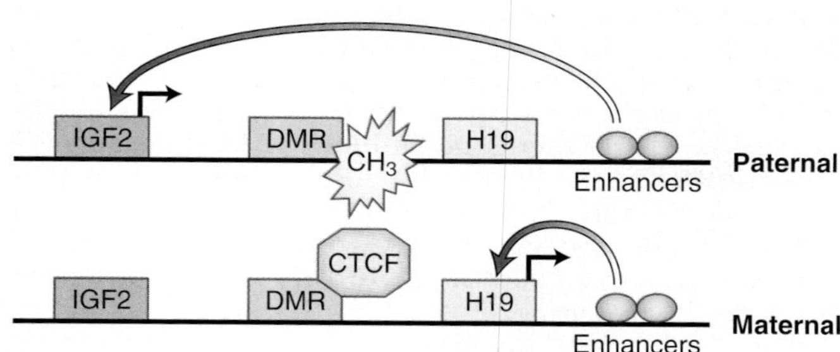

Figure 24-23 Schematic of the imprinted region of the insulin-like growth factor 2 (*IGF2*)-*H19* locus. CTCF, CCCTC binding factor; CH_3, methylation; DMR, differentially methylated region. (Adapted from Chao W, D'Amore P. IGF2: epigenetic regulation and role in development and disease. *Cytokine Growth Factor Rev.* 2008;19:111-120.)

constitutively expressed *IGF2* mRNA and excessive IGF2. *IGF2* mRNA is expressed constitutively in a number of mesenchymal and embryonic tumors, including Wilms' tumor,[245,246] rhabdomyosarcoma, neuroblastoma, pheochromocytoma, hepatoblastoma, leiomyoma, leiomyosarcoma, liposarcoma, and colon carcinoma.[247-251] Loss of imprinting has been demonstrated as the cause for dysregulated expression in some of these tumors. Production of *IGF2* variants by these tumors can cause non–islet cell tumor hypoglycemia (NICTH).[252] Loss of imprinting of *IGF2* resulting in biallelic gene expression has also been found in Beckwith-Weidemann syndrome (BWS), which is characterized by fetal and neonatal overgrowth and an increased risk of childhood cancers. Loss of imprinting in BWS can result from mutations that effect imprinting in the region of chromosome 11 that contains *IGF2*,[253] methylation defects that cause hypermethylation of the region or duplication of the expressed paternal allele resulting in increased *IGF2* expression, or paternal uniparental disomy (i.e., inheritance of only the expressing paternal allele).

Variant peptides of IGF2 have been identified in normal human serum, the significance of which is uncertain. Up to one quarter of the IGF2 isolated from normal human plasma lacked the amino-terminal alanine.[212] Another variant peptide with the Ser29 replaced by Arg-Leu-Pro-Gly has also been identified in human plasma,[254] presumably from the liver.[255] Other IGF2 variants have been identified that are longer than the predominant IGF2 species.[256] The significance of these larger forms of IGF2 is uncertain. In general, these variants appear capable of binding to IGF and insulin receptors and to IGFBPs, and they can participate in formation of the 150-kd IGF–IGFBP3–acid-labile subunit (ALS) ternary complex (discussed later). Large IGF2 variants have been shown to be produced by mesenchymal tumors and cause NICTH. In a patient with leiomyosarcoma and recurrent hypoglycemia, 70% of serum IGF2 consisted of the higher-molecular-weight forms.[252] Removal of the tumor decreased the fraction of the large IGF2 forms and serum and corrected the hypoglycemia. It has been documented that the total serum IGF2 in NICTH is normal, yet the fraction of the larger forms is larger. Zapf [257] proposed that NICTH occurs when secretion of large IGF2 forms results in suppression of GH, insulin, and the normal 7-kd IGF2, leading to decreased production of IGF1, IGFBP3, and the ALS and increased production of IGFBP2. This produces a shift in the distribution of IGF2 from the IGF2-IGFBP ternary complex to the lower-molecular-weight complex. The results is increased bioavailability of IGF2 to target tissues, enhanced glucose consumption, and decreased hepatic glucose production.

Serum Levels. Human newborn levels of IGF2 are typically 50% of adult levels. By 1 year of age, adult levels are attained, and there is little, if any, subsequent decline, even up to the seventh or eighth decade.[258]

Insulin-Like Growth Factor Receptors

There are two types of IGF receptors, type I and type II (Fig. 24-24). Structural characterization of these receptors has provided documentation of the differences between these two forms.[259,260] The type I IGF receptor is closely related to the insulin receptor; both are heterotetramers comprising two membrane-spanning α-subunits and two intracellular β-subunits. The α-subunits contain the binding sites for IGF1 and are linked by disulfide bonds. The β-subunits contain a transmembrane domain, an adenosine triphosphate (ATP)-binding site, and a tyrosine kinase domain, which constitute the presumed signal transduction mechanism for the receptor. One mole of the full heterotetrameric receptor appears to bind 1 mole of ligand.

Although the type I IGF receptor has been commonly termed the "IGF1 receptor," this receptor binds both IGF1 and IGF2 with high affinity, and both IGF peptides can activate tyrosine kinase by binding to the type I receptor. In studies involving transfection and overexpression of the type I IGF receptor complementary DNA (cDNA), the dissociation constant for IGF1 is typically 0.2 to 1.0 nmol/L, whereas the affinity for IGF2 is usually slightly less, although it varies from study to study.[260] The affinity of the type I IGF receptor for insulin is usually 100-fold less, explaining the relatively weak mitogenic effect of insulin.

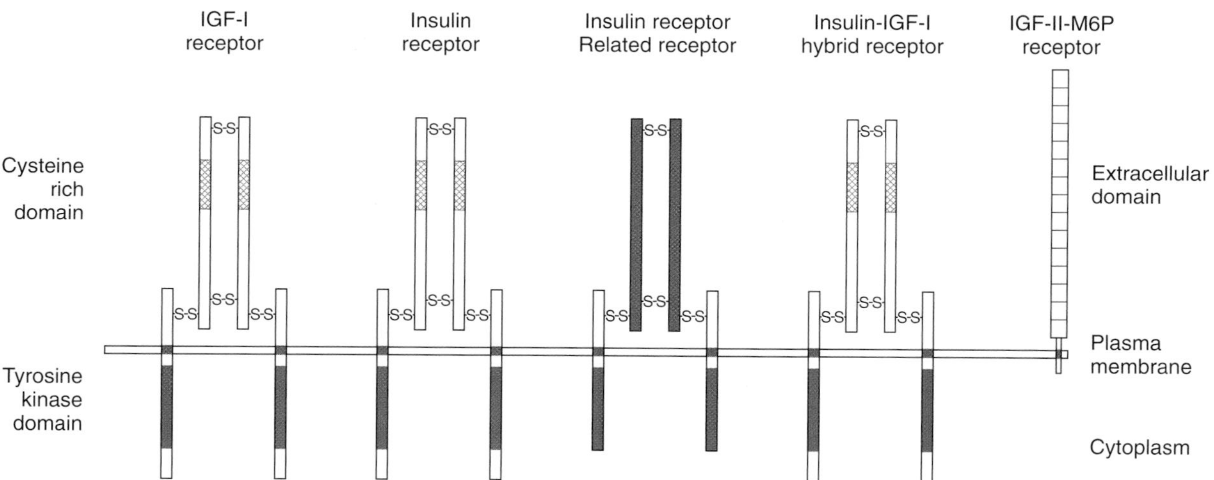

Figure 24-24 Structure of the insulin-like growth factor (IGF) receptors. The insulin receptor and the IGF1 receptor are both heterotetrameric complexes composed of extracellular α-subunits that bind the ligands and β-subunits that anchor the receptor in the membrane and contain tyrosine kinase activity in their cytoplasmic domains. The tyrosine kinase domain of the insulin receptor–related receptor (IRR) is homologous to the tyrosine kinase domains of the insulin and IGF1 receptors. The carboxyl-terminal domain is deleted in the IRR. Hybrids consist of a hemireceptor from both insulin and IGF1 receptors. The IGF2/mannose-6-phosphate (M6P) receptor is not structurally related to the IGF1 and insulin receptors or to the IRR, having a short cytoplasmic tail and no tyrosine kinase activity. (From LeRoith D, Werner H, Geitner-Johnson D, et al. Molecular and cellular aspects of the insulin-like growth factor I receptor. *Endocr Rev.* 1995;16:143-163.)

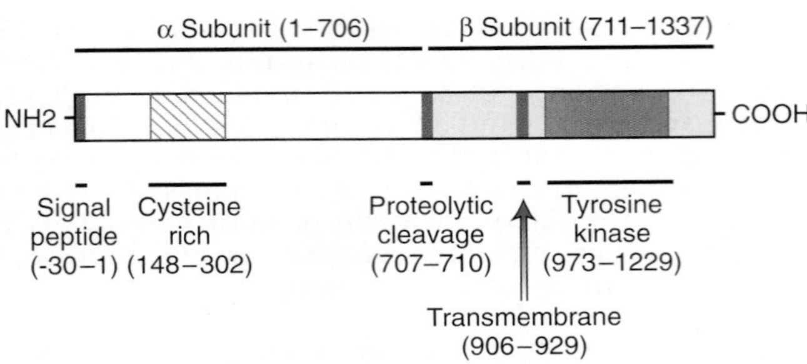

Figure 24-25 Structure of the human insulin-like growth factor type I (IGFI) receptor precursor. Molecular cloning of human IGFI receptor complementary DNAs isolated from a placental library revealed the presence of an open reading frame of 4101 nucleotides. The 1367-amino-acid polypeptide contains, at its amino terminus, a 30-amino-acid hydrophobic signal peptide that is responsible for the transfer of the nascent protein chain into the endoplasmic reticulum. After digestion by endopeptidases at a proteolytic cleavage site (Arg-Lys-Arg-Arg) located at residues 707 through 710, α- and β-subunits are released and linked by disulfide bonds to yield the configuration of the mature heterotetrameric receptor. Also shown are the cysteine-rich domain of the α-subunit and the transmembrane and tyrosine kinase domains of the β-subunit. (From LeRoith D, Werner H, Beitner-Johnson D, et al. Molecular and cellular aspects of the insulin-like growth factor I receptor. *Endocr Rev.* 1995;16:143-163.)

The structure of the human type I IGF receptor has been deduced from cDNA.[261] The mature peptide has 1337 amino acids with a predicted molecular mass of 151,869 kd (Fig. 24-25). The translated αβ heterodimer is cleaved at an Arg-Lys-Arg-Arg sequence at positions 707 through 710. The released α- and β-subunits, linked by disulfide bonds, then form the mature $(\alpha\beta)_2$ receptor, in which two α chains are joined by secondary disulfide bonds. The α-subunits are extracellular and contain a cysteine-rich domain that is critical for IGF binding. The β-subunit has a short extracellular domain, a hydrophobic transmembrane domain, and the intracellular tyrosine kinase domain with the ATP-binding site.

The gene for the type I IGF receptor (*IGF1R*) spans more than 100 kb of genomic DNA, with 21 exons; the genomic organization resembles that of the insulin receptor gene.[261-263] Exons 1 through 3 encode for the 5′ untranslated region and the cysteine-rich domain of the α-subunit that is involved in ligand binding. The remainder of the α-subunit is encoded by exons 4 through 10. The peptide cleavage site involved in generation of the α- and β-subunits is encoded by exon 11, and the tyrosine kinase domain of the β-subunit is encoded by exons 16 through 20. It is in the latter region that *IGF1R* and the insulin receptor gene share the greatest sequence homology, ranging from 80% to 95%. Exon 21 encodes the 3′ untranslated sequences.

IGF1R mRNA has been identified in virtually every tissue except liver.[264,265] The mRNA is most abundant in embryonic tissues and appears to decrease with age. *IGF1R* expression is present at the embryonic 8-cell stage, whereas expression of the type II IGF receptor gene is first demonstrable at the 2-cell stage. *IGF1R* becomes widely expressed after implantation, consistent with the observation that this receptor is essential for normal fetal growth.

As with other growth factor receptor tyrosine kinases, binding of ligand (IGF1 or IGF2) induces receptor autophosphorylation of critical tyrosine residues in the type I IGF receptor.[266-269] Specifically, ligand binding to the α-subunits leads to activation of the tyrosine kinase domain of the β-subunits. Mutations of the ATP-binding site or of critical tyrosine residues (Tyr1131, Tyr1135, and Tyr1136)[266-269] in the tyrosine kinase domain of the β-subunit result in loss of IGF-stimulated thymidine incorporation and glucose uptake. Autophosphorylation appears to occur by transphosphorylation of sites on the opposite β-subunit.[270,271] A tyrosine proximal to the tyrosine kinase domain, Tyr 950, is part of a motif that, when deleted, reduces receptor autophosphorylation, affects receptor internalization, and inhibits postreceptor signaling. The adapter proteins Shc and insulin receptor substrate 1 (IRS1) bind to this domain.

Autophosphorylation and activation of the cytoplasmic region of the IGF type I receptor promotes recruitment or activation of several docking proteins, each of which activate distinct signaling pathways, with some overlap (Fig. 24-26). Proteins that can dock onto the activated IGF type I receptor include members of the IRS family, Shc, 14-3-3e, p85 subunit of PI3 kinase, tyrosine phosphatase PTP1D, and mGRB10. Of these docking proteins, the pathways involving IRS and Shc are best characterized. IRS1 is a 185-kd protein[272] that, when phosphorylated, contains specific phosphotyrosine motifs that can associate with proteins containing SRC homology 2 (SH2) domains such as the p85 subunit of PI3 kinase,[273] growth factor receptor–bound protein 2 (Grb2),[274] Syp (a phosphotyrosine phosphatase),[273] and Nck (an oncogenic protein).[275] Activation of Shc[276] and Grb2 results in activation of the Ras, Raf, MAP kinase kinase, and S6 kinase pathways.[277-279]

Phosphorylation of IRS1 by either the type I IGF receptor or the insulin receptor activates multiple signaling cascades that ultimately influence nuclear transcription and gene expression. Mice with a null deletion for the IRS1 gene have poor growth in addition to insulin resistance.[280] Binding of the p85 subunit of PI3 kinase leads to activation of the p110 subunit of PI3 kinase. This process then activates downstream phospholipid signal transduction pathways that includes Akt. Activation of Akt leads to regulation of diverse cellular processes including apoptosis, glucose transport and metabolism, protein synthesis, mitosis, and differentiation.[281] Activation of the type I IGF receptor leads to phosphorylation of Shc, which then acts as a docking site for the Sh2 domain of Grb2. Grb2 then binds SOS, a guanine nucleotide exchange factor that converts inactive Ras guanosine diphosphate (GDP) into guanosine triphosphate (GTP). GTP-bound Ras then recruits Raf, and Raf subsequently activates MAP kinase and mitogen and extracellular signal-related kinases (MEK) 1 and 2. Activation of these proteins ultimately regulates gene transcription. Given that insulin and IGF peptides activate similar signaling pathways through their own specific receptors, it is unclear how the cell distinguishes among these overlapping ligands. Whether the consequences merely reflect the relative levels of receptors or whether divergent downstream pathways exist for insulin and IGF action remain questions for future investigation.[282]

Although targeted disruption *Igf1r* causes fetal growth retardation, a clear role for this receptor in the cell cycle has not been established. Fibroblast cell lines derived from mouse embryos homozygous for the type I IGF receptor null mutation still undergo cell cycle–dependent division, although at a slower rate.[283-285] However, the transformed nature of some cells in culture may be critically depend on expression of the type I IGF receptor. The simian virus SV40Tg is capable of inducing a transformed phenotype in a cell only in the presence of intact type I IGF receptors.[285] NIH3T3 cells that are made to overexpress the type I IGF receptor develop IGF1-dependent neoplastic transformation with tumor formation in nude rats.[286]

Variants of the α- and β-subunits are present in placenta,[287] muscle,[287,288] and brain.[289] These variants may explain seemingly anomalous competitive binding sites.[290-292] The molecular mechanisms for the formation of

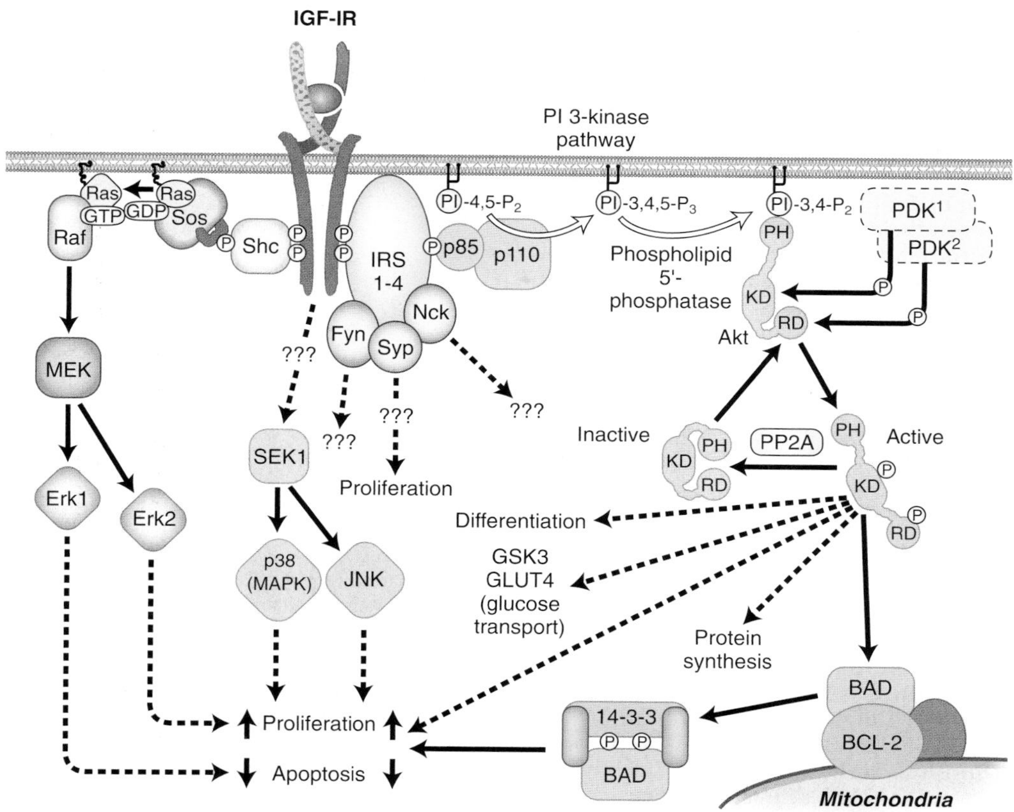

Figure 24-26 Schematic representation of intracellular signaling pathways of the insulin-like growth factor type I (IGF1) receptor. On binding of IGF1, the IGF receptor undergoes autophosphorylation at multiple tyrosine residues. The intrinsic kinase activity of the receptor also phosphorylates IRS1 at multiple tyrosine residues. Various SH domain–containing proteins, including phosphatidylinositol 3 (PI 3) kinase, Syp, Fyn, and Nck associate with specific phosphotyrosine-containing motifs within IRS1. These docking proteins recruit diverse other intracellular substrates, which then activate a cascade of protein kinases including Raf-1 and one or more related kinases including mitogen-activated protein kinase (MAPK), mitogen and extracellular signal-related kinase (MEK), and others. These protein kinases, in turn, activate various other elements, including nuclear transcription factors. Alterations in expression of various IGF1-responsive genes result in longer-term effects of IGF1, including growth and differentiation. This model of signal transduction cascades also shows a potential mechanism for inhibition of apoptosis. BAD, BCL2-associated agonist of cell death; Erk, Extracellular signal-regulated kinase; GDP, guanosine diphosphate; GLUT4, glucose transporter 4; GTP, guanosine triphosphate; JNK, c-Jun N-terminal kinase; KD, catalytic kinase domain of Akt; MEK, mitogen-activated protein kinase; P, phosphorylation; PH, pleckstrin homology domain of Akt; PP2A, protein phosphatase 2A; RD, regulatory C-terminal tail of Akt; SEK1, Serum- and glucocorticoid-inducible proteinn kinase 1. (From Le Roith D, Bondy C, Yakar S, et al. The somatomedin hypothesis: 2001. *Endocr Rev.* 2001;22:53-74.)

such receptor variants have not been identified, nor is it known whether they differentially bind IGF1, IGF2, or insulin. The formation of IGF-insulin receptor hybrids that contain an α-IGF hemireceptor disulfide-linked to an α-insulin hemireceptor (see Fig. 24-24)[293-295] appears to be ligand dependent,[296] and studies with monoclonal antibodies specific for the insulin receptor or the type I IGF receptor suggest that such receptors develop in cells with abundant native receptors, such as muscle or placenta.[297,298] Such hybrids have near-normal affinity for IGF1 but decreased affinity for insulin. The physiologic significance of such hybrid receptors is unknown. Studies in cells are complicated by simultaneous variable expression of insulin receptors, IGF type I receptors, and hybrid receptors. The lack of specific antibodies to hybrid receptors also hinders investigation.

The type II IGF receptor bears no structural homology with either the insulin receptor or type I IGF receptors (see Fig. 24-24). The receptor does not contain an intrinsic tyrosine kinase domain or any other recognized signal transduction mechanism. The type II IGF receptor is identical to the cation-independent mannose-6-phosphate (M6P) receptor, a protein involved in the intracellular lysosomal targeting of acid hydrolases and other mannosylated proteins.[299,300] This common receptor is often referred to as the IGF2/M6P receptor. The gene for the IGF2/M6P receptor (*IGF2R*) is located on the long arm of chromosome 6.[301] Exons 1 through 46 encode the extracellular region of the receptor, which contains 15 repeat sequences of 147 residues each. Exons 47 and 48 encode the 23-residue transmembrane domain and a small cytoplasmic domain consisting of only 164 residues.[302] In mice, gene expression is maternally imprinted, but for humans the expression is bialleic.[303] Like *IGF2*, the *IGF2R* gene is expressed at highest levels early in fetal development and declines to lower levels postnatally.[304]

The IGF2/M6P receptor has an apparent molecular weight of 220,000 under nonreducing conditions and 250,000 after reduction, indicating that it is a monomeric protein.[305] The 15 repeat sequences contain cysteines to form intramolecular disulfide bonds necessary for receptor folding.[306,307] Repeat 11 binds IGF2, whereas repeats 3, 5, and 9 bind M6P.[306,308-310] Because of receptor folding, it appears that the IGF2 binding site is on the opposite face to the M6P binding site.[311] A truncated form of the receptor, missing the cytoplasmic domain, has been observed to be soluble in serum.[312-314] The soluble form is able to bind IGF2[315,316] and is able to inhibit cell responses to IGF2 in vitro.[317,318]

The IGF2/M6P receptor binds a variety of M6P-containing proteins, including lysosomal enzymes, transforming growth factor-β (TGF-β),[319] and leukemia inhibitory factor (LIF).[320] Unlike the type I IGF receptor, which binds both IGF peptides with high affinity and insulin with 100-fold lower affinity, the IGF2/M6P receptor binds only IGF2 with high affinity, the dissociation constant ranging from 0.017 to 0.7 nmol/L; IGF1 binds to this receptor with lower affinity, and insulin does not bind at all.[321] One mole of IGF2 binds 1 mole of receptor. It participates in lysosomal enzyme trafficking between the trans-Golgi network and the extracellular space, regulates extracellular IGF2 and LIF levels, and plays a role in TGF-β activation (reviewed by El-Shewy and colleagues[322]). In addition, the IGF2/M6P binds retinoic acid and may mediate some of the growth-inhibitory effects of retinoids.[323] Mice null for the type II IGF receptor have macrosomia and fetal death, consistent with a potential role in IGF2 degradation.[324]

The mitogenic and metabolic actions of IGF1 and IGF2 appear to be mediated through the type I IGF receptor, because monoclonal antibodies directed against the IGF1 binding site on the type I IGF receptor inhibit the ability of both IGF1 and IGF2 to stimulate thymidine incorporation and cell replication.[325,326] Polyclonal antibodies that block IGF2 binding to the IGF2/M6P receptor do not block IGF2 actions.[327-329] IGF2 analogs with decreased affinity for the type I IGF receptor but reserved affinity for the IGF2/M6P receptor are less potent than IGF2 in stimulating DNA synthesis.[211] However, there is evidence that some of the mitogenic actions of IGF2 may be mediated by the IGF2/M6P receptor.[322] The IGF2/M6P receptor may be involved in production of inositol triphosphate and diacylglycerol in proximal tubules and canine kidney membranes.[330] IGF2 may stimulate the growth of a human erythroleukemia cell line, an action not duplicated by either IGF1 or insulin.[290] IGF2 may be able to act as an autocrine growth factor and cell motility factor for human rhabdomyosarcoma cells, actions apparently mediated through the type II receptor.[291] Additionally, it has been reported that IGF2 activates a calcium-permeable cation channel via the IGF2/M6P receptor, perhaps through coupling to a pertussis toxin–sensitive guanine nucleotide binding protein (G_i protein).[292,296,331-334]

Insights into Function-Targeted Disruption of IGF and IGF Receptor Genes

The role of the IGF axis in prenatal and postnatal growth was firmly established by a series of studies involving IGF and IGF receptor gene null mutations.[335] Unlike *Gh* or *Ghr* null mice[194,336] which are near-normal at size at birth, mice with deletions of *Igf1* or *Igf2* have birth weights approximately 60% of normal.[337-339] Fetal size is proportionately reduced, but mice with deletion of *Igf1* have a higher neonatal death rate. *Igf2* null mice also exhibit smaller placentas. Growth delay begins on day E11 for mice with deletion of *Igf2* and on day E13.5 for mice with deletion of *Igf1*. Postnatally, mice with deletion of *Igf1* who survive the neonatal period continue to have growth failure, with weights 30% of normal by 2 months of age. A similar prenatal and postnatal growth phenotype was observed in the reported case of an *Igf1* deletion[340] and in the case of a bioinactive IGF1 molecule resulting from a missense mutation.[341] When both *Igf1* and *Igf2* were disrupted, weight at birth was only 30% of normal and all animals died shortly after birth, apparently from respiratory insufficiency secondary to muscular hypoplasia (Fig. 24-27).

Mice lacking *Igf1* and the *Ghr* are only 17 % of normal size.[198] Therefore, both IGF1 and IGF2 are important in fetal growth, but GHR signaling may have IGF-independent actions on growth as well. The postnatal growth of *Igf1*$^{-}$/$^{-}$ mice was poorer than that observed in mice with *Ghr* or *Ghrh* receptor mutations, indicating that both GH-dependent and GH-independent effects of IGF1 are necessary for normal growth.

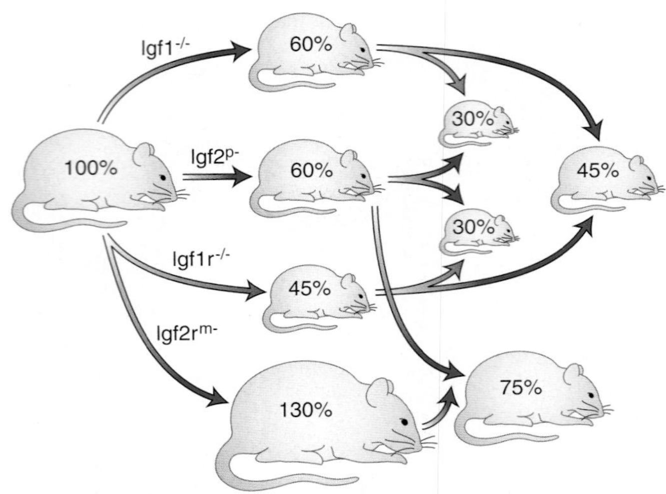

Figure 24-27 Effects of the disruption of one or more genes of the insulin-like growth factor (Igf) system on fetal growth in mice, expressed as percentage of normal body weight. Igfl -/-, Igfl gene null mice; Igf2p-, Igf2 paternal allele null mice; Igflr -/-, Igf2 gene null mice: Igf2rm-, Igf2r maternal allele null mice. Mice with two source arrows are the combined genotype of the source arrow mice. (Reproduced from Giquel and LeBouc. Hormonal regulation of fetal growth. *Horm Res.* 2006;65:28-33.)

Specific ablation of hepatic IGF1 production through the Cre/LoxP recombination system confirmed that the liver is the principal source of circulating IGF1, but the resulting 80% reduction in serum IGF1 levels had no effect on postnatal growth,[199,342-344] suggesting that postnatal growth is relatively independent of hepatic IGF1 production. Presumably, production of IGF1 from local chondrocytes or other tissues maintains adequate endocrine sources of IGF1 to account for growth preservation. Supportive data for the predominant role in growth of locally produced IGF1 include the fact that only modest decrement of postnatal growth is seen in mice null for *Igfals* (the gene encoding ALS).[345] The hormonal profile of the murine models is complex, with reduced IGFBP3 levels despite increased GH. Free IGF1 levels have been reported to be normal in these animals, even though GH levels are elevated.[343,346]

By crossing the liver-derived IGF1 gene–deleted mice with ALS gene–deleted mice, 85% to 90% reduction in serum IGF1 was achieved, and early postnatal growth retardation was observed.[347] These findings suggest that postnatal growth is dependent on both hepatic and tissue IGF1, although definite conclusions are problematic in the face of elevated GH production and perturbations of the IGFBP system observed in these studies.

Deletion of *Igf1r* resulted in birth weights 45% of normal with 100% neonatal lethality.[348] In humans, two cases of mutations in the *IGF1R* gene have been reported; these patients had IUGR and postnatal growth failure with elevated IGF1 levels. One patient had a compound for point mutations in exon 2 of the *IGFR1* gene, leading to decreased receptor affinity for IGF1, whereas the other patient had a nonsense mutation of one allele, resulting in reduced numbers of IGF type I receptors.[349] Concurrent deletion of *Igf1* and the *Igf1r* resulted in no further reduction in birth size compared with deletion of *Igf1r* alone; this is consistent with the hypothesis that all IGF1 actions are mediated via the IGF type I receptor.[335]

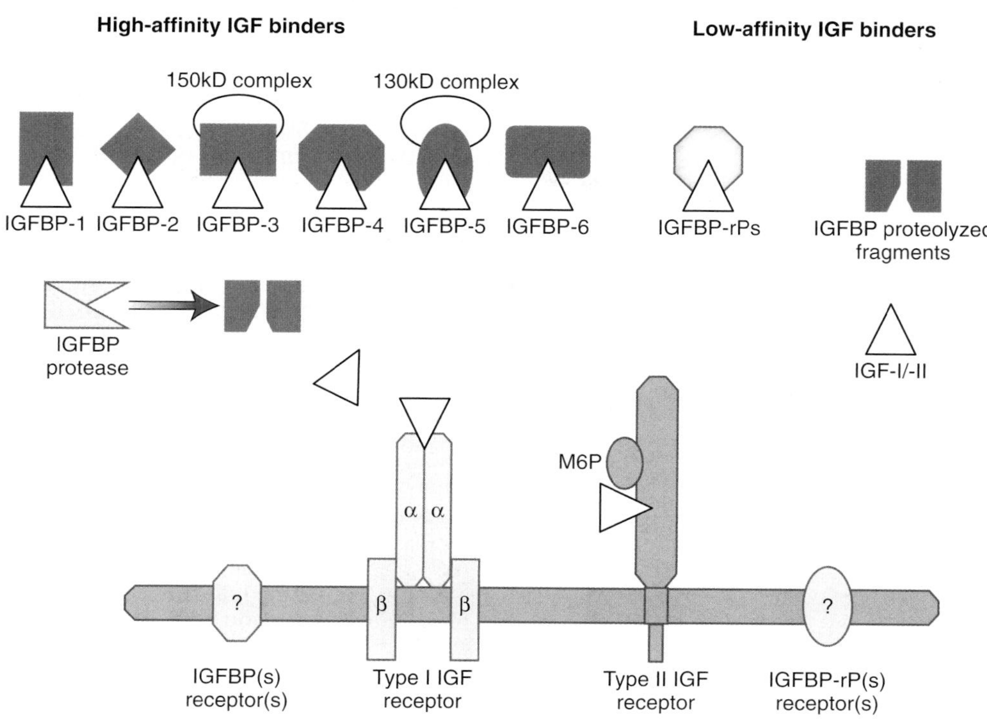

Figure 24-28 Schematic representation of the insulin-like growth factor (IGF) system, including IGF ligands (IGF-I and -II), binding proteins (both high- and low-affinity binders), IGF-binding protein (IGFBP) proteases, type I and type II IGF receptors, and potential receptors for other IGFBPs and IGFBP-related proteins (IGFBP-rPs). MCP, mannose-6-phosphate. (From Hwa V, Oh Y, Rosenfeld RG. The insulin-like growth factor–binding protein [IGFBP] superfamily. *Endocr Rev.* 1999;20:761-787, copyright Endocrine Society.)

Deletion of *Igf2r* in mice causes an increase in birth weight but death in late gestation or at birth.[324] Because this receptor normally degrades IGF2, increased growth reflects excess IGF2 acting through the IGF type I receptor, with variable accumulation of IGF2 in tissues.[350] Deletion of *Igf2r* plus *Igf2* results in a birth weight 60% of normal, similar to the size of mice with knockout of *Igf2* alone, with no effect on neonatal survival.[351] Simultaneous knockout of the genes for *Igf2* and *Igf1r* causes further reduction of birth size to 30% of normal, suggesting that some of the fetal anabolic actions of IGF2 are mediated by another mechanism such as via placental growth or interactions with the insulin receptor. Indeed, specific deletion of *Igf2* in the placenta causes small placenta and growth retardation.[352]

These studies allow the following conclusions: (1) IGF1 is important for both fetal and postnatal growth; (2) IGF2 is a major fetal growth factor but has little, if any, role in postnatal growth; (3) the IGF type I receptor mediates anabolic actions of both IGF1 and IGF2; (4) the IGF type II receptor is bifunctional, serving to target lysosomal enzymes and to enhance IGF2 turnover; (5) IGF2 deletion results in impaired placental growth; (6) IGF1 is the major mediator of GH effects on postnatal growth, although GH and GHR may have small IGF1-independent effects. Whether these effects apply to humans is not yet known.

Insulin-Like Growth Factor–Binding Proteins

In contrast to insulin, the IGFs circulate in plasma complexed to a family of binding proteins that extend the serum half-life of the IGF peptides, transport the IGFs to target cells, and modulate the interactions of the IGFs with surface membrane receptors.[353,354] In addition to these effects, the IGFBPs have been found to have effects on cells independent of IGFs. The presence and various actions of the IGFBPs provide layers of regulation to the GH-IGF axis, greatly increasing its complexity (Fig. 24-28). In the following paragraphs, the structure of the IGFBP family is described first, followed by the role of IGFBPs in IGF physiology and the characteristics of individual IGFBPs.

Structure of IGFBPs. Six distinct human IGFBPs have been cloned, and their highly conserved amino acid sequences have been determined. The six IGFBPs share structural homology in the N-terminal and C-terminal domains but have highly variable midsections, which probably accounts for the more specialized properties of the individual IGFBPs, such as cell dissociation, IGF-binding enhancement, and IGF-independent actions. In each of the conserved N- and C-terminal domains, there are a high number of cysteine-rich residues with a conserved spatial order, implying that the disulfide bond–dependent secondary structure of the IGFBPs is also conserved.[355] Reduction of the disulfide proteins results in loss of IGF binding, further demonstrating the importance of the cysteine-rich region.

The N-terminal domain contains residues that have been shown to be essential for IGF binding to IGFBPs 1, 3, and 4.[356,357] Whether this binding is important for IGF-independent effects of the IGFBPs is unknown. The cysteine-rich C-terminal region also contains regions important in IGFBP binding to proteins such as heparin, fibrinogen, fibrin, and plasminogen.[358,359] The exact sequences in the C-terminal domain that are responsible for binding may differ among the IGFBPs; for example, the arginine-glycine-aspartic acid sequence in the C-terminal of IGFBPs 1 and 2, which is putatively necessary for binding to cellular surfaces,[360,361] is not present on IGFBP3, which

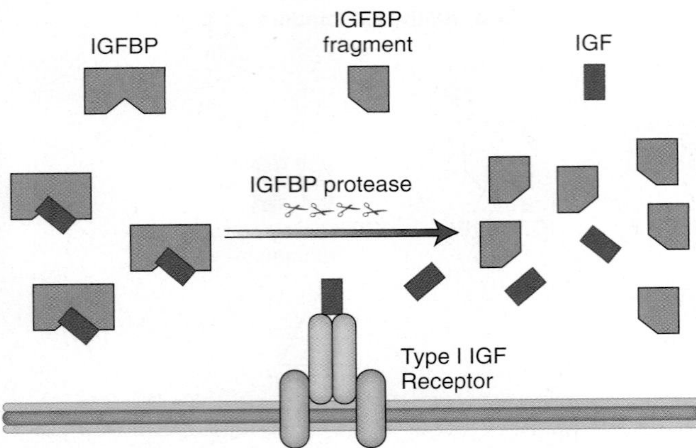

Figure 24-29 Schematic representation of the effect of insulin-like growth factor (IGF)-binding protein (IGFBP) proteases on IGF action. In this model, proteolysis of IGFBPs results in a reduction in their affinity for IGF ligands, leading to enhanced binding of IGF peptides by IGF receptors. (From Cohen P, Rosenfeld RG. The IGF axis. In Rosenbloom AL, ed. *Human Growth Hormone: Basic and Scientific Aspects.* Boca Raton, FL: CRC Press; 1995:43-58.)

can also bind cell membranes.[362,363] The highly variable midregion segment of the IGFBPs is the site of post-translational modifications such as glycosylation and phosphorylation and of proteolysis. Both the primary structure of IGFBPs and their post-translational modifications are responsible for the differential targeting to tissues: glycosylation can affect cell interactions, phosphorylation can affect IGF1 binding affinity and susceptibility to proteases, and proteolysis can affect IGF/IGF receptor–dependent and –independent actions.[364]

The three-dimensional structure of IGFBPs 1, 2, 4, and 5 have been determined, confirming the presence of IGF-binding sites in the N- and C-terminal domains. Crystallography has shown that the structure of the N-terminal domain is critical for IGF binding, whereas the C-terminal domain is important for inhibiting interactions between IGF1 and its receptor.[365-369]

Several groups of cysteine-rich proteins that contain domains similar to the IGFBPs have been discovered, leading to the proposal of an IGFBP superfamily.[370] This superfamily includes the six high-affinity IGFBPs and a number of IGFBP-related proteins (IGFBP-rPs). Three of these proteins—Mac25 (IGFBP-rP1), connective tissue growth factor (CTGF/IGFBP-rP2), and NovH (IGFBP-rP3)—have been shown to bind IGFs, although with considerably lower affinity than the IGFBPs. The role, if any, of IGFBP-rPs in normal IGF physiology is unclear.

Analysis of IGFBPs is complicated by the presence of IGFBP proteases that degrade IGFBP (Fig. 24-29).[371,372] Proteolysis of IGFBPs complicates their assay and must be taken into consideration when measuring the various IGFBPs in biologic fluids.[373] Proteases for IGFBPs 2, 3, 4, and 5 are present in serum, seminal plasma, cerebrospinal fluid, and urine.[374-376] It is likely that multiple IGFBP proteases exist, including calcium-dependent serine proteases, kallikreins, cathepsin, and matrix metalloproteases.[377,378] It is postulated that proteolysis of IGFBPs releases IGFs to interact with cell surface receptors, thereby enhancing the mitogenic and anabolic effects of IGF peptides. There is some evidence that the proteolytic fragments of IGFBP3 and IGFBP5 have IGF1-independent effects.[379,380]

Role of IGFBPs in IGF Physiology

IGFBPs as Carrier Proteins. The IGFBPs complex almost all of the circulating IGF1 and IGF2 secondary to their high affinity for the IGFs (10^{-10} to 10^{-11} mol/L).[381] In adults, 75% to 80% of IGFs are carried in a ternary complex consisting of 1 molecule of IGF plus 1 molecule of IGFBP3 plus 1 molecule of the protein ALS.[382,383] This 150-kd ternary complex is too large to leave the vascular compartment and extends the half-life of IGF peptides from approximately 10 minutes for IGF alone to 12 to 15 hours for IGF in the ternary complex.[384] Binding of IGF to IGFBP3 in a binary complex extends the half-life of IGF to 1 to 2 hours. When IGFs bind as a binary complex to the IGFBPs, diffusion out of the vascular compartment may occur; this has been observed for IGF-binding proteins 1, 2, and 4.[385]

Both IGFBP3 and ALS are GH dependent, providing an additional mechanism for GH regulation of the IGF axis. Whereas GH administration to GH-deficient patients shifts IGF from a 40- to 50-kd form to the ternary complex,[386,387] this shift does not occur after IGF1 treatment. No sustained increase in levels of IGFBP3 occurs after administration of IGF1,[121,388] but ALS levels may decrease after IGF1 administration, possibly reflecting IGF feedback inhibition of pituitary GH secretion.[388,389] In serum of patients with GHD or GH insensitivity, little IGF is present in the 150-kd ternary complex; the IGF present is in the IGF-IGFBP3 binary complex or is bound by other IGFBPs such as IGFBPs 1, 2, 4, or 5.[258,371,386]

IGFBPs as Modulators of IGF Action. IGFBPs also regulate biologic actions by modulating the availability of IGFs (Fig. 24-30). The binding affinity of IGFs for IGFBPs is higher than for IGF receptors, and dissociation of IGFs from IGFBPs is required for IGFs to interact with IGF receptors.[381] Additionally, the concentration of IGFBPs is in excess, compared with IGFs, in many bodily fluids.[390,391] Dissociation of IGFs from IGFBPs is achieved by mass action, proteolysis, or other unknown mechanisms. Alterations in the interaction between IGF1 and its receptor can result in inhibition or potentiation of IGF effects on cell proliferation.[392,393] Inhibition of IGF1 action by the presence of IGFBP4 has been demonstrated in vitro and in vivo,[394,395] because IGF analogs with decreased affinity for IGFBP4 have increased biologic potency. IGFBPs 1, 3, and 5 have been shown to have potentiating effects on IGF action, perhaps by facilitating the delivery of IGF to target receptors, as has been shown for IGFBP3.[396]

The enhancing effects of IGFBP5 were shown to involve binding of IGFBP5 to extracellular matrix proteins, which

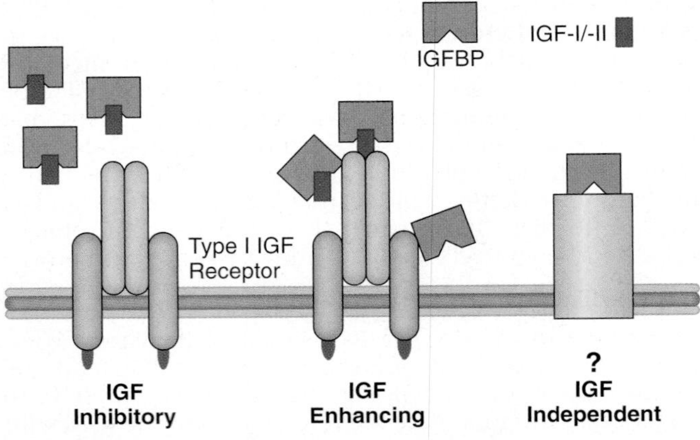

Figure 24-30 Theoretical mechanisms of cellular actions of insulin-like growth factor (IGF)-binding proteins (IGFBPs). See text for details.

reduces the affinity of IGFBP5 for IGF.[397] Possibly, IGFBP5 binding to the extracellular matrix brings IGF close to the cell surface in a low-affinity complex, from which it can be released slowly to bind neighboring IGF receptors.[398] To complicate matters, it appears that the same IGFBP can potentiate or inhibit IGF action in vitro, depending on cell culture conditions, cell type, IGFBP dose, and post-translational modifications such as phosphorylation state.[393] It has been proposed that IGFBP3 and IGFBP5 may have their own receptors that, when activated, interact with IGF receptor signaling pathways.[394]

It has also been proposed that IGFBP-IGF complexes can be stored in tissues to act in a paracrine manner. This has been demonstrated for IGFBP5 and bone matrix. IGFBP5 is produced by osteoblasts, and the IGFBP5-IGF complex can bind hydroxyapatite. It has been proposed that the complex participates in bone turnover.[399]

IGFBP proteases, which degrade IGFBPs, are postulated to play a role in altering IGF availability by lowering affinities of IGFBPs for their ligand, thereby increasing the availability of IGFs to cell membrane receptors.[400,401]

IGF-Independent Actions of IGFBPs. IGFBPs also have IGF-independent actions, such as growth inhibition of certain cell types,[402] growth stimulation of tissues,[403] direct induction of apoptosis,[404] and modulation of the effects of other, non-IGF growth factors. The mechanisms of IGF-independent actions are slowly being unraveled and include binding to IGFBP-specific cell surface receptors, binding to other cell surface receptors, and interaction with nuclear receptors (Fig. 24-31).

IGF-independent actions have been characterized for IGFBPs 1, 3, and 5. IGFBP1 has been shown to increase ovarian cell migration via binding to the fibronectin receptor independent of IGF1.[361] IGFBP3 also appears to have intrinsic inhibitory effects on cells. In in vitro studies, IGFBP3 administration or overexpression inhibits DNA synthesis and cell proliferation in conditions in which IGF1 or the IGF type I receptor is neutralized, suggesting IGF-independent inhibition by IGFBP3.[405] Stimulation of DNA synthesis by basic FGF is inhibited by simultaneous treatment with IGFBP3, even in the presence of insulin, suggesting that sequestration of IGF peptides from IGF receptors is not the only means by which IGFBP3 inhibits cell growth.[406] IGFBP3 is more effective than immunoneutralization of IGF1 in inhibiting serum-stimulated DNA synthesis in cultured ovarian granulosa cells, with or without added IGF.[407] Both overexpression studies and gene knockdown studies suggest that IGFBP3 alone can inhibit DNA synthesis and that it plays a role in the signaling of p53, a potent tumor-suppressor gene. Additionally, IGFBP3 has been demonstrated to induce apoptosis in fibroblasts lacking functional IGF receptors,[379] an IGFBP3 that does not bind IGF stimulates apoptosis in these fibroblasts and in wild-type fibroblasts.[408] IGFBP5 also has IGF-independent effects on osteoblasts. In osteoblasts cultured from mice null for the IGF1 gene, the presence of IGFBP5 increased cell growth, alkaline phosphatase activity, and osteocalcin expression to levels similar to those of wild-type osteoblasts.[409] In additional, IGFBP5 administered to bone of *IGF1* null mice was associated with an increase in markers of bone formation.

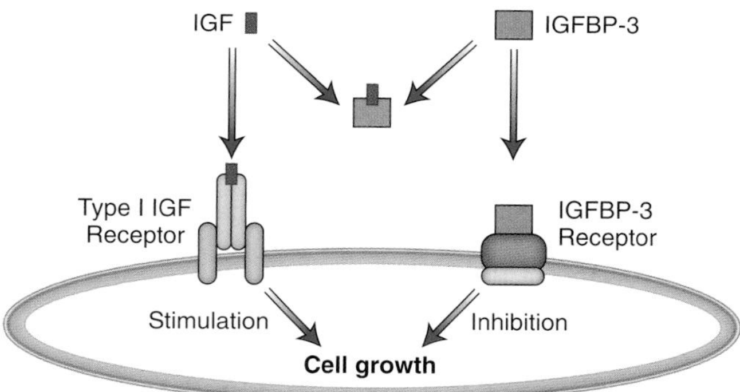

Figure 24-31 Schematic diagram of insulin-like growth factor (IGF)-dependent and IGF-independent actions of IGF-binding protein 3 (IGFBP3), the latter being mediated through a putative membrane-associated IGFBP3 receptor.

The IGFBPs have IGF-independent effects via binding to IGFBP-specific membrane receptors for IGFBP3[405,410] IGFBP5,[411] or other receptors such as the TGF-β receptor type V.[412] The downstream signaling pathways activated by the IGFBP-specific receptors are unknown, as are the possible interactions with IGF receptor signaling. IGFBP3 and IGFBP5 also contain nuclear localization signals, and these proteins have been localized to the nucleus in vitro.[413,414] IGFBP3 has been shown to interact with the retinoic acid receptor-α (RXRα), modulating its ability to act as a transcription factor and ultimately affecting apoptosis in cancer cells.[415] IGFBP proteases can also generate IGFBP3 fragments with enhanced affinity for cell surface IGFBP3 receptors.[416]

Characteristics of IGFBPs 1 through 6. IGFBP1 was the first of the IGFBPs to be purified and to have its cDNA cloned.[417] Its gene is 5.2 kb long, is located on the short arm of chromosome 7, and comprises four exons.[418] The mature protein is 30 kd and is not glycosylated. Messenger RNA is strongly expressed in decidua, liver, and kidney. It is the major IGFBP in fetal serum in early gestation, reaching levels as high as 3000 μg/L by the second trimester. Levels of IGFBP1 in newborn serum are inversely correlated with birth weight, suggesting an inhibitory role on fetal IGF action.

IGFBP1 may be involved in reproductive function, including endometrial cycling,[419] oocyte maturation,[420] and fetal growth.[371,421] It also appears to have an important metabolic role, in that its gene expression is enhanced in catabolic states[258,422,423] and serum levels undergo diurnal variation.[424] Insulin suppresses and glucocorticoids enhance *IGFBP1* mRNA levels.[422,425]

Although most in vitro studies consistently show an inhibitory effect of IGFBP1 on IGF action, presumably reflecting interference with IGF ligand-receptor interactions,[354] IGFBP1 potentiates IGF effects in certain cell systems,[426] possibly as a result of the binding of IGFBP1 to cell membranes through its Arg-Gly-Asp sequence.[361] The ability of IGFBP1 to inhibit or potentiate IGF action may depend on post-translational modifications of IGFBP1, such as phosphorylation, which appears to enhance the affinity of IGFBP1 for IGF1, thereby inhibiting IGF action.[427]

The *IGFBP2* gene is located on the long arm of chromosome 2[428,429] and encodes for a mature protein of 34 kd.[430] Like IGFBP1, IGFBP2 is highly expressed in fetal tissues, particularly in the CNS.[431] It is also expressed in secretory endometrium and endometrial tumors[428] and is the major IGFBP in seminal fluid and in the conditioned media of prostatic epithelial cells.[432] Like IGFBP1, IGFBP2 does not have N-glycosylation and has the amino acid sequence, perhaps allowing association with cell surfaces.[433]

The *IGFBP3* gene is located on chromosome 7.[434] It contains four exons homologous to *IGFBP1* and *IGFBP2* and a fifth exon consisting of 3′ untranslated sequences. Messenger RNA levels are high in the liver, most notably in the hepatic endothelia and Kupffer cells, compared with ALS, which is high in hepatocytes.[435,436] The mature, unglycosylated IGFBP3 protein has a molecular weight of approximately 29 kd and comprises 264 amino acids. IGFBP3 is composed of the conserved N-terminal and C-terminal domains and the variable midsection. The midsection is the site of N-linked glycosylation,[437] which is not present in IGFBP1 or IGFBP2, and this is why it normally migrates as a doublet-triplet of 40 to 46 kd. Glycosylation does not appear to alter its affinity for IGF1 or IGF2.[438] The midsection is also the site of phosphorylation. Studies have shown that this midsection is the site responsible for interaction with cell surfaces.[439] Smaller-molecular-weight fragments of IGFBP3 can be found in patients who are catabolic or have undergone surgery and in patients with non–insulin-dependent diabetes mellitus (NIDDM).[440,441]

IGFBP3 is the predominant IGFBP in adult serum, where it carries approximately 75% of the total IGF, primarily as part of the 150-kd ternary complex consisting of IGF1, IGFBP3, and ALS. IGFBP3 and IGFBP5 are the only IGFBPs to form this complex. It is believed that formation of this ternary complex limits IGF access to target cells, while at the same time prolonging serum half-lives of both the IGF peptide and its binding protein.[442] Serum levels of IGFBP3 and ALS are reduced in patients with GHD or GH insensitivity, conditions in which assays for serum IGFBP3 have important diagnostic value. IGFBP3 is increased in states of GH excess and acromegaly.

IGFBP3 action is GH dependent, either directly or through regulation by IGF. IGF1 administration to hypophysectomized rats increases serum levels of IGFBP3.[443-445] IGF1 treatment of patients with GH insensitivity, however, does not greatly alter serum IGFBP3 levels,[119,361,377] and GH treatment of GH-deficient patients does not increase serum levels. Whether these observations mean that GH has a direct effect on IGFBP3 or reflects GH regulation of ALS and ternary complex formation is unclear, although it appears likely that both factors are contributory.

IGFBP3 associates with cell membrane proteins in a specific, cation-dependent manner and with high affinity.[446] Whether the cell membrane proteins constitute genuine IGFBP3 receptors remains to be determined, although they may mediate IGF-independent actions of IGFBP3. Alternatively, IGFBP3 may associate with heparin-containing proteoglycans in the extracellular matrix and in the cell membrane, because it contains heparin-binding consensus sequences in the C-terminus.[447] It has been suggested that IGFBP3 is a ligand of the serine/theonine kinase type V TGF-β receptor, with the resultant interaction leading to cell growth inhibition.[412,448]

IGFBP3 can also translocate to the cell nucleus from the extracellular compartment. It has a consensus nuclear translocation sequence,[449] and translocation is facilitated by importin-B.[450] IGFBP3 can bind the nuclear RXRα.[451,452] This interaction has been shown to be important in the IGFBP3 effect on apoptosis.[415]

IGFBP3 expression can be induced by cell cycle regulators and growth-inhibitory factors such as TNF-α, TNF-β, retinoic acid, vitamin D, antiestrogens, and antiandrogens.[453] In many cases, modulation of *IGFBP3* expression has been shown to be crucial to the antiproliferative effects of factors in vitro.[453] *IGFBP3* expression is also activated by the tumor suppression gene p53[454,455] in tumor cell lines treated with chemotherapeutic agents.[456] Like many genes, *IGFBP3* expression is affected by methylation and histone modification. Numerous studies have shown that abnormal methylation or histone modification of the *IGFBP3* gene is present in many different types of human cancer (reviewed by Jogie-Brahim and colleagues[453]).

The *IGFBP4* gene is located on chromosome 17 and contains four exons.[457] It is present mostly as a nonglycosylated form of 24 kd, with the glycosylated form being 29 kd. Similar to IGFBP3, its glycosylation site is in the highly variable midregion of the protein. It is widely expressed in embryonic tissues, fibroblasts, osteoblastic cells, prostatic cells, ovarian cells, and liver. The circulating form is derived mostly from the liver. Evidence suggests that IGFBP4 is the only IGFBP that does not have IGF-independent effects. In vitro, IGFBP4 inhibits IGF action, and in vivo studies have demonstrated that the inhibitory action of IGFBP4 on cellular processes is IGF1-dependent.[458] The inhibitory effects of IGFBP4 are reduced by proteolysis, similar to IGFBP3. IGFBP4 proteases are present in a wide variety of cells, including neuroblastoma, smooth muscle, fibroblasts, osteoblasts, and prostatic epithelium.[459-463] Activation of IGFBP4 proteolysis occurs in the presence of IGF1 or IGF2, presumably reflecting a conformational change in IGFBP4 resulting from IGF occupancy.[464,465] The protease pregnancy-associated plasma protein-A (PPAP-A) has been shown to degrade IGFBPs 2, 4, and 5, but not IGFBP3,[466-468] and it has been associated with the decline of IGFBP4 during ovarian follicular growth.[469] Proteolysis of IGFBP4 by PPAP-A in developing ovarian follicles has been postulated to play a role in the development of dominant follicles.[469]

The *IGFBP5* gene is located on chromosome 5 and contains four exons. It is 28 kd and also contains a glycosylation site in the highly variable midregion of the protein.[470-472] In contrast to the other glycosylated IGFBPs, IGFBP5 is *O*-glycosylated rather than *N*-glycosylated. IGFBP5 has been shown to bind extracellular matrix proteins such as types III and IV collagen, laminin, and fibronectin, and it does so in response to binding of IGF1.[397] The affinity of IGFBP5 is reduced about sevenfold when the binding protein is associated with extracellular matrix, providing a potential mechanism for release of IGFs to cell surface receptors. Association of IGFBP5 with extracellular matrix also appears to protect it from proteolysis.[473] Unlike proteolysis of IGFBP4, which is enhanced by the addition of IGFs, degradation of IGFBP5 is inhibited by the binding of IGF peptides.[470,474] Proteolytic fragments of IGFBP5 have been shown to have IGF-independent effects on mitogenesis, possibly by binding an IGFBP5-specific cell surface receptor.[475]

The *IGFBP6* gene is located on chromosome 12 and contains four exons. The mature peptide contains 216 amino acids and is 23 kd, although it may undergo *O*-glycosylation, similar to IGFBP5.[476] Although IGFBP6 binds both IGF1 and IGF2, it has a significantly greater affinity for IGF2.[477] IGFBP6 is found in high levels in cerebrospinal fluid, as is IGFBP2, which also binds IGF2 with high affinity. IGFBP6 may have a role in regulating ovarian activity, perhaps by functioning as an antigonadotropin.[478]

Mice null for the individual IGFBPs have been generated. Only modest, if any, effects on growth have been found. Modest decreases in organ size have been noted in IGFBP2 null mice,[479] whereas growth in IGFBP4 null mice is 85% to 90% of normal. Increases in other IGFBP levels were noted in these mice. Triple knockout mice null for IGFBPs 3, 4, and 5 have been generated,[480] and they exhibit lengths 80% of normal with IGF1 levels 45% that of the wild type. Transgenic mice overexpressing the IGFBPs 1, 2, 3, and 4 have also been generated,[481] and they exhibit growth retardation to varying degrees, demonstrating the role of the IGFBPs in sequestering IGF1 or inhibiting its actions. In addition, mice overexpressing IGFBP1 and IGFBP3 also exhibit impaired glucose tolerance and decreased fertility, further implicating a role for IGF1 or a separate role for these IGFBPs in glucose metabolism and reproduction.

Gonadal Steroids

Androgens and estrogens affect growth predominantly through two mechanisms: regulation of the GH-IGF1 axis and maturation of the epiphyseal growth plates. The adolescent rise in serum gonadal steroid levels is an important part of the pubertal growth spurt. In addition, it is the stimulation of epiphyseal fusion by the pubertal rise of gonadal steroid production that results in the ultimate cessation of linear growth. The details of the roles of androgens and estrogens in enhancing GH secretion and directly stimulating IGF1 production were discussed earlier.

Both androgens and estrogens increase skeletal maturation and accelerate growth plate senescence. However, most of these effects are due to the action of estrogen, with androgens acting indirectly after their conversion to estrogens by aromatase in extraglandular tissues, including locally within the growth plate. The primacy of the role of estrogen comes from animal studies[20] as well as reports of human subjects with mutations. A mutation of the estrogen receptor in a man was associated with tall stature and open epiphyses,[21] and similar findings were reported in patients with mutations of the gene encoding the aromatase enzyme.[22,23] In addition, variants of the estrogen receptor have been associated with height in males[482] and in females,[483] and increased aromatase expression results in short adult stature in males.[484,485]

Whereas most of the effects of androgen on growth are mediated through actions that occur after their aromatization to estrogen, there is evidence of androgen-specific effects. Notably, dihydrotestosterone, a nonaromatizable androgen, can accelerate linear growth in boys. This effect of androgen does not appear to be mediated by either GH or circulating IGF1, but it may be mediated by an increase in local IGF1 production.[486]

Gonadal steroids, along with GH and IGF1, contribute to the attainment of peak bone mass in adults. Again, this sex hormone effect is largely mediated by estrogen action.[487-489]

Thyroid Hormone

Thyroid hormone is of relatively little importance in the growth of the fetus, but it has significant effects on postnatal growth and bone maturation. Patients with hypothyroidism have decreased spontaneous GH secretion and blunted responses to GH provocative tests. Thyroid hormone also has a direct effect on chondrocytes and osteoblasts, which both express thyroid hormone receptors. Thyroid hormone regulates chondrocyte proliferation and stimulates terminal differentiation, mineralization, and angiogenesis.[490,491] In particular, thyroid hormone is essential for hypertrophic chondrocyte differentiation.[492] Postnatally, hypothyroidism can cause growth failure and delayed skeletal maturation, whereas hyperthyroidism can accelerate linear growth and skeletal maturation.

Glucocorticoids

Supraphysiologic doses of glucocorticoids can acutely increase GH secretion.[493] However, prolonged exposure to excess glucocorticoids severely impairs growth. This occurs through multiple mechanisms that act through the GH-IGF1 axis. Chronic glucocorticoid treatment attenuates pituitary secretion of GH through an increase in somatostatin tone.[494,495] Glucocorticoids can also impair growth through direct actions at the growth plate, by inhibiting local IGF1 production through suppression of chondrocyte GHR expression and impairment of chondrocyte IGF1 receptor expression.[496] In addition, IGF1 action at the chondrocyte may be impaired through alterations in IGFBP levels and impairment of intracellular signaling.[497] Finally, glucocorticoids may stimulate apoptosis of growth plate chondrocytes.[486]

Additional indirect effects of excess glucocorticoids on growth can result from glucocorticoid inhibition of calcium absorption and reabsorption, with the development of secondary hyperparathyroidism.[491] In pubertal children, glucocorticoid excess can induce sex hormone deficiency, causing a loss of the normal growth stimulatory effect of these hormones.[491]

PATHOLOGIC BASIS OF GROWTH RETARDATION

A classification of growth retardation is presented in Table 24-1. Growth disorders are subdivided into (1) disorders of the hypothalamic-pituitary axis resulting in deficiency of GH, (2) disorders resulting in deficiency or resistance to the action of IGF1, (3) growth disorders that primarily affect the growth plate or are caused by chronic disease, and (4) idiopathic short stature (ISS), which is considered separately but may have a pathogenic basis in the GH-IGF1 axis or at the growth plate. A schematic diagram of known defects in the GH-IGF1 axis is shown in Fig. 24-32, and the known involved genes are listed in Table 24-2.

Disorders of the GH/IGF1 Axis

Growth Hormone Deficiency

Although it is not always possible to establish definitively whether hypothalamic or pituitary dysfunction is responsible for the hormone deficiency, these compartments are

TABLE 24-1

Classification of Growth Retardation

- I. Disorders of the GH/IGF-1 Axis
  - A. Growth Hormone Deficiency
    - 1. The Hypothalamus
      - a. Congenital Disorders
      - b. Acquired Disorders
    - 2. The Anterior Pituitary
      - a. Congenital Disorders
        - (1) Combined Pituitary Hormone Deficieneies
        - (2) Isolated Growth Hormone Deficiency (IGHD)
      - b. Acquired Disorders
        - (1) Cranyopharyngiomas and Other Tumors
        - (2) Histiocytosis X
  - B. GH Insensitivity
    - 1. Multations in GHR Signaling Proteins and ALS
  - C. Abnormaloties of IGFI and IGFIR Signaling
- II. Growth Disorders Outside the GH/IGF-1 Axis
  - A. Malnutrition
  - B. Chronic Disease
  - C. Endocrine Disorders
  - D. Osteochondrodysplasias
  - E. Chromosomal Abnromalities
  - F. Small for Gestational Age (SGA)
  - G. Maternal and Placental Factors
- III. Idiopathic Short Stature (ISS)

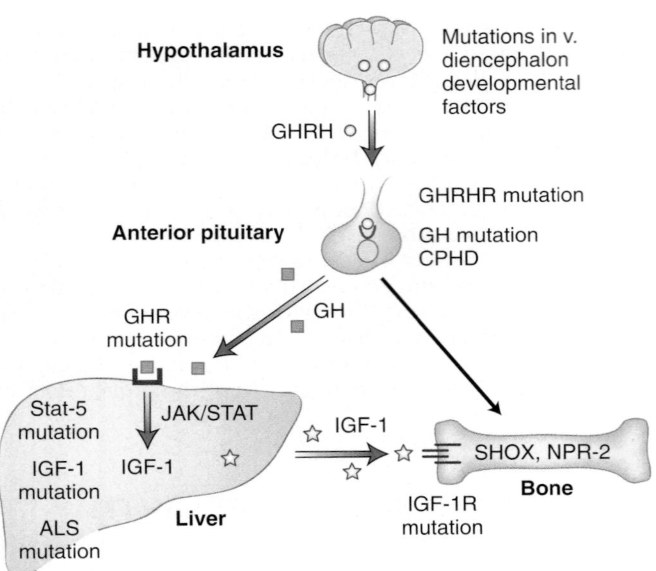

Figure 24-32 The hypothalamic-pituitary-IGF axis: sites of established mutations. ALS, acid-labile subunit; CPHD, combined pituitary hormone deficiency; GH, growth hormone; GHRH, GH-releasing hormone; GHRHR, GHRH receptor; IGF-1, insulin-like growth factor-1, JAK, Janus kinase; NPR-2, natriuretic peptide receptor-2; SHOX, short homoebox; stat, signal transducer and activator of transcription. (Reprinted with permission from Lopez-Bermejo A, Buckway CK, Rosenfeld RG. Genetic defects of the growth hormone-insulin-like growth factor axis. *Trends Endocrinol Metab.* 2000;11:43.)

differentiated to facilitate discussion of the pathology. Table 24-3 indicates possible etiologies for deficiency in the GH-IGF axis. The term *idiopathic* is often used to designate lack of understanding of the basis for the GHD. Developmental or functional abnormalities of the hypothalamus account for most "idiopathic" cases of hypopituitarism, and recent molecular studies have begun to elucidate the molecular bases of these disorders. It is anticipated that most cases of idiopathic hypopituitarism will be defined at the genetic level in the future.

The Hypothalamus

Congenital Disorders. The primary hypothalamic neuropeptide responsible for synthesis and release of GH is GHRH. Somatostatin plays an antagonistic role in GH release. Synthesis of these two hypothalamic proteins is controlled by a series of neurochemicals, and it is the balance between them that is responsible for the tight neuroendocrine control of GH biosynthesis. Mutations of some of the genes encoding hypothalamic peptides explain some cases of GHD due to hypothalamic dysfunction.

As noted earlier, patients with early-diagnosed congenital GHD frequently have an abnormal pituitary stalk, ectopia of the posterior pituitary, and hypoplasia of the anterior pituitary (Fig. 24-33). Anencephaly results in a pituitary gland that is small or abnormally formed and is frequently ectopic.[127,498,499] Despite the loss of hypothalamic regulation, somatotrophs differentiate and proliferate, although in diminished overall mass.[67] During intrauterine life, serum GH and IGF1 levels are 30% to 50% of the normal range,[134] and pituitary GH content at birth is about 15% to 20% of normal,[128,134] with similarly low neonatal plasma GH levels.[129,500,501]

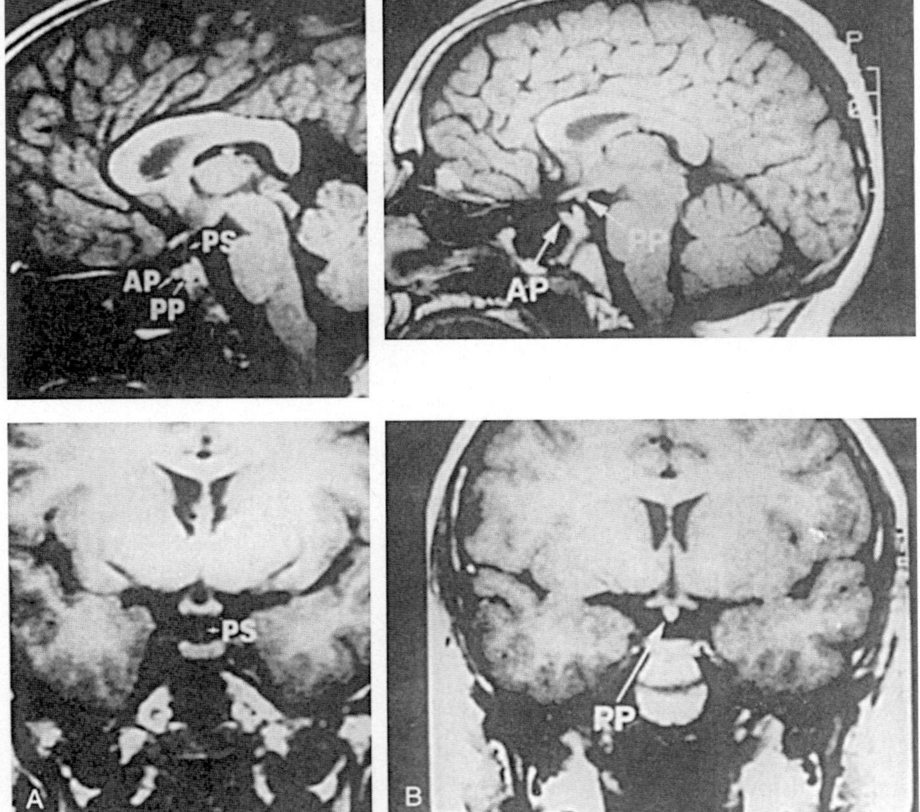

Figure 24-33 Magnetic resonance imaging of infundibular dysgenesis. **A,** T1-weighted sagittal and coronal images of the hypothalamic-pituitary area in a normal 8-year-old girl. The anterior (AP) and posterior pituitary (PP) lobes and the pituitary stalk (PS) are marked. **B,** T1-weighted sagittal and coronal images of the hypothalamic-pituitary area of a 17-year-old boy with isolated growth hormone deficiency. The anterior pituitary lobe (AP) is hypoplastic, the posterior pituitary (PP) is ectopic, and the pituitary stalk is absent. (Reprinted from Root AW, Martinez CR. Magnetic resonance imaging in patients with hypopituitarism. *Trends Endocrinol Metab.* 1992;3:283-287.)

TABLE 24-2

Genetic Defects of the GH-IGF Axis Resulting in Somatotroph Dysfunction and GH Deficiency

Factor	Gene Function	Affected Cell Types	Clinical Phenotype	Mode of Inheritance
Mutations in Factors Resulting in Growth Hormone and Associated Hormone Deficiencies				
Hesx1	• Paired-like homeobox gene • Early marker for pituitary primordium and Rathke's pouch • Requires Lhx3 for maintenance and PROP1 for repression	Somatotrophs, thyrotrophs, gonadotrophs (posterior pituitary may also be affected)	• Isolated GH deficiency or multiple hormone deficiency (including diabetes insipidus) • Puberty may be delayed • Associated with septo-optic dysplasia • Abnormal MRI findings: pituitary hypoplasia, ectopic posterior pituitary, midline forebrain abnormalities	AD, AR
Lhx3 (Lim3, P-LIM)	• Member of LIM-homeodomain family of gene regulatory proteins • Required for survival and proliferation of Rathke's pouch • Activates αGSU promoter • Acts with PIT1 to activate TSHβ gene promoter	Somatotrophs, lactotrophs, thyrotrophs, gonadotrophs, possibly corticotrophs	• Patients may present with rigid cervical spine causing limited neck rotation • Hypoplastic anterior/intermediate pituitary lobe	AR
Lhx4	• An LIM protein with close resemblance to Lhx3 • Important for proliferation and differentiation of cell lineages • May have overlapping function with PROP1 and POU1F1	Somatotrophs, lactotrophs, thyrotrophs, gonadotrophs, corticotrophs	• Combined pituitary hormone deficiencies with predominant GH deficiency • Severe anterior pituitary hypoplasia, ectopic neurohypophysis	AD
SIX6	• Member of the SIX/*sine oculis* family of homeobox genes • Expressed early in hypothalamus, later in Rathke's pouch, neural retina, and optic chiasma	Somatotrophs, gonadotrophs	• Bilateral anophthalmia • Pituitary hypoplasia • Associated with deletion at chromosome 14q22-23	Unknown
PITX2 (RIEG1)	• Bicoid-related homeobox gene expressed early in Rathke's pouch • Important in maintaining expression of Hesx1 and PROP1	Somatotrophs, lactotrophs, thyrotrophs, reduced expression of gonadotrophs	• Associated with Rieger syndrome: • Anterior-chamber eye anomalies • Dental hypoplasia • A protuberant umbilicus • Mental retardation • Pituitary dysfunction	AD
PROP1 (Prophet of PIT1)	• Paired-like homeodomain transcription factor required for PIT1 expression • Coexpressed with Hesx1	Somatotrophs, lactotrophs, thyrotrophs, gonadotrophs, corticotrophs (delayed)	• Combined pituitary deficiencies (GH, TSH, PRL, and late-onset ACTH reported) • Gonadotropin insufficiency or normal puberty with later onset of deficiency • Several mutations noted in nonconsanguineous families.	AR
POU1F1 (PIT1)	• Member of the POU transcription factor family • Important for activation of GH1, PRL, and TSHβ genes	Somatotrophs, lactotrophs, thyrotrophs	• Combined pituitary deficiencies (GH, TSH, PRL, and late-onset ACTH reported); TSH secretion may initially be normal • Pituitary hypoplasia	AD, AR
Otx2	• Bicoid-type homeodomain gene required for forebrain and eye development • Antagonizes *FGF8* and *SHH* expression • May have importance in activation of Hesx1	Somatotrophs, thyrotrophs, corticotrophs, and probably gonadotrophs	• Severe ocular malformation including anophthalmia • Combined pituitary hormone deficiencies with LH/FSH deficiency • Anterior pituitary hypoplasia with ectopic posterior pituitary	Unknown
SOX2	• Member of SOXB1 subfamily as *SOX1* and *SOX3* expressed early in development	Somatotrophs, gonadotrophs (and, in animal models, thyrotrophs)	• Hypogonadotropic hypogonadism • Anterior pituitary hypoplasia • Bilateral anophthalmia/microphthalmia • Midbrain defects including corpus callosum and hippocampus • Sensorineural defects • Esophageal atresia and learning difficulty	De novo
SOX3	• Member of SOX (SRY-related HMG box) • Developmental factor expressed in developing infundibulum and hypothalamus	Somatotrophs and/or additional anterior pituitary cell types	• Duplications of Xq26-27 in affected males (female carriers unaffected) • Variable mental retardation • Hypopituitarism with abnormal MRI • Anterior pituitary hypoplasia • Infundibular hypoplasia • Ectopic/undescended posterior pituitary • Abnormal corpus callosum • Murine studies suggest SOX3 dosage critical for normal pituitary development	X-linked

Table continued on following page

TABLE 24-2

Genetic Defects of the GH-IGF Axis Resulting in Somatotroph Dysfunction and GH Deficiency (Continued)

Factor	Gene Function	Affected Cell Types	Clinical Phenotype	Mode of Inheritance
Isolated Growth Hormone Deficiency				
GLI2	• Member of the GLI gene family; transcription factors that mediate SHH signaling	Somatotrophs	• Heterozygous loss-of-function mutations in patients with holoprosencephaly • Penetrance variable • Pituitary dysfunction accompanied by variable craniofacial abnormalities.	Unknown
GHRHr	• Encodes GHRH receptor	Somatotrophs	• Short stature • Anterior pituitary hypoplasia	AR
GH1	• Encodes GH peptide • Several mutations shown to affect GH secretion or function	Somatotrophs	• Short stature • Abnormal facies • Presentation includes bioinactive GH	AR, AD, or X-linked

ACTH, adrenocorticotropic hormone; AD, autosomal dominant; AR, autosomal recessive; FSH, follicle-stimulating hormone; GH, growth hormone; GHRH, growth hormone–releasing hormone; αGSU, glycoprotein α-subunit; HMG, high mobility group; LH, luteinizing hormone; MRI, magnetic resonance imaging; PRL, prolactin; SHH, Sonic hedgehog; TSH. thyroid-stimulating hormone.

In most patients, so-called idiopathic hypopituitarism or GHD is presumed to be due to abnormalities of synthesis or secretion of hypothalamic hypophysiotropic factors.[97,502,503] In a number of reports, idiopathic GHD is associated with MRI findings of an ectopic neurohypophysis, pituitary stalk dysgenesis, and hypoplasia or aplasia of the anterior pituitary. In series involving 397 children with isolated growth hormone deficiency (IGHD) or with combined pituitary hormone deficiencies (CPHD), 54% had the characteristic MRI findings, and 93% of CPHD patients were abnormal, in contrast to 32% of patients with IGHD.[504-508] Abrahams and colleagues[509] studied 35 patients with idiopathic GHD and found that those with MRI abnormalities could be divided into two groups: (1) 43% had an ectopic neurohypophysis (neurohypophysis located near the median eminence), absent infundibulum, and absence of the normal posterior pituitary bright spot; (2) 43% had a small anterior pituitary, either as an isolated finding or combined with an ectopic neurohypophysis. Overall, those patients with the most striking abnormalities of the hypothalamic-pituitary region, largely those with CPHD, had the smallest anterior pituitary glands.[505,510] Patients with more severe deficiencies of GH have greater frequency of significant morphologic abnormalities.[511,512]

TABLE 24-3

GH/IGF1 Deficiency Syndromes

Congenital Growth Hormone Deficiency
GH deficiency resulting from hypothalamic dysfunction
Holoprosencephaly and septo-optic dysplasia
GH deficiency resulting from pituitary dysfunction
GH deficiency resulting from mutations of the GHRH receptor and GH
GH deficiency resulting from CPHD
Bioinactive GH
Acquired Growth Hormone Deficiency
GH deficiency resulting from CNS tumors, trauma, or inflammation
Circulating antibodies to GH that inhibit GH action
Congenital Igf1 Deficiency
Abnormalities of the GHR
STAT5 mutations
ALS mutations
IGF1 gene mutations
IGF type 1 receptor mutations
Acquired Igf1 Deficiency
Circulating antibodies to the GHR
Chronic disease states

ALS, acid-labile subunit; CHPD, combined pituitary hormone deficiencies; CNS, central nervous system; GHR, growth hormone receptor; GHRH, growth hormone–releasing hormone; IGF1, insulin-like growth factor 1.

Although the increased incidence of breech presentation and birth trauma with neonatal asphyxia in congenital idiopathic hypopituitarism has led some to suggest an etiologic role for these occurrences,[513,514] the syndrome of pituitary stalk dysgenesis with congenital hypopituitarism is probably the result of abnormal development, and the perinatal difficulties are likely the consequence rather than the cause of the abnormalities. Findings of a similar MRI appearance in patients with septo-optic dysplasia,[128,515] in association with type I Arnold-Chiari syndrome and syringomyelia,[128,510,516] and possibly in holoprosencephaly[128] and the occurrence of micropenis with congenital hypopituitarism[128,517-520] all support the concept that congenital hypopituitarism is a genetic or developmental malformation, not a birth injury. A single report of an apparent autosomal dominant mutation of early brain development with infundibular dysgenesis associated with GHD supports the primary nature of the anomaly.[521] Further indirect evidence in studies[522] of isolated, complete anterior pituitary aplasia indicates that hypothalamic hypopituitarism and breech delivery are consequences of congenital midline brain defects, although perinatal residua of breech delivery may exacerbate ischemic damage to the hypothalamic-pituitary unit.

The MRI findings described for early-diagnosed patients with hypopituitarism are also found in children diagnosed at a later age. Most of these children have hypothalamic dysfunction as the cause of diminished pituitary hormone secretion. In the older group, as in the infants, structural, acquired hypothalamic, stalk, or pituitary abnormalities must be considered.

Holoprosencephaly. Holoprosencephaly, which is caused by abnormal midline development of the embryonic forebrain, usually results in hypothalamic insufficiency[523,524] and has been associated with mutations in developmental proteins.[525,526] These mutations are associated with diminished signaling by SHH, a critical factor in forebrain development.[527] Hedgehog ligands bind to and activate the transmembrane receptor Patched (PTCH), which results in release of the coreceptor, Smoothened (SMO), activating GLI transcription factors. SHH and FGF8 play a role in the induction of BMP2 and LHX, which are important for proliferation in the developing pituitary gland and are influenced by loss-of-function mutations of the *GL12* gene.[527,528]

Facial dysmorphism of holoprosencephaly ranges from cyclopia to hypertelorism and is accompanied by absence of the nasal septum, midline clefts of the palate or lip, and sometimes a single central incisor. GHD may be accompanied by other pituitary hormone insufficiencies. The incidence of GHD is increased in cases of simple clefts of the lip or palate (or both),[529,530] and children with cleft palates who grow abnormally require further evaluation.

Septo-Optic Dysplasia. In its complete form, the rare syndrome of *septo-optic dysplasia* combines hypoplasia or absence of the optic chiasm or optic nerves (or both), agenesis or hypoplasia of the septum pellucidum or corpus callosum (or both), and hypothalamic insufficiency.[515,531,532] The extent of the anatomic and functional abnormalities can vary but usually in parallel to each other.[531,532] GHD can occur by itself or in combination with deficiencies of TSH, ACTH, or gonadotropins. About 50% to 70% of children with severe anatomic defects have hypopituitarism or, at least, identifiable abnormalities of the GH-IGF axis,[128,533,534] and the diagnosis should be considered in any child who has growth failure associated with pendular or rotatory nystagmus or impaired vision and a small optic nerve disc. In some patients, a hypoplastic or interrupted pituitary stalk and ectopic posterior pituitary placement have been identified by MRI.[128,515,535] It is not clear whether this disorder is inherited, but there is an increased incidence in offspring of young mothers, in first-born children, in areas of high unemployment, and in babies exposed to intrauterine medications, smoking, alcohol, or diabetes.[536,537]

HESX1. Mutations of *HESX1*, a paired-like homeodomain gene that is expressed early in pituitary and forebrain development, are associated with familial forms of septo-optic dysplasia.[538-540] *HESX1*, also referred to as *RPX* (Rathke's pouch homeobox), is a member of the paired-like class of homeobox genes and is essential for normal forebrain and pituitary formation.[541] It is one of the earliest known specific markers for the pituitary primordium and encodes for a developmental repressor with localization to the Rathke's pouch.[542] TLE1 (the mammalian ortholog of the *Drosophila* protein Groucho) and the nuclear corepressor NCOR1, bind to HESX1 to exert repression.[543,544] *HESX1* downregulation is required for cell determination mediated by PROP1 to occur. The LIM homeodomain proteins LHX1 and LHX3 are required for activation of the HESX1 promoter.[545]

Hesx1 null mutant mice display abnormalities in the forebrain, eyes, and other anterior structures such as the pituitary.[546] Mouse embryos heterozygous for both *Hesx1* and *Six3* null mutations have a mild phenotype, suggesting that these developmental factors control a switch in progenitor proliferation between repression by HESX1 and activation of PROP1.[547] These defects have similarity with human phenotypes such as septo-optic dysplasia and CPHD. Patients with septo-optic dysplasia may present with a wide spectrum of phenotypes associated with congenital hypopituitarism. Several homozygous and heterozygous mutations have been identified in *HESX1* (Online Mendelian Inheritance in Man [OMIM] no. 601802) in patients with hypopituitarism with variable phenotypes.[540,542,546,548-554]

Two siblings (born to consanguineous parents) with a severe septo-optic dysplasia phenotype including anterior pituitary hypoplasia, an ectopic posterior lobe, agenesis of the corpus callosum, absent septum pellucidum, and optic nerve hypoplasia were found to have a homozygous mutation at a highly conserved arginine residue of the homeodomain (p.R160C) that resulted in loss of DNA binding of the mutant protein. Another homozygous mutation, a threonine/isoleucine substitution at residue 26 (p.I26T), was identified in a child with GH and gonadotropin deficiency that later evolved to deficiencies of ACTH and TSH. She had no forebrain abnormalities and normal optic nerves, but on MRI had hypoplasia of the anterior pituitary and an undescended posterior pituitary. This mutation lies in a highly conserved engrailed homology domain that is required for transcriptional repression. Loss of repressor function was found to be caused by impaired interaction with the TLE1 corepressor. To determine the mechanisms by which these mutations cause the disorder, mice homozygous for these mutations were generated.[555] Mice homozygous for the p.R160C mutation displayed pituitary and forebrain defects similar to those in the *Hesx1* null embryos, indicating the critical role of HESX1 interactions with DNA in transcriptional repression during development. Mice homozygous for the p.I26T allele displayed pituitary defects and ocular abnormalities suggestive of a hypomorph allele, indicating the important role of TLE interaction in pituitary and ocular development.

Heterozygous mutations of *HESX1* have been identified in patients with hypopituitarism and septo-optic dysplasia and are usually associated with less affected phenotypes. Approximately 850 patients were studied for mutations in *HESX1,* including more than 300 patients with septo-optic dysplasia; 410 with isolated pituitary dysfunction, optic nerve hypoplasia, or midline neurologic abnormalities; and 126 with familial inheritance. The incidence of coding region mutations in *HESX1* within this population was about 1%, suggesting that mutations in *HESX1* are a rare cause of hypopituitarism and septo-optic dysplasia.[549]

OTX2. Mutations in other genes have been associated with CNS anatomic abnormalities and hypopituitarism. *OTX2* is a homeobox gene that is expressed earliest in the neuroectoderm[556] cells of the forebrain and midbrain and encodes a transcription factor belonging to the orthodenticle family. This factor also plays a role in ocular development. Murine models harboring mutant *Otx2* genes demonstrate abnormal primitive streak organization and a headless phenotype.[556] OTX2 has a role in regulating early expression of HESX1 and is expressed in the pituitary to regulate POU1F1 (PIT1). Dateki and colleagues[557] identified a frameshift *OTX2* mutation in a patient with bilateral anophthalmia and partial IGHD with minimal transactivation activity. A heterozygous *OTX2* mutation was described in two unrelated patients with hypopituitarism; although initial studies demonstrated normal binding to HESX1 binding sites, the mutant *OTX2* gene was demonstrated to have decreased activation of the *HESX1* promoter, suggesting a dominant negative effect leading to CPHD.[558] This relationship between the transcription factors OTX2 and HESX1 emphasizes the complexities of pituitary development and suggests that genetic etiologies may be multifactorial. Further studies have revealed two frameshift mutations, a nonsense mutation in two unrelated patients, and a heterozygous microdeletion in a fifth patient.[557]

SOX3. A syndrome of X-linked hypopituitarism and mental retardation involving duplications of Xq26-27 encompassing *SOX3* (OMIM 313430) has been described in several pedigrees. The affected males have anterior pituitary and infundibular hypoplasia with an undescended posterior pituitary and abnormalities of the corpus callosum. The GHD may also be associated with deficiencies of ACTH, TSH, or gonadotropins. Because *Sox3* is not expressed in Rathke's pouch in the mouse, the anterior pituitary developmental defects are probably secondary to disruption of infundibular development.[559-562] Female carriers appear to be clinically unaffected, and no mutations have been found in patients with sex reversal, gonadal dysgenesis, or infertility.[563,564]

SOX2. Heterozygous mutations within *SOX2* in males have been associated with anophthalmia or microphthalmia and anterior pituitary hypoplasia. The resulting hormonal abnormalities include GH and gonadotropin deficiency. Some patients also present with genital abnormalities.[565-569] A wide variety of additional abnormalities may be present, including hypoplasia of the corpus callosum, hypothalamic hamartoma, hippocampal malformation, esophageal atresia, sensorineural hearing loss, and learning difficulties.[567-576] In addition to de novo heterozygous mutations, nonsynonymous changes have been identified in individuals who inherited the variant from a clinically unaffected parent.[565,577] A perplexing case of a patient with isolated hypogonadotropic hypogonadism but without anterior pituitary hypoplasia suggests that *SOX2* may be independently involved in hypothalamic neuronal development.[569] The expression of *SOX2* has been found to overlap with that of *LHX3* and *HESX1* within Rathke's pouch.[555,566,578,579]

Acquired Disorders

Inflammation of the Brain or Hypothalamus. Bacterial, viral, or fungal infections may result in hypothalamic/pituitary insufficiency,[580,581] and the hypothalamus or pituitary or both may also be involved in sarcoidosis.[582]

Tumors of the Brain or Hypothalamus. Brain tumors are a major cause of hypothalamic insufficiency,[583] especially midline brain tumors such as germinomas, meningiomas, gliomas, ependymomas, and gliomas of the optic nerve. Although short stature and GHD are most often associated with suprasellar lesions in neurofibromatosis, they may also exist without such lesions. Whether growth impairment antedates the pathologic findings is not yet clear.[584,585] Metastases from extracranial carcinomas are rare in children, but hypothalamic insufficiency can result from local extension of craniopharyngeal carcinoma or Hodgkin's disease of the nasopharynx. The laboratory diagnosis of GHD in children with brain tumors can be difficult because levels of IGF1I and IGFBP3 are poor predictors, especially in pubertal patients.[586] Craniopharyngiomas and histiocytosis can cause hypothalamic dysfunction (see later discussion).

Trauma of the Brain or Hypothalamus. Head trauma, resulting from boxing and various injuries, can cause IGHD or multiple anterior pituitary deficiencies.[587-591] Some series of patients with GHD have indicated an increased incidence of birth trauma, such as breech deliveries, extensive use of forceps, prolonged labor, or abrupt delivery. Although GHD can be a consequence of a difficult delivery or hypoxemic perinatal period, it is more commonly associated with developmental deficiencies (discussed previously) or head trauma later in life. In a series of 22 head-injured adolescents and adults, almost 40% had some degree of hypopituitarism.[588]

Psychosocial Dwarfism. An extreme form of failure to thrive is termed *psychosocial dwarfism* or *emptional deprioation dwarfism*.[579a-579c] Most cases of failure to thrive can be traced back to a poor home environment and indadequate parenting, with improved weight gain and growth upon removal of the infant from the dysfunctional home. Some children have been reported, however, to show dramatic behavioral manifestations beyond those in the typical failure-to-thrive infant, namely bizarre eating and drinking habits, such as drinking from toilets, social withdrawal, and primitive speech.[579b] Hyperphagia and abnormalities of GH production may be associated.[579d] GH secretion is low in response to pharmacologic stimuli but returns to normal upon removal from the home. Concomitantly, eating and behavioral habits returned to normal, and a period of catch-up growth ensured. Careful assessment of endogenous GH secretion showed reversal of the GH insufficiency within 3 weeks, including enhancement of GH pulse amplitude and a variable increase of pulse frequency.[579d-579f] The reversibility of GH secretory defects and the later growth increment in the context of the clinical findings described previously confirm the diagnosis of psychosocial dwarfism.[579c,579f-579h]

The neuroendocrinologic mechanisms involved in psychosocial swarfism remain to be elucidated. GH secretion is abnormal and ACTH and TSH levels may also be low, although some patients have high plasma cortisol levels.[579c] Even when GH secretion is reduced, treatment with GH is not usually of benefit unitl the psychosocial situation is improved.[579c] Management of the environmental causes of the growth failure is imperative and often associated with substantial growth. In our experience, although psychosocial dysfunction is a common cause of failure to thrive in infancy, the constellation of bizarre behaviors dexcribed in psychosocial dwarfism is rare.

The fact that GH production is impaired in adults with varied psychiatric disorders[579i,579j] and given the growth aberrations of functional GHD with psychosocial dwarfism together suggest that children with emotional problems may have impaired GH secretion and growth.[579k] Indeed, depression in children, as adults, can lower GH production,[579l] and in girls, anxiety disorders predict a modest height loss in adults.[579k]

The Anterior Pituitary

As discussed earlier, many of the disease processes that impair hypothalamic regulation of GH secretion also impair pituitary function. Another group of abnormalities specifically affect pituitary somatotroph development and function.

Congenital Disorders. As many as 3% to 30% of patients with GHD have an affected parent, sibling, or child.[592-594] Inborn errors of the genes for nuclear transcription factors affecting hypothalamic-pituitary development, the GHRH receptor, or the GH gene can cause GHD and IGF deficiency.

Combined Pituitary Hormone Deficiency. During pituitary development, a series of transcription factors are expressed in a specific timeframe and in a spatial context. The result of cell differentiation and proliferation is a mature anterior pituitary gland with five distinct cell types (see Chapter 8).

PITX2. *PITX2* (also known as *RIEG*) is a member of the bicoid-like homeobox transcription factor family that is closely related to the mammalian OTX genes expressed in the rostral brain during development; it is required at many stages of pituitary development.[595] Studies have shown that activation of the WNT signaling pathway or constitutive activation of β-catenin can induce *PITX2* expression. *PITX2* is expressed in thyrotrophs, gonadotrophs, somatotrophs, and lactotrophs but not in corticotrophs.[596]

PITX2 acts to activate the promoters of pituitary hormone target genes.[597-599] Homozygous loss of *PITX2* results in early embryonic lethality with pituitary development severely affected.[600-603] This is thought to be related to the control of cell cycle regulatory genes by PITX2.[604,605] Furthermore, the lack of *PITX2* also results in excessive cell death during early pituitary development, suggesting a role in cell survival.[606] A mouse line expressing a hypomorphic allele of *Pitx2* provided evidence that the extent of pituitary hypoplasia and cellular differentiation is proportional to the reduced dosage of *Pitx*.[603,607] In this model, the gonadotroph lineage was primarily affected and the numbers of differentiated somatotrophs and thyrotrophs were reduced, but the corticotroph population was unaffected.[607]

In a *Pitx2* overexpression model, the gonadotroph population was expanded, probably because of the role of *Pitx2* in the expression of gonadotroph-specific transcription factors GATA2, EGR1, and NR5A1 (SF1).[606] Mutations of *PITX2* have been described in patients diagnosed with Rieger syndrome, an autosomal dominant condition with variable manifestations including anomalies of the anterior chamber of the eye, dental hypoplasia, a protuberant umbilicus, mental retardation, and pituitary abnormalities. Six point mutations of *PITX2*, located within the homeodomain responsible for DNA binding have been described, and several of these mutations show loss of DNA binding capacity.[608] A heterozygous mutation that changes the lysine at position 50 to glutamic acid in the homeodomain has been found to impart a dominant negative effect leading to a pronounced phenotype.[609]

LHX3. LHX3 is a member of the LIM-type homeodomain protein family of transcription factors that feature two LIM domains in their amino terminus and a centrally located homeodomain used to interact with specific DNA elements on target genes. During development, expression of *LHX3*, which persists in the adult pituitary, is seen in the anterior and intermediate lobes of the pituitary, spinal cord, and medulla.[610] Murine models with targeted disruption of *Lhx3* show depletion of thyrotrophs, gonadotrophs, and somatotrophs, suggesting that *Lhx3* is important for cell specification and proliferation.[611] Three LHX3 isoforms have been identified in humans: LHX3a, LHX3b, and M2-LHX3.[612] Of these, LHX3a displays the greatest ability to activate the promoters of pituitary genes. Patients with reported mutations in *LHX3* have deficits of GH, PRL, TSH, and gonadotropins, as well as abnormal pituitary morphology along with a rigid cervical spine that limits head rotation.[613] *LHX3* mutations are a rare cause of reported hypopituitarism, and one study reported that the incidence of a homozygous *LHX3* mutation in patients studied with CPHD was 2.2%.[613] Several other novel *LHX3* mutations in patients with CPHD demonstrating autosomal recessive inheritance have been reported and characterized.[579,614] There is also evidence to demonstrate that SOX2 is capable of binding and activating transcription of the *LHX3* promoter and therefore may be important in pituitary development.[579]

LHX4. LHX4 is another LIM homeodomain protein with homology to LHX3, and it is also expressed in the developing brain, including the cortex, pituitary, and spinal cord.[615] Despite similarities in protein structure, the role of LHX4 in development is distinct from that of LHX3, as demonstrated by single and combined gene-deletion targeting in mice. Murine models with targeted deletion of *Lhx4* form a definitive Rathke's pouch that arrests and results in a hypoplastic pituitary. In contrast to *Lhx3* gene knockout mice, $Lhx4^{-/-}$ mice contain all five differentiated cell types.[616,617] *Lhx3* expression is impaired in the *Lhx4* mutants, suggesting that *Lhx4* is required for cell survival, expansion of the pouch, and differentiation of pituitary-specific cell lineages.

Several reports have described CPHD patients with evidence of a hypoplastic pituitary who harbored *LHX4* mutations.[618-620] These heterozygous mutations have been shown to result in proteins that are unable to bind DNA and activate pituitary gene expression.[620] Further studies have demonstrated a functional relationship between POU1F1 and LHX4 in the regulation of POU1F1 expression in specific pituitary cell types.[618] Also, several studies have suggested that LHX4 and PROP1 have overlapping functions in pituitary development.[616] Finally, in addition to pituitary hormone deficiencies, *LHX4* mutations have been implicated in structural abnormalities; patients with an *LHX4* mutation have been reported with abnormal MRI findings including a hypoplastic anterior pituitary, ectopic posterior lobe, poorly developed sella turcica, and Chiari malformation.[621]

SIX6. *SIX6* is a member of the SIX/sine oculis family of homeobox genes that is expressed in retina, optic nerve, hypothalamus, and pituitary.[622] Murine expression studies of the TCF/LEF family of transcription factors during pituitary development demonstrated that *Six6* plays a role in proliferation of cells during early formation of Rathke's pouch.[623] SIX6 has also been shown to interact with the Groucho family of transcriptional repressors.[624,625] *SIX6* has been mapped to chromosome 14q22-23, and patients with deletions of this chromosomal region display bilateral anophthalmia and pituitary anomalies.[626] Patients with anophthalmia/microphthalmia were shown to have several frequent polymorphisms of Six6 and one potential causative missense mutation.[622] One case report implicated *SIX6* haploinsufficiency as being responsible for ocular and pituitary maldevelopment. Despite its importance in early development, further studies are required to determine whether *SIX6* mutations are present in patients with pituitary hormone deficiency.

ISL1. ISL1 is a member of the LIM homeodomain family of transcription factors, which are characterized by two tandemly repeated cysteine/histidine-rich LIM domains that are involved in protein-protein interactions. Its expression is restricted to cells that will express *CGA* and subsequently *TSHB*.[627,628] Homozygous loss of *Isl1* in mice results in developmental arrest with no pouch formation.[629] To date, no human mutations in *ISL1* have been identified.

PROP1. Mutations in *PROP1*, a paired-like homeodomain transcription factor with expression restricted to the anterior pituitary during development, have also been found to result in CPHD.[630] Mutation of this gene is responsible for a form of murine pituitary-dependent dwarfism known as the Ames mouse.[55,631,632] The pituitary gland appears to be enlarged in mice bearing mutations in *Prop1*, although the mechanism is unclear.[633-636] In the end, a decrease in proliferation and apoptosis result in pituitary hypoplasia, similar to that seen in humans.[636-638] The switch from repression of target gene expression by HESX1 to activation by PROP1 is important for development of the POU1F1 (GH, PRL, and TSH) and gonadotroph lineages.[544,635,639] PROP1 and β-catenin have been shown to form a complex that represses *Hesx1* while activating *Pou1f1* expression.[640] The gonadotropin deficiency in the Ames dwarf remains unexplained, although treatment with thyroxine (T_4) or GH (or both) restored fertility in some male mice and sexual maturation, but not fertility, in female mice.[641,642]

Mutations of *PROP1* in humans result in GH, PRL, and TSH deficiencies, although failure in all cell lineages, including gonadotrophs and corticotrophs, has been reported.[632,643,644] The characterization of *PROP1* mutations is complex, because the phenotypes are variable and dynamic and hormone deficiencies may develop over time even in patients with similar genetic backgrounds.[643,645,646] Gonadotropin abnormalities are particularly diverse in that approximately 30% of patients have spontaneous pubertal development, including menarche, before ultimately developing hypogonadotropic hypogonadism.[643,647] Apparently normal growth without GH has also been found in a child with PROP1 deficiency.[648,649] The ACTH deficiency may develop in the fourth or fifth decade of life.[650] Striking variability has been described in pituitary size, with very large glands, possibly arising from the intermediate lobe,[651] producing a hyperintense T1 signal occasionally demonstrated by MRI.[632,644,652,653] These glands may undergo involution, leaving a large empty sella in patients with complete anterior hypopituitarism including ACTH deficiency.[654-656]

Many *PROP1* (chromosome 5q35, OMIM 601538) abnormalities have been identified, including missense, frameshift, and splicing mutations. A GA repeat in exon 2 (295-CGA-GAG-AGT-303) has been reported to be a "hot spot" in *PROP1;* any combination of a GA or AG deletion in this repeat region results in a frameshift in the coding sequence and premature termination at codon 109.[647,657] Similar abnormalities result from homozygous lesions at other sites on exon 2 and affect codons 73, 88, and 149.[644,658,659] Compound heterozygosity for two mutations was detected in 36% of children from four families; two different common deletions both led to a stop codon at position 109.[659] These mutations are predicted to result in loss of the DNA-binding and C-terminal transactivating domains of *PROP1*. Some missense mutations have been shown to retain partial activity.[644,660,661]

There does not appear to be strong correlation between phenotype and genotype.[647] A screen of 73 subjects (36 families) diagnosed with CPHD by Deladoey and associates identified 35 patients with *PROP1* gene defects, including three different missense mutations, two frameshift mutations, and one splice site mutation. In 12 of 36 unrelated families, defects were located in the region nt296 through nt302, suggesting a possible hot spot for *PROP1* mutations in CPHD.[647] Although *PROP1* mutations appear to be rare in sporadic cases, their prevalence is 29.5% in familial cases of CHPD, as reported by Turton and colleagues.[662,663]

POU1F1. The *POU1F1* gene (chromosome 3p11, OMIM 173110) encodes PIT1, a member of a large family of transcription factors referred to as POU-domain proteins that is responsible for pituitary-specific transcription of genes for GH, PRL, TSH, and the GHRH receptor.[58,664-667] PIT1, a 290-amino-acid protein, contains two domains, the POU-specific and the POU-homeo domains; both are necessary for DNA binding and activation of GH and PRL genes and for regulation of the PRL, TSH-β, and POU1F1 genes.[668] Its expression is restricted to the anterior pituitary to control differentiation, proliferation, and survival of somatotrophs, lactotrophs, and thyrotrophs.[593,667-670] PIT1 regulates target genes by binding to response elements and recruiting coactivator proteins, such as cAMP response element–binding protein (CREB)-binding protein (CBP).[671]

Two mouse models were first reported to have GH, PRL, and TSH deficiencies associated with mutations or rearrangements of the *Pit1* gene; these were the Snell (dw/dwS) and the Jackson (dw/dwJ) dwarf mice.[672,673] Many different mutations of the *POU1F1* gene have been found internationally in families with GHD and PRL deficiency and variable defects in TSH expression.[631,664,669,674-682] These mutations are transmitted as autosomal recessive or dominant traits and cause variable peptide hormone deficiencies with or without anterior pituitary hypoplasia.[663,664,669,674,676-679,683,684]

The most common mutation is an R271W substitution that affects the POU homeodomain, encoding a mutant protein that binds normally to DNA and acts as a dominant inhibitor of transcription.[663,685-688] Evidence from a patient with the R271W mutation suggests that PIT1 may have a role in cell survival.[689] A patient diagnosed with GHD, along with dysregulation of PRL and TSH was reported to have a lysine-to-glutamic acid mutation at codon 216 (K216E).[668] This mutant PIT1 binds to DNA and appears not to inhibit basal activation of GH and PRL genes; however, the mutant is unable to support retinoic acid induction of *POU1F1* gene expression. Another report suggested that CBP (p300) recruitment and PIT1 dimerization are necessary for target gene activation and that disruption of this process may account for the pathogenesis of CPHD.[690] All of the reported mutations involve sites affecting *POU1F1* DNA-binding, dimerization, or target gene transactivation.

Phenotypic variability occurs among patients with apparently similar genotypes.[684] It does not appear that ACTH or gonadotropin deficiencies occur, as is frequently the case with *PROP1* defects,[663] but adrenarche has been reported to be absent or delayed in patients with a POU1F1 mutation.[691]

Isolated Growth Hormone Deficiency. The incidence of IGHD is estimated to be 1 of every 3,480 to 10,000 live births.[88,692-694] In most children with IGHD, no cause can be identified, and this group is often referred to as having idiopathic GHD. However, there is increasing recognition of genetic defects in idiopathic GHD. Four forms of IGHD have been reported (see Table 24-2).[593,664,695] The classification system is based on clinical characteristics, inheritance patterns, and GH secretion but not necessarily on disease causation.

The gene encoding GH (*GH1*) is located on chromosome 17q23 in a cluster that includes two genes for placental lactogen (hPL), a pseudogene for hPL, and the *GH2* gene that encodes placental GH.[592,594] *GH1* and *GH2* differ in mRNA splicing pattern: *GH1* generates 20- and 22-kd proteins (of approximately equal bioactivity), whereas *GH2* yields a protein that differs from GH1 in 13 amino acid residues.

IGHD Type I. IGHD type IA results primarily from large deletions, with rare microdeletions and single base-pair substitutions of the *GH1* gene that prevent synthesis or secretion of the hormone.[696] IGHD IA is inherited as an autosomal recessive trait, and affected individuals have profound congenital GHD. Because GH is not produced even in fetal life, patients are immunologically intolerant of GH and typically develop anti-GH antibodies when treated with either pituitary-derived or recombinant DNA–derived GH. When antibodies prevent patients from responding to GH, IGHD IA can be viewed as a form of GH insensitivity, and such patients are candidates for IGF1 therapy.

The less severe form of autosomal recessive GHD, termed IGHD type IB, also may result from mutations or rearrangements of the *GH1* gene that cause production of an aberrant GH molecule that retains some function or at least generates immune tolerance. The phenotypic variability is greater than in IGHD IA.[695] These patients usually respond to exogenous GH therapy without antibody production. The very low frequency (1.7%) of *GH1* gene mutations in familial type IB IGHD suggests the importance of studying the *GH1* gene promoter region in patients with unexplained GHD.[664,697] In a group of 65 children with IGHD IB, the GHRH receptor gene *(GHRHR)* was normal in domains coding for the extracellular region,[698] but mutations in transmembrane and intracellular gene domains were found in 10% of families with IGHD IB.[699]

IGHD Type II. IGHD type II is inherited as an autosomal dominant trait. The most common cause appears to be mutations that inactivate the 5′ splice donor site of intron 3 of the *GH1* gene, resulting in skipping of exon 3[631,664] and producing a molecule that cannot fold normally. It is likely that the 17.5-kd GH isoform mutant functions in a dominant-negative manner to suppress intracellular accumulation and secretion of wild-type GH.[700-703] In patients with missense mutations in exon 4 or 5, clinical presentation is quite variable, with some evidence for reversibility of the impairment of intracellular GH storage and secretion by GH treatment.[704] Mullis and coworkers[705] studied 57 subjects from 19 families and found that patients with IGHD type II not only have a variable phenotype in terms of onset, severity, and progression of GHD but also may demonstrate later onset of ACTH or TSH deficiencies and pituitary hypoplasia. An extensive assessment of *GH1* gene mutations in short children with and without GHD did reveal a substantial number of heterozygous mutations.[705] Even though these are not primary explanations for the growth impairment, they may contribute to the observed variation in the growth process.

Mutations in *GHRHR* are also classified as IGHD type IB. The GHRH receptor is G-protein coupled with seven transmembrane domains and is found predominantly in the pituitary gland. Mutation of the gene for *Ghrhr* in its ligand-binding domain has been identified in the *little* mouse *(lit/lit)*[706] and results in dwarfism and decreased numbers of somatotrophs.[667,707,708] In this model, the fetal somatotroph mass is normal, and hypoplasia (but not absence) of the somatotrophs is evident only postnatally.[667,670,707,708] Such data suggest that GHRH is not an essential factor for fetal differentiation of the somatotrophs and that GHRH-independent cells persist or that mutation does not cause total loss of GHRH function. The human *GHRHR* gene is 15 kb with 13 exons. The GHRHR protein is encoded by a 1.3 kb cDNA.[77,709-711]

Wajnrajch and colleagues reported the first human cases of a mutation in the *GHRHR* gene in two cousins in a consanguineous Indian Muslim family with IGF deficiency and profound growth failure.[712] The gene defect, a nonsense mutation that introduced a stop codon at position 72 (E72X), resulted in a markedly truncated GHRHR protein that lacked the membrane-spanning regions and the G-protein–binding site. The affected children had undetectable GH release during standard provocative tests and after exogenous GHRH administration but responded to GH treatment. The same mutation was also identified in a reportedly unrelated Tamoulean kindred in Sri Lanka,[713] in a consanguineous kindred in Pakistan ("dwarfism of Sindh"),[714,715] and in 17 patients from one Muslim and four Hindu families in Western India.[716] The largest kindred with a mutation of *GHRHR* was identified a Brazilian family with a homozygous donor splice mutation (G to A at position +1) of exon 1.[88] This mutation disrupts the highly conserved consensus GT of the 50-donor splice site, generating a truncated GHRHR.[717,718]

A *GHRHR* missense mutation in exon 11 (R357C) was described in two consanguineous Israeli Arab families.[719] Patients in all of the groups had early growth failure with short stature (−4.5 to −8.6 SD), a high-pitched voice, and increased abdominal fat accumulation.[714,718] As expected, all of the patients demonstrated severely reduced or undetectable serum concentrations of GH in response to provocative GH stimulation, as well as very low serum concentrations of IGF1, IGFBP3, and ALS.[718] The adults manifest an unfavorable cardiovascular risk profile, which includes increased levels of low-density lipoprotein cholesterol and total cholesterol, elevated C-reactive protein, elevated blood pressure, and abdominal obesity. However, a perplexing study found no evidence of premature atherosclerosis or premature myocardial ischemia in these patients with *GHRHR* mutations.[720] The patients respond well to exogenous GH without antibody formation. Heterozygotes may have minimal height deficits and may show moderate biochemical deficiencies of the GH-IGF axis.[714] Despite extensive study, the geographic separation and ethnic differences among these patient groups do not suggest recent (>200 years) contact among the families from the Indian subcontinent. At present, the likely explanation for all four families is that of a "founder effect" or one-time mutation in each group followed by propagation within a geographically isolated gene pool.[88] In an analysis of 30 families with IGHD type IB, Salvatori and colleagues[699] found new missense mutations in transmembrane and intracellular domains of the *GHRHR* in three families (10%), with two affected members in each. Transfection experiments indicated normal cellular expression of these mutant receptors.

IGHD Type III. IGHD type III, transmitted as an X-linked trait with associated hypogammaglobulinemia,[721] has not yet been related to a mutation of the *GH1* gene. A large Australian kindred demonstrated GHD with a variable spectrum of pituitary hormonal deficiencies that may have been caused by duplication of the Xq25-Xq28 region.[722]

Bioinactive GH. Serum GH exists in multiple molecular forms, reflecting the consequences of alternative post-transcriptional or post-translational processing of the mRNA or protein, respectively. Some of these forms are presumed to have defects in the amino acid sequences required for binding of GH to its receptor, and different molecular forms of GH may have varying potencies for stimulating skeletal growth, although this remains to be rigorously proved. Short stature with normal GH immunoreactivity but reduced biopotency has been suggested,[723,724] but the molecular abnormalities have been characterized in relatively few patients, and many cases of suspected bioinactive GH have not been rigorously proven.[725,726]

In one child with extreme short stature (−6.1 SDS), a mutant GH caused by a single missense heterozygous mutation (cysteine to arginine, codon 77 of *GH1*) bound with greater affinity than normal to GHBP and the GHR and inhibited the action of normal GH. The child grew more (6 versus 3.9 cm/year) during a period of exogenous GH in moderate dosage. The father was found to have the same genetic abnormality but did not express the mutant hormone. In a second patient[726] with marked short stature (−3.6 SDS), a heterozygous alanine-to-glycine substitution in exon 4 of GH led to a substitution of glycine for arginine. This mutation was located in site 2 of GH molecular binding with its receptor and apparently led to failure of appropriate molecular rotation of the dimerized receptor and subsequent diminished tyrosine phosphorylation and the GH-mediated intracellular cascade of events. Bioactivity determined in a mouse B-cell lymphoma line was about 33% of immunoreactivity.[727] Exogenous GH substantially increased growth velocity (from 4.5 to 11.0 cm/year).

An Ile179Met substitution found in a short child was characterized by normal STAT5 activation but a 50% decrement in ERK activation.[173] This novel finding demonstrated the complexity of the functional interaction of GH with its receptor, but because STAT5B is clearly the major (if not the sole) GH-dependent mediator of IGF1 gene transcription, the role of this mutation is not clear. Six GH heterozygous variants with evidence of impairment of JAK/

STAT activation were found by screening of short children, suggesting that further studies are needed to determine the mechanism of interaction of GH with its receptor.[728] Because these variants occur in heterozygotes, the genotype-phenotype correlations are unclear. In one of the more convincing cases of bioinactive GH reported to date, Besson and associates[729] found a homozygous missense mutation (G705C) in a short child (−3.6 SDS) that resulted in absence of two disulfide bridges. Both GHR binding and JAK2/STAT5 signaling activity were markedly reduced.

Some patients demonstrate a decrease in bioactivity (when measured by sensitive in vitro assays) but not in immunoreactivity. The absence of mutations suggests that abnormal post-translational modifications of GH or other peripheral mechanisms may be responsible.[730,731]

Acquired Disorders

Craniopharyngiomas and Other Tumors. Many tumors that impair hypothalamic function also affect pituitary secretion of GH. In addition, *craniopharyngiomas* are a major cause of pituitary insufficiency.[732-734] These tumors arise from remnants of Rathke's pouch, the diverticulum of the roof of the embryonic oral cavity that normally gives rise to the anterior pituitary. Genetic defects in this condition, although certainly reasonable to suspect, have not yet been identified. This tumor is a congenital malformation present at birth and gradually grows over the ensuing years. The tumor arises from rests of squamous cells at the junction of the adenohypophysis and neurohypophysis and forms a cyst as it enlarges; the cyst contains degenerated cells and may calcify but does not undergo malignant degeneration. The cyst fluid ranges from the consistency of machine oil to a shimmering, cholesterol-laden liquid, and the calcifications may be microscopic or gross.[735] About 75% of craniopharyngiomas arise in the suprasellar region; the remainder resemble pituitary adenomas.[735-740]

Craniopharyngiomas can cause manifestations at any age from infancy to adulthood but usually manifest in middle childhood. The most common presentation results from increased intracranial pressure and includes headaches, vomiting, and oculomotor abnormalities. Visual field defects result from compression of the optic chiasm, and papilledema or optic atrophy may be present. Visual and olfactory hallucinations have been reported, as have seizures and dementia. Most children with craniopharyngiomas have evidence of growth failure at the time of presentation, and they are often found retrospectively to have had reduced growth since infancy.[741] GH and the gonadotropins are the most commonly affected pituitary hormones in children and adults, but deficiency of TSH, ACTH, may also occur, and diabetes insipidus is present in 25% to 50% of patients.[735-737,742] Between 50% and 80% of patients have abnormalities of at least one anterior pituitary hormone at diagnosis.[736,742]

Cystic and solid components can be identified by MRI, and anatomic relationships can be delineated to help plan a rational operative approach. Operative intervention via craniotomy or transsphenoidal resection may result in partial or almost complete removal of the lesion. Postoperative irradiation is commonly used, especially if tumor resection was incomplete. In some patients, particularly those who become obese, a syndrome of normal linear growth without GH may occur. The metabolic syndrome, with evidence of insulin insensitivity and increased body mass index (BMI), is common and is a predictor of potential major long-term morbidity.[741,743,744] The long-term childhood and adolescent consequences of craniopharyngioma are substantial, with many quality-of-life issues exacerbating the hypopituitarism.

Pituitary adenomas (see Chapter 8) are infrequent during childhood and adolescence, accounting for fewer than 5% of patients undergoing surgery at large centers.[739,740,745] Almost two thirds of tumors immunochemically stain for PRL, and a small number stain for GH. GH-secreting pituitary adenomas are exceedingly unusual in youth. There is a variable experience as to the invasive nature of pituitary adenomas, but the prevailing opinion is that they are less aggressive in children than in adults.[739,745] In 56 patients at the Mayo Clinic with non–ACTH-secreting adenomas removed transsphenoidally, macroadenomas were about one third more frequent than microadenomas, with cases in girls outnumbering those in boys 3.3 to 1.[739] The patients with macroadenoma had an approximately 50% incidence of hypopituitarism, compared with zero incidence in those patients with microadenomas; long-term cure rates were between 55% and 65% for both tumor sizes.

Histiocytosis X. The localized or generalized proliferation of mononuclear macrophages (histiocytes) characterizes Langerhans cell histiocytosis, a diverse disorder that occurs in patients of all ages, with a peak incidence at ages 1 to 4 years.[746] Endocrinologists are more familiar with the term *histiocytosis X*, which includes three related disorders: solitary bony disease (eosinophilic granuloma), Hand-Schüller-Christian disease (chronic disease with diabetes insipidus, exophthalmos, and multiple calvarial lesions), and disseminated histiocytosis X (Letterer-Siwe disease, with widespread visceral involvement). These syndromes are characterized by an infiltration and accumulation of Langerhans cells in the involved areas, such as skull, hypothalamic-pituitary stalk, CNS, and viscera. Although these disorders, especially Hand-Schüller-Christian disease, are classically associated with diabetes insipidus, approximately 50% to 75% of patients in selected series have growth failure and GHD at the time of presentation.[747-749] In contrast, a French national registry ($n = 589$) found GHD in 61 subjects, with overall endocrine dysfunction in 148. In the latter group, an evolving neurodegenerative syndrome (identified in 10% of patients with 15-year follow-up) seemed to be associated with pituitary involvement.[750] Only 1% of unselected children with Langerhans cell histiocytosis living in Canada during a 15-year period had GHD.[751]

Growth Hormone Insensitivity

Mutations in GHR Signaling Proteins and ALS. Conditions of GH insensitivity, also referred to as primary IGF1 deficiency, encompass a variety of genetic conditions characterized by growth failure, high serum GH levels, and very low serum IGF1 levels.[752] These findings, first described in siblings in 1966 by Laron and colleagues,[753] are also known collectively as *Laron syndrome*. Fewer than 500 cases of true GH insensitivity have been identified worldwide, with most individuals from pedigrees of Mediterranean or Middle Eastern descent. Members of a well-described pedigree from Ecuador were from an inbred population with Mediterranean origins.[754]

The phenotypic characteristics of GH insensitivity include growth failure evident at birth[753] with postnatal subnormal growth velocities and stature −4 to −10 SD below the mean (Fig. 24-34).[752] Patients also have a subnormal head circumference, protruding forehead, abnormal upper- to lower-body ratio, short extremities, and sparse hair (Table 24-4). There is delayed motor development, indicating the importance of IGF1 in cerebral development. The genitalia are small, and puberty is delayed, but fertility is normal. Metabolically, the most striking feature of IGF1 deficiency is hypoglycemia with later development of obesity, relative hyperinsulinemia, and insulin resistance.[755] Individuals do not respond to exogenous GH, as

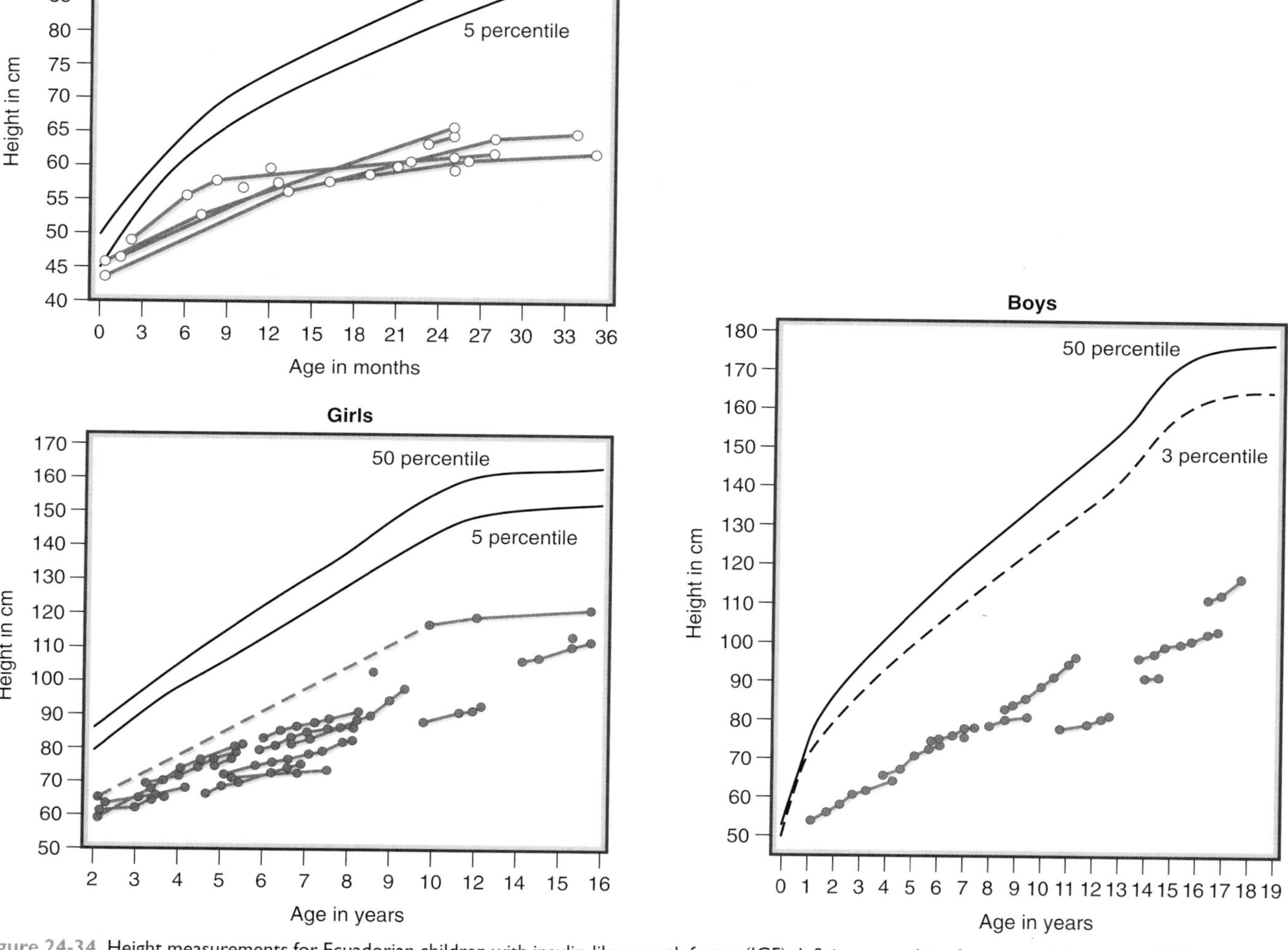

Figure 24-34 Height measurements for Ecuadorian children with insulin-like growth factor (IGF) deficiency resulting from growth hormone (GH) insensitivity. (From Rosenfeld RG, Rosenbloom AL, Guevara-Aguirre J. Growth hormone [GH] resistance due to primary GH receptor deficiency. *Endocr Rev.* 1994;15:369-390.)

determined by growth velocity, hypoglycemia incidence, or serum IGF1 or IGFBP1 levels.[756] In addition, GHBP activity is usually undetectable in sera of these patients,[757,758] but measurable levels correspond to higher final heights.

Almost 20 years after the original description of GH insensitivity, liver biopsy performed on two affected patients demonstrated that microsomal cells did not bind recombinant GH, suggesting a defect in the GHR.[759] Subsequently, both deletions and homozygous point mutations (missense, nonsense, and abnormal splicing) in the GHR were described in persons with GH insensitivity.[702,760,761] The initial described gene deletion involved exons 3, 5, and 6.[762] Deletion of exons 5 and 6 results in a frameshift and a premature translational stop signal with consequent encoding of a receptor lacking most of the extracellular GH-binding domain.

More than 60 distinct mutations of the GHR gene resulting in GH insensitivity have been reported to date.[763] Most of the mutations are in the extracellular (GH-binding) domain of the receptor and result in impaired ability of GH to bind to the receptor; this leads to a deficiency of circulating GHBP, which is derived from the extracellular domain of the receptor. One reported mutation of the extracellular domain does not affect GH binding to the receptor but prevents dimerization of the receptor.[188] Homozygous mutations have also been reported in the transmembrane domain.[189,764] These mutations result in GH insensitivity with normal GH binding but lack of receptor transduction. Because the extracellular domain is intact and the mutant receptor protein apparently becomes detached from the cell receptor surface, GHBP levels are normal to elevated.

Mutations affecting the intracellular domain of the GHR have also been found. Two defects directly involving the intracellular domain have been reported to result in dominantly inherited GH insensitivity.[765-770] In the two heterozygous mutations reported, truncation of the GHR results in absence of the intracellular domain. In vitro, the GHR molecule behaves in a dominant negative manner, presumably by retaining an ability to dimerize with the normal GHR and thereby inhibiting GH-induced tyrosine phosphorylation of STAT5.[769-771] Mutations resulting in C-terminal deletions of the intracellular domain of the GHR have been shown to exhibit normal GH binding and

TABLE 24-4

Clinical Features of Classic Growth Hormone Insensitivity

Parameter	Clinical Finding
Growth and Development	
Birth weight	Near-normal
Birth length	May be slightly decreased
Postnatal growth	Severe growth failure
Bone age	Delayed, but may be advanced relative to height age
Genitalia	Micropenis in childhood; normal for body size in adults
Puberty	Delayed 3 to 7 years
Sexual function and fertility	Normal
Craniofacies	
Hair	Sparse before age 7 years
Forehead	Prominent; frontal bossing
Skull	Normal head circumference; craniofacial disproportion due to small facies
Facies	Small
Nasal bridge	Hypoplastic
Orbits	Shallow
Dentition	Delayed eruption
Sclerae	Blue
Voice	High-pitched
Musculoskeletal/Metabolic/Miscellaneous	
Blood glucose	Hypoglycemia in infants and children; fasting symptoms in some adults
Walking and motor milestones	Delayed
Hips	Dysplasia; avascular necrosis of femoral head
Elbow	Limited extensibility
Skin	Thin, prematurely aged
Bone mineral density	Osteopenia

JAK2 phosphorylation but impaired phosphorylation of STAT5B.[772,773]

That a dominant negative effect has been described for some mutations raises the question of whether heterozygosity for defects of the extracellular domain can also result in short stature. Heterozygosity for defects of the GHR has been reported to cause some degree of relative GH insensitivity, with modest growth improvement occurring only with high doses of GH.[774-777] In addition, a truncated GHR splice variant has been described that functions as a dominant negative inhibitor of the full-length receptor and results in large amounts of GHBP, further downregulating GHR function.[778]

The most extensively studied polymorphism in the GHR gene is the deletion of exon 3 *(GHRd3)*, which is present in up to 50% of Caucasians. It has been proposed that GHRs without exon 3 bind GH with comparable affinity[779,780] but may transduce the signal with a different intensity in vitro.[781] In an observational study, GH treatment of short children with GHD found that those with one or two copies of the *GHRd3* variant grew faster than other children after correction for GH dosing.[781] Similar observations were reported in studies of patients with TS and children with SGA.[782] Different studies reported different findings on whether GH-deficient children with the *GHRd3* variant experience faster growth .[783-785] Different GH dosing between studies and differences among the populations studied could account for the varying results.

Some patients with the phenotype of GH insensitivity but without mutations of the GHR gene have been found to have mutations in downstream GHR signaling molecules. Homozygous mutations in the Stat5B gene have been found to cause GH insensitivity.[786,787] The first mutation characterized was a point mutation that causes a marked decrease in phosphorylation of thyrosine,[699] a critical step in the pathway to STAT activation of IGF1 gene transcription. The mutant Stat5B did not have the ability to dock with phosphotyrosines on GH-activated receptors or to stably bind DNA[788] and exhibited aberrant folding and diminished solubility with aggregation and inclusion body formation.[789] The second characterized mutation was an insertion in exon 10 that leads to early protein termination.[787] Both patients had evidence of immune dysfunction and recurrent pulmonary infections, presumably because Stat5B is involved in downstream signaling for multiple cytokines. To date, no mutations of the genes for JAK2 or MAP kinase have been implicated in GH insensitivity. Deletion of Jak2 in mice is embryonically lethal, as detailed earlier.

Markedly reduced serum concentrations of IGF1 and IGFBP3 have been observed in two cases involving mutations of the ALS gene.[790,791] Even though IGF1 and IGFBP3 were as low as in patients with classic GH insensitivity, the index case attained an adult height within the normal range. Whether the relatively normal growth of these patients reflects the greater importance of locally produced IGF1 or altered kinetics of serum IGF1 in the face of reduced concentrations of binding proteins remains uncertain.

Abnormalities of IGF1 and IGF1 Receptor Signaling. Woods and colleagues[792] described a 15-year-old boy with deletion of exons 4 and 5 of the IGF1 gene that resulted in a truncated IGF1 molecule. The boy exhibited severe prenatal and postnatal (approximately −7 SDS) growth retardation unresponsive to GH in addition to sensorineural deafness, mental retardation, and microcephaly. He had normal IGFBP3 and GHBP levels, undetectable IGF1 levels, and hyperinsulinism. On treatment with IGF1, the child experienced growth and improved metabolic parameters.[793]

Inactivating Mutation of the IGF1 Gene. An adult was identified who had the same phenotype as the boy with the IGF1 deletion but with markedly elevated serum IGF1 levels.[341] A homozygous point mutation in the IGF1 gene was found. This mutation resulted in an IGF1 molecule with markedly reduced affinity for the IGF1 receptor that poorly stimulated autophosphorylation of the IGF1 receptor and activation of AKT or ERK.[794] Family members heterozygous for this mutation were found to have significantly lower birth weight, final height, and head circumference, suggesting an effect of heterozygosity for this mutation on IGF1 function.

Primary Defects of IGF Transport and Clearance. An extremely short boy (−6 SDS) with increased GH, normal IGF1, and 20- to 30-fold elevated IGFBP1 levels had improvement in growth and suppression of IGFBP1 levels with GH administration. The growth failure was hypothesized to result from inhibition of IGF1 action by IGFBP1. Tollefson and colleagues identified a child with growth failure whose fibroblasts were resistant to IGF1.[795] The fibroblasts were able to be stimulated with an IGF variant that exhibited a 600-fold lower binding affinity for IGFBPs and secreted more IGFBPs than normal, suggesting an IGFBP inhibition of IGF1 action.

Primary Defects of IGF1 Receptor Production or Responsiveness. In mouse knockout models, homozygous mutations of the IGF1 receptor resulted in profound growth failure and neonatal mortality, so it is doubtful that significant mutations of the IGF1 receptor will be found in patients. Patients with IUGR and postnatal growth failure, microcephaly, and mental retardation with normal to elevated serum IGF1 levels have been reported to have reduced binding of IGF1 to its receptor.[349,796] Studies in the African Efe pygmies demonstrated extreme insensitivity to the in vitro growth-enhancing effects of IGF1.[797] Explanations for these findings include reduced IGF1 receptor transcripts and sites with resultant diminished tyrosine phosphorylation and postreceptor signaling.

In leprechaunism, a syndrome of growth failure and insulin receptor dysfunction, there is variable IGF1 insensitivity.[798,799] The profound abnormality of the insulin receptor suggests that heterodimeric insulin and IGF1 receptor combinations might lead to failed activation of the IGF1 signaling cascade. The IGF1 receptor gene resides on 15q, so persons with deletions of the distal long arm of chromosome 15 or ring chromosome 15 have heterozygosity of the IGF1 receptor.[798,800] These patients may have IUGR and postnatal growth failure, but lack of a biologic response to IGF1 has not be conclusively demonstrated.[800] Therefore, whether the growth failure is caused by altered levels of IGF1 receptor or is a result of the loss of other genes located on 15q remains to be determined.

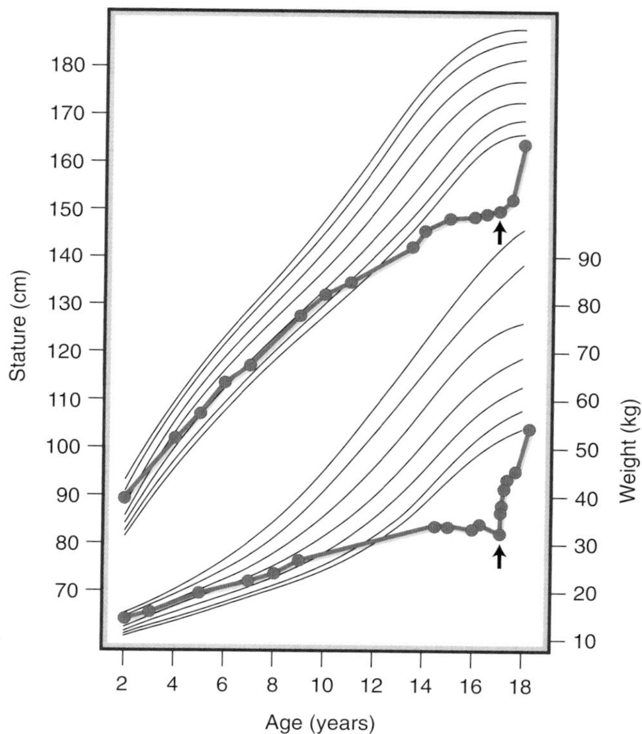

Figure 24-35 Curves of weight and height for a child who had growth failure resulting from prolonged self-imposed caloric restriction due to a fear of becoming obese. Notice that crossing of percentiles on the weight curve preceded that on the height curve, and that, after caloric intake was normalized (*arrow*), gain in weight occurred before improvement in linear growth. At the end of the prolonged period of caloric restriction, weight age (10.2 years) was less than height age (12 years). (From Pugliese MT, Lifshitz F, Grad G, et al. Fear of obesity: a cause of short stature and delayed puberty. *N Engl J Med.* 1983;309:513-518. Reprinted by permission of the *New England Journal of Medicine*.)

Disorders outside the Growth Hormone-IGF Axis

Many systemic disorders, if severe enough, can cause growth failure in children. Those that primarily alter hormones that directly regulate growth (e.g., thyroid hormone, glucocorticoids) can be understood based on the known actions of those hormones. Even in those disorders in which the pathology is not primarily within the endocrine system, there is often an underlying hormonal abnormality contributing to the growth failure. In some cases, the underlying disorder produces a secondary hormone deficiency. Those disorders in which a hormone deficiency cannot be identified may be thought of as demonstrating hormone resistance, because these children have growth failure in the presence of normal GH production.

Malnutrition

Given the worldwide presence of undernutrition, it is not surprising that inadequate intake of energy (calories) or protein or both is the most common cause of growth failure.[801] *Marasmus* refers to an overall deficiency of calories including protein malnutrition. Subcutaneous fat is minimal, and protein wasting is marked. *Kwashiorkor* refers specifically to inadequate protein intake, although it may also be characterized by some caloric undernutrition. In both conditions, multiple deficiencies of vitamins and minerals are apparent.[802] Frequently, the two conditions overlap. Decreased weight growth usually precedes the failure of linear growth by a very short time in the neonatal period and by several years at older ages. Stunting of growth due to caloric or protein malnutrition in early life often has lifelong consequences, including diminished skeletal growth.[803]

Both acute and chronic malnutrition affect the GH/IGF1 system. The impaired growth seen in malnutrition is usually associated with elevated basal or stimulated serum GH levels,[804-806] although in some cases of generalized malnutrition (marasmus) the GH levels are normal or low.[807] In both conditions, serum IGF1 levels are reduced.[808,809] The increase in GH levels is caused by a decrease in negative feedback by IGF1 and a decrease in somatostatin tone.[810] Malnutrition also results in increased ghrelin levels,[811,812] which could also contribute to an increase in GH secretion, although the role of ghrelin in regulating GH secretion remains unclear.[813] With serum IGF1 levels reduced despite normal or elevated GH levels, malnutrition is a form of GH insensitivity. One cause of this insensitivity is a decrease in GHR expression, which is reflected in decreased serum GHBP levels.[423,805] This GH insensitivity may be an adaptive response, diverting scarce energy resources from growth toward use for acute metabolic needs. The low IGF1 minimizes stimulation of anabolism, whereas the direct actions of the elevated GH levels (e.g., lipolysis, insulin antagonism) may increase the availability of energy substrates.[814,815] These adaptive mechanisms are accompanied by changes in serum IGFBPs that further limit IGF action during periods of malnutrition.[805,816]

Inadequate calorie or protein intake complicates many chronic diseases that are characterized by growth failure. Anorexia is a common feature of renal failure and inflammatory bowel disease, and it also occurs with cyanotic heart disease, congestive heart failure, CNS disease, and other illnesses. Some of these conditions may be further characterized by deficiencies of specific dietary components, such as zinc, iron, and vitamins necessary for normal growth and development.

Undernutrition may also be voluntary, as with dieting and food fads (Fig. 24-35).[817] Caloric restriction is especially common in girls during adolescence, in whom it may be associated with anxiety concerning obesity, and in gymnasts and ballet dancers. Anorexia nervosa and bulimia are extremes of "voluntary" caloric deprivation that are commonly associated with impaired growth before epiphyseal fusion, which may result in diminished final adult height.[818-820] Adolescent bone mineral accretion is impaired, and significant osteopenia may persist into adulthood.[821] Later in adolescence, malnutrition may cause delayed puberty or menarche or both, as well as a variety of metabolic alterations. In anorexia nervosa, hormonal profiles are similar to those in protein-energy malnutrition,[818-820,822] with high basal levels of GH. However, in contrast to chronic critical illness, in which there is an increase in nonpulsatile secretion but a decrease in pulsatile GH secretion, in anorexia both nonpulsatile and pulsatile secretion of GH are increased.[810] The GH secretion stimulated by insulin-induced hypoglycemia, dopaminergic agents, or acute administration of dexamethasone is impaired in patients with anorexia nervosa, whereas clonidine and arginine elicit normal GH responses. Finally, a paradoxical increase in GH release to intravenous glucose infusion has been described.[810] As in malnutrition in general, low levels of IGF1 and IGFBP3 are found in anorexia nervosa, indicating GH resistance. Similarly, GHBP levels are decreased,[810] indicating a decrease in GHR expression as a contributing factor to the GH resistance. The hormones of the GH-IGF1 axis return to normal levels with refeeding.[805,818,823]

A rare cause of failure to thrive in infants and young children is the diencephalic syndrome.[824] This syndrome is characterized by a marked impairment of weight gain, or even weight loss, but with normal linear growth (at least initially). It is caused by hypothalamic tumors. Similar to the findings in other causes of low weight for length or height, increased GH levels have been found in patients with diencephalic syndrome. As in patients with anorexia nervosa, GH levels paradoxically increase in response to a glucose load. However, in contrast to the increased GH secretion seen in malnutrition or anorexia nervosa, IGF1 levels are normal rather than decreased.[824] Therefore, diencephalic syndrome does not demonstrate GH resistance in the way that these other disorders do.

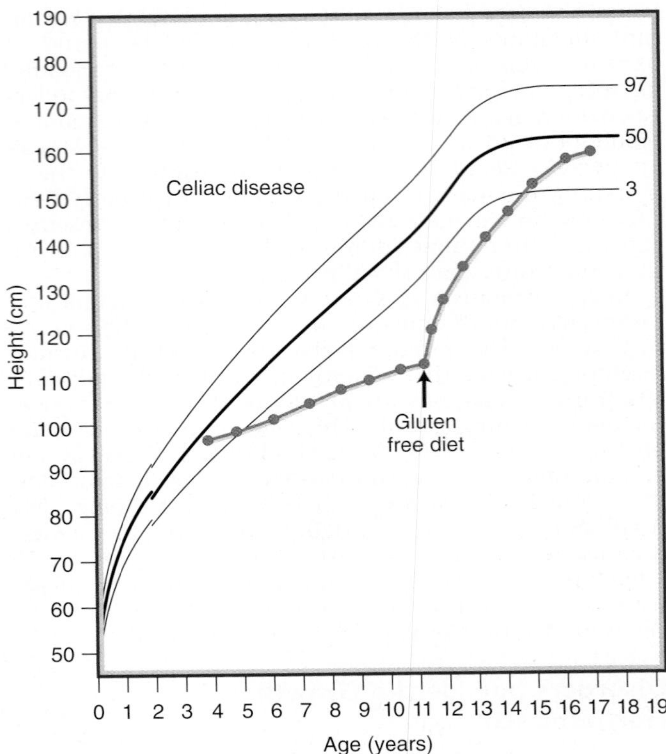

Figure 24-36 Catch-up growth in a girl with gluten-induced enteropathy (celiac disease). After 8 years of growth impairment, the patient was placed on a gluten-free diet and demonstrated substantial catch-up growth, returning to the previous growth percentiles. (Courtesy of J.M. Tanner.)

Chronic Diseases

Malabsorption and Gastrointestinal Diseases. Intestinal disorders that impair absorption of calories or protein cause growth failure, for many of the same reasons as malnutrition per se.[814,825-827] Growth retardation may predate other manifestations of malabsorption or chronic inflammatory bowel disease. Celiac disease (gluten-induced enteropathy) and regional enteritis (Crohn's disease) should be considered in the differential diagnosis of unexplained growth failure. Serum levels of IGF1 may be reduced,[814,828] reflecting the malnutrition, and it is critical to discriminate between these conditions and disorders related to GHD. Documentation of malabsorption requires demonstration of fecal wasting of calories, especially fecal fat, along with other measures of gut dysfunction such as the D-xylose or breath hydrogen studies.

In celiac disease, an immune-mediated disorder in which the intestinal mucosa is damaged by dietary gluten (Fig. 24-36), impaired linear growth may be the first manifestation of disease.[814,829-832] The degree of growth impairment may be similar in patients with or without gastrointestinal symptoms.[814] Celiac disease has an increased incidence in individuals with TS, insulin-dependent (type 1) diabetes mellitus (IDDM), Down syndrome, or Williams' syndrome. In European studies, celiac disease is the cause of unexplained growth impairment in 5% to 20% of unselected patients, although this high frequency does not hold true in many centers and may reflect varying stringency in the diagnostic criteria employed.[830-832] The onset and progression of puberty may be delayed, and menarche may be late.[829] Measurement of an immunoglobulin A (IgA) tissue transglutaminase antibody (tTG-IgA)[833] is the currently recommended screening test. This test has a sensitivity of up to 99%, with much higher specificity than IgA gliadin antibodies (AGA-IgA). However, tTG-IgA has significantly lower sensitivity in children less than 18 months of age,[834] where it may be preferable to also measure AGA-IgA. When measuring IgA antibodies, it is necessary to measure total IgA levels to exclude IgA deficiency, particularly because IgA deficiency has an increased incidence in patients with celiac disease.[835] (In subjects with IgA deficiency, tTG-IgG may be used.[835]) Nonetheless, the diagnosis of celiac disease ultimately requires demonstration of the characteristic mucosal flattening in small bowel biopsy. The incidence of childhood celiac disease in the United States is about 0.9%.[836] Gluten withdrawal is a highly effective treatment for celiac disease and results in rapid catch-up growth and decreased clinical symptoms during the first 6 to 12 months of treatment.[814,829] Low IGF1 and IGFBP3 levels return to normal during this period.[828,837] Most children who receive appropriate dietary management ultimately achieve a normal final height.[838,839]

Growth failure in Crohn's disease, which correlates with disease severity,[840,841] is probably due to a combination of malnutrition from malabsorption, anorexia, nutrient loss, chronic inflammation,[826,827,841] inadequacy of trace minerals in the diet, and use of glucocorticoids. IGF1 levels are low, especially with impaired growth.[814,827] In an animal model, approximately one half of the decrease in IGF1 levels was accounted for by undernutrition, with the other half attributable to the effects of inflammation.[842] One third to two thirds or more of children with Crohn's disease have impaired growth at diagnosis. In some patients, the growth failure precedes clinical symptoms of bowel disease by a few years, with a significant number showing linear growth failure before any weight loss.[814,827,841,843,844] Adequate nutritional supplementation and surgical resection of the diseased intestine can lead to improved growth, but surgery is not always an option.[845-848] Osteopenia is common.[849,850] An elevated erythrocyte sedimentation rate, anemia, and low serum albumin are useful clues, but diagnosis of Crohn's disease ultimately requires colonoscopy and biopsy, along with gastrointestinal imaging studies. Permanent impairment of linear growth and deficits of final height may occur in 30% of patients.[851] Approximately 20% of patients at adult height are more than 8 cm below the midparental target height.[852] Small, mostly uncontrolled trials of GH treatment in children with Crohn's disease have had conflicting results: some have shown improved growth velocity,[853,854] but others have not.[855] Some have shown improved body composition and BMD.[853] None of the reports, however, has extended beyond 2 years of treatment to determine whether there is a long-term benefit.

Chronic Liver Disease. Chronic liver disease in childhood can cause impaired linear growth. Decreased food intake, fat and fat-soluble vitamin malabsorption, and trace element deficiencies contribute to growth failure.[856-860] In addition, these children show evidence of GH resistance, having decreased levels of IGF1 and IGFBP3 and increased GH secretion.[861-864] IGF2 levels are also decreased, and IGFBP1 levels are increased.[861-863] Although the low IGF1 levels might be due to the impaired synthetic capacity of the liver, there is decreased expression of the GHR in cirrhotic liver, just as in malnutrition.[865] However, despite provision of adequate calories, insensitivity to the action of GH persists,[859,862] suggesting that the GH resistance of liver failure is not due solely to malnutrition. Liver transplantation prolongs life expectancy, and linear growth is variably improved in the early post-transplantation years.[858,863,866,867] Exogenous glucocorticoid administration presumably plays a major role in the continued growth retardation[858,867]; GH and IGF1 production are normal, but the amount of "free IGF" may be decreased, because IGFBP3 levels are relatively high.[863,866] Post-transplantation growth is inversely correlated with age and directly correlated with the degree of growth impairment at transplantation.[857,858,866] Exogenous GH treatment enhances growth rates and increases median height SDS by 0.3 to 0.6 units after 1 year of treatment,[868-870] with continued increases in height SDS for up to 5 years during treatment.[868]

Cardiovascular Disease. Congenital heart disease with cyanosis or chronic congestive heart failure can cause growth failure.[871-873] As many as 27% of children with varied cardiac lesions were below the 3rd percentile for height and weight in one survey,[874] and 70% were lower than the 50th percentile in another.[875] Because cardiac defects are usually congenital, many infants have dysmorphic features and IUGR. Inadequate caloric intake is the most common cause of growth impairment in children with congenital heart disease[873,875,876] and is frequently associated with anorexia and vomiting. Chronic congestive heart failure is associated with malabsorption that includes protein-losing enteropathy, intestinal lymphangiectasia, and steatorrhea. Greater cardiac and respiratory work requirement and the relatively higher ratio of metabolically active, energy-utilizing brain and heart tissue to the growth-retarded body mass (cardiac cachexia[877]) cause an increased basal metabolic rate in these children.[878-880] Food intake that appears adequate for the child's weight is often inadequate for normal growth. The degree of cyanosis or hypoxia does correlate with the degree of growth impairment.[873,875,881] Decreased levels of IGF1 and IGFBP3[880,882,883] and normal levels of GH and hepatic GHRs in chronically hypoxemic newborn sheep[883] suggest GH insensitivity distal to the GHR. Linear growth and pubertal maturation depend on left ventricular function in children and adolescents with complicated rheumatic heart disease.[884]

Corrective surgery may restore normal growth, frequently after a phase of catch-up growth with normalization of energy expenditure.[879,885] Surgery must, on occasion, be delayed until the infant reaches an appropriate size, resulting in the conundrum that surgery corrects growth failure but cannot be performed because the infant is too small. In these situations, meticulous attention to caloric support and alleviation of hypoxia and heart failure are necessary to promote growth before surgery. This problem has diminished over time because of operative successes in the neonatal period. The nutritional management of these infants includes calorie-dense feedings because of the need to restrict fluids, calcium supplementation because of the use of diuretics that can cause calcium loss in the urine, and iron to maintain an enhanced rate of erythropoiesis.

Renal Disease. All conditions that impair renal function can impair growth.[886-890] Uremia and renal tubular acidosis can cause growth failure before other clinical manifestations become evident. The growth impairment results from multiple mechanisms, including inadequate formation of 1,25-dihydroxycholecalciferol (1,25-dihydroxyvitamin D_3, calcitriol) with resultant osteopenia, decreased caloric intake, loss of electrolytes necessary for normal growth, metabolic acidosis, protein wasting, insulin resistance, chronic anemia, compromised cardiac function, and impairment of GH and IGF production and action. In nephropathic cystinosis, acquired hypothyroidism contributes to the inadequate growth.[891] Between 60% and 75% of patients with chronic renal failure treated before the GH therapeutic era had final adult heights more than 2 SD below the mean.[892]

The effects of renal failure on the GH-IGF1 axis are complex, and there is evidence for both GH and IGF1 resistance. Children and adolescents have normal or elevated circulating levels of GH, depending on the degree of renal failure.[887,888,893-897] The increased GH levels result from both an increase in GH secretory bursts and a decrease in renal GH clearance.[898] Serum IGF1 and IGF2 levels are usually normal in patients with renal failure.[887,893,894,899,900] Early reports of decreased serum IGF levels in uremia were an artifact caused by inadequate separation of IGF from IGFBPs before assay.[901] However, the normal IGF1 levels in the face of elevated GH levels denotes GH resistance, which is also indicated by the finding of decreased hepatic IGF1 production.[902] The mechanism for GH resistance includes decreased GHR gene expression in the liver and in the growth plate.[899,903] There is also evidence that the uremic state causes a postreceptor defect in GH signal transduction by diminishing phosphorylation and nuclear translocation of GH-activated STAT proteins.[898,904,905] Although a defect in IGF1 receptor signaling has been demonstrated in renal failure,[903] the more important mechanism for decreased IGF1 action in renal failure is alterations in the serum level of IGFBPs that decrease the bioavailability of IGF1. IGFBPs 1, 2, 4, and 6 are increased.[887,888,903,906-910] In addition, low-molecular-weight IGFBP3 fragments, which have decreased affinity for IGF1, accumulate due to reduced renal clearance.[903] In nephrotic syndrome, an additional contribution to growth failure may come from reduced serum levels of IGF1 and IGFBP3 resulting from urinary loss of IGF-IGFBP complexes.[889] Finally, glucocorticoid therapy that may be used for treatment of the renal disease can exacerbate growth retardation by diminishing GH release and blunting IGF1 action at growth plates.[909,911-913]

Even after successful renal transplantation, growth may not be normal.[914-918] In the large cohort of patients in the North American Pediatric Renal Transplant Cooperative Study,[916,918,919] mean height increased after transplantation by only 0.11 SD in the first 4.5 years. The youngest age group (<2 years) had the largest deficit and the most catch-up growth (0.94 SD); children between 6 and 17 years of age had no improvement in height SD score. Although the younger age group had a 16% mortality rate,[916] more recent studies[920,921] suggest that transplantation may have an acceptable high risk in such patients. Growth-retarded post-transplantation children receiving daily or alternate-day glucocorticoid treatment have decreased GH secretion, normal levels of IGF1 and IGFBP1, and elevated levels of IGFBP3. They differ from patients with end-stage renal disease in that IGFBP1 levels are not strikingly elevated, perhaps because of altered glucose tolerance and hyperinsulinism due to chronic glucocorticoid therapy.[909] Overall, height SDS at the time of transplantation and use of alternate-day glucocorticoid therapy after transplant correlate positively with final height, and longer duration of reduced GFR and a higher cumulative dose of prednisone have a negative impact; other factors such as gender, age at transplantation, diagnosis, and number of transplants do not seem to have significant impact on adult height.[914] The importance of height at the time of transplantation in determining final adult height, despite the complex post-transplantation health issues, confirms the value of improving growth velocity and absolute height before transplantation. Children who receive tacrolimus (FK-506)-based immunosuppression, allowing discontinuation of glucocorticoids, have normal growth and absence of obesity.[922]

Although the growth failure of renal disease in the pretransplantation period is not specifically caused by GHD, GH therapy accelerates skeletal growth and is approved by the U.S. Food and Drug Administration (FDA) for use. Such treatment probably increases the molar ratio of IGF peptides to IGFBPs and may override the inhibitory actions of IGFBPs.

Hematologic Disorders. Chronic anemias, such as sickle cell disease, are characterized by growth failure.[923,924] In general, the decrease in height and weight is greater in adolescent years than earlier, because the onset of the adolescent growth spurt is delayed and menarche is late.[923-925] However, the adolescent growth and final adult height in patients with sickle cell disease may be normal.[925] The causes of growth retardation probably include impaired oxygen delivery to tissues, increased work of the cardiovascular system, energy demands of increased hematopoiesis, and impaired nutrition. Long-term chronic transfusion therapy as part of stroke prevention treatment is associated with enhanced growth.[926] The GH/IGF1 system probably does not have an important role in the growth impairment of sickle cell anemia.

In thalassemia, in addition to the consequences of chronic anemia, endocrine deficiencies can result from chronic transfusions and accompanying hemosiderosis.[927] Despite vigorous efforts to maintain hemoglobin levels near normal and to avoid iron overload, growth failure is still a common feature of thalassemia, especially in male adolescents.[928] The patients tend to show body disproportion, with truncal shortening but normal leg length. It is likely that anemia, impaired IGF1 synthesis, hypothyroidism, gonadal failure, and hypogonadotropic hypogonadism all contribute to growth failure in this disorder. GH insensitivity in some cases is suggested by generally adequate GH production with low IGF1 levels.[929,930] Several groups have reported data on treatment of thalassemia patients in whom GH production seemed diminished. In most patients, GH treatment increased growth, at least initially.[929,931] In a longer-term study (average duration, 59 months) starting with young patients (7.2 years of age), an increased growth velocity was maintained throughout the treatment period[932]; when treatment was initiated at an older age (13.6 years), final height was not improved.[933] A small number of adults with thalassemia are found to have continued GHD, so GH treatment for cardiac and bone health reasons may be important in this disease.[934]

About half of the patients in the International Fanconi Anemia Registry have short stature. GHD was demonstrated by provocative testing (22 of 48 patients) or with assessment of endogenous secretion (13 of 13) in a group with a mean height of −2.23 SDS.[935] In pure red-cell aplasia,[936] approximately 30% of patients demonstrated growth retardation. The frequency increased with age (42% in individuals >16 years) and with treatment programs such as chronic transfusions or glucocorticoids.

Inborn Errors of Metabolism. Inborn errors of metabolism are often accompanied by growth failure that may be pronounced. Glycogen storage disease, the mucopolysaccharidoses, glycoproteinoses, and mucolipidoses are characterized by poor growth. Many inborn metabolic disorders are also associated with significant skeletal dysplasia. In a small number of patients with organic acidoses, such as methylmalonic and propionic acidurias, IGF1 levels are low and GH levels are normal, suggesting a possible state of GH insensitivity related to nutritional status.[937] Preliminary data suggest that exogenous GH treatment may improve the metabolic status of such children.[937,938]

Pulmonary Disease. Growth can be retarded in children with asthma who have not received glucocorticoid therapy.[939,940] Mean height and growth velocity and degree of growth failure are related to the severity of the asthma.[939,940] Delayed pubertal maturation in such patients is also associated with growth deceleration in early teenage years.[939,941] Impaired nutrition and increased energy requirements, along with chronic stress, especially with nocturnal asthma and enhanced endogenous glucocorticoid production, cause poor linear growth. The lowered growth in asthmatic children does not appear to be associated with abnormalities of the GH-IGF1 axis.[942] Glucocorticoid therapy, which is typically given to more severely affected patients, further impairs growth throughout childhood.[943-945]

Synthetic glucocorticoids, such as prednisone or dexamethasone, may have a greater growth-suppressive effect than equivalent therapeutic doses of cortisol, presumably because the biopotency of the synthetic agents may be underestimated. Alternate-day or aerosolized glucocorticoid therapy often ameliorates growth retardation and can be associated with an accelerated catch-up phase.[939,944] Intermittent glucocorticoid therapy is usually not associated with impaired final height. The use of spacer devices and effective nebulizer solutions may permit use of inhaled glucocorticoids in young children without growth impairment.[946-948] Clearly, however, sufficient glucocorticoid delivered by any route can diminish growth and impede the function of the adrenal gland.[949] Nonetheless, judicious use of inhaled glucocorticoid results in normal adult height despite long-term exposure and an initial decrement of linear growth velocity.[950,951] Indeed, examination of near-adult heights of Swedish men with asthma demonstrated an improvement in the mean difference between "severe" asthmatics and normal controls in the era of inhaled corticosteroid use.[952] Overall, normal adult height is usually achieved.[953,954]

Bronchopulmonary dysplasia (BPD), a sequela of neonatal respiratory distress syndrome and prematurity, has an incidence as high as 35% in infants with very low birth weight (<1500 g).[955] The use of dexamethasone in the treatment of BPD in neonates causes a transient cessation of growth[956] and has engendered long-term concern for neurodevelopment and somatic growth.[957] Growth in surviving infants is poor through early childhood,[958-960] but the defect usually disappears by 8 years of age.[961-963] Long-term hypoxemia, poor nutrition, chronic pulmonary infections, and reactive airway disease are responsible for the poor early growth.

In patients with cystic fibrosis, chronic pulmonary infection with bronchiectasis, pancreatic insufficiency with exocrine and endocrine inadequacy, malabsorption, and malnutrition all contribute to decreased growth and late sexual maturation. In 17,857 patients with cystic fibrosis, mean height was at the 21st percentile and mean weight was at the 9th percentile.[964] Early impairment of height and weight growth and retardation of skeletal maturation may progress or plateau during middle childhood years but become most marked in the preadolescent period, when growth and maturational changes are frequently delayed.[964-966] The degree of growth retardation is related most closely to the severity and variability of the pulmonary disease rather than to pancreatic dysfunction.[967,968] The degree of steatorrhea does not correlate well with growth impairment, although improved nutrition programs enhance the overall clinical picture.[969,970] Adult heights in surviving patients with cystic fibrosis approach the normal range[825] but remain lower than average.[971] Endocrine abnormalities, such as failure of both alpha and beta islet cells with decreased glucagon and insulin production, do not seem to influence prepubertal growth patterns in children with cystic fibrosis. The incidence of diabetes mellitus increases as patients live past the second decade.[964] Alterations of vitamin D metabolism, while potentially affecting skeletal mineralization, do not diminish growth.[972] Delayed sexual maturation, in which administration of gonadotropin-releasing hormone (GnRH) evokes a prepubertal pattern of pituitary gonadotropin secretion in adolescent patients, is similar to that in patients with CDGD.[973,974]

The GH-IGF1 axis in cystic fibrosis patients shows evidence for some degree of acquired GH insensitivity with lowered mean IGF1 and elevated GH levels.[975] Treatment of prepubertal cystic fibrosis patients with GH for 1 year resulted in an anabolic effect, with greater growth velocity and nitrogen retention and increased protein and decreased fat stores.[976,977] In a separate study, 1 year of GH treatment increased the gain in height, weight, and bone mineral content, improved the clinical status, and decreased hospitalizations.[978] In a 2-year GH treatment program for cystic fibrosis patients who received enteral nutrition before and during GH therapy, auxologic parameters continued to improve.[979] Pulmonary function improved in most patients. A 4-year longitudinal study using the National Cystic Fibrosis Foundation registry found that improved nutrition status and growth were associated with a slower age-related decrement of pulmonary function.[980] Current perspective suggests that GH treatment should be considered for adjunctive use as part of therapy with an aggressive nutritional program, appropriate pulmonary care without glucocorticoid administration, and careful assessment of carbohydrate metabolism.[981]

Chronic Inflammation and Infection. Poor growth is a characteristic feature of chronic inflammatory disease and recurrent serious infection. The impaired growth associated with such disorders as Crohn's disease, cystic fibrosis, and asthma, in which inflammatory processes may be significant, has already been discussed. Inflammatory states are associated with increased levels of numerous cytokines. IL6, specifically, has been implicated in this growth impairment. De Benedetti and colleagues,[982] studying juvenile rheumatoid arthritis in humans and in a transgenic murine model expressing excessive IL6, demonstrated an IL6-mediated decrease in IGF1 production. IL6 has been demonstrated to activate SOCS3; this provides a pathway for inflammation to inhibit IGF1 production, because SOCS3 is a negative regulator of the JAK2/STAT5 GH signal transduction pathway.[159,842,983] IL6 may also cause a decrease in serum IGF1 levels by increasing its clearance through a decrease in IGFBP3 levels.[842] In addition, cytokines can affect the endocrine system at many other levels,[984,985] impairing mineral and nutrient metabolism and the growth and remodeling of bone.[986]

Exposure to human immunodeficiency virus (HIV) in children and adolescents occurs through perinatal transmission, blood transfusions, drug usage, and sexual contact. Growth failure is a cardinal feature of childhood acquired immunodeficiency syndrome (AIDS).[987-992] However, HIV-infected infants and children show growth failure even before demonstrating severe immune dysfunction.[993,994] Weight, length, and head circumference are all affected, although weight-for-height may be normal.[990,992,995] Before the era of highly active antiretroviral therapy (HAART), height growth velocity was associated with survival, independent of either $CD4^+$ T-cell lymphocyte count or viral load, with HAART therapy normalizing growth in most studies.[995] Studies of the GH-IGF1 axis in HIV-infected children have shown evidence of decreased GH secretion, GH resistance, and IGF1 resistance; both normal and low levels of GH and IGF1 are seen.[993] Lipodystrophy associated with HAART therapy occurs in children, although less commonly than in adults, and decreased GH secretion has been demonstrated in HIV-associated lipodystophy,[993] potentially contributing to impaired growth. HIV-infected children frequently have delayed puberty, which could contribute to their linear growth failure. In a short-term treatment trial with standard doses of GH, height and weight growth increased and protein catabolism diminished, without any adverse effect on viral burden.[996]

Endocrine Disorders

Hypothyroidism. Untreated severe congenital hypothyroidism results in profound growth failure. With proper treatment, however, children with congenital hypothyroidism reach a height appropriate for their genetic potential.[997]

Acquired hypothyroidism during childhood may also result in growth failure that can range from subtle to profound, depending on the severity and duration of the hypothyroidism. Growth failure may be the most prominent manifestation of hypothyroidism in children.[998] The poor growth is more apparent in height than in weight gain, so these children tend to be overweight for height. Rivkees and coworkers[998] reported a mean 4.2-year delay between slowing of growth and the diagnosis of hypothyroidism; at diagnosis, girls were 4.04 SD below and boys 3.15 SD below the mean height for their age. Skeletal maturation is delayed in those children in whom the hypothyroidism was sufficient to retard growth, with the bone age at diagnosis corresponding to the age at onset of the hypothyroidism.[998] Body proportion is immature, with an increased upper-to-lower body segment ratio. Although chronic hypothyroidism is usually associated with delayed puberty, precocious puberty and premature menarche can occur in hypothyroid children (see Chapter 13).

In those children with severe growth failure, treatment with thyroid hormone results in rapid catch-up growth. This is typically accompanied by marked skeletal maturation. In cases of prolonged severe hypothyroidism, the advancement of skeletal maturation with treatment can exceed the growth acceleration, resulting in a compromised adult height.[998] The deficit in adult stature correlates with the duration of hypothyroidism before initiation of treatment. Catch-up growth may be particularly compromised if therapy is initiated near puberty.[999]

As expected, hyperthyroidism has effects on growth opposite to those of hypothyroidism: it results in accelerated growth and epiphyseal maturation. Children with hyperthyroidism present with an increased height and advanced bone age. In neonates, hyperthyroidism can result in craniosynostosis. However, despite the advanced bone age at diagnosis, the final height of children treated for hyperthyroidism remains normal in relation to genetic potential.[1000]

Diabetes Mellitus. Although weight loss may occur immediately before the onset of clinically apparent IDDM, children with new-onset diabetes are frequently taller than their peer group, possibly because GH and insulin levels are increased during the preclinical evolution of the disease.[1001-1003] Most children with IDDM, even those with marginal control,[1004] grow quite normally, especially in prepubertal years, although growth velocity may decrease during puberty.[1005] However, growth failure can occur in diabetic children with long-standing poor glycemic control.[1006,1007] The Mauriac syndrome[1008] describes children with poorly regulated IDDM, severe growth failure, and hepatosplenomegaly due to excess hepatic glycogen deposition. This type of growth retardation has become increasingly rare with modern diabetes care.

Many pathophysiologic processes, including malnutrition, chronic intermittent acidosis, increased glucocorticoid production, hypothyroidism, impaired calcium balance, and end-organ unresponsiveness to either GH or IGF, may contribute to growth failure in IDDM.[1001,1009-1011] IGF1 and IGFBP3 levels are diminished in the face of enhanced GH production,[1012-1016] reflecting acquired GH insensitivity. GHBP levels are decreased,[1009,1015] supporting the concept of impaired GHR number or function. Furthermore, IGFBP1 is normally suppressed by insulin, and hypoinsulinemia results in elevated serum IGFBP1 levels that may inhibit IGF action.[1015,1017-1020] In contrast to the situation in adolescents and adults, IGFBP1 levels are not elevated in well-growing prepubertal children.[1019] On the contrary, increased IGFBP3 proteolysis may enhance the bioactivity of the available IGF1.[1016,1021] Most children with IDDM attain normal cellular nutrition and growth factor action despite intermittent hypoinsulinemia and derangements of peripheral indices of the GH/IGF1 system.

Even though glycemic control is inversely correlated with IGF I levels,[1010,1012,1015,1022] the correlation between glycemic control and growth is weak. After conflicting reports as to the influence of glycemic regulation on growth,[1001,1002,1023,1024] a longitudinal study[1024] of 46 children whose diabetes began before age 10 indicated that initial heights at diagnosis were normal and that the final height SDS was minimally reduced from that at onset. In boys, despite a delay of about 2.5 years in onset of puberty, total pubertal height gain was normal. In girls with diabetes, however, total pubertal height gain was diminished and the age at menarche was delayed; the effects of altered insulin and IGF1 levels on ovarian function have not been assessed in such patients. Chronic metabolic control did not correlate with the pubertal height gain or with the normal final height. Nevertheless, good glycemic control may improve growth at certain maturational periods such as puberty.[1001,1014,1025]

Cushing's Syndrome: Glucocorticoid Excess. Glucocorticoid excess impairs skeletal growth, interferes with normal bone metabolism by inhibiting osteoblastic activity, and enhances bone resorption.[1026-1028] These effects are related to the duration of steroid excess,[1029] regardless of whether the Cushing's syndrome is due to ACTH hypersecretion, adrenal tumor, or glucocorticoid administration.

Even modest doses of oral glucocorticoids can inhibit growth; these doses may be as low as 3 to 5 mg/m^2 per day of prednisone or 12 to 15 mg/m^2 per day of hydrocortisone (i.e., only slightly above what is considered physiologic replacement).[1030] The "toxic" effects of glucocorticoids on the epiphysis may persist to some degree after correction of chronic glucocorticoid excess, and patients frequently do not attain their target height.[685,1031] The longer the duration and the greater the intensity of glucocorticoid excess, the less likely is catch-up growth to be completed. Alternate-day glucocorticoid treatment decreases but does not eliminate the risk of growth suppression.[1032-1034] Inhaled glucocorticoids given for the treatment of asthma have an even lower risk of growth suppression, but even at modest doses (e.g., 400 μg/day of beclomethasone,[1035] 200 μg/day of fluticasone,[951,1035] or 400 μg/day of budesonide[951]) they can cause at least temporary slowing of growth. However, inhaled corticosteroids do not appear to impair final height.[950,951]

GH therapy can overcome some of the growth-inhibiting effects of excess glucocorticoids. The GH-induced increase in growth rate is inversely related to the glucocorticoid dose,[1036] with one small study finding no benefit of GH treatment for prednisone doses greater than 0.35 mg/kg per day.[1037] GH or IGF1 administration can diminish many of the catabolic effects of excess glucocorticoids.[1027,1038,1039]

Adrenal tumors secreting large amounts of glucocorticoids can produce excess androgens, which may mask the growth-inhibitory effects of glucocorticoids. In addition, Cushing's syndrome in children may not cause all the clinical signs and symptoms associated with the disorder in adults and may manifest with growth arrest. However, Cushing's syndrome is an unlikely diagnosis in children with obesity, because exogenous obesity is associated with normal or even accelerated skeletal growth and growth deceleration is usually evident by the time other signs of Cushing's syndrome appear (Fig. 24-37). In a series of 10 children and adolescents treated for Cushing's disease with surgery and cranial irradiation, post-therapy GHD was common and mean final height was −1.36 SDS.[1040]

Pseudohypoparathyroidism: Albright's Hereditary Osteodystrophy. Albright's hereditary osteodystrophy (AHO) is caused by mutations in the stimulatory GTP-binding protein, $G_s\alpha$. It exists both with and without multihormone resistance—termed pseudohypoparathyroidism type 1A (PHP-1A) and pseudo-pseudohypoparathyroidism

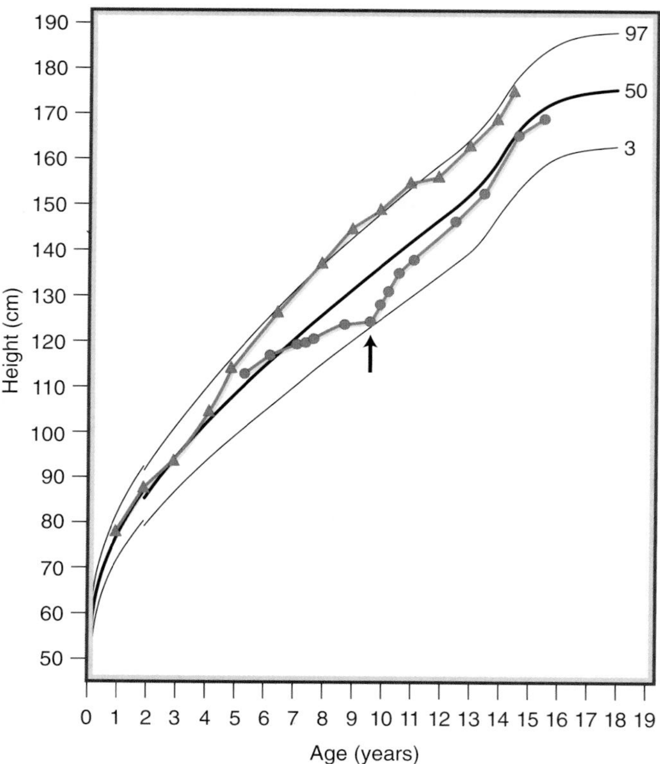

Figure 24-37 Growth curves of two boys with obesity. The boy depicted by the circles had cortisol excess related to Cushing's disease. He had onset of rapid weight gain associated with a decrease in linear growth velocity at age 7. The diagnosis was made, and an adrenalectomy (*arrow*) was performed at age 9½ years, with an almost immediate increase in growth rate and striking catch-up growth. The boy whose growth is depicted by triangles had exogenous obesity. At age 9½, his weight was approximately the same as that of the patient with Cushing's disease, but his height was at the 97th percentile, reflecting the enhancement of linear growth in individuals with exogenous obesity.

(pseudoPHP). This condition is discussed in detail in Chapter 25 but is included here because short adult height is a common feature.[1042] AHO is characterized by obesity (more marked in PHP-1A than in pseudo-PHP[1043]), short metacarpals, subcutaneous ossifications, round facies, and cognitive impairments. Patients with AHO, whether they have PHP-1A or pseudo-PHP, typically have short adult stature. Many patients with PHP-1A demonstrate GHD due to resistance to GHRH.[1044,1045] However, the growth pattern of patients with AHO suggests that there is another contributor to growth failure, because they often have only modest growth failure in early and middle childhood, with early epiphyseal fusion contributing to their short final height.[1046,1047]

Rickets. In the past, hypovitaminosis D was a major cause of short stature and was often associated with other causes of growth failure, such as malnutrition, prematurity, malabsorption, hepatic disease, or chronic renal failure (see Chapter 28). In isolated vitamin D deficiency, breast-fed infants typically have poor exposure to sunlight and are not nutritionally supplemented with vitamin D. Characteristic skeletal manifestations of rickets include frontal bossing, craniotabes, rachitic rosary, and bowing of the legs. Such children usually begin to synthesize 1,25-dihydroxyvitamin D_3 as they become older, broaden their diet, and have increased exposure to sunlight, with amelioration of the transient early decrease of linear growth velocity. The association of vitamin D receptor gene polymorphism with birth length, growth rate, adult stature, and BMD[1048-1052] further emphasizes the importance of vitamin D in normal growth. Additionally, vitamin D and estrogen receptor genotypes appear to interactively affect infant growth, especially in males.[1050,1053] The presence of high-affinity binding sites for the vitamin D receptor DNA-binding domain in the GH promoter suggests that the vitamin D receptor may actually modulate GH expression.[1054]

Hypophosphatemic Rickets. Hypophosphatemic rickets is n X-linked dominant disorder caused by decreased renal tubular reabsorption of phosphate related to mutations in the phosphate regulating endopeptidase gene, *PHEX*, located on chromosome Xp22.1. Other hypophosphatemic syndromes include autosomal-dominant hypophosphatemic rickets, hereditary hypophosphatemic rickets with hypercalciuria, and tumor-induced osteomalacia (see Chapter 28).[1055] In all of these conditions, there are increased levels of FGF23, perhaps a major phosphaturic agent.[1056] The features are usually more severe in boys and include short stature,[936,1057] prominent bowing of the legs, and, sometimes, rachitic signs.[1058] The metabolic and skeletal abnormalities cannot be overcome by vitamin D therapy alone.

Treatment of hypophosphatemic rickets requires oral phosphate replacement, but such therapy may result in poor calcium absorption from the intestine. The addition of calcitriol to oral phosphate increases intestinal phosphate absorption and prevents hypocalcemia and secondary hyperparathyroidism. Such combined therapy improves the rickets but does not necessarily correct growth.[1055,1059,1060,1061] Potential growth-related benefits of this regimen appear to be dependent on the initiation of therapy in early infancy, which leads to achievement of greater childhood and adult height.[1057] There is no clear association between endogenous GH secretion, IGF1, or phosphate levels and height in this disorder.[1062-1064] Nevertheless, GH therapy in eight trials including 83 patients resulted in an enhancement of skeletal growth and improvement in BMD.[1065-1067] In 14 of those patients, treatment for 4 to 5 years resulted in a height gain of up to 1.2 SDS. One report cautioned that GH treatment appeared to exaggerate disproportionate truncal growth.[1068]

Osteochondrodysplasias

The osteochondrodysplasias encompass a heterogeneous group of disorders characterized by intrinsic abnormalities of cartilage and bone.[1069,1070] These disorders include abnormalities in the size or shape of bones in the limbs, spine, or skull, often with abnormalities seen on radiographic evaluation. More than 100 osteochondrodysplasias have been identified based on physical characteristics and radiographic characteristics (Table 24-5). An international classification for the osteochondrodysplasias was developed in 1970[1071] and revised in 1978,[1072] 1992,[1073] 1997,[1074] and 2001.[1075]

Diagnosis of osteochondrodysplasias can be difficult, with clinical and radiologic evaluation central to the diagnosis. The family history is critical, although many cases are caused by de novo mutations, and this is generally the case in autosomal-dominant achondrodysplasia and hypochondrodysplasia. Measurement of body proportions should include arm span, sitting height, upper and lower body segments, and head circumference. Radiologic evaluation should be used to determine whether involvement is of the long bones, skull, or vertebrae and whether abnormalities are primarily at the epiphyses, metaphyses, or diaphyses. The osteochondrodysplasias most commonly encountered in endocrine practice are discussed in the following paragraphs.

TABLE 24-5

Classification of Osteochondrodysplasias

I. Defects of the Tubular (and Flat) Bones and/or Axial Skeleton
A. Achondroplasia group
B. Achondrogenesis
C. Spondylodysplastic group (perinatally lethal)
D. Metatropic dysplasia group
E. Short rib dysplasia group (with or without polydactyly)
F. Atelosteogenesis/diastrophic dysplasia group
G. Kniest-Stickler dysplasia group
H. Spondyloepiphyseal dysplasia congenita group
I. Other spondylo epiphyseal/metaphyseal dysplasias
J. Dysostosis multiplex group
K. Spondylometaphyseal dysplasias
L. Epiphyseal dysplasias
M. Chondrodysplasia punctata (stippled epiphyses) group
N. Metaphyseal dysplasias
O. Brachyrachia (short spine dysplasia)
P. Mesomelic dysplasias
Q. Acro/acromesomelic dysplasias
R. Dysplasias with significant (but not exclusive) membranous bone involvement
S. Bent bone dysplasia group
T. Multiple dislocations with dysplasias
U. Osteodysplastic primordial dwarfism group
V. Dysplasias with increased bone density
W. Dysplasias with defective mineralization
X. Dysplasias with increased bone density
II. Disorganized Development of Cartilaginous and Fibrous Components of the Skeleton
III. Idiopathic Osteolyses

Achondrodysplasia is the most common of the osteochondrodysplasias, with a frequency of 1 in 26,000 individuals. Characteristic abnormalities of the skeleton include megalocephaly, low nasal bridge, lumbar lordosis, short trident hand, and rhizomelia (shortness of the proximal legs and arms) with skin redundancy. Radiologic findings include small, cuboid-shaped vertebral bodies with short pedicles and progressive narrowing of the lumbar interpedicular distance. The small foramen magnum may lead to hydrocephalus, and spinal cord and root compression may result from kyphosis, stenosis of the spinal canal, or disc lesions.[1076,1077] Diminished growth velocity is present from infancy, although short stature may not be evident until after 2 years of age. Mean adult heights in males and females are 130 and 120 cm, respectively.[1078] GH secretion is comparable to that in normal subjects.[1079]

Achondrodysplasia is caused by mutations in the transmembrane domain of the FGF receptor 3 gene (*FGFR3*).[1073,1080-1083] It is transmitted in an autosomal dominant manner, but 80% to 90% of cases are caused by de novo mutations. Most of the cases are the result of activating mutations at nucleotide 1138 of the *FGFR3* gene, which creates new recognition sites for restriction enzymes, thus easing the molecular diagnosis. The mutation rate reported at this site is very high, and *FGFR3* has been labeled the most mutable gene in the genome. As a result of the upregulation of receptor activity, there is abnormal chondrogenesis and osteogenesis during endochondral ossification, leading to the typical phenotypic findings. The homogeneity of the mutation in achondroplasia probably explains the minimal heterogeneity in the phenotype. Infants homozygous for the mutation have severe disease, typically dying in infancy from respiratory insufficiency due to a small thorax. In mice with the equivalent *Fgfr3* mutation, there is ligand-independent dimerization and phosphorylation of Fgfr3 with activation of Stat proteins and upregulation of cell cycle inhibition.[1084] Expression of the Indian hedgehog and parathyroid hormone–related protein (PTHrP) receptor genes is downregulated.[1085]

Hypochondroplasia is also autosomal dominant, and 70% of affected individuals are heterozygous for mutations in the *FGFR3* gene, frequently at amino acid position.[1086] The facial features of achondroplasia are absent, and both short stature and rhizomelia are less pronounced. Adult heights are typically in the 120- to 150-cm range. Poor growth may not by evident until after 2 years of age, but stature then deviates progressively from normal. Occasionally, the disproportionate shorts stature is not apparent until adulthood. Outward bowing of the legs may be accompanied by genu varum. On radiologic evaluation, lumbar interpedicular distances are diminished between L1 and L5, and there may be flaring of the pelvis and narrow sciatic notches. The diagnosis can be difficult to make, with mild variants of the syndrome difficult to distinguish from normal.

The short stature homeobox-containing (SHOX) gene is located in the pseudoautosomal region of distal Xp and Yp. Mutations or deletion of *SHOX* is associated with syndromes of poor growth and skeletal dysplasia, including Léri-Weil dyschondrosteosis (LWD), TS, and Langer mesomelic dysplasia (LMD).[1087] Findings include short stature, Madelung deformity, increased carrying angle, tibial bowing, scoliosis, and high arched palate. The auxologic finding of relatively short limbs suggests a defect in *SHOX*, because the SHOX protein may affect cellular proliferation and apoptosis of chondrocytes at the growth plate.[1088] Indeed, the skeletal manifestations have been associated with areas in which there is intrauterine expression of *SHOX*.[1088,1089] LWD is caused by homozygous gene defects, whereas TS and LMD are caused by haploinsufficency. In LWD, most patients share a distinct 5-kb region for breakpoints, indicating a hot spot for mutations.[1090] The profound findings in LWD, compared with TS, may reflect the impact of pubertal estrogen exposure in LWD.[1091]

Endochondral growth is regulated by multiple endocrine, paracrine, and autocrine factors, and many inborn errors have been identified. In the syndrome of acromesomelic dysplasia, growth is remarkably impaired, leading to adult heights that may be more than 5 SD below the mean. A homozygous mutation in the homodimeric transmembrane natriuretic receptor B (NPR-B) that impairs binding of the ligand C-type natriuretic peptide has been found in some affected individuals.[1091] Obligatory heterozygotes are significantly shorter than normal but have normal skeletal anatomy.[1092] Therefore, heterozygous mutations of NPR-B demonstrate that a subset of children with unexplained short stature may, in fact, have mild forms of osteochondrodysplasias.

Chromosomal Abnormalities

Abnormalities of autosomes or sex chromosomes can cause growth retardation without evidence of skeletal dysplasia, frequently with somatic abnormalities and developmental delay. In many cases, the precise cause of growth failure is not clear because the genetic defects do not affect known components of the GH/IGF1 system. Chromosomal lesions may directly influence normal tissue growth and development or indirectly modulate local responsiveness to IGF or other growth factors at the growth plate.

Down Syndrome. Trisomy 21, or Down syndrome, is probably the most common chromosomal disorder associated with growth retardation, affecting approximately 1 in 600 neonates. On average, newborns with Down syndrome have birth weights 500 g below normal and are 2 to 3 cm shorter than normal. Growth failure continues postnatally and is typically associated with delayed skeletal maturation and a delayed and incomplete pubertal growth spurt. Adult heights range from 135 to 170 cm in men and 127 to 158 cm in women.[12] The etiology of growth failure in Down syndrome is unknown, and attempts to find underlying hormonal explanations for growth retardation have been unsuccessful. Marginal levels of GH secretion and low-normal serum levels of IGF1 has been reported in patients with Down syndrome. Exogenous GH has been tried in some of these patients and have produced short-term increases in growth velocity, but the long-term effects on final adult height have not been studied. In addition, no improvement in gross motor or mental development was noted.[1093,1094] Hashimoto's thyroiditis is common in individuals with Down syndrome and should be sought and treated promptly. Because of the concern for development of leukemia, which is more common in individuals with Down syndrome, GH use is generally not recommended.

Turner Syndrome. In girls with TS, short stature is the single most common feature, occurring more frequently than delayed puberty, cubitus valgus, or webbing of the neck.[1095-1097] Short stature occurs in 95% to 100% of girls with a 45,X karyotype.[1098-1100] Mean adult heights in the United States and Europe range from 142.0 to 146.8 cm, with important genetic and ethnic influences on growth of girls in different regions. Parental height correlates well with final adult height,[1101,1102] and a cross-cultural study in 15 countries demonstrated a very strong correlation between final height in TS and in the normal population, with an approximate 20-cm deficit.[1098] Several distinct phases of growth have been identified in girls with TS[1103-1104]:

1. Mild IUGR with a mean birth weight of 2800 g and a mean birth length of 48.3 cm
2. Slow growth recognized during early infancy and reaching −3 SD by 3 years of age[1106]
3. Delayed onset of the "childhood" phase of growth[26,27,1105] and progressive decline in height velocity from age 3 years until approximately 14 years, resulting in further deviation from normal height percentiles
4. A prolonged adolescent growth phase, characterized by a partial return toward normal height, followed by delayed epiphyseal fusion

These girls have many features of skeletal dysplasia such as Madlung's deformity and are haploinsufficient for the *SHOX* gene, which is located in the pseudoautosomal region of the short arm of the X chromosome.[1107] When heights of girls with TS are compared with those of girls with LWD, which involves a *SHOX* deletion, it appears that the *SHOX* defect may account for about two thirds of the height deficit in TS.[1108] Girls with TS have normal GH and IGF levels during childhood; reports of low levels of GH or IGF, or both, in adolescents are likely due to low serum levels of gonadal steroids.[1109] Multiple studies have shown that GH therapy is capable of accelerating short-term growth and increasing final adult height.[1100,1110,1111] GH treatment in TS is discussed in detail later in the chapter.

Noonan Syndrome. Individuals with Noonan syndrome have postnatal growth failure, right-sided cardiac abnormalities (most often pulmonary valve abnormalities), webbing of the neck, low posterior hairline, ptosis, cubitus valgus, and malformed ears. Microphallus and cryptorchidism are common, and puberty may be delayed or incomplete. Cognitive delay of variable degrees is present in about 25% to 50% of patients. Although this disorder shares phenotypic features with TS, the two are clearly distinct.[1112,1113] Therefore, oft-used terms such as "Turner-like syndrome" or "male Turner syndrome" are misleading. In Noonan syndrome, the sex chromosomes are normal and transmission is autosomal dominant, although about 50% of cases are sporadic. Approximately half of patients have heterozygous missense mutations of *PTPN11* leading to a gain-of-function mutation in a nonreceptor type 2 tyrosine phosphatase (SHP2) that enhances intracellular dephosphorylation.[1114-1116] Through much of childhood, mean growth in length and weight is below the third percentile.[1117-1119] GH secretory abnormalities do not account for the short stature, although endogenous GH production may be slightly reduced.[1119,1120] It is postulated that the enhanced intracellular phosphatase activity diminishes the effectiveness of GH-induced IGF production.[1121-1123] GH therapy has been used in the treatment of patients with Noonan syndrome who have short stature, as discussed in detail later.

Prader-Willi Syndrome. In Prader-Willi syndrome (PWS), growth failure may be evident at birth but is more pronounced postnatally.[1124] This syndrome is discussed at length in a later section of this chapter.

Other Syndromes. Other syndromes associated with moderate to profound growth failure include Bloom's syndrome, de Lange syndrome, leprechaunism, Ellis–van Creveld syndrome, Aarskog's syndrome, Rubenstein-Taybi syndrome, mulibrey nanism, Dubowitz syndrome, progeria, Cockayne's syndrome, and Johanson-Blizzard syndrome.[1125]

Small for Gestational Age

Historically, infants born SGA have comprised a heterogeneous group with birth weight or length below the 3rd, 5th, or 10th percentile for gestational age, depending on the study.[35] As the growth and metabolic consequences of being born SGA have been observed and characterized, studies have more consistently used the definition of SGA as birth weight or length (or both) at least 2 SD below the mean for gestational age (usually at or below the 2.3 percentile for a population). The term IUGR has been used interchangeably with SGA to describe these infants. However, it has been proposed that, because IUGR implies a known underlying pathologic process, that term should be reserved for infants whose abnormal prenatal growth has been confirmed by intrauterine growth assessments and whose growth restriction can be attributed to a specific cause.[1125A] The reason for abnormal fetal growth is unclear in up to 40% of cases[1126]; known underlying reasons are listed in Table 24-6. Accurate assessment of an infant as SGA depends on accurate gestational dating and weight and length measurements, which can be difficult in both developed and developing countries.

Most SGA infants exhibit catch-up growth (as defined by a growth velocity greater than the median for chronologic age and gender) by 2 years of age. Catch-up growth occurs during the first 6 months of life in approximately 80% of infants born SGA.[1127] Approximately 10% to 15% of infants born SGA exhibit slow, attenuated growth with persistent height deficits in childhood and adolescence. The remaining 5% to 10% exhibit a slower catch-up growth pattern, reaching heights 2 SD below the mean between 3 and 5 years of age. These estimations vary by study; in a population of severely affected infants with SGA who required care in a neonatal intensive care unit, 27% had not achieved catch-up growth by 6 years of age.[1128]

TABLE 24-6

Factors Associated with Small for Gestational Age (SGA) Births

I. Intrinsic Fetal Factors
A. Chromosomal Disorders
B. Syndromes
1. Russell-Silver Syndrome
2. Seckel Syndrome
3. Progeria
4. Cockayne Syndrome
5. Bloom Syndrome
6. Rubenstein-Taybi Syndrome
II. Placental Abnormalities
A. Abnormal Implantation of the Placenta
B. Placental Vascular Insufficiency; Infarction
C. Vascular malformations
III. Maternal Disorders
A. Malnutrition
B. Constraints on Uterine Growth
C. Vascular Disorders
1. Hypertension
2. Toxemia
3. Severe Diabetes Mellitus
D. Uterine Malformations
E. Drug Ingestion
1. Tobacco
2. Alcohol
3. Narcotics

Low birth-weight premature babies who are appropriate for gestational age (AGA) invariably experience catch-up growth in the first 2 years of life. Final adult height of all children born SGA is −0.8 to −0.9 SD, a mean deficit of 3.6 to 4 cm when adjusted for family stature.[1129] It has been estimated that the 10% to 15% of SGA children with short stature account for as much as 20% of all short children. In the United States, 2.3% of the population fitting the definition of SGA represents roughly an incidence of 1 in 43 neonates. Therefore, SGA children have a fivefold to sevenfold greater possibility of short stature than AGA children.[35]

Normal fetal growth depends on a complex interplay of maternal and fetal genetic and external environmental influences. Abnormal intrauterine growth can result from pathologic processes in the fetus, the placenta, or the mother. Growth in length occurs early in fetal life, whereas weight gain occurs later in fetal life[1130]; first-trimester growth failure has been closely associated with low birth weight and low birth weight percentile.[1131] Because there is a differential effect on weight and length depending on the fetal period when the pathologic processes occur, IUGR has been subclassified into symmetric and asymmetric types. The symmetric type of IUGR results from an insult early in the pregnancy, often due to fetal genetic factors or syndromes, congenital infections, or toxic effects; asymmetric IUGR results from an insult occurring late in gestation, often due to fetoplacental insufficiency. Historically, it was thought that infants with symmetric IUGR do not experience catch-up growth whereas those with asymmetric IUGR who have normal head circumference and length yet low birth weight usually experience catch-up growth postnatally.[1130] However, studies have suggested that infants with asymmetric IUGR have worse perinatal outcomes than those with symmetric IUGR[1132,1133] and that both types of growth restriction can arise in the second trimester of pregnancy.[1134,1135] Therefore, the subclassification of IUGR, like the term IUGR itself, is controversial.

Endocrine-related causes account for a small fraction of the many contributors to fetal growth abnormalities, but hormonal disorders associated with fetal and neonatal growth restriction shed light on the endocrine mechanisms of growth in the fetus. Although GH plays a major role in postnatal growth, it has a minimal role in fetal growth; infants with neonatal GHD are typically −0.5 to −1.5 SD below the mean in length and are heavy for this length.[518,519,1136] An adequate nutrient supply is the main determinate of fetal growth, but growth factors such as insulin, IGF1, and IGF2 also play a role. Defects of insulin secretion or action are associated with impaired fetal growth.[1130] Congenital defects of insulin secretion such as glucokinase deficiency[1137] or pancreatic agenesis[1138] are associated with severe IUGR. Leprechanism is caused by defects in the insulin receptor and is associated with severe insulin resistance and IUGR.[26] The initial case of a deletion of the IGF1 gene had profound intrauterine growth failure.[340,792] Polymorphisms of the IGF1 gene have also been reported to be associated with IUGR.[340,1139,1140]

Neonates with SGA exhibit hormonal patterns consistent with insensitivity to GH and IGF1 and/or insulin action. In neonates with IUGR, GH levels are elevated[1141] and IGF1 and IGFBP3 levels are low.[134,1142-1144] IGFBP1 and IGFBP2 levels have been reported to be higher than in AGA infants,[371] a pattern seen in individuals with insulin resistance. Similar patterns are found in the first week of life after severe fetal malnutrition.[1145] Exogenous GH treatment has little or no effect on growth, body composition, or energy expenditure[1146,1147] in the neonatal period. In most infants with SGA, normalization of GH, IGF1, and IGFBP3 levels occurs by 3 months of age, with normal response to GH stimulation testing in childhood.[1148] In measurement of spontaneous GH secretion, high pulse frequency with attenuated pulse amplitude and elevated trough values of GH have been noted in SGA children.[1149-1151] Serum IGF1 levels in children with short stature born SGA are slightly but significantly lower than in children with catch-up growth.[1148,1151]

SGA children who have striking weight gain during the first several years of life can develop endocrine disorders later in childhood, including premature adrenarche, insulin resistance, polycystic ovary syndrome, and an attenuated growth spurt.[1152] This subset of SGA children have increased risks of hypertension, maturity-onset diabetes, and cardiovascular disease later in life.[1153-1156] This is consistent with the Barker hypothesis, which states that fetal metabolic responses to a nutritionally hostile intrauterine environment may lead to inappropriate extrauterine consequences.[1157-1159] These problems do not appear to occur in SGA babies without catch-up growth, although insulin resistance has been described.[1160] Whether SGA is causally related to these disorders or is a symptom of an underlying inborn metabolic disorder is not yet known.

Russell-Silver syndrome (RSS) was independently described by Russell[1161] and by Silver and associates.[1162] Findings include IUGR with postnatal growth failure, congenital hemihypertrophy, and small, triangular facies.[1163-1166] Other nonspecific findings include clinodactyly, delayed closure of the fontanelle, delayed bone age, and precocious puberty.[1163-1165] Adults are short, with final heights approximately −4 SD below the mean.[1164,1166] The incidence is between 1 in 50,000 and 1 in 100,000 live births. Endogenous GH secretion in prepubertal RSS children is similar to that in other short IUGR children and less than in AGA short children.[1149,1167] Maternal uniparental disomy of chromosome 7 is present in 7% to 10% of cases.[1168-1171] Although there are a number of imprinted genes or factors involved in growth and development on chromosome 7, numerous studies have not detected any

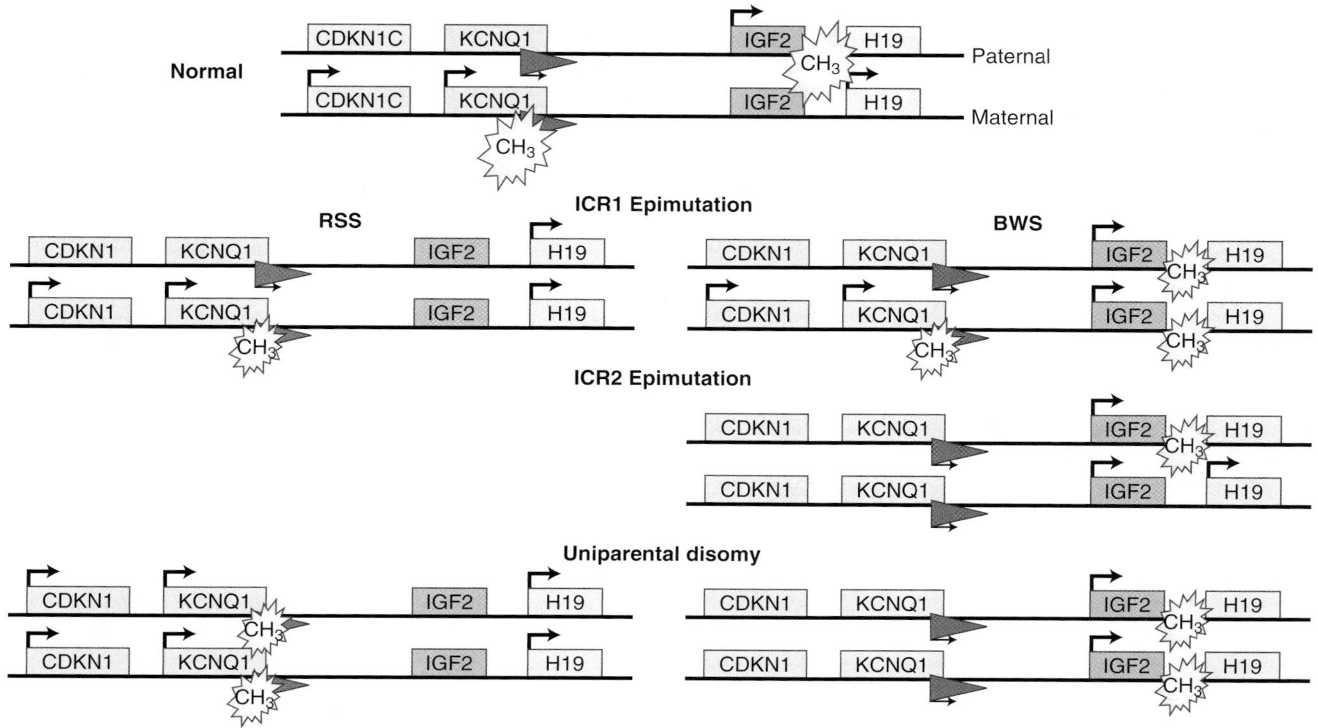

Figure 24-38 Schematic representation of the 11p15 region and the epigenetic mutations associated with Russell Silver syndrome and Beckwith-Weidemann syndrome. Red and pink boxes represent genes of imprinting control region 1 (ICR1), and green boxes represent genes of ICR2. The arrow represents the presence of gene transcription. Dark triangeles represent anti-sense transcripts that can repress transcription of ICR2 genes. When methylated, the transcripts cannot be formed, allowing transcription of ICR2 genes and reciprocal suppression of transcription of downstream genes, (i.e., IGF 2). (Adapted from Eggerman T. Silver-Russell and Beckwith-Weidemann syndromes: opposite (epi)mutations in 11p15 result in opposite clinical pictures. *Horm Res.* 2009;71(suppl 2):30-35.)

pathologic mutations in the candidate genes. A gene on chromosome 7p, *GRB10,* is involved in regulation of insulin and IGF1 receptor signaling and is mainly expressed from the maternal allele; loss of the maternal allele results in fetal and placental overgrowth.[1171,1172] Mutations that could cause overexpression of *GRB10* have not been found in patients with RSS.

A small number of patients with RSS have duplication of the maternal allele of the 11p15 region[1173]; duplication of the paternal allele in this region is associated with BWS and overexpression of IGF2. The 11p15 region contains two imprinting control regions (ICR), ICR1 and ICR2 (Fig. 24-38). ICR1 comprises the *IGF2* and *H19* genes. The noncoding gene *H19* is downstream from *IGF2* and is oppositely imprinted, meaning that only the maternal allele is expressed and the paternal allele is inactive. The promoters of the *IGF2* and *H19* genes share a set of enhancers that act on either gene. On the paternal allele, the *H19* promoter region is methylated and therefore inactivated.[242] Upstream from the *H19* and *IGF2* promoter region is a paternally methylated region that prevents binding of CTCF, allowing enhancers to act on the *IGF2* promoter to activate transcription.[243] On the maternal chromosome, this region is not methylated, allowing CTCF to bind and preventing transcription.[244] In this ICR1 region, mutations causing hypomethylation of the *H19* promoter region has been described in approximately 40% of patients with RSS.[1174] Oppositely, hypermethylation of the ICR1 region has been associated with BWS. Disruption of ICR2 has been described in BWS (described later) but not in RSS. Reduced *IGF2* expression has been demonstrated in fibroblasts of patients with RSS in vitro,[1174] but serum levels of IGF2 in patients with RSS are normal.[1175] Mice with a null mutation of IGF2 have prenatal growth retardation but normal postnatal growth; how reduced expression of IGF2 contributes to postnatal growth failure in RSS has yet to be elucidated.

Maternal and Placental Factors

Maternal factors and placental insufficiency can impair fetal growth and likely account for most cases of asymmetric IUGR. Maternal nutrition is an important contributor to fetal growth and to growth during the first year of life.[1176] Fetal growth retardation may result from use of alcohol,[1177-1179] cocaine,[1180] marijuana,[1180] or tobacco[1181] during pregnancy. The mechanisms for drug-induced fetal growth retardation are unclear but may include uterine vasoconstriction and vascular insufficiency, placental abruption, or premature rupture of membranes. The maternal hormonal milieu is affected by placental steroids and peptides. Maternal IGF1 affects placental function and may facilitate transport of nutrients to the fetus. Maternal IGF1 levels have been found to correlate with fetal growth.[1182,1183] Increased levels of free IGF1 are found during normal human pregnancy.[1184]

The placenta has multiple functions, including the transport of nutrients, oxygen, and waste and the production of hormones. It consumes oxygen and glucose brought by the uterine circulation. Placental GH affects maternal IGF production, which in turn affects placental function. A woman with GHD due to PIT1 mutation exhibited normal levels of placental GH and IGF1, demonstrating the independent production of GH and IGF1 by the placenta.[1185] Human placental lactogen (hPL) is a major regulator of glucose, amino acid, and lipid metabolism in the mother, aiding in the mobilization of nutrients for transport to the fetus. Damage to the placenta resulting from vascular disease, infection, or intrinsic abnormalities of the syncytiotrophoblasts can impair these important functions. At times, examination of the placenta may yield causal information about fetal growth retardation.

An X-linked homeobox gene, *ESX1,* detected only in extraembryonic tissues and human testes, is a chromosomally imprinted regulator of placental morphogenesis.[1186-1188] Heterozygous and homozygous mutant mice are born 20% smaller than normal and have large edematous placentas.[1186] Vasculature is abnormal at the maternal-fetal interface, presumably causing the growth retardation.

PATHOLOGIC BASIS OF EXCESS GROWTH

Although, by definition, there are as many children with heights greater than 2 SD above the mean as with heights less than 2 SD below the mean, tall stature as a chief complaint is encountered much less often in endocrine practice. Nevertheless, it is critical to identify those situations in which tall stature or an accelerated growth rate provides clues of an underlying disorder (Table 24-7).

Statural Overgrowth in the Fetus

Maternal diabetes mellitus is the most common cause of large-for-gestational age (LGA) infants. LGA is defined as length or weight greater than the 90th percentile for gestational age. Even in the absence of clinical symptoms or family history, the birth of an excessively large infant should lead to evaluation for maternal or gestational diabetes.

Two relatively rare syndromes, Sotos syndrome and BWS, can also cause LGA infants.

TABLE 24-7

Differential Diagnosis of Statural Overgrowth

Fetal Overgrowth
Maternal diabetes mellitus Cerebral gigantism (Sotos syndrome) Weaver's syndrome Beckwith-Wiedemann syndrome Other insulin-like growth factor 2 (IGF2) excess syndromes
Postnatal Overgrowth Leading to Childhood Tall Stature
Familial (constitutional) tall stature Cerebral gigantism Beckwith-Wiedemann syndrome Exogenous obesity Excess growth hormone (GH) secretion (pituitary gigantism) McCune-Albright syndrome or multiple endocrine neoplasia (MEN) associated with excess GH secretion Precocious puberty Marfan's syndrome Klinefelter's syndrome (XXY) Weaver's syndrome Fragile X syndrome Homocystinuria XYY Hyperthyroidism
Postnatal Overgrowth Leading to Adult Tall Stature
Familial (constitutional) tall stature Androgen or estrogen deficiency/estrogen resistance (in males) Testicular feminization Excess GH secretion Marfan's syndrome Klinefelter's syndrome (XXY) XYY

Sotos Syndrome

Children with cerebral gigantism (Sotos syndrome) are typically above the 90th percentile for length and weight at birth.[1189-1191] Clinical features also include a prominent forehead; dolichocephaly; macrocephaly; high arched palate; hypertelorism with unusually slanting eyes; prominent ears, jaw, and chin; large hands and feet with thickened subcutaneous tissue; cognitive delay; and motor incoordination. Children continue to grow rapidly during early childhood, but puberty is usually early, with premature epiphyseal fusion. Therefore, most children with Sotos syndrome have a final height within the normal range.[1191] GH secretion and serum IGF levels are normal, and no specific cause of the overgrowth has been identified. About 80% of patients have a loss-of-function mutation in the *NSD1* gene whose product is a nucleus-localized basic transcription factor.[1192]

Beckwith-Weidemann Syndrome

BWS is the most common (1 of every 13,700 live births) of the overgrowth disorders, the group of disorders associated with excessive somatic and specific organ growth. It is characterized by fetal macrosomia with omophalocele[1193] and other clinical features secondary to organomegaly, such as macroglossia, renal medullary hyperplasia, and neonatal hypoglycemia due to islet cell hyperplasia.[1194] Excessive childhood growth ultimately leads to earlier puberty and early epiphyseal fusion with resultant normal adult height.[1195] BWS is postulated to be caused by excess availability of IGF2.[1196] Although an association between BWS and disordered regulation of *IGF2* gene transcription has been documented, no consistent postnatal abnormality of the GH-IGF axis has been identified to date.[1197,1198]

Various lines of evidence have shown that BWS is associated with loss of imprinting of the genes on chromosome 11p15.5, home of the *IGF2* gene (see Fig. 24-38). Under normal conditions, the paternally derived *IGF2* gene is expressed and the maternally transmitted gene is not active, as described in detail earlier in this chapter. BWS has been associated with uniparental disomy or duplication of the paternal 11p15 region and resultant overexpression of the *IGF2* gene.[1199] The ICR1 region of 11p15 contains the *IGF2* and *H19* genes; the noncoding gene *H19* is located downstream from *IGF2* and is oppositely imprinted. The promoters of the *IGF2* and *H19* genes share a set of enhancers that act on either gene. On the paternal allele, the *H19* promoter region is methylated and therefore inactivated.[242] Upstream from the *H19* and *IGF2* promoter region is a paternally methylated region that prevents binding of CTCF, allowing enhancers to act on the *IGF2* promoter to activate transcription.[243] On the maternal chromosome, this region is not methylated, allowing CTCF to bind and preventing transcription.[244] Hypermethylation of the *H19* promoter region with resultant loss of imprinting and biallelic expression of IGF2 has been associated with fewer than 10% of the cases of BWS.[253,1200] Hypomethylation of this region is associated with RSS, a syndrome associated with prenatal and postnatal growth failure (see earlier discussion).

ICR2, located 5′ of *ICR1,* contains the genes for cyclin-dependent kinase inhibitor 1C (CDKN1C) and potassium channel KQT family member 1 (KCNQ1), among others that are methylated on the maternal allele. Associated with these two genes is an antisense transcript with paternal expression that may suppress transcription; it has been postulated that this cluster of genes is in "expression competition" with the IGF2/H19 cluster.[1201] Up to 25% of familial cases of BWS are associated with mutation in the

CDKN1C or *KCNQ1* gene,[1202] but there is debate about whether loss of imprinting of the *IGF2* gene convincingly occurs with most of the mutations. Four children with somatic overgrowth but not the diagnostic features of BWS had *IGF2* gene overexpression.[1196] Additionally, mutations in *GPC3,* a glypican gene that codes for an IGF2 neutralizing membrane receptor, cause the related Simpson-Golabi-Behmel overgrowth syndrome.[1203,1204]

Postnatal Statural Overgrowth

As in the case of the child with growth failure, crossing of height percentiles between infancy and the onset of puberty is an indication for further evaluation because it can indicate serious underlying pathology. As with short stature, children with tall stature must be evaluated in the context of familial growth and pubertal patterns.

Tall Stature

GH secretion and levels of IGF1 and IGFBP3 in familial tall stature are often in the upper-normal range.[1205] Tauber and colleagues[1206] divided 65 children with familial tall stature into a subset with high GH secretion rates and frequent secretory bursts and another subset with lower GH secretion and fewer episodic spikes. IGF1 levels were higher among those producing more GH and normal in the low-GH group. The authors postulated that both enhanced secretion of GH and greater efficiency of GH-mediated IGF1 production might be potential causes of familial tall stature.

Tall stature is also a characteristic of certain syndromes. Marfan syndrome, an autosomal dominant disorder of collagen metabolism, is characterized by hyperextensible joints, dislocation of the lens, kyphoscoliosis, dissecting aortic aneurysm, and long, thin bones that result in arachnodactyly and moderately tall stature. It is caused by mutations in the fibrillin-1 gene *(FBN1)*. The abnormal FBN1 monomers from the mutated gene disrupt the normal aggregation of FBN1, impairing microfibril formation. Homocystinuria is an autosomal recessive disorder that phenotypically resembles Marfan syndrome, but patients also have cognitive disabilities. Tall stature has also been found in patients with familial ACTH resistance due to a defective ACTH receptor.[1207]

Dosage effects of the *SHOX* gene may result in tall stature.[1208] In females with three copies of the *SHOX* gene and gonadal dysgenesis, adult stature was +2 to +2.9 SDS.[1209] In women with 47,XXX karyotype, mean final heights are 5 to 10 cm taller than population means, and men with 47,XXY karyotype (Klinefelter's syndrome) are about 3.5 cm taller than population means.[30,1210,1211] Males with an XYY karyotype may also have moderately tall stature. In addition to SHOX effects, the variable degree of estrogen production in these syndromes may also influence skeletal maturation and final height.[25]

Failure to enter puberty and complete sexual maturation may result in sustained growth during adult life with ultimate tall stature and a characteristic eunuchoid habitus. The description of tall stature with open epiphyses resulting from mutation of the estrogen receptor or from aromatase deficiency[21-23] underscores the fundamental role of estrogen in promoting epiphyseal fusion and termination of normal skeletal growth.

Obesity

Obesity is frequently associated with rapid skeletal growth and early onset of puberty.[1212] Rapid early postnatal weight gain has been associated with taller stature at 8 years of age than that predicted from the midparental target height.[1213] Others have shown that early postnatal growth is associated with altered tempo of development, but sudden weight gain in middle childhood has little effect on height trajectory.[1214] Patients with obesity tend to have diminished overall GH production but normal to high GHBP, and IGF1 levels appear to be capable of maintaining adequate or enhanced linear growth velocity. Bone age is usually modestly accelerated, so that both puberty and epiphyseal fusion occur early and adult height is normal. This association between obesity and rapid growth is so characteristic that a child with obesity and short stature should always be evaluated for underlying pathology, such as hypothyroidism, GHD, Cushing's syndrome, or PWS.

Tumors

Pituitary gigantism is a rare condition, analogous to acromegaly in the adult (see Chapter 9).[1215-1217] GH-secreting tumors of the pituitary are typically eosinophilic or chromophobic adenomas. Their etiology is uncertain, although many result from somatic mutations that generate constitutively activated G proteins with reduced GTPase activity (see Chapter 9).[1218] The resulting increase in intracellular cAMP in the pituitary leads to increased GH secretion. Somatotropic tumors with excess GH secretion may occur in McCune-Albright syndrome, which is caused by mutations resulting in constitutive activation of G proteins.[1219,1220] GH-secreting tumors have also been reported in multiple endocrine neoplasia (MEN) and in association with neurofibromatosis and tuberous sclerosis.[1221]

GH excess that occurs before epiphyseal fusion results in rapid growth and attainment of adult heights above expected adult potential. When GH hypersecretion is accompanied by gonadotropin deficiency, accelerated linear growth may persist for decades, as was the case for the Alton giant, who reached a height of 280 cm by the time of his death in his 20s.[1222] Manifestations typical of acromegaly may also appear, such as soft tissue swelling; enlargement of the nose, ears, and jaw with coarsening of facial features; pronounced increases in hand and foot size; diaphoresis; galactorrhea; and menstrual irregularity.

EVALUATION AND TREATMENT OF GROWTH ABNORMALITIES

Clinical Evaluation of Growth Retardation

The most important parameter in assessing children with growth failure is careful clinical evaluation, including accurate serial assessment of height and height velocity. Consideration of a growth disorder is raised when a child's length or height falls below the normal range (<3rd percentile), the growth velocity is subnormal (indicated by length or height measurements that cross percentiles on the growth curve or by an annual growth velocity less than the 3rd percentile for age), or the child's height is below the range expected based on the parents' heights. To grow along the 3rd percentile for height, a child must maintain a height velocity at the 25th percentile for age.[1223] Therefore, a height velocity below the 25th percentile in a short child suggests abnormal growth. However, because of the greater error intrinsic to assessment of growth velocity compared with height velocity,[1224] a single height velocity measurement above the 25th percentile for age, even based on annual height data, cannot fully exclude a growth abnormality in a short child.[1224]

Figure 24-39 provides an algorithm for evaluation of the child with growth failure. Although one third of healthy

Step 1—Defining the risk of IGF deficiency syndrome

Auxologic abnormalities
- Severe short stature (height SDS <-3 SD)
- Severe growth deceleration (height velocity SDS <-2 SD over 12 months)
- Height <-2 SD and height velocity <-1.0 SD over 12 months
- Height <-1.5 SD and height velocity <-1.5 SD over 2 years

Risk factors
- History of a brain tumor, cranial irradiation, or other documented organic or congenital hypothalamic-pituitary abnormality
- Incidental finding of hypothalamic-pituitary abnormality on MRI
- If any of the above exists, proceed with Step 2; if not, follow clinically and return to Step 1 in 6 months

Step 2—Screening for IGF deficiency and other diseases

A. Order a laboratory panel including a bone age, free T_4, and TSH, chromosomes (in females), and nonendocrine tests; if indicated, refer back to primary care physician or treat diagnosed conditions as appropriate.

and

B. Order an IGF-I and an IGFBP-3 level.
- If IGF-I/IGFBP-3 are both above the -1 SD, follow clinically and return to Step 1 in 6 months.
- If IGF-I/IGFBP-3 are both below -2 SD, proceed to Step 4. If MRI is abnormal, GH provocative testing is optional (Table 23–10).
- Otherwise, proceed to Step 3. If this is a patient with delayed adolescence, consider sex steroid treatment prior to Step 3.

Step 3—Testing GH secretion

This step can be bypassed if a clear GHD risk factor and a severe IGF deficiency are identified.

- Perform two of the following GH stimulation tests (if appropriate, estrogen prime) (see Table 23–8):
  - Clonidine
  - Arginine
  - Insulin
  - Glucagon
  - L-Dopa
  - Propranolol
- If all GH levels are below 10, go to Step 4.
- If peak GH >15 ng/mL, obtain GHBP; if GHBP <-2 SD, consider an IGF-generation test and, if abnormal, IGF treatment.
- If peak GH >15 ng/mL and GHBP is normal, follow clinically and return to Step 1 in 6 months.
- If peak GH is between 10 and 15 ng/mL, go back to Step 2 in 6 months.

Step 4—Evaluating the pituitary

- Perform MRI, with particular emphasis on hypothalamic-pituitary anatomy.
- Test HPA axis, if not already done (CRH stimulation or ITT), and teach cortisol supplementation as needed (must do this if the MRI is abnormal).
- Consider molecular evaluation of GH, GHR, or GHRHR and other potential genetic defects (Fig. 24–2).

Step 5—Treating for growth promotion

- Initiate GH treatment at appropriate dose levels.
- If GHIS is suspected, consider IGF therapy, if available.
- Regularly evaluate growth parameters, IGF-I, and IGFBP-3, as well as compliance and safety (see Table 24–13).
- GH secretion should be retested, according to adult GH assessment protocols, at the end of growth.

Figure 24-39 Clinical and biochemical evaluation of growth failure: evaluating the GH/IGF I axis. CRH, corticotropin-releasing hormone; GH, growth hormone; GHD, growth hormone deficiency; GHIS, growth hormone insensitivity; GHR, growth hormone receptor; GHRHR, growth hormone–releasing hormone receptor; HPA, hypothalamic-pituitary axis; IGF-I, insulin-like growth factor 1; IGFBP-3, IGF-binding protein 3; ITT, insulin tolerance test; MRI, magnetic resonance imaging; SD, standard deviation; SDS, standard deviation score; T_4, thyroxine; TSH, thyroid-stimulating hormone.

infants will cross downward on the length percentile growth curve (discussed previously), this is normal only in relatively large infants born to small parents or in those infants who are following a growth pattern of CDGD (see later discussion). In other situations, the infant who is crossing downward on the length percentile curve should be investigated in the same way as other children with subnormal growth velocities.

History and Physical Examination

The many illness-related causes of diminished growth were discussed in earlier sections of this chapter. A growth pattern in which weight gain is impaired before linear growth or in which there is greater impairment of weight gain than of length/height gain suggests an impairment of nutrition, such as inadequate intake, malabsorption, or increased energy requirements. Nonhormonal causes of growth failure should be investigated based on data obtained from a careful history and physical examination. In addition, careful evaluation of the growth curve in the context of the family history may suggest a normal variant growth pattern, such as crossing linear percentiles of infancy, familial short stature, or CDGD. In such cases, careful observation may be all that is required. One third of all infants have growth parameters that cross percentiles downward on the growth curve, and 3% of the all children have a length or height below the 3rd percentile. Most of these children have no disease or growth disorder and will demonstrate this by having a normal growth velocity on continued observation.

The physical examination should look for evidence of an underlying organ-specific or systemic disease. It should also evaluate for clues specific to growth disorders, such as findings suggestive of genetic disorders such as Noonan syndrome, RSS, or TS. In addition, body proportions should be measured, because skeletal disproportion suggests a skeletal dysplasia.

Findings on the history and examination may point to an increased likelihood of the presence of GHD (Table 24-8). Micropenis in a male newborn should always lead to an evaluation of the GH-IGF1 axis. Nystagmus, indicating neonatal blindness, suggests hypopituitarism due to its association with optic nerve hypoplasia in the syndrome of septo-optic-dysplasia. A history of other midline defects, such as cleft lip and cleft palate,[529] or a single central incisor increases concern for hypopituitarism. Unexplained neonatal hypoglycemia, hepatitis, or prolonged jaundice should prompt an evaluation of pituitary function. Older children with GHD have less impaired weight gain than height gain, resulting in an increased weight for height; they are often described as having a "cherubic" appearance. Increased weight for height with growth failure is also characteristic of hypothyroidism. If the weight gain is dramatic, Cushing's syndrome should be considered. (However, linear growth acceleration with excess weight gain is not consistent with Cushing's syndrome.) Finally, GHD should be suspected in children with known or suspected CNS pathology (e.g., tumors, prior radiation therapy to the CNS, malformations, infection, trauma) or with documented deficiency of TSH, ACTH, antidiuretic hormone, or gonadotropin.

TABLE 24-8

Key History and Physical Examination Findings That Suggest the Diagnosis of Growth Hormone Deficiency (The Growth Hormone Research Society 2000 Criteria)

Findings That Suggest the Diagnosis of GHD
In the Neonate
Hypoglycemia
Prolonged jaundice
Hepatitis
Microphallus
Traumatic delivery
In a Child with Short Stature or Growth Failure
Cranial irradiation
Head trauma or central nervous system infection
Consanguinity and/or an affected family member
Craniofacial midline abnormalities
Findings That Support Immediate Investigation for GHD
In a Child with Short Stature
Signs indicative of an intracranial lesion
Neonatal symptoms and signs of GHD
Auxologic findings
Severe short stature (<−3 SD)
Height <−2 SD and height velocity over 1 yr of <−1 SD
A decrease in height SD of >0.5 over 1 yr in children >2 yr of age
A height velocity below −2 SD over 1 yr
A height velocity >1.5 SD below the mean sustained velocity over 2 yr
Signs of multiple pituitary hormone deficiency (MPHD)

GHD, growth hormone deficiency; SD, standard deviation.

From Growth Hormone Research Society. Consensus guidelines for the diagnosis and treatment of growth hormone (GH) deficiency in childhood and adolescence: summary statement of the GH research society. *J Clin Endocrinol Metab.* 2000;85:3990-3993.

Laboratory Testing

If the history and physical examination do not suggest a specific disorder causing growth failure and the growth pattern and family history do not provide sufficient reassurance that the growth is following a normal variant growth pattern, it is necessary to perform laboratory testing. In many cases, the testing does not identify an abnormality, and the child either is ultimately found to have a normal variant growth pattern or falls into the classification of ISS. The laboratory tests can be divided into those screening for disorders outside the GH-IGF1 axis and those evaluating that axis.

Screening Tests

Because a number of illnesses can cause growth failure either before or in the absence of other signs or symptoms, it is necessary to screen for these disorders in children with abnormal growth. A complete blood count looks for evidence of anemia, chronic infection, or inflammation. A complete blood chemistry panel provides evidence for silent renal disease (including renal tubular acidosis), liver disease, and disorders of calcium and phosphorus. The erythrocyte sedimentation rate is measured to look for evidence of disorders involving chronic inflammation, such as presymptomatic juvenile idiopathic arthritis and inflammatory bowel disease. A urinalysis is obtained to look for renal disease and chronic urinary tract infection. Tissue transglutaminase IgA (and total serum IgA) is measured to screen for celiac disease. In girls in whom no other explanation for short stature is found, a karyotype should be obtained to exclude TS. This is done even in the absence of other physical features of TS, because growth failure may be the only evident feature, particularly in cases of significant mosaicism.

Hypothyroidism should be sought by screening in children with growth failure and may be the cause of the growth failure. Because of the importance of thyroid hormone on brain development in infants, this possibility should be considered early in the evaluation of an infant with growth failure in order to correct identified hypothyroidism quickly. In addition, hypothyroidism results in lower serum IGF1 levels and decreases GH levels during provocative testing.[1225-1227] Therefore, it is necessary to ensure that thyroid function is normal before evaluating for GHD. TSH is measured because it is the most sensitive indicator of primary hypothyroidism. However, because central hypothyroidism must also be considered as a cause for growth failure in children, the thyroxine level should also be measured.

Bone Age. After the neonatal period, a bone age determination can be useful in the evaluation of children with growth disorders. A radiograph of the left hand and wrist is commonly used for comparison with the published standards of Greulich and Pyle.[1228] An alternative method for assessing bone age from radiographs of the left hand involves a scoring system for developmentally identified stages of each of 20 individual bones,[1229] a technique that has been adapted for computerized assessment.[1230,1231] The left hand is used because radiographs of the entire skeleton would be tedious and expensive and would involve additional radiation exposure. However, the hand does not contribute to height, and accurate evaluation of growth potential may require radiographs of the legs and spine.

Although the bone age result does not identify a specific diagnosis in a child with a growth disorder, it can be used to classify the child's growth in relation to groups of diagnoses. Growth disorders caused by an underlying illness or hormone disorder (e.g., renal disease, malnutrition, glucocorticoid excess) are associated with a delayed bone age—that is, a bone age that is younger than the patient's chronologic age. Similarly, hypothyroidism and GHD are associated with a delayed bone age. If short stature is intrinsic to the condition, however, bone age is not delayed and is within the range of normal for the chronologic age. This is true for genetic disorders such as TS, Noonan syndrome, and RSS and also for familial short stature. In CDGD, the bone age is delayed, consistent with the future delay in puberty and late epiphyseal fusion. Given the lack of precise diagnostic laboratory tests for GHD, a lack of bone age delay argues against this diagnosis. On the other hand, the fact that patients with CDGD have a delayed bone age does not help in the sometimes difficult discrimination between this condition and GHD.

A number of important caveats concerning bone age must be considered. Experience in determination of bone age is essential to minimize intraobserver variance, and clinical studies involving bone age benefit from having a single reader perform all interpretations. The normal rate of skeletal maturation differs between boys and girls and among different ethnic groups. The standards of Greulich and Pyle are separable by sex but were developed in American white children between 1931 and 1942. Both those and the Tanner and Whitehouse standards are based on normal children[1232] and may not be applicable to children with skeletal dysplasias, endocrine abnormalities, or other forms of growth retardation or acceleration.

Prediction of Adult Height. The extent of skeletal maturation observed in an individual can be used to predict the ultimate height potential. Such predictions are based on the observation that the more delayed the bone age (relative to the chronologic age), the longer the time before epiphyseal fusion prevents further growth. The most commonly used method for height prediction, based on Greulich and Pyle's *Radiographic Atlas of Skeletal Development,*[1228] was developed by Bayley and Pinneau[1233] and relies on bone age, height, and a semiquantitative allowance for chronologic age (Table 24-9). The system of Tanner and colleagues[1229] uses measurements of height, bone age, chronologic age, and, during puberty, height and bone age increments during the previous year, as well as menarchal status. Roche, Wainer, and Thissen[1234] used the combination of height, bone age, chronologic age, midparental height, and weight (RWT method). Attempts have been made to calculate final height predictions without requiring the determination of skeletal age[1235] by using multiple regression analyses with available data such as height, weight, birth measurements, and midparental stature. All of these systems are, by nature, empiric and are not absolute predictors. Indeed, the 90% confidence intervals for the predictions are approximately ±6 cm at younger ages. The more advanced the bone age, the greater the accuracy of the adult height prediction, because a more advanced bone age places a patient closer to his or her final height.

All methods of predicting adult height are based on data from normal children, and none has been documented to be accurate in children with growth abnormalities. For this kind of precision, it would be necessary to develop disease-specific atlases of skeletal maturation (e.g., for achondroplasia or TS). In addition, height predictions will clearly be inaccurate in predicting the final height in the case of a growth-impairing process that is not adequately treated. In addition, height predictions must be used with care in assessing height outcomes during treatment. For example, in patients with precocious puberty treated with GnRH agonists, height prediction is known to overpredict the actual final height.[1236] It is fair to say that the clinical endocrinologist must not give height predictions a value that is greater than a reasonable estimate.

Tests of the Growth Hormone-IGF1 Axis

In children with growth retardation in whom other causes have been excluded, the possibility of GHD should be considered. However, these tests can have poor specificity, so clinical assessment must always play an important part in the evaluation of abnormalities in the GH-IGF1 axis. For example, a child growing consistently just below the 3rd percentile for height, with a growth rate that is accordingly above the 25th percentile for age, is very unlikely to be GH deficient. Abnormal test results in this situation would most likely represent false-positive results.

Testing of the GH-IGF1 axis begins with "static" testing of GH function, measuring IGF1. It may also be helpful to measure IGFBP3. In some cases—if the clinical presentation is highly suggestive of GHD (see Table 24-8),[1237] and the IGF1 level (and the IGFBP3 level, if obtained) also indicates a high likelihood of GHD—it is appropriate to proceed directly to the dynamic tests of GH secretion. In most cases, however, unless there is an abnormality identified on the screening tests, it is appropriate to monitor the child's growth for a period of 6 to 12 months to accurately assess the child's growth rate. Then, based on the complete clinical picture, including the growth rate and the IGF1 level, the decision is made to proceed with dynamic testing of GH secretion or to continue monitoring the child's growth.

There is no test that definitively diagnoses GHD. Because there is no "gold standard," it is impossible to precisely define the sensitivity or specificity of any test for GHD. Some information on specificity can be obtained by comparing the results with those obtained in normal children, although, for the more complicated tests, these data can be difficult to obtain in children. Sensitivity relies on comparing positive results from one test with those of another—for example, comparing low IGF1 concentrations to failed results on provocative GH tests. Poor sensitivity of IGF1 as an indicator of GHD has been based on results

TABLE 24-9

Prediction of Adult Stature

Bone Age (yr-mo)	FRACTION OF ADULT HEIGHT ATTAINED AT EACH BONE AGE*					
	Girls			Boys		
	Retarded	*Average*	*Advanced*	*Retarded*	*Average*	*Advanced*
6-0	0.733	0.720		0.680		
6-3	0.742	0.729		0.690		
6-6	0.751	0.738		0.700		
6-9	0.763	0.751		0.709		
7-0	0.770	0.757	0.712	0.718	0.695	0.670
7-3	0.779	0.765	0.722	0.728	0.702	0.676
7-6	0.788	0.772	0.732	0.738	0.709	0.683
7-9	0.797	0.782	0.742	0.747	0.716	0.689
8-0	0.804	0.790	0.750	0.756	0.723	0.696
8-3	0.813	0.801	0.760	0.765	0.731	0.703
8-6	0.823	0.810	0.771	0.773	0.739	0.709
8-9	0.836	0.821	0.784	0.779	0.746	0.715
9-0	0.841	0.827	0.790	0.786	0.752	0.720
9-3	0.851	0.836	0.800	0.794	0.761	0.728
9-6	0.858	0.844	0.809	0.800	0.769	0.734
9-9	0.866	0.853	0.819	0.807	0.777	0.741
10-0	0.874	0.862	0.828	0.812	0.784	0.747
10-3	0.884	0.874	0.841	0.816	0.791	0.753
10-6	0.896	0.884	0.856	0.819	0.795	0.758
10-9	0.907	0.896	0.870	0.821	0.800	0.763
11-0	0.918	0.906	0.883	0.823	0.804	0.767
11-3	0.922	0.910	0.887	0.827	0.812	0.776
11-6	0.926	0.914	0.891	0.832	0.818	0.786
11-9	0.929	0.918	0.897	0.839	0.827	0.800
12-0	0.932	0.922	0.901	0.845	0.834	0.809
12-3	0.942	0.932	0.913	0.852	0.843	0.818
12-6	0.949	0.941	0.924	0.860	0.853	0.828
12-9	0.957	0.950	0.935	0.869	0.863	0.839
13-0	0.964	0.958	0.945	0.880	0.876	0.850
13-3	0.971	0.967	0.955		0.890	0.863
13-6	0.977	0.974	0.963		0.902	0.875
13-9	0.981	0.978	0.968		0.914	0.890
14-0	0.983	0.980	0.972		0.927	0.905
14-3	0.986	0.983	0.977		0.938	0.918
14-6	0.989	0.986	0.980		0.948	0.930
14-9	0.992	0.988	0.983		0.958	0.943
15-0	0.994	0.990	0.986		0.968	0.958
15-3	0.995	0.991	0.988		0.973	0.967
15-6	0.996	0.993	0.990		0.976	0.971
15-9	0.997	0.994	0.992		0.980	0.976
16-0	0.998	0.996	0.993		0.982	0.980
16-3	0.999	0.996	0.994		0.985	0.983
16-6	0.999	0.997	0.995		0.987	0.985
16-9	0.9995	0.998	0.997		0.989	0.988
17-0	1.00	0.999	0.998		0.991	0.990
17-3					0.993	
17-6		0.9995	0.9995		0.994	
17-9					0.995	
18-0		1.00			0.996	
18-3					0.998	
18-6					1.00	

*The column headed "Retarded" is used when bone age is >1 yr below chronologic age; the column headed "Advanced" is used when bone age is >1 yr greater than chronologic age.

Table derived from Richman RA, Kirsch LR. Testosterone treatment in adolescent boys with constitutional delay in growth and development. *N Engl J Med* 1988;319:1563-1567. Based on the data of Bayley and Pinneau.[1233] Predicted final height is calculated by dividing the current height by the fraction of adult height achieved determined from the table.

from children with normal IGF1 concentrations who have abnormal results on provocative GH tests. However, because of the known limited specificity of these provocative tests (discussed later), one cannot determine whether the discrepant results are due to the poor sensitivity of the IGF1 test or the poor specificity of the provocative GH test. Again, it is critical to interpret all results together and in the context of the clinical data.

Insulin-Like Growth Factor 1. GHD is associated with a low serum concentrations of IGF1 (Fig. 24-40). Unlike GH

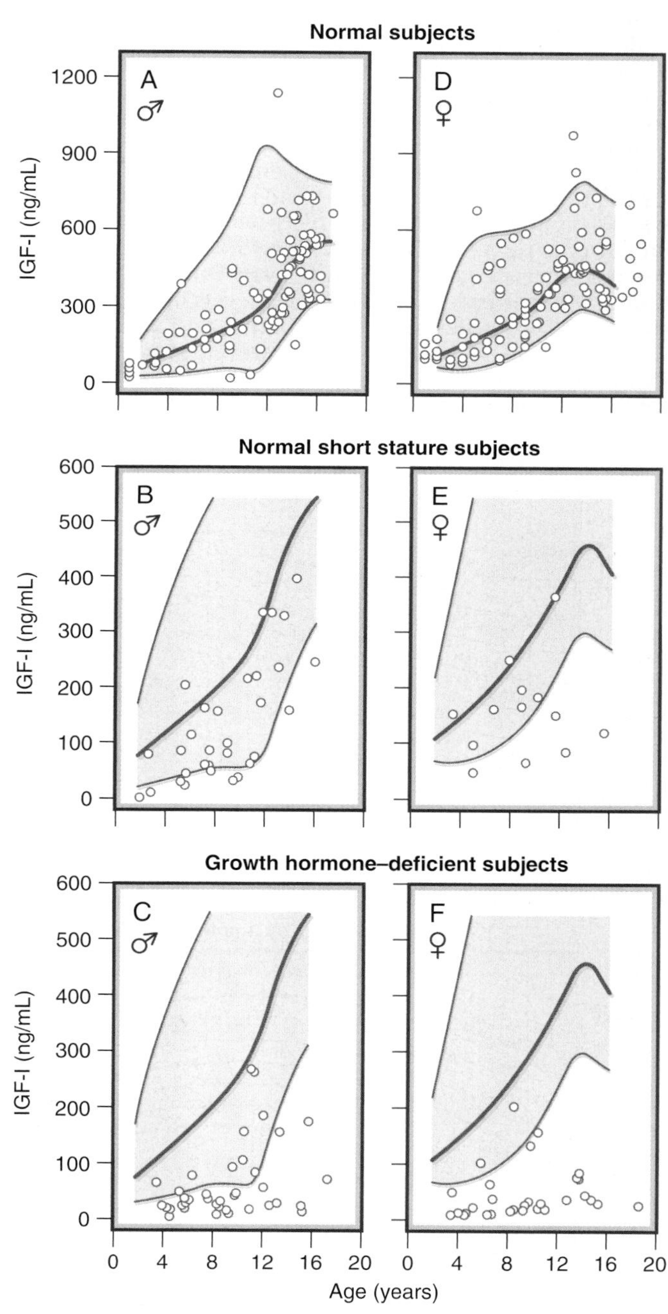

Figure 24-40 Serum levels of insulin-like growth factor I (IGF-I) in normal patients and in patients with growth disorders. Circles represent IGFI levels in normal subjects (A, D), normal short stature subjects (B, E), and growth hormone deficient subjects (C, F). The lines represent the 5th, 50th, 95th percentiles for log-normalized IGFI levels in normal subjects. (From Rosenfeld RG, Wilson DM, Lee PD, et al. Insulin-like growth factors I and II in the evaluation of growth retardation. *J Pediatr.* 1986;109:428-433.)

levels, which rise and fall with its pulsatile secretion, the IGF1 level in blood is stable, with minimal diurnal variation. The GH dependency of the IGFs was established in the initial report from Salmon and Daughaday[200] and was further clarified with the development of sensitive and specific immunoassays that distinguish between IGF1 and IGF2.[1238] IGF1 levels are more GH-dependent than IGF2 levels and are more likely to reflect subtle differences in GH secretory patterns. However, serum IGF1 levels are also influenced by age,[234,235,1239] degree of sexual maturation, and nutritional status. Therefore, IGF1 levels must be compared with age-specific ranges (Fig. 24-41), and with ranges defined by stage of sexual maturation. Some clinicians evaluate IGF1 results against the reference range based on bone age (rather than the chronologic age). This may improve the specificity of this test for GHD, although there are no data to address the validity of this approach.

IGF1 levels in normal children younger than 5 or 6 years of age are low. This leads to poor sensitivity of IGF1 levels for identifying GHD in young children. As few as 40% to 50% of young, short children with evidence of GHD on provocative tests have IGF1 levels below the lower level of the reference range.[1240,1241] IGF1 levels increase with age, resulting in better separation of IGF1 levels in GH-deficient children from those in normal children and a higher sensitivity of IGF1 levels for GHD. However, although sensitivities of 85% to 100% have been reported in some studies,[1241,1242] in others it has averaged approximately

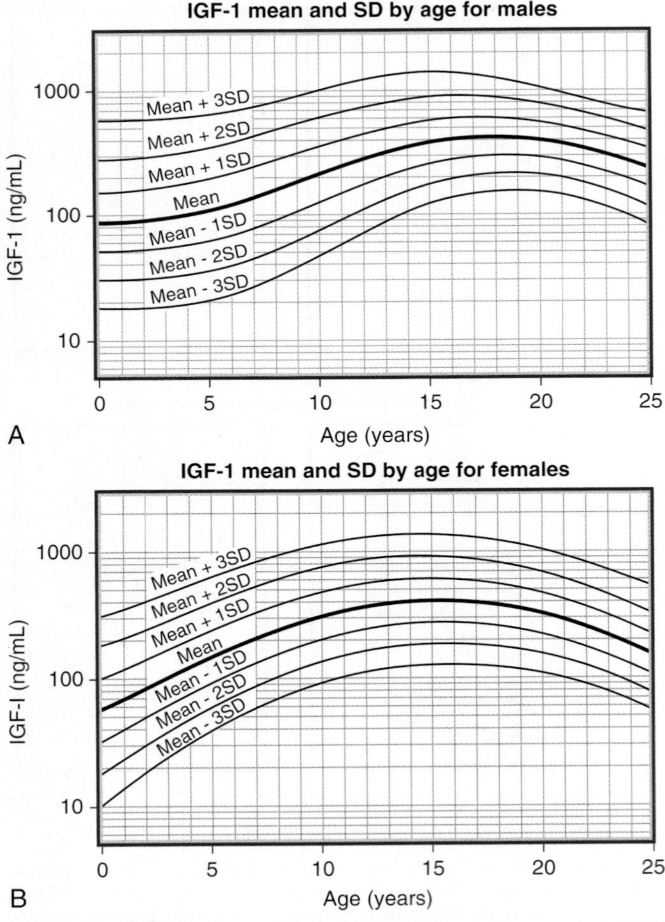

Figure 24-41 Normal serum levels of insulin-like growth factor I (IGF-I) for males **(A)** and females **(B)**. SD, standard deviation. (Data courtesy of Diagnostic Systems Laboratories, Inc., Webster, TX.)

70%.[1225,1242-1245] Again, the lack of a gold standard means that some of the false-negative findings obtained by measurement of IGF1 levels could also represent false-positives on provocative GH testing.

IGF1 levels also suffer from a lack of specificity in diagnosing GHD. In general, IGF1 levels have higher specificity in younger children, with declining specificity in older children. Juul and colleagues[1245] found that IGF1 levels had a specificity for GHD of 98% in children younger than 10 years of age but a specificity of only 67% in those older than 10 years. Similarly, Cianfarani and colleagues[1240] found a sensitivity of 100% in children younger than 9 years of age that dropped to 76% in older children. The overall specificity of a low IGF1 measurement may only be approximately 70%.[1225,1242,1243]

In addition to the specific challenges of accurately quantitating IGF1 levels in serum (see later discussion), the nutritional dependence of IGF1 levels significantly affects the accuracy of this test in evaluating for GHD. Even a few days of decreased caloric intake can lower IGF1 levels.[1225,1246] This probably contributes to the finding that IGF1 levels can vary by as much as 38% from day to day in a given patient.[1246,1247]

Early quantitation of IGFs used bioassays based on [^{35}S]-sulfate incorporation (hence, "sulfation factor" as an early synonym for IGF/somatomedin C); on stimulation of the synthesis of DNA, RNA, or protein; or on glucose uptake.[1248,1249] Development of specific antibodies permitted the development of accurate and specific measurement of IGF1 and IGF2.[1238,1239,1243,1250,1251] However, the presence of IGFBPs results in a significant technical challenge for the accurate quantitation of IGF1 (and IGF2) in serum.[1225,1248,1252] Interference is a particular problem in conditions with a relatively high IGFBP/IGF peptide ratio and at the extremes of the assay (i.e., GHD, acromegaly). In uremia, IGFBPs artifactually lower IGF1 levels and increase IGF2 levels in assays that do not eliminate this interference.[901]

The most effective way to deal with IGFBPs is to separate them from IGF peptides by chromatography under acidic conditions.[1253] This labor-intensive procedure has occasionally been replaced by an acid ethanol extraction procedure.[1254] Although the latter method may be reasonably effective for most serum samples, it is problematic in conditions of high IGFBP/IGF peptide ratios, such as conditioned media from cell lines and sera from newborns or from subjects with GHD or uremia. A number of alternative approaches to addressing the interference from the IGFBs have been developed, including the use of tracers that do not bind to IGFBPs[1255] and "sandwich" assay methods.[1256] Automated IGF1 immunometric (IRMA) or immunochemiluminometric (ICMA) assays typically add an excess of IGF2 to the assay to displace the IGFBPs and use highly specific IGF1 antibodies.[231,1225,1248] Although current IGF1 assays significantly minimize the interference from IGBPs, it is important that each assay develop reference ranges that match the clinical samples to be tested, because ethnic variations and nutritional and environmental factors can affect "normal" serum IGF1 concentrations.

A number of assays have been developed that purport to measure "free" or "free dissociable" IGF1 as a means of assessing concentrations of IGF1 peptides that circulate unbound to IGFBPs.[1257] Both the accuracy and the physiologic relevance of these determinations remain open to debate.[1225]

Insulin-Like Growth Factor–Binding Protein 3. Measurement of the serum level of IGBP3, the major serum carrier of IGF peptides, is a potential additional tool for evaluating GH function.[373,1258,1259] The advantages of assaying IGFBP3 concentration include the following:

1. IGFBP-3 levels are GH dependent.
2. IGFBP3 levels are constant throughout the day.
3. The immunoassay of IGFBP3 is technically simple and does not require separation of the binding protein from IGF peptides.
4. Normal serum levels of IGFBP3 are high, typically in the 1 to 5 mg/L range, so that assay sensitivity is not an issue. (The molar concentration of IGFBP3 approximates the sum of the molar concentration of IGF1 and IGF2.)
5. Serum IGFBP3 levels vary with age to a lesser degree than is the case for IGF1 (Fig. 24-42). Even in infants, serum IGFBP3 levels are sufficiently high to allow discrimination of low values from the normal range.
6. Serum IGFBP3 levels are less dependent on nutrition than serum IGF1, reflecting the "stabilizing" effect of IGF2 levels.

Like IGF1 levels, determination of the sensitivity and specificity of IGBP3 levels for identifying GHD suffers from the lack of a gold standard. With that limitation in mind, Blum and colleagues[1259] initially found that low IGFBP3 levels had both high sensitivity (97%) and high specificity (95%) for GHD. Most subsequent studies confirmed the high specificity, with values generally greater than 80% to 90%.[1225,1240,1242,1244,1260] However, most studies have found that many children diagnosed with GHD on the basis of provocative GH testing actually have normal IGFBP levels, and the sensitivity of this test is less than 60%. In a study by Cianfarani and colleagues,[1240] only 7% (2/28) of children younger than 14 years of age with GHD had an IGFBP3 level more than 1 SD below the mean. Low IGFBP3 levels may be an indicator of more severe GHD. For example, in one study the sensitivity of the IGFBP3 assay if the peak GH was less than 5 μg/L on provocative testing was 93%, but when the peak GH was 5 to 10 μg/L, the sensitivity was only 43%.[1261]

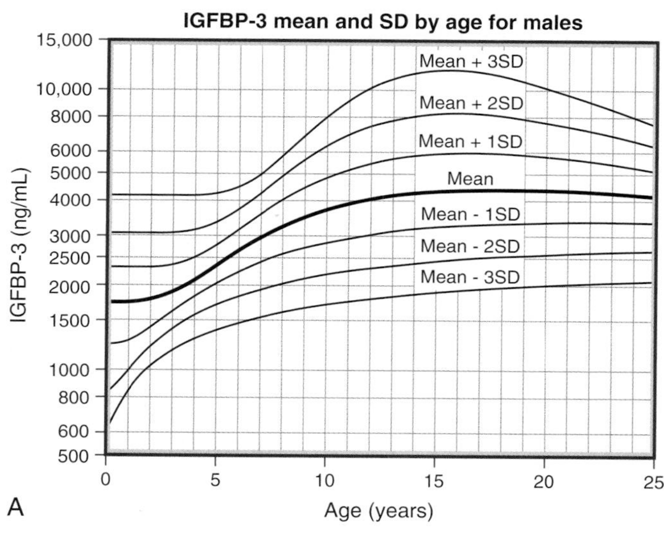

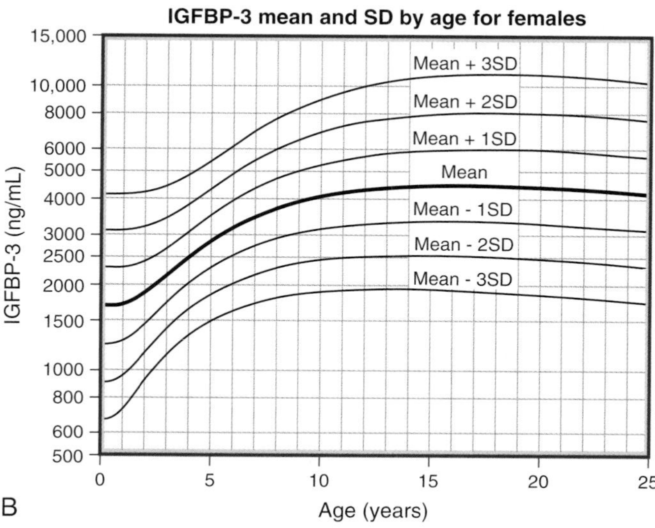

Figure 24-42 Normal serum levels of insulin-like growth factor–binding protein 3 (IGFBP3) for males **(A)** and females **(B)**. (Data courtesy of Diagnostic Systems Laboratories, Inc., Webster, TX.)

Insulin-Like Growth Factor 2. IGF2 levels are higher than those of IGF1. Levels increase rapidly after birth, but thereafter IGF2 levels are less age dependent than those of IGF1. However, although GHD is associated with low IGF2 levels, IGF2 is much less GH dependent than IGF1 (Fig. 24-43). In two studies, IGF2 levels were more than 2 SD below the mean in only 21% and 31% of children defined as GH deficient based on provocative GH testing.[1240,1262]

Rosenfeld and colleagues[1243] found low IGF2 levels in 52% of GH-deficient children and in 35% of normal short children. However, only 4% of GH-deficient children and 11% of normal short children had normal plasma levels of both IGF1 and IGF2, showing a similar sensitivity and specificity to combined IGF1/IGFBP3 testing.

Growth Hormone. Assessment of pituitary GH production is difficult because GH secretion is pulsatile, with the most consistent surges occurring at times of slow-wave electroencephalographic rhythms during stage 3 and stage 4 of sleep. Spontaneous GH secretion varies with gender, age, pubertal stage, and nutritional status, all of which must be factored into the evaluation of GH production.

Between normal pulses of GH secretion, serum GH levels are low (often <0.1 μg/L), below the limits of sensitivity of most conventional assays (typically <0.2 μg/L). Accordingly, measurement of random serum GH concentrations is almost useless in diagnosing GHD but may be useful in the diagnosis of GH insensitivity and GH excess. Measurement of GH "secretory reserve" relies on the use of physiologic or pharmacologic stimuli, and such provocative tests have formed the basis for diagnosis of GHD for more than 30 years.[1263,1264]

Assay Limitations. One of the biggest confounders in the evaluation of GH secretion is the variability of measured GH levels across different assays. Many studies have demonstrated as much as threefold variability in the measurement of serum GH levels among established laboratories.[1265-1268] This is explained, in part, by the presence of several molecular forms of GH in serum. Circulating GH consists of monomers of the two secreted GH isoforms (with approximately 43% existing as the monomeric 22-kd isoform and 8% as the monomeric 20-kd isoform), along with dimers and higher-order oligomers of the two isoforms, acetylated forms of GH, desamidated GH, and peptide fragments of GH.[1225] Therefore, much of the variability in results is due to the use of different monoclonal or polyclonal antibodies, including variability in recognition of the different circulating forms of GH by these antibodies. Additionally, variations in the choice of standards, labeling techniques, and assay buffers (matrix) are also contributory.[1225] Consequently, a child who is determined to have GHD by one assay may be considered

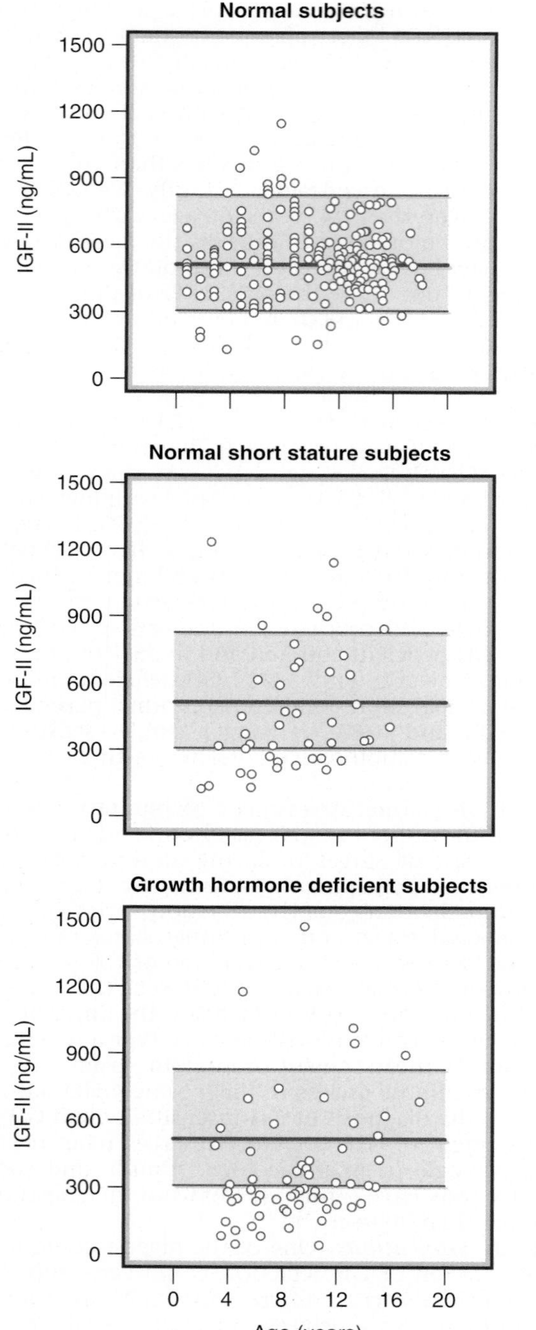

Figure 24-43 Serum insulin-like growth factor 2 (IGF-II) levels in normal patients and in patients with growth disorders. (From Rosenfeld RG, Wilson DM, Lee PD, et al. Insulin-like growth factors I and II in the evaluation of growth retardation. *J Pediatr.* 1986;109:428-433.)

normal by another. This is an unacceptable situation for clinicians, who may be unaware of the type and source of the GH assay being used by a given laboratory.[1269]

Provocative Tests. Because random GH levels cannot be used to diagnose GHD, evaluation of GH secretion requires that samples be obtained after an expected stimulation of GH secretion. Physiologic stimuli include fasting, sleep, and exercise, and pharmacologic stimuli include levodopa, clonidine, glucagon, propranolol, arginine, and insulin. Standard provocative GH tests are summarized in Table 24-10. GH levels are measured on multiple specimens obtained after the stimulus. Failure to increase serum GH above a defined cutoff level is believed to indicate GHD.

Although provocative GH testing has been the foundation for diagnosis of GHD since GH assays first became available, they have a number of weaknesses whey they are used to identify GHD.[1263,1269,1270] Most importantly, there is no clear cutoff level that discriminates a normal response from a deficient response, and secondly, these provocative tests have poor specificity.

Determination of the "Subnormal" Response to Provocative Tests. GH secretion has a continuous distribution; there is not a bimodal distribution of either spontaneous GH secretion or peak GH levels after provocative tests that would clearly separate normal from deficient secretion. The initial levels of GH during provocative testing that were used to define GHD were based on the study of patients with profound classic findings or organic destruction of the adenohypophysis.[1271] In addition, partly because of the limited supply of GH, one goal was to identify the most severely affected children.

Initially, a cutoff level of 2.5 μg/L was used; this was later increased to 5 μg/L and subsequently to 7 μg/L. After the development of recombinant DNA-derived GH eliminated the limits on GH supply, many pediatric endocrinologists considered a peak GH level lower than 10 μg/L to be indicative of GHD. The higher cutoff level can be partially justified by the desire to identify children with GHD that is less complete (i.e., partial GHD). Nonetheless, there have been few data validating the higher cutoff values.[1270,1272]

Further confounding the determination of an evidence-based cutoff level is the variability in GH levels measured across different assays (discussed earlier). Many new GH assays give results that are 33% to 50% lower than earlier assays, but there has not been a systematic reassessment of the "new normal" GH cutoff levels nor a critical evaluation by many endocrinologists of which assay their center might be using.[1273,1274] The same cutoff level has been applied without regard to the stimulus used. However, the peak GH levels obtained are only modestly different for many of these agents, with the exception of GHRH, which leads to substantially higher levels of GH,[1275-1277] indicating a need for a higher cutoff value for such tests.

Specificity of Provocative Tests for Growth Hormone Deficiency. The data that are available suggest a low specificity for the provocative tests, with a substantial number of normal children having peak GH levels lower than 7 to 10 μg/L.[1269] Ghigo and colleagues[1276] studied 472 healthy, normal children, including 296 with normal stature and 177 with normal short stature. Excluding tests that used GHRH (which has generally not been used in the evaluation of GH function in children), they found that between 10% and 25% of their subjects had peak GH levels lower than 7 μg/L and 23% to 49% had peak levels lower than 10 μg/L. Similar results were found in other studies.[1278-1281] Because of this poor specificity, failure on two provocative tests should be obtained before GHD is diagnosed on the basis of provocative testing. This approach significantly improves the specificity of provocative testing, although it remains imperfect. In the study of Ghigo and colleagues,[1276] two tests were performed on 78 children, and 10% had peak GH levels lower than 10 μg/L on both tests (2.6% had peak GH levels <7 μg/L on both tests).

The specificity of provocative GH tests can be increased by using a lower cutoff point to define a normal response. However, this is undesirable if it excludes individuals with less severe degrees of GHD. Because of the continuous nature of GH secretion across individuals and the lack of

TABLE 24-10

Tests to Provoke Growth Hormone Secretion

Stimulus	Dosage	Times Samples Are Taken (min)	Comments
Sleep	Obtain sample from indwelling catheter	60-90 min after onset of sleep	
Exercise	Step climbing; exercise cycle for 10 minutes	0, 10, 20	Observe child closely when on the steps
Levodopa	<15 kg: 125 mg 10-30 kg: 250 mg >30 kg: 500 mg	0, 60, 90	Nausea, rarely emesis
Clonidine	0.15 mg/m^2	0, 30, 60, 90	Tiredness, postural hypotension
Arginine HCl (IV)	0.5 g/kg (max 30 g) 10% arginine HCl in 0.9% NaCl over 30 min	0, 15, 30, 45, 60	
Insulin (IV)*	0.05 to 0.1 unit/kg	0, 15, 30, 60, 75, 90, 120	Hypoglycemia, requires close supervision
Glucagon (IM)	0.03 mg/kg (max 1 mg)	0, 30, 60, 90, 120, 150, 180	Nausea, occasional emesis
GHRH (IV)†	1 μg/kg	0, 15, 30, 45, 60, 90, 120	Flushing, metallic taste

Patients must be euthyroid at the time of testing. Tests should be performed after an overnight fast. For prepubertal children, pretreating with sex hormones increases the specificity of the tests (see text).

†The cutoff used for tests involving GHRH is highter than that for other tests. (Maghnie M et al. J Clin Endocrinol Metab 2002. 87:2740-4 and Pandian R et al. Clin Lab Med 2004. 24:141-74.)

*Insulin-induced hypoglycemia is a potential risk of this procedure, which is designed to lower the blood glucose by at least 50%. Documentation of appropriate lowering of blood glucose is recommended. If GHD is suspected, the lower dosage of insulin is usually administered, especially in infants. $D_{10}W$ and glucagon should be available.

(Table dervived from Post EM, Richman RA. A condensed table for predicting adult stature. *J Pediatr* 1981. 989:440-442 based on the data of Bayley and Pinneau.[1233] Predicted final height is calculated by dividing the current height by the fraction of adult height achieved, determined from the table.)

a gold standard test for GHD, the conflict between specificity and sensitivity cannot be completely resolved. However, two reports have examined multiple clinical and laboratory characteristics of short children who were divided into three groups based on their results on GH stimulation testing: a group whose results were low (<5 or <7 μg/L), fulfilling criteria for GHD; a group whose results were greater than 10 μg and therefore were believed not to have GHD; and a group whose results were intermediate between these high and low cutoff points. In both of these studies, the group with the lowest peak GH levels differed significantly from both the intermediate and the high-GH groups on numerous measures.[1282,1283] However, the intermediate group was indistinguishable from the group without GHD, rather than having characteristics intermediate between the other two groups, as might be expected if they had a less severe degree of GHD.

Sex Hormone Priming. Serum GH levels rise during puberty, with GH secretion stimulated by the rise in estrogen produced from the ovary or from aromatization of testosterone.[135,148] This same process results in higher peak GH levels during provocative testing in pubertal children (compared with prepubertal children)[1279,1284] and in children who have received treatment with estrogen or testosterone.[1279,1284-1288] In a study by Marin and colleagues,[1279] 61% of normal prepubertal children and 44% of normal children in early puberty (Tanner stage I) had GH levels lower than 7 μg/L on provocative testing; based on these results (but not on their heights), they would have met criteria for a diagnosis of GHD. However, after 2 days of treatment with estrogen, 95% of these children had a peak GH level higher than 7 μg/L. Therefore, the specificity of GH provocative tests can be improved by pretreating ("priming") the pediatric patients with exogenous gonadal steroids.[1289,1290] In a placebo-controlled comparison, the specificity of GH provocative tests (using 9 μg/L as a cutoff point on a polyclonal GH assay) increased from 80% to 98% after estrogen priming.[1287] In a study of 50 growth-retarded boys who had subnormal results on provocative GH tests without testosterone priming but normal results after priming, final height (without intervention) was greater than the midparental height, consistent with normal GH function in these children.[1291]

Another factor to consider when evaluating provocative GH testing is the impact of body weight on GH secretion. In both adults[121,156,1292,1293] and children,[152,1294,1295] obese individuals have decreased spontaneous and stimulated GH levels, compared with nonobese individuals. Even within the normal range, the BMI SDS is inversely associated with peak GH level on provocative tests in children.[1296,1297] Therefore, particular care must be taken when interpreting GH stimulation test results in obese individuals.

Although there are limitations to the information gained from provocative GH tests, they continue to be helpful in evaluating a child for GHD. The tests should be performed after an overnight fast, and the patient needs to be euthyroid at the time of testing. Testing should not be performed if the patient is taking supraphysiologic doses of glucocorticoid (i.e., >15 mg/m^2 per day of hydrocortisone or the equivalent of a synthetic glucocorticoid), because these drugs can suppress the GH response. The tests are generally safe, although appropriate precautions must be taken. Specifically, tests involving insulin administration carry the risk of hypoglycemia and seizures, and should be performed only by experienced medical personnel and under appropriate patient supervision. Deaths have been reported from insulin-induced hypoglycemia and from its overly vigorous correction with parenteral glucose.[1297] The specificity of the tests can be increased by pretreating the child with estrogen or testosterone (e.g., 5 mg of conjugated estrogens orally on the night before and the morning of the test, or 50 to 100 μg/day of ethinyl estradiol for 3 consecutive days before testing, or 100 mg of depot testosterone 3 days before testing) and by carefully selecting the lower limit for a normal response.

Tests of Spontaneous Growth Hormone Secretion. Another diagnostic approach to evaluate GH secretion involves measurement of spontaneous GH secretion. This can be done either by multiple sampling (every 5 to 30 minutes) over a 12- to 24-hour period or by continuous blood withdrawal over 12 to 24 hours.[96,1298-1300] The former method allows one to evaluate and characterize GH pulsatility, whereas the latter only permits determination of the mean GH concentration. Both methods are subject to many of the same limitations as provocative GH testing. The problems of expense and discomfort are obvious, and, although it was thought that this approach might be more reproducible than provocative GH tests, variability remains a problem.[1301-1303] The ability of such tests to discriminate between children with GHD and those with normal short stature is very limited due to significant overlap of each of the parameters measured between normal children and children with GHD. Rose and coworkers[1304] reported that measurement of spontaneous GH secretion identified only 57% of children with GHD as defined by provocative testing. Similarly, Lanes[1305] reported that one fourth of normally growing children have low overnight GH levels, and a longitudinal study of normal boys through puberty demonstrated a wide intersubject variance, including many "low" 24-hour GH production rates in children with fully normal growth.[135,136] Therefore, measurement of spontaneous GH secretion does not appear to offer advantages over alternative means of evaluating GH function.

Summary. Despite the many problems associated with GH measurement methods, there continues to be value in determining GH secretory capacity in the diagnostic evaluation of a child with growth failure. Documentation of GH levels as being decreased, normal, or increased helps in discriminating among GHD, non–GH/IGF1-related growth failure (including ISS), and GH insensitivity. Results supporting the presence of GHD alert the clinician to the possibility of other pituitary deficiencies. The presence of pituitary dysfunction mandates clinical and radiologic evaluation for evidence of congenital or acquired structural defects of the hypothalamus or pituitary, including the possibility of intracranial tumors. Finally, documentation of GHD, either alone or combined with other pituitary deficiencies, may warrant evaluation for molecular defects of GH production.

Growth Hormone–Binding Protein. Mutation of the GHR can impair GH signaling, resulting in GH insensitivity. The most severe mutations cause profound growth failure (Laron dwarfism). The extracellular portion of the GHR is cleaved from the remaining portion and circulates in the blood as GHBP. GHBP levels can be measured in serum. Low levels, particularly undetectable levels, may be diagnostic of GH insensitivity due to GHR mutations.

GHBP levels are not low in all forms of GH insensitivity. The levels may be normal, or even increased, with mutations in the GHR that do not alter the GHBP portion of the protein (i.e., mutations in the transmembrane or intracellular domains) or with defects that are downstream of the GHR.

IGF1 and IGFBP Generation Tests. IGF1 and IGFBP3 generation tests are designed to evaluate for the presence of GH insensitivity.[1306] When patients with GH insensitivity are treated with GH for several days, the levels of IGF1 and IGFBP do not increase as they would in normal individuals.[1307-1310] Criteria for a response indicating GH insensitivity have included a rise in IGF1 of less than two times the intra-assay variation (approximately 10%)[755,1311] or a failure to increase IGF1 by at least 15 μg/L.[1312] However, Laron dwarfism is extremely rare outside specific communities, so the role of these tests in clinical practice is limited.

The utility of these tests in identifying more subtle forms of GH insensitivity in children with ISS has been explored,[1307,1313] but at this time additional data are needed to determine the usefulness of this test in such cases. It will also be important to know the limitations of the test in such instances, including understanding of potential confounders. For example, studies have indicated that the IGF1 response to GH is related to BMI and adiposity[1284,1314] and to pubertal stage.[1234]

Interpretation of Tests

Neonate. GH levels in the neonate are much higher than levels seen after this period. Levels are highest in cord blood and within the first days of life.[1315] Cornblath and colleagues reported in 1965 an average GH concentration in cord blood of 66 μg/L; this fell over the first week to an average of 16 to 20 μg/L in infants 7 to 55 days of age.[1315] However, even under the assay conditions used, the range of levels reported included measurements as low as 1 μg/L. Subsequent studies confirmed the high GH levels in neonates, with many documenting cord blood levels in the range of 20 to 40 μg/L,[1316-1319] although other studies using similar assays found levels of 13 to 18 μg/L. Other studies also confirmed that GH levels fall during the first week of life.[1316,1320,1321] GH levels in preterm infants have generally been found to be even higher than those in full-term infants.[1315,1317,1322,1323]

The neonatal period is one period during which random measurement of GH levels may be useful. However, low values can be found in healthy neonates,[1320,1322,1323] so, although a high value can exclude GHD, a single low value is not diagnostic of GHD. There have been no studies reporting GH levels in GH-deficient infants compared with normal infants. However, after the first week of life, if the clinical findings in a neonate raise concern for GHD (see Table 24-8), multiple random GH levels that are all below the cutoff value used to define normal GH secretion during provocative testing would be supportive of the diagnosis of GHD. GH levels that are obtained during an episode of spontaneous hypoglycemia or during a glucagon stimulation test, should also increase at least above the same cutoff value. An IGFBP3 measurement is of value for the diagnosis of neonatal GHD and should be measured in infants with suspected GHD; IGF1 levels are rarely helpful.[1324]

Growth Hormone Deficiency. Both clinical and laboratory evaluation must be utilized when considering the diagnosis of GHD in a child being evaluated because of short stature or growth failure.[1237,1325] As discussed earlier, there is no definitive test for the diagnosis for GHD. In addition, the laboratory tests for GHD have poor specificity and should be performed only in children who have a clinical presentation consistent with GHD. Short children who have well-documented normal height velocities usually do not require evaluation of GH function. Therefore, the evaluation starts with identifying those children who may have GHD based on risk factors or growth parameters (see Table 24-8 and Fig. 24-39).

In a child with a history and growth pattern that indicate a risk for GHD and in whom other causes for growth failure (including hypothyroidism) have been excluded, testing for GHD begins with measurement of the IGF1 level and proceeds to GH provocation tests in selected patients (see Fig. 24-39). In some cases, particularly in younger children, it may also be helpful to measure the IGFBP3 level. If IGHD is suspected, two GH provocation tests (given sequentially or on separate days) are required. A patient is diagnosed with classic GHD when the IGF1 (or IGFBP3) level is below the normal range (i.e., >2 SD below the mean for age and pubertal status) and peak GH levels on two provocative tests are below the cutoff value that supports a diagnosis of GHD. The diagnosis is more firmly established if the child is pretreated with estrogen or testosterone before the provocative GH tests. In a patient with defined CNS pathology, a history of irradiation, CPHD, or a genetic defect, one provocative GH test suffices. In patients who have had cranial irradiation or malformations of the hypothalamic-pituitary unit, GHD may evolve over years, and its diagnosis may require serial testing.

Some patients with auxology suggestive of GHD may have IGF1 and/or IGFBP3 levels below the normal range on repeated tests but GH responses in provocation tests above the cutoff level. Such children do not have classic GHD but may have an abnormality of the GH-IGF1 axis. The child with a history of cranial irradiation, decreased height velocity, and reduced serum levels of IGF1 and IGFBP3 may have GHD (or GH insensitivity) even in the face of normal provocative tests.[1326] Other children may have GHD that is not supported by the results of nonphysiologic provocative tests (perhaps a more mild degree of GHD than in those who fail the provocative tests), or they may have GH insensitivity (discussed later). Systemic disorders affecting the synthesis or action of IGF1 must again be considered and excluded. Such children that continue to show growth failure (i.e., height below the 3rd percentile and growth velocity below the 25th percentile) could be considered for GH treatment.

A difficult clinical situation to resolve is that of the short child with a persistently subnormal growth velocity whose IGF1 and IGFBP3 levels are normal. One can reasonably exclude consideration of GHD if the IGF1 level is higher than 1 SD below the normal mean. However, because up to 30% of children with GHD identified by GH stimulation testing have had IGF1 levels that were not low,[1225,1242-1245] it is appropriate to consider provocative GH testing in those children with persistent growth failure who have an IGF1 level between −1 SD and −2 SD for age and puberty status, with abnormal results on two tests indicating a diagnosis of GHD. In this situation in particular, it would be appropriate to pretreat the child with testosterone or estrogen in order to maximize the specificity of the provocative tests.

A cranial MRI scan with particular attention to the hypothalamic-pituitary region should be carried out in any child who is diagnosed as having GHD. In addition,

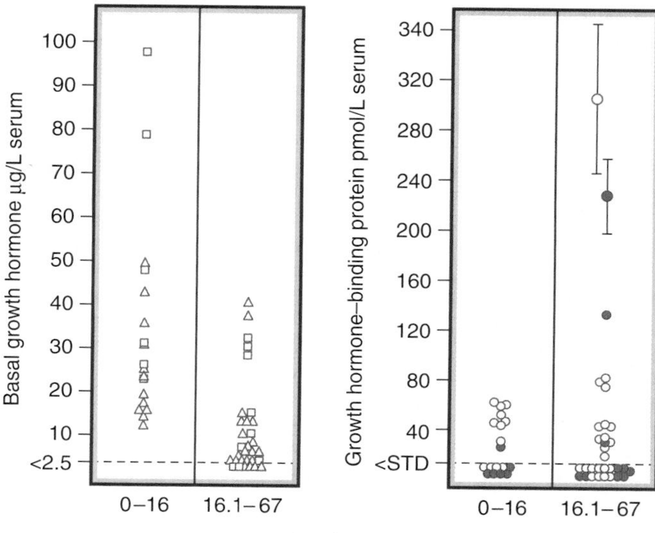

Figure 24-44 GH assays were performed by RIA (*squares*) and by immunoradiometric assay (*triangles*). For GHBP levels, open circles represent females, and closed circles represent males. Mean +/− SEM of GHBP levels in adult Ecuadorian controls are shown. STD, assay standard. (From Rosenfeld RG, Rosenbloom AL, Guevara-Acquirre J. Growth hormone [GH] resistance due to primary GH receptor deficiency. *Endocr Rev.* 1994;15:369-390.)

documentation of abnormal pituitary GH secretion should prompt evaluation for other pituitary hormone deficiencies. Based on the clinical scenario, one may also consider molecular evaluation of GH, GHR, GHRHR and other potential genetic defects.

Growth Hormone Insensitivity. GH insensitivity is characterized by low serum IGF1 concentrations in the presence of normal (or increased) production of GH (Figs. 24-44 and 24-45). As discussed earlier, GH insensitivity can

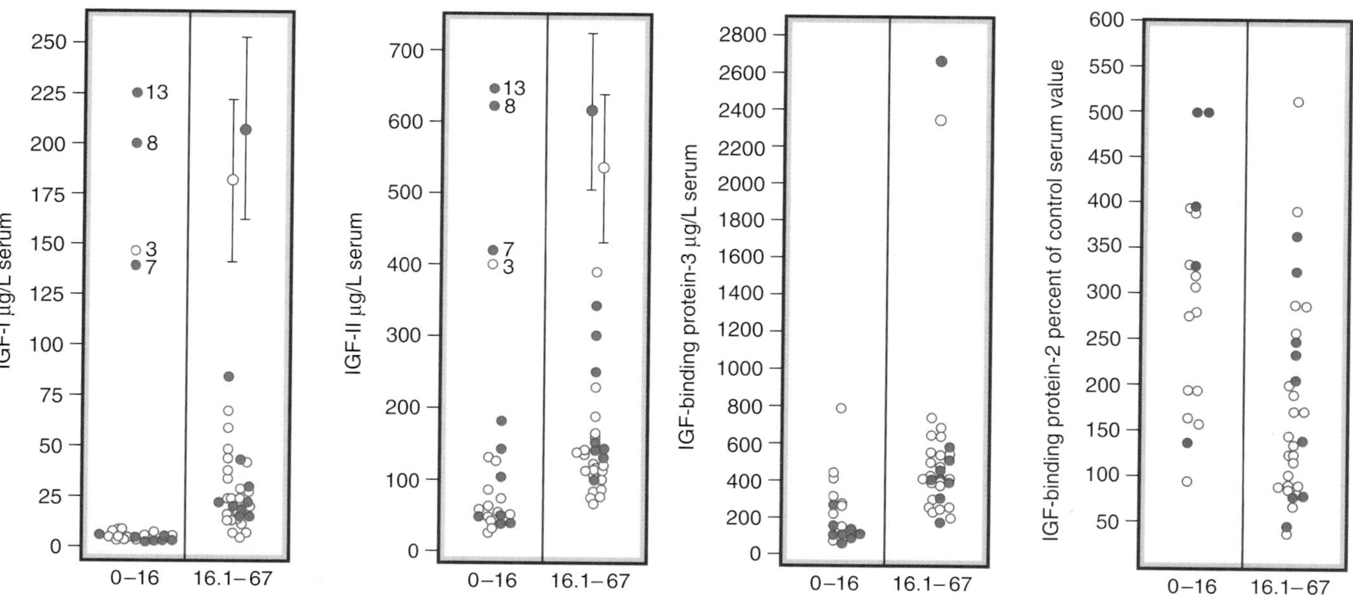

Figure 24-45 Serum levels of insulin-like growth factors (IGF) and IGF-binding proteins in patients from Ecuador with growth hormone receptor deficiency. Open circles represent females, closed circles represent males. Control values for Ecuadorian adults are shown as mean +/−SD for males and females, except for IGFBP-3, where large circles represent pooled male (*closed circle*) and female (*open circle*) control sera. Numbers adjacent to circles represent normal Ecuadorian childred of 3, 7, 8, and 13 yr of age. (From Rosenfeld RG, Rosenbloom AL, Guevara-Acquirre J. Growth hormone [GH] resistance due to primary GH receptor deficiency. *Endocr Rev.* 1994;15:369-390.)

be caused by defects of the GHR (Laron syndrome), the GH signaling cascade, IGFBPs, IGF1, or the IGF1 receptor.[763] If GH insensitivity is defined more broadly as growth failure in the absence of GHD, then defects in IGFBPs, IGF1, and the type I IGF receptor can also be considered forms of "partial" GH insensitivity (i.e., because non–IGF1-mediated growth is not impaired); IGF1 levels may or may not be low in these disorders.[763] GH insensitivity should be considered in a patient with growth failure who has a low IGF1 level but evidence of increased GH secretion based on increased basal or stimulated GH levels (e.g., basal GH levels >5 μg/L or stimulated levels >15 μg/L). This pattern is also seen with malnutrition, a form of physiologic GH insensitivity. If GH insensitivity is suspected, GHBP and ALS can be measured: low values support the diagnosis of GH insensitivity due to mutations in the genes for the GHR or ALS. IGF1/IGFBP3 generation studies may demonstrate GH insensitivity, but they cannot completely discriminate among its various causes. In addition, there is limited normative data or standardization of such tests, so their ability to identify defects other than the severe insensitivity of Laron syndrome is not yet known.

Savage and Rosenfeld[755,1311] devised a scoring system for use in evaluating short children for the diagnosis of GHR deficiency, based on five parameters: (1) basal serum GH level greater than 10 mU/L (approximately 5 μg/L); (2) serum IGF1 level less than 50 μg/L; (3) height SDS less than −3; (4) serum GHBP less than 10% (based on binding of [^{125}I]GH); and (5) a rise in serum IGF1 levels after GH administration of less than two times the intra-assay variation (approximately 10%). Blum and associates[1312] proposed that these criteria could be strengthened by (1) evaluating GH secretory profiles rather than isolated basal levels; (2) employing an age-dependent range and the 0.1 percentile as the cutoff level for evaluation of serum IGF1 concentrations; (3) employing highly sensitive IGF1 immunoassays and defining a failed GH response as the inability to increase serum IGF1 levels by at least 15 μg/L; and (4) measuring both basal and GH-stimulated IGFBP3 levels. These criteria fit well with findings in the population of GHR-deficient patients in Ecuador, but that is a homogeneous population with severe GH insensitivity.[151,1327] The applicability of these criteria elsewhere remains to be evaluated. An important biochemical marker is the response of IGF1 (and possibly, IGFBP3) to GH stimulation.[1313,1328,1329]

Additional considerations related to GH insensitivity include the following:

1. The presence of IUGR (in addition to postnatal growth failure) suggests IGF1 gene deletions, bioinactive IGF1, or IGF type I receptor abnormalities.
2. Low GHBP suggests a defect in the extracellular domain of the GHR, but normal (or increased) GHBP may be seen in some patients with defects of the GHR or the GH signaling cascade.
3. An elevated IGF1 level (in a child with growth failure) may suggest a defect in the IGF type I receptor[1330,1331]; markedly elevated levels suggest bioinactive IGF1.[341]
4. IGFBP3 and ALS concentrations may be increased in patients with molecular defects of IGF1.
5. STAT5B defects should be suspected in a child with evidence of GH insensitivity who has evidence of immune deficiency; an elevated PRL level has also been reported in the presence of STAT5B mutation.[1332]

Constitutional Delay of Growth and Development. The term *CDGD* describes children who have a normal variant of maturational tempo characterized by short stature with relatively normal growth rates during childhood, delayed puberty with a late and attenuated pubertal growth spurt, and attainment of a normal adult height that is also within the target height range based on parental heights (Table 24-11).[38,1333] In childhood, such patients have heights that are lower than expected based on parental heights. CDGD aggregates in families.[1334] The diagnosis of CDGD may be suspected in a child with short stature if one or both parents have a history of a late timing of puberty. Bone age is usually delayed, so the predicted final height is in the normal range and is within the child's target height range, although the correlation between predicted and final height is imperfect and must be viewed with caution.[43,1335,1336] The predicted final height, especially when the skeletal age is extremely delayed, is greater than that usually achieved but is difficult to reliably anticipate.[43,1336,1338] Although the findings described can lead to a presumptive diagnosis of CDGD, the diagnosis can only be made retrospectively, once the child demonstrates a late timing for puberty and completes his or her growth in the normal range and at a height consistent with the parents' heights.

TABLE 24-11

Criteria for Presumptive Diagnosis of Constitutional Delay of Growth and Development

1. No history of systemic illness
2. Normal nutrition
3. Normal physical examination, including body proportions
4. Normal thyroid and growth hormone levels
5. Normal complete blood count, sedimentation rate, electrolytes, blood urea nitrogen
6. Height ≤3rd percentile but with annual growth rate >5th percentile for age
7. Delayed puberty: in males, failure to achieve Tanner G2 stage by age 13.8 yr or P2 by 15.6 yr; in females, failure to achieve Tanner B2 stage by age 13.3 yr
8. Delayed bone age
9. Normal predicted adult height: in males, >163 cm (64"); in females, >150 cm (59")

Because of the estrogen stimulation associated with GH secretion that occurs during puberty, children with CDGD can be expected to have decreased GH secretion and lower IGF1 levels compared with their pubertal, age-matched peers. However, IGF1 levels should be normal for pubertal stage, and GH levels on provocative tests should be normal after pretreatment with gonadal steroids.[122,1289,1338,1339] Overnight GH secretion is usually normal in these children when control groups are carefully matched.[1340]

It is often difficult to differentiate CDGD from GHD. Both groups of patients have height SDS below their target height SDS range, and both have delayed bone ages. As the child with CDGD enters the usual age for puberty, his or her growth rate can be too low to exclude GHD on that basis. (The growth rate normally declines throughout childhood until it increases at the time of the pubertal growth spurt; a child with CDGD and delayed pubertal growth spurt may have an additional 2 or more years of declining growth velocity, which can result in growth velocities <4 cm/year.) If there is a clear family history of CDGD, the likelihood is high that the child also has CDGD, and careful continued observation may be all that is needed. An increase in growth velocity after treatment with a short course of sex hormone can be taken as evidence against the presence of GHD.[1341] In some cases, however, a laboratory investigation to exclude GHD is necessary. In such children, levels of IGF1 and IGFBP3 that are low for pubertal stage or skeletal age and a poor GH response to provocative testing after priming with gonadal steroids would raise concern for GHD and would mandate the appropriate investigation for underlying pathology (e.g., intracranial tumor).

Genetic (Familial) Short Stature. The control of growth in childhood and the final height attained are polygenic in nature. Familial height affects the growth of an individual, and evaluation of a specific growth pattern must be placed in the context of familial growth and stature. As discussed at the beginning of this chapter, calculations can be made to determine whether a child's growth pattern is appropriate based on his or her parents' heights. As a general rule, a child who is growing at a rate that is inconsistent with that of siblings or parents warrants further evaluation.

Genetic short stature (GSS), also called familial short stature, is a normal growth pattern that describes the growth of healthy individuals who fall at the lower extreme of the distribution of height (i.e., below the 3rd percentile). Their height is appropriate for their genetic potential based on the parents' heights; that is, their height SDS is within the target height SDS range. Particularly when the midparental height is significantly above or below the mean, it is important to include adjustment for regression toward the mean when calculating this target height range.

Although the differentiation may not be complete, children with GSS are generally distinguished from children with CDGD: those with GSS will have a final height that is below the 3rd percentile, whereas children with CDGD will achieve a final height in the normal range. The midparental height of children with GSS is lower than that of children with CDGD; often, height in both parents is below the 10th percentile. Growth in children with GSS is at or below the 3rd percentile, but the velocity is usually normal. The onset and progression of puberty are normal, so the skeletal age is concordant with chronologic age. Final heights in these individuals are in the target height range for the family.[42] By definition, the GH/IGF1 system is normal (as are all other systems).

Many diseases characterized by growth retardation are genetically transmitted, including GH insensitivity due to mutations of the *GHR* gene; *GH* gene deletions; mutations of the *PROP1, POUF1,* or *SHOX* genes; pseudohypoparathyroidism; and some forms of hypothyroidism. Inherited nonendocrine diseases characterized by short stature include osteochondrodysplasias and dysmorphic syndromes associated with IUGR (both described earlier), inborn errors of metabolism, renal disease, and thalassemia. Identifying a patient's short stature as inherited does not, by itself, relieve the clinician of responsibility for determining the underlying cause of growth failure. Moreover, a parent's short stature may be the result of an uncharacterized genetic difference that has been transmitted to the child and is causing the child's short stature. Because height is normally distributed in the population, it can be arbitrary whether one characterizes such genetic differences as mutations or as allelic variants. However, the further the parents' and the child's heights are from the mean, the more reasonable it is to consider such genetic alterations as abnormal.

Idiopathic Short Stature. ISS is defined as "a condition in which the height of the individual is more than 2 SD below the corresponding mean height for a given age, sex and population group, and in whom no identifiable disorder is present."[1332] This definition includes children with CDGD, those with GSS, and short children who will not have delayed puberty and whose height is not consistent with parental heights. Therefore, this definition includes both normal, healthy children (those with GSS and CDGD) and children who are presumed to have an unidentified disorder impairing their growth. It is not always a simple matter to distinguish among these possibilities: CDGD can be definitively diagnosed only at the completion of growth, and GSS does not exclude inherited disorders of growth.

Children with ISS may have undiagnosed disorders outside the GH-IGF1 axis (e.g., an uncharacterized chondrodystrophy), or they may have more subtle disorders of the hypothalamic-pituitary-IGF axis than those that are identified by the currently available diagnostics tests.[763,775] Because of the lack of a gold standard for the diagnosis of GHD, the distinction between isolated partial GHD and ISS is somewhat arbitrary, relying heavily on the results of the nonphysiologic provocative stimulation tests. The activity of different GH promoter haplotypes can differ as much as sixfold.[728,1342] Some children with ISS may have GH neurosecretory dysfunction that cannot be detected with current diagnostic tests.[1298,1299] Similarly, although the severe GH insensitivity of Laron syndrome can be identified by laboratory testing, partial GH insensitivity may be an unrecognized cause of ISS.[1343]

Heterozygous mutations in the GHR have been found in significant numbers of children with ISS.[774,777,1344] In heterozygotes, protein from the mutant allele may disrupt the normal dimerization and rotation that is needed for normal GHR activation, leading to diminished GH action and growth impairment.[1345] In addition, GHBP expression may be decreased in patients with ISS, 20% of whom have serum levels of GHBP below the normal range.[1343,1346,1347] Other potential causes for partial GH insensitivity in ISS include heterozygous mutations in other components of the growth system, a relatively greater preponderance of blockers of the GH-signaling cascade (e.g., enhanced intracellular phosphatase activity, production of such signaling factors as SOC2 and CIS), gene-mediated alterations in patterns of GH or IGF production, or other possibilities yet to be discovered.[1348]

Treatment of Growth Retardation

When growth failure is the result of a chronic underlying disease, such as renal failure, CF, or malabsorption, therapy must first be directed at treatment of the underlying condition. Although growth acceleration may occur in such children with GH or IGF1 therapy, complete catch-up requires correction of the primary medical problem. If treatment of the underlying condition involves glucocorticoids, growth failure may be profound and is unlikely to be correctable until steroids are reduced or discontinued.

Correction of growth failure associated with chronic hypothyroidism requires appropriate thyroid replacement. As discussed earlier, thyroid therapy causes dramatic catch-up growth but also markedly accelerates skeletal maturation, potentially limiting adult height.

Treatment of Constitutional Delay

CDGD is a normal growth variant with delayed pubertal maturation and a normal adult height. Most subjects can be managed by careful evaluation to rule out other causes of abnormal growth or delayed puberty combined with appropriate explanation and counseling. A family history of CDGD is frequently a source of reassurance. The skeletal age and Bayley-Pinneau table are often helpful in explaining the potential for normal growth to the patient and parents. The predicted final height is usually greater than that achieved, especially when the skeletal age is extremely delayed, but this is difficult to reliably anticipate.[43,1335,1337]

On occasion, the stigmata of short stature and delayed maturation are psychologically disabling for a preadolescent or teenage patient. Some adolescents with delayed puberty have poor self-image and limited social involvement.[1349] In such patients and in some in whom pubertal delay is predicted based on the overall clinical picture, there may be a role for judicious short-term treatment with androgen.

Androgen (Oxandrolone and Testosterone). Two aspects of CDGD in boys are addressed by androgen treatment: short stature, especially in boys 10 to 14 years of age, and delayed puberty after age 14. In the younger group, in whom CDGD is the presumed cause of short stature, the orally administered synthetic androgen oxandrolone has been used extensively to accelerate growth so that height increases into (or closer to) the normal range sooner than it would without treatment.[1350] In several controlled studies,[1351-1356] oxandrolone therapy for 3 months to 4 years increased linear growth velocity by 3 to 5 cm/year without adverse effects and without decreasing either actual[1356-1358] or predicted[1353,1357,1359] final height. (This treatment does not increase the final height of these boys.) The growth-promoting effects of oxandrolone appear to be related to its androgenic and anabolic effects rather than to augmentation of the GH-IGF1 axis.[1360,1361] The lack of a measurable effect on the GH-IGF1 axis probably reflects the fact that oxandrolone cannot be aromatized to estrogen. Currently recommended treatment is 0.05 to 0.1 mg/kg orally per day.

Oxandrolone is a relatively weak androgen, and its use stimulates only minimal pubertal masculinization. In older boys in whom the delayed pubertal maturation is highly stressful and anxiety-provoking, testosterone enanthate has been administered intramuscularly with success.[1350,1351,1362] Criteria for treatment in such adolescents should include (1) a minimum age of 14 years; (2) height below the 3rd percentile; (3) prepubertal or early Tanner G2 stage with an early-morning serum testosterone level of less than 3.5 nmol/L (<1 ng/mL); and (4) a poor self-image that does not respond to reassurance alone. Therapy consists of intramuscular testosterone enanthate, 50 to 100 mg every 3 to 4 weeks for a total of four to six injections.[1349-1359,1360-1363] Patients typically show early secondary sex characteristics by the fourth injection and grow an average of 10 cm in the ensuing year. Testosterone enhances growth velocity by direct actions, increases GH production, and may have a direct effect on IGF1 secretion.[122,148,149,154,1360,1364] Brief testosterone regimens do not cause overly rapid skeletal maturation, compromise adult height, or suppress pubertal maturation.[1365] It is important to emphasize to the patient that he is normal, that therapy is short-term and is designed to provide some pubertal development earlier than he would on his own, and that treatment will not increase his final adult height. In such situations, the combination of short-term androgen therapy, reassurance, and counseling can help boys with CDGD to cope with a difficult adolescence.

The availability of several new forms of testosterone, which are approved for adults with hypogonadism, provides adolescents with an opportunity for a choice among different androgen replacement therapies. Testosterone gel is painless and easy to apply and has proved popular since its release.[1366] However, there are concerns about environmental contamination, including reports of precocious puberty in children caused by topical testosterone use by an adult in the household.[1367-1369] If topical testosterone is prescribed, careful instruction must be given to avoid such inadvertent exposure of others. Testosterone patches also avoid the need for injections, but they are often poorly tolerated because of local skin reactions. Another disadvantage of topical testosterone and the transdermal patches is the need for daily application. The dosing of these alternative forms of therapy in children and adolescents has not been established, and care must be taken to avoid treating with too high a dose, which risks compromising final height.

Patients must be reevaluated to ensure that they enter "true" puberty. One year after testosterone treatment, boys should have testicular enlargement and a serum testosterone level in the pubertal range. If this is not the case, a diagnosis of hypothalamic-pituitary insufficiency or hypogonadotropic hypogonadism should be considered. Although the diagnosis of constitutional growth delay remains most likely in such patients, some eventually prove to be gonadotropin deficient, especially if they are still prepubertal late in adolescence.

Referrals for CDGD are more common in boys than girls. When CDGD is a problem in girls, short-term estrogen therapy may be employed, but the acceleration of skeletal maturation is a greater hazard at doses that enhance growth velocity and sexual maturation.

Growth Hormone. The final height of a child with CDGD will be in the normal range and appropriate for the child's genetic potential. No treatment is needed for these children to achieve a normal height. However, as discussed earlier, the diagnosis of CDGD cannot be confirmed until a late puberty and normal height are achieved. Therefore, it can be difficult in some cases to distinguish these children from children with ISS or GHD. In such cases, there may be uncertainty about whether the final height will be in the normal range, and treatment to try to increase final height may be considered. If laboratory studies support a diagnosis of GHD, then GH treatment would be appropriate. If there is no evidence of GHD, the consideration regarding treatment with GH would be the same as that regarding the use of GH to treat ISS (discussed later).

The FDA indication for GH treatment includes in its definition of ISS the criterion that the child has "growth rate[s] unlikely to permit attainment of normal adult height." A child with CDGD, who is expected to achieve a normal adult height, would not fit within this definition. Nonetheless, partly because of the uncertainty of the diagnosis and the inability to perfectly predict final height, the database on outcomes of children treated with GH for ISS includes within it data on the treatment of children with CDGD. ISS GH treatment trials may include children with significant bone age delay,[1370,1371] at least some of whom have CDGD. For this reason, the outcome data for GH treatment of ISS (see later) can be taken as an indication of the expected outcome of GH treatment of CDGD. Moreover, because estimated final height gain with GH treatment of ISS is proportional to the bone age delay at the time of initiation of treatment,[1372] height gain with GH treatment of CDGD may be greater than that for treatment of ISS. However, a retrospective study specifically reporting the outcome of GH treatment in CDGD found no difference in adult height between those treated with GH and those receiving either no treatment or testosterone treatment.[1373]

Aromatase Inhibitor. In view of the important role of estrogen in the process of skeletal maturation, aromatase inhibitors could be used in conjunction with androgen therapy to prevent an acceleration of bone age and further enhance final adult height.[1374,1375] The one report of combined use of an aromatase inhibitor (letrozole) and testosterone did not provide a clear answer as to whether the addition of aromatase inhibitor increased final height in boys with CDGD. Whereas the near-final height in the boys treated with letrozole plus testosterone was higher than that of boys treated with testosterone alone, the letrazole-treated boys were a year older at the time of these height measurements and had higher pretreatment and midparental heights.[1375] In addition, the boys treated with testosterone alone achieved a near-final height within the normal range (consistent with the diagnosis of CDGD). Given the lack of long-term safety data on the use of aromatase inhibitors in pubertal boys, there are insufficient data to suggest a role for aromatase inhibitors in CDGD.

Treatment of Growth Hormone Deficiency

Nomenclature and Potency Estimation. The nomenclature for the various biosynthetic GH preparations reflects the source and the chemical composition of the product. *Somatropin* refers to GH of the same amino acid sequence as that in naturally occurring human GH. Somatropin from human pituitary glands is abbreviated *GH* or *pit-GH;* somatropin of recombinant origin is termed *recombinant GH* or *rGH. Somatrem* refers to the methionine derivative of recombinant GH and is abbreviated *met-rGH.* Although the latter is a more antigenic preparation, that propensity is not clinically relevant; despite the presence of anti-GH antibodies, growth responses to met-rGH were similar to those in patients treated with rGH.[1376,1377] This derivative of GH is no longer available for use. In this discussion, we refer to the biosynthetic preparations as GH.

The biopotency of commercially available biosynthetic GH preparations, expressed as international units per milligram of the new World Health Organization (WHO) recombinant GH reference reagent for somatropin 88/624, is 3 IU/mg.[1378] It was necessary to standardize the early GH preparations by bioassay because of variable production techniques (e.g., extraction, column purification). The most common bioassays have been the hypophysectomized rat weight-gain assay, the tibial width assay, and the more sensitive Nb2 rat lymphoma proliferation assay.[1378-1381] With the availability of purified and essentially equivalent recombinant GH products, the requirement for bioassays has become an FDA requisite to substantiate biologic activity rather than to assess potential differences between preparations. The bioassays are likely to be replaced by in vitro binding assays using GHRs or GHBP derived from molecular techniques.[1378]

Historical Perspective. Because untreated patients with GHD have profound short stature (averaging almost −5 SDS,[1382-1385]), the clinical urgency to use GH therapy as soon as it became available is understandable.[1272] The action of GH is highly species-specific, and humans do not respond to animal-derived GH (except that from other primates).[1386] Human cadaver pituitary glands were for many years the only practical source of primate GH for treatment of GHD, and more than 27,000 children with GHD worldwide were treated with pit-GH.[1387] The limited supplies of pit-GH, the low doses used, and interrupted treatment regimens resulted in incomplete growth increments; usually, therapy was discontinued in boys who reached a height of 5 feet 5 inches and in girls who reached 5 feet. Nonetheless, this treatment did increase linear growth and in many patients enhanced final adult height. The dose-response relationship and the relation of age to GH response were recognized during this period.[1388]

Distribution of pit-GH was halted in the United States and most of Europe in 1985 because of concern about a causal relationship with Creutzfeldt-Jakob disease (CJD), a rare and fatal spongiform encephalopathy that had been previously reported to be capable of iatrogenic transmission through human tissue.[1389,1390] In North America and Europe, this disorder has an incidence of approximately 1 case per 1 million in the general population, and it is exceedingly rare before the age of 50 years. To date, more than 200 young adults who had received human cadaver pituitary products have been diagnosed with CJD, with the sad likelihood that all affected patients will die of the disease.[1391-1393] In the United States, the onset of CJD occurred 14 to 33 years after starting treatment, whereas in the large cohort of French patients the median incubation period was approximately 5 years shorter.[1393] No cases of CJD have been identified in Americans who began treatment after new methods of purifying the hormone came into use in the United States in 1977. Although the incubation period is now more than 33 years, vigilant surveillance for this dreadful complication continues; information is available on the website www.niddk.nih.gov/health/endo/pubs/creutz/updatecomp.htm (accessed October 2010).[1394,1395]

By the time the risks of pituitary-derived GH were discovered, biosynthetic GH was being tested for safety and efficacy.[1376,1396,1397] The original recombinant GH mimicked pit-GH in regard to both anabolic and metabolic actions and was scrupulously scrutinized for monoisomerism, antigenic bacterial products, and toxins of any sort. GH has universally replaced pit-GH as the accepted treatment for children with GHD.

Treatment Regimens. The recommended therapeutic starting dose of GH in children with GHD is 0.18 to 0.35 mg/kg body weight per week, administered in seven daily doses, with the mean American dose being 0.3 mg/kg per week.[1398] Alternative regimens include a 6 day/week and a 3 day/week schedule, with the same weekly dosage, but they are not as successful. In general, the growth response to GH is a function of the log-dose given, so increasing dosages further enhance growth velocities,[1387,1388,1399] but daily dosing may be the most important treatment parameter.[1400] Subcutaneous and intramuscular administration have equivalent growth-promoting activity[1401]; the former is now used exclusively. At this time, all of the commercially available GH preparations yield comparable growth outcomes.

Growth responses to exogenous GH vary, depending on the frequency of administration, dosage, age (greater absolute gain in a younger child, although not necessarily greater growth velocity SDS), weight, GHR type and amount (as assessed by serum GHBP levels), and, perhaps, seasonality.[783,1402-1405] Nevertheless, the general regimen of daily GH at the recommended doses typically accelerates growth in a GH-deficient child from a pretreatment rate of 3 to 4 cm/year to 10 to 12 cm/year in year 1 of therapy to 7 to 9 cm/year in years 2 and 3. Progressive waning of GH efficacy occurs and is poorly understood. The importance of dosage frequency is illustrated (Figs. 24-46 and 24-47) by data from a carefully done assessment of growth responses in prepubertal naïve GH-deficient children randomly assigned to receive thrice-weekly or daily GH at the same total weekly dose (0.30 mg/kg per week).[1400] The mean total height gain during this period was 9.7 cm greater in the patients treated daily (38.4 versus 28.7 cm, $P < .0002$), with similar increments in skeletal maturation and no acceleration of the

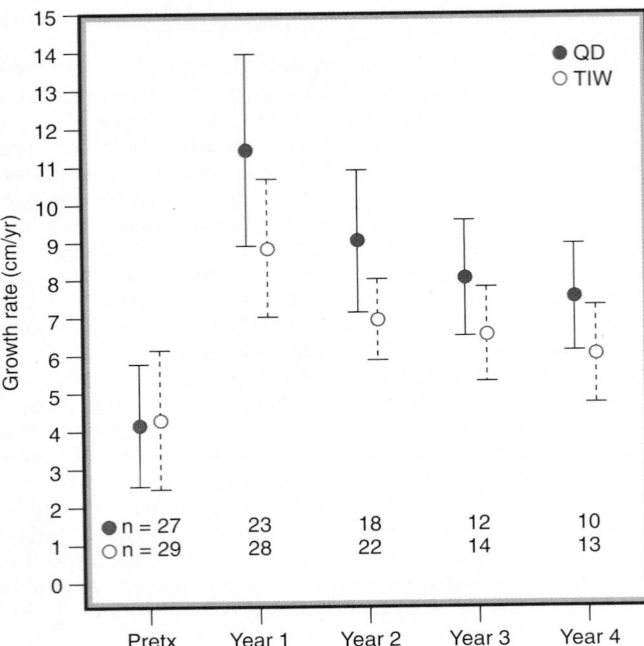

Figure 24-46 Annual growth velocity (mean ± standard deviation) for prepubertal patients with growth hormone (GH) deficiency before and during 4 years of GH treatment, contrasting results from daily (QD) versus thrice-weekly (TIW) injections. The mean annual growth velocity in the QD group was significantly greater than that in the TIW group during each year, although significance diminished from year 1 to year 4. (From MacGillivray MH, Baptista J, Johanson A, et al. Outcome of a four-year randomized study of daily versus three times weekly somatropin treatment in prepubertal naive growth hormone deficient children. *J Clin Endocrinol Metab.* 1996;81:1806-1809. Reproduced by permission of M.H. MacGillivray.)

onset of puberty. Mean height SDS at the end of 4 years was +0.2, or at the midpoint of normal for age. Studies using varying dosing of GH based on gender, growth responsivity, and growth factor concentrations have suggested the need for greater sophistication and individualization of the current treatment regimens.[1406-1407]

Sophisticated mathematical models[1399,1408] have examined many laboratory and auxologic parameters that influence response to GH therapy. Because age at onset of treatment is inversely correlated with growth responses, and because the smaller, lighter child requires less GH (with marked economic benefit), it is important to assess growth data in children treated early. In short-term studies of 134 patients[1409-1411] treated before age 3 years, marked early catch-up growth occurred, with a mean height gain of about 3 SDS by 4 years of therapy, allowing most children to reach their normal height range by middle childhood. Mean height in one study[1409] reached −0.4 SDS after 8 years of treatment. Near-adult height in 13 patients treated before 5 years of age[1412] did not differ significantly from the midparental target height (−0.9 versus −0.7 SDS). In a group of 25 children treated before 12 months of age,[1413] adult height also matched the target height despite low dosage and less frequent administration. In an analysis of postmarketing data for development of a growth prediction model, a greater height gain per GH amount occurred in the very young children, but a seemingly lowered sensitivity to endogenous GH in early infancy adds complexity to interpretation of these data.[1414] If long-term outcome studies continue to show excellent growth responses with achievement of genetic target height and adherence to treatment regimens in very young children, recommendations for early treatment would be appropriate.[1415]

Adult Height Outcomes. Much information on growth has been reported about children treated with pit-GH, usually administered intramuscularly on a thrice-weekly regimen. Five-year data are available from Bundak and colleagues[1416] from a study of 58 prepubertal and 20 pubertal children with GHD. The younger group increased its height from −3.6 SDS to −2 SDS, and the pubertal children grew to −2.3 SDS. However, the height SDS for bone age did not increase. Therefore, further loss of adult height was prevented, but there was no increase in the adult height prediction. The importance of early initiation of treatment is emphasized by such data. Libber and coworkers[1417] similarly found that GH therapy increased mean height from about −4.2 SDS to −2.3 SDS. Bierich[1418] reviewed nine trials of pit-GH to determine effect on final height. Overall, there was a dose-response relationship between doses of 0.11 versus 0.25 mg/kg per week. The greatest SDS increment (2.7) occurred with the highest dosage of pit-GH. The pretreatment heights ranged from −5.6 to −3.6 SDS, with adult heights achieving −3.6 to −1.6 SDS. Final height data from the same large U.S. center permit a comparison of pit-GH and recombinant GH therapeutic results. The mean final height was −2.0 SDS in the group treated with pit-GH, who received only 0.1 mg/kg per week, and −1.5 SDS in the group treated with recombinant GH 0.3 mg/kg per week.[1419]

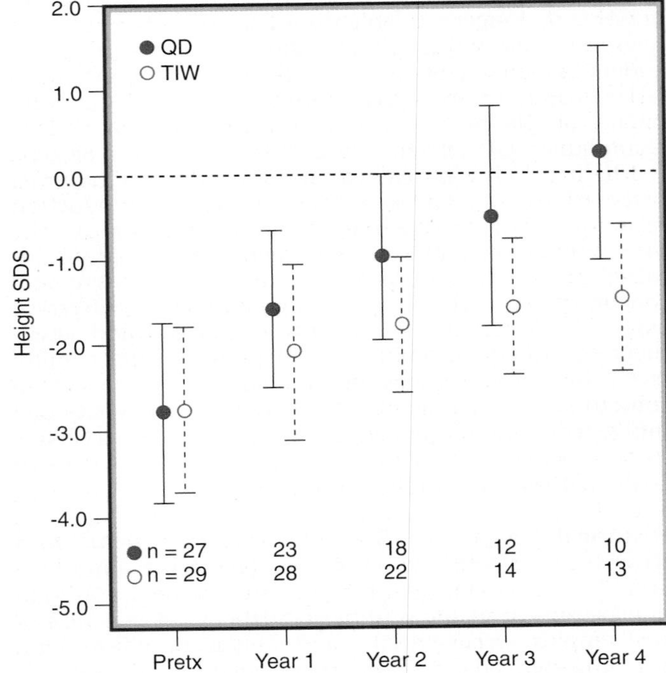

Figure 24-47 Height standard deviation score (SDS) for prepubertal patients with growth hormone (GH) deficiency before and during 4 years of GH treatment, contrasting results (mean ± standard deviation) with daily (QD) versus thrice-weekly (TIW) injections. The mean SDS in the QD group was significantly greater throughout the treatment period. Younger patients had the greatest increase in height SDS, and the effect of age was more marked in the QD group. (From MacGillivray MH, Baptista J, Johanson A, et al. Outcome of a four-year randomized study of daily versus three times weekly somatropin treatment in prepubertal naive growth hormone deficient children. *J Clin Endocrinol Metab.* 1996;81:1806-1809. Reproduced by permission of M.H. MacGillivray.)

TABLE 24-12

Adult Height in Children with Growth Hormone Deficiency Treated with Biosynthetic Growth Hormone

Study	Gender	N	GH Dose (mg/kg/wk)	Duration (yr)	Age (yr)	Height SDS	Change in Height SDS	Height vs MPH
KIGS*								
	M	351	0.22	7.5	18.2	−0.8	+1.6	−0.2
	F	200	0.20	6.9	16.6	−1.0	+1.6	−0.5
KIGS (Sweden)†								
	M	294	0.23	8.4	18.5	−0.9	+1.8	+0.2
	F	107	0.23	8.5	17.4	−0.7	+2.1	+0.2
NCGS†								
	M	2095	0.28	5.2	18.2	−1.1	+1.4	−0.7
	F	1116	0.29	5.0	16.7	−1.3	+1.6	−0.9

GH, growth hormone; KIGS, Pharmacia Kabi International Growth Study; MPH, midparental target height; NCGS, Genentech National Cooperative Growth Study; SDS, standard deviation score.

*Data from Reiter EO, Price DA, Wilton P, et al. Effect of growth hormone (GH) treatment on the near-final height of 1258 patients with idiopathic GH deficiency: analysis of a large international database. *J Clin Endocrinol Metab.* 2006;91:2047-2054.

†Data from Westphal O, Lindberg A, Swedish KIGS National Board. Final height in Swedish children with idiopathic growth hormone deficiency enrolled in KIGS treated optimally with growth hormone. *Acta Paediatr.* 2008 ;97:1698-1706.

†Data from August GP, Julius JR, Blethen SL. Adult height in children with growth hormone deficiency who are treated with biosynthetic growth hormone: The National Cooperative Growth Study experience. *Pediatrics.* 1998;102(2 Pt 3):512-516; updated NCGS data from Dana K, Baptista J, Blethen SL (personal communication, 2001).

Patients treated largely with biosynthetic GH[1272,1412,1419-1428] have improved actual or near-final adult height SDS, with average final height in more than 1400 patients approximating −1.3 SD. Data from the two largest databases,[1420,1422,1427-1429] representing the North American and European experiences as reported by pediatric endocrinologists, are shown in Table 24-12.

Despite the use of GH therapy, long-term studies still show that most patients fail to reach their genetic target heights. Evaluation of adult heights in 121 patients with childhood GHD treated in the Genentech GH research trials indicated a mean adult height in both male and female patients of −0.7 SDS, with 106 patients being within 2 SDS for normal adult Americans.[1425] Even in these closely monitored patients, however, a difference of −0.4 to −0.6 SDS from midparental target height still occurred. The achievement of the genetic target is possible, however: a Swedish subgroup (in the Kabi International Growth Study [KIGS] database) of consistently treated patients reached a median final height SDS of −0.32, which was equivalent to the midparental target height.[1429] A more recent study of the Swedish subgroup actually found a final height SDS greater than midparental target height by +0.2 (see Table 24-12).[1420]

Factors that have been found to correlate with enhanced adult height in GH-treated, GH-deficient children include baseline height, younger age at onset of treatment, longer treatment duration (especially during prepubertal years), and a greater growth velocity during the first year of treatment (Figs. 24-48 and 24-49).[1428] Increased height velocity and subsequent superior adult height outcome, although with considerable overlap, were demonstrated in children with GHD who carried one or both *GHRd3* alleles (i.e., with an exon 3 deletion).[783,1430,1431] Data from National Cooperative Growth Study (NCGS) and KIGS showed that the height gained during puberty in patients with GHD was generally comparable to that in healthy children with delayed bone age.[1427,1432] As might be expected based on that observation, final height correlates with height at the onset of puberty in GHD patients.[1404,1424,1433-1435] Therefore, every effort should be made to enhance growth before puberty, and delays in diagnosis and initiation of therapy probably contribute to the compromised adult heights still reported in many studies.

GH treatment of children who develop GHD as a result of cranial irradiation represents a special case when evaluating final height outcomes. In these children, who have received cranial irradiation for the treatment of malignancy, GH treatment is not initiated until there is no evidence of active tumor; this results in a delay between the diagnosis of GHD and the initiation of treatment. Final height is negatively correlated with the length of that lag time.[1436] In addition, those who have received spinal irradiation in addition to the cranial irradiation have a lower final height due to impairment of spinal growth after irradiation.[1436,1437]

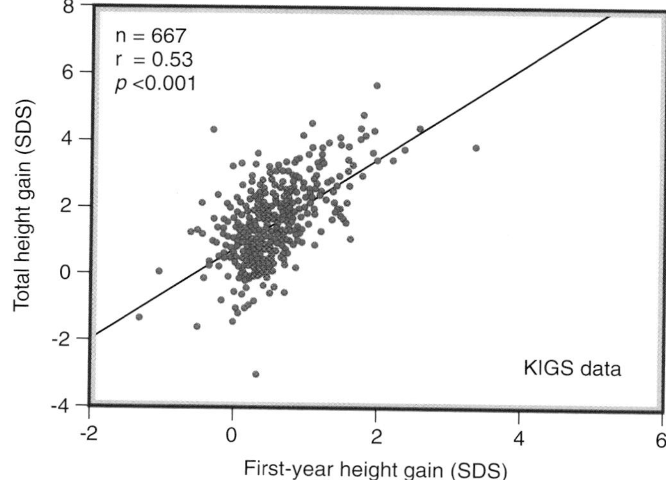

Figure 24-48 Relationship between first-year change in height standard deviation score (SDS) and total change in height SDS between start of growth hormone (GH) treatment and near-final height in children with idiopathic isolated GH deficiency. KIGS, Kabi International Growth Study database. (Modified with permission from Reiter EO, Price DA, Wilton P, et al. Effect of growth hormone [GH] treatment on the final height of 1258 patients with idiopathic GH deficiency: analysis of a large international database. *J Clin Endocrinol Metab.* 2006;91:2047-2054.)

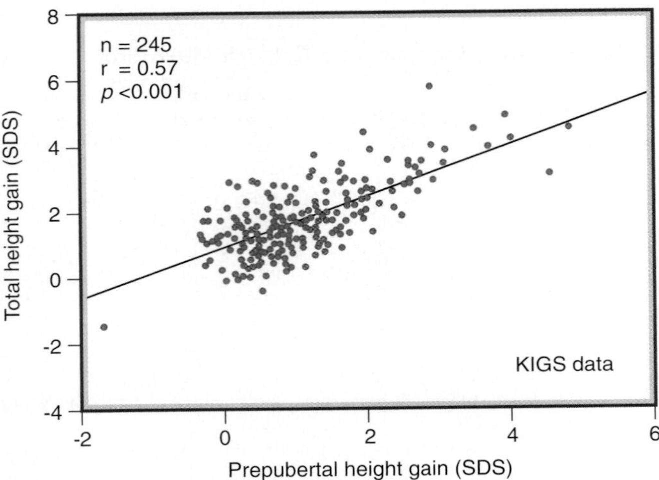

Figure 24-49 Relationship between prepubertal change in height standard deviation score (SDS) and total change in height SDS between start of growth hormone (GH) treatment and near-final height in children with idiopathic isolated GH deficiency. KIGS, Kabi International Growth Study database. (Modified with permission from Reiter EO, Price DA, Wilton P, et al. Effect of growth hormone [GH] treatment on the final height of 1258 patients with idiopathic GH deficiency: analysis of a large international database. *J Clin Endocrinol Metab.* 2006;91:2047-2054.)

In an effort to increase final height in GHD patients, the use of high-dose GH during puberty has been studied, based on the rationale that GH secretion normally rises twofold to fourfold during the pubertal growth spurt, with dramatic concomitant increases in serum IGF1 levels, and the pubertal growth spurt normally accounts for approximately 17% of adult male height and 12% of adult female height. Earlier studies by Stanhope and associates[1438,1439] indicated that little difference in height gain could be observed when adolescent patients were treated with 30 versus 15 IU/m^2 per week of GH (approximately 0.04 versus 0.02 mg/kg per day). Mauras and colleagues[1440] evaluated higher pubertal GH doses (0.1 versus 0.043 mg/kg per day) and found that the higher dosage resulted in a 4.6-cm increase in near-final height. Mean height SDS achieved in the group receiving 0.043 mg/kg per day of GH (as in the earlier report[1425]) was –0.7 ± 0.9, but in the group receiving 0.1 mg/kg per day it was 0.0 ± 1.2. The higher GH dosage did not result in more rapid acceleration of skeletal maturation.

Another approach that has been taken to attempt to increase final height in GH-treated patients has been to adjust the dose of GH to reach a target IGF1 level rather than treating with a fixed, weight-based dose.[1441,1442] A study reported by Cohen and colleagues found that targeting a high IGF1 level (reaching a mean IGF1 SDS of approximately +1.5) resulted in an increase in growth compared with the two comparator groups, which had mean IGF1 SDS of approximately +1.[1441] It required a GH dose approximately three times higher to reach this IGF1 level (0.11 mg/kg per day versus 0.041 and 0.033 mg/kg per day for the comparator groups).[141] In the study reported by Marchisotti and colleagues,[1442] the difference in IGF1 levels between groups (+0.8 SDS versus –0.3 SDS) was even greater than that in the report by Cohen and colleagues,[1441] but the Marchisotti study did not find a difference in growth rate between the two groups. The difference in GH dose was much smaller, however (0.038 versus 0.30 mg/kg per day). Therefore, as would be expected, a higher GH dose results in a higher growth rate, but it is not yet known whether targeting a specific IGF1 level results in an increased final height; nor is it known whether these higher doses have adverse effects not seen with the more usual doses currently used. An interesting finding was the wide range of doses required to reach a given IGF1 level: the high-IGF1 targeted group required GH doses ranging from less than 0.025 mg/kg per day to greater than 0.25 mg/kg per day, whereas the low-IGF1 targeted group required doses ranging from less than 0.025 to 0.15 mg/kg per day.[1441]

The impact of treatments to alter sex hormone levels (e.g., GnRH agonists, aromatase inhibitors) with the aim of improving final height in GHD and other conditions is discussed later.

Combined Pituitary Hormone Deficiencies. If GHD is part of a combined pituitary insufficiency syndrome, it is necessary to address each endocrine deficiency, both for general medical reasons and to ensure maximal effect of GH therapy. TSH deficiency is often "unmasked" during the initial phase of therapy, and thyroid function should be assessed before the onset of therapy, during the first 3 months of GH treatment,[1443] and at least on an annual basis thereafter. The pituitary-adrenal axis can be evaluated during the insulin stimulation test in the workup for GHD or separately if GHD is identified with the use of a different provocative test. If ACTH secretion is impaired, patients should be placed on the lowest safe maintenance dose of glucocorticoids, certainly no more than 10 mg/m^2 per day of hydrocortisone, and less if possible. Higher doses impair the growth response to GH therapy but should be given during times of stress. It is critical to monitor the long-term evolution of glucocorticoid deficiency, especially in those with PROP1 mutations (discussed earlier). However, Lange and colleagues studied 24 adults with a prior history of idiopathic isolated childhood GHD and identified adrenal insufficiency in 10 of them, half of whom did not have evidence of ongoing GHD[1444]; this suggests a need to consider monitoring for impaired ACTH secretion even in those patients with presumed IGHD.

Gonadotropin deficiency may be evident in the infant with microphallus. This can be treated with three or four monthly injections of 25 mg of testosterone enanthate in the first months of life.[1445] Management at puberty can be more complicated, in that the physical and psychological benefits of promoting sexual maturation must be balanced against the effects of epiphyseal fusion. When GH therapy is initiated in childhood and growth is normal before adolescence, it is appropriate to begin gonadal steroid replacement at a normal age (11 to 12 years of age in girls, 12 to 13 years of age in boys). In boys, this can be done by beginning with monthly injections of 50 to 100 mg of testosterone enanthate, gradually increasing to 200 mg per month, and eventually moving to the appropriate adult replacement regimen as determined by monitoring of plasma testosterone levels. In girls, therapy involves the use of conjugated estrogens or ethinyl estradiol and eventual cycling with estrogen and progesterone.

Monitoring Growth Hormone Therapy. Patients treated with GH should be seen every 3 to 6 months to monitor their response to treatment (Table 24-13). An increase in linear growth velocity should be seen within the first 6 months. Height SDS should increase at least 0.25 SDS in the first year.[1446] Treatment models have been developed that predict the expected growth rate in response to GH treatment.[1399,1408,1447-1449] A model[1399] explaining 61% of growth response variability in the first year of therapy includes inverse relationships with maximum GH response

TABLE 24-13

Elements of Monitoring Growth Hormone Therapy

Close follow-up with a pediatric endocrinologist every 3-6 mo
Determination of growth response (change in height SDS)
Evaluation of compliance
Screening for potential adverse effects
Interval measurements of serum IGF1 and IGFBP3
Annual assessment of thyroid function
Consideration of dose adjustment based on IGF values, growth response, and comparison with growth prediction models
Periodic reevaluation of adrenal function

IGF, insulin-like growth factor; IGBP, insulin-like growth factor–binding protein; SDS, standard deviation score.

during provocative testing, age, and height SDS minus midparental height SDS and positive correlation with body weight SDS, GH dose, and birth weight SDS.[1450,1451] The single most important predictive factor for growth in years 2 through 4 is the first-year height velocity. These models can be used to quantify whether the individual patient is responding appropriately to GH treatment. If a patient's initial growth response is lower than predicted, the clinician should consider whether the diagnosis of GHD was correct, whether additional growth disorders (e.g., hypothyroidism) are present, and whether there is lack of compliance with the treatment.[1448]

It is appropriate to monitor the IGF1 and IGFBP3 levels after initiation of GH treatment and perhaps yearly thereafter.[1446,1452] A failure of IGF1 and IGFBP3 levels to increase into the normal range with treatment, together with an inadequate growth response, suggests compliance failure or the presence of GH insensitivity. Because of the association of elevated IGF1 levels with certain cancers (see later discussion), a reduction in GH dose should be considered for patients with serum IGF1 levels substantially above the normal range after the first 2 years of therapy.[1446] Whether the IGF1 level should be used to guide GH dosing awaits additional studies (see earlier discussion).

CPHD may evolve over several years, so children who are initially diagnosed with IGHD may develop CPHD. Thyroxine levels should be assessed after GH treatment has been initiated, and annually thereafter, to identify the development of central hypothyroidism during treatment. Periodic reevaluation for ACTH deficiency should be performed. It is not necessary to routinely monitor fasting insulin and glucose levels, but if impaired glucose control is suspected, a fasting glucose level and glycosylated hemoglobin (HbA_{1c}) should be measured.

The growth response to GH typically attenuates after several years but should continue to be equal to or greater than the normal height velocity for age throughout treatment. Use of statistical growth treatment models can prove valuable in judging therapeutic efficacy.[1399,1408,1448] A suboptimal response to GH can result from several causes: (1) poor compliance, (2) improper preparation of GH for administration or incorrect injection techniques, (3) subclinical hypothyroidism, (4) coexisting systemic disease, (5) excessive glucocorticoid therapy, (6) prior irradiation of the spine, (7) epiphyseal fusion, (8) anti-GH antibodies, or (9) incorrect diagnosis of GHD as the explanation for growth retardation (particularly in a patient with idiopathic IGHD and normal findings on MRI). Although 10% to 20% of recipients of recombinant GH develop anti-GH antibodies, growth failure is rarely caused by such antibodies, except in the case of individuals who have GHD as a result of GH gene deletion.[1376,1377,1453]

Treatment during the Transition to Adulthood and in Adulthood. A growing challenge in the management of patients with GHD has been the issues surrounding their care after the growth process has ceased.[1454] This period, from the middle to late teenage years until the mid-20s, is a normal physiologic phase during which peak bone and muscle mass is achieved and the independence and self-sufficiency characteristic of adulthood are attained. It is also a time during which care of pediatric patients is transferred to endocrinologists who treat adults.

Clinical consequences of GHD in adults and the potential benefits of GH therapy in such patients have already been described.[1455-1458] Signs and symptoms of adult GHD include reduced lean body mass and musculature, increased body fat, reduced BMD, reduced exercise performance, and increased plasma cholesterol. Adults with GHD have a significantly increased risk of death from cardiovascular causes, a finding potentially linked to increased visceral adiposity and other cardiovascular risk factors.[1459,1460] Adults with GHD have been found to have "impaired psychological well-being and quality of life," characterized by depression, anxiety, reduced energy and vitality, and social isolation.[1461] Several placebo-controlled studies have demonstrated that GH therapy for adult GHD results in marked alterations in body composition, fat distribution, bone density, and sense of well-being.[1456,1457,1462,1463]

Based on the adult data, which suggest profound metabolic derangements associated with untreated GHD, continuation of GH treatment in late adolescence in the patient who shows persistent GHD is an important issue. Documentation of persistent GHD is important. Among almost 500 patients with IGHD, 207 (44%) had normal GH levels on provocative retesting.[1464-1471] In contrast, approximately 96% of patients with CPHD, with or without structural abnormalities of the hypothalamic-pituitary area, had sustained GHD.[1465,1466,1468-1472] The presence of multiple anterior pituitary hormone deficiencies or structural disease would seem to obviate the need for retesting. The data are not absolute, so clinical judgment is of paramount importance. The strict pharmacologic definition of GHD in this age group is difficult, as was shown by Maghnie and colleagues,[1473] who demonstrated that the much lower GH responses to testing that characterize older adults should not be used in this population. The issue of testing validity may have influenced the dichotomy observed between the IGD and CPHD patient populations in testing "positive" on the provocative tests. As in the childhood population, it seems reasonable not to rely solely on artificial cutoffs in pharmacologic provocative tests but to include broader clinical and laboratory data.

Many patients do not wish to continue the daily GH regimen, but the data do support strong consideration for sustained treatment. After 1 to 2 years off GH therapy, IGF1 and IGFBP3 levels decrease substantially below baseline levels.[1474-1478] Resumption of GH normalizes these levels, although there is a strong suggestion of a gender-based difference in GH requirements, with females needing higher GH doses.[1476-1478] Loss of energy and strength is a frequent finding,[1479] and some quality-of-life data suggest age-specific psychological issues in patients with untreated severe GHD during the transition to adulthood.[1480,1481] Quality-of-life data with rigorous study designs are lacking in GH-treated childhood GHD.[1482,1483] In untreated patients, total body fat and abdominal fat increase significantly and lean body mass is lost, compared with control subjects, comparable GH-treated patients, or patients who have reinstituted therapy.[1474,1475,1477,1484,1485]

Because bone mass accrual is not completed until the third decade, late adolescence is an important time for GH sufficiency, to prevent later osteopenia.[849,1454] There have been numerous GH treatment studies carried out in the transition age group to assess the impact on bone mineralization.[1476-1478,1486,1487] Differences in age at onset of retreatment, duration of therapy, GH dosage, and gender distribution have led to variations in results. In general, however, the data affirm the concept that reinstitution of treatment with GH enables progression of bone mineralization to appropriate adult levels. Bone density assessment in patients with childhood-onset IGHD who tested negative for GHD in adulthood showed lower bone mineralization than in controls and a correlation with IGF1 levels.[1488]

The cardiovascular risk of stopping GH treatment has also been examined. Colao and associates showed modest left ventricular ejection fraction decrements that paralleled IGF levels when stopping and restarting GH therapy in a group of adolescents with GHD.[1489] The overall IGF levels were rather low, so cardiac changes were relatively modest. It should be recalled that GH treatment during childhood alters cardiac size but does not seem to change cardiac function.[1490] Mauras and associates used a wide array of functional studies in a similar transition-age group and were unable to demonstrate cardiac changes,[1478] but their patients had relatively high IGF1 levels (mean, 427 ng/mL) at GH discontinuation, suggesting a degree of "protectiveness" in the subsequent period off GH treatment. Nonetheless, abnormal cardiovascular risk factors, such as elevated concentrations of lipids, fibrinogen, inflammatory markers, and homocysteine, and platelet hyperactivation may occur in adolescents with untreated GHD.[1491-1493] In prepubertal children with GHD, normalization of homocysteine levels and of markers of oxidative stress is achieved with GH treatment,[1494,1495] buttressing the notion of important effects of GH upon cardiovascular health. Therefore, cardiac function and those factors affecting vascular biology are targets in the spectrum of GH-mediated body compositional changes.

These studies support the continuation of GH treatment in late adolescence, albeit at lower doses than in childhood, to prevent the development of adverse cardiovascular risk, diminished bone mineralization, and an overall lowering of energy level. Whether the diversity of treatment and response data relates to the efficacy of the childhood GH therapeutic process is not clear, but the period of time off GH and the degree of persistent GHD would seem likely predictors of clinical status at the time of reinitiation of GH treatment.

After the adolescent with GHD has completed skeletal growth, the persistence of GHD is evaluated.[1237,1454] If the patient has a high probability of persistent GHD (i.e., CPHD, IGHD with structural abnormalities, or confirmed genetic mutations), a presumption of persistent GHD is made. Otherwise, GH therapy should be halted for 2 to 3 months, followed by a thorough reevaluation. A recommended algorithm for this evaluation is shown in Figure 24-50.[1496]

As in childhood GHD, laboratory testing is imperfectly precise for diagnosis of ongoing GHD. Some patients have results that neither indicate nor eliminate ongoing GHD but are intermediate, suggesting either probable or partial GHD. If ongoing GHD is considered to be present or probable, assessment of body composition, BMD, and fasting lipid levels should be determined. The decision to reinitiate GH treatment is then based on a discussion with the patient and family regarding the risks and benefits in light of the laboratory test results and the risk for metabolic consequences (see Figure 24-50).[1496] In addition, caution should be exercised in considering whether to continue GH therapy when there is a known risk of diabetes or malignancy. This is also an opportunity for a thorough clinical reassessment and a determination of the need for replacement of other hormones. The transition to adult GH replacement should be arranged as a close collaboration between endocrinologists who treat pediatric patients and those who treat adult patients and should include discussion with the patient and family. A discussion of many transition issues was reported by Clayton and associates from a European consensus meeting.[1454]

Growth Hormone Treatment of Other Forms of Short Stature

Prader-Willi Syndrome. Guidelines for the clinical management of PWS were published after an international multidisciplinary expert meeting in 2007.[1497] Short stature due to GH insufficiency is almost always present in children with PWS. In a large cohort of 1135 children with PWS starting GH treatment, median height SDS was −2.2 (range, −4.1 to −0.3) at a median age of 6.4 years (range, 1.3 to 12.9 years).[1498]

Serum levels of IGF1 are reduced in most children with PWS.[1499-1502] Studies have shown that spontaneous GH secretion is reduced, and 70% of children with PWS have GH peaks of less than 10 μg/L during pharmacologic stimulation tests.[1503] Although most experts agree that prior GH testing is not required before GH treatment is initiated, it can be helpful. GH treatment of growth failure in PWS is an FDA-approved indication. GH treatment in children with PWS aims to improve childhood growth, final adult height, and body composition (see review by Burman and associates[1507]). Numerous clinical trials have documented the efficacy of GH therapy. In randomized, controlled studies there were significant increases in height and growth velocity and a significant decrease in percent body fat, as well as increased percentage of fat-free mass, improved muscle strength and agility, and increased fat oxidation during the first year of GH treatment.[1500,1504-1508] Stabilization of these parameters occurs after the second year of therapy. Lean body mass increased significantly during the first 2 years in children with PWS who received GH treatment, compared with no treatment.[1509-1510] GH therapy for 2 additional years resulted in continued beneficial effects on body composition. When the dose of GH was reduced to 0.3 mg/m^2 per day, these improvements were not maintained.[1509]

BMD improves in children with PWS treated with GH. In two German cohorts, the mean spontaneous adult heights were reported in one study as 162 cm in boys and 150 cm in girls[1511] and the other as 159 cm in boys and 149 cm in girls.[1512] In the Kabi International Growth Study database, 33 patients (21 boys and 12 girls) reached adult height, and two thirds of them were above −2 SDS; the median adult height was −1 SDS after a mean duration of 8.4 years.[1513] Another study with 21 adults (13 boys, 8 girls) revealed a mean adult height of 0.3 SDS after a mean duration of 7.9 years of GH treatment.[1514] In this cohort, the strength and agility that were evident during the initial 2 years continued into adulthood. The patients also reported a higher quality of life and reduced depression.[1506] In 55 children monitored during 4 years of continuous GH treatment (1 mg/m^2 per day), body composition was significantly improved, mean height normalized, head

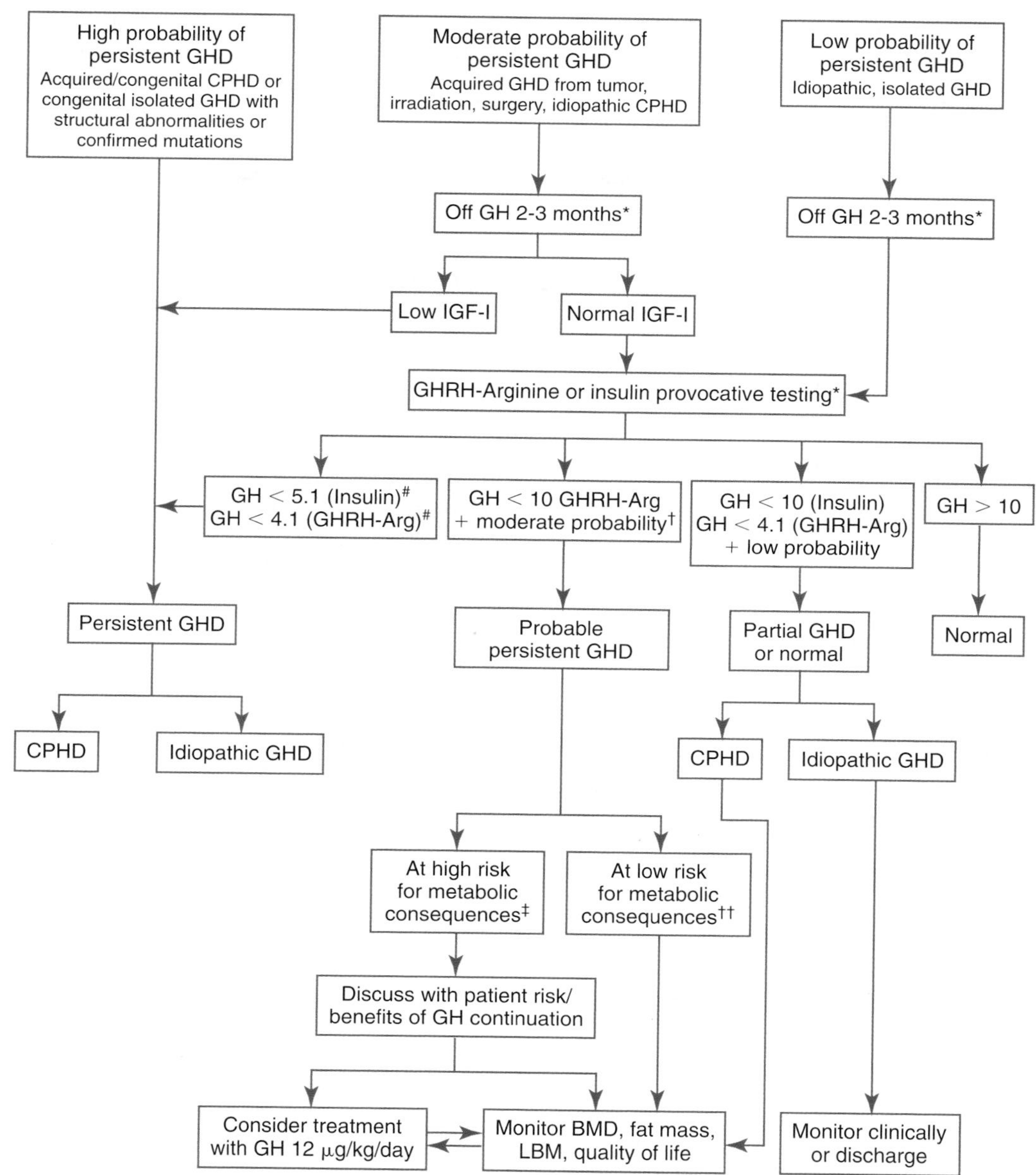

Figure 24-50 Algoritbm for evaluating patients diagnosed with GHD during childhood at the completion of growth. *, Based on consensus and clinical practice guidelines. (From Molitch ME et al. 2006. *J Clin Endocrinol Metab.* 91:1621-1634 and Growth Hormone Research Society 2000. *J Clin Endocrinol Metab,* 85:3990-3993. #, Threshold values that achieve a senstitivity of 95% and specificity 91-92% for diagnosing GHD in adults. (Biller BMK et al. 2002. *J Clin Endocrinol Metab.* 87:2067-2079.) †, Based upon data indicating that patients with irradiation-induced CPHD can have hypothalamic dysfunction causing GHD. (Darzy KH et al. 2003. *J Clin Endocrinol Metab.* 88:95-102.) ‡, Those at high risk for metabolic complications include patients with abnormal BMD, high fat mass, low LBM. ††, Those at low risk for metabolic complications include patients with normal BMD, fat mass, and LBM. GH, growth hormone; GHD, growth hormone deficiency; CPHD, combined pituitary hormone deficencies; BMD. bonemineral density; LBM, lean body mass.

circumference increased, and BMI significantly decreased. GH treatment had no adverse effects on bone maturation, blood pressure, glucose homeostasis, and serum lipids.[1515]

Before GH therapy is begun, screening for hypothyroidism is indicated because of the association with primary and central hypothyroidism.[1516,1517] Continued screening is also recommended. Treatment with GH beginning as early as 2 years of age is recommended, but there may be additional benefits to starting therapy between 6 and 12 months of age. Several studies have found improvements in motor development, muscle tone, head circumference, and, possibly, cognition and behavior.[1518,1519]

Since October 2002, several reports of unexpected deaths in infants and children with PWS have been published.[1520-1522] Between 1985 and 2006, the NCGS monitored the safety and efficacy of recombinant human GH in 54,996 children. Two deaths were reported in patients with PWS.[1523] Although death from presumed obesity-induced hypoventilation or apneic events in PWS without GH treatment is well described, the occurrence of such deaths during GH administration raises the question of whether GH exacerbates this condition.[1524,1525] Tonsillar hypertrophy and fluid retention associated with GH therapy are potential risk factors. Most of the deaths, with or without GH treatment, were related to obesity or to a complicated course of a relatively mild respiratory tract infection, sleep apnea, adenoid or tonsillar hypertrophy (or both), hypoventilation, and aspiration. The obesity-hypoventilation syndrome is the more likely etiologic factor, suggesting that ventilatory and pulmonary function should be assessed with polysomnography studies before and during GH treatment.[1524,1526]

In a recent review that included 64 children (42 boys and 22 girls, 28 receiving GH treatment), the highest death risk occurred during the first 9 months of GH treatment.[1522] Therefore, it is recommended that GH treatment be started at a low dose (e.g., 0.25 to 0.30 mg/m^2 per day or 0.009 to 0.012 mg/kg per day) and increased during the first weeks and months to reach the standard replacement dosage of approximately 1 mg/m^2 per day or 0.24 mg/kg per week. Patients should be monitored for sleep apnea and IGF1 levels. The GH dose should be decreased if there is evidence of high IGF1 levels, especially if associated with edema, worsening or new onset of snoring, headache, or acromegalic clinical features.

Five prospective studies have evaluated the effects of GH treatment on breathing disorders in PWS.[680,1505,1527,1528] Carbon dioxide responsiveness, resting ventilation, and airway occlusion pressure improved during 6 to 9 months of GH treatment,[1528] and the inspiratory and expiratory muscle strength improved during 12 months of GH treatment, compared with controls.[1505] In a double-blind, placebo-controlled, crossover study, the apnea-hypopnea index (AHI) was found to decrease in 12 children with PWS, compared with controls, after 6 months of GH therapy although the difference was not statistically significant.[680] Another study found a decrease in AHI in most of the adults and children studied after 6 weeks of GH therapy.[1529] A subset of patients had an increased AHI with more obstructive events, but most of these latter patients had upper respiratory tract infections and adenoid/tonsil hypertrophy, and two of them had high IGF1 levels. In another study in 35 prepubertal children with PWS, the AHI did not significantly change during 6 months of GH therapy.[1530] However, four of these children had an increase in the number of episodes of obstructive apnea during an upper respiratory illness; these were not present after recovery. Therefore, it is recommended that obesity-related sleep and breathing problems be evaluated before and vigilantly monitored after GH treatment begins. Polysomnography and ear, nose, and throat evaluations should be performed as necessary.

A recent study[1531] showed that 60% of PWS patients had central adrenal insufficiency. This may explain the high rate of sudden death especially during infection- related stress. The authors concluded that patients with PWS should be treated with hydrocortisone during stress until adrenal insufficiency can be ruled out.[1531,1532]

Between 30% and 70% of children with PWS have scoliosis.[1514,1533-1537] Weight control is a vital part of its prevention and management. Therefore, before GH treatment is initiated, spinal radiographs and, if appropriate, orthopedic assessment are recommended. Reports of scoliosis worsening during GH treatment reflect the natural history of this condition rather than a side effect of treatment in most cases, and discontinuation of GH is not indicated.

In view of the childhood findings of low lean body mass and high fat content, osteopenia, and some degree of glucose intolerance ameliorated by GH, the issue of long-term therapy through adulthood must be considered and studied.[1538-1540] After growth is complete, attainment of a normal peak bone mass, continued improvement of muscle mass and strength, reduction of body fat, prevention of cardiovascular morbidity, and improvement in well-being and quality of life are potential benefits of continued GH therapy.[1541] Adult GHD and low IGF1 levels have been reported in patients with PWS.[1502,1542] Short-term GH treatment in GH-naïve adults with PWS has been reported to modestly improve body composition, cognition, motor performance, and social status.[1542] Further long-term studies are needed on adolescents with PWS transitioning to adult therapies.

Chronic Renal Disease. Chronic renal disease (CRD) is regarded as indication for the commencement of GH administration. Short stature is more severe in children with congenital renal disorders than in children with acquired renal diseases.[888,1543,1544] Even after renal transplantation, final height is below the lower limit of normal in about 50% of children.[915,1545] GH treatment is able to increase height velocity and height SDS[900,1546,1547] and significantly improves final height[1548-1550] in patients with CRD (Figs. 24-51 and 24-52). The therapy should be implemented if short stature persists for longer than 6 months and in subjects with marked deceleration of growth velocity, and it should be continued until transplantation is performed.[1551] However, the first-year response to GH is less than in short children with GHD.[1552]

GH accelerates growth in children with CRD, at least over 5 years of therapy.[1553-1556] Using a GH dosage of 0.05 mg/kg per day, Fine and colleagues[1546] reported a mean first-year growth rate of 10.7 cm in GH recipients and 6.5 cm in the placebo group; in the second year, GH-treated patients had a mean growth rate of 7.8 cm/year compared with 5.5 cm/year in placebo recipients, resulting in an improvement of height SDS from −2.9 to −1.5. Twenty patients who were treated for 5 years reached a normal height SDS of −0.7, with a mean height increase of 40 cm.[1556] The youngest patients (<2.5 years of age) had the most impressive growth response to GH therapy (14.1 cm/year). Doses recommended in children with CRD are higher than in GHD patients (i.e., about 0.35 mg/kg per week)[1557] because growth patterns in these patients are dose dependent.[1558] Deleterious effects on renal function and progression of osteodystrophy were not observed.[1559,1560] This treatment regimen does not adversely affect renal graft function after transplantation, nor is there significant

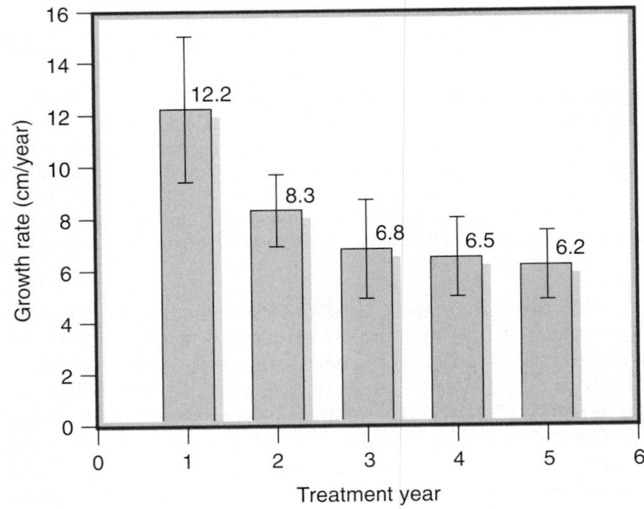

Figure 24-51 Annual growth velocity (mean ± standard deviation) in 20 growth-retarded prepubertal patients with chronic renal insufficiency who were treated with growth hormone. (From Fine RN, Kohaut E, Brown D, et al. Long-term treatment of growth retarded children with chronic renal insufficiency with recombinant human growth hormone. *Kidney Int.* 1996;49:781-785. Reproduced with permission of R.N. Fine.)

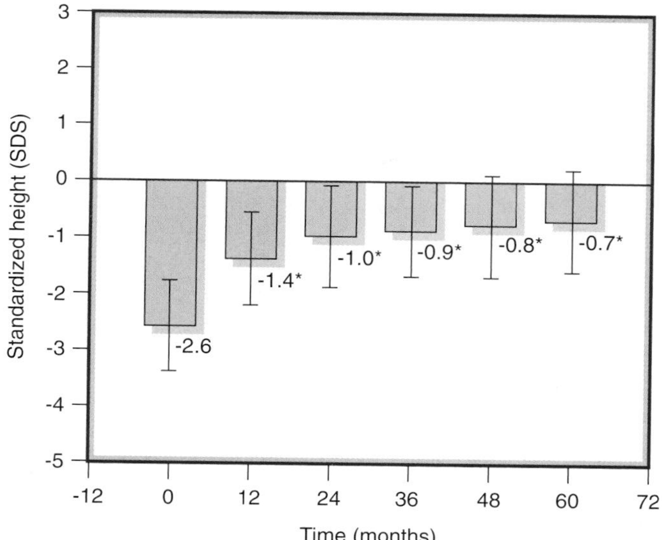

Figure 24-52 Height standard deviation score (SDS) in 20 growth-retarded prepubertal patients with chronic renal insufficiency (mean ± standard deviation). Note that the basal height is outside the normal range (at −2.6 SDS), enters the normal range within 1 year of treatment initiation, and is not different from the mean by the 5th year of growth hormone therapy. (From Fine RN, Kohaut E, Brown D, et al. Long-term treatment of growth retarded children with chronic renal insufficiency with recombinant human growth hormone. *Kidney Int.* 1996;49:781-785. Reproduced with permission of R.N. Fine.)

"catch-down" growth after the transplantation.[1561] The final height in 38 German children treated with GH for an average of 5.3 years was −1.6 ± 1.2 SDS, an increment of 1.4 SDS over the pretreatment baseline. The final height of an untreated control group was −2.1 ± 1.2, or 0.6 SDS below baseline.[1549]

More recently, adult heights of 178 French patients treated with GH were reported. Mean adult height was 162.2 cm in men and 152.9 cm in women, and 46% were more than −2 SDS for height. Adult height SDS was correlated with height SDS and spontaneous height velocity before treatment and with the effect of treatment. These adult heights were significantly better when compared with historical cohorts of patients not treated with GH.[1562]

In 2009, a review of longitudinal data from 7189 patients enrolled in the chronic renal insufficiency registry of the North American Pediatric Renal Trials and Collaborative Studies (NAPRTCS) revealed that 827 patients (11.5%) had received GH. A total of 787 children with CRD who were previously naïve to GH treatment and received recombinant human GH for 1 to 4 years (median, 1.5 years) were paired with 787 control patients and monitored for 4 years. The GH-treated group had a significantly greater height velocity SDS than the control group at 2.5 years. Among 220 pairs evaluated at 2 years, the height SDS of the GH-treated group was 0.56 SDS higher than that of the control group ($P < .05$). Treatment with GH had no significant impact on BMI or estimated glomerular filtration rate (GFR).[1563]

The magnitude of response to GH treatment depends on the GH dosage. A dose of 0.35 mg/kg per week appears to be optimal for short patients with CRD; half of this dose was less effective, and doubling did not significantly improve the response in double-blind studies.[1554,1564] Long-term GH treatment has also been shown to be safe and effective for extremely short (−4.0 SDS) children with nephropathic cystinosis and should be considered if nutrition and cysteamine treatment do not prevent growth failure.[1544] Because children are often short at the time of renal transplantation, have hormone findings of relative GH insensitivity, and receive chronic prednisone therapy, GH is sometimes administered in the post-transplantation period. Data after 1 and 2 years of treatment of such children and adolescents[1564-1567] indicated a large increment of growth velocity at year 1 and a smaller benefit at year 2. As with GH treatment of CRD, the pharmacologic regimen overcomes the relative GH insensitivity. Individual patients show a wide variation in response, and predictors include age, GFR, need for dialysis treatment, target height, and pretreatment growth rate.[9,1568]

A mathematical model for prediction of the individual response to GH in prepubertal children with CRD was developed from the KIGS.[10] Thirty-seven percent of the variation in the first-year growth response was explained by this model, with the greatest first-year response in younger children who had no weight reduction, no hereditary renal disorder, and high residual renal function. There was a small GH dose effect during the first treatment year.[10] Such models, using clinical variables, may allow individualized GH treatment decisions in children with CRD.

Considerable assessment must yet be undertaken to demonstrate whether there is increased growth over a longer term, that renal function does not deteriorate during therapy, and that the risk of rejection is not enhanced. GH treatment does not appear to cause an accelerated decline of allograft function[1569-1571] nor changes in histopathologic findings,[1572] but exacerbation of chronic rejection by GH therapy remains a possibility.[1573] Use of nonsteroid-based immunosuppressive regimens may obviate the need for post-transplantation GH treatment.

A short-term study in chronic well-nourished dialysis patients showed that combined administration of moderate doses of GH with recombinant human IGF1 (rhIGF1) had a complementary effect on protein metabolism.[1574] This approach is theoretically reasonable because GH administration results in an increase in protein synthesis but does not significantly inhibit proteolysis,[1038] whereas the predominant effect of IGF1 is the inhibition of proteolysis.[1575] Confirmation by longer-term studies is needed to assess whether this favorable anabolic effect persists and to determine the safety profile of this intervention.[888,900,915,1543-1552,1554,1557,1558,1564,1576,1577]

Juvenile Idiopathic Arthritis. Juvenile idiopathic arthritis (JIA) is often complicated by growth deficiency. The decrease in linear growth usually correlates with the severity of the disease, although catch-up growth may not occur during remissions. The final height is less than −2 SDS in 11% of patients with polyarticular JIA and in 40% of those with systemic JIA.[1578,1579] Serum GH levels are normal or low, usually with low plasma IGF1 levels.[1580,1581] The pathogenesis of short statue is thought to be GH insensitivity associated with both the inflammatory process and glucocorticoid treatment.[1582,1583] Several trials have been conducted to determine whether GH replacement therapy is effective in patients with JIA.[1583-1588] Trial of GH replacement using GH dosages ranging from 0.1 to 0.46 mg/kg per week increased serum levels of IGF1 and linear growth velocity. However, the trials all had significant interindividual variability.[1589] GH therapy for up to 3 years was notable for a decrease in the loss of growth velocity associated with the active phase of JIA.[1587]

In a randomized, controlled trial of GH therapy (0.33 mg/kg per week for 4 years) in 31 children with JIA, a height increase of 1 SDS was found, compared with a decrease of 0.7 SDS in the untreated control group.[1588] The GH-treated patients had a significantly greater final height compared with untreated control patients (−1.6 ± 0.25 SDS versus −3.4 ± 2.0 SDS; $P < .001$).[1590] As expected, the severity of inflammation negatively affected the efficacy of GH therapy.[1588,1590] In a randomized trial of normal-height children with JIA treated with high-dose GH therapy (0.46 mg/kg per week) starting within 12 to 15 months after initiation of glucocorticoid therapy, the 3 year follow-up showed that the heights of GH-treated children remained normal (−1.1 SDS at baseline and −0.3 SDS after 3 years) while linear growth of the control patients declined from −1.0 SDS to −2.1 SDS.[1591] In the randomized, controlled trials published to date, patients were followed for up to 7 years, and no substantial differences were found in disease activity variables, including worsening of preexisting bone deformities, between GH-treated and control patients.[1582-1588]

Because chronic inflammation, glucocorticoid treatment, and GH therapy are all associated with decreased sensitivity to insulin, children with JIA are at risk for impaired glucose homeostasis.[496,1589,1592] Therefore, monitoring of glucose tolerance using blood glucose, fasting insulin, and HbA_{1c} assays at 6- to 12-month intervals is recommended. More intensive monitoring with oral glucose tolerance tests at baseline and then once yearly during treatment may be indicated.

Turner Syndrome. Patients with TS have a final height averaging 143 cm in the United States,[10,1100] about 20 cm lower than the mean final height of normal women.[1098] The goals of growth-promoting therapies are to attain a normal height for age as early as possible, to progress through puberty at a normal age, and to attain a normal adult height.

Before the availability of recombinant GH, there were conflicting data concerning its efficacy in this disorder,[1593,1594] but the ability of GH to accelerate growth has now been demonstrated in multiple reports. Growth responses are not affected by the karyotype. In 1983, a randomized, controlled North American study of treatment with GH (at a dose of 0.375 mg/kg per week) with or without added oxandrolone was initiated, with a mean age at onset of treatment of approximately 9 years.[1595] Analysis of all 62 girls enrolled in the study at near-final height showed a mean stature of 152.1 cm in the group treated with GH plus oxandrolone (a gain of 10.3 cm compared with the height predictions derived from Lyon and colleagues,[10] whereas girls receiving GH alone averaged 150.4 cm (a gain of 8.4 cm) (Fig. 24-53).[1100] In another arm of this study, addition of estrogen to the GH regimen before age 15 years lowered the final height gain from 8.4 cm to 5.1 cm.[1596] In a reassessment of North American data in the NCGS, early initiation of GH treatment was shown to allow estrogen administration at a physiologic age without loss of adult height.[1597,1598]

Several other studies[1110,1599] using higher doses of GH showed even greater gains in adult height outcomes. In a multicenter trial, Sas and coworkers used a maximum GH dose of approximately 0.63 mg/kg per week for 4.8 estrogen-free GH treatment years beginning at a mean age of 8.1 years, resulting in a gain of 16 cm over the modified Lyon and colleagues' projection.[10,1110] In the same study, the group receiving a GH dose similar to that in the American studies achieved a height gain of 12.5 cm by age 16 with 4.8 estrogen-free GH treatment years starting at 7.9 years. In these girls, induction of puberty at a normal (not delayed) age was associated with these excellent height

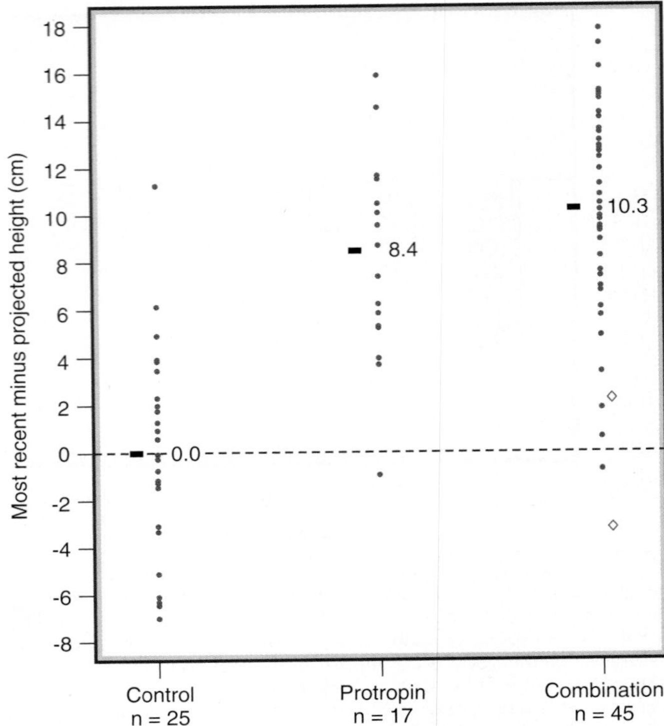

Figure 24-53 Adult heights of patients with Turner syndrome treated with growth hormone (GH) or with a combination GH plus oxandrolone and of historical controls, relative to each subject's projected adult height (indicated by the *dotted zero line*). The mean increments in relative adult height are indicated. The diamond symbols in the combination group indicate two subjects with poor compliance who terminated treatment early. (From Rosenfeld RG, Attie KM, Frane J, et al. Growth hormone therapy of Turner syndrome: beneficial effect on adult height. *J Pediatr.* 1998;132:319-324.)

outcomes.[1600] Carel and colleagues,[1599] using 0.7 mg/kg per week in a group that received 5.1 estrogen-free GH treatment years beginning at 10.2 years, gained 10.6 cm over the projections of Lyon and colleagues.[10] The group receiving a conventional dose (0.3 mg/kg per week) gained only 5.2 cm with 3.0 estrogen-free GH treatment years starting at 11 years. Because girls with TS usually have a normal GH secretory pattern, provocative GH testing should be performed only in those whose growth is clearly abnormal relative to that expected for patients with TS, as determined by plotting lengths and heights on TS-specific growth curves.[10,1103,1107,1601,1602]

Although it was well established that GH therapy was effective in increasing final adult height, the magnitude of the gain in height varied in the earlier studies, depending on study design and treatment parameters. In 2005, in the first randomized, controlled trial to follow GH-treated subjects with TS to final height, the Canadian Growth Hormone Advisory Committee corroborated the increases in adult stature reported by studies with historical controls.[1100,1600,1603,1605] In the Canadian study, girls with TS (age 7 to 13 years) who were randomized to receive GH (0.3 mg/kg per week; maximum weekly dose, 15 mg) achieved a final adult stature 7.2 cm taller than that seen in the control group after an average of 5.7 years. Factors predictive of taller adult stature include a relatively tall height at initiation of therapy, tall parental heights, young age at initiation of therapy, a long duration of therapy, and a high GH dose.[1110,1598,1606-1609]

Although the optimal age for initiation of GH treatment has not been established, preliminary data from the Toddler Turner Study, in which 88 girls between the ages of 9 months and 4 years were randomized to receive GH or no GH therapy, showed that GH therapy is effective beginning as early as 9 months, with a safety profile similar to that in older children with TS.[1610] Treatment with GH should be considered as soon as growth failure is evident. GH therapy in the United States is typically initiated at the FDA-approved dose of 0.375 mg/kg per week. The dose can be changed in response to the patient's growth response and IGF1 levels. Growth prediction models may be helpful in determining the potential effects of changes in dosing.[1606]

Studies have shown that higher doses produce a relatively small gain in final height, although there is no apparent increase in short-term adverse events.[1611] In a study by the Dutch Working Group, the mean gain in final height with 4 IU/m^2 per day (0.045 mg/kg per day), 6 IU/m^2 per day, and 8 IU/m^2 per day averaged 11.9 ± 3.6, 15.7 ± 3.5, and 16.9 ± 5.2 cm, respectively.[1600] However, when GH was given at the higher doses, IGF1 levels were often above the normal range, which theoretically could lead to long-term adverse effects.[1612]

In girls naïve to GH who are older than 9 years of age and in those with extreme short stature, consideration can be given to using higher doses of GH and adding a nonaromatizable anabolic steroid, such as oxandrolone.[1100] The maximum suggested dose of oxandrolone is 0.05 mg/kg per day, because higher doses have been associated with virilization and accelerated skeletal maturation. Liver enzymes should be monitored. Therapy may be continued until a satisfactory height has been attained (bone age >14 years) or until the yearly growth velocity falls to less than 2 cm/year. The children should be monitored at 3- to 6-month intervals.[1613]

The substantial variations in GH-induced growth increments in these studies were presumably related to GH dose, duration of estrogen-free GH treatment years, and age at initiation of GH and estrogen administration, as well as the population and parental adult heights. Additionally, the *GHRd3* polymorphism has been reported to be associated with increased responsivity to GH in girls with TS.[782] Transdermal or depot estrogen administration, as opposed to oral estrogen, may also contribute positively to growth outcomes.[1614,1615] In these higher-dose treatment studies, hyperinsulinism with presumed insulin resistance was evident but reversible.[1599,1616] Other data suggest that impaired insulin secretion may ultimately be the significant issue in patients with TS,[1617,1618] although long-term GH therapy has been well tolerated.

None of these studies was placebo-controlled to adult height, and some studies have yielded much poorer height outcomes,[1111] so some uncertainty existed until the randomized, controlled, multicentered Canadian study, in which the mean height gain ascribed to GH treatment was 7.3 cm at 1 year after cessation of the treatment protocol. Estrogen was initiated at 13 years of age.[1603] Another temporally matched control study from Italy showed a gain of 8.1 cm.[1605] These studies corroborated and supported the information that had accumulated from historical data on natural growth in TS juxtaposed to the available GH treatment results. Such data, in aggregate, provides convincing support that GH can both accelerate growth velocity and increase adult height.

Recommendations include seeking the diagnosis vigorously at any age in every girl with otherwise unexplained short stature and initiating therapy at that young age (i.e., at diagnosis or in early childhood). One must bear in mind that growth velocity in girls with untreated TS can be slowed as early as the 1- to 3-year-old period.[1104,1105] Treatment with the FDA-approved GH dosage of 0.375 mg/kg per week should be initiated and compliance should be monitored with auxologic and IGF1 measurements; continued normal thyroid status should be assured. Oxandrolone may be added to the regimen in the late-diagnosed girl. Estrogen therapy should be initiated at an appropriate physiologic age in girls who started GH therapy at a young age, but it should be delayed as long as clinically reasonable in those whose GH therapy was initiated at a late age. Often, growth-promoting and pubertal needs must be balanced, and the therapeutic approach should be individualized. The diminished areal bone density in TS is enhanced by GH, but estrogen therapy is needed to normalize volumetric density (i.e., not simply size).[1619] Absence of an adverse impact of GH on aortic diameters is reassuring, given the predisposition of such patients for dissecting aneurysms.[691] Use of statistical prediction models for long-term growth in TS may permit a more quantitative assessment of individual therapeutic efficacy.[1606]

Despite evidence for aggressive GH treatment of girls with TS to achieve adequate adult heights and relatively high quality-of-life assessments in adulthood,[589,1620] health-related issues continue to imperil outcomes. Carel and colleagues[1621] reviewed health outcomes of 568 adult French women (in their mid-20s) with GH-treated TS who had a mean height of 150.9 cm (having gained about 9 cm over prediction) and found that neither height nor height gain was associated with quality-of-life scores. Rather, issues regarding cardiologic and otologic health concerns and delay of pubertal initiation beyond 15 years were of greater concern. In contrast, a long-term follow-up assessment of 49 women from the Netherlands who had reached a mean adult height of 160.7 cm (a gain of >15 cm), suggested that the high quality-of-life scores were related to height gain and adequate estrogenization.

The NCGS recently published data on the efficacy and safety of GH therapy in 5220 children with TS treated during the last 20 years. A total of 442 adverse events were reported for these patients, including 117 that were considered to be serious. Seven deaths occurred, including five from aortic dissection or rupture. The incidences of intracranial hypertension, slipped capital femoral epiphysis, scoliosis, and pancreatitis were increased compared with other patients in the registry who did not have TS. Ten new-onset malignancies occurred, including six in patients without known risk factors. The number of patients who developed IDDM also appeared to be increased. It is believed that these adverse events are likely to be unrelated to treatment with GH. The incidence of aortic dissection or rupture reflects the higher baseline risk in TS.[1622]

Two echocardiography studies reported normal left ventricular morphology and function in girls with GH-treated TS[1623,1624] and two MRI studies found no deleterious effect of GH treatment on aortic diameter.[691,1613,1625,1626] Because GH treatment can alter craniofacial proportions, all girls with TS treated with GH should receive periodic orthodontic follow-up.[1627] These studies were not controlled, but their findings emphasize the broad range of health concerns in women with TS and affirm the need for multidisciplinary follow-up care.

Small for Gestational Age. Studies employing GH in short children born SGA have been hampered by the heterogeneity of this group of patients, whose poor growth may reflect maternal factors, chromosomal disorders, dysmorphic syndromes (e.g., RSS, Dubowitz syndrome), toxins, and idiopathic factors.[1632] A 2001 consensus statement recommended that SGA be defined as a birth weight or length at least 2 SD below the mean.[1628] Almost 90% of infants born SGA undergo catch-up growth within the first 2 years of life, and those who do not would then be eligible for GH treatment.[37,1127,1129,1167,1630,1631,1632] Based on these proportions, and because the prevalence of "short SGA" is 2 to 3 per 1000 children, between 1 in 300 and 1 in 500 children are eligible for GH treatment, as approved in the United States in 2001 and in Europe in 2003. It appears that GH mediates the postnatal catch-up growth.[1633] Children born SGA appear to grow at a low-normal growth velocity during childhood,[1634] but puberty tends to occur at a somewhat earlier age and to progress rapidly, resulting in decreased pubertal height gain and an adult height about 1 SD (approximately 7 cm) below the mean[37,1164,1167,1635-1638] and about 4 cm below the midparental target height.[1129]

The impaired postnatal growth observed in children born SGA is probably due to many factors, including generalized cellular hypoplasia,[1639] altered diurnal GH secretion patterns,[232,1149,1151,1634,1640] and, potentially, abnormalities in the GH-IGF axis resulting from GH sensitivity as determined by the presence or absence of exon 3 of the GHR.[1641,1642,1645] Deletions and mutations of the IGF1 gene have been reported in patients with profound IUGR, microcephaly, deafness, and postnatal growth failure.[340,341,1643] SGA patients have also been reported to have IGF1 gene polymorphisms or missense mutations resulting in low serum IGF1 concentrations.[1139,1140,1167,1644-1646] Reduced levels of IGF2 expression, associated with hypomethylation of the telomeric domain of chromosome 11p15 were found in a cohort of SGA patients who had RSS.[1174] Mutations in the type I IGF receptor gene (one compound heterozygous, one nonsense) were found in two patients with IUGR and poor postnatal growth (one with elevated IGF1).[349]

The low levels of IGF1 and IGFBP3 in many infants with IUGR, apparently related to fetal malnutrition, do not seem to predict the degree of subsequent growth impairment,[1148] although continuing low levels are associated with poor catch-up growth.[1647] Short children born SGA make up a substantial portion of growth-retarded patients seen in pediatric endocrine practices.[1129,1167,1648] Because these children may have heights in the range seen in IGF deficiency syndrome, therapeutic attempts are appropriate, assuming that the insulin resistance noted in these thin, small children[1160] does not become a clinical issue. Encouraging growth responses have been obtained with GH treatment.

The FDA approval of GH for the long-term treatment of growth failure in children born SGA who fail to manifest catch-up growth by age 2 was based on data obtained from four randomized, controlled, open-label, clinical trials that enrolled 209 patients between the ages of 2 and 8 years. Height velocity was determined after 1 year without treatment, and then patients were randomized to receive either GH treatment (34 or 69 mg/kg per day [0.24 or 0.48 mg/kg per week]) or no treatment for 2 years, after which a crossover design occurred. Children who received the higher GH dose had an increase of about 0.5 SDS in height after 2 years, compared with the children who received the lower dose, although both treated groups had significant increases in height velocity compared with untreated children (prescribing information for Genotropin somatropin of recombinant DNA origin for injection, Pfizer, Inc., New York, 2006). In Europe, the criteria for treatment differ from those in the United States: height SDS below −2.5, height velocity SDS below 0 during the previous year, and age of greater than 4 years.

The data documenting efficacy in regard to adult height continues to be limited despite European regulatory authorities' requiring this evidence before approval. A meta-analysis of final height data for 56 children born SGA was performed at the request of European authorities and demonstrated a mean height increase of 1.9 SDS for subjects treated with GH at 34 mg/kg per day versus 2.2 SDS for 69 mg/kg per day. A meta-analysis of three randomized studies of 28 patients reported that GH treatment for 7 to 10 years, initiated at doses of 34 to 69 mg/kg per day, can be expected to increase adult height by about 1.0 to 1.4 SDS.[1649] A larger, randomized, controlled study of 91 GH-treated and 33 untreated French adolescents (mean age, 12 years) reported a lower between-group difference of 0.6 SDS in adult height after 2.7 years of treatment.[1650]

The many studies documenting efficacy of GH therapy in thousands of children with SGA are far too numerous to report in detail here and have been reviewed elsewhere.[1649,1651,1652] Although results vary, it appears that GH treatment can be expected to result in a 1-cm increment in height gain each year. The factors that can increase the gain in height include a greater height deficit relative to the midparental height, a higher GH dose, initiation of therapy at an earlier age, longer treatment duration, and the proposed presence of the *GHRd3* allele.[782,1628,1651,1653] In a prediction model derived from KIGS SGA data, Ranke and coworkers[1653] found that age and GH dose were strong predictors of initial growth but that growth achieved during the first year was a powerful predictor of later growth.

Children born SGA, especially those who have rapid postnatal weight gain, have reduced insulin-mediated glucose uptake and are more likely to have insulin resistance.[1160,1654-1659] However, there have been no solid data documenting an increased risk of NIDDM.[1658] There have been reports of several children in GH registration studies who had mild, transient hyperglycemia (prescribing information for Genotropin somatropin of recombinant DNA origin] for injection, Pfizer, Inc., New York, 2006). Insulin resistance during GH treatment in children born SGA has been reported[1611,1660,1661] and typically resolves after discontinuation of GH.[1662] In a large database of children treated with GH, no differences in glucose regulation were found in 1900 children born SGA compared with children with ISS.[1663] With 6000 patient-years of exposure, no cases of diabetes mellitus have been reported during GH treatment.[1663-1666]

The European product labeling for GH treatment of children born SGA reads, "The management of these patients should follow accepted clinical practice and include safety monitoring of fasting insulin and blood glucose before treatment and annually during treatment."[1652] In addition to insulin resistance alone, children born SGA have an increased risk of metabolic syndrome.[1665,1667-1669] The current literature provides no information on whether GH treatment in childhood increases risks for adult metabolic disease. Long-term follow-up studies are needed to determine the metabolic risk associated with GH treatment.

Osteochondrodysplasias. GH therapy has been studied in several skeletal dysplasias. The largest published study in achondroplasia involved 40 children; during the first year of treatment, the height velocity increased from 3.8 to 6.6 cm/year, and in the second year it decreased to approximately 5 cm/year.[1670] A modest improvement was seen in the ratio of lower limb length to height. Although GH was well tolerated, atlantoaxial dislocation during GH therapy was reported in one patient. In another study, normal growth velocity was achieved for up to 6 years in 35 subjects, with a significant increment in height SDS for at least 4 years[1671]; in that study, vertebral growth was disproportionately greater than limb growth.

Bridges and Brook[1672] reported on the effects of GH therapy in 27 patients with hypochondroplasia; response was maximal during the first year of treatment, but substantial benefit was seen through 4 years of treatment in pubertal subjects. Much of the growth response represents an increase of spinal length; with leg-lengthening procedures, some of these patients may achieve adult height within the normal range.[1673]

Experience with GH treatment is limited in other skeletal disorders, such as dyschondrosteosis, hereditary multiple exostoses, osteogenesis imperfecta, and Ellis-van Creveld syndrome.

SHOX Haploinsufficiency and Léri-Weil Syndrome. Patients with mutations or deletions of the *SHOX* gene have variable degrees of short stature with or without mesomelic skeletal dysplasia. If untreated, short patients with SHOX deficiency remain short in adulthood. The *SHOX* gene is located in the pseudoautosomal region 1 (PAR1) on the distal end of the X and Y chromosomes at Xp22.3 and Yp11.3.[1674,1675] Because genes in PAR1 do not undergo X inactivation, normal individuals express two copies of the *SHOX* gene. This gene encodes a homeodomain transcription factor that is expressed during early fetal life in the growth plate and functions in the regulation of chondrocyte differentiation and proliferation.[1088,1676,1677] SHOX haploinsufficiency (or deficiency) is the primary cause of short stature in patients with LWD (see earlier discussion).[1125,1678-1680] *SHOX* mutations and deletions are also found in patients with short stature without clinical evidence of dyschondrosteosis.[1681-1683]

Clinical manifestations of SHOX deficiency include bowing of the forearms and lower legs, cubitus valgus, Madelung deformity or partial dislocation of the ulna at the wrist and elbow, short fourth and fifth metacarpals, and a high-arched palate along with characteristic radiologic signs.[1087,1125,1680,1682,1684,1685,1686] Longitudinal growth data to final height in subjects with SHOX deficiency not treated with GH are lacking. In a randomized 2-year study of 52 prepubertal subjects with a *SHOX* gene defect, the first-year height velocity in the GH-treated group was significantly greater than in the untreated control group (mean ± standard error of the mean [SE], 8.7 ± 0.3 versus 5.2 ± 0.2 cm/year; $P < .001$) and was similar to the first-year height velocity to GH-treated subjects with TS (8.9 ± 0.4 cm/year; $P < .592$). GH-treated subjects with SHOX deficiency also had significantly greater second-year height velocity (7.3 ± 0.2 versus 5.4 ± 0.2 cm/year; $P < .001$), second-year height SDS (−2.1 ± 0.2 versus −3.0 ± 0.2; $P < .001$), and second-year height gain (16.4 ± 0.4 versus 10.5 ± 0.4 cm; $P < .001$) compared with untreated subjects.[1687]

In a more recent retrospective, 2-year study of 14 patients with SHOX deficiency, 13 of whom had LWD, GH treatment improved height velocity and height standard SDS by 1.1, which was sustained over 2 years. This is equivalent to a gain of approximately 7 cm in height.[1688] These results were not different from those achieved with GH therapy in girls with TS, in contrast to the study from Rappold and coworkers,[1687] which revealed a greater height deficit in girls with TS than in those with SHOX deficiency. Therefore, GH treatment is likely to result in significant final height benefit for most patients with SHOX deficiency.

Turner Syndrome and Langer Mesomelic Dysplasia. Homozygous mutation of the *SHOX* gene results in the Langer type of mesomelic dwarfism (i.e., LMD). A child with LMD and TS was found to have a *SHOX* gene abnormality resulting from a downstream allele deletion in her normal X chromosome. Although there have been numerous studies documenting growth improvement with GH therapy in patients with TS[1100,1599,1622,1689] and in those with heterozygous *SHOX* gene deletions,[1680,1690,1691] only one case of growth response to GH therapy in the rare condition of LMD with TS has been found. Growth rates of 3.46, 3.87, 2.3, and 0.7 cm/year were observed in the first, second, third, and fourth years of GH therapy, respectively, and there was no clinical deterioration of the skeletal deformities in this patient. Because there was a failure to achieve growth improvement with GH therapy, the authors concluded that GH therapy was not beneficial in patients with the severe short stature caused by combined TS and LMD resulting from homozygous *SHOX* deficiency.[1692]

Noonan Syndrome. Since 1994, when a gene for Noonan syndrome was mapped to chromosome 12 (12q24.1) and a mutation in the protein tyrosine phosphatase nonreceptor type 11 *(PTPN11)* was identified and characterized in familial cases, at least three other gene mutations have been identified.[1114,1693-1696] While contributing to the broad heterogeneity of NS, these mutations have not completely localized the cause of the short stature. Several studies have reported effects of GH on near-adult height in patients with Noonan syndrome,[1697-1701] but all involved small numbers of patients with varied enrollment ages, treatment durations, GH doses, and responses. The most recent and largest study of the response to GH in children with Noonan syndrome came from the NCGS, a postmarketing observational study of recombinant human GH treatment in children with various disorders. A total of 370 patients with Noonan syndrome (mean enrollment age, 11.6 years) received GH (mean dosage, 0.33 mg/kg per week) for a mean of 5.6 years. In the 65 patients with data to derive near-adult height, the mean gain above the projected height was 10.9 ± 4.9 cm in boys and 9.2 ± 4.0 cm in girls. Duration of prepubertal recombinant human GH therapy and height SDS at puberty were important contributors to the near-adult height. No new adverse events were observed. The authors suggested that greater growth optimization would be possible with earlier initiation of therapy.[1702] This height increase was similar to the change observed in patients with TS but significantly less in those with idiopathic GHD in the same study.

Most experience with GH treatment of short stature in Noonan syndrome has been limited to small, uncontrolled studies in which few patients reached final height.[1113,1703,1704] The clinical diagnosis of a dysmorphic syndrome potentially makes the treatment groups heterogeneous, although identification of a mutant *PTNN11* gene[1114] helps with characterization. Overall, treatment results for 3 to 4 years are similar to those attained in patients with TS; mean growth velocities improve by 2 to 4 cm/year (over baseline rates of approximately 4 cm/year) during the first 4 years of therapy, with patients gaining from about −3.5 to −1.7 SDS of stature without inordinate advancement of bone age.[1113,1121,1123,1703,1704] Those children with identifiable *PTPN11* mutations are reported to have a poorer response to GH treatment in terms of growth and IGF production, suggesting impaired efficiency of phosphorylation-dependent GH signaling pathways.[1121-1123] Although the initial anecdotal experience suggested progression of ventricular hypertrophic cardiomyopathy, this was not confirmed in larger, carefully monitored studies.[1113,1705,1706]

Idiopathic Short Stature (Subtle Errors throughout the Growth Axis). Although children with ISS, by definition, are without an identifiable cause of growth retardation, the term clearly encompasses a heterogeneous group that may include children with constitutional growth delay, genetic short stature, or subtle defects of the GH-IGF axis. Even though they are often grouped in one category, children with ISS have been shown to have a broad range of provocative GH responses, ranging from normal to elevated, and a wide range of serum IGF concentrations, from normal to IGF deficient. This group may also include children with unidentified syndromes or unidentified chronic illnesses or endocrine disorders. Children with ISS may experience stressful behavioral circumstances, but studies suggest that the relationship of psychosocial problems to the short stature is variable.[1707-1711] Nonetheless, hormonal intervention to enhance growth, with the aim of diminishing such difficulties, has been used.

Although the specific etiologies are often unknown, GH treatment has been used widely.[1702] Important questions have been raised about the financial, ethical, and psychosocial impact of GH therapy in "normal" short children.[1705,1712-1715] Given the cost of GH, the financial implications of treating such children are considerable. The point is well taken that 5% of the population will always be below the 5th percentile, whether we treat with GH or not, and that focusing on short stature could potentially handicap an otherwise normal child psychologically and socially. No convincing data have been presented to show that GH treatment of short children definitively improves psychological, social, or educational function.[1715-1717] A possible exception is the improved intellectual function in SGA children treated with GH.[1718] Furthermore, final adult height in the subset of children with CDGD (probably a common inclusion, although not ISS as defined in the FDA approval) may be adequate without any treatment.[40-42]

Finally, the known and unknown treatment risks GH therapy in otherwise apparently normal children, even if exceedingly small, are a legitimate concern.[1719] The failure to report levels of IGF1, IGFBP3, and GHBP in many studies and differing interpretations of endogenous GH secretion studies (e.g., assay variance, control group size), as well as the heterogeneity of the patient groups, confounds assessment of response data. Nevertheless, it is clear that many children who do not meet conventional criteria for the diagnosis of GHD and who fall under the heading of ISS have as great a degree of growth retardation as children with bona-fide GHD and might be considered suitable candidates for growth-promoting therapy.

Members of the Growth Hormone Research Society, the Lawson Wilkins Pediatric Endocrine Society, and the European Society for Pediatric Endocrinology meeting in 2007 published a manuscript detailing their agreement on the evidence-based evaluation and management of ISS in children. They agreed that the primary goal of therapy should be the attainment of normal adult height. They also agreed that the expectation from patients and their families that taller stature is associated with positive changes in quality of life should be discouraged.[1714] Physicians should inform families about the available therapeutic options and provide a realistic expectation for height gain with therapy, including the fact that there may be variability in the outcome and the psychological counseling options should be discussed. In addition, the patient and family should be aware that therapy may be discontinued if the growth response is poor or if the child no longer provides assent. The physician is responsible for continued monitoring of efficacy and safety and should provide flexibility in treatment options.

The studies that ultimately led to approval of GH treatment in the United States included the long-term, randomized, double-blind, placebo-controlled trial at the National Institutes of Health by Leschek and associates[1371] and the randomized dosing trial of the European Idiopathic Short Stature Study Group.[1720] In the former trial, which used a less optimal regimen of 0.22 mg/kg per week given thrice-weekly in subjects with a mean starting height of almost –3 SDS, the treated children had mean final height gain of 3.7 cm over the control group.[1371] In the latter randomized study, GH doses of 0.24 and 0.37 mg/kg per week, given as a regimen of six doses per week in children with a mean starting height of –3.0 to –3.4 SDS, the improvement in the higher-dose group exceeded that in the lower-dose group by 3.6 cm, with subjects achieving a final height of –1.12 SDS.[1720] When the data from the two trials were combined, there was a cumulative gain of 7.3 cm in the group treated with 0.37 mg/kg per week, compared with placebo.

In a meta-analysis looking at an aggregate group of 1089 children, there were four controlled trials that presented adult height data showing treatment benefits ranging from 0.54 to 0.84 SDS, corresponding to a mean effect on growth of 5 to 6 cm.[1721] McCaughey and associates[1722] found that eight prepubertal girls treated with GH at a dose of approximately 0.34 mg/kg per week experienced a mean height SDS of –1.14 after 6.2 years of treatment. This was a 7.6-cm greater gain than that observed in the control groups, whose mean height SDS (–2.55) did not change during the study.

Concerns had been raised that GH treatment might accelerate pubertal onset and progression in children with ISS, resulting in failure to improve height SDS for bone age[1723,1724] and offsetting the positive responses observed during the early years of GH treatment.[1725] In the European ISS study,[1726] there was no evidence of accelerated pubertal or skeletal maturation in the group receiving the higher dose, in contrast to data reported by Kamp and colleagues[1727] with a 30% greater GH dose. This hypothetical effect of advancing maturation has not been substantiated by additional studies.[1398,1722,1728-1730] Taken together, these data show that GH treatment of prepubertal children with ISS increases growth velocity and final height.

The auxologic criteria for GH therapy in the United States are based on FDA approval of GH treatment for children shorter than –2.25 SDS (1.2 percentile). Some believe that children should be treated if their height is below –2.0 SDS and more than 2.0 SDS below their midparental target height or if their predicted height is below –2.0 SDS (or both). Although there is no consensus on the age for initiating treatment, most studies of GH therapy in children with ISS have involved children from 5 years to early puberty. There are no accepted biochemical criteria for initiating GH treatment in ISS. The bone age is used to predict adult height, although in a longitudinal study of ISS subjects, bone age delay had an effect on the precision of the prediction. In children with a bone age delay of about 2 years, the average adult height was almost equal to the predicted height; in children with no bone age delay, the adult height was greater than the initial predicted height; and if the bone age was delayed by more than 2 years, the adult height was significantly below the predicted adult height.[1731] The psychological benefits of GH therapy in children with ISS are unproven,[1732] but medical and psychological intervention should be considered for the child who seems to suffer from his or her short stature.

The clinical trials of the treatment of ISS with GH in the literature often did not contain long-term control groups; hence, the results show variable growth responses.[1719,1733-1737] Most short children treated with GH experience growth acceleration that is usually sustained over the first several years of therapy,[1703] with attenuation of the treatment response over time. In general, a slower pretreatment growth velocity and a higher weight-to-height ratio—factors suggestive of GHD and, to a lesser degree, bone age retardation—are associated with better early growth responses.[1738] Three thousand children were classified as having ISS in the KIGS database, with 153 having reached final height.[1728] GH treatment (0.2 to 0.25 mg/kg per week) resulted in achievement of target height in patients with familial short stature, although they continued to have short stature as adults (−1.7 SDS in males and −2.2 SDS in females), with a mean gain during therapy of 0.6 to 0.9 SDS. In children who did not have familial short stature, the mean final height was greater for males (−1.4 SDS), although not for females (−2.3 SDS), with average gains of 1.3 and 0.9 SDS, respectively. These attained heights were quite different from the midparental target heights, which were near 0 SDS. Hintz and colleagues[1720] assessed adult height in 80 North American children with ISS who were treated for up to 10 years at a GH dose of 0.3 mg/kg per week. At the conclusion of the study, the mean height SDS was −1.4 SDS with a gain of 1.3 SDS, results quite similar to those from the KIGS database. Although the Hintz study was not placebo controlled, the data were compared with predicted and actual final heights in two groups of untreated short children followed for similar periods. Compared to untreated children, treated boys achieved a mean of 9.2 cm and girls 5.7 cm stature above predicted heights.

Several additional studies have documented the increase in final height with GH therapy in children with ISS, although the responses have been highly variable and dose dependent. The mean increase in adult height in children with ISS is 3.5 to 7.5 cm (with an average duration of therapy of 4 to 7 years) when compared with historical controls,[1370,1739] with patients' pretreatment predicted adult heights,[1725] or with nontreatment or placebo control groups.[1371,1721] Multiple factors affect the growth response to GH, and the best response is seen in children who are younger or heavier, those receiving higher GH doses, and those who are shortest relative to their target height. Adult height outcome is influenced negatively by age at initiation of therapy and positively by midparental height, initial height, delayed bone age, and the magnitude of the first-year response to GH.[1731,1740] A 2-year study suggested that an increase in IGF1 correlates with height gain.[1371]

Studies using monotherapy with GnRH agonists have shown only a small and variable effect on final adult height, so GnRH agonist therapy is not recommended. Furthermore, GnRH agonists have been shown to have short-term adverse effects on BMD,[1741] and psychological consequences of delayed puberty have been suggested.[1742] However, combination therapy with a GnRH agonist and GH has potential value in increasing final height, with treatment lasting at least 3 years.[1743,1744]

Monitoring of GH treatment should include height, weight, pubertal development, and adverse effects (scoliosis, tonsillar hypertrophy, papilledema, and slipped capital femoral epiphysis) two to three times per year. After 1 year of therapy, the height velocity SDS and the change in height SDS should be calculated. The bone age may be obtained to reassess height prediction and if one is considering intervention to delay puberty. IGF1 levels may be helpful in guiding GH dose adjustment. Because elevated blood glucose levels in patients with GH-treated ISS have not been reported, routine monitoring of glucose metabolism is not advised.

The FDA-approved dose for GH in ISS is 0.3 to 0.37 mg/kg per week.[1745] The dose may be increased if the growth response is inadequate and compliance was assured. However, there are no data regarding the long-term safety of GH doses higher than 0.5 mg/kg per week in children with ISS. IGF1 levels may be helpful in assessing compliance and GH sensitivity. IGF1 levels that are elevated (>2.5 SDS) should prompt consideration of GH dose reduction. IGF-based dose adjustments in children with ISS increased short-term growth when higher IGF targets were selected, but long-term studies with respect to efficacy, safety, and cost effectiveness have not been done.[1727] If the growth rate continues to be inadequate, GH treatment should be stopped and alternative therapies considered. The duration of treatment is controversial, with consideration given for stopping treatment when near-adult height is achieved (height velocity <2 cm/year or bone age >16 years in boys or >14 years in girls) if height is in the normal adult range (above −2 SDS). Stopping therapy may be influenced by satisfaction of the patient and family with the resulting height, an ongoing cost/benefit analysis, or desire of the child to stop for other reasons (e.g., dissatisfaction with daily injections).

The possible side effects in GH-treated children with ISS are similar to those previously reported in children receiving GH therapy for other indications, with no long-term adverse effects documented.[1746,1747] Post-treatment surveillance with a focus on cancer prevalence and metabolic side effects is advisable.

The average cost of GH treatment of children with ISS is $10,000 to $20,000 per centimeter of growth improvement.[1739] The benefits are less clear,[1739] because it is unknown whether a gain in height improves quality of life. Therefore, recommendations for treatment that increases adult height should be balanced against the high cost of these therapies.

Miscellaneous Causes of Growth Failure. In addition to the clinical conditions described earlier, GH has been employed in the treatment of short stature associated with a variety of other conditions involving postnatal growth failure. In general, such trials have been uncontrolled and have not included sufficient numbers of subjects for efficacy to be evaluated. Examination of such treatments should be continued in the large international databases.

Down Syndrome. The encouraging results of GH trials in TS led to studies of GH therapy in children with Down syndrome. In several preliminary studies, GH accelerated growth in such patients, although ethical issues were raised concerning the appropriateness of such therapy.[1093,1748-1750] In the uncontrolled NCGS experience, 23 children experienced a 1.3 SDS height gain over the first 4 years of GH therapy.[1703] No convincing data exist that GH improves neurologic or intellectual function in such patients. The increased risks of diabetes mellitus and leukemia in children with Down syndrome could be augmented by GH therapy.[1751]

Normal Aging and Other Catabolic States. Detailed consideration of the potential use of GH in normal aging is beyond the scope of this chapter. The rationale for such therapy is based on the concept of the "somatopause," a term that highlights the progressive decline in GH secretion after 30 years of age, as reflected in decreasing IGF1 levels. Aging can be viewed as a catabolic state, with the potential that GH therapy might reverse or retard the loss of muscle mass and strength and the decrease in bone density that occur with aging. Clinical studies are in progress.

Growth failure, often with impaired final adult height, is a characteristic clinical finding in endogenous or exogenous Cushing's syndrome. Excess glucocorticoids cause a catabolic state characterized by increased proteolysis, decreased protein synthesis, lowered osteoblastic and increased osteolytic activity, and insulin resistance.[1752] GH treatment blunts some of these catabolic actions but increases the insulin resistance.[1753] Mauras and Beaufrere[1039] showed that IGF1 therapy similarly induces an anabolic response, despite excess glucocorticoids, but does not cause insulin resistance. GH treatment after transplantation[1569-1571] and in other glucocorticoid-treated children[1028] causes some height increments, but does not produce as good a response as in individuals not taking glucocorticoids. GH does enhance bone formation and increases osteoblastic activity in such children.[1754] The marked increase in IGF1 levels during GH treatment may be sufficient to overcome the local insensitivity to IGF action.[421,910,911,1755]

GH therapy is also being investigated in catabolic states such as burns, tumor cachexia, major abdominal surgery, AIDS, sepsis, metabolic acidosis, and situations requiring total parenteral alimentation. GH should not be used in critically ill patients, because a randomized, controlled trial demonstrated increased morbidity and mortality with GH treatment of such patients.[1756]

The FDA-approved indications for the use of GH for purposes other than stimulation of growth are (1) GHD in adults, (2) AIDS-associated wasting or cachexia, and (3) short-bowel syndrome requiring total parenteral nutrition.

Side Effects of Growth Hormone

Pituitary-derived human GH had an enviable safety record for a quarter of a century but proved to be an agent for transmission of the fatal spongiform encephalopathy, CJD.[1389,1757] Although pit-GH was removed from use in the United States in 1985, and later throughout the world, more than 200 patients with GH-derived CJD have been identified.[1391-1393] Although recombinant DNA–derived GH does not carry this risk, the experience with pit-GH serves as a grim reminder of the potential toxicity that can reside in "normal" products used for physiologic replacement.

Extensive experience with recombinant GH over more than 20 years has been encouraging.[1272,1664,1758,1760] Concerns have been raised about a number of potential complications, which clearly require continued follow-up and assessment. This evaluation has been greatly facilitated by the extensive databases that have been established by GH manufacturers, in particular Genentech (NCGS)[1523] and Pharmacia (KIGS).[1664,1761,1762]

Development of Leukemia. The development of leukemia as a complication of GH therapy was first reported in five cases from Japan in 1988[1763]; to date, more than 50 cases of leukemia have been reported in GH-treated patients. Many of the cases are from Japan,[1764] but some are from the United States.[1390,1759] One difficulty in assessing the role of GH treatment in this disorder is that many GH-deficient children have conditions that predispose to the development of leukemia, such as prior malignancy, a history of irradiation, or concurrent syndromes which themselves are associated with the development of leukemia (e.g., Bloom's syndrome, Down syndrome, Fanconi's anemia). GH-treated patients who develop leukemia do so at a later age than in the normal population. Patients have included recipients of both pit-GH and recombinant GH, and leukemia has occurred both during treatment and after termination of therapy. Calculations of relative risk are imprecise but vary from sevenfold in Japan to twofold to fourfold in the United States. Leukemia also has been reported in GH-deficient individuals without any history of GH therapy, raising the possibility that the GH-deficient state, by itself, may be a predisposing factor.[1762,1765]

It is not possible to be certain whether GH is a causative agent in the development of leukemia. If it is, the increase in risk appears to be modest and may arise from the underlying state rather than from GH therapy. Worldwide, the number of cases of new leukemia in GH-treated children with no known risk factors is approximately what would be expected on a patient-year basis.[1523,1758,1766,1767]

This issue should be discussed with all potential recipients of GH, but it appears that the risk is limited to those children with high risk factors. Particular care should be used in prescribing GH therapy for children with a past history of leukemia or lymphoma or other disorders conveying an increased risk of leukemia. In a study of more than 600 children with prior leukemia who were treated with GH, the relapse rate was within the expected range, consistent with no effect of GH replacement therapy on recurrence of leukemia.[1672,1759,1768]

Data from more than 88,000 GH-treated patients with more than 275,000 patient-years at risk did not reveal an increased risk for nonleukemic extracranial neoplasms.[1523,1672,1758]

Recurrence of Central Nervous System Tumors. Because many recipients of GH have acquired GHD due to CNS tumors or their treatment, the possibility of tumor recurrence with therapy is of obvious importance. Estimates of CNS tumor recurrence rates in non–GH-treated children and adolescents are difficult to obtain, bearing in mind the vast array of treatment programs used in the past 3 decades. In a total of 1083 patients compiled from 11 reports who were not treated with GH, 209 (19.3%) had recurrences.[1768-1778] Such data in a heterogeneous group, including patients with craniopharyngiomas, gliomas, ependymomas, medulloblastomas, and germ cell tumors, provide a background for assessing recurrence rates in GH-treated youth. Reports from nine centers, encompassing 390 patients, indicated recurrence in 64 patients (16.4%) at the time of publication,[1768,1769,1778-1783] which is not much different from the recurrence rate observed in a much larger number of untreated patients. In a particularly well done comparative study at three pediatric neuro-oncology centers comprising 1071 brain tumor patients, 180 patients were treated with GH for a mean of 6.4 years, and 31 of them were monitored for more than 10 years; the relative risk of recurrence or death was similar with and without GH treatment.[1782]

In a study of 361 cancer survivors (including 172 brain tumor patients), disease recurrence of all cancers in GH-treated children did not differ from recurrence in those children not treated with GH. However, there was an overall increased risk of 3.21 (95% confidence interval, 1.88 to 5.46) for second neoplasms, mostly meningiomas.[1784] A follow-up of this study continued to show the increased risk of second neoplasm, but the rate ratio was lower at 2.15.[1785] The decreased rate ratio with longer follow-up raised the possibility that GH treatment may accelerate the manifestation of these tumors, rather than increasing the absolute rate. A similar increased risk for second neoplasms, also largely meningiomas, was found in GH-treated adult patients.[1786]

Cranial irradiation seems to be a most important predisposing factor, but the role of GH remains uncertain. Extensive analysis of 4410 patients with a history of brain tumor or craniopharyngioma before GH therapy in the NCGS and KIGS databases[1664,1758,1787] showed a similar lack of increased tumor recurrence. In the NCGS series, recurrence rates of the most common CNS neoplasms, craniopharyngioma (6.4%), primary neuroectodermal tumors (medulloblastoma, ependymoma; 7.2%), and low-grade glioma (18.1%) were lower than or similar to those reported in non–GH-treated children.[1768,1788,1789]

Despite these comforting data, the relatively short median follow-up times reported, even in the huge international databases, must temper the willingness to eliminate any relationship of GH therapy to recurrence of intracranial neoplasia.

Pseudotumor Cerebri. Pseudotumor cerebri (idiopathic intracranial hypertension) has been reported in GH-treated patients.[1523,1664,1758,1790] The disorder may develop within months after treatment starts or as long as 5 years into the course; it appears to be more frequent in patients with renal failure than in those with GHD.[1758] The mechanism for the effect is unclear but may reflect changes in fluid dynamics within the CNS. Pseudotumor has also been described after thyroid hormone replacement in patients with hypothyroidism. In any case, clinicians should be alert to complaints of headache, nausea, dizziness, ataxia, or visual changes. Significant fluid retention with edema or hypertension is rare.[1791] Because of the possible association of pseudopapilledema with GHD, perhaps representing a variant of optic nerve hypoplasia,[1792] careful ophthalmologic evaluation should be undertaken in patients with suspected GH therapy–associated pseudotumor cerebri to avoid overdiagnosis and invasive treatments.

Slipped Capital Femoral Epiphysis. Slipped capital femoral epiphysis is associated with both hypothyroidism and GHD. Whether GH therapy plays a role in this disorder has been difficult to determine, in part because the incidence of slipped capital femoral epiphysis varies with age, gender, race, and geographic locale. The reported incidence is between 2 and 142 cases per 100,000 population; the data in the KIGS and NCGS studies are in this range.[1523,1664,1758] Accordingly, although slipped capital femoral epiphysis cannot be attributed to GH therapy per se, complaints of hip and knee pain or limp should be evaluated carefully. The occurrence of such pain in a GH-treated child with an exceedingly rapid growth rate should lead to consideration of this diagnosis.

Scoliosis. Both progression of preexisting scoliosis and new-onset scoliosis have been described in children treated with GH.[1523] The numbers are extremely small, with only 238 reported cases among 54,996 patients in the NCGS database. There is specific concern for GH effects on scoliosis in TS and PWS patients, in whom the underlying rate of scoliosis is increased. Although the rate of scoliosis in GH-treated TS patients was higher than in other GH-treated patients, it remained rare, being reported in only 0.69% of patients.[1622] PWS by itself has a rate of scoliosis of 30% to 80%, and GH treatment does not appear to increase the rate or severity of scoliosis in PWS patients.[1537,1793]

Diabetes Mellitus. The association of GH treatment with insulin resistance is well documented.[1794] Data from the KIGS and NCGS databases have been used to estimate the incidence of type 2 diabetes mellitis (T2DM) in GH-treated patients as approximately 14 to 22 cases per 100,000 patient-years.[1523,1664,1758] Although insufficient information is available to determine whether this represents an increased incidence when compared with the baseline risk in similar individuals, it is higher than the overall incidence of T2DM in children (0.8, 8.1, and 11.8 per 100,000 person-years for ages 5 to 9, 10 to 14, and 15 to 19 years, respectively).[1795] An earlier report of the NCGS data indicated that not all of the children with T2DM were obese, because their BMI ranged from 13.2 to 38.1 kg/m^2 (mean, 22.8 kg/m^2).[1758] Therefore, the reduction of insulin sensitivity induced by GH is a concern that demands close assessment in high-risk patients such as those with PWS or TS or a history of IUGR. Studies of the impact of decades of GH therapy on insulin sensitivity are warranted.

Miscellaneous Side Effects.[1523,1664,1758] Other potential side effects of GH therapy include prepubertal gynecomastia,[1796] pancreatitis,[1797] growth of nevi[1798,1799] (although typically without evidence of malignant degeneration[1759]), behavioral changes, worsening of neurofibromatosis, hypertrophy of tonsils and adenoids, and sleep apnea. A report[1800] of reduced testicular volume and elevated gonadotropin levels in four young adult men previously treated with GH for ISS was not confirmed by a double-blind, placebo-controlled study,[1801] nor by the international databases.[1802] This list of side effects is only partial. It is best for the clinician to remember that GH and the peptide growth factors it regulates are potent mitogens with diverse metabolic and anabolic actions. All patients receiving GH treatment, even as replacement therapy, must be carefully monitored for side effects.

For the most part, the side effects of GH are minimal and rare. When they do occur, a careful history and physical examination are adequate to identify their presence. Management of these side effects may include transient reduction of dosage or temporary discontinuation of GH.[1237] In the absence of other risk factors, there is no evidence that the risk of leukemia, brain tumor recurrence, or slipped capital femoral epiphysis is increased in recipients of long-term GH treatment. Any patient receiving GH who has a second major medical condition (e.g., being a tumor survivor) should be followed up in conjunction with an appropriate specialist such as an oncologist or neurosurgeon. Whereas GH has been shown to increase the mortality of critically ill patients in intensive care units,[1803] there is no evidence that GH replacement therapy needs to be discontinued during intercurrent illness in children with GHD.

The Question of Long-Term Cancer Risk. Several epidemiologic studies have suggested an association between high serum IGF1 levels and an increased incidence of malignancies.[1804,1805] The calculated risk of cancer in those studies was also increased for patients with low IGFBP3 levels. Additional studies are being conducted to verify or disprove these associations, but the role of GH also should be carefully examined. Although IGF1 levels were not statistically associated with cancer risk, the combination of high IGF1 and low IGFBP3 was related to a heightened risk.[1806] Because GH positively influences production of both peptides, this finding casts doubt on its role as a driving force in the IGF-cancer relationship. A potential confounder in these studies is the variability of serum IGF1 levels that may be observed normally and the consequent substantial movement of a given individual's risk designation in differing quartiles when multiple samples are obtained.[1247] Additionally, the effects of high IGFBP3 levels on the incidence of premenopausal breast cancer further underscore the complexity of these relationships.[1807] The necessity of long-term, well-designed studies, with a sufficient number of patients to prevent incorrect and inappropriately ominous conclusions, is apparent.[1808]

Epidemiologic studies assessing the risk of malignancy in patients with acromegaly found differing results, with some,[1809-1811] but not others,[1812,1813] identifying significant associations between acromegaly and colon cancer risk. The small size and uncontrolled retrospective nature of these studies and the multiple possible sources of bias make these reports difficult to interpret. The largest study to date, reviewing more than 1000 patients, indicated no overall increased cancer incidence in acromegaly.[1814] Although colon cancer risk was also not increased in that study, the mortality rate was higher, suggesting an effect of GH or IGF on established tumors.[1815] A prospective analysis of colon cancer and colonic polyps in acromegalics did not observe an association between these two diseases when using either autopsy series or prospective colonoscopy screening series for the control population.[1816] Acromegaly is associated with a marked increase in the incidence of benign hyperplasia in several organs, including colonic polyps.[1817] Such findings suggest that the GH-IGF1 axis may lead to symptomatic benign proliferative disease, which could be associated with symptoms, such as rectal bleeding, that would lead to a potential detection (or ascertainment) bias.

Children receiving GH do not appear to have a greater risk of de novo or recurrent tumors.[1272,1664,1758] A cohort of 1848 patients treated with GH in the United Kingdom was assessed after as long as 40 years and found to have increased rates of colorectal cancer and Hodgkin's disease, but the tumor-associated deaths were so few that a single patient death would markedly alter the risk ratios.[1818,1819] No increased incidence of cancer was found in GH recipients among adults who were treated for GHD.[1455,1820] These reports represent imperfect, uncontrolled studies, but the experience gained through them strongly suggests that GH therapy is not associated with future development of neoplasms in the absence of other risk factors.

The use of IGF1 and IGFBP3 in the monitoring of GH recipients, both adult and pediatric, has been recommended and endorsed by international bodies such as the Growth Hormone Research Society[1236] and the Drug and Therapeutics Committees of the Lawson Wilkins Pediatric Endocrine Society and the European Society of Pediatric Endocrinology.[1818,1819] Until the issue of cancer risk in GH therapy is fully resolved, the prudent approach appears to be regular monitoring of both IGF1 and IGFBP3 and alteration of the GH dose to ensure that the theoretical risk profile induced by GH therapy is favorable. This can be done by avoiding the unlikely situation of a GH-treated patient with an IGF1 level at the upper end and a IGFBP3 level at the lower end of the normal range. In the 21st century, many GH-deficient patients will receive lifelong GH replacement, emphasizing the importance of long-term, regular monitoring of IGF1 and IGFBP3.[1820,1821] Although many issues still remain in fully discerning the relationship, if any, between the GH-IGF axis and the risk of cancer, current data strongly suggest the safety of present indications for use of GH in children and adults.[1822,1823]

IGF1 Treatment

In 2005, the FDA approved the use of rhIGF1 for "long term treatment of growth failure in children with severe primary IGF-1 deficiency and in children with GH gene deletions who have developed neutralizing antibodies to GH. Severe primary IGF-1 deficiency is defined by height SD score less than –3.0 and a basal IGF-1 SD score less than –3.0 and normal or elevated GH. Severe primary IGF-1 deficiency includes patients with mutations in the GHR, post-GHR receptor signaling pathway, and IGF-1 gene defects" (Increlex [rhIGF1] prescribing information, 2009, Tercica, Inc.). Clinical trials to study the safety and efficacy of rhIGF1 therapy have been conducted mostly in individuals with proven mutations in the GHR; fewer than 10% of enrollees have had GH insensitivity due to GH antibodies. Because of the rarity of GHR mutations, the clinical trials have been small. When all clinical trials are combined, the total number of children treated to date is less than 200, and relatively few have been treated for longer than 5 years. A discussion of the published clinical trials follows.

When 40 μg/kg of IGF1 was administered every 12 hours to six adults with GHR deficiency, normal serum IGF1 levels were maintained for 2 to 6 hours after injection, followed by a rapid decline because of low serum levels of IGFBP3.[119] Hypoglycemia did not occur, mean 24-hour GH levels were suppressed, and urinary calcium was increased, demonstrating the potential therapeutic utility of subcutaneous IGF1. A number of short-term growth-related studies with subcutaneous IGF1 treatment at varied doses have been reported. Despite slight differences in IGF1 dosage and inclusion criteria, the short-term effects of IGF1 on growth in GH insensitivity were consistent: growth increased from pretreatment rates of 3 to 5 cm/year to 8 to 11 cm/year on average. In five children with GHR deficiency, single daily doses of 150 μg/kg for 3 to 10 months resulted in growth acceleration to rates of 8.8 to 13.6 cm/year.[1824] Twice-daily injections of 120 μg/kg increased the growth rate from 6.5 to 11.4 cm/year in another patient.[1825] Wilton[1826] reported collaborative data on the treatment of 30 patients, ages 3 to 23 years, with GH insensitivity due to GHR deficiency or IGHD 1A with anti-GH antibodies; the dose of IGF1 varied from 40 to 120 μg/kg twice daily. With the exception of the two oldest individuals, growth rates increased in Wilton's subjects by at least 2 cm/year. A mean increment of more than 4 cm/year in growth velocity was found in 11 prepubertal children treated with 80 μg/kg twice daily.[1827] This study also demonstrated a significant inverse relationship between growth response to exogenous IGF1 and the severity of the GH insensitivity phenotype.

Longer-term studies of IGF1 treatment of GH insensitivity demonstrated a progressive waning effect of IGF1 on growth velocity.[1828] Data from 17 patients in a European collaborative trial who were treated for at least 4 years showed an increase in mean height SDS from –6.5 to –4.9, with two adolescents reaching the 3rd percentile. Children who received rhIGF1 for 2 years or less had a higher growth velocity than those children who received rhIGF1 for longer periods. In the longest treatment study,[1829,1830] outcomes were similar to those in the European study, with an initial burst of growth (from 4.0 9.3 cm/year) followed by slowing to just above baseline (4.8 cm/year) by the sixth year of therapy. Height SDS improved from –5.6 to –4.2 by the end of the sixth year.

These limited data indicate that rhIGF1 is effective in increasing statural growth, but the growth response is neither as robust nor as sustained as the growth response to GH among children with GHD. GH treatment of GH-deficient children results in sustained supranormal growth velocity, and children can achieve adult heights in the normal range. In contrast, the near-final height of children with GH insensitivity who received rhIGF1 therapy was below –4 SDS. The suboptimal growth response to rhIGF1 compared with recombinant human GH has been attributed to (1) inability of rhIGF1 to increase IGFBP3 and ALS levels, leading to decreased delivery of IGF1 to target tissues; (2) lack of GH-induced proliferation of prechondrocytes in the growth plate; (3) absence of GH-induced local IGF1 at the growth plate; and (4) difficulty in using higher doses of IGF1 because of the risk of hypoglycemia.[1831]

IGF1 treatment has also been administered to individuals with IGF1 gene deletion[1832] and post-GHR signaling defects with growth patterns similar to those of children with GH insensitivity due to GHR deficiency. Patients with Noonan syndrome and the *PTPN11* gene mutation experience a less robust response to GH therapy than do those without that mutation. Because PTPN11 may play a role in downstream GH signaling, it has been suggested that rhIGF1 therapy may be efficacious in this population.[1833] It has also been suggested that children with renal failure and short stature may benefit from rhIGF1, because there may be diminished GHR signaling.[1834] Limited studies have examined the efficacy of IGF1 therapy in patients with severe insulin resistance due to insulin receptor defects (leprechaunism),[1835] liver disease,[1836] neurologic disorders or injuries,[1837] or critical illnesses.[1838] These studies are investigational, and routine IGF1 therapy in children with these disorders is not indicated.

The most common adverse effect of rhIGF1 is hypoglycemia. In some studies, it occurred in almost half of the patients with GH insensitivity treated with rhIGF1,[1830] usually within the first month of therapy. Importantly, individuals with GHR defects, the highest proportion of enrollees in these treatment studies, have baseline hypoglycemia. In a 6-month, placebo-controlled trial, 67% of children receiving placebo experienced hypoglycemia, compared with 85% of children receiving rhIGF1—a difference that was not statistically significant.[1839] In a study of 23 patients with GH insensitivity, hypoglycemia was noted before the start of treatment; after 3 months, 2.6% of glucose values in those receiving placebo were less than 50 mg/dL, compared with 5.5% of glucose values in those receiving rhIGF1.[1830] The hypoglycemia is avoidable with adequate food intake. In 18 patients with low IGF1 and IGFBP3 levels, blood glucose was monitored after 2 weeks of rhIGF1 in the setting of regular meals, and no levels lower than 60 mg/dL were observed.[1840]

Patients with GH insensitivity treated with rhIGF1 have also experienced lymphoid tissue hypertrophy, encompassing tonsillar/adenoidal growth and associated snoring and sleep apnea, and thymic and splenic enlargement.[1830] The hypertrophy occurred in 22% of patients, with 10% of patients requiring tonsillectomy/adenoidectomy. Acromegaloid coarsening of the face was observed in patients of pubertal age.[1830] Studies have reported an increase in BMI with treatment and a twofold to threefold increase in body fat as assessed by dual-energy x-ray absorptiometry (DEXA).[1841] Intracranial hypertension with associated papilledema as also been observed in as many as 5% of treated patients. Headache is also frequent, but at least one placebo-controlled study found no difference in headache frequency between treatment and placebo groups.[1839] Anti-IGF1 antibodies develop in about half of treated patients during the first year, but they have no effect on the response.[1830,1842] As with recombinant human GH treatment, an increased cancer risk with rhIGF1 treatment is an unknown but legitimate concern, considering the role of IGF1 in neoplasias and the increased cancer risk associated with hypersomatotropism.[1843,1844]

Approval by the FDA and the European Agency for the Evaluation of Medical Products of rhIGF1 has ignited debate about expansion of the diagnosis of severe IGF1 deficiency and consequent expanded use of rhIGF1 beyond those patients with neutralizing GH antibodies or documented mutations in the GHR, GHR signaling pathways, or the IGF1 gene. Some advocate that individuals with ISS, low serum IGF1, or poor response to a GH trial may have unidentified subtle alterations in GHR signaling and could benefit from treatment with rhIGF1.[1845] Others express reservations about expanding the diagnosis of IGF1 deficiency and rhIGF1 use, postulating that the response of children with ISS to rhIGF1 may be minimal considering the lower long-term growth response of children with GHR defects treated with IGF1 compared with GH-deficient children treated with GH. Another theoretical concern regards negative feedback of rhIGF1 on GH secretion, which leads to diminished IGF1-independent effects of GH on growth.[1831,1846]

Other Treatments to Promote Growth

GnRH Agonists

Increasing Adult Height of Children with Idiopathic Short Stature. The effect of GnRH agonist therapy on adult height has been studied in girls with ISS and normal puberty (8 to 10 years of age); there was a mean gain of 0 to 4.2 cm, compared with predicted height.[1741,1847-1858] In boys with rapidly progressing puberty, GnRH agonist therapy increased adult height compared with predicted height,[1859,1860] with mean gains of 4.4 to 10 cm in those receiving the combination therapy, compared with 0.5 to 6.1 cm in untreated controls.[1744,1861]

In these studies, the effects of GH cannot be definitively separated from those of the GnRH agonist. In two randomized studies of adopted girls with normal puberty, treatment with a GnRH agonist plus GH was compared with GnRH agonist alone, and a 3-cm height gain was demonstrated with the combination therapy.[1862,1863]

Disadvantages of the use of GnRH agonists in children with ISS include absence of pubertal growth acceleration, delayed puberty with potential psychosocial disadvantage, and decreased BMD. Long-term follow-up studies are lacking. A panel of experts concluded that GnRH agonist therapy alone in children with ISS and normally timed puberty is minimally effective in increasing adult height, may compromise BMD, and cannot be suggested for routine use.[1864] Combined GnRH agonist and GH therapy leads to a significant height gain but may have adverse effects. Routine use of GnRH agonists in children with ISS being treated with GH cannot be suggested (level of evidence, C-III).

Increasing Adult Height of Children Born Small for Gestational Age. Short children born SGA usually have a normal pubertal timing, although some of them have rapidly progressing puberty, and may be treated with GH.[1629,1865] Data on the additional effect of treatment with GnRH agonists are limited. Routine use of the combination of a GnRH agonist and GH in children born SGA cannot be suggested.

Increasing Adult Height of Children with Growth Hormone Deficiency. Some children with GHD are short at the start of puberty and at risk for short adult stature. Retrospective studies evaluating the addition of GnRH agonists to GH therapy involved a limited number of subjects and provided controversial results.[1866-1868] Three prospective studies that reported near-adult or adult heights showed a height gain of −1 SDS,[1869-1871] possibly without detrimental effect on BMD.[1872] Routine use of combined therapy with a GnRH agonist and GH in GH-deficient children with low predicted adult height at onset of puberty cannot be suggested (level of evidence, C-III).

Aromatase Inhibitors. Men with estrogen deficiency due to aromatase gene defects or estrogen resistance due to inactive estrogen receptors experience growth into the third decade, demonstrating the role of estrogen in growth plate fusion.[21,23] The aromatase enzyme catalyzes aromatization of testosterone and androstenedione to estradiol and estrone, respectively. Various studies have been conducted to explore the efficacy of the aromatase inhibitor class of drugs delaying growth plate fusion and increasing height in disorders associated with short stature in boys. Studies to date have been small, and many have used adjuvant treatments, including GH, GnRH agonist, or testosterone, so the singular effect of the aromatase inhibitor has been unclear. Additionally, most studies to date have been short term and have measured changes in predicted adult height, with only one study investigating the effect on final adult height.

Aromatase inhibitors were first tried in disorders of sex steroid excess and precocious puberty, with only modest, if any, effects on predicted adult height. Treatment of boys with familial male-limited precocious puberty with testolactone, a first-generation aromatase inhibitor, resulted in an improvement in predicted adult height only after 5 to 6 years of treatment.[1873-1875] The improvement in predicted adult height after 6 years was robust, however, at 12.9 cm compared with untreated controls. Case reports using the second-generation aromatase inhibitor, anastrozole, also resulted in modest improvements in predicted adult height.[1876] In contrast, first- and second-generation aromatase inhibitors have not significantly affected predicted adult height in patients with McCune-Albright syndrome.[1877-1879] In children with congenital adrenal hypoplasia, addition of aromatase inhibitors did not significantly affect predicted adult height.[1880,1881]

Aromatase inhibitors have also been used in boys with CDGD. Boys with CDGD who received the second-generation aromatase inhibitor letrozole, in combination with testosterone, for 12 months experienced an increase in predicted adult height of 5.1 cm compared with controls treated with testosterone alone.[1374] When followed to adult height, those boys who received letrozole in addition to testosterone achieved a final adult height 5.7 cm higher than that of boys receiving testosterone alone.[1376] In prepubertal boys with ISS, 2 years of treatment with letrozole increased the predicted adult height by 5.9 cm compared with placebo.[1882] In GH-deficient boys treated with GH, the addition of anastrozole for 3 years increased predicted adult height by 6.7 cm, compared to an increase of 1.0 cm in boys treated with GH alone.[1740] The results of these preliminary, small trials indicate that aromatase inhibitors may be able to increase adult height, but larger, longer trials are needed to determine the optimal conditions and duration of treatment to significantly increase final adult height. In addition, longer follow-up will be needed to demonstrate the safety of such treatments in peripubertal and pubertal boys.

Given the observation of decreased BMD in males with defects in estrogen synthesis or action, the effects of short-term aromatase inhibitor therapy on BMD were investigated in these treatment studies. None of the studies found a difference in BMD as assessed by DEXA scans in patients who received aromatase inhibitor or placebo for up to 3 years.[1740,1883,1884] In boys with CDGD or ISS who received letrozole, serum high-density lipoprotein (HDL)-cholesterol was significantly lower than in placebo-treated boys, but boys with GHD who received anastrozole did not have a significant difference in HDL-cholesterol.[1885] This discrepancy was postulated to be a result of the lower potency of anastrozole compared with letrozole, rather than the underlying disorder. Evidence in animals suggests a role for estrogen and estrogen receptor signaling in spermatogenesis. The one study that examined sperm function after aromatase inhibitor therapy did not find a detrimental effect.[1886] Clearly, longitudinal follow-up is needed to better characterize the safety and efficacy of aromatase inhibitors to promote growth.

Oxandrolone. Oxandrolone, an anabolic steroid, has been used to increase growth velocity in a number of disorders. Because it cannot be aromatized to estrogen, it should not accelerate skeletal maturation. In general, studies evaluating the effect of oxandrolone on growth have found that it increases growth velocity but is not associated with an increase in final height.

Clinical Trials of Efficacy. Numerous studies have investigated oxandrolone therapy in boys with CDGD. The studies have found that oxandrolone increases growth velocity in these boys.[1352,1353,1355-1357,1887] The typical response is an increase in growth velocity from approximately 4 to 4.5 cm/year up to 8 to 9 cm/year. Although treatment does not decrease final height, as might occur with accelerated skeletal maturation from excessive sex hormone exposure, neither does it increase final height.[1353,1357,1887] Therefore, oxandrolone can be used to accelerate the growth of boys with CDGD to allow them to increase their height sooner than they would naturally, but it does not increase their final adult height.

Oxandrolone has been studied in girls with TS, both as a single agent and as combined therapy with GH. As in boys with CDGD, oxandrolone increases the growth rate in girls with TS.[1593,1888,1889] Although some studies found no effect on final height with oxandrolone treatment alone,[1890] others found a mean increase in final height of up to 5.2 cm with oxandrolone treatment.[1888,1889] Studies of oxandrolone in combination with GH treatment of girls with TS have found a modest increase in final height, compared with GH treatment alone.[1601,1604]

Side Effects. No significant side effects have been reported in boys treated with oxandrolone for CDGD. Although oxandrolone has significantly less androgenic effects than testosterone, mild virilization has been reported in girls taking oxandrolone, including clitoromegaly. This is less of a concern at lower doses. Hepatic dysfunction, including hepatic failure, has been reported with oxandrolone treatment.[1891,1892]

Diagnosis and Treatment of Excess Growth and Tall Stature

Diagnosis

The normal distribution of height predicts that 2.5% of the population will be taller than 2 SD above the mean. The most common cause of tall stature is familial, and the diagnostic evaluation centers on distinguishing tall or constitutional stature from rare pathologic causes of tall stature. As with short stature, children with tall stature must be evaluated relative to familial growth patterns and parental target heights.[1893] When a family history of tall stature is available and the growth rate and physical examination findings are normal, support and reassurance are frequently all that is needed without further testing. A careful assessment of pubertal status and bone age facilitates prediction of adult height and discussions with the patient and family. If the history suggests an underlying disorder or growth rate is accelerated, additional testing should be done to investigate the GH-IGF axis, chromosomal disorders, puberty, or other rare causes.

In GH excess, serum IGF1 levels are elevated, although high IGF1 levels may be a normal manifestation of puberty. Basal serum GH levels may be normal to increased, but serum GH is not suppressed by administration of glucose (1.75 g/kg body weight up to a maximum of 100 g). Although abnormalities of the sella turcica can be evident on lateral skull films, the demonstration of increased GH-IGF secretion should lead to radiologic evaluation of the hypothalamus and pituitary by MRI or computed tomography.

Treatment

Definitive treatment of GH-secreting tumors requires surgical ablation, either transsphenoidally or with a more aggressive surgical approach if large. As described in Chapter 9, somatostatin analogs, dopamine agonists, and GH-receptor antagonists are important components of treatment programs for GH excess.

In the past, most patients treated for familial tall stature were females. The numbers of patients treated in the United States has fallen markedly over the past 4 decades as tall stature in girls has become increasing acceptable socially and psychologically. In general, treatment is reserved for extreme cases, for predicted adult heights greater than 198 cm (6 feet 6 inches) in males or 183 cm (6 feet 0 inches) in females. Before deciding on therapy, the risks of therapy (discussed later) should be taken into account, as should the tendency to overestimate height prediction in prepubertal children based on bone age and Bailey-Pinneau tables.[1205,1894,1895] Therapy, when elected, is aimed at acceleration of puberty to cause premature epiphyseal fusion.[1896,1897] Therefore, the optimal time for treatment is before the onset of puberty, and the earlier the age of referral, the more likely it is that treatment will decrease final height.

Typically, ethinyl estradiol at 0.15 to 0.3 mg/day is started, and the dosage is increased, if needed and tolerated, to maximum of 0.5 mg/day. Conjugated estrogens, 7.5 to 10 mg/day, have also been used. Cyclic progestins may be added if breakthrough bleeding occurs. Treatment should be continued until the epiphyses fuse, because post-treatment growth may be substantial if treatment is stopped early.[1895] In prepubertal girls, estrogen therapy can decrease final adult height by as much as 5 to 6 cm relative to predictions; the decrement is lessened if therapy is begun after puberty has started. The use of high-dose estrogen in otherwise normal children must be weighed against the known and unknown toxicity of such therapy[1898] including nausea, weight gain, edema, and hypertension. During the initial phases of therapy, growth is accelerated as the child rapidly progresses through puberty. Other potential problems associated with high-dose estrogen therapy, such as thromboembolism, cystic hyperplasia of the breast, endometrial hyperplasia, and cancer, have not been definitely associated with estrogen therapy in children with tall stature but should be discussed with the patient and family.

In males, estrogen therapy is likely to be most efficacious but undesirable to the patient and family. Androgens have been used to accelerate skeletal maturation via aromatization to estrogen, but virilization is rapid. Benefits must be balanced against risks, and therapy should be individualized.

REFERENCES

1. Heinrichs C, Munson PJ, Counts DR, et al. Patterns of human growth. *Science*. 1995;268:442-447.
2. Lampl M, Veldhuis JD, Johnson ML. Saltation and stasis: a model of human growth. *Science*. 1992;258:801-803.
3. Lampl M, Cameron N, Veldhuis JD, et al. Patterns of human growth: response. *Science*. 1995;268:445-447.
4. Tillmann V, Thalange NK, Foster PJ, et al. The relationship between stature, growth, and short-term changes in height and weight in normal prepubertal children. *Pediatr Res*. 1998;44:882-886.
5. Thalange NK, Foster PJ, Gill MS, et al. Model of normal prepubertal growth. *Arch Dis Child*. 1996;75:427-431.
6. Gelander L, Karlberg J, Albertsson-Wikland K. Seasonality in lower leg length velocity in prepubertal children. *Acta Paediatr*. 1994;83:1249-1254.
7. Hermanussen M, Lange S, Grasedyck L. Growth tracks in early childhood. *Acta Paediatr*. 2001;90:381-386.
8. Ogden CL, Kuczmarski RJ, Flegal KM, et al. Centers for Disease Control and Prevention 2000 growth charts for the United States: improvements to the 1977 National Center for Health Statistics version. *Pediatrics*. 2002;109:45-60.
9. Tanner JM, Davies PS. Clinical longitudinal standards for height and height velocity for North American children. *J Pediatr*. 1985;107:317-329.
10. Lyon AJ, Preece MA, Grant DB. Growth curve for girls with Turner syndrome. *Arch Dis Child*. 1985;60:932-935.
11. Horton WA, Rotter JI, Rimoin DL, et al. Standard growth curves for achondroplasia. *J Pediatr*. 1978;93:435-438.
12. Cronk C, Crocker AC, Pueschel SM, et al. Growth charts for children with Down syndrome: 1 month to 18 years of age. *Pediatrics*. 1988;81:102-110.
13. Bayer LM, Bayley L. *Growth Diagnosis: Selected Methods for Interpreting and Predicting Physical Development from One Year to Maturity*. Chicago: University of Chicago Press; 1959.
14. Tanner JM, Goldstein H, Whitehouse RH. Standards for children's height at ages 2-9 years allowing for heights of parents. *Arch Dis Child*. 1970;45:755-762.
15. Tanner JM. Auxology. In: Kappy MS, Blizzard RM, Migeon CJ, eds. *The Diagnosis and Treatment of Endocrine Disorders*. Springfield, IL: Charles C Thomas; 1994.
16. Wright CM, Cheetham TD. The strengths and limitations of parental heights as a predictor of attained height. *Arch Dis Child*. 1999;81:257-260.
17. Giacobbi V, Trivin C, Lawson-Body E, et al. Extremely short stature: influence of each parent's height on clinical-biological features. *Horm Res*. 2003;60:272-276.
18. Reiter EO, Rosenfeld RG. Normal and aberrant growth. In: Larsen PR, Kronenberg HM, Melmed S, et al. *Williams Textbook of Endocrinology*. Philadelphia, PA: Saunders; 2002.
19. Emons JA, Boersma B, Baron J, et al. Catch-up growth: testing the hypothesis of delayed growth plate senescence in humans. *J Pediatr*. 2005;147:843-846.
20. Weise M, De-Levi S, Barnes KM, et al. Effects of estrogen on growth plate senescence and epiphyseal fusion. *Proc Natl Acad Sci U S A*. 2001;98:6871-6876.
21. Smith EP, Boyd J, Frank GR, et al. Estrogen resistance caused by a mutation in the estrogen-receptor gene in a man. *N Engl J Med*. 1994;331:1056-1061.
22. Conte FA, Grumbach MM, Ito Y, et al. A syndrome of female pseudohermaphrodism, hypergonadotropic hypogonadism, and multicystic ovaries associated with missense mutations in the gene encoding aromatase (P450arom). *J Clin Endocrinol Metab*. 1994;78:1287-1292.
23. Morishima A, Grumbach MM, Simpson ER, et al. Aromatase deficiency in male and female siblings caused by a novel mutation and the physiological role of estrogens. *J Clin Endocrinol Metab*. 1995;80:3689-3698.
24. Bilezikian JP, Morishima A, Bell J, et al. Increased bone mass as a result of estrogen therapy in a man with aromatase deficiency. *N Engl J Med*. 1998;339:599-603.
25. Grumbach MM, Auchus RJ. Estrogen: Consequences and implications of human mutations in synthesis and action. *J Clin Endocrinol Metab*. 1999;84:4677-4694.
26. Karlberg J, Engstrom I, Karlberg P, et al. Analysis of linear growth using a mathematical model: I. From birth to three years. *Acta Paediatr Scand*. 1987;76:478-488.
27. Karlberg J, Fryer JG, Engstrom I, et al. Analysis of linear growth using a mathematical model: II. From 3 to 21 years of age. *Acta Paediatr Scand Suppl*. 1987;337:12-29.
28. Schrier L, Ferns SP, Barnes KM, et al. Depletion of resting zone chondrocytes during growth plate senescence. *J Endocrinol*. 2006;189:27-36.
29. Parfitt AM. Misconceptions (1): epiphyseal fusion causes cessation of growth. *Bone*. 2002;30:337-339.
30. Tanner JM, Whitehouse RH, Takaishi M. Standards from birth to maturity for height, weight, height velocity, and weight velocity: British children, 1965. Part I. *Arch Dis Child*. 1966;41:454-471.

31. Wingerd J, Schoen EJ. Factors influencing length at birth and height at five years. *Pediatrics.* 1974;53:737-741.
32. Smith DW, Truog W, Rogers JE, et al. Shifting linear growth during infancy: illustration of genetic factors in growth from fetal life through infancy. *J Pediatr.* 1976;89:225-230.
33. Knight B, Shields BM, Turner M, et al. Evidence of genetic regulation of fetal longitudinal growth. *Early Hum Dev.* 2005;81:823-831.
34. Mei Z, Grummer-Strawn LM, Thompson D, et al. Shifts in percentiles of growth during early childhood: analysis of longitudinal data from the California Child Health and Development Study. *Pediatrics.* 2004;113:e617-e627.
35. Lee PA, Kendig JW, Kerrigan JR. Persistent short stature, other potential outcomes, and the effect of growth hormone treatment in children who are born small for gestational age. *Pediatrics.* 2003;112(1 Pt 1):150-162.
36. Hokken-Koelega AC, De Ridder MA, Lemmen RJ, et al. Children born small for gestational age: do they catch up? *Pediatr Res.* 1995;38:267-271.
37. Karlberg J, Albertsson-Wikland K. Growth in full-term small-for-gestational-age infants: from birth to final height. *Pediatr Res.* 1995;38:733-739.
38. Horner JM, Thorsson AV, Hintz RL. Growth deceleration patterns in children with constitutional short stature: an aid to diagnosis. *Pediatrics.* 1978;62:529-534.
39. Du Caju MV, Op De Beeck L, Sys SU, et al. Progressive deceleration in growth as an early sign of delayed puberty in boys. *Horm Res.* 2000;54:126-130.
40. Crowne EC, Shalet SM, Wallace WH, et al. Final height in boys with untreated constitutional delay in growth and puberty. *Arch Dis Child.* 1990;65:1109-1112.
41. LaFranchi S, Hanna CE, Mandel SH. Constitutional delay of growth: expected versus final adult height. *Pediatrics.* 1991;87:82-87.
42. Ranke MB, Grauer ML, Kistner K, et al. Spontaneous adult height in idiopathic short stature. *Horm Res.* 1995;44:152-157.
43. Albanese A, Stanhope R. Predictive factors in the determination of final height in boys with constitutional delay of growth and puberty. *J Pediatr.* 1995;126:545-550.
44. Moreira-Andres MN, Canizo FJ, de la Cruz FJ, et al. Bone mineral status in prepubertal children with constitutional delay of growth and puberty. *Eur J Endocrinol.* 1998;139:271-275.
45. Bertelloni S, Baroncelli GI, Ferdeghini M, et al. Normal volumetric bone mineral density and bone turnover in young men with histories of constitutional delay of puberty. *J Clin Endocrinol Metab.* 1998;83:4280-4283.
46. Ruff C. Variation in human size and shape. *Annu Rev Anthropol.* 2002;31:211-232.
47. Tanner JM. *A History of the Study of Human Growth.* Cambridge, UK: Cambridge University Press; 1981.
48. Kioussi C, Carriere C, Rosenfeld MG. A model for the development of the hypothalamic-pituitary axis: transcribing the hypophysis. *Mech Dev.* 1999;81:23-35.
49. Dutour A. A new step understood in the cascade of tissue-specific regulators orchestrating pituitary lineage determination: the Prophet of Pit-1 (Prop-1). *Eur J Endocrinol.* 1997;137:616-617.
50. Gage PJ, Camper SA. Pituitary homeobox 2, a novel member of the bicoid-related family of homeobox genes, is a potential regulator of anterior structure formation. *Hum Mol Genet.* 1997;6:457-464.
51. Rosenfeld RG. Biochemical diagnostic strategies in the evaluation of short stature: the diagnosis of insulin-like growth factor deficiency. *Horm Res.* 1996;46:170-173.
52. Treier M, Gleiberman AS, O'Connell SM, et al. Multistep signaling requirements for pituitary organogenesis in vivo. *Genes Dev.* 1998;12:1691-1704.
53. Ericson J, Norlin S, Jessell TM, et al. Integrated FGF and BMP signaling controls the progression of progenitor cell differentiation and the emergence of pattern in the embryonic anterior pituitary. In: *Development.* 1998;125:1005-1015.
54. Kioussi C, O'Connell S, St-Onge L, et al. Pax6 is essential for establishing ventral-dorsal cell boundaries in pituitary gland development. *Proc Natl Acad Sci U S A.* 1999;96:14378-14382.
55. Sornson MW, Wu W, Dasen JS, et al. Pituitary lineage determination by the prophet of pit-1 homeodomain factor defective in Ames dwarfism. *Nature.* 1996;384:327-333.
56. Dasen JS, O'Connell SM, Flynn SE, et al. Reciprocal interactions of Pit1 and GATA2 mediate signaling gradient-induced determination of pituitary cell types. *Cell.* 1999;97:587-598.
57. Simmons DM, Voss JW, Ingraham HA, et al. Pituitary cell phenotypes involve cell-specific pit-1 mRNA translation and synergistic interactions with other classes of transcription factors. *Genes Dev.* 1990;4:695-711.
58. Li S, Crenshaw 3rd EB, Rawson EJ, et al. Dwarf locus mutants lacking three pituitary cell types result from mutations in the POU-domain gene pit-1. *Nature.* 1990;347:528-533.
59. Ingraham HA, Lala DS, Ikeda Y, et al. The nuclear receptor steroidogenic factor 1 acts at multiple levels of the reproductive axis. *Genes Dev.* 1994;8:2302-2312.
60. Luo X, Ikeda Y, Parker KL. A cell-specific nuclear receptor is essential for adrenal and gonadal development and sexual differentiation. *Cell.* 1994;77:481-490.
61. Bentley CA, Zidehsarai MP, Grindley JC, et al. Pax6 is implicated in murine pituitary endocrine function. *Endocrine.* 1999;10:171-177.
62. Japon MA, Rubinstein M, Low MJ. In situ hybridization analysis of anterior pituitary hormone gene expression during fetal mouse development. *J Histochem Cytochem.* 1994;42:1117-1125.
63. Lamolet B, Pulichino AM, Lamonerie T, et al. A pituitary cell-restricted T box factor, tpit, activates POMC transcription in cooperation with pitx homeoproteins. *Cell.* 2001;104:849-859.
64. Goodyer CG. Ontogeny of pituitary hormone secretion. In: Collu R, Ducharme JR, Guyda HJ, eds. *Pediatric endocrinology.* New York, NY: Raven; 1989.
65. Stanfield JP. The blood supply of the human pituitary gland. *J Anat.* 1960;94:257-273.
66. Gorcyzca W, Hardy J. Arterial supply of the human anterior pituitary gland. *Neurosurgery.* 1987;20:369-378.
67. Pilavdzic D, Kovacs K, Asa SL. Pituitary morphology in anencephalic human fetuses. *Neuroendocrinology.* 1997;65:164-172.
68. Scheithauer BW, Sano T, Kovacs KT, et al. The pituitary gland in pregnancy: a clinicopathologic and immunohistochemical study of 69 cases. *Mayo Clin Proc.* 1990;65:461-474.
69. Thorner MO, Vance ML, Horvath E, et al. The anterior pituitary. In: Wilson JD, Foster DW, eds. *Williams Textbook of Endocrinology.* Philadelphia, PA: Saunders; 1991.
70. Hoyt WF, Kaplan SL, Grumbach MM, et al. Septo-optic dysplasia and pituitary dwarfism. *Lancet.* 1970;1:893-894.
71. Baumann G. Heterogeneity of growth hormone. In: Bercu B, ed. *Basic and Clinical Aspects of Growth Hormone.* New York, NY: Plenum; 1988.
72. Frankenne F, Closset J, Gomez F, et al. The physiology of growth hormones (GHs) in pregnant women and partial characterization of the placental GH variant. *J Clin Endocrinol Metab.* 1988;66:1171-1180.
73. Cooke NE, Ray J, Watson MA, et al. Human growth hormone gene and the highly homologous growth hormone variant gene display different splicing patterns. *J Clin Invest.* 1988;82:270-275.
74. Miller WL, Eberhardt NL. Structure and evaluation of the growth hormone gene family. *Annu Rev Med.* 1983;34:519.
75. Frohman LA, Kineman RD, Kamegai J, et al. Secretagogues and the somatotrope: signaling and proliferation. *Recent Prog Horm Res.* 2000;55:269-290; discussion 290-291.
76. Mayo KE, Cerelli GM, Lebo RV, et al. Gene encoding human growth hormone-releasing factor precursor: structure, sequence, and chromosomal assignment. *Proc Natl Acad Sci U S A.* 1985;82:63-67.
77. Lin C, Lin SC, Chang CP, et al. Pit-1-dependent expression of the receptor for growth hormone releasing factor mediates pituitary cell growth. *Nature.* 1992;360:765-768.
78. Mayo KE, Hammer RE, Swanson LW, et al. Dramatic pituitary hyperplasia in transgenic mice expressing a human growth hormone-releasing factor gene. *Mol Endocrinol.* 1988;2:606-612.
79. Brazeau P, Bohlen P, Esch F, et al. Growth hormone-releasing factor from ovine and caprine hypothalamus: isolation, sequence analysis and total synthesis. *Biochem Biophys Res Commun.* 1984;125:606-614.
80. Guillemin R. Hypothalamic control of pituitary functions: the growth hormone releasing factor. In: *The Sherrington Lectures XVIII.* Liverpool, UK: Liverpool University Press; 1986:1-73.
81. Mayo KE, Miller TL, DeAlmeida V, et al. The growth-hormone-releasing hormone receptor: signal transduction, gene expression, and physiological function in growth regulation. *Ann N Y Acad Sci.* 1996;805:184-203.
82. Vale W, Vaughan J, Yamamoto G, et al. Effects of synthetic human pancreatic (tumor) GH releasing factor and somatostatin, triiodothyronine and dexamethasone on GH secretion in vitro. *Endocrinology.* 1983;112:1553-1555.
83. Barinaga M, Yamonoto G, Rivier C, et al. Transcriptional regulation of growth hormone gene expression by growth hormone-releasing factor. *Nature.* 1983;306:84-85.
84. Frohman LA, Jansson JO. Growth hormone-releasing hormone. *Endocr Rev.* 1986;7:223-253.
85. Miller TL, Godfrey PA, Dealmeida VI, et al. The rat growth hormone-releasing hormone receptor gene: structure, regulation, and generation of receptor isoforms with different signaling properties. *Endocrinology.* 1999;140:4152-4165.
86. Mayo KE, Miller T, DeAlmeida V, et al. Regulation of the pituitary somatotroph cell by GHRH and its receptor. *Recent Prog Horm Res.* 2000;55:237-266; discussion 266-267.
87. Kineman RD, Aleppo G, Frohman LA. The tyrosine hydroxylase-human growth hormone (GH) transgenic mouse as a model of hypothalamic GH deficiency: growth retardation is the result of a selective

reduction in somatotrope numbers despite normal somatotrope function. *Endocrinology*. 1996;137:4630-4636.

88. Salvatori R, Hayashida CY, Aguiar-Oliveira MH, et al. Familial dwarfism due to a novel mutation of the growth hormone-releasing hormone receptor gene. *J Clin Endocrinol Metab*. 1999;84:917-923.
89. Hammer RE, Brinster RL, Rosenfeld MG, et al. Expression of human growth hormone-releasing factor in transgenic mice results in increased somatic growth. *Nature*. 1985;315:413-416.
90. Hartman ML, Faria AC, Vance ML, et al. Temporal structure of in vivo growth hormone secretory events in humans. *Am J Physiol*. 1991;260(1 Pt 1):E101-E110.
91. Deller JJ, Plunket DC, Forsham PH. Growth hormone studies in growth retardation: therapeutic response to administration of androgen. *Calif Med*. 1996;104:359.
92. Zeitler P, Argente J, Chowen-Breed JA, et al. Growth hormone-releasing hormone messenger ribonucleic acid in the hypothalamus of the adult male rat is increased by testosterone. *Endocrinology*. 1990;127:1362-1368.
93. Ho KY, Evans WS, Blizzard RM, et al. Effects of sex and age on the 24-hour profile of growth hormone secretion in man: importance of endogenous estradiol concentrations. *J Clin Endocrinol Metab*. 1987;64:51-58.
94. Katz HP, Youlton R, Kaplan SL, et al. Growth and growth hormone: 3. Growth hormone release in children with primary hypothyroidism and thyrotoxicosis. *J Clin Endocrinol Metab*. 1969;29:346-351.
95. Frantz AG, Rabkin MT. Human growth hormone, clinical measurement, response to hypoglycemia and suppression by corticosteroids. *N Engl J Med*. 1964;271:1375-1381.
96. Thompson RG, Rodriguez A, Kowarski A, et al. Growth hormone: metabolic clearance rates, integrated concentrations, and production rates in normal adults and the effect of prednisone. *J Clin Invest*. 1972;51:3193-3199.
97. Korbonits M, Grossman AB. Growth hormone-releasing peptide and its analogues novel stimuli to growth hormone release. *Trends Endocrinol Metab*. 1995;6:43-49.
98. Smith RG, Palyha OC, Feighner SD, et al. Growth hormone releasing substances: types and their receptors. *Horm Res*. 1999;51(suppl 3):1-8.
99. Kojima M, Hosoda H, Date Y, et al. Ghrelin is a growth-hormone-releasing acylated peptide from stomach. *Nature*. 1999;402: 656-660.
100. Date Y, Kojima M, Hosoda H, et al. Ghrelin, a novel growth hormone-releasing acylated peptide, is synthesized in a distinct endocrine cell type in the gastrointestinal tracts of rats and humans. *Endocrinology*. 2000;141:4255-4261.
101. Malagon MM, Luque RM, Ruiz-Guerrero E, et al. Intracellular signaling mechanisms mediating ghrelin-stimulated growth hormone release in somatotropes. *Endocrinology*. 2003;144:5372-5380.
102. Hataya Y, Akamizu T, Takaya K, et al. A low dose of ghrelin stimulates growth hormone (GH) release synergistically with GH-releasing hormone in humans. *J Clin Endocrinol Metab*. 2001;86:4552.
103. Popovic V, Miljic D, Micic D, et al. Ghrelin main action on the regulation of growth hormone release is exerted at hypothalamic level. *J Clin Endocrinol Metab*. 2003;88:3450-3453.
104. Higgins SC, Gueorguiev M, Korbonits M. Ghrelin, the peripheral hunger hormone. *Ann Med*. 2007;39:116-136.
105. Sun Y, Ahmed S, Smith RG. Deletion of ghrelin impairs neither growth nor appetite. *Mol Cell Biol*. 2003;23:7973-7981.
106. Sun Y, Wang P, Zheng H, et al. Ghrelin stimulation of growth hormone release and appetite is mediated through the growth hormone secretagogue receptor. *Proc Natl Acad Sci U S A*. 2004;101:4679-4684.
107. Savino F, Grassino EC, Fissore MF, et al. Ghrelin, motilin, insulin concentration in healthy infants in the first months of life: relation to fasting time and anthropometry. *Clin Endocrinol (Oxf)*. 2006;65:158-162.
108. Pantel J, Legendre M, Cabrol S, et al. Loss of constitutive activity of the growth hormone secretagogue receptor in familial short stature. *J Clin Invest*. 2006;116:760-768.
109. Wang HJ, Geller F, Dempfle A, et al. Ghrelin receptor gene: identification of several sequence variants in extremely obese children and adolescents, healthy normal-weight and underweight students, and children with short normal stature. *J Clin Endocrinol Metab*. 2004;89:157-162.
110. Muccioli G, Ghe C, Ghigo MC, et al. Specific receptors for synthetic GH secretagogues in the human brain and pituitary gland. *J Endocrinol*. 1998;157:99-106.
111. Akamizu T, Murayama T, Teramukai S, et al. Plasma ghrelin levels in healthy elderly volunteers: the levels of acylated ghrelin in elderly females correlate positively with serum IGF-I levels and bowel movement frequency and negatively with systolic blood pressure. *J Endocrinol*. 2006;188:333-344.
112. Cummings DE, Purnell JQ, Frayo RS, et al. A preprandial rise in plasma ghrelin levels suggests a role in meal initiation in humans. *Diabetes*. 2001;50:1714-1719.
113. Shiiya T, Nakazato M, Mizuta M, et al. Plasma ghrelin levels in lean and obese humans and the effect of glucose on ghrelin secretion. *J Clin Endocrinol Metab*. 2002;87:240-244.
114. Tschop M, Smiley DL, Heiman ML. Ghrelin induces adiposity in rodents. *Nature*. 2000;407:908-913.
115. Jamen F, Persson K, Bertrand G, et al. PAC1 receptor-deficient mice display impaired insulinotropic response to glucose and reduced glucose tolerance. *J Clin Invest*. 2000;105:1307-1315.
116. Rosenfeld RG, Ceda G, Wilson DM, et al. Characterization of high affinity receptors for insulin-like growth factors I and II on rat anterior pituitary cells. *Endocrinology*. 1984;114:1571-1575.
117. Ceda GP, Hoffman AR, Silverberg GD, et al. Regulation of growth hormone release from cultured human pituitary adenomas by somatomedins and insulin. *J Clin Endocrinol Metab*. 1985;60: 1204-1209.
118. Ceda GP, Davis RG, Rosenfeld RG, et al. The growth hormone (GH)-releasing hormone (GHRH)-GH-somatomedin axis: evidence for rapid inhibition of GHRH-elicited GH release by insulin-like growth factors I and II. *Endocrinology*. 1987;120:1658-1662.
119. Vaccarello MA, Diamond Jr FB, Guevara-Aguirre J, et al. Hormonal and metabolic effects and pharmacokinetics of recombinant insulin-like growth factor-I in growth hormone receptor deficiency/Laron syndrome. *J Clin Endocrinol Metab*. 1993;77:273-280.
120. Hartman ML, Veldhuis JD, Thorner MO. Normal control of growth hormone secretion. *Horm Res*. 1993;40:37-47.
121. Veldhuis JD, Liem AY, South S, et al. Differential impact of age, sex steroid hormones, and obesity on basal versus pulsatile growth hormone secretion in men as assessed in an ultrasensitive chemiluminescence assay. *J Clin Endocrinol Metab*. 1995;80:3209-3222.
122. Martha Jr PM, Reiter EO. Pubertal growth and growth hormone secretion. *Endocrinol Metab Clin North Am*. 1991;20:165-182.
123. Veldhuis JD, Johnson ML. Deconvolution analysis of hormone data. *Methods Enzymol*. 1992;210:539-575.
124. Veldhuis JD, Roemmich JN, Rogol AD. Gender and sexual maturation-dependent contrasts in the neuroregulation of growth hormone secretion in prepubertal and late adolescent males and females: a general clinical research center-based study. *J Clin Endocrinol Metab*. 2000;85:2385-2394.
125. Hartman ML, Pincus SM, Johnson ML, et al. Enhanced basal and disorderly growth hormone secretion distinguish acromegalic from normal pulsatile growth hormone release. *J Clin Invest*. 1994;94: 1277-1288.
126. Gill MS, Thalange NK, Foster PJ, et al. Regular fluctuations in growth hormone (GH) release determine normal human growth. *Growth Horm IGF Res*. 1999;9:114-122.
127. Tillmann V, Gill MS, Thalange NK, et al. Short-term changes in growth and urinary growth hormone, insulin-like growth factor-I and markers of bone turnover excretion in healthy prepubertal children. *Growth Horm IGF Res*. 2000;10:28-36.
128. Grumbach MM, Gluckman PD. The human fetal hypothalamic and pituitary gland: the maturation of neuroendocrine mechanisms controlling secretion of fetal pituitary growth hormone, prolactin, gonadotropin, adrenocorticotropin-related peptides and thyrotropin. In: Tulchinsky D, Little AB, eds. *Maternal and Fetal Endocrinology*. Philadelphia, PA: Saunders; 1994.
129. Kaplan SL, Grumbach MM, Aubert ML. The ontogenesis of pituitary hormones and hypothalamic factors in the human fetus: maturation of central nervous system regulation of anterior pituitary function. *Recent Prog Horm Res*. 1976;32:161-243.
130. Siler-Khodr TM, Morgenstern LL, Greenwood FC. Hormone synthesis and release from human fetal adenohypophyses in vitro. *J Clin Endocrinol Metab*. 1974;39:891-905.
131. Thliveris JA, Currie RW. Observations on the hypothalamo-hypophyseal portal vasculature in the developing human fetus. *Am J Anat*. 1980;157:441-444.
132. Puy LA, Asa SL. The ontogeny of pit-1 expression in the human fetal pituitary gland. *Neuroendocrinology*. 1996;63:349-355.
133. Gluckman PD, Grumbach MM, Kaplan SL. The neuroendocrine regulation and function of growth hormone and prolactin in the mammalian fetus. *Endocr Rev*. 1981;2:363-395.
134. Arosio M, Cortelazzi D, Persani L, et al. Circulating levels of growth hormone, insulin-like growth factor-I and prolactin in normal, growth retarded and anencephalic human fetuses. *J Endocrinol Invest*. 1995;18:346-353.
135. Martha Jr PM, Gorman KM, Blizzard RM, et al. Endogenous growth hormone secretion and clearance rates in normal boys, as determined by deconvolution analysis: relationship to age, pubertal status, and body mass. *J Clin Endocrinol Metab*. 1992;74:336-344.
136. Martha Jr PM, Rogol AD, Veldhuis JD, et al. Alterations in the pulsatile properties of circulating growth hormone concentrations during puberty in boys. *J Clin Endocrinol Metab*. 1989;69:563-570.
137. Pincus SM, Veldhuis JD, Rogol AD. Longitudinal changes in growth hormone secretory process irregularity assessed transpubertally in healthy boys. *Am J Physiol Endocrinol Metab*. 2000;279:E417-E424.

138. Martha Jr PM, Rogol AD, Blizzard RM, et al. Growth hormone-binding protein activity is inversely related to 24-hour growth hormone release in normal boys. *J Clin Endocrinol Metab*. 1991;73:175-181.
139. Baumann G, Shaw MA, Amburn K. Circulating growth hormone binding proteins. *J Endocrinol Invest*. 1994;17:67-81.
140. Moran A, Jacobs Jr DR, Steinberger J, et al. Association between the insulin resistance of puberty and the insulin-like growth factor-I/growth hormone axis. *J Clin Endocrinol Metab*. 2002;87:4817-4820.
141. MacGillivray MH, Frohman LA, Doe J. Metabolic clearance and production rates of human growth hormone in subjects with normal and abnormal growth. *J Clin Endocrinol Metab*. 1970;30:632-638.
142. Rudman D, Kutner MH, Rogers CM, et al. Impaired growth hormone secretion in the adult population: relation to age and adiposity. *J Clin Invest*. 1981;67:1361-1369.
143. Van Cauter E, Caufriez A, Kerkhofs M, et al. Sleep, awakenings, and insulin-like growth factor-I modulate the growth hormone (GH) secretory response to GH-releasing hormone. *J Clin Endocrinol Metab*. 1992;74:1451-1459.
144. Veldhuis JD, Iranmanesh A, Ho KK, et al. Dual defects in pulsatile growth hormone secretion and clearance subserve the hyposomatotropism of obesity in man. *J Clin Endocrinol Metab*. 1991;72:51-59.
145. Schalch DS. The influence of physical stress and exercise on growth hormone and insulin secretion in man. *J Lab Clin Med*. 1967;69:256-269.
146. Holl RW, Hartman ML, Veldhuis JD, et al. Thirty-second sampling of plasma growth hormone in man: correlation with sleep stages. *J Clin Endocrinol Metab*. 1991;72:854-861.
147. Jaffe CA, Turgeon DK, Friberg RD, et al. Nocturnal augmentation of growth hormone (GH) secretion is preserved during repetitive bolus administration of GH-releasing hormone: potential involvement of endogenous somatostatin—a clinical research center study. *J Clin Endocrinol Metab*. 1995;80:3321-3326.
148. Mauras N, Blizzard RM, Link K, et al. Augmentation of growth hormone secretion during puberty: evidence for a pulse amplitude-modulated phenomenon. *J Clin Endocrinol Metab*. 1987;64:596-601.
149. Keenan BS, Richards GE, Ponder SW, et al. Androgen-stimulated pubertal growth: the effects of testosterone and dihydrotestosterone on growth hormone and insulin-like growth factor-I in the treatment of short stature and delayed puberty. *J Clin Endocrinol Metab*. 1993;76:996-1001.
150. Veldhuis JD, Metzger DL, Martha Jr PM, et al. Estrogen and testosterone, but not a nonaromatizable androgen, direct network integration of the hypothalamo-somatotrope (growth hormone)–insulin-like growth factor I axis in the human: evidence from pubertal pathophysiology and sex-steroid hormone replacement. *J Clin Endocrinol Metab*. 1997;82:3414-3420.
151. Rosenfeld RG, Rosenbloom AL, Guevara-Aguirre J. Growth hormone (GH) insensitivity due to primary GH receptor deficiency. *Endocr Rev*. 1994;15:369-390.
152. Argente J, Caballo N, Barrios V, et al. Multiple endocrine abnormalities of the growth hormone and insulin-like growth factor axis in prepubertal children with exogenous obesity: effect of short- and long-term weight reduction. *J Clin Endocrinol Metab*. 1997;82:2076-2083.
153. Attia N, Tamborlane WV, Heptulla R, et al. The metabolic syndrome and insulin-like growth factor I regulation in adolescent obesity. *J Clin Endocrinol Metab*. 1998;83:1467-1471.
154. Metzger DL, Kerrigan JR. Estrogen receptor blockade with tamoxifen diminishes growth hormone secretion in boys: evidence for a stimulatory role of endogenous estrogens during male adolescence. *J Clin Endocrinol Metab*. 1994;79:513-518.
155. Martin-Hernandez T, Diaz Galvez M, Torres Cuadro A, et al. Growth hormone secretion in normal prepubertal children: importance of relations between endogenous secretion, pulsatility and body mass. *Clin Endocrinol (Oxf)*. 1996;44:327-334.
156. Iranmanesh A, Lizarralde G, Veldhuis JD. Age and relative adiposity are specific negative determinants of the frequency and amplitude of growth hormone (GH) secretory bursts and the half-life of endogenous GH in healthy men. *J Clin Endocrinol Metab*. 1991;73:1081-1088.
157. Barton DE, Foellmer BE, Wood WI, et al. Chromosome mapping of the growth hormone receptor gene in man and mouse. *Cytogenet Cell Genet*. 1989;50:137-141.
158. Kelly PA, Djiane J, Postel-Vinay MC, et al. The prolactin/growth hormone receptor family. *Endocr Rev*. 1991;12:235-251.
159. Bazan JF. Haemopoietic receptors and helical cytokines. *Immunol Today*. 1990;11:350-354.
160. Pantel J, Machinis K, Sobrier ML, et al. Species-specific alternative splice mimicry at the growth hormone receptor locus revealed by the lineage of retroelements during primate evolution. *J Biol Chem*. 2000;275:18664-18669.
161. Waters MJ, Hoang HN, Fairlie DP, et al. New insights into growth hormone action. *J Mol Endocrinol*. 2006;36:1-7.
162. Fuh G, Cunningham BC, Fukunaga R, et al. Rational design of potent antagonists to the human growth hormone receptor. *Science*. 1992;256:1677-1680.
163. Gent J, van Kerkhof P, Roza M, et al. Ligand-independent growth hormone receptor dimerization occurs in the endoplasmic reticulum and is required for ubiquitin system-dependent endocytosis. *Proc Natl Acad Sci U S A*. 2002;99:9858-9863.
164. Brown RJ, Adams JJ, Pelekanos RA, et al. Model for growth hormone receptor activation based on subunit rotation within a receptor dimer. *Nat Struct Mol Biol*. 2005;12:814-821.
165. Hwa V, Rosenfeld RG. Downstream mechanisms of growth hormone action. In: Carel J-c, Kelly PA, Christen Y, eds. *Deciphering Growth: Research and Perspectives in Endocrine Interactions*. Berlin, Germany: Springer-Verlag; 2005:53-64.
166. Udy GB, Towers RP, Snell RG, et al. Requirement of STAT5b for sexual dimorphism of body growth rates and liver gene expression. *Proc Natl Acad Sci U S A*. 1997;94:7239-7244.
167. Teglund S, McKay C, Schuetz E, et al. Stat5a and Stat5b proteins have essential and nonessential, or redundant, roles in cytokine responses. *Cell*. 1998;93:841-850.
168. Rowland JE, Lichanska AM, Kerr LM, et al. In vivo analysis of growth hormone receptor signaling domains and their associated transcripts. *Mol Cell Biol*. 2005;25:66-77.
169. Woelfle J, Chia DJ, Rotwein P. Mechanisms of growth hormone (GH) action: identification of conserved Stat5 binding sites that mediate GH-induced insulin-like growth factor-I gene activation. *J Biol Chem*. 2003;278:51261-51266.
170. Schindler C, Darnell Jr JE. Transcriptional responses to polypeptide ligands: the JAK-STAT pathway. *Annu Rev Biochem*. 1995;64:621-651.
171. Ihle JN, Kerr IM. Jaks and Stats in signaling by the cytokine receptor superfamily. *Trends Genet*. 1995;11:69-74.
172. Dinerstein-Cali H, Ferrag F, Kayser C, et al. Growth hormone (GH) induces the formation of protein complexes involving Stat5, Erk2, shc and serine phosphorylated proteins. *Mol Cell Endocrinol*. 2000;166:89-99.
173. Lewis MD, Horan M, Millar DS, et al. A novel dysfunctional growth hormone variant (Ile179Met) exhibits a decreased ability to activate the extracellular signal-regulated kinase pathway. *J Clin Endocrinol Metab*. 2004;89:1068-1075.
174. Ling L, Zhu T, Lobie PE. Src-CrkII-C3G-dependent activation of Rap1 switches growth hormone-stimulated p44/42 MAP kinase and JNK/SAPK activities. *J Biol Chem*. 2003;278:27301-27311.
175. Zhu T, Ling L, Lobie PE. Identification of a JAK2-independent pathway regulating growth hormone (GH)-stimulated p44/42 mitogen-activated protein kinase activity. *J Biol Chem*. 2002;277:45592-45603.
176. Jin H, Lanning NJ, Carter-Su C. JAK2, but not src family kinases, is required for STAT, ERK, and akt signaling in response to growth hormone in preadipocytes and hepatoma cells. *Mol Endocrinol*. 2008;22:1825-1841.
177. Hansen JA, Lindberg K, Hilton DJ, et al. Mechanism of inhibition of growth hormone receptor signaling by suppressor of cytokine signaling proteins. *Mol Endocrinol*. 1999;13:1832-1843.
178. Metcalf D, Greenhalgh CJ, Viney E, et al. Gigantism in mice lacking suppressor of cytokine signalling-2. *Nature*. 2000;405:1069-1073.
179. Greenhalgh CJ, Bertolino P, Asa SL, et al. Growth enhancement in suppressor of cytokine signaling 2 (SOCS-2)-deficient mice is dependent on signal transducer and activator of transcription 5b (STAT5b). *Mol Endocrinol*. 2002;16:1394-1406.
180. Colson A, Le Cam A, Maiter D, et al. Potentiation of growth hormone-induced liver suppressors of cytokine signaling messenger ribonucleic acid by cytokines. *Endocrinology*. 2000;141:3687-3895.
181. Mao Y, Ling PR, Fitzgibbons TP, et al. Endotoxin-induced inhibition of growth hormone receptor signaling in rat liver in vivo. *Endocrinology*. 1999;140:5505-5515.
182. Baumann G, Stolar MW, Amburn K, et al. A specific growth hormone-binding protein in human plasma: initial characterization. *J Clin Endocrinol Metab*. 1986;62:134-141.
183. Herington AC, Ymer S, Stevenson J. Identification and characterization of specific binding proteins for growth hormone in normal human sera. *J Clin Invest*. 1986;77:1817-1823.
184. Trivedi B, Daughaday WH. Release of growth hormone binding protein from IM-9 lymphocytes by endopeptidase is dependent on sulfhydryl group inactivation. *Endocrinology*. 1988;123:2201-2206.
185. Holl RW, Snehotta R, Siegler B, et al. Binding protein for human growth hormone: effects of age and weight. *Horm Res*. 1991;35:190-197.
186. Massa G, de Zegher F, Vanderschueren-Lodeweyckx M. Serum growth hormone-binding proteins in the human fetus and infant. *Pediatr Res*. 1992;32:69-72.
187. Buchanan CR, Maheshwari HG, Norman MR, et al. Laron-type dwarfism with apparently normal high affinity serum growth hormone-binding protein. *Clin Endocrinol (Oxf)*. 1991;35:179-185.

188. Duquesnoy P, Sobrier ML, Duriez B, et al. A single amino acid substitution in the exoplasmic domain of the human growth hormone (GH) receptor confers familial GH resistance (Laron syndrome) with positive GH-binding activity by abolishing receptor homodimerization. *EMBO J*. 1994;13:1386-1395.
189. Woods KA, Fraser NC, Postel-Vinay MC, et al. A homozygous splice site mutation affecting the intracellular domain of the growth hormone (GH) receptor resulting in Laron syndrome with elevated GH-binding protein. *J Clin Endocrinol Metab*. 1996;81:1686-1690.
190. Thompson BJL, Shang CA, Waters MJ. Identification of genes induced by growth hormone in rat liver using cDNA arrays. *Endocrinology*. 2000;141:4321-4324.
191. Tollet-Egnell P, Flores-Morales A, Stahlberg N, et al. Gene expression profile of the aging process in rat liver: normalizing effects of growth hormone replacement. *Mol Endocrinol*. 2001;15:308-318.
192. Flores-Morales A, Stahlberg N, Tollet-Egnell P, et al. Microarray analysis of the in vivo effects of hypophysectomy and growth hormone treatment on gene expression in the rat. *Endocrinology*. 2001; 142:3163-3176.
193. Gardmo C, Swerdlow H, Mode A. Growth hormone regulation of rat liver gene expression assessed by SSH and microarray. *Mol Cell Endocrinol*. 2002;190:125-133.
194. Zhou Y, Xu BC, Maheshwari HG, et al. A mammalian model for Laron syndrome produced by targeted disruption of the mouse growth hormone receptor/binding protein gene (the Laron mouse). *Proc Natl Acad Sci U S A*. 1997;94:13215-13220.
195. Fan Y, Menon RK, Cohen P, et al. Liver-specific deletion of the growth hormone receptor reveals essential role of growth hormone signaling in hepatic lipid metabolism. *J Biol Chem*. 2009;284: 19937-19944.
196. Neubauer H, Cumano A, Müller M, et al. Jak2 deficiency defines an essential developmental checkpoint in definitive hematopoiesis. *Cell*. 1998;93:397-409.
197. Levy DE. Physiological significance of STAT proteins: investigations through gene disruption in vivo. *Cell Mol Life Sci*. 1999;55: 1559-1567.
198. Lupu F, Terwilliger JD, Lee K, et al. Roles of growth hormone and insulin-like growth factor 1 in mouse postnatal growth. *Dev Biol*. 2001;229:141-162.
199. Yakar S, Liu JL, Stannard B, et al. Normal growth and development in the absence of hepatic insulin-like growth factor I. *Proc Natl Acad Sci U S A*. 1999;96:7324-7329.
200. Salmon Jr WD, Daughaday WH. A hormonally controlled serum factor which stimulates sulfate incorporation by cartilage in vitro. *J Lab Clin Med*. 1957;49:825-836.
201. Daughaday WH, Rotwein P. Insulin-like growth factors I and II: peptide, messenger ribonucleic acid and gene structures, serum, and tissue concentrations. *Endocr Rev*. 1989;10:68-91.
202. Sherwin RS, Schulman GA, Hendler R, et al. Effect of growth hormone on oral glucose tolerance and circulating metabolic fuels in man. *Diabetologia*. 1983;24:155-161.
203. Rosenfeld RG, Wilson DM, Dollar LA, et al. Both human pituitary growth hormone and recombinant DNA-derived human growth hormone cause insulin resistance at a postreceptor site. *J Clin Endocrinol Metab*. 1982;54:1033-1038.
204. Gerich JE, Lorenzi M, Bier DM, et al. Effects of physiologic levels of glucagon and growth hormone on human carbohydrate and lipid metabolism: studies involving administration of exogenous hormone during suppression of endogenous hormone secretion with somatostatin. *J Clin Invest*. 1976;57:875-884.
205. Kostyo JL, Hotchkiss J, Knobil E. Stimulation of amino acid transport in isolated diaphragm by growth hormone added in vitro. *Science*. 1959;130:1653-1654.
206. Hjalmarson A, Isaksson O, Ahren K. Effects of growth hormone and insulin on amino acid transport in perfused rat heart. *Am J Physiol*. 1969;217:1795-1802.
207. Griffin EE, Miller LL. Effects of hypophysectomy of liver donor on net synthesis of specific plasma proteins by the isolated perfused rat liver: modulation of synthesis of albumin, fibrinogen, alpha 1-acid glycoprotein, alpha 2-(acute phase)-globulin, and haptoglobin by insulin, cortisol, triiodothyronine, and growth hormone. *J Biol Chem*. 1974;249:5062-5069.
208. Daughaday WH, Hall K, Raben MS, et al. Somatomedin: proposed designation for sulphation factor. *Nature*. 1972;235:107.
209. Hall K, Takano K, Fryklund L, et al. Somatomedins. *Adv Metab Disord*. 1975;8:19-46.
210. Van Wyk JJ, Underwood LE, Hintz RL, et al. The somatomedins: a family of insulinlike hormones under growth hormone control. *Recent Prog Horm Res*. 1974;30:259-318.
211. Rinderknecht E, Humbel RE. The amino acid sequence of human insulin-like growth factor I and its structural homology with proinsulin. *J Biol Chem*. 1978;253:2769-2776.
212. Rinderknecht E, Humbel RE. Primary structure of human insulin-like growth factor II. *FEBS Lett*. 1978;89:283-286.
213. Brissenden JE, Ullrich A, Francke U. Human chromosomal mapping of genes for insulin-like growth factors I and II and epidermal growth factor. *Nature*. 1984;310:781-784.
214. Tricoli JV, Rall LB, Scott J, et al. Localization of insulin-like growth factor genes to human chromosomes 11 and 12. *Nature*. 1984;310:784-786.
215. Bell GI, Gerhard DS, Fong NM, et al. Isolation of the human insulin-like growth factor genes: insulin-like growth factor II and insulin genes are contiguous. *Proc Natl Acad Sci U S A*. 1985;82:6450-6454.
216. Adamo ML, Neuenschwander S, LeRoith D, et al. Structure, expression, and regulation of the IGF-I gene. *Adv Exp Med Biol*. 1993;343:1-11.
217. Lund PK. Insulin-like growth factors: gene structure and regulation. In: Conn PM, ed. *Handbook of Physiology—The Endocrine System: Cellular Endocrinology*. Bethesda, MD: American Physiology Society; 1998.
218. Yoon JB, Berry SA, Seelig S, et al. An inducible nuclear factor binds to a growth hormone-regulated gene. *J Biol Chem*. 1990; 265:19947-19954.
219. Lowe Jr WL, Roberts Jr CT, Lasky SR, et al. Differential expression of alternative 5′ untranslated regions in mRNAs encoding rat insulin-like growth factor I. *Proc Natl Acad Sci U S A*. 1987;84:8946-8950.
220. Murphy LJ, Friesen HG. Differential effects of estrogen and growth hormone on uterine and hepatic insulin-like growth factor I gene expression in the ovariectomized hypophysectomized rat. *Endocrinology*. 1988;122:325-332.
221. Bonioli E, Taro M, Rosa CL, et al. Heterozygous mutations of growth hormone receptor gene in children with idiopathic short stature. *Growth Horm IGF Res*. 2005;15:405-410.
222. Duguay SJ, Lai-Zhang J, Steiner DF. Mutational analysis of the insulin-like growth factor I prohormone processing site. *J Biol Chem*. 1995;270:17566-17574.
223. Conover CA, Baker BK, Bale LK, et al. Human hepatoma cells synthesize and secrete insulin-like growth factor Ia prohormone under growth hormone control. *Regul Pept*. 1993;48:1-8.
224. Wilson HE, Westwood M, White A, et al. Monoclonal antibodies to the carboxy-terminal Ea sequence of pro-insulin-like growth factor-IA (proIGF-IA) recognize proIGF-IA secreted by IM9 B-lymphocytes. *Growth Horm IGF Res*. 2001;11:10-17.
225. Goldspink G. Changes in muscle mass and phenotype and the expression of autocrine and systemic growth factors by muscle in response to stretch and overload. *J Anat*. 1999;194:323-334.
226. Hameed M, Orrell RW, Cobbold M, et al. Expression of IGF-I splice variants in young and old human skeletal muscle after high resistance exercise. *J Physiol*. 2003;547:247-254.
227. Owino V, Yang SY, Goldspink G. Age-related loss of skeletal muscle function and the inability to express the autocrine form of insulin-like growth factor-1 (MGF) in response to mechanical overload. *FEBS Lett*. 2001;505:259-263.
228. Goldspink G. Mechanical signals, IGF-I gene splicing, and muscle adaptation. *Physiology*. 2005;20:232-238.
229. Barton ER. Viral expression of insulin-like growth factor-I isoforms promotes different responses in skeletal muscle. *J Appl Physiol*. 2006;100:1778-1784.
230. Bennett A, Wilson DM, Liu F, et al. Levels of insulin-like growth factors I and II in human cord blood. *J Clin Endocrinol Metab*. 1983;57:609-612.
231. Gluckman PD, Johnson-Barrett JJ, Butler JH, et al. Studies of insulin-like growth factor -I and -II by specific radioligand assays in umbilical cord blood. *Clin Endocrinol (Oxf)*. 1983;19:405-413.
232. Lassarre C, Hardouin S, Daffos F, et al. Serum insulin-like growth factors and insulin-like growth factor binding proteins in the human fetus. relationships with growth in normal subjects and in subjects with intrauterine growth retardation. *Pediatr Res*. 1991;29:219-225.
233. Hall K, Hansson U, Lundin G, et al. Serum levels of somatomedins and somatomedin-binding protein in pregnant women with type I or gestational diabetes and their infants. *J Clin Endocrinol Metab*. 1986;63:1300-1306.
234. Luna AM, Wilson DM, Wibbelsman CJ, et al. Somatomedins in adolescence: a cross-sectional study of the effect of puberty on plasma insulin-like growth factor I and II levels. *J Clin Endocrinol Metab*. 1983;57:268-271.
235. Cara JF, Rosenfield RL, Furlanetto RW. A longitudinal study of the relationship of plasma somatomedin-C concentration to the pubertal growth spurt. *Am J Dis Child*. 1987;141:562-564.
236. Cuttler L, Van Vliet G, Conte FA, et al. Somatomedin-C levels in children and adolescents with gonadal dysgenesis: differences from age-matched normal females and effect of chronic estrogen replacement therapy. *J Clin Endocrinol Metab*. 1985;60:1087-1092.
237. Rosenfeld RG, Hintz RL, Johanson AJ, et al. Methionyl human growth hormone and oxandrolone in Turner syndrome: preliminary results of a prospective randomized trial. *J Pediatr*. 1986;109:936-943.
238. Copeland KC. Effects of acute high dose and chronic low dose estrogen on plasma somatomedin-C and growth in patients with Turner's syndrome. *J Clin Endocrinol Metab*. 1988;66:1278-1282.

239. Rudman D, Feller AG, Nagraj HS, et al. Effects of human growth hormone in men over 60 years old. *N Engl J Med*. 1990;323:1-6.
240. Johanson AJ, Blizzard RM. Low somatomedin-C levels in older men rise in response to growth hormone administration. *Johns Hopkins Med J*. 1981;149:115-117.
241. Rappolee DA, Sturm KS, Behrendtsen O, et al. Insulin-like growth factor II acts through an endogenous growth pathway regulated by imprinting in early mouse embryos. *Genes Dev*. 1992;6:939-952.
242. Thorvaldsen JL, Duran KL, Bartolomei MS. Deletion of the H19 differentially methylated domain results in loss of imprinted expression of H19 and Igf2. *Genes Dev*. 1998;12:3693-3702.
243. Bell AC, Felsenfeld G. Methylation of a CTCF-dependent boundary controls imprinted expression of the Igf2 gene. *Nature*. 2000;405:482-485.
244. Ohlsson R, Renkawitz R, Lobanenkov V. CTCF is a uniquely versatile transcription regulator linked to epigenetics and disease. *Trends Genet*. 2001;17:520-527.
245. Reeve AE, Eccles MR, Wilkins RJ, et al. Expression of insulin-like growth factor-II transcripts in Wilms' tumour. *Nature*. 1985;317:258-260.
246. Ogawa O, Eccles MR, Szeto J, et al. Relaxation of insulin-like growth factor II gene imprinting implicated in Wilms' tumour. *Nature*. 1993;362:749-751.
247. Zhan S, Shapiro D, Zhan S, et al. Concordant loss of imprinting of the human insulin-like growth factor II gene promoters in cancer. *J Biol Chem*. 1995;270:27983-27986.
248. El-Badry OM, Helman LJ, Chatten J, et al. Insulin-like growth factor II-mediated proliferation of human neuroblastoma. *J Clin Invest*. 1991;87:648-657.
249. Haselbacher GK, Irminger JC, Zapf J, et al. Insulin-like growth factor II in human adrenal pheochromocytomas and Wilms tumors: expression at the mRNA and protein level. *Proc Natl Acad Sci U S A*. 1987;84:1104-1106.
250. Rainier S, Johnson LA, Dobry CJ, et al. Relaxation of imprinted genes in human cancer. *Nature*. 1993;362:747-749.
251. Tricoli JV, Rall LB, Karakousis CP, et al. Enhanced levels of insulin-like growth factor messenger RNA in human colon carcinomas and liposarcomas. *Cancer Res*. 1986;46(12 Pt 1):6169-6173.
252. Daughaday WH, Emanuele MA, Brooks MH, et al. Synthesis and secretion of insulin-like growth factor II by a leiomyosarcoma with associated hypoglycemia. *N Engl J Med*. 1988;319:1434-1440.
253. Sparago A, Cerrato F, Vernucci M, et al. Microdeletions in the human H19 DMR result in loss of IGF2 imprinting and Beckwith-Wiedemann syndrome. *Nat Genet*. 2004;36:958-960.
254. Zumstein PP, Luthi C, Humbel RE. Amino acid sequence of a variant pro-form of insulin-like growth factor II. *Proc Natl Acad Sci U S A*. 1985;82:3169-3172.
255. Jansen M, van Schaik FM, van Tol H, et al. Nucleotide sequences of cDNAs encoding precursors of human insulin-like growth factor II (IGF-II) and an IGF-II variant. *FEBS Lett*. 1985;179:243-246.
256. Gowan LK, Hampton B, Hill DJ, et al. Purification and characterization of a unique high molecular weight form of insulin-like growth factor II. *Endocrinology*. 1987;121:449-458.
257. Zapf J. Insulinlike growth factor binding proteins and tumor hypoglycemia. *Trends Endocrinol Metab*. 1995;6:37-42.
258. Donovan SM, Oh Y, Pham H, et al. Ontogeny of serum insulin-like growth factor binding proteins in the rat. *Endocrinology*. 1989;125:2621-2627.
259. Oh Y, Muller HL, Neely EK, et al. New concepts in insulin-like growth factor receptor physiology. *Growth Regul*. 1993;3:113-123.
260. LeRoith D, Werner H, Beitner-Johnson D, et al. Molecular and cellular aspects of the insulin-like growth factor I receptor. *Endocr Rev*. 1995;16:143-163.
261. Ullrich A, Gray A, Tam AW, et al. Insulin-like growth factor I receptor primary structure: comparison with insulin receptor suggests structural determinants that define functional specificity. *EMBO J*. 1986;5:2503-2512.
262. Ullrich A, Bell JR, Chen EY, et al. . Human insulin receptor and its relationship to the tyrosine kinase family of oncogenes. *Nature*. 1985;313:756-761.
263. Abbott AM, Bueno R, Pedrini MT, et al. Insulin-like growth factor I receptor gene structure. *J Biol Chem*. 1992;267:10759-10763.
264. Bondy CA, Werner H, Roberts Jr CT, et al. Cellular pattern of insulin-like growth factor-I (IGF-I) and type I IGF receptor gene expression in early organogenesis: comparison with IGF-II gene expression. *Mol Endocrinol*. 1990;4:1386-1898.
265. Werner H, Woloschak M, Adamo M, et al. Developmental regulation of the rat insulin-like growth factor I receptor gene. *Proc Natl Acad Sci U S A*. 1989;86:7451-7455.
266. Kato H, Faria TN, Stannard B, et al. Role of tyrosine kinase activity in signal transduction by the insulin-like growth factor-I (IGF-I) receptor. characterization of kinase-deficient IGF-I receptors and the action of an IGF-I-mimetic antibody (alpha IR-3). *J Biol Chem*. 1993;268:2655-2661.
267. Kato H, Faria TN, Stannard B, et al. Essential role of tyrosine residues 1131, 1135, and 1136 of the insulin-like growth factor-I (IGF-I) receptor in IGF-I action. *Mol Endocrinol*. 1994;8:40-50.
268. Yamasaki H, Prager D, Gebremedhin S, et al. Human insulin-like growth factor I receptor 950tyrosine is required for somatotroph growth factor signal transduction. *J Biol Chem*. 1992;267:20953-20958.
269. Gronborg M, Wulff BS, Rasmussen JS, et al. Structure-function relationship of the insulin-like growth factor-I receptor tyrosine kinase. *J Biol Chem*. 1993;268:23435-23440.
270. Frattali AL, Pessin JE. Relationship between alpha subunit ligand occupancy and beta subunit autophosphorylation in insulin/insulin-like growth factor-1 hybrid receptors. *J Biol Chem*. 1993;268:7393-7400.
271. Treadway JL, Morrison BD, Soos MA, et al. Transdominant inhibition of tyrosine kinase activity in mutant insulin/insulin-like growth factor I hybrid receptors. *Proc Natl Acad Sci U S A*. 1991;88:214-218.
272. Shemer J, Adamo M, Wilson GL, et al. Insulin and insulin-like growth factor-I stimulate a common endogenous phosphoprotein substrate (pp185) in intact neuroblastoma cells. *J Biol Chem*. 1987;262:15476-15482.
273. Kuhne MR, Pawson T, Lienhard GE, et al. The insulin receptor substrate 1 associates with the SH2-containing phosphotyrosine phosphatase syp. *J Biol Chem*. 1993;268:11479-11481.
274. Skolnik EY, Batzer A, Li N, et al. The function of GRB2 in linking the insulin receptor to ras signaling pathways. *Science*. 1993;260:1953-1955.
275. Lee CH, Li W, Nishimura R, et al. Nck associates with the SH2 domain-docking protein IRS-1 in insulin-stimulated cells. *Proc Natl Acad Sci U S A*. 1993;90:11713-11717.
276. Sasaoka T, Rose DW, Jhun BH, et al. Evidence for a functional role of shc proteins in mitogenic signaling induced by insulin, insulin-like growth factor-1, and epidermal growth factor. *J Biol Chem*. 1994;269:13689-13694.
277. Lamphere L, Lienhard GE. Components of signaling pathways for insulin and insulin-like growth factor-I in muscle myoblasts and myotubes. *Endocrinology*. 1992;131:2196-2202.
278. Oemar BS, Law NM, Rosenzweig SA. Insulin-like growth factor-1 induces tyrosyl phosphorylation of nuclear proteins. *J Biol Chem*. 1991;266:24241-24244.
279. Werner H, Le Roith D. The insulin-like growth factor-I receptor signaling pathways are important for tumorigenesis and inhibition of apoptosis. *Crit Rev Oncog*. 1997;8:71-92.
280. Kadowaki T, Tamemoto H, Tobe K, et al. Insulin resistance and growth retardation in mice lacking insulin receptor substrate-1 and identification of insulin receptor substrate-2. *Diabet Med*. 1996;13(9 suppl 6):S103-S108.
281. Marte BM, Downward J. PKB/Akt: connecting phosphoinositide 3-kinase to cell survival and beyond. *Trends Biochem Sci*. 1997;22:355-358.
282. Chao MV. Growth factor signaling: where is the specificity? *Cell*. 1992;68:995-997.
283. Porcu P, Ferber A, Pietrzkowski Z, et al. The growth-stimulatory effect of simian virus 40 T antigen requires the interaction of insulinlike growth factor 1 with its receptor. *Mol Cell Biol*. 1992;12:5069-5077.
284. Baserga R. The double life of the IGF-1 receptor. *Receptor*. 1992;2:261-266.
285. Sell C, Rubini M, Rubin R, et al. Simian virus 40 large tumor antigen is unable to transform mouse embryonic fibroblasts lacking type 1 insulin-like growth factor receptor. *Proc Natl Acad Sci U S A*. 1993;90:11217-11221.
286. Kaleko M, Rutter WJ, Miller AD. Overexpression of the human insulinlike growth factor I receptor promotes ligand-dependent neoplastic transformation. *Mol Cell Biol*. 1990;10:464-473.
287. Alexandrides TK, Chen JH, Bueno R, et al. Evidence for two insulin-like growth factor I receptors with distinct primary structure that are differentially expressed during development. *Regul Pept*. 1993;48:279-290.
288. Alexandrides TK, Smith RJ. A novel fetal insulin-like growth factor (IGF) I receptor. mechanism for increased IGF I- and insulin-stimulated tyrosine kinase activity in fetal muscle. *J Biol Chem*. 1989;264:12922-12930.
289. Garofalo RS, Rosen OM. Insulin and insulinlike growth factor 1 (IGF-1) receptors during central nervous system development: expression of two immunologically distinct IGF-1 receptor beta subunits. *Mol Cell Biol*. 1989;9:2806-2817.
290. Tally M, Li CH, Hall K. IGF-2 stimulated growth mediated by the somatomedin type 2 receptor. *Biochem Biophys Res Commun*. 1987;148:811-816.
291. Minniti CP, Kohn EC, Grubb JH, et al. The insulin-like growth factor II (IGF-II)/mannose 6-phosphate receptor mediates IGF-II-induced motility in human rhabdomyosarcoma cells. *J Biol Chem*. 1992;267:9000-9004.

292. Nishimoto I, Murayama Y, Katada T, et al. Possible direct linkage of insulin-like growth factor-II receptor with guanine nucleotide-binding proteins. *J Biol Chem.* 1989;264:14029-14038.
293. Moxham CP, Duronio V, Jacobs S. Insulin-like growth factor I receptor beta-subunit heterogeneity: evidence for hybrid tetramers composed of insulin-like growth factor I and insulin receptor heterodimers. *J Biol Chem.* 1989;264:13238-13244.
294. Moxham CP, Jacobs S. Insulin/IGF-I receptor hybrids: a mechanism for increasing receptor diversity. *J Cell Biochem.* 1992;48: 136-140.
295. Soos MA, Siddle K. Immunological relationships between receptors for insulin and insulin-like growth factor I: evidence for structural heterogeneity of insulin-like growth factor I receptors involving hybrids with insulin receptors. *Biochem J.* 1989;263:553-563.
296. Misra P, Hintz RL, Rosenfeld RG. Structural and immunological characterization of insulin-like growth factor II binding to IM-9 cells. *J Clin Endocrinol Metab.* 1986;63:1400-1405.
297. Soos MA, Field CE, Siddle K. Purified hybrid insulin/insulin-like growth factor-I receptors bind insulin-like growth factor-I, but not insulin, with high affinity. *Biochem J.* 1993;290:419-426.
298. Kasuya J, Paz IB, Maddux BA, et al. Characterization of human placental insulin-like growth factor-I/insulin hybrid receptors by protein microsequencing and purification. *Biochemistry.* 1993;32: 13531-13536.
299. MacDonald RG, Pfeffer SR, Coussens L, et al. A single receptor binds both insulin-like growth factor II and mannose-6-phosphate. *Science.* 1988;239:1134-1137.
300. Kornfeld S. Trafficking of lysosomal enzymes. *FASEB J.* 1987;1: 462-468.
301. Killian JK, Jirtle RL. Genomic structure of the human M6P/IGF2 receptor. *Mamm Genome.* 1999;10:74-77.
302. Morgan DO, Edman JC, Standring DN, et al. Insulin-like growth factor II receptor as a multifunctional binding protein. *Nature.* 1987;329:301-307.
303. Kalscheuer VM, Mariman EC, et al. The insulin-like growth factor type-2 receptor gene is imprinted in the mouse but not in humans. *Nat Genet.* 1993;5:74-78.
304. Kornfeld S. Structure and function of the mannose 6-phosphate/ insulinlike growth factor II receptors. *Annu Rev Biochem.* 1992;61:307-330.
305. Ludwig T, Tenscher K, Remmler J, et al. Cloning and sequencing of cDNAs encoding the full-length mouse mannose 6-phosphate/ insulin-like growth factor II receptor. *Gene.* 1994;142:311-312.
306. Braulke T. Type-2 IGF receptor: a multi-ligand binding protein. *Horm Metab Res.* 1999;31:242-246.
307. Dahms NM, Hancock MK. P-type lectins. *Biochim Biophys Acta.* 2002;1572:317-340.
308. Brown J, Esnouf RM, Jones MA, et al. Structure of a functional IGF2R fragment determined from the anomalous scattering of sulfur. *EMBO J.* 2002;21:1054-1062.
309. Reddy ST, Chai W, Childs RA, et al. Identification of a low affinity mannose 6-phosphate-binding site in domain 5 of the cation-independent mannose 6-phosphate receptor. *J Biol Chem.* 2004; 279:38658-38667.
310. Schmidt B, Kiecke-Siemsen C, Waheed A, et al. Localization of the insulin-like growth factor II binding site to amino acids 15081566 in repeat 11 of the mannose 6-phosphate/insulin-like growth factor II receptor. *J Biol Chem.* 1995;270:14975-14982.
311. Olson LJ, Hancock MK, Dix D, et al. Mutational analysis of the binding site residues of the bovine cation-dependent mannose 6-phosphate receptor. *J Biol Chem.* 1999;274:36905-36911.
312. Gelato MC, Rutherford C, Stark RI, et al. The insulin-like growth factor II/mannose-6-phosphate receptor is present in fetal and maternal sheep serum. *Endocrinology.* 1989;124:2935-2943.
313. Causin C, Waheed A, Braulke T, et al. Mannose 6-phosphate/insulin-like growth factor II-binding proteins in human serum and urine. their relation to the mannose 6-phosphate/insulin-like growth factor II receptor. *Biochem J.* 1988;252:795-799.
314. MacDonald RG, Tepper MA, Clairmont KB, et al. Serum form of the rat insulin-like growth factor II/mannose 6-phosphate receptor is truncated in the carboxyl-terminal domain. *J Biol Chem.* 1989;264:3256-3261.
315. Bobek G, Scott CD, Baxter RC. Secretion of soluble insulin-like growth factor-II/mannose 6-phosphate receptor by rat tissues in culture. *Endocrinology.* 1991;128:2204-2206.
316. Scott CD, Weiss J. Soluble insulin-like growth factor II/mannose 6-phosphate receptor inhibits DNA synthesis in insulin-like growth factor II sensitive cells. *J Cell Physiol.* 2000;182:62-68.
317. Scott C, Baxter R. Regulation of soluble insulin-like growth factor-II/ mannose 6-phosphate receptor in hepatocytes from intact and regenerating rat liver. *Endocrinology.* 1996;137:3864-3870.
318. Scott C, Ballesteros M, Madrid J, et al. Soluble insulin-like growth factor-II/mannose 6-P receptor inhibits deoxyribonucleic acid synthesis in cultured rat hepatocytes. *Endocrinology.* 1996;137: 873-878.
319. Dennis PA, Rifkin DB. Cellular activation of latent transforming growth factor beta requires binding to the cation-independent mannose 6-phosphate/insulin-like growth factor type II receptor. *Proc Natl Acad Sci U S A.* 1991;88:580-584.
320. Blanchard F, Duplomb L, Raher S, et al. Mannose 6-phosphate/ insulin-like growth factor II receptor mediates internalization and degradation of leukemia inhibitory factor but not signal transduction. *J Biol Chem.* 1999;274:24685-24693.
321. Rosenfeld RG, Conover CA, Hodges D, et al. Heterogeneity of insulin-like growth factor-I affinity for the insulin-like growth factor-II receptor: comparison of natural, synthetic and recombinant DNA-derived insulin-like growth factor-I. *Biochem Biophys Res Commun.* 1987;143:199-205.
322. El-Shewy HM, Luttrell LM. Chapter 24 insulin-like growth factor-2/ mannose-6 phosphate receptors. In: Gerald Litwack, ed. *Vitamins and Hormones.* New York, NY: Academic Press; 2009.
323. Kang JX, Bell J, Beard RL, et al. Mannose 6-phosphate/insulin-like growth factor II receptor mediates the growth-inhibitory effects of retinoids. *Cell Growth Differ.* 1999;10:591-600.
324. Lau MM, Stewart CE, Liu Z, et al. Loss of the imprinted IGF2/ cation-independent mannose 6-phosphate receptor results in fetal overgrowth and perinatal lethality. *Genes Dev.* 1994;8:2953-2963.
325. Beukers MW, Oh Y, Zhang H, et al. [Leu27] insulin-like growth factor II is highly selective for the type-II IGF receptor in binding, cross-linking and thymidine incorporation experiments. *Endocrinology.* 1991;128:1201-1203.
326. Furlanetto RW, DiCarlo JN, Wisehart C. The type II insulin-like growth factor receptor does not mediate deoxyribonucleic acid synthesis in human fibroblasts. *J Clin Endocrinol Metab.* 1987;64: 1142-1149.
327. Mottola C, Czech MP. The type II insulin-like growth factor receptor does not mediate increased DNA synthesis in H-35 hepatoma cells. *J Biol Chem.* 1984;259:12705-12713.
328. Kiess W, Haskell JF, Lee L, et al. An antibody that blocks insulin-like growth factor (IGF) binding to the type II IGF receptor is neither an agonist nor an inhibitor of IGF-stimulated biologic responses in L6 myoblasts. *J Biol Chem.* 1987;262:12745-12751.
329. Adashi EY, Resnick CE, Rosenfeld RG. Insulin-like growth factor-I (IGF-I) hormonal action in cultured rat granulosa cells: mediation via type I but not type II IGF receptors. *Endocrinology.* 1989;126: 216-222.
330. Rogers SA, Hammerman MR. Insulin-like growth factor II stimulates production of inositol trisphosphate in proximal tubular basolateral membranes from canine kidney. *Proc Natl Acad Sci U S A.* 1988;85:4037-4041.
331. Jonas HA, Cox AJ. Insulin-like growth factor binding to the atypical insulin receptors of a human lymphoid-derived cell line (IM-9). *Biochem J.* 1990;266:737-742.
332. Feltz SM, Swanson ML, Wemmie JA, et al. Functional properties of an isolated alpha beta heterodimeric human placenta insulin-like growth factor 1 receptor complex. *Biochemistry.* 1988; 27:3234-3242.
333. Treadway JL, Morrison BD, Goldfine ID, et al. Assembly of insulin/ insulin-like growth factor-1 hybrid receptors in vitro. *J Biol Chem.* 1989;264:21450-21453.
334. Soos MA, Siddle K. Immunological relationships between receptors for insulin and insulin-like growth factor I: Evidence for structural heterogeneity of insulin-like growth factor I receptors involving hybrids with insulin receptors. *Biochem J.* 1989;263:553-563.
335. Efstratiadis A. Genetics of mouse growth. *Int J Dev Biol.* 1998;42:955-976.
336. Sims NA, Clement-Lacroix P, Da Ponte F, et al. Bone homeostasis in growth hormone receptor-null mice is restored by IGF-I but independent of Stat5. *J Clin Invest.* 2000;106:1095-1103.
337. DeChiara TM, Efstratiadis A, Robertson EJ. A growth-deficiency phenotype in heterozygous mice carrying an insulin-like growth factor II gene disrupted by targeting. *Nature.* 1990;345:78-80.
338. Baker J, Liu JP, Robertson EJ, et al. Role of insulin-like growth factors in embryonic and postnatal growth. *Cell.* 1993;75:73-82.
339. Giannoukakis N, Deal C, Paquette J, et al. Parental genomic imprinting of the human IGF2 gene. *Nat Genet.* 1993;4:98-101.
340. Woods KA, Camacho-Hubner C, Savage MO, et al. Intrauterine growth retardation and postnatal growth failure associated with deletion of the insulin-like growth factor I gene. *N Engl J Med.* 1996; 335:1363-1367.
341. Walenkamp MJ, Karperien M, Pereira AM, et al. Homozygous and heterozygous expression of a novel insulin-like growth factor-I mutation. *J Clin Endocrinol Metab.* 2005;90:2855-2864.
342. Sjogren K, Liu JL, Blad K, et al. Liver-derived insulin-like growth factor I (IGF-I) is the principal source of IGF-I in blood but is not required for postnatal body growth in mice. *Proc Natl Acad Sci U S A.* 1999;96:7088-7092.
343. Le Roith D, Bondy C, Yakar S, et al. The somatomedin hypothesis: 2001. *Endocr Rev.* 2001;22:53-74.

344. Butler AA, LeRoith D. Tissue-specific versus generalized gene targeting of the Igr1 and Igf1r genes and their roles in insulin-like growth factor physiology. *Endocrinology*. 2001;142:1685-1688.
345. Ueki I, Ooi GT, Tremblay ML, et al. Inactivation of the acid labile subunit gene in mice results in mild retardation of postnatal growth despite profound disruptions in the circulating insulin-like growth factor system. *Proc Natl Acad Sci U S A*. 2000;97:6868-6873.
346. Le Roith D, Scavo L, Butler A. What is the role of circulating IGF-I? *Trends Endocrinol Metab*. 2001;12:48-52.
347. Yakar S, Rosen CJ, Beamer WG, et al. Circulating levels of IGF-1 directly regulate bone growth and density. *J Clin Invest*. 2002;110:771-781.
348. Liu JP, Baker J, Perkins AS, et al. Mice carrying null mutations of the genes encoding insulin-like growth factor I (Igf1) and type 1 IGF receptor (Igf1r). *Cell*. 1993;75:59-72.
349. Abuzzahab MJ, Schneider A, Goddard A, et al. Intrauterine Growth Retardation (IUGR) Study Group. IGF-I receptor mutations resulting in intrauterine and postnatal growth retardation. *N Engl J Med*. 2003;349:2211-2222.
350. Nolan CM, Lawlor MA. Variable accumulation of insulin-like growth factor II in mouse tissues deficient in insulin-like growth factor II receptor. *Int J Biochem Cell Biol*. 1999;31:1421-1433.
351. Filson AJ, Louvi A, Efstratiadis A, et al. Rescue of the T-associated maternal effect in mice carrying null mutations in Igf-2 and Igf2r, two reciprocally imprinted genes. *Development*. 1993;118:731-736.
352. Constancia M, Hemberger M, Hughes J, et al. Placental-specific IGF-II is a major modulator of placental and fetal growth. *Nature*. 2002;417:945-948.
353. Rechler MM. Insulin-like growth factor binding proteins. *Vitam Horm*. 1993;47:1-114.
354. Jones JI, Clemmons DR. Insulin-like growth factors and their binding proteins: biological actions. *Endocrine Rev*. 1995;16:3-34.
355. Bach LA, Headey SJ, Norton RS. IGF-binding proteins: the pieces are falling into place. *Trends Endocrinol Metab*. 2005;16:228-234.
356. Imai Y, Moralez A, Andag U, et al. Substitutions for hydrophobic amino acids in the N-terminal domains of IGFBP-3 and -5 markedly reduce IGF-I binding and alter their biologic actions. *J Biol Chem*. 2000;275:18188-18194.
357. Buckway CK, Wilson EM, Ahlsen M, et al. Mutation of three critical amino acids of the N-terminal domain of IGF-binding protein-3 essential for high affinity IGF binding. *J Clin Endocrinol Metab*. 2001;86:4943-4950.
358. Campbell PG, Durham SK, Suwanichkul A, et al. Plasminogen binds the heparin-binding domain of insulin-like growth factor-binding protein-3. *Am J Physiol*. 1998;275(2 Pt 1):E321-E331.
359. Campbell PG, Durham SK, Hayes JD, et al. Insulin-like growth factor-binding protein-3 binds fibrinogen and fibrin. *J Biol Chem*. 1999;274:30215-30221.
360. Brewer MT, Stetler GL, Squires CH, et al. Cloning, characterization, and expression of a human insulin-like growth factor binding protein. *Biochem Biophys Res Commun*. 1988;152:1289-1297.
361. Jones JI, Gockerman A, Busby Jr WH, et al. Insulin-like growth factor binding protein 1 stimulates cell migration and binds to the alpha 5 beta 1 integrin by means of its arg-gly-asp sequence. *Proc Natl Acad Sci U S A*. 1993;90:10553-10557.
362. Oh Y, Muller HL, Pham H, et al. Non-receptor mediated, post-transcriptional regulation of insulin-like growth factor binding protein (IGFBP)-3 in Hs578T human breast cancer cells. *Endocrinology*. 1992;131:3123-3125.
363. Oh Y, Muller HL, Lamson G, et al. Insulin-like growth factor (IGF)-independent action of IGF-binding protein-3 in Hs578T human breast cancer cells: cell surface binding and growth inhibition. *J Biol Chem*. 1993;268:14964-14971.
364. Firth SM, Baxter RC. Cellular actions of the insulin-like growth factor binding proteins. *Endocr Rev*. 2002;23:824-854.
365. Kalus W, Zweckstetter M, Renner C, et al. Structure of the IGF-binding domain of the insulin-like growth factor-binding protein-5 (IGFBP-5): implications for IGF and IGF-I receptor interactions. *EMBO J*. 1998;17:6558-6572.
366. Fernández-Tornero C, Lozano RM, Rivas G, et al. Synthesis of the blood circulating C-terminal fragment of insulin-like growth factor (IGF)-binding protein-4 in its native conformation. *J Biol Chem*. 2005;280:18899-18907.
367. Sala A, Capaldi S, Campagnoli M, et al. Structure and properties of the C-terminal domain of insulin-like growth factor-binding protein-1 isolated from human amniotic fluid. *J Biol Chem*. 2005;280:29812-29819.
368. Sitar T, Popowicz GM, Siwanowicz I, et al. Structural basis for the inhibition of insulin-like growth factors by insulin-like growth factor-binding proteins. *Proc Natl Acad Sci U S A*. 2006;103:13028-13033.
369. Kuang Z, Yao S, McNeil KA, et al. Cooperativity of the N- and C-terminal domains of insulin-like growth factor (IGF) binding protein 2 in IGF binding. *Biochemistry*. 2007;46:13720-13732.
370. Hwa V, Oh Y, Rosenfeld RG. The insulin-like growth factor-binding protein (IGFBP) superfamily. *Endocr Rev*. 1999;20:761-787.
371. Giudice LC, de Zegher F, Gargosky SE, et al. Insulin-like growth factors and their binding proteins in the term and preterm human fetus and neonate with normal and extremes of intrauterine growth. *J Clin Endocrinol Metab*. 1995;80:1548-1555.
372. Hossenlopp P, Segovia B, Lassarre C, et al. Evidence of enzymatic degradation of insulin-like growth factor-binding proteins in the 150K complex during pregnancy. *J Clin Endocrinol Metab*. 1990; 71:797-805.
373. Gargosky SE, Pham HM, Wilson KF, et al. Measurement and characterization of insulin-like growth factor binding protein-3 in human biological fluids: discrepancies between radioimmunoassay and ligand blotting. *Endocrinology*. 1992;131:3051-3060.
374. Cohen P, Graves HC, Peehl DM, et al. Prostate-specific antigen (PSA) is an insulin-like growth factor binding protein-3 protease found in seminal plasma. *J Clin Endocrinol Metab*. 1992;75:1046-1053.
375. Muller HL, Oh Y, Gargosky SE, et al. Concentrations of insulin-like growth factor (IGF)-binding protein-3 (IGFBP-3), IGF, and IGFBP-3 protease activity in cerebrospinal fluid of children with leukemia, central nervous system tumor, or meningitis. *J Clin Endocrinol Metab*. 1993;77:1113-1119.
376. Lee DY, Park SK, Yorgin PD, et al. Alteration in insulin-like growth factor-binding proteins (IGFBPs) and IGFBP-3 protease activity in serum and urine from acute and chronic renal failure. *J Clin Endocrinol Metab*. 1994;79:1376-1382.
377. Conover CA, De Leon DD. Acid-activated insulin-like growth factor-binding protein-3 proteolysis in normal and transformed cells: role of cathepsin D. *J Biol Chem*. 1994;269:7076-7080.
378. Fowlkes JL, Enghild JJ, Suzuki K, et al. Matrix metalloproteinases degrade insulin-like growth factor-binding protein-3 in dermal fibroblast cultures. *J Biol Chem*. 1994;269:25742-25746.
379. Zadeh SM, Binoux M. The 16-kDa proteolytic fragment of insulin-like growth factor (IGF) binding protein-3 inhibits the mitogenic action of fibroblast growth factor on mouse fibroblasts with a targeted disruption of the type 1 IGF receptor gene. *Endocrinology*. 1997;138: 3069.
380. Andress DL, Loop SM, Zapf J, et al. Carboxy-truncated insulin-like growth factor-binding protein-5 stimulates mitogenesis in osteoblast-like cells. *Biochem Biophys Res Commun*. 1993;195:25-30.
381. Oh Y, Muller HL, Lee DY, et al. Characterization of the affinities of insulin-like growth factor (IGF)-binding proteins 1-4 for IGF-I, IGF-II, IGF-I/insulin hybrid, and IGF-I analogs. *Endocrinology*. 1993;132: 1337-1344.
382. Leong SR, Baxter RC, Camerato T, et al. Structure and functional expression of the acid-labile subunit of the insulin-like growth factor-binding protein complex. *Mol Endocrinol*. 1992;6:870-876.
383. Baxter RC, Martin JL. Structure of the mr 140,000 growth hormone-dependent insulin-like growth factor binding protein complex: determination by reconstitution and affinity-labeling. *Proc Natl Acad Sci U S A*. 1989;86:6898-6902.
384. Guler HP, Zapf J, Schmid C, et al. Insulin-like growth factors I and II in healthy man: estimations of half-lives and production rates. *Acta Endocrinol (Copenh)*. 1989;121:753-758.
385. Bar RS, Boes M, Clemmons DR, et al. Insulin differentially alters transcapillary movement of intravascular IGFBP-1, IGFBP-2 and endothelial cell IGF-binding proteins in the rat heart. *Endocrinology*. 1990;127:497-499.
386. Gargosky SE, Wilson KF, Fielder PJ, et al. The composition and distribution of insulin-like growth factors (IGFs) and IGF-binding proteins (IGFBPs) in the serum of growth hormone receptor-deficient patients: effects of IGF-I therapy on IGFBP-3. *J Clin Endocrinol Metab*. 1993;77:1683-1689.
387. Gargosky SE, Tapanainen P, Rosenfeld RG. Administration of growth hormone (GH), but not insulin-like growth factor-I (IGF-I), by continuous infusion can induce the formation of the 150-kilodalton IGF-binding protein-3 complex in GH-deficient rats. *Endocrinology*. 1994;134:2267-2276.
388. Wilson KF, Fielder PJ, Guevara-Aguirre J, et al. Long-term effects of insulin-like growth factor (IGF)-I treatment on serum IGFs and IGF binding proteins in adolescent patients with growth hormone receptor deficiency. *Clin Endocrinol (Oxf)*. 1995;42:399-407.
389. Walker JL, Baxter RC, Young S, et al. Effects of recombinant insulin-like growth factor I on IGF binding proteins and the acid-labile subunit in growth hormone insensitivity syndrome. *Growth Regul*. 1993;3:109-112.
390. Malpe R, Baylink DJ, Linkhart TA, et al. Insulin-like growth factor (IGF)-I, -II, IGF binding proteins (IGFBP)-3, -4, and -5 levels in the conditioned media of normal human bone cells are skeletal site-dependent. *J Bone Miner Res*. 1997;12:423-430.
391. Rajaram S, Baylink DJ, Mohan S. Insulin-like growth factor-binding proteins in serum and other biological fluids: regulation and functions. *Endocr Rev*. 1997;18:801-831.
392. Ritvos O, Ranta T, Jalkanen J, et al. Insulin-like growth factor (IGF) binding protein from human decidua inhibits the binding and biological action of IGF-I in cultured choriocarcinoma cells. *Endocrinology*. 1988;122:2150-2157.

393. Mohan S, Baylink D. IGF-binding proteins are multifunctional and act via IGF-dependent and -independent mechanisms. *J Endocrinol.* 2002;175:19-31.
394. Mohan S, Nakao Y, Honda Y, et al. Studies on the mechanisms by which insulin-like growth factor (IGF) binding protein-4 (IGFBP-4) and IGFBP-5 modulate IGF actions in bone cells. *J Biol Chem.* 1995;270:20424-20431.
395. Miyakoshi N, Richman C, Qin X, et al. Effects of recombinant insulin-like growth factor-binding protein-4 on bone formation parameters in mice. *Endocrinology.* 1999;140:5719-5728.
396. Cohen P, Lamson G, Okajima T, et al. Transfection of the human insulin-like growth factor binding protein-3 gene into Balb/c fibroblasts inhibits cellular growth. *Mol Endocrinol.* 1993;7:380-386.
397. Jones JI, Gockerman A, Busby Jr WH, et al. Extracellular matrix contains insulin-like growth factor binding protein-5: potentiation of the effects of IGF-I. *J Cell Biol.* 1993;121:679-687.
398. Clemmons DR, Busby W, Clarke JB, et al. Modifications of insulin-like growth factor binding proteins and their role in controlling IGF actions. *Endocr J.* 1998;45(suppl):S1-S8.
399. Nicolas V, Mohan S, Honda Y, et al. An age-related decrease in the concentration of insulin-like growth factor binding protein-5 in human cortical bone. *Calcif Tissue Int.* 1995;57:206-212.
400. Cohen P, Peehl DM, Graves HC, et al. Biological effects of prostate specific antigen as an insulin-like growth factor binding protein-3 protease. *J Endocrinol.* 1994;142:407-415.
401. Lamson G, Giudice LC, Cohen P, et al. Proteolysis of IGFBP-3 may be a common regulatory mechanism of IGF action in vivo. *Growth Regul.* 1993;3:91-95.
402. Oh Y, Muller HL, Ng L, et al. Transforming growth factor-beta-induced cell growth inhibition in human breast cancer cells is mediated through insulin-like growth factor-binding protein-3 action. *J Biol Chem.* 1995;270:13589-13592.
403. Conover CA, Bale LK, Durham SK, et al. Insulin-like growth factor (IGF) binding protein-3 potentiation of IGF action is mediated through the phosphatidylinositol-3-kinase pathway and is associated with alteration in protein kinase B/AKT sensitivity. *Endocrinology.* 2000;141:3098-3103.
404. Rajah R, Khare A, Lee P, et al. Insulin-like growth factor-binding protein-3 is partially responsible for high-serum-induced apoptosis in PC-3 prostate cancer cells. *J Endocrinol.* 1999;163:487-494.
405. Oh Y, Muller HL, Pham H, et al. Demonstration of receptors for insulin-like growth factor binding protein-3 on Hs578T human breast cancer cells. *J Biol Chem.* 1993;268:26045-26048.
406. Villaudy J, Delbe J, Blat C, et al. An IGF binding protein is an inhibitor of FGF stimulation. *J Cell Physiol.* 1991;149:492-496.
407. Bicsak TA, Shimonaka M, Malkowski M, et al. Insulin-like growth factor-binding protein (IGF-BP) inhibition of granulosa cell function: effect on cyclic adenosine 3′,5′-monophosphate, deoxyribonucleic acid synthesis, and comparison with the effect of an IGF-I antibody. *Endocrinology.* 1990;126:2184-2189.
408. Hong J, Zhang G, Dong F, et al. Insulin-like growth factor (IGF)-binding protein-3 mutants that do not bind IGF-I or IGF-II stimulate apoptosis in human prostate cancer cells. *J Biol Chem.* 2002; 277:10489-10497.
409. Miyakoshi N, Richman C, Kasukawa Y, et al. Evidence that IGF-binding protein-5 functions as a growth factor. *J Clin Invest.* 2001; 107:73-81.
410. Spagnoli A, Hwa V, Horton WA, et al. Antiproliferative effects of insulin-like growth factor-binding protein-3 in mesenchymal chondrogenic cell line RCJ3.1C5.18: relationship to differentiation stage. *J Biol Chem.* 2001;276:5533-5540.
411. Andress DL. Insulin-like growth factor-binding protein-5 (IGFBP-5) stimulates phosphorylation of the IGFBP-5 receptor. *Am J Physiol Endocrinol Metab.* 1998;274:E744-E750.
412. Leal SM, Liu Q, Huang SS, et al. The type V transforming growth factor β receptor is the putative insulin-like growth factor-binding protein 3 receptor. *J Biol Chem.* 1997;272:20572-20576.
413. Radulescu RT. Nuclear localization signal in insulin-like growth factor-binding protein type 3. *Trends Biochem Sci.* 1994;19:278.
414. Amaar YG, Thompson GR, Linkhart TA, et al. Insulin-like growth factor-binding protein 5 (IGFBP-5) interacts with a four and a half LIM protein 2 (FHL2). *J Biol Chem.* 2002;277:12053-12060.
415. Liu B, Lee K, Li H, et al. Combination therapy of insulin-like growth factor binding protein-3 and retinoid X receptor ligands synergize on prostate cancer cell apoptosis in vitro and in vivo. *Clin Cancer Res.* 2005;11:4851-4856.
416. Lalou C, Lassarre C, Binoux M. A proteolytic fragment of insulin-like growth factor (IGF) binding protein-3 that fails to bind IGFs inhibits the mitogenic effects of IGF-I and insulin. *Endocrinology.* 1996;137: 3206-3212.
417. Lee YL, Hintz RL, James PM, et al. Insulin-like growth factor (IGF) binding protein complementary deoxyribonucleic acid from human HEP G2 hepatoma cells: predicted protein sequence suggests an IGF binding domain different from those of the IGF-I and IGF-II receptors. *Mol Endocrinol.* 1988;2:404-411.
418. Brinkman A, Groffen CA, Kortleve DJ, et al. Organization of the gene encoding the insulin-like growth factor binding protein IBP-1. *Biochem Biophys Res Commun.* 1988;157:898-907.
419. Giudice LC, Irwin JC, Dsupin BA, et al. Insulin-like growth factors (IGFs), IGF binding proteins (IGFBPs) and IGFBP protease in human uterine endometrium: their potential relevance to endometrial cyclic function and maternal-embryonic interactions. In: Baxter RC, Gluckman PD, Rosenfeld RG, eds. *The insulin-like growth factors and their regulatory proteins.* Amsterdam, The Netherlands: Elsevier; 1994.
420. Adashi EY. Regulation of intrafollicular IGFBPs: possible relevance to ovarian follicular selection. In: Baxter RC, Gluckman PD, Rosenfeld RG, eds. *The Insulin-Like Growth Factors and Their Regulatory Proteins.* Amsterdam, The Netherlands: Elsevier; 1994.
421. Unterman TG, Simmons RA, Glick RP, et al. Circulating levels of insulin, insulin-like growth factor-I (IGF-I), IGF-II, and IGF-binding proteins in the small for gestational age fetal rat. *Endocrinology.* 1993;132:327-336.
422. Lee PD, Conover CA, Powell DR. Regulation and function of insulin-like growth factor-binding protein-1. *Proc Soc Exp Biol Med.* 1993;204:4-29.
423. Thissen JP, Ketelslegers JM, Underwood LE. Nutritional regulation of the insulin-like growth factors. *Endocr Rev.* 1994;15:80-101.
424. Cotterill AM, Cowell CT, Baxter RC, et al. Regulation of the growth hormone-independent growth factor-binding protein in children. *J Clin Endocrinol Metab.* 1988;67:882-887.
425. Powell DR, Suwanichkul A, Cubbage ML, et al. Insulin inhibits transcription of the human gene for insulin-like growth factor-binding protein-1. *J Biol Chem.* 1991;266:18868-18876.
426. Koistinen R, Itkonen O, Selenius P, et al. Insulin-like growth factor-binding protein-1 inhibits binding of IGF-I on fetal skin fibroblasts but stimulates their DNA synthesis. *Biochem Biophys Res Commun.* 1990;173:408-415.
427. Jones JI, D'Ercole AJ, Camacho-Hubner C, et al. Phosphorylation of insulin-like growth factor (IGF)-binding protein 1 in cell culture and in vivo: effects on affinity for IGF-I. *Proc Natl Acad Sci U S A.* 1991;88:7481-7485.
428. Binkert C, Margot JB, Landwehr J, et al. Structure of the human insulin-like growth factor binding protein-2 gene. *Mol Endocrinol.* 1992;6:826-836.
429. Agarwal N, Hsieh CL, Sills D, et al. Sequence analysis, expression and chromosomal localization of a gene, isolated from a subtracted human retina cDNA library, that encodes an insulin-like growth factor binding protein (IGFBP2). *Exp Eye Res.* 1991;52:549-561.
430. Wood TL, Rogler L, Streck RD, et al. Targeted disruption of IGFBP-2 gene. *Growth Regul.* 1993;3:5-8.
431. Lamson G, Pham H, Oh Y, et al. Expression of the BRL-3A insulin-like growth factor binding protein (rBP-30) in the rat central nervous system. *Endocrinology.* 1989;125:1100-1102.
432. Rosenfeld RG, Pham H, Oh Y, et al. Identification of insulin-like growth factor binding protein-2 (IGF-BP-2) and a low molecular weight IGF-BP in human seminal plasma. *J Clin Endocrinol Metab.* 1989;69:963-965.
433. Bourner MJ, Busby Jr WH, Siegel NR, et al. Cloning and sequence determination of bovine insulin-like growth factor binding protein-2 (IGFBP-2): comparison of its structural and functional properties with IGFBP-1. *J Cell Biochem.* 1992;48:215-226.
434. Cubbage ML, Suwanichkul A, Powell DR. Insulin-like growth factor binding protein-3: organization of the human chromosomal gene and demonstration of promoter activity. *J Biol Chem.* 1990;265: 12642-12649.
435. Arany E, Afford S, Strain AJ, et al. Differential cellular synthesis of insulin-like growth factor binding protein-1 (IGFBP-1) and IGFBP-3 within human liver. *J Clin Endocrinol Metab.* 1994;79:1871-1876.
436. Chin E, Zhou J, Dai J, et al. Cellular localization and regulation of gene expression for components of the insulin-like growth factor ternary binding protein complex. *Endocrinology.* 1994;134:2498-2504.
437. Firth S, Baxter R. Characterisation of recombinant glycosylation variants of insulin-like growth factor binding protein-3. *J Endocrinol.* 1999;160:379-387.
438. Baxter RC. Insulin-like growth factor binding proteins in the human circulation: a review. *Horm Res.* 1994;42:140-144.
439. Yamanaka Y, Fowlkes JL, Wilson EM, et al. Characterization of insulin-like growth factor binding protein-3 (IGFBP-3) binding to human breast cancer cells: kinetics of IGFBP-3 binding and identification of receptor binding domain on the IGFBP-3 molecule. *Endocrinology.* 1999;140:1319-1328.
440. Holly J, Claffey DC, Cwyfan-Hughes SC, et al. Proteases acting on IGFBPs: their occurrence and physiological significance. *Growth Regul.* 1992;3:88-91.
441. Bang P, Brismar K, Rosenfeld RG. Increased proteolysis of insulin-like growth factor-binding protein-3 (IGFBP-3) in noninsulin-dependent diabetes mellitus serum, with elevation of a 29-kilodalton (kDa) glycosylated IGFBP-3 fragment contained in the approximately 130- to

150-kDa ternary complex. *J Clin Endocrinol Metab.* 1994;78: 1119-1127.

442. Janosi JB, Ramsland PA, Mott MR, et al. The acid-labile subunit of the serum insulin-like growth factor-binding protein complexes: structural determination by molecular modeling and electron microscopy. *J Biol Chem.* 1999;274:23328-23332.
443. Zapf J, Hauri C, Waldvogel M, et al. Recombinant human insulin-like growth factor I induces its own specific carrier protein in hypophysectomized and diabetic rats. *Proc Natl Acad Sci U S A.* 1989; 86:3813-3817.
444. Clemmons DR, Thissen JP, Maes M, et al. Insulin-like growth factor-I (IGF-I) infusion into hypophysectomized or protein-deprived rats induces specific IGF-binding proteins in serum. *Endocrinology.* 1989;125:2967-2972.
445. Glasscock GF, Hein AN, Miller JA, et al. Effects of continuous infusion of insulin-like growth factor I and II, alone and in combination with thyroxine or growth hormone, on the neonatal hypophysectomized rat. *Endocrinology.* 1992;130:203-210.
446. Oh Y, Muller HL, Ng L, et al. Transforming growth factor-beta-induced cell growth inhibition in human breast cancer cells is mediated through insulin-like growth factor-binding protein-3 action. *J Biol Chem.* 1995;270:13589-13592.
447. Booth BA, Boes M, Andress DL, et al. IGFBP-3 and IGFBP-5 association with endothelial cells: role of C-terminal heparin binding domain. *Growth Regul.* 1995;5:1-17.
448. Leal SM, Huang SS, Huang JS. Interactions of high affinity insulin-like growth factor-binding proteins with the type V transforming growth factor-β receptor in mink lung epithelial cells. *J Biol Chem.* 1999;274:6711-6717.
449. Jaques G, Noll K, Wegmann B, et al. Nuclear localization of insulin-like growth factor binding protein 3 in a lung cancer cell line. *Endocrinology.* 1997;138:1767.
450. Schedlich LJ, Le Page SL, Firth SM, et al. Nuclear import of insulin-like growth factor-binding protein-3 and -5 is mediated by the importin β subunit. *J Biol Chem.* 2000;275:23462-23470.
451. Liu B, Lee HY, Weinzimer SA, et al. Direct functional interactions between insulin-like growth factor-binding protein-3 and retinoid X receptor-alpha regulate transcriptional signaling and apoptosis. *J Biol Chem.* 2000;275:33607-33613.
452. Schedlich LJ, O'Han MK, Leong GM, et al. Insulin-like growth factor binding protein-3 prevents retinoid receptor heterodimerization: implications for retinoic acid-sensitivity in human breast cancer cells. *Biochem Biophys Res Commun.* 2004;314:83-88.
453. Jogie-Brahim S, Feldman D, Oh Y. Unraveling insulin-like growth factor binding protein-3 actions in human disease. *Endocr Rev.* 2009;30:417-437.
454. Buckbinder L, Talbott R, Velasco-Miguel S, et al. Induction of the growth inhibitor IGF-binding protein 3 by p53. *Nature.* 1995; 377:646-649.
455. Bourdon JC, Deguin-Chambon V, Lelong JC, et al. Further characterisation of the p53 responsive element: identification of new candidate genes for trans-activation by p53. *Oncogene.* 1997;14:85-94.
456. Grimberg A, Coleman CM, Burns TF, et al. P53-dependent and p53-independent induction of insulin-like growth factor binding protein-3 by deoxyribonucleic acid damage and hypoxia. *J Clin Endocrinol Metab.* 2005;90:3568-3574.
457. Gao L, Ling N, Shimasaki S. Structure of the rat insulin-like growth factor binding protein-4 gene. *Biochem Biophys Res Commun.* 1993; 190:1053-1059.
458. Wang J, Niu W, Witte DP, et al. Overexpression of insulin-like growth factor-binding protein-4 (IGFBP-4) in smooth muscle cells of transgenic mice through a smooth muscle α-actin-IGFBP-4 fusion gene induces smooth muscle hypoplasia. *Endocrinology.* 1998;139: 2605-2614.
459. Cheung PT, Wu J, Banach W, et al. Glucocorticoid regulation of an insulin-like growth factor-binding protein-4 protease produced by a rat neuronal cell line. *Endocrinology.* 1994;135:1328-1335.
460. Cohick WS, Gockerman A, Clemmons DR. Vascular smooth muscle cells synthesize two forms of insulin-like growth factor binding proteins which are regulated differently by the insulin-like growth factors. *J Cell Physiol.* 1993;157:52-60.
461. Conover CA, Kiefer MC, Zapf J. Posttranslational regulation of insulin-like growth factor binding protein-4 in normal and transformed human fibroblasts: insulin-like growth factor dependence and biological studies. *J Clin Invest.* 1993;91:1129-1137.
462. Durham SK, Kiefer MC, Riggs BL, et al. Regulation of insulin-like growth factor binding protein 4 by a specific insulin-like growth factor binding protein 4 proteinase in normal human osteoblast-like cells: implications in bone cell physiology. *J Bone Miner Res.* 1994;9:111-117.
463. Lee KO, Oh Y, Giudice LC, et al. Identification of insulin-like growth factor-binding protein-3 (IGFBP-3) fragments and IGFBP-5 proteolytic activity in human seminal plasma: a comparison of normal and vasectomized patients. *J Clin Endocrinol Metab.* 1994;79: 1367-1372.
464. Neely EK, Rosenfeld RG. Insulin-like growth factors (IGFs) reduce IGF-binding protein-4 (IGFBP-4) concentration and stimulate IGFBP-3 independently of IGF receptors in human fibroblasts and epidermal cells. *Endocrinology.* 1992;130:985-993.
465. Fowlkes J, Freemark M. Evidence for a novel insulin-like growth factor (IGF)-dependent protease regulating IGF-binding protein-4 in dermal fibroblasts. *Endocrinology.* 1992;131:2071-2076.
466. Laursen LS, Overgaard MT, Soe R, et al. Pregnancy-associated plasma protein-A (PAPP-A) cleaves insulin-like growth factor binding protein (IGFBP)-5 independent of IGF: implications for the mechanism of IGFBP-4 proteolysis by PAPP-A. *FEBS Lett.* 2001;504:36-40.
467. Rivera GM, Fortune JE. Selection of the dominant follicle and insulin-like growth factor (IGF)-binding proteins: evidence that pregnancy-associated plasma protein A contributes to proteolysis of IGF-binding protein 5 in bovine follicular fluid. *Endocrinology.* 2003;144: 437-446.
468. Laursen LS, Overgaard MT, Nielsen CG, et al. Substrate specificity of the metalloproteinase pregnancy-associated plasma protein-A (PAPP-A) assessed by mutagenesis and analysis of synthetic peptides: substrate residues distant from the scissile bond are critical for proteolysis. *Biochem J.* 2002;367(Pt 1):31-40.
469. Hourvitz A, Kuwahara A, Hennebold JD, et al. The regulated expression of the pregnancy-associated plasma protein-A in the rodent ovary: a proposed role in the development of dominant follicles and of corpora lutea. *Endocrinology.* 2002;143:1833-1844.
470. Conover CA, Kiefer MC. Regulation and biological effect of endogenous insulin-like growth factor binding protein-5 in human osteoblastic cells. *J Clin Endocrinol Metab.* 1993;76:1153-1159.
471. Olney R, Smith R, Kee Y, et al. Production and hormonal regulation of insulin-like growth factor binding proteins in bovine chondrocytes. *Endocrinology.* 1993;133:563-570.
472. Onoda N, Li D, Mickey G, et al. Gonadotropin-releasing hormone overcomes follicle-stimulating hormone's inhibition of insulin-like growth factor-5 synthesis and promotion of its degradation in rat granulosa cells. *Mol Cell Endocrinol.* 1995;110:17-25.
473. Clemmons DR, Nam TJ, Busby WH, et al. Modification of IGF action by insulin-like growth factor binding protein-5. In: Baxter RC, Gluckman PD, Rosenfeld RG, eds. *The Insulin-Like Growth Factors and Their Regulatory Proteins.* Amsterdam, The Netherlands: Elsevier; 1994.
474. Fielder PJ, Pham H, Adashi EY, et al. Insulin-like growth factors (IGFs) block FSH-induced proteolysis of IGF-binding protein-5 (BP-5) in cultured rat granulosa cells. *Endocrinology.* 1993;133:415-418.
475. Andress DL, Birnbaum RS. Human osteoblast-derived insulin-like growth factor (IGF) binding protein-5 stimulates osteoblast mitogenesis and potentiates IGF action. *J Biol Chem.* 1992;5(267): 22467-22472.
476. Bach LA, Thotakura NR, Rechler MM. Human insulin-like growth factor binding protein-6 is O-glycosylated. *Growth Regul.* 1993;3: 59-62.
477. Roghani M, Lassarre C, Zapf J, et al. Two insulin-like growth factor (IGF)-binding proteins are responsible for the selective affinity for IGF-II of cerebrospinal fluid binding proteins. *J Clin Endocrinol Metab.* 1991;73:658-666.
478. Rohan RM, Ricciarelli E, Kiefer MC, et al. Rat ovarian insulin-like growth factor-binding protein-6: a hormonally regulated theca-interstitial-selective species with limited antigonadotropic activity. *Endocrinology.* 1993;132:2507-2512.
479. Wood TL, Rogler LE, Czick ME, et al. Selective alterations in organ sizes in mice with a targeted disruption of the insulin-like growth factor binding protein-2 gene. *Mol Endocrinol.* 2000;14:1472-1482.
480. Ning Y, Schuller AGP, Bradshaw S, et al. Diminished growth and enhanced glucose metabolism in triple knockout mice containing mutations of insulin-like growth factor binding protein-3, -4, and -5. *Mol Endocrinol.* 2006;20:2173-2186.
481. Silha JV, Murphy LJ. Insights from insulin-like growth factor binding protein transgenic mice (minireview). *Endocrinology.* 2002;143: 3711-3714.
482. Lorentzon M, Lorentzon R, Backstrom T, et al. Estrogen receptor gene polymorphism, but not estradiol levels, is related to bone density in healthy adolescent boys: a cross-sectional and longitudinal study. *J Clin Endocrinol Metab.* 1990;84:4597-4601.
483. Lehrer S, Rabin J, Stone J, et al. Association of an estrogen receptor variant with increased height in women. *Horm Metab Res.* 1994;26:486-488.
484. Demura M, Martin RM, Shozu M, et al. Regional rearrangements in chromosome 15q21 cause formation of cryptic promoters for the CYP19 (aromatase) gene. *Hum Mol Genet.* 2007;16:2529-2541.
485. Martin RM, Lin CJ, Nishi MY, et al. Familial hyperestrogenism in both sexes: clinical, hormonal, and molecular studies of two siblings. *J Clin Endocrinol Metab.* 2003;88:3027-3034.
486. Nilsson O, Marino R, De Luca F, et al. Endocrine regulation of the growth plate. *Horm Res.* 2005;64:157-165.
487. Matkovic V. Skeletal development and bone turnover revisited. *J Clin Endocrinol Metab.* 1996;81:2013-2016.

488. Abrams SA, O'Brien KO, Stuff JE. Changes in calcium kinetics associated with menarche. *J Clin Endocrinol Metab.* 1996;81:2017-2020.
489. Slemenda CW, Reister TK, Hui SL, et al. Influences on skeletal mineralization in children and adolescents: evidence for varying effects of sexual maturation and physical activity. *J Pediatr.* 1996;125: 201-207.
490. Wexler JA, Sharretts J. Thyroid and bone. *Endocrinol Metab Clin North Am.* 2007;36:673-705, vi.
491. Robson H, Siebler T, Shalet SM, et al. Interactions between GH, IGF-I, glucocorticoids, and thyroid hormones during skeletal growth. *Pediatr Res.* 2002;52:137-147.
492. Siebler T, Robson H, Shalet SM, et al. Glucocorticoids, thyroid hormone and growth hormone interactions: implications for the growth plate. *Horm Res.* 2001;56(suppl 1):7-12.
493. Veldhuis JD, Lizarralde G, Iranmanesh A. Divergent effects of short term glucocorticoid excess on the gonadotropic and somatotropic axes in normal men. *J Clin Endocrinol Metab.* 1992;74:96-102.
494. Pantelakis SN, Sinaniotis CA, Sbirakis S, et al. Night and day growth hormone levels during treatment with corticosteroids and corticotrophin. *Arch Dis Child.* 1972;47:605-608.
495. Wehrenberg WB, Janowski BA, Piering AW, et al. Glucocorticoids: potent inhibitors and stimulators of growth hormone secretion. *Endocrinology.* 1990;126:3200-3203.
496. Jux C, Leiber K, Hugel U, et al. Dexamethasone impairs growth hormone (GH)-stimulated growth by suppression of local insulin-like growth factor (IGF)-I production and expression of GH- and IGF-I-receptor in cultured rat chondrocytes. *Endocrinology.* 1998;139: 3296-3305.
497. Hochberg Z. Mechanisms of steroid impairment of growth. *Horm Res.* 2002;58(suppl 1):33-38.
498. Ch'in KY. The endocrine glands of anencephalic foetuses. *Chinese Med J* 1938;2(suppl):63-90.
499. Lemire RJ, Beckwith JB, Warkany J. *Anencephaly.* New York, NY: Raven Press; 1978.
500. Grumbach MM, Kaplan SL. Ontogenesis of growth hormone, insulin, prolactin and gonadotropin secretion in the human foetus. In: Cross DW, Nathanielsz P, eds. *Foetal and Neonatal Physiology. Proceedings of the St Joseph Barcroft Centenary Symposium.* Cambridge, UK: Cambridge University Press; 1973.
501. Grumbach MM, Kaplan SL. Fetal pituitary hormones and the maturation of central nervous system regulation of anterior pituitary function. In: Gluck L, ed. *Modern Perinatal Medicine.* Chicago, IL: Year Book Medical Publishers; 1974.
502. Tuilipakov AN, Bulatov AA, Peterkova AV, et al. Growth hormone (GH)-releasing effects of synthetic peptide GH-releasing peptide-2 and GH-releasing hormone (1-29NH2) in children with GH insufficiency and idiopathic short stature. *Metabolism.* 1995;44: 1199-1204.
503. Pombo M, Barreiro J, Penalva A, et al. Absence of growth hormone (GH) secretion after the administration of either GH-releasing hormone (GHRH), GH-releasing peptide (GHRP-6), or GHRH plus GHRP-6 in children with neonatal pituitary stalk transection. *J Clin Endocrinol Metab.* 1995;80:3180-3184.
504. Root AW, Martinez CR. Magnetic resonance imaging in patients with hypopituitarism. *Trends Endocrinol Metab.* 1992;3:283-287.
505. Triulzi F, Scotti G, di Natale B, et al. Evidence of a congenital midline brain anomaly in pituitary dwarfs: a magnetic resonance imaging study in 101 patients. *Pediatrics.* 1994;93:409-416.
506. Nagel BH, Palmbach M, Petersen D, et al. Magnetic resonance images of 91 children with different causes of short stature: pituitary size reflects growth hormone secretion. *Eur J Pediatr.* 1997;156:758-763.
507. Cacciari E, Zucchini S, Carla G, et al. Endocrine function and morphological findings in patients with disorders of the hypothalamo-pituitary area: a study with magnetic resonance. *Arch Dis Child.* 1990;65:1199-1202.
508. Brown RS, Bhatia V, Hayes E. An apparent cluster of congenital hypopituitarism in central Massachusetts: magnetic resonance imaging and hormonal studies. *J Clin Endocrinol Metab.* 1991;72:12-18.
509. Abrahams JJ, Trefelner E, Boulware SD. Idiopathic growth hormone deficiency: MR findings in 35 patients. *AJNR Am J Neuroradiol.* 1991;12:155-160.
510. Argyropoulou M, Perignon F, Brauner R, et al. Magnetic resonance imaging in the diagnosis of growth hormone deficiency. *J Pediatr.* 1992;120:886-891.
511. Hamilton J, Blaser S, Daneman D. MR imaging in idiopathic growth hormone deficiency. *AJNR Am J Neuroradiol.* 1998;19:1609-1615.
512. Kornreich L, Horev G, Lazar L, et al. MR findings in growth hormone deficiency: correlation with severity of hypopituitarism. *AJNR Am J Neuroradiol.* 1998;19:1495-1499.
513. Maghnie M, Larizza D, Triulzi F, et al. Hypopituitarism and stalk agenesis: a congenital syndrome worsened by breech delivery? *Horm Res.* 1991;35:104-108.
514. Kuroiwa T, Okabe Y, Hasuo K, et al. MR imaging of pituitary dwarfism. *AJNR Am J Neuroradiol.* 1991;12:161-164.
515. Hellstrom A, Wiklund LM, Svensson E, et al. Midline brain lesions in children with hormone insufficiency indicate early prenatal damage. *Acta Paediatr.* 1998;87:528-536.
516. Goodman HG, Grumbach MM, Kaplan SL. Growth and growth hormone: II. A comparison of isolated growth-hormone deficiency and multiple pituitary-hormone deficiencies in 35 patients with idiopathic hypopituitary dwarfism. *N Engl J Med.* 1968;278:57-68.
517. Wit JM, van Unen H. Growth of infants with neonatal growth hormone deficiency. *Arch Dis Child.* 1992;67:920-924.
518. Gluckman PD, Gunn AJ, Wray A, et al. Congenital idiopathic growth hormone deficiency associated with prenatal and early postnatal growth failure: the International Board of the Kabi Pharmacia International Growth Study. *J Pediatr.* 1992;121:920-923.
519. DeLuca F, Bernasconi S, Blandino A, et al. Auxological, clinical, and neuroradiological findings in infants with early onset growth hormone deficiency. *Acta Paediatr Scand.* 1995;84:561-565.
520. Lovinger RD, Kaplan SL, Grumbach MM. Congenital hypopituitarism associated with neonatal hypoglycemia and microphallus: four cases secondary to hypothalamic hormone deficiencies. *J Pediatr.* 1975;87(6 Pt 2):1171-1181.
521. Hamilton J, Chitayat D, Blaser S, et al. Familial growth hormone deficiency associated with MRI abnormalities. *Am J Med Genet.* 1998;80:128-132.
522. de Zegher F, Kaplan SL, Grumbach MM, et al. The foetal pituitary, postmaturity and breech presentation. *Acta Paediatr.* 1995;84: 1100-1102.
523. Hintz RL, Menking M, Sotos JF. Familial holoprosencephaly with endocrine dysgenesis. *J Pediatr.* 1968;72:81-87.
524. Lieblich JM, Rosen SE, Guyda H, et al. The syndrome of basal encephalocele and hypothalamic-pituitary dysfunction. *Ann Intern Med.* 1978;89:910-916.
525. Roessler E, Muenke M. Holoprosencephaly: a paradigm for the complex genetics of brain development. *J Inherit Metab Dis.* 1998;21:481-497.
526. Brown SA, Warburton D, Brown LY, et al. Holoprosencephaly due to mutations in ZIC2, a homologue of drosophila odd-paired. *Nat Genet.* 1998;20:180-183.
527. Roessler E, Du YZ, Mullor JL, et al. Loss-of-function mutations in the human GLI2 gene are associated with pituitary anomalies and holoprosencephaly-like features. *Proc Natl Acad Sci U S A.* 2003;100:13424-13429.
528. Treier M, O'Connell S, Gleiberman A, et al. Hedgehog signaling is required for pituitary gland development. *Development.* 2001;128: 377-386.
529. Rudman D, Davis T, Priest JH, et al. Prevalence of growth hormone deficiency in children with cleft lip or palate. *J Pediatr.* 1978;93:378-382.
530. Izenberg N, Rosenblum M, Parks JS. The endocrine spectrum of septo-optic dysplasia. *Clin Pediatr (Phila).* 1984;23:632-636.
531. Wilson DM, Enzmann DR, Hintz RL, et al. Computed tomographic findings in septo-optic dysplasia: discordance between clinical and radiological findings. *Neuroradiology.* 1984;26:279-283.
532. Willnow S, Kiess W, Butenandt O, et al. Endocrine disorders in septo-optic dysplasia (de Morsier syndrome): evaluation and follow-up of 18 patients. *Eur J Pediatr.* 1998;155:179-184.
533. Kaplan SL, Grumbach MM. Pathophysiology of GH deficiency and other disorders of GH metabolism. In: LaCauza C, Root AW, eds. *Problems in Pediatric Endocrinology.* London, UK: Academic Press; 1980.
534. Ahmad T, Garcia-Filion P, Borchert M, et al. Endocrinological and auxological abnormalities in young children with optic nerve hypoplasia: a prospective study. *J Pediatr.* 2006;148:78-84.
535. Stickler GB, Morgenstern BZ. Hypophosphataemic rickets: final height and clinical symptoms in adults. *Lancet.* 1989;2:902-905.
536. Patel L, McNally RJ, Harrison E, et al. Geographical distribution of optic nerve hypoplasia and septo-optic dysplasia in northwest england. *J Pediatr.* 2006;148:85-88.
537. Tornqvist K, Ericsson A, Kallen B. Optic nerve hypoplasia: risk factors and epidemiology. *Acta Ophthalmol Scand.* 2002;80:300-304.
538. Dattani MT, Martinez-Barbera JP, Thomas PQ, et al. HESX1: A novel gene implicated in a familial form of septo-optic dysplasia. *Acta Paediatr Suppl.* 1999;88:49-54.
539. Hermesz E, Mackem S, Mahon KA. Rpx: a novel anterior-restricted homeobox gene progressively activated in the prechordal plate, anterior neural plate and Rathke's pouch of the mouse embryo. *Development.* 1996;122:41-52.
540. Sobrier ML, Netchine I, Heinrichs C, et al. Alu-element insertion in the homeodomain of HESX1 and aplasia of the anterior pituitary. *Hum Mutat.* 2005;25:503.
541. Dattani MT, Robinson IC. HESX1 and septo-optic dysplasia. *Rev Endocr Metab Disord.* 2002;3:289-300.
542. Carvalho LR, Woods KS, Mendonca BB, et al. A homozygous mutation in HESX1 is associated with evolving hypopituitarism due to impaired repressor-corepressor interaction. *J Clin Invest.* 2003;112: 1192-1201.

543. Thomas PQ, Johnson BV, Rathjen J, et al. Sequence, genomic organization, and expression of the novel homeobox gene Hesx1. *J Biol Chem*. 1995;270:3869-3875.
544. Dasen JS, Barbera JP, Herman TS, et al. Temporal regulation of a paired-like homeodomain repressor/TLE corepressor complex and a related activator is required for pituitary organogenesis. *Genes Dev*. 2001;15:3193-3207.
545. Chou SJ, Hermesz E, Hatta T, et al. Conserved regulatory elements establish the dynamic expression of Rpx/HesxI in early vertebrate development. *Dev Biol*. 2006;292:533-545.
546. Dattani MT, Martinez-Barbera JP, Thomas PQ, et al. Mutations in the homeobox gene HESX1/Hesx1 associated with septo-optic dysplasia in human and mouse. *Nat Genet*. 1998;19:125-133.
547. Gaston-Massuet C, Andoniadou CL, Signore M, et al. Genetic interaction between the homeobox transcription factors HESX1 and SIX3 is required for normal pituitary development. *Dev Biol*. 2008; 324:322-333.
548. Wales JK, Quarrell OW. Evidence for possible mendelian inheritance of septo-optic dysplasia. *Acta Paediatr*. 1996;85:391-392.
549. McNay DE, Turton JP, Kelberman D, et al. HESX1 mutations are an uncommon cause of septooptic dysplasia and hypopituitarism. *J Clin Endocrinol Metab*. 2007;92:691-697.
550. Brickman JM, Clements M, Tyrell R, et al. Molecular effects of novel mutations in Hesx1/HESX1 associated with human pituitary disorders. *Development*. 2001;128:5189-5199.
551. Sobrier ML, Maghnie M, Vie-Luton MP, et al. Novel HESX1 mutations associated with a life-threatening neonatal phenotype, pituitary aplasia, but normally located posterior pituitary and no optic nerve abnormalities. *J Clin Endocrinol Metab*. 2006;91:4528-4536.
552. Coya R, Vela A, Perez de Nanclares G, et al. GEDPIT Group. Panhypopituitarism: genetic versus acquired etiological factors. *J Pediatr Endocrinol Metab*. 2007;20:27-36.
553. Tajima T, Hattorri T, Nakajima T, et al. Sporadic heterozygous frameshift mutation of HESX1 causing pituitary and optic nerve hypoplasia and combined pituitary hormone deficiency in a Japanese patient. *J Clin Endocrinol Metab*. 2003;88:45-50.
554. Radovick S, Cohen LE, Wondisford FE. The molecular basis of hypopituitarism. *Horm Res*. 1998;49(suppl 1):30-36.
555. Sajedi E, Gaston-Massuet C, Signore M, et al. Analysis of mouse models carrying the I26T and R160C substitutions in the transcriptional repressor HESX1 as models for septo-optic dysplasia and hypopituitarism. *Dis Model Mech*. 2008;1:241-254.
556. Kurokawa D, Takasaki N, Kiyonari H, et al. Regulation of Otx2 expression and its functions in mouse epiblast and anterior neuroectoderm. *Development*. 2004;131:3307-3317.
557. Dateki S, Kosaka K, Hasegawa K, et al. Heterozygous orthodenticle homeobox 2 mutations are associated with variable pituitary phenotype. *J Clin Endocrinol Metab*. 2010;95:756-764.
558. Diaczok D, Romero C, Zunich J, et al. A novel dominant negative mutation of OTX2 associated with combined pituitary hormone deficiency. *J Clin Endocrinol Metab*. 2008;93:4351-4359.
559. Lagerstrom-Fermer M, Sundvall M, Johnsen E, et al. X-linked recessive panhypopituitarism associated with a regional duplication in Xq25-q26. *Am J Hum Genet*. 1997;60:910-916.
560. Hol FA, Schepens MT, van Beersum SE, et al. Identification and characterization of an Xq26-q27 duplication in a family with spina bifida and panhypopituitarism suggests the involvement of two distinct genes. *Genomics*. 2000;69:174-181.
561. Woods KS, Cundall M, Turton J, et al. Over- and underdosage of SOX3 is associated with infundibular hypoplasia and hypopituitarism. *Am J Hum Genet*. 2005;76:833-849.
562. Laumonnier F, Ronce N, Hamel BC, et al. Transcription factor SOX3 is involved in X-linked mental retardation with growth hormone deficiency. *Am J Hum Genet*. 2002;71:1450-1455.
563. Lim HN, Berkovitz GD, Hughes IA, et al. Mutation analysis of subjects with 46, XX sex reversal and 46, XY gonadal dysgenesis does not support the involvement of SOX3 in testis determination. *Hum Genet*. 2000;107:650-652.
564. Raverot G, Lejeune H, Kotlar T, et al. X-linked sex-determining region Y box 3 (SOX3) gene mutations are uncommon in men with idiopathic oligoazoospermic infertility. *J Clin Endocrinol Metab*. 2004;89:4146-4148.
565. Kelberman D, Rizzoti K, Avilion A, et al. Mutations within Sox2/SOX2 are associated with abnormalities in the hypothalamo-pituitary-gonadal axis in mice and humans. *J Clin Invest*. 2006;116: 2442-2455.
566. Kelberman D, de Castro SC, Huang S, et al. SOX2 plays a critical role in the pituitary, forebrain, and eye during human embryonic development. *J Clin Endocrinol Metab*. 2008;93:1865-1873.
567. Fantes J, Ragge NK, Lynch SA, et al. Mutations in SOX2 cause anophthalmia. *Nat Genet*. 2003;33:461-463.
568. Williamson KA, Hever AM, Rainger J, et al. Mutations in SOX2 cause anophthalmia-esophageal-genital (AEG) syndrome. *Hum Mol Genet*. 2006;15:1413-1422.
569. Sato N, Kamachi Y, Kondoh H, et al. Hypogonadotropic hypogonadism in an adult female with a heterozygous hypomorphic mutation of SOX2. *Eur J Endocrinol*. 2007;156:167-171.
570. Sisodiya SM, Ragge NK, Cavalleri GL, et al. Role of SOX2 mutations in human hippocampal malformations and epilepsy. *Epilepsia*. 2006;47:534-542.
571. Ragge NK, Lorenz B, Schneider A, et al. SOX2 anophthalmia syndrome. *Am J Med Genet A*. 2005;135:1-7, discussion 8.
572. Hagstrom SA, Pauer GJ, Reid J, et al. SOX2 mutation causes anophthalmia, hearing loss, and brain anomalies. *Am J Med Genet A*. 2005;138A:95-98.
573. Zenteno JC, Gascon-Guzman G, Tovilla-Canales JL. Bilateral anophthalmia and brain malformations caused by a 20-bp deletion in the SOX2 gene. *Clin Genet*. 2005;68:564-566.
574. Chassaing N, Gilbert-Dussardier B, Nicot F, et al. Germinal mosaicism and familial recurrence of a SOX2 mutation with highly variable phenotypic expression extending from AEG syndrome to absence of ocular involvement. *Am J Med Genet A*. 2007;143:289-291.
575. Bakrania P, Robinson DO, Bunyan DJ, et al. SOX2 anophthalmia syndrome: 12 new cases demonstrating broader phenotype and high frequency of large gene deletions. *Br J Ophthalmol*. 2007;91: 1471-1476.
576. Guichet A, Triau S, Lepinard C, et al. Prenatal diagnosis of primary anophthalmia with a 3q27 interstitial deletion involving SOX2. *Prenat Diagn*. 2004;24:828-832.
577. Faivre L, Williamson KA, Faber V, et al. Recurrence of SOX2 anophthalmia syndrome with gonosomal mosaicism in a phenotypically normal mother. *Am J Med Genet A*. 2006;140:636-639.
578. Sobrier ML, Attie-Bitach T, Netchine I, et al. Pathophysiology of syndromic combined pituitary hormone deficiency due to a LHX3 defect in light of LHX3 and LHX4 expression during early human development. *Gene Expr Patterns*. 2004;5:279-284.
579. Rajab A, Kelberman D, de Castro SC, et al. Novel mutations in LHX3 are associated with hypopituitarism and sensorineural hearing loss. *Hum Mol Genet*. 2008;17:2150-2159.
579a. Blizzard R. Psychosocial short stature. In: Lifshitz F, ed. *Pediatric Endocrinology*. New York: Marcel Dekker; 1985:87-107.
579b. Powell GF, Brasel JA, Blizzard RM. Emotional deprivation and growth retardation simulating idiopathic hypopituitarism. I. Clinical evaluation of the syndrome. *N Engl J Med*. 1957;276:1271-1278.
579c. Blizzard RM, Bulatovie A. Psychosocial short stanture: a syndrome with many variables. *Vlin Endocrinol Metab*. 1992:6:687-712.
579d. Skuse D, Albanese A, Stanhope R, et al. A new tress-related syndrome of growth failure and hyperphagia in children. associated with reversitbility of growth-hormone insulficiency. *Lancet*. 1996;348:353-358.
579e. Stanhope R, Adlard P, Hamill G, et al. Physiological growth hormone (GH) secretion during the recovery from psychosocial dwarfism: a case report. *Clin Endocrinol*. 1988:28;335-339.
579f. Albanese A, Hamill G, Jones J, et al. Physiological growth hormone secretion in children with psychosocial dwarlism. *Clin Endocrinol*. 1994;40:687-692.
579g. Skuse D. Emotional abuse and delay in growth. *Br Med J*. 1989; 299:113-115.
579h. Miller JD, Tannenbaum GS, Colle E, et al. Daytime pulsatile growth hormone secretion in children with psychosocial dwarfism. *Clin Endocrinol*. 1982;27:581-591.
579i. Brambilla F, Perna G, Garberi A, et al. Alpha-2 adrenergic receptor sensitivity in panic disorder. I. GH response to GHRH and clonidine stimulation in panic disorder. *Psychoneuroendocrinology*. 1995;20:1-9.
579j. Charney DS, Heninger GR, Sternberg DE, et al. Adrenergic receptor sensitivity in depression. Effects of clonidine in depressed patients and healthy subjects. *Arch Gen Psychiatry*. 1982;39:290-291.
579k. Pine DS, Cohen P, Brook J. Emotional problems during youth as predictors of stature during early adulthood: Results from a prospective epidemiologic study. *Pediatrics*. 1996;97:856-863.
579l. Jensen JB, Garfinkel BD. Growth hormone dysregulation in children with major depressive disorder. *J Am Acad Child Adolecs Psychiatry*. 1990;29:295-301.
580. Mayfield RK, Levine JH, Gordon L, et al. Lymphoid adenohypophysitis presenting as a pituitary tumor. *Am J Med*. 1980;69:619-623.
581. Bartsocas CS, Pantelakis SN. Human growth hormone therapy in hypopituitarism due to tuberculous meningitis. *Acta Paediatr Scand*. 1973;62:304-306.
582. Stuart CA, Neelon FA, Lebovitz HE. Hypothalamic insufficiency: the cause of hypopituitarism in sarcoidosis. *Ann Intern Med*. 1978;88: 589-594.
583. Costin G. Endocrine disorders associated with tumors of the pituitary and hypothalamus. *Pediatr Clin North Am*. 1979;26:15-31.
584. Vassilopoulou-Sellin R, Klein MJ, Slopis JK. Growth hormone deficiency in children with neurofibromatosis type 1 without suprasellar lesions. *Pediatr Neurol*. 2000;22:355-358.
585. Carmi D, Shohat M, Metzker A, et al. Growth, puberty, and endocrine functions in patients with sporadic or familial neurofibromatosis type 1: a longitudinal study. *Pediatrics*. 1999;103(6 Pt 1):1257-1262.

586. Weinzimer SA, Homan SA, Ferry RJ, et al. Serum IGF-I and IGFBP-3 concentrations do not accurately predict growth hormone deficiency in children with brain tumours. *Clin Endocrinol (Oxf)*. 1999;51:339-345.
587. Miller WL, Kaplan SL, Grumbach MM. Child abuse as a cause of post-traumatic hypopituitarism. *N Engl J Med*. 1980;302:724-728.
588. Kelly DF, Gonzalo IT, Cohan P, et al. Hypopituitarism following traumatic brain injury and aneurysmal subarachnoid hemorrhage: a preliminary report. *J Neurosurg*. 2000;93:743-752.
589. Carel JC. Growth hormone in Turner syndrome: twenty years after, what can we tell our patients? *J Clin Endocrinol Metab*. 2005;90:3793-3794.
590. Leal-Cerro A, Flores JM, Rincon M, et al. Prevalence of hypopituitarism and growth hormone deficiency in adults long-term after severe traumatic brain injury. *Clin Endocrinol (Oxf)*. 2005;62:525-532.
591. Bondanelli M, Ambrosio MR, Zatelli MC, et al. Hypopituitarism after traumatic brain injury. *Eur J Endocrinol*. 2005;152:679-691.
592. Perez Jurado LA, Argente J. Molecular basis of familial growth hormone deficiency. *Horm Res*. 1994;42:189-197.
593. Parks JS, Pfaffle RW, Brown MR, et al. Growth hormone deficiency. In: Weintraub BD, ed. *Molecular endocrinology: basic concepts and clinical correlations*. New York, NY: Raven; 1995.
594. Phillips 3rd JA, Cogan JD. Genetic basis of endocrine disease: 6. Molecular basis of familial human growth hormone deficiency. *J Clin Endocrinol Metab*. 1994;78:11-16.
595. Suh H, Gage PJ, Drouin J, et al. Pitx2 is required at multiple stages of pituitary organogenesis: pituitary primordium formation and cell specification. *Development*. 2002;129:329-337.
596. Drouin J, Lamolet B, Lamonerie T, et al. The PTX family of homeodomain transcription factors during pituitary developments. *Mol Cell Endocrinol*. 1998;140:31-36.
597. Tremblay JJ, Lanctot C, Drouin J. The pan-pituitary activator of transcription, Ptx1 (pituitary homeobox 1), acts in synergy with SF-1 and Pit1 and is an upstream regulator of the lim-homeodomain gene Lim3/Lhx3. *Mol Endocrinol*. 1998;12:428-441.
598. Tremblay JJ, Goodyer CG, Drouin J. Transcriptional properties of Ptx1 and Ptx2 isoforms. *Neuroendocrinology*. 2000;71:277-286.
599. Quentien MH, Manfroid I, Moncet D, et al. Pitx factors are involved in basal and hormone-regulated activity of the human prolactin promoter. *J Biol Chem*. 2002;277:44408-44416.
600. Lin CR, Kioussi C, O'Connell S, et al. Pitx2 regulates lung asymmetry, cardiac positioning and pituitary and tooth morphogenesis. *Nature*. 1999;401:279-282.
601. Lu MF, Pressman C, Dyer R, et al. Function of Rieger syndrome gene in left-right asymmetry and craniofacial development. *Nature*. 1999;401:276-278.
602. Kitamura K, Miura H, Miyagawa-Tomita S, et al. Mouse Pitx2 deficiency leads to anomalies of the ventral body wall, heart, extra- and periocular mesoderm and right pulmonary isomerism. *Development*. 1999;126:5749-5758.
603. Gage PJ, Suh H, Camper SA. Dosage requirement of Pitx2 for development of multiple organs. *Development*. 1999;126:4643-4651.
604. Kioussi C, Briata P, Baek SH, et al. Identification of a Wnt/Dvl/beta-catenin → Pitx2 pathway mediating cell-type-specific proliferation during development. *Cell*. 2002;111:673-685.
605. Briata P, Ilengo C, Corte G, et al. The Wnt/beta-catenin → Pitx2 pathway controls the turnover of Pitx2 and other unstable mRNAs. *Mol Cell*. 2003;12:1201-1211.
606. Charles MA, Suh H, Hjalt TA, et al. PITX genes are required for cell survival and Lhx3 activation. *Mol Endocrinol*. 2005;19:1893-1903.
607. Suh H, Gage PJ, Drouin J, et al. Pitx2 is required at multiple stages of pituitary organogenesis: pituitary primordium formation and cell specification. *Development*. 2002;129:329-337.
608. Amendt BA, Semina EV, Alward WL. Rieger syndrome: a clinical, molecular, and biochemical analysis. *Cell Mol Life Sci*. 2000;57:1652-1666.
609. Saadi I, Semina EV, Amendt BA, et al. Identification of a dominant negative homeodomain mutation in Rieger syndrome. *J Biol Chem*. 2001;276:23034-23041.
610. Hunter CS, Rhodes SJ. LIM-homeodomain genes in mammalian development and human disease. *Mol Biol Rep*. 2005;32:67-77.
611. Sheng HZ, Zhadanov AB, Mosinger Jr B, et al. Specification of pituitary cell lineages by the LIM homeobox gene Lhx3. *Science*. 1996;272:1004-1007.
612. Sloop KW, Dwyer CJ, Rhodes SJ. An isoform-specific inhibitory domain regulates the LHX3 LIM homeodomain factor holoprotein and the production of a functional alternate translation form. *J Biol Chem*. 2001;276:36311-36319.
613. Pfaeffle RW, Savage JJ, Hunter CS, et al. Four novel mutations of the LHX3 gene cause combined pituitary hormone deficiencies with or without limited neck rotation. *J Clin Endocrinol Metab*. 2007;92:1909-1919.
614. Bhangoo AP, Hunter CS, Savage JJ, et al. Clinical case seminar: a novel LHX3 mutation presenting as combined pituitary hormonal deficiency. *J Clin Endocrinol Metab*. 2006;91:747-753.
615. Mullen RD, Colvin SC, Hunter CS, et al. Roles of the LHX3 and LHX4 LIM-homeodomain factors in pituitary development. *Mol Cell Endocrinol*. 2007;265-266:190-195.
616. Raetzman LT, Ward R, Camper SA. Lhx4 and Prop1 are required for cell survival and expansion of the pituitary primordia. *Development*. 2002;129:4229-4239.
617. Sheng HZ, Moriyama K, Yamashita T, et al. Multistep control of pituitary organogenesis. *Science*. 1997;278:1809-1812.
618. Machinis K, Amselem S. Functional relationship between LHX4 and POU1F1 in light of the LHX4 mutation identified in patients with pituitary defects. *J Clin Endocrinol Metab*. 2005;90:5456-5462.
619. Machinis K, Pantel J, Netchine I, et al. Syndromic short stature in patients with a germline mutation in the LIM homeobox LHX4. *Am J Hum Genet*. 2001;69:961-968.
620. Pfaeffle RW, Hunter CS, Savage JJ, et al. Three novel missense mutations within the LHX4 gene are associated with variable pituitary hormone deficiencies. *J Clin Endocrinol Metab*. 2008;93:1062-1071.
621. Tajima T, Hattori T, Nakajima T, et al. A novel missense mutation (P366T) of the LHX4 gene causes severe combined pituitary hormone deficiency with pituitary hypoplasia, ectopic posterior lobe and a poorly developed sella turcica. *Endocr J*. 2007;54:637-641.
622. Gallardo ME, Rodriguez De Cordoba S, et al. Analysis of the developmental SIX6 homeobox gene in patients with anophthalmia/microphthalmia. *Am J Med Genet A*. 2004;129A:92-94.
623. Brinkmeier ML, Potok MA, Davis SW, et al. TCF4 deficiency expands ventral diencephalon signaling and increases induction of pituitary progenitors. *Dev Biol*. 2007;311:396-407.
624. Zhu CC, Dyer MA, Uchikawa M, et al. Six3-mediated auto repression and eye development requires its interaction with members of the Groucho-related family of co-repressors. *Development*. 2002;129:2835-2849.
625. Lopez-Rios J, Tessmar K, Loosli F, et al. Six3 and Six6 activity is modulated by members of the Groucho family. *Development*. 2003;130:185-195.
626. Nolen LD, Amor D, Haywood A, et al. Deletion at 14q22-23 indicates a contiguous gene syndrome comprising anophthalmia, pituitary hypoplasia, and ear anomalies. *Am J Med Genet A*. 2006;140:1711-1718.
627. Susa T, Ishikawa A, Cai LY, et al. The highly related LIM factors, LMO1, LMO3 and LMO4, play different roles in the regulation of the pituitary glycoprotein hormone alpha-subunit (alpha GSU) gene. *Biosci Rep*. 2009;30:51-58.
628. Cai Y, Xu Z, Nagarajan L, et al. Single-stranded DNA-binding proteins regulate the abundance and function of the LIM-homeodomain transcription factor LHX2 in pituitary cells. *Biochem Biophys Res Commun*. 2008;373:303-308.
629. Takuma N, Sheng HZ, Furuta Y, et al. Formation of Rathke's pouch requires dual induction from the diencephalon. *Development*. 1998;125:4835-4840.
630. Kelberman D, Dattani MT. Hypothalamic and pituitary development: novel insights into the aetiology. *Eur J Endocrinol*. 2007;157(suppl 1):S3-S14.
631. Lopez-Bermejo A, Buckway CK, Rosenfeld RG. Genetic defects of the growth hormone-insulin-like growth factor axis. *Trends Endocrinol Metab*. 2000;11:39-49.
632. Parks JS, Brown MR, Hurley DL, et al. Heritable disorders of pituitary development. *J Clin Endocrinol Metab*. 1999;84:4362-4370.
633. Chen J, Crabbe A, Van Duppen V, et al. The notch signaling system is present in the postnatal pituitary: marked expression and regulatory activity in the newly discovered side population. *Mol Endocrinol*. 2006;20:3293-3307.
634. Kita A, Imayoshi I, Hojo M, et al. Hes1 and Hes5 control the progenitor pool, intermediate lobe specification, and posterior lobe formation in the pituitary development. *Mol Endocrinol*. 2007;21:1458-1466.
635. Gage PJ, Brinkmeier ML, Scarlett LM, et al. The Ames dwarf gene, df, is required early in pituitary ontogeny for the extinction of rpx transcription and initiation of lineage-specific cell proliferation. *Mol Endocrinol*. 1996;10:1570-1581.
636. Ward RD, Raetzman LT, Suh H, et al. Role of PROP1 in pituitary gland growth. *Mol Endocrinol*. 2005;19:698-710.
637. Raetzman LT, Ross SA, Cook S, et al. Developmental regulation of notch signaling genes in the embryonic pituitary: Prop1 deficiency affects Notch2 expression. *Dev Biol*. 2004;265:329-340.
638. Ward RD, Stone BM, Raetzman LT, et al. Cell proliferation and vascularization in mouse models of pituitary hormone deficiency. *Mol Endocrinol*. 2006;20:1378-1390.
639. Andersen B, Pearse 2nd RV, Jenne K, et al. The Ames dwarf gene is required for Pit-1 gene activation. *Dev Biol*. 1995;172:495-503.
640. Olson LE, Tollkuhn J, Scafoglio C, et al. Homeodomain-mediated beta-catenin-dependent switching events dictate cell-lineage determination. *Cell*. 2006;125:593-605.
641. Bartke A. Histology of the anterior hypophysis, thyroid and gonads of two types of dwarf mice. *Anat Rec*. 1964;149:225-235.

642. Bartke A. The response of two types of dwarf mice to growth hormone, thyrotropin, and thyroxine. *Gen Comp Endocrinol*. 1965;5:418-426.
643. Fluck C, Deladoey J, Rutishauser K, et al. Phenotypic variability in familial combined pituitary hormone deficiency caused by a PROP1 gene mutation resulting in the substitution of arg → Cys at codon 120 (R120C). *J Clin Endocrinol Metab*. 1998;83:3727-3734.
644. Osorio MG, Kopp P, Marui S, et al. Combined pituitary hormone deficiency caused by a novel mutation of a highly conserved residue (F88S) in the homeodomain of PROP-1. *J Clin Endocrinol Metab*. 2000;85:2779-2785.
645. Lebl J, Vosahlo J, Pfaeffle RW, et al. Auxological and endocrine phenotype in a population-based cohort of patients with PROP1 gene defects. *Eur J Endocrinol*. 2005;153:389-396.
646. Vieira TC, da Silva MR, Abucham J. The natural history of the R120C PROP1 mutation reveals a wide phenotypic variability in two untreated adult brothers with combined pituitary hormone deficiency. *Endocrine*. 2006;30:365-369.
647. Deladoey J, Fluck C, Buyukgebiz A, et al. "Hot spot" in the PROP1 gene responsible for combined pituitary hormone deficiency. *J Clin Endocrinol Metab*. 1999;84:1645-1650.
648. Dattani MT. GH deficiency might be associated with normal height in PROP1 deficiency. *Clin Endocrinol (Oxf)*. 2002;57:157-158.
649. Arroyo A, Pernasetti F, Vasilyev VV, et al. A unique case of combined pituitary hormone deficiency caused by a PROP1 gene mutation (R120C) associated with normal height and absent puberty. *Clin Endocrinol (Oxf)*. 2002;57:283-291.
650. Pavel ME, Hensen J, Pfaffle R, et al. Long-term follow-up of childhood-onset hypopituitarism in patients with the PROP-1 gene mutation. *Horm Res*. 2003;60:168-173.
651. Voutetakis A, Argyropoulou M, Sertedaki A, et al. Pituitary magnetic resonance imaging in 15 patients with Prop1 gene mutations: pituitary enlargement may originate from the intermediate lobe. *J Clin Endocrinol Metab*. 2004;89:2200-2206.
652. Rosenbloom AL, Almonte AS, Brown MR, et al. Clinical and biochemical phenotype of familial anterior hypopituitarism from mutation of the PROP1 gene. *J Clin Endocrinol Metab*. 1999;84: 50-57.
653. Mendonca BB, Osorio MG, Latronico AC, et al. Longitudinal hormonal and pituitary imaging changes in two females with combined pituitary hormone deficiency due to deletion of A301,G302 in the PROP1 gene. *J Clin Endocrinol Metab*. 1999;84:942-945.
654. Agarwal G, Bhatia V, Cook S, et al. Adrenocorticotropin deficiency in combined pituitary hormone deficiency patients homozygous for a novel PROP1 deletion. *J Clin Endocrinol Metab*. 2000;85:4556-4561.
655. Asteria C, Oliveira JH, Abucham J, et al. Central hypocortisolism as part of combined pituitary hormone deficiency due to mutations of PROP-1 gene. *Eur J Endocrinol*. 2000;143:347-352.
656. Bottner A, Keller E, Kratzsch J, et al. PROP1 mutations cause progressive deterioration of anterior pituitary function including adrenal insufficiency: a longitudinal analysis. *J Clin Endocrinol Metab*. 2004;89:5256-5265.
657. Vallette-Kasic S, Barlier A, Teinturier C, et al. PROP1 gene screening in patients with multiple pituitary hormone deficiency reveals two sites of hypermutability and a high incidence of corticotroph deficiency. *J Clin Endocrinol Metab*. 2001;86:4529-4535.
658. Duquesnoy P, Roy A, Dastot F, et al. Human prop-1: cloning, mapping, genomic structure: mutations in familial combined pituitary hormone deficiency. *FEBS Lett*. 1998;437:216-220.
659. Fofanova O, Takamura N, Kinoshita E, et al. Compound heterozygous deletion of the PROP-1 gene in children with combined pituitary hormone deficiency. *J Clin Endocrinol Metab*. 1998;83:2601-2604.
660. Wu W, Cogan JD, Pfaffle RW, et al. Mutations in PROP1 cause familial combined pituitary hormone deficiency. *Nat Genet*. 1998;18:147-149.
661. Kelberman D, Turton JP, Woods KS, et al. Molecular analysis of novel PROP1 mutations associated with combined pituitary hormone deficiency (CPHD). *Clin Endocrinol (Oxf)*. 2009;70:96-103.
662. Rainbow LA, Rees SA, Shaikh MG, et al. Mutation analysis of POUF-1, PROP-1 and HESX-1 show low frequency of mutations in children with sporadic forms of combined pituitary hormone deficiency and septo-optic dysplasia. *Clin Endocrinol (Oxf)*. 2005;62:163-168.
663. Turton JP, Reynaud R, Mehta A, et al. Novel mutations within the POU1F1 gene associated with variable combined pituitary hormone deficiency. *J Clin Endocrinol Metab*. 2005;90:4762-4770.
664. Procter AM, Phillips 3rd JA, Cooper DN. The molecular genetics of growth hormone deficiency. *Hum Genet*. 1998;103:255-272.
665. Nelson C, Albert VR, Elsholtz HP, et al. Activation of cell-specific expression of rat growth hormone and prolactin genes by a common transcription factor. *Science*. 1988;239:1400-1405.
666. Mangalam HJ, Albert VR, Ingraham HA, et al. A pituitary POU domain protein, pit-1, activates both growth hormone and prolactin promoters transcriptionally. *Genes Dev*. 1989;3:946-958.
667. Lin SC, Lin CR, Gukovsky I, et al. Molecular basis of the little mouse phenotype and implications for cell type-specific growth. *Nature*. 1993;364:208-213.
668. Cohen LE, Zanger K, Brue T, et al. Defective retinoic acid regulation of the pit-1 gene enhancer: a novel mechanism of combined pituitary hormone deficiency. *Mol Endocrinol*. 1999;13:476-484.
669. Parks JS, Kinoshita E, Pfaffle RW. Pit-1 and hypopituitarism. *Trends Endocrinol Metab*. 1993;4:81-85.
670. Montminy M. Cell differentiation: the road not taken. *Nature*. 1993;364:190-191.
671. Xu L, Lavinsky RM, Dasen JS, et al. Signal-specific co-activator domain requirements for pit-1 activation. *Nature*. 1998;395:301-306.
672. Pfaffle RW, DiMattia GE, Parks JS, et al. Mutation of the POU-specific domain of pit-1 and hypopituitarism without pituitary hypoplasia. *Science*. 1992;257:1118-1121.
673. Buckwalter MS, Katz RW, Camper SA. Localization of the panhypopituitary dwarf mutation (df) on mouse chromosome 11 in an intersubspecific backcross. *Genomics*. 1991;10:515-526.
674. Cogan JD, Phillips 3rd JA, Sakati N, et al. Heterogeneous growth hormone (GH) gene mutations in familial GH deficiency. *J Clin Endocrinol Metab*. 1993;76:1224-1228.
675. Wit JM, Drayer NM, Jansen M, et al. Total deficiency of growth hormone and prolactin, and partial deficiency of thyroid stimulating hormone in two Dutch families: a new variant of hereditary pituitary deficiency. *Horm Res*. 1989;32:170-177.
676. Cogan JD, Phillips 3rd JA, Schenkman SS, et al. Familial growth hormone deficiency: a model of dominant and recessive mutations affecting a monomeric protein. *J Clin Endocrinol Metab*. 1994;79: 1261-1265.
677. Cohen LE, Wondisford FE, Salvatoni A, et al. A "hot spot" in the pit-1 gene responsible for combined pituitary hormone deficiency: clinical and molecular correlates. *J Clin Endocrinol Metab*. 1995;80: 679-684.
678. Tatsumi K, Miyai K, Notomi T, et al. Cretinism with combined hormone deficiency caused by a mutation in the PIT1 gene. *Nat Genet*. 1992;1:56-58.
679. Pellegrini-Bouiller I, Belicar P, Barlier A, et al. A new mutation of the gene encoding the transcription factor pit-1 is responsible for combined pituitary hormone deficiency. *J Clin Endocrinol Metab*. 1996;81:2790-2796.
680. Haqq AM, Stadler DD, Jackson RH, et al. Effects of growth hormone on pulmonary function, sleep quality, behavior, cognition, growth velocity, body composition, and resting energy expenditure in Prader-Willi syndrome. *J Clin Endocrinol Metab*. 2003;88:2206-2212.
681. Snabboon T, Plengpanich W, Buranasupkajorn P, et al. A novel germline mutation, IVS4+1G>A, of the POU1F1 gene underlying combined pituitary hormone deficiency. *Horm Res*. 2008;69:60-64.
682. Miyata I, Vallette-Kasic S, Saveanu A, et al. Identification and functional analysis of the novel S179R POU1F1 mutation associated with combined pituitary hormone deficiency. *J Clin Endocrinol Metab*. 2006;91:4981-4987.
683. Radovick S, Nations M, Du Y, et al. A mutation in the POU-homeodomain of pit-1 responsible for combined pituitary hormone deficiency. *Science*. 1992;257:1115-1118.
684. Pfaffle R, Kim C, Otten B, et al. Pit-1: clinical aspects. *Horm Res*. 1996;45(suppl 1):25-28.
685. Mosier Jr HD, Smith Jr FG, Schultz MA. Failure of catch-up growth after Cushing's syndrome in childhood. *Am J Dis Child*. 1972;124:251-253.
686. Cutfield WS, Wilton P, Bennmarker H, et al. Incidence of diabetes mellitus and impaired glucose tolerance in children and adolescents receiving growth-hormone treatment. *Lancet*. 2000;355:610-613.
687. Arnhold IJ, Nery M, Brown MR, et al. Clinical and molecular characterization of a Brazilian patient with pit-1 deficiency. *J Pediatr Endocrinol Metab*. 1998;11:623-630.
688. Kelberman D, Dattani MT. Hypopituitarism oddities: congenital causes. *Horm Res*. 2007;68(suppl 5):138-144.
689. Pellegrini I, Roche C, Quentien MH, et al. Involvement of the pituitary-specific transcription factor pit-1 in somatolactotrope cell growth and death: an approach using dominant-negative pit-1 mutants. *Mol Endocrinol*. 2006;20:3212-3227.
690. Cohen RN, Brue T, Naik K, et al. The role of CBP/p300 interactions and Pit-1 dimerization in the pathophysiological mechanism of combined pituitary hormone deficiency. *J Clin Endocrinol Metab*. 2006;91:239-247.
691. Bondy CA, Van PL, Bakalov VK, et al. Growth hormone treatment and aortic dimensions in Turner syndrome. *J Clin Endocrinol Metab*. 2006;91:1785-1788.
692. Rona RJ, Tanner JM. Aetiology of idiopathic growth hormone deficiency in England and Wales. *Arch Dis Child*. 1977;52:197-208.
693. Vimpani GV, Vimpani AF, Lidgard GP, et al. Prevalence of severe growth hormone deficiency. *Br Med J*. 1977;2:427-430.
694. Lindsay R, Feldkamp M, Harris D, et al. Utah growth study: growth standards and the prevalence of growth hormone deficiency. *J Pediatr*. 1994;125:29-35.
695. Mullis PE. Genetic control of growth. *Eur J Endocrinol*. 2005;152: 11-31.

696. Illig R, Prader A, Ferrandez A, et al. Hereditary prenatal growth hormone deficiency with increased tendency to growth hormone antibody formation ("A-type" of isolated growth hormone deficiency). *Acta Paediatr Scand*. 1971;60:607.
697. Wagner JK, Eble A, Hindmarsh PC, et al. Prevalence of human GH-1 gene alterations in patients with isolated growth hormone deficiency. *Pediatr Res*. 1998;43:105-110.
698. Cao Y, Wagner JK, Hindmarsh PC, et al. Isolated growth hormone deficiency: testing the little mouse hypothesis in man and exclusion of mutations within the extracellular domain of the growth hormone-releasing hormone receptor. *Pediatr Res*. 1995;38:962-966.
699. Salvatori R, Fan X, Phillips 3rd JA, et al. Three new mutations in the gene for the growth hormone (GH)-releasing hormone receptor in familial isolated GH deficiency type Ib. *J Clin Endocrinol Metab*. 2001;86:273-279.
700. Hayashi Y, Yamamoto M, Ohmori S, et al. Inhibition of growth hormone (GH) secretion by a mutant GH-I gene product in neuroendocrine cells containing secretory granules: an implication for isolated GH deficiency inherited in an autosomal dominant manner. *J Clin Endocrinol Metab*. 1999;84:2134-2139.
701. Lee MS, Wajnrajch MP, Kim SS, et al. Autosomal dominant growth hormone (GH) deficiency type II: the Del32-71-GH deletion mutant suppresses secretion of wild-type GH. *Endocrinology*. 2000;141: 883-890.
702. Woods KA, Dastot F, Preece MA, et al. Phenotype: genotype relationships in growth hormone insensitivity syndrome. *J Clin Endocrinol Metab*. 1997;82:3529-3535.
703. Binder G, Keller E, Mix M, et al. Isolated GH deficiency with dominant inheritance: new mutations, new insights. *J Clin Endocrinol Metab*. 2001;86:3877-3881.
704. Deladoey J, Stocker P, Mullis PE. Autosomal dominant GH deficiency due to an Arg183His GH-1 gene mutation: clinical and molecular evidence of impaired regulated GH secretion. *J Clin Endocrinol Metab*. 2001;86:3941-3947.
705. Mullis PE, Robinson IC, Salemi S, et al. Isolated autosomal dominant growth hormone deficiency: an evolving pituitary deficit? A multicenter follow-up study. *J Clin Endocrinol Metab*. 2005;90: 2089-2096.
706. Gaylinn BD, Dealmeida VI, Lyons Jr CE, et al. The mutant growth hormone-releasing hormone (GHRH) receptor of the little mouse does not bind GHRH. *Endocrinology*. 1999;140:5066-5074.
707. Godfrey P, Rahal JO, Beamer WG, et al. GHRH receptor of little mice contains a missense mutation in the extracellular domain that disrupts receptor function. *Nat Genet*. 1993;4:227-232.
708. Mayo KE, Godfrey PA, Suhr ST, et al. Growth hormone-releasing hormone: synthesis and signaling. *Recent Prog Horm Res*. 1995; 50:35-73.
709. Gaylinn BD. Molecular and cell biology of the growth hormone-releasing hormone receptor. *Growth Horm IGF Res*. 1999;9(suppl A):37-44.
710. Mayo KE. Molecular cloning and expression of a pituitary-specific receptor for growth hormone-releasing hormone. *Mol Endocrinol*. 1992;6:1734-1744.
711. Gaylinn BD, Harrison JK, Zysk JR, et al. Molecular cloning and expression of a human anterior pituitary receptor for growth hormone-releasing hormone. *Mol Endocrinol*. 1993;7:77-84.
712. Wajnrajch MP, Gertner JM, Harbison MD, et al. Nonsense mutation in the human growth hormone-releasing hormone receptor causes growth failure analogous to the little (lit) mouse. *Nat Genet*. 1996;12:88-90.
713. Netchine I, Talon P, Dastot F, et al. Extensive phenotypic analysis of a family with growth hormone (GH) deficiency caused by a mutation in the GH-releasing hormone receptor gene. *J Clin Endocrinol Metab*. 1998;83:432-436.
714. Maheshwari HG, Silverman BL, Dupuis J, et al. Phenotype and genetic analysis of a syndrome caused by an inactivating mutation in the growth hormone-releasing hormone receptor: dwarfism of sindh. *J Clin Endocrinol Metab*. 1998;83:4065-4074.
715. Baumann G, Maheshwari H. The Dwarfs of Sindh: severe growth hormone (GH) deficiency caused by a mutation in the GH-releasing hormone receptor gene. *Acta Paediatr Suppl*. 1997;423:33-38.
716. Kamijo T, Hayashi Y, Seo H, et al. A nonsense mutation (E72X) in growth hormone releasing hormone receptor (GHRHR) gene is the major cause of familial isolated growth hormone deficiency in Western region of India: founder effect suggested by analysis of dinucleotide repeat polymorphism close to GHRHR gene. *Growth Horm IGF Res*. 2004;14:394-401.
717. Yokoyama Y, Narahara K, Tsuji K, et al. Growth hormone deficiency and empty sella syndrome in a boy with dup(X) (q13.3-q21.2). *Am J Med Genet*. 1992;42:660-664.
718. Aguiar-Oliveira MH, Gill MS, de A Barretto ES, et al. Effect of severe growth hormone (GH) deficiency due to a mutation in the GH-releasing hormone receptor on insulin-like growth factors (IGFs), IGF-binding proteins, and ternary complex formation throughout life. *J Clin Endocrinol Metab*. 1999;84:4118-4126.
719. Haskin O, Lazar L, Jaber L, et al. A new mutation in the growth hormone-releasing hormone receptor gene in two Israeli Arab families. *J Endocrinol Invest*. 2006;29:122-130.
720. Menezes Oliveira JL, Marques-Santos C, Barreto-Filho JA, et al. Lack of evidence of premature atherosclerosis in untreated severe isolated growth hormone (GH) deficiency due to a GH-releasing hormone receptor mutation. *J Clin Endocrinol Metab*. 2006;91:2093-2099.
721. Fleisher TA, White RM, Broder S, et al. X-linked hypogammaglobulinemia and isolated growth hormone deficiency. *N Engl J Med*. 1980;302:1429-1434.
722. Solomon NM, Nouri S, Warne GL, et al. Increased gene dosage at Xq26-q27 is associated with X-linked hypopituitarism. *Genomics*. 2002;79:553-559.
723. Valenta LJ, Sigel MB, Lesniak MA, et al. Pituitary dwarfism in a patient with circulating abnormal growth hormone polymers. *N Engl J Med*. 1985;312:214-217.
724. Kowarski AA, Schneider J, Ben-Galim E, et al. Growth failure with normal serum RIA-GH and low somatomedin activity: somatomedin restoration and growth acceleration after exogenous GH. *J Clin Endocrinol Metab*. 1978;47:461-464.
725. Takahashi Y, Kaji H, Okimura Y, et al. Brief report: short stature caused by a mutant growth hormone. *N Engl J Med*. 1996;334:432-436.
726. Takahashi Y, Shirono H, Arisaka O, et al. Biologically inactive growth hormone caused by an amino acid substitution. *J Clin Invest*. 1997;100:1159-1165.
727. Ishikawa M, Nimura A, Horikawa R, et al. A novel specific bioassay for serum human growth hormone. *J Clin Endocrinol Metab*. 2000;85:4274-4279.
728. Millar DS, Lewis MD, Horan M, et al. Novel mutations of the growth hormone 1 (GH1) gene disclosed by modulation of the clinical selection criteria for individuals with short stature. *Hum Mutat*. 2003;21:424-440.
729. Besson A, Salemi S, Deladoey J, et al. Short stature caused by a biologically inactive mutant growth hormone (GH-C53S). *J Clin Endocrinol Metab*. 2005;90:2493-2499.
730. Ross M, Francis GL, Szabo L, et al. Insulin-like growth factor (IGF)-binding proteins inhibit the biological activities of IGF-1 and IGF-2 but not des-(1-3)-IGF-1. *Biochem J*. 1989;258:267-272.
731. Radetti G, Bozzola M, Pagani S, et al. Growth hormone immunoreactivity does not reflect bioactivity. *Pediatr Res*. 2000;48:619-622.
732. Jenkins JS, Gilbert CJ, Ang V. Hypothalamic-pituitary function in patients with craniopharyngiomas. *J Clin Endocrinol Metab*. 1976; 43:394-399.
733. Thomsett MJ, Conte FA, Kaplan SL, et al. Endocrine and neurologic outcome in childhood craniopharyngioma: review of effect of treatment in 42 patients. *J Pediatr*. 1980;97:728-735.
734. Lafferty AR, Chrousos GP. Pituitary tumors in children and adolescents. *J Clin Endocrinol Metab*. 1999;84:4317-4323.
735. Laws ER, Thapar K. The diagnosis and management of craniopharyngioma. *Growth Genet Hormones*. 1994;10:6-10.
736. Paja M, Lucas T, Garcia-Uria J, et al. Hypothalamic-pituitary dysfunction in patients with craniopharyngioma. *Clin Endocrinol (Oxf)*. 1995;42:467-473.
737. Rivarola MA, Mendilaharzu H, Warman M, et al. Endocrine disorders in 66 suprasellar and pineal tumors of patients with prepubertal and pubertal ages. *Horm Res*. 1992;37:1-6.
738. Kane LA, Leinung MC, Scheithauer BW, et al. Pituitary adenomas in childhood and adolescence. *J Clin Endocrinol Metab*. 1994;79: 1135-1140.
739. Fraioli B, Ferrante L, Celli P. Pituitary adenomas with onset during puberty: features and treatment. *J Neurosurg*. 1983;59:590-595.
740. Maira G, Anile C. Pituitary tumors in childhood and adolescence. *Can J Neurol Sci*. 1990;65:733-744.
741. Muller HL, Emser A, Faldum A, et al. Longitudinal study on growth and body mass index before and after diagnosis of childhood craniopharyngioma. *J Clin Endocrinol Metab*. 2004;89:3298-3305.
742. DeVile CJ, Grant DB, Hayward RD, et al. Growth and endocrine sequelae of craniopharyngioma. *Arch Dis Child*. 1996;75:108-114.
743. Geffner M, Lundberg M, Koltowska-Haggstrom M, et al. Changes in height, weight, and body mass index in children with craniopharyngioma after three years of growth hormone therapy: analysis of KIGS (Pfizer International Growth Database). *J Clin Endocrinol Metab*. 2004;89:5435-5440.
744. Srinivasan S, Ogle GD, Garnett SP, et al. Features of the metabolic syndrome after childhood craniopharyngioma. *J Clin Endocrinol Metab*. 2004;89:81-86.
745. Richmond IL, Wilson CB. Pituitary adenomas in childhood and adolescence. *J Neurosurg*. 1978;49:163-168.
746. Egeler RM, D'Angio GJ. Langerhans cell histiocytosis. *J Pediatr*. 1996;127:1-11.
747. Braunstein GD, Kohler PO. Pituitary function in Hand-Schuller-Christian disease: evidence for deficient growth-hormone release in patients with short stature. *N Engl J Med*. 1972;286:1225-1229.
748. Broadbent V, Dunger DB, Yeomans E, et al. Anterior pituitary function and computed tomography/magnetic resonance imaging in

patients with Langerhans cell histiocytosis and diabetes insipidus. *Med Pediatr Oncol*. 1993;21:649-654.
749. Maghnie M, Cosi G, Genovese E, et al. Central diabetes insipidus in children and young adults. *N Engl J Med*. 2000;343:998-1007.
750. Donadieu J, Rolon MA, Thomas C, et al. French LCH Study Group. Endocrine involvement in pediatric-onset Langerhans' cell histiocytosis: a population-based study. *J Pediatr*. 2004;144:344-350.
751. Dean HJ, Bishop A, Winter JS. Growth hormone deficiency in patients with histiocytosis X. *J Pediatr*. 1996;109:615-618.
752. Laron Z. The essential role of IGF-I: lessons from the long-term study and treatment of children and adults with Laron syndrome. *J Clin Endocrinol Metab*. 1999;84:4397-4404.
753. Laron Z, Pertzelan A, Mannheimer S. Genetic pituitary dwarfism with high serum concentation of growth hormone: a new inborn error of metabolism? *Isr J Med Sci*. 1966;2:152-155.
754. Rosenbloom AL, Guevara Aguirre J, Rosenfeld RG, et al. The little women of Loja: growth hormone-receptor deficiency in an inbred population of southern Ecuador. *N Engl J Med*. 1990;323:1367-1374.
755. Savage MO, Blum WF, Ranke MB, et al. Clinical features and endocrine status in patients with growth hormone insensitivity (Laron syndrome). *J Clin Endocrinol Metab*. 1993;77:1465-1471.
756. Golde DW, Bersch N, Kaplan SA, et al. Peripheral unresponsiveness to human growth hormone in Laron dwarfism. *N Engl J Med*. 1980;303:1156-1159.
757. Daughaday WH, Trivedi B. Absence of serum growth hormone binding protein in patients with growth hormone receptor deficiency (Laron dwarfism). *Proc Natl Acad Sci U S A*. 1987;84:4636-4640.
758. Baumann G, Shaw MA, Winter RJ. Absence of the plasma growth hormone-binding protein in Laron-type dwarfism. *J Clin Endocrinol Metab*. 1987;65:814-816.
759. Eshet R, Laron Z, Pertzelan A, et al. Defect of human growth hormone receptors in the liver of two patients with Laron-type dwarfism. *Isr J Med Sci*. 1984;20:8-11.
760. Amselem S, Duquesnoy P, Attree O, et al. Laron dwarfism and mutations of the growth hormone-receptor gene. *N Engl J Med*. 1989;321:989-995.
761. Berg MA, Guevara-Aguirre J, Rosenbloom AL, et al. Mutation creating a new splice site in the growth hormone receptor genes of 37 Ecuadorean patients with Laron syndrome. *Hum Mutat*. 1992;1:24-32.
762. Godowski PJ, Leung DW, Meacham LR, et al. Characterization of the human growth hormone receptor gene and demonstration of a partial gene deletion in two patients with Laron-type dwarfism. *Proc Natl Acad Sci U S A*. 1989;86:8083-8087.
763. Rosenfeld RG. Molecular mechanisms of IGF-I deficiency. *Horm Res*. 2006;65(suppl 1):15-20.
764. Silbergeld A, Dastot F, Klinger B, et al. Intronic mutation in the growth hormone (GH) receptor gene from a girl with Laron syndrome and extremely high serum GH binding protein: extended phenotypic study in a very large pedigree. *J Pediatr Endocrinol Metab*. 1997;10:265-274.
765. Kaji H, Nose O, Tajiri H, et al. Novel compound heterozygous mutations of growth hormone (GH) receptor gene in a patient with GH insensitivity syndrome. *J Clin Endocrinol Metab*. 1997;82:3705-3709.
766. Ayling RM, Ross R, Towner P, et al. A dominant-negative mutation of the growth hormone receptor causes familial short stature. *Nat Genet*. 1997;16:13-14.
767. Iida K, Takahashi Y, Kaji H, et al. Growth hormone (GH) insensitivity syndrome with high serum GH-binding protein levels caused by a heterozygous splice site mutation of the GH receptor gene producing a lack of intracellular domain. *J Clin Endocrinol Metab*. 1998;83:531-537.
768. Gastier JM, Berg MA, Vesterhus P, et al. Diverse deletions in the growth hormone receptor gene cause growth hormone insensitivity syndrome. *Hum Mutat*. 2000;16:323-333.
769. Milward A, Metherell L, Maamra M, et al. Growth hormone (GH) insensitivity syndrome due to a GH receptor truncated after Box1, resulting in isolated failure of STAT 5 signal transduction. *J Clin Endocrinol Metab*. 2004;89:1259-1266.
770. Tiulpakov A, Rubtsov P, Dedov I, et al. A novel C-terminal growth hormone receptor (GHR) mutation results in impaired GHR-STAT5 but normal STAT-3 signaling. *J Clin Endocrinol Metab*. 2005;90:542-547.
771. Iida K, Takahashi Y, Kaji H, et al. Functional characterization of truncated growth hormone (GH) receptor-(1-277) causing partial GH insensitivity syndrome with high GH-binding protein. *J Clin Endocrinol Metab*. 1999;84:1011-1016.
772. Horikawa R, Hellmann P, Cella SG, et al. Growth hormone-releasing factor (GRF) regulates expression of its own receptor. *Endocrinology*. 1996;137:2642-2645.
773. Szabo M, Butz MR, Banerjee SA, et al. Autofeedback suppression of growth hormone (GH) secretion in transgenic mice expressing a human GH reporter targeted by tyrosine hydroxylase 5′-flanking sequences to the hypothalamus. *Endocrinology*. 1995;136:4044-4048.
774. Goddard AD, Covello R, Luoh SM, et al. Mutations of the growth hormone receptor in children with idiopathic short stature: the growth hormone insensitivity study group. *N Engl J Med*. 1995;333:1093-1098.
775. Rosenfeld RG. Broadening the growth hormone insensitivity syndrome. *N Engl J Med*. 1995;333:1145-1146.
776. Attie KM. Mutations of the growth hormone receptor: widening the search. *J Clin Endocrinol Metab*. 1996;81:1683-1685.
777. Sanchez JE, Perera E, Baumbach L, et al. Growth hormone receptor mutations in children with idiopathic short stature. *J Clin Endocrinol Metab*. 1998;83:4079-4083.
778. Ross RJ, Esposito N, Shen XY, et al. A short isoform of the human growth hormone receptor functions as a dominant negative inhibitor of the full-length receptor and generates large amounts of binding protein. *Mol Endocrinol*. 1997;11:265-273.
779. Urbanek M, Russell JE, Cooke NE, et al. Functional characterization of the alternatively spliced, placental human growth hormone receptor. *J Biol Chem*. 1993;268:19025-19032.
780. Sobrier M, Duquesnoy P, Duriez B, et al. Expression and binding properties of two isoforms of the human growth hormone receptor. *FEBS Lett*. 1993;319:16-20.
781. Dos Santos C, Essioux L, Teinturier C, et al. A common polymorphism of the growth hormone receptor is associated with increased responsiveness to growth hormone. *Nat Genet*. 2004;36:720-724.
782. Binder G, Baur F, Schweizer R, et al. The D3-growth hormone (GH) receptor polymorphism is associated with increased responsiveness to GH in Turner syndrome and short small-for-gestational-age children. *J Clin Endocrinol Metab*. 2006;91:659-664.
783. Jorge AAL, Marchisotti FG, Montenegro LR, et al. Growth hormone (GH) pharmacogenetics: influence of GH receptor exon 3 retention or deletion on first-year growth response and final height in patients with severe GH deficiency. *J Clin Endocrinol Metab*. 2006;91:1076-1080.
784. Pilotta A, Mella P, Filisetti M, et al. Common polymorphisms of the growth hormone (GH) receptor do not correlate with the growth response to exogenous recombinant human GH in GH-deficient children. *J Clin Endocrinol Metab*. 2006;91:1178-1180.
785. Blum WF, Machinis K, Shavrikova EP, et al. The growth response to growth hormone (GH) treatment in children with isolated GH deficiency is independent of the presence of the exon 3-minus isoform of the GH receptor. *J Clin Endocrinol Metab*. 2006;91:4171-4174.
786. Kofoed EM, Hwa V, Little B, et al. Growth hormone insensitivity associated with a STAT5b mutation. *N Engl J Med*. 2003;349:1139-1147.
787. Hwa V, Little B, Adiyaman P, et al. Severe growth hormone insensitivity resulting from total absence of signal transducer and activator of transcription 5b. *J Clin Endocrinol Metab*. 2005;90:4260-4266.
788. Fang P, Kofoed EM, Little BM, et al. A mutant signal transducer and activator of transcription 5b, associated with growth hormone insensitivity and insulin-like growth factor-I deficiency, cannot function as a signal transducer or transcription factor. *J Clin Endocrinol Metab*. 2006;91:1526-1534.
789. Chia DJ, Subbian E, Buck TM, et al. Aberrant folding of a mutant Stat5b causes growth hormone insensitivity and proteasomal dysfunction. *J Biol Chem*. 2006;281:6552-6558.
790. Domene HM, Bengolea SV, Martinez AS, et al. Deficiency of the circulating insulin-like growth factor system associated with inactivation of the acid-labile subunit gene. *N Engl J Med*. 2004;350:570-577.
791. Hwa V, Haeusler G, Pratt KL, et al. Total absence of functional acid labile subunit, resulting in severe insulin-like growth factor deficiency and moderate growth failure. *J Clin Endocrinol Metab*. 2006;91:1826-1831.
792. Woods KA, Camacho-Hubner C, Barter D, et al. Insulin-like growth factor I gene deletion causing intrauterine growth retardation and severe short stature. *Acta Paediatr Suppl*. 1997;423:39-45.
793. Camacho-Hubner C, Woods KA, Miraki-Moud F, et al. Effects of recombinant human insulin-like growth factor I (IGF-I) therapy on the growth hormone-IGF system of a patient with a partial IGF-I gene deletion. *J Clin Endocrinol Metab*. 1999;84:1611-1616.
794. Denley A, Wang CC, McNeil KA, et al. Structural and functional characteristics of the Val44Met insulin-like growth factor I missense mutation: correlation with effects on growth and development. *Mol Endocrinol*. 2005;19:711-721.
795. Tollefsen SE, Heath-Monnig E, Cascieri MA, et al. Endogenous insulin-like growth factor (IGF) binding proteins cause IGF-1 resistance in cultured fibroblasts from a patient with short stature. *J Clin Invest*. 1991;87:1241-1250.
796. Raile K, Klammt J, Schneider A, et al. Clinical and functional characteristics of the human Arg59Ter insulin-like growth factor I receptor (IGF1R) mutation: implications for a gene dosage effect of the human IGF1R. *J Clin Endocrinol Metab*. 2006;91:2264-2271.
797. Hattori Y, Vera JC, Rivas CI, et al. Decreased insulin-like growth factor I receptor expression and function in immortalized African pygmy T cells. *J Clin Endocrinol Metab*. 1996;81:2257-2263.

798. Jain S, Golde DW, Bailey R, et al. Insulin-like growth factor-I resistance. *Endocr Rev*. 1998;19:625-646.
799. Wertheimer E, Lu SP, Backeljauw PF, et al. Homozygous deletion of the human insulin receptor gene results in leprechaunism. *Nat Genet*. 1993;5:71-73.
800. Siebler T, Lopaczynski W, Terry CL, et al. Insulin-like growth factor I receptor expression and function in fibroblasts from two patients with deletion of the distal long arm of chromosome 15. *J Clin Endocrinol Metab*. 1995;80:3447-3457.
801. Graham GG, Adrianzen B, Rabold J, et al. Later growth of malnourished infants and children: comparison with "healthy" siblings and parents. *Am J Dis Child*. 1982;136:348-352.
802. Allen LH. Nutritional influences on linear growth: a general review. *Eur J Clin Nutr*. 1994;48(suppl 1):S75-S89.
803. Liu Y, Albertsson-Wikland K, Karlberg J. Long-term consequences of early linear growth retardation (stunting) in Swedish children. *Pediatr Res*. 2000;47(4 Pt 1):475-480.
804. Laditan AA. Hormonal changes in severely malnourished children. *Afr J Med Med Sci*. 1983;12:125-132.
805. Zamboni G, Dufillot D, Antoniazzi F, et al. Growth hormone-binding proteins and insulin-like growth factor-binding proteins in protein-energy malnutrition, before and after nutritional rehabilitation. *Pediatr Res*. 1996;39:410-414.
806. Pimstone B, Barbezat G, Hansen JD, et al. Growth hormone and protein-calorie malnutrition: impaired suppression during induced hyperglycaemia. *Lancet*. 1967;2:1333-1334.
807. Beas F, Contreras I, Maccioni A, et al. Growth hormone in infant malnutrition: the arginine test in marasmus and kwashiorkor. *Br J Nutr*. 1971;26:169-175.
808. Grant DB, Hambley J, Becker D, et al. Reduced sulphation factor in undernourished children. *Arch Dis Child*. 1973;48:596-600.
809. Soliman AT, Hassan AE, Aref MK, et al. Serum insulin-like growth factors I and II concentrations and growth hormone and insulin responses to arginine infusion in children with protein-energy malnutrition before and after nutritional rehabilitation. *Pediatr Res*. 1986;20:1122-1130.
810. Scacchi M, Ida Pincelli A, Cavagnini F. Nutritional status in the neuroendocrine control of growth hormone secretion: the model of anorexia nervosa. *Front Neuroendocrinol*. 2003;24:200-224.
811. Altinkaynak S, Selimoglu MA, Ertekin V, et al. Serum ghrelin levels in children with primary protein-energy malnutrition. *Pediatr Int*. 2008;50:429-431.
812. El-Hodhod MA, Emam EK, Zeitoun YA, et al. Serum ghrelin in infants with protein-energy malnutrition. *Clin Nutr*. 2009;28:173-177.
813. Dimaraki EV, Jaffe CA. Role of endogenous ghrelin in growth hormone secretion, appetite regulation and metabolism. *Rev Endocr Metab Disord*. 2006;7:237-249.
814. Mayer E, Stern M. Growth failure in gastrointestinal diseases. *Baillieres Clin Endocrinol Metab*. 1992;6:645-663.
815. Phillips LS. Nutrition, somatomedins, and the brain. *Metabolism*. 1986;35:78-87.
816. Donovan SM, Atilano LC, Hintz RL, et al. Differential regulation of the insulin-like growth factors (IGF-I and -II) and IGF binding proteins during malnutrition in the neonatal rat. *Endocrinology*. 1991;129:149-157.
817. Pugliese MT, Lifshitz F, Grad G, et al. Fear of obesity: a cause of short stature and delayed puberty. *N Engl J Med*. 1983;309:513-518.
818. Golden NH, Kreitzer P, Jacobson MS, et al. Disturbances in growth hormone secretion and action in adolescents with anorexia nervosa. *J Pediatr*. 1994;125:655-660.
819. Root AW, Powers PS. Anorexia nervosa presenting as growth retardation in adolescents. *J Adolesc Health Care*. 1983;4:25-30.
820. Russell GF. Premenarchal anorexia nervosa and its sequelae. *J Psychiatr Res*. 1985;19:363-369.
821. Miller KK, Klibanski A. Clinical review 106: amenorrheic bone loss. *J Clin Endocrinol Metab*. 1999;84:1775-1783.
822. Postel-Vinay MC, Saab C, Gourmelen M. Nutritional status and growth hormone-binding protein. *Horm Res*. 1995;44:177-181.
823. Counts DR, Gwirtsman H, Carlsson LM, et al. The effects of anorexia nervosa and refeeding on growth hormone-binding protein, the insulin-like growth factors (IGFs), and the IGF-binding proteins. *J Clin Endocrinol Metab*. 1992;75:762-766.
824. Fleischman A, Brue C, Poussaint TY, et al. Diencephalic syndrome: a cause of failure to thrive and a model of partial growth hormone resistance. *Pediatrics*. 2005;115:e742-e748.
825. Preece MA, Law CM, Davies PS. The growth of children with chronic paediatric disease. *Clin Endocrinol Metab*. 1986;15:453-477.
826. Sentongo TA, Semeao EJ, Piccoli DA, et al. Growth, body composition, and nutritional status in children and adolescents with Crohn's disease. *J Pediatr Gastroenterol Nutr*. 2000;31:33-40.
827. Savage MO, Beattie RM, Camacho-Hubner C, et al. Growth in Crohn's disease. *Acta Paediatr Suppl*. 1999;88:89-92.
828. Locuratolo N, Pugliese G, Pricci F, et al. The circulating insulin-like growth factor system in children with coeliac disease: an additional marker for disease activity. *Diabetes Metab Res Rev*. 1999;15:254-260.
829. Auricchio S, Greco L, Troncone R. Gluten-sensitive enteropathy in childhood. *Pediatr Clin North Am*. 1988;35:157-187.
830. De Luca F, Astori M, Pandullo E, et al. Effects of a gluten-free diet on catch-up growth and height prognosis in coeliac children with growth retardation recognized after the age of 5 years. *Eur J Pediatr*. 1988;147:188-191.
831. Stenhammar L, Fallstrom SP, Jansson G, et al. Coeliac disease in children of short stature without gastrointestinal symptoms. *Eur J Pediatr*. 1986;145:185-186.
832. Radzikowski T, Zalewski TK, Kapuscinska A, et al. Short stature due to unrecognized celiac disease. *Eur J Pediatr*. 1988;147:334-335.
833. Hill ID, Dirks MH, Liptak GS, et al. North American Society for Pediatric Gastroenterology, Hepatology and Nutrition. Guideline for the diagnosis and treatment of celiac disease in children: recommendations of the North American Society for Pediatric Gastroenterology, Hepatology and Nutrition. *J Pediatr Gastroenterol Nutr*. 2005;40:1-19.
834. Lagerqvist C, Dahlbom I, Hansson T, et al. Antigliadin immunoglobulin A best in finding celiac disease in children younger than 18 months of age. *J Pediatr Gastroenterol Nutr*. 2008;47:428-435.
835. Zawahir S, Safta A, Fasano A. Pediatric celiac disease. *Curr Opin Pediatr*. 2009;21:655-660.
836. Hoffenberg EJ, MacKenzie T, Barriga KJ, et al. A prospective study of the incidence of childhood celiac disease. *J Pediatr*. 2003;143:308-314.
837. Hernandez M, Argente J, Navarro A, et al. Growth in malnutrition related to gastrointestinal diseases: coeliac disease. *Horm Res*. 1992;38(suppl 1):79-84.
838. Bode SH, Bachmann EH, Gudmand-Hoyer E, et al. Stature of adult coeliac patients: no evidence for decreased attained height. *Eur J Clin Nutr*. 1991;45:145-149.
839. Cacciari E, Corazza GR, Salardi S, et al. What will be the adult height of coeliac patients? *Eur J Pediatr*. 1991;150:407-409.
840. Wine E, Reif SS, Leshinsky-Silver E, et al. Pediatric Crohn's disease and growth retardation: the role of genotype, phenotype, and disease severity. *Pediatrics*. 2004;114:1281-1286.
841. Shamir R, Phillip M, Levine A. Growth retardation in pediatric Crohn's disease: pathogenesis and interventions. *Inflamm Bowel Dis*. 2007;13:620-628.
842. Walters TD, Griffiths AM. Mechanisms of growth impairment in pediatric Crohn's disease. *Nat Rev Gastroenterol Hepatol*. 2009;6:513-523.
843. Cezard JP, Touati G, Alberti C, et al. Growth in paediatric Crohn's disease. *Horm Res*. 2002;58(suppl 1):11-15.
844. Kanof ME, Lake AM, Bayless TM. Decreased height velocity in children and adolescents before the diagnosis of Crohn's disease. *Gastroenterology*. 1988;95:1523-1527.
845. Rosenthal SR, Snyder JD, Hendricks KM, et al. Growth failure and inflammatory bowel disease: approach to treatment of a complicated adolescent problem. *Pediatrics*. 1983;72:481-490.
846. Gryboski JD, Spiro HM. Prognosis in children with Crohn's disease. *Gastroenterology*. 1978;74(5 Pt 1):807-817.
847. Homer DR, Grand RJ, Colodny AH. Growth, course, and prognosis after surgery for Crohn's disease in children and adolescents. *Pediatrics*. 1977;59:717-725.
848. Griffiths AM, Nguyen P, Smith C, et al. Growth and clinical course of children with Crohn's disease. *Gut*. 1993;34:939-943.
849. Soyka LA, Fairfield WP, Klibanski A. Clinical review 117: hormonal determinants and disorders of peak bone mass in children. *J Clin Endocrinol Metab*. 2000;85:3951-3963.
850. Cowan FJ, Warner JT, Dunstan FD, et al. Inflammatory bowel disease and predisposition to osteopenia. *Arch Dis Child*. 1997;76:325-329.
851. Kirschner BS. Growth and development in chronic inflammatory bowel disease. *Acta Paediatr Scand Suppl*. 1990;366:98-104, discussion 105.
852. Sawczenko A, Ballinger AB, Savage MO, et al. Clinical features affecting final adult height in patients with pediatric-onset Crohn's disease. *Pediatrics*. 2006;118:124-129.
853. Mauras N, George D, Evans J, et al. Growth hormone has anabolic effects in glucocorticosteroid-dependent children with inflammatory bowel disease: a pilot study. *Metabolism*. 2002;51:127-135.
854. Henker J. Therapy with recombinant growth hormone in children with Crohn disease and growth failure. *Eur J Pediatr*. 1996;155:1066-1067.
855. Calenda KA, Schornagel IL, Sadeghi-Nejad A, et al. Effect of recombinant growth hormone treatment on children with Crohn's disease and short stature: a pilot study. *Inflamm Bowel Dis*. 2005;11:435-441.
856. Wasserman D, Zemel BS, Mulberg AE, et al. Growth, nutritional status, body composition, and energy expenditure in prepubertal children with alagille syndrome. *J Pediatr*. 1999;134:172-177.
857. Viner RM, Forton JT, Cole TJ, et al. Growth of long-term survivors of liver transplantation. *Arch Dis Child*. 1999;80:235-240.
858. Bartosh SM, Thomas SE, Sutton MM, et al. Linear growth after pediatric liver transplantation. *J Pediatr*. 1999;135:624-631.

859. Bucuvalas JC, Cutfield W, Horn J, et al. Resistance to the growth-promoting and metabolic effects of growth hormone in children with chronic liver disease. *J Pediatr*. 1990;117:397-402.
860. Russell WE. Growth hormone, somatomedins, and the liver. *Semin Liver Dis*. 1985;5:46-58.
861. Donaghy A, Ross R, Gimson A, et al. Growth hormone, insulinlike growth factor-1, and insulinlike growth factor binding proteins 1 and 3 in chronic liver disease. *Hepatology*. 1995;21:680-688.
862. Quirk P, Owens P, Moyse K, et al. Insulin-like growth factors I and II are reduced in plasma from growth retarded children with chronic liver disease. *Growth Regul*. 1994;4:35-38.
863. Holt RI, Jones JS, Stone NM, et al. Sequential changes in insulin-like growth factor I (IGF-I) and IGF-binding proteins in children with end-stage liver disease before and after successful orthotopic liver transplantation. *J Clin Endocrinol Metab*. 1996;81:160-168.
864. Maghnie M, Barreca A, Ventura M, et al. Failure to increase insulin-like growth factor-I synthesis is involved in the mechanisms of growth retardation of children with inherited liver disorders. *Clin Endocrinol (Oxf)*. 1998;48:747-755.
865. Shen XY, Holt RI, Miell JP, et al. Cirrhotic liver expresses low levels of the full-length and truncated growth hormone receptors. *J Clin Endocrinol Metab*. 1998;83:2532-2538.
866. Sarna S, Sipila I, Vihervuori E, et al. Growth delay after liver transplantation in childhood: studies of underlying mechanisms. *Pediatr Res*. 1995;38:366-372.
867. Codoner-Franch P, Bernard O, Alvarez F. Long-term follow-up of growth in height after successful liver transplantation. *J Pediatr*. 1994;124:368-373.
868. Puustinen L, Jalanko H, Holmberg C, et al. Recombinant human growth hormone treatment after liver transplantation in childhood: the 5-year outcome. *Transplantation*. 2005;79:1241-1246.
869. Sarna S, Sipila I, Ronnholm K, et al. Recombinant human growth hormone improves growth in children receiving glucocorticoid treatment after liver transplantation. *J Clin Endocrinol Metab*. 1996;81:1476-1482.
870. Rodeck B, Kardorff R, Melter M, et al. Improvement of growth after growth hormone treatment in children who undergo liver transplantation. *J Pediatr Gastroenterol Nutr*. 2000;31:286-290.
871. Bayer LM, Robinson SJ. Growth history of children with congenital heart defects: size according to sex, age decade, surgical status, and diagnostic category. *Am J Dis Child*. 1969;117:564-572.
872. Feldt RH, Strickler GB, Weidman WH. Growth of children with congenital heart disease. *Am J Dis Child*. 1969;117:573-579.
873. Gilger M, Mensen C, Kessler B, et al. Nutrition, growth and the gastrointestinal system: basic knowledge for the pediatric cardiologist. In: Garson Jr A, Bricker JT, McNamara DG, eds. The Science and Practice of Pediatric Cardiology. Philadelphia, PA: Lea & Febiger; 1990.
874. Mehrizi A, Drash A. Growth disturbance in congenital heart disease. *J Pediatr*. 1962;61:418-429.
875. Nadas AS, Rosenthal A, Crigler JF. Nutritional considerations in the prognosis and treatment of children with congenital heart disease. In: Suskind RM, ed. *Textbook of Pediatric Nutrition*. New York, NY: Raven; 1987.
876. McLean WC. Protein energy malnutrition. In: Grand RJ, Sutphen JL, Dietz WH, eds. *Pediatric Nutrition: Theory and Practice*. Stoneham, MA: Butterworths; 1987.
877. Naeye RL. Anatomic features of growth failure in congenital heart disease. *Pediatrics*. 1967;39:433-440.
878. Wahlig TM, Georgieff MK. The effects of illness on neonatal metabolism and nutritional management. *Clin Perinatol*. 1995;22:77-96.
879. Leitch CA, Karn CA, Ensing GJ, et al. Energy expenditure after surgical repair in children with cyanotic congenital heart disease. *J Pediatr*. 2000;137:381-385.
880. Leitch CA, Karn CA, Peppard RJ, et al. Increased energy expenditure in infants with cyanotic congenital heart disease. *J Pediatr*. 1998;133:755-760.
881. Linde LM, Dunn OJ, Schireson R, et al. Growth in children with congenital heart disease. *J Pediatr*. 1967;70:413-419.
882. Barton JS, Hindmarsh PC, Preece MA. Serum insulin-like growth factor 1 in congenital heart disease. *Arch Dis Child*. 1996;75:162-163.
883. Bernstein D, Jasper JR, Rosenfeld RG, et al. Decreased serum insulin-like growth factor-I associated with growth failure in newborn lambs with experimental cyanotic heart disease. *J Clin Invest*. 1992;89:1128-1132.
884. Soliman AT, el Nawawy A, el Azzoni O, et al. Growth parameters and endocrine function in relation to echocardiographic parameters in children and adolescents with compensated rheumatic heart disease. *J Trop Pediatr*. 1997;43:4-9.
885. Schuurmans FM, Pulles-Heintzberger CF, Gerver WJ, et al. Long-term growth of children with congenital heart disease: a retrospective study. *Acta Paediatr*. 1998;87:1250-1255.
886. Holliday MA, Chantler C, Potter DE. Symposium on metabolism and growth in children with kidney disease: introduction. *Kidney Int*. 1978;14:299-300.
887. Kohaut EC. Chronic renal disease and growth in childhood. *Curr Opin Pediatr*. 1995;7:171-175.
888. Mehls O, Blum WF, Schaefer F, et al. Growth failure in renal disease. *Baillieres Clin Endocrinol Metab*. 1992;6:665-685.
889. Lee DY, Park SK, Kim JS. Insulin-like growth factor-I (IGF-I) and IGF-binding proteins in children with nephrotic syndrome. *J Clin Endocrinol Metab*. 1996;81:1856-1860.
890. Kuizon BD, Salusky IB. Growth retardation in children with chronic renal failure. *J Bone Miner Res*. 1999;14:1680-1690.
891. Kimonis VE, Troendle J, Rose SR, et al. Effects of early cysteamine therapy on thyroid function and growth in nephropathic cystinosis. *J Clin Endocrinol Metab*. 1995;80:3257-3261.
892. Warady BA, Jabs K. New hormones in the therapeutic arsenal of chronic renal failure: growth hormone and erythropoietin. *Pediatr Clin North Am*. 1995;42:1551-1577.
893. Tonshoff B, Mehls O. Growth retardation in children with chronic renal insufficiency: current aspects of pathophysiology and treatment. *J Nephrol*. 1955;8:133-142.
894. Tonshoff B, Veldhuis JD, Heinrich U, et al. Deconvolution analysis of spontaneous nocturnal growth hormone secretion in prepubertal children with preterminal chronic renal failure and with end-stage renal disease. *Pediatr Res*. 1995;37:86-93.
895. Ramirez G, O'Neill WM, Bloomer HA, et al. Abnormalities in the regulation of growth hormone in chronic renal failure. *Arch Intern Med*. 1978;138:267-271.
896. Hokken-Koelega AC, Hackeng WH, Stijnen T, et al. Twenty-four-hour plasma growth hormone (GH) profiles, urinary GH excretion, and plasma insulin-like growth factor-I and -II levels in prepubertal children with chronic renal insufficiency and severe growth retardation. *J Clin Endocrinol Metab*. 1990;71:688-695.
897. Schaefer F, Hamill G, Stanhope R, et al. Pulsatile growth hormone secretion in peripubertal patients with chronic renal failure: Cooperative Study Group on Pubertal Development in Chronic Renal Failure. *J Pediatr*. 1991;119:568-577.
898. Mahan JD, Warady BA, Consensus Committee. Assessment and treatment of short stature in pediatric patients with chronic kidney disease: a consensus statement. *Pediatr Nephrol*. 2006;21:917-930.
899. Tonshoff B, Eden S, Weiser E, et al. Reduced hepatic growth hormone (GH) receptor gene expression and increased plasma GH binding protein in experimental uremia. *Kidney Int*. 1994;45:1085-1092.
900. Hokken-Koelega AC, Stijnen T, de Muinck Keizer-Schrama SM, et al. Placebo-controlled, double-blind, cross-over trial of growth hormone treatment in prepubertal children with chronic renal failure. *Lancet*. 1991;338:585-590.
901. Powell DR, Rosenfeld RG, Baker BK, et al. Serum somatomedin levels in adults with chronic renal failure: the importance of measuring insulin-like growth factor I (IGF-I) and IGF-II in acid-chromatographed uremic serum. *J Clin Endocrinol Metab*. 1986;63:1186-1192.
902. Blum WF. Insulin-like growth factors (IGFs) and IGF binding proteins in chronic renal failure: evidence for reduced secretion of IGFs. *Acta Paediatr Scand Suppl*. 1991;379:24-31, discussion 32.
903. Roelfsema V, Clark RG. The growth hormone and insulin-like growth factor axis: its manipulation for the benefit of growth disorders in renal failure. *J Am Soc Nephrol*. 2001;12:1297-1306.
904. Schaefer F, Chen Y, Tsao T, et al. Impaired JAK-STAT signal transduction contributes to growth hormone resistance in chronic uremia. *J Clin Invest*. 2001;108:467-475.
905. Rabkin R, Sun DF, Chen Y, et al. Growth hormone resistance in uremia, a role for impaired JAK/STAT signaling. *Pediatr Nephrol*. 2005;20:313-318.
906. Rees L, Maxwell H. The hypothalamo-pituitary-growth hormone insulin-like growth factor 1 axis in children with chronic renal failure. *Kidney Int Suppl*. 1996;53:S109-S114.
907. Blum WF, Ranke MB, Kietzmann K, et al. Growth hormone resistance and inhibition of somatomedin activity by excess of insulin-like growth factor binding protein in uraemia. *Pediatr Nephrol*. 1991;5:539-544.
908. Saenger P, Wiedemann E, Schwartz E, et al. Somatomedin and growth after renal transplantation. *Pediatr Res*. 1974;8:163-169.
909. Hokken-Koelega AC, Stijnen T, de Muinck Keizer-Schrama SM, et al. Levels of growth hormone, insulin-like growth factor-I (IGF-I) and -II, IGF-binding protein-1 and -3, and cortisol in prednisone-treated children with growth retardation after renal transplantation. *J Clin Endocrinol Metab*. 1993;77:932-938.
910. Hanna JD, Santos F, Foreman JW, et al. Insulin-like growth factor-I gene expression in the tibial epiphyseal growth plate of growth hormone-treated uremic rats. *Kidney Int*. 1995;47:1374-1382.
911. Unterman TG, Phillips LS. Glucocorticoid effects on somatomedins and somatomedin inhibitors. *J Clin Endocrinol Metab*. 1985;61:618-626.
912. Allen DB. Growth suppression by glucocorticoid therapy. *Pediatr Rounds*. 1995;4:1-5.
913. Fine RN, Tejani A. Renal transplantation in children. *Nephron*. 1987;47:81-86.

914. Hokken-Koelega AC, Van Zaal MA, de Ridder MA, et al. Growth after renal transplantation in prepubertal children: impact of various treatment modalities. *Pediatr Res*. 1994;35:367-371.
915. Hokken-Koelega AC, van Zaal MA, van Bergen W, et al. Final height and its predictive factors after renal transplantation in childhood. *Pediatr Res*. 1994;36:323-328.
916. Tejani A, Fine R, Alexander S, et al. Factors predictive of sustained growth in children after renal transplantation: The North American Pediatric Renal Transplant Cooperative Study. *J Pediatr*. 1993;122: 397-402.
917. Schaefer F, Haffner D, Wuhl E, et al. Long-term experience with growth hormone treatment in children with chronic renal failure. *Perit Dial Int*. 1999;19(suppl 2):S467-S472.
918. Fine RN. Growth post renal-transplantation in children: lessons from the North American Pediatric Renal Transplant Cooperative Study (NAPRTCS). *Pediatr Transplant*. 1997;1:85-89.
919. Tejani A, Stablein DM, Donaldson L, et al. Steady improvement in short-term graft survival of pediatric renal transplants: the NAPRTCS experience. *Clin Transpl*. 1999:95-110.
920. Millan MT, Sarwal MM, Lemley KV, et al. A 100% 2-year graft survival can be attained in high-risk 15-kg or smaller infant recipients of kidney allografts. *Arch Surg*. 2000;135:1063-1068, discussion 1068-1069.
921. Kari JA, Romagnoli J, Duffy P, et al. Renal transplantation in children under 5 years of age. *Pediatr Nephrol*. 2000;13:730-736.
922. Ellis D. Growth and renal function after steroid-free tacrolimus-based immunosuppression in children with renal transplants. *Pediatr Nephrol*. 2000;14:689-694.
923. Henderson RA, Saavedra JM, Dover GJ. Prevalence of impaired growth in children with homozygous sickle cell anemia. *Am J Med Sci*. 1994;307:405-407.
924. Modebe O, Ifenu SA. Growth retardation in homozygous sickle cell disease: role of calorie intake and possible gender-related differences. *Am J Hematol*. 1994;44:149-154.
925. Singhal A, Thomas P, Cook R, et al. Delayed adolescent growth in homozygous sickle cell disease. *Arch Dis Child*. 1994;71:404-408.
926. Wang WC, Morales KH, Scher CD, et al. STOP Investigators. Effect of long-term transfusion on growth in children with sickle cell anemia: results of the STOP trial. *J Pediatr*. 2005;147:244-247.
927. Saka N, Sukur M, Bundak R, et al. Growth and puberty in thalassemia major. *J Pediatr Endocrinol Metab*. 1995;8:181-186.
928. Filosa A, Di Maio S, Baron I, et al. Final height and body disproportion in thalassaemic boys and girls with spontaneous or induced puberty. *Acta Paediatr*. 2000;89:1295-1301.
929. Low LC, Kwan EY, Lim YJ, et al. Growth hormone treatment of short Chinese children with beta-thalassaemia major without GH deficiency. *Clin Endocrinol (Oxf)*. 1995;42:359-363.
930. DeLuca G, Maggiolini M, Bria M, et al. GH secretion in thalassemia patients with short stature. *Horm Res*. 1995;44:158-163.
931. Scacchi M, Danesi L, De Martin M, et al. Treatment with biosynthetic growth hormone of short thalassaemic patients with impaired growth hormone secretion. *Clin Endocrinol (Oxf)*. 1991;35:335-339.
932. Masala A, Atzeni MM, Alagna S, et al. Growth hormone secretion in polytransfused prepubertal patients with homozygous beta-thalassemia: Effect of long-term recombinant GH (recGH) therapy. *J Endocrinol Invest*. 2003;26:623-628.
933. Cavallo L, De Sanctis V, Cisternino M, et al. Final height in short polytransfused thalassemia major patients treated with recombinant growth hormone. *J Endocrinol Invest*. 2005;28:363-366.
934. La Rosa C, De Sanctis V, Mangiagli A, et al. Growth hormone secretion in adult patients with thalassaemia. *Clin Endocrinol (Oxf)*. 2005;62:667-671.
935. Wajnrajch MP, Gertner JM, Huma Z, et al. Evaluation of growth and hormonal status in patients referred to the international Fanconi anemia registry. *Pediatrics*. 2001;107:744-754.
936. McNair SL, Stickler GB. Growth in familial hypophosphatemic vitamin-D-resistant rickets. *N Engl J Med*. 1969;281:512-516.
937. Marsden D, Barshop BA, Capistrano-Estrada S, et al. Anabolic effect of human growth hormone: management of inherited disorders of catabolic pathways. *Biochem Med Metab Biol*. 1994;52:145-154.
938. Bain MD, Nussey SS, Jones M, et al. Use of human somatotrophin in the treatment of a patient with methylmalonic aciduria. *Eur J Pediatr*. 1995;154:850-852.
939. Russell G. Asthma and growth. *Arch Dis Child*. 1993;69:695-698.
940. Cohen MB, Abram LE. Growth patterns of allergic children: a statistical study using the grid technique. *J Allergy*. 1948;19:165-171.
941. Balfour-Lynn L. Growth and childhood asthma. *Arch Dis Child*. 1986;61:1049-1055.
942. Crowley S, Hindmarsh PC, Matthews DR, et al. Growth and the growth hormone axis in prepubertal children with asthma. *J Pediatr*. 1995;126:297-303.
943. Ninan TK, Russell G. Asthma, inhaled corticosteroid treatment, and growth. *Arch Dis Child*. 1992;67:703-705.
944. Nassif E, Weinberger M, Sherman B, et al. Extrapulmonary effects of maintenance corticosteroid therapy with alternate-day prednisone and inhaled beclomethasone in children with chronic asthma. *J Allergy Clin Immunol*. 1987;80:518-529.
945. Falliers CJ, Tan LS, Szentivanyi J, et al. Childhood asthma and steroid therapy as influences on growth. *Am J Dis Child*. 1963;105:127-137.
946. Reid A, Murphy C, Steen HJ, et al. Linear growth of very young asthmatic children treated with high-dose nebulized budesonide. *Acta Paediatr*. 1996;85:421-424.
947. Varsano I, Volovitz B, Malik H, et al. Safety of 1 year of treatment with budesonide in young children with asthma. *J Allergy Clin Immunol*. 1990;85:914-920.
948. Volovitz B, Amir J, Malik H, et al. Growth and pituitary-adrenal function in children with severe asthma treated with inhaled budesonide. *N Engl J Med*. 1996;329:1703-1708.
949. Todd G, Dunlop K, McNaboe J, et al. Growth and adrenal suppression in asthmatic children treated with high-dose fluticasone propionate. *Lancet*. 1996;348:27-29.
950. Agertoft L, Pedersen S. Effect of long-term treatment with inhaled budesonide on adult height in children with asthma. *N Engl J Med*. 2000;343:1064-1069.
951. Long-term effects of budesonide or nedocromil in children with asthma: the Childhood Asthma Management Program Research Group. *N Engl J Med*. 2000;343:1054-1063.
952. Norjavaara E, Gerhardsson De Verdier M, et al. Reduced height in Swedish men with asthma at the age of conscription for military service. *J Pediatr*. 2000;137:25-29.
953. Martin AJ, McLennan LA, Landau LI, et al. The natural history of childhood asthma to adult life. *Br Med J*. 1980;280:1397-1400.
954. Shohat M, Shohat T, Kedem R, et al. Childhood asthma and growth outcome. *Arch Dis Child*. 1987;62:63-65.
955. Avery ME, Tooley WH, Keller JB, et al. Is chronic lung disease in low birth weight infants preventable? A survey of eight centers. *Pediatrics*. 1987;79:26-30.
956. Gibson AT, Pearse RG, Wales JK. Growth retardation after dexamethasone administration: assessment by knemometry. *Arch Dis Child*. 1993;69(5 Spec No):505-509.
957. Finer NN, Craft A, Vaucher YE, et al. Postnatal steroids: short-term gain, long-term pain? *J Pediatr*. 2000;137:9-13.
958. Kurzner SI, Garg M, Bautista DB, et al. Growth failure in infants with bronchopulmonary dysplasia: nutrition and elevated resting metabolic expenditure. *Pediatrics*. 1988;81:379-384.
959. Yu VY, Orgill AA, Lim SB, et al. Growth and development of very low birthweight infants recovering from bronchopulmonary dysplasia. *Arch Dis Child*. 1983;58:791-794.
960. Meisels SJ, Plunkett JW, Roloff DW, et al. Growth and development of preterm infants with respiratory distress syndrome and bronchopulmonary dysplasia. *Pediatrics*. 1986;77:345-352.
961. Vrlenich LA, Bozynski ME, Shyr Y, et al. The effect of bronchopulmonary dysplasia on growth at school age. *Pediatrics*. 1995;95:855-859.
962. Ross G, Lipper EG, Auld PA. Growth achievement of very low birth weight premature children at school age. *J Pediatr*. 1990;117(2 Pt 1):307-309.
963. Robertson CM, Etches PC, Goldson E, et al. Eight-year school performance, neurodevelopmental, and growth outcome of neonates with bronchopulmonary dysplasia: a comparative study. *Pediatrics*. 1992;89:365-372.
964. FitzSimmons SC. The changing epidemiology of cystic fibrosis. *J Pediatr*. 1993;122:1-9.
965. Landon C, Rosenfeld RG. Short stature and pubertal delay in male adolescents with cystic fibrosis: androgen treatment. *Am J Dis Child*. 1984;138:388-391.
966. Karlberg J, Kjellmer I, Kristiansson B. Linear growth in children with cystic fibrosis: I—birth to 8 years of age. *Acta Paediatr Scand*. 1991;80:508-514.
967. Lapey A, Kattwinkel J, Di Sant'Agnese PA, et al. Steatorrhea and azotorrhea and their relation to growth and nutrition in adolescents and young adults with cystic fibrosis. *J Pediatr*. 1974;84:328-334.
968. Mearns M. Growth and development. In: Hodson E, Norman A, Batten J, eds. *Cystic Fibrosis*. London, UK: Baillieres Tindall; 1983.
969. Shepherd RW, Holt TL, Thomas BJ, et al. Nutritional rehabilitation in cystic fibrosis: controlled studies of effects on nutritional growth retardation, body protein turnover, and course of pulmonary disease. *J Pediatr*. 1986;109:788-794.
970. Reiter EO, Brugman SM, Pike JW, et al. Vitamin D metabolites in adolescents and young adults with cystic fibrosis: effects of sun and season. *J Pediatr*. 1985;106:21-26.
971. Hardin DS. GH improves growth and clinical status in children with cystic fibrosis: a review of published studies. *Eur J Endocrinol*. 2004;151(suppl 1):S81-S85.
972. Reiter EO, Gerstle RS. Cystic fibrosis in puberty and adolescence. In: Lerner RM, Petersen AC, Brooks-Gunn J, eds. *Encyclopedia of Adolescence*. New York, NY: Garland; 1991.
973. Reiter EO, Stern RC, Root AW. The reproductive endocrine system in cystic fibrosis: 2. Changes in gonadotrophins and sex steroids following LHRH. *Clin Endocrinol (Oxf)*. 1982;16:127-137.

974. Aswani N, Taylor CJ, McGaw J, et al. Pubertal growth and development in cystic fibrosis: a retrospective review. *Acta Paediatr.* 2003;92:1029-1032.
975. Laursen EM, Juul A, Lanng S, et al. Diminished concentrations of insulin-like growth factor I in cystic fibrosis. *Arch Dis Child.* 1995;72:494-497.
976. Huseman CA, Colombo JL, Brooks MA, et al. Anabolic effect of biosynthetic growth hormone in cystic fibrosis patients. *Pediatr Pulmonol.* 1996;22:90-95.
977. Hardin DS, Stratton R, Kramer JC, et al. Growth hormone improves weight velocity and height velocity in prepubertal children with cystic fibrosis. *Horm Metab Res.* 1998;30:636-641.
978. Hardin DS, Adams-Huet B, Brown D, et al. Growth hormone treatment improves growth and clinical status in prepubertal children with cystic fibrosis: results of a multicenter randomized controlled trial. *J Clin Endocrinol Metab.* 2006;91:4925-4929.
979. Hardin DS, Rice J, Ahn C, et al. Growth hormone treatment enhances nutrition and growth in children with cystic fibrosis receiving enteral nutrition. *J Pediatr.* 2005;146:324-328.
980. Zemel BS, Jawad AF, FitzSimmons S, et al. Longitudinal relationship among growth, nutritional status, and pulmonary function in children with cystic fibrosis: analysis of the cystic fibrosis foundation national CF patient registry. *J Pediatr.* 2000;137:374-380.
981. Colombo C, Battezzati A. Growth failure in cystic fibrosis: a true need for anabolic agents? *J Pediatr.* 2005;146:303-305.
982. De Benedetti F, Alonzi T, Moretta A, et al. Interleukin 6 causes growth impairment in transgenic mice through a decrease in insulin-like growth factor-I: a model for stunted growth in children with chronic inflammation. *J Clin Invest.* 1997;99:643-650.
983. Lang CH, Hong-Brown L, Frost RA. Cytokine inhibition of JAK-STAT signaling: a new mechanism of growth hormone resistance. *Pediatr Nephrol.* 2005;20:306-312.
984. McCann SM, Lyson K, Karanth S, et al. Role of cytokines in the endocrine system. *Ann N Y Acad Sci.* 1994;741:50-63.
985. Vassilopoulou-Sellin R. Endocrine effects of cytokines. *Oncology (Williston Park).* 1994;8:(43)46-49, discussion 49-50.
986. Skerry TM. The effects of the inflammatory response on bone growth. *Eur J Clin Nutr.* 1994;48(suppl 1):S190-S197, discussion S198.
987. Abrams EJ, Rogers MF. Pediatric HIV infection. *Baillieres Clin Haematol.* 1991;4:333-339.
988. McKinney Jr RE, Robertson JW. Effect of human immunodeficiency virus infection on the growth of young children: Duke Pediatric AIDS Clinical Trials Unit. *J Pediatr.* 1993;123:579-582.
989. Saavedra JM, Henderson RA, Perman JA, et al. Longitudinal assessment of growth in children born to mothers with human immunodeficiency virus infection. *Arch Pediatr Adolesc Med.* 1995 May; 149(5):497-502.
990. McKinney Jr RE, Wilfert C. Growth as a prognostic indicator in children with human immunodeficiency virus infection treated with zidovudine: AIDS Clinical Trials Group Protocol 043 Study Group. *J Pediatr.* 1994;125(5 Pt 1):728-733.
991. Gertner JM, Kaufman FR, Donfield SM, et al. Delayed somatic growth and pubertal development in human immunodeficiency virus-infected hemophiliac boys: hemophilia growth and development study. *J Pediatr.* 1994;124:896-902.
992. Moye Jr J, Rich KC, Kalish LA, et al. Natural history of somatic growth in infants born to women infected by human immunodeficiency virus: Women and Infants Transmission Study Group. *J Pediatr.* 1996;128:58-69.
993. Majaliwa ES, Mohn A, Chiarelli F. Growth and puberty in children with HIV infection. *J Endocrinol Invest.* 2009;32:85-90.
994. Isanaka S, Duggan C, Fawzi WW. Patterns of postnatal growth in HIV-infected and HIV-exposed children. *Nutr Rev.* 2009;67:343-359.
995. Chantry CJ, Frederick MM, Meyer 3rd WA, et al. Endocrine abnormalities and impaired growth in human immunodeficiency virus-infected children. *Pediatr Infect Dis J.* 2007;26:53-60.
996. Hardin DS, Rice J, Doyle ME, et al. Growth hormone improves protein catabolism and growth in prepubertal children with HIV infection. *Clin Endocrinol (Oxf).* 2005;63:259-262.
997. Chiesa A, Gruneiro de Papendieck L, Keselman A, et al. Growth follow-up in 100 children with congenital hypothyroidism before and during treatment. *J Pediatr Endocrinol.* 1994;7:211-217.
998. Rivkees SA, Bode HH, Crawford JD. Long-term growth in juvenile acquired hypothyroidism: the failure to achieve normal adult stature. *N Engl J Med.* 1988;318:599-602.
999. Boersma B, Otten BJ, Stoelinga GB, et al. Catch-up growth after prolonged hypothyroidism. *Eur J Pediatr.* 1996;155:362-367.
1000. Cassio A, Corrias A, Gualandi S, et al. Influence of gender and pubertal stage at diagnosis on growth outcome in childhood thyrotoxicosis: results of a collaborative study. *Clin Endocrinol (Oxf).* 2006;64: 53-57.
1001. Malone JI. Growth and sexual maturation in children with insulin-dependent diabetes mellitus. *Curr Opin Pediatr.* 1993;5:494-498.
1002. Thon A, Heinze E, Feilen KD, et al. Development of height and weight in children with diabetes mellitus: report on two prospective multicentre studies, one cross-sectional, one longitudinal. *Eur J Pediatr.* 1992 Apr;151:258-262.
1003. Bognetti E, Riva MC, Bonfanti R, et al. Growth changes in children and adolescents with short-term diabetes. *Diabetes Care.* 1998;21: 1226-1229.
1004. Hjelt K, Braendholt V, Kamper J, et al. Growth in children with diabetes mellitus: the significance of metabolic control, insulin requirements and genetic factors. *Dan Med Bull.* 1983;30:28-33.
1005. Jackson RL, Holland E, Chatman ID, et al. Growth and maturation of children with insulin-dependent diabetes mellitus. *Diabetes Care.* 1978;1:96-107.
1006. Vanelli M, de Fanti A, Adinolfi B, et al. Clinical data regarding the growth of diabetic children. *Horm Res.* 1992;37(suppl 3):65-69.
1007. Rogers DG, Sherman LD, Gabbay KH. Effect of puberty on insulinlike growth factor I and HbA1 in type I diabetes. *Diabetes Care.* 1991;14:1031-1035.
1008. Mandell F, Berenberg W. The mauriac syndrome. *Am J Dis Child.* 1974;127:900-902.
1009. Menon RK, Arslanian S, May B, et al. Diminished growth hormone-binding protein in children with insulin-dependent diabetes mellitus. *J Clin Endocrinol Metab.* 1992;74:934-938.
1010. Froesch ER, Hussain M. Metabolic effects of insulin-like growth factor I with special reference to diabetes. *Acta Paediatr Suppl.* 1994;399: 165-170.
1011. Malone JI, Lowitt S, Duncan JA, et al. Hypercalciuria, hyperphosphaturia, and growth retardation in children with diabetes mellitus. *Pediatrics.* 1986;78:298-304.
1012. Clayton KL, Holly JM, Carlsson LM, et al. Loss of the normal relationships between growth hormone, growth hormone-binding protein and insulin-like growth factor-I in adolescents with insulin-dependent diabetes mellitus. *Clin Endocrinol (Oxf).* 1994;41:517-524.
1013. Bereket A, Lang CH, Blethen SL, et al. Effect of insulin on the insulin-like growth factor system in children with new-onset insulin-dependent diabetes mellitus. *J Clin Endocrinol Metab.* 1995;80: 1312-1317.
1014. Rudolf MC, Sherwin RS, Markowitz R, et al. Effect of intensive insulin treatment on linear growth in the young diabetic patient. *J Pediatr.* 1982;101:333-339.
1015. Munoz MT, Barrios V, Pozo J, et al. Insulin-like growth factor I, its binding proteins 1 and 3, and growth hormone-binding protein in children and adolescents with insulin-dependent diabetes mellitus: clinical implications. *Pediatr Res.* 1996;39:992-998.
1016. Bereket A, Lang CH, Wilson TA. Alterations in the growth hormone-insulin-like growth factor axis in insulin dependent diabetes mellitus. *Horm Metab Res.* 1999;31:172-181.
1017. Dunger DB. Insulin and insulin-like growth factors in diabetes mellitus. *Arch Dis Child.* 1995;72:469-471.
1018. Suikkari AM, Koivisto VA, Rutanen EM, et al. Insulin regulates the serum levels of low molecular weight insulin-like growth factor-binding protein. *J Clin Endocrinol Metab.* 1988;66:266-272.
1019. Batch JA, Baxter RC, Werther G. Abnormal regulation of insulin-like growth factor binding proteins in adolescents with insulin-dependent diabetes. *J Clin Endocrinol Metab.* 1991;73:964-968.
1020. Taylor AM, Dunger DB, Preece MA, et al. The growth hormone independent insulin-like growth factor-I binding protein BP-28 is associated with serum insulin-like growth factor-I inhibitory bioactivity in adolescent insulin-dependent diabetics. *Clin Endocrinol (Oxf).* 1990;32:229-239.
1021. Bereket A, Lang CH, Blethen SL, et al. Insulin-like growth factor binding protein-3 proteolysis in children with insulin-dependent diabetes mellitus: a possible role for insulin in the regulation of IGFBP-3 protease activity. *J Clin Endocrinol Metab.* 1995;80: 2282-2288.
1022. Winter RJ, Phillips LS, Klein MN, et al. Somatomedin activity and diabetic control in children with insulin-dependent diabetes. *Diabetes.* 1979;28:952-954.
1023. Clarson D, Daneman D, Ehrlich RM. The relation of metabolic control to growth and pubertal development in children with insulin-dependent diabetes. *Diabetes Res.* 1985;2:237-241.
1024. Du Caju MV, Rooman RP, op de Beeck L. Longitudinal data on growth and final height in diabetic children. *Pediatr Res.* 1995;38: 607-611.
1025. Tamborlane WV, Hintz RL, Bergman M, et al. Insulin-infusion-pump treatment of diabetes: influence of improved metabolic control on plasma somatomedin levels. *N Engl J Med.* 1981;305:303-307.
1026. Reid IR. Pathogenesis and treatment of steroid osteoporosis. *Clin Endocrinol (Oxf).* 1989;30:83-103.
1027. Giustina A, Bussi AR, Jacobello C, et al. Effects of recombinant human growth hormone (GH) on bone and intermediary metabolism in patients receiving chronic glucocorticoid treatment with suppressed endogenous GH response to GH-releasing hormone. *J Clin Endocrinol Metab.* 1995;80:122-129.
1028. Allen DB, Goldberg BD. Stimulation of collagen synthesis and linear growth by growth hormone in glucocorticoid-treated children. *Pediatrics.* 1992;89:416-421.

1029. Schatz M, Dudl J, Zeiger RS, et al. Osteoporosis in corticosteroid-treated asthmatic patients: clinical correlates. *Allergy Proc*. 1993;14:341-345.
1030. Kerrebijn KF, de Kroon JP. Effect of height of corticosteroid therapy in asthmatic children. *Arch Dis Child*. 1968;43:556-561.
1031. Leong GM, Mercado-Asis LB, Reynolds JC, et al. The effect of Cushing's disease on bone mineral density, body composition, growth, and puberty: a report of an identical adolescent twin pair. *J Clin Endocrinol Metab*. 1996;81:1905-1911.
1032. Nassif E, Weinberger M, Sherman B, et al. Extrapulmonary effects of maintenance corticosteroid therapy with alternate-day prednisone and inhaled beclomethasone in children with chronic asthma. *J Allergy Clin Immunol*. 1987;80:518-529.
1033. Reimer LG, Morris HG, Ellis EF. Growth of asthmatic children during treatment with alternate-day steriods. *J Allergy Clin Immunol*. 1975;55:224-231.
1034. Lai HC, FitzSimmons SC, Allen DB, et al. Risk of persistent growth impairment after alternate-day prednisone treatment in children with cystic fibrosis. *N Engl J Med*. 2000;342:851-859.
1035. Sharek PJ, Bergman DA. The effect of inhaled steroids on the linear growth of children with asthma: a meta-analysis. *Pediatrics*. 2000;106:E8.
1036. Allen DB, Julius JR, Breen TJ, et al. Treatment of glucocorticoid-induced growth suppression with growth hormone: National Cooperative Growth Study. *J Clin Endocrinol Metab*. 1998;83:2824-2829.
1037. Rivkees SA, Danon M, Herrin J. Prednisone dose limitation of growth hormone treatment of steroid-induced growth failure. *J Pediatr*. 1994;125:322-325.
1038. Horber FF, Haymond MW. Human growth hormone prevents the protein catabolic side effects of prednisone in humans. *J Clin Invest*. 1990;86:265-272.
1039. Mauras N, Beaufrere B. Recombinant human insulin-like growth factor-I enhances whole body protein anabolism and significantly diminishes the protein catabolic effects of prednisone in humans without a diabetogenic effect. *J Clin Endocrinol Metab*. 1995;80:869-874.
1040. Lebrethon MC, Grossman AB, Afshar F, et al. Linear growth and final height after treatment for Cushing's disease in childhood. *J Clin Endocrinol Metab*. 2000;85:3262-3265.
1041. Savage MO, Lienhardt A, Lebrethon MC, et al. Cushing's disease in childhood: presentation, investigation, treatment and long-term outcome. *Horm Res*. 2001;55(suppl 1):24-30.
1042. Schwindinger WF, Levine MA. Albright hereditary osteodystrophy. *Endocrinologist*. 1994;4:17-27.
1043. Long DN, McGuire S, Levine MA, et al. Body mass index differences in pseudohypoparathyroidism type 1a versus pseudopseudohypoparathyroidism may implicate paternal imprinting of Galpha(s) in the development of human obesity. *J Clin Endocrinol Metab*. 2007;92:1073-1079.
1044. Germain-Lee EL, Groman J, Crane JL, et al. Growth hormone deficiency in pseudohypoparathyroidism type 1a: another manifestation of multihormone resistance. *J Clin Endocrinol Metab*. 2003;88:4059-4069.
1045. Mantovani G, Maghnie M, Weber G, et al. Growth hormone-releasing hormone resistance in pseudohypoparathyroidism type Ia: new evidence for imprinting of the Gs alpha gene. *J Clin Endocrinol Metab*. 2003;88:4070-4074.
1046. Germain-Lee EL. Short stature, obesity, and growth hormone deficiency in pseudohypoparathyroidism type 1a. *Pediatr Endocrinol Rev*. 2006;3(suppl 2):318-327.
1047. Plagge A, Kelsey G, Germain-Lee EL. Physiological functions of the imprinted GNAS locus and its protein variants Galpha(s) and XLalpha(s) in human and mouse. *J Endocrinol*. 2008;196:193-214.
1048. Minamitani K, Takahashi Y, Minagawa M, et al. Difference in height associated with a translation start site polymorphism in the vitamin D receptor gene. *Pediatr Res*. 1998;44:628-632.
1049. Lorentzon M, Lorentzon R, Nordstrom P. Vitamin D receptor gene polymorphism is associated with birth height, growth to adolescence, and adult stature in healthy Caucasian men: a cross-sectional and longitudinal study. *J Clin Endocrinol Metab*. 2000;85:1666-1670.
1050. Suarez F, Zeghoud F, Rossignol C, et al. Association between vitamin D receptor gene polymorphism and sex-dependent growth during the first two years of life. *J Clin Endocrinol Metab*. 1997;82:2966-2970.
1051. Kanan RM, Varanasi SS, Francis RM, et al. Vitamin D receptor gene start codon polymorphism (FokI) and bone mineral density in healthy male subjects. *Clin Endocrinol (Oxf)*. 2000;53:93-98.
1052. Arai H, Miyamoto K, Taketani Y, et al. A vitamin D receptor gene polymorphism in the translation initiation codon: effect on protein activity and relation to bone mineral density in Japanese women. *J Bone Miner Res*. 1997;12:915-921.
1053. Suarez F, Rossignol C, Garabedian M. Interactive effect of estradiol and vitamin D receptor gene polymorphisms as a possible determinant of growth in male and female infants. *J Clin Endocrinol Metab*. 1998;83:3563-3568.
1054. Alonso M, Segura C, Dieguez C, et al. High affinity binding sites to the vitamin D receptor DNA binding domain in the human growth hormone promoter. *Biochem Biophys Res Commun*. 2000;247:882-887.
1055. Cho HY, Lee BH, Kang JH, et al. A clinical and molecular genetic study of hypophosphatemic rickets in children. *Pediatr Res*. 2005;58:329-333.
1056. Shimada T, Hasegawa H, Yamazaki Y, et al. FGF-23 is a potent regulator of vitamin D metabolism and phosphate homeostasis. *J Bone Miner Res*. 2004;19:429-435.
1057. Makitie O, Doria A, Kooh SW, et al. Early treatment improves growth and biochemical and radiographic outcome in X-linked hypophosphatemic rickets. *J Clin Endocrinol Metab*. 2003;88:3591-3597.
1058. Chan JC. Renal hypophosphatemic rickets: a review. *Int J Pediatr Nephrol*. 1982;3:305-310.
1059. Glorieux FH, Marie PJ, Pettifor JM, et al. Bone response to phosphate salts, ergocalciferol, and calcitriol in hypophosphatemic vitamin D-resistant rickets. *N Engl J Med*. 1980;303:1023-1031.
1060. Petersen DJ, Boniface AM, Schranck FW, et al. X-linked hypophosphatemic rickets: a study (with literature review) of linear growth response to calcitriol and phosphate therapy. *J Bone Miner Res*. 1992;7:583-597.
1061. Balsan S, Tieder M. Linear growth in patients with hypophosphatemic vitamin D-resistant rickets: influence of treatment regimen and parental height. *J Pediatr*. 1990;116:365-371.
1062. Jasper H, Cassinelli H. Growth hormone and insulin-like growth factor I plasma levels in patients with hypophosphatemic rickets. *J Pediatr Endocrinol*. 1993;6:179-184.
1063. Saggese G, Baroncelli GI, Bertelloni S, et al. Growth hormone secretion in poorly growing children with renal hypophosphataemic rickets. *Eur J Pediatr*. 1994;153:548-555.
1064. Bistritzer T, Chalew SA, Hanukoglu A, et al. Does growth hormone influence the severity of phosphopenic rickets? *Eur J Pediatr*. 1990;150:26-29.
1065. Wilson DM, Lee PD, Morris AH, et al. Growth hormone therapy in hypophosphatemic rickets. *Am J Dis Child*. 1991;145:1165-1170.
1066. Wilson DM. Growth hormone and hypophosphatemic rickets. *J Pediatr Endocrinol Metab*. 2000;13(suppl 2):993-998.
1067. Baroncelli GI, Bertelloni S, Ceccarelli C, et al. Effect of growth hormone treatment on final height, phosphate metabolism, and bone mineral density in children with X-linked hypophosphatemic rickets. *J Pediatr*. 2001;138:236-243.
1068. Haffner D, Nissel R, Wuhl E, et al. Effects of growth hormone treatment on body proportions and final height among small children with X-linked hypophosphatemic rickets. *Pediatrics*. 2004;113:e593-e596.
1069. Spranger J. International classification of osteochondrodysplasias: The International Working Group on Constitutional Diseases of Bone. *Eur J Pediatr*. 1992;151:407-415.
1070. Pauli RM. Osteochondrodysplasia with mild clinical manifestations: a guide for endocrinologists and others. *Growth Genet Horm*. 1995;11:1-5.
1071. Maroteaux P. Nomenclature internationale des maladies osseuses constitutionnelles. *Ann Radiol*. 1970;13:455-464.
1072. Rimoin DL. International nomenclature of constitutional diseases of bone: revision—May, 1977. *Birth Defects Orig Artic Ser*. 1978;14:39-45.
1073. Shiang R, Thompson LM, Zhu YZ, et al. Mutations in the transmembrane domain of FGFR3 cause the most common genetic form of dwarfism, achondroplasia. *Cell*. 1994;78:335-342.
1074. International nomenclature and classification of the osteochondrodysplasias (1997): International Working Group on Constitutional Diseases of Bone. *Am J Med Genet*. 1998;79:376-382.
1075. Hall CM. International nosology and classification of constitutional disorders of bone (2001). *Am J Med Genet*. 2002;113:65-77.
1076. Hecht JT, Butler IJ. Neurologic morbidity associated with achondroplasia. *J Child Neurol*. 1990;5:84-97.
1077. Hahn YS, Engelhard 3rd HH, Naidich T, et al. Paraplegia resulting from thoracolumbar stenosis in a seven-month-old achondroplastic dwarf. *Pediatr Neurosci*. 1989;15:39-43.
1078. Yamate T, Kanzaki S, Tanaka H, et al. Growth hormone (GH) treatment in achondroplasia. *J Pediatr Endocrinol*. 1993;6:45-52.
1079. Waters KA, Kirjavainen T, Jimenez M, et al. Overnight growth hormone secretion in achondroplasia: deconvolution analysis, correlation with sleep state, and changes after treatment of obstructive sleep apnea. *Pediatr Res*. 1996;39:547-553.
1080. Rousseau F, Bonaventure J, Legeai-Mallet L, et al. Mutations in the gene encoding fibroblast growth factor receptor-3 in achondroplasia. *Nature*. 1994;371:252-254.
1081. Francomano CA. The genetic basis of dwarfism. *N Engl J Med*. 1995;332:58-59.
1082. Bellus GA, Hefferon TW, Ortiz de Luna RI, et al. Achondroplasia is defined by recurrent G380R mutations of FGFR3. *Am J Hum Genet*. 1995;56:368-373.

1083. Vajo Z, Francomano CA, Wilkin DJ. The molecular and genetic basis of fibroblast growth factor receptor 3 disorders: the achondroplasia family of skeletal dysplasias, Muenke craniosynostosis, and Crouzon syndrome with acanthosis nigricans. *Endocr Rev*. 2000;21:23-39.
1084. Chen L, Adar R, Yang X, et al. Gly369Cys mutation in mouse FGFR3 causes achondroplasia by affecting both chondrogenesis and osteogenesis. *J Clin Invest*. 1999;104:1517-1525.
1085. Chen L, Li C, Qiao W, et al. A ser(365) → Cys mutation of fibroblast growth factor receptor 3 in mouse downregulates Ihh/PTHrP signals and causes severe achondroplasia. *Hum Mol Genet*. 2001;10: 457-465.
1086. Ramaswami U, Rumsby G, Hindmarsh PC, et al. Genotype and phenotype in hypochondroplasia. *J Pediatr*. 1998;133:99-102.
1087. Ross JL, Kowal K, Quigley CA, et al. The phenotype of short stature homeobox gene (SHOX) deficiency in childhood: contrasting children with Léri-Weill dyschondrosteosis and Turner syndrome. *J Pediatr*. 2005;147:499-507.
1088. Marchini A, Marttila T, Winter A, et al. The short stature homeodomain protein SHOX induces cellular growth arrest and apoptosis and is expressed in human growth plate chondrocytes. *J Biol Chem*. 2004;279:37103-37114.
1089. Ogata T, Fukami M. Clinical features in SHOX haploinsufficiency: diagnostic and therapeutic implications. *Growth Genet Horm*. 2004;20:17-23.
1090. Schneider KU, Sabherwal N, Jantz K, et al. Identification of a major recombination hotspot in patients with short stature and SHOX deficiency. *Am J Hum Genet*. 2005;77:89-96.
1091. Bartels CF, Bukulmez H, Padayatti P, et al. Mutations in the transmembrane natriuretic peptide receptor NPR-B impair skeletal growth and cause acromesomelic dysplasia, type maroteaux. *Am J Hum Genet*. 2004;75:27-34.
1092. Olney RC, Bukulmez H, Bartels CF, et al. Heterozygous mutations in natriuretic peptide receptor-B (NPR2) are associated with short stature. *J Clin Endocrinol Metab*. 2006;91:1229-1232.
1093. Anneren G, Sara VR, Hall K, et al. Growth and somatomedin responses to growth hormone in Down's syndrome. *Arch Dis Child*. 1986;61:48-52.
1094. Anneren G, Tuvemo T, Gustafsson J. Growth hormone therapy in young children with down syndrome and a clinical comparison of Down and Prader-Willi syndromes. *Growth Horm IGF Res*. 2000;10(suppl B):S87-S91.
1095. Rosenfeld RG, Grumbach MM. *Turner syndrome*. New York, NY: Marcel Dekker; 1990.
1096. Turner syndrome: growth promoting therapies: proceedings of a Workshop on Turner Syndrome. Amsterdam, The Netherlands: Excerpta Medica; 1991.
1097. Basic and clinical approach to Turner syndrome: proceedings of the 3rd International Symposium on Turner Syndrome. Amsterdam, The Netherlands: Excerpta Medica; 1993.
1098. Rochiccioli P, David M, Malpuech G, et al. Study of final height in Turner's syndrome: ethnic and genetic influences. *Acta Paediatr*. 1994;83:305-308.
1099. Nilsson KO, Albertsson-Wikland K, Alm J, et al. Improved final height in girls with Turner's syndrome treated with growth hormone and oxandrolone. *J Clin Endocrinol Metab*. 1996;81:635-640.
1100. Rosenfeld RG, Attie KM, Frane J, et al. Growth hormone therapy of Turner's syndrome: beneficial effect on adult height. *J Pediatr*. 1998;132:319-324.
1101. Brook CG, Gasser T, Werder EA, et al. Height correlations between parents and mature offspring in normal subjects and in subjects with Turner's and Klinefelter's and other syndromes. *Ann Hum Biol*. 1977;4:17-22.
1102. Massa G, Vanderschueren-Lodeweyckx M, Malvaux P. Linear growth in patients with Turner syndrome: influence of spontaneous puberty and parental height. *Eur J Pediatr*. 1990;149:246-250.
1103. Ranke MB, Pfluger H, Rosendahl W, et al. Turner syndrome: spontaneous growth in 150 cases and review of the literature. *Eur J Pediatr*. 1983;141:81-88.
1104. Davenport ML, Punyasavatsut N, Gunther D, et al. Turner syndrome: a pattern of early growth failure. *Acta Paediatr Suppl*. 1999;88: 118-121.
1105. Even L, Cohen A, Marbach N, et al. Longitudinal analysis of growth over the first 3 years of life in Turner's syndrome. *J Pediatr*. 2000;137:460-464.
1106. Davenport ML, Punyasavatsut N, Stewart PW, et al. Growth failure in early life: an important manifestation of Turner syndrome. *Horm Res*. 2002;57:157-164.
1107. Blaschke RJ, Rappold GA. SHOX: growth, Léri-Weill and Turner syndromes. *Trends Endocrinol Metab*. 2000;11:227-230.
1108. Ross JL, Scott Jr C, Marttila P, et al. Phenotypes associated with SHOX deficiency. *J Clin Endocrinol Metab*. 2001;86:5674-5680.
1109. Ross JL, Long LM, Loriaux DL, et al. Growth hormone secretory dynamics in Turner syndrome. *J Pediatr*. 1985;106:202-206.
1110. Sas TC, de Muinck Keizer-Schrama SM, Stijnen T, et al. Normalization of height in girls with Turner syndrome after long-term growth hormone treatment: rsults of a randomized dose-response trial. *J Clin Endocrinol Metab*. 1999;84:4607-4612.
1111. Saenger P. Growth-promoting strategies in Turner's syndrome. *J Clin Endocrinol Metab*. 1999;84:4345-4348.
1112. Collins E, Turner G. The Noonan syndrome: a review of the clinical and genetic features of 27 cases. *J Pediatr*. 1973;83:941-950.
1113. Kelnar CJ. Growth hormone therapy in Noonan syndrome. *Horm Res*. 2000;53(suppl 1):77-81.
1114. Tartaglia M, Mehler EL, Goldberg R, et al. Mutations in PTPN11, encoding the protein tyrosine phosphatase SHP-2, cause Noonan syndrome. *Nat Genet*. 2001;29:465-468.
1115. Kosaki K, Suzuki T, Muroya K, et al. PTPN11 (protein-tyrosine phosphatase, nonreceptor-type 11) mutations in seven Japanese patients with Noonan syndrome. *J Clin Endocrinol Metab*. 2002;87:3529-3533.
1116. Jongmans M, Otten B, Noordam K, et al. Genetics and variation in phenotype in Noonan syndrome. *Horm Res*. 2004;62(suppl 3):56-59.
1117. Patton MA. Noonan syndrome: a review. *Growth Genet Horm*. 1994;10:1-3.
1118. Ranke MB, Heidemann P, Knupfer C, et al. Noonan syndrome: growth and clinical manifestations in 144 cases. *Eur J Pediatr*. 1988;148: 220-227.
1119. Witt DR, Keena BA, Hall JG, et al. Growth curves for height in Noonan syndrome. *Clin Genet*. 1986;30:150-153.
1120. Bernardini S, Spadoni GL, Cianfarani S, et al. Growth hormone secretion in Noonan's syndrome. *J Pediatr Endocrinol*. 1991;4:217-221.
1121. Ferreira LV, Souza SA, Arnhold IJ, et al. PTPN11 (protein tyrosine phosphatase, nonreceptor type 11) mutations and response to growth hormone therapy in children with Noonan syndrome. *J Clin Endocrinol Metab*. 2005;90:5156-5160.
1122. Binder G, Neuer K, Ranke MB, et al. PTPN11 mutations are associated with mild growth hormone resistance in individuals with Noonan syndrome. *J Clin Endocrinol Metab*. 2005;90:5377-5381.
1123. Limal JM, Parfait B, Cabrol S, et al. Noonan syndrome: relationships between genotype, growth, and growth factors. *J Clin Endocrinol Metab*. 2006;91:300-306.
1124. Bray GA, Dahms WT, Swerdloff RS, et al. The Prader-Willi syndrome: a study of 40 patients and a review of the literature. *Medicine (Baltimore)*. 1983;62:59-80.
1125. Jones KL. *Smith's Recognizable Patterns of Human Malformation*. Philadelphia, PA: Saunders; 1988.
1125A. Saenger P, Czernichow, Hughes I, et al. Small for gestational age: short stature and beyond. *Endocr Rev*. 2007;28:219-251.
1126. Lepercq J, Mahieu-Caputo D. Diagnosis and management of intrauterine growth retardation. *Horm Res*. 1998;49(suppl 2):14-19.
1127. Hokken-Koelega AC, De Ridder MA, Lemmen RJ, et al. Children born small for gestational age: do they catch up? *Pediatr Res*. 1995;38:267-271.
1128. Seminara S, Rapisardi G, La Cauza F, et al. Catch-up growth in short-at-birth NICU graduates. *Horm Res*. 2000;53:139-143.
1129. Leger J, Limoni C, Collin D, et al. Prediction factors in the determination of final height in subjects born small for gestational age. *Pediatr Res*. 1998;43:808-812.
1130. Rappaport R. Fetal growth. In: Bertrand J, Rappaport R, Sizonenko PC, eds. *Pediatric Endocrinology: Physiology, Pathophysiology, and Clinical Aspects*, 2nd ed. Baltimore, MD: Williams & Wilkins; 1993.
1131. Smith GC, Smith MF, McNay MB, et al. First-trimester growth and the risk of low birth weight. *N Engl J Med*. 1999;339:1817-1822.
1132. Patterson RM, Pouliot MR. Neonatal morphometrics and perinatal outcome: who is growth retarded? *Am J Obstet Gynecol*. 1987;157:691-693.
1133. Campbell S, Thoms A. Ultrasound measurement of the fetal head to abdomen circumference ratio in the assessment of growth retardation. *Br J Obstet Gynaecol*. 1977;84:165-174.
1134. Hindmarsh PC, Geary MPP, Rodeck CH, et al. Intrauterine growth and its relationship to size and shape at birth. *Pediatr Res*. 2002;52:263-268.
1135. Vik T, Markestad T, Ahlsten G, et al. Body proportions and early neonatal morbidity in small-for-gestational-age infants of successive births. *Acta Obstet Gynecol Scand Suppl*. 1997;165:76-81.
1136. Wit JM, van Unen H. Growth of infants with neonatal growth hormone deficiency. *Arch Dis Child*. 1992;67:920-924.
1137. Hattersley AT, Beards F, Ballantyne E, et al. Mutations in the glucokinase gene of the fetus result in reduced birth weight. *Nat Genet*. 1998;19:268-270.
1138. Warshaw JB. Intrauterine growth restriction revisited. *Growth Genet Horm*. 1992;8:5-8.
1139. Vaessen N, Janssen JA, Heutink P, et al. Association between genetic variation in the gene for insulin-like growth factor-I and low birthweight. *Lancet*. 2002;359:1036-1037.
1140. Arends N, Johnston L, Hokken-Koelega A, et al. Polymorphism in the IGF-I gene: clinical relevance for short children born small for gestational age (SGA). *J Clin Endocrinol Metab*. 2002;87:2720.

1141. de Zegher F, Kimpen J, Raus J, et al. Hypersomatotropism in the dysmature infant at term and preterm birth. *Biol Neonate.* 1990;58:188-191.
1142. Spencer JA, Chang TC, Jones J, et al. Third trimester fetal growth and umbilical venous blood concentrations of IGF-1, IGFBP-1, and growth hormone at term. *Arch Dis Child Fetal Neonatal Ed.* 1995;73:F87-F90.
1143. Leger J, Oury JF, Noel M, et al. Growth factors and intrauterine growth retardation: I. Serum growth hormone, insulin-like growth factor (IGF)-I, IGF-II, and IGF binding protein 3 levels in normally grown and growth-retarded human fetuses during the second half of gestation. *Pediatr Res.* 1996;40:94-100.
1144. Cianfarani S, Germani D, Rossi L, et al. IGF-I and IGF-binding protein-1 are related to cortisol in human cord blood. *Eur J Endocrinol.* 1998;138:524-529.
1145. Cance-Rouzaud A, Laborie S, Bieth E, et al. Growth hormone, insulin-like growth factor-I and insulin-like growth factor binding protein-3 are regulated differently in small-for-gestational-age and appropriate-for-gestational-age neonates. *Biol Neonate.* 1998;73:347-355.
1146. Wollmann HA, Ranke MB. GH treatment in neonates. *Acta Paediatr.* 1996;85:398-400.
1147. van Toledo-Eppinga L, Houdijk EC, Cranendonk A, et al. Effects of recombinant human growth hormone treatment in intrauterine growth-retarded preterm newborn infant on growth, body composition and energy expenditure. *Acta Paediatr.* 1996;85:476-481.
1148. Leger J, Noel M, Limal JM, et al. Growth factors and intrauterine growth retardation: II. Serum growth hormone, insulin-like growth factor (IGF) I, and IGF-binding protein 3 levels in children with intrauterine growth retardation compared with normal control subjects: prospective study from birth to two years of age. study group of IUGR. *Pediatr Res.* 1996;40:101-107.
1149. Boguszewski M, Rosberg S, Albertsson-Wikland K. Spontaneous 24-hour growth hormone profiles in prepubertal small for gestational age children. *J Clin Endocrinol Metab.* 1995;80:2599-2606.
1150. Ackland FM, Stanhope R, Eyre C, et al. Physiological growth hormone secretion in children with short stature and intra-uterine growth retardation. *Horm Res.* 1988;30:241-245.
1151. de Waal WJ, Hokken-Koelega AC, Stijnen T, et al. Endogenous and stimulated GH secretion, urinary GH excretion, and plasma IGF-I and IGF-II levels in prepubertal children with short stature after intrauterine growth retardation: The Dutch Working Group on Growth Hormone. *Clin Endocrinol (Oxf).* 1994;41:621-630.
1152. Ibanez L, Dimartino-Nardi J, Potau N, et al. Premature adrenarche: normal variant or forerunner of adult disease? *Endocr Rev.* 2000;21:671-696.
1153. Barker DJ, Gluckman PD, Godfrey KM, et al. Fetal nutrition and cardiovascular disease in adult life. *Lancet.* 1993;341:938-941.
1154. Barker DJ. Growth in utero and coronary heart disease. *Nutr Rev.* 1996;54(2 Pt 2):S1-S7.
1155. Osmond C, Barker DJ. Fetal, infant, and childhood growth are predictors of coronary heart disease, diabetes, and hypertension in adult men and women. *Environ Health Perspect.* 2000;108(suppl 3):545-553.
1156. Barker DJ, Meade TW, Fall CH, et al. Relation of fetal and infant growth to plasma fibrinogen and factor VII concentrations in adult life. *BMJ.* 1992;304:148-152.
1157. Gluckman PD, Hanson MA. Living with the past: evolution, development, and patterns of disease. *Science.* 2004;305:1733-1736.
1158. Gluckman PD, Hanson MA, Morton SM, et al. Life-long echoes: a critical analysis of the developmental origins of adult disease model. *Biol Neonate.* 2005;87:127-139.
1159. Barker DJ, Bagby SP. Developmental antecedents of cardiovascular disease: a historical perspective. *J Am Soc Nephrol.* 2005;16:2537-2544.
1160. Hofman PL, Cutfield WS, Robinson EM, et al. Insulin resistance in short children with intrauterine growth retardation. *J Clin Endocrinol Metab.* 1997;82:402-406.
1161. Russell A. A syndrome of intra-uterine dwarfism recognizable at birth with cranio-facial dysostosis, disproportionately short arms, and other anomalies (5 examples). *Proc R Soc Med.* 1954;47:1040-1044.
1162. Silver HK. Asymmetry, short stature, and variations in sexual development: a syndrome of congenital malformations. *Am J Dis Child.* 1964;107:495-515.
1163. Angehrn V, Zachmann M, Prader A. Silver-Russell syndrome: observations in 20 patients. *Helv Paediatr Acta.* 1979;34:297-308.
1164. Davies PS, Valley R, Preece MA. Adolescent growth and pubertal progression in the Silver-Russell syndrome. *Arch Dis Child.* 1988;63:130-135.
1165. Saal HM, Pagon RA, Pepin MG. Reevaluation of Russell-Silver syndrome. *J Pediatr.* 1985;107:733-737.
1166. Wollmann HA, Kirchner T, Enders H, et al. Growth and symptoms in Silver-Russell syndrome: review on the basis of 386 patients. *Eur J Pediatr.* 1995;154:958-968.
1167. Albertsson-Wikland K, Boguszewski M, Karlberg J. Children born small-for-gestational age: postnatal growth and hormonal status. *Horm Res.* 1998;49(suppl 2):7-13.
1168. Moore GE, Abu-Amero S, Wakeling E, et al. The search for the gene for Silver-Russell syndrome. *Acta Paediatr Suppl.* 1999;88:42-48.
1169. Eggermann T, Wollmann HA, Kuner R, et al. Molecular studies in 37 Silver-Russell syndrome patients: frequency and etiology of uniparental disomy. *Hum Genet.* 1998;100:415-419.
1170. Hall JG. Russell-Silver syndrome begins to be unraveled. *Growth Genet Horm* 2000;16:35.
1171. Monk D, Wakeling EL, Proud V, et al. Duplication of 7p11.2-p13, including GRB10, in Silver-Russell syndrome. *Am J Hum Genet.* 2000;66:36-46.
1172. Miyoshi N, Kuroiwa Y, Kohda T, et al. Identification of the Meg1/Grb10 imprinted gene on mouse proximal chromosome 11, a candidate for the Silver-Russell syndrome gene. *Proc Natl Acad Sci U S A.* 1998;95:1102-1107.
1173. Eggermann T, Meyer E, Obermann C, et al. Is maternal duplication of 11p15 associated with Silver-Russell syndrome? *J Med Genet.* 2005;42:e26.
1174. Gicquel C, Rossignol S, Cabrol S, et al. Epimutation of the telomeric imprinting center region on chromosome 11p15 in Silver-Russell syndrome. *Nat Genet.* 2005;37:1003-1007.
1175. Binder G, Seidel A, Weber K, et al. IGF-II serum levels are normal in children with Silver-Russell syndrome who frequently carry epimutations at the IGF2 locus. *J Clin Endocrinol Metab.* 2006;91:4709-4712.
1176. Edwards LE, Alton IR, Barrada MI, et al. Pregnancy in the underweight woman: course, outcome, and growth patterns of the infant. *Am J Obstet Gynecol.* 1979;135:297-302.
1177. Ouellette EM, Rosett HL, Rosman NP, et al. Adverse effects on offspring of maternal alcohol abuse during pregnancy. *N Engl J Med.* 1977;297:528-530.
1178. Jones KL, Smith DW, Streissguth AP, et al. Outcome in offspring of chronic alcoholic women. *Lancet.* 1974;1:1076-1078.
1179. Abel EL. Consumption of alcohol during pregnancy: a review of effects on growth and development of offspring. *Hum Biol.* 1982;54:421-453.
1180. Zuckerman B, Frank DA, Hingson R, et al. Effects of maternal marijuana and cocaine use on fetal growth. *N Engl J Med.* 1989;320:762-768.
1181. Abel EL. Smoking during pregnancy: a review of effects on growth and development of offspring. *Hum Biol.* 1980;52:593-625.
1182. Hall K, Enberg G, Hellem E, et al. Somatomedin levels in pregnancy: longitudinal study in healthy subjects and patients with growth hormone deficiency. *J Clin Endocrinol Metab.* 1984;59:587-594.
1183. Mirlesse V, Frankenne F, Alsat E, et al. Placental growth hormone levels in normal pregnancy and in pregnancies with intrauterine growth retardation. *Pediatr Res.* 1993;34:439-442.
1184. Hasegawa T, Hasegawa Y, Takada M, et al. The free form of insulin-like growth factor I increases in circulation during normal human pregnancy. *J Clin Endocrinol Metab.* 1995;80:3284-3286.
1185. Verhaeghe J, Bougoussa M, Van Herck E, et al. Placental growth hormone and IGF-I in a pregnant woman with Pit-1 deficiency. *Clin Endocrinol (Oxf).* 2000;53:645-647.
1186. Li Y, Behringer RR. Esx1 is an X-chromosome-imprinted regulator of placental development and fetal growth. *Nat Genet.* 1998;20:309-311.
1187. Li Y, Lemaire P, Behringer RR. Esx1, a novel X chromosome-linked homeobox gene expressed in mouse extraembryonic tissues and male germ cells. *Dev Biol.* 1997;188:85-95.
1188. Fohn LE, Behringer RR. ESX1L, a novel X chromosome-linked human homeobox gene expressed in the placenta and testis. *Genomics.* 2001;74:105-108.
1189. Sotos JF, Cutler EA, Dodre P. Cerebral gigantism. *Am J Dis Child* 1977;131:625-667.
1190. Wit JM, Beemer FA, Barth PG, et al. Cerebral gigantism (Sotos syndrome)—compiled data of 22 cases: analysis of clinical features, growth and plasma somatomedin. *Eur J Pediatr.* 1985;144:131-140.
1191. Agwu JC, Shaw NJ, Kirk J, et al. Growth in Sotos syndrome. *Arch Dis Child.* 1999;80:339-342.
1192. Waggoner DJ, Raca G, Welch K, et al. NSD1 analysis for Sotos syndrome: insights and perspectives from the clinical laboratory. *Genet Med.* 2005;7:524-533.
1193. Sotelo-Avila C, Gonzalez-Crussi F, Fowler JW. Complete and incomplete forms of Beckwith-Wiedemann syndrome: their oncogenic potential. *J Pediatr.* 1980;96:47-50.
1194. Elliott M, Bayly R, Cole T, et al. Clinical features and natural history of Beckwith-Wiedemann syndrome: presentation of 74 new cases. *Clin Genet.* 1994;46:168-174.
1195. Weng EY, Moeschler JB, Graham Jr JM. Longitudinal observations on 15 children with Wiedemann-Beckwith syndrome. *Am J Med Genet.* 1995;56:366-373.
1196. Morison IM, Becroft DM, Taniguchi T, et al. Somatic overgrowth associated with overexpression of insulin-like growth factor II. *Nat Med.* 1996;2:311-316.
1197. Drummond IA, Madden SL, Rohwer-Nutter P, et al. Repression of the insulin-like growth factor II gene by the Wilms tumor suppressor WT1. *Science.* 1992;257:674-678.

1198. Schofield PN, Nystrom A, Smith J, et al. Expression of a high molecular weight form of insulin-like growth factor II in a Beckwith-Wiedemann syndrome associated adrenocortical adenoma. *Cancer Lett.* 1995;94:71-77.
1199. Kubota T, Saitoh S, Matsumoto T, et al. Excess functional copy of allele at chromosomal region 11p15 may cause Wiedemann-Beckwith (EMG) syndrome. *Am J Med Genet.* 1994;49:378-383.
1200. Prawitt D, Enklaar T, Gartner-Rupprecht B, et al. Microdeletion and IGF2 loss of imprinting in a cascade causing Beckwith-Wiedemann syndrome with Wilms' tumor. *Nat Genet.* 2005;37:785-786, author reply 786-787.
1201. Brannan CI, Bartolomei MS. Mechanisms of genomic imprinting. *Curr Opin Genet Dev.* 1999;9:164-170.
1202. Reik W, Constancia M, Dean W, et al. Igf2 imprinting in development and disease. *Int J Dev Biol.* 2000;44:145-150.
1203. Cano-Gauci DF, Song HH, Yang H, et al. Glypican-3-deficient mice exhibit developmental overgrowth and some of the abnormalities typical of Simpson-Golabi-Behmel syndrome. *J Cell Biol.* 1999;146:255-264.
1204. Veugelers M, Cat BD, Muyldermans SY, et al. Mutational analysis of the GPC3/GPC4 glypican gene cluster on Xq26 in patients with Simpson-Golabi-Behmel syndrome: identification of loss-of-function mutations in the GPC3 gene. *Hum Mol Genet.* 2000;9:1321-1328.
1205. Joss EE, Temperli R, Mullis PE. Adult height in constitutionally tall stature: accuracy of five different height prediction methods. *Arch Dis Child.* 1992;67:1357-1362.
1206. Tauber M, Pienkowski C, Rochiccioli P. Growth hormone secretion in children and adolescents with familial tall stature. *Eur J Pediatr.* 1994;153:311-316.
1207. Elias LL, Huebner A, Metherell LA, et al. Tall stature in familial glucocorticoid deficiency. *Clin Endocrinol (Oxf).* 2000;53:423-430.
1208. Ogata T, Kosho T, Wakui K, et al. Short stature homeobox-containing gene duplication on the der(X) chromosome in a female with 45,X/46,X, der(X), gonadal dysgenesis, and tall stature. *J Clin Endocrinol Metab.* 2000;85:2927-2930.
1209. Nakamura Y, Suehiro Y, Sugino N, et al. A case of 46,X,der(X) (pter→q21::P21→pter) with gonadal dysgenesis, tall stature, and endometriosis. *Fertil Steril.* 2001;75:1224-1225.
1210. Ogata T, Matsuo N. Sex chromosome aberrations and stature: deduction of the principal factors involved in the determination of adult height. *Hum Genet.* 1993;91:551-562.
1211. Tanner JM, Whitehouse RH, Takaishi M. Standards from birth to maturity for height, weight, height velocity, and weight velocity: British children, 1965. Part II. *Arch Dis Child.* 1966;41:613-635.
1212. Forbes GB. Nutrition and growth. *J Pediatr.* 1977;91:40-42.
1213. Ong KK, Ahmed ML, Emmett PM, et al. Association between postnatal catch-up growth and obesity in childhood: prospective cohort study. *BMJ.* 2000;320:967-971.
1214. Cole TJ. The secular trend in human physical growth: a biological view. *Econ Hum Biol.* 2003;1:161-168.
1215. Spence HJ, Trias EP, Raiti S. Acromegaly in a 9 and one-half-year-old boy: pituitary function studies before and after surgery. *Am J Dis Child.* 1972;123:504-506.
1216. AvRuskin TW, Sau K, Tang S, et al. Childhood acromegaly: successful therapy with conventional radiation and effects of chlorpromazine on growth hormone and prolactin secretion. *J Clin Endocrinol Metab.* 1973;37:380-388.
1217. DeMajo SF, Onativia A. Acromegaly and gigantism in a boy: comparison with three overgrown non-acromegalic children. *Pediatrics.* 1960;57:382-390.
1218. Lefkowitz RJ. G proteins in medicine. *N Engl J Med.* 1995;332:186-187.
1219. Lightner ES, Winter JS. Treatment of juvenile acromegaly with bromocriptine. *J Pediatr.* 1981;98:494-496.
1220. Geffner ME, Nagel RA, Dietrich RB, et al. Treatment of acromegaly with a somatostatin analog in a patient with McCune-Albright syndrome. *J Pediatr.* 1987;111:740-743.
1221. Hoffman WH, Perrin JC, Halac E, et al. Acromegalic gigantism and tuberous sclerosis. *J Pediatr.* 1978;93:478-480.
1222. Daughaday WH. Extreme gigantism: analysis of growth velocity and occurrence of severe peripheral neuropathy and neuropathic arthropathy (Charcot joints). *N Engl J Med.* 1977;297:1267-1269.
1223. Hindmarsh PC, Brook CG. Auxological and biochemical assessment of short stature. *Acta Paediatr Scand Suppl.* 1988;343:73-76.
1224. Voss LD, Wilkin TJ, Bailey BJ, et al. The reliability of height and height velocity in the assessment of growth (the Wessex Growth Study). *Arch Dis Child.* 1991;66:833-837.
1225. Pandian R, Nakamoto JM. Rational use of the laboratory for childhood and adult growth hormone deficiency. *Clin Lab Med.* 2004;24:141-174.
1226. Akin F, Yaylali GF, Turgut S, et al. Growth hormone/insulin-like growth factor axis in patients with subclinical thyroid dysfunction. *Growth Horm IGF Res.* 2009;19:252-255.
1227. Purandare A, Co Ng L, Godil M, et al. Effect of hypothyroidism and its treatment on the IGF system in infants and children. *J Pediatr Endocrinol Metab.* 2003;16:35-42.
1228. Greulich WW, Pyle SI. *Radiographic Atlas of Skeletal Development of the Hand and Wrist.* Stanford, CA: Stanford University Press; 1959.
1229. Tanner JM, Whitehouse RH, Cameron N, et al. *Assessment of skeletal maturity and prediction of adult height (TW2 method).* New York: Academic Press; 1983. ID: 255.
1230. Tanner JM, Oshman D, Lindgren G, et al. Reliability and validity of Computer-Assisted Estimates of Tanner-Whitehouse Skeletal Maturity (CASAS): comparison with the manual method. *Horm Res.* 1994;42:288-294.
1231. Van Teunenbroek A, De Waal W, Roks A, et al. Computer-aided skeletal age scores in healthy children, girls with Turner syndrome, and in children with constitutionally tall stature. *Pediatr Res.* 1996;39:360-367.
1232. Roche AF, Davila GH, Eyman SL. A comparison between Greulich-Pyle and Tanner-Whitehouse assessments of skeletal maturity. *Radiology.* 1971;98:273-280.
1233. Bayley N, Pinneau SR. Tables for predicting adult height from skeletal age: revised for use with the Greulich-Pyle hand standards. *J Pediatr.* 1952;40:423-441.
1234. Roche AF, Wainer H, Thissen D. The RWT method for the prediction of adult stature. *Pediatrics.* 1975;56:1027-1033.
1235. Khamis HJ, Roche AF. Predicting adult stature without using skeletal age: the Khamis-Roche method. *Pediatrics.* 1994;94(4 Pt 1):504-507.
1236. Oerter KE, Manasco P, Barnes KM, et al. Adult height in precocious puberty after long-term treatment with deslorelin. *J Clin Endocrinol Metab.* 1991;73:1235-1240.
1237. Growth Hormone Research Society. Consensus guidelines for the diagnosis and treatment of growth hormone (GH) deficiency in childhood and adolescence: summary statement of the GH research society. *J Clin Endocrinol Metab.* 2000;85:3990-3993.
1238. Baxter RC, Axiak S, Raison RL. Monoclonal antibody against human somatomedin-C/insulin-like growth factor-I. *J Clin Endocrinol Metab.* 1982;54:474-476.
1239. Bala RM, Bhaumick B. Radioimmunoassay of a basic somatomedin: comparison of various assay techniques and somatomedin levels in various sera. *J Clin Endocrinol Metab.* 1979;49:770-777.
1240. Cianfarani S, Liguori A, Boemi S, et al. Inaccuracy of insulin-like growth factor (IGF) binding protein (IGFBP)-3 assessment in the diagnosis of growth hormone (GH) deficiency from childhood to young adulthood: association to low GH dependency of IGF-II and presence of circulating IGFBP-3 18-kilodalton fragment. *J Clin Endocrinol Metab.* 2005;90:6028-6034.
1241. Cianfarani S, Boemi S, Spagnoli A, et al. Is IGF binding protein-3 assessment helpful for the diagnosis of GH deficiency? *Clin Endocrinol (Oxf).* 1995;43:43-47.
1242. Cianfarani S, Liguori A, Germani D. IGF-I and IGFBP-3 assessment in the management of childhood onset growth hormone deficiency. *Endocr Dev.* 2005;9:66-75.
1243. Rosenfeld RG, Wilson DM, Lee PD, et al. Insulin-like growth factors I and II in evaluation of growth retardation. *J Pediatr.* 1986;109:428-433.
1244. Cianfarani S, Tondinelli T, Spadoni GL, et al. Height velocity and IGF-I assessment in the diagnosis of childhood onset GH insufficiency: do we still need a second GH stimulation test? *Clin Endocrinol (Oxf).* 2002;57:161-167.
1245. Juul A, Skakkebaek NE. Prediction of the outcome of growth hormone provocative testing in short children by measurement of serum levels of insulin-like growth factor I and insulin-like growth factor binding protein 3. *J Pediatr.* 1997;130:197-204.
1246. Clemmons DR. Commercial assays available for insulin-like growth factor I and their use in diagnosing growth hormone deficiency. *Horm Res.* 2001;55(suppl 2):73-79.
1247. Milani D, Carmichael JD, Welkowitz J, et al. Variability and reliability of single serum IGF-I measurements: impact on determining predictability of risk ratios in disease development. *J Clin Endocrinol Metab.* 2004;89:2271-2274.
1248. Rosenfeld RG, Gargosky SE. Assays for insulin-like growth factors and their binding proteins: practicalities and pitfalls. *J Pediatr.* 1996;128(5 Pt 2):S52-S57.
1249. Daughaday WH, Rotwein P. Insulin-like growth factors I and II: peptide, messenger ribonucleic acid and gene structures, serum, and tissue concentrations. *Endocr Rev.* 1989;10:68-91.
1250. Furlanetto RW, Underwood LE, Van Wyk JJ, et al. Estimation of somatomedin-C levels in normals and patients with pituitary disease by radioimmunoassay. *J Clin Invest.* 1977;60:648-657.
1251. Zapf J, Walter H, Froesch ER. Radioimmunological determination of insulinlike growth factors I and II in normal subjects and in patients with growth disorders and extrapancreatic tumor hypoglycemia. *J Clin Invest.* 1981;68:1321-1330.

1252. Daughaday WH, Kapadia M, Mariz I. Serum somatomedin binding proteins: physiologic significance and interference in radioligand assay. *J Lab Clin Med*. 1986;109:355-363.

1253. Horner JM, Liu F, Hintz RL. Comparison of [125I]somatomedin A and [125I]somatomedin C radioreceptor assays for somatomedin peptide content in whole and acid-chromatographed plasma. *J Clin Endocrinol Metab*. 1978;47:1287-1295.

1254. Daughaday WH, Mariz IK, Blethen SL. Inhibition of access of bound somatomedin to membrane receptor and immunobinding sites: a comparison of radioreceptor and radioimmunoassay of somatomedin in native and acid-ethanol-extracted serum. *J Clin Endocrinol Metab*. 1980;51:781-788.

1255. Bang P, Eriksson U, Sara V, et al. Comparison of acid ethanol extraction and acid gel filtration prior to IGF-I and IGF-II radioimmunoassays: improvement of determinations in acid ethanol extracts by the use of truncated IGF-I as radioligand. *Acta Endocrinol (Copenh)*. 1991;124:620-629.

1256. Khosravi MJ, Diamandi A, Mistry J, et al. Noncompetitive ELISA for human serum insulin-like growth factor-I. *Clin Chem*. 1996;42(8 Pt 1):1147-1154.

1257. Bang P, Ahlsen M, Berg U, et al. Free insulin-like growth factor I: are we hunting a ghost? *Horm Res*. 2001;55(suppl 2):84-93.

1258. Baxter RC, Martin JL. Radioimmunoassay of growth hormone-dependent insulinlike growth factor binding protein in human plasma. *J Clin Invest*. 1986;78:1504-1512.

1259. Blum WF, Ranke MB, Kietzmann K, et al. A specific radioimmunoassay for the growth hormone (GH)-dependent somatomedin-binding protein: its use for diagnosis of GH deficiency. *J Clin Endocrinol Metab*. 1990;70:1292-1298.

1260. Juul A, Skakkebaek NE. Prediction of the outcome of growth hormone provocative testing in short children by measurement of serum levels of insulin-like growth factor I and insulin-like growth factor binding protein 3. *J Pediatr*. 1997;130:197-204.

1261. Hasegawa Y, Hasegawa T, Aso T, et al. Usefulness and limitation of measurement of insulin-like growth factor binding protein-3 (IGFBP-3) for diagnosis of growth hormone deficiency. *Endocrinol Jpn*. 1992;39:585-591.

1262. Rikken B, van Doorn J, Ringeling A, et al. Plasma levels of insulin-like growth factor (IGF)-I, IGF-II and IGF-binding protein-3 in the evaluation of childhood growth hormone deficiency. *Horm Res*. 1998;50:166-176.

1263. Rosenfeld RG, Albertsson-Wikland K, Cassorla F, et al. Diagnostic controversy: the diagnosis of childhood growth hormone deficiency revisited. *J Clin Endocrinol Metab*. 1995;80:1532-1540.

1264. Frasier SD. A review of growth hormone stimulation tests in children. *Pediatrics*. 1974;53:929-937.

1265. Reiter EO, Morris AH, MacGillivray MH, et al. Variable estimates of serum growth hormone concentrations by different radioassay systems. *J Clin Endocrinol Metab*. 1988;66:68-71.

1266. Celniker AC, Chen AB, Wert Jr RM, et al. Variability in the quantitation of circulating growth hormone using commercial immunoassays. *J Clin Endocrinol Metab*. 1989;68:469-476.

1267. Amed S, Delvin E, Hamilton J. Variation in growth hormone immunoassays in clinical practice in Canada. *Horm Res*. 2008;69:290-294.

1268. Wyatt DT, Mark D, Slyper A. Survey of growth hormone treatment practices by 251 pediatric endocrinologists. *J Clin Endocrinol Metab*. 1995;80:3292-3297.

1269. Gandrud LM, Wilson DM. Is growth hormone stimulation testing in children still appropriate? *Growth Horm IGF Res*. 2004;14:185-194.

1270. Reiter EO, Martha Jr PM. Pharmacological testing of growth hormone secretion. *Horm Res*. 1990;33:121-126, discussion 126-127.

1271. Kaplan SL, Abrams CA, Bell JJ, et al. Growth and growth hormone: I. Changes in serum level of growth hormone following hypoglycemia in 134 children with growth retardation. *Pediatr Res*. 1968;2:43-63.

1272. Grumbach MM, Bin-Abbas BS, Kaplan SL. The growth hormone cascade: progress and long-term results of growth hormone treatment in growth hormone deficiency. *Horm Res*. 1998;49(suppl 2):41-57.

1273. Guyda HJ. Growth hormone testing and the short child. *Pediatr Res*. 2000;48:579-580.

1274. Guyda HJ. Four decades of growth hormone therapy for short children: what have we achieved? *J Clin Endocrinol Metab*. 1999;84:4307-4316.

1275. Corneli G, Di Somma C, Prodam F, et al. Cut-off limits of the GH response to GHRH plus arginine test and IGF-I levels for the diagnosis of GH deficiency in late adolescents and young adults. *Eur J Endocrinol*. 2007;157:701-708.

1276. Ghigo E, Bellone J, Aimaretti G, et al. Reliability of provocative tests to assess growth hormone secretory status: study in 472 normally growing children. *J Clin Endocrinol Metab*. 1996;81:3323-3327.

1277. Maghnie M, Cavigioli F, Tinelli C, et al. GHRH plus arginine in the diagnosis of acquired GH deficiency of childhood-onset. *J Clin Endocrinol Metab*. 2002;87:2740-2744.

1278. Tillmann V, Buckler JM, Kibirige MS, et al. Biochemical tests in the diagnosis of childhood growth hormone deficiency. *J Clin Endocrinol Metab*. 1997;82:531-535.

1279. Marin G, Domene HM, Barnes KM, et al. The effects of estrogen priming and puberty on the growth hormone response to standardized treadmill exercise and arginine-insulin in normal girls and boys. *J Clin Endocrinol Metab*. 1994;79:537-541.

1280. Slover RH, Klingensmith GJ, Gotlin RW, et al. A comparison of clonidine and standard provocative agents of growth hormone. *Am J Dis Child*. 1984;138:314-317.

1281. Loche S, Cappa M, Ghigo E, et al. Growth hormone response to oral clonidine test in normal and short children. *J Endocrinol Invest*. 1993;16:899-902.

1282. Nwosu BU, Coco M, Jones J, et al. Short stature with normal growth hormone stimulation testing: lack of evidence for partial growth hormone deficiency or insensitivity. *Horm Res*. 2004;62:97-102.

1283. Smyczynska J, Lewinski A, Hilczer M, et al. Partial growth hormone deficiency (GHD) in children has more similarities to idiopathic short stature than to severe GHD. *Endokrynol Pol*. 2007;58:182-187.

1284. Coutant R, de Casson FB, Rouleau S, et al. Divergent effect of endogenous and exogenous sex steroids on the insulin-like growth factor I response to growth hormone in short normal adolescents. *J Clin Endocrinol Metab*. 2004;89:6185-6192.

1285. Chalew SA, Udoff LC, Hanukoglu A, et al. The effect of testosterone therapy on spontaneous growth hormone secretion in boys with constitutional delay. *Am J Dis Child*. 1988;142:1345-1348.

1286. Moll Jr GW, Rosenfield RL, Fang VS. Administration of low-dose estrogen rapidly and directly stimulates growth hormone production. *Am J Dis Child*. 1986;140:124-127.

1287. Martinez AS, Domene HM, Ropelato MG, et al. Estrogen priming effect on growth hormone (GH) provocative test: a useful tool for the diagnosis of GH deficiency. *J Clin Endocrinol Metab*. 2000;85:4168-4172.

1288. Bonert VS, Elashoff JD, Barnett P, et al. Body mass index determines evoked growth hormone (GH) responsiveness in normal healthy male subjects: diagnostic caveat for adult GH deficiency. *J Clin Endocrinol Metab*. 2004;89:3397-3401.

1289. Gourmelen M, Pham-Huu-Trung MT, Girard F. Transient partial hGH deficiency in prepubertal children with delay of growth. *Pediatr Res*. 1979;13(4 Pt 1):221-224.

1290. Lippe B, Wong SL, Kaplan SA. Simultaneous assessment of growth hormone and ACTH reserve in children pretreated with diethylstilbestrol. *J Clin Endocrinol Metab*. 1971;33:949-956.

1291. Gonc EN, Kandemir N, Ozon A, et al. Final heights of boys with normal growth hormone responses to provocative tests following priming. *J Pediatr Endocrinol Metab*. 2008;21:963-971.

1292. Kopelman PG, Noonan K, Goulton R, et al. Impaired growth hormone response to growth hormone releasing factor and insulin-hypoglycaemia in obesity. *Clin Endocrinol (Oxf)*. 1985;23:87-94.

1293. Williams T, Berelowitz M, Joffe SN, et al. Impaired growth hormone responses to growth hormone-releasing factor in obesity: a pituitary defect reversed with weight reduction. *N Engl J Med*. 1984;311:1403-1407.

1294. Radetti G, Bozzola M, Pasquino B, et al. Growth hormone bioactivity, insulin-like growth factors (IGFs), and IGF binding proteins in obese children. *Metabolism*. 1998;47:1490-1493.

1295. Misra M, Bredella MA, Tsai P, et al. Lower growth hormone and higher cortisol are associated with greater visceral adiposity, intramyocellular lipids, and insulin resistance in overweight girls. *Am J Physiol Endocrinol Metab*. 2008;295:E385-E392.

1296. Stanley TL, Levitsky LL, Grinspoon SK, et al. Effect of body mass index on peak growth hormone response to provocative testing in children with short stature. *J Clin Endocrinol Metab*. 2009;94:4875-4881.

1297. Shah A, Stanhope R, Matthew D. Hazards of pharmacological tests of growth hormone secretion in childhood. *BMJ*. 1992;304:173-174.

1298. Bercu BB, Shulman D, Root AW, et al. Growth hormone (GH) provocative testing frequently does not reflect endogenous GH secretion. *J Clin Endocrinol Metab*. 1986;63:709-716.

1299. Spiliotis BE, August GP, Hung W, et al. Growth hormone neurosecretory dysfunction: a treatable cause of short stature. *JAMA*. 1984;251:2223-2230.

1300. Zadik Z, Chalew SA, Raiti S, et al. Do short children secrete insufficient growth hormone? *Pediatrics*. 1985;76:355-360.

1301. Zadik Z, Chalew SA, Gilula Z, et al. Reproducibility of growth hormone testing procedures: a comparison between 24-hour integrated concentration and pharmacological stimulation. *J Clin Endocrinol Metab*. 1990;71:1127-1130.

1302. Tassoni P, Cacciari E, Cau M, et al. Variability of growth hormone response to pharmacological and sleep tests performed twice in short children. *J Clin Endocrinol Metab*. 1990;71:230-234.

1303. Donaldson DL, Hollowell JG, Pan FP, et al. Growth hormone secretory profiles: variation on consecutive nights. *J Pediatr*. 1989;115:51-56.

1304. Rose SR, Ross JL, Uriarte M, et al. The advantage of measuring stimulated as compared with spontaneous growth hormone levels in the diagnosis of growth hormone deficiency. *N Engl J Med*. 1988; 319:201-207.
1305. Lanes R. Diagnostic limitations of spontaneous growth hormone measurements in normally growing prepubertal children. *Am J Dis Child*. 1989;143:1284-1286.
1306. Blum WF, Cotterill AM, Postel-Vinay MC, et al. Improvement of diagnostic criteria in growth hormone insensitivity syndrome: solutions and pitfalls. Pharmacia Study Group on Insulin-Like Growth Factor I Treatment in Growth Hormone Insensitivity Syndromes. *Acta Paediatr Suppl*. 1994;399:117-124.
1307. Buckway CK, Selva KA, Burren CP, et al. IGF generation in short stature. *J Pediatr Endocrinol Metab*. 2002;15(suppl 5):1453-1454.
1308. Buckway CK, Selva KA, Pratt KL, et al. Insulin-like growth factor binding protein-3 generation as a measure of GH sensitivity. *J Clin Endocrinol Metab*. 2002;87:4754-4765.
1309. Buckway CK, Guevara-Aguirre J, Pratt KL, et al. The IGF-I generation test revisited: a marker of GH sensitivity. *J Clin Endocrinol Metab*. 2001;86:5176-5183.
1310. Rosenfeld RG, Buckway C, Selva K, et al. Insulin-like growth factor (IGF) parameters and tools for efficacy: the IGF-I generation test in children. *Horm Res*. 2004;62(suppl 1):37-43.
1311. Savage MO, Rosenfeld RG. Growth hormone insensitivity: a proposed revised classification. *Acta Paediatr Suppl*. 1999;428:147.
1312. Blum WF, Ranke MB, Savage MO, et al. Insulin-like growth factors and their binding proteins in patients with growth hormone receptor deficiency: suggestions for new diagnostic criteria. The Kabi Pharmacia Study Group on Insulin-Like Growth Factor I Treatment in Growth Hormone Insensitivity Syndromes. *Acta Paediatr Suppl*. 1992;383:125-126.
1313. Buckway CK, Guevara-Aguirre J, Pratt KL, et al. The IGF-I generation test revisited: a marker of GH sensitivity. *J Clin Endocrinol Metab*. 2001;86:5176-5183.
1314. Roman R, Iniguez G, Lammoglia JJ, et al. The IGF-I response to growth hormone is related to body mass index in short children with normal weight. *Horm Res*. 2009;72:10-14.
1315. Cornblath M, Parker ML, Reisner SH, et al. Secretion and metabolism of growth hormone in premature and full-term infants. *J Clin Endocrinol Metab*. 1965;25:209-218.
1316. Miller JD, Esparza A, Wright NM, et al. Spontaneous growth hormone release in term infants: changes during the first four days of life. *J Clin Endocrinol Metab*. 1993;76:1058-1062.
1317. Lanes R, Nieto C, Bruguera C, et al. Growth hormone release in response to growth hormone-releasing hormone in term and preterm neonates. *Biol Neonate*. 1989;56:252-256.
1318. Quattrin T, Albini CH, Mills BJ, et al. Comparison of urinary growth hormone and IGF-I excretion in small- and appropriate-for-gestational-age infants and healthy children. *Pediatr Res*. 1990; 28:209-212.
1319. de Zegher F, Devlieger H, Veldhuis JD. Properties of growth hormone and prolactin hypersecretion by the human infant on the day of birth. *J Clin Endocrinol Metab*. 1993;76:1177-1181.
1320. Shimano S, Suzuki S, Nagashima K, et al. Growth hormone responses to growth hormone releasing factor in neonates. *Biol Neonate*. 1985;47:367-370.
1321. Adrian TE, Lucas A, Bloom SR, et al. Growth hormone response to feeding in term and preterm neonates. *Acta Paediatr Scand*. 1983;72:251-254.
1322. Wright NM, Northington FJ, Miller JD, et al. Elevated growth hormone secretory rate in premature infants: deconvolution analysis of pulsatile growth hormone secretion in the neonate. *Pediatr Res*. 1992;32:286-290.
1323. Samaan NA, Schultz PN, Johnston DA, et al. Growth hormone, somatomedin C, and nonsuppressible insulin-like activity levels compared in premature, small, average birth weight, and large infants. *Am J Obstet Gynecol*. 1987;157:1524-1528.
1324. Bhala A, Harris M, Cohen P. Insulin-like growth factors and their binding proteins in critically ill infants. *J Pediatr Endocrinol*. 1998;11:451-459.
1325. Cohen P, Rogol AD, Deal CL, et al. 2007 ISS Consensus Workshop participants. Consensus statement on the diagnosis and treatment of children with idiopathic short stature: a summary of the Growth Hormone Research Society, the Lawson Wilkins Pediatric Endocrine Society, and the European Society for Paediatric Endocrinology Workshop. *J Clin Endocrinol Metab*. 2008;93:4210-4217.
1326. Stubberfield TG, Byrne GC, Jones TW. Growth and growth hormone secretion after treatment for acute lymphoblastic leukemia in childhood. 18-gy versus 24-gy cranial irradiation. *J Pediatr Hematol Oncol*. 1995;17:167-171.
1327. Guevara-Aguirre J, Rosenbloom AL, Fielder PJ, et al. Growth hormone receptor deficiency in Ecuador: clinical and biochemical phenotype in two populations. *J Clin Endocrinol Metab*. 1993; 76:417-423.
1328. Buckway CK, Selva KA, Pratt KL, et al. Insulin-like growth factor binding protein-3 generation as a measure of GH sensitivity. *J Clin Endocrinol Metab*. 2002;87:4754-4765.
1329. Selva KA, Buckway CK, Sexton G, et al. Reproducibility in patterns of IGF generation with special reference to idiopathic short stature. *Horm Res*. 2003;60:237-246.
1330. Ester WA, van Duyvenvoorde HA, de Wit CC, et al. Two short children born small for gestational age with insulin-like growth factor 1 receptor haploinsufficiency illustrate the heterogeneity of its phenotype. *J Clin Endocrinol Metab*. 2009;94:4717-4727.
1331. Walenkamp MJ, de Muinck Keizer-Schrama SM, de Mos M, et al. Successful long-term growth hormone therapy in a girl with haploinsufficiency of the insulin-like growth factor-I receptor due to a terminal 15q26.2->qter deletion detected by multiplex ligation probe amplification. *J Clin Endocrinol Metab*. 2008;93:2421-2425.
1332. Wit JM, Clayton PE, Rogol AD, et al. Idiopathic short stature: definition, epidemiology, and diagnostic evaluation. *Growth Horm IGF Res* 2008;18:89-110.
1333. Clayton PE, Shalet SM, Price DA. Endocrine manipulation of constitutional delay in growth and puberty. *J Endocrinol*. 1988;116: 321-323.
1334. Sedlmeyer IL, Hirschhorn JN, Palmert MR. Pedigree analysis of constitutional delay of growth and maturation: determination of familial aggregation and inheritance patterns. *J Clin Endocrinol Metab*. 2002;87:5581-5586.
1335. Blethen SL, Gaines S, Weldon V. Comparison of predicted and adult heights in short boys: effect of androgen therapy. *Pediatr Res*. 1984;18:467-469.
1336. Volta C, Ghizzoni L, Buono T, et al. Final height in a group of untreated children with constitutional growth delay. *Helv Paediatr Acta*. 1988;43:171-176.
1337. Krajewska-Siuda E, Malecka-Tendera E, Krajewski-Siuda K. Are short boys with constitutional delay of growth and puberty candidates for rGH therapy according to FDA recommendations? *Horm Res*. 2006;65:192-196.
1338. Eastman CJ, Lazarus L, Stuart MC, et al. The effect of puberty on growth hormone secretion in boys with short stature and delayed adolescence. *Aust N Z J Med*. 1971;1:154-159.
1339. Deller Jr JJ, Boulis MW, Harriss WE, et al. Growth hormone response patterns to sex hormone administration in growth retardation. *Am J Med Sci*. 1970;259:292-297.
1340. Rose SR, Municchi G, Barnes KM, et al. Overnight growth hormone concentrations are usually normal in pubertal children with idiopathic short stature: a Clinical Research Center study. *J Clin Endocrinol Metab*. 1996;81:1063-1068.
1341. Kaplowitz PB. Diagnostic value of testosterone therapy in boys with delayed puberty. *Am J Dis Child*. 1989;143:116-120.
1342. Horan M, Millar DS, Hedderich J, et al. Human growth hormone 1 (GH1) gene expression: complex haplotype-dependent influence of polymorphic variation in the proximal promoter and locus control region. *Hum Mutat*. 2003;21:408-423.
1343. Attie KM, Carlsson LM, Rundle AC, et al. Evidence for partial growth hormone insensitivity among patients with idiopathic short stature: The National Cooperative Growth Study. *J Pediatr*. 1995;127: 244-250.
1344. Goddard AD, Dowd P, Chernausek S, et al. Partial growth-hormone insensitivity: the role of growth-hormone receptor mutations in idiopathic short stature. *J Pediatr*. 1997;131(1 Pt 2):S51-S55.
1345. Brown RJ, Adams JJ, Pelekanos RA, et al. Model for growth hormone receptor activation based on subunit rotation within a receptor dimer. *Nat Struct Mol Biol*. 2005;12:814-821.
1346. Carlsson LM, Attie KM, Compton PG, et al. Reduced concentration of serum growth hormone-binding protein in children with idiopathic short stature: National Cooperative Growth Study. *J Clin Endocrinol Metab*. 1994;78:1325-1330.
1347. Davila N, Moreira-Andres M, Alcaniz J, et al. Serum growth hormone-binding protein is decreased in prepubertal children with idiopathic short stature. *J Endocrinol Invest*. 1996;19:348-352.
1348. Rosenfeld RG. The molecular basis of idiopathic short stature. *Growth Horm IGF Res*. 2005;15(suppl A):S3-S5.
1349. Rosenfeld RG, Northcraft GB, Hintz RL. A prospective, randomized study of testosterone treatment of constitutional delay of growth and development in male adolescents. *Pediatrics*. 1982;69:681-687.
1350. Blizzard RM, Hindmarsh PC, Stanhope R. Oxandrolone therapy: 25 years experience. *Growth Genet Horm*. 1991;7:1-6.
1351. Buyukgebiz A, Hindmarsh PC, Brook CG. Treatment of constitutional delay of growth and puberty with oxandrolone compared with growth hormone. *Arch Dis Child*. 1990;65:448-449.
1352. Clayton PE, Shalet SM, Price DA, et al. Growth and growth hormone responses to oxandrolone in boys with constitutional delay of growth and puberty (CDGP). *Clin Endocrinol (Oxf)*. 1988;29:123-130.
1353. Joss EE, Schmidt HA, Zuppinger KA. Oxandrolone in constitutionally delayed growth, a longitudinal study up to final height. *J Clin Endocrinol Metab*. 1989;69:1109-1115.

1354. Marti-Henneberg C, Niirianen AK, Rappaport R. Oxandrolone treatment of constitutional short stature in boys during adolescence: effect on linear growth, bone age, pubic hair, and testicular development. *J Pediatr.* 1975;86:783-788.
1355. Stanhope R, Buchanan CR, Fenn GC, et al. Double blind placebo controlled trial of low dose oxandrolone in the treatment of boys with constitutional delay of growth and puberty. *Arch Dis Child.* 1988;63:501-505.
1356. Wilson DM, McCauley E, Brown DR, et al. Oxandrolone therapy in constitutionally delayed growth and puberty: Bio-technology General Corporation Cooperative Study Group. *Pediatrics.* 1995;96:1095-1100.
1357. Tse WY, Buyukgebiz A, Hindmarsh PC, et al. Long-term outcome of oxandrolone treatment in boys with constitutional delay of growth and puberty. *J Pediatr.* 1990;117:588-591.
1358. Papadimitriou A, Wacharasindhu S, Pearl K, et al. Treatment of constitutional growth delay in prepubertal boys with a prolonged course of low dose oxandrolone. *Arch Dis Child.* 1991;66:841-843.
1359. Hochberg Z, Korman S. Oxandrolone therapy for short stature. *Pediatri Endocrinol (Israel).* 1987;2:115-120.
1360. Link K, Blizzard RM, Evans WS, et al. The effect of androgens on the pulsatile release and the twenty-four-hour mean concentration of growth hormone in peripubertal males. *J Clin Endocrinol Metab.* 1986;62:159-164.
1361. Malhotra A, Poon E, Tse WY, et al. The effects of oxandrolone on the growth hormone and gonadal axes in boys with constitutional delay of growth and puberty. *Clin Endocrinol (Oxf).* 1993;38:393-398.
1362. Kulin HE, Reiter EO. Managing the patient with delay in puberty development. *Endocrinologist.* 1992;2:231-239.
1363. Richman RA, Kirsch LR. Testosterone treatment in adolescent boys with constitutional delay in growth and development. *N Engl J Med.* 1988;319:1563-1567.
1364. Metzger DL, Kerrigan JR. Androgen receptor blockade with flutamide enhances growth hormone secretion in late pubertal males: evidence for independent actions of estrogen and androgen. *J Clin Endocrinol Metab.* 1993;76:1147-1152.
1365. Wilson DM, Kei J, Hintz RL, et al. Effects of testosterone therapy for pubertal delay. *Am J Dis Child.* 1988;142:96-99.
1366. Wang C, Swerdloff RS, Iranmanesh A, et al. Testosterone Gel Study Group. Transdermal testosterone gel improves sexual function, mood, muscle strength, and body composition parameters in hypogonadal men. *J Clin Endocrinol Metab.* 2000;85:2839-2853.
1367. Stephen MD, Jehaimi CT, Brosnan PG, et al. Sexual precocity in a 2-year-old boy caused by indirect exposure to testosterone cream. *Endocr Pract.* 2008;14:1027-1030.
1368. Franklin SL, Geffner ME. Precocious puberty secondary to topical testosterone exposure. *J Pediatr Endocrinol Metab.* 2003;16:107-110.
1369. Yu YM, Punyasavatsu N, Elder D, et al. Sexual development in a two-year-old boy induced by topical exposure to testosterone. *Pediatrics.* 1999;104:e23.
1370. Hintz RL, Attie KM, Baptista J, et al. Effect of growth hormone treatment on adult height of children with idiopathic short stature: Genentech Collaborative Group. *N Engl J Med.* 1999;340:502-507.
1371. Leschek EW, Rose SR, Yanovski JA, et al. National Institute of Child Health and Human Development-Eli Lilly & Co. Growth Hormone Collaborative Group. Effect of growth hormone treatment on adult height in peripubertal children with idiopathic short stature: a randomized, double-blind, placebo-controlled trial. *J Clin Endocrinol Metab.* 2004;89:3140-3148.
1372. Wit JM, Reiter EO, Ross JL, et al. Idiopathic short stature: management and growth hormone treatment. *Growth Horm IGF Res.* 2008;18:111-135.
1373. Zucchini S, Wasniewska M, Cisternino M, Adult height in children with short stature and idiopathic delayed puberty after different management. *Eur J Pediatr.* 2008;167:677-681.
1374. Wickman S, Sipila I, Ankarberg-Lindgren C, et al. A specific aromatase inhibitor and potential increase in adult height in boys with delayed puberty: a randomised controlled trial. *Lancet.* 2001;357: 1743-1748.
1375. Hero M, Wickman S, Dunkel L. Treatment with the aromatase inhibitor letrozole during adolescence increases near-final height in boys with constitutional delay of puberty. *Clin Endocrinol (Oxf).* 2006;64:510-513.
1376. Kaplan SL, Underwood LE, August GP, et al. Clinical studies with recombinant-DNA-derived methionyl human growth hormone in growth hormone deficient children. *Lancet.* 1986;1:697-700.
1377. Underwood LE, Moore WV. Antibodies to growth hormone: measurement and meaning. *Growth Genet Horm.* 1987;3:1-3.
1378. MacGillivray MH, Blizzard RM. Rationale for dosing recombinant human growth hormone by weight rather than units. *Growth Genet Horm.* 1994;10:7-9.
1379. Marx W, Simpson ME, Evans HM. Bioassay of growth hormone at anterior pituitary. *Endocrinology.* 1942;30:1-10.
1380. Wilhelmi AE. Measurement: Bioassay. In: Berson SA, Yalow RS, eds. *Peptide hormones: methods in investigative and diagnostic endocrinology.* New York, NY: North-Holland Publishing; 1973.
1381. Binder G, Benz MR, Elmlinger M, et al. Reduced human growth hormone (hGH) bioactivity without a defect of the GH-1 gene in three patients with rhGH responsive growth failure. *Clin Endocrinol (Oxf).* 1999;51:89-95.
1382. Wit JM, Kamp GA, Rikken B. Spontaneous growth and response to growth hormone treatment in children with growth hormone deficiency and idiopathic short stature. *Pediatr Res.* 1996;39: 295-302.
1383. Rimoin DL, Merimee TJ, Rabinowitz D, et al. Genetic aspects of clinical endocrinology. *Recent Prog Horm Res.* 1968;24:365-437.
1384. Ranke MB. A note on adults with growth hormone deficiency. *Acta Paediatr Scand Suppl.* 1987;331:80-82.
1385. Rosenfeld RG, Buckway CK. Should we treat genetic syndromes? *J Pediatr Endocrinol Metab.* 2000;13:971-981.
1386. Blizzard RM. Growth hormone as a therapeutic agent. *Growth Genet Horm.* 2005;21:49-54.
1387. Frasier SD. Human pituitary growth hormone (hGH) therapy in growth hormone deficiency. *Endocr Rev.* 1983;4:155-170.
1388. Frasier SD, Costin G, Lippe BM, et al. A dose-response curve for human growth hormone. *J Clin Endocrinol Metab.* 1981;53: 1213-1217.
1389. Fradkin JE. Creutzfeldt-Jakob disease in pituitary growth hormone recipients. *Endocrinologist.* 1993;3:108-114.
1390. Fradkin JE, Mills JL, Schonberger LB, et al. Risk of leukemia after treatment with pituitary growth hormone. *JAMA.* 1993;270:2829-2832.
1391. Tintner R, Brown P, Hedley-Whyte ET, et al. Neuropathologic verification of Creutzfeldt-Jakob disease in the exhumed American recipient of human pituitary growth hormone: epidemiologic and pathogenetic implications. *Neurology.* 1986;36:932-936.
1392. Hintz RL. The prismatic case of Creutzfeldt-Jakob disease associated with pituitary growth hormone treatment. *J Clin Endocrinol Metab.* 1995;80:2298-2301.
1393. Huillard d'Aignaux J, Costagliola D, Maccario J, et al. Incubation period of Creutzfeldt-Jakob disease in human growth hormone recipients in France. *Neurology.* 1999;53:1197-1201.
1394. Swerdlow AJ, Higgins CD, Adlard P, et al. Creutzfeldt-Jakob disease in United Kingdom patients treated with human pituitary growth hormone. *Neurology.* 2003;61:783-791.
1395. Mills JL, Schonberger LB, Wysowski DK, et al. Long-term mortality in the United States cohort of pituitary-derived growth hormone recipients. *J Pediatr.* 2004;144:430-436.
1396. Rosenfeld RG, Aggarwal BB, Hintz RL, et al. Recombinant DNA-derived methionyl human growth hormone is similar in membrane binding properties to human pituitary growth hormone. *Biochem Biophys Res Commun.* 1982;106:202-209.
1397. Hintz RL, Rosenfeld RG, Wilson DM, et al. Biosynthetic methionyl human growth hormone is biologically active in adult man. *Lancet.* 1982;1:1276-1279.
1398. Buchlis JG, Irizarry L, Crotzer BC, et al. Comparison of final heights of growth hormone-treated vs. untreated children with idiopathic growth failure. *J Clin Endocrinol Metab.* 1998;83:1075-1079.
1399. Ranke MB, Lindberg A, Chatelain P, et al. Derivation and validation of a mathematical model for predicting the response to exogenous recombinant human growth hormone (GH) in prepubertal children with idiopathic GH deficiency: KIGS International Board. Kabi Pharmacia International Growth Study. *J Clin Endocrinol Metab.* 1999;84:1174-1183.
1400. MacGillivray MH, Baptista J, Johanson A. Outcome of a four-year randomized study of daily versus three times weekly somatropin treatment in prepubertal naive growth hormone-deficient children: Genentech Study Group. *J Clin Endocrinol Metab.* 1996;81: 1806-1809.
1401. Wilson DM, Baker B, Hintz RL, et al. Subcutaneous versus intramuscular growth hormone therapy: growth and acute somatomedin response. *Pediatrics.* 1985;76:361-364.
1402. Martha Jr PM, Reiter EO, Davila N, et al. The role of body mass in the response to growth hormone therapy. *J Clin Endocrinol Metab.* 1992;75:1470-1473.
1403. Martha Jr PM, Reiter EO, Davila N, et al. Serum growth hormone (GH)-binding protein/receptor: an important determinant of GH responsiveness. *J Clin Endocrinol Metab.* 1992;75:1464-1469.
1404. Price DA, Ranke MB. Final height following growth hormone treatment. In: Ranke MB, Gunnarsson R, eds. *Progress in Growth Hormone Therapy: 5 Years of KIGS.* Mannheim, Germany: J&J Verlag; 1994.
1405. Land C, Blum WF, Stabrey A, et al. Seasonality of growth response to GH therapy in prepubertal children with idiopathic growth hormone deficiency. *Eur J Endocrinol.* 2005;152:727-733.
1406. Cohen P, Bright GM, Rogol AD, et al. American Norditropin Clinical Trials Group. Effects of dose and gender on the growth and growth factor response to GH in GH-deficient children: Implications for efficacy and safety. *J Clin Endocrinol Metab.* 2002;87:90-98.

1407. Cohen P, Rogol AD, Howard C, et al. IGF-based dosing of growth hormone accelerates the growth velocity of children with growth hormone deficiency (GHD) and idiopathic short stature. *Horm Res.* 2005;64(suppl 1):48.
1408. Wikland KA, Kristrom B, Rosberg S, et al. Validated multivariate models predicting the growth response to GH treatment in individual short children with a broad range in GH secretion capacities. *Pediatr Res.* 2000;48:475-484.
1409. Huet F, Carel JC, Nivelon JL, et al. Long-term results of GH therapy in GH-deficient children treated before 1 year of age. *Eur J Endocrinol.* 1999;140:29-34.
1410. Boersma B, Rikken B, Wit JM. Catch-up growth in early treated patients with growth hormone deficiency. Dutch Growth Hormone Working Group. *Arch Dis Child.* 1995;72:427-431.
1411. Rappaport R, Mugnier E, Limoni C, et al. A 5-year prospective study of growth hormone (GH)-deficient children treated with GH before the age of 3 years. French Serono Study Group. *J Clin Endocrinol Metab.* 1997;82:452-456.
1412. De Luca F, Maghnie M, Arrigo T, et al. Final height outcome of growth hormone-deficient patients treated since less than five years of age. *Acta Paediatr.* 1996;85:1167-1171.
1413. Carel JC, Huet F, Chaussain JL. Treatment of growth hormone deficiency in very young children. *Horm Res.* 2003;60(suppl 1): 10-17.
1414. Ranke MB, Lindberg A, Albertsson-Wikland K, et al. Increased response, but lower responsiveness, to growth hormone (GH) in very young children (aged 0-3 years) with idiopathic GH deficiency: analysis of data from KIGS. *J Clin Endocrinol Metab.* 2005;90: 1966-1971.
1415. Saenger P. Growth hormone in growth hormone deficiency. *BMJ.* 2002;325:58-59.
1416. Bundak R, Hindmarsh PC, Smith PJ, et al. Long-term auxologic effects of human growth hormone. *J Pediatr.* 1988;112:875-879.
1417. Libber SM, Plotnick LP, Johanson AJ, et al. Long-term follow-up of hypopituitary patients treated with human growth hormone. *Medicine (Baltimore).* 1990;69:46-55.
1418. Bierich JR. Final height in hypopituitary patients after treatment with HGH. In: Bierch JR, Cacciari E, Raiti S, eds. *Growth abnormalities.* New York, NY: Raven; 1989.
1419. MacGillivray MH, Blethen SL, Buchlis JG, et al. Current dosing of growth hormone in children with growth hormone deficiency: how physiologic? *Pediatrics.* 1998;102(2 Pt 3):527-530.
1420. Westphal O, Lindberg A, Swedish KIGS National Board. Final height in Swedish children with idiopathic growth hormone deficiency enrolled in KIGS treated optimally with growth hormone. *Acta Paediatr.* 2008;97:1698-1706.
1421. Birnbacher R, Riedl S, Frisch H. Long-term treatment in children with hypopituitarism: pubertal development and final height. *Horm Res.* 1998;49:80-85.
1422. Cutfield W, Lindberg A, Albertsson Wikland K, et al. Final height in idiopathic growth hormone deficiency: the KIGS experience. KIGS International Board. *Acta Paediatr Suppl.* 1999;88:72-75.
1423. Bramswig JH, Schlosser H, Kiese K. Final height in children with growth hormone deficiency. *Horm Res.* 1995;43:126-128.
1424. Severi F. Final height in children with growth hormone deficiency. *Horm Res.* 1995;43(4):138-140.
1425. Blethen SL, Baptista J, Kuntze J, et al. Adult height in growth hormone (GH)-deficient children treated with biosynthetic GH. The Genentech Growth Study Group. *J Clin Endocrinol Metab.* 1997;82: 418-420.
1426. Bernasconi S, Arrigo T, Wasniewsk M, et al. Long-term results with growth hormone therapy in idiopathic hypopituitarism. *Horm Res.* 2000;53(suppl 1):55-59.
1427. August GP, Julius JR, Blethen SL. Adult height in children with growth hormone deficiency who are treated with biosynthetic growth hormone: The National Cooperative Growth Study experience. *Pediatrics.* 1998;102(2 Pt 3):512-516.
1428. Reiter EO, Price DA, Wilton P, et al. Effect of growth hormone (GH) treatment on the near-final height of 1258 patients with idiopathic GH deficiency: analysis of a large international database. *J Clin Endocrinol Metab.* 2006;91:2047-2054.
1429. Cutfield WS, Lindberg A, Chatelain P, et al. Final height following growth hormone treatment of idiopathic growth hormone deficiency in KIGS. In: Ranke MB, Wilton P, eds. *Growth Hormone Therapy in KIGS: 10 Years' Experience.* Heidelberg-Leipzig, Germany: Johann Ambrosius Barth Verlag; 1999:93-110.
1430. Wassenaar MJ, Dekkers OM, Pereira AM, et al. Impact of the exon 3-deleted growth hormone (GH) receptor polymorphism on baseline height and the growth response to recombinant human GH therapy in GH-deficient (GHD) and non-GHD children with short stature: a systematic review and meta-analysis. *J Clin Endocrinol Metab.* 2009;94:3721-3730.
1431. Rosenfeld RG. The pharmacogenomics of human growth (editorial). *J Clin Endocrinol Metab.* 2006;91:795-796.
1432. Ranke MB, Price DA, Albertsson-Wikland K, et al. Factors determining pubertal growth and final height in growth hormone treatment of idiopathic growth hormone deficiency: analysis of 195 patients of the Kabi Pharmacia International Growth Study. *Horm Res.* 1997;48:62-71.
1433. Frisch H, Birnbacher R. Final height and pubertal development in children with growth hormone deficiency after long-term treatment. *Horm Res.* 1995;43:132-134.
1434. Burns EC, Tanner JM, Preece MA, et al. Final height and pubertal development in 55 children with idiopathic growth hormone deficiency, treated for between 2 and 15 years with human growth hormone. *Eur J Pediatr.* 1981;137:155-164.
1435. Bourguignon JP, Vandeweghe M, Vanderschueren-Lodeweyckx M, et al. Pubertal growth and final height in hypopituitary boys: a minor role of bone age at onset of puberty. *J Clin Endocrinol Metab.* 1986;63:376-382.
1436. Beckers D, Thomas M, Jamart J, et al. Adult final height after growth hormone therapy for irradiation-induced growth hormone deficiency in childhood survivors of brain tumours: the Belgian experience. *Eur J Endocrinol.* 2010;162:483-490.
1437. Xu W, Janss A, Moshang T. Adult height and adult sitting height in childhood medulloblastoma survivors. *J Clin Endocrinol Metab.* 2003;88:4677-4681.
1438. Stanhope R, Uruena M, Hindmarsh P, et al. Management of growth hormone deficiency through puberty. *Acta Paediatr Scand Suppl.* 1991;372:47-52, discussion 53.
1439. Stanhope R, Albanese A, Hindmarsh P, et al. The effects of growth hormone therapy on spontaneous sexual development. *Horm Res.* 1992;38(suppl 1):9-13.
1440. Mauras N, Attie KM, Reiter EO, et al. High dose recombinant human growth hormone (GH) treatment of GH-deficient patients in puberty increases near-final height: a randomized, multicenter trial. Genentech, Inc., Cooperative Study Group. *J Clin Endocrinol Metab.* 2000;85:3653-3660.
1441. Cohen P, Rogol AD, Howard CP, et al. American Norditropin Study Group. Insulin growth factor-based dosing of growth hormone therapy in children: a randomized, controlled study. *J Clin Endocrinol Metab.* 2007;92:2480-2486.
1442. Marchisotti FG, Jorge AA, Montenegro LR, et al. Comparison between weight-based and IGF-I-based growth hormone (GH) dosing in the treatment of children with GH deficiency and influence of exon 3 deleted GH receptor variant. *Growth Horm IGF Res.* 2009;19: 179-186.
1443. Lippe BM, Van Herle AJ, LaFranchi SH, et al. Reversible hypothyroidism in growth hormone-deficient children treated with human growth hormone. *J Clin Endocrinol Metab.* 1975;40:612-618.
1444. Lange M, Feldt-Rasmussen U, Svendsen OL, et al. High risk of adrenal insufficiency in adults previously treated for idiopathic childhood onset growth hormone deficiency. *J Clin Endocrinol Metab.* 2003;88:5784-5789.
1445. Guthrie RD, Smith DW, Graham CB. Testosterone treatment for micropenis during early childhood. *J Pediatr.* 1973;83:247-252.
1446. Wilson TA, Rose SR, Cohen P, et al. Lawson Wilkins Pediatric Endocrinology Society Drug and Therapeutics Committee. Update of guidelines for the use of growth hormone in children. *J Pediatr.* 2003;143:415-421.
1447. Lechuga-Sancho A, Lechuga-Campoy JL, del Valle-Nunez J, et al. Predicting the growth response of children with idiopathic growth hormone deficiency to one year of recombinant growth hormone treatment: derivation and validation of a useful method. *J Pediatr Endocrinol Metab.* 2009;22:501-509.
1448. Ranke MB, Lindberg A. Predicting growth in response to growth hormone treatment. *Growth Horm IGF Res.* 2009;19:1-11.
1449. de Ridder MA, Stijnen T, Drop SL, et al. Validation of a calibrated prediction model for response to growth hormone treatment in an independent cohort. *Horm Res.* 2006;66:13-16.
1450. Achermann JC, Hamdani K, Hindmarsh PC, et al. Birth weight influences the initial response to growth hormone treatment in growth hormone-insufficient children. *Pediatrics.* 1998;102(2 Pt 1): 342-345.
1451. Cacciari E, Zucchini S, Cicognani A, et al. Birth weight affects final height in patients treated for growth hormone deficiency. *Clin Endocrinol (Oxf).* 1999;51:733-739.
1452. Tillmann V, Patel L, Gill MS, et al. Monitoring serum insulin-like growth factor-I (IGF-I), IGF binding protein-3 (IGFBP-3), IGF-I/IGFBP-3 molar ratio and leptin during growth hormone treatment for disordered growth. *Clin Endocrinol (Oxf).* 2000;53:329-336.
1453. Kristrom B, Carlsson B, Rosberg S, et al. Short-term changes in serum leptin levels provide a strong metabolic marker for the growth response to growth hormone treatment in children. Swedish Study Group for Growth Hormone Treatment. *J Clin Endocrinol Metab.* 1998;83:2735-2741.
1454. Clayton PE, Cuneo RC, Juul A, et al. European Society of Paediatric Endocrinology. Consensus statement on the management of the

GH-treated adolescent in the transition to adult care. *Eur J Endocrinol.* 2005;152:165-170.
1455. Abs R, Bengtsson BA, Hernberg-Stahl E, et al. GH replacement in 1034 growth hormone deficient hypopituitary adults: demographic and clinical characteristics, dosing and safety. *Clin Endocrinol (Oxf).* 1999;50:703-713.
1456. Bengtsson BA, Johannsson G, Shalet SM, et al. Treatment of growth hormone deficiency in adults. *J Clin Endocrinol Metab.* 2000; 85:933-942.
1457. Carroll PV, Christ ER, Bengtsson BA, et al. Growth hormone deficiency in adulthood and the effects of growth hormone replacement: a review. Growth Hormone Research Society Scientific Committee. *J Clin Endocrinol Metab.* 1998;83:382-395.
1458. Attanasio AF, Bates PC, Ho KK, et al. Hypoptiuitary Control and Complications Study International Advisory Board. Human growth hormone replacement in adult hypopituitary patients: long-term effects on body composition and lipid status—3-year results from the HypoCCS database. *J Clin Endocrinol Metab.* 2002;87:1600-1606.
1459. Rosen T, Bengtsson BA. Premature mortality due to cardiovascular disease in hypopituitarism. *Lancet.* 1990;336:285-288.
1460. Maison P, Griffin S, Nicoue-Beglah M, et al. Impact of growth hormone (GH) treatment on cardiovascular risk factors in GH-deficient adults: a metaanalysis of blinded, randomized, placebo-controlled trials. *J Clin Endocrinol Metab.* 2004;89:2192-2199.
1461. Hull KL, Harvey S. Growth hormone therapy and quality of life: possibilities, pitfalls and mechanisms. *J Endocrinol.* 2003;179:311-333.
1462. Salomon F, Cuneo RC, Hesp R, et al. The effects of treatment with recombinant human growth hormone on body composition and metabolism in adults with growth hormone deficiency. *N Engl J Med.* 1989;321:1797-1803.
1463. Bengtsson BA, Eden S, Lonn L, et al. Treatment of adults with growth hormone (GH) deficiency with recombinant human GH. *J Clin Endocrinol Metab.* 1993;76:309-317.
1464. Allen DB, Fost NC. Growth hormone therapy for short stature: panacea or Pandora's box? *J Pediatr.* 1990;117(1 Pt 1):16-21.
1465. Maghnie M, Strigazzi C, Tinelli C, et al. Growth hormone (GH) deficiency (GHD) of childhood onset: reassessment of GH status and evaluation of the predictive criteria for permanent GHD in young adults. *J Clin Endocrinol Metab.* 1999;84:1324-1328.
1466. Longobardi S, Merola B, Pivonello R, et al. Reevaluation of growth hormone (GH) secretion in 69 adults diagnosed as GH-deficient patients during childhood. *J Clin Endocrinol Metab.* 1996;81: 1244-1247.
1467. Cacciari E, Tassoni P, Cicognani A, et al. Value and limits of pharmacological and physiological tests to diagnose growth hormone (GH) deficiency and predict therapy response: first and second retesting during replacement therapy of patients defined as GH deficient. *J Clin Endocrinol Metab.* 1994;79:1663-1669.
1468. Tauber M, Moulin P, Pienkowski C, et al. Growth hormone (GH) retesting and auxological data in 131 GH-deficient patients after completion of treatment. *J Clin Endocrinol Metab.* 1997;82:352-356.
1469. Nicolson A, Toogood AA, Rahim A, et al. The prevalence of severe growth hormone deficiency in adults who received growth hormone replacement in childhood [see comment]. *Clin Endocrinol (Oxf).* 1996;44:311-316.
1470. Rutherford OM, Jones DA, Round JM, et al. Changes in skeletal muscle and body composition after discontinuation of growth hormone treatment in growth hormone deficient young adults. *Clin Endocrinol (Oxf).* 1991;34:469-475.
1471. Clayton PE, Price DA, Shalet SM. Growth hormone state after completion of treatment with growth hormone. *Arch Dis Child.* 1987;62:222-226.
1472. Juul A, Kastrup KW, Pedersen SA, et al. Growth hormone (GH) provocative retesting of 108 young adults with childhood-onset GH deficiency and the diagnostic value of insulin-like growth factor I (IGF-I) and IGF-binding protein-3. *J Clin Endocrinol Metab.* 1997;82:1195-1201.
1473. Maghnie M, Aimaretti G, Bellone S, et al. Diagnosis of GH deficiency in the transition period: accuracy of insulin tolerance test and insulin-like growth factor-I measurement. *Eur J Endocrinol.* 2005;152: 589-596.
1474. Vahl N, Juul A, Jorgensen JO, et al. Continuation of growth hormone (GH) replacement in GH-deficient patients during transition from childhood to adulthood: a two-year placebo-controlled study. *J Clin Endocrinol Metab.* 2000;85:1874-1881.
1475. Johannsson G, Albertsson-Wikland K, Bengtsson BA. Discontinuation of growth hormone (GH) treatment: metabolic effects in GH-deficient and GH-sufficient adolescent patients compared with control subjects. Swedish Study Group for Growth Hormone Treatment in Children. *J Clin Endocrinol Metab.* 1999;84:4516-4524.
1476. Shalet SM, Shavrikova E, Cromer M, et al. Effect of growth hormone (GH) treatment on bone in postpubertal GH-deficient patients: a 2-year randomized, controlled, dose-ranging study. *J Clin Endocrinol Metab.* 2003;88:4124-4129.
1477. Attanasio AF, Shavrikova E, Blum WF, et al. Hypopituitary Developmental Outcome Study Group. Continued growth hormone (GH) treatment after final height is necessary to complete somatic development in childhood-onset GH-deficient patients. *J Clin Endocrinol Metab.* 2004;89:4857-4862.
1478. Mauras N, Pescovitz OH, Allada V, et al. Transition Study Group. Limited efficacy of growth hormone (GH) during transition of GH-deficient patients from adolescence to adulthood: a phase III multicenter, double-blind, randomized two-year trial. *J Clin Endocrinol Metab.* 2005;90:3946-3955.
1479. Hulthen L, Bengtsson BA, Sunnerhagen KS, et al. GH is needed for the maturation of muscle mass and strength in adolescents. *J Clin Endocrinol Metab.* 2001;86:4765-4770.
1480. Attanasio AF, Shavrikova EP, Blum WF, et al. Quality of life in childhood onset growth hormone-deficient patients in the transition phase from childhood to adulthood. *J Clin Endocrinol Metab.* 2005;90:4525-4529.
1481. Stouthart PJ, Deijen JB, Roffel M, et al. Quality of life of growth hormone (GH) deficient young adults during discontinuation and restart of GH therapy. *Psychoneuroendocrinology.* 2003;28:612-626.
1482. Sheppard L, Eiser C, Davies HA, et al. The effects of growth hormone treatment on health-related quality of life in children. *Horm Res.* 2006;65:243-249.
1483. Sandberg DE. Health-related quality of life as a primary endpoint for growth hormone therapy. *Horm Res.* 2006;65:250-252, discussion 252.
1484. Cowan FJ, Evans WD, Gregory JW. Metabolic effects of discontinuing growth hormone treatment. *Arch Dis Child.* 1999;80:517-523.
1485. Tauber M, Jouret B, Cartault A, et al. Adolescents with partial growth hormone (GH) deficiency develop alterations of body composition after GH discontinuation and require follow-up. *J Clin Endocrinol Metab.* 2003;88:5101-5106.
1486. Drake WM, Carroll PV, Maher KT, et al. The effect of cessation of growth hormone (GH) therapy on bone mineral accretion in GH-deficient adolescents at the completion of linear growth. *J Clin Endocrinol Metab.* 2003;88:1658-1663.
1487. Underwood LE, Attie KM, Baptista J; Genentech Collaborative Study Group. Growth hormone (GH) dose-response in young adults with childhood-onset GH deficiency: a two-year, multicenter, multiple-dose, placebo-controlled study. *J Clin Endocrinol Metab.* 2003;88: 5273-5280.
1488. Lange M, Muller J, Svendsen OL, et al. The impact of idiopathic childhood-onset growth hormone deficiency (GHD) on bone mass in subjects without adult GHD. *Clin Endocrinol (Oxf).* 2005;62:18-23.
1489. Colao A, Di Somma C, Salerno M, et al. The cardiovascular risk of GH-deficient adolescents. *J Clin Endocrinol Metab.* 2002;87:3650-3655.
1490. Salerno M, Esposito V, Spinelli L, et al. Left ventricular mass and function in children with GH deficiency before and during 12 months GH replacement therapy. *Clin Endocrinol (Oxf).* 2004;60: 630-636.
1491. Lanes R, Paoli M, Carrillo E, et al. Cardiovascular risk of young growth-hormone-deficient adolescents: differences in growth-hormone-treated and untreated patients. *Horm Res.* 2003;60:291-296.
1492. Lanes R, Paoli M, Carrillo E, et al. Peripheral inflammatory and fibrinolytic markers in adolescents with growth hormone deficiency: relation to postprandial dyslipidemia. *J Pediatr.* 2004;145:657-661.
1493. Reis F, Campos MV, Bastos M, et al. Platelet hyperactivation in maintained growth hormone-deficient childhood patients after therapy withdrawal as a putative earlier marker of increased cardiovascular risk. *J Clin Endocrinol Metab.* 2005;90:98-105.
1494. Mohn A, Marzio D, Giannini C, et al. Alterations in the oxidant-antioxidant status in prepubertal children with growth hormone deficiency: effect of growth hormone replacement therapy. *Clin Endocrinol (Oxf).* 2005;63:537-542.
1495. Esposito V, Di Biase S, Lettiero T, et al. Serum homocysteine concentrations in children with growth hormone (GH) deficiency before and after 12 months GH replacement. *Clin Endocrinol (Oxf).* 2004;61: 607-611.
1496. Radovick S, DiVall S. Approach to the growth hormone-deficient child during transition to adulthood. *J Clin Endocrinol Metab.* 2007;92:1195-1200.
1497. Goldstone AP, Holland AJ, Hauffa BP, et al. contributors at the Second Expert Meeting of the Comprehensive Care of Patients with PWS. Recommendations for the diagnosis and management of Prader-Willi syndrome. *J Clin Endocrinol Metab.* 2008;93:4183-4197.
1498. Fridman C, Kok F, Koiffmann CP. Hypotonic infants and the Prader-Willi syndrome. *J Pediatr (Rio J).* 2000;76:246-250.
1499. Eiholzer U, Stutz K, Weinmann C, et al. Low insulin, IGF-I and IGFBP-3 levels in children with Prader-Labhart-Willi syndrome. *Eur J Pediatr.* 1998;157:890-893.
1500. Lindgren AC, Hagenas L, Muller J, et al. Growth hormone treatment of children with Prader-Willi syndrome affects linear growth and body composition favourably. *Acta Paediatr.* 1998;87:28-31.

1501. Corrias A, Bellone J, Beccaria L, et al. GH/IGF-I axis in Prader-Willi syndrome: evaluation of IGF-I levels and of the somatotroph responsiveness to various provocative stimuli. Genetic Obesity Study Group of Italian Society of Pediatric Endocrinology and Diabetology. *J Endocrinol Invest.* 2000;23:84-89.
1502. Tauber M, Barbeau C, Jouret B, et al. Auxological and endocrine evolution of 28 children with Prader-Willi syndrome: effect of GH therapy in 14 children. *Horm Res.* 2000;53:279-287.
1503. Burman P, Ritzen EM, Lindgren AC. Endocrine dysfunction in Prader-Willi syndrome: a review with special reference to GH. *Endocr Rev.* 2001;22:787-799.
1504. Carrel AL, Myers SE, Whitman BY, et al. Growth hormone improves body composition, fat utilization, physical strength and agility, and growth in Prader-Willi syndrome: a controlled study. *J Pediatr.* 1999;134:215-221.
1505. Myers SE, Carrel AL, Whitman BY, et al. Sustained benefit after 2 years of growth hormone on body composition, fat utilization, physical strength and agility, and growth in Prader-Willi syndrome. *J Pediatr.* 2000;137:42-49.
1506. Whitman BY, Myers MG, Carrel AL, et al. The behavioral impact of growth hormone treatment for children and adolescents with Prader-Willi syndrome: a 2-year controlled study. *Pediatrics.* 2005; 109:308-309.
1507. Davies PS, Evans S, Broomhead S, et al. Effect of growth hormone on height, weight, and body composition in Prader-Willi syndrome. *Arch Dis Child.* 1998;78:474-476.
1508. Lindgren AC, Lindberg A. Growth hormone treatment completely normalizes adult height and improves body composition in Prader-Willi syndrome: experience from KIGS (Pfizer International Growth Database). *Horm Res.* 2008;70:182-187.
1509. Carrel AL, Myers SE, Whitman BY, et al. Benefits of long-term GH therapy in Prader-Willi syndrome: a 4-year study. *J Clin Endocrinol Metab.* 2002;87:1581-1585.
1510. Allen DB, Carrel AL. Growth hormone therapy for Prader-Willi syndrome: a critical appraisal. *J Pediatr Endocrinol Metab.* 2004;17(suppl 4):1297-1306.
1511. Wollmann HA, Schultz U, Grauer ML, et al. Reference values for height and weight in Prader-Willi syndrome based on 315 patients. *Eur J Pediatr.* 1998;157:634-642.
1512. Hauffa BP, Schlippe G, Roos M, et al. Spontaneous growth in German children and adolescents with genetically confirmed Prader-Willi syndrome. *Acta Paediatr.* 2000;89:1302-1311.
1513. Tauber M. Effects of growth hormone treatment in children presenting with Prader-Willi syndrome: the KIGS experience. In: *Growth Hormone Therapy in Pediatrics: 20 Years of KIGS.* Basel, Switzerlans: Karger; 2007.
1514. Angulo MA, Castro-Magana M, Lamerson M, et al. Final adult height in children with Prader-Willi syndrome with and without human growth hormone treatment. *Am J Med Genet A.* 2007;143: 1456-1461.
1515. de Lind van Wijngaarden RF, Siemensma EP, Festen DA, et al. Efficacy and safety of long-term continuous growth hormone treatment in children with Prader-Willi syndrome. *J Clin Endocrinol Metab.* 2009;94:4205-4215.
1516. Miller JL, Goldstone AP, Couch JA, et al. Pituitary abnormalities in Prader-Willi syndrome and early onset morbid obesity. *Am J Med Genet A.* 2008;146:570-577.
1517. Butler MG, Theodoro M, Skouse JD. Thyroid function studies in Prader-Willi syndrome. *Am J Med Genet A.* 2007;143:488-492.
1518. Carrel AL, Moerchen V, Myers SE, et al. Growth hormone improves mobility and body composition in infants and toddlers with Prader-Willi syndrome. *J Pediatr.* 2004;145:744-749.
1519. Festen DA, Wevers M, Lindgren AC, et al. Mental and motor development before and during growth hormone treatment in infants and toddlers with Prader-Willi syndrome. *Clin Endocrinol (Oxf).* 2008;68:919-925.
1520. Bakker B, Maneatis T, Lippe B. Sudden death in Prader-Willi syndrome: brief review of five additional cases. Concerning the article by U. Eiholzer et al.: Deaths in children with Prader-Willi syndrome—a contribution to the debate about the safety of growth hormone treatment in children with PWS (Horm Res 2005;63:33-39). *Horm Res.* 2007;67:203-204.
1521. Whittington JE, Holland AJ, Webb T, et al. Population prevalence and estimated birth incidence and mortality rate for people with Prader-Willi syndrome in one UK health region. *J Med Genet.* 2001;38: 792-798.
1522. Tauber M, Diene G, Molinas C, et al. Review of 64 cases of death in children with Prader-Willi syndrome (PWS). *Am J Med Genet A.* 2008;146:881-887.
1523. Bell J, Parker KL, Swinford RD, et al. Long-term safety of recombinant human growth hormone in children. *J Clin Endocrinol Metab.* 2010;95:167-177.
1524. Eiholzer U. Deaths in children with Prader-Willi syndrome—a contribution to the debate about the safety of growth hormone treatment in children with PWS. *Horm Res.* 2005;63:33-39.
1525. Van Vliet G, Deal CL, Crock PA, et al. Sudden death in growth hormone-treated children with Prader-Willi syndrome. *J Pediatr.* 2004;144:129-131.
1526. Nagai T, Obata K, Tonoki H, et al. Cause of sudden, unexpected death of Prader-Willi syndrome patients with or without growth hormone treatment. *Am J Med Genet A.* 2005;136:45-48.
1527. Festen D, Hokken-Koelega A. Breathing disorders in Prader-Willi syndrome: the role of obesity, growth hormone treatment and upper respiratory tract infections. *Expert Rev Endocrinol Metab.* 2007; 2:529-537.
1528. Lindgren AC, Hellstrom LG, Ritzen EM, et al. Growth hormone treatment increases CO(2) response, ventilation and central inspiratory drive in children with Prader-Willi syndrome. *Eur J Pediatr.* 1999;158:936-940.
1529. Miller J, Silverstein J, Shuster J, et al. Short-term effects of growth hormone on sleep abnormalities in Prader-Willi syndrome. *J Clin Endocrinol Metab.* 2006;91:413-417.
1530. Festen DA, de Weerd AW, van den Bossche RA, et al. Sleep-related breathing disorders in prepubertal children with Prader-Willi syndrome and effects of growth hormone treatment. *J Clin Endocrinol Metab.* 2006;91:4911-4915.
1531. de Lind van Wijngaarden RF, Otten BJ, Festen DA, et al. High prevalence of central adrenal insufficiency in patients with Prader-Willi syndrome. *J Clin Endocrinol Metab.* 2008;93:1649-1654.
1532. de Lind van Wijngaarden RF, Joosten KF, van den Berg S, et al. The relationship between central adrenal insufficiency and sleep-related breathing disorders in children with Prader-Willi syndrome. *J Clin Endocrinol Metab.* 2009;94:2387-2393.
1533. Butler JV, Whittington JE, Holland AJ, et al. Prevalence of, and risk factors for, physical ill-health in people with Prader-Willi syndrome: a population-based study. *Dev Med Child Neurol.* 2002;44:248-255.
1534. Nagai T, Obata K, Ogata T, et al. Growth hormone therapy and scoliosis in patients with Prader-Willi syndrome. *Am J Med Genet A.* 2006;140:1623-1627.
1535. de Lind van Wijngaarden RF, de Klerk LW, Festen DA, et al. Scoliosis in Prader-Willi syndrome: prevalence, effects of age, gender, body mass index, lean body mass and genotype. *Arch Dis Child.* 2008;93: 1012-1016.
1536. Odent T, Accadbled F, Koureas G, et al. Scoliosis in patients with Prader-Willi syndrome. *Pediatrics.* 2008;122:e499-e503.
1537. de Lind van Wijngaarden RF, de Klerk LW, Festen DA, et al. Randomized controlled trial to investigate the effects of growth hormone treatment on scoliosis in children with Prader-Willi syndrome. *J Clin Endocrinol Metab.* 2009;94:1274-1280.
1538. Hoybye C, Thoren M. Somatropin therapy in adults with Prader-Willi syndrome. *Treat Endocrinol.* 2004;3:153-160.
1539. Hoybye C, Frystyk J, Thoren M. The growth hormone–insulin-like growth factor axis in adult patients with Prader-Willi syndrome. *Growth Horm IGF Res.* 2003;13:269-274.
1540. Festen DA, de Lind van Wijngaarden R, van Eekelen M, et al. Randomized controlled GH trial: effects on anthropometry, body composition and body proportions in a large group of children with Prader-Willi syndrome. *Clin Endocrinol (Oxf).* 2008;69:443-451.
1541. Hoybye C, Thoren M, Bohm B. Cognitive, emotional, physical and social effects of growth hormone treatment in adults with Prader-Willi syndrome. *J Intellect Disabil Res.* 2005;49(Pt 4): 245-252.
1542. Partsch CJ, Lammer C, Gillessen-Kaesbach G, et al. Adult patients with Prader-Willi syndrome: clinical characteristics, life circumstances and growth hormone secretion. *Growth Horm IGF Res.* 2000;10(suppl B):S81-S85.
1543. Schaefer F, Wingen AM, Hennicke M, et al. Growth charts for prepubertal children with chronic renal failure due to congenital renal disorders. European Study Group for Nutritional Treatment of Chronic Renal Failure in Childhood. *Pediatr Nephrol.* 1996;10: 288-293.
1544. Wuhl E, Haffner D, Offner G, et al. European Study Group on Growth Hormone Treatment in Children with Nephropathic Cystinosis. Long-term treatment with growth hormone in short children with nephropathic cystinosis. *J Pediatr.* 2001;138:880-887.
1545. Harmon WE, Jabs K. Factors affecting growth after renal transplantation. *J Am Soc Nephrol.* 1992;2(suppl 12):S295-S303.
1546. Fine RN, Kohaut EC, Brown D, et al. Growth after recombinant human growth hormone treatment in children with chronic renal failure: report of a multicenter randomized double-blind placebo-controlled study. Genentech Cooperative Study Group. *J Pediatr.* 1994;124:374-382.
1547. Tonshoff B, Mehls O, Heinrich U, et al. Predicting GH response in short uremic children. *J Clin Endocrinol Metab.* 2010;95:686-692.
1548. Fine RN, Stablein D. Long-term use of recombinant human growth hormone in pediatric allograft recipients: a report of the NAPRTCS transplant registry. *Pediatr Nephrol.* 2005;20:404-408.
1549. Haffner D, Schaefer F, Nissel R, et al. Effect of growth hormone treatment on the adult height of children with chronic renal failure.

German Study Group for Growth Hormone Treatment in Chronic Renal Failure. *N Engl J Med.* 2000;343:923-930.
1550. Hokken-Koelega A, Mulder P, De Jong R, et al. Long-term effects of growth hormone treatment on growth and puberty in patients with chronic renal insufficiency. *Pediatr Nephrol.* 2000;14:701-706.
1551. Wuhl E, Schaefer F. Effects of growth hormone in patients with chronic renal failure: experience in children and adults. *Horm Res.* 2002;58(suppl 3):35-38.
1552. Mehls O. Treatment with growth hormone for growth impairment in renal disorders. In: Ranke MB, Gunnarsson R, eds. *Progress in Growth Hormone Therapy: 5 Years of KIGS.* Mannheim, Germany: J&J Verlag; 1994.
1553. Mardh G, Lundin K, Borg B, et al. Growth hormone replacement therapy in adult hypopituitary patients with growth hormone deficiency: combined data from 12 European placebo-controlled clinical trials. *Endocrinol Metab.* 1994;1(suppl A):43-49.
1554. Hokken-Koelega AC, Stijnen T, De Jong MC, et al. Double blind trial comparing the effects of two doses of growth hormone in prepubertal patients with chronic renal insufficiency. *J Clin Endocrinol Metab.* 1994;79:1185-1190.
1555. Mehls O, Broyer M. Growth response to recombinant human growth hormone in short prepubertal children with chronic renal failure with or without dialysis. The European/Australian Study Group. *Acta Paediatr Suppl.* 1994;399:81-87.
1556. Fine RN, Kohaut E, Brown D, et al. Long-term treatment of growth retarded children with chronic renal insufficiency, with recombinant human growth hormone. *Kidney Int.* 1996;49:781-785.
1557. Vance ML, Mauras N. Growth hormone therapy in adults and children. *N Engl J Med.* 1999;341:1206-1216.
1558. Lanes R. Long-term outcome of growth hormone therapy in children and adolescents. *Treat Endocrinol.* 2004;3:53-66.
1559. Fine RN. Recombinant human growth hormone in children with chronic renal insufficiency—clinical update: 1995. *Kidney Int Suppl.* 1996;53:S115-S118.
1560. Watkins SL. Bone disease in patients receiving growth hormone. *Kidney Int Suppl.* 1996;53:S126-S127.
1561. Fine RN, Sullivan EK, Kuntze J, et al. The impact of recombinant human growth hormone treatment during chronic renal insufficiency on renal transplant recipients. *J Pediatr.* 2000;136:376-382.
1562. Berard E, Andre JL, Guest G, et al. French Society for Pediatric Nephrology. Long-term results of rhGH treatment in children with renal failure: experience of the French Society of Pediatric Nephrology. *Pediatr Nephrol.* 2008;23:2031-2038.
1563. Seikaly MG, Waber P, Warady BA, et al. The effect of rhGH on height velocity and BMI in children with CKD: a report of the NAPRTCS registry. *Pediatr Nephrol.* 2009;24:1711-1717.
1564. Hokken-Koelega AC, Stijnen T, de Ridder MA, et al. Growth hormone treatment in growth-retarded adolescents after renal transplant. *Lancet.* 1994;343:1313-1317.
1565. Van Dop C, Jabs KL, Donohoue PA, et al. Accelerated growth rates in children treated with growth hormone after renal transplantation. *J Pediatr.* 1992;120(2 Pt 1):244-250.
1566. Ingulli E, Tejani A. An analytical review of growth hormone studies in children after renal transplantation. *Pediatr Nephrol.* 1995; 9(suppl):S61-S65.
1567. Van Es A. Growth hormone treatment in short children with chronic renal failure and after renal transplantation: combined data from European clinical trials. The European Study Group. *Acta Paediatr Scand Suppl.* 1991;379:42-48, discussion 49.
1568. Nissel R, Lindberg A, Mehls O, et al. Pfizer International Growth Database (KIGS) International Board. Factors predicting the near-final height in growth hormone-treated children and adolescents with chronic kidney disease. *J Clin Endocrinol Metab.* 2008;93:1359-1365.
1569. Fine RN. Allograft rejection in growth hormone and non-growth hormone treated children. *J Pediatr Endocrinol.* 1994;7:127-133.
1570. Chavers BM, Doherty L, Nevins TE, et al. Effects of growth hormone on kidney function in pediatric transplant recipients. *Pediatr Nephrol.* 1995;9:176-181.
1571. Benfield MR, Parker KL, Waldo FB, et al. Growth hormone in the treatment of growth failure in children after renal transplantation. *Kidney Int Suppl.* 1993;43:S62-S64.
1572. Laine J, Krogerus L, Sarna S, et al. Recombinant human growth hormone treatment: its effect on renal allograft function and histology. *Transplantation.* 1996;61:898-903.
1573. Fine RN. Growth hormone in children with chronic renal insufficiency and end-stage renal disease. *Endocrinologist.* 1998;8:160-169.
1574. Guebre-Egziabher F, Juillard L, Boirie Y, et al. Short-term administration of a combination of recombinant growth hormone and insulin-like growth factor-I induces anabolism in maintenance hemodialysis. *J Clin Endocrinol Metab.* 2009;94:2299-2305.
1575. Jacob R, Barrett E, Plewe G, et al. Acute effects of insulin-like growth factor I on glucose and amino acid metabolism in the awake fasted rat: comparison with insulin. *J Clin Invest.* 1989;83:1717-1723.
1576. Haffner D, Wuhl E, Schaefer F, et al. Factors predictive of the short- and long-term efficacy of growth hormone treatment in prepubertal children with chronic renal failure. The German Study Group for Growth Hormone Treatment in Chronic Renal Failure. *J Am Soc Nephrol.* 1998;9:1899-1907.
1577. Tonshoff B, Mehis O, Heinrich U, et al. Growth-stimulating effects of recombinant human growth hormone in children with end-stage renal disease. *J Pediatr.* 1990;116:561-566.
1578. Zak M, Muller J, Karup Pedersen F. Final height, armspan, subischial leg length and body proportions in juvenile chronic arthritis: a long-term follow-up study. *Horm Res.* 1999;52:80-85.
1579. Simon D, Fernando C, Czernichow P, et al. Linear growth and final height in patients with systemic juvenile idiopathic arthritis treated with longterm glucocorticoids. *J Rheumatol.* 2002;29:1296-1300.
1580. Allen RC, Jimenez M, Cowell CT. Insulin-like growth factor and growth hormone secretion in juvenile chronic arthritis. *Ann Rheum Dis.* 1991;50:602-606.
1581. Bennett AE, Silverman ED, Miller 3rd JJ, et al. Insulin-like growth factors I and II in children with systemic onset juvenile arthritis. *J Rheumatol.* 1988;15:655-658.
1582. Bergad PL, Schwarzenberg SJ, Humbert JT, et al. Inhibition of growth hormone action in models of inflammation. *Am J Physiol Cell Physiol.* 2000;279:C1906-C1917.
1583. Butenandt O. Rheumatoid arthritis and growth retardation in children: treatment with human growth hormone. *Eur J Pediatr.* 1979;130:15-28.
1584. Svantesson H. Treatment of growth failure with human growth hormone in patients with juvenile chronic arthritis: a pilot study. *Clin Exp Rheumatol.* 1991;9(suppl 6):47-50.
1585. Davies UM, Rooney M, Preece MA, et al. Treatment of growth retardation in juvenile chronic arthritis with recombinant human growth hormone. *J Rheumatol.* 1994;21:153-158.
1586. Touati G, Prieur AM, Ruiz JC, et al. Beneficial effects of one-year growth hormone administration to children with juvenile chronic arthritis on chronic steroid therapy: I. Effects on growth velocity and body composition. *J Clin Endocrinol Metab.* 1998;83:403-409.
1587. Simon D, Lucidarme N, Prieur AM, et al. Effects on growth and body composition of growth hormone treatment in children with juvenile idiopathic arthritis requiring steroid therapy. *J Rheumatol.* 2003;30: 2492-2499.
1588. Bechtold S, Ripperger P, Hafner R, et al. Growth hormone improves height in patients with juvenile idiopathic arthritis: 4-year data of a controlled study. *J Pediatr.* 2003;143:512-519.
1589. Simon D. rhGH treatment in corticosteroid-treated patients. *Horm Res.* 2007;68:38-45.
1590. Bechtold S, Ripperger P, Dalla Pozza R, et al. Growth hormone increases final height in patients with juvenile idiopathic arthritis: data from a randomized controlled study. *J Clin Endocrinol Metab.* 2007;92:3013-3018.
1591. Simon D, Prieur AM, Quartier P, et al. Early recombinant human growth hormone treatment in glucocorticoid-treated children with juvenile idiopathic arthritis: a 3-year randomized study. *J Clin Endocrinol Metab.* 2007;92:2567-2573.
1592. Mushtaq T, Farquharson C, Seawright E, et al. Glucocorticoid effects on chondrogenesis, differentiation and apoptosis in the murine ATDC5 chondrocyte cell line. *J Endocrinol.* 2002;175:705-713.
1593. Rudman D, Goldsmith M, Kutner M, et al. Effect of growth hormone and oxandrolone singly and together on growth rate in girls with X chromosome abnormalities. *J Pediatr.* 1980;96:132-135.
1594. Forbes AP, Jacobsen JG, Carroll EL, et al. Studies of growth arrest in gonadal dysgenesis: response to exogenous human growth hormone. *Metabolism.* 1962;11:56-75.
1595. Rosenfeld RG, Hintz RL, Johanson AJ, et al. Three-year results of a randomized prospective trial of methionyl human growth hormone and oxandrolone in Turner syndrome. *J Pediatr.* 1988;113:393-400.
1596. Chernausek SD, Attie KM, Cara JF, et al. Growth hormone therapy of Turner syndrome: the impact of age of estrogen replacement on final height. Genentech, Inc., Collaborative Study Group. *J Clin Endocrinol Metab.* 2000;85:2439-2445.
1597. Reiter EO, Baptista J, Price L, et al. Effect of the age at initiation of GH treatment on estrogen use and near adult height in Turner syndrome. In: Saenger PH, Pasquino AM, eds. *5th International Turner Symposium: Optimizing Health Care for Turner Patients in the 21st Century.* Amsterdam, The Netherlands, 2000.
1598. Reiter EO, Blethen SL, Baptista J, et al. Early initiation of growth hormone treatment allows age-appropriate estrogen use in Turner's syndrome. *J Clin Endocrinol Metab.* 2001;86:1936-1941.
1599. Carel JC, Mathivon L, Gendrel C, et al. Near normalization of final height with adapted doses of growth hormone in Turner's syndrome. *J Clin Endocrinol Metab.* 1998;83:1462-1466.
1600. van Pareren YK, de Muinck Keizer-Schrama SM, Stijnen T, et al. Final height in girls with Turner syndrome after long-term growth hormone treatment in three dosages and low dose estrogens. *J Clin Endocrinol Metab.* 2003;88:1119-1125.

1601. Stahnke N, Keller E, Landy H; Serono Study Group. Favorable final height outcome in girls with Ullrich-Turner syndrome treated with low-dose growth hormone together with oxandrolone despite starting treatment after 10 years of age. *J Pediatr Endocrinol Metab.* 2002;15:129-138.
1602. Rongen-Westerlaken C, Corel L, van den Broeck J, et al. Reference values for height, height velocity and weight in Turner's syndrome. Swedish Study Group for Growth Hormone Treatment. *Acta Paediatr.* 1997;86:937-942.
1603. Stephure DK; Canadian Growth Hormone Advisory Committee. Impact of growth hormone supplementation on adult height in Turner syndrome: results of the Canadian randomized controlled trial. *J Clin Endocrinol Metab.* 2005;90:3360-3366.
1604. Rosenfeld RG, Frane J, Attie KM, et al. Six-year results of a randomized, prospective trial of human growth hormone and oxandrolone in Turner syndrome. *J Pediatr.* 1992;121:49-55.
1605. Pasquino AM, Pucarelli I, Segni M, et al. Adult height in sixty girls with Turner syndrome treated with growth hormone matched with an untreated group. *J Endocrinol Invest.* 2005;28:350-356.
1606. Ranke MB, Lindberg A, Chatelain P, et al. KIGS International Board. Prediction of long-term response to recombinant human growth hormone in Turner syndrome: development and validation of mathematical models. Kabi International Growth Study. *J Clin Endocrinol Metab.* 2000;85:4212-4218.
1607. Quigley CA, Crowe BJ, Anglin DG, et al. Growth hormone and low dose estrogen in Turner syndrome: results of a United States multicenter trial to near-final height. *J Clin Endocrinol Metab.* 2002; 87:2033-2041.
1608. Carel JC, Mathivon L, Gendrel C, et al. Growth hormone therapy for Turner syndrome: evidence for benefit. *Horm Res.* 1997;48(suppl 5):31-34.
1609. Hofman P, Cutfield WS, Robinson EM, et al. Factors predictive of response to growth hormone therapy in Turner's syndrome. *J Pediatr Endocrinol Metab.* 1997;10:27-33.
1610. Davenport ML, Quigley CA, Bryant CG, et al. Effect of early growth hormone (GH) treatment in very young girls with Turner syndrome (TS). Seventh Joint European Society for Paediatric Endocrinology/ Lawson Wilkins Pediatric Endocrine Society Meeting, Lyon, France, 2005.
1611. Sas TC, de Muinck Keizer-Schrama SM, Stijnen T, et al. Carbohydrate metabolism during long-term growth hormone (GH) treatment and after discontinuation of GH treatment in girls with Turner syndrome participating in a randomized dose-response study. Dutch Advisory Group on Growth Hormone. *J Clin Endocrinol Metab.* 2000;85: 769-775.
1612. Park P, Cohen P. The role of insulin-like growth factor I monitoring in growth hormone-treated children. *Horm Res.* 2004;62(suppl 1):59-65.
1613. Bondy CA, Turner Syndrome Study Group. Care of girls and women with Turner syndrome: a guideline of the Turner Syndrome Study Group. *J Clin Endocrinol Metab.* 2007;92:10-25.
1614. Soriano-Guillen L, Coste J, Ecosse E, et al. Adult height and pubertal growth in Turner syndrome after treatment with recombinant growth hormone. *J Clin Endocrinol Metab.* 2005;90:5197-5204.
1615. Rosenfield RL, Devine N, Hunold JJ, et al. Salutary effects of combining early very low-dose systemic estradiol with growth hormone therapy in girls with Turner syndrome. *J Clin Endocrinol Metab.* 2005;90:6424-6430.
1616. Van Pareren YK, De Muinck Keizer-Schrama SM, et al. Effect of discontinuation of long-term growth hormone treatment on carbohydrate metabolism and risk factors for cardiovascular disease in girls with Turner syndrome. *J Clin Endocrinol Metab.* 2002;87:5442-5448.
1617. Radetti G, Pasquino B, Gottardi E, et al. Insulin sensitivity in Turner's syndrome: influence of GH treatment. *Eur J Endocrinol.* 2004; 151:351-354.
1618. Bakalov VK, Cooley MM, Quon MJ, et al. Impaired insulin secretion in the Turner metabolic syndrome. *J Clin Endocrinol Metab.* 2004;89:3516-3520.
1619. Bertelloni S, Cinquanta L, Baroncelli GI, et al. Volumetric bone mineral density in young women with Turner's syndrome treated with estrogens or estrogens plus growth hormone. *Horm Res.* 2000;53:72-76.
1620. Bannink EM, Raat H, Mulder PG, et al. Quality of life after growth hormone therapy and induced puberty in women with Turner syndrome. *J Pediatr.* 2006;148:95-101.
1621. Carel JC, Ecosse E, Bastie-Sigeac I, et al. Quality of life determinants in young women with Turner's syndrome after growth hormone treatment: results of the StaTur population-based cohort study. *J Clin Endocrinol Metab.* 2005;90:1992-1997.
1622. Bolar K, Hoffman AR, Maneatis T, et al. Long-term safety of recombinant human growth hormone in Turner syndrome. *J Clin Endocrinol Metab.* 2008;93:344-351.
1623. Radetti G, Crepaz R, Milanesi O, et al. Cardiac performance in Turner's syndrome patients on growth hormone therapy. *Horm Res.* 2001;55:240-244.
1624. Sas TC, Cromme-Dijkhuis AH, de Muinck Keizer-Schrama SM, et al. The effects of long-term growth hormone treatment on cardiac left ventricular dimensions and blood pressure in girls with Turner's syndrome. Dutch Working Group on Growth Hormone. *J Pediatr.* 1999;135:470-476.
1625. van den Berg J, Bannink EM, Wielopolski PA, et al. Aortic distensibility and dimensions and the effects of growth hormone treatment in the Turner syndrome. *Am J Cardiol.* 2006;97:1644-1649.
1626. Donaldson MD, Gault EJ, Tan KW, et al. Optimising management in Turner syndrome: from infancy to adult transfer. *Arch Dis Child.* 2006;91:513-520.
1627. Russell KA. Orthodontic treatment for patients with Turner syndrome. *Am J Orthod Dentofacial Orthop.* 2001;120:314-322.
1628. Lee PA, Chernausek SD, Hokken-Koelega AC, et al. International Small for Gestational Age Advisory Board consensus development conference statement: management of short children born small for gestational age, April 24-October 1, 2001. *Pediatrics.* 2003;111: 1253-1261.
1629. Clayton PE, Cianfarani S, Czernichow P, et al. Management of the child born small for gestational age through to adulthood: a consensus statement of the International Societies of Pediatric Endocrinology and the Growth Hormone Research Society. *J Clin Endocrinol Metab.* 2007;92:804-810.
1630. Karlberg JP, Albertsson-Wikland K, Kwan EY, et al. The timing of early postnatal catch-up growth in normal, full-term infants born short for gestational age. *Horm Res.* 1997;48(suppl 1):17-24.
1631. Karlberg J, Albertsson-Wikland K, Kwan CW, et al. Early spontaneous catch-up growth. *J Pediatr Endocrinol Metab.* 2002;15(suppl 5):1243-1255.
1632. Albertsson-Wikland K, Karlberg J. Postnatal growth of children born small for gestational age. *Acta Paediatr Suppl.* 1997;423:193-195.
1633. Chatelain P, Job JC, Blanchard J, et al. Dose-dependent catch-up growth after 2 years of growth hormone treatment in intrauterine growth-retarded children. Belgian and French Pediatric Clinics and Sanofi-Choay (France). *J Clin Endocrinol Metab.* 1994;78: 1454-1460.
1634. de Zegher F, Francois I, van Helvoirt M, et al. Clinical review 89. Small as fetus and short as child: from endogenous to exogenous growth hormone. *J Clin Endocrinol Metab.* 1997;82:2021-2026.
1635. Vicens-Calvet E, Espadero RM, Carrascosa A, et al. Spanish SGA Collaborative Group. Small for gestational age: longitudinal study of the pubertal growth spurt in children born small for gestational age without postnatal catch-up growth. *J Pediatr Endocrinol Metab.* 2002;15:381-388.
1636. Job JC, Rolland A. Natural history of intrauterine growth retardation: pubertal growth and adult height. *Arch Fr Pediatr.* 1986;43: 301-306.
1637. Lazar L, Pollak U, Kalter-Leibovici O, et al. Pubertal course of persistently short children born small for gestational age (SGA) compared with idiopathic short children born appropriate for gestational age (AGA). *Eur J Endocrinol.* 2003;149:425-432.
1638. Rogol A. Growth, puberty and therapeutic interventions (abstract S1-15). Presented at the 45th European Society for Pediatric Endocrinology Annual Meeting, Helsinki, Finland, 2006.
1639. Wollmann HA. Intrauterine growth restriction: definition and etiology. *Horm Res.* 1998;49(suppl 2):1-6.
1640. Ogilvy-Stuart AL, Hands SJ, Adcock CJ, et al. Insulin, insulin-like growth factor I (IGF-I), IGF-binding protein-1, growth hormone, and feeding in the newborn. *J Clin Endocrinol Metab.* 1998;83: 3550-3557.
1641. Audi L, Esteban C, Espadero R, et al. D-3 growth hormone receptor polymorphism (D3-GHR) genotype frequencies differ between short small for gestational age children (SGA) (N 1/4 247) and a control population with normal adult height (N 1/4 289) (CPNAH) (abstract S1-15). Presented at the 45th European Society for Pediatric Endocrinology Annual Meeting, Rotterdam, The Netherlands, 2006.
1642. Jensen RB, Vieweth S, Larsen T, et al. High prevalence of D3-growth hormone gene polymorphism in adolescents born SGA/IUGR: association with intrauterine growth velocity, birth weight, postnatal catch-up growth and near-final height (abstract FC1-42). Presented at the 45th European Society for Pediatric Endocrinology Annual Meeting, Rotterdam, The Netherlands, 2006.
1643. Bonapace G, Concolino D, Formicola S, et al. A novel mutation in a patient with insulin-like growth factor 1 (IGF1) deficiency. *J Med Genet.* 2003;40:913-917.
1644. Cianfarani S, Maiorana A, Geremia C, et al. Blood glucose concentrations are reduced in children born small for gestational age (SGA), and thyroid-stimulating hormone levels are increased in SGA with blunted postnatal catch-up growth. *J Clin Endocrinol Metab.* 2003;88:2699-2705.
1645. Tenhola S, Halonen P, Jaaskelainen J, et al. Serum markers of GH and insulin action in 12-year-old children born small for gestational age. *Eur J Endocrinol.* 2005;152:335-340.
1646. Johnston LB, Dahlgren J, Leger J, et al. Association between insulin-like growth factor I (IGF-I) polymorphisms, circulating IGF-I, and

pre- and postnatal growth in two European small for gestational age populations. *J Clin Endocrinol Metab.* 2003;88:4805-4810.

1647. Ali O, Cohen P. Insulin-like growth factors and their binding proteins in children born small for gestational age: implication for growth hormone therapy. *Horm Res.* 2003;60(suppl 3):115-123.
1648. Strauss RS, Dietz WH. Growth and development of term children born with low birth weight: effects of genetic and environmental factors. *J Pediatr.* 1998;133:67-72.
1649. de Zegher F, Hokken-Koelega A. Growth hormone therapy for children born small for gestational age: height gain is less dose dependent over the long term than over the short term. *Pediatrics.* 2005;115:e458-e462.
1650. Carel JC, Chatelain P, Rochiccioli P, et al. Improvement in adult height after growth hormone treatment in adolescents with short stature born small for gestational age: results of a randomized controlled study. *J Clin Endocrinol Metab.* 2003;88:1587-1593.
1651. de Zegher F, Ong KK, Ibanez L, et al. Growth hormone therapy in short children born small for gestational age. *Horm Res.* 2006;65(suppl 3):145-152.
1652. Ong K, Beardsall K, de Zegher F. Growth hormone therapy in short children born small for gestational age. *Early Hum Dev.* 2005;81: 973-980.
1653. Ranke MB, Lindberg A, Cowell CT, et al. KIGS International Board. Prediction of response to growth hormone treatment in short children born small for gestational age: analysis of data from KIGS (Pharmacia International Growth Database). *J Clin Endocrinol Metab.* 2003;88:125-131.
1654. Leger J, Levy-Marchal C, Bloch J, et al. Reduced final height and indications for insulin resistance in 20 year olds born small for gestational age: regional cohort study. *BMJ.* 1997;315:341-347.
1655. Barker DJ, Hales CN, Fall CH, et al. Type 2 (non-insulin-dependent) diabetes mellitus, hypertension and hyperlipidaemia (syndrome X): relation to reduced fetal growth. *Diabetologia.* 1993;36:62-67.
1656. Crowther NJ, Cameron N, Trusler J, et al. Association between poor glucose tolerance and rapid post natal weight gain in seven-year-old children. *Diabetologia.* 1998;41:1163-1167.
1657. Jaquet D, Gaboriau A, Czernichow P, et al. Insulin resistance early in adulthood in subjects born with intrauterine growth retardation. *J Clin Endocrinol Metab.* 2000;85:1401-1406.
1658. Veening MA, Van Weissenbruch MM, Delemarre-Van De Waal HA. Glucose tolerance, insulin sensitivity, and insulin secretion in children born small for gestational age. *J Clin Endocrinol Metab.* 2002;87:4657-4661.
1659. Soto N, Bazaes RA, Pena V, et al. Insulin sensitivity and secretion are related to catch-up growth in small-for-gestational-age infants at age 1 year: results from a prospective cohort. *J Clin Endocrinol Metab.* 2003;88:3645-3650.
1660. de Zegher F, Maes M, Gargosky SE, et al. High-dose growth hormone treatment of short children born small for gestational age. *J Clin Endocrinol Metab.* 1996;81:1887-1892.
1661. de Zegher F, Ong K, van Helvoirt M, et al. High-dose growth hormone (GH) treatment in non-GH-deficient children born small for gestational age induces growth responses related to pretreatment GH secretion and associated with a reversible decrease in insulin sensitivity. *J Clin Endocrinol Metab.* 2002;87:148-151.
1662. van Pareren Y, Mulder P, Houdijk M, et al. Effect of discontinuation of growth hormone treatment on risk factors for cardiovascular disease in adolescents born small for gestational age. *J Clin Endocrinol Metab.* 2003;88:347-353.
1663. Cutfield WS, Lindberg A, Rapaport R, et al. Safety of growth hormone treatment in children born small for gestational age: the US trial and KIGS analysis. *Horm Res.* 2006;65(suppl 3):153-159.
1664. Wilton P. Adverse events during GH treatment: 10 years' experience with KIGS, a pharmacoepidemiological survey. In: Ranke MB, Wilton P, eds. *Growth Hormone Therapy in KIGS: 10 Years' Experience.* Heidelberg-Leipzig, Germany: Johann Ambrosius Barth Verlag; 1999.
1665. Sas T, Mulder P, Hokken-Koelega A. Body composition, blood pressure, and lipid metabolism before and during long-term growth hormone (GH) treatment in children with short stature born small for gestational age either with or without GH deficiency. *J Clin Endocrinol Metab.* 2000;85:3786-3792.
1666. Czernichow P. Treatment with growth hormone in short children born with intrauterine growth retardation. *Endocrine.* 2001;15: 39-42.
1667. Simeoni U, Zetterstrom R. Long-term circulatory and renal consequences of intrauterine growth restriction. *Acta Paediatr.* 2005;94: 819-824.
1668. Chatelain P. Children born with intra-uterine growth retardation (IUGR) or small for gestational age (SGA): long term growth and metabolic consequences. *Endocr Regul.* 2000;34:33-36.
1669. Levy-Marchal C, Czernichow P. Small for gestational age and the metabolic syndrome: which mechanism is suggested by epidemiological and clinical studies? *Horm Res.* 2006;65(suppl 3): 123-130.
1670. Seino Y, Yamate T, Kanzaki S, et al. Achondroplasia: effect of growth hormone in 40 patients. *Clin Pediatr Endocrinol.* 1994;3(suppl 4):41-45.
1671. Ramaswami U, Rumsby G, Spoudeas HA, et al. Treatment of achondroplasia with growth hormone: six years of experience. *Pediatr Res.* 1999;46:435-439.
1672. Bridges NA, Brook CG. Progress report: growth hormone in skeletal dysplasia. *Horm Res.* 1994;42:231-234.
1673. Ramaswami U, Hindmarsh PC, Brook CG. Growth hormone therapy in hypochondroplasia. *Acta Paediatr Suppl.* 1999;88:116-117.
1674. Rao E, Weiss B, Fukami M, et al. Pseudoautosomal deletions encompassing a novel homeobox gene cause growth failure in idiopathic short stature and Turner syndrome. *Nat Genet.* 1997;16:54-63.
1675. Ellison JW, Wardak Z, Young MF, et al. PHOG, a candidate gene for involvement in the short stature of Turner syndrome. *Hum Mol Genet.* 1997;6:1341-1347.
1676. Clement-Jones M, Schiller S, Rao E, et al. The short stature homeobox gene SHOX is involved in skeletal abnormalities in Turner syndrome. *Hum Mol Genet.* 2000;9:695-702.
1677. Munns CJ, Haase HR, Crowther LM, et al. Expression of SHOX in human fetal and childhood growth plate. *J Clin Endocrinol Metab.* 2004;89:4130-4135.
1678. Shears DJ, Vassal HJ, Goodman FR, et al. Mutation and deletion of the pseudoautosomal gene SHOX cause Léri-Weill dyschondrosteosis. *Nat Genet.* 1998;19:70-73.
1679. Belin V, Cusin V, Viot G, et al. SHOX mutations in dyschondrosteosis (Léri-Weill syndrome). *Nat Genet.* 1998;19:67-69.
1680. Binder G, Renz A, Martinez A, et al. SHOX haploinsufficiency and Léri-Weill dyschondrosteosis: prevalence and growth failure in relation to mutation, sex, and degree of wrist deformity. *J Clin Endocrinol Metab.* 2004;89:4403-4408.
1681. Rappold GA, Fukami M, Niesler B, et al. Deletions of the homeobox gene SHOX (short stature homeobox) are an important cause of growth failure in children with short stature. *J Clin Endocrinol Metab.* 2002;87:1402-1406.
1682. Binder G, Ranke MB, Martin DD. Auxology is a valuable instrument for the clinical diagnosis of SHOX haploinsufficiency in school-age children with unexplained short stature. *J Clin Endocrinol Metab.* 2003;88:4891-4896.
1683. Huber C, Rosilio M, Munnich A, et al. French SHOX GeNeSIS Module. High incidence of SHOX anomalies in individuals with short stature. *J Med Genet.* 2006;43:735-739.
1684. Kosho T, Muroya K, Nagai T, et al. Skeletal features and growth patterns in 14 patients with haploinsufficiency of SHOX: implications for the development of Turner syndrome. *J Clin Endocrinol Metab.* 1999;84:4613-4621.
1685. Léri A, Weill J. Une affection congenital et symetrique du developpment osseux: la dyschondrosteose. *Bull Mém Soc Med Paris.* 1929:1491-1494.
1686. Ogata T, Onigata K, Hotsubo T, et al. Growth hormone and gonadotropin-releasing hormone analog therapy in haploinsufficiency of SHOX. *Endocr J.* 2001;48:317-322.
1687. Rappold G, Blum WF, Shavrikova EP, et al. Genotypes and phenotypes in children with short stature: clinical indicators of SHOX haploinsufficiency. *J Med Genet.* 2007;44:306-313.
1688. Blum WF, Cao D, Hesse V, et al. Height gains in response to growth hormone treatment to final height are similar in patients with SHOX deficiency and Turner syndrome. *Horm Res.* 2009;71:167-172.
1689. Plotnick L, Attie KM, Blethen SL, et al. Growth hormone treatment of girls with Turner syndrome: the National Cooperative Growth Study experience. *Pediatrics.* 1998;102(2 Pt 3):479-481.
1690. Munns CF, Berry M, Vickers D, et al. Effect of 24 months of recombinant growth hormone on height and body proportions in SHOX haploinsufficiency. *J Pediatr Endocrinol Metab.* 2003;16: 997-1004.
1691. Blum WF, Crowe BJ, Quigley CA, et al. SHOX Study Group. Growth hormone is effective in treatment of short stature associated with short stature homeobox-containing gene deficiency: two-year results of a randomized, controlled, multicenter trial. *J Clin Endocrinol Metab.* 2007;92:219-228.
1692. Shah BC, Moran ES, Zinn AR, et al. Effect of growth hormone therapy on severe short stature and skeletal deformities in a patient with combined Turner syndrome and Langer mesomelic dysplasia. *J Clin Endocrinol Metab.* 2009;94:5028-5033.
1693. Jamieson CR, van der Burgt I, Brady AF, et al. Mapping a gene for Noonan syndrome to the long arm of chromosome 12. *Nat Genet.* 1994;8:357-360.
1694. Schubbert S, Zenker M, Rowe SL, et al. Germline KRAS mutations cause Noonan syndrome. *Nat Genet.* 2006;38:331-336.
1695. Roberts AE, Araki T, Swanson KD, et al. Germline gain-of-function mutations in SOS1 cause Noonan syndrome. *Nat Genet.* 2007;39:70-74.
1696. Pandit B, Sarkozy A, Pennacchio LA, et al. Gain-of-function RAF1 mutations cause Noonan and LEOPARD syndromes with hypertrophic cardiomyopathy. *Nat Genet.* 2007;39:1007-1012.

1697. Raaijmakers R, Noordam C, Karagiannis G, et al. Response to growth hormone treatment and final height in Noonan syndrome in a large cohort of patients in the KIGS database. *J Pediatr Endocrinol Metab.* 2008;21:267-273.
1698. Kirk JM, Betts PR, Butler GE, et al. Short stature in Noonan syndrome: response to growth hormone therapy. *Arch Dis Child.* 2001;84:440-443.
1699. Osio D, Dahlgren J, Wikland KA, et al. Improved final height with long-term growth hormone treatment in Noonan syndrome. *Acta Paediatr.* 2005;94:1232-1237.
1700. Municchi G, Pasquino AM, Pucarelli I, et al. Growth hormone treatment in Noonan syndrome: report of four cases who reached final height. *Horm Res.* 1995;44:164-167.
1701. Noordam C, Peer PG, Francois I, et al. Long-term GH treatment improves adult height in children with Noonan syndrome with and without mutations in protein tyrosine phosphatase, non-receptor-type 11. *Eur J Endocrinol.* 2008;159:203-208.
1702. Romano AA, Dana K, Bakker B, et al. Growth response, near-adult height, and patterns of growth and puberty in patients with Noonan syndrome treated with growth hormone. *J Clin Endocrinol Metab.* 2009;94:2338-2344.
1703. Rosenfeld RG, Buckway CK. Should we treat genetic syndromes? *J Pediatr Endocrinol Metab.* 2000;13:971-981.
1704. Romano AA, Blethen SL, Dana K, et al. Growth hormone treatment in Noonan syndrome: the National Cooperative Growth Study Experience. *J Pediatr.* 1996;128(5 Pt 2):S18-S21.
1705. Cotterill AM, McKenna WJ, Brady AF, et al. The short-term effects of growth hormone therapy on height velocity and cardiac ventricular wall thickness in children with Noonan's syndrome. *J Clin Endocrinol Metab.* 1996;81:2291-2297.
1706. Rauen KA, Schoyer L, McCormick F, et al. Proceedings from the 2009 Symposium. Genetic Syndromes of the Ras/MAPK Pathway: from bedside to bench and back. *Am J Med Genet A.* 2010;152:4-24.
1707. Pine DS, Cohen P, Brook J. Emotional problems during youth as predictors of stature during early adulthood: results from a prospective epidemiologic study. *Pediatrics.* 1996;97(6 Pt 1):856-863.
1708. Stabler B, Siegel PT, Clopper RR, et al. Behavior changes after growth hormone treatment of children with short stature. *J Pediatr.* 1998;133:366-373.
1709. Voss LD. Growth hormone therapy for the short normal child: who needs it and who wants it? The case against growth hormone therapy. *J Pediatr.* 2000;136:103-106.
1710. Voss LD, Mulligan J. Bullying in school: are short pupils at risk? Questionnaire study in a cohort. *BMJ.* 2000;320:612-613.
1711. Saenger P. The case in support of GH therapy. *J Pediatr.* 2000;136:106-109, discussion 109-110.
1712. Underwood LE, Rieser PA. Is it ethical to treat healthy short children with growth hormone? *Acta Paediatr Scand Suppl.* 1989;362:18-23.
1713. Allen DB, Brook CG, Bridges NA, et al. Therapeutic controversies: growth hormone (GH) treatment of non-GH deficient subjects. *J Clin Endocrinol Metab.* 1994;79:1239-1248.
1714. Allen DB, Fost N. hGH for short stature: Ethical issues raised by expanded access. *J Pediatr.* 2004;144:648-652.
1715. Sandberg DE, Colsman M. Growth hormone treatment of short stature: status of the quality of life rationale. *Horm Res.* 2005;63:275-283.
1716. Ross JL, Sandberg DE, Rose SR, et al. Psychological adaptation in children with idiopathic short stature treated with growth hormone or placebo. *J Clin Endocrinol Metab.* 2004;89:4873-4878.
1717. Voss LD, Sandberg DE. The psychological burden of short stature: evidence against. *Eur J Endocrinol.* 2004;151(suppl 1):S29-S33.
1718. van Pareren YK, Duivenvoorden HJ, Slijper FS, et al. Intelligence and psychosocial functioning during long-term growth hormone therapy in children born small for gestational age. *J Clin Endocrinol Metab.* 2004;89:5295-5302.
1719. Cuttler L. Safety and efficacy of growth hormone treatment for idiopathic short stature. *J Clin Endocrinol Metab.* 2005;90:5502-5504.
1720. Wit JM, Rekers-Mombarg LT, Cutler GB, et al. Growth hormone (GH) treatment to final height in children with idiopathic short stature: evidence for a dose effect. *J Pediatr.* 2005;146:45-53.
1721. Finkelstein BS, Imperiale TF, Speroff T, et al. Effect of growth hormone therapy on height in children with idiopathic short stature: a meta-analysis. *Arch Pediatr Adolesc Med.* 2002;156:230-240.
1722. McCaughey ES, Mulligan J, Voss LD, et al. Randomised trial of growth hormone in short normal girls. *Lancet.* 1998;351:940-944.
1723. de Zegher F, Maes M, Heinrichs C, et al. High-dose growth hormone therapy for short children born small for gestational age. Belgian Study Group for Paediatric Endocrinology. *Acta Paediatr Suppl.* 1994;399:77, discussion 78.
1724. Loche S, Cambiaso P, Setzu S, et al. Final height after growth hormone therapy in non-growth-hormone-deficient children with short stature. *J Pediatr.* 1994;125:196-200.
1725. Cowell CT. Growth hormone therapy in idiopathic short stature in the Kabi International Growth Study. In: Ranke MB, Gunnarsson R, eds. *Progress in Growth Hormone Therapy: 5 Years of KIGS.* Mannheim, Germany: J&J Verlag; 1994.
1726. Crowe BJ, Rekers-Mombarg LT, Robling K, et al. European Idiopathic Short Stature Group. Effect of growth hormone dose on bone maturation and puberty in children with idiopathic short stature. *J Clin Endocrinol Metab.* 2006;91:169-175.
1727. Kamp GA, Waelkens JJ, de Muinck Keizer-Schrama SM, et al. High dose growth hormone treatment induces acceleration of skeletal maturation and an earlier onset of puberty in children with idiopathic short stature. *Arch Dis Child.* 2002;87:215-220.
1728. Wit J. Growth hormone treatment of idiopathic short stature. In: Ranke MB, Wilton P, eds. *Growth Hormone Therapy in KIGS: 10 Years' Experience.* Heidelberg-Leipzig, Germany: Johann Ambrosius Verlag; 1999.
1729. Saenger P, Attie KM, DiMartino-Nardi J, et al. Metabolic consequences of 5-year growth hormone (GH) therapy in children treated with GH for idiopathic short stature. Genentech Collaborative Study Group. *J Clin Endocrinol Metab.* 1998;83:3115-3120.
1730. Kelnar CJ, Albertsson-Wikland K, Hintz RL, et al. Should we treat children with idiopathic short stature? *Horm Res.* 1999;52:150-157.
1731. Wit JM, Rekers-Mombarg LT, Dutch Growth Hormone Advisory Group. Final height gain by GH therapy in children with idiopathic short stature is dose dependent. *J Clin Endocrinol Metab.* 2002;87:604-611.
1732. Visser-van Balen H, Geenen R, Kamp GA, et al. Long-term psychosocial consequences of hormone treatment for short stature. *Acta Paediatr.* 2007;96:715-719.
1733. Van Vliet G, Styne DM, Kaplan SL, et al. Growth hormone treatment for short stature. *N Engl J Med.* 1983;309:1016-1022.
1734. Gertner JM, Genel M, Gianfredi SP, et al. Prospective clinical trial of human growth hormone in short children without growth hormone deficiency. *J Pediatr.* 1984;104:172-176.
1735. Hopwood NJ, Hintz RL, Gertner JM, et al. Growth response of children with non-growth-hormone deficiency and marked short stature during three years of growth hormone therapy. *J Pediatr.* 1993;123:215-222.
1736. Zadik Z, Chalew S, Zung A, et al. Effect of long-term growth hormone therapy on bone age and pubertal maturation in boys with and without classic growth hormone deficiency. *J Pediatr.* 1994;125:189-195.
1737. Weise KL, Nahata MC. Growth hormone use in children with idiopathic short stature. *Ann Pharmacother.* 2004;38:1460-1468.
1738. Spagnoli A, Spadoni GL, Cianfarani S, et al. Prediction of the outcome of growth hormone therapy in children with idiopathic short stature: a multivariate discriminant analysis. *J Pediatr.* 1995;126:905-909.
1739. Bryant J, Baxter L, Cave CB, et al. Recombinant growth hormone for idiopathic short stature in children and adolescents. Cochrane Database Syst Rev. 2007;3:CD004440.
1740. Mauras N, Gonzalez de Pijem L, Hsiang HY, et al. Anastrozole increases predicted adult height of short adolescent males treated with growth hormone: a randomized, placebo-controlled, multicenter trial for one to three years. *J Clin Endocrinol Metab.* 2008;93:823-831.
1741. Yanovski JA, Rose SR, Municchi G, et al. Treatment with a luteinizing hormone-releasing hormone agonist in adolescents with short stature. *N Engl J Med.* 2003;348:908-917.
1742. Mazur T, Clopper RR. Pubertal disorders: Psychology and clinical management. *Endocrinol Metab Clin North Am.* 1991;20:211-230.
1743. Tanaka T. Sufficiently long-term treatment with combined growth hormone and gonadotropin-releasing hormone analog can improve adult height in short children with isolated growth hormone deficiency (GHD) and in non-GHD short children. *Pediatr Endocrinol Rev.* 2007;5:471-481.
1744. van Gool SA, Kamp GA, Visser-van Balen H, et al. Final height outcome after three years of growth hormone and gonadotropin-releasing hormone agonist treatment in short adolescents with relatively early puberty. *J Clin Endocrinol Metab.* 2007;92:1402-1408.
1745. US Food and Drug Administration. Available at: www.accessdata.fda.gov/drugsatfda_docs/label/2008/0202805060Ibl.pdf.
1746. Tanaka T, Cohen P, Clayton PE, et al. Diagnosis and management of growth hormone deficiency in childhood and adolescence: part 2. Growth hormone treatment in growth hormone deficient children. *Growth Horm IGF Res.* 2002;12:323-341.
1747. Quigley CA, Gill AM, Crowe BJ, et al. Safety of growth hormone treatment in pediatric patients with idiopathic short stature. *J Clin Endocrinol Metab.* 2005;90:5188-5196.
1748. Anneren G, Gustafsson J, Sara VR, et al. Normalized growth velocity in children with Down's syndrome during growth hormone therapy. *J Intellect Disabil Res.* 1993;37(Pt 4):381-387.
1749. Neyzi O, Darendelilier F. Growth hormone treatment in syndromes with short stature including Down syndrome, Prader-Labhardt-Willi syndrome, von Recklinghausen syndrome, Williams syndrome, and others. In: Ranke MB, Gunnarsson R, eds. *Progress in Growth Hormone Therapy: 5 Years of KIGS.* Mannheim, Germany: J&J Verlag; 1994.

1750. Torrado C, Bastian W, Wisniewski KE, et al. Treatment of children with Down syndrome and growth retardation with recombinant human growth hormone. *J Pediatr.* 1991;119:478-483.
1751. Allen DB, Frasier SD, Foley Jr TP, et al. Growth hormone for children with Down syndrome. *J Pediatr.* 1993;123:742-743.
1752. Robinson IC, Gabrielsson B, Klaus G, et al. Glucocorticoids and growth problems. *Acta Paediatr Suppl.* 1995;411:81-86.
1753. Reusz GS, Hoyer PF, Lucas M, et al. X linked hypophosphataemia: treatment, height gain, and nephrocalcinosis. *Arch Dis Child.* 1990;65:1125-1128.
1754. Sanchez CP, Goodman WG, Brandli D, et al. Skeletal response to recombinant human growth hormone (rhGH) in children treated with long-term corticosteroids. *J Bone Miner Res.* 1995;10:2-6.
1755. Luo JM, Murphy LJ. Dexamethasone inhibits growth hormone induction of insulin-like growth factor-I (IGF-I) messenger ribonucleic acid (mRNA) in hypophysectomized rats and reduces IGF-I mRNA abundance in the intact rat. *Endocrinology.* 1989;125:165-171.
1756. Takala J, Ruokonen E, Webster NR, et al. Increased mortality associated with growth hormone treatment in critically ill adults. *N Engl J Med.* 1999;341:785-792.
1757. Buchanan CR, Preece MA, Milner RD. Mortality, neoplasia, and Creutzfeldt-Jakob disease in patients treated with human pituitary growth hormone in the United Kingdom. *BMJ.* 1991;302:824-828.
1758. Maneatis T, Baptista J, Connelly K, et al. Growth hormone safety update from the National Cooperative Growth Study. *J Pediatr Endocrinol Metab.* 2000;13(suppl 2):1035-1044.
1759. Blethen SL, Allen DB, Graves D, et al. Safety of recombinant deoxyribonucleic acid-derived growth hormone: the National Cooperative Growth Study experience. *J Clin Endocrinol Metab.* 1996;81:1704-1710.
1760. Cowell CT, Dietsch S. Adverse events during growth hormone therapy. *J Pediatr Endocrinol Metab.* 1995;8:243-252.
1761. Ranke MB, Wilton PM. *Growth Hormone Therapy in KIGS: 10 Years' Experience.* Heidelberg-Leipzig, Germany: Johann Ambrosius Barth Verlag; 1999.
1762. Blethen SL. Complications of growth hormone therapy in children. *Curr Opin Pediatr.* 1995;7:466-471.
1763. Watanabe S, Yamaguchi N, Tsunematsu Y, et al. Risk factors for leukemia occurrence among growth hormone users. *Jpn J Cancer Res.* 1989;80:822-825.
1764. Fisher DA, Job J-C, Preece M, et al. Leukemia in patients treated with growth hormone. *Lancet.* 1988;1:1159-1160.
1765. Wilton P. Adverse events during growth hormone treatment: 5 years' experience. In: Ranke MB, Gunnarsson R, eds. *Progress in Growth Hormone Therapy: 5 Years of KIGS.* Mannheim, Germany: J&J Verlag; 1994.
1766. Blethen SL. Leukemia in children treated with growth hormone. *Trends Endocrinol Metab.* 1999;9:367-370.
1767. Nishi Y, Tanaka T, Takano K, et al. Recent status in the occurrence of leukemia in growth hormone-treated patients in Japan. GH Treatment Study Committee of the Foundation for Growth Science, Japan. *J Clin Endocrinol Metab.* 1999;84:1961-1965.
1768. Ogilvy-Stuart AL, Ryder WD, Gattamaneni HR, et al. Growth hormone and tumour recurrence. *BMJ.* 1992;304:1601-1605.
1769. Arslanian SA, Becker DJ, Lee PA, et al. Growth hormone therapy and tumor recurrence: findings in children with brain neoplasms and hypopituitarism. *Am J Dis Child.* 1985;139:347-350.
1770. Bloom HJ, Glees J, Bell J, et al. The treatment and long-term prognosis of children with intracranial tumors: a study of 610 cases, 1950-1981. *Int J Radiat Oncol Biol Phys.* 1990;18:723-745.
1771. Davis CH, Joglekar VM. Cerebellar astrocytomas in children and young adults. *J Neurol Neurosurg Psychiatry.* 1981;44:820-828.
1772. Halperin EC. Pediatric brain stem tumors: patterns of treatment failure and their implications for radiotherapy. *Int J Radiat Oncol Biol Phys.* 1985;11:1293-1298.
1773. Hoffman HJ, De Silva M, Humphreys RP, et al. Aggressive surgical management of craniopharyngiomas in children. *J Neurosurg.* 1992;76:47-52.
1774. Lapras C, Patet JD, Mottolese C, et al. Craniopharyngiomas in childhood: analysis of 42 cases. *Prog Exp Tumor Res.* 1987;30:350-358.
1775. Nishio S, Fukui M, Takeshita I, et al. Recurrent medulloblastoma in children. *Neurol Med Chir (Tokyo).* 1986;26:19-25.
1776. Schuler D, Somlo P, Borsi J, et al. New drug combination for the treatment of relapsed brain tumors in children. *Pediatr Hematol Oncol.* 1988;5:153-156.
1777. Torres CF, Rebsamen S, Silber JH, et al. Surveillance scanning of children with medulloblastoma. *N Engl J Med.* 1994;330:892-895.
1778. Uematsu Y, Tsuura Y, Miyamoto K, et al. The recurrence of primary intracranial germinomas: special reference to germinoma with STGC (syncytiotrophoblastic giant cell). *J Neurooncol.* 1992;13:247-256.
1779. Clayton PE, Shalet SM, Gattamaneni HR, et al. Does growth hormone cause relapse of brain tumours? *Lancet.* 1987;1:711-713.
1780. Rodens KP, Kaplan SL, Grumbach MM, et al. Does growth hormone therapy increase the frequency of tumor recurrence in children with brain tumors? *Acta Endocrinol.* 1987;28(suppl):188-189.
1781. Moshang Jr T. Is brain tumor recurrence increased following growth hormone treatment? *Trends Endocrinol Metab.* 1995;6:205-209.
1782. Swerdlow AJ, Reddingius RE, Higgins CD, et al. Growth hormone treatment of children with brain tumors and risk of tumor recurrence. *J Clin Endocrinol Metab.* 2000;85:4444-4449.
1783. Karavitaki N, Warner JT, Marland A, et al. GH replacement does not increase the risk of recurrence in patients with craniopharyngioma. *Clin Endocrinol (Oxf).* 2006;64:556-560.
1784. Sklar CA, Mertens AC, Mitby P, et al. Risk of disease recurrence and second neoplasms in survivors of childhood cancer treated with growth hormone: a report from the childhood cancer survivor study. *J Clin Endocrinol Metab.* 2002;87:3136-3141.
1785. Ergun-Longmire B, Mertens AC, Mitby P, et al. Growth hormone treatment and risk of second neoplasms in the childhood cancer survivor. *J Clin Endocrinol Metab.* 2006;91:3494-3498.
1786. Jostel A, Mukherjee A, Hulse PA, et al. Adult growth hormone replacement therapy and neuroimaging surveillance in brain tumour survivors. *Clin Endocrinol (Oxf).* 2005;62:698-705.
1787. Darendeliler F, Karagiannis G, Wilton P, et al. On behalf of the KIGS International, Board. Recurrence of brain tumours in patients treated with growth hormone: analysis of KIGS (Pfizer International Growth Database). *Acta Paediatr.* 2006;95:1284-1290.
1788. Weiss M, Sutton L, Marcial V, et al. The role of radiation therapy in the management of childhood craniopharyngioma. *Int J Radiat Oncol Biol Phys.* 1989;17:1313-1321.
1789. Packer RJ, Sutton LN, Elterman R, et al. Outcome for children with medulloblastoma treated with radiation and cisplatin, CCNU, and vincristine chemotherapy. *J Neurosurg.* 1994;81:690-698.
1790. Malozowski S, Tanner LA, Wysowski D, et al. Growth hormone, insulin-like growth factor I, and benign intracranial hypertension. *N Engl J Med.* 1993;329:665-666.
1791. Ranke MB. Effects of growth hormone on the metabolism of lipids and water and their potential in causing adverse events during growth hormone treatment. *Horm Res.* 1993;39:104-106.
1792. Collett-Solberg PF, Liu GT, Satin-Smith M, et al. Pseudopapilledema and congenital disc anomalies in growth hormone deficiency. *J Pediatr Endocrinol Metab.* 1998;11:261-265.
1793. Fillion M, Deal C, Van Vliet G. Retrospective study of the potential benefits and adverse events during growth hormone treatment in children with Prader-Willi syndrome. *J Pediatr.* 2009;154:230-233.
1794. Alford FP, Hew FL, Christopher MC, et al. Insulin sensitivity in growth hormone (GH)-deficient adults and effect of GH replacement therapy. *J Endocrinol Invest.* 1999;22(suppl 5):28-32.
1795. Dabelea D, Bell RA, D'Agostino Jr RB, et al. Writing Group for the SEARCH for Diabetes in Youth Study Group. Incidence of diabetes in youth in the United States. *JAMA.* 2007;297:2716-2724.
1796. Malozowski S, Stadel BV. Prepubertal gynecomastia during growth hormone therapy. *J Pediatr.* 1995;126:659-661.
1797. Malozowski S, Hung W, Scott DC, et al. Acute pancreatitis associated with growth hormone therapy for short stature. *N Engl J Med.* 1995;332:401-402.
1798. Bourguignon JP, Pierard GE, Ernould C, et al. Effects of human growth hormone therapy on melanocytic naevi. *Lancet.* 1993;341:1505-1506.
1799. Pierard GE, Pierard-Franchimont C. Morphometric evaluation of the growth of nevi. *Ann Dermatol Venereol.* 1993;120:605-609.
1800. Bertelloni S, Baroncelli GI, Viacava P, et al. Can growth hormone treatment in boys without growth hormone deficiency impair testicular function? *J Pediatr.* 1999;135:367-370.
1801. Leschek EW, Troendle JF, Yanovski JA, et al. Effect of growth hormone treatment on testicular function, puberty, and adrenarche in boys with non-growth hormone-deficient short stature: a randomized, double-blind, placebo-controlled trial. *J Pediatr.* 2001;138:406-410.
1802. Frasier SD. A red flag unfurled? growth hormone treatment and testicular function. *J Pediatr.* 1999;135:278-279.
1803. Takala J, Ruokonen E, Webster NR, et al. Increased mortality associated with growth hormone treatment in critically ill adults. *N Engl J Med.* 1999;341:785-792.
1804. Chan JM, Stampfer MJ, Giovannucci E, et al. Plasma insulin-like growth factor-I and prostate cancer risk: a prospective study. *Science.* 1998;279:563-556.
1805. Hankinson SE, Willett WC, Colditz GA, et al. Circulating concentrations of insulin-like growth factor-I and risk of breast cancer. *Lancet.* 1998;351:1393-1396.
1806. Ma J, Pollak MN, Giovannucci E, et al. Prospective study of colorectal cancer risk in men and plasma levels of insulin-like growth factor (IGF)-I and IGF-binding protein-3. *J Natl Cancer Inst.* 1999;91:620-625.
1807. Renehan AG, Zwahlen M, Minder C, et al. Insulin-like growth factor (IGF)-I, IGF binding protein-3, and cancer risk: systematic review and meta-regression analysis. *Lancet.* 2004;363:1346-1353.
1808. Wolk A. The growth hormone and insulin-like growth factor I axis, and cancer. *Lancet.* 2004;363:1336-1337.

1809. Ron E, Gridley G, Hrubec Z, et al. Acromegaly and gastrointestinal cancer. *Cancer*. 1991;68:1673-1677.
1810. Popovic V, Damjanovic S, Micic D, et al. Increased incidence of neoplasia in patients with pituitary adenomas: The Pituitary Study Group. *Clin Endocrinol (Oxf)*. 1998;49:441-445.
1811. Bengtsson BA, Eden S, Ernest I, et al. Epidemiology and long-term survival in acromegaly. *Acta Med Scand*. 1998;223:327-335.
1812. Delhougne B, Deneux C, Abs R, et al. The prevalence of colonic polyps in acromegaly: a colonoscopic and pathological study in 103 patients. *J Clin Endocrinol Metab*. 1995;80:3223-3226.
1813. Ladas SD, Thalassinos NC, Ioannides G, et al. Does acromegaly really predispose to an increased prevalence of gastrointestinal tumours? *Clin Endocrinol (Oxf)*. 1994;41:597-601.
1814. Orme SM, McNally RJ, Cartwright RA, et al. Mortality and cancer incidence in acromegaly: a retrospective cohort study. United Kingdom Acromegaly Study Group. *J Clin Endocrinol Metab*. 1998;83:2730-2734.
1815. Sonksen P, Jacobs H, Orme S, et al. Acromegaly and colonic cancer. *Clin Endocrinol (Oxf)*. 1997;47:647-648.
1816. Renehan AG, O'dwyer ST, Shalet SM. Colorectal neoplasia in acromegaly: the reported increased prevalence is overestimated. *Gut*. 2000;46:440-441.
1817. Colao A, Balzano A, Ferone D, et al. Increased prevalence of colonic polyps and altered lymphocyte subset pattern in the colonic lamina propria in acromegaly. *Clin Endocrinol (Oxf)*. 1997;47:23-28.
1818. Sperling MA, Saenger PH, Ray H, et al. LWPES Executive Committee and the LWPES Drug and Therapeutics Committee. Growth hormone treatment and neoplasia: coincidence or consequence? Lawson Wilkins Pediatric Endocrine Society. *J Clin Endocrinol Metab*. 2002;87:5351-5352.
1819. Swerdlow AJ, Higgins CD, Adlard P, et al. Risk of cancer in patients treated with human pituitary growth hormone in the UK, 1959-1985: a cohort study. *Lancet*. 2002;360:273-277.
1820. Tuffli GA, Johanson A, Rundle AC, et al. Lack of increased risk for extracranial, nonleukemic neoplasms in recipients of recombinant deoxyribonucleic acid growth hormone. *J Clin Endocrinol Metab*. 1995;80:1416-1422.
1821. Juul A, Bernasconi S, Carel JC, et al. Growth hormone treatment and risk of solid tumours: a statement from the Drugs and Therapeutics Committee of the European Society for Paediatric Endocrinology (ESPE). *Horm Res*. 2003;60:103-104.
1822. Wetterau L, Cohen P. Role of insulin-like growth factor monitoring in optimizing growth hormone therapy. *J Pediatr Endocrinol Metab*. 2000;13(suppl 6):1371-1376.
1823. Cohen P, Clemmons DR, Rosenfeld RG. Does the GH-IGF axis play a role in cancer pathogenesis? *Growth Horm IGF Res*. 2000; 10:297-305.
1824. Laron Z, Anin S, Klipper-Aurbach Y, et al. Effects of insulin-like growth factor on linear growth, head circumference, and body fat in patients with Laron-type dwarfism. *Lancet*. 1992;339:1258-1261.
1825. Walker JL, Van Wyk JJ, Underwood LE. Stimulation of statural growth by recombinant insulin-like growth factor I in a child with growth hormone insensitivity syndrome (Laron type). *J Pediatr*. 1992;121: 641-646.
1826. Wilton P. Treatment with recombinant human insulin-like growth factor I of children with growth hormone receptor deficiency (Laron syndrome). Kabi Pharmacia Study Group on Insulin-Like Growth Factor I Treatment in Growth Hormone Insensitivity Syndromes. *Acta Paediatr Suppl*. 1992;383:137-142.
1827. Azcona C, Preece MA, Rose SJ, et al. Growth response to rhIGF-I 80 microg/kg twice daily in children with growth hormone insensitivity syndrome: relationship to severity of clinical phenotype. *Clin Endocrinol (Oxf)*. 1999;51:787-792.
1828. Ranke MB, Savage MO, Chatelain PG, et al. Long-term treatment of growth hormone insensitivity syndrome with IGF-I: results of the European multicentre study. The Working Group on Growth Hormone Insensitivity Syndromes. *Horm Res*. 1999;51:128-134.
1829. Backeljauw PF, Underwood LE. Growth Hormone Insensitivity Syndrome Collaborative Group. Therapy for 6.5-7.5 years with recombinant insulin-like growth factor I in children with growth hormone insensitivity syndrome: a Clinical Research Center study. *J Clin Endocrinol Metab*. 2001;86:1504-1510.
1830. Chernausek SD, Backeljauw PF, Frane J, et al. for the GH Insensitivity Syndrome Collaborative Group. Long-term treatment with recombinant insulin-like growth factor (IGF)-I in children with severe IGF-I deficiency due to growth hormone insensitivity. *J Clin Endocrinol Metab*. 2007;92:902-910.
1831. Collett-Solberg PF, Misra M, on behalf of the Drug and Therapeutics Committee of the Lawson Wilkins Pediatric Endocrine Society. The role of recombinant human insulin-like growth factor-I in treating children with short stature. *J Clin Endocrinol Metab*. 2008;93: 10-18.
1832. Woods KA, Camacho-Hubner C, Bergman RN, et al. Effects of insulin-like growth factor I (IGF-I) therapy on body composition and insulin resistance in IGF-I gene deletion. *J Clin Endocrinol Metab*. 2000;85:1407-1411.
1833. Limal J, Parfait B, Cabrol S, et al. Noonan syndrome: relationships between genotype, growth, and growth factors. *J Clin Endocrinol Metab*. 2006;91:300-306.
1834. Clark RG. Recombinant insulin-like growth factor-1 as a therapy for IGF-1 deficiency in renal failure. *Pediatr Nephrol*. 2005;20:290-294.
1835. Kuzuya H, Matsuura N, Sakamoto M, et al. Trial of insulinlike growth factor I therapy for patients with extreme insulin resistance syndromes. *Diabetes*. 1993;42:696-705.
1836. Conchillo M, de Knegt RJ, Payeras M, et al. Insulin-like growth factor I (IGF-I) replacement therapy increases albumin concentration in liver cirrhosis: results of a pilot randomized controlled clinical trial. *J Hepatol*. 2005;43:630-636.
1837. Saatman KE, Contreras PC, Smith DH, et al. Insulin-like growth factor-1 (IGF-1) improves both neurological motor and cognitive outcome following experimental brain injury. *Exp Neurol*. 1997; 147:418-427.
1838. Carroll PV, Jackson NC, Russell-Jones DL, et al. Combined growth hormone/insulin-like growth factor I in addition to glutamine-supplemented TPN results in net protein anabolism in critical illness. *Am J Physiol Endocrinol Metab*. 2004;286:E151-E157.
1839. Guevara-Aguirre J, Vasconez O, Martinez V, et al. A randomized, double blind, placebo-controlled trial on safety and efficacy of recombinant human insulin-like growth factor-I in children with growth hormone receptor deficiency. *J Clin Endocrinol Metab*. 1995;80: 1393-1398.
1840. Guevara-Aguirre J, Guevara-Aguirre M, Rosenbloom AL. Absence of hypoglycemia in response to varying doses of recombinant human insulin-like growth factor-I (rhIGF-I) in children and adolescents with low serum concentrations of IGF-I. *Acta Paediatr*. 2006;95:199-202.
1841. Laron Z, Ginsberg S, Lilos P, et al. Long-term IGF-I treatment of children with Laron syndrome increases adiposity. *Growth Horm IGF Res*. 2006;16:61-64.
1842. Vasconez O, Martinez V, Martinez AL, et al. Heart rate increases in patients with growth hormone receptor deficiency treated with insulin-like growth factor I. *Acta Paediatr Suppl*. 1994;399:137-139.
1843. Perry JK, Emerald BS, Mertani HC, et al. The oncogenic potential of growth hormone. *Growth Horm IGF Res*. 2006;16:277-289.
1844. Samani AA, Yakar S, LeRoith D, et al. The role of the IGF system in cancer growth and metastasis: overview and recent insights. *Endocr Rev*. 2007;28:20-47.
1845. Bright GM, Mendoza JR, Rosenfeld RG. Recombinant human insulin-like growth factor-1 treatment: ready for primetime. *Endocrinol Metab Clin North Am*. 2009;38:625-638.
1846. Rosenbloom AL. The role of recombinant insulin-like growth factor I in the treatment of the short child. *Curr Opin Pediatr*. 2007;19:458-464.
1847. Lazar L, Padoa A, Phillip M. Growth pattern and final height after cessation of gonadotropin-suppressive therapy in girls with central sexual precocity. *J Clin Endocrinol Metab*. 2007;92:3483-3489.
1848. Arrigo T, Cisternino M, Galluzzi F, et al. Analysis of the factors affecting auxological response to GnRH agonist treatment and final height outcome in girls with idiopathic central precocious puberty. *Eur J Endocrinol*. 1999;141:140-144.
1849. Klein KO, Barnes KM, Jones JV, et al. Increased final height in precocious puberty after long-term treatment with LHRH agonists: the National Institutes of Health experience. *J Clin Endocrinol Metab*. 2001;86:4711-4716.
1850. Carel JC, Lahlou N, Roger M, et al. Precocious puberty and statural growth. *Hum Reprod Update*. 2004;10:135-147.
1851. Pasquino AM, Pucarelli I, Accardo F, et al. Long-term observation of 87 girls with idiopathic central precocious puberty treated with gonadotropin-releasing hormone analogs: impact on adult height, body mass index, bone mineral content, and reproductive function. *J Clin Endocrinol Metab*. 2008;93:190-195.
1852. Mul D, Oostdijk W, Otten BJ, et al. Final height after gonadotrophin releasing hormone agonist treatment for central precocious puberty: the Dutch experience. *J Pediatr Endocrinol Metab*. 2000;13(suppl 1):765-772.
1853. Cassio A, Cacciari E, Balsamo A, et al. Randomised trial of LHRH analogue treatment on final height in girls with onset of puberty aged 7.5-8.5 years. *Arch Dis Child*. 1999;81:329-332.
1854. Antoniazzi F, Cisternino M, Nizzoli G, et al. Final height in girls with central precocious puberty: comparison of two different luteinizing hormone-releasing hormone agonist treatments. *Acta Paediatr*. 1994;83:1052-1056.
1855. Carel JC, Hay F, Coutant R, et al. Gonadotropin-releasing hormone agonist treatment of girls with constitutional short stature and normal pubertal development. *J Clin Endocrinol Metab*. 1996;81: 3318-3322.
1856. Bouvattier C, Coste J, Rodrigue D, et al. Lack of effect of GnRH agonists on final height in girls with advanced puberty: a randomized long-term pilot study. *J Clin Endocrinol Metab*. 1999;84:3575-3578.

1857. Lanes R, Soros A, Jakubowicz S. Accelerated versus slowly progressive forms of puberty in girls with precocious and early puberty: gonadotropin suppressive effect and final height obtained with two different analogs. *J Pediatr Endocrinol Metab.* 2004;17:759-766.
1858. Tuvemo T. Treatment of central precocious puberty. *Expert Opin Investig Drugs.* 2006;15:495-505.
1859. Lazar L, Pertzelan A, Weintrob N, et al. Sexual precocity in boys: accelerated versus slowly progressive puberty gonadotropin-suppressive therapy and final height. *J Clin Endocrinol Metab.* 2001;86:4127-4132.
1860. Carel JC. Management of short stature with GnRH agonist and co-treatment with growth hormone: a controversial issue. *Mol Cell Endocrinol.* 2006;254-255, 226-233.
1861. Pasquino AM, Pucarelli I, Roggini M, et al. Adult height in short normal girls treated with gonadotropin-releasing hormone analogs and growth hormone. *J Clin Endocrinol Metab.* 2000;85:619-622.
1862. Tuvemo T, Jonsson B, Gustafsson J, et al. Final height after combined growth hormone and GnRH analogue treatment in adopted girls with early puberty. *Acta Paediatr.* 2004;93:1456-1462.
1863. Mul D, Oostdijk W, Waelkens JJ, et al. Final height after treatment of early puberty in short adopted girls with gonadotrophin releasing hormone agonist with or without growth hormone. *Clin Endocrinol (Oxf).* 2005;63:185-190.
1864. Carel JC, Eugster EA, Rogol A, et al. ESPE-LWPES GnRH Analogs Consensus Conference Group. Consensus statement on the use of gonadotropin-releasing hormone analogs in children. *Pediatrics.* 2009;123:e752-e762.
1865. Rosenfield RL. Clinical review: identifying children at risk for polycystic ovary syndrome. *J Clin Endocrinol Metab.* 2007;92:787-796.
1866. Carel JC, Ecosse E, Nicolino M, et al. Adult height after long term treatment with recombinant growth hormone for idiopathic isolated growth hormone deficiency: observational follow up study of the French population based registry. *BMJ.* 2002;325:70.
1867. Reiter EO, Lindberg A, Ranke MB, et al. The KIGS experience with the addition of gonadotropin-releasing hormone agonists to growth hormone (GH) treatment of children with idiopathic GH deficiency. *Horm Res.* 2003;60(suppl 1):68-73.
1868. Mul D, Wit JM, Oostdijk W, et al. Dutch Advisory Group on Growth Hormone. The effect of pubertal delay by GnRH agonist in GH-deficient children on final height. *J Clin Endocrinol Metab.* 2001;86:4655-4656.
1869. Mericq MV, Eggers M, Avila A, et al. Near final height in pubertal growth hormone (GH)-deficient patients treated with GH alone or in combination with luteinizing hormone-releasing hormone analog: results of a prospective, randomized trial. *J Clin Endocrinol Metab.* 2000;85:569-573.
1870. Saggese G, Federico G, Barsanti S, et al. The effect of administering gonadotropin-releasing hormone agonist with recombinant-human growth hormone (GH) on the final height of girls with isolated GH deficiency: results from a controlled study. *J Clin Endocrinol Metab.* 2001;86:1900-1904.
1871. Tanaka T, Satoh M, Yasunaga T, et al. When and how to combine growth hormone with a luteinizing hormone-releasing hormone analogue. *Acta Paediatr Suppl.* 1999;88:85-88.
1872. Mericq V, Gajardo H, Eggers M, et al. Effects of treatment with GH alone or in combination with LHRH analog on bone mineral density in pubertal GH-deficient patients. *J Clin Endocrinol Metab.* 2002;87:84-89.
1873. Laue L, Jones J, Barnes KM, et al. Treatment of familial male precocious puberty with spironolactone, testolactone, and deslorelin. *J Clin Endocrinol Metab.* 1993;76:151-155.
1874. Laue L, Kenigsberg D, Pescovitz OH, et al. Treatment of familial male precocious puberty with spironolactone and testolactone. *N Engl J Med.* 1989;320:496-502.
1875. Leschek EW, Jones J, Barnes KM, et al. Six-year results of spironolactone and testolactone treatment of familial male-limited precocious puberty with addition of deslorelin after central puberty onset. *J Clin Endocrinol Metab.* 1999;84:175-178.
1876. Kreher NC, Pescovitz OH, Delameter P, et al. Treatment of familial male-limited precocious puberty with bicalutamide and anastrozole. *J Pediatr.* 2006;149:416-420.
1877. Feuillan PP, Jones J, Cutler Jr GB. Long-term testolactone therapy for precocious puberty in girls with the McCune-Albright syndrome. *J Clin Endocrinol Metab.* 1993;77:647-651.
1878. Nunez SB, Calis K, Cutler Jr GB, et al. Lack of efficacy of fadrozole in treating precocious puberty in girls with the McCune-Albright syndrome. *J Clin Endocrinol Metab.* 2003;88:5730-5733.
1879. Feuillan P, Calis K, Hill S, et al. Letrozole treatment of precocious puberty in girls with the McCune-Albright syndrome: a pilot study. *J Clin Endocrinol Metab.* 2007;92:2100-2106.
1880. Laue L, Merke DP, Jones JV, et al. A preliminary study of flutamide, testolactone, and reduced hydrocortisone dose in the treatment of congenital adrenal hyperplasia. *J Clin Endocrinol Metab.* 1996;81:3535-3539.
1881. Merke DP, Keil MF, Jones JV, et al. Flutamide, testolactone, and reduced hydrocortisone dose maintain normal growth velocity and bone maturation despite elevated androgen levels in children with congenital adrenal hyperplasia. *J Clin Endocrinol Metab.* 2000;85:1114-1120.
1882. Hero M, Norjavaara E, Dunkel L. Inhibition of estrogen biosynthesis with a potent aromatase inhibitor increases predicted adult height in boys with idiopathic short stature: a randomized controlled trial. *J Clin Endocrinol Metab.* 2005;90:6396-6402.
1883. Mauras N, Welch S, Rini A, et al. An open label 12-month pilot trial on the effects of the aromatase inhibitor anastrozole in growth hormone (GH)-treated GH deficient adolescent boys. *J Pediatr Endocrinol Metab.* 2004;17:1597-1606.
1884. Hero M, Makitie O, Kroger H, et al. Impact of aromatase inhibitor therapy on bone turnover, cortical bone growth and vertebral morphology in pre- and peripubertal boys with idiopathic short stature. *Horm Res.* 2009;71:290-297.
1885. Hero M, Ankarberg-Lindgren C, Taskinen M, et al. Blockade of oestrogen biosynthesis in peripubertal boys: effects on lipid metabolism, insulin sensitivity, and body composition. *Eur J Endocrinol.* 2006;155:453-460.
1886. Mauras N, Bell J, Snow BG, et al. Sperm analysis in growth hormone-deficient adolescents previously treated with an aromatase inhibitor: comparison with normal controls. *Fertil Steril.* 2005;84:239-242.
1887. Ferrandez Longas A, Mayayo E, Valle A, et al. Constitutional delay in growth and puberty: a comparison of final height achieved between treated and untreated children. *J Pediatr Endocrinol Metab.* 1996;9(suppl 3):345-357.
1888. Joss E, Zuppinger K. Oxandrolone in girls with Turner's syndrome: a pair-matched controlled study up to final height. *Acta Paediatr Scand.* 1984;73:674-679.
1889. Crock P, Werther GA, Wettenhall HN. Oxandrolone increases final height in Turner syndrome. *J Paediatr Child Health.* 1990;26:221-224.
1890. Sybert VP. Adult height in Turner syndrome with and without androgen therapy. *J Pediatr.* 1984;104:365-369.
1891. Hepatic effects of 17 alpha-alkylated anaboli-androgenic steroids. *HIV Hotline.* 1998;8:2-5.
1892. Salerno M, Di Maio S, Gasparini N, et al. Liver abnormalities in Turner syndrome. *Eur J Pediatr.* 1999;158:618-623.
1893. Dickerman Z, Loewinger J, Laron Z. The pattern of growth in children with constitutional tall stature from birth to age 9 years: a longitudinal study. *Acta Paediatr Scand.* 1984;73:530-536.
1894. Ignatius A, Lenko HL, Perheentupa J. Oestrogen treatment of tall girls: effect decreases with age. *Acta Paediatr Scand.* 1991;80:712-717.
1895. de Waal WJ, Greyn-Fokker MH, Stijnen T, et al. Accuracy of final height prediction and effect of growth-reductive therapy in 362 constitutionally tall children. *J Clin Endocrinol Metab.* 1996;81:1206-1216.
1896. Bierich JR. Estrogen treatment of girls with constitutional tall stature. *Pediatrics.* 1978;62(6 Pt 2):1196-1201.
1897. Sorgo W, Scholler K, Heinze F, et al. Critical analysis of height reduction in oestrogen-treated tall girls. *Eur J Pediatr.* 1984;142:260-265.
1898. Trygstad O. Oestrogen treatment of adolescent tall girls: short term side effects. *Acta Endocrinol Suppl (Copenh).* 1986;279:170-173.

CHAPTER 25

Puberty: Ontogeny, Neuroendocrinology, Physiology, and Disorders

DENNIS M. STYNE • MELVIN M. GRUMBACH

Puberty is not a de novo event but rather a phase in the continuum of development of gonadal function and the ontogeny of the hypothalamic-pituitary-gonadal system from the fetus to full sexual maturation and fertility. During puberty, secondary sexual characteristics appear, and the adolescent growth spurt occurs, resulting in the striking sex dimorphism of mature individuals; fertility is achieved, and profound psychological effects ensue.[1] These changes result from stimulation of the gonads by pituitary gonadotropins and a subsequent increase in gonadal steroid output.

Humans are the most reproductively successful of mammals, and many anthropologists have attributed this success to the prolonged pattern of human growth and development[2] and to the delay in attaining full sexual maturity. The human scheme of growth involves a childhood stage and an adolescent stage that includes an adolescent or pubertal growth spurt (Fig. 25-1). Not even our closest biologic relative, the chimpanzee, which matures twice as rapidly as the human, unequivocally exhibits these two stages, including the unique human adolescent growth spurt. Learning and practice of adult behaviors related to sex and childrearing, particularly provisioning children (not just infants) with food,[3] which is unique to humans,[4] is considered a critical part of human success. Tool making preceded the evolutionary development of adolescence, suggesting that the evolution and value of human childhood and adolescence and this unique pattern of growth and development have had significant roles in the reproductive success of humans.[3,5]

In the developed world, reproductive maturity occurs years earlier than psychosocial maturation, causing a mismatch between biologic stages and psychosocial expectations and roles (Fig. 25-2).[6] In past eras, such as the Neolithic, Greek, or Roman periods, there was not such a mismatch, because menarche occurred at an age similar to today (9 to 14 years), and psychosocial maturation in a simpler world occurred at an age close to that of reproductive maturity. With increased population, the advent of

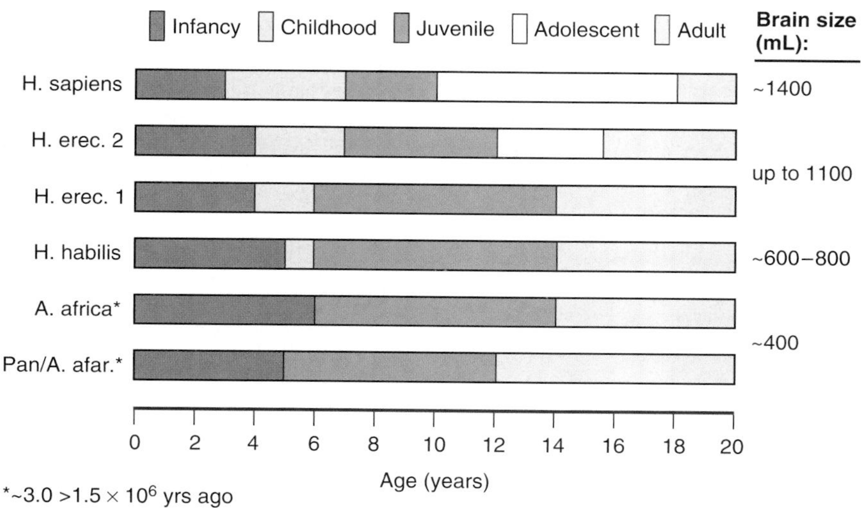

Figure 25-1 Evolution of the human pattern of postnatal growth and development during the first 20 years of life. Specimens include A. afar, *Australopithecus afarensis*, a "bipedal chimpanzee"; A. africa, *Australopithecus africanus;* H. habilis, *Homo habilis,* the toolmaker; H. erec 1, early *Homo erectus;* H. erec 2, late *Homo erectus; H. sapiens, Homo sapiens*. The early hominid australopithecine specimens from South Africa date to about 3.0 to 1.5 million years ago. *H. afarensis*, although a hominid (family of all human species), retained many anatomic features of nonhominid species, such as an adult brain size of about 400 mL compared with *H. habilis* (650 to 800 mL), early *H. erectus* (850 to 900 mL), late *H. erectus* (up to 1100 mL), and modern *H. sapiens* (about 1400 mL). Infancy is the period when the mother's breast milk is the sole or most important source of nutrition, and in preindustrialized societies, it ends at about 36 months. Childhood is the period after weaning, when the child depends on others for food and protection; this period ends when the growth of the brain in weight is almost complete, at about age 7 years. The juvenile stage is defined as prepubertal individuals who are no longer dependent on their parents for survival. The adolescent stage, which begins with the onset of puberty, ends when adult height is attained.[2,5] The pattern in *A. afarensis* is no different from that of the chimpanzee *(Pan troglodytes)*. Notice the first appearance of the childhood stage in *H. habilis* (arising about 2 million years ago) and the first appearance of the adolescent stage in *H. erectus* 2 (about 500,000 years ago); *H. sapiens* arose about 120,000 to 150,000 years ago. (Modified from Bogin B. Growth and development: recent evolutionary and biocultural research. In: Boaz NT, Wolfe LD, eds. *Biological Anthropology: The State of the Science*. Bend, OR: International Institute for Human Evolutionary Research, 1995:49-70.)

agriculture, and the growth of cities and later urban centers, menarche occurred later, and the complexity of life led to a delay in the attainment of an adult role in society. In modern times, the age of menarche has decreased, but the age of social adulthood still occurs later, causing a discrepancy that probably has not occurred previously in human history.

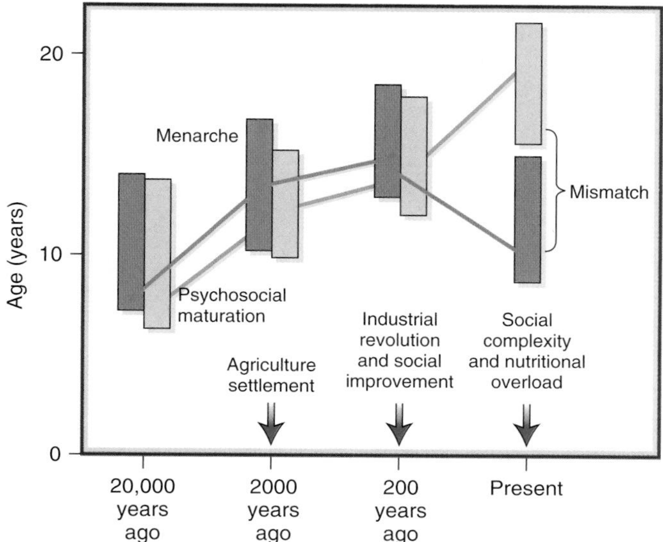

Figure 25-2 The relationship between the likely range of ages of menarche *(green)* and achievement of psychosocial maturity *(pink)* from 20,000 years ago to the current day. The mismatch in timing between these two processes is a novel phenomenon. (From Gluckman PD, Hanson MA. Evolution, development, and timing of puberty. *Trends Endocrinol Metab.* 2006;17:7-12.)

FETAL ORIGINS OF ADULT DISEASE

There are long-lasting effects of abnormalities in fetal and neonatal growth. As seen in longitudinal studies, low birth weight followed by rapid weight gain in infancy (i.e., catch-up growth) leads to tall childhood stature and early pubertal development. Poor prenatal nutrition and small-for-gestational-age (SGA) status tends to advance the age of menarche[7] and the age of adrenarche,[8] and a secondary effect of increased postnatal nutrition, often leading to overweight or obesity, also lowers the age of puberty. Figure 25-3 describes the relationship between excessive adipose tissue and early puberty. A prospective study demonstrated that a lower expected birth weight ratio (i.e., ratio of observed infant's birth weight to median birth weight appropriate for maternal age, weight, height, parity, infant sex, and gestational age) and a higher body mass index (BMI) at 8 years led to an earlier age of menarche.[9] Girls who are longer and lighter at birth and subsequently have greater BMI values at 8 years tend to have earlier menarche.[10] Rapid weight gain in the second to ninth months but not thereafter correlated with a greater BMI at 10 years and with earlier menarche in a longitudinal study.[11]

Many international studies find a relationship between low birth weight or catch-up growth and chronic diseases in adulthood. Birth weight and rate of postnatal growth—not prematurity alone—are inversely related to cardiovascular mortality and prevalence of insulin resistance syndrome (i.e., metabolic syndrome or syndrome X), which consists of hypertension, impaired glucose tolerance, and elevated triglyceride levels, among a growing list of other features. This outcome is attributed to fetal and neonatal *metabolic programming,* in which early adjustments to

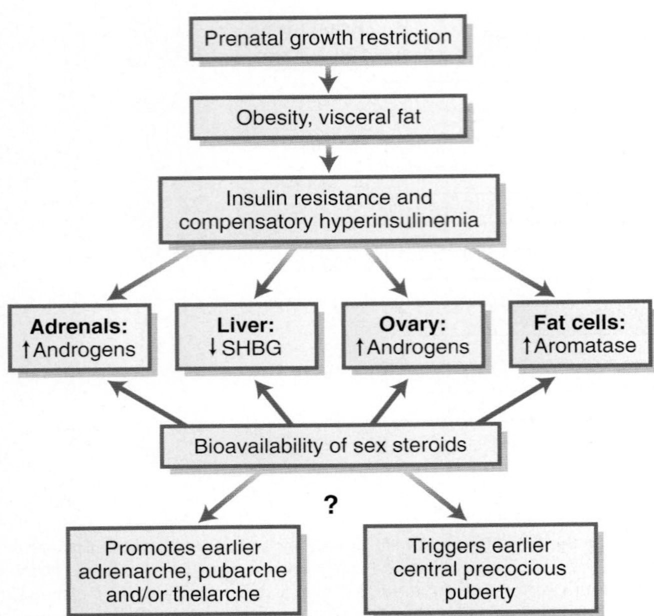

Figure 25-3 Proposed endocrine pathways linking childhood obesity and insulin resistance to early pubertal onset and maturation. Childhood obesity and the predisposition to visceral adiposity after intrauterine growth restraint lead to insulin resistance and peripheral hyperinsulinemia. Insulin acts on various organs, including the adrenals, liver, ovary, and fat cells, to increase sex steroid bioavailability. Elevated circulating and tissue sex steroid levels in obese prepubertal children can have only mild local effects or activate early hypothalamic-pituitary puberty and early reproductive maturation. (From Ahmed ML, Ong KK, Dunger DB. Childhood obesity and the timing of puberty. *Trends Endocrinol Metab.* 2009;20:237-242.)

enhance survival in difficult intrauterine circumstances set the stage for later disorders. Insulin resistance, which may be the basis for most of these complications or may be just one feature of the syndrome, may spare nutrients from use in muscle, leaving them available for the brain. This mechanism can minimize central nervous system (CNS) damage in the fetus during periods of malnutrition.

DETERMINANTS OF THE AGE OF PUBERTY AND MENARCHE

Although historical records show that puberty occurs at an earlier age today, most evidence derives from reports of the age of menarche (Table 25-1). Age of menarche is removed by several years from the first sign of secondary development in girls,[12,13] and modern studies demonstrate correlation coefficients of only 0.37 between age of menarche and age of onset of puberty, suggesting both unique and similar factors exerting effects on these ages.[14] Changes in health and socioeconomic status in regions where data were collected during different decades leads to complexity in the interpretation of modern national data.

Recalled age of menarche is considered to be accurate within 1 year (in 90% of cases) up to 30 years after the event. Contemporaneous recordings are performed with the probit method of asking for a response of "Yes" or "No" to the question, "Are you menstruating?" However, the results are subject to social pressures of the culture and socioeconomic group considered.[15]

The Developed World

The average age of menarche in industrialized European countries has decreased by 2 to 3 months per decade over the past 150 years, and in the United States, the decrease has been approximately 2 to 3 months per decade during the past century (Fig. 25-4).[12,16] However, this secular trend has slowed in developed countries such as the United States, Australia, and Western Europe since approximately 1940, presumably due to improved socioeconomic status, better health, and the benefits of urbanization. There is a relatively small range of ages of menarche in the well-off developed world, where lower socioeconomic classes do not have an increased burden of disease or malnutrition. Chronic diseases previously increased the age of menarche, and delay in menarche is still associated with serious conditions (e.g., celiac disease, asthma) that are not adequately treated. The standard deviation of the mean age of menarche also decreased, suggesting a diminished number of those maturing very late, as might be found among disadvantaged people.[17] Teasing out the various factors involved in any remaining, more subtle secular trends will require further long-term study and newer methodologic approaches in areas where nutrition and health are optimal or close to it.[18] Remarkably, a reverse secular trend is reported in certain areas of Europe, leading to a later age of menarche. This has been attributed to a resurgence of physical and psychological stress, as was seen in previous eras (e.g., World War II).[18]

There are cross-sectional and limited longitudinal data from the 20th century demonstrating a secular trend in the United States, including ethnic influences.[19] The age of menarche in the United States was 12.8 years according to the 1973 U.S. National Center for Health Statistics National Health Education Study,[20] and data from the Third National Health and Nutrition Examination Survey (NHANES III, 1988-1994) indicate that the median age at that time was

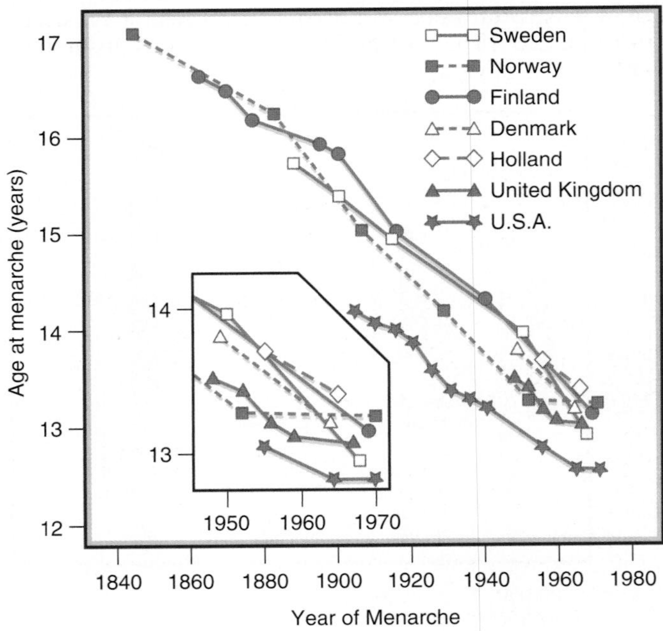

Figure 25-4 The changes in age at menarche between 1840 and 1978 illustrate the advance in the age at menarche in Western Europe and the United States since 1840 and slowing of this trend since about 1965. (Modified from Tanner M, Eveleth PB. Variability between populations in growth and development at puberty. In: Berenberg SR, ed. *Puberty, Biologic and Psychosocial Components.* Leiden, The Netherlands: H.E. Stenfert Kroese, 1975:256-273.)

TABLE 25-1

Comparison of Menarcheal Ages Reported by Various Studies

Study	Year	Plan	Evaluation	*n*	AGE AT MENARCHE (YR) Overall	W	B	M	Comments
Britain	1969	Long	Probit	192 (W)		13.5			
NHES III	1963-1970	Cross	Recalled	3272		Born 1940-1960: 12.8 Born 1890-1910: 13.5	12.52		
NHANES III	1988-1994	Cross	Yes/No Probit	330 (W) 419 (B) 419 (M)		12.7	12.3	12.5	Men. age black < white
NHANES III	1988-1994	Cross	Yes/No Probit	2510 710 (W) 917 (B) 883 (M)	12.43	12.6	12.06	12.3	Men. age black < white
PROS	1992-1993	Cross	Status Quo Probit	17077 (W) 1638 (B)		12.9	12.16		Men. age black < white
NHLB Growth	1987-1997	Long	Recalled	1092 (W) 1164 (B)		12.7	12.1		Men. age black < white BMI inversely proportional to men. age
Bogalusa	1973-1974	Cross		5552		12.7	12.9		
	1992-1994	Cross				12.5	12.1		
	1973-1994	Long		2508		12.6	12.3		Men. age black < white BMI inversely proportional to men. age
NHES	1963-1970	Status Quo	Yes/No Status Quo	3272	12.75	12.8	12.48		
	1988-1994	Status Quo	Median Yes/N	1414	12.54	12.6	12.14		Men. age NHANES III < NHES Growing difference in men. age white-black BMI inversely proportional to men. age

B, black; BMI, body mass index; Cross, cross sectional; Long, longitudinal; M, Mexican American; men., menarcheal; NHANES, National Health and Nutrition Examination Surveys; NHES, National Health Examination Survey; NHLB Growth, National Heart, Lung, and Blood Institute Growth and Health Study; PROS, Pediatric Research in Office Settings; W, white.

From Styne DM. Puberty, obesity and ethnicity. *Trends Endocrinol Metab.* 2004;15:472-478.

12.43 years, 0.37 years earlier than in 1973.[21] During a 20-year period in the Bogalusa Heart Study, the median menarcheal age decreased by approximately 9.5 months among African American girls compared with 2 months among white girls,[22] leading to a 4-month difference. Between the ages of 5 and 9 years, African American girls in the Bogalusa study had taller stature and greater weight, factors that were predictive of menarche before age 11.0 years. African American girls have advanced secondary sexual development compared with white American girls of the same age during the first three stages of puberty,[23] and they have an advanced bone age[24]; this may be related to the higher prevalence of obesity among African American girls and to an ethnic-specific genetic influence.[23,25,26]

Obesity is defined as a BMI (calculated as weight in kilograms divided by height in meters squared) above the 95th percentile for age, and overweight is defined by the Centers for Disease Control and Prevention (CDC) as a BMI greater than the 85th percentile for age. Many studies have reported on the effect of the epidemic of childhood obesity and overweight on age of menarche.[27,28] Most cross-sectional and longitudinal studies[19,25,29] found an inverse relationship between menarcheal age or other stages of puberty and BMI or other reflections of adiposity.[30] If the population in the 1970s had had the same range of BMI values as was found in the 1990s, the projected age of menarche would have been the same in the 1970s as it was in the 1990s.[31] Girls had a greater prevalence of overweight or obesity between the ages of 8 and 10 years if they were in puberty or had advanced breast development.[32] A study of the age at onset of puberty in U.S. boys of various ethnic groups, although controversial because of a lack of physical examination of testicular size, if accurate, indicated a direct relationship between BMI and age at onset of puberty in boys.[33]

International data support the effects of BMI on puberty, but earlier onset of pubertal growth does not lead to a taller adult height.[34] Children in Denmark show no secular trend to earlier pubertal development; there was an effect of increased BMI associated with earlier pubertal development, but this was not sufficient to explain the difference between Danish and U.S. ages at puberty, suggesting genetic or environmental influences.[26]

Longitudinal studies are limited in number but of great importance in the evaluation of a secular trend. The longitudinal National Heart, Lung, and Blood Institute (NHLBI) Growth and Health Study followed 1266 white and 1313 African American girls from 9 or 10 years of age for 10 or more years. The mean age of menarche among whites was 12.7 years, and among African Americans, it was 12.1 years; a direct relationship was found between weight and BMI and the age of menarche.[25] Of these girls, 51.6% started puberty with only one manifestation. Those who experienced breast development first (i.e., thelarche pattern), rather than the appearance of pubic hair (i.e., adrenarche pattern), had an earlier menarche (12.6 versus 13.1 years); this was associated with a greater BMI and body weight, which was not true for those girls manifesting the adrenarche pattern.[35] These findings support the analysis of

NHANES III, in which girls with earlier breast development had greater BMI values at the time of menarche than those with adrenarche occurring first.[36]

African American girls in the National Longitudinal Study of Adolescent Health (Add Health) were 1.55 times more likely than white girls to have menarche before 11 years of age,[37] and Mexican Americans were 1.76 times more likely to do so than whites. Asians were 1.65 more likely than whites to mature later than 14 years. Those undergoing early menarche were twice as likely to be overweight, and African American girls had a 2.57-fold greater risk for overweight if they had menarche before they were 11 years old. Among early-menarcheal African Americans, 57.5% had a BMI greater than the 85th percentile, and 32.5% had a BMI greater than the 95th percentile. A longitudinal study of 180 girls between the ages of 5 and 9 years demonstrated that those with a higher percentage of body fat at 5 years; those with a higher percentage of body fat, higher BMI percentile, or larger waist circumference at 7 years; those with larger increases in the percentage of body fat from 5 to 9 years; and those with larger increases in waist circumference from 7 to 9 years old were more likely to exhibit earlier pubertal development at 9 years.[38]

During the past 40 years, menarcheal age in the white subjects in the Fels Longitudinal Study has remained stable even as BMI has increased, with no relationship shown between the two. Subjects with early menarche had a tendency to increase BMI after menarche,[39] demonstrating that increased weight appears to be a consequence rather than determinant of the age at menarche and that secular changes in BMI and in mean age at menarche may be independent phenomena. There was a rise in BMI, waist circumference, hip circumference, and serum levels of luteinizing hormone (LH), androstenedione, testosterone, and dehydroepiandrosterone sulfate (DHEAS) during the years immediately after menarche in a shorter longitudinal study.[40]

The composition of diet and the amount of calories in the diet may relate to menarche. The prospective, longitudinal Harvard Longitudinal Studies of Childhood Health and Development found that girls had earlier menarche if they were taller and consumed more animal protein and less vegetable protein as early as 3 to 5 years old and that they had earlier peak growth velocity if they had higher dietary fat intake at 1 to 2 years old and higher animal protein intake at 6 to 8 years. Peak height velocity (PHV) increased, controlling for body size, if more calories and animal protein were consumed 2 years before peak growth.[41] A positive relationship between high fiber intake and age of menarche[42] held true in a comparison of 46 countries. On the other hand, lifelong vegetarian dietary intake does not affect the age of menarche,[43] and a low-fat diet in otherwise healthy, prepubertal, 8- to 10-year-old children with elevated low-density lipoprotein (LDL) cholesterol produced no difference in age of menarche or pubertal progression.[44] Phytoestrogen intake delays breast development, particularly in girls with lower BMI values.[45]

The Developing World

The interaction of socioeconomic conditions, nutrition, energy expenditure, states of health, and puberty is of particular importance in areas of the world where nutrition is suboptimal; where the most rapid improvement is found, such as in Oaxaca, Greenland, or South Korea, the age of menarche decreases more rapidly.[46] Where standards of living do not change, neither does the age of menarche. In South America and Africa, some rural children fare better and have earlier puberty and taller stature than urban children, demonstrating a trend of adverse health and nutritional conditions in crowded urban centers. Malnourished individuals have later age of menarche across the world.[47]

As a whole, these reports indicate that populations existing in the most difficult conditions who experience improvement in socioeconomic status demonstrate a greater decrease in the age of menarche. Once a minimum nutritional status or state of health is reached, the effects of socioeconomic status on the age of menarche are minimized or eliminated, but increased BMI can lower the age of menarche further.

Stress and Puberty

Theories aiming to explain influences on the age of puberty address energetics, stress suppression, psychosocial acceleration, paternal investment, and child development, each of which may have various effects on the timing and progression of pubertal development.[47] Evolution optimizes allocation of limited resources to maximize fitness and allow reproductive success.[48]

Stress is variably reported to increase or decrease the age of menarche, depending on the study. The absence of a father or lower parental education increases the likelihood of early menarche and of acceleration of puberty in boys.[49] The question arises of whether psychological stress decreases the age of menarche or stress arises from earlier menarche. War increases the age of voice breaking in boys (e.g., in Bach's choir during the War of Austrian Succession in 1727-1749), and the age of menarche increased during World War II and during more recent hostilities in the former Yugoslavia; poor nutrition, rather than stress, may be a factor in such times.[47,50] Sexual abuse is associated with earlier onset of puberty and earlier menarche compared with a control population.[51,52] In contrast, the age of menarche from the California Childhood Health and Development Study confirmed the mother-daughter association on age of menarche but found no influence of family stress in early life on early menarche.[53]

Short alleles of the GGC-repeat polymorphism of the androgen receptor gene *(AR)* are associated with aggression and impulsivity, increased number of sexual partners, sexual compulsivity, and lifetime number of sex partners of males and with paternal divorce, father absence, and early age of menarche in females.[54] This implies a genetic basis to the relationship between absence of father and early puberty in girls, because this allele can be transferred from the absent father to the daughter who develops early menarche. Other studies have found no relationship between the GGC-repeat polymorphism and aberrant fathering behavior to explain the relationships among adverse early experiences, early menarche, and early sexual activity.[52]

Genetic Effects on Puberty and Menarche

There remains a difference in age at attainment of stages of puberty in different countries even with stability in socioeconomic factors; for example, Japanese boys undergo changes in testicular size about 1 year earlier than Swiss boys do.[55] When socioeconomic and environmental factors lead to good nutrition, general health, and infant care, the age at onset of puberty in normal children appears to be determined largely by genetic factors.

The important role played by genetic factors in the onset of puberty is illustrated by the similar age of menarche in members of an ethnic population and in mother-daughter and sibling or twin pairs.[56-58] The correlation between mother and daughter patterns should theoretically be equal to sister-sister age at menarche if only genetic factors are operative, but because sister-sister correlations are higher than mother-daughter correlations, environmental influences must provide an additional influence beyond genetic factors.[59]

Concordance of ages of pubertal developmental stages and menarche is closer between monozygotic than dizygotic twins, supporting the influence of genetic factors. Monozygotic twins reared together have more similar ages of menarche than those reared apart, and dizygotic twins reared together are less similar than either of the monozygotic groups, pointing to environmental influences on genetic factors. Some twin research suggests that additive genetic factors account for 96% of the variance in the age of puberty in girls and 88% of the variance in boys (although other sources from the United States, Australia, Great Britain, Finland, and Norway have found genetic effects accounting for between 50% and 80% of the variance), with the remainder resulting from shared and nonshared environmental influences.[47,60-62]

Investigations of genes related to the timing of puberty reveal variable results. Gonadotropin-releasing hormone type I (GnRH-I) and its receptor (GnRHR) are only modestly related to the age of menarche.[63] The LEP1875 and XbaI and PvuII polymorphisms of the estrogen receptor α (ERα) gene (*ESR1*) and maternal age at birth (i.e., >30 or <30 years) were associated with age of menarche.[64,65] High-activity *CYP17* alleles involved in estrogen formation and high-activity *CYP1A2* and *CYP1B1* alleles, whose gene products metabolize estradiol, are not associated with pubertal stage, whereas the high activity *CYP3A4** 1B/1B girls had an earlier age of onset of normal puberty alleles.[66] Girls with longer (>8) TAAAA repeats in their sex hormone–binding globulin gene *(SHBG)* have a later age of menarche than those with fewer repeats.[67] A joint analysis of genome-wide association studies enrolling a total of 17,438 women revealed 10 associated single-nucleotide polymorphisms (SNPs) ($P = 1 \times 10^{-7}$ to 3×10^{-13}) for age of menarche; these were clustered at 6q21 (in or near the gene *LIN28B*) and at 9q31.2 (in an intergenic region).[68] Study of 15,297 Icelandic women demonstrated a significant association between rs314280[T] on 6q21, near the *LIN28B* gene, and age of menarche (1.2 months later per allele; $P = 1.8 \times 10^{-14}$); a second SNP within the same linkage disequilibrium (LD) block, rs314277, splits rs314280[T] into two haplotypes with different effects (0.9 months and 1.9 months per allele).[69] A meta-analysis of genome-wide association data for 17,510 women demonstrated the strongest signal related to age of menarche $\times 10^{-9}$, where the nearest genes include *TMEM38B, FKTN, FSD1L, TAL2,* and *ZNF462,* and the next strongest signal near the *LIN28B* gene (rs7759938; $P = 7.0 \times 10^{-9}$), which also influences adult height.[70]

However, in other large studies (e.g., that of Gajdos and colleagues[71]), there was no association of genes with age of menarche. Further study is required to clarify the most important relationships.

Health Effects of Age at Menarche

Many international studies show that earlier age at menarche is associated with a greater risk of development of breast cancer.[72] Menarche at less than 12 years increases the risk by about 50% compared with menarche at 16 years[73]; the risk of premenopausal breast cancer decreases 9% per year of delay in menarche, and the risk for postmenopausal breast cancer decreases 4%.[74] In disease-discordant monozygotic twins, the one with cancer recalled puberty to be earlier, and in disease-concordant twins, the one with earlier menarche had the earlier diagnosis of breast cancer.[75] Women with breast cancer were taller and leaner in childhood and had increased height velocity at age 4 to 7 years and age 11 to 15 years; higher BMI increased this risk. These variables were particularly significant in women with early menarche (at age < 12.5 years),[76] but some studies confirmed the role of childhood growth but not an effect of age of menarche.[77,78] Increased birth weight raises the risk of breast cancer, with no relationship to age of menarche in some studies.[78,79]

There is indirect evidence relating earlier menarche to increasing likelihood of hepatocellular carcinoma.[80] On the other hand, later age of menarche (>14 years) is associated with an increased risk of glioma or non-Hodgkin's lymphoma.[81,82]

Evidence from the Fels Longitudinal Study of white females revealed that girls with self-reported menarcheal age of less than 11.9 years (classified as early menarche; 23% of the sample) had adverse cardiovascular risk factors such as elevated blood pressure and glucose intolerance unrelated to body composition.[83]

Miscellaneous Effects

Seasonality of menarche has been observed. In a U.S. cohort of 3000 college students, those born after 1970 had an earlier age of menarche and a more pronounced frequency peak in July. Factors hypothesized to contribute to seasonality of menarche include stress and the photoperiod.[84] In Peru, puberty begins at a later age, and pubertal development lasts longer at high altitudes than at low altitudes even when nutritional status is similar.[85] There is a north-to-south decrease in the age of menarche in Europe[17] that results from environmental factors or genetic influences. Lefthandedness may increase the age of menarche.

SECONDARY SEXUAL CHARACTERISTICS AND PHYSICAL CHANGES OF PUBERTY

Female Development

Two distinct phenomena occur in the female. The development of the breast and its modified apocrine glands is primarily under the control of estrogens secreted by the ovaries (Fig. 25-5); the growth of pubic and axillary hair (Fig. 25-6) is mainly under the influence of androgens secreted by the adrenal cortex and the ovary. Breast cancer develops in rodents exposed to environmental toxins (e.g., endocrine disruptors) that alter normal mammary development, and this same relationship is postulated to occur in girls exposed to endocrine-disrupting chemicals, especially if development occurs early.[86] Aromatase is present in adipose tissue, and estrogen produced in excess adipose tissue may stimulate breast development at an earlier age in obese girls. Peripubertal girls also demonstrated elevated values of androgens, especially just before the onset of puberty and in the early stages, but there is also decreased LH secretion, suggesting that central pubertal development may not be the cause of the physical signs of pubertal development.[87,88]

The five stages of breast development described by Tanner are the most widely used staging mechanism (see Fig. 25-5). Initial breast development may be unilateral for

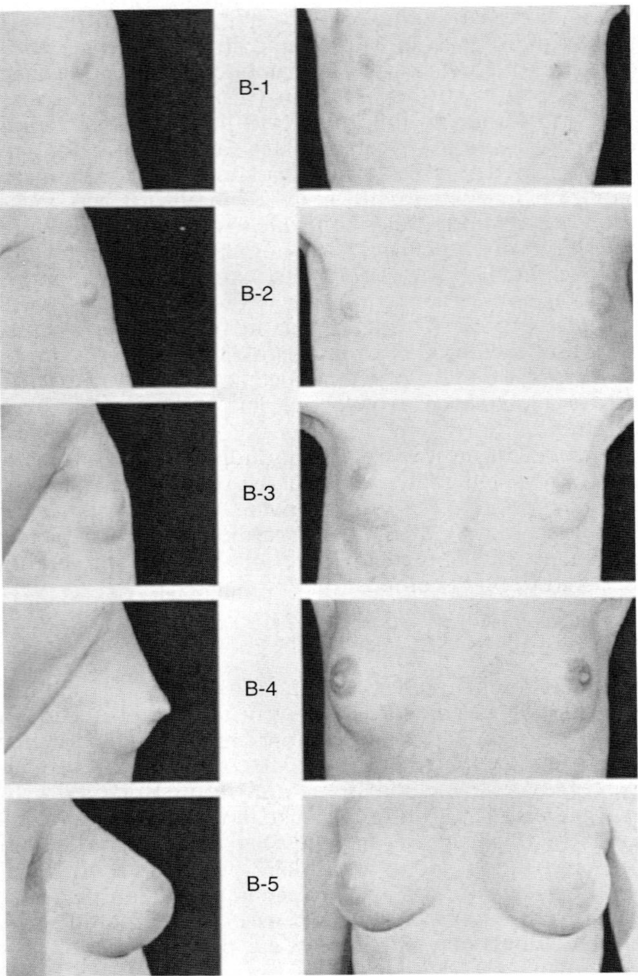

Figure 25-5 Stages of breast development according to Marshall and Tanner.[1076] Stage 1: preadolescent; elevation of papilla only. Stage 2: breast bud stage; elevation of breast and papilla as a small mound, with enlargement of the areolar diameter. Stage 3: further enlargement of the breast and areola, with no separation of their contours. Stage 4: projection of the areola and papilla to form a secondary mound above the level of the breast. Stage 5: mature stage; projection of the papilla only, resulting from recession of the areola to the general contour of the breast. (Photographs from Van Wieringen JD, Wafelbakker F, Verbrugge HP, et al. *Growth Diagrams 1965 Netherlands: Second National Survey on 0-24 Year Olds.* Netherlands Institute for Preventative Medicine TNO. Groningen, The Netherlands: Wolters-Noordhoff, 1971.)

several months, causing unfounded concern by girls or parents. Needless surgical biopsies are carried out for this normal variation, and an ultrasound examination may preempt unfounded concerns about breast cancer. If concern arises about breast cancer during puberty (a rare event), ultrasound evaluation is suggested because of the dense nature of the tissue at this stage. Inherited or sporadic agenesis of the breast allows no glandular or fat enlargement, regardless of the level of estrogen stimulation.[89] Virginal breast hypertrophy, an extreme and rapid increase in breast size at the onset of puberty, is rare but is attributed in part to increased sensitivity to estrogen action or to increased local estrogen synthesis and growth factors.

Changes in the diameter of the papilla of the nipple are sequential and are linked to stages of pubertal development. Nipple papilla diameter (3 to 4 mm) does not increase much during pubic hair stage 1 to 3 or breast stage 1 to 3 but does increase after breast stage 3, providing an objective method of differentiating stage 4 from sage 5 (final diameter, approximately 9 mm).[90] The stage of breast development usually progresses along with the stage of pubic hair development in normal girls, but because different endocrine organs control these two processes, discordance can occur. Therefore, breast and pubic hair developmental stages should be classified separately for greatest accuracy (Table 25-2 and Fig. 25-7). Increase in height velocity (rather than breast development) is usually the first sign of puberty in girls, although breast budding is what most lay or medical observers first notice.

Dulling and thickening of the vaginal mucosa from the prepubertal reddish, glistening appearance occurs as the lining cells cornify and the secretion of clear or whitish discharge increases in the months before menarche as a result of estrogen action. Girls may notice light-colored discharge on their underwear at this stage. The vaginal pH decreases as menarche approaches due to the increase in

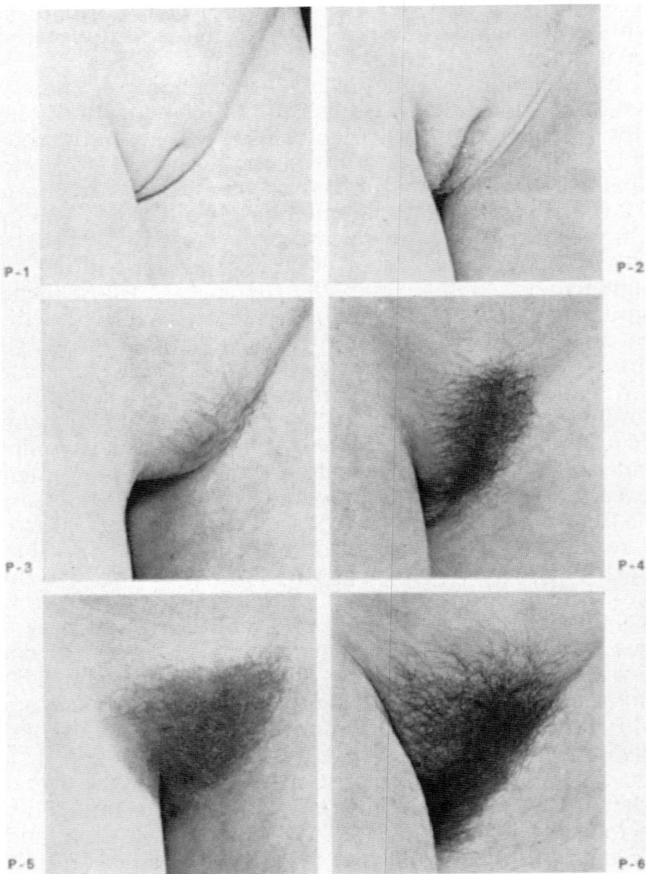

Figure 25-6 Stages of female pubic hair development according to Marshall and Tanner.[1076] Stage 1: preadolescent; the vellus over the pubes is not further developed than that over the anterior abdominal wall; there is no pubic hair. Stage 2: sparse growth of long, slightly pigmented, downy hair that is straight or only slightly curled, appearing chiefly along the labia. This stage is difficult to see on photographs. Stage 3: hair is considerably darker, coarser, and curlier. The hair spreads sparsely over the junction of the pubic region. Stage 4: hair is adult in type, but the area covered by it is still considerably smaller than in most adults. There is no spread to the medial surface of the thighs. Stage 5: hair is adult in quantity and type, distributed as an inverse triangle of the classic feminine pattern. The spread is to the medial surface of the thighs but not up the linea alba or elsewhere above the base of the inverse triangle. (Photographs from Van Wieringen JD, Wafelbakker F, Verbrugge HP, et al. *Growth Diagrams 1965 Netherlands: Second National Survey on 0-24 Year Olds.* Netherlands Institute for Preventative Medicine TNO. Groningen, The Netherlands: Wolters-Noordhoff, 1971.)

TABLE 25-2

Descriptive Statistics for the Timing of Sexual Maturity Stages in Females

BREAST STAGES				
	Onset of Stage		Mean Age for Stage	
Stage	*Mean*	*SD*	*Mean*	*SD*
Stage 2				
Roche et al. (Ohio)	11.2	0.7	11.3	1.1
Herman-Giddens et al. (USA)				
African-American	8.9	1.9		
White	10.0	1.8		
Stage 3				
Roche et al. (Ohio)	12.0	1.0	12.5	1.5
Herman-Giddens et al. (USA)				
African-American	10.2	1.4		
White	11.3	1.4		
Stage 4				
Roche et al. (Ohio)	12.4	0.9		
TANNER PUBIC HAIR				
Tanner Stage 2				
Roche et al. (Ohio)	11.0	0.5		
Herman-Giddens et al. (USA)				
African-American	8.8	2.0		
White	10.5	1.7		
Tanner Stage 3				
Roche et al. (Ohio)	11.8	1.0		
Herman-Giddens et al. (USA)				
African-American	10.4	1.6		
White	11.5	1.2		
Tanner Stage 4				
Roche et al. (Ohio)	12.4	0.8		
MENARCHE				
Herman-Giddes et al. (USA)				
African-American	12.2	1.2		
White	12.9	1.2		
Percent Menstruating	*At Age 11*		*At Age 12*	
African-American	27.9%*		62.1%	
White	13.4%*		35.2%	
Onset of Axillary Hair (Stage 2)				
African-American	10.1 ± 2.0			
White	11.8 ± 1.9			

*African-American girls enter puberty approximately 1 to 1½ years earlier than white girls and begin menses 8½ months earlier.

Mean age for stage 2: 11.3 ± 1.1; mean age for stage 3: 12.5 ± 1.5.

(Data from Roche AF, Weilens R, Attie KM, et al. The timing of sexual maturation in a group of U.S. white youths. *J Pediatr Endocrinol.* 1995;8:11-18; Herman-Giddens ME, Slora EJ, Wasserman RC, et al. Secondary sexual characteristics and menses in young girls seen in office practice: a study from the Pediatric Research in Office Settings network. *Pediatrics.* 1997;99:505-512.)

lactic acid produced by lactobacilli in the vaginal flora. The length of the vagina increases from about 8 cm at onset of puberty to 11 cm at menarche. Thickening, protrusion, and rugation of the labia majora and minora occur. Fat is deposited in the area of the mons pubis, and the appearance of the labia majora becomes wrinkled. Occasionally, the labia minora may enlarge on one or both sides enough to suggest a tumor; childhood asymmetric labium majus enlargement is a disorder of prepuberty or early puberty.[91] The clitoris enlarges slightly, and the urethral opening becomes more prominent. Photographic atlases of normal female prepubertal genitalia are available and include standards for the variation in appearance of the hymenal opening; this information is invaluable in the examination of a victim of suspected child abuse.

Male Development

The growth and maturation of the penis usually correlates closely with pubic hair development, because both features are under androgen control. However, the stages of pubic hair development and genital development should be determined independently, because discordant stages provide clues to potential disease states of the adrenal gland or testes (Figs. 25-8 and 25-9 and Table 25-3).

Growth of the testes is usually the first sign of puberty in the male, and it begins approximately 6 months after the average chronologic age of initiation of breast development in girls (see Fig. 25-4). Pubertal testicular enlargement is indicated when the longitudinal measurement of a testis is greater than 2.5 cm (excluding the epididymis) or the volume is greater than 4 mL. The testicular volume index ([length × width of right testis + length × width of left testis]/2) and testicular volume, measured by comparing the testes with ellipsoids of known volume, correlate with the stages of puberty.[92,93] A longitudinal study supported the utility of adding a stage 2a when testicular volume is 3 mL; further pubertal progression occurred within 6 months in 82% of boys who had reached this 3-mL phase (Table 25-4).[94] The most significant changes in serum testosterone and calculated free testosterone occur at the transitions of testicular volume between 1 and 2 mL, 2 and 3 mL, 6 and 8 mL, and 10 and 15 mL, suggesting the denotation of stages pre-1 (testis, 1 mL), pre-2 (testis, 2 mL), early (testis, 3 to 6 mL), middle (testis, 8 to 12 mL), late-1 (testis, 15 to 25 mL, the boy has not reached final height), and late-2 (testis, 15 to 25 mL, the boy has reached final height).[95] The right testis is normally larger than the left testis, and the left testis is located lower in the scrotum than the right testis.

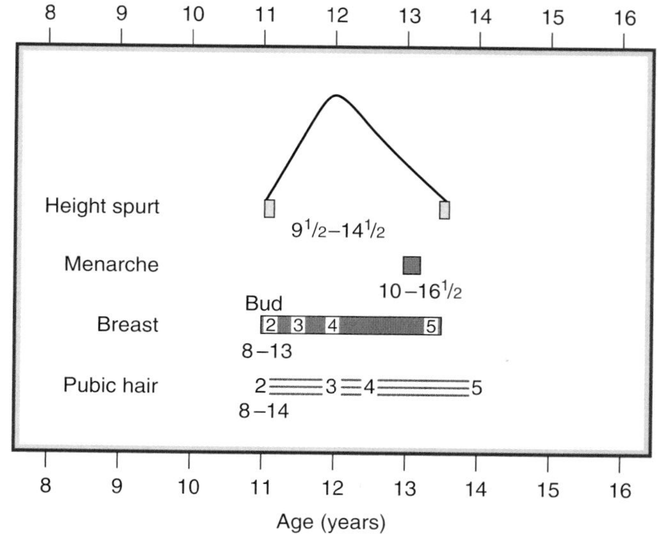

Figure 25-7 The sequence of events at puberty in females. Diagram of the sequence of events at puberty in males. An average is represented in relation to the scale of ages; the range of ages within which some of the changes occur is indicated by the numbers below. The ages are from British girls 40 years in the past, so the sequence of changes, rather than the ages, is the important factor. (From Marshall WA, Tanner JM. Variations in pattern of pubertal changes in girls. *Arch Dis Child.* 1969;44:291-303.)

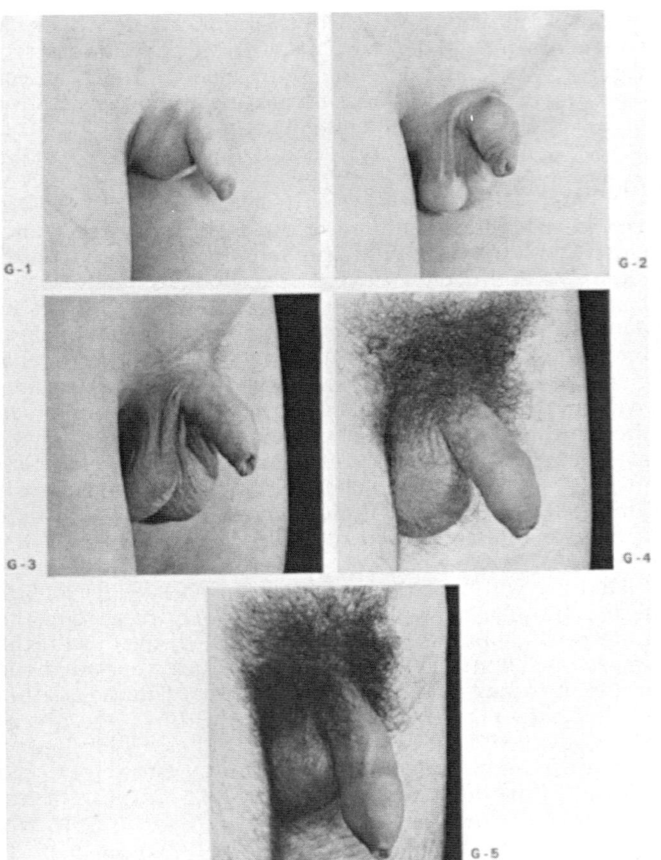

Figure 25-8 Stages of male genital development and pubic hair development according to Marshall and Tanner.[1076] *Genital development:* Stage 1: preadolescent. Testes, scrotum, and penis are about the same size and proportion as in early childhood. Stage 2: the scrotum and testes have enlarged; the scrotal skin shows a change in texture and some reddening. Stage 3: growth of the penis has occurred, at first mainly in length but with some increase in breadth; there is further growth of the testes and scrotum. Stage 4: the penis is further enlarged in length and breadth, along with development of the glans. The testes and scrotum are further enlarged. The scrotal skin has further darkened. Stage 5: genitalia are adult in size and shape. No further enlargement takes place after stage 5 is reached. *Pubic hair development:* Stage 1: preadolescent; the vellus over the pubic region is not further developed than that over the abdominal wall; there is no pubic hair. Stage 2: sparse growth of long, slightly pigmented, downy hair that is straight or slightly curled, appearing chiefly at the base of the penis. Stage 3: hair is considerably darker, coarser, and curlier and spreads sparsely over the junction of the pubes. Stage 4: hair is adult in type, but the area it covers is still considerably smaller than in most adults. There is no spread to the medial surface of the thighs. Stage 5: hair is adult in quantity and type, distributed as an inverse triangle. The spread is to the medial surface of the thighs but not up the linea alba or elsewhere above the base of the inverse triangle. Most men will have further spread of the pubic hair. (Photographs from Van Wieringen JD, Wafelbakker F, Verbrugge HP, et al. *Growth Diagrams 1965 Netherlands: Second National Survey on 0-24 Year Olds.* Netherlands Institute for Preventative Medicine TNO. Groningen, The Netherlands: Wolters-Noordhoff, 1971.)

The phallus should be measured while stretched and in the flaccid state, because there is much variation among individuals in the length of the unstretched penis. The length of the erectile tissue (excluding the foreskin) increases from an average of 6.2 cm in the prepubertal state to 12.4 ±2.7 cm in the white adult. Ethnic differences have been identified; the mean value in African American men is 14.6 cm, and in Asians, it is 10.6 cm.[96]

As in girls, the areolar diameter increases in boys during puberty, with a distinct separation between the sexes

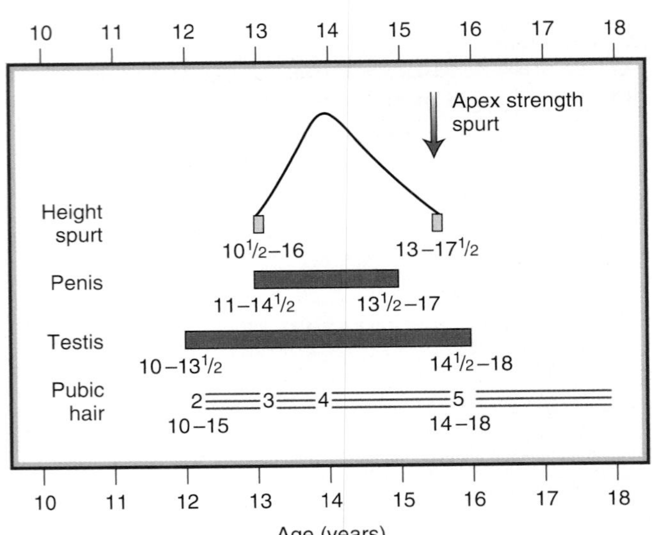

Figure 25-9 Diagram of the sequence of events at puberty in males. An average is represented in relation to the scale of ages, and the range of ages within which some of the changes occur is indicated by the numbers below. The ages are from British boys 40 years in the past, so the sequence of changes, rather than the ages, is the important factor. (From Marshall WA, Tanner JM. Variations in the pattern of pubertal changes in boys. *Arch Dis Child.* 1970;45:13-23.)

occurring in stage 4, when female areolar diameter increases much more than in the male. In gynecomastia, the areolar diameter increases to above-normal values.

Studies of Pubertal Development

National Trends in Pubertal Development

Physical examination with palpation of gonads or breasts by trained observers is the most accurate method of assessment of pubertal development. Detection of the onset of stage 2 breast development in an overweight girl on physical examination may be difficult even for a trained observer (although stage 3 usually is obvious). Visual observation of the stage of development in person (not by photographs)

TABLE 25-3

Descriptive Statistics for the Timing of Sexual Maturity Stages in White Males (Ohio)

	Age at Onset of Stage (Yr)		Age for Stage (Yr)	
Stage	*Mean*	*SD*	*Mean*	*SD*
Genital Stage				
2	11.2	0.7	11.3	1.0
3	12.1	0.8	12.6	1.0
4	13.5	0.7	14.5	1.1
5	14.3	1.1	—	—
Pubic Hair Stages				
2	11.2	0.8	11.3	0.9
3	12.1	1.0	12.4	1.0
4	13.4	0.9	13.7	0.9
5	14.3	0.8	14.8	1.0
6	15.3	0.8	—	—

From Roche AF, Wellens R, Attie KM, et al. The timing of sexual maturation in a group of U.S. white youths. *J Pediatr Endocrinol.* 1995; 8:11-18.

TABLE 25-4

Correlation of Testicular Volume (TV) with Stage of Pubertal Development

Parameter	Pubertal Stage				
	1	*2*	*3*	*4*	*5*
TV Index*					
Burr et al. and August et al.[246,246a]	1.8	4.5	8.2	10.5	—
Volume (cm³)					
Zachmann et al.[93†]	2.5	3.4	9.1	11.8	14
Waaler et al.[‡]	1.8	4.2	10	11	15
Waaler et al.[§]	1.8	5.0	9.5	12.5	17

*TV index calculated as follows: (length × width of right testis + length × width of left testis) ÷ 2.

†Volume estimated by comparison with ellipsoid of known volume (orchidometer) that is equal to or smaller than the testes.

‡Volume by comparison with orchidometer.

§Measurement with calipers and average volume of both testes calculated as follows: 0.52 × longitudinal axis × transverse axis.

is one step removed from physical examination and palpation; errors in the evaluation of breast tissue in obese girls or the stage of testicular enlargement in boys may occur. Visual observation by multiple observers was used in NHANES III (and in the National Health Examination Survey [NHES] that occurred more than 20 years earlier), and visual observation is subject to interobserver variation. In a study by Pediatric Research in the Office Setting (PROS), a network fostered by the American Academy of Pediatrics, specially trained pediatricians, nurse practitioners, or physician assistants (225 offices), used palpation for 30% of the study population and visual inspection for all members of a convenience sample of 17,070 girls across the United States.[97]

The availability of only limited numbers of trained personnel for examination or subjects' refusal of embarrassing examinations sometimes leads to the use of proxy measures. Photographs or drawings of pubertal development allow self-reporting or parental reporting of pubertal progress, but correlations range widely from 0.48 to 0.91 compared with physicians' examinations or visual observation of subjects.[47,98] The answers to self-assessment may be influenced by the subjects' wishes to conform with their understanding of normal development and may be less accurate in some ethnic groups than others, similar to reported menarcheal age. Obese girls may overestimate breast developmental stage, and boys may overestimate pubic hair development. Individuals with learning disabilities, chronic diseases (e.g., cystic fibrosis, Crohn's disease), or psychological conditions (e.g., anorexia nervosa) may have less accurate pubertal staging.[99] Self-report is related to testosterone values for boy and girls and is said to be accurate enough if precision is not needed.[100] With all of its difficulties, physical examination remains the best method to accurately evaluate large populations.

Limits of Normal Pubertal Development

The U.S. Health Examination Survey (HES) enrolled subjects who were 12 years old; although it is useful for defining the upper limits of normal pubertal development, the survey is uninformative about the lower limits of the age at onset of puberty.[20,23,101] A longitudinal study (see Tables 25-2 and 25-3) that enrolled 9.5-year-old white boys and girls added much to the determination of the mean age at attainment of stages of puberty[102]; however, it started too late to include normal children entering puberty at an earlier age. Two studies used data from NHANES III. One[103] found onset of stage 2 breast development for African Americans, Mexican Americans, and whites to occur at 9.5, 9.8, and 10.3 years, respectively, and pubic hair stage 2 to occur at 9.5, 10.3, and 10.5 years, respectively, using a sample of 1623 girls. The other study[104] reported that the ages for onset of stage 2 breast development were 9.5 years for African Americans, 9.8 years for Mexican Americans, and 10.4 years for white Americans, whereas the onset of stage 2 pubic hair occurred at 10.4 years for white Americans, 9.4 years for African Americans, and 10.6 years for Mexican Americans in a sample of 2145 girls.

Because the PROS started at 3 years of age but ended at 12 years of age, it excluded a proportion of normal children who enter puberty at a later age,[97] although the probit statistical method can estimate events even when only a portion of the population has achieved the event. This study was criticized because the subjects were not matched for the many factors considered in a national study such as NHANES. The standard deviation of the longitudinal study described earlier[102] was low, 1.0 years or less in most cases, whereas the cross-sectional study had a larger standard deviation of approximately 2 years.[97] Any study of puberty will demonstrate a limit in the spread of the upper end of the age at onset of puberty curve, because rarely do individuals with the most severe constitutional delay of puberty (CDP) spontaneously enter puberty after 18 years of age. There may be a skewing of the normal age at onset of puberty to an earlier spread of ages.

A study of the age of pubertal stages in children in NHANES revealed that in those with normal BMI values, pubertal signs occurred before 8.0 years of age in fewer than 5% of the non-Hispanic white, female population, although thelarche occurred before age 8.0 in 12% to 19% of normal-BMI, non-Hispanic black and Mexican American girls; the 5th percentile for menarche was 0.8 years earlier for non-Hispanic black than non-Hispanic white subjects.[30] Although the appearance of pubic hair occurred in up to 3% of 8.0-year-old girls with normal BMI values in all ethnicities, it did occur significantly earlier in the minority groups. Girls with the higher BMI values had a significantly higher prevalence of thelarche between the ages of 8.0 and 9.6 years and pubarche from the ages of 8.0 to 10.2 years, compared with girls with normal BMI values. Menarche was significantly more likely to occur in younger girls with elevated BMI values. In boys with normal BMI values, pubic hair appeared in fewer than 2% before 10.0 years. The study authors concluded that pubertal development in girls with normal BMI values before 8 years of age is premature. These data support other analyses of NHANES III, in which the heaviest girls tended to have thelarche before pubarche and the heaviest boys had pubarche before gonadarche.[36]

The latest and largest multiracial and ethnic study of the age at onset of puberty in 2114 American boys between the ages of 8 and 19 years suggested that a decrease has occurred over past decades, but these observations are controversial.[33] Using the NHANES III database, the investigators determined that the onset of pubic hair occurs earlier in African American boys than in white boys, with a tendency to later onset in Mexican American boys. Between the ages of 8 and 9 years, no white boys had pubic hair, whereas 5.3% of African American boys were at least at Tanner stage 2.[33] The age of genital development was based on the visual change in scrotal skin and enlargement of the testes; by the beginning of age 8, the earliest age studied, 29.35% of white boys, 37.8% of African American boys, and 27.3% of Mexican American boys reportedly had genital development. The heights and weights of boys reaching the earlier stages of puberty were greater than reported in the past, although the adult heights and weights were equivalent to the past data. However, several aspects of this study have been questioned.[105] For example, the observers for NHANES III did not physically measure testicular volume, and a one-stage variance was allowed between the observers' findings and the quality control, a variance that is quite significant between stage 1 and 2 of pubertal development in boys because it defines the very onset of puberty. These observations are being further investigated by a PROS project studying pubertal development in boys. If it is confirmed that there is an earlier onset of puberty in a substantial number of boys before the previously accepted lower age limit of 9 years, the guidelines for normal pubertal development in boys will have to be revised downward.

Taking these data as a whole, it seems reasonable to set the lower range of normal puberty at 8 years in girls and 9 years in boys. The influence of BMI must be taken into account. Obese boys characteristically enter puberty early, especially when there is an *MCR4* mutation, but obesity is also associated with delayed puberty.[106] Fröhlich's syndrome (i.e., adiposodysgenesis, originally described in a patient with tuberculosis involving the hypothalamic-pituitary axis), is a constellation of endocrine abnormalities, combining findings of obesity and hypogonadism due to a hypothalamic-pituitary disorder.

The latest comprehensive evaluation of secular changes compared data available from the U.S. HES (3042 white boys, 478 African American boys, 2065 white girls, and 505 African American girls from 1966 to 1970), the Hispanic Health and Nutrition Examination Survey (HHANES: 717 Mexican American boys and 512 Mexican American girls from 1982 to 1984), and NHANES III (259 white boys, 411 African American boys, 291 white girls, 415 African American girls, 576 Mexican American boys, and 512 Mexican American girls from 1988 to 1994).[107] The analysis showed no strong evidence of a secular trend toward earlier puberty between 1966 and 1994 in non-Hispanic black boys and non-Hispanic black and white girls, although there was some evidence of earlier puberty in non-Hispanic white boys between 1966 and 1994 and in Mexican American boys and girls between 1982 and 1994.[104,108]

Spanish investigators demonstrated that the earlier normal girls entered puberty, the longer the duration of puberty before menarche.[109-111] In one of these studies, girls who started puberty at 9, 10, 11, 12, and 13 years of age experienced menarche 2.77, 2.27, 1.78, 1.44, and 0.65 years later, respectively, demonstrating a normalizing trend that keeps the age of menarche relatively stable in the group as a whole.[109] These data may suggest that earlier onset of the first stages of puberty may not exert major effects on the age of menarche. This contrasts with a suggestion of a decrease in the time required to transit puberty from start to end in Dutch and Swedish boys and girls.[17]

In sum, the data show that African American girls develop before white girls, regardless of socioeconomic issues. There is evidence that rising BMI values in childhood are associated with earlier pubertal maturation, which may explain some of the increasing age differences between these ethnic groups. This suggests that an irrefutable decrease in the age at puberty in the overall population of girls may be realized in the future due to the increased BMI percentiles. Environmental disruptors may also play a role. Although there is evidence for earlier menarche, a secular trend toward earlier puberty in girls in the absence of increased BMI cannot be supported from these data because of the different ages studied and lack of comparable studies over past decades.[108,112]

The United States is lacking a comprehensive, large, longitudinal study that would start early enough to include the youngest normal pubertal subjects and last long enough to include the oldest and that would be based on direct physical examination rather than observation. Such a study must be balanced in terms of ethnic groups, and the planners must use the predicted increase of certain ethnic populations in the United States, to avoid the unfortunate position we now have as we look back and try to draw conclusions about secular trends without sufficient data from various ethnic groups.[108]

From all of the longitudinal and some of the cross-sectional data, we may consider the mean age at onset of puberty in boys to be 11 years, with the normal limits being 9 to 14 years.[102] It is possible that some normal boys, especially African American boys, will enter puberty or adrenarche between 8 and 9 years of age.

Guidelines for the normal variation in pubertal development for girls in the United States are controversial. In the cross-sectional, convenience sample study, 3.0% of white girls had stage 2 breast development in their sixth year and 5.0% by the seventh year, whereas 6.4% of African Americans had stage 2 breast development by the sixth year and 15.4% by the seventh year. African American girls have an earlier onset of pubertal development by about 1 year, even though their average age at menarche in the cross-sectional study was only 8.5 months different (12.2 years for African Americans and 12.9 for whites). We may combine these findings and set the normal range for age at puberty in white girls at 7 to 13 years and in African American girls at 6 to 13 years.

These guidelines help the decision of which children with early onset of puberty are candidates for expensive diagnostic tests and for consideration of long-term therapy, because many of those children who appeared to have mild sexual precocity in years past may now be considered to represent normal variation. We emphasize that family history, the rapidity of development of secondary sex characteristics, the rate of growth, and the presence or absence of CNS or other types of disease must enter into the decision to evaluate a child. We recommended these ideas in previous editions of this textbook, and the Drug and Therapeutics and Executive Committees of the Lawson Wilkins Pediatric Endocrine Society support such a revision of the lower limit of the normal age at onset of puberty to age 7 for white girls and age 6 for African American girls, with no changes in the current guidelines for evaluating boys, which target those with signs of puberty developing before 9 years of age.[113]

Several studies indicate the likelihood of missing serious endocrine disorders if the new guidelines are followed.[114-116] With all of these studies, it may be inferred that if the examining physician looks for signs and symptoms of disease rather than just relying on the age criteria, somewhat less than 10% of true precious puberty will be missed; of those cases, some (probably many) will be so mild as to not need intervention and may represent variations of normal. A multinational study from Europe suggested that valid indications for magnetic resonance imaging (MRI) of the CNS in the diagnosis of precocious puberty are puberty onset in girls before 6 years of age, in agreement with our recommendations, and an estradiol value higher than the 45th percentile (in the laboratory performing the diagnostic tests) for girls with central precocious puberty (CPP), a new criterion.[117]

Other Physical and Biochemical Changes of Puberty

The gender difference in voice develops during puberty. In the peripubertal period, the length of the vocal cords in boys and girls is about 12 to 15 mm, of which the membranous portion is 7 to 8 mm.[118] In adult men, the vocal cords attain a length of 18 to 23 mm (membranous portion, 12 to 16 mm), whereas in women, the cords enlarge only slightly (13 to 18 mm). During puberty, the male larynx, cricothyroid cartilage, and laryngeal muscles enlarge, leading to the appearance of an Adam's apple. The largest changes in singing and speaking frequencies occur between Tanner genital stages 3 and 4; breaking of the voice occurs at approximately 13 years, and the adult voice is achieved by about 15 years.

Facial hair in boys is first apparent on the corners of the upper lip and the upper cheeks; it then spreads to the midline of the lower lip and finally to the sides and the lower border of the chin. The first stage of facial hair development usually occurs during pubic hair stage 3 (average age of 14.9 years in the United States), and the last stage occurs after pubic hair stage 5 and genital stage 5.

Axillary hair appears at approximately 14 years in boys. Ninety-three percent of African American girls have axillary hair by age 12, in contrast to 68% of white girls.[97] Axillary sweat glands begin to function as the hair appears. The appearance of circumanal hair slightly precedes that of axillary hair in boys.

Comedones, acne, and seborrhea of the scalp appear as a result of the increased secretion of gonadal and adrenal sex steroids.[119] Early-onset acne correlates with the development of severe acne later in puberty. Acne vulgaris, the most prevalent skin disorder in adolescence, appears at a mean age of 12.2 ± a standard deviation (SD) of 1.4 years (range, 9 to 15 years) in boys and progresses with advancement through puberty. However, acne vulgaris can be the first notable sign of puberty in a girl, preceding pubic hair and breast development.[119] Analysis of the Nurses Study indicates that intake of milk and skim milk is related to the development of acne, an association suggested to reflect the hormone content of milk.[120] At late prepuberty, comedones are present in many boys, and 100% of boys have comedones by genital stage 5.

Facial morphology changes with pubertal development leading to the mature appearance. The mandible and nose enlarge more in boys, but they and the maxilla, brow, frontal sinuses, and middle and posterior fossae enlarge in both sexes, mainly during the pubertal growth spurt. Children with isosexual precocity have the facial appearance of older children, and individuals with delayed puberty have faces of younger children. There is a greater change in various measurements of the face compared with measurements of the skull, with the jaw showing the most increase.[121]

The size of the thyroid gland evaluated by ultrasonography increases roughly 40% to 50% with growth in height, weight, surface area, and fat-free mass during puberty but not with BMI.[122] Lymphoid tissue growth reaches a maximum at about age 12 and thereafter decreases with pubertal progression.

A host of other physiologic and biochemical measurements change with the onset of puberty and must be interpreted in terms of the stage of pubertal development. Age-related standards should be used in all laboratories but often are not, and the interpreting clinician must turn to a textbook of pediatrics or the *Harriet Lane Handbook*. For example, hemoglobin levels increase at puberty in boys; the effect appears to be mediated by androgen, because treatment of boys with CDP with testosterone and letrozole (to block aromatization to estrogen) resulted in increased hemoglobin levels, even in the absence of a rise in insulin-like growth factor type 1(IGF1).[123] The use of biomarkers of pubertal onset and progression will play a role in the upcoming child health study that proposes to longitudinally follow children from conception to adulthood to determine normal changes and the effects of environmental exposures, among other factors.[99]

The peak cohort of germ cells in the fetal ovary is attained at 16 to 20 weeks of gestation.[124-127] Primordial follicles start to appear at 20 weeks of fetal life, and primary follicles soon follow; they constitute the lifelong store of follicles for the individual, which decreases with development and aging. Follicle-stimulating hormone (FSH) receptors have not been detected in midtrimester human fetal ovaries; fetal pituitary FSH is not required for proliferation of oogonia, oocyte differentiation, or formation of primordial follicles.[124] During fetal life and childhood, follicular growth to the large antral stage occurs, but before menarche, all developing follicles are destined to undergo atresia (Fig. 25-10). Large preovulatory follicles are rarely present before puberty.

The ultrasound appearance of the prepubertal ovary changes with pulsatile gonadotropin secretion, and a multicystic appearance occurs with more than six follicles of at least 4 mm in diameter; this appearance differs from that found in the polycystic ovary syndrome (PCOS). During prepuberty, the ovarian volume is 0.2 to 1.6 mL on ultrasound scans, and after the onset of puberty, the volume increases to 2.8 to 15 mL. Tall girls have greater ovarian volume than average-size girls.

The uterus grows until the age of 16 years under the influence of estradiol, progesterone, growth hormone (GH), and IGF1.[128] Ultrasound studies (Fig. 25-11) show that the corpus of the uterus increases during pubertal progression, from an initial tubular shape to a bulbous structure; the length of the uterus increases from 2 to 3 cm to 5 to 8 cm; and the volume increases from 0.4 to 1.6 mL to 3 to 15 mL.[129] Decreased uterine size is found in patients with Turner syndrome, childhood exposure to radiotherapy, abnormalities in *HOX* and *WNT* gene expression, and maternal cigarette smoking can decrease uterine size at adolescence. Smaller uterine size is associated with an increased risk of miscarriage and failed implantation.

Uterine ultrasonography measurements are proposed to aid the clinician in differentiating premature thelarche from precocious puberty. The addition of color Doppler studies may improve accuracy of the diagnosis of precocious puberty and can differentiate the condition from premature thelarche. A Doppler study showed the lowest impedance of the uterine artery to be in girls with established CPP.[130]

Endometriosis is considered to be an estrogen-dependent process, although it has been reported in premenarcheal girls. It was suggested that this cause for chronic abdominal pain is more common than previously considered. One proposed explanation for early-onset endometriosis is that the condition results from müllerian rests.[131]

MENARCHE AND TEENAGE PREGNANCY

Menarche usually occurs in the 6-month period preceding or following the fusion of the second and first distal phalanges and the appearance of the sesamoid bone[132]; this

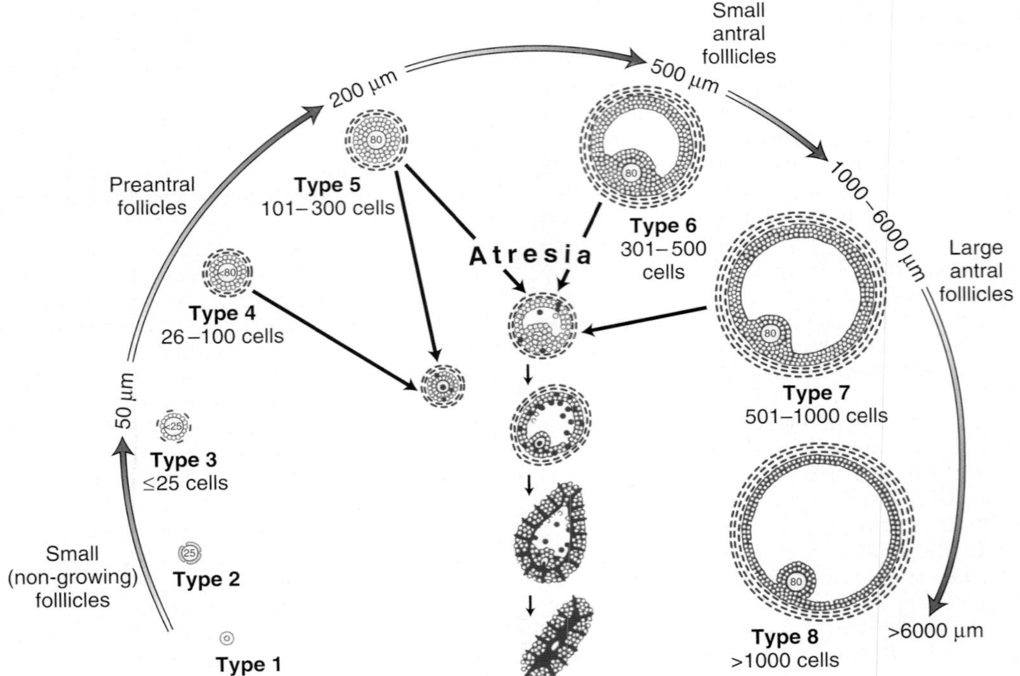

Figure 25-10 Schematic representation of the growth of ovarian follicles during infancy and childhood. Type 1 (primordial follicle) and type 2 (primary follicle) are composed of a small oocyte and a few to a ring of flat granulosa cells. In the diplotene (nesting) stage of prophase, primary follicles are the predominant form of oocyte and constitute the reservoir of cells from which follicular growth occurs. Types 3 to 5 (preantral follicles) are follicles that have entered the growth phase; the oocyte is enlarging and is surrounded by a zona pellucida, and granulosa cells increase in number and differentiate. The growth of the oocyte is complete by the end of the preantral stage, and the increased follicular size is caused by follicular growth and fluid accumulation. Types 6 to 8 represent antral follicles (graafian follicles) and contain a fully grown oocyte, a large number of granulosa cells, a fluid-filled cavity, and a well-developed theca external to the basement membrane. Large preovulatory follicles are absent (10,000 to 15,000 µm). Follicular growth and atresia take place throughout childhood. All follicles that enter the growth phase become atretic, and this can occur at any stage in their development but mainly involves large antral follicles. (From Peters H, Byskov AG, Grinsted J. Follicular growth in fetal and prepubertal ovaries of humans and other primates. *Clin Endocrinol Metab.* 1978;7:469-485.)

corresponds to Tanner stage 4 in most cases. The 95th percentile for menarche is 14.5 years, although many textbooks define primary amenorrhea as absence of menses at 16 years. Reconsideration of the age at onset of female puberty may lead to a reconsideration of the definition of primary amenorrhea. Anovulatory cycles are common in the first years after menarche. There is a reported prevalence of 55% anovulation in the first 2 years after menarche that decreases to 20% anovulatory cycles by the fifth year; others have observed a lower number of ovulatory events shortly after menarche and 5 years after the event. With the high prevalence of PCOS, it is unclear how often delayed regularity is an early sign of PCOS or normal variation. Although the number of pregnancies for U.S. teenagers 15 to 19 years old has been decreasing since 1991, teen childbearing rose 3% in 2006; however, the birth rate fell 2% in 2008 to 41.5 per 1000, reversing this trend,[133] and the birth rate for Hispanic teenagers declined to a historic low.

Male Testicular Development in Puberty

The testes are active during the prepubertal period albeit at a lower level than during pubertal development.[124,134] During pubertal development, the testes increase in size, principally because of the growth of the seminiferous tubules associated with the onset of spermatogenetic activity and mitosis of Sertoli cells, and testosterone production increases (Fig. 25-12 and Table 25-5). The Sertoli cells are the major cell type in the seminiferous cords in prepuberty and early puberty, but in the adult, germ cells predominate. During progression through puberty, the Sertoli cells cease to undergo mitosis, differentiate into adult-type Sertoli cells, and form occlusive junctions with the development of the blood-testes barrier. Although Leydig cells are found in early gestation and during the neonatal period of testosterone secretion, the interstitial tissue is composed principally of undifferentiated mesenchyme-type cells during childhood. With pubertal development and rising serum LH levels, adult-type Leydig cells appear (Table 25-6). It is suggested that three phases of Leydig cell maturation correspond with ages of increased testosterone production: 14 to 18 weeks of fetal life, 2 to 3 months after birth, and puberty through adulthood.[135] The seminal vesicle enlarges through childhood to puberty to hold 3.4 to 4.5 mL, or 70% of the seminal fluid. The mean blood flow in the testes increases to adult values (measured by Doppler sonography) in boys, with a testicular volume greater than 4 cm^3.

Spermatogenesis

The first histologic evidence of spermatogenesis appears between ages 11 and 15 years (see Figs. 25-6, 25-11, and 25-31A). Spermaturia may be the first sign of pubertal development, but the presence of sperm in urine is intermittent and therefore not a reliable indicator in all boys, although in large groups, it holds promise.[99] Spermaturia is more prevalent in early puberty than in late puberty, suggesting that there may be a continuous flow of sperm

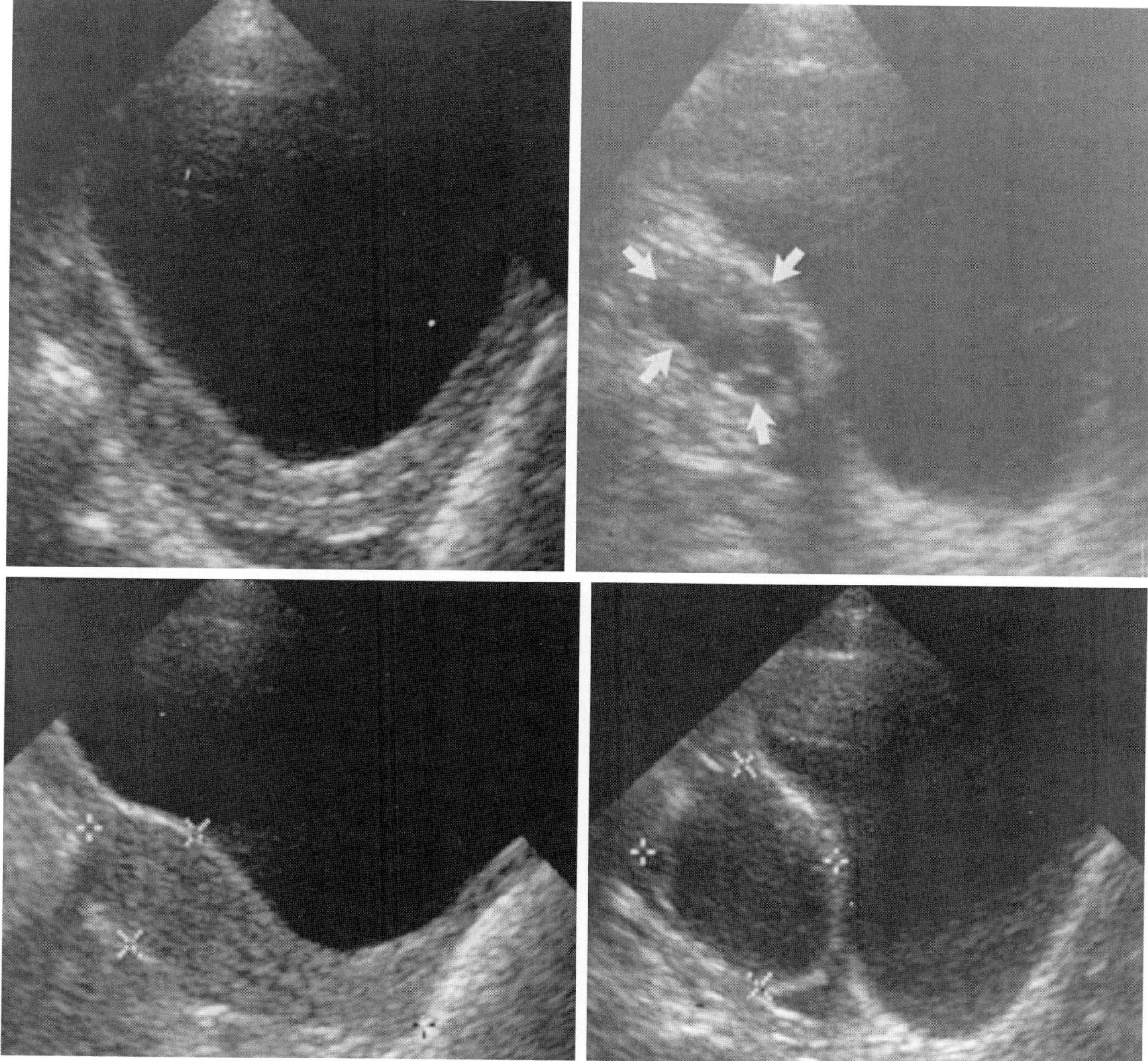

Figure 25-11 High-resolution pelvic ultrasonography. *Top left,* Prepubertal uterus. *Top right,* Prepubertal ovary demonstrating four small follicular cysts *(arrows)*. *Bottom left,* Pubertal postmenarchal uterus. *Bottom right,* Ovarian cyst in a girl with true precocious puberty.

through the urethra in early puberty but that ejaculation is necessary for sperm to appear in the urine in late puberty.[136] Spermaturia in the first morning urine specimen occurs at a mean chronologic age of 13.3 years, and at a mean pubic hair stage 2 to 3 in one study (or 16 years in another study), but may be found in normal boys with bilateral testicular volumes of only 3 mL and no signs of puberty.[137] Normospermia (i.e., normal sperm concentration, morphology, and motility) is not present until a bone age of 17 years.[138] The first conscious ejaculation occurs at a mean chronologic age of 13.5 years in normal boys and at a mean bone age of 13.5 years in boys with delayed puberty.[139] The potential for fertility is reached before an adult phenotype is attained, before adult plasma testosterone concentrations are reached, and before PHV occurs.

Adolescent Growth

Pubertal Growth Spurt

The pubertal growth spurt may be divided for purposes of comparison into three stages: the time of prespurt minimal growth velocity in peripuberty just before the spurt (takeoff velocity); the time of most rapid growth, or PHV; and the stage of decreased velocity and cessation of growth at epiphyseal fusion. The greatest postnatal growth occurs in infancy; growth decreases to the nadir known as the minimal prespurt velocity, the slowest period of growth in childhood, immediately before the pubertal growth spurt.

During puberty, boys and girls experience a growth velocity greater than at any postnatal age since infancy (but paling in comparison to fetal growth, when one fertilized cell grows to 7 pounds in 9 months). Boys reach PHV

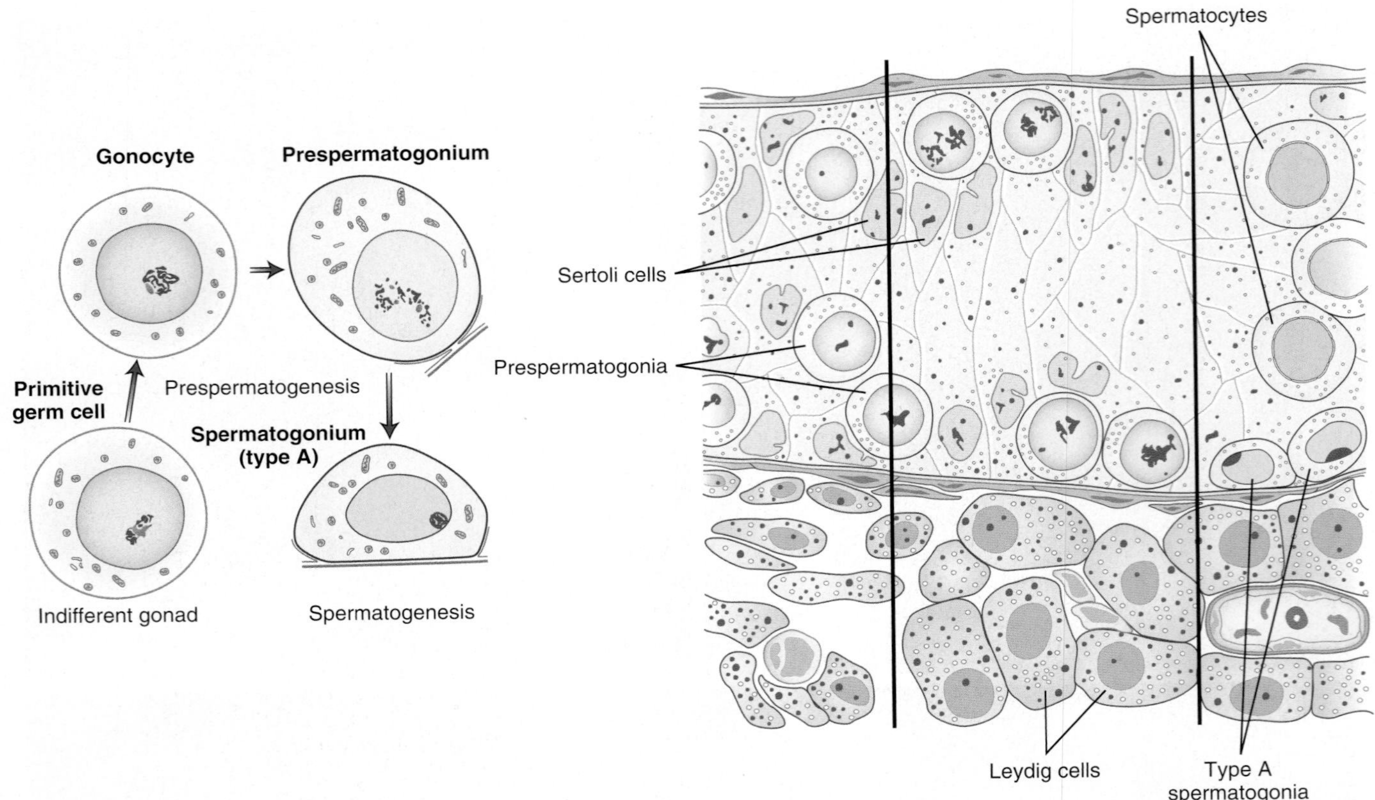

Figure 25-12 *Left,* The diagram shows the developmental stages of testicular germ cells based on electron microscopic findings in the rabbit. Notice the differences between prespermatogonium and spermatogonium. *Right,* The diagram shows maturation of testicular cell types in the rabbit from prepubertal appearance *(left)* to onset of spermatogenesis *(right)*. Interstitial cells undergo changes in shape, size, and arrangement in the process of Leydig cell differentiation. (From Gondos B. Testicular development. In: Johnson AD, Gomes WR, eds. *The Testis,* vol 4. New York, NY; Academic Press, 1977:1-37.)

approximately 2 years later than girls and are taller at takeoff (Fig. 25-13); PHV occurs during stage 3 to 4 of puberty in most boys (see Fig. 25-9) and is completed by stage 5 in more than 95% of boys. Boys achieve a PHV of 9.5 cm/year at a mean of about 13.5 years, with a greater PHV in those who mature earlier than in those who mature later.[140] The pubertal growth spurt in girls (PHV in girls is approximately 8.3 cm/year at a mean chronologic age of 11.5 years) occurs between stages 2 and 3 (see Fig. 25-7). Boys grew a mean of 28 cm, and girls grew 25 cm between takeoff and cessation of growth in a study in the United Kingdom.[141] Although the 8 to 11 cm of increased height gained during the pubertal growth spurt in boys has been held mainly responsible for the difference in adult height between the sexes,[140] twin studies indicate that the difference in adult height results more from the later onset of

TABLE 25-5

Mean Values of Various Body Measurements and Serum Hormone Levels by Pubertal Stage in Boys (Ohio)*

Variable	PS1	PS2a	PS2b	PS3	PS4	PS5
Age (yr)	11.44 (NS)	12.18	12.79	13.74	14.63	15.19
Height (cm)	144.2	149.8	154.6	162.3	169.9	173.3
Weight (kg)	38.18	41.65	47.27	54.67	61.11	66.88
Body mass index (kg/m²)	18.1	18.4	19.5	20.6	21.0	22.2
Testosterone (nmol/L [ng/dL])						
Blacks	0.8 (23)	3.0 (86)	4.9 (141)	11.5 (331)	13.4 (338)	15.5 (449)
Whites	0.6 (16)	2.9 (83)	4.6 (132)	9.7 (281)	13.3 (383)	14.6 (422)
Free testosterone (pmol/L [ng/dL])	11 (0.33)	60 (1.74)	114 (3.28)	294 (8.49)	413 (11.9)	504 (14.5)
DHEAS (μmol/L [μg/dL])	2.71 (99.7)	3.31 (121.8)	4.04 (148.7)	4.75 (175.0)	5.08 (187.0)	5.89 (217.0)
TeBG (nmol/L)	34.6 (NS)	33.3 (NS)	28.4	21.5	14.4	10.7

*Subjects were 515 boys from Ohio, including 237 blacks and 278 whites, aged 10-15 yr at intake, who were monitored every 6 mo for 3 yr. All values were significant by Duncan post-hoc analysis at $P < .01$ except those marked *NS*. Pubertal stages were defined as follows: PS1, absence of pubic hair, testicular volume <3 mL; PS2a, absence of pubic hair, testicular volume ≥3 mL; PS2b, Tanner stage 2 pubic hair; PS3-5, Tanner pubic hair stages 3-5.

DHEAS, dehydroepiandrosterone sulfate; TeBG, testosterone-binding globulin.

Modified from Biro FM, Lucky AW, Hoster GA, et al. Pubertal staging in boys. *J Pediatr.* 1995;127:40-46.

TABLE 25-6

Cellular Activity in Human Testis at Various Stages of Development

Stage	Germ Cells	Sertoli Cells	Leydig Cells
Prepubertal	Prespermatogenic cells are present	Predominant cells in seminiferous cords	Scattered, partially differentiated cells are present
Pubertal	Initiation of spermatogenesis	Increased complexity, formation of occlusive junctions	Fully differentiated cells appear
Adult	Active spermatogenesis, predominant cells	Individual cells associated with groups of germ cells	Groups of fully differentiated cells are present

From Gondos B, Kogan S. Testicular development during puberty. In: Grumbach MM, Sizonenko PC, Aubert ML, eds. *Control of the Onset of Puberty.* Baltimore: Williams & Wilkins, 1990:387-398. © 1990, the Williams & Wilkins Co., Baltimore.)

pubertal growth in boys rather than a difference in growth rate between the genders. The difference in bone widths between boys and girls is in large part established before puberty.[142]

A mathematical model that attempts to define the various stages of the pubertal growth curve based on longitudinal data separates the infancy, childhood, and pubertal phases of growth and allows evaluation of growth despite variation in the age at onset of puberty. A slowly decelerating childhood component is the base, with a sigmoidal pubertal component added during secondary sexual development (see Fig. 25-13C). The infancy-childhood-puberty (ICP) model detected the onset of the pubertal growth spurt, predicted the actual magnitude of the pubertal growth spurt, and predicted adult height using only the age at onset of puberty and a measurement of height.[143] Tanner and Davies[144] constructed growth curves for American children using data from the National Center for Health Statistics, and data calculated from theoretical growth curves can be adjusted for time of PHV.

Daily, meticulous observations of girls during puberty over 120 to 150 days show stasis periods in each girl (three to seven events lasting between 7 and 22 consecutive days); steep changes in each girl (one to four episodes, with the sum of these steep changes calculated as a percentage of total growth during the study period ranging from 15.3% to 42.9%); and continuous growth the remainder of time, with no rhythms or cycles found.[145] Clinicians observe an integrated growth rate during puberty, rather than these various complex patterns occurring during shorter periods of observation.

In a large Swedish registry, faster linear growth during infancy and childhood was associated with earlier PHV during adolescence but less height gain between 8 and 18 years, although greater height and BMI at birth were associated with later PHV in adolescence and more height gain between the ages of 8 and 18 years.[146]

Because girls reach PHV about 1.3 years before menarche, there is limited growth potential after menarche; most girls grow only about 2.5 cm taller after menarche, although there is a variation from 1 to 7 cm. The ages at menarche, takeoff, and PHV are not good predictors of adult height because the duration of pubertal growth is the more important determinant. Later onset of puberty and consequent increase in height at takeoff of the pubertal growth spurt can be balanced by a decrease in actual height achieved during PHV and result in no net change in adult height. However, early onset of puberty can diminish ultimate adult stature,[147] prolonged delay of puberty can increase stature, and an older age at menarche leads to taller adult height in women. The age at PHV and the age at initiation of puberty correlate well with the rate of passage through the stages of pubertal development in normal children. Physical examination of a boy can reveal that he is likely to have significant growth left (if he is in early puberty), whereas limited growth is likely in boys who are in late puberty.

Stature and the upper-to-lower (U/L) segment ratio, defined as the length from the top of the pubic ramus to the top of the head divided by the distance from the top of the pubic ramus to the sole of the foot, change markedly during the peripubertal and early pubertal periods because of the elongation of the extremities.[148] At birth, the U/L ratio is about 1.7; at 1 year, it is 1.4; and at 10 years, it is 1.0 in a normal healthy individual. The legs begin to grow before the trunk, although late in puberty, during the growth spurt, growth of the legs is similar to growth of the upper torso.[149] The mean U/L segment ratio of white adults is 0.92, and that of African American adults is 0.85. There are no differences in U/L segment ratio between the sexes. In general, hypogonadal patients have delayed epiphyseal fusion and lack a pubertal growth spurt; therefore, their extremities grow for a prolonged period, leading to a decreased U/L segment ratio and an increased span for height, a condition known as *eunuchoid proportions*. Eunuchoid proportions are found in subjects with defects in estrogen synthesis and estrogen receptor deficiency, but normal proportions occur in patients with complete androgen insensitivity syndrome, demonstrating the primary role of estrogen in mitigating or establishing these proportions.[150-152] The distal parts of the extremities, the hands and feet, grow before the proximal parts; a rapid increase in shoe size is a harbinger of the pubertal growth spurt. Boys with Klinefelter's syndrome have long legs but not long arms, a physical feature that can assist diagnosis before the onset of puberty. The shoulders become wider in boys, and the hips enlarge more in girls. The female pelvic inlet widens, mainly because of growth of the os acetabuli. The size of the head approaches the adult size by age 10 years, and the brain reaches 95% of adult size by the onset of puberty.

Bone Age. Skeletal maturation is assessed by comparing radiographs of the hand, the knee, or the elbow with standards of maturation in a normal population.[153-155] Ossification centers appear in early life, the bones mature in shape and size and develop articulation of surfaces; ultimately, the epiphyses or growth plates fuse with their shafts. Bone age, an index of physiologic maturation, does not have a well-defined relationship in normal children to the onset of puberty because it appears to be more variable than chronologic age.[156] However, bone age is useful for predicting the age of menarche, and in boys, the onset of normal, premature, and delayed puberty correlates better with the onset of secondary sexual development than does chronologic age. Bone age advancement has no relation to the passage through puberty of normal boys.[156]

Bone age, height, and chronologic age can be used for prediction of adult height from the Bayley-Pinneau tables[157] (or by the use of the Roche-Wainer-Thissen or Tanner-Whitehouse techniques). Skeletal maturation is more advanced in girls than in boys of the same chronologic age

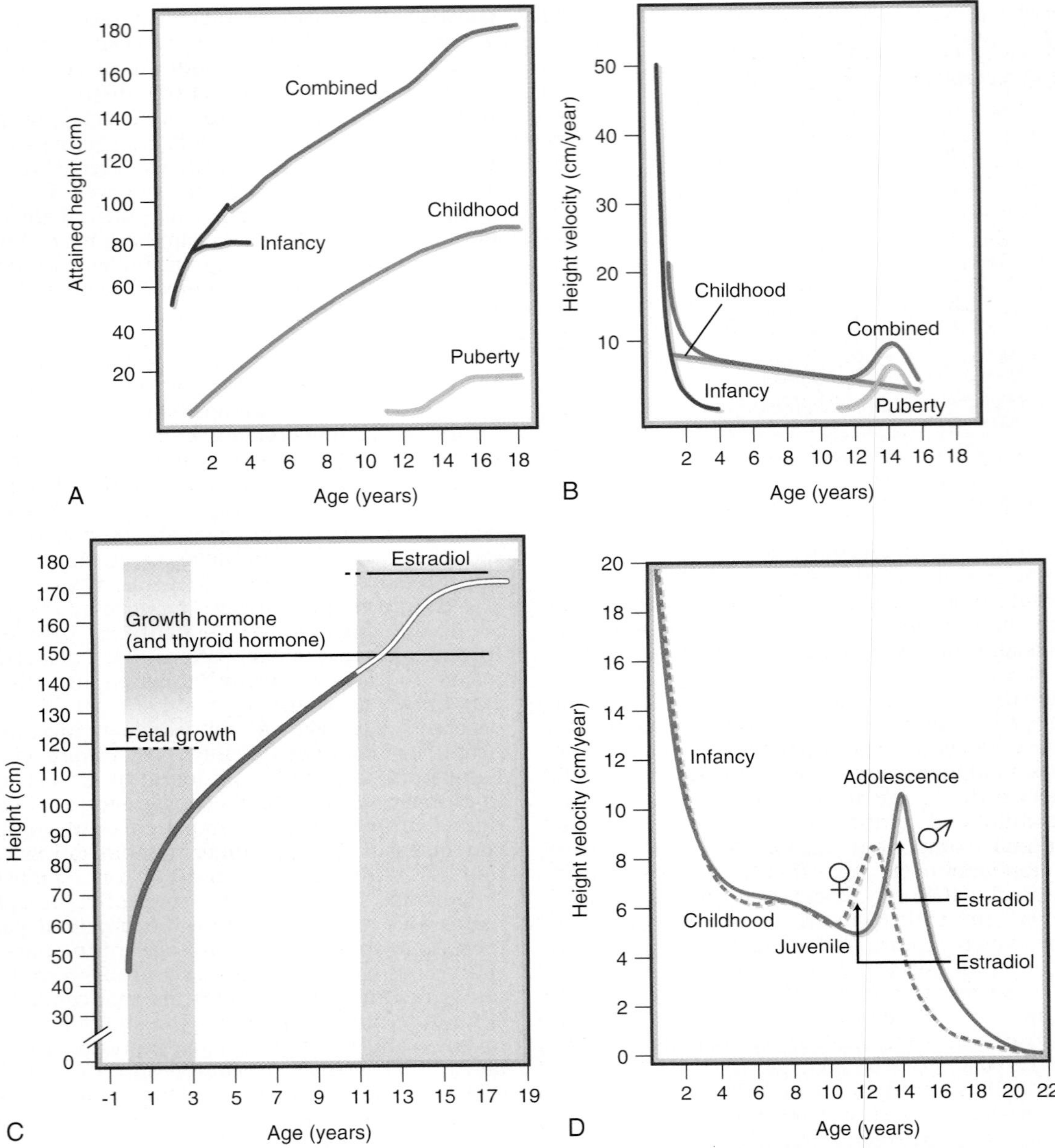

Figure 25-13 The infancy-childhood-puberty (ICP) model of Karlberg for mean attained height (**A**) and height velocity (**B**) for boys. The mean value for each component (infancy, childhood, and puberty) and their sums (combined growth [**A**] and combined velocity [**B**]) are plotted. The growth curve for an individual represents the additive effect of the three biologic phases of the growth process (ICP). Karlberg has provided mathematical functions for each component of his model. *Infancy:* This component starts before birth and falls off by age 3 to 4 years. It can be described by the exponential function $y = a + b[1 - \exp(-ct)]$. Average total gain in height for Swedish boys is 79.0 cm (44.0% of final height) and for girls is 76.8 cm (46.2%). *Childhood:* This phase begins at the end of the first year of life and continues to mature height. A second-degree polynomial function describes this component: $y = a + bt + ct^2$. Average total gain in height for boys is 85.2 cm (47.4%) and for girls is 78.4 cm (47.3%). *Puberty:* The model for the pubertal growth spurt is a logistic function: $y = a/[1 + \exp(-b(t - t_v))]$. Average total gain in height for boys is 15.4 cm (8.6%) and for girls is 10.9 cm (6.5%); y designates attained height at time t in years from birth; a, b, and c are constants; t_v is the age at peak height velocity. **C,** A schematic male growth chart shows the features of the ICP pattern overlaid and illustrates the predominant endocrine mechanisms controlling each phase of growth. The first *shaded area* emphasizes the decreasing velocity of infantile growth as the individual leaves the rapid growth phase of fetal life. The *open area* is the childhood phase, which continues and magnifies the decreased velocity of growth into a plateau of rather constant growth during childhood. These two phases depend largely on the effects of growth hormone (GH) and thyroid hormone, with no or little effect derived from gonadal steroids. In the next period of the pubertal growth spurt, gonadal steroids exert their direct and indirect effects. Gonadal steroids exert direct effects on the bone by stimulating the generation of insulin-like growth factor I (IGF1) and other growth factors locally, and they exert indirect effects by stimulating increased GH secretion, which exerts its own effects on bone and stimulates the production of IGF1. In the female, the major gonadal steroid involved in the pubertal growth spurt is estradiol, whereas in the male, testosterone and estradiol (arising mainly from the aromatization of testosterone) are the major gonadal steroids. **D,** The adolescent growth spurt in girls and boys (growth velocity curves). Notice the later onset of the pubertal growth spurt in boys and the approximately 2-year difference in peak height velocity and the greater magnitude of peak height velocity compared with girls. The timing of the effects of estradiol is indicated. Progressive epiphyseal fusion terminates the growth spurt and leads to final or adult height. (**A** and **B,** Adapted from Karlberg J. On the construction of the infancy-childhood-puberty growth standard. *Acta Paediatr Scand Suppl.* 1989;356:26-37; **C** and **D,** From Grumbach MM. Estrogen, bone, growth, and sex: a sea change in conventional wisdom. *J Pediatr Endocrinol Metab.* 2000;13[suppl 6]:1439-1455.)

because the early pubertal bone ages of 11 years in girls and 13 years in boys are equivalent stages of bone maturation by the hand-wrist method. African American children have slightly more advanced bone ages than do white children of the same chronologic age.[158] A difference between bone age and chronologic age must exceed 2 standard deviations to be of biologic significance. Standard deviations may range from a few months in infancy to 1 year in later adolescence; a 2-year variation of bone age from chronologic age is within normal limits in middle teenage years. As commonly estimated, bone age is imprecise and is a qualitative rather than a quantitative measure.[155] The development of techniques for scanning radiographs coupled with computer analysis may increase the precision of the procedure.[159]

Skeletal Density. Prevailing views locate the determinants of adult bone density in large part in genetic tendencies and the appropriate acquisition of bone mineral in childhood during growth. Osteoporosis and osteopenia are important conditions of the adult that are held to have antecedents in youth, and increasing interest focuses on bone health in children and adolescents, including the effects of age of menarche, nutrition, exercise, and genetics on normal skeletal development.[160,161] However, a contrary view based on other clinical studies and animal models holds that distant-past patterns of bone growth are less important than recent conditions and that childhood bone growth does not exert a strong effect on adult bone density.[162] A relationship of bone density exists between generations if the effects of age and puberty are eliminated: 60% to 80% of variance in peak bone mass is attributed to genetic factors.[163] This controversy is not resolved.

Areal bone mineral density (BMD) represents a two-dimensional image and is a function of the size of bone; this is the measurement most often available clinically with commercial dual-energy x-ray absorptiometry (DEXA) devices. Smaller bones attenuate the radiation beam less than larger bones, and this factor must be considered in the interpretation when measuring bone density using commercial DEXA devices. BMD of the total body, lumbar spine, and femoral neck measured by DEXA increases at a mean annualized rate of 0.047 g/cm^2 for boys and 0.039 g/cm^2 for girls (Fig. 25-14A). Longitudinal studies of total-body DEXA assessments indicate that boys accumulate 407 g/year and girls 322 g/year of mineral (i.e., 359 mg/day for boys and 284 mg/day for girls); 26% of adult calcium is laid down during the adolescent years of peak calcium accretion—14 years (mean) for boys and 12.5 years for girls.[164] BMD approaches a maximum accretion in girls by the age of 16 years, and in boys by about 17 years, with the difference in timing related to the disparity in PHV; the rate then decreases, reaching a plateau in the third decade of life.[165] Although quantitative computed tomography (CT) demonstrates an increase in the cortical bone density of the lumbar spine with age, less increase in cancellous bone density with age occurs until the later stages of puberty. Increased BMD correlates well with height, weight (a main determinant of bone density in adolescent and postpubertal females), age, pubertal development, and BMI but has less relationship with serum IGF1 levels. Some consider that the concept of age at peak bone density attainment is too simplistic and prefer to consider the strength of the bone and its geometry.[166]

Volumetric bone density (bone mineral apparent density [BMAD]) represents the amount of bone within the periosteal envelope and is of more physiologic importance, because it does not rely on the size of the bone that is changing during growth, particularly pubertal growth (see Fig. 25-14A). Volumetric bone density grows in a region-specific pattern, and conditions in childhood and adolescence that affect the accrual of bone mineral have different effects based on the length of time the affected bone has left to achieve its maximum bone mineral content (BMC);

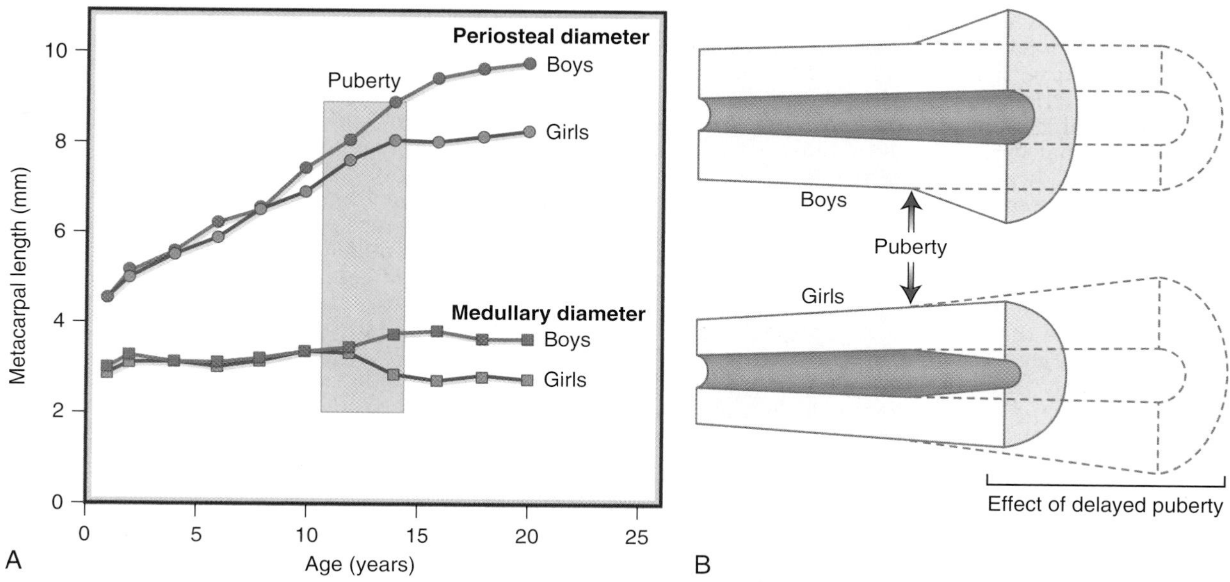

Figure 25-14 **A,** Periosteal diameter of the metacarpal bones does not differ before puberty in boys and girls. During puberty, the periosteal diameter expands in boys and ceases to expand in girls, whereas medullary diameter remains fairly constant in boys throughout growth but contracts in girls. **B,** In boys, delayed puberty may reduce periosteal apposition, leaving a smaller bone with a thinner cortex but normal medullary diameter (*top*). In girls, delayed puberty may result in reduced endocortical apposition, leaving a normal or larger bone (if periosteal apposition continues in absence of the inhibitory effect of estrogen) with a thinner cortex and larger medullary diameter (*bottom*). (**A** and **B,** from Seeman E. Pathogenesis of bone fragility in women and men. *Lancet.* 2002;359:1841-1850.)

deficits may occur in limb dimensions (prepuberty), spine dimensions (early puberty), or volumetric bone density by interference with mineral accrual (late puberty).[167]

Calculations for BMAD are made as follows:

Spine BMAD = spine BMC ÷ (spine area)$^{1.5}$ = spine BMC divided by the square root of (spine area)^3

Femoral neck BMAD = femoral neck BMC divided by (femoral neck area)^2

Whole body BMAD = BMC divided by height (cm) as a means of correcting for bone size

The patterns of areal or volumetric bone density differ during development.[168]

DEXA device manufacturers sometimes provide standards for children and adolescents. Children are often referred for evaluation of osteoporosis because their DEXA results are compared with young adult values although they have not come close to reaching maximal bone density. Bone reaches its adult size and PHV occurs before maximal BMC is reached[169]; these factors may result in a period of increased fragility and susceptibility to trauma characteristic of adolescence. Lean body mass is related to skeletal density (stronger in boys than girls) and fat mass and skeletal density (stronger in girls than in boys).[170] Standards are available to interpret BMC in terms of lean body mass, which appears to be better related to normal bone growth than to chronologic age; muscle stress is an important factor in the development of bone.[171] Normative data for pediatric DEXA studies are available from various centers.[165,171-173]

An applet available on the Stanford University web site (http://www-stat-class.Stanford.EDU/pediatric-bones [accessed February 2011]) generates a Z-score for BMD or BMAD measurements at the lumbar spine (L2-4), hip, or whole body using the Hologic 1000W with respect to the age, gender, and ethnicity of the subject.

Quantitative ultrasound standards are available for children and adolescents.[174] Because they do not require radiation exposure, they may achieve wider use in childhood.

Seeman presented what he considers to be two fallacies in the interpretation of densitometry.[168] The first is the concept that volumetric BMD increases during growth. It does not. Growth builds a bigger, not more dense, skeleton. Second is the idea that peak volumetric BMD is higher in men than in women. It is not. Bone size is greater and is underestimated in patients with larger bones than controls. The misconceptions occur because the result of areal bone density is the BMC per unit projected bone area of bone in the coronal plane, or an areal BMC (g/cm^2). Too often, the "areal" element is deleted, and "content" is replaced by density, so that BMC per unit projected area is called BMD, even though volumetric bone density is the desired measurement. Although BMC may normally be higher in boys than in girls and rises with development, volumetric bone density of the long bones is identical in boys and girls. In contrast to the long bones, volumetric bone density increases at the spine in both sexes.[165,167,168]

The increase in BMD during the prepubertal and pubertal years reflects the increase in the size of the long bones. Legs grow more rapidly than the trunk in prepubertal girls, but during puberty, there is more truncal growth. Boys develop greater bone size due to increased periosteal apposition (increasing bone strength) and endosteal resorption compared with girls; girls add bone on the endocortical surface, which may serve as a reservoir for calcium for later lactation and pregnancy.[175]

Birth weight, weight gain during infancy, and weight gain during the years 9 through 12 influence bone mass achieved at 21 years.[176] The BMD at the beginning of puberty predicted the peak bone mass at sexual maturity and appeared to predict the likelihood of osteoporosis as an adult in longitudinal studies, suggesting a method of identification of those most in need of intervention (see Fig. 25-18).[177] The mechanostat concept posits that developmental changes in bone strength result from the increasing loads imposed by larger muscle forces, which stimulate bone mineral acquisition. In a longitudinal study, a rise in lean body mass occurred before peak BMC, and fat mass later exerted more influence.[178] Increased physical activity is generally beneficial for bone health, but excessive running, gymnastics, and cheerleading are progressively more likely to lead to stress fractures,[179] and excessive exercise can lead to the female athletic triad. Femoral head strength increases markedly during puberty, and the femoral neck increases in density more with impact load sports such as running (compared with active load sports such as swimming); only 3 to 12 minutes of daily exercise increases femoral bone density in early pubertal children,[180] with greater increases occurring during puberty.

Prepubertal girls engaged in gymnastics have increased bone density in the limbs that are more often used, and this occurs in a dose-response manner.[181] A longitudinal study of gymnasts and their mothers found that these effects do not mainly result from genetic influences. Female adolescent athletes have increased bone density, although the effects last only as long as the activity continues.

Calcium intake during puberty has been documented to strongly affect bone density later in life in most studies[163]; the effect of increased ingestion of calcium may last only as long as the calcium is administered. Pubertal girls are estimated to get well below the recommended intake levels, and even recommended levels may be too low for optimal mineralization. Children who avoid dairy products and are without calcium supplementation have an increased prevalence of fractures in the prepubertal period, even with minor trauma.[182] Early pubertal girls cannot increase gastrointestinal calcium absorption enough to compensate for a poor diet, as older individuals may. African American children retain more calcium than white children do, and the bone structure is thicker in African American children; the difference in vertebral bone density between ethnic groups appears to develop by late puberty. Randomized, placebo-controlled clinical trials between 1985 and 2005 that enrolled normal children for at least 3 months revealed a small effect of calcium supplementation in the upper limb, but the increase in BMD was not thought to influence the likelihood of a fracture later in life.[183] However, the lack of effects applies only to normal children, and studies of subjects with disorders of puberty that affect bone development may reveal other findings. Remarkable calcium intake is directly related to the rate of bone age advancement to a degree.[184] Increased sodium intake at the expense of calcium intake adversely affects bone accretion. Adequate zinc intake is another factor related to BMD in puberty.

Vitamin D status is a concern, because 32% of girls with low calcium intake were also vitamin D deficient and had elevated serum concentrations of parathyroid hormone (PTH) and thyroid hormone receptor–associated protein-5b (TRAP-5b), as well as significantly lower cortical volumetric BMD of the distal radius and tibia shaft,[185] and another 46% had low-normal concentrations of vitamin D. Deficient calcium and vitamin D can lead to secondary hyperparathyroidism in adolescence.

Girls with heterozygote ERα genotype (Pp) and high levels of physical activity had significantly higher bone mass, higher BMD, and thicker cortex at loaded bone sites (compared with the distal radius, which is not a weight-bearing bone) than their counterparts with low physical activity.[186] These results suggest that high physical activity benefits those with heterozygous ER genotypes, and the less favorable Pp genotype may be compensated by increasing the amount of leisure-time physical activity at early puberty.

Studies of male athletes are less common than those of girls, but 16- to 19-year-old athletic boys can still gain more bone mass in the spine and femora than nonathletic controls.[187] Abnormalities of puberty impair bone accretion in both sexes and are mainly consequences of estrogen deficiency due to decreased secretion or peripheral aromatization of androgens (see Fig. 25-14B). A 1.9-year increase in mean age at menarche in young women was associated with lower radial areal BMD T-scores; lower trabecular number, thickness, and spacing; and cortical thickness without a reduction in cross-sectional area, a finding compatible with less endocortical accrual and a possible explanation of how late menarche is a risk factor for forearm osteoporosis.[188] Urinary adrenal hormone metabolites are related to the achievement of increased proximal radial diaphyseal bone strength; the level of urinary androstenediol at about 8 years of age is an early predictor of diaphyseal bone strength in late puberty (about 16 years of age).[189] Peripheral conversion of adrenarchal dehydroepiandrosterone by 17β-hydroxysteroid dehydrogenase (17β-HSD) to androstenediol may be associated with radial bone accretion during growth. CDP was thought to lead to decreased areal bone density in adulthood, but normal volumetric bone density was recently found in adults previously affected by CDP,[190] and the same is thought to occur with primary hypogonadism.

Testosterone administration to normal prepubertal boys increases calcium retention and bone growth and also increases bone density in adolescents with CDP, testosterone-deficient Klinefelter's syndrome, or male hypogonadotropic hypogonadism. Bone density is increased in females with excess androgens, whereas girls with anorexia nervosa, hypothalamic amenorrhea, or ovarian failure have decreased bone density.

Serum levels of inorganic phosphate, alkaline phosphatase, serum osteocalcin (Gla-protein level), collagen type I N-telopeptides (NTX),[191] and procollagen type I carboxyl-terminal propeptide (PICP); the cross-linked C-terminal telopeptide of type I collagen (ICTP), procollagen type III amino-terminal propeptide (P3NP), and tartrate-resistant acid phosphatase isoform 5b; and urinary pyridinoline, deoxypyridinoline, and galactosyl-hydroxylysine excretion reflect the increased osteoblastic activity and growth rate during childhood and pubertal growth in both sexes, with values reaching a peak at midpuberty and decreasing thereafter.[192]

Body Composition. Just as endocrine changes bring about remarkable changes in secondary sexual development and growth, body composition is dramatically affected. GH and gonadal steroids play major roles in this process.[193] Lean body mass, skeletal mass, and body fat are equal in prepubertal boys and girls, but by maturity, men have 1.5 times the lean body mass and almost 1.5 times the skeletal mass of women, whereas women have twice as much body fat (25%) as men (13%), producing a gynecoid (woman-like) or android (man-like) appearance.[194] Lean body mass increases by the age of 6 years in girls and 9.5 years in boys. Boys acquire fat-free mass more quickly and for a longer period than girls during puberty; stability is attained by 15 to 16 years in girls and 2 to 3 years later in boys.[140] Fat mass increases in girls at an average rate of 1.14 kg/year, but the fat mass does not change in boys during the pubertal years, leading to the greater fat value in girls than boys with age.[140]

Weight is not an adequate reflection of body fat. The BMI is often invoked in describing the shape of the body in age-adjusted terms and is used as a better, if imperfect, reflection of body fat. BMI changes with age, and there is no specific number indicating normal or abnormal BMI at all stages of development, as there is for adults. Reference charts of BMI compared with age and gender between the 3rd and 97th percentiles are available online (www.CDC.gov/growthcharts/clinical_charts.htm [accessed February 2011]) for interpretation of BMI values.

Increased visceral fat (i.e., intra-abdominal adipose tissue, or IAAT) in obese teenagers is associated with hypertriglyceridemia, decreased high-density lipoprotein (HDL)-cholesterol, and small, dense, cholesterol-laden very-low-density lipoprotein (VLDL) particles. Subcutaneous fat is associated with large, lipid-laden VLDL particles, which are removed directly from the circulation and pose less risk. The subcutaneous adipose tissue that leads to visibly different body forms is only an imperfect reflection of this internal distribution of fat cells, because increased IAAT may cause metabolic derangements without increasing total-body fat. Studies support the role of increased intra-abdominal fat in children as a cause of insulin resistance and dyslipidemia, with small adipocytes demonstrating limited storage ability, leading to increased ectopic fat deposition in myocytes and hepatocytes.[195,196] Waist-to-hip ratios may not reflect IAAT in children and adolescents, because subcutaneous abdominal fat may be low despite increased visceral fat.[195] However, there is renewed interest in waist circumference in children as a reflection of IAAT; standards are available and are being studied to determine clinical implications.[197]

The generalized distribution of fat in males (central fat, apple-shaped, android), which is different from that in females (lower body fat predominance, pear-shaped, gynecoid), develops largely during puberty as males become more android than they were in prepuberty, although girls start and remain gynoid. There are ethnic differences in the pattern of change, and Asians have the most significant changes.[198]

DEXA is used to determine the percentage of body fat, water, and bone mineral with great accuracy but cannot differentiate visceral from subcutaneous adipose tissue. CT was used until the validation of MRI to determine intra-abdominal and subcutaneous fat distribution without the use of radiation.[199]

A *strength spurt* occurs during puberty after the pubertal growth spurt. Muscle mass is 54% of body weight in adolescent boys and 42% of body weight in adolescent girls, with the difference partly due to the presence of more muscle cells and larger muscle cells in men. There is little gender difference before 8 years of age, but by 14 years, boys usually have developed greater lean leg mass and greater power than girls.[200]

Obesity, Puberty, and the Metabolic Syndrome

Between NHANES II and NHANES III, a period of roughly 20 years, there was more than a tripling of the prevalence of children and adolescents above the 95th percentile in weight (denoted by the CDC as *overweight*), to a prevalence of 17.1%, and a 50% increase in those above the 85th percentile (denoted as *at risk for overweight*).[201]

Excessive body fat during childhood and adolescence has significant medical effects early and later in life.[202] Obesity, glucose intolerance, and hypertension in childhood are strongly associated with increased rates of premature death among Native Americans, but childhood hypercholesterolemia is not.[203]

Serum Lipids in Normal Puberty and in Obesity and the Metabolic Syndrome. Testosterone increases serum levels of LDL-cholesterol and decreases HDL-cholesterol concentrations, accounting for the adverse LDL/HDL ratio in men compared with women.[204] Post-heparin hepatic lipase activity is increased by exogenous androgens (and decreased by estrogens), accounting for the decrease in HDL after androgen treatment or after a rise in endogenous androgen secretion.

The epidemic of obesity has led to the advent of the metabolic syndrome in youth. Diagnosis of metabolic syndrome varies among studies, and a generally accepted definition is needed.[205] Elevated cholesterol levels in children and adolescents track to adult values in longitudinal studies.[206] Although familial hypercholesterolemia leads to carotid intimal plaques by puberty, random autopsies demonstrate macroscopic or microscopic evidence of arteriosclerosis in normal youth without familial hypercholesterolemia, and the tendency is increased by obesity. By 15 to 19 years, 2% of autopsied males had advanced (American Heart Association grade 4 or 5) atherosclerotic coronary artery lesions associated with increased serum cholesterol, obesity, and hypertension.[207]

Girls are already expressing dissatisfaction with their weight in the third to the fifth grade, and restrictive dieting begins.[208] Nutrition suffers with dieting because the intake of fruits, vegetables, and calcium is decreased. Some ethnic groups more often try to gain weight, apparently due to parental suggestion that they are too thin.

Insulin and Insulin Resistance. Insulin resistance is a hallmark of obesity and is thought to be the cause of or an associated factor in the metabolic syndrome associated with cardiac disease.[209] Euglycemic clamp techniques are the gold standard for measurement of insulin resistance. Fasting insulin concentrations offer little insight into insulin resistance in an individual, and equations such as the homeostatic model assessment (HOMA) that are based on fasting insulin levels offer little more; however, fasting insulin values[206] are used in epidemiologic studies and offer more useful information. The fasting insulin concentration increases twofold to threefold with peak height velocity, insulin secretion after a glucose load increases over prepubertal levels, and insulin-mediated glucose disposal in peripheral tissues decreases in the hyperinsulinemic euglycemic clamp or the minimal model frequently sampled intravenous glucose tolerance test (IVGTT),[210] showing increased insulin resistance during normal puberty. Insulin sensitivity is inversely related to pubertal stage and BMI.

The response of insulin to an oral glucose tolerance test is greater in African American subjects than in white subjects at all stages of pubertal development; this ethnic difference in insulin resistance is suggested as a cause for the increased incidence of type 2 diabetes among African American adults compared with white adults and appears to offer a similar explanation of the ethnic disparity in youth, with white teenagers having greater insulin sensitivity than African American or Hispanic youth.[211,212] Insulin resistance occurs early in the course of Turner syndrome and thalassemia major, but even in Turner syndrome, in which there is an underlying increase in insulin resistance, there seems to be low or no risk of these conditions developing with GH treatment.

With the increased prevalence of type 2 diabetes (non–insulin-dependent diabetes mellitus, or NIDDM), proposed screening criteria are being evaluated. Currently, children with a BMI higher than the 85th percentile should be screened if they (1) have a family history of type 1 diabetes, (2) have signs of insulin resistance (e.g., acanthosis nigricans, functional ovarian hyperandrogenism, hypertension, dyslipidemia), or (3) belong to one of several specific ethnic groups (e.g., African American, Native American, Hispanic American, Asian American). If a fasting plasma glucose level is higher than 126 mg/dL or a 2-hour postprandial value is higher than 200 mg/dL, or if there are symptoms such as weight loss, polyuria, or polydipsia and a casual plasma glucose level is higher than 200 mg/dL, the diagnosis of diabetes is likely, and determination of the type of diabetes (type 1 or 2) is appropriate.

Patients with type 1 diabetes (insulin-dependent diabetes mellitus, or IDDM) usually require an increase in the dose of insulin for euglycemic control at puberty. The cause of insulin resistance has been attributed in part to increased fat oxidation at puberty, which correlates with rising serum IGF1 levels and may be linked to increased GH secretion. However, there is no evidence that GH treatment alone increases the likelihood of development of type 2 diabetes or impaired glucose tolerance. Weight gain increases in children with type 1 diabetes during puberty, leading to a higher incidence of obesity in children with IDDM than would be expected from family patterns. Some adolescents with IDDM, predominantly girls, reduce their insulin use in order to lose weight, with dire consequences. Retinopathy due to IDDM characteristically appears in the teenage years or later, but duration and control of diabetes in the prepubertal years are contributing factors. The American Diabetes Association recommends screening for microalbuminuria, an indicator of the development of diabetic nephropathy. Microalbuminuria may develop quite early in puberty rather than in the later stages.[213]

A normal individual adapts to the changes in the physiologic rise in pubertal insulin resistance, but an individual at genetic risk for type 2 diabetes, with the accompanying defect in pancreatic beta cell function,[214] may not adapt to the insulin resistance and, with the additional insulin resistance characteristic of obesity, may develop clinical type 2 diabetes during the pubertal years or earlier. Type 2 diabetes in children or adolescents should not be confused with the various forms of monogenetic diabetes (previously called maturity-onset diabetes) or diabetes of the young (MODY), which are inherited as autosomal dominant traits.

Several syndromes of insulin resistance combine hyperglycemia and virilization.[215] The Kahn type A syndrome features include a lean, muscular adolescent female phenotype with acanthosis nigricans, hirsutism, oligomenorrhea or amenorrhea, and ovarian hyperthecosis and stromal hyperplasia associated with abnormalities of the insulin receptor gene. Hyperandrogenism, insulin resistance, acanthosis nigricans (HAIR-AN) syndrome and PCOS are less severe than Kahn type A and usually manifest in adolescent females. Persons with Robson-Mendenhall syndrome have severe insulin resistance (possibly leading to diabetic ketoacidosis), dysmorphic facies, acanthosis nigricans, thickened nails, hirsutism, dental dysplasia, abdominal distention, and phallic or clitoral enlargement. The Robson-Mendenhall syndrome, similar to the Donahue (leprechaunism) syndrome, which shares some of these features, is caused by homozygous or compound heterozygote defects in the insulin receptor gene. Kahn type B syndrome is caused by inhibitory or stimulatory antibodies to the insulin receptor and sometimes occurs with acanthosis nigricans and ovarian hyperandrogenism. This syndrome can occur with ataxia-telangiectasia syndrome or in otherwise normal adolescents. Individuals with the Seip-Berardinelli syndrome combine lipodystrophy and severe insulin resistance and complete or partial absence of subcutaneous fat with increased growth and skeletal maturation, muscle hypertrophy, acanthosis nigricans, hypertrichosis, organomegaly, and mild hypertrophy of the external genitalia.

Most of these NIDDM syndromes can be treated with oral hypoglycemic agents initially; progression of the disorder may require the use of insulin. Several girls with these syndromes of insulin resistance have been described to have low serum gonadotropin values during puberty without response to GnRH but with enlarged ovaries, suggesting a direct role for insulin in stimulating the growth of the ovary. The hypoleptinemic state found in various degrees of lipodystrophy does not appear to affect pubertal progression, but administration of leptin has led to resumption of menstrual periods in some females and adjustment of testosterone production toward normal levels in males.[216]

Obese teenage girls with predominant abdominal adiposity and insulin resistance may have early puberty, early menarche, and longer exposure to an endocrine profile, predisposing to breast cancer.[77] Insulin resistance is characteristic of the state of functional ovarian hyperandrogenism seen after a history of premature pubarche. This constellation is more frequent in children with a history of low birth weight.

Blood Pressure. Blood pressure is related to the age, gender, and height of the child using appropriate standards (available at http://pediatrics.aappublications.org/cgi/content/full/114/2/S2/555 [accessed February 2011]). Blood pressure increases with pubertal maturation, related to increased stature and synchronized with the pubertal growth spurt, suggesting some relationship in the control of the two processes.[217] Hypertension is becoming common in puberty as a comorbidity of obesity. Increased blood pressure at puberty depends on BMI[218] and height, factors that are interrelated. Blood pressure in childhood and adolescence is predictive of adult blood pressure (tracking).[206,219] Blood pressure rises in African American children at lower BMIs than in white children, making the problem worse in the African American population. In sexual precocity, blood pressure rises above prepubertal levels to values commensurate with body size and BMI.

CENTRAL NERVOUS SYSTEM ANATOMY, FUNCTION, PSYCHOLOGY, AND ELECTROENCEPHALOGRAPHIC RHYTHM

Brain anatomy and function change substantially during late childhood and adolescence (Fig. 25-15A). Behavior or psychopathology that becomes evident at this time has its basis in these changes and exposures dating from early life and the prenatal period, all interacting against a genetic background. Puberty is the time of appearance of the ability to solve complex problems in a mature manner. An increase in cortical metabolic rate in infancy is followed by a late childhood decline to adult levels; this decline ceases by the end of the second decade. The prefrontal association cortex, an area of the brain that is concerned with forward planning and regulatory control of emotional behavior, continues to develop until the age of 20 to 25 years.[4] Stress at various stages of development, even in early childhood, may cause psychological manifestations during puberty.[220]

The anatomic changes revealed by functional MRI studies of the prefrontal cortex, an area that is involved with emotional regulation and planning, occur during a time of physical maturation and are likely to relate to many of the characteristic behavior changes of puberty.[4] The volume of white matter increases linearly between 4 and 22 years of age due to an increase in myelination during development, and there are more complex changes in gray matter.[221] A reduction in cortical synaptic density and neuronal density, analogous to programmed cell death, occurs between 2 and 16 years of age, and this pruning of synapses appears to be linked to improved memory.[222] This change in gray matter follows an inverted U-shaped curve of increase from the age of 6 years. Longitudinal studies using dynamic mapping of human cortical development demonstrate that higher-order association cortices (e.g., those involved in executive function, attention, and motor coordination) mature after lower-order somatosensory, motor, and visual cortices mature, and those areas that are phylogenetically older mature before newer ones.[223,224] Intrauterine excess of androgens leads to enlargement of the amygdala, and girls reach greater mass of gray matter 2 years before boys during puberty, demonstrating aspects of the effects of sex steroids on brain growth and remodeling in human beings. Increased LH levels are related to areas of increased white matter density, including the cingulum, middle temporal gyrus, and splenium of the corpus callosum; there is a genetic overlay to this relationship. Gray matter volume, at least in girls, appears to be related to a pubertal increase in estradiol levels.[225]

Brain plasticity decreases during puberty. Examples include the inability to learn to speak a foreign language without an accent after puberty and recovery of a child from the effects of a CNS injury that in an adult might have led to aphasia. Loss of plasticity may be maladaptive to our rapidly changing world and extended life span compared with prehistoric times.[226] Plasticity allowed developmental learning before puberty, but lack of plasticity and a standard response to conditions in the adult allowed success in that static environment of the past.

Mania, depression, obsessive-compulsive disorders, and schizophrenia are more common after puberty. They are postulated to be related to alterations of the normal changes in brain architecture and function that occur during puberty.

Sleep Patterns in Puberty

Increased sleep is characteristic of the period of growth and development across species. Because sleep is a time of vulnerability, threats leading to stress are antithetical to normal sleep, and a feeling of safely is thought to be necessary to allow sleep to proceed normally as the adolescent is preparing for independence and increased self-care in a possibly hostile world. Rising complexity of brain function during puberty is reflected in increases in the amplitude and frequency of delta waves (0- to 3-Hz electroencephalographic waves) found during deep sleep, which appears more related to age than to pubertal development or growth.[227] The function of deep sleep (i.e., slow-wave or

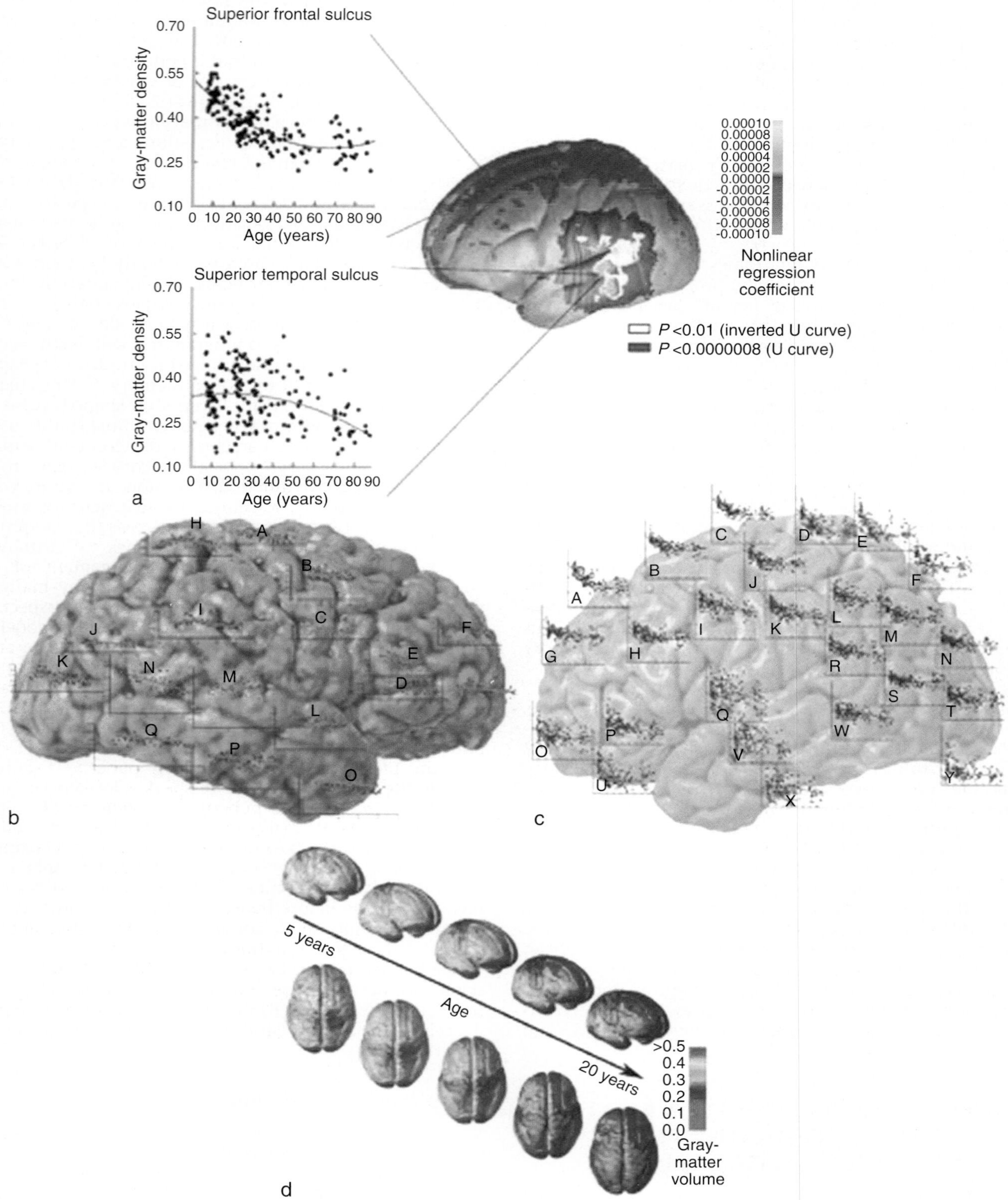

Figure 25-15A Mapping brain change over time. Brain changes in development can be identified by fitting time-dependent statistical models to data collected from subjects cross-sectionally (i.e., across a group of subjects at a particular time) or longitudinally (i.e., following individual subjects as they aged), or both. Measurements such as cortical thickness are then plotted onto the cortex using a color code. Trajectory of gray matter loss over the human life span is based on a cohort of 176 subjects between 7 and 78 years of age.[11] Letter *a* represents a region in which the grey matter density decreases rapidly during adolescence (i.e., superior frontal sulcus in which the decrease in gray matter is described by a quadratic equation represented by an inverted U-shaped curve), or follows a more steadily declining time course during the life span (i.e., superior temporal sulcus in which the decrease in grey matter is described by a quadratic equation represented by a U-shaped curve). In *b* and *c*, plots superimposed on the brain show how gray matter density decreases for particular regions with age, with the regions denoted by different letters. (From Sowell ER, Peterson BS, Thompson PM, Welcome SE, Henkenius AL, Toga AW. Mapping cortical change across the human life span. *Nat Neurosci.* 2003; 6:309-315.) Brain maturation and change in grey matter density is mapped by year of age in *d* with fractional change in grey matter shown by color coding (*c* and *d*). (From Toga AW, Thompson PM, Sowell ER. Mapping brain maturation. *Trends Neurosci.* 2006;29:146-159.)

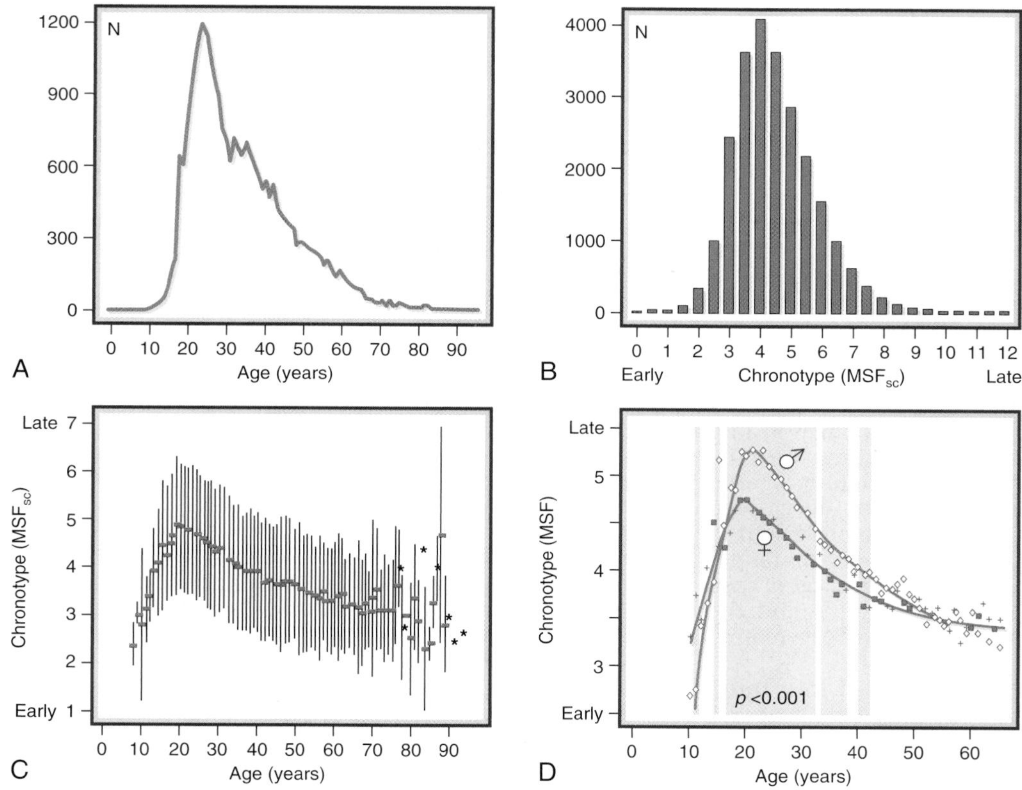

Figure 25-15B Assessment of chronotype (time of awakening in the absence of external cues) using the MCTQ database (N ≈ 25,000). Age distribution within the database **(A)**. Distribution of chronotypes **(B)**. Age-dependent changes **(C)** in average chronotype (± SD) are highly systematic (except for the age groups of 19, 21, 22, and 23, all other age-dependent averages ± SD are significantly different from that of age group 20; *t*-test, $P < .001$). Age-dependent changes of the chronotype **(D)** are different for males and females (*filled circles* and *black line*: females; *open circles* and *gray line*: males). Gray areas indicate significant male-female differences (*t*-test, $P < .001$). (From Roenneberg T, Kuehnle T, Pramstaller PP, et al. A markerfor the end of adolescence. *Curr Biol.* 2004;14:R1038-R1039.)

non–rapid eye movement sleep) is thought to be restorative to learning and other activities of the waking state, and the most restorative portion is high-amplitude delta-wave sleep. During adolescence, the time spent in deep (stage 4) sleep declines by 40% to 50%, and increased (19.7%) stage 2 sleep occurs with pubertal development. The decline of slow-wave sleep during adolescence may reflect developmental changes of the brain.

When an individual is allowed to "run free," the period is entrained (synchronized) to the earth's 24-hour light-dark cycle. Because human beings had little to do after dark, evolution favored an early bedtime, but within this schedule, developmental changes occur. One-year-old infants sleep an average of 11 hours per day, and by age 18, if circumstances permit, the mean is 8 hours. Older people have earlier waking times and rate themselves as more morning-like than adolescents or young adults; because children are also morning-like, there is an inverted U-shaped curve of preferred times of awakening across the span of development. This change to evening from morning alertness during puberty appears to be related to biologic factors, in contrast to social factors; in the past, social factors were thought to be more important.

Without the pressure of work or school, adolescents would stay up longer and awaken hours later than a normal weekday schedule would dictate, a schedule far different from the one they followed at a younger age. Adolescents with early school starts awaken earlier than those with later school starts, but they do not change the time they go to sleep, leading to great variation in the amount of sleep attained. Data from the Add Health study showed decreased self-reported sleep duration during self-reported pubertal development, with girls reporting more problems with sleep (e.g., insomnia, insufficient sleep, awakening tired) as puberty progressed but with no such relationship seen in boys.[228] There is an increase in daytime sleepiness during adolescence, particularly during midpuberty up to stage 3 to 4, even if total sleep time is held constant during longitudinal multiple-year studies.[229] With voluntary sleep deprivation (e.g., with late-night homework habits), sleepiness can reach levels seen in narcolepsy and sleep apnea. Adolescents adapt more poorly to changes in sleep patterns than other age groups; this is manifested in the difference in hours awake between the school week and the weekend. Adolescents are able to shift to a later schedule more easily than to an earlier schedule. When self-selected bedtimes are late during summer but have to be changed to allow school attendance, the adjustment is particularly lengthy and difficult.

After study of 27,000 individuals, it was proposed that the point of inflection from evening alertness during adolescence (after a morning-like pattern in childhood) to morning alertness in adulthood might be used as a marker of the end of adolescence, a sign that developmental remodeling of brain pathways is completed.[230] The age of this inflection point is about 20.9 years in males and 19.5 years in females, who have an earlier change in this and other aspects of puberty than males (see Fig. 25-15B).

Normal Pubertal Behavior and Pathology in Puberty

Most of this chapter deals with the biochemical and physical changes of puberty, but there are also profound psychosocial changes during this period, usually denoted as *adolescence.* Although the attainment of an adult role in society occurs within a few years after achievement of reproductive maturity in non-Western societies, the more technologically advanced the society, the more protracted the time allowed for adolescent psychosocial development. The prolonged period of adolescence in current society, ranging from 11 to 20 years in the United States, arose recently in human history, beginning no more than 100 years ago in Western society.

As expressed by Remschmidt, the most important psychological and psychosocial changes in adolescence are the emergence of abstract thinking, the growing ability to absorb the perspectives or viewpoints of others, an increased capacity for introspection, the development of personal and sexual identity, the establishment of a system of values, increasing autonomy from family and personal independence, greater importance of peer relationships of sometimes subcultural quality, and the emergence of skills and coping strategies to overcome problems and crises.[231]

Adolescence may be divided into three periods (early, middle, and late) by chronologic age. However, these periods may be reached at different maturational ages, because rates of physiologic maturation differ among individuals in these age groups.[232]

Early adolescence (age 11 to 15 years) encompasses most of the physical changes of puberty and in American society includes a profound social change from the sheltered, single-classroom environment of elementary school to the multiple-classroom and multiple-teacher experience of middle school or junior high school. The individual develops a maturing, but not mature, capacity for abstract thought and decision-making processes in contrast to the concrete reasoning of childhood.

Middle adolescence (ages 15 to 17 years) is the period of the high school years, a calmer period than early adolescence. The school experience is not a striking change, and many of the most prominent biologic and physical changes of puberty have been accomplished. There is acceptance of some increased autonomy (e.g., drivers' permits and licenses are allowed), but the individual still lives at home. The individual emotionally moves away from the family and is less influenced by his or her peer group than are early adolescents; friendships assume an increasingly important role.

Late adolescence starts at the senior year of high school and is the age of acceptance of adult roles in work, family, and community. If the individual attends college, this stage is prolonged.

Behavior and Normal Puberty

Almost 100 years ago, Hall, without using what would be considered contemporary research techniques, characterized the maturing child as experiencing *Sturm und Drang* (i.e., storm and stress), which is normally restrained by cultural influences.[233] Contrary to this view, most recent empiric studies describe adolescent development as a continuous, adaptive phase of emotional growth characterized more by stability rather than disorder and more by harmonious relationships between generations rather than conflict. Although mood changes are normally more rapid (occurring over hours or days) and marked in teenagers than in adults, these shifts must be differentiated from long-standing mood and behavior changes associated with serious psychopathology.

Turmoil, or truly tumultuous behavior, in adolescence is not a normal phase but may reflect psychopathology that requires diagnosis and treatment. It is often misdiagnosed as a temporary problem of adjustment reactions of adolescence. When the conditions extend from adolescence to the adult stage, they are more severe. A 4-year longitudinal study of normal first-year U.S. high school students showed that 25% experienced *continuous growth,* characterized by smooth, well-adjusted functioning despite stressful situations; 34% experienced *surgent growth*, demonstrating good adaptation in general and short periods of difficulty and distress after some stressful situations. Twenty-one percent were judged to be in *turmoil*, characterized by mood swings, anxiety, and depression; these teenagers mainly came from homes characterized by conflict, familial mental illness, and socioeconomic distress. Many with adolescent turmoil had not "grown out of it" when studied 5 years later and eventually were diagnosed with unipolar and bipolar depressive disorders. It may be concluded that 80% to 90% of adolescents do well psychologically during puberty and are happy individuals, but 10% to 20% have significant difficulties.[234]

Mood and Self-Image in Puberty

Young girls at the beginning of puberty frequently exhibit a negative self-image but a positive body image; positive peer relationships and superior adjustment improvement are observed with continued breast development. Mood in adolescence is not closely related to stage of puberty, but a significant curvilinear trend is seen for depressive affect (i.e., an increase followed by a decrease), for impulse control (a decrease followed by an increase), and according to the level of serum estradiol. These data suggest that hormonal changes may be more important than physical changes as determinants of certain mood and behavior patterns during adolescence.

Behavior in Variations of the Normal Age at Onset of Puberty

Within the normal limits of pubertal development, early-maturing girls and late-maturing boys have the greatest prevalence of adjustment reactions in puberty and thereafter. Boys and girls who mature earlier are at increased risk for abuse.[235]

Early-developing boys are perceived to be more mature, attractive, and smart and are given more leadership roles; late-developing boys are more insecure, more susceptible to lower levels of self-esteem and body image, and more vulnerable to peer pressure, especially in working-class and minority groups. Most of these difficulties of late maturation focus on the decreased height of the individual rather than the lack of sexual development. Social maturation lags even after androgen treatment in patients with severe CDP. Delayed social maturation may put boys at risk for missing educational opportunities.

In contrast, early-maturing girls tend to experience more difficulty, especially in the junior high school setting, where they may attract the attention of older, more mature boys and have a higher prevalence of internalizing symptoms and disorders. Early puberty may lead to negative body image in girls, compared with boys, in whom the effect is positive. Early maturation may increase a propensity to violent behavior, which is fostered by living in a disadvantaged neighborhood. Early pubertal maturation in girls may be related to a small IQ advantage over late-maturing girls. Late-maturing girls are often more comfortable, remaining with the support of their families longer, and they are less often brought to medical attention than late-maturing boys. Early- and late-maturing girls have a tendency to engage in health-risking behaviors involving strategies to lose weight, strategies to increase muscle, disordered eating, use of food supplements and steroids, and exercise dependence—tendencies not found in boys at the same developmental stages.

Risk-Taking Behavior

Adolescents who function at lower levels of cognitive complexity or concrete thinking and have an early onset of puberty demonstrate an increase in risk-taking behavior. The age at onset of cigarette smoking and alcohol use is proportional to the age at onset of puberty in girls: early-maturing girls partake earlier, and boys may follow the same pattern.

Sexuality during Puberty

By the time they reach age 19 years of age, 7 of 10 teens have engaged in sexual intercourse (data from http://www.guttmacher.org/pubs/fb_sex_ed02.html [accessed February 2011]). Factors such as the onset of puberty, weak self-concept, having tried smoking or drinking, and not being overweight were significantly associated with early sexual activity in girls. For boys, older age, a poor relationship with parents, low household income, and having tried smoking were factors significantly associated with sexual activity. Add Health revealed that adolescents at the upper and lower ends of the intelligence distribution were less likely to have sex.

Fertility is reached well before adult phenotype is acquired. The number of pregnancies for U.S. girls aged 15 to 19 years is 41.5 per 1000.[133] Sexuality appears to be correlated with testosterone production in boys in some studies, but in others, it appears to be modified by the social effects of pubertal maturation. Religious activity may decrease the likelihood of sexual activity.

The social pressures are more mixed in their messages to girls, both encouraging sexuality and restricting it in a way more disparate than that encountered by boys. The earlier onset of puberty today compared with previous centuries has had a profound effect on societal norms of sexual behavior.[6]

A randomized, double-blind, placebo-controlled, crossover clinical trial of boys and girls with delayed puberty addressing the effects of administration of oral conjugated estrogen to girls and testosterone enanthate to boys at three dose levels that were intended to simulate early, middle, and late pubertal levels demonstrated modest or no effects. Boys had increased nocturnal emission and touching behaviors at the middle and high doses but no other effects. Girls demonstrated a significant increase in "necking" related to the administration of estrogen only at the late pubertal dose and no other effects.

HORMONAL AND METABOLIC CHANGES IN PUBERTY

Increased amplitude and alterations of the patterns of GnRH secretion at puberty initiate and regulate the sequential increases in secretion of pituitary gonadotropins and gonadal steroids that culminate in fertility.

Gonadotropins

Because of the pulsatile secretion of GnRH, gonadotropin secretion is also episodic. The newer immunometric supersensitive assays allow accurate measurement in small pediatric samples. The results are lower than previously reported by the older assays.

During the first 2 years after birth, plasma levels of LH and FSH rise intermittently to adult values and occasionally higher but then remain low until puberty. Ultrasensitive assays and third-generation assays for LH and FSH[236-238] confirm earlier evidence of pulsatile secretion of the gonadotropins in prepuberty and indicate that the basal immunoreactive levels of LH are much lower than previously reported.[237,238] The serum FSH level is higher than the LH level in prepubertal boys and girls.[239] There is a more striking rise in serum LH amplitude by at least 1 year before the onset of puberty (i.e., the peripubertal period immediately preceding the appearance of signs of sexual maturation), whereas FSH rises more consistently through male puberty rather than before, with increased pulse amplitude. An increased amplitude of LH and FSH secretion occurs at night in prepubertal boys and girls by 5 years of age[237,238]; the amplitude and frequency of such peaks increase, and daytime secretion increases with the progression of pubertal development.

In girls, FSH levels rise during the early stages of puberty, and LH levels tend to rise in the later stages; from beginning to late puberty, the LH concentration rises more than 100-fold. In boys, FSH levels rise progressively through puberty, and LH levels rise and reach an early plateau (Figs. 25-16 and 25-17).

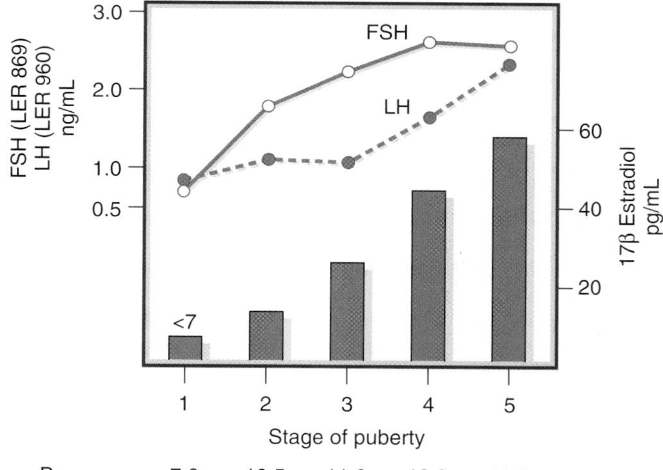

Figure 25-16 Mean plasma estradiol, follicle-stimulating hormone (FSH), and luteinizing hormone (LH) concentrations in prepubertal and pubertal females by pubertal stage of maturation (1, prepubertal; 5, menstruating adolescents) and the mean bone age for each stage. Single daytime values of gonadotropins have limited usefulness because of pulsatility of gonadotropin release and the increased amplitude of LH pulses during sleep throughout puberty. The gonadal steroid values, however, are useful in determining the stage of pubertal development. To convert FSH values (LER-869) to international units per liter, multiply by 8.4. To convert LH values (LER-960) to international units per liter, multiply by 3.8. To convert estradiol values to picomoles per liter, multiply by 3.671. (From Grumbach MM. Onset of puberty. In: Berenberg SR, ed. *Puberty, Biologic and Social Components*. Leiden, The Netherlands: H.E. Stenfert Kroese, 1975:1-21. Reprinted by permission of Kluwer Academic Publishers.)

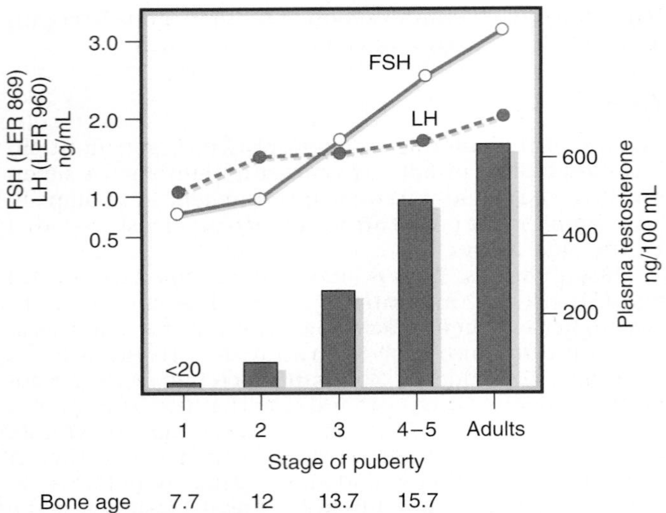

Figure 25-17 Mean plasma testosterone (after solvent extraction and chromatography) and gonadotropin levels in normal boys by stage of maturation (1, prepubertal) and mean bone age for each stage (see Fig. 25-16). To convert testosterone values to nanomoles per liter, multiply by 0.03467. (From Grumbach MM. Onset of puberty. In: Berenberg SR, ed. *Puberty, Biologic and Social Components.* Leiden, The Netherlands: H.E. Stenfert Kroese, 1975:1-21. Reprinted by permission of Kluwer Academic Publishers.)

Disorderly patterns of secretion of LH, but not FSH, were noted just before the onset of puberty; this was followed by, first, increased orderliness in early puberty and, then, increased disorderliness again in later puberty. This suggests that a more integrated feedback system operates in early puberty and is then followed by less stablility.[240]

Doses of exogenous GnRH that are relatively ineffective in stimulating gonadotropin or gonadal steroid secretion before puberty become effective with the onset of puberty; an amplification occurs in the hypothalamic-pituitary-gonadal axis with progression of puberty.[241,242] Although the GnRH test usually requires multiple sampling after the administration of GnRH, a single determination at 30, 45, or 60 minutes may suffice with the new, sensitive assays. Use of a GnRH agonist in a single dose with determination of serum gonadotropins and sex steroids can help to differentiate the pubertal from the prepubertal state. The basal values of serum LH and FSH measured in modern supersensitive assays are reported to predict the onset of pubertal development as well as GnRH testing does; a value of serum LH greater than 4 mIU/mL measured by immunochemiluminometric assay is consistent with the onset of puberty. Moreover, the use of these ultrasensitive assays to determine concentrations of LH and FSH in urine reveals a pattern of a 5-fold rise in urinary FSH in boys and girls, with a 50-fold rise in urinary LH in boys and a 100-fold rise in girls during puberty.[243]

In addition to the well-defined quantitative changes that occur in the pattern of FSH and LH in the pituitary gland, serum, and urine during development, qualitative changes occur. The pattern of glycosylation of the α and the β subunits of the gonadotropins is influenced by maturation, GnRH secretion, and the effects of gonadal steroids on the pituitary gonadotrophs. Variation in glycosylation that affects the size and charge of the hormone is the principal cause of the heterogeneity of FSH and LH and the large number of isoforms that vary according to the more acidic or more basic charge.[244] This pleomorphism has an important effect on biologic half-life and biologic activity and provides an additional mechanism of regulating the biologic activity of the gonadotropins. Discrepancies between serum bioactivity and immunoactivity of LH during pubertal development have been reported by some but not all researchers. However, a change in the isoforms of FSH released during puberty may favor the secretion of increased bioactive FSH, which may favor reproductive development.[244]

Gonadal Steroids

Only recently has it been appreciated that many actions on linear skeletal growth, skeletal maturation, and accretion of bone mass thought to be due to testosterone in the male are mainly attributable to its peripheral aromatization to estrogen (Table 25-7).

Testosterone

The Leydig cells of the testes produce testosterone and, in lesser amounts, androstenedione, α5-androstenediol, dihydrotestosterone, and estradiol, although a small amount of testosterone is derived from extraglandular conversion of androstenedione secreted by the testes and the adrenal. In the female, extraglandular conversion of ovarian and adrenal androstenedione accounts for almost all of the circulating testosterone.

Previous methods of determination of low levels of sex steroids have been demonstrated to be inaccurate.[245,246] This insensitivity is mainly due to the presence of interfering substances and relative insensitivity of antibodies used in assays. Now, larger national laboratories are beginning to use high-performance liquid chromatography tandem mass spectrometry (HPLC-MS/MS), which allows the accurate measurement of extremely low values present in pediatric samples.[247] These newer techniques may lead to

TABLE 25-7

Early Clinical Clues to the Effect of Estrogen on Growth and Skeletal Maturation in the Male

Complete androgen insensitivity (resistance) syndrome (Zachmann M, Prader A, Sobel EH, et al. Pubertal growth in patients with androgen insensitivity: indirect evidence for the importance of estrogen in pubertal growth of girls. *J Pediatr.* 1986;108:694-697)
Short-term estradiol administration increased rate of ulnar growth in prepubertal boys (Caruso-Nicoletti M, Cassorla FG, Skerda MC, et al. Short term, low dose estradiol accelerates ulnar growth in boys. *J Clin Endocrinol Metab.* 1985;61:896-898)
Aromatase inhibitor decreased rapid growth and skeletal maturation in testotoxicosis, whereas antiandrogen had no effect on skeletal maturation (Laue L, Jones J, Barnes K, et al. Treatment of familial male precocious puberty with spironolactone and deslorelin. *J Clin Endocrinol Metab.* 1993;76:151-155)
Aromatase excess syndrome in boys associated with increased rate of growth and skeletal maturation, elevated plasma estrogen concentrations, but prepubertal testosterone values (Stratakis CA, Vottero A, Brodie A, et al. The aromatase excess syndrome is associated with feminization of both sexes and autosomal dominant transmission of aberrant P450 aromatase gene transcription. *J Clin Endocrinol Metab.* 1998;83:1349-1357)
Estrogen-secreting tumors: adrenal and testicular neoplasms (especially Peutz-Jeghers syndrome) (Bulun SE, Rosenthal IM, Brodie AM, et al. Use of tissue-specific promoters in the regulation of aromatase cytochrome P450 gene expression in human testicular and ovarian sex cord tumors, as well as in normal fetal and adult gonads. *J Clin Endocrinol Metab.* 1993;77:1616-1621)

From Grumbach MM. Estrogen, bone, growth, and sex: a sea change in conventional wisdom. *J Pediatr Endocrinol Metab.* 2000;13(suppl 6):1439-1455.

revision of some of the results (described here) obtained by older methods.

Prepubertal boys and girls have plasma testosterone concentrations of less than 0.3 nmol/L (0.1 ng/mL),[236-238,248] except during the first 3 to 5 months of infancy in the male, when pubertal levels are found. Nighttime elevations of serum testosterone levels are detectable in the male by 5 years of age, before the onset of physical signs of puberty, and increase during early puberty after the appearance of sleep-entrained secretion of LH and increased pituitary sensitivity to GnRH. The 60-minute lag between the peak of LH and the increase in testosterone is presumably due to synthesis and secretion of the steroid. In the daytime, increases in testosterone levels are detectable at approximately 11 years in boys after the testis volume is greater than 4 mL, with a consistent increase throughout puberty. The steepest increment in testosterone concentration occurs between pubertal stages 2 and 3 in males (see Fig. 25-17 and Table 25-5). The ratio of testosterone to epitestosterone in the urine, which is used to evaluate "doping" of athletes, may be elevated normally during puberty.

Free testosterone measurements may be determined by dialysis or by calculation using testosterone values and available protein binding sites; the accuracy of the testosterone assay can be problematic.[247] Nonetheless, if the total testosterone concentration on which the free testosterone level is based is measured by a highly specific assay, free or bioavailable testosterone determinations are helpful in evaluation of PCOS or nonclassic congenital adrenal hyperplasia (CAH) in girls.

A sensitive mammalian cell recombinant bioassay for androgen bioactivity strongly correlates with serum immunoreactive testosterone concentration and demonstrates a rise with pubertal development in concert with progression of pubic hair and penile development in patients with CDP.[249] In contrast to this specific bioassay, a novel, highly sensitive transcriptional androgen receptor–mediated bioassay system demonstrated higher circulating values of bioactive androgen in menopausal women and is now being directed toward children.[250]

The values of sex steroids measured in saliva are much lower than in the serum, but trauma (even tooth brushing) that leads to blood in the specimen can influence the results, and the accuracy of the basic assay is critical (see earlier discussion).[247] The steroid level in saliva is not a direct representation of free steroid in the serum, as is often claimed. Testosterone in saliva is said in some reports to correlate well with serum levels of testosterone in normal subjects and in patients with chronic disease (e.g., cystic fibrosis). Salivary progesterone is said to rise with the progression of puberty. Salivary dehydroepiandrosterone (DHEA) is higher after the onset of puberty than before. Salivary steroid measurements, if accurate, can increase the ability of investigators to address the relationship between development and behavior in a noninvasive manner, but it may take the use of LC/MS-MS in salivary assays to achieve such accuracy.

Estrogens

In the female, estradiol is secreted principally (90%) by the ovary; a small fraction of circulating estradiol arises from the extraglandular conversion of testosterone and androstenedione. In the male, approximately 75% of estradiol is derived from extraglandular aromatization of testosterone and (indirectly) androstenedione, and 25% is from testicular secretion.

In the fetus and at term, estrogen is high due to conversion of fetal and maternal adrenal C19-steroids to estrogen by the placenta, but they drop precipitously during the first few days of life. Plasma estradiol levels are so low in prepuberty that detection by standard immunoassays was difficult, but a rise through puberty and a diurnal rhythm were described with a sensitive radioimmunoassay (Table 25-8; see Fig. 25-16).[251] Estrone levels rise early and reach a plateau by midpuberty. A highly sensitive bioassay demonstrated higher estradiol concentrations in girls than in boys before puberty, with a rise through puberty until the pubertal growth spurt and a decrease thereafter. There is a significant correlation between peak growth velocity and the rise in estradiol concentration; the rise is earlier in girls than in boys, but bioactive estradiol levels are equivalent at peak growth velocity.[151,252] The higher estrogen levels in girls may be an important factor in the more advanced levels of skeletal maturation in girls compared with boys and may play a part in their earlier onset of sexual maturation. A new human cell bioassay measuring total estrogenic bioactivity (rather than estradiol alone) in children has an extremely sensitive detection limit of less than 1 pg/mL.[253]

The daily peak of estradiol in early pubertal girls occurs about 6 to 9 hours after the peak of serum LH detected during the night, apparently related to time required for synthesis. In all stages of puberty, boys have higher concentrations of estrone than estradiol, and levels of both estrogens are lower than those measured in girls at comparable stages.

Hormonal Control of the Pubertal Growth Spurt

Postnatal growth follows a specific pattern: a very high growth rate just after birth is followed by a declaration that continues until 3 years of age; next, there is a slower phase of deceleration until puberty. The subsequent pubertal growth spurt, the second greatest period of postnatal growth, is followed by maturation of the spine and long bones until adult height is reached.[140] Many factors influence the growth plate.[254] The adolescent growth spurt in normal girls and boys depends on estradiol and GH levels,[150,255-257] among other factors.

Hormonal control of the pubertal growth spurt is complex (Fig. 25-18; see Fig. 25-14). GH is involved in increasing growth at puberty through stimulation of IGF1 production. Gonadal steroids have two effects on pubertal growth: (1) induction of an increase in GH secretion, with a consequent increase in IGF1 production, thereby indirectly stimulating pubertal growth, and (2) a direct effect on cartilage and bone through stimulation of local production of IGF1 and other local factors.[151,258,259]

Gonadal Steroids

In the developing human skeleton, gonadal steroids have growth-promoting and maturational effects on chondrocytes, osteoblasts, and other bone constituents.[150,151] This action, which eventually leads to epiphyseal fusion and the cessation of longitudinal growth in boys and girls, is mediated mainly by estrogen that is directly secreted (in girls) or arises from the conversion of testosterone and androstenedione to estrogen in peripheral tissues by aromatase (see Table 25-8). Detection of estrogen resistance resulting from a null mutation in the gene encoding the estrogen receptor and from derangements in the *CYP19A1* gene, leading to severe cytochrome P450 aromatase deficiency, has highlighted the cardinal role of estradiol (but not testosterone) in both boys and girls in the pubertal growth spurt, completion of epiphyseal maturation, and normal skeletal proportions and mineralization.[150,151] Individuals

TABLE 25-8

Plasma Gonadal Steroid Values in Children

Steroid and Assay	Age	Normal Values: Males	Normal Values: Females	Sample Volume (Pediatric Minimums)
Testosterone, by LC-MS/MS (ng/dL)	Term infant	75-400	20-64	0.18 mL serum (Quest) 0.5 mL serum (Esoterix) 0.15 mL serum (ARUP)
	1-7 mo	Levels decrease rapidly in first week to 20-50, then increase to 60-400 between 20 and 60 days. Levels then decline to prepubertal range by 7 mo	Levels decrease during the first month to <10 and remain at that level until puberty	
	7-12 mo	<16	<11	
	Tanner stage I	<16	<16	
	Tanner stage II	<167	<40	
	Tanner stage III	7-762*	<60	
	Tanner stage IV	25-912	<62	
	Tanner stage V	110-975	<68*	
Androstenedione, by RIA after extraction (ng/dL)	Term infant	20-290; levels decrease to 10-80 after 1 week	20-290 ng/dL; levels decrease to 10-80 after 1 week	0.25 mL serum (Esoterix) 0.5 mL serum (Quest)
	1-11 mo	6-68	6-68	
	Prepubertal	8-50	8-50	
	Tanner I	8-50	8-50	
	Tanner II	31-65	42-100	
	Tanner III	50-100	80-190	
	Tanner IV	48-140	77-225	
	Tanner V	65-210	80-240	
DHT, by extraction chromatography, RIA (ng/dL)	1-6 mo	12-85	<5	0.5 mL serum (Esoterix) 1.1 mL serum (Quest)
	Prepubertal	<5	<5	
	Tanner II-III	3-33	5-19	
	Tanner IV-V	22-75	3-30	
Estradiol, by LC-MS/MS (ng/dL)	Newborn	Levels are markedly elevated and fall during first week to <1.5	Levels are markedly elevated and fall during first week to <1.5	1.2 mL serum (Esoterix)
	1-11 mo	Levels increase to 1-3.2 between 1-2 mo, then decrease to <1.5 by 6 mo	Levels increase to 0.5-5 between 1 and 2 months, then decrease to <1.5 during the first year	
	Prepubertal	<1.5	<1.5	
	Tanner I	0.5-1.1	0.5-2	
	Tanner II	0.5-1.6	1-2.4	
	Tanner III	0.5-2.5	0.7-6	
	Tanner IV	1-3.6	2.1-8.5	
	Tanner V	1-3.6	3.4-17	
Estradiol, by extraction chromatography, RIA (ng/dL)	Tanner stage I	0.3-1.5	0.5-1	0.6 mL (Quest)
	Tanner stage II	0.3-1	0.5-11.5	
	Tanner stage III	0.5-1.5	0.5-18	
	Tanner stage IV	0.3-4	2.5-34.5	
	Tanner stage V	1.5-4.5	2.5-41	
Estradiol, chemiluminescent immunoassay (ng/dL)	0-8	0.7-0.8	0.7-1.4	0.2 mL serum (ARUP)
	9-10	0.7-1.1	0.7-3.2	
	11-12	0.7-2.2	0.7-3.8	
	13-14	0.7-2.4	1-9.1	
	15-16	1.1-3.3	1.7-18.1	
	17-40	1.8-6.7	2.3-17.0	
Extrone, by LC-MS/MS (ng/dL)		Levels are markedly elevated at birth, then decrease during first week to <1.5	Levels are markedly elevated at birth, then decrease during first week to <1.5	1.2 mL serum (Esoterix)
	Prepubertal	<1.5	<1.5	
	Tanner I	0.5-1.7	0.4-2.9	
	Tanner II	1.0-2.5	1-3.3	
	Tanner III	1.5-2.5	1.5-4.3	
	Tanner IV	1.5-4.5	1.6-7.7	
	Tanner V	2-4.5	2.9-10.5	

*Because this chart combines values from different laboratories, the ranges are larger in the aggregate than would be found in the specific laboratories' standards. Please consult the laboratory being used to interpret results for clinical decisions.

DHT, dihydrotestosterone; LC-MS/MS, liquid chromatography tandem mass spectrometry; RIA, radioimmunoassay.

From Albrecht L, Styne D. Laboratory testing of gonadal steroids in children. *Pediatr Endocrinol Rev.* 2007; 5(suppl 1):599-607.

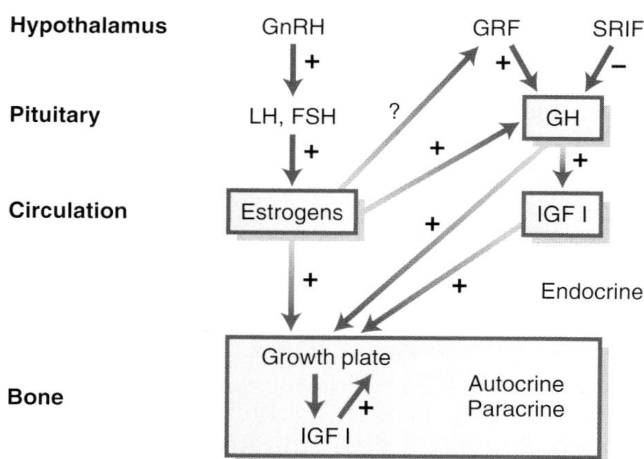

Figure 25-18 Interactions of the major growth-promoting hormones during puberty. Plus (+) indicates stimulatory action; minus (–) indicates inhibitory action. Circulating insulin-like growth factor I (IGFI) arises mainly from liver, but other tissues also contribute (i.e., endocrine action). Growth hormone (GH) and gonadal steroids have a direct stimulatory effect on the generation of IGFI (i.e., paracrine action) locally in bone and cartilage cells. For simplification, the feedback loops for IGFI and gonadal steroids on the hypothalamic pituitary unit are omitted. FSH, follicle-stimulating hormone; GRF, growth hormone–releasing factor; LH, luteinizing hormone; SRIF, somatotropin release–inhibiting factor.

with a mutation in the ERα gene *(ESR1)* or the *CYP19A1* gene encoding aromatase continue to grow, lack a pubertal growth spurt, and have open epiphyses and osteopenia.[150,151,255-257] Estrogen treatment of men with aromatase deficiency leads to epiphyseal closure, cessation of growth, and a striking increase in bone mass.[260-262] Patients with aromatase excess, who produce excess estrogen, have advanced skeletal maturation and rapid growth and ultimately reach short adult stature.[263]

Although estradiol secreted by the ovary has long been recognized as the major sex steroid responsible for the pubertal growth spurt, skeletal maturation, and bone mineral accrual in females, until the detection of the rare human genetic defects in estrogen synthesis or action, conventional wisdom dictated that testosterone mediated these maturational changes during puberty in males. Now it is known that estrogen (not androgen) is the critical sex hormone in males and females in the pubertal growth spurt, skeletal maturation, accrual of peak bone mass, and maintenance of bone mass in the adult. Estrogen stimulates chondrogenesis in the epiphyseal growth plate,[264] increasing pubertal linear growth. At puberty, estrogen promotes skeletal maturation and the gradual progressive closure of the epiphyseal growth plate.[150] The use of a supersensitive assay for plasma estradiol in prepubertal and pubertal boys revealed a high positive correlation between estradiol concentrations and peak growth velocity (but not serum GH level), which was greatest about 3 years after the onset of puberty,[252] further implicating estrogen in the pubertal growth spurt and skeletal maturation of boys and girls.

There are estrogen receptors, both EPα and ERβ, in the growth plate chondrocytes.[254] Histologic studies of the bone and cartilage of rodents treated with corticosteroids or estrogen and clinical evaluations of children with precocious puberty support the theory that senescence of the growth plate occurs because of estrogen exposure in precocious puberty, causing decreased growth during treatment with GnRH agonists.[265]

The high rate of bone turnover in early puberty followed by a decrease in periosteal apposition and endosteal resorption within cortical bone and decreased bone remodeling within cortical and cancellous bone mediated by apoptosis of chondrocytes in the growth plate and osteoclasts within cortical and cancellous bone, is mediated in part by estrogen. This leads to a reduction in bone turnover markers at menarche, reflecting the closure of the epiphyseal growth plates.[266]

Girls with Turner syndrome without estrogen exposure retain elevated markers of bone turnover. Prepubertal girls with Turner syndrome tend to lose bone, but that ceases when estrogen therapy begins; administration of estrogen may best be started earlier in these patients.[267] During puberty and into the third decade, estrogen has an anabolic effect on the osteoblast and an apoptotic effect on the osteoclast, increasing bone mineral acquisition in the axial and appendicular skeletons. Evolutionary theory suggests that positive effects of estrogen on bone density, added to mechanical loading, allow women to carry increased weight for pregnancy and lactation; this process is unnecessary after reproduction, and osteoporosis becomes more common at menopause.[268]

Testosterone may also have a direct action on bone in the human male, because androgen receptors are found in human tibial growth plates in osteoblasts and chondrocytes, osteocytes, mononuclear cells, and endothelial cells of blood vessels in the bone marrow.[269] Androgens that cannot be aromatized to estrogen still cause an increase in growth rate, presumably due to interaction with these receptors. The greater increase in periosteal bone deposition, the resultant thickening of cortical bone and greater bone strength, and the greater bone dimensions[269] in boys probably result from direct effects of testosterone. Androgens may protect men against osteoporosis by maintenance of cancellous bone mass and expansion of cortical bone.

A pubertal growth spurt leading to adult height close to that of genotypic men occurs in individuals with the complete form of androgen resistance, demonstrating the critical role of estrogen rather than androgen in the adolescent growth spurt in boys. A modest decrease in BMD Z-scores occurs in the spine but not in the hip based on age-specific female standard values, but the reductions are greater when male standards are used. Affected women have an increased prevalence of fractures, even with estrogen replacement. This suggests that lack of a direct effect of testosterone on the skeleton, especially the spine, has a part in the defects in bone mineralization observed in women with complete androgen insensitivity (see Table 25-8).[270]

Growth Hormone and Growth Factors

GH secretion approximately doubles during puberty in boys and girls in the basal state or after stimulation but decreases after pubertal development. Remarkably, peak values after hexarelin, a 6-amino-acid GH-releasing peptide (or GH secretagogue) stimulates as much growth hormone secretion in prepuberty as in puberty. The greater elevation in girls starts at an earlier age and pubertal stage than in boys due to the earlier onset of puberty in girls. GH secretion increases coincident with the onset of breast development (Tanner stage 2) and is maximal at Tanner stage 3 to 4 breast development; in boys, GH rises later and peaks at stage 4 genital development. GH secretion and IGF1 levels decrease after late puberty in both sexes. Adolescents of normal height have an inverse relationship between weight and GH levels. Increased GH pulse amplitude and content of GH secreted per pulse (not but frequency, metabolic clearance rate, or intersecretory burst interval and half-life of GH) in the basal state are mainly responsible for the augmented GH levels.[271]

The increase in estradiol at puberty, which in boys results from testicular secretion and extraglandular synthesis from testosterone and androstenedione and in girls from secretion by the ovaries, is the principal mediator of the increase in pulse amplitude and amount of GH secreted per pulse.[272] Administration of exogenous androgens in delayed puberty raises GH secretion. Transdermal application of testosterone increases spontaneous GH secretion overnight independent of growth hormone–releasing hormone (GHRH), because infusion of GnRH antagonist does not affect this phenomenon.[273] The effect of testosterone is mediated mainly through its conversion to estradiol, because treatment of late pubertal boys with tamoxifen, an estrogen receptor blocker, causes smaller GH secretory peaks and fewer GH secretory episodes. Exogenous estrogen increases the peak GH reached after insulin-induced hypoglycemia, exercise, and arginine, a priming effect that is used in clinical practice, because estrogen administered before a provocative test in prepubertal subjects increases the GH response. Androgens that cannot be aromatized to estrogen (e.g., oxandrolone, dihydrotestosterone) have less effect on GH secretion; however, androgen blockade with flutamide increases GH secretion.[274,275] Dihydrotestosterone, which is not aromatized to estrogen, does not increase GH secretion or the plasma concentration of IGF1 and may decrease the integrated GH secretion, but it still stimulates increased growth rate, suggesting a possible direct effect of androgen on pubertal growth independent of GH[258] or estradiol. Increased GH secretion also occurs in sexual precocity. GH secretion decreases with the fall in gonadal steroid levels after treatment of CPP with potent GnRH agonists.[276]

GH deficiency or GH resistance causes an attenuated pubertal growth spurt, indicating the importance of GH and IGF1 in this process. Severe primary or secondary hypogonadism leads to a minimal or absent growth spurt, demonstrating the primary role of gonadal steroids in pubertal growth. Hypopituitary patients deficient in GH and gonadotropins do not have an adolescent growth spurt when GH alone is replaced; gonadal steroids must also be given, substantiating the interaction of GH and gonadal steroids in the pubertal growth spurt. In normal puberty, neither the magnitude of the increase in GH secretion nor the concentration of plasma IGF1 correlates with the PHV of the pubertal growth spurt. Although a threshold level of GH secretion is necessary, the extent of the growth spurt correlates with gonadal sex steroid secretion. Individuals with both CPP and GH deficiency (usually as a consequence of cranial irradiation for a brain tumor) have a growth spurt clinically indistinguishable from that of CPP and normal GH secretion.[258] After treatment with a GnRH agonist for sexual precocity, growth velocity in patients with GH deficiency and CPP is decreased and pubertal progression is suppressed, illustrating the direct effect of gonadal steroids, principally estradiol, on the pubertal growth spurt.

Urinary GH excretion reflects serum levels and changes occurring with pubertal development. A peak is reached at pubertal stage 3 to 4. The level is higher in boys than in girls.

Growth Hormone–Binding Protein

Growth hormone–binding protein (GHBP) has the same amino acid sequence as the extracellular component of the GH receptor, and serum concentrations are directly related to the amount of GH receptors. In normal children, the plasma GHBP level is inversely related to 24-hour GH secretion. The serum GHBP level rises early in childhood and also through puberty in some cross-sectional studies, but not in others. Because plasma GHBP does not change appreciably with the onset of puberty, at the time of the pubertal growth spurt there is a relative increase in unbound (free) GH in relation to GH bound to GHBP. GHBP is related to adiposity, and it may be this factor that accounts for the increased levels of GHBP in girls compared with boys, the rise in GHBP in girls with precocious puberty, and the negative influence of testosterone on GHBP levels.[277]

Insulin-Like Growth Factor Type I

Concentrations of IGF1 rise during puberty to levels higher than those of prepuberty or adulthood; they remain elevated past the time of PHV, with a peak attained 1 or 2 years after the pubertal growth spurt (later in boys than in girls) and then fall to normal adult levels.[276,278] The pattern of the GH-dependent serum levels of IGF-binding protein 3 (IGFBP3) in pubertal development is similar to that of serum IGF1.[279] However, serum IGFBP3 concentrations correlate with BMI even though IGF1 does not. Measurement of free IGF1 shows the same pattern of change with development as the that of total IGF1, a slow rise in serum free IGF1 in prepuberty followed by a steeper rise during puberty. A decrease of free IGF1 is associated with age in the later stages of puberty.[279,280] The increase in the serum ratio of IGF1 to IGFBP3 at the time of the pubertal growth spurt appears to result from production, because proteolysis of IGFBP3 does not change in puberty in normal children. The testosterone level in boys and the estradiol level in girls correlate with the rise in IGF1 concentration, but gonadal steroids are not the direct cause of the increase in circulating IGF1 levels; rather, GH secretion approximately doubles during puberty due to the effect of estrogen causing augmented release of GH.

Plasma IGF1 concentrations are high for chronologic age in sexual precocity and low in delayed puberty. Estrogen mediates the pubertal increase in IGF1 concentration through increased secretion of GH, with an additional effect through the gonadal steroid–induced local generation of IGF1 in cartilage and bone. Treatment with GnRH agonist in a 16-year-old boy with a homozygous mutation in the WSXWS-like motif of the human GH receptor (GHR) causing Laron syndrome led to a further decrease in the already low serum levels of IGF1 and IGFBP3, which did not reverse with dihydrotestosterone treatment, suggesting a direct effect of estradiol on IGF1 production.[281] Children with CPP treated with a GnRH agonist showed suppression of the untreated elevated serum GH concentrations and a decrease in plasma IGF1 concentrations, although not to prepubertal values, supporting the concept that GH is the major (but not the only) factor that raises circulating IGF1 levels in puberty.[276,282]

A confounding factor is the relative roles of hepatic-generated circulating IGF1 (i.e., endocrine role) and of locally produced IGF1 (i.e., paracrine/autocrine role) in linear growth. For example, mice with a totally deleted hepatic IGF1 gene have strikingly reduced circulating levels of IGF1 but normal postnatal body and bone growth.[283]

GH stimulates local IGF1 production in resting zone chondrocytes, located at the epiphyseal end of the growth plate in the area known as the reserve zone or stem cell zone, through GH receptors in the chondrocytes. This IGF1 production stimulates, through autocrine and paracrine effects, the clonal expansion of proliferating chondrocytes derived from the resting chondrocyte or germ cells. GH and IGF1 can reduce the stem cell cycle time, proliferating cell cycle time and duration of the hypertrophic phase, a phase that leads to apoptosis, leaving the cells serving as a scaffold for the mineralization and production of new bone.

Other Hormones

There are glucocorticoid receptors in human growth plates, mostly in hypertrophic chondrocytes. However, children with chronic adrenal insufficiency who receive appropriate replacement therapy have a normal pubertal growth spurt despite deficient adrenal androgen secretion, indicating a minimal impact of these adrenal androgens on normal growth at puberty.[284]

Hypothyroid subjects lack a pubertal growth spurt even when the disorder is accompanied by sexual precocity.[285] Thyroid hormone has a permissive role in the pubertal growth spurt but is a requisite for normal growth. Hypothyroidism decreases GH secretion and affects growth indirectly. However, thyroid hormone also interacts with the thyroid hormone receptors $\alpha1$ and β, whose proteins are found in early proliferating chondrocytes of the human growth plate, and the messenger RNA (mRNA) found in other developing stages of chondrocytes and osteoblasts. Thyroid hormones also interact with the local effects of IGF1 and GH at the growth plate.[254]

Adrenal Androgens. There is a progressive increase in plasma levels of Δ^5-steroids, DHEA, and DHEAS in boys and girls that begins before age 8 (skeletal age of 6 to 8 years) and continues through early adulthood (Table 25-9). The increase in the secretion of adrenal androgen and its precursors is known as *adrenarche*, and the appearance of pubic hair caused by adrenarche is known as *pubarche*. Plasma DHEA levels have a diurnal rhythm similar to that of cortisol, but plasma levels of DHEAS show less variation and are a useful biochemical marker of adrenarche.

DHEA is the predominant precursor to more potent androgens in females, and DHEAS cannot be converted. DHEAS is produced from DHEA by the action of SULT2A1, mainly in the adrenal glands and the liver. The sulfate donor phosphoadenosine phosphosulfate (PAPS) is required by SULT2A1, and in human beings, PAPS is synthesized by the two isoforms of PAPS synthase, PAPSS1 and PAPSS2.[286]

Testosterone-Binding Globulin. Between 97% and 99% of circulating testosterone and estradiol is reversibly bound to testosterone-binding globulin (TeBG) (i.e., sex steroid–binding globulin); prepubertal levels of TeBG are approximately equal in boys and girls, but a decrease in TeBG level occurs with advancing prepubertal age and the concomitant increase in the plasma gonadal steroid levels. At puberty, there is a small decrease in TeBG levels in girls; as a consequence of testosterone, there is a greater decrease in boys, although the drop observed in normal boys is attenuated by treatment with tamoxifen, even with advancing pubertal development.[287] The rise in adrenal androgen levels at adrenarche may explain the early drop in TeBG levels, which allows more circulating free hormone at a given concentration of testosterone. Although the plasma concentration of testosterone is 20 times greater in men than in women, the concentration of free testosterone is 40 times greater.[288] Boys with hypogonadotropic hypogonadism and patients with the androgen resistance syndrome show the same characteristic fall in TeBG levels at puberty, but values are intermediate between those of normal adult males and females.

Prolactin. Prolactin levels rise in girls during puberty. Prepubertal mean (± standard error) plasma prolactin concentrations are 4.0 ± 0.5 μg/L in boys and 4.5 ± 0.6 μg/L in girls. Late pubertal girls and adult women have higher concentrations of prolactin (7.5 ± 0.7 and 8.3 ± 0.7 μg/L, respectively), whereas the mean concentration in adult men is 5.2 ± 0.4 μg/L.[289] This sex difference is probably a consequence of the higher estradiol levels during puberty in girls and in women.

Inhibin, Activin, and Follistatin. Inhibin and follistatin inhibit and activin stimulates FSH β-subunit expression and therefore affect FSH biosynthesis and secretion. Inhibin may also be an inhibitor of LH release in the follicular phase.[290] These hormones are synthesized in a variety of tissues in addition to the gonads and have diverse activities apart from those on the reproductive apparatus.[291]

Two distinct binding proteins for inhibin and activin are present in the circulation, the gonads, and other tissues: α_2-macroglobulin, a high-capacity, low-affinity binding protein and follistatin, a glycosylated, single-peptide chain that functions as a high-affinity binding protein and as a regulator of activin bioactivity (e.g., in the pituitary gland, a site of synthesis of activin and follistatin).[291] Inhibin, a heterodimeric glycoprotein product of the Sertoli cell of the testes and the ovarian granulosa cell (as well as the placenta and other tissues), exerts negative feedback action on the secretion of FSH from the pituitary. Inhibin is composed of an α-subunit and one of two β-subunits, β_A or β_B, which respectively form inhibin A or inhibin B, dimers with apparently identical function. Inhibin is a member of the transforming growth factor-β (TGF-β) superfamily that includes anti-müllerian hormone (AMH, also called müllerian-inhibiting factor) and the dimers of two inhibin

TABLE 25-9

Mean Serum Concentrations (mmol/L [ng/mL]) of DHEAS during Childhood

	6-8 yr	8-10 yr	10-12 yr	12-14 yr	14-16 yr	16-20 yr
By Chronologic Age						
Boys	0.5 (188)	1.6 (586)	3.4 (1260)	3.6 (1330)	7.2 (2640)	7.2 (2640)
Girls	0.8 (306)	3.2 (1170)	3.1 (1130)	4.6 (1690)	6.9 (2540)	6.3 (2320)
By Bone Age						
Boys	0.98 (360)	1.6 (574)	3.4 (1250)	5.8 (2150)	10.9 (4030)	
Girls	0.73 (276)	3.1 (1130)	4.33 (1560)	7.1 (2610)	3.9 (1450)	

DHEAS, dehydroepiandrosterone sulfate.

Modified from Reiter EO, Fuldauer VG, Root AW. Secretion of the adrenal androgen, dehydroepiandrosterone sulfate, during normal infancy, childhood, and adolescence, in sick infants, and in children with endocrinologic abnormalities. *J Pediatr.* 1977;90:766-770.

subunits, activin A and activin B, which stimulate the release of FSH from pituitary cells.[291] Synthesis and secretion of gonadal inhibin is induced by FSH. Inhibin plays a role in the feedback regulation of FSH secretion during puberty in males and females.[291]

During pregnancy, the placenta secretes inhibin A, and the fetal membranes secrete inhibin A and inhibin B, but for at least the first 20 weeks of gestation, only inhibin A is detected in maternal serum. In umbilical cord serum from term female newborn infants, no inhibin dimer was detected, whereas cord serum from male newborns contained inhibin B, the only inhibin detected in adult males.[292] In the human fetal testis, α and β_B (but not β_A) subunits were present in Sertoli and Leydig cells at 16 weeks' gestation; by 24 weeks' gestation, immunoexpression of both subunits was greater in the Sertoli cells. Postnatally, the expression of both subunits was decreased by 4 months of age. Inhibin subunits were not detected in the fetal ovary, nor was immunoreactive follistatin present in fetal or neonatal gonads.[293]

In large cross-sectional studies using highly specific inhibin B and inhibin A immunoassays that correlate with the bioactivity of inhibin and distinguish inhibin B from inhibin A, the mean concentration of serum inhibin B in males increased between prepuberty (a stage when it is higher than the undetectable levels in castrate men)[294] and the first stage of puberty; when the strong correlation with chronologic age was taken into account, a correlation with LH and testosterone values remained. From genital stage 2 of puberty on, inhibin B levels were relatively constant, despite a rise in the mean concentration of serum FSH between stages 2 and 3, after which the FSH value was relatively unchanged. By genital stage 3, a negative partial correlation between inhibin B and FSH was found that persisted as puberty advanced, and by genital stage 4, there was a clear negative correlation of inhibin with serum FSH. Dimeric inhibin B rises twice during development, reflecting the two periods of Sertoli cell proliferation in infancy and in early puberty, whereas an inverse relationship between inhibin and FSH is seen at midpuberty and thereafter, indicating the development of negative feedback inhibition. In the early stages of puberty, inhibin B values are closely related to LH and testosterone levels, but in stage 3, when inhibin B values peak, this relationship is lost, and inhibin B values become more closely related to FSH levels.[295]

Serum levels of inhibin A and B increase early in puberty in girls, although there are individual increases in the prepubertal period directly related to FSH levels demonstrating sporadic follicular development in the infant and child due to FSH stimulation. Inhibin B is predominant in the follicular phase, as is inhibin A during the luteal phase. Inhibin A and inhibin B peak in midpuberty, and inhibin B is thereafter decreased. During the early stages of puberty, inhibin B values are related to estradiol and FSH values, but these relationships diminish with the progression of puberty.[296] Although there is no significant change in activin during female puberty, follistatin decreases from a midpuberty peak to later values that fall below prepubertal values.

Serum values of FSH regulating proteins follow circadian patterns, with higher values of LH and FSH overnight, just after a nadir of inhibin B. Follistatin concentrations were found to reach their greatest value in early morning, and activin A concentrations declined coincident with the nighttime increase in FSH levels in pubertal girls.[297] Diurnal variation of inhibin B in boys in the peripubertal or early pubertal period demonstrates a fall in inhibin during the night as LH and, subsequently, testosterone rise, showing the negative feedback effect of testosterone on inhibin B secretion.[298] Recombinant FSH treatment, which raises testosterone secretion, suppresses inhibin B, demonstrating the ability of testosterone to negatively influence inhibin B secretion.[299] Administration of a GnRH agonist led to an increase in the FSH level by 30 minutes as well as an increase in the inhibin B level in girls older than 5 years of age by 8 hours and in boys by 20 hours.[300] The baseline inhibin B concentration was greater in boys than in girls, baseline activin A concentrations were greater in girls, and activin did not changes with GnRH administration. Testosterone administration to boys in Tanner stage 2 led to decreased FSH and LH, increased activin, and decreased inhibin B levels but caused no change in follistatin. Estradiol administered to girls in Tanner stage 1 or 2 led to decreased LH and FSH and increased activin A levels but no change in inhibin B or follistatin concentrations, whereas administration of estradiol to girls with Tuner syndrome led to decreased serum levels of FSH, although the effectively nondetectable levels of activin and inhibin did not change.[301]

A low concentration of inhibin B in men and pubertal boys is an indicator of impaired seminiferous tubule function.[302] Early pubertal boys with testicular defects have higher FSH concentrations and low inhibin levels. Inhibin B is the form most closely related to testicular function, and it is absent in orchidectomized men. Inhibin B is related to Sertoli cell function in prepuberty, but a developmental change occurs during puberty so that later in life, inhibin B concentration is related to spermatogenesis. Prepubertal boys with the Sertoli cell–only syndrome had normal inhibin B levels, whereas postpubertal affected boys and men with Sertoli cell–only syndrome and early-stage spermatogenic arrest had undetectable or low levels of inhibin B, whereas those with late-stage spermatogenic arrest or obstructive azoospermia had normal or near-normal levels of serum inhibin B.[294] In prepuberty, the α and the β_B inhibin subunits are expressed in Sertoli cells, but during puberty and in men, fully differentiated Sertoli cells express only the α-subunit; the β-subunit is expressed in germ cells. Inhibin B in the adult appears to be a product of germ and Sertoli cells. In prepubertal boys, basal plasma inhibin B concentrations have a high correlation with the incremental testosterone response to administration of human chorionic gonadotropin (hCG), and they provide a useful assessment of the presence of testes and their function.[303]

Anti-müllerian Hormone. AMH, a 14-kd glycoprotein dimer that is structurally related to the subunit of inhibin and TGF-β, is produced by the Sertoli cell of the fetal testis and later in gestation by granulosa cells of the fetal ovary. Immunoassayable concentrations of AMH[304] rise from birth to relatively high levels during the first year of life in males, decrease by age 10 years, and decrease further during puberty. Newborn females have low or nondetectable serum levels of AMH, which rise only slightly thereafter; serum AMH concentrations are virtually nondetectable in most girls just before puberty.[304,305] Serum levels of AMH and of estradiol after GnRH analogue stimulation are increased in low-birth-weight and high-birth-weight female infants, suggesting altered follicular development.[306] Increased post-stimulation FSH levels and low adiponectin concentrations are observed only in high-birth-weight infants, indicating that altered ovarian function occurs by a different mechanism than that found in low-birth-weight infants.

Serum levels of AMH and inhibin B are inversely related to androgen concentrations in pubertal boys, and values in boys with CPP are appropriate for pubertal stage rather than chronologic age. Elevated serum AMH concentrations occur in the newborn period, at puberty, and thereafter in androgen resistance.[304] Treatment with recombinant FSH and hCG in hypogonadotropic hypogonadism increases testosterone and decreases the elevated levels of serum AMH (due to immature Sertoli cells) and inhibin B, further demonstrating this relationship.[299] AMH is slightly higher in boys with delayed puberty than in pubertal age-matched controls and lower in those with testicular dysgenesis associated with impaired virilization than in normal boys. Boys with isolated cryptorchidism have normal values of AMH, and AMH and inhibin B are absent in anorchia, allowing a differential diagnosis[304,307] during the first month after birth.[308] Dysgenetic testes secrete only low serum AMH levels; the testosterone response to hCG indicates the presence of testicular tissue.[307]

AMH is elevated in girls with PCOS and in girls with oligomenorrhea without classic AMH. This finding suggests that oligomenorrheic adolescents may have increased antral follicle number, similar to that observed in girls with PCOS.[309] AMH is a useful gonadal tumor marker because values are elevated in males with primitive Sertoli-like tumors and in girls and women with granulosa cell tumors.

Insulin-Like 3. During puberty, serum levels of insulin-like 3 (INSL3), a protein produced by the Leydig cell, rise in normal boys under LH stimulation and in those in whom increased secretion is induced by letrozole treatment. Values do not increase in Klinefelter's syndrome, in which the initial rise levels off during midpuberty.[310] INSL3 may serve as another indication of Leydig cell function.

Prostate-Specific Antigen. Prostate-specific antigen (PSA) is detectable in male and female cord blood and in the serum of infants, but PSA concentrations decrease to undetectable levels during childhood. PSA concentrations rise to the measurable range with the onset of puberty in the male and correlate with the progression of pubertal stage, the size of the testes, serum LH and testosterone concentrations, and, presumably, the size of the prostate.[311,312] PSA values are increased to the pubertal range in boys with idiopathic CPP, and they decrease with GnRH agonist treatment.

CENTRAL NERVOUS SYSTEM AND PUBERTY

Two independent but associated processes (controlled by different mechanisms but closely linked temporally) are involved in the increased secretion of sex steroids in the peripubertal and pubertal period. In the first process, adrenarche, the increase in adrenal androgen secretion[284,313] precedes by approximately 2 years the second process, gonadarche, which is a consequence of the pubertal reactivation of the hypothalamic-pituitary gonadotropin-gonadal apparatus.[314,315]

The onset of puberty is a consequence of maturational changes, including the development of secondary sexual characteristics, the adolescent growth spurt, the attainment of fertility, and psychosocial changes, all emanating from the disinhibition or reaugmentation of the hypothalamic GnRH pulse generator and gonadotropin secretion, causing an increase in gonadal steroid secretion (Table 25-10).[241,314] The events characterizing the development of gonadal function can be viewed as a continuum extending from sexual differentiation and the ontogenesis of the hypothalamic-pituitary gonadotropin-gonadal system during fetal life and early infancy,[124,239,314-317] through a juvenile pause (in which the system is suppressed to a low level of activity, discussed later),[314,315] to the attainment of full sexual maturation and fertility during puberty, leading to the ability to procreate (Fig. 25-19). In this light, puberty does not represent the initiation or first occurrence of pulsatile secretion of GnRH or pituitary gonadotropins but the reactivation or disinhibition of GnRH neurosecretory neurons in the medial basal hypothalamus and the endogenous, apparently self-sustaining oscillatory secretion of GnRH after the period of quiescent activity during childhood. An increase in the pulsatile release of GnRH heralds the onset of puberty in primates and other mammals.[124,315-319] The CNS, and not the hypothalamic GnRH pulse generator, pituitary gland, gonads, or gonadal steroid target tissues, restrains activation of the hypothalamic-pituitary-gonadal system during the prepubertal years.[241,314,318,319]

Certain CNS lesions involving the hypothalamus and nearby structures can advance or delay the onset of human puberty.[241,314,320] CPP, including cyclic ovulation in girls and spermatogenesis in boys, can result from a variety of CNS disorders. Several regulatory systems control puberty (Fig. 25-20):

1. In primates, the neural component controlling gonadotropin secretion resides in the medial basal hypothalamus, including the arcuate region. There are about 1500 to 2000 transducer GnRH neurosecretory neurons, which are not segregated into a specific nucleus but are functionally interconnected. These GnRH neurons comprise the GnRH pulse generator, which drives and controls the pituitary gonadal components, stimulates the release of LH and FSH, and translates neural signals into a periodic, oscillatory

TABLE 25-10

Hypothesis of the Control of the Onset of Human Puberty

1. *Central Dogma:* The CNS exercises the only major restraint on the onset of puberty. The neuroendocrine control of puberty is mediated by the hypothalamic GnRH-secreting neurosecretory neurons in the medial basal hypothalamus, which act as an endogenous pulse generator (oscillator).
2. The development of reproductive function is a continuum extending from sexual differentiation and the ontogeny of the hypothalamic-pituitary-gonadal system in the fetus to the attainment of full sexual maturation and fertility.
3. In the prepubertal child the GnRH pulse generator, operative in the fetus and infant, functions at a low level of activity (the juvenile pause) because of steroid-independent and steroid-dependent inhibitory mechanisms.
4. Puberty represents the *reactivation* (disinhibition) of the CNS suppressed GnRH pulse generator characteristic of late infancy and childhood, leading to increased amplitude and frequency of GnRH pulsatile discharges, to increased stimulation of the pituitary gonadotropes, and finally to gonadal maturation. Hormonally, puberty is initiated by the recrudescence of augmented pulsatile GnRH and gonadotropin secretion, mainly at night.

CNS, central nervous system; GnRH, luteinizing hormone–releasing hormone.
From Grumbach MM, Kaplan SL. The neuroendocrinology of human puberty: an ontogenetic perspective. In Grumbach MM, Sizonenko PC, Aubert ML, eds. *Control of the Onset of Puberty.* Baltimore, MD: Williams & Wilkins, 1990:1-68.

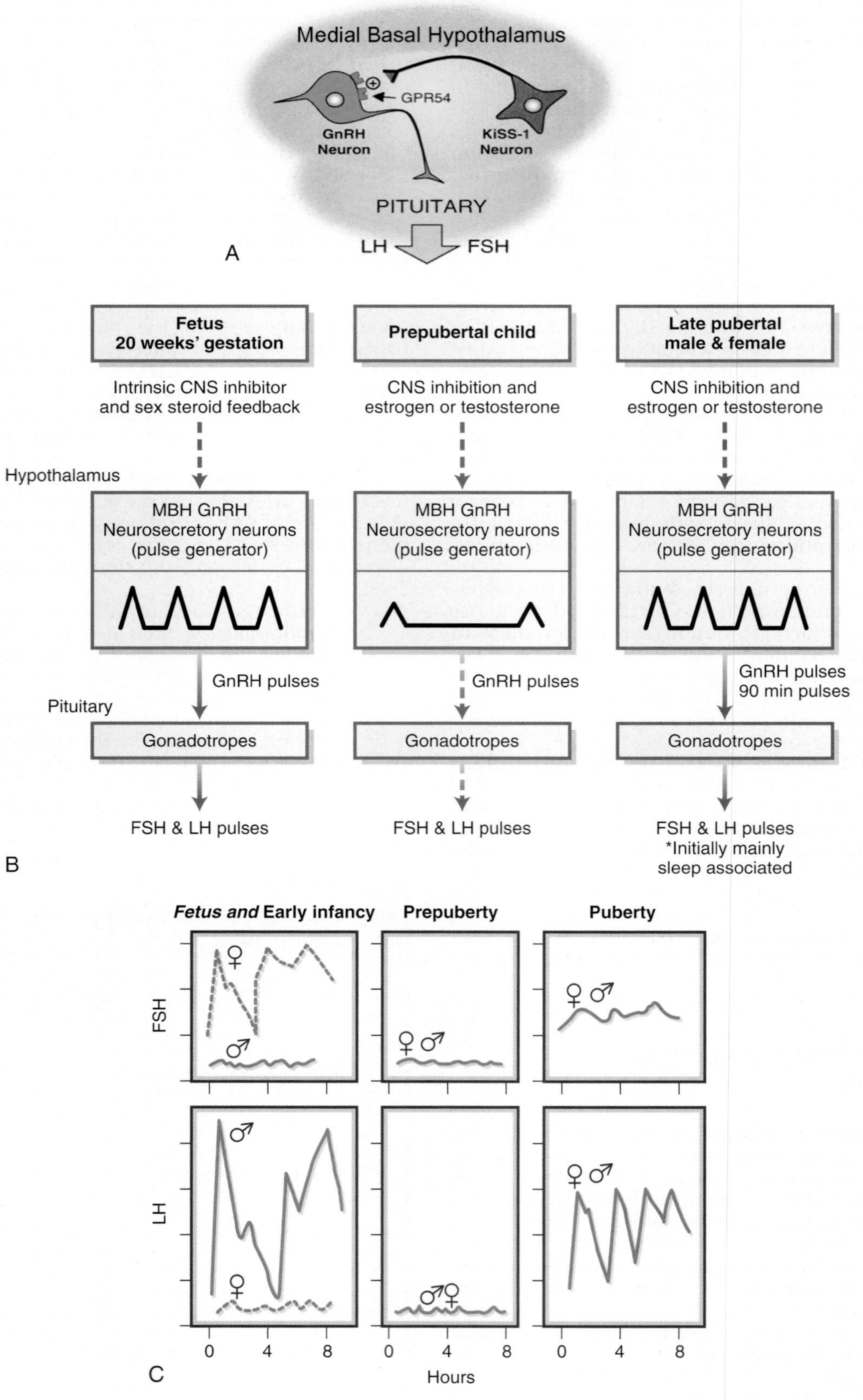

Medial Basal Hypothalamus

GPR54

GnRH Neuron

KiSS-1 Neuron

PITUITARY

LH FSH

A

Fetus 20 weeks' gestation	Prepubertal child	Late pubertal male & female
Intrinsic CNS inhibitor and sex steroid feedback	CNS inhibition and estrogen or testosterone	CNS inhibition and estrogen or testosterone
Hypothalamus: MBH GnRH Neurosecretory neurons (pulse generator)	MBH GnRH Neurosecretory neurons (pulse generator)	MBH GnRH Neurosecretory neurons (pulse generator)
GnRH pulses	GnRH pulses	GnRH pulses 90 min pulses
Pituitary: Gonadotropes	Gonadotropes	Gonadotropes
FSH & LH pulses	FSH & LH pulses	FSH & LH pulses *Initially mainly sleep associated

B

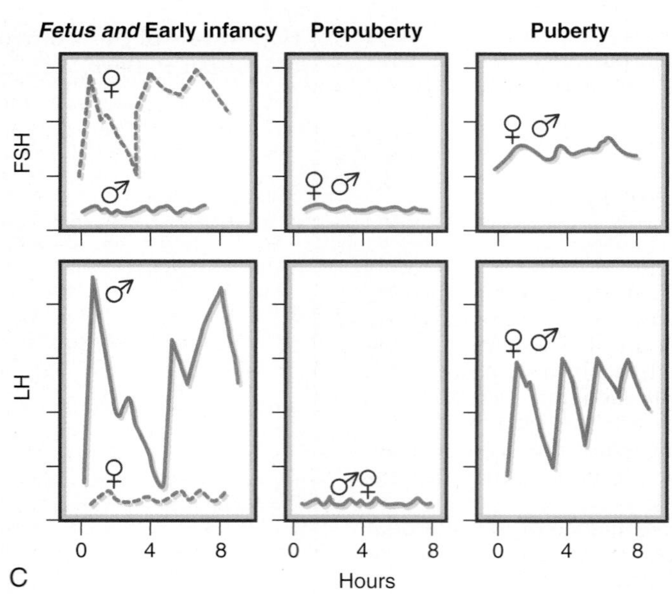

C

Figure 25-19 **A,** Kisspeptin receptor (KISS1R, formerly called GPR54) and the gonadotropin-releasing hormone (GnRH) neuron. KISS1 messenger RNA–expressing neurons in the medial basal hypothalamus synapse with GnRH neurons. Activation of the kisspeptin receptor on the GnRH neuron entrains the release of GnRH into the portal circulation, which induces the gonadotropes to release luteinizing hormone (LH) and follicle-stimulating hormone (FSH). **B,** Postulated ontogeny of the dual mechanism for the inhibition of puberty. *Dashed arrows* indicate inhibition. Notice the action of both components during the juvenile pause (i.e., prepuberty) (see Fig. 25-38 for the relative roles of these two mechanisms during development). MBH, medial basal hypothalamus. **C,** Change in the pattern of pulsatile FSH and LH secretion in the fetus and early infancy, prepuberty, and puberty (data from Waldhauser et al.[1077]). Notice the pulsatile secretion in the fetus and infant and the striking difference in the amplitude of FSH and LH pulses between male and female infants. After infancy, the amplitude and frequency of gonadotropin pulses decrease greatly for almost a decade (i.e., juvenile pause) until the onset of puberty. (**A,** Diagram modified from Smith JT, Clifton DK, Steiner RA. Regulation of the neuroendocrine reproductive axis by kisspeptin-GPR54 signaling. *Reproduction.* 2006;131:623-630; **B** and **C,** Modified from Grumbach MM, Kaplan SL. The neuroendocrinology of human puberty: an ontogenetic perspective. In: Grumbach MM, Sizonenko PC, Aubert ML, eds. *Control of the Onset of Puberty.* Baltimore, MD: Williams & Wilkins, 1990:1-68.)

chemical signal, GnRH, in a coordinated manner. These pulses appear to be generated by a propagated depolarization, the firing of action potentials in individual cells, and the resulting influx of calcium through L-type calcium channels.[321]

2. In response to the GnRH rhythmic signal, the pituitary gonadotrophs, which contain the seven-transmembrane domain G_s-coupled LH/hCG receptors (LHCGRs),[322] release LH and FSH in a pulsatile manner. Each LH and FSH pulse is induced by a pulse of GnRH.
3. The gonads, which are modulated primarily by the amplitude of the gonadotropin pulse, transmit the episodic gonadotropin signal into pulsatile secretion of gonadal steroids.[323]

This control mechanism is common to all mammalian species. At the last two levels—the pituitary gland and the gonad—the target cells contain receptors for the peptide hormones that mediate the cellular response to the signal.[322,323] Diverse adaptive mechanisms and strategies have evolved among species and between the sexes that influence the biology and timing of puberty. Photoperiodicity and seasonal breeding, biologic clocks, and pheromones are integral parts of the pubertal process in some species but not humans. The most enlightening studies on the neuroendocrinology of human puberty have emerged from studies of humans and nonhuman primates.

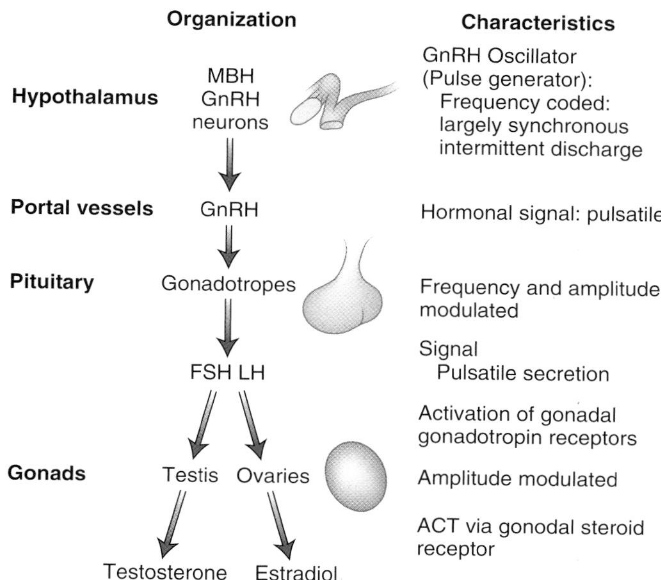

Figure 25-20 Organization and characteristics of the hypothalamic-pituitary gonadotroph-gonadal system. The medial basal hypothalamus (MBH) contains the transducer gonadotropin-releasing hormone (GnRH) neurosecretory neurons. These neurons translate neural signals into a periodic, oscillatory chemical signal, GnRH. This MBH complex functions as an GnRH pulse generator (oscillator), which is frequency coded and releases GnRH from its axon terminals at the median eminence as a largely synchronous, intermittent discharge into the primary capillary plexus of the hypothalamicohypophysial portal circulation. The GnRH pulse generator is influenced by biogenic amine neurotransmitters, peptidergic neuromodulators, neuroexcitatory amino acids, and neural pathways. During the follicular phase in women and men, a GnRH pulse (estimated indirectly by monitoring luteinizing hormone [LH] pulses in peripheral blood) occurs approximately every 90 to 120 minutes throughout the day. Changes in the frequency and probably in the amplitude of the GnRH secretory episodes modulate the pattern of LH and follicle-stimulating hormone (FSH). The major site of action of testosterone and progesterone is on the GnRH pulse generator, because these two classes of steroids decrease LH pulse frequency, but a pituitary site of action has also been described. Estrogens have major direct inhibitory and stimulatory effects on the GnRH-primed pituitary gonadotroph; the inhibitory or negative feedback action is associated with a decrease in the frequency and the amplitude of pituitary LH secretion. Evidence supports the negative and positive feedback action of estrogen on the GnRH pulse generator. Inhibin has a direct inhibitory effect on the pituitary gland and the secretion of FSH. The secretion of gonadal steroids by the gonads is controlled mainly by the amplitude of the gonadotropin signal. (Adapted from Grumbach MM, Kaplan SL. The neuroendocrinology of human puberty: an ontogenetic perspective. In: Grumbach MM, Sizonenko PC, Aubert ML, eds. *Control of the Onset of Puberty.* Baltimore, MD: Williams & Wilkins, 1990:1-68.)

Pattern of Gonadotropin Secretion

Tonic Secretion

Tonic, or basal, secretion is regulated by a negative, or inhibitory, feedback mechanism in which changes in the concentration of circulating gonadal steroids and inhibin result in reciprocal changes in the secretion of pituitary gonadotropins. This is the pattern of secretion in the male and one of the control mechanisms in the female. Clinical studies reveal that testosterone and estradiol in the male have independent effects on LH secretion, Inhibition of LH by testosterone requires aromatization for its pituitary but not its hypothalamic effects, and estradiol-induced negative feedback on LH occurs at the level of the hypothalamus.[324]

In the female, cyclic secretion involves a positive, or stimulatory, feedback mechanism in which an increase in circulating estrogens, to a critical level and of sufficient duration, initiates the synchronous release of LH and FSH (i.e., preovulatory LH surge) that is characteristic of the normal adult woman before menopause.

Pulsatile Secretion

Generation of the GnRH pulse is an intrinsic property of the GnRH neurosecretory neuronal network, and other factors modulate the fundamental autorhythmicity of the GnRH neuron, including the downstream effects of cyclic adenosine monophosphate (cAMP)-gated cation channels on the regulation of pulsatility by cAMP.[325] The immortalized GnRH neurosecretory neuronal cell line and cultured monkey GnRH-I neurons exhibit spontaneous pulsatile release of GnRH at a frequency similar to that observed in vivo. Patch-clamped primary GnRH neurons show disordered patterns of release that are sensitive to increased extracellular potassium; firing activity can be stimulated by exposure to estrogen in a manner that appears to function through the estrogen receptor.[326]

The secretion of FSH and LH is always pulsatile or episodic, regardless of developmental stage, due to the pulsatility of the GnRH pulse generator. The pulsatile secretion of immunoreactive FSH in normal adults is less prominent than that of LH; this is attributed in part to the longer half-life of FSH compared with LH, to differences in the factors that modulate the action of GnRH on FSH and LH release by the gonadotrophs (especially gonadal steroids, inhibin, and possibly activin and follistatin), and to intrinsic differences in the secretory pattern of the two gonadotropins. For example, a change in the frequency of GnRH pulses can modify the ratio of FSH to LH released; midfollicular-phase concentrations of estradiol and adult male concentrations of plasma testosterone have a greater inhibitory effect on the response of FSH to pulsatile injections of GnRH, compared with that of LH.[327]

Intermittent or pulsatile administration (e.g., GnRH, 1 μg/minute for 6 minutes every hour) induces pulsatile release of LH and FSH in adult monkeys in which hypothalamic lesions have obliterated the arcuate nucleus region and eliminated endogenous GnRH secretion.[328] Continuous infusion of GnRH inhibits gonadotropin secretion because of desensitization of GnRH receptors on the gonadotroph. Pulsatile GnRH administration reestablished gonadotropin secretion in animals in which gonadotropin secretion was suppressed by the continuous infusion of GnRH (Fig. 25-21). The GnRH signal to the pituitary gonadotrophs of the adult is frequency coded.

The GnRH neurosecretory neurons of the hypothalamic GnRH pulse generator that arise in the olfactory placode exhibit spontaneous autorhythmicity and function intrinsically as a neuronal oscillator for entrainment of the repetitive release of GnRH. The autorhythmicity in the GnRH neurosecretory neurons[329,330] involves cAMP and cyclic nucleotide-gated cation channels associated with oscillatory increases in intracellular calcium ions (Ca^{2+}), a hallmark of neurosecretion and gap junctional communication. Moreover, the immortalized GnRH neuronal cell line contains neuronal nitric oxide (NO) synthase, and NO generated by GnRH neurons may act as an intercellular or intracellular messenger.[331] GnRH acting as an autocrine factor may play a role in the synchronization mechanism. GnRH is synthesized in these neurons and released episodically from axon terminals at the median eminence into the primary plexus of the hypothalamic-hypophyseal portal circulation; it is then transported by the portal vessels to the anterior pituitary gland to produce the pulsatile LH and FSH secretion.

Ontogeny

In all vertebrates examined, GnRH neurons arise in the embryo from the epithelium of the olfactory placode and migrate in a rostrocaudal direction by an ordered spatiotemporal course along the pathway of the nervous

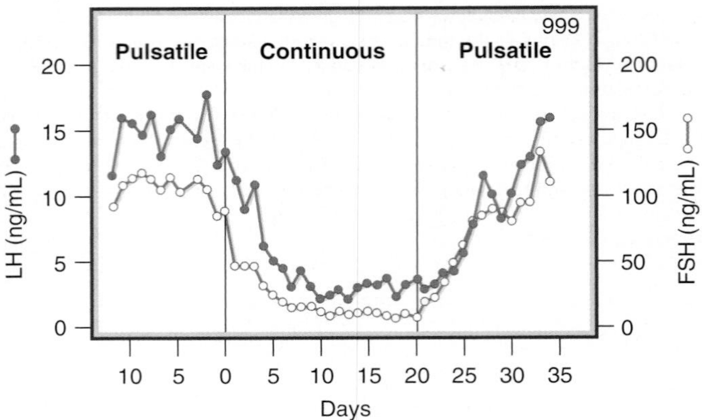

Figure 25-21 The Knobil paradigm. Effect of pulsatile administration of gonadotropin-releasing hormone (GnRH) in contrast to continuous infusion of GnRH in adult oophorectomized rhesus monkeys in which gonadotropin secretion has been abolished by lesions that ablated the medial basal hypothalamic GnRH pulse generator. Notice the high concentrations of plasma luteinizing hormone (LH) and follicle-stimulating hormone (FSH) in monkeys given one GnRH pulse per hour, the suppression of gonadotropin secretion by continuous infusion of GnRH even though the total dose of GnRH was the same, and the restoration of FSH and LH secretion when the pulsatile mode of GnRH administration was reinitiated. (From Belchetz PE, Plant TM, Nakai Y, et al. Hypophysial responses to continuous and intermittent delivery of hypothalamic gonadotropin releasing hormone. *Science.* 1978;202: 631-633.)

terminalis-vermonasal complex to the forebrain.[319,332] The terminalis-vermonasal complex also originates in the olfactory placode and forms a connection between the nasal septum and the forebrain. This contrasts to the pattern of growth hormone–releasing factor (GRF), thyrotropin-releasing factor (TRF), or corticotropin-releasing factor (CRF) neurosecretory neurons, which originate from ventricular zones within the embryonic forebrain.[333]

The GnRH green fluorescent protein model demonstrates an increase in dendritic and somal spines in adult mice compared with juveniles, suggesting an increase in direct excitatory inputs to GnRH neurons and increased glutamatergic stimulation of GnRH neurons across the time of puberty.[334] Embryonic GnRH neurons of the olfactory placode and the hypothalamus coexpress mRNAs for GnRH and the type 1 GnRH receptor. These neurons demonstrate spontaneous electrical pulsatile activity, which can be stimulated by GnRH agonist and abolished by GnRH antagonist in the same pattern as GnRH pulses, all in a calcium-dependent manner (i.e., the intracellular calcium responses are stimulated by the agonist and inhibited by the antagonist).[335]

Human Fetus

GnRH immunoreactivity was observed in the epithelium of the medial aspect of the olfactory placode of the normal human fetus by 42 days of gestation but not at 28 to 32 days (Table 25-11).[332] No GnRH neurosecretory neurons were found in the brain, including the hypothalamus, of a 19-week gestational male human fetus with Kallmann's syndrome,[336] and the olfactory bulbs were absent. However, dense clusters of GnRH cells and fibers were present in the nose, including the nasal septum and cribriform plate, and within the dural layers of the meninges under the forebrain. The GnRH neurosecretory neurons migrate from the olfactory placode to the hypothalamus in normal humans and other mammals.

TABLE 25-11

Early Development of the Human Fetal Pituitary and Hypothalamus

Gestational Age (wk)	Hypothalamus	Pituitary	Portal Circulation
3	Forebrain appears		
4		Rathke's pouch in contact with stomodeum	
5	Diencephalon differentiated	Rathke's pouch separated from stomodeum and in contact with infundibulum; pituitary in culture can secrete corticotropin, prolactin, GH, FSH	
6	Premammillary preoptic nucleus; GnRH detected	Intermediate-lobe primordia; cell cords penetrate mesenchyme around Rathke's pouch	
7	Arcuate, supraoptic nucleus	Sphenoidal plate forms	
8	Median eminence differentiated: TRH detected	Basophils appear	Capillaries in mesenchyme
9	Paraventricular nucleus; dorsal medial nucleus	Pars tuberalis formed: β-endorphin detected*	
10	Serotonin and norepinephrine detected*	Acidophils appear	
11	Mammillary nucleus; primary (hypothalamic) portal plexus present; β-endorphin and opioidergic neurons detected*	Secondary (pituitary) portal plexus present; catecholamines detected by IF	Functional hypothalamic hypophyseal portal system
12	Dopamine present		
13	Corticotropin-releasing hormone detected*	α-Melanocyte–stimulating hormone detected	
14	Fully differentiated hypothalamus	Adult form of hypophysis developed	

*Hormone is detected at this gestational age but may be present earlier.

FSH, follicle-stimulating hormone; GH, growth hormone; GnRH, luteinizing hormone–releasing hormone; IF, immunofluorescence; TRH, thyrotropin-releasing hormone.

Modified from Gluckman P, Grumbach MM, Kaplan SL. The human fetal hypothalamus and pituitary gland. In: Tulchinsky D, Ryan KJ, eds. *Maternal-Fetal Endocrinology.* Philadelphia, PA: WB Saunders, 1980:196-232.

Aberrant migration of the GnRH neurons leads to delayed or absent pubertal development due to hypogonadotropic hypogonadism, and anosmia or hyposmia is a cardinal feature of Kallmann's syndrome and the CHARGE syndrome (see later discussion).

The number of the GnRH neurons and the GnRH mRNA levels in nonhuman primates and mice do not appear to change during pubertal development. The ability of the GnRH neuron to respond to electrical or neurochemical (e.g., glutamatergic, kisspeptinergic) stimuli does not change with pubertal development.[337]

GnRH has been detected in human embryonic brain extracts by 4.5 weeks and in the fetal hypothalamus by 6 weeks (see Table 25-11); the fetal pituitary gonadotrophs are responsive to GnRH.[239] The hypothalamic-hypophyseal portal system is functional by 11.5 weeks' gestation,[338] and by 16 weeks, axon fibers that contain GnRH are present in the median eminence and terminate in contact with capillaries of the portal system.[124,239,314,316]

In fetal sheep, the hypothalamus secretes GnRH in a pulsatile manner.[339,340] The available data are consistent with the development of a human fetal hypothalamic GnRH pulse generator by at least the end of the first trimester.

The human fetal gonad is affected by placental gonadotropins and by fetal pituitary FSH and LH.[124,316] The placental gonadotropin hCG may play an important role in the secretion of testosterone by the Leydig cells of the fetal testes during masculinization of the wolffian ducts and the external genitalia at 8 to 13 weeks' gestation. However, it is uncertain whether functional hCG/LH and FSH receptors are present in the fetal testis by 12 weeks of gestation and whether the early fetal testis responds to hCG. Fetal Leydig cells are a unique population of Leydig cells limited to the fetus and infant, which regress to be followed by the differentiation of adult-type Leydig cells in the peripubertal period.[124,316,341] Fetal testosterone and hCG levels, but not LH levels, were decreased in fetuses studied after elective second-trimester abortions between 11 and 19 weeks' gestation, with no significant change in testicular responsiveness.[128] The proportion of nonfunctional LHCGR transcripts in fetal testes was 2.3-fold lower than in adults, so that available ligand may exert a greater effect. Fetal hCG was reduced, and the ratio of inactive to active LHCGR isoforms was lowered by maternal smoking. Second-trimester fetal testosterone levels appear to decrease due to decreasing maternal hCG, because Leydig cell LH/hCG responsiveness remains constant. Even with the decrease of fetal hCG caused by maternal cigarette smoking, because the ratio of inactive to active LHCGR isoforms is reduced, testosterone remains normal due to fetal gonadotropin stimulation.

Compared with the adult type, fetal Leydig cells form tightly opposed clusters joined by gap junctions and lack Reinke crystals; they are resistant to hCG/LH-induced desensitization (hCG/LH produce upregulation of LHCGRs); and they contain little aromatase activity and few estradiol receptors. In contrast to the fetal testis, FSH receptors in the fetal ovary appear only late in the second trimester, well after completion of male phenotypic differentiation, demonstrating a sex difference in the stage of gestation at which fetal pituitary gonadotropins have an important effect on the development of the fetal gonad. In the anencephalic fetus (which is deficient in hypothalamic GHRH, resulting in deficiency of pituitary gonadotropins), the testes appear hypoplastic by early in the third trimester; however, the ovaries in this disorder are normal until at least 32 weeks' gestation.[124,316,320] Androgen receptor (AR) mRNA expression is lower, and AMH mRNA expression is higher in fetal testicular Sertoli cells than in adult testes. This may explain the failure of testicular testosterone to support spermatogenesis and to suppress AMH at that stage. AR was expressed in peritubular and Leydig cells.[342] Patients with androgen insensitivity syndrome have an increase in circulating testosterone and AMH and have combined gonadotropin stimulation that is consistent with a failure of testosterone to repress AMH in the absence of AR signaling.

The human fetal pituitary gland contains FSH and LH by 10 weeks, secretion begins by 11 to 12 weeks, and the gonadotropin content increases until approximately 25 to 29 weeks of gestation.[124,239,316,317,320] Fetal serum LH and FSH concentrations rise to peak levels by midgestation and then decrease to low values in umbilical venous blood at term. The serum concentrations of FSH and LH and of bioactive FSH at 17 to 24 weeks' gestation are strikingly higher in female than in male fetuses, and in both sexes, they decrease remarkably between 25 and 40 weeks of gestation. Mean FSH and LH concentrations are elevated at the beginning of the third trimester and decrease with advancing gestational age to undetectable values in term fetuses. Mean FSH values are higher in female fetuses between 26 and 36 weeks, whereas the mean LH level is higher in males. In the ovine fetus, LH and FSH are secreted in a pulsatile manner in response to the episodic secretion of fetal hypothalamic GnRH; human fetal pituitary gonadotropins are probably released in the same mode. The mean FSH and LH content of fetal pituitary glands is greater in female than in male fetuses at midgestation. This difference has been ascribed to the higher concentration of plasma testosterone between 11 and 24 weeks in the male fetus (the only major difference in gonadal steroids between the male and female fetus) and to fetal testicular inhibin.[124,316] The decrease in serum FSH and LH concentrations during late gestation and near term is attributed to maturation of the negative feedback mechanism, the development of gonadal steroid receptors in the hypothalamic-pituitary unit,[239,317,343] and the effect of inhibin.[124,316]

In vitro studies indicate that the human fetal pituitary gland is responsive to GnRH as early as 10 weeks' gestation; the GnRH-stimulated release of LH is greater in second-trimester fetal pituitary cells cultured from females than in those cultured from males and is augmented by estradiol in both sexes.[344] In vivo studies during middle and late gestation demonstrate the stimulating action of exogenous GnRH on fetal FSH and LH release by 16 weeks, with a striking sex difference in the FSH response and a fall in responsiveness to GnRH in late gestation. Anencephalic infants and some infants with neonatal hypothalamic hypopituitarism[124,316] have an absent or diminished gonadotropin response to GnRH,[124,239] in contrast to the brisk increase demonstrated in the normal infant.

A pattern of increasing synthesis and secretion of FSH and LH leading to peak serum concentrations at castrate levels, probably the result of relatively autonomous, unrestrained activity of the fetal hypothalamic GnRH pulse generator and subsequent stimulation of the fetal gonadotrophs by GnRH, is followed by a decline after midgestation that persists to term, probably due to maturation of the negative feedback mechanism[343] and increasing sensitivity of the GnRH pulse generator to the inhibitory effects of the high concentration of sex steroids (estrogens and progesterone from the placenta and, in the male, testosterone from the fetal testes) in the fetal circulation[239,314]; in the male fetus, there is also a contributory effect on the decrease in FSH by testicular inhibin in late gestation.[124,316] The increasing CNS control of gonadotropin secretion seems to require the maturation of gonadal steroid receptors (intracellular or on the cell surface, or both) in the fetal hypothalamus and in the pituitary gonadotrophs.[239]

Sheep Fetus

By 0.6 gestation, the secretion of fetal LH and FSH is pulsatile,[339] mediated by the hypothalamic GnRH pulse generator.[314,340,343] A sex difference in gonadotropin secretion occurs in ovine and human fetuses,[314] and orchiectomy (but not oophorectomy) in the ovine fetus leads to increased pulsatile secretion of LH and, to a lesser degree, of FSH.[345] Opioidergic neurons have a tonic suppressive effect on the pulsatile release of GnRH in the ovine fetus,[314,346] and the excitatory amino acid analogue *N*-methyl-D-aspartate (NMDA) evokes an LH pulse mediated by GnRH. The excitatory amino acids, glutamate and aspartate, can stimulate the GnRH pulse generator directly or indirectly.[347] Glutamate is present in abundance in the hypothalamus and is released from glutamatergic neurons by exocytosis in an ATP- and calcium-dependent process.[348] FSH stimulates inhibin synthesis by the ovine fetal testis and ovary, and administration of an inhibin-rich extract inhibits fetal FSH but not LH secretion, evidence of the functional capacity of the FSH-fetal gonadal inhibin feedback system.[349,350] These observations provide support for the central role of this process in the regulation of the CNS in hypothalamic GnRH-pituitary gonadotropin unit.

Human Neonate and Infant

In both sexes, the concentration of plasma FSH and LH is low in cord blood as a consequence of the inhibitory effect of the high levels of placental derived estrogens, but within a few minutes after birth, the concentration of LH increases abruptly in peripheral blood (about 10-fold) in the male neonate, but not in the female; this is followed by an increase in serum testosterone concentration during the first 3 hours that persists for 12 hours or longer.[314,351] After the fall in circulating levels of steroids of placental origin (especially estrogens) during the first few days after birth, the serum concentrations of FSH and LH increase and exhibit a pulsatile pattern with wide perturbations during the first few months of life. FSH pulse amplitude is much greater in the female infant and is associated with a larger FSH response to GnRH throughout childhood; LH pulses are of greater magnitude in the male. This striking sex difference also is present in agonadal male and female infants[314,352] and in infant rhesus monkeys.[353] This sex difference may in part be related to the effect of testosterone in the male fetus on the development and function of the hypothalamic-pituitary apparatus.[124,316]

The high gonadotropin concentrations are associated with a proliferation of Sertoli cells and gonocytes (and their transformation into spermatogonia) and with a transient second wave of differentiation of fetal-type Leydig cells and increased serum testosterone levels in male infants during the first few postnatal months[341] and increased estradiol levels intermittently during the first year of life and part of the second year in females.[354] The mean FSH concentration is higher in females than in males during the first few years of life. By approximately 6 months of age for boys and 2 to 3 years for girls, the concentration of plasma gonadotropins decreases to the low levels that are present until the onset of puberty (earlier in boys than girls) in the juvenile pause.[314,355]

The neonatal-to-midinfancy surge in pulsatile gonadotropin secretion, sex hormones, and inhibin—the so-called postnatal surge (i.e., mini-puberty)—is attributable to an increase in GnRH pulse amplitude and is associated in the male infant with the following[316]:

1. Increase in testicular volume (by direct measurement) due to increased seminiferous tubule length (about a sixfold increase in year 1)
2. Rapid expansion of the Sertoli cell population (which makes up 85% to 95% of seminiferous tubular cell mass)

3. High concentration of circulating inhibin B (low in hypogonadotropic hypogonadism)
4. Sertoli cell number, including postnatal proliferation, as a determinant of spermatogenic function

The increase in circulating testosterone in the normal male infant may lead to facial comedones and even to acneiform lesions, and the increase in gonadotropins may lead to a transient increase in testicular size, but there may be more subtle changes. An LH and testosterone surge is absent in those with the complete androgen insensitivity syndrome. In the McCune-Albright syndrome, an activating mutation in the $G_s\alpha$ gene primarily expressed in the Sertoli cell can cause macroorchidism due to Sertoli cell proliferation and hyperfunction with increased concentration of serum inhibin B and AMH but without increased testosterone levels due to Leydig cell hyperplasia, elevated gonadotropins, or signs of puberty.[316]

The postnatal surge apparently is not essential for masculine-typical psychosexual development. The brain in patients with congenital hypogonadotropic hypogonadism, including Kallmann's syndrome, is masculinized by testosterone therapy at puberty despite the lack of an infantile surge in gonadotropins and testosterone.

The transient postnatal to midinfancy function of the GnRH pulse generator in the male infant may be related to future spermatogenic function and fertility.[356,357] Sertoli cells and germ cells proliferate for about 100 days after birth (indicating mitotic activity and the transformation of gonocytes into adult dark [Ad] spermatogonia, the stem cells for spermatogenesis), with a subsequent decrease, mainly by apoptosis, after about 6 months of age, coincident with the waning of gonadotropins and testosterone.

Neural Control

Maturation of the CNS is the outcome or consequence of the totality of environmental and genetic factors that retard or accelerate the onset of puberty. It is a provocative but unproven hypothesis that a metabolic signal related to body composition is an important factor in the maturation or activation of the hypothalamic GnRH pulse generator and not a result of the early hormonal and body composition changes in human puberty. In either event, clinical and experimental data support the contention that the factors influencing the timing of puberty are expressed finally through CNS regulation of the onset of puberty.[241,314] In humans, the pineal gland and melatonin do not appear to have a major effect on this control system.[314,358]

Timing and Onset of Puberty

Genetic Neural Control

Because many levels control the onset of pubertal development, a systems biology approach holds promise in characterizing the complex components of this neural and neuroendocrine network. It appears that normal and some types of abnormal puberty are under polygenic control.[359] Although the increased pulsatile release of GnRH is most frequently considered, this change is caused by a balance in the inhibitory and excitatory factors through coordinated changes in transsynaptic and glial-neuronal communication, increased stimulatory factors (most prominently glutamate and kisspeptin), and decreased inhibitory tone, mostly through GABAergic neurons (i.e., those secreting γ-aminobutyric acid [GABA]) and opioidergic neurons and ultimately controlled by gene expression. Glial cells affect GnRH secretion through growth factor–dependent cell-cell signaling coordinated by numerous unrelated genes. A second level of genes is postulated to control cell-cell interaction. The third-highest level of control occurs through transcriptional regulation of the subordinate genes by other higher-level genes that maintain the function and integration of the network. New genomic and metabolomic methods should illuminate these complex processes.

Although the action of multiple genes (i.e., quantitative or polygenic inheritance) on the time of onset of puberty (e.g., on stature) has long been recognized, little is known about the gene loci involved in this complex quantitative trait or the effect of gene interactions (i.e., epistaxis) on this paradigm of complex traits. Genetic factors are estimated to account for 50% to 80% of the variation in the onset of normal puberty. These complex traits have been analyzed by linkage analyses (in which quantitative trait loci have been shown to relate to the age of menarche) and by large-scale haplotype-based association studies. Pedigree analyses have revealed relative risks for delay of puberty in kindreds with histories of CDP compared with those without such a history; for example, for first-degree relatives, the risk for a 2-SD delay in the onset of puberty is 4.8. There are clear genetic influences on the time of onset of puberty in monogenetic disorders, such as *KAL1* or *KISS1R (GRP54)* mutations, that can prevent pubertal development (see later discussion).

Nutrition and Metabolic Control

The genetic effects on the time of onset of puberty and its course are influenced by environmental factors (e.g., socioeconomic factors, nutrition, general health, geography) operating through the CNS. It has long been postulated that some alteration of body metabolism linked to energy metabolism may affect the CNS restraints on pubertal onset and progression, because of the earlier age of menarche in moderately obese girls, delayed menarche in states of malnutrition and chronic disease and with early rigorous athletic or ballet training, and changes in gonadotropin secretion and amenorrhea in girls with anorexia nervosa, voluntary weight loss, and strenuous physical conditioning.[360]

An *invariant mean weight* (48 kg) for initiation of the pubertal spurt in weight, the maximal rate of weight gain, and menarche in healthy girls regardless of chronologic age was proposed in the 1970s, but the concept generated controversy and criticism, in part because the empiric estimations and the equations used to determine fat mass were challenged and because no direct measurements supported the theory.[361] A more recent, 5-year longitudinal study of 469 girls revealed that there was a similar percentage of body fat associated with the onset of puberty, although there was a spread of chronologic ages at onset.[362] Body composition in the 2 years before puberty had a modest impact on the age of pubertal growth, but higher fat mass led to more rapid progress through pubertal stages.[363]

The relationships of adipose tissue mass, fat metabolism, and energy balance to reproduction were illuminated by the discovery of the genes encoding leptin, an adipocyte satiety factor,[364,365] and its receptor.[366] Considerable interest has focused on the potential role of leptin in the control of the onset of puberty—from a proposal that it was an essential, if not a key, factor in triggering the onset of puberty to one in which it had a more subsidiary role. Leptin is a well-established afferent satiety factor in humans; it acts on the hypothalamus, including nuclei controlling appetite, to suppress appetite.[124,316,367] Leptin reflects body fat and therefore energy stores and has an important role in the control of body weight and the regulation of metabolism.[365]

Ob/ob mice (which lack leptin) and db/db mice (which lack leptin receptors) are obese and exhibit hypogonadotropic hypogonadism, providing evidence for an important role of leptin in reproduction. Administration of recombinant leptin to hypogonadal ob/ob mice and to rats experiencing pubertal delay associated with food restriction in the rat partially reverses the hypogonadism. However, leptin administration to normal prepubertal rats did not advance the time of onset of puberty. A critical threshold level of leptin was necessary for puberty to begin and advance, but leptin alone (as in administration to normal rodents) was insufficient to promote puberty; it was but one among several permissive factors.[368]

The site of action of leptin in its effect on the hypothalamic GnRH-pituitary gonadotropin apparatus that was uncertain is clarified by experiments in the mouse by the Elias group.[368] Even though leptin receptors (LepR) were reported to be expressed in immortalized mouse GnRH (GT1) cells, leptin receptors are not expressed on GnRH neurons in vivo. Mice with selective deletion of the long form (signaling) of the leptin receptor underwent normal puberty and fertility. Kiss1 neurons express the leptin receptor (Ob-Rb isoform), and the suggestion was advanced that the effect of leptin on puberty onset and fertility was mediated through the Kiss1/Kiss1n complex. Mice with selective deletion of the leptin receptor from Kiss1 neurons underwent normal puberty and fertility, strongly suggesting that the action of leptin on hypothalamic GnRH-pituitary gonadotropin system is not mediated through Kiss1 neurons.[368,369] The Elias group obtained evidence that the leptin receptor is expressed at a high level in ventral premammillary neurons (PMV). The PMV neurons express the excitatory neurotransmitter glutamate which stimulate either GnRH neurons or GnRH terminals in the median eminence or both sites.[368] These observations dissociate the action of leptin on reproductive function and on nutrition (Fig. 25-22).

Leptin levels in the male rhesus monkey were similar during the advancement of prepuberty to puberty. In peripubertal 3- to 5-year-old rhesus monkeys fasted for 2 days, the administration of leptin prevented the decrease in plasma gonadotropins detected in the untreated animals. Continuous infusion of leptin into the lateral ventricle of agonadal male monkeys failed to evoke an increase in GnRH on gonadotropin secretion.[318]

Is leptin the peripheral, somatic trigger for the onset of puberty to the CNS, or does it have a permissive role, signaling the hypothalamus and the GnRH pulse generator that a critical energy store has been attained? A longitudinal study of serum leptin levels in prepubertal and pubertal boys and girls showed leptin to increase gradually during the prepubertal years, with similar levels in the two sexes.[370] During puberty, leptin continued to rise in girls, whereas in boys, the leptin mean levels peaked at Tanner stage 2[371] and decreased to prepubertal concentrations by genital stage 5. This decrease is attributed to the effect of testosterone on leptin secretion.[372] Adipose tissue mass, percentage of body fat, and age correlated with leptin levels, among other variables,[370,373] but there was no correlation between 24-hour serum estradiol and leptin concentrations in nonobese and obese prepubertal and early pubertal girls. Serum leptin levels rose after administration of pulsatile GnRH administration for 36 hours to children with delayed puberty but not after a single dose of buserelin, a GnRH agonist, suggesting that, rather than puberty's being triggered by leptin, pubertal increase in GnRH pulsatility increases leptin.[374]

Leptin circulates in both a free form and a high-molecular-weight, bound form. Leptin-binding activity in serum is highest in childhood and decreases to relatively low levels during puberty. Free leptin is postulated to have more relevance to reproductive development than total

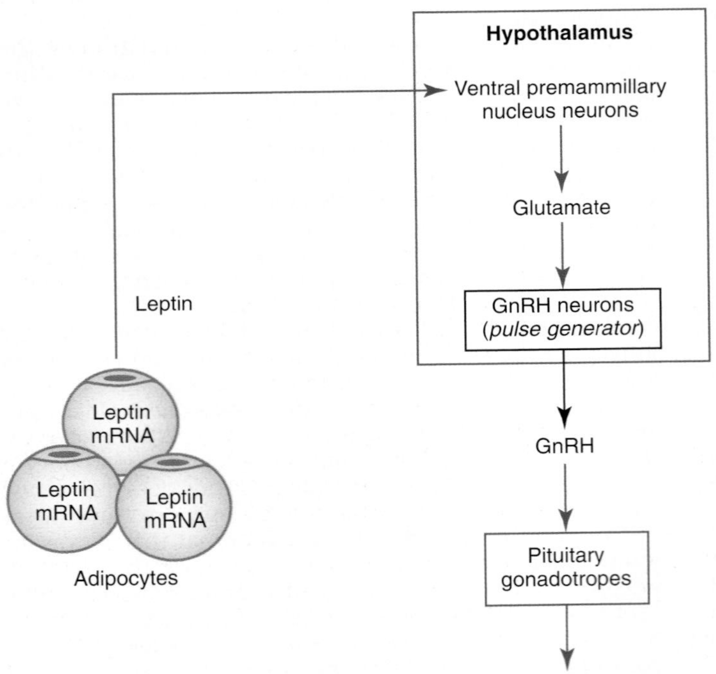

Figure 25-22 The leptin receptor is expressed in ventral premammillary neurons (PMV). Leptin secreted by adipocytes evokes release of the excitatory neurotransmitter glutamate from the PMV leading to activation of GnRH neurons. Leptin functions as a permissive factor, not a trigger, in the onset of human puberty. In rodents, leptin advances the onset of puberty and plays a key role in initiating puberty and infertility. The hypothalamic pathway that regulates energy expenditure and food intake by leptin is independent of the effect of leptin on reproduction.

leptin measured in the circulation; the soluble leptin receptor appears to be higher in males than in females and is inversely related to leptin levels later in development in females.[375] A study of a 132 monozygotic female twin pairs and 48 dizygotic female twin pairs demonstrated a rise in leptin throughout puberty and a decrease in the soluble leptin receptor between stages 1 to 2, leading to a rise in the free leptin index between stages 1 and 2; there was greater hereditability for the soluble leptin receptor than leptin,[376] and there was also high hereditability of free IGF1 values. There is no known relationship between leptin and leptin receptor gene polymorphism and CDP; however, the presence of a short allele of leptin was associated with heavier weight, whereas those who were thin, had significant bone age delay, and had increased frequency of parental pubertal delay were less likely to have this leptin short allele.[377]

As in the ob/ob mouse, human beings with a homozygous mutation in the leptin gene[378] or the leptin receptor[379] have morbid obesity and a striking delay in puberty because of hypogonadotropic hypogonadism. In a pedigree affected by a stop codon mutation in the gene encoding leptin, a 23-year-old man failed to attain puberty because of hypogonadotropic hypogonadism,[378] and two affected women were prepubertal and amenorrheic, one until 29 years of age, after which she began to have irregular, scanty periods, and the other until age 36 years, at which time she began to menstruate monthly. A 9-year-old girl with a bone age of 13 years who was affected with congenital leptin deficiency lost weight and had an early pubertal pattern of LH release in response to the administration of GnRH after treatment with recombinant leptin.[380] A 4-year-old affected relative of this 9-year-old girl benefited from the metabolic improvement that occurred with leptin administration but did not undergo early pubertal development, indicating the permissive nature of leptin on puberty.[318]

Boys with CDP have lower mean levels of leptin than expected and can enter puberty without an increase in circulating leptin. Two women with congenital lipoatrophic diabetes (Berardinelli-Seip syndrome), which is associated with absence of subcutaneous and visceral adipose tissue, did not have a delay in menarche despite severe hypoleptinemia, and one of the women had three unaffected children.[381] Severe leptin deficiency causes hypogonadotropic hypogonadism, suggesting that a critical level of leptin and a leptin signal are required to achieve puberty, but a rise in leptin is not required to trigger puberty.[370,373] In summary, leptin is a permissive factor (tonic mediator) and not a trigger (phasic mediator) in the onset of human puberty (Table 25-12).

In a longitudinal study of boys leading up to an increase in morning salivary testosterone concentrations, they had a relatively constant ratio of basal metabolic rate (BMR) to lean body mass (LBM) but an increase in the ratio of BMR to total daily energy expenditure. A subtle energy-dependent process is in play, possibly related to an increase in brain BMR as a secondary phenomenon at the initiation of puberty or indicating that a central rise in BMR is a signal for the onset of puberty.[382]

Ghrelin is the natural ligand for the GH secretagogue receptor but also serves as an orexigenic signal that is increased after food deprivation; ghrelin is usually negatively correlated with BMI. Ghrelin administration delays pubertal development in rats due to gonadal and central effects, suggesting a link between malnutrition and the decrease in reproductive development or function.[383]

Adiponectin is an adipocytokine produced in fat cells that has antidiabetic, antiatherogenic effects, and anti-inflammatory effects. Adiponectin decreases in the face of excess fat mass in obesity and is suppressed by rising testosterone and DHEAS levels. The concentration of adiponectin falls during pubertal development in males but remains rather stable in females with advancing Tanner stage.[384]

Resistin is an adipocytokine belonging to the resistin-like molecular family of cysteine-rich molecules (RELMs). Values increase with pubertal development in boys, and this appears to be true in girls as well, although the evidence is weaker. Because resistin serum levels were elevated in mouse models of obesity, it was considered to be a potential link between insulin resistance and obesity, but serum resistin levels appear to relate more to pubertal development than to insulin resistance.[385]

TABLE 25-12

Leptin and Puberty: A Permissive Factor, Not a Trigger for the Onset of Puberty

Pro-Trigger Evidence
Congenital leptin deficiency or congenital leptin resistance related to mutations is associated with delayed puberty and gonadotropin deficiency, evidence that the virtual absence of leptin or the leptin signal leads to severe hypogonadotropic hypogonadism.
In congenital leptin deficiency, administration of leptin led to a reduction in weight and an early pubertal pattern of luteinizing hormone release in an affected prepubertal girl.
Pro-Permissive Evidence
A sharp rise in circulating leptin does not occur at the onset of puberty.
In prepubertal and early pubertal girls, the rise in serum leptin did not correlate with the increase in serum estradiol.
In constitutional delay in growth and adolescence, an increase in prepubertal leptin levels is not essential for the onset of puberty.
In congenital lipoatrophic diabetes, despite the absence of subcutaneous and visceral adipose tissue and, as a consequence, severe hypoleptinemia, puberty can occur at the usual age and fertility is reported.
Supportive experimental data exist in rodents, sheep, and nonhuman primates.

From Grumbach MM. The neuroendocrinology of human puberty revisited. *Horm Res.* 2002;57(suppl 2):2-14.

Mechanisms of Control

Diverse strategies and adaptive mechanisms have evolved to control puberty in different species.[315,318,319] In rodents, exteroceptive factors and cues, including light, olfaction, and pheromones, have an important influence by way of the CNS on gonadotropin secretion. In seasonal-breeding species such as sheep, the length of the light-dark cycle is critical, and the pattern of gonadotropin secretion is different. In contrast, male and female primates exhibit an estrogen-provoked LH surge.

In humans and nonhuman primates, after the initial development and function in the fetus, the infantile surge of increased LH and FSH secretion occurs; this is followed by a decade of suppression (but not absence) of activity of the hypothalamic GnRH pulse generator and the resulting quiescence of the pituitary gonadotropin-gonadal axis, known as the prepubertal period or juvenile pause (Table 25-13).[124,314,315,318,319] Then there is gradual disinhibition and reactivation, mainly at night during late childhood,[314,315,318,319,386,387] and, finally, the increased amplitude of the GnRH pulses, reflected in the progressively increased and changing pattern of circulating LH pulses, that occurs with the approach of and during puberty. Two interacting mechanisms have been proposed to explain the juvenile pause (Fig. 25-23).[314,386]

Gonadal Steroid–Dependent Negative Feedback Mechanism. There are three lines of evidence for an operative negative feedback mechanism in prepubertal children[241,314]:

1. The pituitary of the prepubertal child secretes small amounts of FSH and LH, showing a low level of activity of the hypothalamic-pituitary-gonadal complex.
2. In agonadal infants and prepubertal children (e.g., in Turner syndrome), secretion of FSH and, to a lesser degree, LH is increased, suggesting that even low levels of hormones secreted by the normal prepubertal gonad inhibit gonadotropin secretion by a sensitive, functional, tonic, negative feedback mechanism (Fig. 25-24).[241,314,354,386,387]
3. The low level of gonadotropin secretion in childhood is shut off by administration of small amounts of gonadal steroids, showing that the hypothalamic-pituitary gonadotropin unit is highly sensitive (approximately 6 to 15 times more sensitive than in the adult) to the feedback effect of gonadal steroids.[241,314,388]

Gonadal Steroid–Independent (Intrinsic) Central Nervous System Inhibitory Mechanism. The diphasic pattern of basal and GnRH-induced FSH and LH secretion from infancy to adulthood is similar in normal individuals and in agonadal patients, but in the latter, gonadotropin concentrations are higher, except during the middle childhood nadir.[386,387] The high plasma concentrations of FSH and LH in agonadal children between infancy and about 4 years of age and the increased gonadotropin reserve reflect the absence of gonadal steroid inhibition (see Fig. 25-24) of the hypothalamic-pituitary unit by the low plasma levels of gonadal steroids.[314] However, the striking fall in gonadotropin secretion between the ages of 4 and 11 years suggests the presence of a CNS inhibitory mechanism that restrains the hypothalamic GnRH pulse generator, independent of gonadal steroid secretion. The resulting fall in gonadotropin secretion in agonadal children does not result from gonadal steroid feedback (because functional gonads are lacking) nor from increased secretion of adrenal steroids (because concentrations are low and glucocorticoid suppression of the adrenal does not augment the concentration of circulating gonadotropins).[314] A CNS steroid-independent inhibitory mechanism for suppression of the hypothalamic GnRH pulse generator seems to be the dominant factor in restraint of puberty between the ages of 4 and 11 years,[314,389] and a gradual loss of this intrinsic CNS inhibitory mechanism leads to disinhibition or reactivation of the GnRH pulse generator at puberty.

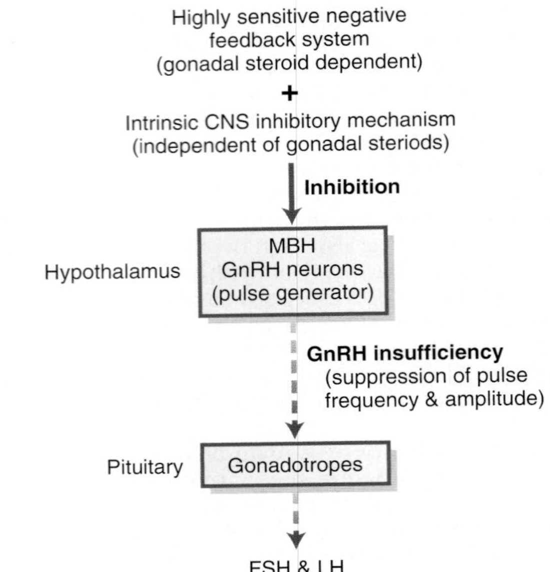

Figure 25-23 Postulated dual mechanism of restraint of puberty involves gonadal steroid-dependent and gonadal steroid-independent processes (i.e., intrinsic central nervous system [CNS] inhibitory mechanism). MBH, medial basal hypothalamus. FSH, follicle-stimulating hormone; GnRH, gonadotropin-releasing hormone; LH, luteinizing hormone. (Modified from Grumbach MM, Kaplan SL. The neuroendocrinology of human puberty: an ontogenetic perspective. In: Grumbach MM, Sizonenko PC, Aubert ML, eds. *Control of the Onset of Puberty.* Baltimore, MD: Williams & Wilkins, 1990:1-68.)

Interaction of the Negative Feedback Mechanism and the Intrinsic Central Nervous System Inhibitory Mechanism. The negative feedback mechanism and the intrinsic CNS inhibitory mechanism appear to interact in restraining puberty (see Fig. 25-24). During the first 2 to 3 years of life, the gonadal-steroid negative feedback mechanism seems to be dominant, but beginning at about 3 years of age, the intrinsic CNS inhibitory mechanism becomes dominant and remains so during the rest of the juvenile pause, as evidenced by the fall in FSH and LH levels between the ages of 3 and 10 years despite the lack of functional gonads. The negative feedback mechanism remains operative during the juvenile pause; agonadal patients in this age group have higher mean plasma FSH levels than normal prepubertal children and a greater FSH and LH response to the acute administration of GnRH.[386,387] As puberty approaches, the CNS inhibitory mechanism gradually wanes, initially during nighttime sleep, and the hypothalamic GnRH pulse generator becomes less sensitive to gonadal steroid negative feedback (see Fig. 25-24).[314] After the onset of puberty, gonadal-steroid negative feedback becomes the dominant mechanism in restraining gonadotropin secretion (along with inhibin), as reflected in the

TABLE 25-13

Potential Components of the Intrinsic Central Nervous System Inhibitory Mechanism ("Juvenile Pause")

- I. Inhibitory
  - A. Inhibitory central neurotransmitter-neuromodulatory pathways
    - 1. γ-Aminobutyric acid (the main inhibitory factor)
    - 2. Endogenous opioid peptides
- II. Stimulatory
  - A. Stimulatory central neurotransmitter-neuromodulatory pathways
    - 1. Excitatory amino acids
    - 2. Calcium-mobilizing agonists
    - 3. Noradrenergic
    - 4. Dopaminergic
    - 5. Neuropeptide Y
    - 6. Nitric oxide
    - 7. Prostaglandins (PGE2)
  - B. Other brain peptides
    - 1. Neurotrophic and growth peptides
    - 2. Activin A
    - 3. Endothelins-1, -2, -3

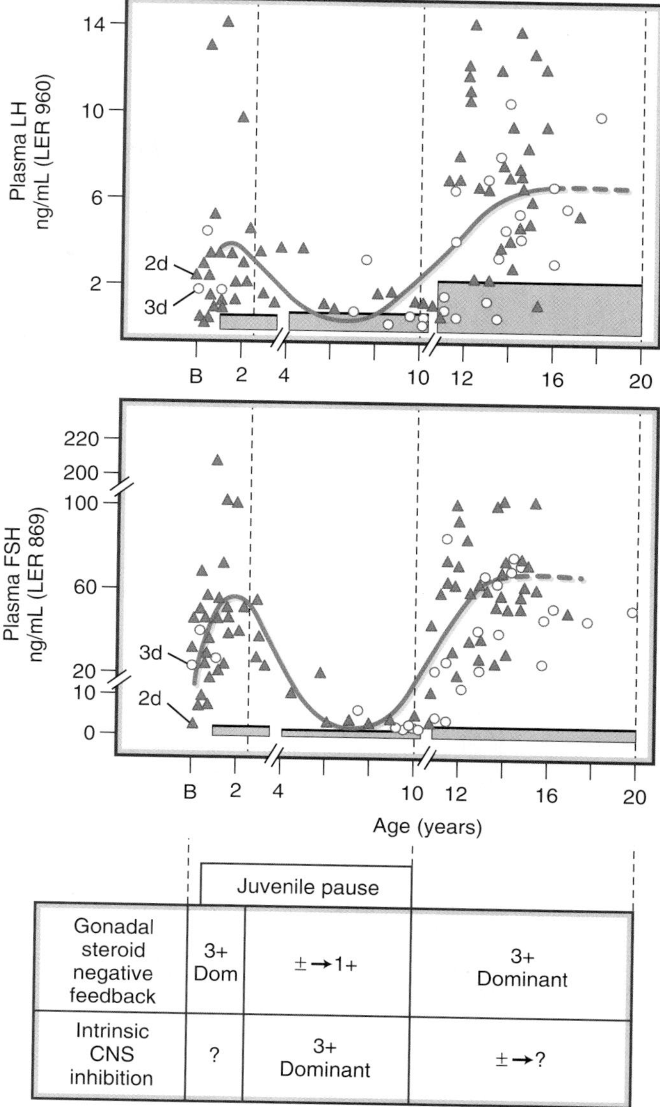

Figure 25-24 Interaction of the negative feedback mechanism and the putative intrinsic central nervous system (CNS) inhibitory mechanism in restraining puberty as extrapolated from the pattern of change in the concentrations of follicle-stimulating hormone (FSH) and luteinizing hormone (LH) in agonadal infants, children, and adolescents. *Triangles* designate patients with the 45,X karyotype. *Circles* indicate Turner syndrome patients with X chromosome mosaicism or structural abnormalities of the X chromosome, or both. Notice the values for the 2- and 3-day-old infants. The *solid line* represents a regression line of best fit. The *hatched area* indicates the mean plasma values for normal females. To convert FSH values to international units per liter, multiply by 8.4. For about the first 3 years of life, the sensitive gonadal steroid negative feedback mechanism has a dominant role in restraining gonadotropin secretion, as exemplified by the high gonadotropin concentrations in this age group in the absence of gonads (and gonadal steroid feedback). A major role of the intrinsic CNS inhibitory mechanism in this age group is unlikely in light of the rise in gonadotropins to castrate levels in the absence of functional gonads. From 4 to 6 years of age, the postulated intrinsic CNS inhibitory mechanism is dominant, as indicated by the fall in FSH and LH concentrations in the absence of gonads. Even in this age group, the augmented gonadotropin response evoked by GnRH and the slightly higher mean basal gonadotropin concentrations in agonadal individuals support a role, although a subsidiary one, for gonadal steroid negative feedback in the suppression of gonadotropin secretion during this period of the juvenile pause. The investigators suggested that the intrinsic CNS inhibitory mechanism suppresses the functional GnRH pulse generator. After about 10 years of age, the CNS inhibition gradually wanes, resulting in disinhibition of the GnRH pulse generator. The gonadal steroid negative feedback mechanism with an adult-type set point and inhibin play a dominant role in regulating the GnRH pulse generator and pituitary gonadotropin system. For conversion to SI units, see Figure 25-16. (Modified from Grumbach MM, Kaplan SL. The neuroendocrinology of human puberty: an ontogenetic perspective. In: Grumbach MM, Sizonenko PC, Aubert ML, eds. *Control of the Onset of Puberty.* Baltimore, MD: Williams & Wilkins, 1990:1-68; and Conte FA, Grumbach MM, Kaplan SL. A diphasic pattern of gonadotropin secretion in patients with the syndrome of gonadal dysgenesis. *J Clin Endocrinol Metab.* 1975;40:670-674. Copyright by The Endocrine Society.)

increased gonadotropin concentrations that are characteristic of the adolescent with severe primary hypogonadism.[318] The postulated ontogeny of this dual mechanism of restraint of puberty is illustrated in Figure 25-24.

The intrinsic CNS inhibitory mechanism remains elusive.[319] In the rhesus monkey, despite the damping of the GnRH pulse generator during the juvenile pause, the content of hypothalamic GnRH and GnRH mRNA during this phase is similar to that in the infant or the adult monkey. Low-amplitude LH and FSH pulses are detectable by sensitive and specific immunoradiometric assays in the juvenile pause, demonstrating a low level of activity of the GnRH pulse generator.[319] The end of the juvenile pause is marked by an increase in LH pulse amplitude that is most evident during the early hours of sleep.

Potential Components of the Intrinsic Central Nervous System Inhibitory Mechanism. Children with CPP associated with posterior hypothalamic neoplasms (usually a pilocytic astrocytoma), irradiation of the CNS, midline CNS developmental abnormalities such as septo-optic dysplasia with deficiency of one or more pituitary hormones, or other CNS lesions provide indirect evidence for an inhibitory neural component located in or projecting through the posterior hypothalamus. These lesions compromise the neural pathway, which inhibits the hypothalamic GnRH pulse generator and results in its disinhibition and activation leading to CPP.[314] For example, a suprasellar arachnoid cyst can cause CPP by compressing and distorting the hypothalamus,[314] but the puberty is reversed with regression of the hormonal and physical features of puberty after decompression of the cyst due to reversal of the disinhibition of the CNS inhibitory mechanism of the posterior pituitary (Fig. 25-25). Precocious sexual maturation can be induced in the juvenile female rhesus monkey by posterior hypothalamic lesions; such lesions advance the age at onset of a pubertal increase in LH secretion and the time of the first positive feedback effects of estrogen.[319]

The GnRH-secreting hypothalamic hamartoma, a heterotypic mass of nervous tissue that contains GnRH neurosecretory neurons[390] attached to the tuber cinereum or the floor of the third ventricle, can cause CPP.[391] The GnRH

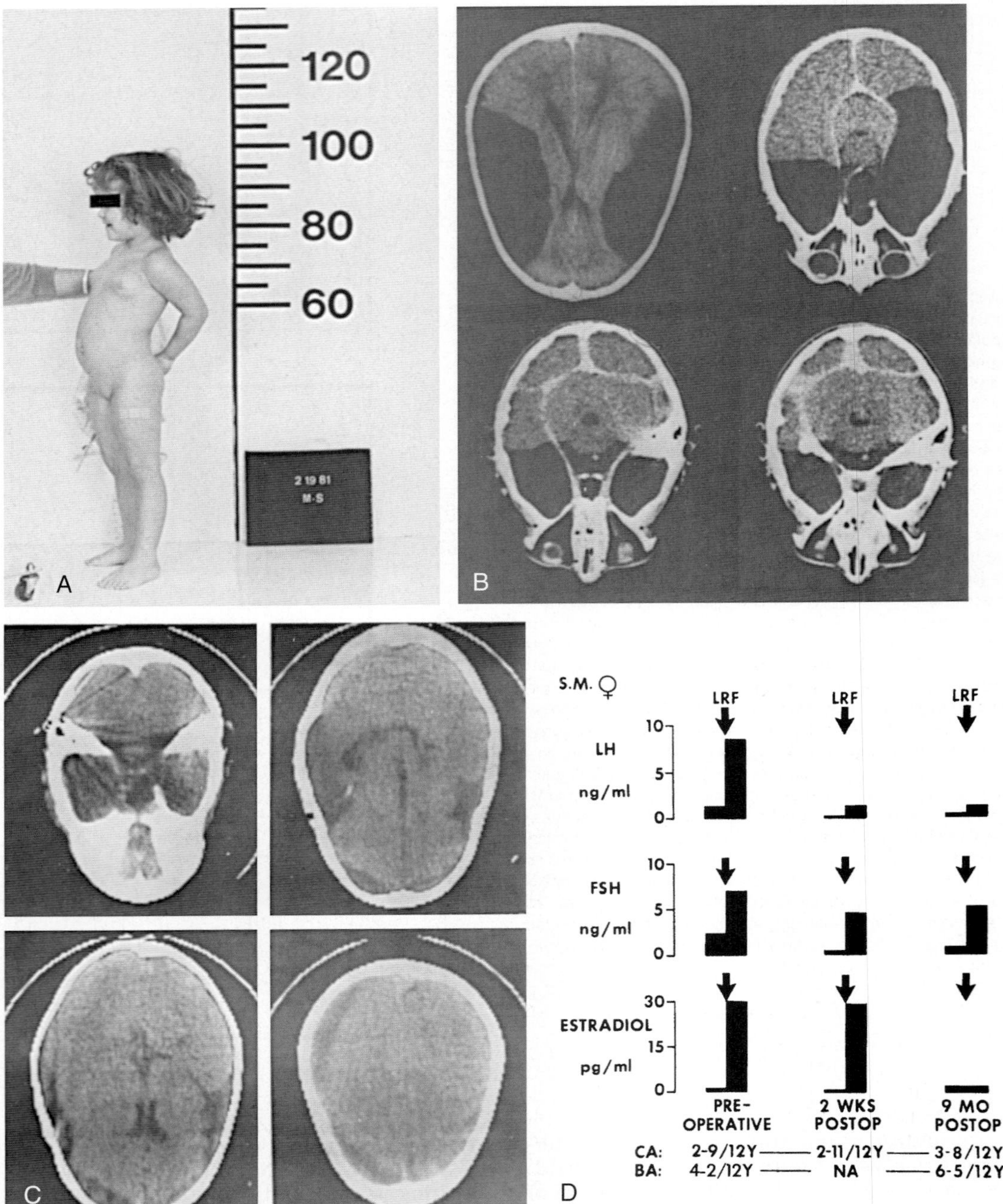

Figure 25-25 A, True precocious puberty in a 2.75-year-old girl is caused by a large, bilateral, congenital suprasellar arachnoid cyst. Signs of sexual precocity were observed during the preceding year. The head circumference was +5 SD above the mean value for age, and frontal bossing was present. Breasts were Tanner stage 3. The serum estradiol level was 26 pg/mL, the estrone level was 38 pg/mL, and the dehydroepiandrosterone sulfate (DHEAS) level was less than 3 μg/dL. The serum luteinizing hormone (LH) concentration rose from 1.4 to 8.7 ng/mL (LER-960) after intravenous administration of gonadotropin-releasing hormone (GnRH), which constitutes a pubertal response. Bone age was 3.5 years. Pelvic ultrasonography showed pubertal-size uterus and ovaries. To convert estrone values to picomoles per liter, multiply by 3.699. To convert DHEAS values to micromoles per liter, multiply by 0.02714. For other conversions, see Figure 25-16. **B,** Cranial computed tomography (CT) scans show a low-density fluid collection in the middle cranial fossa, thinning of the cortex, and striking compression of the lateral and third ventricles. **C,** Cranial CT scans 8 months later, after decompression of the arachnoid cyst and creation of a communication between the cyst and the basal cerebrospinal fluid cisterns and a cystoperitoneal shunt. Notice the striking decrease in size of the fluid collections and expansion of the cerebral cortex. **D,** Basal and peak LH and follicle-stimulating hormone (FSH) concentrations after GnRH administration in SM and serum estradiol values before surgical decompression and 2 weeks and 9 months after surgical decompression of the arachnoid cyst. Notice the prepubertal LH response to GnRH and fall in serum estradiol level by 9 months after surgery. The bone age had increased by 3 years over an 11-month period, but the velocity returned to normal. The patient remained prepubertal during follow-up. (From Grumbach MM, Kaplan SL. The neuroendocrinology of human puberty: an ontogenetic perspective. In: Grumbach MM, Sizonenko PC, Aubert ML, eds. *Control of the Onset of Puberty.* Baltimore, MD: Williams & Wilkins, 1990:1-68.)

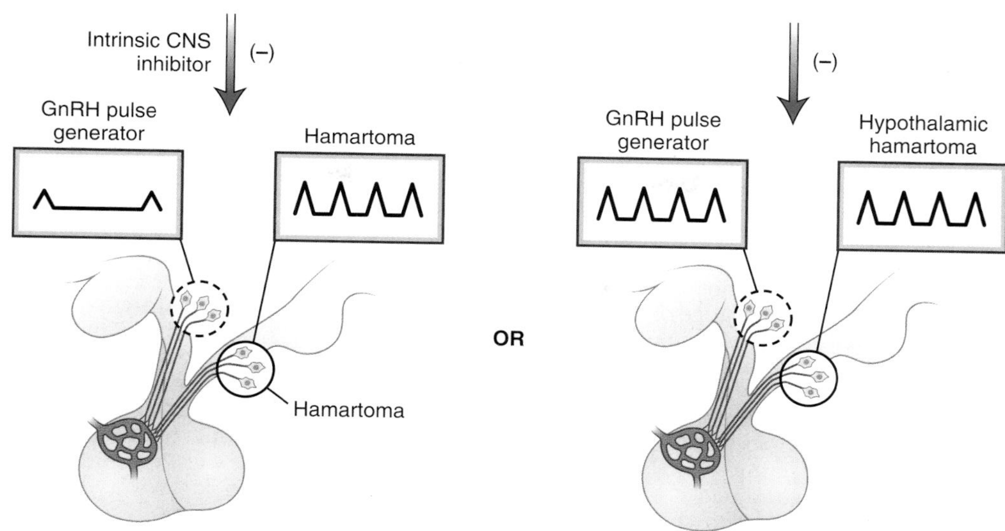

Figure 25-26 Hypothalamic hamartoma as an ectopic gonadotropin-releasing hormone (GnRH) pulse generator that escapes the intrinsic central nervous system (CNS) inhibitory mechanism and results in true precocious puberty. Two possible mechanisms are proposed. *Left,* The GnRH neurosecretory neurons in the hamartoma are functioning as a GnRH pulse generator without activation of the suppressed, normally located GnRH pulse generator. *Right,* The hamartoma acts as an ectopic GnRH pulse generator but communicates with and activates (possibly through axonic connections or by GnRH itself) the normally located hypothalamic GnRH pulse generator, which then functions synchronously with the hamartoma.

neurons within the hamartoma with their axon fibers projecting to the median eminence secrete GnRH in pulsatile fashion. We consider the hypothalamic hamartoma to be an ectopic GnRH pulse generator that functions independently of the CNS inhibitory mechanism, which normally restrains the hypothalamic GnRH pulse generator (Fig. 25-26).[314,391] An analogy can be drawn between the GnRH-secreting hypothalamic hamartoma and the rescue of fertility in GnRH-deficient hypogonadal (hyp/hyg) mice by transplantation of fetal or neonatal hypothalamic tissue into the third ventricle.[392] Some rare, large hypothalamic hamartomas that cause CPP contain TGF-α, an astroglia-derived growth factor, with few or no GnRH neurosecretory neurons, raising the possibility that the secretion of TGF-α may interact directly or indirectly to stimulate GnRH release.

Noradrenergic, dopaminergic, serotoninergic, and opioidergic pathways; inhibitory neurotransmitters (e.g., GABA); excitatory amino acids (e.g., glutamic acid, aspartic acid); nitrergic transmitters; other brain peptides, including neurotrophic and growth factors; and corticotropin-releasing hormone (CRH) affect the hypothalamic GnRH pulse generator (see Table 25-13).[347] Melatonin is not a critical restraining factor in primates, nor are endogenous opioid peptides.[314,318]

The GnRH pulse generator is inhibited by GABA (the most important inhibitory neurotransmitter in the primate brain) and GABAergic neurons during prepuberty, but exogenous administration of GABA in prepuberty is ineffective because of the high local endogenous GABA levels (Fig. 25-27).[319] Both GAD65 and GAD67 forms of glutamic acid decarboxylase (GAD), the enzyme that catalyzes the conversion of glutamate to GABA, are present in the mediobasal hypothalamus, the site of the GnRH pulse generator. Antisense oligodeoxynucleotides for GAD67 and GAD65 mRNAs infused into the stalk median eminence of prepubertal monkeys induced a striking increase in GnRH release, whereas nonsense D-oligos did not. These studies provided additional support for GABA arising from interneurons as the intrinsic CNS inhibitor during the juvenile pause of prepuberty.

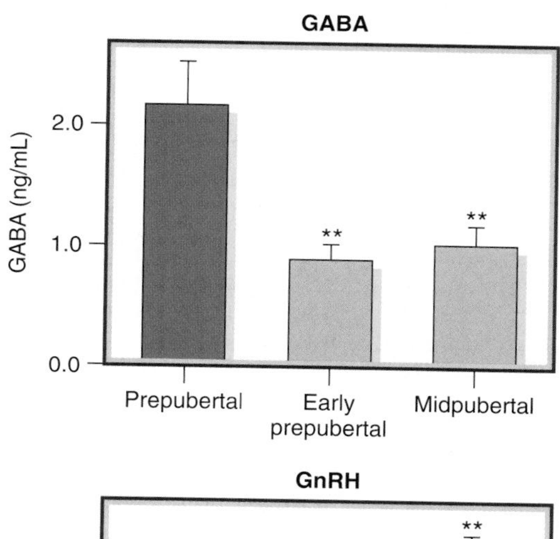

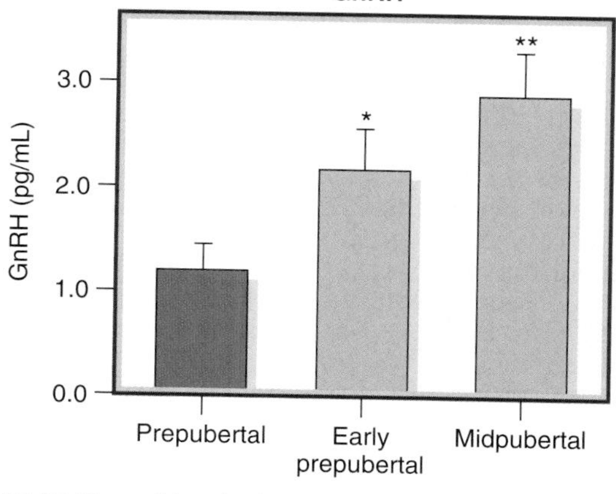

Figure 25-27 The striking developmental changes in γ-aminobutyric acid (GABA) and gonadotropin-releasing hormone (GnRH) release between the prepubertal and the pubertal rhesus monkey as measured in 10-minute perfusate samples from the stalk of the median eminence. Multiple samples were obtained from each animal. Mean ± SEM; $^{**}P < .01$; $^{*}P < .05$ versus prepubertal monkeys. (From Mitsushima D, Hei DL, Terasawa E. γ-Aminobutyric acid is an inhibitory neurotransmitter restricting the release of luteinizing hormone-releasing hormone before the onset of puberty. *Proc Natl Acad Sci U S A.* 1994;91:395-399.)

GABA acting through $GABA_A$ and $GABA_B$ receptors affects GnRH secretion in the perifused mouse GT1 GnRH-releasing neuronal cell line.[393] Conversely, chronic, repetitive administration of bicuculline, a GABA inhibitor, into the base of the third ventricle of a prepubertal monkey caused premature menarche and the onset of the first ovulation.[319] Although GABA is inhibitory in the juvenile and adult brain it is excitatory early in brain development through the postnatal period, increasing the intracellular Ca^{2+} concentration.[394] The switch from dominance of the gonadal steroid-dependent negative feedback mechanism in infancy and early childhood to dominance of the intrinsic CNS inhibitory mechanism may be associated with the developmental switch of GABAergic synaptic transmission from excitatory to inhibitory.

The onset of puberty in the rhesus monkey is characterized by a decrease in GABAergic (and possibly neuropeptide Y [NPY]) inhibition of the hypothalamic GnRH pulse generator and increased release of glutamate,[319] the major excitatory amino acid neurotransmitter in the hypothalamus. The sensitivity to the stimulatory glutamatergic input into the GnRH pulse generator increases strikingly after the onset of puberty, but it is the reduction in GABAergic inhibition that is the critical factor in disinhibition of the GnRH pulse generator.[319]

A persistent question has been how a single central signal can activate GnRH neurons to cause LH release and bring about ovulation by simultaneous suppression of GABA and stimulation of glutamate release, both of which converge in the anteroventral periventricular nucleus (AVPV). Most neurons in the AVPV of female rats express both vesicular glutamate transporter 2 (VGLUT2), a marker of hypothalamic glutamatergic neurons, and glutamic acid decarboxylase and vesicular GABA transporter (VGAT), markers of GABAergic neurons. These dual-phenotype neurons are twice as prevalent in females than in males and are the main targets of the E2 binding site in the region.[395] Moreover, dual-phenotype synaptic terminals contact GnRH neurons, and at the time of the surge, VGAT-containing vesicles decrease and VGLUT2-containing vesicles increase in these terminals. Dual-phenotype GABA/glutamate neurons may act as central transducers of hormonal and neural signals to GnRH neurons to simultaneously decrease GABA and increase glutamate release.

NELL2, a protein containing epidermal growth factor (EGF)-like repeats, is selectively expressed in the glutamatergic neurons containing VGLUT1 and in those expressing VGLUT2 in the postnatal rodent brain. NELL2 mRNA abundance increases selectively in the medial basal hypothalamus of the female rat, reaching a peak at the end of the juvenile period, and declines at the time of puberty with less change observed in the preoptic area. Intraventricular administration of antisense oligodeoxynucleotides to NELL2 reduced GnRH release from the medial basal hypothalamus and delayed the initiation of female puberty. Therefore, NELL2 plays an important role in glutamate-dependent processes of neuroendocrine regulation in puberty.[396]

Excitatory NMDA stimulates LH release in neonatal[397] and adult rats, fetal sheep,[347] and prepubertal[318] and adult rhesus monkeys, and its receptors are widely distributed throughout the CNS, including the hypothalamus.[398] NMDA evoked GnRH secretion from rat hypothalamic explants[399] from a GnRH neuronal cell line and acutely stimulated the GnRH pulse generator in the ovine fetus but did not have a direct effect on pituitary gonadotrophs.[347] Immortalized GnRH neurons contain inotropic NMDA receptors that mediate the release of GnRH by NMDA.[400] The prepubertal male rhesus monkey may be forced to enter puberty by repetitive intravenous administration of NMDA; in the prepubertal and pubertal female rhesus monkey, NMDA administered centrally and peripherally induced the release of GnRH.[319,401]

Description of the role of kisspeptins and their receptors (KISS1R or GRP54) in the CNS hypothalamic-pituitary-gonadal axis led to a flurry of investigation (Figs. 25-28 and 25-29; see Fig. 25-19).[402,403] *KISS1* is a human metastasis suppressor gene at gene map locus 19p13.3, and KISS1 mRNA is found in placenta, testes, pancreas, liver, small intestine, and the brain, mainly in the hypothalamus and basal ganglion.[404,405] KISS1 mRNA is present in the primate in the medial arcuate nucleus only, but in the mouse, it occurs in the arcuate, periventricular, and anteroventral periventricular nuclei, regions important in reproductive function.[406,407] The product of the *KISS1* gene is a 145-amino-acid peptide, but the cleaved and secreted product is a 54-amino-acid protein known as metastin or kisspeptin, which binds to an endogenous receptor.

The KISS1 receptor, KISS1R (formerly called GPR54), is a G protein–coupled receptor found in the brain, mainly in the hypothalamus and basal ganglia, and in the placenta, from which it was first isolated and sequenced. KISS1R is coexpressed within GnRH neurons in the rat, in the medial and lateral sections of the arcuate nucleus and the ventral aspect of the ventromedial hypothalamus in mice,[408] and in primates.[406] Although the expression of KISS1R mRNA does not increase with development in the mouse, kisspeptin mRNA increases dramatically in the AVPV nucleus, and the number of receptors responsive to kisspeptin increase with development.[409] Activation of GnRH neurons by kisspeptin at puberty in the mouse reflects a dual process involving an increase in kisspeptin input from the AVPV and a post-transcriptional change in KISS1R signaling within the GnRH neuron. Increases in kisspeptin lead to increased GnRH release by means of an interneuron, rather than acting directly on the GnRH-secreting neurons.[410]

Mice transfected with mutant *KISS1R* genes exhibited hypogonadotropic hypogonadism, although they had normal content of GnRH in their hypothalamus[411] and were responsive to GnRH or gonadotropin administration,

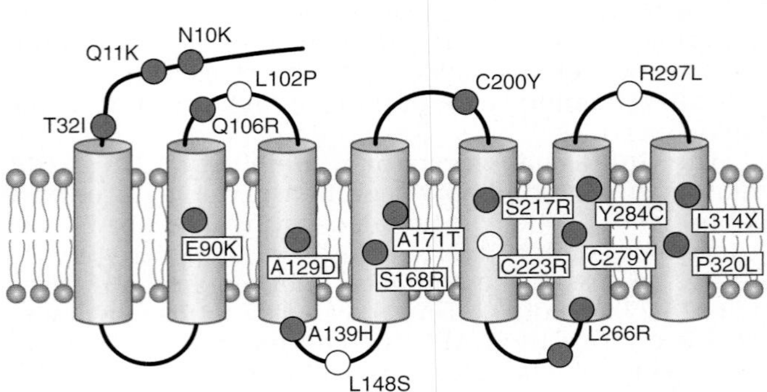

Figure 25-28 Inactivating mutations of the gonadotropin-releasing hormone receptor GnRHR *(closed circles)* and the kisspeptin receptor (KISS1R, formerly GPR54) *(open circles)* were identified in patients with isolated hypogonadotropic hypogonadism. The *dashed line* indicates the intracellular domain of KISS1R. The seven-transmembrane G protein–coupled receptor model is used for illustration of both receptors. (From de Roux N. GnRH receptor and GPR54 inactivation in isolated gonadotropic deficiency. *Best Pract Res Clin Endocrinol Metab.* 2006;20:515-528.)

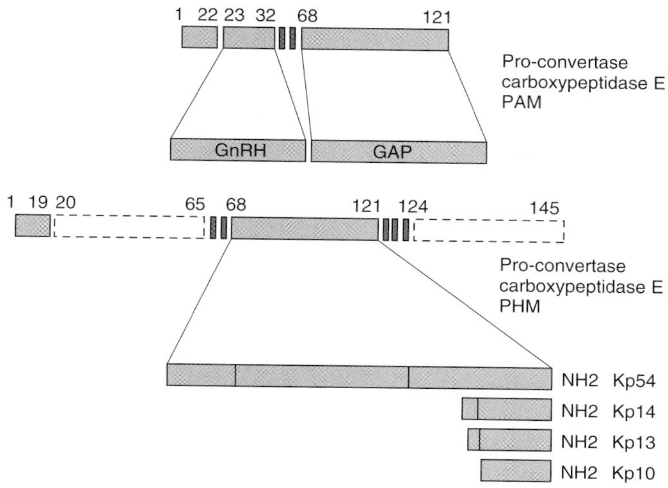

Figure 25-29 Post-translational maturation of gonadotropin-releasing hormone (GnRH) *(top)* and kisspeptins (Kp). Doublets of basic residues and glycine are indicated by *shaded vertical bars*. Enzymes involved in the normal maturation are indicated. PAM, peptidyl glycine α-amidating monooxygenase; PHM, peptidyl α-hydroxylating monooxygenase. (From de Roux N. GnRH receptor and GPR54 inactivation in isolated gonadotropic deficiency. *Best Pract Res Clin Endocrinol Metab.* 2006;20:515-528.)

suggesting normal function of the gonadotroph GnRH receptors and the gonadal LH and FSH receptors despite the mutation. The intact mouse also releases significant LH boluses after kisspeptin administration, an effect that is abolished in the KISS1R$^{-/-}$ mouse, which lacks the receptor.[408] Underfed prepubertal mice have decreased hypothalamic KISS1, but kisspeptin administration leads to increases in KISS1R mRNA, which in turn leads to increased in vivo LH secretion and in vitro GnRH secretion.[335] Chronic kisspeptin administration to these underfed mice restores vaginal opening and enhances gonadotropin and estrogen responses.

Administration of kisspeptin into the rostral preoptic area (RPOA), medial preoptic area (MPOA), paraventricular nuclei (PVN), and arcuate nuclei of the hypothalamus of male adult rats increased plasma LH and testosterone substantially,[412] and intracerebral kisspeptin administration stimulated the release of FSH, albeit at a far higher dose than needed to stimulate LH release.[413,414] Because the release of FSH is abolished with blockade of GnRH, GnRH modulates the central actions of kisspeptin in the rodent. In the rat, the mRNA for kisspeptin and its receptor increase at puberty, and administration of intracerebral injection of kisspeptin in prepubertal female rats caused large peaks of LH and advanced vaginal opening as a sign of pubertal development and premature ovulation.[415,416] The ovulation elicited by peripheral kisspeptin in the prepubertal female rat is abolished by blockade of GnRH.[417]

KISS1 and KISS1R mRNA expression is found in the posterior two thirds of the arcuate nucleus of the monkey.[418] Kisspeptin-beaded axons make only infrequent contacts with GnRH neurons in the medial basal hypothalamus, whereas in the median eminence, kisspeptin and GnRH axons were found in extensive and intimate association with GnRH contacts on kisspeptin perikarya and dendrites were observed. Nonsynaptic pathways of communication in the median eminence may offer a possible mechanism of kisspeptin regulation of GnRH release and provide an anatomic basis for reciprocal control of kisspeptin neuronal activity by GnRH.[419] Although KISS1 increases with puberty in intact male and female monkeys, KISS1R mRNA levels increase in intact females but not in agonadal male monkeys. Administration of KISS1 through intracerebral catheters to GnRH-primed juvenile female rhesus monkeys stimulates GnRH release, but this release is abolished by infusion of GnRH antagonist. These findings have led to the postulation that KISS1 signaling through the KISS1R of primate hypothalamus may be activated at the end of the juvenile pause and may contribute to the pubertal resurgence of pulsatile GnRH release at puberty.[406] Short-term administration of kisspeptin raises gonadotropin secretion in men and nonhuman primates (Fig. 25-30A). Just as continuous infusion of GnRH suppresses GnRH release, continuous infusion of kisspeptin decreased the response of gonadotrophs in the agonadal male monkey to boluses of kisspeptin. However, the release of FSH and LH after a bolus of NMDA or GnRH was maintained, demonstrating that the desensitization of the KISS1Rs was selective for kisspeptin administration (see Fig. 25-30B).[420] This down-sensitization of the KISS1Rs after continuous kisspeptin infusion may have a therapeutic function in CPP in the future, similarly to how GnRH agonists are used.

Administration of testosterone to castrated young male monkeys led to decreased kisspeptin mRNA in the mediobasal hypothalamus, but not in the preoptic area. There was no change in KISS1R expression. This suggests that feedback inhibition of gonadotropin secretion by testosterone is mediated by kisspeptin upstream of the GnRH network.[421]

KISS1R mRNA is expressed in the pituitary gland, and there is evidence that kisspeptin can act directly on the gonadotroph to prompt LH secretion.[413] In sheep, kisspeptin colocalizes to a high proportion of GnRH receptor cells in the preoptic area, as well as various neuronal fibers within the external neurosecretory zone of the median eminence. This raises the possibility that both kisspeptin and GnRH are secreted into the pituitary portal system to affect the pituitary gland.[422] There are also single-labeling KISSP1R cells in the preoptic area, and the number rises with ovariectomy.

Spontaneous mutations in the KISS1/KISS1R axis are rare but instructive in elucidating the role of KISS1 in pubertal development; hypogonadotropic hypogonadism and CPP occur with different mutations of KISS1R. These cases, augmented with studies of various animal species, suggest that kisspeptin acting through the KISS1R stimulates GnRH secretion.

NPY has been suggested as a component of the central restraint mechanism[318] in the male rhesus monkey. A small study of girls demonstrated higher NPY concentrations in those with CDP than in those with normal onset of puberty, supporting this relationship.[423]

These observations provide additional evidence that the hypothalamic GnRH neurosecretory neuron is not a limiting factor in puberty, as is the GnRH pulse generator; the anterior pituitary gland, gonads, and gonadal steroid end organs are functionally intact in the fetus and prepubertally and can be fully activated by the appropriate stimulus. CNS restraint of puberty lies therefore above the level of the autorhythmic GnRH neurosecretory neurons in the hypothalamus. Figure 25-31 contrasts the direct and indirect effects of the GABA inhibitory and excitatory amino-acid stimulatory neurotransmitters (as represented by NMDA and other glutamate receptors) on GnRH release. In the primate, the GABA hypothalamic neural network

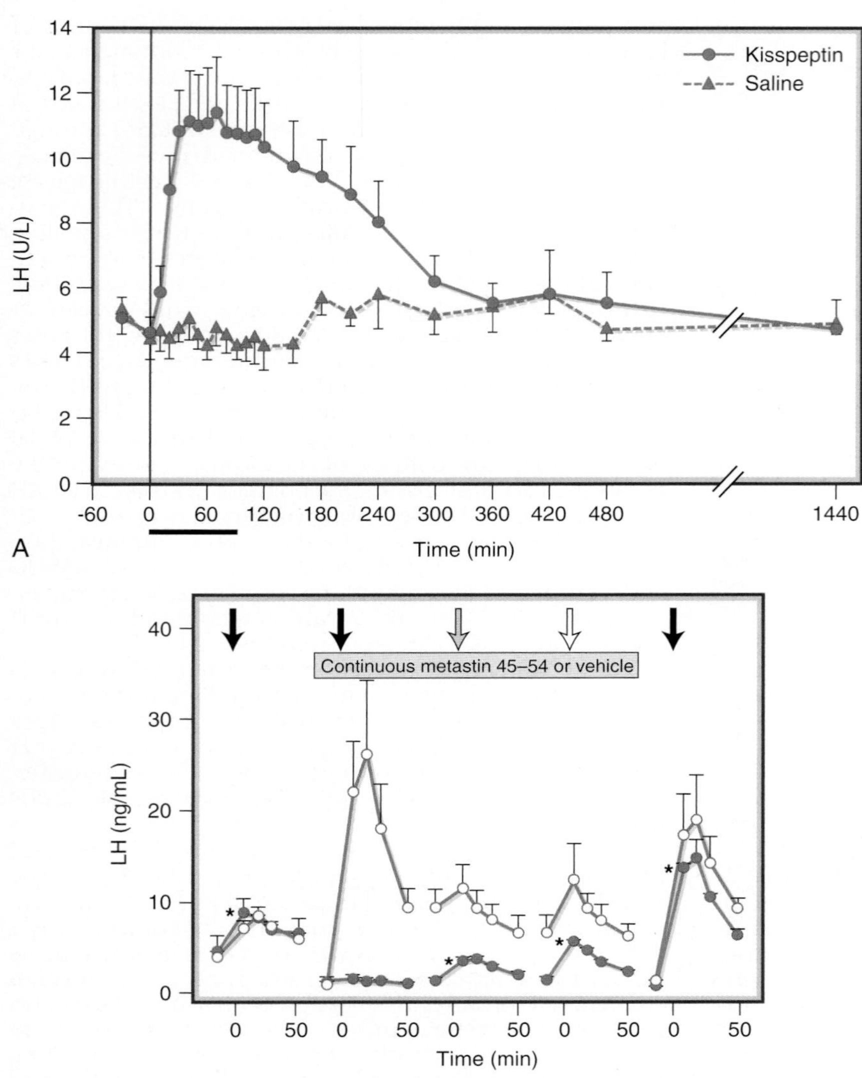

Figure 25-30 A, Effects of kisspeptin-54 (4 pmol/kg/min) or saline infusion in male volunteers (n = 6) on mean plasma. Each volunteer received both kisspeptin-54 and saline infusions and acted as their own controls. **B,** Effect of single sequential boluses of human metastin 45-54 (Met-Kisspeptin 10) *(black arrow)*, *N*-methyl-D-aspartate (NMDA) *(gray arrow)*, and gonadotropin-releasing hormone (GnRH) *(white arrow)* on plasma luteinizing hormone (LH) concentrations (mean ± SEM) during the last 3 hours of the 98-hour intravenous infusion *(shaded box)* of human metastin 45-54 at a dose of 100 μg/hr *(closed circles)* or vehicle compared with the LH response to the same bolus of human metastin 45-54 1 hour before (day 1) and 21 hours after (day 5) the termination of continuous human metastin 45-54 or vehicle infusion. Infusion of human metastin 45-54 *(asterisk)* was significantly different ($P < .05$) from the preinjection mean; n = 3. (**A,** From Dhillo WS, Chaudhri OB, Patterson M, et al. Kisspeptin-54 stimulates the hypothalamic-pituitary gonadal axis in human males. *J Clin Endocrinol Metab.* 2005;90:6609-6615; **B,** from Seminara SB, Dipietro MJ, Ramaswamy S, et al. Continuous human metastin 45-54 infusion desensitizes G protein-coupled receptor 54-induced gonadotropin-releasing hormone release monitored indirectly in the juvenile male rhesus monkey (*Macaca mulatta*): a finding with therapeutic implications. *Endocrinology.* 2006;147[5]:2122-2126.)

seems to be the major component of the intrinsic CNS inhibitory mechanism during the juvenile pause.

Sleep-Associated Luteinizing Hormone Release and Onset of Puberty

In sensitive radioimmunoassays, a diurnal rhythm of serum LH, FSH, and testosterone is already demonstrable in 5- to 6-year-olds, short but otherwise normal girls, demonstrating that preparation for the changes of puberty starts long before the physical features and classic endocrine markers of puberty appear.[237,314,424] Although adult men and women during most phases of the menstrual cycle have little difference in the amplitude or frequency of LH pulses over a 24-hour period, sleep-associated pulsatile release of LH is prominent in early and midpuberty; only in late puberty are prominent LH-secretory episodes detected during the day, but they are still less than during sleep until the adult pattern is achieved. Augmented LH release during sleep leads to a rise in the plasma concentration of testosterone at night in boys, in children with CPP, in glucocorticoid-treated children with CAH who have an advanced bone age and early onset of true puberty, and in agonadal patients during the pubertal age period, suggesting that it does not depend on gonadal function. There is significantly increased excretion of urinary LH in prepubertal children at night compared with the day.

Sleep-enhanced LH secretion can be viewed as a maturational phenomenon related to changes in the CNS and in the hypothalamic restraint of GnRH release. Episodic release of gonadotropins is suppressed by anti-GnRH antibodies and by the administration of gonadal steroids or certain catecholaminergic agonists and antagonists and is augmented by the opioid antagonist naloxone. Naloxone does not alter the testosterone-mediated suppression of LH, nor does it alter the testosterone effect on LH pulsatility in boys in early to middle puberty.[425] We have suggested that an increase in endogenous GnRH secretion at puberty has a priming effect on the gonadotroph[241] and leads to increased sensitivity of the pituitary to endogenous or exogenous GnRH. In monkeys, a striking increase in pulse amplitude and a lesser increase in pulse frequency occurs between prepuberty and puberty.[318,319] Sleep-associated LH

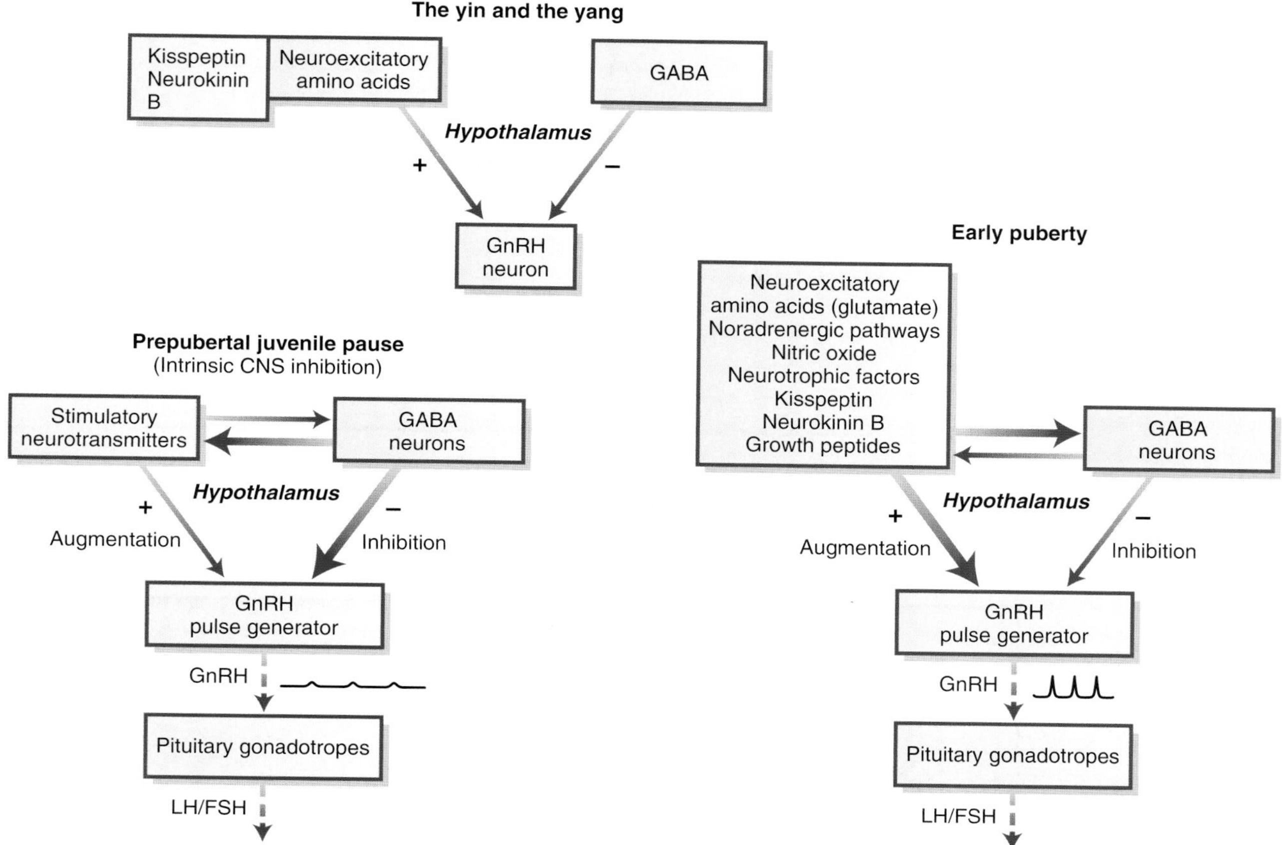

Figure 25-31 The yin and yang of the neuroendocrinology of the prepubertal juvenile pause and its intrinsic central inhibition of the gonadotropin-releasing hormone (GnRH) pulse generator and the reversal of this inhibition and termination of the juvenile pause, which leads to the onset of puberty. The GABAergic neuronal network and its neurotransmitter γ-aminobutyric acid (GABA) constitute the most ubiquitous inhibitory transmitter in the hypothalamus and the brain. During the prepubertal juvenile pause, this neurotransmitter system appears to play the major neural role in inhibiting the GnRH pulse generator. Suppression of GABA inhibition during this period promptly results in reactivation of the suppressed GnRH pulse generator in the rhesus monkey. With the approach of puberty, GABA inhibition of the GnRH pulse generator wanes, and its reactivation gradually occurs. This reactivation likely is augmented by stimulatory neurotransmitters (e.g., kisspeptin excitatory amino acids), some of which depend on increased gonadal steroids for their activation, and by neurotrophic factors and growth peptides. A critical component of the reawakening of the GnRH neuronal network is the increase, independent of sex steroids, in KISS1 mRNA expression in kisspeptinergic neurons in the medial basal hypothalamus and the secretion of kisspeptins, the cognate ligands for the kisspeptin receptor (KISS1R, formerly GPR54) on the surface of the GnRH neuron.[406] As a consequence, the amplitude and, to a lesser extent, the frequency of GnRH pulses increase, which leads to increased pulsatile secretion of follicle-stimulating hormone (FSH) and LH and the activation of the ovary and testis. As shown experimentally in monkeys, the GnRH pulse generator can function in the absence of hypothalamic stimulatory factors. The nature of and factor or factors responsible for this transition from central inhibition and the postulated dominance of GABA in the release of inhibition and reactivation of the GnRH pulse generator are unknown.

release in the peripubertal period correlates with increased sensitivity of the pituitary gonadotrophs to administration of GnRH in the peripubertal period and in puberty and is an indication that the hypothalamic GnRH pulse generator initially is less inhibited during sleep, even in prepubertal children.

Pituitary and Gonadal Sensitivity to Tropic Stimuli

Endogenous GnRH secretion is estimated indirectly and qualitatively by determining the pulsatile pattern of LH and by the gonadotropin response to exogenous GnRH at different stages[426] and in disorders of the hypothalamic-pituitary-gonadal system. The release of LH after administration of GnRH is minimal in prepubertal children beyond infancy, increases during the peripubertal period and puberty[241,314] (Fig. 25-32), and is still greater in adults (depending on the phase of the menstrual cycle in women).[427] These results support the concept that the prepubertal state is characterized by functional GnRH deficiency.[241,314,315,428] FSH release after the administration of GnRH is comparable in prepubertal, pubertal, and adult males, indicating similar pituitary sensitivity to GnRH, but females release more FSH than males at all stages of sexual maturation.[241,426] There is a striking reversal of the FSH/LH ratio after administration of GnRH to males or females between prepuberty and puberty (see Fig. 25-32).[241]

These observations suggest a striking change in pituitary sensitivity to GnRH in prepubertal and pubertal individuals and indicate a sex difference in the "dynamic reserve" of pituitary FSH[241] because the pituitary gonadotrophs of prepubertal females are more sensitive to GnRH than those of prepubertal males, even though the concentration of circulating gonadal steroids is very low in both sexes at that stage of maturation. Prepubertal girls have a larger readily releasable pool of pituitary FSH than prepubertal or pubertal males, possibly related in part to

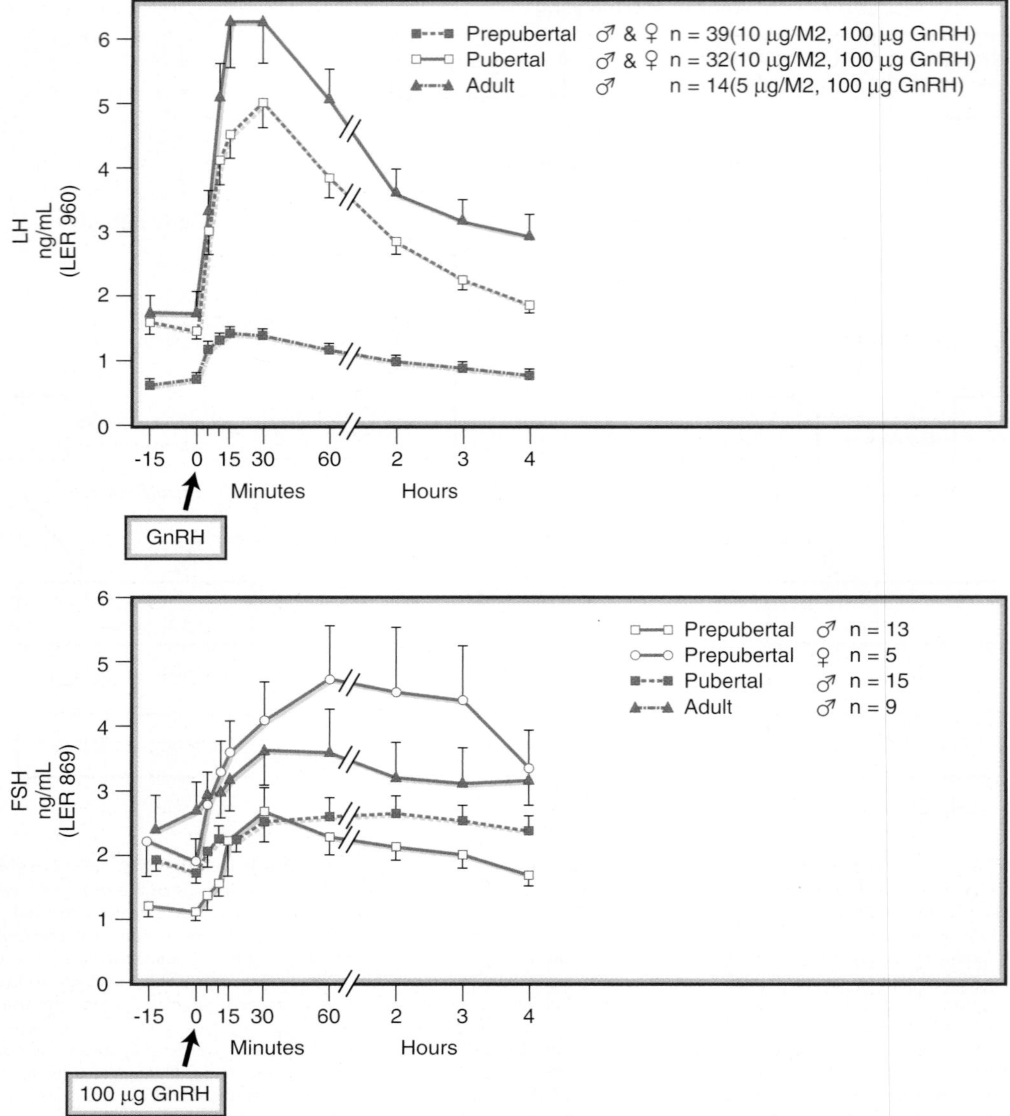

Figure 25-32 Changes in plasma luteinizing hormone (LH) *(top)* and follicle-stimulating hormone (FSH) *(bottom)* levels in prepubertal, pubertal, and adult individuals. Notice the limited LH response in prepubertal children compared with that of pubertal and adult subjects. The FSH response to gonadotropin-releasing hormone (GnRH) is similar in prepubertal, pubertal, and adult males. In females, the FSH response is significantly greater than that of prepubertal, pubertal, or adult males. For conversion to SI units, see Figure 25-16. (Modified from Grumbach MM, Roth JC, Kaplan SL, et al. Hypothalamic pituitary regulation of puberty in man: evidence and concepts derived from clinical research. In: Grumbach MM, Grave GD, Mayer FE, eds. *Control of the Onset of Puberty.* New York, NY: John Wiley & Sons, 1974:115-166.)

the higher concentration of inhibin B in prepubertal boys (see Fig. 25-32). These may be factors in the higher frequency of idiopathic CPP in girls and in the occurrence of premature thelarche.[429] The available data are consistent with the hypothesis that less GnRH is required for FSH than for LH release.

This change in responsiveness of the gonadotrophs is apparently mediated by increased pulsatile secretion of GnRH[241,314]; the increased LH response to synthetic GnRH is one of the earliest hormonal markers of puberty onset. Studies of the effects of acute and chronic administration of synthetic GnRH in hypergonadotropic hypogonadism, hypogonadotropic hypogonadism, constitutionally delayed growth and adolescence, and idiopathic precocious puberty indicate that the degree of previous exposure of gonadotrophs to endogenous GnRH appears to affect both the magnitude and the quality of LH responses—a self-priming phenomenon.[241,242,430] With the approach of puberty, the derepression of the hypothalamic GnRH pulse generator and the increased pulsatile secretion of GnRH augment pituitary sensitivity to GnRH and enlarge the reserve of LH.[431] Reduction in the frequency of exogenous GnRH pulses (from one per hour to one every 3 hours) in adult rhesus monkeys with ablative hypothalamic lesions that eliminated endogenous GnRH secretion increased the FSH/LH ratio,[432] suggesting that GnRH pulse frequency is one factor affecting relative secretion of FSH and LH. Inhibin and endogenous gonadal steroids may also affect this ratio through action on the hypothalamus or the pituitary, or both.

Pulsatile administration of GnRH to prepubertal monkeys promptly initiates puberty (and ovulatory menstrual cycles in females) and restores complete gonadal function in adult monkeys with hypothalamic lesions.[318,433] Similar studies in humans yielded comparable results for prepubertal children, patients with anorexia nervosa, and adults with hypothalamic-hypogonadotropic hypogonadism.[424,434-436] These results provide further support for reactivation of the hypothalamic GnRH pulse generator as the first hormonal change in the onset of puberty.

Responsiveness of the gonads to gonadotropins increases during puberty. For example, the augmented testosterone secretion in response to administration of hCG at puberty in boys is probably a consequence of the priming effect of the increase in endogenous secretion of LH (in the presence of FSH)[437] on the Leydig cell.

Maturation of Positive Feedback Mechanism

Estrogen exerts suppressive effects from late fetal life to peripuberty, when the positive action of endogenous (or exogenous) estradiol on gonadotropin release is not demonstrated.[241,314,438] A positive feedback effect, which is required for ovulation, is a late maturational event in puberty and probably does not occur before midpuberty in normal girls.[241,314,438] The positive feedback effect requires an increased concentration of plasma estradiol for a sufficient length of time during the latter part of the follicular phase in later pubertal and adult women.[328,427]

Among the requirements for the positive feedback action of estradiol on gonadotropin release at puberty[241] are ovarian follicles that are primed by FSH to secrete sufficient estradiol to reach and maintain a critical level in the circulation; a pituitary gland that is sensitized to GnRH and contains a large enough pool of releasable LH to support an LH surge; and sufficient GnRH stores for the GnRH neurosecretory neurons to respond with an acute increase in GnRH release in addition to the usual adult pattern of pulsatile GnRH secretion (this last requirement is controversial in humans but not in lower animals).

Estrogen exerts effects at the anterior pituitary and the hypothalamus.[439] In the rhesus monkey, positive and negative feedback can occur in adult ovariectomized females in whom the medial basal hypothalamus is surgically disconnected from the remainder of the CNS.[318] In monkeys with hypothalamic lesions, unvarying, intermittent GnRH administration leads to sufficient estradiol release from the ovary to induce an ovulatory LH surge in the absence of an increase in the dose of the GnRH pulses.[328,433] Estradiol has a positive feedback effect directly on the pituitary gland in normal women, and prolonged administration of estradiol is accompanied by an augmented LH response to GnRH administration. The fact that the major positive feedback action on the pituitary gland is demonstrable in the absence of an increase in pulsatile GnRH secretion suggests that the failure to elicit positive feedback action with administration of estradiol to prepubertal girls may be related to the inadequate GnRH pulses or insufficient LH reserve, or both.

Gonadotropin cyclicity and estradiol-induced positive feedback can be demonstrated by midpuberty and before menarche but may be insufficient to induce an ovulatory LH surge even when there is an adequate pituitary store of readily releasable LH and FSH.[1,241,355,438] The ovary does not secrete estradiol at a high level or long enough to induce an ovulatory LH surge. We visualize the process leading to ovulation as a gradual one in which the ovary (i.e., the *zeitgeber* for ovulation[328]) and the hypothalamic-pituitary-gonadal complex become progressively more integrated and synchronous until an ovary primed for ovulation secretes sufficient estradiol to induce an ovulatory LH surge.[355]

As many as 55% to 90% of cycles are anovulatory during the first 2 years after menarche, but the proportion decreases to less than 20% of cycles by 5 years after menarche.[440] The mechanism of ovulation seems unstable and immature, and it does not appear to have attained the fine tuning and synchronization that are requisite for maintenance of regular ovulatory cycles. However, the prevalence of PCOS adds to the irregularity of menses and anovulation in puberty.

Overview of Current Concept

Puberty is not an immutable process; it can be arrested or reversed. Environmental factors and certain disorders that affect the onset or progression of puberty mediate their effects by direct or indirect suppression of the hypothalamic GnRH pulse generator and its periodic oscillatory signal, GnRH. Table 25-14 lists some of these factors.

ADRENAL ANDROGENS AND ADRENARCHE

Speculation has focused on the mechanism of adrenarche (the adrenal component of pubertal maturation), the fact that adrenarche occurs earlier than gonadarche (the maturation of the hypothalamic-pituitary-gonadal system), and the interaction between adrenal and gonadal hormones at puberty.[284,441,442]

Nature and Regulation of Adrenal Androgens

The major adrenal androgen precursors secreted by the adrenal cortex are DHEA, DHEAS, and androstenedione, which can undergo extraglandular metabolism to produce physiologically active testosterone and estradiol[150]; however, adrenal androgens do not directly activate the androgen receptor. DHEA and especially DHEAS (which binds avidly to serum proteins, particularly albumin) are useful biochemical markers of adrenal androgen secretion and the onset of adrenarche. Androstenedione is the major androgen secreted by the ovary during and after puberty, and it is more readily converted to potent androgens than DHEA or DHEAS.

Cross-sectional and longitudinal studies have demonstrated a progressive increase in the plasma concentration of DHEA and DHEAS in boys and girls approximately 2 years before the increase in gonadotropin and gonadal steroid secretion that continues through puberty (13 to 15 years),[284,443,444] reaches a peak at age 20 to 30 years, and then gradually decreases (Fig. 25-33).[442] The increase is not associated with increased sensitivity of the pituitary gonadotrophs to GnRH[429] or with sleep-associated LH secretion and occurs at an age when the hypothalamic-pituitary-gonadal complex is functioning at a low level.[284] The importance of adrenarche is a matter of long-term debate. DHEA is a neurosteroid with parallel patterns of increase along with cortical maturation from approximately age 6 years to the middle 20s, suggesting that adrenarche affects brain development. DHEAS may increase activity of the amygdala and hippocampus and promote synaptogenesis within the cortex, with effects on fearfulness, anxiety, and memory that increase social interaction with unfamiliar individuals and shape cognitive development.[445]

Associated with the increase in adrenal secretion of DHEA and DHEAS (and independent of a change in the secretion of cortisol or aldosterone) is the appearance and growth of the zona reticularis (i.e., the principal source of

TABLE 25-14

Postulated Ontogeny of the Hypothalamic-Pituitary-Gonadal Circuit

Fetus
Medial basal hypothalamic GnRH neurosecretory neurons (pulse generator) operative by 80 days of gestation Pulsatile secretion of FSH and LH by 80 days of gestation Initially unrestrained secretion of GnRH (100 to 150 days of gestation) Maturation of negative gonadal steroid feedback mechanism by 150 days of gestation—sex difference Low level of GnRH secretion at term
Early Infancy
Hypothalamic GnRH pulse generator highly functional after 12 days of age Prominent FSH and LH episodic discharges until approximately age 6 mo in males and 18 mo in females, with transient increases in plasma levels of testosterone in males and estradiol in females
Late Infancy and Childhood
Intrinsic CNS inhibition of hypothalamic GnRH pulse generator operative; predominant mechanism in childhood; maximal sensitivity by approximately 4 yr of age Negative feedback control of FSH and LH secretion highly sensitive to gonadal steroids (low set point) GnRH pulse generator inhibited; low amplitude and frequency of GnRH discharges Low secretion of FSH, LH, and gonadal steroids
Late Prepubertal Period
Decreasing effectiveness of intrinsic CNS inhibitory influences and decreasing sensitivity of hypothalamic-pituitary unit to gonadal steroids (increased set point) Increased amplitude and frequency of GnRH pulses, initially most prominent with sleep (nocturnal) Increased sensitivity of gonadotrophs to GnRH Increased secretion of FSH and LH Increased responsiveness of gonad to FSH and LH Increased secretion of gonadal hormones
Puberty
Further decrease in CNS restraint of hypothalamic GnRH pulse generator and in the sensitivity of negative feedback mechanism to gonadal steroids Prominent sleep-associated increase in episodic secretion of GnRH gradually changes to adult pattern of pulses about every 90 min Pulsatile secretion of LH follows pattern of GnRH pulses Progressive development of secondary sexual characteristics Spermatogenesis in males Middle to late puberty—operative positive feedback mechanism and capacity to exhibit an estrogen-induced LH surge Ovulation in females

CNS, central nervous system; FSH, follicle-stimulating hormone; LH, luteinizing hormone; GnRH, LH-releasing hormone.

Modified from Grumbach MM, Roth JC, Kaplan SL, et al. Hypothalamic-pituitary regulation of puberty in man: evidence and concepts derived from clinical research. In: Grumbach MM, Grave GD, Mayer FE, eds. *Control of the Onset of Puberty.* New York, NY: John Wiley & Sons, 1974:115-166.

DHEA and DHEAS) that occurs coincidently with adrenarche (Fig. 25-34).

In contrast to the zona glomerulosa and fasciculata, four main features distinguish the zona reticularis:

1. There is a low level of expression of 3β-HSD/$\Delta^{4,5}$-isomerase type 2 and CYP21 mRNAs and enzyme activities.[446]
2. Abundant dehydroepiandrosterone (hydroxysteroid) sulfotransferase activity is found.[447]
3. There is a relative increase in 17,20-lyase versus 17α-hydroxylase activity of CYP17, the enzyme that catalyzes both activities.[447] These characteristics are shared by the fetal zone of the fetal adrenal cortex.[447]
4. There is expression of major histocompatibility complex (MHC) class II (HLA-DR) antigens,[448] which are not expressed in the fetal zone of the fetal adrenal cortex.

In contrast to the zona fasciculata, the zona reticularis has an increased ratio of 17,20-lyase to 17α-hydroxylase. An Arg347Ala mutation in human CYP17 resulted in

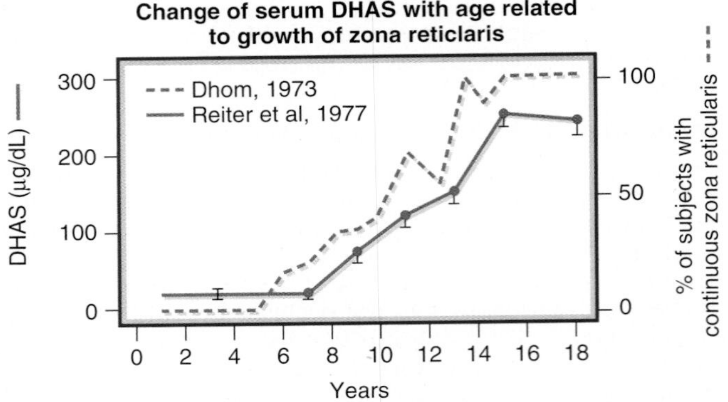

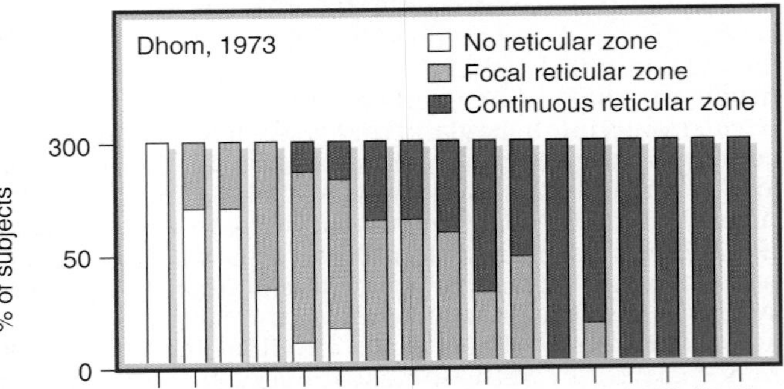

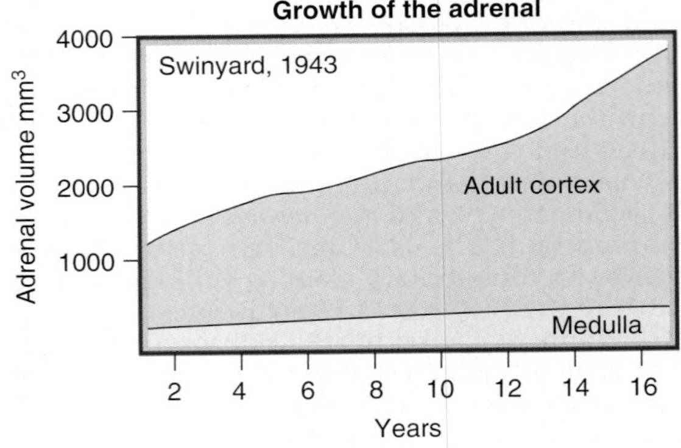

Figure 25-33 Relation of plasma dehydroepiandrosterone sulfate (DHEAS [DHAS]) levels to growth of the zona reticularis and increase in adrenal volume with age. *Top,* The close correlation between the development of the zona reticularis and the increase in the plasma DHEAS level. *Middle,* The age at which focal islands of reticular tissue or a continuous reticular zone was found in a series of patients with sudden death who had not had an antecedent illness. *Bottom,* The increase in adrenal volume at the time of puberty. For conversion to SI units, see Figure 25-26. (From Grumbach MM, Richards HE, Conte FA, et al. Clinical disorders of adrenal function and puberty: assessment of the role of the adrenal cortex and abnormal puberty in man and evidence for an ACTH-like pituitary adrenal androgen stimulating hormone. In: James VHT, Serio M, Giusti G, et al., eds. *The Endocrine Function of the Human Adrenal Cortex.* New York, NY: Academic Press, 1978:583-612.)

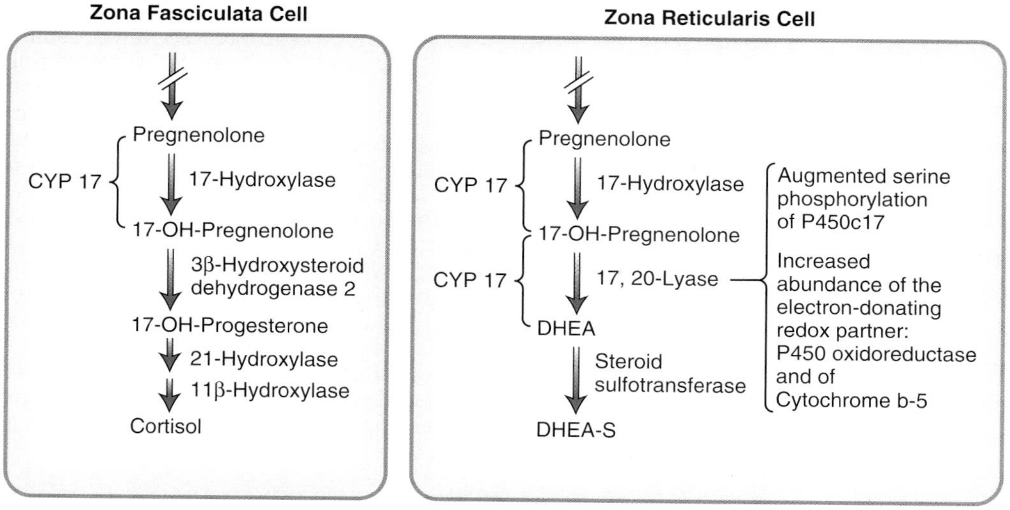

Zona Fasciculata Cell

Pregnenolone
CYP 17 — 17-Hydroxylase
17-OH-Pregnenolone
3β-Hydroxysteroid dehydrogenase 2
17-OH-Progesterone
21-Hydroxylase
11β-Hydroxylase
Cortisol

Zona Reticularis Cell

Pregnenolone
CYP 17 — 17-Hydroxylase — Augmented serine phosphorylation of P450c17
17-OH-Pregnenolone
CYP 17 — 17, 20-Lyase — Increased abundance of the electron-donating redox partner: P450 oxidoreductase and of Cytochrome b-5
DHEA
Steroid sulfotransferase
DHEA-S

Figure 25-34 Adrenarche and the zona reticularis. The rise in circulating dehydroepiandrosterone sulfate (DHEAS) levels is the biochemical hallmark of adrenarche. The diagram compares and contrasts the major steroidogenic pathway in the zona fasciculata with that in the zona reticularis. In contrast to the zona fasciculata, the expression of 3β-hydroxysteroid, $\Delta^{4,5}$ isomerase type 2 messenger ribonucleic acid (mRNA), and its activity (the enzyme that irreversibly traps Δ^5 precursors into Δ^4 steroids) is very low in the zona reticularis, whereas the expression of and activity of steroid sulfotransferase is high. A single gene, *CYP17* (now designated *CYP17A1*), encodes a single enzyme that has 17α-hydroxylase and 17,20-lyase activity, but the ratio of 17,20-lyase to 17α-hydroxylase activity is relatively high in the zona reticularis compared with that in the zona fasciculata. Some of the factors that seem to amplify the increased 17,20-lyase activity of *CYP17* are the augmented serine phosphorylation of the enzyme and the apparent increased abundance of the electron-donating redox partner, including P450 reductase and of cytochrome b_5.

strikingly decreased 17,20-lyase activity but retention of 17α-hydroxylase activity.[449,450] Two XY phenotypic females with hypergonadotropic hypogonadism and normal mineralocorticoid and glucocorticoid function had isolated 17,20-lyase deficiency due to homozygous mutations at the Arg347 or the Arg358 residue in CYP17.[450]

In contrast to these observations of loss of 17,20-lyase activity with retention of 17α-hydroxylase activity, the ratio of human 17,20-lyase to 17α-hydroxylase activities was increased by increased phosphorylation of serine and threonine residues on the CYP17enzyme[451] and by the increased abundance of redox partners such as cytochrome P450 oxidoreductase and by cytochrome b_5, which preferentially promotes 17,20-lyase activity by allosterically affecting the interaction between cyp17 and P450 oxidoreductase.[449,452] These studies provided a provisional hypothesis of the mechanisms that appear to be involved in the relatively increased 17,20-lyase activity of the zona reticularis, although not its regulation (see Fig. 25-34).

Regulation of adrenal androgen secretion in the zona reticularis is postulated to be based on a dual-control mechanism. First, corticotropin (ACTH, adrenocorticotropin) is obligatory, as evidenced by the findings in cases of ACTH deficiency or resistance.[453] Second, the mechanism requires the action of an unidentified adrenal androgen-stimulating factor, possibly pituitary in origin or from a nonadrenal source, or an intra-adrenal event.[284] This concept is illustrated in Figure 25-35.[284,313,441,449,454]

CRH has been advanced as an adrenal androgen secretagogue that has stimulatory action on the zona reticularis. The intravenous infusion of human CRH into dexamethasone-suppressed young men increased DHEA, DHEAS, and androstenedione secretion within 3 hours. Similar results were obtained in adolescent girls with hyperandrogenism and a history of premature adrenarche.[455] CRH directly stimulates DHEAS secretion and the expression of CYP17 by the fetal adrenal cortical cells.[456] Leptin in vitro vigorously stimulates 17,20-lyase activity and transiently stimulates 17α-hydroxylase activity of the microsomal enzyme CYP17, implying a role in adrenarche,[457] but no clinical evidence suggests a pivotal role of leptin in adrenarche. Therefore, a distinct hormone or factor that in addition to ACTH stimulates the zona reticularis and adrenal androgen secretion has not been isolated, and the mechanism regulating adrenarche remains unknown.[458]

A distinct adrenal androgen-stimulating factor, whether of pituitary, intra-adrenal, or other origin, may explain the following observations[284]:

1. The spurt in adrenal growth and the differentiation and growth of the zona reticularis at adrenarche occur independently of an increase in ACTH or cortisol secretion but correlate with the increase in plasma levels of DHEAS (see Fig. 25-34).
2. Cortisol and adrenal androgen secretions vary independently with age, during normal and premature adrenarche, and in Cushing's disease, starvation, malnutrition, anorexia nervosa, and chronic disease.
3. Unlike cortisol secretion, the secretion of DHEA and DHEAS in response to ACTH administration varies with age.
4. Dissociation of adrenarche and gonadarche occurs in a variety of disorders of sexual maturation (see Fig. 25-35), including premature adrenarche (i.e., onset of pubic or axillary hair before 8 years of age), chronic adrenal insufficiency, CPP (when the onset is before age 6 years), primary hypogonadism, isolated gonadotropin deficiency, and anorexia nervosa.[442]

A longitudinal study of 42 children demonstrated that an increase in BMI (but not the value itself at any age) was related to the rise in urinary excretion of DHEAS, suggesting that a change in nutritional status is one physiologic regulator of adrenarche.[459]

Adrenal Androgens and Puberty

The earlier onset of adrenarche than gonadarche and the contribution of adrenal androgens to the growth of pubic and axillary hair have led some to suggest that adrenal

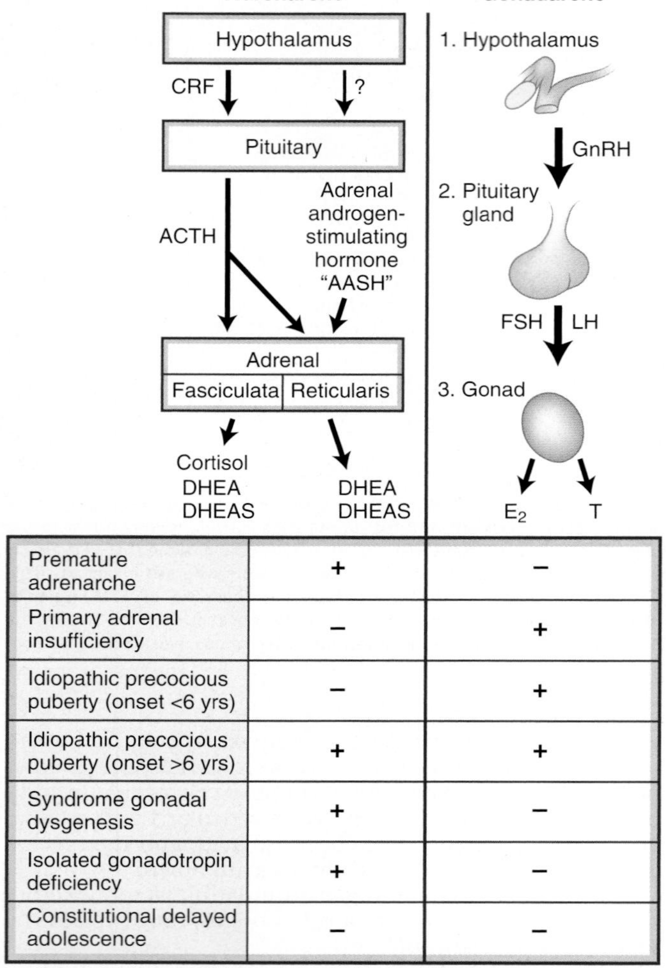

	Adrenarche	Gonadarche
Premature adrenarche	+	−
Primary adrenal insufficiency	−	+
Idiopathic precocious puberty (onset <6 yrs)	−	+
Idiopathic precocious puberty (onset >6 yrs)	+	+
Syndrome gonadal dysgenesis	+	−
Isolated gonadotropin deficiency	+	−
Constitutional delayed adolescence	−	−

Figure 25-35 Hypothesis of the control of pituitary adrenal androgen secretion by a putative separate adrenal androgen-stimulating hormone acting on a corticotropin (ACTH)-primed adrenal cortex. Although this diagram suggests that adrenal androgen-stimulating hormone (AASH) arises from the pituitary gland, a distinct pituitary factor with AASH activity has not been isolated; an extrapituitary factor is not excluded. The lower part of the diagram shows the relationship of adrenarche to gonadarche, including dissociation in various clinical disorders of sexual development (+, present; −, absent). (Modified from Sklar CA, Kaplan SL, Grumbach MM. Evidence for dissociation between adrenarche and gonadarche: studies in patients with idiopathic precocious puberty, gonadal dysgenesis, isolated gonadotropin deficiency, and constitutionally delayed puberty. *J Clin Endocrinol Metab.* 1980;51:548-556. Copyright by The Endocrine Society.)

androgens in normal children are an important factor in the onset of puberty and the maturation of the hypothalamic-pituitary-gonadal complex.

Although CPP may occur when the prepubertal child has previously been exposed to excessive levels of androgens from an endogenous or exogenous source (e.g., after the initiation of glucocorticoid therapy in congenital virilizing adrenal hyperplasia, after removal of a sex steroid–secreting adrenal or gonadal neoplasm),[284,460] there is little evidence that adrenal androgens play an important qualitative or rate-limiting role in the onset of puberty in normal children.[284] Most patients with premature adrenarche, who secrete excessive amounts of adrenal androgens for their age, enter puberty and experience menarche within the normal age range.[284] Moreover, prepubertal children who have congenital or acquired chronic adrenal insufficiency (i.e., Addison's disease) and consequently have deficient or absent adrenal androgen secretion usually have a normal onset and normal progression through puberty when given appropriate glucocorticoid and mineralocorticoid replacement therapy.[284] Studies of children with chronic adrenal insufficiency, isolated gonadotropin deficiency, hypergonadotropic hypogonadism, or androgen resistance suggest that adrenal androgens in girls and boys are not essential for the adolescent growth spurt, whereas gonadal steroids secreted by the testis and ovary are essential and act in concert with GH.[284] The transient increase in height velocity (about 1.5 cm/year in both sexes) that occurs in middle childhood (6 to 7 years) and lasts about 2 years terminates while the serum DHEAS level continues to increase. This increase in height velocity is related to the cyclic pattern of prepubertal growth and to genetic regulation of growth rather than to an increase in adrenal androgen or GH secretion.[451,461]

DISORDERS OF PUBERTY

Delayed Puberty and Sexual Infantilism

The upper limits of the normal age of onset of puberty are 14 years for boys and 13 years for girls (Table 25-15). Functionally, delayed puberty can be divided into disorders that affect the operation of the GnRH pulse generator, the pituitary gland, or the gonad.

Idiopathic or Constitutional Delay in Growth and Puberty

Otherwise healthy girls who spontaneously enter puberty after the age of 13 years and boys who begin after 14 years have constitutional delay in growth and adolescence, the most common diagnosis for delayed puberty. Affected individuals usually are short (2 SD below the mean value of height for age) at evaluation and have been shorter than their classmates for years, although growth velocity and height are usually appropriate for bone age (Fig. 25-36 and Table 25-16). Family history in as many as 77% of cases reveals a mother who had delayed menarche or a father (or sibling) who entered puberty late (i.e., age 14 to 18 years), and the pattern in some cases suggests dominant inheritance with incomplete penetrance.[462,463] Constitutional delay in development is physiologic immaturity with a slow tempo of maturation; full sexual maturity will be reached, but the process takes longer than usual. Because of delay in reactivation of the GnRH pulse generator, there is functional deficiency of GnRH for chronologic age but not for the stage of physiologic development. Adrenarche and gonadarche occur later in individuals with constitutional (idiopathic) delay in growth and adolescence,[462] whereas adrenarche usually occurs at a normal age in patients with isolated gonadotropin deficiency.[442] Bone age is delayed at presentation, but after a bone age of approximately 12 to 14 years for boys or 11 to 13 years for girls is achieved, sexual maturation begins, although bone age is not a fully reliable indicator.

Most of these patients with CDP are thin, but 25% are above the 85th percentile in BMI for age, and their bone age is less delayed than in classic thin patients (i.e., they tend to achieve taller adult stature).[462] There is no impairment of olfaction, as in Kallmann's syndrome, and undescended testes are uncommon. Plasma gonadal steroid levels are low in pediatric assays at the time of presentation, but as bone age advances, the serum gonadotropin

TABLE 25-15

Classification of Delayed Puberty and Sexual Infantilism

IDIOPATHIC (CONSTITUTIONAL) DELAY IN GROWTH AND PUBERTY (DELAYED ACTIVATION OF HYPOTHALAMIC LRF PULSE GENERATOR)	
HYPOGONADOTROPIC HYPOGONADISM: SEXUAL INFANTILISM RELATED TO GONADOTROPIN DEFICIENCY	
CNS Disorders	**HYPERGONADOTROPIC HYPOGONADISM**
Tumors	***Males***
Craniopharyngiomas	The syndrome of seminiferous tubular dysgenesis and its variants (Klinefelter's syndrome)
Germinomas	Other forms of primary testicular failure
Other germ cell tumors	Chemotherapy
Hypothalamic and optic gliomas	Radiation therapy
Astrocytomas	Testicular steroid biosynthetic defects
Pituitary tumors (including MEN-1, prolactinoma)	Sertoli-only syndrome
Other Causes	LH receptor mutation
Langerhans' histiocytosis	Anorchia and cryptorchidism
Postinfectious lesions of the CNS	Trauma/surgery
Vascular abnormalities of the CNS	***Females***
Radiation therapy	The syndrome of gonadal dysgenesis (Turner's syndrome) and its variants
Congenital malformations especially associated with craniofacial anomalies	XX and XY gonadal dysgenesis
Head trauma	Familial and sporadic XX gonadal dysgenesis and its variants
Lymphocytic hypophysitis	Familial and sporadic XY gonadal dysgenesis and its variants
Isolated Gonadotropin Deficiency	Aromatase deficiency
Kallmann's syndrome	Other forms of primary ovarian failure
With hyposmia or anosmia	Premature menopause
Without anosmia	Radiation therapy
LHRH receptor mutation	Chemotherapy
Congenital adrenal hypoplasia (*DAX1* mutation)	Autoimmune oophoritis
Isolated LH deficiency	Galactosemia
Isolated FSH deficiency	Glycoprotein syndrome type 1
Prohormone convertase 1 deficiency (PC1)	Resistant ovary
Idiopathic and Genetic Forms of Multiple Pituitary Hormone Deficiencies Including PROP1 Mutation	FSH receptor mutation
Miscellaneous Disorders	LH/hCG resistance
Prader-Willi syndrome	Polycystic ovarian disease
Laurence-Moon and Bardet-Biedl syndromes	Trauma/surgery
Functional gonadotropin deficiency	Noonan's or pseudo-Turner's syndrome
Chronic systemic disease and malnutrition	Ovarian steroid biosynthetic defects
Sickle cell disease	
Cystic fibrosis	
Acquired immunodeficiency syndrome (AIDS)	
Chronic gastroenteric disease	
Chronic renal disease	
Malnutrition	
Anorexia nervosa	
Bulimia	
Psychogenic amenorrhea	
Impaired puberty and delayed menarche in female athletes and ballet dancers (exercise amenorrhea)	
Hypothyroidism	
Diabetes mellitus	
Cushing's disease	
Hyperprolactinemia	
Marijuana use	
Gaucher's disease	

CNS, central nervous system; hCG, human chorionic gonadotropin; LHRH, luteinizing hormone–releasing hormone; LRF, luteinizing hormone–releasing factor; MEN, multiple endocrine neoplasia.

concentration and the amplitude of LH pulses increase (initially at night); the basal serum gonadotropin concentrations measured by third-generation assays and the LH response to GnRH or GnRH agonists reflect maturation of the hypothalamic-pituitary system.

The first signs of secondary sexual development occur within 1 year after LH rises to pubertal levels in response to administration of 100 μg of intravenous synthetic GnRH or subcutaneous GnRH agonist or within 1 year after gonadotropin and testosterone or estradiol concentrations begin to increase spontaneously above prepubertal values.[241,314] An 8 a.m. serum testosterone value of 0.7 nmol/L (20 ng/dL) heralds the development of phenotypic puberty in boys within 12 to 15 months.[464] CDP is more common in boys and may be a counterpart of idiopathic CPP, a condition that is many times more common in girls. Familial short stature is a physiologic variant of growth in which the velocity of development and bone age

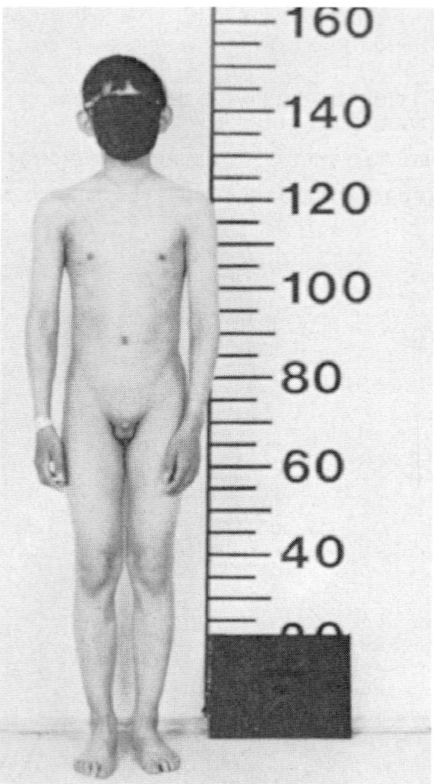

Figure 25-36 A boy age 16 years and 2 months has constitutional delay in growth and puberty. His height is 149.5 cm (4 SD below the mean value for age); upper-to-lower body ratio is 1.1 (retarded for age); phallus is 6.0 × 1.6 cm; testes are 2.5 × 1.4 cm; and the scrotum showed early thinning. At a chronologic age of 15 years and 4 months, the bone age was 11 years and the sella turcica was normal. The plasma concentration of luteinizing hormone (LH) was 0.7 ng/mL (LER-960); the concentration of follicle-stimulating hormone (FSH) was 0.5 ng/mL (LER-869). On gonadotropin-releasing hormone (GnRH) testing, the plasma concentration of LH increased to 2.2 ng/mL (an increment of 1.5 ng/mL), and the testosterone level rose from 52 to 77 ng/dL. The testes subsequently spontaneously enlarged, and the patient progressed through puberty. For conversion to SI units, see Figures 25-16 and 25-17. (From Styne DM, Grumbach MM. Puberty in the male and female: its physiology and disorders. In: Yen SCC, Jaffe RB, eds. *Reproductive Endocrinology,* 2nd ed. Philadelphia, PA: Saunders, 1986:313-384.)

are normal but stature is decreased, in contrast to CDP, which is a disorder of tempo that secondarily impairs growth. The combination of CDP and familial short stature leads to conspicuous shortness during adolescence, especially when other children increase their growth velocity, and referrals occur more often with this combination than with either condition alone. Because no single test reliably distinguishes between CDP and isolated hypogonadotropic hypogonadism (IHH), watchful waiting is usually in order.

TABLE 25-16

Constitutional Delay in Growth and Adolescence

- A variation of normal
- Males more often seek assistance
- Family history of delayed menarche or delayed secondary sexual characteristics
- Height is often below the 5th percentile, but growth rate is normal for skeletal age
- Onset of adrenarche is delayed
- The combination of genetic short stature and constitutional delay leads to more profound short stature
- Final height is less than predicted

The growth rate before the actual onset of puberty in constitutional delay is often suboptimal for chronologic age, but growth velocity usually increases to normal levels after puberty begins.[465] Affected boys seem to be more distressed by short stature than by delay in sexual development.

GH release in the basal state and in response to GH secretagogues, including the administration of GHRH, is low for age and may be decreased further in children with CDP, but the amplitude of GH secretion and the GH response to GHRH is greater after administration of exogenous (aromatizable) androgens or estrogens. Therefore, CDP may constitute a temporary state of functional GH insufficiency for chronologic age but not for bone age. IGF1 interacts with gonadotropins in the ovary and testis, and the relatively low secretion of GH (and presumably intragonadal IGF1) in CDP may impair the gonadal response to gonadotropins.[466]

Patients with constitutional delay in adolescence and growth do not reach their predicted height in some reports,[467] especially if the family is tall. Girls with CDP[468] have a mean deficit in adult height of 2.4 cm below the mean predicted height, although the range of adult height varies about 10 cm above or below predictions. An alternative explanation for reduced adult stature is that the patients most likely to be referred are those that combine genetic short stature with CDP.[467] The magnitude of the catch-up in linear growth during puberty in boys is a major determinant of adult height.[469] Heavier individuals with CDP reach greater height than those who are thinner.[462] When the genetic tendency for growth is greater, subjects with CDP reach taller adult stature. The role of bone density in CDP was discussed earlier.

Because 15% to 20% of adult height is gained during puberty, many approaches have been tried to increase stature in otherwise normal, short children. Delaying the onset or progression with puberty by the use of GnRH agonists was suggested by some, but a decrease in bone density 1 year after cessation led to warnings that routine administration of this treatment carries substantial risk.[470] The additional psychological risk of delaying puberty in otherwise normal children should also be considered, and this treatment is neither established nor recommended.

Although GH therapy seemed likely to increase adult height in CDP, results from initial clinical trials were disappointing.[471]

The U.S. Food and Drug Administration (FDA) approved GH treatment for children who are predicted to reach an adult height less than the 1st percentile (160 cm), which includes some children with CDP, and some studies reported an increase in adult height with this treatment. The GH level rises during pubertal development, and the FDA approved GH therapy in larger doses for subjects with GH deficiency during puberty. However, there are only moderate effects of increased GH doses during puberty on adult height, and both overshadow, although male gender has a positive effect and age at onset of puberty has a negative effect, the effects of the change in dose on adult height.[472]

The combination of GnRH agonist therapy with GH treatment in attempts to increase adult height in children who were normal except for genetic short stature and in SGA children led to inconclusive results or to increased predicted or near-final height, which does not necessarily translate into increased adult height. This approach to treatment remains experimental. Review of a large database from a postmarketing survey did not support the efficacy of this approach,[473] and there was no good follow-up evaluation of adult height. This combination therapy cannot be supported by substantial evidence.[474]

The cost of GH for treatment of non–GH-deficient short stature is exceptionally high: $14,000 per cm or $35,000 per inch gained.[475] Payers are reluctant in many cases to cover the cost of the GH therapy for those without confirmed GH deficiency. There are few controlled studies of adult height, but more such studies are strongly recommended to determine the efficacy of this treatment in short, normal children.[476]

Because the critical role of estradiol in skeletal maturation was appreciated, treatment with a potent aromatase inhibitor to increase adult height by inhibiting skeletal maturation aroused interest.[150,151,257] A double-blind, randomized, placebo-controlled study enrolled boys with CDP who were treated with 6 months of monthly testosterone or testosterone plus an added 12-month trial of daily oral letrozole (a potent fourth-generation aromatase inhibitor). The results revealed a mean increase in predicted adult height of 5.1 cm in the letrozole plus testosterone group[477]; a subsequent study supported these promising effects on increasing the time of pubertal growth height without affecting the development of male secondary sex characteristics, but there are few data on actual adult height.[477] The boys in the group treated with testosterone and letrozole developed increased bioactive testosterone, analyzed by a cellular assay, compared with control boys.[249] Serum testosterone measured by HPLCMS/MS can reach levels of more than 1000 ng/dL. However, markers of bone turnover decrease, and vertebral abnormalities may develop with the use of these agents in idiopathic short stature.[478] A 1-year study of the aromatase inhibitor anastrazole plus GH, compared with GH treatment alone, in boys demonstrated no ill effects on body composition, plasma lipids, bone metabolism, or the tempo of puberty (although estrogen decreased, as expected with the use of anastrozole), and the predicted height was increased.[479] This treatment has not been supported by long-term studies observing patients up to adult height, and concerns about possible effects on bone density must be addressed, probably until the patients are at least 20 to 25 years old, before this off-label therapy can be recommended.[480]

Hypogonadotropic Hypogonadism: Sexual Infantilism Related to Gonadotropin Deficiency

Insufficient pulsatile secretion of GnRH and the resulting FSH and LH deficiency lead to delayed sexual maturation. The phenotype in hypogonadotropic hypogonadism can vary from severe sexual infantilism to apparent CDP (both conditions may be found in the same family[481]). There may be an absolute or relative quantitative deficiency of pulsatile GnRH, or the deficiency may be qualitative, especially in females; it may involve abnormalities in amplitude or frequency of GnRH pulses or in both components (Fig. 25-37).

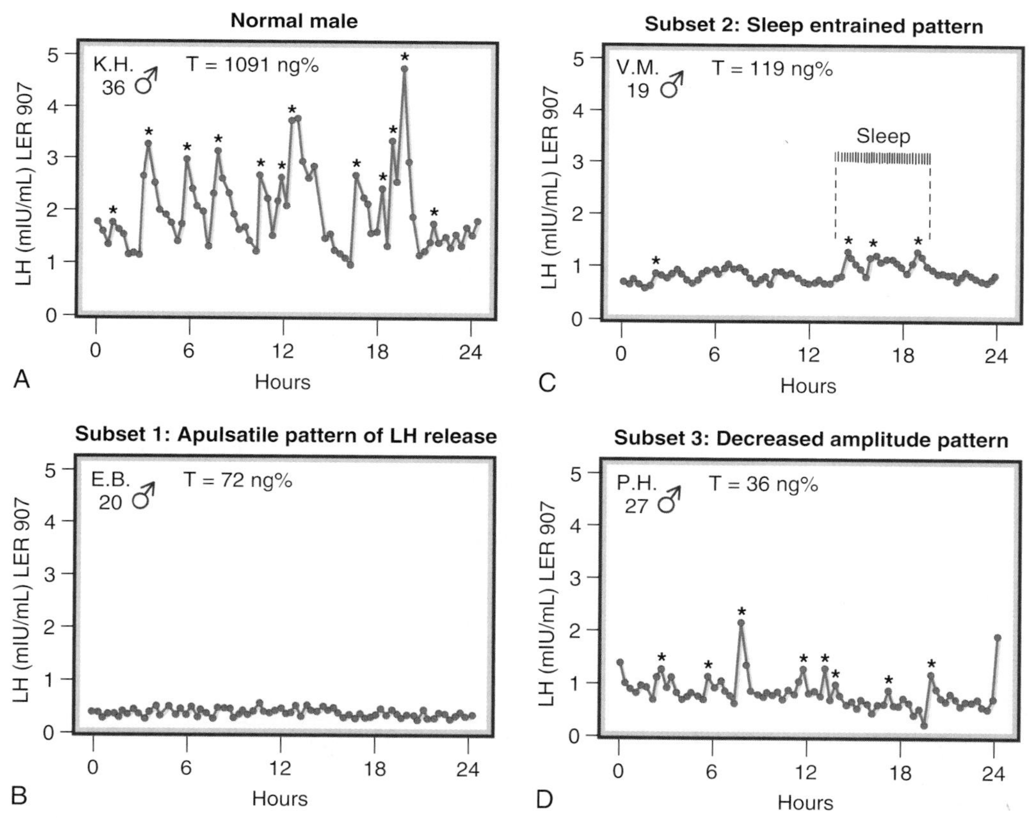

Figure 25-37 Various patterns of pulsatile luteinizing hormone (LH) secretion that can occur in isolated hypogonadotropic hypogonadism (**B** to **D**) are compared with LH secretion in a normal man (**A**). **A,** Discrete LH pulses occur about every 2 hours in a normal 36-year-old man. **B,** Typical apulsatile LH pattern is associated with a low testosterone concentration usually found in isolated hypogonadotropic hypogonadism. **C,** Pattern of developmental arrest with low-amplitude nocturnal LH pulses is apparent only during sleep. **D,** Low-amplitude LH pulse pattern occurs during sleep and wake periods. To convert LH values to international units per liter, multiply by 1.0. (From Spratt DI, Crowley WF. Hypogonadotropic hypogonadism: GnRH therapy. In: Krieger DT, Bardin CW, eds. *Current Therapy in Endocrinology and Metabolism, 1985-1986.* Toronto, Canada: BC Decker, 1985:155-159.)

Patients with IHH usually are of normal height in early or middle adolescent years, whereas patients with CDP usually have a normal growth rate for bone age but are short for chronologic age. In contrast to CDP patients, those with hypogonadotropic hypogonadism usually do not respond to GnRH stimulation, nor do they have a pulsatile LH profile commensurate with bone age. Although serum concentrations of plasma FSH and LH and urinary gonadotropins are low, the differences are relative rather than absolute and are not diagnostic for an individual.

Hypogonadotropic hypogonadism may result from a genetic or developmental defect present at birth but remain undetected until the age of expected puberty, or it may be caused by a tumor, inflammatory process, vascular lesion, irradiation, or trauma to the hypothalamus. Similarly, hypogonadotropic hypogonadism may arise from lesions or defects that involve the pituitary gland directly. When GH is affected as well as gonadotropins, impaired growth is manifested by decreased growth velocity, especially during the expected pubertal growth spurt, and short stature.

Central Nervous System Tumors

Extrasellar masses may interfere with GnRH synthesis, secretion, or stimulation of pituitary gonadotrophs. Most patients with hypothalamic-pituitary tumors causing gonadotropin deficiency have one or more additional pituitary hormone deficiencies (or an increased serum prolactin level with prolactinomas). Those with GH deficiency due to a neoplasm have late onset of growth failure compared with those who have idiopathic and familial hypopituitarism, in which growth failure starts early in life. The presence of anterior and posterior pituitary deficiencies in infancy suggests a midline developmental defect, but the development of this combination after infancy ominously suggests an expanding CNS lesion.

Craniopharyngioma. Craniopharyngioma is a common CNS neoplasm of nonglial origin. It is the most common brain tumor associated with hypothalamic-pituitary dysfunction and sexual infantilism and comprises 80% to 90% of neoplasms found in the pituitary and up to 15% of all intracranial tumors in childhood.[482] This tumor of the Rathke pouch originates from epithelial rests along the pituitary stalk that extend superiorly to the hypothalamus. Craniopharyngiomas may reside within or above the sella turcica, or, more rarely, they may be found in the nasopharynx or the third ventricle. Craniopharyngioma appears to be a monoclonal tumor, and about 50% have cytogenetic abnormalities such as gains in 1q, 12q, and 17q or β-catenin gene mutations in the case of the uncommon adamantinomatous craniopharyngioma.[482]

Craniopharyngiomas are usually symptomatic before age 20 years, with the peak incidence occurring between the ages of 6 and 14 years. CNS signs develop as the tumor encroaches on surrounding structures. Symptoms of craniopharyngioma include headache, visual disturbances, short stature, diabetes insipidus, vomiting, and weakness of one or more limbs. Visual defects (including bilateral temporal field deficits), optic atrophy or papilledema, and signs of GH deficiency, delayed puberty, and hypothyroidism are features of craniopharyngiomas.[483] Although most patients are below the mean in height and height velocity at diagnosis, a long, indolent course is possible. Deficiencies of gonadotropins, GH, thyrotropin (TSH), ACTH, and arginine vasopressin are common. The serum concentration of prolactin is normal or increased. Delayed bone age is common and may point to the onset of tumor growth.

About 70% of patients with a craniopharyngioma have suprasellar or intrasellar calcification (found in fewer than 1% of normal individuals) and an abnormal sella turcica, which are sometimes found on radiographs taken for other indications, including orthodontia.[483] CT (but not MRI) reveals fine calcifications that are not apparent on lateral skull radiographs, and CT or MRI with contrast (the diagnostic procedure of choice) can determine whether the tumor is cystic or solid and indicate the presence of hydrocephalus (Fig. 25-38).[484]

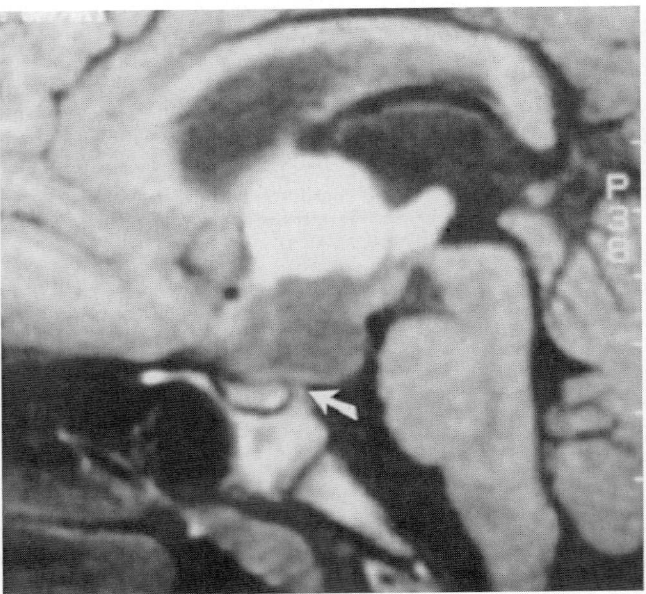

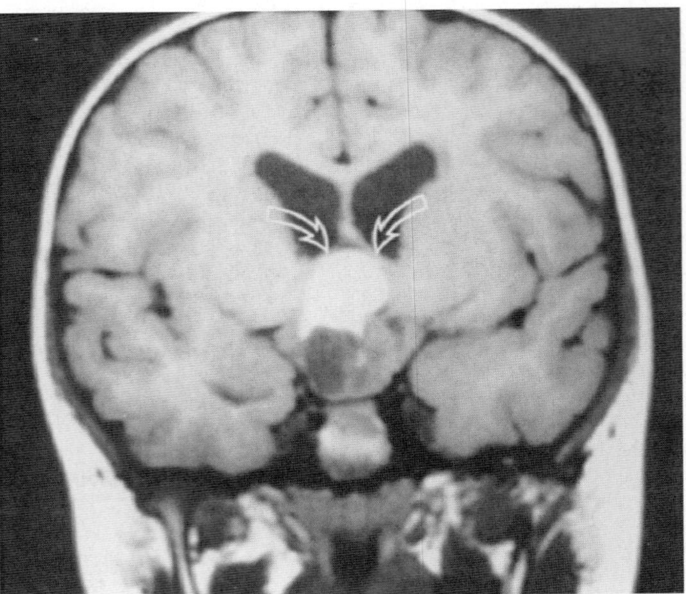

Figure 25-38 Craniopharyngioma in a short 5-year-old girl with a history of frontal headaches, impaired vision, and poor growth. *Left,* Midline, sagittal, T1-weighted image shows a hyperintense region superiorly and an inferior hypointense region. The combination of hyperintense and hypointense areas in a non–contrast-enhanced examination is the most characteristic finding for craniopharyngioma. Notice the erosion of dorsum sellae *(solid arrow)* and posterior pituitary bright spot. *Right,* Coronal, T1-weighted image shows tumor extending upward to the inferior frontal horns, narrowing the foramen of Monro, and causing mild hydrocephalus. The *open arrows* indicate the upper border of the hyperintense area of the tumor.

Smaller craniopharyngiomas, usually intrasellar, can be treated by transsphenoidal microsurgery, but larger or suprasellar masses usually require craniotomy, and the approach must be individualized. The combination of limited tumor removal and radiation therapy leads to a satisfactory neurologic prognosis, better cognitive outcome, and better endocrine outcome compared with attempts at complete surgical extirpation.[483] Frequent and early tumor relapse after apparently complete resection and tumor progression after incomplete resection suggest the wisdom of radiation therapy after surgery.[484] Postoperative hyperphagia and obesity (BMI >5 SD above normal) can be striking and correlate with the magnitude of hypothalamic damage on cranial MRI. Injury to the hypothalamic ventromedial nuclei (associated with increased parasympathetic activity and hyperinsulinemia) or to the paraventricular nuclei may cause these findings, and insulin suppression may be helpful.[485] Aberrant sleep patterns and even narcolepsy and daytime somnolence may follow surgical treatment of craniopharyngiomas, with melatonin improving sleep patterns in some.[486] Although the endocrine complications are more manageable, the combination of antidiuretic hormone insufficiency (i.e., diabetes insipidus) and impaired sense of thirst remains a complex management problems.

A Rathke-cleft cyst is often discovered as an incidental finding on MRI, but it can produce symptoms and signs indistinguishable from those of a craniopharyngioma, such as precocious or delayed puberty.[487] Surgical drainage and excision of the cyst wall are customary.

Other Extrasellar Tumors. Germinomas (i.e., pinealomas, ectopic pinealomas, atypical teratomas, or dysgerminomas) and other germ cell tumors of the CNS are the most common extrasellar tumors that arise in the suprasellar hypothalamic region and in the pineal region that commonly cause sexual infantilism. Peak incidences occur in the second decade and during infancy. They are found more often in males.[488] Polydipsia and polyuria are the most common symptoms, followed by visual difficulties and abnormalities of growth and puberty[489] or movement disorders. Diagnosis is often delayed for months to years because the findings are attributed to psychiatric disorders. Deficiencies of vasopressin and GH are most common, but other anterior pituitary hormone deficiencies (including gonadotropin deficiency) and elevated serum prolactin levels are also frequent. Determination of the concentration of hCG in spinal fluid and in serum and assessment of α-fetoprotein levels provide useful tumor markers in children and adolescents with germ cell tumors. Germ cell tumors in boys cause isosexual GnRH-independent sexual precocity by secretion of hCG (see "Sexual Precocity"). Tumors secreting hCG cause precocious puberty in boys, and there has been one case report of an affected girl.

Subependymal spread of germ cell tumors along the lining of the third ventricle is common, and seeding may involve the lower spinal cord and corda equina. MRI with contrast enhancement is useful in the detection of isolated enlargement of the pituitary stalk, an early finding that requires periodic MRI monitoring, especially in patients with diabetes insipidus.[489,490] The size of the pituitary gland increases by 100% between year 1 and year 15, but the pineal gland does not normally change in size after the first year of life; any later enlargement indicates a mass lesion.[491] Pineal cysts are a rare cause of CPP.

Irradiation is the preferred treatment for pure germ cell tumors such as germinomas; surgery is rarely indicated, except for biopsy to establish a tissue diagnosis.[490] Chemotherapy alone is inadequate, but the combination of chemotherapy and radiation therapy can be successful,[492,493] and both treatment methods are recommended for a mixed germ cell tumor. Because testicular germ cell tumors are occasionally found years after successful therapy for CNS germ cell tumors, long-term surveillance is indicated.[494,495] Hypothalamic and optic gliomas or astrocytomas, occurring as part of neurofibromatosis (von Recklinghausen disease) or arising independently, can also cause sexual infantilism.

Only 2% to 6% of all surgically treated pituitary tumors occur in childhood and adolescence, with about 1 in 1,000,000 children affected.[482] Most functional pituitary adenomas are ACTH secreting, with prolactinomas secreting GH or nonfunctioning adenomas occurring less commonly, although prolactinomas manifest most often in adolescence. Most pituitary tumors are monoclonal lesions caused by mutations of *GNAS*.

A survey of 44 cases reported that 61% of prolactinomas were macroadenomas (more often in boys; hypopituitarism and growth failure were common) and 39% were microadenomas (more often in girls; delayed puberty was common).[496,497] Only 2 of these 29 patients had delayed onset of puberty,[497] although primary amenorrhea was the presenting symptom in 13 of 20 pubertal females. Presenting symptoms included oligomenorrhea and galactorrhea in the girls and headache in the boys. Galactorrhea may be demonstrable only by manual manipulation of the nipples (blood samples for prolactin should be obtained before examination or many hours later, because manipulation of the nipples raises prolactin levels).

Dopaminergic therapy is often successful in decreasing prolactin values.[498] Transsphenoidal resection of microprolactinomas in children and adolescents is an effective treatment.[497] The dopamine agonist bromergocriptine may decrease serum prolactin concentrations and decrease tumor size, which is a useful approach before surgery of large macroprolactinomas is undertaken and when resection of the adenoma is incomplete. Pubertal progression and normal menstrual function in girls usually follows reduction of serum prolactin levels. Pituitary apoplexy followed cabergoline treatment of a macroprolactinoma in a 16-year-old girl; this complication has been seen in adults treated with bromocryptine,[499] and tricuspid regurgitation may be a cumulative effect.[500] High serum levels of macroprolactin, a complex of immunoglobulin G and monomeric prolactin with little biologic activity in vivo, cross-react in commercial prolactin assays, leading to a finding of pseudohyperprolactinaemia.[501]

Other Central Nervous System Disorders Leading to Delayed Puberty

Langerhans Cell Histiocytosis. Langerhans cell histiocytosis (i.e., Hand-Schüller-Christian disease or histiocytosis X) is a clonal proliferative disorder of Langerhans histiocytes or their precursors. It is characterized by the infiltration of lipid-laden histiocytic cells or foam cells in skin, viscera, and bone.[502] The cause is not clear, because there are features of a neoplasm and features of a reactive immunologic disorder. Diabetes insipidus, caused by infiltration of the hypothalamus or the pituitary stalk, is the most common endocrine manifestation, with GH deficiency and delayed puberty possible. The lung, liver, and spleen, cyst-like areas in flat and long bones, and the dorsolumbar spine may be involved. "Floating teeth" within rarefied bone of the mandible, absent or loose teeth, and exophthalmos due to infiltration of the orbit are seen. Mastoid or temporal bone involvement may lead to chronic otitis media. Treatment with glucocorticoids, antineoplastic agents, and radiation therapy is promising in terms of survival, but more than 50% of patients have late sequelae or disease progression. The natural waxing and waning course of this rare disease makes evaluation of therapy difficult and highlights the importance of national treatment protocols.[502]

Postinfectious Inflammatory Lesions of the Central Nervous System, Vascular Abnormalities, and Head Trauma. Tuberculous or sarcoid granulomas of the CNS are associated with delayed puberty. The original case of adiposogenital dystrophy, or Fröhlich's syndrome, is thought to have been caused by tuberculosis rather than a neoplasm. Hydrocephalus may cause delayed puberty that can be reversed with decompression, as may pressure from a subarachnoid cyst.

Irradiation of the Central Nervous System. Irradiation of the CNS for treatment of tumors, leukemia, or neoplasms of the head and face may result in the gradual onset of hypothalamic-pituitary failure.[503,504] Although GH deficiency is the most common hormone disorder resulting from irradiation, gonadotropin deficiency, hypothyroidism, and decreased bone density also occur.[505] Self-reported fertility was reported to be lower in women who received CNS radiotherapy for acute lymphoblastic leukemia at about the time of menarche,[506] although the average age of women in this long-term study was in the early 20s, and longer follow-up of fertility may change the results.

Isolated Hypogonadal Hypogonadism

A defect involving the GnRH pulse generator or gonadotrophs without an anatomic lesion causes selective deficiency of gonadotropins, producing IHH (Tables 25-17 and 25-18).[507,508] Puberty fails to begin by 14 years in boys and 13 years in girls, or pubertal maturation is incomplete or transient. In boys, micropenis or undescended testes or both signs are evidence of a fetal testosterone deficiency caused by gonadotropin deficiency. Prepubertal concentration of gonadal sex steroid values (testosterone in boys; estradiol in girls) and low serum gonadotropin levels or values within the normal range (i.e., normal in the basal state but not in the secretory state) are characteristic. Concentrations of gonadal sex steroids and gonadotropins are low, pulsatile LH secretion is virtually absent, and the LH response to GnRH or GnRH agonist administration is deficient in the severe form. The testes are small and may be hard to find, and serum inhibin B, an estimate of seminiferous tubule function, is low.[509,510]

TABLE 25-17

Isolated Gonadotropin Deficiency

- Males more commonly affected
- Familial (more common in females) or sporadic (more common in males)
- Height normal for age; tall adult height if untreated
- Eunuchoid skeletal proportions
- Delayed bone age
- Small, often cryptorchid testes: diameter <2.5 cm prepubertal size; phallus may be small
- Normal adrenarche
- Examine for anosmia or hyposmia (Kallmann's syndrome)
- Look for associated malformations (facial, central nervous system, skeletal, renal)

TABLE 25-18

Features of Kallmann's Syndrome

Clinical

- GnRH deficiency: absent or arrested puberty
- Anosmia or hyposmia
- In infancy: microphallus; cryptorchidism
- Normal stature and growth in childhood
- Normal adrenarche
- Eunuchoid proportions
- Associated midline defects (e.g., cleft lip, cleft palate, midline cranial anomalies)
- MRI: aplasia or hypoplasia of olfactory bulbs and/or sulci

Prevalence

- Approximately 1 in 7500 males, 1 in 50,000 females; 10% prevalence of Klinefelter's syndrome

Inheritance

- Sporadic and familial cases; genetic heterogeneity
- X linked
  - X-lined recessive (Kallmann et al.)
  - X chromosome deletion: Xp22.3 (Meitinger T et al.)
- Autosomal
  - Dominant (sex limitation) (Santen and Paulsen; Merriam et al.)
  - Recessive (White et al.)

Anatomy

- Developmental field defect
- Aplasia or hypoplasia of olfactory bulb and sulcus
- Arrested migration of GnRH neurosecretory neurons from olfactory placode to medial basal hypothalamus

GnRH, luteinizing hormone-releasing hormone; MRI, magnetic resonance imaging.

(From Meitinger T, Heye B, Petit C, et al. Definitive localization of X-linked Kallmann's syndrome (hypogonadotropic hypogonadism and anosmia) to Xp22.3: close linkage to the hypervariable repeat sequence CRI-S232. *Am J Hum Genet.* 1990; 47:664-669; Merriam GR, Beitins IZ, Bode HH. Father-to-son transmission of hypogonadism with anosmia: Kallmann's syndrome. *Am J Dis Child.* 1977; 131:1216-1219; Santen RJ, Paulsen CA. Hypogonadotropic eunuchoidism. I. Clinical study of the mode of inheritance. *J Clin Endocrinol Metab.* 1973;36:47-54; White BJ, Rogal AD, Brown KS, et al. The syndrome of anosmia with hypogonadotropic hypogonadism: a genetic study of 18 new families and a review. *Am J Heel Genet.* 1983; 15:417-435.)

IHH may occur in families (about 20% to 30% of patients), or it may occur sporadically. In contrast to CNS tumors (in which patients usually have GH deficiency and growth failure) and to CDP (in which patients are short for chronologic age), height is appropriate for age in patients with IHH (Fig. 25-39). Because the levels of gonadal steroids, particularly estradiol, are too low to cause epiphyseal fusion at the normal age, increased arm span for height and a decreased ratio of upper to lower body segments (i.e., eunuchoid body proportions) are present. If the condition is left untreated, growth continues, and adult height is tall.[509,511]

Kallmann's Syndrome

Anosmia or hyposmia resulting from agenesis or hypoplasia of the olfactory lobes or sulci is associated with GnRH deficiency in Kallmann's syndrome, the most common form of IHH (see Table 25-18).[507,512] The condition was first observed in 1856, in the autopsy of a 40-year-old man with micropenis, small cryptorchid testes, and absence of the olfactory bulbs, but Kallmann described a familial pattern in 1944 (Fig. 25-40). The prevalence is 1 of every 10,000 males and 1 of every 5000 females. Although the loss of olfaction usually correlates with the degree of GnRH deficiency, even in complete anosmia, the GnRH deficiency

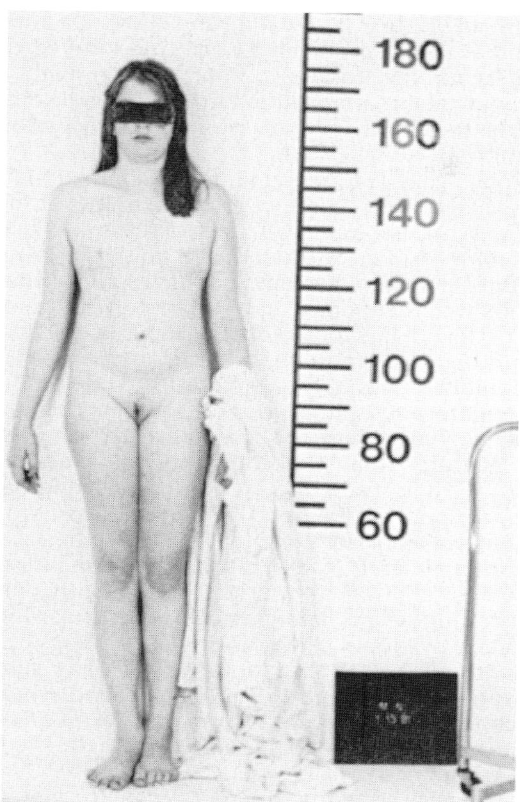

Figure 25-39 A girl aged 18 years and 8 months has isolated gonadotropin deficiency (i.e., sexual infantilism and primary amenorrhea). Her height is 173 cm (+1 SD), weight was 66.5 kg (+1 SD), and the skeletal age was 13 years. Adrenarche with pubic hair development occurred at age 13.5 years. At the time of the photograph, pubic hair was in stage 3, and there was slight breast and nipple development resulting from a previous short course of estrogen therapy. Immature labia minora and majora were observed, and no estrogen effect was seen on the vaginal mucosa. Olfactory testing results were normal. The plasma luteinizing hormone (LH) (LER-960) level after gonadotropin-releasing hormone (GnRH) administration rose from 0.5 to 1.8 ng/mL (a prepubertal response). Serum estradiol was undetectable. The dehydroepiandrosterone sulfate (DHEAS) level was 92 µg/dL (appropriate for pubic hair stage 2). Notice the discrepancy between adrenarche and gonadarche. For conversion to SI units, see Figures 25-16 and 25-25. (From Styne DM, Grumbach MM. Puberty in the male and female: its physiology and disorders. In: Yen SCC, Jaffe RB, eds. *Reproductive Endocrinology*, 2nd ed. Philadelphia, PA: Saunders, 1986:313-384.)

may be partial (see "Isolated Luteinizing Hormone Deficiency").[510] Because affected individuals often do not notice impaired olfaction; testing with graded dilutions of pure scents is necessary. Rarely, affected males with severe delay of puberty spontaneously increase their testicular size and enter full puberty.[513] Patients with Kallmann's syndrome have no or diminished nocturnal pulses of gonadotropins found in normal prepubertal boys, although daytime values are equal. Undescended testes and gynecomastia are common in this and all types of hypogonadotropic hypogonadism in boys.[509] The magnitude of the GnRH deficiency correlates with the size of the testes. Micropenis occurs in about one half of males with Kallmann's syndrome (Fig. 25-41).

Associated defects that are inconstantly present include cleft lip, cleft palate, imperfect facial fusion, seizure disorders, short metacarpals, pes cavus, neurosensory hearing loss (rarely found in the X-linked form[514]), cerebellar ataxia and nystagmus, ocular motor abnormalities, unilateral or rarely bilateral renal aplasia or dysplasia, and mirror movements of the upper extremities (i.e., bimanual synkinesia), limited to the X-linked form (see Table 25-18). Genetic details can be fond in the *Online Mendelian Inheritance in Man* (OMIM) catalog (available at http://www.ncbi.nlm.nih.gov/sites/entrez?db=omim [accessed February 2011]).

A variety of deletions and mutations of the *KAL1* gene have been described, including large and small (exon) deletions, point mutations, and a variety of nonsense mutations leading to frameshift and premature stop codons.[514,515] The *KAL1* mutations are more prevalent in Japanese than in white patients, and they can be associated with normal olfactory function.[516] The defect in some rare patients with no *KAL1* mutation but X-linked inheritance may be located in the promoter region of the *KAL1* gene. Kallmann's syndrome associated with X-linked ichthyosis caused by steroid sulfatase deficiency, mental retardation, and chondroplasia punctata occurs in a contiguous gene syndrome.[517] Only 14% of familial cases and 11% of sporadic cases

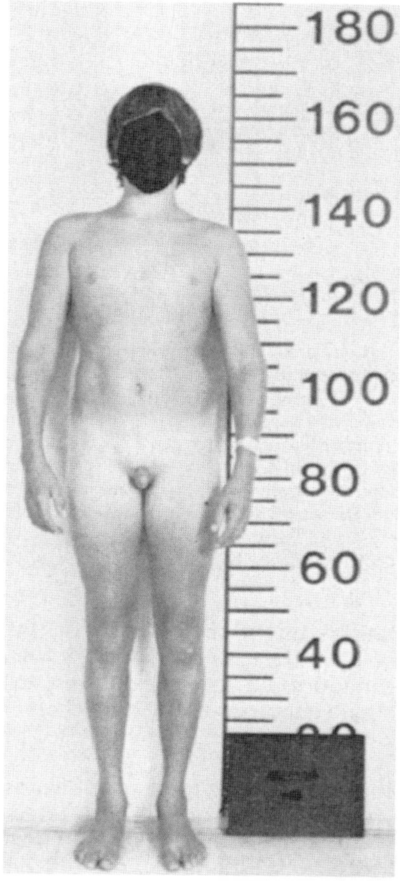

Figure 25-40 A boy aged 15 years and 10 months had isolated gonadotropin deficiency and anosmia (Kallmann's syndrome). He had undescended testes, but after administration of 10,000 U of human chorionic gonadotropin (hCG), the testes descended and were palpable in the scrotum. His height was 163.9 cm (+1.5 SD); the upper-to-lower body ratio was 0.86, which is eunuchoid. The phallus measured 6.3 × 1.8 cm, and the testes were 1.2 × 0.8 cm. The concentration of plasma luteinizing hormone (LH) was less than 0.3 ng/mL; the follicle-stimulating hormone (FSH) level was 1.2 ng/mL; and the testosterone level was 16 ng/dL. After 100 µg of gonadotropin-releasing hormone (GnRH), the plasma LH level (LER-960) was 0.7 ng/mL, and the FSH level (LER-869) was 2.4 ng/mL. For conversion to SI units, see Figures 25-16 and 25-17. (From Styne DM, Grumbach MM. Puberty in the male and female: its physiology and disorders. In: Yen SCC, Jaffe RB, eds. *Reproductive Endocrinology*, 2nd ed. Philadelphia, PA: Saunders, 1986:313-384.)

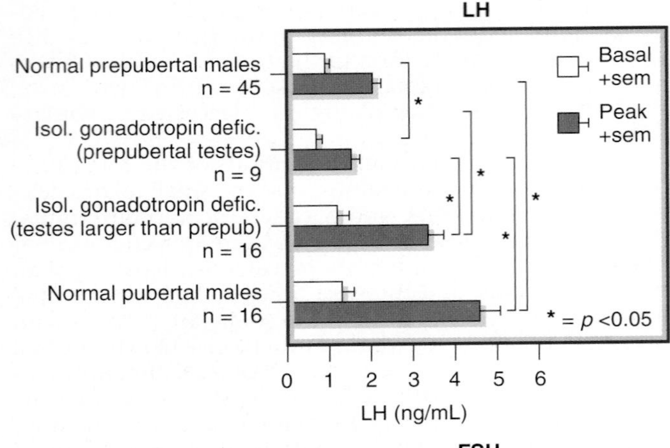

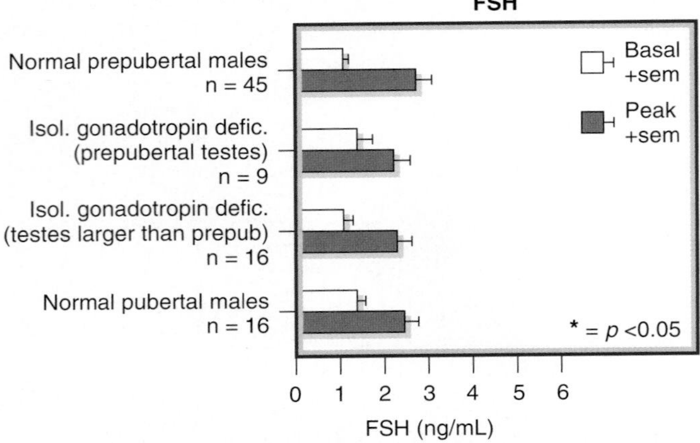

Figure 25-41 Serum luteinizing hormone (LH) and follicle-stimulating hormone (FSH) responses to the administration of gonadotropin-releasing hormone (GnRH) in 25 males with an isolated gonadotropin deficiency with or without anosmia were segregated according to whether the volume of the testes was prepubertal or greater than 2.5 cm^3. Testicular volume in those with testes larger than 2.5 cm^3 was as large as 4 cm^3. Basal and GnRH-stimulated gonadotropin levels after the intravenous injection of 100 μg GnRH (peak value) are shown (P <.05). For conversion to SI units, see Figure 25-16. (From Van Dop C, Burstein S, Conte FA, et al. Isolated gonadotropin deficiency in boys: clinical characteristics and growth. *J Pediatr.* 1987;111:684-692.)

involve mutations in the *KAL1* gene on the X chromosome, but these patients are more likely to have complete absence of gonadotropin secretory pulses and absence of migration of GnRH neurons to the hypothalamus.[518] Hypogonadotropic hypogonadism is rarely caused by a mutation in the *KAL1* gene in females.

The autosomal dominant form is known as Kallmann's syndrome type 2 (KAL2), and the associated gene is the fibroblast growth factor receptor 1 gene, *FGFR1* (previously called *KAL2*) with a gene map locus of 8p11.2-p11.1. Mutations result in autosomal dominant Kallmann's syndrome, autosomal dominant normosmic hypogonadotropic hypogonadism, or delayed puberty. KAL2 is associated with mental retardation, choanal atresia, short stature, congenital heart defects, and sensorineural hearing loss, and its presentations are more varied than those of KAL1.

The loss-of-function mutation of the *FGFR1* gene interferes with migration of the olfactory cells to the olfactory bulb.[519] Anosmin 1, a neuronal protein, may act through FGFR1 to bring about fibroblast growth factor (FGF) signaling. KAL1 partially escapes inactivation in females, and it is postulated that enough KAL1 may be produced in affected females, despite FGFR1 haploinsufficiency, to maintain adequate FGF signaling and allow olfactory function and GnRH neuron migration. One kindred of Kallmann's syndrome contained four women with *FGFR1* mutations that were transmitted to affected male offspring, although the mothers had normal reproduction and olfaction.[519]

Although gain-of-function mutations of the *FGFR1* gene are associated with craniosynostosis, a loss-of-function mutation is not associated with lack of fusion of the cranial sutures. One kindred with an *FGFR1* mutation (Arg622X) in the tyrosine kinase domain, in which some of the manifestations were temporary, has been reported; the mother of the proband had delayed puberty, and the maternal grandmother had anosmia, whereas the proband with KAL2 exhibited normal LH levels, testosterone production, and spermatogenesis after prior testosterone therapy.[520]

Studies of mice revealed that the early emergence of GnRH neurons from the embryonic olfactory placode requires FGF8 signaling as a ligand mediated through FGFR1.[521] About 30% of FGF8/FGFR1 loss-of-function mutations are associated with cleft palate, whereas FGFR1 mutations may rarely lead to cartilage abnormalities in the ears, nose, or digits.[522] An unusual kindred with a proband demonstrating severe ear anomalies, mandibular hypoplasia, thoracic dystrophia, and other usual findings was associated with an Arg622 mutation in the *FGFR1* gene, and investigation for hypogonadism is indicated when such facial abnormalities occur.[523] Prevalence of *FGFR1* mutations in the Japanese population is equal to the prevalence among whites.[516]

Knockout mice lacking the *PROK2* gene (formerly called *KAL4*), which encodes prokineticin 2, an 81-amino-acid peptide that signals through the G protein–coupled product of the *PROKR2* gene (formerly called *KAL3*), had defective development of the olfactory bulbs and failed migration of GnRH neurons.[524] This model led to demonstration of loss-of-function mutations in PROKR2 or PROK2 in 9% of patients with Kallmann's syndrome,[525] who were mostly heterozygous, although homozygous and compound heterozygous mutations were also described. Fibrous dysplasia, sleep disorder, severe obesity, synkinesia, and epilepsy have been described in patients with *PROK2* or *PROKR2* mutations, and 3% of IHH patients were affected in one study.

The CHARGE syndrome (*c*olobomata, *h*eart *a*nomalies, choanal *a*tresia, *r*etardation, *g*enital and *e*ar anomalies) includes IHH and hyposmia, including absent olfactory bulbs. In autosomal dominant familial cases, causative mutations were found in *CHD7*, which encodes a chromatin-remodeling factor, which in a small percentage of cases were found in patients with Kallmann's syndrome and in some patients with IHH due to apparent loss-of-function mutations. Patients with CHARGE syndrome should be evaluated for hypogonadotropic hypogonadism, especially if there is deafness and hypoplasia of the semicircular canals.[526]

Apparent autosomal recessive inheritance characterizes other kindreds with Kallmann's syndrome type 3 (KAL3), for which the affected gene is *PROKR2*. Unilateral renal agenesis, hypotelorism, cleft lip and palate, and a midline cranial fusion defect occur. Although renal aplasia is characteristic of *KAL1* mutations and cleft palate and dental agenesis are characteristic of *FGFR1* mutations in KAL2, these findings can occur in Kallmann's patients without *KAL1* or *FGFR1* mutations.[516]

Therefore, the various forms of Kallmann's syndrome result from heterogeneous mutations in which the phenotype can vary. For example, a 20-year-old man with the

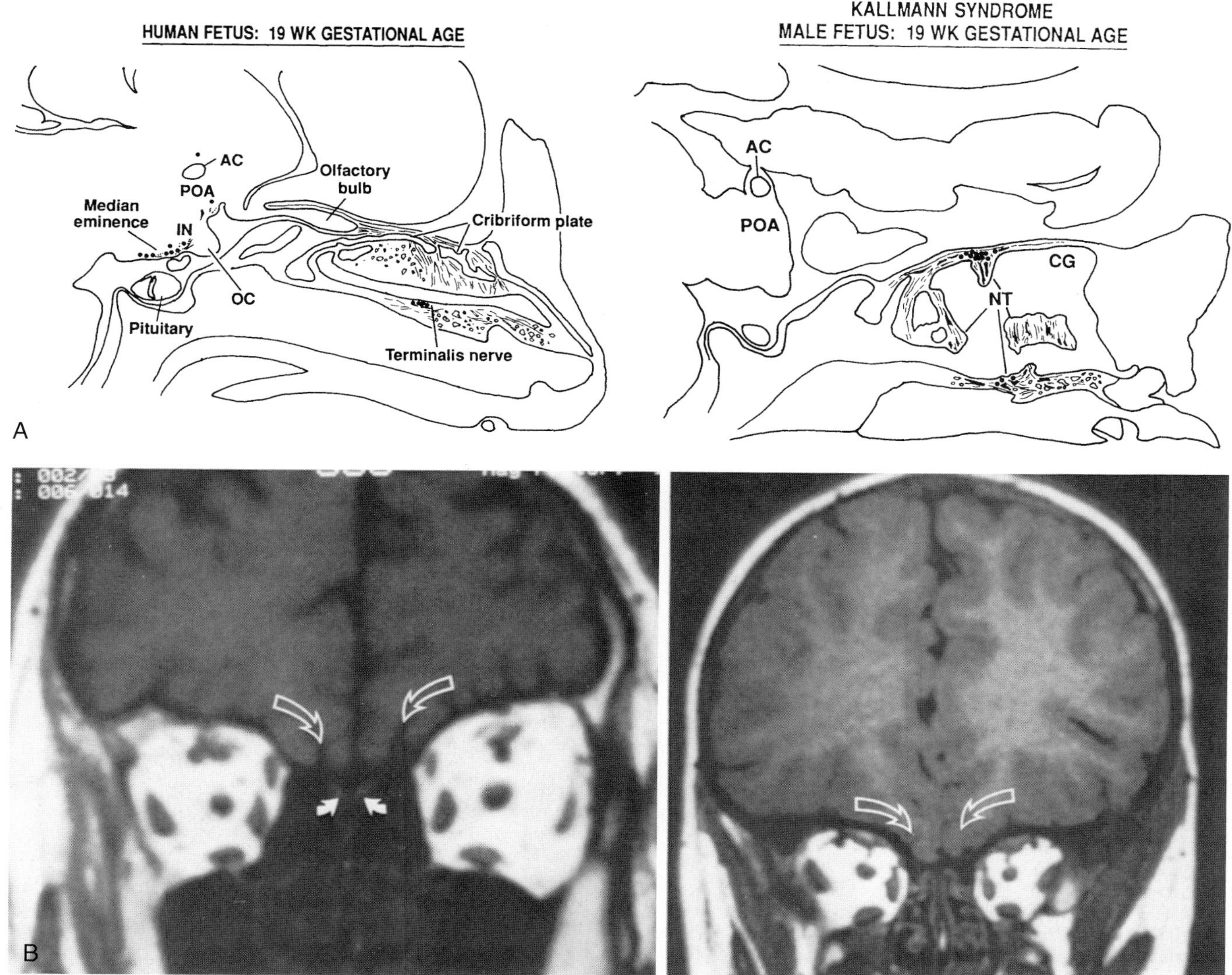

Figure 25-42 Comparison of the brain and nasal cavities of a normal 19-week-old male fetus *(upper left)* and those of a male fetus of similar age with Kallmann's syndrome caused by an X chromosome deletion at Xp22.3 *(upper right)*. In the normal fetal brain, the gonadotropin-releasing hormone (GnRH) neurosecretory neurons *(black dots)* are located in the hypothalamic area, including the medial basal hypothalamus, the anterior hypothalamic area, and of interest regarding hypothalamic hamartoma as an ectopic GnRH pulse generator, the premammillary and retromammillary areas. A small cluster of GnRH neurons exists among the fibers of the terminalis nerve on the floor of the nasal septum. In the male fetus with Kallmann's syndrome, no GnRH neurons were detected in the hypothalamic region, including the basal hypothalamus, median eminence, and preoptic area. The GnRH cells fail to migrate to and enter the brain from their origin in the nose; these cells end in a tangle beneath the forebrain on the dorsal surface of the cribriform plate and in the nasal cavity. AC, anterior commissure; CG, crista galli; IN, infundibular nucleus; NT, terminalis nerve; OC, optic chiasm; POA, preoptic area. Lower panels show magnetic resonance imaging scans of brain (coronal section, TI-weighted image). *Lower left,* Normal olfactory sulci *(open arrows)* and bulbs *(solid arrows)* in a 15-year-old boy. *Lower right,* Absent olfactory sulci *(open arrows)* and bulbs in a 17-year-old, anosmic, sexually infantile boy with Kallmann's syndrome.

complete picture of Kallmann's syndrome had an identical twin brother (proved by genetic fingerprinting) with anosmia but a normal adult phenotype and normal plasma testosterone and gonadotropin concentrations.[527]

Other postulated defects that may interfere with GnRH neuron migration are mutations in the genes for neural cell adhesion molecules (NCAM) and related proteins, such as tenascin, laminin, and phosphacan. Various glycoconjugates may also be involved.

In classic, X-linked KAL1, fetal GnRH neurosecretory neurons do not migrate from the olfactory placode to the medial basal hypothalamus, where they should constitute the GnRH pulse generator, but instead end in a tangle around the cribriform plate and in the dural layers adjacent to the meninges beneath the forebrain.[336] Abnormal or absent olfactory bulbs or folds are seen on MRI scans. Coronal and axial cranial MRI scans of the olfactory bulbs and sulci, unilaterally or bilaterally, reflect this defect in about 90% of cases and can point to the diagnosis,[528] especially in affected infants and prepubertal-age children (Fig. 25-42).[528]

Other Forms of Isolated Hypogonadotropic Hypogonadism

Inheritance of hypogonadotropic hypogonadism (Table 25-19) with none of the other features of Kallmann's syndrome may be found in autosomal dominant (gene map

TABLE 25-19

Molecular Basis for Developmental Disorders Associated with Hypogonadotropic Hypogonadism

Gene	Phenotype	Complex Phenotype
	ISOLATED HYPOGONADOTROPIC HYPOGONADISM	
Kallmann's Syndrome or Normosmic IHH (with the Same Mutant Gene)		
KAL1 (Xp22.3)	X-linked Kallmann's syndrome	Anosmia/hyposmia, renal agenesis, dyskinesia
FGFR1 (KAL2) (8p11.2)	Autosomal dominant Kallmann's syndrome (± recessive)	Anosmia/hyposmia, cleft lip/palate
FGF8 (ligand for FGFR1)(10q25)		
NELF (9p34.3)	Autosomal dominant (?) Kallmann's syndrome	
PROK2 (3p21.1)	Autosomal recessive Kallmann syndrome	
*PROKR2** (20p12.3)		
CHD7 (8p12.1)	Autosomal dominant (some)	CHARGE syndrome includes hyposmia
Normosmic Isolated Hypogonadotropic Hypogonadism		
GNRH1 (8p21-11.2)	Autosomal recessive	
*GNRHR** (4q13.2-3)	Autosomal recessive (± dominant)	
*GPR54** (19p13.3)	Autosomal recessive	
SNRPN		Prader-Willi syndrome
Lack of function of paternal 15q11-q13 region or maternal uniparental disomy		Obesity
LEP (7q31.3)	Autosomal recessive	Obesity
LEPR (1p31)	Autosomal recessive	Obesity
NR0B1 (DAX1) (X21.3-21.2)	X-linked recessive	Adrenal hypoplasia
TAC3 (12q13-12)	Autosomal recessive	
TACR3 (4q25)	Autosomal recessive	
Multiple Pituitary Hormone Deficiencies		
PROP1 (POU1F1)	Autosomal recessive GH, PRL, TSH, and LH/FSH (less commonly, later-onset ACTH deficiency)	
HESX1 (RPX)	Autosomal recessive; and heterozygous mutations	Septo-optic dysplasia
	Multiple pituitary deficiencies including diabetes insipidus, but LH/FSH uncommon	
LHX3	Autosomal recessive GH, PRL, TSH, FSH/LH	Rigid cervical spine
PHF6	X-linked; GH, TSH, ACTH, LH/FSH	Borjeson-Lehmann syndrome: mental retardation; facies

*A G-protein–coupled receptor.

ACTH, corticotropin; CHD7, chromatin-remodeling factor; DAX1, dosage-sensitive sex reversal-adrenal hyperplasia congenita critical region on the X chromosome, gene 1; FGF, fibroblast growth factor; FSH, follicle-stimulating hormone; GH, growth hormone; GNRH, gonadotropin–releasing hormone; GPR54, kisspeptin G-protein–coupled receptor 54; HESX1, homeobox gene expressed in ES cells; IHH, idiopathic hypogonadotropic hypogonadism; LEP, leptin; LH, luteinizing hormone; LHX3, lim homeobox gene 3; NELF, nasal embryonic luteinizing hormone–releasing factor; NR0B1, nuclear receptor family 0, group B, member 1; PHF6, plant homeodomain–like finger gene; PRL, prolactin; PROK2, prokineticin 2; PROP1, prophet of Pit-1; R, receptor; SNRPN, small nuclear ribonucleoprotein polypeptide SmN; TAC3, neurokinin3; TSH, thyroid-stimulating hormone.

locus 19p13.3, 9q34.3), autosomal recessive (8p21-p11.2), or X-linked recessive (Xp21) disorders.[529-531] Males with cerebellar ataxia and deficient gonadotropin production are reported in kindreds with X-linked inheritance (possibly a variant form of Kallmann's syndrome), and hypogonadotropic hypogonadism may be associated with the multiple lentigenes and basal cell nevus syndromes.

Only about 15% of normosmic hypogonadotropic patients have a definable genetic defect. The combination of human genetic studies and mouse models has led to the discovery of many genes involved in gonadotropin regulation.[532] The human equivalent of the mouse nasal embryonic GnRH factor gene *(Nelf)* is *NELF*; a mutation of this gene was found in 1 of 65 patients with IHH but in none of 100 controls, suggesting an etiologic role for this mutation.[533]

Gonadotropin-Releasing Hormone Gene Mutations. The GnRH gene *(GNRH1)* would seem a likely candidate for the cause of hypogonadotropic hypogonadism, but although mutations of the GnRH receptor gene *(GNRHR)* were identified years ago, mutations in the *GNRH1* gene were not demonstrated until 2009. An autosomal recessive form had been described in the mouse (hyg/hyg), in which there is a deletion of part of the GnRH gene. A homozygous *GNRH1* frameshift mutation in human beings, characterized by the insertion of an adenine at nucleotide position 18 (c.18-19insA) in the sequence encoding the N-terminal region of the signal peptide–containing protein precursor of GnRH (prepro-GnRH), was found in a teenage brother and sister who had normosmic IHH.[534] When expressed in vitro, the mutant peptide did not demonstrate immunoreactive GnRH. One patient of 310 with severe, congenital, normosmic IHH (with micropenis, bilateral cryptorchidism, and absent puberty) had a homozygous frameshift mutation that is predicted to disrupt the three C-terminal amino acids of the GnRH decapeptide and to produce a premature stop codon.[535] Of four patients with normosmic IHH, one had a nonsynonymous missense mutation in the eighth amino acid of the GnRH decapeptide; one had a nonsense mutation that causes premature termination within the GnRH-associated peptide (GAP), which lies

C-terminal to the GnRH decapeptide within the GnRH precursor; and two had sequence variants that cause nonsynonymous amino acid substitutions in the signal peptide and GnRH-associated peptide.

KISS1/KISS1R Axis. The KISS1/KISS1R axis plays a role in the increased amplitude of GnRH signaling in puberty. KISS/KISS1R axis mutations are rare. Of 30 normosmic subjects with hypogonadotropic hypogonadism who were evaluated, 1 person had two missense mutations in KISS1R (Cys223Arg in the fifth transmembrane helix and Arg297Leu in the third extracellular loop); the former had no activity, and the latter manifested as mildly decreased signaling ability.[536] Homozygous deletions of 155 nucleotides in the *KISS1R* gene encompassing the splicing acceptor site of the intron 4–exon 5 junction and part of exon 5 were found in all affected family members with IHH,[537] but unaffected family members had no deletion or only one mutant allele. Another kindred had a Leu48Ser mutation in the second intracellular loop (IL2) of KISS1R, and another had two separate mutations in the gene, Arg331Xaa and Xaa399Arg.[411] The latter patient had decreased secretion of GnRH and decreased response to GnRH administration. A line of mice transfected with the affected gene exhibited hypogonadotropic hypogonadism with decreased GnRH in the hypothalamus but were responsive to GnRH or gonadotropin administration. Agonist stimulation may stabilize the switch II region of Gα to promote opening of Gα switch II to facilitate exchange of guanosine diphosphate (GDP) and guanosine triphosphate (GTP).[538] The Leu148Ser mutation does not affect the expression, ligand-binding properties, or protein interaction network of KISS1R, but diverse KISS1R functional responses are markedly inhibited.

Gonadotropin-Releasing Hormone Receptor Mutations. Mutations of the gene encoding the type 1 GnRH receptor (*GNRHR,* gene map locus 4q21.2) that affect the G protein–coupled, seven-transmembrane segments lead to various degrees of familial and sporadic hypogonadotropic hypogonadism with normosmia.[529,531,539,540] A *GNRHR* mutation is found in about 40% to 50% of cases of familial, autosomal recessive, normosmic IHH and in about 17% of sporadic cases of normosmic IHH.

Mutations in hypogonadal hypogonadism with amino acid substitutions in the extracellular N-terminal domain (Thr32Ile), the second extracellular loop (Cys200Tyr), the third intracellular loop (Leu266Arg), and the sixth transmembrane helix (Cys279Tyr) were found to affect specific GnRH binding.[541,542] Except for Thr32Ile, there was no significant inositol phosphate accumulation after GnRH stimulation, demonstrating loss of function even if binding was accomplished. However, an increased dose of GnRH allowed stimulation of the gonadotropin subunit and GnRHR promoters and the ability to partially activate extracellular signal-regulated kinase 1 and stimulate cAMP response element (CRE)–luciferase activity. A higher dose of GnRH caused the Cys200Tyr mutant to stimulate gonadotropin subunit and GnRHR promoter activity because this mutant reduces cell surface receptor expression.

Another human GnRH receptor *(GNRHR)* gene mutation of a highly conserved sequence located in the second-transmembrane helix impairs GNRHR effector coupling due to loss of surface expression of the receptor and leads to a severe manifestation of IHH.[543]

Certain GnRH receptor defects may be rescued by pharmacologic agents that can act as a folding template, correcting the structural defects caused by the mutations and allowing function to occur. A small, membrane-permeant molecule demonstrated pharmacologic rescue (i.e., ligand binding and restoration of receptor coupling to effector) of five naturally occurring missense mutations of the GnRH receptor in families with IHH.[544] These molecules also allowed rescue of intentionally manufactured defective receptors with internal or terminal deletions or substitutions at sites expected to be involved in the establishment of tertiary receptor structure. This approach may allow a therapeutic approach to conditions caused by mutations that result in protein misfolding.

The clinical presentation of patients with mutations in the GnRH receptor is heterogeneous, and impairment of signal transmission is highly variable (e.g., severe features of IHH, sexual infantilism, long-delayed puberty with reversal in adulthood, relatively mild hypogonadism and infertility), even within the same pedigree and especially in patients with compound heterozygous mutations.[545] In all types of congenital gonadotropin deficiency, male patients are likely to manifest micropenis (penile length <2.0 cm at birth and in infancy) due to lack of fetal gonadotropin stimulation of fetal testes during the last half of gestation. Rarely, boys with congenital GH deficiency have micropenis even if gonadotropin function is normal.[546] Because testosterone therapy is effective in increasing penile size (see later discussion), sex reversal is not indicated in these cases of microphallus.

X-Linked Congenital Adrenal Hypoplasia and Hypogonadotropic Hypogonadism. A rare deletion or mutation in the dosage sensitive sex reversal-A (DSS) adrenal hypoplasia congenita gene on the X chromosome gene 1 (*NR0B1,* formerly called *DAX1;* gene map locus Xp21.3-p21.2)[547-549] leads to an X-linked recessive disorder of adrenocortical organogenesis. The gene encodes an orphan receptor, a member of the nuclear receptor superfamily, that is a putative transcriptional repressor mapping to the Xp21 locus. A double dose of *NR0B1* is associated with a female phenotype or ambiguous genitalia in 46XY males. The NR0B1 protein has a novel domain in the N-terminus that contains two putative unique zinc finger motifs, and the C-terminus contains a conserved ligand-binding domain that binds DNA, localizes in the nucleus, and contains a transcriptional silencing domain that antagonizes the steroidogenic factor 1 (SF1, also called NR5A1) transactivation function.[550] NR0B1 has an SF1 response element in the 5′-promoter region that is another orphan member of the nuclear hormone receptor superfamily. Both NR0B1 and SF1 are expressed in the adrenals, gonads, pituitary, and hypothalamus, raising the possibility of an important interaction between these two genes and their products.

Rare abnormalities of *NR0B1* are characterized by severe glucocorticoid, mineralocorticoid, and at puberty, androgen deficiency.[551,552] The abnormal structure of the adrenal cortex resembles that of the fetal zone because it consists of disorganized, vacuolated, cytomegalic cells with a normal mature cortex.[551] The severe primary adrenal insufficiency with hyponatremia, hyperkalemia, acidosis, and hypoglycemia is characterized by failure to thrive, vomiting, poor feeding, dehydration, circulatory collapse, and increased pigmentation, and is lethal if not treated early in life in affected boys.[551]

Adrenoleukodystrophy may manifest with adrenal failure long before neurologic symptoms develop, and some cases of X-linked Addison's disease may represent this diagnosis. This condition is in the differential diagnosis of adrenal hypoplasia. Plasma renin activity, plasma cortisol, and aldosterone levels are low. Symptomatic adrenal insufficiency may first manifest in later childhood. In male infants, signs of salt-wasting are usually the most prominent feature, but cortisol deficiency is detectable, and adrenal insufficiency includes deficient secretion of the zona reticularis steroids, DHEA, and DHEAS. An early sign of elevated ACTH is increased skin pigmentation. The testes are undescended in fewer than one half of patients; micropenis is rare, but urogenital abnormalities and hearing loss occasionally are present. Boys who do not present with clinical evidence of adrenal insufficiency in infancy often have a more insidious onset during childhood or adulthood.[553,554]

In a pedigree in which two affected boys had a hemizygous *NROB1* nonsense mutation and neonatal onset of adrenal insufficiency, a maternal aunt who was homozygous for the mutation had sexual infantilism and primary amenorrhea, but even after decades of follow-up, she maintained normal adrenal function. A maternal grandfather who carried the same mutation was asymptomatic.[555] This pedigree highlights the limitations and complexities of genotype and phenotype correlations. Most commonly, due to hypogonadotropic hypogonadism, signs of sexual maturation at the age of puberty (e.g., pubic and axillary hair, testicular enlargement) are lacking, and the concentrations of serum FSH, LH, and testosterone are low.[551] Delayed puberty is a manifestation in some female carriers of a *NROB1* mutation.

Intragenic mutations in *NROB1* (i.e., frameshift mutations, nonsense mutations, and missense mutations) indicate that the hypogonadotropic hypogonadism is an intrinsic characteristic of the disorder, a manifestation of the single-gene mutation and not a result of involvement of a contiguous gene.[556] The *NROB1* gene is expressed in the adrenal cortex, in testes (and weakly in the ovary), and in the hypothalamus and pituitary. There is evidence of GnRH deficiency and an abnormality in the gonadotrophs, yielding a mixed picture of hypothalamic and intrinsic gonadotroph defects[551] with absent or erratic pulsatile secretion of LH. Even if basal immunoreactive LH and FSH levels are normal, gonadotropins seem to lack bioactivity. In some affected boys, the GnRH pulse generator and pituitary gonadotropin apparatus is intact and functional in infancy and early childhood, and the GnRH-gonadotroph defects do not manifest until later in childhood or during the peripubertal period.[557] Azoospermia unresponsive to gonadotropin treatment was detected in a few affected men.[554,558]

A deletion of the adrenal hypoplasia congenita locus (at Xp21) can include the glycerol kinase *(GK)* and Duchenne muscular dystrophy *(DMD)* genes if it extends centromerically or produce mental retardation if there is extension toward the telomere, leading to contiguous gene syndromes.

Other mutations of the X chromosome may be associated with IHH. Two brothers were reported who had hypogonadotropic hypogonadism, obesity, and short stature associated with a maternally inherited pericentric inversion, (X)(p11.4q11.2). Because the breakpoint is not related to other genes associated with pubertal disorders, it is not clear whether this is a functional relationship or a coincidence.[559]

Other Presentations of Hypogonadotropic Hypogonadism

Neurokinin B (encoded by *TAC3*) is a member of the tachykinin superfamily of 127 neuropeptides that includes substance P and neurokinin A. Its cognate G protein–coupled receptor 126 is NK3R, which is encoded by *TACR3*. Studies demonstrate loss-of-function mutations in this system in familial, congenital hypogonadotropic hypogonadism; administration of pulsatile GnRH caused resumption of gonadotropin secretion (Fig. 25-43).[560,561] A survey of 345 patients with normosmic hypogonadotropic hypogonadism found 13 rare, distinct nucleotide sequence coding variants (three 108 nonsense, six nonsynonymous, and four synonymous mutations [one predicted to affect splicing]) in *TACR3* and one 109 homozygous single-base-pair deletion, resulting in complete loss of neurokinin B. Of the 16 males for whom phenotype information was available, 15 had microphallus, and none of the females had spontaneous thelarche. When subjects were assessed after discontinuation of therapy, 6 of 7 males and 4 of 5 females demonstrated evidence for reversibility of their hypogonadotropism.[562]

Mutations in the prohormone convertase 1 gene (*PCSK1*, also called *PC1*) led to extreme childhood obesity, hypocortisolemia, defects in conversion of proinsulin to insulin leading to hypoglycemia, and isolated partial hypogonadotropic hypogonadism allowing spontaneous pubertal development but primary amenorrhea. The hypogonadal hypogonadism probably resulted from impaired processing of GnRH or neuropeptides involved in its secretion. Findings in another subject extended to gastrointestinal disturbance, small intestinal malabsorption related to monosaccharide and fats, and elevation in progastrin and proglucagon levels, showing that prohormone processing in enteroendocrine cells was abnormal.[563]

Isolated Luteinizing Hormone Deficiency. Isolated LH deficiency (fertile eunuch syndrome) is associated with deficient testosterone production (which responds to hCG administration) in the presence of variable spermatogenesis; the disorder may be idiopathic or may result from a hypothalamic pituitary neoplasm. A homozygous Gln106Arg mutation in the first extracellular loop of the GnRH receptor at gene map locus 4q21.2 was associated with normal testicular volume (17 mL) but with apulsatile, low gonadotropin values and low testosterone values[545] in one subject. After hCG stimulation, he developed adequate spermatogenesis to father a child, and after cessation of hCG treatment, he demonstrated adult testosterone values and pulsatile gonadotropin secretion, an example of reversibility of the syndrome.

Isolated Bioinactive Luteinizing Hormone. A 17-year-old boy with a history of delayed puberty, the only known patient with isolated bioinactive LH, had a striking discrepancy between elevated immunoactive and absent bioactive LH due to a mutation in the gene encoding the LH β-subunit.[530] The subject had a homozygous mutation in exon 3 of the LH β-subunit gene (Glx54Arg). Apparently absent Leydig cells and arrested spermatogenesis improved with hCG treatment. The heterozygote mother exhibited only 50% of normal binding of serum LH to the LH receptor. The patient's normal male sex differentiation most likely resulted from the action of hCG. The absence of a micropenis, as found in male infants with congenital GnRH deficiency, suggests the possibility of initially bioactive LH in utero.

Isolated Follicle-Stimulating Hormone Deficiency. Homozygous or compound heterozygous mutations in the FSH β-subunit have been reported in three females and two males[323,530,564] with delayed puberty or poorly developed

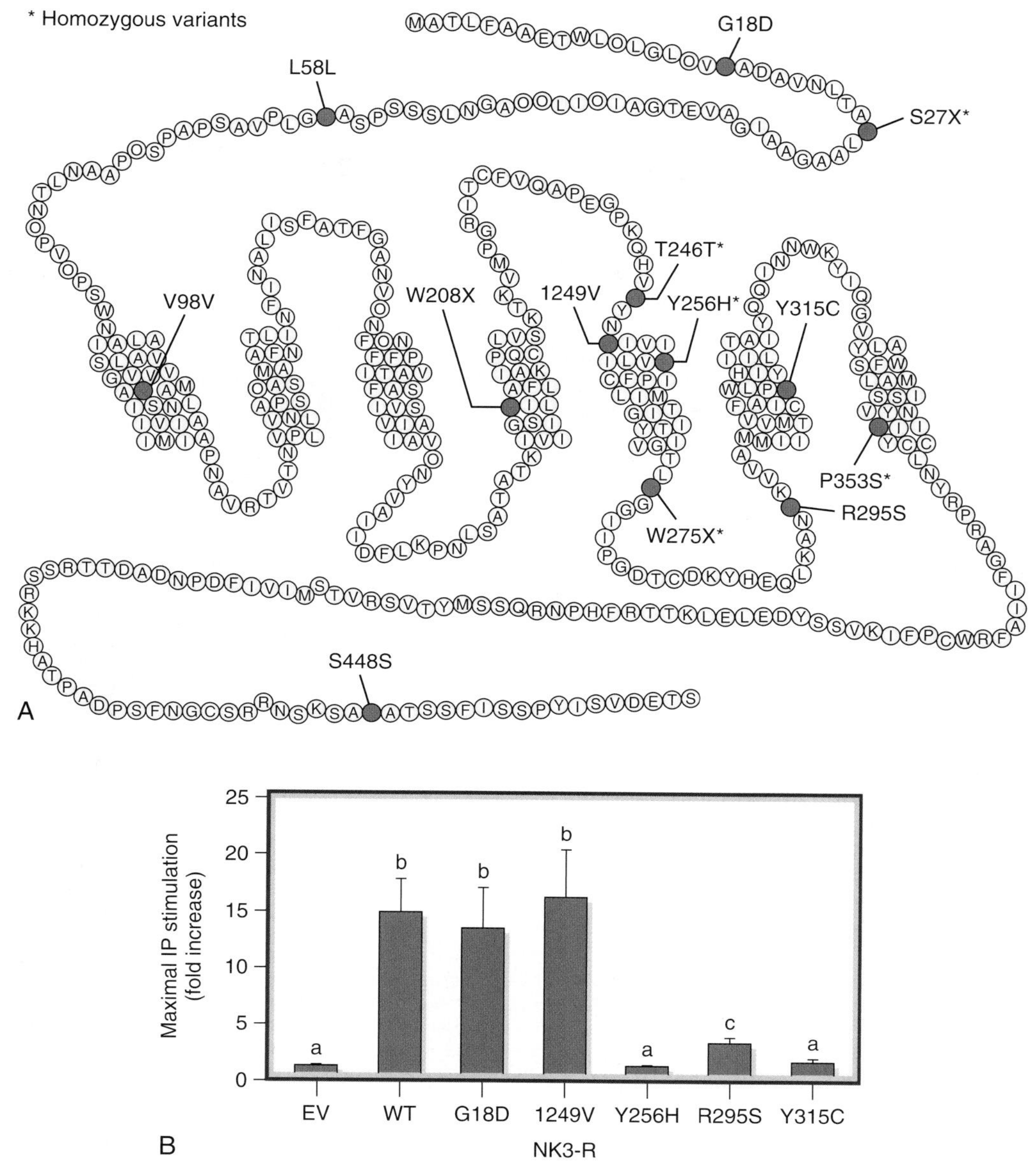

Figure 25-43 **A,** Schematic of mutations in the NK3-R, which is encoded by *TAC3*. **B,** Effects of mutations in *TACR3* on neurokinin B (NKB)-mediated activation of signal transduction. COS-7 cells transfected with wild-type (WT) G18D, I249V, Y256H, R295S, and Y315C NK3-R or empty vector (EV) were treated with NKB (10^{-7} M) for 1 hour. A significant increase in inositol phosphate (IP) accumulation occurred in cells transfected with WT, G18D, or I249V NK3-R. In contrast, there was a marked reduction in NKB-stimulated IP production in cells transfected with Y256H, R295S, or Y315C NK3-R, or with EV. *a*, *b*, and *c* denote significantly different fold increases in IP accumulation. (From Gianetti E, Tusset C, Noel SD, et al. *TAC3/TACR3* mutations reveal preferential activation of gonadotropin-releasing hormone release by neurokinin B in neonatal life followed by reversal in adulthood. *J Clin Endocrinol Metab.* 2010;95:2857-2867.)

secondary sex characteristics and with primary amenorrhea but normal adrenarche in the women. The LH concentration was elevated, the serum level of estradiol was low, and immunoactive FSH was absent. Two of the three women had a homozygous nonsense mutation (Val61X) in the FSH β-subunit gene at gene map locus 11p13, and the other was a compound heterozygote (Cys51Gly/Val61X). The two men had azoospermia; small, soft testes; and absence of serum FSH. One had normal puberty and normal LH and testosterone values, with a missense mutation (Cys82Arg), and the other had slightly delayed puberty, low testosterone and inhibin B levels, high LH levels, and a nonsense mutation (Val61X).

Developmental Defect of the Midline

Septo-optic or optic dysplasia is caused by abnormal development of the prosencephalon leading to small, dysplastic, pale optic discs with a double outline and pendular (evenly moving side to side) nystagmus; blindness may occur. A midline hypothalamic defect may cause GH deficiency, diabetes insipidus, and ACTH, TSH, and gonadotropin deficiency. Short stature and delayed puberty may result, although CPP is an alternative.[565] The septum pellucidum is often absent in association with optic hypoplasia or dysplasia, which is readily demonstrable by imaging techniques.[566] In the University of California at San Francisco

(UCSF) series, the syndrome was associated with decreased maternal age. The pituitary may be hypoplastic due to the lack of hypothalamic stimulatory factors, and the neurohypophysis may have an ectopic location identified by the location of the posterior pituitary hot spot on MRI. The condition is usually sporadic, but one brother and sister were affected from a consanguineous union, and a mutation in *HESX1* at gene map locus 3p21.2-p21.1 is rarely found.[567] Abnormalities of the corpus callosum and cerebellum are common on MRI. Four groups are described: those with normal MRI results, those with abnormalities of the septum pellucidum and with a normal hypothalamic pituitary area, those with abnormalities of the hypothalamic pituitary area and a normal septum pellucidum, and those with abnormalities in both areas.[568] No endocrine abnormalities were described in the first group, but the others had progressively more endocrine abnormalities, with precocious puberty most common in the second group. Early diagnosis is important because of the risk of sudden death associated with adrenal insufficiency.

The solitary median maxillary incisor syndrome is associated with the eponymous midline defect and with a prominent midpalatal ridge (torus palatinus) and hypopituitarism. The defect in this autosomal dominant condition is in the sonic hedgehog gene *(SHH)* at gene map locus 7q3.[569]

Other congenital midline defects ranging from complete dysraphism and holoprosencephaly to cleft palate or lip are associated with hypothalamic-pituitary dysfunction. Delayed puberty is rarely described in duplication of the hypophysis. Myelomeningocele (myelodysplasia) is associated with endocrine abnormalities, including hypothalamic hypothyroidism, hyperprolactinemia, and elevated gonadotropin concentrations, and with CPP.

Long-term follow-up of hypogonadotropic hypogonadism or partial pubertal development revealed that even with defined genetic defects, interruption of androgen treatment for several weeks (mean, 6 weeks) revealed restoration of normal gonadal function, including pulsatile LH secretion and spermatogenesis in adulthood.[513] Of the 15 patients described, 4 had anosmia, 6 had absent puberty, 9 had partial puberty at first, and all had abnormal GnRH-induced LH secretion. Three of 13 evaluated with genetic analysis who reversed their hypogonadotropic hypogonadism had mutations in *FGFR1* or *GNRHR*. Long-term follow-up is necessary, even for patients with established genetic defects.

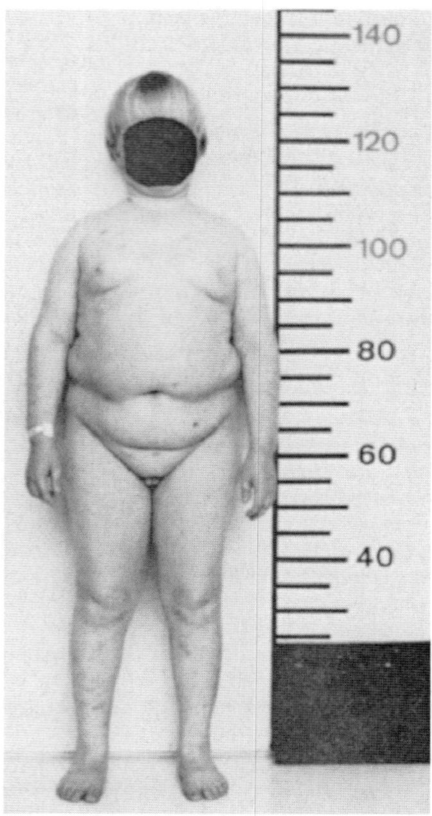

Figure 25-44 A 20-year-old man with idiopathic hypopituitary dwarfism and deficiencies of gonadotropins, thyrotropin, corticotropin, and growth hormone had a history of arrested hydrocephalus. His height was 129 cm (−8 SD), the phallus was 2 cm long, and the testes measured 1.5 × 1 cm. He had received thyroid hormone and glucocorticoid replacement. The basal luteinizing hormone (LH) level was less than 0.2 ng/mL (LER-960), follicle-stimulating hormone (FSH) level was 0.5 ng/mL (LER-869), and testosterone level was less than 0.1 ng/mL. In response to 100 μg of gonadotropin-releasing hormone (GnRH), the plasma LH concentration increased slightly to 0.6 ng/mL, and there was no increase in the plasma testosterone level. The excretion of urinary 17-ketosteroids was 1.1 mg/24 hours. The bone age was 10 years, and the volume of the sella turcica was small on skull radiographs. For conversion to SI units, see Figures 25-16 and 25-17. (From Styne DM, Grumbach MM. Puberty in the male and female: its physiology and disorders. In: Yen SCC, Jaffe RB, eds. *Reproductive Endocrinology*, 2nd ed. Philadelphia, PA: Saunders, 1986:313-384.)

Idiopathic Hypopituitary Dwarfism

In addition to *HESX1* mutations, autosomal recessive mutations in homeobox genes encoding transcription factors involved in the early aspects of pituitary development lead to hypogonadotropic hypogonadism and other pituitary hormone deficiencies.[570] *PROP1* mutations at gene map locus 5q cause GH and TSH deficiency and produce delayed puberty or late onset of secondary hypogonadism in adulthood and rarely cause ACTH deficiency (Fig. 25-44).[571] In one study of 73 patients with idiopathic multiple pituitary hormone deficiencies, 35 had a mutation in *PROP1*.[572] Homozygous Arg73Cys mutation of PROP1 allowed spontaneous puberty in 2 of 10 affected family members.[573] ACTH deficiency is more rarely a feature of PROP1 deficiency.

Homozygous mutations occur in the *LHX3* gene at gene map locus 9q34.3. It encodes a member of the LIM class of homeodomain proteins, which are associated with multiple pituitary hormone deficiencies, including LH and FSH, and with severe restriction of head rotation.[574]

The familial forms of multiple pituitary hormone deficiencies with autosomal recessive or X-linked inheritance are less common. The degree of hormone deficit and the age at onset of pituitary hormone deficiencies may vary within a single kindred having the same genetic defect.

The X-linked form of hypopituitarism can be associated with duplication of the *SOX3* gene.[575] Deficiency of SOX2, a transcription factor involved in early hypothalamic-pituitary embryonic development, leads to anterior pituitary hypoplasia. Patients with *SOX2* mutations have major eye abnormalities, including anophthalmia, microphthalmia, and coloboma. They also have hypogonadotropic hypogonadism as the most common pituitary defect, in contrast to most other types of pituitary hypoplasia, demonstrating GH deficiency most frequently.[576]

There is an association between breech delivery (especially for male infants), perinatal distress, and idiopathic hypopituitarism.[124,577] Malformations of the pituitary stalk demonstrable by MRI are common in these patients.[124] Common to many patients with idiopathic hypopituitary dwarfism is early onset of growth failure; late onset of diminished growth is an ominous finding, suggesting the presence of a CNS tumor.

Isolated GH deficiency allows spontaneous pubertal development when the bone age reaches the pubertal stage of 11 to 13 years, usually after the corresponding chronologic age is reached. Associated gonadotropin deficiency does not allow spontaneous puberty, even when the bone age advances to the pubertal stage during GH therapy.

Miscellaneous Conditions

Prader-Willi Syndrome

Prader-Willi syndrome is an autosomal dominant disorder that combines a tendency for intrauterine growth retardation, delayed onset and poor fetal activity, infantile central hypotonia, and lethargy, followed by early-onset childhood hyperphagia, pathologic obesity, and carbohydrate intolerance (leading to type 2 diabetes in 25% of patients at a mean age of 20 years). Features include short stature, small hands and feet, mild to moderate mental retardation, and emotional instability, including perseveration, obsessions, and compulsions. Almond-shaped eyes, a triangular mouth, and narrow bifrontal diameter combined with delayed puberty and hypogonadotropic hypogonadism caused by hypothalamic dysfunction are characteristic. Despite the late or absent puberty, there is a tendency to early adrenarche[578,579] or even precocious puberty in a few cases.

Affected boys usually have a micropenis and cryptorchidism, and an underdeveloped scrotum is common. In a study of 37 adults with Prader-Willi syndrome, none achieved full genital development, and primary testicular defects were suggested.[580] Serum AMH levels were near the lower limits of normal, inhibin B levels were consistently low or undetectable, and in the adults, FSH levels were high, although LH levels were normal. Two adults had undetectable levels of LH and FSH, but in contrast to the others, they had high AMH levels. Female subjects exhibit underdevelopment of the labia majora, labia minora, or clitoris. Amenorrhea occurs in about one half of cases, and irregular menses are common in others. Weight reduction may lead to menarche in some females, because severe obesity may play a role in the impaired puberty in some patients. Dietary therapy during years 2 through 10 can provide effective treatment of obesity but may decrease growth, although contemporaneous GH therapy may overcome slow growth.[581]

The role of relative GH deficiency in this disorder is uncertain and controversial. The FDA approved Prader-Willi syndrome as an indication for recombinant human GH treatment without a requirement for assessing GH secretion. Genetic testing is used to confirm the clinical diagnosis of the syndrome. GH treatment in a dose of (0.24 mg/kg/wk subcutaneously given 6 to 7 times per week) was shown in long-term, randomized, controlled trials to decrease body fat, increase fat utilization, lean body mass, linear growth, and energy expenditure and possibly to improve physical strength and motor development.[582] Children with Prader-Willi syndrome are at risk for sudden death due to gastrointestinal, respiratory, or cardiac complications.[583] However, the report of sudden deaths due to respiratory complications during GH treatment led to a recommendation for evaluation for sleep apnea or respiratory difficulties before instituting GH therapy. More recent data cast doubt on the beneficial effects of GH on body composition and BMI, but higher parental educational status was correlated with better clinical outcome.[584]

This distinct genetic disorder, with a frequency of about 1 case in 15,000 to 30,000 people, is rarely familial (i.e., the recurrence risk depends on the type of the genetic defect). It is caused by abnormalities involving the long arm of chromosome 15 in the q11-q13 region. Approximately 70% of Prader-Willi cases are caused by a paternal deletion of 15q11-q13 (commonly 3 to 5 mega-base pairs long); 20% to 25% of cases involve maternal uniparental disomy (isodisomy or heterodisomy) in which both chromosomes 15 are derived from the mother, possibly by nondisjunction during maternal meiosis, representing a striking example of genomic imprinting.[578] In 2% to 5% of cases, an imprinting center defect has been detected. Lack of a functional paternal 15q11-q13 region, caused by any of a variety of genetic mechanisms, can result in the syndrome. One imprinted gene, that for small nuclear ribonucleoprotein associated polypeptide SmN (SNRPN), which is implicated in splicing pre-mRNA, is expressed in the brain, including the hypothalamus, and has been advanced as one explanation of the syndrome.

Elevated serum concentrations of the GH secretagogue and orexigenic gastrointestinal hormone ghrelin are found in the basal state in Prader-Willi syndrome. Increased levels are identified after meals, when values should be suppressed, and are a possible cause of the insatiable appetite. Administration of the somatostatin analogue octreotide leads to a decrease in basal ghrelin values and some decrease in values after meals,[585] but no change in appetite was demonstrated in preliminary study.

Laurence-Moon and Bardet-Biedl Syndromes

The Laurence-Moon syndrome has frequently been combined with the Bardet-Biedl syndrome; both are rare autosomal recessive traits, and both combine retinitis pigmentosum and hypogonadism of various causes. Many Bardet-Biedl patients have developmental delay, as do all of the Laurence-Moon patients. The Laurence-Moon syndrome was considered to be associated with spastic paraplegia, whereas the features of Bardet-Biedl syndrome included postaxial polydactyly, onset of obesity (usually in early infancy), and renal dysplasia, and it had a relatively high prevalence among the Bedouin of the Middle East. The genetically and phenotypically heterogenous Bardet-Biedl syndrome is linked to multiple loci that map to, for example, 20p12, 16q21, 15q22.3-q23, 14q32.1, 11q13, 4q27, 3p12-q13, and 2q31. In most cases, three mutant genes are required for the phenotype.[586] However, a 22-year study of 26 families in Newfoundland revealed lack of correlation of the phenotype with the genotype, and the study authors stated that there is no justification for continuing to separate Bardet-Biedl syndrome from Laurence-Moon syndrome.[587] The Biemond syndrome II has similar features, with iris coloboma, hypogenitalism, obesity, polydactyly, and developmental delay, but it is a distinct entity.

Functional Gonadotropin Deficiencies

The effects of malnutrition, which can lead to functional hypogonadotropic hypogonadism, should be separated from the primary effects of chronic systemic disease, some of which have direct effects on the function of the hypothalamic-pituitary unit or the gonads. Even if nutrition is adequate, puberty may be affected. Weight loss of any cause to less than 80% of ideal weight for height can lead to gonadotropin deficiency and low serum leptin levels; weight regain usually restores hypothalamic-pituitary gonadal function over a variable period, although the weight needed to restart menstrual periods varies among individuals and is related to the weight at which menstruation first ceased.[588]

If adequate nutrition and body weight are maintained in patients with regional enteritis or chronic pulmonary disease, gonadotropin secretion is usually adequate. Cystic fibrosis also delays puberty and the age of PHV, in large part through malnutrition.[589] The age of menarche in girls with cystic fibrosis is related to maternal age, as expected, but it is delayed by approximately 1 year compared with menarche in the mother, an effect that is mainly related to nutritional status.[590] However, even with normal pubertal progression, boys with cystic fibrosis almost universally have oligospermia caused by obstruction of the spermatic ducts, which is unrelated to nutritional status. The greater prevalence of reproductive difficulties in male patients with cystic fibrosis compared with female patients may reflect the greater prevalence of the cystic fibrosis transmembrane regulator (CFTR) in male reproductive tissues (e.g., epididymis, vas deferens), and more viscid luminal contents, which ultimately damage the testes and can lead to absence of the epididymides and the vas differentia.[591] Normal ovaries do not express CFTR, and endometrial tissue expresses it only after puberty, with variable levels found in cervical epithelium and the fallopian tubes. Even though the *CFTR* gene and its protein are expressed in the human hypothalamus, mutations in the corresponding gene did not appear to affect LH and FSH secretion in an immortalized mouse hypothalamic GnRH-secreting cell line.

Jamaican boys and girls with sickle cell disease had delayed pubertal growth spurt and PHV, although adult height was comparable to that of normal adults; girls were said to have a marginally to significantly delayed onset of menstruation.[592] Boys with sickle cell anemia often exhibit impaired Leydig cell function caused by ischemia of the testes or gonadotropin deficiency, or both.

Thalassemia carries the risk of hemochromatosis due to transfusional iron deposition in the pituitary and hypothalamus; as a consequence, patients may have hypogonadotropic hypogonadism[593] and impairment of testicular function.[594] Primary hypothyroidism is prevalent in this condition, but it is only part of the problem of sexual maturation and growth failure due to GH deficiency.[595] Before the advent of subcutaneous chelation therapy (with monitoring of serum ferritin), complete absence of pubertal development occurred in more than 40% of patients with thalassemia. The gonads can be stimulated by exogenous gonadotropins, and satisfactory sexual development, including fertility, can be promoted by the use of hCG and human FSH in many patients without gonadal damage,[596] although pituitary and gonadal damage may be severe in children with poorly controlled disease. Desferrioxamine therapy may cause skeletal dysplasia and compromise pubertal growth.[597] Decreased BMD in thalassemia makes early recognition and treatment of the problem all the more important.

Cytotoxic effects of the alkylating agents used to prepare patients for bone marrow transplantation in this condition add to the problem. Treatment after the onset of puberty is safer for gonadal function in boys but not necessarily in girls. Girls with early bone marrow transplantation and apparently normal pubertal development have elevated serum FSH levels and menstrual abnormalities ranging up to amenorrhea,[598] suggesting that gonadal impairment is universal in girls with thalassemia major after bone marrow transplantation.

Growth in stature was delayed in boys with acute immunodeficiency syndrome (AIDS), even when the weight for height was equal to that of normal boys. AIDS did not affect serum testosterone concentrations, but bone age was delayed, as was the progression through the stages of puberty. Because GH secretion is rarely affected by AIDS, poor growth appeared more related to the delay in pubertal development. These concerns also apply to children with prenatally acquired human immunodeficiency virus (HIV) infection. Prepubertal children with HIV infection had lower IGFBP3 levels than case controls, and the DHEAS-to-cortisol ratio was also higher in infected children.[599]

Chronic gastrointestinal disease (e.g., Crohn's disease) is often accompanied by delayed puberty, and therapy to restore nutrition, if successful, enables puberty to progress. The pubertal growth spurt is compromised by active inflammatory bowel disease, especially if glucocorticoid therapy is necessary. Celiac disease decreases the growth rate in childhood and adolescence, but with appropriate dietary restrictions, final adult height appears to be normal.

Chronic renal disease is associated with delayed pubertal development and decreased pulsatile gonadotropin secretion due to a decrease in the mass of bioactive and immunoactive LH secreted rather than an alteration of the frequency. Successful renal transplantation usually restores gonadotropin secretion and improves growth. Immunoreactive gonadotropin concentrations may be elevated, presumably because of impaired renal clearance, but the response to GnRH is blunted in severe renal impairment. TeBG is elevated in chronic renal failure, and the level of free testosterone is low. Survivors of renal transplantation who are undergoing immune suppression and alternate-day steroid treatment often have delayed onset of puberty and decreased pulsatility of GH and gonadotropins at night.

Patients with nephrotic syndrome have poor pubertal growth, poor secondary sexual development, and deficient gonadotropin secretion in a pattern resembling CDP. Glomerulonephritis treated with alternate-day glucocorticoid therapy leads to a late, diminished, but prolonged pubertal growth spurt that can result in a normal final height.

Children with early onset of leukemia and long-term remission experience puberty at an appropriate age or with only a slight delay, whereas patients with initial symptoms of leukemia in late childhood may have considerable delay of pubertal development. Radiation treatment to the CNS may cause hypogonadotropic hypogonadism or GH deficiency, or both, and irradiation of the abdomen or pelvis and certain types of chemotherapy, especially if administered during puberty, may impair gonadal function and cause primary hypogonadism, although ovarian function may return even in the face of elevated serum gonadotropin levels.[600] Total-body irradiation for bone marrow transplantation exerts the most significant effects, such as severe GH deficiency in 50%, hypothyroidism in 56%, and hypogonadism in 83% of males, and 100% of women had ovarian failure; insulin resistance was found in 83% and dyslipidemia in 61%.[601] Children with leukemia treated with CNS irradiation had a diminished pubertal growth spurt and diminished final height. Long-term follow-up studies demonstrate the rising incidence of the metabolic syndrome in childhood cancer survivors,[505,602,603] and data indicate GH deficiency with chemotherapy in the absence of radiation therapy.

Hypothyroidism may delay the onset of puberty or menarche (except in extreme cases in which puberty starts early); treatment with levothyroxine reverses this pattern, but there is likely to be a permanent loss of height if the diagnosis is delayed. Poorly controlled diabetes mellitus can lead to poor growth, fatty infiltration of the liver, and sexual infantilism (i.e., Mauriac syndrome), which is probably related to poor nutritional status. Prepubertal children are most vulnerable to poor glycemic control, and pubertal subjects exhibit normal growth unless severe hyperglycemia occurs. The degree of control necessary to avoid these complications cannot be exactly quantified, but adolescents with even moderately poor control frequently manifest some degree of growth impairment and delayed puberty or irregular menses. Cushing's disease can be associated with delayed onset or arrest of gonadarche, which usually is corrected by transsphenoidal removal of an ACTH-secreting pituitary adenoma.[604,605]

Anorexia Nervosa and Variants

Anorexia Nervosa. Anorexia nervosa, a common cause of gonadotropin deficiency in adolescence, is a functional disorder. Prevalence is increased among girls (it is the third most common chronic disease of adolescent girls),[606] and it starts at ever-younger ages, but it is rare in boys. It is characterized by a distorted body image, obsessive fear of obesity, and food avoidance that can cause severe self-induced weight loss (to less than 85% of normal weight for age and height or a BMI <17.5 kg/m^2 after cessation of growth), primary or secondary amenorrhea in affected females, widespread endocrine disorders, and even death. Specific diagnostic details are provided in the *Diagnostic and Statistical Manual of Mental Disorders,* fourth edition [DSM-IV] criteria of the American Psychiatric Association.[607] The onset of amenorrhea precedes the onset of severe weight loss. Controversy exists regarding inclusion of amenorrhea in the DSM-V, because some individuals with classic psychological profiles still have menses.[608]

Other common features include onset in middle adolescence, hyperactivity, defective thermoregulation with hypothermia and sensitivity to cold, constipation, bradycardia and hypotension, decreased basal metabolic rate, dry skin, fine or downy hypertrichosis, peripheral edema, and parotid enlargement. The pathogenesis is multifactorial and includes a genetic factor and a well-characterized psychological component.[609] Before the diagnosis of anorexia nervosa is made, organic disease must be excluded; a girl with macroprolactinoma may present with signs consistent with anorexia nervosa. The prevalence of anorexia nervosa is increased among individuals with Turner syndrome.

Anorexia nervosa has considerable endocrine ramifications.[610] The concentrations of plasma FSH, LH, leptin, and estradiol and the excretion of urinary gonadotropins are characteristically low. There may be a reversion to a circadian rhythm of LH secretion and to the sleep-associated increase in episodic LH secretion or LH response to GnRH characteristic of early puberty, or the amplitude of the pulsatile episodes may be diminished, as in the pattern of prepubertal children, if onset occurs during puberty. Pulsatile administration of intravenous GnRH at 90- to 120-minute intervals can produce LH pulses that are indistinguishable from the normal pubertal pattern, demonstrating functional GnRH deficiency. Serum leptin levels are low, consistent with the strikingly decreased mass of adipose tissue, and increase with regain of weight.[611,612] Other hormonal changes include increased mean concentrations of plasma GH and plasma cortisol; low levels of plasma IGF1, DHEAS, and T_3 with normal levels of T_4 (unless the low thyroxine syndrome is present) and TSH; a decreased rise in serum prolactin after administration of thyrotropin-releasing hormone (TRH) or insulin-induced hypoglycemia; and a diminished capacity to concentrate urine. This condition must be considered in the differential diagnosis of growth failure in younger subjects.

Lower heart rates, lower systolic blood pressure, lower body temperature, anemia, and leukopenia are found in persons with anorexia nervosa.[613] The ratio of bone age to chronologic age is significantly lower in girls with anorexia nervosa and correlates positively with duration of illness and markers of nutritional status. All measures of BMD are lower, and the most significant predictors of bone density are lean body mass, BMI, and age at menarche. Because treatment of decreased bone density in these individuals has not been proved to be effective, prevention is paramount.[614]

Normal endocrine and metabolic function may follow weight gain, but amenorrhea may persist for months, suggesting persistent hypothalamic dysfunction. Free leptin was an important determinant of menstrual recovery in one longitudinal study.[615] In view of the associated mortality rate, parenteral alimentation may be indicated in resistant patients with severe weight loss, especially in those with infection or an electrolyte imbalance. Treatment of this disorder requires skillful management, understanding, patience, and psychiatric consultation.[609]

Functional amenorrhea can occur in women with normal weight but decreased percentage of body fat, and it is characterized by normal basal levels of gonadotropin and normal gonadotropin response to GnRH stimulation but lack of or an inadequate midcycle LH surge and a decrease in normal pulsatile secretion (amplitude or frequency, or both) of gonadotropins.[616] These patients have higher than average cortisol values; decreased levels of free thyroxine (T_4), free triiodothyronine (T_3), and total T_4 with normal TSH levels; and decreased leptin concentrations that are probably caused by subtle dysfunction of eating patterns and altered energy expenditure.[617] The consequences range from severe estrogen deficiency to anovulation to a short luteal phase. Reduced bone density is a concern.

Bulimia nervosa is thought to be a variant of anorexia nervosa,[609] but separation into two conditions is an approach favored by some.[618] Bulimia occurs in about 1.5% of young women. In this disorder, the individual consumes large amounts of food, but induced vomiting follows food gorging. A hand lesion from the induced vomiting (i.e., Russell's sign) and an abnormal level of serum electrolytes are useful clinical markers. Abuse of laxatives, diet pills, and diuretics is frequent. Although weight loss is not frequent, amenorrhea is common. Bulimia is especially prevalent in high school and college female students. A history of childhood sexual abuse is more common than in unaffected adolescents.

Cessation of growth can occur in infants and young children with psychosocial dwarfism. Stressful social situations can also inhibit growth and physical pubertal development at adolescence.

Exercise, Hypo-Ovarianism, and Amenorrhea: The Female Athlete Triad. In 1992, the American College of Sports Medicine defined the female athletic triad as primary or secondary amenorrhea, disordered eating, and osteoporosis.[619,620] Although there are substantial endocrine effects of excessive athletic training in girls, elite prepubertal and pubertal female athletes suffer relatively few physical injuries. Because there is no demonstrable effect on pubertal development from moderate exercise in subelite female runners, moderate exercise should not be discouraged during adolescence.

Bulimia, anorexia nervosa, or anorexia athletica is most often found in girls engaged in sports that emphasize weight.[621] Teenage ballet dancers are lighter, have less body fat, and have a high incidence of delayed puberty and of primary and secondary amenorrhea than less physically active girls. Factors other than decreased body weight can impair pubertal progression and delay menarche through inhibition of the hypothalamic GnRH pulse generator in healthy ballet dancers and female athletes.

Athletes who began strenuous training before menarche have a delay in menarcheal age.[622] However, genetic influences overlie changes due to weight or activity because there is a positive correlation between the delayed menarche found in athletic girls and the age of menarche of their mothers. Artistic and rhythmic gymnasts have delay in menarche when compared with their mothers and sisters,[623] and the former have a more significant delay.[624,625]

Higher bone density is reported in the femurs of gymnasts compared with those of ballet dancers and controls, but lower radial bone density in the gymnasts and ballet dancers reflects the effect of the application of force on bone remodeling; a positive relationship between serum leptin and tibial bone density is found.[626] The bone density of female long distance runners is greater in those with regular menses than those with menstrual irregularities. Osteopenia in later life may result from amenorrhea in ballet dancers, even with estrogen replacement, and nutrition therapy is considered important to improve outcome.[627]

Thinness and strenuous physical activity appear to act synergistically, but strenuous exercise training by itself may inhibit the GnRH pulse generator, mediated in part by endogenous opioidergic pathways involving β-endorphin. When the strenuous physical activity is interrupted (e.g., by injury), puberty advances, and menarche often occurs within a few months in those with amenorrhea, in some cases before a significant change in body composition or weight. Even though gonadarche is retarded, adrenarche is not delayed.

Female athletes of normal weight who have less fat and more muscle than nonathletic girls (e.g., ice skaters, swimmers) are also at risk for delayed puberty and for primary and secondary amenorrhea. However, the mechanism apparently is different from the hypothalamic amenorrhea in runners and ballet dancers. In swimmers, menstrual cycles frequently are irregular and anovulatory rather than absent, and the plasma concentrations of DHEAS and LH were higher than normal, but plasma estrogen levels were normal.[628]

Prospective study of gymnasts contrasted with swimmers demonstrated decreased growth velocity, stunting in leg length growth, and in some studies, decreased height prediction in the gymnasts.[629] Extensive training (10 to 12 hours/week) may be excessive for prepubertal girls.

Prolactin levels may be elevated in women athletes and may contribute to the delayed menarche found in this group.[497] Osteopenia can result from the associated chronic hypoestrogenism.[630]

Scoliosis in girls usually develops during the pubertal growth spurt and more often occurs in girls with a more rapid pubertal growth spurt. Ballet dancers have a higher incidence of scoliosis than the general population and often have delayed puberty. Idiopathic scoliosis in the general population is associated with a statistically earlier age of menarche and an early adolescent growth spurt. The strongest association with scoliosis is taller stature at the time of the pubertal growth spurt. Adult height in familial constellations of scoliosis does not vary from the family norm.

Although men are less affected than women, men may also be affected by rigorous physical training. They may have decreased LH response to GnRH and decreased spontaneous LH pulse frequency and amplitude; the serum testosterone level is normal or low with extreme activity levels.

Other Causes of Delayed Puberty

Marijuana use has been associated with gynecomastia and is a putative cause of pubertal delay. Gaucher disease caused delay in pubertal development in two thirds of patients in one study. Girls with familial dysautonomia have delayed menarche and often have a severe premenstrual syndrome. The condition is ultimately compatible with pregnancy. Chronic infections may delay the onset of puberty.

Diabetes mellitus type 1 is associated with delayed menarche.[631] Remarkably, this may occur no matter the degree of glycemic control.

Hypergonadotropic Hypogonadism: Sexual Infantilism Caused by Primary Gonadal Disorders

The most common forms of primary gonadal failure are associated with sex chromosome abnormalities and characteristic physical findings.[632] Testicular or ovarian dysfunction as an isolated finding is less commonly a cause of pubertal hypergonadotropic hypogonadism.

Boys

Klinefelter's Syndrome and Its Variants. Klinefelter's syndrome (i.e., syndrome of seminiferous tubular dysgenesis) and its variants occur in approximately 1 in 1000 males, and they are the most common forms of male hypogonadism.[632,633] However, less than 10% are diagnosed before puberty, leaving those with decreased androgen production and no treatment susceptible to decreased bone mass.[634] The invariable clinical features include small, firm testes as an adult (<3.5 cm long); impaired spermatogenesis; and a male phenotype, usually with gynecomastia and long legs but not long arms (Fig. 25-45).[632] Prepubertally, patients can be detected by the disproportionate length of the extremities, decreased upper-to-lower body ratio without an increase in arm span rather than eunuchoid proportions, in which arm span and leg length are increased. Tall stature for family size is common in this disorder due to the disproportionate growth of the legs.

Infants with Klinefelter's syndrome have early evidence of testicular failure because testicular volume and penile length are decreased and the neonatal surge in testosterone is decreased. Muscle tone is also lower in some.[635] Before the age of 12 years, gonadotropin concentrations are in the prepubertal range, but levels usually rise with pubertal progression. Rarely, low gonadotropin concentrations occur when hypogonadotropic hypogonadism is associated with 47,XXY Klinefelter's syndrome or coexisting constitutional delay.

Hyalinization and fibrosis of the seminiferous tubules and pseudoadenomatous changes of the Leydig cells develop after puberty; prepubertal testes show only subtle histologic changes, although the testes are small, and the germ cell content is reduced, whereas Sertoli cells are normal in abundance and appearance before 2 years of age. Older prepubertal subjects have normal seminiferous tubules. Adult-type spermatogonia are found in peripubertal boys, and older boys had no germ cells; the testes degenerate in an accelerated manner at the onset of puberty.[636] However, there is a 44% success rate for sperm

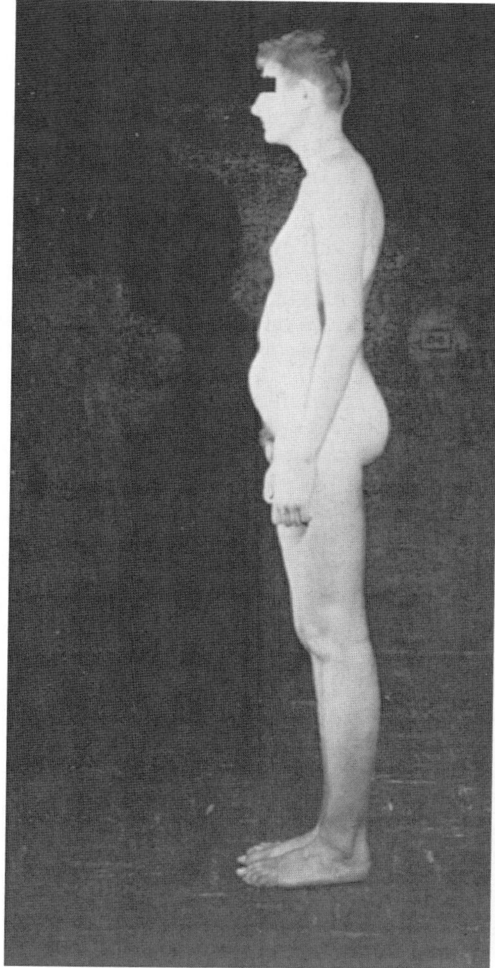
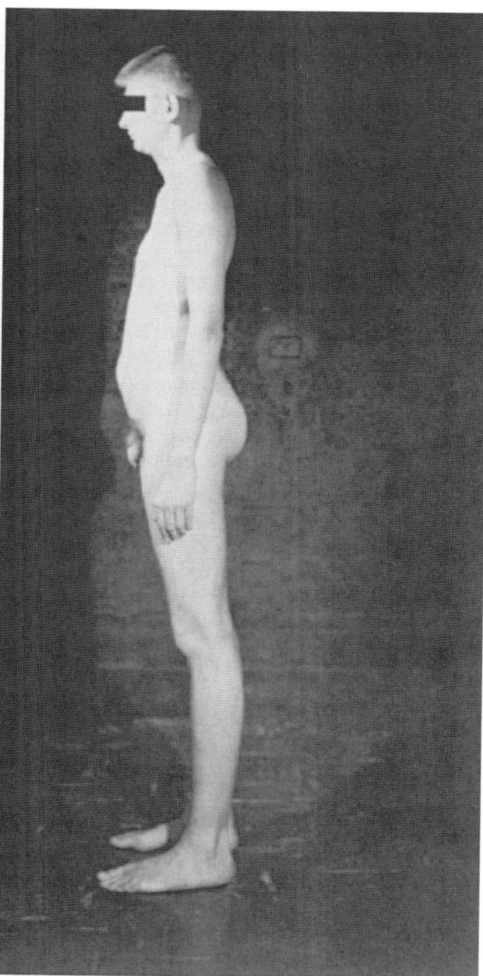

Figure 25-45 47,XXY Klinefelter's syndrome in 17-year-old identical twins. At age 15, gynecomastia was observed. The twins had a eunuchoid habitus and poorly developed male secondary sexual characteristics. Both were 187 cm tall; arm spans were 187 cm and 189.5 cm; the voices were high pitched; the testes measured 1.8 × 1.5 cm; and penis length was 7.5 cm. Gynecomastia and signs of androgen deficiency were more evident in the twin on the left. Urinary gonadotropin levels were greater than 50 mU/24 hours. The testes exhibited extensive tubular fibrosis, small dysgenetic tubules, and clumping or pseudoadenomatous formation of Leydig cells; germ cells were rare. The microscopic appearance was typical of seminiferous tubule dysgenesis. (Patient data from Grumbach MM, Barr ML. Cytologic tests of chromosome sex in relation to sexual anomalies in man. *Recent Prog Horm Res.* 1958;14:255-324.)

retrieval from testicular tissues and a 55% success rate for use of microdissection testicular sperm aspiration. Intracytoplasmic sperm injection led to the birth of 101 children, in whom there was no apparent increase in congenital or genetic defects.[637]

Serum FSH, LH, inhibin B, and AMH levels in nonmosaic XXY infants did not differ from those of control infants. Serum testosterone levels during the first 3 months followed the normal rise in infancy but were lower than those of controls. However, AMH levels were undetectable in XXY adolescents, and inhibin B levels decreased from normal to the low levels characteristic of adult Klinefelter's syndrome during late puberty[638] after an unequivocal increase in serum testosterone (>2.5 nmol/L) levels and degeneration of Sertoli cells.

There is variation in Leydig cell function among childhood and pubertal subjects, but the plasma concentration of testosterone fails to rise to normal adult levels. The onset of puberty usually is not delayed, but impaired Leydig cell reserve and low testosterone levels may lead to slow progression or arrest of pubertal changes. Testosterone replacement should be considered when the LH level rises above the normal range of values but is not necessary in all subjects in early puberty.[639] Serum estradiol-to-testosterone ratios and TeBG levels are higher than those in normal males, which indicates an increased estrogen effect and decreased testosterone effect that may account in part for the gynecomastia characteristic of Klinefelter's syndrome. Testosterone administration does not appear to reduce the gynecomastia, but dihydrotestosterone may help. Aromatase inhibitors or estrogen receptor antagonists initially held promise but do not seem to be effective after longer trials. If the gynecomastia does not regress within 2 years, reduction mammoplasty is required. Breast cancer may develop in these individuals, and monitoring for this possibility is important.

The androgen receptor gene is located on the X chromosome and encodes a ligand-dependent transcription factor with highly polymorphic CAGn trinucleotide repeats in the coding sequence of the first exon. The length of the translated polyglutamate tract in the N-terminal transactivation domain of the resulting protein and the length of this polyglutamate tract is inversely proportional to receptor transactivation activity. The shorter the repeat sequence within the range of normal variation, the more active the androgen receptor, and small changes in this activity may result in more significant effects in Klinefelter's syndrome, in which testosterone secretion may already be impaired. A negative correlation between CAGn repeat length and penile length, but not testicular size, in children has been reported.[640] Another study found a positive association between CAGn repeat length and body height, an inverse relationship to bone density and arm span to body height, and the presence of longer CAGn repeats for gynecomastia and smaller testes in adults.[641] A paternal origin of the extra X chromosome is associated with later onset of puberty and longer CAG repeats.[636]

Behavior and Development in Klinefelter's Syndrome. Neurobehavioral abnormalities, primarily in language, speech, learning, and frontal executive functions, are common, even universal, in Klinefelter's syndrome, but severe retardation is uncommon.[233] These problems may lead to evaluation in childhood and the prepubertal recognition of the syndrome. The prevalence of adjustment problems in adolescence is increased. Psychopathology is a rare finding in most studies, and a 20-year follow-up of 47,XXY individuals showed little or no variation from nonaffected controls in employment, social status, mental or physical health, and criminality.[642] Because patients with clinical or psychological problems are referred more often for evaluation, some earlier studies may be skewed to suggest more significant deficits than is prevalent in an unselected population of XXY individuals.

The global IQ in unselected populations of Klinefelter's syndrome subjects is normal or near normal, but verbal IQ, in contrast to that of patients with Turner syndrome, is usually lower (e.g., 10 to 20 points) than performance IQ.[643]

Prepubertal Klinefelter's syndrome patients have reduced left hemisphere specialization for verbal tasks and enhanced right hemisphere specialization for nonverbal tasks. However, these abnormalities tended to normalize after puberty began, suggesting hemispheric reorganization during puberty. Hypotheses are advanced supporting the effect of prenatal testosterone on cerebral dominance and on language and reading pathology.

There is controversy about the indication for testosterone treatment of infants or adolescents with Klinefelter's syndrome. Although there is a growing feeling among parents that testosterone treatment in the early pubertal period improves language, reading, behavior, and self-image in boys with Klinefelter's syndrome, no well-controlled studies supporting this contention are available, and long-term studies are needed.

Other Aspects of Klinefelter's Syndrome. Conditions associated with Klinefelter's syndrome include aortic valvular disease and ruptured berry aneurysms (six times the normal rate); breast carcinoma (20 times the rate in normal men and one fifth that of women); other malignancies such as acute leukemia, lymphoma, and germ cell tumors at any midline site; systemic lupus erythematosus; and osteoporosis in about 25% of affected adults. There is an increased risk of diabetes mellitus, thyroid disease, fatigue, varicose veins, and essential tremor.

About 20% of mediastinal germ cell tumors are associated with Klinefelter's syndrome, and they occur at a younger age than the mediastinal germ cell tumors that are not associated with the syndrome.[644] With rare exceptions, these germ cell tumors, which may be located in the midline anywhere from the CNS to the pelvis, secrete hCG and induce sexual precocity. Klinefelter's syndrome needs to be considered in boys with hCG-secreting germ cell tumors, especially if the tumor is located in the mediastinum or CNS.

Other Forms of Primary Testicular Failure

Chemotherapy. Cancer therapy, especially irradiation of the gonads or the use of alkylating chemotherapeutic agents, affects testicular function and can lead to adult infertility.[645,646] Chemotherapeutic agents used in the treatment of nephrotic syndrome or leukemia, such as cyclophosphamide or chlorambucil, have led to Sertoli cell, Leydig cell, and germ cell damage in prepubertal patients; these effects are sometimes reversible. Chemotherapy for childhood Hodgkin's disease, including chlorambucil, vinblastine, Mustargen, Oncovin, procarbazine, and prednisone, may allow spontaneous progression through puberty, but FSH and LH concentrations may be elevated, and the inhibin B concentrations decrease during puberty, indicative of gonadal damage. Normal basal LH values may raise hope that Leydig cell function is normal, but if there is an exaggerated rise of the LH level after GnRH, compensated Leydig cell damage is present. The basal serum FSH level and rise in LH and FSH levels after GnRH correlate with the dose of cyclophosphamide. COPP/MOPP chemotherapy for Hodgkin's disease can cause severe damage to Sertoli and germinal cells, but it has less effect on Leydig cells, even if therapy occurred in the prepubertal period. Lower dosing or limiting therapy to less than three courses is suggested to decrease these complications.[647] The combination of Adriamycin, bleomycin, vinblastine, and dacarbazine (ABVD regimen) can cause germ cell depletion. Although initially it was thought that some degree of prepubertal gonadal maturation was necessary before these drugs could cause gonadal damage, gonadal damage can occur earlier as a result of therapy in the prepubertal period but may not be demonstrable until the age of puberty.[648]

Radiation Therapy. Radiotherapy of the gonads can cause primary testicular failure, usually resulting in azoospermia, although normal testosterone secretion may occur with elevated LH and FSH values (i.e., compensated Leydig cell failure). The gonads must be shielded from the treatment unless they are the focus of therapy.

Sperm Preservation. Sperm preservation by cryopreservation is an option for a boy who will undergo chemotherapy or radiation therapy. Alternatively, testicular tissue can be preserved frozen, later to be reimplanted in the subject's own testis or to be stimulated to maturity for use in intracytoplasmic sperm injection. Other methods of preserving fertility years after treatment for childhood cancers are under consideration. This is not established clinical care, but initial study suggests the technique is acceptable to parents and safe.[649]

Testicular Biosynthetic Defects. The 46,XY disorder of sex development is caused by 17α-hydroxylase/17,20-lyase deficiency resulting from mutations in *CYP17A1* at gene map locus 10q24.3; it is associated with sexual infantilism and a female phenotype. The testosterone biosynthetic defect blocks the synthesis of testosterone and adrenal androgens, impairing masculinization at all stages of development.[650] Associated cortisol deficiency and increased mineralocorticoid secretion in this condition lead to hypertension, decreased serum potassium levels, and metabolic alkalosis. Elevated serum progesterone levels and decreased plasma renin activity are helpful diagnostic features.[651] Glucocorticoid replacement suppresses ACTH and mineralocorticoid excess and corrects the electrolyte abnormalities, but no sexual development occurs unless exogenous gonadal steroids are administered. Less-severe deficiencies are associated with ambiguous genitalia. *CYP17A1* mutations leading to isolated 17,20-lyase deficiency are rare.

A rare autosomal recessive condition is steroidogenic acute regulatory protein (StAR) deficiency, in which the ability to produce C21-, C19-, and C18-steroids is lost; severely affected patients have lipid-laden adrenal glands. The adrenals and gonads have a severe impairment of the conversion of cholesterol to pregnenolone.[652] The large adrenal glands may be visualized on ultrasound, CT, or MRI. Death often occurs in infancy because of unrecognized glucocorticoid and mineralocorticoid deficiencies. Affected individuals physically appear to be sexually infantile females, whether their karyotype is 46,XY or 46,XX; because of the absence of gonadal or adrenal androgen production, the affected XY phenotypic females do not develop secondary sexual characteristics, including pubic hair.[633] However, XX females with a null mutation[653] develop female sex characteristics at puberty, including pubic hair and multicystic ovaries, but they also have primary or secondary amenorrhea. In contrast to the fetal testis, the fetal ovary, which is insensitive to FSH and steroidogenically inactive, is undamaged in fetal life and remains so until the onset of puberty. Under FSH stimulation during puberty and with recruitment of ovarian follicles, the ovaries undergo progressive damage and cyst formation. Ovarian damage and impairment of ovarian StAR-independent steroidogenesis appears to be related to lipid deposition in the ovary.[654]

Luteinizing Hormone Resistance. Presumptive evidence of LH resistance caused by an LH receptor[655] abnormality on the Leydig cell was reported in an 18-year-old boy with a male phenotype, no male secondary sexual development, gynecomastia, elevated plasma LH levels, and early pubertal plasma testosterone concentrations that did not increase after hCG administration; there was no elevation of testosterone precursor levels. The testes were prepubertal in size and had the microscopic appearance of normal prepubertal testes. Plasma membrane receptor preparations from the testes bound only one half as much radiolabeled hCG as control testes.

In affected males, this autosomal recessive disorder is caused by a mutation in *LHCGR,* the gene encoding the G protein–coupled, seven-transmembrane LH/hCG cell receptor[323] at gene map locus 2p21. Mutations that cause a more severe compromise in LHCGR function are associated with XY disorders of sex development. Homozygous deletion of exon 10 or the homozygous missense mutations Ser616Tyr and Ile625Lys of the LH receptor are associated with micropenis (but not hypospadias) due to partial impairment of LH receptor function, leading to a discordance with a poor response to LH but not to hCG. Nephropathic cystinosis in boys leads to hypergonadotropic hypogonadism.

Anorchia and Cryptorchidism. A 46,XY male without palpable testes may have intra-abdominal testes, which carry an increased risk of malignant degeneration; anorchia (i.e., vanishing testes syndrome, caused by perinatal torsion), in which no testes are found at laparotomy; or retractile testes, a variation of normal.[352,632,656] About 50% of bilateral, nonpalpable testes are undescended, and the other 50% are testicular remnants from vanishing testes that usually do not contain germ cells, are found in the scrotum, are not at risk for carcinoma, and need not be removed if the history is certain.[657] The prevalence of undescended testes is between 3% and 4% at birth, but it is higher in low-birth-weight, preterm, and SGA males, and the prevalence of these conditions is also increasing. More than two thirds of these descend by 3 months, but there remains a prevalence of undescended testes of about 1% after age 12 months.[657] If at one time there was a male phenotype and male internal ducts, functioning fetal testes capable of secreting testosterone and AMH were present early during fetal life but degenerated thereafter. Administration of 2000 U of hCG (3000 U/m^2) intramuscularly usually evokes an increased concentration of plasma testosterone after 72 hours when functional Leydig cells are present. The lack of a rise in testosterone concentration, in conjunction with an increased plasma concentration of FSH and LH or an augmented gonadotropin response to GnRH, is evidence for the diagnosis of bilateral anorchia. Alternatively, measurement of plasma AMH can indicate the presence of testicular tissue in a range of suspected conditions in prepubertal boys, from presumed anorchia to male pseudohermaphrodism and true hermaphrodism.[305] The serum inhibin B level is a useful indicator of the presence of functional testicular tissue; values correlated with the testosterone response to hCG administration, and values less than 15 pg/mL indicated anorchia.[303]

Discovery of unilateral cryptorchidism may represent the presence of a descended testis on one side and none on the other side, and this presents a diagnostic dilemma. In 90% of cases,[658] there is testicular compensatory hypertrophy of the descended testis if there is absence of the contralateral testis, probably due to elevation of FSH secretion. Because the finding does not universally predict monorchia, laparoscopy is recommended for diagnosis of this condition if ultrasound is unsuccessful. Although there are many statements in the literature that the contralateral descended testis has increased risk of carcinoma in an individual with unilateral undescended testes, analysis suggests the risk is the same as that in the general population.[657]

Studies of cryptorchidism may include all of the conditions mentioned earlier, ranging from retractile testes to unilateral or bilateral cryptorchidism, and conclusions may vary because of the heterogenous data. A recent review of the international literature on cryptorchidism updated conventional wisdom on the subject.[657]

Cryptorchid testes may demonstrate congenital abnormalities and may not function normally even if brought into the scrotum early in life. The descended testis in a unilaterally cryptorchid boy may show abnormal histologic features; these patients have a 69% incidence of decreased sperm counts. Unilateral cryptorchid patients can be infertile even if they received early treatment of unilateral cryptorchism. Because descended and undescended testes may be affected, there may be preexisting disease that is manifested by the lack of descent of one testis. Patients undergoing orchiopexy may sustain subtle damage to the vas deferens, leading to the later production of antibodies to sperm that may result in infertility.

Cryptorchid testes may descend into the scrotum during more prolonged treatment with hCG (3000 U/m^2 of surface area, given intramuscularly every other day for six doses) or with intranasal GnRH or a combination of hCG and GnRH treatment.[659,660] Although such descent occurs in retractile testes, it can occur in true cryptorchid testes but only when descent is not prevented by local anatomic obstructions. One theory posits that hormonal treatment may decrease the number of spermatogonia compared with individuals who had only orchiopexy. Because testicular descent normally occurs by 1 year of age, orchidopexy is recommended between 12 and 18 months in those whose testes are not expected to descend spontaneously. One study linked testicular descent to an adequate neonatal surge of LH and testosterone by 4 months in AGA infants and by 6 months in premature infants; the study authors recommended treatment be considered earlier than at 1 year.[661]

Two critical steps in the maturation of germ cells are described in the normal prepubertal testis that do not occur in the unilaterally undescended testes. First, at 2 to 3 months of age, the gonocytes (primitive spermatogonia) in the fetal stem cell pool transform into the adult dark spermatogonia, which become the adult stem pool (possibly related to the early infancy surge in LH, FSH, and testosterone. Second, at 4 to 5 years of age, meiosis begins, and primary spermatocytes appear.[662] The contralateral descended testis is affected but less so than the undescended testis. Identification of the gonocyte transformation has influenced recommendations on the timing of orchidopexy. Postpubertal orchidopexy is associated with a greater than 85% prevalence of azoospermia or oligospermia. It has been surmised that cryptorchid testes, even if replaced in the scrotum, may never have normal spermatogenic function as a consequence of an early abnormality in germ cell maturation, vascular damage to the testicular circulation during orchidopexy, or an intrinsic testicular defect. However, in a later study of men with cryptorchidism, the paternity rate was 65% for men who had had bilateral cryptorchidism, compared with 90% for the formerly unilateral cryptorchid men and 93% for control men. The reduction in fertility was supported by semen and hormone analyses.[656] Successful fertilization was reported by the use of intracytoplasmic injection of sperm extracted from the testes of cryptorchid men who had orchiopexy after puberty.[663]

The incidence of testicular carcinoma in England at all ages increased from 2 per 100,000 in 1909 to 4.4 per 100,000 in 1999, with a rise noticed during puberty,[664] although the data are nation specific, and there is an approximately 10-fold range between countries.[657] The most contemporary careful studies indicate an overall relative risk of testicular carcinoma in cryptorchidism of 2.5 to 8, with the highest risk associated with intra-abdominal rather than inguinal testes and higher risks observed for those with abnormal chromosomes, syndromes, or late or no orchiopexy. Adverse environmental factors may be important in the apparent increase in testis cancer, cryptorchidism, hypospadia, and low semen quality, and related factors may be explained by the testicular dysgenesis synrome.[665]

Early orchidopexy seems to reduce the risk of carcinoma of the testes,[666] although dysgenetic testes, even if located in the scrotum, carry an increased risk of malignant transformation.[632] Undescended testes remain at a higher temperature than descended testes, and undescended testes have a maturation arrest at the conversion of the gonocytes to spermatogonia, which appears to direct the testes toward malignant degeneration.[666] Orchiopexy before 12 years of age (considered as the age of puberty and therefore an appropriate cutoff for analysis although 10 years is considered in the same manner by some) usually is considered to decrease the risk of cancer, but later orchiopexy must balance the risk of anesthesia with the risk of cancer.[657] There is a very small risk of carcinoma of the testes in prepuberty, but the absence of carcinoma in situ in prepuberty is not an assurance that carcinoma will not develop in adult life. Periodic sonography of the testis of affected patients is recommended after the onset of puberty.

Retractile testes can descend into the scrotum but then reascend. They are considered a normal variation, but a requirement for orchiopexy was reported for 22.7% in a series of 150. The finding of one case of testicular carcinoma in a boy with spontaneous descent in this series led to a suggestion of following such cases in the long term.[667] The risk of breast cancer associated with gynecomastia is increased in men with a history of undescended testes, orchiopexy, orchitis, testicular injury, infertility, or any cause of delayed puberty.

Small for Gestational Age. SGA predisposes males to reproductive problems and is associated with the testicular dysgenesis syndrome. Males born SGA tend to have smaller testes and lower testosterone and higher LH levels,[668] suggesting an impairment of fertility, as is found in SGA females. Adult males born SGA have increased aromatase and 5α-reductase activities, leading to elevated levels of estradiol and dihydrotestosterone.[669] Of most concern is the fact that elevated estradiol levels in males increase the risk of testicular cancer and do not provide the protective effect on cardiovascular health as found in females. The level of inhibin B is elevated in significantly SGA boys (i.e., mean birth weights >2 SD below the mean for gestational age), although other studies with higher-birth-weight SGA boys demonstrated no such chages.[670]

Girls

Syndrome of Gonadal Dysgenesis and Its Variants. The most common form of hypergonadotropic hypogonadism in the female is the syndrome of gonadal dysgenesis (Turner syndrome and its variants), a sporadic disorder with an incidence of 1 per 2500 liveborn girls in which all (i.e., X chromosome monosomy with haploinsufficiency) or part of the second sex chromosome (i.e., partial sex chromosome monosomy) is absent.[632,671] About 99% of 45,X conceptuses abort spontaneously, and 1 in 15 spontaneous abortions has a 45,X karyotype. The 45,X karyotype is associated with female phenotype, short stature, sexual infantilism, and various somatic abnormalities.

Sex chromosome mosaicism or structural abnormalities of an X or Y chromosome (affects about 40% of individuals with Turner syndrome) may modify the features of this syndrome. The syndrome of gonadal dysgenesis and its variants are found in a continuum ranging from the typical 45,X phenotype to a normal male or female phenotype.[632] Comprehensive recommendations for the diagnosis and management of Turner syndrome were presented by an international committee.[672]

45,X Turner Syndrome. Short stature and sexual infantilism are typical features of sex chromatin–negative 45,X gonadal dysgenesis (Turner syndrome), which is the karyotype found in approximately 60% of cases (Fig. 25-46).[632] The short stature is caused by loss of a homeobox-containing gene that is located on the pseudoautosomal region (PAR1) of the short arms of the X (p22) and Y (p11.3) chromosomes[673,674] and encodes an osteogenic factor. This short stature homeobox-containing gene *(SHOX)*[673] was previously called the pseudoautosomal homeobox osteogenic gene *(PHOG)*. Because it is located on the PAR1 of the short arm of the X and Y chromosomes, it escapes X-chromosome inactivation. *SHOX* haploinsufficiency is responsible for, in addition to abnormal growth, mesomelic growth retardation, and Madelung deformity of the wrist (i.e., bilateral bowing of the radius with a dorsal subluxation of the distal ulna)[674,675,676] in Leri-Weill dyschondrosteosis (i.e., *SHOX* haploinsufficiency). Langer mesomelic dysplasia, which includes severe dwarfism with striking hypoplasia or aplasia of the ulnar and fibula, is caused by *SHOX* nullizygosity. *SHOX* haploinsufficiency appears to be responsible for 2.0 SD of the approximately 3.0 SD deficit in stature and the skeletal abnormalities in Turner syndrome.[676-679] On the other hand, patients with complete gonadal dysgenesis and tall stature had a 45,X/46,X der(X) and three doses of the *SHOX* gene due to the *SHOX* duplication on the der(X) chromosome. A method of relating the SHOX genotype to phenotypic manifestations has been developed.[680]

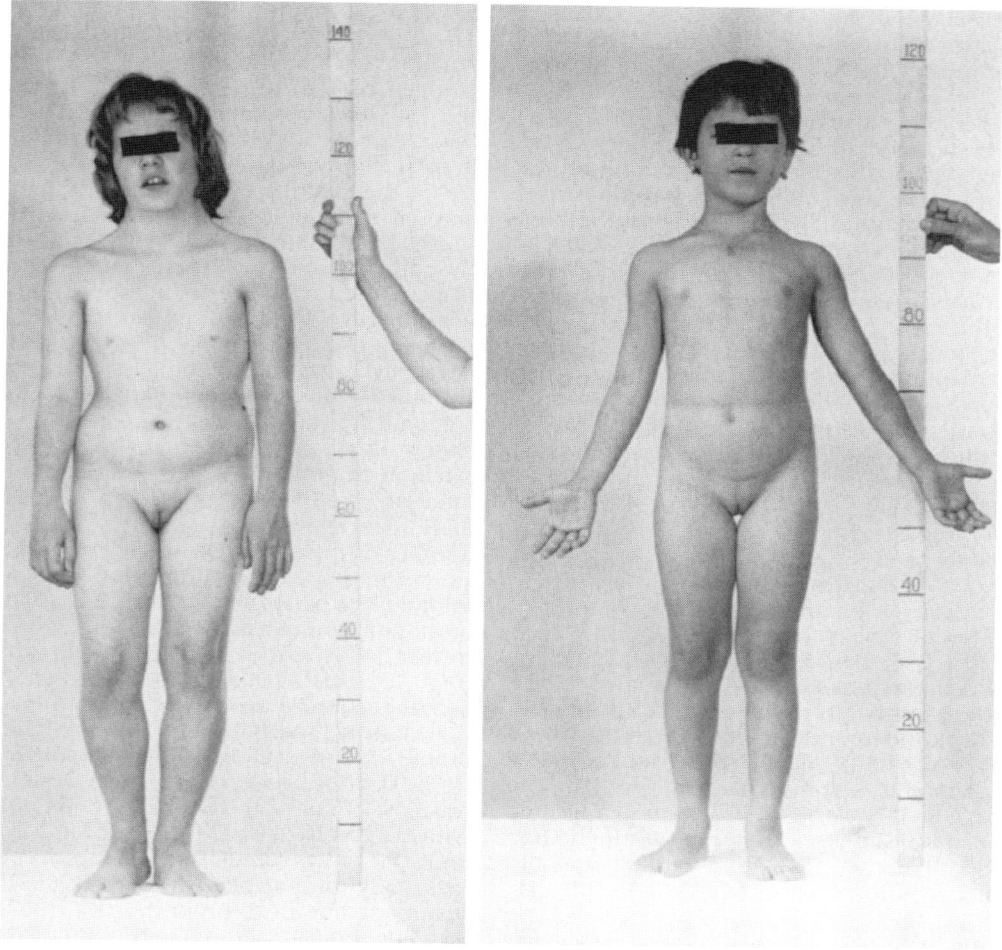

Figure 25-46 *Left,* A girl aged 14 years and 10 months with the typical form of the syndrome of gonadal dysgenesis (Turner syndrome). The X chromatin pattern was negative, and the karyotype was 45,X. She was short (height, 134.5 cm; height age, 9 years and 5 months) and sexually infantile except for the appearance of sparse pubic hair. She exhibited characteristic stigmata of the syndrome: a short, webbed neck; shield-like chest with widely separated nipples; bilateral metacarpal signs; puffiness over the dorsum of the fingers; cubitus valgus; increased number of pigmented nevi; characteristic facies; and low-set ears. The bone age was 13.5 years; the urinary 17-ketosteroid level was 5.1 mg/day; and the urinary gonadotropin level was greater than 100 mU/day. Vaginal smears and the urocytogram showed an immature pattern in which cornified squamous cells were absent. Female secondary sexual characteristics were induced with estrogen therapy, and the cyclic administration resulted in periodic estrogen withdrawal bleeding. *Right,* A 45,X girl aged 9 years and 11 months with Turner syndrome. Apart from short stature (height, 118 cm; height age, 6 years and 11 months), increased pigmented nevi, and subtle changes in the fingers and toes, she had few somatic anomalies. In contrast to the patient on the left, the main clinical feature was short stature.

Turner syndrome may be recognized in the newborn period or before. The 45,X abortuses have edema and large hygromas of the neck that may be seen on prenatal ultrasound studies. This lymphatic defect is the basis for the loose skinfolds that ultimately form the webbed neck (i.e., pterygium colli). Affected newborn infants may also have lymphedema of the extremities; the term *Bonnevie-Ullrich syndrome* has been applied to newborn infants with these features of Turner syndrome.

Frequent features are distinct facies with micrognathia, a fish-mouth appearance, high-arched palate with dental abnormalities, epicanthal folds, ptosis, low-set or deformed ears, short neck with low hairline, webbing (i.e., pterygium colli), and recurrent otitis media, often leading to impaired hearing (25% of affected adults require hearing aids).[632] A broad, shieldlike chest leads to the appearance of widely spaced nipples, and the areolae are often hypoplastic. Skeletal defects include short fourth metacarpals and cubitus valgus (which may develop after birth), Madelung deformity of the wrist (in about 7%), genu valgum, and scoliosis. There are extensive pigmented nevi, a tendency to keloid formation, and hypoplastic nails.[632] Lymphatic obstruction leads to the infantile puffiness of extremities and pterygium colli and to a distinctive shape of the ears. Cardiovascular anomalies affect the left side of the heart and include coarctation of the aorta in about 10% (40% of these have associated webbing of the neck), aortic stenosis, and bicuspid aortic valves; the latter individuals are at risk for a dissecting aortic aneurysm. An echocardiogram of the cardiovascular system must be performed, and prophylactic antibiotics are indicated if an anatomic abnormality is demonstrated. Elevated values on the ambulatory arterial stiffness index (AASI) may be another risk factor for later serious cardiac disease.[681] Abnormal pelvocaliceal collecting systems, abnormal position or alignment of the kidneys, and an abnormal vascular supply to the kidney are encountered in 30% to 60% of patients. Recurrent urinary tract infections are common. Defects of the gastrointestinal system include intestinal telangiectasias and hemangiomatoses that rarely can lead to massive gastrointestinal bleeding. The prevalence of inflammatory bowel disease, chronic liver disease, and colon cancer is increased.[671,682] Autoimmune diseases, such as Hashimoto thyroiditis (16-fold relative risk) and Graves' disease, are common, and an association with juvenile rheumatoid arthritis and psoriatic arthritis has been described.[671,682]

The age of diagnosis of Turner syndrome continues to be delayed, with the exception of newborns with the striking phenotype of the Bonnevie-Ullrich syndrome. It is recommended that all prepubertal age girls below −2.0 SD who have at least two somatic stigmata of the syndrome have a karyotype analysis; early diagnosis is key for optimal management of the growth failure and the detection of occult features of the syndrome.[683]

Pelvic ultrasonography or MRI usually permits the detection of even a small, infantile uterus and reveals streak gonads. Ultrasensitive estrogen bioassays can confirm decreased ovarian function in girls with Turner syndrome because estradiol values are significantly lower than those found in average girls. Long-term follow-up of affected women previously treated with GH and estrogen demonstrated normal adult uterine length only in those with 45,X/46,XX karyotypes, whereas those with pure 45,X karyotypes had a smaller uterus length and volume.[684] The streak gonads result in sexual infantilism, but in about 10% of cases, puberty, menarche, and rarely, pregnancy may occur.[632] Women with some of the variants have been able to achieve fertility and deliver normal infants. Affected adults can undergo hormone replacement to prepare the uterus to receive a donated embryo and proceed to delivery. Unfortunately, some patients receiving a donated ovum have died because of dissection or rupture of the aorta, and caution should be used in recommending this technique.[685] Long-term regular follow-up of adults with Turner syndrome with echocardiography is recommended.

Intrauterine growth retardation with a mean deficit in birth length of 2.6 cm (−1.24 SD) and a slow childhood growth rate result in a loss of about 8 to 9 cm (−3.0 SD) by age 3 years in girls with Turner syndrome.[686] A major portion of the height deficit occurs during the first 3 years of life. Decreased growth rate occurs at the time of expected puberty, and the pubertal growth spurt is absent in those without pubertal development. Subjects who undergo spontaneous puberty have decreased growth in the first year after birth and another decrease at 7 to 8 years. This may reflect a suppressive effect of estrogen on growth in those retaining some ovarian function.[687] Untreated individuals with Turner syndrome in the United Kingdom and United States have a mean final height of approximately 142 to 143 cm, which is about 20 cm less than the average height of normal women; the adult stature of these patients correlates with midparental height and with the height of unaffected women of the same ethnic group. Haploinsufficiency of the *SHOX* gene is estimated to contribute two thirds of the height deficit. It is postulated that a second gene on the short arm of the X chromosome that does not undergo X-chromosome inactivation contributes the other one third of the deficit. In girls with Turner syndrome with spontaneous puberty, pubertal height velocity was transiently higher than in girls with amenorrhea, but adult height was not different.[632] Specific growth curves are available for plotting the growth of affected children.[688]

GH treatment is approved by the FDA for Turner syndrome to increase height. The addition of estrogen therapy at low doses has exerted no effect on adult height or actually reduced the adult height obtained with GH therapy administered alone. The length of GH exposure before estrogen treatment was the major determinant of whether GH and estrogen treatment increased final height.[689,690] With an early age of initiation of GH therapy, low-dose estrogen can be introduced at an appropriate age (about age 13) without compromising adult height. However, if GH is started early enough (e.g., 2 to 8 years old), estrogen therapy may be added at an age (about 13 years) appropriate for the institution of puberty.[670] Percutaneous estrogen may be more beneficial than oral estrogen therapy. An adult height of 149 to 155 cm was achieved compared with an untreated control group, which reached a height of 142 cm even if estrogen administration started at the normal age of puberty or GH administration was started at a later age.[691] The average height gain in various studies has varied from 4 to 16 cm, and a systematic review of the literature shows a 5-cm gain to be the most likely outcome.[692] This variability in gain in height is incompletely understood, but many factors have been implicated, including the age of initiation of therapy, dose duration, age (especially number of years from beginning hGH treatment) at beginning estrogen replacement, number of injections per week, compliance, and whether the last measured height represented the final height. Early initiation of hGH therapy (e.g., 2 to 8 years of age) and a mean duration of treatment of about 7 years can lead most treated Turner patients to achieve an adult height greater than 150 cm; a Dutch study reported the mean adult height was 162.3 ± 6.1 cm.[693] Evaluation of bone density is technique specific, but GH treatment of Turner syndrome for at least 1 year showed no difference in volumetric BMD, although lean body mass was higher and fat mass was lower than in the controls.[694] GH treatment of Turner patients has been safe, and untoward events are uncommon.[692] There is some degree of improvement of the abnormal body proportions of Turner syndrome with hGH treatment, but the disproportionate growth of the foot may dissuade some girls from continuing treatment to maximal benefit on height. Five-year follow-up of young adults with Turner syndrome demonstrated continued beneficial effects of GH on blood pressure, lipid levels, and increased adult height.[695,696]

A nationwide survey of 632 Danish girls with Turner syndrome demonstrated an increased prevalence of fractures, mainly in the forearm, compared with controls. The prevalence was higher still in the absence of ovarian function and in girls with family history of fractures and presumed familial disorders of bone density.[697] It appears that estrogen therapy is critical for the prevention and repair of osteoporosis, but for adolescents and adults, the optimal dose preparation and site of delivery for the prevention of osteoporosis is not known.

About 50% of patients with Turner syndrome have a tendency toward impaired glucose tolerance without GH treatment; in some, this may be caused by associated obesity, and risk of type 2 diabetes mellitus is increased. Although glucose values do not change with GH therapy, insulin levels reversibly rise during treatment, indicating an additional degree of insulin resistance caused by the GH.[698] Turner syndrome patients as young as 11 years can already have elevated serum cholesterol concentrations before treatment with GH or estrogen. The biphasic pattern of gonadotropin secretion in normal infancy and childhood is exaggerated in Turner syndrome (see Fig. 25-22).[386,387]

The appearance of pubic hair (i.e., pubarche) is often delayed in the syndrome of gonadal dysgenesis, even though adrenarche, as assessed by the increase in concentration of plasma DHEAS, occurs at the normal age.[442] Girls with ovarian failure demonstrate early adrenarche, and therefore higher serum values of DHEAS but later pubarche, whereas those who demonstrate at least beginning breast development follow a course of adrenarche similar to that of unaffected girls.[699] This suggests that ovarian function is necessary to convert DHEA to the active androgens responsible for the appearance of pubic hair in normal girls. The pubic hair of affected individuals is sparse, but estrogen therapy increases the growth of pubic hair despite a lack of increase in adrenal androgen secretion, and estrogen affects pubic hair appearance.[700]

Behavior and Development of Turner Syndrome. Counseling and a peer support group are exceedingly important components of long-term management. Girls with Turner syndrome younger than 6 years did not perceive that they had a problem with height, but by 7 to 12 years and especially by 13 to 15 years, affected Turner girls have a strong desire for GH therapy and even unrealistic expectations of what GH therapy can accomplish in terms of adult height. GH therapy improved self-esteem even if there remained a significant difference in height between Turner girls and the normal range. Height gained with GH therapy did not affect quality of life, although cardiac defects and otologic complications did.[701] Girls who have discontinued GH therapy after reaching adult height showed no evidence of depression but still had remaining problems with self-perception and bodily attitude despite significant height gains.[702] Psychological problems in Turner syndrome are not necessarily diminished with GH treatment and an increase in adult height.

Turner syndrome girls resemble normal girls in verbal and language skills, and IQ is normal when verbal ability, including comprehension and vocabulary, are considered, but visual-constructional or visual-perceptual spatiotemporal processing, visuomotor coordination, and mathematical ability (particularly in geometry) may be impaired, leading to a decrease in the performance of IQ tests due to mistakes on operation and alignment processes. Girls with 45,X mosaicism associated with a 46,XX cell line, 45,X/46,XX, scored closer to normal than those with other types of mosaicisms. Only 3.3% of girls with Turner syndrome have developmental delay in the absence of a variant of Turner syndrome caused by a ring X chromosome. It is useful to monitor the patient's progress in high school mathematics. There are consistent MRI abnormalities in the right parietal lobe and the occipital lobes, and decreased volumes in these areas are implicated in defects in visual-spatial processing. Using positron emission tomography, decreased glucose metabolism is found in the right parietal and occipital lobes.[703] These anatomic data relate to the difficulties in visual-spatial skills found in most studies of girls with Turner syndrome, because these problems are most closely linked to the right parietal region.

There is an increased risk of impaired social adjustment in Turner syndrome. Those with the 45,X pattern demonstrate a significant decrease in social competence scores; have an increase in total behavior problems; have increased attention problems, with difficulty in schooling, peer relationships, and concentration; and exhibit immaturity, hyperactivity, nervousness, and withdrawn behaviors. Structural abnormalities of the X chromosome were associated with more behavior problems than a missing X chromosome or mosaicism of the X chromosomes. Mental retardation and a severe phenotype are associated with small ring X chromosomes that undergo X inactivation, resulting in X chromosome disomy for genes that are affected by X inactivation. The 45,X individuals in whom the X is of paternal origin (X^p) show better adjustment and social cognition as a group than X^m individuals. Documented mental health problems may be rooted in the increased peer ridicule experienced by girls with Turner syndrome rather than a biologic abnormality.[704]

Transition of girls with Turner syndrome to adult care is best carried out by an experienced team, which is ideally composed of an endocrinologist; cardiologist; nephrologist; reproductive endocrinologist; audiologic physician; ear, nose, and throat surgeon; plastic surgeon; dentist; and psychologist because of the multiplicity of complications that affected individuals may encounter in the areas of growth failure, cardiovascular disease, gonadal failure, and learning disabilities.[705]

Sex Chromatin–Positive Variants of the Syndrome of Gonadal Dysgenesis. Mosaicism of 45,X/46,XX; 45,X/47,XXX; or 45,X/46,XX/47,XXX chromosomes is associated with a chromatin-positive buccal smear and usually with fewer manifestations of the syndrome of gonadal dysgenesis. Likewise, structural abnormalities of the X chromosome can be associated with fewer phenotypic features of the syndrome. Lack of genetic material on the long or the short arm of the second X chromosome can cause decreased gonadal function; loss of all or part of the short arm of the X leads to the physical findings of Turner syndrome.[632] Depending on the location and extent of the deletion on the short arm of the X chromosome, these patients may be more likely to have modest pubertal growth and some spontaneous pubertal development.

Sex Chromatin–Negative Variants of Gonadal Dysgenesis. These variants include 45,X/46,XY mosaicism and structural abnormalities of the Y chromosome. Affected individuals have phenotypes that vary from that of classic gonadal dysgenesis to that of ambiguous genitalia to phenotypic males.[632] Patients may present with short stature, delayed puberty, and a history of hypospadias repair. There is variable testicular differentiation, ranging from a streak gonad to functioning testes. Patients with mosaicism involving a Y cell line or abnormalities of the Y chromosome are at risk for neoplastic transformation of the dysgenetic testes. Gonadoblastomas, which are benign, nonmetastasizing tumors, may arise within the gonad and produce testosterone or estrogens. The neoplasm may become calcified sufficiently to be detected on an abdominal radiograph. The appearance of feminization or virilization in a patient with dysgenetic gonads and a Y cell line may indicate gonadoblastoma formation. Of greater significance is the increased prevalence of malignant germ cell tumors, arising within the dysgenetic gonad or gonadoblastoma. Examples are dysgerminomas, mature teratomas, and testicular intraepithelial neoplasia.[706] These tumors occur more often in postpubertal subjects and rarely in children.[632]

46,XX and 46,XY Gonadal Dysgenesis. The term *pure gonadal dysgenesis* refers to phenotypic females with sexual infantilism and a 46,XX or 46,XY karyotype without chromosomal abnormalities.[632]

Familial and Sporadic 46,XX Gonadal Dysgenesis and Its Variants. The usual phenotype of 46,XX gonadal dysgenesis includes normal stature, sexual infantilism, bilateral streak gonad, normal female internal and external genitalia, and primary amenorrhea. The streak gonad occasionally produces estrogens or androgens, but malignant transformation is rare. Incomplete forms of this condition may result in hypoplastic ovaries that produce enough estrogen to cause some breast development and a few menstrual periods, followed by secondary amenorrhea. This heterogeneous syndrome occurs sporadically or with autosomal recessive inheritance, and in some instances, it is associated with other congenital malformations. Some familial cases have been associated with sensorineural deafness (i.e., Perrault syndrome).[632]

Familial and Sporadic 46,XY Gonadal Dysgenesis and Its Variants. A phenotype that includes female genitalia with or without clitoral enlargement, normal or tall stature, bilateral streak gonads, normal müllerian structures, sexual infantilism, and a eunuchoid habitus is typical of 46,XY gonadal dysgenesis. About 15% of the patients have a deletion or mutation in the *SRY* gene. If the dysgenetic testes produce significant amounts of testosterone, slight clitoral enlargement may occur at birth, and virilization may ensue at puberty. The incomplete form of 46,XY gonadal dysgenesis may involve any degree of ambiguity of the external genitalia and internal ducts. The risk of neoplastic transformation of the streak gonads or dysgenetic testes is increased, and gonadectomy is indicated. The disorder is usually transmitted as an X-linked or sex-limited autosomal dominant trait or less commonly as an autosomal recessive trait.[632]

Other Causes of Primary Ovarian Failure. The prevalence of primary ovarian failure is increasing as a consequence of the long-term effects of cytotoxic chemotherapy and radiation therapy as these agents prolong the lives of children and adolescents with cancer..[645] The same pattern occurs for males with testes that have been treated with these modalities.

Radiation Therapy. Radiation therapy that includes the ovaries within the field can cause primary ovarian failure. It is useful to surgically move the ovaries out of the radiation field if they are not the target of therapy, thereby greatly decreasing the dose of radiation to them. Ovarian transposition before radiation therapy is compatible with normal menses, pubertal development, and pregnancy in most cases. The uterus may be affected by radiation and may not expand normally during pregnancy.

Chemotherapy. Successful treatment of childhood acute lymphoblastic leukemia has become commonplace. In a large study by Quigley and colleagues, boys and girls after cytotoxic chemotherapy had extensive germ cell damage, as evidenced by increased FSH secretion, and boys had decreased testicular size for the stage of puberty. The concentration of plasma inhibin B is usually decreased, providing a sensitive indicator of damage to the germinal epithelium. Many of the girls at puberty had evidence of a compensated decrease in ovarian follicular function. Quite likely as a result of cranial irradiation, the mean age of menarche was advanced about 12 months despite the ovarian damage; puberty was not advanced in the boys. The type of chemotherapy determines the effects on the gonads. The ovary is less vulnerable to the effects of irradiation and chemotherapy than the testis. The prevalence of ovarian damage does not appear to be high, because fertility and regular menses are reported in most females treated as children.[707] Nevertheless, age at treatment has a significant role. Treatment between 13 and 19 years was associated with a more than twofold increase in premature ovarian failure during the third decade. Attempts to protect the gonads by suppressing the pituitary-gonadal axis with gonadal steroids or GnRH agonists are probably ineffective.[708] Careful endocrine follow-up of children and adolescents treated with chemotherapy or radiation therapy is essential.

Autoimmune Oophoritis. Premature menopause may occur at any age before the normal climacteric and has been reported in adolescent girls. Cessation of ovarian function usually manifests as secondary amenorrhea.[709] Autoimmune oophoritis can cause ovarian failure leading to primary amenorrhea, oligomenorrhea, arrest of puberty, and occasionally cystic enlargement of the ovaries. Most often, it is associated with other autoimmune endocrinopathies, especially autoimmune Addison's disease, in which it may precede the onset of adrenal insufficiency, but it rarely occurs in isolated premature ovarian failure. Glucocorticoid therapy may improve, at least temporarily, ovarian function.

Type I autoimmune polyglandular insufficiency, also known as autoimmune polyendocrinopathy-candidiasis-ectodermal dystrophy (APECED), is a rare systemic autoimmune disorder with an array of clinical features, including hypoparathyroidism, adrenal insufficiency, gonadal failure, diabetes mellitus, pernicious anemia, hypothyroidism, chronic hepatitis, mucocutaneous candidiasis, dystrophic nail hypoplasia, vitiligo, alopecia, keratinopathy, and intestinal malabsorption. Thirty-six percent of women with APECED exhibited ovarian failure before age 20, whereas only 4% of affected men had testicular failure by that age. This autosomal recessive disorder is caused by more than 42 mutations in the *CDK14* (AIRE-1) gene at gene map locus 21q22.3. A study of genotype and phenotype correlations demonstrated a higher prevalence of candidiasis in the patients with the most common mutation, R257X, although HLA class II is a significant determinant.[710] This contrasts with earlier studies, which suggested a phenotype-genotype correlation for other features.

Autoimmune oophoritis occurs in more than 20% of patients with autoimmune adrenal insufficiency. Various autoantibodies have been detected in autoimmune oophoritis, including autoantibodies to cytochrome P450 steroidogenic enzymes; some are organ specific, whereas others react with antigens in more than one tissue and more than one cell type.

Homozygous Galactosemia. Homozygous galactosemia due to mutation in the galactose-1-phosphate uridylyltransferase gene *(GALT)* is commonly associated with primary ovarian failure, from failure to develop puberty to primary or secondary amenorrhea and premature menopause, but puberty is usually normal in males, and the risk of testicular dysfunction is low; compound heterozygotes have normal onset of puberty. Dietary restriction programs have not prevented the ovarian failure, nor are other means of avoiding ovarian failure effective. The pathogenesis of galactose-induced ovarian toxicity remains unclear but probably involves galactose itself and its metabolites, such as galactitol and UDP-galactose.[711] Most cases are detected by newborn screening programs.

Haploinsufficiency of the FOXL2 Gene. A rare autosomal dominant disorder involving eyelid dysplasia and premature ovarian failure is caused by haploinsufficiency of the *FOXL2* gene, a member of the winged helix/forkhead family of transcription factors.[712] The eyelid abnormalities include small palpebral fissures, ptosis, and a small skinfold extending inward and upward from the lower lid (i.e., epicanthus inversus). The gene is expressed in the follicular cells, and the mutations that lead to haploinsufficiency are associated with an increased rate of follicular atresia. The degree of ovarian failure varies from primary amenorrhea to irregular menses and premature ovarian failure, with ultrasound findings ranging from normal-appearing ovaries to streak gonads with an inconsistent number of primordial follicles found on ovarian biopsy.[713] The infertility component of the syndrome is limited to females. Animal studies provide insights into other genetic mutations that may cause premature ovarian failure in humans, including mutations of *BMP15*, *FMR1*, *POF1B*, and *FOXO3A*.[714]

Congential Disorders of Glycosylation-1: Carbohydrate-Deficient Glycoprotein Syndrome Type Ia. The congential disorders of glycosylation-1 (i.e., carbohydrate-deficient glycoprotein syndrome type Ia) include an autosomal recessive disorder associated with circulating glycoproteins deficient in their terminal carbohydrate moieties, including a wide range of glycoproteins, enzymes, binding proteins, and coagulation factors.[715] A typical isoform pattern of serum transferrin detected by isoelectric focusing is used as a diagnostic test. The dominant clinical feature is the neurologic manifestations of involvement of the central and peripheral nervous system. Among the other organ systems affected is the pituitary-gonadal system.

The hypergonadotropic-hypogonadism is more severe in females because males virilize at puberty. The ovary and the pituitary are affected. Affected girls have sexual infantilism; the ovaries are hypoplastic or atrophic. High serum FSH and LH levels exhibited normal electrophoretic isoform patterns, but they appeared to have decreased but not absent FSH bioactivity in an FSH bioassay. However, in the only three girls tested, a response to the administration of human menopausal gonadotropin was indicated by an increase in serum estradiol and, in one patient, by ovarian follicular growth. These observations suggest an abnormality in the FSH molecule and the ovary, which in the latter case was a defect in the configuration and activation of the FSH receptor itself and the binding of ligand, or a post-receptor defect.

Resistant Ovary. The resistant ovary is a heterogeneous cause of primary hypogonadism, a syndrome associated with elevated concentrations of plasma FSH and LH and ovaries that contain primordial follicles. The syndrome is usually idiopathic, but an increasing number of genetic abnormalities are described in addition to the more common X-chromosomal defects.[716]

Follicle-Stimulating Hormone Receptor Resistance: Gene Mutations and Hypergonadotropic Hypogonadism. The FSH receptor is a member of the G protein–linked receptor, seven-transmembrane superfamily. It has a large, extended extracellular ligand-binding domain.[323] An autosomal recessive disorder due to a mutation in the extracellular ligand-binding domain of the FSH receptor in affected females in six Finnish families mainly from the north central region[655] resulted in delayed (40%) or normal puberty but primary amenorrhea, elevated gonadotropin levels, and hypergonadotropic ovarian dysgenesis with arrest of ovarian follicular development at the primary follicle stage and continued atresia. The clinical features are very similar to the findings in FSH-deficient mice generated by targeted disruption of the gene encoding the FSH β-subunit. This disorder likely is responsible for most cases of the "resistant" ovary syndrome. The FSH receptor gene contains 9 small exons (1 through 9) that encode the extracellular ligand-binding domain and one large exon[10] that designates the remainder of the receptor, including the seven-transmembrane and intracellular domains. The Finnish mutation, an Ala1989Val substitution, is in the extracellular domain. Expression of the mutation in transfected cells indicated a small FSH effect on cAMP production, a striking reduction of FSH-binding capacity, but apparently normal binding affinity.

The FSH receptor mutation in the Finnish patients is not a null mutation. It remains to be determined whether the loss or complete inactivation of the FSH receptor leads to failure of puberty and sexual infantilism or to estrogen synthesis by the immature ovarian follicles described in the FSH β-subunit knockout mouse. Affected males in these families are normally masculinized at puberty but tend to have small testes. They have a variable degree of spermatogenic insufficiency, but not azoospermia, increased plasma concentrations of FSH and LH, decreased inhibin B levels, and normal plasma testosterone values.[717]

Luteinizing Hormone and Human Chorionic Gonadotropin Resistance. LH/hCG resistance due to mutations in the gene encoding the seven-transmembrane LHCGR is discussed in Chapter 23. In the affected XY individual, this autosomal recessive disorder leads to various degrees of male pseudohermaphrodism; the mildest form is represented by an isolated micropenis.[718] Less severe mutations of the LHCGR may be associated with delayed puberty. In affected females, LH/hCG resistance does not affect pubertal maturation but does lead to amenorrhea with high serum LH levels but normal FSH and estradiol concentrations.[719]

Polycystic Ovary Syndrome. PCOS, or functional ovarian hyperandrogenism, does not delay the onset of puberty but often delays menarche or causes menstrual abnormalities. It can have serious long-term metabolic consequences such as dyslipidemia and insulin resistance over and above androgen excess and reproductive difficulties.[720]

Noonan Syndrome. Individuals with Noonan syndrome (i.e., pseudo-Turner syndrome, Ullrich syndrome) have webbed neck, ptosis, down-slanting palpebral fissures, low-set ears, short stature, cubitus valgus, and lymphedema, and which explains why this phenotype has been called pseudo-Turner syndrome.[632] Features that differentiate these individuals from those with Turner syndrome include triangular facies, pectus excavatum, right-sided heart disease (e.g., pulmonic stenosis, often with valve dysplasia; atrial septal defect) compared with the left-sided heart disease in Turner syndrome, hypertrophic cardiomyopathy, varied blood clotting defects, and an increased incidence of mental retardation. Females with Noonan syndrome have normal ovarian function. Males have normal differentiation of external genitalia but may have undescended testes; germinal aplasia or hypoplasia and impaired Leydig cell function may be present. Puberty may be delayed by an average of 2 years. Stature is decreased after normal birth length and weight, with a mean adult height of 162.5 cm (63.9 inches) for men and 152.7 cm (60.1 inches) for women, usually following the −2 SD curve. The pubertal growth spurt is often delayed or attenuated, but final height usually is at the low limits of normal.

Administration of hGH is approved by the FDA for use in Noonan syndrome. GH increased the growth rate, with a mean gain in near-adult height above the projected value of 10.9 cm (males) and 9.2 cm (females), which is less than in patients with GH deficiency.[721] Men with Noonan syndrome may have osteopenia, which has been attributed to estrogen deficiency because estrogen administration improves the decreased bone mineral content.[722]

Noonan syndrome is inherited as an autosomal dominant trait.[632] A gene implicated in Noonan syndrome has been localized to the long arm of chromosome 12 (12q24.2-q24.31), and a mutation in *PTPN11* was identified, but at least three other gene mutations have been identified. The incidence is estimated at 1 case in 1000 to 1 in 2500 people. One parent may have features of the syndrome in 40% to 60% of cases. About 50% of patients are thought to have new mutations.

Frasier Syndrome. Chronic renal failure is combined with gonadal dysgenesis in the Frasier syndrome. Although most patients present with ambiguous genitalia, this diagnosis should be considered for any phenotypic female with end-stage renal disease (due to focal segmental glomerulosclerosis) and sexual infantilism. The karyotype may be 46,XY or 46,XX.

Diagnosis of Delayed Puberty and Sexual Infantilism

When girls remain prepubertal at 13 years or boys remain prepubertal at 14 years, the physician must make a clinical judgment about who are variants of the norm and who require extensive evaluation and treatment (Figs. 25-47 and 25-48; Tables 25-20 and 25-21). A boy who has not completed secondary sexual maturation within 4.5 years after onset of puberty or a girl who does not menstruate within 5 years after onset may have a hypothalamic, pituitary, or gonadal disorder. The diagnosis of hypergonadotropic hypogonadism is readily established by elevation of random plasma LH and FSH concentrations. However, differentiating the diagnosis of hypogonadotropic hypogonadism from constitutional delay in growth and adolescence is more difficult because of the overlap in physical and laboratory findings for the two conditions, including an inability to differentiate normal from low concentrations of serum gonadotropins (see Table 25-21). Most boys with pubertal delay have a self-limited variant in the tempo of growth and pubertal-onset CDP.

History taking must elicit all symptoms of chronic or intermittent illnesses and all details pertaining to growth and development, as well as questioning about the patient's sense of smell. Has puberty failed to occur, or did it begin but failed to progress or even regressed? Disorders of pregnancy, abnormalities of labor and delivery, and birth trauma, if part of the patient's history, suggest that a congenital or neonatal event may be related to the delay in puberty. Poor linear growth and poor nutritional status during the neonatal period and childhood may reflect long-standing abnormalities of development. Family history may reveal disorders of puberty or infertility, anosmia, or hyposmia in relatives and delay in the age at onset of puberty in parents or siblings. Recalled age of pubertal onset is relatively reliable in women but less often accurate in men. A history of consanguinity is important in the detection of autosomal recessive disorders.

The physical examination starts with determination of height and weight. The upper-to-lower segment ratio or sitting height is calculated, and the arm span is measured and compared with the height. A growth chart is plotted to represent graphically the increase in stature and to assess growth velocity from birth (see Chapter 42). Late-onset growth failure usually indicates a serious condition requiring immediate evaluation. Weight is plotted to determine states of malnutrition. BMI should be calculated and plotted by age and gender in this era of epidemic obesity or to further determine nutritional status. The height velocity should be documented over a period of at least 6 months, preferably 12 months. The signs of puberty are assessed, and the stage of secondary sexual development is determined by physical examination according to the standards presented earlier (see Figs. 25-5, 26-6, and 25-8). Questionnaires with pictures are used to allow a child to determine his or her own stage of puberty in some studies but do not replace the physical examination, and there is a tendency to overestimate development early in puberty

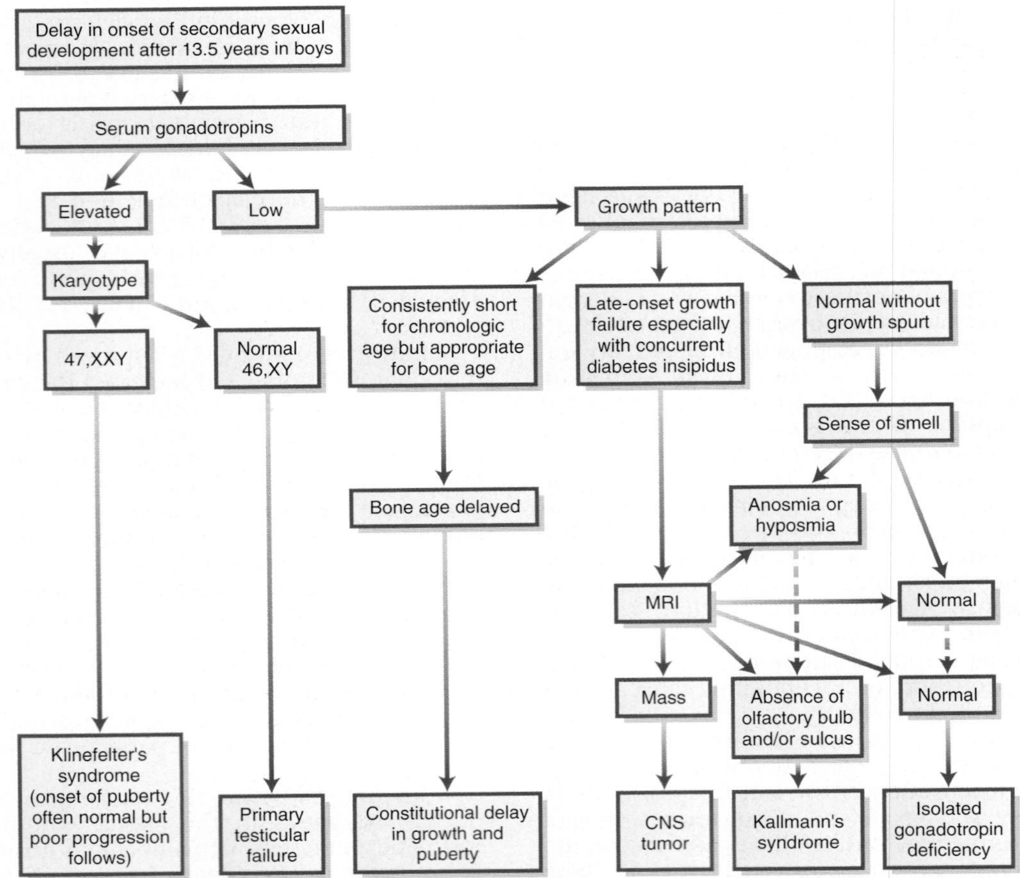

Figure 25-47 Flow chart for the evaluation of delayed puberty in boys.

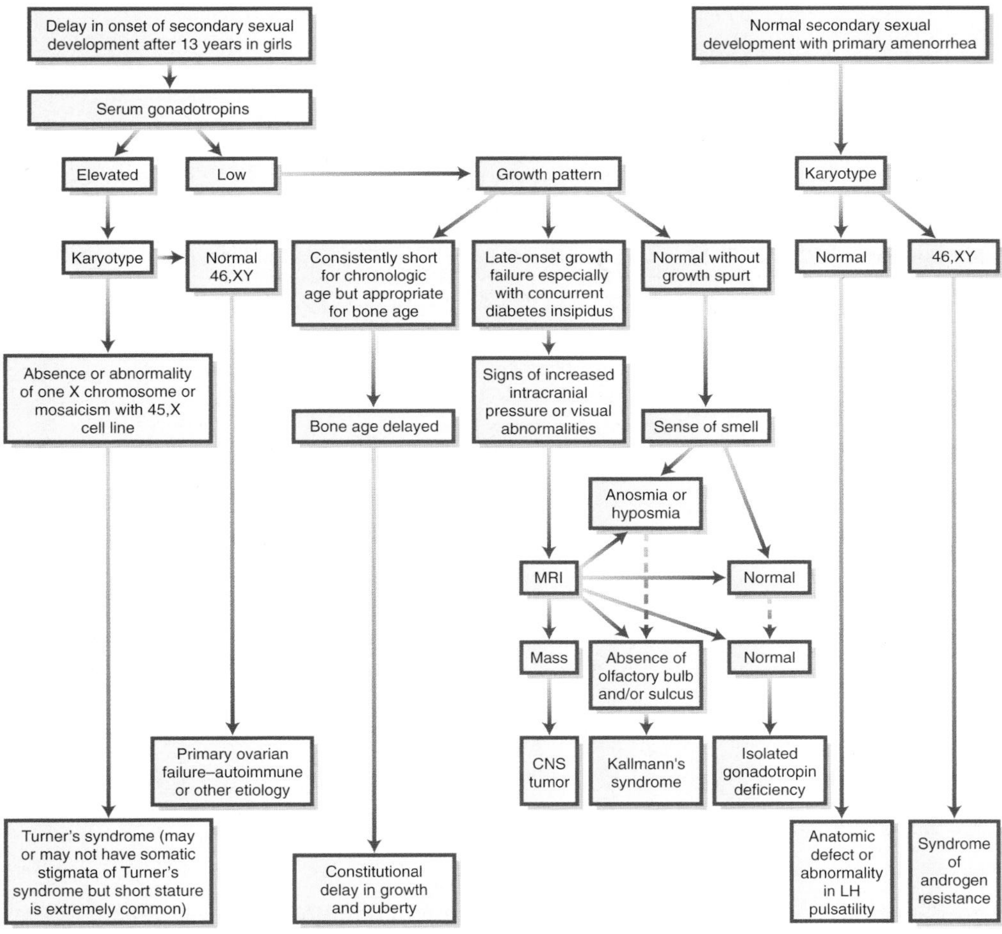

Figure 25-48 Flow chart for the evaluation of delayed puberty in girls.

and underestimate it late in puberty. The length and width of the testes is measured in boys, or the volume is assessed using an orchidometer. The length and diameter of the stretched penis are determined in boys, and the diameter of glandular breast tissue and areolar size are determined in girls. The presence or absence of galactorrhea is documented. Obese boys often appear to have a small penis because of excessive adipose tissue surrounding the phallus; only when the fat is retracted can the full extent of phallic development be assessed. This is among the most common causes of inappropriate referral for hypogonadism. The extent of pubic and axillary hair is assessed, as is the degree of acne or comedones. The possibility of cryptorchidism or retractile testes should be determined if no testes are palpated in the scrotum. Neurologic examination, including examination of the optic discs and visual fields by frontal confrontation perimetry, may reveal findings, suggesting the presence of a CNS neoplasm or a developmental defect. Determination of olfaction is important because many patients with Kallmann's syndrome wait years for the correct diagnosis to be made even in the presence of classic findings; physicians must remain alert to the possibility of this diagnosis. The stigmata of gonadal dysgenesis (i.e., Turner syndrome) or the small testes and gynecomastia of Klinefelter's syndrome may suggest a karyotypic abnormality. Complete physical examination, including the lungs, heart, kidney, and the gastrointestinal tract, is important in the search for a chronic disorder that may delay puberty.

Laboratory studies (Table 25-22) include determination of plasma LH and FSH concentrations by sensitive third-generation assays in pediatric endocrine laboratories, measurement of the rise in the LH level after GnRH or GnRH agonist administration, determination of testosterone concentrations in boys and estradiol levels in girls in pediatric endocrine laboratories using HPLC-MS/MS, all with pediatric standards for that laboratory, and measurements of T_4 and prolactin concentrations in boys and girls if the clinical features warrant. One of the few national endocrine laboratories should be used for determinations of the hormones of puberty, because most local laboratories are interested only in differentiating the normally higher adult values from inappropriately low levels, and they cannot determine the gradations of the low levels found in puberty. Results of commercial immunochemiluminometric (ICMA) LH and FSH assays are reported to be more sensitive for use in pediatrics than immunofluorometric (IFMA) assays.[723] Several national laboratories began using liquid chromatography with tandem mass spectrometry methods for improved sensitivity and specificity and determinations in children (and women) for increased accuracy.[247] Newer ultrasensitive bioassays may be made available commercially for the determination of low values of testosterone and estradiol or for total androgen or estrogen.

Radiographic examination may include bone age determination and, if the history or physical examination is consistent with a CNS lesion, an MRI of the brain, with

TABLE 25-20

Differential Diagnostic Features of Delayed Puberty and Sexual Infantilism

Condition	Stature	Plasma Gonadotropins	GnRH Test LH Response	Plasma Gonadal Steroids	Plasma DHEAS	Karyotype	Olfaction
Constitutional delay in growth and adolescence	Short for chron. age, usually appropriate for bone age	Prepubertal, later pubertal	Prepubertal, later pubertal	Low, later normal	Low for chron. age, appropriate for bone age	Normal	Normal
Hypogonadotropic Hypogonadism							
Isolated gonadotropin deficiency	Normal, absent pubertal growth spurt	Low	Prepubertal or no response	Low	Appropriate for chron. age	Normal	Normal
Kallmann's syndrome	Normal, absent	Low	Prepubertal or no response	Low	Appropriate for chron. age	Normal	Anosmia; pubertal growth spurt or hyposmia
Idiopathic multiple pituitary hormone deficiencies	Short stature and poor growth since early childhood	Low	Prepubertal or no response	Low	Usually low	Normal	Normal
Hypothalamic-pituitary tumors	Late-onset decrease in growth velocity	Low	Prepubertal or no response	Low	Normal or low for chron. age	Normal	Normal
Primary Gonadal Failure							
Syndrome of gonadal dysgenesis (Turner's syndrome) and variants	Short stature since childhood	High	Hyperresponse for age	Low	Normal for chron. age	45,X or variant	Normal
Klinefelter's syndrome and variants	Normal to tall	High	Hyperresponse at puberty	Low or normal	Normal for chron. age	47,XXY or variant	Normal
Familial XX or XY gonadal dysgenesis	Normal for age	High	Hyperresponse	Low	Normal for chron. age	46,XX or46,XY	Normal

chron., chronologic; DHEAS, dehydroepiandrosterone sulfate; GnRH, gonadotropin-releasing hormone; LH, luteinizing hormone.

specific attention to the pituitary and hypothalamic area using contrast. CT can detect calcification, in contrast to MRI scans or plain radiographs, in most cases. Ultrasound evaluation of the uterus and ovaries provides useful information about the state of development of these structures but only if the uiltrasonographer has experience with children and young adolescents.

Assessment of karyotype should be considered for all short girls, even in the absence of somatic signs of Turner syndrome and especially if puberty is delayed or unexplained short stature is involved. Karyotype assessment should be performed for boys with suspected Klinefelter's syndrome stigmata or behavior.

A presumptive diagnosis of constitutional delay in growth and adolescence is made if the history and growth chart reveal a history of short stature but a consistent growth rate for skeletal age (and no signs or symptoms of hypothalamic lesions), if the family history includes parents or siblings with delayed puberty, if the physical examination (including assessment of the olfactory threshold) is normal, if optic discs and visual fields are normal, and if the bone age is significantly delayed. In classic cases, MRI of the hypothalamic-pituitary region may not be necessary. The rate of growth in these patients is usually appropriate for bone age; a decrease in growth velocity occurs in some normal children just before the appearance of secondary sexual characteristics and may awaken concerns if such a pattern occurs in these subjects. The onset at puberty correlates better with bone age than with chronologic age, although bone age is not any better at estimating the onset of puberty in normal boys than is chronologic age.[156]

TABLE 25-21

Endocrine Diagnosis of Constitutional Delayed Adolescence and Hypogonadotropic Hypogonadism

No single test reliably discriminates between the two diagnoses.
Onset of puberty in boys is indicated by
- Testes >2.5 cm in diameter
- Serum testosterone concentration >50 ng/dL
- Pubertal LH response to GnRH bolus
- Pubertal pattern of LH pulsatility

LH, luteinizing hormone; GnRH, LH-releasing hormone.

TABLE 25-22

Endocrine and Imaging Studies in Delayed Adolescence

Initial assessment
- Plasma testosterone or estradiol
- Plasma FSH and LH
- Plasma thyroxine (and prolactin)
- Bone age and lateral skull roentgenograph
- Test of olfaction

Follow-up studies
- Karyotype (short, phenotypic females)
- MRI with contrast enhancement
- Pelvic ultrasonography (females)
- GnRH test
- hCG test (males)
- Pattern of pulsatile LH secretion
- Visual acuity and visual fields

FSH, follicle-stimulating hormone; hCG, human chorionic gonadotropin; LH, luteinizing hormone; MRI, magnetic resonance imaging.

Elevated concentrations of gonadotropins and gonadal steroids to early pubertal levels precede secondary sexual development by several months; measurements of serum LH, FSH, estradiol, or testosterone levels in appropriate assays may help to predict future development. The third-generation LH assays are sufficiently sensitive to allow in most boys the determination of the onset of endocrine puberty with a single blood sample, but a dynamic GnRH test is still often performed using GnRH agonists. The use of 10 μg of GnRH instead of 100 μg can differentiate constitutional delay from hypogonadotropic hypogonadism, but the virtual absence of synthetic native GnRH supplies means that this is not practical for clinical use.[724] The measurement of gonadotropins 40 minutes to 1 hour after a subcutaneous injection of GnRH agonist is the current method of testing dynamic secretion of gonadotropins in the absence of native GnRH supplies.

Measurement of an 8 a.m. serum testosterone level provides an accurate indication of impending pubertal development; a value of greater than 0.7 nmol/L (20 ng/dL) predicts enlargement of testes to greater than 4 mL by 12 months in 77% of cases and in 15 months in 100% of cases, whereas of those with a value less than 0.7 nmol/L, only 12% entered puberty in 12 months and only 25% entered puberty in 15 months. This technique may help predict spontaneous pubertal development, but it still requires considerable watching and waiting.[464] A 5-year longitudinal study of boys with delay of pubertal onset aimed to determine indicators of CDP and those of hypogonadal hypogonadism.[725] An initial basal morning testosterone level of more than 1.7 nmol/L was observed in 55% of patients with constitutional delay exclusively (predictive positive value [PPV] = 100%; predictive negative value [PNV] = 59%). For those with a basal morning testosterone level of less than 1.7 nmol/L, a measurement of the LH peak 3 hours after the GnRH agonist Triptorelin had a PPV of 100% if the upper threshold was set at 14 IU/L, and the PNV was 72%. Because no lower threshold could discriminate hypogonadotropic hypogonadism from constitutional delay if the LH peak 3 hours after Triptorelin was <14 IU/L, hCG stimulation was invoked. In constitutional delay, the PPV of a serum testosterone increment of more than 9 nmol/L (PNV = 72%) after hCG stimulation was 100%, and in isolated hypogonadal hypogonadism patients, the PPV of a rise in testosterone of less than 3 nmol/l (PNV = 82%) after hCG was 100%. However, 29% of the studied population had an increase in testosterone levels after hCG between these thresholds and could not be classified by testing alone, limiting the use of these techniques. Another study suggests that a ratio of peak to basal free α-gonadotropin subunit after GnRH ranging from more than 3.7 to 4.8 can differentiate constitutional delay from hypogonadotropic hypogonadism.[726] These methods require continued evaluation before they become standard clinically, and there does not appear to be a practical and reliable endocrine test for indisputably differentiating constitutional delay in growth and adolescence from hypogonadotropic hypogonadism. Watchful waiting remains the procedure of choice when a patient does not fulfill the delineated criteria and fall into a diagnosable grouping.

A typical patient with isolated gonadotropin deficiency is of average height for age and has eunuchoid proportions; has low plasma concentrations of gonadal steroids, LH, and FSH; and has no increase or a blunted response of LH after GnRH or GnRH agonist administration. The amplitude and usually the frequency of LH pulses are decreased when serial blood samples are studied over a 24-hour period. In some forms of Kallmann's syndrome, the sense of smell is absent or impaired. However, as stated, differentiation of isolated gonadotropin deficiency in the absence of hyposmia or anosmia from CDP may be difficult at initial study. Gonadotropin-deficient patients may be as short as those with constitutional delay in growth and adolescence, and concentrations of LH and FSH in hypogonadotropic hypogonadism may be indistinguishable from those of normal prepubertal children or children with constitutional delay. Sometimes, years of observation are necessary to detect the appearance of spontaneous and progressive signs of secondary sexual development or to document rising concentrations of gonadotropins or gonadal steroids before the diagnosis is clear. There is a tendency for hypogonadotropic patients to undergo adrenarche at a normal age and to have higher DHEAS concentrations than those with constitutional delay in growth, and this pattern is helpful in making the differential diagnosis.[442] In most cases, absence of the first signs of sexual maturation or failure of a rise in gonadotropins or gonadal steroid levels by age 18 years in the presence of a normal concentration of serum DHEAS for chronologic age supports the diagnosis of isolated gonadotropin deficiency.

Patients with deficiency of gonadotropins combined with deficiency of other pituitary hormones require careful evaluation for a CNS neoplasm. Visual field or optic disc abnormalities support the diagnosis of CNS tumor; even if these tests are normal, cranial MRI should be done to evaluate the pituitary gland and stalk and the hypothalamic region. MRI appears superior to CT for detecting mass lesions and developmental abnormalities of the hypothalamic-pituitary region.

Treatment of Delayed Puberty and Sexual Infantilism

Patients with constitutional delay in growth and adolescence ultimately have spontaneous onset and progression through puberty. Often, reassurance and continued observation to ensure that the expected sexual maturation occurs are sufficient. However, the stigma of appearing less mature than one's peers can cause psychological stress. These individuals may be unable to participate in the dating activities their friends are starting; smaller size may lead them to avoid participation in athletics; immature appearance may lead to ridicule, especially in the locker room; and schoolwork may suffer because of their poor self-image. Some children feel such intense peer pressure and low self-esteem that only the appearance of signs of puberty can reassure them and enable them to participate in sports and social activities with their peers. Poor self-image in late-maturing boys may carry into adulthood, even after normal puberty ensues. Growth retardation appears more often responsible for most of the stress rather than the delay in pubertal development itself.

For psychological reasons, for boys 14 years old or older who show no signs of puberty, a 3- to 6-month course of testosterone enanthate, cypionate, or cyclopropionate (50 mg is the safest starting dose, but some suggest up to 100 mg given intramuscularly every 4 weeks) may be helpful. Because starting with the higher dose of 100 mg can lead to priapism in treatment-naïve boys, care, lower dosage, and short-acting preparations are advisable. Decades of experience confirm no effect on adult height of low dosages in the short term.[727,728] The low dose of testosterone enanthate is considered to be safe but can raise apolipoprotein B (apoB) and decrease HDL-cholesterol and apoAI levels (estradiol increases HDL-cholesterol and decreases triglycerides, LDL-cholesterol, and apoB).[204]

Although the use of exogenous androgens may improve self-image and start the secondary sexual changes of puberty, low-dose androgen use does not improve final height.

Alkylated testosterone preparations should be avoided because of the risk of peliosis hepatitis (i.e., hemorrhagic liver cysts), which is not related to dose or duration of treatment. Although regression is possible with discontinuation of testosterone treatment, progression to liver failure can occur.

A course of low-dose oxandrolone (2.5 mg/day orally) is sometimes used as an oral alternative to intramuscular testosterone enanthate; this agent increases growth through androgenic effects reflected by suppression of LH and FSH but does not stimulate GH secretion, because it is not aromatized to estrogen. The temporary increase in growth velocity found with oxandrolone does not affect adult height in most studies. Oral treatment with 2.5 mg of fluoxymesterone (Halotestin) for 6 to 60 months allows increased pubertal development without adverse effect on adult height, although the necessity to take a daily dose may decrease compliance. Testosterone undecanoate at 40 mg/day is likewise an effective but expensive treatment for those opting for an oral therapy (not FDA approved for this use). This treatment can increase the growth rate but does not result in a change in LH pulsatility; mean overnight LH, testosterone, or SHBG levels; or free androgen index, PSA, and testicular volume values. Transdermal testosterone may be applied as a daily patch or a gel (not FDA approved for this use), although experience with these forms of androgen is more limited than with the other forms. Preliminary experience suggests that overnight (about 8 to 9 hours) or every-other-night use of a 2.5-mg Androderm patch can achieve physiologic testosterone levels, produce lower SHBG levels, promote growth and virilization, and increase BMD in hypogonadal teenagers without significant side effects. An overnight study of transdermal testosterone (5 mg of Virormone) applied overnight (8 to 12 hours) for 4-week periods in boys with delayed puberty and short stature raised salivary testosterone levels, stimulated leg growth measured by knemometry (i.e., sensitive short-term measurements of leg growth), and stimulated bone turnover, as reflected by increased serum alkaline phosphatase levels.[729] Testosterone cream is approved for adults and is undergoing clinical trials for use in teenagers with delayed puberty.

For girls 13 years of age or older, a 3- to 4-month course of ethinyl estradiol (5 μg/day orally) or conjugated estrogens (0.3 mg/day orally) may be used to initiate maturation of the secondary sexual characteristics without unduly advancing bone age or limiting final height. Transdermal estrogen has been used in clinical trials for decades in the treatment of delayed puberty or hypogonadism with beneficial results on physical development and bone density and is entering widespread use.[730] However, there is new support for such therapy based on understanding the adverse effects of oral estrogen that enters the portal circulation initially at a high dose (first pass) and stimulates the production of proteins such as C reactive protein, angiotensin precursor, and activated protein C, which are involved in cardiac complications. This contrasts with dermal estrogen, which is administered in lower dosages and reaches its therapeutic targets relatively unchanged and in lower, more physiologic concentrations; there is no change in the listed proteins with dermal estrogen administration.[731] Estrogen patches are undergoing clinical testing for use in initiating or promoting pubertal development in hypogonadal or delayed pubertal girls.

The long-term safety and effects on bone density of aromatase inhibitor therapy remains unknown, and this therapy cannot be recommended for routine use for increasing adult height. GnRH agonists cannot be recommended to prolong growth due to concerns about bone density.

If during the 3 to 6 months after discontinuing gonadal steroid therapy spontaneous puberty does not ensue or the concentrations of plasma gonadotropins and plasma testosterone in boys or plasma estradiol in girls do not increase, the treatment may be repeated. Only one or two courses of therapy usually are necessary. When treatment is discontinued after bone age has advanced, for example, to 12 to 13 years in girls or 13 or 14 years in boys, patients with constitutional delay usually continue pubertal development on their own, whereas those with gonadotropin deficiency do not progress and may regress.

Functional hypogonadotropic hypogonadism associated with chronic disease is treated by alleviating the underlying problem. Delayed puberty in this situation is usually a result of inadequate nutrition and low weight or excessive energy expenditure. When weight returns to normal values, puberty usually occurs spontaneously. Treatment with T_4 allows normal pubertal development in hypothyroid patients with delayed puberty.

Permanent hypogonadism of any cause leads to lifelong therapy. The transition of care from the range of age normally considered to be adolescence, administered by a pediatric practitioner, to adult life, administered by a practitioner experienced in adult endocrinology, presents important implications for a change in the manner medical care is presented. Changes in the individual's autonomy and implications of legal distinctions arise, and some have suggested that this transition period should be considered another stage of the life span.[732]

Congenital or acquired gonadotropin deficiency as a result of a lesion or surgery requires replacement therapy with gonadal steroids at an age approximating the normal age of onset of puberty (Tables 25-23 and 25-24). An exception may occur when GH deficiency coexists with gonadotropin deficiency; if bone age advancement and epiphyseal

TABLE 25-23

Management and Treatment of Delayed Puberty

OBJECTIVE
Determine site and etiology of abnormality Induce and maintain secondary sexual characteristics Induce pubertal growth spurt Prevent the potential short-term and long-term psychological, personality, and social handicaps of delayed puberty Ensure normal libido and potency Attain fertility
THERAPY
Concerned But Not Anxious or Socially Handicapped Adolescent
Reassurance and follow-up (tincture of time) Repeat evaluation (including serum testosterone or estradiol) in 6 mo
Psychosocial Handicaps, Anxiety, Highly Concerned
Therapy for 4 mo *Boys:* testosterone enanthate 100 mg IM q4wk at 14-14.5 yr of age, or overnight transdermal testosterone patch *Girls:* ethinyl estradiol 5-10 mg/day PO or conjugated estrogens 0.3 mg/day PO or overnight ethinyl estradiol patch at 13 yr of age No therapy for 4-6 mo; reevaluate status including serum testosterone or estradiol; if indicated repeat treatment regimen

TABLE 25-24

Hormonal Substitution Therapy in Hypogonadism

Boys

Goal: to approximate normal adolescent development *when diagnosis is established*
Initial therapy: at 13 yr of age, testosterone enanthate (or other long-acting testosterone ester) 50 mg IM every month for about 9 mo (6-12 mo)
Over the next 3-4 yr: gradually increase dose to adult replacement dose of 200 mg q2-3 wk
Testosterone gel is coming into widespread use as discussed in the text
Begin *replacement therapy in boys with suspected hypogonadotropic hypogonadism* by bone age ≤14 yr
To induce fertility at appropriate time in hypogonadotropic hypogonadism: pulsatile GnRH or FSH and hCG therapy

Girls

With a firmly established diagnosis of hypogonadism (e.g., girls with 45,X gonadal dysgenesis), begin hormonal substitution therapy at 12-13 yr of age
Goal: to approximate normal adolescent development
Initial therapy: ethinyl estradiol 5 mg by mouth or conjugated estrogen 0.3 mg (or less) by mouth daily for 4-6 mo or preferably estradiol transdermally
After 6 mo of therapy (or sooner if breakthrough bleeding occurs), begin cyclic therapy:
Estrogen: first 21 days of month
Progestagen: (e.g., medroxyprogesterone acetate 5 mg PO) 12th to 21st day of month
Gradually increase dose of estrogen over next 2-3 yr to conjugated estrogen 0.6-1.25 mg or ethinyl estradiol 10-20 mg daily for first 21 days of month or estradiol patch
In hypogonadotropic hypogonadism, to induce ovulation at appropriate time: pulsatile GnRH or FSH and hCG therapy

FSH, follicle-stimulating hormone; GnRH, luteinizing hormone–releasing hormone; hCG, human chorionic gonadotropin.

fusion are brought about by testosterone or estradiol replacement before therapy with GH causes adequate linear growth, adult height will be compromised. However, if puberty is not initiated early enough, the patient may suffer psychological damage. It is advisable to initiate puberty in these patients with low-dose gonadal steroids by age 14 in boys and age 13 in girls, regardless of the definitive diagnosis of gonadotropin deficiency. Isolated GH-deficient patients may have a delayed onset of puberty; with GH administration, puberty usually occurs at an appropriate age but may progress faster than in normal individuals. Children with GH deficiency showed a correlation between the age of onset of induced puberty and adult height for those who were also gonadotropin deficient, whereas those who underwent spontaneous puberty, which occurred earlier than the age of hormone-induced puberty in the gonadotropin-deficient children, had a decreased final height. This supports the advisability of waiting to initiate puberty in GH- and gonadotropin-deficient children. Height at the onset of puberty is also correlated with adult height in GH-deficient children. However, artificially delaying puberty with a GnRH analogue to attempt to achieve a greater final height has been attempted in isolated cases of GH deficiency or with normal-variant short stature, but concern over decreased bone density seen in subjects treated with GnRH analogues led to warnings about the use of this agent in GH-deficient patients. There is inadequate evidence to recommend this therapy.[474]

Microphallus due to hypothalamic deficiencies[316] may be treated with one or two 3-month courses of testosterone enanthate, with 25 mg per month given intramuscularly to enlarge the size of the penis.[733] Although concern was raised that early testosterone therapy might not allow the attainment of a normal adult penile size, experience has shown otherwise. The concern that the penis might not respond to androgens later in life if exposed to testosterone in childhood, a pattern observed in the rat, proved incorrect. Positive psychological outcomes and attainment of normal stretched penile length have been reported.[546,734] It is appropriate to treat male infants and children with micropenis due to gonadotropin or GH deficiency with short courses of androgens to enlarge the penis into the normal childhood range. Patients with isolated congenital GH deficiency occasionally have micropenis that may be successfully treated with GH replacement alone. It is not appropriate to sex reverse a male infant because of microphallus caused by fetal testosterone or GH deficiency.

Episodic administration of GnRH elicits pulsatile LH and FSH release and gonadal stimulation in prepubertal children or hypogonadotropic patients. Portable pumps are used to administer episodic GnRH over prolonged periods. Pulsatile GnRH therapy can induce puberty and promote the development of secondary sexual characteristics and spermatogenesis in men[735] and ovulation in women, but it is not practical for the routine induction of puberty in adolescent boys and girls with gonadotropin deficiency. Pregnancy can be achieved with this regimen in women and spermatogenesis in men with hypogonadotropic hypogonadism. A lower frequency of GnRH administration favors FSH secretion, whereas a faster frequency favors LH secretion and ultimately has been associated with a PCOS-like picture, although the hypothalamic-pituitary-gonadal axis usually is sufficiently robust to accommodate various frequencies of GnRH secretion.

Human menopausal gonadotropin and hCG can be used as effective substitutes for recombinant human pituitary LH and FSH to produce full gonadal maturation, but this regimen is cumbersome and expensive. Long-term gonadal steroid replacement therapy is the treatment of choice for hypothalamic or pituitary gonadotropin deficiency until fertility is desired.[736]

Hypergonadotropic hypogonadism is treated by replacement of testosterone in boys and estradiol in girls. For treatment of gonadal dysgenesis, estrogen therapy should be initiated when the patient is age 13 (bone age > 11 years) to allow secondary sexual development at an appropriate chronologic age. The Klinefelter's syndrome is compatible with various degrees of masculinization at puberty; some patients require testosterone replacement. The concentration of plasma testosterone and LH should be monitored every 6 months during puberty and yearly thereafter. If the LH level rises more than 2.5 SD above the mean value or the testosterone level decreases below the normal range for age, testosterone replacement therapy is indicated. FSH is increased due to lack of inhibin from affected testes.

Patients receiving gonadal steroid replacement follow the same treatment regimen whether the diagnosis is hypogonadotropic hypogonadism or hypergonadotropic hypogonadism (see Table 25-24). Various testosterone preparations are available with several routes of administration. Alkylated testosterone preparations should be avoided because of the risk of peliosis hepatitis (i.e., hemorrhagic liver cysts), which is not related to dose or duration of treatment; although regression is possible with discontinuation of testosterone treatment, progression to liver failure can occur. Males may receive testosterone enanthate, propionate, or cypionate (50 to 100 mg every 4 weeks intramuscularly) at the start, although priapism has been reported with the higher starting dose in a testosterone-naïve boy; later, the dosage is gradually increased to 200 to 300 mg every 2 to 3 weeks. Low-dose replacement therapy is appropriate until well into the pubertal growth spurt. Testosterone may be administered by cutaneous patch on scrotal skin or nonsexual skin to cause secondary sexual development in hypogonadal adolescents; patches may be given at night to recreate the diurnal variation of testosterone seen in early puberty. Physiologic values of serum testosterone may be reached with these patches, along with secondary sexual development. A teenage boy may be less likely to apply a patch daily, and biweekly or monthly injections may allow better compliance; nonetheless, 2.5- and 5-mg dermal testosterone patches may be useful in motivated teenagers. New testosterone gel preparations, usually rubbed onto the forearms, are approved for adults but not for adolescents. Testosterone ointment may be used as therapy for microphallus to enlarge the size of the phallus intentionally, but a normal infant or child contacting the skin of an individual treated with testosterone gel (before it is absorbed) runs the risk of unplanned testosterone effects.[737]

Initially, girls 12 to 13 years old are given ethinyl estradiol (5 μg/day orally) or conjugated estrogens (0.3 mg/day orally) on the first 21 days of the month. The dose is gradually increased over the next 2 to 3 years to 10 μg of ethinyl estradiol or 0.6 to 1.25 mg of conjugated estrogen for the first 21 days of the month. The maintenance dose should be the minimal amount to maintain secondary sexual characteristics, sustain withdrawal bleeding, and prevent osteoporosis. After breakthrough bleeding occurs, or no later than 6 months after the start of cyclic therapy, a progestagen (e.g., 5 mg/day of medroxyprogesterone acetate) is added on days 12 through 21 of the month. Undesirable effects are uncommon but may include weight gain, headache, nausea, peripheral edema, and mild hypertension. The benefits of transdermal estrogen treatment were discussed earlier. Application of portions of transdermal 17β-estradiol patches at night (not FDA-approved for this use) were shown to mimic levels of estrogen produced in early puberty and to slowly bring about breast development[730]; other therapeutic schedules are possible. Estradiol gel (not FDA approved for this use) in an increasing dose from 0.1 to 1.5 mg given over a 5-year period is reported to be safe and effective as replacement therapy in girls with Turner syndrome.[738] As with testosterone, children must not be in contact with the preparation because untoward estrogen effects may occur. Patches and gels are not approved for use in adolescents.

There is a concern about the increased risk of endometrial and breast carcinoma in patients receiving chronic estrogen replacement therapy, including patients with Turner syndrome.[739] The use of progestational agents to antagonize the effect of estrogens reduces the risk of endometrial cancer, but the best answer about the optimal dose of estrogen and progesterone to enhance development without unduly increasing the risk of cancer must come from future studies. Estrogen replacement is important for its anti-osteoporosis action on bone. Bone density is decreased in Turner syndrome in part because of hypogonadism at puberty, and this tendency becomes more severe with age in patients who discontinue or do not receive estrogen replacement therapy. Transdermal estrogen can increase bone density in subjects with Turner syndrome who have finished statural growth.[740] We lack adequate controlled studies on optional sex steroid replacement regimens in young adolescent women. Biosynthetic hGH therapy in Turner syndrome causes an increase in growth rate, with an increase in adult height approaching or reaching the lower range of the normal growth curves possible.

Patients with hypopituitarism may complain of sparse pubic hair growth or, in girls, total absence of pubic hair. Pubic hair thickens further in affected males with hCG treatment, which adds the testicular contribution of testosterone to the exogenous testosterone therapy. GH therapy in GH- and gonadotropin-deficient males enhances the steroidogenic response of the testes to hCG administration. Adolescent or young adult women have been given a low dose (25 mg) of long-acting intramuscular testosterone every 4 weeks to stimulate the growth of pubic hair without virilization. Oral DHEAS treatment is suggested to improve pubic hair growth in hypopituitary girls.[741]

Sexual Precocity

Sexual precocity (Table 25-25) is the appearance of any sign of secondary sexual maturation before the lower limit of the normal age at onset of puberty (i.e., 9 years for boys, 7 years for white girls, and 6 years for African American girls). These cutoffs assume that there are no signs or symptoms of CNS disorders or other serious diseases that might cause sexual precocity; evaluation is indicated in those cases regardless of age. Careful evaluation is essential at these lower age ranges in girls who have only minimal, relatively nonprogressive signs of sexual precocity. These newer limits are controversial, but if the cautions described are heeded, the limits are appropriate.

If sexual precocity results from premature reactivation of the hypothalamic GnRH pulse generator/pituitary gonadotropin-gonadal axis, the condition is GnRH dependent and is termed *central precocious puberty* (CPP), complete precocious puberty, or true (complete) isosexual precocity (ISP). Pulsatile LH release has a pubertal pattern, and the rise in the concentration of LH after GnRH administration is indistinguishable from the normal pubertal pattern of serum LH. If extrapituitary secretion of gonadotropins or secretion of gonadal steroids independent of pulsatile GnRH stimulation leads to virilization in boys or feminization in girls, the condition is termed *incomplete ISP*, pseudoprecocious puberty, or GnRH-independent sexual precocity. The production of excessive estrogens in males leads to inappropriate feminization, and the production of increased androgen levels in females leads to inappropriate virilization; these conditions are termed *contrasexual precocity* or heterosexual precocity. Disorders causing sexual precocity are therefore separated into those in which the increased secretion of gonadal steroids depends on GnRH stimulation of pituitary gonadotropins and those in which it is unrelated to activation of the hypothalamic GnRH pulse generator.

In all forms of sexual precocity, increased gonadal steroid secretion increases height velocity, somatic development, and the rate of skeletal maturation; because of premature epiphyseal fusion, sexual precocity can lead to the paradox of tall stature in childhood but short adult height (Table 25-26). Untreated females with idiopathic CPP demonstrated a mean adult height of 151 to 155 cm.[742-746] In the few reports of adult height in boys with untreated precocious puberty, mean adult stature was 155.4 cm ± 8.3 SD, with all subjects well below midparental height and far below the father's height from the data available.[743,747]

Serum alkaline phosphatase reflects growth, and IGF1 concentrations reflect the degree of sexual development rather than chronologic age, as do most chemistry and hematology values. The serum concentrations of the propeptide of type III procollagen (P-III-NP) in normal

TABLE 25-25

Classification of Sexual Precocity

TRUE PRECOCIOUS PUBERTY OR COMPLETE ISOSEXUAL PRECOCITY (GNRH-DEPENDENT SEXUAL PRECOCITY OR PREMATURE ACTIVATION OF THE HYPOTHALAMIC GNRH PULSE GENERATOR)

Idiopathic true precocious puberty
CNS tumors
- Optic glioma associated with neurofibromatosis type 1
- Hypothalamic astrocytoma

Other CNS disorders
- Developmental abnormalities including hypothalamic hamartoma of the tuber cinereum
- Encephalitis
- Static encephalopathy
- Brain abscess
- Sarcoid or tubercular granuloma
- Head trauma
- Hydrocephalus
- Arachnoid cyst
- Myelomeningocele
- Vascular lesion
- Cranial irradiation

True precocious puberty after late treatment of congenital virilizing adrenal hyperplasia or other previous chronic exposure to sex steroids
True precocious puberty due to gain of function mutations:
- in KISS1R/GRP54 gene
- in KISS1 gene

INCOMPLETE ISOSEXUAL PRECOCITY (HYPOTHALAMIC GNRH-INDEPENDENT)

Males

Gonadotropin-secreting tumors
- hCG-secreting CNS tumors (e.g., chorioepitheliomas, germinoma, teratoma)
- hCG-secreting tumors located outside the CNS (hepatoma, teratoma, choriocarcinoma)

Increased androgen secretion by adrenal or testis
- Congenital adrenal hyperplasia (CYP21 and CYP11B1 deficiencies)
- Virilizing adrenal neoplasm
- Leydig cell adenoma
- Familial testotoxicosis (sex-limited autosomal dominant pituitary gonadotropin-independent precocious Leydig cell and germ cell maturation)
- Cortisol resistance syndrome

Females

Ovarian cyst
Estrogen-secreting ovarian or adrenal neoplasm
Peutz-Jeghers syndrome

Both Sexes

McCune-Albright syndrome
Hypothyroidism
Iatrogenic or exogenous sexual precocity (including inadvertent exposure to estrogens in food, drugs, or cosmetics)

VARIATIONS OF PUBERTAL DEVELOPMENT

Premature thelarche
Premature isolated menarche
Premature adrenarche
Adolescent gynecomastia in boys
Macroorchidism

CONTRASEXUAL PRECOCITY

Feminization in Males

Adrenal neoplasm
Chorioepithelioma
CYP11B1 deficiency
Late-onset adrenal hyperplasia
Testicular neoplasm (Peutz-Jeghers syndrome)
Increased extraglandular conversion of circulating adrenal androgens to estrogen
Iatrogenic (exposure to estrogens)

Virilization in Females

Congenital adrenal hyperplasia
- CYP21 deficiency
- CYP11B1 deficiency
- 3β-HSD deficiency

Virilizing adrenal neoplasm (Cushing's syndrome)
Virilizing ovarian neoplasm (e.g., arrhenoblastoma)
Iatrogenic (exposure to androgens)
Cortisol resistance syndrome
Aromatase deficiency

CNS, central nervous system; CYP11B1, 11-hydroxylase; CYP21, 21-hydroxylase; GNRH, luteinizing hormone–releasing hormone; hCG, human chorionic gonadotropin; 3β-*HSD,* 3β-hydroxysteroid dehydrogenase 4,5-isomerase; KISS14/GPR54, kisspeptin G-protein–coupled receptor 54.
Modified from Grumbach MM. True or central precocious puberty. In: Kreiger DT, Bardin CW, eds. *Current Therapy in Endocrinology and Metabolism, 1985-1986.* Toronto, Canada: BC Decker, 1985:4-8.

puberty and in CPP parallel the normal pubertal growth curve and also parallel the changes in growth rate in children treated with GnRH agonists.[748] Blood pressure matches that of normal subjects of the same height and gender after correcting for bone age rather than chronologic age according to the latest standards for blood pressure.[749]

True or Central Precocious Puberty: Complete Isosexual Precocity

In the UCSF series of more than 200 patients with CPP,[742] girls had true precocious puberty (i.e., GnRH-dependent CPP) five times more commonly than boys, and idiopathic CPP was eight times more common in girls than in boys (Table 25-27). Others reported a 10-fold increased prevalence of precocious puberty in girls compared with boys.[750] CNS abnormalities occurred at least as often as idiopathic CPP in boys, whereas in girls neurologic lesions were one fifth as common as idiopathic disorders. Therefore, it is essential to search for a CNS cause for CPP, especially in

TABLE 25-26

Historical Controls of Untreated Children with True Precocious Puberty

Study	No. Patients (Women/Men)	Final Height (cm)*	
		Women	*Men*
Thamdrup[747]			
Sigurjonsdottir and Hayles[1062]	26/8	151.3 ± 8.8	155.4 ± 8.3
	40/11	152.7 ± 8.0	156.0 ± 7.3
Werder et al.[1063]	4/0	150.9 ± 5.0	
Lee[745]	15/0	155.3 ± 9.6	
University of California, San Francisco[743]	8/4	153.8 ± 6.8	159.6 ± 8.7
TOTAL	93/23	152.7 ± 8.6	155.6 ± 7.7

*Mean ± 1 SD.
From Paul D, Conte FA, Grumbach MM, et al. Long-term effect of gonadotropin-releasing hormone agonist therapy on final and near-final height in 26 children with true precocious puberty treated at a median age of less than 5 years. *J Clin Endocrinol Metab.* 1995;80:546-551.

TABLE 25-27

Distribution by Sex of Children with Idiopathic and Neurogenic Precocious Puberty

	Idiopathic		Neurogenic	
Series	*Male*	*Female*	*Male*	*Female*
Thamdrup[747] (1961)	4	34	7	11
Wilkins[1064] (1965)	13	67	10	5
Sigurjonsdottir and Hayles[1062] (1968)	8	54	16	16
University of California, San Francisco (1981)*	13	121	26	45

*Unpublished data.

boys, because sexual precocity may be the only manifestation of a CNS tumor (Tables 25-28 and 25-29).[389,742] However, most children referred for evaluation have the benign variants leading to premature thelarche or premature adrenarche.[115]

Idiopathic True or Central Precocious Puberty. In otherwise healthy girls, those with onset of puberty at 6 to 8 years of age represent one end of the normal range of age at puberty onset[97]; those with constitutional delay in growth and adolescence fall at the opposite end of the normal range of variation. The nature of the striking sex difference in the prevalence of idiopathic CPP (females » males), compared with that of constitutional delay in growth and puberty (males » females) is poorly understood. There may be a history of early maturation in families of affected subjects[750]; rarely, CPP is transmitted as an autosomal recessive trait in boys and girls.[742] A familial pattern is far more likely to occur in girls than in boys.[751] However, most children develop CPP with no familial tendency and no signs of organic disease; these children have *idiopathic* CPP. This condition, which may manifest in infancy (see Table 25-27), is commonly associated with electroencephalographic abnormalities.[752] The age at onset is 6 to 7 years for about 50% of affected girls, 2 to 6 years for about 25%, and during infancy for 18% (Fig. 25-49).[742] Patients with organic forms of CPP, especially if associated with hypothalamic hamartoma, have an earlier mean age at onset than those with the idiopathic form.[391,742]

In boys (Fig. 25-50), the testes usually enlarge under gonadotropin stimulation before any other signs of puberty are seen; in girls, an increase in the rate of growth, the appearance of breast development, enlargement of the labia minora, and maturational changes in the vaginal mucosa are the usual presenting signs, with variable manifestations of pubic hair depending on the age at onset. Progression of secondary sexual maturation may be more rapid than normal, but a waxing and waning course of development may occur.[755] Spermatogenesis in males and ovulation in females often occur, and fertility is possible. The rapid growth is associated with the increased GH secretion and elevation of serum IGF1 levels resulting from stimulation by estradiol.[150,151,276,756] The ratio of bone age to chronologic age and the rise of IGF1 above normal values

TABLE 25-28

Etiology of True Precocious Puberty*

Etiology	No. Females	No. Males
Idiopathic	121	13
CNS: hypothalamic tumors including hamartomas	11	15
Arachnoid cyst	2	1
Hydrocephalus	6	1
Head trauma (child abuse)	1	
Perinatal asphyxia, cerebral palsy	3	1
Encephalitis or meningitis	3	1
Sex chromosome abnormalities (47,XXY; 48,XXXY)		2
Nonspecific seizure disorder or mental retardation	26	16
Degenerative CNS disease		3
Congenital virilizing adrenal hyperplasia with secondary true precocious puberty		3

*Data from University of California, San Francisco, Pediatric Endocrine Clinic.
CNS, central nervous system.
From Kaplan SL, Grumbach MM. Pathogenesis of sexual precocity. In Grumbach MM, Sizonenko PC, et al, eds. *Control of the Onset of Puberty.* Baltimore, MD: Williams & Wilkins, 1990:620-660. © 1990, The Williams & Wilkins Co., Baltimore.)

TABLE 25-29

Classification of CNS Tumors Associated with Isosexual Precocity at UCSF

10% of all true precocious puberty patients: CNS tumors, hypothalamic (*n* = 26)
Males—IPP/organic precocious puberty = 13/15 (0.9:1)
Females—IPP/organic precocious puberty = 121/11 (12:1)
GnRH-dependent true precocious puberty
  Astrocytoma 3 M, 5 F
  Hamartomas 3 M, 3 F
  Neurofibromatosis 5 M, 1 F
  Craniopharyngioma 2 F
GnRH-independent incomplete sexual precocity
  hCG-secreting tumor* 4 M

*CNS and extra-CNS neoplasms.
CNS, central nervous system; F, female; GnRH, luteinizing hormone–releasing hormone; IPP, idiopathic true or central precocious puberty; M, male; UCSF, University of California, San Francisco.

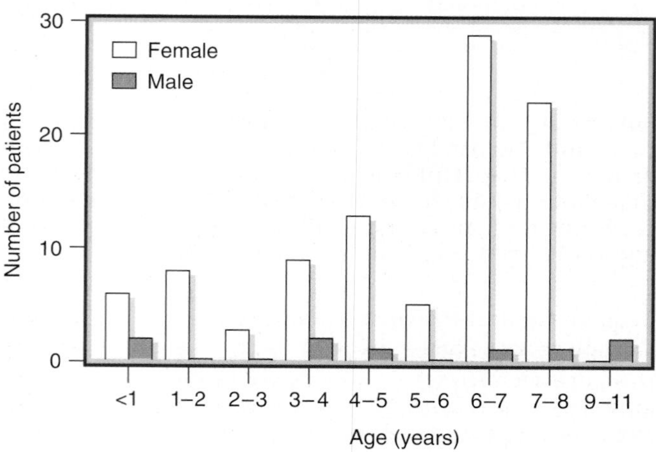

Figure 25-49 Age at onset of idiopathic true precocious puberty in 106 children. At all ages, the frequency is greater in females than in males. The peak prevalence in girls is between ages 6 and 8 years. (From Kaplan SL, Grumbach MM. The neuroendocrinology of human puberty: an ontogenetic perspective. In: Grumbach MM, Sizonenko PC, Aubert ML, eds. *Control of the Onset of Puberty.* Baltimore, MD: Williams & Wilkins, 1990:1-68.)

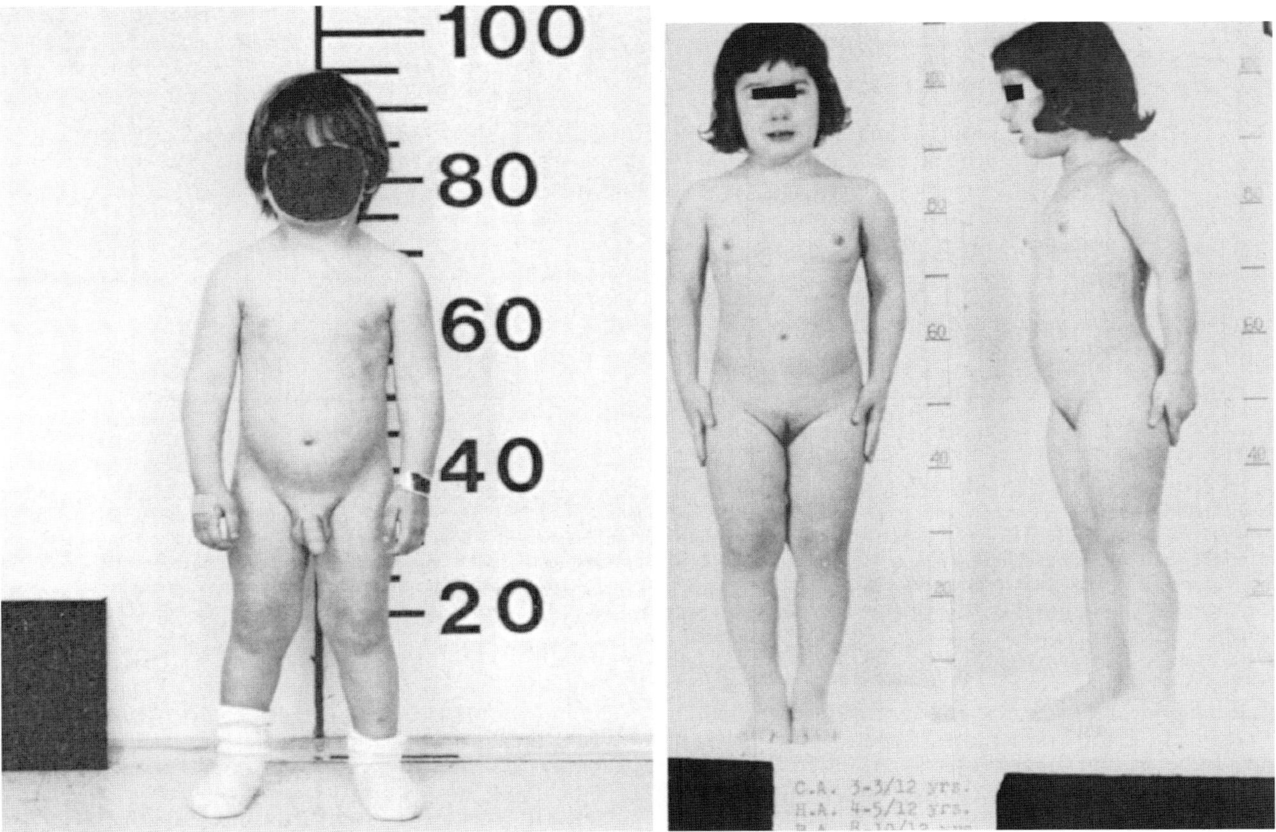

Figure 25-50 *Left,* A boy aged 2 year 5 months with idiopathic precocious puberty. He had pubic hair and phallic and testicular enlargement by 10 months of age. At 1 year, his height was 86 cm (+4 SD); the phallus measured 10 × 3.5 cm, and the testes measured 2.5 × 1.5 cm. The plasma luteinizing hormone (LH) level was 1.9 ng/mL (LER-960); the follicle-stimulating hormone (FSH) level was 1.2 ng/mL (LER-869); and the testosterone level was 416 ng/dL. After 100 µg of gonadotropin-releasing hormone (GnRH), the plasma LH level increased to 8.4 ng/mL, and the FSH level increased to 1.8 ng/mL, a pubertal response. When photographed, the patient had been treated with medroxyprogesterone acetate for 1.5 years. His height was 95.2 cm (+1 SD), the phallus was 6 × 3 cm, and the testes were 2.4 × 1.3 cm. Basal concentrations of LH (LER-960) were 0.9 ng/mL; the FSH (LER-869) level was 0.8 ng/mL; and the testosterone level was 7 ng/dL. After 100 µg of GnRH, LH concentrations rose to 2.3 ng/mL, whereas FSH concentrations did not change when he was on treatment with medroxyprogesterone acetate. For conversion to SI units, see Figures 25-16 and 25-17. *Right,* A girl aged 3 years and 3 months with idiopathic true precocious puberty had recurrent vaginal bleeding since she was 9 months old. Her height age was 4 years and 5 months; bone age was 8 years and 10 months. (*Left,* From Styne DM, Grumbach MM. Puberty in the male and female: its physiology and disorders. In: Yen SCC, Jaffe RB, eds. *Reproductive Endocrinology,* 2nd ed. Philadelphia, PA: Saunders, 1986:313-384.)

for age are predictive of outcome: more mildly affected children progress less rapidly and tend to maintain their target height, and this may represent a benign entity.[757]

Before beginning treatment, it is essential to establish the rapidly progressive nature of the sexual precocity.[758,759] In a subset of girls, the tempo is relatively slow and the sexual precocity may not be sustained.[742,755,760] The growth rate slows to normal for age, skeletal maturation progresses in accordance with chronologic age, and there is little to no risk of impairment of final height[755]; estrogen and IGF1 concentrations are normal or only slightly elevated.[757] If height prediction is normal at the time of diagnosis rather than reduced, the patient does not require therapy[759,761]; the efficacy of treatment with GnRH in those with onset after 6 years of age is inconsistent.[474] In some girls, we have observed within a period of 1 to 2 months the return of a prepubertal pattern of LH pulsatility during sleep, a prepubertal LH response to GnRH, and a concentration of plasma estradiol equivalent to the prepubertal state. Unlike typical patients, such girls do not exhibit the initial hyperresponse of plasma estradiol and LH to the GnRH agonist or the physical changes of the estrogen effect, and they tend to have lower serum IGF1.

Many girls in this subset have clinical and hormonal features that fall between those of premature thelarche and CPP and are typical of neither condition[762]; this is denoted *exaggerated thelarche.* About 10% of girls with apparently classic premature thelarche progress to definite CPP, but there are no signs at the time of first presentation to differentiate them from girls who continue with the pattern of premature thelarche. In most patients in this situation, the onset of breast development was first noticed after 2 years of age.[556] Therapy is not indicated if a pubertal pattern of pulsatile LH secretion during sleep is not present or if the basal LH measured by ultrasensitive assay or the LH response to exogenous GnRH or GnRH agonist is prepubertal. The most severely affected girls are the ones who respond best to GnRH agonist therapy.[758,763]

The uterus and ovaries increase in size in CPP. The ovaries also may develop a multicystic appearance (but not a polycystic appearance) that may remain even after successful treatment with a GnRH agonist.[764] CPP in females does not lead to premature menopause. However, there is increased risk in girls for the development of carcinoma of the breast[72,73,765] in adulthood. Psychosexual development is advanced modestly in patients with sexual

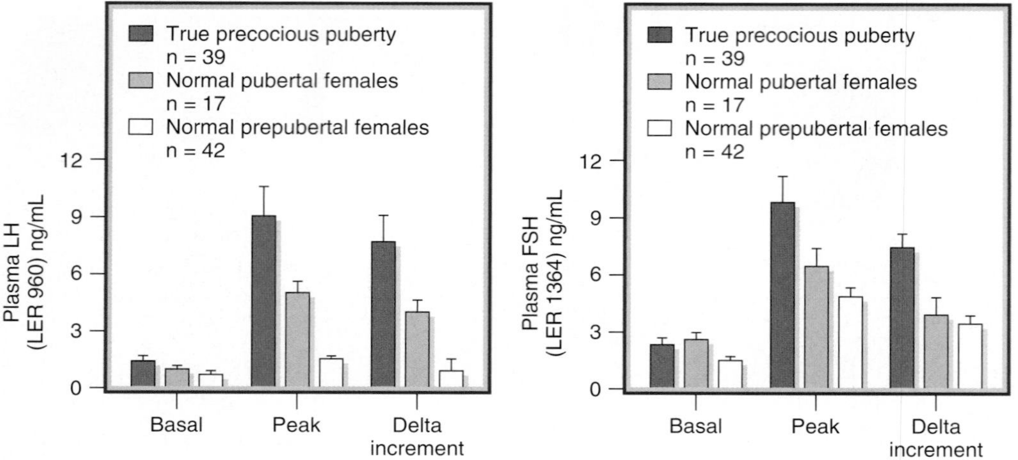

Figure 25-51 *Left*, Mean basal plasma luteinizing hormone (LH) level (LER-960) and mean peak and increment after intravenous gonadotropin-releasing hormone (GnRH) (100 μg) in normal prepubertal and pubertal females and in females with idiopathic true precocious puberty. The mean peak and increments of plasma LH are higher in true precocious puberty than in normal puberty. *Right*, Basal follicle-stimulating hormone (FSH) level (LER-1364) and mean peak and increment after intravenous GnRH (100 μg) in normal prepubertal and pubertal females with true precocious puberty. The concentration of FSH and the response to GnRH were greater in females with true precocious puberty and normal puberty than in prepubertal females. (From Kaplan SL, Grumbach MM. Pathogenesis of sexual precocity. In: Grumbach MM, Sizonenko PC, Aubert ML, eds. *Control of the Onset of Puberty*. Baltimore, MD: Williams & Wilkins, 1990:620-660.)

precocity (about 1.5 years in girls with idiopathic CPP). The pituitary gland undergoes hypertrophy in early infancy, puberty, and pregnancy and also increases in size on MRI imaging in patients with CPP.[766] T1-weighted images indicate a convex upper border of the pituitary gland in both normal patients and those with CPP, indicating the similarity in the physiologic changes in both conditions. Pituitary gland hyperplasia (height >1 cm) is a rare finding reported in CPP. The empty sella syndrome is less frequently observed in patients with CPP than in patients with pituitary hypofunction. Empty sella is found in 10% of children who are imaged for suspected hypothalamic-pituitary disorders including hypogonadotropic hypogonadism.[767,768]

The gonadotropin and gonadal steroid concentrations in plasma, the LH response to GnRH administration, and the amplitude and frequency of LH pulses are in the normal pubertal range (Figs. 25-51 and 25-52).[429,769] The third-generation gonadotropin assays allow diagnosis of CPP by the determination in a single serum sample of LH in the basal state in most (but not all) girls.[770] Gonadotropin determination 30 to 60 minutes after a single subcutaneous dose of GnRH or GnRH agonist can diagnose CPP with high specificity and sensitivity.[771-773] Adrenarche usually does not accompany gonadarche in girls with CPP who are younger than 5 or 6 years of age[442]: pubic hair is sparse or absent initially in such girls. When the onset of CPP occurs after age 6 years, it is usually associated with adrenarche that is early for chronologic age but not for bone age.

A small proportion of patients with CPP proven by a pubertal response of LH to GnRH and increased pulsatile LH secretion at night may revert spontaneously to a more immature pubertal state, persist without further progression, or fluctuate between progression and regression.[742,755,774] There is a continuum in girls with CPP from premature thelarche, through unsustained or slowly progressive precocious puberty, to the relatively rapid progression of sexual maturation once it has begun.[750]

In the UCSF experience and that of others, normal pregnancies have occurred in women with idiopathic CPP, CPP triggered by a CNS abnormality,[742] or premature menarche. Pregnancy has occurred in patients with CPP as early as 5 years of age (an unfortunate result of childhood sexual abuse).

Central Nervous System Tumors Causing True Precocious Puberty. Sexual precocity may be the first manifestation of a hypothalamic tumor of any cell type when it arises in or impinges on the posterior hypothalamus. Neurologic symptoms such as headaches and visual disturbances may develop, and children may have diabetes insipidus, hydrocephalus, or optic atrophy caused by an enlarging tumor in addition to precocious puberty.[742] CPP resulting from CNS tumors (see Table 25-29) has about the same prevalence in boys and in girls in the population; however boys have a lower overall prevalence of precocious puberty, and neurologic abnormalities account for two thirds of those with CPP. In the UCSF experience, a CNS tumor was present in at least half of this group.[742]

A CNS neoplasm must be considered in the differential diagnosis of any patient with CPP.[389,775] The location of CNS tumors causing CPP makes surgical removal difficult. A conservative approach calls for biopsy of the neoplasm and radiation or chemotherapy or both, depending on the pathologic findings. Optic and hypothalamic glioma (often associated with neurofibromatosis), astrocytoma, ependymoma, and, rarely, craniopharyngioma may cause CPP by impinging on the neural pathways that inhibit the GnRH pulse generator in childhood or as a consequence of cranial irradiation for treatment of a brain tumor. Pineal neoplasms are associated with loss of upward gaze (Parinaud's syndrome) due to brain stem compression.

The prevalence of CPP is increased after cranial irradiation for local tumors or leukemia[258,776,777,778] even if radiotherapy targets the pituitary gland.[779] The combination of GH deficiency and CPP can occur in children previously subjected to therapeutic irradiation of the CNS in association with a CNS neoplasm and in those with a variety of other CNS abnormalities, including developmental malformations and head trauma.[258] The lack of GH may not be apparent because of increased growth resulting from the elevated gonadal steroid levels; GH-deficient children with

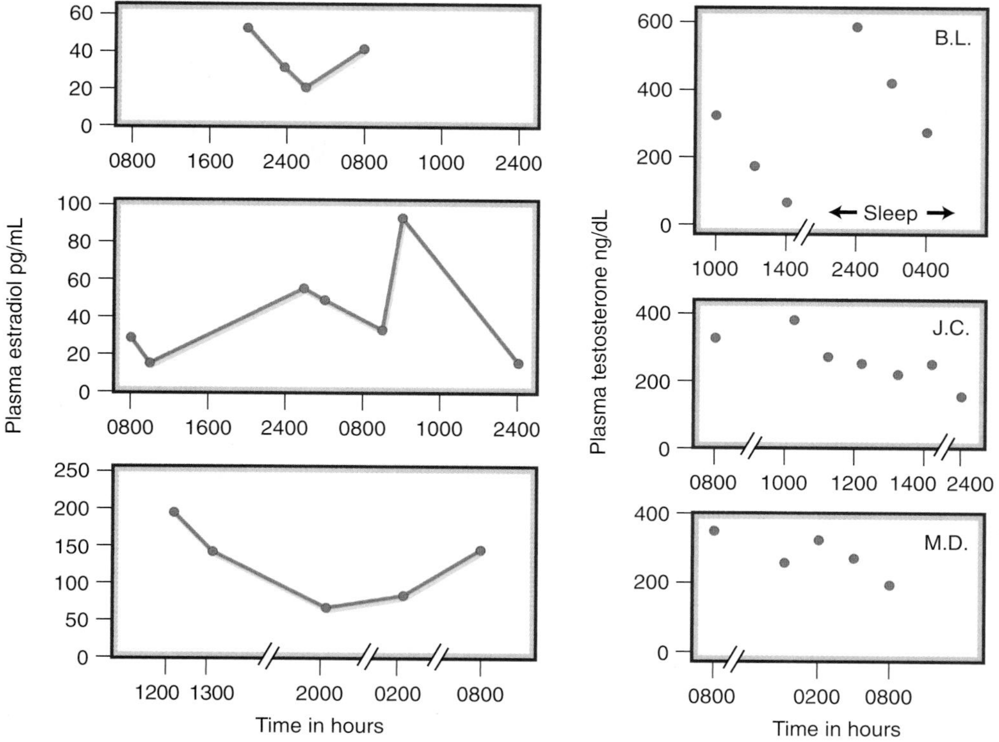

Figure 25-52 *Left,* Serial determinations of plasma estradiol in three girls with idiopathic true precocious puberty. Notice the striking fluctuations in values. *Right,* Serial determinations of plasma testosterone in three boys with true precocious puberty (B.L. and J.C. have a hypothalamic hamartoma; M.D. has the idiopathic form). For conversion to SI units, see Figures 25-16 and 25-17. (From Kaplan SL, Grumbach MM. Pathogenesis of sexual precocity. In: Grumbach MM, Sizonenko PC, Aubert ML, eds. *Control of the Onset of Puberty.* Baltimore, MD: Williams & Wilkins, 1990:620-660.)

CPP grow more slowly than GH-sufficient children with CPP but faster than GH-deficient children without sexual precocity. GH-deficient children with CPP have IGF1 concentrations that are intermediate between the higher levels found in GH-sufficient children with sexual precocity and the lower levels found in prepubertal GH-deficient children.[258]

GH deficiency and CPP can occur with CNS radiation doses of only 18 to 47 Gy, whereas gonadotropin deficiency, TSH deficiency, ACTH deficiency, and hypoprolactinemia usually occur with doses greater than 40 Gy.[258,779,780] The advance in the age of onset of puberty is reported to be positively correlated with the age of diagnosis of the condition for which the radiation therapy was given (i.e., earlier age at onset of puberty with earlier age at diagnosis) and is also positively correlated with BMI at diagnosis.[777] Newer radiation treatment regimens using lower doses of radiation for various malignancies may have less influence on advancing the age of menarche and may lead to less long-term morbidity.[781,782] Treatment with a combination of GH and GnRH agonist is indicated in these patients and results in better growth and improved height prognosis when compared with the use of GnRH agonist alone. Because GH secretion is related to BMI, it is important to rule out a decrease in GH secretion caused by increased BMI in CPP before interpreting the decrease as evidence of GH deficiency.

Hamartomas of the Tuber Cinereum. Hamartomas are congenital malformations composed of a heterotopic mass of nervous tissue containing GnRH neurosecretory neurons, fiber bundles, and glial cells; they are frequently associated with CPP (Fig. 25-53), which usually manifests before the patient is 3 years of age (Table 25-30).[742,783] Hypothalamic hamartomas may be sessile or pedunculated and are usually attached to the posterior hypothalamus between the tuber cinereum and the mamillary bodies. These masses project into the suprasellar cistern, and the pedunculated hamartoma has a distinct stalk. They present a characteristic appearance that does not change with time. Hamartomas of the tuber cinereum are not true neoplasms,[390,391,783] as long-term follow-up demonstrated lack of growth on monitoring by periodic CT or MRI.[391,784,785] Hamartomas appear

TABLE 25-30

Clinical and Laboratory Characteristics of Children with True Precocious Puberty Caused by Hypothalamic Hamartoma

Characteristic	UCSF (6 M, 6 F)	Hochman et al.* (18 M, 9 F)
Age at Onset of Pubertal Signs		
Birth to 1 yr	4	6
1-2 yr	4	17
2-4 yr	3	6
7 yr	1	1
Neurologic Signs		
Seizures including gelastic type	3/12	11/24
Headache and visual symptoms	1/12	5/24
None	7/12	7/24

*Hochman HI, Judge DM, Reichlin S. Precocious puberty and hypothalamic hamartoma [literature review]. *Pediatrics.* 1981;67:236-244.

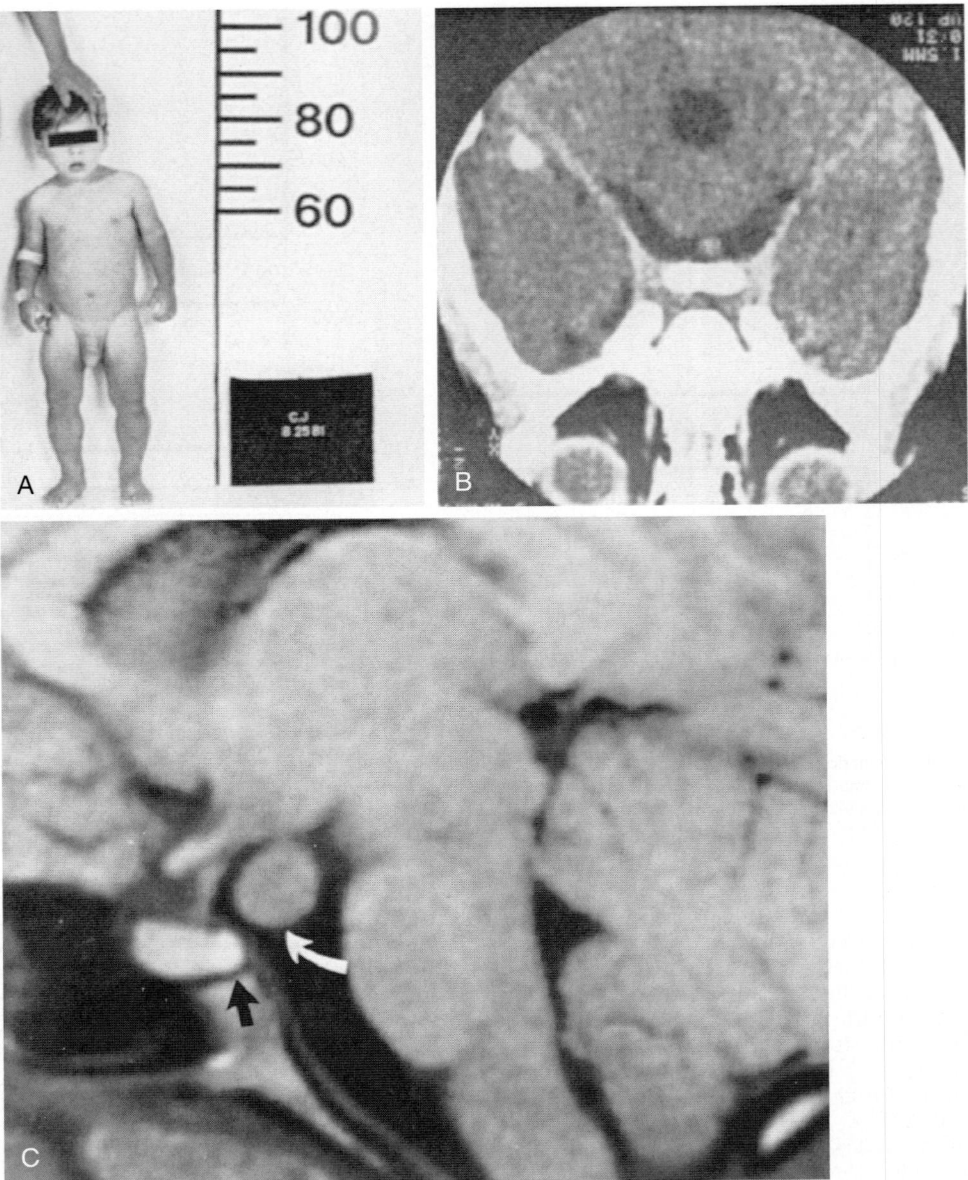

Figure 25-53 **A,** A 17-month-old male infant with hamartoma of the tuber cinereum and true precocious puberty. When the patient was 8 months of age, secondary sexual development was observed, and the patient was misdiagnosed as having congenital virilizing adrenal hyperplasia. He was treated with glucocorticoids, which slowed his growth but did not affect his sexual development and bone age advancement. When he was first seen at 17 months, his height was 84.2 cm, his weight was 14.8 kg, pubic hair stage was stage 2, penis was 10.4 × 2.2 cm, testes were 1.5 × 2.8 cm, and the scrotum was thinned and rugated. The bone age was 4.25 years. After gonadotropin-releasing hormone (GnRH) administration, the LH level rose from 0.5 to 3.1 ng/dL (LER-960), the follicle-stimulating hormone (FSH) level rose from 0.5 to 1.2 ng/mL (LER-869), and the testosterone level rose from 409 to 450 ng/dL. The dehydroepiandrosterone sulfate (DHEAS) was 17 μg/dL (preadrenarchal value). The patient was treated with a potent, long-acting LHRH agonist, deslorelin (D-Trp^{6}Pro^{9}NEt-GnRH), which resulted in arrest of his pubertal advancement and a striking decrease in the plasma concentration of testosterone, LH pulses, and the response to exogenous GnRH. **B,** Computed tomography demonstrated a 1.5-cm mass posterior and rostral to the dorsum sella, which depressed the flow of the third ventricle. For conversion to SI units, see Figures 25-16, 25-17, and 25-25. **C,** Sagittal, T1-weighted magnetic resonance image shows a hypothalamic hamartoma *(white arrow)* in a 4-year-old boy with true precocious puberty. The posterior pituitary hot spot is designated by the *black arrow*. (**B,** From Styne DM, Grumbach MM. Puberty in the male and female: its physiology and disorders. In: Yen SCC, Jaffe RB, eds. *Reproductive Endocrinology,* 2nd ed. Philadelphia, PA: Saunders, 1986:313-384.)

on CT or MRI scans as an isodense, abnormal fullness of the interpeduncular, prepontine, and posterior suprasellar cisterns, occasionally with distortion of the anterior third ventricle. Their appearance and location are related to the clinical manifestation, with distortion of the third ventricle more closely associated with the occurrence of seizures.[786] There is no enhancement with contrast material. T2-weighted MRIs provide the best visualization of the lesion (Fig. 25-54).[391] However, the solid component of hamartomas may be missed when associated with a subarachnoid cyst if lower-resolution MRI studies are invoked.[787]

The etiologic development of the hypothalamic hamartoma may be the converse of the lack of migration of GnRH neurons in Kallmann's syndrome due to absent production of adhesion molecules coded by the *KAL1* gene. We may postulate that in hypothalamic hamartoma, the KAL1

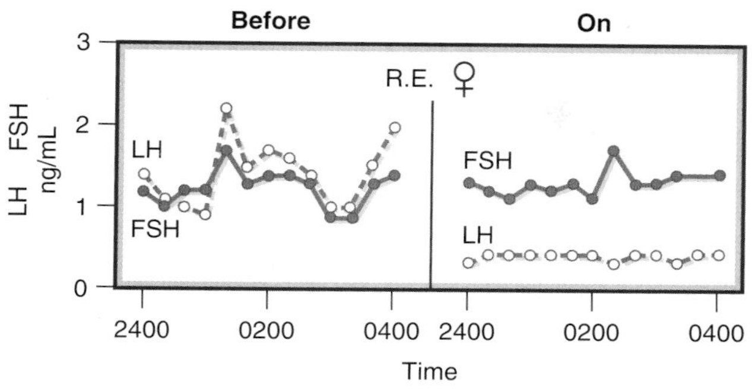

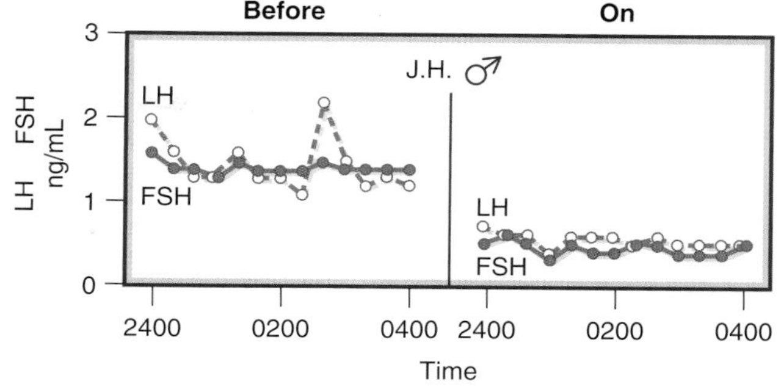

Figure 25-54 Pulsatile luteinizing hormone (LH) secretion before and during gonadotropin-releasing hormone (GnRH) agonist therapy in a boy *(right)* and a girl *(left)* with true precocious puberty resulting from a hypothalamic hamartoma. For conversion to SI units, see Figure 25-16.

protein, among other axon-guiding factors, may cause most of the total complement of about 1500 GnRH neurons to migrate to the hamartoma; alternatively, there may be a stimulus to progenitor cells that are capable of synthesizing GnRH to do so while located in the hamartoma.

Hamartomas associated with CPP contain ectopic GnRH neurosecretory cells that are similar to the GnRH-containing neurons in the medial basal hypothalamus. This developmental abnormality exerts its endocrine effects through elaboration and pulsatile release of GnRH.[389,742] GnRH-containing fibers have been identified passing from the hamartoma toward the median eminence.[742] We have suggested that the GnRH-containing neurosecretory neurons in the tumor are unrestrained by the intrinsic CNS mechanism that inhibits the normal GnRH pulse generator and act as an ectopic GnRH pulse generator,[314] either independently or in synchrony with the GnRH neurosecretory neurons in the medial basal hypothalamus, to produce intermittent secretory bursts of GnRH (see Fig. 25-24).[314] The GnRH is transported to the pituitary by way of the portal circulation and elicits pulsatile release of LH. If the hamartoma were to secrete GnRH in a continuous fashion, CPP would not occur, because the GnRH receptors would be desensitized. About 10% of hypothalamic hamartomas are not associated with CPP.

The hypothalamic hamartoma in two young girls with rapidly progressive CPP did not contain immunoreactive GnRH neurons, but the mass showed a network of astroglial cells containing TGF-α, a member of the EGF family.[788] This suggests that some hypothalamic hamartomas, by virtue of increased production of TGF-α and of neuregulins synthesized by hypothalamic and astroglial cells through paracrine mechanisms, effect the release of bioactive factors, including prostaglandin E_2, that act on GnRH neurons to increase GnRH secretion. However, these hamartomas were much larger than the typical hypothalamic hamartoma associated with CPP[391,783]; the mass bulged into the third ventricle in one girl, and in the other, the pituitary gland was hypertrophic and bulged through the diaphragm sellae.[788] Activation of the GnRH pulse generator through a mass effect and compromise of restraint mechanisms may be the mechanism of CPP, rather than TGF-α signaling. Hypothalamic hamartomas are postulated to elicit their effects via neurons that are able to produce GnRH within the tumor, through the ability to control neurons synaptically connected to GnRH neurons, or through neuronal networks that include GnRH neurons in the hypothalamic hamartoma itself or signaling-competent astrocytic and ependymoglial cells.[789] The precocious sexual development can be controlled by treatment with GnRH agonist therapy.[785,790,791]

Before 1980, only 37 patients were in the literature with hamartomas of the tuber cinereum, but many more have been reported since the advent of CT and MRI brain scans (see Fig. 25-53 and Table 25-30).[792] Of girls with CPP studied at the National Institutes of Health, 16% had a hypothalamic hamartoma, 40% had other CNS abnormalities, and 60% had idiopathic CPP. Among boys with CPP, 10% had idiopathic CPP, 50% had a hypothalamic hamartoma, and the rest had other CNS abnormalities including hypothalamic neoplasms.

Hypothalamic hamartomas that cause CPP can be associated with laughing (gelastic), petit mal, or generalized tonic-clonic seizures; mental retardation; behavioral disturbances; and dysmorphic syndromes beginning as early as the neonatal period.[391,793] Males are more likely to have seizures with these lesions. Seizures can be caused by a hamartoma in the absence of precocious puberty.[786] The occurrence of seizure is uncommon when the mass diameter of the hamartoma is less than 10 mm, whereas a larger mass is associated with a higher risk.[391] Larger hamartomas are also associated with precocious puberty.[794]

Although some have advocated neurosurgical removal of these hamartomas because of the occurrence of precocious puberty alone, we do not recommend neurosurgical extirpation in the absence of strong evidence of growth of the mass or of an associated complication such as intractable seizures or hydrocephalus.[389,391,742,795,796] Gelastic seizures are less amenable to antiepileptic therapy than other hamartoma-related seizures and may require surgical treatment; endoscopic technique is increasingly employed,[797,798] and gamma knife procedures are used, especially for small lesions.[799] Refractory seizures have replaced precocious puberty as the main reason to perform surgery in cases of hamartoma of the tuber cinerium. The endocrine result of surgery on these lesions is rarely reported, but in one series of 29 subjects, hypernatremia, low T_4, low GH, and weight gain were encountered.[800] Prior, unsuccessful surgery may increase the risk for endocrinopathy in these patients. The postoperative endocrine disturbances appear to be transient and mild or asymptomatic, but increased appetite and weight gain appeared in 25% of the subjects and may present an enduring problem. Although there are cases in which removal of a hypothalamic hamartoma led to reversal of the pubertal process,[783,801] deaths have been reported after attempted operative removal.[783] We strongly recommend medical therapy with GnRH agonist in lieu of surgery for the treatment of precocious puberty associated with these hamartomas if seizures are absent or under control.

The Pallister-Hall syndrome is associated with polydactyly, imperfect anus, bifid epiglottis, and hypopituitarism with seizures. This syndrome is not usually associated with precocious puberty, but one apparent case has been reported.

Other Central Nervous System Conditions. CPP may occur secondary to encephalitis, static cerebral encephalopathy, brain abscess, or sarcoid or tuberculous granulomas of the hypothalamus, with or without tuberculous meningitis.[503,802,803] CPP can occur after severe head trauma (usually in girls), and it has been associated with cerebral atrophy or focal encephalomalacia occurring after cerebral edema complicating the treatment of severe diabetic ketoacidosis. Children with nontumor hydrocephalus, even if shunted, experience earlier pubertal development, and those who have not been adequately treated may develop CPP.[742] Delayed puberty is an alternative outcome in a minority of affected children. The growth pattern of children with severe hydrocephalus often includes poor prepubertal growth and an early pubertal growth spurt leading to decreased final height.

Arachnoid Cysts. Arachnoid cysts arising de novo, after infection, or after surgery can cause premature sexual development, possibly with associated GH deficiency.[314,742] Head nodding, abnormal gait, and abnormalities of visual fields are reported in 30% to 40% of cases. Erosion or enlargement of the sella turcica into a J shape may occur. Decompression and extirpation of a suprasellar arachnoid cyst can reverse the sexual precocity (see Fig. 25-25).[314,804]

Neurofibromatosis Type 1. Neurofibromatosis type 1 (NF1 or von Recklinghausen's disease) is associated with a propensity to develop the optic chiasmal tumors that are the most common cause[805] (but not the only cause) of development of CPP in a child with neurofibromatosis. Most optic gliomas appear during the first decade of life, but only 20% to 30% become symptomatic; these tumors rarely progress in the years after diagnosis.[805-807] The tumor suppressor *NF1* gene, located on the long arm of chromosome 17 (q11.2), which has a high mutation rate, encodes a 327-kd protein, neurofibromin, that is widely expressed even though NF1 involves mainly tissues derived from the neural crest. A wide variety of mutations of the *NF1* gene have been reported, especially deletions, nonsense mutations, and truncating mutations distributed over the coding region. In sporadic cases, the new mutation originates in the paternally derived *NF1* allele in most instances, suggesting a role for genomic imprinting. Concentrations of midkine (MK) and stem cell factor, but not EGF, were found to be substantially increased in the serum of NF1 patients compared with healthy controls and serve as a diagnostic feature.[808] Serum MK levels increase dramatically in patients older than 18 years of age, apparently as a feature of pubertal development. Because serum from patients with NF1 enhances proliferation of human neurofibroma-derived primary Schwann cells and endothelial cells, enhanced levels of circulating growth factors contribute to diffuse tumorigenesis in NF1.

NF1 is characterized by multiple pigmented areas and overgrowth of nerve sheaths and fibrous tissue elements (Fig. 25-55). Multiple café au lait spots are frequent and are smoother in outline (coast of California appearance) than those of the McCune-Albright syndrome (coast of Maine appearance). The diagnosis is made if two or more of the following are observed:

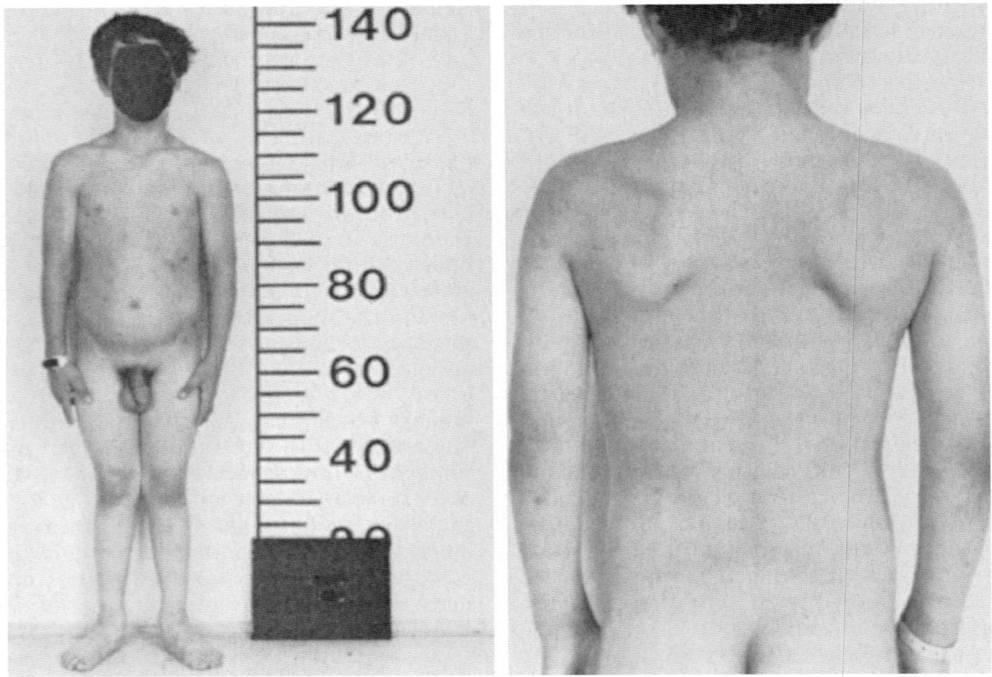

Figure 25-55 A boy aged 8 years and 8 months with neurofibromatosis and precocious puberty resulting from a hypothalamic glioma. He had tonic-clonic seizures at 2.5 years and rapid growth starting at 4 years; an enlarged penis and testes and the presence of pubic hair were first noticed at 7.5 years. At this time, his height was 139.9 cm (+1.4 SD); the phallus was 9 × 3 cm, the right testis measured 5.5 × 3.2 cm, and the left measured 5.4 × 2.9 cm. He had stage 3 pubic hair and 24 large café au lait spots. Computed tomography and pneumoencephalography revealed a 1.5 × 2.5 cm, hypothalamic mass, which was treated with irradiation. The plasma concentration of luteinizing hormone (LH) was 0.5 ng/mL (LER-960); the follicle-stimulating hormone (FSH) level was 0.4 ng/mL (LER-869); and the testosterone level was 221 ng/dL. After 100 μg of intravenous LH-releasing hormone (LHRH), the peak concentration of LH was 4.9 ng/mL, and that of FSH was 1.4 ng/mL, a pubertal response. For conversion to SI units, see Figures 25-16 and 25-17. (From Styne DM, Grumbach MM. Puberty in the male and female: its physiology and disorders. In: Yen SCC, Jaffe RB, eds. *Reproductive Endocrinology,* 2nd ed. Philadelphia, PA: Saunders, 1986:313-384.)

1. Six or more café au lait macules, the greatest diameter being more than 5 mm in prepubertal subjects or more than 12.5 mm in postpubertal subjects
2. Two or more neurofibromas of any type or one plexiform neurofibroma
3. Freckling in the axillae or inguinal region
4. Optic glioma
5. Two or more iris Lisch nodules (ophthalmic hamartomas that occur more frequently after the onset of puberty)
6. A distinctive osseous lesion such as sphenoid dysplasia or pseudoarthrosis
7. A first-degree relative with NF1 according to the criteria described previously

Neurofibromas of the skin in neurofibromatosis may be subcutaneous, sessile or deep, plexiform masses in children; pedunculated lesions develop in later childhood. Internal neurofibromas cause most of the complications. Bone abnormalities such as cysts and pseudoarthrosis, hemihypertrophy, bowing, scoliosis, and skull and facial defects are common (20% of patients); dumbbell-shaped tumors of spinal nerve roots may cause pain, sensory and motor dysfunction, and bone erosions; gliomas or neurofibromas of any part of the CNS, including the optic nerves and the hypothalamus, may calcify. Lisch nodules of the iris are frequent, particularly in adults. Sarcomatous degeneration occurs in 5% to 15% of patients. Other neoplasms include CNS astrocytomas that often involve the visual pathways, ependymomas, meningiomas, neurofibrosarcomas, rhabdomyosarcomas, and nonlymphocytic leukemias. Pheochromocytoma may develop in affected adults.

The clinical manifestations of neurofibromatosis include seizures, visual defects, and either delayed puberty or CPP. Although some manifestations of NF1 are quite common (e.g., café au lait spots, which were found in 99% of a series of 297 subjects), precocious puberty is rarer (found in 3.2% of that same series).[809] GH deficiency is possible at presentation, but after radiation therapy for associated optic glioma, GH, TSH, ACTH, and gonadotropin deficiency may develop. Developmental delay occurs more often in this population but usually is not severe; there is also an increased incidence of psychiatric disease. Most affected children have some manifestations of the disease by 1 year of age. Screening MRI scans are recommended for early detection of CNS tumors.

Other Central Nervous System Abnormalities. Other CNS abnormalities associated with CPP but without demonstrable lesions on imaging study include epilepsy,[752] laughing seizures, developmental delay, and the post-traumatic state. Septo-optic dysplasia (described earlier) may be associated not only with multiple pituitary hormone deficiencies and delayed puberty but also, rarely, with CPP.[565] There may be coexisting deficiencies of some pituitary hormones and excessive secretion of others, including prolactin.

Patients with myelomeningocele (myelodysplasia) have an increased prevalence of endocrine abnormalities, including hypothalamic hypothyroidism, hyperprolactinemia, and elevated gonadotropin concentrations, which in some patients is associated with CPP.

Central Precocious Puberty in Children Adopted from Developing Countries. There was a 15- to 20-fold increased prevalence of CPP among children (with established birth dates) from developing countries who were adopted into Denmark, and other countries have reported similar tendencies. In Sweden, adopted Indian children had pubertal growth spurts similar to those of Swedish children, but adult height was decreased, with the loss of height in childhood and the early puberty apparently being responsible. Environmental influences, many related to the present obesity epidemic, are posited to exert effects in the reported decrease in age at menarche among children from the developing world. These children, who suffer poor prenatal nutrition and often are SGA, are adopted into families in developed countries,[810] and in that environment of affluence they experience precocious puberty.[6]

A confounding factor in the study of adopted children is the finding that children of immigrant groups who were born in their new country may have earlier puberty than children of the predominant ethic group of that country; these influences might be genetic, or they might be related to cultural and dietary differences but could complicate the analysis.[17] Foreign children who immigrated to Belgium with their biologic families from developing countries had greatly elevated concentrations of P,P′-DOE, a derivative of the organochlorine pesticide, dichlorodiphenyltrichloroethane (DDT), raising the possibility of a role for endocrine disrupters in their CPP, although this is unproven. Older age at adoption and immigration is a risk factor for precocious puberty.[811] Remarkably, children adopted from South Korea do not appear to have this tendency.[811]

The use of GnRH agonist in addition to GH treatment to increase adult height is reported in affected children, but the combination is not supported by adequate evidence to recommend this combination in adopted children or any children with CPP.[474] The combination of adoption, living in a culture foreign to the background at birth, and precocious puberty makes these children vulnerable to psychic trauma, which must always be considered.

True Precocious Puberty after Virilizing Disorders. Correction of long-standing virilization may be followed by development of CPP with activation of the hypothalamic-pituitary gonadotropin-gonadal system. This secondary CPP occurs in congenital virilizing adrenal hyperplasia with advanced bone age when glucocorticoid replacement therapy starts after 4 to 8 years.[284,429] CPP has also been documented in children who received or were exposed to androgens or estrogens for long periods during early childhood for a variety of medical conditions.

Gain of Function Mutations as Cause of CPP

KISSIR/GRP54. Whereas inactivating mutations in the KISS1R receptor cause hypogonadotropic hypogonadism, an autosomal dominant *KISS1R* mutation causing an Arg-386Pro substitution was reported to be associated with CPP. The mutation leads to prolonged activation of intracellular signaling pathways in response to kisspeptin and was speculated to desensitize the receptor to its ligand. The 8-year-old patient had had slowly progressing thelarche since birth, but acceleration of growth, bone age maturation, and secondary sexual development occurred at 7 years of age and was reversed with GnRH agonist treatment. Because the girl was adopted, family studies could not be done.[753] It isunclear how many children with apparent idiopathic CPP have such a mutation.

KISS Mutations. Recently, the first detected mutations in the gene encoding *KISS* associated with precocious puberty were reported.[754] Two novel *KISS1* missense mutations were discovered in three children with idiopathic CPP; these mutations were absent in 400 control alleles. The P74S mutation was identified in the heterozygous state in a boy who developed CPP at 1 year of age.

This variant was resistant to kisspeptin degradation, suggesting more bioavailable peptide to stimulate KISS1R; there was no indication of a change of affinity for the receptor. The other variant, the H90D mutation, was identified in the homozygous state in two unrelated girls with CPP manifesting from about 6 years of age. It was not clear what biologic changes this mutation brought about to cause the precocious puberty. Heterozygous H90D mutations were previously found in rare patients with isolated hypogonadotropic hypogonadism. The prevalence of *KISS* mutations causing CPP in children previously thought to have "idiopathic" CPP remains to be determined.

Marfan Syndrome. Marfan syndrome may be associated with tall stature and early PHV and menarche[812] compared with North American averages.

Management of Central Precocious Puberty. Table 25-31 addresses the major psychosocial and clinical goals of therapy for CPP.[795] Three principal agents have been used in the medical treatment of idiopathic or neurologic CPP: medroxyprogesterone acetate, cyproterone acetate, and superactive GnRH agonists.

Medroxyprogesterone Acetate and Cyproterone Acetate. Medroxyprogesterone and cyproterone reversed or arrested the progression of secondary sexual characteristics but had no apparent effect or only a small effect on final height, especially in affected girls.[633] Medroxyprogesterone acetate inhibits gonadotropin secretion by its action on the hypothalamic GnRH pulse generator/pituitary gonadotropin unit and has a direct suppressive effect on gonadal steroidogenesis through 3β-HSD2. Medroxyprogesterone acetate has glucocorticoid action and can suppress ACTH and cortisol secretion, increase appetite and lead to excessive weight gain, and induce hypertension and a cushingoid facies and appearance.[389,742,813]

Cyproterone acetate has been used outside the United States for the treatment of CPP with advantages and disadvantages similar to those of medroxyprogesterone acetate.[389] Cyproterone acetate has antiandrogenic, antigonadotropic, and progestational properties. Cyproterone acetate suppresses the secretion of ACTH and the plasma concentration of cortisol. Fatigue and weakness are common side effects, probably as a consequence of secondary adrenal insufficiency. This agent lacks gluconeogenic activity and does not appear to produce cushingoid features.

The long-term effects of these agents on fertility is not known. For the treatment of CPP, medroxyprogesterone acetate and cyproterone acetate have now been replaced by the much more effective GnRH agonists; however, they may be used as back-up agents for the occasional patients who develop untoward effects from GnRH agonist therapy.

TABLE 25-31

Objectives for the Management and Treatment of True Precocious Puberty

Detection and treatment of an expanding intracranial lesion
Arrest of premature sexual maturation until the normal age at onset of puberty
Regression of secondary sexual characteristics already present
Attainment of normal mature height; suppression of the rapid rate of skeletal maturation
Prevention of emotional disorders and handicaps and alleviation of parental anxiety; promotion of understanding by counseling, early sex education, and acceleration of social age
Reduction of risk of sexual abuse and early sexual debut
Prevention of pregnancy in girls
Preservation of future fertility
Diminishment of the increased risk of breast cancer associated with early menarche

From Grumbach MM. True or central precocious puberty. In: Krieger DT, Bardin CW, eds. *Current Therapy in Endocrinology and Metabolism, 1985-1986.* Toronto, Canada: BC Decker, 1989:4-8.

TABLE 25-32

Action of Gonadotropin-Releasing Hormone Agonists in True Precocious Puberty

A selective, highly specific pharmacologic clamp on the secretion of gonadotropin that produces a "medical gonadectomy"
- Chronic administration induces desensitization of the pituitary gonadotroph to the action of endogenous GnRH

As a consequence:
- Inhibition of pulsatile secretion of LH and FSH
- Inhibition of gonadotropin secretion results in a striking decrease in gonadal steroid output by testes or ovaries and reduction in gonadal size

FSH, follicle-stimulating hormone; GnRH, gonadotropin-releasing hormone; LH, luteinizing hormone.

Superactive Gonadotropin-Releasing Hormone Agonists. The GnRH agonists, synthetic analogues of the amino acid sequence of the natural GnRH decapeptide, are the treatment of choice for CPP of any cause (Tables 25-32 and 25-33).

After initial stimulation, these pharmacologic agents suppress pulsatile LH and FSH release, gonadal steroid output, and gametogenesis, similar to the effects of continuous administration of natural GnRH, which suppresses gonadotropin secretion[328,814,815] after an initial, brief stimulation of gonadotropin release. The agonist binds to the GnRH receptor on gonadotrophs, and this is followed by desensitization of the gonadotroph to GnRH and down-regulation and loss of receptors. Desensitization persists after receptor levels return to normal as a result of uncoupling of the receptors from the intracellular signaling effector pathway.[816] This regimen functions as a selective, highly specific pharmacologic clamp on the secretion of gonadotropins without interfering directly with release of the other pituitary hormones. In essence, the regimen produces a reversible medical gonadectomy (see Table 25-32).

The superactive agonist analogues of GnRH have about 15 to 200 times the potency of the natural GnRH decapeptide, prolonged action, and low toxicity (see Table 25-33). Replacing the glycine-amide terminus of GnRH with alkyl amines (i.e., ethylamide [NEt]), as in [Pro^9-NEt]GnRH; substituting certain D-amino acids at position 6, as in [D-Trp^6] GnRH; or making bulky hydrophobic alterations at position 6, as in [D-Nal(2)^6]GnRH increases the potency and duration of action.[817] These changes make the molecule more resistant to enzymatic degradation, increase the binding affinity of the analogue for the receptor on the pituitary gonadotroph, increase hydrophobicity, and, with some analogues, increase binding to plasma proteins.[389,817,818]

The suppressive effects of the GnRH agonists on gonadotropin secretion make them useful in the treatment of CPP[389,760,819-823] and they are also used in endometriosis and prostatic carcinoma. Although an every-12-week formulation of leuprorelin (leuprolide acetate) has shown success in clinical trials as treatment for CPP and has been FDA-approved for adults,[824] the pediatric depot preparation of leuprorelin is currently the only one that has FDA approval for administration every 4 weeks to children; long-term studies have established its efficacy and safety.[825,826] The bioavailability of agonists given intranasally is much reduced,[389,827] as reflected in the need to use a high dose at more frequent intervals. Recently, a subcutanesus implant of histrelin was approved for 12-month treatment of CPP.

TABLE 25-33

Gonadotropin-Releasing Hormone Agonists: Pharmacologic Treatment of True Precocious Puberty*

	Potency	Formula	Dosage Form	Dose	References
Structure of Natural GnRH					
GnRH (potency 1): <Glu-His-Pro-Ser-Trip-Gly-Leu-Arg-Pro-Gly-NH_2> 1 2 3 4 5 6 7 8 9 10					
Substitutions in GnRH Agonist Analogues					
Deslorelin: D-Trp^6, -Net	150	[D- Trp^{6}Pro^{9}NEt]GnRH	SQ Depot-IM	4-8 μg/kg/day	389, 760, 790, 792, 819, 822, 1065, 1066
Nafarelin: D-Nal(2)^6	150	[D- Nal(2)^{6}Pro^{9}NEt]GnRH	SQ Intranasal	4 μg/kg/day 800-1600 μg/day	389, 760, 1065
Leuprolide: D-Leu^6, -Net	20	[D- Leu^6-Pro^{9}NEt]GnRH	SQ Depot-IM	20-50 μg/kg/day 140-300 μg/kg/mo	1067, 1068, Kaplan and Grumbach 1991†
Buserlin: D-Ser(tBu)^6, -Net	20	[D- Ser(tBu)^{6}Pro^{9}NEt]GnRH	SQ Intranasal	20-40 μg/kg/day 1200-1800 μg/day	820, 823, 827, 1069, 1070, 1071, 1072, 1073
Tryptorelin: D-Trp^6	35	[D-Trp^6]GnRH	SQ Depot-IM	20-40 μg/kg/day 60 μg/kg/mo	1074, 1075
Histerelin: D-His(Bzt)^6, -Net	150	[D- His(Bzt)^{6}NEt]GnRH	SQ implant	12-mo pellet	

*Superscripted numbers indicate substitution at that position of the specified amino acid; -NEt indicates replacement of the terminal glycine-amide with ethylamide.

†Unpublished data.

GnRH, luteinizing hormone–releasing hormone; IM, intramuscular; SQ, subcutaneous.

Modified from Grumbach MM, Kaplan SL. Recent advances in the diagnosis and management of sexual precocity. *Acta Paediatr Jpn.* 1988;30(suppl):155-175.

The effectiveness of GnRH agonists in the treatment of CPP varies with the potency of the analogue, dose, route of administration, and compliance.[389,760,816,828]

Treatment of CPP with a potent GnRH agonist results in 1 to 3 days of increased FSH and LH release and a rise in circulating gonadal steroid levels, followed after 7 to 14 days of treatment by suppression of pulsatile secretion of LH and FSH and of the pubertal LH response to the administration of native GnRH (Figs. 25-56 and 25-57). The isoforms of gonadotropins tend toward a more basic charge. A plasma estradiol concentration of less than 18 pmol/L (5 pg/mL) in girls or a plasma testosterone level of less than 0.7 nmol/L (20 ng/dL) in boys indicates adequate gonadal suppression; this occurs within about 2 to 4 weeks in girls and 6 weeks in boys. GnRH agonist therapy does not affect the secretion of adrenal androgens.[389,790,819]

Changes in secondary sexual characteristics within the first 6 months of therapy (Fig. 25-58) include reduction in breast size and decrease in pubic hair, cessation of menses if present before treatment, and decreased size of the uterus and ovaries as assessed by pelvic sonography in girls. Some girls have recurrent episodes of hot flushes and moodiness. In boys, pubic hair thins, the testes decrease in size, acne and seborrhea regress, penile erections and masturbation become much less frequent, the high energy level and aggressive behavior diminish, and self-esteem improves.

Height velocity decreases by about 60% during the first year of therapy, with greater decreases found in those with the most advanced bone age and taller relative height.[829] Skeletal maturation slows dramatically during the first 3 years, to a rate that often is less than the progression in chronologic age. From the second year on, height velocity for bone age is usually appropriate (Fig. 25-59). Bone age is suggested to represent a surrogate for growth plate senescence due to prior exposure to estrogens. Those with the longest courses before treatment, the most advanced physical findings, and the most rapid bone age advancement before therapy have the lowest growth velocities on treatment.

The rate of growth during treatment with GnRH agonists is inversely related to the bone age at the start of therapy[265]; best results occur when treatment is begun soon after the onset of precocity and when the bone age is advanced by only a few years.[830] There is a striking benefit for those children treated before 5 years of age (girls' height, 164.3 ± 7.7 cm) compared with those treated after age 5 years (157.6 ± 6.6 cm) or with untreated patients (152.7 ± 8.6 cm).[743] Adult height in children treated with GnRH agonists is improved, especially when therapy starts before 6 years of age rather than after 8 years of age (Table 25-34).[474,743,831] Treatment in children with onset of puberty after 6 years of age is not of proven efficacy in increasing adult height. An adult height within the target height occurs with therapy in about 90% of girls and boys.[832] We recommend treatment of all affected children with onset of puberty before 6 years of age to ensure an optimal prognosis for adult height. The optimal age at which to discontinue therapy is undetermined because the post-treatment growth spurt is important in determining adult height.[474]

The addition of hGH treatment to the GnRH regimen is a consideration when growth velocity is reduced sufficiently over a 6-month period to compromise predicted final height.[833] This is in contrast to the concern raised regarding therapy with GnRH agonist and GH in normal variant short stature of CDP. This combination is not proven by evidence-based study.[474]

In a preliminary study, the GnRH antagonist, cetrorelix, appeared to bring about more rapid suppression of gonadotropin secretion and to eliminate the flare-up of gonadotropin secretion after administration of GnRH agonist. There are no reports at present concerning the use of cetrorelix as a sole treatment of precocious puberty, but in one unusual case, a girl with purported gonadotropin-independent precocious puberty responded to this treatment, bringing up a possible direct effect of the agent on ovarian function.[834] This agent suppresses ovarian but not adrenal function and was proposed to be useful as a test to differentiate the origin of severe hyperandrogenism in adolescence.[835]

Girls with CPP have a tendency toward obesity that is unrelated to treatment with GnRH agonist[474,785,836,837]; there is no substantial evidence that GnRH treatment fosters the development of obesity. The BMI before therapy predicts

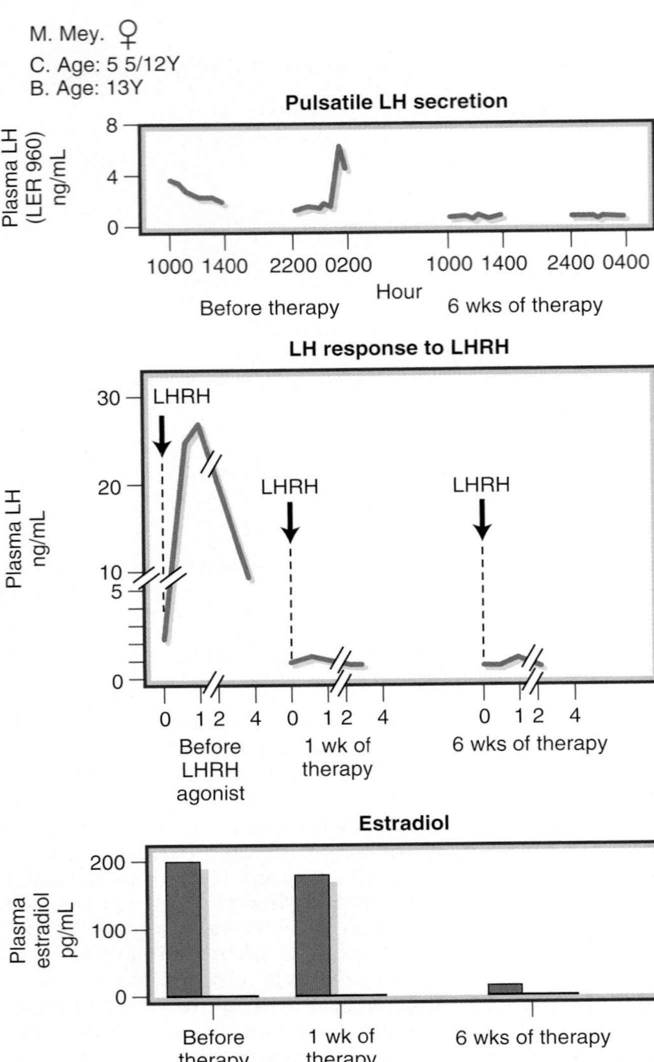

Figure 25-56 Effect of administration of the gonadotropin-releasing hormone (GnRH) agonist deslorelin (4 μg/kg/day subcutaneously) on pulsatile secretion of luteinizing hormone (LH) *(top)*, LH response to GnRH *(middle)*, and plasma concentration of estradiol *(bottom)* in a 5-year, 1-month-old girl with idiopathic true precocious puberty. This patient, who had a bone age of 13 years when treatment was begun, has been administered deslorelin for 7 years. During this period, the estimated predicted final height increased by 15 cm. Surprisingly, the bone age advanced by only about 6 months on serial examinations for several years. (Modified from Grumbach MM, Kaplan SL. Recent advances in the diagnosis and management of sexual precocity. *Acta Paediatr Jpn.* 1988;30[suppl]:155-175.)

the BMI value after cessation.[837-839] However, a recent longitudinal study suggested that, with adequate gonadotropin suppression, BMI for age may improve after at least 2 years of therapy.[840] Serum leptin values in patients with precocious puberty remains in line with the average for children of similar BMI and pubertal development.[841]

The IGF1 concentration in CPP correlates best with the stage of puberty and the plasma concentration of testosterone or estradiol.[276] Treatment with GnRH agonist reduces the level of IGF1 to the normal range for bone age but not for chronologic age.[276] Gonadal steroids increase plasma IGF1 concentrations in CPP, as in normal puberty. Secretion of GH is increased in CPP to a level comparable to that observed in normal puberty.[756] Treatment with GnRH agonist usually results in decreased secretion of GH, most strikingly during sleep, and in a decreased GH response to provocative stimuli.

The depot formulations of GnRH agonists provide continuous exposure to the drug with a single intramuscular injection every 4 weeks (as described earlier) and minimize the problem of compliance.[743,842] However, irregular or inadequate treatment or poor compliance results in persistent or intermittent increase in the concentration of plasma gonadal steroids, leading to decreased growth but advancing bone age.

Regular assessment is essential, initially at intervals of 1 to 3 months, and should include periodic determinations of plasma testosterone levels in boys and estradiol levels in girls; change in basal concentrations of LH and FSH as measured by third-generation assays or in the LH and FSH response to exogenous GnRH or GnRH agonists; growth, bone age, and secondary sexual characteristics; and, in girls, serial evaluations of ovarian morphology and uterine size by pelvic sonography. A decrease in the size of the ovaries and uterus on pelvic sonography occurs with successful GnRH agonist treatment.[790,843] Because GnRH is not available, the rise in serum LH and FSH is evaluated 30 to 120 minutes after administration of the GnRH agonist.[844,845] The LH and FSH responses to GnRH agonist are suppressed with effective therapy, but because standards differ between laboratories, actual cutoff values may differ in clinical practice, depending on location. A 1-year Silastic implant of the histrelin GnRH agonist, although it involves a surgical procedure, eliminates the need to titrate the dose and repeat testing for maximal effect; a second treatment year is reported to be effective.[846]

Whereas urinary excretion of LH correlates with the stage of pubertal development in normal subjects, urinary gonadotropin determinations are not sufficiently sensitive to be used for monitoring purposes in children with CPP.

TABLE 25-34

Effect of GnRH Agonist Treatment on Adult or Near-Adult Height and Height Gain

Chronologic Age at Start of Therapy	No. Patients	Mean Current Height (cm)		Mean Height Gain (cm)*
		Female	*Male*	
Untreated†				
Total	116	152.7 ± 8.6	155.6 ± 7.7	
<5 yr	41	150.2 ± 7.6	153.3 ± 7.1	
>5 yr	75	153.4 ± 8.4	161.3 ± 6.0	
GnRH-Treated‡				
UCSF	26	160.5 ± 6.6	166.3 ± 12.2	
<5 yr	11	164.3 ± 7.7	172.1	10.0 F; 11.1 M
>5 yr	15	157.6 ± 6.6	163.3 ± 13.0	4.0 F; 6.0 M
Reference Untreated Study				
Oerter	40	157.8 ± 5.9	168.8 ± 8.3	5.2 F; 6.7 M
Kauli	8	151.2 ± 5.9		5.8 F
Boepple	26	154.4		4.1 F

*Final predicted height minus initial predicted height (Bayley-Pinneau method).
†Final height.
‡Final or near-final height.
F, female; GnRH, gonadotropin-releasing hormone; M, male; UCSF, University of California, San Francisco.
From Paul D, Conte FA, Grumbach MM, et al. Long-term effect of gonadotropin-releasing hormone agonist therapy on final and near-final height in 26 children with true precocious puberty treated at a median age of less than 5 years. *J Clin Endocrinal Metab.* 1995;80:546-551.

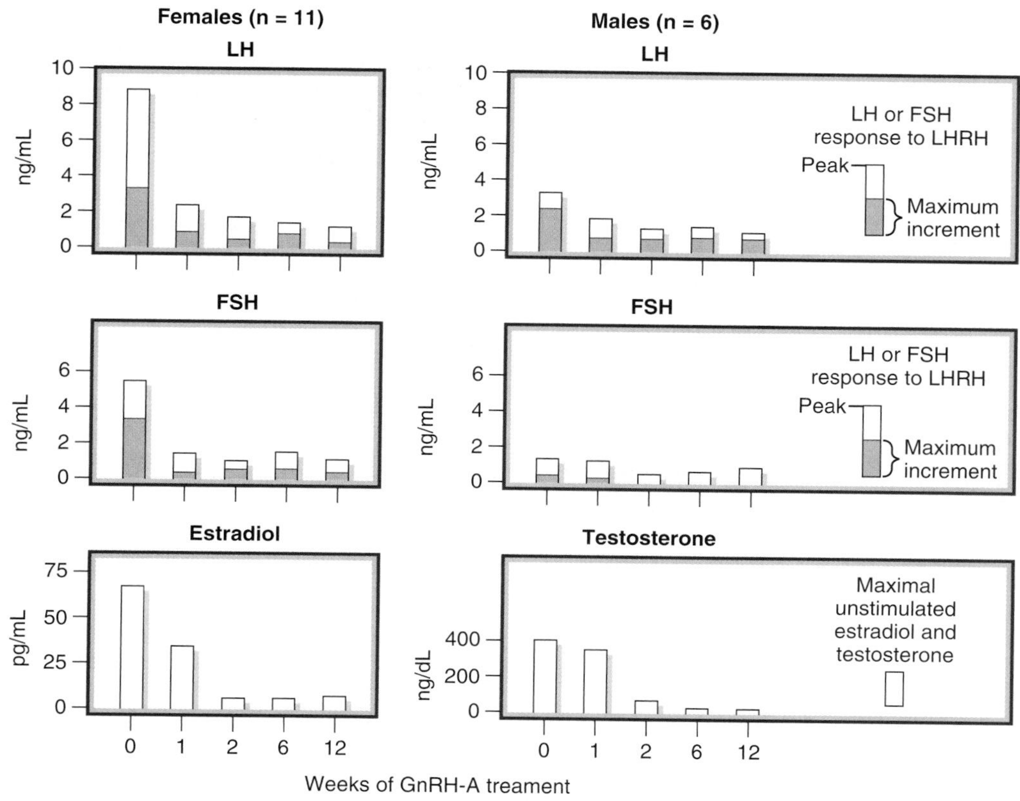

Figure 25-57 Deslorelin treatment (4 μg/kg/day subcutaneously) of girls and boys with true precocious puberty. Effects were seen during the first 12 weeks of treatment on the luteinizing hormone (LH) and follicle-stimulating hormone (FSH) response to a challenge with gonadotropin-releasing hormone (GnRH) (mean peak response and maximum increment) and on the maximal unstimulated concentration of plasma estradiol in the girls and of plasma testosterone in the boys. Notice the relatively rapid change from pubertal values to prepubertal values. For conversion to SI units, see Figures 25-16 and 25-17. (From Styne DM, Harris DA, Egli CA, et al. Treatment of true precocious puberty with a potent luteinizing hormone releasing factor agonist: effect on growth, sexual maturation, pelvic sonography, and the hypothalamic pituitary gonadal axis. *J Clin Endocrinol Metab.* 1985;61:142-181. Copyright by The Endocrine Society.)

When treatment is discontinued, even after 8 years, gonadal suppression is reversed within a few weeks to months, as manifested by a rise in the concentration of plasma gonadal steroids, progression of sexual maturation, and return of menses.[785,847,848] Menarche occurred at an average of 1.2 to 1.5 years after discontinuation of therapy (range, 0 to 60 months). Ovulation had occurred in 50% of girls by 1 year after menarche and in 90% of those studied 2 or more years after menarche.[849] Mean ovarian volume was found to remain greater than in normal subjects, and the LH response to GnRH was less than the normal response.[785,832]

The reversible nature of the therapy has also been confirmed in boys with CPP, because gonadotropins in the basal or GnRH-stimulated state return to normal pubertal values by 1 year after cessation of therapy.[791] Testicular size may take longer to reach normal values.

A report of 46 women studied 12.5 years after cessation of treatment with GnRH agonist revealed an adult height 1.6 cm, or 0.3 SD, below target height, with no evidence of reproductive impairment nor apparent PCOS or hirsutism.[850] However, an increased prevalence of PCOS has been reported in young women (mean age, 18.1 years) with a history of CPP, with onset at a mean age of 7.65 years.[851] Thirty-two percent of the patients had PCOS according to the Rotterdam definition, and 30% had PCOS according to the Androgen Excess Society; the most common presentation was clinical or biochemical hyperandrogenism, or both, and polycystic ovarian morphology. The study authors did not find any other predictive factors for the development of PCOS when the diagnosis of CPP was made. These girls would not have qualified for the diagnosis of CPP based on the newest criteria, so it is of concern that these girls with early rather than precocious puberty had such a high prevalence of PCOS.

An international consensus conference convened by the Lawson Wilkins Pediatric Endocrine Society and the European Society for Pediatric Endocrinology reviewed all the world literature on the use of GnRH to determine, in an evidence-based approach, the appropriate use of the agent in precocious puberty. However, few controlled prospective studies have been performed with gonadotropin-releasing hormone analogues in children, so many of the conclusions relied in part on collective expert opinion. The major conclusions were as follows[474]:

- GnRH analogues exert benefit in increasing adult height in children with early-onset CPP (<6 years in girls) and are not routinely recommended after that age.
- The psychosocial effects of CPP and their alteration by GnRH analogues require additional study.
- The use of GnRH analogues does not appear to cause weight gain or long-term diminution of BMD.
- The use of GnRH analogues for conditions other than CPP, such as to increase adult height in children with idiopathic short stature or SGA, or with GH treatment in children, is not recommended.

Although psychosocial factors and parental anxiety that adversely affect the well-being of the child need to be assessed in the decision to initiate GnRH agonist treatment,

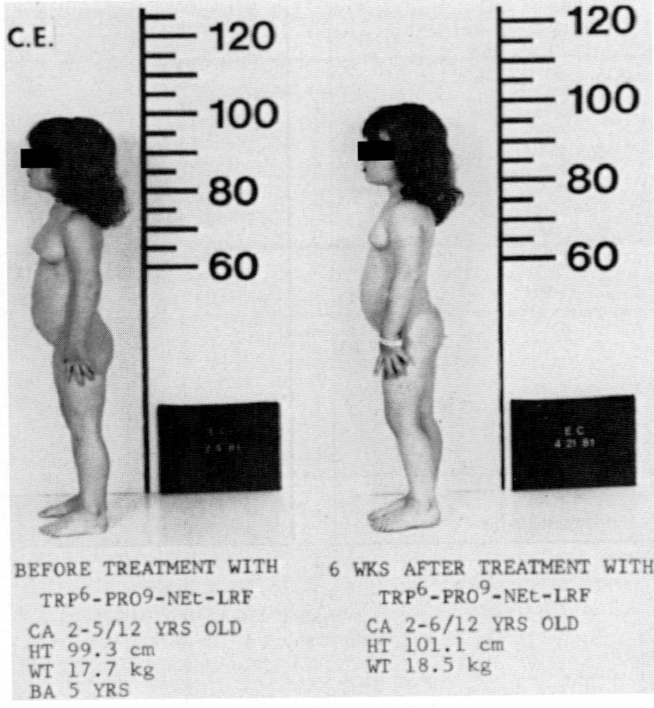

Figure 25-58 A girl aged 2 years and 5 months with true precocious puberty after 6 weeks of deslorelin therapy (4 μg/day subcutaneously). Notice the regression in the size of the breasts; however, the rapid rate of growth had not decreased. At the end of 1 year of therapy, the growth rate was suppressed to 4 cm/year, and bone age advanced only 1 year. BA, bone age; CA, chronologic age; HT, height; WT, weight. (From Styne DM, Grumbach MM. Puberty in the male and female: its physiology and disorders. In: Yen SCC, Jaffe RB, eds. *Reproductive Endocrinology,* 2nd ed. Philadelphia, PA: Saunders, 1986:313-384.)

this therapy cannot be routinely recommended for such concerns (Table 25-35).

Adverse Effects. Rare reactions to GnRH agonists include local and systemic allergic reactions, including asthmatic episodes when the agent is given intranasally. The prevalence of a sterile abscess at the site of intramuscular injection of long-acting repository preparations, including leuprorelin and triptorelin, is clearly increased (5% to 10%); these reactions are unpredictable and intermittent and in most instances are related to the polylactic and polyglycolic polymer and not to the GnRH agonist itself.[826] Switching to daily subcutaneous injections of non-depot preparations or to intranasal preparations is rarely associated with a recurrence. A small increase in serum prolactin above normal limits was described in girls after treatment with GnRH agonist, but galactorrhea was not observed.[852] Volumetric BMD and peak bone mass are normal during and after discontinuation of GnRH therapy.[474] Calcium and vitamin D intake must be ensured during treatment to achieve optimal skeletal health.[853] However, high fruit and vegetable intake (defined as more than three servings per day, lower than the U.S. government recommended intake) is desirable in all children and may serve in early puberty as a factor to increase bone density, possibly because of decreasing calcium excretion in the urine.[854]

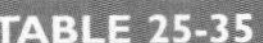

TABLE 25-35

Indications for Therapy with Gonadotropin-Releasing Hormone Agonists in True or Central Precocious Puberty

In children with clinical and unequivocal endocrine features of idiopathic true precocious puberty:
- Rapid advancement over a period of 6-12 mo of secondary sex characteristics, height, height velocity, and bone age (increased >2.5 SD for chronologic age) in affected boys and girls
- A plasma testosterone concentration sustained >2.5 nmol/L (>75 ng/dL) in boys <8 yr of age determined by sensitive, specific immunoassay
- A plasma estradiol concentration, recurrently ≥36 pmol/L (≥10 pg/mL) determined by a sensitive, specific assay capable of quantifying low concentrations of estradiol
- Onset of menarche (and recurrent menses) in girls <9 yr of age
- Psychosocial factors and parental anxiety, including evidence that the child's psychosocial well-being is adversely affected

In children with neurogenic or organic true precocious puberty, especially those with associated GH deficiency, the course is almost invariably progressive and LHRH treatment should not be delayed

LHRH, luteinizing hormone–releasing hormone; SD, standard deviation.

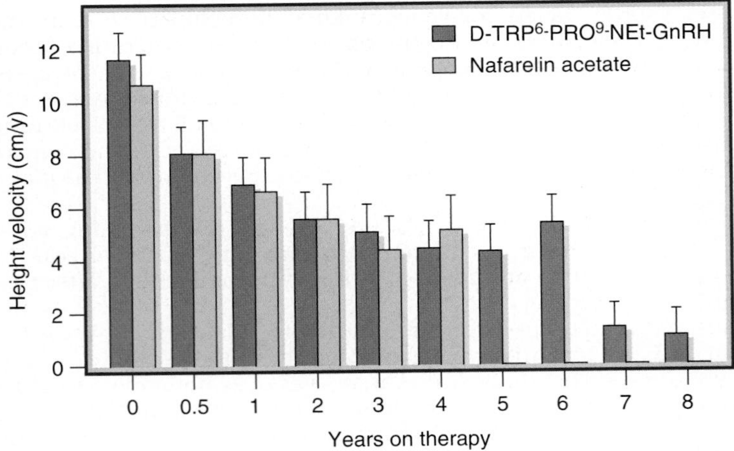

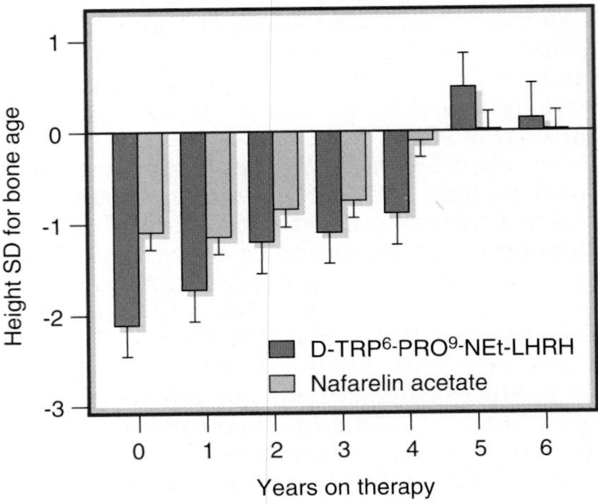

Figure 25-59 Effect of gonadotropin-releasing hormone (GnRH) agonist therapy in true precocious puberty on growth. *Left,* Changes in mean height velocity (cm/year ± 1 SE) after the initiation of GnRH agonist therapy with DTrp^{6}Pro^{9}Net (deslorelin) *(darker bars)* or with nafarelin *(lighter bars).* A sharp decrease in height velocity occurred within 1 year. *Right,* Mean (±1 SE) height for bone age before and during GnRH agonist treatment. The discrepancy between height and the more advanced bone age decreases (reverts to normal) with chronic GnRH agonist treatment. (From Kaplan SL, Grumbach MM. True precocious puberty: treatment with GnRH agonists. In: Delemarre-Van de Waal H, Plant TM, van Rees GP, et al, eds. *Control of the Onset of Puberty,* 3rd ed. Amsterdam, The Netherlands: Elsevier, 1989:357-373.)

Four patients were reported to have developed slipped capital femoral epiphyses during or just after treatment of CPP with GnRH agonist.[855] Slipped capital epiphyses occur mostly during the earliest phase of puberty, when growth is beginning to increase, and not after fusion of the triradiate cartilage, so these cases may have a different etiologic course than that found in average pubertal children.

Psychosocial Aspects. Psychological management is a critical aspect of the care of children with CPP.[389,795,856,857] With the advanced physical maturation for chronologic age, these children tend to seek friends closer to their size, strength, and physical development. Difficulties may arise because they lack the social skills of older children. Sex education of the child and the family is essential and must be given in a skillful, sensitive, and explicit manner; the risks of sexual abuse (in both sexes) and of pregnancy need to be discussed. The parents need to be informed about the management of menses. The onset of sexual activity may be earlier than average but usually remains within the normal range.

It is imperative to provide support in handling the increased height, the advanced sexual maturation, and the effects of gonadal steroids on behavior, activity, and emotional stability. The unrealistic demands and expectations that arise from the discrepancy between the child's physique and his or her chronologic, mental, and psychosexual age require wise counseling, as do the reactions to ridicule by peers and the concern about being different from age-mates. Some of these problems have been mitigated by school acceleration, in which the child is advanced by one or two grades, if this is consistent with the mental and emotional development. These comments are applicable to children with all forms of sexual precocity; the effectiveness of GnRH agonists has reduced but not eliminated many of these issues in CPP.[795]

The GnRH agonists are useful in conjunction with GH in the management of organic or neurogenic CPP with associated GH deficiency (usually as a result of irradiation of the brain), and their use has been advocated even in the absence of precocious puberty to allow a longer period of GH treatment before epiphyseal fusion. A few, usually short-term, studies have evaluated the combination, with variable results. This regimen is experimental, and its cost-effectiveness needs to be considered (see earlier discussion).[474]

Aromatase inhibitors (e.g., letrozole) decrease or eliminate the effect of estrogen on bone age advancement. They may be useful to improve height prognosis in sexual precocity in boys,[150,151,477,858] but no controlled studies are available, and there has been mixed success with aromatase inhibitors in the treatment of incomplete ISP.[859,860] Controlled studies are necessary to establish the safety and efficacy and, especially, the effects on adult bone density, which remains a worrisome subject (Table 25-36).

TABLE 25-36

Potential Use of Aromatase Inhibitors or Estrogen Receptor Antagonists in Disorders of Growth and Sexual Maturation

Growth Disorders or Variants of Normal Growth
Isolated growth hormone deficiency • To restrain epiphyseal maturation Genetic short stature/constitutional delay in growth • To restrain epiphyseal maturation
Sexual Precocity
Congenital virilizing adrenal hyperplasia in male and female • To reduce dose of glucocorticoid • To inhibit conversion of C19 steroids to estrogens (or estrogen action) • With or without use of 17,20-lyase inhibitor of anti-androgen Testotoxicosis • To inhibit conversion of C19 steroids to estrogens McCune-Albright syndrome • To inhibit conversion of C19 steroids to estrogens (or estrogen action)
Adolescent Gynecomastia
• To inhibit estrogen synthesis (or estrogen action)

From Grumbach MM. Estrogen, bone, growth, and sex: a sea change in conventional wisdom. *J Pediatr Endocrinol Metab.* 2000;13(suppl 6):1439-1455.

Incomplete Isosexual Precocity: Gonadotropin-Releasing Hormone–Independent Sexual Precocity

In incomplete forms of ISP, such as GnRH-independent sexual precocity (GISP), the secretion of testosterone in boys and estrogen in girls is independent of the hypothalamic GnRH pulse generator (see Table 25-25). There is no pubertal LH response to GnRH or GnRH, and there is no pubertal pattern of pulsatile LH secretion. Patients do not respond to chronic GnRH agonist therapy with suppression of gonadal steroid output. ISP is a consequence of gonadal or adrenal steroid secretion that is independent of GnRH, iatrogenic exposure to gonadal steroids, or, in boys, rare hCG- or LH-secreting tumors.

Boys

Chorionic Gonadotropin–Secreting Tumors. Several types of germ cell tumors secrete hCG, which may cross-react in some polyclonal LH assays (although they are rarely used presently) and will lead to a positive pregnancy screen. Boys with hCG-secreting neoplasms have slightly enlarged testes (although not to a size consistent with the size of the phallus and other male secondary sex characteristics, because the seminiferous tubules are not affected), and it may be difficult to differentiate these patients from boys in the early stages of CPP on the basis of physical examination alone.[741,861] However, plasma hCG levels are elevated without an increase in the concentration of FSH or LH measured in specific assays.

Boys with hepatoma or hepatoblastoma present with hepatomegaly or firm, irregular liver nodules, anemia, and precocious puberty[862]; these are among the most serious of hCG-secreting tumors (Fig. 25-60). hCG is localized to multinucleated tumor giant cells; α-fetoprotein was found in the embryonal-type tumor cells of the hepatoblastoma in one case. The mean age at onset is 2 years, 8 months, but average survival is only 10.7 months after diagnosis.[863]

Infantile choriocarcinoma is also associated with elevated hCG and is thought to originate in the placenta; infants may be diagnosed at 1 month of age, with a survival time of only 3 months.[864] About 20% of mediastinal germ cell tumors occur in boys with 47,XXY or mosaic Klinefelter's syndrome, a prevalence 30 to 50 times more common than in unaffected boys. Plasma α-fetoprotein is a useful additional marker for yolk sac (endodermal sinus) or mixed germ cell tumors[865]; the cells in the tumor that secrete α-fetoprotein appear to differ from those that secrete hCG. Rarely, the germ cells contain enough aromatase activity to convert circulating C19 precursors (of adrenal origin after adrenarche) to estradiol, which in some instances is sufficient to induce breast development.[866,867]

Some teratomas, chorioepitheliomas, and mixed germ cell tumors in the hypothalamic region (or in the mediastinum, lungs, gonads, or retroperitoneum); certain pineal

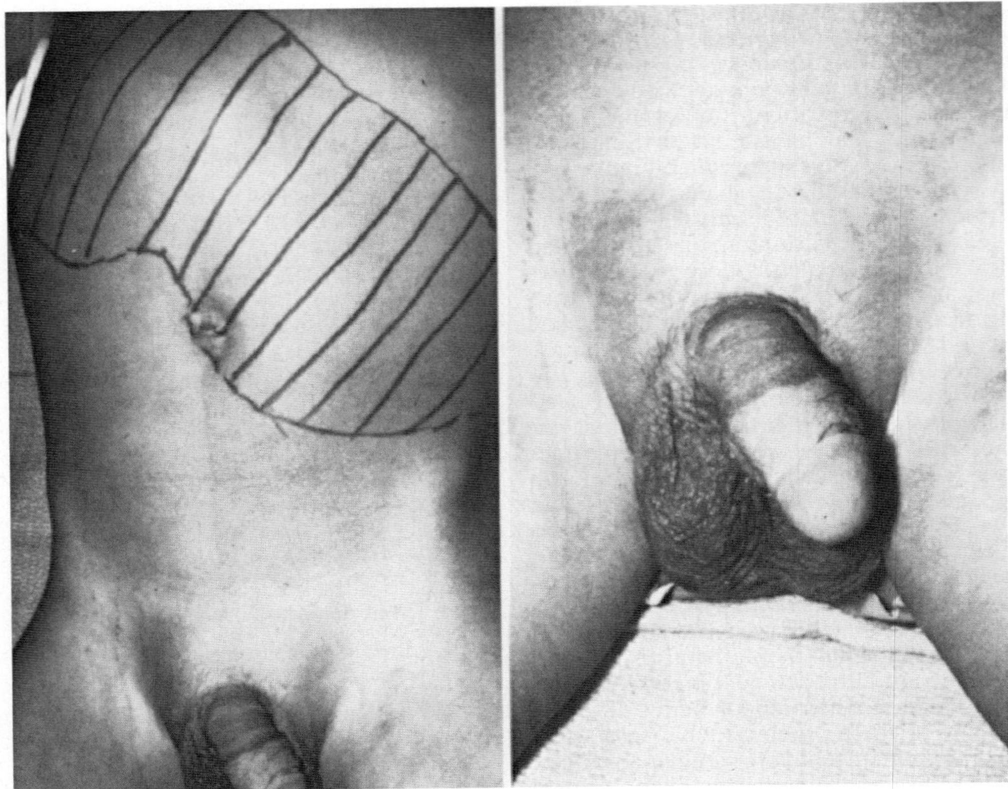

Figure 25-60 A boy aged 1 years and 5 months with a human chorionic gonadotropin (hCG)–secreting hepatoblastoma. Notice the outline of the large liver *(left)* and the penile enlargement *(right)*. The testes were 2 × 1 cm, and pubic hair was stage 2. The plasma hCG level was 50 mIU/mL; the plasma testosterone level was 168 ng/dL; and the plasma α-fetoprotein level was 160,000 ng/mL. Metastatic lesions in both lungs were seen on the chest radiograph. To convert testosterone values to SI units, see Figure 25-26. To convert hCG values to international units per liter, multiply by 1.0. To convert α-fetoprotein values to micrograms per liter, multiply by 1.0. (From Kaplan SL, Grumbach MM. Pathogenesis of sexual precocity. In: Grumbach MM, Sizonenko PC, Aubert ML, eds. *Control of the Onset of Puberty.* Baltimore, MD: Williams & Wilkins, 1990:620-660.)

tumors (usually a germ cell tumor or mixed germ cell tumor)[861,868]; and, less commonly, a chorioepithelioma or its variants cause sexual precocity in boys by secreting hCG rather than by activating the pituitary gonadotropin-gonadal axis via the hypothalamic GnRH pulse generator.

Calcification of the pineal is found in 8% to 11% of 8- to 11-year-old children and by itself is not indicative of a tumor. Intracranial germ cell tumors account for 3% to 11% of malignant CNS tumors in children and adolescents, with a predominance in the Far East.[869] Germ cell tumors of the hypothalamus or pineal region constitute fewer than 1% of primary CNS tumors in Western countries but account for 4.5% of such tumors in Japan. The prevalence of intracranial germ cell tumors is 2.6 times greater in males than in females, but germ cell tumors in the suprasellar-hypothalamic region do not exhibit a sex predominance and are generally associated with pituitary hormone deficiencies including diabetes insipidus and delayed puberty.[490] Germ cell tumors do not cause gonadotropin-induced ISP in females because of the paucity of effects of hCG in prepubertal females. However, CPP may occur through disinhibition of the hypothalamic GnRH pulse generator by local mass effects.

Germ cell tumors that secrete hCG are rarely located in the thalamus and basal ganglia. In "true" pure CNS germ cell tumors (germinomas), hCG cannot be readily detected in the circulation but may be detected in the cerebrospinal fluid.[490] In mixed germ cell tumors, hCG is commonly found in the blood as well as in cerebrospinal fluid. Extremely elevated levels of hCG in a CNS tumor suggest a primary intracranial choriocarcinoma or germ cell tumor with a high risk of tumor hemorrhage during biopsy, and surgical removal or debulking rather than diagnostic biopsy may be the initial operative approach.[870]

Mixed germ cell tumors and especially "pure" germinomas are radiosensitive, and if the bone age is less than 11 years, sexual precocity may regress, only to progress later into normal puberty.[861] Long-term survival is reported in 88% of patients with CNS germ cell tumors after appropriate therapy.[871] However, testicular germ cell tumors are occasionally found years after successful therapy for CNS germ cell tumors, so long-term surveillance is always indicated.[495]

Pineal cysts are a rare cause of CPP.[872]

All pituitary adenomas, including gonadotropin-secreting pituitary adenomas, are exceedingly rare in children. An LH-secreting pituitary adenoma (basal serum LH of 900 IU/L with no rise after GnRH) and a prolactin-secreting pituitary adenoma (215 μg/L) caused sexual precocity in two boys with serum testosterone levels of 7 nmol/L (200 ng/dL).[873] Prepubertal values returned after removal of these "chromophobe" adenomas with suprasellar extension.

Precocious Androgen Secretion Caused by the Adrenal Gland

Virilizing Congenital Adrenal Hyperplasia. Virilizing CAH caused by a defect in 21-hydroxylation (CYP21 deficiency) leads to elevated androgen concentrations and masculinization and is a common cause of GnRH-independent sexual precocity in boys.[874] Approximately 75% of patients with

CYP21 deficiency have salt loss resulting from impaired aldosterone secretion as well as low serum sodium and high serum potassium concentrations. Increased plasma concentrations of 17-hydroxyprogesterone, increased levels of urinary 17-ketosteroids and pregnanetriol, and advanced bone age and rapid growth are characteristic.

Treatment with glucocorticoids suppresses the abnormal androgen secretion and arrests virilization; treatment with mineralocorticoids, when necessary, corrects the electrolyte imbalance. Virilizing CAH accompanied by hypertension occurs in 11β-hydroxylase deficiency; the progressive virilization ceases and the blood pressure falls to normal with glucocorticoid therapy. All forms of CAH are inherited as autosomal recessive traits. Untreated virilizing CAH causes anovulatory amenorrhea in females and oligospermia in males; these conditions are reversible with treatment. Delayed treatment of virilizing CAH may reveal GnRH-dependent CPP (secondary CPP) as a consequence of the advanced somatic and hypothalamic maturation resulting from long exposure to adrenal androgen. Further difficulty is presented in the treatment of CAH during the pubertal years, when androgen secretion normally increases and increased clearance of glucocorticoids at puberty in girls may alter dosing requirements.

Virilizing Adrenal Tumor. Virilizing adrenal carcinomas or adenomas secrete large amounts of DHEA and DHEAS and, on occasion, testosterone. Glucocorticoids do not suppress the increased secretion of adrenal androgens to the normal range for age in carcinoma, as they do in CAH. Cushing's syndrome resulting from adrenal carcinoma may cause ISP and growth failure in boys. Rarely, an adrenal adenoma produces both testosterone and aldosterone, leading to sexual precocity and hypertension with hypokalemia.[875,876]

Adrenal rests, or heterotopic adrenal tissue in the testes, may enlarge (sometimes to massive size) with endogenous ACTH stimulation in boys who have untreated or inadequately treated CAH and may mimic bilateral or unilateral interstitial cell tumors. MRI sonography, including Doppler flow studies of the testes, is useful to define the extent and nature of the testicular masses. In boys in whom the testicular tumors are autonomous and unresponsive to glucocorticoid therapy or improved compliance, surgical management, including enucleation of the tumor or tumors, has been useful to prevent further damage to the testes and improve the potential for fertility.[877] LH receptors have been detected on adrenal/cortical cells,[878,879] so LH may stimulate the testes in some patients.

NROB1 (DAX1) Gene Mutations. Two cases of *NROB1* frameshift mutations demonstrated adrenal failure and GnRH-independent sexual precocity that was suppressible by glucocorticoid therapy but not by GnRH agonist. The exceedingly high ACTH levels, possibly acting through the human melanocortin 1 receptor present in human Leydig cells, may have been the underlying cause of the increased steroidogenesis and testosterone secretion that were reversed by glucocorticoid treatment. Because NR0B1 inhibits transactivation of SF1, a regulator of steroidogenic genes, loss of NR0B1 inhibition of SF1 transcriptional activity also may have had a role.[880,881]

Leydig Cell Tumor. Testicular tumors are rare in childhood, representing 1% to 2% of all pediatric solid tumors, and Leydig cell tumors make up only 1.5% of those.[882] Androgen-producing Leydig cell tumors are rare causes of sexual precocity in boys. They rarely are malignant and are slow growing but must be treated or epiphyseal fusion will limit height and precocious puberty will affect social development. They derive from primordial mesenchyme, are classified as interstitial cell tumors, and occur most frequently around the age of 4 to 5 years. Unilateral enlargement (often nodular) of the testis usually occurs in boys with this neoplasm (although 5% to 10% of cases are bilateral); in contrast, both testes are usually of normal size (small) for chronologic age in boys with CAH or a virilizing adrenal tumor.[883] Although LH receptor–activating mutations were detected in several boys with sporadic Leydig cell adenomas,[884] an absence of known mutations occurs in some cases.[882]

Women with a previous history of CAH or a virilizing tumor may exhibit ovarian hyperandrogenism associated with persistent elevation of LH despite successful treatment of their initial virilizing condition in childhood; this is not usually the case in women who have late-onset CAH.[885]

Familial or Sporadic Testotoxicosis. Pituitary gonadotropin–independent familial premature Leydig cell and germ cell maturation, or testotoxicosis,[886-891] causes boys to develop secondary sexual characteristics with penile enlargement, which may be present at birth,[887] and bilateral enlargement of testes to the early or midpubertal range, although the testes often are smaller than expected in relation to penile growth and pubertal maturation (Fig. 25-61). Premature maturation of Leydig and Sertoli cells and spermatogenesis occur.[886,887,889] Leydig cell hyperplasia may occur; the Leydig cells in affected boys produce dimeric inhibin B as well as tesoterone,[892] and Leydig cells and spermatogonia stain positively for the α and $β_B$ segments of inhibin. The rate of linear growth is rapid, skeletal maturation is advanced, and muscular development is prominent. The presence of prepubertal basal and GnRH-stimulated gonadotropin concentrations, lack of a pubertal pattern of LH pulsatility (as measured by immunologic or bioassay techniques), and normal pubertal or adult testosterone levels and clearance of testosterone are characteristic (Table 25-37).[887] The onset of adrenarche and its biochemical marker, serum DHEAS, correlate with bone age rather than chronologic age.

Treatment with an GnRH agonist does not suppress testicular function or maturation.[887,890] In late childhood or early adolescence, fertility is achieved and an adult pattern of LH secretion and response to GnRH is demonstrable[888]; secondary GnRH-dependent CPP may be superimposed on the substrate of testotoxicosis.[888,889,893] In some adults, impaired spermatogenic function is associated with elevated concentrations of plasma FSH.[888] Testotoxicosis may occur sporadically, probably as a consequence of a germline mutation or even a postzygotic one, but it is usually inherited as a sex-limited autosomal dominant trait[888]; this probably accounts for the earlier descriptions of "true"

TABLE 25-37

Testotoxicosis: Clinical and Laboratory Characteristics

Sex-limited autosomal dominant inheritance; activating mutation in the gene encoding the LH receptor
Early onset of sexual precocity in boys, with bilateral testicular enlargement
Prepubertal immunologic and biologic LH response to GnRH; prepubertal LH pulse secretory pattern
Concentration of plasma testosterone in pubertal range
Premature Leydig cell and seminiferous tubule maturation
No CNS, adrenal, or testicular abnormalities demonstrable by radiologic or hormonal studies
Lack of suppression of plasma testosterone or physical signs of puberty by GnRH agonist

CNS, central nervous system; LH, luteinizing hormone; GnRH, gonadotropin-releasing hormone.

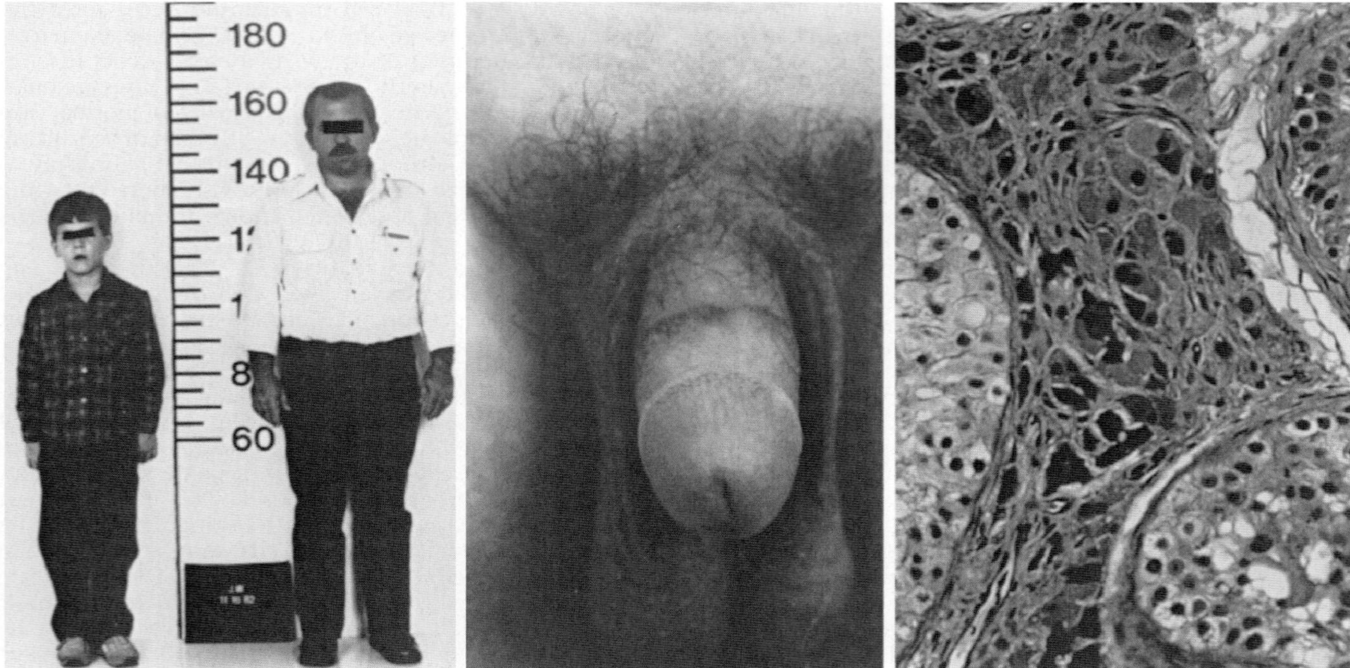

Figure 25-61 *Left,* A boy aged 5.5 years and his 28-year-old father with familial testotoxicosis. The boy exhibited signs of sexual precocity by 3 years of age. His height was 130.6 cm (+4.8 SD), and his bone age was 12.5 years. The plasma testosterone level was 267 ng/dL; the dihydrotestosterone level was 46 ng/dL; and the dehydroepiandrosterone sulfate (DHEAS) level was 23 µg/dL. The plasma luteinizing hormone (LH) and follicle-stimulating hormone (FSH) levels were low, and neither rose after treatment. Pulsatile LH secretion was not demonstrable. Treatment with deslorelin, a gonadotropin-releasing hormone (GnRH) agonist, had no effect. The father had begun sexual maturation by 3 years of age and had reached a final height of 162.6 cm in his early teens. The plasma testosterone level was 294 ng/dL; the LH level was 0.5 ng/mL (LER-960); and the FSH level was 0.5 ng/mL (LER-869). The father had an adult-type LH and FSH response to GnRH; the LH level increased to 7.5 ng/mL, and the FSH level increased to 2 ng/mL. At least 28 male family members over nine generations are affected. To convert dihydrotestosterone values to nanomoles per liter, multiply by 0.03467. For other conversions to SI units, see Figures 25-16 and 25-17. *Center,* External genitalia of the 5.5-year-old boy. The penis measured 12 × 2.8 cm,; the right testis was 4 × 2 cm, and the left testis was 3.5 × 2.5 cm. *Right,* Testis of the boy showed Leydig cell maturation without Reinke crystalloids and spermatogenesis (Mallory trichome stain).

precocious puberty in families in which only males were affected. A kindred with nine generations of affected males has been reported[888]; obligatory female carriers of the trait were unaffected, because constitutional activation of the LH receptor on the ovary causes no ill effects.[888,893]

Heterozygous activating mutations of the heterotrimeric G_s protein-coupled LHCGR that in concert transduce the LH/hCG signal to the main effector, adenyl cyclase, are the cause of testotoxicosis (Fig. 25-62).[893,894] The LH receptor cloned from the human[895] is a glycoprotein of 80 to 90 kd that belongs to a subfamily of the seven transmembrane–spanning, G protein–coupled receptors. The gene is localized to chromosome 2p21 (the same as for the FSH receptor); it spans at least 70 kilobases and contains 11 exons separated by 10 introns. The large glycosylated N-terminal extracellular hormone binding domain of the 701-amino-acid LHCGR[897] is encoded by exons 1 through 10. A single exon, the large exon 11, encodes the entire G protein–linked transmembrane domain with its seven α-helical segments connected by alternating extracellular and intracellular loops; the intracellular domain; and the three untranslated regions—almost two thirds of the receptor.[898]

Thirteen constitutive activating heterozygous missense mutations, all residing within exon 11, have been reported in more than 60 patients (see Fig. 25-62). Six of these mutations involved the transmembrane helix VI, two the flanking third cytoplasmic loop, one helix V, and one helix II; less commonly, mutations occurred in the first transmembrane helix.[894,895,899] Nine mutations were located between amino acid residues 542 and 581, suggesting a mutation hot spot. There appears to be a limited repertoire of mutations in American boys, consistent with a founder effect. European pedigrees are more diverse.[900] A model of the transmembrane domain of the receptor provides novel suggestions for the structural and functional effects of these activating mutations.[901] Transfected cultured cells with these mutations exhibited increased basal cAMP production in the absence of agonist, observations consistent with a constitutive activating mutation.[902] Various possibilities for the conformational changes in the LH receptor that lead to its constitutive activation have been considered.[903] Inactivating mutations of the LHCGR and their clinical consequences are discussed earlier in this chapter.

In one Polish family, the disorder, a Met298Thr mutation in the second transmembrane domain of the LH receptor, led to sexual precocity in one boy but not in the mother, who carried the same mutation, nor in her father (the maternal grandfather) or his son (the maternal uncle), suggesting the involvement of epigenetic factors.[904] Three boys with sexual precocity due to a sporadic Leydig cell adenoma had an Asp578His mutation in the tumor.[323,884]

Although affected boys do not respond to chronic administration of an GnRH agonist with suppression of testosterone secretion, testosterone secretion, height velocity and rate of bone maturation, and aggressive and hyperactive behavior have reportedly been decreased by treatment with oral medroxyprogesterone acetate (Table 25-38).[389,887]

Ketoconazole, an orally active substituted imidazole derivative, suppresses gonadal and adrenal biosynthesis by

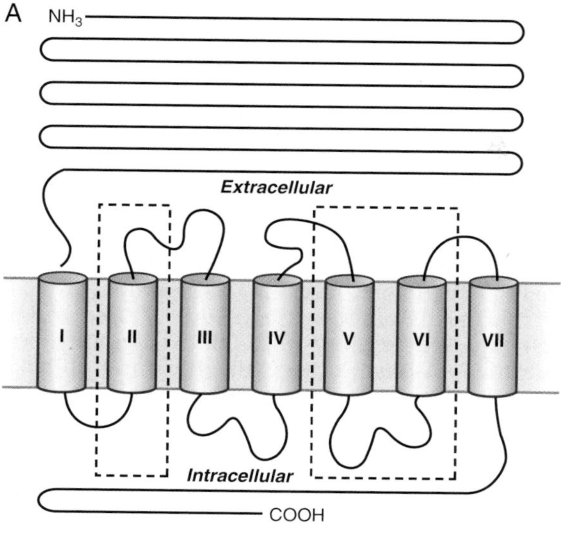

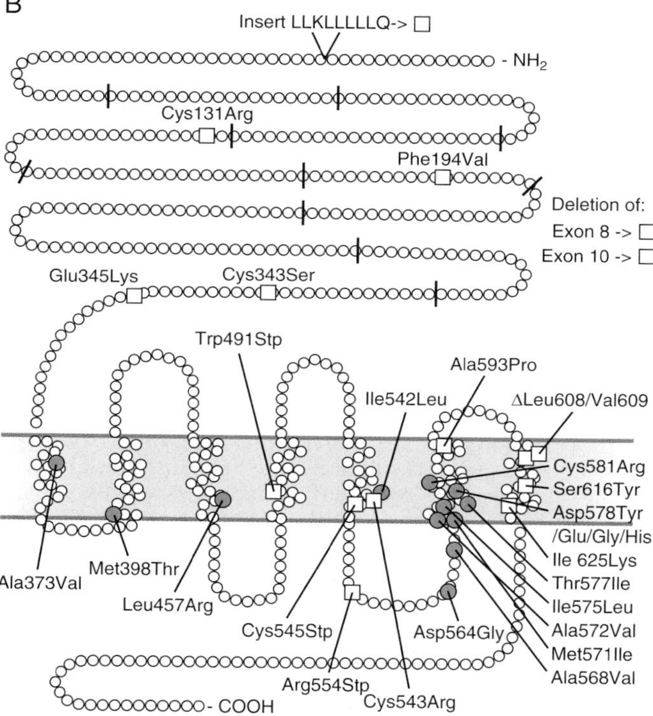

Figure 25-62 **A,** The serpentine, seven-transmembrane, G_s protein–coupled human luteinizing hormone/human chorionic gonadotropin (hLH/hCG) receptor with its large extracellular domain and the intracellular domain. The seven helical transmembrane domains are indicated by roman numerals. **B,** Mutations in the LH receptor protein are shown in the schematic structure of the LH receptor protein and localization of the inactivating *(open squares)* and activating *(solid circles)* mutations in the human LH receptor. Notice the cluster of mutations in the VI transmembrane helix and third cytoplasmic loop. The Asx578Gly mutation is the most common activating mutation. The short lines across the amino acid chain separate the 11 exons. (**A,** Redrawn from Yano K, Kohn LD, Saji M, et al. A case of male limited precocious puberty caused by a point mutation in the second transmembrane domain of the luteinizing hormone choriogonadotropin receptor gene. *Biochem Biophys Res Commun.* 1996;220:1036-1042.); **B,** from Themmen APN, Huhtaniemi IT. Mutations of gonadotropins and gonadotropin receptors. *Endocr Rev.* 2000;21:551-583.)

inhibiting the enzyme CYP17, which regulates both 17-hydroxylation and the scission (17,20-lyase) of 17α-hydroxypregnenolone (Δ^5-17P) to DHEA (see "Nature and Regulation of Adrenal Androgens"). In the dosage used for treatment of testotoxicosis (200 mg every 8 to 12 hours, given orally),[905] the agent produces a mild transient decrease in cortisol secretion and interferes with binding of testosterone to TeBG. Secondary CPP often occurs when the bone age advances to or has already reached the pubertal range (usually >11.5 years), at which time the addition of an GnRH agonist is appropriate.[905] Ketoconazole can cause hepatic injury, which is usually mild and reversible, but in rare cases hepatotoxicity is severe. Reversible renal injury, rash, and interstitial pneumonia were reported in a patient who tolerated lower doses, suggesting a dose-response effect.[906] Nonetheless, five patients treated with ketoconazole experienced no side effects other than one mild and transient elevation of liver enzymes; they had appropriate age of onset of true puberty and reached an adult height almost identical to the target height (a mean increase of 8 cm over the initially predicted height), suggesting great benefit of this therapy in this condition.[907]

TABLE 25-38

Pharmacologic Therapy for Sexual Precocity

Disorder	Treatment	Action and Rationale
GnRH Dependent		
True or central precocious puberty	GnRH agonists	Desensitization of gonadotropes; blocks action of endogenous GnRH
GnRH Independent		
Incomplete sexual precocity		
Girls		
Autonomous ovarian cysts	Medroxyprogesterone acetate	Inhibition of ovarian steroidogenesis; regression of cyst (inhibition of FSH release)
McCune-Albright syndrome	Medroxyprogesterone acetate*	Inhibition of ovarian steroidogenesis; regression of cyst (inhibition of FSH release)
	Third-generation aromatase inhibitor (e.g., letrozole)	Inhibition of P450 aromatase; blocks estrogen synthesis
Boys		
Familial testotoxicosis	Ketoconazole*	Inhibition of CYP17 (mainly 17,20-lyase activity)
	Flutamide or bicalatamide and letrozole or anactrozole	Anti-androgen Inhibition of aromatase; blocks estrogen synthesis
	Medroxyprogesterone acetate*	Inhibition of testicular steroidogenesis

*If true precocious puberty develops, an LHRH agonist can be added.

CYP17, cytochrome P450 17α-hydroxylase/17,20-lyase; LHRH, luteinizing hormone–releasing hormone; FSH, follicle-stimulating hormone; GnRH, luteinizing hormone–releasing hormone.

Modified from Grumbach MM, Kaplan SL. Recent advances in the diagnosis and management of sexual precocity. *Acta Paediatr Jpn.* 1988:30(suppl):155-175.

The antiandrogen (and antimineralocorticoid) spironolactone, in combination with testolactone, an inhibitor of aromatase (CYP19), the key enzyme in the conversion of androgens to estrogens, is also used to treat testotoxicosis.[908] The addition of a GnRH agonist is a useful step to suppress pituitary gonadotropin secretion and secondary CPP that may later develop.[902] More potent nonsteroidal antiandrogens (e.g., flutamide, nilutamide) and aromatase inhibitors (e.g., letrozole) inhibit the rate of skeletal maturation and linear growth by suppressing estradiol synthesis, potentially with greater therapeutic efficacy.[150,151] The combination of bicalutamide and anastrozole is proposed as another approach.[859] Table 25-38 lists the various agents used in the treatment of testotoxicosis; which of these agents or combination of agents will be effective and safe for long-term treatment remains to be determined.

A study of an untreated boy with testotoxicosis (GnRH-independent sexual precocity) had the expected pattern of rapid growth and early cessation, and the adult height of 174 cm was within target height range (171.5 to 188.5 cm), indicating the critical importance of individual approaches to affected boys when considering treatment to maximize height.[908]

Follow-up of boys with testotoxicosis indicates an increased risk of seminoma in adult life and Leydig cell adenoma in later childhood.[909,910] One boy with testotoxicosis developed nodular Leydig cell hyperplasia at 10 years of age.[911] These cases support a relationship between an activating mutation of the gene encoding the LH receptor and of Leydig cell tumors.

Gonadotropin-Independent Sexual Precocity and Pseudohypoparathyroidism Type Ia. A mutation in $G_s\alpha$ can constitutively activate or inactivate adenyl cyclase.[912] Two boys who presented in infancy with classic pseudohypoparathyroidism type Ia (PHPIa), a disorder characterized by resistance to hormones whose action is mediated by cAMP, developed signs of sexual precocity with the hormonal characteristics of testotoxicosis (i.e., gonadotropin-independent sexual precocity) at about 24 months of age.[913] Whereas the alanine residue is usually absolutely conserved in all heterotrimeric G proteins, both of these patients had a unique Ala366Ser mutation[913] in one allele of the $G_s\alpha$ gene. PHPIa is caused by a wide variety of inactivating mutations in $G_s\alpha$ that lead to an approximately 50% reduction in $G_s\alpha$ activity in functional assays.

The paradox of a $G_s\alpha$ mutation causing both inactivation with PHP and constitutive activation with testotoxicosis was resolved by the in vitro demonstration[914] that, unlike other activating mutations of $G_s\alpha$ which involve mutations inhibiting its intrinsic GTPase activity and decreasing the rate of hydrolysis of GTP to GDP, the mutation in these two boys caused accelerated dissociation of GDP at 33° C in transfected Leydig cells but was rapidly degraded at 37° C in a lymphoma cell line[914] and at 33° C and 37° C in skin fibroblasts transfected with the mutation.[913] These observations explain the clinical consequences of increased $G_s\alpha$ activity in the testis, which are 3° to 5° C cooler than the body, and the tissue specificity and temperature dependency of the mutation.[914] The mother of one patient appeared to be a mosaic for the $G_s\alpha$ mutation; in the other boy, a germline mutation was likely.[913]

Girls. GnRH-independent sexual precocity (GISP) in girls (see Table 25-25) is caused by autonomous estrogen secretion by an ovarian cyst or tumor or an adrenal neoplasm or by inadvertent exposure to estrogen. Girls harboring a teratoma or teratocarcinoma (or a CNS germ cell tumor) that secretes hCG have experienced sexual precocity caused by concurrent estrogen secretion by the tumor but no effect from the hCG alone; these girls also may have galactorrhea, especially if chorionic somatomammotropin (hCS or hPL) is also secreted.

Autonomous Ovarian Follicular Cysts. The most common childhood estrogen-secreting ovarian mass and ovarian cause of sexual precocity is the follicular cyst.[915] Antral follicles up to about 8 mm in diameter are common in the ovaries of normal prepubertal girls[916] and may be seen in third-trimester fetuses and newborn infants.[917,918] They may appear and regress spontaneously. Larger follicular cysts may be discovered because of the presence of an abdominal mass or abdominal pain, especially after torsion or as an unexpected finding on pelvic sonography performed for other reasons. Occasionally, the antral follicles secrete estrogen and may form large masses, or the follicular cysts may recur and cause recurrent signs of sexual precocity and acyclic vaginal bleeding. Enlarged antral follicles or cysts occur in premature thelarche, CPP, and transient or incomplete sexual precocity.[742] In some patients with ovarian follicular cysts, the transient or recurrent sexual precocity is GnRH independent (Fig. 25-63). The concentration of estradiol fluctuates, usually correlating with changes in the size of the follicular cyst or cysts when monitored by pelvic sonography, and may increase to levels found in granulosa cell tumors, although values may also be in the pubertal range.

These patients do not have increased plasma granulosa cell tumor markers such as AMH or inhibin.[742,769] The concentration of LH is suppressed, a pubertal pattern of pulsatile LH secretion is absent, and the LH rise induced by GnRH is prepubertal.[742] A constitutive activating mutation of the FSH receptor has not been described in a female, but a heterozygous mutation, Asp567Gly, was detected in the third intracellular loop of the FSH receptor in a hypophysectomized man who, despite the gonadotropin deficiency, was fertile and had normal-sized testes.[919] Accordingly, the possibility that some girls with recurrent ovarian cysts harbor an activating mutation of the FSH receptor seems worthy of study. The McCune-Albright syndrome may lead to recurrent ovarian cysts even in the apparent initial absence of other features of this disorder due to somatic activating mutations in the gene encoding the α-subunit of the heterotrimeric G_s protein. The luteinization of follicular cysts may be related to subtle elevations and increased pulses of plasma FSH. Ovarian cysts and sexual precocity have been associated with the fragile X syndrome in girls.[920]

Estradiol-secreting ovarian cysts occur in preterm infants born before 30 weeks' gestation; they are associated with edema of the labia majora and, in some instances, of the lower abdominal wall.[921] The LH and FSH response to GnRH in these patients suggests GnRH dependence, and treatment with medroxyprogesterone acetate is associated with regression of the cysts. A case of massive ovarian edema associated with ovarian cysts found in a 6-month-old with breast and pubic hair development has been reported.[922]

GnRH agonists are useful in the treatment of ovarian follicular cysts associated with CPP (GISP) but not of so-called autonomous cysts. However, autonomously functioning ovarian follicular cysts, whether recurrent or manifesting in an isolated episode, often respond to treatment with oral medroxyprogesterone acetate, which seems to prevent recurrence, to accelerate involution of the follicular cysts,[742,923] and to reduce the risk of torsion. The use of a potent aromatase inhibitor such as letrozole to reduce estradiol secretion is another potential approach to

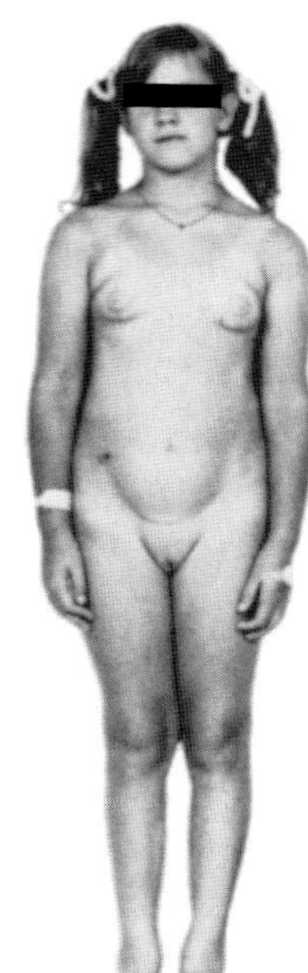

FOLLICULAR CYST OF OVARY
(Pt. G.B.)
AGE OF ONSET: 2 10/12 Y
P.E. AT AGE 4 10/12 Y
HT: 122.8 cm (+3.2 SD)
BREASTS: III, PH: 2
LAB: LRF: LH: 0.4 to 0.7 ng/ml, FSH: 0.4 to 0.8 ng/ml
E2: 180 pg/ml
BA: 6 Y, CA: 4 10/12
Rx: 5 3/12: REMOVAL OF OVARIAN CYST
CYST FLUID: 25,000 pg/ml E1
>34,000 pg/ml E2
MPA: AGE 5 5/12 to 9 0/12 Y
LRF: PREPUBERTAL LH RESPONSE
E2: <10 pg/ml
REMISSION WITH NO PROGRESSION OF PUBERTAL SIGNS
6 11/12 Y, ON MPA

Figure 25-63 A girl aged 4 years and 10 months with recurrent, "autonomous" follicular cysts of the ovary. For conversion to SI units, see Figure 25-16. FSH, follicle-stimulating hormone; LH, luteinizing hormone; MPA, medroxyprogesterone acetate (oral). (From Kaplan SL, Grumbach MM. Pathogenesis of sexual precocity. In: Grumbach MM, Sizonenko PC, Aubert ML, eds. *Control of the Onset of Puberty.* Baltimore, MD: Williams & Wilkins, 1990:620-660.)

treatment.[924] Surgical intervention is rarely indicated; a large or persistent cyst can be reduced by puncture at laparoscopy and the size of the cyst can be monitored readily by pelvic sonography.

Ovarian Tumors. Ovarian tumors are the most common genitourinary tumors of girls,[925] accounting for about 1% of all tumors in girls younger than 17 years of age, but they are rare in the prepubertal period. Most are benign according to some,[926] but not all, studies.[927] Discrepancy among studies may be due to the method of classification of cysts and potentially malignant lesions. Most ovarian tumors arise from germ cells or sex cord–stromal cells in childhood with fewer than 20% being of epithelial origin, whereas in adults, most are of epithelial origin.[928] Early diagnosis of most childhood tumors of the ovary allows successful cure, unlike ovarian cancer in adult women. Most of these girls present with pain or an abdominal mass. Tumors smaller than 5 cm at diagnosis are more likely to be non-neoplastic, and those larger than 10 cm are more likely to be neoplastic.[915] Ultrasonography is helpful in evaluation but does not usually lead to the correct histologic diagnosis. The successful use of tumor markers for diagnosis varies by cause. For example, in one series, cystic teratomas resulted in lactate dehydrogenase (LDH) elevation and an increased erythrocyte sedimentation rate; immature teratomas produced elevated levels of LDH, α-fetoprotein, and cancer antigen 125 (CA125); and granulosa cell tumors had elevated sex steroids (estradiol or testosterone or both).[927]

Granulosa cell tumor of the ovary is rare in childhood, although theca cell tumors are even less common.[929] Characteristic histologic features of juvenile granulosa cell tumors include nodular architecture, follicle formation, abundant interstitial and intrafollicular acid mucopolysaccharide-rich fluid, irregular microcysts, individual cell necrosis, and high mitotic activity (mean activity, 11 mitotic figures per 10 high-power fields). Size can vary from 2.5 to 25 cm, with a mean diameter of 12 cm. The interstitial mucinous fluid consists predominantly of hyaluronic acid. Prognosis is good, the mortality rate being about 3%. However, the age at diagnosis is related to prognosis, and delay leads to substantial complications. In one series, girls who presented with ISP and were correctly diagnosed had no intra-abdominal spread and had Federation of Gynecology and Obstetrics (FIGO) stage IA disease, whereas those who presented with acute abdominal symptoms had 50% prevalence of intra-abdominal spread and two recurrences after surgery. When the diagnosis was made after normal puberty had begun, some girls experienced virilization or abdominal symptoms; 80% had intra-abdominal spread, and 30% had recurrence with FIGO stage IIC.

Approximately 80% of granulosa cell tumors can be palpated on bimanual examination, whereas fewer than 5% are bilateral or clinically malignant. The concentration of plasma estradiol may increase to high levels, but serum FSH and LH concentrations are usually suppressed. AMH and inhibin are sensitive tumor markers[930-932] and are used to screen for metastases; an elevated estradiol concentration in a patient younger than 9 years of age or an abnormal rise in concentration of plasma AMH or inhibin at any age suggests recurrence or metastasis.

Occasionally, gonadoblastomas in streak gonads, rare lipoid tumors, cystadenomas, and ovarian carcinomas secrete estrogens, androgens, or both. Even with successful resection of a gonadal sex steroid–secreting neoplasm, the child is at risk for secondary CPP in the future. Gonadal tumors composed of a mixture of germ cells and sex cord–stromal cells that are distinct from gonadoblastoma are usually benign when discovered in female infants or children with 46,XX karyotypes,[933] although neoplastic transformation is a risk,[934] because two cases of metastasizing malignant mixed germ cell/sex cord–stromal cell tumors have been described in prepubertal girls with ISP. α-Fetoprotein and other tumor markers aid in diagnosis.

Peutz-Jeghers Syndrome. Peutz-Jeghers syndrome is an autosomal dominant syndrome characterized by mucocutaneous pigmentation of the lips, buccal mucosa, fingers, and toes; gastrointestinal hamartomatous polyposis; and a predisposition to malignancy. It is associated with a rare, distinctive sex cord tumor with annular tubules in both boys and girls.[935,936] Estrogen secretion by the tumor may lead to feminization and incomplete sexual precocity in boys and girls. Less frequently, an epithelial tumor of the ovary, a dysgerminoma, or a feminizing Sertoli-Leydig cell tumor has been found in patients with Peutz-Jeghers syndrome.[937] Children with this disorder should be examined at regular intervals for the presence of gonadal tumors by pelvic sonography. The syndrome is caused by mutations in the gene located on 9p13.3 that encodes a serine/threonine protein kinase, STK11, leading to haploinsufficiency of this novel tumor-suppressing gene.[938]

Sex cord–stromal cell tumors derive from the celomic epithelium or mesenchymal cells of the embryonic gonads and are composed of granulosa, theca, Leydig, and Sertoli cells. Estrogen secretion from these tumors can cause ISP, and androgen secretion can cause virilization. Inhibin A and B activin are produced, as is AMH; all serve as useful tumor markers. Sex cord–stromal cell tumors not associated with Peutz-Jeghers syndrome are malignant in 25% of cases; these tumors can grow quite large, but those associated with Peutz-Jeghers syndrome are often small and multiple, and they contain calcifications.[939]

Adrenal Adenomas. Adrenocortical tumors are rare in childhood (0.6% of all childhood tumors and 0.3% of all malignant childhood tumors), but most produce steroid hormones, whereas those in adults usually do not. The median age at diagnosis is 4 years, but 41% of these tumors manifest before 2 years and 71% before 5 years of age. Most cause virilization or Cushing's syndrome, but adrenal tumors may produce estrogen as well as androgens and can cause sexual precocity in a girl or gynecomastia in a boy. One adrenal adenoma found in a 7-year-old girl expressed the gene for aromatase, demonstrating that the tumor could directly produce estrogen[940] to a level of 145 pg/mL, within the range found in adrenal carcinomas.

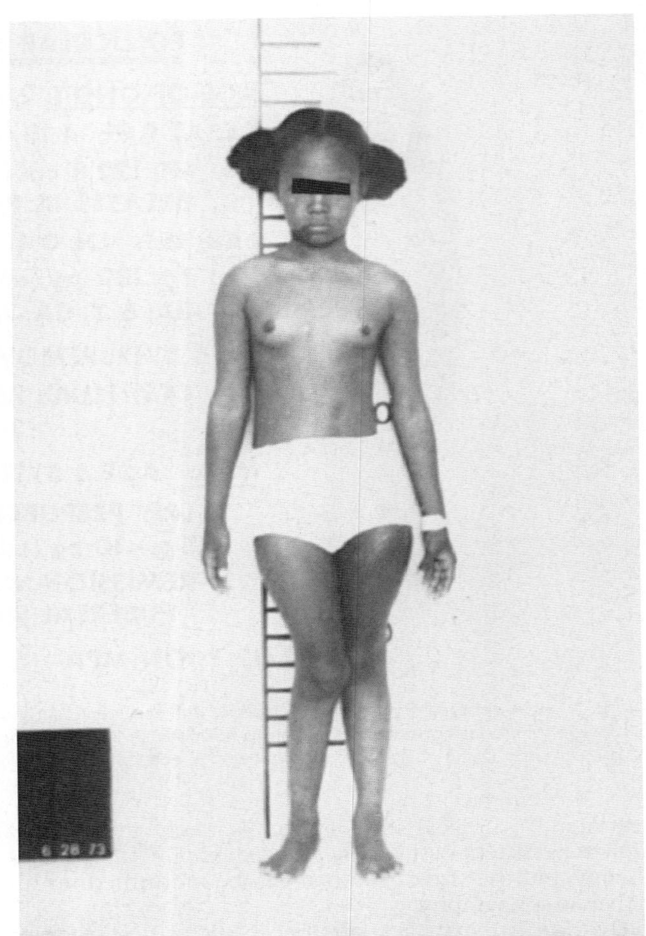

Figure 25-64 A girl aged 7 years and 4 months with gonadotropin-releasing hormone (GnRH)–independent sexual precocity associated with McCune-Albright syndrome. She had breast development since infancy, and it increased noticeably at about 3 years of age; 6 months later, episodes of recurrent vaginal bleeding began. Growth of pubic hair was noticed at about 4 to 5 years. At age 5.5 years, the bone age was 6 years and 11 months; height was +1 SD above the mean value for age. By 6.5 years, when she was seen at the University of California, San Francisco, the bone age had advanced to 9 years, and height was at +1 SD. Breasts were at Tanner stage 4, and pubic hair at stage 3. Extensive, irregular café au lait macules cover the right side of the face, left lower abdomen and thigh, and both buttocks. A bone survey showed widespread involvement of the long bones with typical polyostotic fibrous dysplasia, the floor of the anterior fossa of the skull was sclerotic, and the diploetic space had widened. She has had two pathologic fractures through bone cysts in the right upper femur. Notice the osseous deformities. Plasma estradiol concentrations were consistently in the pubertal range; the LH response to GnRH was prepubertal. Results of thyroid function studies were normal, including the thyrotropin response to thyrotropin-releasing hormone administration, and antithyroid antibodies were not detected. Treatment with oral medroxyprogesterone acetate suppressed menses and arrested pubertal development but did not slow skeletal maturation. Her final height is 142 cm (−2.5 SD). Menstrual cycles are regular.

Boys and Girls

McCune-Albright Syndrome. McCune-Albright syndrome is sporadic and occurs about twice as often in girls than in boys; it is caused by somatic activating mutations in the gene *(GNAS1)* encoding the α-subunit of the trimeric GTP-binding protein ($G_s\alpha$) that stimulates adenyl cyclase.[941] It is characterized by the triad of irregularly edged hyperpigmented macules (café au lait spots of the coast of Maine type); a slowly progressive bone disorder, polyostotic fibrous dysplasia, that can involve any bone and is frequently associated with facial asymmetry and hyperostosis of the base of the skull; and, more commonly in girls, GnRH-independent sexual precocity (Fig. 25-64 and Table 25-39).[942] At least two of the features must be present to consider the diagnosis.

Autonomous hyperfunction most commonly involves the ovary, but other endocrine involvement includes thyroid (nodular hyperplasia with thyrotoxicosis or, remarkably, with euthyroid status[943]); adrenal (multiple hyperplastic nodules with Cushing's syndrome that may occur in the neonatal period[944]), pituitary (adenoma or mammosomatotroph hyperplasia with gigantism, acromegaly, and hyperprolactinemia), and parathyroid (adenoma or hyperplasia with hyperparathyroidism).[942] Hypophosphatemic vitamin D–resistant rickets or osteomalacia occurs, either because of overproduction of a phosphaturic factor, phosphatonin,[945] that is secreted by the bone lesions or because of an intrinsic renal abnormality leading to the excess generation of nephrogenous cAMP in the proximal tubule and, as a result, decreased reabsorption of phosphate.[946] Hepatocellular dysfunction may occur due to expression of the mutant activating gene in liver cells, which leads to jaundice associated with hepatobiliary disease, and pancreatitis.[947] Another nonendocrine manifestation is cardiac disease, and patients carry the risk of cardiac arrhythmia and sudden death. This

TABLE 25-39

Clinical Manifestations of McCune-Albright Syndrome in 158 Reported Patients*

Manifestation	% of Patients			Mean Age at Diagnosis (yr) and Range	Comments
	Total (N = *158)*	*Male* (n = *53)*	*Female* (n = *105)*		
Fibrous dysplasia	97	51	103	7.7 (0-52)	Polystotic more common than monostotic
Café au lait lesion	85	49	86	7.7 (0-52)	Variable size and number of lesions, irregular border ("coast of Maine")
Sexual precocity	52	8	74	4.9 (0.3-9)	Common initial manifestation
Acromegaly/gigantism	27	20	22	14.8 (0.2-42)	17/26 of patients with adenoma on MRI/CT
Hyperprolactinemia	15	9	14	16.0 (0.2-42)	23/42 of acromegalic patients with PRL
Hyperthyroidism	19	7	23	14.4 (0.5-37)	Euthyroid goiter is common
Hypercortisolism	5	4	5	4.4 (0.2-17)	All primary adrenal
Myxomas	5	3	5	34 (17-50)	Extremity myxomas
Osteosarcoma	2	1	2	36 (34-37)	At site of fibrous dysplasia, not related to prior radiation therapy
Rickets/osteomalacia	3	1	3	27.3 (8-52)	Responsive to phosphorus plus calcitriol
Cardiac abnormalities	11	8	9	(0.1-66)	Arrhythmias and CHF reported
Hepatic abnormalities	10	6	10	1.9 (0.3-4)	Neonatal icterus is most common

*Evaluations include clinical and biochemical data; other rarely described manifestations include metabolic acidosis, nephrocalcinosis, developmental delay, thymic and splenic hyperplasia, and colonic polyps.

CHF, congestive heart failure; CT, computed tomography; MRI, magnetic resonance imaging; PRL, prolactin.

Modified from Ringel MD, Schwindinger WF, Levine MA. Clinical implication of genetic defects in G proteins: the molecular basis of McCune-Albright syndrome and Albright hereditary osteodystrophy. *Medicine (Baltimore).* 1996;75:171-184.

is a sporadic condition that can be concordant or discordant in monozygotic twins.[948]

Considering children with at least one of the signs of McCune-Albright syndrome, 24% had the classic triad, 33% had two signs, and 40% had only one classic sign. The mutation was detected in 46% of blood samples from patients presenting the classic triad, but in only 21% and 8% of samples from patients with two signs or one sign, respectively. If an affected tissue was available, the mutation was found in more than 90% of the patients no matter what the number of signs. The mutation was found in 33% of the 39 cases of isolated peripheral precocious puberty. Patients with monostotic fibrous dysplasia, isolated peripheral precocious puberty, neonatal liver cholestasis, or the classic McCune-Albright syndrome all had the same molecular defect.[949] Whereas most endocrine organs involved in McCune-Albright syndrome were not associated with parent specificity,[950] pituitary adenomas secreting GH expressed NESP55 transcripts, which are mono-allelically expressed from the maternal alleles rather than from the exon 1A paternal allele. Mutation of *GNAS1* involving Arg201His replacement is associated with apparent premature or exaggerated thelarche and early menarche.[951]

Most patients have pigmented skin lesions in infancy which usually increase in size along with body growth.[952] The irregularly bordered, café au lait macules usually do not cross the midline, but they may; they often are located on the same side as the main bone lesions and have a segmented distribution.

The skeletal lesions in the cortex are dysplastic and are filled with spindle cells with poorly organized collagen support; they take the form of scattered cystic areas of rarefaction on radiography and often result in pathologic fractures and progressive deformities (Fig. 25-65). Technetium bone scintigraphy has been the most sensitive approach to the detection of bone lesions before they are visible radiographically. Fractures are most common between the sixth and the tenth year but decline thereafter, and they are more frequent if phosphaturia is present.[953] Patients referred for fibrous dysplasia of the bone in one or more locations are often found to have endocrine or dermatologic manifestations of McCune-Albright syndrome as well as *GNAS1* mutations, so suspicion should be kept high when evaluating fibrous lesions.[954] If the skull is involved, there may be entrapment and compression of optic or auditory nerve foramina, which can lead to blindness, deafness, facial asymmetry, and ptosis. Assymetria of the jaw is another manifestation of McCune-Albright syndrome. Fifty percent of affected children in one series manifested bone abnormalities by 8 years of age.[952] Increased serum GH levels have an adverse effect on the skull deformities, depending on the age at onset; somatostatin analogues have variable efficacy. Irradiation of the hypothalamic-pituitary area may be invoked, but it carries a risk of later occurrence of sarcoma. Rapid control of elevated GH can be achieved by the use of long-acting somatostatin agonists such as pagvisomant.[955]

The sexual precocity often begins during the first 2 years of life and is frequently heralded by menstrual bleeding; the cause is autonomously functioning luteinized follicular cysts of the ovary in girls (Table 25-40).[742,942] The ovaries contain no corpora lutea and commonly exhibit asymmetric enlargement as a result of a large solitary follicular cyst that characteristically enlarges and then spontaneously regresses, only to recur (Fig. 25-66).[740,890,942] Serum estradiol is elevated (at times to extraordinarily levels); in contrast, the LH response to GnRH is prepubertal, and the pubertal pattern of nighttime LH pulses is absent at the onset and during the initial years.[742,956,957] Later in the course of the sexual precocity, when the bone age approaches 12 years, the GnRH pulse generator becomes operative and ovulatory cycles ensue.

An affected girl may progress from GnRH-independent puberty to GnRH-dependent puberty (see Table 25-40).[742,956,958] GnRH agonists are not effective for treatment in the GnRH-independent stage. Testolactone, a relatively weak aromatase inhibitor, Fadrazole, and anastrazole have been equivocal or not effective. The new, highly potent, specific, third-generation aromatase inhibitors (e.g., letrozole) may be more effective.[150,151,959] After a single case report of treatment with tamoxifen, an anti-estrogen, showed decreases in bone age advancement, growth rate,

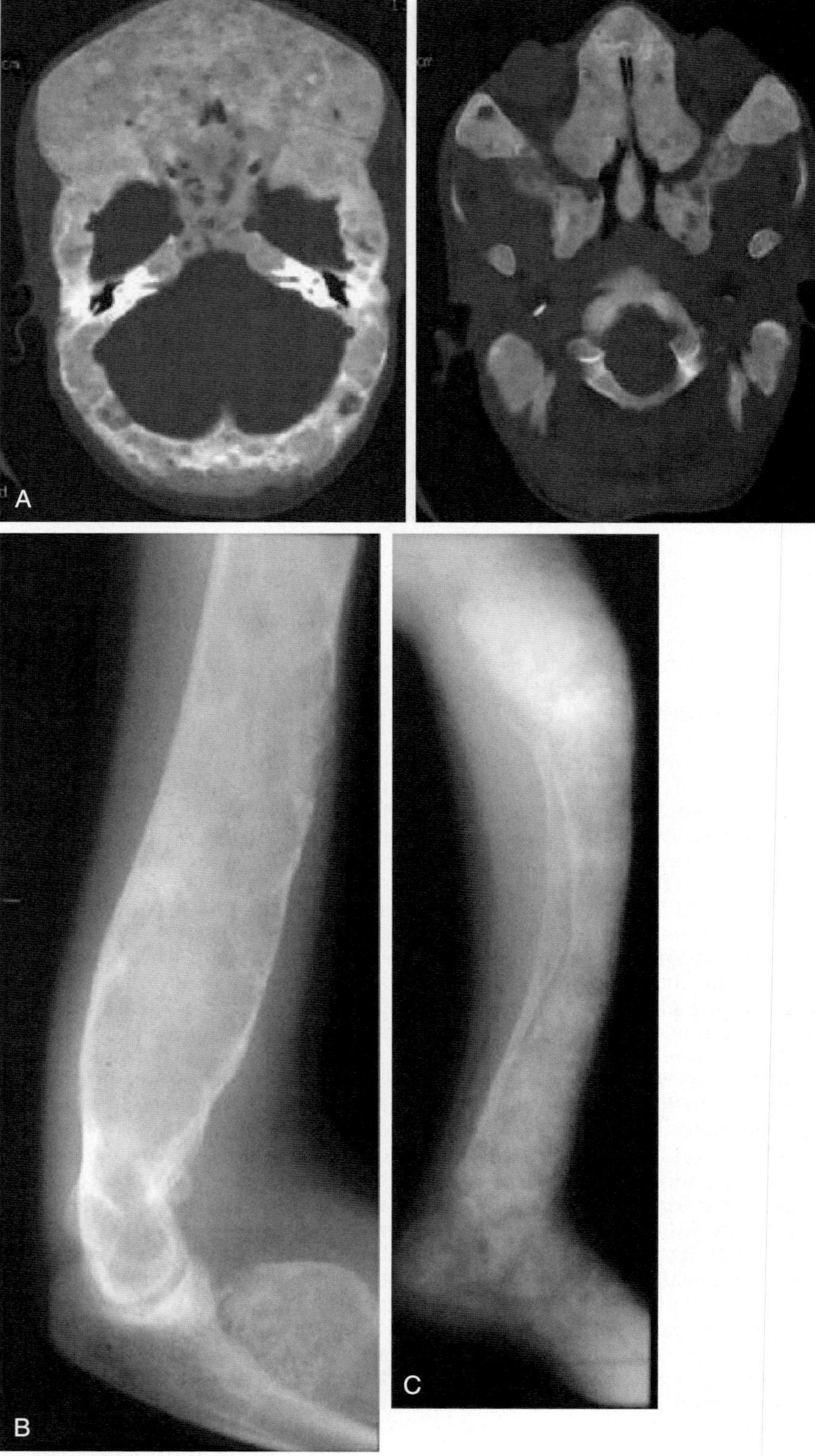

Figure 25-65 Bone lesions in McCune-Albright syndrome. **A,** The skull has severe thickening primarily at the base due to fibrous dysplasia. The auditory and optic nerves can be caught in narrowed foramina, but that is not the case in these patients. **B** and **C,** Distortions of the long bones can develop into a "shepherd's crook" appearance. Notice the multiple bone cysts.

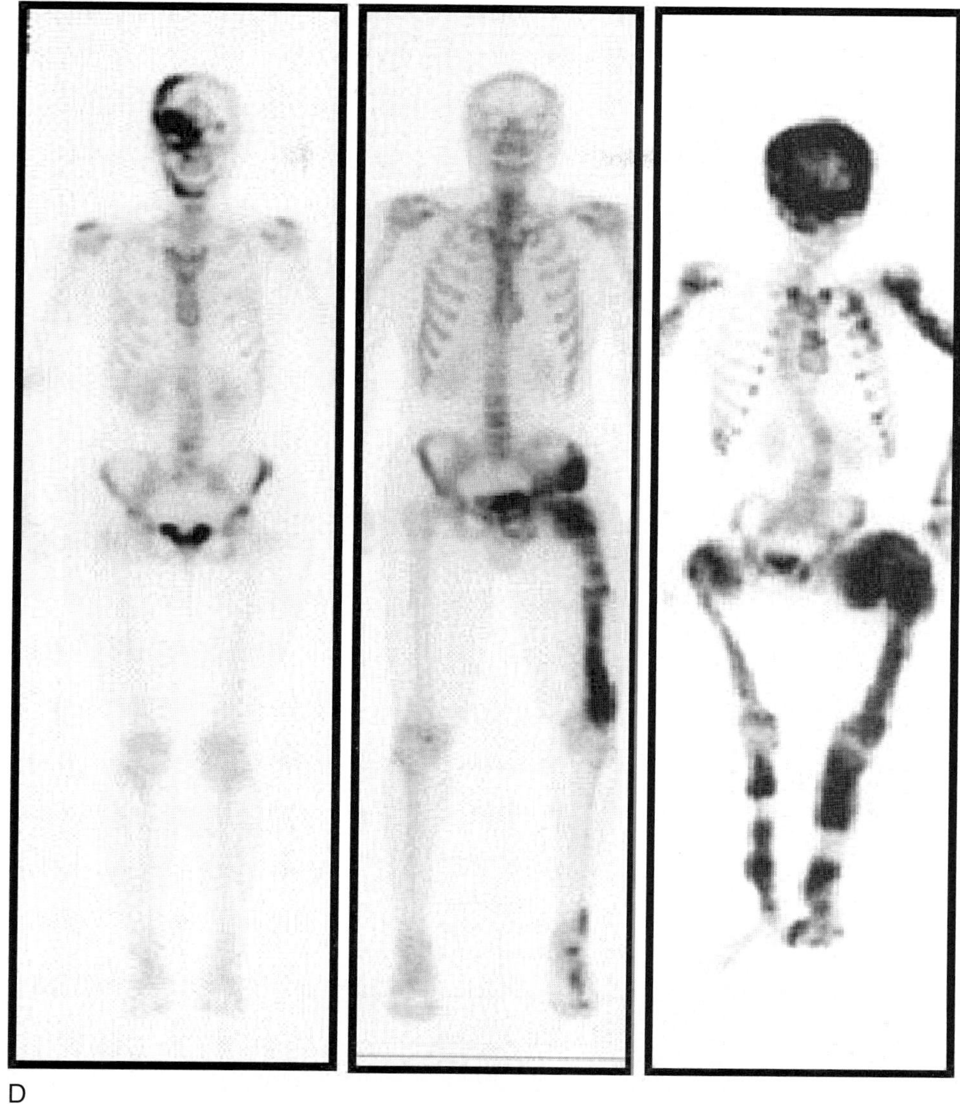

Figure 25-65, cont'd **D,** Bone scan shows the areas of remodeling that "light up," depending on the area affected in individual patients. There are examples of patients primarily affected in the craniofacial area or in the appendicular area, or both areas, and the axial skeleton. (Courtesy of Michael T. Collins, M.D., National Institutes of Health, Bethesda, MD, and Sandra Gorges, M.D., University of California, Davis.)

menses, and pubertal development, a multicenter trial demonstrated the utility of this agent in decreasing vaginal bleeding and decreasing the rate of bone age advancement and growth rate in affected girls.[960] However, ovarian and uterine volumes remained elevated.

Sexual precocity is rare in boys with McCune-Albright syndrome.[942,961] Affected boys may have asymmetric enlargement of the testes in addition to signs of sexual precocity. The histologic changes and hormonal findings are reminiscent of those observed in testotoxicosis: the seminiferous tubules are enlarged and exhibit spermatogenesis, and Leydig cells may be hyperplastic.[942] A 3.8-year-old boy with McCune-Albright syndrome (several café au lait lesions on the back and polyostotic fibrous dysplasia) had an Arg201His mutation detected in bone and testis tissue and the unusual feature of macroorchidism (right testis, 9 mL; left testis, 7 mL), but sexual precocity was absent. Basal and GnRH-stimulated gonadotropins and sex steroid levels were prepubertal, but serum inhibin B and AMH concentrations were strikingly elevated. On histologic examination of the testes, most of the seminiferous tubules were slightly increased in diameter and filled with Sertoli cells but lacked a lumen. The tubules stained intensively for inhibin β_B subunit; mature Leydig cells were absent.[962] An increased incidence of the rare condition, testicular microlithiasis, was described in boys with McCune-Albright syndrome evaluated by ultrasonography.[963]

McCune-Albright syndrome may occur concordantly or discordantly in monozygotic twins; familial cases have not been described. In 1986, Happle[964] posited that the disorder is caused by an autosomal "dominant" lethal gene that results in loss of the zygote in utero and that cells bearing this mutation survive only in embryos mosaic for the lethal gene. Early somatic mutation would lead to a mosaic cell pattern of the distribution of cells containing the mutation. The severity of the disorder would depend on the proportion of mutant cells in various embryonic tissues. The description of somatic mutations in human endocrine tumors that convert the peptide chain of the G_s protein

TABLE 25-40

A Patient with McCune-Albright Syndrome and Recurrent Ovarian Cysts

Chronologic Age (yr)	Bone Age (yr)	Height (cm)	Physical Signs	Basal and Post-LHRH (ng/mL)*†	Plasma Estradiol (pmol/L [pg/mL])	Radiography (Long Bones)
1 4/12	1 3/12	81.1	Café au lait pigmentation, B2, PH1 Vaginal bleeding (×2 mo)	LH 0.6-1.3 FSH 1.9-3.2 DHEAS <50 ng/mL (<0.14 mmol/L)	40 (11)	Normal
1 8/12			B1, PH1			
2 6/12	2 6/12	92.4	B2, PH2 Vaginal bleeding	LH 0.6-1.1 FSH 1.9-3.2 DHEAS <50 ng/mL (<0.14 mmol/L)	55-66 (15-18)	Normal
3 3/12		98.3	B1, PH1			
3 10/12	3 10/12		B2, PH1	LH 1.1-2.0 FSH 1-1.7	51-95 (14-26)	Normal
4 3/12			B1, PH1		7.3-7.3 (20-20)	Polyostotic fibrous dysplasia of femurs
5 1/12	6	123.4	B3, PH2 Vaginal bleeding (×2 mo)	LH 1.1-4.3 FSH 1.0-2.0		
6 6/12	7 10/12	128.5	B3, PH2 Oral medroxyprogesterone acetate, 10 mg bid stated		<5	
7 10/12	8 10/12	136.8				
8 7/12		142.2				

*Matched standard reagents were LER-960 for LH and LER-869 for FSH. To convert ng/mL to IU/L, multiply LH value by 3.8 and FSH value by 8.4.

†Note the prepubertal LH response to GnRH consistent with GnRH-independent sexual precocity until age 5 1/12 yr and the pubertal LH response at 5 1/12 yr, consistent with the development of secondary true precocious puberty (GnRH-dependent). Note discrepancy between gonadarche and adrenarche as evidenced by preadrenarchal concentration of DHEAS.

B, breast stage; DHEAS, dehydroepiandrosterone sulfate; FSH, follicle-stimulating hormone; GnRH, gonadotropin-releasing hormone; LER, matched standard reagent; LH, luteinizing hormone; LHRH, luteinizing hormone–releasing hormone; PH, pubic hair stage.

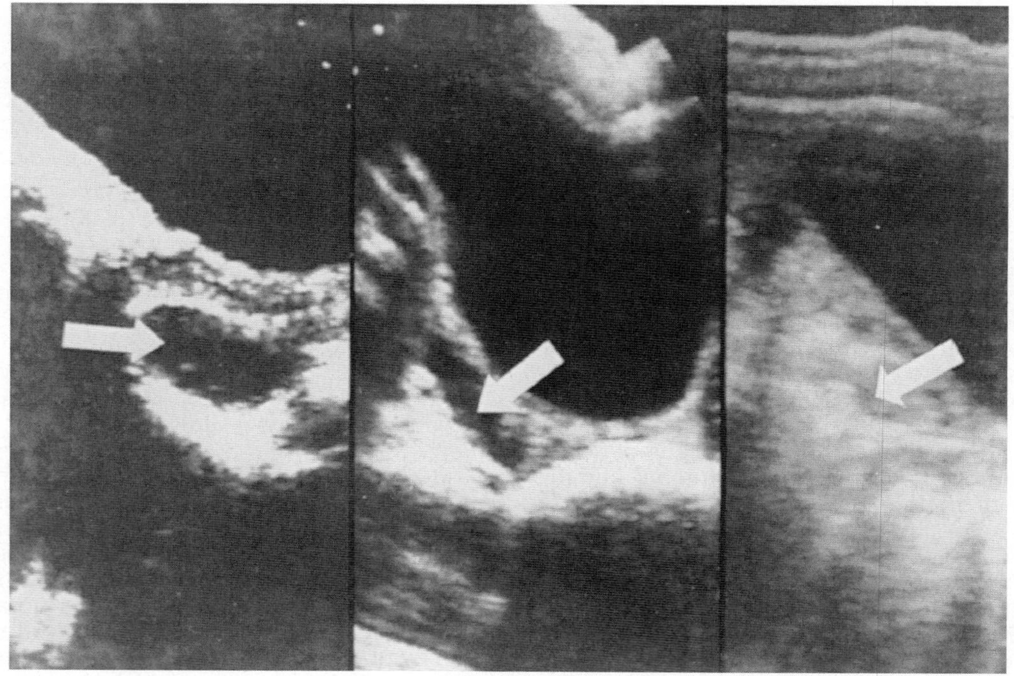

Figure 25-66 Serial pelvic ultrasonograms at 2-week intervals of a 6-year-old girl with McCune-Albright syndrome. Breast development and vaginal bleeding coincided with the enlargement of the ovarian cyst; white arrows denote the decreasing size of the cyst. With the spontaneous regression of the large ovarian cyst, the breasts regressed in size, and vaginal bleeding ceased. (From Kaplan SL, Grumbach MM. Pathogenesis of sexual precocity. In: Grumbach MM, Sizonenko PC, Aubert ML, eds. *Control of the Onset of Puberty.* Baltimore, MD: Williams & Wilkins, 1990:620-660.)

into a putative oncogene (referred to as a *gsp* mutation)[965] raised the possibility of a similar defect in McCune-Albright syndrome that both affects a differentiated function such as a signaling pathway and mediates the regulation of proliferation. These hypotheses are now established, because mutations in the gene encoding the α-subunit of the stimulatory G protein for adenyl cyclase was identified in the tissues of children with the McCune-Albright syndrome.

The heterotrimeric guanine nucleotide–binding proteins (G proteins) are a subfamily within the large superfamily of GTP-binding proteins and serve to transduce signals from a large number of cell surface receptors with a common structural motif of seven-membrane–spanning domains to their intracellular effector molecules, including enzymes and ion channels; in essence, they couple serpentine cell surface receptors to effectors (Fig. 25-67). For G_s, the stimulatory G-protein, the effector is adenyl cyclase, which is controlled by G_s and an inhibitory G protein, G_i.[966] The heterotrimer is composed of an α-subunit (39 to 45 kd) that binds GTP, has intrinsic GTPase activity, and converts GTP to GDP; a β-subunit (35 to 36 kd); and a smaller β-subunit (7 to 8 kd). The latter two subunits are tightly but noncovalently associated with each other. Each of the subunits is encoded by a distinct gene. The G proteins function as conformational switches. The GDP-liganded α-subunit is bound to the βγ-subunits and is in an inactivated state. When the cell surface receptor is activated by its ligand or agonists, the GDP is catalytically released from the α-subunit, enabling GTP to bind. This leads to dissociation of the GTP-activated α-subunit from the bound βγ-subunits and activation of the effector, adenyl cyclase. When GTP is hydrolyzed by the intrinsic GTPase activity of $G_s\alpha$, the α- and βγ-subunits reassociate, and the α-subunit is in the "off" or inactive conformation. The three-dimensional structure of the heterotrimeric G proteins has been determined.[967-969]

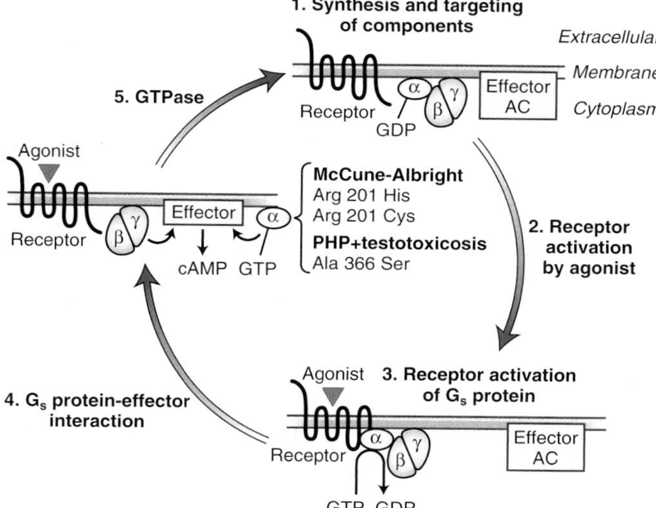

Figure 25-67 The G protein guanosine triphosphatase (GTPase) cycle. The heterotrimeric guanine nucleotide-binding proteins (G proteins), which are composed of three subunits (α, β, γ), couple cell surface receptors consisting of a single serpentine polypeptide having seven helical membrane-spanning domains with an effector. In this instance, adenylate cyclase (AC) catalyzes the transformation of adenosine triphosphate (ATP) to cyclic adenosine monophosphate (cAMP). The G protein stimulation subunit α (G_s) mediates the stimulation of cAMP generation. In the inactive, unstimulated state, the G protein is a heterotrimer, and GDP is tightly bound to the α-subunit. When the cell surface receptor is activated by its cognate agonist, the receptor catalyzes the release of the tightly bound GDP, which enables GTP to bind to the α-subunit. The GTP-bound α-subunit (α-GTP) dissociates from the tightly bound βγ dimer, and both play a role in the G protein activation of the effector, adenylate cyclase. The intrinsic GTPase activity of the α-subunit ends the stimulation of the effector by converting the bound α-GTP to α-GDP; as a consequence, the α-subunit again returns to its inactive state and reassociates with high affinity with the βγ subunit, yielding the α, β, γ heterotrimer. Disorders of signal transduction can arise from germ cell or somatic mutations at any of the five stages of the cycle. The gain-of-function, activating somatic mutations in the *GNAS1* gene that encodes the G $G_s\alpha$-subunit and leads to McCune-Albright syndrome (shown in the bracket), involves the highly conserved arginine 201 residue. These mutations inhibit the intrinsic GTPase activity of the α-subunit and therefore the conversion of the bound GTP to GDP. The Ala366Ser mutation (shown in the bracket) was detected in two boys, both of whom had pseudohypothyroidism Ia (PHPIa) and testotoxicosis. The mutant protein was constitutively activated in the Leydig cells at the scrotal temperature (32° to 33° C), leading to testotoxicosis, but it was rapidly degraded at body temperature, 37° C, which led to PHPIa. (Modified from Spiegel AM. Mutations in G proteins and G protein-coupled receptors in endocrine disease. *J Clin Endocrinol Metab.* 1996;81:2434-2442.)

Activating heterozygous mutations in the $G_s\alpha$-subunit that occurred as an early postzygotic event are described in the McCune-Albright syndrome. The somatic constitutive activating mutation, which leads to excess cAMP production and, in some tissues, cAMP-induced hyperplasia, has a mosaic pattern; the proportion of the hyperactive mutant compared with normal cells varies in different tissues, contributing, at least in part, to the varied clinical findings, the severity, the sporadic nature of the syndrome, and the discordant occurrence in monozygotic twins. A germline mutation is presumed to be lethal to the embryo. Two gain-of-function somatic missense mutations have been described in this disorder, both of which involve the arginine201 residue of the α-subunit.[912] This is the site of covalent modification by cholera toxin: either a cysteine or a histidine is substituted for arginine 201 (see Fig. 25-67).[961,966,970,971] The arginine 201 residue is critical for α-subunit GTPase activity, and each of these two mutations decreases the GTPase activity of the $G_s\alpha$-subunit, leading to constitutive activation. These activating mutations have been found in all tissues affected by the syndrome,[972,973] including bone lesions. There are reports of fertility in adults with McCune-Albright syndrome.

Juvenile Hypothyroidism. Long-standing untreated primary hypothyroidism, usually a consequence of Hashimoto's thyroiditis, is an uncommon cause of incomplete ISP[285,974,975] in both girls and boys and occurs in association with impaired growth and delayed skeletal maturation. If the concentration of plasma prolactin is elevated, galactorrhea may be demonstrable, more commonly in affected girls than boys (Figs. 25-68 and 25-69). Girls have breast development, enlarged labia minora, and estrogenic changes in the vaginal smear, usually without the appearance of pubic hair[285,976]; some girls have irregular vaginal bleeding[285] which could proceed to metrorrhagia, and solitary or multiple ovarian cysts may be demonstrable by pelvic sonography or on physical examination.[285] It is important to recognize the condition to avoid unnecessary surgery, which would be a tragic mistake in view of the success of medical management.[977] In about 80% of boys with juvenile hypothyroidism, the testes are enlarged because of an increase in the size of the seminiferous tubules, but signs of virilization and Leydig cell maturation are absent,[978] and the plasma concentration of testosterone is prepubertal. Enlargement of the sella turcica and the pituitary gland in the face of hypersecretion of TSH (see Fig. 25-69) has led to the misdiagnosis of a pituitary neoplasm. The hypothyroidism, incomplete sexual maturation, galactorrhea, and pituitary

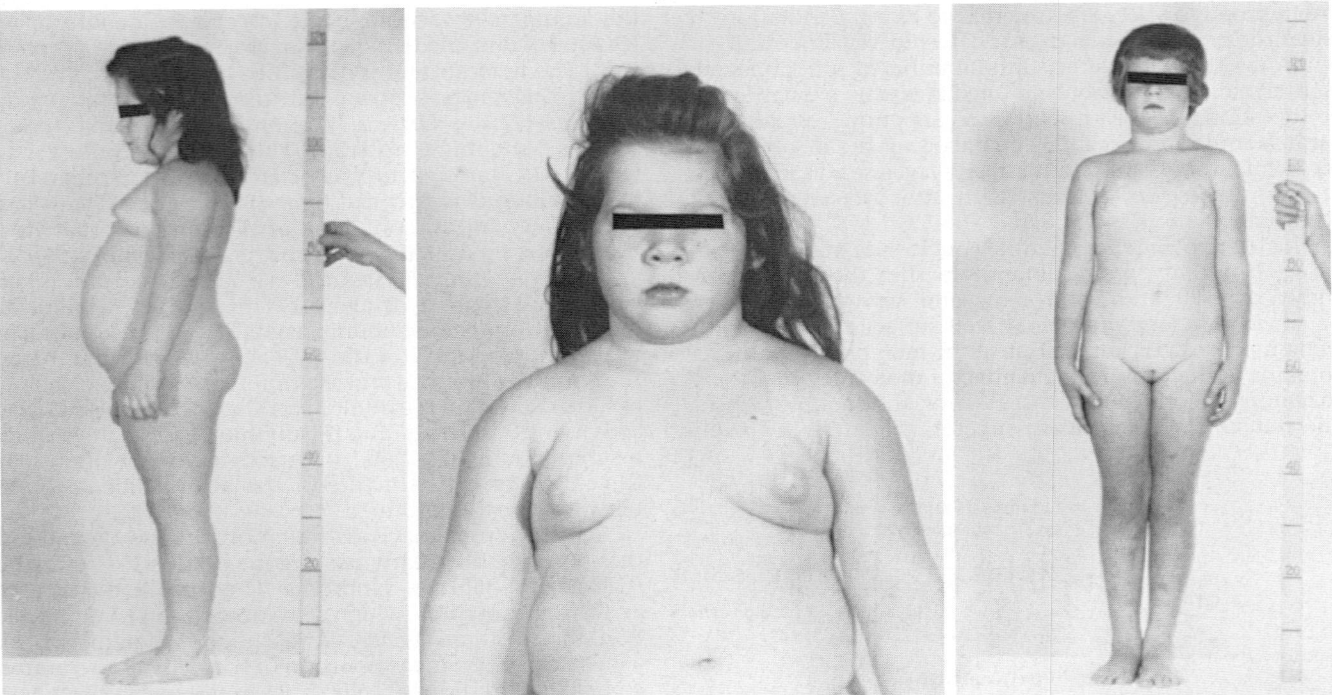

Figure 25-68 *Left* and *center,* Severe, chronic hypothyroidism of Hashimoto's thyroiditis in a girl aged 7 years and 1 month with sexual precocity (without pubic or axillary hair), episodic vaginal bleeding, and galactorrhea. She had symptoms of hypothyroidism and a sharply decreased rate of growth over the previous 2 years (height, −1 SD; bone age, 5 years and 3 months). Breast development was Tanner stage 3, the labia minora were enlarged, and the vaginal mucosa was dull pink, thickened, and rugated, with evidence of an estrogenic effect. No acne, seborrhea, or hirsutism was present. The uterus was of adolescent size, and the endometrial mucosa was in a proliferative phase. Urinary gonadotropins were barely detectable by bioassay. *Right,* Striking change in appearance after 8 months of thyroid hormone treatment. She had grown 7 cm in height and lost 8.1 kg in weight. The breasts had decreased in size, galactorrhea was no longer demonstrable, the labia minora had regressed, and the vaginal mucosa was pink and glistening (no estrogen effect). Ten weeks after the initiation of thyroid hormone replacement therapy, she developed a right slipped capital femoral epiphysis that was repaired surgically; recovery was uneventful.

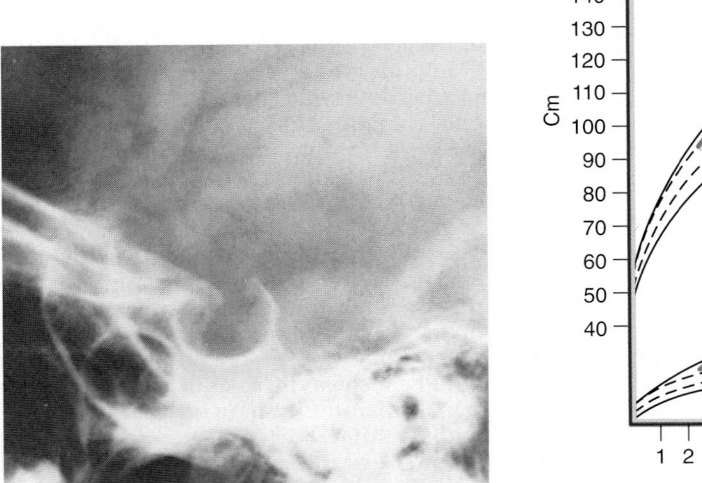

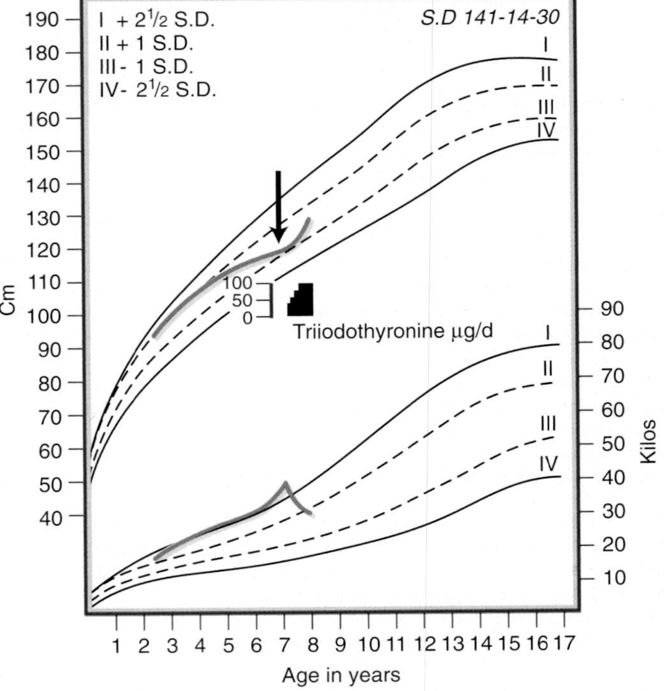

Figure 25-69 *Left,* Radiograph of the skull of a patient with hypothyroidism shows an enlarged pituitary fossa in the lateral view. The dorsum sellae was thin and demineralized, and the floor had a double contour line. The area of the sella turcica was 150 mm². Pneumoencephalography showed a suprasellar mass impinging on the cisterna chiasmatica. After thyroid hormone treatment for 8 months, the volume of the sella had decreased 30% to 100 mm², the dorsum sellae had remineralized, and the double floor was no longer evident. *Right,* Growth curve illustrates the decrease in growth rate despite sexual precocity and the catch-up growth induced by thyroid hormone therapy. (From Van Wyk JJ, Grumbach MM. Syndrome of precocious menstruation and galactorrhea in juvenile hypothyroidism: an example of hormonal overlap in pituitary feedback. *J Pediatr.* 1960;57:416-435.)

enlargement are reversed or corrected by levothyroxine therapy within a few months.[285]

In 1960, Van Wyk and Grumbach[285] suggested that the syndrome resulted from hormonal overlap in negative feedback regulation with increased secretion of gonadotropins, prolactin, and TSH as a consequence of the chronic hypothyroidism. With the advent of radioimmunoassays for pituitary hormones, increased prolactin secretion was documented in children[975] and adults with primary hypothyroidism and in affected girls with the syndrome. GH release is usually decreased, as in uncomplicated primary hypothyroidism.

However, the explanation for the sexual maturation remains uncertain. Pubertal development in primary hypothyroidism is usually delayed and is only rarely advanced for chronologic age. By the use of radioimmunoassays for FSH and LH in which the cross-reaction with TSH is negligible, an increased (pubertal) concentration of plasma immunoreactive and bioactive FSH, but not LH, has been detected.[979] Bioactive LH activity is also low. Increased FSH pulsatility, mainly at night, but not LH release was demonstrated in patients with the syndrome and in some children with primary hypothyroidism who did not exhibit premature sexual maturation.[979,980] The increased FSH release and the high FSH/LH ratio (in contrast to that observed in normal puberty) seem to account for the increased ovarian estrogen secretion in girls and for the enlarged testes without signs of virilization in affected boys; the suggestion here is that FSH-induced Sertoli cell proliferation is an important determinant of mature testis size.[981-983]

A GnRH-independent mechanism is likely, because GnRH did not suppress the pubertal LH levels.[979] Pulsatile TSH release is increased at night, and administration of TRH appears to increase FSH release in normal children (but not in adults). Moreover, the FSH response to TRH, but not GnRH, is augmented in primary hypothyroidism, and this response can occur in gonadotropin-secreting pituitary adenomas. If the latter observations are confirmed, it is likely that the incomplete sexual precocity and the increased prolactin secretion and galactorrhea are a consequence of the increased release of TRH, the increased sensitivity of the mammotrophs and gonadotroph to TRH, or both. This mechanism,[285] which has gained support,[979] would explain the relatively rapid and complete reversal of the syndrome by levothyroxine treatment. Human recombinant TSH at a dose about 1000-fold greater than that of human FSH evoked a dose-dependent cAMP response in COS7 cells transfected with the human FSH receptor, which suggests another possible but less likely mechanism for the FSH-dependent (or FSH-like–dependent) but GnRH-independent sexual precocity.[984] A direct effect of severe hypothyroidism on the prepubertal testis that leads to overproliferation of Sertoli cells also has been advanced as an explication of the macroorchidism.[978]

Diagnosis of Sexual Precocity

The separation of patients with self-limited benign disorders, such as premature adrenarche, premature thelarche, or normal but early puberty, from those with serious or even potentially fatal disorders is the first step in evaluation (Figs. 25-70 through 25-72 and Table 25-41). The history may reveal symptoms suggesting perinatal abnormalities or injuries, previous infections, adventitious ingestion of or exposure to gonadal steroids, or the presence of similar conditions in family members. Previous measurements should be plotted on a growth chart to determine height velocity and the age at onset of any increase in the rate of growth.

Important aspects of the physical examination include description of the secondary sexual development according to Tanner stages; measurement of the penis and the testes in boys and of the breast tissue in girls; and examination for acne, oily skin, facial and body hair, pubic and axillary hair development, apocrine gland odor, muscular development, and galactorrhea. A careful examination of the external genitalia should be done with a nonrelated chaperone present, because the performance of such an examination has been interpreted by patients as sexual abuse in some cases.[985] A thorough neurologic examination is indicated, with emphasis on assessment of the visual fields and optic discs and a search for signs of increased intracranial pressure; evaluation for skin lesions associated with the McCune-Albright syndrome or neurofibromatosis; and examination for abdominal, gonadal, or adnexal masses and for coexisting endocrine disease. Bone age is determined in all cases, although it is an imperfect measure.

Ultrasonography of the ovary and uterus is exceedingly useful in the evaluation of affected girls, because standards are available for shape and volume of the uterus and the ovaries.[986] The largest measurements of uterine size by sonography in infants and children are found at puberty and in the neonatal period. The upper limit of uterine length in the prepubertal state is 3.5 cm. A uterine volume of greater than 1.8 mL is specific for the onset of puberty, but increased ovarian volume is less specific. Patients with premature thelarche were indistinguishable from age-matched controls when this sonographic standard was used.[129] The presence of microcysts and macrocysts of the ovary also can be detected on ultrasound examination. Cysts may be found in the ovaries in patients with CPP or GnRH-independent ISP; they usually are smaller than 9 mm in the former and larger than 9 mm in the latter condition.[763] Ovarian volume is reportedly the best indicator of precocious puberty, and uterine length was best for the differentiation of premature thelarche from premature puberty.[986] The presence of an endometrial stripe was indicative of precocious puberty.[129] Ultrasonography of the breast is suggested as a method of determining rapidly progressive versus slowly progressive or transient precocious puberty; accuracy is increased when breast ultrasound findings are added to those of uterine ultrasound and the other factors discussed previously.[987]

Measurements of basal plasma gonadotropin concentrations and the LH response to administration of GnRH or GnRH agonist or the amplitude and frequency of LH pulses, especially at night, using third-generation assays, as well as measurements of the plasma concentration of testosterone in boys or of estradiol in girls using LC/MS-MS assays, are of primary importance in diagnosis. Standards for pubertal development must be available in the laboratories chosen. Girls early in the course of CPP have elevation of estradiol associated with increasing LH levels but not necessarily an increase in the concentration of FSH. Determination of T_4 concentration is indicated when hypothyroidism is suspected. CPP in males usually begins with enlargement of the testes, followed by other signs of secondary sexual maturation. A Leydig cell tumor usually causes asymmetric enlargement of the testes, whereas an extragonadal hCG-secreting tumor is associated with less marked testicular enlargement than occurs at the same stage of masculinization in CPP. Adrenal rests in the testes may enlarge under chronic stimulation from ACTH in boys with inadequately treated CAH or noncompliant boys and may be bilateral, although they are unlikely to closely mimic normal pubertal testicular development. An elevated hCG level with a

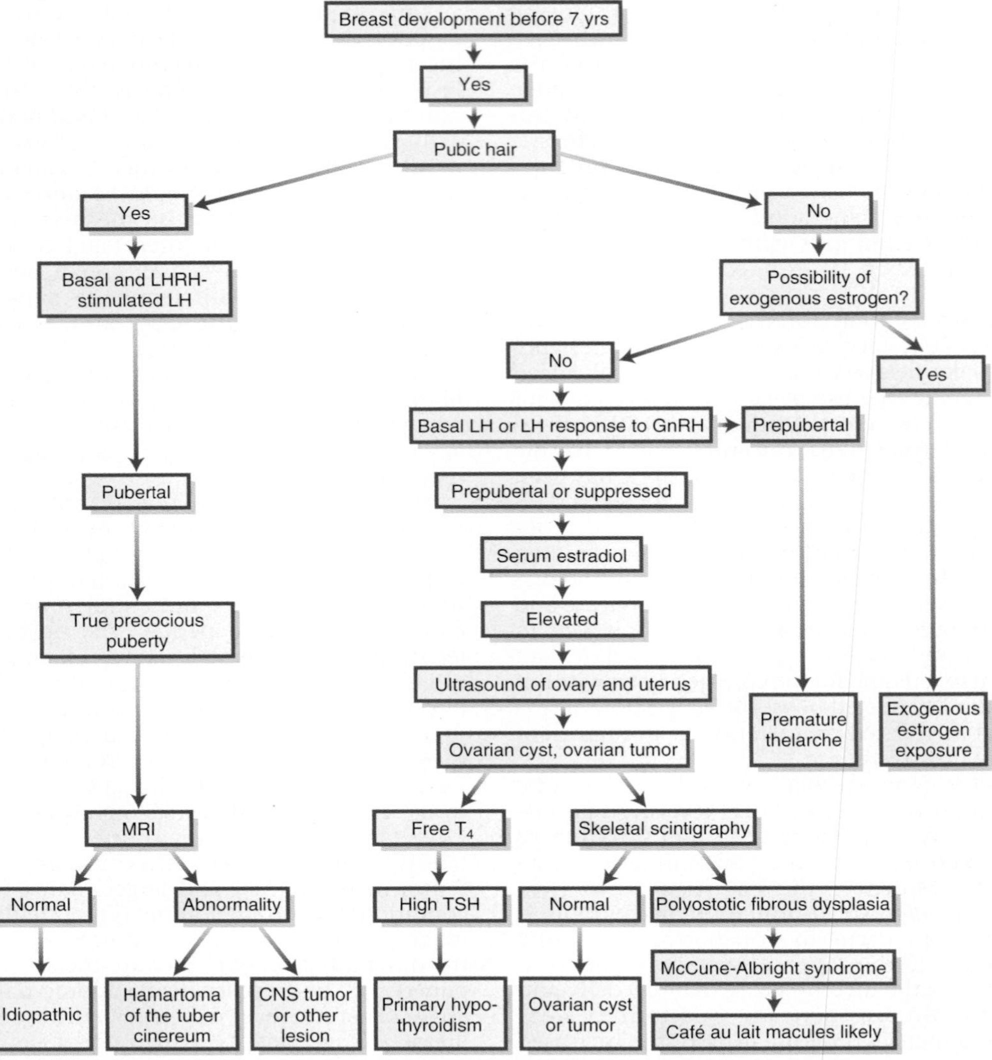

Figure 25-70 Flow chart for diagnosing sexual precocity in girls. CNS, central nervous system; FSH, follicle-stimulating hormone; LH, luteinizing hormone; T_4, thyroxine; TSH, thyroid-stimulating hormone.

prepubertal GnRH test indicates an ectopic, autonomous, gonadotropin-secreting tumor. If this tumor is in the CNS, abnormalities will be present on MRI or CT brain scans. Enlargement of the liver or a mediastinal, retroperitoneal mass in boys with sexual precocity suggests an hCG-producing hepatic or germ cell tumor; the possibility of Klinefelter's syndrome needs to be considered in the latter case.

Pubertal concentrations of LH and FSH, a pubertal mode of pulsatile LH secretion (initially during sleep), or pubertal LH response to GnRH or GnRH agonist confirms the diagnosis of CPP (and in boys differentiates CPP from familial testotoxicosis). A CNS tumor must be considered as a potential cause of this premature activation of the hypothalamic GnRH pulse generator, especially in boys. The evaluation for a CNS tumor as a cause of CPP is similar to the investigation of an hCG-secreting tumor of the CNS. Although CT scanning is now a well established procedure for determining the presence of a CNS abnormality, MRI with contrast is more sensitive for the detection of small tumors in the hypothalamus, such as a hamartoma of the tuber cinereum (see Fig. 25-54). The use of contrast adds to diagnostic certainty and is recommended for MRI of the CNS. All boys with CPP should have CNS MRI evaluation, but girls do not always receive the same recommendation, because a CNS tumor is less likely in girls than in boys to be the cause of CPP. However, studies using MRI or CT brain scans indicate that the hypothalamic hamartoma is more prevalent in both boys and girls with so-called idiopathic CPP than was previously suspected. An unselected group of girls with precocious puberty and no other symptoms underwent CNS MRI; 15% were found to have intracranial pathology, and the investigators found no clinical difference between those girls and the other 85% of girls studied,[988] suggesting that CNS MRI is indicated for girls with precocious puberty.

The height of the pituitary gland on MRI correlates with advancing age and with pubertal development; patients with CPP and higher peak LH/FSH ratios had pituitary heights exceeding 6 mm on average, whereas those with a lower LH/FSH ratio or precocious thelarche had lower heights of approximately 5 mm.[989] The shape of the pituitary gland is also of importance: a convex appearance rather than a flat top is associated with CPP of any cause.[766] The size and shape of the pituitary gland do not decrease with successful GnRH therapy.

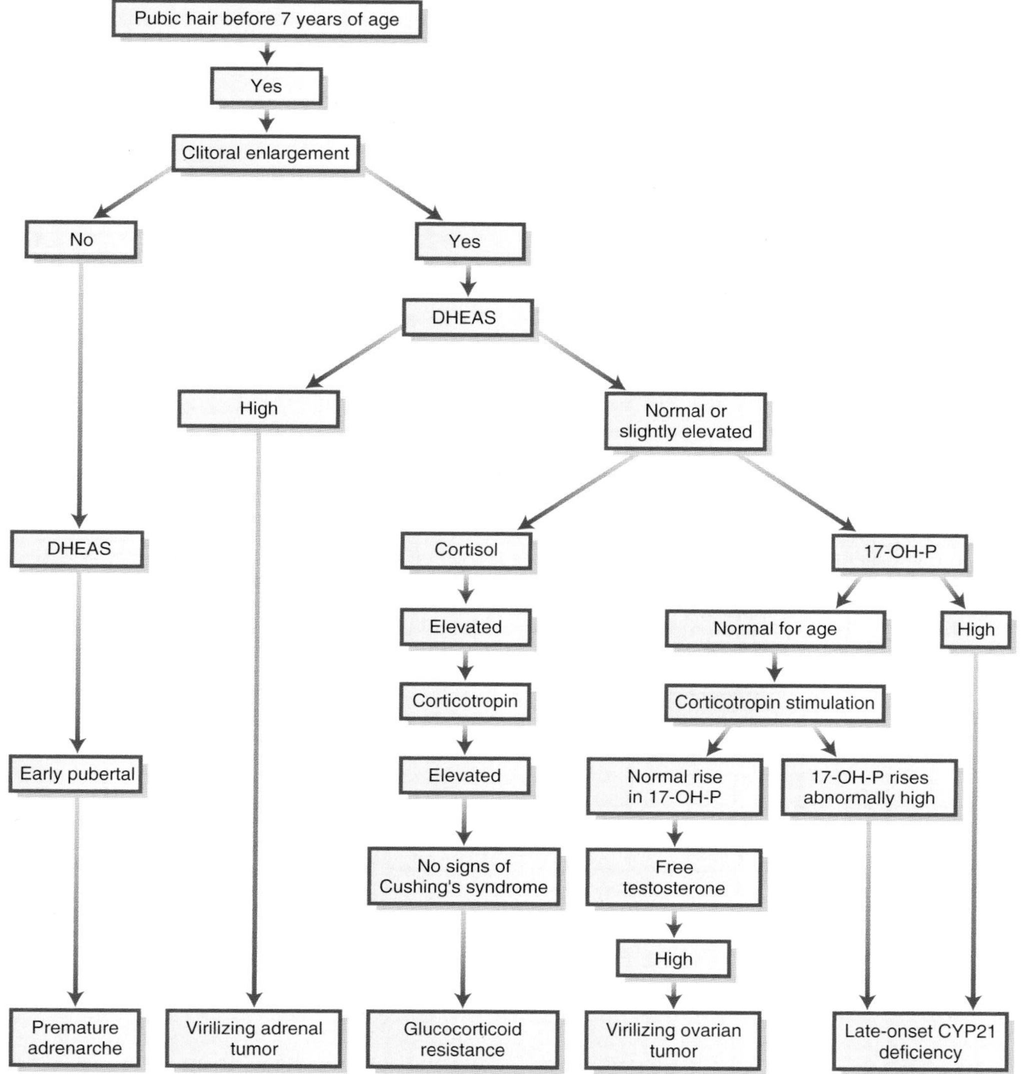

Figure 25-71 Flow chart for the evaluation of pubic hair in normal phenotypic girls before 7 years. DHEAS, dehydroepiandrosterone sulfate; 17-OH-P, 17-hydroxyprogesterone.

The premature appearance of pubic hair, phallic enlargement, and other signs of virilization in a male without enlargement of the testes or the liver suggests the diagnosis of congenital virilizing CAH, virilizing adrenal tumor, or, rarely, Cushing's syndrome. Measurement of plasma 17-hydroxyprogesterone and DHEAS concentrations and their suppressibility with glucocorticoids will distinguish CAH from a virilizing adrenal tumor. If growth rate is suppressed, the possibility of primary hypothyroidism or Cushing's syndrome is raised; elevated plasma concentrations of cortisol, urinary free cortisol, 17-hydroxycorticosteroid, or salivary cortisol after suppression with dexamethasone confirm the latter diagnosis. The appearance in a girl of pubic hair and other signs of virilization, such as clitoral enlargement, acne, deepening voice, muscular development, or growth spurt, is caused by CAH, virilizing adrenal tumor, or virilizing ovarian tumor. Cushing's syndrome caused by an adrenocortical carcinoma can result in virilization associated with growth failure, and a virilizing adrenocortical carcinoma can manifest with so much androgen effect that the Cushing's syndrome is not apparent but rapid growth and virilization are noted; estradiol may be secreted by these tumors as well as androgens. Virilizing ovarian tumors may be detected by pelvic ultrasonography.

The appearance of pubic hair without other signs of puberty in boys or girls, increased growth, or bone age advancement is usually a result of premature adrenarche but may be the first sign of sexual precocity or of adrenal virilism from other causes.

In a girl, breast development associated with dulling and thickening of the vaginal mucosa and enlargement of the labia minora indicates significant estrogen secretion or iatrogenic exposure to estrogen. The differential diagnosis includes CPP, an estrogen-secreting neoplasm, and a cyst of the ovary. If the plasma concentrations of gonadotropins are in the pubertal range, if LH pulses of pubertal amplitude are detected, or if a pubertal LH response to GnRH or GnRH agonist is elicited, CPP is present. In one report, a child had pubertal-level serum LH due to heterophile antibodies that interfered with the LH assay and fallaciously elevated the values in the basal and stimulated state; after addition of anti-mouse antibody, LH values decreased. As always, clinical observation should be congruent with laboratory findings, and the assays should be

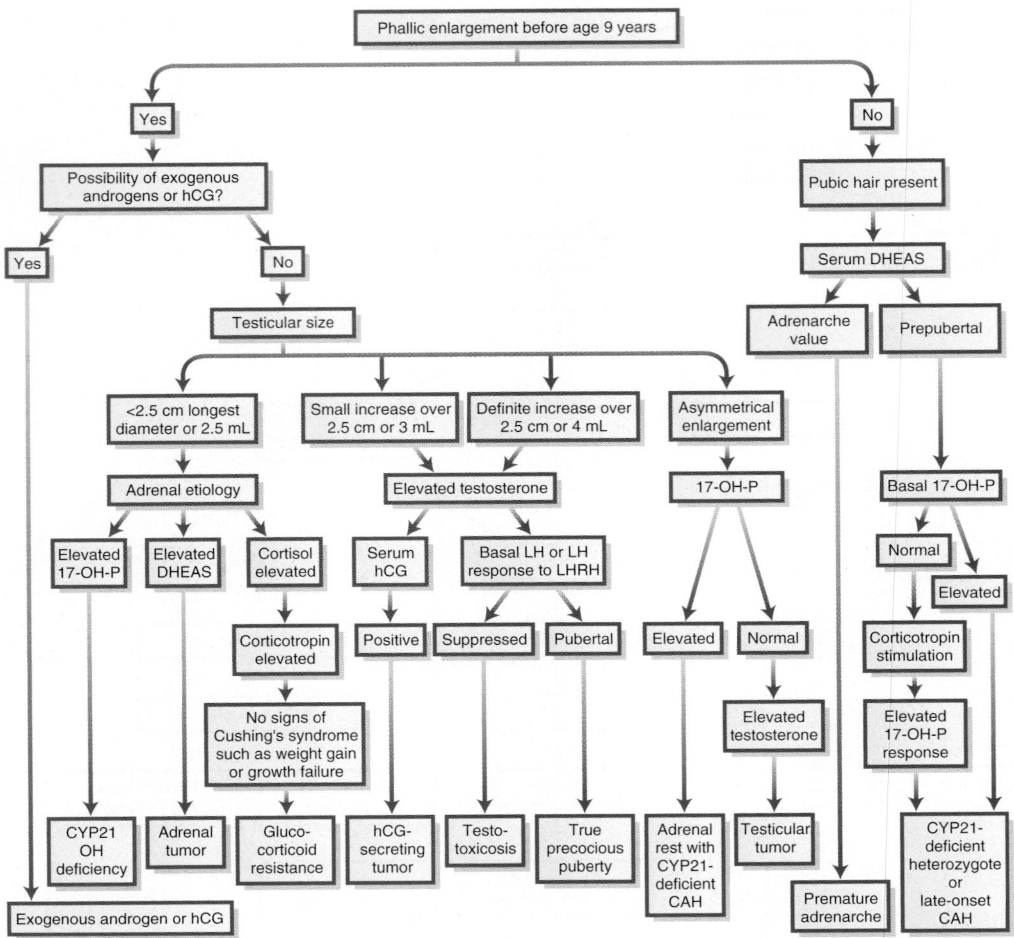

Figure 25-72 Flow chart for diagnosing sexual precocity in a phenotypic male. CAH, congenital adrenal hyperplasia; DHEAS, dehydroepiandrosterone sulfate; hCG, human chorionic gonadotropin; 17-OH-P, 17-hydroxyprogesterone.

highly sensitive and associated with valid pediatric standards.[990] Estradiol concentrations in girls early in normal puberty or CPP are in the prepubertal range for much of the day, and a single determination may be inadequate to reflect ovarian function.[151,742]

If the concentration of plasma estradiol is elevated but gonadotropin levels are low, an estrogen-secreting cyst or neoplasm is present or exogenous estrogens are the cause. Ovarian tumors of moderate size can be palpated by bimanual examination. Advances in pelvic sonography allow the delineation of ovarian cysts or tumors and the determination of uterine size, and this procedure has become an essential component of the diagnostic evaluation.[129] An estrogen-secreting neoplasm of the ovary is usually accompanied by high estradiol concentrations, but some ovarian cysts are associated with concentrations of estradiol as high as those in granulosa cell tumors; the differential diagnosis between these cysts and ovarian neoplasms rarely requires exploratory laparotomy or laparoscopy and usually can be resolved by pelvic sonography and the use of tumor markers. Breast development in the absence of other estrogen effects is almost always a result of premature thelarche.

Iatrogenic Sexual Precocity and Endocrine Disruptors. Prepubertal children are remarkably sensitive to exogenous gonadal steroids and may show signs of sexual maturation resulting from overlooked sources of androgens or estrogens, such as ingested or absorbed tonics, lotions, or hair creams or straighteners that contain or are inadvertently contaminated with an estrogen.[991] Dermal exposure to estrogen may add up to more than 300 µg, far in excess of a therapeutic dose and possibly greater in infants and children exposed to estrogen dermal gel. Oils containing tea tree and lavender oils were reported to cause gynecomastia in three prepuberal boys and demonstrated estrogenic activity in vitro.[992] A short course of application of estrogen cream is used to treat labial adhesions, but long courses may lead to breast development or even withdrawal bleeding. In addition to breast development, pigmentation of the areolae and the linea alba and the appearance of pubic hair may be seen in children exposed to dermal estrogen. Children who touch the skin or the towels of men using androgen gel therapy may themselves develop virilization.[993] The administration of hCG to boys with undescended testes may induce secretion of testosterone sufficient to cause incomplete sexual precocity.

FDA guidelines define a limit of not more that 1% of normal daily estrogen production in prepubertal children as a safe intake of estrogen[994]; this is equivalent to 0.43 ng/day for boys and 3.24 ng/day for girls, based on the most recent data from extremely sensitive estrogen assays, but food is still a suspected source of endocrine disruption.[991,995]

TABLE 25-41

Differential Diagnosis of Sexual Precocity

	Plasma Gonadotropins	LH Response to GnRH	Serum Sex Steroid Concentration	Gonadal Size	Miscellaneous
Gonadotropin-Dependent					
True precocious puberty	Prominent LH pulses (premature reactivation of GnRH pulse generator)	Pubertal LH response initially during sleep	Pubertal values of testosterone or estradiol	Normal pubertal testicular enlargement or ovarian and uterine enlargement	MRI of brain to rule out CNS tumor or other abnormality; skeletal survey for McCune-Albright syndrome (by US)
Incomplete Sexual Precocity (Pituitary Gonadotropin-Independent)					
Males					
Chorionic gonadotropin-secreting tumor in males	High hCG, low LH	Prepubertal LH response	Pubertal value of testosterone	Slight to moderate uniform enlargement of testes	Hepatomegaly suggests hepatoblastoma; CT scan of brain if chorionic gonadotropin-secreting CNS tumor suspected
Leydig cell tumor in males	Suppressed	No LH response	Very high testosterone	Irregular, asymmetric enlargement of testes	
Familial testotoxicosis	Suppressed	No LH response	Pubertal values of testosterone	Testes symmetric and >2.5 cm but smaller than expected for pubertal development; spermatogenesis occurs	Familial; probably sex-limited, autosomal dominant trait
Virilizing congenital adrenal hyperplasia	Prepubertal	Prepubertal LH response	Elevated 17-OHP in CYP21 deficiency or elevated11-deoxycortisol in CYP11B1 deficiency	Testes prepubertal	Autosomal recessive, may be congenital or late-onset form, may have salt loss in CYP21 deficiency or hypertension in CYP11B1 deficiency
Virilizing adrenal tumor	Prepubertal	Prepubertal LH response	High DHEAS and androstenedione values	Testes prepubertal	CT, MRI, or US of abdomen
Premature adrenarche	Prepubertal	Prepubertal LH response	Prepubertal testosterone, DHEAS, or urinary17-ketosteriod values appropriate for pubic hair stage 2	Testes prepubertal	Onset usually after 6 yr of age; more frequent in CNS-injured children
Females					
Granulosa cell tumor (follicular cysts may present similarly)	Suppressed	Prepubertal LH response	Very high estradiol	Ovarian enlargement on physical examination, CT, or US	Tumor often palpable on physical examination
Follicular cyst	Suppressed	Prepubertal LH response	Prepubertal to very high estradiol	Ovarian enlargement on physical examination, CT, or US	Single or recurrent episodes of menses and/or breast development; exclude McCune-Albright syndrome
Feminizing adrenal tumor	Suppressed	Prepubertal LH response	High estradiol and DHEAS values	Ovaries prepubertal	Unilateral adrenal mass
Premature thelarche	Prepubertal	Prepubertal LH, pubertal	Prepubertal or early estradiol response	Ovaries prepubertal	Onset usually before 3 yr of age
Premature adrenarche	Prepubertal	Prepubertal LH response	Prepubertal estradiol; DHEAS or urinary 17-ketosteriod values appropriate for pubic hair stage 2	Ovaries prepubertal	Onset usually after 6 yr of age; more frequent in brain-injured children
Late-onset virilizing congenital adrenal hyperplasia	Prepubertal	Prepubertal LH response	Elevated 17-OHP in basal or corticotropin-stimulated state	Ovaries prepubertal	Autosomal recessive
In Both Sexes					
McCune-Albright syndrome	Suppressed	Suppressed	Sex steroid pubertal or higher	Ovarian (on US); slight testicular enlargement	Skeletal survey for polyostotic fibrous dysplasia and skin examination for café au lait spots
Primary hypothyroidism	LH prepubertal; FSH may be slightly elevated	Prepubertal FSH may be increased	Estradiol may be pubertal	Testicular enlargement; ovaries cystic	TSH and prolactin elevated; T_4 low

CNS, central nervous system; CT, computed tomography; CYP, P450 cytochrome isoenzyme; DHEAS, dehydroepiandrosterone sulfate; GnRH, gonadotropin-releasing hormone; hCG, human chorionic gonadotropin; LH, luteinizing hormone; MRI, magnetic resonance imaging; 17-OHP, 17-hydroxyprogesterone; T_4, thyroxine; TSH, thyrotropin; US, ultrasonography.

Epidemics of gynecomastia in boys and thelarche in girls among schoolchildren in Italy were suspected to be caused by contaminated meat. During a 10-year period, more than 600 cases of gynecomastia in boys and premature thelarche or incomplete sexual precocity in girls were discovered in Puerto Rico; this is the highest prevalence reported in the world, about 10 to 15 times higher than that measured in a survey in Olmsted, Minnesota.[996,997] Maternal ovarian cysts were demonstrated in two thirds of affected Puerto Rican girls. The clandestine use of estrogen preparations in animals to stimulate weight gain, leading to ingestion of estrogen-contaminated meat from these animals, was raised as an possible cause, but this was neither confirmed nor excluded by selected analyses of meat, poultry, and milk in Puerto Rico by the U.S. Department of Agriculture. Significantly elevated concentrations of phthalate and its major metabolites, plasticizers with documented estrogenic and anti-androgenic activity, were found in 28 girls (68%) from a cohort of girls with premature breast development in Puerto Rico,[998] although methodologic criticism of the study arose. One study found no difference between phthalate concentrations in serum between a cohort of girls with CPP and age-matched (nonpubertal) controls.[999]

Endocrine disruptors clearly affect other species, including vertebrates,[1000] but they must be studied in more detail in human beings before specific effects are established. There is convincing evidence for effects of environment on pubertal development when industrial accidents release large amounts of substances but only suggestive epidemiologic evidence that environmental agents are affecting pubertal development in most other situations.[1001] Girls who were breast-fed or exposed during intrauterine life to polybrominated biphenyls (PBBs) after an accidental exposure of their mothers in Michigan experienced early menarche (by about 1 year of age) and early appearance of pubic hair but not breast development, compared with girls who were not exposed or breast-fed.[1002] There was a 9.56 increase in relative risk for precocious puberty treated by GnRH agonist in a localized area in Italy, compared with surrounding areas, suggesting the presence of an endocrine disruptor in the area.[103] Widespread exposure to 2,3,7,8-tetrachlorodibenzo-*p*-dioxin (TCDD), an extremely potent antiestrogenic xenobiotic, in Italy revealed that girls younger than 8 years of age at the time of exposure, who presumably had the highest dose per BMI compared with older girls, showed a tendency for a decrease in age at menarche, suggesting that age of exposure to environmental endocrine disruptors modulates their effects.[1004] Exposure in rodents actually causes a delay in vaginal opening and other reproductive effects. Follow-up of adolescents who were exposed to di-(2-ethylhexyl)-phthalate (DEHP), a component of polyvinyl chloride (PVC) that is used in plastic tubing and medical devices, when they underwent extracorporal membrane oxygenation (ECMO) as neonates demonstrated no effects on pubertal development despite findings of disruption of development in animals exposed to this substance.[1005]

Increased lead levels in Mohawk girls living near the border of New York and Canada delayed the age of menarche, whereas increased levels of polychlorinated biphenyl (PCB) promoted it[1006]; surprisingly, variations in BMI exerted no effect of these toxic substances which are concentrated in adipose tissue. In the NHANES III survey, a serum lead level of 0.7 to 2.0 μg/dL delayed menarche and pubic hair development, and African Americans exposed to 3 μg/dL also experienced delay in breast development.[1007] A long-term study of puberty in Chapaevsk, Russia, an area highly contaminated with industrial waste, demonstrated 43% reduced odds of entering stage 2 genitalia among 8- to 9-year-old boys with serum lead levels equal to or greater than 5 μg/dL.[1008]

There is a high frequency of reproductive problems among adult Danish men, including impaired semen quality, testicular cancer, and increased rate of infantile testicular cancer; these disorders occur in a pattern that is attributed to environmental disruptors, described in the testicular dysgenesis syndrome.[664] A higher rate of hypospadias in Danish newborns and smaller testes with lower serum inhibin B, compared with Finish infants, suggested that environmental agents, rather than genetic influences, were responsible. Phthalates were found in the breast milk of mothers from both countries, and although there was no relationship to the finding of hypospadias, there was an indication of altered reproductive hormones in the boys in a pattern suggesting effects on Leydig cells.

Longitudinal observation of girls in Copenhagen, Denmark, using physical examination of breast tissue showed a significant decline in the age of Tanner stage 2 breast development (estimated mean age, 9.86 years in 2006-2008 versus 10.88 years in 1991) and the age at menarche (13.13 versus 13.42 years, respectively); there was no change in serum gonadotropins, but the serum estradiol concentration was decreased in 2006.[1009] Changes in BMI did not occur in this study between the cohorts, leaving open the possibility of endocrine-disrupting chemicals as an explanation.

Boys exposed to PCBs and polychlorinated dibenzofurans (PCDFs) in utero from contamination of rice ingested by their mothers had decreased testosterone and defects in postpubertal sperm production in a preliminary study, as well as increased estrogen compared with controls, although there was no difference on physical examination or in age at onset of puberty.[1010] Boys exposed to DDT in utero did not demonstrate any abnormalities in puberty in a study from Philadelphia, Pennsylvania.[1011] Exposure to PCBs in inner-city girls with reduced BMI values reportedly delayed thelarche.[45]

The study of endocrine disruptors is active, but the ultimate effects of environmental agents on reproductive development are not yet clear. The complexities of type, amount, developmental age at exposure, and other factors are difficult to tease apart. In the United States, chemicals can enter the environment before their safety is proved, whereas in Norway, all new substances must be proved safe before they can enter the environment. Well-designed longitudinal studies are needed in this area.[1012]

Contrasexual Precocity: Feminization in Boys and Virilization in Girls

Boys. Feminization in a boy before the age of puberty is rare. Rarely, an estrogen-secreting adrenal adenoma or a chorionepithelioma causes gynecomastia. Gynecomastia has been reported in a 1-year-old boy with 11β-hydroxylase deficiency and in boys with late-onset CAH.[1012a]

Aromatase Excess Syndrome. Gynecomastia in prepubertal boys can be caused by increased extraglandular aromatization of C19 steroids of adrenal origin, such as androstenedione, and subsequent increased extraglandular estrogen production in sporadic or familial cases.[257] The autosomal dominant form leads to excess estrogen synthesis from C19 precursors due to aromatase overexpression, especially in fat and skin; it is a consequence of gain-of-function mutations of CYP19, the gene that encodes aromatase, resulting from a chromosome arrangement that gives rise to a cryptic promoter.[1013] An autosomal dominant pattern of prepubertal gynecomastia and adult hypogonadism but not short stature in the presence of elevated serum estrone (with little or no elevation of estradiol) has been reported; the mutations in the CYP19 gene in these patients appeared to be different from those in the families described earlier with gain-of-function mutations resulting from gene inversions.[1014] In a Turkish kindred, there was a potential rearrangement between CYP19 and TRPM7 genes on chromosome 15q21.2 as a cause of aromatase excess syndrome.[1015]

Feminizing Testicular Tumors. Feminizing testicular tumors may cause gynecomastia in boys younger than 6 years of age who have the Peutz-Jeghers syndrome.[936] Aromatase is absent or is present in barely detectable amounts in prepubertal testes, but maximal amounts appear in late puberty. In normal testes, aromatase is predominantly present in the Leydig cells, but in testicular tumors of Sertoli cells or Leydig cells (e.g., associated with the Peutz-Jeghers syndrome), the Sertoli cells of the tumor express aromatase. Both testes may be enlarged, and the histology indicates sex cord or Sertoli cell tumors that form annular tubules and often have areas of calcification; increased estradiol secretion is noted in the basal state, and a further rise occurs after hCG administration. Otherwise, feminizing Sertoli cell tumors are very rare in boys.[937] Sonography or MRI of the testes may be useful in making the diagnosis.

In one series, 5% of 581 boys referred for evaluation of gynecomastia were prepubertal at diagnosis (mean age, 9 years) and in 93% no underlying cause was identified.[1016] Spontaneous resolution was recorded in 6 boys, no change in 15, and further breast enlargement in 6. Prepubertal gynecomastia can be caused by neurofibromatosis.

Girls

Adrenal Causes of Virilization. Virilization in a girl indicates organic disease except for premature adrenarche. CAH resulting from 21-hydroxylase or 11β-hydroxylase deficiency or from androgen-producing tumors of the adrenal can cause virilization (see earlier discussion of their occurrence in males). Nonclassic or late-onset forms of CAH do not demonstrate ambiguous genitalia, but there is evidence of androgen effect in prepuberty or the teenage years. 3β-HSD/$\Delta^{4,5}$-isomerase deficiency is a rare type of CAH characterized by elevated levels of Δ^5-17P, DHEA, and DHEAS, as well as decreased secretion of aldosterone and cortisol in the severe form. Severely affected patients have mineralocorticoid and glucocorticoid deficiencies and may die in infancy. Excess adrenal androgens lead to virilization in utero and to ambiguous external genitalia, including clitoral enlargement in females with continued virilization after birth. Milder forms of this disorder can cause hirsutism in women. Women with a 46,XY phenotype and incomplete forms of androgen resistance syndrome or 17β-HSD type 3 deficiency may have virilization as well as breast development at the time of expected puberty. Mutations in the *CYP19* gene, which encodes aromatase, is associated with intrauterine masculinization of the external genitalia in affected 46XX individuals and also with progressive virilization, lack of female secondary sex characteristics, multicystic ovaries at the age of puberty, tall stature, and osteopenia.[255,257]

Cushing's syndrome resulting from adrenal carcinoma usually manifests as growth failure with or without virilization, obesity, and moon facies; striae may not appear until months to years later.

Syndrome of Glucocorticoid Resistance. The syndrome of glucocorticoid resistance has variable manifestations. Some patients demonstrate hyperandrogenic signs such as acne, hirsutism, male-type baldness, menstrual irregularities, and oligoanovulation and infertility.[1017] Dexamethasone decreases the excessive adrenal androgen secretion, virilization, and advancing bone age found in general glucocorticoid resistance.

Virilizing Ovarian Tumors. Arrhenoblastoma, also called Sertoli tumor of the ovary, is the most common virilizing ovarian tumor, but it is rare in children. Lipoid-cell tumors of the ovary and gonadoblastomas or Sertoli-cell tumors of the ovary are even more unusual sources of androgens.[1018,1019]

Variations of Pubertal Development

Premature Thelarche. Unilateral or bilateral breast enlargement without other signs of sexual maturation (e.g., sexual hair, growth of the labia minora, growth of the uterus) is not uncommon in infancy and childhood and is termed *premature thelarche*. The disorder usually occurs by age 2 (>80% of cases) and rarely after age 4.[1020] In a retrospective study in Minnesota, the incidence of premature thelarche was 21.2 per 100,000 patient-years, 60% of cases were identified in patients between 6 months and 2 years of age, and most cases regressed within 6 months to 6 years after diagnosis, although a few persisted until puberty. When 10- to 35-year follow-up was available, no untoward effects on later health, growth, or fertility were evident.[997] Breast enlargement usually regresses after a few months[1020] but occasionally persists for years or until the onset of normal puberty; in about half of affected girls, the breast development, which is characteristically cyclic, lasts 3 to 5 years. Usually, significant nipple and areolae development is absent, and estrogen-induced thickening and dulling of the vaginal mucosa is uncommon. Enlargement of the uterus on ultrasonography (volume >1.8 mL, length >36 mm) is rare. Measurement of the ellipsoid volume of the uterus (V = longitudinal diameter × anteroposterior diameter × transverse diameter × 0.523) is the most sensitive and specific discriminator between premature thelarche and early CPP[129] and provides better early discrimination than the LH response to GnRH or GnRH agonist. Growth in stature is normal.

This is a benign, self-limited disorder that is compatible with normal pubertal development at an appropriate age; usually, only reassurance and follow-up are necessary. However, the appearance of premature thelarche can be the harbinger of further sexual maturation in a minority of cases, as discussed elsewhere in this chapter.[763,1021] If onset occurs soon after birth and before 2 years of age, the prognosis for regression is better.[129] Because the development may be unilateral, it is important to consider the condition in girls who have unilateral breast development so that needless worry about a breast neoplasm is not stimulated in the parents and no unnecessary surgical procedure is carried out, because removal of tissue in premature thelarche may leave the child with no possibility of future breast development. In selected instances, sonography of the breast is useful to distinguish unilateral premature thelarche from less benign conditions. The most common cause of a breast mass in a pubertal girl is fibroadenoma, and although metastatic disease may locate in the pubertal breast, breast carcinoma is exceedingly rare in young patients.

Plasma estradiol levels are slightly higher for age in patients with premature thelarche determined by a highly sensitive estrogen assay.[1021] However, there is usually no significant increase in plasma levels of TeBG or in thyroxine-binding globulin, which are indicators of estrogen action on circulating plasma proteins, although a modest increase of TeBG for age has been reported. The urocytogram often reveals an estrogen effect on squamous epithelial cells in the urine.[769,1022]

The concentration of serum FSH may be in the pubertal range, nocturnal FSH pulsatility has been detected, and the rise in FSH elicited by administration of GnRH may be augmented for chronologic age, with an FSH/LH ratio higher in precocious thelarche than in normal individuals or in girls with CPP.[429,774] However, the results overlap those in normal prepubertal girls.

As postulated for some recurrent ovarian cysts, premature thelarche appears to result from the ovarian response to transient increases in FSH levels and possibly from variations in ovarian sensitivity to FSH.[429,1022] The LH response to GnRH is prepubertal in all cases.[429] Plasma inhibin B and FSH levels are higher in girls with precocious thelarche than in control subjects, in a range similar to that observed in patients with precocious puberty.[1023] Activin concentrations have not been reported. The possible role of a paracrine-acting pituitary factor in stimulating FSH independent of GnRH is not known.

Sonograms of the ovary often show one or several cysts larger than 0.5 cm that disappear and reappear, usually correlating with changes in the size of the breasts, but the volume of the ovary and uterus is prepubertal.[129] In clinical practice, it is rare to find a cyst at the time of presentation and on ultrasonic study.

Exaggerated thelarche is described as premature thelarche with the added findings of advanced bone age and increased growth rate, which are estrogen effects. The endocrine measurements in the basal state are in the normal prepubertal range, but after GnRH agonist stimulation, the level of FSH (but not of LH) rose higher than in controls or in patients with CPP.[762] Mutation of *GNAS1* involving Arg201His is associated with apparent premature or exaggerated thelarche and early menarche.[951]

Premature Isolated Menarche. Rarely, girls begin periodic vaginal bleeding at between 1 and 9 years of age without any other signs of secondary sexual development. The bleeding can recur for 1 to 6 years and then cease. At the normal age of puberty (3 to 11 years later), secondary sexual development and menses ensue and follow a normal pattern, as does stature. Fertility was later demonstrated after a normal onset of puberty in women with this variant of pubertal development. The cause is uncertain, but it may be a counterpart of premature thelarche. There is a predominance of FSH secretion, but the gonadotropin secretion pattern is not characteristic of CPP.[1024] Isolated menarche may appear before other manifestations of sexual precocity in patients with the McCune-Albright syndrome and in those with the premature sexual maturation that can occur in juvenile hypothyroidism.

Before the diagnosis of premature menarche is accepted, all other causes of vaginal bleeding and precocious estrogen secretion and of exposure to exogenous estrogens should be excluded, including neoplasms, granulomas, infection of the vagina or cervix, and presence of a foreign body. A careful examination for trauma, such as that caused by sexual abuse, is indicated. Urethral prolapse may be misdiagnosed as vaginal bleeding.

Premature Adrenarche. Premature adrenarche (i.e., pubarche) is the precocious appearance of pubic hair or axillary hair or both and, less commonly, an apocrine odor, comedones, and acne, without other signs of puberty or virilization. It is characterized by premature and mild adrenal hyperandrogenism.[313] The term *premature adrenarche* refers to the rise in serum concentrations of adrenal androgens that causes the appearance of the pubic hair. In the past, this designation was assigned when these clinical features appeared before age 8 years in girls or 9 years in boys. Although in boys the 9 years still seems appropriate as a cutoff point, the age of 8 years can no longer be used for American girls, according to the results of the in the PROS study described earlier[97] (mean ages are shown in Table 25-1). We recommend that the diagnosis of premature pubarche should be limited to African American girls younger than 6 years of age and white American girls younger than 7 years, which should affect the age at which laboratory studies are initiated unless there are other signs of virilization, such as clitoromegaly or rapid growth.

Premature adrenarche is about 10 times more common in girls than in boys. The prevalence is increased in children with CNS abnormalities without a clear sex difference; the electroencephalogram may be abnormal[752] in the absence of other neurologic findings. Familial transmission is uncommon.[1025] Premature adrenarche is commonly slowly progressive and does not have an untoward effect on either the onset or the normal progression of gonadarche or final adult height.[284] Nonetheless, there is a relationship between reduced fetal growth leading to intrauterine growth retardation and subsequent SGA and the increased prevalence of premature adrenarche, hyperinsulinism, and ovarian hyperandrogenism in life.[313]

Plasma concentrations of DHEA, DHEAS, androstenedione, testosterone, 17-hydroxyprogesterone, and Δ^5-17P are comparable to values normally found in pubic hair stage 2.[443,1026,1027] ACTH stimulation increases serum DHEA and DHEAS concentrations and the excretion of urinary 17-ketosteroids, but the concentrations of plasma 17-hydroxyprogesterone and Δ^5-17P do not increase to the levels found in individuals with virilizing forms of CAH.[1028] Shorter androgen receptor gene CAG number, indicative of increased androgen sensitivity, is reported in some girls with precocious adrenarche.[1029] As in CAH, dexamethasone suppresses adrenal androgen and androgen precursor secretion. Serum gonadotropin levels in the basal state and after GnRH are in the prepubertal range in patients with premature adrenarche.[429] Premature adrenarche occurs independently of gonadarche and results from some factor other than increased secretion of GnRH or ACTH.[442] Bone age, height, and weight gain are slightly advanced for chronologic age, but normal adult height is commonly achieved,[1030,1031] except, rarely, in some individuals with unusually high levels of adrenal androgens, hirsutism, acne, and a bone age more than 2.5 SD above the mean value for chronologic age. In a follow-up study of 20 girls, the functional adrenal hyperandrogenism in premature adrenarche was limited to childhood.

Premature adrenarche may be considered to be a developmentally regulated, normal variation in the differentiation, growth, and function of the zona reticularis of the adrenal cortex, marked biochemically by the precocious increase in the concentration of plasma DHEAS to more than 40 μg/dL.[284] The latter is probably related to the independent increase of 17,20-lyase activity in the developing zona reticularis, which is mediated by increased phosphorylation of serine and threonine residues on the CYP17 enzyme, and the increased abundance of cytochrome *b*5 and of electron-donating redox partners such as cytochrome P450 oxidoreductase and cytochrome *b*5, which are essential for the 17,20-lyase activity of this functional microsomal enzyme (see Fig. 25-35).[1028] Nonetheless, the factor stimulating development and function of the zona reticularis, independent of ACTH, remains elusive. In the past, failure to recognize the earlier onset of normal adrenarche, and particularly the striking ethnic differences in African American, Hispanic, and Latin populations, contributed to the overdiagnosis of premature adrenarche[313,1032-1034] and, in some instances, to needless laboratory studies.

The appearance of premature pubarche can be a manifestation of nonclassic CAH caused by homozygous or compound heterozygous missense mutations in the *CYP21* gene.[1036] This condition can readily be detected by a plasma 17-hydroxyprogesterone response to ACTH that is at least 6 SD above the mean value. The prevalence of 21-hydroxylase deficiency in children with premature adrenarche is low[1036,1037] except in some ethnic groups[1038,1039] (e.g., Hispanics, Italians, Ashkenazi Jews), in which the prevalence may be as high as 20% to 30%.[1039,1040] The phenotype of premature pubarche is also associated with the rarer nonclassic 11β-hydroxylase deficiency.

There has been controversy about the prevalence and significance of 3β-HSD deficiency and a pervasive belief that a mutation in the gene encoding this enzyme is a common cause of premature adrenarche and nonclassic 3β-HSD deficiency. The possibility of a mutation in the open receding frame of the 3β-HSD type 2 or type 1 gene (i.e., *HSD3B2* or *HSD3B1*) has been excluded as an uncommon cause of this condition.[1041-1043] Mutations in *HSD3B2* have been associated with a Δ^5-17P response to ACTH that exceeds or equals the mean normal value by 6 SD. Of 26 families studied, only 1 family with a mutation (Ala82Thr) had affected females who exhibited premature pubarche; in this family, the affected male was a male pseudohermaphrodite.[1044] Therefore, mutation of *HSD3B2* or *HSD3B1* is an uncommon cause of premature pubarche, exaggerated adrenarche, and hirsutism in adolescent girls and women.

The cause of the observed mild deficiency in 3β-HSD activity is unknown, but it may be multifactorial and may lead to a wide range in secretory capacity of the zona reticularis. A family constellation was described with a dominant pattern of inheritance[1025] of elevated adrenal androgens and androgen precursors that manifested as premature pubarche; later-affected individuals developed hirsutism and anovulation. Several investigators joined to propose hormonal standards for the diagnosis of 3β-HSD deficiency in cases of apparent premature pubarche and stated that ACTH-stimulated Δ^5-17P values must exceed 294 nmol/L or 54 SD above the mean for Tanner stage 2 (17 ± 5 nmol/L) or the ratio of Δ^5-17P to cortisol (F) must be at least 363, which is 3.0 SD above the mean ratio of 20 ± 5. Studies relating genotype and hormonal analyses in basal and ACTH-stimulated conditions have confirmed that significant elevations of the Δ^5-17P-to-F ratio are necessary to prove true 3β-HSD deficiency in genetically proven disease[1045] and that this is a rare disorder in patients presenting with putative premature adrenarche. However, patients with a constellation of findings indicating PCOS may have more subtle elevations of these values and present a picture of adrenal impairment of 3β-HSD activity in the absence of mutations in the gene coding for the enzyme; these children presenting with premature pubarche are postulated to develop clinical PCOS at a later age.[1045]

DHEA stimulates sebaceous gland activity,[1046] and prepubertal acne or comedones may appear in association with elevated serum DHEAS concentrations in some children without the appearance of pubic hair, suggesting that a variant of premature adrenarche may manifest in this manner.[119] More significant androgen effects (e.g., clitoral or penile enlargement, rapid growth, hirsutism, deepening of the voice) exclude premature adrenarche and indicate a more severe form of hyperandrogenism.

Although premature adrenarche was usually considered to be a benign condition with no substantial long-term risk, accumulating observations indicate that girls with premature adrenarche are at increased risk of developing functional ovarian hyperandrogenism and PCOS, hyperinsulinism, acanthosis nigricans, and dyslipidemia in adolescence and adult life, especially if fetal growth was reduced and the birth weight was low.[313] Affected girls have BMI values similar to those of controls but differing distribution of fat; they are more likely to have increased waist circumference along with measures of insulin resistance.[1047] The concept of *exaggerated adrenarche*[1036] was first advanced in relation to a postulated childhood antecedent of PCOS. It has been extended to include rare instances of premature adrenarche associated with excessive responses of Δ^5-17P, DHEAS, and androstenedione to ACTH found in women with functional adrenal hyperandrogenism.

A recent report of a patient with premature adrenarche, advanced bone age, excessive acne, hyperandrogenic anovulation, very low DHEAS levels, and increased androgen levels demonstrated a mutation in PAPSS2, an enzyme that generates the sulfate donor 3′-phosphoadenosine-5′-phosphosulfate (PAPS), which is required for conversion of DHEA to DHEAS by the enzyme SULT2A1. Although the child was described as having premature pubarche, the androgen effects were greater than those usually encountered in this condition. The DHEA level was not elevated for age, but androstenedione was high due to inadequate formation of DHEAS that decreases the conversion of DHEA to androstenedione. This presentation would ordinarily suggest an ovarian cause of the virilization. This monogenetic defect must be added to the differential diagnosis of premature adrenarche.[286]

Polycystic Ovarian Disease. PCOS is the most common endocrine disease; it is estimated to affect 10% of women.[1048,1049] The hallmarks of this condition are hyperandrogenism, hirsutism, anovulation, amenorrhea or oligomenorrhea, and insulin resistance; there is compensatory hyperinsulinemia, with its attendant risk of major metabolic sequelae including type 2 diabetes mellitus, dyslipidemia, an increased propensity to coronary heart disease, and, in about 50% of affected women, obesity. PCOS is considered to be equivalent to the metabolic syndrome in its many manifestations in females. A 2004 review of diagnostic criteria supported most of the original 1990 recommendations.[1050] Premature adrenarche is an risk factor for the later development of the PCOS and functional ovarian hyperandrogenism in adolescent and adult women; the magnitude of this risk is unknown, but it appears to be rare, except in girls with a history of SGA.[7,313,1036,1051] However, catch-up growth after SGA may be as important a factor in the development of PCOS, and even prematurity may be a risk. In an 880-member cohort of 8-year-olds, serum androstenedione and DHEAS levels were directly related to weight gain between 1 and 3 years and current weight and inversely related to birth weight.[8] However, a Dutch study could not confirm such a relationship between increase in premature adrenarche and SGA birth weight in 181 subjects born with SGA compared with 170 subjects born with appropriate weight for gestational age (AGA).[1052]

Plasma plasminogen activator inhibitor 1 (PAI-1), a marker of risk for cardiovascular disease including in women with PCOS, was increased in girls with premature adrenarche, and especially in those with low birth weight, and may be useful in the identification of girls who have an increased risk of developing PCOS.[1053] In certain ethnic groups, and especially in African American and Hispanic girls, there is a greater association of premature adrenarche with the metabolic syndrome (obesity, hyperinsulinism, dyslipidemia, and other factors that increase the risk of later coronary heart disease) and the development of PCOS in late adolescence and early adulthood,[313,313,1054,1055] especially if decreased insulin sensitivity and acanthosis nigricans accompany the premature adrenarche. The adrenal steroid pattern in black and Hispanic patients in one of these studies[1055] did not differ from that in children with uncomplicated premature adrenarche.

As discussed earlier, hyperinsulinism is associated with many metabolic and endocrine conditions and functional ovarian hyperandrogenism which, in some cases, is heralded by premature adrenarche. Therapeutic approaches to reduce insulin resistance, especially the use of insulin sensitizers, have been introduced into the therapy for PCOS. The most widely used drug is metformin because of its low prevalence of adverse effects and therapeutic efficacy, although its major effect is in decreasing gluconeogenesis from the liver rather than insulin sensitizing. In early studies, this agent resulted in decreased insulin resistance, ovarian hyperandrogenism, and hirsutism in obese and nonobese patients in the treatment of PCOS. A short-term, randomized trial[1056] of metformin in 82 children and adolescents with type 2 diabetes mellitus (10 to 16 years of age) provided useful preliminary data to support the safety and efficacy of its use in adolescents with insulin resistance and functional ovarian hyperandrogenism, although metformin is not FDA-approved for such use.

In a trial involving girls just past menarche who had a history of low birth weight and premature adrenarche and were therefore at risk for development of PCOS, metformin prevented this predicted course.[7] Treatment of 8-year-old girls who had similar risk factors appeared to diminish the risk during short-term studies. The beneficial effects on body composition, dyslipidemia, insulin resistance, and other parameters were present only during therapy; they reverted to increased risk factors after discontinuation of metformin.

In an in vitro study, troglitazone, but not metformin, directly inhibited the steroidogenic enzymes CYP17 and 3β-HSD,[1057] and clinical study suggested that this medication may be efficacious in the treatment of PCOS even though it is not approved for this use by the FDA. These are promising approaches to a still poorly understood syndrome that often manifests during adolescence. Many aspects need to be addressed in the management of this heterogeneous disorder, including, apart from pharmacologic agents, concern about nutrition and physical activity, which are also shown to improve the findings of PCOS.

Adolescent Gynecomastia. Normal boys, usually in the early stages of puberty, may have either unilateral breast enlargement (approximately 25% of boys)[1058] or bilateral breast enlargement (approximately 50% to 65% of boys to varying degrees); this commonly occurs between chronologic ages 14 and 14.5 years or with pubic hair stages 3 and 4. In these boys, the plasma concentrations of testosterone and estrogen are normal for their stage of puberty. Some have suggested that the ratio of estrogen to androgen or an increase in the ratio of testosterone to dihydrotestosterone is a cause. In a prospective study, adolescent boys with gynecomastia had a lower mean free testosterone concentration, lower weight, higher plasma TeBG levels, and a tendency toward earlier onset of puberty and more rapid progression through puberty.[1058] In one study, a significant decrease in the concentration ratio of plasma androstenedione to estrone and estradiol and a similarly low ratio of DHEAS to estrone and estradiol were described in boys with pubertal gynecomastia who had normal ratios of plasma estrone and estradiol to testosterone. It was postulated that decreased adrenal production of androgens or (more likely) increased peripheral conversion of adrenal androgens to estrogens was a factor in the development of pubertal gynecomastia.[1059]

Trials of estrogen receptor antagonists (e.g., tamoxifen, raloxifene) or exogenous androgens have had mixed results in gynecomastia, and more study is required. One study of boys (average age, 13 years) with gynecomastia involving a mean of 7 months of treatment with anastrazole demonstrated a substantial decrease in breast area (63%) and volume (53%), as measured manually and by ultrasonography,[1060] compared with watchful waiting; however, larger studies are recommended to prove the utility of this approach.

Pubertal gynecomastia usually resolves spontaneously within 1 to 2 years after onset, and reassurance and continued observation are often adequate treatment. Nevertheless, some boys have conspicuous gynecomastia, and if it lasts longer than 2 years, it is likely to become permanent. These children may have sufficient psychological distress to warrant a reduction mammoplasty. Liposuction is an alternative approach, but its efficacy in adolescent gynecomastia remains to be established. Rarely, untreated gynecomastia persists into adulthood.

Gynecomastia is a component of Klinefelter's syndrome, anorchia, primary and secondary hypogonadism, biosynthetic defects in testosterone synthesis, increased aromatase activity in adipose and other tissues (aromatase excess syndrome), Sertoli cell tumors, adventitious exposure to estrogens in meat or cosmetics, and variants of the androgen resistance syndromes, including Rosewater syndrome (familial hypogonadism and gynecomastia) and Reifenstein syndrome (hypospadias, hypogonadism, and gynecomastia). These disorders usually have characteristic findings or environmental circumstances that allow ready differentiation from the normal gynecomastia of puberty.[633] Gynecomastia has been described in association with the administration of drugs such as cimetidine, spironolactone, digitalis, and phenothiazines, with GH therapy, and with the use of marijuana. The aromatase excess syndrome was described earlier.

Macroorchidism. Macroorchidism, without androgenization, is a rare manifestation of the McCune-Albright syndrome[962] and an occasional finding in prepubertal boys with long-standing primary hypothyroidism. This form of testicular enlargement appears to result from increased FSH secretion, independent of a pubertal increase in LH secretion or a pubertal LH response to GnRH. Testicular adrenal rests in CAH and lymphoma can cause bilateral macroorchidism. It is a feature of severe aromatase deficiency in young male adults[257] and in men with an FSH-secreting pituitary macroadenoma. Bilateral megalotestis (testicular volume, 26 mL) in adults can occur as a normal variant.[1061] One may speculate that some instances of bilateral macroorchidism are the result of a heterozygous constitutive activating mutation of the FSH receptor. As noted earlier, prepubertal enlargement of the testes was reported with a single-base-pair deletion at codon 434 (1301delT) of the *NR0B1/DAX1* gene and led to prepubertal testosterone and gonadotropin values.[881]

The fragile X syndrome is associated with developmental delay, a long face and large prominent ears, and macroorchidism in 80% of affected pubertal boys. Macroorchidism may be evident only after careful measurements. The enlarged testes are caused by increased interstitial volume and excessive connective tissue, including increased peritubular collagen fibers, rather than by an increase in the seminiferous tubules. Enlargement of the testes is demonstrable in the prepubertal period in most patients with fragile X syndrome, but the onset of true macroorchidism (>4 cm) occurs only in the later prepubertal period.[1062]

REFERENCES

1. Grumbach MM. Onset of puberty. In: Berenberg SR, ed. *Puberty: Biologic and Social Components*. Leiden, The Netherlands: H.E. Stenfert Kroese; 1975:1-21.
2. Moggi-Cecchi J. Questions of growth. *Nature*. 2001;414:595-597.
3. Bogin B. Growth and development: recent evolutionary and biocultural research. In: Boaz NT, Wolfe DL, eds. Bend, OR: International Institute for Human Evolutionary Research; 1995:49-70.
4. Keverne EB. Understanding well-being in the evolutionary context of brain development. *Philos Trans R Soc Lond B Biol Sci*. 2004;359: 1349-1358.
5. Conroy GC, Kuykendall K. Paleopediatrics: or when did human infants really become human? *Am J Phys Anthropol*. 1995; 98:121-131.
6. Gluckman PD, Hanson MA. Changing times: the evolution of puberty. *Mol Cell Endocrinol*. 2006;254-255:26-31.
7. Ibanez L, de Zegher F. Puberty and prenatal growth. *Mol Cell Endocrinol*. 2006;254-255:22-25.
8. Ong KK, Potau N, Petry CJ, et al. Opposing influences of prenatal and postnatal weight gain on adrenarche in normal boys and girls. *J Clin Endocrinol Metab*. 2004;89:2647-2651.
9. Sloboda DM, Hart R, Doherty DA, et al. Age at menarche: Influences of prenatal and postnatal growth. *J Clin Endocrinol Metab*. 2007; 92:46-50.
10. Tam CS, de Zegher F, Garnett SP, et al. Opposing influences of prenatal and postnatal growth on the timing of menarche. *J Clin Endocrinol Metab*. 2006;91:4369-4373.
11. Ong KK, Emmett P, Northstone K, et al. Infancy weight gain predicts childhood body fat and age at menarche in girls. *J Clin Endocrinol Metab*. 2009;94:1527-1532.
12. Tanner JM. *A History of the Study of Human Growth*. Cambridge, UK: Cambridge University Press; 1981.
13. Wyshak G, Frisch RE. Evidence for a secular trend in age of menarche. *N Engl J Med*. 1982;306:1033-1035.
14. Biro FM, Huang B, Crawford PB, et al. Pubertal correlates in black and white girls. *J Pediatr*. 2006;148:234-240.
15. Artaria MD, Henneberg M. Why did they lie? Socio-economic bias in reporting menarcheal age. *Ann Hum Biol*. 2000;27:561-569.
16. Marshall WA, Tanner JM. Puberty. In: Falkner F, Tanner JM, eds. *Human Growth*. New York, NY: Plenum; 1986:171-209.
17. Parent AS, Teilmann G, Juul A, et al. The timing of normal puberty and the age limits of sexual precocity: variations around the world, secular trends, and changes after migration. *Endocr Rev*. 2003;24: 668-693.
18. Ong KK, Ahmed ML, Dunger DB. Lessons from large population studies on timing and tempo of puberty (secular trends and relation to body size): the European trend. *Mol Cell Endocrinol*. 2006;254-255: 8-12.
19. Freedman DS, Khan LK, Serdula MK, et al. Relation of age at menarche to race, time period, and anthropometric dimensions: the Bogalusa Heart Study. *Pediatrics*. 2002;110:e43.
20. MacMahon B. Age at menarche: National Health Survey. DHEW Publication No. (HRA) 74-1615, Series 11, No. 133. Washington, DC: 1973.
21. Chumlea WC, Schubert CM, Roche AF, et al. Age at menarche and racial comparisons in US girls. *Pediatrics*. 2003;111:110-113.
22. Himes JH. Examining the evidence for recent secular changes in the timing of puberty in US children in light of increases in the prevalence of obesity. *Mol Cell Endocrinol*. 2006;254-255:13-21.
23. Harlan WR, Harlan EA, Grillo GP. Secondary sex characteristics of girls 12 to 17 years of age: the U.S. Health Examination Survey. *J Pediatr*. 1980;96:1074-1078.
24. Russell DL, Keil MF, Bonat SH, et al. The relation between skeletal maturation and adiposity in African American and Caucasian children. *J Pediatr*. 2001;139:844-848.
25. Biro FM, McMahon RP, Striegel-Moore R, et al. Impact of timing of pubertal maturation on growth in black and white female adolescents: The National Heart, Lung, and Blood Institute Growth and Health Study. *J Pediatr*. 2001;138:636-643.
26. Juul A, Teilmann G, Scheike T, et al. Pubertal development in Danish children: comparison of recent European and US data. *Int J Androl*. 2006;29:247-255.
27. Krebs NF, Himes JH, Jacobson D, et al. Assessment of child and adolescent overweight and obesity. *Pediatrics*. 2007;120(suppl 4):S193-S228.
28. August GP, Caprio S, Fennoy I, et al. Prevention and treatment of pediatric obesity: an Endocrine Society clinical practice guideline based on expert opinion. *J Clin Endocrinol Metab*. 2008; 93:4576-4599.
29. Kaplowitz PB, Slora EJ, Wasserman RC, et al. Earlier onset of puberty in girls: relation to increased body mass index and race. *Pediatrics*. 2001;108:347-353.
30. Rosenfield RL, Lipton RB, Drum ML. Thelarche, pubarche, and menarche attainment in children with normal and elevated body mass index. *Pediatrics*. 2009;123:84-88.
31. Anderson SE, Dallal GE, Must A. Relative weight and race influence average age at menarche: results from two nationally representative surveys of US girls studied 25 years apart. *Pediatrics*. 2003;111 (4 Pt 1):844-850.
32. Himes JH, Obarzanek E, Baranowski T, et al. Early sexual maturation, body composition, and obesity in African-American girls. *Obes Res*. 2004;12(suppl):64S-72S.
33. Herman-Giddens ME, Wang L, Koch G. Secondary sexual characteristics in boys. *Arch Pediatr Adolesc Med*. 2001;155:1022-1028.
34. He Q, Karlberg J. BMI in childhood and its association with height gain, timing of puberty, and final height. *Pediatr Res*. 2001;49: 244-251.
35. Biro FM, Lucky AW, Simbartl LA, et al. Pubertal maturation in girls and the relationship to anthropometric changes: pathways through puberty. *J Pediatr*. 2003;142:643-646.
36. Schubert CM, Chumlea WC, Kulin HE, et al. Concordant and discordant sexual maturation among U.S. children in relation to body weight and BMI. *J Adolesc Health*. 2005;37:356-362.
37. Adair LS, Gordon-Larsen P. Maturational timing and overweight prevalence in US adolescent girls. *Am J Public Health*. 2001;91:642-644.
38. Davison KK, Susman EJ, Birch LL. Percent body fat at age 5 predicts earlier pubertal development among girls at age 9. *Pediatrics*. 2003;111(4 Pt 1):815-821.
39. Demerath EW, Towne B, Chumlea WC, et al. Recent decline in age at menarche: the Fels Longitudinal Study. *Am J Hum Biol*. 2004;16: 453-457.
40. van Hooff MH, Voorhorst FJ, Kaptein MB, et al. Insulin, androgen, and gonadotropin concentrations, body mass index, and waist to hip ratio in the first years after menarche in girls with regular menstrual cycles, irregular menstrual cycles, or oligomenorrhea. *J Clin Endocrinol Metab*. 2000;85:1394-1400.
41. Berkey CS, Gardner JD, Frazier AL, et al. Relation of childhood diet and body size to menarche and adolescent growth in girls. *Am J Epidemiol*. 2000;152:446-452.
42. Koo MM, Rohan TE, Jain M, et al. A cohort study of dietary fibre intake and menarche. *Public Health Nutr*. 2002;5:353-360.
43. Rosell M, Appleby P, Key T. Height, age at menarche, body weight and body mass index in life-long vegetarians. *Public Health Nutr*. 2005;8:870-875.
44. Dorgan JF, Hunsberger SA, McMahon RP, et al. Diet and sex hormones in girls: findings from a randomized controlled clinical trial. *J Natl Cancer Inst*. 2003;95:132-141.
45. Wolff MS, Britton JA, Boguski L, et al. Environmental exposures and puberty in inner-city girls. *Environ Res*. 2008;107:393-400.
46. Malina RM, Pena Reyes ME, Tan SK, et al. Secular change in age at menarche in rural Oaxaca, southern Mexico: 1968-2000. *Ann Hum Biol*. 2004;31:634-646.
47. Ellis BJ. Timing of pubertal maturation in girls: an integrated life history approach. *Psychol Bull*. 2004;130:920-958.
48. Sloboda DM, Beedle AS, Cupido CL, et al. Impaired perinatal growth and longevity: a life history perspective. *Curr Gerontol Geriatr Res* 2009:608-740. (Epub 2009 Sep 6.)
49. Maestripieri D, Roney JR, DeBias N, et al. Father absence, menarche and interest in infants among adolescent girls. *Dev Sci*. 2004;7: 560-566.
50. Prebeg Z, Bralic I. Changes in menarcheal age in girls exposed to war conditions. *Am J Human Biol*. 2000;12:503-508.
51. Brown J, Cohen P, Chen H, et al. Sexual trajectories of abused and neglected youths. *J Dev Behav Pediatr*. 2004;25:77-82.
52. Jorm AF, Christensen H, Rodgers B, et al. Association of adverse childhood experiences, age of menarche, and adult reproductive behavior: does the androgen receptor gene play a role? *Am J Med Genet B Neuropsychiatr Genet*. 2004;125:105-111.
53. Campbell BC, Udry JR. Stress and age at menarche of mothers and daughters. *J Biosoc Sci*. 1995;27:127-134.
54. Westberg L, Eriksson E. Sex steroid-related candidate genes in psychiatric disorders. *J Psychiatry Neurosci*. 2008;33:319-330.
55. Matsuo N, Anzo M, Sato S, et al. Testicular volume in Japanese boys up to the age of 15 years. *Eur J Pediatr*. 2000;159:843-845.
56. Moisan J, Meyer F, Gingras S. A nested case-control study of the correlates of early menarche. *Am J Epidemiol*. 1990;132:953-961.
57. Zacharias L, Wurtman RJ. Age at menarche. *N Engl J Med*. 1969;280:868-875.

58. Palmert MR, Hirschhorn JN. Genetic approaches to stature, pubertal timing, and other complex traits. *Mol Genet Metab.* 2003;80:1-10.
59. Malina RM, Ryan RC, Bonci CM. Age at menarche in athletes and their mothers and sisters. *Ann Hum Biol.* 1994;21:417-422.
60. Eaves L, Silberg J, Foley D, et al. Genetic and environmental influences on the relative timing of pubertal change. *Twin Res.* 2004;7:471-481.
61. Kaprio J, Rimpela A, Winter T, et al. Common genetic influences on BMI and age at menarche. *Hum Biol.* 1995;67:739-753.
62. Towne B, Czerwinski SA, Demerath EW, et al. Heritability of age at menarche in girls from the Fels Longitudinal Study. *Am J Phys Anthropol.* 2005;128:210-219.
63. Sedlmeyer IL, Pearce CL, Trueman JA, et al. Determination of sequence variation and haplotype structure for the gonadotropin-releasing hormone (GnRH) and GnRH receptor genes: investigation of role in pubertal timing. *J Clin Endocrinol Metab.* 2005;90:1091-1099.
64. Comings DE, Gade R, Muhleman D, et al. The LEP gene and age of menarche: maternal age as a potential cause of hidden stratification in association studies. *Mol Genet Metab.* 2001;73:204-210.
65. Stavrou I, Zois C, Ioannidis JP, et al. Association of polymorphisms of the oestrogen receptor alpha gene with the age of menarche. *Hum Reprod.* 2002;17:1101-1105.
66. Kadlubar FF, Berkowitz GS, Delongchamp RR, et al. The CYP3A4*1B variant is related to the onset of puberty, a known risk factor for the development of breast cancer. *Cancer Epidemiol Biomarkers Prev.* 2003;12:327-331.
67. Xita N, Tsatsoulis A, Stavrou I, et al. Association of SHBG gene polymorphism with menarche. *Mol Hum Reprod.* 2005;11:459-462.
68. He C, Kraft P, Chen C, et al. Genome-wide association studies identify loci associated with age at menarche and age at natural menopause. *Nat Genet.* 2009;6:724-728.
69. Sulem P, Gudbjartsson DF, Rafnar T, et al. Genome-wide association study identifies sequence variants on 6q21 associated with age at menarche. *Nat Genet.* 2009;6:734-738.
70. Perry JR, Stolk L, Franceschini N, et al. Meta-analysis of genome-wide association data identifies two loci influencing age at menarche. *Nat Genet.* 2009;6:648-650.
71. Gajdos ZK, Butler JL, Henderson KD, et al. Association studies of common variants in 10 hypogonadotropic hypogonadism genes with age at menarche. *J Clin Endocrinol Metab.* 2008;93:4290-4298.
72. Gao YT, Shu XO, Dai Q, et al. Association of menstrual and reproductive factors with breast cancer risk: results from the Shanghai Breast Cancer Study. *Int J Cancer.* 2000;87:295-300.
73. Persson I. Estrogens in the causation of breast, endometrial and ovarian cancers: evidence and hypotheses from epidemiological findings. *J Steroid Biochem Mol Biol.* 2000;74:357-364.
74. Clavel-Chapelon F, Gerber M. Reproductive factors and breast cancer risk: do they differ according to age at diagnosis? *Breast Cancer Res Treat.* 2002;72:107-115.
75. Hamilton AS, Mack TM. Puberty and genetic susceptibility to breast cancer in a case-control study in twins. *N Engl J Med.* 2003; 348:2313-2322.
76. De Stavola BL, dos SS I, McCormack V, et al. Childhood growth and breast cancer. *Am J Epidemiol.* 2004;159:671-682.
77. Tehard B, Kaaks R, Clavel-Chapelon F. Body silhouette, menstrual function at adolescence and breast cancer risk in the E3N cohort study. *Br J Cancer.* 2005;92:2042-2048.
78. Ahlgren M, Melbye M, Wohlfahrt J, et al. Growth patterns and the risk of breast cancer in women. *N Engl J Med.* 2004;351:1619-1626.
79. dos SS I, De Stavola BL, Hardy RJ, et al. Is the association of birth weight with premenopausal breast cancer risk mediated through childhood growth? *Br J Cancer.* 2004;91:519-524.
80. Mucci LA, Kuper HE, Tamimi R, et al. Age at menarche and age at menopause in relation to hepatocellular carcinoma in women. *Br J Obstet Gynecol.* 2001;108:291-294.
81. Hatch EE, Linet MS, Zhang J, et al. Reproductive and hormonal factors and risk of brain tumors in adult females. *Int J Cancer.* 2005;114:797-805.
82. Zhang Y, Holford TR, Leaderer B, et al. Menstrual and reproductive factors and risk of non-Hodgkin's lymphoma among Connecticut women. *Am J Epidemiol.* 2004;160:766-773.
83. Remsberg KE, Demerath EW, Schubert CM, et al. Early menarche and the development of cardiovascular disease risk factors in adolescent girls: the Fels Longitudinal Study. *J Clin Endocrinol Metab.* 2005;90:2718-2724.
84. Matchock RL, Susman EJ, Brown FM. Seasonal rhythms of menarche in the United States: correlates to menarcheal age, birth age, and birth month. *Womens Health Issues.* 2004;14:184-192.
85. Gonzales GF, Villena A. Body mass index and age at menarche in Peruvian children living at high altitude and at sea level. *Hum Biol.* 1996;68:265-275.
86. Fenton SE. Endocrine-disrupting compounds and mammary gland development: early exposure and later life consequences. *Endocrinology.* 2006;147(6 suppl):S18-S24.
87. McCartney CR, Prendergast KA, Blank SK, et al. Maturation of luteinizing hormone (gonadotropin-releasing hormone) secretion across puberty: evidence for altered regulation in obese peripubertal girls. *J Clin Endocrinol Metab.* 2009;94:56-66.
88. McCartney CR, Blank SK, Prendergast KA, et al. Obesity and sex steroid changes across puberty: evidence for marked hyperandrogenemia in pre- and early pubertal obese girls. *J Clin Endocrinol Metab.* 2007;92:430-436.
89. Lin KY, Nguyen DB, Williams RM. Complete breast absence revisited. *Plast Reconstr Surg.* 2000;106:98-101.
90. Rohn RD. Nipple (papilla) development in puberty: longitudinal observations in girls. *Pediatrics.* 1987;79:745-747.
91. Vargas SO, Kozakewich HP, Boyd TK, et al. Childhood asymmetric labium majus enlargement: mimicking a neoplasm. *Am J Surg Pathol.* 2005;29:1007-1016.
92. Taskinen S, Taavitsainen M, Wikstrom S. Measurement of testicular volume: comparison of 3 different methods. *J Urol.* 1996; 155:930-933.
93. Zachmann M, Prader A, Kind HP, et al. Testicular volume during adolescence: cross-sectional and longitudinal studies. *Helv Paediatr Acta.* 1974;29:61-72.
94. Biro FM, Lucky AW, Huster GA, et al. Pubertal staging in boys. *J Pediatr.* 1995;127:40-46.
95. Ankarberg-Lindgren C, Norjavaara E. Changes of diurnal rhythm and levels of total and free testosterone secretion from pre to late puberty in boys: testis size of 3 ml is a transition stage to puberty. *Eur J Endocrinol.* 2004;151:747-757.
96. Sutherland RS, Kogan BA, Baskin LS, et al. The effect of prepubertal androgen exposure on adult penile length. *J Urol.* 1996;156: 783-787.
97. Herman-Giddens ME, Slora EJ, Wasserman RC, et al. Secondary sexual characteristics and menses in young girls seen in office practice: a study from the Pediatric Research in Office Settings network. *Pediatrics.* 1997;99:505-512.
98. Coleman L, Coleman J. The measurement of puberty: a review. *J Adolesc.* 2002;25:535-550.
99. Rockett JC, Lynch CD, Buck GM. Biomarkers for assessing reproductive development and health: part 1. Pubertal development. *Environ Health Perspect.* 2004;112:105-112.
100. Shirtcliff EA, Dahl RE, Pollak SD. Pubertal development: correspondence between hormonal and physical development. *Child Dev.* 2009;80:327-337.
101. Harlan WR, Grillo GP, Cornoni-Huntley J, et al. Secondary sex characteristics of boys 12 to 17 years of age: the U.S. Health Examination Survey. *J Pediatr.* 1979;95:293-297.
102. Roche AF, Wellens R, Attie KM, et al. The timing of sexual maturation in a group of U.S. white youths. *J Pediatr Endocrinol.* 1995;8:11-18.
103. Wu T, Mendola P, Buck GM. Ethnic differences in the presence of secondary sex characteristics and menarche among US girls: the Third National Health and Nutrition Examination Survey, 1988-1994. *Pediatrics.* 2002;110:752-757.
104. Sun SS, Schubert CM, Chumlea WC, et al. National estimates of the timing of sexual maturation and racial differences among US children. *Pediatrics.* 2002;110:911-919.
105. Reiter EO, Lee PA. Have the onset and tempo of puberty changed? *Arch Pediatr Adolesc Med.* 2001;155:988-989.
106. Kaplowitz P. Delayed puberty in obese boys: comparison with constitutional delayed puberty and response to testosterone therapy [see comments]. *J Pediatr.* 1998;133:745-749.
107. Sun SS, Schubert CM, Liang R, et al. Is sexual maturity occurring earlier among U.S. children? *J Adolesc Health.* 2005;37:345-355.
108. Styne DM. Puberty, obesity and ethnicity. *Trends Endocrinol Metab.* 2004;15:472-478.
109. Marti-Henneberg C, Vizmanos B. The duration of puberty in girls is related to the timing of its onset. *J Pediatr.* 1997;131:618-621.
110. de Ridder CM, de Boer RW, Seidell JC, et al. Body fat distribution in pubertal girls quantified by magnetic resonance imaging. *Int J Obes Relat Metab Disord.* 1992;16:443-449.
111. Bourguignon JP. Variations in duration of pubertal growth: a mechanism compensating for differences in timing of puberty and minimizing their effects on final height. Belgian Study Group for Paediatric Endocrinology. *Acta Paediatr Scand Suppl.* 1988;347:16-24.
112. Lee PA, Guo SS, Kulin HE. Age of puberty: data from the United States of America. *APMIS.* 2001;109:81-88.
113. Kaplowitz PB, Oberfield SE. Reexamination of the age limit for defining when puberty is precocious in girls in the United States: implications for evaluation and treatment. Drug and Therapeutics and Executive Committees of the Lawson Wilkins Pediatric Endocrine Society. *Pediatrics.* 1999;104(4 Pt 1):936-941.
114. Midyett LK, Moore WV, Jacobson JD. Are pubertal changes in girls before age 8 benign? 5050. *Pediatrics.* 2003;111:47-51.
115. Kaplowitz P. Clinical characteristics of 104 children referred for evaluation of precocious puberty. *J Clin Endocrinol Metab.* 2004; 89:3644-3650.

116. De Vries L, Phillip M. Children referred for signs of early puberty warrant endocrine evaluation and follow-up. *J Clin Endocrinol Metab.* 2005;90:593-594.
117. Chalumeau M, Hadjiathanasiou CG, Ng SM, et al. Selecting girls with precocious puberty for brain imaging: validation of European evidence-based diagnosis rule. *J Pediatr.* 2003;143:445-450.
118. Amir O, Biron-Shental T. The impact of hormonal fluctuations on female vocal folds. *Curr Opin Otolaryngol Head Neck Surg.* 2004;12:180-184.
119. Lucky AW, Biro FM, Simbartl LA, et al. Predictors of severity of acne vulgaris in young adolescent girls: results of a five-year longitudinal study. *J Pediatr.* 1997;130:30-39.
120. Adebamowo CA, Spiegelman D, Danby FW, et al. High school dietary dairy intake and teenage acne. *J Am Acad Dermatol.* 2005; 52:207-214.
121. Cozza P, Stirpe G, Condo R, et al. Craniofacial and body growth: a cross-sectional anthropometric pilot study on children during prepubertal period. *Eur J Paediatr Dent.* 2005;6:90-96.
122. Boyanov MA, Temelkova NL, Popivanov PP. Determinants of thyroid volume in schoolchildren: fat-free mass versus body fat mass—a cross-sectional study. *Endocr Pract.* 2004;10:409-416.
123. Hero M, Wickman S, Hanhijarvi R, et al. Pubertal upregulation of erythropoiesis in boys is determined primarily by androgen. *J Pediatr.* 2005;146:245-252.
124. Grumbach MM, Gluckman PD. The human fetal hypothalamus and pituitary gland: the maturation of neuroendocrine mechanisms controlling the secretion of fetal pituitary growth hormone, prolactin, gonadotropin, and adrenocorticotropin-related peptides and thyrotropin. In: Tulchinsky D, Little AB, eds. *Maternal-Fetal Endocrinology.* Philadelphia, PA: Saunders; 1994:193-261.
125. Rabinovici J, Jaffe RB. Development and regulation of growth and differentitated function in human and subhuman primate fetal gonads. *Endocr Rev.* 1990;11:532-551.
126. Ross GT. Follicular development: the life cycle of the follicle and puberty. In: Grumbach MM, Sizonenko PC, Aubert MI, eds. *Control of the Onset of Puberty.* Baltimore, MD: Williams & Wilkins; 1990:376-386.
127. Gougeon A. Regulation of ovarian follicular development in primates: facts and hypotheses. *Endocr Rev.* 1996;17:121-155.
128. Hart R, Sloboda DM, Doherty DA, et al. Prenatal determinants of uterine volume and ovarian reserve in adolescence. *J Clin Endocrinol Metab.* 2009;94:4931-4937.
129. De Vries L, Horev G, Schwartz M, et al. Ultrasonographic and clinical parameters for early differentiation between precocious puberty and premature thelarche. *Eur J Endocrinol.* 2006;154:891-898.
130. Battaglia C, Mancini F, Regnani G, et al. Pelvic ultrasound and color Doppler findings in different isosexual precocities. *Ultrasound Obstet Gynecol.* 2003;22:277-283.
131. Batt RE, Mitwally MF. Endometriosis from thelarche to midteens: pathogenesis and prognosis, prevention and pedagogy. *J Pediatr Adolesc Gynecol.* 2003;16:337-347.
132. Onat J, Ertem B. Age at menarche: relationship to socioeconomic status, growth rate in stature and weight, and skeletal and sexual maturation. *Am J Hum Biol.* 1995;7:741-750.
133. Hamilton BH, Martin JA, Ventura SJ. *Births: Preliminary Data for 2008. National Vital Statistics Reports, vol. 58, no. 16.* Hyattsville, MD: National Center for Health Statistics; Released April 6, 2010.
134. Gondos B, Kogan SJ. Testicular development during puberty. In: Grumbach MM, Sizonenko PC, Aubert ML, et al., eds. *Control of the Onset of Puberty.* 1990:387-402.
135. Prince FP. The triphasic nature of Leydig cell development in humans, and comments on nomenclature. *J Endocrinol.* 2001;168:213-216.
136. Pedersen JL, Nysom K, Jorgensen M, et al. Spermaturia and puberty. *Arch Dis Child.* 1993;69:384-387.
137. Nysom K, Pedersen JL, Jorgensen M, et al. Spermaturia in two normal boys without other signs of puberty. *Acta Paediatr.* 1994;83:520-521.
138. Janczewski Z, Bablok L. Semen characteristics in pubertal boys: II. Semen quality in relation to bone age. *Arch Androl.* 1985;15:207-211.
139. Laron Z, Arad J, Gurewitz R, et al. Age at first conscious ejaculation: a milestone in male puberty. *Helv Paediatr Acta.* 1980;35:13-20.
140. Veldhuis JD, Roemmich JN, Richmond EJ, et al. Endocrine control of body composition in infancy, childhood, and puberty. *Endocr Rev.* 2005;26:114-146.
141. Tanner JM, Whitehouse RH, Marubini E, et al. The adolescent growth spurt of boys and girls of the Harpenden growth study. *Ann Hum Biol.* 1976;3:109-126.
142. Iuliano-Burns S, Hopper J, Seeman E. The age of puberty determines sexual dimorphism in bone structure: a male/female co-twin control study. *J Clin Endocrinol Metab.* 2009;94:1638-1643.
143. Karlberg J, Kwan CW, Gelander L, et al. Pubertal growth assessment. *Horm Res.* 2003;60(suppl 1):27-35.
144. Tanner JM, Davies PSW. Clinical longitudinal standards for height and height velocity for North American children. *J Pediatr.* 1985;107:317-329.
145. Caino S, Kelmansky D, Lejarraga H, et al. Short-term growth at adolescence in healthy girls. *Ann Hum Biol.* 2004;31:182-195.
146. Luo ZC, Cheung YB, He Q, et al. Growth in early life and its relation to pubertal growth. *Epidemiology.* 2003;14:65-73.
147. Bourguignon JP. Linear growth as a function of age at onset of puberty and sex steroid dosage: therapeutic implications. *Endocr Rev.* 1988;9:467-488.
148. McKusick VA. *Heritable Disorders of Connective Tissue.* St. Louis, MO: Mosby; 1972.
149. Tanner JM, Whitehouse RH, Hughes PCR, et al. Relative importance of growth hormone and sex steroids for the growth at puberty of trunk length, limb length, and muscle width in growth hormone-deficient children. *J Pediatr.* 1976;89:1000-1008.
150. Grumbach MM, Auchus RJ. Estrogen: consequences and implication of human mutations in synthesis and action. *J Clin Endocrinol Metab.* 1999;84:4677-4694.
151. Grumbach MM. Estrogen, bone, growth, and sex: a sea change in conventional wisdom. *J Pediatr Endocrinol Metab.* 2000;13(suppl 6):1439-1455.
152. Rochira V, Balestrieri A, Faustini-Fustini M, et al. Role of estrogen on bone in the human male: insights from the natural models of congenital estrogen deficiency. *Mol Cell Endocrinol.* 2001;178: 215-220.
153. Greulich WS, Pyle SI. *Radiographic Atlas of Skeletal Development of the Hand and Wrist.* Stanford, CA: Stanford University Press; 1959.
154. Tanner JM, Whitehouse RH, Marshall WA, et al. *Assessment of Skeletal Maturity and Prediction of Adult Height: TW 2 Method.* New York, NY: Academic Press; 1975.
155. Aicardi G, Vignolo M, Milani S, et al. Assessment of skeletal maturity of the hand-wrist and knee: a comparison among methods. *Am J Hum Biol.* 2000;12:610-615.
156. Flor-Cisneros A, Roemmich JN, Rogol AD, et al. Bone age and onset of puberty in normal boys. *Mol Cell Endocrinol.* 2006;254-255: 202-206.
157. Bayley N, Pinneau SR. Tables for predicting adult height from skeletal age: revised for use with the Greulich-Pyle hand standards. *J Pediatr.* 1952;40:423-441.
158. Roche AF, Roberts J, Hamill PV. Skeletal maturity of children 6-11 years: racial, geographic area, and socioeconomic differentials, United States. *Vital Health Stat.* 1975;11(149):1-81.
159. Thodberg HH. Clinical review: an automated method for determination of bone age. *J Clin Endocrinol Metab.* 2009;94:2239-2244.
160. Seeman E. Pathogenesis of bone fragility in women and men. *Lancet.* 2002;359:1841-1850.
161. Seeman E. Periosteal bone formation: a neglected determinant of bone strength. *N Engl J Med.* 2003;349:320-323.
162. Gafni RI, Baron J. Childhood bone mass acquisition and peak bone mass may not be important determinants of bone mass in late adulthood. *Pediatrics.* 2007;119(suppl 2):S131-S136.
163. Bachrach LK. Acquisition of optimal bone mass in childhood and adolescence. *Trends Endocrinol Metab.* 2001;12:22-28.
164. Bailey DA, Martin AD, McKay HA, et al. Calcium accretion in girls and boys during puberty: a longitudinal analysis. *J Bone Miner Res.* 2000;15:2245-2250.
165. Bachrach LK, Hastie T, Wang M, et al. Bone mineral acquisition in healthy Asian, Hispanic, Black and Caucaisan youth: a longitudinal study. *J Clin Endocrinol Metab.* 1999;84:4702-4712.
166. Schonau E. The peak bone mass concept: is it still relevant? *Pediatr Nephrol.* 2004;19:825-831.
167. Bass S, Delmas PD, Pearce G, et al. The differing tempo of growth in bone size, mass, and density in girls is region-specific [see comments]. *J Clin Invest.* 1999;104:795-804.
168. Seeman E. Clinical review 137: sexual dimorphism in skeletal size, density, and strength. *J Clin Endocrinol Metab.* 2001;86:4576-4584.
169. Bradney M, Karlsson MK, Duan Y, et al. Heterogeneity in the growth of the axial and appendicular skeleton in boys: implications for the pathogenesis of bone fragility in men. *J Bone Miner Res.* 2000;15:1871-1878.
170. Arabi A, Tamim H, Nabulsi M, et al. Sex differences in the effect of body-composition variables on bone mass in healthy children and adolescents. *Am J Clin Nutr.* 2004;80:1428-1435.
171. Crabtree NJ, Kibirige MS, Fordham JN, et al. The relationship between lean body mass and bone mineral content in paediatric health and disease. *Bone.* 2004;35:965-972.
172. Lu PW, Cowell CT, LLoyd-Jones SA, et al. Volumetric bone mineral density in normal subjects, aged 5-27 years. *J Clin Endocrinol Metab.* 1996;81:1586-1590.
173. Binkley TL, Specker BL, Wittig TA. Centile curves for bone densitometry measurements in healthy males and females ages 5-22 yr. *J Clin Densitom.* 2002;5:343-353.

174. Baroncelli GI. Quantitative ultrasound methods to assess bone mineral status in children: technical characteristics, performance, and clinical application. *Pediatr Res*. 2008;63:220-228.
175. Wang Q, Alen M, Nicholson P, et al. Growth patterns at distal radius and tibial shaft in pubertal girls: a 2-year longitudinal study. *J Bone Miner Res*. 2005;20:954-961.
176. Saito T, Nakamura K, Okuda Y, et al. Weight gain in childhood and bone mass in female college students. *J Bone Miner Metab*. 2005; 23:69-75.
177. Loro ML, Sayre J, Roe TF, et al. Early identification of children predisposed to low peak bone mass and osteoporosis later in life. *J Clin Endocrinol Metab*. 2000;85:3908-3918.
178. Rauch F, Bailey DA, Baxter-Jones A, et al. The "muscle-bone unit" during the pubertal growth spurt. *Bone*. 2004;34:771-775.
179. Loud KJ, Gordon CM, Micheli LJ, et al. Correlates of stress fractures among preadolescent and adolescent girls. *Pediatrics*. 2005;115:e399-e406.
180. McKay HA, MacLean L, Petit M, et al. "Bounce at the Bell": a novel program of short bouts of exercise improves proximal femur bone mass in early pubertal children. *Br J Sports Med*. 2005;39: 521-526.
181. Laing EM, Wilson AR, Modlesky CM, et al. Initial years of recreational artistic gymnastics training improves lumbar spine bone mineral accrual in 4- to 8-year-old females. *J Bone Miner Res*. 2005;20: 509-519.
182. Goulding A, Rockell JE, Black RE, et al. Children who avoid drinking cow's milk are at increased risk for prepubertal bone fractures. *J Am Diet Assoc*. 2004;104:250-253.
183. Winzenberg TM, Shaw K, Fryer J, et al. Calcium supplementation for improving bone mineral density in children. Cochrane Database Syst Rev. 2006;(2):CD005119.
184. Chevalley T, Rizzoli R, Hans D, et al. Interaction between calcium intake and menarcheal age on bone mass gain: an eight-year follow-up study from prepuberty to postmenarche. *J Clin Endocrinol Metab*. 2005;90:44-51.
185. Cheng S, Tylavsky F, Kroger H, et al. Association of low 25-hydroxyvitamin D concentrations with elevated parathyroid hormone concentrations and low cortical bone density in early pubertal and prepubertal Finnish girls. *Am J Clin Nutr*. 2003;78:485-492.
186. Suuriniemi M, Mahonen A, Kovanen V, et al. Association between exercise and pubertal BMD is modulated by estrogen receptor alpha genotype. *J Bone Miner Res*. 2004;19:1758-1765.
187. Gustavsson A, Thorsen K, Nordstrom P. A 3-year longitudinal study of the effect of physical activity on the accrual of bone mineral density in healthy adolescent males. *Calcif Tissue Int*. 2003;73:108-114.
188. Chevalley T, Bonjour JP, Ferrari S, et al. Influence of age at menarche on forearm bone microstructure in healthy young women. *J Clin Endocrinol Metab*. 2008;93:2594-2601.
189. Remer T, Manz F, Hartmann MF, et al. Prepubertal healthy children's urinary androstenediol predicts diaphyseal bone strength in late puberty. *J Clin Endocrinol Metab*. 2009;94:575-578.
190. Krupa B, Miazgowski T. Bone mineral density and markers of bone turnover in boys with constitutional delay of growth and puberty. *J Clin Endocrinol Metab*. 2005;90:2828-2830.
191. Bollen AM. A prospective longitudinal study of urinary excretion of a bone resorption marker in adolescents. *Ann Hum Biol*. 2000;27:199-211.
192. Calvo MS, Eyre DR, Gundberg CM. Molecular basis and clinical application of biologic markers of bone turnover. *Endocr Rev*. 1996;17:333-368.
193. Loomba-Albrecht LA, Styne DM. Effect of puberty on body composition. *Curr Opin Endocrinol Diabetes Obes*. 2009;16:10-15.
194. Rogol AD. Sex steroids, growth hormone, leptin and the pubertal growth spurt. *Endocr Dev*. 2010;17:77-85.
195. Taksali SE, Caprio S, Dziura J, et al. High visceral and low abdominal subcutaneous fat stores in the obese adolescent: a determinant of an adverse metabolic phenotype. *Diabetes*. 2008;57:367-371.
196. Liska D, Dufour S, Zern TL, et al. Interethnic differences in muscle, liver and abdominal fat partitioning in obese adolescents. *PLoS One*. 2007;2:e569.
197. Fernandez JR, Redden DT, Pietrobelli A, et al. Waist circumference percentiles in nationally representative samples of African-American, European-American, and Mexican-American children and adolescents. *J Pediatr*. 2004;145:439-444.
198. He Q, Horlick M, Thornton J, et al. Sex-specific fat distribution is not linear across pubertal groups in a multiethnic study. *Obes Res*. 2004;12:725-733.
199. Fox KR, Peters DM, Sharpe P, et al. Assessment of abdominal fat development in young adolescents using magnetic resonance imaging. *Int J Obes Relat Metab Disord*. 2000;24:1653-1659.
200. Dore E, Martin R, Ratel S, et al. Gender differences in peak muscle performance during growth. *Int J Sports Med*. 2005;26:274-280.
201. Ogden CL, Carroll MD, Curtin LR, et al. Prevalence of overweight and obesity in the United States, 1999-2004. *JAMA*. 2006; 295:1549-1555.
202. Styne DM. Childhood and adolescent obesity: prevalence and significance. *Pediatr Clin North Am*. 2001;48:823-854, vii.
203. Franks PW, Hanson RL, Knowler WC, et al. Childhood obesity, other cardiovascular risk factors, and premature death. *N Engl J Med*. 2010;362:485-493.
204. Morrison JA, Barton BA, Biro FM, et al. Sex hormones and the changes in adolescent male lipids: longitudinal studies in a biracial cohort. *J Pediatr*. 2003;142:637-642.
205. Lee S, Bacha F, Gungor N, et al. Comparison of different definitions of pediatric metabolic syndrome: relation to abdominal adiposity, insulin resistance, adiponectin, and inflammatory biomarkers. *J Pediatr*. 2008;152:177-184.
206. Sinaiko AR, Steinberger J, Moran A, et al. Influence of insulin resistance and body mass index at age 13 on systolic blood pressure, triglycerides, and high-density lipoprotein cholesterol at age 19. *Hypertension*. 2006;48:730-736.
207. McGill HJ, McMahan CA, Zieske AW, et al. Association of coronary heart disease risk factors with microscopic qualities of coronary atherosclerosis in youth. *Circulation*. 2000;102:374-379.
208. Neumark-Sztainer D, Hannan PJ. Weight-related behaviors among adolescent girls and boys: results from a national survey. *Arch Pediatr Adolesc Med*. 2000;154:569-577.
209. Reaven GM. The metabolic syndrome: is this diagnosis necessary? *Am J Clin Nutr*. 2006;83:1237-1247.
210. Goran MI, Gower BA. Longitudinal study on pubertal insulin resistance. *Diabetes*. 2001;50:2444-2450.
211. Cruz ML, Weigensberg MJ, Huang TT, et al. The metabolic syndrome in overweight Hispanic youth and the role of insulin sensitivity. *J Clin Endocrinol Metab*. 2004;89:108-113.
212. Goran MI, Bergman RN, Gower BA. Influence of total vs. visceral fat on insulin action and secretion in African American and white children. *Obes Res*. 2001;9:423-431.
213. Janner M, Knill SE, Diem P, et al. Persistent microalbuminuria in adolescents with type I (insulin-dependent) diabetes mellitus is associated to early rather than late puberty: results of a prospective longitudinal study. *Eur J Pediatr*. 1994;153:403-408.
214. Gungor N, Bacha F, Saad R, et al. Youth type 2 diabetes: insulin resistance, beta-cell failure, or both? *Diabetes Care*. 2005;28: 638-644.
215. Glaser NS. Non-insulin-dependent diabetes mellitus in childhood and adolescence. *Pediatr Clin North Am*. 1997;44:307-337.
216. Musso C, Cochran E, Javor E, et al. The long-term effect of recombinant methionyl human leptin therapy on hyperandrogenism and menstrual function in female and pituitary function in male and female hypoleptinemic lipodystrophic patients. *Metabolism*. 2005;54:255-263.
217. Tu W, Eckert GJ, Saha C, et al. Synchronization of adolescent blood pressure and pubertal somatic growth. *J Clin Endocrinol Metab*. 2009;94:5019-5022.
218. Voors AW, Webber LS, Frerichs RR, et al. Body height and body mass as determinants of basal blood pressure in children: the Bogalusa Heart Study. *Am J Epidemiol*. 1977;106:101-108.
219. Pankow JS, Jacobs DR Jr, Steinberger J, et al. Insulin resistance and cardiovascular disease risk factors in children of parents with the insulin resistance (metabolic) syndrome. *Diabetes Care*. 2004;27:775-780.
220. Charmandari E, Kino T, Souvatzoglou E, et al. Pediatric stress: hormonal mediators and human development. *Horm Res*. 2003; 59:161-179.
221. Sowell ER, Thompson PM, Toga AW. Mapping changes in the human cortex throughout the span of life. *Neuroscientist*. 2004;10: 372-392.
222. Sowell ER, Delis D, Stiles J, et al. Improved memory functioning and frontal lobe maturation between childhood and adolescence: a structural MRI study. *J Int Neuropsychol Soc*. 2001;7:312-322.
223. Gogtay N, Giedd JN, Lusk L, et al. Dynamic mapping of human cortical development during childhood through early adulthood. *Proc Natl Acad Sci U S A*. 2004;101:8174-8179.
224. Thompson PM, Sowell ER, Gogtay N, et al. Structural MRI and brain development. *Int Rev Neurobiol*. 2005;67:285-323.
225. Peper JS, Brouwer RM, Schnack HG, et al. Sex steroids and brain structure in pubertal boys and girls. *Psychoneuroendocrinology*. 2009;34:332-342.
226. Yun AJ, Bazar KA, Lee PY. Pineal attrition, loss of cognitive plasticity, and onset of puberty during the teen years: is it a modern maladaptation exposed by evolutionary displacement? *Med Hypotheses*. 2004;63:939-950.
227. Feinberg I, Higgins LM, Khaw WY, et al. The adolescent decline of NREM delta, an indicator of brain maturation, is linked to age and sex but not to pubertal stage. *Am J Physiol Regul Integr Comp Physiol*. 2006;291:R1724-R1729.

228. Knutson KL. The association between pubertal status and sleep duration and quality among a nationally representative sample of U. S. adolescents. *Am J Hum Biol*. 2005;17:418-424.
229. Dahl RE, Lewin DS. Pathways to adolescent health sleep regulation and behavior. *J Adolesc Health*. 2002;31(6 suppl):175-184.
230. Roenneberg T, Kuehnle T, Pramstaller PP, et al. A marker for the end of adolescence. *Curr Biol*. 2004;14:R1038-R1039.
231. Remschmidt H. Psychosocial milestones in normal puberty and adolescence. *Horm Res*. 1994;41(suppl 2):19-29.
232. Steinberg L, Morris AS. Adolescent development. *Annu Rev Psychol*. 2001;52:83-110.
233. Styne DM, Grumbach MM. Puberty in boys and girls. In: Pfaff DW, ed. *The Brain, Hormones and Behaviors*. New York, NY: Academic Press; 2002:661-716.
234. Offer D, Schonert-Reichl KA. Debunking the myths of adolescence: findings from recent research. *J Am Acad Child Adolesc Psychiatry*. 1992;31:1003-1014.
235. Patton GC, McMorris BJ, Toumbourou JW, et al. Puberty and the onset of substance use and abuse. *Pediatrics*. 2004;114:e300-e306.
236. Albertsson-Wikland K, Rosberg S, Lannering B, et al. Twenty-four-hour profiles of luteinizing hormone, follicle-stimulating hormone, testosterone, and estradiol levels: a semilongitudinal study throughout puberty in healthy boys. *J Clin Endocrinol Metab*. 1997; 82:541-549.
237. Mitamura R, Yano K, Suzuki N, et al. Diurnal rhythms of luteinizing hormone, follicle-stimulating hormone, and testosterone secretion before the onset of male puberty. *J Clin Endocrinol Metab*. 1999; 84:29-37.
238. Mitamura R, Yano K, Suzuki N, et al. Diurnal rhythms of luteinizing hormone, follicle-stimulating hormone, testosterone, and estradiol secretion before the onset of female puberty in short children. *J Clin Endocrinol Metab*. 2000;85:1074-1080.
239. Kaplan SL, Grumbach MM, Aubert ML. The ontogenesis of pituitary hormones and hypothalamic factors in the human fetus: maturation of central nervous system regulation of anterior pituitary function. *Recent Prog Horm Res*. 1976;32:161-243.
240. Veldhuis JD, Pincus SM, Mitamura R, et al. Developmentally delimited emergence of more orderly luteinizing hormone and testosterone secretion during late prepuberty in boys. *J Clin Endocrinol Metab*. 2001;86:80-89.
241. Grumbach MM, Roth JC, Kaplan SL, et al. Hypothalamic-pituitary regulation of puberty in man: evidence and concepts derived from clinical research. In: Grumbach MM, Grave GD, Mayer FE, eds. *Control of the Onset of Puberty*. New York, NY: John Wiley & Sons; 1974:115-166.
242. Roth JC, Kelch RP, Kaplan SL, et al. FSH and LH response to luteinizing hormone-releasing factor in prepubertal and pubertal children, adult males and patients with hypogonadotropic and hypertropic hypogonadism. *J Clin Endocrinol Metab*. 1972;35:926-930.
243. Demir A, Voutilainen R, Juul A, et al. Increase in first morning voided urinary luteinizing hormone levels precedes the physical onset of puberty. *J Clin Endocrinol Metab*. 1996;81:2963-2967.
244. Olivares A, Soderlund D, Castro-Fernandez C, et al. Basal and gonadotropin-releasing hormone-releasable serum follicle-stimulating hormone charge isoform distribution and in vitro biological-to-immunological ratio in male puberty. *Endocrine*. 2004;23: 189-198.
245. Wang C, Catlin DH, Demers LM, et al. Measurement of total serum testosterone in adult men: comparison of current laboratory methods versus liquid chromatography-tandem mass spectrometry. *J Clin Endocrinol Metab*. 2004;89:534-543.
246. Taieb J, Mathian B, Millot F, et al. Testosterone measured by 10 immunoassays and by isotope-dilution gas chromatography-mass spectrometry in sera from 116 men, women, and children. *Clin Chem*. 2003;49:1381-1395.
246a. Waaler PE, Thorsen T, Stoa KF, Aarskog D. Studies in normal male pubenty. *Acta Paediatr Scand Suppl*. 1974;249:1-36.
247. Albrecht L, Styne D. Laboratory testing of gonadal steroids in children. *Pediatr Endocrinol Rev*. 2007;5(suppl 1):599-607.
248. August GP, Grumbach MM, Kaplan SL. Hormonal changes in puberty: 3. Correlation of plasma testosterone, LH, FSH, testicular size, and bone age with male pubertal development. *J Clin Endocrinol Metab*. 1972;34:319-326.
249. Raivio T, Dunkel L, Wickman S, et al. Serum androgen bioactivity in adolescence: a longitudinal study of boys with constitutional delay of puberty. *J Clin Endocrinol Metab*. 2004;89:1188-1192.
250. Chen J, Sowers MR, Moran FM, et al. Circulating bioactive androgens in mid-life women. *J Clin Endocrinol Metab*. 2006;91:4387-4394.
251. Norjavaara E, Ankarberg C, Albertsson-Wikland K. Diurnal rhythm of 17 beta-estradiol secretion throughout pubertal development in healthy girls: evaluation by a sensitive radioimmunoassay. *J Clin Endocrinol Metab*. 1996;81:4095-4102.
252. Klein KO, Martha PMJ, Blizzard RM, et al. A longitudinal assessment of hormonal and physical alterations during normal puberty in boys: II. Estrogen levels as determined by an ultrasensitive bioassay. *J Clin Endocrinol Metab*. 1996;81:3203-3207.
253. Paris F, Servant N, Terouanne B, et al. A new recombinant cell bioassay for ultrasensitive determination of serum estrogenic bioactivity in children. *J Clin Endocrinol Metab*. 2002;87:791-797.
254. van der Eerden BC, Karperien M, Wit JM. Systemic and local regulation of the growth plate. *Endocr Rev*. 2003;24:782-801.
255. Conte FA, Grumbach MM, Ito Y, et al. A syndrome of female pseudohermaphrodism, hypergonadotropic hypogonadism and multicystic ovaries associated with missence mutations in the gene encoding aromatase (P450 arom). *J Clin Endocrinol Metab*. 1994;78:1287-1292.
256. Smith EP, Boyd J, Frank GR, et al. Estrogen resistance caused by a mutation by the estrogen-receptor in a man. *N Engl J Med*. 1994;331:1056-1061.
257. Morishima A, Grumbach MM, Simpson ER, et al. Aromatase deficiency in male and female siblings caused by a novel mutation and the physiological role of estrogens. *J Clin Endocrinol Metab*. 1995;80:3689-3698.
258. Attie KM, Ramirez NR, Conte FA, et al. The pubertal growth spurt in eight patients with true precocious puberty and growth hormone deficiency: evidence for a direct role of sex steroids. *J Clin Endocrinol Metab*. 1990;71:975-983.
259. Van Wyk JJ, Smith EP. Insulin-like growth factors and skeletal growth: possibilities for therapeutic interventions. *J Clin Endocrinol Metab*. 1999;84:4349-4354.
260. Bilezikian JP, Morishima A, Bell J, et al. Increased bone mass as a result of estrogen therapy in a man with aromatase deficiency. *N Engl J Med*. 1998;339:599-603.
261. Carani C, Qin K, Simoni M, et al. Effect of testosterone and estradiol in a man with aromatase deficiency. *N Engl J Med*. 1997;337:91-95.
262. Rochira V, Faustini-Fustini M, Balestrieri A, et al. Estrogen replacement therapy in a man with congenital aromatase deficiency: effects of different doses of transdermal estradiol on bone mineral density and hormonal parameters. *J Clin Endocrinol Metab*. 2000;85:1841-1845.
263. Stratakis CA, Vottero A, Brodie A, et al. The aromatase excess syndrome is associated with feminization of both sexes and autosomal dominant transmission of aberrant P450 aromatase gene transcription. *J Clin Endocrinol Metab*. 1998;83:1348-1357.
264. Weise M, De Levi S, Barnes KM, et al. Effects of estrogen on growth plate senescence and epiphyseal fusion. *Proc Natl Acad Sci U S A*. 2001;98:6871-6876.
265. Weise M, Flor A, Barnes KM, et al. Determinants of growth during gonadotropin-releasing hormone analog therapy for precocious puberty. *J Clin Endocrinol Metab*. 2004;89:103-107.
266. Eastell R. Role of oestrogen in the regulation of bone turnover at the menarche. *J Endocrinol*. 2005;185:223-234.
267. Hogler W, Briody J, Moore B, et al. Importance of estrogen on bone health in Turner syndrome: a cross-sectional and longitudinal study using dual-energy X-ray absorptiometry. *J Clin Endocrinol Metab*. 2004;89:193-199.
268. Jarvinen TL, Kannus P, Sievanen H. Estrogen and bone: a reproductive and locomotive perspective. *J Bone Miner Res*. 2003;18:1921-1931.
269. Vanderschueren D, Vandenput L, Boonen S, et al. Androgens and bone. *Endocr Rev*. 2004;25:389-425.
270. Marcus R, Leary D, Schneider DL, et al. The contribution of testosterone to skeletal development and maintenance: lessons from the androgen insensitivity syndrome. *J Clin Endocrinol Metab*. 2000;85:1032-1037.
271. Veldhuis JD, Roemmich JN, Rogol AD. Gender and sexual maturation-dependent contrasts in the neuroregulation of growth hormone secretion in prepubertal and late adolescent males and females: a general clinical research center-based study. *J Clin Endocrinol Metab*. 2000;85:2385-2394.
272. Veldhuis JD, Roemmich JN, Rogol AD. Gender and sexual maturation-dependent contrasts in the neuroregulation of growth hormone secretion in prepubertal and late adolescent males and females: a general clinical research center-based study. *J Clin Endocrinol Metab*. 2000;85:2385-2394.
273. Racine MS, Symons KV, Foster CM, et al. Augmentation of growth hormone secretion after testosterone treatment in boys with constitutional delay of growth and adolescence: evidence against an increase in hypothalamic secretion of growth hormone-releasing hormone. *J Clin Endocrinol Metab*. 2004;89:3326-3331.
274. Kerrigan JR, Veldhuis JD, Rogol AD. Androgen-receptor blockade enhances pulsatile luteinizing hormone production in late pubertal males: evidence for a hypothalamic site of physiologic androgen feedback action. *Pediatr Res*. 1994;35:102-106.
275. Keenan BS, Richards GE, Ponder SW, et al. Androgen-stimulated pubertal growth: the effects of testosterone and dihydrotestosterone on growth hormone and insulin-like growth factor-I in the treatment of short stature and delayed puberty. *J Clin Endocrinol Metab*. 1993;76:996-1001.
276. Harris DA, Van Vliet G, Egli CA, et al. Somatomedin-C in normal puberty and in true precocious puberty before and after treatment

with a potent luteinizing hormone-releasing hormone agonist. *J Clin Endocrinol Metab*. 1985;61:152-159.

277. Juul A, Fisker S, Scheike T, et al. Serum levels of growth hormone binding protein in children with normal and precocious puberty: relation to age, gender, body composition and gonadal steroids. *Clin Endocrinol*. 2000;52:165-172.
278. Lofqvist C, Andersson E, Gelander L, et al. Reference values for IGF-I throughout childhood and adolescence: a model that accounts simultaneously for the effect of gender, age, and puberty. *J Clin Endocrinol Metab*. 2001;86:5870-5876.
279. Lofqvist C, Andersson E, Gelander L, et al. Reference values for insulin-like growth factor-binding protein-3 (IGFBP-3) and the ratio of insulin-like growth factor-I to IGFBP-3 throughout childhood and adolescence. *J Clin Endocrinol Metab*. 2005;90:1420-1427.
280. Juul A, Dalgaard P, Blum WF, et al. Serum levels of insulin-like growth factor (IGF)-binding protein-3 (IGFBP-3) in healthy infants, children, and adolescents: the relation to IGF-I, IGF-II, IGFBP-1, IGFBP-2, age, sex, body mass index, and pubertal maturation. *J Clin Endocrinol Metab*. 1995;80:2534-2542.
281. Jorge AA, Souza SC, Arnhold IJ, et al. The first homozygous mutation (S226I) in the highly-conserved WSXWS-like motif of the GH receptor causing Laron syndrome: supression of GH secretion by GnRH analogue therapy not restored by dihydrotestosterone administration. *Clin Endocrinol (Oxf)*. 2004;60:36-40.
282. Mansfield MJ, Rudlin CR, Crigler JF Jr, et al. Changes in growth and serum growth hormone and plasma somatomedin-C levels during suppression of gonadal sex steroid secretion in girls with central precocious puberty. *J Clin Endocrinol Metab*. 1988;66:3-9.
283. Sjögren K, Liu JL, Blad K, et al. Liver-derived insulin-like growth factor I (IGF-I) is the principal source of IGF-I in blood but is not required for postnatal body growth in mice. *Proc Natl Acad Sci U S A*. 1999;96:7088-7092.
284. Grumbach MM, Richards GE, Conte FA, et al. Clinical disorders of adrenal function and puberty: an assessment of the role of the adrenal cortex in normal and abnormal puberty in man and evidence for an ACTH-like pituitary adrenal androgen stimulating hormone. In: James VHT, Serio M, Giusti G, et al., eds. *The Endocrine Function of the Human Adrenal Cortex: Serono Symposium*. New York, NY: Academic Press; 1977:583-612.
285. Van Wyk JJ, Grumbach MM. Syndrome of precocious menstruation and galactorrhea in juvenile hypothyroidism: an example of hormonal overlap in pituitary feedback. *J Pediatr*. 1960;57:416-435.
286. Noordam C, Dhir V, McNelis JC, et al. Inactivating PAPSS2 mutations in a patient with premature pubarche. *N Engl J Med*. 2009;360:2310-2318.
287. Derman O, Kanbur NO, Tokur TE. The effect of tamoxifen on sex hormone binding globulin in adolescents with pubertal gynecomastia. *J Pediatr Endocrinol Metab*. 2004;17:1115-1119.
288. August GP, Tkachuk M, Grumbach MM. Plasma testosterone-binding affinity and testosterone in umbilical cord plasma, late pregnancy, prepubertal children and adults. *J Clin Endocrinol Metab*. 1969;29:891-899.
289. Aubert ML, Sizonenko PC, Kaplan SL, et al. The ontogenesis of human prolactin from fetal life to puberty. In: Crosignani PG, Robyn C, eds. *Prolactin and Human Reproduction*. New York, NY: Academic Press; 1977:9-20.
290. Robertson DM, Hale GE, Jolley D, et al. Interrelationships between ovarian and pituitary hormones in ovulatory menstrual cycles across reproductive age. *J Clin Endocrinol Metab*. 2009;94:138-144.
291. Vale W, Bilezikjian LM, Rivier C. Reproductive and other roles of inhibins and activins. In: Knobil E, Neil JD, eds. *Physiology of Reproduction*. New York, NY: Raven; 1994:1861-1878.
292. Wallace E, Riley SM, Crossley JA, et al. Dimeric inhibins in amniotic fluid, maternal serum, and fetal serum in human pregnancy. *J Clin Endocrinol Metab*. 1997;82:218-222.
293. Majdic G, McNeilly AS, Sharpe RM, et al. Testicular expression of inhibin and activin subunits and follistatin in the rat and human fetus and neonate and during postnatal development in the rat. *Endocrinology*. 1997;138:2136-2147.
294. Andersson A, Skakkebaek NE. Serum inhibin B levels during male childhood and puberty. *Mol Cell Endocrinol*. 2001;180: 103-107.
295. Chada M, Prusa R, Bronsky J, et al. Inhibin B, follicle stimulating hormone, luteinizing hormone and testosterone during childhood and puberty in males: changes in serum concentrations in relation to age and stage of puberty. *Physiol Res*. 2003;52:45-51.
296. Chada M, Prusa R, Bronsky J, et al. Inhibin B, follicle stimulating hormone, luteinizing hormone, and estradiol and their relationship to the regulation of follicle development in girls during childhood and puberty. *Physiol Res*. 2003;52:341-346.
297. Foster CM, Olton PR, Padmanabhan V. Diurnal changes in FSH-regulatory peptides and their relationship to gonadotrophins in pubertal girls. *Hum Reprod*. 2005;20:543-548.
298. Crofton PM, Evans AE, Wallace AM, et al. Nocturnal secretory dynamics of inhibin B and testosterone in pre- and peripubertal boys. *J Clin Endocrinol Metab*. 2004;89:867-874.
299. Young J, Chanson P, Salenave S, et al. Testicular anti-mullerian hormone secretion is stimulated by recombinant human FSH in patients with congenital hypogonadotropic hypogonadism. *J Clin Endocrinol Metab*. 2005;90:724-728.
300. Elsholz DD, Padmanabhan V, Rosenfield RL, et al. GnRH agonist stimulation of the pituitary-gonadal axis in children: age and sex differences in circulating inhibin-B and activin-A. *Hum Reprod*. 2004;19:2748-2758.
301. Foster CM, Olton PR, Racine MS, et al. Sex differences in FSH-regulatory peptides in pubertal age boys and girls and effects of sex steroid treatment. *Hum Reprod*. 2004;19:1668-1676.
302. Lee PA, Coughlin MT, Bellinger MF. No relationship of testicular size at orchiopexy with fertility in men who previously had unilateral cryptorchidism. *J Urol*. 2001;166:236-239.
303. Kubini K, Zachmann M, Albers N, et al. Basal inhibin B and the testosterone response to human chorionic gonadotropin correlate in prepubertal boys. *J Clin Endocrinol Metab*. 2000;85:134-138.
304. Josso N. Paediatric applications of anti-mullerian hormone research. *Horm Res*. 1995;43:243-248.
305. Lee MM, Donahoe PK, Hasegawa T, et al. Mullerian inhibiting substance in humans: normal levels from infancy to adulthood. *J Clin Endocrinol Metab*. 1996;81:571-576.
306. Sir-Petermann T, Marquez L, Carcamo M, et al. Effects of birth weight on anti-müllerian hormone serum concentrations in infant girls. *J Clin Endocrinol Metab*. 2010;95:903-910.
307. Lee MM, Donahoe PK, Silverman BL, et al. Measurements of serum müllerian inhibiting substance in the evaluation of children with nonpalpable gonads. *N Engl J Med*. 1997;336:1480-1486.
308. Bergada I, Milani C, Bedecarras P, et al. Time course of the serum gonadotropin surge, inhibins, and anti-müllerian hormone in normal newborn males during the first month of life. *J Clin Endocrinol Metab*. 2006;91:4092-4098.
309. Park AS, Lawson MA, Chuan SS, et al. Serum anti-mullerian hormone concentrations are elevated in oligomenorrheic girls without evidence of hyperandrogenism. *J Clin Endocrinol Metab*. 2010;95:1786-1792.
310. Wikstrom AM, Bay K, Hero M, et al. Serum insulin-like factor 3 levels during puberty in healthy boys and boys with Klinefelter syndrome. *J Clin Endocrinol Metab*. 2006;91:4705-4708.
311. Randell EW, Diamandis EP, Ellis G. Serum prostate-specific antigen measured in children from birth to age 18 years. *Clin Chem*. 1996;42:420-423.
312. Vieira JG, Nishida SK, Pereira AB, et al. Serum levels of prostate-specific antigen in normal boys throughout puberty. *J Clin Endocrinol Metab*. 1994;78:1185-1187.
313. Ibanez L, DiMartino-Nardi J, Potau N, et al. Premature adrenarche: normal variant or forerunner of adult disease? *Endocr Rev*. 2000;21:671-696.
314. Grumbach MM, Kaplan SL. The neuroendocrinology of human puberty: an ontogenetic perspective. In: Grumbach MM, Sizonenko PC, Aubert ML, eds. *Control of the Onset of Puberty*. Baltimore, MD: Williams & Wilkins; 1990:1-68.
315. Reiter EO, Grumbach MM. Neuroendocrine control mechanisms and the onset of puberty. *Annu Rev Physiol*. 1982;44:595-613.
316. Grumbach MM. A window of opportunity: the diagnosis of gonadotropin deficiency in the male infant. *J Clin Endocrinol Metab*. 2005;90:3122-3127.
317. Grumbach MM, Kaplan SL. Fetal pituitary hormones and the maturation of central nervous system regulation of anterior pituitary function. In: Gluck L, ed. *Modern Perinatal Medicine*. Chicago, IL: Year Book Medical; 1974:247-271.
318. Plant TM. Hypothalamic control of the pituitary-gonadal axis in higher primates: key advances over the last two decades. *J Neuroendocrinol*. 2008;20:719-726.
319. Terasawa E, Fernandez DL. Neurobiological mechanisms of the onset of puberty in primates. *Endocr Rev*. 2001;22:111-151.
320. Kaplan SL, Grumbach MM. Pituitary and placental gonadotropins and sex steroids in the human and sub-human primate fetus. *Clin Endocrinol Metab*. 1978;7:487-511.
321. Martinez de la Escalera G, Clapp C. Regulation of gonadotropin-releasing hormone secretion: insights from GT1 immortal GnRH neurons. *Arch Med Res*. 2001;32:486-498.
322. Shacham S, Harris D, Ben-Shlomo H, et al. Mechanism of GnRH receptor signaling on gonadotropin release and gene expression in pituitary gonadotrophs. *Vitam Horm*. 2001;63:63-90.
323. Themmen APN, Huhtaniemi IT. Mutations of gonadotropins and gonadotropin receptors: elucidating the physiology and pathophysiology of pituitary-gonadal function. *Endocr Rev*. 2000;21:551-583.
324. Pitteloud N, Dwyer AA, DeCruz S, et al. Inhibition of luteinizing hormone secretion by testosterone in men requires aromatization for its pituitary but not its hypothalamic effects: evidence from the

tandem study of normal and gonadotropin-releasing hormone-deficient men. *J Clin Endocrinol Metab*. 2008;93:784-791.

325. Blackman BE, Yoshida H, Paruthiyil S, et al. Frequency of intrinsic pulsatile gonadotropin-releasing hormone secretion is regulated by the expression of cyclic nucleotide-gated channels in GT1 cells. *Endocrinology*. 2007;148:3299-3306.
326. Abe H, Terasawa E. Firing pattern and rapid modulation of activity by estrogen in primate luteinizing hormone releasing hormone-1 neurons. *Endocrinology*. 2005;146:4312-4320.
327. Finkelstein JS, Budger TM, O'Dea LS, et al. Effects of decreasing the frequency of gonadotropin-releasing hormone stimulation on gonadotropin secretion in gonadotropin-releasing hormone-deficient men and perfused rat pituitary cells. *J Clin Invest*. 1988;81:1725-1733.
328. Knobil E. The neuroendocrine control of the menstrual cycle. *Recent Prog Horm Res*. 1980;36:53-88.
329. Grumbach MM. The neuroendocrinology of human puberty revisited. *Horm Res*. 2002;57(suppl 2):2-14.
330. Reference deleted in proofs.
331. Mahachoklertwattana P, Black SM, Kaplan SL, et al. Nitric oxide synthesized by gonadotropin-releasing hormone neurons is a mediator of N-methyl-D-aspartate (NMDA)-induced GnRH secretion. *Endocrinology*. 1994;135:1709-1712.
332. Schwanzel-Fukuda M, Crossin KL, Pfaff DW, et al. Migration of luteinizing hormone-releasing hormone (LHRH) neurons in early human embryos. *J Comp Neurol*. 1996;366:547-557.
333. Tobet SA, Schwarting GA. Minireview: recent progress in gonadotropin-releasing hormone neuronal migration. *Endocrinology*. 2006;147:1159-1165.
334. Clarkson J, Herbison AE. Development of GABA and glutamate signaling at the GnRH neuron in relation to puberty. *Mol Cell Endocrinol*. 2006;254-255:32-38.
335. Castellano JM, Navarro VM, Fernandez-Fernandez R, et al. Changes in hypothalamic KiSS-1 system and restoration of pubertal activation of the reproductive axis by kisspeptin in undernutrition. *Endocrinology*. 2005;146:3917-3925.
336. Schwanzel-Fukuda M, Bick D, Pfaff DW. Luteinizing hormone-releasing hormone (LHRH)-expressing cells do not migrate normally in an inherited hypogonadal (Kallmann) syndrome. *Mol Brain Res*. 1989;6:311-326.
337. Terasawa E. Postnatal remodeling of gonadotropin-releasing hormone I neurons: toward understanding the mechanism of the onset of puberty. *Endocrinology*. 2006;147:3650-3651.
338. Gluckman PD, Grumbach MM, Kaplan SL. The neuroendocrine regulation and function of growth hormone and prolactin in the mammalian fetus. *Endocr Rev*. 1981;2:363-395.
339. Clark SJ, Ellis N, Styne DM, et al. Hormone ontogeny in the ovine fetus: XVII. Demonstration of pulsatile luteinizing hormone secretion by the fetal pituitary gland. *Endocrinology*. 1984;115:1774-1779.
340. Clark SJ, Hauffa BP, Rodens KP, et al. Hormone ontogeny in the ovine fetus: XIX. The effect of a potent luteinizing hormone-releasing factor agonist on gonadotropin and testosterone release in the fetus and neonate. *Pediatr Res*. 1989;25:347-352.
341. Habert R, Lejeune H, Saez JM. Origin, differentiation and regulation of fetal and adult Leydig cells. *Mol Cell Endocrinol*. 2001;179:47-74.
342. Boukari K, Meduri G, Brailly-Tabard S, et al. Lack of androgen receptor expression in Sertoli cells accounts for the absence of anti-müllerian hormone repression during early human testis development. *J Clin Endocrinol Metab*. 2009;94:1818-1825.
343. Gluckman PD, Marti Henneberg C, Kaplan SL, et al. Hormone ontogeny in the ovine fetus: XIV. The effect of 17β-estradiol infusion on fetal plasma gonadotropins and prolactin and the maturation of sex steroid-dependent negative feedback. *Endocrinology*. 1983;112:1618-1623.
344. Jaffe AB, Mulcahey JJ, DiBabio AM, et al. Peptide regulation of pituitary and target tissue function and growth in the primate fetus. *Recent Prog Horm Res*. 1988;44:431-544.
345. Mesiano S, Hart CS, Heyer BW, et al. Hormone ontogeny in the ovine fetus: XXVI. A sex difference in the effect of castration on the hypothalamic-pituitary gonadotropin unit in the ovine fetus. *Endocrinology*. 1991;129:3073-3079.
346. Cuttler L, Egli CA, Styne DM, et al. Hormone ontogeny in the ovine fetus: XVIII. The effect of an opioid antagonist on luteinizing hormone secretion. *Endocrinology*. 1985;116:1997-2002.
347. Bettendorf M, de Zegher F, Albers N, et al. Acute N-methyl-D,L-aspartate administration stimulates the luteinizing hormone releasing hormone pulse generator in the ovine fetus. *Horm Res*. 1999;51:25-30.
348. Dhandapani KM, Brann DW. The role of glutamate and nitric oxide in the reproductive neuroendocrine system. *Biochem Cell Biol*. 2000;78:165-179.
349. Albers N, Bettendorf M, Hart CS, et al. Hormone ontogeny in the ovine fetus: XXIII. Pulsatile administration of follicle-stimulating hormone stimulates inhibin production and decreases testosterone synthesis in the ovine fetal gonad. *Endocrinology*. 1989;124:3089-3094.
350. Albers N, Hart CS, Kaplan SL, et al. Hormone ontogeny in the ovine fetus: XXIV. Porcine follicular fluid "inhibins" selectively suppress plasma follicle-stimulating hormone in the ovine fetus. *Endocrinology*. 1989;125:675-678.
351. Corbier P, Dehenin L, Castanier M, et al. Sex differences in serum luteinizing hormone and testosterone in the human neonate during the first few hours after birth. *J Clin Endocrinol Metab*. 1990;71:1347-1348.
352. Lustig RH, Conte FA, Kogan BA, et al. Ontogeny of gonadotropin secretion in congenital anorchism: sexual dimorphism versus syndrome of gonadal dysgenesis and diagnostic considerations. *J Urol*. 1987;138:587-591.
353. Terasawa E, Fernandez DL. Neurobiological mechanisms of the onset of puberty in primates. *Endocr Rev*. 2001;22:111-151.
354. Forest MG. Pituitary gonadotropin and sex steroid secretion during the first two years of life. In: Grumbach MM, Sizonenko PC, Aubert AU, eds. *Control of the Onset of Puberty*. Baltimore, MD: Williams & Wilkins; 1990:451-478.
355. Grumbach MM. The central nervous system and the onset of puberty. In: Falkner F, Tanner JM, eds. *Human Growth*. New York, NY: Plenum; 1978:215-238.
356. Sharpe RM, Fraser HM, Brougham MF, et al. Role of the neonatal period of pituitary-testicular activity in germ cell proliferation and differentiation in the primate testis. *Hum Reprod*. 2003;18:2110-2117.
357. Sharpe RM, McKinnell C, Kivlin C, et al. Proliferation and functional maturation of Sertoli cells and their relevance to disorders of testis function in adulthood. *Reproduction*. 2003;125:769-784.
358. Salti R, Galluzzi F, Bindi G, et al. Nocturnal melatonin patterns in children. *J Clin Endocrinol Metab*. 2000;85:2137-2144.
359. Ojeda SR, Lomniczi A, Mastronardi C, et al. Minireview. The neuroendocrine regulation of puberty: is the time ripe for a systems biology approach? *Endocrinology*. 2006;147:1166-1174.
360. McArthur JW, Bullen BA, Beitins IZ, et al. Hypothalamic amenorrhea in runners of normal body composition. *Endocr Res Commun*. 1980;7:13-25.
361. Johnston FE, Roche AF, Schell LM, et al. Critical weight at menarche. *Am J Dis Child*. 1975;129:19-23.
362. Vizmanos B, Marti-Henneberg C. Puberty begins with a characteristic subcutaneous body fat mass in each sex. *Eur J Clin Nutr*. 2000;54:203-208.
363. Buyken AE, Karaolis-Danckert N, Remer T. Association of prepubertal body composition in healthy girls and boys with the timing of early and late pubertal markers. *Am J Clin Nutr*. 2009;89:221-230.
364. Zhang Y, Proenca R, Maffel M, et al. Positional cloning of the mouse obese gene and its human analogue. *Nature*. 1994;372:425-432.
365. Spiegelman BM, Flier JS. Adipogenesis and obesity: rounding out the big picture. *Cell*. 1996;87:377-389.
366. Tartaglia LA, Dembski M, Weng X, et al. Identification and expression cloning of a leptin receptor, OB-R. *Cell*. 1995;83:1263-1271.
367. Ahima RS, Saper CB, Flier JS, et al. Leptin regulation of neuroendocrine systems. *Front Neuroendocrinol*. 2000;21:263-307.
368. Donato JJ, Cravo RM, Frazão, et al. Leptin's effect on puberty in mice is relayed by the ventral premammillary nuclens and does not reguice signaling in Kiss1 neurons. *J Clin Invest*. 2001;121:355-368.
369. Ahima RS. No Kissing by leptin during puberty? *J Clin Invest*. 2011;121:34-36.
370. Ahmed ML, Ong KK, Morrell DJ, et al. Longitudinal study of leptin concentrations during puberty: sex differences and relationship to changes in body composition. *J Clin Endocrinol Metab*. 1999;84:899-905.
371. Horlick MB, Rosenbaum M, Nicolson M, et al. Effect of puberty on the relationship between circulating leptin and body composition. *J Clin Endocrinol Metab*. 2000;85:2509-2518.
372. Palmert MR, Radovick S, Boepple PA. The impact of reversible gonadal sex steroid suppression on serum leptin concentrations in children with central precocious puberty [see comments]. *J Clin Endocrinol Metab*. 1998;83:1091-1096.
373. Clayton PE, Trueman JA. Leptin and puberty. *Arch Dis Child*. 2000;83:1-4.
374. Grasemann C, Wessels HT, Knauer-Fischer S, et al. Increase of serum leptin after short-term pulsatile GnRH administration in children with delayed puberty. *Eur J Endocrinol*. 2004;150:691-698.
375. Mann DR, Bhat GK, Ramaswamy S, et al. Regulation of circulating leptin and its soluble receptor during pubertal development in the male rhesus monkey (*Macaca mulatta*). *Endocrine*. 2007;31:125-129.
376. Li HJ, Ji CY, Wang W, et al. A twin study for serum leptin, soluble leptin receptor, and free insulin-like growth factor-I in pubertal females. *J Clin Endocrinol Metab*. 2005;90:3659-3664.
377. Banerjee I, Trueman JA, Hall CM, et al. Phenotypic variation in constitutional delay of growth and puberty: relationship to specific leptin

and leptin receptor gene polymorphisms. *Eur J Endocrinol.* 2006;155:121-126.

378. Ozata M, Ozdemir IC, Licinio J. Human leptin deficiency caused by a missense mutation: multiple endocrine defects, decreased sympathetic tone, and immune system dysfunction indicate new targets for leptin action, greater central than peripheral resistance to the effects of leptin, and spontaneous correction of leptin-mediated defects. *J Clin Endocrinol Metab.* 1999;84:3686-3695.
379. Clement K, Vaisse C, Lahlou N, et al. A mutation in the human leptin receptor gene causes obesity and pituitary dysfunction. *Nature.* 1998;392:398-401.
380. Farooqi IS, Jebb SA, Langmack G, et al. Effects of recombinant leptin therapy in a child with congenital leptin deficiency. *N Engl J Med.* 1999;341:879-884.
381. Andreelli F, Hanaire-Broutin H, Laville M, et al. Normal reproductive function in leptin-deficient patients with lipoatropic diabetes. *J Clin Endocrinol Metab.* 2000;85:715-719.
382. Brown DC, Kelnar CJ, Wu FC. Energy metabolism during male human puberty: I. Changes in energy expenditure during the onset of puberty in boys. *Ann Hum Biol.* 1996;23:273-279.
383. Fernandez-Fernandez R, Martini AC, Navarro VM, et al. Novel signals for the integration of energy balance and reproduction. *Mol Cell Endocrinol.* 2006;254-255:127-132.
384. Bottner A, Kratzsch J, Muller G, et al. Gender differences of adiponectin levels develop during the progression of puberty and are related to serum androgen levels. *J Clin Endocrinol Metab.* 2004;89:4053-4061.
385. Gerber M, Boettner A, Seidel B, et al. Serum resistin levels of obese and lean children and adolescents: biochemical analysis and clinical relevance. *J Clin Endocrinol Metab.* 2005;90:4503-4509.
386. Conte FA, Grumbach MM, Kaplan SL, et al. Correlation of luteinizing hormone-releasing factor-induced luteinizing hormone and follicle-stimulating hormone release from infancy to 19 years with the changing pattern of gonadotropin secretion in agonadal patients: relation to the restraint of puberty. *J Clin Endocrinol Metab.* 1980;50:163-168.
387. Conte FA, Grumbach MM, Kaplan SL. A diphasic pattern of gonadotropin secretion in patients with the syndrome of gonadal dysgenesis. *J Clin Endocrinol Metab.* 1975;40:670-674.
388. Kelch RP, Kaplan SL, Grumbach MM. Suppression of urinary and plasma follicle-stimulating hormone by exogenous estrogens in prepubertal and pubertal children. *J Clin Invest.* 1973;52:1122-1128.
389. Grumbach MM, Kaplan SL. Recent advances in the diagnosis and management of sexual precocity. *Acta Paediatr Jpn (Overseas Ed).* 1988;30:155-175.
390. Judge DM, Kulin HE, Santen R, et al. Hypothalamic hamartoma: a source of luteinizing-hormone-releasing factor in precocious puberty. *N Engl J Med.* 1977;296:7-10.
391. Mahachoklertwattana P, Kaplan SL, Grumbach MM. The luteinizing hormone-releasing hormone-secreting hypothalamic hamartoma is a congenital malformation: natural history. *J Clin Endocrinol Metab.* 1993;77:118-124.
392. Silverman AJ, Gibson M. Hypothalamic transplantation: repair of defects in hypogonadal mice. *Trends Endocrinol Metab.* 1990; 1:403-408.
393. Martinez de la Escalera G, Choi ALH, Weinter RI. Biphasic gabaergic regulation of GnRH secretion in GT1 cell lines. *Neuroendocrinology.* 1994;59:420-425.
394. Ganguly K, Schinder AF, Wong ST, et al. GABA itself promotes the developmental switch of neuronal GABAergic responses from excitation to inhibition. *Cell.* 2001;105:521-532.
395. Ottem EN, Godwin JG, Krishnan S, et al. Dual-phenotype GABA/glutamate neurons in adult preoptic area: sexual dimorphism and function. *J Neurosci.* 2004;24:8097-8105.
396. Ha CM, Choi J, Choi EJ, et al. NELL2, a neuron-specific EGF-like protein, is selectively expressed in glutamatergic neurons and contributes to the glutamatergic control of GnRH neurons at puberty. *Neuroendocrinology.* 2008;88:199-211.
397. Urbanski HF, Ojeda SR. Activation of luteinizing hormone-releasing hormone release advances the onset of female puberty. *Neuroendocrinology.* 1987;46:273-276.
398. Van den Pol AN, Wuarin JP, Dudek FE. Glutamate, the dominant excitatory transmitter in neuroendocrine regulation. *Science.* 1990;250:1276-1278.
399. Bourguignon JP, Gerard A, Mathieu J, et al. Pulsatile release of gonadotropin-releasing hormone from hypothalamic explants is restrained by blockade of N-methyl-D,L-aspartate receptors. *Endocrinology.* 1989;125:1090-1096.
400. Mahachoklertwattana P, Sanchez J, Kaplan SL, et al. N-methyl-D-aspartate (NMDA) receptors mediate the release of hormone (GnRH) by NMDA in a hypothalamic neuronal cell line (GT1- 1). *Endocrinology.* 1994;134:1023-1030.
401. Terasawa E, Luchansky LL, Kasuya E, et al. An increase in glutamate release follows a decrease in gamma aminobutyric acid and the pubertal increase in luteinizing hormone releasing hormone release in the female rhesus monkeys. *J Neuroendocrinol.* 1999;11:275-282.
402. Seminara SB, Crowley WF Jr. Kisspeptin and GPR54: discovery of a novel pathway in reproduction. *J Neuroendocrinol.* 2008;20:727-731.
403. Smith JT, Clifton DK, Steiner RA. Regulation of the neuroendocrine reproductive axis by kisspeptin-GPR54 signaling. *Reproduction.* 2006;131:623-630.
404. Muir AI, Chamberlain L, Elshourbagy NA, et al. AXOR12, a novel human G protein-coupled receptor, activated by the peptide KiSS-1. *J Biol Chem.* 2001;276:28969-28975.
405. Ohtaki T, Shintani Y, Honda S, et al. Metastasis suppressor gene KiSS-1 encodes peptide ligand of a G-protein-coupled receptor. *Nature.* 2001;411:613-617.
406. Shahab M, Mastronardi C, Seminara SB, et al. Increased hypothalamic GPR54 signaling: a potential mechanism for initiation of puberty in primates. *Proc Natl Acad Sci U S A.* 2005;102:2129-2134.
407. Gottsch ML, Cunningham MJ, Smith JT, et al. A role for kisspeptins in the regulation of gonadotropin secretion in the mouse. *Endocrinology.* 2004;145:4073-4077.
408. Messager S, Chatzidaki EE, Ma D, et al. Kisspeptin directly stimulates gonadotropin-releasing hormone release via G protein-coupled receptor 54. *Proc Natl Acad Sci U S A.* 2005;102:1761-1766.
409. Han SK, Gottsch ML, Lee KJ, et al. Activation of gonadotropin-releasing hormone neurons by kisspeptin as a neuroendocrine switch for the onset of puberty. *J Neurosci.* 2005;25:11349-11356.
410. Nazian SJ. Role of metastin in the release of gonadotropin-releasing hormone from the hypothalamus of the male rat. *J Androl.* 2006;27:444-449.
411. Seminara SB, Messager S, Chatzidaki EE, et al. The GPR54 gene as a regulator of puberty. *N Engl J Med.* 2003;349:1614-1627.
412. Patterson M, Murphy KG, Thompson EL, et al. Administration of kisspeptin-54 into discrete regions of the hypothalamus potently increases plasma luteinising hormone and testosterone in male adult rats. *J Neuroendocrinol.* 2006;18:349-354.
413. Navarro VM, Castellano JM, Fernandez-Fernandez R, et al. Characterization of the potent luteinizing hormone-releasing activity of KiSS-1 peptide, the natural ligand of GPR54. *Endocrinology.* 2005;146:156-163.
414. Navarro VM, Castellano JM, Fernandez-Fernandez R, et al. Effects of KiSS-1 peptide, the natural ligand of GPR54, on follicle-stimulating hormone secretion in the rat. *Endocrinology.* 2005;146:1689-1697.
415. Navarro VM, Castellano JM, Fernandez-Fernandez R, et al. Developmental and hormonally regulated messenger ribonucleic acid expression of KiSS-1 and its putative receptor, GPR54, in rat hypothalamus and potent luteinizing hormone-releasing activity of KiSS-1 peptide. *Endocrinology.* 2004;145:4565-4574.
416. Navarro VM, Fernandez-Fernandez R, Castellano JM, et al. Advanced vaginal opening and precocious activation of the reproductive axis by KiSS-1 peptide, the endogenous ligand of GPR54. *J Physiol.* 2004;561(Pt 2):379-386.
417. Matsui H, Takatsu Y, Kumano S, et al. Peripheral administration of metastin induces marked gonadotropin release and ovulation in the rat. *Biochem Biophys Res Commun.* 2004;320:383-388.
418. Plant TM, Ramaswamy S. Kisspeptin and the regulation of the hypothalamic-pituitary-gonadal axis in the rhesus monkey (*Macaca mulatta*). *Peptides.* 2009;30:67-75.
419. Ramaswamy S, Guerriero KA, Gibbs RB, et al. Structural interactions between kisspeptin and GnRH neurons in the mediobasal hypothalamus of the male rhesus monkey (*Macaca mulatta*) as revealed by double immunofluorescence and confocal microscopy. *Endocrinology.* 2008;149:4387-4395.
420. Seminara SB, Dipietro MJ, Ramaswamy S, et al. Continuous human metastin 45-54 infusion desensitizes G protein-coupled receptor 54-induced gonadotropin-releasing hormone release monitored indirectly in the juvenile male rhesus monkey (*Macaca mulatta*): a finding with therapeutic implications. *Endocrinology.* 2006;147:2122-2126.
421. Shibata M, Friedman RL, Ramaswamy S, et al. Evidence that down regulation of hypothalamic KiSS-1 expression is involved in the negative feedback action of testosterone to regulate luteinising hormone secretion in the adult male rhesus monkey (*Macaca mulatta*). *J Neuroendocrinol.* 2007;19:432-438.
422. Pompolo S, Pereira A, Estrada KM, et al. Colocalization of kisspeptin and gonadotropin-releasing hormone in the ovine brain. *Endocrinology.* 2006;147:804-810.
423. Blogowska A, Rzepka-Gorska I, Krzyzanowska-Swiniarska B. Is neuropeptide Y responsible for constitutional delay of puberty in girls? A preliminary report. *Gynecol Endocrinol.* 2004;19:22-25.
424. Kelch RP, Marshall JC. Pulsatile gonadotropin-releasing hormone and the induction of puberty in human beings. In: Grumbach MM, Sizonenko PC, Aubert ML, eds. *Control of the Onset of Puberty.* Baltimore, MD: Williams & Wilkins; 1990:82-107.

425. Kletter GB, Foster CM, Brown MB, et al. Nocturnal naloxone fails to reverse the suppressive effects of testosterone infusion on luteinizing hormone secretion in pubertal boys. *J Clin Endocrinol Metab.* 1994;79:1147-1151.
426. Roth JC, Grumbach MM, Kaplan SL. Effect of synthetic luteinizing hormone-releasing factor on serum testosterone and gonadotropins in prepubertal, pubertal, and adult males. *J Clin Endocrinol Metab.* 1973;37:680-686.
427. Yen SSC, Lasley BL, Wang FC, et al. The operating characteristics of the hypothalamic-pituitary system during the menstrual cycle and observations of biological action of somatostatin. *Recent Prog Horm Res.* 1975;31:321-363.
428. Watanabe G, Terasawa E. In vivo release of luteinizing hormone releasing hormone increases with puberty in the female rhesus monkey. *Endocrinology.* 1989;125:92-99.
429. Reiter EO, Kaplan SL, Conte FA, et al. Responsivity of pituitary gonadotropes to luteinizing hormone-releasing factor in idiopathic precocious puberty, precocious thelarche, precocious adrenarche, and in patients treated with medroxyprogesterone acetate. *Pediatr Res.* 1975;9:111-116.
430. Spratt DI, Crowley WFJ. Pituitary and gonadal responsiveness is enhanced during GnRH-induced puberty. *Am J Physiol.* 1988;254: E652-E657.
431. Germak JA, Knobil E. Control of puberty in the rhesus monkey. In: Grumbach MM, Sizonenko PC, Aubert ML, eds. *Control of the Onset of Puberty.* Baltimore, MD: Williams & Wilkins; 1990:69-81.
432. Wildt L, Hausler A, Marshall G, et al. Frequency and amplitude of gonadotropin-releasing hormone stimulation and gonadotropin secretion in the rhesus monkey. *Endocrinology.* 1981;109:376-385.
433. Wildt L, Marshall G, Knobil E. Experimental induction of puberty in the infantile female rhesus monkey. *Science.* 1980;207:1373-1375.
434. Marshall JC, Kelch RP. Low dose pulsatile gonadotropin-releasing hormone in anorexia nervosa: a model of human pubertal development. *J Clin Endocrinol Metab.* 1979;49:712-718.
435. Crowley WF Jr, McArthur JW. Stimulation of the normal menstrual cycle in Kallmann's syndrome by pulsatile administration of luteinizing hormone-releasing hormone (LHRH). *J Clin Endocrinol Metab.* 1980;51:173-175.
436. Valk TW, Corley KP, Kelch RP, et al. Hypogonadotropic hypogonadism: hormonal responses to low dose pulsatile administration of gonadotropin-releasing hormone. *J Clin Endocrinol Metab.* 1980;51: 730-737.
437. Sizonenko PC, Cuendet A, Paunier L. FSH: 1. Evidence for its mediating role on testosterone secretion in cryptorchidism. *J Clin Endocrinol Metab.* 1973;37:68-73.
438. Reiter EO, Kulin HE, Hamwood SM. The absence of positive feedback between estrogen and luteinizing hormone in sexually immature girls. *Pediatr Res.* 1974;8:740-745.
439. Hayes FJ, Seminara SB, DeCruz S, et al. Aromatase inhibition in the human male reveals a hypothalamic site of estrogen feedback. *J Clin Endocrinol Metab.* 2000;85:3027-3035.
440. Apter D, Vihko R. Serum pregnenolone, progesterone, 17-hydroxyprogesterone, testosterone and 5 alpha-dihydrotestosterone during female puberty. *J Clin Endocrinol Metab.* 1977;45:1039-1048.
441. Cutler GBJ, Loriaux DL. Andrenarche and its relationship to the onset of puberty. *Fed Proc.* 1980;39:2384-2390.
442. Sklar CA, Kaplan SL, Grumbach MM. Evidence for dissociation between adrenarche and gonadarche: studies in patients with idiopathic precocious puberty, gonadal dysgenesis, isolated gonadotropin deficiency, and constitutionally delayed growth and adolescence. *J Clin Endocrinol Metab.* 1980;51:548-556.
443. Sizonenko PC, Paunier LC. Correlation of plasma dehydroepiandrosterone, testosterone, FSH, and LH with stages of puberty and bone age in normal boys and girls and in patients with Addison's disease or hypogonadism or with premature or late adrenarche. *J Clin Endocrinol Metab.* 1975;41:894-904.
444. Reiter EO, Fuldauer VG, Root AW. Secretion of the adrenal androgen, dehydroepiandrosterone sulfate, during normal infancy, childhood, and adolescence, in sick infants, and in children with endocrinologic abnormalities. *J Pediatr.* 1977;90:766-770.
445. Campbell B. Adrenarche and the evolution of human life history. *Am J Hum Biol.* 2006;18:569-589.
446. Gell JS, Carr BR, Sasano H, et al. Adrenarche results from development of a 3beta-hydroxysteroid dehydrogenase-deficient adrenal reticularis. *J Clin Endocrinol Metab.* 1998;83:3695-3701.
447. Endoh A, Kristiansen SB, Casson PR, et al. The zona reticularis is the site of biosynthesis of dehydroepiandrosterone and dehydroepiandrosterone sulfate in the adult human adrenal cortex resulting from its low expression of 3 beta-hydroxysteroid dehydrogenase. *J Clin Endocrinol Metab.* 1996;81:3558-3565.
448. Marx C, Bornstein SR, Wolkersdorfer GW. Relevance of MHC class II expression as a hallmark for the cellular differentiation in the human adrenal cortex. *J Clin Endocrinol Metab.* 1997;82:3136-3140.
449. Miller WL, Auchus RJ, Geller DH. The regulation of 17,20 lyase activity. *Steroids.* 1997;62:133-142.
450. Geller DH, Auchus RJ, Mendonca BB, et al. The genetic and functional basis of isolated 17,20-lyase deficiency. *Nat Genet.* 1997;17:201-205.
451. Zhang L, Rodriguez H, Ohno S, et al. Serine phosphorylation of human P450c17 increases 17,20 lyase activity: implications for adrenarche and for the polycystic ovary syndrome. *Proc Natl Acad Sci USA.* 1995;92:10619-10623.
452. Auchus RJ, Miller WL. Molecular modeling of human P450c17 (17alpha-hydroxylase/17,20-lyase): insights into reaction mechanisms and effects of mutations. *Mol Endocrinol.* 1999;13:1169-1182.
453. Weber A, Clark AJ, Perry LA, et al. Diminished adrenal androgen secretion in familial glucocorticoid deficiency implicates a significant role for ACTH in the induction of adrenarche. *Clin Endocrinol.* 1997;46:431-437.
454. Miller WL. The molecular basis of premature adrenarche: an hypothesis. *Acta Paediatr Suppl.* 1999;88:60-66.
455. Ibanez L, Potau N, Marcos MV, et al. Corticotropin-releasing hormone: a potent androgen secretagogue in girls with hyperandrogenism after precocious pubarche. *J Clin Endocrinol Metab.* 1999;84:4602-4606.
456. Karteris E, Randeva HS, Grammatopoulos DK, et al. Expression and coupling characteristics of the CRH and orexin type 2 receptors in human fetal adrenals. *J Clin Endocrinol Metab.* 2001;86:4512-4519.
457. Biason-Lauber A, Zachmann M, Schoenle EJ. Effect of leptin on CYP17 enzymatic activities in human adrenal cells: new insight in the onset of adrenarche. *Endocrinology.* 2000;141:1446-1454.
458. Auchus RJ, Rainey WE. Adrenarche: physiology, biochemistry and human disease. *Clin Endocrinol (Oxf).* 2004;60:288-296.
459. Remer T, Manz F. Role of nutritional status in the regulation of adrenarche. *J Clin Endocrinol Metab.* 1999;84:3936-3944.
460. Reiter EO, Grumbach MM, Kaplan SL, et al. The response of pituitary gonadotropes to synthetic LRF in children with glucocorticoid-treated congenital adrenal hyperplasia: lack of effect of intrauterine and neonatal androgen excess. *J Clin Endocrinol Metab.* 1975;40:318-325.
461. Remer T, Manz F. The midgrowth spurt in healthy children is not caused by adrenarche. *J Clin Endocrinol Metab.* 2001;86:4183-4186.
462. Sedlmeyer IL, Palmert MR. Delayed puberty: analysis of a large case series from an academic center. *J Clin Endocrinol Metab.* 2002;87:1613-1620.
463. Sedlmeyer IL, Hirschhorn JN, Palmert MR. Pedigree analysis of constitutional delay of growth and maturation: determination of familial aggregation and inheritance patterns. *J Clin Endocrinol Metab.* 2002;87:5581-5586.
464. Wu FC, Brown DC, Butler GE, et al. Early morning plasma testosterone is an accurate predictor of imminent pubertal development in prepubertal boys. *J Clin Endocrinol Metab.* 1993;76:26-31.
465. Du Caju MV, op de Beeck L, Sys SU, et al. Progressive deceleration in growth as an early sign of delayed puberty in boys. *Horm Res.* 2000;54:126-130.
466. Cara JF, Rosenfield RL. Insulin-like growth factor I and insulin potentiate luteinizing hormone-induced androgen synthesis by rat ovarian theca-interstitial cells. *Endocrinology.* 1988;123:733-739.
467. LaFranchi S, Hanna CE, Mandel SH. Constitutional delay of growth: expected versus final adult height. *Pediatrics.* 1991;87:82-87.
468. Crowne EC, Shalet SM, Wallace WH, et al. Final height in girls with untreated constitutional delay in growth and puberty. *Eur J Pediatr.* 1991;150:708-712.
469. Rensonnet C, Kanen F, Coremans C, et al. Pubertal growth as a determinant of adult height in boys with constitutional delay of growth and puberty. *Horm Res.* 1999;51:223-229.
470. Yanovski JA, Rose SR, Municchi G, et al. Treatment with a luteinizing hormone-releasing hormone agonist in adolescents with short stature. *N Engl J Med.* 2003;348:908-917.
471. Carel JC, Ecosse E, Nicolino M, et al. Adult height after long term treatment with recombinant growth hormone for idiopathic isolated growth hormone deficiency: observational follow up study of the French population based registry. *BMJ.* 2002;325:70.
472. Ranke MB, Lindberg A, Martin DD, et al. The mathematical model for total pubertal growth in idiopathic growth hormone (GH) deficiency suggests a moderate role of GH dose. *J Clin Endocrinol Metab.* 2003;88:4748-4753.
473. Reiter EO. A brief review of the addition of gonadotropin-releasing hormone agonists (GnRH-Ag) to growth hormone (GH) treatment of children with idiopathic growth hormone deficiency: previously published studies from America. *Mol Cell Endocrinol.* 2006;254-255:221-225.
474. Carel JC, Eugster EA, Rogol A, et al. Consensus statement on the use of gonadotropin-releasing hormone analogs in children. *Pediatrics.* 2009;123:e752-e762.
475. Finkelstein BS, Imperiale TF, Speroff T, et al. Effect of growth hormone therapy on height in children with idiopathic short stature: a meta-analysis. *Arch Pediatr Adolesc Med.* 2002;156:230-240.

476. Bryant J, Cave C, Milne R. Recombinant growth hormone for idiopathic short stature in children and adolescents. Cochrane Database Syst Rev. 2003;(4):CD004440.
477. Wickman S, Sipila I, Ankarberg-Lindgren C, et al. A specific aromatase inhibitor and potential increase in adult height in boys with delayed puberty: a randomised controlled trial. *Lancet.* 2001;357:1743-1748.
478. Hero M, Toiviainen-Salo S, Wickman S, et al. Vertebral morphology in aromatase inhibitor treated males with idiopathic short stature or constitutional delay of puberty. *J Bone Miner Res.* 2010; 25:1536-1543.
479. Mauras N, Gonzalez de Pijem L, Hsiang HY, et al. Anastrozole increases predicted adult height of short adolescent males treated with growth hormone: a randomized, placebo-controlled, multicenter trial for one to three years. *Obstet Gynecol Surv.* 2008; 93:823-831.
480. Dunkel L. Use of aromatase inhibitors to increase final height. *Mol Cell Endocrinol.* 2006;254-255:207-216.
481. Lin L, Conway GS, Hill NR, et al. A homozygous R262Q mutation in the gonadotropin-releasing hormone receptor (GNRHR) presenting as constitutional delay of growth and puberty with subsequent borderline oligospermia. *J Clin Endocrinol Metab.* 2006;91:5117-5121.
482. Keil MF, Stratakis CA. Pituitary tumors in childhood: update of diagnosis, treatment and molecular genetics. *Expert Rev Neurother.* 2008;8:563-574.
483. Thomsett MJ, Conte FA, Kaplan SL, et al. Endocrine and neurologic outcome in childhood craniopharyngioma: review of effect of treatment in 42 patients. *J Pediatr.* 1980;97:728-735.
484. Muller HL. Childhood craniopharyngioma: recent advances in diagnosis, treatment and follow-up. *Horm Res.* 2008;69:193-202.
485. Preeyasombat C, Bacchetti P, Lazar AA, et al. Racial and etiopathologic dichotomies in insulin hypersecretion and resistance in obese children. *J Pediatr.* 2005;146:474-481.
486. Muller HL, Handwerker G, Gebhardt U, et al. Melatonin treatment in obese patients with childhood craniopharyngioma and increased daytime sleepiness. *Cancer Causes Control.* 2006;17:583-589.
487. Cohan P, Foulad A, Esposito F, et al. Symptomatic Rathke's cleft cysts: a report of 24 cases. *J Endocrinol Invest.* 2004;27:943-948.
488. Schneider DT, Calaminus G, Koch S, et al. Epidemiologic analysis of 1,442 children and adolescents registered in the German germ cell tumor protocols. *Pediatr Blood Cancer.* 2004;42:169-175.
489. Sklar CA, Grumbach MM, Kaplan SL, et al. Hormonal and metabolic abnormalities associated with central nervous system germinoma in children and adolescents and the effect of therapy: report of 10 patients. *J Clin Endocrinol Metab.* 1981;52:9-16.
490. Mootha SL, Barkovich AJ, Grumbach MM, et al. Idiopathic hypothalamic diabetes insipidus, pituitary stalk thickening and the occult intracranial germinoma in children and adolescents. *J Clin Endocrinol Metab.* 1997;82:1362-1367.
491. Schmidt F, Penka B, Trauner M, et al. Lack of pineal growth during childhood. *J Clin Endocrinol Metab.* 1995;80:1221-1225.
492. Khatua S, Dhall G, O'Neil S, et al. Treatment of primary CNS germinomatous germ cell tumors with chemotherapy prior to reduced dose whole ventricular and local boost irradiation. *Pediatr Blood Cancer.* 2010;55:42-46.
493. da Silva NS, Cappellano AM, Diez B, et al. Primary chemotherapy for intracranial germ cell tumors: results of the third international CNS germ cell tumor study. *Pediatr Blood Cancer.* 2010;54:377-383.
494. Maity A, Shu HK, Judkins AR, et al. Testicular seminoma 16 years after treatment for CNS germinoma. *J Neurooncol.* 2004;70:83-85.
495. Rothman J, Greenberg RE, Jaffe WI. Nonseminomatous germ cell tumor of the testis 9 years after a germ cell tumor of the pineal gland: case report and review of the literature. *Can J Urol.* 2008; 15:4122-4124.
496. Cannavo S, Venturino M, Curto L, et al. Clinical presentation and outcome of pituitary adenomas in teenagers. *Clin Endocrinol (Oxf).* 2003;58:519-527.
497. Mahachoklertwattana P, Conte FA, Grumbach MM, et al. Prolactinomas in children and adolescents: effect on pubertal onset and long term outcome following selective transsphenoidal adenomectomy. *Pediatr Res.* 1994;35:A103.
498. Fideleff HL, Boquete HR, Suarez MG, et al. Prolactinoma in children and adolescents. *Horm Res.* 2009;72:197-205.
499. Knoepfelmacher M, Gomes MC, Melo ME, et al. Pituitary apoplexy during therapy with cabergoline in an adolescent male with prolactin-secreting macroadenoma. *Pituitary.* 2004;7:83-87.
500. Colao A, Galderisi M, Di Sarno A, et al. Increased prevalence of tricuspid regurgitation in patients with prolactinomas chronically treated with cabergoline. *J Clin Endocrinol Metab.* 2008;93:3777-3784.
501. Yuen YP, Lai JP, Au KM, et al. Macroprolactin: a cause of pseudohyperprolactinaemia. *Hong Kong Med J.* 2003;9:119-121.
502. Abla O, Egeler RM, Weitzman S. Langerhans cell histiocytosis: current concepts and treatments. *Cancer Treat Rev.* 2010;36:354-359.
503. Richards GE, Wara WM, Grumbach MM, et al. Delayed onset of hypopituitarism: sequelae of therapeutic irradiation of central nervous system, eye, and middle ear tumors. *J Pediatr.* 1976;89: 553-559.
504. Frisk P, Arvidson J, Gustafsson J, et al. Pubertal development and final height after autologous bone marrow transplantation for acute lymphoblastic leukemia. *Bone Marrow Transplant.* 2004;33:205-210.
505. Gurney JG, Kadan-Lottick NS, Packer RJ, et al. Endocrine and cardiovascular late effects among adult survivors of childhood brain tumors: Childhood Cancer Survivor Study. *Cancer.* 2003;97:663-673.
506. Byrne J, Fears TR, Mills JL, et al. Fertility in women treated with cranial radiotherapy for childhood acute lymphoblastic leukemia. *Pediatr Blood Cancer.* 2004;42:589-597.
507. Seminara SB, Hayes FJ, Crowley WFJ. Gonadotropin-releasing hormone deficiency in the human (idiopathic hypogonadotropic hypogonadism and Kallmann's syndrome): pathophysiological and genetic considerations. *Endocr Rev.* 1999;19:521-539.
508. Layman LC. Mutations in human gonadotropin genes and their physiologic significance in puberty and reproduction. *Fertil Steril.* 1999;71:201-218.
509. Van Dop C, Burstein S, Conte FA, et al. Isolated gonadotropin deficiency in boys: clinical characteristics and growth. *J Pediatr.* 1987;111:684-692.
510. Pitteloud N, Hayes FJ, Boepple PA, et al. The role of prior pubertal development, biochemical markers of testicular maturation, and genetics in elucidating the phenotypic heterogeneity of idiopathic hypogonadotropic hypogonadism. *J Clin Endocrinol Metab.* 2002; 87:152-160.
511. Uriarte MM, Baron J, Garcia HB, et al. The effect of pubertal delay on adult height in men with isolated hypogonadotropic hypogonadism [published erratum appears in *J Clin Endocrinol Metab.* 1992;75:1009]. *J Clin Endocrinol Metab.* 1992;74:436-440.
512. Kallmann F, Schonfeld WA, Barrera SW. Genetic aspects of primary eunuchoidism. *Am J Ment Defic.* 1944;48:203-236.
513. Raivio T, Falardeau J, Dwyer A, et al. Reversal of idiopathic hypogonadotropic hypogonadism. *N Engl J Med.* 2007;357:863-873.
514. Massin N, Pecheux C, Eloit C, et al. X chromosome-linked Kallmann syndrome: clinical heterogeneity in three siblings carrying an intragenic deletion of the KAL-1 gene. *J Clin Endocrinol Metab.* 2003;88:2003-2008.
515. Hardelin JP, Dode C. The complex genetics of Kallmann syndrome: KAL1, FGFR1, FGF8, PROKR2, PROK2, et al. *Sex Dev.* 2008;2: 181-193.
516. Sato N, Katsumata N, Kagami M, et al. Clinical assessment and mutation analysis of Kallmann syndrome 1 (KAL1) and fibroblast growth factor receptor 1 (FGFR1, or KAL2) in five families and 18 sporadic patients. *J Clin Endocrinol Metab.* 2004;89:1079-1088.
517. Maya-Nuanez G, Torres L, Ulloa-Aguirre A, et al. An atypical contiguous gene syndrome: molecular studies in a family with X-linked Kallmann's syndrome and X-linked ichthyosis. *Clin Endocrinol.* 1999;50:157-162.
518. Oliveira LM, Seminara SB, Beranova M, et al. The importance of autosomal genes in Kallmann syndrome: genotype-phenotype correlations and neuroendocrine characteristics. *J Clin Endocrinol Metab.* 2001;86:1532-1538.
519. Dode C, Levilliers J, Dupont JM, et al. Loss-of-function mutations in FGFR1 cause autosomal dominant Kallmann syndrome. *Nat Genet.* 2003;33:463-465.
520. Pitteloud N, Acierno JS Jr, Meysing AU, et al. Reversible Kallmann syndrome, delayed puberty, and isolated anosmia occurring in a single family with a mutation in the fibroblast growth factor receptor 1 gene. *J Clin Endocrinol Metab.* 2005;90:1317-1322.
521. Chung WC, Moyle SS, Tsai PS. Fibroblast growth factor 8 signaling through fibroblast growth factor receptor 1 is required for the emergence of gonadotropin-releasing hormone neurons. *Endocrinology.* 2008;149:4997-5003.
522. Semple RK, Kemal TA. The recent genetics of hypogonadotrophic hypogonadism: novel insights and new questions. *Clin Endocrinol.* 2009;72:427-435.
523. Zenaty D, Bretones P, Lambe C, et al. Paediatric phenotype of Kallmann syndrome due to mutations of fibroblast growth factor receptor 1 (FGFR1). Hormone Research. *Mol Cell Endocrinol.* 2006;254-255: 78-83.
524. Matsumoto S, Yamazaki C, Masumoto KH, et al. Abnormal development of the olfactory bulb and reproductive system in mice lacking prokineticin receptor PKR2. *Proc Natl Acad Sci U S A.* 2006;103: 4140-4145.
525. Pitteloud N, Zhang C, Pignatelli D, et al. Loss-of-function mutation in the prokineticin 2 gene causes Kallmann syndrome and normosmic idiopathic hypogonadotropic hypogonadism. *Proc Natl Acad Sci U S A.* 2007;104:17447-17452.
526. Jongmans MC, Ravenswaaij-Arts CM, Pitteloud N, et al. CHD7 mutations in patients initially diagnosed with Kallmann syndrome: the clinical overlap with CHARGE syndrome. *Clin Genet.* 2009;75:65-71.
527. Hipkin LJ, Casson IF, Davis JC. Identical twins discordant for Kallmann's syndrome. *J Med Genet.* 1990;27:198-199.

528. Truwit CL, Barkovich AJ, Grumbach MM, et al. Magnetic resonance imaging of Kallmann syndrome, a genetic disorder of neuronal migration affecting the ofactory and genital systems. *Am J Neuroradiol.* 1993;14:827-838.
529. Layman LC. Genetics of human hypogonadotropic hypogonadism. *Am J Med Genet.* 1999;89:240-248.
530. Achermann JC, Weiss J, Lee EJ, et al. Inherited disorders of the gonadotropin hormones. *Mol Cell Endocrinol.* 2001;179:89-96.
531. de Roux N, Milgrom E. Inherited disorders of GnRH and gonadotropin receptors. *Mol Cell Endocrinol.* 2001;179:83-87.
532. Beier DR, Dluhy RG. Bench and bedside: the G protein-coupled receptor GPR54 and puberty. *N Engl J Med.* 2003;349:1589-1592.
533. Miura K, Acierno JS Jr, Seminara SB. Characterization of the human nasal embryonic LHRH factor gene, NELF, and a mutation screening among 65 patients with idiopathic hypogonadotropic hypogonadism (IHH). *J Hum Genet.* 2004;49:265-268.
534. Bouligand J, Ghervan C, Tello JA, et al. Isolated familial hypogonadotropic hypogonadism and a GNRH1 mutation. *N Engl J Med.* 2009;360:2742-2748.
535. Chan YM, de Guillebon A, Lang-Muritano M, et al. GNRH1 mutations in patients with idiopathic hypogonadotropic hypogonadism. *Proc Natl Acad Sci U S A.* 2009;106:11703-11708.
536. Semple RK, Achermann JC, Ellery J, et al. Two novel missense mutations in g protein-coupled receptor 54 in a patient with hypogonadotropic hypogonadism. *J Clin Endocrinol Metab.* 2005;90:1849-1855.
537. de Roux N, Genin E, Carel JC, et al. Hypogonadotropic hypogonadism due to loss of function of the KiSS1-derived peptide receptor GPR54. *Proc Natl Acad Sci U S A.* 2003;100:10972-10976.
538. Wacker JL, Feller DB, Tang XB, et al. Disease-causing mutation in GPR54 reveals the importance of the second intracellular loop for class A G-protein-coupled receptor function. *J Biol Chem.* 2008;283:31068-31078.
539. de Roux N, Young J, Brailly-Tabard S, et al. The same molecular defects of the gonadotropin-releasing hormone receptor determine a variable degree of hypogonadism in affected kindred. *J Clin Endocrinol Metab.* 1999;84:567-572.
540. Pralong FP, Gomez F, Castillo E, et al. Complete hypogonadotropic hypogonadism associated with a novel inactivating mutation of the gonadotropin-releasing hormone receptor. *J Clin Endocrinol Metab.* 1999;84:3811-3816.
541. Bedecarrats GY, Linher KD, Janovick JA, et al. Four naturally occurring mutations in the human GnRH receptor affect ligand binding and receptor function. *Mol Cell Endocrinol.* 2003;205:51-64.
542. Janovick JA, Maya-Nunez G, Conn PM. Rescue of hypogonadotropic hypogonadism-causing and manufactured GnRH receptor mutants by a specific protein-folding template: misrouted proteins as a novel disease etiology and therapeutic target. *J Clin Endocrinol Metab.* 2002;87:3255-3262.
543. Maya-Nunez G, Janovick JA, Ulloa-Aguirre A, et al. Molecular basis of hypogonadotropic hypogonadism: restoration of mutant (E(90)K) GnRH receptor function by a deletion at a distant site. *J Clin Endocrinol Metab.* 2002;87:2144-2149.
544. Leanos-Miranda A, Janovick JA, Conn PM. Receptor-misrouting: an unexpectedly prevalent and rescuable etiology in gonadotropin-releasing hormone receptor-mediated hypogonadotropic hypogonadism. *J Clin Endocrinol Metab.* 2002;87:4825-4828.
545. Pitteloud N, Boepple PA, DeCruz S, et al. The fertile eunuch variant of idiopathic hypogonadotropic hypogonadism: spontaneous reversal associated with a homozygous mutation in the gonadotropin-releasing hormone receptor. *J Clin Endocrinol Metab.* 2001;86:2470-2475.
546. Bin-Abbas B, Conte FA, Grumbach MM, et al. Congenital hypogonadotropic hypogonadism and micropenis: effect of testosterone treatment on adult penile size—why sex reversal is not indicated. *J Pediatr.* 1999;134:579-583.
547. Zanarla E, Muscatelli F, Bardoni B, et al. An unusual member of the nuclear hormone receptor superfamily responsible for X-linked adrenal hypoplasia congenita. *Nature.* 1994;372:635-641.
548. Muscatelli F, Strom TM, Walker AP, et al. Mutations in the DAX-1 gene give rise to both X-linked adrenal hypoplasia congenita and hypogonadotropic hypogonadism. *Nature.* 1994;372:672-676.
549. Guo W, Burris TP, Zhang Y-H, et al. Genomic sequence of the DAX1 gene: an orphan nuclear receptor responsible for X-linked adrenal hypoplasia congenita and hypogonadotropic hypogonadism. *J Clin Endocrinol Metab.* 1996;81:2481-2486.
550. Lalli E, Bardoni B, Zazopoulos E, et al. A transcriptional silencing domain in DAX-1 whose mutation causes adrenal hypoplasia congenita. *Mol Endocrinol.* 1997;11:1950-1960.
551. Kletter GB, Gorski JL, Kelch RP. Congenital adrenal hypoplasia and isolated gonadotropin deficiency. *Trends Endocrinol Metab.* 1991;2:123-128.
552. Achermann JC, Wen-xia G, Kotlar J, et al. Mutational analysis of DAX1 in patients with hypogonadotropic hypogonadism or pubertal delay. *J Clin Endocrinol Metab.* 1999;84:4497-4500.
553. Mantovani G, Ozisik G, Achermann JC, et al. Hypogonadotropic hypogonadism as a presenting feature of late-onset X-linked adrenal hypoplasia congenita. *J Clin Endocrinol Metab.* 2002;87:44-48.
554. Tabarin A, Achermann JC, Recan D, et al. A novel mutation in DAX1 causes delayed-onset adrenal insufficiency and incomplete hypogonadotropic hypogonadism. *J Clin Invest.* 2000;105:321-328.
555. Merke DP, Tajima T, Baron J, et al. Hypogonadotropic hypogonadism in a female caused by an X-linked recessive mutation in the DAX1 gene. *N Engl J Med.* 1999;340:1248-1252.
556. Pasquino AM, Pucarelli I, Passeri F, et al. Progression of premature thelarche to central precocious puberty. *J Pediatr.* 1995;126:11-14.
557. Kaiserman KB, Nakamoto JM, Geffner ME, et al. Minipuberty of infancy and adolescent pubertal function in adrenal hypoplasia congenita. *J Pediatr.* 1998;133:300-302.
558. Seminara SB, Achermann JC, Genel M, et al. X-linked adrenal hypoplasia congenita: a mutation in DAX1 expands the phenotypic spectrum in males and females. *J Clin Endocrinol Metab.* 1999;84:4509.
559. Talaban R, Sellick GS, Spendlove HE, et al. Inherited pericentric inversion (X) (p11.4q11.2) associated with delayed puberty and obesity in two brothers. *Cytogenet Genome Res.* 2005;109:480-484.
560. Topaloglu AK, Reimann F, Guclu M, et al. TAC3 and TACR3 mutations in familial hypogonadotropic hypogonadism reveal a key role for neurokinin B in the central control of reproduction. *Nat Genet.* 2009;41:354-358.
561. Young J, Bouligand J, Francou B, et al. TAC3 and TACR3 defects cause hypothalamic congenital hypogonadotropic hypogonadism in humans. *J Clin Endocrinol Metab.* 2010;95:2287-2295.
562. Gianetti E, Tusset C, Noel SD, et al. *TAC3/TACR3* mutations reveal preferential activation of GnRH release by neurokinin B in neonatal life followed by reversal in adulthood. *J Clin Endocrinol Metab.* 2010;95:2857-2867.
563. Jackson RS, Creemers JW, Farooqi IS, et al. Small-intestinal dysfunction accompanies the complex endocrinopathy of human proprotein convertase 1 deficiency. *J Clin Invest.* 2003;112:1550-1560.
564. Layman LC, Lee EJ, Peak DB, et al. Delayed puberty and hypogonadism caused by mutations in the follicle-stimulating hormone beta-subunit gene. *N Engl J Med.* 1997;337:607-611.
565. Hanna CE, Mandel SH, LaFranchi SH. Puberty in the syndrome of septo-optic dysplasia. *Am J Dis Child.* 1989;143:186-189.
566. Kaplan SL, Grumbach MM, Hoyt WF. A syndrome of hypopituitary dwarfism, hypoplasia of optic nerves, and malformation of prosencephalon: report of 6 patients (Abstract). *Pediatr Res.* 1970;4:480-481.
567. Dattani MT, Martinez-Barbera JP, Thomas PQ, et al. Mutations in the homeobox gene HESX1/Hesx1 associated with septo-optic dysplasia in human and mouse. *Nat Genet.* 1998;19:125-133.
568. Birkebaek NH, Patel L, Wright NB, et al. Endocrine status in patients with optic nerve hypoplasia: relationship to midline central nervous system abnormalities and appearance of the hypothalamic-pituitary axis on magnetic resonance imaging. *J Clin Endocrinol Metab.* 2003;88:5281-5286.
569. Nanni L, Ming JE, Du Y, et al. SHH mutation is associated with solitary median maxillary central incisor: a study of 13 patients and review of the literature. *Am J Med Genet.* 2001;102:1-10.
570. Davis SW, Castinetti F, Carvalho LR, et al. Molecular mechanisms of pituitary organogenesis: in search of novel regulatory genes. *Mol Cell Endocrinol.* 2010;323:4-19.
571. Fluck C, Deladoey J, Rutishauser K, et al. Phenotypic variability in familial combined pituitary hormone deficiency caused by a PROP1 gene mutation resulting in the substitution of Arg→Cys at codon 120 (R120C). *J Clin Endocrinol Metab.* 1998;83:3727-3734.
572. Deladoey J, Fluck C, Buyukgebiz A, et al. "Hot spot" in the PROP1 gene responsible for combined pituitary hormone deficiency. *J Clin Endocrinol Metab.* 1999;84:1645-1650.
573. Reynaud R, Chadli-Chaieb M, Vallette-Kasic S, et al. A familial form of congenital hypopituitarism due to a PROP1 mutation in a large kindred: phenotypic and in vitro functional studies. *J Clin Endocrinol Metab.* 2004;89:5779-5786.
574. Netchine I, Sobrier ML, Krude H, et al. Mutations in LHX3 result in a new syndrome revealed by combined pituitary hormone deficiency. *Nat Genet.* 2000;25:182-186.
575. Solomon NM, Ross SA, Morgan T, et al. Array comparative genomic hybridisation analysis of boys with X linked hypopituitarism identifies a 3.9 Mb duplicated critical region at Xq27 containing SOX3. *J Med Genet.* 2004;41:669-678.
576. Tziaferi V, Kelberman D, Dattani MT. The role of SOX2 in hypogonadotropic hypogonadism. *Sex Dev.* 2008;2:194-199.
577. Goodman HG, Grumbach MM, Kaplan SL. Growth and growth hormone: II A comparison of isolated growth-hormone deficiency and multiple pituitary-hormone deficiencies in 35 patients with idiopathic hypopituitary dwarfism *N Engl J Med.* 1968;278:57-68.
578. Cassidy SB, Driscoll DJ. Prader-Willi syndrome. *Eur J Hum Genet.* 2009;17:3-13.
579. Prader A, Labhart A, Willi H. Ein syndrom von Adipositas, Kleinwuchs, Kryptorchidismus und Oligophrenie nach Myatonieartigem

Zustad im Neugeborenalter. *Schweiz Med Wochenschr.* 1956;86: 1260-1261.
580. Hirsch HJ, Eldar-Geva T, Benarroch F, et al. Primary testicular dysfunction is a major contributor to abnormal pubertal development in males with Prader-Willi syndrome. *J Clin Endocrinol Metab.* 2009;94:2262-2268.
581. Schmidt H, Pozza SB, Bonfig W, et al. Successful early dietary intervention avoids obesity in patients with Prader-Willi syndrome: a ten-year follow-up. *J Pediatr Endocrinol Metab.* 2008;21:651-655.
582. Carrel AL, Myers SE, Whitman BY, et al. Sustained benefits of growth hormone on body composition, fat utilization, physical strength and agility, and growth in Prader-Willi syndrome are dose-dependent. *J Pediatr Endocrinol Metab.* 2001;14:1097-1105.
583. Zaglia F, Zaffanello M, Biban P. Unexpected death due to refractory metabolic acidosis and massive hemolysis in a young infant with Prader-Willi syndrome. *Am J Med Genet A.* 2005;132:219-221.
584. Fillion M, Deal C, Van Vliet G. Retrospective study of the potential benefits and adverse events during growth hormone treatment in children with Prader-Willi syndrome. *J Pediatr.* 2009;154:230-233.
585. Haqq AM, Stadler DD, Rosenfeld RG, et al. Circulating ghrelin levels are suppressed by meals and octreotide therapy in children with Prader-Willi syndrome. *J Clin Endocrinol Metab.* 2003;88:3573-3576.
586. Katsanis N, Ansley SJ, Badano JL, et al. Triallelic inheritance in Bardet-Biedl syndrome, a Mendelian recessive disorder. *Science.* 2001;293:2256-2259.
587. Moore SJ, Green JS, Fan Y, et al. Clinical and genetic epidemiology of Bardet-Biedl syndrome in Newfoundland: a 22-year prospective, population-based, cohort study. *Am J Med Genet A.* 2005;132: 352-360.
588. Swenne I. Weight requirements for return of menstruations in teenage girls with eating disorders, weight loss and secondary amenorrhoea. *Acta Paediatr.* 2004;93:1449-1455.
589. Aswani N, Taylor CJ, McGaw J, et al. Pubertal growth and development in cystic fibrosis: a retrospective review. *Acta Paediatr.* 2003;92:1029-1032.
590. Arrigo T, De Luca F, Lucanto C, et al. Nutritional, glycometabolic and genetic factors affecting menarcheal age in cystic fibrosis. *Diabetes Nutr Metab.* 2004;17:114-119.
591. Tizzano EF, Silver MM, Chitayat D, et al. Differential cellular expression of cystic fibrosis transmembrane regulator in human reproductive tissues: clues for the infertility in patients with cystic fibrosis. *Am J Pathol.* 1994;144:906-914.
592. Johannesson M, Gottlieb C, Hjelte L. Delayed puberty in girls with cystic fibrosis despite good clinical status. *Pediatrics.* 1997;99: 29-34.
593. Chatterjee R, Katz M. Evaluation of gonadotrophin insufficiency in thalassemic boys with pubertal failure: spontaneous versus provocative test. *J Pediatr Endocrinol Metab.* 2001;14:301-312.
594. Shalitin S, Carmi D, Weintrob N, et al. Serum ferritin level as a predictor of impaired growth and puberty in thalassemia major patients. *Eur J Haematol.* 2005;74:93-100.
595. Chern JP, Lin KH, Tsai WY, et al. Hypogonadotropic hypogonadism and hematologic phenotype in patients with transfusion-dependent beta-thalassemia. *J Pediatr Hematol Oncol.* 2003;25:880-884.
596. Sklar CA, Lew LQ, Yoon DJ, et al. Adrenal function in thalassemia major following long-term treatment with multiple transfusions and chelation therapy: evidence for dissociation of cortisol and adrenal androgen secretion. *Am J Dis Child.* 1987;141:327-330.
597. Caruso-Nicoletti M, De Sanctis V, Raiola G, et al. No difference in pubertal growth and final height between treated hypogonadal and non-hypogonadal thalassemic patients. *Horm Res.* 2004;62:17-22.
598. Hovi L, Saarinen-Pihkala UM, Taskinen M, et al. Subnormal androgen levels in young female bone marrow transplant recipients with ovarian dysfunction, chronic GVHD and receiving glucocorticoid therapy. *Bone Marrow Transplant.* 2004;33:503-508.
599. Chantry CJ, Frederick MM, Meyer WA III, et al. Endocrine abnormalities and impaired growth in human immunodeficiency virus-infected children. *Pediatr Infect Dis J.* 2007;26:53-60.
600. Wikstrom AM, Hovi L, Dunkel L, et al. Restoration of ovarian function after chemotherapy for osteosarcoma. *Arch Dis Child.* 2003;88:428-431.
601. Steffens M, Beauloye V, Brichard B, et al. Endocrine and metabolic disorders in young adult survivors of childhood acute lymphoblastic leukaemia (ALL) or non-Hodgkin lymphoma (NHL). *Clin Endocrinol (Oxf).* 2008;69:819-827.
602. Follin C, Thilen U, Ahren B, et al. Improvement in cardiac systolic function and reduced prevalence of metabolic syndrome after two years of growth hormone (GH) treatment in GH-deficient adult survivors of childhood-onset acute lymphoblastic leukemia. *J Clin Endocrinol Metab.* 2006;91:1872-1875.
603. Jarfelt M, Lannering B, Bosaeus I, et al. Body composition in young adult survivors of childhood acute lymphoblastic leukaemia. *Eur J Endocrinol.* 2005;153:81-89.
604. Styne DM, Grumbach MM, Kaplan SL, et al. Treatment of Cushing's disease in childhood and adolescence by transsphenoidal microadenomectomy. *N Engl J Med.* 1984;310:889-893.
605. Devoe DJ, Miller WL, Conte FA, et al. Long-term outcome in children and adolescents after transsphenoidal surgery for Cushing's disease. *J Clin Endocrinol Metab.* 1997;82:3196-3202.
606. Halmi KA. Anorexia nervosa: an increasing problem in children and adolescents. *Dialogues Clin Neurosci.* 2009;11:100-103.
607. Diagnostic and Statistical Manual of Mental Disorders: *DSM-IV*. Washington, DC: American Psychiatric Association; 1994.
608. Attia E, Roberto CA. Should amenorrhea be a diagnostic criterion for anorexia nervosa? *Int J Eat Disord.* 2009;42:581-589.
609. Kaye WH, Klump KL, Frank GK, et al. Anorexia and bulimia nervosa. *Annu Rev Med.* 2000;51:299-313.
610. Usdan LS, Khaodhiar L, Apovian CM. The endocrinopathies of anorexia nervosa. *Endocr Pract.* 2008;14:1055-1063.
611. Ferron F, Considine RV, Peino R, et al. Serum leptin concentrations in patients with anorexia nervosa, bulimia nervosa and non-specific eating disorders correlate with the body mass index but are independent of the respective disease. *Clin Endocrinol.* 1997;46:289-293.
612. Casanueva FF, Dieguez C, Popovic V, et al. Serum immunoreactive leptin concentrations in patients with anorexia nervosa before and after partial weight recovery. *Biochem Mol Med.* 1997;60: 116-120.
613. Misra M, Aggarwal A, Miller KK, et al. Effects of anorexia nervosa on clinical, hematologic, biochemical, and bone density parameters in community-dwelling adolescent girls. *Pediatrics.* 2004;114:1574-1583.
614. Mehler PS, MacKenzie TD. Treatment of osteopenia and osteoporosis in anorexia nervosa: a systematic review of the literature. *Int J Eat Disord.* 2009;42:195-201.
615. Misra M, Miller KK, Almazan C, et al. Hormonal and body composition predictors of soluble leptin receptor, leptin, and free leptin index in adolescent girls with anorexia nervosa and controls and relation to insulin sensitivity. *J Clin Endocrinol Metab.* 2004;89:3486-3495.
616. Couzinet B, Young J, Brailly S, et al. Functional hypothalamic amenorrhoea: a partial and reversible gonadotrophin deficiency of nutritional origin. *Clin Endocrinol (Oxf).* 1999;50:229-235.
617. Warren MP, Voussoughian F, Geer EB, et al. Functional hypothalamic amenorrhea: hypoleptinemia and disordered eating. *J Clin Endocrinol Metab.* 1999;84:873-877.
618. Birmingham CL, Touyz S, Harbottle J. Are anorexia nervosa and bulimia nervosa separate disorders? Challenging the "transdiagnostic" theory of eating disorders. *Eur Eat Disord Rev.* 2009;17:2-13.
619. Warren MP, Shantha S. The female athlete. *Baillieres Best Pract Res Clin Endocrinol Metab.* 2000;14:37-53.
620. Warren MP, Perlroth NE. The effects of intense exercise on the female reproductive system. *J Endocrinol.* 2001;170:3-11.
621. Torstveit MK, Sundgot-Borgen J. Participation in leanness sports but not training volume is associated with menstrual dysfunction: a national survey of 1276 elite athletes and controls. *Br J Sports Med.* 2005;39:141-147.
622. Claessens AL, Bourgois J, Beunen G, et al. Age at menarche in relation to anthropometric characteristics, competition level and boat category in elite junior rowers. *Ann Hum Biol.* 2003;30:148-159.
623. Markou KB, Mylonas P, Theodoropoulou A, et al. The influence of intensive physical exercise on bone acquisition in adolescent elite female and male artistic gymnasts. *J Clin Endocrinol Metab.* 2004;89:4383-4387.
624. Theodoropoulou A, Markou KB, Vagenakis GA, et al. Delayed but normally progressed puberty is more pronounced in artistic compared with rhythmic elite gymnasts due to the intensity of training. *J Clin Endocrinol Metab.* 2005;90:6022-6027.
625. Klentrou P, Plyley M. Onset of puberty, menstrual frequency, and body fat in elite rhythmic gymnasts compared with normal controls. *Br J Sports Med.* 2003;37:490-494.
626. Munoz MT, de la Piedra C, Barrios V, et al. Changes in bone density and bone markers in rhythmic gymnasts and ballet dancers: implications for puberty and leptin levels. *Eur J Endocrinol.* 2004;151: 491-496.
627. Fenichel RM, Warren MP. Anorexia, bulimia, and the athletic triad: evaluation and management. *Curr Osteoporos Rep.* 2007;5: 160-164.
628. Constantini NW, Warren MP. Menstrual dysfunction in swimmers: a distinct entity. *J Clin Endocrinol Metab.* 1995;80:2740-2744.
629. Georgopoulos NA, Theodoropoulou A, Leglise M, et al. Growth and skeletal maturation in male and female artistic gymnasts. *J Clin Endocrinol Metab.* 2004;89:4377-4382.
630. Eliakim A, Beyth Y. Exercise training, menstrual irregularities and bone development in children and adolescents. *J Pediatr Adolesc Gynecol.* 2003;16:201-206.
631. Picardi A, Cipponeri E, Bizzarri C, et al. Menarche in type 1 diabetes is still delayed despite good metabolic control. *Fertil Steril.* 2008;90:1875-1877.

632. Grumbach MM, Conte FA. Disorders of sexual differentiation. In: Wilson JD, Foster DW, Kroneberg HM, et al., eds. *Willliams Textbook of Endocrinology*. Philadelphia, PA: Saunders; 1998:1509-1626.
633. Klinefelter HF Jr, Reifenstein EC Jr, Albright F. Syndrome characterized by gynecomastia, aspermatogenesis without A-leydigism, and increased excretion of follicle-stimulating hormone. *J Clin Endocrinol*. 1942;2:615-627.
634. Bojesen A, Juul S, Gravholt CH. Prenatal and postnatal prevalence of Klinefelter syndrome: a national registry study. *J Clin Endocrinol Metab*. 2003;88:622-626.
635. Ross JL, Samango-Sprouse C, Lahlou N, et al. Early androgen deficiency in infants and young boys with 47,XXY Klinefelter syndrome. *Horm Res*. 2005;64:39-45.
636. Wikstrom AM, Painter JN, Raivio T, et al. Genetic features of the X chromosome affect pubertal development and testicular degeneration in adolescent boys with Klinefelter syndrome. *Clin Endocrinol (Oxf)*. 2006;65:92-97.
637. Fullerton G, Hamilton M, Maheshwari A. Should non-mosaic Klinefelter syndrome men be labelled as infertile in 2009? *Hum Reprod*. 2010;25:588-597.
638. Christiansen P, Andersson AM, Skakkebaek NE. Longitudinal studies of inhibin B levels in boys and young adults with Klinefelter syndrome. *J Clin Endocrinol Metab*. 2003;88:888-891.
639. Wikstrom AM, Dunkel L, Wickman S, et al. Are adolescent boys with Klinefelter syndrome androgen deficient? A longitudinal study of Finnish 47,XXY boys. *Pediatr Res*. 2006;59:854-859.
640. Zinn AR, Ramos P, Elder FF, et al. Androgen receptor CAGn repeat length influences phenotype of 47,XXY (Klinefelter) syndrome. *J Clin Endocrinol Metab*. 2005;90:5041-5046.
641. Zitzmann M, Depenbusch M, Gromoll J, et al. X-chromosome inactivation patterns and androgen receptor functionality influence phenotype and social characteristics as well as pharmacogenetics of testosterone therapy in Klinefelter patients. *J Clin Endocrinol Metab*. 2004;89:6208-6217.
642. Kleczkowska A, Fryns JP, Van den Berghe H. X-chromosome polysomy in the male: the Leuven experience 1966-1987. *Hum Genet*. 1988;80:16-22.
643. Boone KB, Swerdloff RS, Miller BL, et al. Neuropsychological profiles of adults with Klinefelter syndrome. *J Int Neuropsychol Soc*. 2001;7:446-456.
644. Billmire D, Vinocur C, Rescorla F, et al. Malignant mediastinal germ cell tumors: an intergroup study. *J Pediatr Surg*. 2001;36:18-24.
645. Afify Z, Shaw PJ, Clavano-Harding A, et al. Growth and endocrine function in children with acute myeloid leukaemia after bone marrow transplantation using busulfan/cyclophosphamide. *Bone Marrow Transplant*. 2000;25:1087-1092.
646. Zaletel LZ, Bratanic N, Jereb B. Gonadal function in patients treated for leukemia in childhood. *Leuk Lymphoma*. 2004;45:1797-1802.
647. van den BH, Furstner F, van den BC, et al. Decreasing the number of MOPP courses reduces gonadal damage in survivors of childhood Hodgkin disease. *Pediatr Blood Cancer*. 2004;42:210-215.
648. Ben Arush MW, Solt I, Lightman A, et al. Male gonadal function in survivors of childhood Hodgkin and non-Hodgkin lymphoma. *Pediatr Hematol Oncol*. 2000;17:239-245.
649. Ginsberg JP, Carlson CA, Lin K, et al. An experimental protocol for fertility preservation in prepubertal boys recently diagnosed with cancer: a report of acceptability and safety. *Hum Reprod*. 2010;25:37-41.
650. Huhtaniemi I. The Parkes lecture. Mutations of gonadotrophin and gonadotrophin receptor genes: what do they teach us about reproductive physiology? *J Reprod Fertil*. 2000;119:173-186.
651. Martin RM, Lin CJ, Costa EM, et al. P450c17 deficiency in Brazilian patients: biochemical diagnosis through progesterone levels confirmed by CYP17 genotyping. *J Clin Endocrinol Metab*. 2003;88:5739-5746.
652. Bose HS, Sugawara T, Strauss JF 3rd, et al. The pathophysiology and genetics of congenital lipoid adrenal hyperplasia. International Congenital Lipoid Adrenal Hyperplasia Consortium. *N Engl J Med*. 1996;335:1870-1878.
653. Bose HS, Pescovitz OH, Miller WL. Spontaneous feminization in a 46,XX female patient with congenital lipoid adrenal hyperplasia due to a homozygous frameshift mutation in the steroidogenic acute regulatory protein. *J Clin Endocrinol Metab*. 1997;82:1511-1515.
654. Kaku U, Kameyama K, Izawa M, et al. Ovarian histological findings in an adult patient with the steroidogenic acute regulatory protein (StAR) deficiency reveal the impairment of steroidogenesis by lipoid deposition. *Endocr J*. 2008;55:1043-1049.
655. Huhtaniemi I, Alevizaki M. Gonadotrophin resistance. *Best Pract Res Clin Endocrinol Metab*. 2006;20:561-576.
656. Lee PA, Coughlin MT. Fertility after bilateral cryptorchidism: evaluation by paternity, hormone, and semen data. *Horm Res*. 2001;55:28-32.
657. Wood HM, Elder JS. Cryptorchidism and testicular cancer: separating fact from fiction. *J Urol*. 2009;181:452-461.
658. Hurwitz RS, Kaptein JS. How well does contralateral testis hypertrophy predict the absence of the nonpalpable testis? *J Urol*. 2001;165:588-592.
659. Bertelloni S, Baroncelli GI, Ghirri P, et al. Hormonal treatment for unilateral inguinal testis: comparison of four different treatments. *Horm Res*. 2001;55:236-239.
660. Esposito C, De Lucia A, Palmieri A, et al. Comparison of five different hormonal treatment protocols for children with cryptorchidism. *Scand J Urol Nephrol*. 2003;37:246-249.
661. Hamza AF, Elrahim M, Elnagar O, et al. Testicular descent: when to interfere? *Eur J Pediatr Surg*. 2001;11:173-176.
662. Huff DS, Fenig DM, Canning DA, et al. Abnormal germ cell development in cryptorchidism. *Horm Res*. 2001;55:11-17.
663. Giwercman A, Hansen LL, Skakkebaek NE. Initiation of sperm production after bilateral orchiopexy: clinical and biological implications. *J Urol*. 2000;163:1255-1256.
664. Moller H, Evans H. Epidemiology of gonadal germ cell cancer in males and females. *APMIS*. 2003;111:43-46.
665. Main KM, Skakkebaek NE, Toppari J. Cryptorchidism as part of the testicular dysgenesis syndrome: the environmental connection. *Endocr Dev*. 2009;14:167-173.
666. Hutson JM, Hasthorpe S, Heyns CF. Anatomical and functional aspects of testicular descent and cryptorchidism. *Endocr Rev*. 1997;18:259-280.
667. La Scala GC, Ein SH. Retractile testes: an outcome analysis on 150 patients. *J Pediatr Surg*. 2004;39:1014-1017.
668. Cicognani A, Alessandroni R, Pasini A, et al. Low birth weight for gestational age and subsequent male gonadal function. *J Pediatr*. 2002;141:376-379.
669. Allvin K, Ankarberg-Lindgren C, Fors H, et al. Elevated serum levels of estradiol, dihydrotestosterone, and inhibin B in adult males born small for gestational age. *J Clin Endocrinol Metab*. 2008;93:1464-1469.
670. Jensen RB, Vielwerth S, Larsen T, et al. Pituitary-gonadal function in adolescent males born appropriate or small for gestational age with or without intrauterine growth restriction. *J Clin Endocrinol Metab*. 2007;92:1353-1357.
671. Elsheikh M, Dunger DB, Conway GS, et al. Turner's syndrome in adulthood. *Endocr Rev*. 2002;23:120-140.
672. Saenger P, Wikland KA, Conway GS, et al. Recommendations for the diagnosis and management of Turner syndrome. *J Clin Endocrinol Metab*. 2001;86:3061-3069.
673. Roa E, Weiss B, Fukami M, et al. Pseudoautosomal deletions encompassing a novel homeobox gene cause growth failure in idiopathic short stature and Turner syndrome. *Nature Genet*. 1997;16:54-62.
674. Ellison JW, Wardak Z, Young M, et al. PHOG, a candidate gene for involvement in the short stature of Turner syndrome. *Hum Mol Genet*. 1997;6:1341-1347.
675. Belin V, Cusin V, Viot G, et al. SHOX mutations in dyschondrosteosis (Leri-Weill syndrome). *Nat Genet*. 1998;19:67-69.
676. Kosho T, Muroya K, Nagai T, et al. Skeletal features and growth patterns in 14 patients with haploinsufficiency of SHOX: implications for the development of Turner syndrome. *J Clin Endocrinol Metab*. 1999;84:4613-4621.
677. Blaschke RJ, Rappold GA. SHOX: growth, Leri-Weill and Turner syndromes. *Trends Endocinol Metab*. 2000;11:227-230.
678. Ogata T, Muroya K, Matsuo N, et al. Turner syndrome and Xp deletions: clinical and molecular studies in 47 patients. *J Clin Endocrinol Metab*. 2001;86:5498-5508.
679. Clement-Jones M, Schiller S, Rao E, et al. The short stature homeobox gene SHOX is involved in skeletal abnormalities in Turner syndrome. *Hum Mol Genet*. 2000;9:695-702.
680. Rappold G, Blum WF, Shavrikova EP, et al. Genotypes and phenotypes in children with short stature: clinical indicators of SHOX haploinsufficiency. *J Med Genet*. 2006;44:306-313.
681. Mortensen KH, Hansen KW, Erlandsen M, et al. Ambulatory arterial stiffness index in Turner syndrome: the impact of sex hormone replacement therapy. *Horm Res*. 2009;72:184-189.
682. Gravholt CH, Juul S, Naeraa RW, et al. Morbidity in Turner syndrome. *J Clin Epidemiol*. 1998;51:147-158.
683. Savendahl L, Davenport ML. Delayed diagnoses of Turner's syndrome: proposed guidelines for change. *J Pediatr*. 2000;137:455-459.
684. Doerr HG, Bettendorf M, Hauffa BP, et al. Uterine size in women with Turner syndrome after induction of puberty with estrogens and long-term growth hormone therapy: results of the German IGLU Follow-up Study 2001. *Hum Reprod*. 2005;20:1418-1421.
685. Karnis MF, Zimon AE, Lalwani SI, et al. Risk of death in pregnancy achieved through oocyte donation in patients with Turner syndrome: a national survey. *Fertil Steril*. 2003;80:498-501.
686. Even L, Cohen A, Marbach N, et al. Longitudinal analysis of growth over the first 3 years of life in Turner's syndrome. *J Pediatr*. 2000;137:460-464.

687. Hochberg Z, Khaesh-Goldberg I, Partsch CJ, et al. Differences in infantile growth patterns in Turner syndrome girls with and without spontaneous puberty. *Horm Metab Res*. 2005;37:236-241.
688. Ranke MB, Stubbe P, Majewski F, et al. Spontaneous growth in Turner's syndrome. *Acta Paediatr Scand Suppl*. 1988;343:22-30.
689. Chernausek SD, Attie KM, Cara JF, et al. Growth hormone therapy of Turner syndrome: the impact of age of estrogen replacement on final height. Genentech, Inc., Collaborative Study Group. *J Clin Endocrinol Metab*. 2000;85:2439-2445.
690. Reiter EO, Blethen SL, Baptista J, et al. Early initiation of growth hormone treatment allows age-appropriate estrogen use in Turner's syndrome. *J Clin Endocrinol Metab*. 2001;86:1936-1941.
691. van Pareren YK, de Muinck Keizer-Schrama SM, Stijnen T, et al. Final height in girls with Turner syndrome after long-term growth hormone treatment in three dosages and low dose estrogens. *J Clin Endocrinol Metab*. 2003;88:1119-1125.
692. Baxter L, Bryant J, Cave CB, et al. Recombinant growth hormone for children and adolescents with Turner syndrome. Cochrane Database Syst Rev 207(1):CD003887.
693. Sas TC, Gerver WJ, De Bruin R, et al. Body proportions during long-term growth hormone treatment in girls with Turner syndrome participating in a randomized dose-response trial. *J Clin Endocrinol Metab*. 1999;84:4622-4628.
694. Ari M, Bakalov VK, Hill S, et al. The effects of growth hormone treatment on bone mineral density and body composition in girls with Turner syndrome. *J Clin Endocrinol Metab*. 2006;91:4302-4305.
695. Bannink EM, van der Palen RL, Mulder PG, et al. Long-term follow-up of GH-treated girls with Turner syndrome: metabolic consequences. *Horm Res*. 2009;71:343-349.
696. Bannink EM, van der Palen RL, Mulder PG, et al. Long-term follow-up of GH-treated girls with Turner syndrome: BMI, blood pressure, body proportions. *Horm Res*. 2009;71:336-342.
697. Gravholt CH, Vestergaard P, Hermann AP, et al. Increased fracture rates in Turner's syndrome: a nationwide questionnaire survey. *Clin Endocrinol (Oxf)*. 2003;59:89-96.
698. Sas TC, de Muinck Keizer-Schrama S, Stijnen T, et al. Carbohydrate metabolism during long-term growth hormone (GH) treatment and after discontinuation of GH treatment in girls with Turner syndrome participating in a randomized dose-response study. Dutch Advisory Group on Growth Hormone. *J Clin Endocrinol Metab*. 2000; 85:769-775.
699. Martin DD, Schweizer R, Schwarze CP, et al. The early dehydroepiandrosterone sulfate rise of adrenarche and the delay of pubarche indicate primary ovarian failure in Turner syndrome. *J Clin Endocrinol Metab*. 2004;89:1164-1168.
700. Sklar CA, Kaplan SL, Grumbach MM. Lack of effect of oestrogens on adrenal androgen secretion in children and adolescents with a comment on oestrogens and pubic hair growth. *Clin Endocrinol*. 1981;14:311-320.
701. Carel JC, Ecosse E, Bastie-Sigeac I, et al. Quality of life determinants in young women with Turner's syndrome after growth hormone treatment: results of the StaTur population-based cohort study. *J Clin Endocrinol Metab*. 2005;90:1992-1997.
702. van Pareren YK, Duivenvoorden HJ, Slijper FM, et al. Psychosocial functioning after discontinuation of long-term growth hormone treatment in girls with Turner syndrome. *Horm Res*. 2005;63:238-244.
703. Reiss AL, Mazzocco MM, Greenlaw R, et al. Neurodevelopmental effects of X monosomy: a volumetric imaging study. *Ann Neurol*. 1995;38:731-738.
704. Rickert VI, Hassed SJ, Hendon AE, et al. The effects of peer ridicule on depression and self-image among adolescent females with Turner syndrome. *J Adolesc Health*. 1996;19:34-38.
705. Davenport ML. Approach to the patient with Turner syndrome. *J Clin Endocrinol Metab*. 2010;95:1487-1495.
706. Hoepffner W, Horn LC, Simon E, et al. Gonadoblastomas in 5 patients with 46,XY gonadal dysgenesis. *Exp Clin Endocrinol Diabetes*. 2005;113:231-235.
707. Paulino AC, Wen BC, Brown CK, et al. Late effects in children treated with radiation therapy for Wilms' tumor. *Int J Radiat Oncol Biol Physics*. 2000;46:1239-1246.
708. Hughes EG, Neal MS. Ovulation suppression to protect against chemotherapy-induced ovarian toxicity: helpful or just hopeful? *Hum Reprod Update*. 2008;14:541-542.
709. Welt CK. Primary ovarian insufficiency: a more accurate term for premature ovarian failure. *Clin Endocrinol (Oxf)*. 2008;68: 499-509.
710. Halonen M, Eskelin P, Myhre AG, et al. AIRE mutations and human leukocyte antigen genotypes as determinants of the autoimmune polyendocrinopathy-candidiasis-ectodermal dystrophy phenotype. *J Clin Endocrinol Metab*. 2002;87:2568-2574.
711. Forges T, Monnier-Barbarino P, Leheup B, et al. Pathophysiology of impaired ovarian function in galactosaemia. *Hum Reprod Update*. 2006;12:573-584.
712. Crisponi L, Deiana M, Loi A, et al. The putative forkhead transcription factor FOXL2 is mutated in blepharophimosis/ptosis/epicanthus inversus syndrome. *Nat Genet*. 2001;27:159-166.
713. Nicolino M, Bost M, David M, et al. Familial blepharophimosis: an uncommon marker of ovarian dysgenesis. *J Pediatr Endocrinol Metab*. 1995;8:127-133.
714. Skillern A, Rajkovic A. Recent developments in identifying genetic determinants of premature ovarian failure. *Sex Dev*. 2008;2: 228-243.
715. Jaeken J, Matthijs G. Congenital disorders of glycosylation. *Annu Rev Genomics Hum Genet*. 2001;2:129-151.
716. Davis CJ, Davison RM, Payne NN, et al. Female sex preponderance for idiopathic familial premature ovarian failure suggests an X chromosome defect: opinion. *Hum Reprod*. 2000;15:2418-2422.
717. Tapanainen JS, Aittomaki K, Min J, et al. Men homozygous for an inactivating mutation of the follicle-stimulating hormone (FSH) receptor gene present variable suppression of spermatogenesis and fertility. *Nature Genet*. 1997;15:205-206.
718. Martens JW, Verhoef-Post M, Abelin N, et al. A homozygous mutation in the luteinizing hormone receptor causes partial Leydig cell hypoplasia: correlation between receptor activity and phenotype. *Mol Endocrinol*. 1998;12:775-784.
719. Latronico AC, Anasti J, Arnhold IJ, et al. Brief report: testicular and ovarian resistance to luteinizing hormone caused by inactivating mutations of the luteinizing hormone-receptor gene. *N Engl J Med*. 1996;334:507-512.
720. Dunaif A. Insulin resistance in women with polycystic ovary syndrome. *Fertil Steril*. 2006;86(suppl 1):S13-S14.
721. Romano AA, Dana K, Bakker B, et al. Growth response, near-adult height, and patterns of growth and puberty in patients with Noonan syndrome treated with growth hormone. *J Clin Endocrinol Metab*. 2009;94:2338-2344.
722. Takagi M, Miyashita Y, Koga M, et al. Estrogen deficiency is a potential cause for osteopenia in adult male patients with Noonan's syndrome. *Calcif Tissue Int*. 2000;66:200-203.
723. Resende EA, Lara BH, Reis JD, et al. Assessment of basal and gonadotropin-releasing hormone-stimulated gonadotropins by immunochemiluminometric and immunofluorometric assays in normal children. *J Clin Endocrinol Metab*. 2007;92:1424-1429.
724. Zevenhuijzen H, Kelnar CJ, Crofton PM. Diagnostic utility of a low-dose gonadotropin-releasing hormone test in the context of puberty disorders. *Horm Res*. 2004;62:168-176.
725. Degros V, Cortet-Rudelli C, Soudan B, et al. The human chorionic gonadotropin test is more powerful than the gonadotropin-releasing hormone agonist test to discriminate male isolated hypogonadotropic hypogonadism from constitutional delayed puberty. *Eur J Endocrinol*. 2003;149:23-29.
726. Mainieri AS, Elnecave RH. Usefulness of the free alpha-subunit to diagnose hypogonadotropic hypogonadism. *Clin Endocrinol (Oxf)*. 2003;59:307-313.
727. Kelly BP, Paterson WF, Donaldson MD. Final height outcome and value of height prediction in boys with constitutional delay in growth and adolescence treated with intramuscular testosterone 125 mg per month for 3 months. *Clin Endocrinol (Oxf)*. 2003;58:267-272.
728. Lampit M, Hochberg Z. Androgen therapy in constitutional delay of growth. *Horm Res*. 2003;59:270-275.
729. Mayo A, Macintyre H, Wallace AM, et al. Transdermal testosterone application: pharmacokinetics and effects on pubertal status, short-term growth, and bone turnover. *J Clin Endocrinol Metab*. 2004;89:681-687.
730. Ankarberg-Lindgren C, Elfving M, Wikland KA, et al. Nocturnal application of transdermal estradiol patches produces levels of estradiol that mimic those seen at the onset of spontaneous puberty in girls. *J Clin Endocrinol Metab*. 2001;86:3039-3044.
731. Turgeon JL, McDonnell DP, Martin KA, et al. Hormone therapy: physiological complexity belies therapeutic simplicity. *Science*. 2004;304:1269-1273.
732. Rosenfeld RG, Nicodemus BC. The transition from adolescence to adult life: physiology of the "transition" phase and its evolutionary basis. *Horm Res*. 2003;60(suppl 1):74-77.
733. Burstein S, Grumbach MM, Kaplan SL. Early determination of androgen-responsiveness is important in the management of microphallus. *Lancet*. 1979;2:983-986.
734. Lee PA, Houk CP. Outcome studies among men with micropenis. *J Pediatr Endocrinol Metab*. 2004;17:1043-1053.
735. Delemarre-van de Waal HA. Application of gonadotropin releasing hormone in hypogonadotropic hypogonadism: diagnostic and therapeutic aspects. *Eur J Endocrinol*. 2004;151(suppl 3): U89-U94.
736. Buchter D, Behre HM, Kliesch S, et al. Pulsatile GnRH or human chorionic gonadotropin/human menopausal gonadotropin as effective treatment for men with hypogonadotropic hypogonadism: a review of 42 cases. *Eur J Endocrinol*. 1998;139:298-303.

737. Kunz GJ, Klein KO, Clemons RD, et al. Virilization of young children after topical androgen use by their parents. *Pediatrics*. 2004; 114:282-284.
738. Piippo S, Lenko H, Kainulainen P, et al. Use of percutaneous estrogen gel for induction of puberty in girls with Turner syndrome. *J Clin Endocrinol Metab*. 2004;89:3241-3247.
739. Hindmarsh PC. How do you initiate oestrogen therapy in a girl who has not undergone puberty? *Clin Endocrinol (Oxf)*. 2009;71: 7-10.
740. Gussinye M, Terrades P, Yeste D, et al. Low areal bone mineral density values in adolescents and young adult Turner syndrome patients increase after long-term transdermal estradiol therapy. *Horm Res*. 2000;54:131-135.
741. Wit JM, Langenhorst VJ, Jansen M, et al. Dehydroepiandrosterone sulfate treatment for atrichia pubis. *Horm Res*. 2001;56:134-139.
742. Kaplan SL, Grumbach MM. Pathogenesis of sexual precocity. In: Grumbach MM, Sizonenko PC, Aubert ML, eds. *Control of the Onset of Puberty*. Baltimore, MD: Williams & Wilkins; 1990:620-660.
743. Paul D, Conte FA, Grumbach MM, et al. Long-term effect of gonadotropin-releasing hormone agonist therapy on final and near-final height in 26 children with true precocious puberty treated at a median age of less than 5 years. *J Clin Endocrinol Metab*. 1995;80:546-551.
744. Kaplan SL, Grumbach MM. Clinical review 14: pathophysiology and treatment of sexual precocity. *J Clin Endocrinol Metab*. 1990;71:785-789.
745. Lee PA. Medroxyprogesterone therapy for sexual precocity in girls. *Am J Dis Child*. 1981;135:443-445.
746. Sorgo W, Kiraly E, Homoki J, et al. The effects of cyproterone acetate on statural growth in children with precocious puberty. *Acta Endocrinol (Copenh)*. 1987;115:44-56.
747. Thamdrup E. *Precocious Sexual Development: A Clinical Study of 100 Patients*. Springfield, IL: Charles C Thomas; 1961.
748. Hertel NT, Stoltenberg M, Juul A, et al. Serum concentrations of type I and III procollagen propeptides in healthy children and girls with central precocious puberty during treatment with gonadotropin-releasing hormone analog and cyproterone acetate. *J Clin Endocrinol*. 1993;76:924-927.
749. National High Blood Pressure Education Program Working Group on High Blood Pressure in Children and Adolescents. The fourth report on the diagnosis, evaluation, and treatment of high blood pressure in children and adolescents. *Pediatrics*. 2004;114(2 suppl 4th report):555-576.
750. Palmert MR, Boepple PA. Variation in the timing of puberty: clinical spectrum and genetic investigation. *J Clin Endocrinol Metab*. 2001;86:2364-2368.
751. De Vries L, Kauschansky A, Shohat M, et al. Familial central precocious puberty suggests autosomal dominant inheritance. *J Clin Endocrinol Metab*. 2004;89:1794-1800.
752. Liu N, Grumbach MM, De Napoli RA, et al. Prevalence of electroencephalographic abnormalities in idiopathic precocious puberty and premature pubarche: bearing on pathogenesis and neuroendocrine regulation of puberty. *J Clin Endocrinol Metab*. 1965; 25:1296-1308.
753. Teles MG, Bianco SD, Brito VN, et al. A GPR54-activating mutation in a patient with central precocious puberty. *N Engl J Med*. 2008; 358:709-715.
754. Silveira LG, Noel SD, Silveira-Neto AP, et al. Mutations of the KISS1 gene in disorders of puberty. *J Clin Endocrinol Metab*. 2010; 95:2276-2280.
755. Palmert MR, Malin HV, Boepple PA. Unsustained or slowly progressive puberty in young girls: initial presentation and long-term follow-up of 20 untreated patients [see comments]. *J Clin Endocrinol Metab*. 1999;84:415-423.
756. Ross JL, Pescovitz OH, Barnes K, et al. Growth hormone secretory dynamics in children with precocious puberty. *Ann Hum Biol*. 1989;16:397-406.
757. Fontoura M, Brauner R, Prevot C, et al. Precocious puberty in girls: early diagnosis of a slowly progressing variant. *Arch Dis Child*. 1989;64:1170-1176.
758. Oerter KE, Manasco PK, Barnes KM, et al. Effects of luteinizing hormone-releasing hormone agonists on final height in luteinizing hormone-releasing hormone-dependent precocious puberty. *Acta Paediatr Suppl*. 1993;388:62-68; discussion 69.
759. Rosenfield RL. Selection of children with precocious puberty for treatment with gonadotropin releasing hormone analogs. *J Pediatr*. 1994;124:989-991.
760. Kaplan SL, Grumbach MM. True precocious puberty: treatment with GnRH-agonists. In: Delemarre-Van de Waal H, Plant TM, van Rees GP, et al, eds. *Control of the Onset of Puberty*. Amsterdam, The Netherlands: Elsevier; 1989:357-373.
761. Kreiter M, Burstein S, Rosenfield RL, et al. Preserving adult height potential in girls with idiopathic true precocious puberty. *J Pediatr*. 1990;117:364-370.
762. Garibaldi LR, Aceto TJ, Weber C. The pattern of gonadotropin and estradiol secretion in exaggerated thelarche. *Acta Endocrinol (Copenh)*. 1993;128:345-350.
763. Brauner R, Malandry F, Rappaport R. Predictive factors for the effect of gonadotrophin releasing hormone analogue therapy on the height of girls with idiopathic central precocious puberty. *Eur J Pediatr*. 1992;151:728-730.
764. Bridges NA, Cooke A, Healy MJ, et al. Ovaries in sexual precocity. *Clin Endocrinol (Oxf)*. 1995;42:135-140.
765. Morabia A, Costanza MC. Reproductive factors and incidence of breast cancer: an international ecological study. *Soz Praventivmed*. 2000;45:247-257.
766. Sharafuddin MJ, Luisiri A, Garibaldi LR, et al. MR imaging diagnosis of central precocious puberty: importance of changes in the shape and size of the pituitary gland. *AJR Am J Roentgenol*. 1994;162:1167-1173.
767. Cacciari E, Zucchini S, Ambrosetto P, et al. Empty sella in children and adolescents with possible hypothalamic-pituitary disorders. *J Clin Endocrinol Metab*. 1994;78:767-771.
768. Zucchini S, Ambrosetto P, Carla G, et al. Primary empty sella: differences and similarities between children and adults. *Acta Paediatr*. 1995;84:1382-1385.
769. Jenner MR, Kelch RP, Kaplan SL, et al. Hormonal changes in puberty: IV. Plasma estradiol, LH, and FSH in prepubertal children, pubertal females, and in precocious puberty, premature thelarche, hypogonadism, and in a child with a feminizing ovarian tumor. *J Clin Endocrinol Metab*. 1972;34:521-530.
770. Houk CP, Kunselman AR, Lee PA. Adequacy of a single unstimulated luteinizing hormone level to diagnose central precocious puberty in girls. *Pediatrics*. 2009;123:e1059-e1063.
771. Neely EK, Wilson DM, Lee PA, et al. Spontaneous serum gonadotropin concentrations in the evaluation of precocious puberty. *J Pediatr*. 1995;127:63-67.
772. Lawson ML, Cohen N. A single sample subcutaneous luteinizing hormone (LH)-releasing hormone (LHRH) stimulation test for monitoring LH suppression in children with central precocoius puberty recieving LHRH agonists. *J Clin Endocrinol Metab*. 1999; 84:4536-4540.
773. Brito VN, Batista MC, Borges MF, et al. Diagnostic value of fluorometric assays in the evaluation of precocious puberty. *J Clin Endocrinol Metab*. 1999;84:3539-3544.
774. Pescovitz OH, Hench KD, Barnes KM, et al. Premature thelarche and central precocious puberty: the relationship between clinical presentation and the gonadotropin response to luteinizing hormone-releasing hormone. *J Clin Endocrinol Metab*. 1988;67:474-479.
775. Bridges NA, Christopher JA, Hindmarsh PC, et al. Sexual precocity: sex incidence and aetiology. *Arch Dis Child*. 1994;70:116-118.
776. Rappaport R, Brauner R. Growth and endocrine disorders secondary to cranial irradiation. *Pediatr Res*. 1989;25:561-567.
777. Oberfield SE, Soranno D, Nirenberg A, et al. Age at onset of puberty following high-dose central nervous system radiation therapy. *Arch Pediatr Adolesc Med*. 1996;150:589-592.
778. Nicholl RM, Kirk JM, Grossman AB, et al. Acceleration of pubertal development following pituitary radiotherapy for Cushing's disease. *Clin Oncol (R Coll Radiol)*. 1993;5:393-394.
779. Sklar CA, Constine LS. Chronic neuroendocrinological sequelae of radiation therapy. *Int J Radiat Oncol Biol Phys*. 1995;31:1113-1121.
780. Armstrong GT, Whitton JA, Gajjar A, et al. Abnormal timing of menarche in survivors of central nervous system tumors: a report from the Childhood Cancer Survivor Study. *Cancer*. 2009;115:2562-2570.
781. Bath LE, Anderson RA, Critchley HO, et al. Hypothalamic-pituitary-ovarian dysfunction after prepubertal chemotherapy and cranial irradiation for acute leukaemia. *Hum Reprod*. 2001;16:1838-1844.
782. Xu W, Janss A, Packer RJ, et al. Endocrine outcome in children with medulloblastoma treated with 18 Gy of craniospinal radiation therapy. *Neuro-oncol*. 2004;6:113-118.
783. Hochman HI, Judge DM, Reichlin S. Precocious puberty and hypothalamic hamartoma. *Pediatrics*. 1981;67:236-244.
784. Turjman F, Xavier JL, Froment JC, et al. Late MR follow-up of hypothalamic hamartomas. *Childs Nerv Syst*. 1996;12:63-68.
785. Feuillan PP, Jones JV, Barnes K, et al. Reproductive axis after discontinuation of gonadotropin-releasing hormone analog treatment of girls with precocious puberty: long term follow-up comparing girls with hypothalamic hamartoma to those with idiopathic precocious puberty. *J Clin Endocrinol Metab*. 1999;84:44-49.
786. Jung H, Neumaier PE, Hauffa BP, et al. Association of morphological characteristics with precocious puberty and/or gelastic seizures in hypothalamic hamartoma. *J Clin Endocrinol Metab*. 2003;88:4590-4595.
787. Booth TN, Timmons C, Shapiro K, et al. Pre- and postnatal MR imaging of hypothalamic hamartomas associated with arachnoid cysts. *AJNR Am J Neuroradiol*. 2004;25:1283-1285.
788. Jung H, Carmel P, Schwartz MS, et al. Some hypothalamic hamartomas contain transforming growth factor alpha, a puberty-inducing

growth factor, not luteinizing hormone releasing hormone neurons. *J Clin Endocrinol Metab*. 1999;84:4695-4701.
789. Jung H, Parent AS, Ojeda SR. Hypothalamic hamartoma: a paradigm/model for studying the onset of puberty. *Endocr Dev*. 2005;8:81-93.
790. Styne DM, Harris DA, Egli CA, et al. Treatment of true precocious puberty with a potent luteinizing hormone-releasing factor agonist: effect on growth, sexual maturation, pelvic sonography, and the hypothalamic-pituitary-gonadal axis. *J Clin Endocrinol Metab*. 1985;61:142-151.
791. Feuillan PP, Jones JV, Barnes KM, et al. Boys with precocious puberty due to hypothalamic hamartoma: reproductive axis after discontinuation of gonadotropin-releasing hormone analog therapy. *J Clin Endocrinol Metab*. 2000;85:4036-4038.
792. Pescovitz OH, Comite F, Hench K, et al. The NIH experience with precocious puberty: diagnostic subgroups and response to short-term luteinizing hormone releasing hormone analogue therapy. *J Pediatr*. 1986;108:47-54.
793. Deonna T, Ziegler AL. Hypothalamic hamartoma, precocious puberty and gelastic seizures: a special model of "epileptic" developmental disorder. *Epileptic Disord*. 2000;2:33-37.
794. Freeman JL, Coleman LT, Wellard RM, et al. MR imaging and spectroscopic study of epileptogenic hypothalamic hamartomas: analysis of 72 cases. *AJNR Am J Neuroradiol*. 2004;25:450-462.
795. Grumbach MM. True or central precocious puberty. In: Kreiger DT, Bardin CW, eds. *Current Therapy in Endocrinology and Metabolism*. Toronto, Canada: B.C. Decker; 1985:4-8.
796. Rosenfeld JV, Harvey AS, Wrennall J, et al. Transcallosal resection of hypothalamic hamartomas, with control of seizures, in children with gelastic epilepsy. *Neurosurgery*. 2001;48:108-118.
797. Brandberg G, Raininko R, Eeg-Olofsson O. Hypothalamic hamartoma with gelastic seizures in Swedish children and adolescents. *Eur J Paediatr Neurol*. 2004;8:35-44.
798. Fohlen M, Lellouch A, Delalande O. Hypothalamic hamartoma with refractory epilepsy: surgical procedures and results in 18 patients. *Epileptic Disord*. 2003;5:267-273.
799. Barajas MA, Ramirez-Guzman MG, Rodriguez-Vazquez C, et al. Gamma knife surgery for hypothalamic hamartomas accompanied by medically intractable epilepsy and precocious puberty: experience in Mexico. *J Neurosurg*. 2005;102(suppl):53-55.
800. Freeman JL, Zacharin M, Rosenfeld JV, et al. The endocrinology of hypothalamic hamartoma surgery for intractable epilepsy. *Epileptic Disord*. 2003;5:239-247.
801. Starceski PJ, Lee PA, Albright AL, et al. Hypothalamic hamartomas and sexual precocity: evaluation of treatment options. *Am J Dis Child*. 1990;144:225-228.
802. Lopponen T, Saukkonen AL, Serlo W, et al. Accelerated pubertal development in patients with shunted hydrocephalus. *Arch Dis Child*. 1996;74:490-496.
803. Robertson CM, Morrish DW, Wheler GH, et al. Neonatal encephalopathy: an indicator of early sexual maturation in girls. *Pediatr Neurol*. 1990;6:102-108.
804. Clark SJ, Van Dop C, Conte FA, et al. Reversible true precocious puberty secondary to a congenital arachnoid cyst. *Am J Dis Child*. 1988;142:255-256.
805. Habiby R, Silverman B, Listernick R, et al. Precocious puberty in children with neurofibromatosis type 1. *J Pediatr*. 1995;126:364-367.
806. Listernick R, Charrow J, Greenwald M, et al. Natural history of optic pathway tumors in children with neurofibromatosis type 1: a longitudinal study [see comments]. *J Pediatr*. 1994;125:63-66.
807. Malina RM. Menarche in athletes: a synthesis and hypothesis. *Ann Hum Biol*. 1983;10:1-24.
808. Mashour GA, Driever PH, Hartmann M, et al. Circulating growth factor levels are associated with tumorigenesis in neurofibromatosis type 1. *Clin Cancer Res*. 2004;10:5677-5683.
809. Boulanger JM, Larbrisseau A. Neurofibromatosis type 1 in a pediatric population: Ste-Justine's experience. *Can J Neurol Sci*. 2005;32:225-231.
810. Teilmann G, Petersen JH, Gormsen M, et al. Early puberty in internationally adopted girls: hormonal and clinical markers of puberty in 276 girls examined biannually over two years. *Horm Res*. 2009;72:236-246.
811. Teilmann G, Pedersen CB, Skakkebaek NE, et al. Increased risk of precocious puberty in internationally adopted children in Denmark. *Pediatrics*. 2006;118:e391-e399.
812. Erkula G, Jones KB, Sponseller PD, et al. Growth and maturation in Marfan syndrome. *Am J Med Genet*. 2002;109:100-115.
813. Sadeghi-Nejad A, Kaplan SL, Grumbach MM. The effect of medroxyprogesterone acetate on adrenocortical function in children with precocious puberty. *J Pediatr*. 1971;78:616-624.
814. Belchetz PE, Plant TM, Nakai Y, et al. Hypophyseal responses to continuous and intermittent delivery of hypothalamic gonadotropin-releasing hormone. *Science*. 1978;202:631-633.
815. Knobil E, Plant TM, Wildt L, et al. Control of the rhesus monkey menstrual cycle: permissive role of the hypothalamic gonadotropin-releasing hormone. *Science*. 1980;207:1371-1373.
816. Conn PM, Crowley WFJ. Gonadotropin-releasing hormone and its analogs. *Annu Rev Med*. 1994;45:391-405.
817. Karten MJ, Rivier JE. Gonadotropin-releasing hormone analog design: structure-function studies toward the development of agonists and antagonists: rationale and perspective. *Endocr Rev*. 1986;7:44-66.
818. Handelsman DJ, Swerdloff RS. Pharmacokinetics of gonadotropin-releasing hormone and its analogs. *Endocr Rev*. 1986;7:95-105.
819. Boepple PA, Mansfield MJ, Wierman ME, et al. Use of a potent, long acting agonist of gonadotropin-releasing hormone in the treatment of precocious puberty. *Endocr Rev*. 1986;7:24-33.
820. Drop SL, Odink RJ, Rouwe C, et al. The effect of treatment with an LH-RH agonist (Buserelin) on gonadal activity growth and bone maturation in children with central precocious puberty. *Eur J Pediatr*. 1987;146:272-278.
821. Crowley WF Jr, Comite F, Vale W, et al. Therapeutic use of pituitary desensitization with a long-acting LHRH agonist: a potential new treatment for idiopathic precocious puberty. *J Clin Endocrinol Metab*. 1981;52:370-372.
822. Comite F, Cassorla F, Barnes KM, et al. Luteinizing hormone releasing hormone analogue therapy for central precocious puberty: long term effect on somatic growth, bone maturation, and predicted height. *JAMA*. 1986;255:2613-2616.
823. Bourguignon JP, Van Vliet G, Vandeweghe M, et al. Treatment of central precocious puberty with an intranasal analogue of GnRH (buserelin). *Eur J Pediatr*. 1987;146:555-560.
824. Mericq V, Lammoglia JJ, Unanue N, et al. Comparison of three doses of leuprolide acetate in the treatment of central precocious puberty: preliminary results. *Clin Endocrinol (Oxf)*. 2009;71:686-690.
825. Neely EK, Hintz RL, Parker B, et al. Two-year results of treatment with depot leuprolide acetate for central precocious puberty. *J Pediatr*. 1992;121:634-640.
826. Carel JC, Lahlou N, Guazzarotti L, et al. Treatment of central precocious puberty with depot leuprorelin. French Leuprorelin Trial Group. *Eur J Endocrinol*. 1995;132:699-704.
827. Holland FJ, Fishman L, Costigan DC, et al. Pharmacokinetic characteristics of the gonadotropin-releasing hormone analog D-Ser (tBU) 6Pro9NEt luteinizing hormone-releasing hormone (buserelin) after subcutaneous and intranasal administration in children with central precocious puberty. *J Clin Endocrinol Metab*. 1986;63:1065-1070.
828. Partsch CJ, Hummelink R, Peter M, et al. Comparison of complete and incomplete suppression of pituitary-gonadal activity in girls with central precocious puberty: influence on growth and predicted final height. The German-Dutch Precocious Puberty Study Group. *Horm Res*. 1993;39:111-117.
829. Mouat F, Hofman PL, Jefferies C, et al. Initial growth deceleration during GnRH analogue therapy for precocious puberty. *Clin Endocrinol (Oxf)*. 2009;70:751-756.
830. Sklar CA, Rothenberg S, Blumberg D, et al. Suppression of the pituitary-gonadal axis in children with central precocious puberty: effects on growth, growth hormone, insulin-like growth factor-I, and prolactin secretion. *J Clin Endocrinol Metab*. 1991;73:734-738.
831. Pasquino AM, Pucarelli I, Accardo F, et al. Long-term observation of 87 girls with idiopathic central precocious puberty treated with gonadotropin-releasing hormone analogs: impact on adult height, body mass index, bone mineral content, and reproductive function. *J Clin Endocrinol Metab*. 2008;93:190-195.
832. Tanaka T, Niimi H, Matsuo N, et al. Results of long-term follow-up after treatment of central precocious puberty with leuprorelin acetate: evaluation of effectiveness of treatment and recovery of gonadal function. The TAP-144-SR Japanese Study Group on Central Precocious Puberty. *J Clin Endocrinol Metab*. 2005;90:1371-1376.
833. Pasquino AM, Pucarelli I, Segni M, et al. Adult height in girls with central precocious puberty treated with gonadotropin-releasing hormone analogues and growth hormone. *J Clin Endocrinol Metab*. 1999;84:449-452.
834. Wu MH, Lin SJ, Wu LH, et al. Clinical suppression of precocious puberty with cetrorelix after failed treatment with GnRH agonist in a girl with gonadotrophin-independent precocious puberty. *Reprod Biomed Online*. 2005;11:18-21.
835. de Man M, Derksen E, Pieters G, et al. Cetrorelix suppression test in the diagnostic work-up of severe hyperandrogenism in adolescence. *J Pediatr Endocrinol Metab*. 2008;21:905-909.
836. Boot AM, De Muinck K, Pols HA, et al. Bone mineral density and body composition before and during treatment with gonadotropin-releasing hormone agonist in children with central precocious and early puberty. *J Clin Endocrinol Metab*. 1998;83:370-373.
837. Palmert MR, Mansfield MJ, Crowley WFJ, et al. Is obesity an outcome of gonadotropin-releasing hormone agonist administration? Analysis of growth and body composition in 110 patients with central precocious puberty. *J Clin Endocrinol Metab*. 1999;84:4480-4488.

838. Paterson WF, McNeill E, Young D, et al. Auxological outcome and time to menarche following long-acting goserelin therapy in girls with central precocious or early puberty. *Clin Endocrinol (Oxf)*. 2004;61:626-634.
839. Unal O, Berberoglu M, Evliyaoglu O, et al. Effects on bone mineral density of gonadotropin releasing hormone analogs used in the treatment of central precocious puberty. *J Pediatr Endocrinol Metab*. 2003;16:407-411.
840. Arrigo T, De Luca F, Antoniazzi F, et al. Reduction of baseline body mass index under gonadotropin-suppressive therapy in girls with idiopathic precocious puberty. *Eur J Endocrinol*. 2004;150:533-537.
841. Verrotti A, Basciani F, Trotta D, et al. Serum leptin levels in girls with precocious puberty. *Diabetes Nutr Metab*. 2003;16:125-129.
842. Chaussain JL, Roger M, Couprie C, et al. Treatment of precocious puberty with a long-acting preparation of D-Trp6-LHRH. *Horm Res*. 1987;28:155-163.
843. Ambrosino MM, Hernanz-Schulman M, Genieser NB, et al. Monitoring of girls undergoing medical therapy for isosexual precocious puberty. *J Ultrasound Med*. 1994;13:501-508.
844. Bhatia S, Neely EK, Wilson DM. Serum luteinizing hormone rises within minutes after depot leuprolide injection: implications for monitoring therapy. *Pediatrics*. 2002;109:E30.
845. Brito VN, Latronico AC, Arnhold IJ, et al. A single luteinizing hormone determination 2 hours after depot leuprolide is useful for therapy monitoring of gonadotropin-dependent precocious puberty in girls. *J Clin Endocrinol Metab*. 2004;89:4338-4342.
846. Rahhal S, Clarke WL, Kletter GB, et al. Results of a second year of therapy with the 12-month histrelin implant for the treatment of central precocious puberty. *Int J Pediatr Endocrinol*. 2009;81:2517.
847. Manasco PK, Pescovitz OH, Feuillan PP, et al. Resumption of puberty after long term luteinizing hormone-releasing hormone agonist treatment of central precocious puberty. *J Clin Endocrinol Metab*. 1988;67:368-372.
848. Heger S, Partsch CJ, Sippell WG. Long-term outcome after depot gonadotropin-releasing hormone agonist treatment of central precocious puberty: final height, body proportions, body composition, bone mineral density, and reproductive function. *J Clin Endocrinol Metab*. 1999;84:4583-4590.
849. Jay N, Mansfield MJ, Blizzard RM, et al. Ovulation and menstrual function of adolescent girls with central precocious puberty after therapy with gonadotropin-releasing hormone agonists. *J Clin Endocrinol Metab*. 1992;75:890-894.
850. Heger S, Muller M, Ranke M, et al. Long-term GnRH agonist treatment for female central precocious puberty does not impair reproductive function. *Mol Cell Endocrinol*. 2006;254-255:217-220.
851. Franceschi R, Gaudino R, Marcolongo A, et al. Prevalence of polycystic ovary syndrome in young women who had idiopathic central precocious puberty. *Fertil Steril*. 2010;93:1185-1191.
852. Kauschansky A, Nussinovitch M, Frydman M, et al. Hyperprolactinemia after treatment of long-acting gonadotropin-releasing hormone analogue Decapeptyl in girls with central precocious puberty. *Fertil Steril*. 1995;64:285-287.
853. Antoniazzi F, Zamboni G, Bertoldo F, et al. Bone development during GH and GnRH analog treatment. *Eur J Endocrinol*. 2004;151(suppl 1):S47-S54.
854. Tylavsky FA, Holliday K, Danish R, et al. Fruit and vegetable intakes are an independent predictor of bone size in early pubertal children. *Am J Clin Nutr*. 2004;79:311-317.
855. van Puijenbroek E, Verhoef E, de Graaf L. Slipped capital femoral epiphyses associated with the withdrawal of a gonadotrophin releasing hormone. *BMJ*. 2004;328:1353.
856. Ehrhardt AA, Meyer-Bahlburg HF. Psychosocial aspects of precocious puberty. *Horm Res*. 1994;41(suppl 2):30-35.
857. Mouridsen SE, Larsen FW. Psychological aspects of precocious puberty: an overview. *Acta Paedopsychiatr*. 1992;55:45-49.
858. Stanhope R. Use of a specific aromatase inhibitor in delayed puberty. *Lancet*. 2001;357:1723-1724.
859. Kreher NC, Pescovitz OH, Delameter P, et al. Treatment of familial male-limited precocious puberty with bicalutamide and anastrozole. *J Pediatr*. 2006;149:416-420.
860. Mieszczak J, Lowe ES, Plourde P, et al. The aromatase inhibitor anastrozole is ineffective in the treatment of precocious puberty in girls with McCune-Albright syndrome. *J Clin Endocrinol Metab*. 2008;93:2751-2754.
861. Sklar CA, Conte FA, Kaplan SL, et al. Human chorionic gonadotropin-secreting pineal tumor; relation to pathogenesis and sex limitation of sexual precocity. *J Clin Endocrinol Metab*. 1981;53:656-660.
862. van der HM, Niggli FK, Willi UV, et al. Solitary infantile choriocarcinoma of the liver: MRI findings. *Pediatr Radiol*. 2004;34:820-823.
863. Heimann A, White PF, Riely CA, et al. Hepatoblastoma presenting as isosexual precocity: the clinical importance of histologic and serologic parameters. *J Clin Gastroenterol*. 1987;9:105-110.
864. Blohm ME, Gobel U. Unexplained anaemia and failure to thrive as initial symptoms of infantile choriocarcinoma: a review. *Eur J Pediatr*. 2004;163:1-6.
865. Englund AT, Geffner ME, Nagel RA, et al. Pediatric germ cell and human chorionic gonadotropin-producing tumors: clinical and laboratory features. *Am J Dis Child*. 1991;145:1294-1297.
866. Starzyk J, Starzyk B, Bartnik-Mikuta A, et al. Gonadotropin releasing hormone-independent precocious puberty in a 5-year-old girl with suprasellar germ cell tumor secreting beta-hCG and alpha-fetoprotein. *J Pediatr Endocrinol Metab*. 2001;14:789-796.
867. O'Marcaigh AS, Ledger GA, Roche PC, et al. Aromatase expression in human germinomas with possible biological effects. *J Clin Endocrinol Metab*. 1995;80:3763-3766.
868. Cohen AR, Wilson JA, Sadeghi-Nejad A. Gonadotropin-secreting pineal teratoma causing precocious puberty. *Neurosurgery*. 1991;28:597-602; discussion 602-603.
869. Kretschmar CS. Germ cell tumors of the brain in children: a review of current literature and new advances in therapy. *Cancer Invest*. 1997;15:187-198.
870. Shinoda J, Sakai N, Yano H, et al. Prognostic factors and therapeutic problems of primary intracranial choriocarcinoma/germ-cell tumors with high levels of HCG. *J Neurooncol*. 2004;66:225-240.
871. Haupt C, Ancker U, Muller M, et al. Intracranial germ-cell tumours: treatment results and residuals. *Eur J Pediatr*. 1996;155:230-236.
872. Dickerman RD, Stevens QE, Steide JA, et al. Precocious puberty associated with a pineal cyst: is it disinhibition of the hypothalamic-pituitary axis? *Neuro Endocrinol Lett*. 2004;25:173-175.
873. Ambrosi B, Bassetti M, Ferrario R, et al. Precocious puberty in a boy with a PRL-, LH- and FSH-secreting pituitary tumour: hormonal and immunocytochemical studies. *Acta Endocrinol (Copenh)*. 1990;122:569-576.
874. White PC, Speiser PW. Congenital adrenal hyperplasia due to 21-hydroxylase deficiency. *Endocr Rev*. 2000;21:245-291.
875. Schmitt K, Frisch H, Neuhold N, et al. Aldosterone and testosterone producing adrenal adenoma in childhood. *J Endocrinol Invest*. 1995;18:69-73.
876. Makino S, Oda S, Saka T, et al. A case of aldosterone-producing adrenocortical adenoma associated with preclinical Cushing's syndrome and hypersecretion of parathyroid hormone. *Endocr J*. 2001;48:103-111.
877. Walker BR, Skoog SJ, Winslow BH, et al. Testis sparing surgery for steroid unresponsive testicular tumors of the adrenogenital syndrome. *J Urol*. 1997;157:1460-1463.
878. Pabon JE, Li X, Lei ZM, et al. Novel presence of luteinizing hormone/chorionic gonadotropin receptors in human adrenal glands. *J Clin Endocrinol Metab*. 1996;81:2397-2400.
879. Lacroix A, Ndiaye N, Tremblay J, et al. Ectopic and abnormal hormone receptors in adrenal Cushing's syndrome. *Endocr Rev*. 2001;22:75-110.
880. Domenice S, Latronico AC, Brito VN, et al. Adrenocorticotropin-dependent precocious puberty of testicular origin in a boy with X-linked adrenal hypoplasia congenita due to a novel mutation in the DAX1 gene. *J Clin Endocrinol Metab*. 2001;86:4068-4071.
881. Argente J, Ozisik G, Pozo J, et al. A novel single base deletion at codon 434 (1301delT) of the DAX1 gene associated with prepubertal testis enlargement. *Mol Genet Metab*. 2003;78:79-81.
882. Petkovic V, Salemi S, Vassella E, et al. Leydig-cell tumour in children: variable clinical presentation, diagnostic features, follow-up and genetic analysis of four cases. *Horm Res*. 2007;67:89-95.
883. Leung AC, Kogan SJ. Focal lobular spermatogenesis and pubertal acceleration associated with ipsilateral Leydig cell hyperplasia. *Urology*. 2000;56:508-509.
884. Liu G, Duranteau L, Carel JC, et al. Leydig-cell tumors caused by an activating mutation of the gene encoding the luteinizing hormone receptor [see comments]. *N Engl J Med*. 1999;341:1731-1736.
885. Barnes RB, Rosenfield RL, Ehrmann DA, et al. Ovarian hyperandrogynism as a result of congenital adrenal virilizing disorders: evidence for perinatal masculinization of neuroendocrine function in women. *J Clin Endocrinol Metab*. 1994;79:1328-1333.
886. Schedewie HK, Reiter EO, Beitins IZ. Testicular Leydig cell hyperplasia as a cause of familial sexual precocity. *J Clin Endocrinol Metab*. 1981;52:271-278.
887. Rosenthal SM, Grumbach MM, Kaplan SL. Gonadotropin-independent familial sexual precocity with premature Leydig and germinal cell maturation (familial testotoxicosis): effects of a potent luteinizing hormone-releasing factor agonist and medroxyprogesterone acetate therapy in four cases. *J Clin Endocrinol Metab*. 1983;57:571-579.
888. Egli CA, Rosenthal SM, Grumbach MM, et al. Pituitary gonadotropin-independent male-limited autosomal dominant sexual precocity in nine generations: familial testotoxicosis. *J Pediatr*. 1985;106:33-40.
889. Gondos B, Egli CA, Rosenthal SM, et al. Testicular changes in gonadotropin-independent familial male sexual precocity: familial testotoxicosis. *Arch Pathol Lab Med*. 1985;109:990-995.

890. Wierman ME, Beardsworth DE, Mansfield MJ, et al. Puberty without gonadotropins: a unique mechanism of sexual development. *N Engl J Med*. 1985;312:65-72.
891. Soriano-Guillen L, Mitchell V, Carel JC, et al. Activating mutations in the luteinizing hormone receptor gene: a human model of non-follicle-stimulating hormone-dependent inhibin production and germ cell maturation. *J Clin Endocrinol Metab*. 2006;91:3041-3047.
892. Rosenthal IM, Refetoff S, Rich B, et al. Response to challenge with gonadotropin-releasing hormone agonist in a mother and her two sons with a constitutively activating mutation of the luteinizing hormone receptor: a clinical research center study. *J Clin Endocrinol Metab*. 1996;81:3802-3806.
893. Shenker A, Laue L, Kosugi S, et al. A constitutively activating mutation of the luteinizing hormone receptor in familial male precocious puberty. *Nature*. 1993;365:652-654.
894. Kremer H, Mariman E, Otten BJ, et al. Cosegregation of missense mutations of the luteinizing hormone receptor gene with familial male-limited precocious puberty. *Hum Mol Genet*. 1993;2:1779-1783.
895. Minegishi T, Nakamura K, Takakura Y, et al. Cloning and sequencing of porcine LH-hCG receptor cDNA. *Biochem Biophys Res Comm*. 1990;172:1049-1054.
896. Atger M, Misrahi M, Sar S, et al. Structure of the human luteininzing hormone/choriogonadotropin receptor gene:unusual promoter and 5′ non-coding regions. *Mol Cell Biol*. 1995;111:113-123.
897. Dufau ML. The luteinizing hormone receptor. *Annu Rev Physiol*. 1998;60:461-496.
898. Latronico AC, Segaloff DL. Naturally occurring mutations of the luteinizing-hormone receptor: lessons learned about reproductive physiology and G protein-coupled receptors. *Am J Hum Genet*. 1999;65:949-958.
899. Kremer H, Martens JW, van Reen M, et al. A limited repertoire of mutations of the luteinizing hormone (LH) receptor gene in familial and sporadic patients with male LH-independent precocious puberty. *J Clin Endocrinol Metab*. 1999;84:1136-1140.
900. Lin Z, Shenker A, Pearlstein R. A model of the lutropin/choriogonadotropin receptor: insights into the structural and functional effects of constitutively activating mutations. *Protein Eng*. 1997;10:501-510.
901. Laue L, Chan WY, Hsueh AJ, et al. Genetic heterogeneity of constitutively activating mutations of the human luteinizing hormone receptor in familial male-limited precocious puberty. *Proc Natl Acad Sci U S A*. 1995;92:1906-1910.
902. Wu SM, Leschek EW, Rennert OM, et al. Luteinizing hormone receptor mutations in disorders of sexual development and cancer. *Front Biosci*. 2000;5:D343-D352.
903. Ignacak M, Hilczer M, Zarzycki J, et al. Substitution of M398T in the second transmembrane helix of the LH receptor in a patient with familial male-limited precocious puberty. *Endocr J*. 2000;47:595-599.
904. Holland FJ, Fishman L, Bailey JD, et al. Ketoconazole in the management of precocious puberty not responsive to LHRH-analogue therapy. *N Engl J Med*. 1985;312:1023-1028.
905. Babovic-Vuksanovic D, Donaldson MD, Gibson NA, et al. Hazards of ketoconazole therapy in testotoxicosis. *Acta Paediatr*. 1994;83:994-997.
906. Soriano-Guillen L, Lahlou N, Chauvet G, et al. Adult height after ketoconazole treatment in patients with familial male-limited precocious puberty. *J Clin Endocrinol Metab*. 2005;90:147-151.
907. Laue L, Kenigsberg D, Pescovitz OH, et al. The treatment of familial male precocious puberty with spironolactone and testolactone. *N Engl J Med*. 1989;320:496-502.
908. Partsch CJ, Krone N, Riepe FG, et al. Long-term follow-up of spontaneous development in a boy with familial male precocious puberty. *Horm Res*. 2004;62:177-181.
909. Liu G, Duranteau L, Carel JC, et al. Leydig-cell tumors caused by an activating mutation of the gene encoding the luteinizing hormone receptor. *N Engl J Med*. 1999;341:1731-1736.
910. Leschek EW, Chan WY, Diamond DA, et al. Nodular Leydig cell hyperplasia in a boy with familial male-limited precocious puberty. *J Pediatr*. 2001;138:949-951.
911. Spiegel AM, Shenker A, Weinstein LS. Receptor-effector coupling by G proteins: implications for normal and abnormal signal transduction. *Endocr Rev*. 1992;13:536-565.
912. Nakamoto JM, Zimmerman D, Jones EA, et al. Concurrent hormone resistance (pseudohypoparathyroidism type Ia) and hormone independence (testotoxicosis) caused by a unique mutation in the G alpha s gene. *Biochem Mol Med*. 1996;58:18-24.
913. Iiri T, Herzmark P, Nakamoto JM, et al. Rapid GDP release from Gs alpha in patients with gain and loss of endocrine function. *Nature*. 1994;371:164-167.
914. de Silva KS, Kanumakala S, Grover SR, et al. Ovarian lesions in children and adolescents: an 11-year review. *J Pediatr Endocrinol Metab*. 2004;17:951-957.
915. Peters H, Byskov AG, Grinsted J. Follicular growth in fetal and prepubertal ovaries of humans and other primates. *Clin Endocrinol Metab*. 1978;7:469-485.
916. Zachariou Z, Roth H, Boos R, et al. Three years' experience with large ovarian cysts diagnosed in utero. *J Pediatr Surg*. 1989;24:478-482.
917. Arisaka O, Hosaka A, Shimura N, et al. Effect of neonatal ovarian cysts on infant growth. *Clin Pediatr Endocrinol*. 1995;4:155-162.
918. Tonetta SA, di Zerega GS. Intragonadal regulation of follicular maturation. *Endocr Rev*. 1989;10:205-229.
919. Butler MG, Najjar JL. Do some patients with fragile X syndrome have precocious puberty. *Am J Med Genet*. 1988;31:779-781.
920. Sedin G, Bergquist C, Lindgren PG. Ovarian hyperstimulation syndrome in preterm infants. *Pediatr Res*. 1985;19:548-551.
921. Natarajan A, Wales JK, Marven SS, et al. Precocious puberty secondary to massive ovarian oedema in a 6-month-old girl. *Eur J Endocrinol*. 2004;150:119-123.
922. Richards GE, Kaplan SL, Grumbach MM. Sexual precocity associated with functional follicular cysts, prepubertal gonadotropins and LRF response and fluctuating estrogen levels (Abstract). *Pediatr Res*. 1977;11:431.
923. Feuillan PP, Jones J, Oerter KE, et al. Luteinizing hormone-releasing hormone (LHRH)–independent precocious puberty unresponsive to LHRH agonist therapy in two girls lacking the features of the McCune-Albright syndrome. *J Clin Endocrinol Metab*. 1991;73:1370-1373.
924. Hassan E, Creatsas G, Michalas S. Genital tumors during childhood and adolescence: a clinical and pathological study of 71 cases. *Clin Exp Obstet Gynecol*. 1999;26:20-21.
925. Cass DL, Hawkins E, Brandt ML, et al. Surgery for ovarian masses in infants, children, and adolescents: 102 consecutive patients treated in a 15-year period. *J Pediatr Surg*. 2001;36:693-699.
926. Schultz KA, Sencer SF, Messinger Y, et al. Pediatric ovarian tumors: a review of 67 cases. *Pediatr Blood Cancer*. 2005;44:167-173.
927. Shankar KR, Wakhlu A, Kokai GK, et al. Ovarian adenocarcinoma in premenarchal girls. *J Pediatr Surg*. 2001;36:511-515.
928. Young RH, Dickersin GR, Scully RE. Juvenile granulosa cell tumor of the ovary: a clinicopathologic analysis of 125 cases *Am J Surg Pathol*. 1984;8:575-596.
929. Lee MM, Donahoe PK, Hasegawa T, et al. Müllerian inhibiting substance in humans: normal levels from infancy to adulthood. *J Clin Endocrinol Metab*. 1996;81:571-576.
930. Silverman LA, Gitelman SE. Immunoreactive inhibin, mullerian inhibitory substance, and activin as biochemical markers for juvenile granulosa cell tumors. *J Pediatr*. 1996;129:918-921.
931. Burger HG, Fuller PJ. The inhibin/activin family and ovarian cancer. *Trends Endocinol Metab*. 1996;7:197-202.
932. Talerman A. The pathology of gonadal neoplasm composed of germ cells and sex cord stroma derivatives. *Pathol Res Pract*. 1980;170:24-38.
933. Lacson AG, Gillis DA, Shawwa A. Malignant mixed germ-cell-sex cord-stromal tumors of the ovary associated with isosexual precocious puberty. *Cancer*. 1988;61:2122-2133.
934. Solh HM, Azoury RS, Najjar SS. Peutz-Jeghers syndrome associated with precocious puberty. *J Pediatr*. 1983;103:593-595.
935. Coen P, Kulin H, Ballantine T, et al. An aromatase-producing sex-cord tumor resulting in prepubertal gynecomastia. *N Engl J Med*. 1991;324:317-322.
936. Berensztein E, Belgorosky A, de Davila MT, et al. Testicular steroid biosynthesis in a boy with a large cell calcifying Sertoli cell tumor producing prepubertal gynecomastia. *Steroids*. 1995;60:220-225.
937. Abed AA, Gunther K, Kraus C, et al. Mutation screening at the RNA level of the STK11/LKB1 gene in Peutz-Jeghers syndrome reveals complex splicing abnormalities and a novel mRNA isoform (STK11 c.597(insertion mark)598insIVS4). *Hum Mutat*. 2001;18:397-410.
938. Zumkeller W, Krause U, Holzhausen HJ, et al. Ovarian sex cord tumor with annular tubules associated with precocious puberty. *Med Pediatr Oncol*. 2000;35:144-146.
939. Phornphutkul C, Okubo T, Wu K, et al. Aromatase p450 expression in a feminizing adrenal adenoma presenting as isosexual precocious puberty. *J Clin Endocrinol Metab*. 2001;86:649-652.
940. Dumitrescu CE, Collins MT. McCune-Albright syndrome. *Orphanet J Rare Dis*. 2008;3:12.
941. Horvath A, Stratakis CA. Clinical and molecular genetics of acromegaly: MEN1, Carney complex, McCune-Albright syndrome, familial acromegaly and genetic defects in sporadic tumors. *Rev Endocr Metab Disord*. 2008;9:1-11.
942. Lair-Milan F, Blevec GL, Carel JC, et al. Thyroid sonographic abnormalities in McCune-Albright syndrome. *Pediatr Radiol*. 1996;26:424-426.
943. Paris F, Philibert P, Lumbroso S, et al. Isolated Cushing's syndrome: an unusual presentation of McCune-Albright syndrome in the neonatal period. *Horm Res*. 2009;72:315-319.
944. Eons MJ, Drezner MK. Tumor-induced osteomalacia: unveiling a new hormone. *N Engl J Med*. 1994;330:1679-1681.

945. Zung A, Chalew SA, Schwindinger WF, et al. Response to PTH(1-34) is altered in patients with McCune-Albright syndrome. *J Bone Miner Res*. 1993;8:S228.
946. Shenker A, Weinstein LS, Moran A, et al. Severe endocrine and non-endocrine manifestations of the McCune-Albright syndrome associated with activating mutations of stimulatory G protein Gs. *J Pediatr*. 1993;123:509-518.
947. Endo M, Yamada Y, Matsuura N, et al. Monozygotic twins discordant for the major signs of McCune-Albright syndrome. *Am J Med Genet*. 1991;41:216-220.
948. Lumbroso S, Paris F, Sultan C. Activating Gsalpha mutations: analysis of 113 patients with signs of McCune-Albright syndrome. A European Collaborative Study. *J Clin Endocrinol Metab*. 2004;89:2107-2113.
949. Mantovani G, Bondioni S, Lania AG, et al. Parental origin of Gsalpha mutations in the McCune-Albright syndrome and in isolated endocrine tumors. *J Clin Endocrinol Metab*. 2004;89:3007-3009.
950. Roman R, Johnson MC, Codner E, et al. Activating GNAS1 gene mutations in patients with premature thelarche. *J Pediatr*. 2004;145:218-222.
951. De Sanctis C, Lala R, Matarazzo P, et al. McCune-Albright syndrome: a longitudinal clinical study of 32 patients. *J Pediatr Endocrinol Metab*. 1999;12:817-826.
952. Leet AI, Chebli C, Kushner H, et al. Fracture incidence in polyostotic fibrous dysplasia and the McCune-Albright syndrome. *J Bone Miner Res*. 2004;19:571-577.
953. Hannon TS, Noonan K, Steinmetz R, et al. Is McCune-Albright syndrome overlooked in subjects with fibrous dysplasia of bone? *J Pediatr*. 2003;142:532-538.
954. Galland F, Kamenicky P, Affres H, et al. McCune-Albright syndrome and acromegaly: effects of hypothalamo-pituitary radiotherapy and/or pegvisomant in somatostatin analogue-resistant patients. *J Clin Endocrinol Metab*. 2006;91:4957-4961.
955. Foster CM, Comite F, Pescovitz OH, et al. Variable response to a long-acting agonist of luteinizing hormone-releasing hormone in girls with McCune-Albright syndrome. *J Clin Endocrinol Metab*. 1984;59:801-805.
956. Foster CM, Ross JL, Shawker T, et al. Absence of pubertal gonadotropin secretion in girls with McCune-Albright syndrome. *J Clin Endocrinol Metab*. 1984;58:1161-1165.
957. Pasquino AM, Tebaldi L, Cives C, et al. Precocious puberty in the McCune-Albright syndrome: progression from gonadotrophin-independent to gonadotrophin-dependent puberty in a girl. *Acta Paediatr Scand*. 1987;76:841-843.
958. Feuillan P, Calis K, Hill S, et al. Letrozole treatment of precocious puberty in girls with the McCune-Albright syndrome: a pilot study. *J Clin Endocrinol Metab*. 2007;92:2100-2106.
959. Eugster EA, Rubin SD, Reiter EO, et al. Tamoxifen treatment for precocious puberty in McCune-Albright syndrome: a multicenter trial. *J Pediatr*. 2003;143:60-66.
960. Ringel MD, Schwindinger WF, Levine MA. Clinical implications of genetic defects in G proteins. *Medicine (Baltimore)*. 1996;75:171-184.
961. Coutant R, Lumbroso S, Rey R, et al. Macroorchidism due to autonomous hyperfunction of Sertoli cells and G (s) alpha gene mutation: an unusual expression of McCune-Albright syndrome in a prepubertal boy. *J Clin Endocrinol Metab*. 2001;86:1778-1781.
962. Wasniewska M, De Luca F, Bertelloni S, et al. Testicular microlithiasis: an unreported feature of McCune-Albright syndrome in males. *J Pediatr*. 2004;145:670-672.
963. Happle R. The McCune-Albright syndrome: a lethal gene surviving by mosaicism. *Clin Genet*. 1986;29:321-324.
964. Lyons J, Landis CA, Harsh G, et al. Two G protein oncogenes in human endocrine tumors. *Science*. 1990;249:655-659.
965. Spiegel AM. Mutations in G proteins and G protein-coupled receptors in endocrine disease. *J Clin Endocrinol Metab*. 1996;81:2434-2442.
966. Bourne HR. Trimeric G proteins: surprise witness tells a tale. *Science*. 1995;270:933-934.
967. Clapham DE. The G-protein nanomachine. *Nature*. 1996; 379:297-299.
968. Dhanasekaran N, Heasley LE, Johnson GL. G protein-coupled receptor systems involved in cell growth and oncogenesis. *Endocr Rev*. 1995;16:259-270.
969. Weinstein LS, Shenker A, Gejman PV, et al. Activating mutations of the stimulatory G protein in the McCune-Albright syndrome. *N Engl J Med*. 1991;325:1688-1695.
970. Schwindinger WF, Francomano CA, Levine MA. Identification of a mutation in the gene encoding the alpha subunit of the stimulatory G protein of adenylyl cyclase in McCune-Albright syndrome. *Proc Natl Acad Sci U S A*. 1992;89:5152-5156.
971. Shenker A, Weinstein LS, Sweet DE, et al. An activating Gs alpha mutation is present in fibrous dysplasia of bone in the McCune-Albright syndrome. *J Clin Endocrinol Metab*. 1994;79:750-755.
972. Candeliere GA, Glouеux FH, Prud'homme J, et al. Increased expression of the C-fos proto-oncogene in bone from patients with fibrous dysplasia. *N Engl J Med*. 1995;332:1546-1551.
973. Kendle FW. Case of precocious puberty in a female cretin. *Br Med J*. 1905;1:246.
974. Suter SN, Kaplan SL, Aubert ML, et al. Plasma prolactin and thyrotropin and the response to throtropin-releasing factor in children with primary and tertiary hypothyroidism. *J Clin Endocrinol Metab*. 1978;47:1015-1020.
975. Wood LC, Olichney M, Locke H, et al. Syndrome of juvenile hypothyroidism associated with advanced sexual development: report of two new cases and comment on the management of an associated ovarian mass. *J Clin Endocrinol Metab*. 1965;25:1289-1295.
976. Chattopadhyay A, Kumar V, Marulaiah M. Polycystic ovaries, precocious puberty and acquired hypothyroidism: the Van Wyk and Grumbach syndrome. *J Pediatr Surg*. 2003;38:1390-1392.
977. Jannini EA, Ulisse S, D'Aromiento M. Thyroid hormone and male gonadal function. *Endocrine Rev*. 1995;16:443-459.
978. Bruder JM, Samuels MH, Bremner WJ, et al. Hypothyroidism-induced macroorchidism: use of a gonadotropin-releasing hormone agonist to understand its mechanism and augment adult stature. *J Clin Endocrinol Metab*. 1995;80:11-16.
979. Buchanan CR, Stanhope R, Adlard P, et al. Gonadotropin, growth hormone and prolactin secretion in children with primary hypothyroidism. *Clin Endocrinol*. 1988;29:427-436.
980. Hess RA, Cooke PS, Bunick D, et al. Adult testicular enlargement induced by neonatal hypothyroidism is accompanied by increased Sertoli and germ cell numbers. *Endocrinology*. 1993;132:2607-2613.
981. Marshall GR, Plant TM. Puberty occurring either spontaneously or induced precociously in rhesus monkey (*Macaca mulatta*) is associated with a marked proliferation of Sertoli cells. *Biol Reprod*. 1996;54:1192-1199.
982. Cortes D, Muller J, Skakkebaek NE. Proliferation of Sertoli cells during development of the human testis assessed by stereological methods. *Int J Androl*. 1987;10:589-596.
983. Anasti JN, Flack MR, Froehlich J, et al. A potential novel mechanism for precocious puberty in juvenile hypothyroidism [see comments]. *J Clin Endocrinol Metab*. 1995;80:276-279.
984. Money J, Lamacz M. Genital examination and exposure experienced as nosocomial sexual abuse in childhood. *J Nerv Ment Dis*. 1987;175: 713-721.
985. Badouraki M, Christoforidis A, Economou I, et al. Evaluation of pelvic ultrasonography in the diagnosis and differentiation of various forms of sexual precocity in girls. *Ultrasound Obstet Gynecol*. 2008;32: 819-827.
986. Calcaterra V, Sampaolo P, Klersy C, et al. Utility of breast ultrasonography in the diagnostic work-up of precocious puberty and proposal of a prognostic index for identifying girls with rapidly progressive central precocious puberty. *Ultrasound Obstet Gynecol*. 2009;33:85-91.
987. Ng SM, Kumar Y, Cody D, et al. Cranial MRI scans are indicated in all girls with central precocious puberty. *Arch Dis Child*. 2003;88:414-418.
988. Perignon F, Brauner R, Argyropoulou M, et al. Precocious puberty in girls: pituitary height as an index of hypothalamo-pituitary activation. *J Clin Endocrinol Metab*. 1992;75:1170-1172.
989. Segal DG, DiMeglio LA, Ryder KW, et al. Assay interference leading to misdiagnosis of central precocious puberty. *Endocrine*. 2003;20:195-199.
990. Partsch CJ, Sippell WG. Pathogenesis and epidemiology of precocious puberty: effects of exogenous oestrogens. *Hum Reprod Update*. 2001; 7:292-302.
991. Henley DV, Lipson N, Korach KS, et al. Prepubertal gynecomastia linked to lavender and tea tree oils. *N Engl J Med*. 2007;356: 479-485.
992. Yu YM, Punyasavatsu N, Elder D, et al. Sexual development in a two-year-old boy induced by topical exposure to testosterone. *Pediatrics*. 1999;104:e23.
993. US Food and Drug Administration. *Guideline 3, part 2: Guideline for toxicological testing*. Silver Spring, MD: FDA; 1999.
994. Andersson AM, Skakkebaek NE. Exposure to exogenous estrogens in food: possible impact on human development and health. *Eur J Endocrinol*. 1999;140:477-485.
995. Larriuz-Serrano MC, Perez-Cardona CM, Ramos-Valencia G, et al. Natural history and incidence of premature thelarche in Puerto Rican girls aged 6 months to 8 years diagnosed between 1990 and 1995. *P R Health Sci J*. 2001;20:13-18.
996. Van Winter JT, Noller KL, Zimmerman D, et al. Natural history of premature thelarche in Olmsted County, Minnesota, 1940 to 1984. *J Pediatr*. 1990;116:278-280.
997. Colon I, Caro D, Bourdony CJ, et al. Identification of phthalate esters in the serum of young Puerto Rican girls with premature breast development. *Environ Health Perspect*. 2000;108:895-900.
998. Lomenick JP, Calafat AM, Melguizo Castro MS, et al. Phthalate exposure and precocious puberty in females. *J Pediatr*. 2010; 156:221-225.

999. Patisaul HB, Adewale HB. Long-term effects of environmental endocrine disruptors on reproductive physiology and behavior. *Front Behav Neurosci*. 2009;3:10.
1000. Den Hond E, Schoeters G. Endocrine disrupters and human puberty. *Int J Androl*. 2006;29:264-271.
1001. Blanck HM, Marcus M, Tolbert PE, et al. Age at menarche and Tanner stage in girls exposed in utero and postnatally to polybrominated biphenyl. *Epidemiology*. 2000;11:641-647.
1002. Massart F, Seppia P, Pardi D, et al. High incidence of central precocious puberty in a bounded geographic area of northwest Tuscany: an estrogen disrupter epidemic? *Gynecol Endocrinol*. 2005;20:92-98.
1003. Wolff MS, Britton JA, Russo JC. TCDD and puberty in girls. *Environ Health Perspect*. 2005;113:A17.
1004. Rais-Bahrami K, Nunez S, Revenis ME, et al. Follow-up study of adolescents exposed to di (2-ethylhexyl) phthalate (DEHP) as neonates on extracorporeal membrane oxygenation (ECMO) support. *Environ Health Perspect*. 2004;112:1339-1340.
1005. Denham M, Schell LM, Deane G, et al. Relationship of lead, mercury, mirex, dichlorodiphenyldichloroethylene, hexachlorobenzene, and polychlorinated biphenyls to timing of menarche among Akwesasne Mohawk girls. *Pediatrics*. 2005;115:e127-e134.
1006. Wu T, Buck GM, Mendola P. Blood lead levels and sexual maturation in U.S. girls: the Third National Health and Nutrition Examination Survey, 1988-1994. *Environ Health Perspect*. 2003;111:737-741.
1007. Hauser R, Sergeyev O, Korrick S, et al. Association of blood lead levels with onset of puberty in Russian boys. *Environ Health Perspect*. 2008;116:976-980.
1008. Aksglaede L, Sorensen K, Petersen JH, et al. Recent decline in age at breast development: the Copenhagen Puberty Study. *Pediatrics*. 2009;123:e932-e939.
1009. Hsu PC, Lai TJ, Guo NW, et al. Serum hormones in boys prenatally exposed to polychlorinated biphenyls and dibenzofurans. *J Toxicol Environ Health A*. 2005;68:1447-1456.
1010. Gladen BC, Klebanoff MA, Hediger ML, et al. Prenatal DDT exposure in relation to anthropometric and pubertal measures in adolescent males. *Environ Health Perspect*. 2004;112:1761-1767.
1011. Buck Louis GM, Gray LE Jr, Marcus M, et al. Environmental factors and puberty timing: expert panel research needs. *Pediatrics*. 2008;121(Suppl 3):S192-S207.
1012. Shozu M, Sebastian S, Takayama K, et al. Estrogen excess associated with novel gain-of-function mutations affecting the aromatase gene. *N Engl J Med*. 2003;348:1855-1865.
1012a. Wasniewska M, Raiola G, Galati MC, et al. Non-classical 21-hxdroxylase deficiency in boys with prepubertal or pubertal gynecomastia. *Eur J Pediatr*. 2008;167:1083-1084.
1013. Binder G, Iliev DI, Dufke A, et al. Dominant transmission of prepubertal gynecomastia due to serum estrone excess: hormonal, biochemical, and genetic analysis in a large kindred. *J Clin Endocrinol Metab*. 2005;90:484-492.
1014. Tiulpakov A, Kalintchenko N, Semitcheva T, et al. A potential rearrangement between CYP19 and TRPM7 genes on chromosome 15q21.2 as a cause of aromatase excess syndrome. *J Clin Endocrinol Metab*. 2005;90:4184-4190.
1015. Harigopal M, Murray MP, Rosen PP, et al. Prepubertal gynecomastia with lobular differentiation. *Breast J*. 2005;11:48-51.
1016. Arai K, Chrousos GP. Syndromes of glucocorticoid and mineralocorticoid resistance. *Steroids*. 1995;60:173-179.
1017. Young RH, Scully RE. Ovarian Sertoli cell tumors: a report of 10 cases. *Int J Gynecol Pathol*. 1984;2:349-363.
1018. Tavassoli FA, Norris HJ.Sertoli tumors of the ovary: a clinicopathologic study of 28 cases with ultrastructural observations. *Cancer*. 1980;46:2282-2297.
1019. Volta C, Bernasconi S, Cisternino M, et al. Isolated premature thelarche and thelarche variant: clinical and auxological follow-up of 119 girls. *J Endocrinol Invest*. 1998;21:180-183.
1020. Klein KO, Mericq V, Brown-Dawson JM, et al. Estrogen levels in girls with premature thelarche compared with normal prepubertal girls as determined by an ultrasensitive recombinant cell bioassay. *J Pediatr*. 1999;134:190-192.
1021. Collett-Solberg PR, Grumbach MM. A simplified procedure for evaluating estrogenic effects and the sex chromatin pattern in exfoliated cells in urine: studies in premature thelarche and gynecomastia of adolescence. *J Pediatr*. 1965;66:883-890.
1022. Crofton PM, Evans NE, Wardhaugh B, et al. Evidence for increased ovarian follicular activity in girls with premature thelarche. *Clin Endocrinol (Oxf)*. 2005;62:205-209.
1023. Saggese G, Ghirri P, Del Vecchio A, et al. Gonadotropin pulsatile secretion in girls with premature menarche. *Horm Res*. 1990; 33:5-10.
1024. Lee PA, Migeon CJ, Bias WB, et al. Familial hypersecretion of adrenal androgens transmitted as a dominant, non-HLA linked trait. *Obstet Gynecol*. 1987;69:259-264.
1025. Korth-Schutz S, Levine LS, New MI. Serum androgens in normal prepubertal and pubertal children and in children with precocious adrenarche. *J Clin Endocrinol Metab*. 1976;42:117-124.
1026. Rosenfield RL. Plasma 17-ketosteroids and 17-beta-hydroxysteroid in girls with premature development of sexual hair. *J Pediatr*. 1971;79:260-266.
1027. Miller WL, Auchus RJ, Geller DH. The regulation of 17,20 lyase activity. *Steroids*. 1997;62:133-142.
1028. Ibanez L, Ong KK, Mongan N, et al. Androgen receptor gene CAG repeat polymorphism in the development of ovarian hyperandrogenism. *J Clin Endocrinol Metab*. 2003;88:3333-3338.
1029. Utriainen P, Voutilainen R, Jaaskelainen J. Girls with premature adrenarche have accelerated early childhood growth. *J Pediatr*. 2009;154:882-887.
1030. Accetta SG, Di Domenico K, Ritter CG, et al. Anthropometric and endocrine features in girls with isolated premature pubarche or nonclassical congenital adrenal hyperplasia. *J Pediatr Endocrinol Metab*. 2004;17:767-773.
1031. Ibanez L, Virdio R, Potau N, et al. Natural history of premature pubarche: an auxological study. *J Clin Endocrinol Metab*. 1992;74:254-257.
1032. Oberfield SE, Mayes DM, Levine LS. Adrenal steroidogenic function in a Black and Hispanic population with precocious pubarche. *J Clin Endocrinol Metab*. 1990;70:76-82.
1033. Sam S, Dunaif A. Polycystic ovary syndrome: syndrome XX? *Trends Endocrinol Metab*. 2003;14:365-370.
1034. Wilson R, Mercado A, Cheng K, et al. Steroid 21-hydroxylase deficiency: genotype may not predict phenotype. *J Clin Endocrinol Metab*. 1995;80:2322-2329.
1035. Likitmaskul S, Cowell CT, Donaghue K, et al. "Exaggerated adrenarche" in children presenting with premature adrenarche. *Clinical Endocrinol*. 1995;42:265-272.
1036. Morris AH, Reiter EO, Geffner ME, et al. Absence of nonclassical congenital adrenal hyperplasia in patients with precocious adrenarche. *J Clin Endocrinol Metab*. 1989;69:709-715.
1037. Speiser PW, Dupont B, Rubenstein P, et al. High frequency of nonclassical steroid 21-hydroxylase deficiency. *Am J Hum Genet*. 1985;35:650-667.
1038. Balducci R, Boscherini B, Mangiantini A, et al. Isolated precocious pubarche: an approach. *J Clin Endocrinol Metab*. 1994;79:582-589.
1039. Temeck JW, Pang S, Nelson C, et al. Genetic defects of steroidogenesis in premature pubarche. *J Clin Endocrinol Metab*. 1987;64:609-617.
1040. Zerah M, RhJaume E, Mani P, et al. No evidence of mutations in the genes for type I and type II 38-hydroxysteroid dehydrogenase (38-HSD) in nonclassical 38-HSD deficiency. *J Clin Endocrinol Metab*. 1994;79:1811-1817.
1041. Chang YT, Zhang L, Alkaddour HS, et al. Absence of molecular defect in type II 38-hydroxysteroid dehydrogenase (38-HSD) gene in premature pubarche children and hirsute female patients with moderately decreased adrenal 38-HSD activity. *Pediatr Res*. 1995;37:820-824.
1042. Morel Y, MJbarki F, RhJaume E, et al. Structure-function relationships of 38-hydroxysteroid dehydrogenase: contribution made by the molecular genetics of 38-hydroxysteroid dehydrogenase deficiency. *Steroids*. 1997;62:176-184.
1043. Mendonca BB, Russell AJ, Vasconcelos-Leite M, et al. Mutation in 3 beta-hydroxysteroid dehydrogenase type II associated with pseudohermaphroditism in males and premature pubarche or cryptic expression in females. *J Mol Endocrinol*. 1994;12:119-122.
1044. Carbunaru G, Prasad P, Scoccia B, et al. The hormonal phenotype of nonclassic 3 beta-hydroxysteroid dehydrogenase (HSD3B) deficiency in hyperandrogenic females is associated with insulin-resistant polycystic ovary syndrome and is not a variant of inherited HSD3B2 deficiency. *J Clin Endocrinol Metab*. 2004;89:783-794.
1045. Deplewski D, Rosenfield RL. Role of hormones in pilosebaceous unit development. *Endocr Rev*. 2000;21:363-392.
1046. Ibanez L, Ong K, de Zegher F, et al. Fat distribution in non-obese girls with and without precocious pubarche: central adiposity related to insulinaemia and androgenaemia from prepuberty to postmenarche. *Clin Endocrinol (Oxf)*. 2003;58:372-379.
1047. Biro FM. Body morphology and its impact on adolescent and pediatric gynecology, with a special emphasis on polycystic ovary syndrome. *Curr Opin Obstet Gynecol*. 2003;15:347-351.
1048. Driscoll DA. Polycystic ovary syndrome in adolescence. *Semin Reprod Med*. 2003;21:301-307.
1049. Azziz R, Carmina E, Dewailly D, et al. Position statement: criteria for defining polycystic ovary syndrome as a predominantly hyperandrogenic syndrome—an Androgen Excess Society guideline. *J Clin Endocrinol Metab*. 2006;91:4237-4245.
1050. Veening MA, van Weissenbruch MM, Roord JJ, et al. Pubertal development in children born small for gestational age. *J Pediatr Endocrinol Metab*. 2004;17:1497-1505.
1051. Boonstra VH, Mulder PG, De Jong FH, et al. Serum dehydroepiandrosterone sulfate levels and pubarche in short children born small for gestational age before and during growth hormone treatment. *J Clin Endocrinol Metab*. 2004;89:712-717.
1052. Ibanez L, Aulesa C, Potau N, et al. Plasminogen activator inhibitor-1 in girls with precocious pubarche: a premenarcheal marker for polycystic ovary syndrome? *Pediatr Res*. 2002;51:244-248.

1053. Ibaenez L, Potau N, Zampolli M, et al. Source localization of androgen excess in adolescent girls. *J Clin Endocrinol Metab.* 1994; 79:1778-1784.
1054. Ibaenez L, Potau N, Zampolli M, et al. Hyperinsulinemia in postpubertal girls with a history of premature pubarche and functional ovarian hyperandrogenism. *J Clin Endocrinol Metab.* 1996; 81:1237-1243.
1055. Jones KL, Arslanian S, Peterokova VA, et al. Effect of metformin in pediatric patients with type 2 diabetes: a randomized controlled trial. *Diabetes Care.* 2002;25:89-94.
1056. Arlt W, Auchus RJ, Miller WL. Thiazolidinediones but not metformin directly inhibit the steroidogenic enzymes P450c17 and 3beta-hydroxysteroid dehydrogenase. *J Biol Chem.* 2001;276:16767-16771.
1057. Biro FM, Lucky AW, Huster GA, et al. Hormonal studies and physical maturation in adolescent gynecomastia. *J Pediatr.* 1990; 116:450-455.
1058. Moore DC, Schlaepfer LV, Punier L, et al. Hormonal changes during puberty: V. Transient pubertal gynecomastia: abnormal androgen-estrogen ratios. *J Clin Endocrinol Metab.* 1997;58:492-499.
1059. Mauras N, Bishop K, Merinbaum D, et al. Pharmacokinetics and pharmacodynamics of anastrozole in pubertal boys with recent-onset gynecomastia. *J Clin Endocrinol Metab.* 2009;94:2975-2978.
1060. Meschede D, Behre HM, Nieschlag E. Endocrine and spermatologic characteristics of 135 patients with bilateral megalotestis. *Andrologia.* 1995;27:207-212.
1061. Lachiewicz AM, Dawson DV. Do young boys with fragile X syndrome have macroorchidism? *Pediatrics.* 1994;93:992-995.
1062. Sigurjonsdottir TJ, Hayles AB. Precocious puberty: a report of 96 cases. *Am J Dis Child.* 1968;115:309-321.
1063. Werder EA, Murset G, Zachmann M, et al. Treatment of precocious puberty with cyproterone acetate. *Pediatr Res.* 1974;8:248-256.
1064. Wilkins L. *The Diagnosis and Treatment of Endocrine Disorders in Childhood and Adolescence.* Springfield, IL: Charles C Thomas; 1965.
1065. Comite F, Cutler GBJ, Rivier J, et al. Short-term treatment of idiopathic precocious puberty with a long-acting analogue of luteinizing hormone-releasing hormone: a preliminary report. *N Engl J Med.* 1981;305:1546-1550.
1066. Oerter KE, Manasco P, Barnes KM, et al. Adult height in precocious puberty after long-term treatment with deslorelin. *J Clin Endocrinol Metab.* 1991;73:11235-11240.
1067. Boepple PA, Crowley WFJ. Gonadotrophin-releasing hormone analogues as therapeutic probes in human growth and development: evidence from children with central precocious puberty. *Acta Paediatr Scand Suppl.* 1991;372-333-38.
1068. Eshet R, Duz Z, Silbergeld A, et al. Erythrocytes from patients with low concentrations of IGF1 have an increase in receptor sites of IGF1. *Acta Endocrinol.* 1991;125:354-358.
1069. Rappaport R, Fontoura M, Brauner R. Treatment of central precocious puberty with an LHRH agonist (buserelin): effect on growth and bone maturation after three years of treatment. *Horm Res.* 1987;28:149-154.
1070. Suwa S, Hibi I, Kato K, et al. LH-RH agonistic analog (buserelin) treatment of precocious puberty: collaborative study in Japan. *Acta Paediatr Jph.* 1988;30(suppl):176-184.
1071. Luder AS, Holland FJ, Costigan DC, et al. Intranasal and subcutaneous treatment of central precocious puberty in both sexes with a long-acting analog of luteinizing hormone-releasing hormone. *J Clin Endocrinol Metab.* 1984;58:966-972.
1072. Donaldson MD, Stanhope R, Lee TJ, et al. Gonadotrophin responses to GnRH in precocious puberty treated with GnRH analogue. *Clin Endocrinol (Oxf).* 1984;21:499-503.
1073. Rime JL, Zumsteg U, Blumberg A, et al. Long-term treatment of central precocious puberty with an intranasal HLRH analogue: control of pituitary function by urinary gonadotrophins. *Eur J Pediatr.* 1988;147:263-269.
1074. Kauli R, Pertzelan A, Ben-Zeev A, et al. Treatment of precocious puberty with LHRH analogue in combination with cyproterone acetate: further experience. *Clin Edocrinol (Oxf).* 1984;20: 377-387.
1075. Roger M, Chaussain JL, Berlier P, et al. Long term treatment of male and female precocious puberty by periodic administration of a long-acting preparation of D-Trp6-luteinizing hormone-releasing hormone microcapsules. *J Clin Endocrinol Metab.* 1986;62:670-677.
1076. Marshall WA, Tanner JM. Variations in pattern of pubertal changes in girls. *Arch Dis Child.* 1969;44:291-303.
1077. Waldhauser F, Weissenbacher G, Frisch H, Pollak A. Pulsatile secretion of gonadotropins in early infancy. *Eur J Pediatr.* 1981;137:71-74.

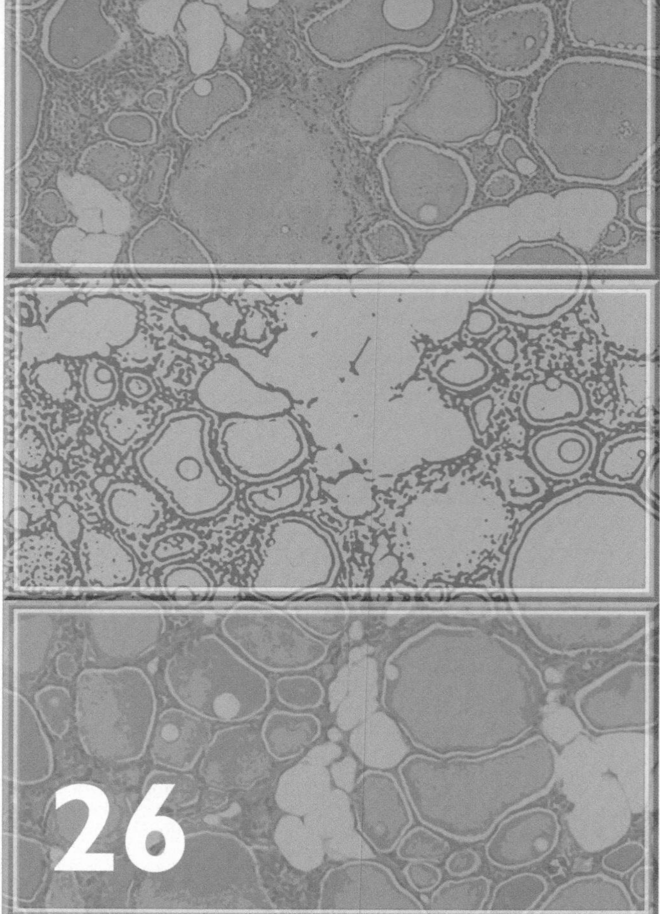

CHAPTER 26

Hormones and Athletic Performance

FABIO LANFRANCO • EZIO GHIGO • CHRISTIAN J. STRASBURGER

EFFECT OF ATHLETIC PERFORMANCE ON HORMONAL SYSTEMS

Catecholamines

The catecholamines norepinephrine and epinephrine are closely coupled in their actions, and they respond rapidly to exercise. Norepinephrine increases from a resting level of 1.2 to 3.0 nmol/L to levels as high as 12.0 nmol/L at maximal exercise.[1] Resting concentrations of epinephrine are 380 to 655 pmol/L. With maximal exercise, epinephrine concentrations can increase up to 3300 pmol/L. Levels of both hormones progressively increase as workload increases. Resting concentrations are achieved within 30 minutes after exercise.[1]

Mild exercise produces little or no catecholamine response, whereas at moderate exercise levels, norepinephrine significantly increases with minimal change in circulating epinephrine. At intense or prolonged exercise levels, levels of both hormones increase significantly.[2] Acute, short-duration, maximal exercise can significantly increase norepinephrine and epinephrine levels. This rapid response suggests that the levels are primarily regulated through neural release mediated by activation of the sympathetic nervous system. Spillover from active muscle during exercise appears to be the primary contributor, but the kidneys also are a possible source.[1] Moreover, alteration in the ratio of norepinephrine to epinephrine, with a greater increase in the release of epinephrine from the adrenal medulla during exercise, suggests possible hypothalamic mediation in the response to exercise.

Graded exercise produces a lower catecholamine response than continuous, prolonged exercise. The responses are directly related to workload and oxygen uptake and are greater with small muscle groups than with large muscle groups.

Many studies report a higher epinephrine response to exercise in endurance-trained compared with untrained subjects at the same relative intensity as all-out exercise. This higher capacity to secrete epinephrine was observed in response to both physical exercise and other stimuli such as hypoglycemia and hypoxia.[3] For some, this phenomenon partly explains the higher physical performance observed in trained versus untrained subjects. These findings have also been reported for anaerobically trained subjects in response to supramaximal exercise. Studies assessing women remain scarce; the results are less consistent than those for men, and the effects of aerobic versus anaerobic training on the catecholamine response need to be specified.[3]

Epinephrine and norepinephrine are responsible for many adaptations at rest and during exercise, including cardiovascular and respiratory adjustments and substrate mobilization and use.[3] Redistribution of circulation to working muscles and to the skin for heat loss and sweating is mediated by changes in catecholamines directly or indirectly through other intermediate hormones. Moreover, catecholamines may mediate the improvement of mental performance that occurs with exercise.[3,4]

Fluid Homeostasis and the Vasopressin–Renin-Angiotensin-Aldosterone System

During physical exercise, there is considerable loss of water and electrolytes in sweat, which maintains body temperature by dissipating heat generated from muscle use. The rate of fluid loss due to sweating may be as high as 1500 mL/hour.[5] Lost fluids are replaced by subsequent ingestion of liquids, modulated by thirst. Replacement of electrolytes is the result of normal food intake. Renal function is the major mechanism by which electrolytes are conserved after exercise.

Fluid and electrolyte homeostasis depends on the action of arginine vasopressin (AVP), natriuretic peptides, the renin-angiotensin-aldosterone (RAA) axis, and catecholamines. These hormonal systems are modified in response to exercise, with different patterns depending on the amount of relative work performed, the duration of exercise, and the training status. Other factors influencing the hormonal response to exercise include the mode of exercise, environmental factors, age and gender of the subjects, and several medical or physiologic conditions.[1] Hormones involved in the regulation of fluid and electrolyte homeostasis show relatively consistent responses among individuals.

AVP concentrations increase during exercise and persist at elevated levels for more than 60 minutes after maximal exercise. The increase in AVP levels during exercise is stimulated by increased plasma osmolality and reduced blood volume.[6]

Atrial natriuretic peptide (ANP) and brain natriuretic peptide (BNP), which may be altered by exercise,[1] also elicit a natriuretic effect. ANP increase is transitory in response to exercise of extended duration, with hormonal values returning to resting levels over time.[7] Sodium intake may affect the ANP response to exercise; the ANP increase is higher with a high-sodium diet (300 mmol/day) than in the same subjects with a low-sodium regimen (40 mmol/day).[8] BNP response to exercise is modulated by sodium intake and hydration status.[1] In several study protocols, BNP levels increased in hypertensive subjects during exercise but no changes occurred in normal subjects.[9,10]

The RAA system is closely coupled and responds to exercise. Increased values of plasma renin activity (PRA) are reported after maximal exercise.[1] The increase in PRA occurs at submaximal workloads of 60% to 70%. With the increase in PRA during exercise, there is a concomitant increase in angiotensin II, which partially mediates the increase in circulating aldosterone concentrations.[1] Elevated levels of aldosterone may persist for days after the end of exercise, depending on water and sodium intake.[1] The primary activator of the RAA system during exercise is the sympathetic nervous system. Release of renin is modulated by changes in renal sympathetic nerve activity that increase local norepinephrine levels.[11] During exercise, increased renin activity correlates with increased norepinephrine concentration in the renal vein.[11] The increase in aldosterone with exercise is assumed to be mediated by the increase in angiotensin II in response to activation of the RAA system. However, inhibition of angiotensin-converting enzyme does not attenuate the increase in aldosterone with maximal exercise in healthy subjects.[12] Other factors involved in the activation of aldosterone production include sodium intake, potassium balance, and levels of adrenocorticotropic hormone (ACTH). The persistent increase in aldosterone long after exercise ceases may be associated with reductions in plasma osmolality and sodium concentrations due to ingestion of water to replace total body water losses.[1] In this way, the interaction of a number of regulating factors is involved in mediating the response of aldosterone.

Hypothalamic-Pituitary-Adrenal Axis

Glucocorticoids

Since the pioneering studies of Davies and Few, it has been known that exercise of an appropriate intensity is a potent stimulus for cortisol secretion.[13] Glucocorticoids exert many beneficial effects in exercising humans, increasing the availability of metabolic substrates to supply energy for muscles, maintaining normal vascular integrity and responsiveness, and protecting the organism from an overreaction of the immune system in the face of exercise-induced muscle damage.[14]

During acute (short-term) exercise, the hypothalamic-pituitary-adrenal (HPA) axis responds to numerous stimuli, demonstrating the regulatory and integrative functions of the HPA axis. These stimuli include neuronal homeostatic signals (i.e., chemoreceptor, baroreceptor, and osmoreceptor stimulation), circulating homeostatic signals (e.g., glucose, leptin, ANP), and inflammatory signals such as interleukin-1 (IL-1), IL-6, and tumor necrosis factor-α (TNF-α).[15]

In humans, physical exercise has a greater effect on ACTH and cortisol secretion than can be accounted for by corticotropin-releasing hormone (CRH) alone. Exercise is accompanied by increased AVP release into the systemic circulation, which occurs in proportion to the intensity of the exercise. In humans, pulses of ACTH and AVP secretion are concordant during exercise.[16]

Cortisol response depends on the relative exercise workload for both aerobic and strength exercise, and the rise in plasma cortisol levels is associated with an increase in ACTH concentrations.[17] Moderate- to high-intensity exercise—60% and 80% of maximum oxygen consumption ($\dot{V}O_2max$), respectively—has been shown to provoke increases in circulating cortisol levels, which seemed to result from a combination of hemoconcentration and HPA axis stimulus (i.e., ACTH). In contrast, low-intensity exercise (40%) did not result in significant increases in cortisol levels.[18]

Prolonged submaximal physical activity and very brief high-intensity exercise can activate the HPA axis.[19,20] Duration of physical activity may be important in determining the response of plasma cortisol to exercise. Plasma cortisol increases more after a 42-km kayak race than after a 19-km race.[21] During a 6-day Nordic ski race, plasma ACTH levels increased and then remained at similar levels throughout the race, whereas the plasma cortisol concentration was highest during the initial 2 days.[22]

The type of exercise influences the cortisol response. In contrast to sustained aerobic activity, intermittent exercise of varying intensities, such as in match-play tennis, does not appear to induce activation of the HPA axis.[23] Isometric exercise activates the HPA axis in an intensity-dependent manner.[24] Anaerobic exercise induces a greater increase in plasma cortisol than aerobic exercise with the same total work output.[25]

Response of the HPA axis to physical activity is independent of age. In elderly men, the cortisol response to heavy-resistance exercise is diminished,[26] although a reduced effort may be involved. Earlier activation of the HPA axis, accompanied by a more pronounced increase in the activity of the sympathetic nervous system, has been demonstrated in elderly subjects during submaximal aerobic exercise.[27] However, no significant difference in cortisol response to aerobic exercise at the same relative intensity has been observed in young and elderly subjects.[28]

Gender does not affect cortisol response to physical activity. Although men show predominantly increased autonomic, cardiovascular, and carbohydrate oxidation counterregulatory responses to exercise and women have predominantly increased lipolytic and ketogenic responses, plasma cortisol levels respond similarly in men and women.[29]

Compared with sedentary women, amenorrheic athletic women and athletic women with regular menstrual cycles have blunted cortisol responses to CRH.[30] Female sex steroids may play a crucial role in mediating the adrenocortical response to external stimulation; estradiol may impair the glucocorticoid receptor–mediated, slow, negative feedback. A reduction in free cortisol levels after physical exercise was demonstrated in women who used an estrogen-containing contraceptive, compared with women who did not.[31] Kirschbaum and coworkers[32] found that short-term estradiol administration resulted in hyperresponsiveness of the HPA axis to a standardized psychosocial stress task in healthy men. Altogether, estrogens are potent regulators of the HPA axis.[33]

Other factors modify the response of the HPA axis to physical activity. The cortisol response to exercise is modulated by hypohydration, meals, and time of day. Independent of external thermal stress, hypohydration (up to 4.8% loss of body mass) greatly amplifies the exercise-induced responses to cortisol. This enhancement probably results from an increased core temperature and cardiovascular demand caused by decreased plasma volume.[34] Meals stimulate cortisol release in humans, and exercise performed immediately after food ingestion results in a blunted cortisol response to the stimulus. The cortisol response to exercise also is significantly modulated by time of day. The incremental response of cortisol to exercise is enhanced during evening exercise compared with morning exercise.[14]

Repeated acute or chronic stress reduces the sensitivity of the rat HPA axis to glucocorticoid negative feedback.[35] Endurance training has been compared with chronic stress in humans.[36] When the HPA axis is repeatedly challenged by exercise, humans demonstrate modifications in the activity of the HPA axis, suggesting adaptation to endurance training. During the past decade, several studies have shown that HPA axis activity in resting conditions is similar in endurance-trained subjects and in healthy sedentary subjects.[33,37,38] However, when the HPA axis is challenged, endurance-trained subjects demonstrate a decreased pituitary sensitivity to the negative feedback of glucocorticoids, which explains their capacity to successfully achieve a second bout of exercise after a short rest period.[33] Different mechanisms may be involved in this adaptation. At the central nervous system level, neuropeptides and corticosteroid receptors (e.g., glucocorticoid receptors, mineralocorticoid receptors) in the brain and anterior pituitary play a major role in the regulation of circulating cortisol levels. At the peripheral level, tissue sensitivity to glucocorticoids may be different in endurance-trained and sedentary subjects.[39] These adaptation processes are finalized to protect the body from the severe metabolic and immune consequences of increased cortisol levels.

Mineralocorticoids

The RAA system components are closely coupled and respond to exercise. PRA values increase after maximal exercise.[1] Progressively higher increases in aldosterone levels have been observed with increasing degrees of exertion. Increased levels of aldosterone may persist for days after the end of exercise, depending on water and sodium intake.[1]

Several regulating factors interact to mediate the response of aldosterone. They include the sympathetic nervous system, renin activity, angiotensin II levels, sodium intake, potassium balance, blood volume reductions, and levels of ACTH.[1]

Endorphins

Exercise can influence the release of β-endorphin, depending on the intensity and duration of physical activity. If a threshold intensity is exceeded, endogenous opiate levels start to increase. Incremental graded exercise tests elevate β-endorphin levels 1.5- to 7-fold. Short bouts of anaerobic exercise induce a twofold to fourfold increase in β-endorphin levels, depending on the duration of exercise stress.[40] Lactate and catecholamine concentrations are the main factors correlated with these responses. Duration of aerobic exercise seems to be an independent factor that stimulates β-endorphin release after about 1 hour if a threshold intensity—approximately 55% to 60% of $\dot{V}O_2max$—is reached.

The psychological and physiologic stresses related to competitive activities are thought to stimulate the secretion of endorphins to counter these negative effects.[41] Little is known about the influence of training status on the release of β-endorphin, and study results are often inconsistent.

Increased endogenous opiate levels in athletes may modulate pain and improve mood.[42] Sudden cessation of regular training can generate a depressed mood, which is considered to be part of the "detraining syndrome."[40] Overall, the action of endogenous opiates can be described as a reward system that makes the athlete continue physical activity.

Hypothalamic-Pituitary-Gonadal Axis

Male Gonadal Axis

The effects of physical activity on the male reproductive system vary with the intensity and duration of exercise, the fitness level of the individual, and his nutritional-metabolic status. Relatively short, intense exercise usually increases serum testosterone levels, and more prolonged exercise usually decreases these concentrations. Endurance and other forms of training can induce subclinical inhibition of normal reproductive function, although clinical expression of reproductive dysfunction with exercise is uncommon in men.[43]

Increased serum testosterone levels have been reported during relatively strenuous free and treadmill running, weight training, and ergometer cycling.[43] The testosterone response increases with increased exercise load.[44] Similar workloads produce similar responses, regardless of whether the load is aerobic or anaerobic.[25] Increased and decreased ambient temperature, altitude, and dehydration have no effect on testosterone response to intense exercise.[45,46] Acute exercise-induced testosterone increments also are seen in older men, despite their different hormonal profiles.[26]

Evidence about the gonadotropin response to exercise is inconsistent, because luteinizing hormone (LH) and follicle-stimulating hormone (FSH) levels have been reported to be unchanged, increased, or decreased by short-term strenuous exercise.[43] Because the LH response to exercise is inconsistent and because testosterone levels increase in response to exercise more quickly than in their response to LH, it is accepted that the exercise-associated increment in circulating testosterone is not mediated by LH. Possible mechanisms, such as hemoconcentration, reduced clearance, or increased testosterone synthesis, may be involved. If nonspecific mechanisms were responsible for the acute increase in serum testosterone levels, a similar increase would be expected for all circulating steroids.[43] However, timing of the testosterone increase differs from that of androstenedione and dehydroepiandrosterone,[47] suggesting that specific testicular mechanisms are involved.

In contrast to the short-term testosterone increment, suppression of serum testosterone levels occurs during and after more prolonged exercise and to some extent in the hours after intense, short-term exercise. During past decades, many investigative studies demonstrated that chronic exposure to endurance exercise training can result in a dysfunction within the reproductive-focused components of the neuroendocrine system. Most studies concentrated on women, but the effects of endurance exercise training on the male reproductive neuroendocrine system were also investigated, beginning in the 1980s.[48] Research in exercising men demonstrates the existence of a select group who, through chronic exposure to endurance exercise training, have developed alterations in their reproductive hormonal profile (i.e., persistently low basal resting testosterone concentrations).[49] Most of these men have clinically normal testosterone concentrations, but these concentrations are at the low end of the normal range or even reach subclinical status. The health consequences of such hormonal changes are increased risk of abnormal spermatogenesis, male infertility, and compromised bone mineralization.[49-51] The prevalence of these health problems seems to be low, but there have been few investigative studies examining this condition and its consequences.[49,50]

The specific terminology used to refer to this condition has not been universally accepted. In 2005, Hackney and associates proposed *the exercise-hypogonadal male* as a label for this condition.[52]

A variety of systems may influence the decrease in testosterone synthesis during and after prolonged exercise. Exercise-hypogonadal men frequently display a lack of significant elevation in basal LH that corresponds with the reduced testosterone concentration, reflecting hypogonadotropic-hypogonadal characteristics.[48,49,53] These LH abnormalities may involve disparities in LH pulsatility (i.e., pulse frequency and amplitude), although evidence for altered LH pulsatile release is inconsistent.[54] Moreover, the gonadotropin response to gonadotropin-releasing hormone (GnRH) may be reduced or increased after prolonged, exhaustive exercise.[55]

Exercise-hypogonadal men have altered basal prolactin levels.[49] At excessively low or high circulating levels, prolactin suppresses testosterone levels in men.[56] It has been speculated that the absence of prolactin at the testicle alters the ability of LH to stimulate testosterone production. This theory is based on the proposed synergistic effects of prolactin on testicular LH receptors.[48] However, not all investigators reporting low resting testosterone levels in endurance-trained men have reported the concomitant existence of low resting prolactin levels.[56] Some studies have focused on a potential relationship between high prolactin levels and low testosterone concentrations, speculating that any "stressful" situation may provoke disproportionate prolactin responses in exercise-hypogonadal men and that this may ultimately promote a reproductive axis disruption.[57]

Leptin is an adipocyte-released hormone associated in part with communicating hypothalamic satiety and the status of energy reserves.[58] It is also linked to reproductive function in women and men. Acute and chronic exercise can affect resting leptin concentrations, independent of changes in body adiposity.[59] However, no studies have examined whether leptin concentrations are altered in exercise-hypogonadal men.

Ghrelin is another hormone associated with appetite regulation. Emerging evidence from animal and human experiments suggests that ghrelin may function as a metabolic modulator of the gonadotropic axis, with predominant inhibitory effects in line with its role as a signal of energy deficit.[60,61] Acute and chronic exercise can influence ghrelin concentration levels.[62] However, no studies have examined whether ghrelin levels in exercise-hypogonadal men are normal.

Investigations of peripheral mechanisms have focused on alterations in the testicular ability to produce and secrete testosterone and to respond to exogenous stimuli (i.e., LH or human chorionic gonadotropin [hCG]). Animal studies have demonstrated that exercise training compromises testicular enzymatic activity,[63] but data for exercise-hypogonadal men are contradictory. Some investigations suggest that testicular steroidogenesis is normal, whereas others indicate it is marginally impaired when challenged with exogenous stimuli.[49]

Cortisol is another potentially disruptive hormone for the gonadal axis. Cumming and associates[64] demonstrated that the direct infusion of cortisol in men resulted in concurrent declines in testosterone levels. However, among the hormonal profile studies reporting the existence of low testosterone in trained men, none has reported elevated resting cortisol levels.[48,65,66] The role of cortisol in the gonadal axis changes observed in trained men requires further study.

Female Gonadal Axis

The endocrine equilibrium that regulates female reproductive function can be affected by physical and psychological factors. Women who engage in regular, high-intensity exercise may be at risk for menstrual disturbances such as delayed menarche, oligomenorrhea, amenorrhea, and luteal-phase defects.[67] Impaired production of gonadotropins, which leads to luteal-phase deficiency and anovulation, is a common hormonal finding in women with exercise-induced menstrual disturbances, but several other hormones may also show significant alterations.[68]

Although factors such as the physical or psychological stress of competition have been postulated to underlie exercise-induced reproductive disorders, accumulated evidence indicates that negative energy balance is the primary cause of the impairment of normal reproductive function commonly observed in female athletes.[69-72] In 1939, Hans Selye reported that "the ovaries undergo atrophy and more or less permanent anestrus ensues" when young female rats are forced to exercise for prolonged periods.[73] Selye observed a *general adaptation syndrome* that involved hypertrophy of the adrenal glands, cessation of growth and lactation, liver shrinkage, loss of muscular tone, decreased body temperature, and disappearance of adipose tissue.[74] In 1980, Warren was the first to suggest that menstrual cycles in dancers are disrupted by an "energy drain."[69] In 1984, Winterer and colleagues hypothesized that a lack of sufficient metabolic fuels to meet the energy requirements of the brain causes an alteration in brain function that disrupts the GnRH pulse generator, through an unknown mechanism.[75] The energy availability hypothesis was supported by endocrine observations of athletes. Amenorrheic athletes have low 24-hour blood glucose levels, low 24-hour insulin levels, and high 24-hour levels of insulin-like growth factor–binding protein 1 (IGFBP1),[76] as well as loss of the leptin diurnal rhythm[77] and low T3 levels in the morning.[78] Loucks and coworkers[70] found that low energy availability reduced LH pulse frequency and increased LH pulse amplitude and that exercise stress had no suppressive effect on LH pulsatility beyond the impact of the energy cost of exercise on energy availability. LH pulsatility was disrupted regardless of whether energy availability was reduced by extreme energy restriction alone, by extreme exercise energy expenditure alone, or by a combination of moderate dietary energy restriction and moderate exercise energy expenditure. Dietary supplementation prevented the suppression of LH pulsatility by exercise energy expenditure. Later experiments on female monkeys induced amenorrhea by increasing the volume of exercise training without increasing dietary energy intake[79] and then restored ovulation by increasing dietary energy intake without moderating the exercise regimen.[80]

To investigate the dose-response relationship between energy availability and LH pulsatility in exercising women, Loucks and associates[81] administered balanced energy intake or one of three low-energy availabilities (45 and 10, 20, or 30 kcal/kg fat-free mass [FFM] per day, respectively) to healthy, habitually sedentary, regularly menstruating, older adolescent women for 5 days. LH pulsatility was disrupted only with energy availabilities below 30 kcal/kg FFM per day. This finding was consistent with the results of many studies of amenorrheic runners, all of which indicated disruption at energy availabilities of less than 30 kcal/kg FFM per day.[82] Only one prospective study showed that refeeding of amenorrheic runners restored menstrual cycles by increasing energy availability from 25 to 31 kcal/kg FFM per day.[83]

The discovery of leptin in 1994 was fundamental in clarifying the relationship between negative energy balance and reproductive dysfunction.[84] Various data sets suggest that leptin may provide the central nervous system with information on the critical amount of adipose tissue stores necessary for GnRH secretion and pubertal activation of the hypothalamic-pituitary-gonadal axis. Several unfavorable metabolic situations are associated with low levels of plasma leptin, increased secretion of hypothalamic neuropeptide Y (NPY), and hypogonadism, and a causal relationship has been suggested. Severe dietary restriction in juvenile female rats is associated with low plasma leptin concentrations and sexual immaturity. Cessation of food restriction leads to an immediate increase in plasma leptin levels followed by sexual maturation.[85] Leptin administration for the relative leptin deficiency in women with hypothalamic amenorrhea improves reproductive, thyroid, and growth hormone (GH) axes and markers of bone formation, confirming that leptin is required for normal reproductive and neuroendocrine function.[86,87]

HPA axis activation may be involved in the functional disruption of the gonadal axis during physical exercise. The so-called stress hypothesis proposes that exercise activates the HPA axis, which disrupts the GnRH pulse generator by another, unknown mechanism. Central and peripheral factors may be involved in this dysregulation. Amenorrheic athletes may have mildly elevated cortisol levels,[76,88] and this observation is the basis for attributing their amenorrhea to stress. Mild hypercortisolism is also associated with amenorrhea in patients with functional hypothalamic amenorrhea and anorexia nervosa.[89] However, because cortisol is a glucoregulatory hormone activated by low blood glucose levels, the mild hypercortisolism observed in amenorrheic athletes may reflect a chronic energy deficiency rather than exercise-induced stress.[90]

Some investigators think that endogenous opioid peptides and catecholestrogens are involved in provoking menstrual irregularities in women athletes.[91] In basal circumstances, β-endorphin may decrease LH levels by suppressing hypothalamic GnRH; some catecholestrogens may suppress LH levels, and others seem to potentiate and induce an LH surge. The activities of β-endorphin and catecholestrogens depend on a sufficiently estrogenic environment. Endogenous opioid peptides and some of the catecholestrogens can suppress prolactin release, probably by interfering with its inhibiting factor dopamine. Increased plasma concentrations of β-endorphin, which are found after physical exercise, suggest their involvement in the common menstrual irregularities of women athletes.[91]

Circulating levels of testosterone, dehydroepiandrosterone, dehydroepiandrosterone sulfate, estradiol, GH, and cortisol increase in women in response to an acute bout of endurance exercise. However, only GH, estradiol, and cortisol increase after resistance exercise.[92]

Hyperandrogenism has been suggested as an alternative mechanism underlying oligomenorrhea or amenorrhea in some female athletes with menstrual disturbances.[93] Sports that emphasize strength over leanness, such as swimming and rowing, are not associated with low weight and restrictive eating patterns, but athletes engaged in these sports are vulnerable to menstrual irregularities. The endocrine profile of athletes engaged in these sports is characterized by mildly elevated LH levels, elevated LH/FSH ratios, and mild hyperandrogenism rather than hypoestrogenism. Hyperandrogenic female athletes have a more anabolic body composition and higher $\dot{V}O_2max$ and performance values compared with female athletes with menstrual disturbances but normal androgen concentrations.[93]

Prolactin

Blood prolactin levels transiently increase during exercise, and this response appears proportional to exercise intensity.[2,56] Provided the intensity is adequate, the increase in prolactin is quite rapid. Nonetheless, short-term, graded exercise may result in a peak hormonal response after the exercise ends. In some situations, excessive emotional stress can cause an anticipatory increase in prolactin levels even before exercise begins.[94]

During prolonged exercise, the prolactin response is proportional to the intensity at which exercise is performed. However, extending the duration of exercise can augment the magnitude of the prolactin response.[95]

The chronic effects of exercise training on basal, resting prolactin levels are unclear and need further research.

Some studies have found increases in resting levels, but others have found decreased levels.[48,57] These contradictions reflect differences in training protocols (i.e., intensity, frequency, and duration of training sessions). McMurray and Hackney showed that the prolactin response to submaximal exercise in men was attenuated after training, but the maximal exercise response was augmented.[94] In men and women who have undergone a training program, the drug-stimulated prolactin response is enhanced.[65,96]

The mechanisms of prolactin increase with exercise are unclear. Prolactin levels may increase when the anaerobic threshold is reached, perhaps concomitantly with a GH increase.[97] Even prolonged (i.e., 90 minutes) exercise below this threshold fails to elicit a response.[98] Prolactin increments with exercise appear to be correlated with proopiomelanocortin derivatives, ACTH, and β-endorphins.[99] Moreover, increased prolactin levels can be related to changes in body temperature and dehydration, are exaggerated by stress, are reduced with habituation and hypoxia, and are unresponsive to metabolic events.[2,100]

Growth Hormone and Insulin-Like Growth Factor I Axis

In 1963, Roth and colleagues[101] demonstrated that plasma levels of GH increase during exercise, and it was later shown that exercise is the most potent physiologic stimulus to GH release.[102] The GH response to exercise depends on the duration and intensity of exercise, the fitness level of the exercising subject, the refractoriness of pituitary somatotroph cells to the exercise stimuli, and other environmental factors.[103-105]

Lactate and nitric oxide may provide afferent stimulation for the exercise-induced GH response.[106] Several investigators have demonstrated that circulating GH levels increase above the lactate/anaerobic threshold (LAT) but not below it.[103] In other reports, loads of 75% to 90% of maximal aerobic power yielded a greater GH rise than milder loads.[102] Pritzlaff and coworkers[107] carried out tests at five exercise intensities normalized to each subject's lactate threshold. A linear dose-response relationship between exercise intensity and the GH secretory response was demonstrated, with escalating GH release across the range of exercise intensities (25% to 175% of the lactate threshold). Deconvolution analysis revealed that increased GH levels resulted from an increase in the mass of GH secreted per pulse, with no change in pulse frequency or the half-life of elimination. Later studies by the same group demonstrated that GH secretion positively correlated with the duration of exercise when intensity remained constant,[108] was augmented by repetitive bouts of exercise,[109] but was not influenced by the time of day that exercise was performed.[38]

Given the influence of intensity of exercise, few studies have investigated the effect of duration of exercise on the GH response, although longer duration of exercise was found to increase the GH response.[110] The exercise duration should be at least 10 minutes,[111] because exercise of shorter duration below and above the lactate threshold was not accompanied by increases in circulating GH levels.[103] The exercise-induced GH peak occurs 25 to 30 minutes after the start of exercise, regardless of exercise duration.[103,112] When the task is brief, a peak may be reached after its cessation, but when the task is long (e.g., 45 minutes), the GH peak occurs while the individual is still exercising.[104,113]

The interaction between duration and intensity of exercise influences GH responses to endurance-type exercise. Short-duration, high-intensity exertion (e.g., 7 minutes of rowing races for Olympic athletes) provoked remarkable GH responses.[114]

The nature of the exercise may also influence the GH response. Whereas continuous exercise protocols may be comparable to competition events, the endurance-type training undertaken by many athletes involves intermittent or interval exertion. Comparing exercise at equivalent total workloads, GH levels are lower with continuous exercise (40% to 45% of $\dot{V}O_2max$) than with interval protocols, with twice the work rate for one half of the time, reflecting the greater metabolic stress and lactate levels in the latter situation.[115] Incremental GH responses also have been described for resistance exercise.[116] The important determinants appear to be the relationship between load and frequency of individual repetitions. Greater GH increments have been reported after so-called hypertrophy protocols (i.e., moderate loads and high number of repetitions) than after strength protocols (i.e., heavy loads and low repetitions) in both men and women.[110]

There is conflicting evidence regarding the neuroendocrine pathways that regulate GH secretion during exercise. Mechanisms involving cholinergic, serotoninergic, α-adrenergic, dopaminergic, and opioidergic pathways have been proposed.[2,117,118] There may be interactions among the pathways, and they may operate at different exercise intensities.

In young men and boys, regular but not sporadic exercise is associated with higher GH production, and it augments GH release by GHRH.[109] This effect may be caused by decreased hypothalamic somatostatinergic activity and higher growth hormone pulsatility.

Fluid intake influences exercise-induced GH release. The increased rate of sweating during physical activity performed without water ingestion results in dehydration and lower GH response to exercise.[119]

Environmental elements, nutritional factors, and some pathologic states may interfere with the GH response to exercise. Cappon and associates[120] showed that a high-fat meal inhibits the magnitude of GH response to exercise, and inhibition of the exercise-induced GH response is correlated with circulating levels of somatostatin.

High ambient temperature alone may increase circulating GH levels,[121] whereas low temperature attenuates GH release.[122] Obesity and polycystic ovarian syndrome are characterized by attenuated GH response to exercise.[123]

Gender governs the relationship between exercise intensity and GH release. For each incremental increase in exercise intensity, the fractional stimulation of GH secretion is greater in women than in men. Moreover, women have greater basal (nonpulsatile) GH secretion across all conditions, more frequent GH secretory pulses, a greater GH secretory pulse amplitude, a greater production rate, and a trend for a greater mass of GH secreted per pulse than men.[124] The more intense GH secretion in women is related to estrogens. Oral and transdermal estrogen administration increase GH release in postmenopausal women,[125] and younger women receiving oral contraceptive therapy exhibit greater GH responses to exercise than nontreated women.[126]

The GH response to exercise (e.g., the 24-hour GH secretion rate) declines with age.[118] Even those in early middle age (mean age, 42 years) had greatly attenuated GH responses to exhaustive exercise compared with younger subjects (mean age, 21 years).[127] However, it is difficult to separate the effects of aging from changes in body composition, because body fat increases with age, and GH secretory rates are reduced in overweight subjects.[128]

Kelley and colleagues[129] found a significant positive correlation between $\dot{V}O_2$max and circulating levels of GH and IGF type 1 in healthy premenopausal and postmenopausal women. They found that $\dot{V}O_2$max and IGF1 concentrations decline with age. However, when the influence of age and fitness was analyzed using multiple regression, $\dot{V}O_2$max remained the only independent predictor of IGF1 concentrations. The investigators concluded that the decrease in serum IGF1 levels with age is not related directly to aging but probably to an age-related decline in physical activity and fitness.

Exercise exerts acute effects on other components of the GH/IGF1 axis. The effect of exercise on circulating IGF1 has been examined by several investigators with differing results. Wilson and Horowitz[130] reported no increase in serum IGF1 levels in children after 15 minutes of a cycle ergometer exercise protocol. Hagberg and coworkers[131] did not find an increase in IGF1 levels after 60 minutes of treadmill exercise at 70% of subjects' $\dot{V}O_2$max in young and old adults. Moreover, the effect of exercise on IGF1 appears to depend on the type of exercise performed.[104] Schwarz and coworkers[132] showed that IGF1 increases after 10 minutes of exercise both below and above the LAT. This study suggested that the increase in IGF1 accompanying exercise is not related to GH.

The transient nature of IGF increases suggests that hemodynamic or metabolic effects of exercise may play a role. Exercise in humans is accompanied by the rapid "hemotransfusion" of hemoconcentrated blood from the spleen into the circulation by increased blood flow to the exercising muscle and by loss of plasma water. These phenomena may explain in part an increased IGF concentration by changes in IGF flux or volume of distribution.

Longer periods of exercise training stimulate *IGF1* gene expression in both central neuroendocrine and local tissue components of the GH/IGF1 system. Zanconato and associates[133] found that 4 weeks of endurance training by young rats increased hepatic and muscle *IGF1* gene expression and muscle IGF1 protein levels. Eliakim and coworkers[134] showed that muscle IGF1 protein concentrations in rats increased with endurance training, despite lack of change in muscle IGF1 mRNA or serum IGF1 levels.

Few studies have investigated the response of insulin-like growth factor–binding proteins (IGFBPs) to exercise. IGFBP1 levels did not to change during 30 minutes of moderate exercise,[110] but increased transiently after short-term exercise.[135] The physiologic role of the postexercise increase in IGFBP1, given the IGFBP1 inhibition of IGF1's metabolic actions, may be to prevent late hypoglicemia.[135]

Schwarz and colleagus[132] demonstrated that IGFBP3 levels increased with low- and high-intensity exercise and that high-intensity exercise increased IGFBP3 proteolysis. A transient increase in IGFBP3 levels in response to short-term exercise was confirmed by Wallace and coworkers,[135] who described an immediate increase of all components of the ternary complex: IGF1, IGFBP3, and the acid-labile subunit (ALS) of the IGF-binding protein complex.

Eliakim and associates[136] correlated functional and structural indices of fitness with mean overnight GH levels, growth hormone–binding protein (GHBP), and serum IGF1 levels in late-pubertal adolescent girls. Moreover, thigh muscle volume was inversely correlated with IGFBP2 and IGFBP4.

Wallace and colleagues described an acute increase in serum GHBP in response to short-term exercise.[135] In a person at rest, GHBP dampens GH oscillation, and the study authors speculated that the postexercise increase in GHBP levels may prolong the GH signal, increasing the GH-mediated signal for postexercise protein synthesis, tissue repair, and muscle glycogen replenishment. The increment in the serum GHBP concentration may represent increased synthesis by the liver or reduced clearance.[135]

Hypothalamic-Pituitary-Thyroid Axis

Exercise has effects on thyroid function, which can be viewed as an adaptive mechanism associated with enhanced performance, possibly providing a better balance between energy consumption and expenditure. Short-term, incremental exercise (≥20 minutes) increases blood thyroid-stimulating hormone (TSH) levels, with a critical intensity threshold of approximately 50% or more of maximal oxygen uptake ($\dot{V}O_2$max) necessary to induce significant changes.[94,137] Even when the TSH level is elevated, most research involving short-term exercise indicates total and free thyroxine (T_4) and triiodothyronine (T_3) are not immediately affected.[94] On the other hand, total T_4 and T_3 levels can increase after short-term exercise, although these findings are primarily linked to exercise-induced hemoconcentration.[138]

The influence of prolonged, submaximal exercise (approaching 60 minutes) on thyroid hormones is controversial. Some investigations have found no effect on blood TSH levels,[94,137] whereas others have reported that TSH, free T_3 (fT_3), or both increase progressively with high-intensity, steady-state workloads.[139] Conversely, Hackney and Gulledge[140] found total T_3 was unchanged but that total T_4 was increased by 60 minutes into a prolonged, steady-state, submaximal exercise session. However, Galbo[137] reported highly strenuous, prolonged exercise to exhaustion increased only circulating fT_4 levels. Some investigators reported that repeated days of stressful, demanding physical activity substantially reduced T_4, T_3, and TSH levels.[94] These divergent findings are difficult to interpret because of the different durations and intensities of exercise and the various blood sampling protocols employed.[141]

The effects of chronic exercise on thyroid hormone parameters have been studied in endurance athletes, with conflicting results about whether baseline hormonal levels are shifted in well-trained athletes. Regular bicycle ergometry training in recreational athletes over 6 weeks did not change the TSH or TSH response to TRH stimulation.[142] Other studies indicate that intensive anaerobic exercise (e.g., cycling interval training) increases total T_4 levels for several hours after the exercise but do not affect T_3.[94,140] These changes appear not to depend on hemoconcentration alone, but to what extent they result from increased T_4 secretion versus a suppressed metabolic clearance rate is unclear.[141] Research is sparse on the effects of resistance exercise, which tends to be anaerobic in nature, on the thyroid.

Several procedural limitations exist in many exercise studies. In some situations, influential factors such as environment, dietary practices, and diurnal hormonal secretion patterns are not controlled effectively and therefore cannot be separated from the influence of exercise alone.[141] For example, variations in ambient temperature appear to alter the thyroid hormone response to exercise. TSH and fT_4 levels rose in swimmers exercising in cold (22° C) water, were unchanged at 26° C, and fell at warm (32° C) water temperatures.[143]

Energy balance plays an important role in the body's thyroid hormone response to exercise. Loucks and coworkers[144] found a decrease in T_3 and fT_3, along with an increase in reverse T_3 (rT_3) in healthy women undergoing aerobic exercise testing with low caloric intake. This low-T_3 syndrome was not seen in individuals receiving a higher caloric diet. Even mild energy deficiencies may influence thyroid hormone levels. Female gymnasts with borderline energy deficit had a decrease in T_3 and increase in T_4 levels during 3 days of heavy workouts.[145] Energy balance has also been investigated in women runners. Those with negative energy balance had a decrease in T_3 and fT_3 but had an increase in rT_3 levels.[144]

Overall, exercise-induced thyroid function changes are influenced by many factors. In various studies, TSH, T_4, fT_4, T_3, and fT_3 levels have been unaffected, increased, or decreased, depending on the type and duration of exercise, ambient temperature, and energy intake. One of the more consistent findings is an increase in rT_3, particularly when a caloric energy deficiency is associated with exercise.

Insulin and Glucose Metabolism

Physical activity affects the metabolism of glucose and other intermediate substrates in normal persons and in those with diabetes mellitus.[146] The effects of exercise on carbohydrate metabolism are complex and involve type, intensity, and duration of exercise; changes in body composition; alterations in other behaviors, such as food intake; degree of insulin deficiency; and the time course of the glucose-insulin response.[147]

During moderate exercise, insulin levels remain unchanged over the first 40 to 60 minutes of exercise. More prolonged or strenuous exercise causes a decline in insulin levels.[148] Counterregulatory hormones, such as catecholamines, glucagon, GH, and cortisol, tend to increase, inducing hepatic glycogenolysis, gluconeogenesis, and lipolysis to provide increased free fatty acids for use as a metabolic fuel.

During short-term, strenuous exercise, when levels of the counterregulatory hormones increase, glucose levels may be elevated transiently. After exercise, insulin levels may rapidly return to baseline. Glucose uptake by exercising muscles is remarkably increased due an increase in blood flow to the muscle during activity, in the number of insulin receptors, and in the number and intrinsic activity of glucose transporter proteins in the plasma membrane of skeletal muscle.[149] The muscle glucose uptake, which is not directly mediated by insulin, requires at least basal levels of insulin.[150] Increased insulin availability above basal levels has little effect on glucose transport, and the supply of glucose to the muscle is maintained during exercise despite decreased insulin levels.

Insulin also plays a role in controlling the sensitivity of hepatic glucose production.[151] Changes in insulin and glucose levels are needed for optimal activity to occur.[2]

Glucagon levels increase during strenuous exercise, whereas the response varies at lesser intensities.[2] During prolonged, mild-intensity exercise by healthy persons, the rise in glucagon is essential for increased hepatic glucose production and increased gluconeogenesis.[152] Decreasing blood glucose levels stimulate glucagon, and the glucagon response usually is blunted by preloading with glucose. Levels of glucagon usually correspond significantly with epinephrine and norepinephrine levels, although the sympathoadrenal system seems to be more important in maintaining euglycemia and enhanced hepatic production of glucose.[153]

In normal individuals, major alterations in blood glucose levels usually do not occur, despite the increase in glucose use by skeletal muscle. With the onset of activity, activation of the α-adrenergic system inhibits insulin release from the pancreas. This results in an increased rate of lipolysis in the periphery and stimulation of hepatic glucose output. As glucose levels begin to fall, glucagon levels rise, further stimulating hepatic glucose output. As the plasma glucose concentration drops toward hypoglycemic levels, epinephrine is released, further stimulating hepatic glucose production and increasing lipolysis in the periphery. The increased availability of free fatty acids for muscle metabolism helps to restrain the rate of glucose use. When one of these mechanisms fails, the others can largely compensate, avoiding hypoglycemia.[147]

Training reduces basal insulin levels and exercise-associated changes in glucagon and insulin levels. Training increases insulin sensitivity at rest and in response to a glucose load, and it reduces the rate of insulin decline during short-term exercise.[2,154]

Regular exercise has become an integral part of the treatment recommendations for type 2 diabetic patients, because it improves insulin sensitivity and reduces average blood glucose concentrations.[155] Physical training increases insulin-stimulated glucose disposal and improves glucose control in type 2 diabetes. However, the increase in insulin sensitivity is rapidly lost if exercise is not performed on a regular basis. Exercise also may be effective in delaying or preventing the development of type 2 diabetes.[155]

USE OF PERFORMANCE-ENHANCING HORMONES

Anabolic Steroids

Anabolic-androgenic steroids (AASs) are chemically modified analogues of testosterone. First isolated in 1935, AASs have been modified many times to maximize the anabolic effects of the drug and to minimize the androgenic effects by alkylation of the 17α position or carboxylation of the 17β-hydroxyl group on the sterol D ring. These analogues are degraded much more slowly than endogenous testosterone, resulting in a higher prolonged concentration of the analogue.[156,157] The AASs used for nontherapeutic purposes are endogenous androgens (e.g., androstenedione, dehydroepiandrosterone [DHEA]); 17-esters of testosterone (e.g., cypionate, enanthate, heptylate, propionate, undecanoate, bucyclate); 17α-alkyl derivatives of testosterone (e.g., methyltestosterone, fluoxymesterone, oxandrolone, stanozolol); 19-nortestosterone (e.g., nandrolone); 17β-esters of 19-nortestosterone (e.g., decanoate, phenylpropionate); 19-norandrostenedione and 19-norandrostenediol; and tetrahydrogestrinone. More than 100 different AASs have been developed, with most of them being used illegally, synthesized in clandestine laboratories, commercialized without medical prescription or safety controls, and sometimes unknown to the scientific world (Table 26-1).[157]

AASs have been used in sports for more than 50 years and represent the class of substances most frequently detected in human sports doping control analyses.[158] Although their use is most common among weight lifters and heavy throwers, almost all types of athletes whose event requires explosive strength, including football players, swimmers, and track and field athletes, have been known to use steroids. Steroid hormones or synthetic analogues of steroid hormones promote tissue growth and masculinization; the androgenic compounds are widely used to enhance lean body mass and to improve sport performance. The anabolic-androgenic activity of each

TABLE 26-1

Performance-Enhancing Hormones

Anabolic Androgenic Steroids
17β-Esters of testosterone (cypionate, enanthate, heptylate, propionate, oxandrolone, bucyclate)
17α-Alkyl derivatives of testosterone (methyltestosterone, fluoxymesterone, oxadroline, stanozolol)
19-Nortestosterone (nandrolone)
17β-Esters of 19-nortestosterone (decanoate, phenpropionate)
19-Norandrostenedione
19-Norandrostenediol
Tetrahydrogestrinone
Peptide Hormones
Growth hormone
Insulin-like growth factor I
Insulin
Erythropoietin

steroid compound is a function of its chemical structure and metabolites, and its activity can vary considerably. These drugs may act by binding with androgen and glucocorticoid receptors, by exerting central and peripheral effects on neurotransmitters, and by interacting with IGF1 or its binding proteins in the circulation or in the muscles.[157]

Surveys of AAS abuse by gymnasia users in the United Kingdom found that about 5% were using these drugs, whereas among people attending gyms equipped for competitive bodybuilding, the proportion of current or previous users was between 25% and 50%.[159,160] Similar surveys indicate a high prevalence of use in the United States.[161] Current estimates indicate that there are as many as 3 million AAS users in the United States and that 2.7% to 2.9% of U.S. young adults have taken an AAS at least once in their lives.[162] Two thirds of AAS users are noncompetitive recreational body builders or nonathletes, who use these drugs for cosmetic purposes rather than to enhance sports performance.[157,163,164]

During the past decade, careful scientific study of supra-pharmacologic doses supports the anabolic efficacy of AAS regimens. Medical use of AAS for the treatment of hypogonadal men, age-related sarcopenia, and HIV-related muscle wasting has gained interest.[163,165]

The positive effects of steroids on body composition include increased FFM, decreased total body fat, and a decrease in the percentage of body fat located in the gluteal, femoral, and triceps regions in women.[164,166] The effects of anabolic steroids on lipolysis and skeletal muscle mass are potentiated by caloric restriction[166] and mechanical loading.[167]

Skeletal muscle is a primary target tissue for the anabolic effects of AAS. The action of AAS in stimulating growth of skeletal muscles in subjects with low circulating testosterone levels, such as women and children, is undisputed. However, an early and comprehensive review of previous results concluded that there was little evidence for supraphysiologic doses of testosterone or synthetic AAS having any appreciable effect on muscle size or strength in healthy men.[168] Even so, many of the studies reviewed lacked adequate controls and standardization. Conclusions from later reviews suggested that the administration of AASs could consistently result in significant increases in strength if male athletes satisfied certain criteria, including the timing of doses and dietary factors.[169,170] In 1996, Bhasin and associates[167] demonstrated that the administration of supraphysiologic doses of testosterone in combination with exercise in male weight lifters increased muscle size and strength compared with exercise alone or testosterone treatment alone (i.e., the effects of combining supraphysiologic doses of testosterone with exercise are additive). Subsequent work showed that increases in FFM, muscle size, strength, and power are highly dose dependent and correlated with serum testosterone concentrations.[171,172]

The anabolic effect of testosterone is dose dependent, and significant increases in muscle size and strength occur with doses of 300 mg per week or higher.[171,173] Muscle size increases because of hypertrophy that results from an increase in cross-sectional area in both type I and type II muscle fibers and an increase in myonuclear number.[173]

In postmenopausal women undergoing caloric restriction, administration of 30 mg of nandrolone decanoate every 2 weeks for 9 months increased FFM, decreased body fat, redistributed abdominal body fat from subcutaneous to visceral stores, and increased thigh muscle cross-sectional area compared with measurements in a control group.[166] Evidence of the effects of anabolic steroids on body fat distribution in young adult females has been accumulated from studies of women undergoing gender reassignment and women athletes. Women ingesting high doses of androgens experience a shift of body fat from a gynoid to an android distribution and a decrease of subcutaneous body fat in the abdomen, hip, and thigh regions.[174] In contrast, postmenopausal women treated with estrogens maintain a gynoid fat pattern, suggesting that fat distribution patterns are controlled by the ratio of circulating estrogens to androgens.

Investigations into the performance-enhancing effects of anabolic steroids began in the late 1960s and continued into the early 1980s. Some studies demonstrated a positive effect of steroids on strength when drug abuse was combined with resistance training, but others did not.

Since 1994, a few studies have documented the performance-enhancing effects of anabolic steroids in athletes and healthy men.[167,175] AASs have improved exercise tolerance and the adaptability of muscle to overload by protecting against muscle fiber damage and increasing the rate of protein synthesis during recovery.[176] However, several issues remain unresolved regarding the use of AASs for athletic enhancement. The minimal dose of a steroid or combination of steroids needed to produce significant increases in strength and muscle mass in healthy, resistance-trained men and women are unknown. Moreover, the theory that several different anabolic steroids used concurrently can elicit a significantly greater anabolic effect than any single drug has not been evaluated in controlled studies. It has been speculated that gains in lean mass and strength acquired while using steroids are maintained indefinitely after cessation of drug treatment, but supportive studies are lacking.[157]

The types and doses of AASs used by athletes are not easy to define, because it is difficult to obtain accurate drug-use information from athletes. In a survey conducted in Great Britain, most male anabolic steroid users reported that testosterone or nandrolone esters were the drugs of choice, whereas women preferred oxandrolone, stanozolol, and methandienone.[160] Testing by International Olympic Committee laboratories in 1993 revealed that the most commonly detected steroids were testosterone (32.5%), nandrolone (23.9%), stanozolol (11.4%), metandienone (10.7%), and methenolone preparations (7.7%).[177] Another study suggested that methyltestosterone and norethandrolone were the drugs most commonly used by athletes.[178]

The dose of AAS used by athletes varies considerably and is often thought to exceed 10 to 40 times the recommended therapeutic dose.[178] In a survey of 100 male AAS users, the drug dosages ranged from 250 to 3200 mg per week of testosterone or its equivalent.[179] Fifty percent of the AAS users in this sample reported using a weekly dose of at least 500 mg. To achieve these supraphysiologic doses, 88% of AAS users in this sample combined two or more types of AAS, a process known as *stacking*.

In most surveys, the duration of steroid administration (i.e., steroid cycle) lasts between 4 and 12 weeks.[163] The time interval between steroid cycles is more variable. Regular users allow a 4- to 6-week drug holiday, whereas less frequent users may remain drug free for months.[163] In one survey, approximately one half of the sample reported that their total annual AAS use was less than 6 months, whereas the other half used AASs for more than 6 months each year.[179] Three of the 100 AAS users surveyed admitted to continuous use of steroids for 52 weeks of the year.

The numerous side effects associated with AAS use involve multiple organ systems.[157,164,180] With the exception of the association between hepatic dysfunction and the use of some oral AASs,[181] many of the reports of serious side effects in otherwise healthy individuals have come from anecdotal case studies.[182] Confounding factors, such as undiagnosed preexisting conditions, family history, and concurrent use of other drugs, further dampen the credibility of case reports. Moreover, because most anabolic steroids are obtained on the black market and are of dubious quality, there is potential for adverse medical events to occur independent of steroid use. However, data from larger observational studies[179,183] suggest that most (88% to 96%) AAS users experience at least one minor subjective side effect, including acne (40% to 54%), testicular atrophy (40% to 51%), gynecomastia (10% to 34%), cutaneous striae (34%), and injection-site pain (36%) (Table 26-2). However, many of the adverse effects can be difficult to recognize without a thorough medical examination, and other damaging effects, such as the potential harmful changes in the cardiovascular system, are insidious and often unrecognized by the athletes themselves.[164]

Dyslipidemia and cardiovascular disease have been linked with the use of AASs. In general, the ingestion of oral C17α-alkylated anabolic steroids causes an average 30% decrease in high-density lipoprotein (HDL) cholesterol and an average 30% increase in low-density lipoprotein (LDL) cholesterol.[184] The mechanisms for this effect are unknown, but they apparently include increased activity of hepatic triglyceride lipase, which catabolizes HDL particles. Most studies indicate that injectable non–C17α-alkylated anabolic steroids, such as testosterone and nandrolone esters, exert minimal adverse effects on blood lipids.[167,184] AASs may influence platelet aggregation and the myocardium, although the relationship between these effects and cardiovascular disease is unclear.[185] Occasional reports of cardiomyopathies and arrhythmias associated with steroid use have been published, and several mechanisms have been proposed.[185] It is unclear whether the adverse changes in blood lipids as a function of testosterone use lead to an increase in the incidence of coronary artery disease.

Liver disease is a well-documented side effect of most C17α-alkylated AASs, the exception being oxandrolone. In contrast, most non–C17α-alkylated steroids exert minimal hepatotoxicity. Liver pathologies associated with anabolic steroids include cholestasis, peliosis hepatis, hepatocellular adenoma and carcinoma, and hepatic angiosarcoma and cholangiocarcinoma.[163,181]

Potential effects on the reproductive system include infertility and testicular atrophy in men and menstrual and genital tract alterations in women.[163] Although all AASs suppress the hypothalamic-pituitary axis to some extent, the resulting infertility in males usually is reversible. There are concerns about potential effects of androgens on the risk of prostrate disease. The long-term effects of supraphysiologic doses of androgens on the risk of prostrate cancer, benign prostatic hyperplasia, and lower urinary tract symptoms are unknown.[186] The effects on the prostate likely depend on the chemical structure and androgenicity of the drugs.

The effects of AAS use on fertility in women are unknown. High doses of androgens decrease circulating FSH and sex hormone–binding globulin concentrations in eugonadal women,[187] whereas no changes are observed in mean nadir and LH pulse amplitude and in circulating concentrations of estradiol, estrone, and adrenal steroids.[188]

TABLE 26-2

Side Effects of Anabolic Androgenic Steroids

Side Effects of Anabolic Androgenic Steroids
Cardiovascular
Cardiomyopathy
Lipid disorders (decreased HDL, increased LDL)
Increased platelet aggregation
Increased hematocrit
Elevated blood pressure
Cosmetic
Gynecomastia
Acne
Hair loss
Cutaneous striae
Reproductive-Endocrine
Libido changes
Subfertility
In Males
Testicular atrophy
Impaired spermatogenesis
Erectile dysfunction
Prostate diseases
In Females
Hirsutism
Breast atrophy
Voice-deepening
Virilization (clitoromegaly)
Menstrual disturbances
Hepatic
Cholestasis
Steatosis
Tumors
Hepatocellular adenoma and carcinoma
Hepatic angiosarcoma and cholangiocarcinoma
Psychological
Aggression
Mood swings
Anxiety
Psychosis
Irritability
Dependence
Withdrawal
Depression
Injection-Related
Infection
Bruising
Fibrosis
Injection site pain

HDL, high-density lipoprotein; LDL, low-density lipoprotein.

Menstruation is diminished or absent in steroid users, but ovulation may occur.[189]

All AASs may cause some degree of acne if taken in high doses.[186] This is particularly true for strong androgen preparations, which may cause severe, scarring acne.

With the exception of oxandrolone and perhaps of methenolone, if used intermittently in modest doses, AAS use by most women will cause some form of permanent virilization. The degree of virilization depends on the drug, the dose, the duration of use, and the individual response. Body composition changes during steroid use are similar to those experienced in young boys during puberty. In addition to irreversible side effects, such as deepened voice, increased terminal facial hair, and a hypertrophied clitoris, some of the hypertrophic effects of anabolic steroids on skeletal muscle in women may be permanent. Balding is common in those who use AASs that undergo 5α-reduction to potent androgens.

In some male steroid users, gynecomastia may be caused by increased circulating estrogen levels associated with the use of aromatizable androgens or hCG, or both. Decreased clearance of circulating estrogens is a result of impaired hepatic function, and a temporary state of hypotestosteronemia may occur after AAS withdrawal.[163]

Ruptured tendons have been associated with AAS use on the basis of a small number of published case reports, and it has been suggested that these drugs predispose to tendon rupture by altering collagen structure.[190] It is possible that the rapid strength adaptations produced by AASs in skeletal muscle are not simultaneously matched by slower-adapting, less-vascular tendon structures, making tendons the weakest link in the chain.

Several studies have suggested that anabolic steroid use may lead to significant psychological morbidity. Psychological pathologies associated with anabolic steroids include anxiety, psychosis, irritability, increased aggression, and antisocial and violent behavior.[191] In addition to behavioral problems, dependence, withdrawal symptoms, and depression have been reported during and after the nonmedical use of anabolic steroids.[179,192]

All known AAS can be detected by urinalysis (i.e., gas chromatography–mass spectrometry) for some period after the last dose.[193,194] The detection of these drugs depends on their chemical structures, metabolism, the form in which they were administered, pattern of dosing, and concomitant use of other drugs. Doping by testosterone can be indirectly tested by measuring the ratio of urinary testosterone to epitestosterone (T/E).[195] In normal, healthy individuals, testosterone and epitestosterone are produced in a ratio of 1 : 1. It is assumed that the urinary T/E ratio increases in athletes taking exogenous testosterone. If an athlete has a T/E of more than 4 : 1, the sample is submitted to further evaluations, such as gas chromatography–combustion–isotope ratio mass spectrometry. However, the T/E ratio is characterized by a larger inter-individual than intra-individual variability.[196] This suggests that a population-based T/E reference is not sensitive to individual variations. According to Sottas and colleagues,[196] the problem can be statistically defined as the detection of an outlier out of series of individual test results using a Bayesian analysis of the T/E ratio (i.e., comparing a value to a population-based reference range and a subject reference range).

Growth Hormone

GH has been used as a drug of abuse in sports since the early 1980s. The first scientific studies demonstrating a clearcut physiologic role for GH in adults were not published in the peer-reviewed medical literature until 1989.[197,198]

There are no well-designed scientific studies providing evidence that GH has performance-enhancing effects in normal individuals, but GH has been shown to have an important role in regulating body composition in adult humans and other species. In cattle, GH is known as a *partitioning agent*; it specifically diverts calories in food toward protein synthesis and away from fat synthesis. Animals made transgenic for GH have greatly increased lean tissues and reduced fat. Similar changes in body composition are seen in humans with acromegaly. GH-deficient adults have reduced lean body mass and increased fat mass, especially in the abdominal region. Physiologic replacement therapy with recombinant human GH (rhGH) in GH-deficient adults results in significant changes in body composition, with an average increase in lean body mass of 5 kg within the first month[198] and a comparable loss of 5 kg of fat.

GH-deficient adults have significantly reduced muscle mass, strength, and exercise performance.[199] Discontinuation of GH supplementation in patients with GH deficiency leads to a 5% reduction in isometric muscle strength and muscle size after 1 year.[200]

Investigators do not agree about whether GH replacement improves physical performance in GH-deficient patients. Exercise capacity is reported to increase in some[197,201] but not all placebo-controlled trials enrolling hypopituitary adult patients.[202] Moreover, GH replacement therapy in GH-deficient patients has been shown to increase lean body mass but not aerobic capacity,[203] whereas $\dot{V}O_2max$ was found to be significantly improved.[204,205] The mechanisms through which GH acts on exercise performance are more complex than the simple increase in lean body mass. For instance, GH stimulates erythropoiesis under various conditions[206] and exerts significant cardiovascular effects, increasing plasma volume and peripheral blood flow and enhancing left ventricular stroke volume and cardiac output.[207,208] All these factors may contribute to improved aerobic capacity. Evidence suggests that GH therapy alone, in the absence of some form of exercise program, may increase lean body mass but not functional capacity, indicating that training may have to be combined with GH replacement in these patients to increase physical performance.[203]

The only controlled studies on the effects of GH on muscle function in experienced weight lifters or power athletes have not shown a significant positive effect of GH on muscular protein biosynthesis or strength.[209-211] Only one study has demonstrated an increase in FFM and a decrease in fat mass in healthy men and women undergoing intensive exercise.[212] Two studies in obese men[213] and women[214] found that GH treatment augmented fat loss in conjunction with dietary restriction or exercise, or both.

Lange and coworkers demonstrated that rhGH combined with endurance training in healthy elderly women increased the activity of muscle oxidative enzymes compared with exercise alone.[215] GH administration for 3 to 6 months to healthy elderly individuals increased IGF1 levels to those observed in younger individuals (controls); muscle mass, skin thickness, and bone mineral content significantly increased, and fat mass decreased.[216] Physiologic doses of GH given for 6 months to healthy older men with well-preserved functional abilities have improved body composition by increasing lean tissue mass and decreasing fat mass. However, functional ability was not improved, and side effects were frequently reported.[217]

Two strategies have been proposed to detect GH doping in sports. Using the marker method, which focuses on pharmacodynamic end points of GH use, the GH-Consortium 2000 identified biochemical parameters of the IGF system, such as IGF1, IGFBP3, and ALS, as suitable markers of GH use in combination with procollagen cleavage products, which also show a clearcut increase after GH use.[218a] The combination of IGF1 and the procollagen type III amino-terminal extension peptide (PIIIP)[218] has been proposed to provide a set of markers that allow detection of GH abuse in athletes for up to 2 weeks after the last injection. During the initial phase of GH application, however, these pharmacodynamic markers are not expected to indicate GH abuse by athletes. The second method, known as the GH-isoform method,[219,220] exploits the difference in isoform composition between rhGH (which consists mostly of monomeric 22-kd hGH) and a variety of GH isoforms secreted by the pituitary, including a 20-kd form lacking 14 amino acids and amidated and acylated isoforms. After peripheral injection of 22-kd rhGH, the pituitary's production of GH isoforms is reduced by negative feedback through IGF1. Subjecting serum samples to two immunoassay analyses, one that is specific for 22-kd monomeric hGH and one that recognizes most isoforms released from the pituitary, allows calculation of an isoform ratio (Fig. 26-1). This approach for the detection of GH doping has been applied since the 2004 Olympic Games, but no case of GH doping has been declared based on this method. Both strategies may be used side by side in the future, and they may primarily have their place in unannounced sampling outside of competition. The isoform test can detect GH abuse during the first 36 hours after the last injection, and the pharmacodynamic end point method provides a longer window of opportunity.

Erythropoietin and the Erythropoietin System

Erythropoietin (EPO), a glycoprotein hormone naturally produced in the kidney and liver, is an essential growth factor for the erythrocytic progenitors in the bone marrow. Tissue hypoxia is the physiologic stimulus for EPO expression and erythropoiesis. After release, EPO stimulates an increase in hemoglobin, thereby increasing the oxygen-carrying capacity of the blood.[221]

The effects of physical exercise on circulating EPO levels have been studied in various sports, including cross-country skiing, cycling, long-distance running, and biathlon.[221] The results indicate that the level of EPO is not significantly affected by single bouts of strenuous exercise, although slight increases were occasionally observed a few hours after long-distance running.[222] Despite the lack of EPO response to short-term physical exercise, the number of reticulocytes may increase within 1 or 2 days after exercise.[223] It is likely that stress hormones such as catecholamines and cortisol stimulate the release of young red blood cells from bone marrow, and sustained training is associated with increased reticulocyte counts.[223] Hemoglobin levels and the hematocrit may nevertheless be below normal. This so-called sports anemia is a pseudoanemia, because the plasma volume is increased.[221]

Successful cloning of the human *EPO* gene[224] allowed production of recombinant human erythropoietin (rhEPO), which was later approved for treating patients with anemia. Unfortunately, some athletes and their coaches were eager to abuse rhEPO because it increases the oxygen supply to

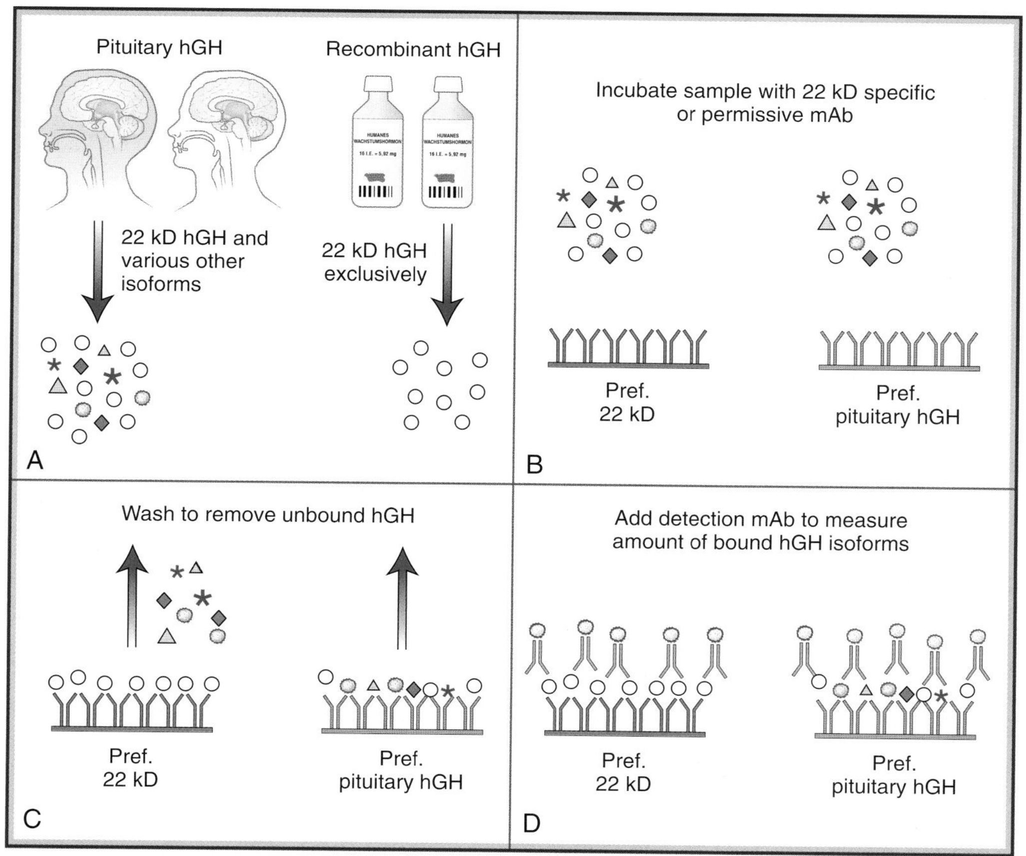

Figure 26-1 Differential immunoassays for growth hormone isoform composition. mAb, monoclonal antibody; hGH, human growth hormone.

the muscles and boosts performance in endurance sports such as skiing, running, and cycling.[225]

Because endurance athletes are particularly sensitive to the oxygen-carrying capacity of their blood, any substance that increases this capacity provides a tremendous aerobic advantage. This advantage is evidenced by the long-recognized practices of living at altitude and sleeping in altitude tents.[156] Another method of achieving this effect is through blood doping, which involves an autologous transfusion of previously donated blood after a period of hematocrit recovery or a homologous transfusion from a crossmatched donor. These transfusions artificially increase the hematocrit mass and oxygen-carrying capacity of blood.

Although few studies on the ergogenic potential of rhEPO have been done, some investigations have come to conclusions similar to those achieved in studies of blood doping. Birkeland and coworkers[226] performed a double-blind, placebo-controlled study for 4 weeks of rhEPO supplementation using a cycle ergometer to measure effects. The investigators reported that in rhEPO subjects, hematocrit increased from 42.7% to 50.8%. The $\dot{V}O_2$max significantly increased from 63.6 to 68.1 mL/kg per minute, a 7% increase. Neither outcome measure showed a significant increase in the placebo group. Similar results were found by Ekblom and Berglund.[227] They reported a 6% to 11% increase in hematocrit and increases in $\dot{V}O_2$max in time to exhaustion after 7 weeks of rhEPO administration.

Williams and Branch[228] reported that an increase of 1 g/dL of hemoglobin in an athlete with an exercise cardiac output of 25 L/min would increase oxygen transport by 335 mL, which extrapolates to an 8% increase for a normal $\dot{V}O_2$max of 4000 mL of oxygen per minute. In male endurance athletes, the treatment with rhEPO (3×50 IU • kg^{-1} • wk^{-1} for 4 weeks, followed by 3×20 IU • kg^{-1} • wk^{-1} for 2 weeks) increased aerobic physical fitness and perceived physical strength scores.[229]

Apart from rhEPO, several other erythropoiesis-stimulating agents (ESAs) have been developed. Darbepoetin alfa is an rhEPO glycosylation analogue that was approved for use in 2002 in the European Union and United States. It has the same mechanism of action as rhEPO—binding and activation of the EPO receptor—but it has a longer serum half-life and increased in vivo potency.[225] Additional ESAs are in various stages of clinical development and may appear in the athletic arena. They include polyethylene glycol (PEG)–conjugated epoetin beta and an EPO mimetic peptide, hematide. PEG epoetin beta has been approved by regulators in the European Union.[225] ESAs include the EPO fusion proteins: rhEPO-IL3, EPO albumin, rhEPO-PAI1, rhEPO-Fc, and rhEPO dimers.[225]

Artificially raising hemoglobin levels can have dangerous consequences. In 1987, the first year of EPO release in Europe, five Dutch cyclists died of unexplained causes. Between 1997 and 2000, 18 cyclists died of stroke, myocardial infarction, or pulmonary embolism.[156] In contrast to the effect of endurance training, which increases plasma volume, the administration of rhEPO produces a selective increase in red cell mass. If the hematocrit exceeds 0.50, blood viscosity and cardiac afterload increase significantly. The main risks of erythrocytosis with a hematocrit greater than 0.55 include heart failure, myocardial infarction, seizures, peripheral thromboembolic events, and pulmonary embolism.[221]

Since the 1996 Atlanta Olympic Games, gas chromatography–mass spectrometry evaluations have been used for screening exogenous EPO in the urine.[156] High-performance liquid chromatography has also been used to detect subtle peptides in the urine.[194] Despite these advances, exogenous EPO remains a particularly difficult substance to detect through tests.

Two teams of scientists developed tests for EPO that were used at the 2000 Sydney Olympic Games. Parisotto and coworkers developed an indirect test based on the measurement of five blood parameters, including reticulocyte hematocrit, serum EPO, hematocrit, soluble transferrin receptor, and the percentage of macrocytes.[230] Two models were developed: the *on model* used all parameters to detect recent use of EPO, whereas the *off model* used three parameters to detect EPO use over a longer period. The on model was used as a screening test at the Sydney Olympics. Confirmation of rhEPO use was accomplished with an isoelectric focusing/immunoblotting/chemiluminescence technique that was able to detect the different glycoforms of recombinant versus native EPO.[231] This method can also detect the use of the novel erythropoiesis-stimulating drug darbepoetin alfa.[232] The limitation of this technique is that it allows detection of EPO for only a few days after use. In Sydney, both tests were required to be positive to confirm EPO use, and no positive cases were detected.

Despite the availability of a test for rhEPO, numerous questions remain. Additional rhEPO products may have different and indistinguishable glycoforms and isoforms. Other approaches to improving oxygen transport can be envisioned, including polymerized and cross-linked hemoglobins (i.e., hemoglobin-based oxygen carriers), blood substitutes such as perfluorohydrocarbons, and 2,3-diphosphoglycerate (2,3-DPG) mimetics. The latter group, including efaproxiral (RSR13), shift the oxygen saturation curve to the left and deliver more oxygen to the tissue per molecule of hemoglobin.[233] Advances in science related to doping require further research.

REFERENCES

1. Wade CE. Hormonal regulation of fluid homeostasis during and following exercise. In: Warren MP, Constantini NW, eds. *Contemporary Endocrinology: Sports Endocrinology*. Totowa, NJ: Humana Press; 2000:207-225.
2. Cumming DC. Hormones and athletic performance. In: Felig P, Baxter JD, Frohman LA, eds. *Endocrinology and metabolism*. 3rd ed. New York: McGraw-Hill; 1995:1837-1885.
3. Zouhal H, Jacob C, Delamarche P, et al. Catecholamines and the effects of exercise, training and gender. *Sports Med*. 2008;38:401-423.
4. Peyrin L, Pequignot JM, Lacour JR, et al. Relationships between catecholamine or 3-methoxy 4-hydroxy phenylglycol changes and the mental performance under submaximal exercise in man. *Psychopharmacology*. 1987;93:188-192.
5. Rogers G, Goodman C, Rosen C. Water budget during ultra-endurance exercise. *Med Sci Sports Exerc*. 1997;29:1477-1481.
6. Wade CE, Claybaugh J. Renin activity, vasopressin concentration, and urinary excretory responses to exercise in men. *J Appl Physiol*. 1980;49:930-936.
7. Nose H, Takamata A, Mack GW, et al. Right atrial pressure and ANP release during prolonged exercise in a hot environment. *J Appl Physiol*. 1994;76:1882-1887.
8. Cuneo RC, Espiner EA, Nicholls MG, et al. Renal, hemodynamic, and hormonal responses to atrial natriuretic peptide infusions in normal man, and effect of sodium intake. *J Clin Endocrinol Metab*. 1986;63:946-953.
9. Mudambo KS, Coutie W, Rennie MJ. Plasma arginine vasopressin, atrial natriuretic peptide and brain natriuretic peptide responses to long-term field training in the heat: effects of fluid ingestion and acclimatization. *Eur J Appl Physiol Occup Physiol*. 1997;75:219-225.
10. Nishikimi T, Morimoto A, Ishikawa K, et al. Different secretion patterns of adrenomedullin, brain natriuretic peptide, and atrial natriuretic peptide during exercise in hypertensive and normotensive subjects. *Clin Exp Hypertens*. 1997;19:503-518.
11. Tidgren B, Hjemdahl P, Theodorsson E, et al. Renal neurohormonal and vascular responses to dynamic exercise in humans. *J Appl Physiol*. 1991;70:2279-2286.

12. Wade CE, Ramee SR, Hunt MM, et al. Hormonal and renal responses to converting enzyme inhibition during maximal exercise. *J Appl Physiol.* 1987;63:1796-1800.
13. Davies CT, Few JD. Effects of exercise on adrenocortical function. *J Appl Physiol.* 1973;35:887-891.
14. Duclos M, Guinot M, Le Bouc Y. Cortisol and GH: odd and controversial ideas. *Appl Physiol Nutr Metab.* 2007;32:895-903.
15. Sapolsky RM, Romero M, Munck AU. How do glucocorticoids influence stress responses? Integrating permissive, suppressive, stimulatory, and preparative actions. *Endocr Rev.* 2000;21:55-89.
16. Wittert GA, Stewart DE, Graves MP, et al. Plasma corticotrophin releasing factor and vasopressin responses to exercise in normal man. *Clin Endocrinol.* 1991;35:311-317.
17. Raastad T, Bjoro T, Hallen J. Hormonal responses to high- and moderate-intensity strength exercise. *Eur J Appl Physiol.* 2000;82:121-128.
18. Hill EE, Zack E, Battaglini C, et al. Exercise and circulating cortisol levels: the intensity threshold effect. *J Endocrinol Invest.* 2008;31:587-591.
19. Farrell PA, Garthwaite TL, Gustafson AB. Plasma adrenocorticotropin and cortisol responses to submaximal and exhaustive exercise. *J Appl Physiol.* 1983;55:1441-1444.
20. Buono MJ, Yeager JE, Hodgdon JA. Plasma adrenocorticotropin and cortisol responses to brief high-intensity exercise in humans. *J Appl Physiol.* 1986;61:1337-1339.
21. Lutoslawska G, Obminski Z, Krogulski A, et al. Plasma cortisol and testosterone following 19-km and 42-km kayak races. *J Sports Med Phys Fitness.* 1991;31:538-542.
22. Fellmann N, Bedu M, Boudet G, et al. Inter-relationships between pituitary-adrenal hormones and catecholamines during a 6-day Nordic ski race. *Eur J Appl Physiol Occup Physiol.* 1992;64:258-265.
23. Bergeron MF, Maresh CM, Kraemer WJ, et al. Tennis: a physiological profile during match play. *Int J Sports Med.* 1991;12:474-479.
24. Häkkinen K, Pakarinen A. Acute hormonal responses to two different fatiguing heavy-resistance protocols in male athletes. *J Appl Physiol.* 1993;74:882-887.
25. Hackney AC, Premo MC, McMurray RG. Influence of aerobic versus anaerobic exercise on the relationship between reproductive hormones in men. *J Sports Sci.* 1995;13:305-311.
26. Häkkinen K, Pakarinen A. Acute hormonal responses to heavy resistance exercise in men and women at different ages. *Int J Sports Med.* 1995;16:507-513.
27. Korkushko OV, Frolkis MV, Shatilo VB, et al. Hormonal and autonomic reactions to exercise in elderly healthy subjects and patients with ischemic heart disease. *Acta Clin Belg.* 1990;45:164-175.
28. Silverman HG, Mazzeo RS. Hormonal responses to maximal and submaximal exercise in trained and untrained men of various ages. *J Gerontol A Biol Sci Med Sci.* 1996;51:B30-B37.
29. Davis SN, Galassetti P, Wasserman DH, et al. Effects of gender on neuroendocrine and metabolic counterregulatory responses to exercise in normal man. *J Clin Endocrinol Metab.* 2000;85:224-230.
30. Loucks AB, Mortola JF, Girton L, et al. Alterations in the hypothalamic-pituitary-ovarian and the hypothalamic-pituitary-adrenal axes in athletic women. *J Clin Endocrinol Metab.* 1989;68:402-411.
31. Bonen A, Haynes FW, Graham TE. Substrate and hormonal responses to exercise in women using oral contraceptives. *J Appl Physiol.* 1991;70:1917-1927.
32. Kirschbaum C, Schommer N, Federenko I, et al. Short-term estradiol treatment enhances pituitary-adrenal axis and sympathetic responses to psychosocial stress in healthy young men. *J Clin Endocrinol Metab.* 1996;81:3639-3643.
33. Duclos M, Corcuff J-B, Rashedi M, et al. Trained versus untrained men: different immediate post-exercise responses of pituitary-adrenal axis. A preliminary study. *Eur J Appl Physiol.* 1997;75:343-350.
34. Judelson DA, Maresh CM, Yamamoto LM et al. Effect of hydration state on resistance exercise-induced endocrine markers of anabolism, catabolism, and metabolism. *J Appl Physiol.* 2008;105:816-824.
35. Akana SF, Dallman MF. Feedback and facilitation in the adrenocortical system: unmasking facilitation by partial inhibition of the glucocorticoid response to prior stress. *Endocrinology.* 1992;131:57-68.
36. Heuser IJE, Wark HJ, Keul J, et al. Hypothalamic-pituitary-adrenal axis function in elderly endurance athletes. *J Clin Endocrinol Metab.* 1991;73:485-488.
37. Gouarne C, Groussard C, Duclos M. Overnight urinary cortisol and cortisone add new insights into adaptation to training. *Med Sci Sports Exerc.* 2005;37:1157-1167.
38. Kanaley JA, Weltman JY, Pieper KS, et al. Cortisol and growth hormone responses to exercise at different times of day. *J Clin Endocrinol Metab.* 2001;86:2881-2889.
39. Duclos M, Gouarne C, Bonnemaison D. Acute and chronic effects of exercise on tissue sensitivity to glucocorticoids. *J Appl Physiol.* 2003;94:869-875.
40. Meyer T, Schwarz L, Kindermann W. Exercise and endogenous opiates. In: Warren MP, Constantini NW, eds. *Contemporary Endocrinology: Sports Endocrinology.* Totowa, NJ: Humana Press; 2000:31-42.
41. Carrasco L, Villaverde C, Oltras CM. Endorphin responses to stress induced by competitive swimming event. *J Sports Med Phys Fitness.* 2007;47:239-245.
42. Allen M. Activity-generated endorphins: a review of their role in sports science. *Can J Appl Sport Sci.* 1983;8:115-133.
43. Cumming DC. The male reproductive system, exercise, and training. In: Warren MP, Constantini NW, eds. *Contemporary Endocrinology: Sports Endocrinology.* Totowa, NJ: Humana Press; 2000:119-131.
44. Gotshalk LA, Loebel CC, Nindl BC, et al. Hormonal responses of multiset versus single-set heavy-resistance exercise protocols. *Can J Appl Physiol.* 1997;22:244-255.
45. Hoffman JR, Falk B, Radom-Isaac S, et al. The effect of environmental temperature on testosterone and cortisol responses to high intensity, intermittent exercise in humans. *Eur J Appl Physiol Occup Physiol.* 1997;75:83-87.
46. Hoffman JR, Maresh CM, Armstrong LE, et al. Effects of hydration state on plasma testosterone, cortisol and catecholamine concentrations before and during mild exercise at elevated temperature. *Eur J Appl Physiol Occup Physiol.* 1994;69:294-300.
47. Cumming DC, Brunsting 3rd LA, Strich G, et al. Reproductive hormone increases in response to acute exercise in men. *Med Sci Sports Exerc.* 1986;18:369-373.
48. Wheeler GD, Wall SR, Belcastro AN, et al. Reduced serum testosterone and prolactin levels in male distance runners. *JAMA.* 1984;252:514-516.
49. Hackney AC. Effects of endurance exercise on the reproductive system of men: the "exercise-hypogonadal male condition." *J Endocrinol Invest.* 2008;31:932-938.
50. Arce JC, DeSouza MJ. Exercise and male factor infertility. *Sports Med.* 1993;15:146-169.
51. Bennell KL, Brukner PD, Malcolm SA. Effect of altered reproductive function and lowered testosterone levels on bone density in male endurance athletes. *Br J Sports Med.* 1996;30:205-208.
52. Hackney AC, Moore AW, Brownlee KK. Testosterone and endurance exercise: development of the "exercise-hypogonadal male condition." *Acta Physiol Hung.* 2005;92:121-137.
53. MacConnie S, Barkan A, Lampman RM, et al. Decreased hypothalamic gonadotropin-releasing hormone secretion in male marathon runners. *N Engl J Med.* 1986;315:411-417.
54. McColl EM, Wheeler GD, Gomes P, et al. The effects of acute exercise on pulsatile LH release in high-mileage male runners. *Clin Endocrinol.* 1989;31:617-621.
55. Kujala UM, Alen M, Huhtaniemi IT. Gonadotrophin-releasing hormone and human chorionic gonadotrophin tests reveal that both hypothalamic and testicular endocrine functions are suppressed during acute prolonged physical exercise. *Clin Endocrinol.* 1990;33:219-225.
56. Hackney AC. The male reproductive system and endurance exercise. *Med Sci Sports Exerc.* 1996;28:180-189.
57. Hackney AC, Sharp RL, Runyan WS, et al. Relationship of resting prolactin and testosterone in males during intensive training. *Br J Sports Med.* 1989;23:194.
58. Blueher S, Mantzoros CS. Leptin in reproduction. *Curr Opin Endocrinol Diabetes Obes.* 2007;14:458-464.
59. Baylor LS, Hackney AC. Resting thyroid and leptin hormone changes in women following intense, prolonged exercise training. *Eur J Appl Physiol.* 2003;88:480-484.
60. Lanfranco F, Bonelli L, Baldi M, et al. Acylated ghrelin inhibits spontaneous LH pulsatility and responsiveness to naloxone, but not that to GnRH in young men: evidence for a central inhibitory action of ghrelin on the gonadal axis. *J Clin Endocrinol Metab.* 2008;93:3633-3639.
61. Tena-Sempere M. Ghrelin and reproduction: ghrelin as novel regulator of the gonadotropic axis. *Vitam Horm.* 2008;77:285-300.
62. Jürimäe J, Cicchella A, Jürimäe T, et al. Regular physical activity influences plasma ghrelin concentration in adolscent girls. *Med Sci Sports Exerc.* 2007;39:1736-1741.
63. Hu Y, Asano K, Kim S, et al. Relationship between serum testosterone and activities of testicular enzymes after continuous and intermittent training in male rats. *Int J Sports Med.* 2004;25:99-102.
64. Cumming DC, Quigley ME, Yen SS. Acute suppression of circulating testosterone levels by cortisol in men. *J Clin Endocrinol Metab.* 1983;57:671-673.
65. Hackney AC, Sinning WE, Bruot BC. Hypothalamic-pituitary-testicular function of endurance-trained and untrained males. *Int J Sports Med.* 1990;11:298-303.
66. Wheeler GD, Singh M, Pierce WD, et al. Endurance training decreases serum testosterone levels in men without change in luteinizing hormone pulsation release. *J Clin Endocrinol Metab.* 1991;72:422-425.
67. Loucks AB, Vaitukaitis J, Cameron JL, et al. The reproductive system and exercise in women. *Med Sci Sports Exerc.* 1992;24:288-293.
68. Arena B, Maffulli N, Maffulli F, et al. Reproductive hormones and menstrual changes with exercise in female athletes. *Sports Med.* 1995;19:278-287.
69. Warren MP. The effects of exercise on pubertal progression and reproductive function in girls. *J Clin Endocrinol Metab.* 1980;51:1150-1157.

70. Loucks AB, Verdun M, Heath EM. Low energy availability, not stress of exercise, alters LH pulsatility in exercising women. *J Appl Physiol.* 1998;84:37-46.
71. Stafford DE. Altered hypothalamic-pituitary-ovarian axis function in young female athletes: implications and recommendations for management. *Treat Endocrinol.* 2005;4:147-154.
72. Loucks A. Is stress measured in joules? *Military Psychology.* 2009;21:S101-S107.
73. Selye H. The effect of adaptation to various damaging agents on the female sex organs in the rat. *Endocrinology.* 1939;25:615-624.
74. Selye H. A syndrome produced by diverse nocuous agents. *Nature.* 1936;138:32.
75. Winterer J, Cutler Jr GB, Loriaux DL. Caloric balance, brain to body ratio, and the timing of menarche. *Med Hypotheses.* 1984;15:87-91.
76. Laughlin GA, Yen SS. Nutritional and endocrine-metabolic aberrations in amenorrheic athletes. *J Clin Endocrinol Metab.* 1996;81:4301-4309.
77. Laughlin GA, Yen SS. Hypoleptinemia in women athletes: absence of a diurnal rhythm with amenorrhea. *J Clin Endocrinol Metab.* 1997;82:318-321.
78. Loucks AB, Laughlin GA, Mortola JF, et al. Hypothalamic-pituitary-thyroidal function in eumenorrheic and amenorrheic athletes. *J Clin Endocrinol Metab,* 1992;75:514-518.
79. Williams NI, Caston-Balderrama AL, Helmreich DL, et al. Longitudinal changes in reproductive hormones and menstrual cyclicity in cynomolgus monkeys during strenuous exercise training: abrupt transition to exercise-induced amenorrhea. *Endocrinology.* 2001;142:2381-2389.
80. Williams NI, Helmreich DL, Parfitt DB, et al. Evidence for a causal role of low energy availability in the induction of menstrual cycle disturbances during strenuous exercise training. *J Clin Endocrinol Metab.* 2001;86:5184-5193.
81. Loucks AB, Thuma JR. Luteinizing hormone pulsatility is disrupted at a threshold of energy availability in regularly menstruating women. *J Clin Endocrinol Metab.* 2003;88:297-311.
82. Loucks AB. Low energy availability in the marathon and other endurance sports. *Sports Med.* 2007;37:348-352.
83. Kopp-Woodroffe SA, Manore MM, Dueck CA, et al. Energy and nutrient status of amenorrheic athletes participating in a diet and exercise training intervention program. *Int J Sport Nutr.* 1999;9:70-88.
84. Zhang Y, Proenca R, Maffei M, et al. Positional cloning of the mouse obese gene and its human homologue. *Nature.* 1994;372: 425-432.
85. Aubert ML, Pierroz DD, Gruaz NM, et al. Metabolic control of sexual function and growth: role of neuropeptide Y and leptin. *Mol Cell Endocrinol.* 1998;140:107-113.
86. Welt CK, Chan JL, Bullen J, et al. Recombinant human leptin in women with hypothalamic amenorrhea. *N Engl J Med.* 2004;351: 987-997.
87. Chan JL, Mantzoros CS. Role of leptin in energy-deprivation states: normal human physiology and clinical implications for hypothalamic amenorrhoea and anorexia nervosa. *Lancet.* 2005;366:74-85.
88. De Souza MJ, Maguire MS, Maresh CM, et al. Adrenal activation and the prolactin response to exercise in eumenorrheic and amenorrheic runners. *J Appl Physiol.* 1991;70:2378-2387.
89. Stoving RK, Hangaard J, Hagen C. Update on endocrine disturbances in anorexia nervosa. *J Pediatr Endocrinol Metab.* 2001;14:459-480.
90. Loucks AB. Exercise training in the normal female: effects of exercise stress and energy availability on metabolic hormones and LH pulsatility. In: Warren MP, Constantini NW, eds. *Contemporary Endocrinology: Sports Endocrinology.* Totowa, NJ: Humana Press; 2000:165-180.
91. De Cree C. The possible involvement of endogenous opioid peptides and catecholestrogens in provoking menstrual irregularities in women athletes. *Int J sports Med.* 1990;11:329-348.
92. Consitt LA, Copeland JL, Tremblay MS. Endogenous anabolic hormone responses to endurance versus resistance exercise and training in women. *Sports Med.* 2002;32:1-22.
93. Rickenlund A, Carlstrom K, Ekblom B, et al. Hyperandrogenicity is an alternative mechanism underlying oligomenorrhea or amenorrhea in female athletes and may improve physical performance. *Fertil Steril.* 2003;79:947-955.
94. McMurray RG, Hackney AC. The endocrine system and exercise. In: Garrett W, Kirkendahl D, eds. *Exercise and Sports Science.* New York: Williams & Wilkins; 2000:135-162.
95. Hackney AC. Characterization of the prolactin response to prolonged endurance exercise. *Acta Kinesiologiae (University of Tartu).* 2008; 13:31-38.
96. Boyden TW, Pamenter RW, Grosso D, et al. Prolactin responses, menstrual cycles, and body composition of women runners. *J Clin Endocrinol Metab.* 1982;54:711-714.
97. De Meirleir KL, Baeyens L, L'Hermite-Baleriaux M, et al. Exercise-induced prolactin release is related to anaerobiosis. *J Clin Endocrinol Metab.* 1985;60:1250-1252.
98. Mastrogiacomo I, Toderini D, Bonanni G, et al. Gonadotropin decrease induced by prolonged exercise at about 55% of the VO_2max in different phases of the menstrual cycle. *Int J Sports Med.* 1990;11:198-203.
99. Oleshansky MA, Zoltick JM, Herman RH, et al. The influence of fitness on neuroendocrine responses to exhaustive treadmill exercise. *Eur J Appl Physiol Occup Physiol.* 1990:59:405-410.
100. Benso A, Broglio F, Aimaretti G, et al. Endocrine and metabolic responses to extreme altitude and physical exercise in climbers. *Eur J Endocrinol.* 2007;157:733-740.
101. Roth J, Glick SM, Yalow RS. Hypoglycemia: a potent stimulus to the secretion of growth hormone. *Science.* 1963;140:987-988.
102. Sutton JR, Lazarus L. Growth hormone and exercise comparison of physiological and pharmacological stimuli. *J Appl Physiol.* 1976;41:523-527.
103. Felsing NE, Brasel JA, Cooper DM. Effect of low and high intensity exercise on circulating growth hormone in men. *J Clin Endocrinol Metab.* 1992;75:157-162.
104. Eliakim A, Brasel JA, Cooper DM. Exercise and the growth hormone-insulin-like growth factor-1 axis. In: Warren MP, Constantini NW, eds. *Contemporary Endocrinology: Sports Endocrinology.* Totowa, NJ: Humana Press; 2000:77-95.
105. Gibney J, Healy ML, Sönksen PH. The growth hormone/insulin-like growth factor-I axis in exercise and sport. *Endocr Rev.* 2007;28: 603-624.
106. Godfrey R, Madgwick Z, Whyte G. The exercise-induced growth hormone response in athletes. *Sports Med.* 2003;33:599-613.
107. Pritzlaff CJ, Wideman L, Weltman JY, et al. Impact of acute exercise intensity on pulsatile growth hormone release in men. *J Appl Physiol.* 1999;87:498-504.
108. Wideman L, Consitt L, Patrie J, et al. The impact of sex and exercise duration on growth hormone secretion. *J Appl Physiol.* 2006; 101:1641-1647.
109. Kanaley JA, Weltman JY, Veldhuis JD, et al. Human growth hormone response to repeated bouts of aerobic exercise. *J Appl Physiol.* 1997;83:1756-1761.
110. Cuneo RC, Wallace JD. Growth hormone, insulin-like growth factors and sport. *Endocrinol Metab.* 1994;1:3-13.
111. Bar-Or O. Growth hormone deficiency: using exercise in the diagnosis. In: Bar-Or O, ed. *Pediatric Sports Medicine for the Practitioner.* New York: Springer-Verlag; 1983:182-191.
112. Eliakim A, Brasel JA, Cooper DM. GH response to exercise: assessment of the pituitary refractory period, and relationship with circulating components of the GH-IGF-I axis in adolescent females. *J Pediatr Endocrinol Metab.* 1999;12:47-55.
113. Ehrnborg C, Lange KHW, Dall R, et al. The growth hormone/insulin-like growth factor-I axis hormones and bone markers in elite athletes in response to a maximum exercise test. *J Clin Endocrinol Metab.* 2003;88:394-401.
114. Snegovskeya V, Viru A. Elevation of cortisol and growth hormone levels in the courses of further improvement of performance capacity in trained rowers. *Int J Sports Med.* 1993;14:202-206.
115. Karagiorgos A, Garcia JF, Brooks GA. Growth hormone response to continuous and intermittent exercise. *Med Sci Sports.* 1979;11: 302-307.
116. Häkkinen K, Pakarinen A, Alen M, et al. Neuromuscular and hormonal responses in elite athletes to two successive strength training sessions in one day. *Eur J Appl Physiol.* 1988;57:133-139.
117. Weltman A, Weltman JY, Womack CJ, et al. Exercise training decreases the growth hormone (GH) response to acute constant-load exercise. *Med Sci Sports Exerc.* 1997;29:669-676.
118. Wideman L, Weltman JY, Hartman ML, et al. Growth hormone release during acute and chronic aerobic and resistance exercise: recent findings. *Sports Med.* 2002;32:987-1004.
119. Peyreigne C, Bouix D, Fedou C, Mercier J. Effect of hydration on exercise-induced growth hormone response. *Eur J Endocrinol.* 2001;145: 445-450.
120. Cappon JP, Ipp E, Brasel JA, Cooper DM. Acute effect of high-fat and high-glucose meals on the growth hormone response to exercise. *J Clin Endocrinol Metab.* 1993;76:1418-1422.
121. Okada Y, Hikita T, Ishitobi K, et al. Human growth hormone secretion during exposure to hot air in normal adult male subjects. *J Clin Endocrinol Metab.* 1972;34:759-763.
122. Christensen SE, Jorgensen OL, Moller N, et al. Characterization of growth hormone release in response to external heating: comparison to exercise induced release. *Acta Endocrinol (Copenh).* 1984;107: 295-301.
123. Wilkinson PW, Parkin JM. Growth hormone response to exercise in obese children. *Lancet.* 1974;2:55.
124. Pritzlaff-Roy CJ, Widemen L, Weltman JY, et al. Gender governs the relationship between exercise intensity and growth hormone release in young adults. *J Appl Physiol.* 2002;92:2053-2060.
125. Friend KE, Hartman ML, Pezzoli SS, et al. Both oral and transdermal estrogen increase growth hormone release in postmenopausal women: a clinical research center study. *J Clin Endocrinol Metab.* 1996; 81:2250-2256.
126. Bernardes RP, Radomski MW. Growth hormone responses to continuous and intermittent exercise in females under oral contraceptive therapy. *Eur J Appl Physiol Occup Physiol.* 1998;79:24-29.

127. Zaccaria M, Varnier M, Piazza P, et al. Blunted growth hormone response to maximal exercise in middle-aged versus young subjects and no effect of endurance training. *J Clin Endocrinol Metab.* 1999;84: 2303-2307.
128. Veldhuis JD, Liem AY, South S, et al. Differential impact of age, sex steroid hormones, and obesity on basal versus pulsatile growth hormone secretion in men as assessed in an ultrasensitive chemiluminescence assay. *J Clin Endocrinol Metab.* 1995;80:3209-3222.
129. Kelley PJ, Eisman JA, Stuart MC, et al. Somatomedin-C, physical fitness, and bone density. *J Clin Endocrinol Metab.* 1990;70:718-723.
130. Wilson DP, Horowitz JL. Exercise-induced changes in growth hormone and somatomedine-C. *Am J Med Sci.* 1987;293:216-217.
131. Hagberg JM, Seals DR, Yerg JE, et al. Metabolic responses to exercise in young and older athletes and sedentary men. *J Appl Physiol.* 1988;65:900-908.
132. Schwarz AJ, Brasel JA, Hintz RL, et al. Acute effect of brief low- and high-intensity exercise on circulating IGF-1, II, and IGF binding protein-3 and its proteolysis in young healthy men. *J Clin Endocrinol Metab.* 1996;81:3492-3497.
133. Zanconato S, Moromisato DY, Moromisato MY, et al. Effect of training and growth hormone suppression on insulin-like growth factor-I mRNA in young rats. *J Appl Physiol.* 1994;76:2204-2209.
134. Eliakim A, Moromisato M, Moromisato D, et al. Increase in muscle IGF-I protein but not IGF-I mRNA after 5 days of endurance training in young rats. *J Appl Physiol.* 1997;42:1557-1561.
135. Wallace JD, Cuneo RD, Baxter R, et al. Responses of the growth hormone (GH) and insulin-like growth factor axis to exercise, GH administration, and GH withdrawal in trained adult males: a potential test for GH abuse in sport. *J Clin Endocrinol Metab.* 1999;84: 3591-3601.
136. Eliakim A, Brasel JA, Mohan S, et al. Physical fitness, endurance training, and the GH-IGF-1 system in adolescent females. *J Clin Endocrinol Metab.* 1996;81:3986-3992.
137. Galbo H. The hormonal response to exercise. *Diabetes Metab Rev.* 1986;1:385-408.
138. McMurray RG, Eubanks TE, Hackney AC. Nocturnal hormonal responses to weight training exercise. *Eur J Appl Physiol.* 1995;72:121-126.
139. Moore AW, Timmerman S, Brownlee KK, et al. Strenuous, fatiguing exercise: relationship of cortisol to circulating thyroid hormones. *Int J Endocrinol Metab.* 2005;1:18-24.
140. Hackney AC, Gulledge TP. Thyroid responses during an 8 hour period following aerobic and anaerobic exercise. *Physiol Res.* 1994; 43:1-5.
141. Hackney AC, Viru A. Research methodology: issues with endocrinological measurements in exercise science and sport medicine. *J Athletic Training.* 2008;43:631-639.
142. Lehmann M, Knizia K, Gastmann U, et al. Influence of 6-week, 6 days per week, training on pituitary function in recreational athletes. *Br J Sports Med.* 1993;27:186-192.
143. Deligiannis A, Karamouzis M, Kouidi E, et al. Plasma TSH, T3, T4 and cortisol responses to swimming at varying water temperatures. *Br J Sports Med.* 1993;27:247-250.
144. Loucks AB, Heath EM. Induction of low-T3 syndrome in exercising women occurs at a threshold of energy availability. *Am J Physiol.* 1994;266:R817-R823.
145. Jahreis G, Kauf E, Frohner G, et al. Influence of intensive exercise on insulin-like growth factor I, thyroid and steroid hormones in female gymnasts. *Growth Regul.* 1991;1:95-99.
146. Task Force on Community Preventive Services. Increasing Physical Activity: A Report on Recommendations of the Task Force on Community Preventive Services. *MMWR Morb Mortal Wkly Rep.* 2001;50:RR-18.
147. Schneider SH, Guleria PS. Diabetes and exercise. In: Warren MP, Constantini NW, eds. *Contemporary Endocrinology: Sports Endocrinology.* Totowa, NJ: Humana Press; 2000:227-238.
148. Felig P, Wahren J. Fuel homeostasis in exercise. *N Engl J Med.* 1975;293:1078-1084.
149. Rodnick KJ, Henriksen EJ, James DE, et al. Exercise training, glucose transporters, and glucose transport in rat skeletal muscles. *Am J Physiol.* 1992;262:C9-C14.
150. DeFronzo RA, Ferrannini E, Sato Y, et al. Synergistic interaction between exercise and insulin on peripheral glucose uptake. *J Clin Invest.* 1981;68:1468-1474.
151. Jenkins AB, Furler SM, Chisholm DJ, et al. Regulation of hepatic glucose output during exercise by circulating glucose and insulin in humans. *Am J Physiol.* 1986;250:R411-R417.
152. Lavoie C, Ducros F, Bourque J, et al. Glucose metabolism during exercise in man: the role of insulin and glucagon in the regulation of hepatic glucose production and gluconeogenesis. *Can J Physiol Pharmacol.* 1997;75:26-35.
153. Naveri H, Kuoppasalmi K, Harkonen M. Plasma glucagon and catecholamines during exhaustive short-term exercise. *Eur J Appl Physiol Occup Physiol.* 1985;53:308-311.
154. O'Rahilly SO, Hosker JP, Rudenski AS, et al. The glucose stimulus-response curve of the beta-cell in physically trained humans, assessed by hyperglycemic clamps. *Metabolism.* 1988;37:919-923.
155. Roberts CK, Barnard RJ. Effects of exercise and diet on chronic disease. *J Appl Physiol.* 2005;98:3-30.
156. Tokish JM, Kocher MS, Hawkins RJ. Ergogenic aids: a review of basic science, performance, side effects, and status in sports. *Am J Sports Med.* 2004;32:1543-1553.
157. Di Luigi L, Romanelli F, Lenzi A. Androgenic-anabolic steroids abuse in males. *J Endocrinol Invest.* 2005;28:81-84.
158. World Anti-Doping Agency. Adverse Analytical Findings Reported by Accredited Laboratories. Laboratory Statistics Report. 2008. Available at http://www.wada-ama.org (accessed July 2010).
159. Lenehan P, Bellis M, McVeigh J. A study of anabolic steroid use in the northwest of England. *J Perform Enhancing Drugs.* 1996;1:57-71.
160. Korkia P, Stimson GV. Indications of prevalence, practice and effects of anabolic steroid use in Great Britain. *Int J Sports Med.* 1997;18:557-562.
161. Yesalis III CE, Kennedy NJ, Kopstein AN, et al. Anabolic-androgenic steroid use in the United States. *JAMA.* 1993;270:1217-1221.
162. National Institute on Drug Abuse. About anabolic steroid abuse. *NIDA Notes.* 2000;15:15.
163. Evans NA. Current concepts in anabolic-androgenic steroids. *Am J Sports Med.* 2004;32:534-542.
164. Kicman AT. Pharmacology of anabolic steroids. *Br J Pharmacol.* 2008;154:502-521.
165. Johns K, Beddall MJ, Corrin RC. Anabolic steroids for the treatment of weight loss in HIV-infected individuals. Cochrane Database Syst Rev. 2005;19(4):CD005483.
166. Lovejoy JC, Bray GA, Bourgeois MO, et al. Exogenous androgens influence body composition and regional body fat distribution in obese postmenopausal women: a clinical research center study. *J Clin Endocrinol Metab.* 1996;81:2198-2203.
167. Bhasin S, Storer TW, Berman N, et al. The effects of supraphysiological doses of testosterone on muscle size and strength in normal men. *N Engl J Med.* 1996;335:1-7.
168. Ryan AJ. Athletics. In: Kochakian CD, ed. Anabolic-Androgenic Steroids. vol 43. Berlin: Springer-Verlag; 1976:515-534.
169. Haupt HA, Rovere GD. Anabolic steroids: a review of the literature. *Am J Sports Med.* 1984;12:469-484.
170. Strauss RH, Yesalis CE. Anabolic steroids in the athlete. *Annu Rev Med.* 1991;42:449-457.
171. Bhasin S, Woodhouse L, Casaburi R, et al. Testosterone dose-response relationships in healthy young men. *Am J Physiol Endocrinol Metab.* 2001;281:E1172-E1181.
172. Woodhouse LJ, Reisz-Porszasz S, Javanbakht M, et al. Development of models to predict anabolic response to testosterone administration in healthy young men. *Am J Physiol Endocrinol Metab.* 2003;284: E1009-E1017.
173. Sinha-Hikim I, Artaza J, Woodhouse L, et al. Testosterone-induced increase in muscle size in healthy young men is associated with muscle fiber hypertrophy. *Am J Physiol Endocrinol Metab.* 2002;283:E154-E164.
174. Elbers JMH, Asscheman H, Seidell JC, et al. Effects of sex steroid hormones on regional fat depots as assessed by magnetic resonance imaging in transexuals. *Am J Physiol.* 1999;276:E317-E325.
175. Alway SE. Characteristics of the elbow flexors in women bodybuilders using androgenic-anabolic steroids. *J Strength Cond Res.* 1994;8: 161-169.
176. Tamaki T, Uchiyama S, Uchiyama Y, et al. Anabolic steroids increase exercise tolerance. *Am J Physiol Endocrinol Metab.* 2001;280:E973-E981.
177. Catlin DH. Androgen abuse by athletes. In: Bhasin S, Gabelnick HL, Spieler JM, et al., eds. *Pharmacology, Biology, and Clinical Applications of Androgens.* New York, NY: Wiley-Liss; 1996:289-295.
178. Bronson FH, Matherne CM. Exposure to anabolic-androgenic steroids shortens life span of male mice. *Med Sci Sports Exerc.* 1997;29: 615-619.
179. Evans NA. Gym and tonic: a profile of 100 male steroid users. *Br J Sports Med.* 1997;31:54-58.
180. Hall RC, Hall RC. Abuse of supraphysiologic doses of anabolic steroids. *South Med J.* 2005;98:550-555.
181. Ishak KG, Zimmerman HJ. Hepatotoxic effects of the anabolic/androgenic steroids. *Semin Liver Dis.* 1987;7:230-236.
182. Street C, Antonio J, Cudlipp D. Androgen use by athletes: a reevaluation of the health risks. *Can J Appl Physiol.* 1996;21:421-440.
183. Bolding G, Sherr L, Elford J. Use of anabolic steroids and associated health risks among gay men attending London gyms. *Addiction.* 2002;97:195-201.
184. Thompson PD, Cullinane EM, Sady SP, et al. Contrasting effects of testosterone and stanozolol on serum lipoprotein levels. *JAMA.* 1989;261:1165-1168.
185. Parssinen M, Seppala T. Steroid use and long term health risks in former athletes. *Sports Med.* 2002;32:83-94.
186. Choong K, Jasuja R, Basaria S, et al. Androgen Abuse. In: Ghigo E, Lanfranco F, Strasburger CJ, eds. Hormone use and abuse by athletes. New York: Springer; 2011:63-88.
187. Malarkey WB, Strauss RH, Leizman DJ, et al. Endocrine effects in female weight lifters who self-administer testosterone and anabolic steroids. *Am J Obstet Gynecol.* 1991;165:1385-1390.

188. Spinder T, Spijkstra JJ, Van Den Tweel JG, et al. The effects of long term testosterone administration on pulsatile luteinizing hormone secretion and on ovarian histology in eugonadal female to male transsexual subjects. *J Clin Endocrinol Metab.* 1989;69:151-157.
189. Strauss RH, Liggett M, Lanese RR. Anabolic steroid use and perceived effects in ten weight-trained women athletes. *JAMA.* 1985;253: 2871-2873.
190. Lasseter JT, Russell JA. Anabolic steroid induced tendon pathology: a review of the literature. *Med Sci Sports Exerc.* 1991;23:1-3.
191. Pope HG, Katz DL. Psychiatric and medical effects of anbolic-androgenic steroid use. *Arch Gen Psychiatry.* 1998;51:375-382.
192. Brower KJ, Eliopulos GA, Blow FC, et al. Evidence for physical and psychological dependence on anabolic androgenic steroids in eight weight lifters. *Am J Psychiatry.* 1990;147:510-512.
193. Catlin DH, Hatton CK, Starcevic SH. Issues in detecting abuse of xenobiotic anabolic steroids and testosterone by analysis of athletes' urine. *Clin Chem.* 1997;43:1280-1288.
194. Bowers LD. Analytical advances in detection of performance-enhancing compounds. *Clin Chem.* 1997;43:1299-1304.
195. World Anti-Doping Agency (WADA). Technical document: reporting and evaluation guidance for testosterone, epitestosterone, T/E ratio and other endogenous steroids. 2004. Available at http://www.wada-ama.org (accessed July 2010).
196. Sottas PE, Saudan C, Schweizer C, et al. From population- to subject-based limits of T/E ratio to detect testosterone abuse in elite sports. *Forensic Sci Int.* 2008;174:166-172.
197. Jorgensen JOL, Pedersen SA, Thuesen L, et al. Beneficial effects of growth hormone treatment in GH deficient adults. *Lancet.* 1989;1: 1221-1225.
198. Salomon F, Cuneo RC, Hesp R, et al. The effects of treatment with recombinant human growth hormone on body composition and metabolism in adults with growth hormone deficiency. *N Engl J Med.* 1989;321:1797-1803.
199. De Boer H, Blok GJ, van der Veen EA. Clinical aspects of growth hormone deficiency in adults. *Endocr Rev.* 1995;16:63-86.
200. Rutherford OM, Jones DA, Round JM, et al. Changes in skeletal muscle after discontinuation of growth hormone treatment in young adults with hypopituitarism. *Acta Paediatr Scand Suppl.* 1989;356:61-63.
201. Svensson J, Stibrant Sunnerhagen K, Johannsson G. Five years of growth hormone replacement therapy in adults: age- and gender-related changes in isometric and isokinetic muscle strength. *J Clin Endocrinol Metab.* 2003;88:2061-2069.
202. Degerblad M, Almkvist O, Grunditz Hall K, et al. Physical and psychological capabilities during substitution therapy with recombinant growth hormone deficiency. *Acta Endocrinol.* 1990;123:185-193.
203. Rodriguez-Arnao J, Jabbar A, Fulcher K, et al. Effects of growth hormone replacement on physical performance and body composition in GH deficient adults. *Clin Endocrinol.* 1999;51:53-60.
204. Nass R, Huber RM, Klauss V, et al. Effect of growth hormone (hGH) replacement therapy on physical work capacity and cardiac and pulmonary function in patients with hGH deficiency acquired in adulthood. *J Clin Endocrinol Metab.* 1995;80:552-557.
205. Hartman ML, Weltman A, Zagar A, et al. Growth hormone replacement therapy in adults with growth hormone deficiency improves maximal oxygen consumption independently of dosing regimen or physical activity. *J Clin Endocrinol Metab.* 2008;93:125-130.
206. Christ ER, Cummings MH, Westwood NB, et al. The importance of growth hormone in the regulation of erythropoiesis, red cell mass, and plasma volume in adults with growth hormone deficiency. *J Clin Endocrinol Metab.* 1997;82:2985-2990.
207. Thuesen L, Jorgensen JOL, Muller JR, et al. Short and long term cardiovascular effects of growth hormone therapy in growth hormone deficient adults. *Clin Endocrinol.* 1994;41:615-620.
208. Boger RH, Skamira C, Bode-Boger SM, et al. Nitric oxide may mediate the hemodynamic effects of recombinant growth hormone in patients with acquired growth hormone deficiency: a double-blind, placebo-controlled study. *J Clin Invest.* 1996;98:2706-2713.
209. Yarasheski KE, Zachwieja JJ, Angelopoulos TJ, et al. Short-term growth hormone treatment does not increase muscle protein synthesis in experienced weightlifters. *J Appl Physiol.* 1993;74:3073-3076.
210. Deyssig R, Frisch H, Blum WF, et al. Effect of growth hormone treatment on hormonal parameters, body composition and strength in athletes. *Acta Endocrinol.* 1993;128:313-318.
211. Ehrnborg C, Bengtsson BA, Rosen T. Growth hormone abuse. *Best Pract Res Clin Endocrinol Metab.* 2000;14:71-77.
212. Crist DM, Peake GT, Egan PA, et al. Body composition response to exogenous GH during training in highly conditioned adults. *J Appl Physiol.* 1988;65:579-584.
213. Johannsson G, Mårin P, Lönn L, et al. Growth hormone treatment of abdominally obese man reduces abdominal fat mass, improves glucose and lipoprotein metabolism, and reduces diastolic blood pressure. *J Clin Endocrinol Metab.* 1997;82:727-734.
214. Thompson JL, Butterfield GE, Gylfadottir UK, et al. Effects of human growth hormone, insulin-like growth factor I, and diet and exercise on body composition of obese postmenopausal women. *J Clin Endocrinol Metab.* 1998;83:1477-1484.
215. Lange KH, Isaksson F, Juul A, et al. Growth hormone enhances effects of endurance training on oxidative muscle metabolism in elderly women. *Am J Physiol Endocrinol Metab.* 2000;279:E989-E996.
216. Rudman D, Feller AG, Nagraj HS, et al. Effects of human growth hormone in men over 60 years old. *N Engl J Med.* 1990;323:1-6.
217. Papadakis MA, Grady D, Black D, et al. Growth hormone replacement in healthy older men improves body composition but not functional ability. *Ann Intern Med.* 1996;124:708-716.
218. Wallace JD, Cuneo RD, Lundberg PA, et al. Responses of markers of bone and collagen turnover to exercise, growth hormone (GH) administration and GH withdrawal in trained adult males. *J Clin Endocrinol Metab.* 1999;85:124-133.
218a. Powrie JK, Bassett EE, Rosen T, et al. Detection of growth hormone abuse in sport. *Growth Horm IGF Res.* 2007;17:220-226.
219. Wu Z, Bidlingmaier M, Dall R, et al. Detection of doping with human growth hormone. *Lancet.* 1999;353:895.
220. Bidlingmaier M, Suhr J, Ernst A, et al. High-sensitivity chemiluminescence immunoassays for detection of growth hormone doping in sports. *Clin Chem* 2009;55:445-453.
221. Jelkmann W. Erythropoietin. *J Endocrinol Invest.* 2003;26:832-837.
222. Schobersberger W, Hobisch-Hagen P, Fries P, et al. Increase in immune activation, vascular endothelial growth factor and erythropoietin after an ultramarathon run at moderate altitude. *Immunobiology.* 2000;201:611-620.
223. Schmidt W, Maassen N, Trost F, et al. Training induced effects on blood volume, erythrocyte turnover and haemoglobin oxygen binding properties. *Eur J Appl Physiol Occup Physiol.* 1988;57:490-498.
224. Lin FK, Suggs S, Lin CH, et al. Cloning and expression of the human erythropoietin gene. *Proc Natl Acad Sci U S A.* 1985;82:7580-7584.
225. Elliott S. Erythropoiesis-stimulating agents and other methods to enhance oxygen transport. *Br J Pharmacol.* 2008;154:529-541.
226. Birkeland KI, Stray-Gundersen J, Hemmersbach P, et al. Effect of rhEPO administration on serum levels of sTfR and cycling performance. *Med Sci Sports Exerc.* 2000;32:1238-1243.
227. Ekblom B, Berglund B. Effect of erythropoietin administration on maximal aerobic power. *Scand J Med Sci Sports.* 1991;1:88-93.
228. Williams MH, Branch JD. Ergogenic aids for improved performance. In: Garrett WE, Kirkendall DT, eds. *Exercise and Sport Science. Philadelphia,* Lippincott: Williams & Wilkins; 2000:373-384.
229. Ninot G, Connes P, Caillaud C. Effects of recombinant human erythropoietin injections on physical self in endurance athletes. *J Sports Sci.* 2006;24:383-391.
230. Parisotto R, Gore CJ, Emslie KR, et al. A novel method utilising markers of altered erythropoiesis for the detection of recombinant human erythropoietin abuse in athletes. *Hematologica.* 2000;85:564-572.
231. Lasne J, de Ceaurriz J. Recombinant erythropoietin in urine. *Nature.* 2000;405:635.
232. Egrie JK, Browne JK. Development and characterization of novel erythropoiesis stimulating protein (NESP). *Br J Cancer.* 2001;84:3-10.
233. Bowers LD. Abuse of performance-enhancing drugs in sport. *Ther Drug Monit.* 2002;24:178-181.

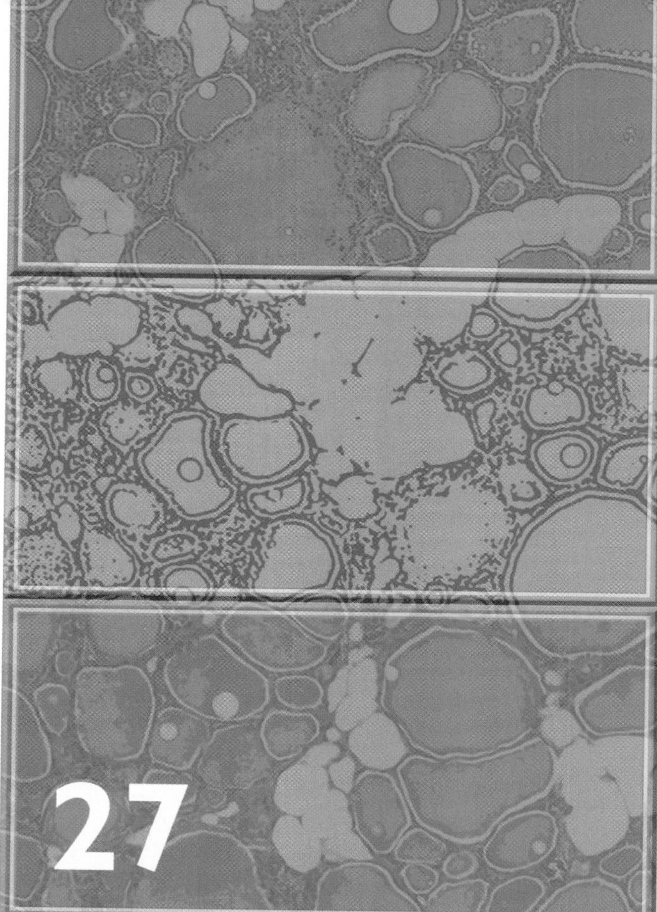

CHAPTER 27

Endocrinology and Aging

STEVEN W. J. LAMBERTS

The average length of human life has increased to 75 to 78 years, and to almost 85 years for Japanese women.[1] The data indicate that the linear climb of recorded life expectancy will continue in the next decade.[1] It is not clear, however, whether these additional years will be satisfactory.

Most data indicate a modest gain in the number of healthy years lived but a far greater increase in years of compromised physical, mental, and social function.[2] The number of days with restricted activity and admissions to hospitals and nursing homes increase sharply after 70 years of age.[3] The compression-of-morbidity hypothesis[4] suggests that it may be possible to reduce cumulative lifetime morbidity. Because chronic illness and disability usually occur late in life, cumulative lifetime disability could be reduced if primary prevention measures postponed the onset of chronic illness. Smoking, body mass index (BMI), and exercise patterns in midlife and late adulthood are important predictors of subsequent disability.[5] Persons with better health habits live longer, with disability postponed and compressed into fewer years at the end of life.

AGING AND PHYSICAL FRAILTY

Throughout adult life, all physiologic functions decline gradually.[6] A diminished capacity for cellular protein synthesis, a decline in immune function, an increase in fat mass, a loss of muscle mass and strength, and a decrease in bone mineral density contribute to declining health status.[6] Most older adults die of atherosclerosis, cancer, or dementia, but in an increasing number of the "healthy" oldest old, loss of muscle strength is the limiting factor that determines their chances of an independent life until death.

Age-related disability is characterized by generalized weakness, impaired mobility and balance, and poor endurance. In the oldest old, this state is called *physical frailty*, defined as a state of reduced physiologic reserves associated with increased susceptibility to disability.[7] Clinical correlates of physical frailty include falls, fractures, impairment in activities of daily living, and loss of independence. Falls contribute to 40% of admissions to nursing homes.[8]

Loss of muscle strength is an important factor in the development of frailty. Muscle weakness can be caused by aging of muscle fibers and their innervation, osteoarthritis, or chronic debilitating diseases.[9] However, a sedentary lifestyle, decreased physical activity, and disuse are also important determinants of the decline in muscle strength.

In a study of 100 frail nursing home residents (average age, 87 years), lower-extremity muscle mass and strength were closely related.[10] Supervised resistance exercise training (45 minutes three times per week for 10 weeks) doubled muscle strength and significantly increased gait velocity and stair-climbing power. This finding demonstrates that frailty in the elderly population is not an irreversible effect of aging and disease but can be influenced and perhaps prevented.[10] In nondisabled elderly persons living in the community, objective measures of lower-extremity function are highly predictive of subsequent disability.[11] Prevention of frailty can be achieved only through work (i.e., training). However, exercise is difficult to implement in the daily routine of the aging population, and the number of dropouts from exercise programs is very high.

Part of the aging process involving body composition—that is, loss of muscle (strength) and bone and increase in fat mass—may also be related to changes in the endocrine system.[6] Current knowledge has shed light on the effects of long-term hormonal replacement therapy on body composition and on atherosclerosis, cancer formation, and cognitive function.

ENDOCRINOLOGY OF AGING

The two most important clinical changes in endocrine activity during aging involve the pancreas and the thyroid gland. Approximately 40% of individuals between the ages of 65 and 74 years and 50% of those older than 80 years have impaired glucose tolerance or diabetes mellitus, and in almost 50% of elderly adults with diabetes the disease is undiagnosed.[12] These adults are at risk for secondary, mainly macrovascular complications occurring at an accelerated rate. Pancreatic, insulin receptor, and postreceptor changes associated with aging are critical components of the endocrinology of aging. Apart from relatively decreased insulin secretion by the beta cells, peripheral insulin resistance related to poor diet, physical inactivity, increased abdominal fat mass, and decreased lean body mass contribute to the deterioration of glucose metabolism.[12] Dietary management, exercise, oral hypoglycemic agents, and insulin are the four components of treatment for these patients, whose medical care is costly and intensive (see Chapter 27).

Age-related thyroid dysfunction is common.[13] Lowered plasma thyroxine (T_4) and increased thyrotropin concentrations occur in 5% to 10% of elderly women.[13] These abnormalities are primarily caused by autoimmunity and are an expression of age-associated disease rather than a consequence of the aging process. Normal aging is accompanied by a slight decrease in pituitary thyrotropin release and especially by decreased peripheral degradation of T_4, which results in a gradual age-dependent decline in serum triiodothyronine (T_3) concentrations without changes in T_4 levels.[13] This slight decrease in plasma T_3 concentrations occurs largely within the broad normal range of the healthy elderly population and has not been convincingly related to functional changes during the aging process.

The detrimental effects of overt thyroid dysfunction in elderly individuals are clearly recognized, but the clinical relevance of mild forms of hypothyroidism and hyperthyroidism are a matter of debate. Subclinical hypothyroidism is present in about 4% to 8.5% of adults in the United States who are without known thyroid disease.[14] Subtle thyroid dysfunction often affects the oldest-old fraction of the elderly population (i.e., those >85 years). In 85-year-old healthy individuals, hypothyroidism was in the subsequent 4 years associated with lower all-cause and cardiovascular mortality rates compared with euthyroid individuals.[15] In a group of 400 men with a mean age of 78 years, Van den Beld and colleagues[16] showed that low serum levels of free T_4 and T_3 (with normal reverse T_3 [rT_3]) concentrations were associated with better physical performance and 4-year survival, whereas subjects with low serum levels of T_3 and high rT_3 concentrations (i.e., fulfilling the criteria for the low T_3 syndrome) did not show a survival advantage and had lower levels of physical activity. These two studies support the concept that some degree of physiologically decreased thyroid activity at the tissue level may have favorable effects in the oldest-old subjects, but caution should be exercised when interpreting the predictive value of thyroid dysfunction in the elderly, which may produce contradictory results if not considered in the appropriate context.[17,18]

Three other hormonal systems exhibit lowered circulating hormone concentrations during normal aging, and these changes have been considered mainly physiologic (Figs. 27-1 and 27-2). Hormone replacement strategies have

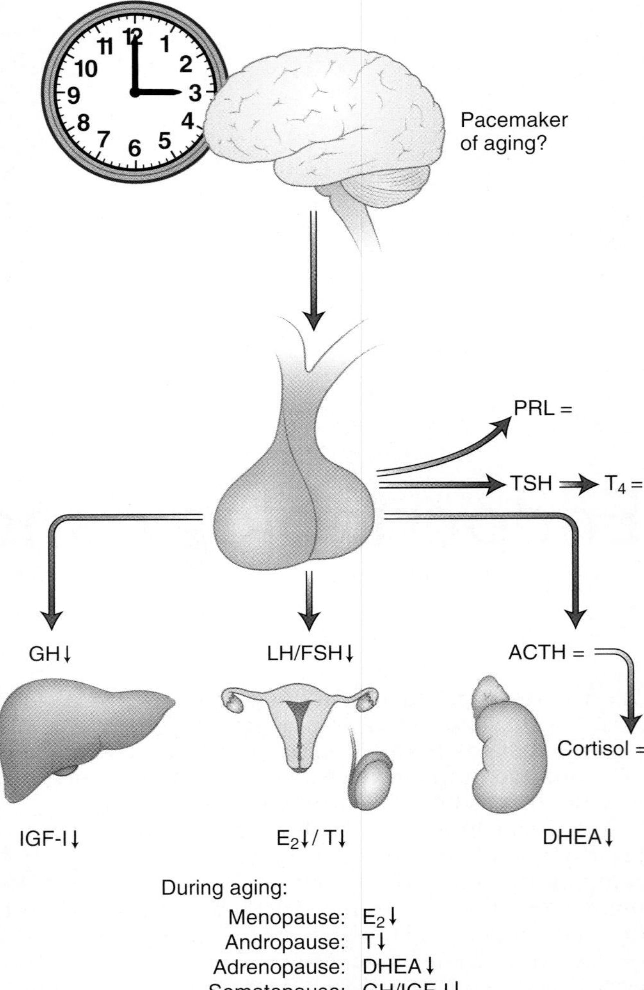

Figure 27-1 During aging, declines in the activities of a number of hormonal systems occur. *Left*, A decrease in growth hormone (GH) release by the pituitary gland causes a decrease in the production of insulin-like growth factor type I (IGF-I) by the liver and other organs (somatopause). *Middle*, A decrease in release of the gonadotropins luteinizing hormone (LH) and follicle-stimulating hormone (FSH) results in menopause, and decreased secretion at the gonadal level from the ovaries, decreased estradiol (E_2) from the testicle, and decreased testosterone (T) cause andropause. (Immediately after the initiation of menopause, serum LH and FSH levels increase sharply.) *Right*, The adrenocortical cells responsible for the production of dehydroepiandrosterone (DHEA) decrease in activity (adrenopause) without clinically evident changes in the secretion of corticotropin (ACTH) and cortisol. A central pacemaker in the hypothalamus or higher brain areas (or both) is hypothesized, which together with changes in the peripheral organs (ovaries, testicles, and adrenal cortex) regulates the aging process of these endocrine axes. PRL, prolactin; T_4, thyroxine; TSH, thyrotropin.

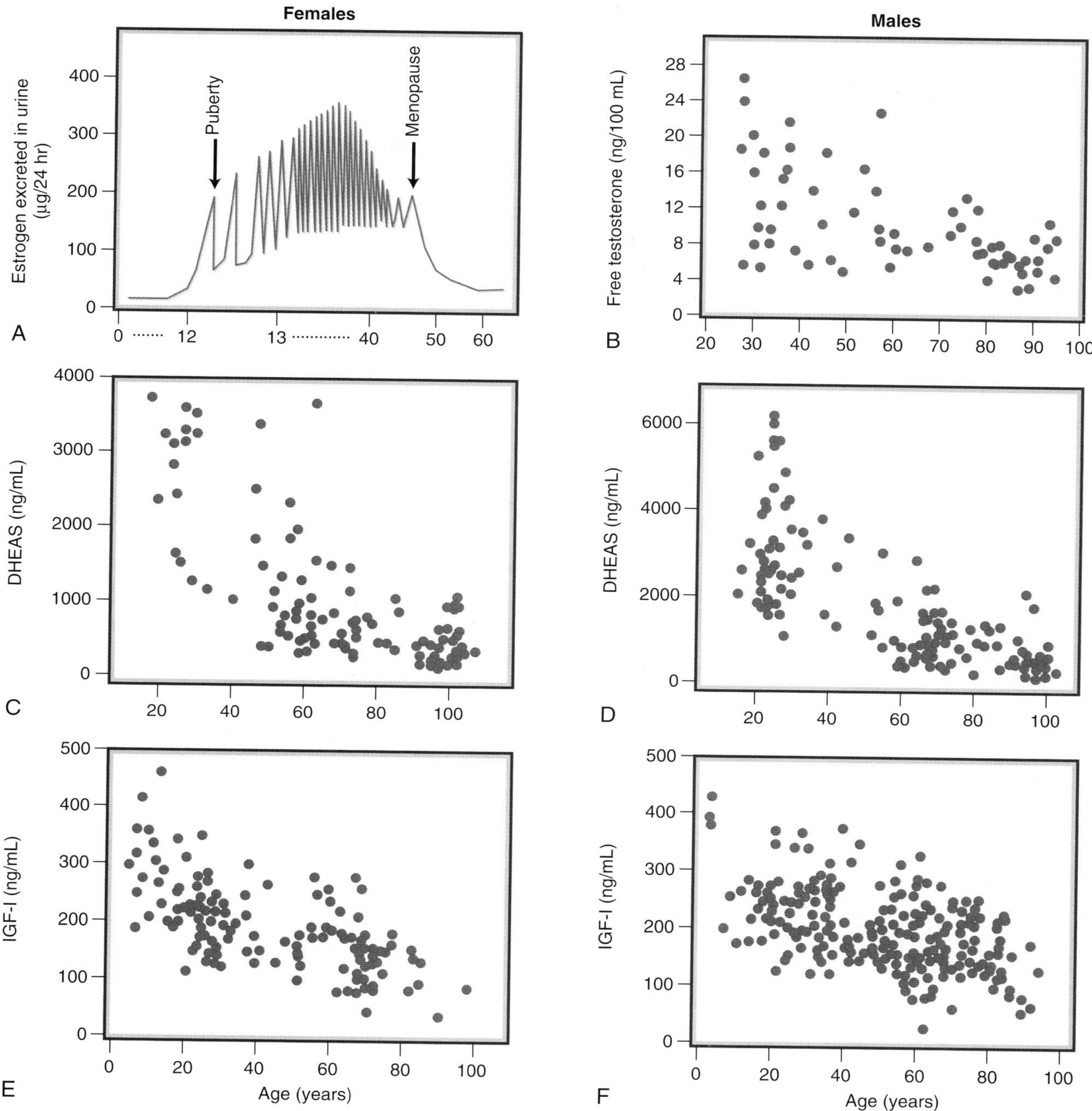

Figure 27-2 Changes in the hormone levels of normal women *(left)* and men *(right)* during the aging process. **A,** Estrogen secretion throughout an individual normal woman's life (expressed as urinary estrogen excretion). **B,** Mean free testosterone (T) index (ratio of serum total T to sex hormone-binding globulin levels) during the life span of healthy men. (From Guyton A. *Textbook of Medical Physiology,* 8th ed. Philadelphia, PA. Saunders; 1991:899.) Serum dehydroepiandrosterone sulfate (DHEAS) concentrations in 114 healthy women **(C)** and 163 healthy men **(D)** during aging. (Adapted from Ravaglia G, Forti P, Maioli F, et al. The relationship of dehydroepiandrosterone sulfate (DHEAS) to endocrine-metabolic parameters and functional status in the oldest-old: results from an Italian study on healthy free-living over-ninety-year-olds. *J Clin Endocrinol Metab.* 81:1173, 1996.) The course of serum insulin-like growth factor I (IGF-I) concentrations in 131 healthy women **(E)** and 223 healthy men **(F)** during aging. Note the difference in the distribution of ages in the different panels. (Adapted from Corpas E, Harman SM, Blackman MR. Human growth hormone and human aging. *Endocr Rev.* 14:20, 1993.)

been developed, but many aspects remain controversial, and replenishing blood hormone levels to those found in 30- to 50-year-old patients has not uniformly proved beneficial and safe.

The most dramatic and rapidly occurring change in women at about the age of 50 years is *menopause.*[19] Cycling estradiol production during the reproductive years is replaced by very low, constant estradiol levels. For many years, the prevailing view was that menopause resulted from exhaustion of ovarian follicles. An alternative perspective is that age-related changes in the central nervous system and the hypothalamic-pituitary unit initiate the menopausal transition. Evidence that both ovary and brain are key pacemakers in menopause is compelling.[19]

Changes in the activity of the hypothalamic-pituitary-gonadal axis in men are slower and more subtle. During aging, a gradual decline in serum total and free testosterone levels occurs.[20] *Andropause* is characterized by a decrease in testicular Leydig cell numbers and their secretory capacity and by an age-related decrease in episodic and stimulated gonadotropin secretion.[21,22] The primary site of the aging effect appears to be the Leydig cell's ability to respond to luteinizing hormone (LH) with increased testosterone production.

The second demonstration of age-related changes in a hormonal system is *adrenopause*, a term that describes the gradual decline in circulating levels of dehydroepiandrosterone (DHEA) and its sulfate (DHEAS).[23,24] Adrenal secretion of DHEA gradually decreases over time, while corticotropin secretion, which is physiologically linked to plasma cortisol levels, remains largely unchanged. The decline in DHEA and DHEAS levels in both sexes contrasts with the maintenance of plasma cortisol levels and seems to be caused by a selective decrease in the number of functional zona reticularis cells in the adrenal cortex rather than regulation by a central (hypothalamic) pacemaker of aging.[25]

The third endocrine system that gradually declines in activity during aging is the growth hormone (GH)–insulin-like growth factor type 1 (IGF1) axis (see Fig. 27-2).[6,26] Mean pulse amplitude and duration and the fraction of GH secreted, but not pulse frequency, gradually decrease during aging. In parallel, a progressive drop in circulating IGF1 levels occurs in both sexes.[26,27] There is no evidence for a peripheral factor in this process of *somatopause*, and its triggering pacemaker seems to be localized mainly in the hypothalamus, because pituitary somatotropes, even of the oldest old, can be restored to their youthful secretory capacity by treatment with GH-releasing peptides (discussed later).

It is unclear whether changes in gonadal function (e.g., menopause, andropause) are interrelated with the processes of adrenopause and somatopause, which occur in both sexes. Functional correlates, such as decrease in muscle size and function, decrease in fat and bone mass, progression of atherosclerosis, and decline of cognitive function, have not been directly causally related to these changes in endocrine activity. However, several effects of normal aging closely resemble features of (isolated) hormonal deficiency (e.g., hypogonadism, GH deficiency), which in subjects in middle adulthood are successfully reversed by replacement of the appropriate hormone.[28,29] Although aging does not simply result from a variety of hormone deficiency states, medical intervention in the processes of menopause, andropause, adrenopause, or somatopause may prevent or delay some aspects of the aging process.

MENOPAUSE

Menopause is the permanent cessation of menstruation that results from the loss of ovarian follicular function. It is diagnosed retrospectively after 12 months of amenorrhea.

In most women, vasomotor reactions, depressed mood, and urogenital complaints accompany this period of estrogen decline. In subsequent years, the loss of estrogens is followed by a high incidence of cardiovascular disease, loss of bone mass, and cognitive impairment. The average age at menopause (51.4 years) has not changed over time and seems to be largely determined by genetic factors.

Perimenopausal Use of Hormone Therapy

Typical symptoms that result from the sudden decrease in estrogen production around menopause are menstrual cycle disorders, vasomotor changes (e.g., hot flashes, night sweats), and urogenital complications (e.g., atrophic vaginal irritation and dryness, dyspareunia, atrophic urethral epithelium leading to micturition disorders). Additional symptoms include irritability, mood swings, joint pain, and sleep disturbances. Frequency, severity, onset, and duration of symptoms vary widely among individuals and ethnic groups. About 75% of women in Western societies experience so few troublesome symptoms during the menopausal transition that hormone therapy (HT) is not needed or requested.[30]

HT quickly alleviates the symptoms of menopause. Hot flashes, vasomotor instability, and symptoms of urogenital atrophy rapidly disappear with the start of HT.

Long-Term Hormone Replacement Therapy

Because life expectancy is increasing, the time a woman spends after menopause constitutes more than one third of her life. Until recently, long-term use of HT (5 to 10 years) was considered to offer advantages with regard to prevention of the three chronic disorders most common in the elderly: cardiovascular diseases, osteoporosis, and dementia. In the early 1990s, a number of cross-sectional and prospective studies demonstrated a statistically significant reduction in coronary heart disease in menopausal women taking HT. Grady and colleagues[31] presented a meta-analysis of published observational studies and reported that HT was associated with one-third less fatal coronary heart disease. A meta-analysis of 25 observational studies conducted between 1976 and 1996 showed that the relative risk for coronary heart disease in women who had ever used HT compared with never-users was 0.70.[32]

The Nurse's Health Study was a comprehensive investigation conducted in 121,700 female nurses between the ages of 30 and 55 years. In the 2000 report, compiled with data from 70,533 postmenopausal nurses followed for 20 years, the overall risk of coronary heart disease in current users of HT was found to be reduced, with a relative risk of 0.61.[33]

Over the past 10 years, findings from a number of prospective, randomized, controlled trials have radically changed the attitudes concerning benefits and harms of HT. The Women's Health Initiative (WHI) trial comprised two large, randomized, placebo-controlled clinical trials, including estrogen-only and combined estrogen-progestin studies in more than 161,000 healthy postmenopausal women between the ages of 50 and 79 years.[34] The WHI was expected to definitively answer whether estrogen was cardioprotective. However, the estrogen-progestin versus placebo trial, which involved more than 16,000 women, was discontinued early because of an increase in cardiovascular complications (i.e., coronary heart disease, stroke, and venous thromboembolism) and an increased incidence of breast cancer in the treatment group.[34] Although important benefits were also seen (i.e., risk reduction for fractures and colon cancer), there was concern that the risks of combined estrogen-progestin therapy outweighed the benefits. The estrogen-only versus placebo trial included almost 11,000 women who had undergone hysterectomy and therefore did not require a progestin. This trial was also stopped early because a small increase in the risk of breast cancer and coronary heart disease risk was seen, but hip fracture risk was reduced.[35]

Three other randomized, controlled trials supported the absence of benefit of HT for prevention of coronary heart disease and ischemic stroke.[36-38] These studies were carried out in postmenopausal women with documented ischemic stroke or transient ischemic attack,[36] in women after documented myocardial infarction,[37] or in women with documented coronary heart disease.[38]

Taken together, the WHI, which studied women presumed healthy at recruitment, and the three other trials enrolling women with documented cardiovascular disorders argued strongly against the earlier assumptions made on the basis of observational studies that estrogen users had a 30% to 40% reduced risk of coronary heart disease mortality and morbidity relative to nonusers.

A series of commentaries has addressed the differences in outcome between the observational studies and the randomized trials.[39,40] Healthy user bias, the age at which study participants started HT, and the different estrogen and progestin preparations and doses have been mentioned as possible confounders.

Subsequently, reassessment of the data from the WHI and other studies has led to a different interpretation of the data, that groups of perimenopausal and early postmenopausal women may derive cardiovascular benefits from HRT. In this regard, much interest has focused on the timing hypothesis, which states that estrogens are atheroprotective if used in an early phase of atherosclerosis development. In an arm of the WHI in which 50- to 59-year-old women were treated with conjugated estrogens, only coronary artery calcium scores were significantly lower than in nontreated controls.[41]

Several studies have confirmed the risk of breast cancer, which increases with longer duration of HT.[42-44] In the Million Women Study, current users of estrogen had an increased risk of incident invasive breast cancer of 30%, whereas in women using estrogen plus progestin, this risk had doubled. Breast cancer risk was unchanged in both the older and younger women with a prior hysterectomy treated with estrogen only. Past users of HT had also no increased risk.[45]

The earlier expectations from observational studies that estrogen use might prevent cognitive decline were not confirmed by randomized, placebo-controlled trials. Estrogen therapy alone did not reduce dementia or mild cognitive impairment in women 65 years old or older, and the estrogen-progestin combination resulted in slightly increased risks for both end points.[46] The efficacy of HT in the prevention of osteoporotic fractures remains undisputed in regard to hip and other fractures (see Table 27-1).[47]

The findings of the WHI trial are so important and have been so broadly publicized that they have created the perception that HT always carries risks that exceed its benefits. Given the described uncertainties, HT is only recommended in the perimenopausal period for women suffering from menopausal symptoms. HT is highly effective in alleviating hot flashes and night sweats. An association between endometrial cancer and estrogen use was observed many years ago. Ten years of unopposed estrogen use increases the risk for endometrial cancer 10-fold.[31] For that reason, the HT regimens were supplemented with progestagens, which almost completely prevented this excess risk of endometrial cancer.

Currently advised doses of estrogen were originally designed to prevent bone loss, and opposing progestagen regimens were added to prevent endometrial cancer. Several estrogen and progestagen preparations are available for HT.[30] Components of available preparations vary in their effects on various target tissues. Commercial preparations differ in their clinical effect by design, and individual women differ in their responses. HT can be administered orally, transdermally, topically, intranasally, or as subcutaneous implants.

TABLE 27-1

Clinical Event Risks and Benefits of Hormone Therapy with Estrogen-Progestin or Estrogen Only in the Women's Health Initiative Trial*

	ESTROGEN-PROGESTIN THERAPY		ESTROGEN THERAPY	
Health Event	**Risk**	**Benefit**	**Risk**	**Benefit**
Coronary heart disease	8	—	—	3
Stroke	8	—	11	—
Breast cancer	8	—	—	8
Venous thromboembolism	18	—	8	—
Colorectal cancer	—	7	1	—
Hip fracture	—	5	—	6
Any fracture	—	47	—	56
New-onset diabetes	—	15	—	14

*Absolute risk or benefit per 10,000 women per year, compared with placebo. For overall hazard ratio, 95% confidence interval, and adjustments, see original paper.

After Hodis HN. Assessing benefits and risks of hormone therapy in 2008: new evidence, especially with regard to the heart. *Cleve Clin J Med.* 2008;75(suppl 4):S3.

Although HT in the perimenopausal state can cause some symptoms (e.g., vaginal discharge, uterine bleeding, breast tenderness), it relieves many others, including hot flashes and the severity of night sweats.[48] Grady estimated that about one serious adverse event will occur among every 1000 50-year-old women using HT for 1 year. The HT regimen used in the WHI trial combined 0.625 mg/day of conjugated equine estrogen and 2.5 mg/day of medroxyprogesterone acetate.[31] However, the dose of estrogen necessary to diminish perimenopausal symptoms can be lower in many women. A dose of 0.3 or 0.45 mg/day of conjugated equine estrogen is effective at diminishing the number and intensity of hot flashes.[49]

Selective Estrogen Receptor Modulators

In the search for optimal HT during menopause, it was observed that tamoxifen has variable antiestrogenic and estrogenic actions in different tissues.[50,51] Tamoxifen suppresses the growth of estrogen receptor–positive breast cancer cells. Long-term treatment of breast cancer in menopausal patients with tamoxifen also lowered the incidence of new (contralateral) breast cancer by 40%. The number of cardiovascular incidents decreased by 70%, and the age-related decrease in bone mineral density was partially prevented.[52]

These initially puzzling observations were explained by the fact that tamoxifen and other compounds such as raloxifene have selective estrogen receptor–modulating effects, exerting antiestrogenic actions on normal and cancerous breast tissue but agonistic actions on bone, lipids, and the blood vessel walls.[53] The effects of tamoxifen and raloxifene may be explained by differential stabilization of the conformation of the estrogen receptor, which facilitates interactions with coactivator or corepressor proteins and subsequently initiates or suppresses transcription of target genes. These specific interactions in the target cell lead to tissue-selective actions.[54]

The efficacy and safety of raloxifene for the prevention of osteoporosis in postmenopausal women were demonstrated in a study that found a 2.5% increase in bone mineral density in the lumbar spine and hip in a group of postmenopausal, non-osteoporotic women treated with raloxifene for 2 years.[55] A significant reduction of vertebral fracture risk by raloxifene was subsequently demonstrated.[56] A total of 7705 postmenopausal women with existing osteoporosis were studied. After 36 months, bone mineral density at the hip and spine increased in the women treated with 60 mg of raloxifene by 2.1% and 2.6%, respectively, compared with those receiving placebo. At 36 months, 7.4% of women had at least one new vertebral fracture, including 10.1% of women receiving placebo and 6.6% of those receiving raloxifene at 60 mg/day. Compared with the placebo group, those receiving 60 mg of raloxifene had a relative risk for fracture of 0.7 ($P < .001$). Forty-six subjects needed raloxifene at 60 mg for 3 years to prevent one vertebral fracture in menopausal women without an existing fracture; for those with an existing fracture, 16 subjects required treatment. A meta-analysis confirmed the effects of raloxifene treatment on reduction of vertebral fracture risk in postmenopausal women without an effect on nonvertebral fracture risk.[57]

In a placebo-controlled clinical trial of 10,000 postmenopausal women with an increased risk of coronary heart disease who were monitored for 5 to 6 years, raloxifene had an overall neutral effect on the incidence of cardiovascular events.[58] The incidence of all strokes was not different in the raloxifene- and the placebo-treated groups. However, among raloxifene-treated individuals, there was a higher incidence of fatal stroke, especially in smokers (incidence rates per 100 women-years, 0.22 versus 0.15 [$P < .0499$]), and a higher incidence of venous thromboembolic events (0.39 versus 0.27 incidents per 100 women-years [$P = .02$]).[59]

Raloxifene, in contrast to tamoxifen and estrogen, does not stimulate endometrial thickness or vaginal bleeding.[55] With regard to side effects, raloxifene causes an increased incidence of leg cramps and hot flashes.[60]

Endocrine approaches to breast cancer prevention have become increasingly successful. Four trials of tamoxifen administration for 5 years or longer in women at increased risk for breast cancer showed an approximately 50% reduction in breast cancer, but only for estrogen receptor–positive disease.[61] (See Fig. 27-3.) Follow-up indicates that there was a carryover effect of tamoxifen after completion of treatment at 5 years so that the preventive effect at 10 years was significantly greater than at 5 years.

Raloxifene has been compared with placebo in three trials: one in women with osteoporosis,[56,62] one in women with or at risk for cardiac disease,[58] and one in which raloxifene was compared with tamoxifen in women at high risk for breast cancer.[63] Reductions of 66%, 44%, and 50% in breast cancer risk were observed after 4 to 5 years of raloxifene therapy, respectively. The last trial showed that raloxifene was as effective as tamoxifen.[63] As with the previous tamoxifen studies, raloxifene reduced the risk only of estrogen receptor α–positive tumors.

In the United States, the 60-mg dose of raloxifene is indicated for the treatment and prevention of osteoporosis in postmenopausal women and for reduction in the risk of invasive breast cancer in postmenopausal women with osteoporosis, and in postmenopausal women at high risk for invasive breast cancer.[64,65]

Tibolone is a compound that regulates estrogen activity selectively in different tissues. It has a high efficacy in the treatment of climacteric symptoms and the prevention of bone loss. The compound is approved in many countries but not in the United States. In a 5-year trial, tibolone (1.5 mg/day) was associated with a 45% decrease in vertebral fractures, a 26% decrease in nonvertebral fractures, a 68% decrease in invasive breast cancer, and a 69% decreased risk of colon cancer.[66] However, the tibolone-treated group had an increased risk of stroke (relative hazard = 2.19; $P = .02$).

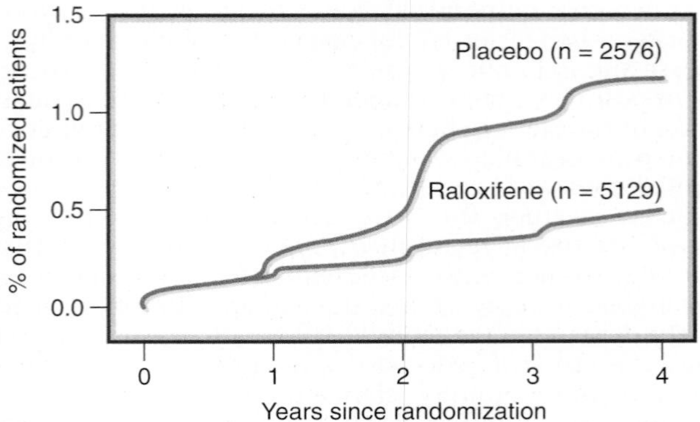

Figure 27-3 Effect of raloxifene administration (60 to 120 mg/day) on the cumulative incidence of breast cancer in 7705 postmenopausal women (mean age, 66.5 years) with osteoporosis. Statistical significance of the difference between the groups was $P < .001$. (From Cummings SR, Eckert S, Krueger KA, et al. The effect of raloxifene on risk of breast cancer in postmenopausal women: results from the MORE randomized trial. Multiple Outcomes of Raloxifene Evaluation. *JAMA.* 281:2189, 1999.)

Androgen Replacement

In premenopausal women, androgen production originates equally from the adrenal glands and the ovaries. Androgen production in women declines with age. After menopause, circulating androgen levels decrease by more than 50%.

There is increasing awareness of the effect of low androgen levels on the emotional and sexual well-being of perimenopausal women. No single androgen level is predictive of low female sexual function, and in one study, most of 1423 women between the ages of 18 and 75 years with low DHEAS levels were found to have normal sexual function.[67]

The efficacy and safety of testosterone treatment for hypoactive sexual desire disorder in postmenopausal women was studied in a double-blind, placebo-controlled, 52-week trial in which more than 800 women participated.[68] Treatment with a patch delivering 300 µg of testosterone per day resulted in a modest but meaningful improvement in sexual function. The long-term effects of testosterone, including effect on the breast, remain uncertain.

Hormone Therapy, Selective Estrogen Receptor Modulators, or No Treatment

The issue of HT in postmenopausal women is controversial, and many aspects remain unresolved. The idea that HT is a global risk reduction strategy has been abandoned. Although the general benefits of HT in the short term during and after the menopausal transition are evident in women suffering from estrogen-withdrawal symptoms, the balance of the effects of long-term HT after menopause points to a negative outcome, with more harm than benefit. Evolution of the association of HT and cardiovascular risk, from protection to harm and now to possible protection again, has resulted in controversy and confusion.[69,70]

HT is usually prescribed for women between the ages of 45 and 60 years who are experiencing vasomotor symptoms. HT is not indicated for cardioprotection for women in their 70s or for women who do not suffer from vasomotor symptoms or urogenital atrophy. Data clearly demonstrate, however, that clinicians can prescribe and women can use low-dose HT confidently during the time when therapy is most needed. The debate regarding the potential benefits of HT on cardiovascular risk and mortality for women who start therapy close to the menopausal transition is not resolved. The benefit and risk of any therapy, including HT, should be reassessed periodically for each individual based on future scientific evidence.[70]

A vast armamentarium of other pharmacologic treatments to reduce cardiovascular and bone risks is available. Agents include cholesterol-lowering statins, β-blockers, selective estrogen receptor modulators (SERMs), and bisphosphonates. An optimal choice of these different lifestyle drugs for menopausal women requires individualization of the treatment decision. Coronary artery disease, for example, is a complex disorder resulting from an interaction of genetic predisposition and environmental factors. Risk factor modification (e.g., diet, smoking, physical activity) should be advised. Secondary prevention of coronary artery disease and atherosclerosis includes the use of lipid-lowering drugs, aspirin, nitrates, and β-blockers.[71]

For women with existing osteoporosis, HT is effective. However, SERMs and especially bisphosphonates come close or are better in their fracture-reducing effects. Recognition of an increased risk of breast cancer in menopausal women is an important consideration in the choice of SERMs. Chemoprevention of breast cancer with raloxifene has become a major consideration in the pharmacologic choice for risk reduction in the long-term preventive treatment of postmenopausal women.

ANDROPAUSE AND PARTIAL ANDROGEN DEFICIENCY

Role of Testosterone during Aging

Age-associated hypogonadism does not develop as clearly in men at andropause as in women at menopause. The key difference is the gradual, often subtle change in androgen levels in men compared with the precipitate fall of estrogen production in women. As men age, there is a decline in serum total testosterone concentrations that begins after the age of 40 years. In cross-sectional studies, the annual decline in total and free testosterone is 1.0%, and 1.2%, respectively. The higher decline in free testosterone levels is related to the increase in the levels of sex hormone–binding globulin (SHBG) with age.[20,72]

It remains unclear whether the well-known biologic changes that occur during aging in men (e.g., reduced sexual activity, muscle mass and strength, skeletal mineralization) are causally related to the changes in testosterone bioactivity. The decline in testosterone levels, when associated with signs and symptoms of androgen deficiency, has been called *andropause*, but this term may be better replaced by (partial) androgen deficiency of the aging male, or (P)ADAM, because androgen production in the elderly male does not cease, but instead gradually decreases.

There has been major disagreement on how to define androgen deficiency in the elderly man. Investigators have initially taken two different approaches; one is purely biochemical, the other clinical. The biochemical approach consists of defining (partial) androgen deficiency by measuring morning serum total testosterone levels or determining, by additionally measuring SHBG levels, a "free" testosterone concentration. Most elderly men have testosterone levels within the normal range; prevalence estimates of low serum testosterone concentrations (<10.4 nmol/L or <300 ng/dL) are usually between 10% and 25%.[73,74] Most men with low testosterone levels do not come to clinical attention, because testosterone levels are not routinely measured in clinical practice.[75] An important problem with a biochemical approach to the diagnosis of (P)ADAM is that men with low testosterone may not exhibit clinically significant symptoms, raising the possibility that large numbers of men may be diagnosed as needing testosterone replacement therapy simply by virtue of falling below an arbitrary threshold.

The clinical approach to the diagnosis of (P)ADAM has important drawbacks.[76] All symptoms and signs of androgen deficiency are nonspecific and readily accounted for by comorbidities. Lethargy, reduced concentration, sleep disturbance, irritability, and depressed mood may relate to physical illness (and side effects of treatment), obesity, or lack of physical exercise and other lifestyle issues (e.g., alcohol or drug use); relationship difficulties; or occupational or financial stresses. Existing screening tools for androgen deficiency lack adequate specificity and sensitivity to be reliably employed in directing clinical diagnosis and treatment.

Araujo and coworkers[75] defined the prevalence of symptomatic androgen deficiency in men by studying the association between symptoms of androgen deficiency (i.e., low libido, erectile dysfunction, osteoporosis or fracture, or two of the following symptoms: sleep disturbance, depressed mood, lethargy, or diminished physical performance) and low serum total testosterone (<10.4 nmol/L or <300 ng/dL) and free testosterone (<0.17 nmol/L or <5 ng/dL) concentrations. Applying these criteria to almost 1500 men 30 to 79 years old, they found 24% with total testosterone levels and 11% with low free testosterone levels. Symptoms included low libido (12% prevalence), erectile dysfunction (16%), osteoporosis or fracture (1%), and two or more of the nonspecific symptoms (20%). Although low testosterone levels were associated with symptoms, many men with low testosterone levels were asymptomatic (e.g., 47.6% of men older than 50 years). In Figure 27-4 the interrelationships are shown; symptomatic androgen deficiency with low serum testosterone (<10.4 nmol/L) was observed in 4.2% of men younger than 50 years old and in 8.4% of men older than 50 years. This prevalence rapidly increases with age, reaching 18.4% among 70-year-olds.

Low testosterone concentrations are especially prevalent among obese men.[77] Although much of the effect of obesity was explained by a decrease in SHBG, the serum free testosterone concentration was especially lower in men with a BMI of 30 kg/m^2 or greater. Lower total testosterone levels are associated with comorbidities, including the presence and degree of atherosclerosis.[78] In line with these observations, men with total testosterone levels in the lowest quartile had a 40% increased risk of death during the next 20 years after testing, independent of multiple risk factors and several preexisting health conditions.[79]

Testosterone Replacement Therapy

Many persuasive reports in the literature demonstrate that testosterone replacement in young, adult, and old men with clear clinical and severe biochemical hypogonadism instantly reverses vasomotor activity (i.e., flashes and sweats); improves libido, sexual activity, and mood;

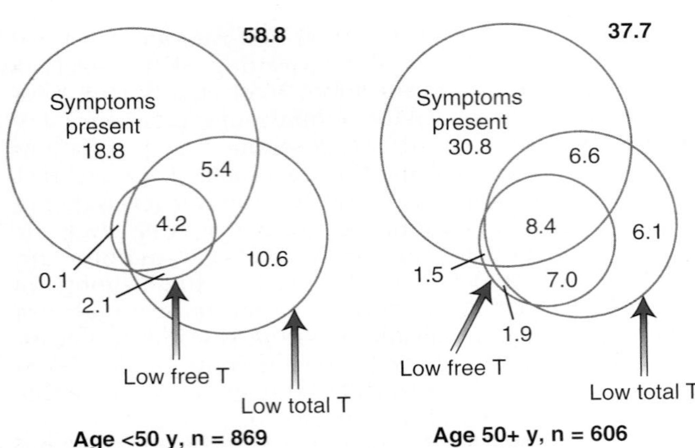

Figure 27-4 Venn diagrams showing the interrelationships among symptoms, low total testosterone (total T <10.4 nmol/L or <300 ng/dL), and low free testosterone (free T <0.17 nmol/L or <5 ng/dL) among men younger than 50 years *(left)* and 50 years or older *(right)*. Circles for the Venn diagrams are proportional within age strata. Numbers displayed are percentages observed within each area. Positive symptom reports and low total T and free T levels were more common among older men. The presence of symptoms was related more strongly to T levels in older than in younger men, as indicated by a greater degree of overlap between symptom presence and low T levels among older subjects (52.4% of men with low total T or free T had symptoms) compared with younger ones (43.1% of men with low total T or free T had symptoms). The intersection of symptoms and low total T and free T levels was more common in older men: prevalence of symptomatic androgen deficiency was 4.2% among men younger than 50 years of age and 8.4% among men 50 years or older). (From Araujo AB, Esche GR, Kupelian V, et al. Prevalence of symptomatic androgen deficiency in men. *J Clin Endocrinol Metab.* 92:4241, 2007.)

increases muscle mass, strength, and bone mineralization; prevents fractures; decreases fat mass; and decreases fatigue and poor concentration.[28,72,80] Treatment of normal adult men with supraphysiologic doses of testosterone, especially when combined with resistance exercise training, increased fat-free mass and muscle size and strength.[81]

Many studies reporting the results of androgen therapy in older men have been small, short-term, not controlled, and without uniform end points. The results of a large, randomized study in healthy elderly men were published in 1999 and seem to be representative for effects expected of androgen therapy.[82,83] Ninety-six men (mean age, 73 years) wore a testosterone patch on their scrotum (6 mg of testosterone/24 hours) or a placebo patch for 36 months. Mean serum testosterone concentrations in the men treated with testosterone increased from 12.7 ± 2.9 nmol/L (367 ± 7.9 ng/dL) before treatment to 21.7 ± 8.6 nmol/L (625 ± 249 ng/dL, $P < .001$) after 6 months of treatment and remained at that level for the duration of the study. The decrease in fat mass (–3.0 ± 0.5 kg) in the testosterone-treated men during the 36 months of treatment was significantly different from the decrease in the placebo-treated men (–0.7 ± 0.5 kg; $P < .001$) (Fig. 27-5). The increase in lean mass (1.9 ± 0.3 kg) with testosterone treatment was also significantly different from that observed with placebo (0.2 ± 0.2 kg, $P < .001$).

Changes in knee extension and flexion strength, hand grip, walking speed, and other parameters of muscle strength and function were not significantly different in the two groups. Bone mineral density in the lumbar spine increased in both groups (4.2% ± 0.8% and 2.5% ± 0.6%, respectively), but mean changes did not differ between groups (see Fig. 27-5). However, the lower the pretreatment serum testosterone concentration, the greater the effects of testosterone treatment on lumbar spine bone density after 36 months ($P = .02$). A minimal effect (0.9 ± 1.0%) of testosterone treatment on bone mineral density was observed in men with a pretreatment serum testosterone concentration of 13.9 nmol/L (400 ng/dL), but an increase of 5.9% ± 2.2% was found in men with a pretreatment testosterone concentration of 6.9 nmol/L (200 ng/dL).

The subjective perception of physical functioning decreased significantly during the 36 months of treatment

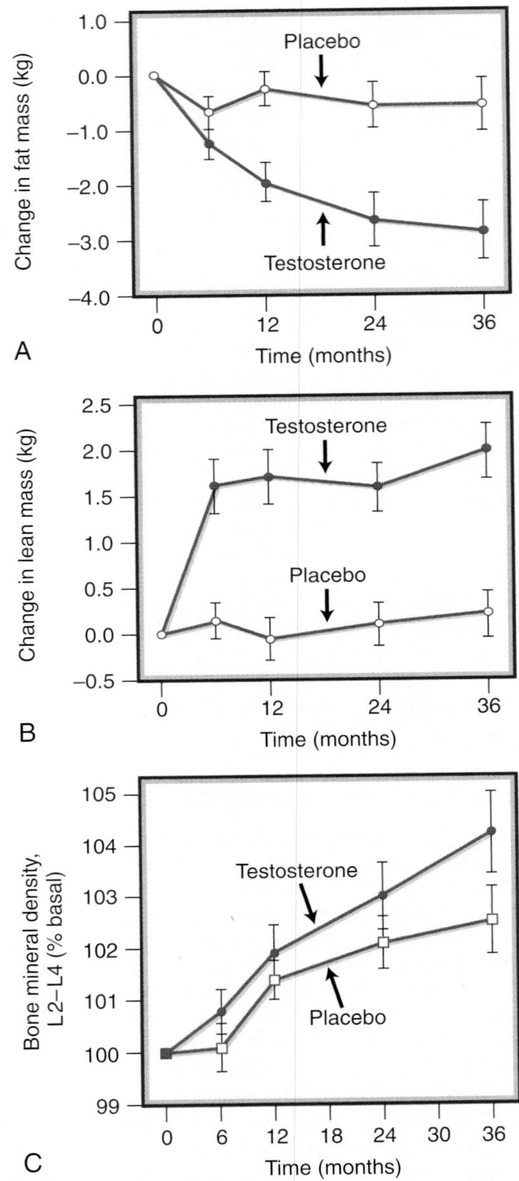

Figure 27-5 **A** through **C**, Mean (± standard error) changes from baseline in fat mass, lean mass, and bone mineral density of the lumbar spine (L2 to L4) as determined by dual-energy x-ray absorptiometry in 108 men older than 65 years who were treated with either testosterone or placebo (54 men each). The decrease in fat mass (P < .005) and the increase in lean mass (P < .01) in the testosterone-treated subjects were significantly different from those in placebo-treated subjects at 36 months. Bone mineral density increased significantly in both groups. (**A** and **B** from Snyder PJ, Peachey H, Hannoush P, et al. Effect of testosterone treatment on bone mineral density in men over 65 years of age. *J Clin Endocrinol Metab.* 84:1966, 1999. **C** from Snyder PJ, Peachey H, Hannoush P, et al. Effect of testosterone treatment on body composition and muscle strength in men over 65 years of age. *J Clin Endocrinol Metab.* 84:2647, 1999.)

in the placebo-treated ($P < .001$) but not in the testosterone-treated group. The effect of testosterone treatment on the perception of physical functioning varied inversely with the pretreatment serum testosterone concentration ($P < .01$). There was no significant difference between the two treatment groups with regard to the subjective perception of energy or sexual function.

With regard to the potential adverse effects of testosterone treatment in healthy elderly men, the study by Snyder and colleagues[82] seems representative. The mean serum prostate-specific antigen (PSA) concentration did not change during the 36 months of treatment in the placebo-treated group, but it increased by a relatively small but statistically significant ($P < .001$) amount by 6 months of treatment in the testosterone-treated group and remained relatively stable for the remainder of the study. The urine flow rate, volume of urine in the bladder after voiding, and number of clinically significant prostate events during the 3 years of the study were similar in the two groups. Hemoglobin and hematocrit levels did not change in the placebo-treated group during treatment, but both increased significantly ($P < .001$) in the testosterone-treated group within 6 months and remained relatively stable for the remainder of the study. Three men treated with testosterone developed persistent erythrocytosis (hemoglobin > 17.5 g/dL; hematocrit > 52%) during treatment.

Numerous studies of large populations of healthy men have shown a marked rise in the incidence of impotence to more than 50% in men 60 to 70 years old.[84] Although this increased rate occurs in the same age group who show a clear decline in serum (free) testosterone levels, no causal relationships have been demonstrated. A systematic review and meta-analysis of randomized, placebo-controlled trials concluded that testosterone use in normal men is associated with a small improvement in satisfaction with erectile function and moderate improvements in libido.[85] Other factors, such as atherosclerosis, alcohol consumption, smoking, and the quality of personal relationships, seem to be more important.[86,87] Only in the case of clear hypogonadism is the decrease in libido and potency restored by testosterone therapy.[28,80]

An Endocrine Society Clinical Practice Guideline on testosterone therapy in adult men with androgen deficiency syndromes summarized the observed effects of randomized, placebo-controlled trials of testosterone administration with 1- to 3-year-old duration in older men with low-normal to low testosterone concentrations.[88] There was a moderate effect on lumbar bone mineral density but no reports on bone fracture rate; a significant increase in lean body mass (+2.7 kg on average) and a reduction in fat mass (−2.0 kg) without a change in body weight; a greater improvement in grip strength than placebo (3.3 kg), without consistent effects on lower extremity muscle strength and unequivocal effects on physical function; and inconsistent or insignificant effects on sexual function, quality of life, depression, and cognition.

In the Guidelines, all reported adverse outcomes with testosterone therapy in elderly men were summarized[88] from a systematic review of 19 randomized trials,[89] and the combined rate of all prostate events was significantly greater in testosterone-treated men than in placebo-treated men (odds ratio = 1.78; 95% confidence level [CI], 1.07 to 2.95). Rates of prostate cancer, PSA greater than 4 ng/mL, and prostate biopsies were not significantly higher for the testosterone group than the placebo group. Testosterone-treated men were almost four times more likely than placebo-treated men to have hematocrits greater than 50% (odds ratio = 3.69; 95% CI, 1.82 to 7.51). The frequency of cardiovascular events, sleep apnea, or death did not differ significantly between groups. Nonsignificant changes in lipids were observed. Compared with placebo, testosterone therapy for older men was associated with a higher risk of detecting prostate events and a hematocrit greater than 50%.

Which Elderly Men Should Be Treated?

A key lesson from the Heart and Estrogen/Progestin Replacement and WHI studies was that conventional medical use of these agents should not precede substantiation with reliable clinical evidence of safety and efficacy.[90] Androgen replacement in older men is the male counterpart of HT in postmenopausal women, but it differs crucially in that a clear syndrome of androgen deficiency is lacking. On the basis of a number of suggestive clinical features collected from the history, symptoms, or signs of an elderly man, the biochemical confirmation of androgen deficiency is sought.

In previous discussions of testosterone replacement in older men,[86,91] it was suggested that the biochemical diagnosis of true hypogonadism seems certain if the serum total testosterone concentration is less than 6.9 nmol/L (200 ng/dL). This cutoff remains arbitrary and does not answer the question of whether healthy elderly men with testosterone levels between 6.9 and 10.4 nmol/L are hypogonadal and would benefit from replacement therapy with testosterone. Intercurrent diseases frequently result in a transient, sharp drop in serum testosterone concentrations,[92] whereas frail, elderly men tend to have testosterone levels 10% to 15% lower than those of healthy, age-matched control subjects.[93] When a serum testosterone concentration is below 6.9 nmol/L (200 ng/dL), an additional evaluation with measurements of serum gonadotropins and prolactin is mandatory to exclude pituitary pathology.

The current recommendation[88] is not to treat asymptomatic older men with age-related decline in testosterone levels. If the decision is made to start testosterone replacement, the major goal of therapy is to return testosterone levels to values as close to physiologic levels in age-matched controls as possible. The dose should be titrated according to serum levels. Considerations concerning the choice of testosterone preparation and the route of administration (i.e., oral, injectable, implantable, or transdermal) are discussed in Chapter 8.

The recommended duration of testosterone administration is uncertain. Control of prostate size, PSA levels, and hematocrit is mandatory. The identification of elderly men who may benefit most from testosterone treatment remains uncertain, and the risks to the prostate and increased blood viscosity require further study. The development of androgenic compounds with variable biologic action in different organs (i.e., selective androgen receptor modulation) is being pursued.[94]

Testosterone's effects are mediated through the androgen receptor, and the considerable variation in testosterone responsiveness that is observed between aging men receiving therapy may be related to variations in the androgen receptor gene. A candidate for this variability is the CAG repeat polymorphism in exon 1 of the androgen receptor gene, which is located on the X chromosome.[95] The CAG repeat encodes for a polyglutamine tract in the androgen receptor protein, and ranges normally form about 6 to 37 repeats, with an average of between 20 and 22. The number of CAG repeats is inversely associated with the transcriptional activity in testosterone target genes.[95] Krithivas and associates[96] demonstrated that the CAG repeat in the androgen receptor gene is associated with the age-related decline in serum testosterone levels in men; the lower the number of repeats, the sharper the decline in serum testosterone concentrations. The lower the number of CAG repeats in normal healthy men, the earlier and higher the degree of prostate hyperplasia during the aging process.[97] For testosterone substitution in hypogonadal adult men for 36 months with a fixed dose, prostate size increased significantly more if the number of CAG repeats in the androgen receptor gene was lower.[95] This first pharmacogenetic study demonstrating that the effect of androgen replacement therapy on prostate growth in hypogonadal men is greatly influenced by the genetic background has important implications for its use in otherwise healthy elderly men. It is assumed that androgen sensitivity as determined by variations in the androgen receptor gene in muscle, fat, brain, vessel walls, and prostate will be similar within one individual. In future selection of aging men for testosterone therapy, the genetic background should probably be taken into account. The same applies to the androgen dose prescribed. Correlation of the CAG repeat in the androgen receptor with the serum testosterone level was confirmed in a population survey involving almost 3000 men.[98] Weaker transcriptional activity of the androgen receptor with longer CAG-encoded polyglutamine repeats appeared to be compensated for by higher testosterone levels. The investigators suggested that the phenotypic correlations may reflect differences in estrogen levels or actions after aromatization of the higher testosterone levels.[98]

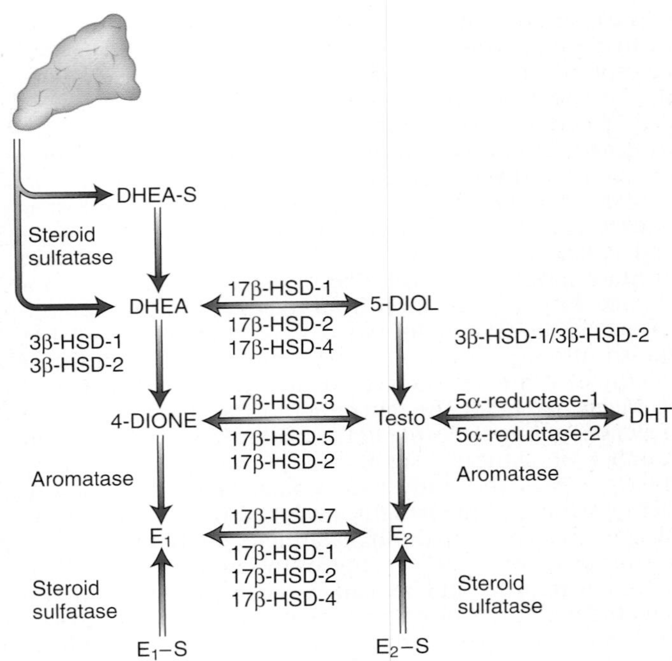

Figure 27-6 Human steroidogenic enzymes in peripheral intracrine tissues. DHEA, dehydroepiandrosterone; DHEA-S, DHEA sulfate; DHT, dihydrotestosterone; 5-DIOL, androsterone-5-ene-3β,17β-diol; 4-DIONE, androstenedione; E_1, estrone; E_2, estradiol; 3β-HSD, 3β-hydroxysteroid dehydrogenase; 17β-HSD, 17β-hydroxysteroid dehydrogenase; S, sulphate; testo, testosterone. (Modified and adapted from Labrie F, Luu-The V, Lin SX, et al. Intracrinology: role of the family of 17 beta-hydroxysteroid dehydrogenases in human physiology and disease. *J Mol Endocrinol.* 25:1, 2000.)

ADRENOPAUSE

Role of Dehydroepiandrosterone during Aging

Humans are unique among primates and rodents because the human adrenal cortex secretes large amounts of the steroid precursor DHEA and its sulfate derivative DHEAS.[99] Serum DHEAS concentrations in adult men and women are 100 to 500 times higher than those of testosterone and 1000 to 10,000 times higher than those of estradiol. In normal subjects, serum concentrations of DHEA and DHEAS are highest in the third decade of life, after which the concentrations of both gradually decrease, and by age 70 to 80 years, the values are about 20% of peak values in men and 30% of peak values in women (see Fig. 27-2).[24]

DHEA and DHEAS seem to be inactive precursors that are transformed within human tissues by a complicated network of enzymes into androgens or estrogens, or both (Fig. 27-6). The key enzymes are aromatase, steroid sulfatase, 3β-hydroxysteroid dehydrogenases (3β-HSD1 and 3β-HSD2), and at least seven organ-specific 17β-hydroxysteroid dehydrogenases (17β-HSD1 to 17β-HSD7). Labrie and colleagues[99] introduced the term *intracrinology* to describe this synthesis of active steroids in peripheral target tissues in which the action is exerted in the same cells in which synthesis takes place and without release into the extracellular space and general circulation.

In postmenopausal women, almost 100% of sex steroids are synthesized in peripheral tissues from precursors of adrenal origin, except for a small contribution from ovarian or adrenal testosterone and androstenedione. In postmenopausal women, virtually all active sex steroids are made in target tissues by an intracrine mechanism. In elderly men, the intracrine production of androgens is also important; less than 50% of the androgen supply is derived from testicular production.

The high secretion rate of adrenal precursor sex steroids in men and women differs from that in laboratory animal models, in which the secretion of sex steroids occurs exclusively in the gonads. In rats and mice, long-term administration of DHEA prevented obesity, diabetes mellitus, cancer, and heart disease and enhanced immune function.[23,25,100]

These experimental animal data have been used to argue that DHEA administration in adult or elderly individuals prolongs the life span and may be an "elixir of youth." Supportive data in humans are few, however, and highly controversial. Epidemiologic studies point to a mild cardioprotective effect of higher DHEAS levels in men and women.[101] Functional parameters of activities of daily living in men older than 90 years were lowest in those with the lowest serum DHEAS concentrations,[24] and in healthy elderly individuals, there was an association between the ratio of cortisol to DHEAS levels and cognitive impairment.[102]

CYP3A7, expressed in the human fetal liver and normally silenced after birth, plays a major role in the 16α-hydroxylation of DHEA, DHEAS, and estrone. A common polymorphism in the *CYP3A7* gene *(CYP3A7*1C)* causes persistence of the enzymatic activity encoded by the gene during adult life. Between 6% and 8% of the population are heterozygous carriers of this polymorphism, resulting in almost 50% lower DHEAS levels compared with homozygous carriers of the reference allele.[103] No evidence was found that such lowered levels are associated with an acceleration of the aging process.

Dehydroepiandrosterone Replacement Therapy

A physiologic functional role of DHEA in women was ascertained in a carefully designed, double-blind study. In women with adrenal insufficiency,[104] DHEA administration (50 mg/day) normalized serum concentrations of DHEA, DHEAS, androstenedione, and testosterone. DHEA significantly improved overall well-being, the scores for depression and anxiety, and the frequency of sexual thoughts, sexual interest, and satisfaction with both mental and physical aspects of sexuality.

A number of short-duration, controlled trials with DHEA in small groups of elderly individuals provided ambiguous results.[105,106] A 2-year placebo-controlled trial showed no effect of the oral administration of DHEA (at a dose of 75 mg/day in men and 50 mg/day in women) on body composition, muscle strength, or insulin sensitivity compared with placebo.[107] In this study involving 87 elderly men with low levels of DHEAS and bioavailable testosterone and 57 elderly women with low levels of DHEAS, DHEA levels increased in both sexes during DHEA administration by about 9.5 µmol/L.

These results are in line with those of a previous study[108] of 280 healthy subjects between 60 and 79 years old, in whom 50 mg of DHEA daily for 1 year did not improve body composition or muscle strength, whereas an increase in libido was observed in women. A double-blind, randomized, controlled trial with 50 mg of DHEA each day for 36 weeks in 50 elderly men 70 years old or older with low scores on muscle strength tests did not improve isometric grip strength, leg extensor power, or physical performance.[109]

With regard to one beneficial effect of DHEA administration, the results seem rather consistently positive: Increases in bone mineral density were repeatedly reported.[107,108,110] These positive effects, however, were very small and not more than approximately one half of those observed with current osteoporosis therapies, such as estrogens and bisphosphonates. They are therefore unlikely to have a significant effect on the risk of fracture.[107]

Conclusions and Recommendations

DHEAS is a universal precursor for peripheral local production and action of estrogens and androgens in target tissues such as brain, bone, skin, and adipose tissue. However, the importance of these pathways remains undefined, particularly in men, who have a relatively much higher production of testosterone from testicular origin. DHEA administration in the elderly, compared with placebo, increases serum DHEAS, testosterone, free testosterone, estrone, estradiol, and IGF1 concentrations and lowers SHBG levels.[107,109,110] It is not known whether this increase in sex steroid levels induced by DHEA administration in the long-term is safe with regard to the development or growth of ovarian, prostate, or other types of steroid-dependent cancers. The addition of DHEA (50 mg/day) to the existing large pool of DHEA and DHEAS in elderly individuals, even if they have been selected on the basis of low circulating levels of these steroids, has very limited or no clinically meaningful effects.

DHEA, which is available as a dietary supplement, is widely used within the United States as an unapproved preventive treatment against aging. There are no convincing arguments to recommend the routine use of DHEA for delaying or preventing the physiologic consequences of aging, and its safety is unknown.[111,112]

SOMATOPAUSE

Role of Growth Hormone and Insulin-Like Growth Factor Type I during Aging

Elderly men and women secrete GH less frequently and at lower amplitude than do young people.[21] GH secretion declines approximately 14% per decade in normal individuals.[113,114] In parallel, serum levels of IGF1 (see Fig. 27-2) are 20% to 80% lower in healthy elderly individuals than in healthy young adults.[115] The concept that the decline in GH and IGF1 secretion contributes to the decline of functional capacity in elderly people (i.e., somatopause) is mainly derived from studies in which GH replacement therapy in GH-deficient adults increased muscle mass, muscle strength, bone mass, and quality of life. A beneficial effect on the lipid profile and an important decrease in fat mass were also observed in these patients.[29,116,117] As in hypogonadal individuals, adult GH deficiency can be considered a model of normal aging because a number of catabolic processes that are central in the biology of aging can be reversed by GH replacement.

Growth Hormone Replacement Therapy

Rudman and colleagues,[118] after a groundbreaking, randomized, controlled trial enrolling healthy men 61 to 81 years old with serum IGF1 concentrations in the lower third for their age, reported in 1990 that GH treatment (30 µg/kg three times weekly for 6 months) restored the men's IGF1 levels to normal. In the treatment group, lean body mass rose by 8.8%, and lumbar vertebral density increased by 1.6%. The magnitudes of these initial changes were equivalent to a reversal of the age-related changes by 10 to 20 years. However, during continuation of this study to 12 months, the significant positive effect on bone mineral density at any site was lost.[119]

In the subsequent years, it became clear that GH administration in healthy elderly individuals frequently caused acute adverse effects, such as carpal tunnel syndrome, gynecomastia, fluid retention, and hyperglycemia, which were severe enough for an appreciable number of individuals to drop out of these studies. The most disappointing aspect, however, was that no positive effects of GH administration were observed on muscle strength, maximal oxygen consumption, or functional capacity. In contrast, when GH was administered in combination with resistance exercise training, a significant positive effect on muscle mass and muscle strength was recorded that did not differ from that seen with placebo treatment, which suggests that GH does not add to the beneficial effects of exercise.[120,121] A representative sample from a well-controlled study[122] of GH administration in unselected elderly men is given in Table 27-2.

In a systematic study of 31 articles describing 18 unique, well-defined study populations the safety and efficacy of GH in the healthy elderly were reviewed.[123] A total of 220 participants who received GH for 107 person-years completed their studies. The mean age was 69 years, and they were overweight (mean BMI, 28 kg/m^2). Initial daily GH dose (mean, 14 µg/kg of body weight), and treatment duration (mean, 27 weeks) varied. Overall fat mass decreased by 2.1 kg, and lean body mass increased by 2.1 kg in those treated with GH; total cholesterol levels decreased by 0.29 mmol/L. Disappointingly, no consistent changes in muscle strength, physical activity, or psychosocial outcomes were observed.

TABLE 27-2

Effects of Growth Hormone (GH) Administration in Healthy Older Men with Low Levels of Insulin-Like Growth Factor Type I (IGF1)*

Parameter	MEAN CHANGE IN VARIABLE GH (n = 26)	Placebo (n = 26)	P Value
IGF1 (ng/mL)	119.2	7.6	<.0001
Body Weight and Composition			
Weight (kg)	0.5	1.0	>.2
Lean mass (%)	4.3	−0.1	<.001
Fat mass (%)	−13.1	−0.3	<.001
Bone mineral content (%)	0.9	−0.1	.05
Skin thickness (%)	13.4	1.1	.09
Muscle Strength (%)			
Knee extension	3.8	1.3	>.2
Knee flexion	10.0	8.2	>.2
Hand grip	−1.5	3.8	.11
Maximum Oxygen Consumption (%)	2.5	−2.0	>.2

*GH, 30 μg/kg three times a week, was administered for 6 months to 52 healthy 69-year-old men with well-preserved functional ability but low levels of IGF1.
(From Papadakis MA, Grady D, Black D, et al. Growth hormone replacement in healthy older men improves body composition but not functional ability. *Ann Intern Med.* 1996;124:708-716.)

GH is associated with substantial adverse effects.[123] To obtain insights into what can be expected, the details of one particularly well-conducted, placebo-controlled study enrolling healthy women (n = 57) and men (n = 74) aged 65 to 88 years is described here[124]: GH administered subcutaneously at an initial dose of 30 μg/kg three times per week and then reduced to 20 μg/kg for 26 weeks was associated with carpal tunnel syndrome in 38% of women (versus 7% for placebo) and in 24% of men (0% for placebo); edema in 39% of women (0% for placebo) and 30% of men (12% for placebo); and arthralgias in 46% of women (7% for placebo) and 41% of men (0% for placebo). Eighteen men treated with GH developed glucose intolerance or diabetes, compared with only seven men in the nontreatment group.[124]

Blackman and colleagues[124] studied in a randomized, controlled trial the synergetic effects of a combination of GH and sex steroids in healthy elderly women and men. A slight increase in lean body mass and muscle strength was observed in elderly men treated with GH and testosterone, but the effects were not seen in women who received GH and estrogen. In a study in healthy elderly men, coadministration of low-dose GH with testosterone resulted in slightly beneficial changes (e.g., muscle strength, quality of life), compared with GH or testosterone alone.[125]

Earlier studies demonstrated that pharmacologic doses of GH prevent the *autocannibalistic* effects of acute diseases on muscle mass.[126] Confirmation is needed, however, before GH can gain a place in the treatment of acute catabolic states in frail elderly people.

Other components in the regulation of the GH-IGF1 axis are effective in activating GH and IGF1 secretion. Long-acting derivatives of the hypothalamic peptide growth hormone–releasing hormone (GHRH), given twice daily subcutaneously for 14 days to healthy 70-year-old men, increased GH and IGF1 levels to those encountered in 35-year-olds.[26] These studies suggest that somatopause is driven primarily by the hypothalamus and that pituitary somatotropes retain their capacity to synthesize and secrete high levels of GH.

Two ghrelin-mimetic GH secretagogues (GHSs) can restore levels of GH and IGF1 in elderly individuals to levels seen in young adults.[127,128] Ghrelin, an octanoylated 28-amino-acid peptide, stimulates GH secretion through a distinct, endogenous GHS receptor, but it also has appetite-stimulating activity.[129]

In a 2-year, double-blind, randomized, placebo-controlled, modified-crossover clinical trial enrolling 65 healthy adults aged 60 to 81 years, the orally active GHS and ghrelin mimetic MK-677 increased GH and IGF1 levels to those of healthy young adults, with a slightly increased fat-free mass but without changing fat mass, muscle strength and function, or quality of life. No important adverse effects were observed, apart from a transient increase in appetite and slight decrease in insulin sensitivity.[130] In a preliminary report of 12-month data from a multicenter study that used a different orally active GHS, capromorelin, in older persons with mild functional decline, dose-responsive increases in IGF1 and changes in body composition were accompanied by small but significant improvements in some measures of physical function (Fig. 27-7).[131] Capromorelin-treated subjects exhibited greater increases in appetite (14 versus 4.9%), insomnia (30.3 versus 17.3%), and higher fasting glucose concentrations at 12 months (+5.4 versus +0.8 mg/dL). Although these results support the hypothesis that endogenous stimulation of GH release may benefit physical performance and delay functional decline in older adults, the magnitude of improvement observed was modest.[131] Stair climbing is a sensitive measure of lower extremity power. In one exercise trial enrolling frail nursing home residents, stair climbing improved by 23% to 34% after 10 weeks of high-intensity resistance training,[10] but only a modest 7% improvement in stair climbing was seen after 2 years of treatment with capromorelin (see Fig. 27-7).

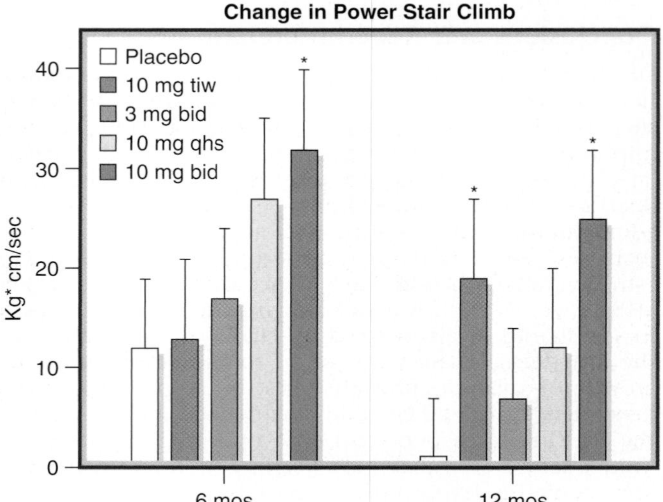

Figure 27-7 Change in power stair climb in elderly individuals (aged 65 to 84 years) with mild functional limitations after 6 and 12 months of therapy with placebo or one of four doses of the oral growth hormone secretagogue/ghrelin memetic, capromorelin. *, $P < .05$ in comparison with placebo group. (Reproduced from White HK, Petrie CD, Landschulz W, et al. Effects of an oral growth hormone secretagogue in older adults. *J Clin Endocrinol Metab.* 94:1198, 2009.)

The long-term safety of activating GH and IGF1 levels in older people has become a concern because of reports of an association between serum IGF1 concentrations and cancer risk. Individuals with high IGF1 levels (or low IGF-binding protein 3 levels) within the broad normal range have an increased risk of prostate, colon, and breast cancer.[132-134] These epidemiologic studies together with experimental data suggest that the IGF1 system is involved in tumor development and progression. However, no causal relationship between IGF1 levels and cancer risk has been established, and possible medical intervention directed at increasing IGF1 bioactivity in elderly people will in most instances be given toward the end of life, presumably not allowing enough time to affect tumor development or progression.

Conclusions and Recommendations

During the aging process, GH-IGF1 axis activity declines. It is unclear whether changes in body composition and functional capacity are directly related. GH administration in older adults causes an increase in lean body mass and an appreciable loss of fat mass. However, GH treatment does not improve muscle strength and functional capacity in elderly people, despite restoration of circulating IGF1 concentrations to young adult levels. Most dose regimens of GH cause appreciable adverse effects, and long-term safety with regard to tumor development and progression remains uncertain. Oral ghrelin mimetics are also capable of restoring GH and IGF1 levels in the elderly population, together with an increase in appetite. Modest functional improvement was observed in one study after 2 years' administration.

In the near future, clinical trials of orally active molecules in frail elderly people or in elderly individuals with clearly lowered IGF1 levels, or both, should be able to delineate the precise role of the GH-IGF1 axis in the aging process. In these trials, safety must be emphasized. There is no evidence to support recommending medical intervention in the GH-IGF1 axis as an anti-aging effort, to prolong life, or to rejuvenate healthy elderly people.[135,136] Only elderly patients with GH deficiency caused by organic diseases, such as pituitary adenomas, benefit from GH replacement therapy.[137]

CONCEPT OF SUCCESSFUL AGING

There is considerable variation in the effects of aging on healthy individuals, with some people exhibiting greater, and others few or no, age-related alterations in physiologic functions. It may be useful to distinguish between usual and successful patterns of aging.[138] Genetic factors, lifestyle, and societal investments in a safe and healthful environment are important aspects of successful aging.[139]

Traditionally, the aging process, including the development of physical frailty toward the end of life, has been considered physiologic and unavoidable, but it may not be necessary to accept the grim stereotype of aging as an unalterable process of decline and loss.[138] As life expectancy increases during the coming decades, the overarching goal should be "an increase in years of healthy life with a full range of functional capacity at each stage of life."[140] Compression of morbidity can be achieved by adapting healthy lifestyle measures, and several aspects of the aging process of the endocrine system invite the development of routine medical intervention programs offering long-term replacement therapy with one or more hormones to delay the aging process and to allow humans to live for a longer period in a relatively intact state.[141] However, current hormonal interventions with sex steroids, DHEA, GH, and oral ghrelin agonists have had very limited effects on physical capacity in elderly individuals but often produced considerable adverse effects.

REFERENCES

1. Oeppen J, Vaupel JW. Demography: broken limits to life expectancy. *Science*. 2002;296:1029.
2. Campion EW. The oldest old. *N Engl J Med*. 1994;330:1819.
3. Kosorok MR, Omenn GS, Diehr P, et al. Restricted activity days among older adults. *Am J Public Health*. 1992;82:1263.
4. Fries JF. Aging, natural death, and the compression of morbidity. *N Engl J Med*. 1980;303:130.
5. Vita AJ, Terry RB, Hubert HB, et al. Aging, health risks, and cumulative disability. *N Engl J Med*. 1998;338:1035.
6. Rudman D, Rao MP. Serum insulin-like growth factor I in healthy older men in relation to physical activity. In: Morley JE, Korenman SG, eds. *Endocrinology and Metabolism in the Elderly*. Oxford: Blackwell Scientific; 1992:50.
7. Buchner DM, Wagner EH. Preventing frail health. *Clin Geriatr Med*. 1992;8:1.
8. Tinetti ME, Speechley M, Ginter SF. Risk factors for falls among elderly persons living in the community. *N Engl J Med*. 1988;319:1701.
9. Kallman DA, Plato CC, Tobin JD. The role of muscle loss in the age-related decline of grip strength: cross-sectional and longitudinal perspectives. *J Gerontol*. 1990;45:M82.
10. Fiatarone MA, O'Neill EF, Ryan ND, et al. Exercise training and nutritional supplementation for physical frailty in very elderly people. *N Engl J Med*. 1994;330:1769.
11. Guralnik JM, Ferrucci L, Simonsick EM, et al. Lower-extremity function in persons over the age of 70 years as a predictor of subsequent disability. *N Engl J Med*. 1995;332:556.
12. Peters AL, Davidson MB. Aging and diabetes. In: Alberti KGMM, Zimmet P, Defrozo RA, Keen H, eds. *International Textbook of Diabetes Mellitus*. Chichester, UK: John Wiley & Sons; 1997:1151.
13. Mariotti S, Franceschi C, Cossarizza A, Pinchera A. The aging thyroid. *Endocr Rev*. 1995;16:686.
14. Surks MI, Ortiz E, Daniels GH, et al. Subclinical thyroid disease: scientific review and guidelines for diagnosis and management. *JAMA*. 2004;291:228.
15. Gussekloo J, van Exel E, de Craen AJ, et al. Thyroid status, disability and cognitive function, and survival in old age. *JAMA*. 2004;292:2591.
16. van den Beld AW, Visser TJ, Feelders RA, et al. Thyroid hormone concentrations, disease, physical function, and mortality in elderly men. *J Clin Endocrinol Metab*. 2005;90:6403.
17. Mariotti S. Thyroid function and aging: do serum 3,5,3′-triiodothyronine and thyroid-stimulating hormone concentrations give the Janus response? *J Clin Endocrinol Metab*. 2005;90:6735.
18. Mariotti S. Mild hypothyroidism and ischemic heart disease: is age the answer? *J Clin Endocrinol Metab*. 2008;93:2969.
19. Wise PM, Krajnak KM, Kashon ML. Menopause: the aging of multiple pacemakers. *Science*. 1996;273:67.
20. Vermeulen A. Clinical review 24: androgens in the aging male. *J Clin Endocrinol Metab*. 1991;73:221.
21. Harman SM, Tsitouras PD. Reproductive hormones in aging men: I. Measurement of sex steroids, basal luteinizing hormone, and Leydig cell response to human chorionic gonadotropin. *J Clin Endocrinol Metab*. 1980;51:35.
22. Harman SM, Tsitouras PD, Costa PT, et al. Reproductive hormones in aging men: II. Basal pituitary gonadotropins and gonadotropin responses to luteinizing hormone-releasing hormone. *J Clin Endocrinol Metab*. 1982;54:547.
23. Herbert J. The age of dehydroepiandrosterone. *Lancet*. 1995;345:1193.
24. Ravaglia G, Forti P, Maioli F, et al. The relationship of dehydroepiandrosterone sulfate (DHEAS) to endocrine-metabolic parameters and functional status in the oldest-old: results from an Italian study on healthy free-living over-ninety-year-olds. *J Clin Endocrinol Metab*. 1996;81:1173.
25. Hornsby PJ. Biosynthesis of DHEAS by the human adrenal cortex and its age-related decline. *Ann N Y Acad Sci*. 1995;774:29.
26. Corpas E, Harman SM, Pineyro MA, et al. Growth hormone (GH)-releasing hormone-(1-29) twice daily reverses the decreased GH and insulin-like growth factor-I levels in old men. *J Clin Endocrinol Metab*. 1992;75:530.
27. Blackman MR. Pituitary hormones and aging. *Endocrinol Metab Clin North Am*. 1987;16:981.
28. Wang C, Swedloff RS, Iranmanesh A, et al. Transdermal testosterone gel improves sexual function, mood, muscle strength, and body composition parameters in hypogonadal men. Testosterone Gel Study Group. *J Clin Endocrinol Metab*. 2000;85:2839.

29. Attanasio AF, Lamberts SW, Matranga AM, et al. Adult growth hormone (GH)-deficient patients demonstrate heterogeneity between childhood onset and adult onset before and during human GH treatment. Adult Growth Hormone Deficiency Study Group. *J Clin Endocrinol Metab.* 1997;82:82.
30. Barrett-Connor E. Hormone replacement therapy. *BMJ.* 1998;317:457.
31. Grady D, Rubin SM, Petitti DB, et al. Hormone therapy to prevent disease and prolong life in postmenopausal women. *Ann Intern Med.* 1992;117:1016.
32. Barrett-Connor E, Grady D. Hormone replacement therapy, heart disease, and other considerations. *Annu Rev Public Health.* 1998;19:55.
33. Grodstein F, Manson JE, Colditz GA, et al. A prospective, observational study of postmenopausal hormone therapy and primary prevention of cardiovascular disease. *Ann Intern Med.* 2000;133:933.
34. Rossouw JE, Anderson GL, Prentice RL, et al. Risks and benefits of estrogen plus progestin in healthy postmenopausal women: principal results from the Women's Health Initiative randomized controlled trial. *JAMA.* 2002;288:321.
35. Anderson GL, Limacher M, Assaf AR, et al. Effects of conjugated equine estrogen in postmenopausal women with hysterectomy: the Women's Health Initiative randomized controlled trial. *JAMA.* 2004;291:1701.
36. Viscoli CM, Brass LM, Kernan WN, et al. A clinical trial of estrogen-replacement therapy after ischemic stroke. *N Engl J Med.* 2001;345:1243.
37. Cherry N, Gilmour K, Hannaford P, et al. Oestrogen therapy for prevention of reinfarction in postmenopausal women: a randomised placebo controlled trial. *Lancet.* 2002;360:2001.
38. Hulley S, Grady D, Bush T, et al. Randomized trial of estrogen plus progestin for secondary prevention of coronary heart disease in postmenopausal women. Heart and Estrogen/Progestin Replacement Study (HERS) Research Group. *JAMA.* 1998;280:605.
39. Dubey RK, Imthurn B, Zacharia LC, et al. Hormone replacement therapy and cardiovascular disease: what went wrong and where do we go from here? *Hypertension.* 2004;44:789.
40. Peterson HB, Thacker SB, Corso PS, et al. Hormone therapy: making decisions in the face of uncertainty. *Arch Intern Med.* 2004;164:2308.
41. Manson JE, Allison MA, Rossouw JE, et al. Estrogen therapy and coronary-artery calcification. *N Engl J Med.* 2007;356:2591.
42. Weiss LK, Burkman RT, Cushing-Haugen KL, et al. Hormone replacement therapy regimens and breast cancer risk. *Obstet Gynecol.* 2002;100:1148.
43. Li CI, Malone KE, Porter PL, et al. Relationship between long durations and different regimens of hormone therapy and risk of breast cancer. *JAMA.* 2003;289:3254.
44. Chlebowski RT, Hendrix SL, Langer RD, et al. Influence of estrogen plus progestin on breast cancer and mammography in healthy postmenopausal women: the Women's Health Initiative Randomized Trial. *JAMA.* 2003;289:3243.
45. Beral V. Breast cancer and hormone-replacement therapy in the Million Women Study. *Lancet.* 2003;362:419.
46. Shumaker SA, Legault C, Kuller L, et al. Conjugated equine estrogens and incidence of probable dementia and mild cognitive impairment in postmenopausal women: Women's Health Initiative Memory Study. *JAMA.* 2004;291:2947.
47. Hodis HN. Assessing benefits and risks of hormone therapy in 2008: new evidence, especially with regard to the heart. *Cleve Clin J Med.* 2008;75(suppl 4):S3.
48. Hays J, Ockene JK, Brunner RL, et al. Effects of estrogen plus progestin on health-related quality of life. *N Engl J Med.* 2003;348:1839.
49. Utian WH, Shoupe D, Bachmann G, et al. Relief of vasomotor symptoms and vaginal atrophy with lower doses of conjugated equine estrogens and medroxyprogesterone acetate. *Fertil Steril.* 2001;75:1065.
50. Santen RJ. Long-term tamoxifen therapy: can an antagonist become an agonist? *J Clin Endocrinol Metab.* 1996;81:2027.
51. Grainger DJ, Metcalfe JC. Tamoxifen: teaching an old drug new tricks? *Nat Med.* 1996;2:381.
52. Grey AB, Stapleton JP, Evans MC, et al. The effect of the antiestrogen tamoxifen on bone mineral density in normal late postmenopausal women. *Am J Med.* 1995;99:636.
53. Draper MW, Flowers DE, Huster WJ, et al. A controlled trial of raloxifene (LY139481) HCl: impact on bone turnover and serum lipid profile in healthy postmenopausal women. *J Bone Miner Res.* 1996;11:835.
54. Palacios S. The future of the new selective estrogen receptor modulators. *Menopause Int.* 2007;13:27.
55. Delmas PD, Bjarnason NH, Mitlak BH, et al. Effects of raloxifene on bone mineral density, serum cholesterol concentrations, and uterine endometrium in postmenopausal women. *N Engl J Med.* 1997;337:1641.
56. Ettinger B, Black DM, Mitlak BH, et al. Reduction of vertebral fracture risk in postmenopausal women with osteoporosis treated with raloxifene: results from a 3-year randomized clinical trial. Multiple Outcomes of Raloxifene Evaluation (MORE) Investigators. *JAMA.* 1999;282:637.
57. Seeman E, Crans GG, Diez-Perez A, et al. Anti-vertebral fracture efficacy of raloxifene: a meta-analysis. *Osteoporos Int.* 2006;17:313.
58. Barrett-Connor E, Mosca L, Collins P, et al. Effects of raloxifene on cardiovascular events and breast cancer in postmenopausal women. *N Engl J Med.* 2006;355:125.
59. Mosca L, Grady D, Barrett-Connor E, et al. Effect of raloxifene on stroke and venous thromboembolism according to subgroups in postmenopausal women at increased risk of coronary heart disease. *Stroke.* 2009;40:147.
60. Davies GC, Huster WJ, Lu Y, et al. Adverse events reported by postmenopausal women in controlled trials with raloxifene. *Obstet Gynecol.* 1999;93:558.
61. Howell A. The endocrine prevention of breast cancer. *Best Pract Res Clin Endocrinol Metab.* 2008;22:615.
62. Martino S, Cauley JA, Barrett-Connor E, et al. Continuing outcomes relevant to Evista: breast cancer incidence in postmenopausal osteoporotic women in a randomized trial of raloxifene. *J Natl Cancer Inst.* 2004;96:1751.
63. Vogel VG, Costantino JP, Wickerham DL, et al. Effects of tamoxifen vs raloxifene on the risk of developing invasive breast cancer and other disease outcomes: the NSABP Study of Tamoxifen and Raloxifene (STAR) P-2 trial. *JAMA.* 2006;295:2727.
64. Shelly W, Draper MW, Krishnan V, et al. Selective estrogen receptor modulators: an update on recent clinical findings. *Obstet Gynecol Surv.* 2008;63:163.
65. Moen MD, Keating GM. Raloxifene: a review of its use in the prevention of invasive breast cancer. *Drugs.* 2008;68:2059.
66. Cummings SR, Ettinger B, Delmas PD, et al. The effects of tibolone in older postmenopausal women. *N Engl J Med.* 2008;359:697.
67. Davis SR, Davison SL, Donath S, et al. Circulating androgen levels and self-reported sexual function in women. *JAMA.* 2005;294:91.
68. Davis SR, Moreau M, Kroll R, et al. Testosterone for low libido in postmenopausal women not taking estrogen. *N Engl J Med.* 2008;359:2005.
69. Rossouw JE. Postmenopausal hormone therapy for disease prevention: have we learned any lessons from the past? *Clin Pharmacol Ther.* 2008;83:14.
70. Tannen RL, Weiner MG, Xie D, et al. Perspectives on hormone replacement therapy: the Women's Health Initiative and new observational studies sampling the overall population. *Fertil Steril.* 2008;90:258.
71. Nabel EG. Coronary heart disease in women: an ounce of prevention. *N Engl J Med.* 2000;343:572.
72. Tenover JS. Androgen administration to aging men. *Endocrinol Metab Clin North Am.* 1994;23:877.
73. Vermeulen A, Kaufman JM. Diagnosis of hypogonadism in the aging male. *Aging Male.* 2002;5:170.
74. Harman SM, Metter EJ, Tobin JD, et al. Longitudinal effects of aging on serum total and free testosterone levels in healthy men. Baltimore Longitudinal Study of Aging. *J Clin Endocrinol Metab.* 2001;86:724.
75. Araujo AB, Esche GR, Kupelian V, et al. Prevalence of symptomatic androgen deficiency in men. *J Clin Endocrinol Metab.* 2007;92:4241.
76. McLachlan RI, Allan CA. Defining the prevalence and incidence of androgen deficiency in aging men: where are the goal posts? *J Clin Endocrinol Metab.* 2004;89:5916.
77. Wu FC, Tajar A, Pye SR, et al. Hypothalamic-pituitary-testicular axis disruptions in older men are differentially linked to age and modifiable risk factors: the European Male Aging Study. *J Clin Endocrinol Metab.* 2008;93:2737.
78. Jones RD, Nettleship JE, Kapoor D, et al. Testosterone and atherosclerosis in aging men: purported association and clinical implications. *Am J Cardiovasc Drugs.* 2005;5:141.
79. Laughlin GA, Barrett-Connor E, Bergstrom J. Low serum testosterone and mortality in older men. *J Clin Endocrinol Metab.* 2008;93:68.
80. Wang C, Eyre DR, Clark R, et al. Sublingual testosterone replacement improves muscle mass and strength, decreases bone resorption, and increases bone formation markers in hypogonadal men: a clinical research center study. *J Clin Endocrinol Metab.* 1996;81:3654.
81. Bhasin S, Storer TW, Berman N, et al. The effects of supraphysiologic doses of testosterone on muscle size and strength in normal men. *N Engl J Med.* 1996;335:1.
82. Snyder PJ, Peachey H, Hannoush P, et al. Effect of testosterone treatment on bone mineral density in men over 65 years of age. *J Clin Endocrinol Metab.* 1999;84:1966.
83. Snyder PJ, Peachey H, Hannoush P, et al. Effect of testosterone treatment on body composition and muscle strength in men over 65 years of age. *J Clin Endocrinol Metab.* 1999;84:2647.
84. Pearlman CK, Kobashi LI. Frequency of intercourse in men. *J Urol.* 1972;107:298.
85. Bolona ER, Uraga MV, Haddad RM, et al. Testosterone use in men with sexual dysfunction: a systematic review and meta-analysis of randomized placebo-controlled trials. *Mayo Clin Proc.* 2007;82:20.
86. Bhasin S, Bremner WJ. Clinical review 85. Emerging issues in androgen replacement therapy. *J Clin Endocrinol Metab.* 1997;82:3.
87. Bagatell CJ, Bremner WJ. Androgens in men: uses and abuses. *N Engl J Med.* 1996;334:707.

88. Bhasin S, Cunningham GR, Hayes FJ, et al. Testosterone therapy in adult men with androgen deficiency syndromes: an Endocrine Society clinical practice guideline. *J Clin Endocrinol Metab.* 2006;91:1995.
89. Calof OM, Singh AB, Lee ML, et al. Adverse events associated with testosterone replacement in middle-aged and older men: a meta-analysis of randomized, placebo-controlled trials. *J Gerontol A Biol Sci Med Sci.* 2005;60:1451.
90. Liu PY, Swerdloff RS, Veldhuis JD. Clinical review 171. The rationale, efficacy and safety of androgen therapy in older men: future research and current practice recommendations. *J Clin Endocrinol Metab.* 2004;89:4789.
91. Bhasin S, Bagatell CJ, Bremner WJ, et al. Issues in testosterone replacement in older men. *J Clin Endocrinol Metab.* 1998;83:3435.
92. Morley JE, Melmed S. Gonadal dysfunction in systemic disorders. *Metabolism.* 1979;28:1051.
93. Gray A, Feldman HA, McKinlay JB, et al. Age, disease, and changing sex hormone levels in middle-aged men: results of the Massachusetts Male Aging Study. *J Clin Endocrinol Metab.* 1991;73:1016.
94. Negro-Vilar A. Selective androgen receptor modulators (SARMs): a novel approach to androgen therapy for the new millennium. *J Clin Endocrinol Metab.* 1999;84:3459.
95. Zitzmann M, Nieschlag E. The CAG repeat polymorphism within the androgen receptor gene and maleness. *Int J Androl.* 2003;26:76.
96. Krithivas K, Yurgalevitch SM, Mohr BA, et al. Evidence that the CAG repeat in the androgen receptor gene is associated with the age-related decline in serum androgen levels in men. *J Endocrinol.* 1999;162:137.
97. Giovannucci E, Platz EA, Stampfer MJ, et al. The CAG repeat within the androgen receptor gene and benign prostatic hyperplasia. *Urology.* 1999;53:121.
98. Huhtaniemi IT, Pye SR, Limer KL, et al. Increased estrogen rather than decreased androgen action is associated with longer androgen receptor CAG repeats. *J Clin Endocrinol Metab.* 2009;94:277.
99. Labrie F, Luu-The V, Lin SX, et al. Intracrinology: role of the family of 17 beta-hydroxysteroid dehydrogenases in human physiology and disease. *J Mol Endocrinol.* 2000;25:1.
100. Labrie F, Belanger A, Simard J, et al. DHEA and peripheral androgen and estrogen formation: intracinology. *Ann N Y Acad Sci.* 1995;774:16.
101. Barrett-Connor E, Goodman-Gruen D. The epidemiology of DHEAS and cardiovascular disease. *Ann N Y Acad Sci.* 1995;774:259.
102. Kalmijn S, Launer LJ, Stolk RP, et al. A prospective study on cortisol, dehydroepiandrosterone sulfate, and cognitive function in the elderly. *J Clin Endocrinol Metab.* 1998;83:3487.
103. Smit P, van Schaik RH, van der Werf M, et al. A common polymorphism in the CYP3A7 gene is associated with a nearly 50% reduction in serum dehydroepiandrosterone sulfate levels. *J Clin Endocrinol Metab.* 2005;90:5313.
104. Arlt W, Callies F, van Vlijmen JC, et al. Dehydroepiandrosterone replacement in women with adrenal insufficiency. *N Engl J Med.* 1999; 341:1013.
105. Morales AJ, Nolan JJ, Nelson JC, et al. Effects of replacement dose of dehydroepiandrosterone in men and women of advancing age. *J Clin Endocrinol Metab.* 1994;78:1360.
106. Yen SS, Morales AJ, Khorram O. Replacement of DHEA in aging men and women:. potential remedial effects. *Ann N Y Acad Sci.* 1995; 774:128.
107. Nair KS, Rizza RA, O'Brien P, et al. DHEA in elderly women and DHEA or testosterone in elderly men. *N Engl J Med.* 2006;355:1647.
108. Baulieu EE, Thomas G, Legrain S, et al. Dehydroepiandrosterone (DHEA), DHEA sulfate, and aging: contribution of the DHEAge Study to a sociobiomedical issue. *Proc Natl Acad Sci U S A.* 2000;97:4279.
109. Muller M, van den Beld AW, van der Schouw YT, et al. Effects of dehydroepiandrosterone and atamestane supplementation on frailty in elderly men. *J Clin Endocrinol Metab.* 2006;91:3988.
110. Jankowski CM, Gozansky WS, Kittelson JM, et al. Increases in bone mineral density in response to oral dehydroepiandrosterone replacement in older adults appear to be mediated by serum estrogens. *J Clin Endocrinol Metab.* 2008;93:4767.
111. Skolnick AA. Scientific verdict still out on DHEA. *JAMA.* 1996;276:1365.
112. Stewart PM. Aging and fountain-of-youth hormones. *N Engl J Med.* 2006;355:1724.
113. Toogood AA, O'Neill PA, Shalet SM. Beyond the somatopause: growth hormone deficiency in adults over the age of 60 years. *J Clin Endocrinol Metab.* 1996;81:460.
114. Toogood AA, Jones J, O'Neill PA, Thorner MO, et al. The diagnosis of severe growth hormone deficiency in elderly patients with hypothalamic-pituitary disease. *Clin Endocrinol (Oxf).* 1998;48:569.
115. Borst SE, Millard WJ, Lowenthal DT. Growth hormone, exercise, and aging: the future of therapy for the frail elderly. *J Am Geriatr Soc.* 1994;42:528.
116. Nass R, Huber RM, Klauss V, et al. Effect of growth hormone (hGH) replacement therapy on physical work capacity and cardiac and pulmonary function in patients with hGH deficiency acquired in adulthood. *J Clin Endocrinol Metab.* 1995;80:552.
117. Salomon F, Cuneo RC, Hesp R, et al. The effects of treatment with recombinant human growth hormone on body composition and metabolism in adults with growth hormone deficiency. *N Engl J Med.* 1989;321:1797.
118. Rudman D, Feller AG, Nagraj HS, et al. Effects of human growth hormone in men over 60 years old. *N Engl J Med.* 1990;323:1.
119. Rudman D, Feller AG, Cohn L, et al. Effects of human growth hormone on body composition in elderly men. *Horm Res.* 1991;36(suppl 1): 73.
120. Taaffe DR, Pruitt L, Reim J, et al. Effect of recombinant human growth hormone on the muscle strength response to resistance exercise in elderly men. *J Clin Endocrinol Metab.* 1994;79:1361.
121. Yarasheski KE, Zachwieja JJ, Campbell JA, et al. Effect of growth hormone and resistance exercise on muscle growth and strength in older men. *Am J Physiol.* 1995;268(2 Pt 1):E268.
122. Papadakis MA, Grady D, Black D, et al. Growth hormone replacement in healthy older men improves body composition but not functional ability. *Ann Intern Med.* 1996;124:708.
123. Liu H, Bravata DM, Olkin I, et al. Systematic review: the safety and efficacy of growth hormone in the healthy elderly. *Ann Intern Med.* 2007;146:104.
124. Blackman MR, Sorkin JD, Munzer T, et al. Growth hormone and sex steroid administration in healthy aged women and men: a randomized controlled trial. *JAMA.* 2002;288:2282.
125. Giannoulis MG, Sonksen PH, Umpleby M, et al. The effects of growth hormone and/or testosterone in healthy elderly men: a randomized controlled trial. *J Clin Endocrinol Metab.* 2006;91:477.
126. Herndon DN, Barrow RE, Kunkel KR, et al. Effects of recombinant human growth hormone on donor-site healing in severely burned children. *Ann Surg.* 1990;212:424.
127. Chapman IM, Hartman ML, Pezzoli SS, et al. Enhancement of pulsatile growth hormone secretion by continuous infusion of a growth hormone-releasing peptide mimetic, L-692,429, in older adults: a clinical research center study. *J Clin Endocrinol Metab.* 1996;81:2874.
128. Chapman IM, Bach MA, Van Cauter E, et al. Stimulation of the growth hormone (GH)-insulin-like growth factor I axis by daily oral administration of a GH secretogogue (MK-677) in healthy elderly subjects. *J Clin Endocrinol Metab.* 1996;81:4249.
129. Smith RG, Jiang H, Sun Y. Developments in ghrelin biology and potential clinical relevance. *Trends Endocrinol Metab.* 2005;16:436.
130. Nass R, Pezzoli SS, Oliveri MC, et al. Effects of an oral ghrelin mimetic on body composition and clinical outcomes in healthy older adults: a randomized trial. *Ann Intern Med.* 2008;149:601.
131. White HK, Petrie CD, Landschulz W, et al. Effects of an oral growth hormone secretagogue in older adults. *J Clin Endocrinol Metab.* 2009;94:1198.
132. Chan JM, Stampfer MJ, Giovannucci E, et al. Plasma insulin-like growth factor-I and prostate cancer risk: a prospective study. *Science.* 1998;279:563.
133. Hankinson SE, Willett WC, Colditz GA, et al. Circulating concentrations of insulin-like growth factor-I and risk of breast cancer. *Lancet.* 1998;351:1393.
134. Ma J, Pollak MN, Giovannucci E, et al. Prospective study of colorectal cancer risk in men and plasma levels of insulin-like growth factor (IGF)-I and IGF-binding protein-3. *J Natl Cancer Inst.* 1999;91:620.
135. Perls TT, Reisman NR, Olshansky SJ. Provision or distribution of growth hormone for "antiaging": clinical and legal issues. *JAMA.* 2005;294:2086.
136. Olshansky SJ, Perls TT. New developments in the illegal provision of growth hormone for "anti-aging" and bodybuilding. *JAMA.* 2008; 299:2792.
137. Shalet SM. GH deficiency in the elderly: the case for GH replacement. *Clin Endocrinol (Oxf).* 2000;53:279.
138. Rowe JW, Kahn RL. Human aging: usual and successful. *Science.* 1987;237:143.
139. Hazzard WR. Weight control and exercise: cardinal features of successful preventive gerontology. *JAMA.* 1995;274:1964.
140. Healthy People 2000: National and Health Promotion and Disease Prevention Objectives. Washington DC: Government Printing Office; 1991.
141. Lamberts SW, van den Beld AW, van der Lely AJ. The endocrinology of aging. *Science.* 1997;278:419.
142. Reference deleted in proofs.
143. Reference deleted in proofs.
144. Reference deleted in proofs.

SECTION VII

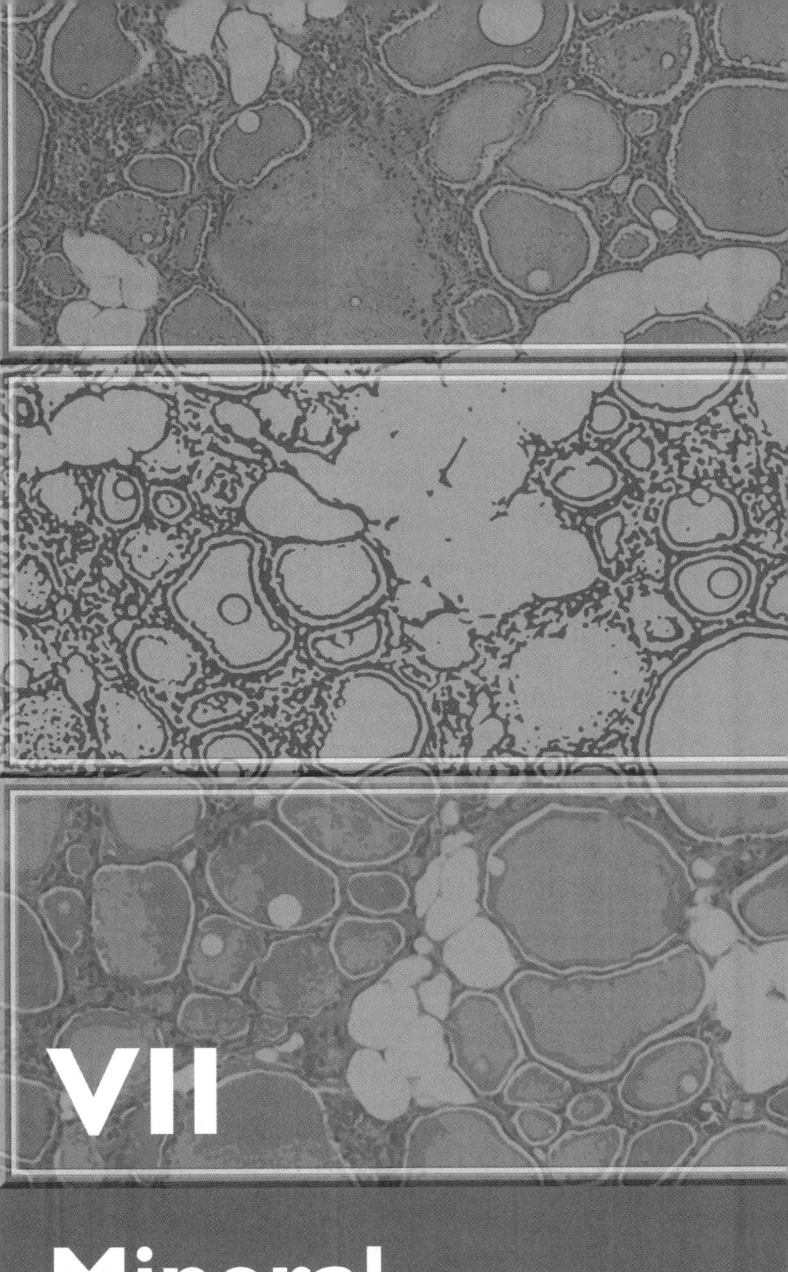

Mineral Metabolism

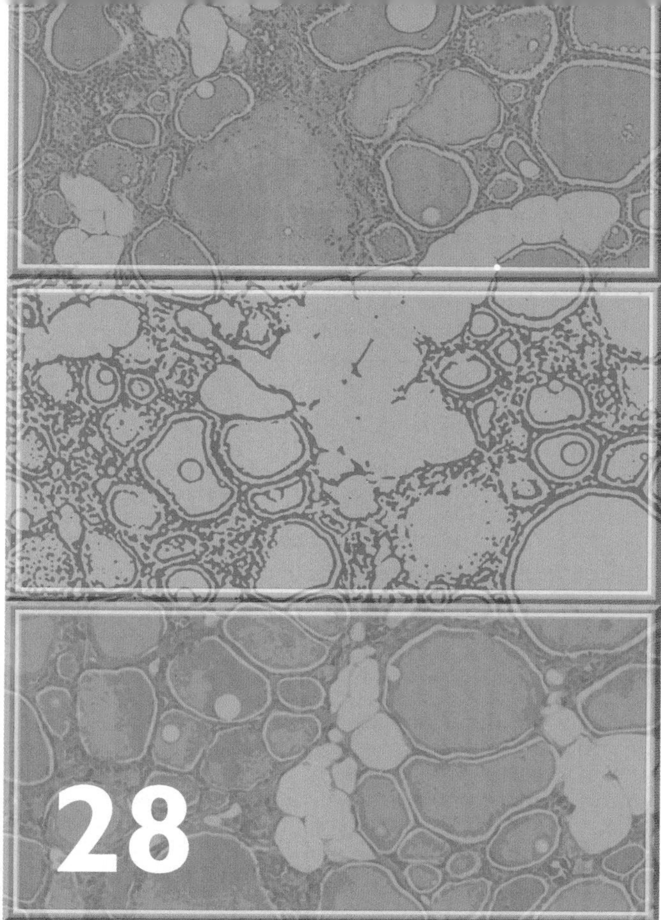

CHAPTER 28

Hormones and Disorders of Mineral Metabolism

F. RICHARD BRINGHURST • MARIE B. DEMAY • HENRY M. KRONENBERG

MINERAL METABOLISM: BASIC BIOLOGY AND ROLES OF THE MINERAL IONS

Calcium (Ca) and phosphorus (P) are the principal constituents of bone, and together they comprise 65% of its weight. Bone, in turn, contains almost all of the calcium and phosphorus and more than half of the magnesium in the human body. The quantitatively minor amounts of each of these ions in the extracellular fluid (ECF) and within cells play crucial roles in normal physiology (Fig. 28-1).

Ninety-nine percent of total body calcium resides in bone, of which 99% is located within the crystal structure of the mineral phase. The remaining 1% of bone calcium is rapidly exchangeable with extracellular calcium; this calcium is equally distributed between the intracellular and extracellular fluids. Extracellular calcium is the principal substrate for the mineralization of cartilage and bone. It also serves as a cofactor for many extracellular enzymes, most notably the enzymes of the coagulation cascade, and as a source of calcium ions that function as signaling molecules for a great diversity of intracellular processes. These processes include automaticity of nerve and muscle; contraction of cardiac, skeletal, and smooth muscle; neurotransmitter release; and various forms of endocrine and exocrine secretion.

In blood, approximately 50% of total calcium is bound to proteins, mainly albumin and globulins. The ionized calcium concentration in serum is approximately 1.2 mmol/L (5 mg/dL), and this ionized fraction is biologically active and tightly controlled by hormonal mechanisms. Because intracellular cytosolic free calcium concentrations typically are in the range of only 100 nmol/L, a very large chemical gradient (i.e., 10,000 : 1), augmented by the large negative electrical potential, favors calcium entry into cells through calcium channels. This gradient is maintained by the limited conductance of resting calcium channels and by the energy-dependent extrusion of calcium into the ECF via high-affinity Ca^{2+}- and H^+-adenosine triphosphatases (ATPases) and low-affinity sodium-calcium (Na^+/Ca^{2+}) exchangers.

More than 99% of intracellular calcium exists in the form of complexes within the mitochondrial compartment,

	Calcium ions	Phosphate ions
Extracellular		
Concentration		
total, in serum	2.5×10^{-3} M	1.00×10^{-3} M
free	1.2×10^{-3} M	0.85×10^{-3} M
Functions	Bone mineral Blood coagulation Membrane excitability	Bone mineral
Intracellular		
Concentration	10^{-7} M	$1–2 \times 10^{-3}$ M
Functions	**Signal for:** • Neuron activation • Hormone secretion • Muscle contraction	• Structural role • High energy bonds • Regulation of proteins by phosphorylation

Figure 28-1 Distribution and function of calcium and phosphate. Note the remarkable difference between intracellular and extracellular concentrations of calcium ion and the dramatically different functions of calcium and phosphate inside cells.

bound to the inner plasma membrane, or associated with the inner membranes of the endoplasmic reticulum and other compartments. Release of calcium from membrane-bound compartments transduces cellular signals and is tightly regulated. The mechanisms responsible for translocations of intracellular calcium between the cytosol and these sequestered regions have become better understood with the identification of specific receptors for calciotropic signaling molecules such as the inositol triphosphate (IP_3) receptor and the ryanodine receptors.

Phosphate is more widely distributed to non-osseous tissues than is calcium. Eighty-five percent of body phosphate is in the mineral phase of bone, and the remainder is located in inorganic or organic form throughout the extracellular and intracellular compartments. In human serum, inorganic phosphate (P_i) is present at a concentration of approximately 1 mmol/L and exists almost entirely in ionized form as either $H_2PO_4^-$ or HPO_4^{2-}. Only 12% of serum phosphate is protein bound, and an additional small fraction is loosely complexed with calcium, magnesium, and other cations. Intracellular free phosphate concentrations are comparable to those in the ECF (i.e., 1 to 2 mmol/L), although the inside-negative electrical potential of the cell creates a significant energy requirement for translocation of phosphate into cells. This process generally is accomplished through sodium-phosphate (NaPi) cotransport driven by the transmembrane sodium gradient. A number of NaPi cotransporters have been cloned; various cells and tissues employ different species of such transporters with distinctive regulatory characteristics.

Organic phosphate is a key component of almost all classes of structural, informational, and effector molecules that are essential for normal genetic, developmental, and physiologic processes. Phosphate is an integral constituent of nucleic acids; phospholipids; complex carbohydrates; glycolytic intermediates; structural, signaling, and enzymatic phosphoproteins; and nucleotide cofactors for enzymes and G proteins. The need for the large amounts of phosphate incorporated into cellular constituents during cell proliferation explains why phosphate levels in the blood are regulated by insulin-like growth factor 1, in addition to regulation by hormones of bone mineralization. Of particular importance are the high-energy phosphate ester bonds present in molecules such as ATP, diphosphoglycerate, and creatine phosphate that store chemical energy. Phosphate plays a particularly prominent role as the key substrate or recognition site in numerous kinase and phosphatase regulatory cascades. Cytosolic phosphate per se also directly regulates a number of crucial intracellular reactions, including those involved in glucose transport, lactate production, and synthesis of ATP. In light of these diverse roles, it is not surprising that disorders of phosphate homeostasis associated with severe depletion of intracellular phosphate lead to profound and global impairment of organ function. (Note that none of these roles for intracellular phosphate involve actions of intracellular calcium; the reason we are discussing these together solely results from their intimate relationship in regulating bone mineralization outside of cells.)

Magnesium is the fourth most abundant cation in the body. Roughly half is found in bone and half in muscle and other soft tissues. As much as half of the magnesium in bone is not sequestered in the mineral phase but is freely exchangeable with the ECF and, therefore, may serve as a buffer against changes in extracellular magnesium concentration. Less than 1% of all magnesium in the body is present in the ECF, where the magnesium concentration is approximately 0.5 mmol/L. The concentration of magnesium in serum normally is 0.7 to 1.0 mmol/L, of which roughly one third is protein bound, 15% is loosely complexed with phosphate or other anions, and 55% is present as the free ion. More than 95% of intracellular magnesium is bound to other molecules, most notably ATP, the concentration of which is approximately 5 mmol/L. The intracellular cytosolic free magnesium concentration is approximately 0.5 mmol/L (i.e., 1000-fold higher than that of calcium) and is maintained by an active sodium-magnesium antiporter. The mechanisms whereby magnesium enters cells, presumably down a favorable electrochemical gradient, are unknown, although some evidence for regulated channels has been obtained.[1]

Intracellular magnesium, like phosphate, is necessary for a wide range of cellular functions. It is an essential cofactor in enzymatic reactions, including most of the same glycolytic, kinase, and phosphatase pathways that also involve phosphate. Magnesium serves to directly stabilize the structures of a variety of macromolecules and complexes, including deoxyribonucleic acid (DNA), ribonucleic acid (RNA), and ribosomes; it is also a key activator of the many ATPase-coupled ion transporters and plays a direct role in mitochondrial oxidative metabolism. As a result, magnesium is critical for energy metabolism and the maintenance of a normal intracellular environment. Extracellular magnesium is crucial for normal neuromuscular excitability and nerve conduction, and many of the clinical consequences of magnesium deficiency or excess reflect abnormalities in this sphere.

The levels of extracellular calcium and phosphate are regulated in a coordinated way that reflects the roles of calcium and phosphate in mineralization of bone. The concentrations of these ions in body fluids are, together, close to the concentrations that could lead to spontaneous precipitation in soft tissues. In fact, elaborate mechanisms, most poorly understood, have evolved to prevent precipitation of calcium phosphate in tissues and yet allow the controlled deposition of calcium and phosphate in bone.[2] The importance of the mineral ions for normal cellular physiology as well as skeletal integrity is reflected in the powerful endocrine control mechanisms that have evolved to maintain their extracellular concentrations within relatively narrow limits. The following sections describe the structures, secretory controls, actions, and interactions of parathyroid hormone (PTH), calcitonin, $1,25(OH)_2D_3$

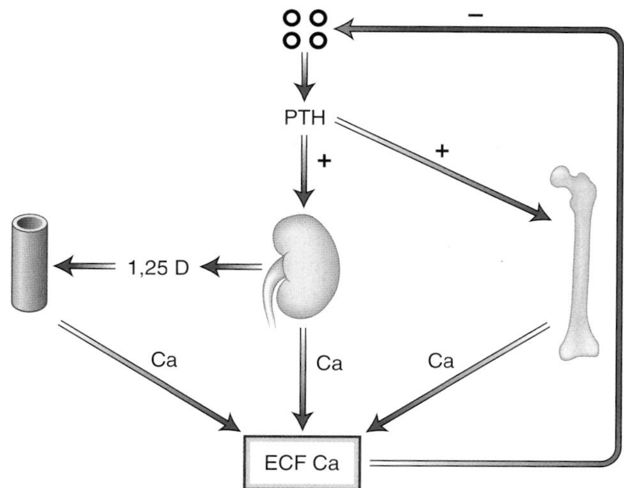

Figure 28-2 Parathyroid hormone (PTH)-calcium feedback loop that controls calcium homeostasis. Four organs—the parathyroid glands, intestine, kidney, and bone—together determine the parameters of calcium homeostasis. +, positive effect; −, negative effect; 1,25 D, 1,25-dihydroxyvitamin D_3; ECF, extracellular fluid.

(1,25-dihydroxyvitamin D or calcitriol), and fibroblast growth factor 23 (FGF23)—the major hormones involved in mineral ion homeostasis. Subsequent sections cover the wide variety of clinical disorders that accompany abnormalities in this hormonal network.

PARATHYROID HORMONE

PTH is the peptide hormone that controls the minute-to-minute level of ionized calcium in the blood and ECF. PTH binds to cell surface receptors in bone and kidney, triggering responses that increase blood calcium (Fig. 28-2). PTH also increases renal synthesis of calcitriol, the hormonally active form of vitamin D, which then acts on the intestine to augment absorption of dietary calcium, in addition to promoting calcium fluxes into blood from bone and kidney. The resulting increase in blood calcium (and in calcitriol) feeds back on the parathyroid glands to decrease the secretion of PTH. The parathyroid glands, bones, kidney, and gut are thus the crucial organs that participate in PTH-mediated calcium homeostasis.

Parathyroid Gland Biology

Parathyroid glands first appeared in evolutionary history with the exit of amphibians from the sea and a switch from dependence on gills to sole dependence on bone, intestine, and kidney to maintain extracellular calcium homeostasis. Reptiles, birds, and mammals all have parathyroid glands that develop as epithelial specializations from the endoderm of the pharyngeal pouches. Although fish have no discrete parathyroid glands, they do synthesize PTH.[3] The physiologic role of this PTH in fish is not yet defined.

Parathyroid chief cells have three properties that are vital to their homeostatic function. First, they rapidly secrete hormone in response to changes in blood calcium. Second, they can synthesize, process, and store large amounts of PTH in a regulated manner. Third, parathyroid cells replicate when chronically stimulated. These functional attributes allow, respectively, for short-term, intermediate-term, and long-term adaptation to changes in calcium availability.

Parathyroid Hormone Biosynthesis

PTH, a protein of 84 amino acids in mammals, is synthesized as a larger precursor, called pre-proparathyroid hormone (pre-pro-PTH); the gene has been sequenced in 11 species ranging from fish to humans.[4] Figure 28-3 illustrates representative pre-pro-PTH sequences. These sequences share a 25-residue "pre" or signal sequence and a 6-residue "pro" sequence. The signal sequence, along with the short pro sequence, functions to direct the protein into the secretory pathway (Fig. 28-4). During transit across the membrane of the endoplasmic reticulum, the signal sequence is cleaved off and rapidly degraded. The importance of the signal sequence for normal secretion of PTH is illustrated by the hypoparathyroidism inherited in families that carry mutations in the signal sequence of pre-pro-PTH.[5,6]

The role of the short pro sequence is not completely understood; it may help the signal sequence to work

```
                         PRE                  ↓ PRO ↓    PTH
          -31                      -6      +1       +10
Human     MIPAKDMAKVMIVMLAICFLTKSDG KSVKKR SVSEIQLMHN
Bovine    MMSAKDMVKVMIVMLAICFLARSDG KSVKKR AVSEIQFMHN
Porcine   MMSAKDTVKVMVVMLAICFLARSDG KPIKKR SVSEIQFMHN
Rat       MMSASTMAKVMILMLAVCFLTQADG KPVKKR AVSEIQLMHN
Canine    MMSAKDMVKVMIVMFAICFLAKSDG KPVKKR SVSEIQFMHN
Chicken   MTSTKNLAKAIVILYAICFFTNSDG RPMMKR SVSEMQLMHN

                   +20       +30       +40       +50
Human     LGKHLNSMERVEWLRKKLQDVHNFVALGAPLAPRDAGSQRPRK
Bovine    LGKHLSSMERVEWLRKKLQDVHNFVALGASIAYRDGSSQRPRK
Porcine   LGKHLSSLERVEWLRKKLQDVHNFVALGASIVHRDGGSQRPRK
Rat       LGKHLASVERMQWLRKKLQDVHNFVSLGVQMAAREGSYQRPTK
Canine    LGKHLSSMERVEWLRKKLQDVHNFVALGAPIAHRDGSSQRPLK
Chicken   LGEHRHTVERQDWLQMKLQDVH..SALE......DARTQRPRN

                +60        +70                   +80
Human     KEDNVLVE...SHEKSLGEA..........DKADVNVLTKAKSQ
Bovine    KEDNVLVE...SHQKSLGEA..........DKADVDVLIKAKPQ
Porcine   KEDNVLVE...SHQKSLGEA..........DKAAVDVLIKAKPQ
Rat       KEENVLVD...GNSKSLGEG..........DKADVDVLVKAKSQ
Canine    KEDNVLVE...SYQKSLGEA..........DKADVDVLTKAKSQ
Chicken   KEDIVLGEIRNRRLLPEHLRAAVQKKSIDLDKAYMNVLFKTKP.
```

Figure 28-3 Sequences of pre-proparathyroid hormone from six species. Completely conserved residues are in boldface. Arrows indicate the sites of signal sequence ("pre") and "pro" sequence cleavage. Numbers start at residue +1 of mature parathyroid hormone (PTH); because of gaps, the numbers correspond only to the mammalian and not to the chicken sequence. Amino acids are indicated by single-letter codes: A, Ala; R, Arg; N, Asn; D, Asp; C, Cys; Q, Gln; E, Glu; G, Gly; H, His; I, Ile; L, Leu; K, Lys; M, Met; F, Phe; P, Pro; S, Ser; T, Thr; W, Trp; Y, Tyr; V, Val.

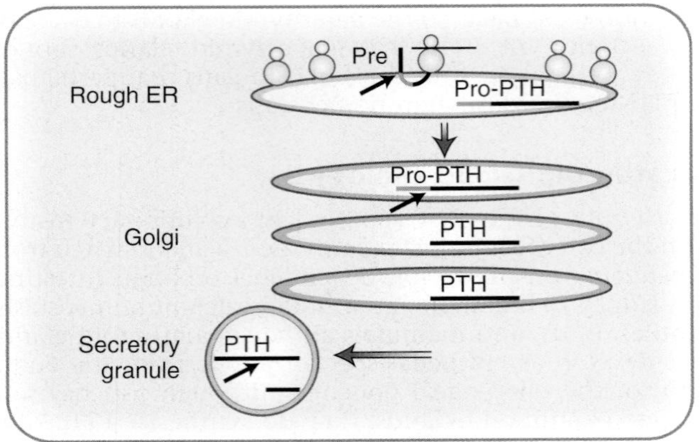

Figure 28-4 Intracellular processing of pre-proparathyroid hormone (pre-pro-PTH). Diagonal arrows indicate sites of cleavage by enzymes that generate pro-PTH in the rough endoplasmic reticulum (ER), PTH in the Golgi apparatus, and carboxy-terminal fragments of PTH in the secretory granule.

efficiently and ensure accurate cleavage of the precursor.[7] After cleavage of the pro sequence, the mature PTH(1-34) is concentrated in secretory vesicles and granules. One morphologically distinct subtype of granule contains both PTH and the proteases cathepsin B and cathepsin H. This co-localization of proteases and PTH in secretory granules probably explains the observation that a portion of the PTH secreted from parathyroid glands consists of carboxy-terminal PTH fragments. No amino-terminal fragments of PTH are secreted. Although the possible functions of carboxy-terminal fragments of PTH are still poorly characterized, they do not activate the receptor for PTH and parathyroid hormone-related protein (PTHrP) and may even block bone resorption (see later discussion).[8] The intracellular degradation of newly synthesized PTH therefore provides an important regulatory mechanism. Under conditions of hypercalcemia, the secretion of PTH is substantially decreased, and most of what is secreted consists of carboxy-terminal fragments.[9]

Parathyroid Hormone Secretion

Although catecholamines, magnesium, and other stimuli can affect PTH secretion, the major regulator of PTH secretion is the concentration of ionized calcium in blood. Increased serum ionized calcium leads to a decrease in PTH secretion (Fig. 28-5A). The shape of the dose-response curve is sigmoid. Properties of the parathyroid cell determine the conformation of the sigmoidal curve but do not alone determine the point on the curve that represents a physiologic steady state for an individual. This point, which is usually between the midpoint and the bottom of the curve, is determined by how vigorously target organs respond to PTH.[10] Figure 28-5C (*solid line*) shows how an individual's calcium level rises in response to increases in PTH; the parathyroid gland's sigmoidal curve is the *dotted line*. In the steady state, the blood levels of PTH and calcium are represented by the intersection of the two lines.

The sigmoidal curve reveals several important physiologic properties of the parathyroid gland. The minimal secretory rate is low, but not zero. The maximal secretory rate represents the reserve of the parathyroid's capacity to respond to hypocalcemia. Because values from normal persons in the steady state are located in the lower portion of the sigmoidal curve, the system seems designed to respond more dramatically to hypocalcemia than to hypercalcemia.

Physiologic studies in humans have confirmed this sigmoidal relationship and have also revealed that the parathyroid cell responds both to the absolute level of blood calcium and to the rate of fall of the calcium level. For example, PTH levels briefly rise higher during a sudden drop in blood calcium than they do during a more gradual fall in calcium. This property of the parathyroid cell offers an additional protection against sudden hypocalcemia.

The biochemical and cellular determinants of the parathyroid gland's sigmoidal response curve are beginning to be defined. A parathyroid calcium-sensing receptor (CASR)[11] on the parathyroid cell surface is a member of the G protein–coupled family of receptors. The sequence of the receptor suggests that it spans the plasma membrane seven times, like other receptors in the G protein–linked receptor family (Fig. 28-6). A large extracellular domain resembles similar domains in brain metabotropic glutamate receptors as well as bacterial periplasmic proteins designed to bind small ligands, including cations. The receptor is expressed in a number of cell types and has been shown to activate phospholipase C and to block stimulation of cyclic adenosine monophosphate (cAMP) production, just as it does in normal parathyroid cells.

The most convincing proof of the identity of the parathyroid CASR has been the observation that mutations in the receptor gene cause characteristic human diseases. Inactivating mutations cause familial hypocalciuric hypercalcemia (FHH), a disease of defective calcium sensing (see later discussion),[12] whereas activating mutations cause familial hypoparathyroidism with hypercalciuria.[13] Furthermore, mice that have been genetically engineered to have only one functioning copy of the CASR gene also have the expected defects in parathyroid calcium sensing. Of importance, calcimimetic compounds that activate the cloned CASR have been shown to inhibit PTH secretion in humans and are useful in the treatment of secondary hyperparathyroidism.[14,15] Despite the enormous increase in understanding of how extracellular calcium activates the parathyroid CASR, the mechanism by which this activation leads to a decrease in PTH secretion is poorly understood.

The CASR is expressed widely. Expression in the renal tubules and in the calcitonin-producing cells of the thyroid contributes to calcium homeostasis, whereas expression in organs such as the brain points to multiple roles for calcium signaling. The observation that the CASR also responds to physiologic levels of certain amino acids[16] suggests that its expression in the gut, parathyroid, and other sites may facilitate the assimilation of multiple nutrients.

Regulation of the Parathyroid Hormone Gene

The minute-to-minute regulation of PTH blood levels can be explained by the two mechanisms already discussed: regulation of PTH secretion by the CASR and amplification of this regulation by intracellular degradation of stored hormone. Over a longer time frame, the parathyroid cell regulates the expression of the PTH gene as well.

Although calcitriol, the active form of vitamin D, has no direct effect on PTH secretion, it dramatically suppresses PTH gene transcription.[17] This suppression of transcription does not occur when calcitriol is administered to chronically hypocalcemic animals, however, perhaps because hypocalcemia leads to a fall in the number of parathyroid cell vitamin D receptors (VDRs) or because hypocalcemia increases the expression of calreticulin in the parathyroid.[18] The capability of hypocalcemia to override the effects of high levels of calcitriol represents an important defense, because it provides a way for the parathyroid cell to

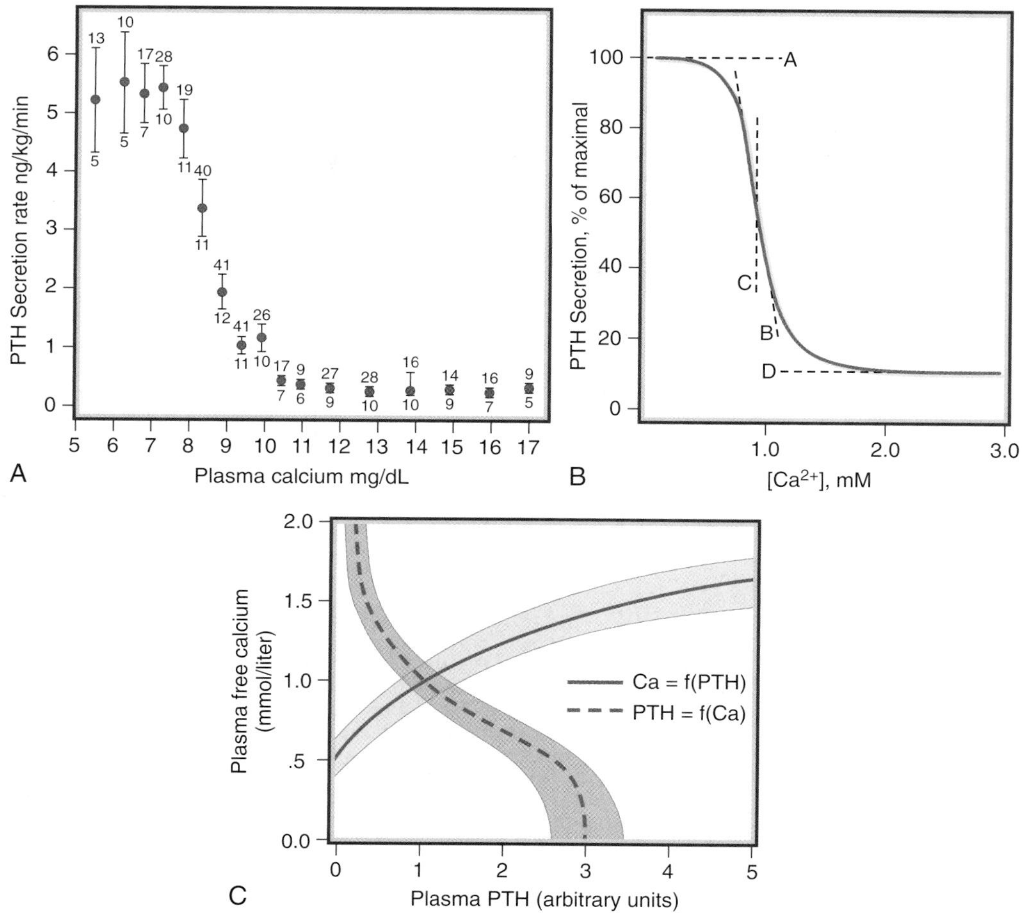

Figure 28-5 Parathyroid hormone (PTH) secretion. **A,** Secretory response of bovine parathyroid glands to induced alterations of plasma calcium concentration. Calves were infused with calcium chloride or ethylenediaminetetra-acetic acid (EDTA), and PTH secretion was assessed by measuring PTH levels in the parathyroid venous effluent. The circles and vertical bars indicate the secretory rate (mean ± SE) in calcium concentration ranges of 1.0 or 0.5 mg/100 mL. The number of calves and samples are indicated, respectively, by numbers below and above the bars. (From Mayer GP, Hurst JG. Sigmoidal relationship between parathyroid hormone secretion rate and plasma calcium concentration in calves. *Endocrinology.* 1978;10:1037-1042.) **B,** Sigmoidal curve generated by the equation $Y = \{[A - D]/[1 + (X/C)^B]\} + D$. Such a curve can be defined by four parameters: the maximal secretory rate (A), the slope of the curve at its midpoint (B), the level of calcium at the midpoint (often called the setpoint) (C), and the minimal secretory rate (D). The significance of A, B, C, and D is described in the text. (Modified from Brown EM. Four-parameter model of the sigmoidal relationship between parathyroid hormone release and extracellular calcium concentration in normal and abnormal parathyroid tissue. *J Clin Endocrinol Metab.* 1983;56:572-581.) **C,** Relationships between calcium and PTH levels when each in turn is treated as an independent variable. The dashed line represents the sigmoidal relationship between calcium and PTH when calcium is the independent variable. This curve is the same as that in **A** and **B**, but it is turned on its side, because the axes are reversed. The solid line represents the relationship between calcium and PTH when PTH is considered the independent variable; values for this curve result from measurements made during PTH infusion into parathyroidectomized animals. Actual data are limited, so the curves should be viewed as illustrative. (From Parfitt AM. Calcium homeostasis. In Mundy GR, Martin TJ, eds. *Physiology and Pharmacology of Bone: Handbook of Experimntal Pharmacology,* vol 107. Berlin: Springer-Verlag; 1993:1-65.)

synthesize large amounts of PTH and calcitriol at the same time, when both are needed.

Calcium also regulates the biosynthesis of PTH. In vivo studies show that acute hypocalcemia in rats leads, within 1 hour, to an increase in PTH messenger RNA (mRNA). In contrast, hypercalcemia leads to little or no change in PTH mRNA. Therefore, under normal conditions, the inhibition by calcium of PTH biosynthesis already is almost maximal, just as it is for PTH secretion. The parathyroid gland is poised to respond to a fall in calcium much more readily than to a rise. The mechanism for the increase in PTH mRNA in response to hypocalcemia is uncertain; differing experimental paradigms suggest regulation at the levels of gene transcription, mRNA translation, and mRNA stability. The latter mechanism is the one best understood at the molecular level.[19,20] In the parathyroid cell, the peptidyl-prolyl isomerase Pin1 binds to and leads to the activation of K-homology splicing regulator protein (KSRP), an RNA-binding protein that destabilizes PTH mRNA. Mice without Pin1 have high PTH and PTH mRNA levels, and hypocalcemic rats and rats with chronic kidney disease have low levels of Pin1. Therefore, Pin1 and KSRP regulate PTH mRNA levels in normal physiology and disease.

For decades it has been known that phosphate elevation stimulates PTH secretion, largely by lowering the levels of blood calcium and calcitriol. More recently, a series of studies in vitro[21,22] and in vivo[23] demonstrated that phosphate can increase PTH secretion directly, independent of effects on blood calcium and calcitriol. Phosphate increases PTH secretion acutely only after a delay, and it probably works largely through regulation of PTH mRNA levels. The mechanisms that phosphate uses to regulate parathyroid

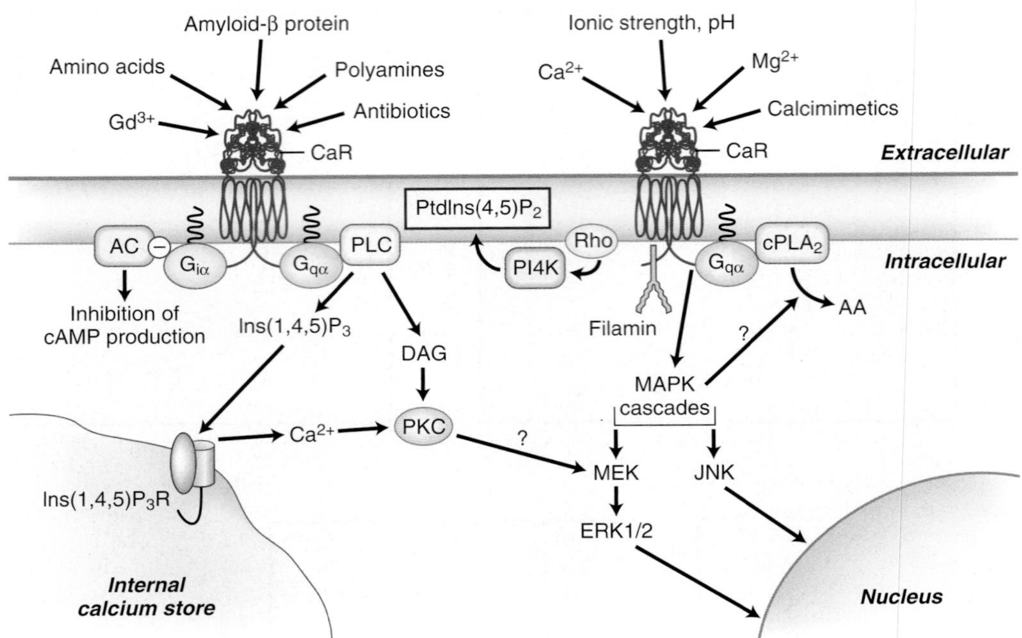

Figure 28-6 Signaling by the calcium-sensing receptor. Numerous agonists activate the calcium-sensing receptor (CaR) and trigger intracellular pathways. AA, arachidonic acid; AC, adenylate cyclase; cAMP, cyclic adenosine monophosphate; cPLA$_2$, cytosolic phospholipase A$_2$; DAG, diacylglycerol; Giα and Gqα, α-subunits of the i- and q-type heterotrimeric G proteins, respectively; Ins(1,4,5)P$_3$, inositol-1,4,5-trisphosphate; Ins(1,4,5)P$_3$R, inositol-1,4,5-trisphosphate receptor; JNK, Jun amino-terminal kinase; MAPK, mitogen-activated protein kinase; MEK, MAPK kinase; PI4K, phosphatidylinositol 4-kinase; PKC, protein kinase C; PLC, phospholipase C; PtdIns(4,5)P$_2$, phoshatidylinositol-4,5-bisphosphate; ERK, extracellular-signal–regulated kinase. (From Hofer AM, Brown EM. Extracellular calcium sensing and signaling. *Nat Rev Molec Cell Biol.* 2003;4:530-538.)

cells are unknown. It is intriguing to speculate that these mechanisms may interact with the pathways regulated by FGF23[24] and Klotho,[25] mediators of phosphate action in other settings, and act directly on parathyroid cells (see later discussion of FGF23).

The regulation of the PTH gene has particular clinical relevance in patients with renal failure. Hypocalcemia, low levels of calcitriol, hyperphosphatemia, FGF23 (see later discussion) and, possibly, uremic toxins disrupt normal calcium homeostasis in this setting. Therapy with calcitriol and calcium increases calcium absorption and also inhibits PTH synthesis by direct effects on the parathyroid gland. Cinacalcet, an activator of the CASR, lowers PTH secretion and thereby lowers both calcium and phosphorus levels.[14] (In renal failure, the role of PTH to increase release of phosphorus from bone dominates over any action of PTH to increase phosphaturia.) Prevention of hyperphosphatemia avoids the direct and indirect actions of phosphate in stimulating PTH secretion.

Regulation of Parathyroid Cell Number

Parathyroid cells divide during the growth of young animals but replicate little in adulthood.[26] Parathyroid cell number can dramatically increase, however, in the setting of hypocalcemia, low levels of calcitriol, hyperphosphatemia, or uremia and during neoplastic growth.

Calcium, acting through the parathyroid CASR, restrains parathyroid proliferation. This effect has been demonstrated clinically in patients who lack both copies of the CASR gene. These neonates exhibit severe primary hyperparathyroidism with large, diffusely hyperplastic glands that presumably have developed because of insufficient activation of the parathyroid CASR by extracellular calcium. Furthermore, administration of the calcimimetic compound NPS R-568, which activates the CASR directly, prevents parathyroid cell proliferation in experimental uremia.

The role of calcitriol, independent of blood calcium, in regulating parathyroid cell proliferation is less well established than that of calcium. That calcitriol can dramatically affect parathyroid cell number has been shown in vivo in many settings, but such studies cannot rigorously eliminate effects of transient changes in blood calcium. The suppression of proliferation of cultured parathyroid cells by calcitriol[27] suggests that it can directly inhibit parathyroid cell replication. In experimental renal failure, the action of calcitriol to decrease parathyroid cell expression of transforming growth factor may partly explain the dampening of parathyroid cell proliferation.[28] Nevertheless, vitamin D action through the VDR is not essential for control of parathyroid cell number, because calcium alone can prevent parathyroid cell hyperplasia in mice engineered to lack VDRs.[29]

Although the ability to increase parathyroid cell number in response to physiologic challenge represents an important defense against hypocalcemia, it is a slow response that is not easily reversible. When the need for an increased number of parathyroid cells disappears (e.g., after renal transplantation for uremia), persistent hyperparathyroidism can cause vexing clinical problems for months and years afterward. The mechanisms for decreasing parathyroid cell number, if they exist, are poorly understood. Apoptosis of normal parathyroid cells in response to experimental manipulation has not been demonstrated.

Parathyroid Gland Development

Genes involved in making parathyroid cells during development may also regulate PTH synthesis and parathyroid cell number throughout life; therefore, understanding of parathyroid cell development could have broad clinical implications. Although the genetic mechanisms used to generate parathyroid chief cells during development are largely unknown, the importance of several specific genes has become clear.

Studies of gene knockout mice have shown that the hoxa3,[30] pax1,[31] pax9,[32] and Eya1[33] transcription factors are needed to form parathyroid glands, as are many other pharyngeal pouch derivatives, such as the thymus (reviewed by Liu and colleagues[34]). Another transcription factor, Tbx1, which is regulated by the developmental paracrine factor, sonic hedgehog, is expressed early in parathyroid development and is essential for parathyroid cell development. In humans and mice, haploinsufficiency for the transcription factor Tbx1 is likely to be responsible for many of the abnormalities found in DiGeorge syndrome, including hypoparathyroidism.[35] Whereas these transcription factors together are essential for the early generation of parathyroid cells, another transcription factor, called "glial cell missing" or GCM2, is needed for the continuing survival of parathyroid cells.[34] Furthermore, mice or humans[36] missing this gene have no parathyroid glands. In both species, deletion of the gene is very specific for controlling parathyroid development, because no abnormalities in other tissues have been noted. Mice, which have only two parathyroid glands normally, still make PTH in a small number of cells in the thymus after *Gcm2* gene ablation, and they secrete this PTH into the circulation. Humans without *GCM2* have little detectable circulating PTH at birth and low levels of PTH several years later.

Studies of human hypoparathyroidism have led to the discovery of the likely roles of other transcription factors in parathyroid development. Sox3 is a transcription factor expressed in the pharyngeal pouches that give rise to parathyroid cells. Humans with X-linked hypoparathyroidism manifest a deletion-insertion near the end of the *SOX3* gene, a finding that suggests an important role for Sox3 in parathyroid development.[37] People with mutations in the gene encoding the transcription factor GATA3 exhibit a syndrome of hypoparathyroidism, sensorineural deafness, and renal anomalies when only one copy of the gene is mutated.[38]

Metabolism of Parathyroid Hormone

The earliest radioimmunoassays for PTH demonstrated that the molecular forms of PTH in the circulation differ from those in the parathyroid gland. Characterization of the metabolism of PTH and its fragments has clarified the origins and significance of immunoreactive PTH molecules in the bloodstream.[39] As noted previously, both PTH(1-84) and carboxy-terminal fragments of PTH are secreted from the parathyroid gland; the ratio of inactive PTH to active PTH secretion increases with increasing blood calcium. Secreted intact PTH(1-84) is extensively metabolized by liver (70%) and kidney (20%) and disappears from the circulation with a half-life of 2 minutes. This rapid peripheral metabolism of PTH is unaffected by widely varying levels of blood calcium or calcitriol. Less than 1% of the secreted hormone finds its way to PTH receptors on physiologic target organs. These features of PTH metabolism ensure that the blood level of PTH is determined principally by the activity of the parathyroid glands and that the PTH level can respond rapidly to small changes in the rate of secretion of the hormone.

In the liver, a small amount of PTH binds to physiologically relevant PTH receptors, but most of the intact PTH is cleaved, initially after residues 33 and 36, probably by cathepsins. In the kidney, a small amount of intact PTH binds to physiologic PTH receptors, but most of the intact PTH is filtered at the glomerulus and subsequently bound by a large, membrane-bound luminal protein, megalin.[40] This binding leads to internalization and degradation of PTH by the tubules.[41] Carboxy-terminal fragments are also cleared efficiently by glomerular filtration. In fact, the kidney is the only known site of clearance of carboxy-terminal PTH fragments, and these fragments accumulate dramatically when the glomerular filtration rate (GFR) falls. Even in the presence of normal renal function, the half-life of carboxy-terminal fragments of PTH exceeds that of PTH^{1-84} by several-fold. Consequently, the concentration of carboxy-terminal fragments in the circulation exceeds that of intact PTH, even though intact PTH usually is the major form of PTH secreted from the parathyroid gland.

Careful analysis of PTH fragments using high-performance liquid chromatography (HPLC) and immunologic methods has revealed almost full-length PTH fragments that are missing the first several amino acids of the hormone but contain most or all of the remaining hormone sequence.[42] These still incompletely characterized fragments are both secreted from the parathyroid gland and generated by peripheral metabolism of the hormone. Because they are missing the amino-terminal portion of PTH, they cannot stimulate cAMP production by the PTH/PTHrP receptor, and they circulate in small amounts except in renal failure. Nevertheless, the possible biologic activity of these and other PTH fragments, possibly through novel receptors, remains an area of active investigation. Experiments with PTH(7-84) suggest that such extended carboxyl fragments may exert potent effects in vivo, opposing those of intact PTH (see later discussion).[8,43,44]

Actions of Parathyroid Hormone

Actions of Parathyroid Hormone on the Kidney

Stimulation of Calcium Reabsorption. Almost all of the calcium in the initial glomerular filtrate is reabsorbed by the renal tubules. Sixty-five percent or more is reabsorbed by the proximal convoluted and straight tubules via a passive, paracellular route.[45] Changes in the transepithelial voltage gradient, determined largely by the rate of sodium reabsorption, control the rate of calcium transport in the proximal tubule, and PTH does little to affect calcium flux in this region. The remaining calcium is largely reabsorbed more distally—20% of the initial filtrate in the cortical thick ascending limb (cTAL) of Henle's loop and 10% in the distal convoluted and connecting tubules.

In the cTAL, calcium reabsorption also is mainly passive and paracellular, although some transcellular, active calcium transport may occur as well. Efficient paracellular calcium and magnesium movement requires expression of a unique tight-junction protein, paracellin-1; mutant paracellin-1 genes underlie a rare renal calcium- and magnesium-wasting disorder.[46] Because paracellular cation transport in the cTAL is driven by the lumen-positive transepithelial voltage gradient that is established by active sodium reabsorption, calcium reabsorption there is strongly inhibited by loop diuretics such as furosemide. The CASR, initially characterized in the parathyroid, also is expressed in the cTAL. When activated by high blood levels of calcium or magnesium, this receptor inhibits $Na/K/Cl_2$ reabsorption in the cTAL and, consequently, paracellular calcium reabsorption as well. This provides a parathyroid-independent mechanism for controlling renal calcium handling in direct response to changes in blood calcium concentration.

Although PTH modestly stimulates paracellular calcium reabsorption in the cTAL, the primary site for hormonal regulation of renal calcium reabsorption is the distal nephron, which normally reabsorbs almost all of the remaining 10% of filtered calcium by a unique transcellular active transport mechanism. As depicted in Figure 28-1, the intracellular level of calcium is extremely low, about 150 nmol/L, compared with the millimolar levels in the glomerular filtrate and the blood. Calcium enters distal tubular cells from the tubular lumen down a highly favorable electrochemical gradient via selective Ca^{2+} channels (TRPV5 and TRPV6) that are present on the apical membrane of cells in the distal convoluted tubule and connecting tubule. Intracellular calcium inhibits the activity of these channels, but this is minimized by the avid binding of calcium to calbindin-D28K, which effectively buffers cytosolic calcium and transports it to the basolateral membrane. There, calcium is ejected via active processes involving mainly the sodium-calcium exchanger NCX1 and an ATP-driven calcium pump (PMCA).[47] PTH stimulates active calcium transport in the distal convoluted tubule and connecting tubule by upregulating several of these components, including TRPV5, calbindin-D28K and NCX1, both directly and indirectly, via increased synthesis of calcitriol.[47,48]

The amount of calcium in the final urine reflects all of the tubular reabsorption processes just enumerated but also depends crucially on the initial filtered load of calcium. All of PTH's actions serve to raise the blood calcium level, so the filtered load of calcium is high in states of PTH excess. In that setting, even though the rate of distal tubular calcium reabsorption is increased by PTH, the total amount of calcium in the final urine is likely to be high, because of the high initial filtered load.

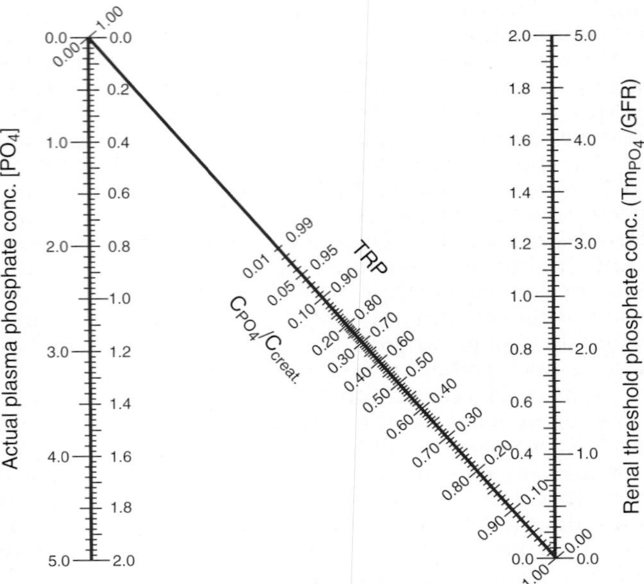

Figure 28-7 Nomogram for determining renal threshold phosphate concentration (Tm_{PO_4}/GFR) from the plasma phosphate concentration [PO_4] and the fractional reabsorption of filtered phosphate (TRP) or fractional excretion of filtered phosphate (1 − TRP, or C_{PO_4}/C_{creat}). Because the blood level of phosphate influences the renal handling of phosphate, the Tm_{PO_4}/GFR best separates normal from abnormal renal phosphate handling. C, clearance; creat, creatinine; GFR, glomerular filtration rate; TRP, tubular resorption of phosphate. (From Walton RJ, Bijvoet OLM. Nomogram of derivation of renal threshold phosphate concentration. *Lancet.* 1975;2:309-310.)

Inhibition of Phosphate Transport. Phosphate reabsorption occurs mainly in the proximal renal tubules, which reclaim roughly 80% of the filtered load. Some additional phosphate (8% to 10%) is reabsorbed in the distal tubule (but not in Henle's loop), leaving about 10% to 12% for excretion in the urine. The normal overall fractional tubular reabsorption of phosphate (TRP), therefore, is about 90%, although a more reliable measure of renal phosphate handling is the *phosphate threshold* (Tm_{PO4}/GFR), which can be derived from the TRP through the use of a nomogram (Fig. 28-7) based on studies of experimental phosphate infusions in healthy persons and in patients with a variety of diseases that affect phosphate excretion.[49]

Phosphate reabsorption in both proximal and distal tubules is strongly inhibited by PTH, although the proximal effect is quantitatively more important. Phosphate is reabsorbed by a transepithelial route. Transport from the glomerular filtrate into the cell is mediated by specific NaPi cotransporters, several types of which have been cloned and extensively characterized.[50] The low level of sodium within the cell drives the cotransport of sodium and phosphate, even though the phosphate travels up an electrochemical gradient. In response to PTH, the maximum velocity (V_{max}) for NaPi cotransport decreases because NaPi cotransporters (both NaPi-IIa and NaPi-IIc) are rapidly (15 minutes) sequestered within subapical endocytic vesicles, after which they are delivered to lysosomes and undergo proteolysis.[51] This response to PTH is dependent on Na^+/H^+ exchange regulatory factors (NHERFs) that physically interact with both the PTH/PTHrP receptor and the NaPi type II cotransporters and control the pattern of PTH receptor signaling.[52] Conversely, in hypoparathyroidism, expression of NaPi protein and mRNA is strongly upregulated.

Dietary intake of phosphate also reciprocally regulates the expression and activity of NaPi cotransporters and, consequently, the proximal tubular absorption of phosphate by a mechanism that is independent of PTH. Dietary deprivation of phosphate, for example, leads to a stimulation of phosphate reabsorption that can override the effects of PTH on the proximal tubule. It is likely that this dietary regulation of NaPi expression is mediated by FGF23[53] (see later discussion).

Other Renal Effects of Parathyroid Hormone. PTH stimulates the synthesis of $1,25(OH)_2D_3$ (calcitriol) in the proximal tubule by rapidly inducing transcription of the 25(OH)D 1α-hydroxylase gene, an effect that can be overridden by hypercalcemia or by calcitriol. The interactions of calcitriol and PTH in regulating the 25(OH)D 1α-hydroxylase gene involve both protein kinase A–mediated phosphorylation of an activating transcription factor and protein kinase C–mediated demethylation of DNA upstream of the 25(OH)D 1α-hydroxylase gene.[54] PTH inhibits proximal tubular transcription of the 25(OH)D 24-hydroxylase gene and antagonizes the upregulation of 24-hydroxylase activity by calcitriol (see "Vitamin D Metabolism"). PTH inhibits proximal tubular sodium, water, and bicarbonate reabsorption, mainly via inhibition of the apical Na^+/H^+ exchanger (NHE3) and the basolateral Na^+,K^+-ATPase. PTH also stimulates proximal tubular gluconeogenesis and acts directly on glomerular podocytes to decrease both the single-nephron and the whole-kidney GFR.

Actions of Parathyroid Hormone on Bone

The actions of PTH on bone are complicated because PTH acts on a number of cell types, both directly and indirectly. For years, the release of calcium from bone through stimulation of bone resorption has been considered to be the major action of PTH on bone. This is only part of the story, however. In fact, PTH administration by any route increases both bone resorption and bone formation. Which action dominates depends on the dose of PTH and the route of administration. When PTH is administered continuously, the effect of PTH on bone resorption dominates, and the net result is release of calcium from bone and a decrease in bone mass. This action of PTH therefore contributes to the increase in blood calcium seen on administration of PTH. In contrast, administration of low doses of PTH or of active, amino-terminal fragments of PTH by once-daily subcutaneous injection leads to a net increase in bone mass, with only transient effects on the blood calcium level. Mechanisms for these divergent effects of PTH are incompletely understood but certainly reflect the variety of cell types in bone that respond directly to PTH, the varying time courses of these responses, and the indirect effects caused by autocrine and paracrine responses to PTH.[55]

Figure 28-8 illustrates the cells of the osteoblast lineage (see also Chapter 29). Osteoblasts are probably derived from pluripotent mesenchymal stem cells that, at least in vitro, can differentiate into chondrocytes, adipocytes, osteoblasts, and other cell types.[56] Perivascular cells within human bone can reconstitute bone that supports hematopoiesis after subcutaneous transplantation in mice[57]; these cells may well represent one group of osteoblast stem cells in vivo. Within the osteoblast lineage, committed osteoprogenitor cells divide, become preosteoblastic stromal cells (which can divide further), and then become osteoblasts. Osteoblasts no longer divide and are cuboidal cells found on the bone surface actively laying down new bone. When these cells become surrounded by bone, they become stellate osteocytes. If, instead, osteoblasts stop synthesizing matrix and remain on the bone surface, they flatten out as bone lining cells. Not all preosteoblasts and osteoblasts mature; a variable number die by apoptotic, programmed cell death.[58]

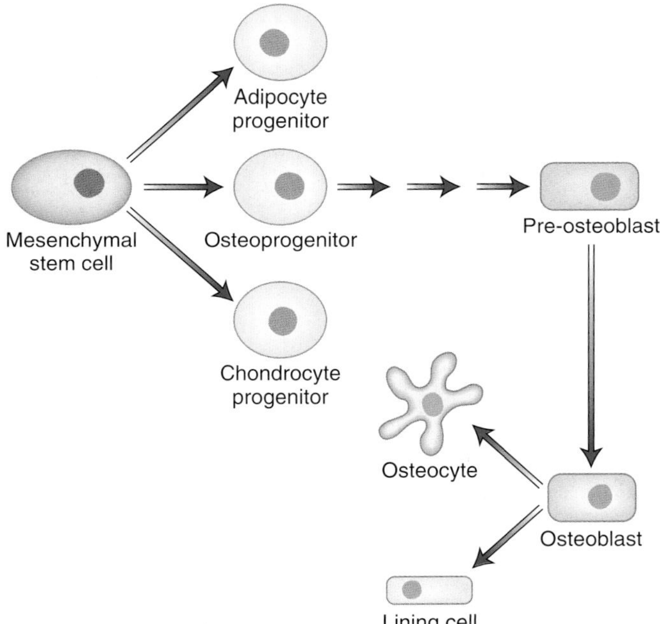

Figure 28-8 Osteoblast lineage. All precursors of osteoblasts can proliferate; osteoblasts are transformed to osteocytes and lining cells without further proliferation. Some data suggest that lining cells may revert to osteoblast function after parathyroid hormone stimulation. At each stage in the lineage, apoptotic cell death is probably an alternative fate.

PTH administration can influence movement of cells through the osteoblast lineage.[55] PTH administration in vivo, whether administered continuously or intermittently, increases osteoblast surface and number and the rate of bone formation. With intermittent PTH administration, the number of bone lining cells decreases as the number of active osteoblasts increases, without an increase in the percentage of osteoblasts incorporating precursors into DNA; these observations suggest that lining cells might be converted to osteoblasts in response to PTH.[59] An alternative, and not mutually exclusive, explanation for the increase in osteoblast number after intermittent PTH administration is the observed decrease in the rate of osteoblast apoptosis after PTH administration.[58] PTH administration in vivo also probably increases the number of early osteoblast precursors. For example, both the number of total stromal cell colonies (CFU-F) generated and the number of CFU-F expressing alkaline phosphatase, were increased when bone marrow cells were plated in vitro after treatment of rats with PTH(1-34) intermittently.[60] This increase in osteoblast precursors may correlate with the in vivo phenomenon of "osteofibrosis," with large numbers of alkaline phosphatase–positive fibroblastic cells present in marrow after prolonged, continuous activation of the PTH receptor in vivo.[61] The effect of PTH administration on osteoblast differentiation after plating of calvarial or marrow cells in vitro has also been studied extensively. For example, when PTH is administered to calvarial cells plated in vitro, bone nodule formation is suppressed, probably by late actions that slow the conversion of preosteoblasts to mature osteoblasts.[62] The precise timing of the addition of PTH in this system has disparate effects, partly through activation of distinct second messenger pathways and stimulation of secretion of other signaling molecules. These in vivo and in vitro studies therefore suggest effects of PTH on movement through the osteoblast lineage at multiple steps.

In addition to changing osteoblast numbers, PTH changes the activity of mature osteoblasts by a variety of mechanisms. When PTH is added to calvariae in vitro, the osteoblasts decrease their synthesis of collagen I and other matrix proteins. This action may reflect, in part, the action of PTH to steer the essential osteoblast transcription factor Runx2 toward proteosomal destruction.[63] In vivo, however, the most obvious effects of PTH are to increase bone formation by osteoblasts, probably by indirect actions of PTH on autocrine and paracrine pathways. PTH stimulation of osteoblastic cells leads to the release of growth factors such as insulin-like growth factor 1, FGF2, and amphiregulin from these cells.[64] PTH also decreases the synthesis of dickkopf-1[65] and SOST,[66] inhibitors of Wnt signaling[67]; these actions are expected to increase the anabolic actions of Wnt proteins on osteoblasts. These paracrine actions of PTH may not only stimulate osteoblastic cells with PTH receptors but might well activate, indirectly, osteoblast precursors that are too immature to express PTH receptors. Further, because bone matrix is a rich source of osteoblast growth factors, the release of these growth factors from this matrix after PTH-induced bone resorption may increase bone formation and bring osteoblastic cells to sites of bone formation.[68] Therefore, a variety of both direct and indirect actions of PTH can lead to the increased production of bone.

Surprisingly, osteoclasts, the bone-resorbing cells derived from hematopoietic precursors, have no PTH receptors on their surfaces. Instead, preosteoblasts and osteoblasts signal to osteoclast precursors to cause them to fuse and form mature osteoclasts. This signaling also serves to stimulate mature osteoclasts to resorb bone and to avoid apoptosis (Fig. 28-9). Two osteoblast surface proteins, macrophage

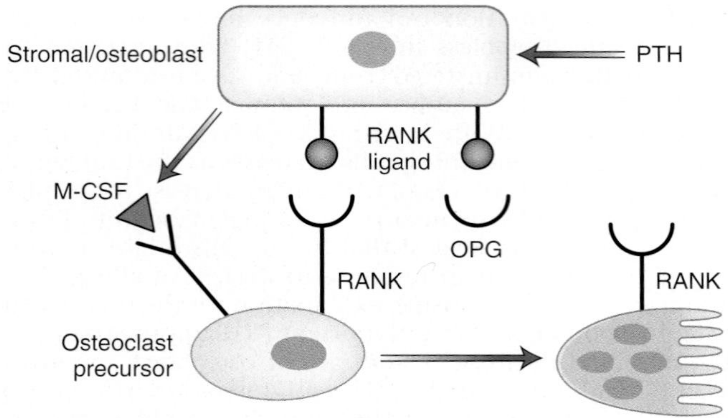

Figure 28-9 Stromal cell control of osteoclastogenesis and osteoclast activity. Parathyroid hormone (PTH) acts on PTH/PTH-related protein (PTHrP) receptors on precursors of osteoblasts to increase the production of macrophage colony-stimulating factor (M-CSF) and receptor activator for nuclear factor κB (RANK) ligand and to decrease the production of osteoprotegerin (OPG). M-CSF and RANK ligand stimulate the production of osteoclasts and increase the activity of mature osteoclasts by binding to the receptor RANK. OPG blocks the interaction of RANK ligand and RANK.

colony-stimulating factor and receptor activator for nuclear factor κB (RANK) ligand, or RANKL, are essential for stimulation of osteoclastogenesis,[69] and RANKL is essential for the activation of mature osteoclasts. Macrophage colony-stimulating factor, a growth factor encoded by *CSF1*, is expressed both as a secreted protein and as a cell surface protein; the production of both forms is stimulated by PTH.[70] RANKL—also called osteoprotegerin (OPG) ligand, osteoclast-differentiating factor, and TRANCE—is a membrane-bound member of the tumor necrosis factor (TNF) family; its synthesis is also increased by PTH. RANKL binds to its receptor, RANK, a member of the TNF receptor family. RANK is found on both osteoclast precursors and mature osteoclasts. The binding of RANKL to RANK can be blocked by osteoprotegerin (OPG), another member of the TNF receptor family. OPG (also called OCIF, TR1, or TNFRSF11B) circulates and is also secreted by cells of the osteoblastic lineage. PTH decreases the synthesis and secretion of OPG from these cells. Therefore, PTH, by increasing RANK and decreasing OPG locally in bone, serves to increase bone resorption.

Because PTH can both increase bone formation and increase resorption, the net effect of PTH on bone mass varies from one part of bone to another and also varies strikingly according to whether PTH is administered continuously or intermittently. Intermittent administration of low doses of PTH causes dramatic net increase in trabecular bone mass with little effect on cortical bone mass in humans. Continuous administration of PTH, in contrast, leads to a decrease in cortical bone mass; the net effect of PTH on trabecular bone depends on the dose. In mild primary hyperparathyroidism, there is little net effect of PTH on trabecular bone and a decrease in cortical bone. In all of these settings, the rate of bone formation is increased; the varying rate of osteoclastic resorption determines the net effect of PTH on bone mass.

Molecular Basis of Parathyroid Hormone Action

Ever since the discovery that PTH stimulates the secretion of cAMP into the urine,[71] PTH has been thought to act by triggering a cascade of intracellular second messengers. This guiding hypothesis, in its current form, postulates that all of the actions of PTH result from binding of the hormone to a receptor on the plasma membrane of target tissues. This receptor is a member of a large family of G protein–linked receptors that span the plasma membrane seven times (Fig. 28-10). The binding of hormone on the outside of the membrane causes conformational changes in the disposition of the seven transmembrane helices that activate the receptor's ability to release guanosine diphosphate (GDP) from the α-subunit of a G protein bound to the receptor. The G protein then binds guanosine triphosphate (GTP) in place of GDP. The GTP-binding α-subunit of the G protein then separates from the βγ-subunits, and the separate subunits of the G protein modulate the activity of enzymes and channels, affecting proteins further downstream and eventually leading to the physiologic responses of bone and kidney cells.

Parathyroid Hormone and Parathyroid Hormone-Related Protein Receptors. DNA encoding a PTH/PTHrP receptor has been isolated from rat, opossum, human, pig, *Xenopus* (toad), and zebrafish cells and tissues.[72] The receptor mediates actions of both PTH and PTHrP (see discussion of PTHrP later in this chapter). The predicted amino acid sequence of the receptor and direct mapping of inserted epitopes suggest that the receptor spans the plasma membrane seven times, but the sequence does not closely resemble those of most known G protein–linked receptors. Instead, it is a member of a distinct subfamily of closely related receptors. Most of these receptors bind peptides that are 30 to 40 amino acids long. Known members include receptors for the secretin family of peptides (secretin, vasoactive intestinal peptide VIP, glucagon, glucagon-like peptide, growth hormone-releasing hormone, pituitary adenylate cyclase–activating peptide, gastric inhibitory peptide), corticotropin-releasing hormone, calcitonin, and insect diuretic hormones related to corticotropin-releasing hormone. The PTH/PTHrP receptor most closely resembles receptors of the secretin group. The gene encoding the PTH/PTHrP receptor has a complicated structure, with 13 introns interrupting the coding sequence.

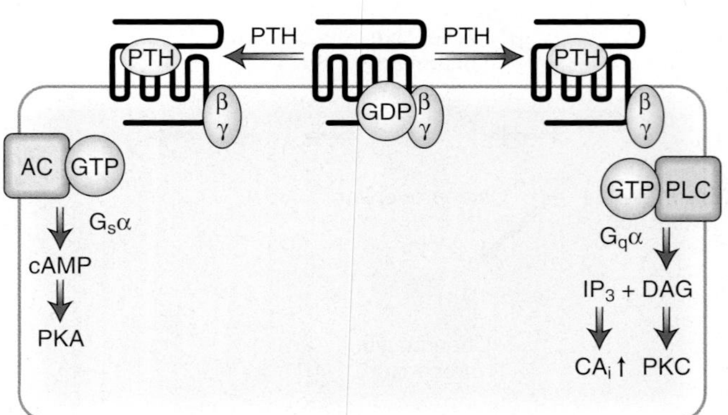

Figure 28-10 Parathyroid hormone (PTH)/PTH-related protein (PTHrP) receptors act as nucleotide exchangers. PTH binding to the receptor leads to exchange of guanosine triphosphate (GTP) for guanosine diphosphate (GDP) bound to stimulatory G protein (G_s) α-subunits. $G_s\alpha$-subunits bound to GTP are released from the receptor and from the βγ-subunits and then activate effectors. $G_s\alpha$ activates adenylate cyclase (AC), leading to the formation of cyclic adenosine monophosphate (cAMP), which then activates protein kinase A (PKA). $G_q\alpha$ and related α-subunits activate phospholipase C (PLC). PLC hydrolyzes phosphatidylinositol 1,4,5-trisphosphate to generate diacylglycerol (DAG) and inositol 1,4,5-trisphosphate (IP_3). The DAG then activates protein kinase C (PKC), and the IP_3 activates a receptor on microsomal vesicles that directs the movement of calcium (CA_i) from microsomal vesicles into the cytosol.

The cloned PTH/PTHrP receptor binds amino-terminal fragments of PTH and PTHrP with equal affinity. The receptor is expressed at high levels in kidney and in osteoblasts of bone but is also expressed in many other tissues, including smooth muscle, brain, and a variety of fetal tissues, which are thought to be target tissues more for PTHrP than for PTH. The interactions of the PTH/PTHrP receptor with its two ligands are similar but do differ in ways that have physiologic significance.[73] After binding to the receptor, PTH continues to interact with the receptor for much longer than does PTHrP.[74] This more stable binding mode of PTH involves interactions with the receptor that allow the ligand to remain receptor bound even when G molecules are not interacting with the receptor. More stable binding results in a different intracellular fate for PTH compared with PTHrP and leads to more prolonged activation of the receptor by PTH.[75] In response to binding of PTH or PTHrP, the receptor activates several G proteins, including G_s, G_q, G_{11}, G_i, G_{12}, and G_{13}.

The PTH/PTHrP receptor mediates many of the actions of PTH and PTHrP. The ligand-binding and signaling properties of the receptor, the pattern of expression of the receptor, and the consequences of mutation of the receptor sequence (see later discussion) are persuasive evidence in this regard. Nevertheless, the scheme of PTH action illustrated in Figure 28-10 should be considered a simplified outline. It is unlikely that all of the actions of PTH can be explained by interactions with the cloned PTH/PTHrP receptor. Fragments of PTH that seem not to bind the receptor may be biologically active,[76] and some cells respond to PTH in ways not mimicked by the cloned receptor.[77] Furthermore, the carboxyl-terminal portion of PTH(1-84) binds a cell surface protein distinct from the PTH/PTHrP receptor.

A second PTH receptor, which can be activated by PTH but not by PTHrP, has been cloned; it is called the PTH2 receptor (PTH2R). This receptor is expressed in multiple tissues, including brain, vascular endothelium and smooth muscle, endocrine cells of the gastrointestinal tract, and sperm. Expression is not seen in osteoblasts or renal tubules, however. Although PTH activates the human PTH2R well, PTH only poorly activates PTH2R in the rat and other species. Furthermore, a novel ligand called TIP39 has been characterized and shown to be a potent activator of PTH2R. TIP39 bears only a weak resemblance to PTH or PTHrP and is likely to be a physiologically relevant activator of the PTH2. The functional role of the PTH2R is unknown, but it appears to mediate many actions of TIP39 in the brain and testis; studies of knockout mice implicate TIP39 in regulation of anxiety reactions[78] and germ cell development.[79] The two cloned PTH receptors, as well as distinct receptors for fragments of PTHrP (see later discussion), probably are part of a complex network of ligands and receptors (Fig. 28-11).

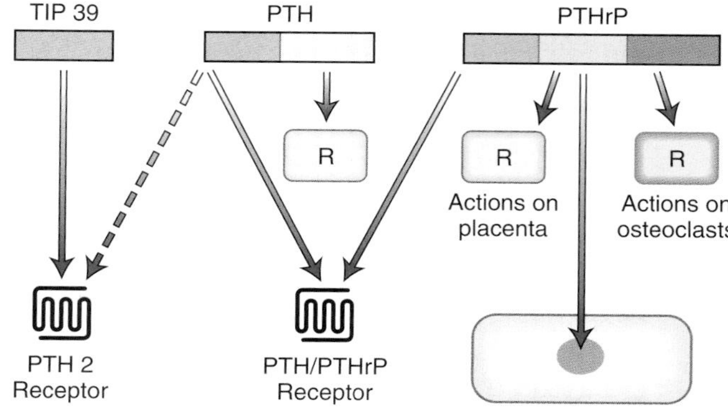

Figure 28-11 Network of parathyroid hormone (PTH) ligands and receptors (R). PTH and PTH-related protein (PTHrP) closely resemble each other at the amino-terminal region; TIP39 is more distantly related. Although only the PTH/PTHrP receptor and the PTH2 receptor have been cloned, biologic actions suggest that there are receptors specific for the carboxy-terminal portion of PTH, as well as distinct receptors for the midregion of PTHrP and for a more distal region of PTHrP. PTHrP is also found in nuclei and may act directly there.

Functional Implications of Parathyroid Hormone Structure. Amino-terminal fragments of PTH as short as the PTH(1-34) peptide have potency at least as great as that of the full-length PTH(1-84). Several discrete portions of PTH(1-34) interact with the receptor. The first several residues of PTH are particularly important for triggering the conformational change in the receptor that results in activation of G_s and adenylate cyclase. Sequences responsible for transmembrane activation of G_s make up most of the first 13 residues of PTH; it is these residues that are highly conserved between PTH and PTHrP. At high concentrations, PTH(1-14) by itself can activate the PTH/PTHrP receptor. This activation domain interacts with the receptor's transmembrane domains and extracellular loops. When the first nine residues of PTH are covalently linked to the receptor's transmembrane domains and extracellular loops, they can activate the receptor. An analogue of PTH(1-14) can trigger G_q activation, thus activating phospholipase C.[80] These data, plus the observation that a PTH analogue modified at position 1 selectively loses its ability to activate phospholipase C,[81] demonstrate that the amino-terminal portion of PTH is essential for activation of both G_s and G_q. More distal regions of PTH(1-34) can activate protein kinase C and can raise intracellular calcium levels by mechanisms that have not been fully clarified. Remarkably, a PTH analogue that is missing the first six residues and cannot activate G proteins can still activate the PTH/PTHrP receptor and increase bone mass in vivo.[82] This analogue can activate mitogen-activated protein kinase (MAPK) signaling through interactions of the receptor with β-arrestin. These studies illustrate how the PTH/PTHrP receptor can signal intracellularly without activating G proteins.

The more carboxy-terminal portions of PTH(1-34) contribute importantly to the specificity and tight binding of PTH to the PTH/PTHrP receptor, at least partly through interactions with the receptor's amino-terminal extracellular domain (Fig. 28-12). A variety of studies of genetically altered receptors, biochemical studies using photoactivated cross-links between PTH and the receptor, and studies of co-crystals of the receptor's amino-terminal domain and PTH/PTHrP fragments[73,83] have reinforced each other and show that the carboxy-terminal portion of PTH makes multiple contacts with the amino-terminal extension of the receptor and with its extracellular loops. This interaction of PTH with the amino-terminal portion of the receptor occurs extremely rapidly, with a time constant of 140 milliseconds.[84] In contrast, the subsequent interaction of the amino-terminal portion of PTH with the so-called J domain of the receptor (the transmembrane domains and associated extracellular loops) occurs more slowly, with a time constant of 1 second. Presumably, this extra time is needed for the amino-terminus of PTH to form a helix and for the receptor to attain an optimal conformation for binding. When this slow interaction occurs, the receptor changes the relationships of its transmembrane domains and activates G proteins.[85]

Studies of the structure of PTH by nuclear magnetic resonance spectroscopy suggest that the activation domain and

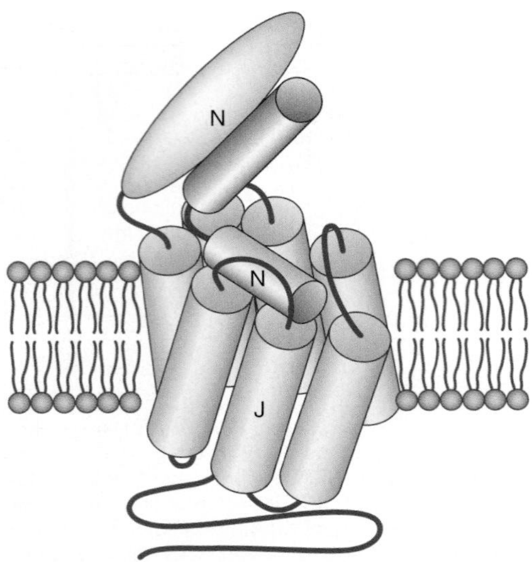

Figure 28-12 Binding of the PTH(1-34) peptide of the parathyroid hormone (PTH) to the PTH/PTH-related protein (PTHrP) receptor. The amino-terminal extracellular domain of the receptor binds rapidly to the carboxy-terminal portion of the ligand. The "J domain" of the receptor, containing the transmembrane domains and associated loops, binds to the amino-terminal domain of the ligand. This binding is slower and may require conformational changes in both the ligand and the receptor. These changes then trigger G protein activation, receptor internalization, and other actions. (Courtesy of Tom Gardella.)

the carboxy-terminal domain are discrete entities dominated by α-helices separated by a flexible loop of variable size, depending on the hydrophobicity of the solvent. In the crystal structure of human PTH(1-34), the flexible loop is entirely replaced by a helical structure.[86] Taken together, these studies suggest that the carboxy-terminal portion of PTH(1-34) makes multiple contacts with the receptor that allow high-affinity binding and positioning of the amino-terminal portion of PTH to activate the receptor through contacts with transmembrane domains and associated loops.

Activation of Second Messengers. Precisely how binding of PTH to the extracellular domains of the PTH/PTHrP receptor leads to activation of G proteins is not understood. The crystal structure of rhodopsin, another member of the seven-transmembrane receptor family, as well as the behavior of certain mutant PTH/PTHrP receptors,[87,88] suggest that the seven transmembrane domains of the PTH/PTHrP receptors form a ring, with the seventh transmembrane domain adjacent to the first and second domains. Presumably, binding of PTH to several different regions of the receptor changes the relationships of the transmembrane domains[85] such that the receptor's three intracellular loops and carboxy-terminal tail interact with G proteins in an altered way.

Receptors with certain point mutations in the second, sixth, and seventh transmembrane domains can activate G_s even without stimulation by hormone. These mutant receptors were discovered by analyzing the PTH/PTHrP receptors in patients with Jansen's metaphyseal chondrodystrophy.[89] Patients with this disorder have signs of parathyroid overactivity (hypercalcemia, hypophosphatemia, high levels of calcitriol, and urinary cAMP) but low PTH and PTHrP levels. The mutations must change the conformation of the intracellular face of the receptor in a way that resembles the effect of binding of PTH to the normal receptor. The observation that inappropriate activation of the PTH/PTHrP receptor in Jansen's chondrodystrophy leads to all of the metabolic abnormalities found in primary hyperparathyroidism is one of the most persuasive pieces of evidence that the cloned PTH/PTHrP receptor does, in fact, mediate the actions of PTH in bone and kidney in humans in vivo.

Second Messengers and Distal Effects of Parathyroid Hormone. The activation of multiple G proteins by PTH raises questions about the individual roles of each second messenger and their possible interactions. The importance of cAMP as a mediator of the physiologic actions of PTH has been demonstrated by studies in vivo[71] and in vitro.[90] Furthermore, patients with pseudohypoparathyroidism type I, who cannot increase urinary cAMP levels in response to PTH, show clear renal resistance to PTH (see later discussion).

Activation of phospholipase C, with concomitant activation of protein kinase C and synthesis of IP_3, may also contribute to physiologic actions of PTH such as inhibition of NaPi cotransport[91] and stimulation of the renal 25(OH) D 1α-hydroxylase.[92] Mice with mutant PTH/PTHrP receptors that cannot activate phospholipase C have a mild delay in bone development[93] and abnormalities of phosphate handling by the kidney when challenged with a low-calcium diet.[94] Some actions of PTH may require activation of both adenylate cyclase and phospholipase C for optimal activity.

The stimulation of one G protein or another by the PTH/PTHrP receptor can vary in different types of cells and even in differing regions of the same cell.[91] In some settings, this choice may be influenced by the interactions of the PTH/PTHrP receptor with intracellular scaffolding proteins such as NHERF1 and NHERF2. Binding of the PTH/PTHrP receptor to NHERFs is directed by the last four amino acids in the receptor sequence. This binding, which is particularly prominent, for example, at the apical surface of the proximal tubular cells of the kidney, may change the G protein activated by the PTH/PTHrP receptor from predominantly G_s to predominantly G_i.[95]

Target Cell Responsiveness to Parathyroid Hormone. Physiologic responses to PTH depend not only on the concentration of PTH in blood but also on the responsiveness of target cells to PTH. This responsiveness can be modified by previous exposure to PTH or by exposure to a variety of other hormones and paracrine factors. Responsiveness can be changed by alterations at virtually every step in the cellular response to PTH.

Major regulators of PTH/PTHrP receptor gene expression include, not surprisingly, PTH and calcitriol, both of which can decrease PTH/PTHrP receptor mRNA in certain target cells. In some settings, PTH decreases the amount of immunoreactive and functional receptor on the cell surface without changing the levels of PTH/PTHrP receptor mRNA. This decrease reflects ligand-induced internalization and degradation of receptors. Internalization of receptor is stimulated by PTH binding, which leads to phosphorylation of specific serines found in the receptor's cytoplasmic tail and subsequent internalization directed by binding of arrestin to the receptor.[96,97] Even without a change in receptor number, the binding of arrestin to the PTH/PTHrP receptor decreases the efficiency of activation of G proteins (desensitization).

Parathyroid Hormone–Related Protein

PTHrP was discovered because its secretion by a wide variety of tumors contributes to the humoral hypercalcemia of malignancy. For this reason, the initial studies of PTHrP in humans and animals stressed the PTH-like structure and properties of the molecule. However, subsequent studies soon showed that PTHrP, unlike PTH, is made by a wide variety of tissues, in which it acts locally in ways that may have little relevance to the control of blood calcium.

Gene and Protein Structure

PTHrP sequences from 10 species, ranging from fish to humans, have been identified (Fig. 28-13).[4] In humans, alternative RNA splicing yields transcripts that encode three distinct proteins, of 139, 141, and 173 residues, which differ only after residue 139.

Inspection of these sequences suggests that PTHrP has several functionally distinct domains. Eight or nine of the first 13 residues of PTHrP are identical to those in known mammalian PTH sequences. These sequences encompass the known "activation" domain of PTH (see earlier discussion) and are instrumental in the ability of PTHrP to activate PTH/PTHrP receptors. The conserved histidine at position 5 of all PTHrP molecules (except those of fish) differs from the hydrophobic residue found at the corresponding position of all PTHs and allows PTHrP to activate the PTH/PTHrP receptor but not the PTH2 receptor.

The sequences in PTHrP(14-34) are also highly conserved. Although these sequences little resemble the corresponding region of PTH, they can displace PTH from the PTH/PTHrP receptor. Studies of the secondary and tertiary structures of PTHrP(1-34) and PTH(1-37) suggest that they have similar structures dominated by α-helices connected by a flexible hinge.

The remaining portion of the PTHrP molecule bears no resemblance to corresponding sequences in PTH. Nevertheless, residues 35 to 111 of PTHrP are strikingly well conserved, with only nine residues differing between mammalian and chicken PTHrP sequences. This sequence conservation is considerably greater than that found in the carboxyl-terminal portion of PTH, suggesting that this region of PTHrP has unique and important functions. After residue 111, the PTHrP sequences vary considerably from species to species.

Interspersed within the PTHrP sequences are multiple sites containing one or several basic residues that might serve as post-translational cleavage sites[98] (see Fig. 28-13). Extensive analysis of PTHrP fragments in tumors, cell lines, and transfected cells has shown that several of these sites are, in fact, functional cleavage signals. PTHrP is cleaved[99] after the arginine at residue 37; this cleavage, followed by carboxypeptidase cleavage, generates a PTH-like PTHrP(1-36) fragment as well as the fragments PTHrP(38-94) amide, PTHrP(38-95), and PTHrP(38-101). More carboxy-terminal fragments of PTHrP have been detected in cells as well.

In the blood of patients with humoral hypercalcemia of malignancy, multiple immunoreactive species of PTHrP have been found that may well correspond to the fragments of PTHrP in cells and tissue culture media, although precise characterization of these various immunoreactive species is incomplete (see later discussion). Full-length PTHrP may not circulate, because an amino-terminal–specific immunoaffinity column was unable to extract carboxy-terminal immunoreactivity from the serum of patients with malignant hypercalcemia.[100]

Functions of Parathyroid Hormone-Related Protein

The first actions of PTHrP to be defined were the PTH-like actions associated with the humoral hypercalcemia of malignancy. In this pathologic entity, PTHrP acts as a hormone; it is secreted from the tumor into the bloodstream and then acts on bone and kidney to raise calcium levels (see "Hypercalcemia of Malignancy").[101] Whether PTHrP circulates at high enough levels in normal adults to contribute to normal calcium homeostasis is an unanswered question. With metastases of breast cancer to bone, locally produced PTHrP can raise serum calcium without necessarily raising blood levels of PTHrP.

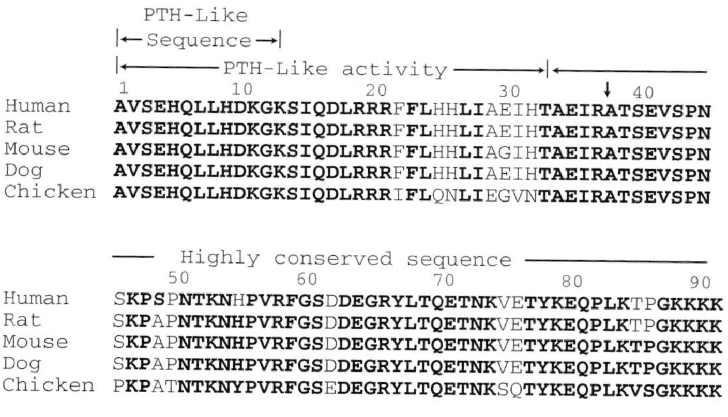

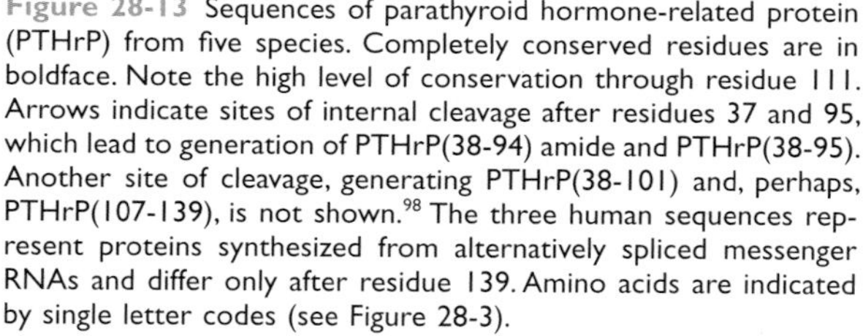

Figure 28-13 Sequences of parathyroid hormone-related protein (PTHrP) from five species. Completely conserved residues are in boldface. Note the high level of conservation through residue 111. Arrows indicate sites of internal cleavage after residues 37 and 95, which lead to generation of PTHrP(38-94) amide and PTHrP(38-95). Another site of cleavage, generating PTHrP(38-101) and, perhaps, PTHrP(107-139), is not shown.[98] The three human sequences represent proteins synthesized from alternatively spliced messenger RNAs and differ only after residue 139. Amino acids are indicated by single letter codes (see Figure 28-3).

PTHrP acts as a calciotropic hormone during fetal life and in lactation. Fetal mice missing the PTHrP gene transport calcium 45 (^{45}Ca) across the placenta inefficiently. This action of PTHrP requires only the midregion of PTHrP and probably involves a receptor distinct from the PTH/PTHrP receptor. Amino-terminal portions of PTHrP and PTH may also be able to increase placental calcium transport, because PTH(1-84) can increase placental calcium transport in mice missing the PTH gene.[102]

The second setting for humoral actions of PTHrP is lactation. In mice, secretion of PTHrP from the breast into the bloodstream leads to an increase in bone resorption.[103] Calcium then activates the CASR in breast tissue, increases the movement of calcium into milk, and downregulates expression of PTHrP in the breast.[104] PTHrP, therefore, probably contributes to the dramatic but largely reversible bone loss that occurs during lactation in humans, which is only minimally affected by calcium supplementation.[105] An exaggeration of this lactational role of PTHrP may explain the rare presentation of hypercalcemia and high PTHrP levels in pregnant and lactating women.[106] Large amounts of PTHrP are also secreted into breast milk, although the role of PTHrP in milk is unknown.

Most of the actions of PTHrP are likely to be paracrine or autocrine.[107] PTHrP is synthesized at one time or another during fetal life in virtually every tissue. Its role in the development of fetal bone has been demonstrated through the striking abnormalities found in genetically engineered mice missing the PTHrP gene. These abnormalities suggest that PTHrP normally keeps chondrocytes proliferating in orderly columns, thereby delaying chondrocyte differentiation.[108] The role of PTHrP in many other fetal tissues may analogously involve regulation of proliferation and differentiation. The widespread expression of PTHrP in fetal life probably underlies the expression of PTHrP in a wide variety of malignancies. As is often the case in malignancy, the expression of PTHrP represents the re-initiation of a fetal pattern of gene expression.

PTHrP is synthesized by many adult tissues. In tissues such as skin, hair, and breast, it is likely that PTHrP regulates cell proliferation and differentiation. PTHrP is also synthesized in response to stretch in the smooth muscle of blood vessels, gastrointestinal tract, uterus, and bladder, and it acts in an autocrine fashion to relax the smooth muscle.[109] PTHrP is also widely expressed in neurons of the central nervous system; its function in the brain is unknown, but it may protect neurons from excitotoxicity by decreasing flux through voltage-gated calcium channels. An analogous mechanism may explain the role of PTHrP in smooth muscle relaxation.

Many of the actions of PTHrP are mediated by the PTH/PTHrP receptor. Others, such as the activation of placental calcium transport, are probably mediated in part by a distinct receptor, and other actions on bone cells probably involve yet another receptor responsive to more distal portions of PTHrP. Increasing evidence also suggests that some actions of PTHrP involve direct nuclear actions of PTHrP.[110] Therefore, both PTH and PTHrP are likely to use multiple mechanisms to stimulate cells (see Fig. 28-11).

CALCITONIN

Calcitonin has an important role in regulating blood calcium in fish and a demonstrable role in rodents; however, the importance of calcitonin in human calcium homeostasis remains uncertain.

The existence of a second calcium-regulating hormone, in addition to PTH, was first demonstrated during perfusion studies of the thyroid/parathyroid glands of dogs.[111] High calcium perfusion resulted in a rapid decrease in plasma calcium, even more rapid than after parathyroidectomy. This suggested that calcium had stimulated the secretion of a hormone that lowered blood calcium. It was subsequently demonstrated that this missing hormone, named calcitonin for its role in regulating the "tone" or level of calcium, was elaborated by the thyroid gland, not the parathyroids. Calcitonin is found in the nonfollicular cells of the thyroid, called C cells, which originate from the neural crest.

In fish, the location of the C cells in discrete organs led to the rapid isolation of calcitonin from these ultimobranchial bodies in dogfish, salmon, and several other species. The identification of the glandular origin of calcitonin enabled the isolation of sufficient quantities of calcitonin for sequence analysis and studies of its structure and biologic function.

Synthesis and Secretion

Calcitonin consists of a 32-amino-acid polypeptide with an intrachain disulfide bond provided by the cysteines at positions 1 and 7 (Fig. 28-14). These two cysteine residues,

Peptide	Species	Sequence	
CT	Human	**C**GNLST**C**MLGTYTQDFNKFHTFPQTAIGVGAP	-NH2
	Salmon-1	**C**S----**C**V--KLS-ELH-LQTY-R-NT-SGT-	-NH2
	Salmon-2	**C**S----**C**V--KLS-DLH-LQTF-R-NT-AGV-	-NH2
	Salmon-3	**C**S----**C**M--KLS-DLH-LQTF-R-NT-AGV-	-NH2
CGRP	Human α	A**C**DTAT**C**VTHRLAGLLSRSGGVVKNNFVPTNVGSKAF	-NH2
	Human β	-**C**N---**C**-----------------S------------	-NH2
	Salmon	-**C**N---**C**------DF-N-----GNS------------	-NH2
Amylin	Human	A**C**DTAT**C**VTHRLAGLLSRSGGVVKNNFVPTNVGSKAF	-NH2
ADM	Human	YRQSMNNFQGLRSFG**C**RFGT**C**TVQKLAHQIYQFTDKDKDNVAPRSKISPQGY	-NH2
IMD	Human	TQAQLLRVG**C**VLGT**C**QVQNLSHRLWQLMGPAGRQDSAPVDPSSPHSYG	-NH2
CRSP-1	Porcine	S**C**NTAT**C**MTHRLVGLLSRSGSMVRSNLLPTKMGFKVFG	-NH2
CRSP-2	Porcine	-**C**---S**C**V--KMT-W------VAKN-FM--NVDS-IL	-NH2
CRSP-3	Porcine	-**C**---I**C**V--KMA-W------V-KN-FM-IN--S-VL	-NH2

Figure 28-14 The amino acid sequences of calcitonin (CT), calcitonin gene–related peptide (CGRP), amylin, adrenomedullin (ADM), intermedin (IDM), and calcitonin receptor–stimulating proteins (CSRP) from selected species. The letters "C" in boldface represent the cysteine residues that form the disulfide linkages critical for the secondary structure of these peptides. The other conserved residues are indicated by a dashed line (see Figure 28-3 for the single-letter amino acid codes).

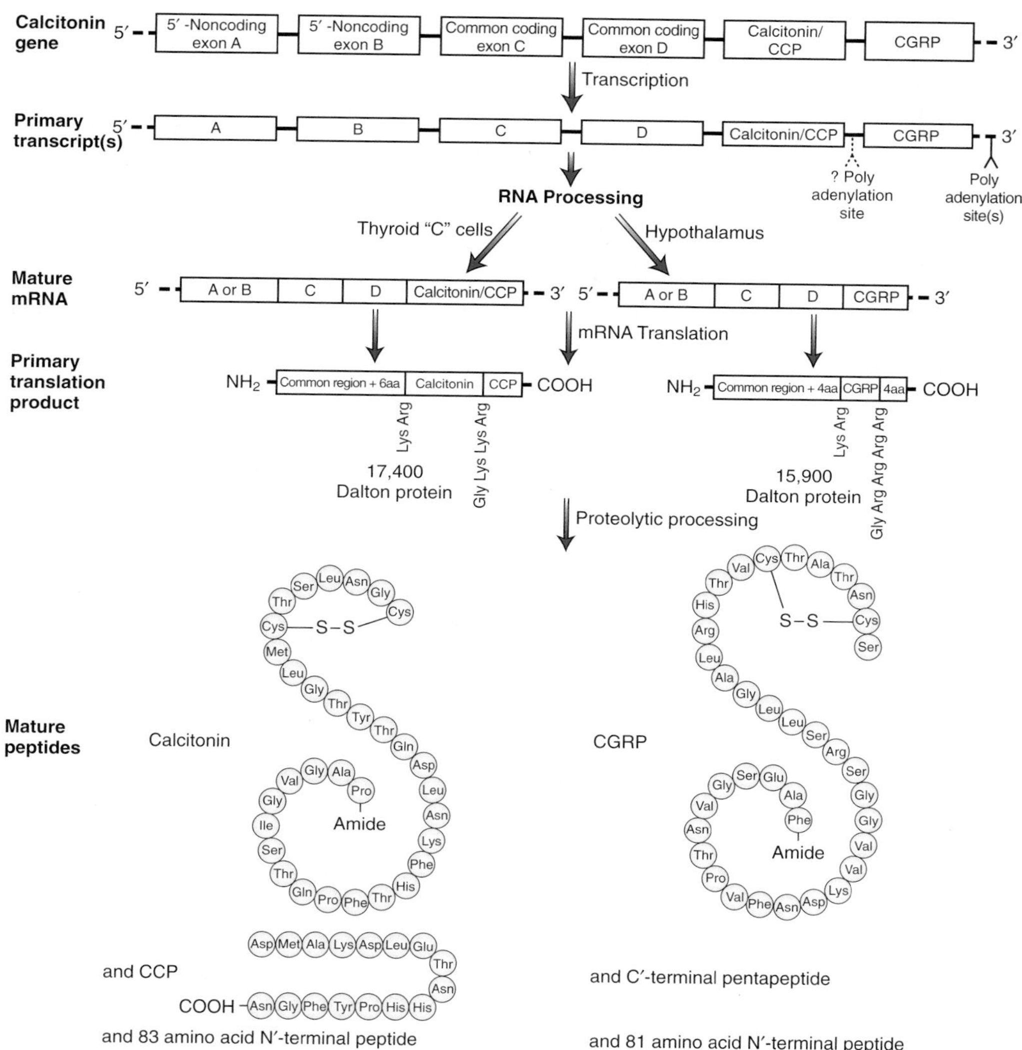

Figure 28-15 Tissue-specific expression of the calcitonin gene. Splicing of alternative exons leads to two different messenger RNAs (mRNAs). The mRNA encoding calcitonin is found predominantly in the thyroid C cell; the mRNA encoding calcitonin gene–related peptide (CGRP) is found predominantly in the hypothalamus and other nervous tissue. aa, amino acids; CCP, calcitonin carboxy-terminal peptide. (From Amara SG, Jonas V, Rosenfeld MG, et al. Alternative RNA processing in calcitonin gene expression generates mRNAs encoding different polypeptide products. *Nature.* 1982;298:240-244.)

along with the carboxy-terminal proline-amide and six additional residues, are the only amino acids conserved among the calcitonins isolated from various species. The disulfide linkage and proline-amide residues are important for the function of the molecule, although biologically active analogues lacking disulfide bonds have been developed.

Interestingly, fish calcitonin is more potent in mammals than the mammalian hormone itself. The mature peptide is derived from the middle of a 136-amino-acid precursor. The human calcitonin gene, located on the short arm of chromosome 11, contains six exons which are alternatively spliced in a tissue-specific manner to yield the mRNAs encoding calcitonin or calcitonin gene–related peptide (CGRP) (Fig. 28-15). The mRNA encoding calcitonin is derived by splicing together the first four exons, and it represents more than 95% of mature transcripts in the thyroid C cells. The splicing of the first three exons to exons 5 and 6 results in an mRNA that encodes the 37-amino-acid α-CGRP peptide. The mRNA encoding α-CGRP is expressed in multiple tissues and is the only mature transcript of the calcitonin gene detected in neural tissue. A second CGRP gene encodes the closely related β-CGRP. In humans, the predicted sequence of the mature peptide differs from that of α-CGRP by only three amino acids (see Fig. 28-14). The β-CGRP gene is also found on chromosome 11, and its tissue distribution is the same as that of α-CGRP.

The synthesis and secretion of calcitonin are tightly regulated. Studies in a porcine model revealed a linear relationship between the secretion of calcitonin and ambient calcium levels. Cell culture studies with calcium ionophores and calcium channel blockers demonstrated that the calcium ion concentration within the C cell determines this secretion rate. The CASR cloned from parathyroid cells is also expressed in C cells and contributes to the regulation of calcitonin secretion.[112] Other calcitonin secretagogues include glucocorticoids, CGRP, glucagon, enteroglucagon, gastrin, pentagastrin, pancreozymin, and β-adrenergic agents.[113] The physiologic role of the gastrointestinal hormones in regulating calcitonin remains unclear; however, they have been postulated to play a role in the regulation of postprandial hypercalcemia. The secretion of calcitonin is inhibited by somatostatin, which is also secreted by the thyroidal C cells. In vivo and in vitro studies have demonstrated that calcitriol decreases calcitonin mRNA levels by a transcriptional mechanism.

Calcitonin, when administered acutely, decreases tubular reabsorption of calcium[114] and impairs osteoclast-mediated bone resorption by a direct action on osteoclasts.[115] In rodents, calcitonin has been shown to play a role in the regulation of postprandial hypercalcemia.[116] Studies in calcitonin/CGRP knockout mice revealed a doubling of the bone formation rate in the absence of hormone, accompanied by resistance to ovariectomy-induced bone loss.[117] A similar increase in bone formation was found in mice heterozygous for ablation of the calcitonin receptor.[118] Recent studies have emphasized a dramatic increase in bone resorption caused by the knockout of calcitonin/CGRP, demonstrating an important physiologic role for calcitonin in normally suppressing osteoclast activity.[119]

The physiologic role of calcitonin in humans, however, remains elusive. The effect of calcitonin on bone density was examined in patients with long-term hypercalcitoninemia secondary to medullary carcinoma of the thyroid and in patients with subtotal thyroidectomy resulting in lack of calcitonin secretory reserve.[120] Bone density at the lumbar spine and distal radius were not influenced by the abnormal calcitonin levels. Furthermore, no physiologic abnormalities have been reported with long-term, high-dose administration of exogenous calcitonin.

Many of the effects of calcitonin are mediated by a G protein–coupled cell surface receptor in the PTH/secretin receptor family.[121] The mRNA encoding this receptor has been found in multiple tissues including kidney, brain, and osteoclasts. The coupling of this receptor to different G proteins results in the activation of either adenylate cyclase or phospholipase C; in some settings, this action is cell cycle dependent.[122]

Calcitonin Family: Calcitonin Gene-Related Peptide, Amylin, Adrenomedullin, and Intermedin

CGRP, amylin, adrenomedullin, calcitonin receptor–stimulating peptide 1 (CRSP1), and intermedin have all been shown to have high-affinity binding sites on cell membranes, and displacement studies suggest that several receptor subtypes for these related ligands are present. However, cloning of specific receptors for these ligands has proved difficult, because the functional receptors consist of heterodimers between G protein–coupled receptors and single transmembrane proteins of the RAMP (receptor activity–modifying proteins) family.[123] Interaction of the calcitonin receptor–like receptor, a relative of the calcitonin receptor, with RAMP1 results in a CGRP receptor, whereas RAMP2 and RAMP3 interactions with the same calcitonin receptor–like receptor generate adrenomedullin receptors. Interaction of RAMP1 with the calcitonin receptor creates an amylin receptor.[124]

CGRP is thought to act as a neurotransmitter and vasodilator rather than as a hormone. In support of this hypothesis, mice lacking α-CGRP have been shown to have an increase in mean arterial pressure.[125] Immunohistochemical studies of CGRP in the brain and in the peripheral nervous system suggest that this neuropeptide also plays an important role in sensory and integrative motor functions.

Three structurally related peptides have been isolated from porcine brain (see Fig. 28-14). These CRSPs, found in many mammals but not in primates,[126] are also expressed in the thyroid gland. CRSP1, which is 60% homologous to α-CGRP at the amino acid level, binds to the calcitonin receptor and dose-dependently stimulates cAMP production. Consistent with this observation, administration of CRSP1, like that of calcitonin, results in a decrease in serum calcium. The receptors for CRSP2 and CRSP3 have not been identified.

Amylin is highly homologous to CGRP and calcitonin (see Fig. 28-14). Although amylin has been shown to have skeletal actions, the presence of amylin in the pancreas of patients with type 2 diabetes mellitus suggests an etiologic role for this peptide in this disorder.[127] Analogues of this peptide are currently being explored as therapeutic agents for type 1 diabetes in children.[128] Amylin administration inhibits bone loss associated with ovariectomy and streptozotocin-induced diabetes mellitus in rats. Targeted ablation of amylin in mice results in low bone mass due to an increase in bone resorption.[118] Amylin has also been shown to decrease food intake and inhibit gastric acid secretion, protecting against ulcer development in numerous models.

Adrenomedullin (see Fig. 28-14) has vasodilatory effects similar to those of CGRP. In addition to activating CGRP receptors, adrenomedullin binds to specific receptors in the vascular system. Mice that lack the DNA coding adrenomedullin die in midgestation.[129] The physiologic roles of adrenomedullin in adults remain to be clarified.

Intermedin, the newest member of this family (see Fig. 28-14), was identified by homology screening of expressed sequence tags. It is expressed primarily in the pituitary and the gastrointestinal tract. Intermedin is able to signal through CGRP receptors and competes with CGRP for receptor binding.[130] However, unlike CGRP and adrenomedullin, intermedin is a nonselective agonist for the RAMP coreceptors.

Calcitonin in Human Disease

Calcitonin is secreted by several endocrine malignancies and, therefore, can serve as a tumor marker. Basal and pentagastrin-stimulated calcitonin levels have been used to identify and monitor patients who are at risk for, or affected by, medullary carcinoma of the thyroid (see Chapter 41), although abnormal basal and stimulated levels may be observed in patients undergoing chronic hemodialysis. Calcitonin may also be ectopically secreted by other tumors, including insulinomas, VIPomas, and lung cancers. Severely ill patients, including those with burn inhalation injury, toxic shock syndrome, or pancreatitis may also have elevated calcitonin levels.

Therapeutic Uses

The observation that calcitonin inhibits osteoclastic bone resorption has led to its therapeutic use for the treatment of several disorders associated with excess bone resorption, including osteoporosis and Paget's disease (see Chapter 29). Calcitonin has also been used for its analgesic effect, in the treatment of patients with vertebral crush fractures, osteolytic metastases, or phantom limb.

VITAMIN D

Metabolism of Vitamin D

Vitamin D is not a true vitamin, because nutritional supplementation is not required in humans who have adequate sun exposure. When exposed to ultraviolet irradiation,

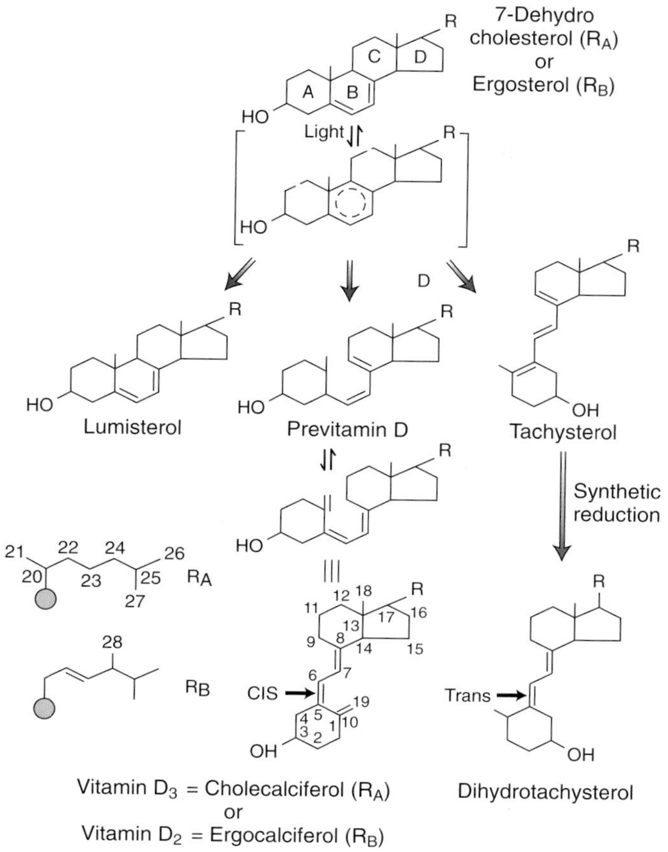

Figure 28-16 Vitamin D precursors and alternative reaction products. The numbering system for vitamin D carbons and the distinct structures of vitamin D_2 (ergocalciferol) and D_3 (cholecalciferol) are noted, as is the structure of dihydrotachysterol, a synthetic product not produced in vivo. Note that the 3-hydroxyl group of dihydrotachysterol is in a pseudo-1-hydroxyl configuration. This may explain the relatively high potency of dihydrotachysterol in conditions associated with low 1α-hydroxylase activity.

the cutaneous precursor of vitamin D, 7-dehydrocholesterol, undergoes photochemical cleavage of the carbon bond between carbons 9 and 10 of the steroid ring (Fig. 28-16). The resultant product, previtamin D, is thermally labile and over a period of 48 hours undergoes a temperature-dependent molecular rearrangement that results in the production of vitamin D. Alternatively, this thermally labile product can isomerize to two biologically inert products, luminosterol and tachysterol. This alternative photoisomerization prevents production of excessive amounts of vitamin D with prolonged sun exposure. The degree of skin pigmentation, which increases in response to solar exposure, also regulates the conversion of 7-dehydrocholesterol to vitamin D by blocking the penetration of ultraviolet rays.

The alternative source of vitamin D is dietary. Elderly people, institutionalized individuals, and those living in northern climates probably obtain most of their vitamin D from dietary sources. However, with increasing avoidance of sun exposure by the general population, ensuring adequate dietary intake of vitamin D has become important for the population at large. Vitamin D deficiency is prevalent and has been shown to contribute significantly to osteopenia and fracture risk. The major dietary sources of vitamin D are fortified dairy products, although lack of monitoring of this supplementation results in marked variation in the amount of vitamin D provided.[131] Other dietary sources include egg yolks, fish oils, and fortified cereal products. Vitamin D provided by plant sources is in the form of vitamin D_2, whereas that provided by animal sources is in the form of vitamin D_3 (see Fig. 28-16). These two forms have equivalent biologic potencies and are activated equally efficiently by the hydroxylases in humans.

Vitamin D is absorbed into the lymphatics and enters the circulation bound primarily to vitamin D–binding protein (VDBP), although a fraction of vitamin D circulates bound to albumin. The human VDBP is a 52-kd α-globulin that is synthesized in the liver. The protein has a high affinity for 25(OH)D (25-hydroxyvitamin D) but also binds vitamin D and calcitriol. Approximately 88% of 25(OH)D circulates bound to the VDBP, 0.03% is free, and the rest circulates bound to albumin. In contrast, 85% of circulating calcitriol is bound to the VDBP, 0.4% is free, and the rest is bound to albumin. Mice lacking the vitamin D–binding protein have increased susceptibility to calcitriol toxicity and to dietary vitamin D deficiency.[132] Therefore, the role of VDBP is to maintain a serum reservoir and to modulate the activity of vitamin D metabolites. Studies in megalin-null mice suggest that vitamin D–binding protein is filtered by the glomerulus and reabsorbed by a megalin-dependent pathway in the proximal renal tubule.[133] Further investigations will be required to determine the importance of this pathway in vitamin D metabolism and the tissues in which megalin-dependent endocytosis plays an important role.[134]

In the liver, vitamin D undergoes 25-hydroxylation by a cytochrome P450–like enzyme present in the mitochondria and microsomes. The half-life of 25(OH)D is approximately 2 to 3 weeks. The 25-hydroxylation of vitamin D is not tightly regulated; therefore, the blood levels of 25(OH)D reflect the amount of vitamin D entering the circulation. When levels of VDBP are low, such as in nephrotic syndrome, circulating levels of 25(OH)D are also reduced. The half-life of 25(OH)D is shortened by increases in levels of its active metabolite, calcitriol.

The final step in the production of the active hormone is the renal 1α-hydroxylation of 25(OH)D to $1,25(OH)_2D_3$ (calcitriol). The half-life of this hormone is approximately 6 to 8 hours. Like the 25-hydroxylase, the 1α-hydroxylase in the proximal convoluted tubule is a cytochrome P450–like mixed-function oxidase, but unlike the 25-hydroxylase, the 1α-hydroxylase is tightly regulated. PTH and hypophosphatemia are the major inducers of this microsomal enzyme, whereas calcium and the enzyme's product, calcitriol, repress it.[135] FGF23 (see later discussion) also represses 1α-hydroxylase mRNA production.[136] In animal models and in vitro studies, other hormones such as estrogen, calcitonin, growth hormone, and prolactin have been shown to increase 1α-hydroxylase activity; however, the clinical importance of these observations has not been established. Ketoconazole has been shown to decrease levels of calcitriol in a dose-dependent manner, presumably by interfering with 1α-hydroxylase activity.

The 1α-hydroxylase enzyme is also expressed in keratinocytes, in the trophoblastic layer of the placenta, and in the activated macrophages that are present in granulomata, including sarcoid granulomata, among many other tissues. In granulomatous tissue, the 1α-hydroxylase gene that is expressed is identical to that expressed in the kidney but is not regulated by PTH, phosphate, calcium, or vitamin D metabolites in these cells. However, activation of macrophages with interferon-γ[137] or with ligands that activate the heterodimer of toll-like receptors 1 and 2[138] increases expression of the 1α-hydroxylase in macrophages, whereas treatment of sarcoidosis-associated hypercalcemia with glucocorticoids, ketoconazole,[139] or chloroquine[140] has been shown to lower serum calcitriol levels. Activation of the VDR in human macrophages induces the antimicrobial peptide, cathelicidin, and increases killing of intracellular *Mycobacterium tuberculosis*.[138] Therefore, the pathologic excess of calcitriol in sarcoidosis may represent an exaggeration of a healthy paracrine response of tissue macrophages. This action can be viewed as a paradigm for many other actions of vitamin D that are mediated more by the local production of calcitriol than by circulating calcitriol.

Both 25(OH)D and calcitriol can also be hydroxylated by the vitamin D 24-hydroxylase that is present in most tissues, including kidney, cartilage, and intestine. Calcitriol increases the activity of 24-hydroxylase, thereby inducing its own metabolism. The 24-hydroxylated vitamin D metabolites, $24,25(OH)_2D_3$ and $1,24,25(OH)_3D_3$, are not thought to play major biologic roles. Mice null for the 24-hydroxylase gene demonstrate hypercalcemia, hypercalciuria, and nephrocalcinosis due to vitamin D toxicity.[141] Although $24,25(OH)_2D_3$ has been shown to have unique actions in a number of biologic systems,[142] no unique receptor for this metabolite has been identified, and the physiologic role of $24,25(OH)_2D_3$ is unclear.

Calcitriol is also metabolized to several inactive products by 23- or 26-hydroxylation and side chain oxidation and cleavage. This latter side chain cleavage, resulting in the formation of calcitroic acid, occurs in the liver and intestine, whereas inactivation of calcitriol by 24-hydroxylation occurs in a wide variety of target tissues. In addition, polar metabolites of calcitriol are excreted in the bile. Some of these metabolites are deconjugated in the intestine and reabsorbed into the enterohepatic circulation.

Actions of Vitamin D

Vitamin D Receptors

Calcitriol exerts its biologic functions by binding to a nuclear receptor, which then regulates transcription of DNA into RNA. Among the other nuclear receptors, the VDR most closely resembles the retinoic acid, triiodothyronine, and retinoid-X receptors (RXRs). The affinity of the receptor for calcitriol is approximately three orders of magnitude greater than that for other vitamin D metabolites (Fig. 28-17). Although 25(OH)D is less potent on a molar basis, its concentration in the serum is approximately three orders of magnitude greater than that of calcitriol. However, its free concentration is only two orders of magnitude greater. Therefore, under normal circumstances it is unlikely that 25(OH)D contributes importantly to calcium homeostasis. As a substrate for local 1α-hydroxylases in many tissues, however, 25(OH)D may contribute to local tissue homeostasis.

Because the affinity of the VDBP for 25(OH)D is greater than for calcitriol, in states of vitamin D intoxication (with its associated high levels of 25(OH)D), the free levels of calcitriol increase[143] because 25(OH)D displaces it from the VDBP. Therefore, 25(OH)D may play a role in the clinical syndrome of vitamin D intoxication both by its direct biologic effects, when it is present at toxic levels, and by increasing the free levels of calcitriol.

The VDR acts by forming a heterodimer with the RXR, binding to DNA elements, and recruiting coactivators in a ligand-dependent fashion. These coactivators link the receptor complex to the basal transcription apparatus, thereby regulating transcription of target genes. In most cases, the upregulatory response elements for vitamin D contain hexameric repeats separated by three bases (Fig. 28-18). However, vitamin D also promotes the DNA-protein interactions of other transcription factors, such as SP1 and NF-Y, in genes lacking classic response elements, by

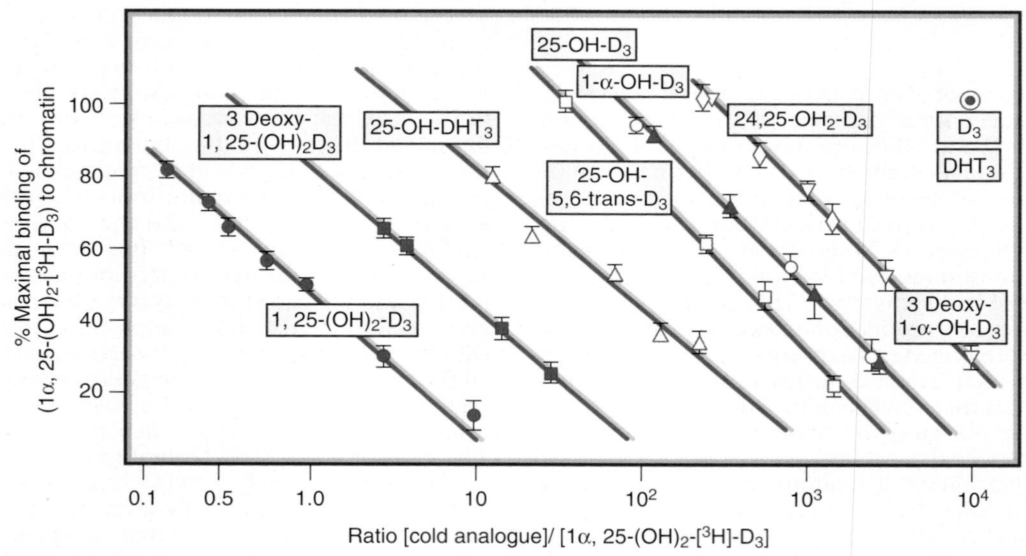

Figure 28-17 Relative potency of analogues of $1,25(OH)_2D_3$ (calcitriol) in competitive binding to vitamin D receptors of chick intestinal mucosa. Slopes are plotted (*left to right*) for $1,25(OH)_2D_3$ (1,25-dihydroxyvitamin D_3); 3-deoxy-$1,25(OH)_2D_3$ (3-deoxy-1,25-dihydroxyvitamin D_3); 25-OH-DHT_3 (25-hydroxydihydrotachysterol); 25-OH-5,6-trans-D_3 (25-hydroxy-5,6-transvitamin D_3); 25-OH-D_3 (25-hydroxyvitamin D_3); 1-α-OH-D_3 (1α-hydroxyvitamin D_3); 24,25-OH_2-D_3 (24,25-dihydroxyvitamin D_3); and 3-deoxy-1α-OH-D_3 (3-deoxy-1α-hydroxyvitamin D_3). D_3, vitamin D_3; DHT_3, dihydrotachysterol. (From Proscal DA, Okamura WH, Norman AW. Structural requirements for the interaction of 1α,25-(OH)2-vitamin D3 with its chick intestinal system. *J Biol Chem.* 1975;250:8382-8388.)

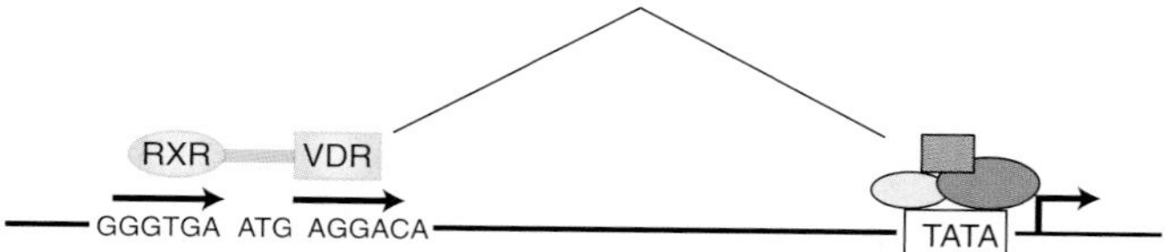

Figure 28-18 Transcriptional activation by 1,25(OH)$_2$D$_3$ (1,25-dihydroxyvitamin D$_3$ or calcitriol). A heterodimer of retinoid-X receptor (RXR) and vitamin D receptor (VDR) binds to a pair of hexameric sequences separated by three intervening bases (ATG). Arrows indicate that the hexamers found in the upregulated rat osteocalcin gene are variants of a consensus sequence, repeated here with identical orientations (direct repeats). On binding to DNA, the RXR-VDR heterodimer facilitates formation of a transcription initiation complex, which binds to DNA at and near the TATA sequence.

uncertain mechanisms.[144] The mechanism of transcriptional repression by vitamin D is varied. For example, VDR-RXR heterodimers repress the 1α-hydroxylase and renin genes by blocking the function of other transcription factors,[145,146] whereas interaction of the VDR with the Ku antigen, acting as a transcription factor, is required for transcriptional repression of the human PTHrP gene.[147]

Glucocorticoids have been shown to decrease the expression of the VDR gene in osteosarcoma cell lines, whereas calcitriol increases its expression in many cells. In the renal proximal convoluted tubule, however, calcitriol decreases the VDR levels. This decrease has been postulated to lead to decreased activation of the renal 24-hydroxylase by calcitriol, thereby protecting the newly synthesized calcitriol from local inactivation.[148]

Calcitriol also has some biologic effects which occur too rapidly for transcriptional mechanisms to be implicated. These "nongenomic actions," including a rapid increase in intracellular calcium, activation of phospholipase C, and opening of calcium channels, are observed in several cell types within minutes of exposure to calcitriol. Additional data supporting the hypothesis that nongenomic actions are not dependent on the classic receptor include the identification of specific binding sites for calcitriol on the antiluminal surface of intestinal cells[149] and a disparity between the affinity of the various vitamin D analogues for the nuclear receptor and their potency in these nongenomic actions. However, both the rapid intracellular accumulation of cyclic guanosine monophosphate in association with the VDR and the rapid increase in intracellular calcium in response to calcitriol depend on the presence of an intact nuclear receptor, because these effects are not observed in cells derived from patients and mice with VDR mutations.[150] The physiologic importance of the nongenomic actions of vitamin D metabolites has not yet been established.

The VDR is expressed in most tissues and has been shown to regulate cellular differentiation and function in many cell types. Nevertheless, the most dramatic physiologic effects of vitamin D, acting through the VDR, involve regulation of intestinal calcium transport. This is most clearly demonstrated by the phenotype of patients and mice with mutant VDRs (hereditary vitamin D–resistant rickets)[151,152]: dramatic abnormalities in bone mineralization can be reversed by bypassing the defect in intestinal calcium absorption.[153-155]

Intestinal Calcium Absorption

Under normal dietary conditions, calcium intake is in the range of 700 to 900 mg daily. Approximately 30% to 35% of this calcium is absorbed; however, losses from intestinal secretion of calcium lead to a net daily uptake of approximately 200 mg. Although vitamin D is the major hormonal determinant of intestinal calcium absorption, the bioavailability of mineral ions in the intestinal lumen may be affected by a number of local factors and dietary constituents. Absorption of calcium and magnesium is impaired by bile salt deficiency, unabsorbed free fatty acids in steatorrheic states, and high dietary content of fiber or phytate. Gastric acid is needed to promote dissociation of calcium from anionic components of food or therapeutic preparations of calcium salts. Administration of calcium salts with meals, especially in achlorhydrics, and use of divided doses or more soluble salts such as calcium citrate are commonly employed strategies to increase calcium bioavailability.

Calcium is thought to be absorbed by three pathways: the transcellular route, vesicular calcium transport, and paracellular transport. The first two pathways have been shown to be dependent on calcitriol. Although the necessity of vitamin D for paracellular calcium absorption remains controversial, substantial evidence exists that the hormone enhances this pathway as well.[156] Notably, the expression of claudin 2 and claudin 12, which contribute to intestinal calcium absorption and are thought to form paracellular channels between neighboring cells, has been shown to be induced by calcitriol.[157]

The most extensively studied mechanism of intestinal calcium absorption is the transcellular route. This pathway is thought to involve three steps: entry of calcium into the enterocyte (which is the rate-limiting step), transport across the cell, and extrusion across the basolateral membrane.

Entry into the Enterocyte. A number of brush border proteins, including the intestinal membrane calcium-binding protein, brush border alkaline phosphatase, and low-affinity Ca^{2+},Mg^{2+}-ATPase have been shown to be induced by calcitriol. The activity of these proteins correlates with active calcium transport; however, a causal relationship remains to be established. Two calcium channels, TRPV5 and TRPV6, members of the transient receptor potential vanilloid receptor subfamily containing six membrane-spanning domains, are expressed in the duodenum, the jejunum, and the kidney as well as other tissues. TRPV6 is thought to play a critical role in intestinal calcium absorption, and its expression is increased by calcitriol, as is that of TRPV5.[158] Studies in mice lacking TRPV5 demonstrate that this channel is primarily responsible for renal calcium reabsorption; mice lacking TRPV5 have enhanced, rather than impaired, intestinal calcium absorption, because of their high circulating levels of calcitriol.[159] In contrast, mice missing TRPV6 do exhibit a decrease in intestinal calcium transport and the stimulation of this transport by vitamin D. Nevertheless, these knockout mice retain some responsiveness of intestinal calcium transport to calcitriol, emphasizing our still incomplete understanding of this process.[160]

On entering the enterocyte, calcium binds to components of the brush border complex subjacent to the plasma membrane. Calmodulin is redistributed to the brush border in response to calcitriol and may play a role in this process, as may the calcitriol-inducible calcium-binding protein, calbindin-D9K .

Transcellular Transport. The best-studied effect of vitamin D on the enterocyte is the induction of synthesis of the intestinal calcium-binding protein, calbindin-D9K. This protein has an EF hand structure, which permits the binding of two calcium ions per molecule. The affinity of calbindin for calcium is approximately four times that of the brush border calcium-binding components, so calcium is preferentially transferred to calbindin. Calbindin serves to buffer the intracellular free calcium concentration during calcium absorption. It associates with microtubules and may play a role in the transport of calcium across the enterocyte. Nevertheless, mice without calbindin-D9K exhibit normal vitamin D–mediated intestinal calcium transport; this demonstrates that the role of calbindin-D9K is not rate-limiting for this activity.[160] Organelles such as the mitochondria, Golgi apparatus, and endoplasmic reticulum also serve as repositories for intracellular calcium.

Exit from the Enterocyte. The transport of calcium across the antiluminal surface of the enterocyte, the final process involved in intestinal calcium absorption, is dependent on calcitriol. The main mechanism of calcium extrusion is the calcitriol-inducible, ATP-dependent plasma membrane Ca^{2+} pump (PMCA1b). The affinity of the pump for calcium is approximately 2.5 times that of calbindin. With high calcium intake, a calcitriol-independent Na^+/Ca^{2+} exchanger may also play a role in the transfer of calcium across the basolateral membrane.

Actions on the Parathyroid Gland

Calcitriol has been shown to regulate gene transcription and cell proliferation in the parathyroids. The hormone also inhibits the proliferation of dispersed parathyroid cells in culture, although the relative contributions of calcium and calcitriol in the regulation of parathyroid cell proliferation in vivo have not been established. Normocalcemic mice lacking functional VDRs have normal serum PTH levels and normal-sized parathyroid glands, demonstrating that the genomic actions of calcitriol are not essential for parathyroid cellular homeostasis.[155] However, calcitriol has been shown to decrease transcription of the PTH gene both in vivo and in vitro. This action has been exploited in the use of calcitriol for treatment of the secondary hyperparathyroidism associated with chronic renal failure (see "Parathyroid Hormone Biosynthesis" and "Vitamin D Deficiency"). Nevertheless, the VDR in parathyroid cells has a modest role in normal physiology. When the receptor is removed specifically from parathyroid cells in genetically manipulated mice, the resultant mice have modest decreases in the levels of CASRs in their parathyroids, accompanied by modest elevations of blood PTH levels and evidence of increased resorption of bone.[161]

Actions on Bone

The effects of calcitriol on bone are numerous. Calcitriol is a major transcriptional regulator of the two most abundant bone matrix proteins: it represses the synthesis of type I collagen and induces the synthesis of osteocalcin. Calcitriol promotes the differentiation of osteoclasts from monocyte-macrophage stem cell precursors in vitro and also increases osteoclastic bone resorption in high doses in vivo, by stimulating production of RANKL (osteoclast-differentiating factor) by osteoblasts.[162] Despite the multiple effects of calcitriol on the biology of bone in vitro, in vivo studies in calcitriol-deficient rats and in mice lacking functional VDRs[152,153] suggest that the major osseous consequences of hormone and receptor deficiency can be reversed after mineral ion homeostasis is normalized. In addition, parenteral calcium infusions have been shown to heal the osteomalacic lesions in children with mutant VDRs.[154] These observations suggest that the major role of calcitriol in bone is to provide the proper microenvironment for bone mineralization through stimulation of the intestinal absorption of calcium and phosphate.

Other Actions of Vitamin D

The effects of calcitriol on phosphate transport are less well studied than the effects on calcium transport. However, vitamin D has been shown to promote the already efficient intestinal phosphate absorption. Importantly, calcitriol also induces expression of the phosphaturic hormone FGF23.[53]

One of the striking clinical features of profound vitamin D deficiency that is poorly understood is severe proximal myopathy. Muscle cells express VDRs, and calcitriol has nongenomic effects on muscle. Further, calcitriol increases amino acid uptake and alters phospholipid metabolism in vitro in muscle cells. Vitamin D administration has been shown to increase the concentration of troponin C, a calcium-binding protein that plays a role in excitation coupling and increases the rate of uptake of calcium by the sarcoplasmic reticulum. VDR knockout mice demonstrate a delay in myoblast differentiation.[163] However, little is known regarding the direct role of vitamin D in normal muscle physiology. The myopathy that accompanies vitamin D deficiency is characterized by normal levels of creatine phosphokinase, a myopathic electromyogram, and biopsy findings of loss of myofibrils, fatty infiltration, and interstitial fibrosis. The myopathy resolves within days to weeks on vitamin D replacement and is not related to normalization of mineral ion homeostasis.

Vitamin D Analogues

The recognition that calcitriol promotes cellular differentiation and inhibits cellular proliferation has led to efforts directed at producing new analogues that retain these effects but do not cause hypercalcemia. Several analogues have been shown to have antiproliferative effects on normal and malignant cells in vitro and in xenografts in immunosuppressed mice.[164] In addition, analogues of vitamin D have been shown to synergize with cyclosporine in preventing rejection of transplanted islet cells in a murine model.[165] One nonhypercalcemic analogue, 22-oxacalcitriol, has been shown to suppress PTH synthesis and secretion in rats,[166] at doses that stimulate intestinal calcium absorption less than calcitriol does. This suggests that such analogues may be useful in the prevention and treatment of hyperparathyroidism. The antiproliferative effects of vitamin D have been exploited clinically in the treatment of psoriasis.[167] Although analogues with reduced calcemic activity are predominantly used, hypercalcemic crisis can occur after excessive topical use of such compounds.

The physiology underlying the various biologic effects of these analogues is not completely understood. Altered affinity for VDBP, metabolism by target tissues,[168] and effects on recruitment of coactivators by the VDR may contribute to the unique properties of vitamin D analogues.[169]

FIBROBLAST GROWTH FACTOR 23

FGF23 in Human Disease

A new era in the understanding of phosphate metabolism was ushered in with the identification of the molecular basis for the human disorder, autosomal dominant hypophosphatemic rickets (ADHR).[170] Linkage analyses of affected kindreds identified mutation of the gene encoding FGF23 as the basis for ADHR. The mutation in affected individuals abolishes an RXXR protease recognition motif that is thought to be responsible for the cleavage and inactivation of FGF23.[171,172] The complementary DNA encoding FGF23 predicts a peptide of 251 amino acids, the first 24 of which comprise a signal peptide. Studies using recombinant FGF23 demonstrate that the full-length mature peptide is required for its biologic activity and that mutation of the cleavage site in the patients with ADHR is responsible for its inactivation. Cleavage of FGF23 is inhibited by furin inhibition, suggesting that the enzyme responsible is a subtilisin-like proprotein convertase.

Analyses of tumors isolated from patients with tumor-induced osteomalacia revealed a dramatic increase in levels of mRNA encoding FGF23.[173] Serum levels of FGF23 are elevated in patients with tumor-induced osteomalacia and have been shown to normalize after removal of the tumor, correlating with resolution of the hypophosphatemia that characterizes this disorder.[174-176] Conversely, patients with the rare syndrome known as tumoral calcinosis present with hyperphosphatemia and soft tissue calcium phosphate deposits. Some of these patients have point mutations in the FGF23 gene that cause abnormal processing of the protein, with low serum levels of the active hormone and high levels of inactive fragments.[177-179] Yet others have mutations in the FGF23 coreceptor Klotho or in GALNT3 which normally *O*-glycosylates FGF23.[180,181] Therefore, human diseases of both increased and decreased FGF23 activity suggest that this "new" factor represents an important regulator of phosphate metabolism.

Actions of FGF23

Evidence that FGF23 is a novel hormone that plays a key role in normal phosphate homeostasis has been obtained in murine models of overexpression and ablation. Overexpression of FGF23 or administration of FGF23 to animals results in the development of hypophosphatemia[172] and impaired 1α-hydroxylation of 25(OH)D,[136,182] recapitulating the findings observed in patients affected by tumor-induced osteomalacia. Investigations in mice with targeted ablation of FGF23 have proven that endogenous production of this hormone is critical for normal phosphate homeostasis and the regulation of vitamin D metabolism.[183,184] Absence of FGF23 results in impaired renal phosphate excretion, leading to the development of hyperphosphatemia within the first 2 weeks of life. Affected mice also develop hypercalcemia due to high levels of calcitriol, a result of the lack of the normal suppressive effect of FGF23 on the renal 25(OH)D 1α-hydroxylase.[136] Ablation of FGF23 results in premature death associated with ectopic mineralization of soft tissues, including the kidney. Impairing calcitriol action in these animals prevents the development of hypercalcemia and improves survival, suggesting that the premature death is a direct consequence of impaired mineral ion homeostasis rather than a specific developmental or maturational effect of FGF23.[185]

FGF23 impairs Na^+-dependent phosphate transport in both intestinal and renal brush border membrane vesicles.[186] It has been shown to decrease the levels of type IIa, IIb, and IIc NaPi transporters, thereby regulating both intestinal and renal phosphate transport.[187-189] FGF23 decreases circulating levels of calcitriol, both by decreasing mRNA levels for the renal 25(OH)D 1α-hydroxylase and by increasing expression of 24-hydroxylase, the key enzyme involved in inactivation of calcitriol.[136] FGF23 activates FGF receptor 1 in the presence of Klotho, a single-pass transmembrane protein that acts as a coreceptor.[190] Klotho knockout mice exhibit the same hyperphosphatemia and high calcitriol levels seen in FGF23 knockout mice,[191] demonstrating that Klotho plays a critical role in mediating the actions of FGF23.

Regulation of FGF23

Circulating FGF23 levels are increased by dietary phosphorus, serum phosphorus and calcitriol.[53,192,193] Precisely how phosphate is sensed to regulate FGF23 production is unknown. Studies in mice with mutations in the *Phex* or *Dmp1* gene suggest that these genes are upstream of FGF23 and suppress its expression.[184,194] The products of these genes, as well as FGF23 itself, are synthesized primarily by osteocytes, cells derived from osteoblasts, that reside in the bone matrix. Interestingly, studies in mice with chondrocyte-specific ablation of the VDR suggest that this receptor regulates a factor elaborated by chondrocytes that suppresses FGF23 production.[195] In patients with chronic renal failure, an increase in FGF23 levels has been shown to antedate the development of secondary hyperparathyroidism and thus may be beneficial in predicting which individuals will develop this disorder.[196]

Treatment of dialysis patients with sevelamer hydrochloride and calcium carbonate decreases levels of phosphate and FGF23 in parallel, implicating increases in serum phosphate or in intestinal absorption of phosphate as the pathophysiologic basis for the increased FGF23 levels in this population.[197] Thus, FGF23 has emerged as an essential regulator of normal phosphate and calcitriol homeostasis. Phosphate and calcitriol increase FGF23 levels; this FGF23 then acts on the renal proximal tubule to suppress synthesis of calcitriol and decrease the reabsorption of phosphate.

CALCIUM AND PHOSPHATE HOMEOSTASIS

The cytosolic concentrations of intracellular calcium, phosphorus, and magnesium differ markedly, as reviewed previously, and their physiologic roles within cells are diverse and largely unrelated (see Fig. 28-1). In contrast, the concentrations of these mineral ions in ECF are quite comparable (i.e., 1 to 2 mmol/L), and it is here that they exert important interactions, both with cells and with one another, that are critical for bone mineralization, neuromuscular function, and normal mineral ion homeostasis. Extracellular calcium and phosphate, in particular, exist so close to the limits of their mutual solubility that stringent regulation of their concentrations is required to avoid diffuse precipitation of calcium phosphate crystals in tissues.

Serum concentrations and total body balances of the mineral ions are maintained within narrow limits by powerful, interactive homeostatic mechanisms. PTH, calcitriol, and FGF23 regulate mineral ion levels; mineral ion levels, in turn, regulate PTH, calcitriol, and FGF23 secretion, and these hormones may regulate the production of one another. Calcium sensors in the parathyroid glands control PTH secretion by monitoring the blood concentration of ionized calcium, whereas those in the kidney act to adjust tubular calcium reabsorption independently of PTH or calcitriol. However, the mechanisms of phosphate sensing needed for normal homeostasis are not understood. The operation of these homeostatic mechanisms can be

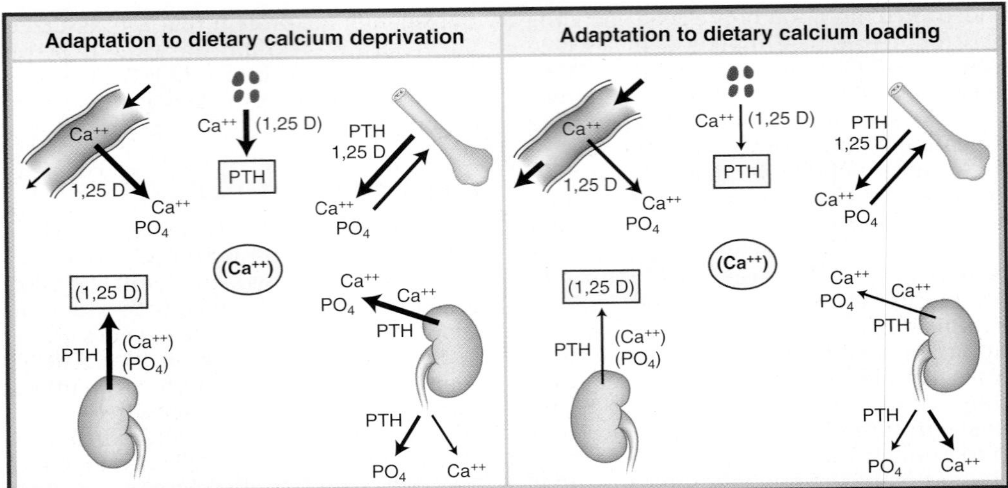

Figure 28-19 Homeostatic responses to variations in dietary calcium content. Major homeostatic responses to dietary calcium deprivation or loading are depicted. Arrow thickness indicates relative activity of transport or secretory mechanisms, and the amounts of hormones or transported ions are indicated by the size of their notations. Parentheses indicate an inhibitory regulation. Note that the extracellular calcium concentration is well maintained, although different underlying mechanisms are involved in the two circumstances (see text for details). 1,25 D, calcitriol; PTH, parathyroid hormone.

appreciated by considering the following examples of how the organism adapts to changes in calcium loads (Fig. 28-19).

Dietary calcium restriction leads to an increase in the efficiency of intestinal calcium absorption. This increased efficiency results from a sequence of homeostatic responses in which the lowered concentration of ionized calcium in blood activates secretion of PTH, PTH augments synthesis of calcitriol by the proximal tubules of the kidney, and calcitriol then acts directly on enterocytes to increase active transcellular transport of calcium. Enhanced intestinal calcium absorption is quantitatively the most important response to calcium deprivation, but a series of other homeostatic events also occur that limit the impact of this stress. Renal tubular calcium reabsorption is increased by PTH, an effect that is enhanced by increased calcitriol-stimulated expression of calbindin-D28K in the distal tubules. Calcium reabsorption is also enhanced directly by any tendency to hypocalcemia, which is detected by CASRs in Henle's loop (and possibly also in the distal nephron) that control transepithelial calcium movements independent of PTH or calcitriol.

The impact of dietary calcium deprivation is reduced by approximately 15% through release of calcium from bone in response to PTH and calcitriol. The concomitant increase in net bone resorption causes release of phosphate as well as calcium into the ECF. Intestinal phosphate absorption also is increased by calcitriol. These phosphate loads are problematic, in that phosphate directly lowers ionized calcium in ECF, suppresses renal synthesis of calcitriol, and directly inhibits bone resorption. These potentially negative effects of phosphate are obviated by the powerful phosphaturic actions of PTH and FGF23, the secretion of which is promoted by phosphate, calcium and calcitriol.

Finally, the possibility of unrestrained secretion of PTH, which would lead to excessive bone resorption and severe hypophosphatemia, is prevented by the effects of calcium on PTH secretion and by the direct suppressive effect of calcitriol on the synthesis of PTH and PTH receptors. As a result of these homeostatic responses, calcium-deprived people maintain near-normal serum calcium and phosphate concentrations but display increased intestinal calcium absorption, increased bone resorption and progressive osteopenia, increased renal tubular calcium reabsorption, decreased renal TRP, low urinary calcium excretion, elevated urinary phosphate excretion, and high serum concentrations of PTH and calcitriol.

Calcium loads induce an opposite series of adaptations: parathyroid suppression, inhibition of renal calcitriol synthesis, decreased intestinal active transport of calcium, increased renal excretion of calcium and decreased renal excretion of phosphate (secondary to functional hypoparathyroidism), and decreased bone resorption sufficient to allow a positive skeletal calcium balance. The decline in intestinal calcium absorption is the major safeguard against calcium overload, although this mechanism may be overridden with extraordinarily high intakes of calcium because of the persistence of the passive, non–vitamin D-dependent mode of calcium absorption. Moreover, nonenteral sources of calcium, such as intravenous calcium infusion or excessive net bone resorption (as from immobilization or malignancy), may readily overwhelm the limited homeostatic adaptations that remain once the capacity of suppressed intestinal calcium absorption is exceeded. In such situations, the kidney rather than the intestine becomes the principal defense against hypercalcemia, and calcium homeostasis becomes critically dependent on adequate renal function. If renal function is impaired in these settings, as frequently occurs clinically, severe hypercalcemia and pathologic calcium deposition in extraskeletal sites may ensue.

LABORATORY ASSESSMENT OF MINERAL METABOLISM

Parathyroid Hormone

The major challenges in the measurement of blood PTH have been the low levels of circulating PTH and the presence of inactive PTH fragments in far greater abundance than the intact, biologically active PTH molecule. The measurement of inactive fragments would not be a concern if the ratio of inactive to active PTH molecules remained constant. However, this ratio changes in response to changes in GFR or in parathyroid gland secretory activity (see "Parathyroid Hormone Secretion" and "Metabolism of Parathyroid Hormone"). Consequently, radioimmunoassays of PTH have suffered from lack of sensitivity and from inability to measure the biologically active hormone directly.

For these reasons, two-site assays, which require the presence of amino-terminal and carboxy-terminal sequences of full-length PTH(1-84) on the same molecule, have replaced older radioimmunoassays.[198] The assays are sensitive enough to detect PTH in all normal persons. The assays have demonstrated modest circadian variation in PTH levels and some pulsatility in PTH secretion, but these variations have not interfered with the diagnostic usefulness of randomly drawn PTH measurements. Some studies have reported modest increases in PTH levels with age, although others have not. Unlike older radioimmunoassays, the two-site assays demonstrate virtually no overlap in PTH levels between patients with primary hyperparathyroidism and those with nonparathyroid hypercalcemia (Fig. 28-20). Because this distinction represents the most important challenge in the clinical setting, the use of the two-site assay has dramatically facilitated the clinician's task.

This straightforward picture has been complicated by the realization that most two-site assays detect small amounts of PTH fragments that are large but do not extend to the hormone's amino-terminus.[199] These fragments accumulate in significant amounts in patients with renal failure. These observations have prompted the development of two-site PTH assays that use antibodies specific for the first four amino acids of PTH and therefore do not detect large fragments of PTH. Although it seems plausible that such assays might prove particularly useful in some clinical situations, their role is presently unclear. They offer no advantage over older two-site assays, for example, in diagnosing primary hyperparathyroidism.[200]

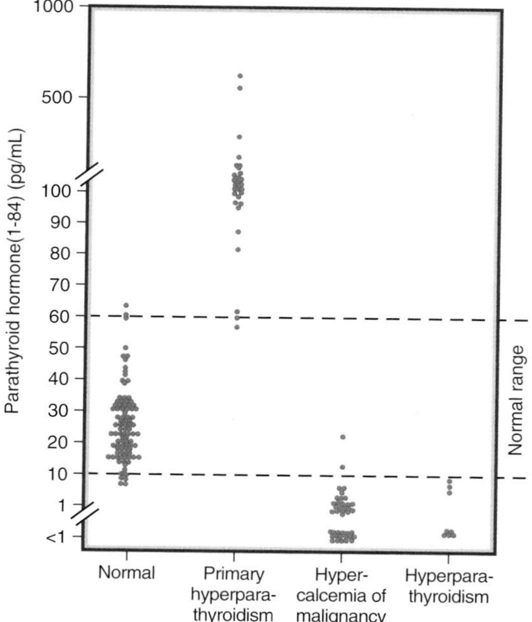

Figure 28-20 Intact immunoreactive parathyroid hormone (PTH) determined using a two-site immunoradiometric assay in normal subjects and in three different patient groups. Note that there is some overlap between normal people and patients with primary hyperparathyroidism but no overlap between hypercalcemic patients with primary hyperparathyroidism and those with hypercalcemia of malignancy. (From Segre GV. Advances in techniques for measurement of parathyroid hormone: current applications in clinical medicine and directions for future research. *Trends Endocrinol Metab.* 1990;1:243-247.)

Parathyroid Hormone–Related Protein

The measurement of PTHrP in serum presents a series of challenges. The concentration of PTHrP in the bloodstream, even in some patients with PTHrP-mediated malignant hypercalcemia, is not high, and the molecular definition of circulating, biologically active fragments is incomplete. Despite these problems, several groups of investigators have developed assays for PTHrP that can be helpful in the evaluation of hypercalcemia in a subset of patients. Radioimmunoassays for amino-terminal portions of PTHrP and two-site assays for amino-terminal and midregion PTHrP[201] separate healthy persons and patients with nonmalignant hypercalcemia from most patients with the humoral hypercalcemia of malignancy (Fig. 28-21). When measured with the most recently developed assays, PTHrP levels are found to be elevated in almost all patients with malignant hypercalcemia without bone metastases and in most patients with hypercalcemia and bone metastases.

Occasionally, the PTHrP assay has helped distinguish an occult malignancy from other causes of non–PTH-dependent hypercalcemia. Nevertheless, because the diagnosis of malignancy as the cause of hypercalcemia is usually clinically obvious and the PTH assay can be used to diagnose primary hyperparathyroidism, the role of PTHrP assays in clinical practice is limited.[202]

Calcitonin

Several assays for measuring serum calcitonin are commercially available. The measurements are based on single- or double-antibody radioimmunoassays or enzyme immunoassays, several of which are sufficiently sensitive to detect calcitonin deficiency.[203,204] The calcitonin monomer is thought to be the biologically active molecule; therefore, some investigators believe that extraction of the multimeric forms before radioimmunoassay provides a more sensitive and more specific measurement of serum calcitonin levels. However, the double-antibody radioimmunoassay is thought by others to provide the same information with less sample manipulation. The only clinical use of the calcitonin assay is as a tumor marker, primarily in medullary carcinoma of the thyroid.

Vitamin D Metabolites

The radioligand assays for determining the levels of vitamin D metabolites require fractionation and extraction of the hormone from serum proteins by HPLC or silica cartridges. These assays are sufficiently sensitive to detect subnormal values. Because the assays measure both protein-bound and unbound vitamin D metabolites, results may not always reflect the levels of biologically relevant ("free") metabolites. This limitation may lead to misleading results in patients with nephrotic syndrome or vitamin D intoxication. With the move away from using radioligand-based assays, other methods for measuring vitamin D metabolites, including chemiluminescent assays, have been pioneered.[205] Although these assays have not withstood the test of time, they have been proven to be as accurate as the currently available radioimmunoassay. Mass spectrometry is being increasingly used for measuring levels of 25(OH) D. Regardless of the method used, it has been recognized

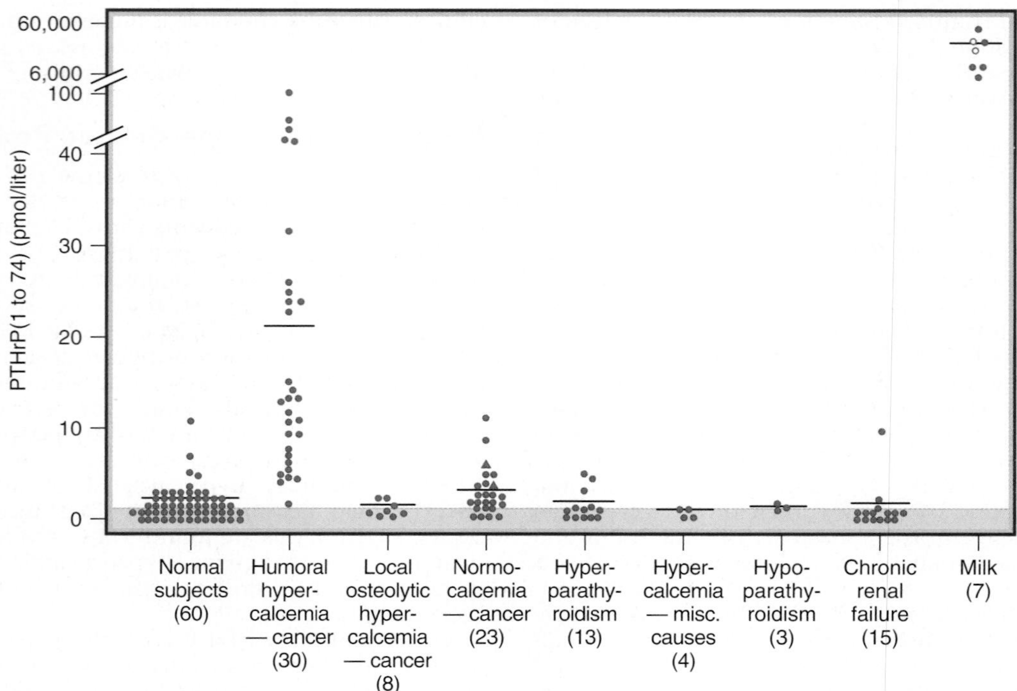

Figure 28-21 Plasma PTHrP(1-74) determined by two-site immunoradiometric assay in selected patient groups and normal subjects. Also shown are concentrations of PTHrP in human milk *(filled circles)* and in bovine milk *(open circles)*. Two normocalcemic patients with cancer *(filled triangles)* subsequently became hypercalcemic. The number of samples in each category is shown in parentheses. Hatched area denotes levels too low to detect with this assay. PTHrP, parathyroid hormone–related protein. (Adapted from Burtis WJ, Brady TG, Orloff JJ, et al. Immunochemical characterization of circulating parathyroid hormone-related protein in patients with humoral hypercalcemia of cancer. *N Engl J Med.* 1990;322:1106-1112.)

that a central repository for uniform standards is required for validation of these assays and of the laboratories performing them. The National Institute of Standards and Technology in the United States has developed standard reference materials for this purpose.[206]

The levels of 25(OH)D correlate better with the clinical signs and symptoms of vitamin D deficiency than do the levels of calcitriol. Because the 25-hydroxylation of vitamin D is not tightly regulated, measurements of 25(OH)D more accurately reflect body stores of vitamin D. Measurement of this metabolite should, therefore, be performed if vitamin D deficiency is suspected.

Measurements of calcitriol should be reserved for cases in which excessive or impaired 1α-hydroxylation is suspected. High calcitriol levels can be seen in sarcoidosis, lymphomas, Williams' syndrome, and intoxication with 1α-hydroxylated metabolites (see "Parathyroid-Independent Hypercalcemia"). Impaired 1α-hydroxylation can contribute to the hypocalcemia of patients with renal dysfunction, increasead FGF23 levels, or hereditary defects of vitamin D metabolism (see "Hypocalcemic Disorders").

Fibroblast Growth Factor 23

Currently, two types of immunoassays are available for the measurement of serum FGF23 in humans. An assay using two polyclonal antibodies directed against carboxyl-terminal epitopes[207] detects most, if not all, circulating forms of FGF23 but does not discriminate between the intact active hormone and the cleaved fragment, which is not thought to have biologic activity. One assay for the intact hormone is a classic sandwich assay with antibodies directed against both the amino- and the carboxyl-terminus of the hormone.[208] This assay has been shown to be more useful than others for studying the effects of dietary phosphate on FGF23 levels in humans thought to provide a more precise determination of the biologically active levels of the hormone in the circulation, particularly when such levels may be changing.[209]

HYPERCALCEMIC DISORDERS

Parathyroid-Dependent Hypercalcemia

It is useful to delineate two categories of hypercalcemia: that associated with dysfunction of the parathyroid cell and that in which hypercalcemia occurs despite appropriate suppression of PTH secretion by the parathyroid. This distinction is particularly useful clinically because it emphasizes the centrality of the PTH assay in the diagnostic approach to the patient with hypercalcemia. Abnormal parathyroid glands are associated with hypercalcemia in three settings: primary hyperparathyroidism, familial hypocalciuric hypercalcemia (FHH), and lithium-induced hypercalcemia.

Primary Hyperparathyroidism

In primary hyperparathyroidism, a primary abnormality of parathyroid tissue leads to inappropriate secretion of PTH. In contrast, increased secretion of PTH that is an appropriate response to hypocalcemia is called *secondary hyperparathyroidism*. The inappropriately high serum concentration of PTH in primary hyperparathyroidism sustains excessive renal calcium reabsorption, phosphaturia, and calcitriol synthesis, as well as increased bone resorption. These actions of PTH produce the characteristic biochemical phenotype of hypercalcemia and hypophosphatemia, loss of cortical bone, hypercalciuria, and the various clinical sequelae of chronic hypercalcemia.

Primary hyperparathyroidism results most often (75% to 80%) from the occurrence of one or more adenomas in previously normal parathyroid glands; in 20% of cases diffuse hyperplasia of all parathyroid glands may be present, and, rarely, parathyroid carcinoma may be found (<1% to 2%).[210-213]

Classic Primary Hyperparathyroidism. The bone disease called osteitis fibrosa cystica was first described by von Recklinghausen in 1891, but the etiologic link between this disease and parathyroid neoplasms was not established until 1925, when Mandl observed clinical improvement after removal of a parathyroid adenoma from a young man with severe bone disease. In early clinical descriptions of primary hyperparathyroidism, the disease emerged as a distinctly uncommon disorder, with significant morbidity and mortality, in which almost all affected patients manifested radiographically significant or symptomatic skeletal or renal involvement, or both.

The skeletal involvement seen in classic primary hyperparathyroidism reflects a striking and generalized increase in osteoclastic bone resorption, which is accompanied by fibrovascular marrow replacement and increased osteoblastic activity. The radiographic appearance (Fig. 28-22) is characterized by the following features:

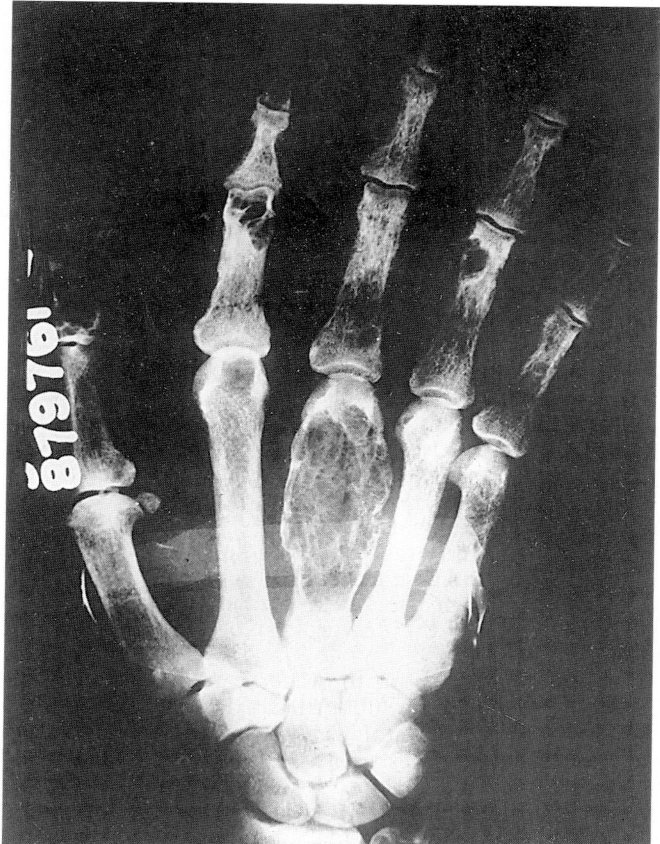

Figure 28-22 Radiograph of the hand of a patient with severe primary hyperparathyroidism. Note the dramatic remodeling associated with the intense region of high bone turnover in the third metacarpal and the widespread evidence of subperiosteal, endosteal, and trabecular resorption. (Courtesy of Fuller Albright Collection, Massachusetts General Hospital.)

- Generalized demineralization of bone, with coarsening of the trabecular pattern (due to osteoclastic resorption of the smaller trabeculae)
- Subperiosteal resorption, often most evident in the phalanges of the hands, which gives an irregular, serrated appearance to the outer, subperiosteal cortex and may progress to extensive cortical resorption
- Bone cysts, usually multiple, which contain a brownish serous or mucoid fluid; tend to occur in the central medullary portions of the shafts of the metacarpals, ribs, or pelvis; and may expand into and disrupt the overlying cortex
- Osteoclastomas, or "brown tumors," composed of numerous multinucleated osteoclasts ("giant cells") admixed with stromal cells and matrix, which are found most often in trabecular portions of the jaw, long bones, and ribs
- Pathologic fractures

The skull may exhibit a finely mottled, salt-and-pepper radiographic appearance, with loss of definition of the inner and outer cortices. Dental radiographs typically show erosion or disappearance of the lamina dura due to subperiosteal resorption, often with extension into the adjacent mandibular bone. The erosion and demineralization of cortical bone may lead to radiographic disappearance of some bones, most notably the tufts of the distal phalanges of the hands, the inferolateral cortex of the distal third of the clavicles, the distal ulna, the inferior margin of the femoral neck and pubis, and the medial aspect of the proximal tibia. The clinical correlates of these changes may include aching bone pain and tenderness, "bowing" of the shoulders, kyphosis and loss of height, and collapse of lateral ribs and pelvis with "pigeon breast" and triradiate deformities, respectively.

The renal manifestations of classic severe primary hyperparathyroidism include recurrent calcium nephrolithiasis, nephrocalcinosis, and renal functional abnormalities that range from impaired concentrating ability to end-stage renal failure. Associated signs and symptoms include recurrent flank pain, polyuria, and polydipsia. No unique features of the stone disease seen in primary hyperparathyroidism serve to distinguish it from that associated with other, more common causes of calcium kidney stones. It may more often be recurrent and severe, and in some patients the stones may be composed entirely of calcium phosphate, instead of the pure oxalate or mixed oxalate and phosphate stones more commonly encountered in other disorders. In patients diagnosed before 1965, the frequency with which nephrolithiasis complicated primary hyperparathyroidism was reportedly as high as 60% to 80% (currently, it is less than 25%), yet in studies of unselected patients conducted throughout the past 50 years, primary hyperparathyroidism has accounted for fewer than 5% of all calcium kidney stones.

Other clinical features that have been reported in association with classic severe primary hyperparathyroidism are conjunctival calcifications, band keratopathy, hypertension (50%), gastrointestinal signs and symptoms (anorexia, nausea, vomiting, constipation, or abdominal pain), peptic ulcer disease, and acute or chronic pancreatitis. The issue of whether primary hyperparathyroidism increases the risk for peptic ulcer disease and pancreatitis remains controversial. Although hyperparathyroidism is associated with a higher risk of hypertension, successful parathyroidectomy has not been shown to correct the hypertension.

Signs and symptoms in primary hyperparathyroidism may result from the involvement of bone (fracture, bone pain) or kidneys (renal colic, renal failure), peptic ulcer disease, pancreatitis, or hypercalcemia per se (weakness, apathy, depression, polyuria, constipation, coma). The presence and severity of neuropsychiatric symptoms, in particular, correlate poorly with the serum calcium concentration, although few patients with severe hypercalcemia are entirely asymptomatic. Elderly persons are most likely to exhibit such symptoms. A peculiar neuromuscular syndrome, first described in 1949 but rarely encountered now, includes symmetric proximal weakness and gait disturbance, with muscle atrophy, characteristic electromyographic abnormalities, generalized hyperreflexia and tongue fasciculations.[214]

Contemporary Primary Hyperparathyroidism. The clinical spectrum of primary hyperparathyroidism was changed dramatically in the early 1970s by the introduction of routine multichannel serum chemistry screening, which unearthed a large population of patients with previously unsuspected, asymptomatic disease. In Rochester, Minnesota, for example, the annual incidence of the disease increased abruptly, from 0.15 to 1.12 per 1000 persons, between the prescreening era (1965-1974) and 1975, the year after routine screening was introduced.[215] The peak incidence occurs in the sixth decade of life, and the disease rarely is encountered in patients younger than 15 years of age. It is twofold to threefold more common in women, who also tend to be slightly older at diagnosis than men.

Annual incidence rates were widely reported to be 0.1 to 0.3 per 1000 persons in the wake of this surge of ascertainment in Europe and the United States, but they appear to have declined substantially since then, to levels as low as 0.04 per 1000.[215] This may represent a true decline in disease incidence or simply the residual effect of "sweeping" the population of prevalent subclinical disease over the previous 3 decades. Ascertainment of mild or asymptomatic disease may decline even further in the future because of prevalent economic disincentives to routine serum chemistry screening in the primary care setting.

On the other hand, insistence on overt hypercalcemia as a diagnostic criterion may underestimate the true incidence of the disease. For example, when serum calcium and immunoreactive PTH (iPTH) were measured in a large population of Swedish women undergoing routine mammographic screening, the prevalence of unsuspected primary hyperparathyroidism, defined by criteria that included the combination of high-normal serum calcium plus elevated or high-normal iPTH, was 2.1%.[216] Two thirds of these women (72/109) were normocalcemic (10.0 to 10.4 mg/dL), yet bone density was reduced in the group as a whole, and the disease was confirmed histologically in 98% of the 61 who had surgery. Furthermore, the widespread practice of evaluating PTH levels in patients with osteoporosis has led to the identification of patients with high PTH levels and normocalcemia.[217] Many of these patients become hypercalcemic during follow-up.

Not surprisingly, given that primary hyperparathyroidism now usually is diagnosed incidentally, few patients are found to have overt signs or symptoms of the classic disease, and most therefore are considered to be "asymptomatic." For example, only 2% of patients with primary hyperparathyroidism residing in Olmsted County, Minnesota, and only 17% of 121 patients studied at an academic referral center in New York City had classic disease symptoms[215,218]; in most of cases, the relevant symptom was urolithiasis. Many clinicians argue, however, that most of the patients who are regarded as having asymptomatic primary hyperparathyroidism and who have only minimally elevated serum calcium actually suffer from various neuropsychiatric or other symptoms that may improve after curative surgery.[219] Nonetheless, these symptoms—which include fatigability, weakness, forgetfulness, depression, somatization, polydipsia, polyuria, and bone and joint pain—are also common in otherwise normal persons.

In the small randomized studies of surgery for primary hyperparathyroidism (discussed later), the effects of surgery on measures of quality of life have been conflicting.[217,220-222] This remains a critical issue, because the advent of less invasive operative approaches and concerns regarding fracture, cancer, and mortality risk have lowered the threshold for consideration of surgery in many patients with the disease (see later discussion). Throughout this chapter, the term *asymptomatic primary hyperparathyroidism* refers to patients who lack signs or symptoms of the classic disease, whether or not they experience any of the subtle symptoms mentioned previously.

The natural history of untreated asymptomatic primary hyperparathyroidism, as currently detected, remains incompletely understood. Few patients seem to experience progression of the disease, as measured by extreme elevations of serum or urinary calcium or by the advent of renal dysfunction, nephrocalcinosis, or worsening osteopenia over many years of observation.[218] On the other hand, late cortical bone loss observed at the femoral neck and distal radius in a small number of patients who were observed without surgery for 15 years points to the potential importance of continued monitoring in such patients.[226] Also, an excess risk of mortality, mainly from cardiovascular disease, has been noted during extended follow-up of large cohorts of patients with chronic hypercalcemia (and presumed primary hyperparathyroidism) identified by population health screening in Sweden,[223] and similar observations have been made during extended follow-up of postsurgical patients with hyperparathyroidism.[224] Associations of hypertension, hyperuricemia, and glucose intolerance with primary hyperparathyroidism have been implicated, together with hypercalcemia per se, as contributors to this elevated risk.[225]

Abnormal cardiac calcification and left ventricular hypertrophy (reversible by successful parathyroidectomy) have also been reported in primary hyperparathyroidism.[227] Increased cardiovascular mortality may be a feature only of severe hyperparathyroidism, because it was restricted to those in the highest quartile of serum calcium in the Olmsted County study, which otherwise showed an overall decreased risk of death.[228] A 40% excess risk of malignancy also was reported among 4163 Swedish patients who had undergone surgery more than a year earlier for (presumably symptomatic) primary hyperparathyroidism.[229] It has been argued that these increased risks for mortality and malignancy, even if confirmed, may apply only to those with primary hyperparathyroidism that is more severe than the "asymptomatic" version typically encountered today.[225]

Abnormalities of bone in modern, mild primary hyperparathyroidism are far subtler than those associated with the classic disease. Histologically, the rate at which new bone remodeling cycles are activated is increased. Because the phase of restorative bone formation at each remodeling site takes much more time than does the initial resorptive phase, such an increase in remodeling rate inevitably increases the ambient volume of the "remodeling space" and, thus, the porosity of bone. Depending on the rate and extent of the accompanying increase in osteoblastic activity and the resulting local balance between net bone formation and resorption, mineralized bone volume may decrease

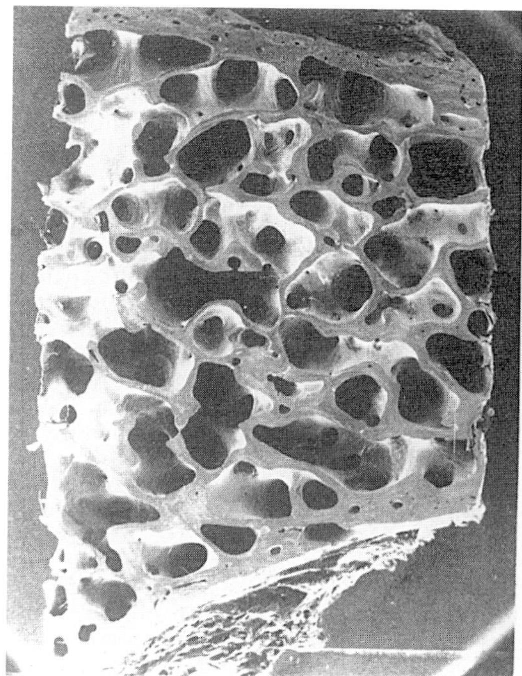
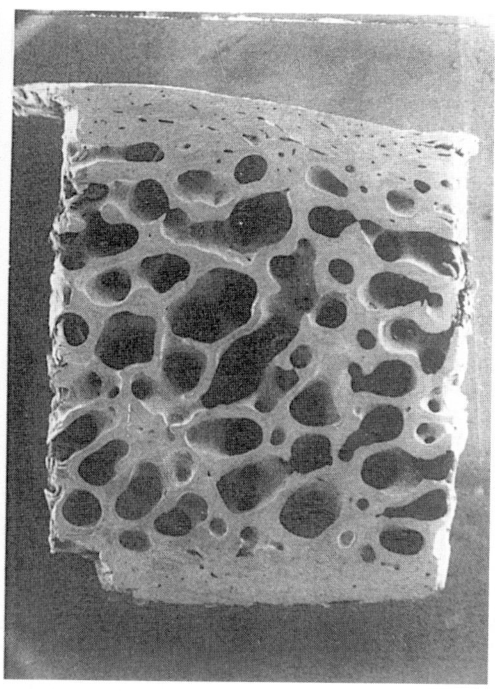

Figure 28-23 Iliac crest biopsy specimens from a patient with primary hyperparathyroidism *(left)* and a normal control *(right)*, viewed by scanning electron microscopy. Note the thin cortices and contrasting maintenance of trabecular bone in the patient. (From Parisien M, Silverberg SJ, Shane E, et al. The histomorphometry of bone in primary hyperparathyroidism: preservation of cancellous bone structure. *J Clin Endocrinol Metab.* 1990;70:930-938.)

further, remain stable, or even increase (despite an increased remodeling space). For reasons not yet understood, the balance achieved between increased resorption and formation of bone in primary hyperparathyroidism depends not only on the severity of the hyperparathyroidism but also on skeletal location: Net resorption of endosteal bone may predominate in cortical sites, whereas net apposition of mineral may occur in trabecular bone (Fig. 28-23).[230]

In mild primary hyperparathyroidism, osteopenia usually is not evident radiographically, although bone mineral density may be reduced by as much as 10% to 20%, particularly at sites of predominantly cortical bone such as the midradius.[231] The mass of trabecular or cancellous bone, as represented in the vertebral bodies, is preferentially preserved and often is normal.[232] Curiously, the reduced cortical bone density at the forearm is not improved by successful parathyroidectomy, whereas density at trabecular-rich sites such as the hip and spine may increase by 10% to 15% over several years postoperatively.[218]

The critical issue of whether fracture risk is increased in patients with primary hyperparathyroidism was addressed by a retrospective analysis of fracture incidence within a cohort of 407 residents of Rochester, Minnesota, who were diagnosed with the disease between 1965 and 1992.[233] Compared to the expected age- and sex-adjusted rates of incident fractures in that community, the relative risk among those with hyperparathyroidism was significantly elevated at the vertebrae (3.2-fold), distal forearm (2.2-fold) and ribs (2.7-fold), although not at the hip (1.4-fold). Overall risk of fracture at any site was significantly increased as well (1.3-fold) and was as high in those diagnosed incidentally, after the institution of automated chemistry screening in 1974, as in those diagnosed before that time. Similar findings were reported in 674 Danish patients who were scheduled to undergo parathyroidectomy.[234] These results are consistent with those of several previous studies involving smaller cohorts of patients and, absent data from an appropriately controlled prospective study, strongly support the conclusion that patients with primary hyperparathyroidism should be considered to be at increased risk for fracture. This presumably is true in both symptomatic and asymptomatic disease, because less than 10% of the post-screening Rochester cohort had symptoms or complications of primary hyperparathyroidism.[215] What is not yet known is whether fracture risk is reduced by successful parathyroidectomy, although in the Danish series the risk for vertebral and lower-extremity fractures was no longer increased postoperatively.[234]

Kidney stones now are reported in only 10% to 25% of patients with primary hyperparathyroidism, although some degree of renal dysfunction—either a significant reduction in creatinine clearance (Cl_{Cr}) or impaired concentrating or acidifying ability—may be found in up to one third of those with asymptomatic disease. These renal abnormalities are not progressive in the majority of affected patients.[218,235] The association of kidney stones with primary hyperparathyroidism generally is viewed as an indication for parathyroidectomy, however, because successful surgery usually prevents further symptomatic stone disease.[218,224] On the other hand, it is not possible at present to confidently predict, from biochemical measurements in blood or urine, which asymptomatic patients with hyperparathyroidism will go on to develop new stone disease. Stone-formers are more likely to be hypercalciuric than not, but fewer than one third of hypercalciuric patients with hyperparathyroidism actually develop stones.

Etiology and Pathogenesis. Parathyroid adenomas are caused by mutations in the DNA of parathyroid cells; these mutations confer a proliferative or survival advantage for affected cells compared with their normal neighbors.[236,237] As a consequence of this advantage, the descendants of one particular parathyroid cell, a clone of cells, undergo clonal expansion to produce an adenoma.

Multiple chromosomal regions are missing in the parathyroid cells of individual parathyroid adenomas, probably reflecting the deletion of tumor suppressor genes. These chromosomal loci include portions of chromosome 1p-pter (in 40% of adenomas), 6q (in 32% of adenomas), 15q (in 30% of adenomas), and 11q (in 25% to 30% of adenomas). Many of the 11q deletions are associated, in the undeleted chromosome 11, with mutations in the gene encoding the transcription factor menin, the gene that is mutated in multiple endocrine neoplasia type 1 (MEN1). This gene is also commonly involved in somatic mutations in patients with sporadic parathyroid adenomas. Somatic mutations have also been found in the mitochondrial genomes of a fraction of chief cell adenomas and have been found even more frequently in so-called oxyphil adenomas, which are known to exhibit mitochondria with abnormal morphology.[238] The widespread presence of somatic mutations in sporadic parathyroid adenomas, which are detectable only because large numbers of cells in any one tumor contain the same deletion, constitutes the strongest evidence that parathyroid adenomas are clonal expansions of mutant cells.

One parathyroid proto-oncogene has been identified: the cyclin D1 gene (*CCND1*, also called parathyroid adenomatous 1 or *PRAD1*).[239] This gene was discovered at the breakpoint of an inversion on chromosome 11 in a parathyroid adenoma. This inversion led to juxtaposition of the PTH gene's regulatory region and the DNA encoding cyclin D1. As a consequence, the cyclin D1 gene was overexpressed. Cyclin D1 is an important regulator of the transition from the G_1 phase of the cell cycle (which follows mitosis) to the S phase (associated with DNA synthesis), and it is mutated or amplified in a wide variety of malignancies. Cyclin D1 is overexpressed in about 20% of parathyroid adenomas, although cyclin D1 gene rearrangements have been documented in only 5% of adenomas. Overexpression of cyclin D1 in the parathyroids of transgenic mice leads to formation of parathyroid adenomas and hypercalcemia over many months.[240] The phenotype of these mice demonstrates that cyclin D1 overexpression can cause primary hyperparathyroidism.

As expected for a disease caused by mutations in DNA, parathyroid adenomas occur more frequently in patients who underwent neck irradiation decades earlier, with greater radiation exposure leading to higher risk. Most patients have no definite history of exposure to specific mutagens, however. An intriguing clue that abnormalities of vitamin D physiology may predispose to primary hyperparathyroidism has come from the observation that patients with parathyroid adenomas are more likely than others to have inherited a particular allele of the VDR gene.[241] These patients have tumors with particularly low levels of mRNA encoding the VDR. Nevertheless, no mutations in the coding regions of the gene encoding the VDR have been found in parathyroid adenomas.[242]

The cause of sporadic primary parathyroid hyperplasia is unknown. The known stimulus for parathyroid cell proliferation—low levels of blood calcium or calcitriol—is not present in this disease. Presumably, some other stimulus outside the parathyroid glands, or a genetic abnormality present in all four parathyroid glands, leads to inappropriate cell proliferation. Such abnormalities have been found in several inherited forms of parathyroid hyperplasia (see later discussion), but most cases of parathyroid hyperplasia do not occur as part of familial clusters.

The theoretical distinction between adenoma as a clonal proliferation and hyperplasia as a polyclonal growth is clearcut. In some settings, however, clonal expansion can occur in the context of preexisting nonclonal proliferation. The clearest example of this complication has been found in the large parathyroid glands associated with severe renal failure. In many such glands removed surgically because of hypercalcemia or severe parathyroid-dependent bone disease, evidence for clonal proliferation complicating secondary hyperplasia has been found. Interestingly, the pattern of chromosomal abnormalities in these clonal tumors differs from that found in parathyroid adenomas in patients without renal failure.[243] Analogous mechanisms may be operative in a number of settings associated with stimuli to parathyroid cell proliferation, such as X-linked hypophosphatemia and long-term lithium therapy. Furthermore, just as clonal tumors can arise in the setting of secondary parathyroid hyperplasia, they can also arise in the setting of sporadic primary parathyroid hyperplasia[244] and in MEN1.[245]

The distinction between adenoma and hyperplasia is clinically important, because removal of the one gland that is abnormal can be expected to cure a parathyroid adenoma, whereas removal of multiple glands is required to cure parathyroid hyperplasia. However, differentiating adenoma from hyperplasia and from normal parathyroid tissue at pathologic examination is not straightforward. Pathologists distinguish normal from abnormal parathyroid glands by the increase in size and the paucity of fat in abnormal glands. Attempts have been made to distinguish an adenoma from an individual hyperplastic gland on the basis of morphologic features, but no criteria have proved completely reliable.[246] The formation of clonal neoplasms in originally hyperplastic tumors may explain some of the difficulty encountered in pathologic diagnosis.

An increase in cell number is not the only abnormality in primary hyperparathyroidism. The ability of the normal parathyroid cell to suppress PTH secretion in response to hypercalcemia might be expected to protect an individual from sustained hypercalcemia even if the number of parathyroid cells increases moderately. However, parathyroid cells in parathyroid adenomas usually demonstrate abnormalities in their responsiveness to calcium, with a shift in setpoint to the right (Fig. 28-24). This setpoint shift, combined with the nonsuppressible component of PTH secretion, leads to a new steady state in which both the PTH level and the blood calcium level are higher than normal.

The molecular underpinning of the abnormal parathyroid cell responsiveness is beginning to be understood. Parathyroid cells from adenomas respond to changes in extracellular calcium with smaller than normal increases in intracellular calcium, and the amount of CASR protein on the cell surface is reduced.[247] Perhaps surprisingly, no mutations in the gene encoding the CASR have been found in parathyroid adenomas. In the experimental model in which overexpression of cyclin D1 results in primary hyperparathyroidism,[240] reduced expression of the CASR occurs only after cell proliferation has been increased for some time. Therefore, the decreased expression of the CASR in parathyroid adenomas is likely to be a secondary response that occurs during tumor formation. One demonstrated regulator of expression of the CASR gene in parathyroid cells is the developmental regulator, GCM2.[248]

Inherited Primary Hyperparathyroidism. Although inherited forms of primary hyperparathyroidism are uncommon, they are clinically important for several reasons. Management of the parathyroid tumors found in familial parathyroid syndromes often differs from that of sporadic primary hyperparathyroidism. Furthermore,

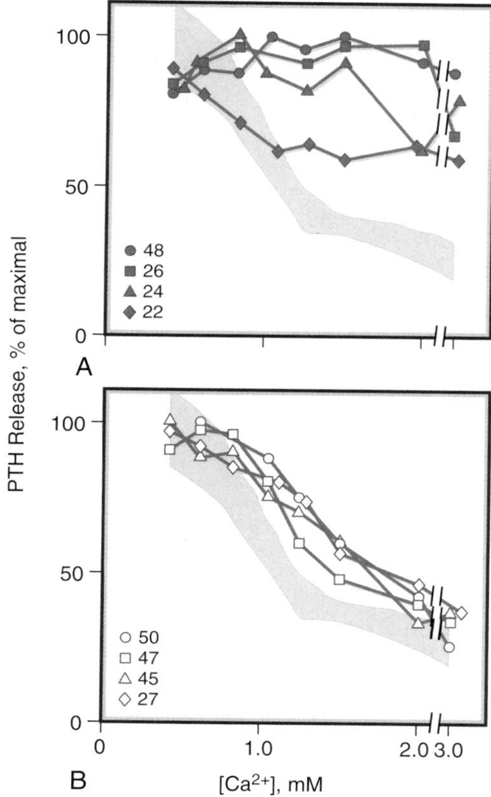

Figure 28-24 Abnormal patterns of parathyroid hormone (PTH) secretion from cells prepared from adenomatous glands and stimulated with varying levels of calcium in tissue culture. The shaded area shows the pattern of PTH release (±1 standard deviation) from normal human parathyroid cells. Panel **A** illustrates the pattern from four patients with little suppression of PTH secretion by calcium. Panel **B** illustrates the pattern from four patients with relatively intact mechanisms of suppression of PTH secretion by calcium. Even in this group, the setpoint for calcium suppression is shifted to the right. (From Brown EM. Calcium-regulated parathyroid hormone release in primary hyperparathyroidism: studies in vitro with dispersed parathyroid cells. *Am J Med.* 1979;66:923-931.)

extraparathyroidal manifestations of inherited syndromes may need treatment, and awareness of familial clustering should prompt systematic family screening.

Multiple Endocrine Neoplasia Type 1. MEN1 (see also Chapter 41) is caused by inactivitating mutations in the tumor suppressor gene encoding menin.[249] Menin is a ubiquitously expressed transcription factor that is part of a complex that targets histone H_3 for methylation[250] and thereby leads to expression of cell cycle inhibitors in pancreatic islets and other tissues.[251] Rarely, mutations in genes encoding cyclin-dependent kinase inhibitors such as p27 (CDKN1B) are found in MEN1 patients without menin mutations.[252] Although MEN1 includes tumors of the parathyroid, anterior pituitary, and pancreatic islets, the parathyroid tumors are far more prevalent than the others; 95% of affected patients eventually develop hyperparathyroidism. Most of the parathyroid tumors harbor mutations in both copies of the menin gene; one mutation is inherited, and the second occurs in the parathyroid cell whose progeny form the tumor.

The onset of hypercalcemia occurs in the second and third decades of life, although occasionally a patient presents in the first decade. Hypercalcemia never manifests at birth or in infancy. The disease involves all four parathyroid glands, although the involvement can be asymmetric and apparently asynchronous. Apart from the earlier age at diagnosis, the presenting clinical picture resembles that of sporadic primary hyperparathyroidism, perhaps with somewhat greater loss of bone density.[253] One common complicating feature of hypercalcemia is that it can dramatically increase the gastrin levels and symptomatology in those patients who also have gastrinomas. Treatment of the parathyroid disease in this setting can greatly simplify management of the gastric hyperacidity.

After parathyroid surgery, hypoparathyroidism and recurrent hyperparathyroidism are more common than in other forms of hyperparathyroidism.[254] The timing and type of surgery are therefore more complicated issues than in sporadic primary hyperparathyroidism. Most authorities agree that parathyroid disease recurs eventually, particularly if fewer than three glands are removed. Some surgeons prefer subtotal parathyroidectomy, whereas others prefer total parathyroidectomy with forearm implantation of a small amount of parathyroid tissue.

Multiple Endocrine Neoplasia Type 2a. Parathyroid disease is usually a late and infrequent (5% to 20%) occurrence in patients with MEN type 2a (see also Chapter 41), a disease defined by the clustering of medullary carcinoma of the thyroid, pheochromocytoma, and hyperparathyroidism. In some families, hyperparathyroidism is more common; however, these families have the same mutations in the *RET* proto-oncogene that are found in families without frequent hyperparathyroidism. Both parathyroid hyperplasia and adenoma have been noted at surgery. Because asymptomatic parathyroid hyperplasia has been observed at the time of thyroid surgery, a progression from hyperplasia to adenoma in MEN2a has been suggested. The approach to diagnosis and treatment of hyperparathyroidism is similar to that for sporadic primary hyperparathyroidism, but hyperplasia is more frequently the underlying disorder. The pathogenesis of the hyperparathyroidism is uncertain, but the *RET* gene, which is mutated in almost all cases of MEN2a, is expressed in parathyroid cells,[255] so abnormal RET expression in parathyroid cells may directly cause parathyroid tumor formation. Hyperparathyroidism does not occur in MEN2b, the variant associated with mucosal neuromas.

Hyperparathyroidism–Jaw Tumor Syndrome. Patients with hereditary hyperparathyroidism–jaw tumor syndrome[256] present with parathyroid adenomas that can be multiple and are usually cystic. These tumors are often but not invariably associated with fibrous jaw tumors that are unrelated to the hyperparathyroidism. Importantly, the parathyroid tumors are frequently malignant, in contrast to the findings in MEN1 and MEN2a. Wilms' tumor and polycystic renal disease also have occurred in affected families. The gene mutated in this syndrome, *HRPT2* (now called *CDC73*), encodes the nuclear protein, parafibromin.[257] Parafibromin is part of the evolutionarily highly conserved PAF complex, which binds RNA polymerase II, regulates chromatin structure, and regulates gene expression.[258-260] Parafibromin binds β-catenin and can mediate Wnt pathway signaling and Notch signaling, although it is not known whether these properties of parafibromin are related to its tumor suppressor function.[261] Inactivating mutations in parafibromin are found in a high number of patients with apparently sporadic parathyroid cancer.[262] Because some of these patients have subsequently proved to be members of families with inherited *CDC73* mutations, perhaps all patients with parathyroid cancer should be screened for germline mutations in *CDC73*.

Management of Primary Hyperparathyroidism. The strategy for management of primary hyperparathyroidism has evolved in parallel with the changing presentation of the disease. The only opportunity for permanent cure is surgical removal of the abnormal gland or glands, an approach that clearly was appropriate for virtually all patients in whom the classic, severe form of the disease was diagnosed 4 to 5 decades ago and that still is the treatment of choice for those patients who do present with recurrent kidney stones, nephrocalcinosis, clinically overt bone disease, or severe hypercalcemia.

In contrast, the choice of surgical versus medical management for patients with asymptomatic primary hyperparathyroidism remains an open and hotly debated question. Those who favor surgery point to the expected improvement in bone mineral density (at the hip and spine) and left ventricular hypertrophy after successful surgical intervention; evidence of increased risk for fracture, cardiovascular mortality, malignancy, and neuropsychiatric symptoms associated with primary hyperparathyroidism; and the recent successful development of effective minimally invasive surgical procedures (discussed later). Those who favor an observational approach emphasize the evidence for lack of disease progression in most asymptomatic patients; the small but finite risk of surgical failure and postoperative complications; the probability that excess mortality and cancer risks documented in patients with relatively severe disease may not apply to those with mild, asymptomatic primary hyperparathyroidism; the difficulty in assigning vague neuropsychiatric symptoms to the parathyroid disorder; the lack of evidence (or negative evidence) that hypertension and increased risk of cancer, fracture, or cardiovascular mortality, even if present, are improved by successful parathyroidectomy; and the availability of sensitive techniques for monitoring disease status in patients who do not undergo surgery.[225]

No large prospective studies powered to compare clinical outcomes in patients with asymptomatic primary hyperparathyroidism randomly assigned to surgery versus medical management have been conducted. Nevertheless, three valuable smaller, randomized controlled trials of surgery versus observation have been conducted that allow some conclusions about surrogate markers of disease.[220-222] All three trials demonstrated increased bone density in the spine and hip in those treated surgically; the increases were similar to those produced with bisphosphonate therapy in patients with primary hyperparathyroidism (see later discussion). Two of the three studies showed modest improvements in some quality-of-life measures, although the unblinded nature of the studies limits interpretation of these findings. All of the findings reported so far have been after 2 years or less. As useful as these studies have been, their limitations have forced the field to tap observational studies to draw tentative recommendations based on limited data.

Such provisional recommendations have emanated from a series of conferences. A Consensus Conference sponsored by the National Institutes of Health (NIH) was held in 1990, followed by a more informal update in 2002 and, most recently, in 2008.[263] The major conclusion of that group was that, although surgery is indicated for symptomatic hyperparathyroidism and always should be considered an appropriate option in patients with asymptomatic hyperparathyroidism, many patients with asymptomatic disease can be safely monitored without surgery. Those suitable for medical observation should have no evidence of significant compromise of skeletal integrity or renal function and no history of urolithiasis or gastrointestinal or neuropsychiatric symptoms, and they should meet the criteria listed in Table 28-1. Such patients comprise at least 50% of those who currently present with primary hyperparathyroidism.

TABLE 28-1

Indications for Surgery in Primary Hyperparathyroidism

Overt clinical manifestations of disease
Kidney stones or nephrocalcinosis
Fractures or classic radiographic findings of osteitis fibrosa
Classic neuromuscular disease
Symptomatic or life-threatening hypercalcemia
Serum calcium >1 mg/dL above the upper limit of normal
Creatinine clearance <60 mL/min
Bone mineral density low (T score ≤−2.5) at any site*
History of fragility fracture
Young age (<50 yr)
Uncertain prospects for adequate medical monitoring

*Z score ≤−2.5 in premenopausal women and in men <50 years old.

Modified from Bilezikian JP, Khan AA, Potts JT Jr. Third International Workshop on the Management of Asymptomatic Primary Hyperparathyroidism. Guidelines for the management of asymptomatic primary hyperparathyroidism: summary statement from the Third International Workshop. *J Clin Endocrinol Metab.* 2009;94:335-339. Based on recommendations of the 2008 National Institutes of Health–sponsored "Workshop on the Management of Asymptomatic Primary Hyperparathyroidism.")

On the other hand, the conferences concluded, surgery may be preferable if the patient desires surgery even when asymptomatic, if the probability of consistent monitoring seems low, if concomitant illness seems likely to complicate management or obscure significant disease progression, or if the patient is relatively young (less than 50 years of age). The last recommendation reflects the absence of reliable information about the natural history of the disease over many decades of follow-up; the cumulative cost of medical monitoring, which begins to exceed that of surgery by 5 to 10 years; and some data suggesting that young people are more likely than others to have progressive disease.[264] However, age alone is not viewed as a contraindication to parathyroidectomy, because the procedure has been accomplished with excellent results, with a perioperative mortality rate of 1% to 3%, in large numbers of appropriately selected patients older than 75 years of age. Because hypertension is not thought to be a feature of mild primary hyperparathyroidism, and because hypertension generally is not improved by parathyroidectomy, hypertension is not viewed as an indication for surgery.

Although the Consensus Conference recommendations and subsequent modifications provide a useful framework for decision-making, supporting data from large clinical trials are lacking. In a series of 52 asymptomatic patients who were selected for nonoperative management mainly on the basis of the 1990 Consensus Conference criteria and whose course was followed for 10 years, approximately 25% developed one or more new indications for surgery.[218] Patients who do not meet the Consensus Conference criteria for surgery may nevertheless experience the same postsurgical increase in bone density as those who do.[265] Some have emphasized that evidence of baseline vertebral osteopenia, an unusual finding in primary hyperparathyroidism, should be considered among the criteria for surgery[232] and that surgery also should be considered for postmenopausal women who exhibit vertebral bone loss in the setting of primary hyperparathyroidism.[218,225]

A common dilemma is the inability to ascertain whether vague but troublesome symptoms such as fatigue, lethargy, weakness (without objective muscle weakness), or depression are caused by the hyperparathyroidism and therefore qualify as "significant" in the context of considering the decision for surgery. Most clinicians do not routinely recommend parathyroidectomy on the basis of such symptoms alone, although dramatic responses to surgery are occasionally seen. With the availability of improved, minimally invasive surgical approaches, the threshold for considering surgery in patients who are significantly disabled by such symptoms clearly is lower now than in the past. Some have advocated, in selected cases, a limited trial of medical therapy (i.e., calcimimetics) to reduce serum calcium levels (see later discussion) and thereby attempt to predict the symptomatic response to surgical cure.

Medical Monitoring of Primary Hyperparathyroidism. The updated NIH Consensus Conference recommendations suggest that patients not treated surgically should be monitored carefully, with annual measurement of serum calcium and calculation of Cl_{Cr} and serial determinations of bone mineral density at 1- to 2-year intervals. The most appropriate bone densitometric site is considered to be one that reflects mainly changes in cortical bone (e.g., distal forearm), although the importance of monitoring vertebral bone density as well has been emphasized,[218] and current criteria acknowledge the importance of significant bone loss at any site.[263]

Patients undergoing nonoperative medical management must be cautioned to maintain adequate hydration, to avoid diuretics and prolonged immobilization, and to seek prompt medical attention in the event of illnesses accompanied by significant vomiting or diarrhea. Dietary calcium should not be restricted.

The goal of an effective pharmacologic therapy for primary hyperparathyroidism remains elusive, although study of sex hormones and selective estrogen receptor modulators, bisphosphonates, and calcimimetics continue. Estrogens and progestins may reduce serum calcium and phosphorus, urinary calcium and hydroxyproline, and histologic evidence of active bone resorption in women with primary hyperparathyroidism, although safety concerns have limited these therapeutic options in postmenopausal women. Limited data with raloxifene suggest that this drug may be useful in controlling serum calcium and lowering bone turnover in women with primary hyperparathyroidism.[266]

Intravenous bisphosphonates have been employed successfully in the urgent treatment of hypercalcemia caused by primary hyperparathyroidism, and several trials have shown that treatment with oral alendronate for 1 year or longer improves bone density at the spine and hip, with only transient effects on serum calcium and PTH.[267,268] The calcimimetics represent a new class of agents that, by sensitizing the CASR to extracellular calcium, can reduce PTH secretion. Cinacalcet, the first calcimimetic approved for control of secondary hyperparathyroidism in renal disease, was shown to lower serum calcium and PTH in patients with primary hyperparathyroidism (and in some patients with parathyroid carcinoma), although improvement in bone density has not been documented in this population.[269] Therefore, in patients for whom surgery for asymptomatic primary hyperparathyroidism is not an option, therapy with oral bisphosphonates can improve bone density without worsening other features of the disease, at least over 2 years of follow-up. Whether this or any other medical therapy offers a beneficial long-term alternative to surgery is unknown.

Surgical Treatment of Primary Hyperparathyroidism. Parathyroidectomy is a safe and highly effective approach for definitive treatment of primary hyperparathyroidism. The most serious potential complications of parathyroid surgery are vocal cord paralysis and permanent hypoparathyroidism, which occur after fewer than 1% and 4%, respectively, of procedures performed by highly skilled surgeons, although these rates can be much higher in less experienced hands. Such complications occur most often in patients who require subtotal parathyroid resections for hyperplasia or resection of carcinoma. The surgical cure rate for primary hyperparathyroidism in the best hands is at least 95%.[270,271]

Apart from operator inexperience, the usual cause of initial surgical failure ("persistent disease") is the presence of either unrecognized (often very asymmetric) parathyroid hyperplasia or ectopic parathyroid tissue (i.e., intrathyroidal, undescended, retroesophageal, or mediastinal glands) (Fig. 28-25).[272] Up to one in five parathyroid glands may be located ectopically, and this is especially true of supernumerary glands. Recurrent disease, defined as that occurring after an interval of at least 6 to 12 months of normocalcemia, varies in incidence from 2% to 16%. Recurrent hyperparathyroidism usually arises in unresected hyperplastic glands, but rarely it may be caused by parathyroid carcinoma, a second adenoma, or a multicentric or miliary "parathyromatosis" engendered by inadvertent local seeding of parathyroid tissue (usually hyperplastic) into the neck during previous parathyroid surgery.[210,273]

In the past, there was broad agreement that the best approach is a bilateral neck exploration in which all four parathyroids are identified and all enlarged glands are removed. With this procedure, preoperative parathyroid localization studies before initial cervical exploration are superfluous, because the positive predictive value of even the best current technique (i.e., technetium 99m [^{99m}Tc]-sestamibi scanning) falls well short of the success rate of experienced surgeons unaided by prior imaging.[210,274]

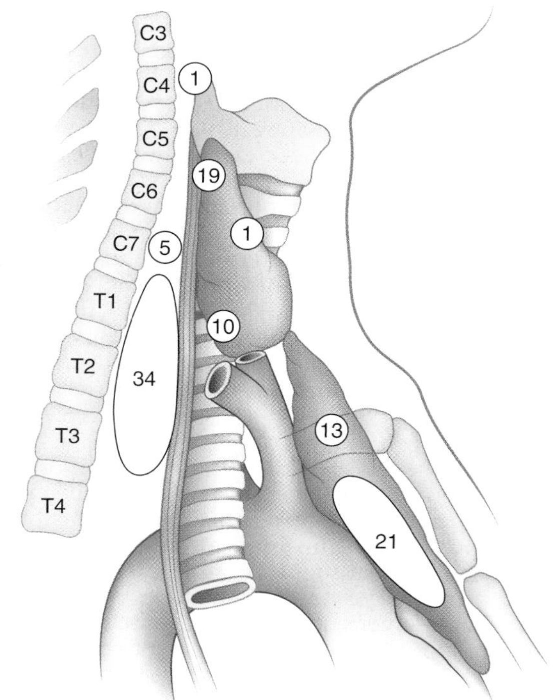

Figure 28-25 Sites of ectopic location of 104 parathyroid glands found at reoperation for primary hyperparathyroidism. (From Wang C-A. A clinical and pathological study of 112 cases. *Ann Surg.* 1977;186:140-145.)

Preoperative ^{99m}Tc-sestamibi scanning, however, can accurately localize 80% to 90% of the single adenomas that account for 75% to 85% of cases, and since it became available there has been renewed interest in the performance of directed unilateral explorations, which reduce operative and recovery room time, minimize the number of frozen sections required, are associated with significantly fewer postoperative complications, and can more readily be performed using minimally invasive techniques (including local anesthesia and intravenous sedation), enabling same-day discharge.[275] Sestamibi scanning also can identify the occasional mediastinal adenoma, allowing the surgeon to avoid an unnecessary neck exploration. On the other hand, the sensitivity and positive predictive value of sestamibi scanning is poor (<50%) in the presence of multiglandular disease (hyperplasia or double adenomas), so the test may frequently miss the presence of bilateral disease.[271] To reduce this failure rate, which is unacceptably high in comparison to bilateral exploration, supplemental preoperative ultrasonic imaging (with or without needle biopsy) is often employed, and rapid intraoperative PTH assays have been developed to verify successful excision.[276] Because the half-life of intact PTH in blood is very short (<2 min), a decline of 50% or more from baseline within approximately 10 minutes can signal successful removal of all hyperfunctioning parathyroid tissue. This approach has functioned well in patients with single adenomas but can be misleading in those with multiglandular disease unless more stringent criteria for cure are applied (i.e., >90% decline, or even normalization, of iPTH).[277]

At present, preoperative imaging enables consideration of a minimally invasive unilateral parathyroidectomy in approximately 70% of those patients thought preoperatively to have sporadic primary hyperparathyroidism due to a solitary adenoma. Surgical cure rates in appropriately selected patients are comparable to those achieved after bilateral neck exploration (i.e., 95% to 97%),[271] although a recent study in which all patients selected for minimally invasive surgery were also subjected to immediate bilateral neck dissection demonstrated a failure to recognize multiglandular disease in 16% of the subjects.[278] Patients with known or suspected multiglandular disease, such as those with MEN1 and those younger than 30 years of age, should undergo bilateral neck exploration.[279] Options for patients with hyperplasia include resection limited to visibly abnormal glands, subtotal parathyroidectomy with cryopreservation of tissue, and total parathyroidectomy with immediate autotransplantation (i.e., in the forearm) of some excised tissue. In patients with MEN1, considerations of the rate (30% to 50% or higher with long-term follow-up) and the timing of recurrences versus the potential morbidity of surgical hypoparathyroidism tend to favor subtotal parathyroidectomy as the preferred approach at present.

The incidence of parathyroid carcinoma in primary hyperparathyroidism is less than 1%,[213] but this possibility should be strongly considered in patients with unusually severe hyperparathyroidism, a palpable neck mass, hoarseness, evidence of local invasion at surgery, or recurrent hypercalcemia.[280] Even so, parathyroid carcinoma rarely is suspected preoperatively and often eludes diagnosis at the time of initial surgery. When the disease is recognized, vigorous attempts should be made to remove the tumor en bloc. The incidence of local recurrence approaches 50%, however, and distant metastases, particularly to lung, may be heralded by recurrent, severe hyperparathyroidism.[281] Because apparently sporadic and isolated parathyroid cancer can occur in families with parafibromin mutations, a search for such mutations in all patients with parathyroid cancer can facilitate family counseling.[262]

The immediate postoperative management of parathyroidectomy focuses on establishing the success of the surgery and monitoring the patient closely for symptomatic hypocalcemia and for uncommon but potentially serious acute complications such as bleeding, vocal cord paralysis, and laryngospasm. After successful resection of a parathyroid adenoma, serum levels of intact PTH decline rapidly, often to undetectable concentrations, with a disappearance half-time of about 2 minutes. Serum calcium typically reaches a nadir between 24 and 36 hours after surgery. Serum PTH returns to the normal range within 30 hours, although measurements of the parathyroid secretory response to hypocalcemia suggest that it does not fully normalize for at least several weeks.[282]

In the past, patients usually were maintained on a low-calcium diet until normalization of serum calcium was clearly documented. Ampoules of injectable calcium and other seizure precautions were maintained at the bedside, serum calcium was measured at least every 12 hours until stable, and symptomatic hypocalcemia was promptly treated with calcium, either intravenously (90-mg bolus, then 50 to 100 mg/hour) or orally (1.5 to 3.0 g/day). This approach is no longer appropriate for most patients, who are discharged within a few hours after limited surgery. Instead, oral calcium supplements routinely are provided as soon as oral intake is reestablished. Moderate doses of calcitriol (0.5 to 1.0 μg daily) are added for those with large adenomas and severe hyperparathyroidism and for those in whom alkaline phosphatase had been elevated preoperatively—that is, patients in whom an impressive calcium requirement can be anticipated, often for many weeks postoperatively, as they remineralize their skeletons. This so-called hungry bone syndrome is associated with hypocalcemia, hypophosphatemia, and low urinary calcium excretion.

Serum calcium should be checked at intervals of several days initially to guide adjustment of calcium and vitamin D therapy as needed to achieve a stable result. In those in whom hypocalcemia persists for more than several days, serum PTH should be measured to exclude the possibility of postoperative hypoparathyroidism. Given evidence that bone mineral density continues to increase for at least 1 year after successful parathyroidectomy,[218] it is prudent to continue calcium supplementation for at least that long.

The approach to patients with persistent or recurrent hyperparathyroidism is informed by the recognition that parathyroid hyperplasia or carcinoma, ectopic or supernumerary parathyroid tissue, and postoperative hypoparathyroidism and other complications of further surgery all are more common in this population.[272,274] The first issue to address is whether surgery is indicated. If a presumed adenoma was not identified initially, the original indications for surgery usually still exist, although some patients may not be suitable candidates for more extensive surgery (e.g., median sternotomy) because of concurrent medical illness. Patients with parathyroid hyperplasia may have experienced significant clinical improvement, even after incomplete parathyroidectomy, although those with MEN1 are very likely to experience further progression of their disease.

Preoperative localization studies are recommended for patients with persistent or recurrent disease after a first operation. Scanning with ^{99m}Tc-sestamibi offers the highest sensitivity and accuracy, although other studies (ultrasonography, computed tomography [CT], magnetic resonance imaging) may provide additional or confirmatory

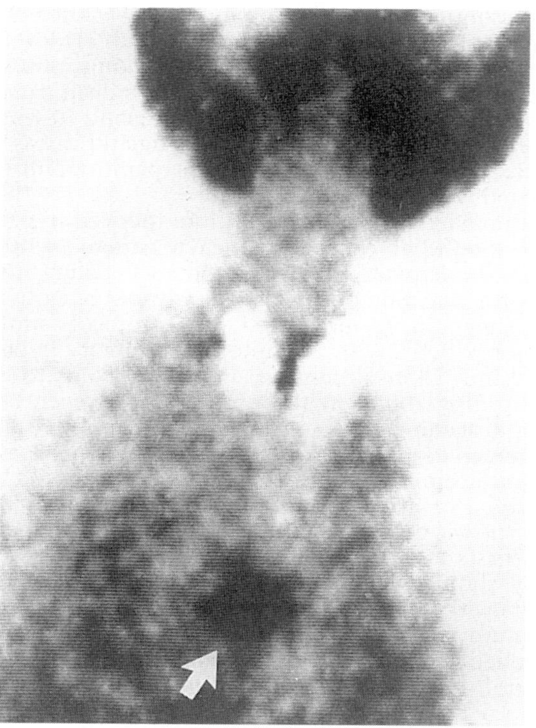

Figure 28-26 Technetium 99m (^{99m}Tc) sestamibi, iodine 123 (^{123}I) subtraction scanning of a patient with persistent hyperparathyroidism after two previous unsuccessful operations. The arrow points to parathyroid adenoma, shown as increased tracer uptake in the aortopulmonary window. (From Thule P, Thakore K, Vansant J, et al. Preoperative localization of parathyroid tissue with technetium-99m sestamibi 123I subtraction scanning. *J Clin Endocrinol Metab.* 1994;78:77-82.)

information.[283] Sestamibi does localize to thyroid nodules, which may accompany parathyroid disease in 20% to 40% of patients, although it tends to wash out from thyroid tissue much more rapidly than from parathyroids. ^{99m}Tc-sestamibi can be combined with iodine 123 (^{123}I) scanning to improve distinction of parathyroids from thyroid nodules or with single-photon emission computed tomographic (SPECT) imaging to achieve accuracy in localization not possible with planar imaging (Fig. 28-26). On the other hand, sestamibi scanning may fail to reveal small glands (uptake is related to gland size and PTH levels[284] or to demonstrate multiple abnormal glands in cases of parathyroid hyperplasia, the most common cause of persistent postoperative hyperparathyroidism.[271,285] Recently, the use of so-called four-dimensional CT with synchronous contrast-enhanced multiplanar anatomic reconstruction was shown in one study to provide sensitivity superior to sestamibi scanning alone for localizing functioning parathyroid tissue in candidates for reoperation.[286]

More invasive techniques have been used, including angiography and selective venous sampling for measurement of PTH.[287,288] Ultrasound- or CT-guided fine-needle aspiration of suspected parathyroid tissue may be used to obtain cytologic or immunochemical confirmation before surgery, and intraoperative ultrasonography has been useful in some cases to locate cervical or intrathyroidal glands.[274] Video-assisted thoracoscopic resection of documented mediastinal lesions has been successful[262,289] and offers a less invasive alternative to median sternotomy for this relatively common cause of persistent hyperparathyroidism.

The need for these procedures depends on the experience of the original surgeon and the confidence that the neck was adequately explored initially. For example, among reoperations at one center, more than half of the "missed" hyperplastic parathyroid glands in cases previously explored by a highly experienced parathyroid surgeon were found in the mediastinum or another ectopic location, whereas more than 90% of cases referred by less experienced surgeons were discovered in a normal anatomic location in the neck.[210]

After successful surgery for primary hyperparathyroidism, bone mass typically improves by as much as 5% to 10% during the first year at sites rich in trabecular bone (spine, femoral neck), whereas improvement at cortical sites (distal radius) is less predictable.[218,290] Increases at trabecular sites may continue for several years, to as much as 12% to 15% after 10 years, although normal bone mineral density may not be achieved. This improvement, which is most apparent in those with the greatest preoperative reductions in bone mass, may be related in part to rapid remineralization of the previously enlarged bone remodeling volume,[265] but the continued improvement over years suggests a more sustained increase in net bone formation and total bone volume as well.[218]

Familial Hypocalciuric Hypercalcemia

FHH, also appropriately called *familial benign hypercalcemia*, is, in most families, a disorder of autosomal dominant inheritance caused by mutations of the CASR gene found in parathyroid glands, kidney, and other organs (see earlier discussion of calcium sensing). The mutations, which cause complete or partial loss of function of the CASR, lead to a shift in the parathyroid cell's setpoint for calcium.[291] As a consequence, higher than normal levels of blood calcium are needed to suppress PTH secretion. Furthermore, abnormal function of the CASR in the renal thick ascending limb leads to increased PTH-independent calcium reabsorption and consequent hypocalciuria.

The presence of one normal sensing receptor gene with the abnormal one usually leads to a very mild clinical disorder, although the receptor functions as a dimer, and certain mutations can worsen the function of the normal allele. Rare patients who inherit mutant CASR genes from both parents present at birth with severe, life-threatening, primary hyperparathyroidism and almost always require immediate parathyroid surgery. In another genetic variation, a familial form of CASR-dependent hypercalcemia has been described in association with other autoimmune disorders such as Hashimoto's hypothyroidism and celiac sprue, in which autoantibodies directed against the sensor apparently antagonize calcium recognition by the parathyroids and renal tubules.[292,293]

FHH is manifested at birth by hypercalcemia. Although some controversy exists, most observers have concluded that the condition is asymptomatic and that apparent symptoms represent ascertainment bias. Possible exceptions include the occurrence of chondrocalcinosis and perhaps pancreatitis. The blood calcium level is usually less than 12 mg/dL but can be higher. Phosphate measurements are low, as in primary hyperparathyroidism. Blood magnesium levels are high-normal or slightly elevated. PTH levels are inappropriately normal for the degree of hypercalcemia and are occasionally modestly elevated. Urine calcium is usually low, although one novel mutation in the receptor's intracellular tail has been associated with hypercalciuria, possibly because of only mild dysfunction in the kidney.[294]

When patients present as adults, the distinction between FHH and mild primary hyperparathyroidism can be

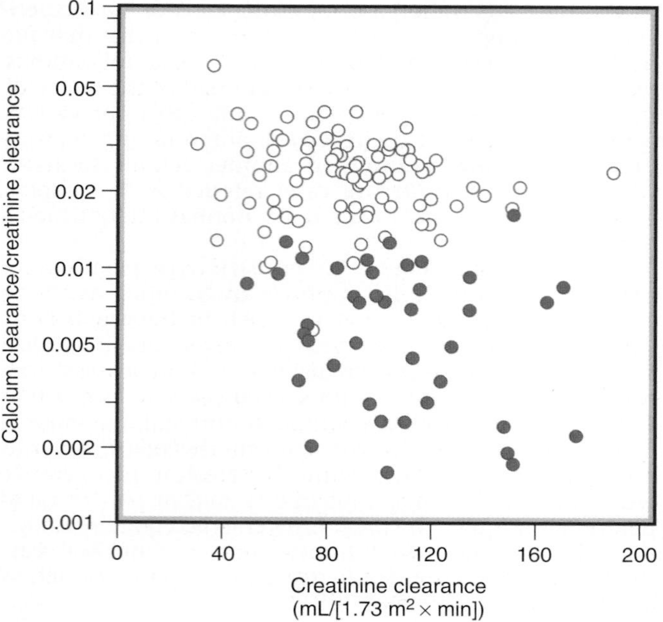

Figure 28-27 Index of urinary excretion rate for calcium as a function of creatinine clearance. Each point represents the mean of multiple determinations for a hypercalcemic patient with either familial hypocalciuric hypercalcemia *(filled circles)* or typical primary hyperparathyroidism *(open circles)*. The data are based on average 24-hour urinary excretion values and average fasting serum samples. (From Marx SJ, Attie MF, Levine M, et al. The hypocalciuric or benign variant of familial hypercalcemia: clinical and biochemical features in fifteen kindreds. *Medicine [Baltimore].* 1981;60:397-412.)

difficult. However, this distinction is crucial. Young patients with primary hyperparathyroidism are usually treated surgically and cured. In contrast, hypercalcemia always recurs after surgery for FHH, unless the patient is rendered hypoparathyroid by the removal of all parathyroid tissue. Therefore, surgery is contraindicated as therapy for FHH, except in the very rare patient with severe, symptomatic hypercalcemia. No blood or urine measurements are completely reliable for distinguishing between the two conditions, although the ratio of calcium clearance (Cl_{Ca}) to Cl_{Cr} differentiates most patients with FHH from those with primary hyperparathyroidism.[295] However, although this ratio separates the two groups with modest overlap (Fig. 28-27), primary hyperparathyroidism is much more common than FHH, so most patients with values near the cutoff Cl_{Ca}/Cl_{Cr} ratio of 0.01 have primary hyperparathyroidism and not FHH. Consequently, a case can be made[296] that many such patients, particularly before parathyroid surgery, should undergo sequencing of their CASR gene, a procedure that is now available commercially. The most helpful diagnostic information is the presence of hypercalcemia in an infant relative; such early hypercalcemia does not occur in MEN1. Furthermore, a past history of clearly normal blood calcium concentrations, considerably lower than current measurements, makes FHH unlikely in the absence of another reason for a change in blood calcium levels.

Lithium Toxicity

Treatment of bipolar affective disorders with lithium commonly leads to mild, persistent increases in blood calcium,[297] occasionally out of the normal range, in affected persons. After several years of therapy, clear elevations of PTH levels and modest increases in parathyroid gland size, detected by ultrasonography, often occur. Usually, after lithium therapy is stopped, the blood calcium and PTH levels normalize within several months. Uncommonly, substantial hypercalcemia and clear hyperparathyroidism ensue. At surgery, both single-gland and multigland disease are found, with a higher fraction of multigland disease than in patients who have primary hyperparathyroidism not associated with lithium therapy.[298]

The management of mild, lithium-induced hypercalcemia is somewhat complicated. Like patients with mild primary hyperparathyroidism, patients taking lithium usually tolerate mild hypercalcemia without obvious symptoms. They can be monitored with protocols similar to those for patients with asymptomatic primary hyperparathyroidism. Close attention must be paid to urine-concentrating ability in these patients, however, because the nephrogenic diabetes insipidus associated with lithium therapy can lead to dehydration and sudden worsening of hypercalcemia. Substantial hypercalcemia should lead to withdrawal of lithium therapy, if possible, with substitution of newer psychopharmacologic agents. If hypercalcemia persists after withdrawal of lithium, decisions about surgery should follow the same guidelines as for those patients with primary hyperparathyroidism.

Lithium increases the setpoint for PTH secretion when it is added to isolated parathyroid cells in vitro, and the setpoint for PTH secretion in vivo is shifted to the right in patients who have received lithium for several years. A corresponding shift in the concentration of extracellular calcium needed to raise intracellular calcium levels[299] suggests that lithium interferes with the action of the parathyroid CASR.

Parathyroid-Independent Hypercalcemia

In parathyroid-independent hypercalcemia, PTH secretion is appropriately suppressed. PTH levels, measured with the use of two-site assays, are invariably lower than 25 pg/mL and are usually lower than normal or undetectable. Most affected patients have malignant hypercalcemia, although parathyroid-independent hypercalcemia occurs in a number of other settings as well.[300]

Hypercalcemia of Malignancy

The presentation of malignant hypercalcemia is seldom a subtle one.[101] Most malignancies produce hypercalcemia only when they are far advanced; the diagnosis becomes evident after routine studies, guided by the history and physical examination. Patients with malignant hypercalcemia usually die within 1 or 2 months after hypercalcemia is discovered. Patients present with the classic signs and symptoms of hypercalcemia: confusion, polydipsia, polyuria, constipation, nausea, and vomiting. Perhaps because of the acuteness of the hypercalcemia and the elderly patient population involved, dramatic changes in mental status, culminating in coma, are relatively common. The diagnosis can be missed because the manifestations often overlap those of the underlying malignancy and because low blood albumin may lead to an apparently normal total blood calcium value despite an elevated blood ionized calcium concentration. Even though the overall prognosis is grim, the diagnosis of malignant hypercalcemia is important to make.

Treatment is usually simple and effective in the short term; such treatment can importantly reverse the patient's symptoms for several weeks and can even provide time for a fundamental attack on the underlying tumor, if it is treatable. Only effective treatment of the underlying neoplasm can significantly influence the long-term prognosis for patients with malignant hypercalcemia.

Although mechanisms in a given patient may be multiple, it is still useful to distinguish hypercalcemia associated with local involvement of bone from that caused by humoral mechanisms. In all cases, resorption of bone plays a pivotal role in the pathogenesis.

Local Osteolytic Hypercalcemia. Hypercalcemia resulting from tumors invading bone occurs most clearly in multiple myeloma and in some cases of breast cancer. There is little evidence that the tumor cells themselves resorb bone. Instead, active osteoclasts found near the tumor cells are thought to be the proximate mediators of bone resorption.[301] Myeloma cells and marrow cells associated with myeloma cells secrete numerous cytokines and chemokines that are capable of stimulating bone resorption, including MIP1, lymphotoxin (TNF-β), and interleukins 1β, 3, and 6. These factors lead to increased expression of RANKL (see Fig. 28-9) on the surface of marrow stromal cells and to stimulation of osteoclast formation and activity. RANKL is also found on the surface of myeloma cells, so these cells may directly stimulate the production and activity of osteoclasts. The increased bone resorption not only releases calcium into the circulation but also weakens the bone structurally. Bone is further weakened by the suppression of bone formation resulting from secretion of dickkopf-1, an inhibitor of Wnt signaling, by myeloma cells.[302,303] In patients with myeloma, treatment with intermittent intravenous bisphosphonates inhibits bone resorption and reduces the incidence of bone pain, fracture, and hypercalcemia.

The pathogenesis of hypercalcemia in breast cancer is not completely understood. Extensive metastases to bone are detected in most patients with hypercalcemia and breast cancer; this finding suggests that factors produced in bone by the metastatic tumor cells may be important. Breast cancer cells make a host of cytokines that are capable of resorbing bone. The role of tumor-produced PTHrP may be particularly important.[303] A majority of breast cancer patients with hypercalcemia have elevated blood levels of PTHrP. This circulating PTHrP, as well as PTHrP produced in bone by metastatic tumor cells, may generate the hypercalcemia. Primary breast tumors that stain for PTHrP are more likely to result in bone metastases than are those that do not stain for PTHrP; this PTHrP may be instrumental in the establishment of lytic metastases. Animal models indicate that transforming growth factor-β, released from bone matrix by PTHrP-stimulated osteoclastic resorption, may augment PTHrP secretion by the tumor cells. The latter may be further promoted by estrogen, which may explain the occasional occurrence of hypercalcemia after institution of estrogen or tamoxifen therapy in this disease.[304]

Humoral Hypercalcemia of Malignancy. Albright, in 1941, was the first to propose that a PTH-like humoral factor caused the hypercalcemia observed in patients with malignancy but few or no bone metastases.[305] Four decades later, biochemical analysis demonstrated that such patients have high blood calcium levels, low blood phosphate levels, and high urinary cAMP levels, similar to those found in primary hyperparathyroidism, but no elevation in iPTH levels.[306] The stimulation of cAMP production was used as an assay to eventually purify PTHrP from human tumors associated with the humoral hypercalcemia of malignancy.[307]

The evidence that PTHrP mediates the humoral hypercalcemia of malignancy in most patients is substantial. As noted previously, PTHrP binds to the PTH/PTHrP receptor and mimics all of the actions of amino-terminal fragments of PTH. Blood levels of PTHrP are elevated in most patients with solid tumors and hypercalcemia. In animal models of the humoral hypercalcemia of malignancy, antibodies against PTHrP can reverse the hypercalcemia.[308]

The acute actions of PTHrP cannot explain all of the findings in patients with the hypercalcemia of malignancy, however. Acutely administered PTHrP increases blood levels of calcitriol by stimulating the renal 1α-hydroxylase, although the stimulation is less than that induced by PTH.[309] Nevertheless, patients with the humoral hypercalcemia of malignancy usually have low levels of calcitriol.[306] This finding is particularly puzzling, because human tumors associated with low calcitriol levels stimulate calcitriol synthesis after they are transplanted into nude mice.[310] Possible explanations for the low calcitriol levels observed in patients include the weak activation of the renal 1α-hydroxylase in humans by PTHrP, combined with inhibition of the 1α-hydroxylase by hypercalcemia[311] or by tumor products.

A second disparity between the acute actions of PTHrP and the findings in patients with malignant hypercalcemia involves the rate of bone formation. Acutely, PTHrP infused in rats, like PTH, leads to increased bone formation.[312] However, in patients with malignant hypercalcemia, bone formation is markedly lower than normal. The explanation for this effect may well lie in the action of other cytokines, immobilization, or particular fragments of PTHrP with novel properties.

The tumors most commonly associated with humoral hypercalcemia include squamous cell cancers of the lung, head and neck, esophagus, cervix, vulva, and skin; breast cancer; renal cell cancer; and bladder cancer. Benign or malignant pheochromocytomas, islet cell tumors, and carcinoids can also overproduce PTHrP, causing hypercalcemia. The aggressive T-cell lymphoma associated with human T-cell lymphotropic virus 1 (HTLV-1) infection is the only hematologic malignancy commonly associated with PTHrP overproduction and hypercalcemia.

It is unlikely that PTHrP is the sole cause of the humoral hypercalcemia of malignancy. As noted previously, many cytokines produced by tumors can stimulate bone resorption. The actions of these cytokines have been shown to synergize with those of PTHrP in a number of experimental models. Furthermore, in hypercalcemic patients with non-Hodgkin's lymphoma, blood levels of calcitriol were found to be higher than otherwise expected,[313] and such patients show abnormal sensitivity to 25(OH)D administration.[314] In these hypercalcemic patients, the relative importance of calcitriol cytokines, PTHrP, and immobilization needs to be clarified.

In a few reported cases, malignant tumors secrete PTH and not PTHrP.[101] Although this phenomenon has now been well documented, it should be stressed that in almost all patients with cancer and high PTH levels, concurrent primary hyperparathyroidism, not ectopic PTH production, is the cause of the hyperparathyroidism.

Vitamin D Intoxication

Because the synthesis of calcitriol is so tightly regulated, extremely large doses of vitamin D, on the order of 100,000 units per day, are required to cause hypercalcemia. Such doses are available in the United States only by prescription; therefore, most cases of vitamin D intoxication are iatrogenic. Occasionally, inadvertent ingestion occurs. Patients present with nausea, vomiting, weakness, and altered level of consciousness. Hypercalcemia can be severe and prolonged because of the storage of vitamin D in fat. As expected, PTH levels are suppressed, and levels of 25(OH)D, which are poorly regulated and reflect levels of ingested vitamin D, are dramatically elevated. In contrast, the levels of calcitriol are only modestly elevated, and they can be normal or even low. The modest changes in calcitriol levels result from downregulation of the renal 1α-hydroxylase by low levels of PTH and high levels of phosphate, calcium, FGF23, and calcitriol itself. The cause of the hypercalcemia, when it occurs in the face of normal levels of calcitriol, is uncertain but may reflect the direct action of 25(OH)D and possibly other vitamin D metabolites that are capable of binding the calcitriol receptor weakly or that may be locally 1α-hydroxylated by nonrenal 1α-hydroxylases. Also, the weaker vitamin D metabolites may displace calcitriol from the circulating VDBP and increase the concentration of active, free calcitriol.[143,315]

The hypercalcemia of vitamin D intoxication results from both increased intestinal absorption of calcium and the direct effect of calcitriol to increase resorption of bone. Therefore, in severe cases, bisphosphonate therapy can be usefully added to the therapeutic regimen of hydration and omission of dietary calcium.

Sarcoidosis and Other Granulomatous Diseases

Sarcoidosis may be associated with hypercalcemia and, even more commonly, with hypercalciuria.[316] Hypercalcemic patients have high levels of calcitriol; this probably causes the hypercalcemia, although overproduction of bone-resorbing cytokines and PTHrP may contribute in some patients. As expected in calcitriol-dependent hypercalcemia, intestinal absorption of calcium is increased and PTH levels are suppressed. The hypercalcemia and the high levels of calcitriol fall after treatment with glucocorticoids. The unregulated synthesis of calcitriol, found even in anephric patients, occurs not in the kidney but rather in the sarcoid granulomas. Removal of a large amount of granulomatous tissue can reverse hypercalcemia. Furthermore, isolated sarcoid macrophages can synthesize calcitriol from 25(OH)D, as can normal macrophages after stimulation with interferon-γ or after activation of toll-like receptors. Such macrophages express the gene encoding the identical 25(OH)D 1α-hydroxylase found in the kidney. Local synthesis of calcitriol by activated macrophages and activation of VDRs in those cells represents a paracrine system that activates antibacterial mechanisms as part of the normal action of macrophages.[138]

The unusual increase in the numbers of activated macrophages in sarcoidosis leads to elevations of blood calcium. These patients have unusual sensitivity to vitamin D and can become hypercalcemic in response to ultraviolet radiation or oral vitamin D intake. Abnormalities in calcium metabolism are usually found only in patients with active disease and large, clinically obvious total-body burdens of granulomas. Nevertheless, hypercalcemia can manifest in patients without obvious pulmonary disease. Furthermore, subtle abnormalities of vitamin D metabolism can be demonstrated even in patients with only mildly active sarcoidosis.

Hypercalcemia is also associated with other granulomatous diseases, such as tuberculosis, fungal infections, and berylliosis, and has been reported in Wegener's granulomatosis, in acquired immunodeficiency syndrome (AIDS)-related *Pneumocystis jiroveci (Pneumocystis carinii)* infection, in fat necrosis of the newborn,[317] and even in association with extensive granulomatous foreign-body reactions.[300] Patients with Crohn's disease occasionally have hypercalcemia with elevations of calcitriol, but often they have elevated calcitriol levels with normal calcium levels and low bone mass, associated with increased production of calcitriol in intestinal macrophages.[318]

Hyperthyroidism

Mild hypercalcemia can result from thyrotoxicosis.[319] Blood calcium levels seldom exceed 11 mg/dL, but mild elevations are found in a quarter of patients. Patients have low PTH levels, low calcitriol levels, and hypercalciuria. The hypercalcemia is caused by a direct action of thyroid hormone to stimulate bone resorption.[320] β-Adrenergic blocking agents can reverse the hypercalcemia.[321]

Vitamin A Intoxication

Excess ingestion of vitamin A (retinol) results in a syndrome of dry skin, pruritus, headache from pseudotumor cerebri, bone pain, and, occasionally, hypercalcemia. Hypercalcemia occurs only with the ingestion of 10 times the Recommended Dietary Allowance (RDA) of 5000 IU/day. The identical syndrome can result from ingestion of the vitamin A derivatives isotretinoin (13-*cis*-retinoic acid [Accutane]) and tretinoin (all-*trans*-retinoic acid [Retin-A]), which are used to treat acne and acute promyelocytic leukemia.[322,323] Bones can show characteristic periosteal calcification on radiographs. The hypercalcemia is probably caused by the action of retinoids to stimulate bone resorption. The diagnosis is made by association of a history of excess ingestion of retinoids with the characteristic syndrome and abnormal results of liver function tests; elevated vitamin A levels confirm the diagnosis. Treatment involves hydration and, if necessary, glucocorticoids or bisphosphonates.

Adrenal Insufficiency

Hypercalcemia occurs in the setting of adrenal insufficiency. Blood calcium is elevated partly as a result of hemoconcentration and increased albumin levels, but the level of ionized calcium can also be increased.[324] PTH and calcitriol levels are low to low-normal.[325] The hypercalcemia in this study resulted from a combination of influx of calcium into the vascular space, probably from bone, and low renal clearance.

Thiazide Diuretics

Thiazide diuretics do not cause hypercalcemia by themselves, but they can exacerbate the hypercalcemia of primary hyperparathyroidism or any other cause of increased input of calcium into the bloodstream that is not suppressed by hypercalcemia. The mechanism of the hypercalcemia may involve the action of thiazide diuretics to increase proximal tubular calcium reabsorption as a secondary consequence of direct action of thiazides on the distal tubule.[326] Decreased renal clearance of calcium alone would be expected to raise blood calcium in the normal human only transiently because the transient hypercalcemia should suppress PTH secretion and lead to return of the blood calcium to normal. However, in the presence of primary hyperparathyroidism, sarcoidosis, excess calcium intake, or any other cause of high, fixed calcium load, thiazide administration will increase the level of calcium in blood.

As predicted by this model, thiazide administration leads to chronic hypercalcemia in patients with abnormal parathyroid physiology but not in normal individuals.[327] In primary hyperparathyroidism, thiazide administration exacerbates the hypercalcemia; in hypoparathyroidism, thiazide administration facilitates the maintenance of normocalcemia when given in conjunction with calcitriol and calcium.

Milk-Alkali Syndrome

The triad of hypercalcemia, metabolic alkalosis, and renal failure can be the consequence of massive ingestion of calcium and absorbable alkali. This syndrome was first described when milk and sodium bicarbonate were used in large amounts to treat peptic ulcer disease. With the change in ulcer treatment to nonabsorbable antacids and suppression of acid secretion, milk-alkali syndrome became rare. In the last several years, however, the increased use of calcium carbonate to treat dyspepsia and osteoporosis has led to the reappearance of milk-alkali syndrome.[328] In most cases, a history of ingestion of several grams per day of calcium in the form of calcium carbonate can be elicited. The pathogenesis of the syndrome is not understood in detail but may well involve a vicious circle in which alkalosis decreases renal calcium clearance and hypercalcemia helps maintain alkalosis. Nephrocalcinosis, nephrogenic diabetes insipidus, decreased GFR associated with hypercalcemia, and hypovolemia from vomiting all lead to renal failure, which can be severe. PTH levels, measured with currently available two-site assays, are invariably low in hypercalcemic patients, as are levels of calcitriol. After clearance of the calcium by hydration or by dialysis, if necessary, renal function usually returns to normal, unless the disorder has been severe and long-standing.

Immobilization

Immobilization can lead to bone resorption sufficient to cause hypercalcemia. The immobilization is usually caused by spinal cord injury or extensive casting after fractures, although it can occur in settings such as Parkinson's disease.[329] Hypercalcemia of immobilization occurs predominantly in the young and in patients with other reasons for a high rate of bone turnover, such as Paget's disease or extensive fractures. Hypercalciuria and substantial bone loss are more common than hypercalcemia. After spinal cord injury, the hypercalciuria is maximal at 4 months and can persist for longer than 1 year. PTH and calcitriol levels are suppressed, and bone biopsies show increased resorption and decreased formation of bone. Osteocytes are essential mediators of the bone loss associated with immobilization.[330] Bisphosphonates have been used to reverse the hypercalcemia and hypercalciuria of spinal cord injury.

Renal Failure

After rhabdomyolysis, during the oliguric phase of acute renal failure, severe hypocalcemia can result from acute hyperphosphatemia and calcium deposition in muscle.[331] PTH levels are high. In the diuretic phase that follows, hypercalcemia can occur. The hypercalcemia results from the high calcitriol levels observed in some patients and from mobilization of the calcium deposits.[332]

In chronic renal failure, hypercalcemia can result from tertiary hyperparathyroidism, or it may appear during therapy for aplastic bone disease associated with low PTH levels and sometimes with aluminum toxicity.

Williams' Syndrome

Williams' syndrome is a developmental disorder in which supravalvular aortic stenosis is associated with elfin facies and mental retardation.[333] Hypercalcemia can occur transiently in the first 4 years of life. Affected hypercalcemic infants have been found to have increased intestinal absorption of calcium and associated elevations of calcitriol that fall to normal as the blood calcium level normalizes.[334] Levels of 25(OH)D are normal. The hypercalcemia can usually be controlled by dietary manipulation and, if needed, bisphosphonates.[335]

Molecular analysis has clarified the origin of the connective tissue component of Williams' syndrome. Isolated supravalvular aortic stenosis is associated with deletion or translocation of the distal portion of the elastin gene. Williams' syndrome, with more protean connective tissue abnormalities and mental retardation, is associated with large deletions that include the elastin gene and a gene encoding the protein kinase, LIM-kinase 1. A gene within the Williams' syndrome deletion region encodes a nuclear protein, Williams' syndrome transcription factor, that is part of a large chromatin-remodeling complex that can bind the VDR and influence the transcription of VDR-responsive genes.[336] This makes the gene a strong candidate for the gene associated with transient hypercalcemia in this disorder. However, genetic proof that this gene is responsible for the hypercalcemia is still lacking.

Jansen's Metaphyseal Chondrodysplasia

Jansen's metaphyseal chondrodysplasia is a rare disease in which affected persons present in childhood with short stature and hypercalcemia (Fig. 28-28). Blood chemistry studies suggest hyperparathyroidism, with high calcium, low-normal phosphate, high calcitriol, high alkaline phosphatase, and high urinary hydroxyproline, but PTH levels are suppressed.[337] A generalized defect in endochondral bone formation results from abnormally organized chondrocytes in growth plates. Metaphyses appear disordered and rachitic on radiographs. The bones may show signs of osteitis fibrosa cystica. Constitutive activation of the PTH/PTHrP receptor, caused by point mutations in the transmembrane domains of the receptor, explains the findings in this disorder.[89,338] The abnormalities on serum chemistry studies result from PTH-like actions of the receptor in bone and kidney. The growth plate disorder results from PTHrP-like actions of the receptor on the growth plate.

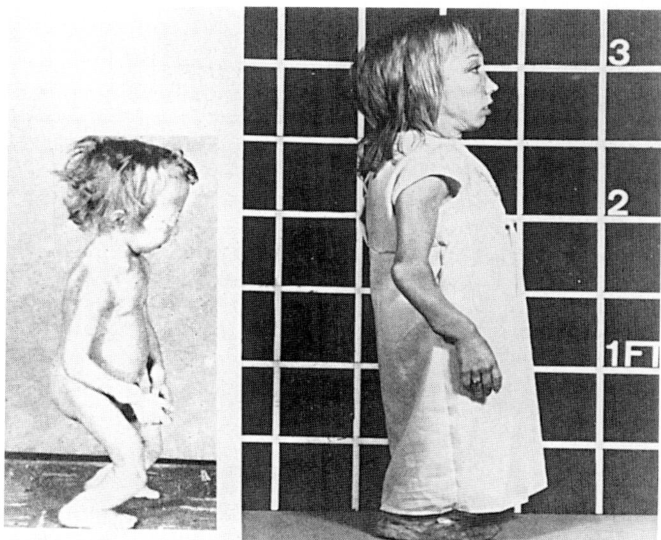

Figure 28-28 A patient with Jansen's metaphyseal chondrodysplasia at ages 5 years and 22 years. Note the short stature, characteristic facies, and misshapen metaphyseal region of long bones. (From Frame B, Poznanski AK. Conditions that may be confused with rickets. In DeLuca HF, Anastas CS, eds. *Pediatric Diseases Related to Calcium.* New York: Elsevier; 1980:269-289.)

Approach to the Hypercalcemic Patient

The diagnostic approach to the hypercalcemic patient is strongly influenced by the clinical setting and the knowledge that primary hyperparathyroidism is at least twice as common as all other causes combined (Table 28-2). These considerations are particularly significant in the patient who seems otherwise well and in whom the hypercalcemia is detected incidentally or is mild, stable, or known to be of long duration (i.e., years). Among outpatients referred to endocrinologists for evaluation of hypercalcemia, more than 90% are found to have primary hyperparathyroidism. Among ill or hospitalized patients, malignant disease is the cause in more than 50% of cases. The differential diagnosis is seldom complicated, however, because malignant hypercalcemia usually manifests in the context of advanced, clinically obvious disease.

Because hypercalcemia usually is first detected as an elevation of total serum calcium, it is important to distinguish hemoconcentration or rare instances of calcium-binding paraproteinemia or thrombocythemia-associated hypercalcemia (due to release of intracellular calcium in vitro) from a true increase in serum ionized calcium (Fig. 28-29). The presence of hypercalcemia should be confirmed by direct measurement of ionized calcium, and the total calcium measurement should be repeated, together with albumin, globulin electrolytes, blood urea nitrogen, creatinine, and phosphate. Especially when hypercalcemia is mild, it is prudent to repeat the serum total or ionized calcium measurement at least twice, preferably fasting and without venous occlusion, before proceeding with more costly studies directed at its etiology.

A careful history and physical examination, combined with efforts to assess chronicity by seeking prior results of routine multichannel serum chemistry determinations, most often will point to the likely diagnosis. Serum phosphate is frequently low in hyperparathyroidism, but this often is true also of PTHrP-secreting malignancies, so the presence of hypophosphatemia is not helpful in distinguishing these two possibilities. If serum phosphate is normal or high despite correction of dehydration, the possibility of PTH- or PTHrP-independent hypercalcemia should be considered more strongly. Elevations in serum chloride and alkaline phosphatase, often observed in primary hyperparathyroidism, cannot be reliably employed in the differential diagnosis of hypercalcemia. Important elements in the medical history of hypercalcemic patients include inquiries about kidney stones or fractures; weight loss; back or bone pain; fatigue or weakness; cough or dyspnea; ulcer disease or pancreatitis; ingestion of vitamins, calcium preparations, lithium, or thiazides; dates of most recent mammograms and chest radiographs; and a family history of hypercalcemia, kidney stones, ulcer disease, endocrinopathy, or tumors of the head or neck. Because malignancy is a common cause of hypercalcemia and may occur concomitantly with primary hyperparathyroidism, clinical findings strongly suggestive of malignancy should be acted upon by proceeding directly to a search for an underlying tumor, regardless of serum PTH.

The single most important test in the differential diagnosis of hypercalcemia is the measurement of serum PTH, preferably in a two-site assay specific for the intact, biologically active molecule (see Fig. 28-20). New PTH assays have been introduced that ignore long circulating fragments of the hormone, which lack the amino-terminal residues required for activity at the PTH/PTHrP receptor, but whether these will be more useful than standard "intact PTH" assays remains to be established.[339,340] A consistently elevated serum PTH in the presence of true hypercalcemia always is abnormal and almost always indicates the presence of primary hyperparathyroidism. The exceptions that also can be associated with elevated PTH levels are FHH, autonomous parathyroid secretion complicating secondary hyperparathyroidism (so-called tertiary hyperparathyroidism), lithium-associated hyperparathyroidism, and, very rarely, ectopic PTH secretion by a malignant neoplasm or the presence of antagonizing autoantibodies directed against the CASR in patients with another autoimmune disease—an acquired condition that mimics FHH.[341,342]

Diagnosis of primary hyperparathyroidism is complicated by the fact that some patients fail to exhibit both hypercalcemia and elevated iPTH. In up to 10% of patients with hypercalcemia and primary hyperparathyroidism, PTH levels fall within the high-normal range with current PTH assays. However, in the face of hypercalcemia, such PTH levels are inappropriate and support the diagnosis of PTH-dependent hypercalcemia. In fact, many such patients will manifest frankly elevated serum PTH if retested, especially if dietary calcium is restricted beforehand. As noted earlier, some patients present with serum calcium in the high-normal range (>10.0 mg/dL) and an elevated or high-normal PTH. This may be discovered incidentally in an otherwise asymptomatic patient or in the course of evaluation of recurrent urolithiasis or osteopenia. Those with persistently high-normal serum calcium and high-normal iPTH should be retested at intervals and, meanwhile, given a provisional diagnosis of hyperparathyroidism and evaluated accordingly.

In patients with PTH-dependent hypercalcemia (Fig. 28-30), calcium and creatinine should be measured in a 24-hour urine collection with a simultaneous serum sample to determine total urinary calcium output (milligrams per

TABLE 28-2

Causes of Hypercalcemia

Causes of Hypercalcemia
Parathyroid-Dependent Hypercalcemia
Primary hyperparathyroidism
Tertiary hyperparathyroidism
Familial hypocalciuric hypercalcemia
Lithium-associated hypercalcemia
Antagonistic autoantibodies to the calcium-sensing receptor
Parathyroid-Independent Hypercalcemia
Neoplasms
PTHrP-dependent
Other humoral syndromes
Local osteolytic disease (including metastases)
PTHrP excess (non-neoplastic)
Excess vitamin D action
Ingestion of excess vitamin D or vitamin D analogues
Topical vitamin D analogues
Granulomatous disease
Williams' syndrome
Thyrotoxicosis
Adrenal insufficiency
Renal failure
Acute renal failure
Chronic renal failure with aplastic bone disease
Immobilization
Jansen's disease
Drugs
Vitamin A intoxication
Milk-alkali syndrome
Thiazide diuretics
Theophylline

PTHrP, parathyroid hormone–related protein.

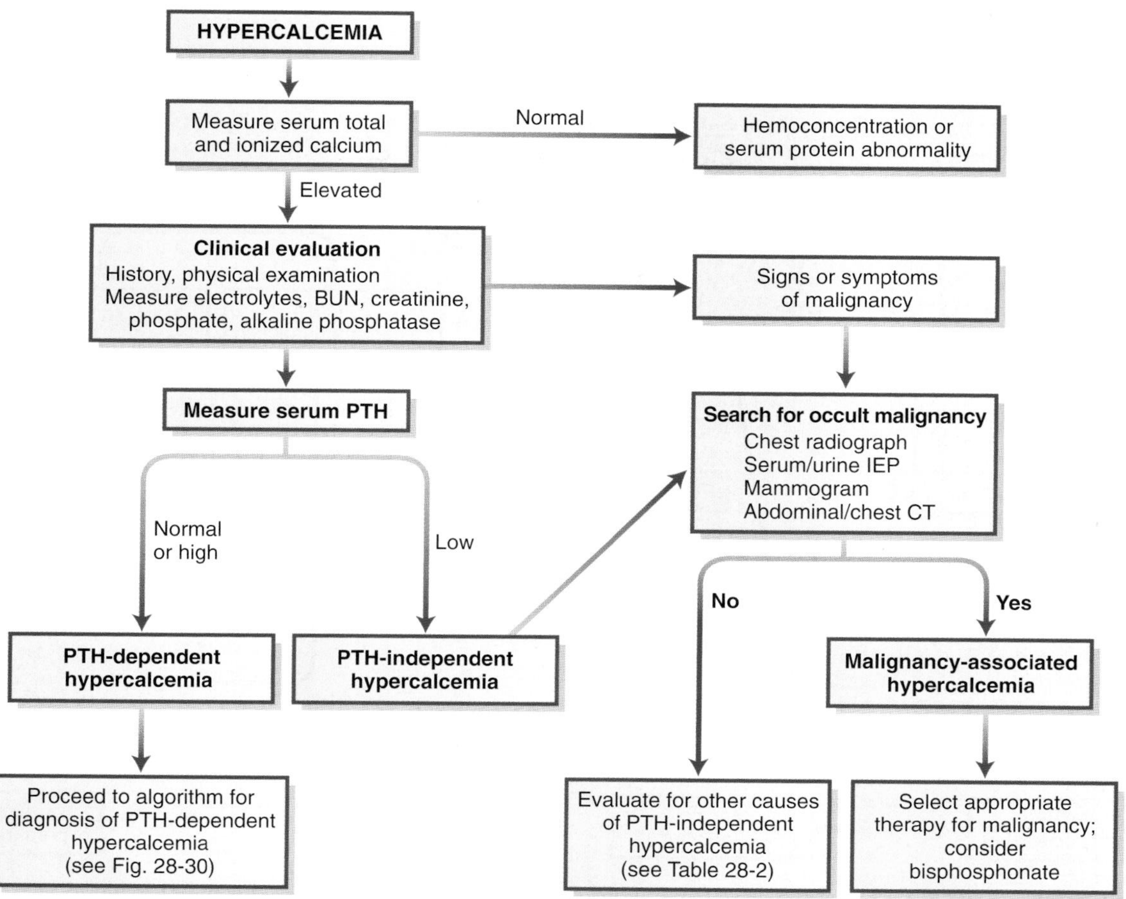

Figure 28-29 Approach to the management of hypercalcemia. BUN, blood urea nitrogen; CT, computed tomography; IEP, immunoelectrophoresis; PTH, parathyroid hormone.

day) and the clearance rates of calcium and creatinine (Cl_{Ca} and Cl_{Cr}, respectively). A calcium excretion rate of less than 100 mg/day or a Cl_{Ca}/Cl_{Cr} ratio of less than 0.01 should prompt consideration of FHH, especially in patients who are younger than 40 years of age, have a family history of FHH, or have serum iPTH levels within the normal range. A urinary calcium excretion rate greater than 4 mg/kg per day or a Cl_{Ca}/Cl_{Cr} ratio greater than 0.02 effectively excludes FHH. In FHH, serum phosphate is normal or slightly low, serum magnesium may be slightly high, and serum calcitriol is normal or low (unlike in primary hyperparathyroidism).

A definite diagnosis of FHH, as in the MEN syndromes, may be provided by confirming the presence of mutations in the relevant genes; however, such studies are not invariably informative, presumably because of mutations in introns and other unchecked regions, and they are usually unnecessary. The identification of *RET* gene mutations is now an essential part of the management in families with MEN2, because this information most effectively guides the decision for preventive thyroidectomy to prevent medullary cancer of the thyroid. In contrast, the identification of mutations in the menin gene has not yet led to any effective preventive strategies, so genetic analysis may be useful only for genetic counseling in families with MEN1. Even for this purpose, however, the incomplete ascertainment of mutations limits the effectiveness of such analysis.

In patients with suspected lithium-induced hyperparathyroidism, a trial off lithium, if feasible clinically, may confirm the diagnosis or indicate the presence of persistent primary hyperparathyroidism. Patients with primary hyperparathyroidism should undergo bone densitometry, preferably at both cortical- and trabecular-rich sites (i.e., forearm or hip and lumbar spine, respectively) to assist in the decision about surgery. Those who are younger than 40 years of age or have a family history of hypercalcemia (or other MEN manifestations) should be evaluated for these syndromes as well. Patients not meeting criteria for parathyroidectomy should be monitored medically, as should those with FHH. In the rare patients with CASR-blocking autoantibodies, hypercalcemia may respond to glucocorticoids.[342]

A low or undetectable serum PTH level signifies the presence of nonparathyroid hypercalcemia and should prompt a detailed evaluation for malignancy or other causes of PTH-independent hypercalcemia (see Table 28-2). Breast and lung cancers alone account for more than 50% of all cases of malignancy-associated hypercalcemia. Mammography, chest radiography with or without CT, abdominal CT, and serum and urinary immunoelectrophoresis are among the more useful tests for detecting the cause of nonparathyroid hypercalcemia. Although humoral mechanisms, especially secretion of PTHrP, are implicated in the pathogenesis of most cancer-associated hypercalcemias, bone metastases are common, particularly in breast cancer. Technetium 99m bone scanning is useful for detecting this syndrome and identifying bones vulnerable to fracture. The utility of serum PTHrP measurements probably is limited to the unusual situation in which serum PTH is

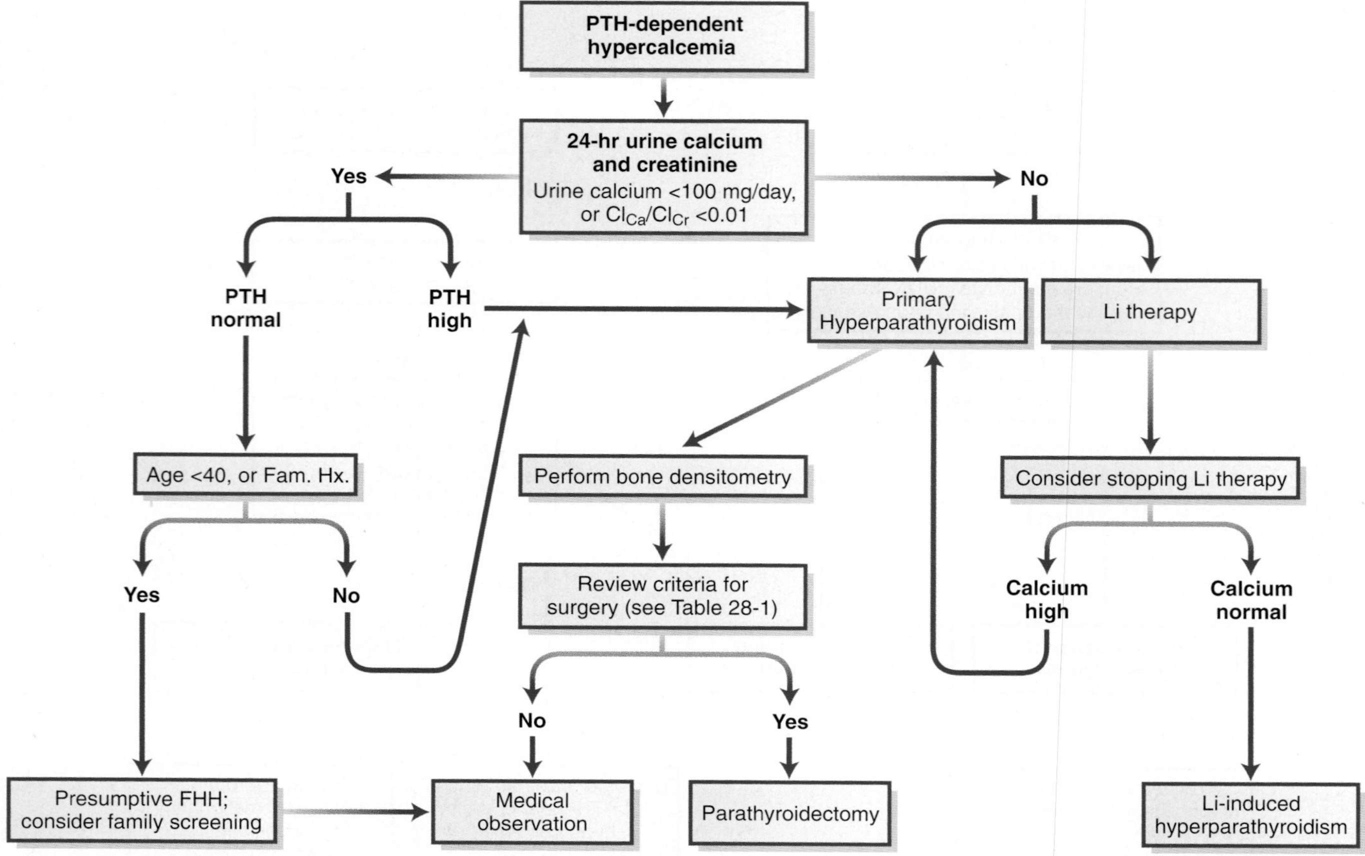

Figure 28-30. Approach to the management of hypercalcemia in patients with parathyroid hormone–dependent hypercalcemia. Cl, clearance; Fam. Hx., family history; FHH, familial hypocalciuric hypercalcemia; Li, lithium; PTH, parathyroid hormone.

suppressed but an underlying malignancy cannot readily be demonstrated. PTHrP-associated hypercalcemia can occur rarely during pregnancy and lactation, via secretion from benign neoplasms or in association with lymphoid hyperplasia in patients with lupus erythematosus or human immunodeficiency virus (HIV) infection.[343]

In the absence of evident malignancy, unusual causes of hypercalcemia should be sought.[343] Intoxication with vitamin D and vitamin A can be excluded by measurement of serum 25(OH)D and retinoids, respectively. Elevated calcitriol and hypercalcemia may occur in several settings, including sarcoidosis and other granulomatous diseases, B-cell and T-cell lymphomas (including AIDS-associated lymphomas), and, uncommonly, Crohn's disease, neonatal subcutaneous fat necrosis syndrome, and epithelial neoplasms such as lung cancer. Very rarely, patients with severe idiopathic hypercalciuria and excessive absorption of dietary calcium may manifest mild, dietary-dependent hypercalcemia. Overtreatment of hypoparathyroidism or other conditions with oral calcitriol or topical use of analogues of the active metabolite in psoriasis should be obvious from the history. Because hypercalcemia and hypercalciuria are observed in up to 10% and 30%, respectively, of patients with thyrotoxicosis, measurement of serum thyroid-stimulating hormone may be helpful, especially in older patients, who may be less overtly symptomatic. Adrenal insufficiency and pheochromocytoma usually are accompanied by characteristic clinical features, but a definite diagnosis may be sought with appropriate studies. Granulomatous diseases are among the more common disorders that underlie initially unexplained hypercalcemia.

Management of Severe Hypercalcemia

Causes of Severe Hypercalcemia

The need for urgent treatment of acute, severe hypercalcemia, usually defined as a serum calcium concentration greater than 14 mg/dL (3.5 mmol/L), is unusual. This is because most patients with hypercalcemia have primary hyperparathyroidism, in which hypercalcemia is typically chronic and mild. Episodes of acute, severe hypercalcemia may occur occasionally in primary hyperparathyroidism ("parathyroid crisis"), usually in patients with large parathyroid adenomas and very high PTH levels. The severe hypercalcemia in this setting may be triggered by dehydration resulting from diarrheal illness, protracted vomiting, or diuretic therapy; recovery from major surgery; immobilization; ingestion of large amounts of oral calcium salts; hemorrhage or rupture of a cystic parathyroid neoplasm; or parathyroid carcinoma.

Most often, acute, severe hypercalcemia is encountered in patients with underlying malignancy, in whom accelerated bone resorption dramatically increases the filtered load of calcium. The ensuing profound hypercalciuria impairs renal tubular sodium reabsorption, which induces progressive extracellular volume depletion, reduces GFR, impairs renal calcium clearance, and further aggravates the hypercalcemia. In many such patients, elevated circulating levels of PTHrP compound the problem by mimicking the action of PTH to enhance distal tubular calcium reabsorption.

Clinical Features of Severe Hypercalcemia

The indications for urgent treatment of hypercalcemia usually relate more to the presence of clinical symptoms of hypercalcemia than to the absolute level of serum calcium, although few clinicians would hesitate to treat patients in whom total serum calcium exceeded 14 mg/dL (3.5 mmol/L). Many patients with previously mild hypercalcemia become symptomatic when serum calcium concentrations exceed 12 mg/dL (3.0 mmol/L). It is important to remember that hypoalbuminemia can mask significant elevations of ionized calcium. The most common symptoms of severe hypercalcemia are referable to disturbances of nervous system and gastrointestinal function: fatigue, weakness, lethargy, confusion, coma (rarely), anorexia, nausea, abdominal pain (rarely due to pancreatitis), and constipation. Polyuria, nocturia, and polydipsia commonly are present also.

Bone pain is often present but is usually a result of the underlying metastatic disease. Cardiac arrhythmias may occur, particularly bradyarrhythmias or heart block; digitalis toxicity may be potentiated, and ST-segment elevation responsive to treatment of the hypercalcemia may be seen. Patients who suffer a fatal outcome from acute severe hypercalcemia may manifest coma, hypotension, acute pancreatitis, acute renal failure, widespread soft tissue calcification, heart failure, or venous thrombosis, particularly of the renal veins.

Treatment of Severe Hypercalcemia

The first decision to be made in the management of acute, severe hypercalcemia is whether to treat the problem at all. This may become an issue for the patient with an untreatable, widely disseminated malignancy if all other approaches to controlling the neoplasm have been exhausted and the patient has chosen not to have complications treated. Otherwise, as noted earlier, patients who are symptomatic or have serum calcium levels greater than 14 mg/dL ordinarily should be treated aggressively. Treatment most often entails rehydration and administration of a bisphosphonate intravenously (Table 28-3). Calcitonin can be useful as a temporary measure early in therapy, and glucocorticoids or dialysis may be indicated in some patients.[344]

Volume Repletion. When treatment is indicated, the first priority is to correct the extracellular volume depletion that almost invariably is present, usually by infusing isotonic saline at a rate of 2 to 4 L/day. The aggressiveness with which the individual patient is rehydrated must be considered in relation to both the patient's volume status and the risk of precipitating or aggravating congestive heart failure or ascites. Diuretics, particularly thiazides, should be discontinued. The use of furosemide or other potent loop diuretics to promote calciuresis may exacerbate extracellular volume depletion if used too early in the course of treatment. In light of the availability of highly effective alternatives for the treatment of hypercalcemia, such drugs probably are best avoided, except in circumstances in which vigorous rehydration fails to improve severe hypercalcemia or might precipitate congestive heart failure. In any case, prolonged use of saline-induced calciuresis without the early introduction of an effective antiresorptive agent is ill-advised and ultimately futile.

Bisphosphonates. Intravenous bisphosphonates rapidly inhibit bone resorption and currently are the agents of first choice in managing severe hypercalcemia that is known or suspected to be driven mainly by osteoclastic bone resorption.[344] Bisphosphonates should not be used in patients with milk-alkali syndrome, in whom they are likely to induce post-treatment hypocalcemia.[345] Pamidronate and zoledronate are approved by the U.S. Food and Drug Administration for treatment of malignant hypercalcemia and are the most widely used agents in the United States, although ibandronate and clodronate have been successfully deployed elsewhere. These drugs generally are well tolerated, although local pain or swelling at the infusion site, low-grade fever lasting 1 to 2 days after the infusion, transient lymphopenia, and mild hypophosphatemia or hypomagnesemia may occur. Serum calcium usually declines within 24 hours and reaches a nadir within 1 week after a single infusion, at which point calcium levels may be normal in 70% to 90% of treated patients. Intravenous bisphosphonates may be nephrotoxic, but clinical data to guide their use in patients with renal insufficiency are not yet available. Most clinicians employ the standard dose (see Table 28-3), perhaps at half or less of the usual rate of administration, in patients with moderate renal insufficiency (GFR >30 mL/min), which is common in the setting of severe hypercalcemia. In patients with more severe renal insufficiency, bisphosphonates probably are best avoided, and dialysis may be a more appropriate alternative (see later discussion). The duration of the response to intravenous bisphosphonate treatment is quite variable, ranging from a week or two to several months. Depending on the clinical circumstances, repeated courses of therapy may be indicated and effective.

Calcitonin. Calcitonin, which directly inhibits osteoclast function, may be used with other antiresorptive agents to achieve more rapid control of severe hypercalcemia. However, calcitonin rarely produces a decline in serum calcium of more than 1 to 2 mg/dL, and its efficacy typically is limited to a few days at most, possibly because of receptor downregulation in target cells of bone and kidney. Its major advantages are a more rapid onset of action than bisphosphonates (several hours) and the potential to augment renal calcium excretion directly. Calcitonin usually is well tolerated, although transient nausea, vomiting, abdominal cramps, flushing, and local skin reactions may occur.

Other Approaches to Treatment of Severe Hypercalcemia. Because of their potential toxicity, other antiresorptive agents such as gallium nitrate, plicamycin (mithramycin), and intravenous phosphate (in patients with severe hypophosphatemia) have largely been abandoned in the treatment of severe hypercalcemia, although

TABLE 28-3

Management of Severe Hypercalcemia

Therapy	Usual Dose	Frequency
Rehydration	2-4 L/day of 0.9% NaCl IV	qd × 1-5 days
Furosemide	20-40 mg IV (after rehydration)	q12-24hr
Pamidronate	60-90 mg IV over 2-4 hr	Once
Zoledronate	4 mg IV over 15-30 min	Once
Calcitonin	4-8 IU/kg SC	q12-24hr
Gallium nitrate	200 mg/m^2 IV over 24 hr	qd × 5 days
Glucocorticoids	200-300 mg hydrocortisone IV	qd × 3-5 days
	40-60 mg prednisone PO	qd × 3-5 days
Dialysis		

a recent randomized trial demonstrated that gallium nitrate may be more effective than bisphosphonate in controlling hypercalcemia of malignancy.[346] Oral or enteral phosphate repletion is appropriate for patients with significant hypophosphatemia (<2.5 mg/dL), provided that serum phosphate and renal function are closely monitored. Intravenous or oral glucocorticoids should be considered early in patients with suspected vitamin D–dependent hypercalcemia, including those with lymphoma or granulomatous disease. The response to glucocorticoids may be more delayed than that to bisphosphonates. Successful treatment of hypercalcemia in Crohn's disease with infliximab has been reported.[347]

In patients with severe renal insufficiency with or without complicating heart disease, in whom saline rehydration and associated calciuresis may not be feasible and bisphosphonates probably are best avoided, dialytic therapy against a low- or zero-calcium dialysate may be the most appropriate tactic. In patients with known primary hyperparathyroidism and intercurrent severe hypercalcemia ("parathyroid storm"), urgent parathyroidectomy (after initial medical stabilization) should be considered.

Novel approaches to the treatment of severe hypercalcemia are in development. One available therapy for parathyroid carcinoma is the calcimimetic cinacalcet, which may be effective in some patients.[348] Monoclonal antibodies directed against PTHrP could prove useful in controlling PTHrP-dependent hypercalcemia,[349] and other novel antiresorptives (monoclonal antibodies against the osteoclastogenic factor RANKL or recombinant OPG, which neutralizes RANKL) are on the horizon.

HYPOCALCEMIC DISORDERS

Clinical Presentation

The predominant clinical symptoms and signs of hypocalcemia are those of neuromuscular irritability, including perioral paresthesias, tingling of the fingers and toes, and spontaneous or latent tetany. Tetany can be elicited by percussion of the facial nerve below the zygoma, resulting in ipsilateral contractions of the facial muscle (Chvostek's sign), or by 3 minutes of occlusive pressure with a blood pressure cuff resulting in carpal spasm, which on occasion can be very painful (Trousseau's sign) (Fig. 28-31). The usefulness of these signs in diagnosing hypocalcemia and in monitoring therapeutic responses cannot be overemphasized.

Electrocardiographic abnormalities also result from hypocalcemia, including prolonged QT intervals and marked QRS and ST-segment changes that may mimic acute myocardial infarction or conduction abnormalities. Ventricular arrhythmias are a rare complication of hypocalcemia, although congestive heart failure, corrected by normalization of serum calcium, has been reported.

In profound hypocalcemia or during acute falls in serum calcium, grand mal seizures or laryngospasm also may be observed. Chronic hypocalcemia is associated with milder symptoms and signs of neuromuscular irritability and may even be asymptomatic. Long-standing hypocalcemia associated with hyperphosphatemia (observed in PTH deficiency or resistance) may lead to calcification of the basal ganglia and occasional extrapyramidal disorders. In addition, mineral ion deposits in the lens may lead to cataract formation.

Chronic hypocalcemia, particularly when associated with hypophosphatemia as in vitamin D deficiency, is associated with growth plate abnormalities in children (rickets) and defects in the mineralization of new bone (osteomalacia) (see Chapter 29). Severe symptomatic hypocalcemia constitutes an emergency that requires immediate attention to prevent seizures and death from laryngospasm or cardiac causes.

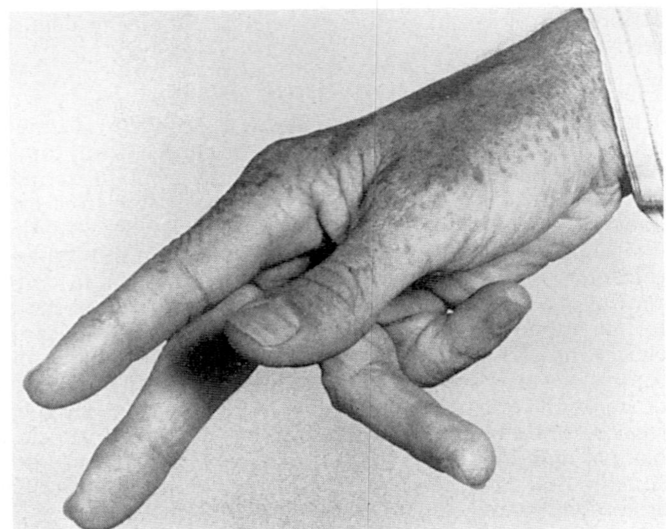

Figure 28-31 Trousseau's sign. (From Burnside JW, McGlynn TJ. *Physical Diagnosis*, 17th ed. Baltimore: Williams & Wilkins; 1987:63.)

Total calcium in serum includes both the free (biologically active) and the protein-bound components; the major binding protein is albumin (see earlier discussion). Therefore, measurements of total calcium cannot be interpreted without concurrent measurement of albumin. Studies of hypoalbuminemic patients with cirrhosis have led to a formula for correction of total calcium based on concurrent albumin levels: Calcium is decreased by 0.8 mg/dL for every 1 g/dL decrease in albumin. However, no formula has proved accurate for assessment of calcium in acutely ill patients. This probably relates to the variety of factors that can increase protein binding and decrease the fraction of total calcium present as the free ion, including alkalosis, elevated circulating free fatty acids, and lipid infusions. Consequently, ionized calcium should be measured when the diagnosis of hypocalcemia is considered in the setting of acute illness or severe hypoalbuminemia.

Chronic hypocalcemia is most often caused by deficiency of PTH or calcitriol or by resistance to the biologic effects of these calcium-regulating hormones (Table 28-4).

Parathyroid-Related Disorders

Hypocalcemia associated with parathyroid dysfunction can be differentiated from other causes of hypocalcemia by routine laboratory tests. Serum calcium is low due to lack of PTH-mediated bone resorption and urinary calcium reabsorption. Serum phosphate is increased owing to impaired renal clearance. Serum calcitriol is low because PTH and hypophosphatemia stimulate the renal 25(OH)D 1α-hydroxylase. Consequently, calcitriol-mediated intestinal calcium absorption is markedly decreased, further exacerbating the hypocalcemia. PTH levels as measured by sensitive two-site PTH assays (see Fig. 28-20) are usually low or undetectable but may be inappropriately normal if some degree of PTH production is preserved. Elevated levels of PTH are found in syndromes associated with resistance to the biologic effects of PTH.

TABLE 28-4

Causes of Hypocalcemia

Parathyroid-Related Disorders
Absence of the Parathyroid Glands or of PTH
Congenital
DiGeorge's syndrome
X-linked or autosomally inherited hypoparathyroidism
Autoimmune polyglandular syndrome type I
PTH gene mutations
Postsurgical hypoparathyroidism
Infiltrative disorders
Hemochromatosis
Wilson's disease
Metastases
Hypoparathyroidism following radioactive iodine thyroid ablation
Impaired Secretion of PTH
Hypomagnesemia
Respiratory alkalosis
Activating mutations of the calcium sensor
Target Organ Resistance
Hypomagnesemia
Pseudohypoparathyroidism
Type I
Type 2
Vitamin D–Related Disorders
Vitamin D deficiency
Dietary absence
Malabsorption
Accelerated loss
Impaired enterohepatic recirculation
Anticonvulsant medications
Impaired 25-hydroxylation
Liver disease
Isoniazid
Impaired 1α-hydroxylation
Renal failure
Vitamin D–dependent rickets type I
Oncogenic osteomalacia
Target organ resistance
Vitamin D–dependent rickets type II
Phenytoin
Other Causes
Excessive deposition into the skeleton
Osteoblastic malignancies
Hungry bone syndrome
Chelation
Foscarnet
Phosphate infusion
Infusion of citrated blood products
Infusion of EDTA-containing contrast reagents
Fluoride
Neonatal hypocalcemia
Prematurity
Asphyxia
Diabetic mother
Hyperparathyroid mother
HIV infection
Drug therapy
Vitamin D deficiency
Hypomagnesemia
Impaired PTH responsiveness
Critical illness
Pancreatitis
Toxic shock syndrome
Intensive care unit patients

EDTA, ethylenediaminetetra-acetic acid; HIV, human immunodeficiency virus; PTH, parathyroid hormone.

Congenital or Inherited Parathyroid Disorders

Several rare syndromes associated with congenital or inherited hypoparathyroidism appear sporadically or in a variety of inheritance patterns suggesting multiple etiologies. Mutation of the transcription factor GCM2 (chromosome 6p23), which is expressed in the PTH-secreting cells of the developing parathyroids, has been shown to be a cause of familial hypoparathyroidism in humans and mice.[36] Although it is usually inherited in an autosomal recessive fashion, GCM2-associated hypoparathyroidism can be autosomal dominant through expression of a dominant-negative mutant GCM2 gene.[551] The genetic abnormality responsible for X-linked, recessive hypoparathyroidism has been identified as a deletion/insertion of DNA near the *SOX3* gene at Xq26-q27.[37]

In a number of diseases, hypoparathyroidism is associated with multiple abnormalities in embryonic development in the neck and chest region. DiGeorge's syndrome occurs sporadically and is associated with an embryologic defect in the formation of the third, fourth, and fifth branchial pouches, resulting in the absence of parathyroid glands. DiGeorge's syndrome may, in fact, be a neurocrestopathy, because ablation of the premigratory cephalic neural crest in chick embryos produces the same phenotype.[350] The contribution of homeobox genes to parathyroid development and their potential relationship to DiGeorge's syndrome is also demonstrated by the absence of thymic and parathyroid tissue, accompanied by cardiac and craniofacial abnormalities, in mice lacking the homeobox gene *Hoxa3*.[351] DiGeorge's syndrome is often associated with other congenital abnormalities in a syndrome referred to by the acronym CATCH 22 (*c*ardiac defects, *a*bnormal facies, *t*hymic hypoplasia, *c*left palate, *h*ypocalcemia, and *22*q11 deletions).[352] Microdeletion of 22q11.21-q11.23[353] and a t(2;22)(q14;q11) balanced translocation suggest that a gene at chromosome 22q11 may be pathogenetic in this syndrome.[354] Hypoparathyroidism also has been reported in two patients with a 22q11 deletion.[355] Although deletion of the *TBX1* gene has been shown to be responsible for the cardiovascular defects in this syndrome,[356] the molecular basis for impaired parathyroid gland development has not yet been elucidated. A number of cases of DiGeorge's syndrome and velocardiofacial syndrome have been shown to have no detectable abnormality at 22q11, but rather terminal 10p deletions or interstitial 10p13/10p14 deletions, suggesting that two loci may be critical for the development of branchial pouch structures.[357] Terminal deletions of 10p accompanied by hypoparathyroidism can be further subdivided into the second DiGeorge critical region (10p13-p14) and a more telomeric region (10p14-10pter). In the latter region, mutation of the transcription factor GATA3 causes the HDR syndrome (*h*ypoparathyroidism, sensorineural *d*eafness, and *r*enal anomaly).[358] The genetic basis for HDR (hypoparathyroidism, retardation, dysmorphism) or the related disorder known as Kenny-Caffey syndrome, which is additionally associated with recurrent bacterial infections, has been shown to be linked to 1q43-q44; it involves mutations in the chaperone protein, TBCE, which is required for the proper folding of α-tubulin and formation of αβ-tubulin heterodimers.[359]

Familial hypoparathyroidism is seen in conjunction with mucocutaneous candidiasis, Addison's disease, and other immune disorders in autosomal recessive autoimmune polyglandular syndrome type 1, which is caused by mutations in the autoimmune regulatory gene, *AIRE*.[360,361] NALP5 (encoded by *NLRP5*) has been identified as a parathyroid-specific antigen in affected patients.[362]

Hypoparathyroidism may also be observed in association with mitochondrial myopathies such as mitochondrial trifunctional protein deficiency[363] and the Kearns-Sayre syndrome.[364] Other inherited forms of hypoparathyroidism may be observed as isolated defects[365] or in association with other features such as lymphedema, dysmorphism, and renal and cardiac abnormalities.[366,367]

Abnormalities in the Parathyroid Hormone Gene

Specific defects have been found in the PTH gene in a small number of kindreds affected by congenital hypoparathyroidism. These include point mutations in the signal peptide[368,369] and in an intron border, leading to aberrant splicing.[370] No abnormalities in the sequences encoding PTH^{1-84} have been discovered in familial hypoparathyroidism.

Destruction of the Parathyroid Glands

The most common cause of chronic hypocalcemia is postsurgical hypoparathyroidism. This may occur after removal of all parathyroid tissue during thyroidectomy and radical neck dissection for malignancies, or after inadvertent interruption of the blood supply to the parathyroid glands during head and neck surgery. Transient hypoparathyroidism, attributed to reversible damage to the remaining normal glands, is common after parathyroidectomy; permanent hypoparathyroidism may occur after vascular or surgical injury or inadvertent removal of all parathyroid tissue. Rarely, transient hypoparathyroidism may follow spontaneous infarction of autonomous tissue in primary hyperparathyroidism.[371] Hypoparathyroidism is a rare complication of radioactive iodine ablation of the thyroid gland in patients with Graves' disease.[372]

Hypoparathyroidism also can occur as a result of infiltrative diseases of the parathyroids. This is seen in diseases of iron overload such as hemochromatosis and in patients with thalassemia major who have been heavily transfused.[373] Copper deposition in Wilson's disease[374] may also cause parathyroid dysfunction. Metastatic disease to the parathyroids can cause hypoparathyroidism, but rarely, presumably because of the need for four-gland involvement before significant hypoparathyroidism is observed.

Impaired Parathyroid Hormone Secretion

Impaired secretion of PTH from the parathyroid glands can lead to functional hypoparathyroidism. This is commonly seen in profound hypomagnesemia,[375] in which target organ resistance to PTH can also occur. Both of these abnormalities are reversible on magnesium repletion (see "Disorders of Magnesium Metabolism").[376,377]

Chronic respiratory alkalosis leads to hyperphosphatemia and decreased ionized calcium levels accompanied by impaired renal calcium resorption and inappropriately normal PTH levels.[378] This biochemical phenotype suggests both an abnormality of PTH secretion and renal resistance to PTH. Acute alkalosis in dogs also suppresses PTH secretion.[379]

Activating mutations in the CASR cause autosomal dominant hypocalcemia associated with inappropriately normal PTH levels. The clinical syndrome is variable; patients present with hypocalcemia and seizures, but their affected relatives may be only later diagnosed with asymptomatic hypocalcemia.[380] Unlike patients with inactivating mutations of the CASR, homozygously affected individuals do not appear to have a more severe phenotype.[381] The presence of hypercalciuria in these patients makes medical management uniquely challenging. Treatment with vitamin D metabolites often results in a marked increase in renal calcium excretion, associated with renal calcification and resultant renal impairment. Based on these observations, it has been suggested that asymptomatic individuals should be left untreated and that the goal of therapy in patients with symptomatic hypocalcemia should be solely to relieve symptoms, not to achieve normocalcemia. Treatment with calcium and vitamin D metabolites should be accompanied by the use of thiazide diuretics to decrease urinary calcium excretion and ensure a urinary volume that is adequate to decrease the urinary calcium concentration.

Pseudohypoparathyroidism

The idiopathic and inherited forms of PTH resistance are referred to as pseudohypoparathyroidism (PHP). The first cases of documented PTH resistance were described by Albright in 1942.[382] The patients were hypocalcemic and hyperphosphatemic and they also exhibited a number of features that are characteristic of the disorder now called *Albright's hereditary osteodystrophy* (AHO). These features include short stature, rounded face, foreshortened fourth and other metacarpals, obesity, and subcutaneous calcifications (Figs. 28-32 and 28-33).

PTH administration to these patients failed to provoke a phosphate diuresis or an increase in serum calcium. It was subsequently demonstrated that hypocalcemic patients with features of AHO had elevated PTH levels and that PTH infusions failed to stimulate renal production of cAMP. Failure of stimulation of cAMP production suggested a defect in the PTH receptor or in its cAMP-mediated signal transduction.[383] The measurement of cAMP in the urine after an infusion of synthetic PTH^{1-34} is now used to establish the diagnosis of PTH resistance.[384]

The variable presence of AHO and renal resistance to PTH in PHP has led to subclassification of PHP (Table 28-5). PHP type 1A is characterized by AHO and diminished activity (approximately 50% of normal) of $G_s\alpha$, the α-subunit

TABLE 28-5

Types of Pseudohypoparathyroidism (PHP)

Disorder	Urinary cAMP Response to PTH	Urinary PO_4 Response to PTH	Other Hormonal Resistance	AHO	Pathophysiology
PHP type 1A	Decreased	Decreased	Yes	Yes	$G_s\alpha$ mutation
Pseudo-PHP	Normal	Normal	No	Yes	$G_s\alpha$ mutation
PHP type 1B	Decreased	Decreased	No	No	*GNAS1* imprinting mutations
PHP type 1C	Decreased	Decreased	Yes	Yes	$G_s\alpha$ activity normal
PHP type 2	Normal	Decreased	No	No	Vitamin D deficiency or myotonic dystrophy in some cases

AHO, Albright's hereditary osteodystrophy; cAMP, cyclic adenosine monophosphate; *GNAS1*, portion of the *GNAS* complex locus encoding $G_s\alpha$; $G_s\alpha$, α-subunit of the stimulatory G protein; PO_4, phosphate; PTH, parathyroid hormone.

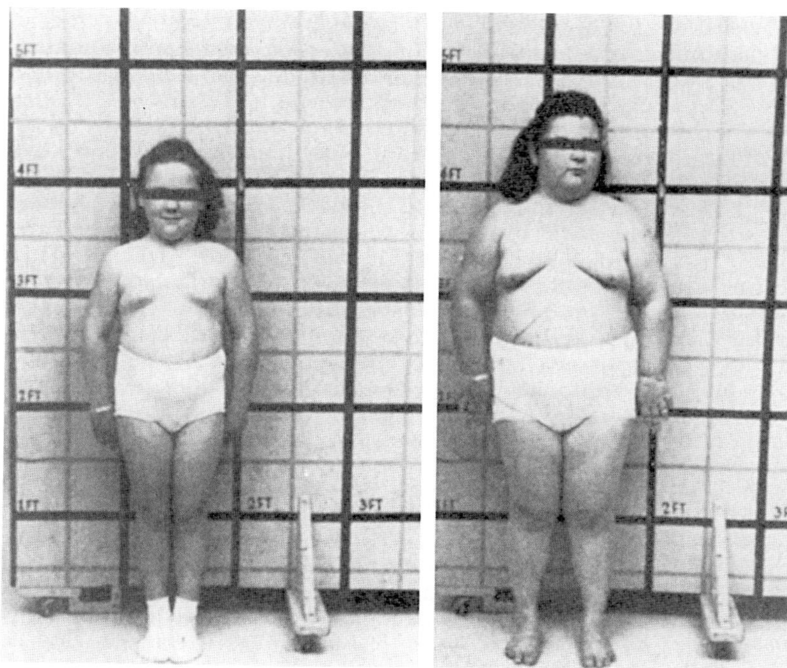

Figure 28-32 Daughter *(left)* and mother *(right)* with pseudohypoparathyroidism and Albright's hereditary osteodystrophy.

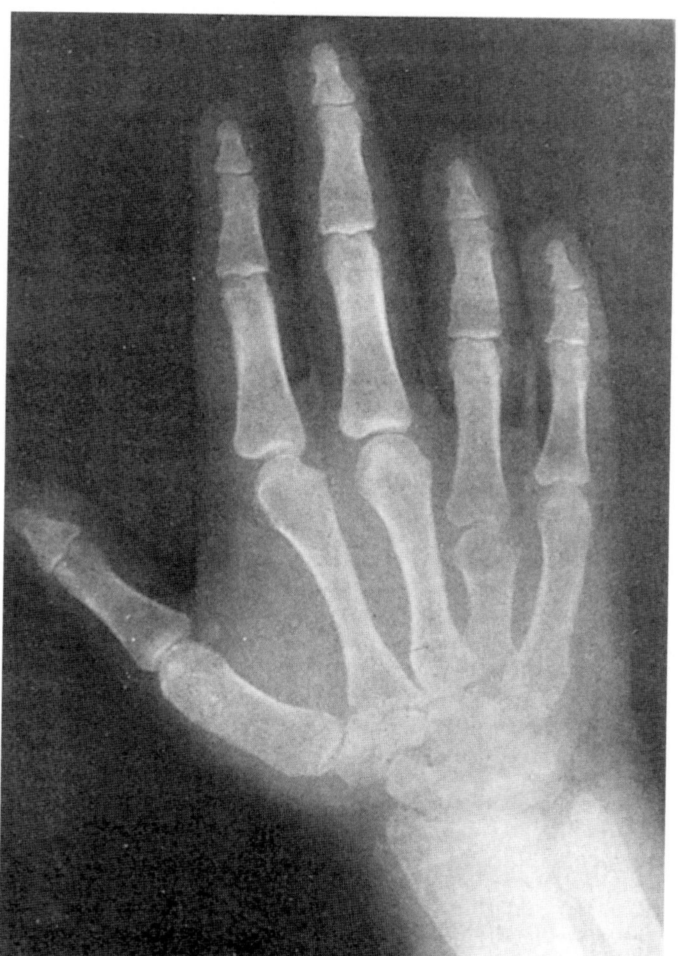

Figure 28-33 Radiograph of hand from a patient with pseudohypoparathyroidism and Albright's hereditary osteodystrophy. Note the shortened fourth metacarpal.

of the stimulatory G protein, G_s. These patients have mutations that inactivate one allele of the $G_s\alpha$ gene, through a variety of mechanisms, including missense mutations, chain-terminating mutations, changes that induce abnormal splicing, small insertions, deletions, and inversions.[385] The resultant diminished $G_s\alpha$ activity has been demonstrated in several tissues, including kidney, fibroblasts, transformed lymphocytes, platelets, and erythrocytes.

Impaired mentation is seen in approximately half of patients with PHP-1A and appears to be related to the $G_s\alpha$ deficiency rather than to chronic hypocalcemia, because patients with other forms of PHP and hypocalcemia have normal mentation. The $G_s\alpha$ deficiency in PHP-1A may be associated not only with PTH resistance but also with resistance to other hormones such as thyroid-stimulating hormone, glucagon, and gonadotropins, resulting in thyroidal and gonadal dysfunction. Paradoxically, two unrelated male patients with both PHP-1A and gonadotropin-independent precocious puberty have been described. The $G_s\alpha$ point mutation found in these individuals is thought to lead to a protein that is unstable at 37° C and, therefore, to confer renal resistance to PTH. In the testes, however, the temperature is lower and the protein is not degraded. In this setting, the stable but mutated protein is constitutively active and stimulates the Leydig cell, in a manner similar to the skeletal effects of the G_s mutations in McCune-Albright syndrome (see Chapter 25).[386]

The term *pseudo-pseudohypoparathyroidism*, or pseudo-PHP, is used to refer to individuals with the phenotype of AHO who are without evidence of PTH resistance. Patients with pseudo-PHP often are found in the same kindreds as those with PHP-1A, and they invariably inherit the same abnormal $G_s\alpha$ gene found in their PTH-resistant relatives.[387] People who inherit the mutant $G_s\alpha$ gene from their father exhibit pseudo-PHP, whereas those who inherit it from their mother exhibit PHP.[388,389] This pattern, in which the renal hormone resistance phenotype depends on the parent of origin, is considered a form of tissue-specific genetic imprinting. Mice with targeted ablation of the gene that encodes $G_s\alpha$ *(Gnas1)* also display such imprinting.[390] Notably, mice with targeted ablation of one *Gnas1* gene fail to express $G_s\alpha$ mRNA in the renal cortex when the mutant gene is inherited from the mother but have normal expression in the cortex when it is inherited from the father. No such imprinting pattern is seen in the inner medulla. This correlates with the findings in mice (and patients) exhibiting resistance to PTH but not to vasopressin[390] and emphasizes the cell type–specific nature of the imprinting. The parental origin of the $G_s\alpha$ mutation affects certain other features of the clinical presentation of these patients: obesity is often seen in patients with PHP-1A and not in those with pseudo-PHP.[391] In a mouse model of PHP-1A, this obesity was traced to imprinting of *Gnas* in the hypothalamus.[392] Further, whereas subcutaneous ossification is seen in patients with both PHP-1A and pseudo-PHP, extension of this ossification deep into muscle (called *progressive osseous heteroplasia*) is seen almost exclusively in patients with pseudo-PHP.[393]

Pseudohypoparathyroidism type 1B (PHB-1B) manifests with hypocalcemia, high PTH levels, and failure of PTH infusions to increase urinary cAMP production. However, PHP-1B is not accompanied by any of the clinical features of AHO, nor is it associated with abnormal $G_s\alpha$ levels in fibroblasts. As in PHP-1A, mild resistance to thyroid-stimulating hormone has been reported.[394-396] The PTH target organ manifestations of PHP-1B are variable, with some affected individuals having manifestations of PTH overactivity in bone and PTH resistance in kidney, a pattern that resembles PHP-1A. Cultured osteoblast-like cells from a patient with PHP-1B demonstrated normal cAMP responsiveness to PTH despite the lack of renal responsiveness.[397]

When inherited, PHP-1B has been found to map to chromosome 20q13.3,[398] the same region that contains the *GNAS1* gene. Although the disease is inherited with the imprinting characteristics of PHP-1A, mapping studies suggest that the disease-causing mutations are close to, but distinct from, the $G_s\alpha$ coding region. Affected individuals have imprinting abnormalities of the *GNAS* complex locus that lead to abnormal patterns of expression of $G_s\alpha$ without effects on the $G_s\alpha$ coding sequence.[395,399,400] The discovery that PHP-1B is a disease of imprinting may explain why these patients exhibit PTH resistance but not AHO: Presumably, the normal structure of the $G_s\alpha$ gene allows normal expression of $G_s\alpha$ in most tissues, which do not exhibit tissue-specific imprinting. In the renal proximal tubule, where $G_s\alpha$ is expressed only from the maternal allele, abnormal imprinting leads to no expression of $G_s\alpha$ and to PTH resistance in those cells.

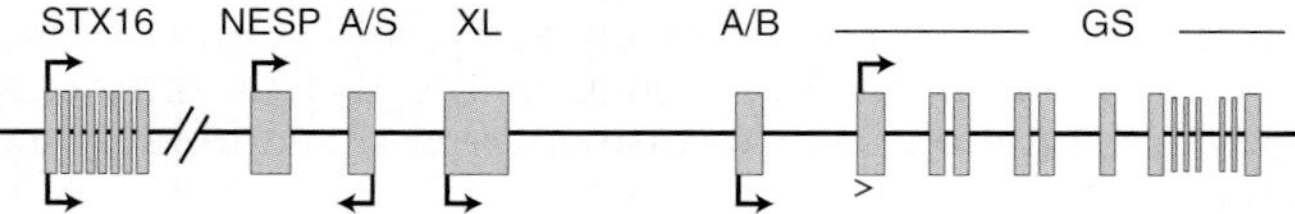

Figure 28-34 The *GNAS* complex locus and the adjacent syntaxin *(STX16)* locus. A schematic representation of the *GNAS* complex locus is shown, with the black boxes indicating exons for STX16, neuroendocrine secretory protein 55 (NESP), the antisense NESP55 transcript (A/S), the $G_s\alpha$ isoforms XLαs (XL), loss-of-methylation locus A/B, and $G_s\alpha$ (GS). The start site and the direction of transcription (sense versus antisense) are indicated by the arrows. Genes that are maternally transcribed are indicated by arrows above the relevant exons, whereas those that are paternally transcribed are indicated below. The expression of XLαs, A/B, and A/S is through the paternal allele, whereas it is the maternal NESP55 transcript that is expressed. Expression of STX16 is biallelic. The arrowhead below the GS locus indicates that only the maternal allele is expressed in certain tissues (e.g., the renal tubules). $G_s\alpha$, α-subunit of the stimulatory G protein.

The *GNAS* complex locus gives rise to multiple transcripts (Fig. 28-34), including $G_s\alpha$. $G_s\alpha$ is biallelically expressed in most tissues, but only the maternal transcript is expressed in the renal proximal tubules, thyroid, gonads, and pituitary. In contrast, the XLαs, A/B, and antisense (A/S) transcripts are expressed only paternally, and the (NESP55) transcript only maternally. These patterns of expression involve differential methylation of DNA sequences associated with each transcript. All patients with PHP-1B exhibit loss of methylation at exon A/B, which results in biallelic expression of the transcript. This abnormality may play a role in the hormone resistance observed.[400] The methylation defect in exon A/B, when found in families with PHP-1B, is most often caused by 3-kilobase deletions of DNA—not in exon A/B but instead 200 kilobases upstream of *GNAS*.[401,402] How these deletions lead to methylation abnormalities in exon A/B is unknown. In sporadic cases of PHP-1B, deletions within *GNAS* also cause abnormal methylation of exon A/B and an abnormal expression pattern of $G_s\alpha$.

Several patients with AHO and PTH resistance have been found to have normal $G_s\alpha$ activity, and this subgroup of the disorder has been designated pseudohypoparathyroidism type 1C (PHP-1C). Biochemical characterization in one case[403] revealed a significant decrease in the manganese-stimulated adenylate cyclase activity in fibroblast membranes, raising the possibility that a second defect in the cAMP pathway may lead to the phenotype of PHP-1C. Another PCP-1C patient, studied after $G_s\alpha$ sequencing became easier, was found to have a short deletion at the carboxy-terminus of G_s, which resulted in normal levels of G_s activity when assayed in erythrocytes but defective activation by receptors.[404]

In pseudohypoparathyroidism type 2 (PHP-2), PTH infusions increase urinary cAMP normally, but PTH does not elicit a phosphaturic response.[405] Patients with this syndrome, like those with PHP-1B, lack signs of AHO or resistance to other hormones, but PHP-2, unlike PHP-1B, is not familial in origin. The age at onset of patients with this disorder is variable, ranging from infancy to senescence, suggesting that it is an acquired defect or that the biochemical phenotype may be unmasked by intercurrent abnormalities. A subset of patients with myotonic dystrophy display the biochemical features of PHP-2, with the degree of PTH resistance correlating with the degree of expansion of the pathogenetic CTG repeats in the myotonin protein kinase gene.[406] A similar biochemical phenotype can also be observed in vitamin D deficiency,[407] and some authors have suggested that PHP-2 is a manifestation of vitamin D deficiency rather than a distinct clinical entity.[408] Minagawa and colleagues reported on three neonates who had no signs of rickets and normal levels of vitamin D but presented with transient PHP-2 that resolved at about 6 months of age.[409] They postulated that PTH responsiveness is subject to maturation during fetal and neonatal development. PHP-2, therefore, seems to reflect a heterogeneous clinical disorder associated with defects in PTH responsiveness distal to cAMP or involving a separate signal transduction pathway.[410]

The specificity of PTH resistance for the proximal tubule has implications for the management of PHP. Because bone is not resistant to PTH, hyperparathyroid bone disease may occur.[411,412] Patients with PHP have lower bone density than normal subjects or hypoparathyroid controls. Basal urinary hydroxyproline excretion in patients with PHP is twice that of hypoparathyroid controls, and they have similar increases in response to parathyroid extract.[413] Further, the renal resistance to PTH is limited to the proximal tubule, where the 1α-hydroxylase activates 25(OH)D, and the normal distal tubular reabsorption of calcium keeps the urinary calcium excretion low in comparison to that in patients with primary hypoparathyroidism.[414] Therefore, therapy with calcitriol can be used, with the goal of normalizing PTH levels to avoid bone disease, with less concern that urinary calcium excretion might be excessive.

Vitamin D–Related Disorders

Hypocalcemia secondary to vitamin D deficiency or resistance to the biologic effects of calcitriol is easily differentiated from the hypocalcemia of hypoparathyroidism by routine clinical and laboratory evaluations. The primary cause of hypocalcemia in vitamin D deficiency is decreased intestinal absorption of calcium. In the setting of normal renal function, the hypocalcemia of vitamin D deficiency, unlike that of hypoparathyroidism, is accompanied by hypophosphatemia and increased renal phosphate clearance. This increase in phosphate clearance is a direct result of compensatory (secondary) hyperparathyroidism. The hyperparathyroidism is a consequence of the hypocalcemic stimulus to PTH secretion and the stimulation of PTH gene expression and parathyroid cell proliferation caused by hypocalcemia (see "Parathyroid Hormone Biosynthesis"). Therefore, measurements of serum phosphate and PTH are very useful in distinguishing these disorders from hypoparathyroidism. The secondary hyperparathyroidism results in increased calcium mobilization from the skeleton, increased renal reabsorption of calcium, and increased renal 1α-hydroxylation of 25(OH)D. In severe vitamin D deficiency, the increased levels of PTH no longer lead to increased bone resorption, perhaps because osteoclasts appear not to resorb unmineralized osteoid.

In profound vitamin D deficiency, the level of calcitriol is usually low; in moderate vitamin D deficiency, the stimulation of the renal 1α-hydroxylase by PTH can result in a normal or even elevated calcitriol level. These high levels of calcitriol reflect the action of PTH on the renal 1α-hydroxylase. The ineffectiveness of the high levels of total calcitriol in normalizing serum calcium may be explained by increased binding of this metabolite to VDBP when the levels of 25(OH)D are very low.

Vitamin D Deficiency

Because the two sources of vitamin D are the diet and cutaneous synthesis after ultraviolet irradiation, lack of solar irradiation and decreased intake or impaired absorption of vitamin D can lead to vitamin D deficiency. As the population has become increasingly educated about the risks of skin cancer from solar irradiation, the avoidance of long periods of intense sun exposure and the use of sun blocks with high solar protective factor (SPF) values have resulted in increased reliance on dietary sources of vitamin D. The RDA for vitamin D is 400 IU; however, this level of intake is lower than that required to prevent vitamin D deficiency in the absence of solar exposure especially in elderly or housebound individuals.[415]

Vitamin D is present in many food sources, both vegetable and animal. In addition, many prepared foods, especially cereal products, are fortified with vitamin D. Although dairy products have been fortified with vitamin D as well, the actual amount of vitamin D provided does not correlate well with the purported content.[131] The vitamin D derived from vegetable sources is vitamin D_2, and that derived from animal sources is vitamin D_3. These two forms of vitamin D are metabolized identically and have equivalent biologic potency in humans. Both forms have been used to fortify foods.

Early vitamin D deficiency can be detected when the serum level of 25(OH)D falls to less than 15 ng/dL, because this level has been shown to be associated with the development of secondary hyperparathyroidism. Although elderly, homebound individuals in particular are at high risk, several studies have demonstrated that vitamin D deficiency is prevalent in the general population (reviewed by Thomas and associates in 2000[416]). The clinical relevance of this vitamin D deficiency was confirmed by a study demonstrating that administration of vitamin D (800 IU/day) to an ambulatory elderly population decreased serum PTH levels as well as the incidence of hip fracture.[417]

Malabsorption also remains an important cause of vitamin D deficiency in all age groups. Because vitamin D is a fat-soluble vitamin, its absorption depends on emulsification by bile acids. Any cause of fat malabsorption or short-bowel syndrome can result in vitamin D deficiency; therefore, malabsorption should be ruled out in patients with very low 25(OH)D levels (<8 ng/dL).

Accelerated Loss of Vitamin D

Both 25(OH)D and calcitriol are secreted with bile salts and undergo enterohepatic circulation; therefore, intestinal disease may also result in vitamin D deficiency due to excessive losses. Increased metabolism of vitamin D, leading to low blood levels of 25(OH)D, is seen in individuals given anticonvulsant medications or anti-tuberculosis therapy. Phenobarbital, primidone, phenytoin,[418] rifampin, and glutethimide[419] have all been reported to accelerate the hepatic inactivation of vitamin D.

Impaired 25-Hydroxylation of Vitamin D

The vitamin D that is absorbed undergoes 25-hydroxylation in the liver; therefore, severe hepatic parenchymal damage can result in 25(OH)D deficiency. Clinically, severe vitamin D deficiency as a consequence of liver disease is rare, because the degree of hepatic destruction necessary to impair 25-hydroxylation is incompatible with long-term survival. However, isoniazid has been shown to decrease the 25-hydroxylation of vitamin D.[420] Two kindreds have been described in whom the clinical and biochemical presentations and therapeutic responses suggest an inherited 25-hydroxylation defect.[421]

Impaired 1α-Hydroxylation of 25-Hydroxyvitamin D

The final step in the activation of vitamin D is hydroxylation of 25(OH)D by the renal 1α-hydroxylase to yield $1,25(OH)_2D_3$ (calcitriol). Renal parenchymal damage, therefore, can result in deficiency of the active metabolite of vitamin D. Impaired 1α-hydroxylation is observed once the creatinine clearance decreases to approximately 30 to 40 mL/minute. In contrast to the situation with liver failure, dialysis permits long-term survival of patients with renal failure; therefore, deficiency of calcitriol as a result of impaired renal 1α-hydroxylation is a common and important clinical entity.

The metabolic consequences of chronic renal failure on the parathyroid glands and the skeleton are complex (see Chapter 29). Impaired renal 1α-hydroxylation leads to decreased intestinal absorption of calcium, resulting in hypocalcemia. The diminished phosphate clearance associated with renal failure leads to elevated levels of blood phosphate and, consequently, increases in circulating FGF23; this, in turn, further lowers levels of calcitriol and calcium. The resultant secondary hyperparathyroidism increases the release of calcium and phosphate from bone; however, because of the renal insufficiency, PTH does not have a phosphaturic effect. As a result, the increased serum phosphate level rises further.

Oral phosphate binders are used to lower blood phosphate. Calcium-containing antacids, which replaced the more toxic aluminum-containing antacids (see Chapter 29), are being supplemented or replaced with the phosphate-binding exchange resin, sevelamer. Calcium administration also attenuates the hypocalcemic stimulus to parathyroid secretion. Calcitriol therapy is critical for the absorption of this calcium and should be administered early in the course of renal failure (when the Cl_{Cr} falls to less than 30 to 40 mL/minute), to avoid the development of secondary hyperparathyroidism, and with careful monitoring to avoid hypercalcemia. Once secondary hyperparathyroidism has developed, pharmacologic doses of intravenous or oral calcitriol or calcimimetics[422] may be required to suppress PTH gene transcription and parathyroid cellular proliferation. Efforts are currently under way to develop nonhypercalcemic analogues of calcitriol that maintain their PTH-suppressing and antiproliferative effects. Such analogues would be invaluable for the prevention and treatment of secondary hyperparathyroidism in the setting of chronic renal failure and perhaps in the treatment of malignancies whose proliferation may be inhibited by pharmacologic doses of calcitriol.

Decreased levels of calcitriol may also be observed in patients taking ketoconazole[139] and those with X-linked hypophosphatemia or tumor-induced osteomalacia, diseases associated with high levels of FGF23 (see Chapter 29).[136]

A rare heritable defect of vitamin D activation has been described in several kindreds. Biochemically, pseudo–vitamin D deficiency rickets is characterized by hypocalcemia and secondary hyperparathyroidism. The only metabolic abnormalities that differentiate it from dietary vitamin D deficiency are the presence of normal or elevated levels of vitamin D and 25(OH)D accompanied by low levels of calcitriol.[423,424] The disease is inherited in an autosomal recessive fashion and manifests in infancy with rickets, osteomalacia, and seizures. Cloning of the 1α-hydroxylase gene has confirmed that mutation of this gene is the molecular basis for the disorder[425,426] and that, as expected, physiologic replacement doses of 1α-hydroxylated metabolites of vitamin D results in clinical remission.[427]

Target Organ Resistance to 1,25-Dihydroxyvitamin D_3

A second rare inherited disorder, characterized by resistance to the biologic actions of calcitriol, has been described in several kindreds. This disorder, referred to as hereditary vitamin D–resistant rickets (HVDRR), is also characterized by autosomal recessive inheritance. Its biochemical presentation, with hypocalcemia, hypophosphatemia, and secondary hyperparathyroidism, resembles that of vitamin D deficiency, but it is accompanied by elevated levels of calcitriol. The molecular basis for this disease is mutation of the VDR gene, which results in impaired target organ responsiveness. Most of the mutations that have been described involve the DNA-binding domain of the receptor. These mutations cause a decreased affinity of the receptor for its response elements on target genes, leading to impaired regulation of these genes. Mutations in the hormone-binding and nuclear receptor coactivator-binding domains of the receptor have also been described in kindreds with HVDRR.[428]

The clinical presentation of HVDRR is variable; however, most patients present in infancy with rickets, hypophosphatemia, and seizures, although presentation in late adolescence has also been described. Alopecia totalis, developing in the first 2 years of life, is present in some kindreds.[429] The finding of alopecia in mice with VDR mutations[150,152] confirms the association of alopecia with disruption of the VDR gene.

Because of target organ resistance to the active metabolite of vitamin D, there is no ideal treatment for HVDRR. Pharmacologic doses of vitamin D, 25(OH)D, 24,25$(OH)_2D_3$, and 1,25$(OH)_2D_3$ (calcitriol) have been administered in an attempt to overcome this target organ resistance,[430] with variable effects. For those patients in whom the hypocalcemia and osteomalacia are resistant to such therapeutic interventions, parenteral calcium infusions have been used to heal osteomalacic lesions.[154] Studies in VDR-ablated mice have demonstrated that maintenance of normal mineral ion homeostasis prevents all the complications of VDR ablation except alopecia.[153,155] Based on these observations, patients with VDR mutations should be treated early and aggressively to prevent skeletal abnormalities and parathyroid hyperplasia. Lifelong therapy is usually required, although spontaneous remissions off therapy have been described.[431] The pathophysiology of the spontaneous remissions is not well understood, because the underlying genetic defect still exists. It is likely that these "remissions" reflect compensated calcium homeostasis once the needs of the growing skeleton are met. In support of this hypothesis is a report of a relapse in a pregnant woman, followed by a postpartum remission.[432]

Phenytoin causes target organ resistance to the biologic effects of calcitriol, in addition to its acceleration of the hepatic catabolism of vitamin D metabolites. Phenytoin has been shown to impair intestinal calcium absorption in vivo in rats[433] and to impair PTH- and calcitriol-mediated bone resorption in vitro. Combination chemotherapy with 5-fluorouracil and low-dose leucovorin has been reported to cause hypocalcemia in 65% of patients, associated with an acute decrease in plasma calcitriol levels.[434]

Other Causes of Hypocalcemia

Excessive Deposition into the Skeleton

Excessive deposition of calcium into the skeleton can occur in association with osteoblastic metastases, with chondrosarcomas,[435] or in the hungry bone syndrome. This last syndrome manifests with prolonged hypocalcemia, hypocalciuria, and hypophosphatemia after parathyroidectomy for primary hyperparathyroidism (see "Primary Hyperparathyroidism"). The hypocalcemia is a consequence of remineralization of a skeleton that has been subjected to the bone-resorbing effects of PTH for a prolonged period. Hungry bone syndrome can also be observed after treatment of other diseases that are associated with excessive bone resorption. It has been described after radioactive iodine treatment of a patient with Graves' disease.[436]

Chelation

Decreases in ionized calcium have been reported with foscarnet, a pyrophosphate analogue that is used as an antiviral agent,[437] perhaps because of the formation of complexes between ionized calcium and the drug.

Hyperphosphatemia caused by phosphate administration or rapid destruction of soft tissue (e.g., rhabdomyolysis, chemotherapy for hematologic malignancies) may produce profound hypocalcemia by directly complexing and precipitating calcium in bone or soft tissues, by inhibiting bone resorption, and by blocking renal synthesis of calcitriol (see "Hyperphosphatemia").

Massive infusions of citrated blood products may cause hypocalcemia, presumably because citrate complexes with calcium in the recipient's plasma.[438] Large doses of ethylenediaminetetra-acetic acid (EDTA)-containing radiographic contrast dyes have also been reported to cause hypocalcemia.

Hypocalcemia resulting from complexes of calcium and fluoride has been reported with hydrofluoric acid burns[439] or ingestion.[440]

Neonatal Hypocalcemia

Neonatal hypocalcemia is seen in infants of hyperparathyroid mothers, infants of diabetic mothers, premature infants, and infants with birth asphyxia. The cause of hypocalcemia in infants of diabetic mothers is likely multifactorial. Prematurity per se does not account for the higher incidence.[441] The response of premature infants and infants of diabetic mothers to exogenous PTH suggests that functional hypoparathyroidism may, in part, account for the increased hypocalcemia in these two populations.[441,442] The hypocalcemia in infants of hyperparathyroid mothers is presumably secondary to the maternal hypercalcemia that, in turn, suppresses fetal parathyroid function.[443]

Human Immunodeficiency Virus Infection

Hypocalcemia is sixfold more prevalent in HIV-infected patients than in the general population.[444] Although hypocalcemia is often a consequence of antiretroviral and antibiotic/antimycotic therapy, vitamin D deficiency and hypomagnesemia are also common in patients with AIDS. Impaired parathyroid responsiveness to hypocalcemia has also been documented (see Chapter 38).

Critical Illness

Hypocalcemia is commonly seen in critically ill patients and is thought to be a reflection of parathyroid gland suppression, failure to activate vitamin D, calcium chelation or sequestration, hypomagnesemia, or some combination of these. However, an increased basal level and secretory response of PTH to lowering of serum calcium has been observed in some septic and nonseptic patients in intensive care units, emphasizing the multifactorial origin of the hypocalcemia.[445] There was a correlation between cytokine levels and hypocalcemia in this study, as in others, suggesting that these inflammatory agents may play a role in redistribution of calcium to the intracellular or other pools. Interleukins 1 and 6 have been shown to increase the expression of the CASR on parathyroid cells and to lower PTH secretion and blood calcium levels in rats injected with the cytokine.[446,447]

Severe acute pancreatitis is often associated with hypocalcemia, and this association is a negative prognostic indicator. The hypocalcemia occurs shortly after the onset of the pancreatitis and is associated with an increase in PTH levels, suggesting that parathyroid function is normal. It has long been thought that this hypocalcemia is secondary to the deposition of "calcium soaps" consisting of calcium and fatty acids. Supporting this hypothesis, studies in a patient with a pancreatic fistula demonstrated hypocalcemia (4.3 mg/dL) in the setting of high levels of calcium (26 mg/dL) and fatty acids in ascitic fluid.[448] Subsequent studies in a rat model supported this finding and demonstrated that oleate has a high binding capacity for calcium.[449] However, other investigations in a porcine model of experimental pancreatitis demonstrated that hypocalcemia does not occur if the animals are subjected to thyroidectomy before the induction of pancreatitis.[450] This finding suggests a role for calcitonin in the development of hypocalcemia with acute pancreatitis, although several clinical studies have documented normal calcitonin levels in hypocalcemic individuals with pancreatitis.[451]

Severe hypocalcemia with hypercalcitoninemia and hypophosphatemia has been reported in the patients with toxic shock syndrome sepsis and in critically ill patients.[452] As in acute pancreatitis, this hypocalcemia is usually accompanied by increased serum levels of PTH, and the degree of hypocalcemia is a negative prognostic indicator. The mechanism of hypocalcemia in these patients is likely to be heterogeneous and has not been clearly defined.

Treatment of Hypocalcemia

Acute hypocalcemia is an emergency that requires prompt attention. If symptoms of neuromuscular irritability are present and carpopedal spasm is elicited on physical examination, treatment with intravenous calcium is indicated until the signs and symptoms of hypocalcemia subside. Approximately 100 mg of elemental calcium should be infused over a period of 10 to 20 minutes (Table 28-6). If this is not sufficient to alleviate the clinical findings of hypocalcemia, an infusion of 100 mg/hour can be given to adults for several hours, with close monitoring of calcium levels. In hypocalcemia associated with hypomagnesemia, magnesium replacement also is required. Magnesium should be given intravenously, 100 mEq over 24 hours in the acute setting. Because most of the parenteral magnesium is excreted in the urine, oral magnesium oxide should be instituted as soon as possible to replete body stores. Special caution and reduced doses are necessary when administering magnesium to patients in renal failure (see "Disorders of Magnesium Metabolism").

The treatment of hypocalcemia should be directed at the underlying disorder. In all cases, replacement with exogenous calcium (1 to 3 g of elemental calcium daily, given orally) should be instituted. Calcium carbonate is the least expensive formulation, but it requires acidification for efficient absorption. This becomes important for patients with achlorhydria and for those in whom gastric acid production is being suppressed with pharmacologic agents. Notable in this respect is the acid-buffering capacity of calcium carbonate. It is recommended that patients take their calcium carbonate supplements in divided doses of 1 g or less. The calcium should be taken with food or citrus drinks to promote maximal absorption.

In cases of vitamin D deficiency or resistance, the metabolite of vitamin D chosen depends on the underlying disorder. If impaired renal 1α hydroxylation is present, such as in renal failure, hypoparathyroidism (or PTH resistance), or the vitamin D–dependent rickets syndromes, metabolites that do not require this modification should be administered (calcitriol 0.25 to 1 μg/day or dihydrotachysterol 0.2 to 1 mg/day). If decreased intake or increased losses are the problem, vitamin D should be administered and the treatment directed at the underlying disorder. Initial repletion of stores can be undertaken with 50,000 IU of vitamin D daily for 2 to 3 weeks, followed by weekly or bimonthly administration until the underlying disorder has been treated. In patients with resistance to vitamin D, such as those taking phenytoin, high doses (50,000 IU one to three times weekly) should be used as maintenance therapy. In other patients, once treatment of

TABLE 28-6

Therapeutic Mineral Ion Preparations

				AVAILABLE FORMULATIONS					
		Mineral Ion Content		Oral Preprations			Parenteral Preparations		
					Mineral Ion Content			Mineral Ion Content	
Compound	*MW**	*mg/g*	*mmol/g*	*Compound*	*mg/g*	*mmol/g*	*Compound*	*mg/g*	*mmol/g*
Calcium									
Ca carbonate	100	400	10.0	1250 mg†	500 mg	12.5 mmol			
Ca phosphate	310	383	9.6	1565 mg	600 mg	15.0 mmol			
Ca acetate	158	253	6.3	668 mg†	167 mg	4.2 mmol			
Ca citrate	498	210	6.0	950 mg†	200 mg	5.0 mmol			
Ca lactate	218	130	4.6	650 mg†	84 mg	2.1 mmol			
Ca glubionate		64	1.7	5 mL	115 mg	2.0 mmol			
Ca gluconate	430	93	2.3	1000 mg†	93 mg	2.3 mmol	10% soln	93 mg/10 mL	2.3 mmol/10 mL
Ca gluceptate	488	82	2.0				22% soln	90 mg/5 mL	2.3 mmol/10 mL
Ca chloride	147	273	6.8				10% soln	273 mg/10 mL	11.2 mmol/mL
Magnesium									
Mg oxide	40	603	24.8	400 mg†	241 mg	9.9 mmol			
Mg gluconate	450	54	2.2	500 mg	27 mg	1.1 mmol			
Mg chloride	203	120	4.9	535 mg	64 mg	2.6 mmol	20% soln	24 mg/mL	1.0 mmol/mL
Mg sulfate	246	99	4.1				50% soln†	49 mg/mL	2.0 mmol/mL
Phosphorus‡									
Na/K phosphate (neutral)				Capsule	250 mg	8.1 mmol			
K phosphate (neutral)				Capsule	250 mg	8.1 mmol	soln	94 mg/mL	3.0 mmol/mL
Na phosphate (neutral)							soln	94 mg/mL	3.0 mmol/mL

*Molecular weights (MW) shown are for the usual chemical form, including water molecules (e.g., $MgSO_4 \cdot 7\ H_2O$).
†Other formulations exist. Those shown are among those approved in the United States.
‡Phosphate preparations contain buffered mixtures of monobasic ($H_2PO_4^-$) and dibasic (HPO_4^-) ions; the phosphorus content therefore is specified in millimoles. Oral phosphates contain 7 mEq sodium and potassium per capsule (Na/K form) or 14 mEq potassium per capsule (K form). Parenteral solutions typically contain 4 mEq of sodium or potassium per milliliter.
MW, molecular weight; soln, solution.
Data from *Drug Facts and Comparisons*, 1995 ed. St. Louis: Facts and Comparisons.

the underlying disorder and repletion of body stores have been addressed, two multivitamins (i.e., 800 IU) per day should provide sufficient maintenance therapy. In cases of severe malabsorption, vitamin D can be administered parenterally.

Patients should be monitored closely, both to assess response to therapy and to prevent therapeutic complications. Serum calcium should be monitored frequently (daily in profound hypocalcemia, weekly in moderate hypocalcemia) for the first month of therapy. Concomitant with resolution of the hypocalcemia, a decline in serum PTH should be observed as the secondary hyperparathyroidism resolves. Measurement of serum PTH and assessment of 24-hour urinary calcium excretion should be performed within 2 to 4 weeks after institution of therapy. The urinary calcium measurement reflects the effect of therapy on the patient's ability to absorb calcium and the net uptake of calcium by bone. A low urine calcium concentration indicates poor adherence to a regimen, poor absorption of calcium, or increased uptake by bone. In addition, the urine calcium level provides important information on which to base therapeutic modifications to avoid nephrolithiasis.

Once normalization of serum and urinary calcium and a decrease in PTH levels have been observed, a transition from aggressive replacement therapy to maintenance therapy should be undertaken to prevent hypercalcemia and nephrolithiasis. These same parameters should be monitored at 1 and 3 months after a dose change to assess the effect of the therapeutic intervention. Monitoring of the alkaline phosphatase concentration can also be performed at this time. Alkaline phosphatase levels may actually increase soon after treatment is started, because of healing of the osteomalacic lesions; however, by 3 to 4 months after institution of therapy, a clear downward trend should be observed. Alkaline phosphatase and PTH values may remain elevated for 6 to 12 months after therapy begins; this should not be a cause for alarm, provided that the levels are declining and that monitoring of the other parameters indicates that therapy is effective.

The treatment of hypoparathyroidism is similar to that of vitamin D deficiency, with the exception that these patients have impaired renal 1α hydroxylation of 25(OH)D and therefore require treatment with 1α-hydroxylated metabolites. PTH has been used experimentally for the treatment of hypoparathyroidism, with twice-daily injections providing a better result than once-daily administration.[453] This therapy controls hypocalcemia with lower urine calcium excretion compared with calcium and calcitriol therapy, but it is expensive and requires parenteral administration. Therefore, oral calcium and 1α-hydroxylated vitamin D metabolites remain the mainstay of therapy. Monitoring of serum and urinary calcium should be performed as in the treatment of vitamin D deficiency.

Therapy in these patients is lifelong, and careful monitoring is required to avoid renal or hypercalcemic complications. The aim of therapy should be to maintain serum calcium in the low-normal range without causing frank hypercalciuria, to avoid nephrolithiasis and decrease in GFR. Because PTH plays an important role in renal calcium reabsorption, difficulties are often encountered in attaining these therapeutic goals. In such cases, renal calcium losses can be minimized by the addition of a thiazide diuretic to the treatment regimen. As stated earlier, in patients with PHP, the intact distal tubular reabsorption of calcium leads less often to hypercalciuria and allows more aggressive treatment aimed at normalizing PTH levels, to protect bones from the hyperparathyroid bone disease sometimes seen in PHP.

One of the frustrations often encountered in treating patients with hypoparathyroidism is the fluctuating response to a seemingly stable therapeutic regimen. Episodes of hypercalcemia are occasionally observed without any discernible cause. Because of this, serum calcium should be monitored every 3 months to permit temporary withdrawal of calcitriol, should a hypercalcemic trend be observed. The half-life of this metabolite is short, so that discontinuation for a few days to 1 week, with subsequent resumption at a lower dose, is usually efficacious.

All patients receiving vitamin D metabolites and calcium need to be aware of potential therapeutic complications. Importantly, the mild symptoms of hypercalcemia should be emphasized to the patient. It is essential that these patients be aware that their calcium level should be monitored more frequently during intercurrent illnesses that may affect their absorption of calcium or their hydration status, and also on introduction of drugs such as thiazides or loop diuretics that might change the dosing requirement, to prevent the development of hypocalcemia or severe hypercalcemia.

DISORDERS OF PHOSPHATE METABOLISM

Hyperphosphatemia

Serum phosphate levels are controlled primarily by the rate of proximal renal phosphate reabsorption, which is due, in turn, to the integrated activity of the major sodium-dependent cotransporters (NaPi-IIa and NaPi-IIc). This activity is strongly downregulated by PTH and FGF23, both of which are stimulated by phosphate. Therefore, absent extraordinary filtered loads of phosphate, the capacity of normal kidneys to excrete phosphate is not easily exceeded. Consequently, the occurrence of hyperphosphatemia usually signifies impaired renal function, hypoparathyroidism, defective FGF23 action, a huge flux of phosphate into the ECF, or some combination of these factors (Table 28-7).

The most common cause of hyperphosphatemia is acute or chronic renal failure in which the GFR is so reduced that the usual daily load of phosphate cannot be excreted at a normal level of serum phosphate, despite maximal inhibition of phosphate reabsorption in the remaining functional nephrons. In hypoparathyroidism (or PHP), the serum phosphate level may rise to as high as 6 to 8 mg/dL because of loss of the tonic inhibitory effect of PTH on phosphate reabsorption, although increased FGF23 levels may prevent even further increases in serum phosphate.[454] The hyperphosphatemia of hypoparathyroidism is only partly caused by the absence of PTH per se. Hypocalcemia may further impair phosphate clearance in this setting, and correction of hypocalcemia by treatment with vitamin D metabolites and oral calcium may reduce serum phosphate even if PTH levels remain low.[455]

TABLE 28-7

Causes of Hyperphosphatemia

Impaired Renal Phosphate Excretion
Renal insufficiency
Familial tumoral calcinosis
Endocrinopathies
Acromegaly
Hypoparathyroidism
Pseudohypoparathyroidism
Heparin
Increased Extracellular Phosphate
Rapid Administration of Phosphate (Intravenous, Oral, Rectal)
Phosphate salts
Fosphenytoin
Liposomal amphotericin B
Rapid Cellular Catabolism or Lysis
Catabolic states
Tissue injury
Hyperthermia
Crush injuries
Fulminant hepatitis
Cellular lysis
Hemolytic anemia
Rhabdomyolysis
Tumor lysis syndrome
Transcellular Shifts of Phosphate
Metabolic acidosis
Respiratory acidosis

Other circumstances in which renal tubular phosphate excretion is decreased, in the absence of renal failure, include acromegaly,[456] chronic therapy with heparin, and familial tumoral calcinosis.[457] Familial tumoral calcinosis can result from inactivating mutations in either FGF23 or the *O*-linked glycosyl transferase GALNT3, which may glycosylate and activate FGF23.[458,459] The choice of FGF23 assay is important, because the responsible FGF23 mutations may render the molecule more susceptible to proteolytic degradation, such that the blood levels of (inactive) carboxyl fragments may be quite high in contrast to low levels of (bioactive) intact FGF23.[458] Affected patients may display focal hyperostosis; large, lobulated periarticular ectopic calcifications, especially around the shoulders or hips; hyperphosphatemia due to increased renal TRP; increased serum calcitriol despite normal or low serum PTH; and increased intestinal calcium absorption, consistent with the elevated serum calcitriol concentration. The disorder may manifest in childhood or adulthood, is more common among blacks, and is lifelong, with a tendency for the tumoral calcifications to progress at affected sites. In contrast to the elevated serum calcitriol, hyperphosphatemia is not a constant feature of tumoral calcinosis, although it tends to be most severe in those with prominent calcifications. Despite their chronic hyperphosphatemia, secondary hyperparathyroidism does not develop in these patients, presumably because of the high levels of calcitriol and intestinal hyperabsorption of calcium. Treatment is problematic, although some success has been reported with phosphate-binding antacids, calcium deprivation, and calcitonin therapy.

Hyperphosphatemia may result from overly rapid administration of therapeutic phosphate preparations or phosphate-rich drugs (fosphenytoin, liposomal amphotericin B), especially if renal function is compromised,[460] or from rapid shifts of phosphate out of cells, most often provoked by mechanical injury or metabolic insult. Most cases of hyperphosphatemia associated with intestinal phosphate loads have involved children who received phosphate-containing laxatives or enemas or older adults with impaired renal function receiving phosphate-based cathartics in preparation for colonoscopy.[461] Hyperphosphatemia due to cytolytic release of intracellular phosphate can be quite dramatic, with serum phosphate concentrations up to or exceeding 20 mg/dL. This was described initially as a complication of rapid induction chemotherapy for certain hematologic malignancies ("tumor lysis syndrome"), although it also may occur from cellular injury associated with trauma, hyperthermia, overwhelming infection, hemolysis, rhabdomyolysis, or metabolic acidosis.[462] Rarely, apparent hyperphosphatemia reflects measurement artifact caused by paraproteins in myeloma.[463]

Most often, hyperphosphatemia is mild and asymptomatic, although chronic hyperphosphatemia is an important factor in the development of secondary hyperparathyroidism in progressive renal failure. The clinical manifestations of acute, severe hyperphosphatemia are related mainly to those of the accompanying hypocalcemia, caused by formation of insoluble calcium phosphate precipitates. Tetany, muscle cramps, paresthesias, and seizures may occur, and these may be compounded by other metabolic disturbances (e.g., hyperkalemia, acidosis, hyperuricemia) that frequently coexist. Generalized precipitation of calcium phosphate into soft tissues may produce organ dysfunction, notably renal failure.[461]

Therapeutic options for hyperphosphatemia are limited. Volume expansion may be helpful to improve GFR in acute syndromes. Identification and removal of any exogenous sources of phosphate is important, and phosphate-binding aluminum hydroxide antacids may be useful in limiting intestinal phosphate absorption and chelating phosphate secreted into the intestine. Hemodialysis is the most effective approach and should be considered early in severe hyperphosphatemia, especially in the tumor lysis syndrome and particularly if symptomatic hypocalcemia cannot be adequately treated for fear of inducing widespread soft tissue calcification.

Hypophosphatemia

Etiology

Hypophosphatemia may result from one or more of three general mechanisms (Table 28-8): increased urinary losses due to decreased net renal TRP; rapid shifts of phosphate from ECF into the intracellular space or the mineral phase of bone; or, rarely, severe and selective deprivation of dietary phosphate, as may occur with chronic ingestion of large amounts of nonabsorbable aluminum-containing antacids. Fasting or starvation does not lead directly to hypophosphatemia, apparently because phosphate is mobilized from catabolized bone and soft tissue in amounts sufficient to maintain serum phosphate, even during prolonged caloric deprivation.[464] Starvation does induce phosphate deficiency and, therefore, predisposes to subsequent hypophosphatemia.[465]

Chronic hypophosphatemia usually can be traced to ongoing renal phosphate wasting. Elevation of serum PTH for any reason (other than renal failure), as in primary hyperparathyroidism or secondary hyperparathyroidism due to vitamin D or calcium deficiency, results in inhibition of TRP and fasting hypophosphatemia. Phosphate

TABLE 28-8

Causes of Hypophosphatemia

Reduced Renal Tubular Phosphate Reabsorption

Excess PTH or PTHrP
- Primary hyperparathyroidism
- PTHrP-dependent hypercalcemia of malignancy
- Secondary hyperparathyroidism
  - Vitamin D deficiency/resistance
  - Calcium starvation or malabsorption
  - Imatinib
  - Rapid, selective correction of severe hypomagnesemia

Excess FGF23 or Other "Phosphatonins"
- Familial hypophosphatemic rickets (XLH)
- Autosomal dominant hypophosphatemic rickets (ADHR)
- Autosomal recessive hypophosphatemia (ARHP)
- Tumor-induced osteomalacia syndrome (TIO)
- McCune-Albright syndrome (fibrous dysplasia)
- Epidermal nevus syndrome
- Idiopathic hypercalciuria

Intrinsic Renal Disease
- Fanconi syndromes, other renal tubular disorders
  - Cystinosis
  - Amyloidosis
  - Hemolytic uremic syndrome
  - Magnesium deficiency
  - Wilson's disease
  - Multiple myeloma
  - Heavy metal toxicity
  - Rewarming or hyperthermia
- NaPi-IIa mutations
- NaPi-IIc mutations (HHRH)

Other
- Poorly controlled diabetes, alcoholism
- Hyperaldosteronism
- Post-partial hepatectomy
- Post-renal transplantation
- Drugs or toxins
  - Ethanol
  - Acetazolamide, other diuretics
  - High-dose glucocorticoids
  - Bicarbonate
  - Toluene
  - Heavy metals (Pb, Cd)
  - Calcitonin
  - Tenofovir
  - High-dose estrogens
  - Ifosfamide
  - Cisplatin
  - Suramin
  - Foscarnet
  - *N*-methyl formamide
  - Bisphosphonates
  - Paraquat

Shifts of Extracellular Phosphate into Cells or Bone

Acute Intracellular Shifts
- Intravenous glucose, fructose, glycerol
- Insulin therapy for hyperglycemia, diabetic ketoacidosis
- Catecholamines (epinephrine, albuterol, terbutaline, dopamine)
- Thyrotoxic periodic paralysis
- Acute respiratory alkalosis, salicylate intoxication, acute gout
- Gram-negative sepsis, toxic shock syndrome
- Recovery from acidosis, starvation, anorexia nervosa, hepatic failure
- Rapid cellular proliferation
  - Leukemic blast crisis
  - Intensive erythropoetin, G-CSF therapy

Accelerated Net Bone Formation
- Post-parathyroidectomy
- Osteoblastic metastases
- Treatment of vitamin D deficiency
- Antiresorptive therapy for severe Paget's disease

Impaired Intestinal Phosphate Absorption
- Aluminum-containing antacids

FGF23, fibroblast growth factor 23; G-CSF, granulocyte colony-stimulating factor; PTH, parathyroid hormone; PTHrP, parathyroid hormone–related hormone.

clearance also is increased in PTHrP-associated hypercalcemia of malignancy, although when such patients develop severe hypercalcemia, hypophosphatemia may be masked initially by underlying volume depletion and compromised GFR. Therapy with the tyrosine kinase inhibitor imatinib appears to cause hypophosphatemia, at least in part by inhibiting bone turnover, lowering serum calcium, and stimulating secondary hyperparathyroidism.[466] When PTH secretion is compromised by severe hypomagnesemia, rapid intravenous administration of magnesium alone, without concurrent attention to coexisting hypocalcemia, can provoke massive phosphaturia and hypophosphatemia in patients with underlying phosphate depletion.

The discovery that gain-of-function mutations in FGF23 cause rickets (i.e., ADHR) inaugurated a new era in the understanding of phosphate homeostasis.[467-469] Elevated FGF23 also occurs in autosomal recessive hypophosphatemia, which is caused by mutations in the gene encoding dentin matrix protein-1 (DMP1). DMP1 is expressed in osteocytes and presumably regulates local production of FGF23.[470] Immunoassays for FGF23[471] have pointed to elevated circulating FGF23 as at least one "phosphatonin" responsible for the reduction of phosphate reabsorption and serum calcitriol levels observed in the more common disorder, X-linked hypophosphatemic rickets, in the rare but distinctive tumor-induced osteomalacia and epidermal nevus syndromes, and in the approximately 50% of patients with McCune-Albright syndrome (fibrous dysplasia of bone) who manifest hypophosphatemia.[467-469,472-474] These disorders share a common biochemical phenotype, which may include a more generalized proximal tubular dysfunction, with modest proteinuria and aminoaciduria. Serum calcium usually is normal or low-normal, urinary calcium often is low, PTH is normal or only slightly elevated, and calcitriol is inappropriately normal. The clinical picture is dominated by weakness, bone pain, and other features attributable to the associated rickets or osteomalacia (see Chapter 29). Increased FGF23 also may play a role in impaired phosphate reabsorption, which is seen in the 20% or so of patients with calcium kidney stones and idiopathic hypercalciuria who exhibit fasting hypophosphatemia,[475] although a few such patients may harbor mutations in the NaPi-IIa cotransporter.[476]

Renal phosphate clearance may be impaired in the context of a more generalized renal tubular disorder such as the Fanconi syndromes or others associated with systemic diseases such as amyloidosis, Wilson's disease, or cystinosis (see Table 28-8). In addition to NaPi-IIa mutations, inactivating mutations in the NaPi-IIc cotransporter, also expressed in the proximal tubule and known to be regulated by both PTH and FGF23, have been shown to account for the rare disorder known as hereditary hypophosphatemic rickets with hypercalciuria, in which primary renal tubular phosphate wasting causes appropriate elevation of serum calcitriol and resulting hypercalciuria.[477,478] Other causes of impaired renal TRP include the osmotic diuresis associated with poorly controlled diabetes, alcoholism, hyperaldosteronism, or exposure to any of a wide variety of drugs or toxins (see Table 28-8). The pathogenesis of phosphate wasting that often follows partial hepatectomy or renal transplantation remains unclear, but humoral mechanisms seem to be involved.[479,480]

Rapid egress of extracellular phosphate into cells is the cause of the hypophosphatemia that develops acutely during administration of intravenous glucose, insulin therapy for hyperglycemia, administration of catecholamines (pressors or bronchodilators), thyrotoxic periodic paralysis, profound respiratory alkalosis, refeeding syndrome in the wake of severe acidosis or starvation, recovery from acute hepatic failure (in which hypophosphatemia is a recognized favorable prognostic factor[481]), or other circumstances involving rapid cellular proliferation, such as leukemic blast crisis or responsiveness to hematopoietic growth factors. Hypophosphatemia in these situations is most pronounced when there is underlying phosphate depletion, as in hyperparathyroidism or vitamin D deficiency, or after prolonged malnutrition, alcoholism, or glycosuria. Accelerated uptake of phosphate into cells is particularly common in patients who have experienced surgery, burns, or trauma, in whom it may be promoted by high levels of circulating catecholamines and exacerbated by concurrent respiratory alkalosis, fever, volume expansion, sepsis, and hypokalemia. Situations of greatly accelerated net bone formation—such as in hungry bone syndrome occurring immediately after parathyroidectomy for primary or tertiary hyperparathyroidism; during initial treatment of severe vitamin D deficiency or Paget's disease; or occasionally in patients with extensive osteoblastic bone metastases—may manifest hypophosphatemia as well as hypocalcemia.

Clinical Features

The clinical significance of hypophosphatemia depends on the presence and severity of underlying phosphate depletion. The status of the total-body phosphorus pool, and more particularly the critical intracellular pool, is reflected only indirectly by the concentration of phosphate in the ECF, which contains less than 0.5% of body phosphorus. Therefore, although serum phosphate concentrations generally are used to characterize hypophosphatemia as severe (<1 to 1.5 mg/dL or <0.3 to 0.5 mmol/L), moderate (1.5 to 2.2 mg/dL or 0.5 to 0.7 mmol/L), or mild (2.2 to 3.0 mg/dL or 0.75 to 1.0 mmol/L), serum phosphate may be normal or even high (depending on renal function) in the presence of profound intracellular phosphate deficiency. Conversely, it may be low when intracellular phosphate is relatively normal, such as after a sudden movement of extracellular phosphate into cells.

The prevalence of severe hypophosphatemia among hospitalized patients overall is less than 1%, whereas mild or moderate hypophosphatemia may be detected in 2% to 5% of these patients.[482] Hypophosphatemia is recognized most often in critically ill patients, alcoholics or other malnourished individuals, decompensated diabetics, and those with acute infectious or pulmonary disorders.[482]

The clinical manifestations of severe hypophosphatemia are protean. Among the most common are various neuromuscular symptoms, ranging from progressive lethargy, muscle weakness, and paresthesias to paralysis, coma, and even death, depending on the severity of the phosphate depletion. Confusion, profound weakness, paralysis, seizures, and other major sequelae usually are limited to those patients with serum phosphate concentrations lower than 0.8 to 1.0 mg/dL.[483] Biochemical evidence of muscle injury is observed within 1 to 2 days in more than one third of patients whose serum phosphate concentrations fall to less than 2 mg/dL.[484] Overt rhabdomyolysis also may occur, especially in the setting of chronic alcoholism with underlying malnutrition and phosphate depletion.[485,486] However, by the time this is recognized, the serum phosphate level often has been raised by the large amounts of cellular phosphate released from damaged muscle. Reversible respiratory failure due to respiratory muscle weakness may preclude successful weaning from ventilatory support.[487,488] Left ventricular dysfunction, heart failure, and ventricular arrhythmias may result from profound hypophosphatemia but may not be significant if the serum phosphate concentration is greater than 1.5 mg/dL.[489] Correction of moderate hypophosphatemia (<2 mg/dL) in patients with septic shock led to a significant increase in blood pressure as well as left ventricular function and arterial pH.[489] Hematologic sequelae of severe hypophosphatemia include hemolysis, platelet dysfunction with bleeding, and impaired leukocyte function (phagocytosis and killing).[490] Erythrocytes demonstrate increased fragility; altered membrane composition, rigidity, and microspherocytosis; and reduced levels of ATP and 2,3-diphosphoglycerate.[490] The reduction in erythrocyte 2,3-diphosphoglycerate impairs oxyhemoglobin dissociation and may thereby reduce oxygen delivery to tissues. This problem, together with accelerated hemolysis, may provoke a substantial increase in cardiac output. The blockade in cellular glycolysis becomes demonstrable at levels of serum phosphate between 1 and 2 mg/dL.[491] Glucose intolerance and insulin resistance also have been demonstrated in these patients.[492]

Treatment

Hypophosphatemia appears most often in acutely or critically ill individuals. Accordingly, it often is difficult to discern whether hypophosphatemia is responsible for features of the multiple organ dysfunction commonly encountered in this population. For example, although depression of intracellular high-energy organophosphates has been demonstrated during treatment of diabetic ketoacidosis and phosphate repletion leads to more rapid recovery of erythrocyte 2,3-diphosphoglycerate concentrations, opinion is divided as to whether phosphate therapy in this setting hastens recovery, prevents complications, or improves mortality.[493,494] Nevertheless, because severe hypophosphatemia has been associated, in a variety of clinical settings, with serious neuromuscular, cardiovascular, and hematologic dysfunction that is at least partially reversible with phosphate repletion, most now agree that a relatively low threshold for treatment should be adopted.[489]

The decision to correct hypophosphatemia urgently should be guided by the estimated severity of the cellular phosphate deficit, the presence of signs or symptoms suggestive of phosphate depletion, and the overall clinical status of the patient. The presence of renal insufficiency (a risk for iatrogenic hyperphosphatemia), concomitant administration of intravenous glucose (alone or as a component of hyperalimentation solutions), and the potential for aggravating coexistent hypocalcemia also should be considered.

Limited data are available from clinical trials to predict the appropriate dose and rate of phosphate administration. In patients without severe renal insufficiency or hypocalcemia, administration of intravenous phosphate at rates of 2 to 8 mmol/hour of elemental phosphorus over 4 to 8 hours frequently corrects hypophosphatemia without provoking hyperphosphatemia or hypocalcemia.[482,495-497] Suggested guidelines based on serum phosphate are shown in Table 28-9. It is essential that serum calcium and phosphate be monitored every 6 to 12 hours during and after phosphate therapy, both to detect untoward consequences and because many patients require additional infusions for recurrent hypophosphatemia within 24 to 48 hours after apparently successful repletion.[496] Less acute or severe hypophosphatemia should be managed with oral (or enteral) phosphate supplements if possible, usually given as a total of 1.0 to 2.0 g/day (as elemental phosphate) of neutral sodium or potassium phosphate in divided doses three to four times a day (see Table 28-6). In many patients, however, oral phosphate therapy is limited by gastrointestinal symptoms such as nausea or diarrhea.

TABLE 28-9

Guidelines for Urgent Treatment of Hypophosphatemia*

Serum PO_4 (mg/dL)	Rate of Infusion (mmol/hr)	Duration (hr)	Total PO_4 (mmol)
<2.5	2.0	6	12
<1.5	4.0	6	24
<1.0	8.0	6	48

*Rates shown are normalized for a 70-kg person. Most formulations available in the United States provide 3 mmol/mL of sodium or potassium phosphate. The following factors should be considered: severity of hypophosphatemia, likelihood of underlying phosphate depletion, clinical condition of the patient, renal function, serum calcium, and concurrent parenteral therapy (glucose, hyperalimentation).

DISORDERS OF MAGNESIUM METABOLISM

The fourth most abundant extracellular cation, magnesium, like calcium, plays a critical physiologic role, particularly in neuromuscular function but also as a component of the mineral phase of bone. Intracellular magnesium is crucial for normal energy metabolism, as a cofactor for ATP and numerous enzymes and transporters, and this is reflected in the rather global clinical effects that accompany disorders of magnesium homeostasis. Hypomagnesemia and hypermagnesemia are among the most common electrolyte disturbances; one or the other of these abnormalities is observed in as many as 20% of hospitalized patients and even more frequently (30% to 40%) among those admitted to intensive care units.[498]

Hypermagnesemia

Magnesium homeostasis is achieved mainly through highly efficient regulation of tubular magnesium reabsorption in the loop of Henle.[1] Because normal kidneys can readily excrete even large amounts of magnesium (i.e., 500 mEq/day), high filtered loads of magnesium rarely cause hypermagnesemia except in patients with significant renal insufficiency.[499] Increased magnesium loads in such cases may arise from ingestion of large amounts of oral magnesium salts, typically given as cathartics or antacids, or from extensive soft tissue ischemia or necrosis in patients with trauma, sepsis, cardiopulmonary arrest, burns, or shock (Table 28-10).[499] Hypermagnesemia may result from parenteral administration of magnesium salts, such as when magnesium is used to treat preeclampsia or as a tocolytic.[500] The infants of such hypermagnesemic mothers may manifest transient hypermagnesemia as well, along with parathyroid suppression and neurobehavioral symptoms.[501,502] The use of oral magnesium preparations as laxatives may lead to hypermagnesemia if absorption is increased by intestinal ileus, obstruction, or perforation.[503]

The most prominent clinical manifestations of hypermagnesemia are vasodilatation and neuromuscular blockade, which may involve both presynaptic and postsynaptic inhibition of neuromuscular transmission.[504] Signs and symptoms usually do not appear unless the serum magnesium concentration exceeds 4 mEq/L.[499] Hypotension, often refractory to pressors and volume expansion, may be one of the earliest signs of progressive hypermagnesemia.[504,505] Lethargy, nausea, and weakness, accompanied by reduction or loss of deep tendon reflexes, may progress to stupor or coma with respiratory insufficiency or

TABLE 28-10

Causes of Hypermagnesemia

Excessive Magnesium Intake
Cathartics, antacids, enemas
Dead Sea drowning
Parenteral magnesium administration
Magnesium-rich urologic irrigants
Intestinal obstruction or perforation after magnesium ingestion
Rapid Mobilization from Soft Tissues
Trauma
Shock, sepsis
Cardiac arrest
Burns
Impaired Magnesium Excretion
Renal failure
Familial hypocalciuric hypercalcemia
Other
Adrenal insufficiency
Hypothyroidism
Hypothermia

quadriparesis at serum concentrations in excess of 8 to 10 mEq/L. Gastrointestinal hypomotility or ileus is common. Facial flushing and pupillary dilatation may be observed. Hypotension may be complicated by a paradoxical relative bradycardia, and other cardiac effects may be evident, including prolongation of the PR, QRS, and QTc intervals, appearance of heart block, and, ultimately, asystole as serum concentrations approach 20 mEq/L.

Hypermagnesemia activates CASRs in the parathyroids, thereby suppressing PTH secretion,[506] and in the renal distal tubules, thereby reducing tubular calcium and magnesium reabsorption. Severe hypocalcemia opposes the effect of hypermagnesemia on PTH secretion, so that serum PTH may remain within the normal range but still be inappropriate for the level of serum calcium.[507]

Successful treatment of hypermagnesemia requires identification and interruption of the source of magnesium and measures to increase clearance of magnesium from the ECF. Use of magnesium-free cathartics or enemas to accelerate clearance of ingested magnesium from the gastrointestinal tract, together with vigorous intravenous hydration, usually is successful in reversing hypermagnesemia. Refractory cases, especially those with advanced renal insufficiency, may require hemodialysis. Infusions of intravenous calcium (100 to 200 mg) have been advocated as an effective antidote to hypermagnesemia, and there are examples in which this therapy has apparently been successful, at least in the short run.[499,504,508]

Hypomagnesemia

Hypomagnesemia may occur because of impaired intestinal magnesium absorption or, more commonly, because of excessive gastrointestinal losses due to diarrhea, preprocedural bowel preparation, or prolonged drainage. Most often, hypomagnesemia reflects defective renal tubular reabsorption of magnesium, although rapid shifts into cells, other extrarenal losses, or incorporation into new bone may occur (Table 28-11). Because only 1% of the body's magnesium content is present in ECF, measurements of serum total or ionized magnesium may not adequately reflect total-body magnesium or the magnesium status of the intracellular compartment in critical tissues such as muscle.[509] Therefore, patients with deficiency of tissue magnesium may fail to manifest overt hypomagnesemia[510] while exhibiting abnormal retention (i.e., >50% in 24 hours) of infused magnesium, a maneuver that may be employed to assess magnesium status.[511]

Etiology

Intestinal Causes of Hypomagnesemia. Selective dietary magnesium deficiency does not occur, and in fact it is remarkably difficult to induce magnesium depletion experimentally by feeding magnesium-deficient diets, probably because renal magnesium conservation is so efficient. Large amounts of magnesium may be lost in chronic diarrheal states (this fluid may contain more than 10 mEq/L of magnesium) or via intestinal fistulae or prolonged gastrointestinal drainage.[512] More commonly, magnesium becomes trapped within fatty acid soaps in disorders associated with chronic malabsorption.[513] Investigation of a rare autosomal recessive disorder, hypomagnesemia with secondary hypocalcemia, has led to identification of the transient receptor potential channel protein TRPM6, in the form of a hetero-oligomer with the closely related channel protein TRPM7, as a key molecular mediator of intestinal (and renal tubular) transepithelial magnesium transport.[514]

Renal Causes of Hypomagnesemia. Roughly 60% of renal magnesium reabsorption occurs in the thick ascending limb of Henle's loop, and another 5% to 10% is reabsorbed in the distal tubules.[1] Investigations of the pathogenesis of several genetic disorders associated with renal magnesium wasting have identified key pathways of magnesium reabsorption at these sites (see Table 28-11).

In familial hypomagnesemia with hypercalciuria and nephrocalcinosis, loss-of-function mutations in the claudin 16 gene *(CLDN16)* that encodes the paracellin-1 protein, a component of the tight junctions between adjacent epithelial cells (or in the related gene, *CLDN19*), selectively impair paracellular reabsorption of magnesium (and calcium) in response to the (lumen-positive) transepithelial voltage gradient.[515,516]

In Bartter's syndromes, inactivating mutations in any of several transporters involved in sodium chloride reabsorption in the ascending limb cause salt wasting, compromise the voltage gradient, and similarly impair paracellular magnesium and calcium reabsorption.[517-519] In autosomal dominant hypocalcemia, mutations causing increased sensitivity of CASRs to cationic agonists may cause hypomagnesemia, as well as hypocalcemia, through inappropriate CASR-dependent suppression of PTH secretion and of renal tubular cation reabsorption.[520]

In Gitelman's syndrome, inactivating mutations in the gene encoding the luminal thiazide-sensitive sodium-chloride cotransporter (NCC), which is expressed in the distal convoluted tubules, leads to sodium chloride and magnesium wasting, in this case with hypocalciuria.[517-519,521] The mechanisms by which impaired NCC activity compromises (transcellular) magnesium reabsorption in this segment are unclear, although NCC-knockout mice (or normal mice treated with thiazides) display reduced distal tubular expression of the TRPM6 channel protein required for normal magnesium transport across the apical membrane.[329]

Mutations in the FXYD2 γ-subunit of the distal tubular basolateral Na^+,K^+-ATPase similarly impair salt and magnesium reabsorption at that site and account for some, but not all, cases of isolated renal magnesium wasting.[522,523] An autosomal recessive form of renal hypomagnesemia is caused by inactivating mutations in the epidermal growth factor gene; this likely also explains why hypomagnesemia

TABLE 28-11

Causes of Hypomagnesemia

Causes of Hypomagnesemia	
Impaired Intestinal Magnesium Absorption	
Hypomagnesemia with secondary hypocalcemia Malabsorption syndromes	
Increased Intestinal Magnesium Losses	
Protracted vomiting or diarrhea Bowel preparation (procedures, surgery) Intestinal drainage or fistula	
Impaired Renal Tubular Magnesium Reabsorption	
Genetic Magnesium-Wasting Syndromes Bartter's syndromes Familial hypomagnesemia with hypercalciuria and nephrocalcinosis Autosomal dominant hypocalcemia Gitelman's syndrome Isolated renal magnesium wasting Hypomagnesmia with hypertension and hypercholesterolemia Hypomagnesemia with secondary hypocalcemia *Acquired Renal Disease* Tubulointerstitial disease Postobstruction, acute tubular necrosis (diuretic phase) Renal transplantation *Drugs and Toxins* Ethanol Digoxin Diuretics (loop, thiazide, osmotic) *cis*-Platinum Cyclosporine Tacrolimus Cetuximab	Interleukin 2 Pentamidine Aminoglycosides Foscarnet Amphotericin B *Endocrine and Metabolic Abnormalities* Extracellular fluid volume expansion Hyperaldosteronism (primary, secondary) Inappropriate ADH secretion Diabetes mellitus Hypercalcemia Phosphate depletion Metabolic acidosis Hyperthyroidism *Other* Hypothermia Sezary syndrome Acute brain injury Hydrogen fluoride burns
Rapid Shifts of Magnesium out of Extracellular Fluid	
Intracellular Redistribution Recovery from diabetic ketoacidosis Refeeding syndrome Correction of respiratory acidosis Catecholamines Thyrotoxic periodic paralysis *Accelerated Net Bone Formation* Post-parathyroidectomy Osteoblastic metastases	Treatment of vitamin D deficiency Calcitonin therapy *Other Losses* Pancreatitis Blood transfusions Extensive burns Excessive sweating Pregnancy (third trimester) and lactation

may complicate the use of cetuximab, a monoclonal antibody directed against the epidermal growth factor receptor.[524] Another genetic syndrome that, like Gitelman's syndrome, features renal magnesium wasting and hypocalciuria (and therefore presumably a defect in distal tubular function) in association with hypertension and hypercholesterolemia, is linked to a mutation in mitochondrial transfer RNA DNA.[525]

Most often, renal magnesium wasting is attributable to an acquired abnormality in tubular magnesium reabsorption. In normal subjects, magnesium reabsorption is virtually complete within several days after institution of experimental dietary magnesium deficiency, even before the serum magnesium level has declined substantially.[526] Therefore, the finding of more than 1 mEq/day of urinary magnesium in a frankly hypomagnesemic patient indicates a defect in renal tubular magnesium reabsorption. The causes of acquired primary tubular magnesium wasting include various tubulointerstitial disorders, recovery from acute tubular necrosis or obstruction, renal transplantation, various endocrinopathies, alcoholism, and exposure to certain drugs (see Table 28-11).

Hypomagnesemia or magnesium depletion due to subnormal renal reabsorption may complicate a variety of endocrinopathies, including hyperaldosteronism, hyperthyroidism, and disorders associated with hypercalcemia, hypercalciuria, or phosphate depletion.[511] In primary hyperparathyroidism, PTH stimulates increased tubular magnesium reabsorption, but this is opposed by a direct tubular effect of hypercalcemia. As a result, the serum magnesium level in patients with primary hyperparathyroidism usually is normal or only slightly reduced.[527] In hypoparathyroidism, serum and urinary magnesium concentrations are low. The magnesium depletion in hypoparathyroidism is consistent with loss of both the magnesium-retaining renal action of PTH and the stimulatory effect of calcitriol on intestinal magnesium absorption.[528]

Diabetes is among the disorders most commonly associated with hypomagnesemia.[529,530] The severity of the hypomagnesemia in diabetics correlates with indices of glycosuria and poor glycemic control,[531] suggesting that urinary losses of magnesium on the basis of glycosuria may partly explain the magnesium depletion. Rapid correction of hyperglycemia with insulin therapy causes magnesium to enter cells and may further lower the extracellular magnesium concentration during treatment.

Alcoholism is another very common clinical setting in which hypomagnesemia occurs. Magnesium depletion in alcoholism may result in part from nutritional deficiency of magnesium, overall caloric starvation and ketosis, and gastrointestinal losses due to vomiting or diarrhea, but an acute magnesuric effect of alcohol ingestion most likely plays the major role.[532] This effect of alcohol is most evident during the rising limb of the blood ethanol curve and may be related to transient suppression of PTH secretion.[532] Other factors that may contribute to hypomagnesemia in alcoholism include pancreatitis, malabsorption, secondary hyperaldosteronism, respiratory alkalosis, and elevated plasma catecholamines, which increase intracellular sequestration of magnesium.[511]

A number of drugs have been identified as causes of defective renal tubular magnesium reabsorption and hypomagnesemia.[511] These include diuretics (especially loop diuretics), digoxin, cisplatin, cetuximab, pentamidine, cyclosporine, tacrolimus, interleukin 2, aminoglycosides, foscarnet, and amphotericin B. Most often, drug-induced hypomagnesemia is mild and reversible, particularly when it is associated with diuretic therapy. In more than half of patients treated with cisplatin, hypomagnesemia occurs within days or weeks, and roughly half of those who develop it exhibit persistent hypomagnesemia many months or even years later. The median duration of hypomagnesemia in cisplatin-treated patients is about 2 months, but recovery has been observed for up to 2 years after treatment.[533] Cisplatin may induce a more global nephropathy and azotemic renal failure, but the magnesium wasting appears to be an isolated functional abnormality.

Other Causes of Hypomagnesemia. Magnesium, like phosphate, is a major intracellular ion, and significant shifts of magnesium from the extracellular compartment may occur during recovery from chronic respiratory acidosis or acute ketoacidosis, refeeding, or administration of hyperalimentation solutions and in response to elevations of circulating catecholamines.[511] Other rapid losses of extracellular magnesium may occur during periods of greatly accelerated net bone formation (after parathyroidectomy, during recovery from vitamin D deficiency, or with osteoblastic metastases) or with large losses due to pancreatitis, cardiopulmonary bypass surgery,[534] massive transfusion,[535] extensive burns, excessive sweating, or pregnancy or lactation.

Consequences of Hypomagnesemia

Most of the signs and symptoms of hypomagnesemia reflect alterations in neuromuscular function: tetany, hyperreflexia, positive Chvostek and Trousseau signs, tremors, fasciculations, seizures, ataxia, nystagmus, vertigo, choreoathetosis, muscle weakness, apathy, depression, irritability, delirium, and psychosis.[511] Patients usually are not symptomatic unless the serum magnesium concentration falls to less than 1 mEq/L, although the occurrence of symptoms, like the intracellular magnesium concentration, may not correlate well with serum magnesium levels. Atrial or ventricular arrhythmias may occur, as may various electrocardiographic abnormalities such as prolonged PR or QT intervals, T-wave flattening or inversion, and ST-segment straightening.[511] Hypomagnesemia also increases myocardial sensitivity to digitalis intoxication.[536]

Hypomagnesemia evokes important alterations in mineral ion and potassium homeostasis that frequently aggravate the clinical syndrome. Magnesium-deprived humans or animals develop hypocalcemia, hypocalciuria, hypokalemia (due to impaired tubular reabsorption of potassium), and positive calcium and sodium balances.[526,537] Sustained correction of hypocalcemia or hypokalemia cannot be achieved by administration of calcium or potassium alone, but both abnormalities respond to administration of magnesium.[513,538]

The mechanism of hypocalcemia in this setting may be multifactorial. Inappropriately normal or low serum PTH, despite hypocalcemia, is common and indicates a defect in PTH secretion[539] that is caused by augmented signaling by CASR-associated G proteins (normally inhibited by magnesium) within the parathyroid cell.[540] Other evidence indicates that hypomagnesemia also may impair PTH action on target cells in bone and kidney, although some have observed normal responsiveness, and the issue remains controversial.[375,376,538,539,541]

Vitamin D resistance also is a feature of hypomagnesemic states.[542,543] This appears to be caused mainly by impaired renal 1α-hydroxylation of 25(OH)D, although tissue resistance to calcitriol also may play a role.[528,544] The serum calcitriol concentration usually is low during hypomagnesemia; this may result from magnesium depletion per se, from parathyroid insufficiency, or from coexistent vitamin D deficiency.[545-547] Deficiency of calcitriol probably is not the main cause of hypocalcemia in these patients, however, because hypocalcemia can be rapidly corrected (within hours to days) by magnesium therapy alone, well in advance of any increase in the serum calcitriol concentration.[545,546]

Therapy of Hypomagnesemia

Patients with mild, asymptomatic hypomagnesemia may be treated with oral magnesium salts—$MgCl_2$, MgO, or $Mg(OH)_2$—usually given in divided doses totaling 40 to 60 mEq (480 to 720 mg) per day (see Table 28-6). Diarrhea sometimes occurs with larger doses but usually is not a problem. The gluconate form (54 mg magnesium per gram) is said to cause less diarrhea.[511] Patients with malabsorption or ongoing urinary magnesium losses may require chronic oral therapy to avoid recurrent magnesium depletion. Although intestinal magnesium absorption is severely impaired in renal failure,[548] oral magnesium must be administered with great caution in this setting, especially in patients receiving concomitant therapy with calcitriol.

Symptomatic or severe (<1 mEq/L) hypomagnesemia, especially if complicated by hypocalcemia, usually signifies magnesium deficits of at least 1 to 2 mEq/kg and is best treated promptly with parenteral magnesium salts. The use of intramuscular $MgSO_4$ is to be discouraged, because the injections are painful and provide relatively little magnesium (e.g., 2 mL of 50% $MgSO_4$ supplies only 8 mEq of magnesium, compared with typical magnesium deficits in excess of 100 mEq). Moreover, because unretained sulfate ions also may increase urinary calcium excretion, intravenous magnesium chloride or gluconate probably is the most logical initial parenteral therapy for patients who also may be hypocalcemic. In adult hypomagnesemic patients with normal renal function, rates of infusion of 2 to 4 mEq/hour (50 to 100 mEq/day) usually are needed to maintain serum magnesium in the range of 2 to 3 mEq/L.[513,545,549] Up to 100 mEq/day for 2 days can be safely administered without elevating the serum magnesium concentration above 4 mEq/L, whereas doses of 200 mEq/day may increase serum magnesium to 4.5 to 5.5 mEq/L and therefore are excessive.[549] In patients with active seizures or other urgent indications, the infusion may be preceded by a slowly administered bolus of 10 to 20 mEq, followed by a higher rate of infusion (10 to 15 mEq/hour) for the first 1 to 2 hours only. Patients with normal renal function can readily excrete more than 400 mEq/day of magnesium in the urine without becoming hypermagnesemic, but even mild renal failure may greatly limit magnesium excretion. Therefore, doses of magnesium supplements should be reduced twofold to threefold, and careful serial monitoring of serum magnesium should be performed in patients with compromised renal function.

It is important to appreciate that a large fraction of parenterally administered magnesium may be excreted in the urine, even in patients with profound magnesium deficiency. Many such patients excrete as much as 50% to 75% of infused magnesium, and in normal subjects excretion approaches 100%.[513] Moreover, because equilibration of the intracellular and extracellular magnesium pools is relatively slow, it is usually necessary to continue magnesium therapy for 3 to 5 days to achieve adequate repletion of the typical 1 to 2 mEq/kg deficit. Because serum magnesium may become normal well before tissue stores are repleted, monitoring of urinary magnesium excretion is a more reliable measure of the approach to full repletion, especially after patients are switched to oral therapy.

The need for calcium, potassium, and phosphate supplementation should be considered in the usual clinical setting of hypomagnesemia. Vitamin D deficiency also frequently coexists and should be treated with oral or parenteral vitamin D or 25(OH)D. Use of calcitriol is not necessary, does not hasten recovery, and may actually worsen hypomagnesemia by suppressing PTH secretion and thereby promoting renal magnesium excretion.[550] Initial parenteral magnesium therapy in hypocalcemic patients may produce a dramatic hypophosphatemia via the rapid stimulation of PTH secretion. This is most likely to be problematic in those patients with underlying phosphate depletion (e.g., malabsorption, alcoholism, diabetes), in whom it may provoke acute neuromuscular dysfunction, and it may be avoided by concomitant intravenous calcium therapy.

REFERENCES

1. de Rouffignac C, Quamme G. Renal magnesium handling and its hormonal control. *Physiol Rev*. 1994;74:305-322.
2. Murshed M, Harmey D, Millan JL, et al. Unique coexpression in osteoblasts of broadly expressed genes accounts for the spatial restriction of ECM mineralization to bone. *Genes Dev*. 2005;19:1093-1104.
3. Gensure RC, Ponugoti B, Gunes Y, et al. Identification and characterization of two parathyroid hormone-like molecules in zebrafish. *Endocrinology*. 2004;145:1634-1639.
4. Canario AV, Rotllant J, Fuentes J, et al. Novel bioactive parathyroid hormone and related peptides in teleost fish. *FEBS Lett*. 2006;580:291-299.
5. Arnold A, Horst SA, Gardella TJ, et al. Mutation of the signal peptide-encoding region of the preproparathyroid hormone gene in familial isolated hypoparathyroidism. *J Clin Invest*. 1990;86:1084-1087.
6. Sunthornthepvarakul T, Churesigaew S, Ngowngarmratana S. A novel mutation of the signal peptide of the preproparathyroid hormone gene associated with autosomal recessive familial isolated hypoparathyroidism. *J Clin Endocrinol Metab*. 1999;84:3792-3796.
7. Wiren KM, Potts Jr JT, Kronenberg HM. Importance of the propeptide sequence of human preproparathyroid hormone for signal sequence function. *J Biol Chem*. 1988;263:19771-19777.
8. Divieti P, John MR, Juppner H, et al. Human PTH-(7-84) inhibits bone resorption in vitro via actions independent of the type 1 PTH/PTHrP receptor. *Endocrinology*. 2002;143:171-176.
9. D'Amour P, Rakel A, Brossard JH, et al. Acute regulation of circulating PTH molecular forms by calcium: utility of PTH fragments/PTH(1-84) ratios derived from three generations of PTH assays. *J Clin Endocrinol Metab*. 2006;91:283-289.
10. Parfitt AM. Calcium homeostasis. In: Mundy GR, Martin TJ, eds. *Physiology and Pharmacology of Bone*. Berlin: Springer-Verlag; 1993:1-65.
11. Hofer AM, Brown EM. Extracellular calcium sensing and signalling. *Nat Rev Mol Cell Biol*. 2003;4:530-538.
12. Pollak MR, Brown EM, WuChou YH, et al. Mutations in the human Ca^{2+}-sensing receptor gene cause familial hypocalciuric hypercalcemia and neonatal severe hyperparathyroidism. *Cell*. 1993;75:1297-1303.
13. Pearce SHS, Williamson C, Kifor O, et al. A familial syndrome of hypocalcemia with hypercalciuria due to mutations in the calcium-sensing receptor. *N Engl J Med*. 1996;335:1115-1122.
14. Drueke TB, Ritz E. Treatment of secondary hyperparathyroidism in CKD patients with cinacalcet and/or vitamin D derivatives. *Clin J Am Soc Nephrol*. 2009;4:234-241.
15. Moe SM, Cunningham J, Bommer J, et al. Long-term treatment of secondary hyperparathyroidism with the calcimimetic cinacalcet HCl. *Nephrol Dial Transplant*. 2005;20:2186-2193.
16. Conigrave AD, Mun HC, Delbridge L, et al. L-Amino acids regulate parathyroid hormone secretion. *J Biol Chem*. 2004;279:38151-38159.
17. Silver J, Naveh-Many T, Mayer H, et al. Regulation by vitamin D metabolites of parathyroid hormone gene transcription in vivo in the rat. *J Clin Invest*. 1986;78:1296-1301.
18. Sela-Brown A, Russell J, Koszewski NJ, et al. Calreticulin inhibits vitamin D's action on the PTH gene *in vitro* and may prevent vitamin D's effect *in vivo* in hypocalcemic rats. *Mol Endocrinol*. 1998;12:1193-1200.
19. Nechama M, Uchida T, Mor Yosef-Levi I, et al. The peptidyl-prolyl isomerase Pin1 determines parathyroid hormone mRNA levels and stability in rat models of secondary hyperparathyroidism. *J Clin Invest*. 2009;119:3102-3114.
20. Bell O, Gaberman E, Kilav R, et al. The protein phosphatase calcineurin determines basal parathyroid hormone gene expression. *Mol Endocrinol*. 2005;19:516-526.
21. Almaden Y, Canalejo A, Hernandez A, et al. Direct effect of phosphorus on PTH secretion from whole rat parathyroid glands in vitro. *J Bone Min Res*. 1996;11:970-976.
22. Slatopolsky E, Finch J, Denda M, et al. Phosphorus restriction prevents parathyroid gland growth. *J Clin Invest*. 1996;97:2534-2540.
23. Kilav R, Silver J, Naveh-Many T. Parathyroid hormone gene expression in hypophosphatemic rats. *J Clin Invest*. 1995;96:327-333.
24. Ben-Dov IZ, Galitzer H, Lavi-Moshayoff V, et al. The parathyroid is a target organ for FGF23 in rats. *J Clin Invest*. 2007;117:4003-4008.
25. Imura A, Tsuji Y, Murata M, et al. Alpha-Klotho as a regulator of calcium homeostasis. *Science*. 2007;316:1615-1618.
26. Parfitt AM. Parathyroid growth: normal and abnormal. In: Bilezikian JP, ed. *The Parathyroids*. 2nd ed. San Diego: Academic Press; 2001: 293-329.
27. Kremer R, Bolivar I, Goltzman D, et al. Influence of calcium and 1,25-dihydroxycholecalciferol on proliferation and proto-oncogene expression in primary cultures of bovine parathyroid cells. *Endocrinology*. 1989;125:935-941.
28. Dusso A, Cozzolino M, Lu Y, et al. 1,25-Dihydroxyvitamin D downregulation of TGFalpha/EGFR expression and growth signaling: a mechanism for the antiproliferative actions of the sterol in parathyroid hyperplasia of renal failure. *J Steroid Biochem Mol Biol*. 2004;89-90:507-511.
29. Li YC, Pirro AE, Amling M, et al. Targeted ablation of the vitamin D receptor: an animal model of vitamin D-dependent rickets type II with alopecia. *Proc Natl Acad Sci U S A*. 1997;94:9831-9835.
30. Manley NR, Capecchi MR. Hox group 3 paralogs regulate the development and migration of the thymus, thyroid, and parathyroid glands. *Dev Biol*. 1998;195:1-15.
31. Su D, Ellis S, Napier A, et al. Hoxa3 and pax1 regulate epithelial cell death and proliferation during thymus and parathyroid organogenesis. *Dev Biol*. 2001;236:316-329.
32. Peters H, Neubuser A, Kratochwil K, et al. Pax9-deficient mice lack pharyngeal pouch derivatives and teeth and exhibit craniofacial and limb abnormalities. *Genes Dev*. 1998;12:2735-2747.
33. Xu PX, Zheng W, Laclef C, et al. Eya1 is required for the morphogenesis of mammalian thymus, parathyroid and thyroid. *Development*. 2002;129:3033-3044.
34. Liu Z, Yu S, Manley NR. Gcm2 is required for the differentiation and survival of parathyroid precursor cells in the parathyroid/thymus primordia. *Dev Biol*. 2007;305:333-346.
35. Baldini A. Dissecting contiguous gene defects: TBX1. *Curr Opin Genet Dev*. 2005;15:279-284.
36. Ding C, Buckingham B, Levine MA. Familial isolated hypoparathyroidism caused by a mutation in the gene for the transcription factor GCMB. *J Clin Invest*. 2001;108:1215-1220.
37. Bowl MR, Nesbit MA, Harding B, et al. An interstitial deletion-insertion involving chromosomes 2p25.3 and Xq27.1, near SOX3, causes X-linked recessive hypoparathyroidism. *J Clin Invest*. 2005;115: 2822-2831.
38. Ali A, Christie PT, Grigorieva IV, Harding B, et al. Functional characterization of GATA3 mutations causing the hypoparathyroidism-deafness-renal (HDR) dysplasia syndrome: insight into mechanisms of DNA binding by the GATA3 transcription factor. *Hum Mol Genet*. 2007;16:265-275.

39. Bringhurst FR. Circulating forms of parathyroid hormone: peeling back the onion. *Clin Chem.* 2003;49:1973-1975.
40. Hilpert J, Nykjaer A, Jacobsen C, et al. Megalin antagonizes activation of the parathyroid hormone receptor. *J Biol Chem.* 1999;274: 5620-5625.
41. Martin KJ, Hruska KA, Freitag JJ, et al. The peripheral metabolism of parathyroid hormone. *N Engl J Med.* 1979;301:1092-1098.
42. D'Amour P, Brossard JH, Rousseau L, et al. Structure of non-(1-84) PTH fragments secreted by parathyroid glands in primary and secondary hyperparathyroidism. *Kidney Int.* 2005;68:998-1007.
43. Slatopolsky E, Finch J, Clay P, et al. A novel mechanism for skeletal resistance in uremia. *Kidney Int.* 2000;58:753-761.
44. D'Amour P, Brossard JH. Carboxyl-terminal parathyroid hormone fragments: role in parathyroid hormone physiopathology. *Curr Opin Nephrol Hypertens.* 2005;14:330-336.
45. Friedman PA, Gesek FA. Calcium transport in renal epithelial cells. *Am J Physiol.* 1993;264:F181-F198.
46. Simon DB, Lu Y, Choate KA, et al. Paracellin-1, a renal tight junction protein required for paracellar Mg2+ resorption. *Science.* 1999;285: 103-106.
47. Hoenderop JG, Nilius B, Bindels RJ. Calcium absorption across epithelia. *Physiol Rev.* 2005;85:373-422.
48. van Abel M, Hoenderop JG, van der Kemp AW, et al. Coordinated control of renal Ca(2+) transport proteins by parathyroid hormone calcium absorption across epithelia: characterization of a murine renal distal convoluted tubule cell line for the study of transcellular calcium transport. *Kidney Int.* 2005;68:1708-1721.
49. Walton RJ, Bijvoet OL. Nomogram for derivation of renal threshold phosphate concentration. *Lancet.* 1975;2:309-310.
50. Murer H, Forster I, Biber J. The sodium phosphate cotransporter family SLC34. *Pflugers Arch.* 2004;447:763-767.
51. Segawa H, Yamanaka S, Onitsuka A, et al. Parathyroid hormone-dependent endocytosis of renal type IIc Na-Pi cotransporter. *Am J Physiol Renal Physiol.* 2007;292:F395-F403.
52. Capuano P, Bacic D, Roos M, et al. Defective coupling of apical PTH receptors to phospholipase C prevents internalization of the Na+-phosphate cotransporter NaPi-IIa in Nherf1-deficient mice. *Am J Physiol Cell Physiol.* 2007;292:C927-C934.
53. Saito H, Maeda A, Ohtomo S, et al. Circulating FGF-23 is regulated by 1alpha,25-dihydroxyvitamin D3 and phosphorus in vivo. *J Biol Chem.* 2005;280:2543-2549.
54. Kim MS, Kondo T, Takada I, et al. DNA demethylation in hormone-induced transcriptional derepression. *Nature.* 2009;461:1007-1012.
55. Jilka RL. Molecular and cellular mechanisms of the anabolic effect of intermittent PTH. *Bone.* 2007;40:1434-1446.
56. Aubin J. Mesenchymal stem cells and osteoblast differentiation. In: Bilezikian J, Raisz L, Martin T, eds. *Principles of Bone Biology.* 3rd ed. Amsterdam: Elsevier; 2008:85-108.
57. Sacchetti B, Funari A, Michienzi S, et al. Self-renewing osteoprogenitors in bone marrow sinusoids can organize a hematopoietic microenvironment. *Cell.* 2007;131:324-336.
58. Jilka RL, Weinstein RS, Parfitt AM, et al. Quantifying osteoblast and osteocyte apoptosis: challenges and rewards. *J Bone Miner Res.* 2007;22:1492-1501.
59. Dobnig H, Turner RT. Evidence that intermittent treatment with parathyroid hormone increases bone formation in adult rats by activation of bone lining cells. *Endocrinology.* 1995;136:3632-3638.
60. Nishida S, Yamaguchi A, Tanizawa T, et al. Increased bone formation by intermittent parathyroid hormone administration is due to the stimulation of proliferation and differentiation of osteoprogenitor cells in bone marrow. *Bone.* 1994;15:717-723.
61. Lotinun S, Sibonga JD, Turner RT. Evidence that the cells responsible for marrow fibrosis in a rat model for hyperparathyroidism are preosteoblasts. *Endocrinology.* 2005;146:4074-4081.
62. Bellows CG, Ishida H, Aubin JE, et al. Parathyroid hormone reversibly suppresses the differentiation of osteoprogenitor cells into functional osteoblasts. *Endocrinology.* 1990;127:3111-3116.
63. Bellido T, Ali AA, Plotkin LI, et al. Proteasomal degradation of Runx2 shortens parathyroid hormone-induced anti-apoptotic signaling in osteoblasts: a putative explanation for why intermittent administration is needed for bone anabolism. *J Biol Chem.* 2003;278: 50259-50272.
64. Qin L, Tamasi J, Raggatt L, Li X, et al. Amphiregulin is a novel growth factor involved in normal bone development and in the cellular response to parathyroid hormone stimulation. *J Biol Chem.* 2005;280:3974-3981.
65. Kulkarni NH, Halladay DL, Miles RR, et al. Effects of parathyroid hormone on Wnt signaling pathway in bone. *J Cell Biochem.* 2005;95:1178-1190.
66. Bellido T, Ali AA, Gubrij I, et al. Chronic elevation of parathyroid hormone in mice reduces expression of sclerostin by osteocytes: a novel mechanism for hormonal control of osteoblastogenesis. *Endocrinology.* 2005;146:4577-4583.
67. Semenov M, Tamai K, He X. SOST is a ligand for LRP5/LRP6 and a Wnt signaling inhibitor. *J Biol Chem.* 2005;280:26770-26775.
68. Tang Y, Wu X, Lei W, et al. TGF-beta1-induced migration of bone mesenchymal stem cells couples bone resorption with formation. *Nat Med.* 2009;15:757-765.
69. Teitelbaum SL, Ross FP. Genetic regulation of osteoclast development and function. *Nat Rev Genet.* 2003;4:638-649.
70. Yao GQ, Sun B, Hammond EE, et al. The cell-surface form of colony-stimulating factor-1 is regulated by osteotropic agents and supports formation of multinucleated osteoclast-like cells. *J Biol Chem.* 1998;273:4119-4128.
71. Chase LR, Aurbach GD. Parathyroid function and the renal excretion of 3'5'-adenylic acid. *Proc Natl Acad Sci U S A.* 1967;58:518-525.
72. Gensure RC, Gardella TJ, Juppner H. Parathyroid hormone and parathyroid hormone-related peptide, and their receptors. *Biochem Biophys Res Commun.* 2005;328:666-678.
73. Pioszak AA, Parker NR, Gardella TJ, et al. Structural basis for parathyroid hormone-related protein binding to the parathyroid hormone receptor and design of conformation-selective peptides. *J Biol Chem.* 2009;284:28382-28391.
74. Okazaki M, Ferrandon S, Vilardaga JP, et al. Prolonged signaling at the parathyroid hormone receptor by peptide ligands targeted to a specific receptor conformation. *Proc Natl Acad Sci U S A.* 2008;105:16525-16530.
75. Ferrandon S, Feinstein TN, Castro M, et al. Sustained cyclic AMP production by parathyroid hormone receptor endocytosis. *Nat Chem Biol.* 2009;5:734-742.
76. Murray TM, Rao LG, Divieti P, et al. Parathyroid hormone secretion and action: evidence for discrete receptors for the carboxyl-terminal region and related biological actions of carboxyl-terminal ligands. *Endocr Rev.* 2005;26:78-113.
77. Gaich G, Orloff JJ, Atillasoy EJ, et al. Amino-terminal parathyroid hormone-related protein: specific binding and cytosolic calcium responses in rat insulinoma cells. *Endocrinology.* 1993;132:1402-1409.
78. Fegley DB, Holmes A, Riordan T, et al. Increased fear- and stress-related anxiety-like behavior in mice lacking tuberoinfundibular peptide of 39 residues. *Genes Brain Behav.* 2008;7:933-942.
79. Usdin TB, Paciga M, Riordan T, et al. Tuberoinfundibular peptide of 39 residues is required for germ cell development. *Endocrinology.* 2008;149:4292-4300.
80. Shimizu M, Potts Jr JT, Gardella TJ. Minimization of parathyroid hormone. *J Biol Chem.* 2000;275:21836-21843.
81. Takasu H, Gardella TJ, Luck MD, et al. Amino-terminal modifications of human parathyroid hormone (PTH) selectively alter phospholipase C signaling via the type 1 PTH receptor: implications for design of signal-specific PTH ligands. *Biochemistry.* 1999;38:13453-13460.
82. Gesty-Palmer D, Flannery P, Yuan L, et al. A β-arrestin-biased agonist of the parathyroid hormone receptor (PTH1R) promotes bone formation independent of G protein activation. *Sci Transl Med.* 2009;1:1ra1.
83. Pioszak AA, Xu HE. Molecular recognition of parathyroid hormone by its G protein-coupled receptor. *Proc Natl Acad Sci U S A.* 2008; 105:5034-5039.
84. Castro M, Nikolaev VO, Palm D, et al. Turn-on switch in parathyroid hormone receptor by a two-step parathyroid hormone binding mechanism. *Proc Natl Acad Sci U S A.* 2005;102:16084-16089.
85. Vilardaga JP, Bunemann M, Krasel C, et al. Measurement of the millisecond activation switch of G protein-coupled receptors in living cells. *Nat Biotechnol.* 2003;21:807-812.
86. Jin L, Briggs SL, Chandrasekhar S, et al. Crystal structure of human parathyroid hormone 1-34 at 0.9-A resolution. *J Biol Chem.* 2000;275:27238-27244.
87. Gardella TJ, Luck MD, Fan MH, et al. Transmembrane residues of the parathyroid hormone (PTH)/PTH-related peptide receptor that specifically affect binding and signaling by agonist ligands. *J Biol Chem.* 1996;271:12820-12825.
88. Sheikh SP, Vilardarga JP, Baranski TJ, et al. Similar structures and shared switch mechanisms of the beta2-adrenoceptor and the parathyroid hormone receptor. Zn(II) bridges between helices III and VI block activation. *J Biol Chem.* 1999;274:17033-17041.
89. Bastepe M, Raas-Rothschild A, Silver J, et al. A form of Jansen's metaphyseal chondrodysplasia with limited metabolic and skeletal abnormalities is caused by a novel activating parathyroid hormone (PTH)/PTH-related peptide receptor mutation. *J Clin Endocrinol Metab.* 2004;89:3595-3600.
90. Bringhurst FR, Zajac JD, Daggett AS, et al. Inhibition of parathyroid hormone responsiveness in clonal osteoblastic cells expressing a mutant form of 3',5'-cyclic adenosine monophosphate-dependent protein kinase. *Mol Endocrinol.* 1989;3:60-67.
91. Traebert M, Volkl H, Biber J, et al. Luminal and contraluminal action of 1-34 and 3-34 PTH peptides on renal type IIa Na-P(i) cotransporter. *Am J Physiol Renal Physiol.* 2000;278:F792-F798.
92. Janulis M, Tembe V, Favus MJ. Role of protein kinase C in parathyroid hormone stimulation of renal 1,25-dihydroxyvitamin D3 secretion. *J Clin Invest.* 1992;90:2278-2283.
93. Guo J, Chung UI, Kondo H, et al. The PTH/PTHrP receptor can delay chondrocyte hypertrophy in vivo without activating phospholipase C. *Dev Cell.* 2002;3(2):183-194.

94. Guo J, Liu M, Thomas CC, et al. Phospholipase C signaling via the PTH/PTHrP receptor is essential for normal full response to PTH in both bone and kidney. *J Bone Miner Res*. 2007;22(suppl): 1119 (Abstract).
95. Mahon MJ, Segre GV. Stimulation by parathyroid hormone of a NHERF-1-assembled complex consisting of the parathyroid hormone I receptor, phospholipase Cβ, and actin increases intracellular calcium in opossum kidney cells. *J Biol Chem*. 2004;279:23550-23558.
96. Vilardaga JP, Krasel C, Chauvin S, et al. Internalization determinants of the parathyroid hormone receptor differentially regulate beta-arrestin/receptor association. *J Biol Chem*. 2002;277:8121-8129.
97. Tawfeek HA, Qian F, Abou-Samra AB. Phosphorylation of the receptor for PTH and PTHrP is required for internalization and regulates receptor signaling. *Mol Endocrinol*. 2002;16:1-13.
98. Orloff JJ, Reddy D, de Papp AE, et al. Parathyroid hormone-related protein as a prohormone: posttranslational processing and receptor interactions. *Endocr Rev*. 1994;15:40-60.
99. Wu TL, Vasavada RC, Yang KH, et al. Structural and physiologic characterization of the mid-region secretory species of parathyroid hormone-related protein. *J Biol Chem*. 1996;271:24371-24381.
100. Burtis WJ, Brady TG, Orloff JJ, et al. Immunochemical characterization of circulating parathyroid hormone related protein in patients with humoral hypercalcemia of cancer. *N Engl J Med*. 1990;322: 1106-1112.
101. Stewart AF. Clinical practice: hypercalcemia associated with cancer. *N Engl J Med*. 2005;352:373-379.
102. Simmonds CS, Karsenty G, Karaplis AC, et al. Parathyroid hormone regulates fetal-placental mineral homeostasis. *J Bone Miner Res*. 2010;25:594-605.
103. VanHouten JN, Dann P, Stewart AF, et al. Mammary-specific deletion of parathyroid hormone-related protein preserves bone mass during lactation. *J Clin Invest*. 2003;112:1429-1436.
104. VanHouten J, Dann P, McGeoch G, et al. The calcium-sensing receptor regulates mammary gland parathyroid hormone-related protein production and calcium transport. *J Clin Invest*. 2004;113:598-608.
105. Kalkwarf HJ, Specker BL, Ho M. Effects of calcium supplementation on calcium homeostasis and bone turnover in lactating women. *J Clin Endocrinol Metab*. 1999;84:464-470.
106. Khosla S, Johansen KL, Ory SJ, et al. Parathyroid hormone-related peptide in lactation and in umbilical cord blood. *Mayo Clin Proc*. 1990;65:1408-1414.
107. Strewler GJ. The physiology of parathyroid hormone-related protein. *N Engl J Med*. 2000;342:177-185.
108. Kronenberg HM. Developmental regulation of the growth plate. *Nature*. 2003;423:332-336.
109. Maeda S, Sutliff RL, Qian J, et al. Targeted overexpression of parathyroid hormone-related protein (PTHrP) to vascular smooth muscle in transgenic mice lowers blood pressure and alters vascular contractility. *Endocrinology*. 1999;140:1815-1825.
110. Miao D, Su H, He B, et al. Severe growth retardation and early lethality in mice lacking the nuclear localization sequence and C-terminus of PTH-related protein. *Proc Natl Acad Sci U S A*. 2008;105:20309-20314.
111. Copp DH, Cameron EC, Cheney B, et al. Evidence for calcitonin—a new hormone from the parathyroid that lowers blood calcium. *Endocrinology*. 1962;70:638-649.
112. Garrett JE, Tamir H, Kifor O, et al. Calcitonin-secreting cells of the thyroid express and extracellular calcium receptor gene. *Endocrinology*. 1995;136:5202-5211.
113. Care AD. The regulation of the secretion of calcitonin. *Bone Miner*. 1992;16:182-185.
114. Friedman PA, Gesek FA. Cellular calcium transport in renal epithelia: measurement, mechanisms and regulation. *Physiol Rev*. 1995;75: 429-471.
115. Chambers TJ, McSheehy PM, Thomson BM, et al. The effect of calcium-regulating hormones and prostaglandins on bone resorption by osteoclasts disaggregated from neonatal rabbit bones. *Endocrinology*. 1985;116:234-239.
116. Talmage RV, Vanderwiel CJ, Decker SA, et al. Changes produced in postprandial urinary calcium excretion by thyroidectomy and calcitonin administration in rats on different calcium regimes. *Endocrinology*. 1979;105:459-464.
117. Hoff AO, Catala-Lehnen P, Thomas PM, et al. Increased bone mass is an unexpected phenotype associated with deletion of the calcitonin gene. *J Clin Invest*. 2002;110:1849-1857.
118. Dacquin R, Davey RA, Laplace C, et al. Amylin inhibits bone resorption while the calcitonin receptor controls bone formation in vivo. *J Cell Biol*. 2004;164:509-514.
119. Gagel R, Hoff A, Huang S, et al. Deletion of the calcitonin/CGRP gene causes a profound cortical resorption phenotype in mice. *J Bone Miner Res*. 2007;22(suppl 1): 1120 (Abstract).
120. Hurley DL, Tiegs RD, Wahner HW, et al. Axial and appendicular bone mineral density in patients with long-term deficiency or excess of calcitonin. *N Engl J Med*. 1987;317:537-541.
121. Purdue BW, Tilakaratne N, Sexton PM. Molecular pharmacology of the calcitonin receptor. *Receptors Channels*. 2002;8:243-255.
122. Chakraborty M, Chatterjee D, Kellokumpu S, et al. Cell cycle-dependent coupling of the calcitonin receptor to different G proteins. *Science*. 1991;251:1078-1082.
123. Udawela M, Hay DL, Sexton PM. The receptor activity modifying protein family of G protein coupled receptor accessory proteins. *Semin Cell Dev Biol*. 2004;15:299-308.
124. Zumpe E, Tilakaratne N, Fraser N, et al. Multiple ramp domains are required for generation of amylin receptor phenotype from the calcitonin receptor gene product. *Biochem Biophys Res Commun*. 2000;267:368-372.
125. Gangula P, Zhao H, Supowit S, et al. Increased blood presure in alpha-calcitonin gene-related peptide/calcitonin gene knockout mice. *Hypertension*. 2000;35(1 Pt 2):470-475.
126. Katafuchi T, Yasue H, Osaki T, et al. Calcitonin receptor-stimulating peptide: its evolutionary and functional relationship with calcitonin/calcitonin gene-related peptide based on gene structure. *Peptides*. 2009;30:1753-1762.
127. Lorenzo A, Razzaboni B, Weir GC, et al. Pancreatic islet cell toxicity of amylin associated with type-2 diabetes mellitus. *Nature*. 1994;368: 756-757.
128. Chase HP, Lutz K, Pencek R, et al. Pramlintide lowered glucose excursions and was well-tolerated in adolescents with type 1 diabetes: results from a randomized, single-blind, placebo-controlled, crossover study. *J Pediatr*. 2009;155:369-373. Epub 2009 May 21.
129. Shimosawa T, Shibagaki Y, Ishibashi K, et al. Adrenomedullin, an endogenous peptide, counteracts cardiovascular damage. *Circulation*. 2002;105:106-111.
130. Roh J, Chang CL, Bhalla A, et al. Intermedin is a calcitonin/calcitonin gene-related peptide family peptide acting through the calcitonin receptor-like receptor/receptor activity-modifying protein receptor complexes. *J Biol Chem*. 2004;279:7264-7274.
131. Holick MF, Shao Q, Liu WW, et al. The vitamin D content of fortified milk and infant formula. *N Engl J Med*. 1992;326:1178-1181.
132. Safadi F, Thornton P, Magiera H, et al. Osteopathy and resistance to vitamin D toxicity in mice null for vitamin D binding protien. *J Clin Invest*. 1999;103:239-251.
133. Nykjaer A, Dragun D, Walther D, et al. An endocytic pathway essential for renal uptake and activation of the steroid 25-(OH) vitamin D3. *Cell*. 1999;96:507-515.
134. Saito A, Iino N, Takeda T, et al. Role of megalin, a proximal tubular endocytic receptor, in calcium and phosphate homeostasis. *Ther Apher Dial*. 2007;11(suppl 1):S23-S26.
135. Murayama A, Takeyama K, Kitanaka S, et al. Positive and negative regulations of the renal 25-hydroxyvitamin D_3 1a-hydroxylase gene by parathyroid hormone, calcitonin, and 1α, $25(OH)_2D_3$ in intact animals. *Endocrinology*. 1999;140:2224-2231.
136. Shimada T, Hasegawa H, Yamazaki Y, et al. FGF-23 is a potent regulator of vitamin D metabolism and phosphate homeostasis. *J Bone Miner Res*. 2004;19:429-435.
137. Overbergh L, Decallonne B, Valckx D, et al. Identification and immune regulation of 25-hydroxyvitamin D-1-alpha-hydroxylase in murine macrophages. *Clin Exp Immunol*. 2000;120:139-146.
138. Liu PT, Stenger S, Li H, et al. Toll-like receptor triggering of a vitamin D-mediated human antimicrobial response. *Science*. 2006;311: 1770-1773.
139. Adams JS, Sharma OP, Diz MM, et al. Ketoconazole decreases the serum 1,25-dihydroxyvitamin D and calcium concentration in sarcoidosis-associated hypercalcemia. *J Clin Endocrinol Metab*. 1990;70: 1090-1095.
140. Adams JS, Diz MM, Sharma OP. Effective reduction in the serum 1,25-dihydroxyvitamin D and calcium concentration in sarcoidosis-associated hypercalcemia with short-course chloroquine therapy. *Ann Intern Med*. 1989;111:437-438.
141. St-Arnaud R, Arabian A, Travers R, et al. Deficient mineralization of intramembranous bone in vitamin D-24-hydroxylase-ablated mice is due to elevated 1,25-dihydroxyvitamin D and not to the absence of 24,25-dihydroxyvitamin D. *Endocrinology*. 2000;141:2658-2666.
142. Schwartz Z, Brooks B, Swain L, et al. Production of 1,25-dihydroxyvitamin D_3 and 24,25-dihydroxyvitamin D_3 by growth zone and resting zone chondrocytes is dependent on cell maturation and is regulated by hormones and growth factors. *Endocrinology*. 1992;130:2495-2504.
143. Pettifor JM, Bikle DD, Cavaleros M, et al. Serum levels of free 1,25-dihydroxyvitamin D in vitamin D toxicity. *Ann Intern Med*. 1995;122:511-513.
144. Inoue T, Kamiyama J, Sakai T. Sp1 and NF-Y synergistically mediate the effect of vitamin D_3 in the $p27^{Kip1}$ gene promotor that lacks vitamin D response elements. *J Biol Chem*. 1999;274:32309-32317.
145. Kim MS, Fujiki R, Murayama A, et al. 1Alpha,25(OH)2D3-induced transrepression by vitamin D receptor through E-box-type elements in the human parathyroid hormone gene promoter. *Mol Endocrinol*. 2007;21:334-342.
146. Yuan W, Pan W, Kong J, et al. 1,25-Dihydroxyvitamin D3 suppresses renin gene transcription by blocking the activity of the cyclic AMP response element in the renin gene promoter. *J Biol Chem*. 2007;282:29821-29830.

147. Nishishita T, Okazaki T, Ishikawa T, et al. A Negative vitamin D response DNA element in the human parathyroid hormone-related peptide gene binds to vitamin D receptor along with Ku antigen to mediate negative gene regulation by vitamin D. *J Biol Chem.* 1998;273:10901-10907.
148. Iida K, Shinki T, Yamaguchi A, et al. A possible role of vitamin D receptors in regulating vitamin D activation in the kidney. *Proc Natl Acad Sci U S A.* 1995;92:6112-6116.
149. Nemere I, Dormanen MC, Hammond MW, et al. Identification of a specific binding protein for 1α,25-dihydroxyvitamin D_3 in basal-lateral membranes of chick intestinal epithelium and relationship to transcaltachia. *J Biol Chem.* 1994;269:23750-23756.
150. Erben RG, Soegiarto DW, Weber K, et al. Deletion of deoxyribonucleic acid binding domain of the vitamin D receptor abrogates genomic and nongenomic functions of vitamin D. *Mol Endocrinol.* 2002;16:1524-1537.
151. Hughes MR, Malloy PJ, Kieback DG, et al. Point mutations in the human vitamin D receptor gene associated with hypocalcemic rickets. *Science.* 1988;242:1702-1705.
152. Li YC, Pirro AE, Amling M, et al. Targeted ablation of the vitamin D receptor: an animal model of vitamin D-dependent rickets type II with alopecia. *Proc Natl Acad Sci U S A.* 1997;94:9831-9835.
153. Amling M, Priemel M, Holzmann T, et al. Rescue of the skeletal phenotype of vitamin D receptor-ablated mice in the setting of normal mineral ion homeostasis: formal histomorphometric and biomechanical analyses. *Endocrinology.* 1999;140:4982-4987.
154. Balsan S, Garabedian M, Larchet M, et al. Long-term nocturnal calcium infusions can cure rickets and promote normal mineralization in hereditary resistance to 1,25-dihydroxyvitamin D. *J Clin Invest.* 1986;77:1661-1667.
155. Li YC, Amling M, Pirro AE, et al. Normalization of mineral ion homeostasis by dietary means prevents hyperparathyroidism, rickets, and osteomalacia, but not alopecia in vitamin D receptor-ablated mice. *Endocrinology.* 1998;139:4391-4396.
156. Karbach U. Paracellular calcium transport across the small intestine. *J Nutr.* 1992;122:672-677.
157. Fujita H, Sugimoto K, Inatomi S, et al. Tight junction proteins claudin-2 and -12 are critical for vitamin D-dependent Ca2+ absorption between enterocytes. *Mol Biol Cell.* 2008;19:1912-1921.
158. van de Graaf SF, Boullart I, Hoenderop JG, et al. Regulation of the epithelial Ca2+ channels TRPV5 and TRPV6 by 1alpha,25-dihydroxy vitamin D3 and dietary Ca2+. *J Steroid Biochem Mol Biol.* 2004;89-90:303-308.
159. Hoenderop JG, van Leeuwen JP, van der Eerden BC, et al. Renal Ca2+ wasting, hyperabsorption, and reduced bone thickness in mice lacking TRPV5. *J Clin Invest.* 2003;112:1906-1914.
160. Benn BS, Ajibade D, Porta A, et al. Active intestinal calcium transport in the absence of transient receptor potential vanilloid type 6 and calbindin-D9k. *Endocrinology.* 2008;149:3196-3205.
161. Meir T, Levi R, Lieben L, et al. Deletion of the vitamin D receptor specifically in the parathyroid demonstrates a limited role for the receptor in parathyroid physiology. *Am J Physiol Renal Physiol.* 2009;297:F1192-F1198.
162. Yasuda H, Shima N, Nakagawa N, et al. Osteoclast differentiation factor is a ligand for osteoprotegerin/osteoclastogenesis-inhibitory factor and is identical to TRANCE/RANKL. *Proc Natl Acad Sci U S A.* 1998;95:3597-3602.
163. Endo I, Inoue D, Mitsui T, et al. Deletion of vitamin D receptor gene in mice results in abnormal skeletal muscle development with deregulated expression of myoregulatory transcription factors. *Endocrinology.* 2003;144:5138-5144.
164. Zhou JY, Norman AW, Chen DL, et al. 1,25-Dihydroxy-16-ene-23-yne-vitamin D_3 prolongs survival time of leukemic mice. *Proc Natl Acad Sci U S A.* 1990;87:3929-3932.
165. Mathieu C, Laureys J, Waer M, et al. Prevention of autoimmune destruction of transplanted islets in spontaneously diabetic NOD mice by KH1060, a 20-epi analog of vitamin D: synergy with cyclosporine. *Transplant Proc.* 1994;26:3128-3129.
166. Brown AJ, Ritter CR, Finch JL, et al. The noncalcemic analogue of vitamin D, 22-oxacalcitriol, suppresses parathyroid hormone synthesis and secretion. *J Clin Invest.* 1989;84:728-732.
167. Holick MF, Smith E, Pincus S. Skin as the site of vitamin D synthesis and target tissue for 1,25-dihydroxyvitamin D_3: use of calcitriol (1,25-dihydroxyvitamin D_3) for treatment of psoriasis. *Arch Dermatol.* 1987;123:1677-1683.
168. Kamimura S, Gallieni M, Kubodera N, et al. Differential catabolism of 22-oxacalcitriol and 1,25-dihydroxyvitamin D_3 by normal human peripheral monocytes. *Endocrinology.* 1993;133:2719-2722.
169. Peleg S, Sastry M, Collins ED, et al. Distinct conformational changes induced by 20-epi analogues of 1α,25-dihydroxyvitamin D_3 are associated with enhanced activation of the vitamin D receptor. *J Biol Chem.* 1995;270:10551-10558.
170. ADHR Consortium. Autosomal dominant hypophosphataemic rickets is associated with mutations in FGF23. *Nat Genet.* 2000;26:345-348.
171. White KE, Carn G, Lorenz-Depiereux B, et al. Autosomal-dominant hypophosphatemic rickets (ADHR) mutations stabilize FGF-23. *Kidney Int.* 2001;60:2079-2086.
172. Shimada T, Muto T, Urakawa I, et al. Mutant FGF-23 responsible for autosomal dominant hypophosphatemic rickets is resistant to proteolytic cleavage and causes hypophosphatemia in vivo. *Endocrinology.* 2002;143:3179-3182.
173. Shimada T, Mizutani S, Muto T, et al. Cloning and characterization of FGF23 as a causative factor of tumor-induced osteomalacia. *Proc Natl Acad Sci U S A.* 2001;98:6500-6505.
174. White KE, Jonsson KB, Carn G, et al. The autosomal dominant hypophosphatemic rickets (ADHR) gene is a secreted polypeptide overexpressed by tumors that cause phosphate wasting. *J Clin Endocrinol Metab.* 2001;86:497-500.
175. Ward LM, Rauch F, White KE, et al. Resolution of severe, adolescent-onset hypophosphatemic rickets following resection of an FGF-23-producing tumour of the distal ulna. *Bone.* 2004;34:905-911.
176. Endo I, Fukumoto S, Ozono K, et al. Clinical usefulness of measurement of fibroblast growth factor 23 (FGF23) in hypophosphatemic patients: proposal of diagnostic criteria using FGF23 measurement. *Bone.* 2008;42(6):1235-1239.
177. Araya K, Fukumoto S, Backenroth R, et al. A novel mutation in fibroblast growth factor 23 gene as a cause of tumoral calcinosis. *J Clin Endocrinol Metab.* 2005;90:5523-5527.
178. Chefetz I, Heller R, Galli-Tsinopoulou A, et al. A novel homozygous missense mutation in FGF23 causes familial tumoral calcinosis associated with disseminated visceral calcification. *Hum Genet.* 2005;118:261-266.
179. Larsson T, Yu X, Davis SI, et al. A novel recessive mutation in fibroblast growth factor-23 causes familial tumoral calcinosis. *J Clin Endocrinol Metab.* 2005;90:2424-2427.
180. Garringer HJ, Fisher C, Larsson TE, et al. The role of mutant UDP-*N*-acetyl-alpha-D-galactosamine-polypeptide *N*-acetylgalactosaminyltransferase 3 in regulating serum intact fibroblast growth factor 23 and matrix extracellular phosphoglycoprotein in heritable tumoral calcinosis. *J Clin Endocrinol Metab.* 2006;91:4037-4042.
181. Ichikawa S, Imel EA, Kreiter ML, et al. A homozygous missense mutation in human KLOTHO causes severe tumoral calcinosis. *J Clin Invest.* 2007;117:2684-2691.
182. Larsson T, Marsell R, Schipani E, et al. Transgenic mice expressing fibroblast growth factor 23 under the control of the alpha1(I) collagen promoter exhibit growth retardation, osteomalacia, and disturbed phosphate homeostasis. *Endocrinology.* 2004;145:3087-3094.
183. Shimada T, Kakitani M, Yamazaki Y, et al. Targeted ablation of Fgf23 demonstrates an essential physiological role of FGF23 in phosphate and vitamin D metabolism. *J Clin Invest.* 2004;113:561-568.
184. Sitara D, Razzaque MS, Hesse M, et al. Homozygous ablation of fibroblast growth factor-23 results in hyperphosphatemia and impaired skeletogenesis, and reverses hypophosphatemia in Phex-deficient mice. *Matrix Biol.* 2004;23:421-432.
185. Razzaque M, Sitara D, Taguchi T, et al. Premature ageing-like phenotype in fibroblast growth factor 23 null mice is a vitamin-D mediated process. *FASEB.* 2006;20:720-722.
186. Saito H, Kusano K, Kinosaki M, et al. Human fibroblast growth factor-23 mutants suppress Na+-dependent phosphate co-transport activity and 1alpha,25-dihydroxyvitamin D3 production. *J Biol Chem.* 2003;278:2206-2211.
187. Segawa H, Kawakami E, Kaneko I, et al. Effect of hydrolysis-resistant FGF23-R179Q on dietary phosphate regulation of the renal type-II Na/Pi transporter. *Pflugers Arch.* 2003;446:585-592.
188. Yan X, Yokote H, Jing X, et al. Fibroblast growth factor 23 reduces expression of type IIa Na+/Pi co-transporter by signaling through a receptor functionally distinct from the known FGFRs in opossum kidney cells. *Genes Cells.* 2005;10:489-502.
189. Miyamoto K, Ito M, Kuwahata M, et al. Inhibition of intestinal sodium-dependent inorganic phosphate transport by fibroblast growth factor 23. *Ther Apher Dial.* 2005;9:331-335.
190. Kurosu H, Ogawa Y, Miyoshi M, et al. Regulation of fibroblast growth factor-23 signaling by klotho. *J Biol Chem.* 2006;281:6120-6123.
191. Yoshida T, Fujimori T, Nabeshima Y. Mediation of unusually high concentrations of 1,25-dihydroxyvitamin D in homozygous klotho mutant mice by increased expression of renal 1alpha-hydroxylase gene. *Endocrinology.* 2002;143:683-689.
192. Yu X, Sabbagh Y, Davis SI, et al. Genetic dissection of phosphate- and vitamin D-mediated regulation of circulating Fgf23 concentrations. *Bone.* 2005;36:971-977.
193. Perwad F, Azam N, Zhang MY, et al. Dietary and serum phosphorus regulate fibroblast growth factor 23 expression and 1,25-dihydroxyvitamin D metabolism in mice. *Endocrinology.* 2005;146:5358-5364.
194. Ye L, Mishina Y, Chen D, Huang H, et al. Dmp1-deficient mice display severe defects in cartilage formation responsible for a chondrodysplasia-like phenotype. *J Biol Chem.* 2005;280:6197-6203.

195. Masuyama R, Stockmans I, Torrekens S, et al. Vitamin D receptor in chondrocytes promotes osteoclastogenesis and regulates FGF23 production in osteoblasts. *J Clin Invest.* 2006;116:3150-3159.
196. Nakanishi S, Kazama JJ, Nii-Kono T, et al. Serum fibroblast growth factor-23 levels predict the future refractory hyperparathyroidism in dialysis patients. *Kidney Int.* 2005;67:1171-1178.
197. Koiwa F, Kazama JJ, Tokumoto A, et al. Sevelamer hydrochloride and calcium bicarbonate reduce serum fibroblast growth factor 23 levels in dialysis patients. *Ther Apher Dial.* 2005;9:336-339.
198. Nussbaum SR, Zahradnik RJ, Lavigne JR, et al. Highly sensitive two-site immunoradiometric assay of parathyrin and its clinical utility in evaluating patients with hypercalcemia. *Clin Chem.* 1987;33:1364-1367.
199. Gao P, D'Amour P. Evolution of the parathyroid hormone (PTH) assay: importance of circulating PTH immunoheterogeneity and of its regulation. *Clin Lab.* 2005;51:21-29.
200. Boudou P, Ibrahim F, Cormier C, et al. Third- or second-generation parathyroid hormone assays: a remaining debate in the diagnosis of primary hyperparathyroidism. *J Clin Endocrinol Metab.* 2005;90: 6370-6372.
201. Burtis WJ, Brady TG, Orloff JJ, et al. Immunochemical characterization of circulating parathyroid hormone-related protein in patients with humoral hypercalcemia of cancer. *N Engl J Med.* 1990;322:1106-1112.
202. Fritchie K, Zedek D, Grenache DG. The clinical utility of parathyroid hormone-related peptide in the assessment of hypercalcemia. *Clin Chim Acta.* 2009;402:146-149.
203. Isomura M, Honda N, Kawada A, et al. Development of a highly sensitive enzyme immunoasay for human calcitonin using solid phase coupled with multiple antibodies. *Ann Clin Biochem.* 1999;36: 629-635.
204. Lavigne JR, Zahradnik RJ, Conklin RL, et al. Stimulation of calcitonin secretion by calcium receptor activators: evaluation using a new, highly sensitive, homologous immunoradiometric assay for rat calcitonin. *Endocrine.* 1998;9:293-301.
205. Ersfeld DL, Rao DS, Body JJ, et al. Analytical and clinical validation of the 25-OH vitamin D assay for the LIAISON automated analyzer. *Clin Biochem.* 2004;37:867-874.
206. Phinney KW. Development of a standard reference material for vitamin D in serum. *Am J Clin Nutr.* 2008;88:511S-512S.
207. Jonsson KB, Zahradnik R, Larsson T, et al. Fibroblast growth factor 23 in oncogenic osteomalacia and X-linked hypophosphatemia. *N Engl J Med.* 2003;348:1656-1663.
208. Yamazaki Y, Okazaki R, Shibata M, et al. Increased circulatory level of biologically active full-length FGF-23 in patients with hypophosphatemic rickets/osteomalacia. *J Clin Endocrinol Metab.* 2002;87: 4957-4960.
209. Burnett S, Gunawardene S, Bringhurst R, et al. Regulation of C-terminal and intact FGF-23 by dietary phosphate in men and women. *J Bone Miner Res.* 2006;21:1187-1196.
210. Weber CJ, Sewell CW, McGarity WC. Persistent and recurrent sporadic primary hyperparathyroidism: histopathology, complications, and results of reoperation. *Surgery.* 1994;116:991-998.
211. LiVolsi VA. Embryology, anatomy, and pathology of the parathyroids. In: Bilezikian JP, ed. *The Parathyroids.* New York: Raven Press; 1994:1-14.
212. Rosen IB, Young JEM, Archibald SD, et al. Parathyroid cancer: clinical variations and relationships to autotransplantation. *Can J Cancer.* 1994;37:465-469.
213. Shane E, Bilezikian JP. Parathyroid carcinoma: a review of 62 patients. *Endocr Rev.* 1982;3:218-226.
214. Patten BM, Bilezikian JP, Mallette LE, et al. Neuromuscular disease in hyperparathyroidism. *Ann Intern Med.* 1974;80:182-193.
215. Wermers RA, Khosla S, Atkinson EJ, et al. The rise and fall of primary hyperparathyroidism: a population-based study in Rochester, Minnesota, 1965-1992. *Ann Intern Med.* 1997;126:433-440.
216. Lundgren E, Rastad J, Thrufjell E, et al. Population-based screening for primary hyperparathyroidism with serum calcium and parathyroid hormone values in menopausal women. *Surgery.* 1997;121:287-294.
217. Lowe H, McMahon DJ, Rubin MR, et al. Normocalcemic primary hyperparathyroidism: further characterization of a new clinical phenotype. *J Clin Endocrinol Metab.* 2007;92:3001-3005.
218. Silverberg SJ, Shane E, Jacobs TP, et al. A 10-year prospective study of primary hyperparathyroidism with or without parathyroid surgery [see comments]. *N Engl J Med.* 1999;341:1249-1255.
219. Walgenbach S, Hommel G, Junginger T. Outcome after surgery for primary hyperparathyroidism: ten-year prospective follow-up study. *World J Surg.* 2000;24:564-569.
220. Rao DS, Phillips ER, Divine GW, et al. Randomized controlled clinical trial of surgery versus no surgery in patients with mild asymptomatic primary hyperparathyroidism. *J Clin Endocrinol Metab.* 2004;89: 5415-5422.
221. Ambrogini E, Cetani F, Cianferotti L, et al. Surgery or surveillance for mild asymptomatic primary hyperparathyroidism: a prospective, randomized clinical trial. *J Clin Endocrinol Metab.* 2007;92:3114-3121.
222. Bollerslev J, Jansson S, Mollerup CL, et al. Medical observation, compared with parathyroidectomy, for asymptomatic primary hyperparathyroidism: a prospective, randomized trial. *J Clin Endocrinol Metab.* 2007;92:1687-1692.
223. Palmer M, Adami HO, Bergstrom R, et al. Mortality after surgery for primary hyperparathyroidism: a followup of 441 patients operated on from 1956-1979. *Surgery.* 1987;102:1-7.
224. Walgenbach S, Hommel G, Junginger T. Outcome after surgery for primary hyperparathyroidism: ten-year prospective follow-up study. *World J Surg.* 2000;24:564-569; discussion 569-570.
225. Silverberg SJ, Bilezikian JP, Bone HG, et al. Therapeutic controversies in primary hyperparathyroidism. *J Clin Endocrinol Metab.* 1999;84: 2275-2285.
226. Rubin MR, Bilezikian JP, McMahon DJ, et al. The natural history of primary hyperparathyroidism with or without parathyroid surgery after 15 years. *J Clin Endocrinol Metab.* 2008;93:3462-3470.
227. Stefenelli T, Abela C, Frank H, et al. Cardiac abnormalities in patients with primary hyperparathyroidism: implications for follow-up. *J Clin Endocrinol Metab.* 1997;82:106-112.
228. Wermers RA, Khosla S, Atkinson EJ, et al. Survival after the diagnosis of hyperparathyroidism: a population-based study. *Am J Med.* 1998;104:115-122.
229. Palmer M, Adami HO, Krusemo UB, et al. Increased risk of malignant diseases after surgery for primary hyperparathyroidism: a nationwide cohort study. *Am J Epidemiol.* 1988;127:1031-1040.
230. Parisien M, Silverberg SJ, Shane E, et al. The histomorphometry of bone in primary hyperparathyroidism: preservation of cancellous bone structure. *J Clin Endocrinol Metab.* 1990;70:930-938.
231. Silverberg SJ, Gartenberg F, Jacobs TP, et al. Longitudinal measurements of bone density and biochemical indices in untreated primary hyperparathyroidism. *J Clin Endocrinol Metab.* 1995;80:723-728.
232. Silverberg SJ, Locker FG, Bilezikian JP. Verterbral osteopenia: a new indication for surgery in primary hyperparathyroidism. *J Clin Endocrinol Metab.* 1996;81:4007-4012.
233. Khosla S, Melton LJI, Wermers RA, et al. Primary hyperparathyroidism and the risk of fracture: a population-based study. *J Bone Miner Res.* 1999;14:1700-1707.
234. Vestergaard P, Mollerup CL, Frokjaer VG, et al. Cohort study of risk of fracture before and after surgery for primary hyperparathyroidism. *BMJ.* 2000;321:598-602.
235. Rao DS, Wilson RJ, Kleerekoper M, et al. Lack of biochemical progression or continuation of accelerated bone loss in mild asymptomatic primary hyperparathyroidism: evidence for biphasic disease course. *J Clin Endocrinol Metab.* 1988;67:1294-1298.
236. Arnold A, Staunton CE, Kim HG, et al. Monoclonality and abnormal parathyroid hormone genes in parathyroid adenomas. *N Engl J Med.* 1988;318:658-662.
237. Arnold A, Shattuck TM, Mallya SM, et al. Molecular pathogenesis of primary hyperparathyroidism. *J Bone Miner Res.* 2002;17(suppl 2):N30-N36.
238. Costa-Guda J, Tokura T, Roth SI, et al. Mitochondrial DNA mutations in oxyphilic and chief cell parathyroid adenomas. *BMC Endocr Disord.* 2007;7:8.
239. Motokura T, Bloom T, Kim HG, et al. A BCL1-linked candidate oncogene which is rearranged in parathyroid tumors encodes a novel cyclin. *Nature.* 1991;350:512-515.
240. Mallya SM, Gallagher JJ, Wild YK, et al. Abnormal parathyroid cell proliferation precedes biochemical abnormalities in a mouse model of primary hyperparathyroidism. *Mol Endocrinol.* 2005;19:2603-2609.
241. Carling T. Molecular pathology of parathyroid tumors. *Trends Endocrinol Metab.* 2001;12:53-58.
242. Samander EH, Arnold A. Mutational analysis of the vitamin D receptor does not support its candidacy as a tumor suppressor gene in parathyroid adenomas. *J Clin Endocrinol Metab.* 2006;91:5019-5021.
243. Imanishi Y, Tahara H, Palanisamy N, et al. Clonal chromosomal defects in the molecular pathogenesis of refractory hyperparathyroidism of uremia. *J Am Soc Nephrol.* 2002;13:1490-1498.
244. Arnold A, Brown MF, Urena P, et al. Monoclonality of parathyroid tumors in chronic renal failure and in primary parathyroid hyperplasia. *J Clin Invest.* 1995;95:2047-2053.
245. Friedman E, Sakaguchi K, Bale AE, et al. Clonality of parathyroid tumors in familial multiple endocrine neoplasia type I. *N Engl J Med.* 1989;321:213-218.
246. Livolsi V. Parathyroids: morphology and pathology. In: Bilezikian J, ed. *The parathyroids: basic and clinical concepts.* 2nd ed. San Diego: Academic Press; 2001:1-16.
247. Kifor O, Moore FD, Wang P, et al. Reduced immunostaining for the extracellular Ca2+-sensing receptor in primary and uremic secondary hyperparathyroidism. *J Clin Endocrinol Metab.* 1996;81:1598-1606.
248. Mizobuchi M, Ritter CS, Krits I, et al. Calcium-sensing receptor expression is regulated by glial cells missing-2 in human parathyroid cells. *J Bone Miner Res.* 2009;24:1173-1179.
249. Marx SJ. Molecular genetics of multiple endocrine neoplasia types 1 and 2. *Nat Rev Cancer.* 2005;5:367-375.
250. Hughes CM, Rozenblatt-Rosen O, Milne TA, et al. Menin associates with a trithorax family histone methyltransferase complex and with the hoxc8 locus. *Mol Cell.* 2004;13:587-597.

251. Karnik SK, Hughes CM, Gu X, et al. Menin regulates pancreatic islet growth by promoting histone methylation and expression of genes encoding p27Kip1 and p18INK4c. *Proc Natl Acad Sci U S A*. 2005;102:14659-14664.
252. Agarwal SK, Mateo CM, Marx SJ. Rare germline mutations in cyclin-dependent kinase inhibitor genes in multiple endocrine neoplasia type 1 and related states. *J Clin Endocrinol Metab*. 2009;94:1826-1834.
253. Eller-Vainicher C, Chiodini I, Battista C, et al. Sporadic and MEN1-related primary hyperparathyroidism: differences in clinical expression and severity. *J Bone Miner Res*. 2009;24:1404-1410.
254. Norton JA, Venzon DJ, Berna MJ, et al. Prospective study of surgery for primary hyperparathyroidism (HPT) in multiple endocrine neoplasia-type 1 and Zollinger-Ellison syndrome: long-term outcome of a more virulent form of HPT. *Ann Surg*. 2008;247:501-510.
255. Pausova Z, Soliman E, Amizuka N, et al. Role of the RET proto-oncogene in sporadic hyperparathyroidism and in hyperparathyroidism of multiple endocrine neoplasia type 2. *J Clin Endocrinol Metab*. 1996;81:2711-2718.
256. Haven CJ, Wong FK, van Dam EW, et al. A genotypic and histopathological study of a large Dutch kindred with hyperparathyroidism-jaw tumor syndrome. *J Clin Endocrinol Metab*. 2000;85:1449-1454.
257. Carpten JD, Robbins CM, Villablanca A, et al. HRPT2, encoding parafibromin, is mutated in hyperparathyroidism-jaw tumor syndrome. *Nat Genet*. 2002;32:676-680.
258. Rozenblatt-Rosen O, Hughes CM, Nannepaga SJ, et al. The parafibromin tumor suppressor protein is part of a human Paf1 complex. *Mol Cell Biol*. 2005;25:612-620.
259. Yart A, Gstaiger M, Wirbelauer C, et al. The HRPT2 tumor suppressor gene product parafibromin associates with human PAF1 and RNA polymerase II. *Mol Cell Biol*. 2005;25:5052-5060.
260. Newey PJ, Bowl MR, Thakker RV. Parafibromin: functional insights. *J Intern Med*. 2009;266:84-98.
261. Mosimann C, Hausmann G, Basler K. Parafibromin/Hyrax activates Wnt/Wg target gene transcription by direct association with beta-catenin/Armadillo. *Cell*. 2006;125:327-341.
262. Shattuck TM, Valimaki S, Obara T, et al. Somatic and germ-line mutations of the HRPT2 gene in sporadic parathyroid carcinoma. *N Engl J Med*. 2003;349:1722-1729.
263. Bilezikian JP, Khan AA, Potts Jr JT. Third International Workshop on the Management of Asymptomatic Primary Hyperthyroidism. Guidelines for the management of asymptomatic primary hyperparathyroidism: summary statement from the Third International Workshop. *J Clin Endocrinol Metab*. 2009;94:335-339.
264. Silverberg SJ, Brown I, Bilezikian JP. Age as a criterion for surgery in primary hyperparathyroidism. *Am J Med*. 2002;113:681-684.
265. Nakaoka D, Sugimoto T, Kobayashi T, et al. Prediction of bone mass change after parathyroidectomy in patients with primary hyperparathyroidism. *J Clin Endocrinol Metab*. 2000;85:1901-1907.
266. Rubin MR, Lee KH, McMahon DJ, et al. Raloxifene lowers serum calcium and markers of bone turnover in postmenopausal women with primary hyperparathyroidism. *J Clin Endocrinol Metab*. 2003;88:1174-1178.
267. Khan AA, Bilezikian JP, Kung AW, et al. Alendronate in primary hyperparathyroidism: a double-blind, randomized, placebo-controlled trial. *J Clin Endocrinol Metab*. 2004;89:3319-3325.
268. Chow CC, Chan WB, Li JK, et al. Oral alendronate increases bone mineral density in postmenopausal women with primary hyperparathyroidism. *J Clin Endocrinol Metab*. 2003;88:581-587.
269. Peacock M, Bilezikian JP, Klassen PS, et al. Cinacalcet hydrochloride maintains long-term normocalcemia in patients with primary hyperparathyroidism. *J Clin Endocrinol Metab*. 2005;90:135-141.
270. Grant CS, Thompson G, Farley D, et al. Primary hyperparathyroidism surgical management since the introduction of minimally invasive parathyroidectomy: Mayo Clinic experience. *Arch Surg*. 2005;140:472-478; discussion 478-479.
271. Ruda JM, Hollenbeak CS, Stack Jr BC. A systematic review of the diagnosis and treatment of primary hyperparathyroidism from 1995 to 2003. *Otolaryngol Head Neck Surg*. 2005;132:359-372.
272. Akerstrom G, Rundberg C, Grimelius L, et al. Causes of failed primary exploration and technical aspects of reoperation in primary hyperparathyroidism. *World J Surg*. 1992;16:562-569.
273. Kollmorgen CF, Aust MR, Ferreiro JA, et al. Parathyromatosis: a rare yet important cause of persistent or recurrent hyperparathyroidism. *Surgery*. 1994;116:111-115.
274. Mitchell BK, Merrell RC, Kinder BK. Localization studies in patients with hyperparathyroidism. *Surg Clin North Am*. 1995;75:483-498.
275. Udelsman R, Donovan PI. Open minimally invasive parathyroid surgery. *World J Surg*. 2004;28:1224-1226.
276. Inabnet WB. Intraoperative parathyroid hormone monitoring. *World J Surg*. 2004;28:1212-1215.
277. Weber KJ, Misra S, Lee JK, et al. Intraoperative PTH monitoring in parathyroid hyperplasia requires stricter criteria for success. *Surgery*. 2004;136:1154-1159.
278. Siperstein A, Berber E, Barbosa GF, et al. Predicting the success of limited exploration for primary hyperparathyroidism using ultrasound, sestamibi, and intraoperative parathyroid hormone: analysis of 1158 cases. *Ann Surg*. 2008;248:420-428.
279. Lambert LA, Shapiro SE, Lee JE, et al. Surgical treatment of hyperparathyroidism in patients with multiple endocrine neoplasia type 1. *Arch Surg*. 2005;140:374-382.
280. Marcocci C, Cetani F, Rubin MR, et al. Parathyroid carcinoma. *J Bone Miner Res*. 2008;23:1869-1880.
281. Oertli D, Richter M, Kraenzlin M, et al. Parathyroidectomy in primary hyperparathyroidism: preoperative localization and routine biopsy of unaltered glands are not necessary. *Surgery*. 1995;117:392-396.
282. Bergenfelz A, Valdermarsson S, Ahren B. Functional recovery of the parathyroid glands after surgery for primary hyperparathyroidism. *Surgery*. 1994;116:827-836.
283. Gross ND, Weissman JL, Veenker E, et al. The diagnostic utility of computed tomography for preoperative localization in surgery for hyperparathyroidism. *Laryngoscope*. 2004;114:227-231.
284. Biertho LD, Kim C, Wu HS, et al. Relationship between sestamibi uptake, parathyroid hormone assay, and nuclear morphology in primary hyperparathyroidism. *J Am Coll Surg*. 2004;199(2):229-233.
285. Milas M, Wagner K, Easley KA, et al. Double adenomas revisited: nonuniform distribution favors enlarged superior parathyroids (fourth pouch disease). *Surgery*. 2003;134:995-1003; discussion 1003-1004.
286. Mortenson MM, Evans DB, Lee JE, et al. Parathyroid exploration in the reoperative neck: improved preoperative localization with 4D-computed tomography. *J Am Coll Surg*. 2008;206:888-895; discussion 895-886.
287. Estella E, Leong MS, Bennett I, et al. Parathyroid hormone venous sampling prior to reoperation for primary hyperparathyroidism. *A N Z J Surg*. 2003;73:800-805.
288. Chaffanjon PC, Voirin D, Vasdev A, et al. Selective venous sampling in recurrent and persistent hyperparathyroidism: indication, technique, and results. *World J Surg*. 2004;28:958-961.
289. Smythe WR, Bavaria JE, Hall RA, et al. Thoracoscopic removal of mediastinal parathyroid adenoma. *Ann Thorac Surg*. 1995;59:236-238.
290. Nomura R, Sugimoto T, Tsukamoto T, et al. Marked and sustained increase in bone mineral density after parathyroidectomy in patients with primary hyperparathyroidism: a six-year longitudinal study with or without parathyroidectomy in a Japanese population. *Clin Endocrinol*. 2004;60:335-342.
291. Khosla S, Ebeling PR, Firek AF, et al. Calcium infusion suggests a "set-point" abnormality of parathyroid gland function in familial benign hypercalcemia and more complex disturbances in primary hyperparathyroidism. *J Clin Endocrinol Metab*. 1993;76:715-720.
292. Kifor O, Moore Jr FD, Delaney M, et al. A syndrome of hypocalciuric hypercalcemia caused by autoantibodies directed at the calcium-sensing receptor. *J Clin Endocrinol Metab*. 2003;88:60-72.
293. Pallais JC, Kifor O, Chen YB, et al. Acquired hypocalciuric hypercalcemia due to autoantibodies against the calcium-sensing receptor. *N Engl J Med*. 2004;351:362-369.
294. Carling T, Szao E, Bai M, et al. Familial hypercalcemia and hypercalciuria caused by a novel mutation in the cytoplasmic tail of the calcium receptor. *J Clin Endoceinol Metab*. 2000;85:2042-2047.
295. Marx SJ, Attie MF, Levine MA, et al. The hypocalciuric or benign variant of familial hypercalcemia: clinical and biochemical features in fifteen kindreds. *Medicine (Baltimore)*. 1981;60:397-412.
296. Christensen SE, Nissen PH, Vestergaard P, et al. Discriminative power of three indices of renal calcium excretion for the distinction between familial hypocalciuric hypercalcaemia and primary hyperparathyroidism: a follow-up study on methods. *Clin Endocrinol (Oxf)*. 2008;69:713-720.
297. Mallette LE, Khouri K, Zengotita H, et al. Lithium treatment increases intact and midregion parathyroid hormone and parathyroid volume. *J Clin Endocrinol Metab*. 1989;68:654-660.
298. Saunders BD, Saunders EF, Gauger PG. Lithium therapy and hyperparathyroidism: an evidence-based assessment. *World J Surg*. 2009;33:2314-2323.
299. McHenry CR, Racke F, Meister M, et al. Lithium effects on dispersed bovine parathyroid cells grown in tissue culture. *Surgery*. 1991;110:1061-1066.
300. Jacobs TP, Bilezikian JP. Clinical review: rare causes of hypercalcemia. *J Clin Endocrinol Metab*. 2005;90:6316-6322.
301. Ehrlich LA, Roodman GD. The role of immune cells and inflammatory cytokines in Paget's disease and multiple myeloma. *Immunol Rev*. 2005;208:252-266.
302. Tian E, Zhan F, Walker R, et al. The role of the Wnt-signaling antagonist DKK1 in the development of osteolytic lesions in multiple myeloma. *N Engl J Med*. 2003;349:2483-2494.
303. Gavriatopoulou M, Dimopoulos MA, Christoulas D, et al. Dickkopf-1: a suitable target for the management of myeloma bone disease. *Expert Opin Ther Targets*. 2009;13:839-848.
304. Guise TA. Molecular mechanisms of osteolytic bone metastases. *Cancer*. 2000;88(12 Suppl):2892-2898.

305. Case records of the Massachusetts General Hospital (case 27461). *N Engl J Med*. 1941;225:789-791.
306. Stewart AF, Horst R, Deftos LJ, et al. Biochemical evaluation of patients with cancer-associated hypercalcemia: evidence for humoral and non-humoral groups. *N Engl J Med*. 1980;303:1377-1383.
307. Suva LJ, Winslow GA, Wettenhall RE, et al. A parathyroid hormone-related protein implicated in malignant hypercalcemia: cloning and expression. *Science*. 1987;237:893-896.
308. Kukreja SC, Shevrin DH, Wimbiscus SA, et al. Antibodies to parathyroid hormone-related protein lower serum calcium in athymic mouse models of malignancy-associated hypercalcemia due to human tumors. *J Clin Invest*. 1988;82:1798-1802.
309. Horwitz MJ, Tedesco MB, Sereika SM, et al. Continuous PTH and PTHrP infusion causes suppression of bone formation and discordant effects on 1,25(OH)2 vitamin D. *J Bone Miner Res*. 2005;20:1792-1803.
310. Strewler GJ, Wronski TJ, Halloran BP. Pathogenesis of hypercalcemia in nude mice bearing a human renal carcinoma. *Endocrinology*. 1986;119:303-309.
311. Bushinsky DA, Riera GS, Favus MJ, et al. Evidence that blood ionized calcium can regulate serum $1,25(OH)_2D_3$ independently of parathyroidhormone and phosphorus in the rat. *J Clin Invest*. 1985;76: 1599-1604.
312. Kitazawa R, Imai Y, Fukase M, et al. Effects of continuous infusion of parathyroid hormone and parathyroid hormone-related peptide on rat bone in vivo: comparative study by histomorphometry. *Bone Miner*. 1991;12:157-166.
313. Seymour JF, Gagel RF, Hagemeister FB, et al. Calcitriol production in hypercalcemic and normocalcemic patients with non-hodgkin lymphoma. *Ann Intern Med*. 1994;121:633-640.
314. Davies M, Hayes ME, Yin JA, et al. Abnormal synthesis of 1,25-dihydroxyvitamin D in patients with malignant lymphoma. *J Clin Endocrinol Metab*. 1994;78:1202-1207.
315. Jones G. Pharmacokinetics of vitamin D toxicity. *Am J Clin Nutr*. 2008;88:582S-586S.
316. Conron M, Young C, Beynon HL. Calcium metabolism in sarcoidosis and its clinical implications. *Rheumatology (Oxf)*. 2000;39:707-713.
317. Farooque A, Moss C, Zehnder D, et al. Expression of 25-hydroxyvitamin D3-1alpha-hydroxylase in subcutaneous fat necrosis. *Br J Dermatol*. 2009;160:423-425.
318. Abreu MT, Kantorovich V, Vasiliauskas EA, et al. Measurement of vitamin D levels in inflammatory bowel disease patients reveals a subset of Crohn's disease patients with elevated 1,25-dihydroxyvitamin D and low bone mineral density. *Gut*. 2004;53:1129-1136.
319. Auwerx J, Bouillon R. Mineral and bone metabolism in thyroid disease: a review. *Q J Med*. 1986;60:737-752.
320. Bassett JH, Williams GR. The molecular actions of thyroid hormone in bone. *Trends Endocrinol Metab*. 2003;14:356-364.
321. Mallette LE, Rubenfeld S, Silverman V. A controlled study of the effects of thyrotoxicosis and propranolol treatment on mineral metabolism and parathyroid hormone immunoreactivity. *Metabolism*. 1985;34: 999-1006.
322. Valentic JP, Elias AN, Weinstein GD. Hypercalcemia associated with oral isotretinoin in the treatment of severe acne. *J Am Med Assoc*. 1986;250:1899-1900.
323. Bennett MT, Sirrs S, Yeung JK, et al. Hypercalcemia due to all trans retinoic acid in the treatment of acute promyelocytic leukemia potentiated by voriconazole. *Leuk Lymphoma*. 2005;46:1829-1831.
324. Muls E, Bouillon R, Boelaert J, et al. Etiology of hypercalcemia in a patient with Addison's disease. *Calcif Tissue Int*. 1982;34: 523-526.
325. Katahira M, Yamada T, Kawai M. A case of Cushing syndrome with both secondary hypothyroidism and hypercalcemia due to postoperative adrenal insufficiency. *Endocr J*. 2004;51:105-113.
326. Nijenhuis T, Vallon V, van der Kemp AW, et al. Enhanced passive Ca2+ reabsorption and reduced Mg2+ channel abundance explains thiazide-induced hypocalciuria and hypomagnesemia. *J Clin Invest*. 2005;115: 1651-1658.
327. Wermers RA, Kearns AE, Jenkins GD, et al. Incidence and clinical spectrum of thiazide-associated hypercalcemia. *Am J Med*. 2007;120: 911.e919-911.e15.
328. Medarov BI. Milk-alkali syndrome. *Mayo Clin Proc*. 2009;84:261-267.
329. Nijenhuis T, Vallon V, van der Kemp AW, et al. Enhanced passive Ca2+ reabsorption and reduced Mg2+ channel abundance explains thiazide-induced hypocalciuria and hypomagnesemia. *J Clin Invest*. 2005;115: 1651-1658.
330. Tatsumi S, Ishii K, Amizuka N, et al. Targeted ablation of osteocytes induces osteoporosis with defective mechanotransduction. *Cell Metab*. 2007;5:464-475.
331. Llach F, Felsenfeld AJ, Haussler MR. The pathophysiology of altered calcium metabolism in rhabdomyolysis-induced acute renal failure. *N Engl J Med*. 1981;305:117-123.
332. Shrestha SM, Berry JL, Davies M, et al. Biphasic hypercalcemia in severe rhabdomyolysis: serial analysis of PTH and vitamin D metabolites. A case report and literature review. *Am J Kidney Dis*. 2004;43:e31-e35.
333. Williams JCP, Barratt-Boyes BG, Lowe JB. Supravalvular aortic stenosis. *Circulation*. 1961;24:1311-1318.
334. Garabedian M, Jacqz E, Guillozo H, et al. Elevated plasma 1,25-dihydroxyvitamin D concentrations in infants with hypercalcemia and an elfin facies. *N Engl J Med*. 1985;312:948-952.
335. Cagle AP, Waguespack SG, Buckingham BA, et al. Severe infantile hypercalcemia associated with Williams syndrome successfully treated with intravenously administered pamidronate. *Pediatrics*. 2004;114:1091-1095.
336. Kitagawa H, Fujiki R, Yoshimura K, et al. The chromatin-remodeling complex WINAC targets a nuclear receptor to promoters and is impaired in Williams syndrome. *Cell*. 2003;113:905-917.
337. Kruse K, Schutz C. Calcium metabolism in the Jansen type of metaphyseal dysplasia. *Eur J Pediatr*. 1993;152:912-915.
338. Schipani E, Kruse K, Juppner H. A constitutively active mutant PTH-PTHrP receptor in Jansen-type metaphyseal chondrodysplasia. *Science*. 1995;268:98-100.
339. Silverberg SJ, Gao P, Brown I, et al. Clinical utility of an immunoradiometric assay for parathyroid hormone (1-84) in primary hyperparathyroidism. *J Clin Endocrinol Metab*. 2003;88:4725-4730.
340. Carnevale V, Dionisi S, Nofroni I, et al. Potential clinical utility of a new IRMA for parathyroid hormone in postmenopausal patients with primary hyperparathyroidism. *Clin Chem*. 2004;50:626-631.
341. Kifor O, Moore Jr FD, Delaney M, et al. A syndrome of hypocalciuric hypercalcemia caused by autoantibodies directed at the calcium-sensing receptor. *J Clin Endocrinol Metab*. 2003;88:60-72.
342. Pallais JC, Kifor O, Chen YB, et al. Acquired hypocalciuric hypercalcemia due to autoantibodies against the calcium-sensing receptor [see comment]. *N Engl J Med*. 2004;351:362-369.
343. Jacobs TP, Bilezikian JP. Clinical review: rare causes of hypercalcemia. *J Clin Endocrinol Metab*. 2005;90:6316-6322.
344. Stewart AF. Clinical practice: hypercalcemia associated with cancer. *N Engl J Med*. 2005;352:373-379.
345. Picolos MK, Lavis VR, Orlander PR. Milk-alkali syndrome is a major cause of hypercalcaemia among non-end-stage renal disease (non-ESRD) inpatients. *Clin Endocrinol*. 2005;63:566-576.
346. Cvitkovic F, Armand JP, Tubiana-Hulin M, et al. Randomized, double-blind, phase II trial of gallium nitrate compared with pamidronate for acute control of cancer-related hypercalcemia [see comment]. *Cancer J*. 2006;12:47-53.
347. Ioachimescu AG, Bauer TW, Licata A. Active Crohn disease and hypercalcemia treated with infliximab: case report and literature review. *Endocr Pract*. 2008;14:87-92.
348. Barman Balfour JA, Scott LJ. Cinacalcet hydrochloride. *Drugs*. 2005;65:271-281.
349. Onuma E, Sato K, Saito H, et al. Generation of a humanized monoclonal antibody against human parathyroid hormone-related protein and its efficacy against humoral hypercalcemia of malignancy. *Anticancer Res*. 2004;24:2665-2673.
350. Bockman DE, Kriby ML. Dependence of thymus development on derivatives of the neural crest. *Science*. 1984;223:498-500.
351. Chisaka O, Capecchi MR. Regionally restricted developmental defects resulting from targeted disruption of the mouse homeobox gene hox-1.5. *Nature*. 1991;350:473-479.
352. Garabedian M. Hypocalcemia and chromosome 22q11 microdeletion. *Genet Couns*. 1999;10:389-394.
353. Karayiorgou M, Morris MA, Morrow B, et al. Schizophrenia susceptibility associated with interstitial deletions of chromosome 22q11. *Proc Natl Acad Sci U S A*. 1995;92:7612-7616.
354. Budarf ML, Collins J, Gong W, et al. Cloning a balanced translocation associated with DiGeorge syndrome and identfication of a disrupted candidate gene. *Nat Genet*. 1995;10:269-278.
355. Scire G, Dallapiccola B, Iannetti P, et al. Hypoparathyroidism as the major manifestation in two patients with 22q11 deletions. *Am J Med Genet*. 1994;52:478-482.
356. Merscher S, Funke B, Epstein JA, et al. TBX1 is responsible for cardiovascular defects in velo-cardio-facial/DiGeorge syndrome. *Cell*. 2001;104:619-629.
357. Daw S, Taylor C, Kraman M, et al. A common region of 10p deleted and velocardiofacial syndromes. *Nat Genet*. 1996;13:458-460.
358. Van Esch H, Groenen P, Nesbit MA, et al. GATA3 haplo-insufficiency causes human HDR syndrome. *Nature*. 2000;406:419-422.
359. Parvari R, Hershkovitz E, Grossman N, et al. Mutation of TBCE causes hypoparathyroidism-retardation-dysmorphism and autosomal recessive Kenny-Caffey syndrome. *Nat Genet*. 2002;32:448-452.
360. Su MA, Anderson MS. Aire: an update. *Curr Opin Immunol*. 2004;16(6):746-752.
361. Gardner JM, Fletcher AL, Anderson MS, et al. AIRE in the thymus and beyond. *Curr Opin Immunol*. 2009;21:582-589.
362. Alimohammadi M, Bjorklund P, Hallgren A, et al. Autoimmune polyendocrine syndrome type 1 and NALP5, a parathyroid autoantigen. *N Engl J Med*. 2008;358:1018-1028.
363. Dionisi-Vici C, Garavaglia B, Burlina A, et al. Hypoparathyroidism in mitochondrial trifunctional protein deficiency. *J Pediatr*. 1996; 129:159-162.

364. Papadimitriou A, Hadjigeorgiou G, Divari R, et al. The influence of coenzyme Q10 on total serum calcium concentration in two patients with Kearns-Sayre syndrome and hypoparathyroidism. *Neuromuscul Disord*. 1996;6:49-53.
365. Ahn TG, Antonarakis SE, Kronenberg HM, et al. Familial isolated hypoparathyroidism: a molecular genetic analysis of 8 families with 23 affected persons. *Medicine (Baltimore)*. 1986;65:73-81.
366. Baldellou A, Bone J, Tamparillas M, et al. Congenital hypoparathyroidism, ocular colobomata, unilateral renal agenesis and dysmorphic features. *Genet Couns*. 1991;2:245-247.
367. Dahlberg PJ, Borer WZ, Newcomer KL, et al. Autosomal or X-linked recessive syndrome of congenital lymphedema, hypoparathyroidism, nephropathy, prolapsing mitral valve, and brachytelephalangy. *Am J Med Genet*. 1983;16:99-104.
368. Arnold A, Horst SA, Gardella RJ, et al. Mutation of the signal peptide-encoding region of the preproparathyroid hormone gene in familial isolated hypoparathyroidism. *J Clin Invest*. 1990;86:1084-1087.
369. Sunthornthepvarakul T, Churesigaew S, Ngowngarmratana S. A novel mutation of the signal peptide of the preporparathyroid hormone gene associated with autosomal recessive familial isolated hypoparathyroidism. *J Clin Endocrinol Metab*. 1999;84:3792-3796.
370. Parkinson DB, Thakker RV. A donor splice site mutation in the parathyroid hormone gene is associated with autosomal recessive hypoparathyroidism. *Nat Genet*. 1992;2:149-152.
371. Hammes M, DeMory A, Sprague SM. Hypocalcemia in end-stage renal disease: a consequence of spontaneous parathyroid gland infarction. *Am J Kidney Dis*. 1994;24:519-522.
372. Burch WM, Posillico JT. Hypoparathyroidism after I-131 therapy with subsequent return of parathyroid function. *J Clin Endocrinol Metab*. 1983;57:398-401.
373. Gertner JM, Broadus AE, Anast CS, et al. Impaired parathyroid response to induced hypocalcemia in thalassemia major. *J Pediatr*. 1979;95:210-213.
374. Carpenter TO, Carnes DL, Anast CS. Hypoparathyroidism in Wilson's disease. *N Engl J Med*. 1983;309:873-877.
375. Suh SM, Tashjian AH, Matsuo N, et al. Pathogenesis of hypocalcemia in primary hypomagnesemia: normal end-organ responsiveness to parathyroid hormone, impaired parathyroid gland function. *J Clin Invest*. 1973;52:153-160.
376. Estep H, Shaw WA, Watlington C, et al. Hypocalcemia due to hypomagnesemia and reversible parathyroid hormone unresponsiveness. *J Clin Endocrinol Metab*. 1969;29:842-848.
377. Rude RK, Oldham SB, Singer FR. Functional hypoparathyroidism and parathyroid hormone end-organ resistance in human magnesium deficiency. *Clin Endocrinol*. 1976;5:209-224.
378. Krapf R, Jaeger P, Hulter HN, et al. Chronic respiratory alkalosis induces renal PTH-resistance, hyperphosphatemia and hypocalcemia in humans. *Kidney Int*. 1992;42:727-734.
379. Lopez I, Rodriguez M, Felsenfeld AJ, et al. Direct suppressive effect of acute metabolic and respiratory alkalosis on parathyroid hormone secretion in the dog. *J Bone Miner Res*. 2003;18:1478-1485.
380. Pearce S, Williams C, Kifor O, et al. A familial syndrome of hypocalcemia with hypercalciuria due to mutations in the calcium-sensing receptor. *N Engl J Med*. 1996;335:1115-1122.
381. Leinhardt A, Garabédian M, Bai M, et al. A large homozygous or heterozygous in-frame deletion within the calcium-sensing receptor's carboxylterminal cytoplasmic tail that causes autosomal dominant hypocalcemia. *J Clin Endocrinol Metab*. 2000;85:1695-1702.
382. Albright F, Aub J, Bauer W. Hyperparathyroidism: a common and polymorphic condition as illustrated by seventeen proved cases from one clinic. *J Am Med Assoc*. 1934;102:1276-1287.
383. Chase LR, Melson GL, Aurbach GD. Pseudohypoparathyroidism: defective excretion of 3′,5′-AMP in response to parathyroid hormone. *J Clin Invest*. 1969;48:1832-1844.
384. Mallette LE, Kirkland JL, Gagel RF, et al. Synthetic human parathyroid hormone-(1-34) for the study of pseudohypoparathyroidism. *J Clin Endocrinol Metab*. 1988;67:964-972.
385. Bastepe M. The GNAS locus and pseudohypoparathyroidism. *Adv Exp Med Biol*. 2008;626:27-40.
386. Iiri T, Herzmark P, Nakamoto JM, et al. Rapid GDP release from Gsα in patients with gain and loss of endocrine function. *Nature*. 1994;371:164-168.
387. Levine MA, Ahn TG, Klupt SF, et al. Genetic deficiency of the α subunit of the guanine nucleotide-binding protein Gs as the molecular basis for Albright hereditary osteodystrophy. *Proc Natl Acad Sci U S A*. 1988;85:617-621.
388. Davies SJ, Hughes HE. Imprinting in Albright's hereditary osteodystrophy. *J Med Genet*. 1993;30:101-103.
389. Wilson LC, Oude Luttikhuis ME, Clayton PT, et al. Parental origin of Gs alpha gene mutations in Albright's hereditary osteodystrophy. *J Med Genet*. 1994;31:835-839.
390. Yu S, Yu D, Lee E, et al. Variable and tissue-specific hormone resistance in heterotrimeric G_s protein α-subunit ($G_s\alpha$) knockout mice is due to tissue-specific imprinting of the $G_s\alpha$ gene. *Proc Natl Acad Sci U S A*. 1998;95:8715-8720.
391. Long DN, McGuire S, Levine MA, et al. Body mass index differences in pseudohypoparathyroidism type 1a versus pseudopseudohypoparathyroidism may implicate paternal imprinting of Galpha(s) in the development of human obesity. *J Clin Endocrinol Metab*. 2007;92:1073-1079.
392. Chen M, Wang J, Dickerson KE, et al. Central nervous system imprinting of the G protein G(s)alpha and its role in metabolic regulation. *Cell Metab*. 2009;9:548-555.
393. Adegbite NS, Xu M, Kaplan FS, et al. Diagnostic and mutational spectrum of progressive osseous heteroplasia (POH) and other forms of GNAS-based heterotopic ossification. *Am J Med Genet A*. 2008;146A:1788-1796.
394. Bastepe M, Lane AH, Juppner H. Paternal uniparental isodisomy of chromosome 20q—and the resulting changes in GNAS1 methylation—as a plausible cause of pseudohypoparathyroidism. *Am J Hum Genet*. 2001;68:1283-1289.
395. Bastepe M, Pincus JE, Sugimoto T, et al. Positional dissociation between the genetic mutation responsible for pseudohypoparathyroidism type Ib and the associated methylation defect at exon A/B: evidence for a long-range regulatory element within the imprinted GNAS1 locus. *Hum Mol Genet*. 2001;10:1231-1241.
396. Liu J, Erlichman B, Weinstein LS. The stimulatory G protein alpha-subunit Gs alpha is imprinted in human thyroid glands: implications for thyroid function in pseudohypoparathyroidism types 1A and 1B. *J Clin Endocrinol Metab*. 2003;88:4336-4341.
397. Murray TM, Rao LG, Wong MM, et al. Pseudohypoparathyroidism with osteitis fibrosa cystica: direct demonstration of skeletal responsiveness to parathyroid hormone in cells cultured from bone. *J Bone Miner Res*. 1993;8:83-91.
398. Jüppner H, Schipani E, Bastepe M, et al. The gene responsible for pseudohypoparathyroidism type Ib is paternally imprinted and maps in four unrelated kindreds to chromosome 20q13.3. *Proc Natl Acad Sci U S A*. 1998;95:11798-11803.
399. Jan de Beur S, Ding C, Germain-Lee E, et al. Discordance between genetic and epigenetic defects in pseudohypoparathyroidism type 1b revealed by inconsistent loss of maternal imprinting at GNAS1. *Am J Hum Genet*. 2003;73:314-322.
400. Liu J, Litman D, Rosenberg MJ, et al. A GNAS1 imprinting defect in pseudohypoparathyroidism type IB. *J Clin Invest*. 2000;106:1167-1174.
401. Bastepe M, Frohlich LF, Hendy GN, et al. Autosomal dominant pseudohypoparathyroidism type Ib is associated with a heterozygous microdeletion that likely disrupts a putative imprinting control element of GNAS. *J Clin Invest*. 2003;112:1255-1263.
402. Linglart A, Gensure RC, Olney RC, et al. A novel STX16 deletion in autosomal dominant pseudohypoparathyroidism type Ib redefines the boundaries of a cis-acting imprinting control element of GNAS. *Am J Hum Genet*. 2005;76:804-814.
403. Barrett D, Breslau NA, Wax MB, et al. New form of pseudohypoparathyroidism with abnormal catalytic adenylate cyclase. *Am J Physiol*. 1989;257:E277-E283.
404. Linglart A, Carel JC, Garabedian M, et al. GNAS1 lesions in pseudohypoparathyroidism Ia and Ic: genotype phenotype relationship and evidence of the maternal transmission of the hormonal resistance. *J Clin Endocrinol Metab*. 2002;87:189-197.
405. Drezner M, Neelon FA, Lebovitz HE. Pseudohypoparathyroidism type II: a possible defect in the reception of the cyclic amp signal. *N Engl J Med*. 1973;289:1056-1060.
406. Konoshita M, Komori T, Ohtake T, et al. Abnormal calcium metabolism in myotonic dystrophy as shown by the Ellsworth-Howard test and its relation to CTG triplet repeat length. *J Neurol*. 1997;244:613-622.
407. Rao DS, Parfitt AM, Kleerekoper M, et al. Dissociation between the effects of endogenous parathyroid hormone on adenosine 3′,5′-monophosphate generation and phosphate reabsorption in hypocalcemia due to vitamin D depletion: an acquired disorder resembling pseudohypoparathyroidism type II. *J Clin Endocrinol Metab*. 1985;61:285-290.
408. Koo BB, Schwindinger WF, Levine MA. Characterization of Albright hereditary osteodystrophy and related disorders. *Acta Pediatr Sin*. 1995;36:3-13.
409. Minagawa M, Yasuda T, Kobayashi Y, et al. Transient pseudohypoparathyroidism of the neonate. *Eur J Endocrinol*. 1995;133:151-155.
410. Silve C. Pseudohypoparathyroidism syndromes: the many faces of parathyroid hormone resistance. *Eur J Endocrinol*. 1995;133:145-146.
411. Kidd GS, Schaaf M, Adler RA, et al. Skeletal responsiveness in pseudohypoparathyroidism. *Am J Med*. 1980;68:772-781.
412. Kruse K, Kracht U, Wohlfart K, et al. Biochemical markers of bone turnover, intact serum parathyroid hormone and renal calcium excretion in patients with pseudohypoparathyroidism and hypoparathyroidism before and during vitamin D treatment. *Eur J Pediatr*. 1989;148:535-539.
413. Breslau NA, Moses AM, Pak CYC. Evidence for bone remodeling but lack of calcium mobilization response to parathyroid hormone in

pseudohypoparathyroidism. *J Clin Endocrinol Metab.* 1983;57: 638-644.

414. Yamamoto M, Takuwa Y, Masuko S, et al. Effects of endogenous and exogenous parathyroid hormone on tubular reabsorption of calcium in pseudohypoparathyroidism. *J Clin Endocrinol Metab.* 1988;66: 618-625.
415. Thomas M, DM L-J, Thadhani R, et al. Hypovitaminosis D in medical patients. *N Engl J Med.* 1998;338:777-783.
416. Thomas M, Demay M. Vitamin D deficiency and disorders of vitamin D metabolism. *Endocrinol Metab Clin North Am.* 2000;29:611-627.
417. Chapuy MC, Arlot ME, Duboeuf F, et al. Vitamin D_3 and calcium to prevent hip fractures in elderly women. *N Engl J Med.* 1992;327: 1637-1642.
418. Hahn TJ, Hendin BA, Scharp CR, et al. Effect of chronic anticonvulsant therapy on serum 25-hydroxycalciferol levels in adults. *N Engl J Med.* 1972;287:900-904.
419. Greenwood RH, Pruntz FTG, Silver J. Osteomalacia after prolonged glutethimide administration. *Br Med J.* 1973;1:643-645.
420. Brodie MJ, Boobis AR, Hillyard CJ, et al. Effect of rifampicin and isoniazid on vitamin D metabolism. *Clin Pharmacol Ther.* 1982;32: 525-530.
421. Casella SJ, Reiner BJ, Chen TC, et al. A possible genetic defect in 25-hydroxylation as a cause of rickets. *J Pediatr.* 1994;124: 929-932.
422. Goodman WG. Calcimimetic agents for the treatment of secondary hyperparathyroidism. *Semin Nephrol.* 2004;24:460-463.
423. Delvin EE, Glorieux FH, Marie PJ, et al. Vitamin D dependency: replacement therapy with calcitriol. *Pediatrics.* 1981;99:26-34.
424. Scriver CR, Reade TM, DeLuca HF, et al. Serum 1,25-dihydroxyvitamin D levels in normal subjects and in patients with hereditary rickets or bone disease. *N Engl J Med.* 1978;299:976-979.
425. Kitnaka S, Takeyama K-I, Muryama A, et al. Inactivating mutations in the 25-hydroxyvitamin D, 1α-hydroxylase gene in patients with pseudovitamin d-deficiency rickets. *N Engl J Med.* 1998;338:653-661.
426. Wang J, Lin C-J, Burridge S, et al. Genetics of Vitamin D 1α-hydroxylase deficiency in 17 families. *Am J Hum Gen.* 1998;63:1694-1702.
427. Glorieux FH. Calcitriol treatment in vitamin D-dependent and vitamin D-resistant rickets. *Metabolism.* 1990;39:10-12.
428. Malloy PJ, Pike JW, Feldman D. The vitamin D receptor and the syndrome of hereditary 1,25-dihydroxyvitamin D-resistant rickets. *Endocr Rev.* 1999;20:156-188.
429. Fraher LJ, Karmali R, Hinde FRJ, et al. Vitamin D-dependent rickets type II: extreme end organ resistance to 1,25-dihydroxy vitamin D_3 in a patient without alopecia. *Eur J Pediatr.* 1986;145:389-395.
430. Bell NH. Vitamin D-dependent rickets type II. *Calcif Tissue Int.* 1980;31:89-91.
431. Takeda E, Yokota I, Kawakami I, et al. Two siblings with vitamin-D-dependent rickets type II: no recurrence of rickets for 14 years after cessation of therapy. *Eur J Pediatr.* 1989;149:54-57.
432. Marx SJ, Liberman UA, Eil C, et al. Hereditary resistance to 1,25-dihydroxyvitamin D. *Recent Prog Horm Res.* 1984;40:589-615.
433. Harrison HC, Harrison HE. Inhibition of vitamin D-stimulated active transport of calcium of rat intestine by diphenylhydantoin-phenobarbital treatment. *Proc Soc Exp Biol Med.* 1976;153:220-224.
434. Kido Y, Okamura T, Tomikawa M, et al. Hypocalcemia associated with 5-fluorouracil and low dose leucovorin in patients with advanced colorectal or gastric carcinomas. *Cancer.* 1996;78:1794-1797.
435. Relkin R. Hypocalcemia resulting from calcium accretion by a chondrosarcoma. *Cancer.* 1974;34:1834-1837.
436. Dembinski TC, Yatscoff RW, Blandford DE. Thyrotoxicosis and hungry bone syndrome—a cause of posttreatment hypocalcemia. *Clin Biochem.* 1994;27:69-74.
437. Jacobson MA, Gambertoglio JG, Aweeka FT, et al. Foscarnet-induced hypocalcemia and effects of foscarnet on calcium metabolism. *J Clin Endocrinol Metab.* 1991;72:1130-1135.
438. Aggeler PM, Perkins HA, Watkins HB. Hypocalcemia and defective hemostasis after massive blood transfusion: report of a case. *Transfusion.* 1967;7:35-39.
439. Greco RJ, Hartford CE, Haith LR, et al. Hydrofluroic acid-induced hypocalcemia. *J Trauma.* 1988;28:1593-1596.
440. Kao W, Dart R, Kuffner E, et al. Ingestion of low-concentration hyrofluoric acid: an insidious and potentially fatal poisoning. *Ann Emerg Med.* 1999;34:35-41.
441. Tsang RC, Kleinman LI, Sutherland JM, et al. Hypocalcemia in infants of diabetic mothers. *J Pediatr.* 1972;80:384-395.
442. Tsang RC, Light IJ, Sutherland JM, et al. Possible pathogenetic factors in neonatal hypocalcemia of prematurity. *J Pediatr.* 1973;82:423-429.
443. Kaplan EL, Burrington JD, Klementschitsch P, et al. Primary hyperparathyroidism, pregnancy and neonatal hypocalcemia. *Surgery.* 1984;96:717-722.
444. Kuehn E, Anders H, Bogner J, et al. Hypocalcemia in HIV infection and AIDS. *J Intern Med.* 1999;247:69-73.
445. Lind L, Carlstedt F, Rastad J, et al. Hypocalcemia and parathyroid hormone secretion in critically ill patients. *Crit Care Med.* 2000;28:93-99.
446. Canaff L, Hendy GN. Calcium-sensing receptor gene transcription is up-regulated by the proinflammatory cytokine, interleukin-1beta: role of the NF-kappaB PATHWAY and kappaB elements. *J Biol Chem.* 2005;280:14177-14188.
447. Canaff L, Zhou X, Hendy GN. The proinflammatory cytokine, interleukin-6, up-regulates calcium-sensing receptor gene transcription via Stat1/3 and Sp1/3. *J Biol Chem.* 2008;283:13586-13600.
448. Stewart AF, Longo W, Kreutter D, et al. Hypocalcemia associated with calcium-soap formation in a patient with a pancreatic fistula. *N Engl J Med.* 1986;315:496-498.
449. Dettelbach MA, Deftos LJ, Stewart AF. Intraperitoneal free fatty acids induce severe hypocalcemia in rats: a model for the hypocalcemia of pancreatitis. *J Bone Miner Res.* 1990;5:1249-1255.
450. Norberg HP, DeRoos J, Kaplan EL. Increased parathyroid hormone secretion and hypocalcemia in experimental pancreatitis: necessity for an intact thyroid gland. *Surgery.* 1975;77:773-779.
451. Weir GC, Lesser PB, Drop LJ, et al. The hypocalcemia of acute pancreatitis. *Ann Intern Med.* 1975;83:185-189.
452. Desai TK, Carlson RW, Geheb MA. Prevalence and clinical implications of hypocalcemia in acutely ill patients in a medical intensive care setting. *Am J Med.* 1988;84:209-214.
453. Winer KK, Sinaii N, Peterson D, et al. Effects of once versus twice-daily parathyroid hormone 1-34 therapy in children with hypoparathyroidism. *J Clin Endocrinol Metab.* 2008;93:3389-3395.
454. Gupta A, Winer K, Econs MJ, et al. FGF-23 is elevated by chronic hyperphosphatemia. *J Clin Endocrinol Metab.* 2004;89:4489-4492.
455. Okano K, Furukawa Y, Hirotoshi M, et al. Comparative efficacy of various vitamin D metabolites in the treatment of various types of hypoparathyroidism. *J Clin Endocrinol Metab.* 1982;55:238-242.
456. Corvilain J, Abramow M. Growth and renal control of plasma phosphate. *J Clin Endocrinol Metab.* 1972;34:452-459.
457. Lyles KW, Halsey DL, Friedman NE, et al. Correlations of serum concentrations of 1,25-dihydroxyvitamin D, phosphorous, and parathyroid hormone in tumoral calcinosis. *J Clin Endocrinol Metab.* 1988;67:88-92.
458. Larsson T, Davis SI, Garringer HJ, et al. White KE. Fibroblast growth factor-23 mutants causing familial tumoral calcinosis are differentially processed. *Endocrinology.* 2005;146:3883-3891.
459. Topaz O, Shurman DL, Bergman R, et al. Mutations in GALNT3, encoding a protein involved in O-linked glycosylation, cause familial tumoral calcinosis. *Nature Genetics.* 2004;36:579-581.
460. McBryde KD, Wilcox J, Kher KK. Hyperphosphatemia due to fosphenytoin in a pediatric ESRD patient. *Pediatr Nephrol.* 2005;20: 1182-1185.
461. Markowitz GS, Stokes MB, Radhakrishnan J, et al. Acute phosphate nephropathy following oral sodium phosphate bowel purgative: an underrecognized cause of chronic renal failure. *J Am Soc Nephrol.* 2005;16:3389-3396.
462. Miller PD, Heinig RE, Waterhouse C. Treatment of alcoholic ketoacidosis. *Arch Intern Med.* 1978;138:57-72.
463. Marcu CB, Hotchkiss M. Pseudohyperphosphatemia in a patient with multiple myeloma. *Conn Med.* 2004;68:71-72.
464. Spencer H, Lewin I, Samachson J, et al. Changes in metabolism in obese persons during starvation. *Am J Med.* 1966;40:27-37.
465. Silvis SE, Paragas Jr PU. Paresthesias, weakness, seizures and hypophosphatemia in patients receiving hyperalimentation. *Gastroenterology.* 1972;62:513-520.
466. Berman E, Nicolaides M, Maki RG, et al. Altered bone and mineral metabolism in patients receiving imatinib mesylate. *N Engl J Med.* 2006;354:2006-2013.
467. Quarles LD. FGF23, PHEX, and MEPE regulation of phosphate homeostasis and skeletal mineralization. *Am J Physiol Endocrinol Metab.* 2003;285:E1-E9.
468. Schiavi SC, Kumar R. The phosphatonin pathway: new insights in phosphate homeostasis. *Kidney Int.* 2004;65:1-14.
469. Berndt TJ, Schiavi S, Kumar R. "Phosphatonins" and the regulation of phosphorus homeostasis. *Am J Physiol Renal Physiol.* 2005;289: F1170-F1182.
470. Lorenz-Depiereux B, Bastepe M, Benet-Pages A, et al. DMP1 mutations in autosomal recessive hypophosphatemia implicate a bone matrix protein in the regulation of phosphate homeostasis [see comment]. *Nat Genet.* 2006;38:1248-1250.
471. Ito N, Fukumoto S, Takeuchi Y, et al. Comparison of two assays for fibroblast growth factor (FGF)-23. *J Bone Miner Metab.* 2005;23: 435-440.
472. Yamamoto T, Imanishi Y, Kinoshita E, et al. The role of fibroblast growth factor 23 for hypophosphatemia and abnormal regulation of vitamin D metabolism in patients with McCune-Albright syndrome. *J Bone Miner Metab.* 2005;23:231-237.
473. Riminucci M, Collins MT, Fedarko NS, et al. FGF-23 in fibrous dysplasia of bone and its relationship to renal phosphate wasting [see comment]. *J Clin Invest.* 2003;112:683-692.
474. Hoffman WH, Jueppner HW, Deyoung BR, et al. Elevated fibroblast growth factor-23 in hypophosphatemic linear nevus sebaceous syndrome. *Am J Med Genet.* 2005;134:233-236.

475. Rendina D, Mossetti G, De Filippo G, et al. Fibroblast growth factor 23 is increased in calcium nephrolithiasis with hypophosphatemia and renal phosphate leak. *J Clin Endocrinol Metab*. 2006;91:959-963.
476. Prie D, Huart V, Bakouh N, et al. Nephrolithiasis and osteoporosis associated with hypophosphatemia caused by mutations in the type 2a sodium-phosphate cotransporter [see comment]. *N Engl J Med*. 2002;347:983-991.
477. Bergwitz C, Roslin NM, Tieder M, et al. SLC34A3 mutations in patients with hereditary hypophosphatemic rickets with hypercalciuria predict a key role for the sodium phosphate cotransporter NaPi IIc in maintaining phosphate homeostasis. *Am J Hum Genet*. 2006;78:179-192.
478. Lorenz Depiereux B, Benet Pages A, Eckstein G, et al. Hereditary hypophosphatemic rickets with hypercalciuria is caused by mutations in the sodium phosphate cotransporter gene SLC34A3. *Am J Hum Genet*. 2006;78:193-201.
479. Green J, Debby H, Lederer E, et al. Evidence for a PTH-independent humoral mechanism in post-transplant hypophosphatemia and phosphaturia. *Kidney Int*. 2001;60:1182-1196.
480. Salem RR, Tray K. Hepatic resection-related hypophosphatemia is of renal origin as manifested by isolated hyperphosphaturia. *Ann Surg*. 2005;241:343-348.
481. Chung PY, Sitrin MD, Te HS. Serum phosphorus levels predict clinical outcome in fulminant hepatic failure [see comment]. *Liver Transplant*. 2003;9:248-253.
482. Daily WH, Tonnesen AS, Allen SJ. Hypophosphatemia: incidence, etiology and prevention in the trauma patient. *Crit Care Med*. 1990;18:1210-1214.
483. Vanneste J, Hage J. Acute severe hypophosphatemia mimicking Wernicke's encephalopathy. *Lancet*. 1986;1:44.
484. Singhal PC, Kumar A, Desroches L, et al. Prevalence and predictors of rhabdomyolysis in patients with hypophosphatemia. *Am J Med*. 1992;92:458-464.
485. Gabow PA, Kaehny WD, Kelleher SP. The spectrum of rhabdomyolysis. *Medicine (Baltimore)*. 1982;61:141-152.
486. Knochel JR, Bilbrey GL, Fuller TJ, et al. The muscle cell in chronic alcoholism: the possible role of phosphate depletion in alcoholic myopathy. *Ann N Y Acad Sci*. 1975;252:274-286.
487. Agusti AG, Torres A, Estopa R, et al. Hypophosphatemia as a cause of failed weaning: the importance of metanolic factors. *Crit Care Med*. 1984;12:142-143.
488. Aubier M, Murciano D, Lecocguic Y, et al. Effect of hypophosphatemia on diaphragmatic contractility in patients with acute respiratory failure. *N Engl J Med*. 1985;3131:420-424.
489. Bollaert PE, Levy B, Nace L, et al. Hemodynamic and metabolic effects of rapid correction of hypophosphatemia in patients with septic shock. *Chest*. 1995;107:1698-1701.
490. Lichtman MA, Miller DR, Cohen J, et al. Reduced red cell glycolysis, 2,3-diphosphoglycerate and adenosine triphosphate concentration and increased hemoglobin oxygen affinity caused by hypophosphatemia. *Ann Intern Med*. 1971;74:562-568.
491. Travis SF, Sugerman HJ. Alterations in red-cell glycolytic intermediates and oxygen transport as a consequence of hypophosphatemia in patients receiving intravenous hyperalimentation. *N Engl J Med*. 1971;285:763-768.
492. DeFronzo RA, Lang R. Hypophosphatemia and glucose intolerance: evidence for tissue insensitivity to insulin. *N Engl J Med*. 1980;202:1259-1263.
493. Wilson HK, Keuer SP, Lea AS, et al. Phosphate therapy in diabetic ketoacidosis. *Arch Intern Med*. 1982;142:517-520.
494. Keller U, Berger W. Prevention of hypophosphatemia by phosphate infusion during treatment of diabetic ketoacidosis and hypersmolar coma. *Diabetes*. 1980;29:87-95.
495. Rosen GH, Boullata JI, O'Rangers EA, et al. Intravenous phosphate repletion regimen for critically ill patients with moderate hypophosphatemia. *Crit Care Med*. 1995;23:1204-1210.
496. Charron T, Bernard F, Skrobik Y, et al. Intravenous phosphate in the intensive care unit: more aggressive repletion regimens for moderate and severe hypophosphatemia. *Intensive Care Med*. 2003;29:1273-1278.
497. Taylor BE, Huey WY, Buchman TG, et al. Treatment of hypophosphatemia using a protocol based on patient weight and serum phosphorus level in a surgical intensive care unit [see comment]. *J Am Coll Surg*. 2004;198:198-204.
498. Broner CW, Stidham GL, Westenkirchner DF, et al. Hypermagnesemia and hypocalcemia as predictors of high mortality in critically ill pediatric patients. *Crit Care Med*. 1990;18:921-928.
499. Mordes JP, Wacker WE. Excess magnesium. *Pharmacol Rev*. 1978;29:273-300.
500. Cao Z, Bideau R, Valdes Jr R, et al. Acute hypermagnesemia and respiratory arrest following infusion of MgSO4 for tocolysis. *Clin Chim Acta*. 1999;285:191-193.
501. Rasch DK, Huber PA, Richardson CJ, et al. Neurobehavioral effects of neonatal hypermagnesemia. *J Pediatr*. 1982;100:272-276.
502. Donovan EF, Tsang RC, Steichen JJ, et al. Neonatal hypermagnesemia: effect on parathyroid hormone and calcium homeostasis. *J Pediatr*. 1980;96:305-310.
503. Brand JM, Greer FR. Hypermagnesemia and intestinal perforation following antacid administration in a premature infant [see comments]. *Pediatrics*. 1990;85:121-124.
504. Mordes JP, Swartz R, Arky RA. Extreme hypermagnesemia as a cause of refractory hypotension. *Ann Intern Med*. 1975;83:657-658.
505. Ferdinandus J, Pederson JA, Whang R. Hypermagnesemia as a cause of refractory hypotension, respiratory depression, and coma. *Arch Intern Med*. 1981;141:669-670.
506. Cholst IN, Steinberg SF, Tropper PJ, et al. The influence of hypermagnesemia on serum calcium and parathyroid hormone levels in human subjects. *N Engl J Med*. 1984;310:1221-1225.
507. Cruikshank DP, Pitkin RM, Donnelly E, et al. Urinary magnesium, calcium, and phosphate excretion during the magnesium sulfate infusion. *Obstet Gynecol*. 1981;58:430-434.
508. Fassler CA, Rodriguez RM, Badesch DB, et al. Magnesium toxicity as a cause of hypotension and hypoventilation: occurrence in patients with normal renal function. *Arch Intern Med*. 1985;145:1604-1606.
509. Alfrey AC, Miller NL, Butkus D. Evaluation of body magnesium stores. *J Lab Clin Med*. 1974;84:153-162.
510. Lim P, Jacob E. Magnesium status of alcoholic patients. *Metabolism*. 1972;21:1045-1051.
511. Al-Ghamdi SMG, Cameron EC, Sutton RAL. Magnesium deficiency: pathophysiologic and clinical overview. *Am J Kidney Dis*. 1994;24:737-752.
512. Barnes BA. Magnesium conservation: a study of surgical patients. *Ann N Y Acad Sci*. 1969;162:786-801.
513. Rude RK, Singer FR. Magnesium deficiency and excess. *Ann Rev Med*. 1981;32:245-259.
514. Schmitz C, Perraud AL, Fleig A, et al. Dual-function ion channel/protein kinases: novel components of vertebrate magnesium regulatory mechanisms. *Pediatr Res*. 2004;55:734-737.
515. Simon DB, Lu Y, Choate KA, et al. Paracellin-1, a renal tight junction protein required for paracellular Mg2+ resorption [see comment]. *Science*. 1999;285:103-106.
516. Konrad M, Schaller A, Seelow D, et al. Mutations in the tight-junction gene claudin 19 (CLDN19) are associated with renal magnesium wasting, renal failure, and severe ocular involvement. *Am J Hum Genet*. 2006;79:949-957.
517. Ellison DH. Divalent cation transport by the distal nephron: insights from Bartter's and Gitelman's syndromes. *Am J Physiol Renal Physiol*. 2000;279:F616-F625.
518. Konrad M, Schlingmann KP, Gudermann T. Insights into the molecular nature of magnesium homeostasis. *Am J Physiol Renal Physiol*. 2004;286:F599-F605.
519. Schlingmann KP, Konrad M, Seyberth HW. Genetics of hereditary disorders of magnesium homeostasis. *Pediatr Nephrol*. 2004;19:13-25.
520. Nagase T, Murakami T, Tsukada T, et al. A family of autosomal dominant hypocalcemia with a positive correlation between serum calcium and magnesium: identification of a novel gain of function mutation (Ser(820)Phe) in the calcium-sensing receptor. *J Clin Endocrinol Metab*. 2002;87:2681-2687.
521. Simon DB, Nelson-Williams C, Bia MJ, et al. Gitelman's variant of Bartter's syndrome, inherited hypokalaemic alkalosis, is caused by mutations in the thiazide-sensitive Na-Cl cotransporter. *Nat Genet*. 1996;12:24-30.
522. Meij IC, Koenderink JB, De Jong JC, et al. Dominant isolated renal magnesium loss is caused by misrouting of the Na+,K+-ATPase gamma-subunit. *Ann N Y Acad Sci*. 2003;986:437-443.
523. Kantorovich V, Adams JS, Gaines JE, et al. Genetic heterogeneity in familial renal magnesium wasting. *J Clin Endocrinol Metab*. 2002;87:612-617.
524. Groenestege WM, Thebault S, van der Wijst J, et al. Impaired basolateral sorting of pro-EGF causes isolated recessive renal hypomagnesemia [see comment]. *J Clin Invest*. 2007;117:2260-2267.
525. Wilson FH, Hariri A, Farhi A, et al. A cluster of metabolic defects caused by mutation in a mitochondrial tRNA. *Science*. 2004;306:1190-1194.
526. Shils ME. Experimental human magnesium depletion. *Medicine (Baltimore)*. 1969;48:61-85.
527. King RG, Stanbury SW. Magnesium metabolism in primary hyperparathyroidism. *Clin Sci*. 1970;39:281-303.
528. Jones KH, Fourman P. Effects of infusions of magnesium and of calcium in parathyroid insufficiency. *Clin Sci*. 1966;30:139-150.
529. Jackson CE, Meier DW. Rotuine serum magnesium analysis. *Ann Intern Med*. 1968;69:743-748.
530. Mather HM, Nisbet JA, Burton GH, et al. Hypomagnesemia in diabetes. *Clin Chim Acta*. 1979;95:235-242.
531. Martin HE. Clinical magnesium deficiency. *Ann N Y Acad Sci*. 1969;162:891-900.
532. Laitinen K, Lamberg-Allardt C, Tunninen R, et al. Transient hypoparathyroidism during acute alcohol intoxication. *N Engl J Med*. 1991;324:721-727.

533. Schilsky RI, Anderson T. Hypomagnesemia and renal magnesium wasting in patients receiving cisplatin. *Ann Intern Med.* 1979;90:929-931.
534. England MR, Gordon G, Salem M, et al. Magnesium administration and dysrhythmias after cardiac surgery: a placebo-controlled, double-blind, randomized trial [see comments]. *J Am Med Assoc.* 1992;268:2395-2402.
535. McLellan BA, Reid SR, Lane PL. Massive blood transfusion causing hypomagnesemia. *Crit Care Med.* 1984;12:146-147.
536. Beller GA, Hood DB, Smith TW, et al. Correlation of serum magnesium levels and cardiac digitalis intoxication. *Am J Cardiol.* 1974;33:225-229.
537. Whang R, Morosi HJ, Rodgers D, et al. The influence of sustained magnesium deficiency on muscle potassium repletion. *J Lab Clin Med.* 1967;70:895-902.
538. Muldowney FP, McKenna TJ, Kyle LH, et al. Parathormone-like effect of magnesium replenishment in steatorrhea. *N Engl J Med.* 1970;281:61-68.
539. Allgrove J, Adami S, Fraher L, et al. Hypomagnesemia: studies of parathyroid hormone secretion and function. *Clin Endocrinol.* 1984;21:435-449.
540. Quitterer U, Hoffmann M, Freichel M, et al. Paradoxical block of parathormone secretion is mediated by increased activity of G alpha subunits. *J Biol Chem.* 2001;276:6763-6769.
541. Johannesson AJ, Raisz LG. Effects of low media magnesium concentration on bone resorption in response to parathyroid hormone and 1,25-dihydroxyvitamin D in organ culture. *Endocrinology.* 1983;113:2294-2298.
542. Medalle R, Waterhouse C, Hahn TJ. Vitamin D resistance in magnesium deficiency. *Am J Clin Nutr.* 1976;29:854-858.
543. Heaton FW, Fourman P. Magnesium deficiency and hypocalcaemia in intestinal malabsorption. *Lancet.* 1965;2:50-52.
544. Rosler A, Rabinowitz D. Magnesium induced reversal of vitamin D resistance in hypoparathyroidism. *Lancet.* 1973;1:803-805.
545. Rude RK, Adams JS, Ryzen E, et al. Low serum concentrations of 1,25-dihydroxyvitamin D in human magnesium deficiency. *J Clin Endocrinol Metab.* 1985;61:933-940.
546. Fuss M, Cogan E, Gillet C, et al. Magnesium administration reverses the hypocalcemia secondary to hypomagnesemia despite low circulating levels of 25-hydroxyvitamin D and 1,25-dihydroxyvitamin D. *Clin Endocrinol.* 1985;22:807-815.
547. Fuss M, Bergmann P, Bergans A, et al. Correction of low circulating levels of 1,25-dihydroxyvitamin D by 25-hydroxyvitamin D during reversal of hypomagnesaemia. *Clin Endocrinol.* 1989;31:31-38.
548. Brannan PG, Vergne-Marini P, Pak CYC, et al. Magnesium absorption in the human small intestine. *J Clin Invest.* 1976;57:1412-1418.
549. Flink EB. Therapy of magnesium deficiency. *Ann N Y Acad Sci.* 1969;162:901-905.
550. Sutton RAL, Walker VR, Halabe A, et al. Chronic hypomagnesemia caused by cisplatin: effect of calcitriol. *J Lab Clin Med.* 1991;117:40-43.
551. Mannstadt M, Bertrand G, Muresan M, et al. Dominant-negative GCMB mutations cause an autosomal dominant form of hypoparathyroidism. *J Clin Endocrinol Metab.* 2008;93:3568-3576.

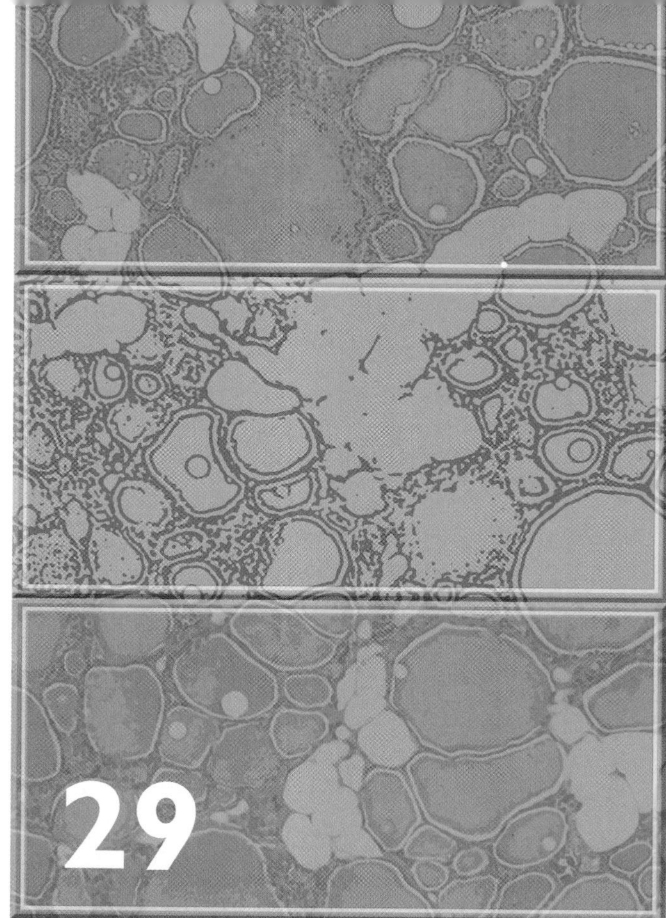

CHAPTER 29

Metabolic Bone Disease

JOSEPH A. LORENZO • ERNESTO CANALIS • LAWRENCE G. RAISZ

STRUCTURE AND FUNCTION OF THE SKELETON

The skeleton, one of the largest organ systems in the body, consists of a mineralized matrix and a highly active cellular fraction. Its multiple functions include providing structural integrity to the body, serving as a storehouse of minerals, playing an essential role in the maintenance of serum calcium and phosphate levels, and being the site of hematopoiesis. Imbalances between the structural and metabolic functions of the skeleton appear to be important in the pathogenesis of bone diseases.[1]

Embryology and Anatomy

In the embryo, skeletal development begins with the condensation of mesenchyme into cartilage. Bone formation then occurs through endochondral or intramembranous bone formation.[2] The growth of long bones and of the vertebrae involves endochondral bone formation (Fig. 29-1). The cartilage cells in the growth plate proliferate and undergo hypertrophy; this is followed by partial degradation of the matrix, which then mineralizes. The cartilage is invaded by vessels, and the spicules of mineralized cartilage are covered by osteoblasts to form a cancellous or trabecular bone called *primary spongiosa*. These structures are resorbed and replaced by trabecular plates made up entirely of bone, called *secondary spongiosa*. This process is most abundant at the ends of the long bones and in the bodies of the vertebrae.

Intramembranous bone formation occurs adjacent to the cartilage template, typically in flat bones, such as the skull, scapula, and ileum, and on the outer surfaces of long bones, leading to periosteal apposition. Initially, relatively disorganized woven bone is formed, but this rapidly converts into more organized lamellar bone produced by oriented layers of osteoblasts. The main difference between endochondral and intramembranous bone formation is that the latter does not use calcified cartilage as a direct template for osteoblasts.

Cortical bone is dense bone found in the shafts of long bones. It makes up 80% of the mass of the skeleton, determines its shape, and provides much of its strength. During longitudinal skeletal growth, endochondral and periosteal appositional bone formation determine the length and width of the bones.[3] As new bone is formed, it is shaped by a process called *modeling*, which is carried out by uncoupled osteoblasts and osteoclasts. Modeling of cortical bone alters skeletal shape (see Fig. 29-1). Modeling is influenced

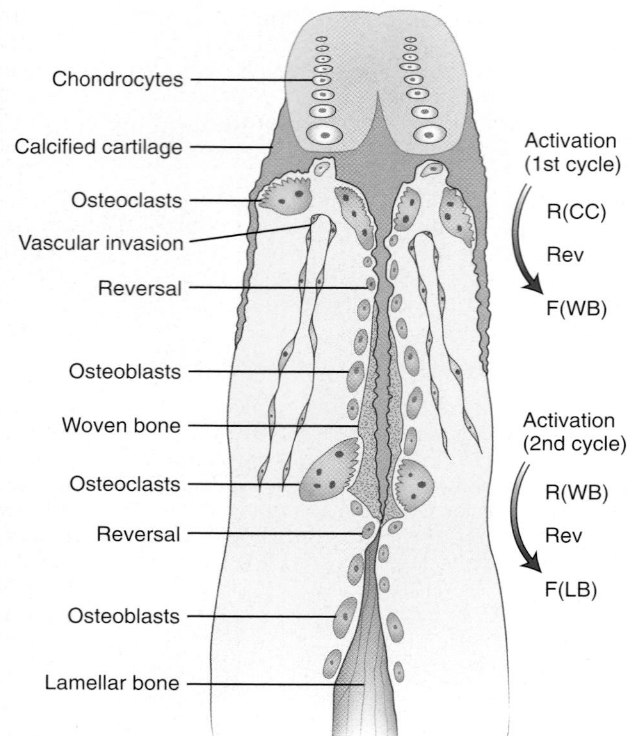

Figure 29-1 Steps in endochondral bone formation. CC, calcified cartilage; F, formation; LB, lamellar bone; R, resorption; Rev, reversal; WB, woven bone. (Redrawn from Baron R. Anatomy and ultrastructure of bone. In Favus MJ, ed. *Primer on the Metabolic Bone Diseases and Disorders of Mineral Metabolism*, 2nd ed. New York, NY: Lippincott-Raven; 1993:3-9. Copyright 1993, American Society for Bone and Mineral Research.)

by mechanical forces and is increased during the adolescent growth spurt.[4] The wide cortex at the epiphyseal plate of long bones must be resorbed by the modeling process because these bones elongate to maintain the narrow tubular structure of the diaphysis.

In contrast to bone modeling, bone remodeling is a temporally regulated process, which results in the coordinated resorption and formation of bone. It is carried out in basic multicellular units throughout life. Remodeling is more active in cancellous or trabecular bone than in cortical bone.[5] In smaller animals, such as rodents, cortical bone can remain lamellar. In large animals and humans, lamellar cortical bone is gradually replaced through haversian remodeling to form cylindrical osteons.

Chemistry of Bone Matrix and Mineral

The bone matrix consists of fibers of type I collagen laid down in layers that have various orientations, which may add to the strength of the matrix. The matrix contains many additional proteins, including small amounts of other collagen types that may be important in the interaction of type I collagen with noncollagen proteins. The noncollagen proteins represent about 10% of the total protein in bone and may direct the formation of fibers, mineralize bone, regulate the attachment of bone cells to its matrix, and play a role in the function of bone forming and resorbing cells (Table 29-1).

Protein composition of the matrix may vary, particularly between woven and lamellar bone.[6] These proteins range from the large cell-attachment proteins (e.g., thrombospondin, fibronectin), which have molecular masses higher than 400 kd, to the small, vitamin K–dependent γ-carboxylated proteins (e.g., matrix Gla protein, osteocalcin), which are 6-kd calcium-binding proteins. Some noncollagen proteins (e.g., biglycan, decorin, bone sialoprotein, osteopontin, osteoadherin) are highly acidic. In addition to cell-attachment sequences, these proteins contain various amounts of carbohydrate and are called *glycoproteins* or *proteoglycans*. Noncollagen proteins of bone are often highly phosphorylated, which enables them to bind calcium, and they may regulate mineralization. The use of targeted gene deletion in experimental murine models has provided important information on the function of noncollagenous proteins. For example, null mutations of the osteonectin gene lead to osteopenia, indicating that this matrix protein is important for the maintenance of a normal bone structure.[7]

Collagen Synthesis

Type I collagen is the most abundant protein of the bone matrix. It is a rigid, rodlike, insoluble molecule composed of two α1 chains and one α2 chain.[8,9] Collagen chains consist of repeating triplets of amino acids, with glycine in every third position and a high content of proline and lysine (Fig. 29-2). The two α1 and the α2 collagen chains form a triple helix that is stabilized by the hydroxylation

TABLE 29-1

Noncollagen Proteins of Bone

Name	Possible Function
γ-Carboxyglutamic Acid-Containing Proteins	
Osteocalcin	May regulate bone mineral maturation; negative regulator of bone formation and osteoblast function
Matrix Gla protein	Inhibits mineralization
Rgd-Containing Glycoproteins	
Fibronectin	Binds to cells; binds to gelatin and collagen
Thrombospondins	Cell attachment; binds to heparin, type I collagen, thrombin, laminin
Vitronectin	Cell attachment; binds to collagen and heparin
Fibrillin	May regulate elastic fiber formation
Osteopontin	Binds to cells; mediates effect of mechanical stress on osteoclasts and osteoblasts
Bone sialoprotein	Binds cells, binds calcium; may initiate mineralization
Glycoproteins	
Alkaline phosphatase	Hydrolyzes mineralization inhibitors
Osteonectin	Binds to growth factors; may regulate mineralization
Tetranectin	May regulate mineralization
GAG-Containing	
Biglycan	May bind to collagen and TGF-β
Decorin	Binds to collagen and may regulate fibril diameter; binds to TGF-β
Fibromodulin	Binds to collagen and may regulate fibril diameter; binds to TGF-β
Osteoadherin	Promotes integrin-mediated cell attachment
Hyaluronan	Synthesized during early bone formation; may capture space destined to become bone

GAG, glycosaminoglycan; RGD, arginine-glycine-aspartate; TGF-β, Transforming growth factor-β.

Adapted from Liam JB, Stein GS, Canalis E, et al. Bone formation osteoblast lineage cells, growth factors, matrix proteins, and the mineralization process. In Favus MJ, ed. *Primer on the Metabolic Bone Disorders of Mineral Metabolism*, 4th ed. Philadelphia, PA: Lippincott Williams & Wilkins, 1999:14-29.

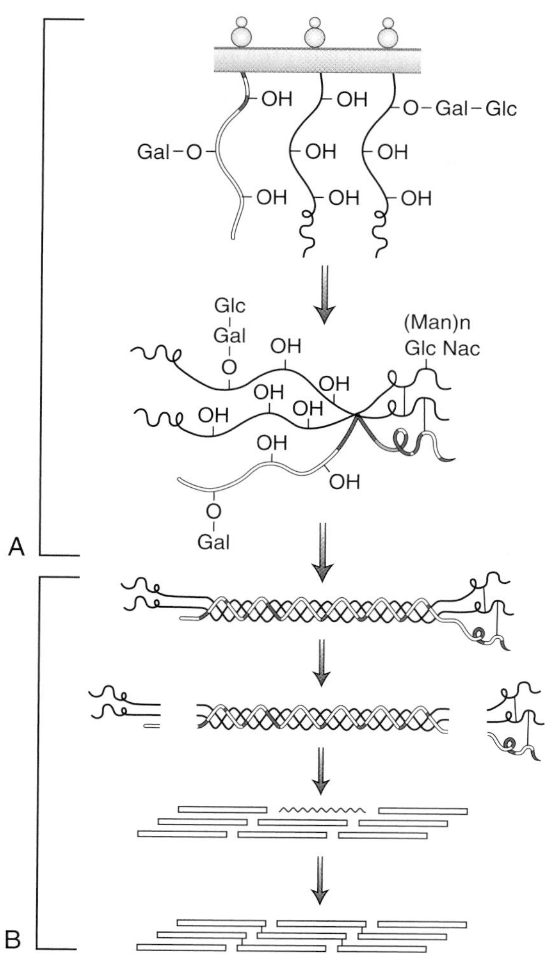

Figure 29-2 Synthesis and assembly of collagen fibrils. **A,** Intracellular post-translational modifications of pro-alpha chains, association of propeptide domains, and folding into triple-helical conformation. Gal, galactose; Glc, glucose; (Man)n, mannose; Nac, *N*-acetylglucosamine. **B,** Enzymatic cleavage of procollagen to collagen, self-assembly of collagen monomers into fibrils, and cross-linking of fibrils. (Modified from Prockop DJ, Kivirikko K. Heritable diseases of collagen. *N Engl J Med.* 1984;311:376-386.)

of proline and lysine residues, which requires ascorbic acid. Collagen is synthesized as a soluble propeptide with large nonhelical extensions at the carboxyl- and amino-terminal ends. Procollagen also contains C-terminal interchain disulfide bonds that help to initiate formation of the triple helical structure. Procollagen is released into the cisternae of the rough endoplasmic reticulum, packaged in the Golgi vesicles, and secreted extracellularly. The procollagen peptide ends are then removed by specific peptidases to produce mature insoluble collagen molecules, which are further stabilized by intramolecular and intermolecular cross-links. The major cross-links are formed by lysine and hydroxylysine residues that ultimately form pyridinium ring structures.

Mineralization

Bone mineral is formed by small, imperfect hydroxyapatite crystals, which contain carbonate, magnesium, sodium, and potassium. Mineralization occurs by two distinct mechanisms. The initial mineralization of calcified cartilage and woven bone probably occurs by means of matrix vesicles.[10] These membrane-bound bodies are released from chondrocytes and osteoblasts, contain alkaline phosphatase, and can form a nidus for crystallization. In contrast, in lamellar bone, the collagen fibers are tightly packed, and matrix vesicles are rarely seen. Mineralization does not occur immediately after collagen deposition, and there is a layer of 10 to 100 μm of unmineralized osteoid between the mineralization front and the osteoblast. Changes in the packing of the fibrils and in the composition of the noncollagen proteins may be required for mineralization. Mineralization of collagen fibrils begins in the *hole zones*, where there is more room for inorganic ions to accumulate (Fig. 29-3). Mineralization requires calcium, phosphate, and alkaline phosphatase. This process is impaired in vitamin D deficiency and hypophosphatasia.

Collagen Degradation

As part of the bone remodeling process, collagen is cleaved and degraded by a group of proteases called *collagenases*. They are matrix metalloproteases (MMPs) that can initiate cleavage of collagen fibrils at neutral pH, and they are central to the process of collagen degradation, matrix breakdown, and bone remodeling. Three collagenases have been described: collagenase 1 (MMP1), 2 (MMP8), and 3 (MMP13).[11,12] Human osteoblasts express the collagenase 1 and 3 genes (*MMP1* and *MMP13*). Unstimulated osteoblasts

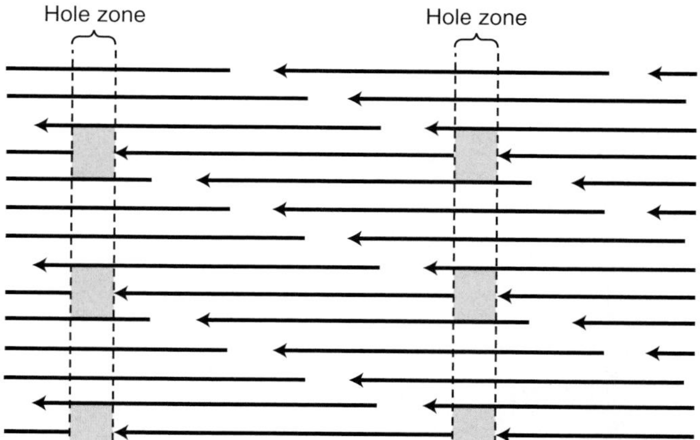

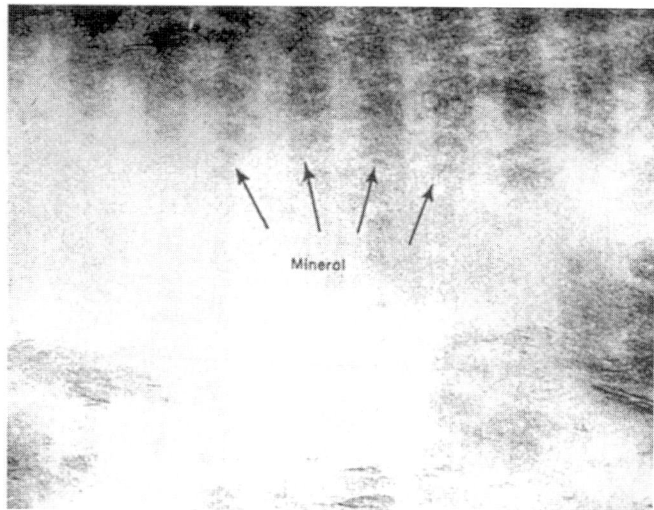

Figure 29-3 The staggered arrangement of individual molecules in collagen fibers results in hole zones between the head of one molecule and the tail of the next. Mineral deposition (*bottom*) begins within the hole zones. (From Glimcher MJ, Krane SM. *Treatise on Collagen 2: Part B.* New York, NY: Academic Press, 1968:67-251.)

secrete limited amounts of collagenase, and changes in the synthesis of collagenase correlate with changes in bone resorption. Collagenase plays a critical function in bone remodeling. Mice with deletions of the collagenase 3 gene or mutations of the $\alpha 1^1$ type I collagen gene have resistance to collagenase 3 cleavage and fail to resorb bone after exposure to parathyroid hormone (PTH).[13] The synthesis of collagenase by osteoblasts is regulated by hormones and by cytokines in the bone microenvironment that act by transcriptional and post-transcriptional mechanisms.[14]

Osteoblast Differentiation and Function

Bone is formed by *osteoblasts*, which are highly differentiated cells with many unique features (Fig. 29-4).[15] Osteoblasts are derived from mesenchymal cells in the skeletal microenvironment.[16] Osteogenic precursors may appear in the circulation, but they originate from skeletal tissue, and their contribution to bone formation is not well documented.[17] Osteoprogenitor cells, or preosteoblasts, replicate and differentiate into active osteoblasts that exhibit various phenotypic characteristics.[15] For example, osteoblasts in early development and during repair produce woven bone, whereas more mature osteoblasts produce lamellar bone. Osteoblast activity varies during bone formation. Some cells are tall and closely packed and produce a large amount of matrix in a small area; others are flatter and produce matrix at a slower rate over a larger area. Nevertheless, all differentiated osteoblasts share certain features. They are connected by gap junctions and contain a dense network of rough endoplasmic reticulum and a large Golgi complex, and they secrete collagen and noncollagen proteins in an oriented fashion. Some products, such as osteocalcin, are produced almost uniquely by osteoblasts, and changes in serum levels of osteocalcin directly reflect changes in osteoblast activity.

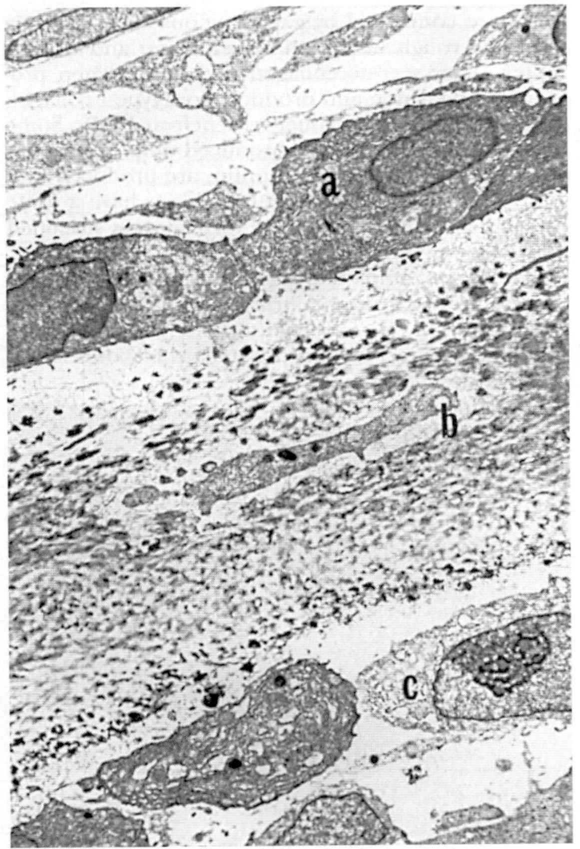

Figure 29-4 Electron micrograph of rat calvarial bone shows mature osteoblasts with their dense, rough endoplasmic reticulum and large Golgi apparatus (a), an osteocyte embedded in the bone (b), and a less differentiated cell that may represent a preosteoblast (c). (Courtesy of Dr. Marijke E. Holtrop.)

Mature osteoblasts have a finite capacity to produce matrix, and bone formation is sustained by the arrival of new populations of cells at the bone surface. The number and the function of osteoblasts are determined by hormones and local signals. Some act as classic cell mitogens and increase the population of preosteoblastic cells, some determine their differentiation into mature osteoblasts, and others modify the function of mature cells.[18] The ultimate fate of mature osteoblasts varies. They may die by apoptosis, they may become embedded in the matrix and become an osteocyte, or they may be converted to flattened lining cells, which cover a large percentage of the surface of bone with a thin cytoplasmic layer.

Bone marrow stroma contain pluripotential cells with the potential to differentiate into diverse cells of mesenchymal lineage, including osteoblasts, chondrocytes, and adipocytes.[16] The ultimate cellular phenotype depends on factors present in the cellular microenvironment and their effects on intracellular signals and gene expression. Transcription factors are nuclear proteins that bind to DNA to regulate gene transcription. Some play a role in determining the fate of undifferentiated cells.

CCAAT/enhancer binding proteins (CEBPs) β and δ play an essential role in the differentiation of cells toward adipocytes, whereas runt-related transcription factor (RUNX2) plays a central role in the differentiation of cells toward osteoblasts.[19,20] Targeted disruption of the *RUNX2* gene results in disorganized chondrocyte maturation and a complete lack of bone formation due to an arrest of osteoblast development.[21]

Osterix is another transcription factor that is required for endochondral and intramembranous bone formation. O*sterix*-null mice fail to develop a mineralized skeleton because of an arrest of late stages of osteoblast differentiation. Interactions between nuclear factors are common steps in the regulation of transcription and differentiation.[22] Osterix associates and acts cooperatively with nuclear factor of activated T cells (NFAT), a transcription factor that regulates osteoblastogenesis and osteoclastogenesis.[23] CEBPs can interact with RUNX2 and with the activator of transcription (ATF)/cyclic adenosine monophosphate (cAMP) response element–binding protein (CREB) family of proteins. ATF4 plays a central role in osteoblastic function, and its activity is regulated by a nuclear matrix attachment region binding protein, SATB2, which interacts with ATF4 and RUNX2 to regulate osteoblast differentiation.[24]

The conversion of osteoblasts to osteocytes involves a reduction but not a complete loss of metabolic activity.[25] A critical feature is the development of an extensive network of cytoplasmic connections. The osteoblasts have multiple cell processes that are connected to underlying osteocytes through small canaliculi. After mineralization is complete and the osteocyte is encased in mineralized bone, these processes maintain connections among osteocytes (Fig. 29-5). This extended syncytium is probably important for maintaining the viability of the osteocytes, which otherwise would be separated from the extracellular fluid.

Initially, osteocytes may continue to synthesize collagen and play a role in mineralization. Later, the major role of the osteocyte-osteoblast syncytium may be to sense mechanical forces.[26] Osteocytes probably sense bone

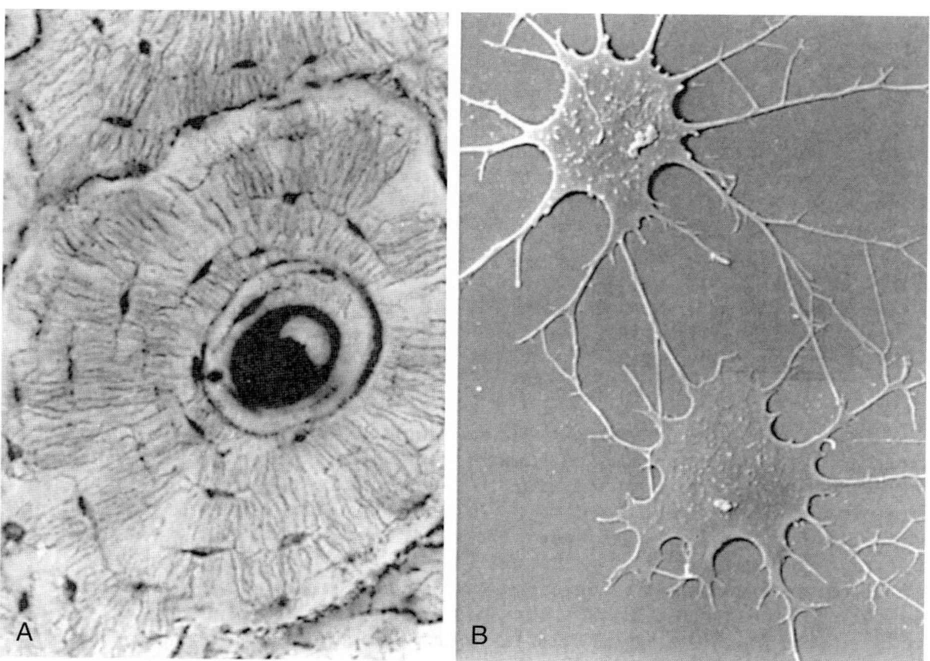

Figure 29-5 **A,** Cross-section of an osteon. **B,** Cultured cells from avian bone, showing osteocytes and their cytoplasmic connections. (From Aarden EM, Burger EH, Nijweide PJ. Function of osteocytes and bone. *J Cell Biochem.* 1994;55:287-299. Reprinted by permission of Wiley-Liss, Inc., a subsidiary of John Wiley & Sons, Inc.)

deformation and provide signals for the adaptive remodeling of bone size and shape.[27] One hypothesis is that small strains produce fluid shear stress in the canaliculi between osteocytes. This effect may result in intracellular signaling through changes in ion channels or in the production of biologically active molecules. Regions of bone microdamage contain apoptotic osteocytes, which may provide signals for the initiation of bone remodeling by osteoclasts and the consequent removal of damaged bone.[8]

Cells of the osteoblastic lineage are important for forming bone and for initiating bone resorption. Both mature osteoblasts and osteocytes may play a role in activating resorption. Most of the hormonal factors that stimulate bone resorption act on cells of the osteoblastic lineage. They release receptor activator for nuclear factor κB ligand (RANKL) and colony-stimulating factor 1 (CSF1), which are essential for osteoclastogenesis. Osteoblasts also produce additional factors that regulate bone resorption, including cytokines, prostaglandins, and local growth factors. In cell culture, contact between osteoblastic cells and hematopoietic cells appears to be necessary for osteoclast formation (Fig. 29-6). Osteoblasts may also play a role in initiating bone resorption by releasing collagenases, other metalloproteinases, and plasminogen activator. These enzymes may remove the surface proteins of bone, which prevent the access of osteoclasts to the mineralized matrix. Osteoblasts also influence the development and maintenance of the marrow through their production of growth factors, cytokines, and chemokines that regulate the growth and development of hematopoietic cells.

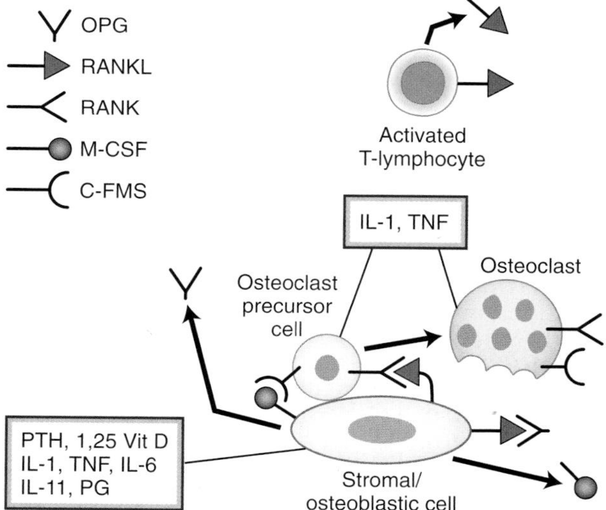

Figure 29-6 Osteoclast formation. Osteoclasts form from osteoclast precursor cells, which are derived from hematopoietic-lineage cells. They express C-FMS (CSF1R, the receptor for M-CSF) and RANK and attach to stromal/osteoblastic cells, which express membrane-bound and soluble M-CSF, membrane-bound RANKL, and OPG under the influence of stimulators of resorption (i.e., PTH, 1,25-Vit D, IL-1, TNF, IL-6, IL-11, or PGs). If stromal or osteoblastic cells produce more RANKL than OPG, osteoclasts are formed and activated, which increases bone resorption. If stromal or osteoblastic cells produce more OPG than RANKL, OPG binds the available RANKL, and new osteoclast formation is prevented. During states of inflammation, T lymphocytes are activated and produce membrane-bound and soluble RANKL, which can stimulate osteoclast-mediated bone resorption. IL-1 and TNF can augment the effects of RANKL and M-CSF on osteoclast formation and bone resorption by directly stimulating osteoclast precursor cells and mature osteoclasts. IL, interleukin; M-CSF, macrophage colony-stimulating factor; OPG, osteoprotegerin; PG, prostaglandin; PTH, parathyroid hormone; RANK, receptor activator of nuclear factor κB; RANKL, RANK ligand; TNF, tumor necrosis factor; 1,25 Vit D, 1,25-dihydroxyvitamin D.

Osteoclast Differentiation and Function

Osteoclasts are derived from hematopoietic progenitors and appear to be myeloid in origin. Hematopoietic stem cells under the direction of cytokines and possibly cell-cell interactions express transcription factors that define their commitment to the osteoclast lineage. Colony-stimulating factor 1 (i.e., macrophage colony-stimulating factor [M-CSF]) appears to be the major cytokine, which regulates the replication and development in bone marrow of progenitor cells that are capable of differentiating into osteoclasts. Expression of the transcription factor SPI1 (formerly called PU.1) is also necessary for the osteoclast precursor cell to develop.[28] In bone marrow the osteoclast precursor cell is multipotent and can differentiate into monocyte-macrophages, dendritic cells, or preosteoclasts.[29] The latter fuse to form highly differentiated, multinucleated osteoclasts that resorb bone (see Fig. 29-6). Progression through the osteoclast pathway probably involves multiple local and systemic hormones that may include 1,25-dihydroxyvitamin D [1,25$(OH)_2$D], prostaglandins, and the cytokines interleukin-1 (IL-1), IL-6, and tumor necrosis factor (TNF).

The nature of the osteoblast-lineage cell products, which directly regulate osteoclast formation and function, has been clarified.[30] The principal stimulator of osteoclast formation is RANKL, a member of the TNF protein superfamily. This protein was originally identified as a product of activated T lymphocytes, but it is also recognized as a critical stimulator of osteoclastogenesis.

Production of RANKL in osteoblast-lineage cells is stimulated by essentially all agents that enhance osteoclast formation, including PTH, 1,25$(OH)_2$D, prostaglandins, and many cytokines. Mice that are deficient in RANKL do not form osteoclasts and have osteopetrosis. In contrast, injection of RANKL into mice stimulates osteoclast formation and bone resorption. RANKL is produced as a membrane protein. In activated T lymphocytes, RANKL is cleaved from the cell membrane and is released as a soluble factor.[31] It is unclear whether similar events occur in osteoblast-lineage cells, although there is some evidence that cleavage and release of soluble RANKL occurs in malignant cells that metastasize to bone.

Osteoprotegerin (OPG) is an inhibitor of osteoclastogenesis. OPG is a soluble receptor for RANKL that binds this ligand and prevents interaction of RANKL with its cognate receptor, RANK. OPG is produced widely. In bone marrow cultures, a number of stimulators of resorption, including PTH, 1,25$(OH)_2$D, and prostaglandin E_2 (PGE_2), inhibit OPG production. For these factors, there is a reciprocal relationship between RANKL stimulation and OPG inhibition that causes activation of osteoclastogenesis and enhanced resorption. Mice that are deficient in OPG have osteoporosis, whereas mice that overexpress OPG have increased bone mass. These results, together with those for RANKL-deficient mice and mice injected with RANKL, demonstrate that osteoclast-mediated bone resorption is tightly regulated by the combined actions of RANKL and OPG.

The active receptor for RANKL is RANK, a member of the TNF receptor superfamily. Osteoclasts and their immediate precursor cells express RANK, and this expression is induced by M-CSF.[32] Binding of RANKL to RANK activates a series of intracellular pathways that activate NF-κB and mitogen-activated protein (MAP) kinases, as well as NFAT and the activator protein-1 (AP1) family of transcription factors. The TNF receptor-associated factors (TRAFs), and particularly TRAF-6, bind RANK intracellularly and are involved in RANK responses. Mice deficient in TRAF-6, like those deficient in RANK, develop osteopetrosis. In addition to its effects on bone, the RANKL/RANK system is involved in lymphocyte function and in breast and lymph node development. Mature osteoclasts express RANK, and treatment of these cells with RANKL inhibits apoptosis and stimulates resorptive activity.[33]

In addition to RANKL, M-CSF is essential for osteoclast formation. Mice that are deficient in M-CSF have osteopetrosis and few osteoclasts.[34] In cultures of isolated osteoclast precursor cells, both M-CSF and RANKL must be present for mature osteoclasts to form. M-CSF enhances RANK production in osteoclast precursors and inhibits apoptosis of osteoclast precursors and mature osteoclasts. The receptor for M-CSF, CSF1R (formerly designated C-FMS), is present on osteoclast precursors and mature osteoclasts.[32,35] Binding of CSF1R by M-CSF activates tyrosine kinase activity in the receptor, which initiates a series of intracellular downstream events.

A series of coactivator molecules is critical for osteoclast development. These molecules include members of the cytoplasmic immunoreceptor tyrosine-based activation motif (ITAM) family, namely FC-receptor common γ subunit (FCRγ) and DNAX activator protein 12 (DAP12). ITAM proteins interact with receptor proteins in the cell membrane of osteoclast precursor cells. The search for receptors associated with these ITAM adaptors in myeloid cells has identified at least two candidates that associate with FCRγ—osteoclast-associated receptor (OSCAR) and PIR—and two that associate with DAP12—the triggering receptor expressed by myeloid cells-2 (TREM2) and the signal regulatory protein-β1 (SIRPB1). Mice that are deficient in FCRγ and DAP12 have osteopetrosis and deficient osteoclast formation despite their ability to express RANKL, RANK, M-CSF, and CSF1R.[23,36] This signaling pathway responds to ligands that have not yet been established genetically; together with RANK, it stimulates the accumulation of intracellular calcium, which is required for NFAT activity in the nucleus.

The formation of multinucleated osteoclast-like cells in vitro requires hematopoietic precursors and cells of the mesenchymal/osteoblast lineage. In vivo and in cultures with devitalized bone, mononuclear preosteoclasts attach to the bone surface and form multinucleated osteoclasts by fusion. The accumulation of additional nuclei into osteoclasts by fusion probably continues while the cell is actively resorbing. The life span of the osteoclast is limited. As osteoclasts become inactive, they die by apoptosis. Hormones that enhance bone resorption may delay apoptosis, and inhibitors of resorption probably accelerate it. The mechanisms that limit the extent of osteoclastic resorption are incompletely understood and may involve inhibition by calcium ions, which accumulate under the osteoclast resorbing surface, or by local inhibitory factors, such as transforming growth factor-β (TGF-β), which are released and activated during resorption.

The mature osteoclast is a unique and highly specialized cell (Fig. 29-7). It usually contains 10 to 20 nuclei, but giant osteoclasts with up to 100 nuclei can be seen in Paget's disease and in giant cell tumors of bone. The large size of osteoclasts is probably essential for their resorptive function. The best evidence for this comes from studies of dendritic cell–specific transmembrane protein (DC-STAMP), because inhibition of this protein or its complete deficiency in mouse models results in the generation of only mononuclear osteoclasts that have impaired resorptive activity.[37,38]

The capacity of osteoclasts to resorb bone depends on their ability to isolate a region of the bone surface from the extracellular fluid and produce a local environment that can dissolve bone mineral and degrade matrix. The osteoclast must polarize and produce a basolateral membrane opposite the resorption space, which facilitates the excretion of resorption products. The resorbing apparatus consists of a central ruffled border area, which secretes

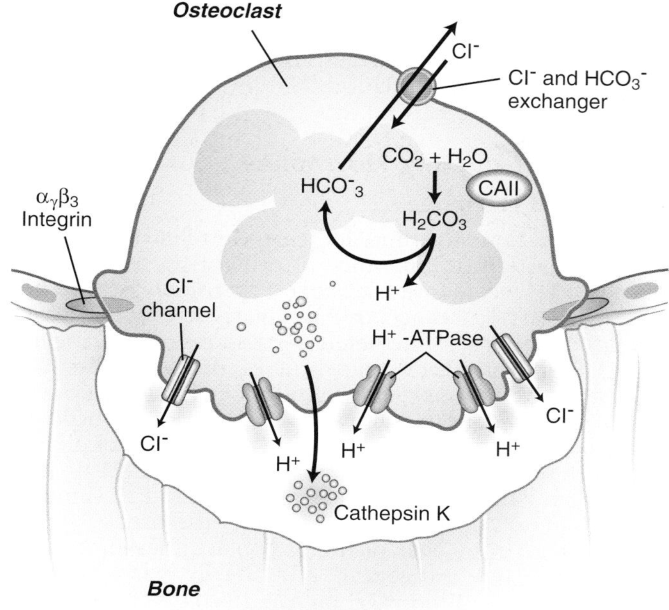

Figure 29-7 Functional elements of the fully differentiated osteoclast. Osteoclasts attach to bone by means of podosomes containing $\alpha_\gamma\beta_3$ integrin. Protons are generated through the actions of carbonic anhydrase II (CAII), which is transported into the resorption space by the vacuolar-type H^+-ATPase proton pump. A chloride channel coupled to the proton pump facilitates charge neutrality across the membrane while passive exchange of chloride (Cl^-) for bicarbonate (HCO_3^-) in the basolateral membrane removes excess bicarbonate. Cathepsin K is an important enzyme for the removal of the organic components of bone in the acid environment of the resorption space. (Redrawn from Tolar J, Teitelbaum SL, Orchard PJ. Osteopetrosis. *N Engl J Med.* 2004;351:2839-2849.)

hydrogen ions and proteolytic enzymes, surrounded by a clear or sealing zone in a structure called the *podosome*. The podosome contains filamentous actin linked to $\alpha_v\beta_3$ integrin, and it anchors the cell to the bone surface. The osteoclast attaches to bone through the interaction of integrins in the podosome with noncollagenous proteins such as vitronectin and osteopontin in the matrix.

Acidification of the resorption space adjacent to the ruffled border membrane requires that osteoclasts have a vacuolar proton pump (H^+-ATPase) and a chloride channel that is charged coupled to H^+ secretion across the ruffled membrane to preserve electron neutrality. These osteoclast H^+-ATPase pumps are similar to the vacuolar proton pumps that acidify intracellular organelles, but in the osteoclast they are exteriorized to increase the extracellular hydrogen ion concentration in the resorption space.[39] The hydrogen ions dissociate from carbonic acid, which is synthesized by carbonic anhydrase II; the bicarbonate generated by this dissociation is removed from the cell by chloride-bicarbonate exchange at the basolateral membrane of the osteoclast. Ion pumps can transport the dissolved calcium from the bone surface through the cell to the extracellular fluid.

However, calcium can also reach the extracellular fluid directly if the sealing zone is disrupted. The proteolytic enzymes produced by the osteoclast include lysosomal enzymes and metalloproteinases. Lysosomal proteases can degrade collagen at the low pH present in the ruffled border area. Cathepsin K is probably the most important of these.[40] Metalloproteinases, which are active at neutral pH, have also been detected at the resorption site.[41] The products of resorption are transported across the ruffled border membrane and excreted through the basolateral membrane of the osteoclast by a process called *transcytosis*.[42] In trabecular bone, osteoclasts characteristically resorb to a limited depth and then move laterally to produce irregular, plate-like resorption areas called *Howship's lacunae*. In cortical remodeling, the path of directed resorption is longer, possibly because of renewal of osteoclasts from hematopoietic cells brought to the site through the haversian canal.

BONE REMODELING AND ITS REGULATION

Bone remodeling is a temporally regulated process that results in the coordinated resorption and formation of skeletal tissue carried out in basic multicellular units.[5] Bone remodeling occurs throughout life. Signals determining the fate, function, and death of cells of the osteoclast, and osteoblast lineages define the populations of cells that resorb and form bone in basic multicellular units. Osteoblasts appear at sites vacated by osteoclasts, a process called *coupling*. As resorption by osteoclasts is terminated, the resorptive surface is covered by a thin layer of cement, where osteoblasts assemble to form bone and fill the cavity.[3,5] The remodeling cycle has four steps: activation, resorption, reversal, and formation (Figs. 29-8 and 29-9). Cells of the osteoblast and osteoclast lineages produce factors that regulate each other's function.[43,44]

Similar sequences are seen in trabecular and cortical remodeling, although remodeling is more active in trabecular bone.[8] In young adults, this cycle is tightly coupled and the amount of new bone formed by osteoblasts is equal to the amount resorbed by osteoclasts. However, during the menopausal years, remodeling of bone occurs at a higher rate than in the premenopause, and rates of resorption exceed formation, which results in a net loss of bone and an increased risk of developing osteoporosis.[45]

Although 80% of skeletal mass is cortical bone, the surface area of cortical bone is only about one fifth that of cancellous bone. Moreover, more osteoclast precursor cells are available in cancellous bone and on the endosteal surfaces of cortical bone. Consequently, turnover is greater on these surfaces than on those of periosteal bone, which normally undergoes little remodeling. However, subperiosteal resorption can be activated in hyperparathyroidism, and the periosteal surface contains preosteoblasts that may become active late in life and cause an age-related increase in the periosteal diameter of long bones. This periosteal expansion may maintain bone strength and compensate for losses at the endosteal surfaces and in cancellous bone.

Remodeling can be activated by systemic and local factors, and it is necessary to maintain skeletal strength and the serum levels of calcium. Changes in mechanical force can activate remodeling to improve skeletal strength, and remodeling removes and repairs bone that has undergone microdamage. This occurs particularly in cortical bone and may explain the fact that remodeling is sustained in the aging skeleton.[46] However, loss of osteocytes with age may impair this response.[47] Systemic hormones influence bone remodeling to regulate the movement of mineral from bone to the extracellular fluid to maintain serum calcium levels and as part of their overall effects on growth. During pubertal growth, bone modeling and remodeling

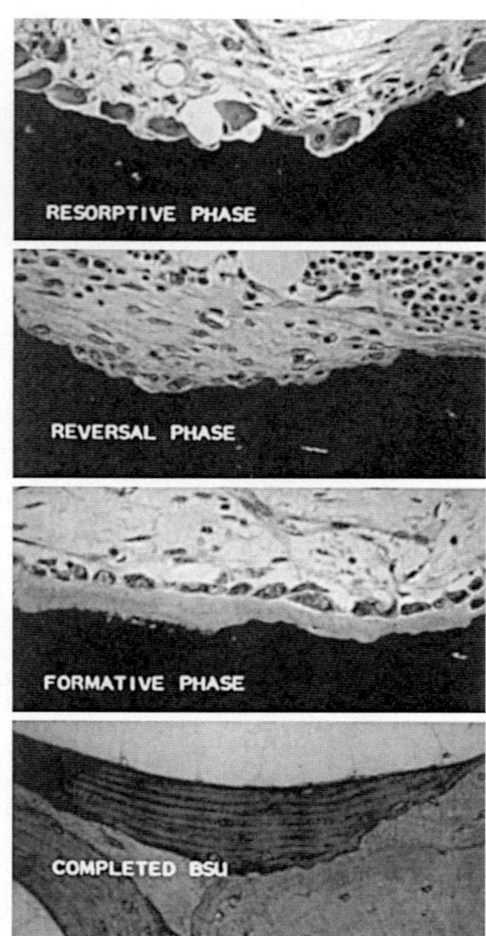

Figure 29-8 Stages of bone remodeling. The resorptive, reversal, and formative phases of bone remodeling and a completed bone structural unit (BSU) on a trabecular surface are shown. The morphologic features of the activation step have not been defined. (Courtesy of Dr. Robert E. Schenk, University of Berne, Switzerland.)

intensify and correlate with serum levels of insulin-like growth factor 1 (IGF1).[4] Studies performed in mice lacking molecular clock genes suggest that bone remodeling is subject to circadian regulation.[48]

Calcium-Regulating Hormones

Parathyroid Hormone

PTH acts on bone to stimulate resorption but does not act on osteoclasts in the absence of cells of the osteoblastic lineage. PTH receptors are abundant on osteoblasts but not on osteoclasts.[49] PTH acts on osteoblasts to cause cell contraction; to induce immediate-early response genes, including FOS and the inducible form of prostaglandin G/H synthase (i.e., cyclooxygenase), and to increase the synthesis of local mediators, IGF1 and IL-6.[49,50] High concentrations of PTH in vitro inhibit the expression of type I collagen, but intermittent administration of PTH in vivo or in vitro can stimulate bone formation.[50] PTH induces the production of RANKL and inhibits the production of osteoprotegerin by cells of the osteoblast lineage, thereby increasing osteoclastogenesis and the activity of osteoclasts. In some settings, PTH increases proliferation of cells of the osteoblast lineage and decreases their death by apoptosis.[51]

Vitamin D

The hormonal form of vitamin D, $1,25(OH)_2D_3$, is necessary for intestinal calcium and phosphorus absorption and therefore for mineralization. This form of vitamin D also has effects on the skeleton, but its physiologic role in bone remodeling is not clear.[52] By increasing RANKL production on osteoblasts or osteoblast progenitor cells, vitamin D is a potent stimulator of osteoclast formation in cell culture. High concentrations increase osteocalcin synthesis by osteoblasts and inhibit collagen synthesis. Lower concentrations may increase bone formation, although not to the extent seen with intermittent administration of PTH.

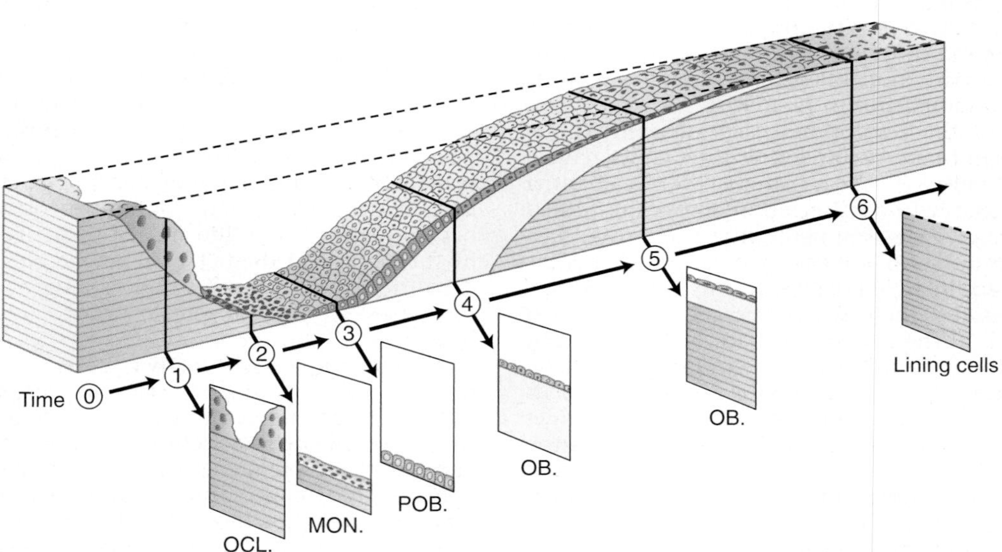

Figure 29-9 Three-dimensional reconstruction of the remodeling sequence in human trabecular bone. 1, Early bone resorption with osteoclasts (OCL); 2, late bone resorption with mononuclear cells (MON); 3, reversal phase with preosteoblasts (POB); 4, early matrix formation by osteoblasts (OB); 5, late bone formation with mineralization; 6, completed remodeling cycle with reversion to lining cells. (From Eriksen EF. Normal and pathological remodeling of human trabecular bone: three dimensional reconstruction of the remodeling sequence in normals and in metabolic bone disease. *Endocr Rev.* 1986;7:379-408. Copyright 1986 by The Endocrine Society.)

Calcitonin

Calcitonin inhibits bone resorption by acting directly on the osteoclast, but it appears to play a small role in the regulation of bone turnover in adults. Bone mass is not greatly altered in patients with medullary thyroid carcinoma, who have an excess of calcitonin production, or in athyreotic patients receiving adequate thyroid hormone replacement, who have low calcitonin levels.[53] Bone turnover is increased in patients with medullary thyroid carcinoma.[54] Mice with a deletion of the gene for calcitonin/calcitonin-related polypeptide-α *(CALCA)*, which is responsible for the production of calcitonin and its alternate transcript calcitonin gene–related peptide, have increased bone mass and enhanced rates of bone formation.[55] In contrast, mice with a deletion of only the calcitonin gene–related peptide have decreased bone mass.[56] These results imply that calcitonin influences bone formation and bone resorption. However, the mechanisms by which calcitonin affects bone formation are unknown.

Other Systemic Hormones

Growth Hormone

Deficiency and excess of growth hormone have marked effects on skeletal growth.[57] Growth hormone increases circulating and local levels of IGF1, which mediates many of the skeletal effects of growth hormone. Exogenous growth hormone and IGF1 increase bone remodeling. Growth hormone also stimulates cartilage growth, probably through an increase in local and systemic IGF1 production and possibly by direct stimulation of cartilage cell proliferation, because low levels of growth hormone receptors are present in skeletal cells.

Glucocorticoids

Glucocorticoids exert profound effects on bone remodeling.[58] Glucocorticoids decrease the intestinal absorption of calcium and have the potential to induce osteoclastogenesis and bone resorption because they increase the expression of RANKL and CSF1 in osteoblasts.[59] However, the most significant effect of glucocorticoids is their ability to suppress bone remodeling through depletion of the osteoblastic cell population.[60] Glucocorticoids inhibit the replication of osteoblast precursors and their differentiation into mature osteoblasts. This occurs in part because they suppress Wnt signaling, factors necessary for osteoblastic differentiation.[61] Glucocorticoids induce the apoptosis of osteoblasts and osteocytes, contributing to the decrease in bone forming cells.[62] Glucocorticoids inhibit the differentiated function of the osteoblast and bone formation. This results from direct effects of glucocorticoids on the osteoblast and suppression of IGF1 transcription.[63]

Thyroid Hormones

In children, hyperthyroidism is associated with increased skeletal growth, and hypothyroidism results in decreased growth.[64] Thyroid hormones are crucial for cartilage growth and differentiation and enhance the response to growth hormone. Thyroid hormones increase bone resorption and turnover, although their effects on bone formation are less clear.[65] Coupled with their effects on bone resorption, thyroid hormones increase the transcription of collagenase and gelatinase by osteoblasts.[66] As thyroid hormones increase bone remodeling, they may also increase bone formation. Thyroid hormones also have indirect effects on skeletal metabolism by suppressing the synthesis of thyroid-stimulating hormone (TSH), which can inhibit osteoclast formation and survival and as a consequence bone resorption.[67,68]

Insulin

Normal skeletal growth depends on an adequate amount of insulin.[69] Excess insulin production by the fetuses of mothers with uncontrolled diabetes results in excessive growth of the skeleton and other tissues, and undertreated diabetes mellitus impairs skeletal growth and mineralization. Children and adolescents with type 1 diabetes are at increased risk for decreased bone mineral acquisition.[70] In vitro, insulin at physiologic concentrations selectively stimulates osteoblastic collagen synthesis by a pretranslational mechanism. Insulin can mimic the effects of IGF1, although only at supraphysiologic levels.[71] Mice deficient in insulin receptor substrate 1, a major substrate of insulin and IGF1 receptor tyrosine kinases, exhibit impaired osteoblastic function and low-bone-turnover osteopenia, documenting the central role of insulin and IGF1 signaling in the maintenance of bone remodeling.[72]

Gonadal Hormones

Estrogens and androgens are critical for skeletal development and maintenance. Bone cells contain estrogen and androgen receptors, but it has been difficult to demonstrate direct effects of gonadal steroids on bone formation or resorption in cell and organ culture. Gonadal hormones are crucial for the pubertal growth spurt, and estrogen is necessary for epiphyseal closure.[73] Deficiency of estrogen or androgen increases bone resorption in vivo, possibly by increasing the local synthesis or sensitivity to cytokines, such as IL-1 and IL-6 or TNF-α, and to prostaglandins. Androgens can increase bone formation in vivo.[74] The effect of estrogens on bone formation is less clear. The absolute rate of bone formation is increased in estrogen deficiency states because of an increase in bone remodeling. However, estrogen deficiency causes bone loss, implying a relative deficiency in bone formation that is not sufficient to compensate for the increased resorption.[45]

Local Regulators

Characterization of local regulators produced within the bone itself represents a major advance in bone biology.[75,76] These local factors can be synthesized by bone cells or by adjacent hematopoietic cells and can interact with each other and with systemic hormones. They are critical in the repair of skeletal damage and in the response to mechanical forces.

Cytokines

The proinflammatory cytokines IL-1α, IL-1β,TNF-α, and TNF-β are potent stimulators of bone resorption and inhibitors of bone formation, which may play a role in the bone loss after estrogen withdrawal.[77,78] IL-6 increases osteoclastogenesis in cell cultures and may mediate some of the resorbing activity of PTH. IL-6 is produced by osteoblasts, and its production is stimulated by PTH,[79] PGE_2, and other factors that increase bone resorption. IL-11, another member of the IL-6 cytokine family, also stimulates resorption. Colony-stimulating factors regulate the early stages of osteoclast precursor cell development.

IL-4 and IL-13 inhibit resorption and prostaglandin synthesis in bone cells,[80] and leukemia inhibitory factor has biphasic effects on bone formation.[81] IL-7 stimulates B lymphopoiesis, which may be involved in osteoclastogenesis.[82] IL-10[83] is an inhibitor of osteoclastogenesis and bone resorption. IL-15 and IL-17 stimulate resorption, whereas IL-18 is inhibitory through its ability to increase production of granulocyte-macrophage colony-stimulating factor (GM-CSF).[84]

Interferon-β and interferon-γ inhibit resorption by blocking RANK signaling pathways.[85] In addition to direct effects, responses to cytokines can be blocked by inhibitors, such as the IL-1 receptor antagonist and the soluble TNF receptor, or they can be enhanced by activators such as the soluble IL-6 receptor.

Transforming Growth Factor-α and Epidermal Growth Factor

These peptides stimulate bone resorption through the same receptor and act by prostaglandin-dependent and prostaglandin-independent pathways. TGF-α and epidermal growth factor (EGF) are potent mitogens in bone that probably act on mesenchymal and hematopoietic precursors.[86,87] TGF-α is produced by neoplasms and may play a role in the increased bone resorption that occurs in certain malignancies.

Prostaglandins

Prostaglandins are potent regulators of bone cell metabolism and are synthesized by many cell types in the skeleton.[88] Prostaglandin production in bone is regulated by the effects on the inducible cyclooxygenase 2 (COX2) of local and systemic hormones and mechanical forces. Increased prostaglandin production may contribute to the increase in bone resorption that occurs with immobilization, the enhanced bone formation seen with impact loading, and the bone loss after estrogen withdrawal. Many of the hormones, cytokines, and growth factors that stimulate bone resorption also increase prostaglandin production.

Prostaglandins have biphasic effects on bone formation. Stimulation of bone formation is seen in vivo, and inhibition of collagen synthesis occurs in osteoblast cultures. Bone cells produce PGE_2, $PGF_{2\alpha}$, prostacyclin, and lipoxygenase products (e.g., leukotriene B_4), which may also stimulate bone resorption.

Growth Factors

Skeletal cells synthesize a variety of growth factors that regulate the replication, differentiation, and function of bone cells. These growth factors are not synthesized specifically by skeletal cells, and some are present in the systemic circulation and can act as local and systemic regulators of bone remodeling. Skeletal cells also synthesize growth factor binding proteins. These regulate the activity and storage of a specific factor and its interactions with other proteins in the extracellular matrix.[75]

Fibroblast Growth Factors

Fibroblast growth factors (FGFs) form a large family of polypeptides characterized by their affinity to glycosaminoglycan heparin binding sites.[89] FGF1 and FGF2, which have been studied extensively, have mitogenic properties for cells of the osteoblastic lineage, which eventually differentiate into mature osteoblasts, but FGFs do not stimulate osteoblast differentiation or function.[71] FGF2 inhibits Wnt signaling and the synthesis of IGF1, which results in a decrease in osteoblastogenesis and in osteoblastic function.[90,91] In vivo experiments have confirmed this action of FGF, and mice overexpressing FGF2 are osteopenic.[92] However, studies in *Fgf2*-null mice indicate that FGF is necessary for osteoblast formation, possibly because of its effects on cell replication.[93] FGF can stimulate bone resorption by prostaglandin-dependent and independent pathways.[94]

Platelet-Derived Growth Factors, Vascular Endothelial Growth Factors, Hypoxia-Inducible Factors, and Reactive Oxygen Species

Platelet-derived growth factor (PDGF) was originally isolated from human platelets, and four members of the *PDGF* gene family have been identified: *PDGFA, PDGFB, PDGFC,* and *PDGFD*.[95] Vascular endothelial growth factor (VEGF) shares a high degree of sequence homology with PDGF, and these factors are often referred to as members of the PDGF/VEGF family.[96]

PDGFs must form homodimers or heterodimers to exhibit activity. PDGF-AA, -AB, and -BB are the isoforms studied more extensively in skeletal cells, and they exert similar biologic actions. The primary function of PDGF in bone is the stimulation of cell replication, and PDGF impairs osteoblast differentiation and function.[97] PDGF also stimulates bone resorption. In mice, null mutations of *Pdfga* or *Pdfgb* and their receptors cause embryonic lethality or perinatal death, not allowing the study of the function of PDGF in the postnatal skeleton.[98] Although skeletal cells express products of the *Pdfga, Pdfgb,* and *Pdfgc* genes, the major source of PDGF is the systemic circulation and skeletal cells become exposed to PDGF after platelet aggregation.

Vascular endothelial growth factor A (VEGFA) is essential for angiogenesis, and *VEGFA* and VEGF receptor genes are expressed by chondrocytes and osteoblasts.[99] VEGFA is required for blood vessel formation and vessel invasion into cartilage during the process of endochondral bone formation and for chondrocyte survival during skeletal development.[100] VEGFA is required for intramembranous bone formation and osteoblastic maturation.[101] Osteoblast expression of PDGF and VEGF is regulated by other growth factors.

Hypoxia-inducible factors (HIFs) are produced locally in response to low oxygen tension and mediate pathways that lead to angiogenesis, including production of VEGF. It was shown that more bone was produced during fracture repair in a mouse model with constitutively active HIF-1α in osteoblasts. Conversely, mice deficient in HIF-1α in osteoblasts had defective bone healing.[102]

Reactive oxygen species (ROS), which are free radicals that include peroxides, are products of cell metabolism that are normally inactivated to prevent cell damage. In a mouse model, some changes that occur in bone turnover and cell metabolism with aging and the loss of sex steroid were associated with increases in the levels of ROS in bone cells.[103] The study authors found that the effects on bone of the loss of sex steroids could be reversed by antioxidant treatment of the mice.

Insulin-Like Growth Factors

IGFs increase the differentiated function of the osteoblast, and bone formation.[104] The systemic circulating and locally synthesized IGF1 contribute to bone formation.[105] Transgenic mice overexpressing IGF1 have increased bone mass, whereas *Igf1*-null mice exhibit decreased bone formation and decreased cortical bone.[106,107] IGF1 increases osteoclastogenesis and bone remodeling.[108] IGF1 and IGF2 are synthesized by bone cells and are stored in the bone matrix, but IGF1 is a more potent stimulator of osteoblastic function.[104] Six IGF-binding proteins have been identified in bone. IGF-binding proteins can inhibit or enhance IGF responses. PTH and PGE_2 are major inducers of skeletal IGF1 synthesis and glucocorticoids suppress IGF1 transcription.[104] IGFs mediate selected effects of these hormones on bone formation.

Transforming Growth Factor-β

TGF-β belongs to a family of closely related polypeptides with various degrees of structural homology and important effects on cell function.[109] Skeletal cells express TGF-β1, TGF-β2, and TGF-β3. TGF-β has complex and somewhat contradictory actions in bone cells. TGF-β can stimulate osteoblastic cell replication and bone formation, but it does not favor osteoblastic cell differentiation.[110,111] The effects of TGF-β depend on the target cell and experimental conditions. The actions of TGF-β on bone resorption have been a source of controversy. TGF-β has a biphasic effect on osteoclastogenesis, but it decreases bone resorption.[112] Targeted disruption of the mouse *Tgfb1* gene is lethal but does not result in abnormal skeletal development.[113] TGF-β is secreted as a latent high-molecular-weight complex consisting of the C-terminal remnant of the TGF-β precursor and a TGF-β-binding protein.[114] The biologically active levels of TGF-β depend on changes in its synthesis and in its activation from its latent form.

Bone Morphogenetic Proteins and WNTs

Bone morphogenetic proteins (BMPs) are members of the TGF-β superfamily of polypeptides, and they were originally identified because of their ability to induce endochondral bone formation. BMPs are expressed by osteoblasts and play an autocrine role in osteoblastic differentiation and function.[75] The fundamental function of BMPs is the induction of osteoblastic cell differentiation, endochondral ossification, and chondrogenesis.[75,115] The genesis and differentiation of osteoblasts and osteoclasts are coordinated events, and BMPs also induce osteoclastogenesis and osteoclast survival.[116]

BMP activity is regulated by a large group of secreted polypeptides that bind and limit BMP action. These extracellular BMP antagonists prevent BMP signaling. Extracellular BMP antagonists include noggin, follistatin, twisted gastrulation, the chordin family, and the Dan/Cerberus family of proteins.[75]

The Wnt family of secreted glycoproteins, like BMPs, plays a critical role in directing osteoblastogenesis. In skeletal cells, many Wnt family members use the canonical Wnt/β-catenin signaling pathway.[117] In the absence of Wnt, the proteins axin, adenomatous polyposis coli (APC), and β-catenin form a complex that facilitates the phosphorylation and degradation of β-catenin. Binding of Wnt family proteins to specific frizzled membrane receptors and their coreceptors (typically, lipoprotein receptor–related protein [LRP] family members), leads to the stabilization of β-catenin. This allows β-catenin to be translocated to the nucleus, where it can regulate the transcription of target genes. The Wnt/β-catenin signaling pathway is central to osteoblastogenesis and bone formation, and Wnt and BMPs act in concert to regulate cell differentiation. Deletions of Wnt or β-catenin genes result in the absence of osteogenesis and of skeletal tissue, and inactivating mutations of Wnt coreceptors result in osteopenia.[118] Wnt/β-catenin signaling induces osteoprotegerin, and through this mechanism, Wnts are negative regulators of osteoclastogenesis.[119,120] Wnt activity, like that of BMPs, is controlled by extracellular antagonists and intracellular signaling proteins.[76] Extracellular antagonists such as sclerostin and dickkopf-1 (DKK1) prevent interactions between Wnt family members and their receptors and coreceptors. This limits Wnt signaling, which decreases osteoblast function and bone mass.[117,121] Conversely, deletion of sclerostin in mice produces a high bone mass phenotype.[122] Sclerostin, made predominantly by osteocytes, is regulated by systemic factors such as PTH and by mechanical forces on bone. Precisely how sclerostin, an osteocyte product, regulates bone formation and resorption, is an important unanswered question.

CLINICAL EVALUATION OF METABOLIC BONE DISEASE

Bone Densitometry

The most widely used procedure for measuring bone mass is dual-energy x-ray absorptiometry (DEXA).[123] Other methods include quantitative computed tomography (QCT), quantitative radiography, single-energy x-ray absorptiometry, and ultrasonography.[124-127] Correlations among these methods vary broadly.

Densitometry and ultrasound data are reported in terms of *T-scores* (i.e., standard deviations from the young adult norm for that instrument) or *Z-scores* (i.e., standard deviations from the expected value for individuals of the same sex, age, and body size). These values depend on the normative data that have been obtained for each instrument. Moreover, the normative data are likely to be different for men and women and for members of different racial and ethnic groups. The combination of BMD measurements with other risk factors using a computer algorithm (FRAX) has probably strengthened the utility of BMD measurements and diagnosis[128] (the osteoporosis diagnosis is discussed later). Further enhancement could occur if practical methods for measuring changes in microarchitecture were developed using magnetic resonance imaging (MRI) or quantitative high-resolution QCT.[122,129,130]

Dual-Energy X-Ray Absorptiometry

DEXA can provide accurate and reproducible values for *bone mineral content* (BMC) and *bone mineral density* (BMD) in the lumbar spine, the proximal femur, the distal radius, and the whole body. BMD is calculated from the BMC and the area of bone scanned (g/cm^2); it represents a real bone density rather than true volumetric density.

DEXA has many advantages. Radiation exposure is minimal (<10 mrem), and scanning time is short (5 to 20 minutes). If quality control is maintained, variability of repeated readings is less than 1% for phantom standards; less than 2% for lumbar spine, total body, and radius; and less than 3% for proximal femur.

DEXA has some major disadvantages. Changes with disease progression or therapy are small in relation to the variability of the measurement.[131] The test is moderately expensive. Anteroposterior measurements of the lumbar spine in older patients are subject to errors caused by aortic calcification and osteoarthritic changes. The latter disadvantage can be overcome by performing lateral densitometry of the lumbar spine, but this measurement is less precise. Newer DEXA systems may have sufficient resolution to measure changes in vertebral body height in the thoracic and lumbar vertebrae. Detection of new vertebral compressions by this method may be particularly useful in patients with prior vertebral fractures, height loss, or thoracic back pain (Fig. 29-10).[132] Although there is agreement that BMD measurements are useful in diagnosis, there is debate about whether both spine and hip should be measured initially.[133] Although there is evidence that follow-up

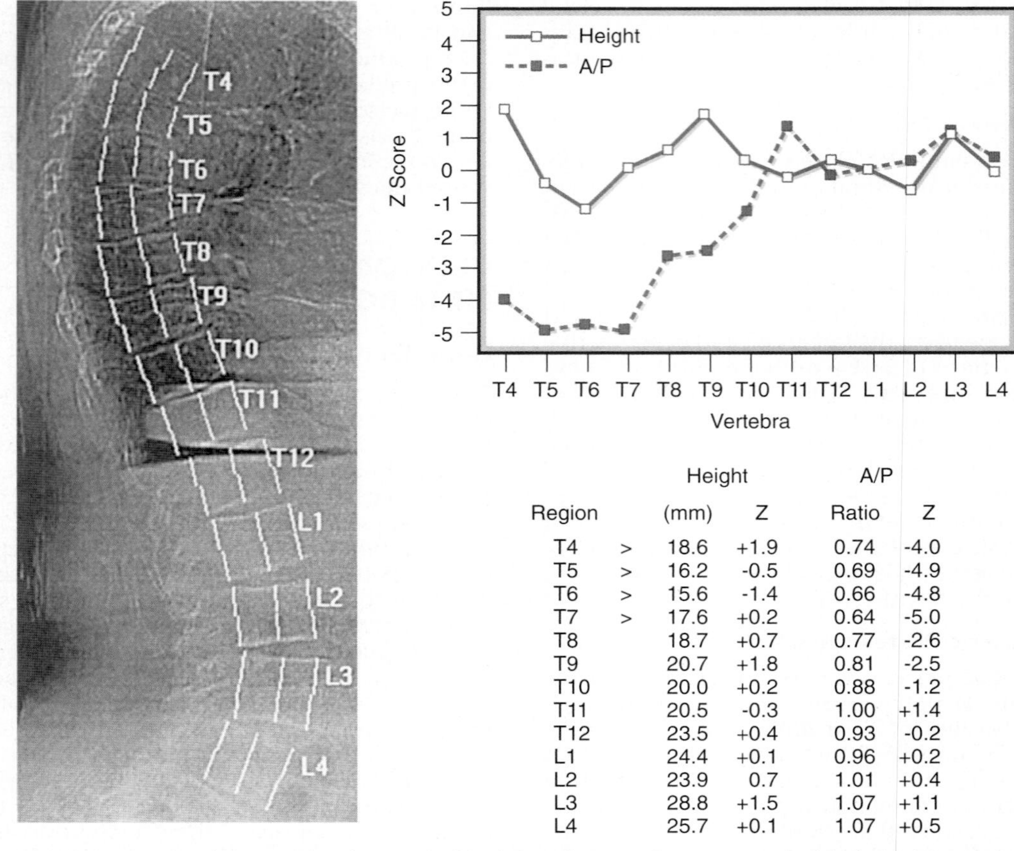

Region		Height (mm)	Height Z	A/P Ratio	A/P Z
T4	>	18.6	+1.9	0.74	-4.0
T5	>	16.2	-0.5	0.69	-4.9
T6	>	15.6	-1.4	0.66	-4.8
T7	>	17.6	+0.2	0.64	-5.0
T8		18.7	+0.7	0.77	-2.6
T9		20.7	+1.8	0.81	-2.5
T10		20.0	+0.2	0.88	-1.2
T11		20.5	-0.3	1.00	+1.4
T12		23.5	+0.4	0.93	-0.2
L1		24.4	+0.1	0.96	+0.2
L2		23.9	0.7	1.01	+0.4
L3		28.8	+1.5	1.07	+1.1
L4		25.7	+0.1	1.07	+0.5

Figure 29-10 Use of dual-energy x-ray absorptiometry for vertebral body morphometry. Posterior vertebral body heights and the ratio of anterior to posterior (A/P) height are presented in terms of standard deviation scores. Minor anterior wedging alone may not indicate an osteoporotic fracture. (Courtesy of Dr. Richard B. Mazess.)

BMD measurements are useful in predicting clinical response, there is debate about its cost-effectiveness.[134,135]

Quantitative Computed Tomography

QCT, which employs instruments available in most radiology departments, can be used to assess true bone density (g/cm^3) and to separate cancellous and cortical bone in the vertebral body. It can measure trabecular BMD in the presence of osteoarthritis.[136] QCT has also been used to measure cortical and trabecular bone density in the appendicular skeleton. The radiation exposure (100 to 300 mrem) is larger than for DEXA, and the precision and accuracy are lower but within the acceptable range. A major disadvantage may be cost, although it varies widely.

Peripheral Densitometry

Several methods to measure bone mass and density in the appendicular skeleton have been developed that are less expensive, faster, and more portable than DEXA or QCT.[137] Measurement of cortical bone in the shaft of the radius and ulna and trabecular bone in the distal radius or calcaneus by radiography, x-ray absorptiometry, or CT scanning is precise and can be used to predict fracture risk in populations, but it cannot predict BMD of the spine and hip in individual patients. The advantages of ultrasonography, particularly of the calcaneus, are that it does not use x-rays, it is rapid and portable, and it can predict fracture risk.[138] These measurements may be particularly useful for large-scale screening programs.

Biochemical Measurements

One of the most important advances in metabolic bone disease has been development of more accurate biochemical measurements that can assess rates of bone formation and resorption. In population studies, these methods have been used to show that increased turnover (i.e., high rates of resorption and formation) correlates inversely with bone mass and may predict a high rate of bone loss and an increased risk of fracture.[139-141] However, the available markers are characterized by a wide normal range and considerable variability, which limit their use in individual patients.[142] Efforts to standardize these measurements should improve their utility.[143] The most common clinical use of these assays in patient care is as a rapid assessment of the response to antiresorptive agents. Typically, decreases in resorption markers as a result of therapy can be detected at 3 to 6 months, which is before changes in BMD are measurable by DEXA.[144,145]

Markers of Bone Formation

Alkaline Phosphatase

Total serum alkaline phosphatase is measured to assess osteoblastic activity in Paget's disease, primary hyperparathyroidism, osteomalacia, and rickets.[146,147] An immunoassay that selectively measures the bone isoenzyme may increase the usefulness of this test for osteoporosis, in which changes in osteoblastic activity are smaller. High serum bone-specific alkaline phosphatase values in postmenopausal women have been shown to predict bone loss and fracture incidence.[148]

Osteocalcin

Osteocalcin, a bone carboxyglutamic acid–containing protein, is one of the few proteins that are relatively specific for skeletal tissue. A fraction of the osteocalcin synthesized by osteoblasts is released into the circulation. C-terminal cleavage of the molecule may occur after release, but the intact and N-terminal portions can be measured by specific immunoassays. Serum osteocalcin correlates with skeletal growth rates in childhood and puberty and is increased when bone turnover is accelerated (e.g., hyperparathyroidism, hyperthyroidism).[146,147] In Paget's disease, the osteocalcin level is elevated to a lesser degree than alkaline phosphatase.

Because osteocalcin production is increased by $1,25(OH)_2D$, its levels may be low in osteomalacia and rickets, even when the alkaline phosphatase level is elevated. Conversely, osteocalcin levels may be selectively reduced in patients given glucocorticoids to a greater degree than other formation markers. Undercarboxylated osteocalcin is present in patients with vitamin K and vitamin D deficiency and older patients, and it is associated with increased fracture risk.[149] Osteocalcin has been implicated in energy metabolism, but the utility of serum measurements in assessing diabetes, obesity, and arthrosclerosis has not been established.[150,151]

Procollagen Peptides

The N-terminal and C-terminal extension peptides of procollagen (see Fig. 29-2), which are removed during processing of collagen, are released into the circulation. Their measurement is an index of total-body synthesis of collagen, the bulk of which is derived from bone. Procollagen peptide levels correlate with histologic measures of bone formation.[152] Levels of procollagen peptides are high in infants and may provide a clinically useful index of growth. Increases in N-terminal procollagen peptide levels (P1NP) can predict the BMD response to intermittent PTH therapy.[152] High levels of P1NP can predict bone loss and fracture risk[153] and bone metastases in cancer.[154]

Markers of Bone Resorption

Calcium

Measurement of fasting urinary calcium excretion is convenient but shows wide variation, reflecting the net result of intestinal absorption, bone resorption, and mineralization and the renal tubular handling of calcium. Increased urinary calcium occurs when there is a marked increase in osteoclastic activity without a change in formation, as in some patients with osteolytic bone metastases. The association of hypercalciuria with or without nephrolithiasis and low bone mass makes this an important measurement. A new experimental approach has been the measurement of urinary excretion of the stable isotope ^{41}Ca as a measure of bone resorption.[155] Although the assay is highly accurate, it is currently too expensive for clinical use.

Hydroxyproline

Collagen degradation releases hydroxyproline into the circulation in free and peptide-bound forms. Because bone resorption is by far the largest contributor to collagen breakdown, urinary hydroxyproline excretion has been used as a measure of bone resorption. However, 80% to 90% of the released hydroxyproline is metabolized, and hydroxyproline from collagen or gelatin in the diet is also excreted in urine. Because cross-link excretion can also be used in these conditions, hydroxyproline assays are used infrequently in clinical assessment.

Collagen Cross-Links

Unlike hydroxyproline, the pyridinoline and deoxypyridinoline cross-links that stabilize collagen in the extracellular matrix (Fig. 29-11) are not metabolized but are excreted in the urine in a free or peptide-bound form. The deoxypyridinoline cross-link is largely derived from skeletal tissue and therefore is a more sensitive indicator of bone resorption than pyridinoline, which is also found in skin and other connective tissues.

Measurement of total urinary pyridinoline and particularly deoxypyridinoline by high-performance liquid chromatography (HPLC) probably provides the best measure of bone resorption, but this assay is expensive and time-consuming. Immunoassays have been developed for free pyridinoline and deoxypyridinoline and for peptides that include these cross-links, such as C-terminal telopeptide (CTX) and N-terminal telopeptide (NTX), which are released during resorption. These assays can be carried out in serum or urine, which may increase precision.[156,157] Measurements correlate with bone turnover and change in response to agents that affect resorption. They are useful in assessing changes in resorption in the course of disease or in response to therapy. They may also be valuable in identifying patients with high bone turnover, who have low bone mass, lose bone rapidly, and are more likely to develop osteoporosis.

All of these assays have shown diurnal variation and may be affected by meals.[158] Fasting serum or fasting, second-voided morning urine samples are probably the most reliable assays.

Other Assays

Tartrate-resistant acid phosphatase 5b is secreted by osteoclasts into serum and may be useful as a measure of bone resorption.[159,160] Measurements of enzymes such as cathepsin K and other degradation products of bone matrix are being developed.[161]

Bone Biopsy

Transiliac bone biopsy can provide direct information about cancellous bone volume, the density of connections between trabecular plates (connectivity), and the function of bone cells.[162] The rate of bone formation and mineralization can be measured by this technique with the use of dynamic histomorphometry after tetracycline labeling (Fig. 29-12), but bone resorption is more difficult to assess by bone biopsy. Bone biopsy necessitates the use of a large needle with a 7- to 9-mm internal bore and the technical skill to obtain a sample that is not crushed or distorted. The sample must be processed without decalcification and stained appropriately. Unstained sections are needed to see fluorescent tetracycline labels. Special stains may be used to identify mast cells in mastocytosis or aluminum in renal osteodystrophy.

Bone biopsies are critical for the assessment of therapeutic responses in clinical trials.[163] They are rarely indicated in the clinical care of patients with osteoporosis, but they may be indicated for patients with unusual skeletal lesions or for young men or women who have fragility fractures with no evident secondary cause. Therapeutic decisions usually can be made without performing biopsies; but they

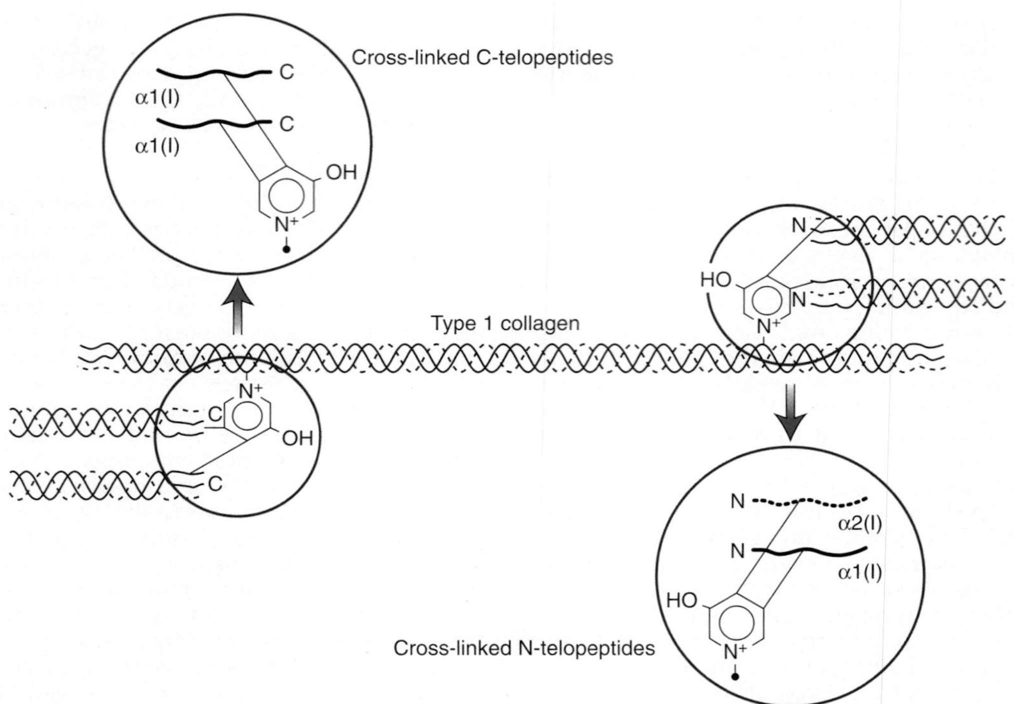

Figure 29-11 Collagen cross-links. Cross-links are formed between the COOH-terminal and NH_2-terminal nonhelical portions of collagen and adjacent helical molecules. Immunoassays are available for the pyridinoline and deoxypyridinoline molecules and for the adjacent nonhelical peptides. (Redrawn from Eyre DR. The specificity of collagen crosslinks as markers of bone and connective tissue degradation. *Acta Orthop Scand.* 1995;266:166-170.)

may be indicated in renal osteodystrophy because the different forms of this disorder are managed differently.[164]

Skeletal Imaging

The use of radiographs, CT, bone scans, and MRI in diagnosis is discussed with specific disorders throughout this chapter. All of these methods are useful in detecting fractures.[165] Methods for assessing microarchitectural changes in the skeleton using high-resolution CT or MRI are rapidly being developed[122,129,130] but are not ready for general clinical use. High-resolution radiographs and CT images have also been used to assess cortical porosity.

Bone scans using technetium 99m linked to a bisphosphonate are useful in localization of bone lesions. Uptake is a function of blood flow to the region and the amount of mineralizing bone. The test does not give information about the nature of the lesion but may serve as a guide for further studies. Radiographs or CT scans cannot differentiate old from new fractures, but increased uptake on bone scan or edema on MRI can indicate that the fracture is relatively recent.

OSTEOPOROSIS

Primary Osteoporosis

Definition

Osteoporosis is by far the most common metabolic bone disease. One of two white and Asian postmenopausal women and at least one of eight older men and women of other racial backgrounds are likely to have an osteoporotic fracture at some time during their lifetimes (Fig. 29-13). However, osteoporosis should not be defined simply by the occurrence of fractures. An international Consensus Development Conference[166] more correctly labeled it as "a disease characterized by low bone mass and microarchitectural deterioration of bone tissue, leading to enhanced bone fragility and a consequent increase in fracture risk."

Diagnostic categories for postmenopausal women are based on measurements of BMD (Table 29-2). Although these categories are arbitrary and do not define distinct clinical processes, they do give some indication of fracture risk. However, the risk of fracture at any given BMD increases markedly with age and can be affected by a number of other factors.[167,168]

A more rational approach to diagnosis and management is to obtain an estimate of fracture risk based on all factors

TABLE 29-2

Diagnostic Categories for Osteoporosis Based on Measurements of Bone Mineral Density (BMD) and Bone Mineral Content (BMC)

Category	Definition
Normal	BMD or BMC ± 1 SD of the young adult reference mean
Low bone mass (osteopenia)	BMD or BMC > 1 SD and < 2.5 SD lower than the young adult mean
Osteoporosis	BMD or BMC > 2.5 SD lower than the young adult mean
Severe osteoporosis (established osteoporosis)	BMD or BMC > 2.5 SD lower than the young adult mean in the presence of one or more fragility fractures

BMC, Bone mineral content; BMD, bone mineral density; SD, standard deviation.

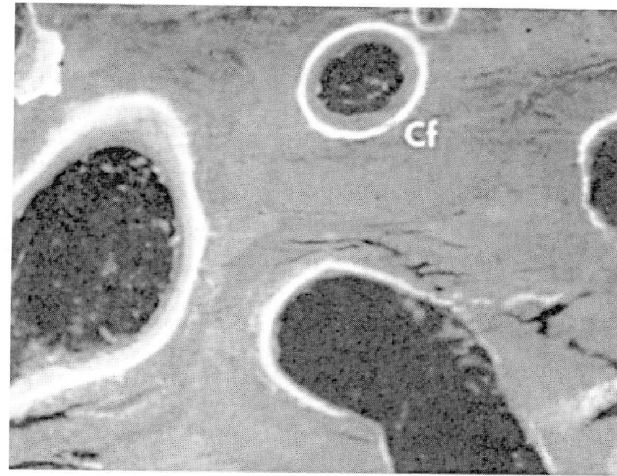

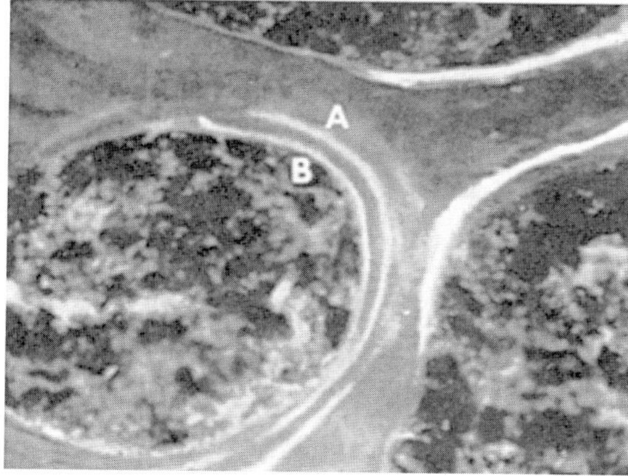

Figure 29-12 Tetracycline labels sites of active mineralization and is deposited at the calcification front (Cf) (*top*). A double-label technique can be used to measure the rate of mineralization; label A was administered about 10 days before label B (*bottom*). The undecalcified iliac crest is seen under ultraviolet light (original magnification, ×113). (From Aaron J. Histology and microanatomy of bone. In Nordin BEC, ed. *Calcium, Phosphate and Magnesium Metabolism*. Edinburgh, UK: Churchill Livingstone; 1976:298-356.)

TABLE 29-3

Estimated Lifetime Fracture Risk in Women and Men from Rochester, Minnesota, at Age 50 Years

Fracture Site	Women (% [95% CI])	Men (% [95% CI])
Proximal femur	17.5 (16.8-18.2)	6.0 (5.6-6.5)
Vertebra*	15.6 (14.8-16.3)	5.0 (4.6-5.4)
Distal forearm	16.0 (15.7-16.7)	2.5 (2.2-3.1)
Any of the above	39.7 (38.7-40.6)	13.1 (12.4-13.7)

*Clinically diagnosed fractures.
95% CI, 95% confidence interval.
From Melton LJ III, Chrischilles EA, Cooper C, et al. How many women have osteoporosis? *J Bone Miner Res*. 1992;7:1005-1010.

in individual patients. The use of T-scores and FRAX analysis (discussed later) to categorize BMD measurements as indicating the presence or absence of osteoporosis is complicated by the fact that the estimation of fracture risk is site and method specific.[169]

Epidemiology

Osteoporosis was once considered a disorder of postmenopausal women of Northern European descent because they have high rates of fractures.[170,171] However, the frequency of fragility fractures is high in men and women throughout the world[172,173] and is likely to increase further as life expectancy increases. Moreover, the age-adjusted incidence of hip fractures in many parts of the world is rising, possibly because of increased industrialization and decreased physical activity. Most of the epidemiologic data are for hip fractures, but vertebral fractures are equally common. In one study, the lifetime risk of osteoporotic fractures of the hip, spine, or wrist after age 50 years was about 40% in women and 13% in men (Table 29-3). The temporal pattern of the increase in fracture incidence differs for the hip, spine, and wrist (Fig. 29-14).

Pathogenesis

Understanding of the pathogenesis of primary osteoporosis remains largely descriptive.[174] Decreased bone mass and increased fragility can occur because of failure to achieve optimal peak bone mass, bone loss caused by increased bone resorption, or inadequate replacement of lost bone as

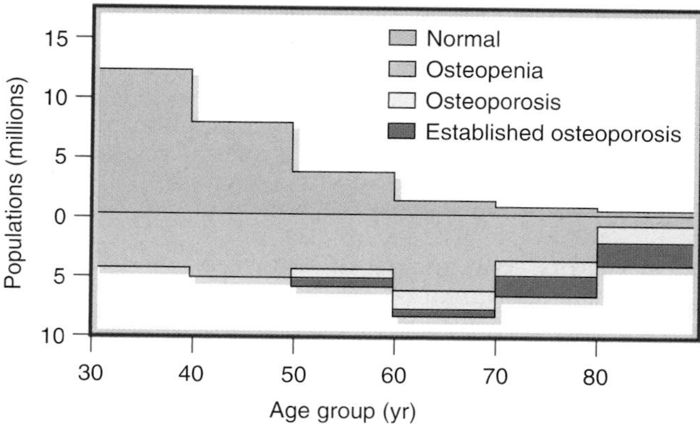

Figure 29-13 Estimated prevalence of osteoporosis in the United States. On the basis of World Health Organization criteria, more than 9 million U.S. women have osteoporosis; more than one half of these women have established osteoporosis with fractures. Seventeen million postmenopausal women have osteopenia (i.e., low bone mass) and are at risk for osteoporosis. (From Melton LJ. How many women have osteoporosis now? *J Bone Miner Res*. 1995;10:175-177.)

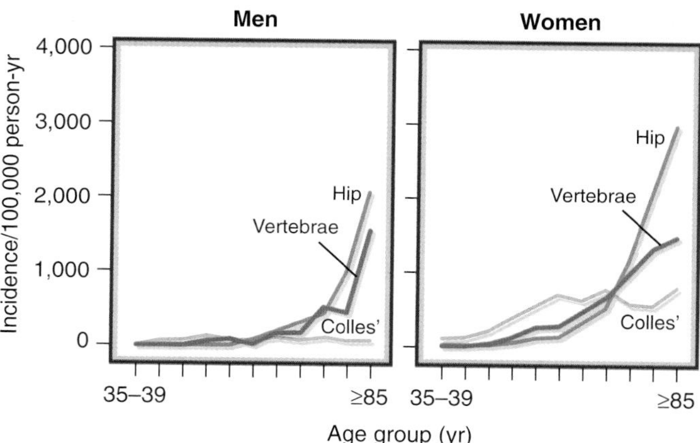

Figure 29-14 Age-specific incidence rates for hip, vertebral, and Colles' fractures in Rochester, Minnesota. (From Cooper C, Melton LJ. Epidemiology of osteoporosis. *Trends Endocrinol Metab*. 1992;3:224. Copyright 1992 by Elsevier Science Inc.)

a result of decreased bone formation. Moreover, an analysis of the pathogenesis of osteoporosis must take into account the heterogeneity of clinical expression.

Inadequate Peak Bone Mass and Strength. Studies of twins suggest that genetic determinants are responsible for up to 85% of the variation in peak bone mass and may also determine bone turnover and fracture risk.[175] Polymorphisms of candidate genes, including vitamin D and estrogen receptors, collagen, cytokines, neurotransmitters and growth regulators, have been analyzed to assess their possible roles in determining peak bone mass, remodeling, and fracture risk.[176-180] Larger populations have been studied, but the results usually show small effects. This may reflect the fact that it is difficult to determine the appropriate control population or that these polymorphisms may reflect effects of linked genes.[181] Moreover, gene effects may be influenced by environmental factors.

A broader search for quantitative trait loci associated with differences in bone mass has identified a number of chromosomes that may be involved in determining peak bone mass, architecture, and turnover. These loci may be different in men and women.[182-184] Genome-wide association studies have identified a series of genes that make contributions to bone mass (reviewed by Ralston and Uitterlinden[185]).

Although the major determinants of peak bone mass and strength are genetic, factors during childhood and adolescence can affect the ability to achieve optimal peak bone mass.[186] These factors include nutrition (particularly of calcium), physical activity, and a wide variety of intercurrent illnesses. Estrogen plays a critical role in men and women in regulating bone remodeling and in determining the time of epiphyseal closure.[187]

Increased Resorption. Peak bone mass is probably achieved in the 20s. Over the next 3 decades, there is some bone loss, but fragility fractures are rare, even in those who have low peak bone mass.[188,189] An increase in the rate of Colles' fractures occurs before menopause in women, whereas the increase in vertebral and hip fractures begins after menopause in women and in men in their 80s (see Fig. 29-14). Increased bone resorption is the major mechanism for increased skeletal fragility. The time required for resorption is much shorter than that for formation in the bone remodeling cycle; any increase in the number of resorption sites produces decreased bone mass and changes in microarchitecture, which lead to a more fragile skeleton.[190] High rates of bone remodeling, as reflected by high values for the biochemical markers of bone turnover, persist into old age and are associated with an increased risk of fracture, independent of BMD.[191]

Decreased Bone Formation. Skeletal bone mass increases during puberty and young adult life, even though the rate of resorption is high. Menopausal and age-related bone loss must involve an impairment of bone formation relative to resorption. With age, the amount of bone formed decreases with each bone structural unit, as evidenced by a decrease in mean wall thickness. This decrease may be due to an age-related decline in skeletal growth factors.[192] Biopsies of patients with established osteoporosis often show decreased bone formation.[193]

Biochemical Abnormalities. Classically, osteoporosis is differentiated from disorders such as osteomalacia and osteogenesis imperfecta by the fact that there is no obvious defect in mineralization or the structure of collagen. However, polymorphisms in the collagen gene *COL1A*, glycation end products, or differences in circulating homocysteine levels may result in an increased risk of fracture independent of BMD.[194-197] This may reflect subtle alterations in the collagenous matrix.[198,199] Differences in crystal structure and alignment have also been described, but they may be the consequence of differences in turnover.[200] The further possibility that one or more of the many noncollagen proteins in bone is abnormal in osteoporosis has not been adequately explored.

Pathogenetic Factors

Systemic Hormones. In the past, the search for pathogenetic factors in osteoporosis focused primarily on systemic hormones. A critical role for estrogen deficiency is supported by the fact that postmenopausal women have the highest incidence of osteoporosis and the lowest levels of estradiol. Moreover, estrogen levels correlate strongly with BMD in elderly men, and low estrogen levels are associated with increased fracture risk in men.[201-203]

Osteoporosis can occur, albeit rarely, in the absence of any evidence of gonadal hormone deficiency, but defects in receptors for these hormones and other downstream events may be involved. Low BMD and osteoporosis are also associated with high levels of sex hormone–binding globulin (SHBG).[204,205] This association may reflect decreased availability of sex hormones to the tissues when SHBG levels are high. Follicle-stimulating hormone (FSH) has been implicated as a mediator of increased turnover, but it does not appear to play a central role.[206-208]

Other systemic hormones may be involved in age-related bone loss. PTH levels increase with age, and fracture risk is increased in hyperparathyroidism.[209] The increase is probably caused by decreased dietary intake and impaired intestinal absorption of calcium, which is often associated with vitamin D deficiency. Secondary hyperparathyroidism and vitamin D deficiency accelerate bone loss and impair neuromuscular functions. This increases the risk of falls and fractures.[210,211] However, PTH levels in patients with vertebral fractures are not different from those in age-matched control subjects. The 25(OH) vitamin D levels are often decreased in the elderly and particularly in osteoporotic patients.[212] Calcitonin deficiency does not appear to play a role in osteoporosis,[213] although pharmacologic doses of calcitonin can prevent bone loss or increase bone mass in patients with high bone turnover.

Glucocorticoid excess can produce secondary osteoporosis but does not appear to play a major role in primary osteoporosis. Growth hormone secretion and circulating IGF1 levels decrease with age, and differences in IGF1 levels have been associated with fracture risk and bone cell function.[192,214] Thyroid hormone excess may exacerbate bone loss, and hyperthyroidism and hypothyroidism are associated with increased fracture risk.[215,216]

Local Factors. Two features of osteoporosis suggest a role for local factors in pathogenesis. Systemic hormones that influence the skeleton, including estrogen and PTH, alter the production of local factors (e.g., cytokines, prostaglandins, growth factors)[217] and the differential bone loss that occurs in different parts of the skeleton.

Limited genetic and biochemical data support a role for cytokines in human osteoporosis.[218-220] The most striking evidence for the role of cytokines in the bone loss of estrogen deficiency comes from rodent models. The loss of bone after ovariectomy in rats can be blocked by inhibiting the activity of IL-1 and TNF-α.[221] Ovariectomy does not cause bone loss in mice lacking the receptor for IL-1.[222] PGE_2

production is increased in bones from oophorectomized animals and decreased by estrogen administration.[223] Studies in rodent models suggest the existence of an important interaction between cytokines produced by cells in the marrow (possibly hematopoietic and mesenchymal) and osteoblasts.[218] These local factors act through the RANKL-RANK system, including OPG, but defects in this system have not been identified in osteoporotic patients.[224,225] OPG levels in the blood are positively rather than negatively associated with BMD and fracture risk.[226,227]

It is likely that skeletal and systemic production of IGF or IGF-binding proteins plays a role in osteoporosis.[214] Other growth factors, including BMP2, have been implicated in genetic studies.

Nutrition and Lifestyle

Calcium or vitamin D deficiency and decreased physical activity in early life can contribute to a failure to achieve optimal peak bone mass, accelerated bone loss later in life, and increased fracture risk.[186,228,229] Calcium and vitamin D supplementation can slow bone loss and reduce fractures in elderly people.[230-232]

Low protein intake is associated with increased fracture in the United States, although in worldwide epidemiologic studies, high animal protein intakes are associated with increased risk.[233,234] Vitamin K deficiency is associated with increased hip fracture risk.[235] There are also positive correlations among body fat, lean body mass, and bone density. One mechanism for the relatively high bone density of overweight people may be conversion of adrenal androgens to estrogens in fat. Another pathway may be the decrease in SHBG associated with increased body mass index.[236] Increased fat and muscle mass can lead to increased impact loading and mechanical stress on bone. Through a variety of mechanisms, smoking significantly increases the risk of osteoporosis.[237-239]

Nonskeletal Factors

Low body weight and weight loss are important risk factors for osteoporotic fractures. Nonskeletal effects, such as decreased padding of the hip and decreased muscle strength, likely play a role. Neuromuscular factors, such as loss of muscle strength, impaired balance, and impaired vision, are important, particularly by increasing the risk of falls that result in hip fracture.[240] Drugs that affect the central nervous system or decrease vascular volume and cause postural hypotension also are likely to increase this risk, particularly in older adults.

Clinical Features

Vertebral Crush Fractures. Compression fractures of the vertebrae, which occur spontaneously or with minimal trauma, are the most common manifestation of osteoporosis. The terms *postmenopausal osteoporosis* and *type 1 osteoporosis* have been applied to vertebral crush fractures at a younger age, which occur mainly in women, whereas *senile osteoporosis* and *type 2 osteoporosis* have been used for hip fractures in older women and men.[241] However, these distinctions may not be helpful clinically. These groups overlap, and patients with any type of osteoporotic fracture are more likely to have subsequent fractures of the spine or the hip.

The clinical course of the vertebral crush fracture syndrome varies. Some patients exhibit compression of only one vertebra, but others show collapse of multiple vertebrae. Nevertheless, the risk of additional fractures is high.[242] Vertebrae may show extensive loss of trabecular structure before they collapse (Fig. 29-15). Radiologically, fractures can vary from mild end-plate deformities or anterior wedging to complete vertebral collapse (Fig. 29-16). They may be unstable, particularly at the thoracolumbar junction.[243] The most common fractures are in the thoracic vertebrae below T6 and in the lumbar vertebrae.

Patients with vertebral crush fractures often have back pain that leads to radiologic assessment. Pain in the lumbar or sacral area, compared with pain in the thoracic area, is less likely to be associated with vertebral compression. Height loss is a sensitive indicator of compression, but height loss can occur without fractures as a result of narrowing of vertebral disks and postural changes.[244] Many patients are asymptomatic. Silent vertebral fractures are still an indication of increased risk and can be assessed by DEXA or radiographs.[245-248] However, anterior wedging in the upper thoracic vertebrae (T5 to T8) is common in older men and women and is not necessarily caused by compression fractures. Bone density measurements can help predict

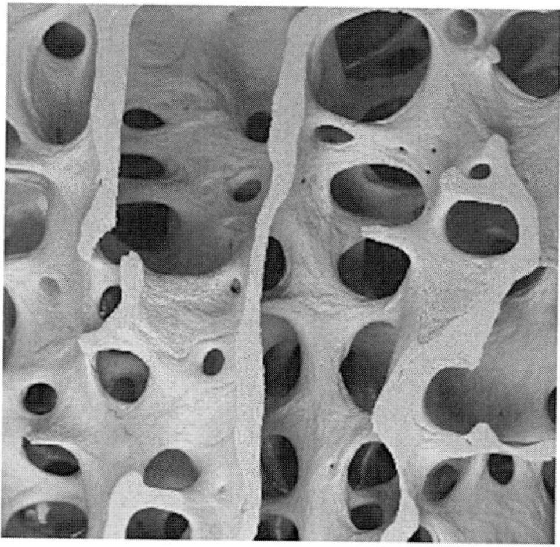

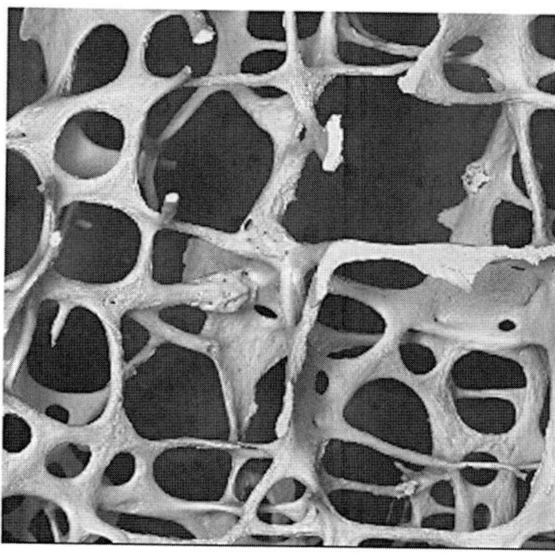

Figure 29-15 Scanning electron micrographs of a normal vertebra from a 31-year-old man and an osteoporotic vertebra from an 89-year-old woman show extensive loss of trabecular bone architecture with conversion of plates to rods and a microfracture. (From Boyd A. Morphologic detail of aging bone in human vertebrae. *Endocrine.* 2002;17:5-14.)

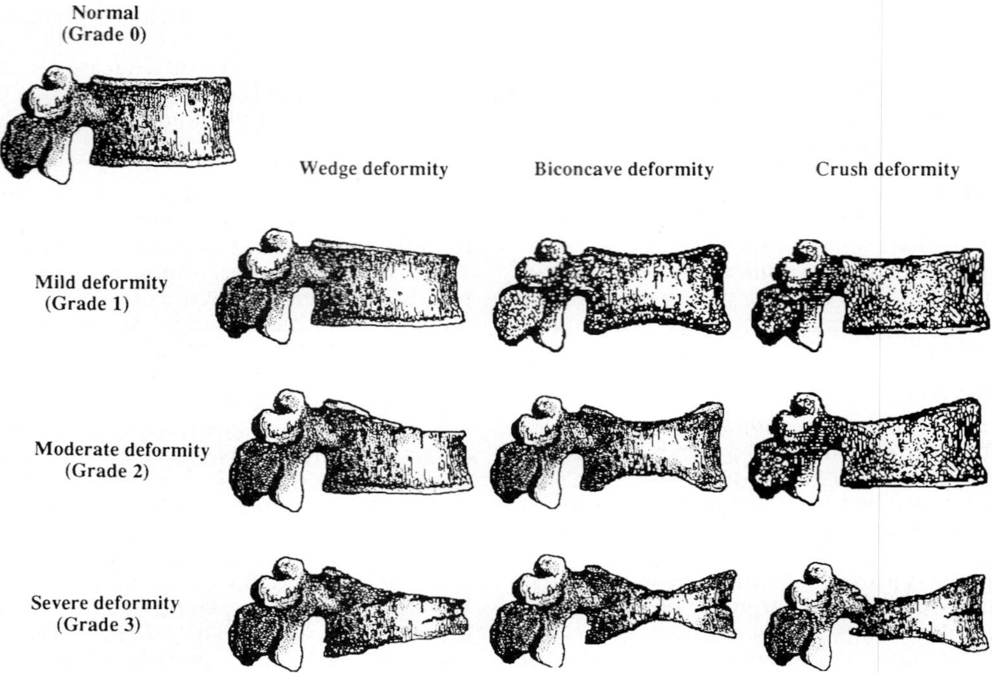

Figure 29-16 Types of vertebral compression fractures. Changes in vertebral height can be quantitated by measuring percent change or standard deviations from expected normal heights. (From Genant HK, Wu CY, van Kuijk C, et al. Vertebral fracture assessment using a semiquantitative technique. *J Bone Miner Res.* 1993;8:1137-1148.)

fracture risk in these patients. Anterior wedging may also develop early in life, probably during pubertal growth, because of a genetic disorder called *Scheuermann's disease.*[249]

Multiple vertebral crush fractures cause severe impairment. Kyphosis and loss of the lumbar lordosis are deforming and can exacerbate back pain. Impairment of chest wall function may reduce vital capacity.[250] Compression of abdominal contents may be disfiguring and uncomfortable. Ultimately, impingement of the ribs on the iliac crest is another source of pain. Many patients have additional spinal abnormalities, including spondylolisthesis, intervertebral disk disease, and osteoarthritis, particularly in the spinal facets. Osteoporosis itself rarely compresses nerve roots or the spinal cord. Although patients with severe osteoarthritis are somewhat less likely to have osteoporosis, these two common disorders often occur in the same patient.[251,252]

Hip Fracture. Fractures of the proximal femur are a major cause of morbidity and mortality in older people. Most fractures are in the femoral neck or at the base of the greater trochanter and are associated with trauma, although the trauma may be minimal. The risk is influenced by factors that increase the risk of falling and by the type of fall, as well as the structure of the skeleton and surrounding soft tissue. The increased incidence of hip fractures with age is caused by increased falls and by continued bone loss.[253]

Hip fracture is usually treated surgically, and the costs are substantial. Perioperative and postoperative complications are associated with a 5% to 20% mortality rate. Many elderly patients cannot return to their previous level of activity after hip fracture and require long-term nursing home care. It is important to perform a diagnostic evaluation and to develop a prevention and treatment plan for these patients because a second hip fracture or a fragility fracture at another site is likely to occur.[254] Unfortunately, most patients with hip fractures do not undergo evaluation or treatment to prevent progression of osteoporosis and the development of additional fractures.[255]

Colles' Fracture. Colles' fractures of the distal radius, which is composed largely of trabecular bone, are caused by falling on an outstretched hand. The incidence among women begins to increase after age 40 years and may be associated with premenopausal and perimenopausal bone loss and with genetic factors.[256,257] Unlike vertebral and hip fractures, the incidence of Colles' fractures in men does not increase with age. Colles' fractures usually heal well and only occasionally result in long-term morbidity. Patients with a Colles' fracture should be assessed for osteoporosis so that an appropriate treatment plan can be provided.[258]

Other Fractures. Fractures at any site, with the possible exception of the face and skull, can be associated with osteoporosis. Measurements of bone mass and further diagnostic workup are indicated for all fractures that occur with minimal trauma and for older patients with high-trauma fractures.[259]

Osteoporosis in Men

The incidence of hip and spine fractures for men increases with age and is about one third that for women.[203] Men often have vertebral deformities associated with trauma earlier in life, whereas increases in hip fractures tend to occur later in life, and a higher proportion of men have definable secondary causes.[260] Bone histomorphometry in typical patients shows increased resorption and decreased formation.[261]

Osteoporosis in men is associated with low androgen and estrogen and high SHBG levels.[262,263] Abnormalities of the IGF system and polymorphism of the *LRP5* gene are also implicated.[264,265] A diagnostic workup and therapeutic plan should be provided for men with fragility fractures, but this is rarely carried out in practice. Screening for osteoporosis in older men who do not have fractures has not been evaluated but may be justified now that preventive therapy is available.

Juvenile Osteoporosis

Juvenile osteoporosis is a rare, self-limiting disease that can begin between the ages of 8 and 14 years with back pain and vertebral compression.[266,267] Antiresorptive agents may be beneficial.[266] However, deficient bone formation may be the critical defect leading to fractures in these children.[268] Mutations in type I collagen and LRP5 have been reported in this disorder.[269,270] Spontaneous remission usually occurs, and the disorder usually does not lead to permanent deformity.

Idiopathic Osteoporosis

Osteoporosis with no obvious secondary cause in premenopausal women or younger men is called *idiopathic osteoporosis*. The term is not used consistently, and patients so defined include individuals with high and low bone turnover.[271,272] Some patients have a transient, self-limited condition, whereas others have a progressive and disabling disease. Idiopathic osteoporosis can be associated with nonspecific inflammatory changes, and these cases may be caused by abnormal cytokine activity.[273] A careful evaluation, including consideration of bone biopsy, should be made to search for secondary causes.

Osteoporosis in Pregnancy

Osteoporosis in pregnancy is rare and may represent a genetically determined bone disease that was present before pregnancy.[274] Bone loss can occur during pregnancy and lactation, but this is transient and ordinarily not a risk factor for osteoporosis.[275]

Localized Osteoporosis

Immobilization is the most common cause of localized osteoporosis (discussed later). Transient osteoporosis of the hip has been reported in middle-aged men and in pregnant women.[276] Regional migratory osteoporosis can occur without immobilization, particularly in the lower extremities.[277] This phenomenon may be associated with local inflammation or autonomic dysfunction with vasomotor changes and hyperesthesia, a syndrome called *reflex sympathetic dystrophy* (RSD) or complex regional pain syndrome.[278]

TABLE 29-4

Causes of Secondary Osteoporosis

Endocrine Disorders
Hyperparathyroidism
Cushing's syndrome
Hypogonadism
Hyperthyroidism
Prolactinoma
Diabetes mellitus
Acromegaly
Pregnancy and lactation
Hematopoietic Disorders
Plasma cell dyscrasias: multiple myeloma and macroglobulinemia
Systemic mastocytosis
Leukemias and lymphomas
Sickle cell disease and thalassemia minor
Lipidoses: Gaucher's disease
Myeloproliferative disorders: polycythemia
Connective Tissue Disorders
Osteogenesis imperfecta
Ehlers-Danlos syndrome
Marfan's syndrome
Homocystinuria and lysinuria
Menkes' syndrome
Scurvy
Drug-Induced Disorders
Glucocorticoids
Heparin
Anticonvulsants
Methotrexate, cyclosporine
Luteinizing hormone-releasing hormone (LHRH) agonist or antagonist therapy
Aluminum-containing antacids
IMMOBILIZATION
Renal Disease
Chronic renal failure
Renal tubular acidosis
Nutritional and Gastrointestinal Disorders
Malabsorption
Total parenteral nutrition
Gastrectomy
Hepatobiliary disease
Chronic hypophosphatemia
Miscellaneous
Familial dysautonomia (Riley-Day syndrome)
Reflex sympathetic dystrophy

Secondary Osteoporosis

The division of osteoporosis into primary and secondary forms is somewhat arbitrary. For example, patients with diseases that lead to hypogonadism early in life are considered to have *secondary* osteoporosis, whereas osteoporosis in women with natural menopause and older men with low sex hormone levels is called *primary*. Moreover, patients may have a combination of primary and secondary causes. Although most postmenopausal women and older men do not have a definable secondary cause, those who do can be treated more effectively. This possibility should be considered for every patient. There are many causes of secondary osteoporosis (Table 29-4), only a few of which are discussed here.[279]

Glucocorticoid-Induced Osteoporosis

The most common form of secondary osteoporosis is that induced by exogenous glucocorticoids.[280] Cushing's syndrome, caused by an excess of endogenous glucocorticoids, is less common but may also involve osteoporosis at presentation. Patients with rheumatoid arthritis, chronic pulmonary disease, or inflammatory bowel disease who receive exogenous glucocorticoids are at additional risk, because disease-associated inflammation, poor nutrition, and immobilization can worsen bone loss. Glucocorticoid-induced osteoporosis is particularly common in postmenopausal women, presumably because they also have primary osteoporosis. However, fragility fractures can occur in any patient receiving chronic glucocorticoids. The increased fracture risk appears within a few months of initiating therapy and rapidly declines after cessation of treatment.[184]

Glucocorticoid-induced osteoporosis is a result of increased bone resorption and decreased bone formation. Increased resorption may be related to the induction of RANKL and M-CSF by bone marrow stromal cells and osteoblastic cells. Glucocorticoids decrease the intestinal absorption of calcium and increase urinary calcium and phosphate excretion, but they do not appear to cause secondary hyperparathyroidism.[58,60] Decreased bone formation is caused by an inhibition of cell replication, differentiation of osteoblast precursors, and suppression of osteoblastic function.[58] Even at low doses, glucocorticoids can affect bone remodeling. For example, as little as 2.5 mg of prednisone given at bedtime can block the normal nocturnal rise in osteocalcin levels.[281] Glucocorticoids can decrease osteoblast and osteocyte number by increasing apoptosis[282] and may increase osteoclast number by preventing apoptosis.[283] Glucocorticoids inhibit gonadal hormone production by blocking gonadotropin release. Levels of testosterone are low in men receiving glucocorticoids.[284] Exogenous glucocorticoids decrease secretion of corticotrophin, thereby decreasing the production of adrenal androgens, which are the major precursors for estrogen formation in postmenopausal women.

Clinically, glucocorticoid-induced osteoporosis has some similarities to postmenopausal osteoporosis, but at comparable levels of BMD, the risk of fractures is higher in glucocorticoid-induced osteoporosis than in postmenopausal osteoporosis.[285] Initial bone loss is predominantly trabecular and is best assessed in the spine or distal radius. However, rib fractures and aseptic necrosis of the femoral or humeral heads or the vertebrae are common in glucocorticoid-induced osteoporosis. In contrast, they are rare in primary osteoporosis. Glucocorticoid-induced osteoporosis can be reversible, particularly in young patients who are cured of Cushing's syndrome.[286] In patients who cannot discontinue glucocorticoid therapy, early preventive therapy may be effective. Bisphosphonates and teriparatide prevent bone loss and decrease fracture risk in patients with glucocorticoid-induced osteoporosis.[287-291]

Hypogonadism

Hypogonadism, which can occur in men or women, has multiple causes. Patients with primary hypogonadism related to ovarian or testicular failure or secondary hypogonadism related to hypothalamic or pituitary disease lose bone rapidly and often have fragility fractures. The hypogonadotropic group includes patients with anorexia nervosa, athletic amenorrhea, prolactinoma, or lesions of the pituitary gland or hypothalamus, including tumors. Undernutrition and hypercortisolism may also contribute to bone loss in anorexia nervosa and athletes who develop amenorrhea.[292-294] Loss of growth hormone and consequently IGF1 may play a role in the osteoporosis of pituitary tumors.

The frequency of drug-induced hypogonadism is increasing. Long-acting progestins used for contraception in young women cause bone loss that is usually reversible.[295] Gonadotropin-releasing hormone (GnRH) analogues and aromatase inhibitors, which are used to block sex hormone production in women with breast cancer or endometriosis and men with prostate cancer, can cause rapid bone loss.[296-299]

Other Endocrine Causes

Thyroid hormone excess or deficiency may increase the risk of fractures.[215,216] In young women with hyperthyroidism who are treated early, only small changes in bone mass may occur because increases in formation rates match those of resorption.[300] In individuals at risk for osteoporosis, primary hyperthyroidism may be missed, or excessive amounts of exogenous thyroid hormone may be administered for many years. Osteoporosis can occur in patients with growth hormone deficiency and can respond to growth hormone replacement.[76,301] Active acromegaly also is associated with an increased risk of osteoporotic fractures in postmenopausal women and in men.[302,303] A large pituitary tumor may cause gonadotropin deficiency and bone loss.[304] Decreased estradiol levels may be the main determinant of low BMD in both sexes.

Patients with insulin-dependent diabetes mellitus often have low bone mass and diminished bone formation, perhaps because they lack an anabolic effect of insulin.[305] The role of non–insulin-dependent (type 2) diabetes mellitus in the pathogenesis of osteoporosis is unclear. BMD and structural parameters of bone strength are usually normal or high in type 2 diabetes mellitus, but they do not confer fracture protection because bone load to strength ratios are higher in diabetic patients, and the incidence of fractures may be increased in these individuals.[306-308] The frequency of falls may also be increased, and contribute to the risk of fractures.

Malignancy

Multiple myeloma and other lymphoproliferative malignancies can produce a clinical picture that resembles primary osteoporosis. It is particularly important to exclude myeloma in patients with rapidly progressive vertebral crush fracture syndrome. Myeloma may cause rapid bone loss because the malignant cells produce stimulators of resorption and inhibitors of formation.[309,310] One of these formation inhibitors has been identified as DKK1, which blocks Wnt signaling and impairs osteoblastogenesis.[310] Metastases to the spine may also cause vertebral compression and should be considered in the differential diagnosis, particularly for patients with normal bone density. These lesions can usually be differentiated from osteoporotic fractures by MRI.[311]

Other Diseases

The incidence and severity of osteoporosis are increased in patients with chronic hepatic and inflammatory bowel diseases. This is related to poor nutrition, the use of glucocorticoids and other drugs that affect the skeleton, and increased cytokine production.[312,313] The cause of osteoporosis in patients with celiac disease is complex. Calcium and vitamin D absorption may be impaired, but a chronic inflammatory component also contributes to the bone disorder.[314,315] Although it was initially thought that impairment of vitamin D function in hepatic and intestinal disease would cause osteomalacia, the most common lesion in such patients is osteoporosis, and these patients often do not respond to vitamin D supplementation. People with severe alcoholism also can have osteoporosis; however, lower intakes of ethanol may be associated with increased bone mass and a decreased fracture risk.[316]

Mastocytosis causes osteoporosis and osteosclerosis, and the number of mast cells may be increased in the marrow of patients with primary osteoporosis.[317-319] The functional significance of the mast cells is unknown, although they do produce heparin, which can cause bone loss. Hyperplastic anemias, such as thalassemia, can also cause bone loss,[320] partly because of bone erosion by the marrow and partly because of hypogonadism associated with transfusion-induced hemochromatosis.[321] Osteoporosis after organ transplantation is common and results from the underlying disease and from the drugs used to prevent graft rejection.[322]

Drugs

Several drugs can produce osteoporosis.[279,323] Heparin stimulates bone resorption and inhibits bone formation and can cause osteoporosis. Patients receiving anticonvulsants, including phenytoin, barbiturates, and carbamazepine, often have low bone mass. Impairment of vitamin D metabolism has been described, but most patients have osteoporosis with normal mineralization. Patients receiving selective serotonin reuptake inhibitors have increased risk of fractures and serotonin inhibits osteoblastic cell replication and bone formation.[178,324] Immunosuppressive agents, such as cyclosporine, FK506, and glucocorticoids are associated with bone loss. GnRH analogues, which decrease production of gonadal hormones, and aromatase inhibitors, which block formation of estrogen from androgen, can lead to osteoporosis.[325,326] Long-acting progestins can cause hypogonadism and bone loss. Some agents used in cancer chemotherapy probably act by inhibiting osteoblasts and by suppressing gonadal hormones. Long-term use of proton pump inhibitors, frequently prescribed for the prevention and treatment of gastroesophageal disorders, is associated with bone loss and increased risk of fractures.[327,328] In contrast, histamine H_2-receptor antagonists are not associated with increased risk of fractures.[329] Thiazolidinedione (TZD) use for the treatment of type 2 diabetes is associated with bone loss.[330-332] The mechanism involves the activation of peroxisome proliferator activated receptor-γ (PPARγ), which inhibits osteoblastogenesis and favors adipogenesis.[262,333-335]

Diagnosis

As indicated by the World Health Organization (WHO), osteoporosis can be diagnosed before fracture occurs by measuring bone density. The frequency of diagnosis therefore depends on the frequency, site, and timing of bone density measurements.[336,337] Although there is not complete agreement about who should be screened or when screening should be done, a suggested approach is illustrated in Figure 29-17.

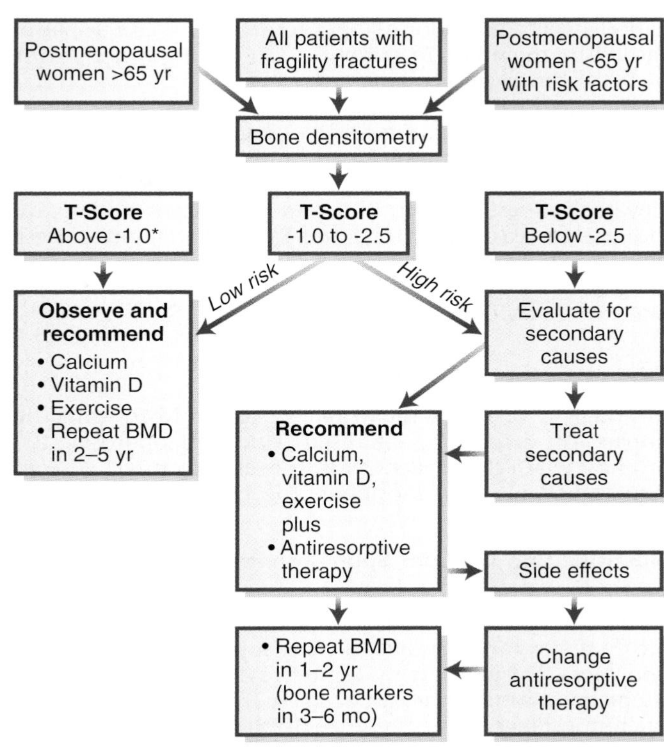

*Patients with fragility fractures and a T-score above -1.0 should be evaluated for other causes of pathologic fracture.

Figure 29-17 Diagnosis and management of osteoporosis. The diagram outlines an approach based largely on evidence from studies of postmenopausal white women, with dual-energy x-ray absorptiometry used to measure bone mineral density (BMD). Its application to other populations, including patients with secondary osteoporosis and other methods of assessing BMD, is not established.

Because the goal of diagnosis in patients who have no fractures is to predict fracture and decide about preventive therapy, BDM alone is insufficient; age and other risk factors can be added to BMD or used separately for this purpose based on the WHO fracture risk assessment test FRAX (http://www.shef.ac.uk/FRAX/ [accessed February 2011]).[128] Although it is based on a limited number of factors, it does provide an estimate of the 10-year probability of a fragility fracture and a separate estimate for hip fracture. FRAX scores without BMD values can be used for treatment decisions, but they may be misleading in some groups.[338]

Universal screening of postmenopausal women after age 65 years has been recommended as cost-effective.[339,340] Earlier screening is recommended for women who have multiple risk factors, such as low body weight or a personal or family history of fragility fractures (defined as appendicular or axial fractures after a fall from a standing height or less). Bone density should also be measured in men and premenopausal women with fragility fractures. BMD measurements may be useful in early postmenopausal women under consideration for hormone replacement therapy (HRT). Bone density measurements can establish the severity of bone loss, which can further predict risk,[341] and may be used to monitor therapeutic response.[342,343] The test may also enhance health-related behavior.[344,345]

The subsequent workup should be the same whether osteoporosis is diagnosed on the basis of screening or after the finding of a fragility fracture. The history should include a detailed analysis of calcium intake and nutrition, changes in height or weight, physical activity and lifestyle, smoking history, menstrual and reproductive history, and personal or family history of fragility fractures or other metabolic or endocrine disorders that may affect the skeleton. Physical examination should include a careful height measurement, assessment of the spine, and evaluation for thyroid or adrenal disease.

Radiologic assessment of spine fractures (many of which are silent) should be considered using DEXA and ordinary radiographs.[132] MRI or CT may be indicated if there are neurologic changes or there are fractures associated with normal bone density, which raises the possibility of malignancy.

A minimal laboratory screen should include measurement of serum calcium as ionized calcium or with albumin to permit correction for protein-bound calcium and urinary 24-hour or fasting calcium (most easily measured as the calcium-to-creatinine ratio in the second-voided morning specimen). Routine measurement of 25-hydroxyvitamin D may be indicated. Appropriate tests to exclude secondary causes of osteoporosis should be based on the history and physical findings. Serum phosphorus and alkaline phosphatase are useful in ruling out hyperparathyroidism and osteomalacia. Measurements of 1,25-dihydroxyvitamin D and PTH are indicated if the screening test results are abnormal. Serum electrophoresis, complete blood cell count, and erythrocyte sedimentation rate can help to rule out myeloma, and thyroid function should be assessed. Laboratory studies for Cushing's syndrome are indicated in patients with suggestive clinical features. Measurements of gonadal and pituitary hormones are indicated for younger patients with osteoporosis. Gluten-sensitive enteropathy should be ruled out in patients with low body weight or frequent bowel movements.

Despite the inverse correlation between markers of bone resorption and formation and bone mass, these measurements have wide variations and cannot substitute for measurements of BMD in the diagnosis of osteoporosis. Because elevated values of resorption and formation markers do indicate increased risk for bone loss and fractures, these measurements may become useful in determining the need for and response to therapy, particularly if they can be made more accurate and less expensive.[346]

Prevention and Therapy

Although it is important to relieve pain and to limit the impact of deformities in established osteoporosis, the primary goal of treatment is to prevent fractures. Prevention and therapy are considered together in the following sections.

Nutrition and Calcium Supplementation

The calcium intakes recommended for prevention and treatment of osteoporosis range from 1 to 2 g/day.[347,348] Most studies indicate that calcium supplementation slows bone loss,[349] but there is limited evidence that calcium supplementation alone can decrease fracture risk.[350,351] Low calcium intakes in the presence of low calcium absorption increases the risk of hip fractures.[352]

The Institute of Medicine (IOM) of the United States National Academy of Sciences released a report in November 2010 on dietary reference intake recommendations for calcium and vitamin D (1). The IOM report set the recommended dietary allowance (RDA) for calcium to between 700 mg per day for individuals 1 to 3 years old and 1200 mg per day for 51 to 70-year-old females and all individuals older than 71 years of age. Pregnant or lactating females aged 14 to 18 years were assigned an RDA of 1300 mg per day. The RDA is an estimation of the minimum amount of supplement that needs to be consumed to fully meet the needs of 97.5% of the population. The report stated that the upper safe level of intake for calcium ranged from 2000 to 3000 mg per day.

There is no clear advantage for any particular calcium formulation. *Calcium carbonate* is inexpensive and, when taken with meals, is usually well absorbed, even in patients with achlorhydria.[353] *Calcium citrate* and other salts may be absorbed better than calcium carbonate in the fasting state or in patients who do not produce gastric acid.[354] It is also worthwhile to include foods high in calcium in the diet. Patients should be informed about the calcium content of the major food sources, such as dairy products.

The IOM report on dietary reference intake recommendations for calcium and vitamin D set the RDA for vitamin D supplementation as 600 international units (IUs) per day for all groups except individuals older than 71 years of age who were given an RDA of 800 IUs per day. The report stated that the upper safe daily level of intake for vitamin D was 4000 IUs for all individuals older than 9 years of age. Vitamin D3 (cholecalciferol) usually is regarded as preferable over vitamin D2 (ergocalciferol) for supplementation.[355,356]

The question of how much vitamin D supplementation is optimal is not firmly resolved. Measurement of serum total 25(OH) vitamin D (D3 + D2) provides an accurate estimate of overall vitamin D status. The IOM report concluded that individuals were at risk of vitamin D deficiency if their serum 25 (OH) vitamin D levels were below 30 nmol/L (12 ng/mL). Some, but not all, individuals were potentially at risk for inadequacy at serum 25 (OH) vitamin D levels between 30 and 50 nmol/L (12 and 20 ng/mL). Practically all persons were sufficient if their serum 25 (OH) vitamin D levels were at least 50 nmol/L (20 ng/mL). The report concluded that there may be reason for concern if serum 25 (OH) vitamin D levels exceeded 125 nmol/L (50 ng/mL). In the past, the variability of the serum 25 (OH)D assay has limited its utility. However, the use of a standardized reference source and newer technologies such as HPLC appears to have reduced assay variability.[358]

High levels of oral intake of vitamin D with calcium may produce hypercalciuria or hypercalcemia, but they have not been adequately defined.[359] In the Women's Health Initiative (WHI) clinical trial, healthy postmenopausal women given 1000 mg of elemental calcium as calcium carbonate with 400 IU of vitamin D_3 daily had an increased risk of kidney stones (hazard ratio of 1.17) compared with placebo controls.[360] Calcium and vitamin D increase bone mass, decrease seasonal bone loss,[349] and can decrease the incidence of fractures, particularly in populations likely to have deficient intakes or limited sun exposure.[361] Other forms of vitamin D have been used, including calcidiol [25(OH)D], calcitriol [$1,25(OH)_2D$], and $1\alpha(OH)D$, but there is little direct evidence that, except in renal disease or hypoparathyroidism, these forms are superior to ordinary vitamin D, which is less expensive.[362,363] Dietary intake of protein, minerals, and vitamins C and K, which are important for bone matrix synthesis, should be adequate.

Exercise, Lifestyle, and Prevention of Falls

The role of exercise in treatment of osteoporosis has not been fully defined.[364] On the basis of limited data, 0.5 hour of weight-bearing exercise per day is recommended for patients who can tolerate it.[365] Epidemiologic data suggest that lifetime leisure exercise is associated with higher BMD at the hip but may have no effect on fracture incidence.[366] Patients are often better able to develop and maintain a suitable exercise program under the supervision of a physical therapist. Patients should also be instructed in body mechanics and posture to minimize musculoskeletal damage and the likelihood of falls. They should also stop smoking and limit their intake of alcohol.

Medicines that cause prolonged sedation[367] or postural hypertension should be avoided in elderly people. Help should be provided for coping with osteoporosis and for designing a lifestyle that maintains function and minimizes fracture risk.[368,369] Excessive sodium and protein intake should be avoided because they can increase urinary calcium excretion.[234] Hip protectors may reduce fractures in high-risk populations.[370]

Management of Fractures

Fractures of the hip and other appendicular fractures usually are treated surgically. Vertebral fractures may require transient bed rest. A careful but intensive program of rehabilitation is critical in patients with fractures of the hip and spine.[365] Pain relief for patients with vertebral crush fractures can usually be achieved with mild analgesics and local physical therapy. Calcitonin has analgesic effects and may be useful in patients with severe pain.

Surgical treatment of individual vertebral fractures by injection of methacrylate has been used to relieve pain and expand the compressed vertebral body. Kyphoplasty employs a balloon to create a space for the resin, whereas in vertebroplasty the resin is injected directly.[371] Controlled trials have cast doubt on the efficacy of vertebroplasty.[372,373]

Hormone Replacement Therapy

The role of HRT for the prevention and treatment of osteoporosis has been altered substantially by the findings of the large WHI clinical trial and several other controlled trials. The finding that the risks of cardiovascular disease and breast cancer were increased, although fracture risk was decreased, has shifted the risk/benefit ratio and substantially decreased the use of HRT.[374-377] Although HRT may still be appropriate for the treatment of menopausal symptoms, prevention of osteoporosis is no longer considered an appropriate primary indication. An approach that deserves further exploration is the use of much lower doses of estrogen, which have been shown to prevent bone loss with minimal side effects.[378,379] Oral and transdermal ultra-low-dose estrogen produce minimal stimulation of the uterus and breast, but their effects on cardiovascular disease and on fracture risk have not been assessed. In contrast to bisphosphonate therapy, there is often accelerated bone loss after withdrawal of estrogen therapy.[380] Patients who have discontinued estrogen need to be carefully monitored, and alternative therapy should be considered.

Bisphosphonates

Bisphosphonates are pyrophosphate analogues that bind to bone mineral, are then taken up by osteoclasts, and rapidly inhibit resorption.[381,382] The first compound available for clinical use, etidronate, inhibits bone mineralization at high doses but increases bone mass without impairing mineralization when given intermittently.[383] Another first-generation compound, clodronate, may be more effective but is not marketed in the United States.[384] Second-generation amino-bisphosphonates, such as alendronate, risedronate, ibandronate, and zoledronic acid, do not impair mineralization and are more potent. The inhibitory effects on osteoclast function differ for the first-generation compounds, which lower adenosine triphosphate levels at high concentrations. Second-generation compounds impair isoprenylation of proteins at low concentrations by blocking the enzyme farnesyl diphosphate synthase (FPPS) in the HMG-CoA reductase pathway.[385]

Alendronate, risedronate, ibandronate, and zoledronic acid are approved for prevention and treatment of osteoporosis in the United States on the basis of evidence that they decrease bone resorption, increase bone mass in the spine and hip, and decrease the incidence of fractures.[386-388] Bisphosphonates can prevent bone loss in patients receiving glucocorticoids[389] and in men.[390] There is no consensus on the duration of therapy, but continued benefit has been observed in patients treated for up to 10 years.[391]

Bisphosphonates are poorly absorbed orally and must be taken on an empty stomach with no food or other medication. The major side effects are gastrointestinal, particularly esophageal irritation. Gastrointestinal side effects may also be reduced by giving bisphosphonates weekly instead of daily.[392] This problem may be circumvented by using parenteral bisphosphonates. Pamidronate, ibandronate, and zoledronic acid are available for intravenous use. Annual use of intravenous zoledronic acid has been approved for use in osteoporosis.[254,393,394] Another concern is the development of osteonecrosis of the jaw in bisphosphonate-treated patients. This syndrome appears to be most prevalent in individuals who have received high-dose intravenous bisphosphonate therapy for treatment of malignant disease and is rare in osteoporotic patients.[395-397]

Side effects of bisphosphonates have been of increasing concern. Although gastrointestinal side effects can be circumvented by intravenous therapy, there may be long-term adverse effects on bone remodeling and strength, leading to atypical poorly healing fractures, particularly of the shaft of the femur.[398,399] These fractures are sufficiently uncommon that the association with bisphosphonate therapy is unsettled.[400]

Calcitonin

Calcitonin, an inhibitor of osteoclasts and bone resorption, can increase bone mass, particularly in association with high turnover rates. Calcitonin also has some analgesic properties and may be useful in patients with recent painful vertebral fractures.[401] It is available for subcutaneous injection or as a nasal spray. The former preparation is probably more effective but is less well tolerated, often producing gastrointestinal side effects. In a 3-year randomized trial, nasal calcitonin at 200 U/day was found to decrease fracture incidence significantly, although the effects on bone turnover and bone mass were diminished by the end of the study.[402] However, the fact that doses of 100 or 400 U/day did not significantly decrease fractures in another study and other concerns have raised questions about the efficacy of calcitonin.[403] Nasal calcitonin is less effective in increasing BMD than alendronate.[404] New approaches to calcitonin therapy are being tested.[405]

Selective Estrogen Receptor Modulators

Several compounds have effects similar to those of estrogen on bone, but they act as antagonists in the breast and therefore have been called selective estrogen receptor modulators (SERMs).

Tamoxifen can diminish bone loss in women with breast cancer.[406] Another SERM, raloxifene, can prevent bone loss and reduce the risk of vertebral fracture in osteoporotic patients.[407] Its effects on bone turnover and mass are somewhat less than those of estrogen.[408] Raloxifene has minimal effects on the breast or uterus and appears to decrease the risk of breast cancer.[409] It reduces low-density lipoprotein levels but does not increase high-density lipoprotein.[410] However, it is associated with an increased risk of thromboembolism and may produce hot flashes. New SERMS with potentially greater effects in bone are being studied, including combined therapy with estrogen.[411,412]

Anabolic Therapy

Parathyroid Hormone. Many years ago, PTH given intermittently in low doses was shown to increase bone mass in animals. The use of intermittent low-dose synthetic PTH (teriparatide) in men and women with osteoporosis has produced a substantial increase in trabecular bone mass with little loss or even a gain in cortical bone in the femur and has reduced the incidence of fractures.[413,414] Treatment with PTH is likely to be the most effective approach in patients who lose bone or continue to have fractures on antiresorptive therapy. PTH may be particularly useful in glucocorticoid-induced osteoporosis.[289,291] PTH must be given by once daily injection, and patients must be monitored carefully for hypercalcemia and hypercalciuria. Prior or concomitant therapy with bisphosphonates may blunt or delay the anabolic response to PTH but certainly does not abrogate it.[415,416] Treatment with bisphosphonates after a course of PTH may help maintain the gains of PTH therapy.[417,418]

Strontium Ranelate. Strontium ranelate has been proposed as an anabolic agent that also may be antiresorptive. It has reduced the incidence of vertebral and nonvertebral fractures in large clinical trials.[200,419] Although side effects are minimal, there are reports of rare but severe allergic reactions.[420,421] It has not been approved for the treatment of osteoporosis in the United States.

Anabolic Steroids. Anabolic androgenic steroids (e.g., testosterone) may increase bone and muscle mass. However, high doses produce unacceptable androgenic side effects in many women. Testosterone therapy can increase bone mass and improves trabecular architecture in hypogonadal men.[422-425] Selective androgen receptor modulators are being tested in both sexes.[426,427]

Diuretics. Thiazides and indapamide can decrease urinary calcium excretion and increase bone mass in patients with hypercalciuria and may reduce cortical bone loss in normal postmenopausal women and decrease the incidence of hip fractures.[428-431] Thiazide therapy is particularly appropriate in patients with osteoporosis who have high fasting urinary calcium excretion due to a renal leak.

Denosumab. Injections of denosumab, a human monoclonal antibody to RANKL, can increase BMD, reduce fractures, and markedly inhibit bone resorption.[432,433] Denosumab may also be effective in preventing bone loss in malignancy.[434,435]

Other Osteoclast Inhibitors. Several critical aspects of osteoclast function, including the secretion of acid and of proteolytic enzymes (particularly cathepsin K), and the expression of integrins may be potential sites for effective intervention in osteoporosis. Selective antagonists for these processes have been developed and are being explored in the laboratory and the clinic.[436-438]

Other Anabolic Agents. Wnt signaling can have anabolic and anti-catabolic effects on bone. This pathway is tonically inhibited by proteins that block Wnt receptors (e.g., sclerostin, DKK) or Wnt ligands (e.g., secreted frizzled receptor [SFR]). Disinhibition using antibodies to sclerostin can increase bone mass in animal models.[439] Increased levels of DKK1 in myeloma, which produces a bone disease characterized by increased bone resorption and decreased formation, suggest this may also be a target for antibody therapy.[440] Activins and inhibins can affect bone formation and a soluble activin receptor can increase bone formation in mice.[441,442]

Activation of the calcium sensing receptor in bone may be anabolic. This may account in part for the effect of strontium.[443]

RICKETS AND OSTEOMALACIA

Rickets and osteomalacia are disorders of the mineralization of newly synthesized organic matrix. In adults, the disorder involves only bone. However, in children, abnormalities also occur in the growth plate and in the mineralization of cartilage, leading to characteristic deformities.

Pathogenesis

To understand the pathogenesis of rickets and osteomalacia, we should recognize that vitamin D is a prohormone that can be synthesized in the skin or supplied in the diet. Vitamin D deficiency is usually the combined result of deficient sun exposure and decreased dietary intake or intestinal malabsorption. Rickets and osteomalacia can also be caused by metabolic defects in the vitamin D hormone system, including inadequate activation in the liver and kidney and abnormalities of the vitamin D receptor (see Chapter 28). Mineralization can be incomplete when the supply or transport of mineral, particularly phosphate, is impaired in renal, intestinal, or bone cell disorders.[444]

Nutritional and Gastrointestinal Disorders

Inadequate vitamin D intake is less common in the United States than in other countries because many foods are supplemented with this vitamin. However, the combination of reduced amounts of exposure to appropriate ultraviolet wavelengths (UVB) during the winter in the northern half of the United States and inadequate vitamin D supplements in the diet can lead to rickets in infants and osteomalacia in older persons. Individuals with darker pigmentation of the skin are more susceptible to vitamin D deficiency because they are less efficient in converting 7-dehydrocholesterol to vitamin D.[445,446] For example, nutritional rickets occurs in black infants who are breastfed without vitamin D supplementation. Adult Asiatic Indians in the United States and Europe have low 25(OH) vitamin D levels and are more likely to have osteomalacia. Intestinal malabsorption of fat can also cause deficiency of vitamin D and of other fat-soluble vitamins.[447] Inability to produce adequate amounts of 25(OH) vitamin D can occur in advanced liver disease and with the use of antiepileptic drugs.

Calcium deficiency rickets may differ from other forms of rickets and osteomalacia, particularly in adolescents, who may have genu valgum without end-plate deformities.[448,449] In contrast, phosphate deficiency causes typical rickets. Because most foods contain phosphate, this form of rickets requires markedly unbalanced nutrition, such as can occur with prolonged intravenous feeding, removal of phosphate by dialysis with a low-phosphate solution, or use of aluminum-containing antacids, which bind phosphate in the intestine.

Renal Defects

Impairment of 1α-hydroxylase can occur because of loss of renal mass or in renal tubular disorders such as the Fanconi syndrome. A hereditary deficiency of 1α-hydroxylase—vitamin D–dependent rickets type I or pseudo-vitamin D deficiency—is a rare autosomal recessive disorder in which rickets develops during the first year of life. It occurs in rodents with homozygous inactivating mutations of the 1α-hydroxylase gene and responds to physiologic doses of calcitriol.[450,451]

Hereditary Resistance to Vitamin D: Vitamin D–Dependent Rickets Type II

Vitamin D–dependent rickets type II occurs in members of families who are homozygous for defects in the vitamin D receptor gene. These patients also often have alopecia. They show improvement in mineralization in response to high doses of calcium and phosphorus, but this does not reverse the alopecia.[452]

Familial X-Linked Hypophosphatemia

Originally called vitamin D–resistant rickets, familial X-linked hypophosphatemia (XLH) is caused by a defect in renal phosphate transport, with a resultant inappropriate excess excretion of phosphate in the urine. Although the most apparent abnormality is decreased renal tubular reabsorption of phosphate, phosphate transport may be impaired in other cells, particularly osteoblasts. Inactivating mutations in the gene *PHEX* (phosphate regulating gene with homologies to endopeptidases on the X chromosome), which encodes a protein that is a member of the MMP13 family of membrane-bound metalloproteases, have been found in this disorder.[453-455]

The exact mechanism by which *PHEX* mutations mediate this condition is unknown. One hypothesis is that *PHEX* normally directly or indirectly modifies one or more hormones that regulate renal phosphate transport. These substances, which have been called *phosphatonins*, consist of a family of four proteins: fibroblast growth factor-23 (FGF23), FGF7, secreted frizzle–related protein-4 (SFRP4), and matrix extracellular phosphoglycoprotein (MEPE). All decrease renal sodium phosphate transport, and FGF23 and SFRP4 inhibit syntheses of 1,25-dihydroxy vitamin D.[453]

In support of the hypothesis that XLH results from abnormal circulating levels of phosphatonins, the serum level of FGF23, which is produced by osteocytes, is elevated in most patients with this condition.[456] XLH patients frequently have some impairment in 1α-hydroxylase activity, which is consistent with the known ability of FGF23 to inhibit this enzyme.

XLH exhibits genetic and phenotypic heterogeneity. Autosomal dominant, autosomal recessive, and X-linked forms of transmission have been described.[457] Treatment involves a combination of calcitriol and phosphate.[458] However, it is difficult to achieve normal growth rates in this disorder.

Oncogenic Osteomalacia

Oncogenic osteomalacia is a severe form of osteomalacia that is presumably caused by production of one or more phosphatonins by fibrous and mesenchymal tumors, which are often small and difficult to identify. Removal of the tumor causes rapid reversal of the osteomalacia. The phosphatonin that has been most frequently identified is FGF23, but FGF7 and MEPE may also be involved.[459,460]

Hypophosphatasia

A rare autosomal recessive disorder, hypophosphatasia is characterized by mutations in the gene for the tissue-nonspecific (liver, bone, and kidney) isoenzyme of alkaline phosphatase.[461] The six recognized clinical forms depend on the age at diagnosis and the severity of the symptoms: perinatal lethal, infantile, childhood, adult, odontohypophosphatasia, and perinatal benign.[462] Clinical manifestations vary from death in utero related to severe deformities to infantile and childhood rickets to adult-onset osteomalacia.[463] Premature loss of deciduous teeth and impaired dentition in adults are common. Plasma levels of organic phosphate compounds, such as pyridoxal 5-phosphate, are increased.[464] Infusion of normal alkaline phosphatase has provided only temporary improvement, but prolonged response has been observed after transplantation of marrow cells, which express the normal enzymes.[465]

Drug-Induced Osteomalacia

High doses of sodium fluoride or of first-generation bisphosphonates (e.g., etidronate) can produce osteomalacia. Anticonvulsant therapy in patients with a marginal vitamin D supply can cause osteomalacia by decreasing 25(OH)D levels.[466]

Clinical Features

Rickets differs from osteomalacia in that it occurs before closure of the epiphyses. Enlargement of cartilage at the growth plate causes the so-called rachitic rosary at the costochondral junctions of the ribs and widening of the cartilaginous ends of the long bones. Impaired mineralization results in bowing of long bones. Radiologically, widening, cupping, and fraying of the metaphyses are seen (Fig. 29-18). Severe vitamin D deficiency causes muscle weakness, and this weakness, combined with the deformity of the chest wall, causes an increased incidence of pneumonia. The clinical expression of osteomalacia in adults varies widely. The most common deformity is bowing of the legs, and in severe cases, bone pain and weakness may cause the patient to be bedridden.[467]

Radiographic changes include subperiosteal erosions caused by marked secondary hyperparathyroidism and a virtually pathognomonic but relatively uncommon

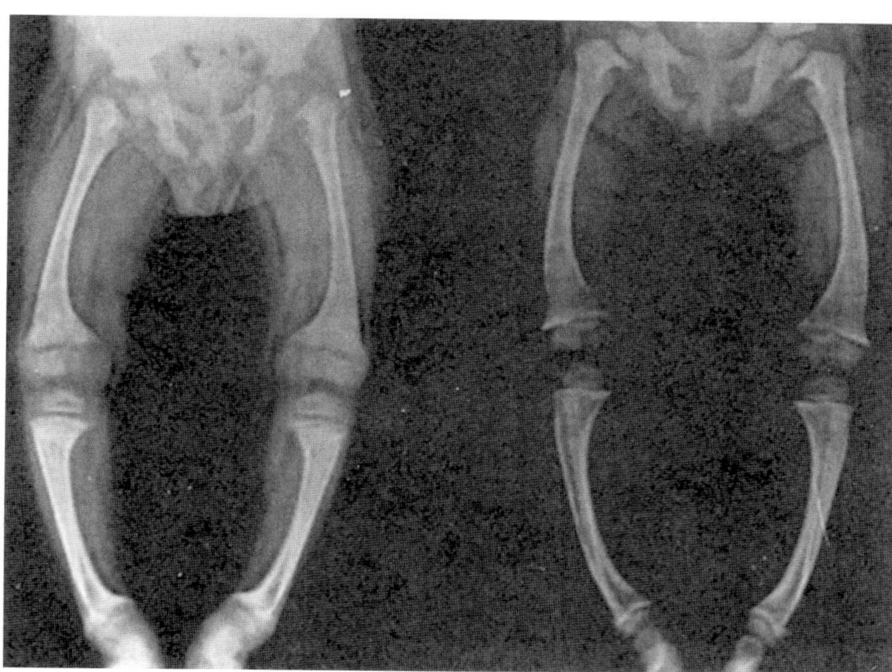

Figure 29-18 Rickets. *Left,* Active rickets in a patient with tissue resistance to 1,25-dihydroxyvitamin D at age 21 months with genu varum, irregular metaphyses, and widened growth plates. *Right,* Inactive rickets in the same patient at age 27 months after treatment with massive doses of ergocalciferol. (From Marx SJ, Spiegel AM, Brown EM, et al. Familial syndrome of decrease in sensitivity to 1,25-hydroxyvitamin D. *J Clin Endocrinol Metab.* 1978;47:1303-1310. Copyright © 1978 by The Endocrine Society.)

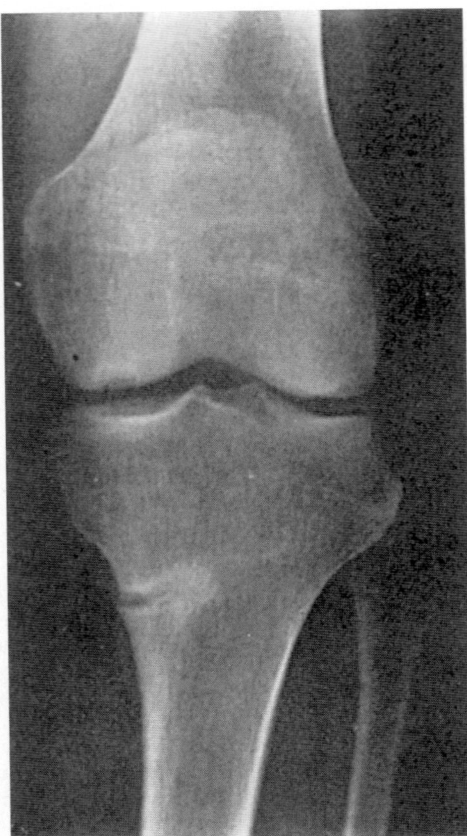

Figure 29-19 Active osteomalacia in a patient (sibling of the patient in Fig. 29-18) with hereditary tissue resistance to 1,25-dihydroxyvitamin D at age 18 with pseudofracture of the left tibia. (From Marx SJ, Spiegel AM, Brown EM, et al. Familial syndrome of decrease in sensitivity to 1,25-hydroxyvitamin D. *J Clin Endocrinol Metab.* 1978;47:1303-1310. Copyright © 1978 by The Endocrine Society.)

lesion, the so-called pseudofracture (Looser's zones or Milkman's syndrome) of the long bones, ribs, scapulae, or pubic rami (Fig. 29-19). Coarsening of the trabecular pattern in the spine may be present, but it is also seen in osteoporosis.

Diagnosis

Although clinical features may point to rickets or osteomalacia, the diagnosis depends on laboratory studies. The biochemical picture can vary with different pathogenetic mechanisms and with different stages of disease. In infants with vitamin D deficiency, serum calcium may be low and the serum phosphorus concentration may be normal initially; as secondary hyperparathyroidism develops, however, calcium concentrations usually return to the low-normal range, and serum phosphorus levels fall further. In advanced stages, the serum calcium concentration may fall again. This fall has been attributed to the inability of secondary hyperparathyroidism to maintain the serum calcium level when the bone surface is covered by osteoid and is resistant to attack by osteoclasts.

In adults, the characteristic picture is a low-normal or slightly decreased serum calcium level, a decreased urinary calcium level, and a low serum phosphate level. Increased alkaline phosphatase levels reflect the activity of the osteoblasts, which form unmineralized matrix. PTH levels may be markedly increased. The key diagnostic test in vitamin D deficiency is demonstration of a decreased serum 25(OH) D value. The 25(OH)D levels may also be decreased in severe hepatic disease or with drugs that impair 25-hydroxylase. The $1,25(OH)_2D$ levels may be normal in vitamin D deficiency, presumably because of a maximal stimulation of 1α-hydroxylase by the low serum phosphorus and high PTH levels. Nevertheless, the amount of this hormone is inadequate to activate the receptors in intestine and bone. Because of the high activity of 1α-hydroxylase, administration of vitamin D to these patients causes a further increase in $1,25(OH)_2D$ to supranormal levels.

The diagnosis of other forms of rickets and osteomalacia can be made by measuring vitamin D metabolite levels. For example, low values of $1,25(OH)_2D$ and normal levels of 25(OH)D suggest a defect in 1α-hydroxylase that may be genetic or acquired as a result of loss of renal function or tumor-induced osteomalacia. High levels of $1,25(OH)_2D$ and normal levels of 25(OH)D are seen in patients with vitamin D receptor defects. In X-linked hypophosphatemia, serum phosphorus levels are low, and levels of serum calcium and vitamin D metabolites are normal. If alkaline phosphatase levels are low, a definitive diagnosis of hypophosphatasia should be sought by measuring pyridoxal 5-phosphate; elevated levels are relatively specific for hypophosphatasia and correlate with clinical severity.

Although the diagnosis of osteomalacia can usually be made on the basis of clinical findings and laboratory studies, a bone biopsy is sometimes needed for a definitive diagnosis. The characteristic finding is markedly widened osteoid seams and impaired mineralization with diffuse or absent tetracycline labeling. The bone also shows great variation in trabecular width and resorption lacunae resulting from secondary hyperparathyroidism. A modest increase in osteoid width can occur in a high-turnover state, such as hyperparathyroidism, thyrotoxicosis, or Paget's disease; however, tetracycline labeling shows a normal mineralization front in these conditions.

Therapy

Vitamin D is effective in the treatment of nutritional and malabsorptive rickets and osteomalacia. High doses may be given initially, but it is important not to overtreat patients because vitamin D is stored in the fat and excessive amounts can cause prolonged hypercalcemia and hypercalciuria. Monitoring of urinary calcium excretion is useful to determine when the vitamin D dose should be decreased. Patients with malabsorption may require large doses or parenteral vitamin D. Patients with defects in 1α-hydroxylase can be treated with calcitriol. If the cause is tumor-induced osteomalacia, the treatment is to find and remove the lesion. However, oral or intravenous phosphate and calcitriol can be used to heal the skeletal lesions, but this may lead to tertiary hyperparathyroidism.[468]

Severe defects in the vitamin D receptor are most difficult to treat. Massive doses of calcium and phosphorus have been given to these patients, but normal growth is rarely achieved, and alopecia persists.[452,469] Intravenous calcium therapy may be necessary and is effective in restoring bone mineralization. Similarly, normal growth may not occur despite repletion of phosphorus and administration of calcitriol in patients with X-linked hypophosphatemia, although bone mineralization can be restored. Growth hormone has been used to help achieve normal height.[470] Careful monitoring of levels of calcium, phosphorus, and vitamin D metabolites is important to prevent impairment of renal function. There is no effective therapy for hypophosphatasia.

HYPERPARATHYROID BONE DISEASE

In the past, severe cases of primary hyperparathyroidism showed osteitis fibrosa cystica generalisata, manifested by generalized bone loss with increased bone resorption, including subperiosteal and endosteal surfaces.[471] The formation of fibrotic cystic lesions (i.e., brown tumors) in the long bones and jaw caused swelling, pathologic fractures, and bone pain. This bone disease is now rarely seen in primary hyperparathyroidism but may occur in poorly managed secondary hyperparathyroidism.

With the common forms of relatively mild, asymptomatic hyperparathyroidism, the major finding is an increased rate of remodeling in bone. Bone density is low in the cortical bone of the radius, but bone density in the metaphyses and vertebrae, which represent largely trabecular bone, may be normal or only moderately decreased.[472] Vitamin D insufficiency is common and associated with lower BMD.[473] Patients with mild to moderate disease may have cortical bone loss.[474] When these patients' hyperparathyroidism is cured surgically, bone density in the spine can increase by as much as 15%,[475] even in postmenopausal women who are at the highest risk for fracture. Bone density also increases in the radius and hip. Moreover, bone loss is attenuated in postmenopausal women with hypoparathyroidism.[476] On the basis of these results, patients with primary hyperparathyroidism and low bone density who are at risk for fractures, are candidates for parathyroid surgery.[477]

Renal Osteodystrophy

The bone disease associated with chronic and end-stage kidney disease is renal osteodystrophy (ROD), which is a subset of a spectrum of mineral metabolism, vascular, and skeletal complications seen in the syndrome of chronic kidney disease–mineral bone disorder (CKD-MBD). In view of the central role of the kidney in regulating mineral metabolism, it is not surprising that patients with chronic renal failure frequently have skeletal abnormalities. The most frequent form of osteodystrophy in renal failure is caused by the decreased capacity to synthesize $1,25(OH)_2D$ and to excrete phosphate. Lowering of serum calcium by phosphate, impairment of calcium absorption in the intestine, and loss of the feedback inhibitory effect of $1,25(OH)_2D$ on PTH production produce severe secondary hyperparathyroidism and can in certain individuals produce osteitis fibrosis cystica. Circulating levels of the phosphatonin FGF23 are also increased in chronic kidney disease, likely because of hyperphosphatemia. This further compromises the ability of the kidney to synthesize $1,25(OH)_2D$. Chronic kidney disease directly inhibits osteoblast function and bone formation.

In addition to the high turnover bone disease of osteitis fibrosis cystica, which is typically seen with serum intact PTH values of greater than 500 pg/mL, some patients present with low to absent turnover and the syndrome of adynamic bone disorder. These individuals typically have serum intact PTH values of less than 100 pg/mL. Certain individuals with high turnover may have a mineralization defect, which leads to very wide osteoid seam width as measured by bone biopsy. Serum intact PTH values in this "mixed uremic osteodystrophy syndrome" are typically between 100 and 500 pg/mL.[478-481]

Development of bone disease can be slowed or prevented by phosphate restriction or by treatment with phosphate binders and calcitriol or analogues of calcitriol that are less likely to cause hypercalcemia.[482] When this fails, it is possible to reduce PTH levels with a calcimimetic agent such as cinacalcet.[483] In the past, aluminum hydroxide was used to bind phosphate, a therapy that sometimes caused aluminum-induced adynamic bone disease. This condition is less common with use of calcium salts, sevelamer, or lanthanum to decrease phosphate absorption. Adynamic bone disease can occur without aluminum excess, particularly in patients in whom secondary hyperparathyroidism has been reversed. However, the relation of serum intact PTH levels and bone turnover varies, and biopsies are needed in most patients for a definitive diagnosis.[484] Osteomalacia can occur in patients receiving dialysis if they have an inadequate supply of vitamin D and calcium, but this is unusual. Osteoporosis is common in chronic renal failure and is often aggravated after transplantation.[485]

Renal osteodystrophy causes growth retardation and skeletal deformities in children, and children and adults have bone pain and muscle weakness. Soft tissue calcifications are particularly dangerous when they occur in blood vessels and lead to ischemia and gangrene. Calcification may be the result of a high calcium-phosphorus product and of vessel wall changes resulting from renal failure or the direct effects of PTH. To prevent calcification, it is important to avoid a high serum level of a calcium-phosphorus ion product and to minimize secondary hyperparathyroidism.[484]

Diagnosis

The diagnosis of a specific form of renal osteodystrophy can be aided by biochemical measurements. Levels of PTH can help to differentiate osteitis fibrosa cystica from adynamic bone disorder or mixed uremic osteodystrophy. Plasma aluminum levels may be elevated in patients with aluminum-induced osteodystrophy but do not necessarily reflect the stores in bone. Deferoxamine chelates aluminum, and this agent can be used to measure the body burden and to treat aluminum overload. The interpretation of biochemical markers of bone turnover is difficult in renal disease because their clearance may be altered.

A bone biopsy often is needed to clarify the pathogenesis of renal osteodystrophy.[486] Using tetracycline labeling, it is possible to determine whether mineralization is impaired. Sections that have not been decalcified show the extent of osteoid seams and resorption surfaces. Aluminum can be identified by special stains. Amyloid deposits, which consist largely of β_2-microglobulin, may be seen in the bone. Amyloidosis of the bone is associated with cystic lesions but not necessarily with bone pain.

Therapy

The treatment of renal osteodystrophy can be highly successful if it is correctly focused on specific pathogenetic mechanisms. The goal should be to maintain normal serum calcium and phosphorus levels and to minimize exposure to aluminum. Phosphate restriction should be instituted relatively early in renal failure, but diets low in phosphorus are difficult to achieve. After the filtration rate is reduced below 25% of normal, it is usually necessary to administer phosphate binders such as calcium salts, sevelamer, or lanthanum. The ability of citrate to increase aluminum absorption is a concern. Correction of acidosis is also important in preventing bone disease.

Early in renal failure, modest supplementation with vitamin D may be sufficient to maintain $1,25(OH)_2D$ levels, but calcitriol itself should be administered eventually. Low doses (0.25 to 0.5 μg/day) are well tolerated, but higher doses can lead to hypercalcemia and hypercalciuria. Vitamin

D analogues, which produce less hypercalcemia, such as paricalcitol and doxercalciferol, are frequently employed for the control of secondary hyperparathyroidism.[164,480,481]

In some cases, parathyroidectomy may be required. Persistent hypercalcemia in patients with renal failure, intractable pruritus, extracellular calcifications, or severe skeletal lesions is an indication for surgery. However, parathyroidectomy should be avoided in patients with adynamic bone disease because symptoms may be worsened.

Renal transplantation corrects many of the biochemical disturbances that lead to renal osteodystrophy, but bone disease may progress. Usually, secondary hyperparathyroidism slowly resolves, but patients with persistent hypercalcemia or autonomy of the parathyroid glands (i.e., tertiary hyperparathyroidism) may require surgery. A major concern, particularly in older patients, is progressive osteoporosis because glucocorticoids and immunosuppressants, which are needed to control transplant rejection, can worsen bone loss in these patients. Optimal therapy has not been defined, but bisphosphonates and vitamin D analogues may slow the bone loss that is associated with renal transplantation.[482,485] Osteonecrosis or avascular necrosis, particularly of the proximal femur, is common after renal transplantation.

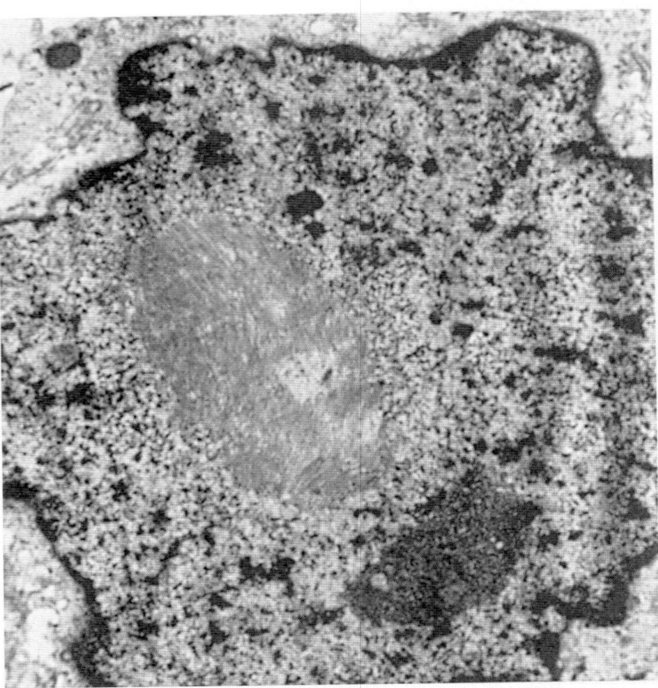

Figure 29-20 Electron micrograph of an osteoclast nucleus from a patient with Paget's disease shows a characteristic intranuclear inclusion, consisting of microfilaments that are 125 nm in diameter. Decalcified bone can be seen (original magnification, ×32,400). (Courtesy of Dr. Barbara G. Mills and Dr. Frederick R. Singer.)

PAGET'S DISEASE

Paget's disease may affect up to 3% of adults older than 40 years. It is often asymptomatic and usually progresses slowly.[487]

Pathogenesis

The primary abnormality in Paget's disease is the localized, uncontrolled formation of large, highly active osteoclasts. The initial lesion is an increase in bone resorption. The response to this resorption, particularly in bones that are subject to mechanical force, is an intense but chaotic increase in osteoblastic activity. The characteristic histologic appearance is of focal lesions with many giant osteoclasts and active osteoblasts. The bone that forms in the lesions is disorganized and has a mosaic pattern with loss of the usual lamellar structure. The marrow shows a pattern of fibrosis and increased vascularity.[488]

The concept that there is a viral origin to Paget's disease is controversial. It is based on the finding of nuclear inclusion bodies in osteoclasts (Fig. 29-20) and the detection of viral transcripts in hematopoietic cells from patients with the disease. Several paramyxoviruses have been suggested, including measles and canine distemper virus.[489] Expression of the measles virus nucleocapsid protein gene in osteoclast precursor cells was found to enhance the ability of these cells to form osteoclasts.[490] However, similar nuclear structures have been found in the osteoclasts of patients with unrelated illnesses, and a number of investigators have failed to detect evidence of a viral infection in pagetic bone or peripheral blood cells from pagetic patients.[491] Further work is needed to establish pathogenetic links between viral sequences and the production of abnormal osteoclasts in this condition. Pagetic osteoclasts differ from normal osteoclasts in their greater size, the presence of viral inclusions, and expression of IL-6, which may play a role in pathogenesis.[492] Expression of resorption stimulators by osteoblast-lineage cells is probably also involved in the development of Paget's disease.

Pagetic bone often distributes in a heterogeneous pattern throughout the skeleton. When lesions appear, they remain stationary within a particular bone over many years, although they may advance within an involved bone over time. A description of the pathogenetic mechanisms in Paget's disease must elucidate how the spotty distribution of this condition develops. Some insight into this puzzle was provided by studies of osteoblasts and bone marrow stromal cells from pagetic lesions. These cells, which are believed to be stationary in bone, produce enhanced RANKL, IL-1, IL-6, and DKK1 mRNA.[493,494]

There appears to be a genetic component to Paget's disease for many patients.[495] Between 15% and 30% of patients have a positive family history, and first-degree relatives of patients with Paget's disease have a sevenfold greater relative risk of having the disorder than individuals with no affected relatives. Ethnic and geographic clustering exists. The incidence is high in some areas of northern Europe, particularly in northern England, but it is low in Norway and Sweden. Mutations in four genes have been linked to Paget's disease and illnesses with pagetoid features in humans. Perhaps the most frequently identified mutations are found in the sequestosome 1 (p62) gene *(SQSTM1)*, which has been identified in 20% to 50% of patients with familial Paget's disease and in 5% to 20% of patients with sporadic Paget's disease.[496-498] Multiple mutations in *SQSTM1* have been identified as predisposing individuals to Paget's disease. Most are in the ubiquitin-associated (UBA) domain, but others are in areas outside the UBA domain that also regulate the binding of SQSTM1 to ubiquitin. SQSTM1 appears involved in RANK signaling through its role in the activation of NF-κB, but the exact mechanism by which mutations in this gene predispose individuals to the development of Paget's disease is unknown.

Mutations in other genes can lead to pagetoid bone lesions. These occur in a number of rare diseases, including familial expansile osteolysis, expansile skeletal hyperphosphatasia, and early-onset familial Paget's disease (all caused by mutations of the RANK gene [*TNFRSF11A*]); idiopathic hyperphosphatasia, also known as juvenile Paget's disease (caused by mutations in the gene for osteoprotegerin [*TNFRSF11B*]); and the syndrome of hereditary inclusion-body myopathy, Paget's disease, and frontotemporal dementia (IBMPFD) (caused by mutations in the gene for valosin-containing protein [*VCP*]).

Clinical Features

Paget's disease affects men and women, with a somewhat higher prevalence among men. The disease usually is not clinically apparent until age 50 to 60 years. It typically progresses slowly and does not usually develop at new bone sites after it is identified. Many different bones can be affected, and the lesions can vary from single, monostotic lesions to involvement of almost the entire skeleton. The pelvis, femur, spine, skull, and tibia are most commonly involved, whereas hands and feet are rarely affected.

Paget's disease is often discovered in asymptomatic patients because of an elevated serum alkaline phosphatase measurement obtained on routine screening or because of a radiograph taken for an unrelated problem. The most common symptom is bone pain at the site of pagetic involvement. Pain also commonly occurs in adjacent joints as a result of secondary degenerative arthritis. Bowing of the legs (Fig. 29-21) and pathologic fractures can also occur. Vertebral involvement can cause kyphosis and compression of the spinal cord. Neural changes can also result from vascular steal because of the high blood flow to the lesion. The most common consequence of Paget's disease of the skull is hearing loss, which can be conductive and neurosensory. Extensive involvement of the base of the skull can produce basilar impression and rarely cause brain stem compression (Fig. 29-22). Dental problems and facial and skull deformities can occur.

The incidence of osteosarcoma is increased but is less than 1%. When osteosarcoma does occur, it is highly malignant. Most patients do not live longer than 1 to 3 years. Fibrosarcomas, chondrosarcomas, and benign giant cell tumors are occasionally seen. The giant cell tumors, called *reparative granulomas,* may represent an extension of pagetic tissue outside the skeleton.

Patients with Paget's disease may have an increased incidence of primary hyperparathyroidism. Hypercalcemia also has been reported in immobilized patients. Angioid streaks are often seen in the fundus. Pseudogout, gout, and osteoarthritis occur. Patients with underlying heart disease may show worsening of heart failure, which has been attributed to increased blood flow in pagetic bone.

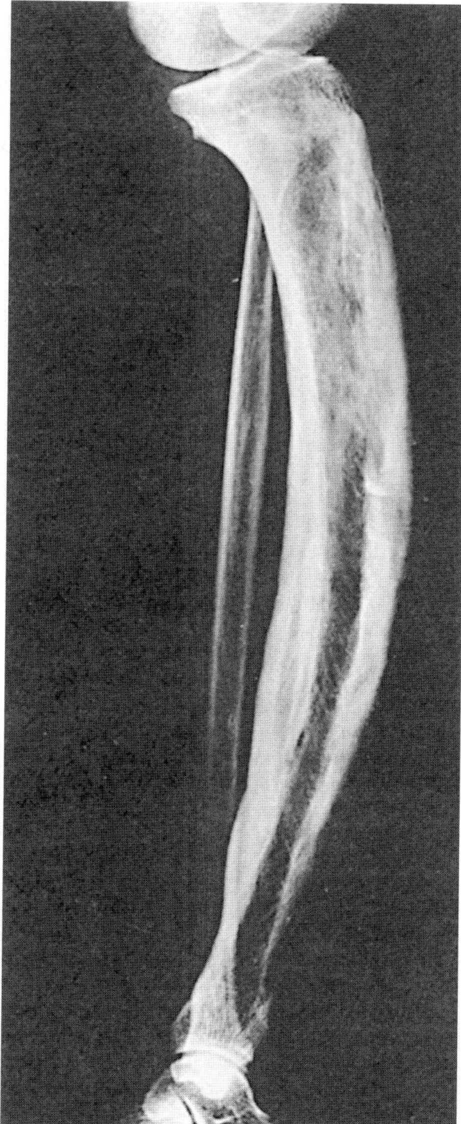

Figure 29-21 Paget's disease of the tibia. Notice the bowing, marked irregularity of the anterior cortex and the flame-shaped lytic lesion of the posterior cortex. (Courtesy of Dr. Ethel S. Siris.)

Diagnosis

The diagnosis of Paget's disease may be made by the finding of an elevated serum alkaline phosphatase concentration or after a routine radiograph. In older persons with deformities or bone pain, the diagnosis should be considered and a careful family history and review of the musculoskeletal system by history and physical examination obtained. A bone scan should be carried out to localize possible pagetic sites. Positive scans do not necessarily indicate Paget's disease, and radiographs should be obtained to confirm that Paget's disease is the cause of the increased uptake. Radiographs typically show irregular areas of osteosclerosis with adjacent areas of osteolysis. Rarely, pagetic sites in bone are not evident on bone scan because there is a minimal formation response in the lesion. Such primarily resorptive lesions in the skull are called *osteoporosis circumscripta*.

An audiogram should be obtained for patients with involvement of the petrous bone or those with complaints of hearing loss. Because of the possible increased incidence of hyperparathyroidism, ionized calcium levels should be measured in the initial workup. Monostotic Paget's disease, particularly in the vertebrae, may be difficult to distinguish from metastatic disease. In males, it is prudent to rule out the diagnosis of metastatic prostate cancer, which can mimic many of the laboratory, radiographic, and bone scan findings of Paget's disease. Some patients with vertebral disease may have impingement on the spinal canal. In these individuals, the area should be examined by CT or MRI. Bone biopsies can be useful in atypical cases. An ordinary aspiration biopsy sometimes yields the giant osteoclasts that are pathognomonic of Paget's disease. Samples of bone that show the irregular *marble bone pattern* can also be diagnostic.

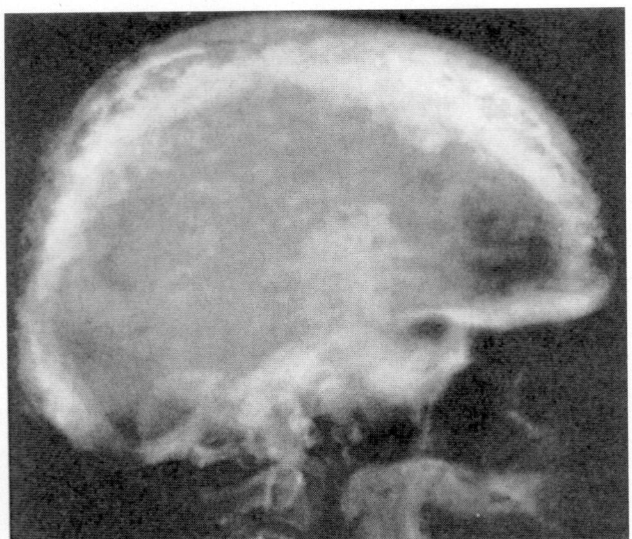

Figure 29-22 Radiograph of the skull of a patient with advanced Paget's disease shows thickening, disordered new bone formation (cotton-wool patches), and basilar impression. (From Singer FR. *Paget's Disease of Bone*. New York, NY: Plenum, 1977.)

After the initial evaluation has been completed, the patient can usually be monitored biochemically by serial measurements of serum total or bone-specific alkaline phosphatase and a marker of bone resorption.[499] Urinary hydroxyproline measurements may be used, as may serum or urinary levels of type I collagen breakdown products such as C-terminal telopeptide or N-terminal telopeptide or measurements of pyridinoline or deoxypyridinoline in the urine.

Therapy

In the past, patients with Paget's disease were often observed until symptoms were clearcut or until there was evidence of progression in critical areas of the skeleton. With the newer bisphosphonates, treatment is instituted earlier. The bisphosphonates zoledronic acid and pamidronate are available for intravenous use. Patients with more extensive disease may require retreatment and should be evaluated by measuring levels of bone turnover markers at regular intervals. Intravenous bisphosphonates are associated with a transient fever and a transient increase in bone pain in 10% to 25% of patients.[498,500] Rare idiosyncratic reactions include uveitis.

Other bisphosphonates are given orally. Alendronate, risedronate, and tiludronate are approved in the United States. As with pamidronate, patients may require repeated therapy with oral bisphosphonates after a drug-free period that varies with each agent. Oral bisphosphonates need to be taken in a manner that minimizes the development of esophagitis or interactions with food and other therapeutics in the stomach. Osteonecrosis of the jaw has been detected occasionally in this condition in patients treated with any of the bisphosphonates. Treatments with the newer bisphosphonates have largely replaced therapy with calcitonin, etidronate, or plicamycin. All of these agents act by inhibiting osteoclastic activity, and the earliest indication of therapeutic response is a drop in resorption markers followed by a decrease in formation markers.

The indications for treatment are pain that can be attributed to Paget's disease and deformities that may produce neurologic changes or are likely to lead to fracture, such as the osteolytic flame lesion or blade of grass lesion in weight-bearing bones (see Fig. 29-20). Hearing loss may be an indication for therapy, although most patients do not show major improvement after treatment.

Patients with heart disease and extensive Paget's disease should be treated in the hope that decreased pagetic activity will improve management. With the advent of safe and effective therapy, patients with mild to moderate disease, particularly those with the potential for complications (i.e., those with lesions in weight-bearing bone, the vertebral bodies, or the base of the skull), can be considered for treatment before symptoms develop. Early treatment is logical in young patients with Paget's disease because it is hoped that therapy may prevent progression. However, proof of this hypothesis is not conclusive.

Many patients with Paget's disease have pain associated with joint damage that does not respond to antipagetic therapy. These patients may respond to anti-inflammatory drugs. If osteoarthritis is advanced, knee and hip replacement may be appropriate, but biochemical remission of the Paget's disease should be obtained before surgery.

A high calcium intake may be useful in Paget's disease. Bisphosphonate therapy can lower the serum calcium level and cause secondary hyperparathyroidism, which is probably not advantageous; increased calcium intake may prevent this development. Moreover, calcium loading can increase endogenous calcitonin secretion, which may have beneficial effects. It is important to monitor serum 25(OH)D levels periodically in patients with Paget's disease who are treated with bisphosphonates, because osteomalacia is not uncommon in the elderly population who are at risk for this condition and low serum vitamin D levels may exacerbate the potential of bisphosphonates to cause hypocalcemia. Urinary calcium should be checked before calcium or vitamin D supplementation is given, because an increase in the incidence of renal stones has been reported in pagetic patients.

Hereditary Hyperphosphatasia

Although hereditary hyperphosphatasia has been called *juvenile Paget's disease*, it involves all of the skeleton and develops in infants.[501] Serum alkaline phosphatase levels are very high, and there are severe bone deformities. The histologic appearance resembles that of Paget's disease with high bone turnover, although the osteoclasts are not enlarged. Treatment with bisphosphonates or calcitonin may be effective in reducing bone turnover and improving bone lesions. A familial form with expansile long bone lesions has been described.[502,503] The disease has been associated with mutations in the gene for osteoprotegerin *(TNFRSF11B)* in some affected individuals.[504]

OSTEOGENESIS IMPERFECTA

Osteogenesis imperfecta, or brittle bone disease, is a heterogeneous, congenital disorder in which increased bone fragility leads to fractures and deformity.[505] It ranges in severity from a lethal perinatal form to a mild disorder that results only in increased fractures.

Pathogenesis

Most patients with osteogenesis imperfecta have defects in one of the two genes for type I collagen (*COL1A1* and

TABLE 29-5

Classification of Osteogenesis Imperfecta

Type	Clinical Features	Inheritance	Common Biochemical Abnormality
I	Normal stature, little or no deformity, blue sclerae, hearing loss in 50% of families Dentinogenesis imperfecta may distinguish a subset.	AD	Nonfunctional allele of the α1(I) procollagen gene *(COL1A1)*
II	Lethal in the perinatal period; minimal calvarial mineralization, beaded ribs, compressed femurs, marked long bone deformity, platyspondyly	AD (new mutations) AR (rare)	Substitution of glycine in triple helix of *COL1A1* or *COL1A2*
III	Progressively deforming bones, usually with moderate deformity at birth Scleral hue varies, often lightening with age Dentinogenesis imperfecta common, hearing loss common Stature very short	AD AR (uncommon)	Substitution of glycine in triple helix of *COL1A1* or *COL1A2*
IV	Normal sclerae, mild to moderate bone deformity, and variable short stature; dentinogenesis imperfecta is common and hearing loss occurs in some families	AD	Substitution of glycine in triple helix of *COL1A1* or *COL1A2*; exon skipping in *COL1A2*

AD, Autosomal dominant; AR, autosomal recessive.
Classification by Sillence and Rimoin, as modified by Byers PH. Osteogenesis imperfecta. In: Royce PM, Steinman B, eds. *Connective Tissue and Its Heritable Disorders: Molecular, Genetic and Medical Aspects*. New York, NY: Wiley-Liss, 1993:317-350.

COL1A2). Bones, ligaments, skin, sclerae, and teeth are affected. The incidence of osteogenesis imperfecta is estimated to be 1 in 25,000 to 1 in 100,000 persons. The heterogeneity of the features is caused by the variety of genetic defects, although phenotypic variation occurs even with the same genetic abnormality (Table 29-5). The more severe forms, type II and type III, involve mutations in the helical portion of the collagen molecule that prevent normal assembly and produce unstable triple helices. Point mutations in this portion of the collagen gene can be associated with mild disease (type IV). Genetically engineered mouse models of type IV osteogenesis imperfecta exhibit decreased bone mass caused by increased osteoclastic bone resorption and decreased osteoblastic function.[506]

Type I osteogenesis imperfecta differs from the other forms in that there is usually a deletion of one allele of the α1(I) procollagen gene *(COL1A1)*, resulting in decreased collagen production but a normal molecular structure.[507] This disorder is of particular interest because familial osteoporosis may also exhibit such defects.[508,509] Bone biopsies show decreased cortical width and trabecular bone volume, increased turnover, and decreased bone formation in patients with type I disease.[510] In a subgroup of patients with low turnover and ligamentous calcifications, the disorder has been named type V osteoporosis imperfecta.[401] Autosomal recessive osteogenesis imperfecta is caused by mutations in any of three proteins that form a complex that 3-hydoxylates proline 396 in collagen α1(I) and α1(II) (reviewed by Chang and colleagues[511]).

Classification and Clinical Features

The classification devised by Sillence and Rimoin, which was modified by Byers,[505] is summarized in Table 29-5. In addition to bone involvement, patients may have ligament laxity, joint hypermobility, and easy bruising. Dentin formation is often abnormal, and the teeth are fragile and discolored. Blue sclerae are a variable manifestation and do not correlate with severity. Because of the thoracic deformities, patients with severe manifestations are predisposed to pulmonary infections and usually have a shortened life span. Intelligence is not affected, and individuals with marked deformities can be highly productive if appropriate conditions are provided.

Diagnosis

In patients with moderate to severe disease, the clinical features make the diagnosis relatively straightforward. In patients with the milder forms, however, the diagnosis may be missed. In children without deformities, multiple fractures are usually attributed to trauma. In infants, the presence of such fractures may lead to an accusation of parental abuse. In the absence of typical clinical features, the diagnosis can be made only biochemically. Culture of fibroblasts from skin biopsies and analysis of the collagen by gel electrophoresis can point to a defect, and gene sequencing of the *COL1A1* and *COL1A2* genes identifies 80% to 85% of mutations. In individuals without identifiable mutations of the type I collagen genes, sequencing of the genes for cartilage-associated protein (CRTAP) and prolyl-3-hydroxylase (LEPREI), which are involved in stabilizing collagen, have identified additional mutations. These analyses are useful for families because specific DNA polymorphisms may allow prenatal diagnosis if the mutation has already been identified in other affected family members.

In children and adolescents with multiple fractures but no deformity, measurements of bone density and turnover may point toward the diagnosis. In the type I disorder, bone density and serum type I procollagen peptide levels are likely to be decreased. However, because excretion of collagen cross-links is increased in most types of osteogenesis imperfecta, increased bone resorption may play a role in pathogenesis.[512]

Therapy

Antiresorptive therapy with intravenous bisphosphonates has decreased fractures in children with severe osteogenesis imperfecta, even before 3 years of age.[513,514] Oral bisphosphonates may also be effective in older children and adults.[515] However, the efficacy of bisphosphonate therapy to prevent fractures in this disease is controversial and not evident in all studies.[516] Supportive treatment is important. The Osteogenesis Imperfecta Foundation works with patients and families to improve quality of life. Orthopedic and rehabilitation services can be helpful in dealing with deformities. Genetic counseling and prenatal diagnosis, including ultrasound examination and testing for informative DNA polymorphisms, are important for the family. Gene therapy is being explored.[517]

Other Connective Tissue Disorders Affecting the Skeleton

Other inherited disorders of connective tissue with impairment of skeletal development or increased bone fragility include Ehlers-Danlos syndrome, Menkes' disease, lysinuric protein intolerance, and homocystinuria.[279] In these disorders, abnormalities of collagen cross-linking can affect bone and other connective tissues. In Ehlers-Danlos syndrome, the cross-linking enzyme lysyl oxidase is deficient, and in Menkes' disease, copper deficiency impairs the function of this enzyme. Lysinuric protein intolerance and homocystinuria probably also impair collagen cross-linking.

OSTEOPETROSIS

Osteopetrosis, or marble bone disease, is a heterogeneous group of disorders that are characterized by a generalized increase in bone density. They are predominantly caused by defective osteoclastic bone resorption.[518] However, rates of resorption and formation in bone are coupled through poorly understood mechanisms, and it is likely that bone resorption and formation rates are altered in most cases of this disease.

Osteopetrosis is divided by the severity of the clinical presentation into autosomal recessive osteopetrosis (ARO), intermediate autosomal recessive osteopetrosis (IARO) and benign autosomal dominant osteopetrosis (ADO), which is further divided into type I and type II. Type I ADO results from mutations of the *LRP5* gene, which are not thought to directly influence osteoclast function.

A variety of genetic mutations have been identified in humans with osteopetrosis. Mutations in the *TCIRG1, CLCN7,* and *OSTM1* genes, which influence acid generation in the resorption lacuna of osteoclasts, are found in most ARO patients, whose bones contain dysfunctional osteoclasts. In contrast, mutations in the RANK and RANKL genes (*TNFRSF11A* and *TNFS11*) are associated with ARO in patients whose bones are without osteoclasts.

CLCN7 mutations are also found in IARO and ADO type II patients. IARO is also associated with mutations in the gene for carbonic anhydrase II *(CA2)*, which catalyzes acid generation, and in *PLEKHM1,* which is involved in vesicular trafficking.

Additional cases of osteopetrosis are caused by mutations in the gene for the inhibitor of kappa light polypeptide gene enhancer in B cells *(IKBKG)*, which encodes the protein NF-κB essential modulator (IKBKG, formerly designated NEMO) that is involved in RANK signaling, and by mutations in the gene for integrin-β_3 *(ITGB3)*, which is involved in the attachment of osteoclasts to bone.

Osteopetrotic rats and mice with specific defects in osteoclasts have been found as a result of spontaneous mutations and targeted gene deletion techniques. The *op/op* mouse has a genetic defect in the production of M-CSF that results in failure of osteoclast formation, which can be corrected by treatment with M-CSF.[519] Knockouts of the proto-oncogenes *src* and *fos*; of TRAF6, a mediator of RANK action; and of tartrate-resistant acid phosphatase also cause osteopetrosis.[520-524]

Clinical Presentations in Specific Conditions

Autosomal Recessive Osteopetrosis

ARO or malignant infantile osteopetrosis is a rare, autosomal recessive disorder in which failure to resorb bone and calcified metaphyseal cartilage causes near obliteration of the marrow spaces.[454,525-529] Extramedullary hematopoiesis occurs in the liver and spleen. The cranial nerve foramina do not form normally, causing optic atrophy and other cranial nerve defects. The bones, although dense, are brittle, and pathologic fractures can occur.

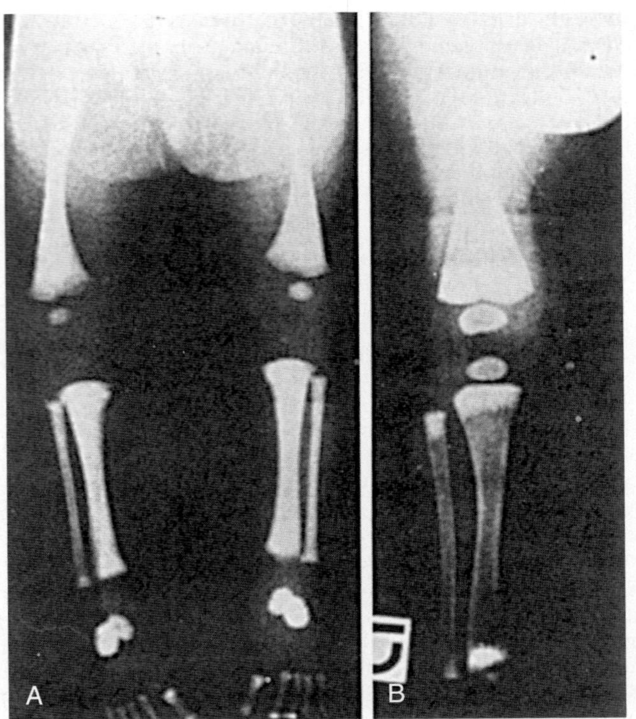

Figure 29-23 Radiographs of the lower limb of a patient with osteopetrosis at age 2 months **(A)** before bone marrow transplantation and at age 9 months after transplantation **(B)** show formation of normal medullary bone. (From Ballet JJ, Griscelli C. Lymphoid cell transplantation in human osteopetrosis. In Horton JE, Tarpley TM, Davis WF, eds. *Mechanisms of Localized Bone Loss.* London, UK: IRI, 1978:399-414, by permission of Oxford University Press.)

The impaired function of the hematopoietic system causes death in the first decade from hemorrhage or infection. On the basis of studies in animal models in which transfer of hematopoietic tissue resulted in cure, patients have been treated with total-body irradiation and grafting of marrow from human leukocyte antigen–identical donors (Fig. 29-23).[526] When suitable donors cannot be found, therapy with high doses of interferon have improved bone resorption.[530]

Carbonic Anhydrase II Deficiency

Carbonic anhydrase II deficiency, a nonlethal autosomal recessive disorder, is associated with a complete deficiency of the type II carbonic anhydrase that provides carbonic acid for hydrogen ion secretion by osteoclasts and by the distal tubules.[531] In this condition, osteopetrosis is accompanied by renal tubular acidosis that may involve distal and proximal lesions. Affected individuals are shorter than their normal siblings and may have calcification of the basal ganglia. Bone marrow transplantation can correct the skeletal abnormalities.[532]

Autosomal Dominant Osteopetrosis Type II

ADO II (Albers-Schönberg disease) is characterized by generalized osteosclerosis with thickening of the vertebral end plates (i.e., sandwich vertebrae) and bone within bone in the pelvis. Although ADO II has been called *benign osteoporosis*, most patients have clinical problems, presumably related to impaired bone remodeling, that include fractures, osteoarthritis, skeletal deformities, and cranial nerve involvement.[533] Most patients with ADO II have a milder form of mutation in the chloride transport gene *ClCN7* than that seen in the more severe forms of infantile osteopetrosis, although other genes may be involved. Decreased bone resorption presumably results from impaired acidification, and tartrate-resistant acid phosphatase activity in the serum is actually increased.[534-536]

OTHER SCLEROSING BONE DISORDERS

Several rare skeletal disorders cause irregular bone structure and various degrees of sclerosis. Some are associated with increased bone formation rather than decreased resorption, although both processes may be affected. Acquired osteosclerosis related to increased bone formation occurs in fluorosis[537] and in rare cases of hepatitis C virus infection,[538] and a localized form is seen in certain metastatic malignancies, particularly cancers of the prostate and breast.

Pyknodysostosis

Pyknodysostosis is an autosomal recessive disorder characterized by short stature, a large cranium, small facies, and skeletal fragility.[539] Unlike patients with osteopetrosis, these patients do not have loss of the marrow cavity and are not anemic. Histologically, trabecular bone volume is increased despite an increase in the number of osteoclasts. There is a defect in osteoclast function due to a mutation of the cathepsin K gene, which is the principal acid-active protease that is secreted by osteoclasts into the resorption space.[540-542]

Progressive Diaphyseal Dysplasia

Known as Camurati-Engelmann disease, progressive diaphyseal dysplasia consists of patchy thickening of the bone on periosteal and endosteal surfaces, and it is associated with pain in the extremities, gait abnormalities, and muscle wasting. The histologic picture is one of increased bone formation rather than decreased resorption.[543] The disease can be inherited as an autosomal dominant disorder, and it is associated with mutations in the TGF-β1 gene *(TGFB1)*, mainly in the latency-associated peptide region.[544,545] Expression in the osteoblasts of mice of a mutated form of TGF-β1 that is identical to that found in some patients with Camurati-Engelmann disease increased the levels of active TGF-β1 in the bone microenvironment and produced bone lesions that were similar to those seen in humans with this condition.[546] In some cases, glucocorticoid therapy relieves the bone pain and reverses the histologic abnormalities of this condition.

Autosomal Dominant Osteopetrosis Type I

After initial identification of an activating mutation of *LRP5* in two families with autosomal dominant high bone mass (HBM)[547,548] several other families were found to have missense mutations in the *LRP5* gene and increased canonical Wnt/β-catenin signaling with somewhat variable phenotypic expression.[549] In the original families, there was little evidence of deformity, but in other families, a picture described as autosomal dominant osteopetrosis type I was found, which can have cranial nerve involvement. The increase in bone mass appears to be attributable to increased bone formation as a result of enhanced canonical Wnt/β-catenin signaling in patients and in a mouse model of this disorder.[550] Abnormal regulation of intestinal serotonin production may be involved in the pathogenesis of HBM.[324] There may also be an abnormality of osteoclast function in vivo, although isolated osteoclasts from these patients are still active in vitro.[551]

Sclerosteosis and van Buchem's Disease

Sclerosteosis and van Buchem's disease are rare, autosomal recessive disorders that are associated with progressive bone thickening due to increased bone formation and sclerosis of the skeleton. Comparison of bone biopsy specimens in these patients with those of normal controls demonstrated activated osteoblasts.[552,553] Both conditions are caused by homozygous mutations in the *SOST* gene, which result in decreased expression of its protein product sclerostin. In sclerosteosis, the mutation causes an improperly spliced SOST mRNA.[554]

In van Buchem's disease, an enhancer element is deleted.[555] Lifelong sclerostin deficiency in both conditions leads to progressive increases in bone mass from childhood to adulthood. Sclerostin is a secreted Wnt antagonist. Several studies have demonstrated that sclerostin binds to LRP5 and LRP6 and inhibits downstream signaling events in the canonical Wnt/β-catenin pathway.[556-558] A decrease in sclerostin in these conditions is thought to increase canonical Wnt/β-catenin signaling and produce an increased bone mass in a manner similar to that seen in HBM patients.

Other Disorders of Bone Density

Three disorders characterized by irregular increases in bone density—osteopoikilosis, the Buschke-Ollendorff syndrome, and melorheostosis—may represent different phenotypes of a common genetic abnormality. A loss of function mutation of *LEMD3*, a gene that encodes an inner nuclear membrane protein, has been found in families with these disorders,[559] although the evidence that isolated melorheostosis is caused by mutations in *LEMD3* is less clear.[560]

Osteopathia striata with cranial sclerosis is a rare syndrome characterized by longitudinal striations in metaphyses of long bones. It is more common in females and may have an X-linked dominant inheritance pattern.[561] Axial osteomalacia is a disorder characterized by back pain and osteosclerosis of the spine and pelvis, which may respond to anti-inflammatory agents.[562,563] Fibrogenesis imperfecta ossium is another rare condition characterized by increased bone density and patchy areas of bone loss, which may represent a defect in bone matrix synthesis.[564]

More localized periosteal new bone formation can occur in a number of different syndromes. Caffey disease or cortical hyperostosis can vary from a severe and lethal disorder to mild increases in periosteal bone formation.[565] A mutation in the *COL1A1* gene has been identified in multiple families with an autosomal dominant form of this disorder.[566-568] However, this disorder can be mimicked by prolonged infusion of PGE_1 in neonates, and such infusions can also cause hypertrophic osteoarthropathy in adults.[569,570] Pachydermoperiostosis is a rare congenital disorder with skin changes and digital hypertrophic osteoarthropathy (i.e., clubbing).[571] Secondary hypertrophic osteoarthropathy and clubbing can occur with pulmonary disease or as a paraneoplastic syndrome, possibly related to overproduction of multiple vascular growth factors.[572-575] If the underlying disorder cannot be treated effectively, bisphosphonates may provide relief from pain.[572]

FIBROUS DYSPLASIA

Clinical Features

Fibrous dysplasia is characterized by expanding lesions within the bone that contain fibroblastic and osteoblastic elements. The disorder can occur as a monostotic lesion without any associated abnormalities or in a polyostotic form, which may occur as part of the McCune-Albright syndrome, associated with functional abnormalities of one or more endocrine glands and irregular hyperpigmented macules called café au lait spots.

The most common endocrine manifestation is precocious puberty, particularly in girls.[576] The molecular defect in the McCune-Albright syndrome is somatic mosaicism for an activating mutation of the $G_s\alpha$ subunit of the nucleotide-binding regulatory protein that couples receptors to adenylyl cyclase. Similar defects have been found in bone lesions in the absence of McCune-Albright syndrome.[577] Local production of PTH-related peptide (PTHrP) may also be involved in pathogenesis.[578] Hypophosphatemia can occur and is associated with increased FGF23 production.[579,580]

Diagnosis

Monostotic fibrous dysplasia is usually diagnosed in the second or third decade of life as an expanding bone lesion that can cause fracture, deformity, or nerve entrapment. Sarcomatous degeneration can occur. In fibrous dysplasia, any skeletal site can be affected, but the femur, tibia, ribs, and face are most often involved. Histologically, the lesions contain many spindle-shaped fibroblasts and islands of woven bone. Bone lesions can worsen during pregnancy, and estrogen receptors have been identified in the bone lesions of patients with McCune-Albright syndrome.[581]

Therapy

The course of monostotic and polyostotic fibrous dysplasia varies. Patients who show progression, nerve compression, or pathologic fractures may require surgery. Careful assessment of the endocrine system is critical in the McCune-Albright syndrome because early intervention can prevent irreversible changes, resulting from precocious puberty. The bone lesions may respond to bisphosphonate.[582] Treatment with $1{,}25(OH)_2D$ may reduce PTHrP production and decrease activity of the bone lesions.[578]

EXTRASKELETAL CALCIFICATION AND OSSIFICATION

Mineral deposition in soft tissues is a common consequence of tissue damage and of a local elevation of the extracellular calcium-phosphate product. Ectopic or heterotopic bone formation can occur at sites of injury or surgical trauma and may be related to the presence of an inductive protein matrix.[583] This form of bone induction stimulated the search for BMPs. The frequency of heterotopic ossification after hip replacement or spinal cord injury can be decreased by treatment with local irradiation or nonsteroidal anti-inflammatory drugs that inhibit prostaglandin synthesis.[584] Extensive subcutaneous calcium deposition may be crippling in inflammatory disorders such as dermatomyositis.

The term *myositis ossificans* is used when bone formation occurs in traumatized muscle. Similar masses can be formed in tendon, ligaments, joint capsules, and fascia without trauma.[583]

Tumoral Calcinosis

Primary tumoral calcinosis is an inherited disorder characterized by periarticular calcification and hyperphosphatemia. It is associated with defective phosphate transport and sometimes with excessive activity of renal 1α-hydroxylase. Multiple missense mutations in the *FGF23* gene have been associated with this disorder,[585] as have mutations in the *GALNT3* gene, whose product *O*-glycosylates FGF23.[586] Primary tumoral calcinosis must be differentiated from secondary tumoral calcinosis, which occurs in association with renal failure and with hypercalcemic disorders.

Treatment with phosphate depletion, using phosphate-binding antacids or with diuretics, parathyroidectomy, and dialysis has been attempted.[587]

Fibrodysplasia Ossificans Progressiva

This rare congenital disorder is most often sporadic but can be transmitted as an autosomal dominant disorder.[588] Characteristic short phalanges and soft tissue swelling can be detected at birth. Abnormal regulation of BMPs has been implicated.[589] Painful, tender lesions caused by true ectopic bone can develop in connective tissues. Severe progressive deformities may include scoliosis and ankylosis of the spine and rib cage. There is no known therapy. However, in the classic and atypical forms of the disease, activating mutations have been identified in the gene for BMP type 1 receptor *(ACVR1)*.[590,591]

Progressive osseous heteroplasia is another genetic disorder in which ossification occurs largely in the skin but extends into the underlying muscle. It may be caused by an inactivating mutation of $G_s\alpha$.[588]

REFERENCES

1. Raisz L, Shoukri KC. *Pathogeneis of Osteoporosis in Physiology and Pharmacology of Bone.* New York, NY: Springer-Verlag; 1993.
2. Baron R. *Anatomy and Ultrastructure of Bone.* New York, NY: Lippincott Williams & Wilkins; 1999.
3. Parfitt AM. The mechanism of coupling: a role for the vasculature. *Bone* 2000:26:319-323.
4. Canalis E. The fate of circulating osteoblasts. *N Engl J Med.* 2005;352:2014-2016.
5. Parfitt AM. The bone remodeling compartment: a circulatory function for bone lining cells. *J Bone Miner Res.* 2001;16:1583-1585.
6. Gorski JP. Is all bone the same? Distinctive distributions and properties of non-collagenous matrix proteins in lamellar vs. woven bone imply the existence of different underlying osteogenic mechanisms. *Crit Rev Oral Biol Med.* 1998;9:201-223.
7. Delany AM, Amling M, Priemel M, et al. Osteopenia and decreased bone formation in osteonectin-deficient mice. *J Clin Invest.* 2000;105:1325.
8. Seeman E, Delmas PD. Bone quality: the material and structural basis of bone strength and fragility. *N Engl J Med.* 2006;354:2250-2261.
9. Viguet-Carrin S, Garnero P, Delmas PD. The role of collagen in bone strength. *Osteoporos Int.* 2006;17:319-336.
10. Anderson HC. Molecular biology of matrix vesicles. *Clin Orthop Relat Res.* 1995;314;266-280.
11. Mauviel A. Cytokine regulation of metalloproteinase gene expression. *J Cell Biochem.* 1993;53:288-295.
12. Rajakumar RA, Quinn CO. Parathyroid hormone induction of rat interstitial collagenase mRNA in osteosarcoma cells is mediated through an AP-1-binding site. *Mol Endocrinol.* 2006;10:867-878.

13. Zhao W, Byrne MH, Boyce BF, et al. Bone resorption induced by parathyroid hormone is strikingly diminished in collagenase-resistant mutant mice. *J Clin Invest.* 1999;103:517-524.
14. Rydziel S, Delany AM, Canalis E. AU-rich elements in the collagenase 3 mRNA mediate stabilization of the transcript by cortisol in osteoblasts. *J Biol Chem.* 2004;279:5397-5404.
15. Liu F, Malaval L, Aubin JE. The mature osteoblast phenotype is characterized by extensive plasticity. *Exp Cell Res.* 1997;232:97-105.
16. Bianco P, Gehron Robey P. Marrow stromal stem cells. *J Clin Invest.* 2000;105:1663-1668.
17. Eghbali-Fatourechi GZ, Lamsam J, Fraser D, et al. Circulating osteoblast-lineage cells in humans. *N Engl J Med.* 2005;352:1959-1966.
18. Canalis E, Deregowski V, Pereira RC, et al. Signals that determine the fate of osteoblastic cells. *J Endocrinol Invest.* 2005;28:3-7.
19. Karsenty G Minireview: transcriptional control of osteoblast differentiation. *Endocrinology.* 2001;142:2731-2733.
20. Tanaka T, Yoshida N, Kishimoto T, et al. Defective adipocyte differentiation in mice lacking the C/EBPbeta and/or C/EBPdelta gene. *EMBO J* 1997:16:7432-7443.
21. Ducy P, Zhang R, Geoffroy V, et al. Osf2/Cbfa1: a transcriptional activator of osteoblast differentiation. *Cell.* 1997;89:747-754.
22. Nakashima K, Zhou X, Kunkel G, et al. The novel zinc finger-containing transcription factor osterix is required for osteoblast differentiation and bone formation. *Cell.* 2002;108:17-29.
23. Koga T, Inui M, Inoue K, et al. Costimulatory signals mediated by the ITAM motif cooperate with RANKL for bone homeostasis. *Nature* 2004:428:758-763.
24. Dobreva G, Chahrour M, Dautzenberg M, et al. SATB2 is a multifunctional determinant of craniofacial patterning and osteoblast differentiation. *Cell.* 2006;125:971-986.
25. Aarden EM, Burger EH, Nijweide PJ. Function of osteocytes in bone. *J Cell Biochem.* 1994;55:287-299.
26. Burger EH, Klein-Nulend J. Mechanotransduction in bone: role of the lacuno-canalicular network. *FASEB J* 1959;13(suppl):S101-S112.
27. Han Y, Cowin SC, Schaffler MB, et al. Mechanotransduction and strain amplification in osteocyte cell processes. *Proc Natl Acad Sci U S A.* 2004;101:16689-16694.
28. Tondravi MM, McKercher SR, Anderson K, et al. Osteopetrosis in mice lacking haematopoietic transcription factor PU.1. *Nature.* 1997;386:81-84.
29. Miyamoto T, Ohneda O, Arai F, et al. Bifurcation of osteoclasts and dendritic cells from common progenitors. *Blood.* 2001;98:2544-2554.
30. Suda T, Takahashi N, Udagawa N, et al. Modulation of osteoclast differentiation and function by the new members of the tumor necrosis factor receptor and ligand families. *Endocr Rev.* 1999;20:345-357.
31. Lorenzo J. Interactions between immune and bone cells: new insights with many remaining questions. *J Clin Invest.* 2000;106:749-752.
32. Arai F, Miyamoto T, Ohneda O, et al. Commitment and differentiation of osteoclast precursor cells by the sequential expression of c-Fms and receptor activator of nuclear factor kappaB (RANK) receptors. *J Exp Med.* 1999;190:1741-1754.
33. Lacey DL, Tan HL, Lu J, et al. Osteoprotegerin ligand modulates murine osteoclast survival in vitro and in vivo. *Am J Pathol.* 2000;157:435-448.
34. Yoshida H, Hayashi S, Kunisada T, et al. The murine mutation osteopetrosis is in the coding region of the macrophage colony stimulating factor gene. *Nature.* 1990;345:442-444.
35. Hofstetter W, Wetterwald A, Cecchini MG, et al. Detection of transcripts and binding sites for colony-stimulating factor-1 during bone development. *Bone.* 1995;17:145-151.
36. Mocsai A, Humphrey MB, Van Ziffle JA, et al. The immunomodulatory adapter proteins DAP12 and Fc receptor gamma-chain (FcRgamma) regulate development of functional osteoclasts through the Syk tyrosine kinase. *Proc Natl Acad Sci U S A.* 2004;101:6158-6163.
37. Kukita T, Wada N, Kukita A, et al. RANKL-induced DC-STAMP is essential for osteoclastogenesis. *J Exp Med.* 2004;200:941-946.
38. Yagi M, Miyamoto T, Sawatani Y, et al. DC-STAMP is essential for cell-cell fusion in osteoclasts and foreign body giant cells. *J Exp Med.* 2005;202:345-351.
39. Ravesloot JH, Eisen T, Baron R, et al. Role of Na-H exchangers and vacuolar H+ pumps in intracellular pH regulation in neonatal rat osteoclasts. *J Gen Physiol.* 1995;105:177-208.
40. Blair HC, Sidonio RF, Friedberg RC, et al. Proteinase expression during differentiation of human osteoclasts in vitro. *J Cell Biochem.* 2000;78:627-637.
41. Delaisse JM, Eeckhout Y, Neff L, et al. (Pro)collagenase (matrix metalloproteinase-1) is present in rodent osteoclasts and in the underlying bone-resorbing compartment. *J Cell Sci.* 1993;106(Pt 4): 1071-1082.
42. Salo J, Lehenkari P, Mulari M, et al. Removal of osteoclast bone resorption products by transcytosis. *Science.* 1997;276:270-273.
43. Martin T, Gooi JH, Sims NA. Molecular mechanisms in coupling of bone formation to resorption. *Crit Rev Eukaryot Gene Expr.* 2009;19:73-88.
44. Pederson L, Ruan M, Westendorf JJ, et al. Regulation of bone formation by osteoclasts involves Wnt/BMP signaling and the chemokine sphingosine-1-phosphate. *Proc Natl Acad Sci U S A.* 2008;105:20764-20769.
45. Recker R, Lappe J, Davies KM, et al. Bone remodeling increases substantially in the years after menopause and remains increased in older osteoporosis patients. *J Bone Miner Res.* 2004;19:1628-1633.
46. Hirano T, Turner CH, Forwood MR, et al. Does suppression of bone turnover impair mechanical properties by allowing microdamage accumulation? *Bone.* 2000;27:13-20.
47. Verborgt O, Gibson GJ, Schaffler MB. Loss of osteocyte integrity in association with microdamage and bone remodeling after fatigue in vivo. *J Bone Miner Res.* 2000;15:60-67.
48. Fu L, Patel MS, Bradley A, et al. The molecular clock mediates leptin-regulated bone formation. *Cell.* 2005;122:803-815.
49. Dempster DW, Cosman F, Parisien M, et al. Anabolic actions of parathyroid hormone on bone. *Endocr Rev.* 1993;14:690-709.
50. Canalis E, Centrella M, Burch W, et al. Insulin-like growth factor I mediates selective anabolic effects of parathyroid hormone in bone cultures. *J Clin Invest.* 1989;83:60-65.
51. Manolagas SC. Birth and death of bone cells: basic regulatory mechanisms and implications for the pathogenesis and treatment of osteoporosis. *Endocr Rev.* 2000;21:115-137.
52. Shiraishi A, Takeda S, Masaki T, et al. Alfacalcidol inhibits bone resorption and stimulates formation in an ovariectomized rat model of osteoporosis: distinct actions from estrogen. *J Bone Miner Res.* 2000;15:770-779.
53. Hurley DL, Tiegs RD, Wahner HW, et al. Axial and appendicular bone mineral density in patients with long-term deficiency or excess of calcitonin. *N Engl J Med.* 1987;317:537-541.
54. Eriksen EF, Kudsk H, Emmertsen K, et al. Bone remodeling during calcitonin excess: reconstruction of the remodeling sequence in medullary thyroid carcinoma. *Bone.* 1993;14:399-401.
55. Hoff AO, Catala-Lehnen P, Thomas PM, et al. Increased bone mass is an unexpected phenotype associated with deletion of the calcitonin gene. *J Clin Invest.* 2002;110:1849-1857.
56. Schinke T, Liese S, Priemel M, et al. Decreased bone formation and osteopenia in mice lacking alpha-calcitonin gene-related peptide. *J Bone Miner Res.* 2004;19:2049-2056.
57. Giustina A, Mazziotti G, Canalis E. Growth hormone, insulin-like growth factors, and the skeleton. *Endocr Rev.* 2008;29:535-559.
58. Canalis E, Mazziotti G, Giustina A, et al. Glucocorticoid-induced osteoporosis: pathophysiology and therapy. *Osteoporos Int.* 2007;18:1319-1328.
59. Hofbauer LC, Gori F, Riggs BL, et al. Stimulation of osteoprotegerin ligand and inhibition of osteoprotegerin production by glucocorticoids in human osteoblastic lineage cells: potential paracrine mechanisms of glucocorticoid-induced osteoporosis. *Endocrinology.* 1999;140:4382-4389.
60. Canalis E, Bilezikian JP, Angeli A, et al. Perspectives on glucocorticoid-induced osteoporosis. *Bone.* 2004;34:593-598.
61. Smith E, Frenkel B. Glucocorticoids inhibit the transcriptional activity of LEF/TCF in differentiating osteoblasts in a glycogen synthase kinase-3beta-dependent and -independent manner. *J Biol Chem.* 2005; 280:2388-2394.
62. Weinstein RS, Jilka RL, Parfitt AM, et al. Inhibition of osteoblastogenesis and promotion of apoptosis of osteoblasts and osteocytes by glucocorticoids: potential mechanisms of their deleterious effects on bone. *J Clin Invest.* 1998;102:274-282.
63. Delany AM, Durant D, Canalis E. Glucocorticoid suppression of IGF I transcription in osteoblasts. *Mol Endocrinol.* 2001;15:1781-1789.
64. Greenspan SL, Greenspan FS. The effect of thyroid hormone on skeletal integrity. *Ann Intern Med.* 1999;130:750-758.
65. Engler H, Oettli RE, Riesen WF. Biochemical markers of bone turnover in patients with thyroid dysfunctions and in euthyroid controls: a cross-sectional study. *Clin Chim Acta.* 1999;289:159-172.
66. Pereira RC, Jorgetti V, Canalis E. Triiodothyronine induces collagenase-3 and gelatinase B expression in murine osteoblasts. *Am J Physiol.* 1999;277:E496-E504.
67. Abe E, Marians RC, Yu W, et al. TSH is a negative regulator of skeletal remodeling. *Cell.* 2003;115:151-162.
68. Sun L, Vukicevic S, Baliram R, et al. Intermittent recombinant TSH injections prevent ovariectomy-induced bone loss. *Proc Natl Acad Sci U S A.* 2008;105:4289-4294.
69. Bex M, Bouillon R. Growth hormone and bone health. *Horm Res.* 2003;60(suppl 3):80-86.
70. Moyer-Mileur LJ, Slater H, Jordan KC, et al. IGF-1 and IGF-binding proteins and bone mass, geometry, and strength: relation to metabolic control in adolescent girls with type 1 diabetes. *J Bone Miner Res.* 2008;23:1884-1891.
71. Canalis E. Effect of insulinlike growth factor I on DNA and protein synthesis in cultured rat calvaria. *J Clin Invest.* 1980;66:709-719.
72. Ogata N, Chikazu D, Kubota N, et al. Insulin receptor substrate-1 in osteoblast is indispensable for maintaining bone turnover. *J Clin Invest.* 2000;105:935-943.

73. Bilezikian JP, Morishima A, Bell J, et al. Increased bone mass as a result of estrogen therapy in a man with aromatase deficiency. *N Engl J Med.* 1998;339:599-603.
74. Falahati-Nini A, Riggs BL, Atkinson EJ, et al. Relative contributions of testosterone and estrogen in regulating bone resorption and formation in normal elderly men. *J Clin Invest.* 2000;106:1553-1560.
75. Canalis E, Economides AN, Gazzerro E. Bone morphogenetic proteins, their antagonists, and the skeleton. *Endocr Rev.* 2003;24:218-235.
76. Canalis E, Giustina A, Bilezikian JP. Mechanisms of anabolic therapies for osteoporosis. *N Engl J Med.* 2007;357:905-916.
77. Lorenzo JA. The role of cytokines in the regulation of local bone resorption. *Crit Rev Immunol.* 1991;11:195-213.
78. Pacifici R. Cytokines, estrogen, and postmenopausal osteoporosis: the second decade. *Endocrinology.* 1998;139:2659-2661.
79. Grey A, Mitnick MA, Masiukiewicz U, et al. A role for interleukin-6 in parathyroid hormone-induced bone resorption in vivo. *Endocrinology.* 1999;140:4683-4690.
80. Onoe Y, Miyaura C, Kaminakayashiki T, et al. IL-13 and IL-4 inhibit bone resorption by suppressing cyclooxygenase-2-dependent prostaglandin synthesis in osteoblasts. *J Immunol.* 1996;156:758-764.
81. Malaval L, Gupta AK, Aubin JE. Leukemia inhibitory factor inhibits osteogenic differentiation in rat calvaria cell cultures. *Endocrinology.* 1995;136:1411-1418.
82. Miyaura C, Onoe Y, Inada M, et al. Increased B-lymphopoiesis by interleukin 7 induces bone loss in mice with intact ovarian function: similarity to estrogen deficiency. *Proc Natl Acad Sci U S A.* 1997;94:9360-9365.
83. Owens J, Chambers TJ. Differential regulation of osteoclast formation: interleukin 10 (cytokine synthesis inhibitory factor) suppresses formation of osteoclasts but not machrophages in murine bone marrow cultures. *J Bone Miner Res.* 1995;10:S220.
84. Horwood NJ, Udagawa N, Elliott J, et al. Interleukin 18 inhibits osteoclast formation via T cell production of granulocyte macrophage colony-stimulating factor. *J Clin Invest.* 1998;101:595-603.
85. Takayanagi H, Ogasawara K, Hida S, et al. T-cell-mediated regulation of osteoclastogenesis by signalling cross-talk between RANKL and IFN-gamma. *Nature.* 2000;408:600-605.
86. Guise TA, Yoneda T, Yates AJ, et al. The combined effect of tumor-produced parathyroid hormone-related protein and transforming growth factor-alpha enhance hypercalcemia in vivo and bone resorption in vitro. *J Clin Endocrinol Metab.* 1993;77:40-45.
87. Lorenzo JA, Quinton J, Sousa S, et al. Effects of DNA and prostaglandin synthesis inhibitors on the stimulation of bone resorption by epidermal growth factor in fetal rat long-bone cultures. *J Clin Invest.* 1986;77:1897-1902.
88. Pilbeam CC, Harrision JR, Raisz LG. Prostaglandins and bone metabolism. In: Billezikian JP, Raisz LG, Rodan GA, eds. *Principles of Bone Biology.* San Diego, CA: Academic Press; 1997:715-728.
89. Itoh N, Ornitz DM. Evolution of the Fgf and Fgfr gene families. *Trends Genet.* 2004;20:563-569.
90. Mansukhani A, Ambrosetti D, Holmes G, et al. Sox2 induction by FGF and FGFR2 activating mutations inhibits Wnt signaling and osteoblast differentiation. *J Cell Biol.* 2005;168:1065-1076.
91. Ambrosetti D, Holmes G, Mansukhani A, et al. Fibroblast growth factor signaling uses multiple mechanisms to inhibit Wnt-induced transcription in osteoblasts. *Mol Cell Biol.* 2008;28:4759-4771.
92. Sobue T, Naganawa T, Xiao L, et al. Over-expression of fibroblast growth factor-2 causes defective bone mineralization and osteopenia in transgenic mice. *J Cell Biochem.* 2005;95:83-94.
93. Montero A, Okada Y, Tomita M, et al. Disruption of the fibroblast growth factor-2 gene results in decreased bone mass and bone formation. *J Clin Invest.* 2000;105:1085-1093.
94. Okada Y, Montero A, Zhang X, et al. Impaired osteoclast formation in bone marrow cultures of Fgf2 null mice in response to parathyroid hormone. *J Biol Chem.* 2003;278:21258-21266.
95. Fredriksson L, Li H, Eriksson U. The PDGF family: four gene products form five dimeric isoforms. *Cytokine Growth Factor Rev.* 2004; 15:197-204.
96. Ferrara N, Davis-Smyth T. The biology of vascular endothelial growth factor. *Endocr Rev.* 1997;18:4-25.
97. Hock JM, Canalis E. Platelet-derived growth factor enhances bone cell replication, but not differentiated function of osteoblasts. *Endocrinology.* 1994;134:1423-1428.
98. Betsholtz C. Insight into the physiological functions of PDGF through genetic studies in mice. *Cytokine Growth Factor Rev.* 2004;15: 215-228.
99. Zelzer E, Olsen BR. Multiple roles of vascular endothelial growth factor (VEGF) in skeletal development, growth, and repair. *Curr Top Dev Biol.* 2005;65:169-187.
100. Gerber HP, Vu TH, Ryan AM, et al. VEGF couples hypertrophic cartilage remodeling, ossification and angiogenesis during endochondral bone formation. *Nat Med.* 1999;5:623-628.
101. Street J, Bao M, deGuzman L, et al. Vascular endothelial growth factor stimulates bone repair by promoting angiogenesis and bone turnover. *Proc Natl Acad Sci U S A.* 2002;99:9656-9661.
102. Wan C, Gilbert SR, Wang Y, et al. Activation of the hypoxia-inducible factor-1alpha pathway accelerates bone regeneration. *Proc Natl Acad Sci U S A.* 2008;105:686-691.
103. Almeida M, Han L, Martin-Millan M, et al. Skeletal involution by age-associated oxidative stress and its acceleration by loss of sex steroids. *J Biol Chem.* 2007;282:27285-27297.
104. Gazzerro E, Canalis E. Skeletal actions of insulin-like growth factors. *Expert Rev Endocrinol Metab.* 2006;1:47-56.
105. Yakar S, Bouxsein ML, Canalis E, et al. The ternary IGF complex influences postnatal bone acquisition and the skeletal response to intermittent parathyroid hormone. *J Endocrinol.* 2006;189:289-299.
106. Bikle D, Majumdar S, Laib A, et al. The skeletal structure of insulin-like growth factor I-deficient mice. *J Bone Miner Res.* 2001;16:2320-2329.
107. Zhao G, Monier-Faugere MC, Langub MC, et al. Targeted overexpression of insulin-like growth factor I to osteoblasts of transgenic mice: increased trabecular bone volume without increased osteoblast proliferation. *Endocrinology.* 2000;141:2674-2682.
108. Hill PA, Reynolds JJ, Meikle MC. Osteoblasts mediate insulin-like growth factor-I and -II stimulation of osteoclast formation and function. *Endocrinology.* 1995;136:124-131.
109. Barnard JA, Lyons RM, Moses HL. The cell biology of transforming growth factor beta. *Biochim Biophys Acta.* 1990;1032:79-87.
110. Hock JM, Canalis E, Centrella M. Transforming growth factor-beta stimulates bone matrix apposition and bone cell replication in cultured fetal rat calvariae. *Endocrinology.* 1990;126:421-426.
111. Spinella-Jaegle S, Roman-Roman S, Faucheu C, et al. Opposite effects of bone morphogenetic protein-2 and transforming growth factor-beta1 on osteoblast differentiation. *Bone.* 2001;29:323-330.
112. Pfeilschifter J, Seyedin SM, Mundy GR. Transforming growth factor beta inhibits bone resorption in fetal rat long bone cultures. *J Clin Invest.* 1988;82:680-685.
113. Shull MM, Ormsby I, Kier AB, et al. Targeted disruption of the mouse transforming growth factor-beta 1 gene results in multifocal inflammatory disease. *Nature.* 1992;359:693-699.
114. Centrella M, McCarthy TL, Canalis E. Transforming growth factor-beta and remodeling of bone. *J Bone Joint Surg Am.* 1991;73:1418-1428.
115. Leboy P, Grasso-Knight G, D'Angelo M, et al. Smad-Runx interactions during chondrocyte maturation. *J Bone Joint Surg Am.* 2001;83A(suppl 1):S15-S22.
116. Kaneko H, Arakawa T, Mano H, et al. Direct stimulation of osteoclastic bone resorption by bone morphogenetic protein (BMP)-2 and expression of BMP receptors in mature osteoclasts. *Bone.* 2000;27:479-486.
117. Johnson ML, Harnish K, Nusse R, et al. LRP5 and Wnt signaling: a union made for bone. *J Bone Miner Res.* 2004;19:1749-1757.
118. Glass DA 2nd, Karsenty G. Molecular bases of the regulation of bone remodeling by the canonical Wnt signaling pathway. *Curr Top Dev Biol.* 2006;73:43-84.
119. Glass DA 2nd, Bialek P, Ahn JD, et al. Canonical Wnt signaling in differentiated osteoblasts controls osteoclast differentiation. *Dev Cell.* 2005;8:751-764.
120. Holmen SL, Zylstra CR, Mukherjee A, et al. Essential role of beta-catenin in postnatal bone acquisition. *J Biol Chem.* 2005; 280:21162-21168.
121. Baron R, Rawadi G. Targeting the Wnt/beta-catenin pathway to regulate bone formation in the adult skeleton. *Endocrinology.* 2007;148:2635-2643.
122. Diederichs G, Link T, Marie K, et al. Feasibility of measuring trabecular bone structure of the proximal femur using 64-slice multidetector computed tomography in a clinical setting. *Calcif Tissue Int.* 2008;83:332-341.
123. Cummings SR, Bates D, Black DM. Clinical use of bone densitometry: scientific review. *JAMA.* 2002;288:1889-1897.
124. Bauer DC, Gluer CC, Genant HK, et al. Quantitative ultrasound and vertebral fracture in postmenopausal women. Fracture Intervention Trial Research Group. *J Bone Miner Res.* 1995;10:353-358.
125. Williams ED, Daymond TJ. Evaluation of calcaneus bone densitometry against hip and spine for diagnosis of osteoporosis. *Br J Radiol.* 2003;76:123-128.
126. Kroger H, Lunt M, Reeve J, et al. Bone density reduction in various measurement sites in men and women with osteoporotic fractures of spine and hip: the European quantitation of osteoporosis study. *Calcif Tissue Int.* 1999;64:191-199.
127. Faulkner KG, von Stetten E, Miller P. Discordance in patient classification using T-scores. *J Clin Densitom.* 1999;2:343-350.
128. Kanis JA, Johnell O, Oden A, et al. FRAX and the assessment of fracture probability in men and women from the UK. *Osteoporos Int.* 2008;19:385-397.
129. Kazakia GJ, Hyun B, Burghardt AJ, et al. In vivo determination of bone structure in postmenopausal women: a comparison of HR-pQCT and high-field MR imaging. *J Bone Miner Res.* 2008;23:463-474.
130. Wehrli FW, Ladinsky GA, Jones C, et al. In vivo magnetic resonance detects rapid remodeling changes in the topology of the trabecular bone network after menopause and the protective effect of estradiol. *J Bone Miner Res.* 2008;23:730-740.

131. Cummings SR, Palermo L, Browner W, et al. Monitoring osteoporosis therapy with bone densitometry: misleading changes and regression to the mean. Fracture Intervention Trial Research Group. *JAMA*. 2000;283:1318-1321.
132. McCloskey EV, Vasireddy S, Threlkeld J, et al. Vertebral fracture assessment (VFA) with a densitometer predicts future fractures in elderly women unselected for osteoporosis. *J Bone Miner Res*. 2008; 23:1561-1568.
133. El Maghraoui A, Mouinga Abayi DA, et al. Discordance in diagnosis of osteoporosis using spine and hip bone densitometry. *J Clin Densitom*. 2007;10:153-156.
134. Compston J. Monitoring bone mineral density during antiresorptive treatment for osteoporosis. *BMJ*. 2009;338:b1276.
135. Compston J, Cooper A, Cooper C, et al. Guidelines for the diagnosis and management of osteoporosis in postmenopausal women and men from the age of 50 years in the UK. *Maturitas*. 2009;62: 105-108.
136. Guglielmi G, Floriani I, Torri V, et al. Effect of spinal degenerative changes on volumetric bone mineral density of the central skeleton as measured by quantitative computed tomography. *Acta Radiol*. 2005;46:269-275.
137. Masud T, Francis RM. The increasing use of peripheral bone densitometry. *BMJ*. 2000;321:396-398.
138. Siris ES, Miller PD, Barrett-Connor E, et al. Identification and fracture outcomes of undiagnosed low bone mineral density in postmenopausal women: results from the National Osteoporosis Risk Assessment. *JAMA*. 2001;286:2815-2822.
139. Chapurlat RD, Garnero P, Breart G, et al. Serum type I collagen breakdown product (serum CTX) predicts hip fracture risk in elderly women: the EPIDOS study. *Bone*. 2000;27:283-286.
140. Brown JP, Albert C, Nassar BA, et al. Bone turnover markers in the management of postmenopausal osteoporosis. *Clin Biochem*. 2009;42:929-942.
141. Ivaska KK, Lenora J, Gerdhem P, et al. Serial assessment of serum bone metabolism markers identifies women with the highest rate of bone loss and osteoporosis risk. *J Clin Endocrinol Metab*. 2008; 93:2622-2632.
142. Rogers A, Hannon RA, Eastell R. Biochemical markers as predictors of rates of bone loss after menopause. *J Bone Miner Res*. 2000;15:1398-1404.
143. Glover SJ, Gall M, Schoenborn-Kellenberger O, et al. Establishing a reference interval for bone turnover markers in 637 healthy, young, premenopausal women from the United Kingdom, France, Belgium, and the United States. *J Bone Miner Res*. 2009;24:389-397.
144. Eastell R, Barton I, Hannon RA, et al. Relationship of early changes in bone resorption to the reduction in fracture risk with risedronate. *J Bone Miner Res*. 2003;18:1051-1056.
145. Greenspan SL, Rosen HN, Parker RA. Early changes in serum N-telopeptide and C-telopeptide cross-linked collagen type 1 predict long-term response to alendronate therapy in elderly women. *J Clin Endocrinol Metab*. 2000;85:3537-3540.
146. Gundberg CM. Biochemical markers of bone formation. *Clin Lab Med*. 2000;20:489-501.
147. Gundberg CM, Looker AC, Nieman SD, et al. Patterns of osteocalcin and bone specific alkaline phosphatase by age, gender, and race or ethnicity. *Bone*. 2002;31:703-708.
148. Ross PD, Kress BC, Parson RE, et al. Serum bone alkaline phosphatase and calcaneus bone density predict fractures: a prospective study. *Osteoporos Int*. 2000;11:76-82.
149. Booth SL, Broe KE, Peterson JW, et al. Associations between vitamin K biochemical measures and bone mineral density in men and women. *J Clin Endocrinol Metab*. 2004;89:4904-4909.
150. Kanazawa I, Yamaguchi T, Sugimoto T. Relationships between serum osteocalcin vs. serum glucose and lipids levels and atherosclerosis in type 2 diabetes mellitus. *J Bone Miner Res*. 2009;160:265-273.
151. Confavreux CB, Levine RL, Karsenty G. A paradigm of integrative physiology, the crosstalk between bone and energy metabolisms. *Mol Cell Endocrinol*. 2009;310:21-29.
152. Chen P, Satterwhite JH, Licata AA, et al. Early changes in biochemical markers of bone formation predict BMD response to teriparatide in postmenopausal women with osteoporosis. *J Bone Miner Res*. 2005; 20:962-970.
153. Bauer DC, Garnero P, Harrison S, et al., For the Osteoporotic Fractures in Men (MrOS) Research Group. Biochemical markers of bone turnover, hip bone loss and fracture in older men: The MrOS Study. *J Bone Miner Res*. 2009;12:2032-2038
154. Klepzig M, Jonas D, Oremek GM. Procollagen type 1 amino-terminal propeptide: a marker for bone metastases in prostate carcinoma. *Anticancer Res*. 2009;29:671-673.
155. Denk E, Hillegonds D, Hurrell RF, et al. Evaluation of 41calcium as a new approach to assess changes in bone metabolism: effect of a bisphosphonate intervention in postmenopausal women with low bone mass. *J Bone Miner Res*. 2007;22:1518-1525.
156. Fall PM, Kennedy D, Smith JA, et al. Comparison of serum and urine assays for biochemical markers of bone resorption in postmenopausal women with and without hormone replacement therapy and in men. *Osteoporos Int*. 2000;11:481-485.
157. Huber F, Traber L, Roth HJ, et al. Markers of bone resorption: measurement in serum, plasma or urine? *Clin Lab*. 2003;49:203-207.
158. Henriksen DB, Alexandersen P, Bjarnason NH, et al. Role of gastrointestinal hormones in postprandial reduction of bone resorption. *J Bone Miner Res*. 2003;18:2180-2189.
159. Obrant KJ, Ivaska KK, Gerdhem P, et al. Biochemical markers of bone turnover are influenced by recently sustained fracture. *Bone*. 2005;36:786-792.
160. Halleen JM, Tiitinen SL, Ylipahkala H, et al. Tartrate-resistant acid phosphatase 5b (TRACP 5b) as a marker of bone resorption. *Clin Lab*. 2006;52:499-509.
161. Meier C, Meinhardt U, Greenfield JR, et al. Serum cathepsin K concentrations reflect osteoclastic activity in women with postmenopausal osteoporosis and patients with Paget's disease. *Clin Lab*. 2006; 52:1-10.
162. Trueba D, Sawaya BP, Mawad H, et al. Bone biopsy: indications, techniques, and complications. *Semin Dial*. 2003;16:341-345.
163. Recker RR, Bare SP, Smith SY, et al. Cancellous and cortical bone architecture and turnover at the iliac crest of postmenopausal osteoporotic women treated with parathyroid hormone 1-84. *Bone*. 2009; 44:113-119.
164. Martin KJ, Olgaard K, Coburn JW, et al. Diagnosis, assessment, and treatment of bone turnover abnormalities in renal osteodystrophy. *Am J Kidney Dis*. 2004;43:558-565.
165. Lenchik L, Rogers LF, Delmas PD, et al. Diagnosis of osteoporotic vertebral fractures: importance of recognition and description by radiologists. *AJR Am J Roentgenol*. 2004;183:949-958.
166. Consensus development conference: diagnosis, prophylaxis, and treatment of osteoporosis. *Am J Med*. 1993;94:646-650.
167. Kanis JA, Melton LJ 3rd, Christiansen C, et al. The diagnosis of osteoporosis. *J Bone Miner Res*. 1994;9:1137-1141.
168. Kanis JA, Borgstrom F, De Laet C, et al. Assessment of fracture risk. *Osteoporos Int*. 2005;16:581-589.
169. Melton LJ 3rd, Khosla S, Achenbach SJ, et al. Effects of body size and skeletal site on the estimated prevalence of osteoporosis in women and men. *Osteoporos Int*. 2000;11:977-983.
170. Johnell O, Kanis JA. An estimate of the worldwide prevalence, mortality and disability associated with hip fracture. *Osteoporos Int*. 2004;15:897-902.
171. Kannus P, Palvanen M, Niemi S, et al. Osteoporotic fractures of the proximal humerus in elderly Finnish persons: sharp increase in 1970-1998 and alarming projections for the new millennium. *Acta Orthop Scand*. 2000;71:465-470.
172. Burge R, Dawson-Hughes B, Solomon DH, et al. Incidence and economic burden of osteoporosis-related fractures in the United States, 2005-2025. *J Bone Miner Res*. 2007;22:465-475.
173. Johnell O, Kanis JA. An estimate of the worldwide prevalence and disability associated with osteoporotic fractures. *Osteoporos Int*. 2006;17:1726-1733.
174. Raisz L. Pathogenesis of osteoporosis: concepts, conflicts, and prospects. *J Clin Invest*. 2005;115:3318-3325.
175. Ralston SH, Galwey N, MacKay I, et al. Loci for regulation of bone mineral density in men and women identified by genome wide linkage scan: the FAMOS study. *Hum Mol Genet*. 2005;14:943-951.
176. Jin H, Van't Hof RJ, Albagha OM, et al. Promoter and intron 1 polymorphisms of COL1A1 interact to regulate transcription and susceptibility to osteoporosis. *Hum Mol Genet*. 2009;18:2729-2738.
177. Langdahl BL, Uitterlinden AG, Ralston SH, et al. Large-scale analysis of association between polymorphisms in the transforming growth factor beta 1 gene *(TGFB1)* and osteoporosis: the GENOMOS study. *Bone*. 2008;42:969-981.
178. Richards JB, Papaioannou A, Adachi JD, et al. Effect of selective serotonin reuptake inhibitors on the risk of fracture. *Arch Intern Med*. 2007;167:188-194.
179. Styrkarsdottir U, Halldorsson BV, Gretarsdottir S, et al. Multiple genetic loci for bone mineral density and fractures. *N Engl J Med*. 2008; 358:2355-2365.
180. van Meurs JB, Trikalinos TA, Ralston SH, et al. Large-scale analysis of association between LRP5 and LRP6 variants and osteoporosis. *JAMA*. 2008;299:1277-1290.
181. Shen H, Liu Y, Liu P, et al. Nonreplication in genetic studies of complex diseases: lessons learned from studies of osteoporosis and tentative remedies. *J Bone Miner Res*. 2005;20:365-376.
182. Kaufman JM, Ostertag A, Saint-Pierre A, et al. Genome-wide linkage screen of bone mineral density (BMD) in European pedigrees ascertained through a male relative with low BMD values: evidence for quantitative trait loci on 17q21-23, 11q12-13, 13q12-14, and 22q11. *J Clin Endocrinol Metab*. 2008;93:3755-3762.
183. Peacock M, Koller DL, Lai D, et al. Bone mineral density variation in men is influenced by sex-specific and non sex-specific quantitative trait loci. *Bone*. 2009;45:443-448.
184. Van Staa TP, Leufkens HG, Abenhaim L, et al. Use of oral corticosteroids and risk of fractures. *J Bone Miner Res*. 2000;15:993-1000.

185. Ralston SH, Uitterlinden AG. Genetics of osteoporosis. *Endocr Rev*. 2010;31:629-662.
186. Heaney RP, Abrams S, Dawson-Hughes B, et al. Peak bone mass. *Osteoporos Int*. 2000;11:985-1009.
187. Kuchuk NO, van Schoor NM, Pluijm SM, et al. The association of sex hormone levels with quantitative ultrasound, bone mineral density, bone turnover and osteoporotic fractures in older men and women. *Clin Endocrinol (Oxf)*. 2007;67:295-303.
188. Riggs BL, Melton LJ 3rd, Robb RA, et al. Population-based study of age and sex differences in bone volumetric density, size, geometry, and structure at different skeletal sites. *J Bone Miner Res*. 2004; 19:1945-1954.
189. Riggs BL, Melton LJ, Robb RA, et al. A population-based assessment of rates of bone loss at multiple skeletal sites: evidence for substantial trabecular bone loss in young adult women and men. *J Bone Miner Res*. 2008;23:205-214.
190. Aaron JE, Shore PA, Shore RC, et al. Trabecular architecture in women and men of similar bone mass with and without vertebral fracture: II. Three-dimensional histology. *Bone*. 2000;27:277-282.
191. Sornay-Rendu E, Munoz F, Garnero P, et al. Identification of osteopenic women at high risk of fracture: the OFELY study. *J Bone Miner Res*. 2005;20:1813-1819.
192. Perrini S, Natalicchio A, Laviola L, et al. Abnormalities of insulin-like growth factor-I signaling and impaired cell proliferation in osteoblasts from subjects with osteoporosis. *Endocrinology*. 2008;149:1302-1313.
193. Parfitt AM, Villanueva AR, Foldes J, et al. Relations between histologic indices of bone formation: implications for the pathogenesis of spinal osteoporosis. *J Bone Miner Res*. 1995;10:466-473.
194. Mann V, Ralston SH. Meta-analysis of COL1A1 Sp1 polymorphism in relation to bone mineral density and osteoporotic fracture. *Bone*. 2003;32:711-717.
195. van Meurs JB, Dhonukshe-Rutten RA, Pluijm SM, et al. Homocysteine levels and the risk of osteoporotic fracture. *N Engl J Med*. 2004;350:2033-2041.
196. Leboff MS, Narweker R, LaCroix A, et al. Homocysteine levels and risk of hip fracture in postmenopausal women. *J Clin Endocrinol Metab*. 2009;94:1207-1213.
197. McLean RR, Jacques PF, Selhub J, et al. Plasma B vitamins, homocysteine, and their relation with bone loss and hip fracture in elderly men and women. *J Clin Endocrinol Metab*. 2008;93:2206-2212.
198. Herrmann M, Tami A, Wildemann B, et al. Hyperhomocysteinemia induces a tissue specific accumulation of homocysteine in bone by collagen binding and adversely affects bone. *Bone*. 2009;44: 467-475.
199. Viguet-Carrin S, Roux JP, Arlot ME, et al. Contribution of the advanced glycation end product pentosidine and of maturation of type I collagen to compressive biomechanical properties of human lumbar vertebrae. *Bone*. 2006;39:1073-1079.
200. Seeman E, Devogelaer JP, Lorenc R, et al. Strontium ranelate reduces the risk of vertebral fractures in patients with osteopenia. *J Bone Miner Res*. 2008;23:433-438.
201. Khosla S, Melton LJ 3rd, Robb RA, et al. Relationship of volumetric BMD and structural parameters at different skeletal sites to sex steroid levels in men. *J Bone Miner Res*. 2005;20:730-740.
202. Van Pottelbergh I, Goemaere S, Zmierczak H, et al. Perturbed sex steroid status in men with idiopathic osteoporosis and their sons. *J Clin Endocrinol Metab*. 2004;89:4949-4953
203. Khosla S, Amin S, Orwoll E. Osteoporosis in men. *Endocr Rev*. 2008;29:441-464.
204. Lormeau C, Soudan B, d'Herbomez M, et al. Sex hormone-binding globulin, estradiol, and bone turnover markers in male osteoporosis. *Bone*. 2004;34:933-939.
205. Rapuri PB, Gallagher JC, Haynatzki G. Endogenous levels of serum estradiol and sex hormone binding globulin determine bone mineral density, bone remodeling, the rate of bone loss, and response to treatment with estrogen in elderly women. *J Clin Endocrinol Metab*. 2004;89:4954-4962.
206. Gao J, Tiwari-Pandey R, Samadfam R, et al. Altered ovarian function affects skeletal homeostasis independent of the action of follicle-stimulating hormone. *Endocrinology*. 2007;148:2613-2621.
207. Iqbal J, Sun L, Kumar TR, et al. Follicle-stimulating hormone stimulates TNF production from immune cells to enhance osteoblast and osteoclast formation. *Proc Natl Acad Sci U S A*. 2006;103:14925-14930.
208. Karim N, MacDonald D, Dolan AL, et al. The relationship between gonadotrophins, gonadal hormones and bone mass in men. *Clin Endocrinol (Oxf)*. 2008;68:94-101.
209. Mosekilde L. Primary hyperparathyroidism and the skeleton. *Clin Endocrinol (Oxf)*. 2008;69:1-19.
210. Bischoff-Ferrari HA, Dawson-Hughes B, Willett WC, et al. Effect of vitamin D on falls: a meta-analysis. *JAMA*. 2004;291:1999-2006.
211. Sambrook PN, Chen JS, March LM, et al. Serum parathyroid hormone is associated with increased mortality independent of 25-hydroxy vitamin D status, bone mass, and renal function in the frail and very old: a cohort study. *J Clin Endocrinol Metab*. 2004;211;89:5477-5481.
212. Gaugris S, Heaney RP, Boonen S, et al. Vitamin D inadequacy among post-menopausal women: a systematic review. *QJM*. 2005;98: 667-676.
213. Tiegs RD, Body JJ, Wahner HW, et al. Calcitonin secretion in postmenopausal osteoporosis. *N Engl J Med*. 1985;312:1097-1100.
214. Niu T, Rosen CJ. The insulin-like growth factor-I gene and osteoporosis: a critical appraisal. *Gene*. 2005;361:38-56.
215. Murphy E, Williams GR. The thyroid and the skeleton. *Clin Endocrinol (Oxf)*. 2004;61:285-298.
216. Vestergaard P, Rejnmark L, Mosekilde L. Influence of hyper- and hypothyroidism, and the effects of treatment with antithyroid drugs and levothyroxine on fracture risk. *Calcif Tissue Int*. 2004;74:486-491.
217. Mundy GR. Osteoporosis and inflammation. *Nutr Rev*. 2007; 65:S147-S151.
218. Teitelbaum SL. Postmenopausal osteoporosis, T cells, and immune dysfunction. *Proc Natl Acad Sci U S A*. 2004;101:16711-16712.
219. Ferrari SL, Karasik D, Liu J, et al. Interactions of interleukin-6 promoter polymorphisms with dietary and lifestyle factors and their association with bone mass in men and women from the Framingham Osteoporosis Study. *J Bone Miner Res*. 2004;19:552-559.
220. Moffett SP, Zmuda JM, Oakley JI, et al. Tumor necrosis factor-alpha polymorphism, bone strength phenotypes, and the risk of fracture in older women. *J Clin Endocrinol Metab*. 2005;90:3491-3497.
221. Kimble RB, Matayoshi AB, Vannice JL, et al. Simultaneous block of interleukin-1 and tumor necrosis factor is required to completely prevent bone loss in the early postovariectomy period. *Endocrinology*. 1995;136:3054-3061.
222. Lorenzo JA, Naprta A, Rao Y, et al. Mice lacking the type I interleukin-1 receptor do not lose bone mass after ovariectomy. *Endocrinology*. 1998;139:3022-3025.
223. Kawaguchi H, Pilbeam CC, Vargas SJ, et al. Ovariectomy enhances and estrogen replacement inhibits the activity of bone marrow factors that stimulate prostaglandin production in cultured mouse calvariae. *J Clin Invest*. 1995;96:539-548.
224. Hofbauer LC, Heufelder AE. Role of receptor activator of nuclear factor-kappaB ligand and osteoprotegerin in bone cell biology. *J Mol Med*. 2001;79:243-253.
225. Stern A, Laughlin GA, Bergstrom J, et al. The sex-specific association of serum osteoprotegerin and receptor activator of nuclear factor kappaB legend with bone mineral density in older adults: the Rancho Bernardo study. *Eur J Endocrinol*. 2007;156:555-562.
226. Rogers A, Eastell R. Circulating osteoprotegerin and receptor activator for nuclear factor kappaB ligand: clinical utility in metabolic bone disease assessment. *J Clin Endocrinol Metab*. 2005;90:6323-6331.
227. Mezquita-Raya P, de la Higuera M, Garcia DF, et al. The contribution of serum osteoprotegerin to bone mass and vertebral fractures in postmenopausal women. *Osteoporos Int*. 2005;16:1368-1374.
228. Garnero P, Munoz F, Sornay-Rendu E, et al. Associations of vitamin D status with bone mineral density, bone turnover, bone loss and fracture risk in healthy postmenopausal women: the OFELY study. *Bone*. 2007;40:716-722.
229. van Schoor NM, Visser M, Pluijm SM, et al. Vitamin D deficiency as a risk factor for osteoporotic fractures. *Bone*. 2008;42:260-266.
230. Chapuy MC, Pamphile R, Paris E, et al. Combined calcium and vitamin D3 supplementation in elderly women: confirmation of reversal of secondary hyperparathyroidism and hip fracture risk. The Decalyos II study. *Osteoporos Int*. 2002;13:257-264.
231. Lilliu H, Pamphile R, Chapuy MC, et al. Calcium-vitamin D3 supplementation is cost-effective in hip fractures prevention. *Maturitas*. 2003;44:299-305.
232. Bischoff-Ferrari HA, Willett WC, Wong JB, et al. Fracture prevention with vitamin D supplementation: a meta-analysis of randomized controlled trials. *JAMA*. 2005;293:2257-2264.
233. Wengreen HJ, Munger RG, West NA, et al. Dietary protein intake and risk of osteoporotic hip fracture in elderly residents of Utah. *J Bone Miner Res*. 2004;19:537-545.
234. Frassetto LA, Todd KM, Morris RC Jr, et al. Worldwide incidence of hip fracture in elderly women: relation to consumption of animal and vegetable foods. *J Gerontol A Biol Sci Med Sci*. 2000;55:M585-M592.
235. Bugel S. Vitamin K and bone health. *Proc Nutr Soc*. 2003;62:839-843.
236. Heiss CJ, Sanborn CF, Nichols DL, et al. Associations of body fat distribution, circulating sex hormones, and bone density in postmenopausal women. *J Clin Endocrinol Metab*. 1995;80:1591-1596.
237. Tziomalos K, Charsoulis F. Endocrine effects of tobacco smoking. *Clin Endocrinol (Oxf)*. 2004;61:664-674.
238. Kapoor D, Jones TH. Smoking and hormones in health and endocrine disorders. *Eur J Endocrinol*. 2005;152:491-499.
239. Bjarnason NH, Nielsen TF, Jorgensen HL, et al. The influence of smoking on bone loss and response to nasal estradiol. *Climacteric*. 2009;12:59-65.
240. Tinetti ME, Williams CS. Falls, injuries due to falls, and the risk of admission to a nursing home. *N Engl J Med*. 1997;337:1279-1284.
241. Riggs BL, Melton LJ 3rd. Involutional osteoporosis. *N Engl J Med*. 1986;314:1676-1686.

242. Lindsay R, Silverman SL, Cooper C, et al. Risk of new vertebral fracture in the year following a fracture. *JAMA*. 2001;285:320-323.
243. McKiernan F, Jensen R, Faciszewski T. The dynamic mobility of vertebral compression fractures. *J Bone Miner Res*. 2003;18:24-29.
244. Siminoski K, Warshawski RS, Jen H, et al. The accuracy of historical height loss for the detection of vertebral fractures in postmenopausal women. *Osteoporos Int*. 2006;17:290-296.
245. Binkley N, Krueger D, Gangnon R, et al. Lateral vertebral assessment: a valuable technique to detect clinically significant vertebral fractures. *Osteoporos Int*. 2005;16:1513-1518.
246. Fuerst T, Wu C, Genant HK, et al. Evaluation of vertebral fracture assessment by dual X-ray absorptiometry in a multicenter setting. *Osteoporos Int*. 2009;20:1199-1205.
247. Schousboe JT, Debold CR. Reliability and accuracy of vertebral fracture assessment with densitometry compared to radiography in clinical practice. *Osteoporos Int*. 2006;17:281-289.
248. Rea JA, Li J, Blake GM, et al. Visual assessment of vertebral deformity by X-ray absorptiometry: a highly predictive method to exclude vertebral deformity. *Osteoporos Int*. 2000;11:660-668.
249. Axenovich TI, Zaidman AM, Zorkoltseva IV, et al. Segregation analysis of Scheuermann disease in ninety families from Siberia. *Am J Med Genet*. 2001;100:275-279.
250. Lombardi I Jr, Oliveira LM, Mayer AF, et al. Evaluation of pulmonary function and quality of life in women with osteoporosis. *Osteoporos Int*. 2005;16:1247-1253.
251. Makinen TJ, Alm JJ, Laine H, et al. The incidence of osteopenia and osteoporosis in women with hip osteoarthritis scheduled for cementless total joint replacement. *Bone*. 2007;40:1041-1047.
252. Yoshimura N, Muraki S, Oka H, et al. Prevalence of knee osteoarthritis, lumbar spondylosis, and osteoporosis in Japanese men and women: the research on Osteoarthritis/Osteoporosis Against Disability study. *J Bone Miner Metab*. 2009;27:620-628.
253. Nguyen ND, Pongchaiyakul C, Center JR, et al. Identification of high-risk individuals for hip fracture: a 14-year prospective study. *J Bone Miner Res*. 2005;20:1921-1928.
254. Lyles KW, Colon-Emeric CS, Magaziner JS, et al. Zoledronic acid in reducing clinical fracture and mortality after hip fracture. *N Engl J Med*. 2007;357:nihpa40967.
255. Solomon DH, Finkelstein JS, Katz JN, et al. Underuse of osteoporosis medications in elderly patients with fractures. *Am J Med*. 2003;115:398-400.
256. Deng HW, Chen WM, Recker S, et al. Genetic determination of Colles' fracture and differential bone mass in women with and without Colles' fracture. *J Bone Miner Res*. 2000;15:1243-1252.
257. Hung LK, Wu HT, Leung PC, et al. Low BMD is a risk factor for low-energy Colles' fractures in women before and after menopause. *Clin Orthop Relat Res*. 2005;435:219-225.
258. Majumdar SR, Beaupre LA, Harley CH, et al. Use of a case manager to improve osteoporosis treatment after hip fracture: results of a randomized controlled trial. *Arch Intern Med*. 2007;167:2110-2115.
259. Mackey DC, Lui LY, Cawthon PM, et al. High-trauma fractures and low bone mineral density in older women and men. *JAMA*. 2007;298:2381-2388.
260. Orwoll ES, Klein RF. Osteoporosis in men. *Endocr Rev*. 1995;16:87-116.
261. Chavassieux P, Meunier PJ. Histomorphometric approach of bone loss in men. *Calcif Tissue Int*. 2001;69:209-213.
262. Meier C, Nguyen TV, Handelsman DJ, et al. Endogenous sex hormones and incident fracture risk in older men: the Dubbo Osteoporosis Epidemiology Study. *Arch Intern Med*. 2008;168:47-54.
263. Mellstrom D, Vandenput L, Mallmin H, et al. Older men with low serum estradiol and high serum SHBG have an increased risk of fractures. *J Bone Miner Res*. 2008;23:1552-1560.
264. Rucker D, Ezzat S, Diamandi A, et al. IGF-I and testosterone levels as predictors of bone mineral density in healthy, community-dwelling men. *Clin Endocrinol (Oxf)*. 2004;60:491-499.
265. Ferrari SL, Deutsch S, Baudoin C, et al. LRP5 gene polymorphisms and idiopathic osteoporosis in men. *Bone*. 2005;37:770-775.
266. Bachrach LK. Osteoporosis and measurement of bone mass in children and adolescents. *Endocrinol Metab Clin North Am*. 2005;34:521-535, vii.
267. Bianchi ML. Osteoporosis in children and adolescents. *Bone*. 2007;41:486-495.
268. Rauch F, Travers R, Norman ME, et al. Deficient bone formation in idiopathic juvenile osteoporosis: a histomorphometric study of cancellous iliac bone. *J Bone Miner Res*. 2000;15:957-963.
269. Dawson PA, Kelly TE, Marini JC. Extension of phenotype associated with structural mutations in type I collagen: siblings with juvenile osteoporosis have an alpha2(I)Gly436 → Arg substitution. *J Bone Miner Res*. 1999;14:449-455.
270. Hartikka H, Makitie O, Mannikko M, et al. Heterozygous mutations in the LDL receptor-related protein 5 (LRP5) gene are associated with primary osteoporosis in children. *J Bone Miner Res*. 2005;20:783-789.
271. Khosla S, Lufkin EG, Hodgson SF, et al. Epidemiology and clinical features of osteoporosis in young individuals. *Bone*. 1994;15:551-555.
272. Peris P, Ruiz-Esquide V, Monegal A, et al. Idiopathic osteoporosis in premenopausal women: clinical characteristics and bone remodelling abnormalities. *Clin Exp Rheumatol*. 2008;26:986-991.
273. Pernow Y, Granberg B, Saaf M, et al. Osteoblast dysfunction in male idiopathic osteoporosis. *Calcif Tissue Int*. 2006;78:90-97.
274. Peris P, Guanabens N, Monegal A, et al. Pregnancy associated osteoporosis: the familial effect. *Clin Exp Rheumatol*. 2002;20:697-700.
275. Karlsson MK, Ahlborg HG, Karlsson C. Maternity and bone mineral density. *Acta Orthop*. 2005;76:2-13.
276. Schapira D, Braun Moscovici Y, Gutierrez G, et al. Severe transient osteoporosis of the hip during pregnancy: successful treatment with intravenous biphosphonates. *Clin Exp Rheumatol*. 2003;21:107-110.
277. Toms AP, Marshall TJ, Becker E, et al. Regional migratory osteoporosis: a review illustrated by five cases. *Clin Radiol*. 2005;60:425-438.
278. Manicourt DH, Brasseur JP, Boutsen Y, et al. Role of alendronate in therapy for posttraumatic complex regional pain syndrome type I of the lower extremity. *Arthritis Rheum*. 2004;50:3690-3697.
279. Stein E, Shane E. Secondary osteoporosis. *Endocrinol Metab Clin North Am*. 2003;32:115-134, vii.
280. Shaker JL, Lukert BP. Osteoporosis associated with excess glucocorticoids. *Endocrinol Metab Clin North Am*. 2005;34:341-356, viii-ix.
281. Nielsen HK, Charles P, Mosekilde L. The effect of single oral doses of prednisone on the circadian rhythm of serum osteocalcin in normal subjects. *J Clin Endocrinol Metab*. 1988;67:1025-1030.
282. O'Brien CA, Jia D, Plotkin LI, et al. Glucocorticoids act directly on osteoblasts and osteocytes to induce their apoptosis and reduce bone formation and strength. *Endocrinology*. 2004;145:1835-1841.
283. Weinstein RS, Chen JR, Powers CC, et al. Promotion of osteoclast survival and antagonism of bisphosphonate-induced osteoclast apoptosis by glucocorticoids. *J Clin Invest*. 2002;109:1041-1048.
284. Reid IR, Heap SW. Determinants of vertebral mineral density in patients receiving long-term glucocorticoid therapy. *Arch Intern Med*. 1990;150:2545-2548.
285. Van Staa TP, Laan RF, Barton IP, et al. Bone density threshold and other predictors of vertebral fracture in patients receiving oral glucocorticoid therapy. *Arthritis Rheum*. 2003;48:3224-3229.
286. Hermus AR, Smals AG, Swinkels LM, et al. Bone mineral density and bone turnover before and after surgical cure of Cushing's syndrome. *J Clin Endocrinol Metab*. 1995;80:2859-2865.
287. Saag KG, Emkey R, Schnitzer TJ, et al. Alendronate for the prevention and treatment of glucocorticoid-induced osteoporosis: Glucocorticoid-Induced Osteoporosis Intervention Study Group. *N Engl J Med*. 1998;339:292-299.
288. Lane NE, Sanchez S, Modin GW, et al. Parathyroid hormone treatment can reverse corticosteroid-induced osteoporosis: results of a randomized controlled clinical trial. *J Clin Invest*. 1998;102:1627-1633.
289. Lane NE, Sanchez S, Modin GW, et al. Bone mass continues to increase at the hip after parathyroid hormone treatment is discontinued in glucocorticoid-induced osteoporosis: results of a randomized controlled clinical trial. *J Bone Miner Res*. 2000;15:944-951.
290. Wallach S, Cohen S, Reid DM, et al. Effects of risedronate treatment on bone density and vertebral fracture in patients on corticosteroid therapy. *Calcif Tissue Int*. 2000;67:277-285.
291. Saag KG, Shane E, Boonen S, et al. Teriparatide or alendronate in glucocorticoid-induced osteoporosis. *N Engl J Med*. 2007;357:2028-2039.
292. Misra M. Long-term skeletal effects of eating disorders with onset in adolescence. *Ann N Y Acad Sci*. 2008;1135:212-218.
293. Grinspoon S, Thomas E, Pitts S, et al. Prevalence and predictive factors for regional osteopenia in women with anorexia nervosa. *Ann Intern Med*. 2000;133:790-794.
294. Birch K. Female athlete triad. *BMJ*. 2005;330:244-246.
295. Scholes D, LaCroix AZ, Ichikawa LE, et al. Change in bone mineral density among adolescent women using and discontinuing depot medroxyprogesterone acetate contraception. *Arch Pediatr Adolesc Med*. 2005;159:139-144.
296. Hoff AO, Gagel RF. Osteoporosis in breast and prostate cancer survivors. *Oncology (Williston Park)*. 2005;19:651-658.
297. Eastell R, Hannon R. Long-term effects of aromatase inhibitors on bone. *J Steroid Biochem Mol Biol*. 2005;95:151-154.
298. Rabaglio M, Sun Z, Price KN, et al. Bone fractures among postmenopausal patients with endocrine-responsive early breast cancer treated with 5 years of letrozole or tamoxifen in the BIG 1-98 trial. *Ann Oncol*. 2009;20:1489-1498.
299. Saad F, Adachi JD, Brown JP, et al. Cancer treatment-induced bone loss in breast and prostate cancer. *J Clin Oncol*. 2008;26:5465-5476.
300. Karga H, Papapetrou PD, Korakovouni A, et al. Bone mineral density in hyperthyroidism. *Clin Endocrinol (Oxf)*. 2004;61:466-472.
301. Biermasz NR, Hamdy NA, Pereira AM, et al. Long-term skeletal effects of recombinant human growth hormone (rhGH) alone and rhGH combined with alendronate in GH-deficient adults: a seven-year follow-up study. *Clin Endocrinol (Oxf)*. 2004;60:568-575.
302. Bonadonna S, Mazziotti G, Nuzzo M, et al. Increased prevalence of radiological spinal deformities in active acromegaly: a cross-sectional

study in postmenopausal women. *J Bone Miner Res.* 2005;20:1837-1844.

303. Mazziotti G, Bianchi A, Bonadonna S, et al. Prevalence of vertebral fractures in men with acromegaly. *J Clin Endocrinol Metab.* 2008;93:4649-4655.
304. Colao A, Loche S, Cappa M, et al. Prolactinomas in children and adolescents: clinical presentation and long-term follow-up. *J Clin Endocrinol Metab.* 1998;83:2777-2780.
305. Thrailkill KM, Lumpkin CK Jr, Bunn RC, et al. Is insulin an anabolic agent in bone? Dissecting the diabetic bone for clues. *Am J Physiol Endocrinol Metab.* 2005;289:E735-E745.
306. Strotmeyer ES, Cauley JA, Schwartz AV, et al. Nontraumatic fracture risk with diabetes mellitus and impaired fasting glucose in older white and black adults: the health, aging, and body composition study. *Arch Intern Med.* 2005;165:1612-1617.
307. de Liefde II, van der Klift M, de Laet CEDH, et al. Bone mineral density and fracture risk in type-2 diabetes mellitus: the Rotterdam Study. *Osteoporos Int.* 2005;16:1713-1720.
308. Melton LJ 3rd, Riggs BL, Leibson CL, et al. A bone structural basis for fracture risk in diabetes. *J Clin Endocrinol Metab.* 2008;93:4804-4809.
309. Oyajobi BO, Mundy GR. Receptor activator of NF-kappaB ligand, macrophage inflammatory protein-1alpha, and the proteasome: novel therapeutic targets in myeloma. *Cancer.* 2003;97:813-817.
310. Tian E, Zhan F, Walker R, et al. The role of the Wnt-signaling antagonist DKK1 in the development of osteolytic lesions in multiple myeloma. *N Engl J Med.* 2003;349:2483-2494.
311. Tehranzadeh J, Tao C. Advances in MR imaging of vertebral collapse. *Semin Ultrasound CT MRI.* 2004;25:440-460.
312. Hay JE, Guichelaar MM. Evaluation and management of osteoporosis in liver disease. *Clin Liver Dis.* 2005;9:747-766.
313. Sylvester FA. IBD and skeletal health: children are not small adults! *Inflamm Bowel Dis.* 2005;11:1020-1023.
314. Bianchi ML, Bardella MT. Bone in celiac disease. *Osteoporos Int.* 2008;19:1705-1716.
315. Collin P. Should adults be screened for celiac disease? What are the benefits and harms of screening? *Gastroenterology.* 2005; 128:S104-S108.
316. Cauley JA, Fullman RL, Stone KL, et al. Factors associated with the lumbar spine and proximal femur bone mineral density in older men. *Osteoporos Int.* 2005;16:1525-1537.
317. Brumsen C, Papapoulos SE, Lentjes EG, et al. A potential role for the mast cell in the pathogenesis of idiopathic osteoporosis in men. *Bone.* 2002;31:556-561.
318. Chines A, Pacifici R, Avioli LV, et al. Systemic mastocytosis presenting as osteoporosis: a clinical and histomorphometric study. *J Clin Endocrinol Metab.* 1991;72:140-144.
319. Pardanani A. Systemic mastocytosis: bone marrow pathology, classification, and current therapies. *Acta Haematol.* 2005;114:41-51.
320. Wonke B, Jensen C, Hanslip JJ, et al. Genetic and acquired predisposing factors and treatment of osteoporosis in thalassaemia major. *J Pediatr Endocrinol Metab.* 1998;11(suppl 3):795-801.
321. Diamond T, Stiel D, Posen S. Effects of testosterone and venesection on spinal and peripheral bone mineral in six hypogonadal men with hemochromatosis. *J Bone Miner Res.* 1991;6:39-43.
322. Maalouf NM, Shane E. Osteoporosis after solid organ transplantation. *J Clin Endocrinol Metab.* 2005;0:2456-2465.
323. Tannirandorn P, Epstein S. Drug-induced bone loss. *Osteoporos Int.* 2000;11:637-659.
324. Yadav VK, Ryu JH, Suda N, et al. Lrp5 controls bone formation by inhibiting serotonin synthesis in the duodenum. *Cell.* 2008;135:825-837.
325. Shahinian VB, Kuo YF, Freeman JL, et al. Risk of fracture after androgen deprivation for prostate cancer. *N Engl J Med.* 2005;352:154-164.
326. Lester J, Coleman R. Bone loss and the aromatase inhibitors. *Br J Cancer.* 2005;93(suppl 1):S16-S22.
327. Roux C, Briot K, Gossec L, et al. Increase in vertebral fracture risk in postmenopausal women using omeprazole. *Calcif Tissue Int.* 2009;84:13-19.
328. Targownik LE, Lix LM, Metge CJ, et al. Use of proton pump inhibitors and risk of osteoporosis-related fractures. *CMAJ.* 2008;179:319-326.
329. Vestergaard P, Rejnmark L, Mosekilde L. Proton pump inhibitors, histamine H2 receptor antagonists, and other antacid medications and the risk of fracture. *Calcif Tissue Int.* 2006;79:76-83.
330. Schwartz AV, Sellmeyer DE, Vittinghoff E, et al. Thiazolidinedione use and bone loss in older diabetic adults. *J Clin Endocrinol Metab.* 2006;91:3349-3354.
331. Grey A. Skeletal consequences of thiazolidinedione therapy. *Osteoporos Int.* 2008;19:129-137.
332. Watts NB, D'Alessio DA. Type 2 diabetes, thiazolidinediones: bad to the bone? *J Clin Endocrinol Metab.* 2006;91:3276-3278.
333. Rzonca SO, Suva LJ, Gaddy D, et al. Bone is a target for the antidiabetic compound rosiglitazone. *Endocrinology.* 2004;145:401-406.
334. Akune T, Ohba S, Kamekura S, et al. PPARgamma insufficiency enhances osteogenesis through osteoblast formation from bone marrow progenitors. *J Clin Invest.* 2004;113:846-855.
335. Meier C, Kraenzlin ME, Bodmer M, et al. Use of thiazolidinediones and fracture risk. *Arch Intern Med.* 2008;168:820-825.
336. Hannan MT, Felson DT, Dawson-Hughes B, et al. Risk factors for longitudinal bone loss in elderly men and women: the Framingham Osteoporosis Study. *J Bone Miner Res.* 2000;15:710-720.
337. Raisz LG. Clinical practice: screening for osteoporosis. *N Engl J Med.* 2005;353:164-171.
338. Hamdy RC, Kiebzak GM. Variance in 10-year fracture risk calculated with and without T-scores in select subgroups of normal and osteoporotic patients. *J Clin Densitom.* 2009;12:158-161.
339. Baim S, Binkley N, Bilezikian JP, et al. Official positions of the International Society for Clinical Densitometry and executive summary of the 2007 ISCD Position Development Conference. *J Clin Densitom.* 2008;11:75-91.
340. Liu H, Paige NM, Goldzweig CL, et al. Screening for osteoporosis in men: a systematic review for an American College of Physicians guideline. *Ann Intern Med.* 2008;148:685-701.
341. Berger C, Langsetmo L, Joseph L, et al. Association between change in bone mineral density (BMD) and fragility fracture in women and men. *J Bone Miner Res.* 2009;24:361-370.
342. Watts NB, Ettinger B, LeBoff MS. FRAX facts. *J Bone Miner Res.* 2009;24:975-979.
343. Watts NB, Michael Lewiecki E, Bonnick SL, et al. Clinical value of monitoring bone density in patients treated with bisphosphonates for osteoporosis. *J Bone Miner Res.* 2009;24:1643-1646.
344. Marci CD, Anderson WB, Viechnicki MB, et al. Bone mineral densitometry substantially influences health-related behaviors of postmenopausal women. *Calcif Tissue Int.* 2000;66:113-118.
345. Cadarette SM, Gignac MA, Jaglal SB, et al. Access to osteoporosis treatment is critically linked to access to dual-energy x-ray absorptiometry testing. *Med Care.* 2007;45:896-901.
346. Szulc P, Delmas PD. Biochemical markers of bone turnover: potential use in the investigation and management of postmenopausal osteoporosis. *Osteoporos Int.* 2008;19:1683-1704.
347. Heaney RP, Weaver CM. Calcium and vitamin D. *Endocrinol Metab Clin North Am.* 2003;32:181-194, vii-viii.
348. Heaney RP. The vitamin D requirement in health and disease. *J Steroid Biochem Mol Biol.* 2005;97:13-19.
349. Storm D, Eslin R, Porter ES, et al. Calcium supplementation prevents seasonal bone loss and changes in biochemical markers of bone turnover in elderly New England women: a randomized placebo-controlled trial. *J Clin Endocrinol Metab.* 1998;83:3817-3825.
350. Dawson-Hughes B, Bischoff-Ferrari HA. Therapy of osteoporosis with calcium and vitamin D. *J Bone Miner Res.* 2007;22(suppl 2):V59-V63.
351. Dawson-Hughes B, Chen P, Krege JH. Response to teriparatide in patients with baseline 25-hydroxyvitamin D insufficiency or sufficiency. *J Clin Endocrinol Metab.* 2007;92:4630-4636.
352. Ensrud KE, Duong T, Cauley JA, et al. Low fractional calcium absorption increases the risk for hip fracture in women with low calcium intake. Study of Osteoporotic Fractures Research Group. *Ann Intern Med.* 2000;132:345-353.
353. Recker RR. Calcium absorption and achlorhydria. *N Engl J Med.* 1985;313:70-73.
354. Wright MJ, Proctor DD, Insogna KL, et al. Proton pump-inhibiting drugs, calcium homeostasis, and bone health. *Nutr Rev.* 2008; 66:103-108.
355. Holick MF. Vitamin D deficiency. *N Engl J Med.* 2007;357:266-281.
356. Holick MF. Vitamin D status: measurement, interpretation, and clinical application. *Ann Epidemiol.* 2009;19:73-78.
357. Binkley N, Krueger D, Cowgill CS, et al. Assay variation confounds the diagnosis of hypovitaminosis D: a call for standardization. *J Clin Endocrinol Metab.* 2004;89:3152-3157.
358. Binkley N, Krueger D, Gemar D, et al. Correlation among 25-hydroxy-vitamin D assays. *J Clin Endocrinol Metab.* 2008;93:1804-1808.
359. Vieth R. Vitamin D toxicity, policy, and science. *J Bone Miner Res.* 2007;22(suppl 2):V64-V68.
360. Jackson RD, LaCroix AZ, Gass M, et al. Calcium plus vitamin D supplementation and the risk of fractures. *N Engl J Med.* 2006;354: 669-683.
361. Chapuy MC, Arlot ME, Delmas PD, et al. Effect of calcium and cholecalciferol treatment for three years on hip fractures in elderly women. *BMJ.* 1994;308:1081-1082.
362. Andress DL. Vitamin D treatment in chronic kidney disease. *Semin Dial.* 2005;18:315-321.
363. Avenell A, Gillespie W, Gillespie L, et al. Vitamin D and vitamin D analogues for preventing fractures associated with involutional and post-menopausal osteoporosis. Cochrane Database Syst Rev. 2005; (3):CD000227.
364. Schmitt NM, Schmitt J, Doren M. The role of physical activity in the prevention of osteoporosis in postmenopausal women: an update. *Maturitas.* 2009;63:34-38.
365. Bonner FJ Jr, Sinaki M, Grabois M, et al. Health professional's guide to rehabilitation of the patient with osteoporosis. *Osteoporos Int.* 2003;14(suppl 2):S1-S22.

366. Bonaiuti D, Shea B, Iovine R, et al. Exercise for preventing and treating osteoporosis in postmenopausal women. Cochrane Database Syst Rev. 2002(3):CD000333.
367. Pierfitte C, Macouillard G, Thicoipe M, et al. Benzodiazepines and hip fractures in elderly people: case-control study. *BMJ*. 2001;322: 704-708.
368. Gold DT. Osteoporosis and quality of life psychosocial outcomes and interventions for individual patients. *Clin Geriatr Med*. 2003;19:271-280, vi.
369. Gold DT, Shipp KM, Pieper CF, et al. Group treatment improves trunk strength and psychological status in older women with vertebral fractures: results of a randomized, clinical trial. *J Am Geriatr Soc*. 2004;52:1471-1478.
370. Koike T, Orito Y, Toyoda H, et al. External hip protectors are effective for the elderly with higher-than-average risk factors for hip fractures. *Osteoporos Int*. 2009;20:1613-1620.
371. Mathis JM, Ortiz AO, Zoarski GH. Vertebroplasty versus kyphoplasty: a comparison and contrast. *AJNR Am J Neuroradiol*. 2004;25: 840-845.
372. Buchbinder R, Osborne RH, Ebeling PR, et al. A randomized trial of vertebroplasty for painful osteoporotic vertebral fractures. *N Engl J Med*. 2009;361:557-568.
373. Kallmes DF, Comstock BA, Heagerty PJ, et al. A randomized trial of vertebroplasty for osteoporotic spinal fractures. *N Engl J Med*. 2009;361:569-579.
374. Nelson HD, Humphrey LL, Nygren P, et al. Postmenopausal hormone replacement therapy: scientific review. *JAMA*. 2002;288:872-881.
375. Anderson GL, Limacher M, Assaf AR, et al. Effects of conjugated equine estrogen in postmenopausal women with hysterectomy: the Women's Health Initiative randomized controlled trial. *JAMA*. 2004;291:1701-1712.
376. Majumdar SR, Almasi EA, Stafford RS. Promotion and prescribing of hormone therapy after report of harm by the Women's Health Initiative. *JAMA*. 2004;292:1983-1988.
377. Lindsay R. Hormones and bone health in postmenopausal women. *Endocrine*. 2004;24:223-230.
378. Prestwood KM, Kenny AM, Kleppinger A, et al. Ultralow-dose micronized 17beta-estradiol and bone density and bone metabolism in older women: a randomized controlled trial. *JAMA*. 2003;290:1042-1048.
379. Ettinger B, Ensrud KE, Wallace R, et al. Effects of ultralow-dose transdermal estradiol on bone mineral density: a randomized clinical trial. *Obstet Gynecol*. 2004;104:443-451.
380. Greenspan SL, Emkey RD, Bone HG, et al. Significant differential effects of alendronate, estrogen, or combination therapy on the rate of bone loss after discontinuation of treatment of postmenopausal osteoporosis: a randomized, double-blind, placebo-controlled trial. *Ann Intern Med*. 2002;137:875-883.
381. Leu CT, Luegmayr E, Freedman LP, et al. Relative binding affinities of bisphosphonates for human bone and relationship to antiresorptive efficacy. *Bone*. 2005;38:628-636.
382. Raisz L, Smith JA, Trahiotis M, et al. Short-term risedronate treatment in postmenopausal women: effects on biochemical markers of bone turnover. *Osteoporos Int*. 2000;11:615-620.
383. Kherani RB, Papaioannou A, Adachi JD. Long-term tolerability of the bisphosphonates in postmenopausal osteoporosis: a comparative review. *Drug Saf*. 2002;25:781-790.
384. Frediani B, Cavalieri L, Cremonesi G. Clodronic acid formulations available in Europe and their use in osteoporosis: a review. *Clin Drug Investig*. 2009;29:359-379.
385. Russell RG, Watts NB, Ebetino FH, et al. Mechanisms of action of bisphosphonates: similarities and differences and their potential influence on clinical efficacy. *Osteoporos Int*. 2008;19:733-759.
386. Harris ST, Watts NB, Genant HK, et al. Effects of risedronate treatment on vertebral and nonvertebral fractures in women with postmenopausal osteoporosis: a randomized controlled trial. Vertebral Efficacy with Risedronate Therapy (VERT) Study Group. *JAMA*. 1999;282:1344-1352.
387. McClung MR, Geusens P, Miller PD, et al. Effect of risedronate on the risk of hip fracture in elderly women. Hip Intervention Program Study Group. *N Engl J Med*. 2001;344:333-340.
388. Felsenberg D, Miller P, Armbrecht G, et al. Oral ibandronate significantly reduces the risk of vertebral fractures of greater severity after 1, 2, and 3 years in postmenopausal women with osteoporosis. *Bone*. 2005;37:651-654.
389. Reid DM, Hughes RA, Laan RF, et al. Efficacy and safety of daily risedronate in the treatment of corticosteroid-induced osteoporosis in men and women: a randomized trial. European Corticosteroid-Induced Osteoporosis Treatment Study. *J Bone Miner Res*. 2000;15:1006-1013.
390. Orwoll E, Ettinger M, Weiss S, et al. Alendronate for the treatment of osteoporosis in men. *N Engl J Med*. 2000;343:604-610.
391. Bone HG, Hosking D, Devogelaer JP, et al. Ten years' experience with alendronate for osteoporosis in postmenopausal women. *N Engl J Med*. 2004;350:1189-1199.
392. Schnitzer T, Bone HG, Crepaldi G, et al. Therapeutic equivalence of alendronate 70 mg once-weekly and alendronate 10 mg daily in the treatment of osteoporosis. Alendronate Once-Weekly Study Group. *Aging (Milano)*. 2000;12:1-12.
393. Black DM, Delmas PD, Eastell R, et al. Once-yearly zoledronic acid for treatment of postmenopausal osteoporosis. *N Engl J Med*. 2007;356: 1809-1822.
394. Grey A, Bolland MJ, Wattie D, et al. The antiresorptive effects of a single dose of zoledronate persist for two years: a randomized, placebo-controlled trial in osteopenic postmenopausal women. *J Clin Endocrinol Metab*. 2009;94:538-544.
395. Khan AA, Sandor GK, Dore E, et al. Bisphosphonate associated osteonecrosis of the jaw. *J Rheumatol*. 2009;36:478-490.
396. Khosla S, Burr D, Cauley J, et al. Bisphosphonate-associated osteonecrosis of the jaw: report of a task force of the American Society for Bone and Mineral Research. *J Bone Miner Res*. 2007;22:1479-1491.
397. Silverman SL, Landesberg R. Osteonecrosis of the jaw and the role of bisphosphonates: a critical review. *Am J Med*. 2009;122:S33-S45.
398. Odvina CV, Levy S, Rao S, et al. Unusual mid-shaft fractures during long term bisphosphonate therapy. *Clin Endocrinol (Oxf)*. 2009;72:161-168.
399. Solomon DH, Hochberg MC, Mogun H, et al. The relation between bisphosphonate use and non-union of fractures of the humerus in older adults. *Osteoporos Int*. 2009;20:895-901.
400. Black DM, Kelly MP, Genant HK, et al. Bisphosphonates and fractures of the subtrochanteric or diaphyseal femur. *N Engl J Med*. 2010;362:1761-1771.
401. Glorieux FH, Rauch F, Plotkin H, et al. Type V osteogenesis imperfecta: a new form of brittle bone disease. *J Bone Miner Res*. 2000;15: 1650-1658.
402. Chesnut CH 3rd, Silverman S, Andriano K, et al. A randomized trial of nasal spray salmon calcitonin in postmenopausal women with established osteoporosis: the Prevent Recurrence of Osteoporotic Fractures study. PROOF Study Group. *Am J Med*. 2000;109:267-276.
403. Cummings SR, Chapurlat RD. What PROOF proves about calcitonin and clinical trials. *Am J Med*. 2000;109:330-331.
404. Downs RW Jr, Bell NH, Ettinger MP, et al. Comparison of alendronate and intranasal calcitonin for treatment of osteoporosis in postmenopausal women. *J Clin Endocrinol Metab*. 2000;85:1783-1788.
405. Karsdal MA, Henriksen K, Arnold M, et al. Calcitonin: a drug of the past or for the future? Physiologic inhibition of bone resorption while sustaining osteoclast numbers improves bone quality. *BioDrugs*. 2008;22:137-144.
406. Baum M, Buzdar A, Cuzick J, et al. Anastrozole alone or in combination with tamoxifen versus tamoxifen alone for adjuvant treatment of postmenopausal women with early-stage breast cancer: results of the ATAC (Arimidex, Tamoxifen Alone or in Combination) trial efficacy and safety update analyses. *Cancer*. 2003;98:1802-1810.
407. Ettinger B, Black DM, Mitlak BH, et al. Reduction of vertebral fracture risk in postmenopausal women with osteoporosis treated with raloxifene: results from a 3-year randomized clinical trial. Multiple Outcomes of Raloxifene Evaluation (MORE) Investigators. *JAMA*. 1999;282:637-645.
408. Prestwood KM, Gunness M, Muchmore DB, et al. A comparison of the effects of raloxifene and estrogen on bone in postmenopausal women. *J Clin Endocrinol Metab*. 2000;85:2197-2202.
409. Martino S, Cauley JA, Barrett-Connor E, et al. Continuing outcomes relevant to Evista: breast cancer incidence in postmenopausal osteoporotic women in a randomized trial of raloxifene. *J Natl Cancer Inst*. 2004;96:1751-1761.
410. Johnston CC Jr, Bjarnason NH, Cohen FJ, et al. Long-term effects of raloxifene on bone mineral density, bone turnover, and serum lipid levels in early postmenopausal women: three-year data from 2 double-blind, randomized, placebo-controlled trials. *Arch Intern Med*. 2000;160:3444-3450.
411. Lindsay R, Gallagher JC, Kagan R, et al. Efficacy of tissue-selective estrogen complex of bazedoxifene/conjugated estrogens for osteoporosis prevention in at-risk postmenopausal women. *Fertil Steril*. 2009;92:1045-1052.
412. Rogers A, Glover SJ, Eastell R. A randomised, double-blinded, placebo-controlled, trial to determine the individual response in bone turnover markers to lasofoxifene therapy. *Bone*. 2009;45:1044-1052.
413. Neer RM, Arnaud CD, Zanchetta JR, et al. Effect of parathyroid hormone (1-34) on fractures and bone mineral density in postmenopausal women with osteoporosis. *N Engl J Med*. 2001;344:1434-1441.
414. Kurland ES, Cosman F, McMahon DJ, et al. Parathyroid hormone as a therapy for idiopathic osteoporosis in men: effects on bone mineral density and bone markers. *J Clin Endocrinol Metab*. 2000;85:3069-3076.
415. Boonen S, Marin F, Obermayer-Pietsch B, et al. Effects of previous antiresorptive therapy on the bone mineral density response to two years of teriparatide treatment in postmenopausal women with osteoporosis. *J Clin Endocrinol Metab*. 2008;93:852-860.
416. Miller PD, Delmas PD, Lindsay R, et al. Early responsiveness of women with osteoporosis to teriparatide after therapy with alendronate or risedronate. *J Clin Endocrinol Metab*. 2008;93:3785-3793.

417. Black DM, Bilezikian JP, Ensrud KE, et al. One year of alendronate after one year of parathyroid hormone (1-84) for osteoporosis. *N Engl J Med.* 2005;353:555-565.
418. Eastell R, Nickelsen T, Marin F, et al. Sequential treatment of severe postmenopausal osteoporosis after teriparatide: final results of the randomized, controlled European Study of Forsteo (EUROFORS). *J Bone Miner Res.* 2009;418;24:726-736.
419. Meunier PJ, Roux C, Seeman E, et al. The effects of strontium ranelate on the risk of vertebral fracture in women with postmenopausal osteoporosis. *N Engl J Med.* 2004;350:459-468.
420. Jonville-Bera AP, Crickx B, Aaron L, et al. Strontium ranelate-induced DRESS syndrome: first two case reports. *Allergy.* 2009;64:658-659.
421. Pernicova I, Middleton ET, Aye M. Rash, strontium ranelate and DRESS syndrome put into perspective: European Medicine Agency on the alert. *Osteoporos Int.* 2008;19:1811-1812.
422. Snyder PJ, Peachey H, Berlin JA, et al. Effects of testosterone replacement in hypogonadal men. *J Clin Endocrinol Metab.* 2000;85:2670-2677.
423. Kenny AM, Prestwood KM, Gruman CA, et al. Effects of transdermal testosterone on bone and muscle in older men with low bioavailable testosterone levels. *J Gerontol A Biol Sci Med Sci.* 2001;56:M266-M272.
424. Snyder PJ, Peachey H, Hannoush P, et al. Effect of testosterone treatment on bone mineral density in men over 65 years of age. *J Clin Endocrinol Metab.* 1999;84:1966-1972.
425. Tuck SP, Francis RM. Testosterone, bone and osteoporosis. *Front Horm Res.* 2009;37:123-132.
426. Allan G, Sbriscia T, Linton O, et al. A selective androgen receptor modulator with minimal prostate hypertrophic activity restores lean body mass in aged orchidectomized male rats. *J Steroid Biochem Mol Biol.* 2008;110:207-213.
427. Kearbey JD, Gao W, Fisher SJ, et al. Effects of selective androgen receptor modulator (SARM) treatment in osteopenic female rats. *Pharm Res.* 2009;26:2471-2477.
428. Schoofs MW, van der Klift M, Hofman A, et al. Thiazide diuretics and the risk for hip fracture. *Ann Intern Med.* 2003;139:476-482.
429. Reid IR, Ames RW, Orr-Walker BJ, et al. Hydrochlorothiazide reduces loss of cortical bone in normal postmenopausal women: a randomized controlled trial. *Am J Med.* 2000;109:362-370.
430. Bolland MJ, Ames RW, Horne AM, et al. The effect of treatment with a thiazide diuretic for 4 years on bone density in normal postmenopausal women. *Osteoporos Int.* 2007;18:479-486.
431. Giusti A, Barone A, Pioli G, et al. Alendronate and indapamide alone or in combination in the management of hypercalciuria associated with osteoporosis: a randomized controlled trial of two drugs and three treatments. *Nephrol Dial Transplant.* 2009;24:1472-1477.
432. Bone HG, Bolognese MA, Yuen CK, et al. Effects of denosumab on bone mineral density and bone turnover in postmenopausal women. *J Clin Endocrinol Metab.* 2008;93:2149-2157.
433. Cummings SR, San Martin J, McClung MR, et al. Denosumab for prevention of fractures in postmenopausal women with osteoporosis. *N Engl J Med.* 2009;361:756-765.
434. Smith MR, Egerdie B, Hernandez Toriz N, et al. Denosumab in men receiving androgen-deprivation therapy for prostate cancer. *N Engl J Med.* 2009;361:745-755.
435. Vij R, Horvath N, Spencer A, et al. An open-label, phase 2 trial of denosumab in the treatment of relapsed or plateau-phase multiple myeloma. *Am J Hematol.* 2009;84:650-656.
436. Murphy MG, Cerchio K, Stoch SA, et al. Effect of L-000845704, an alphaVbeta3 integrin antagonist, on markers of bone turnover and bone mineral density in postmenopausal osteoporotic women. *J Clin Endocrinol Metab.* 2005;90:2022-2028.
437. Rodan GA, Martin TJ. Therapeutic approaches to bone diseases. *Science.* 2000;289:1508-1514.
438. Gauthier JY, Chauret N, Cromlish W, et al. The discovery of odanacatib (MK-0822), a selective inhibitor of cathepsin K. *Bioorg Med Chem Lett.* 2008;18:923-928.
439. Li X, Ominsky MS, Warmington KS, et al. Sclerostin antibody treatment increases bone formation, bone mass, and bone strength in a rat model of postmenopausal osteoporosis. *J Bone Miner Res.* 2009;24:578-588.
440. Kaiser M, Mieth M, Liebisch P, et al. Serum concentrations of DKK-1 correlate with the extent of bone disease in patients with multiple myeloma. *Eur J Haematol.* 2008;80:490-494.
441. Nicks KM, Perrien DS, Akel NS, et al. Regulation of osteoblastogenesis and osteoclastogenesis by the other reproductive hormones, activin and inhibin. *Mol Cell Endocrinol.* 2009;310:11-20.
442. Pearsall RS, Canalis E, Cornwall-Brady M, et al. A soluble activin type IIA receptor induces bone formation and improves skeletal integrity. *Proc Natl Acad Sci U S A.* 2008;105:7082-7087.
443. Fromigue O, Hay E, Barbara A, et al. Calcium sensing receptor-dependent and -independent activation of osteoblast replication and survival by strontium ranelate. *J Cell Mol Med.* 2009;13:2189-2199.
444. Godsall JW, Baron R, Insogna KL. Vitamin D metabolism and bone histomorphometry in a patient with antacid-induced osteomalacia. *Am J Med.* 1984;77:747-750.
445. Awumey EM, Mitra DA, Hollis BW, et al. Vitamin D metabolism is altered in Asian Indians in the southern United States: a clinical research center study. *J Clin Endocrinol Metab.* 1998;83:169-173.
446. Kreiter SR, Schwartz RP, Kirkman HN Jr, et al. Nutritional rickets in African American breast-fed infants. *J Pediatr.* 2000;137:153-157.
447. Basha B, Rao DS, Han ZH, et al. Osteomalacia due to vitamin D depletion: a neglected consequence of intestinal malabsorption. *Am J Med.* 2000;108:296-300.
448. Schnitzler CM, Pettifor JM, Patel D, et al. Metabolic bone disease in black teenagers with genu valgum or varum without radiologic rickets: a bone histomorphometric study. *J Bone Miner Res.* 1994;9:479-486.
449. Pettifor JM. Rickets and vitamin D deficiency in children and adolescents. *Endocrinol Metab Clin North Am.* 2005;34:537-553, vii.
450. Kitanaka S, Takeyama K, Murayama A, et al. Inactivating mutations in the 25-hydroxyvitamin D3 1alpha-hydroxylase gene in patients with pseudovitamin D-deficiency rickets. *N Engl J Med.* 1998;338:653-661.
451. Kato S, Yoshizazawa T, Kitanaka S, et al. Molecular genetics of vitamin D-dependent hereditary rickets. *Horm Res.* 2002;57:73-78.
452. Kruse K, Feldmann E. Healing of rickets during vitamin D therapy despite defective vitamin D receptors in two siblings with vitamin D-dependent rickets type II. *J Pediatr.* 1995;126:145-148.
453. Berndt TJ, Schiavi S, Kumar R. "Phosphatonins" and the regulation of phosphorus homeostasis. *Am J Physiol Renal Physiol.* 2005;289:F1170-F1182.
454. Quarles LD. FGF23, PHEX, and MEPE regulation of phosphate homeostasis and skeletal mineralization. *Am J Physiol Endocrinol Metab.* 2003;285:E1-E9.
455. Dixon PH, Christie PT, Wooding C, et al. Mutational analysis of PHEX gene in X-linked hypophosphatemia. *J Clin Endocrinol Metab.* 1998;83:3615-3623.
456. Yamazaki Y, Okazaki R, Shibata M, et al. Increased circulatory level of biologically active full-length FGF-23 in patients with hypophosphatemic rickets/osteomalacia. *J Clin Endocrinol Metab.* 2002;87:4957-4960.
457. ADHR Consortium. Autosomal dominant hypophosphataemic rickets is associated with mutations in FGF23. *Nat Genet.* 2000;26:345-348.
458. Petersen DJ, Boniface AM, Schranck FW, et al. X-linked hypophosphatemic rickets: a study (with literature review) of linear growth response to calcitriol and phosphate therapy. *J Bone Miner Res.* 1992;7:583-597.
459. Carpenter TO, Ellis BK, Insogna KL, et al. Fibroblast growth factor 7: an inhibitor of phosphate transport derived from oncogenic osteomalacia-causing tumors. *J Clin Endocrinol Metab.* 2005;90:1012-1020.
460. Jonsson KB, Zahradnik R, Larsson T, et al. Fibroblast growth factor 23 in oncogenic osteomalacia and X-linked hypophosphatemia. *N Engl J Med.* 2003;348:1656-1663.
461. Whyte MP. Hypophosphatasia and the role of alkaline phosphatase in skeletal mineralization. *Endocr Rev.* 1994;15:439-461.
462. Mornet E. Hypophosphatasia. *Best Pract Res Clin Rheumatol.* 2008;22:113-127.
463. Pauli RM, Modaff P, Sipes SL, et al. Mild hypophosphatasia mimicking severe osteogenesis imperfecta in utero: bent but not broken. *Am J Med Genet.* 1999;86:434-438.
464. Iqbal SJ, Brain A, Reynolds TM, et al. Relationship between serum alkaline phosphatase and pyridoxal-5′-phosphate levels in hypophosphatasia. *Clin Sci (Lond).* 1998;94:203-206.
465. Whyte MP, Kurtzberg J, McAlister WH, et al. Marrow cell transplantation for infantile hypophosphatasia. *J Bone Miner Res.* 2003;18:624-636.
466. Xu Y, Hashizume T, Shuhart M, et al. Intestinal and hepatic CYP3A4 catalyze hydroxylation of 1α,25-dihydroxyvitamin D3: implications for drug-induced osteomalacia. *Mol Pharmacol.* 2006;69:56-65.
467. Reginato AJ, Falasca GF, Pappu R, et al. Musculoskeletal manifestations of osteomalacia: report of 26 cases and literature review. *Semin Arthritis Rheum.* 1999;28:287-304.
468. Huang QL, Feig DS, Blackstein ME. Development of tertiary hyperparathyroidism after phosphate supplementation in oncogenic osteomalacia. *J Endocrinol Invest.* 2000;23:263-267.
469. Li YC, Amling M, Pirro AE, et al. Normalization of mineral ion homeostasis by dietary means prevents hyperparathyroidism, rickets, and osteomalacia, but not alopecia in vitamin D receptor-ablated mice. *Endocrinology.* 1998;139:4391-4396.
470. Wilson DM. Growth hormone and hypophosphatemic rickets. *J Pediatr Endocrinol Metab.* 2000;13(suppl 2):993-998.
471. Albright F, Reifenstein EC Jr. *The Parathyroid Glands and Metabolic Bone Disease: Selected Studies.* Baltimore, MD: Williams & Wilkins; 1948.
472. Bilezikian JP, Silverberg SJ. Clinical practice: asymptomatic primary hyperparathyroidism. *N Engl J Med.* 2004;350:1746-1751.
473. Moosgaard B, Vestergaard P, Heickendorff L, et al. Vitamin D status, seasonal variations, parathyroid adenoma weight and bone mineral density in primary hyperparathyroidism. *Clin Endocrinol (Oxf).* 2005;63:506-513.

474. Rubin MR, Bilezikian JP, McMahon DJ, et al. The natural history of primary hyperparathyroidism with or without parathyroid surgery after 15 years. *J Clin Endocrinol Metab.* 2008;93:3462-3470.
475. Silverberg SJ, Gartenberg F, Jacobs TP, et al. Increased bone mineral density after parathyroidectomy in primary hyperparathyroidism. *J Clin Endocrinol Metab.* 1995;80:729-734.
476. Chan FK, Tiu SC, Choi KL, et al. Increased bone mineral density in patients with chronic hypoparathyroidism. *J Clin Endocrinol Metab.* 2003;88:3155-3159.
477. Bilezikian JP, Khan AA, Potts JT Jr. Guidelines for the management of asymptomatic primary hyperparathyroidism: summary statement from the third international workshop. *J Clin Endocrinol Metab.* 2009;94:335-339.
478. Mathew S, Lund R, Hruska KA. The mechanism of skeletal involvment in cardiovascular mortality in chronic kidney disease (CKD). *J Bone Miner Res.* 2007;22:S354.
479. Mathew S, Lund RJ, Strebeck F, et al. Reversal of the adynamic bone disorder and decreased vascular calcification in chronic kidney disease by sevelamer carbonate therapy. *J Am Soc Nephrol.* 2007;18:122-130.
480. Hruska KA, Mathew S, Lund R, et al. Hyperphosphatemia of chronic kidney disease. *Kidney Int.* 2008;74:148-157.
481. Hruska KA, Mathew S, Lund RJ, et al. The pathogenesis of vascular calcification in the chronic kidney disease mineral bone disorder: the links between bone and the vasculature. *Semin Nephrol.* 2009;29:156-165.
482. Palmer S, McGregor DO, Strippoli GF. Interventions for preventing bone disease in kidney transplant recipients. Cochrane Database Syst Rev. 2005;(3):CD005015.
483. Lindberg JS. Calcimimetics: a new tool for management of hyperparathyroidism and renal osteodystrophy in patients with chronic kidney disease. *Kidney Int Suppl.* 2005;(95):S33-S36.
484. Gal-Moscovici A, Popovtzer MM. New worldwide trends in presentation of renal osteodystrophy and its relationship to parathyroid hormone levels. *Clin Nephrol.* 2005;63:284-289.
485. Cunningham J, Sprague SM, Cannata-Andia J, et al. Osteoporosis in chronic kidney disease. *Am J Kidney Dis.* 2004;43:566-571.
486. Hughes AE, Ralston SH, Marken J, et al. Mutations in TNFRSF11A, affecting the signal peptide of RANK, cause familial expansile osteolysis. *Nat Genet.* 2000;24:45-48.
487. Siris ES. Extensive personal experience: Paget's disease of bone. *J Clin Endocrinol Metab.* 1995;80:335-338.
488. Singer FR. Paget's disease of bone: classical pathology and electron microscopy. *Semin Arthritis Rheum.* 1994;23:217-218.
489. Reddy SV, Singer FR, Roodman GD. Bone marrow mononuclear cells from patients with Paget's disease contain measles virus nucleocapsid messenger ribonucleic acid that has mutations in a specific region of the sequence. *J Clin Endocrinol Metab.* 1995;80:2108-2111.
490. Kurihara N, Reddy SV, Menaa C, et al. Osteoclasts expressing the measles virus nucleocapsid gene display a pagetic phenotype. *J Clin Invest.* 2000;105:607-614.
491. Ralston SH. Pathogenesis of Paget's disease of bone. *Bone.* 2008;43:819-825.
492. Roodman GD, Kurihara N, Ohsaki Y, et al. Interleukin 6: a potential autocrine/paracrine factor in Paget's disease of bone. *J Clin Invest.* 1992;89:46-52.
493. Menaa C, Reddy SV, Kurihara N, et al. Enhanced RANK ligand expression and responsivity of bone marrow cells in Paget's disease of bone. *J Clin Invest.* 2000;105:1833-1838.
494. Naot D, Bava U, Matthews B, et al. Differential gene expression in cultured osteoblasts and bone marrow stromal cells from patients with Paget's disease of bone. *J Bone Miner Res.* 2007;22:298-309.
495. Siris ES. Epidemiological aspects of Paget's disease: family history and relationship to other medical conditions. *Semin Arthritis Rheum.* 1994;23:222-225.
496. Laurin N, Brown JP, Morissette J, et al. Recurrent mutation of the gene encoding sequestosome 1 (SQSTM1/p62) in Paget disease of bone. *Am J Hum Genet.* 2002;70:1582-1588.
497. Layfield R, Ciani B, Ralston SH, et al. Structural and functional studies of mutations affecting the UBA domain of SQSTM1 (p62) which cause Paget's disease of bone. *Biochem Soc Trans.* 2004;32:728-730.
498. Ralston SH, Langston AL, Reid IR. Pathogenesis and management of Paget's disease of bone. *Lancet.* 2008;372:155-163.
499. Alvarez L, Guanabens N, Peris P, et al. Discriminative value of biochemical markers of bone turnover in assessing the activity of Paget's disease. *J Bone Miner Res.* 1995;10:458-465.
500. Siris ES, Lyles KW, Singer FR, et al. Medical management of Paget's disease of bone: indications for treatment and review of current therapies. *J Bone Miner Res.* 2006;21(suppl 2):P94-P98.
501. Chosich N, Long F, Wong R, et al. Post-partum hypercalcemia in hereditary hyperphosphatasia (juvenile Paget's disease). *J Endocrinol Invest.* 1991;14:591-597.
502. Demir E, Bereket A, Ozkan B, et al. Effect of alendronate treatment on the clinical picture and bone turnover markers in chronic idiopathic hyperphosphatasia. *J Pediatr Endocrinol Metab.* 2000;13:217-221.
503. Whyte MP, Mills BG, Reinus WR, et al. Expansile skeletal hyperphosphatasia: a new familial metabolic bone disease. *J Bone Miner Res.* 2000;15:2330-2344.
504. Whyte MP, Obrecht SE, Finnegan PM, et al. Osteoprotegerin deficiency and juvenile Paget's disease. *N Engl J Med.* 2002;347:175-184.
505. Byers PH. Osteogenesis imperfecta. In: Royce PM, Steinmann B, eds. *Connective Tissue and Its Heritable Disorders: Molecular, Genetic, and Medical Aspects.* New York: Wiley-Liss; 1993:317-350.
506. Uveges TE, Collin-Osdoby P, Cabral WA, et al. Cellular mechanism of decreased bone in Brtl mouse model of OI: imbalance of decreased osteoblast function and increased osteoclasts and their precursors. *J Bone Miner Res.* 2008;23:1983-1994.
507. Redford-Badwal DA, Stover ML, Valli M, et al. Nuclear retention of COL1A1 messenger RNA identifies null alleles causing mild osteogenesis imperfecta. *J Clin Invest.* 1996;97:1035-1040.
508. Spotila LD, Colige A, Sereda L, et al. Mutation analysis of coding sequences for type I procollagen in individuals with low bone density. *J Bone Miner Res.* 1994;9:923-932.
509. Spotila LD, Constantinou CD, Sereda L, et al. Mutation in a gene for type I procollagen (COL1A2) in a woman with postmenopausal osteoporosis: evidence for phenotypic and genotypic overlap with mild osteogenesis imperfecta. *Proc Natl Acad Sci U S A.* 1991;88:5423-5427.
510. Rauch F, Travers R, Parfitt AM, et al. Static and dynamic bone histomorphometry in children with osteogenesis imperfecta. *Bone.* 2000;26:581-589.
511. Chang W, Barnes AM, Cabral WA, et al. Prolyl 3-hydroxylase 1 and CRTAP are mutually stabilizing in the endoplasmic reticulum collagen prolyl 3-hydroxylation complex. *Hum Mol Genet.* 2010;19:223-234.
512. Braga V, Gatti D, Rossini M, et al. Bone turnover markers in patients with osteogenesis imperfecta. *Bone.* 2004;34:1013-1016.
513. Glorieux FH, Bishop NJ, Plotkin H, et al. Cyclic administration of pamidronate in children with severe osteogenesis imperfecta. *N Engl J Med.* 1998;339:947-952.
514. Munns CF, Rauch F, Travers R, et al. Effects of intravenous pamidronate treatment in infants with osteogenesis imperfecta: clinical and histomorphometric outcome. *J Bone Miner Res.* 2005;20:1235-1243.
515. Vyskocil V, Pikner R, Kutilek S. Effect of alendronate therapy in children with osteogenesis imperfecta. *Joint Bone Spine.* 2005;72:416-423.
516. Basel D, Steiner RD. Osteogenesis imperfecta: recent findings shed new light on this once well-understood condition. *Genet Med.* 2009;11:375-385.
517. Chamberlain JR, Schwarze U, Wang PR, et al. Gene targeting in stem cells from individuals with osteogenesis imperfecta. *Science.* 2004;303:1198-1201.
518. Tolar J, Teitelbaum SL, Orchard PJ. Osteopetrosis. *N Engl J Med.* 2004;351:2839-2849.
519. Abboud SL, Woodruff K, Liu C, et al. Rescue of the osteopetrotic defect in op/op mice by osteoblast-specific targeting of soluble colony-stimulating factor-1. *Endocrinology.* 2002;143:1942-1949.
520. Gowen M, Lazner F, Dodds R, et al. Cathepsin K knockout mice develop osteopetrosis due to a deficit in matrix degradation but not demineralization. *J Bone Miner Res.* 1999;14:1654-1663.
521. Grigoriadis AE, Wang ZQ, Cecchini MG, et al. c-Fos: a key regulator of osteoclast-macrophage lineage determination and bone remodeling. *Science.* 1994;266:443-448.
522. Hollberg K, Hultenby K, Hayman A, et al. Osteoclasts from mice deficient in tartrate-resistant acid phosphatase have altered ruffled borders and disturbed intracellular vesicular transport. *Exp Cell Res.* 2002;279:227-238.
523. McHugh KP, Hodivala-Dilke K, Zheng MH, et al. Mice lacking beta3 integrins are osteosclerotic because of dysfunctional osteoclasts. *J Clin Invest.* 2000;105:433-440.
524. Naito A, Azuma S, Tanaka S, et al. Severe osteopetrosis, defective interleukin-1 signalling and lymph node organogenesis in TRAF6-deficient mice. *Genes Cells.* 1999;4:353-362.
525. Chalhoub N, Benachenhou N, Rajapurohitam V, et al. Grey-lethal mutation induces severe malignant autosomal recessive osteopetrosis in mouse and human. *Nat Med.* 2003;9:399-406.
526. Fasth A, Porras O. Human malignant osteopetrosis: pathophysiology, management and the role of bone marrow transplantation. *Pediatr Transplant.* 1999;3(suppl 1):102-107.
527. Frattini A, Orchard PJ, Sobacchi C, et al. Defects in TCIRG1 subunit of the vacuolar proton pump are responsible for a subset of human autosomal recessive osteopetrosis. *Nat Genet.* 2000;25:343-346.
528. Frattini A, Pangrazio A, Susani L, et al. Chloride channel ClCN7 mutations are responsible for severe recessive, dominant, and intermediate osteopetrosis. *J Bone Miner Res.* 2003;18:1740-1747.
529. Ramirez A, Faupel J, Goebel I, et al. Identification of a novel mutation in the coding region of the grey-lethal gene OSTM1 in human malignant infantile osteopetrosis. *Hum Mutat.* 2004;23:471-476.
530. Key LL Jr, Rodriguiz RM, Willi SM, et al. Long-term treatment of osteopetrosis with recombinant human interferon gamma. *N Engl J Med.* 1995;332:1594-1599.
531. Cotter M, Connell T, Colhoun E, et al. Carbonic anhydrase II deficiency: a rare autosomal recessive disorder of osteopetrosis, renal

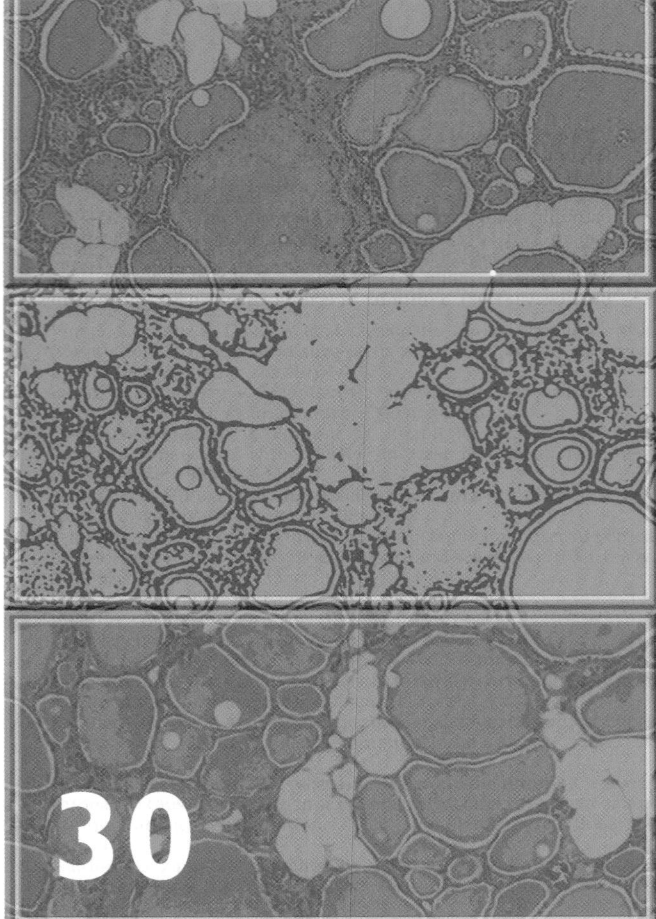

CHAPTER 30

Kidney Stones

REBECA D. MONK • DAVID A. BUSHINSKY

Nephrolithiasis is a common disorder with an incidence greater than 1 case per 1000 patients per year. The prevalence in industrialized nations is approximately 6% in women and 12% in men and appears to be rising over time.[1] The incidence peaks in the third and fourth decades, and prevalence increases with age until approximately age 70 years.[1-4]

In general, stones may be composed of calcium oxalate, calcium phosphate, uric acid, magnesium ammonium phosphate (struvite), or cystine, alone or in combination. A variety of pathogenic mechanisms determine the type of stone formed. Symptomatic stones tend to localize in the renal tubules and collecting system but are also commonly found within the ureters and bladder.[5]

Kidney stones result in substantial morbidity. The severe pain of renal colic can lead to frequent hospitalization, shock wave lithotripsy, or invasive surgical procedures. Although rarely a cause of end-stage renal disease, nephrolithiasis has been associated with chronic kidney disease (CKD) in various populations,[6-10] and even mild CKD is associated with significant adverse cardiovascular events.[11-13] Insight into the mechanisms involved in stone formation can help direct appropriate therapy, which is known to significantly decrease the incidence of stone formation and its associated morbidity. If this morbidity also includes cardiovascular disease, then stone prevention may have more significant overall health benefits for patients than merely controlling the pain and consequences of renal colic.

STONE FORMATION

Epidemiology

Numerous factors determine the prevalence of stones, including gender, age, race, and geographic distribution. Nephrolithiasis is more common in men than in women, the ratio being between 2:1 and 4:1.[1-4] In the United States, Blacks, Latin Americans, and Asian Americans are much less likely to have stones than whites. Geography also appears to influence stone formation in the United States, with a decreasing prevalence from south to north and, to some degree, from east to west.

The greater exposure to sunlight in the southeastern United States may be responsible for the increased rates of nephrolithiasis in that area. Sun exposure can lead to more concentrated urine by increasing insensible fluid losses due to sweating.[14-16] Although the increased sun exposure should increase levels of vitamin D and measured 25-hydroxyvitamin D_3, there is no evidence that this will increase levels of 1,25-dihydroxyitamin D_3 (calcitriol) or cell-mediated calcium absorption.

TABLE 30-1

Percentage of Patients with Various Stone Types in the United States

Type	Percentage
Mixed calcium oxalate and calcium phosphate	37
Calcium oxalate	26
Calcium phosphate	7
Uric acid	5
Struvite	22
Cystine	2

Adapted from Bushinsky DA. Renal lithiasis. In: Humes HD, ed: *Kelly's Textbook of Medicine*. Philadelphia, PA: Lippincott Williams & Wilkins, 2000:1243-1248.

Geographic location and genetic predisposition can also influence the type of stones formed.[14,17] Uric acid stones, for example, predominate in Mediterranean and Middle Eastern countries, where they constitute up to 75% of all the stones formed. In the United States, fewer than 10% of kidney stones are pure uric acid stones, and more than 70% are composed of calcium and an associated anion. Less common are magnesium ammonium phosphate (struvite or infection) stones, which account for 10% to 15% of stones formed, and cystine stones, which form as a result of an autosomal recessive disorder and constitute only about 1% of all stones formed (Table 30-1).[2,17,18]

Diet and pharmacologic agents can also significantly affect stone formation. A recent outbreak of nephrolithiasis in Chinese infants was attributed to ingestion of melamine in infant formula and milk powder. The large melamine particles, intentionally added to raise the apparent protein content of the concentrates, led in many cases to nephrolithiasis and in some cases to renal failure due to obstructive uropathy.[19-21] A variety of dietary factors can have a significant impact on both formation and prevention of kidney stones (see later discussion).

PATHOGENESIS OF STONE FORMATION

Physiology

Kidney stones form when urine becomes oversaturated with respect to the specific components of the stone. Saturation depends on the chemical free ion activities of the stone constituents. Factors that affect chemical free ion activity include urinary ion concentration, pH, and combination with other substances. For example, an increase in the urinary calcium concentration or a decrease in urine volume increases the free ion activity of calcium ions in the urine. Urinary pH can also modify chemical free ion activity. A low urinary pH increases the free ion activity of uric acid ions but decreases the activity of calcium and phosphate ions. Citrate combines with calcium ions to form soluble complexes and decreases their free ion activity. When the chemical free ion activities are increased, the urine becomes oversaturated (also termed *supersaturated*). In this setting, new stones may form, and established stones may grow. In the setting of decreased free ion activity, urine becomes undersaturated; stones do not grow and can even dissolve. The *equilibrium solubility product* is the degree of chemical free ion activity of stone components in a solution in which the stone neither grows nor dissolves.

Formation of stones occurs through homogeneous or heterogeneous nucleation. In *homogeneous nucleation*, progressive supersaturation can eventually result in complexation of identical ions into small clusters; these clusters grow to form a permanent solid phase, or crystals. *Heterogeneous nucleation* refers to crystal formation on the surface of a different crystal type or on other dissimilar substances, such as cells. In vivo, this type of nucleation is more common than homogeneous nucleation, because crystals form at a lower level of supersaturation in the presence of a solid phase.

The crystals must then aggregate into clinically significant stones, a process that may take longer than the passage of urine through the renal tubules. For stone formation to occur before the crystals are eliminated, the crystals must anchor themselves to the renal tubular epithelium to allow more time for growth. This anchoring of crystals occurs at the renal papillae, over areas of interstitial calcium phosphate (in the form of apatite) termed *Randall's plaques*.[22-24] The apatite crystals appear to originate at the basement membrane of tubular cells in the thin loop of Henle and to extend into the interstitium without damaging the cells themselves or filling the tubular lumens. A combination of apatite crystal and organic material extends from the loop of Henle tubular basement membrane to the papillary uroepithelial surface, where calcium oxalate crystals or other crystals can adhere and form stones.

An important factor in the development of kidney stones may be the absence of adequate levels or activity of crystallization inhibitors in patients with stones. Uropontin, pyrophosphate, and nephrocalcin are endogenously produced substances that have been shown to inhibit calcium crystallization. Differences in the amount or activity of inhibitors might account for the variability in stone formation among people with similar degrees of urinary supersaturation.[18,25]

Clinically, most physicians evaluate the lithogenic potential of urine from stone formers by measuring the rates of excretion of the principal stone-forming elements in terms of mass per unit time (e.g., milligrams or millimoles per 24 hours). It is clear, however, that the lithogenic potential of urine is better determined by the degree of supersaturation. Computer programs that calculate saturation from concentrations of various elements in the urine and the urinary pH are now available and more accurately determine the risk of stone formation. Any calculation of mean saturation underestimates the maximum supersaturation because of hourly variations in water and solute excretion throughout the day.

Diet

Dietary factors have a great influence on the concentration of excreted ions. Simply advising patients to increase fluid intake can have a great impact on reducing stone growth and formation.[26-28] Renal calcium excretion is augmented by increased sodium excretion,[29] and hypercalciuric patients tend to have a greater calciuric response to a sodium load than control subjects.[30] Dietary sodium restriction, with the consequent decrease in urinary sodium, thus reduces calcium excretion. Patients are counseled to limit their daily sodium intake to a maximum of 3000 mg (approximately 130 mEq) in an attempt to reduce hypercalciuria.[2,29,31]

A moderate reduction in animal protein (to approximately 1.0 mg/kg per day) is beneficial in patients with nephrolithiasis because of the multiple mechanisms by which animal protein can contribute to stone formation.[31]

A mild metabolic acidosis develops when animal proteins are metabolized. To buffer the excess hydrogen ions, calcium is resorbed from bone, increasing the filtered load of calcium.[32] Metabolic acidosis also directly decreases renal tubular calcium reabsorption, which further enhances hypercalciuria.[32] In addition, metabolism of amino acids contained in animal protein generates sulfate ions, which couple with calcium ions to form insoluble complexes.[32,33] Citrate, a base, forms soluble complexes with calcium and is beneficial in lowering calcium oxalate and calcium phosphate supersaturation and in reducing stone formation. During metabolic acidosis, citrate is reabsorbed proximally, reducing the amount of citrate excreted in the urine.[34] Hypokalemia can also lead to reduced citrate excretion. An animal protein–induced reduction in citrate can promote formation of both calcium oxalate and uric acid stones.[30,35]

Fructose has become a ubiquitous sweetener in American processed foods. In large food questionnaire studies, this sugar has been associated with a significant risk of developing nephrolithiasis. Though the mechanism is not known, fructose is the only carbohydrate that can increase uric acid production, and its metabolism may increase stone formation.[36]

Studies have demonstrated the benefits of a diet containing an age- and gender-appropriate amount of calcium in patients with kidney stones.[27,31,37,38] Ingested calcium binds intestinal oxalate, reducing its absorption and consequent renal excretion.[27] In a long-term prospective trial, Borghi and colleagues randomly assigned male patients with hypercalciuric stones to either a low-calcium diet or a diet with a normal amount of calcium but low sodium and low animal protein.[31] Both groups of men were instructed to restrict oxalate intake and to drink 2 to 3 L of water daily. The group of men on the normal-calcium, low-sodium, low–animal protein diet had a significantly lower recurrence of nephrolithiasis and a greater reduction in oxalate excretion and calcium oxalate supersaturation compared with the men on the low-calcium diet.[31]

Therefore, patients should be maintained on an age- and gender-appropriate intake of calcium, and dietary calcium restriction should be strongly discouraged as not only increasing the risk of recurrent stone formation but engendering a significant risk of bone demineralization.[39,40] The recommended dietary intake for men and women is 1000 mg/day of elemental calcium from ages 19 through 50 years and 1200 mg/day of calcium thereafter.[41] Teenagers should consume 1300 mg of calcium per day. Excess calcium should be avoided, because the combination of calcium and vitamin D supplementation has been shown to significantly increase the risk of kidney stones in postmenopausal women.[42]

Pathogenesis of Idiopathic Hypercalciuria

Idiopathic hypercalciuria (IH) is the most common cause of calcium-containing kidney stones. Hypercalciuria is defined as excessive urinary calcium excretion. IH is excessive urinary calcium excretion in the setting of normocalcemia and in the absence of secondary causes of hypercalciuria. The disorder is familial; it was initially thought to exhibit an autosomal dominant pattern of inheritance but is almost certainly polygenetic.[43]

The mechanism by which IH leads to hypercalciuria is not known. It has been postulated that IH comprises three distinct disorders: excessive intestinal calcium absorption, decreased renal tubular calcium reabsorption, and enhanced bone demineralization. Many believe that IH is a systemic disorder of calcium homeostasis with dysregulation of calcium transport at all of these sites.[44] An understanding of calcium homeostasis helps elucidate the potential mechanisms involved in IH.

Calcium Homeostasis

Urinary calcium homeostasis is regulated by the gastrointestinal tract, the kidneys, and bone and by the hormones parathyroid hormone (PTH) and calcitriol. Approximately 99% of the calcium in the body is contained within the bone mineral. Daily bone resorption and bone formation, which in healthy, nonpregnant adults should be equal, allow less than 1% of bone calcium to be exchanged with calcium in the extracellular fluid.

Both PTH and calcitriol, at high concentrations, stimulate release of calcium from the bone mineral through osteoclast-mediated bone resorption. Net calcium influx into the extracellular fluid is achieved by absorption from the gastrointestinal tract, which occurs through calcitriol-dependent and -independent mechanisms. Although PTH appears to have no direct effect on gastrointestinal calcium absorption, increased levels of the hormone can stimulate production of calcitriol, which leads to enhanced absorption. Increased serum levels of calcium and calcitriol provide negative feedback to the parathyroid glands, resulting in reduced PTH secretion.

The roughly 60% of calcium in the extracellular fluid that is not protein bound is freely filtered by the renal glomeruli. Approximately 80% to 85% of this amount is passively reabsorbed in the proximal tubule. Most of the remaining calcium is reabsorbed in the thick ascending limb of Henle's loop and in the distal cortical tubules under PTH stimulation. Ultimately, these reabsorptive mechanisms result in a urinary calcium excretion that is less than 2% of the daily filtered load of calcium.[45] Except during pregnancy and lactation, in healthy, nonosteoporotic adults, urinary calcium excretion (and any calcium lost in sweat) precisely equals net intestinal calcium absorption.

Potential Mechanisms for Development of Idiopathic Hypercalciuria

Dysregulation of calcium transport in the intestine, kidney, or bone can lead to hypercalciuria. For example, excessive calcium absorption by the gastrointestinal tract leads to a transient increase in serum calcium. This suppresses secretion of PTH, which, along with the increased filtered load of calcium to the kidneys, results in hypercalciuria. Excessive calcitriol has a similar effect of increasing intestinal calcium absorption but also results in an influx of calcium into the extracellular fluid because of enhanced bone resorption. The result is hypercalciuria even in the setting of a low-calcium diet or an overnight fast. The excess calcitriol also suppresses PTH secretion, further reducing the renal tubular reabsorption of calcium.

If a primary defect in renal calcium reabsorption has led directly to hypercalciuria, there is a fall in the serum calcium concentration that stimulates synthesis of PTH and calcitriol. Increased calcitriol results in enhanced intestinal calcium absorption and bone resorption. The renal loss of calcium persists even with a low-calcium diet or overnight fast.

Hypercalciuria can also develop as a result of a defect in renal phosphorus reabsorption. The resultant hypophosphatemia leads to enhanced calcitriol production, which stimulates intestinal absorption of phosphorus and calcium. The increased serum calcium and calcitriol suppress PTH synthesis and release. The increased filtered load of calcium in the setting of suppressed PTH leads to hypercalciuria. Enhanced bone resorption increases the serum calcium concentration, which in turn suppresses PTH production further. The increase in the filtered load of calcium in this setting results in hypercalciuria.

Therefore, there are several potential mechanisms for hypercalciuria.[44] Do human or animal data support one mechanism above all others? From a clinical therapeutic standpoint, is it worth differentiating among the various potential mechanisms in each patient with suspected IH?

Human Data

Lemann[46] compiled the results of numerous calcium balance studies of patients with IH and normocalciuric control subjects and normalized the results for calcium intake. He found that intestinal calcium absorption was significantly higher in the subjects with IH.

Coe and colleagues also collected data from published metabolic balance studies, comparing net intestinal calcium absorption and urinary calcium excretion in hypercalciuric and normocalciuric adults.[47] They also noted an increase in intestinal calcium absorption in subjects with IH but found that urinary excretion of calcium was increased to an even greater degree, placing many of these patients in net negative calcium balance. Although these data confirm that enhanced intestinal absorption of calcium probably plays a role in the pathogenesis of IH, the investigators could not clarify whether this condition is the primary defect or is secondary to another lesion, such as a primary dysregulation of renal tubular calcium reabsorption. Others have suggested that the increase in intestinal calcium absorption, in combination with a decrease in renal calcium reabsorption, points to a more generalized defect in calcium homeostasis. Nonetheless, the finding of enhanced calcium absorption makes enhanced bone resorption an unlikely primary mechanism of IH, because the increase in serum calcium concentration resulting from bone resorption would suppress calcitriol-mediated intestinal calcium absorption.

In most published studies, patients with IH have higher serum levels of calcitriol than normocalciuric control subjects.[5,44,48] Kaplan and colleagues[48] determined that calcitriol levels were higher than control values in approximately one third of patients with IH and that intestinal calcium absorption was inappropriately high for the level of calcitriol. These studies support either calcitriol-mediated intestinal calcium absorption or a primary defect in renal tubular calcium reabsorption as a primary mechanism for hypercalciuria in IH.

PTH levels in patients with IH have been reported as normal or slightly lower than those in controls.[35,39] This finding argues against a reduction in renal tubular calcium reabsorption as the primary defect in IH, because with that mechanism the hypercalciuria would lead to low serum calcium levels and stimulation of PTH secretion. This finding also does not support the hypothesis that elevated levels of PTH are the stimulus for the increased levels of serum calcitriol observed in many studies. It is, however, consistent with the other potential mechanisms for IH.

Bone mass in patients with IH has been assessed by a number of methods, including radiologic densitometry, quantitative computed tomography (CT), dual-energy x-ray absorptiometry (DEXA), and single-photon absorptiometry. Studies of patients with IH have generally shown a mild reduction of bone mineral density compared with values in controls.[35,39,49] The studies were unable to reveal a unifying mechanism for the mild reduction in bone mineral density, but primary net bone resorption is unlikely, because a much greater decrease in bone density would be expected in that setting. Altered calcitriol regulation is consistent with this finding, because the effects of calcitriol on bone resorption would be mitigated by the increased intestinal calcium absorption stimulated by the hormone.

Previously it was considered essential to determine whether a patient with IH tended to have excessive gastrointestinal calcium absorption (absorptive hypercalciuria) or excessive renal excretion (renal leak).[50,51] Patients with excessive renal calcium excretion were prescribed thiazide diuretics, and those who were thought to have a predominantly absorptive defect were prescribed a low-calcium diet. Coe and colleagues[39] undermined the validity of this approach in a study in which 24 patients with IH and 9 control subjects were given a low-calcium diet (2 mg/kg per day) for more than 1 week. Urine and blood tests revealed normal serum calcium levels, a mild decrease in PTH levels in the patients with IH, and no difference in calcitriol levels.

The striking finding of Coe's work[39] was that, whereas all the normocalciuric subjects excreted less calcium than they ingested on the low-calcium diet, 16 of the 24 subjects with IH had excreted urinary calcium in amounts that exceeded their calcium intake. Therefore, most of the patients with IH receiving a low-calcium diet were in net negative calcium balance. No clear demarcation was noted between the patients who tended to excrete excessive amounts of calcium and those who did not. Instead, there was a smooth continuum of urinary calcium excretion among patients with IH that appeared not to be influenced by calcemic hormones. From a therapeutic standpoint, these findings have rendered obsolete both the need to clinically distinguish among the various IH mechanisms in humans and the prescription of a low-calcium diet in any of these patients. This changed approach to diet is important, because a low-calcium diet can result in a dangerous reduction in bone mineral density, especially in women.[39,40,44,49] As mentioned earlier, a low-calcium diet appears to increase recurrent stone formation.[27,31] Therefore, advising a low-calcium diet to prevent recurrent stone formation offers no benefit but carries a number of well-documented risks.

Genetic Hypercalciuric Stone-Forming Rats

To explain more fully the mechanism of IH in humans, we developed an animal model of this disorder.[52-57] Through more than 90 generations of successive inbreeding of the most hypercalciuric progeny of hypercalciuric Sprague-Dawley rats, we established a strain of rats that excrete 8 to 10 times as much urinary calcium as control Sprague-Dawley rats (Fig. 30-1).

Compared with control Sprague-Dawley rats, the genetic hypercalciuric rats absorb far more calcium at lower dietary levels of calcitriol.[54,58] When these hypercalciuric rats were fed a diet very low in calcium, their urinary calcium excretion remained elevated, compared with that of similarly treated control rats, indicating a defect in renal calcium reabsorption or an increase in bone resorption, or both[59]—again similar to observations in humans.[39,60] Bone from these hypercalciuric rats released more calcium than the bone of control rats when exposed to increasing amounts of calcitriol[61]; their bone mineral density was lower than that of control rats[62]; and the administration of a bisphosphonate to rats fed a low-calcium diet significantly reduced their urinary calcium excretion.[63] In addition, a primary defect in renal calcium reabsorption was observed during clearance studies.[64] We have shown that, in addition to the intestine, both the bone and the kidney of the

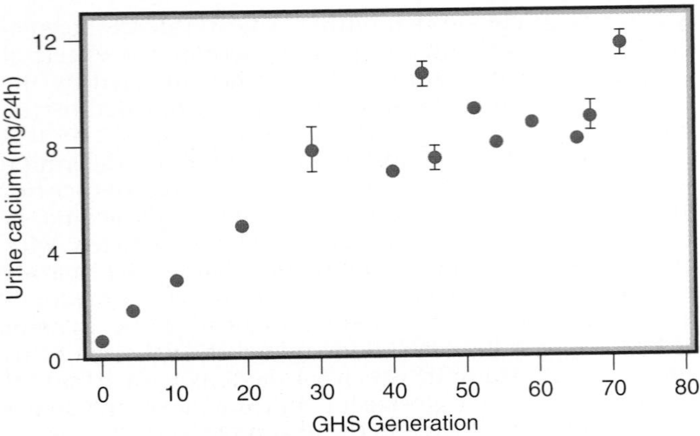

Figure 30-1 Urine calcium levels in genetic hypercalciuric stone-forming (GHS) rats.

hypercalciuric rats have an increased number of vitamin D receptors and calcium receptors.[52,57,61,65,66]

In summary, this strain of hypercalciuric rats appear to have a systemic abnormality in calcium homeostasis: they absorb more intestinal calcium, they resorb more bone, and they do not adequately reabsorb filtered calcium. Because every one of the hypercalciuric rats forms renal stones, we have described them as genetic hypercalciuric stone-forming (GHS) rats.[54,55] These studies suggest that an increased number of vitamin D receptors, or possibly increased calcium receptors, or both, may be the underlying mechanism for hypercalciuria in these rats[66] and perhaps in humans as well.[54,56,65] In a clinical study, circulating monocytes from humans with IH were shown to have an increased number of vitamin D receptors.[67]

Genetics of Idiopathic Hypercalciuria in Humans

The difficulty in ascertaining the genetics of IH arises, in part, from the numerous other factors that influence stone formation, such as diet, environment, and gender. Because half of patients with IH report a family history of stones and male patients often have fathers or sons with the disorder, inheritance is not believed to be recessive or X-linked. A multitude of monogenic hereditary disorders (see later discussion) can lead to hypercalciuria by causing a variety of mutations resulting in changes in calcium handling in kidney, bone, and gut, as well as changes in the calcium-sensing receptor in the kidneys and parathyroid glands. Given the evidence (discussed earlier) that IH is a complex trait that as a phenotype can develop in multiple ways, it is most likely a polygenic disorder, with heterogeneity of loci and polygenic modifiers.

Although attempts at diagnosing the exact cause of IH in a particular patient might not be critical from a therapeutic standpoint, determining the etiology of IH in a particular family is essential for researchers attempting to clarify the genetics of IH.[15,23,43,68] Recently, a team of investigators using the technique of genome-wide association studies found that a member of the claudin family, claudin 14, is associated with stone formation.[69] Whether this association will be found in other populations, supporting its link to stone formation, remains to be determined.

Other Genetic Causes of Stones and Nephrocalcinosis

Numerous monogenic disorders cause hypercalciuria and subsequent nephrolithiasis or nephrocalcinosis.[15,23,43,68,70-72] Disorders that lead to hypercalciuria by augmenting bone resorption include osteogenesis imperfecta type 1, multiple endocrine neoplasia type 1 (MEN1) syndrome with hyperparathyroidism, McCune-Albright syndrome, and infantile hypophosphatemia. Disorders that result in hypercalciuria via intestinal hyperabsorption of calcium include hypophosphatemia, Down syndrome, and congenital lactate deficiency.

The following sections provide a more detailed description of several disorders that result in hypercalciuria via their effect on the kidney. Other disorders in this group include autosomal dominant hypocalcemia (which is caused by an activating mutation of the calcium-sensing receptor), Lowe oculocerebrorenal syndrome, and Wilson's disease.

X-Linked Hypercalciuric Nephrolithiasis (Dent's Disease and Others)

Several families around the world were discovered to have a variable combination of disorders including hypercalciuria, low-molecular-weight proteinuria, nephrocalcinosis or stones, hypophosphatemic rickets, and renal failure.[70,71] Some affected persons demonstrate evidence of defects in proximal tubular reabsorption of amino acids, glucose, or phosphate. PTH tends to be quite low and calcitriol high in the majority of patients. The abnormalities completely resolve in those patients who receive renal transplants, a finding that suggests a renal tubular disorder rather than a systemic process. In all families, the pattern of inheritance is consistent with an X-linked recessive disorder, with male patients affected to a greater extent than female patients. The latter are often minimally affected but transmit the disorder to half of their male offspring.

Over time, the various disorders—X-linked recessive nephrolithiasis in the United States, Dent's disease in the United Kingdom, X-linked recessive hypophosphatemic rickets in Italy, and low-molecular-weight proteinuria with hypercalciuria and nephrocalcinosis in Japan—have all been linked to mutations affecting the *CLCN5* gene on the Xp11.22 locus of the X chromosome. This gene encodes the CLC-5 protein, which is one of the nine members of the CLC family of voltage-gated chloride channels. How defects in this channel lead to the array of disorders listed here, including hypercalciuria, stones, and renal failure, is not yet understood.

Bartter's Syndrome

Bartter's syndrome comprises approximately five genetic mutations, predominantly autosomal recessive, that lead to sodium chloride wasting at the thick ascending limb of the loop of Henle.[23,24,43,72,73]

Defects can arise in the sodium-potassium-chloride cotransporter (NKCC2), the renal outer medullary potassium channel (ROMK), the basolateral chloride channel (CLC-Kb), or in a chloride channel subunit known as barttin. The resultant defect in sodium transport leads to a reduction in the transtubular potential difference, which causes a decrease in paracellular calcium reabsorption in the thick ascending limb. The ensuing reduction in intravascular volume also induces an aldosterone-mediated metabolic alkalosis. Bartter's syndrome, therefore, resembles high-dose furosemide administration and differs from Gitleman's syndrome in that hypercalciuria, nephrocalcinosis, and nephrolithiasis are seen with Bartter's but not with Gitleman's.

An autosomal dominant form of Bartter's results from a gain-of-function mutation in the calcium-sensing receptor in renal tubular cells. This mutation leads to reduced calcium reabsorption, hypocalcemia, and low PTH levels. Therapy with vitamin D and calcium supplementation can exacerbate stone disease in this disorder.

For unknown reasons, the barttin defect leads to deafness but not to nephrocalcinosis or stones.

Familial Hypomagnesemia with Hypercalciuria and Nephrocalcinosis

Familial hypomagnesemia with hypercalciuria and nephrocalcinosis (FHHNC) is an autosomal recessive disorder that results in hypomagnesemia, hypercalciuria, nephrolithiasis, and distal (type 1) renal tubular acidosis (dRTA). Polyuria and severe nephrocalcinosis also ensue, and progressive renal failure is common by late childhood.[23,24] The genetic disorder results in defective production of the tight junction proteins claudin 16 and claudin 19, which facilitate paracellular calcium and magnesium transport in the thick ascending limb as well as renal sodium reabsorption.[74,75]

Distal Renal Tubular Acidosis

dRTA is caused by dysfunctional α-intercalated cells, resulting in defective acid excretion.[23,24,43,68,76] This inability to adequately acidify the urine results in metabolic acidosis, hypocitraturia, hypokalemia, hypercalciuria, and nephrocalcinosis and stones. The metabolic acidosis leads to resorption of calcium and phosphate from bone. The increased filtered load of calcium and phosphate, along with the elevated urine pH and hypocitraturia, results in favorable conditions for calcium phosphate stone formation.

Although there are secondary causes of dRTA, such as Sjögren's syndrome and carbonic anhydrase inhibitors (e.g., acetazolamide), there are also a number of hereditary causes. Some are autosomal recessive and can also result in hearing loss; others are autosomal dominant. One form of dRTA that targets carbonic anhydrase II results in osteopetrosis and brain calcifications. Patients with dRTA fail to lower their urine pH below 5.5 after ingestion of an acid load. Their urine citrate levels are extremely low, despite often mildly reduced or even normal serum bicarbonate levels.

Hereditary Hypophosphatemic Rickets with Hypercalciuria

Hereditary hypophosphatemic rickets with hypercalciuria is an autosomal form of hypophosphatemic rickets that is manifested clinically by hypophosphatemia secondary to renal phosphate wasting.[77,78] In these patients, hypophosphatemia induces increased levels of calcitriol, leading to increased intestinal calcium absorption and hypercalciuria. The bone pain, muscle weakness, limb deformities, and rickets remit completely with administration of oral phosphate. This disorder has been mapped to a region of chromosome 9 that contains the gene for the renal sodium-phosphate cotransporter NaPi-IIc. Mutations of this gene likely result in a complete loss of function of this protein in patients who have a homozygous single-nucleotide deletion.

Primary Hyperoxaluria and Cystinuria

Primary hyperoxaluria (PH) and cystinuria are each discussed later in this chapter (see "Specific Therapy and Etiology").

CLINICAL PRESENTATION AND EVALUATION

Kidney stones vary in clinical presentation from asymptomatic retained stones, to passage, to large, obstructing staghorn calculi that can significantly impair renal function and lead to end-stage renal disease.[4,79] The severity of stone disease depends on the pathogenetic factors contributing to the rate of stone formation in addition to stone type, size, and location.

In its most classic form, nephrolithiasis is manifested as renal colic. This discomfort of abrupt onset intensifies over time into an excruciating, severe flank pain that resolves only with stone passage or removal. The pain often migrates anteriorly along the abdomen and inferiorly to the groin, testicles, or labia majora as the stone moves toward the ureterovesical junction. Gross hematuria, urinary urgency and frequency, nausea, and vomiting may be present. Stones smaller than 5 mm are likely to pass spontaneously with hydration, whereas larger stones often necessitate urologic intervention for removal.

Certain disorders can lead to small, diffuse renal parenchymal calcifications, termed *nephrocalcinosis*.[4,24,76,80] The calcifications, usually calcium phosphate or calcium oxalate, may be present in the cortex or medulla. Among the most common causes of stone-related nephrocalcinosis are PH and medullary sponge kidney.

Metabolic Evaluation of Stone Formers

Although it is uniformly accepted that patients with multiple stones merit a thorough investigation into the cause of their nephrolithiasis, evaluation of the patient with a single stone is controversial. This probably reflects the difficulty in determining the cost-benefit ratio of stone evaluations and the wide differences in reported rates of stone recurrence.

The National Institutes of Health has convened several consensus conferences to resolve such issues related to the prevention and treatment of kidney stones.[3] These panels determined that all patients, even those with a single stone, should undergo at least a basic evaluation to rule out a systemic etiologic mechanism. Patients with an increase in number or size of stones (metabolically active stones), all children, all noncalcium stone formers, and all of those in demographic groups not typically susceptible to stone formation warrant a more complete metabolic evaluation (Fig. 30-2).[3]

The Basic Evaluation

Elements of the basic evaluation are listed in Table 30-2.

History

In addition to the medical history typically obtained from new patients, evaluation of the stone former includes a stone history and a thorough review of diet, fluid intake, and lifestyle. Specific laboratory studies and radiographic tests are also required.

Stone History. The stone history begins with a chronology of stone events: age at incidence of first stone, size and number of stones formed, frequency of passage, stone type if known, and whether the stones occur equally in both kidneys or unilaterally. Also helpful is a report of the patient's symptoms with each episode and the need for and response to surgical intervention.

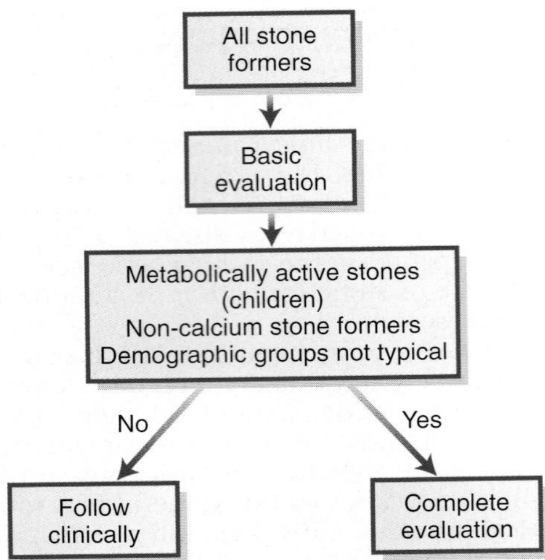

Figure 30-2 Evaluation of stone formers.

This information imparts not only the severity of the stone disease but also clues to the origin of the patient's nephrolithiasis. For example, nephrolithiasis that begins at a young age may be attributable to an inherited metabolic disorder such as PH or cystinuria. Large staghorn calculi that are difficult to eradicate and that recur despite frequent surgical intervention are more likely to be composed of struvite instead of calcium oxalate. Cystine stones are not disintegrated thoroughly with the use of lithotripsy, and alternative surgical modalities are usually required for stone removal. For patients who tend to form stones in only one kidney, the possibility of congenital abnormalities of that kidney, such as megacalyx or medullary sponge kidney, should be explored.

TABLE 30-2

The Basic Evaluation

History
- Stone history
- Medical history
- Family history

Medications
Occupation and Lifestyle
Diet and Fluid Intake
Physical Examination
Laboratory Tests
- Urinalysis
- Urine culture and sensitivity
- Cystine screening

Blood Tests
- Sodium, potassium, chloride, bicarbonate
- Calcium, phosphorus, uric acid, creatinine
- Intact parathyroid hormone if calcium is elevated or at upper limit of normal
- Tetrahydrodeoxycortisol, urinary free cortisol, and 25-hydroxyvitamin D_3 levels as appropriate

Stone Analysis
Radiology*
- Unenhanced helical (spiral) computed tomography
- Kidneys, ureter, and bladder examination
- Intravenous pyelography
- Ultrasonography

*Choose appropriate study as indicated; see text.
Adapted from Monk RD. Clinical approach to adults. *Semin Nephrol.* 1996;16:375-388; Monk RD, Bushinsky DA. Nephrolithiasis and nephrocalcinosis. In: Johnson R, Feehally J, eds. *Comprehensive Clinical Nephrology,* 3rd ed. London, UK: Mosby, 2007:641-655.

Medical History. Systemic disorders that can contribute to nephrolithiasis are sought in the medical history. Any disorder that can result in hypercalcemia, such as sarcoidosis or certain malignancies, may also lead to hypercalciuria. A variety of gastrointestinal disorders associated with malabsorption (e.g., sprue, Crohn's disease) can cause calcium oxalate nephrolithiasis on the basis of enteric hyperoxaluria. Patients with gout or insulin resistance are more likely to have uric acid stones (Tables 30-3 and 30-4).[15,17]

Family History. As noted earlier, a number of stone disorders are inherited, making the family history an important component of the basic evaluation. IH appears to be a familial disorder. Although the exact chromosomes and genes have not yet been identified, the pattern of inheritance is almost certainly polygenic.

Stones arising in childhood or young adulthood can be related to autosomal recessive disorders such as cystinuria and primary oxaluria. These genetic disorders are reviewed in the sections on treatment of cystine and oxalate stones.

The high prevalence of uric acid stones in certain areas of the world is suggestive of genetic as well as environmental risk factors. Genes that cause either excessively acidic urine or hyperuricosuria have been implicated.[2,4,17,23,80-83]

TABLE 30-3

Causes of Calcium Stone Formation

Hypercalciuria
- Cushing's syndrome
- Granulomatous diseases
- Hypercalcemic disorders
- Idiopathic hypercalciuria
- Immobilization
- Malignancy
- Milk-alkali syndrome
- Primary hyperparathyroidism
- Sarcoid
- Thyrotoxicosis

Medications (see Table 30-5)
Hyperoxaluria
- Biliary obstruction
- Chronic pancreatitis
- Crohn's disease
- Dietary hyperoxaluria (urine oxalate 40-60 mg/day)
- Enteric oxaluria (urine oxalate 60-100 mg/day)
- Jejunoileal bypass
- Malabsorptive disorders
- Primary hyperoxaluria types I and 2 (oxalate 80-300 mg/day)
- Sprue (celiac disease)

Hyperuricosuria (see Table 30-4)
Hypocitraturia
- Androgens
- Exercise
- Hypokalemia
- Hypomagnesemia
- Infection
- Metabolic acidosis
- Starvation

Renal tubular acidosis (distal, type I)
Anatomic genitourinary tract abnormalities
- Congenital megacalyx
- Medullary sponge kidney
- Tubular ectasia

Adapted from Monk RD. Clinical approach to adults. *Semin Nephrol.* 1996;16:375-388; Monk RD, Bushinsky DA. Nephrolithiasis and nephrocalcinosis. In: Johnson R, Feehally J, eds. *Comprehensive Clinical Nephrology,* 3rd ed. London, UK: Mosby, 2007:641-655; Bushinsky DA, Monk RD. Calcium. *Lancet.* 1998;352:306-311.

TABLE 30-4

Factors Associated with Noncalcium Stone Formation

Uric Acid Stones
Cushing's syndrome
Diarrhea
Diet high in animal protein
Excessive dietary purine
Excessive insensible losses
Genetic predisposition
Glucose-6-phosphatase deficiency
Gout
Hemolytic anemia
Hyperuricemia
Hyperuricosuria
Inadequate fluid intake
Inborn errors of metabolism
Insulin resistance
Intracellular to extracellular uric acid shift
Lesch-Nyhan syndrome
Low urine pH (<5.5)
Low urine volume
Malabsorptive disorders
Medications (see Table 30-5)
Metabolic syndrome
Myeloproliferative disorders
Obesity
Tumor lysis
Struvite Stones
Urease-producing bacteria
Proteus, Pseudomonas, Haemophilus, Yersinia, Ureaplasma, Klebsiella, Corynebacterium, Serratia, Citrobacter, Staphylococcus, and others
Never *Escherichia coli*—not a urease producer
High urine pH (~6.5)
Indwelling urinary catheter
Neurogenic bladder
Cystine Stones
Autosomal recessive trait
Excessive excretion of cystine, ornithine, lysine, and arginine
Low solubility of cystine (<250 mg/L)

Adapted from Monk RD. Clinical approach to adults. *Semin Nephrol.* 1996;16:375-388; Monk RD, Bushinsky DA. Nephrolithiasis and nephrocalcinosis. In: Johnson R, Feehally J, eds. *Comprehensive Clinical Nephrology,* 3rd ed. London, UK: Mosby, 2007:641-655.

Medications

Medications can contribute to stone formation in several ways. Calcium-containing supplements can increase the amount of calcium absorbed and subsequently excreted.[42] Loop diuretics can directly promote renal tubular excretion of calcium and are associated with nephrocalcinosis in neonates who have received the drug.[84,85] Acetazolamide, a weak diuretic, induces a mild metabolic acidosis and alkaline urine, favorable conditions for the development of calcium phosphate stones. Other medications, such as salicylates and probenecid, are implicated in uric acid lithiasis.

Certain crystals or stones can consist completely of precipitated medication. Such medications include intravenously administered acyclovir, triamterene, indinavir, and various sulfonamides (e.g., sulfadiazine). Oxalate is a metabolic end product of vitamin C, and large doses of vitamin C increase oxalate excretion and may predispose to stone formation (Table 30-5).[86,87]

Lifestyle and Diet

Occupation and lifestyle are aspects of the social history that can be relevant to stone formation. Surgeons and traveling salespeople, for example, tend to minimize fluid intake to avoid frequent micturition throughout the day. Loss of insensible fluid can also exacerbate nephrolithiasis and may be related to employment (e.g., construction work) or hobbies (e.g., running, gardening).

The evaluation proceeds with a thorough review of the patient's diet and fluid intake. Patients are asked to review what they eat at all meals and snacks. Particular attention is paid to ingestion of foods high in sodium (fast foods, canned foods, added salt or soy sauce) and the quantity of animal protein consumed (discussed later). Patients are also asked to list four or five favorite foods or snacks to assess whether they may be consuming foods high in oxalate or purine. Many patients are erroneously counseled by physicians to avoid calcium-containing foods. As discussed earlier, doing so may result in bone demineralization (a grave concern in women with stones) if renal tubular calcium reabsorption is inadequate, and is also associated with increased stone formation.[27,31,37]

Physical Examination

For most patients with nephrolithiasis, physical findings are normal, but in some, the findings reveal a systemic disorder related to the stone disease. For example, an enterocutaneous fistula may be associated with Crohn's disease, a common cause of enteric oxaluria. A paraplegic patient with an indwelling catheter may be susceptible to frequent urinary tract infections with urease-producing organisms and consequent struvite stone formation. Hyperuricosuria and uric acid stone formation may be seen in patients with tophi related to gout.[2,4]

TABLE 30-5

Medications Associated with Renal Lithiasis and Nephrocalcinosis

Medications That Promote Calcium Stone Formation
Acetazolamide
Amphotericin B
Antacids (calcium and noncalcium antacids)
Calcium supplements
Glucocorticoids
Loop diuretics
Theophylline
Vitamin C?
Vitamin D
Medications That Promote Uric Acid Lithiasis
Allopurinol (associated with xanthene stones)
Probenecid
Salicylates
Medications That Can Precipitate into Stones or Crystals
Acyclovir (when infused rapidly intravenously)
Indinavir
Nelfinavir
Sulfonamides
Triamterene

Adapted from Monk RD. Clinical approach to adults. *Semin Nephrol.* 1996;16:375-388; Monk RD, Bushinsky DA. Nephrolithiasis and nephrocalcinosis. In: Johnson R, Feehally J, eds. *Comprehensive Clinical Nephrology,* 3rd ed. London, UK: Mosby, 2007:641-655.

Laboratory Tests

Although valuable information is gleaned from the history and physical examination, it is often difficult to determine the metabolic cause of a patient's nephrolithiasis without laboratory data. The urinalysis is an easy and inexpensive test that provides a great deal of information. Uric acid and calcium oxalate stones grow more favorably at an acidic pH, and a consistently high urinary pH may suggest calcium phosphate or struvite nephrolithiasis. The specific gravity, if high, can confirm the suspicion of inadequate fluid intake.

Hematuria is often present in active stone disease. Microscopic examination of the urine in this case may reveal characteristic crystals. Bacteria and pyuria noted in conjunction with a high urinary pH (approximately 6.5) are characteristic of struvite stone disease. Urine specimens for culture should be obtained in such a setting. Because enough urease may be produced to form struvite stones even when colony counts are low (approximately 50,000 colony-forming units), the microbiology laboratory should be instructed specifically to identify the organism and to check for urease despite low colony counts.[88]

Qualitative cystine screening should be performed on a urine specimen. Urine turns purple-red when sodium nitroprusside is added to a specimen containing cystine at a concentration greater than 75 mg/L.[81]

Recommended blood tests in the basic evaluation include electrolytes (sodium, potassium, chloride, bicarbonate), serum creatinine to determine the overall renal function, uric acid, calcium, and phosphorus.[2,3] If the calcium level is elevated or at the upper limit of normal, or if the serum phosphorus level is reduced or at the lower limit of normal, a serum intact PTH level is also determined to rule out primary hyperparathyroidism. Low serum bicarbonate levels suggest a hypocitraturic disorder such as renal tubular acidosis or acetazolamide ingestion.

Stone Analysis

Stone analysis should be performed, whenever possible, in patients with a new history of nephrolithiasis and in patients with long-standing stone disease who note a difference in clinical presentation or in the color, shape, or texture of any stone passed. Knowing the constituents of a stone can help the physician target certain elements of the medical history and specific urine studies. In most cases, the stone must be sent to an outside laboratory for examination. X-ray diffraction crystallography and infrared spectroscopy are currently the most accurate methods available for stone analysis.[89]

Radiologic Evaluation

Various radiologic tests can help determine the location and extent of the stone burden and may elucidate genitourinary abnormalities contributing to stone formation. For acute renal colic, spiral (or helical) CT without contrast (unenhanced) has replaced intravenous pyelography (IVP) as the optimal modality for detection and localization of kidney stones. Helical CT has proved to be at least as sensitive and specific as IVP in detecting stones of all types in the kidneys and ureters. In addition, it can more accurately reveal causes of flank pain and hematuria not related to stones and requires no exposure to intravenous contrast material. Radiation exposure is a disadvantage of both CT and IVP, and the exposure to patients undergoing helical CT may be triple that of IVP. Therefore, it should be used judiciously, especially in young patients with frequent episodes of renal colic. Helical CT takes less time to perform, which is a potential advantage in an emergency department setting, but it tends to be more costly.[79,90-92]

CT should be followed by a plain film (radiograph) of the abdomen that includes the kidneys, ureter, and bladder (KUB). Plain films can assist in determining stone composition. Stones composed of calcium, cystine, or struvite are radiopaque and visible on KUB, whereas radiolucent stones, such as those composed of uric acid or xanthine, are not.

IVPs are useful in detecting certain genitourinary abnormalities that can predispose to nephrolithiasis, such as medullary sponge kidney and caliceal abnormalities. Another advantage of IVP is that the osmotic diuresis generated by the administered contrast agent may aid in excretion of the offending stone during an episode of acute renal colic. A major disadvantage of IVP is exposure to radiographic contrast material. Administration of contrast should be avoided in patients who are at high risk for development of nephrotoxicity from the contrast agent, such as elderly patients; those with diabetes mellitus, proteinuria, or preexisting kidney disease; and those with significant intravascular volume depletion.

Renal ultrasound is a useful test for patients who must avoid exposure to radiation or contrast agents, such as pregnant women and children. It is fairly specific but not as sensitive as spiral CT for detecting stones within the kidney. Visualization of ureteral stones is poor with ultrasound.

Once a patient is known to have a certain type of stone, specific tests may be used in follow-up. For example, a patient who is known to have asymptomatic calcium stones can have a KUB test 6 to 12 months later to assess for any increase in stone size or number.[2,4] However, radiation exposure should be limited to patients in whom the results of the test will alter treatment. Little is gained in asymptomatic patients by checking for stone growth or movement if maximal dietary and pharmacologic therapy is already being prescribed.

The Complete Evaluation

The complete evaluation comprises the entire basic examination as well as a 24-hour urine collection to determine volume and levels of calcium, oxalate, citrate, sodium, urate, phosphorus, and creatinine and supersaturation with respect to the common solid phases (Table 30-6). Creatinine is used to assess the adequacy of the collection; men should excrete approximately 15 to 20 mg/kg of creatinine per day, and women should excrete 10 to 15 mg/kg of creatinine per day. Cystine should also be measured in patients known to have cystine stones or in whom prior urine studies have not determined whether there is excessive excretion of this amino acid.

Patients should be instructed to collect the urine on a day when they perform usual activities and have their typical fluid and dietary intake. The first morning's urine specimen is discarded, and all urine for the next 24 hours (including the next morning's specimen) is collected in the container. The ideal 24-hour urine collection includes measurement and reporting of the daily excretion of the constituents listed in Table 30-6 and also the presence of supersaturation of calcium oxalate, calcium phosphate, or uric acid. Patients should be instructed to discontinue multivitamins approximately 5 days before the collection to prevent any antioxidant effect of the vitamins on the urine sample. In most cases, an acid or antibiotic is included in the collection container or added with the first urine sample as a preservative. Certain laboratories require various preservatives for the different factors measured.

TABLE 30-6

Optimal 24-Hour Urine Values in Patients with Nephrolithiasis

Parameter	Value
Volume	>2-2.5 L
pH	>5.5 and <7.0 (24-hr specimen not required)
Calcium	>300 mg or >3.5-4.0 mg/kg in men; >250 mg or >3.5-4.0 mg/kg in women
Oxalate	>40 mg
Sodium	>3000 mg or >130 mEq
Uric acid	>800 mg in men; >750 mg in women
Phosphorus	>1100 mg
Citrate	>320 mg
Creatinine	>15 mg/kg in men; >10 mg/kg in women in order to ensure adequacy of collection
Supersaturation of calcium oxalate	>5
Supersaturation of calcium phosphate	0.5-2* (ideally <1)
Supersaturation of uric acid	0-1*

*Ideal values can vary among laboratories that perform supersaturation analysis.

Physicians should ask their laboratory how many 24-hour urine collections and which preservatives are required for the complete evaluation. Several national laboratories simplify this process to a single urine collection on which all of the measurements are preformed and resultant supersaturation is calculated; this almost certainly improves adherence and perhaps the accuracy of the calculation of supersaturation.[2,93]

Patients who require the complete evaluation include all children, nonwhite patients (i.e., demographic groups not typically prone to nephrolithiasis in the United States), noncalcium stone formers, and patients with metabolically active stone disease (i.e., stones that grow in size or number within 1 year).[2-4]

THERAPY

Surgical Treatment

Treatment of an acute episode of renal colic often involves surgical management for large stones that do not pass spontaneously. Stones smaller than 5 mm in largest diameter have a 68% chance of passing spontaneously, whereas those larger than 5 mm but smaller than 10 mm have a spontaneous stone passage rate of less than 50%.[94] Most stones greater than 10 mm, and many of those between 5 and 10 mm in size, require surgical intervention for relief of renal colic, ureteral obstruction, or other symptoms of clinically active stone disease. With the advent of newer, less invasive urologic therapies, open surgical stone extraction is rarely done. Current urologic therapy includes extracorporeal shock-wave lithotripsy (ESWL), ureteroscopic extraction (URS), and percutaneous nephrolithotomy. The exact procedure used varies according to stone location in the kidney or ureter, size, composition, various patient factors, and surgical expertise.[94-97]

ESWL involves focusing sound waves from a machine outside the body onto the kidney stone. The impulses fragment the stone into smaller stones or "gravel" that can more easily be passed spontaneously. Newer-generation lithotripters do not require a water bath and often require less analgesia.[98] Kidney stones smaller than about 15 mm, proximal ureteral stones, upper- and middle-pole kidney stones, and those not composed of cystine or calcium oxalate monohydrate respond best to ESWL.[94,96-98] Because fluoroscopy is typically used to visualize radiopaque stones during the procedure, ESWL may be more complicated in patients with uric acid lithiasis. ESWL is relatively contraindicated in patients with coagulopathy and in pregnant women. It may be less successful in patients with a higher body mass index, because a low skin-to-stone distance is necessary to achieve optimal success.[97,98]

Ureteroscopy, the passage of a semirigid or flexible scope through the bladder and into the ureter, has become a mainstay of surgical stone extraction for most ureteral stones, especially distal ureteral stones, and larger proximal stones. Endocorporeal lithotripsy can be added to URS to directly fragment visualized stones. One of the more commonly used devices is the holmium:yttrium-aluminum-garnet (YAG) laser lithotripter, which combines both pneumatic and ultrasound lithotripsy to fragment stones. This results in high stone-free rates after the procedure.[95,99] Complications of ESWL and URS include urinary tract infection, sepsis, ureteral stricture, ureteral injury, and steinstrasse or "stone street"—the linear accumulation of small stones blocking a ureter after fragmentation of a larger stone.

Percutaneous nephrolithotomy involves placement of a large needle through the flank into the renal collecting system. The tract is dilated, and instruments are used to rupture and remove the stone. Although percutaneous nephrolithotomy is more invasive than ESWL and URS, it is more effective in removing large (>2 cm) or staghorn calculi and stones that do not fragment well with lithotripsy. Large, infected stones such as struvite stones, in which complete removal is desired, are best treated with percutaneous nephrolithotomy.[96,97]

Medical Expulsive Therapy

Another form of therapy that has been shown to reduce the time to stone passage is medical expulsive therapy. Several medications have demonstrated benefit in reducing the time to stone passage and in assisting with passage of larger stones.[100] Most of these, such as the calcium-channel blocker nifedipine (extended-release formulation, 30 mg taken daily or twice daily) and α-adrenergic receptor blockers such tamsulosin (0.4 mg daily by mouth), terazosin, and doxazosin act by reducing spasms of the ureteral smooth muscle and allowing ureteral peristalsis to more effectively move the stone through. The addition of corticosteroids may also assist with stone passage by reducing ureteral inflammation and swelling in the ureter where the stone is lodged.

In several prospective, randomized, controlled trials, calcium channel blockers and α-adrenergic blockers showed significant benefit in both the rate of successful stone passage and the time to passage. In the controlled studies, these therapies were compared with placebo[101] or with standard therapy such as antispasmodic therapy, nonsteroidal anti-inflammatory agents, or analgesics. In a few studies comparing α-adrenergic receptor blockers to calcium channel blockers, the α-blocker tamsulosin was found to result in higher stone passage rates and more rapid stone expulsion than nifedipine.[100,102,103] Both agents were generally well tolerated, although perhaps with less hypotension in the tamsulosin groups.

Medical expulsive therapy may be cautiously attempted for up to 4 weeks as long as pain is well controlled; the patient has normal, stable kidney function; no urinary tract infection is present; and the patient does not have an obstructed solitary kidney or bilateral obstruction. Frequent follow-up and occasional imaging with ultrasound are recommended to ensure that the patient remains free of complications while awaiting stone passage.

Medical Preventive Therapy

Medical preventive therapy is the mainstay of medical management. The remainder of the chapter focuses on this approach.

Nonspecific Therapy

Most patients, irrespective of stone type, are given general advice about fluid and dietary modification to prevent further stone formation. These nonpharmacologic interventions, which include an increase in fluid intake as well as restriction of dietary sodium and animal protein, can reduce the incidence of stone formation, a result termed the *stone clinic effect.*[27,28,104] In one study, such interventions resulted in a 40% decrease in stone recurrence over 5 years.[26]

The mainstay of nonspecific therapy involves dietary measures (see earlier discussion): increased fluid intake to raise urine volume to approximately 2 to 2.5 L, a reduction in sodium intake to less than 3000 mg/day (130 mEq/day), moderate reduction in animal protein ingestion to approximately 1.0 mg/kg per day, and, perhaps, eating certain fruits or juices high in citrate.[2,27-29,104-106] Dietary calcium restriction is no longer recommended because it not only reduces bone mineral content but also increases the rate of stone recurrence, presumably by decreasing intestinal calcium oxalate complexation and increasing urinary oxalate excretion.[27] In retrospective studies of dietary intake, both women and men were found to have reduced stone formation with increased dietary calcium ingestion. However, calcium supplements were associated with an increased risk of stones in women; patients should be advised to maintain an age- and gender-appropriate intake of dietary calcium, preferably without supplements.[27,31,37,42,107]

Specific Therapy and Etiology

The optimal therapy for patients with metabolically active stone disease is directed at the particular metabolic abnormality. Before medications for nephrolithiasis are prescribed, all patients should be treated with the nonspecific measures just noted. Before any therapeutic intervention, some clinicians assess the patient's existing stone burden with a radiologic examination (KUB, spiral CT, IVP, or ultrasonography). If stones are seen, the subsequent passage of stones would not necessarily indicate therapeutic failure. However, this approach must be weighed against the not insignificant cost of these procedures and the radiation exposure. In our practice, we do not obtain baseline radiographs in asymptomatic patients unless the results will alter subsequent therapy. The basic and complete evaluations help direct the clinician to the specific treatments discussed here.

Calcium Stones. Most kidney stones (approximately 70%) contain calcium (see Table 30-1). More than one third of these are composed of calcium oxalate alone, and another 7% are composed of calcium phosphate alone. The remainder are composed of a combination of calcium oxalate and either urate or calcium phosphate. The stones tend to be gray, brown, or tan and rarely grow larger than 1 to 2 cm.[2,25,89]

The main causes of calcium stone formation are hypercalciuria (excessive urinary calcium excretion), hyperoxaluria (excessive oxalate excretion), hyperuricosuria (excessive uric acid excretion), hypocitraturia (insufficient citrate excretion), renal tubular acidosis, congenital abnormalities of the genitourinary tract, and certain medications.

Hypercalciuria. Patients with persistent hypercalciuria often benefit from a thiazide diuretic. This class of drugs is inexpensive and extremely effective at reducing urinary calcium excretion and stone formation.[2,108]

To maximize the efficacy of thiazides, patients must consume a sodium-restricted diet. Whereas hydrochlorothiazide is commonly used for hypertension, chlorthalidone is favored for treatment of hypercalciuria because it has a longer half-life and requires only once-daily dosing. The starting dose is 25 mg and can be increased to 50 mg. In petite patients and in those with low blood pressure, therapy can be initiated with once-daily doses of 12.5 mg.

Side effects of thiazides include an increase in serum lipid levels and hyperglycemia. For patients in whom this is a concern, such as those with hypercholesterolemia, other cardiac risk factors, or elevated blood glucose levels, indapamide (1.25 to 2.5 mg) is an effective alternative.[109] This agent has less of an effect on serum lipids and blood sugar than thiazides.

Hypokalemia is another common side effect of thiazide therapy. Patients should be advised to increase their dietary intake of potassium-rich foods, and the potassium level should be checked 7 to 10 days after the medication is started. Hypokalemia can result not only in cardiac and neuromuscular problems but also in hypocitraturia, another risk factor for stone formation. The supplement of choice is potassium with a base, such as citrate or bicarbonate, as the accompanying anion.

Potassium citrate is available as a liquid or as a wax-matrix tablet. The wax-matrix form is preferable, because patients find the liquid unpalatable. However, patients with malabsorption disorders absorb potassium citrate better in the liquid form. Potassium citrate in the wax-matrix formulation is available in tablets of 5 or 10 mEq. Between 20 and 40 mEq/day in single or divided doses is usually adequate supplementation. Determination of follow-up potassium and bicarbonate levels may be required for further dose adjustment. Because citrate is a base, metabolic alkalosis can result with this medication, especially if it is given with a thiazide diuretic. An alternative potassium supplement (e.g., potassium chloride) may be required. If hypokalemia persists or if large doses of supplemental medication are required, the patient might benefit from the addition of a potassium-sparing diuretic. Triamterene is generally avoided because it can precipitate into stones. Amiloride may be initiated at a starting dose of 5 mg or in a combination tablet with thiazide.

After at least 4 weeks of therapy with the new medication, the 24-hour urine collection should be repeated to assess its efficacy in reducing calcium levels; 24-hour urinary sodium and citrate levels should also be measured. The thiazide dose may need to be increased to decrease calcium excretion to less than 3 to 4 mg/kg per day. If sodium excretion remains high in conjunction with elevated urinary calcium excretion, further dietary counseling aimed at reducing dietary sodium may be required. Additional potassium citrate may be required if urinary citrate or serum potassium levels remain low.[2,110]

Hyperoxaluria. Oxalate is produced predominantly by endogenous metabolism of glyoxylate and, to a lesser extent, by ascorbic acid. Some urinary oxalate is derived from dietary sources, such as rhubarb, cocoa, nuts, tea, and certain leafy green vegetables. Absorbed oxalate is excreted unchanged in the urine and raises urinary supersaturation with respect to calcium oxalate.[5,80,111,112] Hyperoxaluria, as the sole metabolic abnormality, accounts for the formation of only about 5% of all calcium stones.[23,113,114]

The three main causes of hyperoxaluria are excessive oxalate ingestion (dietary oxaluria), malabsorptive gastrointestinal disorders (enteric oxaluria), and excessive endogenous production of oxalate related to a hepatic enzyme deficiency (PH).

Because ethylene glycol (used as antifreeze in automobiles) is metabolized to oxalate, nephrolithiasis, in conjunction with severe metabolic acidosis and renal failure, is often observed in patients after ingestion of ethylene glycol.

Dietary Oxaluria. Dietary oxaluria results in urinary oxalate levels that are mildly elevated (40 to 60 mg/day). Many high-oxalate foods are fruits, vegetables, and nuts that are generally considered beneficial in most diets. In a retrospective analysis, patients consuming diets similar to the Dietary Approaches to Stop Hypertension (DASH) diet had fewer stones than those who consumed markedly different diets, despite the fact that the DASH diet is high in oxalate.[115] The diet is also high in potassium and calcium and low in sodium, factors that may be more preventive in stone formation than oxalate is detrimental. Patients with dietary hyperoxaluria should be provided with a detailed list of high-oxalate foods to review (Table 30-7). How restrictive patients need to be with regard to the list is unclear, and common sense should be used, especially because many patients with stones also have hypertension and diabetes mellitus and benefit from a diet that is high in fruits and vegetables.

Patients are instructed to ingest calcium-containing foods, such as a glass of milk, when eating foods high in oxalate. The calcium in milk binds the dietary oxalate and may prevent its absorption.[23,27] In patients who have severe dietary hyperoxaluria with active stone disease, 2 or 3 tablets of calcium carbonate (500 to 650 mg per tablet) may be prescribed to be taken with high-oxalate meals. This should be done cautiously, however, given the association between calcium supplements and kidney stones in women in the general population (see earlier discussion).

TABLE 30-7

Foods High in Oxalate

Beans (green and dried)
Beer: draft, stout, lager, pilsner
Beets
Berries: blackberries, blueberries, raspberries, strawberries, juice containing berries
Black tea
Black pepper
Celery
Chocolate, cocoa
Eggplant
Figs, dried
Greens: collard greens, dandelion greens, endive, escarole, kale, leeks, mustard greens, parsley, sorrel, spinach, Swiss chard, watercress
Green peppers
Lemon, lime, and orange peel
Nuts
Pecans, peanuts, peanut butter
Okra
Rhubarb
Sweet potato
Tofu

Adapted from Monk RD, Bushinsky DA. Nephrolithiasis and nephrocalcinosis. In: Johnson R, Feehally J, eds. *Comprehensive Clinical Nephrology,* 3rd ed. London, UK: Mosby, 2007:641-655; Wainer L, Resnik BA, Resnik MI. *Nutritional Aspects of Stone Disease.* Boston, MA: Martinus Nijhoff, 1987.

Enteric Oxaluria. Enteric oxaluria results in higher urinary oxalate levels (60 to 100 mg/day) than dietary hyperoxaluria. Gastrointestinal malabsorptive conditions associated with normal colonic function, such as Crohn's disease, celiac sprue, jejunoileal bypass, chronic pancreatitis, and biliary obstruction, can lead to enteric oxaluria. In these disorders, malabsorbed fatty acids bind calcium in the intestinal lumen, making more free oxalate available for absorption in the colon. In addition, the colonic mucosa becomes more permeable to oxalate as a result of exposure to malabsorbed bile salts.[116-118]

The mainstay of treatment, whenever possible, is therapy for the underlying disorder. A gluten-free diet can significantly reduce hyperoxaluria associated with sprue; for other conditions (e.g., surgical short-bowel syndrome), no specific therapy is feasible. In such cases, reduction of malabsorption and oxalate absorption may be achieved by instituting general therapy for steatorrhea, such as a low-fat diet, cholestyramine, and medium-chain triglycerides. As in patients with dietary oxaluria, an oxalate-restricted diet and calcium carbonate with meals should be prescribed (Fig. 30-3).[27,119] Because of chronic diarrhea, these patients are at substantial risk for low urine volumes, hypocitraturia, hypokalemia, and hypomagnesuria. The acidic, concentrated urine also predisposes to development of uric acid stones.[120,121] Additional fluid intake must be stressed, and potassium citrate (the liquid form is usually better absorbed, although poorly tolerated, in these patients) and magnesium supplementation are often prescribed. Magnesium appears to be an inhibitor of stone formation and is supplied as magnesium oxide at 400 mg by mouth twice a day or as magnesium gluconate at 0.5 to 1 g by mouth three times a day.[122]

Primary Hyperoxaluria. PH leads to nephrolithiasis because hepatic enzyme deficiencies in these patients result in massive endogenous oxalate production.[80,82,123] PH results not only in severe hyperoxaluria (80 to 300 mg/day) but also in widespread deposition of oxalate in numerous organs and tissues such as the heart, bone marrow, muscle, and renal parenchyma at a young age. Cardiomyopathy, bone marrow suppression, and renal failure can ensue. In type 1 PH, the deficient hepatic enzyme is alanine-glyoxylate aminotransferase (AGT), and the deficiency is caused by one of several mutations found in the AGT gene, *AGXT*. In type 2 PH, which is an even more uncommon disorder, patients lack D-glycerate reductase and glyoxylate reductase due to mutations in the gene *GRHPR*. In some patients with type 1 PH, pyridoxine (vitamin B_6) can increase enzyme activity, thereby reducing oxalate production.

All patients with PH should be treated with measures that reduce calcium oxalate precipitation, such as ample fluid supplementation, potassium citrate, magnesium, and orthophosphate. Orthophosphate is an effective inhibitor of calcium oxalate crystallization but should be avoided in patients who have a glomerular filtration rate of less than 50 mL/minute. *Oxalobacter forminges* is a bacterium that relies on oxalate for its metabolism.[36,124] In small studies, administration of these bacteria to patients with PH type 1 resulted in a very modest reduction in urinary oxalate excretion.[36] When commercially available, provision of

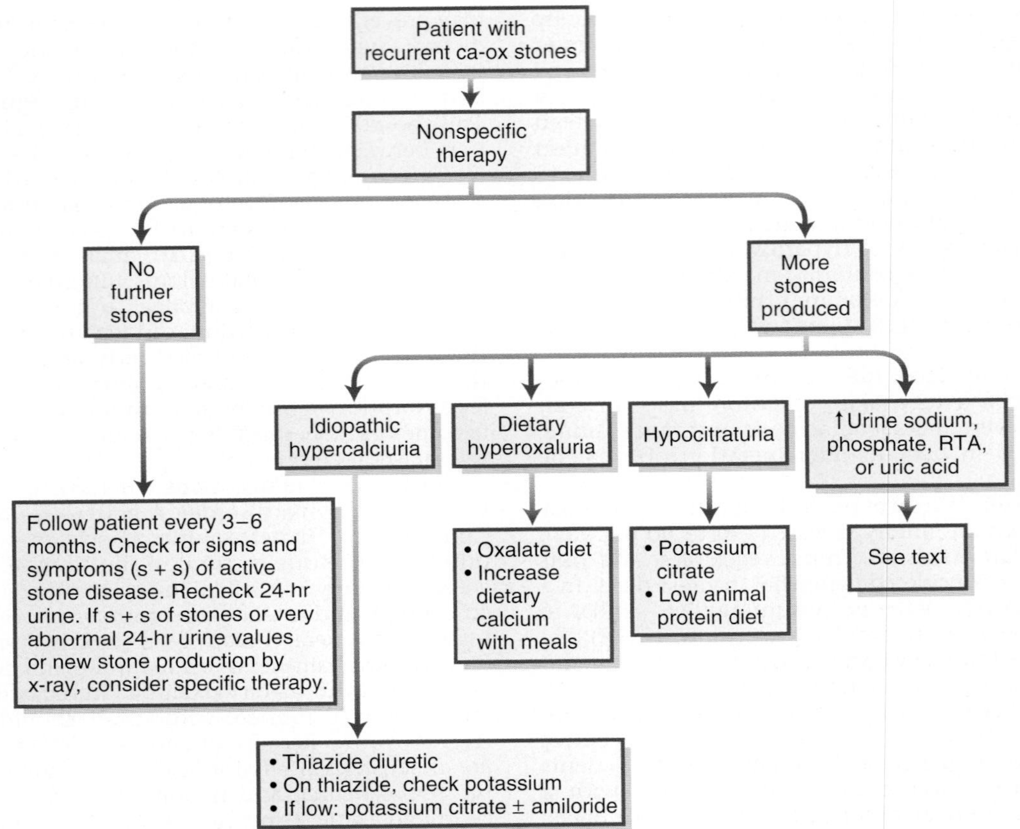

Figure 30-3 Treatment of the patient with recurrent calcium oxalate stones. ca-ox, calcium oxalate; RTA, Renal tubular acidosis.

these bacteria may provide additional therapy in the treatment of PH.

Patients with renal failure might benefit from renal transplantation, because dialysis is not as effective as a functioning kidney in oxalate removal. Measures to reduce calcium oxalate precipitation should be continued after renal transplantation to prevent rapid loss of the allograft from calcium oxalate deposition. Ultimately, for patients with type 1 PH, liver transplantation can supply the missing AGT and may be curative, especially if it is performed before the development of end-stage renal failure. Some patients require combined liver and kidney transplantation.[80,82,125]

Hyperuricosuria. Up to 15% of calcium stones are found in patients with hyperuricosuria. In contrast to patients with pure calcium oxalate stones, these patients typically have elevated urinary uric acid levels but normal urinary calcium and oxalate levels.[126,127] They also differ from patients with pure uric acid stones in that they tend to have a higher urinary pH (approximately 5.5).

The mechanism by which uric acid promotes calcium stone formation is unclear. The term "heterogeneous nucleation" or "epitaxy" has been used to describe the preferential formation of calcium oxalate crystals around a lattice of uric acid crystals present in the urine.[5,128,129] However, this mechanism has come into question. Grover and colleagues showed that the addition of sodium urate to urine or a similar solution increases calcium oxalate crystallization, with denser, more highly aggregated deposits, but no urate crystals form, and there is no increase in calcium oxalate supersaturation. They attributed this result to "salting out," a process in which the solubility of electrolytes (or salts) in a solution is reduced (or ion activity is increased) by the addition of different electrolytes or salts. In this case, the activity coefficients of calcium and oxalate would be increased not only by the concentrations of calcium and oxalate in the urine but also by the urate concentration.[130,131] This theory would explain why allopurinol is often an effective therapy for recalcitrant calcium oxalate nephrolithiasis, even in the absence of hyperuricosuria.[132,133] Another potential mechanism (not borne out by some studies) is that urate may reduce the concentration or the activity of urinary stone inhibitors.[134-136]

Whatever the mechanism, uric acid in the form of sodium urate is important in calcium oxalate crystal formation. Therapy has typically consisted of dietary purine restriction and increased fluid intake. If urinary uric acid levels remain uncontrolled with these measures, allopurinol, 100 to 300 mg/day, may be added.[126,127]

Hypocitraturia. Citrate combines with calcium to form a soluble complex that reduces calcium oxalate and calcium phosphate precipitation. In some patients, hypocitraturia is the principal metabolic abnormality found in the 24-hour urine collection. Risk factors for hypocitraturia include high protein intake, hypokalemia, metabolic acidosis, exercise, infection, starvation, androgens, and acetazolamide. Men tend to have lower urinary citrate concentrations than women, which may explain the higher incidence of stone formation in men. Furthermore, women with nephrolithiasis have lower urinary citrate concentrations than do non–stone-forming women.[137]

Along with therapy for the underlying condition, such as moderating dietary protein intake, potassium citrate is prescribed. This salt is preferable to sodium citrate because sodium excretion promotes calcium excretion. Again, potassium citrate in the wax-matrix formulation is preferred to the liquid preparation because of increased palatability. Large amounts (30 to 75 mEq/day) in divided doses may be required to raise the urinary citrate concentration to more than 320 mg/day. Potassium and bicarbonate levels should be closely monitored, especially in patients with CKD. If metabolic alkalosis or hyperkalemia ensues, reduction of the dose may be necessary.[110,138]

Renal Tubular Acidosis. dRTA is a disorder in which distal tubular hydrogen ion excretion is impaired, resulting in a non-anion gap metabolic acidosis and a persistently alkaline urine. The acidosis leads to calcium and phosphate release from bone as well as enhanced proximal tubular reabsorption of citrate and diminished tubular reabsorption of calcium. The net result is an increased filtered load and excretion of calcium and phosphate, severe hypocitraturia, and an elevated urinary pH, all of which promote calcium phosphate precipitation. Nephrocalcinosis, or renal parenchymal calcification, is frequently seen in this setting.

The 24-hour urinary citrate level is commonly less than 100 mg in patients with dRTA. Therapy consists of potassium citrate or potassium bicarbonate supplementation to treat both the metabolic acidosis and the hypocitraturia. Large doses of these medications are often required: 1 to 3 mEq/kg per day in two or three divided doses.[25,82,126]

Nephrocalcinosis. Nephrocalcinosis is a condition in which calcium is deposited in the renal parenchyma. There are two forms: dystrophic calcification and metastatic calcification.

In dystrophic calcification, calcium deposition arises from tissue necrosis secondary to neoplasm, infarction, or infection. It may be seen in the setting of renal transplant rejection, renal cortical necrosis, chronic glomerulonephritis, ethylene glycol toxicity, acquired immunodeficiency syndrome (AIDS)-related infections, or Alport's syndrome. In general, serum calcium and phosphorus levels are normal, and calcium phosphate deposition occurs predominantly in the renal cortex.

In metastatic calcification, patients often have elevated serum calcium and phosphate levels or an elevated urinary pH. Calcification in this setting occurs more commonly in the renal medulla. Common causes include RTA, primary hyperparathyroidism (or any disorder resulting in elevated serum calcium levels), medullary sponge kidney, papillary necrosis, PH, and administration of acetazolamide, amphotericin B, or triamterene. PH can result in both medullary and cortical calcifications.

Both medullary and cortical parenchymal calcifications are easily identified on ultrasonography and CT scanning, even before they can be detected on plain radiographs. Therapy consists of treatment of the underlying disorder whenever possible. Otherwise, measures aimed at reducing hypercalcemia, oxalosis, and hyperphosphatemia should be attempted.[24,43,139]

Uric Acid Stones. The prevalence of uric acid lithiasis is greater in Mediterranean countries than in the United States, where it accounts for 5% to 10% of all calculi formed, a prevalence that may be rising.[1] The incidence of uric acid stones in the United States appears to be rising in parallel with the epidemic of obesity and consequent insulin resistance, which results in a very low urine pH.[17,140] Uric acid stones tend to be round, smooth, and yellow-orange. Because they are radiolucent, they are not visible on plain films but can be detected by ultrasonography or CT or as filling defects on IVP. Uric acid is a purine metabolite and is also found in large quantities within cells. Most patients with uric acid stones have a reduced urinary pH. Other, less common causes are low urine volume and elevated urinary uric acid levels. Factors associated with uric acid stones are listed in Table 30-4.

Urine Volume and pH. Diarrhea and diets high in animal protein can also contribute to an acidic urinary pH. Any disorder that results in low urine volume (e.g., diarrheal disorders, diaphoresis, reduced fluid intake) can contribute to uric acid lithiasis. Uric acid is increasingly soluble at an alkaline urinary pH; urine with a pH of 6.5 can contain more than five times more uric acid than urine at pH 5.3 without inducing precipitation and can actually dissolve existing stones.[17,127]

There is evidence that uric acid stone formers have greater body weight and a higher incidence of insulin resistance and type 2 diabetes mellitus. Most of these patients have significantly lower urinary pH compared with non–uric acid stone formers. Insulin resistance can lead to impaired ammoniagenesis and ammonium excretion, resulting in excretion of more urinary hydrogen ions with anions other than ammonium and a lower urinary pH.[15,17,140,141]

Hyperuricosuria may be evident in patients who ingest large quantities of dietary purine or animal protein. Foods high in purine include organ meats, shellfish, certain fish, meat extracts, yeast, gravy, and stock (Table 30-8). Hyperuricemic disorders such as gout, myeloproliferative disorders, tumor lysis syndrome, and certain inborn errors of metabolism (e.g., glucose 6-phosphatase deficiency, Lesch-Nyhan syndrome) can also contribute to an increased urinary filtered load of uric acid. Certain medications such as salicylates and probenecid can be hyperuricosuric as well.[4,17,86]

Therapy for uric acid stones begins with nonspecific measures such as increasing fluid intake to maintain urine volume at about 3 L/day. A lowered animal protein diet is generally beneficial because the decreased endogenous acid production raises urinary pH.[32] Ideally, the urinary pH should be elevated to approximately 6.5 to 7.0, a level that can dissolve existing crystals and stones. A urinary pH higher than 7.0 should be avoided, because calcium phosphate deposition can result. A low-fructose diet may also be beneficial in reducing uric acid levels and hyperuricosuria (see earlier discussion).[36]

Potassium citrate at doses of 30 mEq by mouth twice a day or greater may be required to raise the urinary pH sufficiently. (The available potassium citrate preparations are discussed in the sections on Hypercalciuria and Hypocitraturia.) If the urinary pH cannot be raised adequately despite high doses of potassium citrate or if the dose prescribed results in hyperkalemia, the carbonic anhydrase inhibitor acetazolamide may be initiated and added to the treatment. Use of this medication results in an alkaline urine and mild systemic metabolic acidosis, a pattern

TABLE 30-8

Foods High in Purine

Organ meats: brain, heart, kidney, liver, sweetbreads
Meat extracts: bouillon, consommé, stock, gravy
Meat: beef, chicken, goose, lamb, pork
Shellfish: clams, mussels, scallops, shrimp, oysters
Fish: anchovies, fish roe, herring, mackerel, sardines, others
Certain vegetables: asparagus, cauliflower, kidney beans, lentils, lima beans, mushrooms, peas, spinach

Adapted from Monk RD, Bushinsky DA. Nephrolithiasis and nephrocalcinosis. In: Johnson R, Feehally J, eds. *Comprehensive Clinical Nephrology.* London, UK: Mosby, 2000:973-989; Wainer L, Resnik BA, Resnik MI. *Nutritional Aspects of Stone Disease.* Boston, MA: Martinus Nijhoff, 1987.

similar to that seen in dRTA. Again, the urinary pH should be maintained at less than 7.0 to avoid calcium phosphate precipitation.[126] Prescription of Nitrazine paper allows patients to monitor their urinary pH at various times of day and adjust their potassium citrate intake accordingly.

Patients with hyperuricemia are prescribed a low-purine diet to decrease uric acid production. Despite dietary intervention, hyperuricemia often persists, especially in patients with disorders of cellular metabolism. In this setting, allopurinol should be prescribed at a starting dose of 100 mg/day, increasing to 300 mg/day as needed.[5,142]

Although sodium bicarbonate can effectively alkalinize the urine, it should be avoided because the additional sodium excretion encourages sodium urate formation, which may result in further crystal formation (see "Hyperuricosuria").

Struvite Stones. Struvite stones have also been termed triple phosphate stones, magnesium ammonium phosphate stones, and infection stones. Although they make up only about 10% to 15% of all stones formed, most staghorn calculi (large stones that extend beyond a single renal calyx) are composed of struvite. The propensity of these stones to grow rapidly to a large size, to recur despite therapy, and to result in significant morbidity (and potential mortality) has also led to the appellation "stone cancer." Because infection with urease-producing bacteria must be present for these stones to form, severe renal infections as well as sepsis and loss of renal function can develop. Factors associated with struvite stones are listed in Table 30-4.

In contrast to other stone types, struvite stones occur with a higher incidence in women than in men, largely because of women's increased susceptibility to urinary tract infections. Other groups at risk for development of struvite stones because of urinary stasis or infection include elderly people and patients with neurogenic bladders, indwelling urinary catheters, spinal cord lesions, or genitourinary abnormalities. Even in the absence of stone analysis, struvite stones should be suspected in patients who have large stones, an alkaline urinary pH (approximately 7), and the presence of urease-producing urinary bacteria. Early detection and therapy are essential to prevent great potential morbidity.[88]

Urease-Producing Bacteria. The formation of struvite stones depends on the presence of both ammonium ions and an alkaline urinary pH—conditions met clinically only through the actions of urease-producing bacteria. Ammonium, magnesium, and carbonate apatite $[Ca_{10}(PO_4)_6CO_3]$ in the urine combine with phosphate, which is present in this setting in its trivalent form.

Numerous gram-negative and gram-positive bacteria, as well as *Mycoplasma* and yeast species, have been implicated in urease production. Bacterial species in which urease is frequently isolated include *Proteus, Haemophilus, Corynebacterium,* and *Ureaplasma. Escherichia coli,* despite its frequent role as a urinary tract pathogen, has not been shown to produce urease. Urease production adequate to stimulate stone formation may be present despite low bacterial colony counts. For this reason, the microbiology laboratory should be asked specifically to perform bacteria identification and to determine sensitivities even with colony counts lower than 100,000 colony-forming units. If no bacteria are isolated but a urease producer is suspected, special cultures for *Ureaplasma urealyticum,* a mycobacterium, should be ordered.[143]

Therapy for Struvite Stones. To eradicate struvite stones, early and aggressive medical and urologic management is required. Appropriate antibiotic therapy is essential but must be combined with long-term bacterial suppression and complete surgical or medical stone removal. ESWL is often adequate for fragmentation of stones smaller than 2 cm, but percutaneous nephrostolithotomy or a combination of the two procedures is usually required for larger stones. Antibiotics should be continued on the basis of cultures of any stone fragments retrieved. After approximately 2 weeks of antibiotic therapy, when the urine culture is sterile, the dose of antibiotic should be halved. Suppressive antibiotics should continue at this dose until monthly surveillance cultures remain sterile for three consecutive months. At this point, antibiotics may be discontinued as long as surveillance urine cultures are obtained monthly for 1 year.[143,144]

In addition to antimicrobial therapy, medical treatment may involve urease inhibition and chemolysis. In chemolysis, the kidney is irrigated with an acidic solution through a nephrostomy tube or ureteral catheter. Although this procedure is rarely used since the advent of less invasive surgical techniques, it may be useful in the dissolution of residual stone fragments. The solution most commonly used, 10% hemiacidrin, is composed of carbonic acid, citric acid, D-gluconic acid, and magnesium at a pH of 3.9. Chemolysis has been controversial because high mortality rates were reported in the past. The morbidity and mortality were mainly due to sepsis from instrumentation, local bacterial or fungal infections, and uroepithelial irritation rather than toxicity from the agents. With chemolysis used as an adjuvant to surgical removal, lower stone and infection recurrence rates have been reported.[145-147] The safety of the procedure remains in question because of the variety of techniques, stone burden, and comorbidities reported in the older literature, but with close monitoring of serum magnesium levels, intrapelvic pressures, infection, and obstruction to flow, it may have a supporting role in the treatment of large struvite stones.[143,145,148]

Urease inhibition has been shown to retard stone growth and to prevent new stone formation. It does not decrease bacterial counts and cannot eradicate existing stones. Combined with antimicrobial therapy, it serves primarily as palliative care for patients who cannot undergo definitive surgical management. The agent most commonly used is acetohydroxamic acid. These medications require adequate renal clearance for therapeutic efficacy and are contraindicated in patients with a glomerular filtration rate of less than 60 mL/minute. CKD increases the incidence of side effects of these medications, which are numerous and limit their use. Side effects that result in discontinuation of the drug include neurologic symptoms, gastrointestinal upset, hair loss, hemolytic anemia, and rash; these all resolve after discontinuation of the drug. Acetohydroxamic acid is also teratogenic. The starting dose of acetohydroxamic acid is 250 mg by mouth twice a day. If it is well tolerated for about 1 month, the dose is increased to 250 mg by mouth three times a day.[143]

Cystine Stones. Cystinuria is an autosomal disorder that may be recessive or dominant with incomplete penetrance.[149] The disorder is caused by mutations in two members of the solute carrier family, encoded by the *SLC3A1* gene on chromosome 2 and the *SLC7A9* gene on chromosome 19, both of which result in decreased renal tubular reabsorption and excessive urinary excretion of the dibasic amino acids cystine, ornithine, lysine, and arginine. The genetic defect would probably go unnoticed were it not for the low solubility of cystine, approximately 300 mg/L. Factors associated with cystine stones are listed in Table 30-4.

People with no tubular defect in cystine transport excrete approximately 30 to 50 mg of cystine per day; heterozygotes excrete about 400 mg/day, and homozygotes excrete larger amounts, often more than 600 mg/day.[81] Cystinuria should not be confused with cystinosis, a more serious and debilitating disorder that results in extensive intracellular cystine accumulation.

Stones usually develop in patients within the second or third decade. The stones can grow to a large size and can appear as staghorn calculi or multiple stones. They are radiopaque because of the sulfur content of cystine. The disease should be suspected in any patient with stone onset in childhood, frequent recurrence of nephrolithiasis, and a strong family history of the disease. The presence of the classic hexagonal cystine crystals in the urine can verify the diagnosis. Because these crystals might not be evident in dilute or alkaline urine, qualitative screening with the sodium nitroprusside test better confirms the presence of cystinuria at a concentration greater than 75 mg/L. Quantitative cystine measurement with a 24-hour urine sample should follow to determine the risk of stone formation and to guide therapy.

Therapy for Cystine Stones. The aim of treatment is to lower the urinary cystine concentration below the limits of solubility (approximately 300 mg/L). Patients are advised to drink large quantities of fluids. A patient with a cystine excretion of 750 mg/day should drink enough fluid to increase urine output to more than 3 L/day. Large quantities of milk should be avoided, because dairy products and foods high in protein contain large amounts of methionine, an essential amino acid that is a precursor of cystine.[150] Juices are encouraged because they tend to alkalinize the urine and cystine is more soluble at a higher pH. Potassium citrate (see "Hypercalciuria" and "Hypocitraturia" for details) is also prescribed to maintain the urinary pH between 6.5 and 7.0.

Approximately 50% of cystine stones are mixed stones. Patients with cystinuria often have other metabolic defects such as hypercalciuria, hypocitraturia, and hyperuricosuria. Therefore, a complete 24-hour urine collection for all stone-forming elements is necessary to treat nephrolithiasis fully in this setting.

If these measures are inadequate in controlling stone formation, or if the urinary cystine concentration is too high to make adequate fluid intake practical, chelating agents may be added. D-Penicillamine is a chelating agent that reduces the cystine concentration by forming a more soluble compound with cystine. The medication is associated with numerous serious side effects that limit its use. Second-generation and third-generation chelating agents such as α-mercaptoproprionylglycine and bucillamine are now available that reduce the cystine concentration with fewer side effects.[81,151,152]

ACKNOWLEDGMENTS

This work was supported in part by grants RO1 DK 56788 and RO1 AR 46289 from National Institutes of Health and grants from the Renal Research Institute (all to David A. Bushinsky).

REFERENCES

1. Stamatelou KK, Francis ME, Jones CA, et al. Time trends in reported prevalence of kidney stones in the United States: 1976-1994. *Kidney Int.* 2003;63:1817-1823.
2. Monk RD. Clinical approach to adults. *Semin Nephrol.* 1996;16:375-388.
3. Consensus Conference. Prevention and treatment of kidney stones. *JAMA.* 1988;260:977-981.
4. Monk RD, Bushinsky DA. Nephrolithiasis and nephrocalcinosis. In: Frehally J, Floege J, Johnson RJ, eds. *Comprehensive Clinical Nephrology.* London, UK: Mosby; 2007:641-655.
5. Bushinsky DA, Coe FL, Moe OW. Nephrolithiasis. In: Brenner BM, ed. *The Kidney.* Philadelphia, PA: WB Saunders; 2008:1299-1349.
6. Gillen DL, Worcester EM, Coe FL. Decreased renal function among adults with a history of nephrolithiasis: a study of NHANES III. *Kid Int.* 2005;67:685-690.
7. Rule AD, Bergstralh EJ, Melton III LJ, et al. Kidney stones and the risk for chronic kidney disease. *Clin J Am Soc Nephrol.* 2009;4:804-811.
8. Chen N, Wang W, Huang Y, et al. Community-based study on CKD subjects and the associated risk factors. *Nephrol Dial Transplant.* 2009;24:2117-2123.
9. Stankus N, Hammes M, Gillen D, et al. African American ESRD patients have a high pre-dialysis prevalence of kidney stones compared to NHANES III. *Urol Res.* 2007;35:83-87.
10. Sakhaee K. Nephrolithiasis as a systemic disorder. *Curr Opin Nephrol Hypertens.* 2008;17:304-309.
11. Anavekar NS, McMurray JJ, Velazquez EJ, et al. Relation between renal dysfunction and cardiovascular outcomes after myocardial infarction. *N Engl J Med.* 2004;351:1285-1295.
12. Go AS, Chertow GM, Fan D, et al. Chronic kidney disease and the risks of death, cardiovascular events, and hospitalization. *N Engl J Med.* 2004;351:1296-1305.
13. Weiner DE, Tighiouart H, Amin MG, et al. Chronic kidney disease as a risk factor for cardiovascular disease and all-cause mortality: a pooled analysis of community-based studies. *J Am Soc Nephrol.* 2004; 15:1307-1315.
14. Soucie JM, Thun MJ, Coates RJ, et al. Demographic and geographic variability of kidney stones in the United States. *Kidney Int.* 1994;46:893-899.
15. Moe OW. Kidney stones: pathophysiology and medical management. *Lancet.* 2006;367:333-344.
16. Soucie JM, Coates RJ, McClellan W, et al. Relation between geographic variability in kidney stones prevalence and risk factors for stones. *Am J Epidemiol.* 1996;143:487-495.
17. Maalouf NM, Cameron.MA, Moe OW, et al. Novel insights into the pathogenesis of uric acid nephrolithiasis. *Curr Opin Nephrol Hypertens.* 2004;13:181-189.
18. Mandel N. Mechanism of stone formation. *Semin Nephrol.* 1996;16:364-374.
19. Hau AK, Kwan TH, Li PK. Melamine toxicity and the kidney. *J Am Soc Nephrol.* 2009;20:245-250.
20. Bhalla V, Grimm PC, Chertow GM, et al. Melamine nephrotoxicity: an emerging epidemic in an era of globalization. *Kidney Int.* 2009;75:774-779.
21. Guan N, Fan Q, Ding J, et al. Melamine-contaminated powdered formula and urolithiasis in young children. *N Engl J Med.* 2009; 360:1067-1074.
22. Evan AP, Lingeman JE, Coe FL, et al. Randall plaque of patients with nephrolithiasis begins in basement membranes of thin loops of Henle. *J Clin Invest.* 2003;111:607-616.
23. Coe FL, Evan A, Worcester E. Kidney stone disease. *J Clin Invest.* 2005;115:2598-2608.
24. Sayer JA, Carr G, Simmons NL. Nephrocalcinosis: molecular insights into calcium precipitation within the kidney. *Clin Sci.* 2004; 106:549-561.
25. Bushinsky DA. Renal lithiasis. In: Humes HD, ed. *Kelly's Textbook of Medicine.* New York, NY: Lippincott Williams & Wilkens; 2000: 1243-1248.
26. Borghi L, Meschi T, Amato F, et al. Urinary volume, water, and recurrences in idiopathic calcium nephrolithiasis: a 5-year randomized prospective study. *J Urol.* 1996;155:839-843.
27. Lemann Jr J, Pleuss JA, Worcester EA, et al. Urinary oxalate excretion increases with body size and decreases with increasing dietary calcium intake among healthy adults. [Erratum: Kidney Int 50:341,1996.] *Kidney Int.* 1996;49:200-208.
28. Hosking DH, Erickson SB, Van Den Berg CJ, et al. The stone clinic effect in patients with idiopathic calcium urolithiasis. *J Urol.* 1983;130:1115-1118.
29. Muldowney FP, Freaney R, Moloney MF. Importance of dietary sodium in the hypercalciuria syndrome. *Kidney Int.* 1972;22:292-296.
30. Lemann Jr J, Worcester EA, Gray RW. Hypercalciuria and stones. Finlayson Colloquium on Urolithiasis. *Am J Kidney Dis.* 1991;17: 386-391.
31. Borghi L, Schianchi T, Meschi T, et al. Comparison of two diets for the prevention of recurrent stones in idiopathic hypercalciuria. *N Eng J Med.* 2002;346:77-84.
32. Lemann Jr J, Bushinsky DA, Hamm LL. Bone buffering of acid and base in humans. *Am J Physiol Renal Physiol.* 2003;285:F811-F832.
33. Bushinsky DA. Acid-base balance and bone health. In: Holick MF, Dawson-Hughes B, eds. *Nutrition and Bone Health.* Totowa, NJ: Humana; 2004:279-304.

34. Hamm LL. Renal handling of citrate. *Kidney Int.* 1990;38:728-735.
35. Bataille P, Achard JM, Fournier A, et al. Diet, vitamin D and vertebral mineral density in hypercalciuric calcium stone formers. *Kidney Int.* 1991;39:1193-1205.
36. Taylor EN, Curhan GC. Fructose consumption and the risk of kidney stones. *Kidney Int.* 2007;73:207-212.
37. Curhan GC, Willett WC, Rimm EB, et al. A prospective study of dietary calcium and other nutrients and the risk of symptomatic kidney stones. *N Engl J Med.* 1993;328:833-838.
38. Bushinsky DA. Recurrent hypercalciuric nephrolithiasis: does diet help? *N Eng J Med.* 2002;346:124-125.
39. Coe FL, Favus MJ, Crockett T, et al. Effects of low-calcium diet on urine calcium excretion, parathyroid function and serum 1,25(OH)2D3 levels in patients with idiopathic hypercalciuria and in normal subjects. *Am J Med.* 1982;72:25-32.
40. Freundlich M, Alonzo E, Bellorin-Font E, et al. Reduced bone mass in children with idiopathic hypercalciuria and in their asymptomatic mothers. *Nephrol Dial Transplant.* 2002;17:1396-1401.
41. Standing Committee on the Scientific Evaluation of Dietary Reference Intakes, Food and Nutrition Board, Institute of Medicine. *Dietary Reference Intakes for Calcium, Phosphorus, Magnesium, Vitamin D, and Fluoride.* Washington, DC: National Academy Press; 1997.
42. Jackson RD, LaCroix AZ, Gass M, et al. Calcium plus vitamin D supplementation and the risk of fractures. *N Engl J Med.* 2006;354:669-683.
43. Moe OW, Bonny O. Genetic hypercalciuria. *J Am Soc Nephrol.* 2005;16:729-745.
44. Monk RD, Bushinsky DA. Pathogenesis of idiopathic hypercalciuria. In: Coe F, Favus M, Pak C, et al. eds. *Kidney Stones: Medical and Surgical Management.* Philadelphia, PA: Lippincott-Raven; 1996:759-772.
45. Bushinsky DA, Monk RD. Calcium. *Lancet.* 1998;352:306-311.
46. Lemann Jr J. Pathogenesis of idiopathic hypercalciuria and nephrolithiasis. In: Coe FL, Favus MJ, eds. *Disorders of Bone and Mineral Metabolism.* New York, NY: Raven Press, Ltd.; 1992:685-706.
47. Coe FL, Favus MJ, Asplin JR. Nephrolithiasis. In: Brenner BM, Rector Jr FC, eds. *The Kidney.* Philadelphia, PA: WB Saunders; 2004: 1819-1866.
48. Kaplan RA, Haussler MR, Deftos LJ, et al. The role of 1,25 dihydroxyvitamin D in the mediation of intestinal hyperabsorption of calcium in primary hyperparathyroidism and absorptive hypercalciuria. *J Clin Invest.* 1977;59:756-760.
49. Asplin JR, Bauer KA, Kinder J, et al. Bone mineral density and urine calcium excretion among subjects with and without nephrolithiasis. *Kidney Int.* 2003;63:662-669.
50. Pak CYC, Odvina CV, Pearle MS, et al. Effect of dietary modification on urinary stone risk factors. *Kidney Int.* 2005;68:2264-2273.
51. Pak CYC, Ohata M, Lawrence EC, et al. The hypercalciurias: causes, parathyroid functions, and diagnostic criteria. *J Clin Invest.* 1974;54:387-400.
52. Yao J, Karnauskas AJ, Bushinsky DA, et al. Regulation of renal calcium-sensing receptor gene expression in response to 1,25(OH)2D3 in genetic hypercalciuric stone-forming rats. *J Am Soc Nephrol.* 2005;16:1300-1308.
53. Bushinsky DA, Asplin JR. Thiazides reduce brushite, but not calcium oxalate, supersaturation and stone formation in genetic hypercalciuric stone-forming rats. *J Am Soc Nephrol.* 2005;16:417-424.
54. Bushinsky DA, Frick KK, Nehrke K. Genetic hypercalciuric stone-forming rats. *Curr Opinion Nephrol Hyperten.* 2006;15:403-418.
55. Bushinsky DA, Parker WR, Asplin JR. Calcium phosphate supersaturation regulates stone formation in genetic hypercalciuric stone-forming rats. *Kidney Int.* 2000;57:550-560.
56. Bushinsky DA, Asplin JR, Grynpas MD, et al. Calcium oxalate stone formation in genetic hypercalciuric stone-forming rats. *Kidney Int.* 2002;61:975-987.
57. Hoopes Jr RR, Middleton FA, Sen S, et al. Isolation and confirmation of a calcium excretion quantitative trait locus on chromosome 1 in genetic hypercalciuric stone-forming congenic rats. *J Am Soc Nephrol.* 2006;17:1292-1304.
58. Bushinsky DA, Favus MJ. Mechanism of hypercalciuria in genetic hypercalciuric rats: inherited defect in intestinal calcium transport. *J Clin Invest.* 1988;82:1585-1591.
59. Kim M, Sessler NE, Tembe V, et al. Response of genetic hypercalciuric rats to a low calcium diet. *Kidney Int.* 1993;43:189-196.
60. Pak CY. Nephrolithiasis. *Current Ther Endo Metab.* 1997;6:572-576.
61. Krieger NS, Stathopoulos VM, Bushinsky DA. Increased sensitivity to 1,25(OH)2D3 in bone from genetic hypercalciuric rats. *Am J Physiol (Cell Physiol).* 1996;271:C130-C135.
62. Grynpas M, Waldman S, Holmyard D, et al. Genetic hypercaliuric stone-forming rats have a primary decrease in bone mineral density and strength. *J Bone Miner Res.* 2009;24:1420-1426.
63. Bushinsky DA, Neumann KJ, Asplin J, et al. Alendronate decreases urine calcium and supersaturation in genetic hypercalciuric rats. *Kidney Int.* 1999;55:234-243.
64. Tsuruoka S, Bushinsky DA, Schwartz GJ. Defective renal calcium reabsorption in genetic hypercalciuric rats. *Kidney Int.* 1997;51: 1540-1547.
65. Karnauskas AJ, van Leeuwen JP, van den Bemd GJ, et al. Mechanism and function of high vitamin D receptor levels in genetic hypercalciuric stone-forming rats. *J Bone Min Res.* 2005;20:447-454.
66. Li X-Q, Tembe V, Horwitz GM, et al. Increased intestinal vitamin D receptor in genetic hypercalciuric rats: a cause of intestinal calcium hyperabsorption. *J Clin Invest.* 1993;91:661-667.
67. Favus MJ, Karnauskas AJ, Parks JH, et al. Peripheral blood monocyte vitamin D receptor levels are elevated in patients with idiopathic hypercalciuria. *J Clin Endocrinol Metab.* 2004;89:4937-4943.
68. Gambaro G, Vezzoli G, Casari G, et al. Genetics of hypercalciuria and calcium nephrolithiasis: from the rare monogenic to the common polygenic forms. *Am J Kidney Dis.* 2004;44:963-986.
69. Thorleifsson G, Holm H, Edvardsson V, et al. Sequence variants in the CLDN14 gene associate with kidney stones and bone mineral density. *Nat Genet.* 2009;41:926-930.
70. Scheinman SJ, Guay-Woodford LM, Thakker RV, et al. Genetic disorders of renal electrolyte transport. *N Engl J Med.* 1999;340: 1177-1187.
71. Lloyd SE, Pearce SH, Fisher SE, et al. A common molecular basis for three inherited kidney stone diseases. *Nature.* 1996;379:445-449.
72. Frick KK, Bushinsky DA. Molecular mechanisms of primary hypercalciuria. *J Am Soc Nephrol.* 2003;14:1082-1095.
73. Naesens M, Steels P, Verberckmoes R, et al. Bartter's and Gitelmans' syndromes: from gene to clinic. *Nephron Phys.* 2004;96:65-78.
74. Hou J, Renigunta A, Gomes AS, et al. Claudin-16 and claudin-19 interaction is required for their assembly into tight junctions and for renal reabsorption of magnesium. *Proc Natl Acad Sci U S A.* 2009;106: 15350-15355.
75. Hou J, Renigunta A, Konrad M, et al. Claudin-16 and claudin-19 interact and form a cation-selective tight junction complex. *J Clin Invest.* 2008;118:619-628.
76. Nicoletta JA, Schwartz GJ. Distal renal tubular acidosis. *Current Opin Pediatr.* 2004;16:194-198.
77. Bergwitz C, Roslin NM, Tieder M, et al. SLC34A3 mutations in patients with hereditary hypophosphatemic rickets with hypercalciuria predict a key role for the sodium-phosphate cotransporter NaPi-IIc in maintaining phosphate homeostasis. *Am J Hum Genet.* 2006;78:179-192.
78. Levi M, Blaine J, Breusegem S, et al. Renal phosphate-wasting disorders. *Adv Chron Kidney Dis.* 2006;13:155-165.
79. Teichman JMH. Acute renal colic from ureteral calculus. *N Engl J Med.* 2004;350:684-693.
80. Milliner DS. The primary hyperoxalurias: an algorithm for diagnosis. *Am J Nephrol.* 2005;25:154-160.
81. Sakhaee K. Pathogenesis and medical management of cystinuria. *Semin Nephrol.* 1996;16:435-447.
82. Danpure CJ. Molecular etiology of primary hyperoxaluria type 1: new direction for treatment. *Am J Nephrol.* 2005;25:303-310.
83. Nehrke K, Arreola J, Nguyen HV, et al. Loss of hyperpolarization-activated Cl^- current in salivary acinar cells from Clcn2 knockout mice. *J Biol Chem.* 2002;277:23604-23611.
84. Gimpel C, Krause A, Franck P, et al. Exposure to furosemide as the strongest risk factor for nephrocalcinosis in preterm infants. *Pediatr Int.* 2009. 52:51-56.
85. Schell-Feith EA, Kist-van Holthe JE, Conneman N, et al. Etiology of nephrocalcinosis in preterm neonates: association of nutritional intake and urinary parameters. *Kidney Int.* 2000;58:2102-2110.
86. Daudon M, Jungers P. Drug-induced renal calculi: epidemiology, prevention and management. *Drugs.* 2004;64:245-275.
87. Taylor EN, Curhan GC. Determinants of 24-hour urinary oxalate excretion. *Clin J Am Soc Nephrol.* 2008;3:1453-1460.
88. Rodman JS. Struvite stones. *Nephron.* 1999;81(suppl 1):50-59.
89. Mandel GS, Mandel N. Analysis of stones. In: Coe FL, Favus MJ, Pak CYC, et al., eds. *Kidney Stones: Medical and Surgical Management.* Philadelphia, PA: Lippincott-Raven; 1996:323-335.
90. Denton ER, Mackenzie A, Greenwell T, et al. Unenhanced helical CT for renal colic: is the radiation dose justifiable? *Clin Radiol.* 1999;54:444-447.
91. Smith RC, Coll DM. Helical computed tomography in the diagonosis of ureteric colic. *BJU Int.* 2000;86(suppl 1):33-41.
92. Nakada SY, Hoff DG, Attai S, et al. Determination of stone composition by noncontrast spiral computed tomography in the clinical setting. *Urology.* 2000;55:816-819.
93. Parks JH, Coward M, Coe FL. Correspondence between stone composition and urine supersaturation in nephrolithiasis. *Kidney Int.* 1997;51:894-900.
94. Preminger GM, Tiselius HG, Assimos DG, et al. 2007 Guideline for the management of ureteral calculi. *J Urol.* 2007;178:2418-2434.
95. Sofer M, Watterson JD, Wollin TA, et al. Holmium:YAG laser lithotripsy for upper urinary tract calculi in 598 patients. *J Urol.* 2002;167: 31-34.
96. Wignall GR, Canales BK, Denstedt JD, et al. Minimally invasive approaches to upper urinary tract urolithiasis. *Urol Clin North Am.* 2008;35:441-454, viii.
97. Samplaski MK, Irwin BH, Desai M. Less-invasive ways to remove stones from the kidneys and ureters. *Cleve Clin J Med.* 2009;76:592-598.

98. Putman SS, Hamilton BD, Johnson DB. The use of shock wave lithotripsy for renal calculi. *Curr Opin Urol*. 2004;14:117-121.
99. Leveillee RJ, Lobik L. Intracorporeal lithotripsy: which modality is best? *Curr Opin Urol*. 2003;13:249-253.
100. Beach MA, Mauro LS. Pharmacologic expulsive treatment of ureteral calculi. *Ann Pharmacother*. 2006;40:1361-1368.
101. Borghi L, Meschi T, Amato F, et al. Nifedipine and methylprednisolone in facilitating ureteral stone passage: a randomized, double-blind, placebo-controlled study. *J Urol*. 1994;152:1095-1098.
102. Porpiglia F, Ghignone G, Fiori C, et al. Nifedipine versus tamsulosin for the management of lower ureteral stones. *J Urol*. 2004; 172:568-571.
103. Dellabella M, Milanese G, Muzzonigro G. Randomized trial of the efficacy of tamsulosin, nifedipine and phloroglucinol in medical expulsive therapy for distal ureteral calculi. *J Urol*. 2005;174:167-172.
104. Uribarri J, Oh MS, Carroll HJ. The first kidney stone. *Kidney Int*. 1989;111:1006-1009.
105. Meschi T, Schianchi T, Ridolo E, et al. Body weight, diet and water intake in preventing stone disease. *Urol Int*. 2004;72:29-33.
106. Meschi T, Maggiore U, Fiaccadori E, et al. The effect of fruits and vegetables on urinary stone risk factors. *Kidney Int*. 2004;66:2402-2410.
107. Curhan GC, Willett WC, Speizer FE, et al. Comparison of dietary calcium with supplemental calcium and other nutrients as factors affecting the risk for kidney stones in women. *Ann Intern Med*. 1997;126:497-504.
108. Coe FL, Parks JH, Bushinsky DA, et al. Chlorthalidone promotes mineral retention in patients with idiopathic hypercalciuria. *Kidney Int*. 1988;33:1140-1146.
109. Borghi L, Meschi T, Guerra A, et al. Randomized prospective study of a nonthiazide diuretic, indapamide, in preventing calcium stone recurrences. *J Cardiovasc Pharmacol*. 1993;22(suppl 6):S78-S86.
110. Pak CYC, Fuller C, Sakhaee K, et al. Long-term treatment of calcium oxalate nephrolithiasis with potassium citrate. *J Urol*. 1985;134:11-19.
111. Hatch M, Freel RW. Intestinal transport of an obdurate anion: oxalate. *Urol Res*. 2005;33:1-16.
112. Jaeger P, Robertson WG. Role of dietary intake and intestinal absorption of oxalate in calcium stone formation. *Nephron Phys*. 2004;98:64-71.
113. Holmes RP, Goodman HO, Assimos DG. Contribution of dietary oxalate to urinary oxalate excretion. *Kid Int*. 2001;59:270-276.
114. Parks JH, Worcester EM, O'Connor RC, et al. Urine stone risk factors in nephrolithiasis patients with and without bowel disease. *Kid Int*. 2003;63:255-265.
115. McIntyre CW. Calcium balance during hemodialysis. *Semin Dial*. 2008;21:38-42.
116. Barilla DE, Notz C, Kennedy D, et al. Renal oxalate excretion following oral oxalate loads in patients with ileal disease and with renal and absorptive hypercalciurias: effect of calcium and magnesium. *Am J Med*. 1978;64:579-585.
117. Hatch M, Freel RW, Goldner AM, et al. Comparison of effects of low concentrations of ricinoleate and taurochenodeoxycholate on colonic oxalate and chloride absorption. *Gastroenterology*. 1983;84:1181.
118. Hatch M, Freel RW, Goldner AM, et al. Effect of bile salt on active oxalste transport in the colon. In: Kasper H, Goebell H, eds. *Colon and Nutrition*. Lancaster, England: MTP; 1981:299-305.
119. Nordenvall B, Backman L, Larsson L, et al. Effects of calcium, aluminum, magnesium and cholestyramine on hyperoxaluria in patients with jejunoileal bypass. *Acta Chir Scand*. 1983;149:93-98.
120. Clarke AM, McKenzie RG. Ileostomy and the risk of urinary uric acid stones. *Lancet*. 1969;2:395-397.
121. Rudman D, Dedonis JL, Fountain MT, et al. Hypocituria in patients with gastrointestinal malabsorption. *N Engl J Med*. 1980;303:657-661.
122. Worcester EM. Stones due to bowel disease. In: Coe FL, Favus MJ, Pak CYC, et al, eds. *Kidney Stones: Medical and Surgical Management*. Philadelphia, PA: Lippincott-Raven; 1996:883-903.
123. Petrarulo M, Vitale C, Facchini P, et al. Biochemical approach to diagnosis and differentiation of primary hyperoxalurias: an update. *J Nephrol*. 1998;11:23-28.
124. Kwak C, Kim HK, Kim EC, et al. Urinary oxalate levels and the enteric bacterium *Oxalobacter formigenes* in patients with calcium oxalate urolithiasis. *Eur Urol*. 2003;44:475-481.
125. Watts RWE, Danpure CJ, de Pauw L, et al. Combined liver-kidney and isolated liver transplantations for primary hyperoxaluria type 1: the European experience. *Nephrolol Dial Transplant*. 1991;6:502-511.
126. Coe FL, Parks JH, Asplin JR. The pathogenesis and treatment of kidney stones. *N Engl J Med*. 1992;327:1141-1152.
127. Millman S, Strauss AL, Parks JH, et al. Pathogenesis and clinical course of mixed calcium oxalate and uric acid nephrolithiasis. *Kidney Int*. 1982;22:366-370.
128. Grases F, Sanchis P, Isern B, et al. Uric acid as inducer of calcium oxalate crystal development. *Scand J Urol Nephrol*. 2007;41:26-31.
129. Pak CY, Arnold LH. Heterogeneous nucleation of calcium oxalate by seeds of monosodium urate. *Proc Soc Exp Biol Med*. 1975;149: 930-932.
130. Grover PK, Marshall VR, Ryall RL. Dissolved urate salts out calcium oxalate in undiluted human urine in vitro: implications for calcium oxalate stone genesis. *Chem Biol*. 2003;10:271-278.
131. Grover PK, Ryall RL, Marshall VR. Dissolved urate promotes calcium oxalate crystallization: epitaxy is not the cause. *Clin Sci (Lond)*. 1993;85:303-307.
132. Grover PK, Ryall RL. Allopurinol for stones: right drug—wrong reasons. *Am J Med*. 2007;120:380.
133. Coe FL. Treated and untreated recurrent calcium nephrolithiasis in patients with idiopathic hypercalciuria, hyperuricosuria, or no metabolic disorder. *Ann Int Med*. 1977;87:404-410.
134. Zerwekh JE, Holt K, Pak CY. Natural urinary macromolecular inhibitors: attenuation of inhibitory activity by urate salts. *Kidney Int*. 1983;23:838-841.
135. Grover PK, Ryall RL, Marshall VR. Calcium oxalate crystallization in urine: role of urate and glycosaminoglycans. *Kid Int*. 1992;41: 149-154.
136. Ryall RL, Hibberd CM, Marshall VR. The effect of crystalline monosodium urate on the crystallization of calcium oxalate in whole human urine. *Urol Res*. 1986;14:63-65.
137. Pak CY. Citrate and renal calculi. *Miner Electrolyte Metab*. 1987;13:257-266.
138. Pak CYC, Fuller C. Idiopathic hypocitraturic calcium oxalate nephrolithiasis successfully treated with potassium citrate. *Ann Intern Med*. 1986;104:33-37.
139. Ramchandani P, Pollack HM. Radiologic evaluation of patients with urolithiasis. In: Coe FL, Favus MJ, Pak CYC, et al., eds. *Kidney Stones: Medical and Surigical Management*. Philadelphia, PA: Lippincott-Raven; 1996:369-435.
140. Maalouf NM, Sakhaee K, Parks JH, et al. Association of urinary pH with body weight in nephrolithiasis. *Kidney Int*. 2004;65:1422-1425.
141. Sakhaee K, Adams-Huet B, Moe OW, et al. Pathyophysiologic basis for normouricosuric uric acid nephrolithiasis. *Kidney Int*. 2002;62: 971-979.
142. Ettinger B, Tang A, Citron JT, et al. Randomized trial of allopurinol in the prevention of calcium oxalate calculi. *N Engl J Med*. 1986;315:1386-1389.
143. Wong HY, Riedl CR, Griffith DP. Medical management and prevention of struvite stones. In: Coe FL, Favus MJ, Pak CYC, eds. *Kidney Stones: Medical and Surgical Management*. Philadelphia, PA: Lippincott-Raven; 1996:941-950.
144. Michaels EK. Surgical management of struvite stones. In: Coe FL, Favus MJ, Pak CYC, et al, eds. *Kidney Stones: Medical and Surgical Management*. Philadelphia, PA: Lippincott-Raven; 1966:951-970.
145. Bernardo NO, Smith AD. Chemolysis of urinary calculi. *Urol Clin North Am*. 2000;27:355-365.
146. Griffith DP, Moskowitz PA, Carlton Jr CE. Adjunctive chemotherapy of infection-induced staghorn calculi. *J Urol*. 1979;121:711-715.
147. Silverman DE, Stamey TA. Management of infection stones: the Stanford experience. *Medicine (Baltimore)*. 1983;62:44-51.
148. Sant GR, Blaivas JG. Hemiacidrin irrigation in the management of struvite calculi: long-term results. *J Urol*. 1983;130:1048-1050.
149. Font-Llitjos M, Jimenez-Vidal M, Bisceglia L, et al. New insights into cystinuria: 40 new mutations, genotype-phenotype correlation, and digenic inheritance causing partial phenotype. *J Med Genet*. 2005;42:58-68.
150. Kolb FO, Earll JM, Harper HA. "Disappearance" of cystinuria in a patient treated with prolonged low methionine diet. *Metabolism*. 1967;16:378-381.
151. Pak CYC. Prevention of recurrent nephrolithiasis. In: Pak CYC, ed. *Renal Stone Disease: Pathogenesis, Prevention, and Treatment*. Boston, MA: Martinus-Njhoff; 1987:165-199.
152. Pak CYC. Cystine lithiasis. In: Resnick MI, Pak CYC, eds. *Urolithiasis: A Medical and Surgical Reference*. Philadelphia, PA: WB Saunders; 1990:133-143.

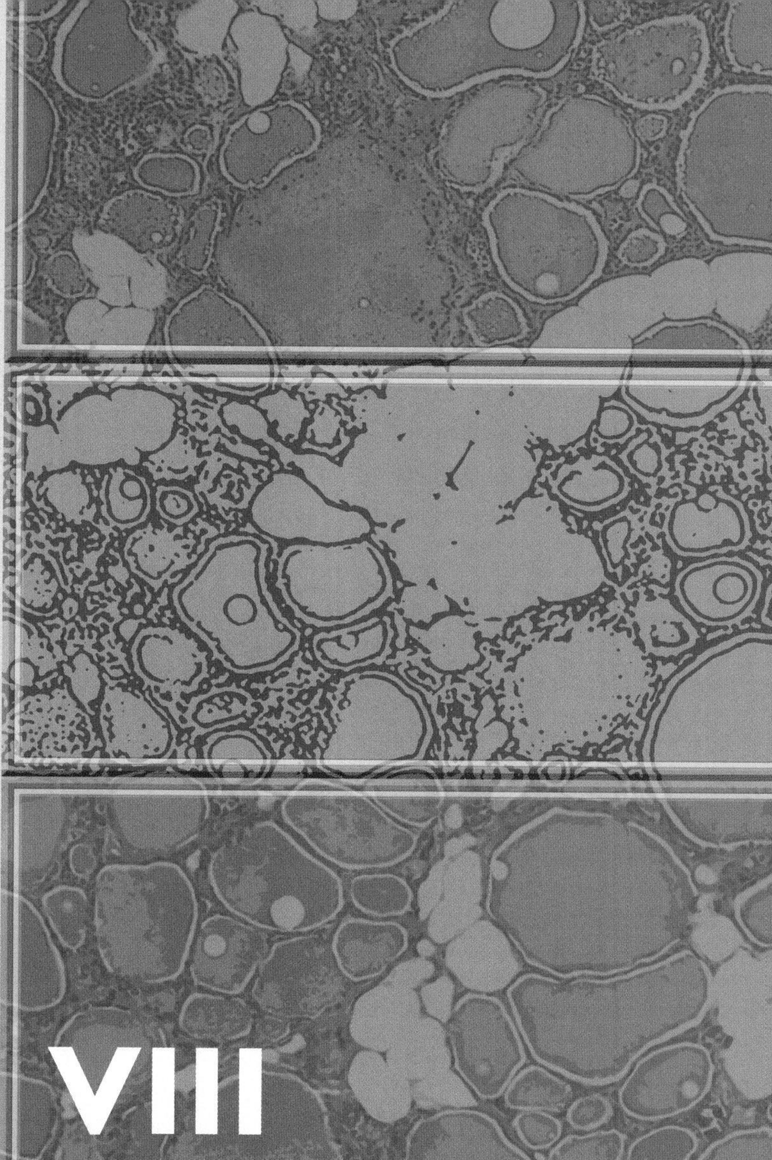

SECTION VIII

Disorders of Carbohydrate and Metabolism

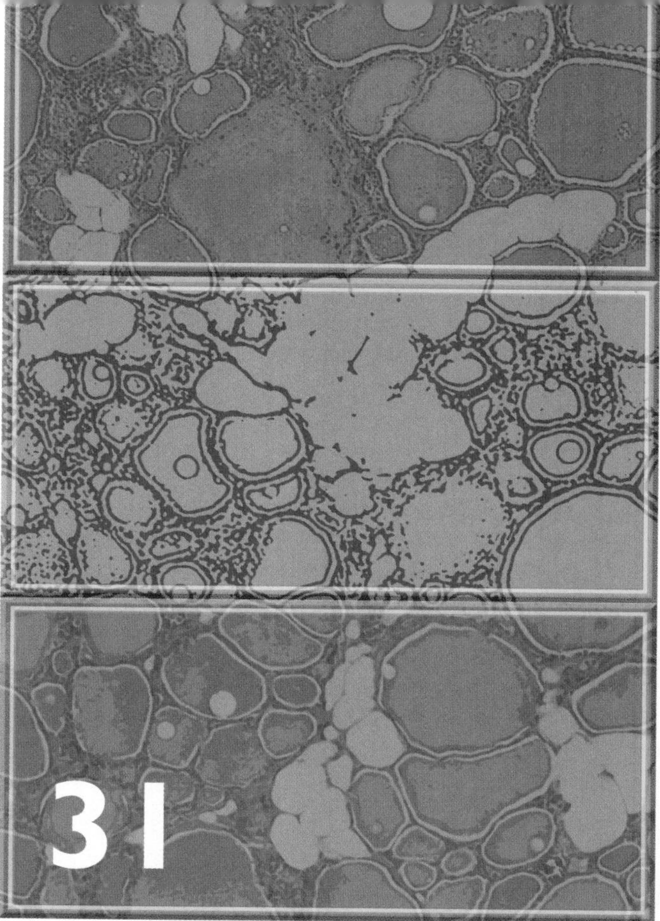

CHAPTER 31

Type 2 Diabetes Mellitus

JOHN B. BUSE • KENNETH S. POLONSKY • CHARLES F. BURANT

EPIDEMIOLOGY AND DIAGNOSIS

Epidemiology

Type 2 diabetes mellitus (T2DM) is the predominant form of diabetes worldwide, accounting for 90% of cases globally.[1,2] An epidemic of T2DM is under way in both developed and developing countries, although the brunt of the disorder is felt disproportionately in non-European populations. In the Pacific island of Nauru, diabetes was virtually unknown 50 years ago and is now present in approximately 40% of adults. Globally, the number of people with diabetes is expected to rise from the current estimate of 285 million in 2010 to 438 million in 2030, both figures substantially higher than even recent estimates. T2DM has become one of the world's most important public health problems.

Considerable information is available on the factors that are responsible for the development of T2DM, and these are summarized in Table 31-1. T2DM is thought to occur in genetically predisposed persons who are exposed to a series of environmental influences that precipitate the onset of clinical disease. The genetic basis of T2DM is discussed in detail later in this chapter, but the syndrome consists of monogenic and polygenic forms that can be differentiated both on clinical grounds and in terms of the genes that are involved in the pathogenesis of these disorders.

Sex, age, and ethnic background are important factors in determining the risk of developing T2DM.[2] The disorder is more common in women, and the increased prevalence in certain racial and ethnic groups has already been alluded to. Age is also a critical factor. T2DM has been viewed in the past as a disorder of aging, and this remains true today. However, a disturbing trend has become apparent in which the prevalence of obesity and T2DM in children is rising dramatically. In the past, it was believed that the overwhelming majority of children with diabetes had type 1 diabetes (T1DM), and only 1% to 2% of diabetic children were considered to have T2DM or other rare forms of diabetes.[3] Later reports suggested that as many as 8% to 45% of children with newly diagnosed diabetes have non–immune-mediated forms of the disease. Most of these children have T2DM, but other types are being increasingly identified. In arguably the most comprehensive study of diabetes in youth in the United States, 15% of diabetic children aged 10 to 19 years had T2DM in 2001. Nevertheless, T2DM in children remains relatively rare, with an estimated prevalence between ages 10 and 19 years of 0.4%.[4]

Data relating to the alarming increase in the prevalence of T2DM in children and adolescents has recently been

TABLE 31-1

Epidemiologic Determinants and Risk Factors of Type 2 Diabetes

Genetic Factors
Genetic markers Family history "Thrifty genes"
Demographic Characteristics
Sex Age Ethnicity
Behavioral and Lifestyle-Related Risk Factors
Obesity (including distribution of obesity and duration) Physical inactivity Diet Stress Westernization, urbanization, modernization
Metabolic Determinants and Intermediate-Risk Categories of Type 2 Diabetes

Impaired glucose tolerance
Insulin resistance
Pregnancy-related determinants
  Parity
  Gestational diabetes
  Diabetes in offspring of women with diabetes during pregnancy
  Intrauterine malnutrition or overnutrition

From Zimmer P, Alberti KG, Shaw J. Global and societal implications of the diabetes epidemic. *Nature.* 2001;414:782-787.

reviewed.[5] The National Health and Nutrition Examination Study (NHANES) data for 1999 to 2008 suggest that 18.1% of 12- to 19-year-olds, 19.6% of 6- to 11-year-olds, and 10.4% of 2- to 5-year-olds have a body mass index (BMI) above the 95th percentile adjusted for age and sex. This represents an increase of more than 30% in obesity over the prevalence previously determined for 1988 to 1994. The increases are particularly striking in Hispanic and African American children. Of even greater concern, impaired glucose tolerance (IGT) and T2DM have now emerged as critical health issues in overweight children, particularly overweight African American, Latin American, and Native American adolescents. In a clinic-based study, 25% of 55 obese children and 21% of 112 obese adolescents had IGT, and 4% of the latter group had undiagnosed T2DM.[6]

Diagnostic Criteria for Diabetes Mellitus

The diagnosis of diabetes rests on the measurement of glycemia. Current criteria for the diagnosis of diabetes and various categories of "prediabetes" or "high risk for diabetes" are shown in Table 31-2.[7]

Because plasma glucose concentrations range as a continuum, the criteria are based on estimates of the threshold for the complications of diabetes. The primary end point used to evaluate the relationship between glucose levels and complications is retinopathy. All three tests—fasting plasma glucose (FPG), 2-hour plasma glucose (2-hour PG), and glycosylated hemoglobin A_{1c} (HbA_{1c})—are able to predict the presence of retinopathy and, by inference, glucose levels that are diagnostic of diabetes[8] (Fig. 31-1). Furthermore, there is a relationship between elevated levels of all three markers and cardiovascular disease, although the relationship is generally stronger for HbA_{1c}.

Whereas previously HbA_{1c} was specifically not recommended for the diagnosis of diabetes and states of high diabetes risk based on poor standardization of assays, the current HbA_{1c} assay has several technical (preanalytic and analytic) advantages over the currently used laboratory measurements of glucose. Furthermore, measures of fasting and postchallenge glucose concentrations in the same individual over time are less reproducible than the HbA_{1c}. The intraindividual coefficient of variation in one study was 6.4% for the FPG and 16.7% for the 2-hour PG value, compared with less than 2% for HbA_{1c}.

Although the oral glucose tolerance test (OGTT) is an invaluable tool in research, it is not recommended for routine use in diagnosing diabetes. It is inconvenient for patients, and in most cases the diagnosis can be made on the basis of either an elevated FPG concentration or an elevated random glucose determination in the presence of hyperglycemic symptoms.

Screening for Type 2 Diabetes

Undiagnosed T2DM is common, accounting for almost 20% of diabetes cases in the United States.[9] Subjects at high risk for diabetes and with undiagnosed T2DM are at significantly increased risk for coronary heart disease, stroke, and peripheral vascular disease. Delay in the diagnosis of T2DM causes an increase in microvascular and macrovascular disease. In addition, affected individuals have a greater likelihood of having dyslipidemia, hypertension, and obesity. Therefore, it is important for the clinician to screen for diabetes in a cost-effective manner in subjects who demonstrate major risk factors for diabetes as summarized

TABLE 31-2

Criteria for the Diagnosis of Diabetes*

		INCREASED RISK*			
Test	**Normoglycemia**	**Impaired Fasting Glucose**	**Impaired Glucose Tolerance**	**High Risk**	**Diabetes**†
PG, fasting (mg/dL)	<100	100-125			≥126
PG, 2-hour (mg/dL)	<140		140-199		≥200
Hemoglobin A_{1c} (%)				5.7-6.4	≥6.5
PG, casual (mg/dL)					>200 mg/dL plus symptoms of diabetes

*Risk for diabetes is continuous, extending below the lower limit and becoming disproportionately greater at the higher end of the ranges shown.
†In the absence of unequivocal hyperglycemia, a diagnostic result should be confirmed by repeat testing.
Adapted from American Diabetes Association. Standards of medical care in diabetes—2010. *Diabetes Care.* 2010;29:s11-s61.

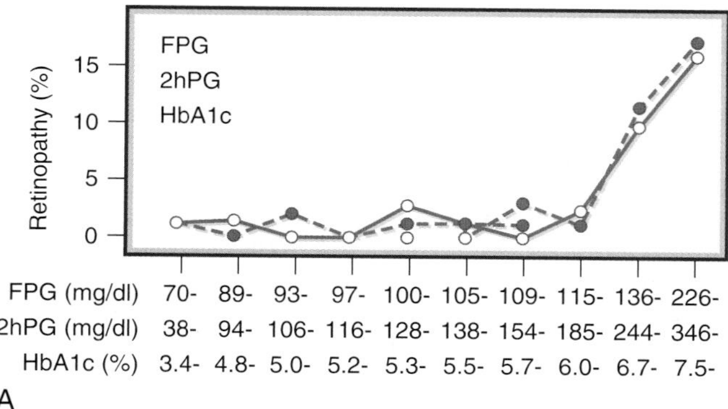

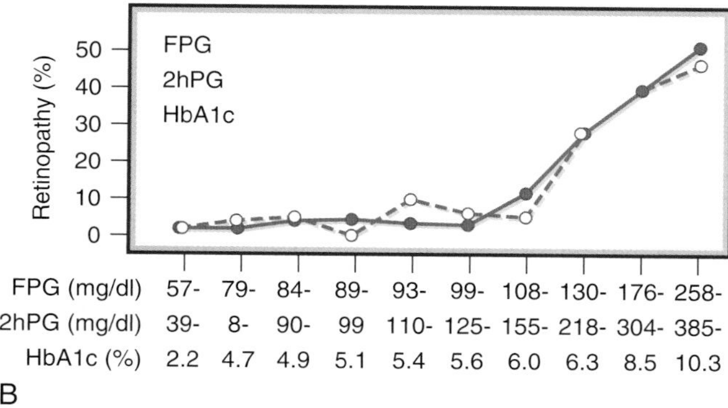

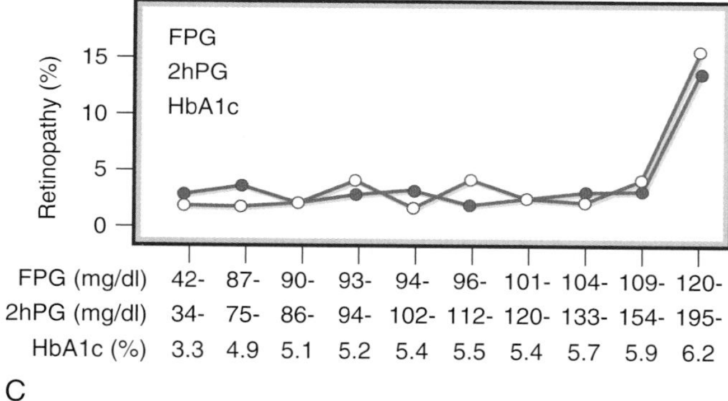

Figure 31-1 Prediction of retinopathy by levels of plasma glucose on standard tests (American Diabetes Association consensus): **A,** Fasting plasma glucose (FPG); **B,** 2-hour plasma glucose (2hPG); **C,** glycosylated hemoglobin (HbA_{1c}).

in Table 31-3. Recent modeling studies based on the U.S. population suggest that universal screening programs coupled with guideline-based therapy for T2DM is cost-effective when initiated between the ages of 30 and 45 and subsequently conducted every 3 to 5 years.[10] Recommendations for screening are summarized in Table 31-4. The pivotal role of screening to identify individuals at high risk in prevention strategies for T2DM is discussed at the end of this chapter.

PATHOGENESIS

The pathogenesis of T2DM is complex and involves the interaction of genetic and environmental factors. A number of environmental factors have been shown to play a critical role in the development of the disease, particularly excessive caloric intake leading to obesity and a sedentary lifestyle. The clinical presentation is also heterogeneous, with a wide range in age at onset, severity of associated hyperglycemia, and degree of obesity. From a pathophysiologic standpoint, persons with T2DM consistently demonstrate three cardinal abnormalities:

- Resistance to the action of insulin in peripheral tissues, particularly muscle and fat but also liver
- Defective insulin secretion, particularly in response to a glucose stimulus
- Increased glucose production by the liver

Recently, it has been suggested that the list of cardinal abnormalities in diabetes should be expanded to eight, adding accelerated lipolysis in the fat cell, incretin hormone deficiency and resistance, hyperglucagonemia, increased renal tubular reabsorption, and the role of the central nervous system in metabolic regulation.[11]

Although the precise way in which genetic, environmental, and pathophysiologic factors interact to lead to the clinical onset of T2DM is not known, understanding of these processes has increased substantially. With the

TABLE 31-3

Major Risk Factors for Type 2 Diabetes

Overweight (BMI ≥25 kg/m^2)
Physical inactivity
First-degree relative with diabetes
Member of a high-risk ethnic population (e.g., African American, Latino, Native American, Asian American, Pacific Islander)
Female with a history of delivering a baby weighing >9 lb or diagnosis of GDM
Hypertension (≥140/90 mm Hg or on therapy for hypertension)
HDL cholesterol level <35 mg/dL (0.90 mmol/L) or triglyceride level >250 mg/dL (2.82 mmol/L) or both
Female with polycystic ovary syndrome
Hemoglobin A_{1c} ≥5.7%, impaired glucose tolerance, or impaired fasting glucose on previous testing
Other clinical conditions associated with insulin resistance (e.g., severe obesity, acanthosis nigricans)
History of cardiovascular disease

BMI, body mass index; GDM, gestational diabetes mellitus; HDL, high-density lipoprotein.

Adapted from American Diabetes Association. Standards of medical care in diabetes—2010. *Diabetes Care.* 2010;29:s11-s61.

TABLE 31-4

Summary of Major Recommendations for T2DM Screening

Testing to detect T2DM and to assess risk for future diabetes should be considered in asymptomatic adults of any age who are overweight or obese (BMI ≥25 kg/m^2) and who have one or more additional risk factors for diabetes (see Table 30-3).
In those without risk factors for T2DM, testing should begin at age 30-45 yr.
If test results are normal, repeat testing should be carried out at 3- to 5-yr intervals.
Any of the following tests is appropriate: HbA_{1c}, FPG, 2-hr 75-g OGTT.
In those found to have increased risk for future diabetes, identify and, if appropriate, treat other CVD risk factors.

BMI, body mass index; CVD, cardiovascular disease; FPG, fasting plasma glucose; HbA_{1c}, glycosylated hemoglobin; OGTT, oral glucose tolerance test; T2DM, type 2 diabetes mellitus.

Adapted from references American Diabetes Association. Standards of medical care in diabetes—2010. *Diabetes Care.*2010;29:s11-s61; and Kahn R, Alperin P, Eddy D, et al. Age at initiation and frequency of screening to detect type 2 diabetes: a cost-effectiveness analysis. *Lancet.* 2010;375:1365-1374.

exception of specific monogenic forms of the disease that might result from defects largely confined to the pathways that regulate insulin action in muscle, liver, and fat or defects in insulin secretory function in the pancreatic beta cell, there is an emerging consensus that the common forms of T2DM are polygenic in nature and are caused by a combination of insulin resistance, abnormal insulin secretion, and other factors.

From a pathophysiologic standpoint, it is the inability of the pancreatic beta cell to adapt to the reductions in insulin sensitivity that occur over a lifetime that precipitates the onset of T2DM. The most common factors that place an increased secretory burden on the beta cell are puberty, pregnancy, a sedentary lifestyle, and overeating leading to weight gain. An underlying genetic predisposition appears to be a critical factor in determining the frequency with which beta cell failure occurs.

Genetic Factors in the Development of Type 2 Diabetes

Genetically, T2DM consists of monogenic and polygenic forms.[12,13] The monogenic forms, although relatively uncommon, are nevertheless important, and a number of the genes involved have been identified and characterized. The genes involved in the common polygenic forms of the disorder have been far more difficult to identify and characterize.

Monogenic Forms of Diabetes

In the monogenic forms of diabetes, the gene involved is both necessary and sufficient to cause disease. In other words, environmental factors play little or no role in determining whether a genetically predisposed person develops clinical diabetes. The monogenic forms of diabetes usually are diagnosed in younger patients, often in the first 2 to 3 decades of life; however, if only mild, asymptomatic elevations in blood glucose occur, the diagnosis may be missed until later in life.

The monogenic forms of diabetes are summarized in Table 31-5 and can be divided into those in which the mechanism is a defect in insulin secretion and those that involve defective responses to insulin or insulin resistance.

TABLE 31-5

Monogenic Forms of Diabetes

Monogenic Forms of Diabetes
Forms Associated with Insulin Resistance
Mutations in the insulin receptor gene
Type A insulin resistance
Leprechaunism
Rabson-Mendenhall syndrome
Lipoatrophic diabetes
Mutations in the PPARγ gene
Forms Associated with Defective Insulin Secretion
Mutations in insulin or proinsulin genes
Mitochondrial gene mutations
Maturity-onset diabetes of the young (MODY)
HNF-4α (MODY 1)
Glucokinase (MODY 2)
HNF-1α (MODY 3)
IPF1 (MODY 4)
HNF-1β (MODY 5)
NeuroD1/BETA2 (MODY 6)

HNF, hepatocyte nuclear factor; IPF, insulin promoter factor; NeuroD1/BETA2, neurogenic differentiation 1/beta cell E-box *trans*-activator 2; PPAR, peroxisome proliferator-activated receptor.

Monogenic Forms of Diabetes Associated with Insulin Resistance

Mutations in the Insulin Receptor. More than 70 mutations have been identified in the insulin receptor gene in various insulin-resistant patients.[14] There are at least three clinical syndromes caused by mutations in the insulin receptor gene. *Type A insulin resistance* is defined by the presence of insulin resistance, acanthosis nigricans, and hyperandrogenism.[15] Patients with *leprechaunism* have multiple abnormalities, including intrauterine growth retardation, fasting hypoglycemia, and death within the first 1 to 2 years of life.[16-18] The *Rabson-Mendenhall syndrome* is associated with short stature, protuberant abdomen, and abnormalities of teeth and nails; pineal hyperplasia was a characteristic in the original description of this syndrome.[19]

These mutations could impair receptor function by a number of different mechanisms, including decreasing the number of receptors expressed on the cell surface, such as by decreasing the rate of receptor biosynthesis (class 1), accelerating the rate of receptor degradation (class 5), or inhibiting the transport of receptors to the plasma membrane (class 2). The intrinsic function of the receptor may be abnormal if the affinity of insulin binding is reduced (class 3) or if receptor tyrosine kinase is inactivated (class 4). The insulin resistance that is associated with insulin receptor mutations can be severe, manifesting in the neonatal period (e.g., leprechaunism, Rabson-Mendenhall syndrome), or it can occur in a milder form in adulthood, leading to insulin-resistant diabetes with marked hyperinsulinemia, acanthosis nigricans, and hyperandrogenism.

Lipoatrophic Diabetes. In another monogenic form of diabetes, lipoatrophic diabetes, severe insulin resistance is associated with lipoatrophy and lipodystrophy. This form of diabetes is characterized by a paucity of fat, insulin resistance, and hypertriglyceridemia.[20] The disease has several genetic forms, including face-sparing partial lipoatrophy (the Dunnigan or Koberling-Dunnigan syndrome), an autosomal dominant form caused by mutations in the lamin A/C gene,[21] and congenital generalized lipoatrophy (the Seip-Berardinelli syndrome), an autosomal recessive form that appears to be due to mutations in either 1-acyl-*sn*-glycerol-3-phosphate acyltransferase-2 (AGPAT2) or in the seipin gene product.[22,23]

Mutations in Peroxisome Proliferator-Activated Receptor-γ. It has been demonstrated that mutations in the transcription factor peroxisome proliferator-activated receptor-γ (PPARγ) can cause T2DM of early onset (familial lipodystrophy type 3).[24] Two different heterozygous mutations were identified in the ligand-binding domain of PPARγ in three subjects with severe insulin resistance. In the PPARγ crystal structure, the mutations destabilize helix 12, which mediates *trans*-activation. Both receptor mutants showed markedly decreased transcriptional activation and inhibited the action of coexpressed wild-type PPARγ in a dominant negative manner. A Dutch kindred with a 14A → G mutation within the promoter of the PPARγ4 isoform, which results in decreased expression but no qualitative protein abnormalities, has been described.[25]

A common amino acid polymorphism (Pro12Ala) in PPARγ has been associated with T2DM. People homozygous for the Pro12 allele are more insulin resistant than those with one Ala12 allele and have a 1.25-fold increased risk of diabetes. There is also evidence for interaction between this polymorphism and fatty acids, linking this locus with diet. A second polymorphism, C161 → T, has been linked to insulin resistance in Hispanic and non-Hispanic white women.[26]

Neonatal Diabetes. Newborns may have permanent or transient neonatal diabetes. The prevalence of all causes of neonatal diabetes has been estimated to be between 1 in 100,000 and 1 in 300,000 live births. Transient neonatal diabetes usually resolves between 6 and 12 months of life. If the onset is before 6 months of age, a genetic cause is the most likely underlying etiology. The presence of hyperglycemia is often undetected, and the diagnosis is then made when the clinical condition deteriorates due to marked hyperglycemia with or without ketoacidosis. Morbidity is high. Associated features include low birth weight below the 10th percentile (especially in the absence of maternal diabetes), developmental delay, learning disorders, speech disorders, muscle weakness especially with climbing stairs, and seizures. Some children have been diagnosed with attention deficit disorder (ADD) as well. Occasionally, multiple family members are also found to have early-onset, relapsing, or nonobese young adult appearance of diabetes, but most cases are sporadic.

Etiology. The most common cause of relapsing transient neonatal diabetes is the uniparental disomy 6 chromosome abnormality (UDP6), which can also be caused by methylation defects in this region of the chromosome. Mutations in the *ABCC8* gene or, less commonly, in *KCNJ11*, both components of the adenosine triphosphate (ATP)-sensitive potassium channel (K_{ATP} channel), may also be responsible. The K_{ATP} channel is well described as a key molecular switch in the beta cell that closes in response to generation of ATP after glucose metabolism. If the channel does not close at physiologic levels of glucose, hypoinsulinism and hyperglycemia result. This causes severe diabetes with low or negative C-peptide and ketosis in the first few weeks of life.

Permanent neonatal diabetes is most often caused by mutations in *KCNJ11*, and less often by mutations in *ABCC8*. The K_{ATP} channel, composed of the beta-cell proteins sulfonylurea receptor (SUR1) and inward-rectifying potassium channel subunit KIR6.2, is a key regulator of insulin release. It is inhibited by the binding of adenine nucleotides to subunit KIR6.2, which closes the channel, and it is activated by nucleotide binding or hydrolysis on SUR1, which opens the channel. The balance of these opposing actions determines the low open-channel probability, P_O, which controls the excitability of pancreatic beta cells.[26a] It has been hypothesized that activating mutations in *ABCC8*, which encodes SUR1, can cause neonatal diabetes. Mutations in these genes that cause the opposite condition, decreased channel function, are a cause of familial hyperinsulinemia with hypoglycemia.[1,19,20]

After *KCNJ11* mutations, the second most common group of causes of permanent neonatal diabetes is mutations in the insulin gene (*INS*) itself. These mutations are also rare causes of young adult–onset T2DM and ketosis-prone type 1b diabetes, usually with negative diabetes-associated autoantibodies.[8] More than 200 cases have been identified worldwide. Rarely, homozygous gene mutations in glucokinase (*GCK*) and transcription factor genes lead to insulin insufficiency or failure of development of the endocrine pancreas or of the entire pancreas.

Therapy. Many of the mutations in *KCNJ11* and *ABCC8* can be treated with a relatively high dose of sulfonylureas. However, it is critical that this be done after a mutation has been documented, because the protocol involves high doses of sulfonylureas (administered in divided doses and off-label in the United States for children) and simultaneous aggressive insulin withdrawal. Collaboration with or referral to a center with experience in this treatment is highly encouraged because of potential side effects and other adverse effects. There is no therapy at this time for either UDP6 or *INS* mutations other than insulin replacement in the manner used for the treatment of type 1 diabetes.

Most of these mutations are heterozygous and dominant (i.e., each child of an affected individual has a 50% chance of having the disease). In the case of unaffected parents with one affected child, several studies have reported germline mosaicism as a known or possible cause of the presence of the syndrome in several siblings in one family. Therefore, the risk that each subsequent child will have neonatal diabetes can range from less than 10% to 50%, depending on the presence of mosaicism in the gametes.

Monogenic Forms of Diabetes Associated with Defects in Insulin Secretion

Mutant Insulin Syndromes. The first syndrome associated with diabetes to be characterized in terms of the clinical picture, genetic mechanisms, and clinical pathophysiology was that associated with mutant insulin or proinsulin.[27] Persons with this disorder present clinically with a mild, non–insulin-dependent form of diabetes. Affected persons characteristically have marked hyperinsulinemia on routine insulin assays. Increases in the concentration of insulin in association with diabetes usually indicate insulin resistance, but in this syndrome, insulin resistance can be easily excluded because the patients respond normally to administration of exogenous insulin. Characterization of the insulin by high-performance liquid chromatography (HPLC) reveals that the hyperinsulinemia results from the presence of the abnormal insulin or proinsulin and related breakdown products. The increased concentrations of insulin appear to be related to the presence of mutations in regions of the insulin molecule that are important for receptor binding, particularly the carboxyl terminus of the insulin B chain.

Because the liver is the major site of insulin clearance and first-pass hepatic insulin uptake and degradation are mediated by the insulin receptor, mutant forms of insulin with diminished insulin receptor binding ability are cleared more slowly from the circulation, and this reduction in insulin clearance leads to hyperinsulinemia. Alternatively, mutations in proinsulin can reduce the conversion of proinsulin to insulin, leading to accumulation of proinsulin.[28,29] Because proinsulin is cleared more slowly from the circulation than insulin, proinsulin levels increase. Proinsulin cross-reacts in most commercially available assays, and this insulin-like immunoreactivity can be characterized as being related to the presence of proinsulin (rather than insulin only) by HPLC or by the use of assays that are specific for insulin and proinsulin.

A patient with a mutation in prohormone convertase 1, one of the enzymes responsible for the conversion of proinsulin to insulin, has been described.[30]

Mitochondrial Diabetes. An A-to-G transition in the mitochondrial transfer RNA Leu(UUR) gene at base pair 3243 has been shown to be associated with maternally transmitted diabetes and sensorineural hearing loss.[31] In other subjects, this mutation is associated with diabetes and the syndrome of mitochondrial myopathy, encephalopathy, lactic acidosis, and stroke-like episodes (MELAS syndrome). The mitochondrion plays a key role in the regulation of insulin secretion, particularly in response to glucose. We have documented abnormal insulin secretion on at least one of a battery of tests in subjects with this mitochondrial mutation, even in subjects with normal glucose tolerance or IGT who have not developed overt diabetes.[32]

Maturity-Onset Diabetes of the Young. Maturity-onset diabetes of the young (MODY) is a genetically and clinically heterogeneous group of disorders characterized by nonketotic diabetes mellitus, an autosomal dominant mode of inheritance, onset usually before 25 years of age and often in childhood or adolescence, and a primary defect in pancreatic beta cell function. A detailed review of MODY has been published,[33] and the information contained in that review is summarized here.

Etiology and Clinical Presentation

MODY can result from mutations in any one of at least six different genes. One of these genes *(GCK)* encodes the glycolytic enzyme glucokinase; mutations in this gene cause MODY2.[34] The other five genes encode transcription factors. MODY1 is associated with mutations in the gene for hepatocyte nuclear factor-4α *(HNF4A)*[35]; MODY3 with mutations in *HNF1A*[36]; MODY4 with mutations in pancreatic and duodenal homeobox 1 *(PDX1),* which encodes insulin promoter factor 1 (IPF1)[37]; MODY5 with mutations in *HNF1B*[38]; and MODY6 with mutations in *NEUROD1*, which encodes the neurogenic differentiation 1/beta cell E-box *trans*-activator 2 (NeuroD1/BETA2).[39] All of these genes are expressed in the insulin-producing pancreatic beta cell, and heterozygous mutations cause diabetes related to beta cell dysfunction. Abnormalities in liver and kidney function occur in some forms of MODY, reflecting expression of the transcription factors in these tissues. Nongenetic factors that affect insulin sensitivity (infection, puberty, pregnancy, and rarely obesity) can trigger diabetes onset and affect the severity of hyperglycemia in MODY but do not play a significant role in the development of MODY.

The most common clinical presentation of MODY is a mild, asymptomatic increase in blood glucose in a child, adolescent, or young adult with a prominent family history of diabetes, often in successive generations, that suggests an autosomal dominant mode of inheritance. Some patients have mild hyperglycemia for many years, whereas others have varying degrees of IGT for several years before the onset of persistent hyperglycemia.[33] The diagnosis may not be made until adulthood even though the elevation in plasma glucose has been present for many years. Prospective testing indicates that in most patients the disease onset occurs in childhood or adolescence. In some patients, there may be a rapid progression to overt asymptomatic or symptomatic hyperglycemia, necessitating therapy with an oral hypoglycemic drug or insulin. The presence of persistently normal plasma glucose levels in subjects with mutations in any of the known MODY genes is unusual, and most eventually experience diabetes (with the exception of many patients with glucokinase mutations; see later discussion).

Although the exact prevalence of MODY is not known, current estimates suggest that MODY might account for 1% to 5% of all cases of diabetes in the United States and other industrialized countries.[33] Several clinical characteristics distinguish patients with MODY from those with T2DM, including a prominent family history of diabetes in three or more generations, young age at presentation, and absence of obesity.

Functional Effects of MODY Genes. The identification of several genes associated with diabetes has provided a unique opportunity to characterize the pathophysiologic mechanisms by which genetic mutations can lead to an increase in the plasma glucose concentration. All the susceptibility genes identified to date cause impaired insulin secretory responses to glucose, although the mechanisms differ.

Glucokinase. Glucokinase is expressed at its highest levels in the pancreatic beta cell and the liver. It catalyzes the transfer of phosphate from ATP to glucose to generate glucose-6-phosphate (Fig. 31-2). This reaction is the first rate-limiting step in glucose metabolism. Glucokinase functions as the glucose sensor in the beta cell by controlling the rate of entry of glucose into the glycolytic pathway (glucose phosphorylation) and its subsequent metabolism. In the liver, glucokinase plays a key role in the ability to store glucose as glycogen, particularly in the postprandial state.

Heterozygous mutations leading to partial deficiency of glucokinase are associated with MODY, and homozygous mutations resulting in complete deficiency of this enzyme lead to permanent neonatal diabetes mellitus.[40] As predicted by the physiologic functions of glucokinase, the increase in plasma glucose concentrations in patients with this form of diabetes results from a combination of reduced glucose-induced insulin secretion from the pancreatic beta cell and reduced glycogen storage in the liver after glucose ingestion.

Liver-Enriched Transcription Factors. The transcription factors HNF-1α, HNF-1β, and HNF-4α play a key role in the

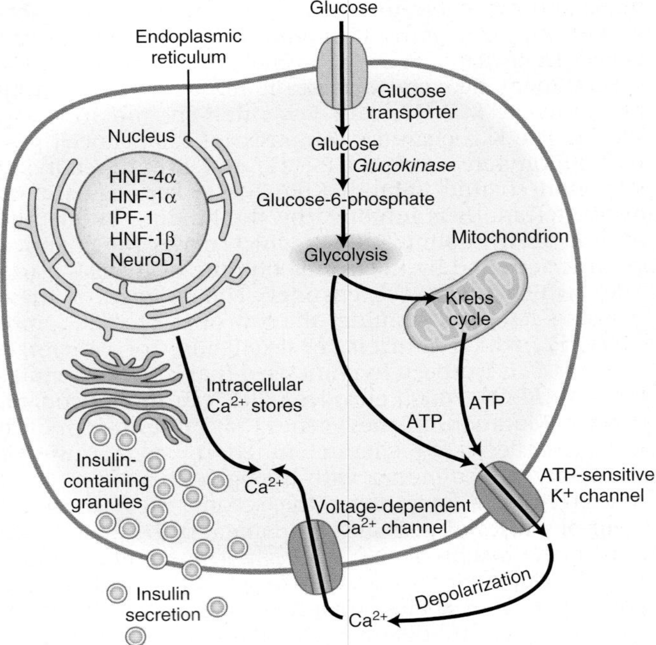

Figure 31-2 Model of a pancreatic beta cell and the proteins implicated in maturity-onset diabetes of the young. ATP, adenosine triphosphate; HNF, hepatocyte nuclear factor, IPF, insulin promoter factor; NeuroD1, neurogenic differentiation 1. (From Fajans SS, Bell GI, Polonsky KS. Molecular mechanisms and clinical pathophysiology of maturity-onset diabetes of the young. *N Engl J Med.* 2001;345:973.)

tissue-specific regulation of gene expression in the liver[41] and are also expressed in other tissues, including pancreatic islets, kidney, and genital tissues. HNF-1α and HNF-1β are members of the homeodomain-containing family of transcription factors, and HNF-4α is an orphan nuclear receptor.[41,42]

HNF-1α, HNF-1β, and HNF-4α make up part of an interacting network of transcription factors that function together to control gene expression during embryonic development and in adult tissues in which they are coexpressed. In the pancreatic beta cell, these transcription factors regulate the expression of the insulin gene as well as proteins involved in glucose transport and metabolism and mitochondrial metabolism (all linked to insulin secretion) and lipoprotein metabolism.[43] The expression of HNF-1α is regulated at least in part by HNF-4α.

Persons with diabetes related to mutations in these genes have defects in insulin secretory responses to a variety of secretagogues, particularly glucose, that are present before the onset of hyperglycemia, suggesting that they represent the primary functional defect in the syndrome. Reduced glucagon responses to arginine have also been observed, suggesting that the pancreatic alpha cell is also involved in a broader pancreatic developmental abnormality.

Insulin Promoter Factor 1. IPF1 is a homeodomain-containing transcription factor that was originally isolated as a transcriptional regulator of the insulin and somatostatin genes. It also plays a central role in the development of the pancreas and in regulation of the expression of a variety of pancreatic islet genes, including (besides insulin) the genes encoding glucokinase, islet amyloid polypeptide, and glucose transporter 2. IPF1 also appears to mediate glucose-induced stimulation of insulin gene transcription.[44]

A child born with pancreatic agenesis was shown to have a mutation in IPF1 that lacked the homeodomain required for DNA binding and nuclear localization. Heterozygous carriers of an IPF1 mutation from the same kindred developed an early-onset autosomal dominant form of diabetes (i.e., MODY) caused by dominant negative inhibition of transcription of the insulin gene and other beta cell–specific genes regulated by the mutant IPF1.[45] Additional IPF1 mutations have been discovered in pedigrees with late-onset T2DM.[46] Therefore, mutations in IPF1 can cause a range of phenotype manifestations, depending on whether the subjects have homozygous or heterozygous mutations and the severity of the functional effects.

Neurogenic Differentiation-1 Transcription Factor. The basic helix-loop-helix transcription factor NeuroD1/BETA2 was isolated on the basis of its ability to activate transcription of the insulin gene, and it is required for normal pancreatic islet development. Two patients with heterozygous mutations in NeuroD1 and diabetes have been described,[39] and a third was identified in an Icelandic population.[47] Studies in other populations have failed to detect mutations in NeuroD1 even in subjects with a MODY phenotype. It therefore appears that mutations in NeuroD1 are a rare cause of MODY.

Genetics of the Polygenic Forms of Type 2 Diabetes

The common polygenic form of T2DM has complex pathophysiology, and genetic and environmental factors play a major role. The phenotypic manifestations of the disease are also complex and include resistance to the action of insulin in muscle, fat, and liver; defects in insulin secretory responses from the pancreatic beta cell; and increases in hepatic glucose production. However, the primary defect or defects responsible for the development of the syndrome remain elusive and are likely not to be defined until more is known about the genes responsible for diabetes and the nature of the gene-environment interactions that are ultimately responsible for development of the disorder in predisposed persons.

Insulin resistance is present in persons predisposed to T2DM before the onset of hyperglycemia, and this finding has been interpreted by some to indicate that insulin resistance is the primary abnormality that is responsible for the development of T2DM. However, defective beta cell function is also present before the onset of T2DM when IGT is present and in first-degree relatives of persons with T2DM who have completely normal plasma glucose concentrations. Therefore, although there is still controversy about whether insulin resistance or abnormal insulin secretion represents the primary defect in T2DM, there is general consensus that both defects are present in essentially all subjects with the disorder, often from an early preclinical stage.

In recent years, and particularly since 2007, there have been dramatic advances in understanding of the genetic basis of T2DM. Earlier genetic studies relied either on the candidate gene approach, in which the search for diabetes genes was dictated by the prevailing understanding of the pathways involved in glucose regulation, or on linkage studies. Linkage studies involve defining regions of chromosomal DNA that are shared to excess by affected family members. Parents are genotyped at a particular marker, and the offspring are scored for sharing of zero, one, or two alleles inherited from their parents. Markers are genotyped in family members in the regions of polymorphic repeats called microsatellites or simple tandem repeats.

Although these two approaches did identify important diabetes genes, the application of genome-wide association studies (GWAS) has led to a dramatic increase in the number of diabetes genes that have been identified. GWAS uses an unbiased interrogation of the entire genome in cases and controls to determine which single-nucleotide polymorphisms (SNPs) are associated with disease. The development of this approach depended on a number of factors including the completion of the Human Genome Project, the genotyping of 3.8 million SNPs and identification of haplotype-tagged SNPs by the International HapMap Project, the development of affordable, high-throughput genotyping technologies, and the availability of multiple analytical tools for the cleaning,[48] mining, and interpretation of very large datasets. The genes that have been implicated in the pathogenesis of T2DM are listed in Table 31-6. This is a rapidly changing field, and it is certain that the list of diabetes genes will increase. A number of excellent reviews have been published. The following sections provide a brief summary of the genes that have been implicated in the pathogenesis of T2DM.[70,795,796]

Calpain-10 Gene

The linkage between calpain-10 and T2DM first observed by a group headed by Graeme Bell[49] was completely unexpected and was based purely on the application of sophisticated methods of analysis in a genetic study rather than on any novel physiologic insights. A number of studies have corroborated the initial observation that genetic variation in *CAPN10,* the calpain-10 gene, increases the risk of T2DM, but others have not. However, two meta-analyses of all the published data supported a role for this gene in diabetes susceptibility. Song's group,[50] after analyzing 11

TABLE 31-6

Polygenic Type 2 Diabetes Genes*

Gene Name	Common Protein Name	Function	Mechanism for Association with Type 2 Diabetes
PPARG	Peroxisome proliferator-activated receptor-γ	Nuclear receptor	Insulin resistance
IGF2BP2	IGF-2 mRNA-binding protein 2 (IMP2)	IGF2 binding protein	Unknown
CDKAL1	CDK5 regulatory subunit associated protein 1-like 1	Presumed regulator of cell cycle through cyclin kinase	Abnormal insulin secretion
SLC30A8	Solute carrier family 30, member 8 (ZNT8)	Zinc transporter 8	Abnormal insulin secretion
CDKN2A	P16(INK4a) and P14(ARF)	Cyclin-dependent kinase inhibitor 2A	Unknown
CDKN2B	P15(INK4b)	Cyclin-dependent kinase inhibitor 2B	
WFS1	Wolframin	Protects against endoplasmic reticulum stress	Abnormal insulin secretion
IDE	Insulin-degrading enzyme	Peptide degradation	Abnormal insulin secretion
HHEX	Hematopoietically expressed homeobox	Homeobox transcription factor important in beta cell function	Abnormal insulin secretion
KIF11	Kinesin family member 11	Kinesin-related motor in microtubule and spindle function	Unknown
TCF7L2	Transcription factor 4 (TCF4)	Transcription factor	Insulin secretion
KCNJ11	Kir6.2	Inward rectifier potassium channel	Insulin secretion
FTO	Fat mass and obesity associated gene	Functions as a DNA demethylase in vitro	Obesity
JAZF1	Juxtaposed with another zinc finger 1	Encodes a transcriptional repressor of a nuclear receptor Nr2c2 that regulates growth, IGF2, and blood sugar	Unknown
CDC123	Cell division cycle protein 123 homolog	Required for S phase entry of the cell cycle	Unknown
CAMK1D	Calcium/calmodulin-dependent protein kinase 1δ	Mediator of chemokine signal transduction in granulocytes	
TSPAN8	Tetraspanin 8	Cell surface glycoprotein	Unknown
LGR5	Leucine-rich repeat-containing G protein-coupled receptor	Orphan G-protein receptor	
THADA	Thyroid adenoma associated protein	Unknown	Unknown
ADAMS TS9	*Cell Metabolism* review[795]	*Cell Metabolism* review	Unknown
NOTCH2/ADAM30	Transmembrane receptor important in pancreas development	Regulator of cell differentiation	Abnormal insulin secretion
ADCY5	Adenylate cyclase 5	Catalyses generation of cAMP and cAMP responses to GLP1 in the beta cell	Unknown? Abnormal insulin secretion
PROX1	Prospero homeobox protein 1	A novel corepressor of HNF-4α that plays a critical role in beta-cell development	Unknown? Abnormal insulin secretion
GCK	Glucokinase	Converts glucose to glucose-6-phosphate, the first rate-limiting step in glucose metabolism	Reduced insulin secretion, reduced liver glycogen storage
GCKR	Glucokinase regulatory protein	Inhibits glucokinase in the liver	Unknown
DGKB	Diacylglycerol kinase β-subunit	Regulation of insulin secretion	Unknown
TMEM195	Transmembrane protein 195	Integral membrane phosphoprotein highly expressed in liver	
MTNR1B	Melatonin receptor type 1B	Expressed in the hypothalamus and human pancreatic islets, where it regulates melatonin action and timing of circadian activity	Unknown. Possibly abnormal insulin secretion
GIPR	Glucose-dependent insulinotropic peptide (GIP) receptor	Regulation of insulin secretion in response to the incretin peptide GIP	Abnormal insulin secretion

cAMP, cyclic adenosine monophosphate; CDK5, cyclin-dependent kinase 5; GLP1, glucagon-like peptide 1; IGF, insulin-like growth factor; *KCNJ11*, potassium inwardly rectifying channel, subfamily J, member 11; Nr2c2, nuclear receptor subfamily 2, group C, member 2; *TCF7L2*, transcription factor 7-like 2 gene; WFS, Wolfram syndrome.

*More information on these genes can be found in recent reviews of diabetes genetics[70,795,796] and in publications of additional diabetes loci.[73,797-799]

studies, showed an odds ratio for T2DM of 1.19 comparing persons with the G/G genotype of UCSNP43 in *CAPN10* with all carriers of the A allele. Weedon's group[51] calculated an odds ratio of 1.17 for UCSNP44.

Calpains are Ca^{2+}-dependent cysteine proteases.[52] The precise physiologic mechanisms by which genetic variation in *CAPN10* leads to altered susceptibility to diabetes is still being characterized. Pharmacologic inhibition of calpain activity results in insulin resistance and impaired insulin secretion.[53,54] Studies in mice have led to similar conclusions.[55,56] Therefore, calpains play a role in regulating insulin secretion and insulin action.

KIR6.2 Gene

The beta cell K_{ATP} channel is composed of two subunits, SUR1 and KIR6.2, as discussed earlier.[57] The missense mutation Glu23Lys (E23K) in *KCNJ11*, the gene encoding KIR6.2, has been associated with increased risk of T2DM in some but not all studies,[51,58-60] similar to what was observed with *CAPN10*. Meta-analyses have shown that the E23K variant affects diabetes risk.[51,61] The study by Love-Gregory's group[61] suggested that the K allele of the E23K polymorphism increases the risk of T2DM by an average of 13% and that the KK homozygote is at greatest risk (relative risk,

1.28). 't Hart and colleagues examined the influence of the E23K variant of KIR6.2 on the insulin secretory responses to glucose and found no effect. However, they did not consider the confounding effect of insulin resistance.[62]

Peroxisome Proliferator-Activated Receptor-γ

PPARγ is a member of the PPAR subfamily of nuclear receptors. It is an important regulator of lipid and glucose homeostasis and cellular differentiation. Although PPARγ is most abundantly expressed in adipose tissue, it is also expressed in the pancreatic beta cell, and targeted elimination of the receptor in the beta cell leads to a blunting of the normal increase in beta cell mass that occurs on a high-fat diet.[63] Meta-analyses of all published studies performed by Altshuler and colleagues[64] in 2000 showed that the missense mutation Pro12Ala (P12A) in *PPARG* (the gene encoding PPARγ2) is associated with decreased risk for T2DM (estimated risk ratio for the alanine allele, 0.79).

Hepatocyte Nuclear Factor-4α Gene

The role of HNF-4α in the development of MODY has been clearly documented. Mutations in this gene lead to abnormalities in insulin secretion. Studies involving various populations[65-67] have demonstrated that genetic variation in the region of an alternative promoter for the *HNF4A* gene is associated with increased risk of T2DM. It is likely that these at-risk polymorphisms alter expression of *HNF4A*, thereby causing increased susceptibility to T2DM.

Transcription Factor 7-Like 2 Gene

Grant and colleagues[68] genotyped 228 microsatellite markers in Icelandic patients with T2DM and in controls. A microsatellite, DG10S478, within intron 3 of the transcription factor 7-like 2 gene (*TCF7L2;* formerly *TCF4)* was associated with T2DM. This was replicated in a Danish cohort and in a U.S. cohort. Compared with noncarriers, heterozygous and homozygous carriers of the at-risk alleles (38% and 7% of the population, respectively) have relative risks of 1.45 and 2.41. This corresponds to a population attributable risk of 21%. The TCF7L2 gene product is a high-mobility group box containing transcription factors previously implicated in blood glucose homeostasis. It is thought to act through regulation of proglucagon gene expression in enteroendocrine cells via the Wnt signaling pathway.

In a follow-up study, Florez and colleagues[69] observed that specific polymorphisms in *TCF7L2* increase the risk of progression from IGT to T2DM, and this effect is mediated through a reduction of glucose-induced insulin secretion.

Diabetes Genes Identified by GWAS

The reader is directed to recent excellent reviews of the results of GWAS for T2DM.[70,71] The first GWAS for T2DM clearly replicated the *TCF7L2* association and also discovered associations with a missense SNP in *SLC30A8* and common variants in *HHEX*.[72] *SLC30A8* encodes a zinc transporter that is expressed in insulin granules in beta cells, and *HHEX* encodes a transcription factor that is involved in early pancreatic development. Although it is not certain that these effects are responsible for the association with diabetes, the findings provided evidence of the relevance of the information uncovered by GWAS. The results of this and subsequently published GWAS[73,74] substantially increased the list of T2DM susceptibility genes as demonstrated in Table 31-7.

Based on these advances, the following general comments can be made regarding the genetics of T2DM:

TABLE 31-7

Glycemic Targets

Parameter	Normal	ADA	ACE
Premeal PG (mg/dL)	<100 (mean, ~90)	70-130	<110
Postprandial PG (mg/dL)	<140	<180	<140
HbA_{1c} (%)	4-6	<7	≤6.5

ACE, American College of Endocrinology; ADA, American Diabetes Association; PG, plasma glucose concentration; HbA_{1c}, glycosylated hemoglobin.

From American Diabetes Association. Standards of medical care in diabetes—2010. *Diabetes Care.* 2010;29:s11-s61; Rodbard HW, Blonde L, Braithwaite SS, et al., AACE Diabetes Mellitus Clinical Practice Guidelines Task Force. American Association of Clinical Endocrinologists medical guidelines for clinical practice for the management of diabetes mellitus. *Endocr Pract.* 2007;13(suppl 1):1-68.

1. A large number of genes are associated with increased susceptibility to this disease. The approximately 30 genes identified to date are thought to account for a small proportion (estimated at no more than 5% to 10%) of the total genetic risk for diabetes in the population.
2. The genes identified to date individually lead to a modest increase in the risk of diabetes. Persons with these individual polymorphisms have odds ratios between 1.10 and 1.45 when compared with individuals who do not have the at-risk polymorphisms.
3. The presence of multiple at-risk polymorphisms in a single individual substantially increases the risk of developing diabetes.
4. A significant proportion of the genetic variants associated with increased risk for diabetes appear to do so by inhibiting insulin secretion. Very few appear to increase insulin resistance or obesity. Whether this is a reflection of the relative importance of the roles of these factors in the pathogenesis of T2DM or whether the design of the GWAS did not allow genetic risk factors for insulin resistance and obesity to be identified is yet to be determined.

The application of additional techniques of exomic and whole genome sequencing will certainly provide additional insights into the genetic architecture of T2DM. Such studies are under way at a number of centers.

Insulin Resistance and the Risk of Type 2 Diabetes

Insulin Resistance

Substantial data indicate that insulin resistance plays a major role in the development of IGT and diabetes. Insulin resistance is a consistent finding in patients with T2DM, and resistance is present years before the onset of diabetes.[75-80] Prospective studies have shown that insulin resistance predicts the onset of diabetes.[76,77]

The term *insulin resistance* indicates the presence of an impaired biologic response to either exogenously administered or endogenously secreted insulin. Insulin resistance is manifested by decreased insulin-stimulated glucose transport and metabolism in adipocytes and skeletal muscle and by impaired suppression of hepatic glucose output.

Insulin sensitivity is influenced by a number of factors, including age,[81] weight, ethnicity, body fat (especially abdominal), physical activity, and medications. Insulin resistance is associated with the progression to IGT and T2DM,[82] although diabetes is rarely seen in insulin-resistant

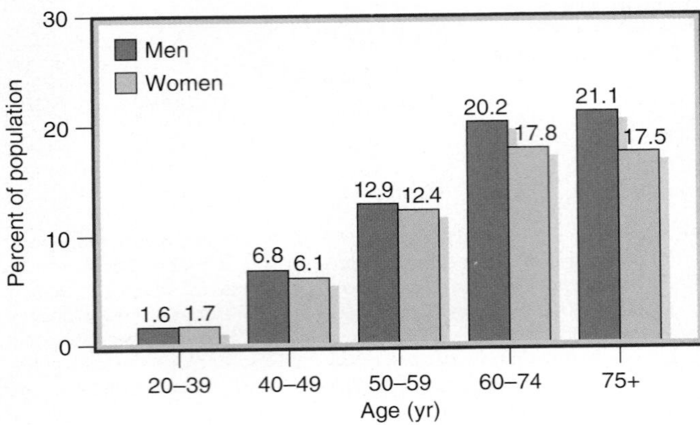

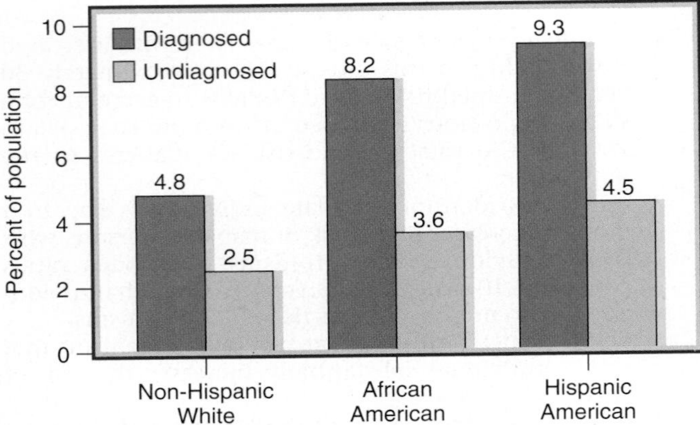

Figure 31-3 Prevalence of diabetes by age *(top panel)* and by ethnicity *(bottom panel).* (From Harris MI, Flegal KM, Cowie CC, et al. Prevalence of diabetes, impaired fasting glucose, and impaired glucose tolerance in U.S. adults. The Third National Health and Nutrition Examination Survey, 1988-1994. *Diabetes Care.* 1998;21:518-524.)

persons without some degree of beta-cell dysfunction.[80] First-degree relatives of type 2 diabetics have insulin resistance even at a time when they are not obese, implying a strong genetic component in the development of insulin resistance.[76,82,83] There is also a strong influence of environmental factors on the genetic predisposition to insulin resistance and therefore to diabetes.[84,85]

Obesity and Type 2 Diabetes

The association of obesity with T2DM has been recognized for decades. A close association between obesity and insulin resistance is seen in all ethnic groups and is found across the full range of body weights, across all ages, and in both sexes (Fig. 31-3).[86-88] A number of large epidemiologic studies have shown that the risk of diabetes, and presumably that of insulin resistance, rises as body fat content increases from the very lean to the very obese, implying that the absolute amount of body fat has an effect on insulin sensitivity across a broad range (Fig. 31-4A).[89-91] However, central (intra-abdominal) adiposity is more strongly linked to insulin resistance (see Fig. 31-4B) and to a number of important metabolic variables, including plasma glucose, insulin, total plasma cholesterol and triglyceride concentrations, and decreased plasma high-density lipoprotein (HDL)-cholesterol concentration, than is total adiposity.[92-98] In addition, the effect of accumulation of abdominal fat on glucose tolerance is independent of total adiposity.[99,100]

The reason for the relationship between intra-abdominal fat and abnormal metabolism is not clearly defined, but a number of hypotheses, which are not mutually exclusive, have been proposed. First, abdominal fat is more lipolytically active than subcutaneous fat, perhaps because of its greater complement of adrenergic receptors.[101,102] In addition, the abdominal adipose store is resistant to the antilipolytic effects of insulin,[103] including alterations in lipoprotein lipase activity; this leads to increased lipase activity and a greater flux of fatty acids into the circulation, with the portal circulation receiving the greatest fatty acid load. Finally, the high levels of 11β-hydroxysteroid dehydrogenase type 1 (HSD11B1) in mesenteric fat could result in enhanced conversion of inactive cortisone to active cortisol, resulting in increased local cortisol production. This might change adipocytes to increase lipolysis and alter the production of adipokines, which might directly modulate glucose metabolism. The roles of the skeletal muscle and liver in insulin resistance and hyperglycemia are discussed later.

Nutrient Overload and Insulin Resistance. Cells have developed a number of ways to sense incoming nutrients, including direct and indirect activation of transcription factors and protein kinases. These pathways integrate with incoming hormonal signals to modulate cellular metabolism, increasing anabolic reactions in times of nutrient surfeit and catabolic reactions in postprandial or nutrient

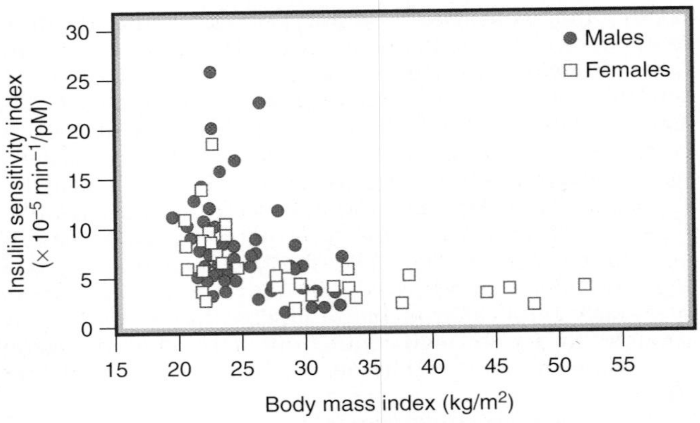

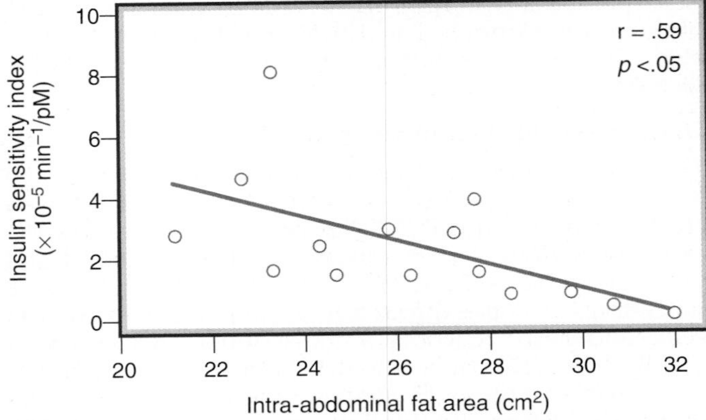

Figure 31-4 Relationship between body mass index *(top panel)* or intra-abdominal fat *(bottom panel)* and insulin sensitivity. (*Top*, From Fujimoto WY, Bergstrom RW, Boyko EJ, et al. Susceptibility to development of central adiposity among populations. *Obesity Res.* 1995;3(suppl 2):179S-186S; *bottom*, from Kahn SE, Prigeon RL, McCulloch DK, et al. Quantification of the relationship between insulin sensitivity and beta-cell function in human subjects: evidence for a hyperbolic function. *Diabetes.* 1993;42:1663-1672.)

deficient states. In a sense, the reaction of different tissues to obesity may be a relatively normal physiologic response to excess nutrient delivery, with prolonged activation leading to unintended and pathologic states that result in insulin resistance, inflammation, and even cell death. A variety of interacting factors functioning within and between tissues determine the final phenotypic response of a person to continued nutrient overload. An individual can be obese with normal objective findings related to glucose and lipid homeostasis or other cardiovascular risk factors, whereas another person can be only slightly above normal weight and yet harbor a distinctly abnormal physiology. Clearly, genetics plays a role in these responses, as demonstrated by the increased burden of metabolic dysfunction in Asians at a much lower BMI than in Caucasians or other ethnic groups.[104]

Adipose Tissue and Insulin Resistance. To maintain metabolic homeostasis, nutrient intake exceeding expenditure must be converted to biologic precursors to increase cellular mass or it must be stored. Most excess nutrients, whether carbohydrate, protein, or lipid, are stored as fatty acids in the form of triglyceride in adipose tissue. This storage segregates the excess nutrients in a form that is mobilizable in times of energy deficit. If the storage capacity of adipose tissue is exceeded, lipids and other nutrients enter nonstorage tissues, such as myocytes, hepatocytes, vascular cells, and beta cells, and trigger a variety of adaptive and nonadaptive cellular responses that lead to insulin resistance and cellular dysfunction.

Adipocytes are more than storage cells; they regulate the uptake and release of fatty acids; participate in the glycerol free fatty acid cycle; release leptin and other hormones that signal the energy status of the body; and secrete an ever-expanding number of cytokines that have hormonal, paracrine, and autocrine actions.[105] The adipocyte itself can be adversely affected by accumulation of excess nutrients, leading to events that can have adverse consequences on the body. As adipocyte surface area increases in obesity, there is increased expression of leptin, interleukin 6 (IL-6), IL-8, monocyte chemoattractant protein 1, and granulocyte colony-stimulating factor. These and possibly other cytokines attract pro-inflammatory macrophages (M1 type), which release factors such as tumor necrosis factor-α (TNF-α) that have local and systemic inflammatory effects.[106]

mTOR. The mammalian target of rapamycin (mTOR) may be part of the integration of excess nutrient accumulation and insulin resistance. mTOR is part of a multisubunit serine/threonine protein kinase complex, called TORC, that integrates signaling from the insulin and other growth factor receptors and regulates many cell processes including growth, autophagy, apoptosis, protein synthesis, and transcription. The TORC1 complex is activated by growth factors, including insulin and insulin-like growth factors, as well as nutrients, primarily the essential branched-chain amino acid leucine and fatty acids, the latter via formation of phosphatidic acid.

Several downstream targets have been identified, with S6 kinase (S6K) and 4E-BP being the best characterized. Phosphorylation of these proteins increase ribosomal protein translation augmenting cellular growth. Mutations in the tuberous sclerosis complex proteins (TSC1 and TSC2), which are inhibitory regulators of the mTOR kinase, result in the formation of hypertrophic tumors. As part of a feedback loop, S6K can phosphorylate insulin receptor substrate 1 (IRS1) on serine and inhibit its activity, resulting in downregulation of insulin signaling.[107]Cells harboring TSC mutations have high levels of IRS1 serine phosphorylation and are extremely insulin resistant. Conversely, mice with ablation of S6K-1 are protected from developing obesity and insulin resistance when given a high-fat diet, indicating a critical role in both growth and insulin resistance.[108]

Unfolded Protein Response. The endoplasmic reticulum (ER) functions in the post-translational processing of protein, including protein folding, maturation, quality control, and trafficking to other cellular compartments. As part of its quality control machinery, when the ER accumulates excess levels of unfolded or malfolded proteins, a distinct series of reactions occurs that slows overall protein synthesis while increasing the production of chaperones and other proteins that increase the fidelity of protein processing. The RNA-dependent protein kinase (PKR)–like eukaryotic initiation factor 2α (eIF2α) kinase known as PKR-like endoplasmic reticulum kinase (PERK), inositol-requiring enzyme 1 (IRE1), and activating transcription factor 6 (ATF6) are ER membrane–associated proteins that are normally complexed to the ER protein BiP/GRP78. Accumulation of unfolded proteins results in dissociation of these proteins from BiP/GRP78. PERK phosphorylates eIF2α, resulting in inhibition of most protein synthesis, IRE1 cleaves X-box binding protein 1 (XBP1), forming a messenger RNA (mRNA) translated into the active transcription factor, and, in combination with ATF6α, activates transcription to produce chaperones and proteins involved in ER biogenesis, phospholipid synthesis, ER-associated protein degradation (ERAD), and secretion.[109]

In states of overfeeding and obesity, evidence for activation of this unfolded protein response (UPR) can be seen in liver, adipose tissue, pancreatic beta cells, and other tissues. The UPR response to overnutrition is thought to have several effects, including activation of the Janus kinase (JNK) and nuclear factor-κB (NF-κB)/inhibitor of κB kinase (IKK) pathways leading to decreased IRS1 activity, increased levels of endogenous inflammatory mediators, alteration in sterol regulatory element–binding protein 1 (SREBP1)-mediated transcription, reduction in hepatic gluconeogenesis, and, after prolonged activation, cellular dysfunction and apoptosis.[110]

Innate Immunity. The innate immune system was originally thought to be a cellular system that allowed discrimination of self and nonself so as to adapt cellular metabolism to fight microbial pathogens. However, this system is now recognized as a general response to cellular stress that activates the inflammation and cellular repair systems. The innate immune system contains a series of pattern-recognition receptor proteins (PRRs) to detect microbial motifs. These proteins, including toll-like receptors (TLRs) and C-type lectins (CTLs), are expressed on a variety of cell types, including macrophages, monocytes, dendritic cells, neutrophils, and epithelial cells and cells of the adaptive immune system. The PRRs detect extracellular and intracellular pathogen-related molecules, including lipids and nucleic acids, and initiate a stereotypical response, including NF-κB activation and activator protein-1 (AP1) transcription, which increases expression of cytokines and chemokines.

Activation of the innate pathway also increases the production of so-called inflammasomes—large, multisubunit protein complexes that are important in the control of caspase 1–mediated, post-translational maturation and secretion of interleukins, primarily IL-1β, that have potent proinflammatory responses and are a risk factor for development of T2DM, perhaps through disruption of beta-cell function.[111]

Activation of the innate immune system in acute infection is associated with significant insulin resistance and likely plays a role in the insulin resistance seen in obesity, mediated by elevated levels of free fatty acids (FFAs). TLRs, especially TLR2 and TLR4, which respond to bacterial cell wall lipids and induce the innate inflammatory response, are activated by saturated fatty acids, whereas polyunsaturated fatty acids inhibit TLR signaling. Activation of TLRs in cells results in insulin resistance, whereas genetic disruption of the TLR4 receptor in mice is protective against fatty acid–induced insulin resistance.[112]

Results of human clinical trials involving disruption of the innate immune system show efficacy in the treatment of T2DM. Treatment of diabetics for 13 weeks with anakinra, a recombinant human IL-1R antagonist, reduced HbA_{1c} and enhanced insulin secretion without effects on insulin sensitivity, suggesting a primary effect on beta-cell function.[113]

Circadian Rhythms, Obesity, and Insulin Resistance. Almost all mammals have a well-developed circadian cycle which is controlled by a complex, integrated network of transcription-translation feedback loops that work in a 24-hour cycle. A defined set of genes establish the circadian cycle, which sets behavioral and physiologic functions, including sleep-wake cycles, feeding behaviors, hormone secretion, and metabolism.

There are significant epidemiologic associations in humans between reduction of sleep and increased obesity and other metabolic disturbances, including T2DM.[114] Experimental sleep disruption can directly impair insulin action, alter secretion of leptin and ghrelin with stimulation of appetite, increase inflammatory cytokine production, and create alterations in other cardiovascular risk factors. Alterations in normal feeding patterns that are attuned to the circadian metabolism can change the relationship between nutrient appearance and nutrient-metabolizing enzymes. For instance, alterations in fatty acid appearance and lipoprotein lipase activity could lead to altered partitioning of lipids to vulnerable tissues, leading to lipotoxicity and decreased secretion of leptin, increasing appetite.[115] These disturbances can be exacerbated by obesity-related sleep apnea. Although the cognitive improvements associated with successful treatment of sleep apnea are clear, the metabolic benefits continue to be debated.[116]

Skeletal Muscle Insulin Resistance

The primary site of glucose disposal after a meal is skeletal muscle, and the primary mechanism of glucose storage is through its conversion to glycogen. Given the relatively limited nutrient storage capacity of skeletal muscle, it is not surprising that, in obesity, insulin resistance in skeletal muscle is manifested before abnormalities in insulin signaling in adipose tissue and liver. Studies using the hyperinsulinemic-euglycemic clamp technique have demonstrated that in insulin-resistant people (with and without T2DM), there is a deficiency in the nonoxidative disposal of glucose related primarily to a defect in glycogen synthesis (Fig. 31-5).[117,118]

Fatty Acids and Insulin Resistance

Free Fatty Acids. Elevated FFAs predict the progression from IGT to diabetes.[119,120] In the periphery, FFAs might not be markedly elevated because of efficient extraction by the liver and skeletal muscle. Therefore, normal or minimally elevated FFA levels might not reflect the true exposure of fatty acids to peripheral tissues. Increased fatty acid flux to

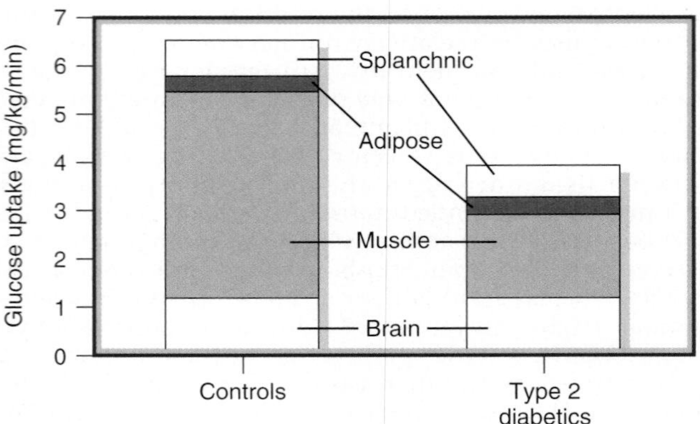

Figure 31-5 Tissue uptake of glucose in nondiabetic and insulin-resistant diabetic subjects during a hyperinsulinemic-euglycemic clamp. (From DeFronzo RA. The triumvirate: beta-cell, muscle, liver—a collusion responsible for NIDDM. Lilly Lecture 1987. *Diabetes.* 1988;37:667-687.)

skeletal muscle related to increased visceral lipolysis has been implicated in the inhibition of muscle glucose uptake.

The Randle hypothesis, or the glucose–fatty acid cycle, was originally proposed to account for the ability of FFAs to inhibit muscle glucose utilization. Randle's group[121] demonstrated that fatty acids compete with glucose for substrate oxidation in isolated muscle. The increase in fatty acid metabolism leads to an increase in the intramitochondrial acetyl coenzyme A (acetyl-CoA)/CoA and reduced nicotinamide adenine dinucleotide (NADH/NAD+) ratios, with subsequent inhibition of pyruvate dehydrogenase. The resulting increased intracellular mitochondrial (and cytosolic) citrate concentrations result in allosteric inhibition of phosphofructokinase, the key rate-controlling enzyme in glycolysis. Subsequent accumulation of glucose-6-phosphate inhibits hexokinase II activity, resulting in an increase in intracellular glucose concentrations and decreased glucose uptake.

Studies in vivo in humans suggest that the primary effect of fatty acids, at least in the presence of elevated insulin levels, is a decrease in glucose transport, as measured by a reduction in the rate of accumulation of intracellular glucose and glycogen using ^{13}C and ^{31}P nuclear magnetic resonance (NMR) spectroscopy. In normal subjects, elevated fatty acids, achieved by infusion of triglyceride emulsions and heparin (to activate lipoprotein lipase), resulted in a fall in intracellular glucose and glucose-6-phosphate concentrations that preceded the fall in glycogen accumulation.[122,123] These results challenge the Randle hypothesis (which predicts a rise in intracellular glucose-6-phosphate concentrations) as the basis of the reduction in insulin sensitivity seen with elevated fatty acids. Similar decreases in glucose transport have been seen in patients with T2DM[124] and in lean, normoglycemic, insulin-resistant offspring of type 2 diabetics.[125,126] These studies also found decreased activity of phosphatidylinositol 3-kinase (PI3K) and increased protein kinase C-θ activity that might, in part, mediate the effect of elevated FFAs.[127,128]

Studies also suggest that PKC-mediated serine phosphorylation of the IKKβ subunit, leading to its degradation and the unregulated translocation of NF-κB into the nucleus, might also be important to fatty acid–induced insulin resistance.[129] This is the mechanism by which high-dose aspirin therapy improves glucose metabolism in T2DM.[129] Disruption of the IKKβ inflammatory pathway by high-dose aspirin therapy in a small human trial resulted in an improvement in insulin sensitivity.

Intramuscular Triglycerides. Insulin-stimulated glucose uptake is inversely related to the amount of intramuscular triglycerides. A strong correlation between intramuscular triglyceride concentration and insulin resistance was demonstrated by evaluation of intramuscular triglyceride with biopsy,[130] computed tomography,[131] and magnetic resonance imaging (MRI).[132] MRI has been a valuable addition because the magnetic resonance signal can distinguish intramyocellular from extramyocellular fat and demonstrates the increased triglyceride accumulation within the myofiber itself.[133] First-degree relatives of type 2 diabetics have an increase in intramyocellular fat, and in this group there is also a correlation with insulin resistance.[132]

The mechanism for accumulation of triglyceride in the skeletal muscle of obese and insulin-resistant persons is probably related to mismatching of FFA uptake and oxidation. During resting postabsorptive conditions, about 30% of fatty acid flux in the plasma pool is accounted for by oxidation, and the remaining 70% of flux is recycled into triglyceride, indicating a physiologic reserve that exceeds immediate tissue needs for oxidative substrates. The equilibrium between oxidation and reesterification within muscle is paramount in determining fatty acid storage within tissue. The uptake, transport, and metabolism of fatty acids are highly regulated processes (Fig. 31-6), and alteration of the balance between uptake and oxidation in skeletal muscle leads to increased intramyocellular triglycerides. The increased lipolysis associated with obesity provides an increased amount of FFA presented to muscle.

Increased muscle triglyceride content is not invariably linked to insulin resistance, because exercise training is associated with increased muscle triglyceride content,[134] and chronic exercise increases insulin sensitivity as well as the capacity for fatty acid oxidation.[135-139] Studies suggest that acute exercise increases intramyocellular triglyceride synthesis, reducing fatty acid oxidation and preventing fatty acid–induced insulin resistance.[140]

Fatty Acid Metabolism in Skeletal Muscle. The uptake of fatty acid from the serum, where it is mostly bound to albumin, is mediated by at least three families of proteins: fatty acid translocase, plasma membrane fatty acid–binding proteins (FABPs), and fatty acid transport proteins.[141-143] The levels of the putative transport proteins are regulated by exercise,[144] are correlated with body weight (at least in women), and can be modulated by insulin infusion.[145]

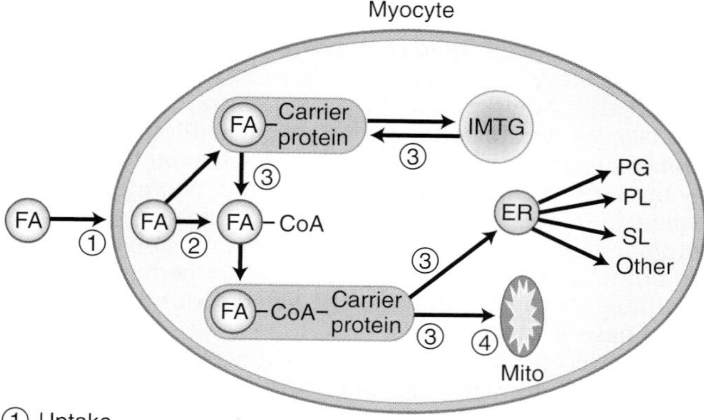

Figure 31-6 Simplified schematic diagram demonstrating fatty acid (FA) uptake, activation (formation of FA-coenzyme A [CoA]), and intracellular transport to organelles within a muscle cell. ER, endoplasmic reticulum; IMTG, intramuscular triglyceride; Mito, mitochondrion; PG, prostaglandin; PL, phospholipid; SL, sphingolipid.

FABPs are capable of binding multiple hydrophobic ligands, including fatty acids, eicosanoids, and retinoids, with high affinity.[146] FABPs are thought to facilitate uptake of fatty acids and to promote subsequent intracellular transport to subcellular organelles.[147] There is a direct correlation between heart-type FABP content and oxidative capacity observed during development and among different muscle types.[148,149] In mice that have a disruption of the heart isoform[150] or the adipocyte isoform[151] of FABP, plasma fatty acid concentrations were significantly elevated and plasma glucose was decreased, suggesting a key role in normal regulation of fatty acid oxidation. Some,[151] but not all,[153] studies have shown a decrease in heart-type FABP in insulin-resistant humans.

Carnitine palmitoyltransferase 1 (CPT1) has been the subject of intense scrutiny for many years because of its central role in the balance between mitochondrial glucose and fatty acid metabolism, and primarily because of inhibition of mitochondrial fatty acid uptake by malonyl-CoA.[154,155] A specific isoform contributes 97% of the CPT1 in muscle and has 100-fold lower sensitivity to inhibition by malonyl-CoA.[156] This lower sensitivity to malonyl-CoA inhibition suggests that the level of CPT1 itself may be important in the balance of uptake and oxidation of fatty acids. Evidence for this in skeletal muscle stems from the finding that, as with other fatty acid–oxidizing enzymes, muscle CPT1 mRNA is regulated by PPARα activators, fat feeding, and exercise in rodents and is inversely correlated with obesity in humans.[157-160]

Long-chain fatty acids, after passing through the inner mitochondrial membrane as acylcarnitines, are metabolized at the surface of the inner mitochondrial membrane by CPT2 and the long chain–specific oxidation system consisting of very-long-chain acyl-CoA dehydrogenase (VLCAD) and the trifunctional protein (TFP) oxidation complex (Fig. 31-7). Transfer of the acyl chain from carnitine to CoA, catalyzed by CPT2, is followed by one cycle of oxidation catalyzed by VLCAD and TFP to yield a chain-shortened acyl-CoA that can recycle through the same oxidation system.[161] In actuality, four different acyl-CoA dehydrogenase enzymes catalyze the initial dehydrogenation of straight-chain fatty acids in mitochondria. Three of them—short-chain acyl-CoA dehydrogenase (SCAD), medium-chain acyl-CoA dehydrogenase (MCAD), and long-chain acyl-CoA dehydrogenase (LCAD)—are soluble enzymes located in the mitochondrial matrix as homotetramers. A fourth, VLCAD, is attached to the inner membrane as a homodimer. Their names derive from the length of the fatty acids that they process. VLCAD and LCAD shorten the long-chain fatty acids into medium-chain fatty acids that can then be processed by MCAD and SCAD.[162] The SCAD, MCAD, and LCAD monomers share a high degree of homology but do not share homology with VLCAD. At least some of these enzymes can be regulated in humans during exercise training.[163]

Uncoupling protein-1 (UCP1) is clearly related to the uncoupling of oxidative phosphorylation in brown adipose tissue.[124] UCP2 and UCP3 have structural similarities to UCP1, but it is not clear that they are actually uncouplers of oxidative phosphorylation.[164] Newer members of the family, such as brain mitochondrial carrier protein 1 (BMCP1) and UCP4, have an even more distant sequence relationship.[165] BMCP1 and UCP4 are predominantly expressed in neural tissues, namely the brain. UCP3 mRNA

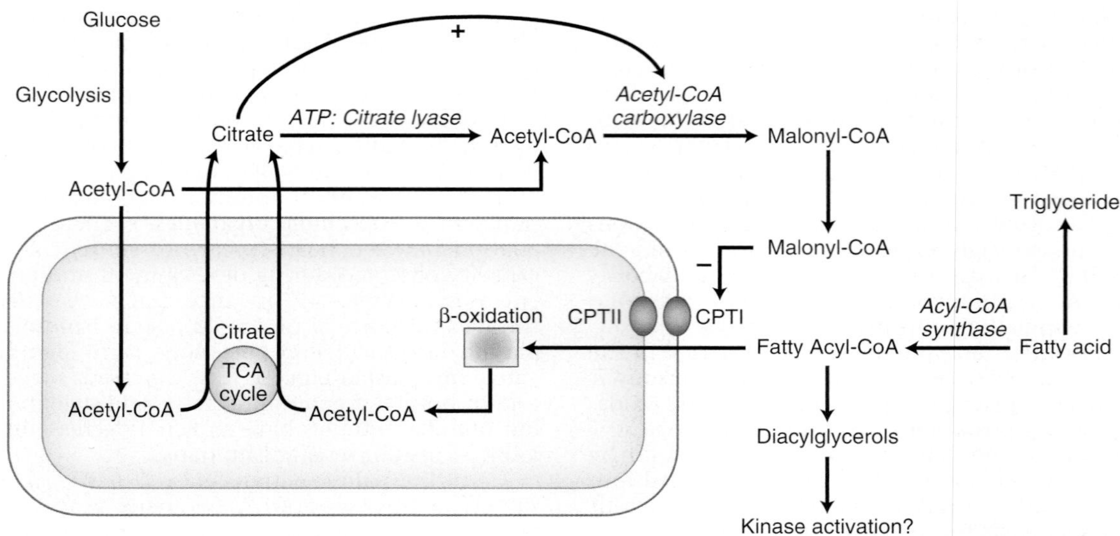

Figure 31-7 Glucose effect on triglyceride metabolism. Increased uptake of glucose results in increased production of acetyl coenzyme A (acetyl-CoA) as a product of glycolysis. The increased tricarboxylic acid (TCA) cycle activity associated with oxidation of triglycerides and glucose increases the production of citrate, which is shuttled to the cytoplasm, activates the enzyme acetyl-CoA carboxylase (ACC) by allosteric mechanisms, and increases the susceptibility of ACC to phosphatases. This leads to increased ACC activity, converting acetyl-CoA to malonyl-CoA. Malonyl-CoA is a potent inhibitor of carnitine palmitoyltransferase (CPT) I on the outer mitochondrial membrane, which leads to accumulation of fatty acyl-CoAs in the cytoplasm. This may result in the production of signaling molecules that can increase the activity of kinases and other enzymes and lead to insulin resistance. ATP, adenosine triphosphate.

is found primarily in skeletal muscle and in brown adipose tissue. UCP2 has a ubiquitous tissue distribution. UCP2 and UCP3 mRNA levels have been correlated with different physiologic states, and numerous studies indicate that expression of UCP2 and UCP3 is stimulated by thyroid hormones and in the presence of high levels of fatty acids.[166] In humans, the levels of UCP2 and UCP3 mRNAs were upregulated by a high-fat diet, and the upregulation was more pronounced in humans with high percentages of type IIA muscle fibers.[167] In a small study, exercise training in humans increased mitochondrial oxidative capacity but did not change UCP2 or UCP3 levels.[168] Obesity itself was shown to be positively correlated with a splice isoform of UCP3.[169] A unique polymorphism in the promoter region of UCP3 correlated with expression of UCP3 in skeletal muscle.[170]

Mitochondrial Abnormalities and Insulin Resistance

A decrease in oxidative capacity is seen in both humans and animals with insulin resistance, obesity, and T2DM.[171,172] Studies have suggested that increases in intramyocellular fat content in skeletal muscle associated with insulin resistance (see earlier discussion) may be caused by alterations in mitochondrial mass. In one study, young insulin-resistant offspring of parents with T2DM demonstrated a 60% reduction in insulin-stimulated skeletal muscle glucose uptake compared with control subjects, and this reduction correlated with an increase of approximately 80% in intramyocellular lipid content.[173] The elevated intramyocellular lipid content was attributable to the 30% reduction in mitochondrial oxidative capacity. The insulin-resistant subjects showed a lower ratio of type I to type II muscle fibers. Type I fibers are mostly oxidative and contain more mitochondria than type II muscle fibers, which are more glycolytic.

Decreased expression of nuclear-encoded genes that regulate mitochondrial biogenesis, such as PPARγ coactivators-1α and -1β (PGC-1α and PGC-1β, respectively), have been shown to be important for mitochondrial biogenesis and for fiber type selection during development.[174] PGC-1α transcriptionally activates the nuclear respiratory factors NRF1 and NRF2, which are known to be important for mitochondrial biogenesis.[175] PGC-1α–responsive genes were found to be downregulated in obese white patients with IGT and T2DM.[176,177] In obese diabetic and nondiabetic Mexican Americans, PGC-1α and PGC-1β expression levels were reduced compared with levels in nonobese persons.[178] The activity of the electron transport chain is reduced and intramyofibrillar mitochondria are smaller in patients with T2DM, and both the size of intramyofibrillar mitochondria and electron transport chain activity in muscle homogenates correlate with severity of insulin resistance.[179]

In one study, rats bred for differences in oxidative capacity (determined by their intrinsic ability to run) were described.[180] The skeletal muscle of the animals with a low capacity for aerobic exercise showed a reduction in mitochondrial gene expression and PGC-1α, similar to that seen in humans. When multiple metabolic parameters were assessed, it was determined that the group with poor aerobic capacity had several significant abnormalities, including obesity, insulin resistance, hypertension, and dyslipidemia, suggesting that the defects found in humans could have a genetic basis.

More recent studies have questioned the cause-effect relationship between alterations in mitochondrial mass and mitochondrial function, suggesting that, rather than being an inherited trait, these observed changes could be acquired. First, because insulin itself can upregulate mitochondrial biogenesis, muscle insulin resistance could provide a mechanism for the reduction in mitochondria. Second, the observed reduction in ATP synthesis and tricarboxylic acid (TCA) cycle activity could be explained by reduced turnover of ATP in relatively sedentary individuals. Persistent delivery of fatty acids to skeletal muscle, seen in obesity and after high-fat feeding, increases fatty acid β-oxidation. In the absence of energy demand (e.g., exercise), the reduction in the adenosine diphosphate (ADP)/ATP ratio would impair electron transport in the mitochondria, increasing NADH levels, which would impair TCA cycle activity. Indicative of impaired oxidation in the mitochondria, mice fed a high-fat diet show a reduction in TCA cycle intermediates and an impairment of adequate β-oxidation of fatty acids marked by increases in even-chained acyl-carnitine levels. Increases in plasma acylcarnitines are found in obese, insulin-resistant individuals.[181] An emerging concept, nonexercise activity thermogenesis (NEAT), which is the energy expended for everything that is not sleeping, eating, or sports-like exercise, suggests that subtle differences in activity throughout the day can result in a difference in caloric expenditure of up to 350 calories per day.[182] Whether long-term differences in NEAT could result in acquired changes in skeletal muscle metabolism remains to be determined.

Glucose Influence on Fatty Acid Metabolism

An emerging concept that could couple increased fatty acid flux into skeletal muscle with impaired insulin action is the central role of malonyl-CoA in regulating fatty acid and glucose oxidation (see Fig. 31-7).[183] Malonyl-CoA is an allosteric inhibitor of CPT1, the enzyme that controls the transfer of long-chain fatty acyl-CoAs into the mitochondria.[154,184,185] Even in insulin-resistant skeletal muscle, glucose uptake into the skeletal muscle is higher than normal especially at the elevated levels of glucose found in T2DM.[186,187] The glucose is shunted toward the glycolytic pathway, generating acetyl-CoA that can be converted to malonyl-CoA in the cytoplasm by the action of the highly regulated enzyme acetyl-CoA carboxylase (ACC).

In humans, an infusion of insulin and glucose at a high rate leads to increases in the concentration of malonyl-CoA in skeletal muscle and to decreases in whole-body and, presumably, muscle fatty acid oxidation.[188] In the presence of elevated glucose and insulin levels, the tricarboxylic acid (TCA) cycle is activated, resulting in an increase in citrate in the cytoplasm through increased malate cycling in the mitochondria. The increased citrate is converted to acetyl-CoA through citrate lyase and thus provides an indirect substrate for ACC. Citrate also allosterically activates ACC and makes ACC a better substrate for phosphatases that activate the enzyme.[189,190] ACC is also regulated by a phosphorylation-dephosphorylation cycle, with the important participation of adenosine monophosphate (AMP)-activated protein kinase (AMPK), which inhibits ACC basal activity and reduces ACC activation by citrate.[191] ACC then generates malonyl-CoA, which in turn allosterically inhibits CPT1 residing on the outer mitochondrial membrane, inhibiting uptake of acyl-CoA. The resulting buildup of long-chain acyl-CoAs and diacylglycerols is proposed to activate one or more PKC isoforms or other lipid-activated proteins, resulting in insulin resistance.[183] Support for this hypothesis is the finding that exercise, which activates AMPK, inactivates ACC, lowers intracellular long-chain acyl-CoA levels, and has an acute insulin-sensitizing effect.[192]

Hyperinsulinemia and Insulin Resistance

Hyperinsulinemia per se has been proposed to cause insulin resistance. Elevated concentrations of insulin can cause insulin resistance by downregulating insulin receptors and desensitizing postreceptor pathways.[193] Del Prato and associates showed that 24 and 72 hours of sustained physiologic hyperinsulinemia in normal persons specifically inhibited the ability of insulin to increase nonoxidative glucose disposal in association with an impaired ability of insulin to stimulate glycogen synthase activity.[194] Suppression of insulin secretion in obese, insulin-resistant persons results in increased insulin sensitivity.[195,196]

Insulin-Signaling Abnormalities in Insulin Resistance

The pathways that are critical for insulin regulation of glucose and lipid metabolism are being clarified. However, the complete cascade of events remains to be determined. Besides intermediary metabolism of glucose and lipid, signaling by insulin affects other cellular processes such as amino acid transport and metabolism, protein synthesis, cell growth, differentiation, and apoptosis.

Insulin Signaling

Insulin signaling is initiated through binding and activation of its cell-surface receptor and initiates a cascade of phosphorylation and dephosphorylation events, second-messenger generation, and protein-protein interactions that result in diverse metabolic events in almost every tissue (Fig. 31-8). The insulin receptor consists of two insulin-binding α-subunits and two catalytically active β-subunits that are disulfide linked into an $\alpha_2\beta_2$ heterotetrameric complex. Insulin binds to the extracellular α-subunits, activating the intracellular tyrosine kinase domain of the β-subunit.[197] One receptor β-subunit phosphorylates its partner on specific tyrosine residues that may have distinct functions such as stimulation of intermolecular association of signaling molecules such as Shc and Grb, IRS1 through IRS4, Shc adapter protein isoforms, and SIRP (signal regulatory protein) family members Gab-1, Cbl, CAP, and APS[198,199]; stimulation of mitogenesis[200]; and receptor internalization.[201]

The insulin receptor β-subunit has also been shown to undergo serine/threonine phosphorylation, which might decrease the ability of the receptor to autophosphorylate. The activities of a number of PKC isoforms that catalyze the serine or threonine phosphorylation of the insulin receptor are elevated in animal models of insulin resistance and in insulin-resistant humans.[202,203] Interventions that decrease serine phosphorylation of the insulin receptor result in increased insulin signaling.[204] Termination of the insulin-signaling event occurs when the receptor is internalized and dephosphorylated by protein tyrosine phosphatases. Increased activity of protein tyrosine phosphatase can attenuate insulin signaling. Two protein tyrosine phosphatases that have been shown to negatively regulate insulin signaling, PTP1B and LAR (leukocyte antigen–related), have been reported to be elevated in insulin-resistant patients.[205,206] Conversely, disruption of PTB1B in mice resulted in a marked increase in insulin sensitivity and resistance to diet-induced obesity.[207]

Mutations in the insulin receptor are associated with rare forms of insulin resistance. These mutations affect insulin receptor number, splicing, trafficking, binding, and phosphorylation. The affected patients demonstrate severe insulin resistance, manifest as clinically diverse syndromes including the type A syndrome, leprechaunism, Rabson-Mendenhall syndrome, and lipoatrophic diabetes.[208,209]

Downstream Events after Insulin Receptor Phosphorylation

The IRSs act as multifunctional docking proteins activated by tyrosine phosphorylation.[210] The IRS proteins have multiple functional domains—including Pleckstrin

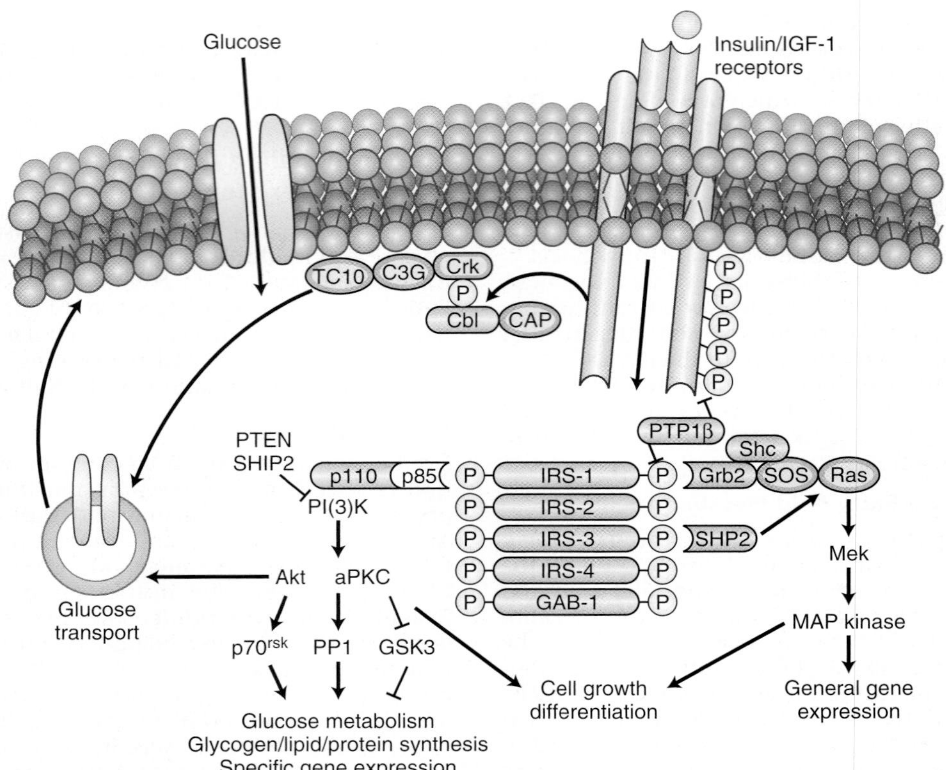

Figure 31-8 Insulin signaling. The insulin receptor is autophosphorylated on multiple tyrosine residues, allowing the docking and activation of multiple signaling molecules that mediate the increases in glucose uptake and metabolism as well as changes in protein and lipid metabolism. aPKC, atypical protein kinase C; C3G, guanine nucleotide exchange factor C3G; CAP, Cbl-associated protein; Cbl, Cas-Br-M (murine) ecotropic retroviral transforming sequence; Crk, CT10 related kinase; GAB, Grb2-associated binding protein; Grb2, growth factor receptor-bound protein 2; GSK3, glycogen synthase kinase-3; IGF, insulin-like growth factor; IRS, insulin receptor substrate; MAP, mitogen-activated protein; mek, MAPK/ERK kinases; P, phosphate; PI(3)K, phosphatidylinositol-3-kinase; PP1, protein phosphatase 1; PTEN, phosphatase and tensin homolog deleted on chromosome 10; PTP, protein tyrosine phosphatase; RAS, Rat sarcoma oncogene; Shc, SH3-containing protein; SHIP2, SH2 domain–containing inositol 5-phosphatase; SHP2, SH2 domain–containing protein-tyrosine phosphatase (now called PTPN11); SOS, son of seven less, TC10, small GTP binding protein TC10. (From Saltiel AR, Kahn CR. Insulin signalling and the regulation of glucose and lipid metabolism. *Nature.* 2001;414:799-806.)

homology (PH) and phosphotyrosine binding (PTB)—and SH domains that interact with other proteins to mediate the insulin-signaling events. Disruption of IRS1 in mice resulted in mild insulin resistance and growth retardation, whereas disruption of IRS2 resulted in beta-cell failure and secondary insulin resistance.[211] Alterations in the phosphorylation and levels of IRS1 and IRS2 are found in many insulin-resistant tissues. Serine phosphorylation on IRS proteins is mediated by a variety of kinases, including PKC isoforms and mTOR/S6K. Serine phosphorylation on appropriate residues might increase ubiquitination and downregulation of the protein, which would result in decreased downstream signaling.[212]

PI3K, which is regulated by interaction with IRS proteins, is necessary but not sufficient for stimulation of glucose transporter 4 (GLUT4)-mediated increase in glucose transport in insulin-sensitive tissues.[213] In addition, inhibition of PI3K activity with the fungal inhibitor wortmannin inhibited insulin-stimulated glucose uptake, glycogen synthesis, triglyceride accumulation, protein synthesis, and modulation of gene expression.[214] PI3K generates 3,4,5-phosphoinositol, which activates several phosphatidylinositol 3,4,5-triphosphate (PIP_3)-dependent serine-threonine kinases, such as PI-dependent protein kinases 1 and 2 (PDK1 and PDK2), which in turn activate Akt, salt- and glucocorticoid-induced kinases,[144] PKC, wortmannin-sensitive and insulin-stimulated serine kinase, and others.

Akt kinase (also known as protein kinase B) exists as three distinct isoforms that are activated by phosphorylation on specific threonine and serine residues.[215,216] Activated Akt has the ability to phosphorylate proteins that regulate lipid synthesis, glycogen synthesis, protein synthesis, and apoptosis. Disruption of Akt2 resulted in insulin resistance and diabetes in mice.[217] Several investigators have examined the role of PI3K and Akt in persons with insulin resistance. Studies have shown a decrease in IRS-associated PI3K[218] and Akt[219] activity in insulin-resistant skeletal muscle; however, in some patients with reduced PI3K activity, there was normal activation of Akt.[220]

A primary effect of insulin is to stimulate translocation of GLUT4 from an intracellular pool to the surface of cells, primarily in skeletal muscle, adipose tissue, and heart.[221] Akt substrate of 160 kd (AS160) and TBC1D1 are paralog Rab family guanosine triphosphatase (GTPase)-activating proteins that have been proposed to inhibit the translocation of GLUT4 to the plasma membrane.[222] On phosphorylation, the inhibition is relieved, contributing to the increased translocation. Although the composition and signaling pathways that converge on the intracellular GLUT4-containing vesicles to cause GLUT4 translocation are still not well understood, it appears that the number of glucose transporters in skeletal muscle of insulin-resistant persons is not changed, but the ability of insulin to effect this translocation is disrupted.[223-225]

Glucocorticoid-Induced Insulin Resistance

Cushing's syndrome and exogenous glucocorticoid treatment have long been known to induce significant insulin resistance in humans. The exact mechanism is unknown, but it is associated with redistribution of fat from the periphery to the central compartment. Elevations in triglyceride and FFA levels also occur. At a molecular level, dexamethasone has differential effects on the proteins involved in the early steps of insulin action in liver and muscle. In both tissues, dexamethasone treatment results in a reduction in insulin-stimulated IRS1-associated PI3K, which may play a role in the pathogenesis of insulin resistance at the cellular level. On the basis of studies performed in mice, it has been suggested that the effects of glucocorticoids to raise glucose concentrations and cause hypertension are mediated through activation of PPARα receptors in the liver[226]; however, the relevance of this observation to humans is not known.

Tumor Necrosis Factor-α

Studies in humans and in animal models of obesity have identified changes in the expression and activity of key molecules involved in the insulin-signaling pathway. Decreases in the number and the kinase activity of insulin receptors[227] and impairment in the activation of IRS1,[228] PI3K,[229,230] and protein kinase B[231] have been observed. Although the basis for the changes is generally unknown, a TNF-α–mediated mechanism for the decreased activity in the initial steps of the insulin-signaling cascade has been proposed. TNF-α, made and secreted by adipocytes, is elevated in a variety of experimental models of obesity.[232] The kinase activity of the insulin receptor in rats[233] or in 3T3-L1 adipocytes[232] treated with TNF-α was reduced, possibly by increased serine phosphorylation.[234] Fat-fed mice with genetic ablation of TNF-α production had increased kinase activity of the insulin receptor compared with control mice and demonstrated increased insulin sensitivity.[235] In addition, rats treated with neutralizing antisera or soluble TNF receptors demonstrated an amelioration of their insulin resistance. As described later, other interventions to decrease TNF-α action result in increased insulin sensitivity.

Glucotoxicity, Glucosamine

Hyperglycemia is a primary factor in the development of diabetes complications, and decreases in average blood glucose have a profound effect to prevent complications in both T1DM[236] and T2DM.[237] Hyperglycemia itself can cause insulin resistance. In Pima Indians, the level of fasting glycemia is the primary determinant of insulin sensitivity.[238] The defect is primarily in skeletal muscle[239] and is related to the degree of hyperglycemia.

Entry of glucose into the cell results in its phosphorylation to glucose-6-phosphate, which has multiple metabolic fates. The hexosamine pathway is a relatively minor branch of the glycolytic pathway, encompassing less than 3% of total glucose used. The first and rate-limiting enzyme glutamine–fructose-6-phosphate (F6P) amidotransferase (GFAT), converts F6P and glutamine to glucosamine-6-phosphate (GlcN6P) and glutamate. Subsequent steps metabolize GlcN6P to uridine diphosphate-*N*-acetylglucosamine (UDP-GlcNAc), UDP-*N*-acetylgalactosamine (UDP-GalNAc), and cytidine monophosphate (CMP)-sialic acid, essential building blocks of the glycosyl side chains of glycoproteins, glycolipids, proteoglycans, and gangliosides.[240] Evidence suggests that the hexosamine pathway underlies the defect in glucose utilization associated with hyperglycemia. Increased flux through the hexosamine pathway appears to be required for some of the metabolic effects of sustained increased glucose flux, which promotes the complications of diabetes including diminished expression of sarcoplasmic reticulum Ca^{2+}-ATPase in cardiomyocytes and induction of TGF-β and plasminogen activator inhibitor 1 (PAI-1) in vascular smooth muscle cells, mesangial cells, and aortic endothelial cells.[241]

Hexosamines, such as glucosamine, when incubated with adipose tissue, induce insulin resistance in fat cells[242] and in skeletal muscle.[243] Infusion of glucosamine into rats resulted in a dose-dependent increase in insulin resistance of skeletal muscle,[243] and transgenic mice that overexpress GFAT specifically in skeletal muscle acquired severe insulin resistance.[244] By a pathway that is unclear, glucosamine overproduction resulted in a disruption of the ability of insulin to cause translocation of GLUT4 to the cell surface.[245] Through its anti-insulin action, the hexosamine pathway has been hypothesized to be a glucose sensor that allows the cell to sense and adapt to the prevailing level of glucose.[239]

Insulin Resistance and Lipodystrophy Associated with Human Immunodeficiency Virus Infection

A syndrome with many of the clinical and metabolic features of insulin resistance is increasingly being recognized in patients with human immunodeficiency virus (HIV) infection.[246] An unusual form of lipodystrophy is observed in certain of these patients in whom there is significant fat redistribution from the extremities and face to the torso with accumulation of intra-abdominal and intrascapular fat. This form of lipodystrophy is associated with significant insulin resistance and T2DM, dyslipidemia with elevated total and low-density lipoprotein (LDL)-cholesterol and suppressed HDL-cholesterol concentrations and a susceptibility to lactic acidemia.[247]

Epidemiologic studies have associated this syndrome with previous or current treatment with antiretroviral protease inhibitors or nucleoside reverse transcriptase inhibitors. There is also an association with increased age.[246] Other possible contributing factors are male sex, diagnosis of the acquired immunodeficiency syndrome (AIDS), responsiveness to antiretroviral treatment, and increases in CD4 T-cell counts. An increased emphasis has been placed on the role of protease inhibitors in the pathogenesis of the syndrome. Administration of these drugs or ritonavir to normal subjects caused increases in plasma triglyceride and very-low-density lipoprotein (VLDL)-cholesterol and decreased plasma HDL-cholesterol levels.[248] Indinavir administration for 4 weeks resulted in small increases in serum glucose and insulin levels and decreased insulin-mediated glucose disposal as assessed with a hyperinsulinemic euglycemic clamp; there were no changes in lipoprotein, triglyceride, or FFA levels.[249]

The molecular basis of the metabolic syndrome is not clear. A number of protease inhibitors can inhibit glucose transport in vitro and in vivo, and there is evidence for a direct interaction with GLUT4[250] that could inhibit glucose uptake specifically in insulin-responsive tissue. Mitochondrial abnormalities have been described in subcutaneous adipose tissue biopsy specimens obtained from HIV-infected patients with lipodystrophy compared with specimens from patients without the syndrome.[251] A direct effect of protease inhibitors on differentiation of adipocytes has also been described.[252-254] Additionally, reductions in mitochondrial number and oxidative function have been described in adipocytes from subcutaneous biopsies obtained from patients treated with highly active antiretroviral therapy (HAART).[255] The precise mechanism for the lipodystrophy associated with HIV infection is not known.

Treatment of HIV-associated lipodystrophy is at present inadequate. Use of alternative protease inhibitors might improve metabolic abnormalities, particularly those induced or increased by protease inhibitor therapy. However, changing protease inhibitors has little impact on body fat. Switching thymidine analogues has been the only intervention to improve lipoatrophy in independent studies.[256] Insulin-sensitizing thiazolidinediones have shown mixed results, with improvement in insulin sensitivity but little alteration in fat distribution.[257] More than 75% of patients with HIV who have acute myocardial infarction (MI) are older than 55 years of age. Because of the increased risk of cardiovascular disease, treatment of hyperlipidemia is essential in these patients, with 3-hydroxy-3-methylglutaryl (HMG)-CoA reductase inhibitors and fibrates, alone or in combination, as first-line drugs.[258,259]

MEASURES TO IMPROVE INSULIN SENSITIVITY

Mechanisms of Reducing Insulin Resistance

The most effective measures to improve insulin sensitivity are weight loss and exercise. Both modalities are effective and can be additive in their ability to improve insulin action. Later in this chapter, the roles of these interventions in the treatment of patients with T2DM are discussed. The scientific basis and molecular mechanisms responsible for the improvements in insulin sensitivity seen with these interventions are summarized in the following paragraphs.

Mechanisms for Improved Insulin Sensitivity with Weight Loss

Weight loss can be a highly effective treatment for overweight patients with T2DM and other cardiovascular risk factors, and it is advocated as the first line of therapy. Weight loss may also play a role in preventing T2DM.[89,260] In overweight patients with T2DM, weight loss can reduce hepatic glucose production, insulin resistance, and fasting hyperinsulinemia and can improve glycemic control. Weight loss in T2DM is also associated with a reduction in blood pressure and an improvement in the lipid profile. These benefits can occur with as little as 5% to 10% weight loss.[261-263] Moreover, preventing obesity in primates with long-term caloric restriction attenuates the development of insulin resistance.

One possible mechanism for improvements in insulin sensitivity through weight loss may be its effects on the pattern of muscle fatty acid metabolism and the accumulation of lipid within muscle. In this context, it would be important to know whether alterations in the pathways of fatty acid utilization in skeletal muscle represent primary defects in obese persons or arise secondarily, after a person has become obese. This question cannot be answered by cross-sectional comparisons of lean and obese subjects. One prospective clinical study indicated that lower rates of lipid oxidation were a predisposing factor for greater weight gain,[170] and collateral studies implicated altered skeletal muscle enzyme activities in impaired lipid oxidation.[183,184] A reduced reliance on lipid oxidation has also been identified as a risk factor for weight regain after weight loss.[185] These data raise the possibility that impairment in the capacity for lipid oxidation may be a primary defect in obesity.

Weight loss can markedly improve insulin-resistant glucose metabolism in skeletal muscle. If the patient's response indicates a substantial acquired or secondary component of obesity-related insulin-resistant glucose metabolism, it is important to determine whether weight loss can modulate patterns of skeletal muscle metabolism of fatty acids, including the content of fat within muscle.

Mechanisms for Improved Insulin Sensitivity with Exercise

Exercise is clearly effective in increasing insulin sensitivity in animals and humans. There appear to be two separable but related effects of exercise on insulin action. A single bout of exercise can result in an acute increase in insulin-independent glucose transport that is measurable during and for a relatively short period after exercise.[264-268] Like insulin, exercise and muscle contractions increase glucose transport by translocation of intracellular GLUT4 to the cell surface.[269-271]

Acute Exercise

The signaling pathway leading to the exercise-induced increase in glucose transporter translocation and glucose transport is unknown, although there is ample evidence that the pathway is independent of the insulin-stimulated, receptor-mediated pathway. The effect of exercise and contractions on translocation and transport is additive to the maximal effect of insulin.[264,271-274] Insulin-stimulated glucose transport in muscle is inhibited by specific inhibitors of PI3K, such as wortmannin, whereas transport or translocation stimulated by muscle contractions is insensitive to these inhibitors.[271-276] Stimulation of muscle contractions in situ and exercise do not increase insulin receptor phosphorylation, tyrosine kinase activity, IRS phosphorylation, or PI3K activity.[270,277] In addition, in many insulin-resistant states, the acute exercise–stimulated (but not insulin-stimulated) glucose transport and GLUT4 translocation are normal. This has been demonstrated in the obese, insulin-resistant Zucker rat[278] and in patients with T2DM.[225] Finally, hypoxia, a stimulus for glucose transport that is also independent of the insulin receptor–mediated pathway, is effective in increasing glucose transport in muscle strips from obese, insulin-resistant patients and in patients with T2DM.[279]

The acute effect of exercise and hypoxia may be mediated by AMPK. AMPK is thought to be a sensor of intracellular energy stores and is activated by increases in intracellular AMP. A stable AMP analog, 5-amino-4-imidazole carboxamide ribotide (ZMP), can be generated intracellularly from 5-aminoimidazole-4-carboxamide ribonucleoside (AICAR) and can activate AMPK in cells, leading to increased phosphorylation of known substrates for AMPK, including HMG-CoA reductase, acyl-CoA carboxylase, and creatine kinase.[280] Treatment of incubated skeletal muscle with AICAR resulted in increased glucose uptake and glucose transporter translocation.[281] Similarly, the inclusion of 2 mmol/L of AICAR in the perfusate of the rat hind limb resulted in inactivation of ACC, decreases malonyl-CoA levels, and a twofold increase in glucose uptake.[282,283]

The euglycemic clamp technique was used in conscious rats to demonstrate that infusion of AICAR results in a greater than twofold increase in glucose utilization.[283a] Uptake of the glucose analog 2-deoxyglucose was also increased twofold in vivo in soleus and gastrocnemius muscles. As with previous studies, this uptake was not associated with PI3K activation, again indicating a separate pathway from that of insulin.

A second effect of exercise, which becomes evident as the acute effect on glucose transport reverses, is a large increase in the sensitivity of glucose transport to stimulation by insulin.[284-287] This effect is due to translocation of a greater amount of GLUT4 to the cell surface for any given dose of insulin.[288,289] As with the acute stimulation of transport by exercise, the cellular mechanisms leading to enhanced translocation in response to submaximally effective stimuli are unknown. However, several studies have shown that steps in the insulin-signaling cascade leading to activation of PI3K are not enhanced after a bout of exercise. There is no change in insulin binding to its receptor,[277,290] insulin stimulation of receptor tyrosine kinase activity,[277,291] increased insulin-stimulated tyrosine phosphorylation of IRS1,[288] or PI3K activity associated with IRS1.[270,291]

Exercise Training

Exercise training also results in increases in insulin sensitivity[292,293] and can delay or prevent the onset of T2DM in those at high risk.[294] Using the hyperinsulinemic-euglycemic clamp, Perseghin and coworkers[295] compared exercise training for 45 minutes on a stair-climbing machine 4 days per week for 6 weeks in normal insulin-sensitive subjects and a group of high-risk, insulin-resistant relatives of T2DM. A 100% increase in insulin sensitivity was seen in both groups without a significant change in body weight. The higher basal and glucose-stimulated insulin release seen in the insulin-resistant subjects was not altered after exercise training. The effect of exercise training on insulin sensitivity has been proposed to be caused by upregulation.

Primary effects of exercise training include increased glucose transporter number, changes in capillary density, increased number of red, glycolytic (type IIa) fibers, and increased density of mitochondria.[296,297] A reduction in mitochondrial oxidative capacity could underlie the dysregulation of lipid metabolism that results in reduced skeletal muscle glucose metabolism. Expression of nuclear-encoded genes that regulate mitochondrial biogenesis, such as the NRFs, PGC-1α, and PGC-1β have been shown to be important for both mitochondrial biogenesis and fiber type selection during development.[174,298] In muscle-specific transgenic mice, PGC-1α promotes muscle fiber-type switching from fast-twitch glycolytic fibers (types IIa and IIb) to slow-twitch oxidative fibers (type I), increases mitochondrial density, and improves oxidative capacity.[299] These changes are also observed after exercise training.

Many of the changes observed after exercise are likely to be mediated in part through PGC-1α levels and activity. Exercise-induced expression of PGC-1α in skeletal muscle is thought to be mediated by myocyte enhancer factor 2 (MEF2),[300] possibly through its interaction with MEF2C[301] and cyclic AMP (cAMP) response element–binding protein (CREB).[300] PGC-1α regulates its own promoter activity in a positive autoregulation loop. Activation of estrogen-related receptor α (Errα) and GA repeat–binding protein-α (Gabpa) by PGC-1α appears to mediate much of the effect to increase oxidative phosphorylation gene expression in muscle.[176] Nitric oxide produced by endothelial nitric oxide synthase controls mitochondrial biogenesis,[302] possibly through increased expression of PGC-1α and other transcription factors. This process is mediated by cyclic guanosine 3′,5′-phosphate, resulting from activation of "soluble" guanylate cyclase.

The pathway from exercise to activation of PGC-1α has been partially elucidated. Increases in calcium levels activate calcium/calmodulin-dependent kinase IV (CaMKIV) and calcineurin. Activated CaMKIV phosphorylates CREB, which increases transcription at CREB-responsive elements in the PGC-1α promoter.[303] Exercise also increases PGC-1α activity via phosphorylation through p38 mitogen-activated protein kinase.[304,305] AMPK, which is activated by exercise-induced changes in AMP levels, also increases mitochondrial biogenesis and PGC-1α activity in skeletal muscle,[306-308] but at present there is no evidence that PGC-1α is an AMPK substrate. Other conditions that induce mitochondrial biogenesis also increase PGC-1α promoter activity.

MECHANISMS THAT LINK CARDIOVASCULAR DISEASE AND INSULIN RESISTANCE

The Metabolic Syndrome or Syndrome X

MI, stroke, or nonischemic cardiovascular disease is the cause of death in up to 80% of patients with T2DM. Independent of other risk factors, T2DM increases the risk of cardiovascular morbidity and mortality but also provides a synergistic interaction with other risk factors such as smoking, hypertension, and dyslipidemia.[309] In a Finnish population, diabetes increased the risk of MI fivefold,[310] and insulin resistance, as measured by elevated fasting insulin levels, increased the risk of death from heart disease.[311] Women are particularly vulnerable to the cardiovascular effects of T2DM, because they appear to lose the protective effects of estrogen in the premenopausal period.[312,313]

A constellation of metabolic derangements often seen in patients with insulin resistance and T2DM are individually associated with an increased risk of cardiovascular disease. These metabolic derangements have been variously designated *syndrome X*; the *dysmetabolic syndrome*; hypertension, obesity, non–insulin-dependent diabetes mellitus (NIDDM), dyslipidemia, and atherosclerotic cardiovascular disease *(HONDA)*; and the *deadly quartet*.[314,315] The syndrome has also been associated with easily oxidized, small LDL particles; heightened blood-clotting activity (e.g., increased PAI-1); and elevated serum uric acid concentrations. The proposed central abnormality associated with syndrome X is insulin resistance. Some of the abnormalities themselves have also been proposed to contribute to insulin resistance.

Controversy surrounding the metabolic syndrome has not called into question the clustering of cardiovascular risk factors such as central obesity, dyslipidemia, and hypertension and the association of this clustering with the risk of developing diabetes and cardiovascular disease. The controversy largely focuses on the etiology of the syndrome, how best to define its presence, how clinical decision making should be modified based on those definitions, and whether there are not more effective ways to screen for diabetes and cardiovascular risk.[316]

Perhaps the overriding risk factor for coronary artery disease in insulin resistance and T2DM is the associated dyslipidemia. The profile includes hypertriglyceridemia, low plasma HDL, and small, dense LDL particle concentrations. The percentage of men with T2DM who have abnormal cholesterol levels is not different from that of nondiabetic men. However, diabetic women, compared with nondiabetic women, have almost double the rate of

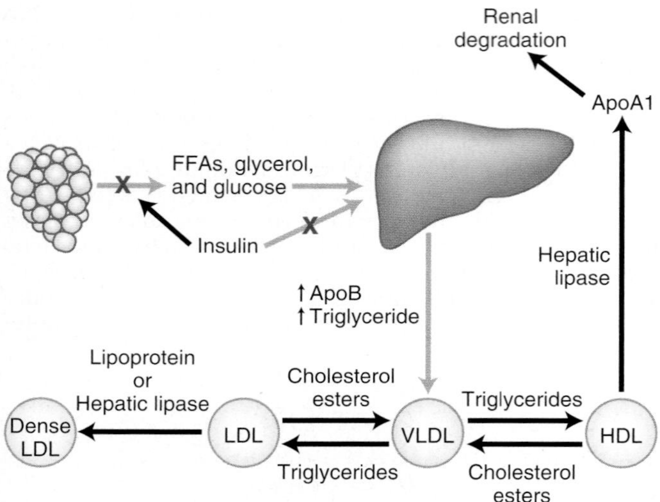

Figure 31-9 Insulin resistance and dyslipidemia. The suppression of lipoprotein lipase and very-low-density lipoprotein (VLDL) production by insulin is defective in insulin resistance, leading to increased flux of free fatty acids (FFAs) to the liver and increased VLDL production, which results in increased circulating triglyceride concentrations. The triglycerides are transferred to low-density lipoprotein (LDL) and high-density lipoprotein (HDL), and the VLDL particles gain cholesterol esters by the action of the cholesterol ester transfer protein (CETP). This leads to increased catabolism of HDL particles by the liver and loss of apolipoprotein (Apo) A, resulting in low HDL concentrations. The triglyceride-rich LDL particle is stripped of its triglycerides, resulting in the accumulation of atherogenic small, dense LDL particles.

hypercholesterolemia[317] and greater changes in other lipid parameters that increase the risk of cardiovascular disease (Fig. 31-9). The physiologic basis for this abnormal lipid profile appears to be overproduction of apolipoprotein B–containing VLDL particles. Production of apolipoprotein B by the liver is primarily post-translational[318] and is augmented by insulin and by the increased availability of FFAs in the portal circulation,[319-323] probably as a result of increased lipolysis in the visceral adipose tissue.[324-326] Part of the post-translational regulation may be due to insulin– and fatty acid–mediated increases in microsomal triglyceride transfer protein levels that catalyze the transfer of lipids to apolipoprotein B and decrease the ubiquitination-dependent degradation of apolipoprotein B.[327-329]

The overproduction of VLDL triglyceride results in increased transfer of VLDL triglyceride to HDL particles in exchange for HDL-cholesterol esters mediated by the cholesterol ester transfer protein.[330] The triglyceride-rich HDL is hydrolyzed by hepatic lipase; this leads to the generation of small HDL, which is degraded more readily by the kidney, resulting in low HDL levels in serum. Cholesterol ester transfer protein–mediated exchange of VLDL triglyceride for LDL-cholesterol esters and subsequent triglyceride hydrolysis by hepatic lipase probably result in generation of the small, dense LDL particles found in insulin-resistant subjects.[331-334]

The increased risk of heart disease in patients with diabetes has prompted the recommendation that persons with diabetes be treated for their dyslipidemia as aggressively as persons who have had a previous MI. In addition, patients with the metabolic syndrome of insulin resistance and obesity are considered to be in a higher risk category and should also be aggressively treated to lower lipids.[335]

The presence of hypertension and overt diabetes doubles the risk of cardiovascular disease. Defects in vasodilation and alterations in blood flow may provide a link to hypertension in insulin-resistant subjects. The normal vasodilative response of insulin is disrupted in obese, insulin-resistant, and diabetic persons,[336] perhaps through insulin's inability to increase the production of the potent vasodilator nitric oxide by endothelial cells.[337,338] The defect may be magnified by increases in plasma FFAs.[339] Other proposed mechanisms for insulin resistance leading to hypertension are activation of the sympathetic nervous system by insulin[340-342] and the intrinsic ability of insulin to cause salt and water readsorption in the kidney, resulting in expanded plasma volume.[343-345]

Hypertension itself, independent of other risk factors, has been associated with the propensity to become diabetic.[346] A prospective cohort study found that T2DM was almost 2.5 times more likely to develop in subjects with hypertension than in subjects with normal blood pressure.[347] A possible mechanism is that an intrinsic defect in vasodilation might contribute to insulin resistance by decreasing the surface area of the vasculature perfusing skeletal muscle, decreasing the efficiency of glucose uptake.[339] Conversely, vasodilative agents might improve glucose uptake and might even prevent the onset of diabetes, as has been observed with angiotensin-converting enzyme (ACE) inhibitor therapy.[348]

Several factors involved in clotting and fibrinolysis, including fibrinogen, factor VII, and PAI-1, have been shown to be increased in persons with insulin resistance.[349-354] PAI-1 has been extensively studied, and there is a clear relationship between elevated PAI-1 levels and risk of coronary artery disease.[355] Insulin increased PAI-1 expression in hepatocytes, endothelial cells, and abdominal adipose tissue,[356-358] and insulin-sensitizing thiazolidinediones decreased PAI-1 activity.[359]

Upper-body rather than lower-body obesity (the apple rather than the pear shape) is highly correlated with insulin resistance and risk for T2DM. Therefore, the anatomic distribution of fat, rather than the overall degree of obesity, appears to determine risk for the metabolic syndrome. The reported association between increased abdominal (upper-body) fat and an increased risk of coronary heart disease is related to visceral fat, for which the waist-to-hip ratio is a convenient index. A waist-to-hip ratio greater than 1.0 in men or greater than 0.8 in women indicates abdominal obesity.[360] The National Cholesterol Education Program (NCEP) has suggested that a waist circumference greater than 40 inches (101.5 cm) in men or greater than 35 inches (89 cm) in women is a marker for the metabolic syndrome.[361]

The Role of Increased Hepatic Glucose Production

The disposal of glucose after meals depends on the ability of insulin to increase peripheral glucose uptake and to simultaneously decrease endogenous glucose production. Although studies have suggested that the kidney can contribute up to 25% of endogenous glucose production,[362,363] the defect in T2DM is primarily in defective regulation of glucose production from the liver (hepatic glucose output). Two routes of glucose production by the liver are glycogenolysis of stored glycogen and gluconeogenesis from two- and three-carbon substrates derived primarily from skeletal muscle.[364,365] Under different conditions and at different times postprandially, the contribution of each of these mechanisms to maintenance of glucose levels varies. In studies using ^{13}C NMR spectroscopy combined with measurement of whole-body glucose production in normal human subjects at different intervals after fasting, it was found that gluconeogenesis accounted for 50% to 96% of glucose production, and the percentage increased with increasing duration of fasting.[366,367]

The production of glucose by the liver is regulated primarily by the relative actions of glucagon and insulin to activate or suppress glucose production, respectively, although the nervous system[368] and glucose autoregulation of hepatic glucose production probably play less important roles.[369] The ability of insulin to reduce hepatic glucose output is an important mechanism for maintaining normal glucose tolerance.[370,371] Under normal circumstances, insulin suppresses up to 85% of glucose production in normal persons by directly inhibiting glycogenolysis, especially at lower insulin concentrations.[372] When glycogenolysis is enhanced by glucagon, the effects of insulin in suppressing hepatic glucose production may be even greater.[373] Glucagon increases glycogenolysis by activation of the classic protein kinase cascade involving AMPK and phosphorylase and also increases gluconeogenesis in part by increasing transcription of phosphoenolpyruvate carboxykinase by means of the binding protein CREB.[371,374,375]

Data suggest that the regulatory mechanisms triggered by cAMP are much more complex, with the CREB transcriptional coactivator, TORC2, playing an important role. TORC2 is specifically dephosphorylated in response to cAMP; this results in translocation of the TORC2 protein to the nucleus, allowing activation of CREB-dependent transcription of gluconeogenic enzymes.[376] In addition, CREB may increase transcription of PGC-1α, which serves as a critical coactivator of the transcription factor forkhead box protein O1 (FOXO1), which also plays a role in the transcriptional activation of various genes associated with gluconeogenesis.[374] Recent data suggest that the NAD+-dependent protein deacetylase, SIRT1, can regulate gluconeogenesis. SIRT1 deacetylates PGC-1α and FOXO1, increasing their nuclear interaction with HNF4A. The PGC-1α/FOXO1/HNF4A complex is a potent activator of gluconeogenic gene transcription.[374]

Insulin decreases endogenous glucose production by direct and indirect mechanisms (Fig. 31-10).[378] In its direct action, portal insulin suppresses glucose production by inhibiting glycogenolysis through an increase in phosphodiesterase activity[379,380] or changes in the assembly of protein phosphatase complexes.[381,382] Insulin can also

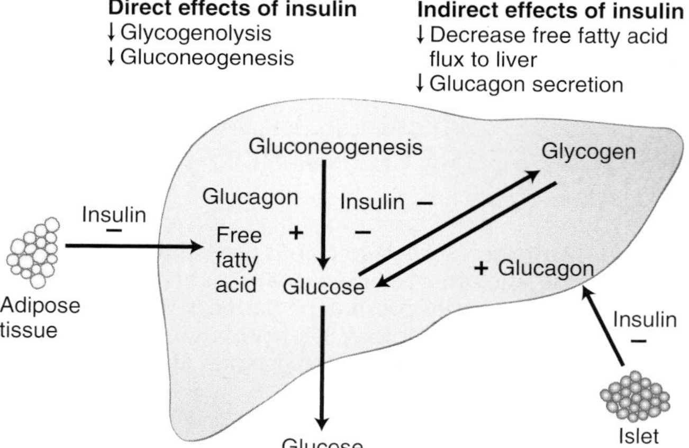

Figure 31-10 Insulin suppresses hepatic glucose production by direct and indirect mechanisms. In insulin resistance, the ability of insulin to suppress lipolysis in adipose tissue and glucagon secretion by alpha cells in the islet results in increased gluconeogenesis. In addition, insulin inhibition of glycogenolysis is impaired. Therefore, both hepatic and peripheral insulin resistance result in abnormal glucose production by the liver.

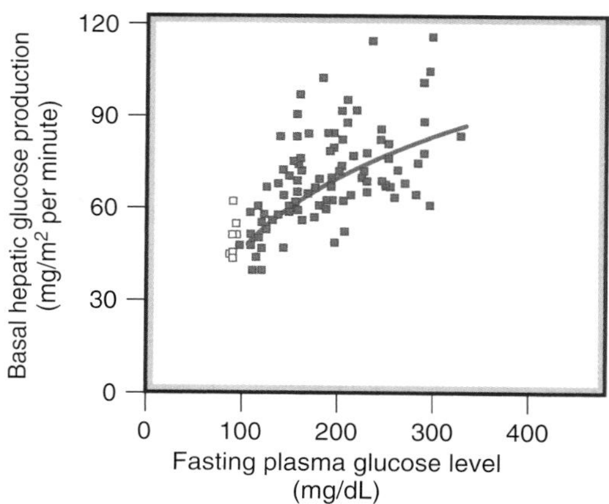

Figure 31-11 Relationship between fasting hepatic glucose output and fasting plasma glucose levels. *Open squares* represent nondiabetic control subjects; *closed squares* represent diabetic subjects. (From Maggs DG, Buchanan TA, Burant CF, et al. Metabolic effects of troglitazone monotherapy in type 2 diabetes mellitus: a randomized, double-blind, placebo-controlled trial. *Ann Intern Med.* 1998;128:176-185.)

directly suppress gluconeogenesis by inhibiting the activation of phosphoenolpyruvate carboxykinase transcription through insulin-dependent phosphorylation of FOXO1 (and perhaps FOXA2), sequestering it in the cytoplasm.[383-386]

The indirect or peripheral effect of insulin in controlling glucose production by the liver is twofold. First, insulin profoundly decreases glucagon secretion by the alpha cell of the pancreas through systemic and paracrine effects.[387,388] The decrease in glucagon secretion decreases the activation of glycogenolysis and gluconeogenesis. The second important peripheral action of insulin is to decrease FFA levels by suppressing lipolysis. FFAs increase hepatic glucose production by stimulating gluconeogenesis.[389] When the reduction in plasma FFAs during a hyperinsulinemic clamp was prevented by infusion of triglyceride emulsions with heparin (which produces increased FFA levels through activation of lipoprotein lipase), insulin-mediated suppression of hepatic glucose output was reduced.[364,390] The suppression of glucagon secretion and the decrease in FFA delivery to the liver are additive in reducing liver glucose production.[391]

Hepatic insulin resistance plays an important role in the hyperglycemia of T2DM,[392-395] and the impaired suppression of hepatic glucose output appears to be quantitatively similar to, or even larger than, the defect in stimulation of peripheral glucose disposal.[393,396] There is a direct relationship between increased hepatic glucose output and fasting hyperglycemia[80] (Fig. 31-11). Insulin-mediated suppression of hepatic glucose output is impaired at both low and high plasma insulin levels in T2DM[396-399]; hepatic glucose production is elevated early in the course of the disease[400] but may be normal in lean, relatively insulin-sensitive type 2 diabetics.[399] Treatment of patients with metformin, which suppresses hepatic glucose production, results in improved glucose tolerance.[401]

Alterations in the direct and indirect effects of insulin in T2DM appear to play a role in the elevation of hepatic glucose production. Defects in the direct effect of insulin to suppress hepatic glucose production that have been demonstrated in humans[402] appear to be caused by a large rightward shift in the steep dose-response curve for insulin's inhibition of glycogenolysis.[403] However, peripheral insulin resistance may play the bigger role in elevated hepatic glucose production in T2DM. The resistance of adipose tissue, especially visceral fat, to suppression of lipolysis by insulin is responsible for part of insulin's inability to suppress hepatic glucose production by the indirect route, resulting in enhanced gluconeogenesis.[404,405] In addition, the suppression of glucagon levels in humans with insulin resistance may be impaired, again leading to an increase in endogenous glucose production.[406]

Central Control of Glucose Metabolism

The hypothalamus and perhaps other brain regions can sense metabolic requirements and change peripheral metabolism. Studies by Rossetti and colleagues suggested that uptake of fatty acids by the mediobasal hypothalamus decreases feeding behavior and decreases hepatic glucose production via central nervous system (CNS) efferents.[407] Inhibition of fatty acid oxidation results in decreased food intake and reduced glucose production, suggesting that buildup of long-chain fatty acids or their derivatives changes feeding and hepatic glucose production.

AMPK may also play a role in integrating CNS nutrient supply. AMPK is activated by cellular AMP levels and therefore is a sensor of energy supply.[408] Higher cellular energy, resulting from glucose or fatty acid surfeit, would lead to decreased activation of AMPK and its downstream target, ACC. ACC generates malonyl-CoA (an allosteric inhibitor of CPT1), which decreases the entry of long-chain fatty acids into the mitochondria, resulting in their buildup in the cytoplasm.

Cytokines and Insulin Sensitivity. Adipose tissue is classically viewed as simply the site for storage of excess energy in the form of triglycerides. However, it is now clear that adipose tissue secretes a variety of endocrine and paracrine factors that have significant effects on metabolism.[409] These adipokines regulate a diverse array of actions, including alterations in feeding behavior; changes in liver, muscle, and adipose tissue insulin sensitivity; vascular reactivity; and atherosclerosis progression.

Leptin. Leptin is a 16-kd protein synthesized mainly in adipose tissue that is mutated in *ob/ob* mice. Leptin suppresses feeding behavior, and humans with mutations in leptin are morbidly obese and insulin resistant. However, studies from a number of laboratories, using in vitro and in vivo models, indicate a direct role for leptin in lipid metabolism, including increased metabolic rate, lipolysis, stimulation of fatty acid oxidation, inhibition of lipogenesis, and increased AMPK activity.

Adiponectin. Adiponectin (also known as ACRP30, adipoQ, apM1, and GBP28) is a 30-kd protein that is synthesized and secreted from adipocytes and circulates as a trimer and in multimeric complexes (called the *HMW form*). The HMW form may be further cleaved to forms that may be the active transducer of signaling. The purported receptor for adiponectin is controversial, so its exact signaling mechanism remains uncertain. In the mouse, adiponectin can increase fatty acid oxidation, perhaps through the activation of AMPK.[410,411] Disruption of adiponectin in mice predisposes them to high-fat diet–induced insulin resistance, although there is little alteration in mice consuming a normal diet.[412] Adiponectin levels are low in humans with obesity and insulin resistance and are increased by insulin-sensitizing PPARγ agonists.

Resistin. Resistin is a 12-kd protein that is synthesized and secreted from adipose tissue and is a member of the FIZZ family of proteins, which are C-terminal cysteine-rich proteins.[413,414] As with adiponectin, resistin circulates in both trimeric and hexameric forms, with the smaller form having greater activity.[149] Resistin levels are elevated in both diet-induced obesity and genetic mouse models of obesity and diabetes. Leptin causes hepatic insulin resistance, and disruption of resitin results in lowered ambient glucose levels. The role of resistin in human physiology remains uncertain.[415]

Tumor Necrosis Factor-α. TNF-α is a 26-kd transmembrane protein that is cleaved and circulates in a 17-kd soluble form. It is elaborated by multiple tissues, including adipocytes, and its role in insulin resistance is unclear. It may work primarily as a paracrine effector to induce tissue insulin resistance.[416] Data suggest that much of TNF-α, along with other inflammatory cytokines associated with adipose tissue, is elaborated by resident macrophages as well as adipocytes.[417,418] TNF-α has two main receptors, type 1 and type 2, that signal through the p44/42 and JNK pathway. Systemic effects on TNF-α include the induction of lipogenesis in the liver and insulin resistance in skeletal muscle.

Monocyte Chemotactic Protein 1. Monocyte chemotactic protein 1 (MCP1), also called C-C motif chemokine ligand 2 (CCL2), is increased in proportion to adipose tissue mass and correlates with insulin resistance.[419] CCL2 inhibits insulin action and adipocyte differentiation.[420] The receptor for MCP1, C-C motif chemokine receptor 2 (CCR2), regulates monocyte and macrophage recruitment and is necessary for macrophage-dependent inflammatory responses. Disruption of CCR2 in mice reduced their food intake, attenuated the development of obesity on a high-fat diet, and attenuated the infiltration of macrophages into adipose tissue, further supporting the concept that adipose-resident macrophages are important for their systemic effect of adipocity.[421]

Interleukin-6. IL-6 is a glycoprotein of 22 to 27 kd that circulates at relatively high concentrations. Circulating levels correlate with the degree of adiposity.[422] Humans receiving IL-6 infusions show increases in insulin resistance, hepatic glucose production, lipolysis, and fatty acid oxidation.[423] About a third of circulating IL-6 is secreted by adipocytes; however, a significant amount is elaborated by skeletal muscle and is increased by exercise. The lipolytic effect of IL-6 might link exercise to the mobilization of fatty acids.[173]

INSULIN SECRETION AND TYPE 2 DIABETES

Normal insulin secretory function is essential for maintaining normal glucose tolerance, and abnormal insulin secretion is invariably present in patients with T2DM. In this section, the physiology of normal insulin and the alterations that are present in persons with T2DM are reviewed.

Quantitation of Beta-Cell Function

The measurement of peripheral insulin concentrations by radioimmunoassay is still the most widely used method for quantifying beta-cell functions in vivo.[424] Although this approach provides valuable information, it is limited because 50% to 60% of the insulin produced by the pancreas is extracted by the liver without ever reaching the systemic circulation.[425,426] The standard radioimmunoassay for measuring insulin concentrations is also unable to distinguish between endogenous and exogenous insulin, making it ineffective as a measure of endogenous beta-cell reserve in the insulin-treated diabetic patient. Anti-insulin antibodies that may be present in patients treated with insulin interfere with the insulin radioimmunoassay, making insulin measurements in insulin-treated patients inaccurate. Conventional insulin radioimmunoassays are also unable to distinguish between levels of circulating proinsulin and true levels of circulating insulin.

Insulin is derived from a single-chain precursor, proinsulin.[427] Within the Golgi apparatus of the pancreatic beta cell, proinsulin is cleaved by convertases to form insulin, C peptide, and two pairs of basic amino acids. Insulin is subsequently released into the circulation at concentrations equimolar with those of C peptide.[428,429] In addition, small amounts of intact proinsulin and proinsulin conversion intermediates are released. Proinsulin and its related conversion intermediates can be detected in the circulation, where they constitute 20% of the total circulating insulin-like immunoreactivity.[430] In vivo, proinsulin has a biologic potency that is only about 10% of that of insulin,[431,432] and the potency of split proinsulin intermediates is between that of proinsulin and that of insulin.[433,434] C peptide has no known conclusive effects on carbohydrate metabolism,[435,436] although certain physiologic effects of C peptide have been proposed.[437] Unlike insulin, C peptide is not extracted by the liver[428,438,439] and is excreted almost exclusively by the kidneys. Its plasma half-life of approximately 30 minutes[440] contrasts sharply with that of insulin, which is approximately 4 minutes.

Because C peptide is secreted in equimolar concentrations with insulin and is not extracted by the liver, many investigators have used levels of C peptide as a marker of beta-cell function. The use of plasma C-peptide levels as an index of beta-cell function depends on the critical assumption that the mean clearance rate of C peptide is constant over the range of C-peptide levels observed under normal physiologic conditions. This assumption has been shown to be valid for both dogs and humans,[426,441] and this approach can be used to derive rates of insulin secretion from plasma concentrations of C peptide under steady-state conditions.[441] However, because of the long plasma half-life of C peptide, under non–steady-state conditions (e.g., after a glucose infusion), peripheral plasma levels of C peptide do not change in proportion to the changing insulin secretion rate.[441,442] Therefore, under such conditions, insulin secretion rates are best calculated with use of the two-compartment model initially proposed by Eaton and coworkers.[443]

Modifications to the C peptide model of insulin secretion have been introduced. They combine the minimal model of insulin action with the two-compartment model of C-peptide kinetics and allow insulin secretion and insulin sensitivity to be derived after intravenous or oral administration of glucose.[444-447]

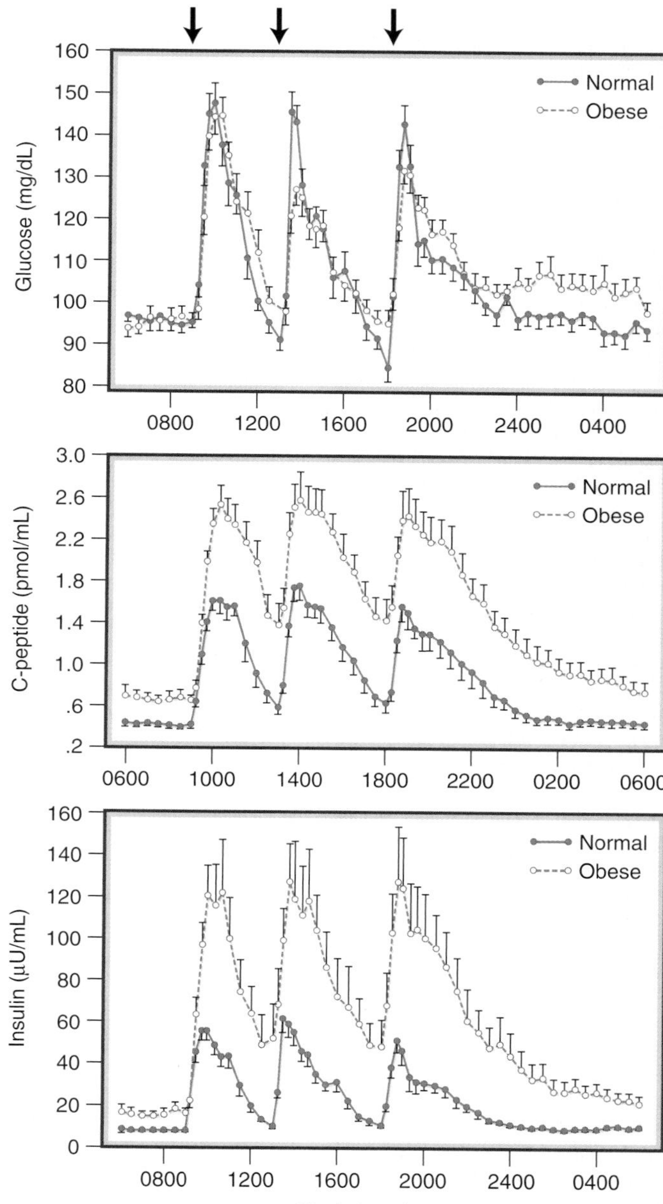

Figure 31-12 Mean 24-hour profiles of plasma concentrations of glucose *(top panel)*, C peptide *(middle panel)*, and insulin *(bottom panel)* in normal and obese subjects. The three arrows above the figure indicate the ingestion of the breakfast, lunch, and dinner meals, respectively. (From Polonsky KS, Given BD, van Cauter E. Twenty-four-hour profiles and pulsatile patterns of insulin secretion in normal and obese subjects. *J Clin Invest.* 1988;81:442-448.)

Signaling Pathways in the Beta Cell and Insulin Secretion

The signaling pathways in the pancreatic beta cell are involved in the stimulus-secretion coupling of insulin release. These pathways provide the mechanism whereby insulin secretion rates respond to changes in blood glucose concentrations (Fig. 31-12). Glucose enters the pancreatic beta cell by a process of facilitated diffusion mediated by the glucose transporter GLUT2. Although levels of GLUT2 on the beta-cell membrane are reduced in diabetic states for various reasons, it is not currently believed that this is a rate-limiting step in the regulation of insulin secretion.

The first rate-limiting step in this process is the phosphorylation of glucose to glucose-6-phosphate. This reaction is mediated by the enzyme glucokinase.[448,449] There is considerable evidence that glucokinase, by determining the rate of glycolysis, functions as the glucose sensor of the beta cell and that this is the primary mechanism by which the rate of insulin secretion adapts to changes in blood glucose. According to this view, as blood glucose levels increase, more glucose enters the beta cell, the rate of glycolysis increases, and the rate of insulin secretion increases. A fall in blood glucose levels results in a fall in the rate of glycolysis and a reduction in the rate of insulin secretion.

Glucose metabolism produces an increase in cytosolic ATP, the key signal that initiates insulin secretion by causing blockade of the K_{ATP} channel on the beta-cell membrane. Blockade of this channel induces membrane depolarization, which leads to an increase in cytosolic Ca^{2+} and insulin secretion. The biochemical events that link the increase in glycolysis to an increase in ATP are complex. Dukes and coworkers[450] proposed that glycolytic production of NADH during the oxidation of glyceraldehyde-3-phosphate is the key process because NADH is subsequently processed into ATP by mitochondria through the operation of specific shuttle systems.

The rate of pyruvate generation has also been proposed as an explanation for the link between glucose metabolism and increased insulin secretion.[451] According to this view, pyruvate generated by the glycolytic pathway enters the mitochondria and is metabolized further in the TCA cycle. Electron transfer from the TCA cycle to the respiratory chain by NADH and the reduced form of flavin adenine dinucleotide ($FADH_2$) promotes the generation of ATP, which is exported into the cytosol. The increase in ATP closes ATP-sensitive K^+ channels, which depolarizes the beta-cell membrane and opens the voltage-dependent Ca^{2+} channels, leading to an increase in intracellular Ca^{2+}. The increase in cytosolic Ca^{2+} is the main trigger for exocytosis, the process by which insulin-containing secretory granules fuse with the plasma membrane, leading to the release of insulin into the circulation. The increase in ATP not only closes K_{ATP} channels but also serves as a major permissive factor for movement of insulin granules and for priming of exocytosis.

Cyclic AMP also plays an important role in beta cell signal transduction pathways. This second messenger is generated at the plasma membrane from ATP and potentiates glucose-stimulated insulin secretion, particularly in response to glucagon, glucagon-like peptide 1 (GLP1), and gastric inhibitory polypeptide (also known as glucose-dependent insulinotropic peptide [GIP]). The cAMP-dependent pathways appear to be particularly important in the exocytotic machinery.

K_{ATP} channels play an essential role in beta cell stimulus-secretion coupling; an excellent review was published by Aguilar-Bryan and colleagues.[452] K_{ATP} channels include sulfonylurea receptors (SURs) and potassium inward rectifiers (KIR6.1 and KIR6.2), which assemble to form a large octameric channel with a (SUR/KIR6.x) stoichiometry. In the pancreatic beta cell, the SUR1/KIR6.2 pairs constitute the K_{ATP} channel. K_{ATP} channels control the flux of potassium ions driven by an electrochemical potential. Opening of these channels can set the resting membrane potential of beta cells below the threshold for activation of voltage-gated Ca^{2+} channels when plasma glucose levels are low, thus reducing insulin secretion. Changes in the cytosolic concentrations of ATP and adenosine diphosphate (ADP) lead to closure of the channels and depolarization of the beta-cell membrane. Mutations in both components of the beta-cell K_{ATP} (i.e., SUR1 and KIR6.2) have been shown to lead to hypersecretion of insulin, resulting clinically in either a recessive form of familial hyperinsulinemia or persistent hyperinsulinemic hypoglycemia of infancy.

Physiologic Factors Regulating Insulin Secretion

Carbohydrate Nutrients

The most important physiologic substance involved in the regulation of insulin release is glucose.[453-455] The effect of glucose on the beta cell is dose related. Dose-dependent increases in concentrations of insulin and C peptide and in rates of insulin secretion have been observed after oral and intravenous glucose loads, with 1.4 units of insulin, on average, being secreted in response to an oral glucose load as small as 12 g.[456-459] The insulin secretory response is greater after oral than after intravenous glucose administration.[460-462] Known as the *incretin effect*,[458,463] this enhanced response to oral glucose has been interpreted as an indication that absorption of glucose by way of the gastrointestinal tract stimulates the release of hormones and other mechanisms that ultimately enhance the sensitivity of the beta cell to glucose (see later discussion). In a study involving nine normal volunteers, glucose was infused at a rate designed to achieve levels previously attained after an oral glucose load. The amount of insulin secreted in response to the intravenous load was 26% less than that secreted in response to the oral load.[462]

Insulin secretion does not respond as a linear function of glucose concentration. The relationship of glucose concentration to the rate of insulin release follows a sigmoidal curve. The threshold corresponds to the glucose levels normally seen under fasting conditions, and the steep portion of the dose-response curve corresponds to the range of glucose levels normally achieved postprandially.[464-466] The sigmoidal nature of the dose-response curve has been attributed to a gaussian distribution of thresholds for stimulation among the individual beta cells.[466-468]

When glucose is infused intravenously at a constant rate, an initial biphasic secretory response is observed that consists of a rapid, early insulin peak followed by a second, more slowly rising peak.[453,459,460] The significance of the first-phase insulin release is unclear, but it might reflect the existence of a compartment of readily releasable insulin within the beta cell or a transient rise and fall of a metabolic signal for insulin secretion.[471] Despite early suggestions to the contrary,[472,473] it has been demonstrated that the first-phase response to intravenous glucose is highly reproducible within subjects.[474] After the acute response, a second phase of insulin release occurs that is directly related to the level of glucose elevation. In vitro studies of isolated islet cells and perfused pancreas have identified a third phase of insulin secretion that commences 1.5 to 3.0 hours after exposure to glucose and is characterized by a spontaneous decline in secretion to 15% to 25% of the amount released during peak secretion. This low level is subsequently maintained for longer than 48 hours.[475-478]

In addition to its acute secretagogue effects on insulin secretion, glucose has intermediate- and longer-term effects that are physiologically and clinically relevant. In the intermediate term, exposure of the pancreatic beta cell to a high concentration of glucose primes its response to a subsequent glucose stimulus, leading to a shift to the left in the dose-response curve relating glucose and insulin secretion.[479,480] However, when pancreatic islets are exposed to high concentrations for prolonged periods, a reduction of insulin secretion is seen. Although all of the precise mechanisms responsible for these adverse effects, termed *glucotoxicity*, are not known, there is evidence that long-term exposure to high glucose reduces the expression of a number of genes that are critical to normal beta-cell function, including the insulin gene.[481,482]

Noncarbohydrate Nutrients

Amino acids have been shown to stimulate insulin release in the absence of glucose, the most potent secretagogues being the essential amino acids leucine, arginine, and lysine.[483,484] The effects of arginine and lysine on the beta cell appear to be more potent than that of leucine. The effects of amino acids on insulin secretion are potentiated by glucose.[485,486]

In contrast to amino acids, various lipids and their metabolites appear to have only minor effects on insulin release in vivo. Although carbohydrate-rich fat meals stimulate insulin secretion, carbohydrate-free fat meals have minimal effects on beta cell function.[487] Ketone bodies and short- and long-chain fatty acids have been shown to stimulate insulin secretion acutely in islet cells and in human subjects.[488-492] The effects of elevated FFAs on the insulin secretory responses to glucose are related to the duration of the exposure. Zhou and Grill[493] first suggested that long-term exposure of pancreatic islets to FFAs inhibited glucose-induced insulin secretion and biosynthesis. This observation was confirmed in rats.[494] In humans, it was demonstrated that the insulin resistance induced by an acute (90-minute) elevation in FFAs was compensated by an appropriate increase in insulin secretion.[495] After chronic elevation of FFAs (48 hours), the beta cell compensatory response for insulin resistance was not adequate. Additional studies demonstrated that the adverse effects of prolonged FFAs on glucose-induced insulin secretion are not seen in subjects with T2DM. From these results, it appears that elevated FFAs might contribute to the failure of beta-cell compensation for insulin resistance.

Hormonal Factors

The release of insulin from the beta cell after a meal is facilitated by a number of gastrointestinal peptide hormones, including GIP, cholecystokinin, and GLP1.[463,496-503] These hormones are released from small-intestinal endocrine cells postprandially and travel in the bloodstream to reach the beta cells, where they act through second messengers to increase the sensitivity of these islet cells to glucose. In general, these hormones are not themselves secretagogues, and their effects are evident only in the presence of hyperglycemia.[496-498] The release of these peptides might explain why the modest postprandial glucose levels achieved in normal subjects in vivo have such a dramatic effect on insulin production, whereas similar glucose concentrations in vitro elicit a much smaller response.[503] Similarly, this incretin effect could account for the greater beta-cell response observed after oral as opposed to intravenous glucose administration.

Whether impaired postprandial secretion of incretin hormones plays a role in the inadequate insulin secretory response to oral glucose and to meals in patients with IGT or diabetes is controversial,[504-511] but pharmacologic doses of these peptides might have future therapeutic benefit. Subcutaneous administration of GLP1, the most potent of the incretin peptides, lowers glucose in patients with T2DM by stimulating endogenous insulin secretion and perhaps by inhibiting glucagon secretion and gastric empyting.[512,513] However, because of the short half-life of GLP1, its longer-acting analog, exendin-4, has greater therapeutic promise.[514] Treatment with supraphysiologic doses of GIP during hyperglycemia has been shown to augment insulin secretion in normal humans[515,516] but not in diabetics.[507,516] Although cholecystokinin has the ability to augment insulin secretion in humans, it is not firmly established whether it is an incretin at physiologic levels.[517-520] Its effects are also seen largely at pharmacologic doses.[521]

The postprandial insulin secretory response may also be influenced by other intestinal peptide hormones, including vasoactive intestinal polypeptide,[522] secretin,[523-526] and gastrin,[523,527] but the precise roles of these hormones remain to be elucidated.

The hormones produced by pancreatic alpha and beta cells also modulate insulin release. Whereas glucagon has a stimulatory effect on the beta cell,[528] somatostatin suppresses insulin release.[529] It is currently unclear whether these hormones reach the beta cell by traveling through the islet cell interstitium (thus exerting a paracrine effect) or through islet cell capillaries. Indeed, the importance of these two hormones in regulating basal and postprandial insulin levels under normal physiologic circumstances is in doubt. Paradoxically, the low insulin levels observed during prolonged periods of starvation have been attributed to the elevated glucagon concentrations seen in this setting.[487,530-533] Other hormones that exert a stimulatory effect on insulin secretion include growth hormone,[534] glucocorticoids,[535] prolactin,[536-538] placental lactogen,[539] and the sex steroids.[540]

Whereas all of the preceding hormones might stimulate insulin secretion indirectly by inducing a state of insulin resistance, some might also act directly on the beta cell, possibly to augment its sensitivity to glucose. Hyperinsulinemia is associated with conditions in which these hormones are present in excess, such as acromegaly, Cushing's syndrome, and the second half of pregnancy. Furthermore, treatments with placental lactogen,[541] hydrocortisone,[542] and growth hormone[542,543] are all effective in reversing the reduction in insulin response to glucose that is observed in vitro after hypophysectomy. Although hyperinsulinemia after an oral glucose load has been observed in patients with hyperthyroidism,[544,545] the increased concentration of immunoreactive insulin in this setting may reflect elevations in serum proinsulin rather than a true increase in serum insulin.[546]

Neural Factors

The islets are innervated by the cholinergic and adrenergic limbs of the autonomic nervous system. Although both sympathetic stimulation and parasympathetic stimulation enhance secretion of glucagon,[547,548] the secretion of insulin is stimulated by vagal nerve fibers and inhibited by sympathetic nerve fibers.[547-552] Adrenergic inhibition of the beta cell appears to be mediated by the α-adrenoceptor, because its effect is attenuated by the α-antagonist phentolamine[548] and reproduced by the α_2-agonist clonidine.[553] There is also considerable evidence that many indirect effects of sympathetic nerve stimulation play a role in regulating beta-cell function through stimulation or inhibition of somatostatin, β_2-adrenoceptors, and the neuropeptides galanin and neuropeptide Y.[554]

Parasympathetic stimulation of islets results in stimulation of insulin, glucagon, and pancreatic polypeptide directly and through the neuropeptides vasoactive intestinal polypeptide, gastrin-releasing polypeptide, and pituitary adenylate cyclase-activating polypeptide.[554] In addition, sensory innervation of islets may play a role in tonic inhibition of insulin secretion through the neuropeptides calcitonin gene-related peptide[555-557] and, less clearly, substance P.[558,559]

The importance of the autonomic nervous system in regulating insulin secretion in vivo is unclear. The neural effects on beta-cell function cannot be entirely dissociated from the hormonal effects because some of the neurotransmitters of the autonomic nervous system are, in fact, hormones. Furthermore, the secretion of insulinotropic hormones such as GIP and GLP1 postprandially has been shown to be under vagal[560,561] and adrenergic[562,563] control.

Temporal Pattern of Insulin Secretion

It has been estimated that 50% of the total insulin secreted by the pancreas in any 24-hour period is secreted under basal conditions, and the remainder is secreted in response to meals.[564,565] The estimated basal insulin secretion rates range from 18 to 32 units (0.7 to 1.3 mg) per 24 hours.[441,443,456,564] After meal ingestion, the insulin secretory response is rapid, and insulin secretion increases approximately fivefold over baseline to reach a peak within 60 minutes (Fig. 31-13; see Fig. 31-12). When study subjects consumed 20% of calories with breakfast and 40% with lunch and dinner, the amount of insulin secreted after each meal did not differ significantly. There was a rapid insulin secretory response to breakfast, with 71.6% ± 1.6% of the insulin secreted in the 4 hours after the meal being produced in the first 2 hours and the remainder in the next 2 hours. Insulin secretion did not decrease as rapidly after lunch and dinner, with, respectively, 62.8% ± 1.6% and 59.6% ± 1.4% of the total meal response secreted during the first 2 hours after the meal.

The normal insulin secretory profile is characterized by a series of insulin secretory pulses. After breakfast, 1.8 ± 0.2 secretory pulses were identified in normal volunteers, and the peaks of these pulses occurred 42.8 ± 3.4 minutes after the meal. Multiple insulin secretory pulses were also identified after lunch and dinner. After these meals, up to four pulses of insulin secretion were identified in both groups of subjects. In the 5-hour time interval between lunch and dinner, an average of 2.5 ± 0.3 secretory pulses were identified, and 2.6 ± 0.2 were identified in the same period after dinner.[565]

Pulses of insulin secretion that did not appear to be meal related were also identified. Between 11:00 p.m. and 6:00 a.m. and in the 3 hours before breakfast, on average 3.9 ± 0.3 secretory pulses were present in normal subjects. Therefore, over the 24-hour period of observation, a total of 11.1 ± 0.5 pulses were identified in normal subjects. Almost 90% (87% ± 3%) of postmeal pulses in insulin secretion, but only 47% ± 8% of non–meal-related pulses, were concomitant with a pulse in glucose.[565]

In vivo studies of beta-cell secretory function have demonstrated that insulin is released in a pulsatile manner. This behavior is characterized by rapid oscillations occurring every 8 to 15 minutes that are superimposed on slower (ultradian) oscillations occurring at a periodicity of 80 to 150 minutes.[566] The rapid oscillations persist in vitro and therefore are likely to be the result of metabolic pathways in the pancreatic beta cell that involve negative feedback loops with time lags.

Rapid Oscillations

The rapid oscillations of insulin are of small amplitude in the systemic circulation, averaging between 0.4 and 3.2 μU/mL in several published human studies.[567-569] Because these values are close to the limits of sensitivity of most standard insulin radioimmunoassays, the characterization of these oscillations is subject to considerable pitfalls,[570] not the least of which is the need to differentiate between true oscillations of small amplitude and random assay noise. The latter problem has been overcome by the development of extremely sensitive enzyme-linked immunosorbent

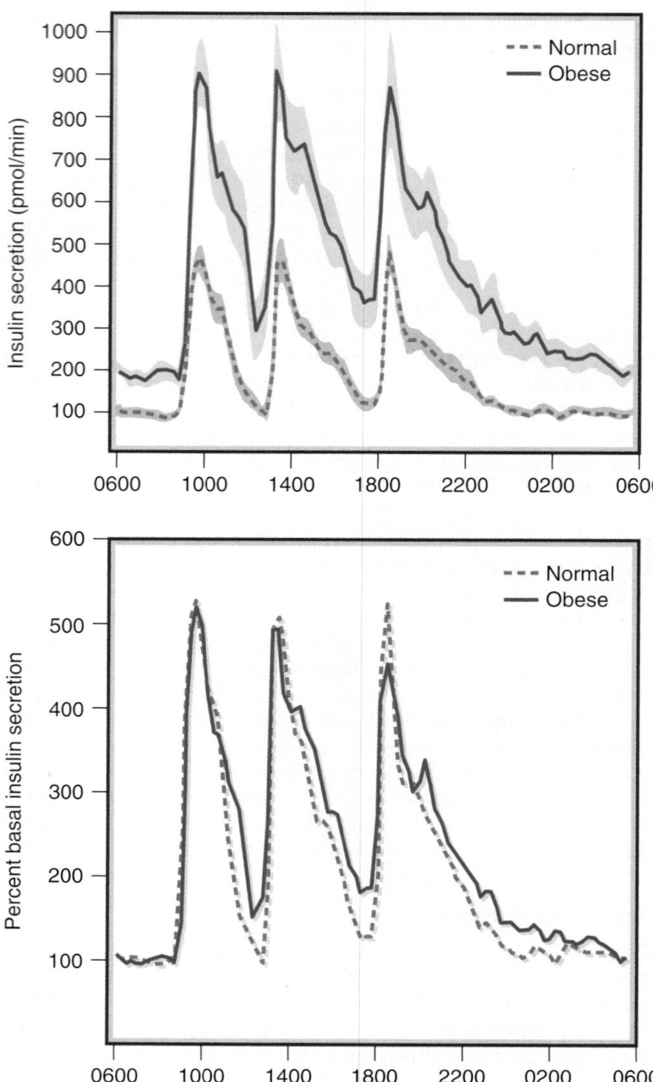

Figure 31-13 Mean 24-hour profiles of insulin secretion rates in normal and obese subjects *(top)*. The *hatched areas* represent ±1 standard error of the mean. The curves in the *lower panel* were derived by dividing the insulin secretion rate measured in each subject by the basal secretion rate derived in the same subject. Mean data for normal *(dashed line)* and obese *(solid line)* subjects are shown. (From Polonsky KS, Given BD, van Cauter E. Twenty-four-hour profiles and pulsatile patterns of insulin secretion in normal and obese subjects. *J Clin Invest.* 1988;81:442-448.)

assays (ELISAs) that allow the detection of extremely small changes in peripheral insulin concentrations. The application of these assays in studies involving frequent sampling from the peripheral circulation has led to a series of studies of the role of these oscillations in the overall regulation of insulin secretion.[571-575]

These investigations suggested that the increases in overall insulin secretion seen in response to a variety of secretagogues in various physiologic and pathophysiologic states result from an increase in the amplitude of the bursts of insulin secretion. The researchers have proposed that 75% of insulin secretion is accounted for by secretory bursts and that the responses to GLP1, sulfonylureas, and oral glucose are all mediated by an increase in the amplitude of insulin secretory pulses. Furthermore, consistent with observations made by O'Rahilly and colleagues,[576] relatives of patients with T2DM demonstrate a disorderly profile of the insulin secretory oscillations. A number of mathematical programs have been developed that allow these insulin secretory oscillations to be evaluated and studied.[577] The latest additions to the list are so-called approximate entropy *(ApEn)* and cross-approximate entropy *(cross-ApEn)*, which are statistics that measure temporal regularity of the oscillations in the insulin secretory profile.[578]

The low amplitude of the rapid oscillations in the systemic circulation contrasts sharply with observations in the portal vein, where pulse amplitudes of 20 to 40 μU/mL have been recorded in dogs.[579] Although the physiologic importance of these low-amplitude rapid pulses in the periphery is unclear, they are likely to be of physiologic importance in the portal vein. It is possible that the liver responds more readily to insulin delivered in a pulsatile fashion than to insulin delivered at a constant rate.[580-582]

Ultradian Oscillations

In contrast to the rapid oscillations, the slower (ultradian) oscillations are of much larger amplitude in the peripheral circulation. They are present under basal conditions but are amplified postprandially (Fig. 31-14), and they have been observed in subjects receiving intravenous glucose, suggesting that they are not generated by intermittent absorption of nutrients from the gut. Furthermore, they do not appear to be related to fluctuations in glucagon or cortisol levels,[475] and they are not regulated by neural factors, because these oscillations are also present in recipients of successful pancreas transplants.[583,584] Many of these ultradian insulin and C-peptide pulses are synchronous with pulses of similar oscillatory periods in glucose, raising the possibility that these oscillations are a product of the insulin-glucose feedback mechanism. Ultradian oscillations are self-sustained during constant glucose infusion at various rates; they are increased in amplitude after stimulation of insulin secretion without change in frequency, and there is a slight temporal advance of the glucose versus the insulin oscillation.

These findings suggest that the ultradian oscillations may be entirely accounted for by the major dynamic characteristics of the insulin-glucose feedback system, with no need to postulate the existence of an intrapancreatic pacemaker.[585] In support of this hypothesis, Sturis and colleagues[586] demonstrated that when glucose is administered in an oscillatory pattern, ultradian oscillations in plasma glucose and insulin secretion are generated that are 100% concordant with the oscillatory period of the exogenous glucose infusion. This close relationship between the ultradian oscillations in insulin secretion and similar oscillations in plasma glucose was further exemplified in a series of dose-response studies in which the largest-amplitude oscillations in insulin secretion were observed in those subjects exhibiting the largest-amplitude glucose oscillations, which in turn were directly related to the infusion dose of glucose. It has been shown that, in normal humans, insulin is more effective in reducing plasma glucose levels when it is administered intravenously as a 120-minute oscillation than when it is delivered at a constant rate. These results indicate that the ultradian oscillations have functional significance.[586]

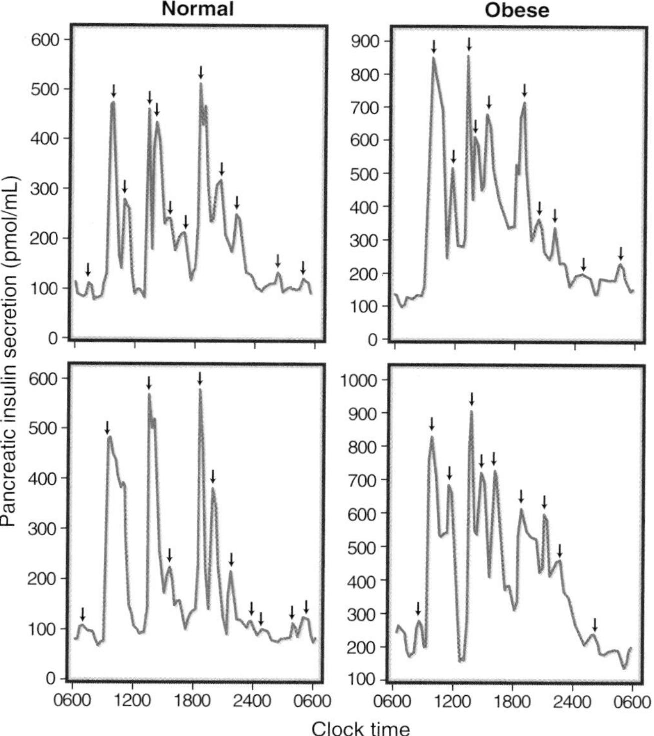

Figure 31-14 Patterns of insulin secretion in normal and obese subjects. Four representative 24-hour profiles are shown from two normal-weight subjects *(left)* and two obese subjects *(right)*. Meals were consumed at 0900, 1300, and 1800 hours. Statistically significant pulses of secretion are shown by the *arrows*. (From Polonsky KS, Given BD, van Cauter E. Twenty-four-hour profiles and pulsatile patterns of insulin secretion in normal and obese subjects. *J Clin Invest.* 1988;81:442-448.)

Circadian Oscillations

Circadian variations in the secretion of insulin have also been reported. When insulin secretory responses were measured for a 24-hour period during which subjects received three standard meals, the maximal postprandial responses were observed after breakfast.[565,567] These findings were mirrored by the results of studies in which subjects were tested for oral glucose tolerance at different times of the day and were found to exhibit maximal insulin secretory responses in the morning and lower responses in the afternoon and evening.[587-589] These diurnal differences were also noted in tests for intravenous glucose tolerance. Furthermore, although ultradian glucose and insulin oscillations are closely correlated during a constant 24-hour glucose infusion, the nocturnal rise in mean glucose levels is not accompanied by a similar increase in the insulin secretory rate.[590] It has been postulated that these diurnal differences reflect diminished responsiveness of the beta cell to glucose in the afternoon and evening.[589]

Insulin Secretion in Obesity and Insulin Resistance

Obesity and other insulin-resistant states are associated with a substantially greater risk of developing T2DM. The ability of the pancreatic beta cell to compensate for insulin resistance determines whether blood glucose levels remain normal in insulin-resistant subjects or whether the subjects develop IGT or diabetes.

The nature of the beta cell's compensation for insulin resistance involves hypersecretion of insulin even in the presence of normal glucose concentrations. This can occur only if beta-cell sensitivity to glucose is increased. The increase in beta-cell sensitivity to glucose in obesity appears to be mediated by two factors. First, increased beta-cell mass is observed in obesity and other insulin-resistant states.[591] Second, insulin resistance appears to be associated with increased expression of hexokinase in the beta cell relative to the expression of glucokinase.[592] Because hexokinase has a significantly lower Michaelis constant (K_m) for glucose than glucokinase does, the functional effect of increased hexokinase expression is to shift the glucose–insulin secretion dose-response curve to the left, leading to increased insulin secretion across a wide range of glucose concentrations.

Assessment of the adequacy of the beta-cell compensation for insulin resistance is important because this is the major determinant of the development of diabetes. In insulin-resistant states, it is important to evaluate beta-cell function in relation to the degree of insulin resistance. Kahn and coworkers[593] studied the relationship between insulin sensitivity and beta-cell function in 93 relatively young, apparently healthy human subjects with varying degrees of obesity. A sensitivity index (SI) was calculated using the minimal model of Bergman as a measure of insulin sensitivity and was then compared with various measures of insulin secretion.[446,594] The relationship between the SI and the beta-cell measures was curvilinear and reciprocal for fasting insulin concentration ($P < .0001$), first-phase (acute) insulin response (AIR glucose; $P < .0001$), glucose potentiation slope ($n = 56$; $P < .005$), and beta-cell secretory capacity (AIR_{max}; $n = 43$; $P < .0001$). The curvilinear relationship between SI and the beta-cell measures could not be distinguished from a hyperbola (i.e., SI × beta cell function = a constant). The nature of this relationship is consistent with a regulated feedback loop control system such that, for any difference in SI, a proportionate reciprocal difference occurs in insulin levels and responses in subjects with similar carbohydrate tolerance. Therefore, in human subjects with normal glucose tolerance and varying degrees of obesity, beta-cell function varies quantitatively with differences in insulin sensitivity. The increase in insulin secretion that is observed with a fall in SI should be viewed as the beta-cell compensation that allows normal glucose tolerance to be maintained in the presence of insulin resistance.

The insulin resistance of obesity is characterized by hyperinsulinemia. Hyperinsulinemia in this setting reflects a combination of increased insulin production and decreased insulin clearance, but most evidence suggests that increased insulin secretion is the predominant factor.[595,596] Both basal and 24-hour insulin secretory rates are three to four times higher in obese subjects and are strongly correlated with BMI. Insulin secretory responses to intravenous glucose have been studied in otherwise healthy insulin-resistant subjects and compared with the responses in insulin-sensitive subjects by means of a graded glucose infusion.

Figure 31-15 depicts insulin concentrations and insulin secretion rates at each level of plasma glucose achieved, outlining the respective dose-response relationships. Both insulin concentrations and insulin secretion rates are increased in insulin-resistant subjects due to a combination of increased insulin secretion and decreased insulin clearance. For each level of glucose, insulin secretion rates are higher in insulin-resistant than in insulin-sensitive subjects, reflecting an adaptive response of the beta cell to peripheral insulin resistance. Similar compensatory hyperinsulinemia has been demonstrated using other clinical techniques, such as the frequently sampled intravenous glucose tolerance test, in obese patients and in those with other insulin-resistant states, such as late pregnancy.[593,597]

The temporal pattern of insulin secretion is unaltered in obese subjects compared with normal subjects. Basal insulin secretion in obese subjects accounts for 50% of the total daily production of insulin, and secretory pulses of insulin occur every 1.5 to 2 hours.[567,595] However, the amplitude of these pulses postprandially is greater in obese subjects. Nevertheless, when these postprandial secretory responses are expressed as a percentage of the basal secretory rate, the postprandial responses in obese and normal subjects are identical.

Insulin Secretion in Subjects with Impaired Glucose Tolerance

It has been suggested that insulin secretion may be normal in subjects with IGT. However, substantial defects in insulin secretion have been demonstrated in people who have normal FPG and normal HbA_{1c} concentrations, with glucose values greater than 140 mg/dL (7.8 mmol/L) 2 hours after oral ingestion of 75 g of glucose. Therefore,

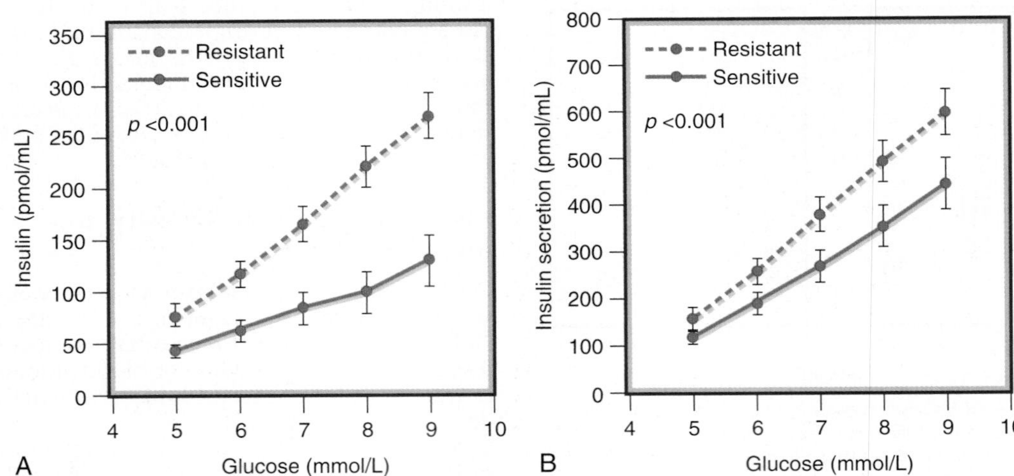

Figure 31-15 Plasma insulin concentrations **(A)** and insulin secretion rates **(B)** in response to molar increments in the plasma glucose concentration during a graded glucose infusion in insulin-resistant *(dotted line)* and insulin-sensitive *(solid line)* groups. (From Jones CNO, Pei D, Staris P, et al. Alterations in the glucose-stimulated insulin secretory dose-response curve and in insulin clearance in nondiabetic insulin-resistant individuals. *J Clin Endocrinol Metab.* 1997;82:1834-1838.)

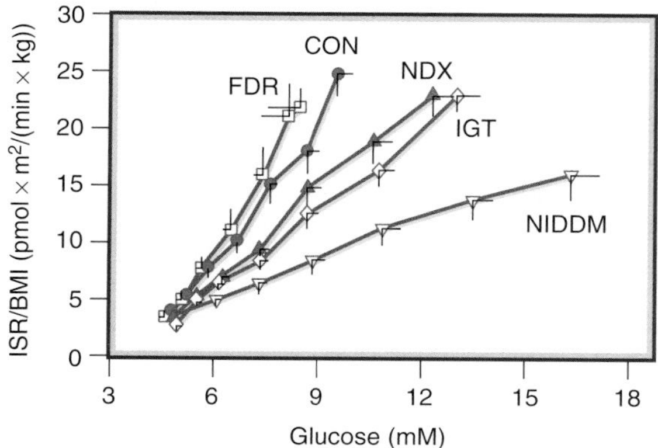

Figure 31-16 Dose-response relationship between glucose and insulin secretory rate (ISR) after an overnight fast in control subjects (CON), normoglycemic subjects with a family history of non–insulin-dependent diabetes mellitus (FDR), subjects with a nondiagnostic oral glucose tolerance test (NDX), subjects with impaired glucose tolerance (IGT), and subjects with non–insulin-dependent diabetes mellitus (NIDDM). BMI, body mass index. (From Byrne MM, Sturis J, Sobel RJ, et al. Elevated plasma glucose 2 h postchallenge predicts defects in beta-cell function. *Am J Physiol.* 1996;270:E572-E579. Copyright 1996, the American Physiological Society.)

defects in insulin secretion can be detected before the onset of overt hyperglycemia.

Detailed study of insulin secretion in patients with IGT has demonstrated consistent quantitative and qualitative defects in this group. During OGTT, there is a delay in the peak insulin response.[79,598,599] The glucose–insulin secretion dose-response relationship is flattened and shifted to the right (Fig. 31-16), and first-phase insulin responses to an intravenous glucose bolus are consistently decreased in relation to ambient insulin sensitivity.[600,601]

The temporal pattern of insulin secretory responses is altered in IGT and is similar to but not as pronounced as that seen in diabetic subjects (see later discussion). There is a loss of coordinated insulin secretory responses during oscillatory glucose infusion, indicating that the ability of the beta cell to sense and respond appropriately to parallel changes in the plasma glucose level is impaired (Fig. 31-17). Abnormalities in rapid oscillations of insulin secretion have also been observed in first-degree relatives of patients with T2DM who have only mild IGT,[576] further suggesting that abnormalities in the temporal pattern of beta-cell function may be an early manifestation of beta-cell dysfunction preceding the development of T2DM.

Because an elevation in serum proinsulin is seen in subjects with diabetes, the contribution of proinsulin to the hyperinsulinemia of IGT has been questioned. The hyperinsulinemia of IGT has not been accounted for by an increase in proinsulin, although elevations in fasting and stimulated proinsulin levels or proinsulin-to-insulin ratios have been found by many (although not all) investigators.[602-607] Correlation of elevated proinsulin levels in IGT as a predictor of future conversion to diabetes has also been observed.[608-610]

Insulin Secretion in Type 2 Diabetes Mellitus

Because of the presence of concomitant insulin resistance, patients with T2DM are often hyperinsulinemic, but the degree of hyperinsulinemia is inappropriately low for the prevailing glucose concentrations. Nevertheless, many of these patients have sufficient beta-cell reserve to maintain a euglycemic state by diet restriction with or without an oral agent. The beta-cell defect in patients with T2DM is characterized by an absent first-phase insulin and C-peptide response to an intravenous glucose load and a reduced second-phase response.[611] Although hyperglycemia can play a role in mediating these changes, the abnormal first-phase response to intravenous glucose persists in patients whose diabetic control has been greatly improved,[612,613] consistent with the idea that patients with T2DM have an intrinsic defect in the beta cell.

Furthermore, abnormalities in first-phase insulin secretion were observed in first-degree relatives of patients with T2DM who exhibited only mild IGT,[614] and an attenuated

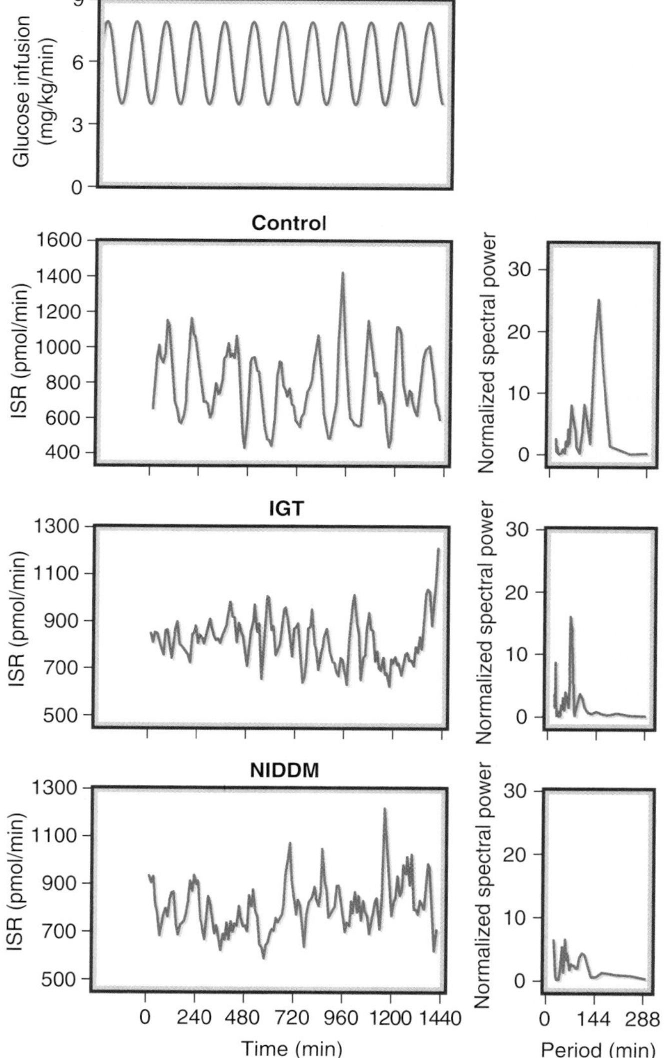

Figure 31-17 Oscillatory glucose infusions *(top panel)* were administered with a periodicity of 144 minutes to representative subjects with normal glucose tolerance (Control), impaired glucose tolerance (IGT), or type 2 diabetes (NIDDM). In the control subject, the insulin secretion rate (ISR) adjusts and responds to the 144-minute oscillations in glucose, resulting in sharp spectral peak at 144 minutes. In the other subjects, the ISR does not respond to the oscillatory glucose stimulus. Although oscillations in insulin secretion are evident, they are irregular, resulting in markedly reduced spectral peaks at 144 minutes and small-amplitude, high-frequency spectral peaks. These results are shown in the curves of normalized spectral power *(right column)* for each subject. (Adapted from O'Meara NM, Sturis J, Van Cauter E, et al. Lack of control by glucose of ultradian insulin secretory oscillations in impaired glucose tolerance and in non-insulin-dependent diabetes mellitus. *J Clin Invest.* 1993;92:262-271.)

insulin response to oral glucose was observed in normoglycemic twins of patients with T2DM,[615] a group at high risk for T2DM and who can legitimately be classified as prediabetic.[616] This pattern of insulin secretion during the prediabetic phase was also seen in subjects with IGT who later developed T2DM[488,617,618] and in normoglycemic obese subjects with a recent history of gestational diabetes,[619] another group at high risk for T2DM.[620] Beta-cell abnormalities can therefore precede the development of overt T2DM by many years.

T2DM also affects proinsulin levels in serum. Increased levels of proinsulin are consistently seen in association with increases in the proinsulin-to-insulin molar ratio.[611] The amount of proinsulin produced in this setting appears to be related to the degree of glycemic control rather than the duration of the diabetic state, and in one series proinsulin levels contributed almost 50% of the total insulin immunoreactivity in T2DM patients who had marked hyperglycemia. In addition to intact proinsulin, the beta cell secretes one or more of the four major proinsulin conversion products (split 32,33-proinsulin, split 65,66-proinsulin, des-31,32-proinsulin, and des-64,65-proinsulin) into the circulation. These conversion products are produced within the secretory granules of the islet as a result of the activity of specific conversion enzymes at the two cleavage sites in proinsulin that link the C peptide to the A and B chains.[602-609]

The composition of the elevated proinsulin-like immunodeficiency in patients with T2DM compared with control subjects has not been fully characterized. Hales and colleagues[621] developed immunoradiometric assays for this purpose. In studies using these assays, split 32,33-proinsulin was reported to be the predominant proinsulin conversion product in the circulation, although des-31,32-proinsulin levels can also be elevated. Insulin, proinsulin, and conversion product concentrations were also measured with these assays 30 minutes after oral glucose administration in patients with T2DM. Insulin was reduced in all patients, with no overlap between patients and controls, and concentrations of proinsulin and conversion products were elevated in the diabetic patients. These data highlight the importance of the potentially confounding effects of proinsulin and proinsulin conversion products in the interpretation of circulating immunoreactive insulin in patients with T2DM and emphasize the need to measure the concentrations of the individual peptides.

Abnormalities in the temporal pattern of insulin secretion have also been demonstrated in patients with T2DM. In contrast to normal subjects, in whom equal amounts of insulin are secreted basally and postprandially in a given 24-hour period, patients with T2DM secrete a greater proportion of their daily insulin under basal conditions (Fig. 31-18).[622] This reduction in the proportion of insulin secreted postprandially appears to be related in part to a reduction in the amplitude of the secretory pulses of insulin occurring after meals, rather than to a reduction in the number of pulses. In contrast to normal subjects, patients with T2DM have ultradian oscillations in insulin secretion that are less tightly coupled with oscillations in plasma glucose (Fig. 31-19). Similar findings were observed in patients with IGT studied under the same experimental conditions and in a further group of T2DM patients studied under fasting conditions. The rapid insulin pulses are also abnormal in patients with T2DM. The persistent regular rapid oscillations present in normal subjects are not observed. Instead, the cycles are shorter and irregular. Similar findings were observed in a group of first-degree relatives of patients with T2DM who had only mild IGT, suggesting that abnormalities in oscillatory activity may be an early manifestation of beta-cell dysfunction.[600]

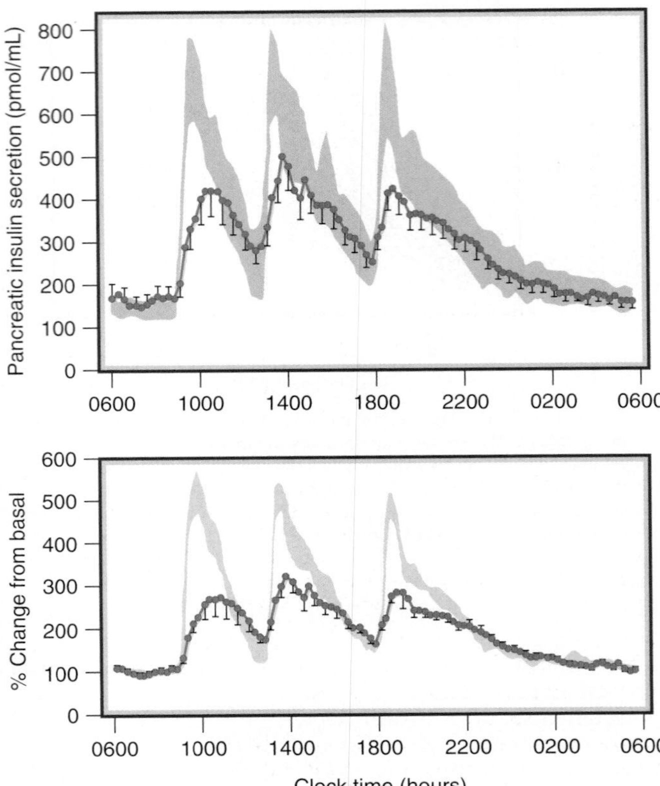

Figure 31-18 Mean rates of insulin secretion in type 2 diabetic patients compared with control subjects *(top panel)*. *Vertical bars* indicate standard error of the mean (SEM). The *shaded area* corresponds to 1 SEM above and below the mean in control subjects. The curves indicating percent change from basal secretion *(lower panel)* were derived by dividing, for each subject, the insulin secretion rate at each sampling time by the average fasting secretion rate measured between 6 a.m. and 9 a.m. in the same subject. (From Polonsky KS, Given BD, Hirsch LJ et al. Abnormal patterns of insulin secretion in non-dependent diabetes mellitus. *N Engl J Med.* 1988;318:1231-1239.)

The effects of therapy on beta-cell function in patients with T2DM have also been investigated. Although interpretation of the results in many instances is limited because beta-cell function was not always studied at comparable levels of glucose before and during therapy, the majority of the studies indicated that improvements in diabetic control are associated with an enhancement of beta-cell secretory activity. This increased endogenous production of insulin appears to be independent of the mode of treatment and is in particular associated with increases in the amount of insulin secreted postprandially.[613,623] The enhanced beta-cell secretory activity after meals reflects an increase in the amplitude of existing secretory pulses rather than an increased number of pulses. Despite improvements in glycemic control, beta-cell function is not normalized after therapy, suggesting that the intrinsic defect in the beta cell persists.

Treatment with the sulfonylurea glyburide increases the amount of insulin secreted in response to meals but does not correct the underlying abnormalities in the pattern of insulin secretion. In particular, the abnormalities in the pulsatile pattern of ultradian insulin secretory oscillations persist on treatment with glyburide despite the increased secretion of insulin.[623a]

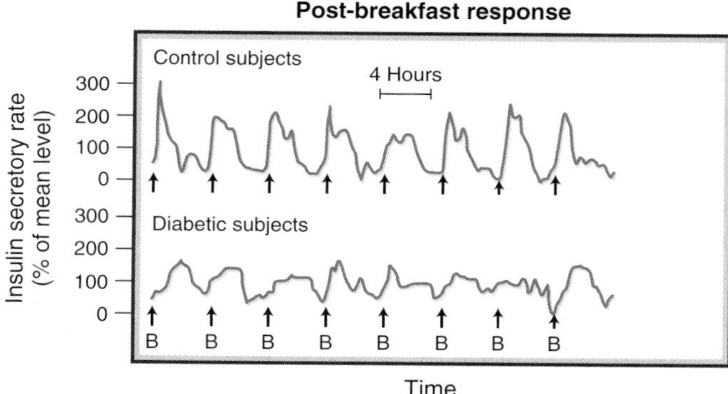

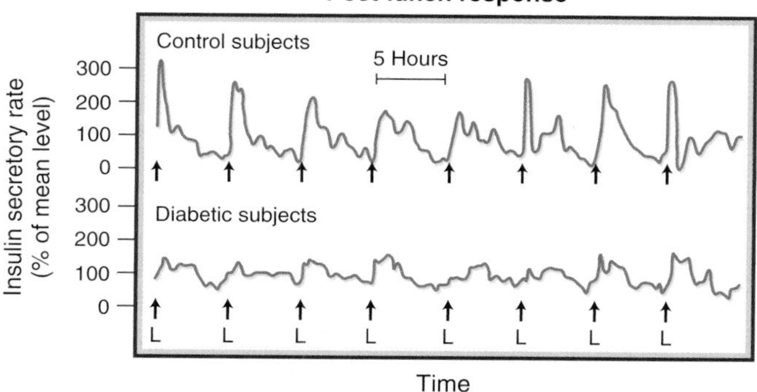

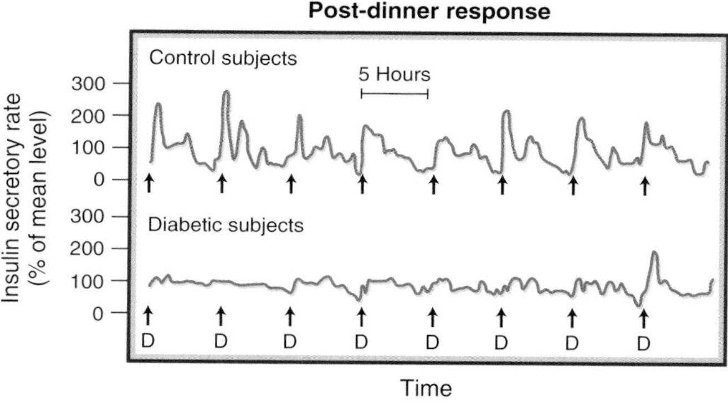

Figure 31-19 Temporal variations in rates of insulin secretion in control and diabetic subjects after breakfast, lunch, and dinner (*top, middle, and bottom panels*, respectively). In each subject, the secretion rates during the 30 minutes before the meal and the 4 hours after breakfast or the 5 hours after lunch or dinner were expressed as a percentage of the mean rate of insulin secretion during that interval. The curves were obtained by concatenating the resulting postmeal profiles in eight representative subjects. The times when the meals were served to the eight successive subjects in the series are indicated by *arrows*. (From Polonsky KS, Given BD, Hirsch LJ, et al. Abnormal patterns of insulin secretion in non-insulin-dependent diabetes mellitus. *N Engl J Med*. 1988;318:1231-1239.)

The effects on insulin secretion of improving insulin resistance in subjects with IGT through the use of the insulin-sensitizing agent troglitazone, a thiazolidinedione, have also been investigated. Troglitazone therapy improved insulin sensitivity, and this was associated with enhanced ability of the pancreatic beta cell to respond to a glucose stimulus, as judged by improvements in the dose-response relationships between glucose and insulin secretion as well as enhanced ability of the pancreatic beta cell to detect and respond to small oscillations in the plasma glucose concentration.[624]

Effects of Genetic Variants on Insulin Secretion

A number of the loci that have been associated with increased risk for T2DM appear to affect insulin secretion. Gene-phenotype studies have involved large numbers of subjects, and, as a consequence, they have generally relied on simple measures of beta cell function (e.g., the early insulin response to oral glucose). This approach has been very successful in identifying variants that primarily reduce insulin levels. More detailed phenotyping studies are now being undertaken in smaller groups of subjects to answer specific questions including the following:

1. Are the risk variants associated with altered clinical and physiologic findings before diabetes onset?
2. Is insulin secretion reduced equally in response to both oral and intravenous glucose?
3. Is the incretin effect reduced?
4. Are the dose-response relationships between glucose and insulin secretion altered?
5. Is there a concomitant change in insulin action?

Studies demonstrate that *KCNJ11* and *TCF7L2* are involved in the regulation of insulin secretion, but their clinical manifestations in humans are different, consistent with different mechanisms for their effects on the beta cell. Nondiabetic subjects with the *KCNJ11* T2DM-associated Lys-variant of E23K showed a significant reduction (approximately 40%) in insulin secretion after both oral and intravenous glucose, compared with subjects who did not carry this variant.[625] Hyperinsulinemic euglycemic clamps demonstrated that hepatic insulin sensitivity is increased in subjects with the Lys-variant and, as a result, normal glucose tolerance is maintained despite reduced insulin secretion. Therefore, the E23K variant appears to affect both insulin secretion and insulin action. The mechanisms responsible for the increase in insulin sensitivity are unclear. One possibility is that they represent a compensatory response to reduced insulin secretion. An increase in insulin sensitivity has also been observed in normoglycemic carriers of HNF1A mutations who have reduced insulin secretion.[626]

In contrast, carriers of risk variants in *TCF7L2* have a different phenotype, with normal insulin secretory responses to intravenous glucose including normal dose-response relationships between glucose and insulin secretion, reduced responses to oral glucose with a reduced incretin effect, and no change in insulin sensitivity. Concentrations of the two major incretins GLP1 and GIP are normal after oral glucose administration, implicating resistance of the pancreatic beta cell to the stimulatory effects of one or both of these incretins. These results are consistent with those of Schafer and associates,[627] who also documented reduced responses to GLP1.

RODENT MODELS OF TYPE 2 DIABETES

A number of spontaneous and genetically selected animal models of T2DM have been identified. Most of the models combine the two main features of T2DM: obesity-associated insulin resistance and beta-cell dysfunction with or without diminished beta-cell mass. As with diabetes in humans, the different rodent models of T2DM have similarities, but a number of overt and subtle differences make them useful surrogates for intensive study of the syndromes associated with T2DM.

An interesting observation is the striking sexual dimorphism in most rodent models of T2DM, with the male being affected exclusively, earlier, or more severely in most instances. This is not like the human situation. The advent of transgenic and knockout technology in mice has produced a wide range of models of insulin resistance and beta-cell dysfunction that result in hyperglycemia. It is beyond the scope of this chapter to review each of these, and the reader is referred to the primary literature for review of these animals. The discussion here is limited to the well-documented spontaneous or derived models of the disease in rodents.

Mouse Models of Type 2 Diabetes

Leptin (Lep^{ob}) and Leptin Receptor (*db*) Mutations

The *ob* mutation, now designated Lep^{ob}, was first described in 1950,[628] but the gene mutation responsible for the syndrome was not described until the *ob* mutation was found to be located in the gene for leptin.[629] Mice homozygous for the *ob* mutation do not produce the satiety factor leptin and become markedly hyperphagic, obese, insulin resistant, and hyperinsulinemic. They have a multitude of other hypothalamic dysfunctions that render them hypometabolic, contribute to the obesity, and also result in infertility.[630,631] Leptin treatment of these mice results in decreased food intake and reverses many of their other metabolic defects.[632-636] The *ob* mice develop obesity at weaning that becomes progressive because of hyperphagia. Insulin resistance is seen in muscle, adipose tissue, and liver, with a variety of signaling defects that are reversible with insulin administration.[637] The *ob* mouse becomes hyperglycemic and has a profound hyperinsulinemia associated with beta-cell hyperplasia, with up to a 10-fold increase in islet mass.[638,639]

Parabiotic experiments between *ob* and *db* mice suggested that the *db* mutation would be found in the receptor for ob. This was confirmed with the identification of multiple mutations in the leptin receptor in *db* mice.[640,641] Like *ob* mice, *db* mice are hyperphagic and begin to surpass their littermates in weight at weaning. They are progressively hyperinsulinemic, become hyperglycemic at 6 to 8 weeks, and, because of a decline in beta-cell function,[642-645] become markedly hyperglycemic at 4 to 6 months. The reason for the more severe diabetes in *db* mice is not clear, but it may be related to background strain differences, because similar defects in insulin signaling are seen in this animal model as well.[646-637] Treatment of both *ob* and *db* mice with insulin-sensitizing agents such as thiazolidinediones reversed the insulin resistance and ameliorated or prevented the onset of diabetes.[649,650]

Agouti Mouse

In mice, dominant "yellow" mutations in the *agouti* gene produce obesity and hyperglycemia. Depending on the background strain, the *agouti* mutation has a variable phenotype. In susceptible strains, the onset of hyperinsulinemia begins at 6 weeks of age, and insulin levels continue to increase with age, along with beta-cell hyperplasia and hypertrophy.[651,652] The *agouti* mutation results in systemic production of a protein normally expressed in the skin, most frequently because of a retrotransposon insertion into the promoter region of the gene.[653] A number of genes, including the fatty acid synthase gene, have both insulin and agouti response elements; this results in a marked increase in expression and leads to increased hepatic fatty acid synthesis and enhanced fat deposition in adipocytes.[641,654,655] The hyperglycemia is postprandial, and the FPG levels are usually normal. The exact function of the *agouti* gene is unknown, but the animals are hyperphagic and show enhanced growth.

KK Mouse

KK mice were originally bred for enhanced size, but they are not as obese as most other obese mice (usually <60 g). Breeding of the KK mouse into various background strains has produced variable insulin resistance, hyperinsulinemia, and hyperglycemia. The most studied strain is the KKA^y, produced in Japan.[656] This mouse has markedly increased insulin levels (>1000 μU/mL) when fed a high-fat diet.[657,658] As the male mouse ages, glucose levels fall toward the normal range. The mutation responsible for the KK phenotype is unknown.

New Zealand Obese Mouse

New Zealand obese (NZO) mice were derived by inbreeding of abdominally obese outbred mice.[639,659-661] NZO neonates have high birth weights, and mice of both sexes are large and at weaning exhibit an elevated carcass fat content.[659] Approximately 40% to 50% of group-caged NZO males, but not females, develop T2DM between 12 and 20 weeks of age when maintained with a chow diet containing 4.5% fat.[662] Obesity in NZO mice is characterized by widespread accumulation of subcutaneous and visceral fat. The obesity in these mice is accompanied by IGT in males, associated with increased hepatic and peripheral insulin resistance. In contrast to those in *ob* and *db* mice, genes encoding certain gluconeogenic and glycolytic enzymes in the liver of NZO mice retain normal responsiveness to insulin, although there is evidence for an inappropriately active fructose-1,6-biphosphatase.[663-665] Defective beta-cell insulin secretion from NZO islets in vitro and in vivo has been described.[659] There appears be a defect in the glycolytic pathway in beta cells that leads to defective glucose-stimulated insulin release.[666]

The genetics of NZO mice show a polygenic disorder, and none of the allelic variants have been discovered. Complicating the analysis of the model is the susceptibility of the mice to autoimmune disorders, including a lupus-like syndrome[667,668] and insulin receptor autoantibodies.[669] There is also a maternal influence in the peripartum period in the development of the disorder, which may reflect substances in the maternal milk.[670]

Gold Thioglucose–Induced Diabetes

Gold thioglucose induces specific lesions in the ventromedial hypothalamus and induces an initial chronic hyperinsulinemia that leads to hypoglycemia, hyperphagia, obesity, and the development of insulin resistance and hyperglycemia.[671] This model has been used as an example of pancreatic dysfunction preceding the induction of insulin resistance as opposed to pancreatic compensation for insulin resistance.

Diabetes Induced by Fat Ablation

Three models of insulin-resistant diabetes have been created in which adipose tissue is genetically eliminated by overproduction of foreign genes using the fat-specific promoter aP2. Expression of an attenuated diphtheria toxin in adipose tissue resulted in an age-dependent loss of fat, progressive insulin resistance, hyperinsulinemia, and significant diabetes.[672,673] Adipose-specific expression of a constitutively active form of the sterol regulatory element-binding protein SREBP1c also resulted in fat ablation.[674] Lipoatrophy was induced by fat-specific overexpression of a dominant-negative form of the transcription factor A-ZIP/F.[675,676] The A-ZIP/F protein heterodimerizes with and inactivates basic zipper (bZIP) transcription factors, including activator protein-1 (AP1) and CCAAT/enhancer binding protein (CEBP) isoforms, probably disrupting normal fat development.

The lack of fat in the various models leads to hepatomegaly, insulin resistance with hyperinsulinemia, hypoleptinemia, and significant IGT and diabetes. These mice represent a model of human lipodystrophic diabetes and demonstrate the importance of fat in normal glucose homeostasis. It has been suggested that the lack of fat depots results in elevated fatty acid delivery to liver and muscle and the development of insulin resistance. The diabetes in these animals can be variously treated by thiazolidinediones,[672] leptin administration,[677] and fat transplantation.[676] Human lipodystrophy also responds to thiazolidinedione treatment,[678] suggesting that some of the effects of these compounds are not wholly dependent on adipose tissue.

C57BL/6J Mouse Fed a High-Fat Diet. Male C57BL/6J (also known as B6) mice that were fed a high-fat, high-carbohydrate diet (a so-called Western diet, 58% fat by kilocalories) developed hyperglycemia, hyperinsulinemia, hyperlipidemia, and increased adiposity.[679,680] Glucose-stimulated insulin secretion was blunted, and there was significant insulin resistance.[681,682] Despite obesity, plasma leptin levels in the Western diet–fed B6 mice were significantly lower than in control mice in the absence of hyperphagia.[679,683] The weight gain is related primarily to an increase in mesenteric adiposity, which makes this a good model for human adult-onset T2DM.

Rat Models of Type 2 Diabetes

Zucker Diabetic Fatty Rat

The ortholog of the *db* mouse, the obese Zucker rat (*fa/fa*), has a mutation in the leptin receptor that results in significant hyperphagia.[686] The *fa* mutation is different from the mutations in *db* in that it does not disrupt leptin receptor gene expression and does not affect ligand binding.[686,687] This mutation results in a constitutive intracellular signaling domain, which may induce a desensitization of the leptin signaling pathways.[688]

The selection of the inbred Zucker diabetic fatty (ZDF) rat strain used Zucker (*fa/fa*) rats that had progressed to a diabetic phenotype. Brother-sister matings resulted in a strain exhibiting development of diabetes in almost 100% of the male rats consuming a 5% fat diet.[689] Hyperglycemia begins to develop in males at 7 weeks of age, with serum glucose levels rising to 500 mg/dL by 12 weeks of age. The hyperinsulinemia precedes hyperglycemia with marked islet hyperplasia and dysmorphogenesis,[690] but by 19 weeks insulin levels drop concomitantly with islet atrophy, in part because of an imbalance of hyperplasia and apoptosis.[591] The islets of prediabetic ZDF rats secrete significantly more insulin in response to glucose, with elevated basal levels of insulin secretion and a leftward shift but a blunted glucose dose-response curve.[592,691] Islets of prediabetic male ZDF rats also have defects in the normal oscillatory pattern of insulin secretion.[692]

In contrast to the male ZDF rat, the female rat has significant insulin resistance but does not become diabetic unless given a proprietary high-fat diet (GMI 13004).[693] The high-fat diet appears to have a direct effect on the beta cell, because there is no change in peripheral insulin sensitivity (P. Hansen and C.F. Burant, unpublished observations). There is a decrease in peripheral triglyceride and FFA levels in the female rat after institution of the high-fat diet.

The underlying genetic defect that results in beta-cell failure in the ZDF rat is unknown. The beta cell number and insulin content are not different from those in homozygous normal animals, but insulin promoter activity is doubled in the ZDF rat.[694] Insulin promoter mapping studies suggest that a critical region in the promoter of the insulin gene is affected. A number of other gene expression differences have been described in ZDF islets, including decreases in the expression of GLUT2[695,696]; increases in glucokinase and hexokinase activity[691]; decreases in mitochondrial metabolism[691]; accumulation of intraislet lipid and long-chain fatty acyl-CoA, which is associated with abnormal beta-cell secretion[692,697,698]; and increased accumulation of nitric oxide and ceramide,[699,700] which is associated with apoptosis. Other gene expression changes are also found in the prediabetic rat islet.[701] Which of these defects are important for the development of the diabetes is not clear.

The fixed genetic defect in the male animal leads to diabetes, but this defect also interacts with the insulin resistance, because treatment with insulin-sensitizing agents can prevent the onset of diabetes in male and female rats.[698,702] These agents are not effective in the male after establishment of diabetes; however, the female rat can respond to thiazolidinediones even after significant hyperglycemia.

Goto-Kakizaki Rat

The Goto-Kakizaki (GK) inbred rat strain was derived from outbred Wistar rats by selection for IGT.[703] Early in the development of diabetes, glucose and insulin are mildly elevated, but as the animals age, reduced beta-cell mass becomes evident, with markedly diminished insulin stores and abnormal secretory responses to glucose.[704,705] A number of biochemical defects have been described in the islets of these animals, including decreased energy production,[706-708] expression of proteins involved in insulin granule movement,[709] and decreased adenylate cyclase activity.[710] Defects in peripheral signaling include decreased maximal and submaximal insulin-stimulated IRS1 tyrosine phosphorylation, IRS1-associated PI3K activity, Akt activation in muscle,[711] and defective regulation of protein phosphatase-1 and -2A, and mitogen-activated protein kinase activation by upstream insulin-signaling components in adipocytes.[712] Some of these defects may be a result of hyperglycemia, because they can be reversed by phlorizin-induced normalization of serum glucose.[711]

BHE/Cdb Rat

The Bureau of Home Economics (BHE/Cdb) rat is a subline of the parent BHE strain that was obtained by selection for hyperglycemia and dyslipidemia without obesity.[713] Glucose-stimulated insulin secretion is markedly diminished in these rats, a trait that is maternally inherited.[714] A significant defect appears to be present in the liver. Increased gluconeogenesis and lipogenesis precede the hyperglycemia, which may be caused by defects in mitochondrial respiration associated with mitochondrial DNA mutations.[715,716]

Psammomys Obesus (Sand Rat)

The sand rat (*Psammomys obesus*) is a nutritionally induced obesity model of T2DM. Genetically, the animal is in reality a gerbil, and it usually lives on a low-calorie vegetable diet.[717] When given a high-carbohydrate diet, the sand rat rapidly becomes hyperglycemic secondary to weight gain associated with significant insulin resistance[718] and enhanced hepatic glucose production.[719] When a relatively hypocaloric diet is restored, the metabolic syndrome reverts to normoglycemia. A subpopulation of the sand rat develops frank beta-cell failure and becomes ketotic.

Otsuka Long-Evans Tokushima Fatty Rat

The Otsuka Long-Evans Tokushima fatty (OLETF) rat strain was derived from the Long-Evans rat with polyuria, polydipsia, and mild obesity.[720] About 90% of the male animals become diabetic by 1 year of age. Statistical tests have determined that the locus containing the cholecystokinin A receptor is responsible for about 50% of the T2DM in the OLETF rats.[721] The receptor is disrupted in the OLETF rat because of a 165-bp deletion in exon 1.[722,723] Genetic segregation analysis has shown interaction with a second locus, *Obd2*, which acts in a synergistic fashion to result in NIDDM, and both of these loci are required in homozygous OLETF rats to cause elevated plasma glucose.[724]

The role of sex hormones is pronounced in this strain. Orchiectomy markedly reduces the incidence of diabetes in the male, and oophorectomy increases the rate of hyperglycemia to 30% in the female. Treatment of castrated males with testosterone restores the incidence of diabetes to 89%. The islets undergo a progressive inflammatory reaction with progressive fibrosis. This reaction is associated with the impairment of beta-cell function.[725] Obesity and insulin resistance appear to precede the development of beta-cell failure.[726] Studies have also shown that obesity is necessary for the development of T2DM in OLETF males and that insulin resistance may be closely related to fat deposition in the abdominal cavity.[727] Troglitazone and metformin have been used successfully to treat diabetes in the OLETF rat, and troglitazone completely prevents the morphologic and functional deterioration of the beta cells.[728]

Neonatal Streptozotocin

Two models have been described in which a single dose of the beta cell toxin, streptozotocin, is given to 2-day-old female Wistar[729,730] or male Sprague-Dawley rats.[731,732] These animals have a transient hyperglycemia but develop IGT at 4 to 6 weeks of age. There is an initial reduction of beta-cell mass, but subsequent regeneration results in restoration of the beta-cell mass to a level approximately 50% lower than the normal adult level.

MANAGEMENT OF TYPE 2 DIABETES

Over the last 15 years, a conceptual transformation in the principles of management of T2DM has occurred. Fundamentally, there has been a change in the level of concern about diabetes as a public health issue and in attitudes about its treatment. Dramatic advances in the spectrum of pharmacologic agents and monitoring technology available for the treatment of diabetes have made it possible to lower glucose levels safely to the near-normal range in most patients. Great strides have been made in establishing an evidence base for guidelines regarding glycemic control and efforts to reduce the risk of complications. Corporate and government health insurance providers have greatly improved the extent to which diabetes equipment and supplies are covered.

A comprehensive review of all the subtleties of diabetes management in the 21st century is beyond the scope of this chapter. Here, we deal with the salient features of the epidemiology of the complications of T2DM, diagnostic strategies, treatment guidelines, lifestyle interventions, and pharmacotherapy before turning briefly to a discussion of preventive measures for T2DM and its complications. An excellent source of information on these issues is *Summary of Revisions for the Clinical Practice Recommendations* of the American Diabetes Association (ADA), which is published as the first supplement to the journal *Diabetes Care* each January and is available online at http://professional.diabetes.org/CPR_search.aspx (accessed December 2010).

Scope of the Problem

In the United States in 2007, the prevalence of diabetes was estimated to be 23.6 million, or 7.8% of the population, including 17.9 million diagnosed cases and 5.7 million undiagnosed cases. More than 1.6 million cases were diagnosed in people older than 20 years in 2007 alone.[733] This increase is driven by population aging; by population growth, particularly among ethnic groups with greater susceptibility to the disease; and by dramatic increases in rates of obesity as a consequence of increasingly sedentary lifestyles and greater consumption of simple sugars and calorie-dense foods. At least in the United States, opportunistic screening for diabetes in high-risk populations is recommended by professional societies and many insurers, and this has resulted in an increase in the fraction of affected persons with diagnosed diabetes, from approximately 50% in the 1990s to more than 80% in 2006.[9]

The morbidity, mortality, and expense associated with diabetes are staggering.[733] In Western society, people with diabetes are three times more likely to be hospitalized than nondiabetic persons. In the United States, diabetes is the leading cause of blindness and accounts for more than 40% of new cases of end-stage renal disease. The risk of heart disease and stroke is two to four times higher, and the risk of lower-extremity amputation is approximately 20 times higher for people with diabetes than for those without diabetes. Life expectancy is reduced by approximately 10 years in people with diabetes, and although diabetes is the seventh leading cause of death in the United States, this is clearly an underestimate. Only about 35% to 40% of those who die with diabetes have the disease listed anywhere on the death certificate, and only 10% to 15% have it listed as the underlying cause of death.[733]

Tragically, though a smaller proportion of people with diabetes are developing end-stage complications of diabetes,[734] the epidemic of diabetes is one of the drivers of increasing health care costs. Current estimates suggest that the diabetes population and associated costs will at least double in the next 25 years.[735] Annual disbursements for people with diabetes are approximately 2.3 times higher per capita than for those persons without diabetes. In the United States, at least 20% of health care expenditures are related to the treatment of people with diabetes.[736]

Glucose Treatment Guidelines

Study Results and Recommendations

Prospective, randomized clinical trials have documented improved rates of microvascular complications in patients with T2DM treated to lower glycemic targets. In the United Kingdom Prospective Diabetes Study (UKPDS),[737,738] patients with new-onset diabetes were treated with diet and exercise for 3 months, with an average reduction in HbA_{1c} from approximately 9% to 7% (upper limit of normal is 6%). Those patients with FPG greater than 108 mg/dL (6 mmol/L) were then randomly assigned to two treatment policies. In the standard intervention, subjects continued the lifestyle intervention. Pharmacologic therapy was initiated only if the FPG reached 15 mmol/L (270 mg/dL) or the patient became symptomatic. In the more intensive treatment program, all patients were randomly assigned and treated with either sulfonylurea, metformin, or insulin as initial therapy, with the dose increased to try to achieve an FPG of less than 108 mg/dL. Combinations of agents were used only if the patient became symptomatic or FPG rose to greater than 270 mg/dL (15 mmol/L).

As a consequence of the design, although the HbA_{1c} fell initially to about 6%, over the average 10 years of follow-up it rose to approximately 8%. The average HbA_{1c} in the standard treatment group was approximately 1 percentage point higher. The risk of severe hypoglycemia was small (on the order of 1% to 5% per year in the insulin-treated group) and weight gain was modest; both were higher in patients randomly assigned to insulin and lower in those receiving metformin.[738] Associated with this improvement in glycemic control, there was a reduction in the risk of microvascular complications (retinopathy, nephropathy, and neuropathy) in the group receiving intensive treatment. Although there was a trend toward reduced rates of macrovascular events in the more intensively treated group, it did not reach statistical significance.[737]

Similar reductions in microvascular events were observed in another trial of entirely different design and much smaller size. In the Kumamoto study, Japanese patients of normal weight with T2DM receiving insulin were randomly assigned to standard treatment or an intensive program of insulin therapy designed to achieve normal glycemia. The control group maintained HbA_{1c} values at approximately 9%, whereas the HbA_{1c} in the intensive therapy group was reduced to approximately 7%, and the separation was maintained for 6 years. Again, there was a modest increased risk of hypoglycemia and weight gain, a reduction in microvascular complications, and a nonstatistically significant trend toward reduced rates of vascular end points.[739]

In 2008, three studies examining the effects of two levels of glycemic control on cardiovascular end points in T2DM were reported. Action to Control Cardiovascular Risk in Diabetes (ACCORD),[740] Action in Diabetes and Vascular Disease—Preterax and Diamicron Modified Release Controlled Evaluation (ADVANCE),[741] and the Veterans Affairs Diabetes Trial (VADT)[742] each randomized middle-aged and older individuals who were at high risk for cardiovascular events. ACCORD and VADT aimed for an HbA_{1c} target of less than 6% using complex combinations of oral agents and insulin. ADVANCE aimed for an HbA_{1c} target of 6.5% or less using a somewhat less intensive approach based on the addition of the sulfonylurea gliclazide. None of the trials demonstrated a statistically significant benefit on combined vascular end points. ACCORD demonstrated a 22% increase in total mortality, whereas VADT had numerically more deaths in the intensively treated group (hazard ratio, 1.07). Modest improvements in some microvascular end points in all three trials were demonstrated. In these studies, there were suggestions that people who were without clinical cardiovascular disease and had shorter duration of disease and lower baseline HbA_{1c} demonstrated greater benefits from the more intensive glucose-lowering strategies.

Furthermore, a 10-year follow-up of the UKPDS cohort demonstrated that the relative benefit of more intensive management of glucose demonstrated at the end of the randomized portion of the trial was maintained, resulting in the emergence of statistically significant benefits on cardiovascular end points and total mortality.[743] Meta-analysis of cardiovascular outcomes in randomized trials suggested that an average HbA_{1c} reduction of 0.9% correlates with a 17% reduction in nonfatal MI and a 15% reduction in coronary heart disease without significant effects on stroke or all-cause mortality; however, as mentioned previously, there is significant heterogeneity in the result with respect to mortality across trials, the etiology of which is completely uncertain.[744]

Blood Glucose Treatment Targets

Guidelines from the ADA and the American College of Endocrinology (ACE) are presented in Table 31-7. The ADA suggests that the goal of treatment in the management of diabetes should be an HbA_{1c} value of less than 7% in general. Furthermore, the ADA suggests that lower targets may be pursued in selected patients, such as those with recent-onset disease, long life expectancy, and no significant cardiovascular disease, if they can be achieved without significant hypoglycemia or other adverse effects of treatment. Conversely, they recommend that less-stringent HbA_{1c} goals "may be appropriate for patients with a history of severe hypoglycemia, limited life expectancy, advanced microvascular or macrovascular complications, and extensive comorbid conditions and those with longstanding diabetes in whom the general goal is difficult to attain despite diabetes self-management education, appropriate glucose monitoring, and effective doses of multiple glucose lowering agents including insulin."[7] ACE has recommended an HbA_{1c} goal of less or equal to 6.5%, again with language suggesting individualization of targets.[745,746]

With respect to fasting, premeal, or postprandial targets, there is little support for any particular level of glycemic control in the management of T2DM because no large-scale outcome study has targeted particular levels of glucose with home glucose monitoring. The ADA target for fasting (and premeal) plasma glucose levels, 70 to 130 mg/dL, was initially developed based on an estimate of the range of average glucose values that would be associated with a low risk of hypoglycemia and an HbA_{1c} of less than 7%. It was later modified based on recognition that in many patients, routine achievement of an HbA_{1c} of less than 7% would lead to moderate hypoglycemic events, with glucose levels in the 70 to 90 mg/dL range.[747] The ACE fasting glucose target of less than 110 mg/dL is an effort to achieve normal levels of glycemia.[746] However, consistent fasting and premeal glucose levels lower than 110 mg/dL would be expected to be associated with an HbA_{1c} of approximately 5.5%.[748]

The ADA treatment target for peak postprandial glucose levels is set at less than 180 mg/dL, in part because such levels would be associated with an HbA_{1c} of approximately 7% and because nondiabetic persons who consume a large evening meal have been demonstrated to exhibit transient elevations of glucose to that level.[749] There are no published studies documenting safety or outcomes for a particular targeted level of postprandial blood glucose. However, there are effective HbA_{1c}-lowering agents that primarily target postprandial glucose levels, and monitoring of postprandial glucose levels may be necessary to optimize dose adjustment of these agents. Furthermore, there are patients with diabetes who have average FPG levels within their target range but whose HbA_{1c} is elevated. In these patients, monitoring and specific treatment of postprandial elevations can provide improvements in HbA_{1c}, perhaps with a lower risk of hypoglycemia and weight gain than has been associated with further lowering of fasting and premeal glucose levels.[750] The ACE has recommended a targeted 2-hour postprandial glucose concentration of less than 140 mg/dL (7.8 mmol/L) in an effort to achieve near-normal glycemia.[746] Consistent postprandial glucose values lower than 140 mg/dL would be associated with an average HbA_{1c} of approximately 5%.[748]

Lifestyle Intervention

The components of lifestyle intervention include medical nutrition counseling, exercise recommendations, and comprehensive diabetes education with the purpose of changing the paradigm of care in diabetes from provider focused to patient focused. Arguably, since the turn of the 21st century, nothing has changed more fundamentally than the emphasis on lifestyle intervention. For decades, physicians and patients have paid lip service to the notion that lifestyle intervention is important. Now we have significant clinical trial evidence that each component of lifestyle intervention, when appropriately administered, can contribute to improved outcomes. Furthermore, since passage of the Balanced Budget Act of 1997 and complementary legislation in most state governments, lifestyle intervention has been a covered benefit for most insured people. Although full implementation of these regulations is still in progress, they have dramatically expanded the fraction of the population with diabetes who can acquire insurance coverage for these essential services.

Patient Education

Diabetes is a lifelong disease, and health care providers have almost no control over the extent to which patients adhere to the day-to-day treatment regimen. The appropriate role of the health care provider is to serve as a coach to the patient, who has primary responsibility for the delivery of daily care. As a result, health care providers must carefully engage patients as partners in the therapeutic process. It is critical for the health care professional to understand the context in which patients are taking care of their disease. A prescriptive approach, in which patients are told what to do, can work in some situations but fails more often than not because of unrecognized barriers to the execution of a particular plan. For long-term success, diabetes self-management education is critical.

As defined by the ADA,[751] diabetes self-management education is the process of providing to the person with diabetes knowledge and skills needed to perform self-care, manage crises, and make lifestyle changes. As a result of this process, the patient must become a knowledgeable and active participant in the management of his or her disease. To achieve this task, patients and providers work together in a long-term, ongoing process. Minimal diabetes education should be universally provided and individualized with emphasis on the core issues highlighted in Table 31-8. There are many more specialized topics relevant to almost all patients, such as how to adjust therapy when eating out or during travel, review of available local health care resources such as support groups, and insurance issues. Although there are only limited studies, they do provide support for the concept that diabetes education can be cost-effective and can improve outcomes.[752]

TABLE 31-8

Curricular Areas That Should Be Addressed in Diabetes Self-Management Education

Pathophysiology of the patient's diabetes and its relationship to treatment options
Incorporating appropriate nutritional management
Incorporating physical activity into lifestyle
Using medications (if applicable) for therapeutic effectiveness
Monitoring blood glucose and (when appropriate) urine ketones and using the results to improve control
Preventing, detecting, and treating acute complications including sick day rules and hypoglycemia
Preventing (through risk detection), detecting, and treating chronic complications
Goal-setting to promote health and problem-solving for daily living
Integrating psychosocial adjustment into daily life
Promoting preconception care, management during pregnancy, and gestational diabetes management (if applicable)

Adapted from Mensing C, Boucher J, Cypress M, et al. National standards for diabetes self-management education. *Diabetes Care.* 2006;29:S78-S85.

A team of providers is usually required to fully implement the process of diabetes self-management education, because the amount of information that needs to be exchanged is large and the needed range of expertise is broad. It is usually not possible to cover the recommended content fully in the context of several or even many brief encounters with a physician in an office setting. Potential providers in a team care approach include nurses, dietitians, exercise specialists, behavioral therapists, pharmacists, and other medical specialists including diabetologists or endocrinologists, podiatrists, medical subspecialists, obstetrician-gynecologists, psychiatrists, and surgeons. The potential role of the community in which the patient lives and works in the diabetes self-care process is enormous; family, friends, employers, and health insurance providers may all be involved. Each potential member of the team has a role to play in the process, which must be reviewed and assessed frequently (Table 31-9). The primary roles of the providers in this process are to supply guidance in goal setting to manage the risk of complications, suggest strategies for achieving goals and techniques to overcome barriers, provide training in skills, and help screen for complications. For this process to be a success, the patient must commit to the principles of self-care, participate fully in the development of a treatment plan, make ongoing decisions regarding self-care from day to day, and communicate honestly and with sufficient frequency with the team.

Fortunately, barriers to providing team care are becoming less daunting. Diabetes education programs are being rapidly established. The American Association of Diabetes Educators (telephone 800-TEAM-UP4) and the ADA (telephone 800-DIABETEs) can provide information regarding diabetes educators and education programs in the local area.

For team care to be most effective, communication, trust, and mutual respect are critical. However, in many communities, the full benefit of consultation and ongoing care with diabetes educators, nurses, dietitians, pharmacists, or others is not achieved because of overly hierarchic approaches to care. Nonphysicians, including patients, ought to provide suggestions regarding medication and lifestyle adjustments and help in the process of identifying barriers to effective management such as lack of

TABLE 31-9

Team Care: Roles of the Players

Primary Care Provider
To be a source of accurate information and to refer to and coordinate with other sources of information as necessary To provide guidance in developing goals of treatment To screen for complications and evaluate progress in meeting treatment goals To help develop strategies for achieving treatment goals and avoiding complications
Other Providers
To be a source of accurate information, to communicate with the primary care provider, and to coordinate with other sources of information as necessary To provide guidance in developing goals of treatment and to help the primary care provider develop strategies to achieve treatment goals and avoid complications
Patient
To commit to diabetes self-management (see Table 31-8) To be an active participant in the process To communicate with other team members when goals are not achieved or barriers or problems are encountered
Community
To provide support to encourage ongoing diabetes self-care

knowledge, lack of time, and lack of resources and strategies to overcome barriers.

Perhaps some of the most overlooked contributors to ineffective care in the setting of T2DM are the relatively common barriers created by psychiatric, neurocognitive function, and adjustment disorders, which are largely responsive to psychosocial therapies.[753]

Nutrition

With respect to self-management education, recent ADA statements document the effect of medical nutrition therapy and offer specific advice on diabetes-related outcomes (e.g., HbA_{1c}, weight, proteinuria).[7,754] These recommendations are summarized in Table 31-10. A comprehensive, individually negotiated nutrition program in which each patient's circumstances, preferences, and cultural background as well as the overall treatment program are considered is most likely to result in optimal outcomes. Because of the complexity of the medical and nutritional issues for most patients, it is recommended that a registered dietitian with specific skill and experience in implementing nutrition therapy in diabetes management work collaboratively with the patient and other health care team members to provide medical nutrition therapy.

Structured programs that emphasize lifestyle changes including education, reduced energy intake (and therefore often fat intake), conscious decisions regarding carbohydrate intake, regular physical activity, and recurring participant contact can produce long-term weight loss of 5% to 7% of starting weight and reduce the risk of developing diabetes. Everyone, especially family members of persons with T2DM, should be encouraged to engage in mindful eating and regular physical activity to decrease the risk of developing T2DM.

Physicians and other members of the health care team need to understand the major issues in diabetes and nutrition and to support the nutritional plan developed

TABLE 31-10

Major Nutrition Recommendations for Diabetes

General
Individuals who have prediabetes or diabetes should receive individualized medical nutrition therapy (MNT) as needed to achieve treatment goals, preferably provided by a registered dietitian familiar with the components of diabetes MNT. Because MNT can result in cost savings and improved outcomes, MNT should be covered by insurance and other payers.
Energy Balance, Overweight, and Obesity
In overweight and obese insulin-resistant individuals, modest weight loss has been shown to reduce insulin resistance; therefore, weight loss is recommended for all overweight or obese individuals who have diabetes or are at risk for diabetes. For weight loss, either a low-carbohydrate diet or a low-fat calorie-restricted diet may be effective in the short-term (up to 1 year). For patients on a low-carbohydrate diet, lipid profiles, renal function, and protein intake (in those patients with nephropathy) should be monitored and hypoglycemic therapy adjusted as needed. Physical activity and behavior modification are important components of weight loss programs and are most helpful in maintenance of weight loss.
Dietary Fat Intake in Diabetes Management
Saturated fat intake should be <7% of total calories. Reducing intake of *trans* fat lowers low-density lipoprotein (LDL)-cholesterol and increases high-density lipoprotein (HDL)-cholesterol; therefore, intake of *trans* fat should be minimized.
Carbohydrate Intake in Diabetes Management
Monitoring of carbohydrate intake by carbohydrate counting, exchanges, or experience-based estimation remains a key strategy in achieving glycemic control. For individuals with diabetes, the use of the glycemic index and glycemic load may provide a modest additional benefit for glycemic control over that observed when total carbohydrate is considered alone.
Other Nutrition Recommendations
Sugar alcohols and nonnutritive sweeteners are safe when consumed within the acceptable daily intake levels established by the U.S. Food and Drug Administration (FDA). If adults with diabetes choose to use alcohol, daily intake should be limited to a moderate amount (i.e., ≤1 drink per day for adult women or ≤2 drinks per day for adult men). Routine supplementation with antioxidants (e.g., vitamin E, vitamin C, carotene) is not advised because of lack of evidence of efficacy and concerns related to long-term safety. Benefit from chromium supplementation in people with diabetes or obesity has not been conclusively demonstrated, and therefore it cannot be recommended. Individualized meal planning should include optimization of food choices to meet recommended dietary allowances (RDAs) or dietary reference intakes (DRIs) for all micronutrients. Lifestyle therapy for hypertension consists of: weight loss (if overweight), a Dietary Approaches to Stop Hypertension (DASH)-style dietary pattern including reduced sodium and increased potassium intake, moderation of alcohol intake, and increased physical activity. Lifestyle modification focusing on reduced saturated fat, *trans* fat, and cholesterol intake; increased n-3 fatty acids, viscous fiber, and plant stanols/sterols; weight loss (if indicated); and increased physical activity should be recommended to improve the lipid profile in patients with diabetes. Reduction of protein intake to 0.8-1.0 g/kg of body weight per day in individuals with diabetes and the earlier stages of chronic kidney disease (CKD) or to 0.8 g/kg per day in those with later stages of CKD may improve measures of renal function (e.g., urine albumin excretion rate, glomerular filtration rate) and is recommended.

Adapted from American Diabetes Association. Standards of medical care in diabetes—2010. *Diabetes Care.* 2010;29:s11-s61.

collaboratively. Individualized dietary advice can be developed by a physician from a brief diet history obtained by asking questions such as the following: What do you eat for breakfast? Lunch? Dinner? Do you have snacks between breakfast and lunch? Lunch and dinner? Dinner and bedtime? and What do you drink during the day? Ideally, this information should be obtained at each visit, with specific suggestions for changes that both patient and provider agree are important and achievable.

Easy issues to address include caloric beverages, which tend to elevate glucose levels dramatically and can usually be replaced quite painlessly by artificially sweetened alternatives. Juices are generally perceived as healthful but can significantly affect glycemic control and total calorie intake. Substituting low-fat products for higher-fat alternatives is often suggested but needs to be done with the recognition that these products are generally higher in carbohydrates. Fat-free and sugar-free foods need to be recognized as food that is not "free." Portion control and recipe modification are excellent techniques, particularly for meats and fried foods.

Adequate spacing between meals is usually good advice for patients with T2DM, because postprandial glucose levels typically peak 2 hours after a meal, when a snack would normally be taken. Eating approximately every 4 hours while awake is the most practical dietary plan for most overweight people. Frequent small meals have been shown to be of benefit when used in a controlled inpatient setting, but overweight patients who are encouraged to eat more frequently often overeat more frequently. At a minimum, avoiding high-calorie snacks is reasonable advice for most people with diabetes. A repeated diet history and additional modest changes negotiated every few weeks to months by all health care providers (i.e., doctor, nurse, or dietitian) allow assessment of whether previously agreed to changes were enacted, reinforcement of the importance of diet efforts, and slow enticement of patients into more healthful dietary choices.

In general, the critical nutrient for glycemic consistency is carbohydrate. Essentially every molecule of carbohydrate consumed is converted to glucose in the gut and requires the action of insulin to be cleared from the circulation. The carbohydrate-counting technique can be used in patients with T2DM to facilitate consistent carbohydrate intake or to allow insulin dose adjustment in response to changes in carbohydrates consumed.[755] Whereas the beta cell in T2DM has usually lost its responsiveness to glucose, the second phase of insulin secretion is largely spared in T2DM and is in part driven by amino acids and fatty acids. Therefore, including some protein and fat in each meal and snack is useful.

Dietary fat is the nutrient that is most closely associated in epidemiologic studies with the risk of developing T2DM. Although dietary fats clearly have an impact on total caloric intake (related to their calore density) and on circulating lipids, they have a minimal impact on glycemia acutely. Fat intake is a contributor to obesity and is the critical nutrient for cardiovascular risk management. It is recommended that people with diabetes (and everyone in general) consume a diet that is modestly restricted in calories (if overweight) and contains less than 10% of total calories as saturated fat and less than 10% as polyunsaturated fat. Some advocate substituting foods high in monounsaturated fatty acids (i.e., seeds, nuts, avocado, olives, olive oil, and canola oil) for carbohydrate, but most patients do not find adequate variety in the monounsaturated fatty acid category and often overeat these high-calorie foods. Higher-carbohydrate diets can raise postprandial glucose and triglycerides but are much less calorically dense than higher-fat diets and have a higher thermic effect, both of which tend to promote weight loss.

Dietary protein similarly has a minimal impact on glucose levels, although amino acids do promote insulin secretion, which may be advantageous in patients with T2DM. Metabolism of protein results in the formation of acids and nitrogenous waste, which can lead to bone demineralization and glomerular hyperfiltration. At least 0.8 g of high-quality dietary protein per kilogram of body weight is generally recommended; restriction of protein intake to 10% to 20% of total calories minimizes potential adverse long-term effects of high protein intake.

The roles of vitamins, trace minerals, and nutritional supplements in the treatment of diabetes are poorly understood. Some clinicians are convinced of the utility of soluble fiber, magnesium, chromium, zinc, folic acid, pyridoxine, cyanocobalamin, vitamin A, vitamin C, vitamin E, vanadium, selenium, garlic, and other micronutrients. Clinical trial data to support their safety and efficacy are inconclusive at best. Many patients are convinced that nutritional supplementation is healthful, and it is often counterproductive to engage in scholarly discussion of the nature of the evidence base for their decision. At a minimum, discussion should include the documented efficacy of more classic lifestyle and pharmacologic interventions and the idea that these efforts should not be left by the wayside when budget constraints affect potentially more effective interventions.[756] In a small randomized, controlled trial, a daily multivitamin and mineral supplement reduced the incidence of participant-reported infection and related absenteeism among patients with T2DM, perhaps related to a high prevalence of subclinical micronutrient deficiency.[757]

Although a wide range of dietary recommendations have their proponents, there are few data to support these suggestions from long-term outcome studies of prescribed diets. Mixed meals containing 10% to 20% of calories from protein, no more than 10% of calories from saturated fat, and the remainder largely from monounsaturated fats and carbohydrates (particularly whole grains, fruits, vegetables, and low-fat milk) are probably most reasonable. There is evidence that a diet rich in complex carbohydrates and low in fat and animal protein is a beneficial component of comprehensive lifestyle management in the setting of cardiovascular disease.[758] On the other hand, a number of studies suggest that diets lower in carbohydrate and higher in protein and fat reduce caloric intake and provide improvements in insulin sensitivity, glycemia, and cardiovascular risk markers.

Weight loss is a goal of many patients with and without diabetes and certainly is associated with improvements in glycemic control, insulin resistance, circulating lipids, and blood pressure. As reviewed previously, numerous studies document that certain changes can result in modest weight loss that can be largely maintained with sustained effort. These changes include intensive lifestyle programs involving frequent contact with patients, individualized counseling, and education aimed at reducing calorie intake. Additional, complementary changes by the patient include regular physical activity and efforts to understand and control behaviors that result in overeating.

Exercise

There is a substantial body of literature supporting exercise as a modality of treatment in T2DM.[7,759] Exercise is perhaps the single most important lifestyle intervention in diabetes because it is associated with improved glycemic control, insulin sensitivity, cardiovascular fitness, and remodeling. Aerobic exercise and resistance (strength) training have positive impacts on glucose control. Improvements in glycemic control are usually apparent immediately and become maximal after a few weeks of consistent exercise. However, they may persist for only 3 to 6 days after cessation of training; hence, the rationale for negotiating a minimum of three exercise sessions per week to maintain the benefit of the intervention.

The key concept is to promote an increase in activity using an approach similar to the one discussed for diet. Goals, methods, intensity, and frequency must be negotiated with patients with great sensitivity to recognizing barriers and helping patients discover solutions. The role of educators, exercise specialists, physical therapists, and social supports in this process is critical. The major role for the physician is to screen for complications (neuropathy, nephropathy, retinopathy, vascular disease) and discover ways for patients to be able to exercise safely. Exercise in the presence of uncontrolled diabetes, hypertension, retinopathy, nephropathy, neuropathy, and cardiovascular disease can create devastating problems. These obstacles can all be addressed creatively and should never present an insurmountable barrier to increasing physical activity.

Some authorities recommend that all patients older than 35 years have a stress test before initiating an exercise program. The utility of stress tests is potentially limited by their poor sensitivity and specificity.[760] If the exercise program contemplated does not involve more strenuous activity (in intensity and duration) than the patient has engaged in recently but merely more frequent activity, screening cardiovascular stress testing is unlikely to be useful. However, when sedentary patients plan to embark on a program of strenuous exercise, stress testing may be prudent to evaluate for subclinical coronary disease. Patients at high risk for coronary artery disease should start with short periods of low-intensity exercise and increase the intensity and duration slowly as tolerated. Patients who develop symptoms of coronary ischemia, including dyspnea out of proportion with activity, should be referred for further evaluation and treatment. Even with negative results on stress testing, it is important to encourage patients not to overexert and to recognize exertional chest, jaw, or arm discomfort as well as palpitations and dyspnea as symptoms of cardiac dysfunction.

Over time, improved exercise tolerance should be viewed as a measure of improved cardiorespiratory function. For aerobic exercise to improve insulin sensitivity, glycemic control, and cardiovascular risk, the patient must engage in at least 150 minutes per week of moderate-intensity aerobic physical activity (50%-70% of maximum heart rate) or 75 minutes per week of vigorous aerobic exercise (>70% of maximum heart rate).[7] Exercise should be regular, at least every 48 hours. Patients with T2DM should be encouraged to perform resistance exercise targeting all major muscle groups three times a week.[7] For the average patient with T2DM starting an exercise program, this equates to quite low-level activity initially, such as walking at a pace of 2 miles/hour. Initially, it may even be advantageous to negotiate once-weekly walks or shorter-duration exercise sessions, or both, and proceed from there. Over time, patients are encouraged to pick up the pace as tolerated and to increase the duration and frequency of exercise sessions slowly to avoid overuse injuries. It is not unreasonable to suggest to patients that if they are going to incorporate exercise into their diabetes management program, they must think of exercise as a treatment that takes the place of a pill and requires adherence to produce benefit.

Self-Monitoring of Blood Glucose

Self-monitoring of blood glucose (SMBG) has not been demonstrated in clinical trials to change outcomes in T2DM when evaluated in isolation.[7] However, many diabetes self-management programs have been demonstrated to help reduce complications. In all of these, SMBG is an integral part of the process, suggesting that SMBG is at least a component of effective therapy. The frequency and type of monitoring in diabetes therapy should be determined in consultation with the patient, taking into account the nature of the diabetes, the overall treatment plan and goals, and the patient's abilities. SMBG is particularly recommended for all patients with T2DM who are taking insulin or sulfonylureas because it allows patients to identify minimal or asymptomatic episodes of hypoglycemia.

Although severe hypoglycemia is relatively rare in T2DM, it can have devastating consequences, such as trauma or self-injury or change in the perceived ability of a patient to continue to live independently as a result of confusion or loss of consciousness. Also, it is essential to have patients critically assess the nature of any hypoglycemic symptoms that may occur. Many patients are fearful or overconcerned about hypoglycemia and routinely consume extra calories in response to a variety of life's circumstances, such as when they are hungry, sweaty, nervous, or upset. Monitoring studies document that most symptoms in patients with T2DM are not related to hypoglycemia and should not be treated with excessive calorie consumption.

Timing of SMBG varies depending on the diabetes therapy. It is important to advise patients to vary the time of the day at which blood glucose levels are checked. For some patients, the highest blood glucose of the day is the morning glucose, whereas for others the highest is before bed. Particularly in early diabetes, gestational diabetes, and well-controlled diabetes, monitoring 1 to 2 hours after meals allows patients to assess the effect of their lifestyle and pharmacologic efforts in controlling postprandial glucose levels, which are usually the only glycemic abnormality present. Monitoring (and thus targeting therapy) at just one time of day can leave the patient with a less than ideal overall response to therapy.

When glucose control is poor, having patients concentrate on premeal glucose levels is adequate. Once the premeal glucose levels reach the low 100s, many advocate that patients switch to checking 1- to 2-hour postprandial glucose levels; the latter approach amplifies the observed effect of diet on glycemic control and enables patients to see that moderate changes in meal plan, activity, and medications have a significant impact on glycemic control. Even after substantial inappropriate changes in food intake, activity, or timing or dose of medication, blood sugar values often return to near-normal levels overnight or by the time of the next meal.

The frequency of glucose monitoring needs to be matched to the individual patient's needs and treatment. Many clinicians ask patients to monitor at least once a day (at varying times before a meal, at bedtime, and at midsleep) as well as with hypoglycemic symptoms. Others ask patients receiving intensive insulin treatment to monitor with an intensity similar to that described for patients with T1DM: four times per day before meals; with weekly checks at least once after breakfast, lunch, dinner, and at midsleep; and with symptoms. Some ask for sets of glycemic readings more infrequently (e.g., fasting and 1 hour after the biggest meal). In the subset of patients who achieve stable blood glucose levels without significant hypoglycemia, it is usually appropriate to decrease the frequency of SMBG to a few times a week. It is critical that SMBG be frequent enough that both patient and provider have a good understanding of the adequacy of the treatment regimen and the stability of glycemic control.

It has been widely assumed that the benefits of SMBG stem from the effect of putting patients in a situation in which they can be in control of their own therapy. If patients are aware of the glycemic targets associated with the outcomes they seek to achieve, SMBG enables them to critically evaluate their response to therapy and assure themselves that they are reaching their goals. It is useful for patients to keep a daily diary of their SMBG results, so that they can assess their results periodically and can share them with the health care team. Many patients faithfully perform daily or more frequent SMBG, record the results as instructed, and discuss them with their health care team only at quarterly or semiannual visits even though their control is inadequate. Unless SMBG results are generally within agreed target ranges, they should be communicated and reviewed at least monthly with a member of the health care team by telephone, fax, mail, or e-mail or at an interim visit to trigger changes in therapy as the need arises. Unfortunately, such services usually are not reimbursed and can become an unsustainable burden on health care teams.

One of the most difficult areas in which to keep current is the area of available equipment and supplies, particularly for glucose monitoring. A useful resource in this regard is the annual *Resource Guide*, which is published as the January issue of *Diabetes Forecast*, a magazine for lay people with diabetes and their families. The most recent issue is available online at www.forecast.diabetes.org (accessed December 2010).

Pharmacotherapy for Type 2 Diabetes

The revolution in the treatment of T2DM since 1995 in the United States has been driven by the release of several new classes of drugs that independently address different pathophysiologic mechanisms that contribute to the development of diabetes. The available oral antihyperglycemic agents can be divided by mechanism of action into several groups: insulin sensitizers with primary action in the liver, insulin sensitizers with primary action in peripheral tissues, insulin secretagogues, agents that slow the absorption of carbohydrates, insulins, agents that increase the activity of the incretin system, and novel agents whose influence on carbohydrate metabolism is still unclear. Insulin therapy in patients with T2DM effectively is a supplement to endogenous insulin secretion. The relative benefits of lifestyle intervention and the 13 classes of drugs available for the management of T2DM are shown in Table 31-11. This area has been the subject of extensive reviews.[745,746,761-763] In the following discussion, the principles outlined in these reviews are summarized, and limited additional references are provided.

Insulin Sensitizers with Predominant Action in the Liver

Metformin is the only biguanide available in the United States. Phenformin was removed from the U.S. market in the 1970s because of deaths associated with lactic acidosis. Phenformin and buformin remain available in some countries. Although metformin has been available in Europe for approximately 40 years, it has been approved in the United States only since 1995. The precise mechanism of action of metformin is unknown; recent studies suggest that it activates AMPK, an intracellular signal of depleted cellular energy stores that has been implicated in stimulation of skeletal muscle glucose uptake and inhibition of hepatic gluconeogenesis.[764] The major clinical activity of metformin is to reduce hepatic insulin resistance and thereby gluconeogenesis and glucose production. It has more inconsistently improved insulin sensitivity in peripheral tissues. Because of its limited duration of action, it is usually taken at least twice daily, although a sustained-release formulation is now available.

Because biguanides do not increase insulin levels, they are not associated with a significant risk of hypoglycemia. The most common adverse events are gastrointestinal: nausea, diarrhea, crampy abdominal pain, and dysgeusia. About one third of patients have some gastrointestinal distress, particularly early in their course of treatment. This distress can be minimized by starting with a low dose once daily with meals and titrating upward slowly (over weeks) to effective doses. Sustained-release metformin is associated with less frequent and less severe upper gastrointestinal symptoms, the more common of the adverse effects of metformin, but it can increase the frequency of diarrhea, a much less common adverse effect overall. Most patients note no adverse effects with metformin therapy, and at least 90% tolerate it adequately with long-term use. Perhaps as a result of clinical or subclinical gastrointestinal effects, metformin is associated with less weight gain than other antihyperglycemic agents, and in some studies it has been associated with a modest weight loss.

Metformin has been said to cause lactic acidosis, which is quite rare and occurs almost exclusively in patients who are at high risk for development of the condition independent of metformin therapy.[765] The package insert states that metformin is contraindicated in patients with renal insufficiency (male patients with a serum creatinine concentration of 1.5 mg/dL or higher or female patients with 1.4 mg/dL or higher). The drug is cleared renally. Because there is a complex relationship between serum creatinine and renal function, reasonable practice might suggest that metformin can safely be used in patients with an estimated glomerular filtration rate (eGFR) based on the Modification of Diet in Renal Disease (MDRD) equation down to 30 mL/min per 1.73 m^2, with dose reduction to a maximum daily dose of 1000 mg when the eGFR falls below about 50 mL/min per 1.73 m^2.[766] Metformin is also contraindicated in patients with hepatic insufficiency and in the setting of alcohol abuse. Some patients taking metformin develop progressive vitamin B_{12} deficiency, which may be prevented with calcium coadministration.[767]

The glucose-lowering efficacy and the prevalence of adverse gastrointestinal effects of metformin increase proportionately in the dose range of 500 to 2000 mg/day. The maximal daily dose of 2550 mg does not generally provide additional benefit beyond that seen at 2000 mg daily. Newer formulations of metformin combined with various classes of oral antihyperglycemic agents have been developed to maximize glucose-lowering effectiveness with a single prescription through the synergy of two classes of agents with different actions.

Arguably, metformin has the best record among oral antihyperglycemic agents in outcome studies. In the UKPDS, among overweight subjects, those randomly assigned to metformin not only had improvements in microvascular complications similar to those of subjects randomly assigned to insulin and sulfonylurea but also demonstrated reduced rates of diabetes-related death and MI.[738] However, the validity of this observation has been challenged because of unusual responses in a subsequent

TABLE 31-11

Comparison of Therapies for Type 2 Diabetes

Property	Lifestyle	Insulins	Sulfonylureas	Metformin	α-Glucosidase Inhibitors	Glitazones	Glinides	Exenatide	Pramlintide
Target tissue	Muscle or fat	Beta cell supplement	Beta cell	Liver	Gut	Muscle	Beta cell	Various	Brain
ΔHbA_{1c} (%) as (monotherapy)	Variable	1->2	1-2	1-2	0.5-1	0.5-2	Re: 1-2 N: 0.5-1	~1	~0.5
Fasting effect	Good	Excellent	Good	Good	Poor	Good	Re: Moderate N: Poor	Poor	Poor
Postprandial effect	Good	Excellent	Good	Good	Excellent	Good	Re: Good N: Excellent	Excellent	Excellent
Severe hypoglycemia	No	Yes	Yes	No	No	No	Re: Yes N: No	No	No
Dosing interval	Continuous	qd to continuous	qd to tid	bid or tid	bid to qid	P: qd Ro: qd or bid	tid to qid with meals	bid	tid
ΔWeight (lb/yr)	+1	+3	+1 to 3	0 to −6	0 to −10	+1 to 13	+1 to 3	−6 to −12	−3 to −6
ΔInsulin	Variable	Increase	Increase	Modest decrease	Modest decrease	Decrease	Increase	Increase	None
ΔLDL	Minimal decrease	Minimal decrease	None	Decrease	Minimal decrease	Increase	None	None	None
ΔHDL	Minimal increase	None	None	Increase	None	Increase	None	Decrease	None
ΔTG	Minimal decrease	Decrease	None	Decrease	Minimal decrease	P: Decrease Ro: None	None	Decrease	None
Common problem	Recidivism, injury	Hypoglycemia, weight gain	Hypoglycemia, weight gain	Transient GI	Flatulence	Weight gain, edema, anemia	Hypoglycemia	GI	GI
Rare problem	—	—	—	Lactic acidosis	—	Hepatotoxicity?	—	—	—
Contraindications	None	None	Allergy	Renal failure, Liver failure, CHF (>80 yr old)	Intestinal disease	Hepatocellular disease	—	None	None
Cost ($/mo)	0-200	30-450	10-15	30-60	40-80	75-180	70-110	170-200	200-400
Maximum effective dose	—	1-2 U/kg per day	½ maximum or double starting	1000 mg bid	50 mg tid	P: 45 mg qd Ro: 4 mg bid	Re: 2 mg tid N: 120 mg tid	10 μg bid	120 μg ac

Δ, change; ac, before food; CHF, congestive heart failure; GI, gastrointestinal disturbance; HbA_{1c}, glycosylated hemoglobin; HDL, high-density lipoprotein; LDL, low-density lipoprotein; N, nateglinide; P, pioglitazone; Re, repaglinide; Ro, rosiglitazone; TG, triglycerides.

subrandomization. The beneficial effect of metformin on macrovascular complications through mechanisms independent of glycemic control is certainly plausible and is supported by such observations as metformin-associated modest reductions in LDL, triglycerides, blood pressure, and procoagulant factors. The ADA has recently published a consensus statement on medical management that suggests initiation of metformin therapy in all patients with T2DM (absent contraindications) at or near the time of diagnosis of diabetes.[747]

Insulin Sensitizers with Predominant Action in Peripheral Insulin-Sensitive Tissues

The thiazolidinedione class of drugs (TZDs or glitazones) has engendered great enthusiasm and controversy since the first agent, troglitazone, was approved in 1997. Rare fatal hepatotoxicity was associated with troglitazone, and it was withdrawn from the U.S. market in 2000, largely because the other TZDs (pioglitazone and rosiglitazone) were thought to be safer. These agents are believed to work through binding and modulation of the activity of a family of nuclear transcription factors termed *peroxisome proliferator-activated receptors* (PPARs). They are associated with slow improvement in glycemic control over weeks to months in parallel with an improvement in insulin sensitivity and a reduction in FFA levels.

Each of these agents varies in important ways with regard to potency, pharmacokinetics, metabolism, binding characteristics, and demonstrated lipid effects. At the same time, all are effective glucose-lowering agents that are generally well tolerated. The only significant early adverse effects are weight gain and fluid retention (and associated edema formation and hemodilution). There is no substantial evidence that these newer agents are associated with hepatotoxicity, but a record of safety has been established in appropriate patients. Patients should have liver function tests before beginning TZD therapy. TZDs are contraindicated in patients with active hepatocellular disease and in patients with unexplained serum alanine aminotransferase (ALT) levels greater than 2.5 times the upper limit of normal.

Pioglitazone and rosiglitazone are equally effective glucose-lowering agents with similar adverse effect profiles. They also provide equivalent improvements in markers of insulin resistance and inflammation. They differ with respect to lipid effects. In a head-to-head study among dyslipidemic patients, pioglitazone reduced triglycerides by approximately 20%, whereas rosiglitazone increased triglycerides on average by 5%. Pioglitazone is associated with a modestly greater improvement in HDL particle number and size and an improvement in LDL particle size and number. Rosiglitazone was associated with an increase in LDL particle number and improved LDL particle size.[768]

The promise of the glitazone class to reverse or prevent the negative cardiovascular associations of insulin resistance, in parallel with its demonstrated effect of improving insulin sensitivity, was suggested by a series of associations: reduced carotid intimal medial thickness, normalization of vascular endothelial function, improvements in dyslipidemia, lower blood pressure, and improved fibrinolytic and coagulation parameters. The PROactive Study was a randomized, double-blind, placebo-controlled trial in 5238 patients with T2DM and documented macrovascular disease. Subjects were randomized to placebo or to 45 mg/day of pioglitazone and otherwise treated according to guidelines for hyperglycemia and major cardiovascular risk factors. The primary end point was the time from randomization to a broad set of macrovascular end points. Pioglitazone was associated with a 10% reduction in the primary end point, but the reduction was not statistically significant. However, for the principal secondary end point, time from randomization to any cause of mortality, nonfatal MI (excluding silent MI), and stroke, pioglitazone therapy was associated with a 16% reduction, which was marginally statistically significant. Subsequent analysis and discussion of this technically negative and somewhat flawed trial has been extensive and supports the notion that pioglitazone therapy is associated with reductions in cardiovascular events that are largely accounted for by improvements in glycemia, lipids, and blood pressure. The benefits were in part mitigated by an increased incidence of heart failure, weight gain, and edema.[769]

The RECORD trial was an open-label study that compared the effect of adding rosiglitazone versus either metformin or sulfonylurea to patients who had T2DM inadequately controlled with sulfonylurea or metformin. There was no difference in cardiovascular hospitalizations or death.[770] There has been a brewing controversy that perhaps rosiglitazone is associated with excess MI, with some calling for its withdrawal from the market.[771] Although there are no definitive data to prove this allegation, it has resulted in dramatic shifts in the marketplace away from rosiglitazone use.

A second attribute of the glitazones that has generated great enthusiasm is an improvement in insulin secretory dynamics in subjects with diabetes and IGT. More importantly, the ADOPT trial in patients with early diabetes demonstrated a lesser rate of secondary glycemic failure in patients treated with rosiglitazone, compared with metformin, and both showed a lesser failure rate than glyburide; these benefits were correlated with indices of beta-cell function.[772] Several trials have demonstrated the remarkable effectiveness of thiazolidinediones to delay or prevent the development of diabetes, with greater magnitude than has been reported for other antihyperglycemic agents.[7]

The glitazones have the best track record in regard to slowing the progressive nature of beta-cell deterioration, and this may have important implications for long-term prognosis. On the other hand, multiple adverse effects of the class have raised concerns; these effects include weight gain, fluid retention, and increased risk of bone fractures. Careful study indicates that the weight gain is a result of both fluid retention and subcutaneous (but not visceral) fat accumulation. There is, in fact, a reduction in visceral fat, hepatic fat, and intramyocellular fat. Therefore, it has been argued that the weight gain observed with glitazones may not have the same negative metabolic consequences that are generally ascribed to overweight and obesity. Nevertheless, weight gain is viewed negatively by most patients and practitioners. All patients prescribed glitazones should be counseled to redouble lifestyle efforts to minimize weight gain.

With regard to edema, with appropriate caution, almost no one should need to withdraw from therapy as a result of fluid retention. The patients most likely to experience edema are those treated with insulin and those with preexisting edema. Therefore, women, overweight patients, and patients with diastolic dysfunction or renal insufficiency are at greatest risk. It is prudent to teach patients with preexisting edema how to assess pitting pretibial edema at home and to suggest that they make a habit of checking nightly. If they note a pattern of increasing edema at home, patients can be instructed to restrict sodium intake, to start a diuretic, or to increase their diuretic dosage by some specified quantity on their own as needed.

In the previously edematous patient and in patients treated with insulin, it is prudent to initiate therapy with the lowest available dose of glitazone. In 1 to 3 months, if the glycemic response has been inadequate and significant edema has not developed, consider increasing the dose of glitazone further, with continued expectant home evaluation for edema. Most patients with mild edema respond to a thiazide diuretic or spironolactone. In patients with more extensive edema, combination therapy with a moderate-dose loop diuretic is sometimes required.[773] Anecdotal reports suggest that avoidance of nonsteroidal anti-inflammatory agents and dihydropyridine calcium channel blockers can reduce the frequency of edema as an adverse event. Fluid retention to the point of congestive heart failure and anasarca has been reported; in the PROactive and RECORD studies, an excess of approximately 2% of patients treated with high-dose glitazones required hospitalization for heart failure. In some patients, edema is refractory to diuretic therapy. Edema resolves with a reduction of glitazone dose is some patients, but some require drug withdrawal.

A more recent safety concern regarding thiazolidinediones is bone health. In pharmacoepidemiologic studies and in randomized, controlled trials, excess fractures have been reported, mainly in older women. Whereas distal sites were primarily affected in these studies, small randomized, controlled trials have identified loss of bone density in the lumbar spine as well. Preclinical studies suggest that activation of PPARγ inhibits bone formation by diverting stem cells from the osteogenic to the adipocytic lineage. No data are available with respect to the prevention or management of thiazolidinedione-related bone loss, but prudent measures would include at a minimum an assessment of risk factors and appropriate bone density screening.[774]

An early and universal role for thiazolidinediones has been advocated by some because of their beta-cell effects.[11] Use of thiazolidinediones early in the natural history of disease creates maximum opportunities for beta-cell benefits, and the risk of heart failure related to fluid retention is also less; however, early use also increases the potential for long-term consequences related to weight gain and bone loss. Efforts to improve safety by creating agents with more selective effects continue.[775]

Insulin Secretagogues

Currently available insulin secretagogues all bind to the sulfonylurea receptor (SUR1), a subunit of the K_{ATP} potassium channel on the plasma membrane of pancreatic beta cells. The SUR1 subunit regulates the activity of the channel and also binds ATP and ADP, effectively functioning as a glucose sensor and trigger for insulin secretion. Sulfonylurea binding leads to closing of the channel, as do increases in intracellular ATP and decreases in ADP resulting from fuel metabolism. The membrane depolarization that ensues causes the opening of voltage-dependent L-type calcium channels. Subsequent calcium influx results in an increase in intracellular calcium, which leads to insulin secretion. Differences in pharmacokinetic and binding properties of the various insulin secretagogues result in the specific responses that each agent produces. The major differences among the insulin secretagogues seem to be related to duration of action and to subtle variations in hypoglycemic potential.

Sulfonylureas. The sulfonylureas have been available since the 1950s. They have a relatively slow onset and a variable duration of action. The numerous choices available (Table 31-12) can be divided into first- and second-generation agents. In general, the second-generation agents are more potent and, as a result, have fewer adverse effects and drug-drug interactions. Extended-release glipizide and glimepiride are preferred agents because they can be given once daily in most patients and involve a relatively low risk of hypoglycemia and weight gain. Gliclazide is not available in the United States but is a similarly preferred agent in much of the world. Nonetheless, glyburide is one of the most commonly prescribed insulin secretagogues, even in the face of concerns about its potential cardiovascular toxicity and higher risks of hypoglycemia compared with other secretagogues.[761,776]

An unusual characteristic of sulfonylureas is that the maximum marketed dose is two to four times higher than the maximum effective dose. There has been concern that sulfonylureas might cause increased arrhythmic cardiovascular events in patients with diabetes as a result of their activity on vascular and cardiac SUR2 receptors that blunts

TABLE 31-12

Characteristics of Sulfonylureas

Drug	Initial Daily Dose	Maximum Daily Dose	Equivalent Doses (mg)	Duration of Action	Comments
Acetohexamide	250 mg	1500 mg, div bid	500	Int: 12-18 hr	Metabolized by liver to active metabolite twice as potent as parent compound. Has diuretic activity. Has uricosuric activity.
Chlorpropamide	100 mg	750 mg (500 mg in older patients)	250	Very long: 60 hr	70% metabolized by liver to less active metabolites; 30% excreted intact by kidneys. Can potentiate ADH. Disulfiram-like reaction with alcohol occurs in almost 1/3 of patients.
Tolazamide	100 mg	1000 mg, div bid	250	Int: 12-24 hr	Metabolized by liver to less active and inactive products. Has diuretic activity.
Tolbutamide	250-500 mg or tid	3000 mg, div bid	1000	Short: 6-12 hr	Metabolized by liver to inactive product.
Glipizide	5 mg	40 mg, div bid	5	Int: 12-24 hr	Metabolized by liver to inactive products that are excreted in the urine and, to a lesser extent, in the bile. Mild diuretic activity.
Glipizide ER	5 mg	20 mg qd	5	Long: >24 hr	
Glyburide	2.5 mg	20 mg, div bid	5	Int: 16-24 hr	Metabolized by liver to weakly active and inactive products, excreted in urine and bile. Mild diuretic activity. Highest risk of hypoglycemia.
Micronized glyburide	3 mg	6 mg bid	3	Shorter	
Glimepiride	1 mg	8 mg qd	2	Long: >24 hr	Metabolized to inactive metabolites by liver, excreted in urine and bile.

div, divided; int, intermediate.

ischemic preconditioning, a protective autoregulatory mechanism in the heart. On the other hand, of the three recent cardiovascular outcome studies examining the effects of more intensive glycemic control on cardiovascular outcomes, only the ADVANCE trial, which employed the sulfonylurea gliclazide as its dominant strategy, did not exhibit any suggestion of cardiovascular toxicity.[741,777]

Sulfonylureas are arguably the most cost-effective glucose-lowering agents. In general, limiting the dose to one fourth of the maximum marketed dose, unless higher doses are clearly demonstrated to provide significant benefits in glycemic control, minimizes costs and adverse events. Small doses of sulfonylurea (e.g., 0.5 to 1 mg of glimepiride or 2.5 mg of extended-release glipizide) are remarkably effective, particularly in patients receiving concomitant insulin-sensitizing therapy, and are almost uniformly well tolerated.

Glinides. Repaglinide is a member of the meglitinide family of insulin secretagogues, distinct from the sulfonylureas. It has a short half-life and a distinct SUR1 binding site. As a result of more rapid absorption, it produces a generally faster and briefer stimulus to insulin secretion. As a result, it is typically taken with each meal and provides better postprandial control and generally less hypoglycemia and weight gain than glyburide. Repaglinide does seem to have a long residence time on the sulfonylurea receptor and a prolonged effect on FPG, even though its pharmacologic half-life is quite short. Repaglinide is available in 0.5-, 1-, and 2-mg tablets. The maximum dose is 4 mg with each meal. As with the sulfonylureas, there is only a modest glucose-lowering advantage of high doses compared with moderate doses of repaglinide.

Nateglinide is a derivative of phenylalanine and is structurally distinct from both sulfonylureas and the meglitinides. It has a quicker onset and a shorter duration of action than repaglinide. Its interaction with SUR1 is fleeting. As a result, its effect in lowering postprandial glucose is quite specific, and it has little effect in lowering FPG. This provides both advantages (less hypoglycemia) and disadvantages (less overall glucose-lowering effectiveness). Nateglinide is most appropriately used when FPG levels are modestly elevated in early diabetes or in combination with insulin sensitizers or long-acting evening insulin. Nateglinide is available as 120-mg tablets and is taken with each meal. A 60-mg tablet is available but is not generally used except in patients with minimal hyperglycemia.

The rationale for stimulating insulin secretion in a way that minimizes fasting hyperinsulinemia and maximizes postprandial control is compelling. Furthermore, these newer agents demonstrate little binding to the vascular smooth muscle and cardiac SUR2 receptors. However, the use in the United States of these newer glinide agents has been modest, in part because of the need for multiple daily doses, greater expense than with sulfonylureas, and lack of head-to-head comparative studies that demonstrate superiority over newer sulfonylureas, which are already perceived as having low potential for producing hypoglycemia and weight gain.

Carbohydrate Absorption Inhibitors: α-Glucosidase Inhibitors

α-Glucosidase inhibitors (AGIs) work to inhibit the terminal step of carbohydrate digestion at the brush border of the intestinal epithelium. As a result, carbohydrate absorption is shifted more distally in the intestine and is delayed, allowing the sluggish insulin secretory dynamics characteristic of T2DM to catch up with carbohydrate absorption.

There are two currently available agents, acarbose and miglitol. Vogliobose is available in other countries. The use of AGIs in the United States has been limited by a number of factors, including the need to administer the medication at the beginning of each meal, flatulence as a common side effect, and only modest reductions in blood glucose levels. These factors should be balanced against the ability of AGIs to lower postprandial glucose, thereby improving glycemia without increasing weight or hypoglycemic risk. Even though they potentially lower glucose in everyone, the extent of the lowering is modest, calling into question the utility of these agents in light of the substantial expense and side effects. On the other hand, there is evidence that acarbose improves cardiovascular outcomes better than most antihyperglycemic agents.[778]

To maximize the potential for these agents to be well tolerated, start with a low dose (e.g., one fourth of the maximum dose) just once daily and increase over a period of weeks or months to one quarter to one half of the maximum dose with each meal.

Insulins

Insulin has been commercially available since the early 1920s and is arguably still the mainstay of therapy for most people with T2DM worldwide. Subcutaneous injection of insulin in T2DM is designed to supplement endogenous production of insulin both in the basal state, to modulate hepatic glucose production, and in the postprandial state, in which a surge in insulin release normally facilitates glucose clearance into muscle and fat for storage to allow intraprandial metabolism. Currently, almost all insulin used worldwide is of recombinant human origin or an analogue. The available formulations largely differ in their pharmacokinetics, as shown in Table 31-13.

Insulin lispro, insulin aspart, and insulin glulisine are rapid-acting insulin analogues that have an onset of action in 5 to 15 minutes, peak activity in approximately 1 hour, and duration of activity of approximately 4 hours. Regular insulin is approximately half as fast as the rapid-acting analogues, with onset in 30 minutes, a peak at 2 to 4 hours, and duration of action of 6 to 8 hours or longer. Regular

TABLE 31-13

Pharmacology of Insulin

Duration	Insulin	Peak (hr)	Duration (hr)	Forms and Modifiers	Variability in Absorption
Rapid	Lispro, aspart, glulisine	~1	3-4	Analogue, monomeric	Minimal
Short	Regular	2-4	6-8	None	Moderate
Intermediate	NPH	4-8	12-16	Protamine	High
Long	Glargine	No distinct peak	~24	Analogue, precipitates at neutral pH	Moderate
	Detemir	No distinct peak	~24 (less at doses <20-30 units)	Analogue with fatty-acid side chain	Minimal

human insulin, when administered intravenously, is instantly effective, with a half-life on the order of 10 minutes. Administered intramuscularly, regular human insulin has a half-life of approximately 20 minutes. Rapid-acting insulin analogues do not exhibit discernible advantages on intravenous or intramuscular administration.

Neutral protamine Hagedorn (NPH) is the only intermediate-acting insulin available since Lente insulin was withdrawn from the market. Onset, peak, and duration are about twofold greater than those of regular insulin, with an onset of action in 1 to 2 hours, a peak at 4 to 8 hours, and a duration of action of 12 to 16 hours.

Ultralente insulin is no longer available as human long-acting insulin. Insulin glargine is a long-acting insulin analogue that is solubilized in acid but precipitates when neutralized in tissues on injection, producing no consistent or distinctive peak in activity and a duration of action of more than 24 hours in most patients. Insulin detemir is a long-acting analogue in which a fatty-acid side chain has been covalently bound to the insulin molecule; it remains soluble both in the vial and in tissues and has a duration of action of approximately 24 hours except at low doses (<20 to 30 units).

Premixed insulin formulations provide greater convenience and accuracy of mixing than those mixed by patients but at the expense of reduced flexibility. Premixed formulations available in the United States are 70/30 and 50/50 mixtures of NPH and regular insulin, a 75/25 and a 50/50 mixture of lispro insulin in its NPH-like formulation with insulin lispro, and a 70/30 mixture of insulin aspart with its NPH-like congener. Premixed insulin provides a profile of activity as expected from the addition of the activities of its components.

The tactics of insulin administration in the setting of T2DM are the focus of great debate and strong opinion. Questions remain regarding the relative benefits of analogue insulins in light of the approximately threefold greater expense and whether the greater convenience of low-complexity regimens is justifiable in comparison with the greater risk associated with lesser flexibility in dosing, particularly in T2DM.[7,779,780] Adverse events associated with insulin are well known and include weight gain and hypoglycemia. Both fast-acting and long-acting insulin analogues have been shown to provide a modest reduction in hypoglycemia. Insulin allergies are rare, as are chronic skin reactions, which include lipodystrophy and lipohypertrophy. The absolute risk of severe hypoglycemia in patients with T2DM is relatively small, approximately one third to one tenth as high as in similarly treated patients with T1DM. This risk can be further minimized with appropriate education of patients and expectant home glucose monitoring at times when unrecognized hypoglycemia is most likely to occur, such as at midsleep or during unplanned or strenuous activity.

Newer insulin needles cause less discomfort than those previously available because of a finer gauge, shorter length, sharper points, and smoother surfaces. Insulin pen technology makes teaching a patient to take insulin much easier and provides greater convenience and accuracy of dosing. Insulin pump therapy has been used in patients with T2DM but is not widely accepted as cost-effective in routine use.

Incretin-Related Therapies

The incretin effect describes the observation that oral glucose has a greater stimulatory effect on insulin secretion than does intravenous glucose at the same circulating glucose concentration. In humans, this effect seems to be primarily mediated by GLP1 and GIP. GLP1 is produced from the proglucagon gene in intestinal L cells and is secreted in response to nutrients. GLP1 stimulates insulin secretion in a glucose-dependent fashion, inhibits inappropriate hyperglucagonemia, slows gastric emptying, reduces appetite and improves satiety, and has beta-cell proliferative, antiapoptotic, and differentiation effects at least in vitro and in preclinical models. GLP1 has a very short half-life in plasma (1 to 2 minutes) due to amino-terminal degradation by the enzyme dipeptidyl peptidase IV (DPP4). A variety of pharmacologic techniques have been developed to harness the potential of GLP1 signaling to treat diabetes, including GLP1 receptor agonists, which are peptides that produce increases of 10-fold or higher in GLP1 activity, and DPP4 inhibitors, which are small-molecule inhibitors of the degradation of GLP1 and GIP as well as other hormones.[781]

GLP1 Receptor Agonists. Exendin-4 is a naturally occurring component of the saliva of the Gila monster *(Heloderma suspectum)* and shares 53% sequence identity with GLP1; it is resistant to DPP4 degradation. Exenatide is synthetic exendin-4 and was the first GLP1-based therapeutic agent to be approved for human use. When injected subcutaneously, it produces the effects listed earlier and has a peak of action and half-life of approximately 2 hours. With twice-daily injection within 1 hour before a meal, it produces a reduction of approximately 1% in HbA_{1c}, driven largely by a reduction in postprandial glucose along with modest weight loss (average, 5 to 10 lb/year). With prolonged use, weight loss has been associated with expected improvements in blood pressure and lipids. The most common adverse effect is nausea, which occurs in 40% to 50% of patients, usually early in the course of therapy. The nausea is mild to moderate in intensity and typically wanes over time. Nausea leads to withdrawal of therapy in about 5% of patients.

Hypoglycemia is not an effect of exenatide, but it can amplify the hypoglycemic effects of other agents. Therefore, for coadministeration with secretagogues, it is recommended that the minimum dose of secretagogue be used when initiating exenatide, uptitrating the secretagogue later if necessary. A concern that emerged from postmarketing reports is pancreatitis. A causal link has not been proven, nor has a mechanism been established. Nevertheless, it is recommended that incretin based therapy be avoided in those with a history of pancreatitis.[781] Exenatide is renally cleared and is not tolerated in the setting of advanced kidney disease (eGFR <30 mL/min per 1.73 m^2). Cases of acute renal failure have been reported in association with exenatide therapy, usually in patients with chronic renal insufficiency who develop superimposed prerenal azotemia in the context of prolonged nausea, anorexia, and/or vomiting.

Newer, longer-acting GLP1 receptor agonists include liraglutide and once-weekly exenatide. In general, these longer-acting agents are associated with greater HbA_{1c}-lowering efficacy due to more predominant effects on FPG. They are also associated with less gastrointestinal adverse effects, probably because they seem to produce little or no gastric emptying effects. Arguably, they are more convenient and therefore promote greater patient adherence. Liraglutide is administered once daily without any restriction as to timing or relation to meals. Once-weekly exenatide requires reconstitution and a somewhat larger bore needle for administration.

Weight loss is similar among the various GLP1 receptor agonists.[782,783] A new safety concerns that arose in preclinical testing with these long-acting agents is medullary thyroid cancer. No signal exists for this problem with GLP1-based therapy in humans, but there is a clear increase in the incidence of these tumors in rodents, although not in other animal models. GLP1 plays a role in regulation of C cells in the rodent but apparently not in the human. Nevertheless, it is suggested that these agents be avoided in those with a personal or family history of medullary thyroid cancer.[781]

DPP4 Inhibitors. Two DPP4 inhibitors, sitagliptin and saxagliptin, are available in the United States. Two more (vildagliptin and alogliptin) are available elsewhere, and numerous others are under development. These agents produce approximately twofold increases in fasting and postprandial GLP1 and GIP levels, with subsequent HbA_{1c} reductions of approximately 0.7%. They are remarkably well tolerated, with an adverse effect profile similar to that of placebo. Specifically, they are not associated with nausea. Probably because of the lesser increase in GLP1 activity than with the GLP1 receptor agonists, there is no weight loss with DPP4 inhibitors; they tend to be weight neutral.

Postmarketing cases of pancreatitis have been reported for the DPP4 inhibitors, and they are contraindicated for use in those with a prior history. Specificity for DPP4 appears to be crucial, because less specific inhibitors have demonstrated adverse effects on immune function and cancer growth in animal studies. Although the currently marketed DPP4 inhibitors are thought to be highly selective, continued long-term surveillance for unexpected adverse events is essential. A nice feature of these agents is that they do not require titration. The usual dose is the maximum marketed dose; because these drugs are cleared renally, smaller doses are recommended in the setting of stage 3 or greater chronic kidney disease. Serious hypersensitivity reactions have been reported, including anaphylaxis, angioedema, and exfoliative skin conditions with sitagliptin, but causality has not been substantiated due to the rarity of events. The weight neutrality, lack of hypoglycemia, broad applicability, tolerability, and ease of use create a unique niche for DPP4 inhibitors.[784]

The precise role of incretin-related therapies in diabetes management has not been established; cost, modest efficacy and uncertain long-term safety remain barriers to use. That said, preclinical and in vitro studies suggest that they may have benefits on the progression of beta-cell failure as well as cardiovascular health. There are no data yet to substantiate those hopes in humans, although long-term outcome studies are under way.[785]

Novel Agents

Amylinomimetics. Amylin is a neuroendocrine hormone that is cosecreted with insulin by pancreatic beta cells. As would be expected, amylin deficiencies are evident in patients with T1DM or T2DM, in parallel with the insulin deficiencies. Amylin and insulin have complementary actions in regulating plasma glucose. Amylin binds to brain nuclei. It promotes satiety and reduces appetite, and through vagal efferents it mediates a decrease in the rate of gastric emptying. It also regulates suppression of glucagon secretion in a glucose-dependent fashion, thus regulating the rate of glucose appearance from the gastrointestinal tract and the liver. Insulin, on the other hand, regulates the rate of glucose disappearance from the circulation by stimulating glucose uptake in muscle and fat.

Amylin is relatively insoluble in aqueous solution and aggregates on plastic and glass. Pramlintide was developed as a soluble, nonaggregating, equipotent amylin analogue. It is indicated for patients with insulin-treated T2DM for mealtime subcutaneous injection. In patients with T2DM, when pramlintide was added to insulin therapy with or without a sulfonylurea or metformin, HbA_{1c} was reduced by about 0.5 to 0.7 percentage points, and weight was reduced by about 0.5 lb/month.[786]

Mild nausea, which wanes with continued therapy, is the most common adverse effect. It is minimized by titrating the dose from 60 µg with meals to the usual 120 µg over 3 to 7 days as tolerated. Hypoglycemia is less frequent in patients with T2DM than in patients with T1DM, who do occasionally exhibit severe hypoglycemia. Prandial insulin should be reduced by 50% when initiating therapy, although subsequent retitration to higher doses is often required.

Oral medications that require rapid absorption for effectiveness should be administered either 1 hour before or 2 hours after injection of pramlintide.

Colesevelam. Colesevelam is a second-generation bile acid sequestrant. It was observed to mediate modest reductions in glucose during the clinical development program. An expanded program in patients with T2DM resulted in approval for marketing of this drug as an adjunct for the treatment of diabetes. It provides an HbA_{1c} reduction of about 0.5% in addition to approximately 15% improvement in LDL. HDL changes tend to be trivial. Triglycerides can increase by 5% to 20%. Gastrointestinal side effects affect 10% or more of patients but lead to withdrawals uncommonly. The mechanisms for the glycemic effects are not definitively known.[787]

Bromocriptine. A quick-release formulation of bromocriptine administered within 2 hours of rising in the morning has been developed and is approved by regulatory authorities in the United States, although it is not yet marketed for the treatment of T2DM. It is suggested that creating a circadian peak in central dopaminergic tone improves insulin sensitivity. Nausea is the most common adverse effect, occurring in about 30% of patients and leading to discontinuation in about 10% at highest doses; lower doses are better tolerated. HbA_{1c} reductions are generally modest but have been reported to be as high as 1.2%. In a 1-year safety study, broad cardiovascular outcomes were improved 40% compared with placebo. Although the formulation examined in these studies is not available currently, bromocriptine remains a possibility for future combination therapy.[788]

Practical Aspects of Initiating and Progressively Managing Type 2 Diabetes

A significant challenge in clinical decision making in diabetes is that the increased availability of therapeutic options for antihyperglycemic therapy is far ahead of adequate prospective outcome studies. Currently available clinical trial data have not identified the preferred agents in T2DM, either as initial therapy or in subsequent care. Each class of drugs and even individual agents within each class have advantages and limitations, and individual issues can significantly affect the appropriate choice of therapy in particular patients. Table 31-14 highlights some of the relative advantages and disadvantages of various agents and classes.

General Approach

A general approach in the absence of any patient-specific factors is suggested in the algorithm presented in Figure 31-20.[7] A growing body of experience suggests that the use

TABLE 31-14

Classes of Antihyperglycemic Therapy

Class	Representative Agents	Major Action	HbA_{1c} Lowering (%)	Fasting or Prandial Effect	Usual Dosing Frequency (Doses/Day)	Route	Hypoglycemia	Weight Effect	CVD Risk Factor Benefits	Important Contraindications	Daily Cost ($)
Lifestyle	—	Broad	>1	Both	—	—	No	Loss	Yes	—	—
Biguanide	Metformin	Liver sensitizer	>1	Fasting	1-2	Oral	No	Neutral	Modest	Renal or hepatic failure	<$1
Sulfonylurea	Glimepiride, glipizide	Insulin secretagogue	>1	Fasting	1-2	Oral	Yes	Gain	Negligible	—	<<$1
Meglitinide	Repaglinide	Insulin secretagogue	>1	Both	With meals	Oral	Yes	Gain	Negligible	—	~$5
Benzoic acid–derived	Nateglinide	Insulin secretagogue	<1	Prandial	With meals	Oral	Minimal	Minimal	Negligible	—	~$5
Basal insulin	NPH, glargine, detemir	Insulin supplement/ substitute	>1	Fasting	1	SQ	Yes++	Gain++	Lowers TG	—	~$5
Bolus insulin	R, lispro, aspart, glulisine	Insulin supplement/ substitute	>1	Prandial	With meals	SQ	Yes++	Gain++	Lowers TG	—	~$5
Thiazolidinediones	Pioglitazone, rosiglitazone	Peripheral sensitizer	>1	Fasting	1	Oral	No	Gain++	Variable (see text)	Heart or liver failure	~$5
α-Glucosidase inhibitors	Acarbose, miglitol	Slow carbohydrate absorption	<1	Prandial	With meals	Oral	No	Neutral	Negligible	—	~$3
Amylinomimetics	Pramlintide	Broad	<1	Prandial	With meals	SQ	No	Loss	Negligible	—	~$10
GLP1 receptor agonists	Exenatide	Broad	~1	Prandial	2	SQ	No	Loss	Modest with weight loss	Pancreatitis, renal failure	~$9
Long-acting GLP1 receptor agonists	Liraglutide	Broad	>1	Both	1	SQ	No	Loss	Lowers BP	Pancreatitis, medullary thyroid cancer	~$13
DPP4 inhibitors	Sitagliptin, saxagliptin	Improved insulin/ glucagon secretion	<1	Both	1	Oral	No	Neutral	Negligible	Pancreatitis	~$7
Bile acid sequestrants	Colesevelam	Uncertain	<1	Prandial	1-2	Oral	No	Neutral	Lowers LDL	Hypertriglyceridemia	~$9
Dopamine agonists	Bromocriptine	Uncertain	<1	Fasting	1	Oral	No	Neutral	Modest	—	NA

BP, blood pressure; CVD, cardiovascular disease; LDL, low-density lipoprotein; SQ, subcutaneous; TG, triglyceride.

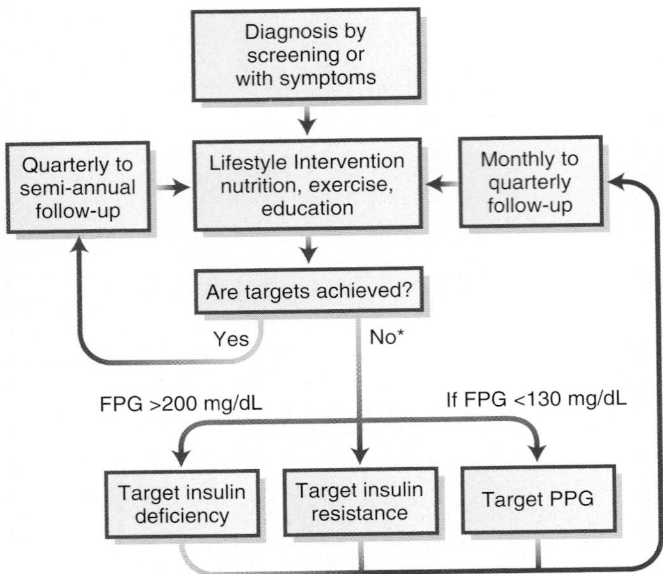

Figure 31-20 Treatment algorithm for type 2 diabetes. Reinforce lifestyle interventions at every visit, and check glycosylated hemoglobin (HbA_{1c}) every 3 months until the HbA_{1c} is less than 7% and then at least every 6 months. The interventions should be changed if the HbA_{1c} is 7% or higher. FPG, fasting plasma glucose; PPG, postprandial plasma glucose. (From American Diabetes Association. Standards of medical care in diabetes—2010. *Diabetes Care*. 2010;29:s11-s61.)

of metformin as initial therapy in combination with diet, exercise, and a comprehensive diabetes education program can provide impressive lowering of glucose with essentially no risk of hypoglycemia. Because metformin is available as a generic preparation, relative cost is low, and if the response is judged to be inadequate, essentially any other agent can be added. There are four potential second-line therapies. Sulfonylurea and insulin are termed "well-validated therapies" but are often complicated by hypoglycemia. The alternative nonhypoglycemic, "less well-validated therapies" are pioglitazone and GLP1 receptor agonists. The latter has the additional advantage of promoting weight loss. Certainly other alternatives exist although they may provide no distinct advantage over these four. The combination of metformin and a DPP4 inhibitor is generally well tolerated, is not associated with weight gain or hypoglycemia, and has become quite popular. Insulin plus metformin is suggested as the final common therapy for most patients with diabetes who do not achieve adequate control otherwise.

Patients with higher levels of glucose (typically HbA_{1c} ≥8.5%) almost always require agents to increase insulin levels. Because insulin, sulfonylureas, and glinides provide much faster improvements in overall control than other agents, they are preferred in patients with higher blood glucose levels, either as monotherapy or as part of initial combined therapy. Starting a patient with a low dose of a sulfonylurea or insulin combined with either metformin or glitazone is a reasonable initial approach to the patient with poor glucose control. Some advocate starting patients who have higher levels of HbA_{1c} with two agents as initial therapy.[745]

In patients who have reasonable control of FPG and preprandial plasma glucose (PPG) levels (i.e., more than 50% of values being <130 mg/dL) whose overall control as assessed by HbA_{1c} is still higher than desired, monitoring may be either inaccurate ineffective, or PPG levels may be elevated. Because it can be more difficult to have patients monitor in the postprandial state, almost all patients with T2DM have elevated PPG in the absence of specific therapy. In such patients, targeting presumed PPG elevations with the use of AGIs, glinides, exenatide, or rapid-acting insulin analogues can theoretically lower average glucose levels with a lower risk of weight gain and hypoglycemia compared with sulfonylureas or long-acting insulin.

The most critical issue in long-term glycemic management is that of continuously reassessing with patients the adequacy of their control, examining glucose monitoring logs and HbA_{1c} values, and refining treatment regimens to achieve optimal control with the lowest doses of the fewest medications. Most patients in specialty care require two or more drugs to achieve recommended targets. Many patients require three or more (particularly if long-acting and short-acting insulin are considered as two agents). Almost all of the possible two-drug combinations and many of the three-drug combinations have been examined in modest-sized studies and have been shown to be safe and effective. In general, it is preferred to add agents if there was an improvement in control with the first agent selected and to continue to add agents as needed to achieve goals. Subsequent back-titration to optimize treatment is often possible after glycemic goals are achieved. The selection of initial therapy should be based on priorities mutually recognized by the patient and provider. Increasingly, practitioners are using combinations of submaximal doses of agents to increase the ratio of efficacy to adverse effects and in recognition of the potential synergy of sensitizers and secretagogues as well as the value of treatment of PPG and FPG with combination therapy.

When adding insulin in the management of inadequately controlled T2DM, some practitioners prefer to stop the oral antihyperglycemic agents and switch to insulin. Most continue the oral agents and add an evening dose of insulin. Classically, bedtime NPH insulin and, more recently, long-acting insulin analogues have been preferred for initiating insulin therapy. There are data suggesting that long-acting analogues can provide for lower morning glucose values with less nocturnal hypoglycemia or weight gain than NPH insulin, particularly in more overweight patients. Many patients eventually require more complex regimens, such as twice-daily injections or multiple-injection regimens, but insulin pump therapy is only rarely required.

Some advocate starting multiple-injection therapy with rapid-acting insulin at each meal if adequate control is not achieved with basal insulin. Although the finding is not intuitive, recent data suggest that adding a single injection of rapid-acting insulin (at the morning meal or at the largest meal) to basal insulin titrated to provide for FPG control provides for a similar level of HbA_{1c} as the multiple-injection regimen with less weight gain and hypoglycemia. As one progresses from an injection of basal insulin plus a single injection of rapid-acting insulin to higher-order regimens, it seems incumbent on the health care team to ensure that improved control develops or to simplify the regimen. Studies suggest that to achieve HbA_{1c} levels lower than 7%, many patients require insulin doses on the order of 1 to 2 units/kg per day in addition to metformin. In the typical patient with insulin-resistant T2DM, there is usually little advantage to splitting basal insulin into two injections; in general, if a second injection is needed it should be prandial insulin.

It is important that both patient and health care provider agree on how to reach the goals of therapy. Therefore, biases and concerns of the patient should be addressed when trying to determine which agent should be prescribed. These biases can be elucidated in interviews with patients through discussions of various strategies.

Strategies

Minimal Cost Strategy. For a large fraction of patients, particularly those who are elderly, the cost of drugs is an overwhelming issue. Diet and exercise can be extremely effective and are almost cost-free. The least expensive drugs for the treatment of diabetes are the sulfonylureas, and metformin and human insulin are relatively inexpensive. Therefore, a minimum-cost strategy could start with a sulfonylurea or metformin or both and progress to the addition of bedtime NPH insulin. Although insulin is relatively inexpensive, at high doses (≥1U/kg) the costs begin to rise and the benefits are modest, creating a rationale for adding a thiazolidinedione. Most pharmaceutical companies have programs to provide no-cost or low-cost medications to the poor. Many of these are listed with links on the NeedyMeds web site (http://www.needymeds.com [accessed December 2010]). For an increasing number of patients, the major driving force in their drug expenses is the number of prescriptions, because each is associated with a copayment. This provides another rationale for the use of combination agents.

Minimal Weight Gain Strategy. Weight gain associated with the treatment of diabetes is of concern to most clinicians and is often an overriding issue with patients. A strategy to minimize weight gain would emphasize diet and exercise and would almost certainly employ metformin as initial therapy. GLP1 receptor agonists are associated with substantial weight loss in most patients with long-term use, and they would almost always be used as second-line therapy if weight were truly the major consideration. AGIs, DPP4 inhibitors, colesevelam, and bromocriptine are all weight neutral.

Minimal Progressive Beta-Cell Loss Strategy. Progressive loss of beta-cell function is the hallmark of diabetes. It results in progressive deterioration of glycemic control and the eventual need for insulin treatment. Thiazolidinediones seem to be associated with the lowest rate of secondary failure and sulfonylurea with the highest, at least in comparison to metformin. Adoption of a strategy to minimize progressive beta-cell loss would lead to the use of a thiazolidinedione with metformin as initial therapies and the avoidance of secretagogues. GLP1 receptor agonists and DPP4 inhibitors have been associated with improvements in beta-cell mass in rodent models, but this is completely unproven in humans.

Minimal Injection Strategy. Too many patients are determined to avoid insulin injections at any cost. The minimal injection strategy could involve the use of almost any combination of oral agents. Metformin and thiazolidinediones in combination with either sulfonylureas or DPP4 inhibitors have been best studied. Injected insulin or a GLP1 receptor agonist would be added only if absolutely necessary. The strategy of using thiazolidinediones early in the course of diabetes, in the hope that this might reduce the rate of progressive beta-cell dysfunction, would be rational in this setting. It is important to try to dispel notions that insulin therapy is difficult, ominous, or fraught with peril by highlighting its efficacy and the great strides that have been made in insulin formulations and delivery devices. Most diabetic patients require insulin at some point in their lifetime. Quite a few patients who have resisted the use of insulin have not balked at GLP1 receptor agonists. This suggests that, although patients may have identified the needle as the predominant barrier to insulin therapy, they really had other biases driving their fears.

Minimal Insulin Resistance Strategy. The possible atherogenic effects of insulin have been widely touted in the lay press and by marketing programs within the pharmaceutical industry. The relationship between circulating insulin levels and cardiovascular risk in nondiabetic populations is incontrovertible but is probably related to the presence of insulin resistance rather than the insulin concentrations per se. Furthermore, in essentially all studies of intensive management with insulin, improved outcomes were observed with insulin treatment. There are no clinical data to suggest that exogenous insulin is associated with adverse side effects or long-term complications beyond its hypoglycemic effects and the associated weight gain. A recent trial compared an insulin-providing strategy and an insulin-sparing strategy in high-risk patients in terms of mortality; there were essentially no differences in cardiovascular outcomes.[789] Adoption of a strategy to minimize insulin resistance would lead to the use of metformin and a thiazolidinedione before consideration of adding an AGI, DPP4 inhibitor, or GLP1 receptor agonist. Nateglinide is associated with more specific stimulation of insulin levels after meals than the other insulin secretagogues, which all increase peripheral insulin levels less than injected insulin does.

Minimal Effort Strategy. Many patients are capable of making only a minimal effort with regard to their diabetes. Questioning patients about their pill-taking history and their realistic ability to comply with a prescribed frequency of therapy is important. Twice-daily therapy is a barrier to metformin use. Taking a once-a-day sulfonylurea, DPP4 inhibitor, or thiazolidinedione requires the least effort by the patient. The use of basal insulin or a GLP1 receptor agonist is relatively well accepted by patients to whom this consideration is important. Developing strategies to improve adherence and increase motivation is a long-term goal in this population.

Hypoglycemia Avoidance Strategy. Hypoglycemia avoidance is another important consideration for many patients. The AGIs and glitazones have been reported in small studies to reduce reactive hypoglycemia. Theoretically, GLP1 receptor agonists, DPP4 inhibitors, and metformin should not be associated with hypoglycemia. Other oral agents could be added in any order, with the exception that insulin secretagogues would be added last, their dose minimized, and glyburide avoided. Nateglinide in particular among the secretagogues is associated with an exceptionally low risk of significant hypoglycemia. Basal insulin strategies seem to be associated with a lower risk of hypoglycemia than prandial insulin.[790] The long-acting insulin analogue detemir seems to be associated with a substantially lower risk of hypoglycemia than NPH and perhaps modestly less hypoglycemic risk than glargine.

Postprandial Targeting Strategy. Achieving postprandial glucose targets is generally associated with better control than just meeting premeal targets.[791] On the basis of epidemiologic studies, it has been suggested that PPG is more highly correlated with cardiovascular disease risk than FPG. However, correction for confounding variables such as components of the multiple metabolic syndrome has not been performed in these studies. Furthermore, there are no outcome studies that have demonstrated the superiority of these approaches in patients with T2DM.

Control of postprandial glycemia can be achieved only with specific lifestyle efforts and pharmacologic agents that target PPG. PPG monitoring is helpful in this regard because it reinforces the goals and is the most effective measure to assess the effectiveness of treatment. Nonpharmacologic techniques that can improve postprandial control include lowering the carbohydrate content of meals, adding fiber, substituting monounsaturated fats for carbohydrates, and encouraging physical activity after meals. The pharmacologic approach includes AGIs, exenatide, and rapid-acting insulin analogues. Nateglinide and repaglinide provide a theoretical advantage in this situation compared with other secretagogues, although formal head-to-head studies comparing the glinides with glimepiride and sustained-release glipizide have not been completed.

Preventing Type 2 Diabetes

The possibility that T2DM can be prevented in high-risk persons has been formally tested in a series of clinical trials reviewed elsewhere.[7] Lifestyle intervention seems to provide for a reduction of 30% to 60% in progression to diabetes over a 3- to 5-year time frame. These benefits seem to be sustained and best correlated with weight loss; however, the average sustained weight loss in these trials was modest, on the order of 5%. Metformin has likewise been associated with a somewhat more modest reduction in the progression of diabetes, although the benefit seemed to be similar to that of lifestyle intervention in those patients younger than 45 years of age, those with BMI greater than 35 kg/m^2, and those with an FPG level greater than 110 mg/dL. On average, metformin was generally without effect in patients older than 60 years of age, those with a BMI of less than 30 kg/m^2, and those with an FPG of less than 100 mg/dl. Acarbose has also been shown to reduce progression to diabetes, without evidence of diminished efficacy in different subgroups. The thiazolidinediones seem to be the most active antihyperglycemic agents tested for prevention, with efficacy as great as or greater than that of lifestyle intervention. However, concern regarding the long-term safety of thiazolidinediones in relation to effects on weight, heart, and bones has limited the enthusiasm for use of this class for prevention.

The success of the lifestyle interventions is impressive, demonstrating conclusively that with a variety of techniques it is possible for patients to achieve physiologically relevant changes in body weight. It is unknown whether lifestyle plus medications provides even greater benefit. The questions that arise are how to screen for people at risk and what intervention should be initiated in those with an interest in prevention. It seems reasonable to screen on the basis of current recommendations, as outlined earlier primarily for case finding, but also recognizing that patients with abnormal glucose values (HbA_{1c} >5.7% and particularly ≥6%, FPG ≥100 mg/dL and particularly ≥110 mg/dL, or IGT) would be ideal candidates for preventive strategies. Certainly, high-risk persons should be counseled about nutritional approaches to achieve weight loss, instructed to increase physical activity, and observed prospectively to determine whether progression of hyperglycemia has occurred. Treatment for other cardiovascular risk factors should also be considered if they are present.

In the absence of outcome studies, it is difficult to strongly advocate for drug therapy to prevent diabetes, because significant diabetes complications are unlikely to develop in the short window of time during which glucose levels increase from an FPG of 100 to 126 mg/dL. On the other hand, metformin therapy seems innocuous enough, and its benefits are broad; therefore, consideration of metformin therapy in patients who are at particularly high risk is recommended.[7] An extension phase of the Diabetes Prevention Program that is under way should provide evidence concerning whether prevention or delay in the development of diabetes will prevent death or disability.

Future Directions

The present-day management of T2DM is significantly more effective and easier for patients than the situation that prevailed even in the 1990s. A better understanding of the barriers to effective diabetes management and how to overcome them would be of great benefit. Changes in the health care system in the United States promise to eradicate access to care as the major barrier to prevention of disabling complications. The epidemic in diabetes and obesity that is under way, coupled with the predicted early death and disability that follow, threatens to overwhelm health care systems globally. Screening for diabetes or prediabetes may be cost-saving.[792] Practical, cost-effective public health approaches to stem this tide are desperately needed.[793] Whether new blockbuster drugs exist in the pipeline of 235 novel pharmaceutical agents for the treatment of diabetes and its complications is uncertain.[794] Although the prognosis for people with diabetes has never been better, the major challenges that they face relate to the complexity and cost of care. The opportunities for therapies that broadly address the metabolic underpinnings and consequences of diabetes are enormous.

REFERENCES

1. Zimmet P, Alberti KG, Shaw J. Global and societal implications of the diabetes epidemic. *Nature*. 2001;414:782-787.
2. Shaw JE, Sicree RA, Zimmet PZ. Global estimates of the prevalence of diabetes for 2010 and 2030. *Diabetes Res Clin Pract*. 2010;87:4-14.
3. American Diabetes Association. Type 2 diabetes in children and adolescents. *Diabetes Care*. 2000;23:381-389.
4. Mayer-Davis EJ. Type 2 diabetes in youth: epidemiology and current research toward prevention and treatment. *J Am Diet Assoc*. 2008;108(4 suppl 1):S45-S51.
5. Ogden CL, Carroll MD, Curtin LR, et al. Prevalence of high body mass index in US children and adolescents, 2007-2008. *JAMA*. 2010;303:242-249.
6. Sinha, R, Fisch G, Teague B, et al. Prevalence of impaired glucose tolerance among children and adolescents with marked obesity. *N Engl J Med*. 2002;346:802-810.
7. American Diabetes Association. Standards of medical care in diabetes—2010. *Diabetes Care*. 2010;29:s11-s61.
8. International Expert Committee. Report on the role of the A1C assay in the diagnosis of diabetes. *Diabetes Care*. 2009;32:1327-1334.
9. Cowie CC, Rust KF, Byrd-Holt DD, et al. Prevalence of diabetes and high risk for diabetes using A1C criteria in the U.S. population in 1988-2006. *Diabetes Care*. 2010;33:562-568.
10. Kahn R, Alperin P, Eddy D, et al. Age at initiation and frequency of screening to detect type 2 diabetes: a cost-effectiveness analysis. *Lancet*. 2010;375:1365-1374.
11. Defronzo RA. From the triumvirate to the ominous octet: a new paradigm for the treatment of type 2 diabetes mellitus. Banting Lecture. *Diabetes*. 2009;58:773-795.
12. Almind K, Doria A, Kahn CR. Putting the genes for type II diabetes on the map. *Nat Med*. 2001;7:277-279.
13. Bell GI, Polonsky KS. Diabetes mellitus and genetically programmed defects in beta-cell function. *Nature*. 2001;414:788-791.
14. Taylor SI, Arioglu E. Genetically defined forms of diabetes in children. *J Clin Endocrinol Metab*. 1999;84:4390-4396.
15. Kahn CR, Flier JS, Bar RS, et al. The syndromes of insulin resistance and acanthosis nigricans: insulin-receptor disorders in man. *N Engl J Med*. 1976;294:739-745.
16. Donohue W. Leprechaunism: a euphemism for a rare familial disorder. *J Pediatr*. 1954;45:505-519.

17. Elders MJ, Schedewie HK, Olefsky J, et al. Endocrine-metabolic relationships in patients with leprechaunism. *J Natl Med Assoc.* 1982;74:1195-1210.
18. Rosenberg AM, Haworth JC, Degroot GW, et al. A case of leprechaunism with severe hyperinsulinemia. *Am J Dis Child.* 1980;134:170-175.
19. Rabson S, Mendenhall E. Familial hypertrophy of pineal body, hyperplasia of adrenal cortex and diabetes mellitus. *Am J Clin Pathol.* 1956;26:283-290.
20. Garg A. Lipodystrophies. *Am J Med.* 2000;108:143-152.
21. Vigouroux C, Magre J, Vantyghem MC, et al. Lamin A/C gene: sex-determined expression of mutations in Dunnigan-type familial partial lipodystrophy and absence of coding mutations in congenital and acquired generalized lipoatrophy. *Diabetes.* 2000;49:1958-1962.
22. Garg A. Acquired and inherited lipodystrophies. *N Engl J Med.* 2004;350:1220-1234.
23. Magre J, Delepine M, Khallouf E, et al. Identification of the gene altered in Berardinelli-Seip congenital lipodystrophy on chromosome 11q13. *Nat Genet.* 2001;28:365-370.
24. Barroso I, Gurnell M, Crowley VE, et al. Dominant negative mutations in human PPARγ associated with severe insulin resistance, diabetes mellitus and hypertension. *Nature.* 1999;402:880-883.
25. Hegele RA, Pollex RL. Genetic and physiological insights into the metabolic syndrome. *Am J Physiol Regul Integr Comp Physiol.* 2005;289:R663-R669.
26. Moffett SP, Feingold E, Barmada MM, et al. The C161→T polymorphism in peroxisome proliferator-activated receptor gamma, but not P12A, is associated with insulin resistance in Hispanic and non-Hispanic white women: evidence for another functional variant in peroxisome proliferator-activated receptor gamma. *Metabolism.* 2005;54:1552-1556.
26a. Hattersley AT, Ashcroft FM. Activating mutations in Kir6.2 and neonatal diabetes: new clinical syndromes, new scientific insights and new therapy. *Diabetes.* 2005;54:2503-2513.
27. Haneda M, Polonsky KS, Bergenstal RM, et al. Familial hyperinsulinemia due to a structurally abnormal insulin: definition of an emerging new clinical syndrome. *N Engl J Med.* 1984;310:1288-1294.
28. Gruppuso PA, Gorden P, Kahn CR, et al. Familial hyperproinsulinemia due to a proposed defect in conversion of proinsulin to insulin. *N Engl J Med.* 1984;311:629-634.
29. Shibasaki Y, Kawakami T, Kanazawa Y, et al. Posttranslational cleavage of proinsulin is blocked by a point mutation in familial hyperproinsulinemia. *J Clin Invest.* 1985;76:378-380.
30. O'Rahilly S, Gray H, Humphreys PJ, et al. Brief report: impaired processing of prohormones associated with abnormalities of glucose homeostasis and adrenal function. *N Engl J Med.* 1995;333:1386-1390.
31. Ballinger SW, Shoffner JM, Hedaya EV, et al. Maternally transmitted diabetes and deafness associated with a 10.4 kb mitochondrial DNA deletion. *Nat Genet.* 1992;1:11-15.
32. Velho G, Byrne MM, Clement K, et al. Clinical phenotypes, insulin secretion, and insulin sensitivity in kindreds with maternally inherited diabetes and deafness due to mitochondrial tRNALeu(UUR) gene mutation. *Diabetes.* 1996;45:478-487.
33. Fajans SS, Bell GI, Polonsky KS. Molecular mechanisms and clinical pathophysiology of maturity-onset diabetes of the young. *N Engl J Med.* 2001;345:971-980.
34. Froguel P, Zouali H, Vionnet N, et al. Familial hyperglycemia due to mutations in glucokinase: definition of a subtype of diabetes mellitus. *N Engl J Med.* 1993;328:697-702.
35. Yamagata K, Furuta H, Oda N, et al. Mutations in the hepatocyte nuclear factor-4α gene in maturity-onset diabetes of the young (MODY1). *Nature.* 1996;384:458-460.
36. Yamagata K, Oda N, Kaisaki PJ, et al. Mutations in the hepatocyte nuclear factor-1α gene in maturity-onset diabetes of the young (MODY3). *Nature.* 1996;384:455-458.
37. Stoffers DA, Ferrer J, Clarke WL, et al. Early-onset type-II diabetes mellitus (MODY4) linked to IPF1. *Nat Genet.* 1997;17:138-139.
38. Horikawa Y, Iwasaki N, Hara N, et al. Mutation in hepatocyte nuclear factor-1β gene (TCF2) associated with MODY. *Nat Genet.* 1997;17:384-385.
39. Malecki MT, Jhala US, Antonellis A, et al. Mutations in NEUROD1 are associated with the development of type 2 diabetes mellitus. *Nat Genet.* 1999;23:323-328.
40. Njolstad PR, Sovik O, Cuesta-Munoz A, et al. Neonatal diabetes mellitus due to complete glucokinase deficiency. *N Engl J Med.* 2001;344:1588-1592.
41. Cereghini S. Liver-enriched transcription factors and hepatocyte differentiation. *FASEB J.* 1996;10:267-282.
42. Duncan SA, Navas MA, Dufort D, et al. Regulation of a transcription factor network required for differentiation and metabolism. *Science.* 1998;281:692-695.
43. Stoffel M, Duncan SA. The maturity-onset diabetes of the young (MODY1) transcription factor HNF4α regulates expression of genes required for glucose transport and metabolism. *Proc Natl Acad Sci U S A.* 1997;94:13209-13214.
44. Edlund H. Factors controlling pancreatic cell differentiation and function. *Diabetologia.* 2001;44:1071-1079.
45. Stoffers DA, Stanojevic V, Habener JF. Insulin promoter factor-1 gene mutation linked to early-onset type 2 diabetes mellitus directs expression of a dominant negative isoprotein. *J Clin Invest.* 1998;102:232-241.
46. Hani EH, Stoffers DA, Chevre JC, et al. Defective mutations in the insulin promoter factor-1 (IPF-1) gene in late-onset type 2 diabetes mellitus. *J Clin Invest.* 1999;104:R41-R48.
47. Kristinsson SY, Thorolfsdottir ET, Talseth B, et al. MODY in Iceland is associated with mutations in HNF-1α and a novel mutation in NeuroD1. *Diabetologia.* 2001;44:2098-2103.
48. Permutt MA, Hattersley AT. Searching for type 2 diabetes genes in the post-genome era. *Trends Endocrinol Metab.* 2000;11:383-393.
49. Horikawa Y, Oda N, Cox NJ, et al. Genetic variation in the gene encoding calpain-10 is associated with type 2 diabetes mellitus. *Nat Genet.* 2000;26:163-175.
50. Song Y, Niu T, Manson JE, et al. Are variants in the CAPN10 gene related to risk of type 2 diabetes? A quantitative assessment of population and family-based association studies. *Am J Hum Genet.* 2004;74:208-222.
51. Gloyn AL, Weedon MN, Owen KR, et al. Large-scale association studies of variants in genes encoding the pancreatic beta-cell KATP channel subunits Kir6.2 (KCNJ11) and SUR1 (ABCC8) confirm that the KCNJ11 E23K variant is associated with type 2 diabetes. *Diabetes.* 2003;52:568-572.
52. Goll DE, Thompson VF, Li H, et al. The calpain system. *Physiol Rev.* 2003;83:731-801.
53. Sreenan SK, Zhou YP, Otani K, et al. Calpains play a role in insulin secretion and action. *Diabetes.* 2001;50:2013-2020.
54. Zhou YP, Sreenan S, Pan CY, et al. A 48-hour exposure of pancreatic islets to calpain inhibitors impairs mitochondrial fuel metabolism and the exocytosis of insulin. *Metabolism.* 2003;52:528-534.
55. Otani K, Han DH, Ford EL, et al. Calpain system regulates muscle mass and glucose transporter GLUT4 turnover. *J Biol Chem.* 2004;279:20915-20920.
56. Johnson JD, Han Z, Otani K, et al. RyR2 and calpain-10 delineate a novel apoptosis pathway in pancreatic islets. *J Biol Chem.* 2004;279:24794-24802.
57. Aguilar-Bryan L, Bryan J. Molecular biology of adenosine triphosphate-sensitive potassium channels. *Endocr Rev.* 1999;20:101-135.
58. Nielsen EM, Hansen L, Carstensen B, et al. The E23K variant of Kir6.2 associates with impaired post-OGTT serum insulin response and increased risk of type 2 diabetes. *Diabetes.* 2003;52:573-577.
59. Gloyn AL, Hashim Y, Ashcroft SJ, et al. Association studies of variants in promoter and coding regions of beta-cell ATP-sensitive K-channel genes SUR1 and Kir6.2 with type 2 diabetes mellitus (UKPDS 53). *Diabet Med.* 2001;18:206-212.
60. Hani EH, Boutin P, Durand E, et al. Missense mutations in the pancreatic islet beta cell inwardly rectifying K^+ channel gene (KIR6.2/BIR): a meta-analysis suggests a role in the polygenic basis of type II diabetes mellitus in Caucasians. *Diabetologia.* 1998;41:1511-1515.
61. Love-Gregory L, Wasson J, Lin J, et al. E23K single nucleotide polymorphism in the islet ATP-sensitive potassium channel gene (Kir6.2) contributes as much to the risk of type II diabetes in Caucasians as the PPARγ Pro12Ala variant. *Diabetologia.* 2003;46:136-137.
62. 't Hart, LM, van Haeften TW, Dekker JM, et al. Variations in insulin secretion in carriers of the E23K variant in the KIR6.2 subunit of the ATP-sensitive K(+) channel in the beta-cell. *Diabetes.* 2002;51:3135-3138.
63. Rosen ED, Kulkarni RN, Sarraf P, et al. Targeted elimination of peroxisome proliferator-activated receptor gamma in beta cells leads to abnormalities in islet mass without compromising glucose homeostasis. *Mol Cell Biol.* 2003;23:7222-7229.
64. Altshuler D, Hirschhorn JN, Klannemark M, et al. The common PPARγ Pro12Ala polymorphism is associated with decreased risk of type 2 diabetes. *Nat Genet.* 2000;26:76-80.
65. Love-Gregory LD, Wasson J, Ma J, et al. A common polymorphism in the upstream promoter region of the hepatocyte nuclear factor-4α gene on chromosome 20q is associated with type 2 diabetes and appears to contribute to the evidence for linkage in an Ashkenazi Jewish population. *Diabetes.* 2004;53:1134-1140.
66. Silander K, Mohlke KL, Scott LJ, et al. Genetic variation near the hepatocyte nuclear factor-4α gene predicts susceptibility to type 2 diabetes. *Diabetes.* 2004;53:1141-1149.
67. Weedon MN, Owen KR, Shields B, et al. Common variants of the hepatocyte nuclear factor-4α P2 promoter are associated with type 2 diabetes in the U.K. population. *Diabetes.* 2004;53:3002-3006.
68. Grant SF, Thorleifsson G, Reynisdottir I, et al. Variant of transcription factor 7-like 2 (TCF7L2) gene confers risk of type 2 diabetes. *Nat Genet.* 2006;38:320-323.
69. Florez JC, Jablonski KA, Bayley N, et al. TCF7L2 polymorphisms and progression to diabetes in the Diabetes Prevention Program. *N Engl J Med.* 2006;355:241-250.

70. Florez JC. Clinical review: the genetics of type 2 diabetes—a realistic appraisal in 2008. *J Clin Endocrinol Metab.* 2008;93: 4633-4642.
71. Ridderstrale M, Groop L. Genetic dissection of type 2 diabetes. *Mol Cell Endocrinol.* 2009;297:10-17.
72. Sladek R, Rocheleau G, Rung J, et al. A genome-wide association study identifies novel risk loci for type 2 diabetes. *Nature.* 2007; 445:881-885.
73. Dupuis J, Langenberg C, Prokopenko I, et al. New genetic loci implicated in fasting glucose homeostasis and their impact on type 2 diabetes risk. *Nat Genet.* 2010;42:105-116.
74. Saxena R, Hivert MF, Langenberg C, et al. Genetic variation in GIPR influences the glucose and insulin responses to an oral glucose challenge. *Nat Genet.* 2010;42:142-148.
75. Himsworth H, Kerr RB. Insulin-sensitive and insulin-insensitive types of diabetes mellitus. *Clin Sci.* 1939;4:119-152.
76. Warram JH, Martin BC, Krowelski AS, et al. Slow glucose removal rate and hyperinsulinemia precede the development of type II diabetes in the offspring of diabetic parents. *Ann Intern Med.* 1990;113:909-915.
77. Lillioija S, Mott DM, Howard BV, et al. Impaired glucose tolerance as a disorder of insulin action: longitudinal and cross-sectional studies in Pima Indians. *N Engl J Med.* 1988;318:1217-1225.
78. Haffner SM, Stern MP, Dunn J, et al. Diminished insulin sensitivity and increased insulin response in nonobese, nondiabetic Mexican Americans. *Metabolism.* 1990;39:842-847.
79. Reaven GM, Bernstein R, Davis B, et al. Nonketotic diabetes mellitus: insulin deficiency or insulin resistance? *Am J Med.* 1976;60: 80-88.
80. DeFronzo RA. The triumvirate: beta-cell, muscle, liver—a collusion responsible for NIDDM. Lilly Lecture 1987. *Diabetes.* 1988;37: 667-687.
81. Paolisso G, Tagliamonte MR, Rizzo MR, et al. Advancing age and insulin resistance: new facts about an ancient history. *Eur J Clin Invest.* 1999;29:758-769.
82. Groop L. Genetics of the metabolic syndrome. *Br J Nutr.* 2000;83(suppl 1):S39-S48.
83. Lehtovirta M, Kaprio J, Forsblom C, et al. Insulin sensitivity and insulin secretion in monozygotic and dizygotic twins. *Diabetologia.* 2000;43:285-293.
84. Mayer EJ, Newman B, Austin MA, et al. Genetic and environmental influences on insulin levels and the insulin resistance syndrome: an analysis of women twins. *Am J Epidemiol.* 1996;143:323-332.
85. Hong Y, Pedersen NL, Brismar K, et al. Genetic and environmental architecture of the features of the insulin-resistance syndrome. *Am J Hum Genet.* 1997;60:143-152.
86. Fujioka S, Matsuzawa Y, Tokunaga K, et al. Contribution of intra-abdominal fat accumulation to the impairment of glucose and lipid metabolism in human obesity. *Metabolism.* 1987;36:54-59.
87. Brambilla P, Manzoni P, Sironi S, et al. Peripheral and abdominal adiposity in childhood obesity. *Int J Obes Relat Metab Disord.* 1994;18:795-800.
88. Berman DM, Rodriguez LM, Nicklas BJ, et al. Racial disparities in metabolism, central obesity, and sex hormone-binding globulin in postmenopausal women. *J Clin Endocrinol Metab.* 2001;86:97-103.
89. Hu FB, Manson JE, Stampfer MJ, et al. Diet, lifestyle, and the risk of type 2 diabetes mellitus in women. *N Engl J Med.* 2001;345: 790-797.
90. Tuomilehto J, Lindstrom J, Eriksson G, et al. Prevention of type 2 diabetes mellitus by changes in lifestyle among subjects with impaired glucose tolerance. *N Engl J Med.* 2001;344:1343-1350.
91. Must A, Spadano J, Coakley EH, et al. The disease burden associated with overweight and obesity. *JAMA.* 1999;282:1523-1529.
92. Cefalu WT, Werbel S, Bell-Farrow AD, et al. Insulin resistance and fat patterning with aging: relationship to metabolic risk factors for cardiovascular disease. *Metabolism.* 1998;47:401-408.
93. Larsson B, Svardsudd K, Welin L, et al. Abdominal adipose tissue distribution, obesity, and risk of cardiovascular disease and death: 13 year follow up of participants in the study of men born in 1913. *Br Med J (Clin Res Ed).* 1984;288:1401-1404.
94. Despres JP, Tremblay A, Perusse L, et al. Abdominal adipose tissue and serum HDL-cholesterol: association independent from obesity and serum triglyceride concentration. *Int J Obes.* 1988;12:1-13.
95. Landin K, Krotkiewski M, Smith U. Importance of obesity for the metabolic abnormalities associated with an abdominal fat distribution. *Metabolism.* 1989;38:572-576.
96. Heitmann BL. The variation in blood lipid levels described by various measures of overall and abdominal obesity in Danish men and women aged 35-65 years. *Eur J Clin Nutr.* 1992;46:597-605.
97. Reeder BA, Senthilselvan A, Despres JP, et al. The association of cardiovascular disease risk factors with abdominal obesity in Canada. Canadian Heart Health Surveys Research Group. *Can Med Assoc J.* 1997;157(suppl 1):S39-S45.
98. Lamarche B. Abdominal obesity and its metabolic complications: implications for the risk of ischaemic heart disease. *Coron Artery Dis.* 1998;9:473-481.
99. Evans DJ, Hoffmann RG, Kalkhoff RK, et al. Relationship of body fat topography to insulin sensitivity and metabolic profiles in premenopausal women. *Metabolism.* 1984;33:68-75.
100. Peiris AN, Mueller RA, Smith GA, et al. Splanchnic insulin metabolism in obesity: influence of body fat distribution. *J Clin Invest.* 1986;78:1648-1657.
101. Arner P, Hellstrom L, Wahrenberg H, et al. Beta-adrenoceptor expression in human fat cells from different regions. *J Clin Invest.* 1990;86:1595-1600.
102. Nicklas BJ, Rogus EM, Colman EG, et al. Visceral adiposity, increased adipocyte lipolysis, and metabolic dysfunction in obese postmenopausal women. *Am J Physiol.* 1996;270:E72-E78.
103. Mittelman SD, Van Citters GW, Kim SP, et al. Longitudinal compensation for fat-induced insulin resistance includes reduced insulin clearance and enhanced beta-cell response. *Diabetes.* 2000;49:2116-2125.
104. Chan JC, Malik V, Jia W, et al. Diabetes in Asia: epidemiology, risk factors, and pathophysiology. *JAMA.* 2009;301:2129-2140.
105. Iyer A, Fairlie DP, Prins JB, et al. Inflammatory lipid mediators in adipocyte function and obesity. *Nat Rev Endocrinol.* 2010;6:71-82.
106. Karastergiou K, Mohamed-Ali V. The autocrine and paracrine roles of adipokines. *Mol Cell Endocrinol.* 2010;318:69-78.
107. Tzatsos A, Kandror KV. Nutrients suppress phosphatidylinositol 3-kinase/Akt signaling via raptor-dependent mTOR-mediated insulin receptor substrate 1 phosphorylation. *Mol Cell Biol.* 2006;26:63-76.
108. Um SH, Frigerio F, Watanabe M, et al. Absence of S6K1 protects against age- and diet-induced obesity while enhancing insulin sensitivity. *Nature.* 2004;431:200-205.
109. Ron D, Walter P. Signal integration in the endoplasmic reticulum unfolded protein response. *Nat Rev Mol Cell Biol.* 2007;8:519-529.
110. Hotamisligil GS. Endoplasmic reticulum stress and the inflammatory basis of metabolic disease. *Cell.* 2010;140:900-917.
111. Schroder K, Tschopp J. The inflammasomes. *Cell.* 2010;140:821-832.
112. Shi H, Kokoeva MV, Inouye K, et al. TLR4 links innate immunity and fatty acid-induced insulin resistance. *J Clin Invest.* 2006;116: 3015-3025.
113. Larsen CM, Faulenbach M, Vaag A, et al. Interleukin-1-receptor antagonist in type 2 diabetes mellitus. *N Engl J Med.* 2007;356:1517-1526.
114. Knutson KL, Van Cauter E. Associations between sleep loss and increased risk of obesity and diabetes. *Ann N Y Acad Sci.* 2008;1129:287-304.
115. Maury E, Ramsey KM, Bass J. Circadian rhythms and metabolic syndrome: from experimental genetics to human disease. *Circ Res.* 2010;106:447-462.
116. Punjabi NM, Workshop Participants. Do sleep disorders and associated treatments impact glucose metabolism? *Drugs.* 2009;69(suppl 2): 13-27.
117. Del Prato S, Bonadonna RC, Bonora E, et al. Characterization of cellular defects of insulin action in type 2 (non-insulin-dependent) diabetes mellitus. *J Clin Invest.* 1993;91:484-494.
118. Freymond D, Bogardus C, Okubo M, et al. Impaired insulin-stimulated muscle glycogen synthase activation in vivo in man is related to low fasting glycogen synthase phosphatase activity. *J Clin Invest.* 1988;82:1503-1509.
119. Charles MA, Eschwege E, Thibult N, et al. The role of non-esterified fatty acids in the deterioration of glucose tolerance in Caucasian subjects: results of the Paris Prospective Study. *Diabetologia.* 1997;40: 1101-1106.
120. Paolisso G, Tataranni PA, Foley JE, et al. A high concentration of fasting plasma non-esterified fatty acids is a risk factor for the development of NIDDM. *Diabetologia.* 1995;38:1213-1217.
121. Garland PB, Newsholme EA, Randle PJ. Regulation of glucose uptake by muscle: 9. Effects of fatty acids and ketone bodies, and of alloxan-diabetes and starvation, on pyruvate metabolism and on lactate-pyruvate and L-glycerol 3-phosphate-dihydroxyacetone phosphate concentration ratios in rat heart and rat diaphragm muscles. *Biochem J.* 1964;93:665-678.
122. Roden M, Price TB, Perseghin G, et al. Mechanism of free fatty acid-induced insulin resistance in humans. *J Clin Invest.* 1996;97:2859-2865.
123. Jucker BM, Rennings AJ, Cline GW, et al. ^{13}C and ^{31}P NMR studies on the effects of increased plasma free fatty acids on intramuscular glucose metabolism in the awake rat. *J Biol Chem.* 1997;272:10464-10473.
124. Adams SH. Uncoupling protein homologs: emerging views of physiological function. *J Nutr.* 2000;130:711-714.
125. Rothman DL, Magnusson I, Cline G, et al. Decreased muscle glucose transport/phosphorylation is an early defect in the pathogenesis of non-insulin-dependent diabetes mellitus. *Proc Natl Acad Sci U S A.* 1995;92:983-987.
126. Price TB, Parseghin G, Duleba A, et al. NMR studies of muscle glycogen synthesis in insulin-resistant offspring of parents with non-insulin-dependent diabetes mellitus immediately after glycogen-depleting exercise. *Proc Natl Acad Sci U S A.* 1996;93:5329-5334.

127. Itani SI, Pories WJ, Macdonald KG, et al. Increased protein kinase C theta in skeletal muscle of diabetic patients. *Metabolism.* 2001;50:553-557.
128. Griffin ME, Marcucci MJ, Cline GW, et al. Free fatty acid-induced insulin resistance is associated with activation of protein kinase C theta and alterations in the insulin signaling cascade. *Diabetes.* 1999;48:1270-1274.
129. Hundal RS, Petersen KF, Mayerson AB, et al. Mechanism by which high-dose aspirin improves glucose metabolism in type 2 diabetes. *J Clin Invest.* 2002;109:1321-1326.
130. Pan DA, Lillioja S, Kriketos AD, et al. Skeletal muscle triglyceride levels are inversely related to insulin action. *Diabetes.* 1997;46:983-988.
131. Goodpaster BH, Thaete FL, Simoneau JA, et al. Subcutaneous abdominal fat and thigh muscle composition predict insulin sensitivity independently of visceral fat. *Diabetes.* 1997;46:1579-1585.
132. Perseghin G, Scifo P, De Cobelli F, et al. Intramyocellular triglyceride content is a determinant of in vivo insulin resistance in humans: a ^{1}H-^{13}C nuclear magnetic resonance spectroscopy assessment in offspring of type 2 diabetic parents. *Diabetes.* 1999;48:1600-1606.
133. Boesch C, Slotboom J, Hoppeler H, et al. In vivo determination of intra-myocellular lipids in human muscle by means of localized ^{1}H-MR-spectroscopy. *Magn Reson Med.* 1997;37:484-493.
134. Carlson LA, Ekelund LG, Froberg SO. Concentration of triglycerides, phospholipids and glycogen in skeletal muscle and of free fatty acids and beta-hydroxybutyric acid in blood in man in response to exercise. *Eur J Clin Invest.* 1971;1:248-254.
135. Laws A, Reaven GM. Effect of physical activity on age-related glucose intolerance. *Clin Geriatr Med.* 1990;6:849-863.
136. Gollnick PD, Saltin B. Significance of skeletal muscle oxidative enzyme enhancement with endurance training. *Clin Physiol.* 1982;2:1-12.
137. Turcotte LP, Richter EA, Kiens B. Increased plasma FFA uptake and oxidation during prolonged exercise in trained vs. untrained humans. *Am J Physiol.* 1992;262:E791-E799.
138. Romijn JA, Klein S, Coyle EF, et al. Strenuous endurance training increases lipolysis and triglyceride-fatty acid cycling at rest. *J Appl Physiol.* 1993;75:108-113.
139. Phillips SM, Green HJ, Tamopolsky MA, et al. Effects of training duration on substrate turnover and oxidation during exercise. *J Appl Physiol.* 1996;81:2182-2191.
140. Schenk S, Horowitz JF. Acute exercise increases triglyceride synthesis in skeletal muscle and prevents fatty acid-induced insulin resistance. *J Clin Invest.* 2007;117:1690-1698.
141. Stremmel W, Strohmeyer G, Borchard F, et al. Isolation and partial characterization of a fatty acid binding protein in rat liver plasma membranes. *Proc Natl Acad Sci U S A.* 1985;82:4-8.
142. Abumrad NA, el-Maghrabi MR, Amri EZ, et al. Cloning of a rat adipocyte membrane protein implicated in binding or transport of long-chain fatty acids that is induced during preadipocyte differentiation: homology with human CD36. *J Biol Chem.* 1993;268: 17665-17668.
143. Stahl A, Gimeno RE, Tartaglia LA, et al. Fatty acid transport proteins: a current view of a growing family. *Trends Endocrinol Metab.* 2001;12:266-273.
144. Luiken JJ, Glatz JF, Bonen A. Fatty acid transport proteins facilitate fatty acid uptake in skeletal muscle. *Can J Appl Physiol.* 2000;25: 333-352.
145. Binnert C, Koistinen HA, Martin G, et al. Fatty acid transport protein-1 mRNA expression in skeletal muscle and in adipose tissue in humans. *Am J Physiol.* 2000;279:E1072-E1079.
146. Veerkamp JH. Fatty acid transport and fatty acid-binding proteins. *Proc Nutr Soc.* 1995;54:23-37.
147. Schaap FG, van der Vusse GJ, Glatz JF. Fatty acid-binding proteins in the heart. *Mol Cell Biochem.* 1998;180:43-51.
148. Van Nieuwenhoven FA, Verstijnen CP, Abumrad NA, et al. Putative membrane fatty acid translocase and cytoplasmic fatty acid-binding protein are co-expressed in rat heart and skeletal muscles. *Biochem Biophys Res Commun.* 1995;207:747-752.
149. Linssen MC, Vork MM, de Jong YF, et al. Fatty acid oxidation capacity and fatty acid-binding protein content of different cell types isolated from rat heart. *Mol Cell Biochem.* 1990;98:19-25.
150. Binas B, Danneberg H, McWhir J, et al. Requirement for the heart-type fatty acid binding protein in cardiac fatty acid utilization. *FASEB J.* 1999;13:805-812.
151. Hotamisligil GS, Johnson RS, Distel RJ, et al. Uncoupling of obesity from insulin resistance through a targeted mutation in aP2, the adipocyte fatty acid binding protein. *Science.* 1996;274:1377-1379.
152. Blaak EE, Wagenmakers AJ, Glatz JF, et al. Plasma FFA utilization and fatty acid-binding protein content are diminished in type 2 diabetic muscle. *Am J Physiol.* 2000;279:E146-E154.
153. Simoneau JA, Veerkamp JH, Turcotte LP, et al. Markers of capacity to utilize fatty acids in human skeletal muscle: relation to insulin resistance and obesity and effects of weight loss. *FASEB J.* 1999;13: 2051-2060.
154. McGarry JD. Glucose-fatty acid interactions in health and disease. *Am J Clin Nutr.* 1998;67(3 suppl):500S-504S.
155. McGarry JD. Malonyl-CoA and satiety? Food for thought. *Trends Endocrinol Metab.* 2000;11:399-400.
156. Zammit VA, Price NT, Fraser F, et al. Structure-function relationships of the liver and muscle isoforms of carnitine palmitoyltransferase I. *Biochem Soc Trans.* 2001;29:287-292.
157. Minnich A, Tian N, Byan L, et al. A potent PPARα agonist stimulates mitochondrial fatty acid beta-oxidation in liver and skeletal muscle. *Am J Physiol.* 2001;280:E270-E279.
158. Power GW, Newsholme EA. Dietary fatty acids influence the activity and metabolic control of mitochondrial carnitine palmitoyltransferase I in rat heart and skeletal muscle. *J Nutr.* 1997;127:2142-2150.
159. Hildebrandt AL, Neufer PD. Exercise attenuates the fasting-induced transcriptional activation of metabolic genes in skeletal muscle. *Am J Physiol.* 2000;278:E1078-E1086.
160. Kim JY, Hickner RC, Cartright RL, et al. Lipid oxidation is reduced in obese human skeletal muscle. *Am J Physiol.* 2000;279:E1039-E1044.
161. Eaton S, Bartlett K, Pourfarzam M. Mammalian mitochondrial beta-oxidation. *Biochem J.* 1996;320:345-357.
162. Nada MA, Rhead WJ, Sprecher H, et al. Evidence for intermediate channeling in mitochondrial beta-oxidation. *J Biol Chem.* 1995;270: 530-535.
163. Horowitz JF, Leone TC, Feng W, et al. Effect of endurance training on lipid metabolism in women: a potential role for PPARα in the metabolic response to training. *Am J Physiol.* 2000;279:E348-E355.
164. Porter RK. Mitochondrial proton leak: a role for uncoupling proteins 2 and 3? *Biochim Biophys Acta.* 2001;1504:120-127.
165. Bouillaud F, Couplan E, Pecqueur C, et al. Homologues of the uncoupling protein from brown adipose tissue (UCP1): UCP2, UCP3, BMCP1 and UCP4. *Biochim Biophys Acta.* 2001;1504:107-119.
166. Boss O, Muzzin P, Giacobino JP. The uncoupling proteins, a review. *Eur J Endocrinol.* 1998;139:1-9.
167. Schrauwen P, Hoppeler H, Billeter R, et al. Fiber type dependent upregulation of human skeletal muscle UCP2 and UCP3 mRNA expression by high-fat diet. *Int J Obes Relat Metab Disord.* 2001;25:449-456.
168. Tonkonogi M, Krook A, Walsh B, et al. Endurance training increases stimulation of uncoupling of skeletal muscle mitochondria in humans by non-esterified fatty acids: an uncoupling-protein-mediated effect? *Biochem J.* 2000;351:805-810.
169. Bao S, Kennedy A, Wojciechowski B, et al. Expression of mRNAs encoding uncoupling proteins in human skeletal muscle: effects of obesity and diabetes. *Diabetes.* 1998;47:1935-1940.
170. Schrauwen P, Xia J, Wakler K, et al. A novel polymorphism in the proximal UCP3 promoter region: effect on skeletal muscle UCP3 mRNA expression and obesity in male non-diabetic Pima Indians. *Int J Obes Relat Metab Disord.* 1999;23:1242-1245.
171. Schrauwen P, Hesselink MK. Oxidative capacity, lipotoxicity, and mitochondrial damage in type 2 diabetes. *Diabetes.* 2004;53:1412-1417.
172. Boirie Y. Insulin regulation of mitochondrial proteins and oxidative phosphorylation in human muscle. *Trends Endocrinol Metab.* 2003;14:393-394.
173. Pedersen BK, Steensberg A, Fischer C, et al. The metabolic role of IL-6 produced during exercise: is IL-6 an exercise factor? *Proc Nutr Soc.* 2004;63:263-267.
174. Puigserver P, Spiegelman BM. Peroxisome proliferator-activated receptor-γ coactivator 1α (PGC-1α): transcriptional coactivator and metabolic regulator. *Endocr Rev.* 2003;24:78-90.
175. Puigserver P, Wu Z, Park CW, et al. A cold-inducible coactivator of nuclear receptors linked to adaptive thermogenesis. *Cell.* 1998;92:829-839.
176. Mootha VK, Handschin C, Arow D, et al. Erralpha and Gabpa/b specify PGC-1α-dependent oxidative phosphorylation gene expression that is altered in diabetic muscle. *Proc Natl Acad Sci U S A.* 2004;101: 6570-6575.
177. Mootha VK, Lindgren CM, Eriksson KF, et al. PGC-1α-responsive genes involved in oxidative phosphorylation are coordinately downregulated in human diabetes. *Nat Genet.* 2003;34:267-273.
178. Patti ME, Butte AJ, Crunkhorn S, et al. Coordinated reduction of genes of oxidative metabolism in humans with insulin resistance and diabetes: potential role of PGC1 and NRF1. *Proc Natl Acad Sci U S A.* 2003;100:8466-8471.
179. Kelley DE, He J, Menshikova EV, et al. Dysfunction of mitochondria in human skeletal muscle in type 2 diabetes. *Diabetes.* 2002;51:2944-2950.
180. Wisløff U, Najjar SM, Ellingsen O, et al. Cardiovascular risk factors emerge after artificial selection for low aerobic capacity. *Science.* 2005;307:418-420.
181. Muoio DM. Intramuscular triacylglycerol and insulin resistance: guilty as charged or wrongly accused? *Biochim Biophys Acta.* 2010; 1801:281-288.
182. Levine JA, Lanningham-Foster LM, McCrady SK, et al. Interindividual variation in posture allocation: possible role in human obesity. *Science.* 2005;307:584-586.
183. Ruderman NB, Saha AK, Vavvas D, et al. Malonyl-CoA, fuel sensing, and insulin resistance. *Am J Physiol.* 1999;276:E1-E18.

184. McGarry JD. Malonyl-CoA and carnitine palmitoyltransferase I: an expanding partnership. *Biochem Soc Trans*. 1995;23:481-485.
185. Swanson ST, Foster DW, McGarry JD, et al. Roles of the N- and C-terminal domains of carnitine palmitoyltransferase I isoforms in malonyl-CoA sensitivity of the enzymes: insights from expression of chimaeric proteins and mutation of conserved histidine residues. *Biochem J*. 1998;335:513-519.
186. Kelley DE, Simoneau JA. Impaired free fatty acid utilization by skeletal muscle in non-insulin-dependent diabetes mellitus. *J Clin Invest*. 1994;94:2349-2356.
187. Kelley DE, Mandarino LJ. Hyperglycemia normalizes insulin-stimulated skeletal muscle glucose oxidation and storage in noninsulin-dependent diabetes mellitus. *J Clin Invest*. 1990;86:1999-2007.
188. Bavenholm PN, Pigon J, Saha AK, et al. Fatty acid oxidation and the regulation of malonyl-CoA in human muscle. *Diabetes*. 2000;49:1078-1083.
189. Jamil H, Madsen NB. Phosphorylation state of acetyl-coenzyme A carboxylase: I. Linear inverse relationship to activity ratios at different citrate concentrations. *J Biol Chem*. 1987;262:630-637.
190. Jamil H, Madsen NB. Phosphorylation state of acetyl-coenzyme A carboxylase: II. Variation with nutritional condition. *J Biol Chem*. 1987;262:638-642.
191. Winder WW, Wilson HA, Hardie DG, et al. Phosphorylation of rat muscle acetyl-CoA carboxylase by AMP-activated protein kinase and protein kinase A. *J Appl Physiol*. 1997;82:219-225.
192. Dean D, Daugaard JR, Young ME, et al. Exercise diminishes the activity of acetyl-CoA carboxylase in human muscle. *Diabetes*. 2000;49:1295-1300.
193. Olefsky JM, Revers RR, Prince M, et al. Insulin resistance in non-insulin dependent (type II) and insulin dependent (type I) diabetes mellitus. *Adv Exp Med Biol*. 1985;189:176-205.
194. Del Prato S, Leonetti F, Simonson DC, et al. Effect of sustained physiologic hyperinsulinaemia and hyperglycaemia on insulin secretion and insulin sensitivity in man. *Diabetologia*. 1994;37:1025-1035.
195. Ratzmann KP, Ruhnke R, Kohnert KD. Effect of pharmacological suppression of insulin secretion on tissue sensitivity to insulin in subjects with moderate obesity. *Int J Obes*. 1983;7:453-458.
196. Alemzadeh R, Langley G, Upchurch L, et al. Beneficial effect of diazoxide in obese hyperinsulinemic adults. *J Clin Endocrinol Metab*. 1998;83:1911-1915.
197. White MF, Kahn CR. The insulin signaling system. *J Biol Chem*. 1994;269:1-4.
198. Ward CW, Gough KH, Rashke M, et al. Systematic mapping of potential binding sites for Shc and Grb2 SH2 domains on insulin receptor substrate-1 and the receptors for insulin, epidermal growth factor, platelet-derived growth factor, and fibroblast growth factor. *J Biol Chem*. 1996;271:5603-5609.
199. Pessin JE, Saltiel AR. Signaling pathways in insulin action: molecular targets of insulin resistance. *J Clin Invest*. 2000;106:165-169.
200. McClain DA, Maegawa H, Thies RS, et al. Dissection of the growth versus metabolic effects of insulin and insulin-like growth factor-I in transfected cells expressing kinase-defective human insulin receptors. *J Biol Chem*. 1990;265:1678-1682.
201. McClain DA. Mechanism and role of insulin receptor endocytosis. *Am J Med Sci*. 1992;304:192-201.
202. Formisano P, Beguinot F. The role of protein kinase C isoforms in insulin action. *J Endocrinol Invest*. 2001;24:460-467.
203. Itani SI, Zhou Q, Pories WJ, et al. Involvement of protein kinase C in human skeletal muscle insulin resistance and obesity. *Diabetes*. 2000;49:1353-1358.
204. Peraldi P, Xu M, Spiegelman BM. Thiazolidinediones block tumor necrosis factor-α-induced inhibition of insulin signaling. *J Clin Invest*. 1997;100:1863-1869.
205. Goldstein BJ, Ahmad F, Ding W, et al. Regulation of the insulin signalling pathway by cellular protein-tyrosine phosphatases. *Mol Cell Biochem*. 1998;182:91-99.
206. Drake PG, Bevan AP, Burgess JW, et al. A role for tyrosine phosphorylation in both activation and inhibition of the insulin receptor tyrosine kinase in vivo. *Endocrinology*. 1996;137:4960-4968.
207. Elchebly M, Payette P, Michaliszyn E, et al. Increased insulin sensitivity and obesity resistance in mice lacking the protein tyrosine phosphatase-1B gene. *Science*. 1999;283:1544-1548.
208. Krook A, O'Rahilly S. Mutant insulin receptors in syndromes of insulin resistance. *Baillieres Clin Endocrinol Metab*. 1996;10:97-122.
209. Taylor SI, Arioglu E. Syndromes associated with insulin resistance and acanthosis nigricans. *J Basic Clin Physiol Pharmacol*. 1998;9:419-439.
210. White MF. The IRS-signaling system: a network of docking proteins that mediate insulin and cytokine action. *Recent Prog Horm Res*. 1998;53:119-138.
211. Previs SF, Withers DJ, Ren JM, et al. Contrasting effects of IRS-1 versus IRS-2 gene disruption on carbohydrate and lipid metabolism in vivo. *J Biol Chem*. 2000;275:38990-38994.
212. White MF. IRS proteins and the common path to diabetes. *Am J Physiol Endocrinol Metab*. 2002;283:E413-E422.
213. Czech MP, Corvera S. Signaling mechanisms that regulate glucose transport. *J Biol Chem*. 1999;274:1865-1868.
214. Kido Y, Nakae J, Accili D. Clinical review 125: the insulin receptor and its cellular targets. *J Clin Endocrinol Metab*. 2001;86:972-979.
215. Kohn AD, Barthel A, Kovacina KS, et al. Construction and characterization of a conditionally active version of the serine/threonine kinase Akt. *J Biol Chem*. 1998;273:11937-11943.
216. Sarbassov DD, Guertin DA, Ali SM, et al. Phosphorylation and regulation of Akt/PKB by the rictor-mTOR complex. *Science*. 2005;307:1098-1101.
217. Cho H, Mu J, Kim JK, et al. Insulin resistance and a diabetes mellitus-like syndrome in mice lacking the protein kinase Akt2 (PKB beta). *Science*. 2001;292:1728-1731.
218. Zierath JR, Krook A, Wallberg-Henriksson H. Insulin action in skeletal muscle from patients with NIDDM. *Mol Cell Biochem*. 1998;182:153-160.
219. Krook A, Roth RA, Jiang XJ, et al. Insulin-stimulated Akt kinase activity is reduced in skeletal muscle from NIDDM subjects. *Diabetes*. 1998;47:1281-1286.
220. Kim YB, Nikoulina SE, Ciaraldi TP, et al. Normal insulin-dependent activation of Akt/protein kinase B, with diminished activation of phosphoinositide 3-kinase, in muscle in type 2 diabetes. *J Clin Invest*. 1999;104:733-741.
221. Zorzano A, Sevilla L, Tomas E, et al. Trafficking pathway of GLUT4 glucose transporters in muscle. *Int J Mol Med*. 1998;2:263-271.
222. Sakamoto K, Holman GD. Emerging role for AS160/TBC1D4 and TBC1D1 in the regulation of GLUT4 traffic. *Am J Physiol Endocrinol Metab*. 2008;295:E29-E37.
223. Davidson MB. Role of glucose transport and GLUT4 transporter protein in type 2 diabetes mellitus. *J Clin Endocrinol Metab*. 1993;77:25-26.
224. Garvey WT, Maianu L, Zhu JH, et al. Multiple defects in the adipocyte glucose transport system cause cellular insulin resistance in gestational diabetes: heterogeneity in the number and a novel abnormality in subcellular localization of GLUT4 glucose transporters. *Diabetes*. 1993;42:1773-1785.
225. Kennedy JW, Hirshman MF, Gervino EV, et al. Acute exercise induces GLUT4 translocation in skeletal muscle of normal human subjects and subjects with type 2 diabetes. *Diabetes*. 1999;48:1192-1197.
226. Bernal-Mizrachi C, Weng S, Feng C, et al. Dexamethasone induction of hypertension and diabetes is PPARα-dependent in LDL receptor-null mice. *Nat Med*. 2003;9:1069-1075.
227. Gumbiner B, Mucha JF, Lindstrom JE, et al. Differential effects of acute hypertriglyceridemia on insulin action and insulin receptor autophosphorylation. *Am J Physiol*. 1996;270:E424-E429.
228. Saad MJ, Araki E, Miralpeix M, et al. Regulation of insulin receptor substrate-1 in liver and muscle of animal models of insulin resistance. *J Clin Invest*. 1992;90:1839-1849.
229. Zierath JR, Houseknecht KL, Gnudi L, et al. High-fat feeding impairs insulin-stimulated GLUT4 recruitment via an early insulin-signaling defect. *Diabetes*. 1997;46:215-223.
230. Anai M, Funaki M, Ogihara T, et al. Altered expression levels and impaired steps in the pathway to phosphatidylinositol 3-kinase activation via insulin receptor substrates 1 and 2 in Zucker fatty rats. *Diabetes*. 1998;47:13-23.
231. Krook A, Kawano Y, Song XM, et al. Improved glucose tolerance restores insulin-stimulated Akt kinase activity and glucose transport in skeletal muscle from diabetic Goto-Kakizaki rats. *Diabetes*. 1997;46:2110-2114.
232. Hotamisligil GS, Spiegelman BM. Tumor necrosis factor alpha: a key component of the obesity-diabetes link. *Diabetes*. 1994;43:1271-1278.
233. Miles PD, Romeo OM, Higo K, et al. TNF-α-induced insulin resistance in vivo and its prevention by troglitazone. *Diabetes*. 1997;46:1678-1683.
234. Hotamisligil GS, Peraldi P, Budavari A, et al. IRS-1-mediated inhibition of insulin receptor tyrosine kinase activity in TNF-α- and obesity-induced insulin resistance. *Science*. 1996;271:665-668.
235. Uysal KT, Wiesbrock SM, Marino MW, et al. Protection from obesity-induced insulin resistance in mice lacking TNF-α function. *Nature*. 1997;389:610-614.
236. The Diabetes Control and Complications Trial Research Group. The effect of intensive treatment of diabetes on the development and progression of long-term complications in insulin-dependent diabetes mellitus. *N Engl J Med*. 1993;329:977-986.
237. Turner RC. The U.K. Prospective Diabetes Study: a review. *Diabetes Care*. 1998;21(suppl 3):C35-C38.
238. Sakul H, Pratley R, Cardon L, et al. Familiality of physical and metabolic characteristics that predict the development of non-insulin-dependent diabetes mellitus in Pima Indians. *Am J Hum Genet*. 1997;60:651-656.
239. Yki-Jarvinen H, Sahlin K, Ren JM, et al. Localization of rate-limiting defect for glucose disposal in skeletal muscle of insulin-resistant type I diabetic patients. *Diabetes*. 1990;39:157-167.

240. Kornfeld R. Studies on L-glutamine D-fructose 6-phosphate amidotransferase: I. Feedback inhibition by uridine diphosphate-N-acetylglucosamine. *J Biol Chem.* 1967;242:3135-3141.
241. Buse MG. Hexosamines, insulin resistance, and the complications of diabetes: current status. *Am J Physiol Endocrinol Metab.* 2006;290:E1-E8.
242. Marshall S, Bacote V, Traxinger RR. Discovery of a metabolic pathway mediating glucose-induced desensitization of the glucose transport system: role of hexosamine biosynthesis in the induction of insulin resistance. *J Biol Chem.* 1991;266:4706-4712.
243. Robinson KA, Weinstein ML, Lindenmayer GE, et al. Effects of diabetes and hyperglycemia on the hexosamine synthesis pathway in rat muscle and liver. *Diabetes.* 1995;44:1438-1446.
244. Hebert Jr LF, Daniels MC, Zhou J, et al. Overexpression of glutamine: fructose-6-phosphate amidotransferase in transgenic mice leads to insulin resistance. *J Clin Invest.* 1996;98:930-936.
245. Baron AD, Zhu JS, Zhu JH, et al. Glucosamine induces insulin resistance in vivo by affecting GLUT 4 translocation in skeletal muscle: implications for glucose toxicity. *J Clin Invest.* 1995;96:2792-2801.
246. Mallon PW, Cooper DA, Carr A. HIV-associated lipodystrophy. *HIV Med.* 2001;2:166-173.
247. Shevitz A, Wanke CA, Falutz J, et al. Clinical perspectives on HIV-associated lipodystrophy syndrome: an update. *AIDS.* 2001;15:1917-1930.
248. Purnell JQ, Zambon A, Knopp RH, et al. Effect of ritonavir on lipids and post-heparin lipase activities in normal subjects. *AIDS.* 2000;14:51-57.
249. Noor MA, Lo JC, Mulligan K, et al. Metabolic effects of indinavir in healthy HIV-seronegative men. *AIDS.* 2001;15:F11-F18.
250. Murata H, Hruz PW, Mueckler M. The mechanism of insulin resistance caused by HIV protease inhibitor therapy. *J Biol Chem.* 2000;275:20251-20254.
251. Shikuma CM, Hu N, Milne C, et al. Mitochondrial DNA decrease in subcutaneous adipose tissue of HIV-infected individuals with peripheral lipoatrophy. *AIDS.* 2001;15:1801-1809.
252. Caron M, Auclair M, Vigouroux C, et al. The HIV protease inhibitor indinavir impairs sterol regulatory element-binding protein-1 intranuclear localization, inhibits preadipocyte differentiation, and induces insulin resistance. *Diabetes.* 2001;50:1378-1388.
253. Dowell P, Flexner C, Kwiterovich PO, et al. Suppression of preadipocyte differentiation and promotion of adipocyte death by HIV protease inhibitors. *J Biol Chem.* 2000;275:41325-41332.
254. Carr A, Samaras K, Chisholm DJ, et al. Pathogenesis of HIV-1-protease inhibitor-associated peripheral lipodystrophy, hyperlipidaemia, and insulin resistance. *Lancet.* 1998;351:1881-1883.
255. Nolan D, Hammond E, Martin A, et al. Mitochondrial DNA depletion and morphologic changes in adipocytes associated with nucleoside reverse transcriptase inhibitor therapy. *AIDS.* 2003;17:1329-1338.
256. Milinkovic A, Martinez E. Current perspectives on HIV-associated lipodystrophy syndrome. *J Antimicrob Chemother.* 2005;56:6-9.
257. Grinspoon SK. Metabolic syndrome and cardiovascular disease in patients with human immunodeficiency virus. *Am J Med.* 2005;118(suppl 2):23S-28S.
258. Mauss S. HIV-associated and antiretroviral-induced hyperlipidaemia: an update. *J HIV Ther.* 2003;8:29-31.
259. Chuck SK, Penzak SR. Risk-benefit of HMG-CoA reductase inhibitors in the treatment of HIV protease inhibitor-related hyperlipidaemia. *Expert Opin Drug Saf.* 2002;1:5-17.
260. Knowler WC, Barrett-Connor E, Fowler SE, et al. Reduction in the incidence of type 2 diabetes with lifestyle intervention or metformin. *N Engl J Med.* 2002;346:393-403.
261. Kelley DE, Mandarino LJ. Fuel selection in human skeletal muscle in insulin resistance: a reexamination. *Diabetes.* 2000;49:677-683.
262. Long SD, O'Brien K, MacDonald Jr KG, et al. Weight loss in severely obese subjects prevents the progression of impaired glucose tolerance to type II diabetes: a longitudinal interventional study. *Diabetes Care.* 1994;17:372-375.
263. Wing RR, Venditti E, Jakicic JM, et al. Lifestyle intervention in overweight individuals with a family history of diabetes. *Diabetes Care.* 1998;21:350-359.
264. Nesher R, Karl IE, Kipnis DM. Dissociation of effects of insulin and contraction on glucose transport in rat epitrochlearis muscle. *Am J Physiol.* 1985;249:C226-C232.
265. Wallberg-Henriksson H, Holloszy JO. Activation of glucose transport in diabetic muscle: responses to contraction and insulin. *Am J Physiol.* 1985;249:C233-C237.
266. Wallberg-Henriksson H, Constable SH, Young DA, et al. Glucose transport into rat skeletal muscle: interaction between exercise and insulin. *J Appl Physiol.* 1988;65:909-913.
267. Young DA, Wallberg-Henriksson H, Sleeper MD, et al. Reversal of the exercise-induced increase in muscle permeability to glucose. *Am J Physiol.* 1987;253:E331-E335.
268. Douen AG, Ramlal T, Rastogi S, et al. Exercise induces recruitment of the "insulin-responsive glucose transporter": evidence for distinct intracellular insulin- and exercise-recruitable transporter pools in skeletal muscle. *J Biol Chem.* 1990;265:13427-13430.
269. Goodyear LJ, Hirshman MF, King PA, et al. Skeletal muscle plasma membrane glucose transport and glucose transporters after exercise. *J Appl Physiol.* 1990;68:193-198.
270. Goodyear LJ, Giorgino F, Balon TW, et al. Effects of contractile activity on tyrosine phosphoproteins and PI3-kinase activity in rat skeletal muscle. *Am J Physiol.* 1995;268:E987-E995.
271. Lund S, Holman GD, Schmitz O, et al. Contraction stimulates translocation of glucose transporter GLUT4 in skeletal muscle through a mechanism distinct from that of insulin. *Proc Natl Acad Sci U S A.* 1995;92:5817-5821.
272. Zorzano A, Balon TW, Goodman MN, et al. Additive effects of prior exercise and insulin on glucose and AIB uptake by rat muscle. *Am J Physiol.* 1986;251:E21-E26.
273. Henriksen EJ, Bourey RE, Rodnick KJ, et al. Glucose transporter protein content and glucose transport capacity in rat skeletal muscles. *Am J Physiol.* 1990;259:E593-E598.
274. Gao J, Ren J, Gulve EA, et al. Additive effect of contractions and insulin on GLUT-4 translocation into the sarcolemma. *J Appl Physiol.* 1994;77:1597-1601.
275. Lee AD, Hansen PA, Holloszy JO. Wortmannin inhibits insulin-stimulated but not contraction-stimulated glucose transport activity in skeletal muscle. *FEBS Lett.* 1995;361:51-54.
276. Yeh JI, Gulve EA, Rameh L, et al. The effects of wortmannin on rat skeletal muscle: dissociation of signaling pathways for insulin- and contraction-activated hexose transport. *J Biol Chem.* 1995;270:2107-2111.
277. Treadway JL, James DE, Burcel E, et al. Effect of exercise on insulin receptor binding and kinase activity in skeletal muscle. *Am J Physiol.* 1989;256:E138-E144.
278. Brozinick JT Jr, Etgen GJ Jr, Yaspelkis BB 3rd, et al. Contraction-activated glucose uptake is normal in insulin-resistant muscle of the obese Zucker rat. *J Appl Physiol.* 1992;73:382-387.
279. Azevedo JL Jr, Carey JO, Pories WJ, et al. Hypoxia stimulates glucose transport in insulin-resistant human skeletal muscle. *Diabetes.* 1995;44:695-698.
280. Winder WW, Hardie DG. AMP-activated protein kinase, a metabolic master switch: possible roles in type 2 diabetes. *Am J Physiol.* 1999;277:E1-E10.
281. Hayashi T, Hirshman MF, Kurth EJ, et al. Evidence for 5′ AMP-activated protein kinase mediation of the effect of muscle contraction on glucose transport. *Diabetes.* 1998;47:1369-1373.
282. Merrill GF, Kurth EJ, Hardie DG, et al. AICA riboside increases AMP-activated protein kinase, fatty acid oxidation, and glucose uptake in rat muscle. *Am J Physiol.* 1997;273:E1107-E1112.
283. Bergeron R, Russell RR 3rd, Young LH, et al. Effect of AMPK activation on muscle glucose metabolism in conscious rats. *Am J Physiol.* 1999;276:E938-E944.
283a. Bergeron R, Previs SF, Cline GW, et al. Effect of 5-aminoimidazole-4-carboxamide-1-beta-D-ribofuranoside infusion on invivo glucose and lipid metabolism in lean and obese Zucker rats. *Diabetes.* 2001 May;50(5):1076-1082.
284. Richter EA, Garetto LP, Goodman MN, et al. Muscle glucose metabolism following exercise in the rat: increased sensitivity to insulin. *J Clin Invest.* 1982;69:785-793.
285. Garetto LP, Richter EA, Goodman MN, et al. Enhanced muscle glucose metabolism after exercise in the rat: the two phases. *Am J Physiol.* 1984;246:E471-E475.
286. Cartee GD, Young DA, Sleeper MD, et al. Prolonged increase in insulin-stimulated glucose transport in muscle after exercise. *Am J Physiol.* 1989;256:E494-E499.
287. Richter EA, Young DA, Sleeper MD, et al. Effect of exercise on insulin action in human skeletal muscle. *J Appl Physiol.* 1989;66:876-885.
288. Hansen PA, Nolte LA, Chen MM, et al. Increased GLUT-4 translocation mediates enhanced insulin sensitivity of muscle glucose transport after exercise. *J Appl Physiol.* 1998;85:1218-1222.
289. Thorell A, Hirshman MF, Nygren J, et al. Exercise and insulin cause GLUT-4 translocation in human skeletal muscle. *Am J Physiol.* 1999;277:E733-E741.
290. Zorzano A, Balon TW, Garetto LP, et al. Muscle α-aminoisobutyric acid transport after exercise: enhanced stimulation by insulin. *Am J Physiol.* 1985;248:E546-E552.
291. Wojtaszewski JF, Hansen BF, Kiens B, et al. Insulin signaling in human skeletal muscle: time course and effect of exercise. *Diabetes.* 1997;46:1775-1781.
292. Oshida Y, Yamanouchi K, Hayamizu S, et al. Long-term mild jogging increases insulin action despite no influence on body mass index or VO_2 max. *J Appl Physiol.* 1989;66:2206-2210.
293. DeFronzo RA, Sherwin RS, Kraemer N. Effect of physical training on insulin action in obesity. *Diabetes.* 1987;36:1379-1385.
294. Helmrich SP, Rayland DR, Leung RW, et al. Physical activity and reduced occurrence of non-insulin-dependent diabetes mellitus. *N Engl J Med.* 1991;325:147-152.

295. Perseghin G, Price TB, Petersen KF, et al. Increased glucose transport-phosphorylation and muscle glycogen synthesis after exercise training in insulin-resistant subjects. *N Engl J Med.* 1996;335:1357-1362.
296. Ebeling P, Bourey R, Koranyi L, et al. Mechanism of enhanced insulin sensitivity in athletes: increased blood flow, muscle glucose transport protein (GLUT-4) concentration, and glycogen synthase activity. *J Clin Invest.* 1993;92:1623-1631.
297. Houmard JA, Egan PC, Neufer PD, et al. Elevated skeletal muscle glucose transporter levels in exercise-trained middle-aged men. *Am J Physiol.* 1991;261:E437-E443.
298. Hood DA. Invited review: contractile activity-induced mitochondrial biogenesis in skeletal muscle. *J Appl Physiol.* 2001;90:1137-1157.
299. Lin J, Wu H, Tarr PT, et al. Transcriptional co-activator PGC-1 alpha drives the formation of slow-twitch muscle fibres. *Nature.* 2002;418:797-801.
300. Handschin C, Rhee J, Lin J, et al. An autoregulatory loop controls peroxisome proliferator-activated receptor γ coactivator 1α expression in muscle. *Proc Natl Acad Sci U S A.* 2003;100:7111-7116.
301. Michael LF, Wu Z, Cheatham RB, et al. Restoration of insulin-sensitive glucose transporter (GLUT4) gene expression in muscle cells by the transcriptional coactivator PGC-1. *Proc Natl Acad Sci U S A.* 2001;98:3820-3825.
302. Nisoli E, Tonello C, Cardile A, et al. Calorie restriction promotes mitochondrial biogenesis by inducing the expression of eNOS. *Science.* 2005;310:314-317.
303. Wu H, Kanatous SB, Thurmond FA, et al. Regulation of mitochondrial biogenesis in skeletal muscle by CaMK. *Science.* 2002;296:349-352.
304. Puigserver P, Rhee J, Lin J, et al. Cytokine stimulation of energy expenditure through p38 MAP kinase activation of PPARγ coactivator-1. *Mol Cell.* 2001;8:971-982.
305. Cao W, Medvedev AV, Daniel KW, et al. β-Adrenergic activation of p38 MAP kinase in adipocytes: cAMP induction of the uncoupling protein 1 (UCP1) gene requires p38 MAP kinase. *J Biol Chem.* 2001;276:27077-27082.
306. Terada S, Tabata I. Effects of acute bouts of running and swimming exercise on PGC-1α protein expression in rat epitrochlearis and soleus muscle. *Am J Physiol Endocrinol Metab.* 2004;286:E208-E216.
307. Terada S, Goto M, Kato M, et al. Effects of low-intensity prolonged exercise on PGC-1 mRNA expression in rat epitrochlearis muscle. *Biochem Biophys Res Commun.* 2002;296:350-354.
308. Zong H, Ren JM, Young LH, et al. AMP kinase is required for mitochondrial biogenesis in skeletal muscle in response to chronic energy deprivation. *Proc Natl Acad Sci U S A.* 2002;99:15983-15987.
309. Stamler J, Vaccaro O, Neaton JD, et al. Diabetes, other risk factors, and 12-yr cardiovascular mortality for men screened in the Multiple Risk Factor Intervention Trial. *Diabetes Care.* 1993;16:434-444.
310. Haffner SM, Lehto S, Ronnemaa T, et al. Mortality from coronary heart disease in subjects with type 2 diabetes and in nondiabetic subjects with and without prior myocardial infarction. *N Engl J Med.* 1998;339:229-234.
311. Fontbonne AM, Eschwege EM. Insulin and cardiovascular disease. Paris Prospective Study. *Diabetes Care.* 1991;14:461-469.
312. Willeit J, Kiechl S, Egger G, et al. The role of insulin in age-related sex differences of cardiovascular risk profile and morbidity. *Atherosclerosis.* 1997;130:183-189.
313. Hu FB, Stampfer MJ, Soloman CG, et al. The impact of diabetes mellitus on mortality from all causes and coronary heart disease in women: 20 years of follow-up. *Arch Intern Med.* 2001;161:1717-1723.
314. Reaven GM. Role of insulin resistance in human disease. Banting Lecture 1988. *Nutrition.* 1997;13:65; discussion 64, 66.
315. Reaven GM. Role of insulin resistance in human disease (syndrome X): an expanded definition. *Annu Rev Med.* 1993;44:121-131.
316. Kahn R, Buse J, Ferrannini E, et al. The metabolic syndrome: time for a critical appraisal: Joint Statement from the American Diabetes Association and the European Association for the Study of Diabetes. *Diabetes Care.* 2005;28:2289-2304.
317. Siegel RD, Cupples A, Schaefer EJ, et al. Wilson PW. Lipoproteins, apolipoproteins, and low-density lipoprotein size among diabetics in the Framingham offspring study. *Metabolism.* 1996;45:1267-1272.
318. Davidson NO, Shelness GS. Apolipoprotein B: mRNA editing, lipoprotein assembly, and presecretory degradation. *Annu Rev Nutr.* 2000;20:169-193.
319. Lewis GF, Steiner G. Acute effects of insulin in the control of VLDL production in humans: implications for the insulin-resistant state. *Diabetes Care.* 1996;19:390-393.
320. Riches FM, Watts GF, Naoumova RP, et al. Hepatic secretion of very-low-density lipoprotein apolipoprotein B-100 studied with a stable isotope technique in men with visceral obesity. *Int J Obes Relat Metab Disord.* 1998;22:414-423.
321. Wang SL, Du EZ, Martin TD, et al. Coordinate regulation of lipogenesis, the assembly and secretion of apolipoprotein B-containing lipoproteins by sterol response element binding protein 1. *J Biol Chem.* 1997;272:19351-19358.
322. Moberly JB, Cole TG, Alpers DH, Schonfeld G. Oleic acid stimulation of apolipoprotein B secretion from HepG2 and Caco-2 cells occurs post-transcriptionally. *Biochim Biophys Acta.* 1990;1042:70-80.
323. Ellsworth JL, Erickson SK, Cooper AD. Very low and low density lipoprotein synthesis and secretion by the human hepatoma cell line Hep-G2: effects of free fatty acid. *J Lipid Res.* 1986;27:858-874.
324. Kobatake T, Matsuzawa Y, Tokunaga K, et al. Metabolic improvements associated with a reduction of abdominal visceral fat caused by a new α-glucosidase inhibitor, AO-128, in Zucker fatty rats. *Int J Obes.* 1989;13:147-154.
325. Matsuzawa Y, Shimomura I, Nakamura T, et al. Pathophysiology and pathogenesis of visceral fat obesity. *Diabetes Res Clin Pract.* 1994;24(suppl):S111-S116.
326. Nguyen TT, Mijares AH, Johnson CM, et al. Postprandial leg and splanchnic fatty acid metabolism in nonobese men and women. *Am J Physiol.* 1996;271:E965-E972.
327. Gordon DA, Jamil H, Sharp D, et al. Secretion of apolipoprotein B-containing lipoproteins from HeLa cells is dependent on expression of the microsomal triglyceride transfer protein and is regulated by lipid availability. *Proc Natl Acad Sci U S A.* 1994;91:7628-7632.
328. Gordon DA, Jamil H. Progress towards understanding the role of microsomal triglyceride transfer protein in apolipoprotein-B lipoprotein assembly. *Biochim Biophys Acta.* 2000;1486:72-83.
329. Liao W, Kobayashi K, Chan L. Adenovirus-mediated overexpression of microsomal triglyceride transfer protein (MTP): mechanistic studies on the role of MTP in apolipoprotein B-100 biogenesis. *Biochemistry.* 1999;38:7532-7544.
330. Horowitz BS, Goldberg IJ, Merab J, et al. Increased plasma and renal clearance of an exchangeable pool of apolipoprotein A-I in subjects with low levels of high density lipoprotein cholesterol. *J Clin Invest.* 1993;91:1743-1752.
331. Lemieux I, Couillard C, Pascot A, et al. The small, dense LDL phenotype as a correlate of postprandial lipemia in men. *Atherosclerosis.* 2000;153:423-432.
332. Tan KC, Cooper MB, Ling KL, et al. Fasting and postprandial determinants for the occurrence of small dense LDL species in non-insulin-dependent diabetic patients with and without hypertriglyceridaemia: the involvement of insulin, insulin precursor species and insulin resistance. *Atherosclerosis.* 1995;113:273-287.
333. Austin MA, Selby JV. LDL subclass phenotypes and the risk factors of the insulin resistance syndrome. *Int J Obes Relat Metab Disord.* 1995;19(suppl 1):S22-S26.
334. Stewart MW, Laker MF, Dyer RG, et al. Lipoprotein compositional abnormalities and insulin resistance in type II diabetic patients with mild hyperlipidemia. *Arterioscler Thromb.* 1993;13:1046-1052.
335. Alexander JK. Obesity and coronary heart disease. *Am J Med Sci.* 2001;321:215-224.
336. Laakso M, Edelman SV, Brechtel G, et al. Impaired insulin-mediated skeletal muscle blood flow in patients with NIDDM. *Diabetes.* 1992;41:1076-1083.
337. Steinberg HO, Brechtel G, Johnson A, et al. Insulin-mediated skeletal muscle vasodilation is nitric oxide dependent: a novel action of insulin to increase nitric oxide release. *J Clin Invest.* 1994;94:1172-1179.
338. Baron AD, Zhu JS, Marshall S, et al. Insulin resistance after hypertension induced by the nitric oxide synthesis inhibitor L-NMMA in rats. *Am J Physiol.* 1995;269:E709-E715.
339. Steinberg HO, Paradisi G, Hook G, et al. Free fatty acid elevation impairs insulin-mediated vasodilation and nitric oxide production. *Diabetes.* 2000;49:1231-1238.
340. Landsberg L. Insulin resistance, energy balance and sympathetic nervous system activity. *Clin Exp Hypertens A.* 1990;12:817-830.
341. Weidmann P, de Courten M, Bohlen L. Insulin resistance, hyperinsulinemia and hypertension. *J Hypertens Suppl.* 1993;11(suppl 5):S27-S38.
342. Masuo K, Mikami H, Itoh M, et al. Sympathetic activity and body mass index contribute to blood pressure levels. *Hypertens Res.* 2000;23:303-310.
343. DeFronzo RA. Insulin and renal sodium handling: clinical implications. *Int J Obes.* 1981;5(suppl 1):93-104.
344. DeFronzo RA, Goldberg M, Agus ZS. The effects of glucose and insulin on renal electrolyte transport. *J Clin Invest.* 1976;58:83-90.
345. DeFronzo RA, Cooke CR, Andres R, et al. The effect of insulin on renal handling of sodium, potassium, calcium, and phosphate in man. *J Clin Invest.* 1975;55:845-855.
346. Welborn TA, Breckenridge A, Rubinstein AH, et al. Serum-insulin in essential hypertension and in peripheral vascular disease. *Lancet.* 1966;1:1336-1337.
347. Gress TW, Nieto FJ, Shahar E, et al. Hypertension and antihypertensive therapy as risk factors for type 2 diabetes mellitus. Atherosclerosis Risk in Communities Study. *N Engl J Med.* 2000;342:905-912.
348. Yusuf S, Sleight P, Pogue J, et al. Effects of an angiotensin-converting-enzyme inhibitor, ramipril, on cardiovascular events in high-risk patients. The Heart Outcomes Prevention Evaluation Study Investigators. *N Engl J Med.* 2000;342:145-153.

349. Sebestjen M, Zegura B, Guzic-Salobir B, et al. Fibrinolytic parameters and insulin resistance in young survivors of myocardial infarction with heterozygous familial hypercholesterolemia. *Wien Klin Wochenschr.* 2001;113:113-118.
350. Juhan-Vague I, Alessi MC, Morange PE. Hypofibrinolysis and increased PAI-1 are linked to atherothrombosis via insulin resistance and obesity. *Ann Med.* 2000;32(suppl 1):78-84.
351. Fujii S, Goto D, Zaman T, et al. Diminished fibrinolysis and thrombosis: clinical implications for accelerated atherosclerosis. *J Atheroscler Thromb.* 1998;5:76-81.
352. Sobel BE. The potential influence of insulin and plasminogen activator inhibitor type 1 on the formation of vulnerable atherosclerotic plaques associated with type 2 diabetes. *Proc Assoc Am Physicians.* 1999; 111:313-318.
353. Festa A, D'Agostino R Jr, Mykkanan L, et al. Relative contribution of insulin and its precursors to fibrinogen and PAI-1 in a large population with different states of glucose tolerance. The Insulin Resistance Atherosclerosis Study (IRAS). *Arterioscler Thromb Vasc Biol.* 1999; 19:562-568.
354. Lormeau B, Aurousseau MH, Valensi P, et al. Hyperinsulinemia and hypofibrinolysis: effects of short-term optimized glycemic control with continuous insulin infusion in type II diabetic patients. *Metabolism.* 1997;46:1074-1079.
355. Hamsten A, Eriksson P, Karpe F, et al. Relationships of thrombosis and fibrinolysis to atherosclerosis. *Curr Opin Lipidol.* 1994;5:382-389.
356. Grenett HE, Benza RL, Li XN, et al. Expression of plasminogen activator inhibitor type I in genotyped human endothelial cell cultures: genotype-specific regulation by insulin. *Thromb Haemost.* 1999;82: 1504-1509.
357. Chomiki N, Henry M, Alessi MC, et al. Plasminogen activator inhibitor-1 expression in human liver and healthy or atherosclerotic vessel walls. *Thromb Haemost.* 1994;72:44-53.
358. Koistinen HA, Dusserre E, Ebeling P, et al. Subcutaneous adipose tissue expression of plasminogen activator inhibitor-1 (PAI-1) in nondiabetic and type 2 diabetic subjects. *Diabetes Metab Res Rev.* 2000;16: 364-369.
359. Kruszynska YT, Yu JG, Olefsky JM, et al. Effects of troglitazone on blood concentrations of plasminogen activator inhibitor 1 in patients with type 2 diabetes and in lean and obese normal subjects. *Diabetes.* 2000;49:633-639.
360. Stunkard AJ. Current views on obesity. *Am J Med.* 1996;100:230-236.
361. Expert Panel on Detection, Evaluation and Treatment of High Blood Cholesterol in Adults. Executive Summary of the Third Report of the National Cholesterol Education Program (NCEP) Expert Panel on Detection, Evaluation and Treatment of High Blood Cholesterol in Adults (Adult Treatment Panel III). *JAMA.* 2001;285:2486-2497.
362. Gerich JE, Meyer C, Woerle HJ, et al. Renal gluconeogenesis: its importance in human glucose homeostasis. *Diabetes Care.* 2001; 24:382-391.
363. Meyer C, Stumvoll M, Nadkami V, et al. Abnormal renal and hepatic glucose metabolism in type 2 diabetes mellitus. *J Clin Invest.* 1998;102:619-624.
364. Rebrin K, Steil GM, Mittelman SD, et al. Causal linkage between insulin suppression of lipolysis and suppression of liver glucose output in dogs. *J Clin Invest.* 1996;98:741-749.
365. Mittelman SD, Fu YY, Rebrin K, et al. Indirect effect of insulin to suppress endogenous glucose production is dominant, even with hyperglucagonemia. *J Clin Invest.* 1997;100:3121-3130.
366. Rothman DL, Magnusson I, Katz LD, et al. Quantitation of hepatic glycogenolysis and gluconeogenesis in fasting humans with ^{13}C NMR. *Science.* 1991;254:573-576.
367. Petersen KF, Price T, Cline GW, et al. Contribution of net hepatic glycogenolysis to glucose production during the early postprandial period. *Am J Physiol.* 1996;270:E186-E191.
368. Nonogaki K. New insights into sympathetic regulation of glucose and fat metabolism. *Diabetologia.* 2000;43:533-549.
369. Moore MC, Connolly CC, Cherrington AD. Autoregulation of hepatic glucose production. *Eur J Endocrinol.* 1998;138:240-248.
370. Bavenholm PN, Pigon J, Ostenson CG, et al. Insulin sensitivity of suppression of endogenous glucose production is the single most important determinant of glucose tolerance. *Diabetes.* 2001;50:1449-1454.
371. Mitrakou A, Kelley D, Mokan M, et al. Role of reduced suppression of glucose production and diminished early insulin release in impaired glucose tolerance. *N Engl J Med.* 1992;326:22-29.
372. McCall RH, Wiesenthal SR, Shi ZQ, et al. Insulin acutely suppresses glucose production by both peripheral and hepatic effects in normal dogs. *Am J Physiol.* 1998;274:E346-E356.
373. Lewis GF, Vranic M, Giacca A. Glucagon enhances the direct suppressive effect of insulin on hepatic glucose production in humans. *Am J Physiol.* 1997;272:E371-E378.
374. Herzig S, Long F, Jhala US, et al. CREB regulates hepatic gluconeogenesis through the coactivator PGC-1. *Nature.* 2001;413:179-183.
375. Yoon JC, Puigserver P, Chen G, et al. Control of hepatic gluconeogenesis through the transcriptional coactivator PGC-1. *Nature.* 2001; 413:131-138.
376. Koo SH, Flechner L, Qi L, et al. The CREB coactivator TORC2 is a key regulator of fasting glucose metabolism. *Nature.* 2005;437: 1109-1111.
377. Reference deleted in proofs.
378. Cherrington AD, Edgerton D, Sindelar DK. The direct and indirect effects of insulin on hepatic glucose production in vivo. *Diabetologia.* 1998;41:987-996.
379. Chiasson JL, Liljenquist JE, Finger FE, et al. Differential sensitivity of glycogenolysis and gluconeogenesis to insulin infusions in dogs. *Diabetes.* 1976;25:283-291.
380. Rossetti L, Giaccari A, Barzilai N, et al. Mechanism by which hyperglycemia inhibits hepatic glucose production in conscious rats: implications for the pathophysiology of fasting hyperglycemia in diabetes. *J Clin Invest.* 1993;92:1126-1134.
381. Gasa R, Jansen PB, Berman HK, et al. Distinctive regulatory and metabolic properties of glycogen-targeting subunits of protein phosphatase-1 (PTG, GL, GM/RGl) expressed in hepatocytes. *J Biol Chem.* 2000;275:26396-26403.
382. Newgard CB, Brady MJ, O'Doherty RM, et al. Organizing glucose disposal: emerging roles of the glycogen targeting subunits of protein phosphatase-1. *Diabetes.* 2000;49:1967-1977.
383. Yeagley D, Guo S, Unterman T, et al. Gene- and activation-specific mechanisms for insulin inhibition of basal and glucocorticoid-induced insulin-like growth factor binding protein-1 and phosphoenolpyruvate carboxykinase transcription: roles of forkhead and insulin response sequences. *J Biol Chem.* 2001;276:33705-33710.
384. Jackson JG, Kreisberg JI, Koterba AP, et al. Phosphorylation and nuclear exclusion of the forkhead transcription factor FKHR after epidermal growth factor treatment in human breast cancer cells. *Oncogene.* 2000;19:4574-4581.
385. Hall RK, Yamasaki T, Kucera T, et al. Regulation of phosphoenolpyruvate carboxykinase and insulin-like growth factor-binding protein-1 gene expression by insulin: the role of winged helix/forkhead proteins. *J Biol Chem.* 2000;275:30169-30175.
386. Wolfrum C, Asilmaz E, Luca E, et al. Foxa2 regulates lipid metabolism and ketogenesis in the liver during fasting and in diabetes. *Nature.* 2004;432:1027-1032.
387. Asplin CM, Paquette TL, Palmer JP. In vivo inhibition of glucagon secretion by paracrine beta cell activity in man. *J Clin Invest.* 1981;68:314-318.
388. Shi ZQ, Wasserman D, Vranic M. Metabolic implications of exercise and physical fitness in physiology and diabetes. In: Porte D, Sherwin R, eds. *Ellenberg and Rifkin Diabetes Mellitus.* Norwalk, CN: Appleton & Lange; 1997:653-687.
389. Chen X, Iqbal N, Boden G. The effects of free fatty acids on gluconeogenesis and glycogenolysis in normal subjects. *J Clin Invest.* 1999;103:365-372.
390. Boden G. Fatty acids and insulin resistance. *Diabetes Care.* 1996;19:394-395.
391. Lewis GF, Vranic M, Giacca A. Role of free fatty acids and glucagon in the peripheral effect of insulin on glucose production in humans. *Am J Physiol.* 1998;275:E177-E186.
392. Perriello G, Pampanelli S, Del Sindaco P, et al. Evidence of increased systemic glucose production and gluconeogenesis in an early stage of NIDDM. *Diabetes.* 1997;46:1010-1016.
393. DeFronzo RA, Bonadonna RC, Ferrannini E. Pathogenesis of NIDDM: a balanced overview. *Diabetes Care.* 1992;15:318-368.
394. DeFronzo RA, Simonson D, Ferrannini E. Hepatic and peripheral insulin resistance: a common feature of type 2 (non-insulin-dependent) and type 1 (insulin-dependent) diabetes mellitus. *Diabetologia.* 1982;23:313-319.
395. Bogardus C, Lillioja S, Howard BV, et al. Relationships between insulin secretion, insulin action, and fasting plasma glucose concentration in nondiabetic and noninsulin-dependent diabetic subjects. *J Clin Invest.* 1984;74:1238-1246.
396. Hother-Nielsen O, Beck-Nielsen H. Insulin resistance, but normal basal rates of glucose production in patients with newly diagnosed mild diabetes mellitus. *Acta Endocrinol (Copenh).* 1991;124:637-645.
397. Hother-Nielsen O, Beck-Nielsen H. On the determination of basal glucose production rate in patients with type 2 (non-insulin-dependent) diabetes mellitus using primed-continuous 3-^{3}H-glucose infusion. *Diabetologia.* 1990;33:603-610.
398. Firth R, Bell P, Rizza R. Insulin action in non-insulin-dependent diabetes mellitus: the relationship between hepatic and extrahepatic insulin resistance and obesity. *Metabolism.* 1987;36:1091-1095.
399. Groop LC, Bonadonna RC, Shank M, et al. Role of free fatty acids and insulin in determining free fatty acid and lipid oxidation in man. *J Clin Invest.* 1991;87:83-89.
400. Pigon J, Giacca A, Ostenson CG, et al. Normal hepatic insulin sensitivity in lean, mild noninsulin-dependent diabetic patients. *J Clin Endocrinol Metab.* 1996;81:3702-3708.
401. Stumvoll M, Nurjhan N, Perriello G, et al. Metabolic effects of metformin in non-insulin-dependent diabetes mellitus. *N Engl J Med.* 1995;333:550-554.

402. Lewis GF, Carpentier A, Vranic N, et al. Resistance to insulin's acute direct hepatic effect in suppressing steady-state glucose production in individuals with type 2 diabetes. *Diabetes*. 1999;48:570-576.
403. Staehr P, Hother-Nielsen O, Levin K, et al. Assessment of hepatic insulin action in obese type 2 diabetic patients. *Diabetes*. 2001;50:1363-1370.
404. Magnusson I, Rothman DL, Gerard DP, et al. Contribution of hepatic glycogenolysis to glucose production in humans in response to a physiological increase in plasma glucagon concentration. *Diabetes*. 1995;44:185-189.
405. Magnusson I, Rothman DL, Katz LD, et al. Increased rate of gluconeogenesis in type II diabetes mellitus: a ^{13}C nuclear magnetic resonance study. *J Clin Invest*. 1992;90:1323-1327.
406. Baron AD, Schaeffer L, Shragg P, et al. Role of hyperglucagonemia in maintenance of increased rates of hepatic glucose output in type II diabetics. *Diabetes*. 1987;36:274-283.
407. Lam TK, Pocai A, Gutierrez-Juarez R, et al. Hypothalamic sensing of circulating fatty acids is required for glucose homeostasis. *Nat Med*. 2005;11:320-327.
408. Minokoshi Y, Alquier T, Furukawa N, et al. AMP-kinase regulates food intake by responding to hormonal and nutrient signals in the hypothalamus. *Nature*. 2004;428:569-574.
409. Yu YH, Ginsberg HN. Adipocyte signaling and lipid homeostasis: sequelae of insulin-resistant adipose tissue. *Circ Res*. 2005;96:1042-1052.
410. Yamauchi T, Kamon J, Minokoshi Y, et al. Adiponectin stimulates glucose utilization and fatty-acid oxidation by activating AMP-activated protein kinase. *Nat Med*. 2002;8:1288-1295.
411. Tomas E, Tsao TS, Saha AK, et al. Enhanced muscle fat oxidation and glucose transport by ACRP30 globular domain: acetyl-CoA carboxylase inhibition and AMP-activated protein kinase activation. *Proc Natl Acad Sci U S A*. 2002;99:16309-16313.
412. Maeda N, Shimomura I, Kishida K, et al. Diet-induced insulin resistance in mice lacking adiponectin/ACRP30. *Nat Med*. 2002;8:731-737.
413. Steppan CM, Brown EJ, Wright CM, et al. A family of tissue-specific resistin-like molecules. *Proc Natl Acad Sci U S A*. 2001;98:502-506.
414. Steppan CM, Bailey ST, Bhat S, et al. The hormone resistin links obesity to diabetes. *Nature*. 2001;409:307-312.
415. Kusminski CM, McTernan PG, Kumar S. Role of resistin in obesity, insulin resistance and type II diabetes. *Clin Sci (Lond)*. 2005;109:243-256.
416. Ruan H, Lodish HF. Insulin resistance in adipose tissue: direct and indirect effects of tumor necrosis factor-α. *Cytokine Growth Factor Rev*. 2003;14:447-455.
417. Weisberg SP, McCann D, Desai M, et al. Obesity is associated with macrophage accumulation in adipose tissue. *J Clin Invest*. 2003;112:1796-1808.
418. Fain JN, Madan AK, Hiler ML, et al. Comparison of the release of adipokines by adipose tissue, adipose tissue matrix, and adipocytes from visceral and subcutaneous abdominal adipose tissues of obese humans. *Endocrinology*. 2004;145:2273-2282.
419. Takahashi K, Mizuarai S, Araki H, et al. Adiposity elevates plasma MCP-1 levels leading to the increased CD11b-positive monocytes in mice. *J Biol Chem*. 2003;278:46654-46660.
420. Sartipy P, Loskutoff DJ. Monocyte chemoattractant protein 1 in obesity and insulin resistance. *Proc Natl Acad Sci U S A*. 2003;100:7265-7270.
421. Weisberg SP, Hunter D, Huber R, et al. CCR2 modulates inflammatory and metabolic effects of high-fat feeding. *J Clin Invest*. 2006;116:115-124.
422. Kern PA, Ranganathan S, Li C, et al. Adipose tissue tumor necrosis factor and interleukin-6 expression in human obesity and insulin resistance. *Am J Physiol Endocrinol Metab*. 2001;280:E745-E751.
423. van Hall G, Steensberg A, Sacchetti M, et al. Interleukin-6 stimulates lipolysis and fat oxidation in humans. *J Clin Endocrinol Metab*. 2003;88:3005-3010.
424. Yalow R, Berson S. Immunoassay of endogenous plasma insulin in man. *J Clin Invest*. 1960;39:1157-1175.
425. Polonsky K, Jaspan J, Emmanouel D, et al. Differences in the hepatic and renal extraction of insulin and glucagon in the dog: evidence for saturability of insulin metabolism. *Acta Endocrinol (Copenh)*. 1983;102:420-427.
426. Polonsky K, Jaspan J, Pugh W, et al. Metabolism of C-peptide in the dog: in vivo demonstration of the absence of hepatic extraction. *J Clin Invest*. 1983;72:1114-1123.
427. Steiner DF, James DE. Cellular and molecular biology of the beta cell. *Diabetologia*. 1992;35(suppl 2):S41-S48.
428. Melani F, Ryan WG, Rubenstein AH, et al. Proinsulin secretion by a pancreatic beta-cell adenoma: proinsulin and C-peptide secretion. *N Engl J Med*. 1970;283:713-719.
429. Horwitz D, Starr JI, Mako ME, et al. Proinsulin, insulin, and C-peptide concentrations in human portal and peripheral blood. *J Clin Invest*. 1975;55:1278-1283.
430. Melani F, Rubenstein A, Steiner D. Human serum proinsulin. *J Clin Invest*. 1970;49:497-507.
431. Bergenstal R, Cohen RM, Lever E, et al. The metabolic effects of biosynthetic human proinsulin in individuals with type I diabetes. *J Clin Endocrinol Metab*. 1984;58:973-979.
432. Revers R, Henry R, Schmeiser L, et al. The effects of biosynthetic human proinsulin on carbohydrate metabolism. *Diabetes*. 1984;33:762-770.
433. Peavy D, Brunner MR, Duckworth W, et al. Receptor binding and biological potency of several split forms (conversion intermediates) of human proinsulin: studies in cultured IM-9 lymphocytes and in vivo and in vitro in rats. *J Biol Chem*. 1985;260:13989-13994.
434. Gruppuso P, Frank B, Schwartz R. Binding of proinsulin and proinsulin conversion intermediates to human placental insulin-like growth factor 1 receptors. *J Clin Endocrinol Metab*. 1988;67:197.
435. Polonsky K, Rubenstein A. C-peptide as a measure of the secretion and hepatic extraction of insulin: pitfalls and limitations. *Diabetes*. 1984;33:486-494.
436. Wojcikowski C, Blackman J, Ostrega D, et al. Lack of effect of high-dose biosynthetic human C-peptide on pancreatic hormone release in normal subjects. *Metabolism*. 1990;39:827-832.
437. Wahren J, Ekberg K, Johansson J, et al. Role of C-peptide in human physiology. *Am J Physiol*. 2000;278:E759-E768.
438. Polonsky K, Pugh W, Jaspan JB, et al. C-peptide and insulin secretion: relationship between peripheral concentrations of C-peptide and insulin and their secretion rates in the dog. *J Clin Invest*. 1984;74:1821-1829.
439. Bratusch-Marrain P, Waldhausl WK, Gasic S, et al. Hepatic disposal of biosynthetic human insulin and porcine C-peptide in humans. *Metabolism*. 1984;33:151-157.
440. Faber O, Hagen C, Binder C, et al. Kinetics of human connecting peptide in normal and diabetic subjects. *J Clin Invest*. 1978;62:197-203.
441. Polonsky K, Licinio-Paixas J, Given BD, et al. Use of biosynthetic human C-peptide in the measurement of insulin secretion rates in normal volunteers and type I diabetic patients. *J Clin Invest*. 1986;77:98-105.
442. Shapiro E, Tillil H, Rubenstein H, et al. Peripheral insulin parallels changes in insulin secretion more closely than C-peptide after bolus intravenous glucose administration. *J Clin Endocrinol Metab*. 1988;67:1094-1099.
443. Eaton R, Allen RC, Schade DS, et al. Prehepatic insulin production in man: kinetic analysis using peripheral connecting peptide behavior. *J Clin Endocrinol Metab*. 1980;51:520-528.
444. Welch S, Gebhart SS, Bergman RN, et al. Minimal model analysis of intravenous glucose tolerance test-derived insulin sensitivity in diabetic subjects. *J Clin Endocrinol Metab*. 1990;71:1508-1518.
445. Breda E, Cavaghan MK, Toffolo G, et al. Oral glucose tolerance test minimal model indexes of beta-cell function and insulin sensitivity. *Diabetes*. 2001;50:150-158.
446. Bergman R, Phillips L, Cobelli C. Physiologic evaluation of factors controlling glucose tolerance in man: measurement of insulin sensitivity and beta-cell glucose sensitivity from the response to intravenous glucose. *J Clin Invest*. 1981;68:1456-1467.
447. Caumo A, Bergman R, Cobelli C. Insulin sensitivity from meal tolerance tests in normal subjects: a minimal model index. *J Clin Endocrinol Metab*. 2000;85:4396-4402.
448. Davis EA, Cuesta-Munoz A, Raoul M, et al. Mutants of glucokinase cause hypoglycaemia and hyperglycaemia syndromes and their analysis illuminates fundamental quantitative concepts of glucose homeostasis. *Diabetologia*. 1999;42:1175-1186.
449. Matschinsky FM, Glaser B, Magnuson MA. Pancreatic beta-cell glucokinase: closing the gap between theoretical concepts and experimental realities. *Diabetes*. 1998;47:307-315.
450. Dukes ID, McIntyre MS, Mertz RJ, et al. Dependence on NADH produced during glycolysis for beta-cell glucose signaling. *J Biol Chem*. 1994;269:10979-10982.
451. Maechler P, Wollheim CB. Mitochondrial function in normal and diabetic beta-cells. *Nature*. 2001;414:807-812.
452. Aguilar-Bryan L, Bryan J, Nakazaki M. Of mice and men: K_{ATP} channels and insulin secretion. *Recent Prog Horm Res*. 2001;56:47-68.
453. Porte DJ, Pupo A. Insulin responses to glucose: evidence for a two-pooled system in man. *J Clin Invest*. 1969;48:2309-2319.
454. Chen M, Porte DJ. The effect of rate and dose of glucose infusion on the acute insulin response in man. *J Clin Endocrinol Metab*. 1976;42:1168-1175.
455. Ward W, Beard JC, Halter JB, et al. Pathophysiology of insulin secretion in non-insulin-dependent diabetes mellitus. *Diabetes Care*. 1984;7:491-502.
456. Waldhäus W, Bratusch-Marrain P, Gasic S, et al. Insulin production rate following glucose ingestion estimated by splanchnic C-peptide output in normal man. *Diabetologia*. 1979;17:221-227.
457. Eaton R, Allen R, Schade D. Hepatic removal of insulin in normal man: dose response to endogenous insulin secretion. *J Clin Endocrinol Metab*. 1983;56:1294-1300.

458. Nauck M, Homberger E, Siegel EG, et al. Incretin effects of increasing glucose loads in man calculated from venous insulin and C-peptide responses. *J Clin Endocrinol Metab*. 1986;63:492-498.
459. Tillil H, Shapiro ET, Miller MA, et al. Dose-dependent effects of oral and intravenous glucose on insulin secretion and clearance in normal humans. *Am J Physiol*. 1988;254:E349-E357.
460. Faber O, Madsbad S, Kehlet H, et al. Pancreatic beta cell secretion during oral and intravenous glucose administration. *Acta Med Scand Suppl*. 1979;624:61-64.
461. Madsbad S, Kehlet H, Hilsted J, et al. Discrepancy between plasma C-peptide and insulin response to oral and intravenous glucose. *Diabetes*. 1983;32:436-438.
462. Shapiro E, Tillil H, Miller MA, et al. Insulin secretion and clearance: comparison after oral and intravenous glucose. *Diabetes*. 1987;93:1120-1130.
463. Creutzfeldt W, Ebert R. New developments in the incretin concept. *Diabetologia*. 1985;28:565-576.
464. Pagliara A, Stillings SN, Hover B, et al. Glucose modulation of amino acid-induced glucagon and insulin release in the isolated perfused rat pancreas. *J Clin Invest*. 1974;54:819-832.
465. Gerich J, Charles M, Grodsky G. Characterization of the effects of arginine and glucose on glucagon and insulin release from the perfused rat pancreas. *J Clin Invest*. 1974;54:833-847.
466. Grodsky G. The kinetics of insulin release. In: Hasselblatt A, Bruchhausen F, eds. *Handbook of Experimental Pharmacology*. Vol 32. Berlin, Germany: Springer-Verlag; 1975:1-19.
467. Salomon D, Meda P. Heterogeneity and contact-dependent regulation of hormone secretion by individual β cells. *Exp Cell Res*. 1986;162:507-520.
468. Schmitz O, Porksen N, Nyholm B, et al. Disorderly and nonstationary insulin secretion in relatives of patients with NIDDM. *Am J Physiol*. 1997;272:E218-E226.
469. Cerasi E, Luft R. The plasma insulin response to glucose infusion in healthy subjects and in diabetes mellitus. *Acta Endocrinol (Copenh)*. 1967;55:278-304.
470. Reference deleted in proofs.
471. Reference deleted in proofs.
472. Smith C, Tam AC, Thomas JM, et al. Between and within subject variation of the first phase insulin response to intravenous glucose. *Diabetologia*. 1988;31:123-125.
473. Bardet S, Pasqual C, Maugendre D, et al. Inter and intra individual variability of acute insulin response during intravenous glucose tolerance tests. *Diabetes Metab*. 1989;15:224-232.
474. Rayman G, Clark P, Schneider AE, et al. The first phase insulin response to intravenous glucose is highly reproducible. *Diabetologia*. 1990; 33:631-634.
475. Bolaffi J, Haldt A, Lewis LD, et al. The third phase of in vitro insulin secretion: evidence for glucose insensitivity. *Diabetes*. 1986; 35:370-373.
476. Curry D. Insulin content and insulinogenesis by the perfused rat pancreas: effects of long term glucose stimulation. *Endocrinology*. 1986;118:170-175.
477. Hoenig M, MacGregor L, Matschinsky F. In vitro exhaustion of pancreatic β-cells. *Am J Physiol*. 1986;250:E502-E511.
478. Grodsky G. A new phase of insulin secretion: how will it contribute to our understanding of β-cell function? *Diabetes*. 1989;38:673-678.
479. Cerasi E. Potentiation of insulin release by glucose in man. *Acta Endocrinol (Copenh)*. 1975;79:511-534.
480. Grill V. Time and dose dependencies for priming effect of glucose on insulin secretion. *Am J Physiol*. 1981;240:E24-E31.
481. Poitout V, Robertson RP. Minireview: secondary beta-cell failure in type 2 diabetes—a convergence of glucotoxicity and lipotoxicity. *Endocrinology*. 2002;143:339-342.
482. Leahy JL. Natural history of beta-cell dysfunction in NIDDM. *Diabetes Care*. 1990;13:992-1010.
483. Levin S, Karam JH, Hane S, et al. Enhancement of arginine-induced insulin secretion in man by prior administration of glucose. *Diabetes*. 1971;20:171-176.
484. Fajans S, Floyd J. Stimulation of islet cell secretion by nutrients and by gastrointestinal hormones released during digestion. In: Steiner D, Freinkel N, eds. *Handbook of Physiology: Section 7. Endocrinology*. Washington, DC: American Physiological Society; 1972:473-493.
485. Ward W, Bolgiano DC, McKnight B, et al. Diminished β-cell secretory capacity in patients with non-insulin dependent diabetes mellitus. *J Clin Invest*. 1984;74:1318-1328.
486. Kadowaki T, Miyake Y, Hagura R, et al. Risk factors for worsening to diabetes in subjects with impaired glucose tolerance. *Diabetologia*. 1984;26:44-49.
487. Muller W, Faloona G, Unger R. The influence of the antecedent diet upon glucagon and insulin secretion. *N Engl J Med*. 1971;285: 1450-1454.
488. Goberna R, Tamarit J Jr, Osorio J, et al. Action of β-hydroxybutyrate, acetoacetate and palmitate on the insulin release from the perfused isolated rat pancreas. *Horm Metab Res*. 1974;6:256-260.
489. Crespin S, Greenough D, Steinberg D. Stimulation of insulin secretion by long-chain free fatty acids. *J Clin Invest*. 1973;52: 1979-1984.
490. Crespin S, Greenough W, Steinberg D. Stimulation of insulin secretion by infusion of fatty acids. *J Clin Invest*. 1969;48:1934-1943.
491. Paolisso G, Gambardella M, Amato L, et al. Opposite effects of short- and long-term fatty acid infusion on insulin secretion in healthy subjects. *Diabetologia*. 1995;38:1295-1299.
492. Boden G, Chen X. Effects of fatty acids and ketone bodies on basal insulin secretion in type 2 diabetes. *Diabetes*. 1999;48:577-583.
493. Zhou Y-P, Grill V. Long term exposure of rat pancreatic islets to fatty acids inhibits glucose-induced insulin secretion and biosynthesis through a glucose fatty acid cycle. *J Clin Invest*. 1994;93:870-876.
494. Mason T, Goh T, Tchipashvili V, et al. Prolonged elevation of plasma free fatty acids desensitizes the insulin secretory response to glucose in vivo in rats. *Diabetes*. 1999;48:524-530.
495. Carpentier A, Mittelman SD, Lamarche B, et al. Acute enhancement of insulin secretion by FFA in humans is lost with prolonged FFA elevation. *Am J Physiol*. 1999;276:E1055-E1066.
496. Dupre J, Ross SA, Watson D, et al. Stimulation of insulin secretion by gastric inhibitory polypeptide in man. *J Clin Endocrinol Metab*. 1973;37:826-828.
497. Andersen D, Elahi D, Brown JC, et al. Oral glucose augmentation of insulin secretion: interactions of gastric inhibitory polypeptide with ambient glucose and insulin levels. *J Clin Invest*. 1978;62:152-161.
498. Schmidt W, Siegel E, Creutzfeldt W. Glucagon-like peptide-2 stimulates insulin release from isolated rate pancreatic islets. *Diabetologia*. 1985;28:704-707.
499. Kreymann B, Williams G, Ghatei MA, et al. Glucagon-like peptide-1 7-36: a physiological incretin in man. *Lancet*. 1987;2:1300-1304.
500. Zawalich W, Diaz V. Prior cholecystokinin exposure sensitizes islets of Langerhans to glucose stimulation. *Diabetes*. 1987;36:118-227.
501. Zawalich W. Synergistic impact of cholecystokinin and gastric inhibitory polypeptide on the regulation of insulin secretion. *Metabolism*. 1988;37:778-781.
502. Weir G, Mojsovs S, Hendrick GK, et al. Glucagon-like peptide 1(7-37) actions on endocrine pancreas. *Diabetes*. 1989;38:338-342.
503. Rasmussen H, Zawalich KC, Ganesan S, et al. Physiology and pathophysiology of insulin secretion. *Diabetes Care*. 1990;13:655-666.
504. Fukase N, Manaka H, Sugiyama K, et al. Response of truncated glucagon-like peptide-1 and gastric inhibitory polypeptide to glucose ingestion in non-insulin dependent diabetes mellitus: effect of sulfonylurea therapy. *Acta Diabetol*. 1995;32:165-169.
505. Groop P. The influence of body weight, age and glucose tolerance on the relationship between GIP secretion and beta-cell function in man. *Scand J Clin Lab Invest*. 1989;49:367-379.
506. Creutzfeldt W, Ebert R, Nauck M, et al. Disturbances of the entero-insulin axis. *Scand J Gastroenterol*. 1983;83(suppl):111-119.
507. Nauck M, Heimesaat MM, Orskov C, et al. Preserved incretin activity of glucagon-like peptide 1(7-36 amide) but not of synthetic human gastric inhibitory polypeptide in patients with type 2 diabetes mellitus. *J Clin Invest*. 1993;91:301-307.
508. Ahrén B, Larsson H, Holst J. Reduced gastric inhibitory polypeptide but normal glucagon-like peptide 1 response to oral glucose in postmenopausal women with impaired glucose tolerance. *Eur J Endocrinol*. 1997;137:127-131.
509. Rushakoff R, Goldfine ID, Beccaria LJ, et al. Reduced postprandial cholecystokinin (CCK) secretion in patients with noninsulin-dependent diabetes mellitus: evidence for a role for CCK in regulating postprandial hyperglycemia. *J Clin Endocrinol Metab*. 1993;76:489-493.
510. Meguro T, Shimosegawa T, Satoh A, et al. Gallbladder emptying and cholecystokinin and pancreatic polypeptide responses to a liquid meal in patients with diabetes mellitus. *J Gastroenterol*. 1997;32:628-634.
511. Hasegawa H, Shirohara H, Okabayashi Y, et al. Oral glucose ingestion stimulates cholecystokinin release in normal subjects and patients with non-insulin-dependent diabetes mellitus. *Metabolism*. 1996;45: 196-202.
512. Nauck M, Wollschlager D, Werner J, et al. Effects of subcutaneous glucagon-like peptide 1 (GLP-1 (7-36 amide)) in patients with NIDDM. *Diabetologia*. 1996;39:1546-1553.
513. Creutzfeldt W, Kleine N, Willms B, et al. Glucagonostatic actions and reduction of fasting hyperglycemia by exogenous glucagon-like peptide I(7-36) amide in type I diabetic patients. *Diabetes Care*. 1996;19:580-586.
514. Young A, Gedulin BR, Bhavsar S, et al. Glucose-lowering and insulin-sensitizing actions of exendin-4: studies in obese diabetic *(ob/ob, db/db)* mice, diabetic fatty Zucker rats, and diabetic rhesus monkeys *(Macaca mulatta)*. *Diabetes*. 1999;48:1026-1034.
515. Nauck M, Bartels E, Orskov C, et al. Additive insulinotropic effects of exogenous synthetic human gastric inhibitory polypeptide and glucagon-like peptide-1-(7-36) amide infused at near-physiological insulinotropic hormone and glucose concentrations. *J Clin Endocrinol Metab*. 1993;76:912-917.

516. Elahi D, McAloon-Dyke M, Fukagawa NK, et al. The insulinotropic actions of glucose-dependent insulinotropic polypeptide (GIP) and glucagon-like peptide-1 (7-37) in normal and diabetic subjects. *Regul Pept*. 1994;51:63-74.
517. Niederau C, Schwarzendrube J, Luthen R, et al. Effects of cholecystokinin receptor blockade in circulating concentrations of glucose, insulin, C-peptide, and pancreatic polypeptide after various meals in healthy human volunteers. *Pancreas*. 1992;7:1-10.
518. Fieseler P, Bridenbaugh S, Nustede R, et al. Physiological augmentation of amino acid-induced insulin secretion by GIP and GLP-I but not by CCK-8. *Am J Physiol*. 1995;268:E949-E955.
519. Reimers J, Nauck M, Creutzfeldt W, et al. Lack of insulinotropic effect of endogenous and exogenous cholecystokinin in man. *Diabetologia*. 1988;31:271-280.
520. Rushakoff R, Goldfine ID, Carter JD, et al. Physiological concentrations of cholecystokinin stimulate amino acid-induced insulin release in humans. *J Clin Endocrinol Metab*. 1987;65:395-401.
521. Ahrén B, Holst J, Efendic S. Antidiabetogenic action of cholecystokinin-8 in type 2 diabetes. *J Clin Endocrinol Metab*. 2000;85:1043-1048.
522. Schebalin M, Said S, Makhlouf G. Stimulation of insulin and glucagon secretion by vasoactive intestinal peptide. *Am J Physiol*. 1977;232: E197-E200.
523. Dupre J, Curtis JD, Unger RH, et al. Effects of secretin, pancreozymin, or gastrin on the response of the endocrine pancreas to administration of glucose or arginine in man. *J Clin Invest*. 1969;48:745-757.
524. Halter J, Porte DJ. Mechanisms of impaired acute insulin release in adult onset diabetes: studies with isoproterenol and secretin. *J Clin Endocrinol Metab*. 1978;46:952-960.
525. Glaser B, Shapiro B, Glowniak J, et al. Effects of secretin on the normal and pathological beta-cell. *J Clin Endocrinol Metab*. 1988;66: 1138-1143.
526. Bertrand G, Puech R, Maisonnasse Y, et al. Comparative effects of PACAP and VIP on pancreatic endocrine secretions and vascular resistance in rat. *Br J Pharmacol*. 1996;117:764-770.
527. Rehfeld J, Stadil F. The effect of gastrin on basal- and glucose-stimulated insulin secretion in man. *J Clin Invest*. 1973;52:1415-1426.
528. Samols E, Marri G, Marks V. Promotion of insulin secretion by glucagon. *Lancet*. 1965;2:15-16.
529. Alberti K, Christensen NJ, Christensen SE, et al. Inhibition of insulin secretion by somatostatin. *Lancet*. 1973;2:1299-1301.
530. Aguilar-Parada E, Eisentraut A, Unger R. Effects of starvation on plasma pancreatic glucagon in normal man. *Diabetes*. 1969;18:717-723.
531. Marliss E, Aoki TT, Unger RH, et al. Glucagon levels and metabolic effects in fasting man. *J Clin Invest*. 1970;49:2256-2270.
532. Malaisse W, Malaisse L, Wright P. Effect of fasting upon insulin secretion in the rat. *Am J Physiol*. 1967;213:843-848.
533. Zawalich W, Dye ES, Pagliara AS, et al. Starvation diabetes in the rat: onset, recovery and specificity of reduced responsiveness of pancreatic β-cells. *Endocrinology*. 1979;104:1344-1351.
534. Felig P, Marliss E, Cahill JG. Metabolic response to human growth hormone during prolonged starvation. *J Clin Invest*. 1971;50: 411-421.
535. Kalhan S, Adam P. Inhibitory effect of prednisone on insulin secretion in man: model for duplication of blood glucose concentration. *J Clin Endocrinol Metab*. 1975;41:600-610.
536. Landgraf R, Landgraf-Luers MM, Weissmann A, et al. Prolactin: a diabetogenic hormone. *Diabetologia*. 1977;13:99-104.
537. Gustafson A, Banasiak MF, Kalkhoff RK, et al. Correlation of hyperprolactinemia with altered plasma insulin and glucagon: similarity to effects of late human pregnancy. *J Clin Endocrinol Metab*. 1980;51:242-246.
538. Brelje T, Sorenson R. Nutrient and hormonal regulation of the threshold of glucose-stimulated insulin secretion in isolated rat pancreases. *Endocrinology*. 1988;123:1582-1590.
539. Beck P, Daughaday W. Human placental lactogen: studies of its acute metabolic effects and disposition in normal man. *J Clin Invest*. 1967;46:103-110.
540. Ensinck J, Williams R. Hormonal and nonhormonal factors modifying man's response to insulin. In: Steiner D, Freinkel N, eds. *Handbook of Physiology: Section 7. Endocrinology*. Washington, DC: American Physiological Society; 1972:665-669.
541. Martin J, Friesen H. Effect of human placental lactogen on the isolated islets of Langerhans in vitro. *Endocrinology*. 1969;84:619-621.
542. Curry D, Bennett L. Dynamics of insulin release by perfused rat pancreases: effects of hypophysectomy, growth hormone, adrenocorticotropic hormone and hydrocortisone. *Endocrinology*. 1973;93:602-609.
543. Malaisse W, Malaisse-Lagae F, King S, et al. Effect of growth hormone on insulin secretion. *Am J Physiol*. 1968;215:423-428.
544. Randin J, Scazziga B, Jequier E, et al. Study of glucose and lipid metabolism by continuous indirect calorimetry in Graves' disease: effect of an oral glucose load. *J Clin Endocrinol Metab*. 1985;61:1165-1171.
545. Foss M, Paccola GM, Saad MJ, et al. Peripheral glucose metabolism in human hyperthyroidism. *J Clin Endocrinol Metab*. 1990;70:1167-1172.
546. Sestoft L, Heding L. Hypersecretion of proinsulin in thyrotoxicosis. *Diabetologia*. 1981;21:103-107.
547. Nishi S, Seino Y, Ishida H, et al. Vagal regulation of insulin, glucagon, and somatostatin secretion in vitro in the rat. *J Clin Invest*. 1987;79:1191-1196.
548. Kurose T, Seino Y, Nishi S, et al. Mechanism of sympathetic neural regulation of insulin, somatostatin, and glucagon secretion. *Am J Physiol*. 1990;251:E220-E227.
549. Woods S, Porte DJ. Neural control of the endocrine pancreas. *Physiol Rev*. 1974;54:596-619.
550. Bloom SR, Edwards A. Certain pharmacological characteristics of the release of pancreatic glucagon in response to stimulation of the splanchnic nerves. *J Physiol (Lond)*. 1978;280:25-35.
551. Porte Jr D, Girardier L, Seydoux J, et al. Neural regulation of insulin secretion in the dog. *J Clin Invest*. 1973;52:210-214.
552. Roy M, Lee KC, Jones MS, et al. Neural control of pancreatic insulin and somatostatin secretion. *Endocrinology*. 1984;115:770-775.
553. Skoglund G, Lundquist I, Ahren B. Selective α_2-adrenoceptor activation by clonidine: effects on $^{45}Ca^{2}+$ efflux and insulin secretion from isolated rat islets. *Acta Physiol Scand*. 1988;132:289-296.
554. Ahrén B. Autonomic regulation of islet hormone secretion: implications for health and disease. *Diabetologia*. 2000;43:393-410.
555. Pettersson M, Ahrén B. Calcitonin gene-related peptide inhibits insulin secretion: studies on ion fluxes and cyclic AMP in isolated rat islets. *Diabetes Res Clin Pract*. 1990;15:9-14.
556. Pettersson M, Ahrén B, Bottcher G, et al. Calcitonin gene-related peptide: occurrence in pancreatic islets in the mouse and the rat and inhibition of insulin secretion in the mouse. *Diabetologia*. 1986;119: 865-869.
557. Ahrén B, Mårtensson H, Nobin A. Effects of calcitonin gene-related peptide (CGRP) on islet hormone secretion in the pig. *Diabetologia*. 1987;30:354-359.
558. Lundquist I, Sundler F, Ahrén B, et al. Somatostatin, pancreatic polypeptide, substance P, and neurotensin: cellular distribution and effects on stimulated insulin secretion in the mouse. *Endocrinology*. 1979; 104:832-838.
559. Hermansen K. Effects of substance P and other peptides on the release of somatostatin, insulin and glucagon in vitro. *Endocrinology*. 1980;107:256-261.
560. Larrimer J, Mazzaferri EL, Cataland S, et al. Effect of atropine on glucose-stimulated gastric inhibitory polypeptide. *Diabetes*. 1978;27: 638-642.
561. Rocca A, Brubaker P. Role of the vagus nerve in mediating proximal nutrient-induced glucagon-like peptide-1 secretion. *Endocrinology*. 1999;140:1687-1694.
562. Flaten O, Sand T, Myren J. β-Adrenergic stimulation and blockade of the release of gastric inhibitory polypeptide and insulin in man. *Scand J Gastroenterol*. 1982;17:283-288.
563. Claustre J, Brechet S, Plaisancie P, et al. Stimulatory effect of β-adrenergic agonists on ileal L cell secretion and modulation by α-adrenergic activation. *J Endocrinol*. 1999;162:271-278.
564. Kruszynska Y, Home PD, Hanning I, et al. Basal and 24-h C-peptide and insulin secretion rate in normal man. *Diabetologia*. 1987;30: 16-21.
565. Polonsky KS, Given BD, Van Cauter E. Twenty-four-hour profiles and pulsatile patterns of insulin secretion in normal and obese subjects. *J Clin Invest*. 1988;81:442-448.
566. Polonsky KS. The beta-cell in diabetes: from molecular genetics to clinical research. Lilly Lecture 1994. *Diabetes*. 1995;44:705-717.
567. Lang DA, Matthews DR, Peto J, et al. Cyclic oscillations of basal plasma glucose and insulin concentrations in human beings. *N Engl J Med*. 1979;301:1023-1027.
568. Hansen BC, Jen KC, Belbez Pek S, et al. Rapid oscillations in plasma insulin, glucagon, and glucose in obese and normal weight humans. *J Clin Endocrinol Metab*. 1982;54:785-792.
569. Matthews DR, Lang DA, Burnett MA, et al. Control of pulsatile insulin secretion in man. *Diabetologia*. 1983;24:231-237.
570. O'Meara NM, Sturis J, Van Cauter E, et al. Lack of control by glucose of ultradian insulin secretory oscillations in impaired glucose tolerance and in non-insulin-dependent diabetes mellitus. *J Clin Invest*. 1993;92:262-271.
571. Porksen N, Grafte B, Nyholm B, et al. Glucagon-like peptide 1 increases mass but not frequency or orderliness of pulsatile insulin secretion. *Diabetes*. 1998;47:45-49.
572. Porksen N, Nyholm B, Veldhuis JD, et al. In humans at least 75% of insulin secretion arises from punctuated insulin secretory bursts. *Am J Physiol*. 1997;273:E908-E914.
573. Porksen N, Hussain MA, Bianda TL, et al. IGF-I inhibits burst mass of pulsatile insulin secretion at supraphysiological and low IGF-I infusion rates. *Am J Physiol*. 1997;272:E352-E358.
574. Porksen NK, Munn SR, Steers JL, et al. Mechanisms of sulfonylurea's stimulation of insulin secretion in vivo: selective amplification of insulin secretory burst mass. *Diabetes*. 1996;45:1792-1797.
575. Porksen N, Munn S, Steers J, et al. Effects of glucose ingestion versus infusion on pulsatile insulin secretion: the incretin effect is achieved by amplification of insulin secretory burst mass. *Diabetes*. 1996; 45:1317-1323.

576. O'Rahilly S, Turner RC, Matthews DR. Impaired pulsatile secretion of insulin in relatives of patients with non-insulin-dependent diabetes. *N Engl J Med*. 1988;318:1225-1230.
577. Van Cauter E. Estimating false-positive and false-negative errors in analyses of hormonal pulsatility. *Am J Physiol*. 1988;254: E786-E794.
578. Pincus SM. Quantification of evolution from order to randomness in practical time series analysis. *Methods Enzymol*. 1994;240:68-89.
579. Jaspan JB, Lever E, Polonsky KS, et al. In vivo pulsatility of pancreatic islet peptides. *Am J Physiol*. 1986;251:E215-E226.
580. Matthews DR, Naylor BA, Jones RG, et al. Pulsatile insulin has greater hypoglycemic effect than continuous delivery. *Diabetes*. 1983;32: 617-621.
581. Bratusch-Marrain PR, Komjati M, Waldhausl WK. Efficacy of pulsatile versus continuous insulin administration on hepatic glucose production and glucose utilization in type I diabetic humans. *Diabetes*. 1986;35:922-926.
582. Ward GM, Walters JM, Aitken PM, et al. Effects of prolonged pulsatile hyperinsulinemia in humans: enhancement of insulin sensitivity. *Diabetes*. 1990;39:501-507.
583. Sonnenberg GE, Hoffmann RG, Johnson CP, et al. Low- and high-frequency insulin secretion pulses in normal subjects and pancreas transplant recipients: role of extrinsic innervation. *J Clin Invest*. 1992;90:545-553.
584. Blackman JD, Polonsky KS, Jaspan JB, et al. Insulin secretory profiles and C-peptide clearance kinetics at 6 months and 2 years after kidney-pancreas transplantation. *Diabetes*. 1992;41:1346-1354.
585. Sturis J, Polonsky KS, Mosekilde E, et al. Computer model for mechanisms underlying ultradian oscillations of insulin and glucose. *Am J Physiol*. 1991;260:E801-E809.
586. Sturis J, Van Cauter E, Blackman JD, et al. Entrainment of pulsatile insulin secretion by oscillatory glucose infusion. *J Clin Invest*. 1991;87:439-445.
587. Jarrett RJ, Baker IA, Keen H, et al. Diurnal variation in oral glucose tolerance: blood sugar and plasma insulin levels morning, afternoon, and evening. *Br Med J*. 1972;1:199-201.
588. Reference deleted in proofs.
589. Aparicio NJ, Puchulu FE, Gagliardino JJ, et al. Circadian variation of the blood glucose, plasma insulin and human growth hormone levels in response to an oral glucose load in normal subjects. *Diabetes*. 1974;23:132-137.
590. Van Cauter E, Desir D, Decoster C, et al. Nocturnal decrease in glucose tolerance during constant glucose infusion. *J Clin Endocrinol Metab*. 1989;69:604-611.
591. Pick A, Clark J, Kubstrup P, et al. Role of apoptosis in failure of beta-cell mass compensation for insulin resistance and beta-cell defects in the male Zucker diabetic fatty rat. *Diabetes*. 1998;47:358-364.
592. Cockburn BN, Ostrega DM, Sturis J, et al. Changes in pancreatic islet glucokinase and hexokinase activities with increasing age, obesity, and the onset of diabetes. *Diabetes*. 1997;46:1434-1439.
593. Kahn SE, Prigeon RL, McCulloch DK, et al. Quantification of the relationship between insulin sensitivity and beta-cell function in human subjects: evidence for a hyperbolic function. *Diabetes*. 1993;42: 1663-1672.
594. Toffolo G, Bergman RN, Finegood DT, et al. Quantitative estimation of beta cell sensitivity to glucose in the intact organism: a minimal model of insulin kinetics in the dog. *Diabetes*. 1980;29:979-990.
595. Polonsky KS, Given BD, Hirsch L, et al. Quantitative study of insulin secretion and clearance in normal and obese subjects. *J Clin Invest*. 1988;81:435-441.
596. Jones CN, Pei D, Staris P, et al. Alterations in the glucose-stimulated insulin secretory dose-response curve and in insulin clearance in non-diabetic insulin-resistant individuals. *J Clin Endocrinol Metab*. 1997;82:1834-1838.
597. Buchanan TA, Metzger BE, Freinkel N, et al. Insulin sensitivity and B-cell responsiveness to glucose during late pregnancy in lean and moderately obese women with normal glucose tolerance or mild gestational diabetes. *Am J Obstet Gynecol*. 1990;162:1008-1014.
598. Bergstrom RW, Wahl PW, Leonetti DL, et al. Association of fasting glucose levels with a delayed secretion of insulin after oral glucose in subjects with glucose intolerance. *J Clin Endocrinol Metab*. 1990;71:1447-1453.
599. Phillips DI, Clark PM, Hales CN, et al. Understanding oral glucose tolerance: comparison of glucose or insulin measurements during the oral glucose tolerance test with specific measurements of insulin resistance and insulin secretion. *Diabet Med*. 1994;11:286-292.
600. Byrne MM, Sturis J, Sobel RJ, et al. Elevated plasma glucose 2 h post-challenge predicts defects in beta-cell function. *Am J Physiol*. 1996;270:E572-E579.
601. Ahrén B, Pacini G. Impaired adaptation of first-phase insulin secretion in postmenopausal women with glucose intolerance. *Am J Physiol*. 1997;273:E701-E707.
602. Yoshioka N, Kuzuya T, Matsuda A, et al. Serum proinsulin levels at fasting and after oral glucose load in patients with type 2 (non-insulin-dependent) diabetes mellitus. *Diabetologia*. 1988;31:355-360.
603. Saad MF, Kahn SE, Nelson RG, et al. Disproportionately elevated proinsulin in Pima Indians with noninsulin-dependent diabetes mellitus. *J Clin Endocrinol Metab*. 1990;70:1247-1253.
604. Reaven GM, Chen YD, Hollenbeck CB, et al. Plasma insulin, C-peptide, and proinsulin concentrations in obese and nonobese individuals with varying degrees of glucose tolerance. *J Clin Endocrinol Metab*. 1993;76:44-48.
605. Larsson H, Ahren B. Relative hyperproinsulinemia as a sign of islet dysfunction in women with impaired glucose tolerance. *J Clin Endocrinol Metab*. 1999;84:2068-2074.
606. Snehalatha C, Ramachandran A, Satyavani K, et al. Specific insulin and proinsulin concentrations in nondiabetic South Indians. *Metabolism*. 1998;47:230-233.
607. Birkeland KI, Torjesen PA, Eriksson J, et al. Hyperproinsulinemia of type II diabetes is not present before the development of hyperglycemia. *Diabetes Care*. 1994;17:1307-1310.
608. Inoue I, Takahashi K, Katayama S, et al. A higher proinsulin response to glucose loading predicts deteriorating fasting plasma glucose and worsening to diabetes in subjects with impaired glucose tolerance. *Diabet Med*. 1996;13:330-336.
609. Kahn SE, Leonetti DL, Prigeon RL, et al. Proinsulin levels predict the development of non-insulin-dependent diabetes mellitus (NIDDM) in Japanese-American men. *Diabet Med*. 1996;13(9 suppl 6):S63-S66.
610. Heine RJ, Nijpels G, Mooy JM. New data on the rate of progression of impaired glucose tolerance to NIDDM and predicting factors. *Diabet Med*. 1996;13(3 suppl 2):S12-S14.
611. Porte Jr D. Clinical importance of insulin secretion and its interaction with insulin resistance in the treatment of type 2 diabetes mellitus and its complications. *Diabetes Metab Res Rev*. 2001;17:181-188.
612. Ferner RE, Ashworth L, Tronier B, et al. Effects of short-term hyperglycemia on insulin secretion in normal humans. *Am J Physiol*. 1986;250:E655-E661.
613. O'Meara NM, Shapiro ET, Van Cauter E, et al. Effect of glyburide on beta cell responsiveness to glucose in non-insulin-dependent diabetes mellitus. *Am J Med*. 1990;89:11S-16S; discussion 51S-53S.
614. O'Rahilly SP, Nugent Z, Rudenski AS, et al. Beta-cell dysfunction, rather than insulin insensitivity, is the primary defect in familial type 2 diabetes. *Lancet*. 1986;2:360-364.
615. Barnett AH, Spiliopoulos AJ, Pyke DA, et al. Metabolic studies in unaffected co-twins of non-insulin-dependent diabetics. *Br Med J (Clin Res Ed)*. 1981;282:1656-1658.
616. Gerich JE. The genetic basis of type 2 diabetes mellitus: impaired insulin secretion versus impaired insulin sensitivity. *Endocr Rev*. 1998;19:491-503.
617. Kosaka K, Hagura R, Kuzuya T. Insulin responses in equivocal and definite diabetes, with special reference to subjects who had mild glucose intolerance but later developed definite diabetes. *Diabetes*. 1977;26:944-952.
618. Efendic S, Luft R, Wajngot A. Aspects of the pathogenesis of type 2 diabetes. *Endocr Rev*. 1984;5:395-410.
619. Ward WK, Johnston CL, Beard JC, et al. Insulin resistance and impaired insulin secretion in subjects with histories of gestational diabetes mellitus. *Diabetes*. 1985;34:861-869.
620. O'Sullivan JB. Body weight and subsequent diabetes mellitus. *JAMA*. 1982;248:949-952.
621. Clark PM, Levy JL, Cox L, et al. Immunoradiometric assay of insulin, intact proinsulin and 32-33 split proinsulin and radioimmunoassay of insulin in diet-treated type 2 (non-insulin-dependent) diabetic subjects. *Diabetologia*. 1992;35:469-474.
622. Polonsky KS, Given BD, Hirsch LJ, et al. Abnormal patterns of insulin secretion in non-insulin-dependent diabetes mellitus. *N Engl J Med*. 1988;318:1231-1239.
623. Block MB, Rosenfield RL, Mako ME, et al. Sequential changes in beta-cell function in insulin-treated diabetic patients assessed by C-peptide immunoreactivity. *N Engl J Med*. 1973;288:1144-1148.
623a. Shapiro ET, Van Cauter E, Tillel H, et al. *J Clin Endocrinol Metab*. 1989 Sep;69(3):571-576.
624. Cavaghan MK, Ehrmann DA, Byrne MM, et al. Treatment with the oral antidiabetic agent troglitazone improves beta cell responses to glucose in subjects with impaired glucose tolerance. *J Clin Invest*. 1997;100:530-537.
625. Villareal DT, Koster JC, Robertson H, et al. Kir6.2 variant E23K increases ATP-sensitive K+ channel activitiy and is associated with impaired insulin release and enhanced insulin sensitivity in adults with normal glucose tolerance. *Diabetes*. 2009;58:1869-1878.
626. Stride A, Ellard S, Clark P, et al. β-Cell dysfunction, insulin sensitivity, and glycosuria precede diabetes in hepatocyte nuclear factor-1α mutation carriers. *Diabetes Care*. 2005;28:1751-1756.
627. Schafer SA, Tschritter O, Machiacao F, et al. Impaired glucagon-like peptide-1-induced insulin secretion in carriers of transcription factor 7-like 2 (TCF7L2) gene polymorphisms. *Diabetologia*. 2007;50: 2443-2450.
628. Ingalls AM, Dickie MM, Snell GD. Obese, a new mutation in the house mouse. *Obes Res*. 1996;4:101.

629. Zhang Y, Proenca R, Maffei M, et al. Positional cloning of the mouse obese gene and its human homologue. *Nature*. 1994;372:425-432.
630. Pelleymounter MA, Cullen MJ, Baker MB, et al. Effects of the obese gene product on body weight regulation in ob/ob mice. *Science*. 1995;269:540-543.
631. Halaas JL, Gajiwala KS, Maffei M, et al. Weight-reducing effects of the plasma protein encoded by the obese gene. *Science*. 1995;269: 543-546.
632. Friedman JM, Halaas JL. Leptin and the regulation of body weight in mammals. *Nature*. 1998;395:763-770.
633. Friedman JM. Leptin and the regulation of body weight. *Harvey Lect*. 1999;95:107-136.
634. Halaas JL, Boozer C, Blair-West J, et al. Physiological response to long-term peripheral and central leptin infusion in lean and obese mice. *Proc Natl Acad Sci U S A*. 1997;94:8878-8883.
635. Friedman JM. The alphabet of weight control. *Nature*. 1997;385:119-120.
636. Friedman JM. Leptin, leptin receptors and the control of body weight. *Eur J Med Res*. 1997;2:7-13.
637. Kerouz NJ, Horsch D, Pons S, et al. Differential regulation of insulin receptor substrates-1 and -2 (IRS-1 and IRS-2) and phosphatidylinositol 3-kinase isoforms in liver and muscle of the obese diabetic (ob/ob) mouse. *J Clin Invest*. 1997;100:3164-3172.
638. Genuth SM, Przybylski RJ, Rosenberg DM. Insulin resistance in genetically obese, hyperglycemic mice. *Endocrinology*. 1971;88:1230-1238.
639. Herberg L, Coleman DL. Laboratory animals exhibiting obesity and diabetes syndromes. *Metabolism*. 1977;26:59-99.
640. Lee GH, Proenca R, Montez JM, et al. Abnormal splicing of the leptin receptor in diabetic mice. *Nature*. 1996;379:632-635.
641. Chen H, Charlat O, Tartaglia LA, et al. Evidence that the diabetes gene encodes the leptin receptor: identification of a mutation in the leptin receptor gene in db/db mice. *Cell*. 1996;84:491-495.
642. Coleman DL, Hummel KP. Hyperinsulinemia in pre-weaning diabetes (db) mice. *Diabetologia*. 1974;10(suppl):607-610.
643. Like AA, Chick WL. Studies in the diabetic mutant mouse. I. Light microscopy and radioautography of pancreatic islets. *Diabetologia*. 1970;6:207-215.
644. Lavine RL, Chick WL, Like AA, et al. Glucose tolerance and insulin secretion in neonatal and adult mice. *Diabetes*. 1971;20:134-139.
645. Like AA, Chick WL. Studies in the diabetic mutant mouse: II. Electron microscopy of pancreatic islets. *Diabetologia*. 1970;6:216-242.
646. Shargill NS, Tatoyan A, el-Rafai MF, et al. Impaired insulin receptor phosphorylation in skeletal muscle membranes of db/db mice: the use of a novel skeletal muscle plasma membrane preparation to compare insulin binding and stimulation of receptor phosphorylation. *Biochem Biophys Res Commun*. 1986;137:286-294.
647. Reference deleted in proofs.
648. Reference deleted in proofs.
649. Cantello BC, Cawthorne MA, Cottam GP, et al. [[omega-(Heterocyclylamino)alkoxy]benzyl]-2,4-thiazolidinediones as potent antihyperglycemic agents. *J Med Chem*. 1994;37:3977-3985.
650. Lohray BB, Bhushan V, Rao BP, et al. Novel euglycemic and hypolipidemic agents: 1. *J Med Chem*. 1998;41:1619-1630.
651. Frigeri LG, Wolff GL, Robel G. Impairment of glucose tolerance in yellow (Avy/A) (BALB/c X VY) F-1 hybrid mice by hyperglycemic peptide(s) from human pituitary glands. *Endocrinology*. 1983;113: 2097-2105.
652. Warbritton A, Gill AM, Yen TT, et al. Pancreatic islet cells in preobese yellow Avy/-mice: relation to adult hyperinsulinemia and obesity. *Proc Soc Exp Biol Med*. 1994;206:145-151.
653. Michaud EJ, Bultman SJ, Klebig ML, et al. A molecular model for the genetic and phenotypic characteristics of the mouse lethal yellow (Ay) mutation. *Proc Natl Acad Sci U S A*. 1994;91:2562-2566.
654. Claycombe KJ, Wang Y, Jones BH, et al. Transcriptional regulation of the adipocyte fatty acid synthase gene by agouti: interaction with insulin. *Physiol Genomics*. 2000;3:157-162.
655. Claycombe KJ, Wang Y, Jones BH, et al. Regulation of leptin by agouti. *Physiol Genomics*. 2000;2:101-105.
656. Kondo ZK, Nozawa K, Tomito T, et al. Inbred strains resulting from Japanese mice. *Bull Exp Anim*. 1957;5:107-116.
657. Iwatsuka H, Shino A, Suzuoki Z. General survey of diabetic features of yellow KK mice. *Endocrinol Jpn*. 1970;17:23-35.
658. Matsuo T, Shino A, Iwatsuka H, et al. Induction of overt diabetes in KK mice by dietary means. *Endocrinol Jpn*. 1970;17:477-488.
659. Veroni MC, Proietto J, Larkins RG. Evolution of insulin resistance in New Zealand obese mice. *Diabetes*. 1991;40:1480-1487.
660. Cameron DP, Opat F, Insch S. Studies of immunoreactive insulin secretion in NZO mice in vivo. *Diabetologia*. 1974;10(suppl):649-654.
661. Bielschowsky M, Bielschowsky F. A new strain of mice with hereditary obesity. *Proc Univ Otago Med Sch*. 1953;31:29-31.
662. Leiter EH, Reifsnyder PC, Flurkey K, et al. NIDDM genes in mice: deleterious synergism by both parental genomes contributes to diabetogenic thresholds. *Diabetes*. 1998;47:1287-1295.
663. Thorburn A, Andrikopoulos S, Proietto J. Defects in liver and muscle glycogen metabolism in neonatal and adult New Zealand obese mice. *Metabolism*. 1995;44:1298-1302.
664. Andrikopoulos S, Proietto J. The biochemical basis of increased hepatic glucose production in a mouse model of type 2 (non-insulin-dependent) diabetes mellitus. *Diabetologia*. 1995;38:1389-1396.
665. Andrikopoulos S, Rosella G, Kacmarczyk SJ, et al. Impaired regulation of hepatic fructose-1,6-biphosphatase in the New Zealand obese mouse: an acquired defect. *Metabolism*. 1996;45:622-626.
666. Larkins RG, Simeonova L, Veroni MC. Glucose utilization in relation to insulin secretion in NZO and C57Bl mouse islets. *Endocrinology*. 1980;107:1634-1638.
667. Melez KA, Harrison LC, Gilliam JN, et al. Diabetes is associated with autoimmunity in the New Zealand obese (NZO) mouse. *Diabetes*. 1980;29:835-840.
668. Melez KA, Reeves JP, Steinberg AD. Regulation of the expression of autoimmunity in NZB × NZW F1 mice by sex hormones. *J Immunopharmacol*. 1978;1:27-42.
669. Harrison LC, Itin A. A possible mechanism for insulin resistance and hyperglycaemia in NZO mice. *Nature*. 1979;279:334-336.
670. Reifsnyder PC, Churchill G, Leiter EH. Maternal environment and genotype interact to establish diabesity in mice. *Genome Res*. 2000;10:1568-1578.
671. Blair SC, Caterson ID, Cooney GJ. Glucose and lipid metabolism in the gold-thioglucose injected mouse model of diabesity. In: Shafir E, ed. *Lessons from Animal Diabetes VI*. Boston, MA: Birkhauser; 1996:239-267.
672. Burant CF, Sreenan S, Hirano K, et al. Troglitazone action is independent of adipose tissue. *J Clin Invest*. 1997;100:2900-2908.
673. Ross SR, Graves RA, Choy L, et al. Transgenic mouse models of disease: altering adipose tissue function in vivo. *Ann NY Acad Sci*. 1995;758:297-313.
674. Shimomura I, Hammer RE, Richardson JA, et al. Insulin resistance and diabetes mellitus in transgenic mice expressing nuclear SREBP-1c in adipose tissue: model for congenital generalized lipodystrophy. *Genes Dev*. 1998;12:3182-3194.
675. Reitman ML, Gavrilova O. A-ZIP/F-1 mice lacking white fat: a model for understanding lipoatrophic diabetes. *Int J Obes Relat Metab Disord*. 2000;24(suppl 4):S11-S14.
676. Gavrilova O, Marcus-Samuels B, Graham D, et al. Surgical implantation of adipose tissue reverses diabetes in lipoatrophic mice. *J Clin Invest*. 2000;105:271-278.
677. Shimomura I, Hammer RE, Ikemoto S, et al. Leptin reverses insulin resistance and diabetes mellitus in mice with congenital lipodystrophy. *Nature*. 1999;401:73-76.
678. Arioglu E, Duncan-Marin J, Sebring N, et al. Efficacy and safety of troglitazone in the treatment of lipodystrophy syndromes. *Ann Intern Med*. 2000;133:263-274.
679. Surwit RS, Feinglos MN, Rodin J, et al. Differential effects of fat and sucrose on the development of obesity and diabetes in C57BL/6J and A/J mice. *Metabolism*. 1995;44:645-651.
680. Rebuffe-Scrive M, Surwit R, Feinglos M, et al. Regional fat distribution and metabolism in a new mouse model (C57BL/6J) of non-insulin-dependent diabetes mellitus. *Metabolism*. 1993;42:1405-1409.
681. Wencel HE, Smothers C, Opara ED, et al. Impaired second phase insulin response of diabetes-prone C57BL/6J mouse islets. *Physiol Behav*. 1995;57:1215-1220.
682. Lee SK, Opara EC, Surwit RS, et al. Defective glucose-stimulated insulin release from perifused islets of C57BL/6J mice. *Pancreas*. 1995;11:206-211.
683. Parekh PI, Petro AE, Tiller JM, et al. Reversal of diet-induced obesity and diabetes in C57BL/6J mice. *Metabolism*. 1998;47:1089-1096.
684. Shibata M, Yasuda B. (Spontaneously occurring diabetes in NSY mice). *Jikken Dobutsu*. 1979;28:584-590.
685. Kim JH, Sen S, Avery CS, et al. Genetic analysis of a new mouse model for non-insulin-dependent diabetes. *Genomics*. 2001;74:273-286.
686. Phillips MS, Liu Q, Hammond HA, et al. Leptin receptor missense mutation in the fatty Zucker rat. *Nat Genet*. 1996;13:18-19.
687. Chua Jr SC, White DW, Wu-Peng XS, et al. Phenotype of fatty due to Gln269Pro mutation in the leptin receptor (Lepr). *Diabetes*. 1996;45:1141-1143.
688. White DW, Wang DW, Chua Jr SC, et al. Constitutive and impaired signaling of leptin receptors containing the Gln → Pro extracellular domain fatty mutation. *Proc Natl Acad Sci U S A*. 1997;94: 10657-10662.
689. Peterson RG, et al. Zucker diabetic fatty rat as a model for non-insulin-dependent diabetes mellitus. *ILAR News*. 1990;32:16-19.
690. Janssen SW, Hermus AR, Lange WP, et al. Progressive histopathological changes in pancreatic islets of Zucker diabetic fatty rats. *Exp Clin Endocrinol Diabetes*. 2001;109:273-282.
691. Zhou YP, Cockburn BN, Pugh W, et al. Basal insulin hypersecretion in insulin-resistant Zucker diabetic and Zucker fatty rats: role of enhanced fuel metabolism. *Metabolism*. 1999;48:857-864.

692. Unger RH. Lipotoxicity in the pathogenesis of obesity-dependent NIDDM: genetic and clinical implications. *Diabetes*. 1995;44: 863-870.
693. Corsetti JP, Sparks JD, Peterson RG, et al. Effect of dietary fat on the development of non-insulin dependent diabetes mellitus in obese Zucker diabetic fatty male and female rats. *Atherosclerosis*. 2000;148:231-241.
694. Griffen SC, Wang J, German MS. A genetic defect in beta-cell gene expression segregates independently from the fa locus in the ZDF rat. *Diabetes*. 2001;50:63-68.
695. Johnson JH, Ogawa A, Chen L, et al. Underexpression of beta cell high K_m glucose transporters in noninsulin-dependent diabetes. *Science*. 1990;250:546-549.
696. Orci L, Ravazzola M, Baetens D, et al. Evidence that down-regulation of beta-cell glucose transporters in non-insulin-dependent diabetes may be the cause of diabetic hyperglycemia. *Proc Natl Acad Sci U S A*. 1990;87:9953-9957.
697. Lee Y, Hirose H, Zhou YT, et al. Increased lipogenic capacity of the islets of obese rats: a role in the pathogenesis of NIDDM. *Diabetes*. 1997;46:408-413.
698. Sreenan S, Keck S, Fuller T, et al. Effects of troglitazone on substrate storage and utilization in insulin-resistant rats. *Am J Physiol*. 1999;276:E1119-E1129.
699. Shimabukuro M, Ohneda M, Lee Y, et al. Role of nitric oxide in obesity-induced beta cell disease. *J Clin Invest*. 1997;100:290-295.
700. Shimabukuro M, Higa M, Zhou YT, et al. Lipoapoptosis in beta-cells of obese prediabetic fa/fa rats: role of serine palmitoyltransferase overexpression. *J Biol Chem*. 1998;273:32487-32490.
701. Tokuyama Y, Sturis J, DePaoli AM, et al. Evolution of beta-cell dysfunction in the male Zucker diabetic fatty rat. *Diabetes*. 1995;44:1447-1457.
702. Sreenan S, Sturis J, Pugh W, et al. Prevention of hyperglycemia in the Zucker diabetic fatty rat by treatment with metformin or troglitazone. *Am J Physiol*. 1996;271:E742-E747.
703. Goto Y, Kakizaki M, Masaki N. Spontaneous diabetes produced by selective breeding of normal Wistar rats. *Proc Jpn Acad*. 1975;51:80-85.
704. Movassat J, Saulnier C, Serradas P, et al. Impaired development of pancreatic beta-cell mass is a primary event during the progression to diabetes in the GK rat. *Diabetologia*. 1997;40:916-925.
705. Movassat J, Saulnier C, Portha B. Beta-cell mass depletion precedes the onset of hyperglycaemia in the GK rat, a genetic model of non-insulin-dependent diabetes mellitus. *Diabet Metab*. 1995;21:365-370.
706. Ostenson CG, Khan A, Abdel-Halim SM, et al. Abnormal insulin secretion and glucose metabolism in pancreatic islets from the spontaneously diabetic GK rat. *Diabetologia*. 1993;36:3-8.
707. Ostenson CG, Abdel-Halim SM, Rasschaert J, et al. Deficient activity of FAD-linked glycerophosphate dehydrogenase in islets of GK rats. *Diabetologia*. 1993;36:722-726.
708. Abdel-Halim SM, Guenifi A, Efendic S, et al. Both somatostatin and insulin responses to glucose are impaired in the perfused pancreas of the spontaneously noninsulin-dependent diabetic GK (Goto-Kakizaki) rats. *Acta Physiol Scand*. 1993;148:219-226.
709. Nagamatsu S, Nakamichi Y, Yamamura C, et al. Decreased expression of t-SNARE, syntaxin 1, and SNAP-25 in pancreatic beta-cells is involved in impaired insulin secretion from diabetic GK rat islets: restoration of decreased t-SNARE proteins improves impaired insulin secretion. *Diabetes*. 1999;48:2367-2373.
710. Guenifi A, Portela-Gomes GM, Grimelius L, et al. Adenylyl cyclase isoform expression in non-diabetic and diabetic Goto-Kakizaki (GK) rat pancreas: evidence for distinct overexpression of type-8 adenylyl cyclase in diabetic GK rat islets. *Histochem Cell Biol*. 2000;113:81-89.
711. Song XM, Kawano Y, Krook A, et al. Muscle fiber type-specific defects in insulin signal transduction to glucose transport in diabetic GK rats. *Diabetes*. 1999;48:664-670.
712. Begum N, Ragolia L. Altered regulation of insulin signaling components in adipocytes of insulin-resistant type II diabetic Goto-Kakizaki rats. *Metabolism*. 1998;47:54-62.
713. Berdanier CD. The BHE strain to rat: an example of the role of inheritance in determining metabolic controls. *Fed Proc*. 1976;35: 2295-2299.
714. Berdanier CD, Tobin RB, DeVore V. Effects of age, strain, and dietary carbohydrate on the hepatic metabolism of male rats. *J Nutr*. 1979;109:261-271.
715. Mathews CE, McGraw RA, Dean R, et al. Inheritance of a mitochondrial DNA defect and impaired glucose tolerance in BHE/Cdb rats. *Diabetologia*. 1999;42:35-40.
716. McCusker RH, Deaver OE Jr, Berdanier CD. Effect of sucrose or starch feeding on the hepatic mitochondrial activity of BHE and Wistar rats. *J Nutr*. 1983;113:1327-1334.
717. Borenshtein D, Ofri R, Werman M, et al. Cataract development in diabetic sand rats treated with alpha-lipoic acid and its gamma-linolenic acid conjugate. *Diabetes Metab Res Rev*. 2001;17:44-50.
718. Ikeda Y, Olsen GS, Ziv E, et al. Cellular mechanism of nutritionally induced insulin resistance in *Psammomys obesus:* overexpression of protein kinase Cepsilon in skeletal muscle precedes the onset of hyperinsulinemia and hyperglycemia. *Diabetes*. 2001;50:584-592.
719. Kanety H, Moshe S, Shafrir E, et al. Hyperinsulinemia induces a reversible impairment in insulin receptor function leading to diabetes in the sand rat model of non-insulin-dependent diabetes mellitus. *Proc Natl Acad Sci U S A*. 1994;91:1853-1857.
720. Kawano K, Hirashima T, Mori S, et al. Spontaneous long-term hyperglycemic rat with diabetic complications: Otsuka Long-Evans Tokushima Fatty (OLETF) strain. *Diabetes*. 1992;41:1422-1428.
721. Moralejo DH, Ogino T, Zhu M, et al. A major quantitative trait locus co-localizing with cholecystokinin type A receptor gene influences poor pancreatic proliferation in a spontaneously diabetogenic rat. *Mamm Genome*. 1998;9:794-798.
722. Takiguchi S, Takata Y, Takahashi N, et al. A disrupted cholecystokinin A receptor gene induces diabetes in obese rats synergistically with *ODB1* gene. *Am J Physiol*. 1998;274:E265-E270.
723. Takiguchi S, Takata Y, Funakoshi A, et al. Disrupted cholecystokinin type-A receptor (CCKAR) gene in OLETF rats. *Gene*. 1997;197:169-175.
724. Hirashima T, Kawano K, Mori S, et al. A diabetogenic gene, ODB2, identified on chromosome 14 of the OLETF rat and its synergistic action with ODB1. *Biochem Biophys Res Commun*. 1996;224:420-425.
725. Shi K, Mizuno A, Sano T, et al. Sexual difference in the incidence of diabetes mellitus in Otsuka-Long-Evans-Tokushima-Fatty rats: effects of castration and sex hormone replacement on its incidence. *Metabolism*. 1994;43:1214-1220.
726. Ishida K, Mizuno A, Murakami T, et al. Obesity is necessary but not sufficient for the development of diabetes mellitus. *Metabolism*. 1996;45:1288-1295.
727. Okauchi N, Mizuno A, Zhu M, et al. Effects of obesity and inheritance on the development of non-insulin-dependent diabetes mellitus in Otsuka-Long-Evans-Tokushima fatty rats. *Diabetes Res Clin Pract*. 1995;29:1-10.
728. Kosegawa I, Chen S, Awata T, et al. Troglitazone and metformin, but not glibenclamide, decrease blood pressure in Otsuka Long Evans Tokushima fatty rats. *Clin Exp Hypertens*. 1999;21:199-211.
729. Triadou N, Portha B, Picon L, et al. Experimental chemical diabetes and pregnancy in the rat: evolution of glucose tolerance and insulin response. *Diabetes*. 1982;31:75-79.
730. Portha B, Picon L, Rosselin G. Chemical diabetes in the adult rat as the spontaneous evolution of neonatal diabetes. *Diabetologia*. 1979;17:371-377.
731. Kodama T, Iwase M, Nunoi K, et al. A new diabetes model induced by neonatal alloxan treatment in rats. *Diabetes Res Clin Pract*. 1993;20:183-189.
732. Iwase M, Nunoi K, Wakisaka M, et al. Spontaneous recovery from non-insulin-dependent diabetes mellitus induced by neonatal streptozotocin treatment in spontaneously hypertensive rats. *Metabolism*. 1991;40:10-14.
733. Centers for Disease Control and Prevention. *National diabetes fact sheet: general information and national estimates on diabetes in the United States, 2007*. Atlanta, GA: U.S. Department of Health and Human Services, Centers for Disease Control and Prevention; 2007.
734. Gregg EW, Albright AL. The public health response to diabetes: two steps forward, one step back. *JAMA*. 2009;301:1596-1598.
735. Huang ES, Basu A, O'Grady M, et al. Projecting the future diabetes population size and related costs for the U.S. *Diabetes Care*. 2009;32:2225-2229.
736. American Diabetes Association. Economic costs of diabetes in the U.S. in 2007. *Diabetes Care*. 2008;31:596-615.
737. U.K. Prospective Diabetes Study (UKPDS) Group. Intensive blood-glucose control with sulphonylureas or insulin compared with conventional treatment and risk of complications in patients with type 2 diabetes (UKPDS 33). *Lancet*. 1998;352:837-853.
738. U.K. Prospective Diabetes Study (UKPDS) Group. Effect of intensive blood-glucose control with metformin on complications in overweight patients with type 2 diabetes (UKPDS 34). *Lancet*. 1998;352:854-865.
739. Ohkubo Y, Kishikawa H, Araki E, et al. Intensive insulin therapy prevents the progression of diabetic microvascular complications in Japanese patients with non-insulin-dependent diabetes mellitus: a randomized prospective 6-year study. *Diabetes Res Clin Pract*. 1995;28:103-117.
740. Action to Control Cardiovascular Risk in Diabetes Study Group, Gerstein HC, Miller ME, Byington RP, et al. Effects of intensive glucose lowering in type 2 diabetes. *N Engl J Med*. 2008;358:2545-2559.
741. ADVANCE Collaborative Group, Patel A, MacMahon S, Chalmers J, et al. Intensive blood glucose control and vascular outcomes in patients with type 2 diabetes. *N Engl J Med*. 2008;358:2560-2572.
742. Duckworth W, Abraira C, Moritz T, et al. Intensive glucose control and complications in American veterans with type 2 diabetes. *N Engl J Med*. 2009;360:129-139.
743. Holman RR, Paul SK, Bethel MA, et al. 10-Year follow-up of intensive glucose control in type 2 diabetes. *N Engl J Med*. 2008;359: 1577-1589.

744. Ray KK, Seshasai SR, Wijesuriya S, et al. Effect of intensive control of glucose on cardiovascular outcomes and death in patients with diabetes mellitus: a meta-analysis of randomised controlled trials. *Lancet.* 2009;373:1765-1772.
745. Rodbard HW, Jellinger PS, Davidson JA, et al. Statement by an American Association of Clinical Endocrinologists/American College of Endocrinology Consensus Panel on Type 2 Diabetes Mellitus: an algorithm for glycemic control. *Endocr Pract.* 2009;15:540-559.
746. Rodbard HW, Blonde L, Braithwaite SS, et al, AACE Diabetes Mellitus Clinical Practice Guidelines Task Force. American Association of Clinical Endocrinologists medical guidelines for clinical practice for the management of diabetes mellitus. *Endocr Pract.* 2007;13(suppl 1): 1-68.
747. Nathan DM, Buse JB, Davidson MB, et al. Management of hyperglycemia in type 2 diabetes mellitus: a consensus algorithm for the initiation and adjustment of therapy. *Diabetes Care.* 2006;29:1963-1972.
748. Rohlfing CL, Wiedmeyer HM, Little RR, et al. Defining the relationship between plasma glucose and HbA_{1c}: analysis of glucose profiles and HbA_{1c} in the Diabetes Control and Complications Trial. *Diabetes Care.* 2002;25:275-278.
749. Service FJ, Hall LD, Westland RE, et al. Effects of size, time of day and sequence of meal ingestion on carbohydrate tolerance in normal subjects. *Diabetologia.* 1983;25:316-321.
750. American Diabetes Association. Postprandial blood glucose. *Diabetes Care.* 2001;24:775-778.
751. Funnell MM, Brown TL, Childs BP, et al. National standards for diabetes self-management education. *Diabetes Care.* 2010;33(suppl 1): S89-S96.
752. Boren SA, Fitzner KA, Panhalkar PS, et al. Costs and benefits associated with diabetes education: a review of the literature. *Diabetes Educ.* 2009;35:72-96.
753. Delamater AM, Jacobson AM, Anderson B, et al. Psychosocial therapies in diabetes: report of the Psychosocial Therapies Working Group. *Diabetes Care.* 2001;24:1286-1292.
754. American Diabetes Association. Nutrition Recommendations and Interventions for Diabetes: A position statement of the American Diabetes Association. *Diabetes Care.* 2008 31:S61-S78.
755. Gillespie SJ, Kulkarni KD, Daly AE. Using carbohydrate counting in diabetes clinical practice. *J Am Diet Assoc.* 1998;98:897-905.
756. Nahas R, Moher M. Complementary and alternative medicine for the treatment of type 2 diabetes. *Can Fam Physician.* 2009;55:591-596.
757. Barringer TA, Kirk JK, Santaniello AC, et al. Effect of a multivitamin and mineral supplement on infection and quality of life: a randomized, double-blind, placebo-controlled trial. *Ann Intern Med.* 2003;138:365-371.
758. Connor WE, Connor SL. Should a low-fat, high-carbohydrate diet be recommended for everyone? The case for a low-fat, high-carbohydrate diet. *N Engl J Med.* 1997;337:562-563; discussion, 566-567.
759. Sigal RJ, Kenny GP, Wasserman DH, et al. Physical activity/exercise and type 2 diabetes: a consensus statement from the American Diabetes Association. *Diabetes Care.* 2006;29:1433-1438.
760. Bax JJ, Young LH, Frye RL, et al, American Diabetes Association. Screening for coronary artery disease in patients with diabetes. *Diabetes Care.* 2007;30:2729-2736.
761. Nathan DM, Buse JB, Davidson MB, et al, European Association for Study of Diabetes. Medical management of hyperglycemia in type 2 diabetes: a consensus algorithm for the initiation and adjustment of therapy. A Consensus Statement of the American Diabetes Association and the European Association for the Study of Diabetes. *Diabetes Care.* 2009;32:193-203.
762. Phung OJ, Scholle JM, Talwar M, et al. Effect of noninsulin antidiabetic drugs added to metformin therapy on glycemic control, weight gain, and hypoglycemia in type 2 diabetes. *JAMA.* 2010;303:1410-1418.
763. Bergenstal RM, Bailey CJ, Kendall DM. Type 2 diabetes: assessing the relative risks and benefits of glucose-lowering medications. *Am J Med.* 2010;123:374.e9-374.e18.
764. Long YC, Zierath JR. AMP-activated protein kinase signaling in metabolic regulation. *J Clin Invest.* 2006;116:1776-1783.
765. Salpeter SR, Greyber E, Pasternak GA, et al. Risk of fatal and nonfatal lactic acidosis with metformin use in type 2 diabetes mellitus. Cochrane Database Syst Rev. 2010;(4):CD002967.
766. George JT, McKay GA. Establishing pragmatic estimated glomerular filtration rate thresholds to guide metformin prescribing: careful assessment of risks and benefits is required. *Diabet Med.* 2008;25: 636-637.
767. de Jager J, Kooy A, Lehert P, et al. Long term treatment with metformin in patients with type 2 diabetes and risk of vitamin B-12 deficiency: randomised placebo controlled trial. *BMJ.* 2010;340:c2181.
768. Goldberg RB, Kendall DM, Deeg MA, et al, GLAI Study Investigators. A comparison of lipid and glycemic effects of pioglitazone and rosiglitazone in patients with type 2 diabetes and dyslipidemia. *Diabetes Care.* 2005;28:1547-1554.
769. Dormandy JA, Charbonnel B, Eckland DJ, et al. Secondary prevention of macrovascular events in patients with type 2 diabetes in the PROactive Study (PROspective pioglitAzone Clinical Trial In macroVascular Events): a randomised controlled trial. *Lancet.* 2005;366: 1279-1289.
770. Home PD, Pocock SJ, Beck-Nielsen H, et al, RECORD Study Team. Rosiglitazone evaluated for cardiovascular outcomes in oral agent combination therapy for type 2 diabetes (RECORD): a multicentre, randomised, open-label trial. *Lancet.* 2009;373:2125-2135.
771. Graham DJ, Ouellet-Hellstrom R, Macurdy TE, et al. Risk of acute nyocardial infarction, stroke, heart failure, and death in elderly Medicare patients treated with rosiglitazone or pioglitazone. *JAMA.* 2010;304:411-418.
772. Kahn SE, Haffner SM, Heise MA, et al, ADOPT Study Group. Glycemic durability of rosiglitazone, metformin, or glyburide monotherapy. *N Engl J Med.* 2006;355:2427-2443.
773. Karalliedde J, Buckingham RE. Thiazolidinediones and their fluid-related adverse effects: facts, fiction and putative management strategies. *Drug Saf.* 2007;30:741-753.
774. Riche DM, Travis King S. Bone loss and fracture risk associated with thiazolidinedione therapy. *Pharmacotherapy.* 2010;30:716-727.
775. Higgins LS, Depaoli AM. Selective peroxisome proliferator-activated receptor gamma (PPARgamma) modulation as a strategy for safer therapeutic PPARgamma activation. *Am J Clin Nutr.* 2010;91:267S-272S.
776. Riddle MC. Sulfonylureas differ in effects on ischemic preconditioning: is it time to retire glyburide? (Editorial). *J Clin Endocrinol Metab.* 2003;88:528-530.
777. Skyler JS, Bergenstal R, Bonow RO, et al, American Diabetes Association; American College of Cardiology Foundation; American Heart Association. Intensive glycemic control and the prevention of cardiovascular events: implications of the ACCORD, ADVANCE, and VA diabetes trials. A position statement of the American Diabetes Association and a scientific statement of the American College of Cardiology Foundation and the American Heart Association. *Diabetes Care.* 2009;32:187-192.
778. Hanefeld M, Schaper F. Acarbose: oral anti-diabetes drug with additional cardiovascular benefits. *Expert Rev Cardiovasc Ther.* 2008;6:153-163.
779. Hirsch IB, Bergenstal RM, Parkin CG, et al. A real-world approach to insulin therapy in primary care practice. *Clin Diabetes.* 2005;23: 78-86.
780. Bergenstal RM. Treatment models from the International Diabetes Center: advancing from oral agents to insulin therapy in type 2 diabetes. *Endocr Pract.* 2006;12(suppl 1):98-104.
781. Drucker DJ, Sherman SI, Gorelick FS, et al. Incretin-based therapies for the treatment of type 2 diabetes: evaluation of the risks and benefits. *Diabetes Care.* 2010;33:428-433.
782. Buse JB, Rosenstock J, Sesti G, et al, LEAD-6 Study Group. Liraglutide once a day versus exenatide twice a day for type 2 diabetes: a 26-week randomised, parallel-group, multinational, open-label trial (LEAD-6). *Lancet.* 2009;374:39-47.
783. Drucker DJ, Buse JB, Taylor K, et al, DURATION-1 Study Group. Exenatide once weekly versus twice daily for the treatment of type 2 diabetes: a randomised, open-label, non-inferiority study. *Lancet.* 2008;372: 1240-1250.
784. Palalau AI, Tahrani AA, Piya MK, et al. DPP-4 inhibitors in clinical practice. *Postgrad Med.* 2009;121:70-100.
785. Fonseca VA, Zinman B, Nauck MA, et al. Confronting the type 2 diabetes epidemic: the emerging role of incretin-based therapies. *Am J Med.* 2010;123:S2-S10.
786. Ryan G, Briscoe TA, Jobe L. Review of pramlintide as adjunctive therapy in treatment of type 1 and type 2 diabetes. *Drug Des Devel Ther.* 2009;2:203-214.
787. Fonseca VA, Handelsman Y, Staels B. Colesevelam lowers glucose and lipid levels in type 2 diabetes: the clinical evidence. *Diabetes Obes Metab.* 2010;12:384-392.
788. Gaziano JM, Cincotta AH, O'Connor CM, et al. Randomized clinical trial of quick-release bromocriptine among patients with type 2 diabetes on overall safety and cardiovascular outcomes. *Diabetes Care.* 2010;33:1503-1508.
789. BARI 2D Study Group, Frye RL, August P, et al. A randomized trial of therapies for type 2 diabetes and coronary artery disease. *N Engl J Med.* 2009;360:2503-2515.
790. Holman RR, Farmer AJ, Davies MJ, et al, 4-T Study Group. Three-year efficacy of complex insulin regimens in type 2 diabetes. *N Engl J Med.* 2009;361:1736-1747.
791. Buse JB, Hroscikoski M. The case for a role for postprandial glucose monitoring in diabetes management. *J Fam Pract.* 1998;47(5 suppl):S29-S36.
792. Chatterjee R, Narayan KM, Lipscomb J, et al. Screening adults for pre-diabetes and diabetes may be cost-saving. *Diabetes Care.* 2010;33:1484-1490.
793. Narayan KM, Gregg EW, Engelgau MM, et al. Translation research for chronic disease: the case of diabetes. *Diabetes Care.* 2000;23: 1794-1798.

794. 2010 Report: Medicines in Development for Diabetes. Available at: http://www.phrma.org/sites/phrma.org/files/attachments/Diabetes_2010.pdf (accessed November 2010).
795. Doria A, Patti ME, Kahn CR. The emerging genetic architecture of type 2 diabetes. *Cell Metab*. 2008;8:186-200.
796. Perry JR, Frayling TM. New gene variants alter type 2 diabetes risk predominantly through reduced beta-cell function. *Curr Opin Clin Nutr Metab Care*. 2008;11:371-377.
797. Stancáková A, Kuulasmaa T, Paananen J, et al. Association of 18 confirmed susceptibility loci for type 2 diabetes with indices of insulin release, proinsulin conversion, and insulin sensivitity in 5,327 nondiabetic Finnish men. *Diabetes*. Jan 2009;58:2129-2136.
798. Simonis-Bik AM, Nijpels G, van Haeften TW, et al. Gene variants in the novel type 2 diabetes loci CDC123/CAMK1D, THADA, ADAMTS9, BCL11A, and MTNR1B affect different aspects of pancreatic beta-cell function. *Diabetes*. 2010;59:293-301.
799. Ingelsson E, Langenberg C, Hivert MF, et al. Detailed physiologic characterization reveals diverse mechanisms for novel genetic loci regulating glucose and insulin metabolism in humans. *Diabetes*. 2010;59:1266-1275.

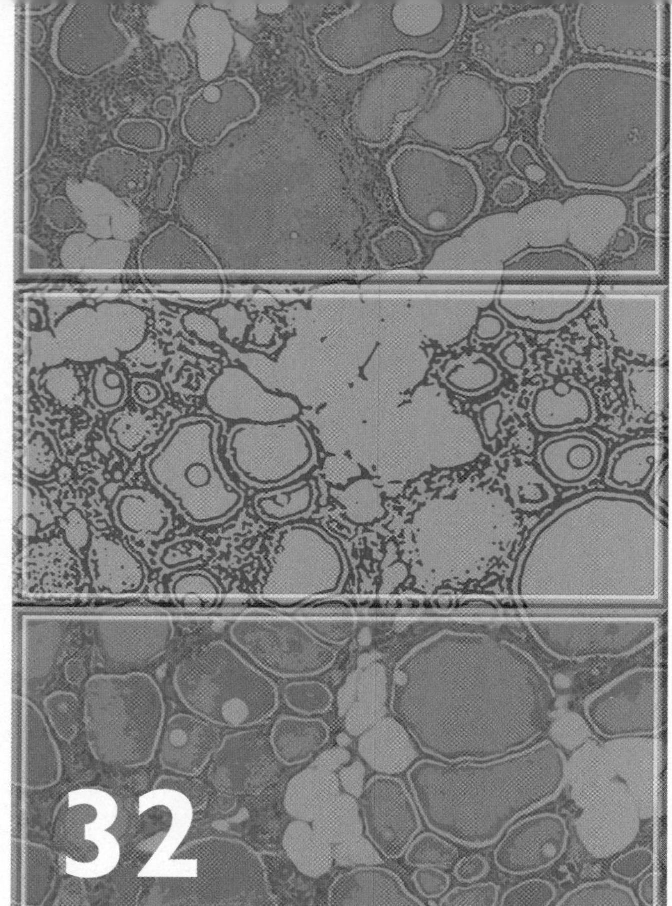

CHAPTER 32

Type 1 Diabetes Mellitus

GEORGE S. EISENBARTH • JOHN B. BUSE

In 1984, Sutherland and coworkers[1] transplanted the tail of the pancreas from nondiabetic identical twins to their twin mates who had type 1 diabetes mellitus (T1DM). In contrast to the transplantation of organs such as kidneys, in which the transplants are accepted between identical twins, the pancreatic islets (but not acinar pancreas) were rapidly destroyed.[1] The diabetes of the twin transplant recipients was cured for only a matter of weeks. In retrospect, these results were predictable, given the autoimmune nature of type 1A diabetes and similar results in animal models of the disorder.[2] Since that time, T1DM became one of the most intensively studied autoimmune disorders, and the National Institutes of Health has designated type 1A diabetes a Priority One target for the development of a preventive immunologic vaccine. Knowledge of the immunogenetics and immunopathogenesis of type 1A diabetes is beginning to influence clinical care,[3] greatly influences current clinical research, and will, we hope, lead to successful strategies for disease prevention.[4]

DIFFERENTIAL DIAGNOSIS OF TYPE 1 DIABETES

An expert committee of the American Diabetes Association (ADA), with its etiologic diagnostic criteria (Table 32-1), has recommended dividing T1DM into type 1A (immune-mediated) and type 1B (other forms of diabetes with severe insulin deficiency).[5] At the onset of diabetes, distinguishing type 1A diabetes from type 2 diabetes (T2DM), let alone type 1B diabetes, is not always a simple task. The best current criterion for diagnosis of type 1A diabetes is the presence of anti-islet autoantibodies measured with highly specific (and reasonably sensitive) autoantibody radioassays.[6]

The presence of autoantibodies with assays defined as positive in fewer than 1 of 100 control subjects (specificity ≥99%) is reasonably diagnostic of type 1A diabetes. Non-Hispanic white children presenting with diabetes usually have type 1A diabetes, whereas adults older than 40 years usually have T2DM.[7] More than 90% of such children presenting with diabetes express one of four measured anti-islet autoantibodies (see later discussion). In contrast, among black or Latin American children, almost one half lack any autoantibody.[8-10] Most of these children appear to have an early age at onset of type 2 diabetes mellitus, many have attendant risk factors such as obesity, and many lack human leukocyte antigen (HLA) alleles associated with type 1A diabetes (discussed later).

Imagawa and coworkers[11] described an unusual form of diabetes in which the patients had a normal glycosylated hemoglobin (HbA_{1c}) level despite severe hyperglycemia,

TABLE 32-1
Differential Diagnosis of Type 1A Diabetes

Diabetes Type	Anti-Islet Autoantibodies	Genetics	Comments
Type 1A	Positive >90%	HLA 30-50% DR3 *and* DR4 HLA 90% DR3 *or* DR4 HLA <3% DQB1*0602	90% non-Hispanic white children 50% black children 50% Latin American children
Type 1B	Negative	Unknown	Rare in whites
Type 2	Negative	Unknown	If Ab⁺, likely LADA, and HLA is similar to type 1A
Other	Negative	MODY mutations, other syndromes	

Ab, antibody; HLA, human leukocyte antigen; LADA, latent autoimmune diabetes adult; MODY, maturity-onset diabetes of the young.

suggesting that the diabetes had been present for only a short time. Histologic examination of pancreatic sections demonstrated pancreatitis but no insulitis, and anti-islet autoantibodies were not detected. It is not clear whether this represents one of the first examples of type 1B diabetes, although a fulminant type 1A is possible and later studies indicated that a large fraction of these patients have HLA alleles associated with type 1A diabetes.

Obesity does not protect a person from developing type 1A diabetes, although it is usually associated with insulin-resistant forms of diabetes. It is also important to realize that patients can have both insulin resistance and type 1A diabetes, and such autoantibody-positive patients with both conditions can present with diabetes with high levels of fasting insulin or C peptide but loss of stimulated insulin secretion. With current assays for anti-islet autoantibodies, a subset of children with type 1A diabetes will test negative for the autoantibodies. Uncommonly, some children, when they progress to diabetes, lose expression of all autoantibodies by the time of diagnosis.[12] Such type 1A autoantibody-negative children typically have HLA alleles associated with type 1A diabetes; are not insulin resistant; may present with ketoacidosis; and, with time, lose C-peptide secretion. However, the diagnosis is not clear at diabetes onset, and with current laboratory tests, designations such as positive or negative for anti-islet autoantibodies are more accurate.

ANIMAL MODELS OF TYPE 1A DIABETES

In relation to other autoimmune disorders, type 1A diabetes is unusual in having a series of spontaneous animal models of the disease.[13-16] These animal models provide clues to potential mechanisms of pathogenesis and allow testing of therapies for disease prevention. As for most animal models, only some therapeutic results translate into efficacy in humans.[14] It should also be recognized that many of the spontaneous animal models are inbred and are not diallelic at any locus, whereas all humans have different alleles at tens of thousands of loci. Therefore, each animal model might or might not provide insights into one of the forms of human diabetes.

Despite these caveats, the animal models are remarkably similar to humans in a number of key immunologic parameters. The most notable include the importance of the major histocompatibility complex (MHC) for disease and the presence of lymphocytic islet invasion followed by specific destruction of islet beta cells. For reasons that are currently unclear given specific HLA molecules, humans, rats, and mice have a marked propensity for autoimmunity directed at islet beta cells. This propensity may be related to a specific lack of tolerance to a single islet molecule such as insulin, to a specific sensitivity of islet beta cells to immune-mediated destruction, or to factors not currently appreciated. It is likely that understanding of this propensity will lead to effective therapies.

Polygenic Spontaneous Animal Models: Nonobese Diabetic Mouse

The nonobese diabetic (NOD) mouse is the most intensively studied animal model.[17] As with type 1A diabetes of humans, specific HLA class II and class I molecules are central for disease pathogenesis (see later discussion).[18,19] The NOD mouse has mutations that cause absence of the I-E (histocompatibility) molecule (similar to human DR) and an unusual I-A molecule (similar to human DQ).[20] The I-A molecule in the NOD mouse is termed I-A^g,[7] which designates a specific amino acid sequence. HLA class II molecules (in humans there are three—DP, DQ, and DR) function to bind peptides and present these peptides to the T-cell receptor of CD4-positive (helper or Th2) T lymphocytes. The HLA genes were termed *immune response genes* because common variations in their sequences (allelic variation) determine the peptides to which an individual mouse or person can mount a T-cell response. Therefore, a central role for these molecules in immune function and autoimmunity is expected.

If the lack of I-E expression is corrected in the NOD mouse with introduction of an I-E transgene, diabetes is prevented.[21] If a different I-A sequence is introduced as a transgene into the NOD mouse, diabetes is also prevented.[22] In addition to these class II molecules determining diabetes susceptibility, more than 15 other genetic loci contribute to disease, each with a relatively small contribution, each neither necessary nor sufficient.[23-26] Therefore, inheritance of diabetes in the NOD mouse is polygenic. One way the NOD mouse differs from humans is that more female than male NOD mice develop diabetes.

NOD mice, like humans, produce anti-insulin autoantibodies before developing diabetes.[27] Autoantibodies usually appear between 6 and 8 weeks of age, and diabetes usually develops after 16 weeks of age. Studies of islet beta-cell mass indicate that islet beta-cell destruction and beta-cell regeneration are present months before the onset of diabetes,[28] although there is convincing evidence of an acceleration of beta-cell destruction at disease onset.[29-31] T cells, and not autoantibodies, mediate islet beta-cell destruction, and clones of T cells that react with several antigens are able to transfer disease.[32-35] A large number of T-cell clones that react with insulin[36] or with other antigens have been characterized. There is debate about whether any given autoantigen is primary, although studies have provided evidence for a central role of T-cell autoimmunity directed at insulin.[36] In addition, lymphocytes and autoantibodies contribute to pathogenesis.

Diabetes can be prevented in the NOD mouse by more than 100 different therapies.[14] Most, but not all, of these therapies target the immune system, and a number of them are now in clinical trials in humans. Consistent with mediation of diabetes by T lymphocytes, immunosuppression or genes that block T-cell function prevent disease.

Some of the most interesting therapies use autoantigens as vaccines; in particular, both glutamic acid decarboxylase (GAD) and insulin, when administered to the NOD mice, prevented diabetes.[37-40] The insulin molecule does not have to be metabolically active, and a dominant insulin peptide, insulin peptide B(9-23), given as a single subcutaneous injection, prevented diabetes in 90% of susceptible NOD mice.[32] It is thought that vaccination prevents diabetes by generating Th2 T lymphocytes that produce transforming growth factor-β (TGF-β); these T cells target an islet molecule (e.g., insulin) but produce protective cytokines (e.g., interleukin 4 [IL4], IL-10, TGF-β) when they home to the islets.

Oligogenic Animal Models

BioBreeding Rat

The BioBreeding (BB) rat was the first intensively studied animal model of type 1A diabetes. The diabetes in this model differs from human diabetes in that diabetes-prone BB rats have an autosomal recessive mutation that produces a severe T-cell lymphopenia.[42] Infection with a number of viruses, presumably activating innate immunity, can induce diabetes in a related strain of rat that does not have lymphopenia, termed the *BB diabetes-resistant* (BB-DR) rat. As in humans and the NOD mouse, the disease depends on specific class II alleles (similar to human HLA-DR and HLA-DQ) of the MHC, in particular RT1-U. Diabetes can be induced to develop in a series of rat strains with RT1-U (see later discussion). Anti-inflammatory drugs given after infection can prevent diabetes, and this might have relevance to humans if the timing of the triggering of autoimmunity could be defined. Additional genes segregate to create diabetes susceptibility in these rat strains, but the number of genes is much less than for NOD mice.[41-43]

Prevention of diabetes in BB rats is more difficult than in NOD mice, possibly related to the severe T-cell lymphopenia, which results from mutation of an *Ian* gene inherited in an autosomal recessive manner.[44] For example, insulin administration to BB rats prevented both diabetes and insulitis, but, in contrast to NOD mice, metabolically active insulin and insulin doses high enough to induce hypoglycemia were usually required for prevention.[45,46]

Long-Evans Tokushima Lean Rat

Like BB rats, the Long-Evans Tokushima Lean (LETL) rat strain has the RT-1U alleles and has an oligogenic inheritance of diabetes with mutation of a gene (*Cbl-b*) that alters T-cell signaling.[47-49]

Induced Models of Type 1A Diabetes

Diabetes or insulitis can be induced in several strains of animals by means of drugs that induce islet destruction and broadly activate immune responses or by specific islet antigens. The drug streptozotocin is directly toxic to islet beta cells. In high doses, it rapidly induces diabetes. In low doses, a more chronic diabetes develops that is likely to have some immunologic derivation.[50,51] Administration of copolymer of polyinosinic and polycytidylic acids (poly-IC), a simple polynucleotide that activates production of interferon-α (IFN-α) when administered to a number of rat strains with the diabetes-susceptible RT1-U alleles, induced insulitis and diabetes.[52] This suggests that many animals are susceptible to diabetes or insulitis given a strong immunologic stimulus. Treatment with IFN-α in humans has been associated with the development of anti-islet autoantibodies and with acceleration of diabetes development in patients with anti-islet autoantibodies.[53]

HISTOPATHOLOGY OF TYPE 1A DIABETES

As in animal models, type 1A diabetes of humans is characterized by selective destruction of the beta cells within islets.[54-57] The non–insulin-producing cells of the islets remain in patients with long-standing T1DM, and these remaining islets, lacking insulitis and beta cells, are termed *pseudoatrophic*. A remarkable feature of the pancreas of patients with new-onset diabetes is heterogeneity of islet lesions. Within the same section of pancreas, a normal islet with no infiltrate can coexist with an islet containing beta cells with intense infiltration and a pseudoatrophic islet that has no infiltrate. This spottiness of the pathologic process is reminiscent of the destruction of areas of the skin in patients with vitiligo, in which melanocytes are destroyed in patches. Such heterogeneity of lesions may underlie the chronic development of type 1A diabetes in humans.

Islets of patients with type 1A diabetes overexpress class I HLA antigens, rarely if ever express class II HLA molecules on beta cells, express IFN-α, and are reported to upregulate Fas molecules on all islet cells.[55,58-60] The hypothesis that class II HLA expression contributes directly to beta-cell autoimmunity is controversial. The specific way in which the immune system destroys beta cells is not known, but molecules such as Fas may be important, because T cells expressing Fas ligand may induce apoptosis of beta cells.[61-63] Cytokines (e.g., IL-1) and CD8+ cytotoxic lymphocytes are also likely to contribute to beta cell destruction.[64-70]

Searches for viral particles and viral RNA within islets of patients with new-onset diabetes have been unrewarding, but newer technologies and concepts should facilitate additional studies, and it is likely that there is heterogeneity among patients.[70,71] In contrast to the islets of patients with new-onset diabetes, the pancreata of identical twin donors have been described as normal, and the pancreata from the few studied patients with long-standing diabetes were composed of pseudoatrophic islets without markers of immune activation, with a subset of patients having retained islet beta cells within patches[54] with relatively little insulitis.

GENETICS OF TYPE 1A DIABETES

It has long been recognized that diabetes is a heterogeneous group of disorders. It is also becoming apparent that type 1A diabetes is heterogeneous. There are probably many genetic forms of type 1A diabetes, and most forms are influenced by HLA class II molecules.[72] This group of disorders is likely to be linked by the presence of immunologic abnormalities that foster loss of tolerance to self-antigens. Patients with specific HLA class I and class II molecules with immune dysfunction are susceptible to target islet autoantigens.

Many of the genes underlying diabetes susceptibility are similar in diverse countries, although specific alleles of those genes differ in their frequency.[73] Several monogenic forms of type 1A diabetes can now be identified. It is not clear whether these genetically characterized forms of diabetes should now be included in the group of other defined causes of diabetes.[5]

Monogenic Forms of Type 1A Diabetes

Autoimmune Polyendocrine Syndrome Type I (AIRE Gene)

The autoimmune polyendocrine syndrome type 1 (APS-1) is rare, with an increased incidence in Finland and Sardinia and among Iranian Jews, but it has a worldwide occurrence. The disorders of the syndrome, such as T1DM, mucocutaneous candidiasis, hypoparathyroidism, Addison's disease, and hepatitis (see Chapter 37 for a more detailed discussion) identify a unique syndrome, and patients with this group of disorders almost always have mutations (usually autosomal recessive, although one family with dominant mutation has been identified) of the autoimmune regulator gene *(AIRE)* on chromosome 21. This gene encodes a DNA-binding protein. Studies of this gene with its expression in the thymus indicate that it may play an important role in maintaining self-tolerance and influences the expression of what are termed *peripheral antigens* (e.g., insulin) in the thymus. It is hypothesized that greater expression of insulin and other tissue-specific antigens leads to tolerance and disease suppression.[74]

There is considerable variability in the diseases expressed even for siblings with the same mutation. Some of this variability is likely to be influenced by genetic loci other than the *AIRE* gene. One example is the observation that although 18% of patients with APS-1 develop T1DM, those with the common diabetes-protective HLA allele DQB*10602 appear to have some protection from diabetes but not from Addison's disease.

X-Linked Polyendocrinopathy, Immune Dysfunction, and Diarrhea (Scurfy Gene)

The syndrome of X-linked polyendocrinopathy, immune dysfunction, and diarrhea (XPID, also termed IPEX) is associated with overwhelming neonatal autoimmunity, and most children die in the first few days of life or in infancy.[75-78] In this syndrome, lymphocytes invade multiple organs. It is associated with insulitis and beta-cell destruction as well as lymphocytic intestinal inflammation with flattened villi and severe malabsorption. It is inherited as an X-linked recessive disease affecting only boys, with a frequent clinical history of lack of male births.

The disease results from mutations of the gene encoding forkhead box P3 *(FOXP3)*, whose function as a transcription factor has been elucidated.[75,79,80] This gene functions as a master switch for regulatory (suppressor) CD4+/CD25+ T lymphocytes. Lack of such regulatory T cells leads to overwhelming autoimmunity in humans and mice. This is an important syndrome to recognize, because bone marrow transplantation with restoration of T-regulatory cells (even with partial chimerism) is therapeutic.

Idiopathic Type 1A Diabetes

Descriptive Genetics

In the United States, the risk of childhood diabetes is approximately 1 in 300.[81] This is 15-fold less than the diabetes risk for a first-degree relative of a patient with T1DM (Table 32-2). It is 150-fold less than the risk for a monozygotic twin of a patient with T1DM.[82,83] Although the population risk of T1DM in Japan is 15-fold less than in the United States, the risk for an identical twin in Japan is similar to that for an identical twin in the United States.[84,85] This suggests that when genetic susceptibility is present, either in Japan or in the United States, the diabetes risk is extremely high.

TABLE 32-2

Risk of Type 1A Diabetes

Proband with DM	% Childhood DM (Annual Incidence)	Anti-Islet Autoantibody	Comment
U.S. general population	0.3% (15-25/100,000)	3% single Ab; 0.3% multiple Abs	Japanese incidence 1/100,000; incidence increasing in United States and many European countries; Colorado now 25/100,000
Offspring	1%		4.1%
Sibling	3.2%; 6% lifetime		7.4%
Dizygotic twin	6%		10%
Mother	2%	5%	Lower risk than offspring of father with DM
Father	4.6%	6.5%	
Both parents	10%?		?
MZT	50%, but incidence varies with age of index twin	50%	MZT in Japan, 40% risk of DM

Ab, antibody; DM, diabetes mellitus; MZT, monozygotic twin.

Although the risk of diabetes is much greater for relatives of patients with type 1A diabetes, it is important to realize that most persons (>85%) in whom type 1A diabetes develops do not have a first-degree relative with the disease. The incidence of sporadic cases results in part because almost 40% of persons in the general population carry high-risk HLA alleles for type 1A diabetes (see "The Major Histocompatibility Complex").

The highest known incidence of type 1A diabetes is found in Finland and Sardinia. Finland now has an annual incidence approaching 50 per 100,000 children. Since the 1960s, the incidence has increased almost threefold, suggesting a dramatic environmental change (either an increase of causative factors or a decrease of protective factors), and it is doubling in many Western countries, including the United States, every 20 years.

Twin Studies

Twin studies of diabetes have an impressive pedigree. The study of monozygotic twins of patients with diabetes by Pyke and coworkers[86] contributed to the recognition of distinct forms of diabetes, initially termed adult-onset and juvenile-onset, later insulin-dependent and non–insulin-dependent, and now type 1 and type 2 diabetes.[5] The concordance rates for monozygotic and dizygotic twins provide important information regarding genetic factors contributing to a given disease, because monozygotic twins share all germline-inherited polymorphisms or mutations, whereas dizygotic twins are similar to siblings of patients with a disease and have only half of their genes in common. For a locus that contributes to disease in a recessive manner, only one quarter of dizygotic twins would be homozygous to a sibling with diabetes at that locus, but all monozygotic twins would be homozygous for all recessive loci of their diabetic twin. Although overall concordance rates of monozygotic twins for T1DM are calculated, it is likely that type 1 diabetes is heterogeneous and that groups of monozygotic twins have different genetic etiologies for their diabetes. With such genetic heterogeneity, one would expect different concordance rates for different genetic etiologies.

Redondo and coworkers[87] analyzed prospective follow-up data from a large series of initially discordant monozygotic twins from Great Britain combined with a series from the United States. Progression to diabetes was identical for both series of twins. There was no length of time of discordance beyond which a monozygotic twin of a patient with T1DM did not have a risk of developing T1DM. Nevertheless, the hazard rate for development of diabetes decreased as the period of discordance increased. There was also a marked variation in the risk of diabetes relative to the age at which diabetes developed in the index twin. With long-term follow-up, the overall rate of concordance for monozygotic twins exceeds 50%.[88] However, if T1DM developed in the index twin after age 25 years, the concordance rate by life table analysis in Redondo's study was less than 10% (Fig. 32-1). If diabetes developed in the index twin before age 5 years, the concordance rate was 70% after 40 years of follow-up. Environmental factors, random factors, and non–germline-inherited variations (e.g., imprinting, T-cell receptor polymorphisms, somatic mutations) contribute to diabetes risk.

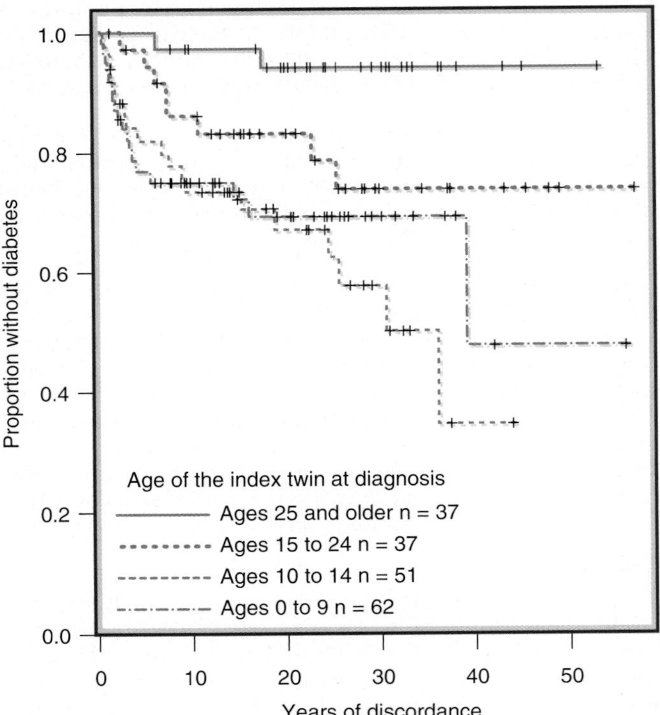

Figure 32-1 Progression to diabetes of initially discordant monozygotic twins of patients with type 1 diabetes subdivided by the age at diabetes onset of the first twin to develop diabetes (proband). Late progression to diabetes is evident, with some twins becoming diabetic more than 20 years after their twin mate. For discordant twins whose twin mate developed diabetes after age 25 years, the risk of diabetes is less than 10%. (From Redondo MJ, Yu L, Hawa M, et al. Heterogeneity of type 1 diabetes: analysis of monozygotic twins in Great Britain and the United States. *Diabetologia.* 2001;44:354-362.)

TABLE 32-3
Associated Autoimmune Diseases

Disease	Autoantibody Type	Autoantibody Percentage	Disease Prevalence (%)
Addison's disease[91]	21-Hydroxylase	1.5	0.5
Celiac disease[90]	Transglutaminase	12	6
Pernicious anemia[92]	Parietal cell	21	2.6
Thyroiditis or Graves' disease	Peroxidase or thyroglobulin	25	4

An important unanswered question (given the limited number and size of studies) is whether dizygotic twins of patients with type 1A diabetes have a diabetes risk greater than that of siblings. If the risk is identical, it suggests that environmental factors whose presence is time-dependent (e.g., uncommon infections) have little influence on the development of diabetes. Dizygotic twins differ from siblings in terms of a greater commonality of environment over time (e.g., common pregnancy). Studies of dizygotic twins suggest that their risk of diabetes may not differ from that of siblings or at most may be increased by a factor of 2 compared with the 10-fold increase for monozygotic twins.[87a]

Genetic factors influence not only the development of diabetes but also the expression of anti-islet autoantibodies. For identical twins, the expression of anti-islet autoantibodies is tightly linked to the eventual progression to overt diabetes, and monozygotic twins have a high prevalence of expression of autoantibodies.[83] Dizygotic twins much less often express anti-islet autoantibodies, and the prevalence is similar to that of siblings.[89]

Associated Autoimmune Disorders

Because type 1A diabetes is an immune-mediated illness that develops in a genetically susceptible person, it is not surprising that most patients with type 1A diabetes have one or more additional autoimmune diseases. The most common associated disorders are thyroid autoimmunity (Graves' disease or Hashimoto's thyroiditis) and celiac disease (Table 32-3).

The Major Histocompatibility Complex

The most important loci determining the risk of T1DM are within the MHC on chromosome 6p21 (Fig. 32-2), in particular the HLA class II molecules (DR, DQ, and DP).[19,93-95] In addition, the standard class I loci (HLA A, B, and C) influence disease, and it is likely that additional loci within or linked to the MHC that influence immune function contribute to diabetes risk.[96] Figure 32-2 illustrates the MHC. The nomenclature for alleles of this region is somewhat daunting, but with definitions of several terms and a description of the basis for classification it is comprehensible.

The function of HLA molecules is to present peptides to T lymphocytes. Each molecule is made up of two chains, and each chain is encoded by a separate gene. These molecules are extremely polymorphic in amino acid sequence. Each polymorphic variant of each chain is designated with a gene locus name (e.g., DRB1) followed by an asterisk (*), followed by two digits referring to the serologic specificity (from the time when typing was performed with antibodies), followed by two digits for the specific allele (now

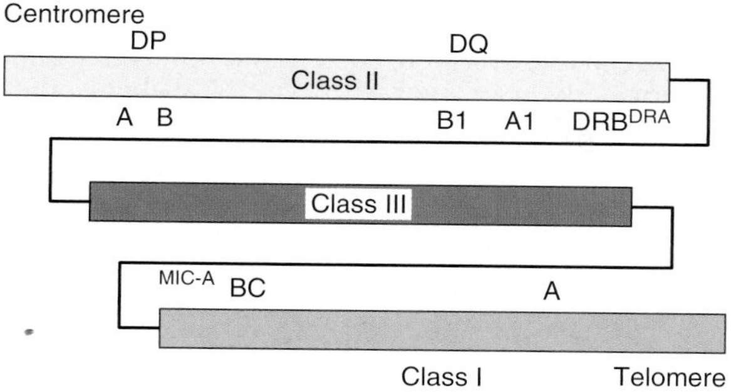

Figure 32-2 Genes within the human leukocyte antigen (HLA) region (major histocompatibility complex) with HLA class I, class II, and class III regions illustrated. Each class II molecule is made up of two chains. DRB alleles are polymorphic; DRA does not vary. DQA and DQB molecules are both polymorphic, as are DPA and DPB. The class III region contains important genes such as complement components and the tumor necrosis factor-α gene. The class I region includes MIC-A and MIC-B genes as well as the classic histocompatibility HLA genes, A, B, and C.

determined with DNA-based typing), followed by a single digit to distinguish silent nucleotide polymorphisms (nucleotide differences that do not change the amino acid sequence). For example, the designated allele DRB1*0405 has DR4 serologic specificity and is associated with high diabetes risk. For DR alleles, usually only the DRB chain is specified, because the DRA chain is not polymorphic. Likewise, for the class I molecules (A, B, and C), only a single chain is specified, because the other chain, β_2-microglobulin, is minimally polymorphic. There are hundreds of known alleles of DRB1. Each person inherits two DRB1 alleles, one from each parent.

Because HLA gene loci are in close proximity to each other on the sixth chromosome, a group of alleles is usually inherited as a unit, and this is termed a *haplotype*. For example, the alleles A*0101, B*0801, DRB1*0301, and DQA1*0501,DQB1*0201 constitute a common haplotype associated with diabetes risk probably related to the presence of DRB1*0301. When specific alleles of different genes are nonrandomly associated with each other on a haplotype (e.g., A1, B8, and DR3), the alleles are said to be in *linkage dysequilibrium*. Linkage dysequilibrium is not the same as linkage, although to have linkage dysequilibrium, genes must be linked. Genes are linked when they are close together on the same chromosome and thus transmitted from parent to child as a haplotype group. If alleles of linked genes are nonrandomly associated with each other in a population, they are in linkage dysequilibrium.

Two MHC haplotypes, one inherited from each parent, constitute an individual's MHC genotype. This genotype ultimately determines the MHC-encoded risk of type 1A diabetes. For DQ molecules, both of the chains (DQA and DQB) are polymorphic. This adds an important level of diversity in that the protein chains encoded by the alleles of one haplotype can combine with the chains encoded by the other haplotype. For example, persons with the highest-risk genotype DRB1*0301,DQA1*0501,DQB1*0201 and DRB1*0405,DQA1*0301,DQB1*0302 can produce four different DQ molecules: the expected DQA1*0501,DQB1*0201 and DQA1*0301,DQB1*0302 but also DQA1*0501,DQB1*0302 and DQA1*0301,DQB1*0201. Studies suggest that the DQA1*0501, DQB1*0302 combination determines enhanced diabetes risk for DR3/4 individuals. The DQ molecule DQA1*0501,DQB1*0201 is also called DQ2, and DQA1*0301,DQB1*0302 is called DQ8. A common DQ molecule, DQA1*0102,DQB1*0602, provides dominant protection from T1DM and is termed DQ6.

The major determinants of diabetes susceptibility are DR and DQ molecules, and specific alleles of both DR and DQ can either increase or decrease the risk of diabetes. Table 32-4 summarizes the diabetes risk associated with a number of DR and DQ haplotypes.[96a]

In a number of studies, children from the general population or relatives of patients with T1DM have been HLA typed at birth.[27,97,98] The typing is relatively straightforward and is based on direct DNA sequencing of polymerase chain reaction (PCR)-amplified DNA fragments or DNA probes that hybridize specifically to different allelic sequences. In Denver, Colorado, 2.4% of newborns have the highest-risk DR-DQ genotype for type 1A diabetes, namely DR3-DQ2 with DR4-DQ8 (DR3/4,DQ8/2 heterozygotes). Fifty percent of children younger than 10 years and approximately 30% of older children who develop diabetes have this highest-risk genotype. Approximately 1 of 16 children with the highest-risk HLA genotype from the general population progresses to diabetes (compared with a population risk of 1 per 300). Alternatively, 15 of 16 children from the general population who are DQ8/DQ2 heterozygotes do not develop diabetes. Studies indicate that newborn siblings of patients with T1DM who have DQ2 and DQ8 have a risk of expressing islet autoantibodies exceeding 40% by age 6 years, and 50% of these newborns will develop diabetes by age 10 years. This suggests that a genetic risk, especially MHC encoded, is extremely high.[99]

Ninety-five percent of persons who develop diabetes have either DR3-DQ2 or DR4-DQ8, as do approximately 40% of the general population. The protective haplotype DRB1*1501,DQA1*0102,DQB1*0602 is present in 20% of the general population and in fewer than 3% of patients with type 1A diabetes. A DR allele, DRB1*1401, also appears to provide dominant protection.[100] There are additional high-risk haplotypes that are not common, such as DQA1*0401,DQB1*0402.[101] It has been proposed as a simple rule that the presence of aspartic acid at position 57 of the DQβ chain and arginine at DQα 52 is associated with

TABLE 32-4

Diabetes Risk of Representative DR and DQ Haplotypes

DRB1	DQA1	DQB1
High Risk		
0401 or 0403 or 0405	0301	0302 (DQ8)
0301	0501	0201 (DQ2)
Moderate Risk		
0801	0401	0402
0404	0301	0302
0101	0101	0501
0901	0301	0303
Moderate Protection		
0403	0301	0302
0701	0201	0201
1101	0501	0301
Strong Protection		
1501	0102	0602 (DQ6)
1401	0101	0503
0701	0201	0303

diabetes risk.[102] There are many exceptions to this rule, and knowledge of the complete sequences (allele) rather than dependence on this rule is essential.

Insulin Locus

In 1984, Bell and colleagues[103] published their discovery that variations in the number of nucleotide repeat elements located 5′ of the insulin gene were associated with the development of type 1A diabetes. The longest group of repeats was associated with decreased diabetes risk. These studies have been replicated, and the locus of importance is clearly limited to the insulin gene.[104] The protective insulin gene polymorphism is associated with greater insulin messenger RNA (mRNA) expression within the thymus.[105,106] Hanahan[107] advanced the hypothesis that within lymphoid organs there are "peripheral antigen expressing cells," which, for example, produce insulin, and that such expression leads to tolerance and thereby decreases the risk of diabetes. Therefore, for both the AIRE mutation of APS-1 and the effect of insulin gene mutations, the level of expression of insulin in the thymus may be critical. Higher levels can lead to deletion of anti-insulin T cells.

PTPN22 Gene

PTPN22, a gene encoding a lymphoid-specific phosphatase that influences T-cell receptor signaling, is the third confirmed gene influencing T1DM risk.[108] This gene influences T-cell receptor signaling, and the polymorphism associated with diabetes (Trp for Arg) blocks binding to a signaling molecule, CSK. Nevertheless, the relative risk associated with this polymorphism for T1DM and other autoimmune disorders, such as rheumatoid arthritis, is only 1.7. The variant associated with disease risk results in gain of function and decreased T cell receptor signaling.[109]

Other Loci

There is an international effort to define additional genes that contribute to the development of type 1A diabetes. Polymorphisms of the cytotoxic T-lymphocyte-associated protein 4 gene (*CTLA4*; formerly called *IDDM12*) contribute to Graves' disease and apparently to diabetes in some but not all populations, with relative risks less than 1.3.[110] A locus associated with the IL-2 receptor has a statistical association based on analysis of thousands of persons.[111]

Recent genome-wide association studies have led to the identification of more than 40 loci having small effects on diabetes risk,[112] and detailed sequencing in one region identified rare mutations of a gene influencing IFN-α induction.[113] At present only HLA typing is being used to define the risk of diabetes at birth. The defined risk can be extremely high, depending on the relationship to a proband with diabetes and the specific HLA genotype. For example, siblings of patients with type 1A diabetes with the DR3-DQ2/DR4-DQ8 genotype appear to have a diabetes risk that exceeds 50%.[114] In contrast, children from the general population with the same HLA DR and DQ genotype have a risk of less than 6%. There is evidence that this extreme additional risk is due to genes linked to DR and DQ alleles, so siblings who can share both HLA haplotypes with a proband in addition to having DQ8-DQ2 alleles have a much higher risk than offspring of patients with T1DM or the general population.[115]

In addition to influencing diabetes risk, specific HLA genotypes contribute to the risk of associated autoimmune disorders. One third of DR3-DQ2 homozygous patients with type 1A diabetes express transglutaminase autoantibodies, and half of them have celiac disease on biopsy.[116]

ENVIRONMENTAL FACTORS

Despite decades of research, there is only one environmental factor clearly associated with type 1A diabetes, namely congenital rubella infection (see later discussion).[117] The association of only one factor is probably related to the long prodromal phase that precedes type 1A diabetes, which makes the discovery of relevant environmental factors particularly difficult.

A number of factors can induce type 1A diabetes in animal models, one of the most interesting being the Kilham rat virus infection of BB-DR rats and other normal rat strains with RT1-U.[118] In this model, which lacks the lymphopenia of the related BB strain, diabetes does not develop unless the animals are infected with Kilham virus (a parvovirus) or injected with poly-IC.[52] Poly-IC mimics double-stranded RNA and induces high levels of IFN-α. The Kilham virus apparently does not directly infect islets and is thought to be an immune activator, similar to poly-IC. Diabetes induction depends on specific class II alleles termed RT1-U, and a number of animal strains with RT1-U are susceptible to diabetes.[52]

In countries throughout the world, the incidence of type 1A diabetes is increasing, particularly for children in whom the disease develops before age 5 years.[119-121] This is strong evidence that environmental factors related to diabetes risk have changed since the 1960s. Factors that increase diabetes risk may be increasing, or, just as likely, factors that suppress the development of diabetes may be decreasing. For example, in animal models of type 1A diabetes (NOD mouse and BB rat), infections with common viruses usually decrease the development of diabetes.

Infections

Congenital rubella, but not noncongenital infection, greatly increases the development of type 1A diabetes.[122] Children with diabetes usually have high-risk HLA alleles,[123] and these children commonly have thyroid autoimmunity.[124] The way in which this congenital infection increases diabetes development is currently unknown. Hypotheses have ranged from potential molecular mimicry[125] to long-term alteration in T-cell function secondary to the congenital insult.[126]

Enteroviruses are small RNA viruses that often infect young children. Initial anecdotal reports that Coxsackievirus infections might cause diabetes involved children who had severe infections and who died at diabetes onset.[127,128] These studies preceded the realization that type 1A diabetes is not an acute disease, and it is likely that viral infection at the onset of T1DM is most often incidental. At the time of presentation with diabetes, almost all children have elevated HbA_{1c}, reflecting probably months of hyperglycemia preceding diagnosis. A description from Japan of persons with acute-onset diabetes and normal HbA_{1c}, elevated amylase, and infiltrates within the exocrine (but not endocrine) pancreas appears to represent a form of type 1B diabetes.[11]

The potential importance of enteroviral infection was emphasized by studies from Scandinavia in which enteroviral infection was evaluated during pregnancy and in infancy. Infection is usually detected by changes in antiviral antibodies or detection of enteroviral RNA by molecular techniques.[117] Although some studies have reported an increased incidence of enteroviral infection during pregnancy among mothers whose children later developed diabetes, others have not.[129,130] As infants with a genetic risk for the development of diabetes are followed from birth, it becomes possible to analyze prospectively the expression of enterovirus RNA. Enteroviral infection was found to be associated with the appearance of anti-islet autoantibodies.[129] However, similar studies from Denver, Colorado, did not find an association.[130] The major difference between the two studies appeared to be the lower rate of enteroviral infection in Finnish control subjects compared with Colorado control subjects.

Other viruses are being evaluated for association with the triggering of autoimmunity. One study from Australia found an association with rotavirus infection.[131] Rotavirus infection is common in young children. The Australian study did not find an increase in rotavirus infection in children with T1DM compared with control subjects, but there was an association of rotavirus infection with increased anti-islet autoantibodies. Studies from Denver did not indicate an increase in rotavirus infection in infants developing autoantibodies.

Vaccination

It has been claimed that the timing of routine childhood vaccinations influences the development of type 1A diabetes.[132] This is an important health concern if parents alter their family's childhood vaccination schedule because of concern about development of diabetes. A series of studies have been carried out[133-135] and did not provide any evidence that childhood vaccinations influence the development of diabetes.

Diet

A disease such as celiac disease is critically dependent on the ingestion of a specific food, namely the wheat protein gliadin.[136] In addition, a number of dietary modifications have been found to alter the development of diabetes in NOD mice and BB rats.[137]

Some investigators have championed the hypothesis that early introduction of bovine milk increases the development of diabetes, based primarily on retrospective studies associating early or increased bovine milk ingestion (or less breast-feeding) with an increased risk of type 1A diabetes.[138] Several prospective studies in which infants were observed until the development of anti-islet autoantibodies failed to find an association or found only a weak association with either breast-feeding or bovine milk ingestion.[139-142] Pilot studies of an infant formula lacking bovine milk proteins have been initiated in Finland. Preliminary data suggest that such a restricted diet might produce a small decrease of cytoplasmic islet cell autoantibodies but not GAD65 autoantibodies.[143]

Studies from Germany and Denver provided evidence that early (<3 months) introduction of cereals may increase the development of islet autoimmunity.[144,145] Both vitamin D and ω-3 fatty acids, which can influence immune function, have been associated with risk of diabetes.[146,147]

NATURAL HISTORY OF TYPE 1A DIABETES

The development of type 1A diabetes is typically divided into a series of stages beginning with genetic susceptibility and ending with essentially complete beta-cell destruction (Fig. 32-3). Mathis and coworkers[148] proposed the existence of checkpoints in the development of diabetes, and such checkpoints may have a strong genetic component. As discussed later, type 1A diabetes is predictable given specific immunologic, genetic, and metabolic characteristics, and it is such characteristics that set the stage for preventive trials.

Genetic and Immunologic Heterogeneity by Age of Onset

Type 1A diabetes can develop at any age, from the neonatal period to the sixth decade of life. Given that identical twins can become concordant as long as 30 years after the first twin develops type 1A diabetes, not all age heterogeneity can be ascribed to different genetic syndromes.[89] Nevertheless, there is an overall correlation between the age at which diabetes develops in one twin or sibling and the age

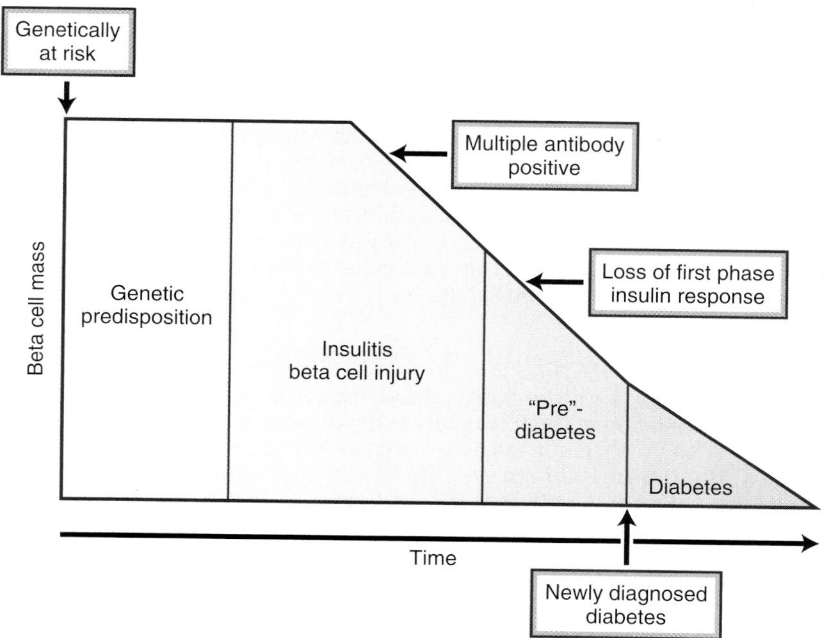

Figure 32-3 Hypothetical stages in the development of type 1A diabetes beginning with genetic susceptibility and ending with complete beta-cell destruction. (Modified from Eisenbarth GS. Type 1 diabetes mellitus: a chronic autoimmune disease. *N Engl J Med.* 1986;314:360-368; modifications by Jay Skyler, University of Miami.)

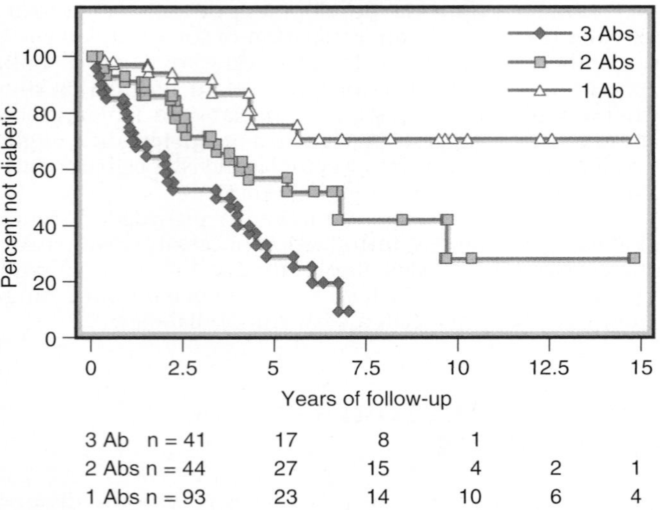

Figure 32-4 Progression to type 1 diabetes of first-degree relatives of patients with diabetes. Patients are subdivided by the number of anti-islet autoantibodies expressed against insulin, glutamic acid decarboxylase (GAD65), and the transmembrane protein tyrosine phosphatase IA-2 (ICA512). Ab, antibody. (From Verge CF, Gianani R, Kawasaki E, et al. Prediction of type 1 diabetes in first-degree relatives using a combination of insulin, GAD, and ICA512 bdc/IA-2 autoantibodies. *Diabetes.* 1996;45:926-933.)

of development of diabetes in his or her relative. Children in whom type 1A diabetes develops at an early age more often are DR3/4,DQ8/2 heterozygotes. In addition, there is evidence that class I HLA alleles (or other non–class II genes within the HLA region) can influence the age at diabetes onset; an example is the A24 allele.[149] At the other end of the age spectrum, there is evidence that the protective HLA allele DQA*10102, DQB1*0602 is not as protective for young adults as it is for children.[150]

The most characteristic difference related to age at diabetes onset is the presence of higher levels of insulin autoantibodies (IAA) in children who develop the disease at an early age (e.g., <5 years).[151,152] The high levels and frequent positivity of IAA make measurement of these autoantibodies the best single marker for diabetes development in young children. In those children in whom autoantibodies arise during the first 3 years of life, IAA often appear first. In contrast, GAD65 autoantibodies are more often positive in adults who develop type 1A diabetes. The correlation of levels of IAA and age at diabetes onset may be related to faster progression to diabetes in children with higher levels.[153] However, such rapid progression occurs only if IAA are present with another anti-islet autoantibody (discussed in the next section) (Fig. 32-4).

Combinatorial Autoantibody Prediction

The most specific anti-islet autoantibody assays are usually set with cutoffs above the 99th percentile of control populations. With four major autoantibody assays measuring GAD65, the transmembrane protein tyrosine phosphatase IA-2 (also called ICA512), ZnT8[154] and insulin, it can be predicted that approximately 4 of 100 normal persons express one or more of the four autoantibodies. Because approximately 3 of 1000 children develop type 1A diabetes, this suggests that diabetes never develops in most antibody-positive persons or develops only late in life.

A relatively low positive predictive value for single antibodies may be related to methodologic limitations (e.g., nonreproducible assay positivity) or to the presence of autoantibodies identical to those in patients with prediabetes but found in some persons who do not progress to diabetes. It is likely that both occur. For example, a low positive (i.e., still above the 99th percentile) autoantibody result in a control subject is often not confirmed on repeated testing. Autoantibodies from prediabetic persons usually react with multiple epitopes of the IA-2 molecule, whereas false-positive autoantibodies often react with only one or no clearly defined epitope of the molecule, suggesting that false-positive and diabetes-associated anti–IA-2 autoantibodies differ. However, there are some persons, usually adult relatives of patients with type 1A diabetes (often with DQB1*0602), who have extremely high levels of GAD65 autoantibodies that react with multiple GAD epitopes but no evidence of progression to diabetes.[155]

Bonifacio and coworkers analyzed the affinity of IAA from children in the BabyDiab study from Germany. High-affinity IAA measured in offspring of patients with T1DM were associated with progression to diabetes.[156]

As for any diagnostic test, assessment of the significance of an autoantibody result is improved by taking into account the prior probability of disease. A patient with overt diabetes and expression of a single anti-islet autoantibody has a high probability of having type 1A diabetes. A person from the general population or even a relative expressing a single autoantibody (and not developing more than that one autoantibody) has a much lower risk of progressing to type 1A diabetes.[157]

Usually, attempts to improve the specificity of a test sacrifice sensitivity. For prediction of type 1A diabetes, the four biochemical autoantibody assays can be combined, and the presence of two or more autoantibodies is associated with a very high risk of diabetes.[158,159] Approximately 1 of 350 persons from the general population express two or more of the GAD65, ICA512, ZnT8, or IAA, approaching population estimates of type 1A diabetes. Among first-degree relatives of patients with type 1A diabetes, the presence of two or more autoantibodies indicates a risk of more than 90% over 10 years, whereas a single autoantibody is associated with a risk of less than 20% over 10 years.[158]

Metabolic Progression before Hyperglycemia

The intravenous glucose tolerance test (GTT) aids in evaluating the time to onset of diabetes among persons expressing anti-islet autoantibodies.[160] Most commonly, glucose is given at 0.5 g/kg over 5 minutes (maximum 35 g, 25 g/dL), and insulin levels are measured before and 1 and 3 minutes after the glucose infusion.[161,162] Most persons who are within 1 year of developing overt diabetes have no first-phase insulin secretion after intravenous glucose administration. A simpler measurement in someone progressing to type 1 diabetes is the HbA_{1c}, which in most prediabetic individuals increases progressively (although in the normal range) 1 or 2 years before overt hyperglycemia develops.

The diagnosis of type 1A diabetes usually relies on the presence of fasting hyperglycemia (≥126 mg/dL), but with prospective evaluation, many persons have diabetes on oral glucose tolerance testing (OGTT) by the 120-minute criterion (≥200 mg/dL), with a nondiagnostic fasting glucose level. Impaired fasting glucose (100 to 125 mg/dL) or impaired glucose tolerance (glucose at 120 minutes on

OGTT, 140 to 199 mg/dL) is usually present within 6 months before the onset of overt diabetes.

C-Peptide Loss after Hyperglycemia

After diabetes is diagnosed, levels of C peptide can be used to assess remaining beta-cell function. C-peptide levels are usually measured in the fasting state or after intravenous glucagon or with a standard liquid meal. Such measurements are primarily of importance for trials of therapies to alleviate loss of insulin secretion after diagnosis. Determination of the C-peptide concentration provides the best current measure for assessing the impact of new therapies. As shown in the Diabetes Control and Complications Trial (DCCT), a small amount of remaining C peptide is associated with impressive metabolic benefit.[163,164]

Type 1A Diabetes with Pregnancy

Approximately 5% of women with gestational diabetes (diabetes diagnosed during pregnancy) have an early form of type 1A diabetes that is discovered during pregnancy.[165] These women express anti-islet autoantibodies and progress to overt diabetes more rapidly after pregnancy.

Latent Autoimmune Diabetes of Adults

Type 1A diabetes can occur at any age. Depending on the population, between 5% and 15% of persons with what appears to be T2DM express anti-islet autoantibodies.[166,167] Multiple studies have demonstrated that such persons progress relatively rapidly (within 3 years) to insulin-requiring diabetes. The HLA alleles of such persons reflect that of type 1A diabetes.[168]

Transient Hyperglycemia

A significant number of children are evaluated by endocrinologists for transient hyperglycemia. The usual history is one of severe stress associated with hyperglycemia that resolves within days to 1 month. Such children may be in the honeymoon phase of type 1A diabetes, or they may truly have a transient episode of hyperglycemia. Rarely, diabetes in children is misdiagnosed. For example, we have seen a child with normal HbA_{1c} values for several years who stopped insulin and was subsequently found to have renal glucosuria and not diabetes. Children without severe stress who have transient hyperglycemia or who have a relative with type 1A diabetes are more likely to have early type 1A diabetes. Absence of anti-islet autoantibodies and a normal intravenous GTT result strongly indicate transient hyperglycemia and not type 1A diabetes.[169] It is not known whether children with transient hyperglycemia are at increased risk for T2DM later in life.

IMMUNOTHERAPY OF TYPE 1A DIABETES

At the onset of type 1A diabetes, a major clinical research goal is the prevention of further beta-cell destruction. At present, there is no proven safe and effective therapy to prevent such further destruction or to prevent the development of type 1A diabetes in those at risk (e.g., genetically at-risk persons with anti-islet autoantibodies). A number of clinical trials have been completed, and a large number of trials are under way or about to be initiated.

Immunosuppression

The earliest studies of therapies to prevent beta-cell destruction used immunosuppressive agents. Large trials of cyclosporine indicated that cyclosporine prevented further loss of C-peptide secretion and improved metabolic function while it was administered.[170-172] It did not, however, maintain a nondiabetic state when therapy was instituted after the onset of diabetes, and with discontinuation of the drug, patients rapidly lost C-peptide reserve. The combination of inability to cure diabetes and toxicities associated with cyclosporine (in particular nephrotoxicity and concern about increased risk of malignancy) has ruled out its use. Other immunosuppressive agents such as prednisone or azathioprine had relatively little effect.[174-176] A small study suggested that methotrexate, another common immunotherapeutic agent, is ineffective.[177] Therefore, at present, although type 1A diabetes is an immune-mediated disorder, it is not treated with common immunotherapeutic agents.

Two studies of modified antibodies to CD3 have been reported, and additional trials are likely.[178] A single course of anti-CD3 therapy decreased loss of C-peptide secretion in new-onset patients, but it appears that after 1 year progressive loss of secretion resumed.[179] Concerns related to the activation of Epstein-Barr virus infection and the lack of information regarding the duration of C-peptide preservation caution against nonresearch application of such therapy at present.[179a] In an oral presentation at the ADA, Dr. Pescovitz reported that a single course of anti-CD20 antibody targeting B lymphocytes delayed loss of C-peptide for approximately 3 months. Neither an anti–IL-2 receptor antibody, nor mycophenolate, nor the combination delayed loss of C-peptide (oral report by Gottlieb-TrialNet).

The TrialNet group has a number of randomized, multicenter trials under way and planned. Subjects for such trials in the setting of new-onset T1DM may be referred by contacting Type 1 TrialNet at 1-800-HALT-DM1 or http://www.diabetestrialnet.org (accessed December 2010).

Immunologic Vaccination

In animal models (especially the NOD mouse), it is relatively easy to prevent T1DM.[14] Potentially the most exciting modalities use forms of immunologic vaccination. Much of the excitement derives from the specificity of the therapy and the relatively low risk compared with immunosuppression, not from demonstrated efficacy in humans. The basic concept behind most such therapies is the induction of lymphocytes that target a given islet antigen and, on encountering the target antigen (e.g., insulin), produce cytokines that suppress autoimmunity and tissue destruction.[38,180]

A Th2 class of T lymphocytes produce the cytokine IL-4 rather than IFN-γ and IL-2 (which are produced by Th1 T cells) and decrease cell-mediated immune destruction. Induction of a protective immune response may depend on the route of administration of the given antigen (e.g., oral tolerance) or on the use of an altered antigen (e.g., altered peptide ligands). For example, insulin given either orally or by subcutaneous injection prevented diabetes in NOD mice.[181,182] Intact insulin is not necessary, because the insulin B chain and an immunodominant B(9-23) peptide of insulin were also effective.[40] The latter molecules have no insulin-like metabolic effect but are able to activate T lymphocytes that target insulin.

The Diabetes Prevention Trial Type 1 studied both oral insulin and parenteral injections of low doses of insulin.

The results of the parenteral trial did not demonstrate a reduction in the risk of developing diabetes.[183] The oral trial did not document an overall benefit of insulin, but in the subgroup with higher levels of IAA at entry, a statistically significant delay in progression to diabetes was observed.[184] Because this was a subgroup analysis, replication of this potentially exciting finding is imperative. Relatives of patients with T1DM can be tested for anti-islet autoantibodies by TrialNet at the telephone number or website given earlier.

Other Therapies

A review by Atkinson and Leiter[184a] pointed out that more than 100 different interventions prevent diabetes in NOD mice. The relative ease of diabetes prevention in this animal model has provided the basis for a number of trials initiated in humans. The largest European trial, the European Nicotinamide Trial (ENDIT), uses nicotinamide in gram doses. Nicotinamide can prevent diabetes induced by the drug streptozotocin and probably acts by preserving nicotinamide adenine dinucleotide levels in islet cells or by blocking cytokine-induced destruction. Nicotinamide did not delay progression to diabetes in humans.[154]

IMMUNOLOGY OF PANCREATIC ISLET TRANSPLANTATION

Pancreatic transplantation for patients requiring a kidney transplant is an accepted clinical procedure.[185] Patients with a kidney transplant receive immunosuppressive drugs, and results for pancreatic transplantation in this setting have progressively improved. With a successful pancreas transplant, hyperglycemia is immediately reversed, and there is some evidence of improved long-term outcomes,[185,186] although there is considerable debate concerning pancreas transplantation without the transplantation of a kidney.[187] Nevertheless, the surgery is extensive, and there are many potential complications associated with the transplant. Diabetes can recur because of recurrent autoimmunity or, more often, allograft rejection.[188] It is difficult to monitor specific islet destruction, and with the development of hyperglycemia it is usually not possible to restore euglycemia.

Up until studies from Edmonton, the results of islet transplantation were poor: fewer than 10% of patients with type 1A diabetes achieved insulin independence at 1 year.[189] In contrast, with autotransplantation of patients with pancreatitis, most patients become insulin independent and remain so.[189] The Edmonton group used meticulous islet isolation techniques, transplantation of islets from multiple pancreata, and an immunosuppressive regimen using the drug rapamycin.

The Edmonton protocol has been tested in a series of specialized centers throughout North America and Europe. It is clear that many centers with varying success rates can successfully transplant islets, and for patients with severe hypoglycemia there is long-term prevention of severe hypoglycemic episodes. For most of the patients who achieve insulin independence, resumption of use of low doses of insulin is necessary within 2 years.[190] Even if the Edmonton results are reproduced at multiple centers, the number of islets available from cadaveric donors for transplantation is limited, and the toxicities of the drugs used probably exceed the level of benefit achieved. Further research to achieve tolerance without long-term immunosuppression with calcineurin inhibitors and rapamycin is essential, as is the development of xenogeneic transplantation or production of islets from stem cells. The increasing use of long-term continuous glucose monitoring in patients with T1DM will almost certainly raise the bar for consideration of the risks and benefits of both islet and pancreatic transplantation.

INSULIN AUTOIMMUNE SYNDROME

The insulin autoimmune syndrome, also termed *Hirata syndrome,* is rare and is typically associated with hypoglycemia.[191] These patients have extremely high concentrations of autoantibodies that react with human insulin. It is thought that inappropriate (nonregulated) release of autoantibody-bound insulin produces the hypoglycemia. The disease occurs most commonly in Asian persons. Among 50 Japanese patients with the syndrome and the typical polyclonal anti-insulin autoantibodies, 96% had a DR4 allele and 84% (42 of 50) had the DRB1*0406 allele.[192] In contrast, patients with monoclonal anti-insulin autoantibodies do not have such a remarkable HLA association. Most patients develop the disease in association with treatment with sulfhydryl-containing medications, in particular methimazole. Treatment usually consists of stopping these medications, and for more than 75% of the patients, the disease remits.[192]

INSULIN ALLERGY

Mild forms of immune reactivity to insulin are not uncommon. Essentially all patients treated with human insulin produce anti-insulin autoantibodies that are measurable with sensitive fluid-phase radioassays. The levels of these autoantibodies are relatively low, and they do not appear to interfere with insulin therapy, although there are reports correlating insulin antibodies with macrosomia.[193] With the introduction of recombinant human insulin replacing animal insulins, symptomatic immune responses to insulin such as immediate hypersensitivity, delayed hypersensitivity, lipoatrophy, and lipohypertrophy have decreased.[194] Allergic reactions can occur with insulin analogues, although this is uncommon. More common are allergies to protamine, which is used to complex insulin in neutral protamine Hagedorn (NPH) formulations, or the lubricants, preservatives, and plastics in bottles, stoppers, syringes, and needles.

The usual therapy consists of switching the type or formulation of insulin followed by oral antihistamines for immunoglobulin E–mediated local reactions, followed by insulin desensitization or addition of small amounts of glucocorticoids to the insulin injected for local delayed hypersensitivity reactions.

ANTI-INSULIN RECEPTOR AUTOANTIBODIES

Anti-insulin receptor autoantibodies (type B insulin resistance) are associated with both hypoglycemia and insulin resistance.[195] It appears that anti-insulin receptor autoantibodies can act as either antagonists or agonists. This syndrome is rare and is often associated with non–organ-specific autoimmunity.[196]

CLINICAL PRESENTATION

The peak age at presentation of T1DM in children is at puberty. The symptoms and signs are related to the presence of hyperglycemia and the resulting effects on fluid and electrolyte balance; they include polyuria, polydipsia, polyphagia, weight loss, and blurred vision. Because infection may have precipitated the initial presentation, symptoms of infection may also be present, such as fever, sore throat, cough, or dysuria. In children in particular, the onset of symptoms can occur over a brief period, and families may be able to date the onset with considerable accuracy. Onset of symptoms can also be insidious, particularly in older persons with T1DM, and can occur over a time frame of weeks or even months.

If onset of T1DM is associated with ketoacidosis, which is not uncommon, additional symptoms related to this acute metabolic complication of diabetes are also present. These symptoms can include abdominal pain, nausea, and vomiting. Variable effects on mental status may be seen, ranging from slight drowsiness to profound lethargy and even coma if the condition has been untreated for a significant period.

LABORATORY FINDINGS

Plasma glucose concentrations at presentation are elevated, usually in the range 300 to 500 mg/dL. If the presentation is uncomplicated, the remainder of the fluid and electrolyte measurements may be completely normal. On the other hand, if diabetic ketoacidosis (DKA) is present, the measurements will reflect the presence of an acidosis as well as more severe dehydration. In DKA, the serum sodium value is often at the lower limit of normal or even mildly reduced, reflecting the osmotic effect of hyperglycemia and, on occasion, the presence of vomiting with continued water intake. A sodium value lower than 120 mmol/L is usually associated with severe hypertriglyceridemia that can lead to spurious hyponatremia.

Despite significant losses of potassium in the urine and total-body potassium deficits, acidosis usually leads to an elevated serum potassium concentration at the time of the initial presentation. Serum bicarbonate concentrations are usually less than 10 mg/dL, and elevations in serum concentrations of triglyceride and free fatty acids are found. Levels of ketone bodies are also elevated. Because dehydration is invariably present, this leads to increases in the concentrations of blood urea nitrogen (BUN) and creatinine. In conjunction with the increase in serum glucose, the increases in BUN invariably increase the serum osmolality, often to greater than 300 mmol/kg.

TREATMENT OF TYPE 1 DIABETES

Importance of Tight Glucose Control

The overriding principle in the treatment of most patients with T1DM is that a health care team that includes a physician, diabetes nurse educator, nutritionist, and other health care professionals as appropriate should work closely with the patient to achieve blood glucose concentrations as close to normal as possible, because these values are associated with a reduced risk of diabetic complications. Although studies in animal models[197-199] and epidemiologic studies[200-202] have suggested that tighter glucose control is associated with better long-term outcomes for the diabetic patient in terms of a reduced risk of complications, the most definitive study in this regard has been the DCCT, which was completed in 1993.[203] This landmark study involved a total of 1441 patients with T1DM—726 with no retinopathy at baseline (the primary prevention cohort) and 715 with mild retinopathy (the secondary intervention cohort)—who were randomly assigned to intensive therapy or conventional therapy.

Intensive therapy consisted of insulin administration by an external pump or by three or more daily insulin injections. The dosage was adjusted according to the results of self-monitoring of blood glucose performed at least four times per day as well as dietary intake and anticipated exercise. The goals of intensive therapy were to achieve blood glucose concentrations between 70 and 120 mg/dL before meals, values less than 180 mg/dL after meals, a weekly 3 a.m. measurement greater than 65 mg/dL, and an HbA_{1c} value within the normal range (≤6.05%). Patients in the intensive treatment group visited their centers each month and had more frequent contacts with a member of the health care team, usually weekly, to review and adjust their regimens.

Conventional therapy consisted of one or two daily injections of insulin, including mixed intermediate and rapid-acting insulins, daily self-monitoring of urine or blood glucose, and education about diet and exercise. The goals of conventional therapy included absence of symptoms of hyperglycemia; absence of ketonuria; maintenance of normal growth, development, and ideal body weight; and freedom from frequent severe hypoglycemia.

The entire cohort of patients was observed for a mean of 6.5 years, and 99% of the patients completed the study. Although only 5% of the subjects in the intensive treatment group were able to sustain the goal of a normal HbA_{1c} over time, they nevertheless did have significantly lower average values (approximately 7%) over time than the subjects in the conventional treatment group (approximately 9%). Average capillary blood glucose profiles in the intensive treatment group were 155 ± 30 mg/dL, compared with 231 ± 55 mg/dL in the conventional therapy group ($P < .0001$). These differences in glucose control formed the basis of analyses to determine the effects of lower levels of glycemia on diabetic complications.

When both the primary prevention and secondary intervention cohorts were considered, intensive therapy was shown to reduce the risk of proliferative or severe nonproliferative retinopathy by 47% and the need for treatment with photocoagulation by 56%. Intensive therapy reduced the mean adjusted risk of microalbuminuria (defined as urinary albumin excretion >40 mg/24 hours) by 34% in the primary prevention cohort and by 43% in the secondary intervention cohort. The risk of albuminuria was reduced by 56% in the secondary intervention cohort. Intensive therapy reduced the appearance of neuropathy by 69% in the primary prevention cohort and by 57% in the secondary intervention cohort.

Some have suggested a potential adverse effect of aggressive insulin therapy in exacerbating the predisposition to macrovascular disease in diabetes. In the DCCT study, intensive insulin therapy reduced the development of macrovascular disease by 41%, although the difference was not statistically significant.[204] Ninety-three percent of DCCT participants were monitored after the randomized portion of the trial in the Epidemiology of Diabetes Interventions and Complications (EDIC) study. Glycemic control in both groups drifted toward an HbA_{1C} value of slightly less than 8% within the first year or so after conclusion of the randomized trial. With 17 years of follow-up after randomization, despite similar glycemic control in both groups for 10 years, cardiovascular disease (defined as nonfatal myocardial infarction, stroke, death from cardiovascular disease, confirmed angina, or the need for coronary-artery revascularization) was reduced by 42% and nonfatal myocardial infarction, stroke, and cardiovascular deaths were reduced by 57%. The authors concluded that "the decrease in glycosylated hemoglobin values during the DCCT was significantly associated with most of the positive effects of intensive treatment on the risk of cardiovascular disease. Intensive diabetes therapy has long-term beneficial effects on the risk of cardiovascular disease in patients with type 1 diabetes."[205]

Were there any adverse events associated with the intensive treatment regimen in the DCCT? Overall mortality did not differ in the two treatment groups and was actually less than expected on the basis of population-based mortality studies. However, the incidence of severe hypoglycemia was approximately three times higher in the intensive therapy group than in the conventional therapy group ($P < .001$). Some of the episodes of hypoglycemia were quite severe, resulting in motor vehicle accidents or need for hospitalization. Severe hypoglycemia occurred more often during sleep,[206] and approximately one third of the episodes that occurred while the patients were awake were not associated with warning symptoms. In intensively treated subjects, predictors of hypoglycemia included a history of severe hypoglycemia, longer duration of diabetes, higher baseline HbA_{1c}, and a lower recent HbA_{1c} value.

Weight gain also occurred in more of the intensively treated patients. Intensive therapy was associated with a 33% increase in risk of becoming overweight, defined as a body weight more than 120% above the ideal. Five years into the trial, patients being treated intensively had gained a mean of 4.6 kg more than patients receiving conventional therapy. Among subjects in the top quartile of weight gain, changes in plasma lipids, blood pressure, and body fat distribution were observed that were similar to those seen in cases of insulin resistance.[207]

Goals of Treatment

On the basis of the results just described, the authors of the DCCT study recommended that most patients with T1DM be treated with an intensive treatment regimen under the close supervision of a health care team consisting of a physician, nurses, nutritionist, and behavioral and exercise specialists as needed. However, for certain groups of patients, this recommendation may need to be modified, because the risk-to-benefit ratio might not be as favorable as it was in the cohorts with mild or no diabetic complications that were studied in the DCCT.

Patients for whom it may be appropriate to be more cautious about instituting intensive treatment regimens include children younger than 13 years of age, elderly people, and patients with advanced complications such as end-stage renal disease or significant cardiovascular or cerebrovascular disease. It has also been reported[208-210] that institution of aggressive insulin therapy in subjects with proliferative or severe nonproliferative retinopathy can lead to accelerated progression of retinopathy. Treatment of the eye disease should be considered before an aggressive insulin regimen is started. Patients who do not experience warning adrenergic symptoms of hypoglycemia (hypoglycemia unawareness) are at significantly greater risk for severe recurrent hypoglycemia, and this may prevent the safe institution of tight glucose control.[211]

TABLE 32-5

Glycemic Targets

Parameter	Normal	ADA	ACE
Premeal PG (mg/dL)	<100 (mean ~90)	70-130	<110
Postprandial PG (mg/dL)	<140	<180	<140
HbA_{1c} (%)	4-6	<7	≤6.5

ACE, American College of Endocrinology; ADA, American Diabetes Association; HbA_{1c}, glycosylated hemoglobin; PG, plasma glucose concentration.

From American Diabetes Association. Standards of medical care in diabetes—2010. *Diabetes Care.* 2010;29:s11-s61; Rodbard HW, Blonde L, Braithwaite SS, et al., AACE Diabetes Mellitus Clinical Practice Guidelines Task Force. American Association of Clinical Endocrinologists medical guidelines for clinical practice for the management of diabetes mellitus. *Endocr Pract.* 2007;13(suppl 1):1-68.

Guidelines from the ADA and the American College of Endocrinology (ACE) are presented in Table 32-5. The ADA suggests that the goal of treatment in the management of diabetes should be an HbA_{1c} value of less than 7% in general. Furthermore, the ADA suggests that lower targets can be pursued in selected patients, such as those with disease of recent onset, long life expectancy, and no significant cardiovascular disease, if they can be achieved without significant hypoglycemia or other adverse effects of treatment. Conversely, they recommend that less-stringent HbA_{1c} goals "may be appropriate for patients with a history of severe hypoglycemia, limited life expectancy, advanced microvascular or macrovascular complications, and extensive comorbid conditions and those with longstanding diabetes in whom the general goal is difficult to attain despite diabetes self-management education, appropriate glucose monitoring, and effective doses of multiple glucose lowering agents including insulin."[212] The ACE has recommended an HbA_{1c} goal of less than 6.5%.[213] It is recognized that to achieve glucose control at this level, patients need to monitor glucose frequently and to receive nutritional counseling and training in self-management of the insulin doses as well as problem solving to allow them to deal with the problems that they encounter in their daily lives.

Team Approach to Treatment

The DCCT trial validated the use of continuous subcutaneous insulin infusion (CSII) with an insulin pump and multiple daily injections (MDI), which are titrated based on frequent glucose monitoring. Several companies have developed continuous glucose sensors, and pramlintide, an amylin analogue, is the first fundamentally new treatment for patients with T1DM to become available since 1922. Because of the complex nature of modern intensive diabetes treatment regimens and the need for regular feedback and modification of the parameters of treatment, it has now become generally accepted that intensive insulin regimens can be instituted more effectively by a health care team than by a physician alone. Members of the team can include diabetes nurse educators, nutritionists, psychologists, medical social workers, and others, such as exercise physiologists, depending on the needs of a particular patient. A critical aspect of intensive diabetes treatment is the need for continuous monitoring of the effectiveness of specific components of the regimen with adjustments in response to changing life circumstances of the patient.

Pharmacokinetics of Available Insulin Preparations

In the past, insulin for human use was obtained from animal sources (i.e., cows and pigs). With advances in recombinant DNA technology, it is now possible to produce large quantities of insulin with an amino acid structure identical to that of human insulin or to modify the human amino acid sequence to produce desirable pharmacodynamic properties. The various formulations of insulin differ in the rapidity of their onset of action, the time from injection to peak action, and the duration of action, depending on the chemical nature of the particular insulin preparation. These data are summarized in Table 32-6. The available insulins can be divided on a pharmacokinetic basis into three broad categories: rapid-acting, intermediate, and long-acting.

Rapid-Acting Insulins

Rapid-acting insulins have an onset of action of 1 hour or less and are used to reduce the peak of glycemia that occurs after meal ingestion.

Regular Insulin. Regular insulin consists of zinc-insulin crystals dissolved in a clear fluid. After subcutaneous injection, regular insulin tends to dissociate from its normal hexameric form, first into dimers and then into monomers; only the monomeric and dimeric forms can pass through the endothelium into the circulation to any appreciable degree.[214] This feature determines the pharmacokinetic profile of regular insulin. The resulting relative delay in onset and duration of action of regular insulin limits its effectiveness in controlling postprandial glucose and results in dose-dependent pharmacokinetics, with a prolonged onset, peak, and duration of action with higher doses.

Insulin Analogues

Insulin Lispro. Insulin lispro, of recombinant DNA origin, is a human insulin analogue created by reversal of the amino acids at positions 28 and 29 on the human insulin B chain. Insulin lispro was the first insulin analogue to receive approval by the U.S. Food and Drug Administration. It is chemically Lys(B28),Pro(B29) insulin and is created in a special, nonpathogenic laboratory strain of *Escherichia coli* that has been genetically altered by the addition of the gene for insulin lispro.

TABLE 32-6

Pharmacokinetic Properties of Insulin Preparations

Preparation	Onset (hr)	Peak (hr)	Duration (hr)
Rapid-Acting			
Regular	0.5-1	2-4	6-8
Lispro	0.25	1	3-4
Aspart	0.25	1	3-4
Glulisine	0.25	1	3-4
Intermediate-Acting			
NPH	1-3	6-8	12-16
Long-Acting			
Glargine	1	NA	11-24
Detemir	1	3-9	6-23

NPH, neutral protamine Hagedorn.

The effect of this amino acid rearrangement is to reduce the capacity of the insulin to self-aggregate in subcutaneous tissues, resulting in behavior similar to that of monomeric insulin. This leads to lispro's more rapid absorption and shorter duration of action compared with regular insulin when given by subcutaneous injection. However, lispro is not intrinsically more active and on a molar basis is equipotent to human insulin. When they are given by intravenous injection, the pharmacokinetic profiles of lispro and human regular insulin are similar. Because of its rapid onset of action (within 5 to 15 minutes after administration) and peak action within 1 to 2 hours, lispro was the first insulin to mimic the time course of the increase in plasma glucose seen after ingestion of a carbohydrate-rich meal.

Insulin Aspart. Insulin aspart differs from human insulin by substitution of aspartic acid for proline in position B28.

Insulin Glulisine. Insulin glulisine involves substitution of lysine for the asparagine at position B3 and of glutamic acid for the lysine in position B29.

Advantages of Analogues. Lispro, aspart, and glulisine seem to have similar pharmacokinetics and clinical effects in the setting of T1DM. Although little difference is observed in most cases by either patients or providers, there certainly may be differences, at least in subsets of patients, that could be exploited to improve glycemic control.

In general, treatment with monomeric insulin analogues (lispro, aspart, and glulisine) is associated with a lower risk of hypoglycemia, particularly in sleep, than treatment with regular insulin. It is quite easy to document improved glycemic control in the postprandial state. Finally, patients may inject these insulin analogues immediately before or after meals instead of 30 to 60 minutes before meals, as is classically recommended with regular insulin, providing greater convenience. These features have been exploited in clinical trials to produce modest improvements in overall control with monomeric insulin analogues compared with regular insulin.

Intermediate and Long-Acting Insulins

Intermediate and long-acting insulins have a significantly longer delay in their onset and duration of action. In the setting of T1DM, they should be always used in combination with a rapid-acting form of insulin. They are usually administered before bedtime and are titrated to produce normal glucose levels through the night and in the fasting state.

NPH Insulin. NPH insulin is a crystalline suspension of insulin with protamine and zinc, providing an intermediate-acting insulin with onset of action in 1 to 3 hours, duration of action up to 24 hours, and peak action from 6 to 8 hours. NPH insulin usually cannot be administered once daily in the setting of T1DM, at least in combination with rapid-acting monomeric analogue insulin. In the pre-analogue era, NPH insulin was used successfully in combination with regular insulin, although this human insulin-based regimen has now been largely supplanted by analogue insulin because of a perceived lower risk of hypoglycemia.[215]

Insulin Glargine. Insulin glargine is a recombinant human insulin analogue that does provide 24-hour duration of action in most, but not all, patients with T1DM. It differs from human insulin in that the amino acid asparagine at position A21 is replaced by glycine, and two arginines are added to the carboxyl-terminus of the B chain. In the injection solution at pH 4, insulin glargine is completely soluble. However, it has low solubility at neutral pH.

After injection into the subcutaneous tissue, the acidic solution is neutralized, leading to the formation of microprecipitates from which small amounts of insulin glargine are slowly released; this results in absorption over a period of approximately 24 hours with no pronounced peak. Insulin glargine thus simulates the basal production of insulin. In other respects, its mechanism of action is similar to that of human insulin, and on a molar basis its glucose-lowering effects are similar to those of human insulin when given intravenously.

Because this insulin is provided in an acid vehicle, it cannot be mixed with other forms of insulin or intravenous fluids, and some patients have greater discomfort with injection at least some of the time. In general, glargine is less variably absorbed than NPH insulin, and in clinical trials in patients with T1DM it has been associated with a reduced risk of hypoglycemia, particularly nocturnal hypoglycemia.

In about 10% of patients, insulin glargine must be taken twice daily to provide 24-hour coverage of basal insulin needs. In a smaller percentage of patients, a modest peak in effect occurs 2 to 6 hours after injection and can result in nocturnal hypoglycemia.

Insulin Detemir. Insulin detemir differs from human insulin in that the threonine in position B30 has been eliminated and a C14 fatty acid chain has been attached to amino acid B29. It is unique among insulins of prolonged duration in that it is soluble both in the vial and under the skin. This may be the cause of its more consistent absorption after subcutaneous injection.[216] In comparison to NPH insulin in the setting of T1DM, detemir is associated with less weight gain (in some trials patients have experienced weight loss) and with reduced risk of hypoglycemia.[215]

Alternative Routes of Insulin Administration

Numerous alternative routes of insulin administration are being examined.[217,218] There is tremendous interest on the part of patients in inhaled insulin. Some studies suggest that there is substantial preference, at least among most research volunteers, for the pulmonary versus the subcutaneous route of insulin administration.

One inhaled insulin product (Exubera) was found to have several limitations in the setting of T1DM. Most importantly, it did not allow for the precise titration employed by many patients. Second, there were concerns that greater variability in absorption from the intrapulmonary rather than the subcutaneous site would amplify the glycemic instability inherent in T1DM, particularly in the setting of intercurrent respiratory illness or exposures such as tobacco smoke. Third, the long-term safety of the pulmonary route of insulin administration is unknown, particularly in the setting of T1DM, in which insulin is likely to be administered three or more times a day potentially for 50 or more years. Exubera was withdrawn from the market due to commercial failure. The development of other inhaled insulin preparations and other alternative routes of administration is proceeding.

Approach to the Treatment of Type 1 Diabetes

Levels of glucose control equivalent to those achieved in the intensive treatment group in the DCCT are not possible in most patients unless an MDI regimen combining rapid- and long-acting insulin or CSII is used. More important than the schedule and method of administration is the need for the patient to adjust the insulin dose depending on the self-monitored glucose levels, dietary intake, and physical activity. The reason is relatively simple. In patients with little or no endogenous insulin production, the exogenous insulin regimen needs to simulate the multiphasic profile of insulin secretory responses to meals and snacks that is present in normal subjects if levels of glycemia approaching normal are to be achieved.

A number of regimens have been used to achieve these ends. Three basic approaches are reviewed here, although others approaches may be effective in individual patients. Achieving the glycemic goals of therapy is far more important than the details of the insulin regimen. Nevertheless, one of the following general approaches to therapy is most likely to lead to the desired outcome.

Combination of Rapid-Acting and Intermediate-Acting Insulin with Breakfast and Dinner and Intermediate-Acting Insulin at Bedtime

The rationale for regimens that use rapid- and intermediate-acting insulin at breakfast and dinner is that the rapid-acting insulin limits the postprandial glucose rise after breakfast and dinner, the intermediate-acting insulin administered before breakfast limits glycemia in the afternoon, and the intermediate-acting insulin before dinner limits glycemia in the early hours of the morning. Although such a regimen may be sufficient to achieve glucose targets in some patients, in many persons the intermediate-acting insulin given before dinner is insufficient to control elevations in blood glucose commonly seen in the early morning (*dawn phenomenon*). Attempts to increase the dose of intermediate-acting insulin at dinner expose the patient to a greater risk of hypoglycemia in the middle of the night; hence, the need for a smaller dose at bedtime to provide sufficient insulin to restrain the dawn phenomenon the following morning while moderating the risk of nocturnal hypoglycemia. This three-injection regimen was the mainstay of therapy in the DCCT but has largely been supplanted by regimens that take greater advantage of the availability of insulin analogues.

Combination of Rapid-Acting Insulin Given with Meals and Long-Acting Insulin at Bedtime

The combination of rapid-acting insulin with means and long-acting insulin at bedtime can also simulate the pattern of insulin production that occurs normally. Use of monomeric insulin analogues provides excellent meal coverage. Use of long-acting insulin at bedtime provides excellent control of the fasting plasma glucose level. This combination of rapid-acting monomeric insulin analogues with long-acting analogues has largely supplanted human insulin-based treatment regimens because it seems to be associated with less variability in glycemic control and with lower risks of hypoglycemia. When long-acting insulin is administered once a day in the evening, an unexplained and consistent rise in glucose can occur just before the evening injection of long-acting insulin because the analogue's duration is less than 24 hours. This is more common in patients who require low doses (<20 units) of long-acting analogue and arguably is more common with detemir than with glargine; it can be remedied by dosing the long-acting insulin twice daily.

Insulin Administration by an External Insulin Pump

An alternative method of delivering insulin is by an external mechanical pump. This approach involves administering a rapid-acting insulin preparation by CSII through a catheter that is usually inserted into the subcutaneous tissues of the anterior abdominal wall. The pump delivers insulin as a preprogrammed basal infusion in addition to patient-directed boluses given before meals or snacks or in response to elevations in the blood glucose concentration outside the desired range. With currently available pumps, the basal insulin infusion rate (usually about 1 U/hour) can be programmed either to continue at a constant rate over the 24-hour period or, more commonly, to increase and decrease at predetermined times of the day to prevent anticipated excursions in the blood glucose concentration (e.g., morning rises in glucose). Newer pumps allow multiple basal profiles to deal with recurrent patterns (e.g., menstruation, weekends, and activity). Protocols for insulin administration by the pump usually provide for approximately half of the insulin to be administered as a basal infusion and the remainder as premeal boluses.

Insulin administration by an external pump has some advantages over regimens that use multiple insulin injections. Only rapid-acting insulin is used in the insulin pump. Consequently, adjustments to the basal insulin infusion rate or changes in the size and timing of the insulin boluses result in more rapid changes in the blood glucose concentration than are possible when adjustments are made to the dose of intermediate- or long-acting insulin. This leads to greater flexibility for the patient. It has been suggested that use of analogue insulin can lead to a lower risk of hypoglycemia.[219,220]

There are also disadvantages of insulin pump therapy. There is a significant initial cost of the pump itself, and the tubing, which needs to be changed every 24 to 72 hours, and other supplies are expensive. The risk of infection at the site of insulin administration is significant. Infections occur on average once per year per patient even in the best of practices; although they can usually be treated by changing the site of infusion and giving a short course of oral antibiotics, surgical drainage may be necessary if an abscess develops. In addition, because only rapid-acting insulin is used, pump failure as a result of mechanical malfunction or catheter-related problems can quickly result in severe hyperglycemia and even ketoacidosis. Patients treated with insulin pump therapy must monitor their glucose level frequently and must always be alert to the possibility of failure of the infusion system.

Controlled clinical trials have indicated that, on average, insulin pump therapy is associated with modest improvements in glycemic control compared with MDI regimens—on the order of 0.2% to 0.3% as assessed by HbA_{1c}, at least in adults. Some patients never achieve adequate control with MDI but experience dramatic improvements with pump therapy. According to the ADA,[212] the insulin pump should be used only by candidates who are strongly motivated to improve glucose control and willing to work with their health care provider in assuming substantial responsibility for their day-to-day care. They must also understand and demonstrate use of the insulin pump and self-monitoring of blood glucose and be able to use the data obtained in an appropriate fashion.

Sensor-Augmented Pump Therapy

Recent studies have examined the use of sensor-augmented pump (SAP) therapy in patients with T1DM who have inadequate control with an MDI regimen.[221] SAP therapy integrates insulin pump therapy with a continuous glucose monitor that transmits to the pump and allows patients and clinicians to monitor treatment (insulin doses, carbohydrate intake, exercise) and response (glucose measured by the continuous monitor and by self-monitoring of blood glucose) through the use of Internet-based software. The Sensor-Augmented Pump Therapy for A1C Reduction (STAR-3) study was a 1-year, multicenter, randomized, controlled comparison of SAP versus MDI in 329 adults and 156 children with inadequately controlled T1DM previously treated in the investigator's practice for at least 6 months with MDI. Patients in both arms received recombinant insulin analogues and were supervised by expert clinical teams. HbA_{1c} was reduced from a baseline of 8.3% to 7.5% in the SAP group, compared with 8.1% in the MDI group ($P < .001$). There was no difference between the randomized therapies in the rates of severe hypoglycemia, ketoacidosis, or weight gain. This 0.6% relative difference is substantial and is of the same range required for approval of an antihyperglycemic medication. This is the first device that has been demonstrated to provide improvements in average glycemic control of that magnitude.

Algorithms of Insulin Administration

An essential component of intensive regimens of insulin replacement is the need to make regular adjustments to the insulin dose depending on the prevailing blood glucose concentration, planned activity, and food intake. Algorithms have been developed to guide these adjustments that aim to simulate the normal feedback control of insulin secretion, whereby hyperglycemia stimulates and hypoglycemia inhibits insulin secretion. They all involve frequent monitoring of the blood glucose concentration, usually four or more times per day; increases in the insulin dose if glucose levels are above the target upper level; reductions in the insulin dose if glucose levels are below the acceptable lower level; and techniques for adjusting insulin doses in relation to changes in diet. Several algorithms are available.[222-224]

Pramlintide

Amylin is a neuroendocrine hormone cosecreted with insulin by pancreatic beta cells. It was originally identified as a major constituent of pancreatic amyloid deposits. Its biologically active form is a 37-amino-acid peptide that undergoes extensive post-translational processing, including C-terminal amidation and glycosylation. As would be expected, amylin deficiency develops in parallel with insulin deficiency in patients with T1DM. Amylin and insulin have complementary actions in regulating plasma glucose. Insulin can be thought of as regulating the rate of glucose disappearance from the circulation. Amylin is thought to exert its major antihyperglycemic actions through central mechanisms after binding to brain nuclei such as the nucleus accumbens, dorsal raphe, and area postrema, promoting satiety and reducing appetite. It also is thought to act via vagal efferents, mediating a decrease in the rate of gastric emptying and a suppression of glucagon secretion in a glucose-dependent fashion. Effectively, amylin plays a role in regulating the rate of glucose appearance from the gastrointestinal tract and the liver.[225,226]

However, amylin is relatively insoluble in aqueous solution and aggregates on plastic and glass. Pramlintide was developed as a soluble, nonaggregating, equipotent amylin analogue. In 2005, pramlintide was approved for human use in the United States. As expected, when pramlintide is injected before meals, it slows gastric emptying, suppresses glucagon, and promotes satiety, with a subsequent reduction in the postprandial glucose level. In T1DM, pramlintide therapy is usually initiated at a dose of 15 μg before meals (0.025 mL or "2.5 units" in a U-100 insulin syringe of the marketed pramlintide acetate 0.6 mg/dL). Slow titration from there to the usual dose in patients with T1DM (60 μg before meals) as tolerated is recommended to minimize nausea and insulin-induced hypoglycemia. The maximally labeled dose in the setting of T2DM is 120 μg before meals.

In T1DM, the addition of pramlintide can be expected to produce modest reductions in HbA_{1c} (0.3 percentage points) and weight (1.5 kg), compared with placebo in controlled trials. Weight loss is more prevalent in overweight patients than in those with normal body weight, and it is generally independent of nausea. Severe insulin hypoglycemia can develop as a complication, particularly on initiation, because the effect of pramlintide on satiety can be robust, effectively stopping some patients from eating midmeal. To minimize this risk, it is suggested that patients reduce rapid-acting insulin at meals by approximately 50% on initiation of pramlintide; this is optimally accomplished by reducing the insulin-to-carbohydrate ratio and in many cases by administering pramlintide before the meal and insulin after the meal so that insulin dose reduction can be accomplished if the meal is not finished. Despite its role in glucagon regulation, pramlintide does not interfere with recovery from insulin-induced hypoglycemia.

Pramlintide is an agent whose role in the routine management of T1DM is evolving. The additional injections and expense certainly constitute a burden to patients and the health care system. Most patients note a dramatic improvement in postprandial glucose. Many find the appetite-suppressing effects quite helpful even in the absence of substantial weight gain. Some report an improvement in sense of well-being and energy. What is certain is that initiating and titrating pramlintide is complex and fraught with potential pitfalls. Perhaps more so than any other treatment for diabetes, it requires careful collaboration of patients and diabetes educators.

Complications of Intensive Management of Type 1 Diabetes

Hypoglycemia

The most serious complication of intensive regimens of insulin replacement is hypoglycemia, and this is usually the factor that limits patients' ability to achieve tight glucose control. In the DCCT, patients in the intensive treatment group had an approximately threefold greater risk of hypoglycemia than those in the conventional treatment group. Hypoglycemia can be life-threatening, leading to motor vehicle accidents, serious falls with fractures, and seizures. Patients with T1DM have serious defects in mechanisms responsible for glucose counterregulation, and this is a major underlying reason for the predisposition to hypoglycemia. Glucose counterregulation is reviewed in detail in Chapter 33.

The risk of hypoglycemia can be reduced if all patients treated with intensive regimens of insulin replacement are carefully educated about recognizing the symptoms of hypoglycemia and about the measures that should be taken to prevent more serious hypoglycemia after symptoms are initially experienced. Certain patients, particularly those with long-standing diabetes and autonomic neuropathy, may not subjectively sense symptoms of hypoglycemia even in the presence of low glucose concentrations. Glycemic targets of therapy should be adjusted upward in these patients, because they are at particularly high risk for hypoglycemia. Similarly, patients with advanced end-stage microvascular or macrovascular diabetic complications, in whom the benefit of intensive glucose control is likely to be less, should not be exposed to the increased risk of hypoglycemia that is inherent in extremely intensive insulin-treatment regimens.

In addition to the availability of glucose tablets, hard candy, or other sources of a readily absorbable form of carbohydrate, almost all patients with T1DM should have emergency glucagon kits at home and at work, assuming that there are people in those settings who can be trained to use them. The administration of 0.5 to 1 mg of glucagon intramuscularly to a severely symptomatic person with hypoglycemia rapidly increases the plasma glucose concentration to an acceptable range and prevents the difficulties and dangers associated with attempting to get a stuporous or disoriented person to ingest glucose by mouth. Nevertheless, because of occasional failures of glucagon to reverse hypoglycemia fully, friends and family members should always be instructed to call for medical assistance as soon as the injection is provided.

The use of continuous glucose sensors with alarms can reduce the time that patients spend with glucose in the hypoglycemic range. Early experience suggests that this can be particularly valuable in the setting of hypoglycemia unawareness.[227]

Weight Gain

Improvement in glucose control with a reduction in glycosuria is invariably associated with weight gain as the leakage of calories into the urine is reduced or eliminated. In addition, increased food intake to treat or prevent hypoglycemia can contribute to weight gain. Insulin itself can stimulate appetite. As a result of the combination of all these effects, weight gain is common, particularly with intensive regimens of insulin replacement. As discussed earlier, weight gain can be minimized or partially reversed with the addition of pramlintide.

Worsening of Retinopathy

The institution of regimens of tight glucose control has been reported to exacerbate underlying retinopathy. Therefore, if a patient with a serious background of proliferative retinopathy presents in poor glucose control, ophthalmologic treatment of the retinopathy should be considered before tight glucose control is instituted.

Insulin Allergy

Insulin allergy has become much less common with the use of human insulin. Most manifestations of allergic reactions to insulin consist of local wheal-and-flare reactions at the site of injection. The allergic reaction can be to the insulin itself or to other components of the insulin preparation, such as the protamine in NPH insulin. Occasionally, more generalized allergic reactions occur, and even more rarely, anaphylactic reactions take place. In general, mild local allergic reactions to insulin can be treated with antihistamines. More severe reactions require desensitization or coadministration of glucocorticoids. Admission to the hospital is necessary. Under close supervision of a physician with access to equipment for emergency resuscitation, a protocol is followed in which the patient is exposed to gradually increasing amounts of insulin administered according to a set schedule.[228]

ACUTE DIABETIC EMERGENCIES: DIABETIC KETOACIDOSIS

DKA is a life-threatening condition in which severe insulin deficiency leads to hyperglycemia, excessive lipolysis, and unrestrained fatty acid oxidation, producing the ketone bodies acetone, β-hydroxybutyrate, and acetoacetate. This results in metabolic acidosis, dehydration, and deficits in fluid and electrolytes. Excess secretion of primarily glucagon, as well as catecholamines, glucocorticoids, and growth hormone, in combination with insulin deficiency produces hyperglycemia by stimulating glycogenolysis and gluconeogenesis and impairing glucose disposal. DKA is a far more characteristic feature of T1DM than of T2DM, but it may be seen in persons with T2DM under conditions of stress such as occur with serious infections, trauma, and cardiovascular or other emergencies.

Clinical Presentation

Patients with uncontrolled diabetes present with nonspecific complaints. If the disease follows an indolent course over months to years, patients can manifest profound wasting, cachexia, and prostration similar in degree to those of patients with long-standing malignancy or chronic infection. With significant physical or emotional stress, sudden metabolic decompensation can occur. The cases of DKA that are misdiagnosed usually occur in patients with new-onset diabetes. Polyuria (or at least nocturia) and weight loss are almost always present, although they are often not reported by the patient. Any patient with severe illness (acute or chronic) or neurologic changes should have glucose and electrolytes measured.

In DKA, metabolic decompensation usually develops over a period of hours to a few days. Patients with DKA classically present with lethargy and a characteristic hyperventilation pattern with deep, slow breaths (Kussmaul respirations) associated with the fruity odor of acetone. They often complain of nausea and vomiting; abdominal pain is somewhat less frequent. The abdominal pain can be quite severe and may be associated with distention, ileus, and tenderness without rebound, but it usually resolves relatively quickly with therapy unless there is underlying abdominal pathology. Most patients are normotensive, tachycardic, and tachypneic and have signs of mild to moderate volume depletion. Hypothermia has been described in DKA, and patients with underlying infection might not manifest fever. Cerebral edema does occur, usually during therapy. Patients with DKA can have stupor and obvious profound dehydration, and they often demonstrate focal neurologic deficits such as Babinski reflexes, asymmetrical reflexes, cranial nerve findings, paresis, fasciculations, and aphasia.

Laboratory Test Results and Differential Diagnosis

Laboratory Tests

Laboratory tests that are routinely monitored in the setting of DKA include hemoglobin, white blood cell and differential count, glucose, electrolytes, BUN, and creatinine. Changes in Na, K, Cl, P, BUN, and creatinine are also monitored.

The *sine qua non* of DKA is acidosis, and the serum bicarbonate (HCO_3^-) concentration is usually less than 10 mEq/L. The acidosis is caused by production and accumulation of ketones in the serum. Three ketones are produced in DKA: two ketoacids (β-hydroxybutyrate and acetoacetate) and the neutral ketone, acetone. Ketones can be detected in serum and urine using the nitroprusside reaction on diagnostic strips for use at the patient's bedside or in the clinical laboratory. This test detects acetoacetate more effectively than acetone and does not detect an increased concentration of β-hydroxybutyrate. Particularly in severe DKA, β-hydroxybutyrate is the predominant ketone, and it is possible, although unusual, to have a negative serum nitroprusside reaction in the presence of severe ketosis. However, under these circumstances the serum bicarbonate is still markedly reduced and the anion gap is increased, indicating metabolic acidosis. The urinary β-hydroxybutyrate measurement can be performed at many centers and commercially but is not usually readily available.

The *anion gap* is a readily available index for unmeasured anions in the blood (normal, ≤14 mEq/L):

$$\text{Anion gap} = \text{sodium} - (\text{chloride} + \text{bicarbonate})$$

Most patients with DKA present with an anion gap greater than 20 mEq/L, and some present with a gap greater than 40 mEq/L. However, patients occasionally have a hyperchloremic metabolic acidosis without a significant anion gap.[229]

Patients with DKA almost invariably have large amounts of ketones in their urine. The serum glucose in DKA is usually in the 500 mg/dL range. However, an entity known as euglycemic DKA has been described, particularly in patients who have decreased oral intake or are pregnant, in which the serum glucose is normal or near normal but the patient requires insulin therapy for clearance of ketoacidosis.[230] The arterial pH is commonly less than 7.3 and can be as low as 6.5. There is partial respiratory compensation with hypocarbia. Patients are often mildly hyperosmolar, although osmolality greater than 330 mOsm/kg is unusual without mental status changes.

Differential Diagnosis

Not all patients with hyperglycemia and an anion gap metabolic acidosis have DKA, and other causes of metabolic acidosis must be considered in these patients, particularly if the serum or urine ketone measurements are not elevated. The following causes of metabolic acidosis need to be considered in the differential diagnosis of DKA.

Lactic acidosis is the most common cause of metabolic acidosis in hospitalized patients and can be seen in patients with uncomplicated diabetes as well as those with DKA. Lactic acidosis usually occurs in the setting of decreased tissue oxygen delivery, which results in the nonoxidative metabolism of glucose to lactic acid. Lactic acidosis complicates other primary metabolic acidoses as a consequence of dehydration or shock, and assessing its relative contribution can be difficult. The presentation is identical to that of DKA. In pure lactic acidosis, the serum glucose and ketones should be normal and the serum lactate concentration should be greater than 5 mmol/L. The therapy for lactic acidosis is directed at the underlying cause and at optimization of tissue perfusion.[231]

Starvation ketosis is caused by inadequate carbohydrate availability, which results in physiologically appropriate lipolysis and ketone production to provide fuel substrates for muscle. The blood glucose concentration is usually normal. Although the urine can have large amounts of ketones, the blood rarely does. Arterial pH is normal, and the anion gap is at most mildly elevated.

Alcoholic ketoacidosis is a more severe form of starvation ketosis wherein the appropriate ketogenic response to poor carbohydrate intake is increased through as yet poorly defined effects of alcohol on the liver. Classically, these patients are long-standing alcoholics for whom ethanol has been the main caloric source for days to weeks. The ketoacidosis occurs when, for some reason, alcohol and caloric intake decreases. In isolated alcoholic ketoacidosis, the metabolic acidosis is usually mild to moderate. The anion gap is elevated. Serum and urine ketones are always present. However, alcoholic ketoacidosis produces an even higher ratio of β-hydroxybutyrate to acetoacetate than DKA does, and negative or weakly positive nitroprusside reactions are common. Respiratory alkalosis associated with delirium tremens, agitation, or pulmonary processes often normalizes the pH but should be evident with careful analysis of acid-base status. Usually, the patient is normoglycemic or hypoglycemic, although mild hyperglycemia is occasionally present. Patients who are significantly hyperglycemic should be treated as if they had DKA. The therapy for alcoholic ketoacidosis consists of thiamine, carbohydrates, fluids, and electrolytes, with special attention to the more severe consequences of alcohol toxicity, alcohol withdrawal, and chronic malnutrition. In more severely ill patients in whom alcoholic ketoacidosis is considered a possibility, there is usually another underlying illness such as pancreatitis, gastrointestinal bleeding, hepatic encephalopathy, delirium tremens, or infection complicated by concomitant lactic acidosis.[232,233]

Uremic acidosis is characterized by extremely large elevations in the BUN (often >200 mg/dL) and creatinine (>10 mg/dL) values with normoglycemia. The pH and anion gap are usually only mildly abnormal. The treatment is supportive, with careful attention to fluid and electrolytes until dialysis can be performed. Rhabdomyolysis is a cause of renal failure in which the anion gap can be significantly elevated and acidosis can be severe. There should be marked elevation of creatine phosphokinase and myoglobin. Mild rhabdomyolysis is not uncommon in DKA, but the presence of hyperglycemia and ketonemia leaves no doubt about the primary etiology of the acidosis.[234]

Toxic ingestions can be differentiated from DKA by history and laboratory investigation. Salicylate intoxication produces an anion gap metabolic acidosis, usually with an accompanying respiratory alkalosis. The plasma glucose level is normal or low, the osmolality is normal, ketones are negative, and salicylates can be detected in the urine or blood. Salicylates can cause a false-positive glucose determination when the cupric sulfate method is used and a false-negative result when the glucose oxidase reaction is used. Methanol and ethylene glycol also produce an anion gap metabolic acidosis without hyperglycemia or ketones, but these toxins need to be kept in mind primarily because they produce an increase in the measured serum osmolality but not in the calculated serum osmolality—an osmolar gap. Their serum levels can also be measured. Isopropyl alcohol does not cause a metabolic acidosis but should be remembered because it is metabolized to acetone, which can produce a positive result in the nitroprusside reaction commonly used for the detection of ketoacids. These intoxications must be appropriately treated.[235-237] Rare cases of anion gap acidoses have been reported with other ingestions, including toluene, iron, hydrogen sulfide, nalidixic acid, papaverine, paraldehyde, strychnine, isoniazid, and outdated tetracycline.

When DKA is considered, the diagnosis can be made quickly with routine laboratory tests. Measurements of blood and urine glucose and ketones can be obtained in minutes, using, respectively, glucose oxidase–impregnated strips and the nitroprusside reaction.

Osmolarity

The increase in osmolarity (in milliosmoles per liter [mOsm/L]) that occurs in DKA must be differentiated from the increase in osmolarity seen in hyperosmolar-hyperglycemic nonketotic (diabetic) coma (HHNC). The osmolarity can be measured by freezing point depression or estimated with the use of the following formula:

$$\text{Osmolarity} = (2 \times \text{sodium}) + (\text{glucose}/18) + (\text{BUN}/2.8) + (\text{ethanol}/4.6)$$

Patients with DKA not uncommonly present with hyperosmolarity and coma. In HHNC, the osmolarity is usually greater than 350 mOsm/L, and it can exceed 400 mOsm/L. The serum sodium and potassium levels can be high, normal, or low and do not reflect total-body levels, which are uniformly depleted. The glucose concentration is usually greater than 600 mg/dL, and levels higher than 1000 mg/dL are common. In pure HHNC, there is no significant metabolic acidosis or anion gap.

Patients often present with combinations of the preceding findings. HHNC can involve mild to moderate ketonemia and acidosis. Alcoholic ketoacidosis can contribute to either DKA or HHNC. Lactic acidosis is common in severe DKA and HHNC. Any patient with hyperglycemia greater than 250 mg/dL and an anion gap metabolic acidosis should be treated by the general principles outlined in the following section, with special consideration for other possible contributing metabolic acidoses.

Therapy

The optimal management of DKA has been a source of considerable controversy since the 1950s. Only recently have prospective studies of various therapeutic approaches been performed. The guidelines we propose rely heavily on prospective studies of DKA by Kitabchi and coworkers.[238,239] The general approach is to provide necessary fluids to restore the circulation, treat insulin deficiency with continuous insulin, treat electrolyte disturbances, observe the patient closely and carefully, and search for underlying causes of metabolic decompensation.

Fluids

Volume contraction is one of the hallmarks of DKA. It can contribute to acidosis through lactic acid production and decreased renal clearance of organic and inorganic acids. It contributes to hyperglycemia by decreasing renal clearance of glucose. Decreased tissue perfusion, if significant, causes insulin resistance by decreasing insulin delivery to the sites of insulin-mediated glucose disposal, namely muscle and adipose tissue, and through stimulation of catecholamine and glucocorticoid secretion. Fluid deficits on the order of 5 to 10 L are common in DKA. The urine produced during the osmotic diuresis of hyperglycemia is approximately half-normal with respect to sodium. Therefore, water deficits are in excess of sodium deficits. Historically, large quantities of isotonic intravenous fluids have been administered rapidly to patients in DKA. For patients with a history of congestive heart failure, chronic or acute renal failure, severe hypotension, or significant pulmonary disease, early invasive hemodynamic monitoring should be considered.

When there is physical evidence of dehydration (i.e., hypotension, decreased skin turgor, or dry mucous membranes), the general treatment is to administer 1 L of normal saline over the first hour and 200 to 500 mL/hour in subsequent hours until hypotension resolves and adequate circulation is maintained. If hypotension is severe, there is clinical evidence of hypoperfusion, and hypotension does not respond to crystalloid, therapy with colloid is considered, often in combination with invasive hemodynamic monitoring. If there is no hypotension and no concern about renal failure, 1 L of half-normal saline is administered over the first hour.

During that first hour, the laboratory data usually return and can be quite helpful in planning further therapy. Despite the excess of water losses over sodium, the measured sodium is usually low because of the osmotic effects of glucose. These osmotic effects can be corrected using a simple formula:

$$\text{Corrected sodium concentration} = \text{measured sodium} + 0.016 \times (\text{glucose} - 100)$$

Severe hypertriglyceridemia, which is common in severe diabetes, can cause a false decrease in the serum sodium concentration by approximately 1.0 mEq/L at a serum lipid concentration of 460 mg/dL.[228] An estimated water deficit can be calculated using the corrected sodium concentration:

$$\text{Water deficit in liters} = 0.6 \times \text{weight in kg} \times [(\text{sodium}/140) - 1]$$

Based on these formulas, a 70-kg patient with a measured sodium level of 140 mEq/L and a glucose concentration of 1000 mg/dL would have a calculated water deficit of 4.3 L. If the patient is normotensive after the first liter of fluids has been administered, it is reasonable to aim to replace urinary losses with one-half normal saline and also to provide approximately one half of the water deficit (in this example, 2 L) as 5% dextrose over the first 12 to 24 hours and the remainder over the subsequent 24 hours. The plan for fluid therapy should be continuously reevaluated in light of the clinical and laboratory response of the patient. When the serum glucose level reaches 250 to 300 mg/dL, all fluids should contain 5% dextrose and therapy should be aimed at maintaining the serum glucose concentration in that range for 24 hours to allow slow equilibration of osmotically active substances across cell membranes.

The primary goal of fluid therapy is to maintain an adequate circulation, and the secondary goal is to maintain a brisk diuresis. Beyond that, pulmonary edema, hyperchloremic metabolic acidosis, and a rapid fall in the serum osmolality should be prevented by frequent monitoring of the patient and administration of glucose and electrolytes. It has been demonstrated that fluid administration and subsequent continued osmotic diuresis are responsible for a large portion of the initial decline in glucose during therapy.

Insulin

Insulin is the mainstay of therapy for DKA, because DKA is essentially an insulin-deficient state. In the past, high doses of insulin (50 U/hour or more) were favored. In later studies, low-dose insulin therapy (0.1 U/kg/hour) has been shown to be as effective as higher doses in producing a decrease in serum glucose and clearance of ketones. Furthermore, low-dose therapy results in a reduction in the major morbidity of intensive insulin therapy, namely hypoglycemia and hypokalemia.

Studies have also shown that intravenous insulin is significantly more effective than intramuscular or subcutaneous insulin in lowering the ketone body concentration over the first 2 hours of therapy. The subcutaneous route is probably inappropriate for the critically ill patient because of the possibility of tissue hypoperfusion and slower kinetics of absorption; however, one study documented that a subcutaneous rapid-acting insulin analogue administered every 1 to 2 hours was as safe and effective as intravenous regular insulin in the treatment of uncomplicated DKA.[240] Numerous studies attest to the efficacy of intramuscular therapy in severe DKA. If there is insufficient nursing monitoring or intravenous access to allow safe intravenous administration, intramuscular therapy is the route of choice.

It has been shown that a 10-U intravenous insulin priming dose given at the initiation of insulin therapy significantly improves the glycemic response to the first hour of therapy. The rationale is to saturate insulin receptors fully before beginning continuous therapy and to avoid the lag time that is necessary to achieve steady-state insulin levels. When insulin is mixed in normal saline, it does not seem to be necessary to add albumin to prevent insulin adsorption to the infusion set. However, the intravenous tubing should be flushed with the insulin infusate before use.

In the rare instances in which the glucose level does not decrease by at least 10% or 50 mg/dL in 1 hour, the insulin infusion rate should be increased by 50% to 100% and a second bolus of intravenous insulin should be administered. As the glucose level decreases, it is usually necessary to decrease the rate of infusion. After the glucose reaches approximately 250 mg/dL, it is prudent to decrease the insulin infusion rate and administer dextrose. It usually takes an additional 12 to 24 hours to clear ketones from the circulation after hyperglycemia is controlled. With resolution of ketosis, the rate of infusion approaches the physiologic range of 0.3 to 0.5 U/kg per day.

When the decision is made to feed the patient, intravenous or intramuscular therapy should be changed to subcutaneous therapy. Subcutaneous insulin should be administered before a meal, and the insulin drip should be discontinued approximately 30 minutes later. The glucose should be checked in 2 hours and at least every 4 hours afterward until a relatively stable insulin regimen is determined. Early conversion to oral feeding and subcutaneous insulin therapy is associated with a shorter hospital stay.

Potassium

Potassium losses during the development of DKA are usually quite high (3-10 mEq/kg) and are mediated by shifts to the extracellular space secondary to acidosis and protein catabolism compounded by hyperaldosteronism and osmotic diuresis. Although most patients with DKA or HHNC have a normal or even high serum potassium level at presentation, the initial therapy with fluids and insulin causes it to fall.

Our approach has been to monitor the electrocardiogram (ECG) for signs of hyperkalemia (peaked T wave, QRS widening) initially and to administer potassium if these signs are absent and the serum potassium level is less than 5.5 mEq/L. If the patient is oliguric, we do not administer potassium unless the serum concentration is less than 4 mEq/L or there are ECG signs of hypokalemia (U wave), and even then potassium is administered with extreme caution. With treatment of DKA, the potassium level always falls, usually reaching a nadir after several hours. We usually replace potassium at 10 to 20 mEq/hour (half as potassium chloride and half as potassium phosphate), monitor serum levels at least every 2 hours initially, and monitor ECG morphology. Occasionally, patients with

DKA who have had protracted courses that include vomiting, hypokalemia, and acidosis require 40 to 60 mEq/hour by central line to prevent further decreases in the serum potassium concentration.

Phosphate

Like potassium, phosphate is depleted in patients with DKA. Although patients usually present with an elevated serum phosphate concentration, the serum level declines with therapy. No well-documented clinical significance of these findings has been determined and no benefit of phosphate administration has been demonstrated, but most authorities recommend phosphate therapy as before and monitoring for its possible complications, which include hypocalcemia and hypomagnesemia.

Bicarbonate

Serum bicarbonate is always low in DKA, but a true deficit is not present because the ketoacids and lactate anions are metabolized to bicarbonate during therapy. The use of bicarbonate in the treatment of DKA is highly controversial. No benefit of bicarbonate therapy has been demonstrated in clinical trials. In fact, in two trials, hypokalemia was more common in bicarbonate-treated patients. There are theoretical considerations against the use of bicarbonate. Cellular levels of 2,3-diphosphoglycerate are depleted in DKA, causing a shift in the oxyhemoglobin dissociation curve to the left and thus impairing tissue oxygen delivery. Acidemia has the opposite effect, and therefore acute reversal of acidosis could decrease tissue oxygen delivery. In addition, in vitro data suggest that pH is a regulator of cellular lactate metabolism, and correction of acidosis could increase lactate production. These observations are of questionable clinical relevance, however.

We reserve bicarbonate therapy for patients with severe acidosis (pH <6.9), patients with hemodynamic instability if the pH is less than 7.1, and patients with hyperkalemia with ECG findings. When bicarbonate is used, it should be used sparingly and considered a temporizing measure while definitive therapy with insulin and fluids is under way. Approximately 1 mEq/kg of bicarbonate is administered as a rapid infusion over 10 to 15 minutes, and further therapy is based on repeated arterial blood gas sampling every 30 to 120 minutes. Potassium therapy should be considered before treatment with bicarbonate is undertaken, because transient hypokalemia is not an uncommon complication of the administration of alkali.

Monitoring

It is possible to manage many cases of mild DKA without admitting the patient to the intensive care unit, depending on staff availability. We routinely admit patients with DKA to the intensive care unit if they have a pH of less than 7.3. If mental status is compromised, prophylactic intubation is considered, and nasogastric suctioning is always performed because of frequent ileus and danger of aspiration. If the patient cannot void at will, bladder catheterization is necessary to monitor urine output adequately. ECG monitoring is continuous, with hourly documentation of QRS intervals and T-wave morphology. Initially, serum glucose, electrolytes, BUN, creatinine, calcium, magnesium, phosphate, ketones, lactate, creatine phosphokinase, and liver function tests as well as urinalysis, ECG, upright chest radiograph, complete blood count, and arterial blood gas analyses are obtained. If there is any concern about possible toxic ingestions, toxicology screening is also performed. Subsequently, glucose and electrolytes are measured at least hourly; calcium, magnesium, and phosphate every 2 hours; and BUN, creatinine, and ketones every 6 to 24 hours.

It is often not necessary to monitor arterial blood gases routinely, because the bicarbonate level and the anion gap are relatively good indices of the response to therapy. Monitoring of venous pH has also been shown to reflect acidemia and response to therapy adequately. Usually, frequent blood work is necessary only for the first 12 hours or so. In the severely ill patient with obvious underlying disease, the course is often more protracted, and, particularly when venous access is a problem, early consideration should be given to placement of an arterial line. A flow sheet tabulating these findings as well as mental status, vital signs, insulin dose, fluid and electrolytes administered, and urine output allows easy analysis of response to therapy. After the acidosis begins to resolve and the response to therapy becomes predictable, it is reasonable to curtail laboratory testing. If the patient's cardiovascular status is unclear or troublesome, invasive hemodynamic monitoring is an appropriate guide for fluid therapy. The goals should be to achieve hemodynamic stability rapidly and to correct DKA fully in 12 to 36 hours.

Search for Underlying Causes

After the patient is stabilized, a careful history and physical examination is performed and a diagnostic strategy is developed that should be aimed at determining the precipitating event. In most inner-city practices, the most common cause of DKA is noncompliance with insulin therapy, which is usually easily treated. The second most common cause is infection, with viral syndromes, urinary tract infection, pelvic inflammatory disease, and pneumonia predominating. It is often difficult to determine initially whether the patient is infected. Fever is absent in a significant fraction of patients with diabetic emergencies. The white blood cell count is not uncommonly elevated in the range of 20,000/μL or higher even in the absence of infection.[241] As a result, cultures should be performed for most patients, and if there is significant concern about infection, empiric broad antibiotic coverage should be considered pending microbiologic findings.

Special consideration should be given to ruling out meningitis in the patient with altered mental status. In this regard, most would perform lumbar puncture in all patients with meningismus and in patients with disproportionate mental status changes. If the index of suspicion is lower, the antibiotic therapy should be geared to cover bacterial meningitis, and a lumbar puncture should be performed if the mental status does not improve quickly with therapy. The cerebrospinal fluid glucose measurement is not particularly useful in determining whether the fluid is infected, and a level lower than 100 mg/dL is unusual when the serum glucose concentration is greater than 250 mg/dL.[242] The relative frequency of sinus infection (particularly with *Mucor*), foot infection, bacterial arthritis, cholecystitis, cellulitis, and necrotizing fasciitis should also be considered.

Pneumonia can be difficult to diagnose in patients with dehydration because the alveolar edema fluid that shows up as an infiltrate on chest radiographs is often not present but develops along with progressive hypoxia during hydration. To prevent this occurrence, we administer intravenous fluid judiciously to patients with suspected pneumonia. Pancreatitis and pregnancy are common precipitants and should be especially considered when assessing the abdominal pain that is almost ubiquitous at presentation. Abdominal guarding and tenderness associated with vomiting are common, and rebound is occasionally present. These symptoms and findings usually resolve quickly with therapy in the absence of intra-abdominal pathology. The serum amylase is often elevated without pathologic significance, although lipase is usually more specific.[243] Acute myocardial infarction, stroke, and thromboembolic phenomena are frequent precipitants and complications of DKA.

The more insulin resistant the patient seems to be, the more likely one is to find a precipitating cause. If a precipitating cause is found, treatment is essential if adequate metabolic control is to be achieved.

Complications and Prognosis

It should now be possible to treat almost all cases of DKA successfully. The most troublesome complication is cerebral edema. It is common particularly in children and can be fatal. In most reported series, specific causes could not be assigned, although aggressive hydration, particularly with hypotonic fluids, can contribute.[244] In 50% of patients who subsequently had a respiratory arrest, there were premonitory symptoms, and despite early intervention only half of them avoided severe or fatal brain damage.

Other complications of life-threatening severity that have been reported include the acute respiratory distress syndrome and bronchial mucous plugging.[245-247] Arterial and venous thromboembolic events are quite common. Standard prophylactic low-dose heparin is certainly reasonable in patients with DKA, but currently no indication exists for full anticoagulation.

Two studies show that specialists (endocrinologists) provide more cost-effective care than nonspecialists. Patients under the care of specialists have a shorter hospital stay, fewer medical procedures, and lower medical costs.[248,249]

REFERENCES

1. Sutherland DE, Sibley R, Xu XA, et al. Twin-to-twin pancreas transplantation: reversal and reenactment of the pathogenesis of type I diabetes. *Trans Assoc Am Physicians*. 1984;97:80-87.
2. Wang YO, Ponteselli RG, Gill RG, et al. The role of CD4 and CD8 T cells in the destruction of islet grafts by diabetic NOD mice. *Proc Natl Acad Sci U S A*. 1991;88:527-531.
3. Devendra D, Liu E, Eisenbarth GS. Type 1 diabetes: recent developments. *Br Med J*. 2004;328:750-754.
4. Glandt M, Herold KC. Treatment of type 1 diabetes with anti-T-cell agents: from T-cell depletion to T-cell regulation. *Curr Diab Rep*. 2004;4:291-297.
5. American Diabetes Association. Clinical practice recommendations 2002. *Diabetes Care*. 2002;25(suppl 1):S1-S147.
6. Leslie RD, Atkinson MA, Notkins AL. Autoantigens IA-2 and GAD in type I (insulin-dependent) diabetes. *Diabetologia*. 1999;42:3-14.
7. Rewers M, Norris JM, Dabela D. Epidemiology of type I diabetes. In: Eisenbarth GS, Lafferty KJ, eds. *Type 1 Diabetes: Molecular, Cellular, and Clinical Immunology*. 2nd ed. New York, NY: Kluwer Academic; 2005:219-246.
8. Pinhas-Hamiel O, Dolan LM, Daniels SR, et al. Increased incidence of non-insulin dependent diabetes mellitus among adolescents. *J Pediatr*. 1996;128:608-615.
9. Pinhas-Haniel O, Dolan LM, Zeitlers PS. Diabetic ketoacidosis among obese African-American adolescents with NIDDM. *Diabetes Care*. 1997;20:484-486.
10. Rosenbloom AL, House DV, Winter WE. Non-insulin dependent diabetes mellitus (NIDDM) in minority youth: research priorities and needs. *Clin Pediatr (Phila)*. 1998;37:143-152.
11. Imagawa A, Hanafusa T, Miyagawa J. A novel subtype of type 1 diabetes mellitus characterized by a rapid onset and an absence of diabetes-related antibodies. *N Engl J Med*. 2000;342:301-307.
12. Ziegler A-G, Hummel M, Schenker M, et al. Autoantibody appearance and risk for development of childhood diabetes in offspring of parents with type 1 diabetes: the 2-year analysis of the German BABYDIAB study. *Diabetes*. 1999;48:460-468.
13. Mordes JP, Bortell R, Doukas J, et al. The BB/Wor rat and the balance hypothesis of autoimmunity. *Diabetes Metab Rev*. 1996;12:1 03-109.
14. Roep BO, Atkinson M, von Herrath M. Satisfaction (not) guaranteed: re-evaluating the use of animal models of type 1 diabetes. *Nat Rev Immunol*. 2004;4:989-997.
15. Thomas HE, Kay TW. Beta cell destruction in the development of autoimmune diabetes in the non-obese diabetic (NOD) mouse. *Diabetes Metab Res Rev*. 2000;16:251-261.
16. Wong FS, Janeway CAJ. Insulin-dependent diabetes mellitus and its animal models. *Curr Opin Immunol*. 1999;11:643-647.
17. Eisenbarth GS. Animal models of type 1 diabetes: genetics and immunological function. In: Eisenbarth GS, Lafferty KJ, eds. *Type 1 Diabetes: Molecular, Cellular, and Clinical Immunology*. 2nd ed. New York, NY: Kluwer Academic; 2005:91-116.
18. Hattori M, Buse JB, Jackson RA, et al. The NOD mouse: recessive diabetogenic gene within the major histocompatibility complex. *Science*. 1986;231:733-735.
19. Noble JA, Valdes AM, Cook M, et al. The role of HLA class II genes in insulin-dependent diabetes mellitus: molecular analysis of 180 Caucasian, multiplex families. *Am J Hum Genet*. 1996;59:1134-1148.
20. Todd JA, Bell JI, McDevitt HO. HLA-DQB gene contributes to susceptibility and resistance to insulin-dependent diabetes mellitus. *Nature*. 1987;329:599-604.
21. Nishimoto H, Kikutani H, Yamamura K, et al. Prevention of autoimmune insulitis by expression of I-E molecules in NOD mice. *Nature*. 1987;328:432-434.
22. Singer SM, Tisch R, Yang XD, et al. Prevention of diabetes in NOD mice by a mutated I-Ab transgene. *Diabetes*. 1998;47:1570-1577.
23. Lyons PA, Hancock WW, Denny P, et al. The NOD Idd9 genetic interval influences the pathogenicity of insulitis and contains molecular variants of Cd30, Tnfr2, and Cd137. *Immunity*. 2000;13:107-115.
24. Mathews CE, Graser RT, Serreze DV, et al. Reevaluation of the major histocompatibility complex genes of the NOD-progenitor CTS/Shi strain. *Diabetes*. 2000;49:131-134.
25. Yui MA, Muralidharan K, Moreno-Altamirano B, et al. Production of congenic mouse strains carrying NOD-derived diabetogenic genetic intervals: an approach for the genetic dissection of complex traits. *Mamm Genome*. 1996;7:331-334.
26. Wicker LS, Miller BJ, Coker LZ, et al. Genetic control of diabetes and insulitis in the nonobese diabetic (NOD) mouse. *J Exp Med*. 1987; 165:1639-1654.
27. Yu L, Robles DT, Abiru N, et al. Early expression of anti-insulin autoantibodies of man and the NOD mouse: evidence for early determination of subsequent diabetes. *Proc Natl Acad Sci U S A*. 2000;97: 1701-1706.
28. Sreenan S, Pick AJ, Levisetti M, et al. Increased β-cell proliferation and reduced mass before diabetes onset in the nonobese diabetic mouse. *Diabetes*. 1999;48:989-996.
29. Dilts SM, Lafferty KJ. Autoimmune diabetes: the involvement of benign and malignant autoimmunity. *J Autoimmun*. 1999;12: 229-232.
30. Shimada A, Charlton B, Taylor-Edwards C, et al. β-Cell destruction may be a late consequence of the autoimmune process in nonobese diabetic mice. *Diabetes*. 1996;45:1063-1067.
31. Chatenoud L, Primo J, Bach JF. CD3 antibody-induced dominant self tolerance in overtly diabetic NOD mice. *J Immunol*. 1997;158: 2947-2954.
32. Wegmann DR, Eisenbarth GS. It's insulin. *J Autoimmun*. 2000; 15:286-291.
33. Nagata M, Santamaria P, Kawamura T, et al. Evidence for the role of $CD8^+$ cytotoxic T cells in the destruction of pancreatic β-cells in nonobese diabetic mice. *J Immunol*. 1994;152:2042-2050.
34. Schmidt D, Amrani A, Verdaguer J, et al. Autoantigen-independent deletion of diabetogenic $CD4^+$ thymocytes by protective MHC class II molecules. *J Immunol*. 1999;162:4627-4636.
35. Haskins K. T cell receptor gene usage in autoimmune diabetes. *Int Rev Immunol*. 1999;18:61-81.
36. Nakayama M, Abiru N, Moriyama H, et al. Prime role for an insulin epitope in the development of type 1 diabetes in NOD mice. *Nature*. 2005;435:220-223.
37. Tian J, Atkinson M, Clare-Salzer M, et al. Nasal administration of glutamate decarboxylase (GAD65) peptides induces Th2 responses and prevents murine insulin-dependent diabetes. *J Exp Med*. 1996;183: 1561-1567.
38. Muir A, Peck A, Clare-Salzler M, et al. Insulin immunization of nonobese diabetic mice induces a protective insulitis characterized by diminished intraislet interferon-gamma transcription. *J Clin Invest*. 1995;95:628-634.
39. Cetkovic-Cvrlje M, Gerling IC, Muir A, et al. Retardation or acceleration of diabetes in NOD/Lt mice mediated by intrathymic administration of candidate β-cell antigens. *Diabetes*. 1997;46:1975-1982.
40. Daniel D, Wegmann DR. Protection of nonobese diabetic mice from diabetes by intranasal or subcutaneous administration of insulin peptide B-(9-23). *Proc Natl Acad Sci U S A*. 1996;93:956-960.

41. Awata T, Guberski DL, Like AA. Genetics of the BB rat: association of autoimmune disorders (diabetes, insulitis, and thyroiditis) with lymphopenia and major histocompatibility complex class II. *Endocrinology*. 1995;136:5731-5735.
42. Achenbach P, Koczwara K, Knopff A, et al. Mature high-affinity immune responses to (pro)insulin anticipate the autoimmune cascade that leads to type 1 diabetes. *J Clin Invest*. 2004;114:589-597.
43. Jacob HJ, Pettersson A, Wilson D, et al. Genetic dissection of autoimmune type I diabetes in the BB rat. *Nat Genet*. 1992;2:56-60.
44. Hornum L, Romer J, Markholst H. The diabetes-prone BB rat carries a frameshift mutation in *Ian4*, a positional candidate of *Iddm1*. *Diabetes*. 2002;51:1972-1979.
45. Gottlieb PA, Handler ES, Appel MC, et al. Insulin treatment prevents diabetes mellitus but not thyroiditis in RT 6-depleted diabetes resistant BB/Wor rats. *Diabetologia*. 1991;34:296-300.
46. Song HY, Abad MM, Mahoney CP, et al. Human insulin B chain but not A chain decreases the rate of diabetes in BB rats. *Diabetes Res Clin Pract*. 1999;46:109-114.
47. Yokoi N, Komeda K, Wang HY, et al. Cblb is a major susceptibility gene for rat type 1 diabetes mellitus. *Nat Genet*. 2002;31:391-394.
48. Kawano K, Hirashima T, Mori S, et al. New inbred strain of Long-Evans Tokushima lean rats with IDDM without lymphopenia. *Diabetes*. 1991;40:1375-1381.
49. Yokoi N, Kanazawa M, Kitada K, et al. A non-MHC locus essential for autoimmune type I diabetes in the Komeda diabetes-prone rat. *J Clin Invest*. 1997;100:2015-2021.
50. Uchigata Y, Yamamoto H, Nagai H, et al. Effect of poly(ADP-ribose) synthetase inhibitor administration to rats before and after injection of alloxan and streptozotocin on islet proinsulin synthesis. *Diabetes*. 1983;32:316-318.
51. Tanaka SI, Nakajima AS, Inoue S, et al. Genetic control by I-A subregion in H-2 complex of incidence of streptozotocin-induced autoimmune diabetes in mice. *Diabetes*. 1990;39:1298-1304.
52. Ellerman KE, Like AA. Susceptibility to diabetes is widely distributed in normal class IIu haplotype rats. *Diabetologia*. 2000;43:890-898.
53. Schreuder TC, et al. High incidence of type 1 diabetes mellitus during or shortly after treatment with pegylated interferon alpha for chronic hepatitis C virus infection. *Liver Int*. 2008;28(1):39-46.
54. Pipeleers D, Ling Z. Pancreatic beta cells in insulin-dependent diabetes. *Diabetes Metab Rev*. 1992;8:209-227.
55. Foulis AK, Clark A. Pathology of the pancreas in diabetes mellitus. In: Kahn CR, Weir GC, eds. *Joslin's Diabetes Mellitus*. 13th ed. Philadelphia, PA: Lea & Febiger; 1994:265-281.
56. Doniach D, Morgan AG. Islets of Langerhans in juvenile diabetes mellitus. *Clin Endocrinol (Oxf)*. 1973;2:233-248.
57. Gepts W, LeCompte PM. The pancreatic islets in diabetes. *Am J Med*. 1981;70:105-115.
58. Foulis AK, Liddle CN, Farquharson MA, et al. The histopathology of the pancreas in type I diabetes (insulin dependent) mellitus: a 25-year review of deaths in patients under 20 years of age in the United Kingdom. *Diabetologia*. 1986;29:267-274.
59. Foulis AK, Farquharson MA, Hardman R. Aberrant expression of class II major histocompatibility complex molecules by β cells and hyperexpression of class I major histocompatibility complex molecules by insulin containing islets in type 1 (insulin dependent) diabetes mellitus. *Diabetologia*. 1987;30:333-343.
60. Huang X, Yuan J, Goddard A, et al. Interferon expression in the pancreases of patients with type I diabetes. *Diabetes*. 1995;44:658-664.
61. Amrani A, Verdaguer J, Thiessen S, et al. IL-1α, IL-1β, and IFN-γ mark beta cells for fas-dependent destruction by diabetogenic CD4+ T lymphocytes. *J Clin Invest*. 2000;105:459-468.
62. Itoh N, Imagawa A, Hanafusa T, et al. Requirement of Fas for the development of autoimmune diabetes in nonobese diabetic mice. *J Exp Med*. 1997;186:613-618.
63. Chervonsky AV, Wang Y, Wong FS, et al. The role of Fas in autoimmune diabetes. *Cell*. 1997;89:17-24.
64. Thomas HE, Kay TW. How beta cells die in type 1 diabetes. *Curr Dir Autoimmun*. 2001;4:144-170.
65. Marleau AM, Sarvetnick N. T cell homeostasis in tolerance and immunity. *J Leukoc Biol*. 2005;78:575-584.
66. Lo D. Immune regulation: susceptibility and resistance to autoimmunity. *Immunol Res*. 2000;21:239-246.
67. Wong FS, Janeway CAJ. The role of CD4 vs. CD8 T cells in IDDM. *J Autoimmun*. 1999;13:290-295.
68. Lieberman SM, Takaki T, Han B, et al. Individual nonobese diabetic mice exhibit unique patterns of CD8+ T cell reactivity to three islet antigens, including the newly identified widely expressed dystrophia myotonica kinase. *J Immunol*. 2004;173:6727-6734.
69. Wong FS, Dittel BN, Janeway CAJ. Transgenes and knockout mutations in animal models of type 1 diabetes and multiple sclerosis. *Immunol Rev*. 1999;169:93-104.
70. Ylipaasto P, Klingel K, Lindberg AM, et al. Enterovirus infection in human pancreatic islet cells, islet tropism in vivo and receptor involvement in cultured islet beta cells. *Diabetologia*. 2004;47:225-239.
71. Foulis AK, McGill M, Farquharson MA, et al. A search for evidence of viral infection in pancreases of newly diagnosed patients with IDDM. *Diabetologia*. 1997;40:53-61.
72. Thorsby E. Invited anniversary review: HLA associated diseases. *Hum Immunol*. 1997;53:1-11.
73. Yu J, Shin CH, Yang SW, et al. Analysis of children with type 1 diabetes in Korea: high prevalence of specific anti-islet autoantibodies, immunogenetic similarities to Western populations with "unique" haplotypes, and lack of discrimination by aspartic acid at position 57 of DQB. *Clin Immunol*. 2004;113:318-325.
74. Anderson MS, Venanzi ES, Klein L, et al. Projection of an immunological self shadow within the thymus by the aire protein. *Science*. 2002;298:1395-1401.
75. Clark LB, Appleby MW, Brunkow ME, et al. Cellular and molecular characterization of the scurfy mouse mutant. *J Immunol*. 1999; 162:2546-2554.
76. Powell BR, Buist NR, Stenzel P. An X-linked syndrome of diarrhea, polyendocrinopathy, and fatal infection in infancy. *J Pediatr*. 1982;100:731-737.
77. Roberts J, Searle J. Neonatal diabetes mellitus associated with severe diarrhea, hyperimmunoglobulin E syndrome, and absence of islets of Langerhans. *Pediatr Pathol Lab Med*. 1995;15:477-483.
78. Cilio CM, Bosco A, Moretti C, et al. Congenital autoimmune diabetes mellitus (Letter). *N Engl J Med*. 2000;342:1529-1531.
79. Kanangat S, Blair P, Reddy R, et al. Disease in the scurfy (sf) mouse is associated with overexpression of cytokine genes. *Eur J Immunol*. 1996;26:161-165.
80. Fontenot JD, Gavin MA, Rudensky AY. Foxp3 programs the development and function of CD4+CD25+ regulatory T cells. *Nat Immunol*. 2003;4:330-336.
81. Rewers M, Norris J, Dabelea D. Epidemiology of type 1 diabetes mellitus. *Adv Exp Med Biol*. 2004;552:219-246.
82. Redondo MJ, Yu L, Hawa M, et al. Late progression to type 1 diabetes of discordant twins of patients with type 1 diabetes: combined analysis of two twin series (United States and United Kingdom) (Abstract). *Diabetes*. 1999;48:780.
83. Kyvik KO, Green A, Beck-Nielsen H. Concordance rates of insulin dependent diabetes mellitus: a population based study of young Danish twins. *BMJ*. 1995;311:913-917.
84. Committee on Diabetic Twins, Japan Diabetes Society. Diabetes mellitus in twins: a cooperative study in Japan. *Diabetes Res Clin Pract*. 1988;5:271-280.
85. Ikegami H, Ogihara T. Genetics of insulin-dependent diabetes mellitus. *Endocr J*. 1996;43:605-613.
86. Barnett AH, Eff C, Leslie RD, et al. Diabetes in identical twins: a study of 200 pairs. *Diabetologia*. 1981;20:87-93.
87. Redondo MJ, Yu L, Hawa M, et al. Heterogeneity of type 1 diabetes: analysis of monozygotic twins in Great Britain and the United States. *Diabetologia*. 2001;44:354-362.
87a. Kaprio J, Tuomilehto J, Koskenvuo M, et al. Concordance for type 1 (insulin-dependent) and type 2 (non-insulin dependent) diabetes mellitus in a population-based cohort of twins in Finland. *Diabetol*. 1992 Nov;35(11):1060.
88. Redondo MJ, et al. Concordance for islet autoimmunity among monozygotic twins. *N Engl J Med*. 2008;359(26):2849-2850.
89. Redondo MJ, Fain PR, Krischer JP, et al. Expression of beta-cell autoimmunity does not differ between potential dizygotic twins and siblings of patients with type 1 diabetes. *J Autoimmun*. 2004 Nov;23(3): 275-279.
90. Bao F, Yu L, Babu S, et al. One third of HLA DQ2 homozygous patients with type 1 diabetes express celiac disease associated transglutaminase autoantibodies. *J Autoimmun*. 1999;13:143-148.
91. Yu L, Brewer KW, Gates S, et al. DRB104 and DQ alleles: expression of 21-hydroxylase autoantibodies and risk of progression to Addison's disease. *J Clin Endocrinol Metab*. 1999;84:328-335.
92. De Block CE, De Leeuw IH, Van Gaal LF. High prevalence of manifestations of gastric autoimmunity in parietal cell antibody-positive type 1 (insulin-dependent) diabetic patients. The Belgian Diabetes Registry. *J Clin Endocrinol Metab*. 1999;84:4062-4067.
93. Nepom GT, Kwok WW. Perspectives in diabetes: molecular basis for HLA-DQ associations with IDDM. *Diabetes*. 1998;47:1177-1184.
94. McDevitt HO. The role of MHC class II molecules in susceptibility and resistance to autoimmunity. *Curr Opin Immunol*. 1998;10:677-681.
95. Eisenbarth GS. Genetic counseling for type 1 diabetes. In: Lebovitz H, ed. *Therapy for Diabetes Mellitus and Related Disorders*. Alexandria, VA: American Diabetes Association; 2004.
96. Nakanishi K, Kobayashi T, Murase T, et al. Human leukocyte antigen-A24 and -DQA10301 in Japanese insulin-dependent diabetes mellitus: independent contributions to susceptibility to the disease and additive contributions to acceleration of beta-cell destruction. *J Clin Endocrinol Metab*. 1999;84:3721-3725.
96a. Erlich H, Valdes AM, Noble J, et al. HLA DR-DQ Haplotypes and genotypes and type 1 diabetes risk: analysis of the type 1 diabetes genetics consortium families. *Diabetes*. 2008 Feb 5;57:1084.

97. Rewers M, Bugawan TL, Norris JM, et al. Newborn screening for HLA markers associated with IDDM: diabetes autoimmunity study in the young (DAISY). *Diabetologia*. 1996;39:807-812.
98. Kulmala P, Savola K, Reijonen H, et al. Genetic markers, humoral autoimmunity, and prediction of type 1 diabetes in siblings of affected children. Childhood Diabetes in Finland Study Group. *Diabetes*. 2000;49:48-58.
99. Aly TA, et al. Extreme genetic risk for type 1A diabetes. *Proc Natl Acad Sci U S A*. 2006;103(38):14074-14079.
100. Redondo MJ, Kawasaki E, Mulgrew CL, et al. DR and DQ associated protection from type 1 diabetes: comparison of DRB11401 and DQA*10102-DQB*10602. *J Clin Endocrinol Metab*. 2000;85:3793-3797.
101. Kawasaki E, Noble J, Erlich H, et al. Transmission of DQ haplotypes to patients with type 1 diabetes. *Diabetes*. 1998;47:1971-1973.
102. Morel PA, Dorman JS, Todd JA, et al. Aspartic acid at position 57 of the HLA-DQ beta chain protects against type I diabetes: a family study. *Proc Natl Acad Sci U S A*. 1988;85:8111-8115.
103. Bell GI, Horita S, Karam JH. A polymorphic locus near the human insulin gene is associated with insulin-dependent diabetes mellitus. *Diabetes*. 1984;33:176-183.
104. Bennett ST, Lucassen AM, Gough SCL, et al. Susceptibility to human type I diabetes at *IDDM2* is determined by tandem repeat variation at the insulin gene minisatellite locus. *Nat Genet*. 1995;9:284-292.
105. Pugliese A, Zeller M, Fernandez A, et al. The insulin gene is transcribed in the human thymus and transcription levels correlate with allelic variation at the INS VNTR-IDDM2 susceptibility locus for type I diabetes. *Nat Genet*. 1997;15:293-297.
106. Vafiadis P, Bennett ST, Todd JA, et al. Insulin expression in human thymus is modulated by INS VNTR alleles at the IDDM2 locus. *Nat Genet*. 1997;15:289-292.
107. Hanahan D. Peripheral-antigen-expressing cells in thymic medulla: factors in self-tolerance and autoimmunity. *Curr Opin Immunol*. 1998;10:656-662.
108. Bottini N, Musumeci L, Alonso A, et al. A functional variant of lymphoid tyrosine phosphatase is associated with type I diabetes. *Nat Genet*. 2004;36:337-338.
109. Vang T, et al. Protein tyrosine phosphatase PTPN22 in human autoimmunity. *Autoimmunity*. 2007;40(6):453-461.
110. Larsen ZM, Kristiansen OP, Mato E, et al. *IDDM12* (CTLA4) on 2q33 and *IDDM13* on 2q34 in genetic susceptibility to type 1 diabetes (insulin-dependent). *Autoimmunity*. 1999;31:35-42.
111. Vella A, Cooper JD, Lowe CE, et al. Localization of a type 1 diabetes locus in the IL2RA/CD25 region by use of tag single-nucleotide polymorphisms. *Am J Hum Genet*. 2005;76(5):773-779.
112. Concannon P, Rich SS, Nepom GT. Genetics of type 1A diabetes. *N Engl J Med*. 2009;360(16):1646-1654.
113. Nejentsev S, et al. Rare variants of IFIH1, a gene implicated in antiviral responses, protect against type 1 diabetes. *Science*. 2009; 324(5925):387-389.
114. Eisenbarth GS, Elsey C, Yu L, Rewers M. Infantile anti-islet autoimmunity: DAISY study (Abstract). *Diabetes*. 1998;47:A210.
115. Stene LC, Joner G. Use of cod liver oil during the first year of life is associated with lower risk of childhood-onset type 1 diabetes: a large, population-based, case-control study. *Am J Clin Nutr*. 2003;78(6): 1128-1134.
116. Schenker M, Hummel M, Ferber K, et al. Early expression and high prevalence of islet autoantibodies for DR3/4 heterozygous and DR4/4 homozygous offspring of parents with type I diabetes: the German BABYDIAB study. *Diabetologia*. 1999;42:671-677.
117. Robles DT, Eisenbarth GS. Type 1A diabetes induced by infection and immunization. *J Autoimmun*. 2001;16:355-362.
118. Ellerman KE, Richards CA, Guberski DL, et al. Kilham rat virus triggers T cell-dependent autoimmune diabetes in multiple strains of rat. *Diabetes*. 1996;45:557-562.
119. Gardner SG, Bingley PJ, Sawtell PA, et al. Rising incidence of insulin dependent diabetes in children aged under 5 years in the Oxford region: time trend analysis. *BMJ*. 1997;315:713-717.
120. Tuomilehto J, Karvonen M, Pitkaniemi J, et al. Record-high incidence of type I (insulin-dependent) diabetes mellitus in Finnish children. The Finnish Childhood Type I Diabetes Registry Group. *Diabetologia*. 1999;42:655-660.
121. Feltbower RG, McKinney PA, Bodansky HJ. Rising incidence of childhood diabetes is seen at all ages and in urban and rural settings in Yorkshire, United Kingdom (Letter). *Diabetologia*. 2000;43:682-684.
122. Shaver KA, Boughman JA, Nance WE. Congenital rubella syndrome and diabetes: a review of epidemiologic, genetic, and immunologic factors. *Am Ann Deaf*. 1985;130:526-532.
123. Rubenstein P. The HLA system in congenital rubella patients with and without diabetes. *Diabetes*. 1982;31:1088-1091.
124. Clarke WL, Shaver KA, Bright GM, et al. Autoimmunity in congenital rubella syndrome. *J Pediatr*. 1984;104:370-373.
125. Ou D, Jonsen LA, Metzger DL, et al. CD4+ and CD8+ T cell clones from congenital rubella syndrome patients with IDDM recognize overlapping GAD65 protein epitopes: implications for HLA class I and II allelic linkage to disease susceptibility. *Hum Immunol*. 1999;60:652-664.
126. Rabinowe SL, George KL, Loughlin R, et al. Congenital rubella: monoclonal antibody-defined T cell abnormalities in young adults. *Am J Med*. 1986;81:779-782.
127. Yoon JW, Austin M, Onodera T, et al. Isolation of a virus from the pancreas of a child with diabetic ketoacidosis. *N Engl J Med*. 1979;300:1173-1179.
128. Nigro G, Pacella ME, Patane E, et al. Multi-system Coxsackie virus B-6 infection with findings suggestive of diabetes mellitus. *Eur J Pediatr*. 1986;145:557-559.
129. Lonnrot M, Korpela K, Knip M, et al. Enterovirus infection as a risk factor for beta-cell autoimmunity in a prospectively observed birth cohort: the Finnish Diabetes Prediction and Prevention Study. *Diabetes*. 2000;49:1314-1318.
130. Graves PM, Rewers M. The role of enteroviral infections in the development of IDDM: limitations of current approaches. *Diabetes*. 1997;46:161-168.
131. Honeyman MC, Coulson BS, Stone NL, et al. Association between rotavirus infection and pancreatic islet autoimmunity in children at risk of developing type 1 diabetes. *Diabetes*. 2000;49:1319-1324.
132. Classen DC, Classen JB. The timing of pediatric immunization and the risk of insulin-dependent diabetes mellitus. *Infect Dis Clin Pract*. 1997;6:449-454.
133. Karvonen M, Cepaitis Z, Tuomilehto J. Association between type 1 diabetes and *Haemophilus influenzae* type b vaccination: birth cohort study. *BMJ*. 1999;318:1169-1172.
134. Lindberg B, Ahlfors K, Carlsson A, et al. Previous exposure to measles, mumps, and rubella—but not vaccination during adolescence—correlates to the prevalence of pancreatic and thyroid autoantibodies. *Pediatrics*. 1999;104:e12.
135. Graves PM, Barriga KJ, Norris JM, et al. Lack of association between early childhood immunizations and beta-cell autoimmunity. *Diabetes Care*. 1999;22:1694-1697.
136. Bao F, Rewers M, Scott F, et al. Celiac disease. In: Eisenbarth GS, ed. *Endocrine and Organ Specific Autoimmunity*. Austin, TX: RG Landes; 1999:85-96.
137. Scott FW, Cloutier HE, Kleemann R, et al. Potential mechanisms by which certain foods promote or inhibit the development of spontaneous diabetes in BB rats. *Diabetes*. 1997;46:589-598.
138. Akerblom HK, Savilahti E, Saukkonen TT, et al. The case for elimination of cow's milk in early infancy in the prevention of type 1 diabetes: the Finnish experience. *Diabetes Metab Rev*. 1993;9:269-278.
139. Virtanen SM, Laara E, Hypponen E, et al. Cow's milk consumption, HLA-DQB1 genotype, and type 1 diabetes: a nested case-control study of siblings of children with diabetes. Childhood Diabetes in Finland Study Group. *Diabetes*. 2000;49:912-917.
140. Virtanen SM, Rasanen L, Aro A, et al. Infant feeding in Finnish children less than 7 yr of age with newly diagnosed IDDM. Childhood Diabetes in Finland Study Group. *Diabetes Care*. 1991;14: 415-417.
141. Couper JJ, Steele C, Beresford S, et al. Lack of association between duration of breast-feeding or introduction of cow's milk and development of islet autoimmunity. *Diabetes*. 1999;48:2145-2149.
142. Norris JM, Beaty B, Klingensmith G, et al. Lack of association between early exposure to cow's milk protein and β-cell autoimmunity: Diabetes Autoimmunity Study in the Young (DAISY). *JAMA*. 1996; 276:609-614.
143. Akerblom HK, Virtanen SM, Ilonen J, et al. Dietary manipulation of beta cell autoimmunity in infants at increased risk of type 1 diabetes: a pilot study. *Diabetologia*. 2005;48:829-837.
144. Norris JM, Barriga K, Klingensmith G, et al. Timing of initial cereal exposure in infancy and risk of islet autoimmunity. *JAMA*. 2003;290:1713-1720.
145. Ziegler AG, Schmid S, Huber D, et al. Early infant feeding and risk of developing type 1 diabetes-associated autoantibodies. *JAMA*. 2003;290:1721-1728.
146. Norris JM, et al. Omega-3 polyunsaturated fatty acid intake and islet autoimmunity in children at increased risk for type 1 diabetes. *JAMA*. 2007;298(12):1420-1428.
147. Wenzlau JM, et al. The cation efflux transporter ZnT8 (Slc30A8) is a major autoantigen in human type 1 diabetes. *Proc Natl Acad Sci U S A*. 2007;104(43):17040-17445.
148. Andre I, Gonzalez A, Wong B, et al. Checkpoints in the progression of autoimmune disease: lessons from diabetes models. *Proc Natl Acad Sci U S A*. 1996;93:2260-2263.
149. Fennessy M, Metcalfe K, Hitman GA, et al. A gene in the HLA class I region contributes to susceptibility to IDDM in the Finnish population. Childhood Diabetes in Finland (DiMe) Study Group. *Diabetologia*. 1994;37:937-944.
150. Kockum I, Sanjeevi CB, Eastman S, et al. Population analysis of protection by HLA-DR and DQ genes from insulin-dependent diabetes mellitus in Swedish children with insulin-dependent diabetes and controls. *Eur J Immunogenet*. 1995;22:443-465.
151. Vardi P, Ziegler AG, Matthews JH, et al. Concentration of insulin autoantibodies at onset of type I diabetes: inverse log-linear correlation with age. *Diabetes Care*. 1988;11:736-739.

152. Arslanian SL, Becker DJ, Rabin B, et al. Correlates of insulin antibodies in newly diagnosed children with insulin-dependent diabetes before insulin therapy. *Diabetes*. 1985;34:926-930.
153. Eisenbarth GS, Gianani R, Yu L, et al. Dual-parameter model for prediction of type 1 diabetes mellitus. *Proc Assoc Am Physicians*. 1998; 110:126-135.
154. Gale EA, et al. European Nicotinamide Diabetes Intervention Trial (ENDIT): a randomised controlled trial of intervention before the onset of type 1 diabetes. *Lancet*. 2004;363(9413):925-931.
155. Pugliese A, Kawasaki E, Zeller M, et al. Sequence analysis of the diabetes-protective human leukocyte antigen-DQB*10602 allele in unaffected, islet cell antibody-positive first degree relatives and in rare patients with type 1 diabetes. *J Clin Endocrinol Metab*. 1999;84: 1722-1728.
156. Achenbach P, Koczwara K, Knopff A, et al. Mature high-affinity immune responses to (pro)insulin anticipate the autoimmune cascade that leads to type 1 diabetes. *J Clin Invest*. 2004;114:589-597.
157. Barker JM, Barriga KL, Yu L, et al. Prediction of autoantibody positivity and progression to type 1 diabetes: Diabetes Autoimmunity Study in the Young (DAISY). *J Clin Endocrinol Metab*. 2004;89:3896-3902.
158. Verge CF, Gianani R, Kawasaki E, et al. Prediction of type I diabetes in first-degree relatives using a combination of insulin, GAD, and ICA512bdc/IA-2 autoantibodies. *Diabetes*. 1996;45:926-933.
159. Bingley PJ, Bonifacio E, Williams AJK, et al. Prediction of IDDM in the general population: strategies based on combinations of autoantibody markers. *Diabetes*. 1997;46:1701-1710.
160. Chase HP, Cuthbertson DD, Dolan LM, et al. First phase insulin release during the intravenous glucose tolerance test as a risk factor for type 1 diabetes. *J Pediatr*. 2001;138:244-249.
161. Bingley PJ, Colman P, Eisenbarth GS, et al. Standardization of IVGTT to predict IDDM. *Diabetes Care*. 1992;15:1313-1316.
162. Bingley PJ. Interactions of age, islet cell antibodies, insulin autoantibodies, and first-phase insulin response in predicting risk of progression to IDDM in ICA$^+$ relatives: the ICARUS data set. *Diabetes*. 1996;45:1720-1728.
163. The DCCT Research Group. Epidemiology of severe hypoglycemia in the diabetes control and complications trial. Diabetes Control and Complications Trial. *Am J Med*. 1991;90:450-459.
164. Palmer JP, Fleming GA, Greenbaum CJ, et al. C-peptide is the appropriate outcome measure for type 1 diabetes clinical trials to preserve beta-cell function: report of an ADA workshop, 21-22 October 2001. *Diabetes*. 2004;53:250-264.
165. Füchtenbusch M, Ferber K, Standl E, et al. Prediction of type I diabetes postpartum in patients with gestational diabetes mellitus by combined islet cell autoantibody screening: a prospective multicenter study. *Diabetes*. 1997;46:1459-1467.
166. Zimmet PZ, Tuomi T, Mackay IR, et al. Latent autoimmune diabetes mellitus in adults (LADA): the role of antibodies to glutamic acid decarboxylase in diagnosis and prediction of insulin dependency. *Diabet Med*. 1994;11:299-303.
167. Turner R, Stratton I, Horton V, et al. UKPDS 25: autoantibodies to islet-cell cytoplasm and glutamic acid decarboxylase for prediction of insulin requirement in type 2 diabetes. UK Prospective Diabetes Study Group. *Lancet*. 1997;350:1288-1293.
168. Horton V, Stratton I, Bottazzo GF, et al. Genetic heterogeneity of autoimmune diabetes: age of presentation in adults is influenced by HLA DRB1 and DQB1 genotypes (UKPDS 43). UK Prospective Diabetes Study (UKPDS) Group. *Diabetologia*. 1999;42:608-616.
169. Ricker AT, Herskowitz R, Wolfsdorf JI, et al. Prognostic factors in children and young adults presenting with transient hyperglycemia or impaired glucose tolerance (Abstract). *Diabetes*. 1986;35(suppl 1):93A.
170. Assan R, Feutren G, Debray-Sachs M, et al. Metabolic and immunological effects of cyclosporine in recently diagnosed type I diabetes mellitus. *Lancet*. 1985;1:67-71.
171. Chase HP, Butler-Simon N, Garg SK, et al. Cyclosporine A for the treatment of new-onset insulin-dependent diabetes mellitus. *Pediatrics*. 1990;85:241-245.
172. Stiller CR, Dupre J, Gent M, et al. Effects of cyclosporine immunosuppression in insulin-dependent diabetes mellitus of recent onset. *Science*. 1984;223:1362-1367.
173. Carel J-C, Boitard C, Eisenbarth G, et al. Cyclosporine delays but does not prevent clinical onset in glucose intolerant pre-type 1 diabetic children. *J Autoimmun*. 1996;9:739-745.
174. Cook JJ, Hudson I, Harrison LC, et al. Double-blind controlled trial of azathioprine in children with newly diagnosed type I diabetes. *Diabetes*. 1989;38:779-783.
175. Silverstein J, Maclaren N, Riley W, et al. Immunosuppression with azathioprine and prednisone in recent-onset insulin-dependent diabetes mellitus. *N Engl J Med*. 1988;319:599-604.
176. Eisenbarth GS, Srikanta S, Jackson R, et al. Anti-thymocyte globulin and prednisone immunotherapy of recent onset type I diabetes mellitus. *Diabetes Res*. 1985;2:271-276.
177. Buckingham BA, Sandborg CI. A randomized trial of methotrexate in newly diagnosed patients with type 1 diabetes mellitus. *Clin Immunol*. 2000;96:86-90.
178. Herold KC, Hagopian W, Auger JA, et al. Anti-CD3 monoclonal antibody in new-onset type 1 diabetes mellitus. *N Engl J Med*. 2002;346:1692-1698.
179. Herold KC, Gitelman SE, Masharani U, et al. A single course of anti-CD3 monoclonal antibody hOKT3γ1(Ala-Ala) results in improvement in C-peptide responses and clinical parameters for at least 2 years after onset of type 1 diabetes. *Diabetes*. 2005;54:1763-1769.
179a. Pescovitz MD, Greenbaum CJ, Krause-Steinrauf H, et al. Ritaximab, B-lymphocyte depletion, and preservation of beta-cell function. *N Engl J Med*. 2009 Nov 26;361(22):2143.
180. Weiner HL, Miller A, Khoury SJ, et al. Suppression of organ-specific autoimmune diseases by oral administration of autoantigens. In: *Proceedings of the 8th International Congress on Immunology*. Heidelberg: Springer-Verlag; 1992:627-634.
181. Zhang ZJ, Davidson L, Eisenbarth G, et al. Suppression of diabetes in nonobese diabetic mice by oral administration of porcine insulin. *Proc Natl Acad Sci U S A*. 1991;88:10252-10256.
182. Atkinson MA, Maclaren NK, Luchetta R. Insulitis and diabetes in NOD mice reduced by prophylactic insulin therapy. *Diabetes*. 1990;39: 933-937.
183. Diabetes Prevention Trial–Type 1 Diabetes Study Group. Effects of insulin in relatives of patients with type 1 diabetes mellitus. *N Engl J Med*. 2002;346:1685-1691.
184. Skyler JS, Krischer JP, Wolfsdorf J, et al. Effects of oral insulin in relatives of patients with type 1 diabetes: The Diabetes Prevention Trial–Type 1. *Diabetes Care*. 2005;28:1068-1076.
184a. Malek R, Chong AY, Lupsa BC, et al. Treatment of type B insulin resistance: a novel approach to reduce insulin receptor autoantibodies. *J Clin Endocrinol Metab*. 2010 Aug;95(8):3641.
185. Robertson RP, Sutherland DER, Kendall DM, et al. Metabolic characterization of long-term successful pancreas transplants in type I diabetes. *J Investig Med*. 1996;44:549-555.
186. Robertson RP, Kendall D, Teuscher A, et al. Long-term metabolic control with pancreatic transplantation. *Transplant Proc*. 1994;26: 386-387.
187. Naftanel MA, Harlan DM. Pancreatic islet transplantation. *PLoS Med*. 2004;1:e58; quiz e75.
188. Nakhleh RE, Gruessner RWG, Swanson PE, et al. Pancreas transplant pathology: a morphologic, immunohistochemical, and electron microscopic comparison of allogeneic grafts with rejection, syngeneic grafts, and chronic pancreatitis. *Am J Surg Pathol*. 1991;15:246-256.
189. Shapiro AM, Lakey JR, Ryan EA, et al. Islet transplantation in seven patients with type 1 diabetes mellitus using a glucocorticoid-free immunosuppressive regimen. *N Engl J Med*. 2000;343:230-238.
190. Nanji SA, Shapiro AM. Advances in pancreatic islet transplantation in humans. *Diabetes Obes Metab*. 2006;8:15-25.
191. Uchigata Y, Kuwata S, Tsushima T, et al. Patients with Graves' disease who developed insulin autoimmune syndrome (Hirata disease) possess HLA-Bw62/Cw4/DR4 carrying DRB*10406. *J Clin Endocrinol Metab*. 1993;77:249-254.
192. Uchigata Y, Hirata Y. Insulin autoimmune syndrome (IAS, Hirata disease). In: Eisenbarth G, ed. *Molecular Mechanisms of Endocrine and Organ Specific Autoimmunity*. Austin, TX: RG Landes; 1999: 133-148.
193. Menon RK, Cohen RM, Sperling MA, et al. Transplacental passage of insulin in pregnant women with insulin-dependent diabetes mellitus: its role in fetal macrosomia. *N Engl J Med*. 1990;323:309-315.
194. Schernthaner G. Immunogenicity and allergenic potential of animal and human insulins. *Diabetes Care*. 1993;16:155-165.
195. Taylor SI, Grunberger G, Marcus-Samuels B, et al. Hypoglycemia associated with antibodies to the insulin receptor. *N Engl J Med*. 1982; 307:1422-1426.
196. Dons RF, Havlik R, Taylor SI, et al. Clinical disorders associated with autoantibodies to the insulin receptor: simulation by passive transfer of immunoglobulins to rats. *J Clin Invest*. 1983;72:1072-1080.
197. Engerman R, Bloodworth Jr JM, Nelson S. Relationship of microvascular disease in diabetes to metabolic control. *Diabetes*. 1977;26: 760-769.
198. Engerman RL, Kern TS. Progression of incipient diabetic retinopathy during good glycemic control. *Diabetes*. 1987;36:808-812.
199. Cohen AJ, McGill PD, Rossetti RG, et al. Glomerulopathy in spontaneously diabetic rat: impact of glycemic control. *Diabetes*. 1987;36: 944-951.
200. Klein R, Klein BE, Moss SE, et al. The Wisconsin epidemiologic study of diabetic retinopathy: II. Prevalence and risk of diabetic retinopathy when age at diagnosis is less than 30 years. *Arch Ophthalmol*. 1984;102:520-526.
201. Klein R, Klein BE, Moss SE, et al. Glycosylated hemoglobin predicts the incidence and progression of diabetic retinopathy. *JAMA*. 1988;260:2864-2871.
202. Chase HP, Jackson WE, Hoops SL, et al. Glucose control and the renal and retinal complications of insulin-dependent diabetes. *JAMA*. 1989; 261:1155-1160.
203. The effect of intensive treatment of diabetes on the development and progression of long-term complications in insulin-dependent diabetes

mellitus. The Diabetes Control and Complications Trial Research Group. *N Engl J Med.* 1993;329:977-986.
204. Effect of intensive diabetes management on macrovascular events and risk factors in the Diabetes Control and Complications Trial. *Am J Cardiol.* 1995;75:894-903.
205. Nathan DM, Cleary PA, Backlund JY, et al. Intensive diabetes treatment and cardiovascular disease in patients with type 1 diabetes. *N Engl J Med.* 2005;353:2643-2653.
206. Sherwin R, Felig P. Hypoglycemia. In: Felig P, ed. *Endocrinology and Metabolism.* 2nd ed. New York, NY: McGraw-Hill; 1987:1043-1178.
207. Purnell JQ, Hokanson JE, Marcovina SM, et al. Effect of excessive weight gain with intensive therapy of type 1 diabetes on lipid levels and blood pressure: results from the DCCT. Diabetes Control and Complications Trial. *JAMA.* 1998;280:140-146.
208. Blood glucose control and the evolution of diabetic retinopathy and albuminuria: a preliminary multicenter trial. The Kroc Collaborative Study Group. *N Engl J Med.* 1984;311:365-372.
209. Lauritzen T, Frost-Larsen K, Larsen HW, et al. Effect of 1 year of near-normal blood glucose levels on retinopathy in insulin-dependent diabetics. *Lancet.* 1983;1:200-204.
210. Dahl-Jorgensen K, Brinchmann-Hansen O, Hansen KF, et al. Rapid tightening of blood glucose control leads to transient deterioration of retinopathy in insulin dependent diabetes mellitus: the Oslo study. *Br Med J (Clin Res Ed).* 1985;290:811-815.
211. Cryer PE. Hypoglycemia-associated autonomic failure in diabetes. *Am J Physiol.* 2001;281:E1115-E1121.
212. American Diabetes Association. Standards of medical care in diabetes—2010. *Diabetes Care.* 2010;29:s11-s61.
213. Rodbard HW, Blonde L, Braithwaite SS, et al; AACE Diabetes Mellitus Clinical Practice Guidelines Task Force. American Association of Clinical Endocrinologists medical guidelines for clinical practice for the management of diabetes mellitus. *Endocr Pract.* 2007;13(suppl 1): 1-68.
214. Hirsch IB. Intensive treatment of type 1 diabetes. *Med Clin North Am.* 1998;82:689-719.
215. Home P, Kurtzhals P. Insulin detemir: from concept to clinical experience. *Expert Opin Pharmacother.* 2006;7:325-343.
216. Heise T, Nosek L, Ronn BB, et al. Lower within-subject variability of insulin detemir in comparison to NPH insulin and insulin glargine in people with type 1 diabetes. *Diabetes.* 2004;53:1614-1620.
217. Cefalu WT. Evolving strategies for insulin delivery and therapy. *Drugs.* 2004;64:1149-1161.
218. Pfizer Labs: Exubera prescribing information. New York, NY: Pfizer; 2007. Available at http://www.pfizer.com/pfizer/download/uspi_exubera.pdf (accessed January 29, 2007).
219. Lougheed WD, Zinman B, Strack TR, et al. Stability of insulin lispro in insulin infusion systems. *Diabetes Care.* 1997;20:1061-1065.
220. Bode BW, Steed RD, Davidson PC. Reduction in severe hypoglycemia with long-term continuous subcutaneous insulin infusion in type I diabetes. *Diabetes Care.* 1996;19:324-327.
221. Bergenstal RM, Tamborlane WV, Ahmann A, et al., for the STAR3 Study Group. Effectiveness of sensor-augmented insulin pump therapy in type 1 diabetes. *N Engl J Med.* 2010;363:311-320.
222. Hirsch IB, Edelman SV. *Practical Management of Type 1 Diabetes.* Caddo, OK: Professional Communications; 2005.
223. American Diabetes Association. *Medical Management of Type 1 Diabetes.* 4th ed. Alexandria, VA: American Diabetes Association; 2003.
224. American Diabetes Association. *Intensive Diabetes Management.* 3rd ed. Alexandria, VA: American Diabetes Association; 2003.
225. Dungan K, Buse J. Amylin and GLP-1-based therapies for the treatment of diabetes. UpToDate, 2006 (subscription required).
226. Young A. Clinical studies. *Adv Pharmacol.* 2005;52:289-320.
227. Garg S, Zisser H, Schwarz S, et al. Improvement in glycemic excursions with a transcutaneous, real-time continuous glucose sensor: a randomized controlled trial. *Diabetes Care.* 2006;29:44-50.
228. Weisberg LS. Pseudohyponatremia: a reappraisal. *Am J Med.* 1989;86: 315-318.
229. Adrogue HJ, Wilson H, Boyd 3rd AE, et al. Plasma acid-base patterns in diabetic ketoacidosis. *N Engl J Med.* 1982;307:1603-1610.
230. Munro JF, Campbell IW, McCuish AC, et al. Euglycaemic diabetic ketoacidosis. *BMJ.* 1973;2:578-580.
231. Madias NE. Lactic acidosis. *Kidney Int.* 1986;29:752-774.
232. Fulop M. Alcoholism, ketoacidosis, and lactic acidosis. *Diabetes Metab Rev.* 1989;5:365-378.
233. Duffens K, Marx JA. Alcoholic ketoacidosis: a review. *J Emerg Med.* 1987;5:399-406.
234. Moller-Petersen J, Andersen PT, Hjorne N, et al. Nontraumatic rhabdomyolysis during diabetic ketoacidosis. *Diabetologia.* 1986;29: 229-234.
235. Brenner BE, Simon RR. Management of salicylate intoxication. *Drugs.* 1982;24:335-340.
236. Turk J, Morrell L. Ethylene glycol intoxication. *Arch Intern Med.* 1986;146:1601-1603.
237. Rich J, Scheife RT, Katz N, et al. Isopropyl alcohol intoxication. *Arch Neurol.* 1990;47:322-324.
238. Kitabchi AE. Low-dose insulin therapy in diabetic ketoacidosis: fact or fiction? *Diabetes Metab Rev.* 1989;5:337-363.
239. Kitabchi AE, Umpierrez GE, Murphy MB, et al. Hyperglycemic crises in diabetes. *Diabetes Care.* 2004;27(suppl 1):S94-S102.
240. Umpierrez GE, Guervo R, Karabell A, et al. Treatment of diabetic ketoacidosis with subcutaneous insulin aspart. *Diabetes Care.* 2004;27:1873-1878.
241. Burris AS. Leukemoid reaction associated with severe diabetic ketoacidosis. *South Med J.* 1986;79:647-648.
242. Powers WJ. Cerebrospinal fluid to serum glucose ratios in diabetes mellitus and bacterial meningitis. *Am J Med.* 1981;71: 217-220.
243. Campbell IW, Duncan LJ, Innes JA, et al. Abdominal pain in diabetic metabolic decompensation: clinical significance. *JAMA.* 1975;233: 166-168.
244. Rosenbloom AL. Intracerebral crises during treatment of diabetic ketoacidosis. *Diabetes Care.* 1990;13:22-33.
245. Brun-Buisson CJ, Bonnet F, Bergeret S, et al. Recurrent high-permeability pulmonary edema associated with diabetic ketoacidosis. *Crit Care Med.* 1985;13:55-56.
246. Brandstetter RD, Tamarin FM, Washington D, et al. Occult mucous airway obstruction in diabetic ketoacidosis. *Chest.* 1987;91: 575-578.
247. Hansen LA, Prakash UB, Colby TV. Pulmonary complications in diabetes mellitus. *Mayo Clin Proc.* 1989;64:791-799.
248. Levetan CS, Salas JR, Wilets JF, Zumoff B. Impact of endocrine and diabetes team consultation on hospital length of stay for patients with diabetes. *Am J Med.* 1995;99:22-28.
249. Levetan CS, Passaro MD, Jablonski KA, et al. Effect of physician specialty on outcomes in diabetic ketoacidosis. *Diabetes Care.* 1999; 22:1790-1795.

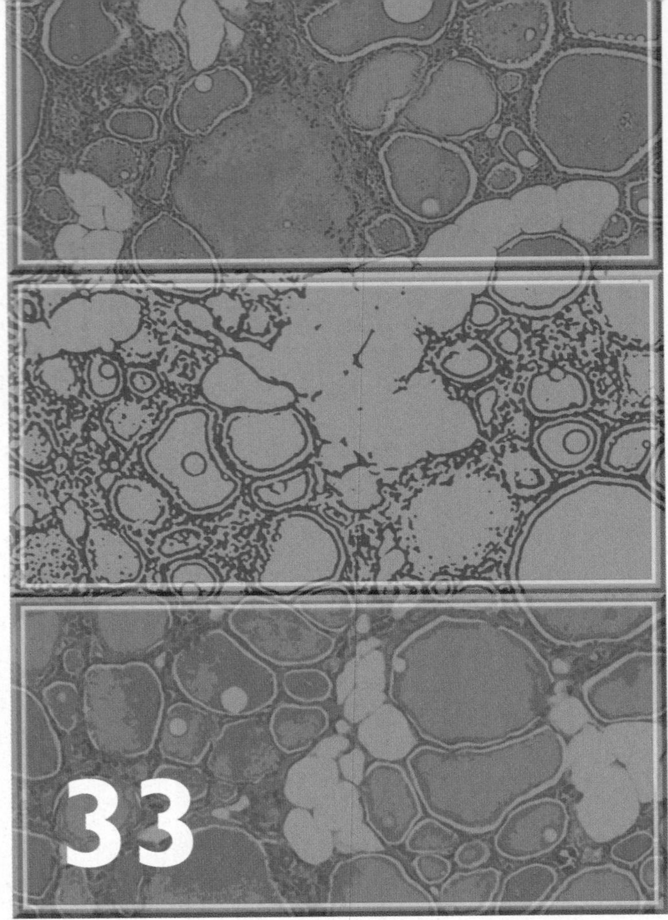

CHAPTER 33

Complications of Diabetes Mellitus

MICHAEL BROWNLEE • LLOYD P. AIELLO • MARK E. COOPER • AARON I. VINIK • RICHARD W. NESTO • ANDREW J.M. BOULTON

BIOCHEMISTRY AND MOLECULAR CELL BIOLOGY

All forms of diabetes, both inherited and acquired, are characterized by hyperglycemia, a relative or absolute lack of insulin, and the development of diabetes-specific microvascular pathology in the retina, renal glomerulus, and peripheral nerve. Diabetes is also associated with accelerated atherosclerotic macrovascular disease affecting arteries that supply the heart, brain, and lower extremities. Pathologically, this condition resembles macrovascular disease in nondiabetic patients, but it is more extensive and progresses more rapidly. As a consequence of its microvascular pathology, diabetes mellitus is now the leading cause of new blindness in people 20 to 74 years of age and the leading cause of end-stage renal disease (ESRD).

People with diabetes mellitus are the fastest growing group of renal dialysis and transplant recipients. The life expectancy of patients with diabetic ESRD is only 3 or 4 years. More than 60% of diabetic patients are affected by neuropathy, which includes distal symmetric polyneuropathy (DSPN), mononeuropathies, and a variety of autonomic neuropathies causing erectile dysfunction, urinary incontinence, gastroparesis, and nocturnal diarrhea. Because of accelerated lower-extremity arterial disease in conjunction with neuropathy, diabetes mellitus accounts for 50% of all nontrauma amputations in the United States. The risk of cardiovascular complications is increased by twofold to sixfold in subjects with diabetes. Overall, life expectancy is about 7 to 10 years shorter than for people without diabetes mellitus because of increased mortality from diabetic complications.[1]

Large prospective clinical studies show a strong relationship between glycemia and diabetic microvascular complications in both type 1 diabetes mellitus (T1DM) and type 2 diabetes (T2DM).[2,3] There is a continuous, although not linear, relationship between the level of glycemia and the risk of development and progression of these complications (Fig. 33-1).[4,5] Hyperglycemia and the consequences of insulin resistance both appear to play important roles in the pathogenesis of macrovascular complications.[6-10]

Shared Pathophysiologic Features of Microvascular Complications

In the retina, glomerulus, and vasa nervorum, diabetes-specific microvascular disease is characterized by similar pathophysiologic features.

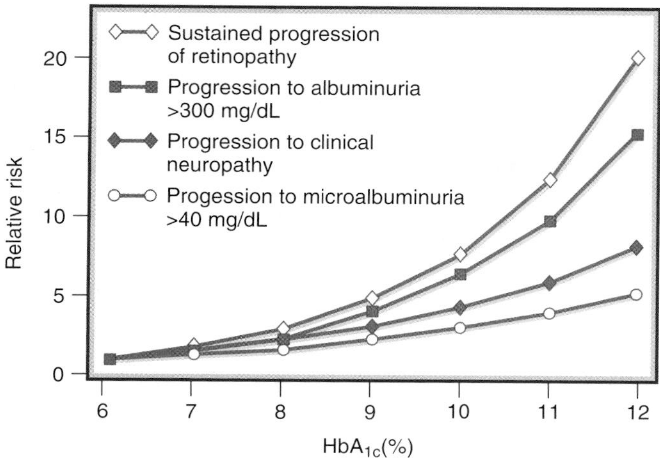

Figure 33-1 Relative risks for the development of diabetic complications at different mean levels of glycosylated hemoglobin (HbA_{1c}) obtained from the Diabetes Control and Complications Trial. (Adapted from Skyler J: Diabetic complications: the importance of glucose control. *Endocrinol Metab Clin North Am.* 1996;25:243-254.)

Requirement for Intracellular Hyperglycemia

Clinical and animal model data indicate that chronic hyperglycemia is the central initiating factor for all types of diabetic microvascular disease. The duration and magnitude of hyperglycemia are strongly correlated with the extent and rate of progression of diabetic microvascular disease. In the Diabetes Control and Complications Trial (DCCT), for example, T1DM patients whose intensive insulin therapy resulted in glycosylated hemoglobin (HbA_{1c}) levels 2% lower than those receiving conventional insulin therapy had a 76% lower incidence of retinopathy, a 54% lower incidence of nephropathy, and a 60% reduction in neuropathy.[2,3] However, further analysis of the DCCT data showed that, although intensive therapy reduced the risk of sustained retinopathy progression by 73% compared with standard treatment, HbA_{1c} and duration of diabetes (glycemic exposure) explained only about 11% of the variation in retinopathy risk for the entire study population, suggesting that the remaining 89% of the variation in risk can be explained by aspects of glycemia not captured by HbA_{1c}.[11]

Although all diabetic cells are exposed to elevated levels of plasma glucose, hyperglycemic damage is limited to those cell types (e.g., endothelial cells) that develop intracellular hyperglycemia. Endothelial cells develop intracellular hyperglycemia because, unlike many other cells, they cannot downregulate glucose transport when exposed to extracellular hyperglycemia. As illustrated in Figure 33-2, vascular smooth muscle cells (VSMC), which are not damaged by hyperglycemia, show an inverse relationship between extracellular glucose concentration and subsequent rate of glucose transport measured as 2-deoxyglucose uptake (Fig. 33-2, *upper part*). In contrast, vascular endothelial cells show no significant change in subsequent rate of glucose transport after exposure to elevated glucose concentrations (see Fig. 33-2, *lower part*).[12] That intracellular hyperglycemia is necessary and sufficient for the development of diabetic pathology is further demonstrated by the fact that overexpression of glucose transporter 1 (GLUT1) in mesangial cells cultured in a normal glucose milieu mimics the diabetic phenotype, inducing the same increases in collagen type IV, collagen type I, and fibronectin gene expression as are observed in diabetic hyperglycemia (Fig. 33-3).[13]

Abnormal Endothelial Cell Function

Early in the course of diabetes mellitus, before structural changes are evident, hyperglycemia causes abnormalities in blood flow and vascular permeability in the retina, glomerulus, and peripheral nerve vasa nervorum.[14,15] The increase in blood flow and intracapillary pressure is thought to reflect a hyperglycemia-induced decrease in nitric oxide (NO) production on the efferent side of capillary beds and possibly an increased sensitivity to angiotensin II. As a consequence of increased intracapillary pressure and endothelial cell dysfunction, retinal capillaries exhibit increased leakage of fluorescein, and glomerular capillaries have an elevated albumin excretion rate (AER). Comparable changes occur in the vasa vasorum of peripheral nerves. Early in the course of diabetes, increased permeability is reversible, but as time progresses, it becomes irreversible.

Increased Vessel Wall Protein Accumulation

The common pathophysiologic feature of diabetic microvascular disease is progressive narrowing and eventual occlusion of vascular lumina, which results in inadequate perfusion and function of the affected tissues. Early hyperglycemia-induced microvascular hypertension and increased vascular permeability contribute to irreversible microvessel occlusion by three processes.

The first process is an abnormal leakage of periodic acid–Schiff (PAS)-positive, carbohydrate-containing plasma proteins, which are deposited in the capillary wall and can stimulate perivascular cells such as pericytes and mesangial cells to elaborate growth factors and extracellular matrix.

The second process is extravasation of growth factors, such as transforming growth factor-β1 (TGF-β1), which

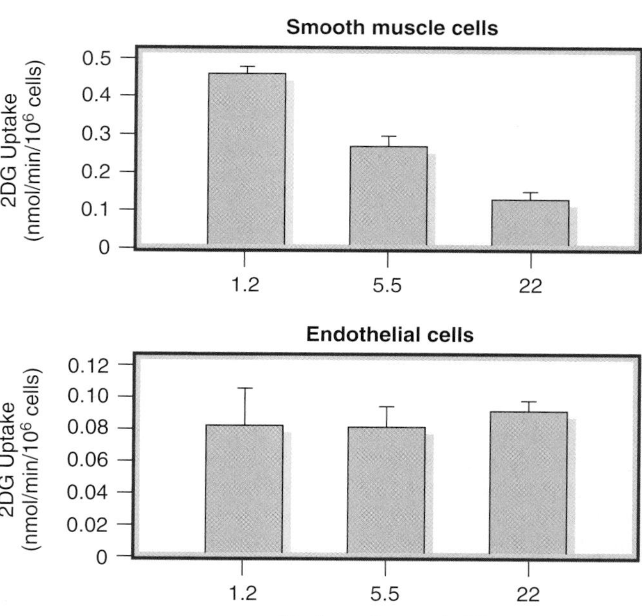

Figure 33-2 Lack of downregulation of glucose transport in cells affected by diabetic complications. *Upper panel,* 2-deoxyglucose (2DG) uptake in vascular smooth muscle cells preexposed to 1.2, 5.5, or 22 mmol/L glucose. *Lower panel,* 2DG uptake in bovine endothelial cells preexposed to 1.2, 5.5, or 22 mmol/L glucose. (From Kaiser N, Feener EP, Boukobza-Vardi N, et al. Differential regulation of glucose transport and transporters by glucose in vascular endothelial and smooth muscle cells. *Diabetes.* 1993;42:80-89.)

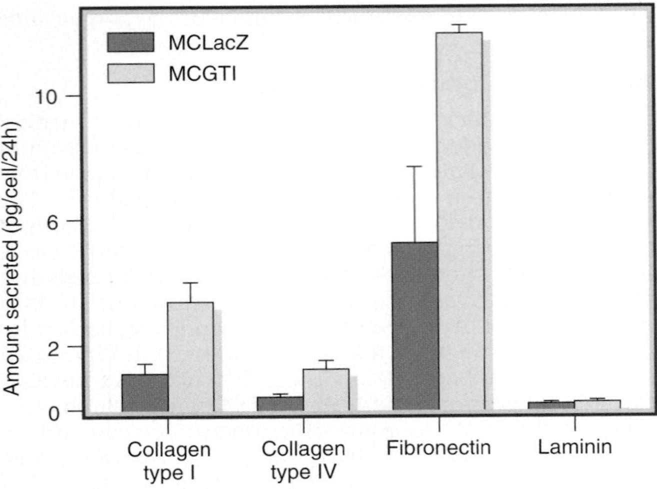

Figure 33-3 Overexpression of glucose transporter 1 (GLUT1) in mesangial cells cultured in normal glucose mimics the diabetic phenotype. Mesangial cells transfected with either LacZ (MCLacZ)-expressing or GLUT1 (MCGT1)-expressing constructs were cultured in 5 mmol/L glucose, and the secreted amounts of the indicated matrix components were determined. (From Heilig CW, Concepcion LA, Riser BL, et al. Overexpression of glucose transporters in rat mesangial cells cultured in a normal glucose milieu mimics the diabetic phenotype. *J Clin Invest.* 1995;96:1802-1814.)

directly stimulates overproduction of extracellular matrix components[16] and can induce apoptosis in certain complication-relevant cell types.

The third process is hypertension-induced stimulation of pathologic gene expression by endothelial cells and supporting cells, which include GLUT1, growth factors, growth factor receptors, extracellular matrix components, and adhesion molecules that can activate circulating leukocytes.[17] The observation that unilateral reduction in the severity of diabetic microvascular disease occurs on the side with ophthalmic or renal artery stenosis is consistent with this concept.[18,19]

Microvascular Cell Loss and Vessel Occlusion

The progressive narrowing and occlusion of diabetic microvascular lumina are also accompanied by microvascular cell loss. In the retina, diabetes mellitus induces programmed cell death of Müller cells and ganglion cells,[20] pericytes, and endothelial cells.[21] In the glomerulus, declining renal function is associated with widespread capillary occlusion and podocyte loss, but the mechanisms underlying glomerular cell loss are not yet known. In the vasa nervorum, degeneration of endothelial cells and pericytes occur,[22] and these microvascular changes appear to precede the development of diabetic peripheral neuropathy.[23] The multifocal distribution of axonal degeneration in diabetes supports a causal role for microvascular occlusion, but hyperglycemia-induced decreases in neurotrophins might contribute by preventing normal axonal repair and regeneration.[24]

Development of Microvascular Complications during Posthyperglycemic Euglycemia

Another common feature of diabetic microvascular disease has been termed *hyperglycemic memory,* or the persistence or progression of hyperglycemia-induced microvascular alterations during subsequent periods of normal glucose homeostasis. The most striking example of this phenomenon is the development of severe retinopathy in histologically normal eyes of diabetic dogs, which occurred entirely during a 2.5-year period of normalized blood glucose that followed 2.5 years of hyperglycemia (Fig. 33-4).[25] Normal dogs were compared to diabetic dogs with either poor control for 5 years, good control for 5 years, or poor control for 2.5 years ($P \rightarrow G_a$) followed by good control for the next 2.5 years ($P \rightarrow G_b$). HbA_{1c} values for both the good control group and the $P \rightarrow G_b$ group were identical to those of the normal group. Hyperglycemia-induced increases in selected matrix gene transcription also persist for weeks after restoration of normoglycemia in vivo, and a less pronounced but qualitatively similar prolongation of hyperglycemia-induced increase in selected matrix gene transcription occurs in cultured endothelial cells.[26]

Data from the DCCT suggested that hyperglycemic memory occurs in patients. In the secondary intervention cohort, there was no difference in the incidence of sustained progression of retinopathy for the first 3 years, no difference in development of clinical albuminuria for 4 years, and no difference in the rate of change in creatinine clearance during the entire study. For neuropathy, the sural nerve sensory conduction velocity did not differ between the groups for 4 years, and intensive therapy did not slow the rate of decline of autonomic function at all.[2,27-29]

Data from the DCCT suggested that hyperglycemic memory occurs in patients. In the secondary intervention cohort, there was no difference in the incidence of sustained progression of retinopathy for the first 3 years, no difference in development of clinical albuminuria for 4 years, and no difference in the rate of change in creatinine clearance during the entire study. For neuropathy, the sural nerve sensory conduction velocity did not differ between the groups for 4 years, and intensive therapy did not slow the rate of decline of autonomic function at all.[2,27-29]

Data from the post-DCCT long-term follow-up study, the Epidemiology of Diabetes, Interventions, and Complications (EDIC) study, proved that the effects of former intensive and conventional therapy persist for 12 years. In the conventional therapy group, the effects of previous high HbA_{1c} on poststudy retinopathy, nephropathy, and cardiovascular disease (CVD) persisted as if there had been no improvement in HbA_{1c} at all. Atherosclerotic changes

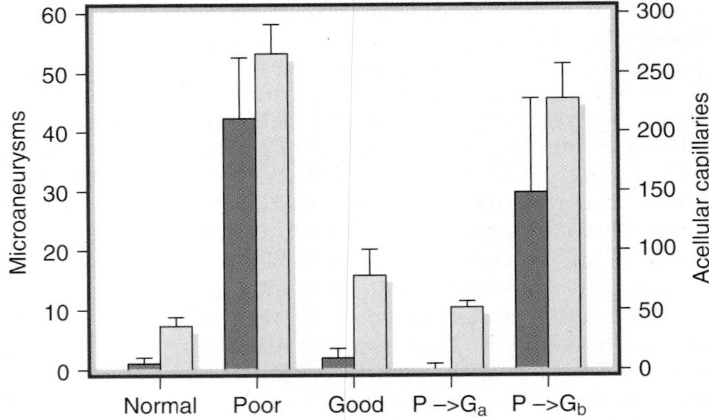

Figure 33-4 Development of retinopathy during posthyperglycemic normoglycemia (hyperglycemic memory). Quantitation of retinal microaneurysms and acellular capillaries in normal dogs (Normal), dogs with poor glycemic control for 5 years (Poor), dogs with good glycemic control for 5 years (Good), dogs with poor glycemic control for 2.5 years ($P \rightarrow G_a$), and the same dogs after a subsequent 2.5 years of good glycemic control ($P \rightarrow G_b$). (Adapted from Engerman RL, Kern TS. Progression of incipient diabetic retinopathy during good glycemic control. *Diabetes.* 1987;36:808-812.)

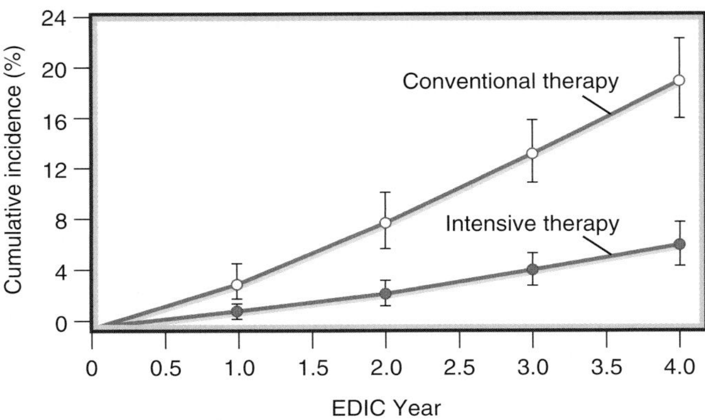

Figure 33-5 Cumulative incidence of further progression of retinopathy 4 years after the end of the Diabetes Control and Complications Trial. The median glycosylated hemoglobin level was 8.2% for the conventional therapy group and 7.9% for the intensive therapy group. EDIC, Epidemiology of Diabetes, Interventions, and Complications [Research Group]. (From Retinopathy and nephropathy in patients with type 1 diabetes four years after a trial of intensive therapy. The Diabetes Control and Complications Trial/Epidemiology of Diabetes Interventions and Complications Research Group. *N Engl J Med.* 2000;342:381-389.)

not even present at the end of the DCCT appeared subsequently in the previously higher HbA_{1c} group, followed by a twofold increase in heart attacks, strokes, and cardiovascular death, even though the HbA_{1c} level in these patients since the end of the DCCT was identical to that of the formerly intensive-control group during the entire time that these arterial changes developed (Fig. 33-5).[30,31] On the other hand, the beneficial effects of previous lower HbA_{1c} also persisted in the intensive treatment group after their HbA_{1c} went up, as if there had been no deterioration in their HbA_{1c}.

Therefore, the phenomenon of hyperglycemic memory presents a paradox: Patients in the DCCT with long-term exposure to a higher level of hyperglycemia became more susceptible to damage from subsequent lower levels of hyperglycemia than they were when they first started the trial. In contrast, lower levels of hyperglycemia made patients more resistant to damage from subsequent higher levels.

Genetic Determinants of Susceptibility to Microvascular Complications

Clinicians have long observed that different patients with similar duration and degree of hyperglycemia differ markedly in their susceptibility to microvascular complications. Such observations suggested that genetic differences exist that affected the pathways by which hyperglycemia damages microvascular cells. The leveling of risk of overt proteinuria after 30 years' duration of T1DM at 27% is evidence that only a subset of patients are susceptible to development of diabetic nephropathy.[32]

A role for a genetic determinant of susceptibility to diabetic nephropathy is most strongly supported by familial clustering, with an estimated heritability of at least 40%.[33] In two studies of families in which two or more siblings had T1DM, the risk of nephropathy in a diabetic sibling was 83% or 72% if the probrand diabetic sibling had advanced diabetic nephropathy, but only 17% or 22% if the index patient did not have diabetic nephropathy (Fig. 33-6),[34,35] or retinopathy. The DCCT reported familial clustering as well, with an odds ratio of 5.4 for the risk of severe retinopathy in diabetic relatives of positive versus negative subjects from the conventional treatment group.[36] Coronary artery calcification, an indicator of subclinical atherosclerosis, also shows familial clustering.

Numerous associations have been made between various genetic polymorphisms and the risk of diabetic complications. Examples include the 5′ insulin gene polymorphism,[37] the G2m23+ immunoglobulin allotype,[38] angiotensin-converting enzyme (ACE) insertion/deletion polymorphisms,[39,40] HLA-DQB10201/0302 alleles,[41] polymorphisms of the aldose reductase gene,[42] and a polymorphic CCTTT(n) repeat of nitric oxide synthase 2A (NOS2A).[43] In all of these studies, there was no indication that the polymorphic gene actually plays a functional role rather than simply being in linkage disequilibrium with the locus encoding the unidentified relevant genes.

A whole-genome linkage analysis using families of Pima Indians showed susceptibility loci for diabetic nephropathy on chromosome 3, 7, and 20. Another linkage analysis using discordant sib-pairs of white families with T1DM identified a critical area on chromosome 3q. Evidence for linkage to kidney disease has been detected and replicated at several loci on chromosomes 3q (T1DM and T2DM nephropathy), 10q (diabetic and nondiabetic kidney disease), and 18q (T2DM nephropathy).[44]

Family-based studies of simple tandem repeat polymorphisms (STRPs) and single-nucleotide polymorphisms (SNPs) in 115 candidate genes for linkage and association with diabetic nephropathy in T1DM families of European descent showed a positive association with polymorphisms in 20 genes, including 12 that had not been studied previously. Three of these genes code for components of the extracellular matrix *(COL4A1, LAMA4,* and *LAMC1),* and two are involved in its metabolism *(MMP9* and *TIMP3).* Five genes code for transcription factors or signaling molecules *(HNF1B1/TCF2, NRP1, PRKCB1, SMAD3,* and *USF1).* Three genes code for growth factors or growth factor receptors *(IGF1, TGFBR2,* and *TGFBR3).* The other genes *(AGTR1, AQP1, BCL2, CAT, GPX1, LPL,* and *p22phox)* code for a variety of products that are likely to be relevant in kidney function.[45]

An individual-based genetic association study of subjects from the DCCT/EDIC found that multiple variations

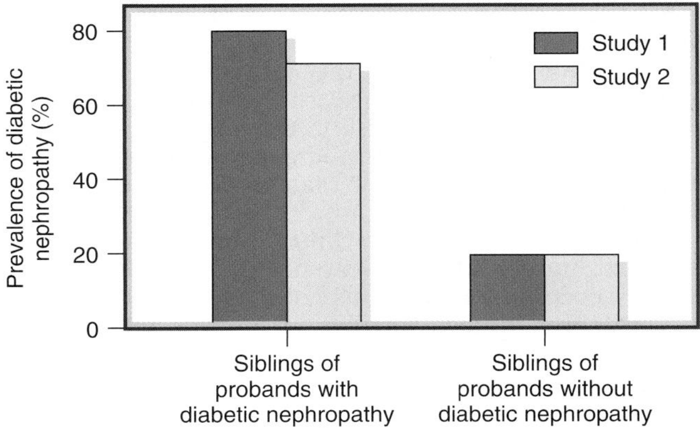

Figure 33-6 Familial clustering of diabetic nephropathy. Prevalence of diabetic nephropathy in two studies of diabetic siblings of probands with or without diabetic nephropathy. (Adapted from Seaquist ER, Goetz FC, Rich S, et al. Familial clustering of diabetic kidney disease: evidence for genetic susceptibility to diabetic nephropathy. *N Engl J Med.* 1989;320:1161-1165; Quinn M, Angelico MC, Warram JH, et al. Familial factors determine the development of diabetic nephropathy in patients with IDDM. *Diabetologia.* 1996;39:940-945.)

in superoxide dismutase 1 were significantly associated with persistent microalbuminuria and severe nephropathy.[46] A combination of case-control association and functional studies demonstrated that the T allele of SNP rs1617640 in the promoter of the erythropoietin gene *(EPO)* was significantly associated with proliferative diabetic retinopathy (PDR) and ESRD in three European-American cohorts, suggesting that rs1617640 in the *EPO* promoter is significantly associated with PDR and ESRD.[47] In addition, a multicenter study based on 518 subjects with long-standing diabetes mellitus showed that three *EPO* SNPs were associated with overall diabetic retinopathy status in the combined T1DM and T2DM groups and in the T2DM-alone group.[48]

As genes are identified that affect susceptibility to diabetic complications, a new area of research has emerged that will make it possible to identify genetic modifiers of the clinical manifestations of complications. With the completion of the genetic map known as the International HapMap Project and new high-throughput genotyping technologies, this promising area of research holds great potential for understanding genetic determinants of the varying clinical severity of diabetic complications. These modifying genes are genetic variants that are distinct from disease-susceptibility genes and that modify the phenotypic and clinical expression of the disease genes.[49] Because complications are likely to result not only from hyperglycemia but also from a susceptibility to later pathophysiologic steps such as inflammation or aberrant angiogenesis, a number of modifier genes may be relevant to diabetic complications.

Pathophysiologic Features of Macrovascular Complications

Unlike microvascular disease, which occurs only in patients with diabetes mellitus, macrovascular disease resembles that in subjects without diabetes. However, subjects with diabetes have more rapidly progressive and extensive CVD, with a greater incidence of multivessel disease and a greater number of diseased vessel segments than nondiabetic persons.[50] Although dyslipidemia and hypertension occur with great frequency in T2DM populations, there is still excess risk in diabetic subjects after adjusting for these other risk factors.[51,52] Diabetes itself can confer 75% to 90% of the excess risk of coronary disease in these diabetic subjects, and it enhances the deleterious effects of the other major cardiovascular risk factors (Fig. 33-7).[53,54] The importance of hyperglycemia in the pathogenesis of diabetic macrovascular disease is suggested by the observation that HbA_{1c} is an independent risk factor for CVD[55] in T1DM, and numerous correlational studies show that hyperglycemia is a continuous risk factor for macrovascular disease.[56-60]

However, data from the United Kingdom Prospective Diabetes Study (UKPDS) show that hyperglycemia is not nearly as central a determinant of diabetic macrovascular disease as it is in microvascular disease. For microvascular disease end points, there is an almost 10-fold increase in risk as HbA_{1c} increases from 5.5% to 9.5%, whereas over the same HbA_{1c} range, macrovascular risk increases only about twofold.[3]

Insulin resistance occurs in most patients with T2DM and in two thirds of subjects with impaired glucose tolerance.[61] Both these groups have a significantly higher risk of developing CVD.[62-65] To isolate the effects of insulin resistance from those of hyperglycemia and diabetes, several studies have evaluated subjects with normal glucose tolerance. In T1DM, hyperglycemia itself causes secondary insulin resistance in almost all patients. In nonobese subjects without diabetes, insulin resistance predicted the development of CVD independently of other known risk factors.[66] In another group of subjects without diabetes or impaired glucose tolerance, those in the highest quintile of insulin resistance had a 2.5-fold increase in CVD risk compared with those in the lowest quintile.[67] These data indicate that insulin resistance itself promotes atherogenesis.

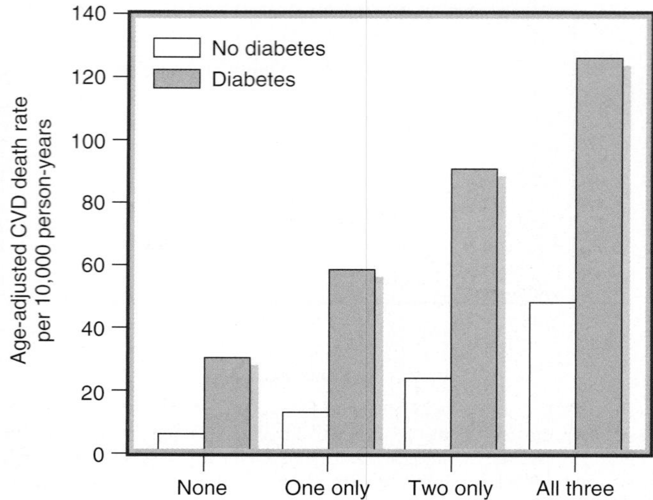

Figure 33-7 Adjusted death rates by number of cardiovascular disease (CVD) risk factors for diabetic and nondiabetic men. Subjects are participants from the Multiple Risk Factor Intervention Trial (MRFIT) study; risk factors are hypercholesterolemia, hypertension, and cigarette smoking. (From Stamler J, Vaccaro O, Neaton JD, et al. Diabetes, other risk factors, and 12-year cardiovascular mortality for men screened in the Multiple Risk Factor Intervention Trial. *Diabetes Care.* 1993;2:434-444.)

Insulin resistance is commonly associated with a proatherogenic dyslipidemia; data from Brown, Goldstein, and colleagues suggested that this dyslipidemia results from hyperinsulinemia-induced activation of sterol regulatory element–binding protein 1c (SREBP-1c) transcription in the liver by a mechanism that is not affected by the defects in hepatic phosphatidylinositol 3 kinase (PI3K)-mediated insulin signaling.[68,69] Insulin resistance is associated with a characteristic lipoprotein profile that includes a high level of very-low-density lipoprotein (VLDL) and low levels of high-density lipoprotein (HDL) and small, dense low-density lipoprotein (LDL). Both low HDL and small, dense LDL are independent risk factors for macrovascular disease. This profile arises as a direct result of increased net free fatty acid (FFA) release by insulin-resistant adipocytes (Fig. 33-8).[10] Increased FFA flux into hepatocytes stimulates VLDL secretion. In the presence of cholesteryl ester transfer protein, excess VLDL transfers significant amounts of triglyceride to HDL and LDL while depleting HDL and LDL of cholesteryl ester. The resultant triglyceride-enriched HDL carries less cholesteryl ester for reverse cholesterol transport to the liver, and loss of apolipoprotein 1A-1 (Apo1A-1) from these particles reduces the total concentration of HDL available for reverse cholesterol transport. The triglyceride-enriched, cholesteryl ester–depleted LDL is smaller and denser than normal LDL, allowing it to penetrate the vessel wall and be oxidized more easily.

In vitro studies suggest that at the level of the vessel wall, insulin has both antiatherogenic and proatherogenic effects (Fig. 33-9).[70,71] One major antiatherogenic effect is the stimulation of endothelial NO production. NO released

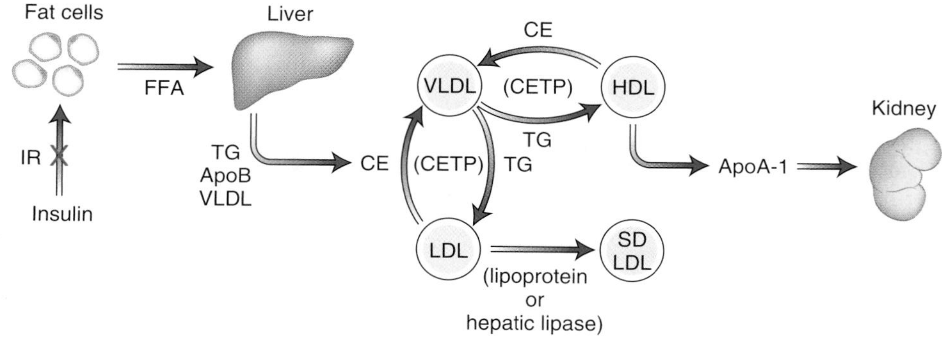

Figure 33-8 Schematic summary relating insulin resistance (IR) to the characteristic dyslipidemia of type 2 diabetes mellitus. IR at the adipocyte results in increased free fatty acid (FFA) release. Increased FFA flux stimulates secretion of very-low-density lipoprotein (VLDL), causing hypertriglyceridemia (TG). VLDL stimulates a reciprocal exchange of TG to cholesteryl ester (CE) from both high-density lipoprotein (HDL) and low-density lipoprotein (LDL), catalyzed by CE transfer protein (CETP). TG-enriched HDL dissociates from apolipoprotein (Apo) A-1, leaving less HDL for reverse cholesterol transport. TG-enriched LDL serves as a substrate for lipases that convert it to atherogenic small, dense LDL particles (SD LDL). (From Ginsberg HN. Insulin resistance and cardiovascular disease. *J Clin Invest.* 2000;106:453-458.)

from endothelial cells is a potent inhibitor of platelet aggregation and adhesion to the vascular wall. Endothelial NO also controls the expression of genes involved in atherogenesis. It decreases expression of monocyte chemoattractant protein 1 (MCP-1) and of surface adhesion molecules such as CD11/CD18, P-selectin, vascular cell adhesion molecule 1 (VCAM-1), and intercellular adhesion molecule 1 (ICAM-1). Endothelial cell NO also reduces vascular permeability and decreases the rate of oxidation of LDL to its proatherogenic form. Finally, endothelial cell NO inhibits proliferation of VSMC.[72]

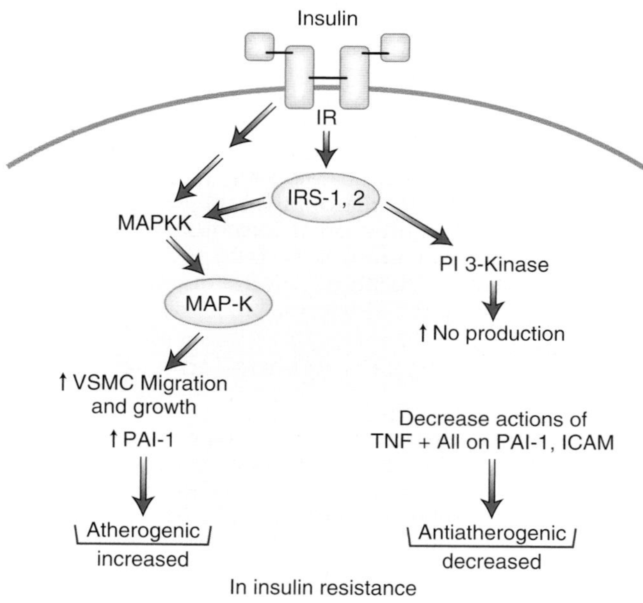

Figure 33-9 Schematic summary of proatherosclerotic and antiatherosclerotic actions of insulin on vascular cells. ICAM, intercellular adhesion molecule; IRS, insulin resistance syndrome; MAP-K, mitogen-activated protein kinase; MAPKK, MAPK kinase; PAI, plasminogen activator inhibitor; PI, phosphatidylinositol; TNF, tumor necrosis factor; VSMC, vascular smooth muscle cell. (Adapted from King G, Brownlee M. The cellular and molecular mechanisms of diabetic complications. *Endocrinol Metab Clin North Am.* 1996;2:255-270; Hsueh WA, Law RE. Cardiovascular risk continuum: implications of insulin resistance and diabetes. *Am J Med.* 1998;105:4S-14S.)

Two major proatherogenic effects of insulin are the potentiation of platelet-derived growth factor (PDGF)-induced VSMC proliferation and the stimulation of VSMC production of plasminogen activator inhibitor 1 (PAI-1).[73,74] Because insulin-induced NO production is mediated by the insulin receptor substrate–PI3K signal transduction pathway and the effects on smooth muscle cells are mediated by the signal transduction pathway involving Ras, Raf, MAPK (mitogen-activated protein kinase), and MEKK (MAPK/extracellular-signal–regulated kinase [ERK] kinase [MEK] kinase),[71,72] it has been proposed that pathway-selective insulin resistance in arterial cells may contribute to diabetic atherosclerosis. Evidence of such selective vascular resistance to insulin has been demonstrated in the obese Zucker rat.[75]

Hyperglycemia also inhibits arterial endothelial NO production, both in vivo and in vitro.[76-79] Similarly, hyperglycemia potentiates PDGF-induced VSMC proliferation and stimulates endothelial cell PAI-1 production.[78,80] In addition, hyperglycemia has a variety of other proatherogenic effects on endothelial cells, platelets, and monocyte/macrophages. These include increased expression of MCP-1,[81] upregulation of adhesion molecules such as ICAM-1 and VCAM-1,[82-84] potentiation of collagen-induced platelet activation, and increased secretion of collagen type IV and fibronectin.[85,86]

Surprisingly, however, in subjects without diabetes or impaired glucose tolerance, after adjustment for 11 known cardiovascular risk factors, including LDL, triglycerides, HDL, systolic blood pressure (BP), and smoking, the most insulin-resistant subjects still have a twofold increase in the risk of CVD.[67] This observation suggests that a significant part of the increased CVD risk due to insulin resistance reflects a consequence of insulin resistance not previously identified as being proatherogenic. Data suggest that increased oxidation of FFAs by insulin-resistant aortic endothelial cells inactivates two important antiatherosclerotic enzymes: prostacyclin synthase and endothelial NOS (eNOS). This inactivation is reversed by inhibition of the rate-limiting enzyme of fatty acid oxidation, carnitine palmitoyltransferase I, through inhibition of FFA release from insulin-resistant adipose tissue and reduction of superoxide levels.[87]

Although the association of insulin resistance with CVD risk is clear, data concerning the relative role of hyperglycemia in promoting CVD in diabetes appear to be somewhat contradictory. In T1DM, in which severe insulin resistance is not a major abnormality, lowering of HbA_{1c} levels with more intensive insulin treatment during the DCCT reduced both atherosclerosis surrogates during the trial and actual CVD events years after the trial had concluded. Intensive treatment reduced the risk of any CVD event by 42% and the risk of nonfatal myocardial infarction (MI), stroke, or death from CVD by 57%.[88] In contrast, intensive insulin treatment during the Action to Control Cardiovascular Risk in Diabetes (ACCORD) trial was associated with an unexpected excess of cardiovascular mortality in the intensive arm that caused the study to end early. Patients in this group were treated with a goal of lowering HbA_{1c} to 6.0%. A higher average on-treatment HbA_{1c} level was a stronger predictor of mortality than the HbA_{1c} for the last interval of follow-up or the decrease in HbA_{1c} during the first year. Of note, the excess risk associated with intensive glycemic treatment occurred among those participants whose average HbA_{1c}, contrary to the intent of the strategy, was greater than 7%.[89]

How might these apparently conflicting results be explained? One possibility is that intensive therapy in extremely insulin-resistant diabetic patients causes proatherogenic effects through overstimulation of insulin signaling pathways not affected by insulin resistance. In the liver, insulin exerts two predominant actions: it reduces glucose production (gluconeogenesis) and it increases the synthesis of fatty acids and triglycerides (lipogenesis). In the insulin-resistant state, only one of these actions is blocked in liver. Insulin loses its ability to reduce gluconeogenesis but it retains its ability to enhance lipogenesis.[90,91]

Therefore, the increase in insulin levels to overcome the hyperglycemia caused by pathway-selective insulin resistance likely overdrives nonresistant pathways of insulin signaling, including MAPK. In arterial endothelial cells, such selective overdrive of the MAPK pathway by insulin would stimulate cellular growth and migration and the production of prothrombotic and profibrotic factors. Insulin stimulates secretion of the vasoconstrictor endothelin-1 and increases cellular adhesion molecule expression. In arterial smooth muscle cells, overdrive of the MAPK pathway by high insulin levels would stimulate VSMC proliferation and migration as well as expression of angiotensinogen and its receptor, AT1R.[75,92]

Impaired Collateral Blood Vessel Formation from Bone Marrow Progenitor Cells

It has become apparent that diabetic complications result not only from damage to vascular cells but also from a defective repair process. Normally, in response to acute ischemia, new blood vessel growth rescues stunned areas of the heart or central nervous system, reducing morbidity and mortality. In response to chronic ischemia, collateral vessel development reduces the size and severity of subsequent infarction. In response to ischemia, circulating endothelial progenitor cells from the bone marrow promote the regeneration of blood vessels, acting in concert with cells and extracellular matrix at the site of injury. In experimental diabetes, however, these circulating endothelial progenitor cells are depleted and dysfunctional. As a result, diabetic animals have decreased vascular density after hind limb ischemia. Similarly, in human diabetes, endothelial progenitor cells are also depleted and dysfunctional.[93]

Clinically, diabetes is associated with poor outcomes after acute vascular occlusive events. This results in part from a failure to form adequate compensatory microvasculature in response to ischemia. Advanced glycation end products (AGEs) appear to play a central role in this failure. High glucose induces a decrease in transactivation by the transcription factor hypoxia-inducible factor-1α (HIF-1α), which mediates production of hypoxia-stimulated chemokine and vascular endothelial growth factor (VEGF) by hypoxic tissue and expression of chemokine receptor and eNOS in endothelial precursor cells in the bone marrow. Decreasing superoxide in diabetic mice, by transgenic expression of manganese superoxide dismutase or by administration of a superoxide dismutase mimetic, corrected postischemic defects in neovascularization, oxygen delivery, and chemokine expression, and normalized tissue survival. Decreased HIF-1α functional activity was specifically caused by impaired formation of the HIF-1α heterodimer with arylhydrocarbon receptor nuclear translocator (ARNT) and by impaired binding of the coactivator p300 to the HIF-1α–ARNT heterodimer. Hyperglycemia-induced covalent modification of p300 by the dicarbonyl metabolite methylglyoxal is responsible for this decreased association (Fig. 33-10). In diabetic mouse models of impaired angiogenesis and wound healing, decreasing mitrochondrial formation of reactive oxygen species (ROS) normalizes both ischemia-induced new vessel formation and wound healing.[94,95]

Many diabetic patients who have impaired blood vessel growth after ischemic events also have increased retinal neovascularization (diabetic retinopathy). This diabetic paradox is at present poorly understood.[96,97] The question of how endothelial progenitor cell dysfunction can participate in diabetic retinopathy is especially intriguing, given the findings by Grant and colleagues[98] that bone marrow–derived endothelial progenitor cells play a role in a model of adult retinal revascularization. A plausible explanation may be that the cells responsible for increased VEGF production in the diabetic retina do not develop intracellular hyperglycemia and consequent HIF-1α dysfunction. They respond normally to ischemia, in contrast to ischemic tissue elsewhere in the body. VEGF is known to be significantly elevated in the ocular fluid of diabetic patients, but it has also been shown to be decreased in ischemic nonretinal tissues.[99] Because VEGF has a stimulatory effect on endothelial progenitor cell proliferation and is a potent stimulator of vasculogenesis,[100] retinal cells whose VEGF expression in response to ischemia is not affected by hyperglycmia may be sufficient to overcome endothelial progenitor cell dysfunction and cause PDR.

Mechanisms of Hyperglycemia-Induced Damage

Four major hypotheses about how hyperglycemia causes diabetic complications have generated a large amount of data as well as several clinical trials based on specific inhibitors of these mechanisms. Until recently, there was no unifying hypothesis linking these four mechanisms together, nor was there an obvious connection between any of these mechanisms, each of which responds quickly to normalization of hyperglycemia, and the phenomenon of hyperglycemic memory (see earlier discussion).

Increased Polyol Pathway Flux

Aldose reductase [alditol:NADP+ 1-oxidoreductase, EC 1.1.1.21] is a cytosolic, monomeric oxidoreductase that catalyzes the reduced nicotinamide adenine dinucleotide phosphate (NADPH)-dependent reduction of a wide variety of carbonyl compounds, including glucose. Triphosphopyridine nucleotide, the reduced form of NADP (NADPH), is the cofactor in this reaction and in the regeneration of

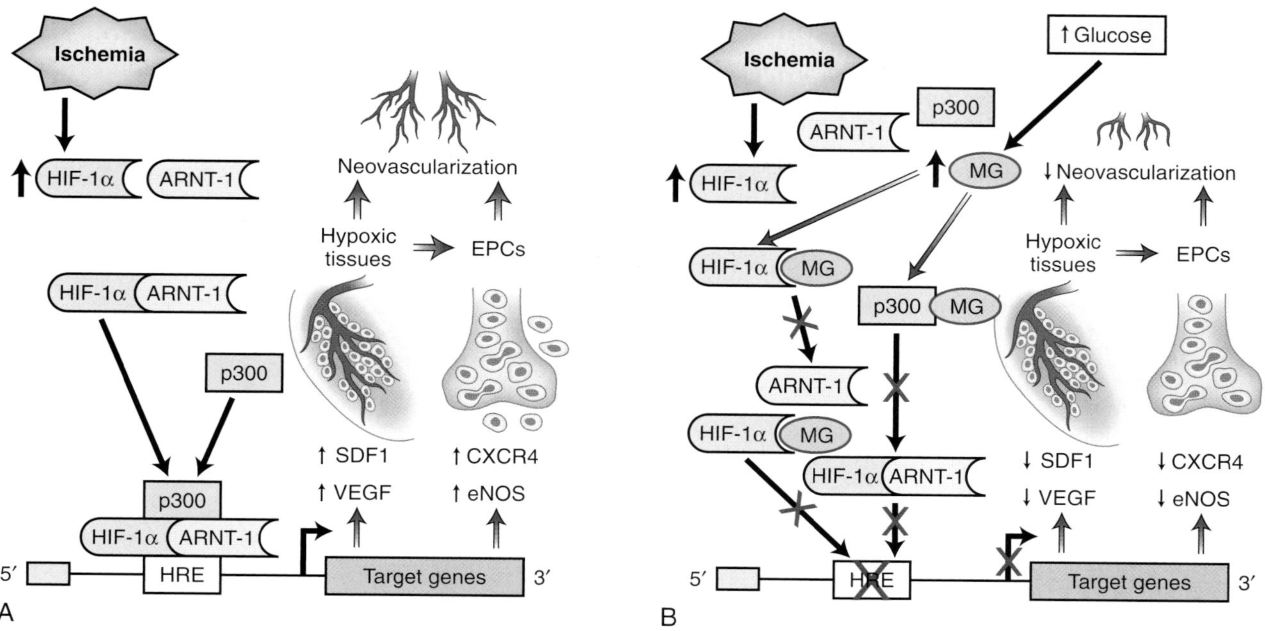

Figure 33-10 Ischemia-induced neovascularization in normal and high glucose. **A,** In the presence of normal glucose concentrations, ischemia-stabilized HIF-1α forms heterodimers with ARNT, which bind the coactivator p300. This complex binds to the hypoxia response element (HRE) and activates expression of genes required for neovascularization. **B,** High glucose–induced methylglyoxal (MG) modifies HIF-1α and p300, inhibiting complex binding to the HREs of genes required for neovascularization.

glutathione by glutathione reductase. Aldose reductase has a low-affinity (high Michaelis constant [K_m]) for glucose, and at the normal glucose concentrations found in nondiabetic patients, the metabolism of glucose by this pathway constitutes a small percentage of total glucose utilization. In a hyperglycemic environment, however, increased intracellular glucose results in increased enzymatic conversion to the polyalcohol sorbitol, with concomitant decreases in NADPH. In the polyol pathway, sorbitol is oxidized to fructose by the enzyme sorbitol dehydrogenase, with nicotinamide adenine dinucleotide (NAD+) reduced to NADH (Fig. 33-11). Flux through this pathway during hyperglycemia varies from 33% of total glucose utilization in the rabbit lens to 11% in human erythrocytes. Therefore, the contribution of this pathway to diabetic complications may be very much species, site, and tissue dependent.

A number of mechanisms have been proposed to explain the potential detrimental effects of hyperglycemia-induced increases in polyol pathway flux. These include sorbitol-induced osmotic stress, decreased activity of the sodium-potassium adenosine triphosphatase (Na^+,K^+-ATPase) pump, increased cytosolic NADH/NAD+, and decreased cytosolic NADPH. Sorbitol does not diffuse easily across cell membranes, and it was originally suggested that this resulted in osmotic damage to microvascular cells. However, sorbitol concentrations measured in diabetic vessels and nerves are far too low to cause osmotic damage.

Another early suggestion was that increased flux through the polyol pathway decreased Na^+,K^+-ATPase activity. Although this was originally thought to be mediated by polyol pathway–linked decreases in phosphatidylinositol synthesis, it has been shown to result from activation of protein kinase C (PKC) (see later discussion). Hyperglycemia-induced activation of PKC increases cytosolic phospholipase A_2 activity, which increases the production of two inhibitors of Na^+,K^+-ATPase, arachidonate and prostaglandin E_2 (PGE_2).[101]

More recently, it has been proposed that oxidation of sorbitol by NAD+ increases the cytosolic NADH/NAD+ ratio, thereby inhibiting activity of the enzyme glyceraldehyde-3-phosphate dehydrogenase (GADPH) and increasing the concentrations of triose phosphate.[102] Elevated triose phosphate concentrations could increase the formation of both methylglyoxal a precursor of AGEs, and (via α-glycerol-3-phosphate) diacylglycerol (DAG), thus activating PKC (discussed later). Although increased NADH

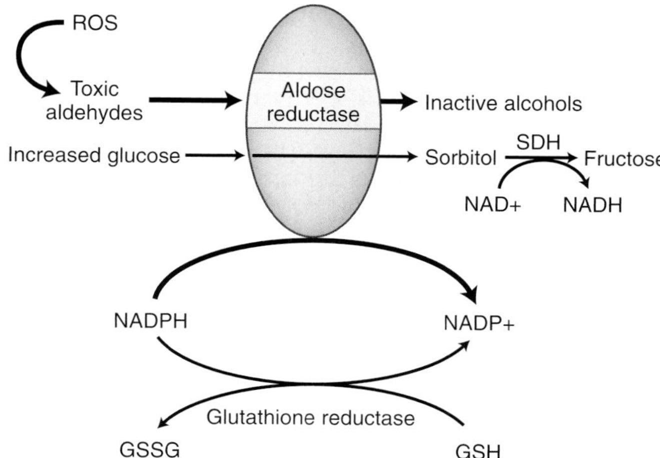

Figure 33-11 Aldose reductase and the polyol pathway. Aldose reductase reduces reactive oxygen species (ROS)-generated toxic aldehydes to inactive alcohols, and glucose to sorbitol, using triphosphopyridine nucleotide (NADPH), the reduced form of nicotinamide adenine dinucleotide phosphate (NADP), as a cofactor. In cells in which aldose reductase activity is sufficient to deplete reduced glutathione (GSH), oxidative stress would be augmented. Sorbitol dehydrogenase (SDH) oxidizes sorbitol to fructose using nicotinamide-adenine dinucleotide (NAD+) as a cofactor. GSSG, oxidized glutathione.

production is supported by the observation that hyperglycemia increases both the lactate concentration and the lactate-to-pyruvate ratio, there is no direct evidence that the concentrations of NADH and NAD+, as opposed to NADH and NAD+ flux, are altered. In endothelial cells, where aldose reductase activity is low, increased NADH production might also reflect hyperglycemia-induced increased flux through glycolysis[103] and through the glucuronic acid pathway.[104]

Other evidence presented in support of this hypothesis includes the observation that administration of pyruvate can prevent diabetes-related endothelial dysfunction in some systems. However, the observed effects of pyruvate on microvascular function may reflect its potent antioxidant properties rather than effects on the NADH/NAD^+ ratio, because ROS also partially inhibit GADPH and increase glyceraldehyde-3-phosphate levels.[105,106] The source of hyperglycemia-induced ROS is discussed later in this section.

It has also been proposed that reduction of glucose to sorbitol by NADPH consumes the cofactor NADPH. Because NADPH is required for regeneration of reduced glutathione, this could induce or exacerbate intracellular oxidative stress. Indeed, overexpression of human aldose reductase increased atherosclerosis in diabetic mice and reduces the expression of genes that regulate regeneration of glutathione.[107] Less reduced glutathione has been found in the lens of transgenic mice that overexpress aldose reductase, and this is the most likely mechanism by which increased flux through the polyol pathway has deleterious consequences.[108] This conclusion is further supported by recent experiments with aldose reductase–deficient homozygous knockout mice, showing that, in contrast to wild-type mice, diabetes neither decreases sciatic nerve content of reduced glutathione nor reduces motor nerve conduction velocity.[109]

Observations suggest that NO maintains aldose reductase in an inactive state and that this repression is relieved in diabetic tissues.[110] Aldose reductase appears to be inhibited by NO-derived adduct formation on active-site Cys-298.[111,112] These observations suggest that diabetes-induced decreases in NO might further activate the polyol pathway.

In vivo studies of polyol pathway inhibition have yielded inconsistent results. In a 5-year study in dogs, aldose reductase inhibition prevented diabetic neuropathy but failed to prevent retinopathy or capillary basement membrane thickening in the retina, kidney, or muscle.[113] Several negative clinical trials have questioned the relevance of this mechanism in humans.[114] However, the positive effect of aldose reductase inhibition on diabetic neuropathy has been confirmed in humans in a rigorous multidose, placebo-controlled trial with the potent aldose reductase inhibitor, zenarestat.[115]

Increased Intracellular Formation of Advanced Glycation End Products

Advanced Glycation End Products Are Formed from Intracellular Dicarbonyl Precursors. AGEs are found in increased amounts in extracellular structures of diabetic retinal vessels[116-118] and renal glomeruli,[119-121] where they can cause damage by mechanisms described later in this section. These AGEs were originally thought to arise from nonenzymatic reactions between extracellular proteins and glucose. However, the rate of AGE formation from glucose is orders of magnitude slower than the rate of AGE formation from glucose-derived dicarbonyl precursors generated intracellularly, and it now seems likely that intracellular hyperglycemia is the primary initiating event in the formation of both intracellular and extracellular AGEs.[122] AGEs can arise from intracellular auto-oxidation of glucose to glyoxal,[123] decomposition of the Amadori product to 3-deoxyglucosone (perhaps accelerated by an amadoriase), and fragmentation of glyceraldehyde-3-phosphate to methylglyoxal (Fig. 33-12).[124] These reactive intracellular dicarbonyls react with amino groups of intracellular and extracellular proteins to form AGEs. Methylglyoxal and glyoxal are detoxified by the glyoxalase system.[124] All three AGE precursors are also substrates for other reductases.[125,126]

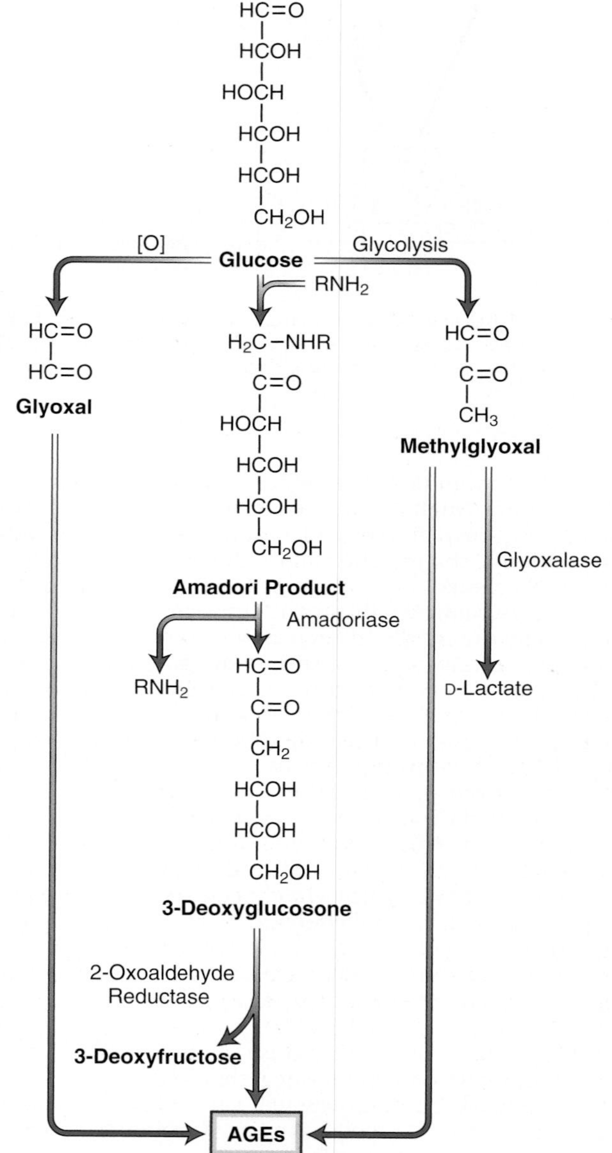

Figure 33-12 Potential pathways leading to the formation of advanced glycation end products (AGEs) from intracellular dicarbonyl precursors. Glyoxal arises from the auto-oxidation of glucose, 3-deoxyglucosone arises from decomposition of the Amadori product, and methylglyoxal arises from fragmentation of glyceraldehyde-3-phosphate. These reactive dicarbonyls react with amino groups of proteins to form AGEs. Methylglyoxal and glyoxal are detoxified by the glyoxalase system. (Adapted from Shinohara M, Thornalley PJ, Giardino I, et al. Overexpression of glyoxalase-I in bovine endothelial cells inhibits intracellular advanced glycation end-product formation and prevents hyperglycemia-induced increases in macromolecular endocytosis. *J Clin Invest.* 1998;101:1142-1147.)

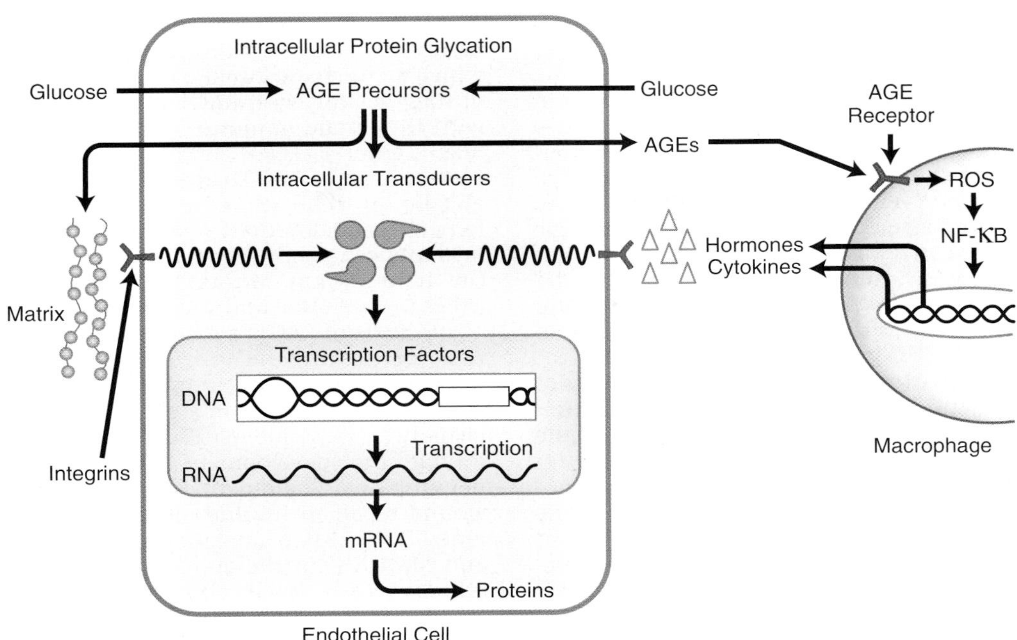

Figure 33-13 Potential mechanisms by which intracellular production of advanced glycation end-product (AGE) precursors damages vascular cells. First, intracellular protein modification alters protein function. Second, extracellular matrix modified by AGE precursors has abnormal functional properties. Third, plasma proteins modified by AGE precursors bind to AGE receptors on adjacent cells such as macrophages, thereby inducing receptor-mediated production of deleterious gene products such as cytokines. mRNA, messenger RNA; NFκB, nuclear factor-κB; ROS, reactive oxygen species. (Adapted from Brownlee M. Lilly Lecture 1993: glycation and diabetic complications. *Diabetes*. 1994;43:836-841.)

In vascular endothelial cells, methylglyoxal accounts for almost all or the hyperglycemia-induced increase in reactive AGE precursors.

The potential importance of AGEs in the pathogenesis of diabetic complications is suggested by the observation in animal models that two structurally unrelated AGE inhibitors partially prevented various functional and structural manifestations of diabetic microvascular disease in retina, kidney, and nerve.[127,128] In the human diabetic retina, AGEs might contribute to both macular edema and retinal neovascularization by increasing expression of VEGF through activation of the MAPK ERK1/2 and concomitant activation of the transcription factor HIF1.[129] In the early phase of diabetic nephropathy, AGEs induce hyperfiltration and microalbuminuria by stimulating the secretion of VEGF and MCP-1.[130] AGEs contribute to more advanced lesions of diabetic nephropathy by inducing apoptosis in glomerular mesangial cells and by inducing epithelial-myofibroblast transdifferentiation via ligation of the receptor for advanced glycation end products (RAGE; see later discussion), ultimately leading to tubulointerstitial fibrosis.[131]

Intracellular production of AGE precursors damages target cells by three general mechanisms (Fig. 33-13): Intracellular proteins modified by AGEs have altered function. Extracellular matrix components modified by AGE precursors interact abnormally with other matrix components and with matrix receptors (integrins) on cells. Plasma proteins modified by AGE precursors bind to AGE receptors on cells such as macrophages, inducing receptor-mediated ROS production. This AGE-receptor ligation activates the pleiotropic transcription factor nuclear factor-κB (NFκB), causing pathologic changes in gene expression.[132]

Advanced Glycation End Products Alter Intracellular Protein Function. It has recently been shown that AGE modification of intracellular proteins can regulate expression of genes involved in the pathogenesis of diabetic retinopathy. In diabetic retinal capillaries, the earliest morphologic changes are pericyte loss and acellular capillary formation. The primary pathologic processes of retinal pericyte loss and acellular capillary formation are regulated by complex context-dependent interactions among a number of proangiogenic and antiangiogenic factors,[133-135] including angiopoietin-2 (Ang-2). When insufficient levels of VEGF and other angiogenic signals are present, Ang-2 causes endothelial cell death and vessel regression.[136-138]

Diabetes induces a significant increase in retinal expression of Ang-2 in rats,[139] and diabetic Ang-2$^{+/-}$ mice have both decreased pericyte loss and reduced acellular capillary formation.[140] In retinal Müller cells, increased glycolytic flux causes increased methylglyoxal modification of the corepressor, mSin3A. Methylglyoxal modification of mSin3A results in increased Ang-2 expression. A similar mechanism involving methylglyoxal modification of other coregulator proteins may play a role in a variety of other diabetes-induced changes in gene expression.[141]

Advanced Glycation End Products Interfere with Normal Matrix-Matrix and Matrix-Cell Interactions. Methylglyoxal also leaks out of cells and is increased threefold to fivefold in the blood of diabetic patients, circulating at a concentration as high as 8 μmol/L.[142] Methylglyoxal at this level greatly enhances apoptosis caused by agents that induce oxidative stress and DNA damage.[143] Methylglyoxal also can act as an antiapoptotic modulator by direct modification of heat shock protein 27 (HSP27) at amino acid Arg-188, which allows HSP27 to repress cytochrome *c*–mediated caspase activation.[144]

AGE formation from circulating methylglyoxal and other AGE precursors alters the functional properties of several important matrix molecules. On type I collagen, this cross-linking induces an expansion of the molecular packing.[145] These AGE-induced cross-links alter the function of intact vessels. For example, AGEs decrease elasticity in large vessels from diabetic rats, even after vascular tone is abolished, and increase fluid filtration across the carotid artery.[146] AGE formation on type IV collagen from basement membrane inhibits lateral association of these molecules into a normal network-like structure by interfering with binding of the noncollagenous NC1 domain to the helix-rich domain.[147] AGE formation on laminin causes decreased polymer self-assembly, decreased binding to type IV collagen, and decreased binding of heparan sulfate proteoglycan.[148] In vitro AGE formation on intact glomerular basement membrane increases its permeability to albumin in a manner that resembles the abnormal permeability of diabetic nephropathy.[149,150]

AGE formation on extracellular matrix interferes not only with matrix-matrix interactions but also with matrix-cell interactions.[151] For example, AGE modification of the cell-binding domains of type IV collagen decreases endothelial cell adhesion, and AGE modification of a 6-amino-acid growth-promoting sequence in the A chain of the laminin molecule markedly reduces neurite outgrowth.[152] AGE modification of vitronectin reduces cell attachment–promoting activity.[153] Research has shown that increased modification of vascular basement membrane type IV collagen by methylglyoxal, at hot spot modification sites in the RGD and GFOGER integrin-binding sites of collagen, causes endothelial cell detachment and inhibition of angiogenesis.[154] In addition, matrix glycation impairs agonist-induced Ca^{2+} increases, and this may adversely affect regulatory functions of the endothelium.[155]

Advanced Glycation End Product Receptors Mediate Pathologic Changes in Gene Expression. Several cell-associated binding proteins for AGEs have been identified, including OST-48, 80K-H, galectin-3, macrophage scavenger receptor type II, and RAGE.[156,160] Some of these are more likely to contribute to clearance of AGEs, whereas others can cause sustained cellular perturbations mediated by AGE ligand binding. In cell culture systems, the receptors identified to date appear to mediate long-term effects of AGEs on key cellular targets of diabetic complications such as macrophages, glomerular mesangial cells, and vascular endothelial cells, although not all of these receptors bind proteins with physiologic AGE-modified levels. These effects include expression of cytokines and growth factors by macrophages and mesangial cells—interleukin 1 (IL-1), insulin-like growth factor type 1 (IGF1), tumor necrosis factor-α (TNF-α), TGF-β, macrophage colony-stimulating factor (M-CSF), granulocyte-macrophage colony-stimulating factor (GM-CSF), and PDGF[161-175]—and expression of procoagulatory or proinflammatory molecules by endothelial cells (i.e., thrombomodulin, tissue factor, and VCAM-1).[176-179] In addition, endothelial AGE receptor binding appears to mediate, in part, the hyperpermeability induced by diabetes, probably through the induction of VEGF.[180-182] RAGE deficiency attenuates the development of atherosclerosis in the diabetic apolipoprotein E (apoE)-null mouse model of accelerated atherosclerosis. Diabetic $RAGE^{-/-}/apoE^{-/-}$ mice had significantly reduced atherosclerotic plaque area. These beneficial effects on the vasculature were associated with attenuation of leukocyte recruitment; decreased expression of proinflammatory mediators, including the NKκB subunit p65, VCAM-1, and MCP-1; and reduced oxidative stress.[183]

More recent studies indicate that AGEs at the concentrations found in diabetic sera are not the major ligand for RAGE. Rather, several proinflammatory protein ligands have been identified that activate RAGE at low concentrations. These include several members of the S100 calgranulin family and high-mobility group box 1 (HMGB1), all of which are increased by diabetic hyperglycemia.[184] Ligation of these ligands with RAGE causes cooperative interaction with the innate immune system signaling molecule, toll-like receptor 4 (TLR4).[185,186] Expressions of RAGE, S100A8, S100A12, and HMGB1 are all increased by high levels of glucose in cell culture and in diabetic animals. This hyperglycemia-induced overexpression is mediated by ROS-induced methylglyoxal, which increases binding of the transcription factors NFκB and activator protein 1 (AP1) to the RAGE and RAGE ligands, respectively.[187]

Blockade of RAGE, a member of the pattern-recognition receptor class of the innate immune system, suppresses macrovascular disease in an atherosclerosis-prone type 1 diabetic mouse model in a glucose- and lipid-independent fashion.[188] Blockade of RAGE has also been shown to inhibit the development of diabetic vasculopathy,[189] nephropathy,[131] and periodontal disease[190] and to enhance wound repair in murine models via suppression of cytokines, TNF-α, IL-6, metalloproteinase 2 (MMP2), MMP3, and MMP9.[191] In the apoE-null mouse model of diabetic atherosclerosis, RAGE plays an important role in accelerated lesion formation and in lesion regression. Blockade of RAGE significantly reduced lesion size and structure and decreased parameters of inflammation as well as mononuclear phagocyte and smooth muscle cell activation.[188,192] In human saphenous vein endothelial cells, engagement of RAGE by heterogeneous AGEs or *N*-(carboxymethyl) lysine (CML)-modified adducts enhanced levels of mRNA and antigen for VCAM-1, ICAM-1, and E-selectin, leading to increased adhesion of polymorphonuclear leukocytes to stimulated endothelial cells. These effects were markedly reduced by blockade of RAGE.[193] RAGE has been shown to mediate signal transduction via generation of ROS, which activates both NFκB, and p21 ras.[194-196] AGE signaling is blocked in cells by expression of RAGE antisense complementary DNA[194,197] or antiRAGE ribozyme.[195,198]

Vascular endothelial cells and pericytes have been demonstrated to express two splice variants of full-length RAGE mRNA. One codes for an isoform that lacks the amino-terminal V-type immunoglobulin-like domain (N-truncated), and one codes for an isoform lacking the carboxyl-terminal transmembrane domain (C-truncated). The C-truncated type lacks the transmembrane domain and is secreted extracellularly and detected in human sera as endogenous secretory RAGE (esRAGE). Circulating esRAGE levels are significantly lower in T1DM patients than in nondiabetic subjects, and plasma esRAGE levels are inversely correlated with carotid intima medial thickness (CIMT) and with increased risk of CVD.[199,200] Therefore, it is possible that individual differences in esRAGE expression influence the development of diabetic vascular complications.

Activation of Protein Kinase C

Mechanism of Hyperglycemia-Induced Protein Kinase C Activation. The PKC family comprises at least 11 isoforms, 9 of which are activated by the lipid second-messenger, DAG. Intracellular hyperglycemia increases DAG content in cultured microvascular cells and in the retina and renal glomeruli of diabetic animals.[201-203] Intracellular hyperglycemia appears to increase DAG content primarily by increasing its de novo synthesis from the glycolytic intermediate glyceraldehyde-3-phosphate via reduction to glycerol-3-phosphate and stepwise acylation.[202,204] Increased de novo synthesis of DAG activates PKC in cultured vascular cells[203,205-207] and in retina and

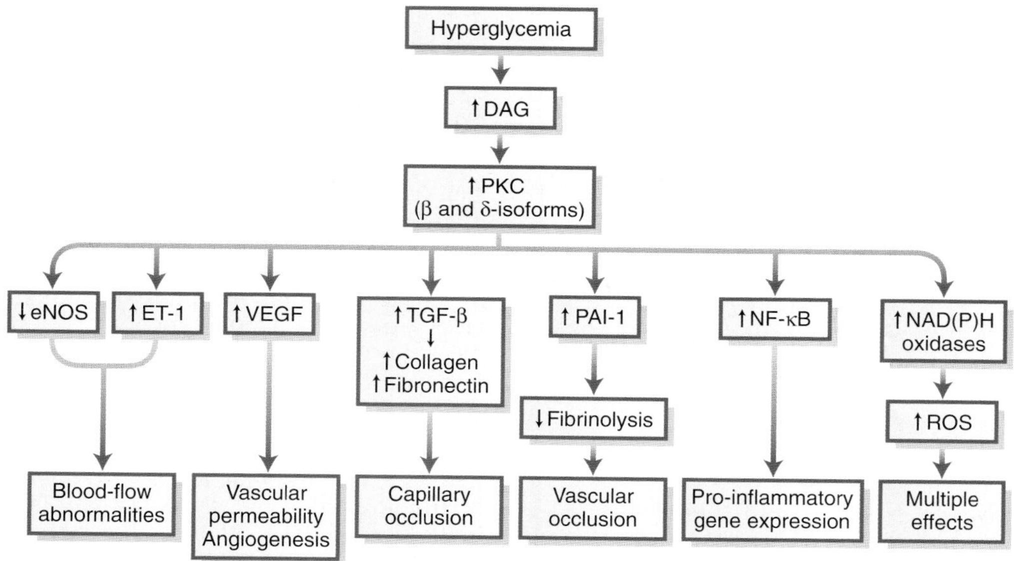

Figure 33-14 Potential consequences of hyperglycemia-induced protein kinase C (PKC) activation. Hyperglycemia increases diacylglycerol (DAG) content, which activates PKC, primarily the β and δ isoforms. Activated PKC has a number of pathogenic consequences. eNOS, endothelial nitric oxide synthase; ET-1, endothelin 1; NAD(P)H, nicotinamide adenine dinucleotide phosphate; NFκB, nuclear factor-κB; PAI, plasminogen activator inhibitor; ROS, reactive oxygen species; TGF, transforming growth factor; VEGF, vascular endothelial growth factor. (Adapted from Koya D, Jirousek MR, Lin YW, et al. Characterization of protein kinase C beta isoform activation on the gene expression of transforming growth factor-beta, extracellular matrix components, and prostanoids in the glomeruli of diabetic rats. *J Clin Invest.* 1997;100:115-126.)

glomeruli of diabetic animals.[202,203,205] Increased DAG primarily activates the β and δ isoforms of PKC, but increases in other isoforms have also been found, such as PKC-α and -ε isoforms in the retina[208] and PKC-α and -δ isoforms in the glomerulus[209,210] of diabetic rats. DAG, its mimetics, the phorbol esters, and ROS all activate PKC isoforms by triggering the release of zinc ions from the cysteine-rich zinc finger of the regulatory domain. PKC isoforms can also be activated through tyrosine phosphorylation in a manner unrelated to receptor-coupled hydrolysis of inositol phospholipids. The effect of hyperglycemia on PKC tyrosine phosphorylation has not yet been examined.[211,212]

Consequences of Hyperglycemia-Induced Protein Kinase C Activation. In early experimental diabetes, activation of PKC-β isoforms has been shown to mediate retinal and renal blood flow abnormalities,[213] perhaps by depressing NO production and increasing endothelin-1 activity (Fig. 33-14). In the diabetic retina, hyperglycemia persistently activates PKC and p38a MAPK to increase the expression of a previously unknown target of PKC signaling, Src homology-2 domain-containing phosphatase-1 (SHP-1), a protein tyrosine phosphatase. This signaling cascade leads to PDGF receptor-β dephosphorylation and a reduction in downstream signaling from this receptor, resulting in pericyte apoptosis.[214] Abnormal activation of PKC also has been implicated in the decreased glomerular production of NO induced by experimental diabetes[215] and in the decreased smooth muscle cell NO production induced by hyperglycemia.[216] PKC activation also mediates glucose-enhanced extracellular matrix accumulation in rat glomerular mesangial cells.[217] Hyperglycemia increases endothelin 1–stimulated MAPK activity in glomerular mesangial cells by activating PKC isoforms.[218] The increased endothelial cell permeability induced by high glucose concentrations in cultured cells is mediated by activation of PKC-α[219] and is independent of the intracellular calcium concentration–NO pathway.[220] Activation of PKC by elevated glucose levels also induces expression of the permeability-enhancing factor VEGF in smooth muscle cells.[221]

In addition to affecting hyperglycemia-induced abnormalities of blood flow and permeability, activation of PKC contributes to increased microvascular matrix protein accumulation by inducing the expression of TGF-β1, fibronectin, and α1 type IV collagen in cultured mesangial cells[217,222] and in glomeruli of diabetic rats.[215] This effect appears to be mediated through PKC's inhibition of NO production.[223] Hyperglycemia-induced expression of laminin C1 in cultured mesangial cells is independent of PKC activation.[224] Hyperglycemia-induced activation of PKC has also been implicated in the overexpression of the fibrinolytic inhibitor PAI-1[225] and in the activation of the pleiotrophic transcription factor NFκB in cultured endothelial cells and VSMC.[226,227] When PKC-β2 is selectively overexpressed in the myocardium of diabetic mice, expression of connective tissue growth factor (CTGF) and TGF-β1 increases, and the mice develop cardiomyopathy and cardiac fibrosis.[228]

In VSMC, activation of PKC by elevated glucose increases p38 MAPK activity and induces expression of the permeability-enhancing factor, VEGF.[222,229] PKC activation also activates various membrane-associated NAD(P)H-dependent oxidases.[230] Ex vivo treatment of human blood vessels from patients with diabetes and coronary artery disease (CAD) with a PKC inhibitor reduced diabetes-induced vascular superoxide production by NAD(P)H oxidases and superoxide-induced uncoupling of eNOS.[231] In normal subjects, the reduction in endothelium-dependent vasodilation induced by acute hyperglycemia is normalized by inhibition of PKC-β, consistent with prevention of hyperglycemia-induced eNOS uncoupling.[232]

Increased Hexosamine Pathway Flux

A fourth hypothesis about how hyperglycemia causes diabetic complications[233-236] states that glucose is shunted into the hexosamine pathway (Fig. 33-15). In this pathway,

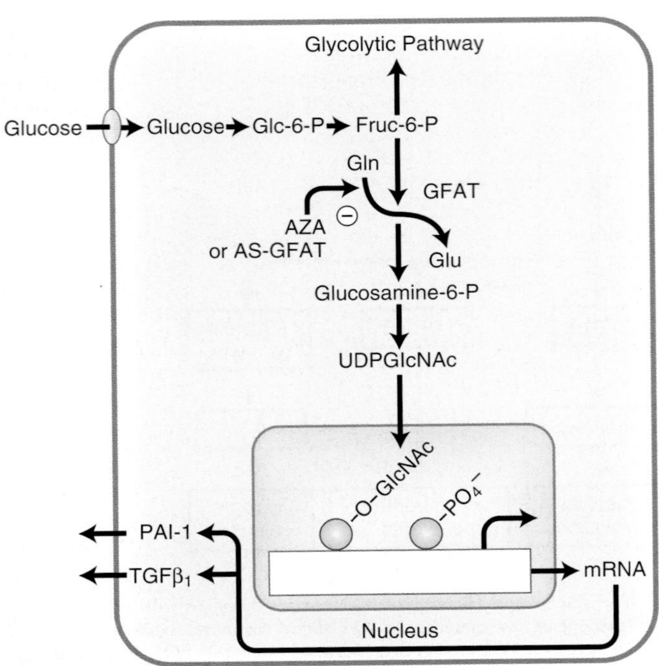

Figure 33-15 Schematic representation of the hexosamine pathway. The glycolytic intermediate, fructose-6-phosphate (Fruc-6-P), is converted to glucosamine-6-phosphate (Glc-6-P) by the enzyme glutamine: fructose 6-phosphate amidotransferase (GFAT). Increased donation of *N*-acetylglucosamine moieties to serine and threonine residues of transcription factors such as Sp1 increases production of such complication-promoting factors as plasminogen activator inhibitor 1 (PAI-1) and transforming growth factor-β1 (TGF-β_1). AS-GFAT, antisense to GFAT; AZA, azaserine; GlcNAc, *N*-acetylglucosamine; mRNA, messenger RNA; UDP, uridine diphosphate. (Adapted from Du XL, Edelstein D, Rossetti L, et al. Hyperglycemia-induced mitochondrial superoxide overproduction activates the hexosamine pathway and induces plasminogen activator inhibitor-1 expression by increasing Sp1 glycosylation. *Proc Natl Acad Sci U S A.* 2000;97:12222-12226.)

fructose-6-phosphate is diverted from glycolysis to provide substrates for reactions that require uridine diphosphate-*N*-acetylglucosamine (UDP-GlcNAc), such as proteoglycan synthesis and the formation of *O*-linked glycoproteins. Inhibition of glutamine:fructose-6-phosphate amidotransferase (GFAT), the rate-limiting enzyme in the conversion of glucose to glucosamine, blocks hyperglycemia-induced increases in the transcription of both TGF-α1[233] and TGF-β1.[234] This pathway has previously been shown to play an important role in hyperglycemia-induced and fat-induced insulin resistance[237-239] by impairing activation of the insulin resistance/insulin resistance syndrome (IRS)/PI3K/Akt pathway.[240]

The mechanism by which increased flux through the hexosamine pathway mediates hyperglycemia-induced increases in gene transcription has not been clear, but the observation that Sp1 sites regulate hyperglycemia-induced activation of the PAI-1 promoter in VSMC[241] suggested that covalent modification of Sp1 by GlcNAc might explain the link between hexosamine pathway activation and hyperglycemia-induced changes in gene transcription. Glucosamine itself subsequently was shown to activate the PAI-1 promoter through Sp1 sites in glomerular mesangial cells.[242] Hyperglycemia has been shown to induce a 2.4-fold increase in hexosamine pathway activity in aortic endothelial cells, resulting in a 1.7-fold increase in Sp1 *O*-linked GlcNAc and a 70% to 80% decrease in Sp1 *O*-linked phosphothreonine and phosphoserine.[79] Concomitantly, hyperglycemia increased expression from an 85-base-pair truncated PAI-1 promoter luciferase reporter containing two Sp1 sites by 3.8-fold but failed to increase expression when the two Sp1 sites were mutated.[79] In endothelial cells, signal transduction by the hexosamine pathway requires PKC-β1 and PKC-δ activation for regulation of the PAI-1 promoter.[243] GlcNAc modification of Sp1 also regulates glucose-responsive expression of the prosclerotic growth factor TGF-β1.

Because virtually every RNA polymerase II transcription factor examined has been found to be *O*-GlcNAcylated,[244] it is possible that reciprocal modification by *O*-GlcNAcylation and phosphorylation of transcription factors other than Sp1 function as a more generalized mechanism for regulating glucose-responsive gene transcription. In addition to transcription factors, many other nuclear and cytoplasmic proteins are dynamically modified by *O*-GlcNAc moieties and might exhibit reciprocal modification by phosphorylation in a manner analogous to Sp1.[192] One example relevant to diabetic complications is the inhibition of eNOS activity by hyperglycemia-induced *O*-GlcNAcylation at the Akt site of the eNOS protein.[80,244] Hyperglycemia-induced activation of the hexosamine pathway increases activation of MMP2 and MMP9 in human coronary artery endothelial cells, and in carotid plaques from patients with T2DM, *O*-GlcNAcylation of endothelial cell proteins is significantly increased.[240]

Hyperglycemia increases GFAT activity in aortic smooth muscle cells, and biochemical analyses show that hyperglycemia qualitatively and quantitatively alters the glycosylation or expression of many *O*-GlcNAc–modified proteins in the nucleus of these cells.[245] Therefore, activation of the hexosamine pathway by hyperglycemia can result in many changes in gene expression and in protein function that together contribute to the pathogenesis of diabetic complications. In addition, it has been shown that *O*-GlcNAc transferase (OGT) harbors a type of phosphoinositide-binding domain. After induction with insulin, phosphatidylinositol 3,4,5-triphosphate recruits OGT from the nucleus to the plasma membrane, where the enzyme catalyzes modification of the insulin signaling pathway by *O*-GlcNAc, leading to attenuation of insulin signal transduction. Hepatic overexpression of OGT reduces the expression of insulin-responsive genes and causes insulin resistance and dyslipidaemia.[246] A similar mechanism could explain pathway-selective insulin resistance in vascular endothelial cells.

Different Hyperglycemia-Induced Pathogenic Mechanisms Reflect a Single Process

Although specific inhibitors of aldose reductase activity, AGE formation, and PKC activation ameliorate various diabetes-induced abnormalities in animal models, there has been no apparent common element linking the four mechanisms of hyperglycemia-induced damage discussed in the preceding section.[113,215,247-249] It has also been conceptually difficult to explain the phenomenon of hyperglycemic memory (discussed earlier) as a consequence of four processes that quickly normalize when euglycemia is restored. These issues have now been resolved by the discovery that each of the four different pathogenic mechanisms reflects a single hyperglycemia-induced process: overproduction of superoxide by the mitochondrial electron transport chain.[79,250,251]

Hyperglycemia increases ROS production inside cultured bovine aortic endothelial cells. To understand how this occurs, a brief overview of glucose metabolism is helpful. Intracellular glucose oxidation begins with glycolysis in the cytoplasm, which generates NADH and pyruvate. Cytoplasmic NADH can donate reducing equivalents to the mitochondrial electron transport chain via two shuttle systems, or it can reduce pyruvate to lactate, which exits the cell to provide substrate for hepatic gluconeogenesis. Pyruvate can also be transported into the mitochondria, where it is oxidized by the tricarboxylic acid (TCA) cycle to produce CO_2, H_2O, four molecules of NADH, and one molecule of reduced flavin adenine dinucleotide ($FADH_2$). Mitochondrial NADH and $FADH_2$ provide energy for ATP production via oxidative phosphorylation by the electron transport chain.

Electron flow through the mitochondrial electron transport chain is carried out by four inner membrane–associated enzyme complexes, plus cytochrome *c* and the mobile carrier, ubiquinone.[252] NADH derived from cytosolic glucose oxidation and mitochondrial TCA cycle activity donates electrons to NADH:ubiquinone oxidoreductase *(complex I)*. Complex I ultimately transfers its electrons to ubiquinone. Ubiquinone can also be reduced by electrons donated from several $FADH_2$-containing dehydrogenases, including succinate:ubiquinone oxidoreductase *(complex II)* and glycerol-3-phosphate dehydrogenase. Electrons from reduced ubiquinone are then transferred to ubiquinol:cytochrome-*c* oxidoreductase *(complex III)* by the ubisemiquinone radical-generating Q cycle.[253] Electron transport then proceeds through cytochrome *c*, cytochrome-*c* oxidase *(complex IV)*, and, finally, molecular oxygen.

Electron transfer through complexes I, III, and IV generates a proton gradient that drives ATP synthase *(complex V)*. When the electrochemical potential difference generated by this proton gradient is high, the life of superoxide-generating electron transport intermediates such as ubisemiquinone is prolonged. There appears to be a threshold value above which superoxide production is markedly increased (Fig. 33-16).[254]

Investigators using inhibitors of both the shuttle that transfers cytosolic NADH into mitochondria and the transporter that transfers cytosolic pyruvate into the mitochondria showed that the TCA cycle is the source of hyperglycemia-induced ROS in endothelial cells. Overexpression of uncoupling protein 1 (UCP-1), a specific protein uncoupler of oxidative phosphorylation capable of collapsing the proton electrochemical gradient,[255] also prevented the effect of hyperglycemia. These results demonstrated that hyperglycemia-induced intracellular ROS are produced by the proton electrochemical gradient generated by the mitochondrial electron transport chain. Overexpression of manganese superoxide dismutase (Mn-SOD), the mitochondrial form of this antioxidant enzyme,[256] prevents the effect of hyperglycemia. Prevention of mitochondrial superoxide production also completely prevents activation of the polyol pathway, AGE formation, PKC, and the hexosamine pathway (Fig. 33-17). In endothelial cells, PKC activates NFκB, a transcription factor that itself activates many proinflammatory genes in the vasculature. As expected, hyperglycemia-induced NFκB activation is also prevented by UCP-1 or Mn-SOD in cells and in animals.

In addition, diabetes-induced loss of vascular cyclic adenosine monophosphate (cAMP)-responsive element–binding protein (CREB) and enhanced expression of PDGFR-α in nonobese diabetic (NOD) mice are both reversed by treatment with an SOD mimetic,[257] and hyperglycemia-mediated interference with neuronal CREB and bcl-2 expression can be restored by treatment of the neurons in vitro with an SOD mimetic.[258]

Therefore, hyperglycemia-induced mitochondrial production of ROS is both necessary and sufficient for activation of each of these pathways.

After hyperglycemia induces mitochondrial ROS production, these ROS can activate a number of other superoxide production pathways that may amplify the original damaging effect of hyperglycemia (M. Brownlee, unpublished observations).

How does hyperglycemia-induced ROS activate AGE formation, PKC, the hexosamine pathway, and the polyol pathway? It does this by inhibiting activity of the key glycolytic enzyme, glyceraldehyde-3-phosphate dehydrogenase (GAPDH) (Fig. 33-18). When GAPDH activity is inhibited, the levels of all the glycolytic intermediates that are upstream of GAPDH increase. An increased level of the upstream glycolytic metabolite glyceraldehyde-3

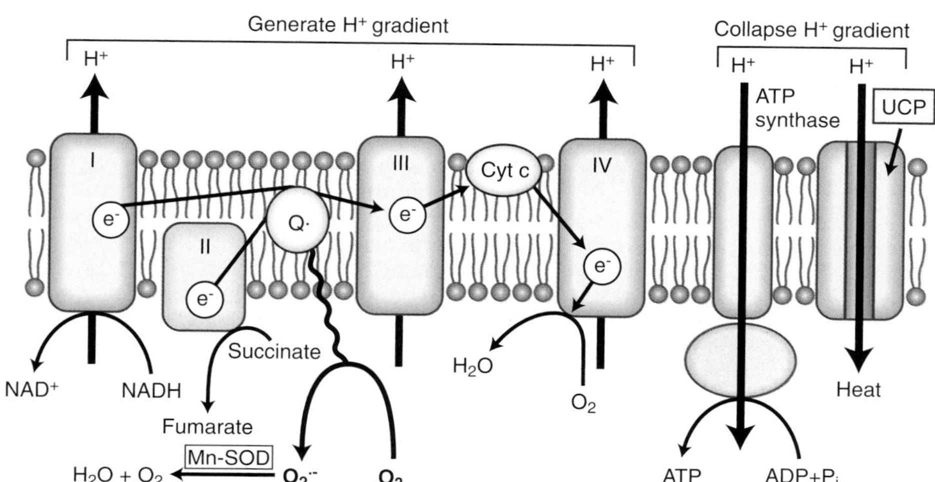

Figure 33-16 Production of superoxide by the mitochondrial electron transport chain. Increased hyperglycemia-derived electron donors from the tricarboxylic acid cycle (NADH and $FADH_2$) generate a high mitochondrial membrane potential ($\Delta\mu$ H^+) by pumping protons across the mitochondrial inner membrane. This inhibits electron transport at complex III and increases the half-life of free radical intermediates of coenzyme Q, which reduce O_2 to superoxide. ADP, adenosine diphosphate; ATP, adenosine triphosphate; Mn-SOD, manganese superoxide dismutase; NAD^+, nicotinamide adenine dinucleotide; NADH, reduced nicotinamide adenine dinucleotide; Pi, inorganic phosphate; UCP, uncoupling protein. (From Boss O, Hagen T, Lowell BB. Uncoupling proteins 2 and 3: potential regulators of mitochondrial energy metabolism. *Diabetes.* 2000;49:143-156.)

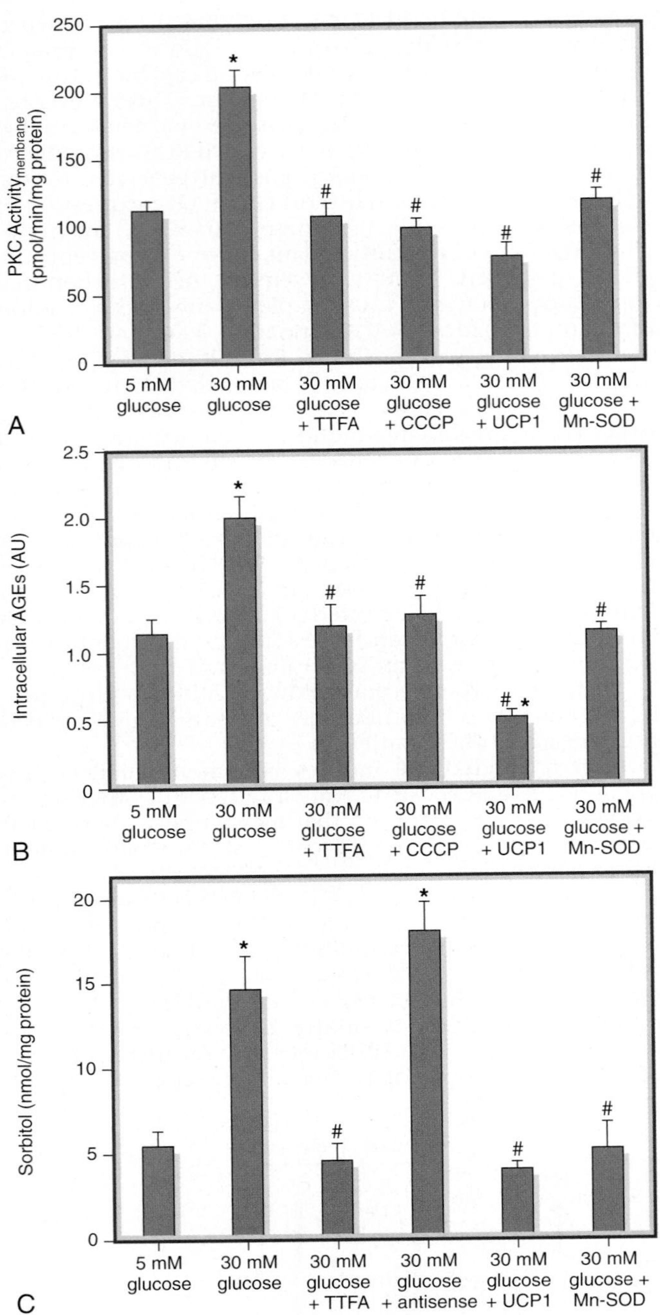

Figure 33-17 Effect of agents that alter mitochondrial electron transport chain function on the three main pathways of hyperglycemic damage. **A,** Hyperglycemia-induced protein kinase C (PKC) activation. **B,** Intracellular advanced glycation end-product (AGE) formation. **C,** Sorbitol accumulation. Cells were incubated in 5-mmol/L glucose, 30-mmol/L glucose alone, and 30-mmol/L glucose plus either agents that uncouple oxidative phosphorylation and reduce the high mitochondrial membrane potential (TTFA, CCCP, UCP-1) or manganese dismutase superoxide (Mn-SOD). CCCP, carbonyl cyanide *m*-chlorophenylhydrazone; TTFA, thenoyltrifluoroacetone; UCP-1, uncoupling protein 1. (From Nishikawa T, Edelstein D, Du XL, et al. Normalizing mitochondrial superoxide production blocks three pathways of hyperglycaemic damage. *Nature.* 2000;404:787-790.)

phosphate activates two of the four pathways, because the major intracellular AGE precursor, methylglyoxal, and the activator of PKC, DAG, are both formed from glyceraldehyde-3 phosphate. Farther upstream, levels of the glycolytic metabolite fructose-6-phosphate increase, which increases flux through the hexosamine pathway, in which fructose-6 phosphate is converted by the enzyme GFAT to UDP-GlcNAc. Finally, inhibition of GAPDH increases intracellular levels of the first glycolytic metabolite, glucose. This increases flux through the polyol pathway, where the enzyme aldose reductase reduces it, consuming NADPH in the process. Therefore, inhibition of GAPDH using DNA antisense activates each of the four pathways, to the same extent as diabetes, when glucose concentrations are physiologic.[259]

Hyperglycemia-induced mitochondrial superoxide itself can directly inactivate GAPDH, but only at concentrations that far exceed levels found in hyperglycemic cells. In vivo, hyperglycemia-induced superoxide inhibits GAPDH activity by modifying the enzyme with polymers of adenosine diphosphate (ADP)-ribose.[260] Inhibition of mitochondrial superoxide production with UCP-1 or Mn-SOD prevents both modification of GAPDH by ADP-ribose and reduction of its activity by hyperglycemia. Most importantly, both the modifications of GAPDH by ADP-ribose and the reduction of its activity by hyperglycemia are prevented by a specific inhibitor of the enzyme poly(ADP-ribose) polymerase (PARP). PARP is a nuclear DNA-repair enzyme that is activated by DNA strand breaks. Increased intracellular glucose generates increased ROS in the mitochondria, and these free radicals cause DNA strand breaks, thereby activating PARP (Fig. 33-19). Once activated, PARP splits the NAD+ molecule into its two component parts: nicotinic acid and ADP-ribose. PARP then generates polymers of ADP-ribose, which accumulate on GAPDH and other nuclear proteins. Although GAPDH is commonly thought to reside exclusively in the cytosol, it normally shuttles in and out of the nucleus, where it plays a critical role in DNA repair.[261,262]

A schematic summary showing the elements of the unified mechanism of hyperglycemia-induced cellular damage is shown in Figure 33-20. When intracellular hyperglycemia develops in target cells of diabetic complications, it causes increased mitochondrial production of ROS. The ROS causes strand breaks in nuclear DNA, which activates PARP. PARP then modifies GAPDH, reducing its activity. Decreased GAPDH activity activates the polyol pathway, increases intracellular AGE formation, activates PKC and subsequently NFκB, and activates hexosamine pathway flux.

In cultured glomerular mesangial cells, overexpression of Mn-SOD suppresses the increase in collagen synthesis induced by high glucose.[262] In dorsal root ganglion (DRG) neurons from both wild-type and Mn-SOD$^{+/-}$ mice, overexpression of Mn-SOD decreases hyperglycemia-induced programmed cell death, and in embryonic rat DRG neurons, overexpression of UCP-1 inhibits cleavage of programmed cell death effector caspases.[263] In aortic endothelial cells, overexpression of UCP-1 or Mn-SOD completely blocks hyperglycemia-induced monocyte adhesion to endothelial cells (J.L. Nadler and C.C. Hedrick, personal communication). Overexpression of UCP-1 or Mn-SOD also prevents hyperglycemia-induced inhibition of the antiatherogenic enzyme, prostacyclin synthase (M. Brownlee, et al., unpublished observation). In diabetes, inhibition of prostacyclin synthase causes accumulation of the precursor (PGI_2), which activates thromboxane receptors that trigger vasoconstriction, platelet aggregation, increased expression of leukocyte adhesion molecules, and apoptosis.[264]

Overexpression of Mn-SOD or UCP-1 also prevents inhibition of eNOS activity by hyperglycemia.[80] In platelets, chemical uncouplers or SOD mimetics prevent potentiation by hyperglycemia of collagen-induced platelet

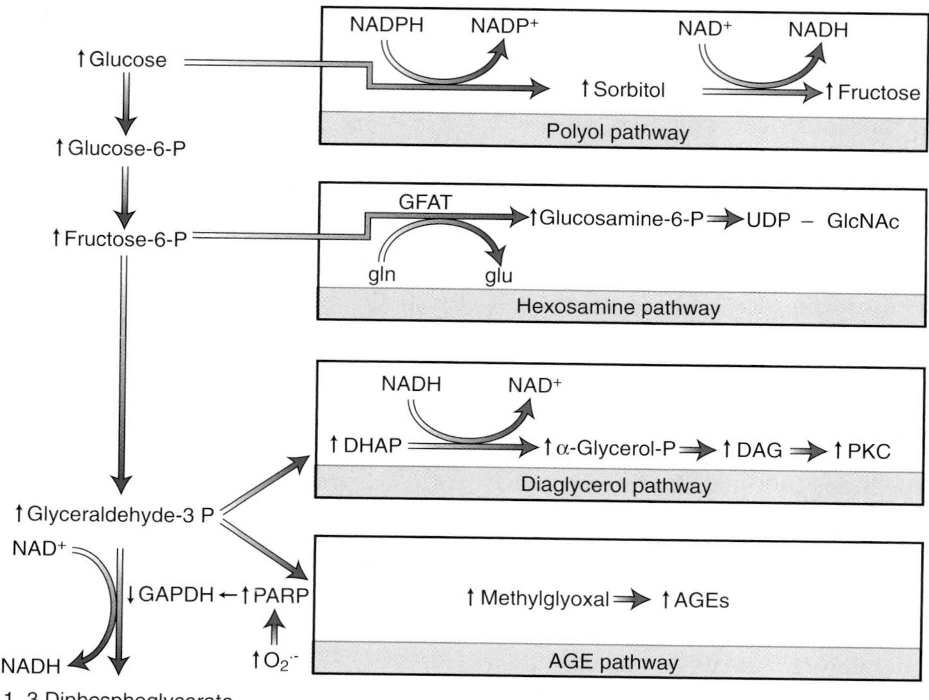

Figure 33-18 Potential mechanism by which hyperglycemia-induced mitochondrial superoxide overproduction activates four pathways of hyperglycemic damage. Excess superoxide partially inhibits the glycolytic enzyme glyceraldehyde-3-phosphate dehydrogenase (GAPDH) by activating PARP and causing ADP-ribosylation of GAPDH. Decreased GAPDH activity increases the concentrations of upstream metabolites and diverts them from glycolysis into pathways of glucose overutilization. This results in increased flux of triose phosphate to diacylglycerol (DAG), an activator of protein kinase C (PKC), and to methylglyoxal, the major intracellular advanced glycation end-product (AGE) precursor. Increased flux of fructose-6-phosphate to uridine diphosphate (UDP)-*N*-acetylglucosamine increases modification of proteins by hexosamine, and increased glucose flux through the polyol pathway consumes NADPH and depletes reduced glutathione (GSH). ADP, adenosine diphosphate; DHAP, dihydroxyacetone phosphate; GFAT, glutamine:fructose-6-phosphate amidotransferase; GlcNAc, -*N*-acetylglucosamine; NAD^+, nicotinamide adenine dinucleotide; NADH, reduced nicotinamide adenine dinucleotide; P, phosphate; PARP, poly(ADP-ribose) polymerase; NADPH, nicotinamide adenine dinucleotide phosphate.

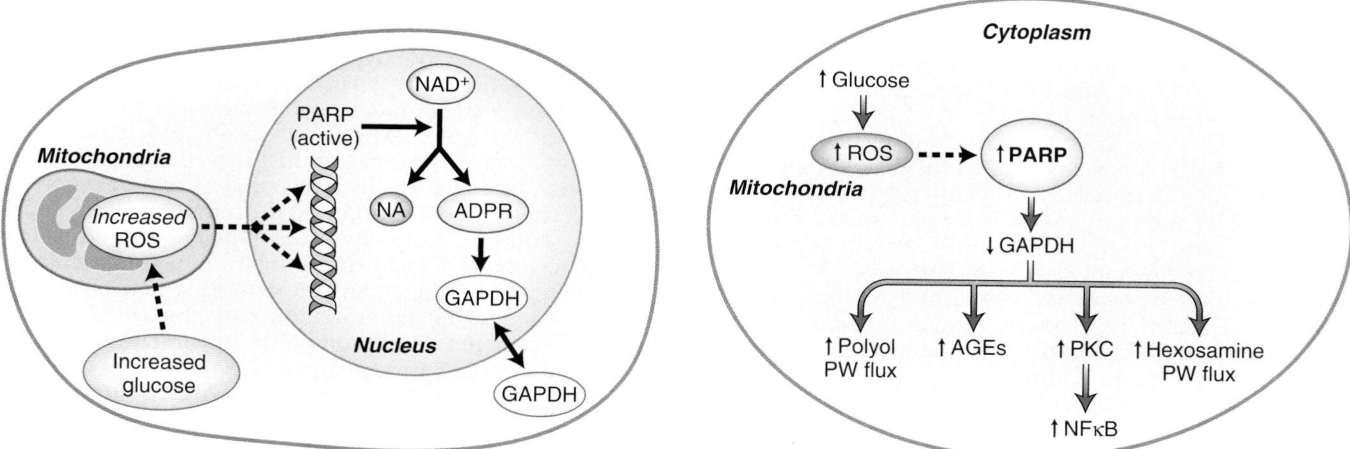

Figure 33-19 Schematic representation of the mechanism by which hyperglycemia-induced mitochondrial superoxide overproduction activates PARP and modifies GAPDH. Hyperglycemia-induced mitochondrial superoxide overproduction causes DNA strand breaks, thereby activating the nuclear DNA-repair enzyme, poly(ADP-ribose) polymerase (PARP). Activated PARP splits the NAD+ molecule into its two component parts: nicotinic acid (NA) and adenosine diphosphate–ribose (ADPR). PARP then generates polymers of ADP-ribose, which accumulate on glyceraldehyde-3-phosphate dehydrogenase, GAPDH, inactivating the enzyme. ROS, reactive oxygen species. (Adapted from Brownlee M. Banting Lecture 2004. The pathobiology of diabetic complications: a unifying mechanism. *Diabetes.* 2005;54:1615-1625.)

Figure 33-20 Unifying mechanism of hyperglycemia-induced cellular damage. Intracellular hyperglycemia causes increased mitochondrial production of reactive oxygen species (ROS). The ROS cause strand breaks in nuclear DNA, which activates poly(ADP-ribose) polymerase (PARP). PARP then modifies glyceraldehyde-3-phosphate dehydrogenase (GAPDH), thereby reducing its activity. Decreased GAPDH activity activates the polyol pathway, increases intracellular formation of advanced glycation end products (AGE), activates protein kinase C (PKC) and subsequently nuclear factor-κB (NFκB), and activates hexosamine pathway (PW) flux. (Adapted from Brownlee M. Banting Lecture 2004. The pathobiology of diabetic complications: a unifying mechanism. *Diabetes.* 2005;54:1615-1625.)

activation and aggregation.[81] Antioxidant treatment prevents hyperglycemia-induced activity of MMP9 in VSMC.[265]

In streptozotocin-diabetic transgenic mice overexpressing human cytoplasmic Cu^{2+}/Zn^{2+}-SOD, albuminuria, glomerular hypertrophy, and glomerular content of TGF-β and α1 type IV collagen were all attenuated compared with wild-type littermates after 4 months of diabetes.[266] Overexpression of the human *SOD1* transgene in db/db diabetic mice similarly normalized the extensive expansion of the glomerular mesangial matrix that was otherwise evident by age 5 months in the nontransgenic db/db littermates.[267] Similarly, transgenic overexpression of the antioxidant enzymes Mn-SOD and catalase reduced ROS and prevented diabetes-induced abnormalities in cardiac contractility in an animal model of diabetic cardiomyopathy.[268,269] In humans, skin fibroblast gene expression profiles from two groups of T1DM patients—20 with very fast (fast-track) and 20 with very slow (slow-track) rates of development of diabetic nephropathy lesions—showed that the fast-track group has increased expression of oxidative phosphorylation genes, mitochondrial electron transport system complex III, and TCA-cycle genes. These associations are consistent with a central role for mitochondrial ROS production in the pathogenesis of diabetic nephropathy.[270]

Human atherosclerotic samples obtained during vascular surgery show greater mitochondrial DNA damage than nonatherosclerotic samples obtained from age-matched transplant donors, consistent with increased ROS production. Mitochondrial damage precedes the development of atherosclerosis and tracks with lesion extent in apoE-null mice, and mitochondrial dysfunction caused by heterozygous deficiency of superoxide dismutase (SOD2) increases atherosclerosis and vascular mitochondrial damage in the same model.[271-273]

Free Fatty Acid–Induced Proatherogenic Changes Are Also Caused by Mitochondrial Production of Reactive Oxygen Species

Insulin resistance causes increased FFA release from adipocytes. In macrovascular, but not microvascular, endothelial cells, the increased flux of FFA results in increased FFA oxidation by the mitochondria. Because both oxidation of fatty acids and oxidation of FFA-derived acetyl coenzyme A by the TCA cycle generate the same electron donors (NADH and $FADH_2$) as are generated by glucose oxidation, increased FFA oxidation causes mitochondrial overproduction of ROS by the same mechanism described for hyperglycemia. As with hyperglycemia, this FFA-induced increase in ROS activates the same damaging pathways: AGEs, PKC, the hexosamine pathway (GlcNAc), and NFκB. Together, they activate a variety of proinflammatory signals previously implicated in hyperglycemia-induced vascular damage (Fig. 33-21). In addition, these ROS directly inactivate two important antiatherogenic enzymes, prostacyclin synthase and eNOS, independent of the pathways just discussed. In two insulin-resistant nondiabetic animal models, inhibition of either FFA release from adipocytes or FFA oxidation in arterial endothelium prevents the increased production of ROS and its damaging effects.[93]

Possible Molecular Basis for Hyperglycemic Memory

Continued mitochondrial superoxide production might explain the occurrence of complications during posthyperglycemic normoglycemia. In the retina of diabetic rats with poor glycemic control for 2 months, subsequent normalization of HbA_{1c} for 7 months lowered elevated retinal lipid peroxides by only about 50% and had no beneficial effects on levels of the oxidative marker 3-nitrotyrosine. In the retinas of diabetic animals with poor glycemic control for 6 months, subsequent normalization of HbA_{1c} for 6 months had no effect on elevated retinal oxidative stress levels and only a small effect on elevated levels of 3-nitrotyrosine.[274]

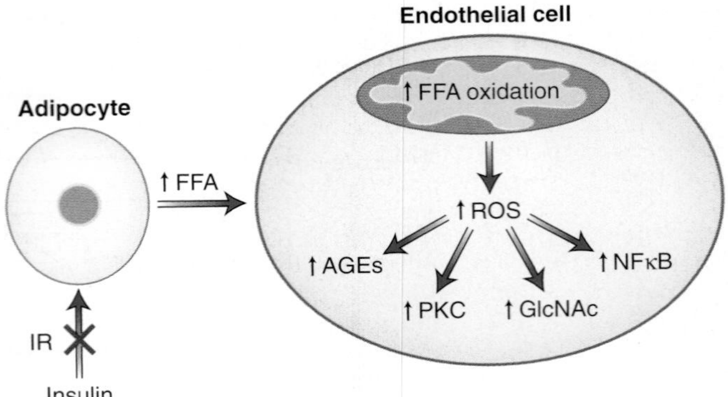

Figure 33-21 Schematic mechanism by which insulin resistance (IR) causes increased oxidation of free fatty acids (FFA) in arterial endothelial cells, which activates proatherogenic signals and inhibits key antiatherogenic enzymes. IR causes increased FFA release from adipocytes. In macrovascular endothelial cells, the increased flux of FFA results in increased FFA oxidation by the mitochondria, thereby causing mitochondrial overproduction of reactive oxygen species (ROS). FFA-induced increase in ROS activates advanced glycation end products (AGEs), protein kinase C (PKC), the hexosamine pathway (GlcNAc), and nuclear factor κB (NFκB), which together activate a variety of proinflammatory signals. In addition, ROS directly inactivate two important antiatherogenic enzymes, prostacyclin synthase and endothelial nitric oxide synthase (eNOS). GlcNAc, -*N*-acetylglucosamine. (Adapted from Du X, Edelstein D, Obici S, et al. Insulin resistance reduces arterial prostacyclin synthase and eNOS activities by increasing endothelial fatty acid oxidation. *J Clin Invest.* 2006;116:1071-1080.)

Although the molecular changes that result in continuous overproduction of ROS in normoglycemic animals and humans have not yet been identified, several hypotheses are being tested. One hypothesis involves induction of stable epigenetic changes such as DNA methylation and histone methylation and acetylation. Such changes can alter levels of gene expression for many years. Posttranslational modifications of histones cause chromatin remodeling and changes in levels of gene expression.[275-277] Because these modifications do not involve differences in DNA sequence, they are called "epigenetic." Transient hyperglycemia, at a level sufficient to increase mitochondrial ROS production, induces long-lasting activating epigenetic changes (increased monomethylation of histone 3 lysine 4) in the proximal promoter of the nuclear factor κB (NFκB) subunit p65 in human aortic endothelial cells (16 hours' exposure) and in aortic cells in vivo in nondiabetic mice (6 hours' exposure). These epigenetic changes cause sustained increases in p65 gene expression and in the expression of p65-dependent proinflammatory genes. Both the epigenetic changes and the gene expression changes persist for at least 6 days of subsequent normal glycemia in cultured cells, and for months in previously diabetic mice whose beta-cell function recovered.[279] Hyperglycemia-induced epigenetic changes and increased p65 expression are prevented by normalizing mitochondrial superoxide production or superoxide-induced methylglyoxal.[279] These results highlight the dramatic and long-lasting effects that short-term hyperglycemic spikes can have on vascular cells and suggest that transient spikes of hyperglycemia may be an HbA_{1c}-independent risk factor for diabetic complications. Demethylation of another histone lysine residue, histone 3 lysine 9, is also induced by hyperglycemia-induced overproduction of ROS. This reduces inhibition of p65 gene expression, and therefore acts synergistically with the activating methylation of histone 3 lysine 4 (Fig. 33-22).[278,279] Consistent with these observations, others have shown similar epigenetic changes in lymphocytes from patients with T1DM[280] and in VSMC derived from db/db mice.[281,282]

Another hypothesis concerns changes in mitochondrial biology. It is now recognized that mitochondria are not all the same but have important functional differences. Furthermore, mitochondria are not static structures in the cell. Rather, they continuously fuse to form larger organelles or pull apart to form smaller organelles. The processes underlying these changes are beginning to be understood, but aberrations induced by diabetes and different degrees of hyperglycemia are important new areas that will likely yield new insights into hyperglycemic memory.[283]

The third hypothesis currently being evaluated is altered regulation of the antioxidant response element. Perhaps not surprisingly, cells have their own protective antioxidant machinery.[283a] Cells responded to oxidative stress by activating a previously sequestered transcription factor (Nrf2) that controls the expression of a diverse set of genes involved in decreasing ROS in the cell. An important research focus is the identification and regulation of proteins in this pathway, including proteins that bind to a special promoter element called the antioxidant response element (ARE) after activation by ROS.

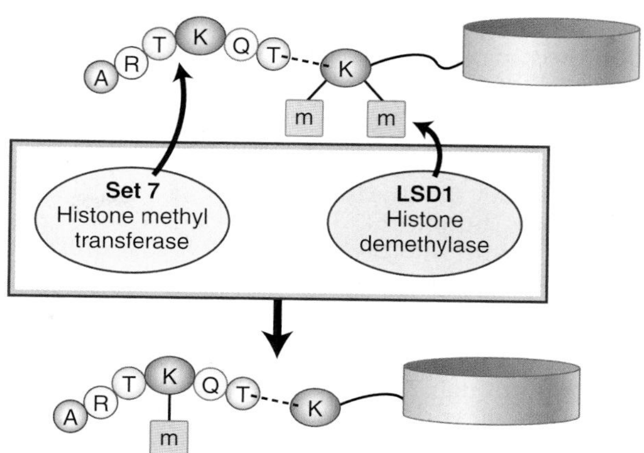

Figure 33-22 Hyperglycemia-induced activating modifications of histone 3 lysine 4 (monomethylation) and derepressing modifications of histone 3 lysine 9 (removal of two methyl groups) at the NFκB p65 proximal promoter. (From Brasacchio D, Okabe J, Tikellis C, et al. Hyperglycemia induces a dynamic cooperativity of histone methylase and demethylase enzymes associated with gene-activating epigenetic marks that co-exist on the lysine tali. *Diabetes.* 2009;58:1229-1236 and El-Osta A, Brasacchio D, Yao D, et al. Transient high glucose causes persistent epigenetic changes and altered gene expression during subsequent normoglycemia. *J Exp Med.* 2008;205:2409-2417.)

RETINOPATHY, MACULAR EDEMA, AND OTHER COMPLICATIONS*

Diabetic retinopathy is a well-characterized, sight-threatening, chronic microvascular complication that eventually afflicts virtually all patients with diabetes mellitus.[64] Diabetic retinopathy is characterized by gradually progressive alterations in the retinal microvasculature that lead to areas of retinal nonperfusion, increased vascular permeability, and pathologic intraocular proliferation of retinal vessels. The complications associated with the increased vascular permeability, termed *macular edema,* and uncontrolled neovascularization, termed *proliferative diabetic retinopathy* (PDR), can result in severe and permanent vision loss.

Despite decades of research, there is currently no known means of preventing diabetic retinopathy, and, despite effective therapies, diabetic retinopathy remains the leading cause of new-onset blindness among working-aged persons in most developed countries of the world.[64] With appropriate medical and ophthalmologic care, however, more than 90% of vision loss resulting from PDR can be prevented. Therefore, until a cure for diabetes is discovered, the primary clinical care emphasis for the prevention of vision loss is appropriately directed at early identification, accurate classification, and timely treatment of retinopathy.

Nevertheless, increased understanding of the mechanistic pathways underlying hyperglycemia-induced retinal changes has provided new targets against which novel therapies have been devised. These novel therapies, such as VEGF inhibitors, corticosteroids, and PKC-β inhibitors,[285-293] have entered clinical trials with promising results and have expanded the therapeutic options for patients with diabetic eye disease. Furthermore, selected systemic medications such as ACE inhibitors and angiotensin II receptor blockers (ARBs) may affect the development and progression of diabetic retinopathy. These developments place further emphasis on the importance of adhering to lifelong routine ophthalmologic follow-up of the diabetic patient and optimization of associated systemic disorders.

Epidemiology and Impact

It is estimated that 489 million persons worldwide will have diabetes by the year 2030.[294] Almost 24 million Americans currently have diabetes mellitus, and, of these, more than 5 million remain unaware that they have the disease.[295] For the past 20 years, diabetic retinopathy has remained the leading cause of new cases of legal blindness among Americans between the ages of 20 and 74 years.[296] There is a higher risk of more frequent and severe ocular complications in T1DM, compared with T2DM.[297] Approximately 25% of patients with T1DM have retinopathy after 5 years, and this figure increases to 60% and 80% after 10 and 15 years, respectively. Because T2DM accounts for 90% to 95% of the diabetic population in the United States, it accounts for a higher fraction of patients with vision loss. The most threatening form of retinopathy (PDR) is present in approximately 67% of T1DM patients who have had diabetes for 35 years.[298]

An estimated 700,000 persons in the United States have PDR; 130,000 have high-risk PDR, 500,000 have macular edema, and 325,000 have *clinically significant macular*

*Portions of this section draw on the following sources, among others: Aiello LM, Cavallerano JD, Aiello LP. Diagnosis, management, and treatment of nonproliferative diabetic retinopathy and diabetic macular edema. In: Albert DM, Jokobiec FA, eds. *Principles and Practice of Ophthalmology,* 2nd ed. Philadelphia, PA: WB Saunders, 2000:1900-1914; Aiello LP, Cavallerano J, Klein R. Diabetic eye disease. In: DeGroot LJ, James JL, eds. *Endocrinology,* 5th ed. Philadelphia, PA: WB Saunders, 2005:1305-1317; Aiello LP, Gardner TW, King GL, et al. Diabetic retinopathy: technical review. American Diabetes Association. *Diabetes Care.* 1998;21:143-156; and Aiello LP, Cavallerano J. Diabetic retinopathy. In: Johnstone MT, Veves A, eds. *Contemporary Cardiology: Diabetes and Cardiovascular Disease.* Totowa, NJ: Humana Press, 2001:385-398.

edema (CSME).[299-303] An estimated 63,000 cases of PDR, 29,000 cases of high-risk PDR, 80,000 cases of macular edema, 56,000 cases of CSME, and 12,000 to 24,000 new cases of legal blindness occur each year as a result of diabetic retinopathy.[299,300,304] Blindness has been estimated to be 25 times more common in persons with diabetes than in those without the disease.[305,306]

The DCCT showed that both the rate of development of any retinopathy and the rate of retinopathy progression once it was present were significantly reduced after 3 years of intensive insulin therapy.[307] The effect of reducing the HbA_{1c} in this group from 9.1% with conventional treatment to 7.3% with intensive treatment resulted in a benefit maintained through 7 years of follow-up, even though the difference in mean HbA_{1c} levels of the two randomized treatment groups was only 0.4% at 1 year ($P < .001$), continued to narrow, and became statistically nonsignificant by 5 years (8.1% versus 8.2%, $P = .09$). The further rate of progression of complications from their levels at the end of the DCCT remained less in the former intensive treatment group. Therefore, the benefits of 6.5 years of intensive treatment extended well beyond the period of its most intensive implementation.[27,30,308,309] Applying DCCT intensive insulin therapy to all persons in the United States with T1DM would result in a gain of 920,000 person-years of sight,[310] although the costs of intensive therapy are three times those of conventional therapy.[311]

Pathophysiology

A detailed discussion of the pathophysiologic mechanisms underlying diabetic retinopathy and other diabetes-related complications has been presented earlier in this chapter. The earliest histologic effects of diabetes mellitus in the eye include loss of retinal vascular pericytes (supporting cells for retinal endothelial cells), thickening of vascular endothelium basement membrane, and alterations in retinal blood flow (Fig. 33-23).[25,312-317] With increasing loss of

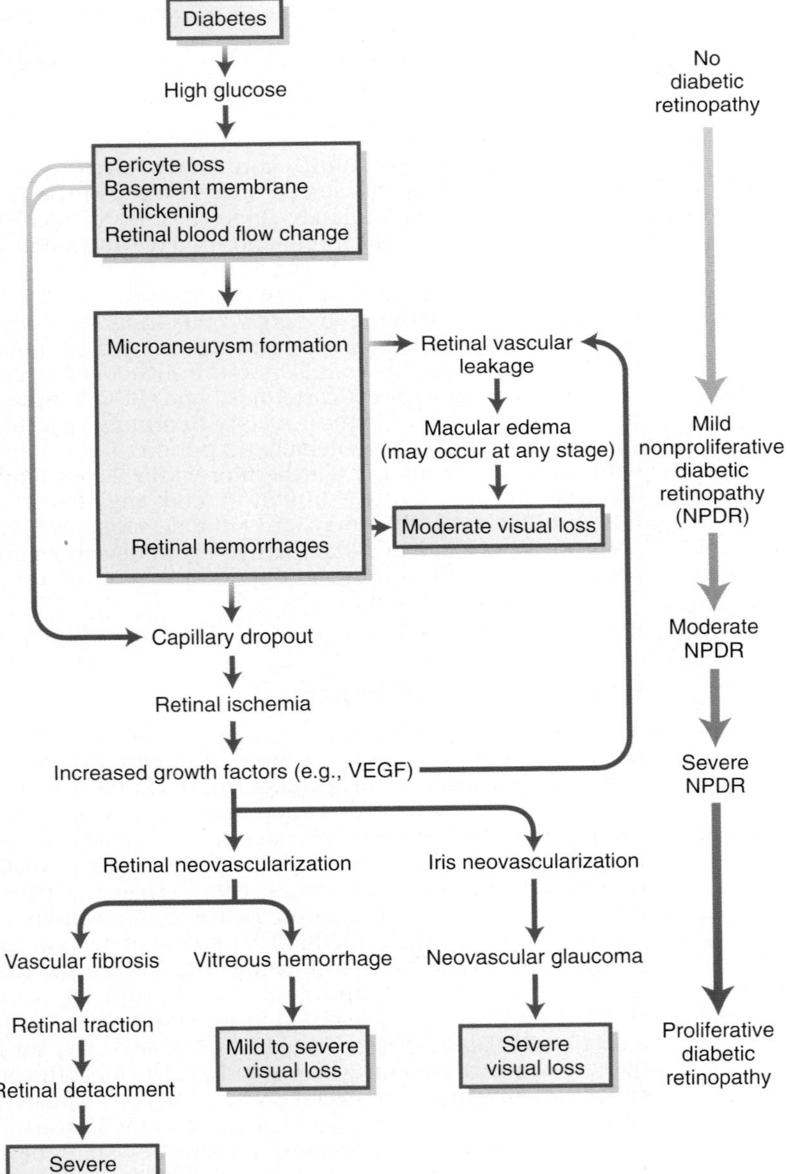

Figure 33-23 Diabetic retinopathy pathogenesis flow chart. The schematic flow chart represents the major preclinical and clinical findings associated with the full spectrum of diabetic retinopathy and macular edema. VEGF, vascular endothelial growth factor.

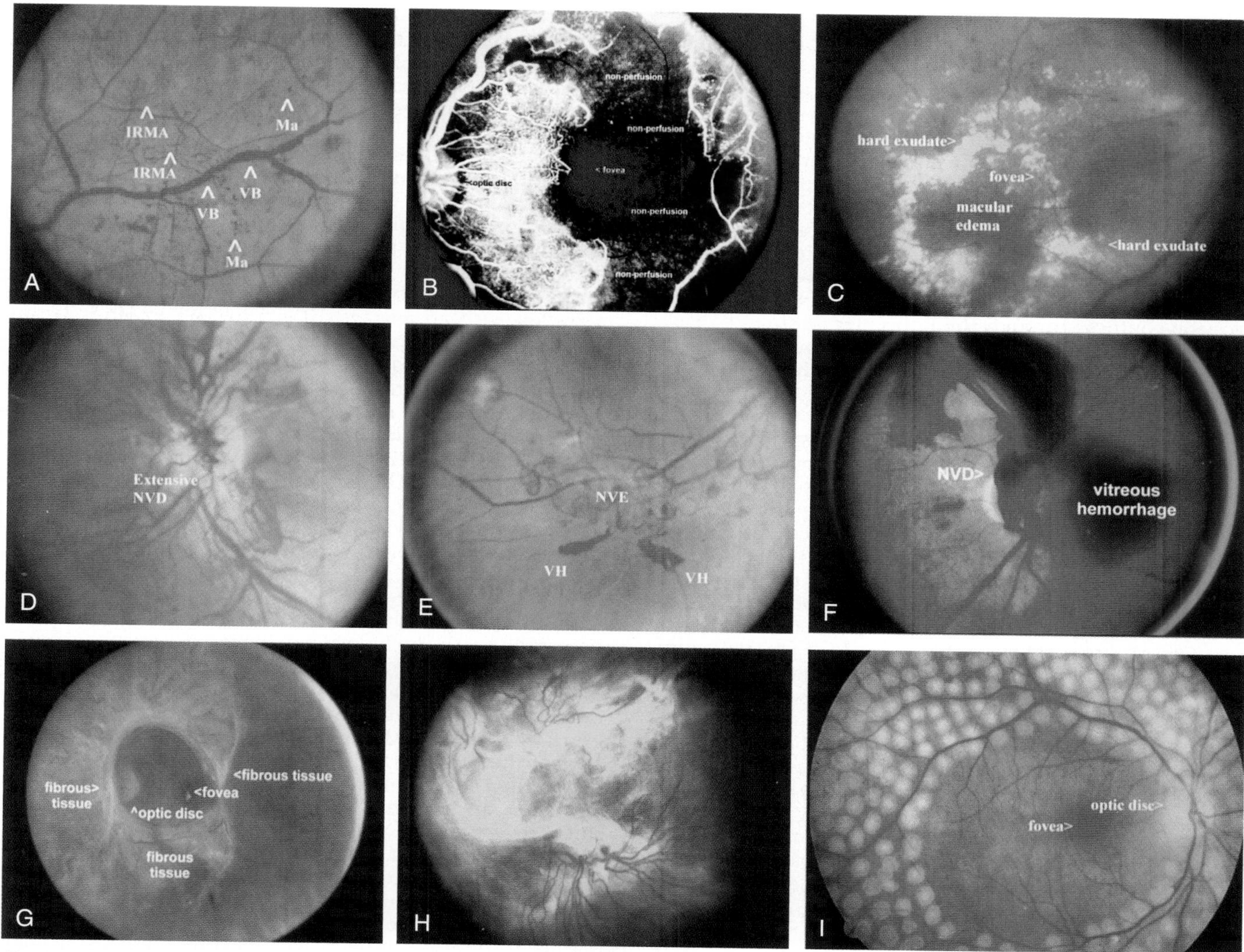

Figure 33-24 Clinical features of diabetic retinopathy: Some typical findings in human diabetic retinopathy. **A,** Findings in severe nonproliferative diabetic retinopathy, including microaneurysms (Ma), venous beading (VB), and intraretinal microvascular abnormalities (IRMA). **B,** Fluorescein angiogram showing marked capillary nonperfusion. **C,** Clinically significant macular edema with retinal thickening and hard exudates involving the fovea. **D,** Extensive neovascularization of the optic disc (NVD), illustrating high-risk proliferative diabetic retinopathy. **E,** Neovascularization elsewhere (NVE) and two small vitreous hemorrhages (VH), also illustrating high-risk proliferative diabetic retinopathy. **F,** Extensive vitreous hemorrhage arising from severe neovascularization of the disc (NVD). **G,** Severe fibrovascular proliferation surrounding the fovea. **H,** Traction retinal detachment from extensive fibrovascular proliferation. **I,** Scars from scatter (panretinal) laser photocoagulation. The macula, fovea, and optic disc are not treated to preserve central vision. Laser burns are evident as white retinal lesions. (Adapted from Aiello LP. Eye complications of diabetes. In Korenman SG, Kahn CR, eds. *Atlas of Clinical Endocrinology. Vol 2: Diabetes.* Philadelphia, PA: Blackwell Scientific, 1999.)

retinal pericytes, the retinal vessel wall develops outpouchings (microaneurysms) and becomes fragile.

Clinically, microaneurysms and small retinal hemorrhages are not always readily distinguishable and are usually evaluated together as "hemorrhages and microaneurysms" (Fig. 33-24A). Rheologic changes occur in diabetic retinopathy as a result of increased platelet aggregation, integrin-mediated leukocyte adhesion, and endothelial damage.[318-320] Disruption of the blood-retina barrier can ensue, characterized by increased vascular permeability.[321,322] The subsequent leakage of blood and serum from the retinal vessels results in retinal hemorrhages, retinal edema, and hard exudates (see Fig. 33-24A and C). Moderate vision loss follows if the fovea is affected by the leakage.[323]

With time, increasing sclerosis and endothelial cell loss lead to narrowing of the retinal vessels, which decreases vascular perfusion and can ultimately lead to obliteration of the capillaries and small vessels (see Fig. 33-24B). The resulting retinal ischemia is a potent inducer of angiogenic growth factors. Several angiogenic growth factors have been isolated from eyes with diabetic retinopathy, including IGFs, basic fibroblast growth factor (bFGF), hepatocyte growth factor (HGF), and VEGF.[324-327] These factors promote the development of new vessel growth and retinal vascular permeability.[328-332] Indeed, inhibition of molecules such as VEGF and their signaling pathways can suppress the development of retinal neovascularization and retinal vascular permeability.[329,333-337] Endogenous inhibitors of angiogenesis and vascular permeability, such as pigment epithelial-derived factor (PEDF), and other VEGF-independent pathways, such as kallikrein and erythropoietin, have also been found in the eye, and these have physiologic and therapeutic potential.[47,338-340]

New vessels tend to grow in regions of strong vitreous adhesion to the retina, such as at the optic disc and major vascular arcades (see Fig. 33-24D and E). The posterior vitreous face also serves as a scaffold for pathologic neovascularization, and the new vessels commonly arise at the junctions between perfused and nonperfused retina. When the retina is severely ischemic, the concentration of angiogenic growth factors can reach sufficient concentration in the anterior chamber to cause abnormal new vessel proliferation on the iris and in the anterior chamber angle.[325,341] Uncontrolled anterior segment neovascularization can result in neovascular glaucoma because the fibrovascular proliferation in the angle of the eye causes blockage of aqueous outflow through the trabecular meshwork.[342]

Proliferating new vessels in diabetic retinopathy are fragile and have a tendency to bleed, which results in preretinal and vitreous hemorrhages (see Fig. 33-24E and F). Although the presence of a large amount of blood in the preretinal space or vitreous cavity per se is not damaging to the retina, these intraocular hemorrhages often cause prolonged vision loss by blocking the visual axis. Membranes on the retinal surface can be induced by blood and result in wrinkling and traction on the retina. Although all retinal neovascularization given sufficient time eventually becomes quiescent, as with most scarring processes there is progressive fibrosis of the new vessel complexes that is associated with contraction. In the eye, such forces can exert traction on the retina, leading to tractional retinal detachment and retinal tears that can result in severe and permanent vision loss if left untreated (see Fig. 33-24G and H).

In short, causes of vision loss from complications of diabetes mellitus include retinal ischemia involving the fovea, macular edema at or near the fovea, preretinal or vitreous hemorrhages, retinal detachment, and neovascular glaucoma. Vision loss can also result from more indirect effects of disease progression in diabetic patients, such as retinal vessel occlusion, accelerated atherosclerotic disease, and embolic phenomena.

Clinical Features

Risk Factors

Duration of diabetes is closely associated with the onset and severity of diabetic retinopathy. Diabetic retinopathy is rare in prepubescent patients with T1DM, but almost all patients with T1DM and more than 60% of patients with T2DM develop some degree of retinopathy after 20 years.[64,298,343] In U.S. reports of patients with T2DM, approximately 20% had retinopathy at the time of diabetes diagnosis,[343] and most had some degree of retinopathy over subsequent decades. In the UKPDS study of T2DM, 35% of female subjects and 39% of male subjects had some level of diabetic retinopathy at the time of diabetes diagnosis.[344]

Diabetic retinopathy is the most common cause of new-onset blindness among American adults aged 20 to 74 years. In the Wisconsin Epidemiologic Study of Diabetic Retinopathy, approximately 4% of patients younger than 30 years of age at diagnosis and almost 2% of patients older than 30 years of age at diagnosis were legally blind. In the younger-onset group, 86% of blindness was attributable to diabetic retinopathy. In the older-onset group, in whom other eye diseases were also common, 33% of the cases of legal blindness were due to diabetic retinopathy.[298,343] Currently, diabetes is thought to account for 12,000 to 24,000 new cases of blindness in the United States each year.[304]

Lack of appropriate glycemic control is another significant risk factor for the onset and progression of diabetic retinopathy. The DCCT demonstrated a clear relationship between hyperglycemia and diabetic microvascular complications, including retinopathy, in 1441 patients with T1DM.[27,28,309,310,345]

In patients monitored for 4 to 9 years, the DCCT showed that intensive insulin therapy reduced or prevented the development of retinopathy by 27%, compared with conventional therapy.[345a] Additionally, intensive insulin therapy reduced the progression of diabetic retinopathy by 34% to 76% and had a substantial beneficial effect over the entire range of retinopathy severity. This improvement was achieved with an average 10% reduction in HbA_{1c}, from 8% to 7.2%. Therefore, although intensive therapy may not prevent retinopathy completely, it reduces the risk of retinopathy onset and progression.

Renal disease, as manifested by microalbuminuria and proteinuria, is yet another significant risk factor for onset and progression of diabetic retinopathy.[346,347] Hypertension is associated with PDR and is an established risk factor for the development of macular edema.[348] Additionally, elevated serum lipid levels are associated with extravasated lipid in the retina (hard exudates) and vision loss.[349]

Clinical Findings

Clinical findings associated with early and progressing diabetic retinopathy include hemorrhages or microaneurysms, cotton-wool spots, hard exudates, intraretinal microvascular abnormalities, and venous caliber abnormalities such as venous loops, venous tortuosity, and venous beading (see Fig. 33-24A and C). Microaneurysms are saccular outpouchings of the capillary walls that can leak fluid and result in intraretinal edema and hemorrhages. The intraretinal hemorrhages can be flame-shaped or dot-blot–like in appearance, reflecting the architecture of the layer of the retina in which they occur. Flame-shaped hemorrhages occur in inner retina closer to the vitreous, and dot-blot hemorrhages occur deeper in the retina. Intraretinal microvascular abnormalities are either new vessel growth within the retinal tissue itself or shunt vessels through areas of poor vascular perfusion. It is common for intraretinal microvascular abnormalities to be located adjacent to cotton-wool spots. Cotton-wool spots are caused by microinfarcts in the nerve fiber layer of the retina. Venous caliber abnormalities are generally a sign of severe retinal hypoxia. In some cases of extensive vascular loss, however, the retina actually appears free of nonproliferative lesions. Such areas are termed *featureless retina* and are a sign of severe retinal hypoxia.

Vision loss from diabetic retinopathy generally results from persistent nonclearing vitreous hemorrhage, traction retinal detachment, or diabetic macular edema (DME) (see Figs. 33-23 and 32-24). Neovascularization with fibrous tissue contraction can distort the retina and lead to traction retinal detachment. The new vessels can bleed, causing preretinal or vitreous hemorrhage. The most common cause of vision loss from diabetes is macular disease and macular edema. Macular edema is more likely to occur in patients with T2DM, who represent 90% to 95% of the diabetic population. In diabetic macular disease, macular edema involving the fovea or nonperfusion of the capillaries in the central macula is responsible for the loss of vision.

Classification Systems

Classification of Diabetic Retinopathy. Diabetic retinopathy is broadly classified into nonproliferative (NPDR) and proliferative (PDR) categories.[350,351] Macular edema

TABLE 33-1

Glossary and Abbreviations Pertinent to Diabetic Eye Disease

Term	Definition
Background diabetic retinopathy (BDR)	An outdated term referring to some stages of NPDR. Because this terminology is not closely associated with disease progression, it has been replaced by the various levels of NPDR.
Clinically significant macular edema (CSME)	Thickening of the retina in the macular region of sufficient extent and location to threaten central visual function
Cotton-wool spot	A gray or white area lesion in the nerve fiber layer of the retina resulting from stasis of axoplasmic flow caused by microinfarcts of the retinal nerve fiber layer
Diabetes Control and Complications Trial (DCCT)	A multicenter, randomized clinical trial designed to address whether intensive insulin therapy could prevent or slow the progression of systemic complications of diabetes mellitus
Diabetic retinopathy (DR)	Retinal pathology related to the underlying systemic disease of diabetes mellitus
Diabetic Retinopathy Study (DRS)	The first multicenter, randomized clinical trial to demonstrate the value of scatter (panretinal) photocoagulation in reducing the risk of vision loss among patients with all levels of diabetic retinopathy
Diabetic Retinopathy Vitrectomy Study (DRVS)	A multicenter clinical trial evaluating early vitrectomy for patients with very advanced diabetic retinopathy or nonresolving vitreous hemorrhage
Early Treatment Diabetic Retinopathy Study (ETDRS)	A multicenter, randomized clinical trial that addressed at what stage of retinopathy scatter (panretinal) photocoagulation was indicated, whether focal photocoagulation was effective for preventing moderate vision loss due to clinically significant macular edema, and whether aspirin therapy altered the progression of diabetic retinopathy
Focal or grid laser photocoagulation	A type of laser treatment whose main goal is to reduce vascular leakage, either by focal treatment of leaking retinal microaneurysms or by application of therapy in a grid-like pattern for patients with clinically significant macular edema
Hard exudate	Lipid accumulation within the retina as a result of increased vasopermeability
High-risk-characteristic proliferative diabetic retinopathy (HRC-PDR)	Proliferative diabetic retinopathy of defined extent, location, and/or clinical findings that is particularly associated with severe vision loss
Microaneurysm	An early vascular abnormality consisting of an outpouching of the retinal microvasculature
Neovascular glaucoma (NVG)	Elevation of intraocular pressure caused by the development of neovascularization in the anterior segment of the eye
Noevascularization at the disc (NVD)	Retinal neovascularization occurring at or within 1500 μm of the optic disc
Neovascularization elsewhere (NVE)	Retinal neovascularization that is located more than 1500 μm away from the optic disc
Neovascularization of the iris (NVI)	Neovascularization occurring on the iris (rubeosis iridis), usually as a result of extensive retinal ischemia
No light perception (NLP)	The inability to perceive light
Nonproliferative diabetic retinopathy (NPDR)	Severities of clinically evident diabetic retinopathy that precede the development of PDR
Preproliferative diabetic retinopathy (PPDR)	An outdated term referring to more advanced levels of NPDR. Because this term is not closely associated with disease progression, it has been replaced by the various levels of NPDR.
Proliferative diabetic retinopathy (PDR)	An advanced level of diabetic retinopathy in which proliferation of new vessels or fibrous tissue occurs on or within the retina
Rubeosis iridis	See NVI

can coexist with either group and is not used in the classification of level of retinopathy. The historical terms *background retinopathy* and *preproliferative diabetic retinopathy* have been replaced to reflect the specific characteristics and risk stratification of the prognostically important subgroups in NPDR (Table 33-1).

Generally, diabetic retinopathy progresses from no retinopathy through mild, moderate, severe, and very severe NPDR and eventually on to PDR. The level of NPDR is determined by the extent and location of clinical manifestations of retinopathy. Mild NPDR is characterized by limited microvascular abnormalities such as hemorrhages or microaneurysms, cotton-wool spots, and increased vascular permeability. Moderate and severe NPDR are characterized by increasing severity of hemorrhages or microaneurysms, venous caliber abnormalities, intraretinal microvascular abnormalities, and vascular closure. The level of NPDR establishes the risk of progression to sight-threatening retinopathy and dictates appropriate clinical management and follow-up.

PDR is characterized by vasoproliferation of the retina and its complications, including new vessels on the optic disc (NVD), new vessels elsewhere on the retina (NVE), preretinal hemorrhage (PRH), vitreous hemorrhage, and fibrous tissue proliferation (FP). On the basis of the extent and location of these lesions, PDR is classified as *early PDR* or *high-risk PDR*. Larger areas of these complications and new vessels that are near the optic disc are associated with greater risks of vision loss.

Classification of Diabetic Macular Edema. DME can be present with any level of diabetic retinopathy. When edema involves or threatens the center of the macula, it is called CSME. CSME exists if there is retinal thickening at or within 500 μm of the fovea; hard exudates with adjacent retinal thickening at or within 500 μm of the fovea; or an area of retinal thickening 1500 μm or more in diameter, any part of which is within 1500 μm of the fovea.[350,352,353] CSME is a clinical diagnosis that is not dependent on visual acuity or results of ancillary testing such as fluorescein angiography, and it can be present even when vision is 20/20 or better.

International Classification of Diabetic Retinopathy. The American Academy of Ophthalmology initiated a project to establish a consensus International Classification of Diabetic Retinopathy and Diabetic Macular Edema in an effort to simplify classification and standardize communication among diabetes health care providers.[354,355] This International Classification describes five clinical

TABLE 33-2

Levels of Diabetic Retinopathy

International Classification Level	ETDRS Level
No apparent retinopathy	Level 10: DR absent
Mild NPDR	Level 20: very mild NPDR
Moderate NPDR	Levels 35, 43, and 47: moderate NPDR
Severe NPDR	Levels 53A-E: severe to very severe NPDR
PDR	Levels 61, 65, 71, 75, 81, 85: PDR, high-risk PDR, very severe or advanced PDR

DR, diabetic retinopathy; ETDRS, Early Treatment Diabetic Retinopathy Study; NPDR, nonproliferative diabetic retinopathy; PDR, proliferative diabetic retinopathy. (From Grading diabetic retinopathy from stereoscopic color fundus photographs—an extension of the modified Airlie House classification. ETDRS report number 10. Early Treatment Diabetic Retinopathy Study Research Group. *Ophthalmology*. 1991;98:786-806.)

levels of diabetic retinopathy: no apparent retinopathy (no abnormalities), mild NPDR (microaneurysms only), moderate NPDR (more than microaneurysms only but less than severe NPDR), severe NPDR (any of the following: more than 20 intraretinal hemorrhages in each of four quadrants, definite venous beading in two or more quadrants, prominent intraretinal microvascular abnormalities in one or more quadrants, and no PDR), and PDR (one or more of the following: retinal neovascularization, vitreous hemorrhage, and preretinal hemorrhage). Table 33-2 compares levels of retinopathy in the international classification to those defined by the landmark Early Treatment Diabetic Retinopathy Study (ETDRS).

In regard to DME, the International Classification identifies two broad categories: macular edema apparently absent (no apparent retinal thickening or hard exudates in the posterior pole) and macular edema apparently present (some apparent retinal thickening or hard exudates in the posterior pole). Macular edema is subclassified as mild (some retinal thickening or hard exudates in the posterior pole but distant from the center of the macula), moderate (retinal thickening or hard exudates approaching the center of the macula but not involving the center), or severe (retinal thickening or hard exudates involving the center of the macula). Table 33-3 compares levels of DME in the international classification to ETDRS levels of DME.

TABLE 33-3

International Classification of Diabetic Macular Edema (DME)

Disease Severity Level	Ophthalmic Findings (Retinal Thickening or Hard Exudates in Posterior Pole)	ETDRS Scale Equivalent
DME apparently absent	None apparent	
DME apparently present	Some apparent	
Mild DME	Some findings present but distant from center of the macula	DME but not CSME
Moderate DME	Findings approaching the center but not involving the center	CSME
Severe DME	Findings involving the center of the macula	CSME

CSME, clinically significant macular edema; ETDRS, Early Treatment Diabetic Retinopathy Study.

Compared with ETDRS retinopathy grading, the International Classification of Diabetic Retinopathy and Diabetic Macular Edema reduces the number of levels of diabetic retinopathy, simplifies descriptions of the categories, and describes the levels without relying on reference to the standard photographs of the Airlie House Classification of diabetic retinopathy. This makes clinical use easier and more uniform among practitioners not versed in the complexities of the ETDRS grading system. However, because of this simplification, the International Classification is not a replacement for ETDRS levels of diabetic retinopathy in large-scale clinical trials or studies where precise retinopathy classification is required.

Other Ocular Manifestations of Diabetes

All structures of the eye are susceptible to complications of diabetes. The consequence of these changes can range from being unnoticed by both patient and physician, to being symptomatic but not sight-threatening, to requiring evaluation to rule out potentially life-threatening underlying causes other than diabetes.

Mononeuropathies of the third, fourth, or sixth cranial nerves can arise in association with diabetes; of these, mononeuropathy of the fourth cranial nerve is least likely to be associated with diabetes.[356-358] Nerve palsies present a significant diagnostic challenge because misdiagnosis can result in a life-threatening lesion's remaining untreated. In one review of cranial nerve palsies treated in a diabetic patient population in 1967, 42% of mononeuropathies were not diabetic in origin.[357] This finding underscores the danger of routinely attributing mononeuropathies to the diabetic condition itself without carefully ruling out other potential causes. The percentage of all extraocular muscle palsies attributable to diabetes mellitus is estimated to be 4.5% to 6%.[358] Mononeuropathies may be the initial presenting sign of new-onset diabetes, and diabetes should therefore be considered in the differential diagnosis of any mononeuropathy affecting the extraocular muscles, even in patients who do not claim a history of diabetes. Diabetes-induced third-, fourth-, and sixth-nerve palsies are usually self-limited and should resolve spontaneously in 2 to 6 months. Palsies can recur or subsequently develop in the contralateral eye.

The optic disc can be affected by diabetes in a variety of ways other than by vasoproliferation. Diabetic papillopathy must be distinguished from other causes of disc swelling, including true papilledema from increased intracranial pressure, pseudopapilledema such as optic nerve head drusen, toxic optic neuropathies, neoplasms of the optic nerve, and hypertension.[359] Optic disc pallor can occur with spontaneous remission of PDR or with remission after scatter (panretinal) laser photocoagulation (see Fig. 33-24I). Because diabetes poses an increased risk for development of open-angle glaucoma, the disc pallor that occurs after remission of retinopathy or laser photocoagulation must be considered when evaluating the optic nerve head for glaucoma.

A potentially serious diabetic ocular complication is neovascularization of the iris. Usually, the new iris vessels are first observed at the pupillary border, followed by a fine network of vessels over the iris tissue progressing into the filtration angle of the eye. Closure of the angle by the fibrovascular network results in neovascular glaucoma.[360] Neovascular glaucoma is difficult to manage and requires aggressive treatment. Diabetes is the second leading cause of neovascular glaucoma, accounting for 32% of cases.[361] Neovascularization of the iris occurs in 4% to 7% of diabetic eyes and may be present in up to 40% to 60% of eyes with PDR.[362,363] When possible, scatter (panretinal) laser photocoagulation is the primary therapy for neovascularization of the iris, although other approaches such as goniophotocoagulation, topical or systemic antiglaucoma medications, and antiglaucomatous filtration surgery are available when needed.[364-366] Intravitreal administration of VEGF inhibitors has been tried in small-scale, uncontrolled studies with remarkably rapid transient regression of the neovascularization.[367]

The cornea of the diabetic person is more susceptible to injury and slower to heal after injury than is the nondiabetic cornea.[359,368] The diabetic cornea is also more prone to infectious corneal ulcers, which can lead to rapid loss of vision, need for corneal transplant, or loss of the eye if it is not treated aggressively. Consequently, diabetic patients using contact lenses should exercise caution and maintain careful monitoring.

Open-angle glaucoma is 1.4 times more common in the diabetic population than in the nondiabetic population.[369] The prevalence of glaucoma increases with age and duration of diabetes, but medical therapy for open-angle glaucoma is generally effective. In a study of 76,318 women enrolled in the Nurses' Health Study, Pasquale and coworkers found that T2DM is associated with an increased risk of primary open-angle glaucoma in women.[370]

The effects of diabetes on the crystalline lens can result in transient refractive changes, alterations in accommodative ability,[371] and cataracts. Refractive change can be significant and is related to fluctuation of blood glucose levels with osmotic lens swelling.[361] Cataracts can occur earlier in life and progress more rapidly in the presence of diabetes.[372,373] Cataracts are 1.6 times more common in people with diabetes than in those without diabetes.[372,373] In patients with earlier-onset diabetes, duration of diabetes, retinopathy status, diuretic use, and HbA_{1c} levels are risk factors.[374] In patients with later-onset diabetes, age of the patient, lower intraocular pressure, smoking, and lower diastolic BP may be additional risk factors.[375,376] Diabetic patients undergoing simultaneous kidney and pancreas transplantation are at increased risk for development of all types of cataract, independent of the use of corticosteroids after transplantation.[377] Both phacoemulsification and extracapsular cataract extraction with intraocular lens implantation are appropriate surgical therapies. The principal determinant of postoperative vision and progression of retinopathy is related to the preoperative presence of DME and the level of NPDR.[378,379]

Other findings with higher incidence among patients with diabetes include xanthelasma,[356] microaneurysms of the bulbar conjunctiva,[380] posterior vitreous detachment,[381] and the rare but often fatal orbital fungal infection *Mucorales* phycomycosis.[362,363] Prompt diagnosis and treatment of phycomycosis caused by *Mucor* species is crucial, although the survival rate is still only 57%.[363,382]

Monitoring and Treatment of Diabetic Retinopathy

Appropriate clinical management of diabetic retinopathy has been defined by results of major randomized, multicenter clinical trials (Fig. 33-25): the Diabetic Retinopathy Study (DRS),[383] the ETDRS,[323] the Diabetic Retinopathy Vitrectomy Study (DRVS),[384] the DCCT,[385] and the UKPDS.[3] These studies have elucidated the progression rates of each level of diabetic retinopathy, guided follow-up intervals, and elucidated the proper delivery, timing, and resulting effectiveness of glycemic control and laser photocoagulation surgery (Figs. 33-26 through 33-29). They have also established recommendations for vitrectomy surgery.

Comprehensive Eye Examination

An accurate ocular examination detailing the extent and location of retinopathy-associated findings is critical for making monitoring and treatment decisions in patients with diabetic retinopathy. As detailed later, most of the blindness associated with advanced stages of retinopathy can be averted with appropriate and timely diagnosis and therapy. Unfortunately, many diabetic patients do not receive adequate eye care at an appropriate stage in their disease.[385,386] In one study, 55% of patients with high-risk PDR or CSME had never had laser photocoagulation.[385] In fact, 11% of T1DM and 7% of T2DM patients with high-risk PDR necessitating prompt treatment had not been examined by an ophthalmologist within the past 2 years.[386]

The comprehensive eye examination is the mainstay of such evaluation and is necessary on a repetitive, lifelong basis for patients with diabetes.[350,387] Such an evaluation has four major components: history, examination, diagnosis, and treatment. Annual retinal evaluation to assess the presence and level of diabetic retinopathy and DME is essential to guide patient care. The fundamentals of a comprehensive eye examination for the nondiabetic patient have been detailed by the American Academy of

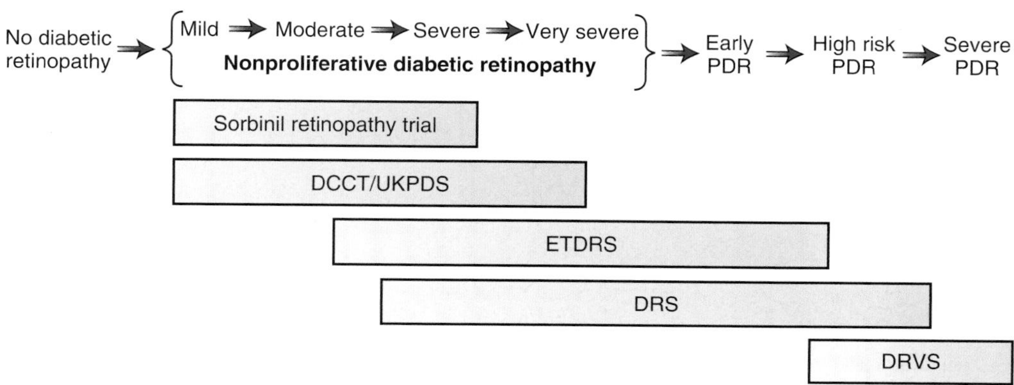

Figure 33-25 Major multicenter clinical trials of diabetic retinopathy. Schematic representation of the major multicenter clinical trials of diabetic retinopathy and the levels of diabetic retinopathy that they primarily addressed. DCCT, Diabetes Control and Complications Trial; DRS, Diabetic Retinopathy Study; DRVS, Diabetic Retinopathy Vitrectomy Study; ETDRS, Early Treatment Diabetic Retinopathy Study; PDR, proliferative diabetic retinopathy; UKPDS, United Kingdom Prospective Diabetes Study.

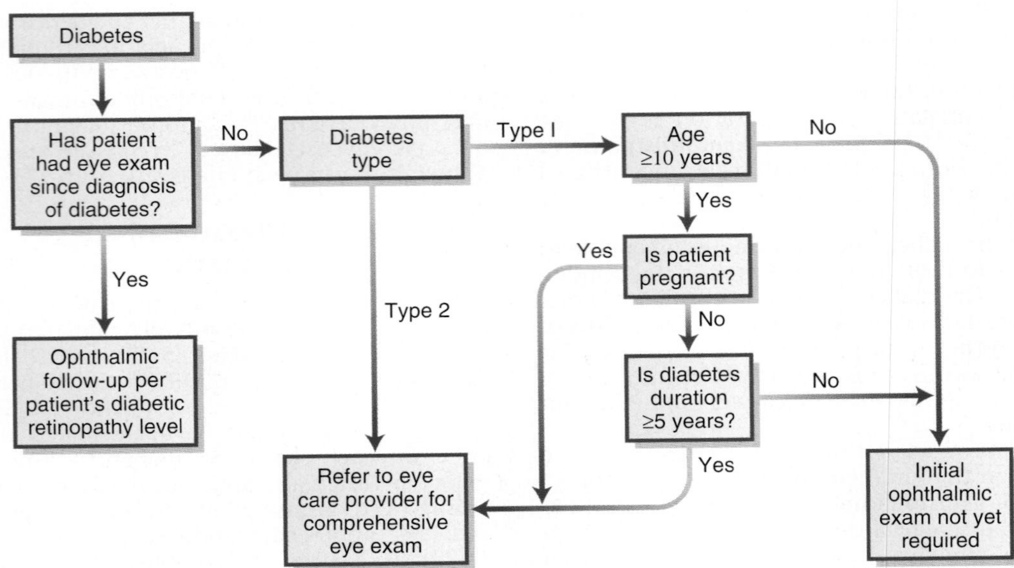

Figure 33-26 Initial ophthalmic examination flow chart. Schematic flow chart of major principles involved in determining the timing of initial ophthalmic examination after a diagnosis of diabetes mellitus. These are minimal recommended times. Ocular symptoms, complaints, or other associated medical issues can necessitate earlier evaluation. Guidelines are regularly reevaluated based on new study results.

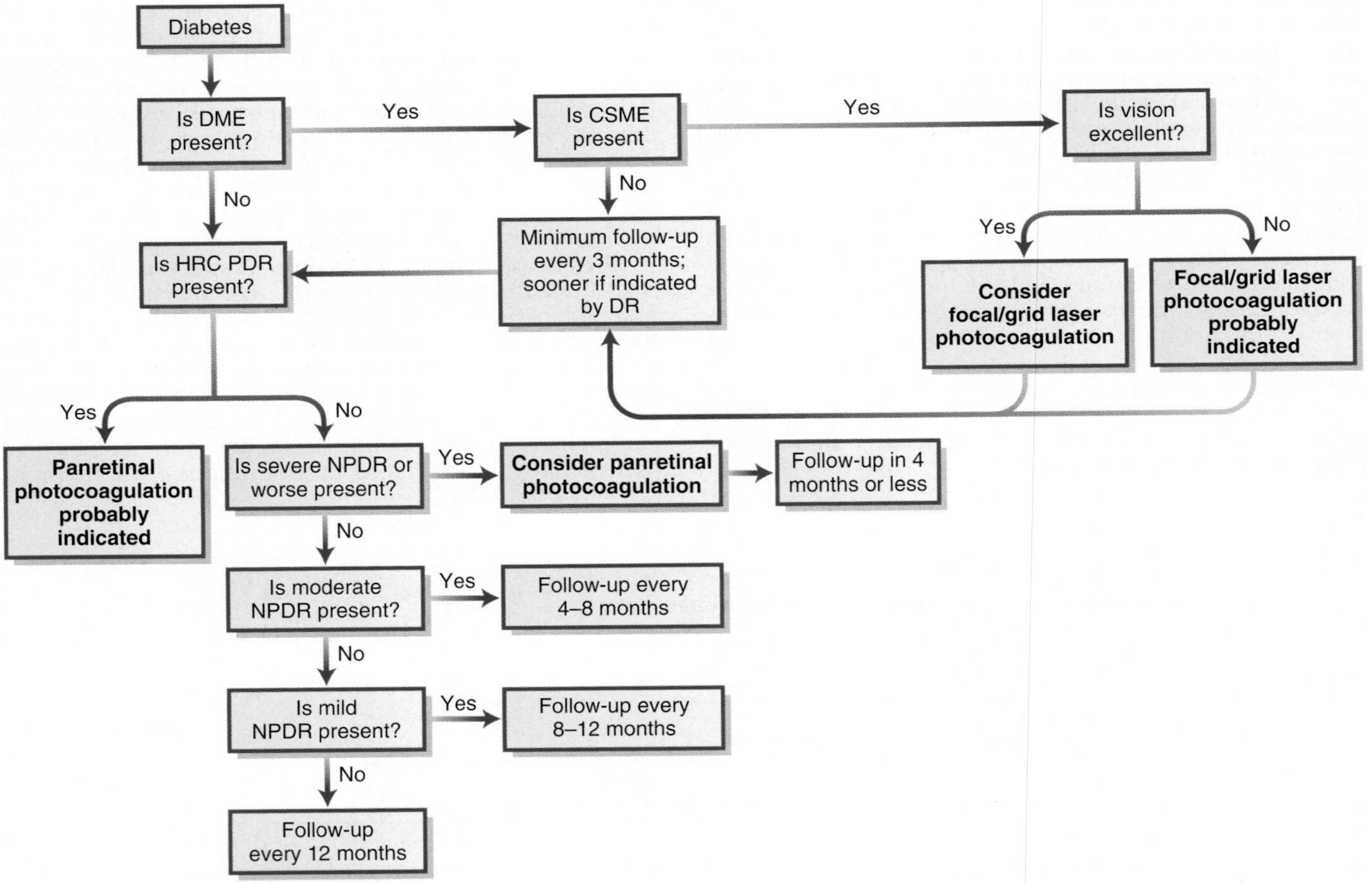

Figure 33-27 Diabetic retinopathy and macular edema examination and treatment flow chart: nonpregnant patients. The schematic flow chart presents major principles involved in determining routine ophthalmic follow-up and indications for treatment in nonpregnant patients with diabetes. These are only general, minimal recommended frequencies. Ocular symptoms, complaints, or other associated ophthalmic or medical issues can necessitate earlier evaluation and/or an altered approach. Guidelines are regularly reevaluated based on new study results. CSME, clinically significant macular edema; DME, diabetic macular edema; DR, diabetic retinopathy; HRC PDR, high-risk characteristic proliferative diabetic retinopathy; NPDR, nonproliferative diabetic retinopathy; PDR, proliferative diabetic retinopathy.

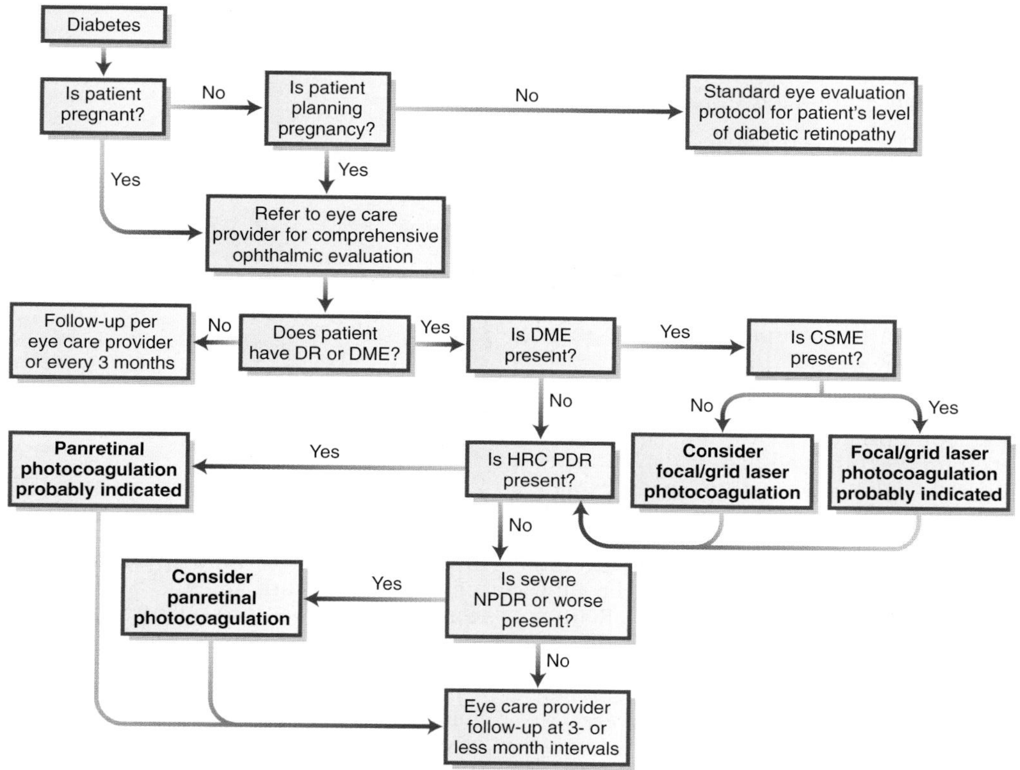

Figure 33-28 Diabetic retinopathy and macular edema examination and treatment flow chart: pregnant patients. The schematic flow chart shows major principles involved in determining routine ophthalmic follow-up and indications for treatment in pregnant patients with diabetes. These are only general, minimal recommended frequencies. Ocular symptoms, complaints, or other associated ophthalmic or medical issues can necessitate earlier evaluation and/or an altered approach. Because retinopathy can progress rapidly in pregnant patients with diabetes, careful and more frequent evaluation is often indicated. Guidelines are regularly reevaluated based on new study results. CSME, clinically significant macular edema; DME, diabetic macular edema; DR, diabetic retinopathy; HRC PDR, high-risk characteristic proliferative diabetic retinopathy; NPDR, nonproliferative diabetic retinopathy.

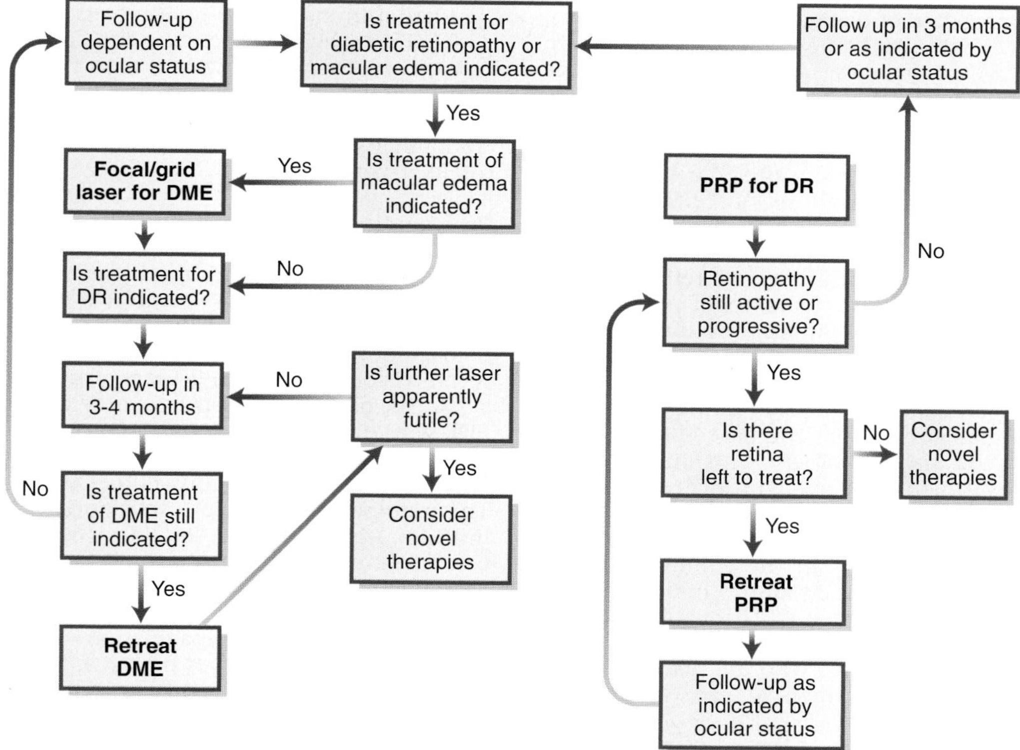

Figure 33-29 Photocoagulation flow chart. The schematic flow chart details general photocoagulation treatment approaches in patients with diabetic retinopathy and/or diabetic macular edema. These are only general guidelines, and actual treatment choices can be affected by numerous other factors, including findings in the same eye or in the contralateral eye and systemic issues. DR, diabetic retinopathy; DME, diabetic macular edema; PRP, scatter (panretinal) photocoagulation.

Ophthalmology[387] and the American Optometric Association.[388] The examination of the patient with diabetes should be similar, with additional emphasis on portions of the examination that relate to problems particularly relevant to diabetes.

Dilated ophthalmic examination is superior to undilated evaluation because only 50% of eyes are correctly classified as to presence and severity of retinopathy through undilated pupils.[389,390] Appropriate ophthalmic evaluation entails pupillary dilation, slit-lamp biomicroscopy, examination of the retinal periphery with indirect ophthalmoscopy or mirrored contact lens, and sometimes gonioscopy.[387,388] Because of the complexities of the diagnosis and treatment of PDR and CSME, ophthalmologists with specialized knowledge and experience in the management of diabetic retinopathy are required to determine and provide appropriate surgical intervention.[391] Therefore, it is recommended that all patients with diabetes should have dilated ocular examinations by an experienced eye care provider (ophthalmologist or optometrist), and diabetic patients should be under the direct or consulting care of an ophthalmologist experienced in the management of diabetic retinopathy at least by the time severe diabetic retinopathy or DME is present.[350] Retinal imaging that has demonstrated equivalency to dilated retinal fundus examination or the accepted standard of seven-standard-field stereoscopic retinal imaging when interpreted by a trained eye care provider can also be appropriate.[392]

Initial Ophthalmic Evaluation

The recommendation for initial ocular examination in persons with diabetes is based on prevalence rates of retinopathy (see Fig. 33-26). Approximately 80% of T1DM patients have retinopathy after 15 years of disease, but only about 25% have any retinopathy after 5 years.[390] The prevalence of PDR is less than 2% at 5 years and 25% by 15 years. For T2DM, the onset date of diabetes is usually unknown, and more severe disease can be observed at diagnosis. Up to 3% of patients whose diabetes is first diagnosed after age 30 years (T2DM) have CSME or high-risk PDR at the time of initial diagnosis of diabetes.[394] Therefore, in patients older than 10 years of age, initial ophthalmic examination is recommended beginning 5 years after the diagnosis of T1DM and at the time of diagnosis of T2DM (see Fig. 33-26).[350,395]

Puberty and pregnancy can accelerate retinopathy progression. The onset of vision-threatening retinopathy is rare in children before puberty, regardless of the duration of diabetes[298,395-397]; however, significant retinopathy can arise within 6 years of disease if diabetes is diagnosed between the ages of 10 and 30 years.[299] Diabetic retinopathy can become particularly aggressive during pregnancy in patients with diabetes.[398,399] In the past, the prognosis for pregnancy in the diabetic patient with microvascular complications was so poor that pregnant diabetic patients were commonly advised to avoid or terminate pregnancies.[400] With recognition of the importance of glycemic control, many diabetic patients in the child-bearing age now experience safe pregnancy and childbirth with minimal risk to mother and baby. There are excellent reviews on this subject.[401]

Ideally, patients with diabetes who are planning pregnancy should have a comprehensive eye examination within 1 year before conception (see Fig. 33-28). Patients who become pregnant should have a comprehensive eye examination in the first trimester of pregnancy. Close follow-up throughout pregnancy is indicated, with subsequent examinations determined by the findings present at the first-trimester examination.[350] This recommendation does not apply to women who develop gestational diabetes, because such women are not at increased risk of developing diabetic retinopathy.

TABLE 33-4

Progression to PDR by Level of NPDR

Retinopathy Level	Chance of High-Risk PDR (%) 1 Year	5 Years
Mild NPDR	1	16
Moderate NPDR	3-8	27-39
Severe NPDR	15	56
Very severe NPDR	45	71
PDR with fewer high-risk characteristics	22-46	64-75

NPDR, nonproliferative diabetic retinopathy; PDR, proliferative diabetic retinopathy.

From Aiello LP, Gardner TW, King GL, et al. Diabetic retinopathy: technical review. *Diabetes Care.* 1998;21:143-156.

Follow-Up Ophthalmic Examination

Follow-up ocular examination is determined from the risk of disease progression at any particular retinopathy level (see Fig. 33-27). NPDR is categorized into four levels of severity based on clinical findings compared with stereo fundus photographic standards: mild, moderate, severe, and very severe.[402] Progression of nonproliferative retinopathy to the visually threatening level of high-risk PDR is closely correlated to NPDR level (Table 33-4). Progression rates from each individual NPDR level to any other retinopathy level are also known. These are used to define standard minimal follow-up intervals, as detailed in Figure 33-27 and Table 33-5. Because significant sight-threatening retinopathy can initially occur with no or minimal symptoms, patients with no clinically evident diabetic retinopathy and no known ocular problems require annual comprehensive ophthalmic examinations even if they are totally asymptomatic.

Proliferative Diabetic Retinopathy. The extent and location of neovascularization determine the level of PDR.[403,404] PDR is best evaluated by dilated examination using slit-lamp biomicroscopy combined with indirect ophthalmoscopy or stereo fundus photography. Without photocoagulation, eyes with high-risk PDR have a 28% risk of severe vision loss within 2 years. This risk compares with a 7% risk of severe vision loss after 2 years for eyes with PDR without high-risk characteristics.[403]

Severe vision loss is defined as best-corrected acuity of 5/200 or worse on two consecutive visits 4 months apart. This represents vision loss substantially worse than the limit for legal blindness, 20/200 or worse. The DRS demonstrated that scatter (panretinal) laser photocoagulation was effective in reducing the risk of severe vision loss from PDR by 50% or more. The ETDRS demonstrated that scatter (panretinal) laser photocoagulation applied when an eye approaches or just reaches high-risk PDR reduces the risk of severe vision loss to less than 4%. Prompt scatter photocoagulation is therefore indicated for all patients with high-risk PDR, usually indicated for patients with PDR less than high risk, and may be advisable for patients with severe or very severe NPDR, especially in the setting of

TABLE 33-5

Recommended General Management of Diabetic Retinopathy

	Risk of Progression (%)		Evaluation		Treatment		
Level of DR	*To PDR (1 yr)*	*To High-Risk PDR (5 yr)*	*Color Photo*	*FA*	*Scatter Laser (PRP)*	*Focal Laser*	**Follow-up (mo)**
Mild NPDR							
All	5	15					
No ME			No	No	No	No	12
ME			Yes	Occ	No	No	4-6
CSME			Yes	Yes	No	Yes	2-4
Moderate NPDR							
All	12-27	33					
No ME			Yes	No	No	No	6-8
ME			Yes	Occ	No	Occ	4-6
CSME			Yes	Yes	No	Yes	2-4
Severe NPDR							
All	52	60					
No ME			Yes	No	Rarely	No	3-4
ME			Yes	Occ	Occ AF	Occ	2-3
CSME			Yes	Yes	Occ AF	Yes	2-3
Very Severe NPDR							
All	75	75					
No ME			Yes	No	Occ	No	2-3
ME			Yes	Occ	Occ AF	Occ	2-3
CSME			Yes	Yes	Occ AF	Yes	2-3
PDR < High Risk							
All	—	75					
No ME			Yes	No	Occ	No	2-3
ME			Yes	Occ	Occ AF	Occ	2-3
CSME			Yes	Yes	Occ AF	Yes	2-3
PDR with High-Risk Characteristics							
All	—	—					
No ME			Yes	No	Yes	No	2-3
ME			Yes	Yes	Yes	Usually	1-2
CSME			Yes	Yes	Yes	Yes	1-2

AF, after focal; CSME, clinically significant macular edema; FA, fluorescein angiography; ME macular edema; NPDR, nonproliferative diabetic retinopathy; Occ, occasionally; PDR, proliferative diabetic retinopathy.
Courtesy of Lloyd M. Aiello, MD. Joslin Diabetes Center, Boston, Mass.

T2DM (see Fig. 33-27).[323,403-406] Recent progression of eye disease, status of the fellow eye, compliance with follow-up, concurrent health concerns such as hypertension or kidney disease, and other factors must be considered in determining whether laser surgery should be performed in these patients. In particular, patients with T2DM should be considered for scatter photocoagulation before high-risk PDR develops, because the risk of severe vision loss and the need for pars plana vitrectomy (PPV) can be reduced by 50% in these patients, especially when macular edema is present.[406]

In scatter photocoagulation, 1200 to 1800 laser burns are applied to the peripheral retinal tissue, actually focally destroying the outer photoreceptor and retinal pigment epithelium of the retina (see Fig. 33-24I). Large vessels are avoided, as are areas of preretinal hemorrhage. The treatment is thought to exert its effect by increasing oxygen delivery to the inner retina, decreasing viable hypoxic growth factor–producing cells, and increasing the relative perfusion per area of viable retina. The total treatment is usually applied over two or three sessions, spaced 1 to 2 weeks apart. Follow-up evaluation usually occurs at 3 months.

The response to scatter photocoagulation varies. The most desirable effect is to see a regression of the new vessels, although stabilization of the neovascularization with no further growth can result. This latter situation requires careful clinical monitoring. In some cases, new vessels continue to proliferate, requiring additional scatter photocoagulation (see Fig. 37-29). As discussed later, novel therapeutic approaches are now being used in some clinical settings, especially in cases in which the response to scatter photocoagulation is inadequate. Initial results from definitive multicenter, randomized, controlled clinical trials will soon be reported, and additional clinical trials using these new therapeutic approaches continue to be performed.

The DRVS, completed in 1989, demonstrated that early PPV in persons with severe fibrovascular proliferation was more likely to result in better vision and less likely to result in poor vision, particularly in patients with T1DM.[384] PPV is surgery within the eye aimed primarily at removing abnormal fibrovascular tissue, alleviating retinal traction, allowing the retina to obtain a more anatomically normal position, and removing vitreous opacities such as vitreous hemorrhage. The actual outcome data from this study may not be entirely applicable today because of the dramatic advances in surgical techniques and the advent of laser endophotocoagulation that have occurred in the intervening years. It is clear that PPV can save and restore vision in many cases of severe retinal disease not amenable or not responsive to laser photocoagulation.

Macular Edema. Untreated CSME is associated with an approximately 25% chance of moderate vision loss after 3 years (defined as at least doubling of the visual angle, such as 20/40 reduced to 20/80).[323] Macular edema is best evaluated clinically by dilated examination using slit-lamp biomicroscopy or stereo fundus photography. The newer diagnostic ophthalmic imaging technique called optical coherence tomography (OCT) has provided a means to objectively quantify retinal thickening and is the objective method of choice currently. OCT has been used in conjunction with visual acuity measurement to monitor response to treatment and help determine timing of intervention.[408,409] Focal laser photocoagulation is generally indicated for patients with CSME (see Figs. 33-24C and 33-27). The ETDRS demonstrated that focal laser photocoagulation for CSME reduced the 5-year risk of moderate vision loss by 50%, but 15% of patients continued to experience vision loss.[353] In focal laser photocoagulation, lesions located 500 to 3000 μm from the center of the macula that are contributing to thickening of the macular area are usually directly photocoagulated. These lesions are identified clinically or by fluorescein angiography and consist primarily of leaking microaneurysms. When leakage is diffuse or microaneurysms are extensive, photocoagulation may be applied to the macula in a grid configuration, avoiding the fovea region.

Although fluorescein angiography is useful for guiding therapy once CSME has been diagnosed, it is not required for the diagnosis of CSME or PDR, because these findings should be clinically evident in most cases (Fig. 33-30). Fluorescein angiography is a valuable test for guiding treatment of CSME, identifying macular capillary nonperfusion, and evaluating unexplained vision loss. Because there are risks associated with fluorescein angiography, including nausea, urticaria, hives, and rarely death (1 in 222,000 patients) or severe medical sequelae (1 in 2000 patients),[407,410,411] fluorescein angiography is not part of the examination of an otherwise normal patient with diabetes, and the procedure is usually contraindicated in patients with known allergy to fluorescein dye or during pregnancy.

Follow-up evaluation of focal laser surgery usually occurs after 3 months (see Fig. 33-27). If macular edema persists, further treatment may be necessary. Patients with severe or very severe NPDR should be considered for focal treatment of macular edema whether or not the macular edema is clinically significant, because they are likely to require scatter laser photocoagulation in the near future and because scatter photocoagulation, although beneficial for PDR, can exacerbate existing macular edema. As discussed later, novel therapeutic approaches are now being used in clinical settings to treat DME, and their benefit, when combined with focal laser therapy, has been confirmed by results from multicenter, randomized clinical trials. However, this approach requires repeated intraocular injections. Additionally, the pathogenesis of DME is highly complex, and a variable response to treatment modalities has been observed in many patients. These observations have prompted the investigation of varying drug dosages to identify the optimal treatment concentration and sustained drug delivery devices to limit repeated intraocular injections. Multicenter, randomized, controlled clinical trials are under way for most of these new approaches.

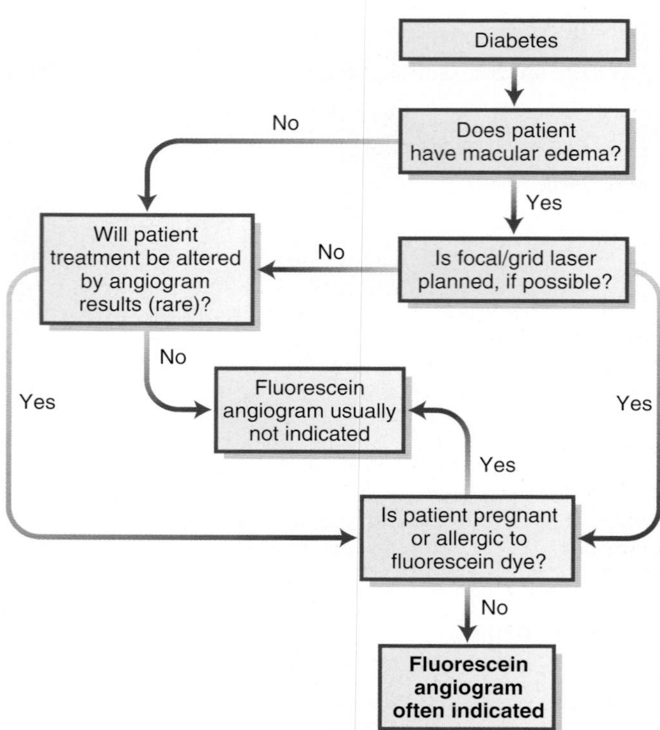

Figure 33-30 Fluorescein angiogram flow chart. The schematic flow chart details a general algorithm for appropriate use of fluorescein angiography in the ocular evaluation of patients with diabetes mellitus. In unusual cases, confounding factors can alter the appropriate approach.

Novel Approaches. Advances in understanding of the pathogenic mechanisms underlying diabetic retinopathy have given rise to the development of novel pharmacologic therapies that may limit the progression of diabetic retinopathy and may be more effective than laser in the treatment of PDR and DME. Laser photocoagulation has shown established effectiveness in the treatment of both PDR and DME, but it is inherently destructive and relies on focal ablation of areas of the retina. Growth factors such as VEGF have been shown to mediate both the neovascularization of PDR and the increased permeability associated with DME. These observations have prompted novel approaches in the management of retinal diseases with pharmacologic agents that modulate the response to these factors to effectively treat PDR and DME without the retinal tissue destruction associated with laser photocoagulation.

Intravitreal injections of anti-VEGF agents, either as an aptamer (pegatanib) or as antibodies (ranibizumab and bevazicumab), have been shown to cause the regression of choroidal and retinal neovascularization and to reduce the amount of vascular leakage. These compounds are injected into the vitreous cavity of the eye on a repetitive basis. Both pegatanib and ranibizumab have been approved by the U.S. Food and Drug Administration for the treatment of neovascular age-related macular degeneration, and all three anti-VEGF agents have been used off-label in the treatment of diabetic retinopathy and DME. Neovascular processes have been shown to be exquisitely sensitive to anti-VEGF agents, and eyes with severe neovascularization of the retina or anterior segment have dramatically and rapidly improved with anti-VEGF treatment.[335,412]

Results from a multicenter, randomized, controlled clinical trial evaluating intravitreal administration of ranibizumab with immediate or deferred laser showed a marked benefit for anti-VEGF agents compared with laser alone.[413] After 1 year, ranibizumab, as applied in the trial, resulted in a mean gain of nine letters of vision ($P < .001$) when combined either with prompt laser or with deferral of laser for at least 24 weeks. Ranibizumab was more effective than prompt laser alone (three-letter gain) for the treatment of center-involving DME in eyes with central thickening and vision reduced to between 20/32 and 20/320. The number of eyes gaining two or more lines of vision were almost doubled in the anti-VEGF groups compared with laser alone. Conversely, eyes losing two or more lines of vision were about one third as many in the anti-VEGF groups compared with laser alone. No increased systemic events or serious ocular adverse events were attributed to the treatment other than the known small risk of endophthalmitis associated with intravitreal injections themselves. Currently, further randomized clinical trials are under way to determine the optimal dosage regimen for anti-VEGF agents. Much work is being done on drug delivery systems so as to eventually reduce the number of intravitreal injections required.

The ophthalmic use of corticosteroids, administered through the periocular or the intravitreal route for the treatment of DME, has gained widespread use over the last 5 years, largely due to early case reports and uncontrolled clinical trials documenting its rapid and often dramatic effect on retinal thickening. Two multicenter, randomized, prospective clinical trials were undertaken to address the effectiveness and safety of both routes of steroid administration. Peribulbar steroid injections were found to have no significant benefit for the treatment of DME, but a beneficial effect of limiting retinopathy progression was observed.[414] The 3-year results of the multicenter, randomized, controlled trial comparing intravitreal steroids to focal laser showed that, despite an initial rapid reduction in retinal thickness and improvement in vision with the intravitreal steroid injection, the results at 1 year were no better than with laser photocoagulation, and after 2 years, the steroid was inferior to the laser treatment in both visual outcome and retinal thickness.[415,416] Intravitreal steroid injection was associated with increases of approximately fourfold in rate of intraocular pressure complications and fourfold in need for cataract surgery, compared with laser treatment. As with peribulbar steroids, intravitreal steroid administration resulted in a 32% reduction in relative risk (RR) for retinopathy progression. When used in combination with laser in patients who have already undergone cataract surgery before initiation of anti-VEGF treatment, vision improvement may be comparable to that achieved with anti-VEGF agents.[413]

Currently, intravitreal steroid alone is not the preferred primary therapy for DME, but it may play a future role in treatment to limit retinopathy progression or in combination with laser in patients who cannot receive anti-VEGF agents or who are pseudophakic before treatment. However, development of cataracts and increases in intraocular pressure may limit its potential benefit.

Control of Systemic Disorders and Effect of Systemic Medications

In addition to the importance of intensive glycemic control in reducing the onset and progression of diabetic retinopathy as discussed earlier, it is critical for optimal ocular health of diabetic patients that several other systemic considerations be optimized.

Patients with diabetes mellitus commonly suffer from concomitant hypertension. Patients with T1DM have a 17% prevalence of hypertension at baseline and a 25% incidence after 10 years.[417] There is a 38% to 68% prevalence in T2DM.[418-420] In most studies, hypertension is correlated with the duration of diabetes, higher HbA_{1c} level, presence of gross proteinuria, and male gender. Elevated BP exacerbates the development and progression of diabetic retinopathy. The risk of PDR is associated with the presence of hypertension at the baseline visit, higher HbA_{1c} levels, and presence of more severe levels of retinopathy at the initial visit.[421] Patients with hypertension are more likely to develop retinopathy, diffuse macular edema, and more severe levels of retinopathy[421-423] and have more rapid progression of retinopathy than diabetic patients who do not have hypertension.[424-426]

The large, randomized, prospective UKPDS in 1148 patients with T2DM demonstrated a 34% ($P = .0004$) reduction in risk of diabetic retinopathy progression and a 47% ($P = .004$) reduction in moderate visual acuity loss in patients assigned to intensive BP control.[427] These effects were independent of glycemic control, and the risk reductions were similar regardless of whether the hypertension was controlled with an ACE inhibitor (captopril) or a β-blocker (atenolol). Overall, hypertension appears to be a significant risk factor in the development and progression of diabetic retinopathy and should be rigorously controlled. Until the results of specific trials investigating the BP levels required to minimize end-organ damage in patients with diabetes are known, target BP should most likely be maintained as low as safely possible.

Associations between renal and retinal angiopathy are numerous. Proteinuria and microalbuminuria are associated with retinopathy.[429-441] The presence and severity of diabetic retinopathy are indicators of the risk of gross proteinuria,[433,442] and, conversely, proteinuria predicts PDR.[431,442,444] Half of all patients who have T1DM with PDR and 10 or more years of diabetes have concomitant proteinuria.[429] In T1DM, the prevalence of PDR increases from 7% at onset of microalbuminuria to 29% 4 years after onset of albuminuria, compared with 3% and 8%, respectively, in patients without persistent microalbuminuria.[432] The Appropriate Blood Pressure Control in Diabetes (ABCD) Trial found that both the severity and the progression of retinopathy were associated with overt albuminuria.[445-447] In patients with T1DM, the presence of gross proteinuria at baseline is associated with 95% increased risk of developing macular edema,[421] and dialysis can improve macular edema in diabetic patients with renal failure.[365]

Despite these associations, the frequent coexistence of retinal and renal microangiopathies and factors such as associated hypertension and disease duration can confound these results.[448] Overall, it is important to carefully consider the renal status of any patient with diabetes mellitus and to ensure that the patient is receiving optimal care in this regard. In addition, rapidly progressive retinopathy, especially in a patient with a long history of diabetes mellitus in whom retinopathy has been previously stable, should suggest the need for renal evaluation.

Low hematocrit was an independent risk factor in the ETDRS analysis of baseline risk factors for development of high-risk PDR and of severe vision loss.[449] A cross-sectional study involving 1691 patients revealed a twofold increased risk of any retinopathy in patients with a hemoglobin level lower than 12 g/dL, compared to those with a higher hemoglobin concentration, using multivariate analyses controlling for serum creatinine, proteinuria, and other factors.[450] Among patients with retinopathy, those with low hemoglobin levels have a fivefold increased risk of severe retinopathy compared to those with higher hemoglobin levels. There have been limited reports of resolution of macular edema and hard exudate with improvement or stabilization of visual acuity in erythropoietin-treated patients after an increase in mean hematocrit.[451] In view of the potential association of low hematocrit and diabetic retinopathy, it is important to ensure that patients with diabetic retinopathy and anemia are receiving appropriate management.

In summary, diabetes is clearly a multisystem disease that requires a comprehensive medical team approach. Even with regard to ocular health, this necessitates the involvement of multiple health care specialists for optimal patient care.

DIABETIC NEPHROPATHY

Diabetic nephropathy remains a major cause of morbidity and mortality for persons with either T1DM or T2DM. In Western countries, diabetes is the leading single cause of ESRD.[452] Indeed, in many countries such as the United States, more than 50% of patients in renal replacement therapy programs have diabetes as the major cause of their renal failure.[453] However, the full impact of diabetic nephropathy is far greater.[454] Globally, most patients with diabetes are in developing countries[455] that do not have the resources or health infrastructure to provide universal renal replacement therapy. Even in developed countries, fewer than 1 in 20 patients with diabetes and chronic kidney disease survive to ESRD, succumbing instead to CVD, heart failure, or infection, to which the presence and severity of diabetic renal disease significantly contribute. For example, almost all of the excess in cardiovascular deaths in persons with diabetes younger than 50 years of age can be attributed to nephropathy.[456] Indeed, in T1DM subjects without nephropathy there is no evidence of premature mortality.[457] In patients with T2DM, microalbuminuria is associated with a twofold to fourfold increase in the risk of death. In patients with overt proteinuria and hypertension, the risk is even higher.[458] Consequently, the goal to reduce ESRD in patients with diabetes is only one component of the overall benefit in preventing diabetic kidney disease.

It is estimated that 25% to 40% of patients with T1DM and 5% to 40% of patients with T2DM ultimately develop diabetic kidney disease.[459,460] Up to 20% of patients with T2DM already have diabetic kidney disease when they are diagnosed with diabetes,[461] and a further 30% to 40% develop diabetic nephropathy, mostly within 10 years of diagnosis.[462] Nephropathy appears be more common in T1DM, but, because of the large and increasing number of persons with T2DM,[463] more than 80% of diabetic patients in renal replacement programs have T2DM.

Natural History of Nephropathy in Type 1 Diabetes

Nephropathy and specifically proteinuria in the setting of diabetes have been known for more than 100 years, and the classic structural features of glomerulosclerosis were described more than 70 years ago.[464] However, it is only since the 1980s that the natural history of this condition has been extensively delineated. This is partly because significantly more patients are surviving to see the full presentation of this condition. For example, in 1971, the median survival time of patients with T1DM and overt nephropathy was 5 years, with fewer than 10% surviving more than 10 years.[465] Consequently, few patients were able to survive the course of their renal disease. By comparison, in 1996, the median survival time in an equivalent population was more than 17 years. Not surprisingly, almost 10 times more patients with T1DM are now entering ESRD programs.

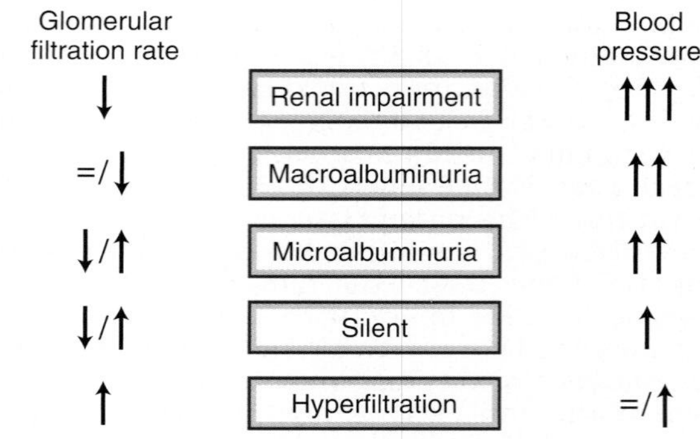

Figure 33-31 The phases (natural history) of diabetic nephropathy.

Diabetic nephropathy is characterized clinically as a triad of hypertension, proteinuria, and, ultimately, renal impairment.[466] The classic five stages of nephropathy as described by Mogensen,[467] although not totally accurate, remain the best way of describing this condition (Fig. 33-31). This description relies on functional evaluation of the renal disease and is based on serial measurements of glomerular filtration rate (GFR) and albuminuria.

Stage 1: Hyperfiltration

The initial phase has been termed the *hyperfiltration* phase. It is associated with an elevation of GFR[468] and an increase in capillary glomerular pressure. Although elevated GFR is invariably present in animal models of T1DM,[469] it occurs in only a significant minority of T1DM patients. Hyperfiltration is considered to occur as a result of concomitant renal hypertrophy[470] and in part because of a range of intrarenal hemodynamic abnormalities that occur in the diabetic milieu and contribute to glomerular hypertension.[471] The pathophysiology of renal hypertrophy associated with diabetes remains unexplained, although specific growth factors such as the growth hormone (GH)-IGF1 system and TGF-β have been implicated.[472,473] There is not only glomerular but also tubular hypertrophy. The tubular hypertrophy explains the increased kidney weight in diabetes, because tubules make up more than 90% of the kidney weight.[474] In addition, increased salt reabsorption associated with proximal tubular hypertrophy can contribute to glomerular hyperfiltration via tubuloglomerular feedback.[470]

The second explanation for the increase in GFR associated with diabetes relates to hemodynamic changes within the kidney. Although not directly tested in humans, micropuncture studies in rodents, particularly by Brenner's group in the 1980s, revealed that experimental diabetes was associated with a range of intrarenal hemodynamic changes.[471] Alongside hyperfiltration, there is an increase in effective renal plasma flow, and some investigators call this the *hyperperfusion-hyperfiltration* phase of diabetic nephropathy. At the same time, increased intraglomerular capillary pressure is increased, reflecting relative efferent versus afferent arteriolar vasoconstriction[471] with activation of the intrarenal renin-angiotensin system and reduced synthesis of the vasodilator NO.

The importance of this hyperfiltration phase as predicting and leading to diabetic nephropathy remains controversial. Several groups have confirmed the initial relationship between elevated GFR and later development of proteinuria described by Mogensen.[475] However, this has not been a universal finding. Nevertheless, later studies with antihypertensive agents, and in particular agents that interrupt the renin-angiotensin system, have shown attenuation of some of these glomerular hemodynamic abnormalities. This provides justification to consider that at least some of these intrarenal hemodynamic changes in diabetes play a role in the development and progression of nephropathy.

Stage 2: The Silent Stage

The next stage is known as the *silent stage*: from a clinical point of view, there is no overt evidence of any form of renal dysfunction. Patients usually have normal GFR with no evidence of albuminuria. However, this phase is associated with significant structural changes, including basement membrane thickening and mesangial expansion. With detailed quantitative studies of renal morphology, it is often possible to detect those patients who will develop renal damage.[476]

This is a very important phase clinically, because it is hoped that investigators will be able to develop new tests, such as biomarkers in plasma or urine or sophisticated assessments from renal biopsy material, to identify which patients will progress to more advanced renal disease. Because overall fewer than 40% of subjects with T1DM will progress, it is critical that the potential progressors, who could be candidates for early prevention and treatment strategies to avoid ESRD, be detected. As yet, no such surrogate markers or predictors have been identified in association with the silent phase of the disease.

Extensive studies using various plasma markers such as prorenin[477] or DNA studies to identify certain gene polymorphisms such as the ACE genotype[39] have been promising. The measurement of albumin fragments (ghost albumin) in the urine of patients with diabetes may be another, albeit unproven, approach.[478] Serial prospective ambulatory BP monitoring studies have also demonstrated modest rises in BP in patients in this silent phase up to 5 years before urinary albumin excretion begins to increase.[479] However, none of these markers has been proven to be sensitive or specific enough on further clinical evaluation for widespread clinical application.

Stage 3: Microalbuminuria

The third phase is known as *microalbuminuria* or the stage of *incipient nephropathy*. At this stage, often 5 to 15 years after the initial diagnosis of T1DM, the urinary albumin excretion rate has increased into the microalbuminuric range of 20 to 200 μg/minute or 30 to 300 mg/24 hours.[480] In the past, microalbuminuria was considered to be a predictor rather than a manifestation of diabetic kidney disease. Increasingly it has been appreciated, particularly based on interpretation of renal morphologic studies, that in the microalbuminuric phase there is already widespread evidence of advanced glomerular structural changes.[481] Concomitant with these changes, systolic and diastolic BP are increased. Furthermore, the nocturnal dip in BP seen in normal persons is often lost with the development of microalbuminuria.[482] Renal function during this phase may be increased, normal, or reduced.

The best approach to screen for microalbuminuria remains controversial. The original studies used 24-hour or overnight urine sampling methods. However, a spot urine albumin-to-creatinine ratio in an early morning urine specimen has been validated as a marker and appears to be a practical option for routine clinical practice.[480] Because persistent microalbuminuria, if left untreated, is often a reliable harbinger of overt nephropathy,[475] it is incumbent on clinicians to perform serial measurements of this parameter and to repeat the measurement if there is an isolated elevation in urinary albumin excretion.

Studies suggest that in many patients with T1DM, microalbuminuria can be transient and can reverse to normoalbuminuria.[483] Therefore, the onset of microalbuminuria does not irrevocably seal the fate of the patient. A study of 386 patients with persistent microalbuminuria showed that regression of microalbuminuria occurred in 58% of patients,[483] although other groups have reported much lower rates of this phenomenon.[484] Notably, in that study, microalbuminuria of short duration, optimal levels of HbA_{1c} (<8%), low systolic BP (<115 mm Hg), and low levels of both cholesterol and triglycerides were independently associated with the regression of microalbuminuria. Therefore, screening of diabetic patients for nephropathy is now recommended to include measurements of urinary albumin concentrations at least twice annually in T1DM patients.

Stage 4: Macroalbuminuria

The next stage is the *macroalbuminuria* phase or *overt nephropathy*. This stage represents the phase that has been previously described as diabetic nephropathy and is highly predictive of subsequent renal failure if left untreated. It is characterized by a urinary albumin excretion rate greater than 300 mg/24 hours (>200 μg/minute). This phase usually occurs after 10 to 15 years of diabetes, but the risk of overt renal disease never truly disappears, and macroalbuminuria can appear after 40 or 50 years of T1DM.

There are at least two peaks of incidence of overt nephropathy, and this has been termed by some investigators as representing slow and fast trackers.[485] The key contributors of this marked variation in the timing of onset of proteinuria, independent of glycemia or BP control, remains elusive, although a range of genetic, molecular, and environmental factors have been proposed. In association with this increase in proteinuria, more than two thirds of patients have overt systemic hypertension.[486] If macroalbuminuria is left untreated, BP continues to rise, accelerating the decline in GFR, which promotes a further rise in BP, creating a vicious cycle of progressive renal impairment that ultimately leads to ESRD.

Stage 5: Uremia

The final *uremic* phase, which can occur in up to 40% of T1DM subjects, requires the institution of renal replacement therapy. As recently as the 1970s, patients with diabetes were not considered candidates for renal replacement therapy because of their abysmal prognosis. However, improvements in the management of CVD and renal replacement options have seen the survival rate of diabetic patients on dialysis approach that of patients with renal disease from other causes. Many patients with diabetes and ESRD are also now considered candidates for renal transplantation, which is associated with better outcomes than remaining on dialysis. However, there is evidence that the renal lesions of diabetes often recur in the transplanted kidney, although the lead time to develop ESRD means that few kidneys are lost through recurrent disease.

Increasingly, single pancreas-kidney (SPK) and pancreas-after-kidney (PAK) transplantation have become therapeutic options for patients with T1DM and ESRD, and they appear to offer advantages over kidney-alone transplantation. In particular, there is some evidence that maintenance of euglycemia after pancreas transplantation can lead to resolution of many diabetes-related renal lesions, such as mesangial expansion.[487] This reversal is often not apparent until after 10 years of euglycemia, emphasizing the slow turnover of matrix and the potential long-term effects of hyperglycemic memory in the kidney.

Natural History of Nephropathy in Type 2 Diabetes

The natural history of diabetic nephropathy in patients with T2DM is less well understood than in patients with T1DM. This partly reflects the fact that T2DM is largely a disease of an older population, with associated obesity, hypertension, and dyslipidemia and high rates of CVD that restrict the manifestation of diabetic renal disease. In addition, approximately 7% of patients with T2DM already have microalbuminuria at the time of diagnosis. This may be partly related to the fact that most of these patients have had untreated diabetes for 10 years (on average) before diagnosis. Within 5 years after a diagnosis of T2DM, up to 18% of patients have microalbuminuria, especially those with poor metabolic control and high BP levels. This has led some investigators to suggest that nephropathy in T2DM is different from that seen in patients with T1DM.

However, the natural history of nephropathy in T2DM has more similarities than differences from that seen in T1DM. Hyperfiltration does occur in T2DM,[488] although it has been reported to be less common than in T1DM. This observation must be interpreted with caution, because GFR normally declines with age, and hyperfiltration can still exist even though the GFR remains in the normal adult range. Microalbuminuria also occurs in T2DM. However, the finding of microalbuminuria in T2DM might not be as specific for diabetic renal disease as described in the seminal studies in T1DM. In the context of a very high prevalence of CVD, microalbuminuria may be more closely associated with nonrenal events such as stroke and MI.[444] Furthermore, incipient or overt cardiac failure, urinary tract infection, and urinary obstruction (e.g., enlarged prostate) can also lead to microalbuminuria.[471]

Many patients with T2DM and microalbuminuria also progress to overt proteinuria. However, it is increasingly appreciated that the situation is much more complex, and many groups have now described subjects with T1DM[489] as well as T2DM[490] who develop renal impairment in the absence of significant proteinuria. The exact explanation for this phenomenon is unknown, and ongoing studies are exploring whether these patients have different renal morphologic changes from those with the more classic syndrome of diabetic nephropathy (i.e., overt proteinuria and declining GFR). Preliminary studies suggest a prominent vascular component for this form of nonproteinuric renal dysfunction. Nonetheless, it appears that the risk of ESRD in patients with T2DM and renal impairment is similar in the presence or absence of microalbuminuria, underlining the importance of an estimated GFR in the management of T2DM. Many of the national and international guidelines now recommend the inclusion of regular measurements of serum creatinine[491] and determination of estimated GFR using a variety of different formulas.

Pathogenesis

It is likely that many of the mechanisms implicated in diabetic microvascular complications, in general, play a central role in the development and progression of diabetic nephropathy (Fig. 33-32).[250] It is clear that hyperglycemia is necessary for the initiation of renal injury, because patients without diabetes do not develop this type of nephropathy. Moreover, intensive therapy designed to achieve improved glycemic control is able to attenuate the development of nephropathy, as assessed by urinary albumin excretion, although it is not fully prevented.[308] However, it is now clear that other factors must also be involved, because continuous florid hyperglycemia is not necessarily required for diabetic hyperfiltration and kidney growth to occur. Indeed, glomerular hyperfiltration and tubular hypertrophy can persist in patients with T1DM even after euglycemia is achieved through aggressive insulin therapy.[492]

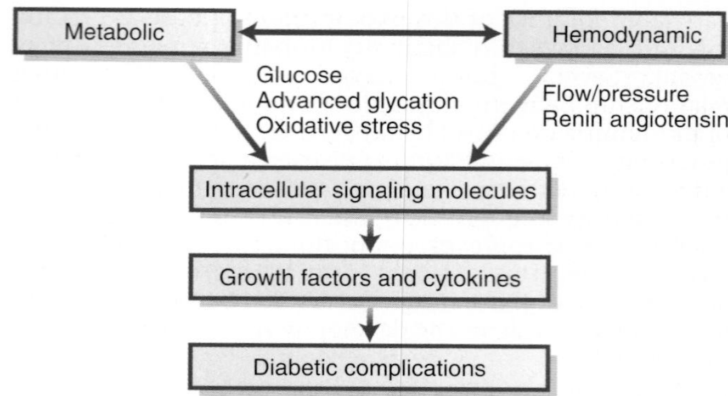

Figure 33-32 Interactions between metabolic and hemodynamic factors in promoting diabetic complications including nephropathy.

Other pathways that may be involved in diabetic nephropathy include generation of mitochondrial ROS, accumulation of AGEs, and activation of intracellular signaling molecules such as PKC.[250] Many of the seminal studies performed in endothelial cells demonstrating a central role of mitochondrial ROS in activating pathways implicated in diabetic vascular complications have been reproduced in mesangial cells.[493] Advanced glycation, which occurs at an accelerated rate in diabetic patients, is a prominent phenomenon in the kidney. Not only is the kidney the major site for excretion of AGEs, but also many of the proteins with a long life, such as collagen, are extensively glycated in patients with diabetes.[494] Furthermore, various AGE receptors (e.g., RAGE) have been described in the kidney and appear to play a role in mediating some of the deleterious effects of AGEs, such as stimulation of growth factor expression and induction of important phenotypic changes within certain renal cell populations to promote scarring.[131]

Preliminary studies have been performed using various approaches to inhibit renal AGE accumulation and action, including the use of a soluble RAGE (sRAGE). A range of pharmacologic agents have shown promising results, but clinical translation of these findings remains to be fully defined.[494] Selective PKC isoform inhibitors have been evaluated in small clinical trials, but their role in renal disease remains to be confirmed.[495] Some exciting pilot studies evaluating a number of cytosolic sources of oxidative stress, such as NADPH oxidase, suggest that certain NADPH oxidase isoforms such as Nox4 may be excellent targets for new renoprotective therapies.[496]

In addition to the mechanisms described earlier, the diabetic kidney appears to be readily modulated by a range of vasoactive hormones. It is increasingly appreciated that there may be important interactions between metabolic pathways and various hemodynamic factors, including vasoactive hormones such as angiotensin II, in mediating renal injury in diabetes (see Fig. 33-32).[497,498] Although many drugs that modulate hormone levels or action are not specific for diabetic kidney disease, interruption of the renin-angiotensin system appears to be an excellent approach, not only for reducing BP but also for correcting many of the cellular, biochemical, hemodynamic, and structural abnormalities seen in the diabetic kidney. These drugs appear to be very powerful antiproteinuric agents, although the exact mechanism of action remains to be fully defined. Based on the discovery in the late 1990s that proteinuria in a range of nephropathies could occur as a result of molecular and structural abnormalities in a highly specialized structure known as the slit diaphragm within the glomerular epithelial cell (podocyte), a number of experimental studies, subsequently confirmed in humans, showed that depletion of one of these slit pore proteins, nephrin, could be attenuated or prevented by agents that interrupt the renin-angiotensin system.[499]

In addition to promoting glomerular nephrin depletion, angiotensin II also appears to have other actions that promote the development of proteinuria, including trophic effects on the kidney and increasing glomerular membrane pore size.[500] Although many investigators have focused on the renin-angiotensin system and, in particular, the vasoconstrictor angiotensin II, it is increasingly appreciated that other vasoconstrictors may be important. These include endothelin and a number of vasodilators such as NO, bradykinin, atrial natriuretic peptide, and vasodilative angiotensins such as angiotensin(1-7).[501] Exploration of the role of vasoactive hormones and their respective receptors in the diabetic kidney is critical for designing new treatments for this condition, because these pathways are ideal targets for drug development. This point has already been demonstrated for agents that interrupt the renin-angiotensin system, including ACE inhibitors and ARBs.

Pathology

Diabetic renal disease was originally described as a glomerulopathy associated with diffuse or nodular glomerulosclerosis.[464] Subsequent studies using electron microscopy revealed that glomerular basement membrane thickening and mesangial expansion are prominent glomerular abnormalities in diabetes (Fig. 33-33).[476] Prospective studies showed that these changes predict, to a certain degree, the development of overt renal disease in patients with T1DM. However, fewer than one third of diabetic patients with microalbuminuria have the typical glomerulopathy described by Kimmelsteil and Wilson in 1936.[464,502] Although initial studies emphasized the mesangial cell changes in the glomerulus, glomerular epithelial cell abnormalities represent a new area of active research.[48] Podocyte dysfunction and subsequent apoptosis ultimately leading to depletion of podocytes within the glomerulus appear to play a pivotal role in the development of proteinuria in diabetes.

Although most of the focus has been on glomerular changes in the diabetic kidney, more recent studies have identified important changes in other sites within the kidney, including the tubules, interstitium, medulla, and papilla.[474] *Diabetic tubulopathy* is characterized by a variety of structural and functional changes including tubuloepithelial cell hypertrophy, tubular basement membrane thickening, epithelial-mesenchymal transition,[131] and the accumulation of glycogen (see Fig. 33-33). There is also an expansion of the interstitial space with infiltration of various cell types, including myofibroblasts and macrophages.

Glomerulopathy

Mesangial expansion
Glomerular hypertension
Diffuse thickening of the GBM
Broadening of foot processes
Podocyte loss
Reduced slit pore proteins
Glomerulomegaly
Kimmelstiel-Wilson lesion
Adhesions to Bowman's capsule
Neovascularization
Nodular and diffuse glomerulosclerosis

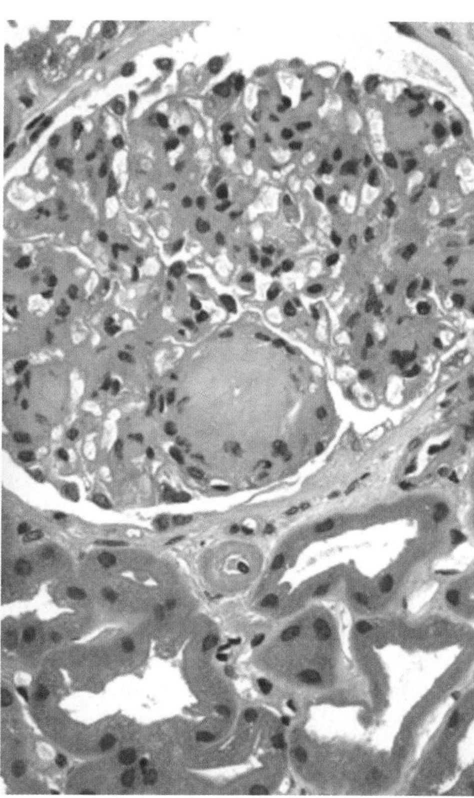

Tubulopathy

Tubular hyperplasia and hypertrophy
Progressive and cumulative atrophy
Thickening of the TBM
Epithelial mesenchymal transition
Accumulation of lysosomal bodies
Armani-Ebstein lesion
Reduced tubular brush border
Increased tubular salt reabsorption
Increased Na^+/H^+ antiporter activity
Impaired tubular acidification
Abnormal tubuloglomerular feedback
Decreased endocytosis of protein
Abnormal lysosomal processing
Impaired uptake of organic ions

Figure 33-33 Glomerular and tubular manifestations of diabetic nephropathy. GBM, glomerular basement membrane; TBM, tubular basement membrane.

These tubular changes represent more than just the aftermath of diabetic nephropathy. The dysregulation of tubular functions in diabetes can precede or accompany the changes in the renal glomerulus and the onset of albuminuria.[502] Indeed, the functional and structural changes in the proximal tubule may be a key contributor to the development and progression of diabetic nephropathy.[474] For example, it has been suggested that tubuloglomerular feedback mechanisms can drive hyperfiltration associated with diabetes[470] and that tubular dysfunction can contribute to albuminuria through defective uptake and lysosomal processing.[478] Renal function and prognosis correlate better with structural lesions in the tubules and cortical interstitium than with classic glomerular changes of diabetic nephropathy.

Renal Artery Stenosis

Because diabetic patients have, in general, an increased burden of atherosclerosis, they appear to have a higher risk of renal artery stenosis. However, although angiographic studies have demonstrated a high prevalence of renal artery stenosis in diabetic patients, these lesions are often of no hemodynamic significance. Nevertheless, a small subgroup have a hemodynamically significant stenosis enhancing hypertension, increasing the risk of acute pulmonary edema, and inducing progressive renal impairment.[503] In such subjects, specific interventions such as surgery or angioplasty need to be considered.[504] Furthermore, some patients have bilateral renal artery stenosis that, on commencement of treatment with an agent such as an ACE inhibitor, can lead to acute renal failure.[505] In most patients in this situation, if the renal failure is diagnosed early, cessation of the ACE inhibitor leads to rapid restoration of renal function.

Renal Papillary Necrosis

Renal papillary necrosis involves a severe destructive process that presumably results from ischemia to the medulla and papilla.[505]Beethoven's final illness might have been papillary necrosis in the context of diabetes.[507] The papilla is very sensitive to these ischemic changes because even in the normal setting it is exposed to a relatively hypoxic environment. Concomitant exacerbating factors include urinary tract infection and analgesic abuse. The importance of ischemia and possibly angiotensin II in this disorder has been suggested in experimental studies using transgenic rats that overexpress renin and angiotensin II in their kidneys after induction of diabetes.[508] In these rats, diabetes was associated with development of papillary necrosis, and development of papillary necrosis was prevented by blockade of the renin-angiotensin system. Clinically, papillary necrosis often manifests as flank pain, hematuria, and fever. Urinalysis reveals red and white blood cells, bacteria, and papillary fragments. Ureteric obstruction can occur as a result of these fragments and must be addressed as an emergency.

Renal Tubular Acidosis

A well-known functional abnormality associated with diabetic tubulopathy is *renal tubular acidosis,* which manifests as hyperkalemia and hyperchloremic metabolic acidosis.[509] This is thought to be a manifestation of hyporeninemic hypoaldosteronism associated with diabetes, which results in reduction of proximal tubule ammonia production to levels that are inadequate to buffer acid in the distal nephron. The precise causes of this abnormality remain to be established. In some patients, there appears to be a defect in the conversion of prorenin to active renin.[510] It has also been suggested that damage to the tubular cells of the juxtaglomerular apparatus associated with diabetes can contribute to impaired renin release, possibly due to reduced renal prostaglandin production and elevated vasopressin levels.[511]

A major risk associated with hyporeninemic hypoaldosteronism is the development of life-threatening hyperkalemia. This is an increasingly important issue because of the widespread use of ACE inhibitors and ARBs, often in combination, in this population. This is further exacerbated by the use of potassium-sparing diuretics (e.g., spironolactone) and β-blockers.

Other Renal Manifestations

Because many diabetic subjects have impaired renal function, they are at high risk for increased renal impairment from certain nephrotoxic agents. One of the most important risks relates to radiocontrast dyes.[512] If possible, patients with diabetes and renal impairment should avoid imaging studies that involve the use of contrast agents and, in particular, multiple studies performed in rapid succession. Where intravenous contrast forms an indispensable tool to management, low-osmolality, nonionic or gadolinium-based contrast media may be less nephrotoxic in patients with renal failure.[513] It is also critical to ensure that patients who require such procedures are well hydrated before, during, and after the procedure. *N*-acetylcysteine, a thiol-containing antioxidant, shows promise to protect against contrast-induced nephropathy.[514] The oral hypoglycemic drug metformin should also be discontinued before contrast procedures to prevent life-threatening lactic acidosis.

Management

Blood pressure and glycemic control represent the major cornerstones for preventing and treating diabetic nephropathy (Figs. 33-34 and 33-35). In the early 1980s a number of Scandinavian researchers found that aggressive BP reduction reduces the rate of progression of diabetic nephropathy,[515,516] and in the 1990s other researchers found that intensified glycemic control has a similar benefit in both T1DM (DCCT)[308] and T2DM (UKPDS) diabetic subjects.[517] These findings have led to the view that optimization of BP and plasma glucose levels should be the mainstay of therapy for diabetic nephropathy.

Glycemic Control

The importance of glucose as a factor in the progression of diabetic kidney disease, as initially suggested from epidemiologic and preclinical studies, was clearly demonstrated in the DCCT study in patients with T1DM.[308] In both the primary and secondary prevention cohorts of the study, any decrease in HbA_{1c} was strongly associated with a reduction in the risk of development of microalbuminuria as well as a decrease in the risk of progression to overt nephropathy. The follow-up EDIC study confirmed long-lasting benefits of this therapeutic approach. The UKPDS clearly demonstrated a role for intensified glycemic control in subjects newly diagnosed with T2DM when treatment led to a reduction in HbA_{1c} from 7.9% to 7.0%.[518] The recent ADVANCE study demonstrated that a further reduction of HbA_{1c} to an average of 6.5% was associated with a further reduction in renal events, as assessed by the development and progression of microalbuminuria.[519] Therefore, despite the ongoing controversy as to the appropriate HbA_{1c} target to reduce macrovascular disease brought about by the findings from the ACCORD study,[520] no such

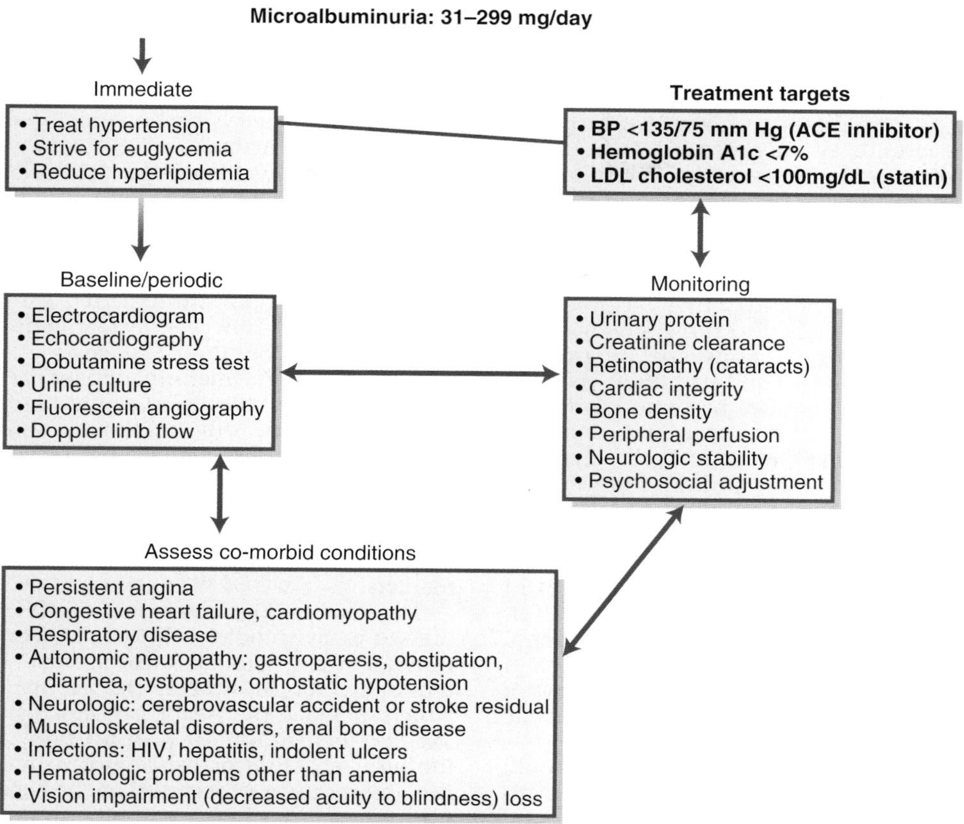

Figure 33-34 Flow chart illustrating the management of diabetic nephropathy before the onset of renal failure. ACE, angiotensin-converting enzyme; BP, blood pressure; HIV, human immunodeficiency virus; LDL, low-density lipoprotein.

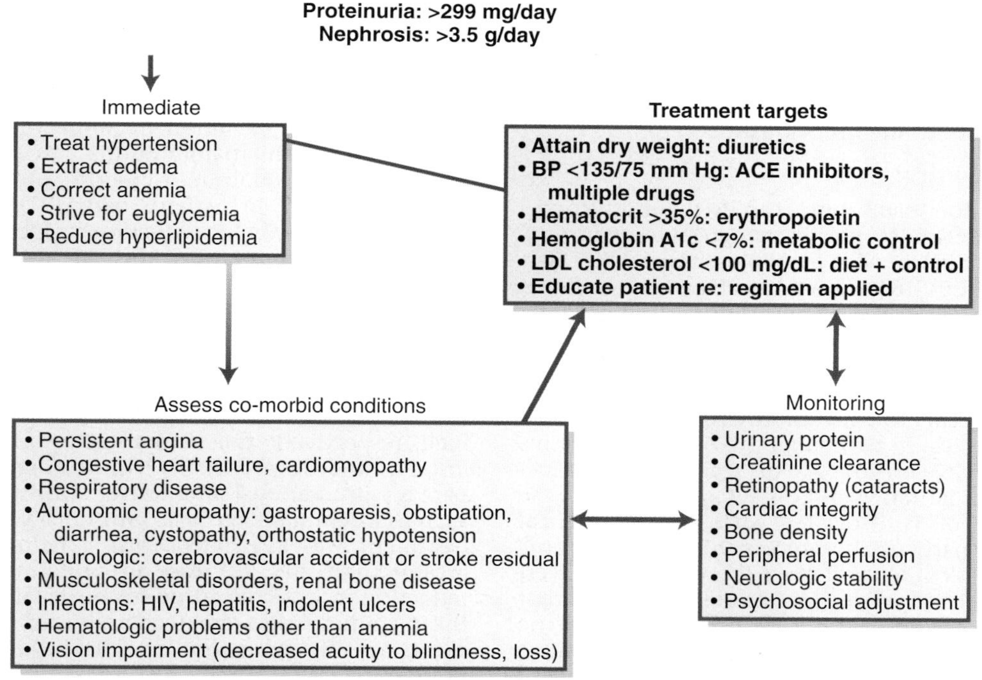

Figure 33-35 Flow chart illustrating the management of diabetic nephropathy after the onset of clinical proteinuria. ACE, angiotensin-converting enzyme; BP, blood pressure; HIV, human immunodeficiency virus; LDL, low-density lipoprotein.

controversy as to a possible deleterious effect of intensified glycemic control has been reported with respect to nephropathy.

It remains to be determined how useful intensification of glycemic control is in the setting of overt nephropathy as a last-ditch strategy to delay the onset of ESRD. Aggressive management of hypertension is clearly more important than glycemic control in reducing cardiovascular events and slowing renal disease progression at this stage of relatively advanced disease, although some studies suggest that poor glycemic control can accelerate the loss of renal function in diabetic nephropathy.[517] However, a number of large studies have failed to show any evidence that strict glycemic control per se retards renal progression once overt nephropathy is present.[521] In addition, as renal function fails, tight glycemic control becomes more hazardous, with an increased risk of hypoglycemia. Nonetheless, because there is sufficient evidence that glycemic control can reduce both macrovascular events and microvascular complications of diabetes at other sites, it is reasonable to suggest that optimization of metabolic control in patients with overt nephropathy remains worthwhile.

Similar benefits on renal disease in the context of T2DM are seen after optimization of glycemic control.[3] However, the choice of agent remains controversial. Certainly, several types of drugs are able to improve glycemic control in patients with T2DM; however, the particular advantages of one class over another for preventing and treating diabetic nephropathy remain to be established.

A number of differences in the side effect profiles should influence prescribing habits. In patients with renal impairment, particular care must be exercised in selecting and dosing oral agents, because an accumulation of the drug or active metabolites can lead to hypoglycemia (e.g., with glyburide) and other serious adverse effects such as lactic acidosis (e.g., with metformin). Thiazolodinediones, such as pioglitazone and rosiglitazone, should be used with caution in patients with advanced nephropathy who have, or are at risk for, heart failure.

Other agents that directly inhibit glucose-induced changes in various biochemical pathways will likely become available. These include benfotiamine, a thiamine alternative that appears to inhibit the downstream effects of mitochondrial ROS generation,[522] and various antiglycation strategies,[523] as outlined previously.

Blood Pressure Control

A sustained reduction in BP appears to be the most important single intervention to prevent progressive nephropathy in T1DM and T2DM. For example, in the UKPDS, a reduction in BP from 154 to 144 mm Hg was associated with a 30% reduction in microalbuminuria.[524] All national and international guidelines now emphasize the importance of BP reduction in the diabetic patient. Although many guidelines suggest specific targets to be achieved, no such threshold appears to exist for any renal end point in patients with diabetes. In particular, the risk of progressive diabetic nephropathy continues to decrease with BP reductions into the normal range and below, meaning that the lowest achievable BP is associated with the best clinical outcomes. This is particularly important in those patients with the greatest risk of renal damage (i.e., those with overt nephropathy). In these patients, it has been suggested that optimal BP control is less than 125/75 mm Hg.[525] In the recent subanalysis from the BP arm of the ADVANCE study, no BP threshold was detected. Specifically, in those subjects in whom BP was reduced to levels even lower than currently recommended in national and international guidelines, there was a further decrease in renal events.[526] Therefore, it may be worth considering treating some patients with T2DM to achieve BP levels below those currently recommended, provided that the patients can tolerate these lower levels without major side effects such as dizziness and syncope.

There is good evidence that tight BP control, no matter how achieved, is associated with a significant reduction in the risk of microalbuminuria (primary prevention). Although BP reduction appears to be paramount, there is also evidence that ACE inhibitors[527] have renoprotective actions beyond their antihypertensive effects for primary prevention.[528-530] However, if treatment should commence in the normoalbuminuric stage, such a strategy would involve treating the majority of patients who are not at risk for nephropathy. Ideally, it would be useful to be able to identify patients, still normoalbuminuric, whose likelihood of progression is increased. As yet, no such markers of predisposition to renal disease are available, although serum prorenin[477] and modest elevations in urinary albumin excretion, albeit still within the normal range (borderline microalbuminuria),[483] might ultimately be such markers.

The issue of primary prevention has recently been readdressed in two studies in which subjects with normoalbuminuria were treated with agents that interrupt the renin-angiotensin system. In the first and smaller trial, which included the performance of sequential renal biopsies, no benefit of early institution of either the ACE inhibitor enalapril or the angiotensin II receptor antagonist losartan was observed (lack of benefit was defined as not only a lack of effect on albuminuria but also no significant retardation in progression of renal morphologic injury).[531] In the second, much larger trial, known as the DIRECT study, the angiotensin II antagonist, candesartan, despite some modest retinoprotective effects, had no major impact on reducing the new onset of microalbuminuria.[531]

In secondary prevention studies, the additional benefits achieved from blockade of the renin-angiotensin system are clearer.[532] A meta-analysis incorporating the findings of more than 10 studies in patients with microalbuminuria demonstrated the ability of ACE inhibitors to retard the development of overt proteinuria and also to decrease urinary albumin excretion by more than 30%. In some patients with microalbuminuria, ACE inhibition can reduce urinary albumin excretion into the normoalbuminuric range.[528] In patients with T1DM and overt proteinuria, aggressive BP reduction reduced proteinuria by up to 50% and retarded the rate of decline in renal function.[515,516]

Similar studies have been performed in patients with T2DM. Two landmark trials, RENAAL (Reduction in Endpoints in patients with Non-insulin-dependent diabetes mellitus with the Angiotensin II Antagonist Losartan) and IDNT (Irbesartan in Diabetic Nephropathy Trial), examined, respectively, the renoprotective effects of the ARBs losartan and irbesartan.[533,534] In both studies, when compared with various alternative antihypertensive agents such as calcium antagonists (but not ACE inhibitors), ARB treatment was associated with a reduction in ESRD, a greater than 30% decrease in proteinuria, and a major reduction in hospitalization for heart failure. As a result of these studies, ARBs are recommended as first-line treatment for BP reduction in T2DM patients with overt proteinuria.[535]

Although ACE inhibitors have not been as extensively studied in this population, the recently reported DETAIL

(Diabetics Exposed to Telmisartan And EnalaprIL) trial suggested similar renoprotective actions of both drug classes.[536] Similar findings comparing the angiotensin II antagonist, telmisartan, to the ACE inhibitor, ramipril, were also reported in the much larger ONTARGET study, although that trial was not performed exclusively in diabetic subjects.[537] Therefore, from a clinical perspective, no clear differences between these two drug classes have been identified. (The one exception is cough, which occurs in 5% to 30% of patients taking ACE inhibitors, depending on ethnicity [higher in Asian subjects].) In microalbuminuric T2DM subjects, ARBs have also been demonstrated to have a role. For example, in the IRMA2 (IRbesartan MicroAlbuminuria type 2) trial, irbesartan dose-dependently reduced the risk of development of macroproteinuria,[538] confirming the findings seen predominantly with ACE inhibitors in microalbuminuric T1DM subjects.[528]

Another approach to inhibit the renin-angiotensin system has involved the use of the recently introduced renin inhibitors such as aliskiren. For example, in the AVOID study in T2DM subjects,[539] this agent appeared to have an additional effect on albuminuria when administered with the angiotensin II antagonist, losartan. The long-term implications of this drug study for renal function and cardiovascular events are as yet unknown and are under active clinical investigation. Other approaches focusing on BP reduction continue to be examined in these populations. These include use of mineralocorticoid receptor antagonists such as spironolactone[540] and the more selective agent, epleronone, which has fewer antiandrogenic side effects.[541] Furthermore, a number of agents at various stages of preclinical and early clinical development are under investigation, including endothelin antagonists and vasopeptidase (dual ACE/neutral endopeptidase [NEP]) inhibitors.[542]

Other Approaches

Low-protein diets (0.75 g/kg per day) have been shown to retard the progression of renal disease, although the data are not totally convincing for diabetic nephropathy per se. A meta-analysis of five studies in T1DM subjects supported a minor renoprotective role for these diets,[543] but this has not been a universal finding.[544] There are even fewer data in regard to T2DM subjects with overt nephropathy.[545] However, the expected benefits that can be achieved through protein restriction in patients with diabetic nephropathy are at best modest in comparison with adequate BP control and blockade of the renin-angiotensin system. Moreover, the nutritional impact of such interventions must be carefully considered, particularly in patients with brittle glycemic control.

The role of lipid-lowering agents as renoprotective drugs remains controversial. Although in rodents a large body of evidence suggests that lipids promote renal injury and that various lipid-lowering drugs reduce nephropathy even in the setting of no or minimal effect on lipids,[546] the data in humans are variable.[547] However, in a study of fenofibrate in T2DM, there was an impressive reduction in albuminuria.[548] Furthermore, in the Heart Protection Study, simvastatin appeared to retard the decline in renal function, although this analysis was not confined to the diabetic subgroup.[549] Another group has also reported a potential renoprotective effect of a statin,[550] although this effect has not been observed in all studies. Nevertheless, because CVD is so prominent in diabetic patients, particularly those with incipient or overt renal disease, lipid-lowering treatment should be considered in most patients independent of its putative renoprotective actions.[551]

Other approaches to consider include correction of anemia with agents such as erythropoietin.[552] The role of these agents as renoprotective drugs remains to be clarified,[553] but the potential benefits in terms of general patient well-being and reduction of left ventricular hypertrophy[554] provide a rationale for the judicious use of such agents in diabetic patients. However, in the recently reported TREAT study, which focused on cardiovascular events and mortality using the erythropoietin analogue, darbopoietin, the drug was not shown to be renoprotective and was unfortunately associated with a twofold increase in cerebrovascular events.[555]

Over the last few years, several clinical trials targeting diabetic nephropathy with novel agents have yielded disappointing results. For example, PKC-β inhibition with ruboxistaurin, which had renal benefits in experimental diabetes, failed to show any major benefits on albuminuria in T2DM subjects.[556] Another promising agent, sulodexide, which was postulated to restore the glomerular charge by repleting the loss of glycosaminoglycans[557] and thereby act as an antiproteinuric and ultimately renoprotective drug, also failed to demonstrate any evidence of renoprotection in several large trials. Finally, a promising endothelin antagonist, avosentan, was assessed in the ASCEND trial.[558] Although this drug was associated with impressive reductions in albuminuria, the associated side effect of fluid retention has reduced the current level of enthusiasm for this agent.

Treatment of the Diabetic Uremic Patient

Renal impairment in a patient with diabetes necessitates changes in therapy. Often, blood glucose control becomes more brittle because the half-life of insulin is prolonged and the renal response to hypoglycemia is impaired. High swinging blood glucose levels in a patient with nephropathy can often mistakenly lead to an increase in oral therapy. However, in patients with renal impairment, particular care must be exercised in the selection and dosing of oral hypoglycemic therapy. Nonsteroidal anti-inflammatory drugs (NSAIDs) and cyclooxygenase-2 (COX2) inhibitors should be avoided if possible, because their use is associated with inadequate BP control, often as a result of reduced efficacy of antihypertensive drug therapy. Patients at high risk for progressive deterioration in their renal function should be considered for early referral to a nephrology service for management of renal failure (Fig. 33-36). This facilitates access to erythropoietin therapy and control of calcium phosphate balance and to planning for renal replacement therapy with the preemptive placement of access catheters and lines. Delay in referral can result in a more precipitous start to renal replacement and usually a bad prognostic outcome.[559]

Many options are now available for the diabetic patient requiring renal replacement therapy.[560] These include home- or facility-based hemodialysis, peritoneal dialysis, renal transplantation (cadaveric or living related donor), and combined pancreas-kidney transplantation. Most patients choose hemodialysis rather than peritoneal dialysis, although the data are conflicting regarding which approach leads to better survival (Table 33-6). Some patients opt for withdrawal of treatment because their quality of life, with advanced CVD, visual impairment, and amputations, is poor.

The Burden of Nephropathy

One must never consider renal disease in a diabetic patient in isolation. Proteinuria per se is strongly associated with

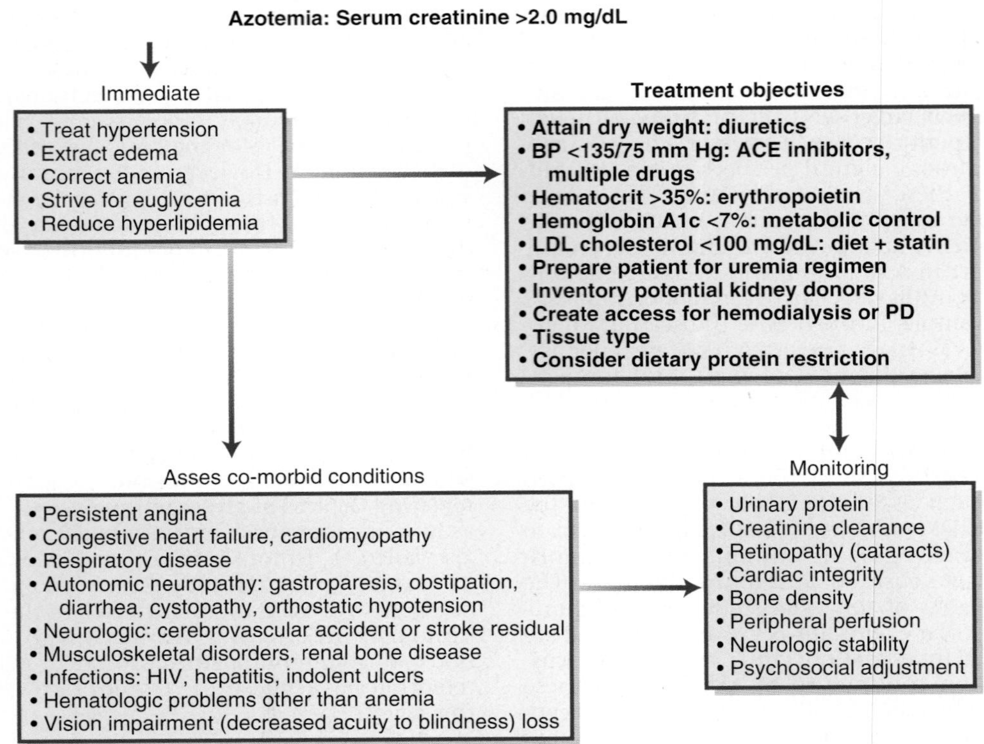

Figure 33-36 Flow chart illustrating the management of diabetic nephropathy after onset of renal failure. ACE, angiotensin-converting enzyme; BP, blood pressure; HIV, human immunodeficiency virus; LDL, low-density lipoprotein; PD, peritoneal dialysis.

TABLE 33-6

Options in Therapy for End-Stage Renal Disease in Diabetic Patients

Variable	Peritoneal Dialysis	Hemodialysis	Kidney Transplantation
Extensive extrarenal disease	No limitation	No limitation except for hypotension	Excluded in cardiovascular insufficiency
Geriatric patients		No limitation	Arbitrary exclusion as determined by program
Complete rehabilitation	Rare, if ever	Very few patients	Common so long as graft functions
Death rate	Much higher than for nondiabetic patients	Much higher than for nondiabetic patients	About the same as for nondiabetic patients
First-year survival	~75%	~75%	>90%
Morbidity during first year	~15 days in hospital	~12 days in hospital	Weeks to months hospitalized
Survival to second decade	Almost never	<5%	~1 in 5
Progression of complications	Usual and unremitting; hyperglycemia and hyperlipidemia	Usual and unremitting; might benefit from metabolic control	Interdicted by functioning pancreas plus kidney; partially ameliorated by correction of azotemia
Special advantage	Can be self-performed; avoids swings in solute and level of intravascular volume	Can be self-performed; efficient extraction of solute and water in hours	Cures uremia; freedom to travel
Disadvantages	Peritonitis; hyperinsulinemia; hyperglycemia, hyperlipidemia; long hours of treatment; more days hospitalized than with either hemodialysis or transplantation	Blood access a hazard for clotting, hemorrhage, and infection; cyclic hypotension, weakness, aluminum toxicity, amyloidosis	Cosmetic disfigurement, hypertension, personal expense for cytotoxic drugs; induced malignancy; HIV transmission
Patient acceptance	Variable, usual compliance with passive tolerance for regimen	Variable; often noncompliant with dietary, metabolic, or antihypertensive components of regimen	Enthusiastic during periods of good renal allograft function; exalted when pancreas proffers euglycemia
Relative cost	Most expensive over long run	Less expensive than kidney transplantation in the first year; subsequent years more expensive	Pancreas plus kidney engraftment most expensive uremia therapy for diabetics; after first year, kidney transplantation alone is lowest-cost option

other complications such as macrovascular disease, heart failure, and retinopathy, and treatments directed toward one complication may be useful for the others. Intensified glycemic control has been shown to be particularly useful for other microvascular complications,[2] and the various antihypertensive regimens, particularly those using agents that interrupt the renin-angiotensin system, also confer important cardiovascular benefits, such as reducing heart failure.[533] Therefore, as clearly expounded in the Steno-2 study, the multifactorial approach in microalbuminuric subjects leads to renal benefits and also confers other advantages to the diabetic patient.[561] Because those patients with renal disease have the greatest risk for nonrenal complications, it stands to reason that they also are likely to have the greatest absolute benefit from risk-reduction strategies.

DIABETIC NEUROPATHIES

Diabetic neuropathies are a heterogeneous group of disorders that cause a wide range of abnormalities. They are among the most common long-term complications of diabetes and are a significant source of morbidity and mortality.[562,563] Estimates of the prevalence of neuropathy vary substantially, depending on specific diagnostic criteria.[564,565] In the United States, prevalence estimates have ranged from 5% to 100%.[562,564,565-567] In Pirart's classic study of a cohort of 4400 diabetic patients, prevalence was found to reach approximately 45% after 25 years.[568] Using this estimate, about 7 million persons in the United States alone have diabetic neuropathy, and about 2.7 million have painful neuropathy.[569] Furthermore, it is now evident that neuropathy can occur with impaired glucose tolerance[570] and with the metabolic syndrome in the absence of hyperglycemia.[571] It is the most common form of neuropathy in the developed countries of the world; it accounts for more hospitalizations than all the other diabetic complications combined; and it is responsible for 50% to 75% of nontrauma amputations.[566,567] Diabetic peripheral neuropathy is also responsible for weakness and ataxia, with an estimated increase in likelihood of falling that is 15 times that of the unaffected population.[572,573]

Diabetic neuropathy is a set of clinical syndromes that affect distinct regions of the nervous system, singly or combined. Clinical signs and symptoms can be nonspecific and insidious, and progression can be slow. Neuropathy can be silent and go undetected while exercising its ravages, or it can manifest with clinical symptoms and signs that mimic those seen in many other diseases. It is, therefore, diagnosed by exclusion.

The true prevalence is not known and depends on the criteria and methods used to define neuropathy. Of patients attending a diabetes clinic, 25% volunteered symptoms, but 50% were found to have neuropathy after a simple clinical test such as eliciting the ankle reflex or vibration perception test. Almost 90% tested positive on sophisticated tests of autonomic function or peripheral sensation.[574] Neuropathy is grossly underdiagnosed by endocrinologists and nonendocrinologists.[575] Neurologic complications occur equally in T1DM and T2DM and additionally in various forms of acquired diabetes.[565]

The major morbidity associated with somatic neuropathy is foot ulceration, the precursor of gangrene and limb loss. Neuropathy increases the risk of amputation 1.7-fold overall, 12-fold if there is deformity (itself a consequence of neuropathy), and 36-fold if there is a history of previous ulceration.[576] There are 96,000 amputations performed in the United States each year, one every 10 minutes, and neuropathy is the major contributor in 87% of cases.[563] It has tremendous negative effects on the quality of life of persons with diabetes.[577] Once autonomic neuropathy is present, life can become quite dismal, and the mortality rate approximates 25% to 50% within 5 to 10 years.[578-581] The presence of neuropathy can severely affect quality of life, causing impaired activities of daily living, compromised physical functioning, and depression.[577,582] Impairment of physical functioning is associated with a 15-fold increase in the likelihood of falling and fractures, particularly in older diabetics.[583] Depression complicates the management of neuropathic pain and is a predictor of progression of neuropathy.[582]

Classification

Diabetic neuropathy is not a single entity but a number of different syndromes with subclinical or clinical manifestations depending on the classes of nerve fibers involved. According to the San Antonio Convention,[584] the main groups of neurologic disturbance in diabetes mellitus include the following:

- Subclinical neuropathy, which is determined by abnormalities in electrodiagnostic and quantitative sensory testing
- Diffuse clinical neuropathy with distal symmetric sensorimotor and autonomic syndromes
- Focal syndromes

Subclinical neuropathy is diagnosed on the basis of abnormal electrodiagnostic tests with decreased nerve conduction velocity (NCV) or decreased amplitudes; abnormal quantitative sensory tests (QST) for vibration, tactile, thermal warming, and cooling thresholds; and quantitative autonomic function tests (QAFT) revealing diminished heart rate variation with deep breathing, Valsalva maneuver, and postural testing. The importance of the skin biopsy as a diagnostic tool for diabetic polyneuropathy (DPN) is now firmly established.[571,585] This technique quantitates small epidermal nerve fibers through antibody staining of the panaxonal marker protein gene product 9.5 (PGP 9.5). It is minimally invasive (3-mm-diameter punch biopsies), yet enables a direct study of small fibers that cannot be evaluated by NCV studies. Intraepidermal nerve fiber density is reduced in approximately 88% of subjects with small-fiber neuropathy, compared with 10% of healthy controls.[586] Skin biopsy with intraepidermal nerve fiber density evaluation may be more sensitive than either clinical examination or quantitative sensory testing for detecting abnormalities in subjects with the small-fiber neuropathy phenotype. In a recent retrospective evaluation of 486 patients referred to neurology or neuromuscular disease clinics, skin biopsy showed a diagnostic efficiency of 88.4%, compared with 54.6% for clinical examination and 46.9% for QSTs.[587] The last evidence-based review on distal symmetric polyneuropathy from the American Academy of Neurology concluded that skin biopsy is a validated technique for determining intraepidermal nerve fiber density and may be considered for the diagnosis of DPN, particularly small-fiber sensory neuropathy.[588]

The different clinical presentations of diabetic neuropathy are schematically illustrated in Figure 33-37.

Natural History

The natural history of neuropathies separates them into two distinct entities: those that progress gradually with

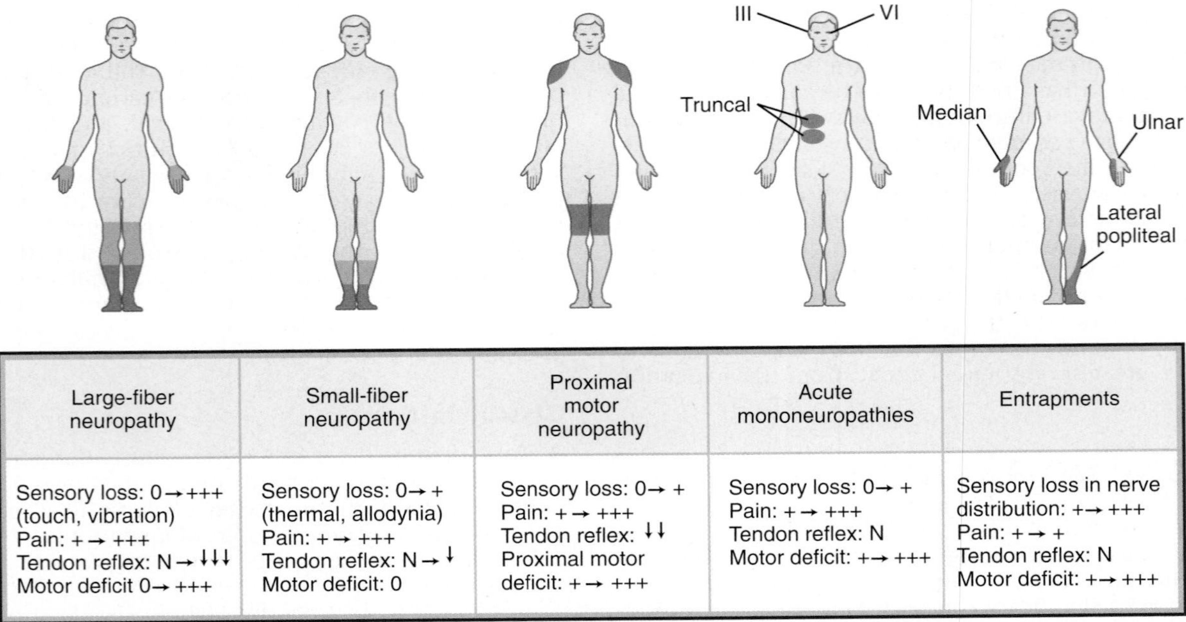

Large-fiber neuropathy	Small-fiber neuropathy	Proximal motor neuropathy	Acute mononeuropathies	Entrapments
Sensory loss: 0→+++ (touch, vibration) Pain: +→ +++ Tendon reflex: N→↓↓↓ Motor deficit 0→ +++	Sensory loss: 0→ + (thermal, allodynia) Pain: +→ +++ Tendon reflex: N→↓ Motor deficit: 0	Sensory loss: 0→ + Pain: +→ +++ Tendon reflex: ↓↓ Proximal motor deficit: +→ +++	Sensory loss: 0→ + Pain: +→ +++ Tendon reflex: N Motor deficit: +→ +++	Sensory loss in nerve distribution: +→ +++ Pain: +→ + Tendon reflex: N Motor deficit: +→ +++

Figure 33-37 **Clinical presentations of diabetic neuropathies.** (Modified from Pickup J, Williams G, eds. *Textbook of Diabetes*, Vol 1. Oxford, UK: Blackwell Scientific, 1997.)

increasing duration of diabetes and those that remit, usually completely. Sensory and autonomic neuropathies typically progress. Although the symptoms of mononeuropathies, radiculopathies, and acute painful neuropathies are severe, they are short-lived, and patients tend to recover.[589]

Progression of neuropathy is related to glycemic control in both T1DM and T2DM.[590,591] The most rapid deterioration of nerve function occurs soon after the onset of T1DM, and within 2 to 3 years the rate of progression slows. In contrast, in T2DM, slowing of NCVs may be one of the earliest neuropathic abnormalities and often is present even at diagnosis.[592] After diagnosis, slowing of NCV usually progresses at a steady rate of approximately 1 m/sec per year, and the level of impairment is positively correlated with duration of diabetes. Although in most studies, symptomatic patients are more likely to have slower NCVs than patients without symptoms, NCVs do not relate to the severity of symptoms. In a long-term follow-up study of T2DM patients,[593] the prevalence of electrophysiologic abnormalities in the lower limb increased from 8% at baseline to 42% after 10 years.

A decrease in sensory and motor amplitudes, indicating axonal destruction, is more pronounced than the slowing of the NCVs. An increase of about 2 points in an 80-point clinical scale can be expected per year. These scales contain information on motor, sensory, and autonomic signs and symptoms. Using objective measures of sensory function, such as the vibration perception threshold test, the rate of decline in function has been reported to be 1 to 2 vibration units per year. However, this rate of evolution may be declining. For example, in a study of nerve growth factor (NGF), the vibration perception threshold in the placebo group was identical to that in the treatment group at the beginning of the study and at the end of 1 year.[594,595]

Host factors pertaining to general health and nerve nutrition are changing. This is particularly important in studies on the treatment of diabetic neuropathy, which have always relied on differences between drug treatment and placebo and have apparently been successful because of the decline in placebo-treated patients.[596] Based on the earlier estimates of change, clinically meaningful loss of vibration perception and conduction velocity was estimated to take at least 3 years, dictating the need for studies to be carried out over a longer period of time.

It is also important to recognize that diabetic neuropathy is a disorder in which the prevailing abnormality is a loss of axons that electrophysiologically translates to a reduction in the amplitude and not the velocity of conduction. Changes in NCV might not be an appropriate means of monitoring progress or deterioration of nerve function. It has always been assumed that diabetes affects the longest fibers first—hence, the increased predisposition in taller persons.[597] Now it seems that small-fiber involvement can herald the onset of neuropathy and even diabetes. Small-fiber function is not detectable by standard electrophysiology and requires measurement of sensory, neurovascular, and autonomic thresholds and cutaneous nerve fiber density.[571,598-600] There are few data on the longitudinal trends in small-fiber dysfunction, although it appears that the nerve fiber loss in prediabetic neuropathy might respond to lifestyle changes.[601]

Much remains to be learned about the natural history of diabetic autonomic neuropathy. Karamitsos and colleagues[602] have reported that the progression of diabetic autonomic neuropathy is significant during the 2 years following its discovery. The mortality rate for diabetic autonomic neuropathy has been estimated to be 44% within 2.5 years after diagnosis of symptomatic autonomic neuropathy.[578] A meta-analysis[603] revealed that the mortality rate after 5.8 years of diabetes with symptomatic autonomic neuropathy was 29%. In a meta-analysis of 12 published studies, reduced cardiovascular function as measured by heart rate variability was shown to be associated with an increased risk of silent MI.[581]

Similarly, a meta-analysis of prospective studies demonstrated increased mortality in patients with cardiac autonomic neuropathy, with the risk ratio increasing in direct proportion to the number of autonomic abnormalities.[580,581] The RR of mortality from 15 studies (N = 2900) was increased in patients with cardiac autonomic neuropathy by 2.14 (95% confidence interval [CI], 1.83 to 2.51).[581] However, if cardiac autonomic neuropathy is defined by the presence of at least two abnormal autonomic function tests, this risk increased to 3.45 (95% CI, 2.66 to 4.47).[580] Probably the greatest justification for carrying out autonomic function tests resides in their predictive capacity for subsequent cardiovascular events and unexplained sudden death. In the ACCORD study, there was a significant increase in mortality in the intensively treated arm of glycemic control. Analysis of the hazard risk of mortality revealed an increase of up to 2.5 with loss of heart rate variability. If symptoms of neuropathy such as numbness were included, the risk rose to 4.33.[604] This is a cogent argument for identifying people at risk and tailoring the management of diabetes accordingly, as well as a serious consideration for study designs estimating cardiovascular risk or benefit for the future.

Clinical Presentation

An international consensus meeting on the outpatient diagnosis and management of diabetic neuropathy agreed on the following as a simple definition of diabetic neuropathy: "the presence of symptoms and/or signs of peripheral nerve dysfunction in people with diabetes after the exclusion of other causes."[588] It was also agreed that neuropathy cannot be diagnosed without a careful clinical examination; absence of symptoms cannot be equated with absence of neuropathy, because asymptomatic neuropathy is common. The American Diabetes Association (ADA) has endorsed these recommendations.[605]

The importance of excluding nondiabetic causes was emphasized in the Rochester Diabetic Neuropathy Study, in which up to 10% of peripheral neuropathy in diabetic patients was deemed to be of nondiabetic etiology.[565] Many conditions need to be excluded before the diagnosis of diabetic neuropathy can be made.[563] A more detailed definition of neuropathy was previously accepted by the San Antonio Consensus Conference: "Diabetic neuropathy is a descriptive term meaning a demonstrable disorder, either clinically evident or sub-clinical, that occurs in the setting of diabetes mellitus without other causes for peripheral neuropathy. The neuropathic disorder includes manifestations in the somatic and/or autonomic parts of the peripheral nervous system."[584] A consensus panel was convened in 2009 and revised some of these definitions, but the information is not as yet in the public domain.

It is generally agreed that diabetic neuropathy should not be diagnosed on the basis of one symptom, sign, or test alone. A minimum of two abnormalities (from symptoms, signs, nerve conduction abnormalities, quantitative sensory tests, or quantitative autonomic tests) is recommended.[606] Diabetic neuropathy is, however, woefully underdiagnosed by endocrinologists as well as nonendocrinologists. In the GOAL A_{1c} study,[575] the absence of neuropathy in 7000 patients could be adequately determined, but the presence of mild neuropathy was detected accurately only one third of the time, and accuracy of detection reached 75% only if neuropathy was severe. Clearly, there is a need for education on methods for detecting neuropathy.

The spectrum of clinical neuropathic syndromes described in patients with diabetes mellitus includes dysfunction of almost every segment of the somatic peripheral and autonomic nervous systems.[607] It has been said that to know neuropathy means to know the whole of medicine. Each syndrome can be distinguished by its pathophysiologic, therapeutic, and prognostic features.

TABLE 33-7

Mononeuritis and Entrapment Syndromes

Feature	Mononeuritis	Entrapment
Onset	Sudden	Gradual
Nerves	Usually single but may be multiple	Single nerves exposed to trauma
Common nerves	C3, C6, C7, ulnar, median, peroneal	Median, ulnar, peroneal, medial and lateral plantar
Progression	Not progressive; resolves spontaneously	Progressive
Treatment	Symptomatic	Rest, splints, diuretics, steroid injections, surgery for paralysis

Adapted from Vinik A, Mehrabyan A. Diabetic neuropathies. *Med Clin North Am.* 2004;88:947-999.

Focal Neuropathies

Mononeuropathies occur primarily in the older population. Their onset is usually acute and associated with pain, and their course is self-limited, resolving within 6 to 8 weeks. Mononeuropathies result from vascular obstruction after which adjacent neuronal fascicles take over the function of those infarcted.[608] Mononeuropathies must be distinguished from entrapment syndromes, which start slowly, progress, and persist without intervention (Table 33-7). Common entrapment sites in diabetic patients involve median, ulnar, and radial nerves; femoral nerves, lateral cutaneous nerves of the thigh, and peroneal nerves; and the medial and lateral plantar nerves.

Carpal tunnel syndrome occurs three times as often in persons with diabetes than in a normal, healthy population,[609,610] and its increased prevalence in diabetes may be related to diabetic cheiroarthropathy,[611] repeated undetected trauma, metabolic changes, or accumulation of fluid or edema within the confined space of the carpal tunnel.[607] It is found in up to one third of patients with diabetes.[612] If carpal tunnel syndrome is recognized, the diagnosis can be confirmed by electrophysiologic study, and therapy is simple, with surgical release. The mainstays of nonsurgical treatment are resting of the wrist, aided by the placement of a wrist splint in a neutral position for day and night use, and the addition of anti-inflammatory medications. Surgical treatment consists of sectioning the volar carpal ligament.[613] The decision to proceed with surgery should be based on several considerations, including severity of symptoms, appearance of motor weakness, and failure of nonsurgical treatment.[614]

Diffuse Neuropathies

Proximal Motor Neuropathies. For many years, proximal neuropathy has been considered to be a component of diabetic neuropathy, although its pathogenesis was ill understood.[615] The condition has a number of synonyms: proximal neuropathy, femoral neuropathy, diabetic amyotrophy, and diabetic neuropathic cachexia.

Proximal motor neuropathy has certain common features. It primarily affects the elderly. Its onset, which can be gradual or abrupt, begins with pain in the thighs and hips or buttocks, followed by significant weakness of the proximal muscles of the lower limbs with inability to rise from the sitting position (positive Gower's maneuver). The neuropathy begins unilaterally, spreads bilaterally, and coexists with DSPN and spontaneous muscle fasciculation. It can be provoked by percussion.

The condition is now recognized as secondary to a variety of causes that are unrelated to diabetes but have a greater incidence in patients with diabetes than in the general population. These include chronic inflammatory demyelinating polyneuropathy (CIDP), monoclonal gammopathy, circulating monosialoganglioside (GM1) antibodies and antibodies to neuronal cells, and inflammatory vasculitis.[616,617] Proximal motor neuropathy was formerly thought to resolve spontaneously in 1.5 to 2 years. However, immune-mediated neuropathy can resolve within days on immunotherapy, such as intravenous immunoglobulin, Etanercept or Immuran.[618]

The condition is readily recognizable clinically; there is prevailing weakness of the iliopsoas, obturator, and adductor muscles, together with relative preservation of function of the gluteus maximus and minimus and hamstrings.[619] Patients have great difficulty rising out of chairs unaided and often use their arms to assist themselves. Heel or toe standing is surprisingly good. In the classic form of diabetic amyotrophy, axonal loss is the predominant process, and the condition coexists with DSPN.[620] Electrophysiologic evaluation reveals lumbosacral plexopathy.[619]

If demyelination predominates and the motor deficit affects proximal and distal muscle groups, a diagnosis of CIDP, monoclonal gammopathy of unknown significance (MGUS), or vasculitis should be considered.[621,622] It seems probable that these conditions occur more commonly in people with diabetes.[623,624] Vinik and colleagues[573,615-627] have pointed out that almost half the patients with proximal neuropathies have a vasculitis and all but 9% have CIDP or MGUS or a ganglioside antibody syndrome.[628] Sharma examined more than 1000 patients with neurologic disorders and found that CIDP was 11 times more common in people with diabetes than in the nondiabetic population.[624]

Biopsy of the obturator nerve reveals demyelination, deposition of immunoglobulin, and inflammatory cell infiltrate of the vasa nervorum (Fig. 33-38).[629] Cerebrospinal fluid protein content is high, and there is an increase in the lymphocyte count. Treatment options include intravenous immunoglobulin for CIDP, plasma exchange for MGUS, steroids and azathioprine for vasculitis, and withdrawal from drugs or other agents that might have caused a vasculitis. It is important to divide proximal syndromes into these subcategories, because the CIDP variant responds dramatically to intervention,[621,630] whereas amyotrophy runs its own course over months to years. Until more evidence is available, they should be considered separate syndromes.

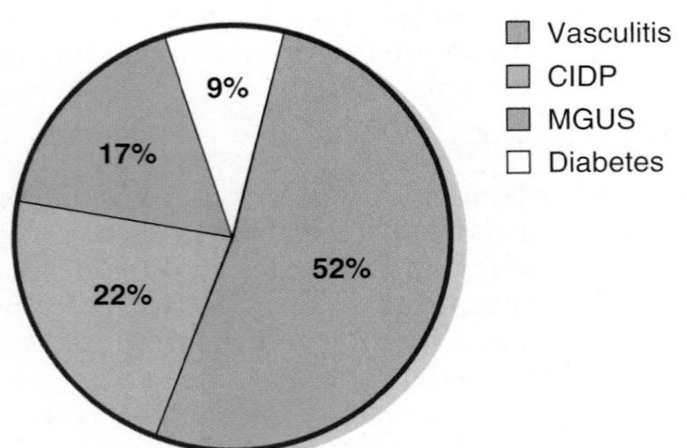

Figure 33-38 Obturator nerve biopsy findings. CIDP, chronic inflammatory demyelinating polyradiculoneuropathy; MGUS, monoclonal gammopathy of undetermined significance. (Adapted from Vinik A: Diagnosis and management of diabetic neuropathy. *Clin Geriatr Med.* 1999;15:293-319.)

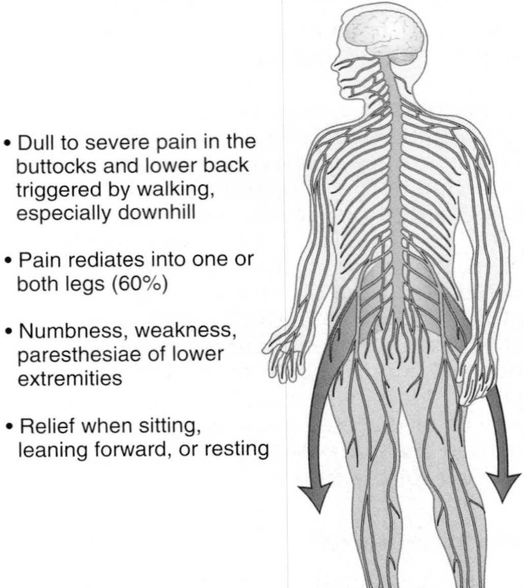

Spinal stenosis/claudication
• Dull to severe pain in the buttocks and lower back triggered by walking, especially downhill
• Pain rediates into one or both legs (60%)
• Numbness, weakness, paresthesiae of lower extremities
• Relief when sitting, leaning forward, or resting

Figure 33-39 Spinal stenosis syndromes.

These conditions need to be distinguished from spinal stenosis syndromes (Fig. 33-39). In spinal stenosis, there is encroachment on nerve roots as they emerge from the spinal cord, and osteophytes can cause compression. With aging, there is hypertrophy of the ligamentum flavum and disk dehydration, and there may even be some form of arachnoiditis. When the compression involves the vascular system, claudication typically occurs on walking downhill, is relieved by bending forward, and originates at the watershed level between T12 and L1-2. Nerve root compression is more typical at L5-S1, and in difficult cases it may be necessary to obtain an magnetic resonance image (MRI) of the lumbosacral spine. Diagnosis is critical, because therapy may range from simple physical therapy to surgical decompression if symptoms are severe or there is motor paralysis.

Distal Symmetric Polyneuropathy. DSPN is the most common and widely recognized form of diabetic neuropathy. The onset is usually insidious but occasionally is acute, occurring after stress or initiation of therapy for diabetes. DSPN may be sensory or motor and can involve small fibers, large fibers, or both.[631] Figure 33-40 is a simplified schematic diagram of the fibers of the peripheral nervous system. Also shown in Figure 33-40 is the usual clinical presentation of the large- and small-fiber neuropathies.

Dysfunction of the small nerve fibers usually occurs early and often is present without objective signs or electrophysiologic evidence of nerve damage.[632] It is manifested early with symptoms of pain and hyperalgesia in the lower limbs, followed by a loss of thermal sensitivity and reduced sensation to light touch and pinprick.[607]

There is evidence that DSPN may be accompanied by loss of cutaneous nerve fibers that stain positive for the neuronal antigen PGP 9.5[633] (Fig. 33-41) and by impaired neurovascular blood flow.[634] The importance of the skin

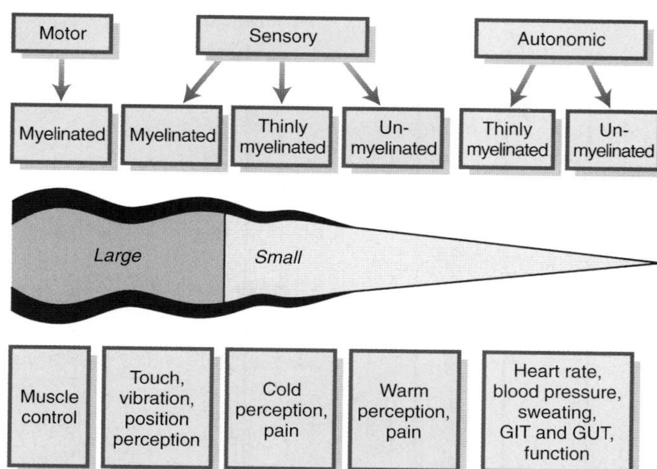

Figure 33-40 Simplified view of the peripheral nervous system (PNS). GIT, gastrointestinal tract; GUT, genitourinary tract. (Vinik A, Ullal J, Parson H, et al. Diabetic neuropathies: clinical manifestations and current treatment options. *Nat Clin Pract Endocrinol Metab.* 2006;2:269-281.)

biopsy as a diagnostic tool for diabetic peripheral neuropathy is increasingly being recognized.[571,598,635,636] This technique quantitates small epidermal nerve fibers through antibody staining of PGP 9.5.[629,637,638] It is minimally invasive (3-mm-diameter punch biopsies) but enables direct study of small fibers that cannot be evaluated by NCV studies (see Fig. 33-37). More recently, assessment of small nerve fiber function has been carried out using corneal confocal microscopy,[2,3] laser doppler flare response to heat or acetylcholine, sudomotor responses to cholinergic stimulaton,[4-6] and Contact Heat Evoked Potentials.[7] However, the sensitivity and specificity of these techniques have not yet been established.

Pain in Diabetic Neuropathies

Overall, approximately 10% of patients with diabetes experience persistent pain from neuropathy.[639] Pain syndromes that last less than 6 to 12 months are classified as acute. These include the insulin neuritis syndrome, which occurs often at the beginning of therapy for diabetes and is self-limited. Pain syndromes lasting longer than 6 to 12 months are classified as chronic.[640] The pain may be ongoing, spontaneous, or hyperalgesic (increased response to a painful stimuli). It can be severe and is sometimes intractable.

Management of painful diabetic neuropathy, as well as other pain syndromes, is changing as research elucidates underlying pathophysiologic mechanisms. The complexities of pain syndromes and advances in basic pain research have contributed to an evolving concept of pain and strategies for its management. Backonja defined neuropathic pain as "a group of disorders characterized by pain due to dysfunction or disease of the nervous system at a peripheral level, a central level, or both."[641]

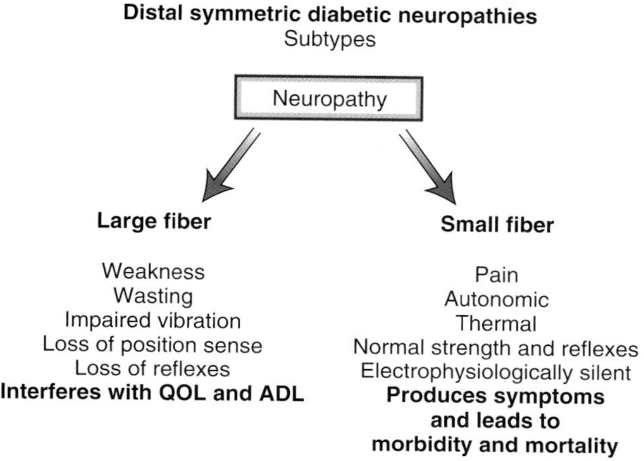

Figure 33-41 Differences in clinical presentations of large- and small-fiber neuropathies. ADL, activities of daily living; QOL, quality of life. (Adapted from Vinik AI, Mehrabyan A. Diabetic neuropathies. *Med Clin North Am.* 2004;88:947-999.)

Acute Painful Neuropathy

Some patients develop a predominantly *small-fiber neuropathy,* which is manifested by pain and paresthesias early in the course of diabetes (Fig. 33-42). It may be associated with the onset of insulin therapy and has been termed *insulin neuritis.*[642] By definition, it has been present for less than 6 months.

Symptoms often are exacerbated at night and are manifested in the feet more than the hands. Spontaneous episodes of pain can be severely disabling. The pain varies in intensity and character. In some patients, this pain has been variably described as burning, lancinating, stabbing, or sharp. Paresthesias or episodes of distorted sensation, such as pins and needles, tingling, coldness, numbness, or burning, often accompany the pain.[631] The lower legs may be exquisitely tender to touch, with any disturbance of the hair follicles resulting in excruciating pain. Because pain can be aggravated by repeated contact of the lower limbs with foreign objects, even basic daily activities such as

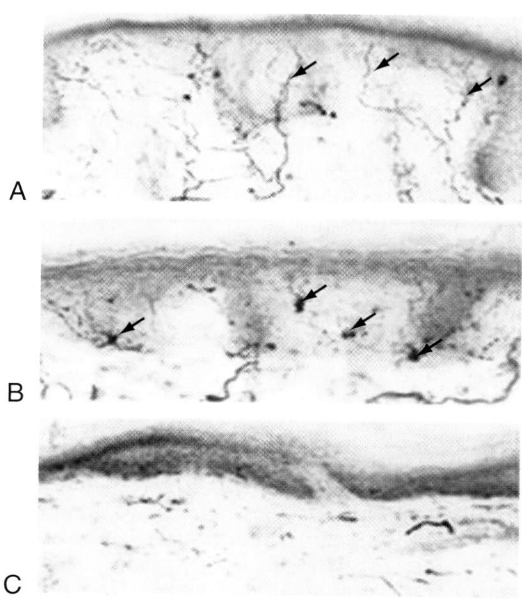

Figure 33-42 Loss of cutaneous nerve fibers that stain positive for the neuronal antigen protein gene product 9.5 (PGP 9.5) in sensory neuropathy. **A,** Normal epidermal fibers in the back. **B,** Slightly reduced density and swelling in the proximal thigh. **C,** Complete clearance in calf. (From McArthur JC, Stocks EA, Hauer P. Epidermal nerve fiber density: normative reference range and diagnostic efficiency. *Arch Neurol.* 1998;55:1513-1520.)

sitting at a desk may be disrupted. Pain often occurs at the onset of the disease and is often worsened by initiation of therapy with insulin or sulfonylureas.[642] Recently, Vinik has provided an outline of the approach to the management of patients with what has been referred to as the "insulin neuritis syndrome."[8]

Neuropathy may be associated with profound weight loss and severe depression that has been termed *diabetic neuropathic cachexia*.[643] This syndrome occurs predominantly in male patients and can occur at any time in the course of T1DM or T2DM. It is self-limited and invariably responds to simple symptomatic treatment. Conditions such as Fabry's disease, amyloid, human immunodeficiency virus (HIV) infection, heavy metal poisoning (e.g., arsenic), and excess alcohol consumption should be excluded. Acute painful neuropathy does overlap with the idiopathic variety of acute painful small-fiber neuropathy that is also a diagnosis by exclusion.[644]

Chronic Painful Neuropathy

Chronic painful neuropathy is another variety of painful polyneuropathy. Onset is later, often years into the course of the diabetes; pain persists for longer than 6 months and becomes debilitating (see Fig. 33-40). This condition can result in tolerance to narcotics and analgesics, finally resulting in addiction. It is extremely resistant to all forms of intervention and is most frustrating to both patient and physician.

Pathophysiologic changes in the nervous system can produce symptoms defined as either negative (e.g., loss of sensory quality) or positive (e.g., spontaneous pain). Patients with neuropathic pain usually present with both positive and negative symptoms. Absence of pain sometimes is not from improvement in neuropathy but is rather a consequence of neuronal loss. Physicians must exclude progression of neuropathy when patients report loss of pain. Neuropathic pain can manifest as stimulus-independent pain or as stimulus-evoked or stimulus-dependent pain, whose underlying mechanisms are likely to differ. A simplified scheme of pain generation is shown in Figure 33-43.

Similarly, the mechanisms responsible for hyperalgesia and allodynia differ. Hyperalgesia is defined as an increased pain response to a normally painful stimulus. Allodynia occurs when pain is provoked by a stimulus that is not normally painful. This difference is related to the different nerve pathways implicated. For example, aberrations of the C and Aδ fibers can result in the burning and prickling sensations of stimulus-independent pain or of hyperalgesia. Under pathologic conditions, touch-sensitive Aβ fibers can cause stimulus-independent dysesthesias or paresthesias or stimulus-evoked allodynia.

Small-Fiber Neuropathies

Symptoms are prominent in small-fiber neuropathies. Pain is of the C-fiber type. It is burning and superficial and is associated with allodynia. Patients have defective autonomic function with decreased sweating, dry skin, impaired vasomotion and blood flow, and cold feet. There are abnormalities in thresholds for warm thermal perception, neurovascular function, pain, quantitative sudorimetry, and QAFTs. Late in the condition, hypoalgesia is present. However, there is remarkable intactness of reflexes and motor strength.

Clinical diagnosis is by reduced sensitivity to 1.0-g Semmes-Weinstein monofilament and a pricking sensation on the Waardenberg wheel or similar instrument. These neuropathies are electrophysiologically silent, but there is loss of cutaneous nerve fibers that stain for PGP 9.5. These

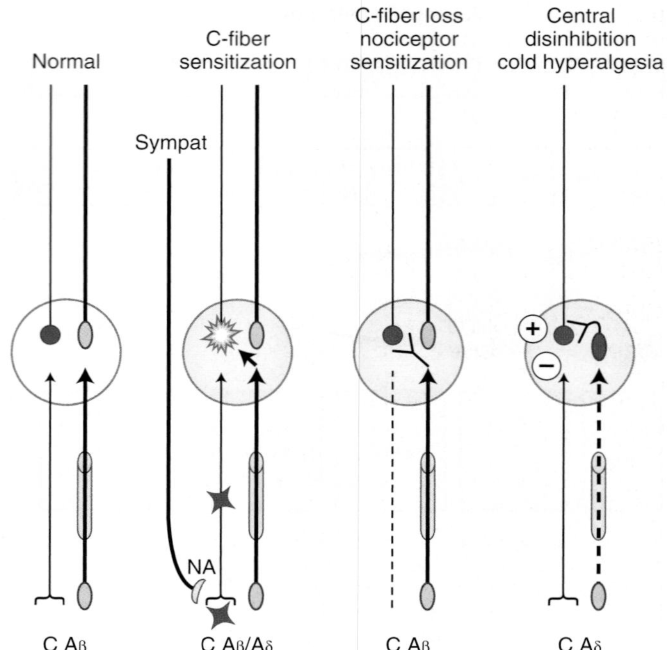

Figure 33-43 Schematic representation of the generation of pain. *Left panel,* Normal situation, no pain. Central terminals of unmyelinated primary C-afferents project into the dorsal horn and make contact with secondary pain-signaling neurons. Low-threshold mechanoreceptive primary Aβ-afferents project without synaptic transmission into the dorsal columns (not shown) and also contact secondary afferent dorsal horn neurons. *Center-left panel,* Peripheral sensitization and central sensitization processes in peripheral nociceptors (peripheral sensitization, star in the periphery) leading to spontaneous burning pain, static mechanical hyperalgesia, and heat hyperalgesia. This spontaneous activity in nociceptors induces secondary changes in central sensory processing, leading to spinal cord hyperexcitability (central sensitization, star in spinal cord) that causes input from mechanoreceptive Aβ fibers (light touching) and Aδ fibers (punctuate stimuli) to be perceived as pain (dynamic and punctuate mechanical allodynia). Moreover, afferent terminals in the periphery or afferent somata in the dorsal root ganglion acquire sensitivity to norepinephrine (noradrenaline, NA) through expression of A-receptors at their membrane. Activity in postganglionic sympathetic neurons is then capable of activating afferent neurons through the release of NA. *Center-right panel,* Synaptic reorganization after C-nociceptor degeneration. Nociceptor function may be selectively impaired and the fibers may degenerate after nerve lesion. Accordingly, the synaptic contacts between central nociceptor terminals and secondary nociceptive neurons are reduced. Central terminals from intact mechanoreceptive Aβ fibers start to sprout to form novel synaptic contacts with the free central nociceptive neurons. This anatomic reorganization in the dorsal horn causes input from mechanoreceptive Aβ fibers (light touching) to be perceived as pain (dynamic mechanical allodynia). In such patients, temperature sensation is profoundly impaired in areas of severe allodynia. *Right panel,* Central disinhibition and cold hyperalgesia. Normally, cold stimuli are conveyed by Aδ fibers and cold pain by C fibers. A selective damage of cold-sensitive Aδ fibers leads to a loss of central inhibition mediated by interneurons (disinhibition), resulting in cold hyperalgesia. (Adapted from Vinik A, Mehrabyan A. Diabetic neuropathies. *Med Clin North Am.* 2004;88:947-999.)

may also be detected by evaluation of corneal confocal microscopy, laser doppler flare reactions, and contact heat-evoked potentials as outlined previously, but sensitivity and specificity of each remain to be defined.

Large-Fiber Neuropathies

Large-fiber neuropathies can involve sensory or motor nerves, or both. These tend to be the neuropathies of signs rather than symptoms. Large fibers subserve motor function, vibration perception, position sense, and cold thermal perception. Unlike the small nerve fibers, these are the myelinated, rapidly conducting fibers that begin in the toes and have their first synapse in the medulla oblongata. They tend to be affected first because of their length and the tendency in diabetes for nerves to die back. Because they are myelinated, they are the fibers represented in the electromyogram, and subclinical abnormalities in nerve function are readily detected. The symptoms may be minimal and include a sensation of walking on cotton, floors feeling strange, inability to turn the pages of a book, or inability to discriminate among coins.

Clinical Presentation

Signs and symptoms of large-fiber neuropathy include impaired vibration perception (often the first objective evidence) and position sense, depressed tendon reflexes, and sensory ataxia (waddling like a duck). Aδ-fiber pain is deep-seated, gnawing, dull, like a toothache in the bones of the feet, or even crushing or cramp-like pain. Signs in the distal lower extremities include wasting of the small muscles of the feet, with hammertoes (intrinsic minus feet and hands) and weakness of the feet; shortening of the Achilles tendon with pes equinus; and increased blood flow (hot foot). Patients also have weakness in the hands.

Most patients with DSPN, however, have a mixed variety of neuropathy, with both large and small nerve fiber damage. In the case of DSPN, a glove-and-stocking distribution of sensory loss is almost universal.[607] Early in the course of the neuropathic process, multifocal sensory loss also may be found. In some patients, severe distal muscle weakness can accompany the sensory loss, resulting in an inability to stand on the toes or heels. Some grading systems use this as a definition of severity.

Diagnosis and Differential Diagnosis of Peripheral Neuropathy

The diagnosis of diabetic neuropathy rests heavily on a careful history, for which a number of questionnaires have been developed by Young and colleagues,[564] Dyck,[645] Vinik,[646] and others.[647,648] The initial neurologic evaluation should be directed toward detecting the specific part of the nervous system affected by diabetes (Fig. 33-44). Bedside neurologic examination is quick and easy but provides nominal or ordinal measures and contains substantial interindividual and intraindividual variation. For example, it is useless to measure vibration perception with a tuning fork other than one that has a frequency of 128 Hz.

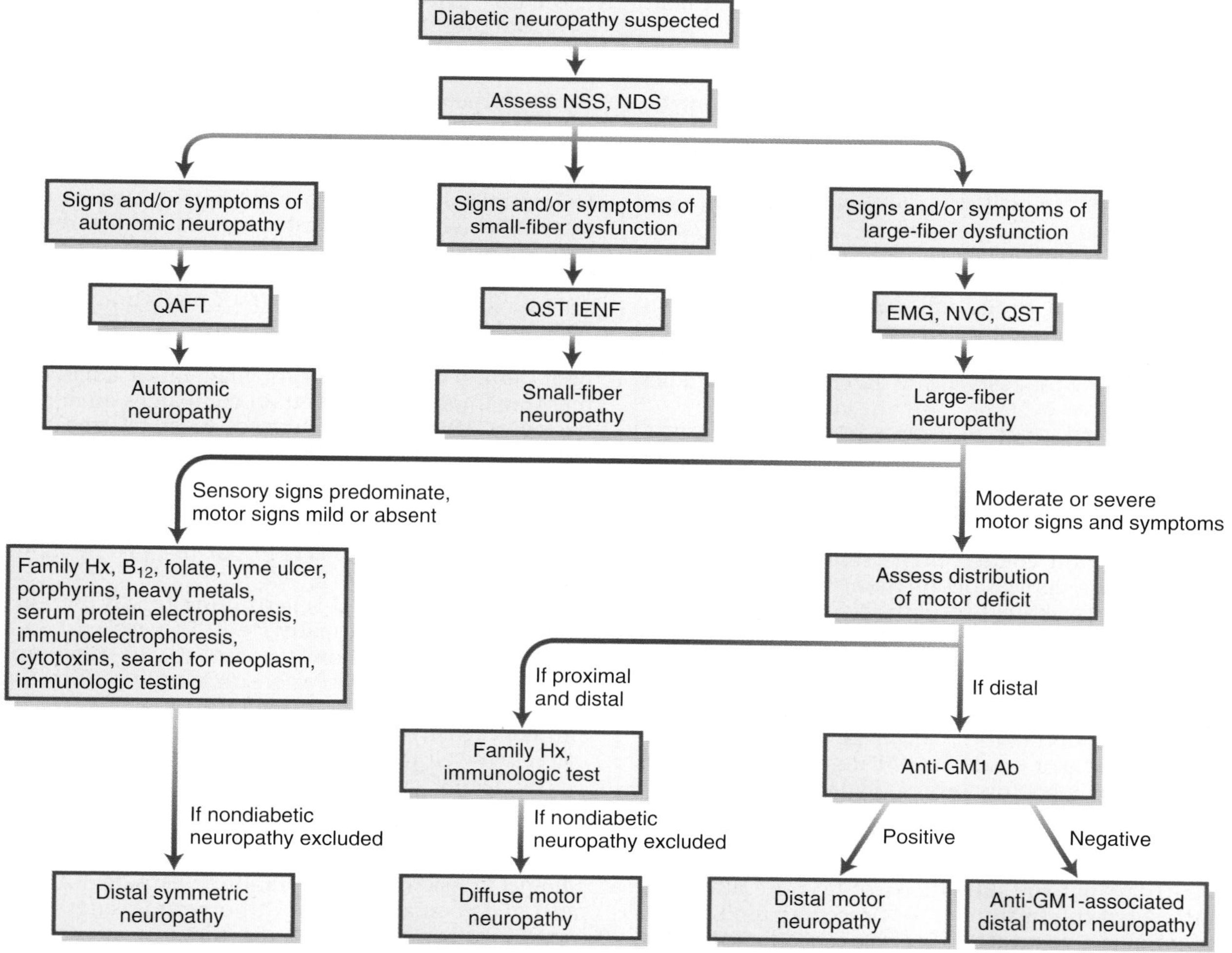

Figure 33-44 A diagnostic algorithm for assessing neurologic deficit and classification of neuropathic syndrome. Ab, antibody; EMG, electromyogram; GM1, monosialoganglioside; Hx, history; IENF, intraepidermal nerve fiber density; MGUS, monoclonal gammopathy of unknown significance; NCV, nerve conduction velocity; NDS, nerve disability (sensory and motor evaluation); NSS, neurologic symptom score; QAFT, quantitative autonomic function tests; QST, quantitative sensory tests. (Adapted with permission from Vinik A, Mehrabyan A. Diabetic neuropathies. *Med Clin North Am.* 2004;88:947-999.)

Similarly, use of a 10-g monofilament is good for predicting foot ulceration, as is the Achilles reflex, but both are insensitive to the early detection of neuropathy; a 1.0-g monofilament increases the sensitivity of detection from 60% to 90%.[649]

Sensory function must be evaluated on both sides of the feet and hands if one wants to be sure not to miss entrapment syndromes.[650] Tinel's sign is not only useful for carpal tunnel problems but can also be applied to the ulnar notch, the head of the fibula, and below the medial tibial epicondyle for ulnar, peroneal, and medial plantar entrapments, respectively.

The 2010 Toronto conference on diabetic neuropathy[1] and the 2009 conference of the American Academy of Neurology[9] recommended that at least one parameter from each of the following five categories be measured to classify diabetic neuropathy: symptom profiles, neurologic examination, QST, nerve conduction study, and autonomic function testing. A number of simple symptom screening questionnaires are available to record symptom quality and severity. A simplified neuropathy symptom score that was used in the European prevalence studies could also be useful in clinical practice.[564,651] The Michigan Neuropathy Screening Instrument (MNSI) is a 15-item questionnaire that can be administered to patients as a screening tool for neuropathy.[648] Other similar symptom-scoring systems have also been described, such as the nerve impairment score of the lower limbs (NIS-LL).[652]

Simple visual analogue or verbal descriptive scales may be used to monitor patients' responses to treatment of their neuropathic symptoms.[213,653,654] However, it must always be remembered that identification of neuropathic symptoms is not useful as a diagnostic or screening tool in assessing diabetic neuropathy, as was shown by Franse and colleagues.[655] The QST and QAFT are objective indices of neurologic functional status. Combined, these tests cover vibratory, proprioceptive, tactile, pain, thermal, and autonomic function. A useful tool that evaluates quality of life in relation to health status and quantifies symptoms of small, large, and autonomic nervous system dysfunction has been validated and translated into 35 different languages and is being used globally as an endpoint in studies on neuropathy.[10]

An international group of experts in diabetic neuropathy held a consensus meeting to develop guidelines for management of diabetic peripheral neuropathy by the practicing clinician.[584] This clinical staging is in general agreement with that proposed by Dyck[606] for use in both clinical practice and epidemiologic studies or controlled clinical trials. The clinical designation, "no neuropathy," is equivalent to Dyck's N0 (no objective evidence of diabetic neuropathy) or N1a (no symptoms or signs but neuropathic test abnormalities). "Clinical neuropathy" is equivalent to N1b (test abnormalities plus neuropathic impairment on neurologic examination), N2a (symptoms, signs, and test abnormalities), and N2b (N2a plus significant ankle dorsiflexor weakness). "Late complications" is equivalent to Dyck N3 (disabling polyneuropathy).

There have been a number of other relevant reports, including two on measures for use in clinical trials to assess symptoms[656] and QST.[657] The strengths of QST are well documented,[657] but the limitations of QST are also clear. No matter what the instrument or procedure used, QST is only a semiobjective measure, because it is affected by the subject's attention, motivation, and cooperation and by anthropometric variables such as age, gender, body mass, and history of smoking and alcohol consumption.[658,659] Expectancy and subject bias are additional factors that can exert a powerful influence on QST findings.[660] Further, QST is sensitive to changes in structure or function along the entire neuroaxis from nerve to cortex; it is not a specific measure of peripheral nerve function.[661] The American Academy of Neurology reported on the use of QST for clinical and research purposes,[657] suggesting that it could be used as an ancillary test but was not sufficiently robust for routine clinical use.

Peripheral Testing Devices

A number of relatively inexpensive devices allow suitable assessment of somatosensory function, including vibration, thermal, light touch, and pain perception.[662] These types of instruments allow cutaneous sensory functions to be assessed noninvasively, and their measurements are correlated with specific neural fiber function.

The most widely used device in clinical practice is the Semmes-Weinstein monofilament.[663-665] The filament assesses pressure perception when gentle pressure is applied to the handle sufficient to buckle the nylon filament. Although filaments of many different sizes are available, the one that exerts 10 g of pressure is most commonly used to assess pressure sensation in the diabetic foot. It is also referred to as the 5.07 monofilament because, during calibration, the filaments are calibrated to exert a force measured in grams that is 10 times the log of the force exerted at the tip: hence, 5.07 exerts 10 g of force.

A number of cross-sectional studies have assessed the sensitivity of the 10-g monofilament to identify feet at risk for ulceration. Sensitivities vary from 86% to 100%,[666,667] although there is no consensus as to how many sites should be tested. The most common algorithm recommends four sites per foot, usually the hallux and the first, third, and fifth metatarsal heads.[664] However, there is little advantage to multiple site assessments.[662] There is also no universal agreement about what constitutes an abnormal result (one, two, three, or four abnormal findings from the sites tested). Despite these problems, the 10-g monofilament is widely used to clinically asses risk of foot ulceration; however, as we pointed out, one needs to use a monofilament of 1 g or less to detect neuropathy with a high sensitivity.[662] A final caution on the use of the filaments is advised[668]: Filaments manufactured by certain companies do not actually buckle at 10 g of force. Indeed, several tested filaments buckled at less than 8 g. In our practice, we use 25-lb strain fishing line and cut it into 1000 pieces at a total cost of $5. We provide patients with these to test themselves at home, which assists in behavior modification. This has reduced the incidence of foot ulcers in our practice by more than 50%.[665]

The graduated Rydel-Seifer tuning fork is used in some centers to assess neuropathy.[669,670] This fork uses a visual optical illusion to allow the assessor to determine the intensity of residual vibration on a scale of 0 to 8 at the point of threshold (disappearance of sensation). Liniger and colleagues reported that results with this instrument correlated well with other QST measures.[669]

The tactile circumferential discriminator assesses the perception of calibrated change in the circumference of a probe (a variation of two-point discrimination).[671] Vileikyte and coworkers reported a 100% sensitivity in identifying patients at risk for foot ulceration.[672] This device also demonstrated good agreement with other measures of QST.

Neuropen is a clinical device that assesses pain using a pin (Neurotip) at one end of the pen and a 10-g monofilament at the other end. This was shown to be a sensitive device for assessing nerve function when compared with the simplified neuropathy disability score.[673]

Newly introduced means of evaluating small-fiber function include the use of corneal confocal microscopy, which allows the identification of unmyelinated axons in the cornea. Early data suggest that there is early loss of these fibers and reduction of their length, which may precede other measures of neuropathy and may predict the development of foot ulceration.[674]

Contact heat-evoked potentials (CHEP) can be elicited by non-noxious heat or painful stimuli from the toe to the dorsum of the back with measurement of negative and positive amplitudes and latencies by recording impulses in the central nervous system. This promises to provide both temporal and spatial resolution of measures of nociception and has the unique ability to measure conduction in C and Aδ fibers, which are normally below the resolution of standard methods. CHEP coupled with functional MRI may lead to an improved understanding of nociceptive pathways and enhance the generation of new therapies directed at the pathways involved.[675]

Cardiovascular Testing Devices

QAFT consists of a series of simple, noninvasive tests for detecting cardiovascular autonomic neuropathy.[632,676] These tests are based on detection of heart rate and BP responses to a series of maneuvers. Specific tests are used in evaluating disordered regulation of gastrointestinal, genitourinary, and sudomotor function and peripheral skin blood flow induced by autonomic diabetic neuropathy.[649]

Biopsy

Biopsy of nerve tissue may be helpful for excluding other causes of neuropathy and for determining predominant pathologic changes in patients with complex clinical findings as a means of dictating choice of treatment.[620,678] Skin biopsy has some clinical advantages in diagnosing small-fiber neuropathies by quantification of PGP 9.5 when all other measures are negative.[598,679]

Differential Diagnosis

Diabetes as the cause of neuropathy is diagnosed by excluding other causes of neuropathy.[607,680] Patients presenting with painful feet might have impaired glucose tolerance[681,682] or the metabolic syndrome.[683] Quantitation of intraepidermal nerve fiber density has also been used to demonstrate the ability to induce nerve regeneration and correlates with indices of neuropathy relevant to function of small unmyelinated C fibers.[684]

More recently, confocal corneal microscopy has been used to assess peripheral neuropathy. This is a completely noninvasive technique that offers the future potential of assessing nerve structure in vivo without the need for biopsy.[685]

Nerve Conduction Studies

Whole-nerve electrophysiologic procedures (e.g., NCV, F waves, sensory amplitudes, motor amplitudes) have emerged as important methods of tracing the onset and progression of peripheral neuropathy.[686] An appropriate battery of electrophysiologic tests supports the measurement of the speed of sensory and motor conduction, the amplitude of the propagating neural signal, the density and synchrony of muscle fibers activated by maximal nerve stimulation, and the integrity of neuromuscular transmission.[687,688] These are objective, parametric, noninvasive, and highly reliable measures. However, standard procedures, such as maximal NCV, reflect only a limited aspect of neural activity, and then only in a small subset of large-diameter and heavily myelinated axons. Even in large-diameter fibers, NCV is insensitive to many pathologic changes known to be associated with peripheral neuropathy.

However, a key role for electrophysiologic assessment is to rule out other causes of neuropathy or to identify neuropathies superimposed on peripheral neuropathy. Unilateral conditions, such as entrapments, are far more common in patients with diabetes than in healthy subjects.[610] The principal factors that influence the speed of NCV are the integrity and degree of myelination of the largest-diameter fibers, the mean cross-sectional diameter of the responding axons, the representative internodal distance in the segment under study, and the microenvironment at the nodes, including the distribution of ion channels.[689] Demyelinating conditions affect conduction velocities, whereas diabetes primarily reduces amplitudes. Therefore, the finding of a profound reduction in conduction velocity strongly supports the occurrence in a diabetic patient of an alternative condition. The odds of occurrence of chronic inflammatory demyelinating polyradiculoneuropathy was found to be 11 times higher among diabetic compared with nondiabetic patients.[690] NCV is only gradually diminished by peripheral neuropathy, with estimates of loss of approximately 0.5 m/sec per year.[686]

In a 10-year natural history study of 133 patients with newly diagnosed T2DM, NCV deteriorated in all six nerve segments evaluated, but the largest deficit was 3.9 m/sec for the sural nerve (48.3 m/sec slowed to 44.4 m/sec); peroneal motor NCV was decreased by 3.0 m/sec over the same period.[593] A similar slow rate of decline was demonstrated in the DCCT. A simple rule is that a decrease in HBA_{1c} of 1 percentage point improves conduction velocity by approximately 1.3 m/sec.[691] There is, however, a strong correlation between myelinated fiber density and whole-nerve sural amplitude ($r = 0.74$; $P < 0.001$).[692]

Management

Once neuropathy has been diagnosed, therapy can be instituted with the goal of ameliorating symptoms and preventing the progression of neuropathy. Successful management of these syndromes must be geared to individual pathogenic processes (Fig. 33-45).

Control of Hyperglycemia

Retrospective and prospective studies have suggested a relationship between hyperglycemia and the development and severity of diabetic neuropathy. Pirart[568] followed 4400 diabetic patients over 25 years and showed an increase in prevalence of clinically detectable diabetic neuropathy from 12% of patients at the time of diagnosis of diabetes to almost 50% after 25 years. The highest prevalence occurred among those patients with the poorest diabetes control.

The DCCT Research Group[590] reported significant effects of intensive insulin therapy on prevention of neuropathy. The prevalence rates for clinical or electrophysiologic evidence of neuropathy were reduced by 50% in those treated by intensive insulin therapy during 5 years. At that stage of the study, only 3% of the patients in the primary prevention cohort treated by intensive insulin therapy showed minimal signs of diabetic neuropathy, compared with 10% of those treated by the conventional regimen. In the secondary prevention cohort, intensive insulin therapy significantly reduced the prevalence of clinical neuropathy by 56% (7% in intensive insulin therapy group versus 16% in conventional therapy group). In the UKPDS, control of

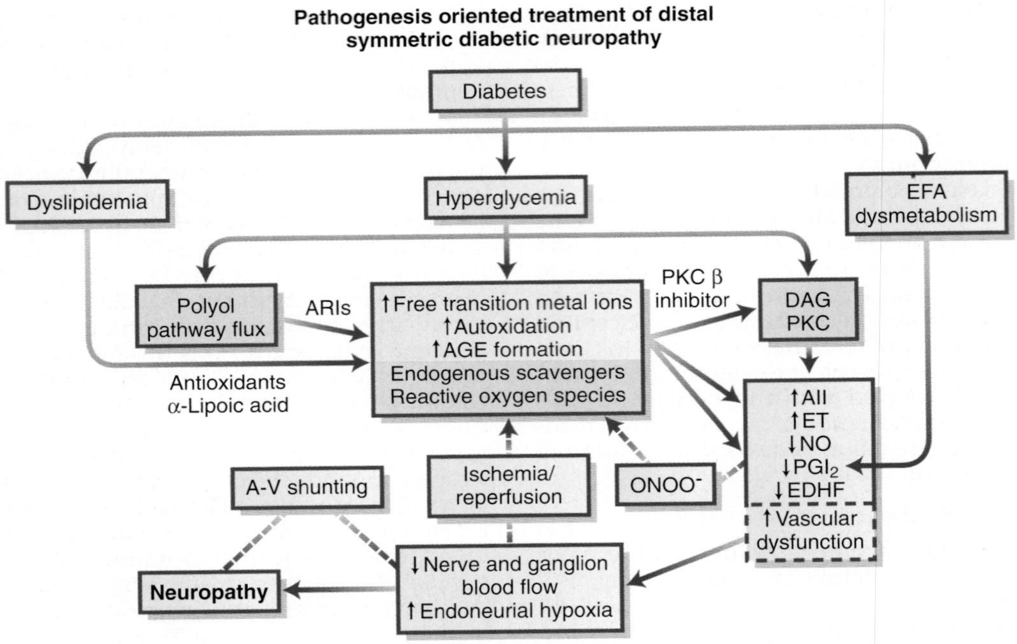

Figure 33-45 Management aimed at pathogenic mechanisms. AII, angiotensin II; AGE, advanced glycation end products; ARIs, aldose reductase inhibitors; A-V, arteriovenous; DAG, diacylglycerol; EDHF, endothelium-derived hyperpolarizing factor; EFA, essential fatty acid; ET, endothelin; NO, nitric oxide; $OONO^-$, peroxynitrite; PGI_2, prostaglandin I_2; PKC, protein kinase C. (Adapted from Vinik A, Mehrabyan A. Diabetic neuropathies. *Med Clin North Am.* 2004;88:947-999.)

blood glucose was associated with improvement in vibration perception.[3,478,635] Similar to what was found in the DCCT trial, despite loss of diabetes control, with time nerve function improved in the formerly well-controlled group in what has now come to be known as legacy effect or good metabolic memory.[12,13]

In the UKPDS, control of blood glucose was associated with improvement in vibration perception.[3,524,693] The follow-up study to the DCCT trial, the EDIC study, has shown that, despite convergence of A1c levels with time, the advantage accrued to the intensively controlled people during the course of the study persists (EDIC). In the Steno trial,[694] a reduction of the odds ratio for the development of autonomic neuropathy to 0.32 was reported. This was a stepwise, progressive study that involved treatment of T2DM patients with hypotensive drugs, including ACE inhibitors, calcium-channel antagonists, hypoglycemic agents, aspirin, hypolipidemic agents, and antioxidants. These findings argue strongly for the multifactorial nature of neuropathy and for the need to address the multiple metabolic abnormalities.

Pharmacologic Therapy

Aldose Reductase Inhibitors. Aldose reductase inhibitors (ARIs) reduce the flux of glucose through the polyol pathway, inhibiting tissue accumulation of sorbitol and fructose and preventing reduction of redox potentials.

In a placebo-controlled, double-blind study of tolrestat, 219 diabetic patients with symmetric polyneuropathy, as defined by at least one pathologic cardiovascular reflex, were treated for 1 year.[695] Patients who received tolrestat showed significant improvement in autonomic function tests and in vibration perception, whereas placebo-treated patients showed deterioration in most of the parameters measured.[696]

There was a dose-dependent improvement in nerve fiber density, particularly in small unmyelinated nerve fibers, in a 12-month study of zenarestat.[115] This was accompanied by an increase in NCV, although the changes in NCV occurred at a dose of the drug that did not change the nerve fiber density. Impaired cardiac ejection fractions can be improved with zopolrestat.[697] Clinical improvement was reported for fidarestat and epalrestat in studies from Japan.[698,699]

The promise shown with the newer ARIs is being exploited by other companies, and promising results have been reported in a phase 2 study of the drug AS-3201 in the United States.[700] This study is now being pursued as a phase 3 study. This ARI is now in phase 3 clinical trials in the United States and Canada. It is also becoming clear that aldose reductase inhibition may be insufficient to achieve the desirable degree of metabolic enhancement in patients with a multitude of biochemical abnormalities. Combinations of therapy with ARIs and antioxidants may become critical to curb the relentless progression of diabetic neuropathy. There is also support for the role of AGE/RAGE interaction in generating inflammation and oxidative and nitrosative stress and promising therapies with compounds that inhibit AGE accumulation and promote a reduction in the aggregation of amyoid fibrils in the nervous system. In addition, it has now been established that sRAGE may act as a decoy in which AGEs and other ligands preferentially bind to sRAGE, thereby precluding access to RAGE and resulting in a net decrease in the inflammation, oxidative, and nitrosative stress effects with salutary effects on the nervous system.[14]

α-Lipoic Acid. Lipoic acid (1,2-dithiolane-3-pentanoic acid), a derivative of octanoic acid, is present in food and is also synthesized by the liver. It is a natural cofactor in the pyruvate dehydrogenase complex, where it binds acyl groups and transfers them from one part of the complex to another. α-Lipoic acid, which is also known as thioctic acid, has generated considerable interest as a thiol-replenishing and redox-modulating agent. It has been shown to be effective in ameliorating the somatic and autonomic neuropathies in patients with diabetes.[701-703] It is undergoing extensive trials in the United States and Europe, and promising results for treating diabetes and diabetic neuropathy are forthcoming.

γ-Linolenic Acid. Linoleic acid, an essential fatty acid, is metabolized to dihomo-γ-linolenic acid, which serves as an important constituent of neuronal membrane phospholipids and as a substrate for the formation of PGE, which appears to be important for preserving nerve blood flow. In diabetes, conversion of linoleic acid to γ-linolenic acid and subsequent metabolites is impaired, possibly contributing to the pathogenesis of diabetic neuropathy.[704] In a recent multicenter, double-blind, placebo-controlled trial, patients using γ-linolenic acid for 1 year showed significant improvements in clinical measures and on electrophysiologic testing.[705]

Protein Kinase C-β Inhibition. Neural vascular insufficiency has been proposed as a contributing factor to development of diabetic neuropathy.[706] PKC activation is a critical step in the pathway to diabetic microvascular complications.[707] It is hyperactivated by hyperglycemia and disordered fatty acid metabolism, resulting in increased production of vasoconstrictive, angiogenic, and chemotactic cytokines including TGF-β, VEGF, endothelin, and ICAMs. Nonselective PKC inhibitors normalize hyperglycemia-induced decreases in endoneurial blood flow and abrogate the neuronal abnormalities seen in diabetic rodents.[66,653,708] Preclinical studies in animal diabetes models using ruboxistaurin mesylate (LY333531), a PKC-β inhibitor, have shown improvement in many diabetes-related changes in vascular function such as retinal blood flow,[213] endoneurial blood flow, and NCV.[709,710]

Preliminary results of a multinational, randomized, double-blind, placebo-controlled phase 2 trial showed a statistically significant improvement in symptoms, measured by the Neuropathy Total Symptom Score 6 (NTSS-6), in ruboxistaurin-treated neuropathy groups compared with placebo treatment.[711] In patients with symptomatic neuropathy (NTSS-6 score >6) and a sural nerve action potential greater than 0 μV at baseline, a measure that has been shown to define a responsive subpopulation of peripheral neuropathy,[605] the frequency and intensity of symptoms and the change from baseline for vibratory detection threshold were statistically significantly improved in the treated groups. Vibratory detection threshold changes correlated well with the improvement in symptoms; the drug was well tolerated, and there were few adverse events.

Aminoguanidine. Animal studies using aminoguanidine, an inhibitor of the formation of AGEs, have shown improvements in nerve conduction velocity in streptozotocin-induced diabetic neuropathy in rats. Controlled clinical trials to determine the efficacy of aminoguanidine in humans[712,713] were discontinued because of toxicity. There are, however, successors to aminoguanidine that hold promise for this approach.[714] Studies outlined previously on AGE/RAGE interactions support the notion that this pathway may contribute significantly to neruopathy and deficiencies in sRAGE may be the hallmark of severity of diabetic neruopathy.[16]

Human Intravenous Immunoglobulin. Immune intervention with intravenous immune globulin (IVIG) has become appropriate in some patients with forms of peripheral diabetic neuropathy associated with signs of antineuronal autoimmunity.[621,630] Treatment with immunoglobulin is well tolerated and is considered safe, especially with respect to viral transmission.[687] The major toxicity of IVIG has been an anaphylactic reaction, but the frequency of these reactions is now low and confined mainly to patients with immunoglobulin (usually immunoglobulin A) deficiency. Patients may experience severe headache due to aseptic meningitis, which resolves spontaneously. In some instances, it may be necessary to combine treatment with prednisone or azathioprine. Relapses can occur, requiring repeated courses of therapy. However, new data support a predictive role of the presence of antineuronal antibodies on the later development of neuropathy[688]; they may not be innocent bystanders but neurotoxins.[715] Some patients, particularly those with autonomic neuropathy, antineuronal autoimmunity, and CIDP, may benefit from IVIG.[619,630] Others may benefit from the use of Etanercept or Immuran.[618,716]

Neurotrophic Therapy

There is now considerable evidence in animal models of diabetes that decreased expression of NGF and its receptors, TrkA and p75, reduces retrograde axonal transport of NGF and diminishes support of small unmyelinated neurons and their neuropeptides, such as substance P and calcitonin gene–related peptide (CGRP), both potent vasodilators.[569,715,717,718] Furthermore, administration of recombinant human NGF (rhNGF) restores these neuropeptide levels toward normal and prevents the manifestations of sensory neuropathy in animals.[719]

In a 15-center, double-blind, placebo-controlled study of the safety and efficacy of rhNGF in 250 subjects with symptomatic small-fiber neuropathy,[594] rhNGF improved the neurologic impairment score of the lower limbs and improved small nerve fiber function, cooling threshold (Aδ fibers), and the ability to perceive heat pain (C fibers) compared with placebo. These results were consistent with the postulated actions of NGF on TrkA receptors present on small-fiber neurons. This led to two large, multicenter studies conducted in the United States and the rest of the world. Subsequently, a phase 3 trial in 1019 diabetic patients with sensory polyneuropathy failed to demonstrate a significant benefit.[720] Results of these NGF studies were presented at the ADA meetings in June 1999.[595] Regrettably, rhNGF was not found to have beneficial effects over placebo. The reason for this dichotomy has not been resolved, but this has somewhat dampened the enthusiasm for growth factor therapy of diabetic neuropathy.

More recently, a randomized, double-blind, placebo-controlled study of brain-derived neurotrophic factor (rhBDNF) in 30 diabetic patients demonstrated no significant improvement in nerve conduction or on quantitative sensory and autonomic function tests, including the cutaneous axon reflex.[721] A small trial of neurotrophin 3 (NT3) for safety was interpreted as negative for efficacy, and IGF1 and IGF11 have not been considered to be safe for administration to humans. A more promising therapy may be found with the proinsulin C-peptide.[722]

Pain Control

Control of pain constitutes one of the most difficult management issues in diabetic neuropathy. In essence, simple measures are tried first. If no distinction is made for pain syndromes, then the number needed to treat (NNT) to reduce pain by 50% is 1.4 for optimal-dose tricyclic antidepressants, 1.9 for dextromethorphan, 3.3 for carbamazepine, 3.4 for tramadol, 3.7 for gabapentin, 5.9 for capsaicin, 6.7 for selective serotonin reuptake inhibitors (SSRIs), and 10.0 for mexiletine.[723] If, however, pain is divided

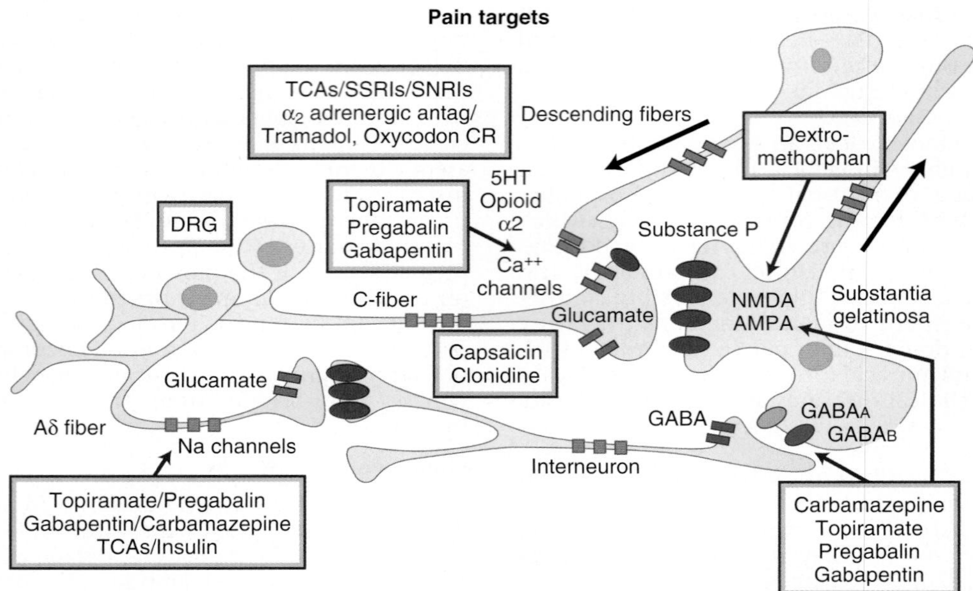

Figure 33-46 Pain response to various therapies. C fibers are modulated by sympathetic input with spontaneous firing of different neurotransmitters to the dorsal root ganglia, spinal cord, and cerebral cortex. Sympathetic blockers (e.g., clonidine) and depletion of axonal substance P used by C fibers as their neurotransmitter (e.g., by capsaicin) can relieve pain. In contrast, Aδ fibers use Na^+ channels for conduction. Agents that inhibit Na^+ exchange, such as antiepileptic drugs, tricyclic antidepressants (TCAs), and insulin, can ameliorate this form of pain. Anticonvulsants (carbamazepine, gabapentin, pregabalin, topiramate) potentiate the activity of γ-aminobutyric acid (GABA), inhibit Na^+ and Ca^{2+} channels, and inhibit *N*-methyl-D-aspartate (NMDA) receptors and α-amino-3-hydroxy-5-methyl-4-isoxazole propionic acid (AMPA) receptors. Dextromethorphan blocks NMDA receptors in the spinal cord. TCAs, selective serotonin reuptake inhibitors (e.g., fluoxetine), and serotonin-norepinephrine reuptake inhibitors (SNRIs) inhibit serotonin and norepinephrine reuptake, enhancing their effect in endogenous pain-inhibitory systems in the brain. Tramadol is a central opioid analgesic. Antag, antagonists; CR, controlled release; 5HT, 5-hydroxytryptamine; DRG, dorsal root ganglia; SSRIs, selective serotonin reuptake inhibitors. (Adapted from Vinik AI, Ullal J, Parson H, et al. Diabetic neuropathies: clinical manifestations and current treatment options. *Nature Clin Pract Endocrinol Metab.* 2006;2:269-281.)

according to its derivation from different nerve fiber types (Aδ versus C fiber), from spinal cord, or from cerebral cortex, then different types of pain respond to different therapies (Fig. 33-46).

C-Fiber Pain. Initially, when there is ongoing damage to the nerves, the patient experiences pain of the burning, lancinating, dysesthetic type, often accompanied by hyperalgesia and allodynia. Because the peripheral sympathetic nerve fibers are also small, unmyelinated C fibers, sympathetic blocking agents (clonidine) can improve the pain. Loss of sympathetic regulation of sweat glands and arteriovenous shunt vessels in the foot creates a favorable environment for bacteria to penetrate, multiply, and wreak havoc with the foot. These fibers use the neuropeptide substance P as their neurotransmitter, and agents that deplete axonal substance P (capsaicin) often lead to amelioration of the pain. However, when the destructive forces persist, the patient becomes pain free and develops impaired warm temperature and pain thresholds. Disappearance of pain in these circumstances should be viewed as a warning that the neuropathy is progressing. Targeting higher levels of pain transmission also helps with C-fiber pain.[724,725]

Capsaicin. Capsaicin is extracted from chili peppers, and a simple, cheap mixture can be made by adding 1 to 3 teaspoons (15 to 45 mL) of cayenne pepper to a jar of cold cream and applying the cream to the area of pain. Capsaicin has high selectivity for a subset of sensory neurons that have been identified as unmyelinated C-fiber afferent or thin-myelinated (Aδ) fibers. Prolonged application of capsaicin depletes stores of substance P, and possibly other neurotransmitters, from sensory nerve endings. This reduces or abolishes the transmission of painful stimuli from the peripheral nerve fibers to the higher centers.[726] Care must be taken to avoid eyes and genitals, and gloves must be worn. Because of capsaicin's volatility, it is safer to cover affected areas with plastic wrap. There is initial exacerbation of symptoms followed by relief in 2 to 3 weeks.

Clonidine. There is an element of sympathetic-mediated C-fiber type pain that can be overcome with clonidine (an α_2-adrenergic agonist) or phentolamine. Clonidine can be applied topically,[727] but the dose titration may be more difficult. If clonidine fails, a trial of the local anesthetic agent, mexiletine, is warranted. If there is no response, treatment can continue as outlined in Figure 33-47.

Aδ-Fiber Pain. Aδ-fiber pain is a more deep-seated, dull, and gnawing ache that often does not respond to the previously described measures. A number of different agents have been used for the pain associated with these fibers with varying success.

Insulin. Continuous intravenous insulin infusion without resort to blood glucose lowering may be useful in patients with Aδ-fiber pain. A response with reduction of pain usually occurs within 48 hours,[728] and the insulin infusion can be discontinued. If this measure fails, several medications are available that might abolish the pain.

Nerve Blocking. Lidocaine given by slow infusion has been shown to provide relief of intractable pain for 3 to 21 days. This form of therapy may be of most use in self-limited forms of neuropathy. If successful, therapy can be continued with oral mexiletine. Because of the cardiac conduction block reported with these drugs when given systemically, this is no longer done, and only the topical agents are still in use. These compounds target the pain

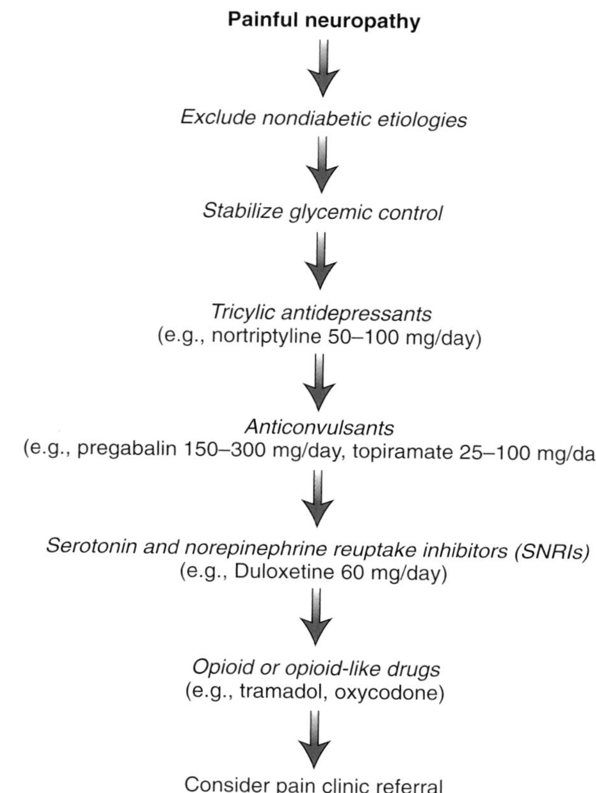

Figure 33-47 Algorithm for managing painful diabetic neuropathy. Nonpharmacologic, topical, or physical therapies (e.g., capsaicin, acupuncture) can be useful at any time. (Modified from Boulton AJ, Vinik AI, Arezzo JC, et al. Diabetic neuropathies: a statement by the American Diabetes Association. *Diabetes Care.* 2005;28:956-962.)

caused by hyperexcitability of superficial free nerve endings.[729]

Tramadol and Dextromethorphan. There are two possible targeted therapies. Tramadol is a centrally acting, weak opioid analgesic that is used to treat moderate to severe pain. Tramadol was shown to be better than placebo in a randomized, controlled trial[730] of only 6 weeks' duration, but a subsequent follow-up study[731] suggested that symptomatic relief could be maintained for at least 6 months. Side effects are relatively common and are similar to those of other opioid-like drugs.

Another spinal cord target for pain relief is the excitatory glutaminergic *N*-methyl-D-aspartate (NMDA) receptor. Blockade of NMDA receptors is believed to be one mechanism by which dextromethorphan exerts analgesic efficacy.[732] The pharmacist can procure a sugar-free solution of dextromethorphan.

Antidepressants. Tricyclic antidepressants are an important component in the treatment of chronic pain syndromes. Imipramine, amitriptyline, and clomipramine induce a balanced reuptake inhibition of both norepinephrine and serotonin, whereas desipramine is a relatively selective norepinephrine reuptake inhibitor. The NNT for greater than 50% pain relief by tricyclic antidepressants is 2.4 (95% CI, 2.0 to 3.0).[67] Amitriptyline is frequently the drug of first choice, but it can alternatively be replaced by nortryptyline, which has less pronounced sedative and anticholinergic effects.

Antidepressants inhibit reuptake of norepinephrine or serotonin, or both. Their use is limited by anticholinergic effects, orthostatic hypotension, and sexual side effects. Clinical trials have focused on interrupting pain transmission with antidepressant drugs that inhibit the reuptake of norepinephrine or serotonin. This central action accentuates the effects of these neurotransmitters in activation of endogenous pain-inhibitory systems in the brain that modulate pain-transmission cells in the spinal cord.[733] Side effects, including dysautonomia and dry mouth, can be troublesome. Switching to nortriptyline can lessen some of the anticholinergic effects of amitriptyline.

Antidepressants remain first-line agents in many centers, but consideration of their safety and tolerability is important to avoid adverse effects, a common result of treatment of neuropathic pain. Dosages must be titrated based on positive responses, treatment adherence, and adverse events.[734] Among the norepinephrine reuptake inhibitors, desipramine, amitriptyline, and imipramine have been shown to be of benefit.[735,736]

SSRIs that have been used for neuropathic pain are paroxetine, fluoxetine, sertraline, and citalopram. Paroxetine appears to be associated with greater pain relief.[737] Fluoxetine failed a placebo-controlled trial.[733]

Recent interest has focused on antidepressants with dual selective inhibition of serotonin and norepinephrine (SNRIs), such as duloxetine and venlafaxine. Duloxetine has recently been approved for neuropathic pain in the United States. The efficacy and safety of duloxetine was evaluated in three controlled studies using doses of 60 and 120 mg/day over 12 weeks.[738] In all three studies, the average 24-hour pain intensity was significantly reduced with either dose, compared with placebo treatment. The response rates, defined as 50% or greater pain reduction, were 48.2% for the 120-mg/day dose, 47.2% for 60 mg/day, and 27.9% for placebo, giving an NNT of 4.9 (95% CI, 3.6 to 7.6) for 120 mg/day and 5.2 (95% CI, 3.8 to 8.3) for 60 mg/day.[738] Patients with higher pain intensity do tend to respond better than those with lower pain levels.[739] The most frequent adverse effects are nausea, somnolence, dizziness, constipation, dry mouth, and reduced appetite. Physicians must be alert to suicidal ideation and exacerbation of autonomic symptoms as well as aggravation of depression in patients with bipolar tendencies. Venlafaxmine (Effexor), another SNRI, has also shown efficacy in the treatment of painful diabetic neuropathy.[740]

Antiepileptic Drugs. For a detailed discussion of the subject of antiepileptic drug therapy for painful diabetic neuropathy, the reader is referred to the review by Vinik.[741]

Anticonvulsants have stood the test of time in the treatment of diabetic neuropathy.[742,743] Principal mechanisms of action include sodium channel blockade (felbamate, lamotrigine, oxcarbazepine, topiramate, zonisamide), potentiation of γ-aminobutyric acid (GABA) activity (pregabalin, tiagabine, topiramate), calcium-channel blockade (felbamate, lamotrigine, topiramate, zonisamide), and antagonism of glutamate at NMDA receptors (felbamate) or α-amino-3-hydroxy-5-methyl-4-isoxazole propionic acid (AMPA) receptors (felbamate, topiramate).[744]

Pregabalin (Lyrica) is a GABA analogue with similar structure and actions to gabapentin, but it is a more specific α2-δ ligand with a higher binding affinity than gabapentin. The efficacy and safety of pregabalin were reported in a pooled analysis of seven studies over 5 to 13 weeks in 1510 patients with DPN. The response rates, defined as 50% or greater pain reduction, were 47% for a dosage of 600 mg/day, 39% for 300 mg/day, 27% for 150 mg/day, and 22% for placebo, giving NNTs of 4.0, 5.9, and 20.0, respectively.[745] The most frequent adverse effects were dizziness,

Autonomic Neuropathies

The autonomic nervous system (ANS) supplies all organs in the body and consists of an afferent and an efferent system, with long efferents in the vagus (cholinergic) system and short postganglionic unmyelinated fibers in the sympathetic (adrenergic) system. A third component is the neuropeptidergic system, with its neurotransmitters, substance P, vasoactive intestinal polypeptide (VIP), and CGRP, among others.

Diabetic autonomic neuropathy can cause dysfunction of every part of the body. Diabetic autonomic neuropathy often goes completely unrecognized by patient and physician alike because of its insidious onset and protean multiple-organ involvement. Alternatively, the appearance of complex and confusing symptoms in a single organ system as a result of diabetic autonomic neuropathy can cause profound symptoms and receive intense diagnostic and therapeutic attention. Subclinical involvement may be widespread, whereas clinical symptoms and signs may be focused within a single organ. The organ systems that most often exhibit prominent clinical autonomic signs and symptoms in diabetes include the ocular pupil, sweat glands, genitourinary system, gastrointestinal system, adrenal medullary system, and cardiovascular system (Table 33-8).

Involvement of the ANS can occur as early as the first year after diagnosis. Major manifestations are cardiovascular, gastrointestinal, and genitourinary system dysfunction.[607,768] Reduced exercise tolerance, edema, paradoxical supine or nocturnal hypertension, and intolerance to heat due to defective thermoregulation are consequences of autonomic neuropathy.

TABLE 33-8

Clinical Manifestations of Autonomic Neuropathy

Cardiovascular
Alterations in skin blood flow
Cardiac denervation, painless myocardial infarction
Heat intolerance
Orthostatic hypotension
Tachycardia, exercise intolerance
Gastrointestinal
Constipation
Diarrhea
Esophageal dysfunction
Fecal incontinence
Gastroparesis diabeticorum
Genitourinary
Cystopathy
Erectile dysfunction
Neurogenic bladder
Retrograde ejaculation
Metabolic
Hypoglycemia unawareness
Hypoglycemia unresponsiveness
Pupillary
Argyll-Robertson pupil
Decreased diameter of dark-adapted pupil
Sweating Disturbances
Areas of symmetric anhidrosis
Gustatory sweating

Defective blood flow in the capillary circulation is found, with decreased responsiveness to mental arithmetic, cold pressor, hand grip, and heating.[634] The defect is associated with a reduction in the amplitude of vasomotion[759] that resembles premature aging.[634] There are differences in the glabrous and hairy skin circulations. In hairy skin, a functional defect is found before neuropathy develops,[769] and it is correctable with antioxidants.[770] The clinical counterpart is skin that is dry and cold, loses the ability to sweat, and develops fissures and cracks that are portals of entry for organisms leading to infectious ulcers and gangrene. Silent MI, respiratory failure, amputations, and sudden death are hazards for diabetic patients with cardiac autonomic neuropathy.[603,771] There is now evidence that the greatest predictor of CVD as well as increased mortality is autonomic nerve dysfunction,[20,21] and the increase in sudden death in the ACCORD study is likely due to the presence of autonomic dysfunction.[22] It has also become apparent that a combination of self-reported somatic neuropathy viz. numbness combined with an index of loss in heart rate variability increase the risk of cardiac events and mortality by a RR of 4.5.[23] Therefore, it is vitally important to make this diagnosis early so that appropriate intervention can be instituted.[603,710,771,772] Furthermore, since the risk factors for CVD in the recent ADVANCE, ACCORD, and VADT trials have been established, the presence of autonomic dysfunction necessitates a modified approach to attempts at intensification of glycemic control and suggests a relaxation of the A1c goals from those recommended by ACE and the ADA to less stringent criteria.

Disturbances in the ANS may be functional and include gastroparesis with hyperglycemia and ketoacidosis. In organic disturbances, nerve fibers are actually lost. This creates inordinate difficulties in diagnosing, treating, and prognosticating as well as establishing true prevalence rates. Tests of autonomic function typically stimulate entire reflex pathways. Furthermore, autonomic control for each organ system is usually divided between opposing sympathetic and parasympathetic innervations, so that heart rate acceleration, for example, could reflect either decreased parasympathetic or increased sympathetic nervous system stimulation.

Because many conditions affect the ANS and autonomic neuropathy is not unique to diabetes, the diagnosis of diabetic autonomic neuropathy rests with establishing the diagnosis and excluding other causes. The best-studied tests, and those for which there are large databases and evidence to support their use in clinical practice, relate to the evaluation of cardiovascular reflexes. Evaluation of orthostasis is fairly straightforward and is readily done in clinical practice, and the same can be said for the establishment of the causes of gastrointestinal symptoms and erectile dysfunction. The evaluation of pupillary abnormalities, hypoglycemia unawareness and unresponsiveness, neurovascular dysfunction, and sweating disturbances is for the most part done only in research laboratories, requires specialized equipment and familiarity with the diagnostic procedures, and is best left in the hands of those who have a special interest in the area.

Tables 33-9 and 33-10 present the diagnostic tests that apply to the diagnosis of cardiovascular autonomic neuropathy. These tests can be used as a surrogate for the diagnosis of autonomic neuropathy of any system, because it is rare (although it does occur) to find involvement of any other division of the ANS in the absence of cardiovascular autonomic dysfunction. For example, if one entertains the possibility that the patient's erectile dysfunction is caused by autonomic neuropathy, then

TABLE 33-9

Differential Diagnosis of Diabetic Autonomic Neuropathy

Clinical Manifestations	Differential Diagnosis
Cardiovascular	
Cardiac denervation	Carcinoid syndrome
Exercise intolerance	Congestive heart disease
Orthostatic hypotension	Hyperadrenergic hypotension
Painless myocardial infarction	Hypovolemia
Tachycardia	Idiopathic orthostatic hypotension
	Multiple system atrophy with parkinsonism
	Panhypopituitarism
	Pheochromocytoma
	Orthostatic tachycardia
	Shy-Drager syndrome
Gastrointestinal	
Constipation	Bezoars
Diarrhea	Biliary disease
Esophageal dysfunction	Medications
Fecal incontinence	Obstruction
Gastroparesis diabeticorum	Psychogenic vomiting
	Secretory diarrhea (endocrine tumors)
Genitourinary	
Cystopathy	Alcohol abuse
Erectile dysfunction	Atherosclerotic vascular disease
Neurogenic bladder	Genital and pelvic surgery
Retrograde ejaculation	Medications
Neurovascular	
Dry skin	Amyloidosis
Gustatory sweating	Arsenic
Heat intolerance	Chagas' disease
Impaired skin blood flow	
Metabolic	
Hypoglycemia-associated autonomic failure	Drugs that mask hypoglycemia
Hypoglycemia unawareness	Other cause of hypoglycemia
Hypoglycemia unresponsiveness	Intensive glycemic control
Pupillary	
Argyll-Robertson pupil	Syphilis
Decreased diameter of dark-adapted pupil	

before embarking on a sophisticated and expensive evaluation of erectile status, one should measure the heart rate and its variability in response to deep breathing. If this measurement is normal, autonomic neuropathy is excluded as a cause of erectile dysfunction, and the cause should be sought elsewhere. Similarly, it is extremely unusual to find gastroparesis secondary to autonomic neuropathy in a patient with normal cardiovascular autonomic reflexes.

Prevention and Reversibility

It has now become clear that strict glycemic control[591] and stepwise progressive management of hyperglycemia, lipids, and BP, together with the use of antioxidants[702] and ACE inhibitors,[773] reduce the odds ratio for autonomic neuropathy to 0.32.[683] It has also been shown that mortality is a function of loss of beat-to-beat variability with MI. This can be reduced by 33% with acute administration of insulin.[774] Kendall and coworkers[775] reported that successful pancreas transplantation improves epinephrine response and normalizes hypoglycemia symptom recognition in patients with long-standing diabetes and established autonomic neuropathy. Burger's group[776] showed a reversible metabolic component in patients with early cardiac autonomic neuropathy (Table 33-11).

Management

Postural Hypotension. The syndrome of postural hypotension consists of posture-related dizziness and syncope

TABLE 33-10

Diagnostic Tests for Cardiovascular Autonomic Neuropathy

Resting Heart Rate
Rate >100 beats/min is abnormal.
Beat-to-Beat Heart Rate Variation*
With the patient at rest and supine (no overnight coffee or hypoglycemic episodes), breathing 6 breaths/min, heart rate monitored by ECG or Anscore device, an HRV of >15 beats/min is normal and <10 beats/min is abnormal, R-R inspiration to R-R expiration >1.17. All indices of HRV are age-dependent.†
Heart Rate Response to Standing*
During continuous ECG monitoring, the R-R interval is measured at beats 15 and 30 after standing. Normally, a tachycardia is followed by reflex bradycardia. The 30:15 ratio is normally >1.03.
Heart Rate Response to Valsalva Maneuver*
The subject forcibly exhales into the mouthpiece of a manometer to 40 mm Hg for 15 seconds during ECG monitoring. Healthy subjects develop tachycardia and peripheral vasoconstriction during strain and an overshoot bradycardia and rise in blood pressure with release. The ratio of longest R-R to shortest R-R should be >1.2.
Systolic Blood Pressure Response to Standing
Systolic blood pressure is measured in the supine subject. The patient stands and the systolic blood pressure is measured after 2 min. Normal response is a fall of <10 mm Hg, borderline is a fall of 10-29 mm Hg, and abnormal is a fall of >30 mm Hg with symptoms.
Diastolic Blood Pressure Response to Isometric Exercise
The subject squeezes a handgrip dynamometer to establish a maximum. Grip is then squeezed at 30% maximum for 5 min. The normal response for diastolic blood pressure is a rise of >16 mm Hg in the other arm.
Electrocardiographic QT/QTc Intervals
The QTc (corrected QT interval on ECG) should be <440 msec.
Spectral Analysis
High-frequency peak ↓ (parasympathetic dysfunction) Low-frequency peak ↓ (sympathetic dysfunction) Low-frequency/high-frequency ratio ↓ (sympathetic imbalance) Very-low-frequency peak ↓ (sympathetic dysfunction)
Neurovascular Flow
Noninvasive laser Doppler measures peripheral sympathetic responses to nociception.

*These can be performed quickly (<15 min) in the practitioner's office, with a central reference laboratory providing quality control and normative values, and are now readily available in most cardiology practices.

†Lowest normal value of E/I ratio: Age 20-24 yr: 1.17; 25-29 yr: 1.15; 30-34 yr: 1.13; 35-30 yr: 1.12; 40-44 yr: 1.10; 45-49 yr: 1.08; 50-54 yr: 1.07; 55-59 yr: 1.06; 60-64 yr: 1.04; 65-69 yr: 1.03; 70-75 yr: 1.02.

ECG, electrocardiogram; HRV, heart rate variation.

TABLE 33-11

Clinical Features, Diagnosis, and Treatment of Diabetic Autonomic Neuropathy

Symptoms	Tests	Treatments
Cardiac		
Resting tachycardia, exercise intolerance	HRV, MUGA thallium scan, MIBG scan	Graded supervised exercise, ACE inhibitors, β-blockers
Postural hypotension, dizziness, weakness, fatigue, syncope	HRV, supine and standing BP, catecholamines	Mechanical measures, clonidine, midodrine, octreotide, erythropoietin
Gastrointestinal		
Gastroparesis, erratic glucose control	Gastric emptying study, barium study	Frequent small meals, prokinetic agents (metoclopramide, domperidone, erythromycin)
Abdominal pain, early satiety, nausea, vomiting, bloating, belching	Endoscopy, manometry, electrogastrogram	Antibiotics, antiemetics, bulking agents, tricyclic antidepressants, pyloric botulinum toxin, gastric pacing
Constipation	Endoscopy	High-fiber diet, bulking agents, osmotic laxatives, lubricating agents
Diarrhea (often nocturnal alternating with constipation)		Soluble fiber, gluten and lactose restriction, anticholinergic agents, cholestyramine, antibiotics, somatostatin, pancreatic enzyme supplements
Sexual Dysfunction		
Erectile dysfunction	H&P, HRV, penile-brachial pressure index, nocturnal penile tumescence	Sex therapy, psychological counseling, phosphodiesterase inhibitors, PGE_1 injections, devices or prostheses
Vaginal dryness		Vaginal lubricants
Bladder Dysfunction		
Frequency, urgency, nocturia, urinary retention, incontinence	Cystometrogram, postvoid sonography	Bethanechol, intermittent catheterization
Sudomotor Dysfunction		
Anhidrosis, heat intolerance, dry skin, hyperhidrosis	Quantitative sudomotor axon reflex, sweat test, skin blood flow	Emollients and skin lubricants, scopolamine, glycopyrrolate, botulinum toxin, vasodilators
Pupillomotor and Visceral Dysfunction		
Blurred vision, impaired adaptation to ambient light, Argyll-Robertson pupil	Pupillometry, HRV	Care with driving at night
Impaired visceral sensation: silent MI, hypoglycemia unawareness		Recognition of unusual presentation of MI, control of risk factors, control of plasma glucose levels

ACE, acetylcholinesterase; BP, blood pressure; H&P, history and physical examination; HRV, heart rate variability; MI, myocardial infarction; MIBG, metaiodobenzylguanidine; MUGA, multigated angiography; PGE_1, prostaglandin E_1.

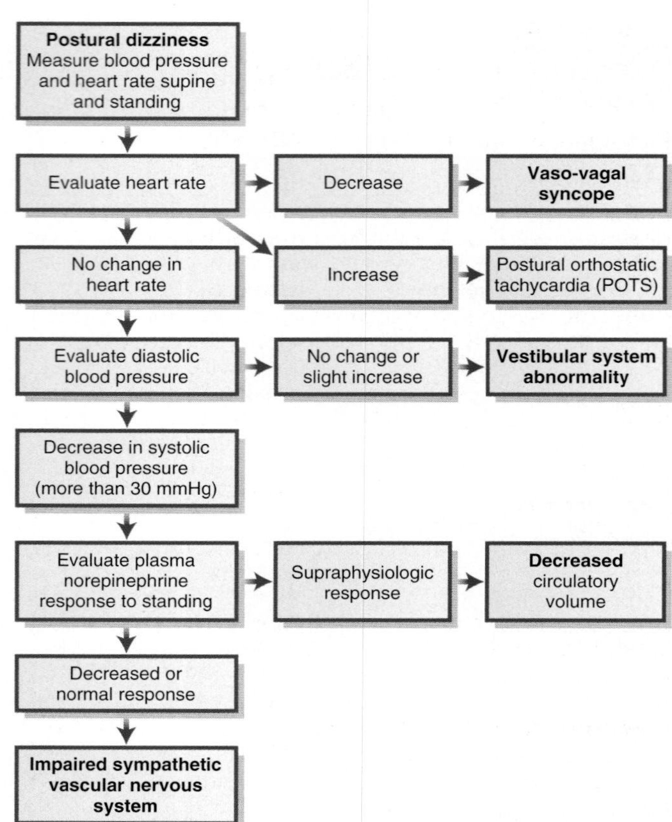

Figure 33-49 Evaluation of postural dizziness in diabetic patients. (Modified from Vinik A, Mehrabyan A. Diabetic neuropathies. *Med Clin North Am.* 2004;88:947-999.)

(Fig. 33-49). Patients who have T2DM and orthostatic hypotension are hypovolemic and have sympathoadrenal insufficiency; both factors contribute to the pathogenesis of orthostatic hypotension.[777] Postural hypotension in the patient with diabetic autonomic neuropathy can present a difficult management problem. Increasing BP in the standing position to avoid symptoms often results in hypertension in the supine position. It is now recognized that symptoms of orthostasis can also result from inappropriate changes in heart rate without a fall in BP (i.e., orthostatic tachycardia or bradycardia without a fall in BP). Devices with algorithms for quantification of sympathetic or parasympathetic function allow the determination of ANS dysfunction in the arm,[779] which may provide a rationale for trying drugs that reduce either sympathetic or parasympathetic activity in these patients.

Supportive Garments. Whenever possible, attempts should be made to increase venous return from the periphery using total body stockings. Leg compression alone is less effective, presumably reflecting the large capacity of the abdomen relative to the legs.[778] Patients should be instructed to put these garments on while lying down and not to remove them until returning to the supine position.

Drug Therapy. Some patients with postural hypotension benefit from treatment with 9-fluorohydrocortisone. However, symptoms do not improve until edema occurs, and there is a significant risk of developing congestive heart failure (CHF) and hypertension. If 9-fluorohydrocortisone does not work satisfactorily, various adrenergic agonists and antagonists may be used.

If the adrenergic receptor status is known, therapy can be guided to the appropriate agent. Metoclopramide may be helpful in patients with dopamine excess or increased sensitivity to dopaminergic stimulation. Patients with α_2-adrenergic receptor excess might respond to the α_2-antagonist, yohimbine. Those few patients in whom β-receptors are increased may be helped with propranolol. α_2-Adrenergic receptor deficiency can be treated with the α_2-agonist, clonidine, which in this setting can paradoxically increase BP. One should start with small doses and gradually increase the dose. If these measures fail, midodrine (an α_1-adrenergic agonist) or dihydroergotamine in combination with caffeine can help.

A particularly refractory form of postural hypotension occurs in some patients postprandially and may respond to therapy with octreotide given subcutaneously in the mornings.

Gastropathy. Gastrointestinal motor disorders (Fig. 33-50) are frequent and widespread in patients with T2DM regardless of symptoms,[780] and there is a poor correlation between symptoms and objective evidence of functional or organic defects. The first step in management of diabetic gastroparesis consists of multiple small feedings. The amount of fat should be decreased, because fat tends to delay gastric emptying. Maintenance of glycemic control is important.[781,782] Metoclopramide may be used. Cisapride and domperidone[783,784] have been shown to be effective in some patients, although probably no more so than metoclopramide. (Cisapride has been withdrawn from the market.) Erythromycin, given as a liquid or as a suppository, also may be helpful. Erythromycin acts on the motilin receptor (the sweeper of the gut) and shortens gastric emptying time.[785] Several novel drugs including ghrelin (an orexigenic hormone) and ghrelin receptor agonists, motilin agonist (mitemcinal), 5HT4-receptor agonists, and a muscarinic antagonist are being investigated for their prokinetic effects. If medications fail and severe gastroparesis persists, jejunostomy placement into normally functioning bowel may be needed. Gastric pacing has not been as rewarding as originally anticipated, but studies are ongoing.

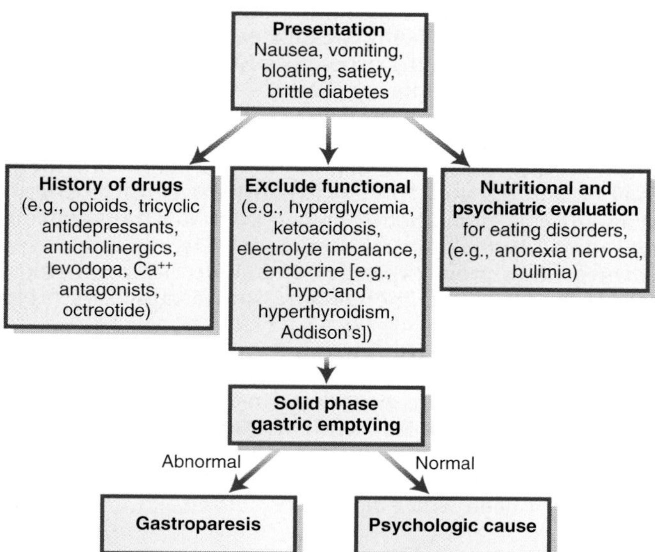

Figure 33-50 Evaluation of the patient with suspected gastroparesis. (Adapted with permission from Vinik A, Mehrabyan A. Diabetic neuropathies. *Med Clin North Am.* 2004;88:947-999.)

Enteropathy. Enteropathy involving the small bowel and colon can produce both chronic constipation and explosive diabetic diarrhea, making treatment of this particular complication difficult.

Antibiotics. Stasis of bowel contents with bacterial overgrowth can contribute to the diarrhea. Treatment with broad-spectrum antibiotics is the mainstay of therapy, including tetracycline or trimethoprim-sulfamethoxazole. Metronidazole appears to be the most effective agent and should be continued for at least 3 weeks.

Cholestyramine. Retention of bile can occur and can be highly irritating to the gut. Chelation of bile salts with cholestyramine, 4 g mixed with fluid three times a day, can relieve symptoms.

Diphenoxylate plus Atropine. Diphenoxylate plus atropine can help to control the diarrhea. However, toxic megacolon can occur, and extreme care should be used.

Diet. Patients with poor digestion can benefit from a gluten-free diet. Beware of certain fibers in the neuropathic patient that can lead to bezoar formation because of bowel stasis in gastroparetic or constipated patients.

Sexual Dysfunction

Male Sexual Dysfunction. Erectile dysfunction (ED) occurs in 50% to 75% of diabetic men, and it tends to occur at an earlier age than in the general population. The incidence of ED in diabetic men aged 20 to 29 years is 9% and increases to 95% by age 70 years. It may be the presenting symptom of diabetes. More than 50% of men who develop ED notice its onset within 10 years after the diagnosis of diabetes, but ED can precede the other complications of diabetes.

The etiology of ED in diabetes is multifactorial. Neuropathy, vascular disease, diabetes control, nutrition, endocrine disorders, psychogenic factors, and drugs used to treat diabetes and its complications play a role.[786,787] The diagnosis of the cause of ED is made by a logical, stepwise progression in all instances.[786,787] An approach to therapy has been presented and is discussed later in this chapter.[786]

Diagnosis. A thorough workup for impotence includes a medical and sexual history; physical and psychological evaluations; blood tests for diabetes and to check levels of testosterone, prolactin, and thyroid hormones; a test for nocturnal erections; tests to assess penile, pelvic, and spinal nerve function; and tests to assess penile blood supply and BP.

The health care provider should initiate questions that will help distinguish the various forms of organic ED from those that are psychogenic. The physical examination must include evaluations of the ANS, vascular supply, and hypothalamic-pituitary-gonadal axis.

Autonomic neuropathy causing ED is almost always accompanied by loss of ankle jerks and absence or reduction of vibration sense over the large toes. More direct evidence of impairment of penile autonomic function can be obtained by demonstrating normal perianal sensation, assessing the tone of the anal sphincter during a rectal examination, and ascertaining the presence of an anal wink when the area of the skin adjacent to the anus is stroked or contraction of the anus when the glans penis is squeezed (bulbo-cavernosus reflex). These measurements are easily and quickly done at the bedside and reflect the integrity of sacral parasympathetic divisions.

Vascular disease is usually manifested by buttock claudication but may be caused by stenosis of the internal pudendal artery. A penile-brachial index of less than 0.7 indicates diminished blood supply. A venous leak

TABLE 33-12

Pharmacologic Treatment of Autonomic Neuropathy

Drug	Class	Dosage	Side Effects
Orthostatic Hypotension			
9α-Fluorohydrocortisone	Mineralocorticoid	0.5-2 mg/day	Congestive heart failure, hypertension
Clonidine	α_2-Adrenergic agonist	0.1-0.5 mg at bedtime	Hypotension, sedation, dry mouth
Octreotide	Somatostatin analogue	0.1-0.5 μg/kg per day	Injection site pain, diarrhea
Gastroparesis			
Metoclopramide	D_2-Receptor antagonist	10 mg 30-60 min before meals and at bedtime	Galactorrhea, extrapyramidal symptoms
Domperidone	D_2-Receptor antagonist	10-20 mg 30-60 min before meals and at bedtime	Galactorrhea
Erythromycin	Motilin receptor agonist	250 mg 30 min before meals	Abdominal cramp, nausea, diarrhea, rash
Levosulfide	D_2-Receptor antagonist	25 mg tid	Galactorrhea
Diabetic Diarrhea			
Metronidazole	Broad-spectrum antibiotic	250 mg tid, minimum 3 wk	Orthostatic hypotension
Clonidine	α_2-Adrenergic agonist	0.1 mg bid or tid	Toxic megacolon
Cholestyramine	Bile acid sequestrant	4 g 1-6 times/day	Aggravates nutrient malabsorption (at higher doses)
Loperamide	Opiate-receptor agonist	2 mg qid	
Octreotide	Somatostatin analogue	50 μg tid	
Cystopathy			
Bethanechol	Acetylcholine receptor agonist	10 mg, 4 times/day	
Doxazosin	α_1-Adrenergic antagonist	1-2 mg, 2-3 times/day	Hypotension, headache, palpitations
Erectile Dysfunction			
Sildenafil	GMP type 5 phosphodiesterase inhibitor	50 mg before sexual activity, only once per day	Hypotension and fatal cardiac event (with nitrate-containing drugs), headache, flushing, nasal congestion, dyspepsia, musculoskeletal pain, blurred vision

D_2, dopamine 2; GMP, guanosine monophosphate.

manifests as unresponsiveness to vasodilators and needs to be evaluated by penile Doppler sonography.

To distinguish psychogenic from organic erectile dysfunction, nocturnal penile tumescence (NPT) can be tested. Normal NPT defines psychogenic ED, and a negative response to vasodilators implies vascular insufficiency. Application of NPT is not so simple. It is much like having a sphygmomanometer cuff inflate over the penis many times during the night while one is trying to have a normal night's sleep. The patient might have to take home the device and become familiar with it over several nights before a reliable estimate of the failure of NPT can be obtained.

Treatment. A number of treatment modalities are available, and each has positive and negative effects. Patients must be made aware of positive and negative aspects before a therapeutic decision is made. Before any form of treatment is considered, every effort should be made to have the patient withdraw from alcohol and eliminate smoking. The patient should be removed, if possible, from drugs that are known to cause ED. Metabolic control should be optimized.

Relaxation of the corpus cavernosa smooth muscle cells is caused by NO and cGMP, and the ability to have and maintain an erection depends on the generation of NO. The peripherally acting phosphodiesterase inhibitors are the major oral medications for erectile dysfunction in diabetic patients. The PDE5 inhibitors block the action of phosphodiesterase and permit cGMP to accumulate. This class of agents consists of sildenafil, vardenafil, and tadafil. These agents enhance blood flow to the corpora cavernosa with sexual stimulation and have been evaluated in diabetic patients with efficacy of about 70%. Generally, people with diabetes and ED require the maximum dose of each drug: sildenafil 100 mg, tadafil 20 mg, and vardenafil 20 mg. Lower doses should be considered in patients with renal failure and hepatic dysfunction. The duration of the drug effect is 4 to 24 hours but may be prolonged. Before these drugs are prescribed, it is important to exclude ischemic heart disease. These drugs are absolutely contraindicated in patients being treated with nitroglycerine or other nitrate-containing drugs because severe hypotension and fatal cardiac events can occur.[725,788]

Direct injection of prostacyclin into the corpus cavernosum induces satisfactory erections in a significant number of men. Also, surgical implantation of a penile prosthesis may be appropriate. The less expensive type of prosthesis is a semirigid, permanently erect type that is embarrassing and uncomfortable for some patients. The inflatable type is three times more expensive and subject to mechanical failure, but it avoids the embarrassment caused by other devices.

Female Sexual Dysfunction. Women with diabetes mellitus can experience decreased sexual desire and more pain on sexual intercourse, but they are also at risk for decreased sexual arousal, with inadequate lubrication.[789] Diagnosis of female sexual dysfunction using vaginal plethysmography to measure lubrication and vaginal flushing has not been well established.

Cystopathy. In diabetic autonomic neuropathy, the motor function of the bladder is unimpaired, but afferent fiber damage results in diminished bladder sensation. The urinary bladder can be enlarged to more than three times its normal size. Patients are seen with bladders filled to their umbilicus, yet they feel no discomfort. Loss of bladder sensation occurs with diminished voiding frequency, and the patient is no longer able to void completely. Consequently, dribbling and overflow incontinence are common complaints. A postvoid residual of greater than 150 mL diagnoses cystopathy. Cystopathy can put patients at risk for urinary infections.

Patients with cystopathy should be instructed to palpate the bladder and, if they are unable to initiate micturition when their bladder is full, to use Crede's maneuver (massage or pressure on the lower portion of the abdomen just above the pubic bone) to start the flow of urine. The principal aim of the treatment should be to improve bladder emptying and to reduce the risk of urinary tract infection. Parasympathomimetics such as bethanechol are sometimes helpful, although often they do not help to fully empty the bladder. Extended sphincter relaxation can be achieved with an α_1-blocker, such as doxazosin.[607] Self-catheterization can be particularly useful in this setting, and the risk of infection generally is low.

Sweating Disturbances

Hyperhidrosis of the upper body, often related to eating (gustatory sweating), is a characteristic feature of autonomic neuropathy. Gustatory sweating accompanies the ingestion of certain foods, particularly spicy foods and cheeses. Gustatory sweating is more common than previously believed, and topically applied glycopyrrolate (an antimuscarinic compound) is a very effective treatment in reducing both severity and frequency.[790,791] Symptoms are avoided by avoiding the inciting food.

Anhidrosis of the lower body is also common in autonomic neuropathy. Loss of lower body sweating can cause dry, brittle skin that cracks easily, predisposing the patient to ulcer formation that can lead to loss of a limb. Special attention must be paid to foot care.

Metabolic Dysfunction

Blood glucose concentration is normally maintained during starvation or increased insulin action by an asymptomatic parasympathetic response that includes bradycardia and mild hypotension, followed by a sympathetic response with glucagon and epinephrine secretion for short-term glucose counterregulation and growth hormone and cortisol for long-term regulation. The release of catecholamine alerts the patient to take the required measures to prevent coma due to low blood glucose. The absence of warning signs of impending neuroglycopenia is known as *hypoglycemic unawareness*. The failure of glucose counterregulation can be confirmed by the absence of glucagon and epinephrine responses to hypoglycemia induced by a standard controlled dose of insulin.[792]

In patients with T1DM, the glucagon response is impaired with diabetes duration of 1 to 5 years, and after 14 to 31 years of diabetes the glucagon response is almost undetectable. It is not present in those with autonomic neuropathy. However, a syndrome of hypoglycemic autonomic failure occurs with intensification of diabetes control and repeated episodes of hypoglycemia. The exact mechanism is not understood, but it does represent a real barrier to physiologic glycemic control. In the absence of severe autonomic dysfunction, hypoglycemic unawareness associated with hypoglycemia is at least in part reversible.

Patients with hypoglycemia unawareness and unresponsiveness pose a significant management problem for the physician. Although autonomic neuropathy can improve with intensive therapy and normalization of blood glucose, there is a risk to the patient, who may become hypoglycemic without being aware of it and who cannot mount a counterregulatory response. It is our recommendation that, if a pump is used, boluses of smaller than calculated amounts should be used. If intensive conventional therapy is used, long-acting insulin with very small boluses should be given. In general, to prevent hypoglycemia in these patients, normal glucose and HbA_{1c} levels should not be goals.[793]

Further complicating management in some diabetic patients is the development of a functional autonomic insufficiency associated with intensive insulin treatment, which resembles autonomic neuropathy in all relevant aspects. In these instances, it is prudent to relax therapy, as for the patient with bona fide autonomic neuropathy. If hypoglycemia occurs in these patients at a certain glucose level, it will take a lower glucose level to trigger the same symptoms in the next 24 to 48 hours. Avoidance of hypoglycemia for a few days results in recovery of the adrenergic response.

CORONARY HEART DISEASE

The last decades have witnessed substantial declines in coronary heart disease (CHD) mortality in the general population in the United States, but the improvement in CHD mortality has been significantly lower in diabetic men and women.[794] More than 90% of all patients with diabetes have T2DM, and it is this population (mostly middle-aged and elderly) that has been evaluated in most of the studies of CHD risk. In these studies, the excess morbidity and mortality associated with diabetes and elevated glucose remained even after adjustment for traditional CHD risk factors.

Effect of Diabetes on Risk of Coronary Heart Disease

The Framingham Study showed a twofold to threefold elevation in the risk of clinically evident atherosclerotic disease in patients with T2DM compared to those without diabetes.[795] Diabetic men in the Multiple Risk Factor Intervention Trial (MRFIT) had an absolute risk of CHD death more than three times higher than that of the nondiabetic cohort, even after adjustment for established risk factors.[51] Seminal work from Finland showed that patients with T2DM without a previous MI have a risk of MI over 7 years as high as that of nondiabetic patients with a history of MI (Fig. 33-51).[62] In this study, the case-fatality rate after MI was also substantially higher in patients with diabetes. In women, diabetes mitigates the cardioprotective effects of the premenopausal period, and women with diabetes had a CHD mortality rate as high as that of diabetic men.

The risk of cardiovascular mortality and events conferred by T2DM has been examined in several prospective and observational trials with varying populations of patients.[796-799] Prospective data from the Organization to Assess Strategies for Ischemic Syndromes (OASIS) registry was analyzed to determine the effect of diabetes on outcomes of patients with unstable angina and non–Q-wave MI.[796] Patients with diabetes had a significantly increased adjusted RR for total mortality (1.57; 95% CI, 1.38 to 1.81; $P < .001$), death due to CVD (1.49; 95% CI, 1.27 to 1.74; $P < .001$), new MI (1.34; 95% CI, 1.14 to 1.57, $P < .001$), stroke (1.45; 95% CI, 1.09 to 1.92, $P = .009$), and new CHF

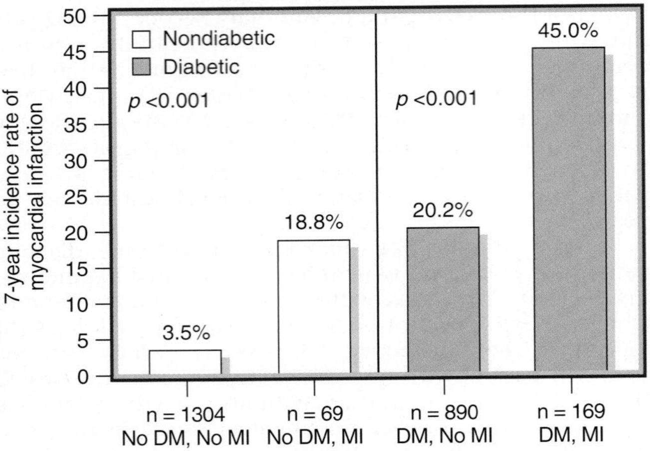

Figure 33-51 Marked increase in the risk of coronary artery disease in patients with type 2 diabetes mellitus (DM) compared with nondiabetic subjects, in a population-based study in Finland, over a 7-year follow-up period. Patients with diabetes who had no previous myocardial infarction (MI) had a risk of first MI approximately equal to that of nondiabetic subjects who had already sustained an MI. These data support recommendations from the American Diabetes Association to treat diabetic subjects as if they already have established coronary artery disease. (From Haffner SM, Lehto S, Ronnemaa T, et al. Mortality from coronary heart disease in subjects with type 2 diabetes and in nondiabetic subjects with and without prior myocardial infarction. *N Engl J Med.* 1998;339:229-234.)

(1.41; 95% CI, 1.24 to 1.60, *P* < .001). Diabetic patients without prior CVD had the same event rates for all outcomes as nondiabetic patients with previous vascular disease.

In another prospective cohort trial,[797] the adjusted hazard ratio (HR) for overall mortality in diabetic patients (*n* = 393) after a first MI was 1.5 (95% CI, 1.1 to 2.0) compared with equivalent nondiabetic patients (*n* = 1132). The HR for cardiovascular mortality in diabetic patients was similar to that in nondiabetic patients who had experienced a previous MI. The risk of mortality from all causes was significantly higher in women than in men (adjusted HR, 2.7 versus 1.3, *P* = .01).

In contrast to these findings, two large observational trials failed to find that diabetes conferred equivalent or greater risk of mortality than previous MI.[799,800] In the cross-sectional study, RR for all-cause mortality was 1.33 (95% CI, 1.14 to 1.55) for patients with MI compared to patients with T2DM. In the cohort study, patients with MI also had a significantly higher risk of all-cause death (adjusted RR, 1.35; 95% CI, 1.25 to 1.44), cardiovascular death (RR, 2.93; 95% CI, 2.54 to 3.41), and hospital admission for MI (RR, 3.1; 95% CI, 2.57 to 3.73). Based on these findings, the authors concluded that established CVD confers greater risk than diabetes.[798]

The risk of mortality conferred by diabetes was also assessed in the Atherosclerosis Risk in Communities (ARIC) study, a population-based cohort study that investigated the etiology of atherosclerosis in a biracial population in the United States.[799] Patients with prior MI had an adjusted RR of 1.9 (95% CI, 1.35 to 2.56; *P* < .001) for fatal CHD or nonfatal MI and adjusted RR of 1.8 (95% CI, 1.22 to 2.72; *P* = .003) for fatal CHD or nonfatal MI, compared to the patients with diabetes and no previous MI. There was no significant difference in the risk of stroke in the two groups.

All of these studies demonstrated that diabetes alone results in a significantly increased risk of CVD. The strategy of considering diabetes as a CHD risk equivalent for purposes of assessing risk and defining a treatment regimen is appropriate.

The risk of CHD has also been evaluated in small subsets of patients with T1DM. In the Framingham Study, the cumulative CAD mortality in patients with T1DM was approximately four times that of nondiabetic patients by age 55 years.[800] As in patients with T2DM, the first deaths related to CAD in patients with T1DM occurred by the fourth decade of life, and the cumulative mortality increased at a similar rate in both groups in the subsequent 20 years. The rise in CAD mortality with age in patients with T1DM is substantially higher in those patients with nephropathy. In these patients, the risk of CAD can be as much as 15 times higher than in patients without persistent proteinuria. Therefore, persistent proteinuria is a strong predictor of the development of CAD in this population. These findings suggest that proteinuria is a marker of generalized vascular damage that predisposes to CVD.

Two prospective epidemiologic studies, the Pittsburgh Epidemiology of Diabetes Complications study (EDC)[801] and Eurodiab,[802] a multicenter, clinic-based study in Europe, confirmed the Framingham findings and reported an incidence of total coronary events of 16% over 10 years and 9% over 7 years of follow-up in patients with T1DM. These incidence rates presumably reflect patients in their late 30s, 10 years beyond baseline age in the studies. In EDC, the total incidence of CAD (including angina and ischemic electrocardiographic changes) was more than 2% per year for those older than 35 years. A more recent report, using 12-year follow-up data,[803] proposed that the annual rate of major CAD events (MI, fatal CAD, or revascularization) is 0.98% for those with diabetes duration of 20 to 30 years (average age, 28 to 38 years). The event rates are identical for both genders, consistent with a loss of the protection from CHD mortality in premenopausal women with diabetes.

The follow-up of the Diabetes UK cohort, a group of 23,751 subjects with insulin-treated diabetes diagnosed before the age of 30 years, also showed similar mortality rates for men and women, and the size of this cohort permitted robust gender-specific estimates of standardized mortality ratios (SMRs).[804] Among those aged 20 to 29 years, the SMRs for ischemic heart disease mortality were 11.8 in men and 44.8 in women; for those aged 30 to 39 years, the SMRs were 8.0 and 41.6, respectively. Other forms of CVD, such as hypertension, valvular disease, cardiomyopathy, heart failure, and stroke, were also increased.

It is unclear whether there has been any recent decline in mortality or morbidity from CHD associated with T1DM. The Pittsburgh EDC reported no difference in the cumulative incidence of CAD with 20, 25, or 30 years' disease duration according to year of diagnosis (1950 through 1980).[803] The benefits of improved diabetes care therefore do not appear to have reduced CAD mortality associated with T1DM.

Aggregation of Traditional Coronary Heart Disease Risk Factors in Diabetes

It is now well established that a number of traditional CHD risk factors (e.g., hypertension, dyslipidemia, obesity, insulin resistance) tend to occur together in patients with diabetes.[805] Approximately 50% of patients with diabetes have hypertension, and more than 30% have hypercholesterolemia at the time of diagnosis. As in nondiabetic

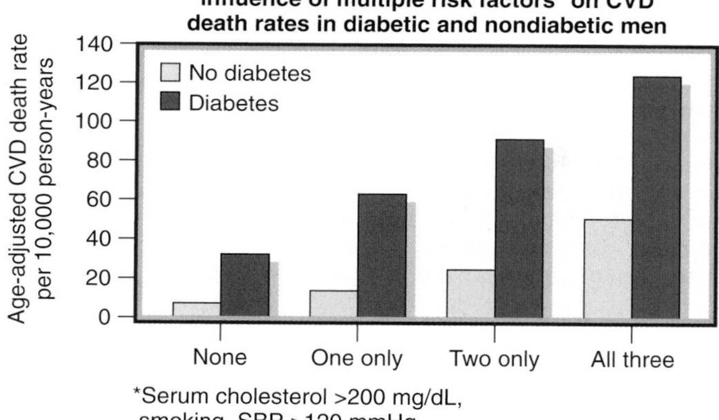

Figure 33-52 Age-adjusted cardiovascular disease (CVD) death rates by number of risk factors for men with and without diabetes at baseline screened for the Multiple Risk Factor Intervention Trial. In the presence of diabetes, the cardiovascular death rate steeply rises at any level of concomitant risk factors. SBP, systolic blood pressure. (From Stamler J, Vaccaro O, Neaton JD, et al. Diabetes, other risk factors, and 12-year cardiovascular mortality for men screened in the Multiple Risk Factor Intervention Trial. *Diabetes Care*. 1993;16:434-444.)

patients, these risk factors independently predict the risk of CVD mortality.[51] However, even in the presence of one or more concomitant risk factors, diabetes increases the CVD death rate (Fig. 33-52). It also appears that diabetes interacts synergistically with other risk factors to more sharply increase risk as the number of total risk factors increases.

There are data suggesting that the cardiovascular risk associated with T2DM is a consequence of insulin resistance during the prediabetic state.[806] A population-based study of diabetes and CVD monitored Mexican American and non–Latin American white subjects for 7 years. Those subjects who converted to diabetes from a prediabetic state and who were insulin resistant had higher BP, higher triglyceride levels, and lower HDL-cholesterol levels. These CVD risk factors suggest that the atherogenic changes seen during the prediabetic state are primarily associated with increased insulin resistance and that treatment strategies that increase insulin secretion in these patients can reduce cardiovascular risk.

Other studies have also concluded that impaired insulin sensitivity during the prediabetic state contributes to atherogenic risk.[807] Prediabetic subjects who were insulin resistant had higher levels of inflammatory markers (C-reactive protein, PAI-1, and fibrinogen) than converters with predominantly low insulin secretion or nonconverters. Therefore, a proinflammatory state can contribute to the atherogenic risk profile in prediabetic patients with increased insulin resistance. Evidence of inflammation is not seen in prediabetic patients with a primary defect in insulin secretion.

The UKPDS further confirmed the importance of risk factor aggregation in diabetic patients. In this large population of patients with newly diagnosed T2DM, the development of CAD during follow-up was significantly associated with increased concentrations of LDL-cholesterol, decreased concentrations of HDL-cholesterol, increased levels of HbA_{1c} and systolic BP, and a history of smoking measured at baseline.[808]

Given the multifactorial nature of atherogenic risk in patients with T2DM, it is reasonable to conclude that an aggressive multifactorial intervention could significantly reduce cardiovascular risk. The value of such a treatment regimen was tested in the Steno-2 study,[561] in which 160 patients with T2DM and microalbuminuria were randomized to receive either conventional treatment in accordance with national guidelines or intensive therapy that included behavior modification and targeted pharmacologic therapy for hyperglycemia, hypertension, dyslipidemia, and microalbuminuria along with secondary prevention of CVD with aspirin. Over a mean follow-up period of 7.8 years, patients who received intensive treatment had greater improvements in HbA_{1c}, BP, fasting serum cholesterol and triglyceride values, and urinary albumin excretion than patients receiving conventional therapy. The greater degree of improvement in risk factors with intensive therapy was also reflected in outcomes. Patients receiving intensive therapy had a significantly lower risk of CVD (HR 0.47; 95% CI, 0.24 to 0.73), nephropathy (HR 0.39; 95% CI, 0.17 to 0.87), retinopathy (HR 0.42; 95% CI, 0.21 to 0.86), and autonomic neuropathy (HR 0.37; 95% CI, 0.18 to 0.79). Overall, long-term intensive treatment of risk factors reduced the risk of CVD and microvascular events by about 50%.[561]

Plasma Glucose and Insulin Resistance as Independent Risk Factors for Atherosclerosis

Hyperglycemia may be responsible for the high excess risk of CHD that cannot be accounted for by the interaction of multiple risk factors alone. This association appears to be graded and continuous, without a clear threshold below which the relationship ends. One study showed that mortality from all causes, CVD, and ischemic heart disease increased progressively across quintiles of fasting blood glucose levels in patients with T2DM (Fig. 33-53).[809] Other data suggest a dose-response relationship between hyperglycemia and CVD mortality in diabetes, with patients with the highest levels of fasting blood glucose having a CVD mortality rate almost five times higher than patients with the two lowest levels combined.[810]

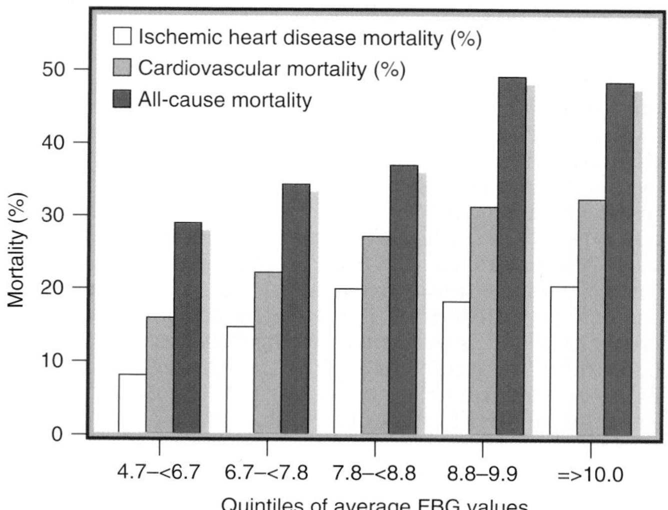

Figure 33-53 All-cause mortality, cardiovascular mortality, and ischemic heart disease mortality in patients with type 2 diabetes mellitus by quintiles of average fasting blood glucose (FBG). Cardiovascular mortality and all-cause mortality increase throughout the range of fasting plasma glucose in a graded fashion. (From Andersson DK, Svardsudd K. Long-term glycemic control relates to mortality in type II diabetes. *Diabetes Care*. 1995;18:1534-1543.)

In a more recent study of the relationship between blood glucose cardiovascular mortality, 17,869 male civil servants enrolled in the Whitehall Study from 1967 to 1969 were monitored, and outcomes were correlated with baseline measurements of the 2-hour postload blood glucose (2hBG) level after a 50-g oral glucose load.[811] In these subjects, the HR for CHD mortality increased as a linear function of 2hBG for all values of 2hBG greater than 83 mg/dL. With 2hBG values between 83 and 200 mg/dL, the age-adjusted HR for CHD was 3.62 (95% CI, 2.3 to 5.6).

Tominaga and colleagues examined survival rates in a cohort of participants in a diabetes prevalence trial in Japan[812] and concluded that the risk of cardiovascular mortality is based on impaired glucose tolerance rather than impaired fasting glucose.

Further substantiation of the role of impaired glucose tolerance in cardiovascular mortality risk was provided by an analysis of data from the Diabetes Epidemiology: Collaborative analysis of Diagnostic criteria in Europe (DECODE) study.[813] In this study, more than 25,000 men and women were monitored for a mean of 7.3 years, and outcomes were correlated with measurements of fasting glucose and 2hBG after a 75-mg glucose load at baseline. The results indicated that the oral glucose tolerance test provides the best index of risk of mortality associated with impaired glucose tolerance.

The Nurses' Health Study also implicated the prediabetic state as a risk factor for CVD.[814] In this large cohort of women, 5894 developed diabetes over a 20-year follow-up. In this group, the age-adjusted RR for MI was 3.75 (95% CI, 3.10 to 4.53) in the period before diagnosis of diabetes and 4.57 (95% CI, 3.87 to 5.39) after diagnosis, compared with women who did not develop diabetes, even after adjustment for other cardiovascular risk factors. The risk of stroke was also increased before onset of diabetes.

The continuum of CVD risk with rising glucose levels has also been identified in patients with T1DM[815] and in subjects without clinically overt diabetes but with varying levels of glucose intolerance.[816] Hyperglycemia also has adverse effects on the vessel wall as judged by objective assessment of CIMT.[6,817-819]

The Metabolic Syndrome

Definitions and Diagnosis

Almost all patients with diabetes and the concomitant CVD risk factors of hypertension, obesity, and dyslipidemia also have insulin resistance.[61] The clustering of these risk factors in a single patient has been termed the *metabolic syndrome*. Although there is general agreement on the components of the metabolic syndrome (i.e., obesity, hypertension, dyslipidemia, and dysfunctional glucose metabolism), the criteria for clinical diagnosis are still under discussion. Separate sets of diagnostic criteria for the metabolic syndrome have been published by the National Cholesterol Education Program (NCEP) Adult Treatment Panel III (ATP III),[820] by the World Health Organization (WHO),[821] and by the International Diabetes Federation (IDF).[822]

According to the NCEP guidelines,[820] the metabolic syndrome is based on the presence of three of the following five risk factors[820]:

- Abdominal obesity (waist circumference <40 inches in men, <35 inches in women)
- Plasma triglycerides 150 mg/dL or higher
- Plasma HDL-cholesterol <40 mg/dL in men, <50 mg/dL in women
- Blood pressure 130/85 mm Hg or higher
- Fasting plasma glucose 110 mg/dL or higher

The NCEP criteria give precedence to obesity as a contributor to the metabolic syndrome and apply cutpoints for triglycerides and HDL that are probably less stringent than would be used to identify a categorical risk factor, reflecting the fact that many marginal risk factors can result in a significant risk for CVD. The NCEP criteria do not require explicit demonstration of insulin resistance for diagnosis of the metabolic syndrome, and patients with diabetes are not excluded from the diagnosis.[821] There are modest differences between the NCEP criteria and those developed by the WHO[821] and the IDF.[822]

Epidemiology

The prevalence of the metabolic syndrome in the Unites States, as defined by the NCEP criteria, has been estimated from the National Health and Nutrition Examination Survey (NHANES) database.[823] Based on data from the third NHANES (1988-1994) survey, the overall age-adjusted prevalence of the metabolic syndrome was 23.7%. The prevalence increased with age, ranging from 6.7% in subjects aged 20 to 29 years to 43.5% in subjects aged 60 to 69 years. There were also differences in prevalence based on ethnicity, with the highest overall prevalence among Mexican Americans (31.9%).

The Metabolic Syndrome and Cardiovascular Disease

The impact of metabolic syndrome on incidence and mortality of CVD has been examined in several studies.[824-826] A Finnish prospective cohort study showed that the age-adjusted RR for CHD mortality was 2.96 (95% CI, 1.30 to 6.76), compared to patients without this condition. Similar increases in risk were also noted for CVD mortality (RR, 2.76; 95% CI, 1.45 to 5.24) and all-cause mortality (RR, 2.05; 95% CI, 1.31 to 3.21). Similar degrees of increase in risk with the metabolic syndrome were also seen when other diagnostic criteria were used.

In the United States, NHANES II studied the impact of the metabolic syndrome on CVD mortality.[827] The HRs for CHD mortality and CVD mortality were 1.65 (95% CI, 1.10 to 2.47; $P = .02$) and 1.56 (95% CI, 1.15 to 2.12, $P = .005$), respectively, compared to subjects without the metabolic syndrome.

The West of Scotland Coronary Prevention Study[826] also demonstrated increased risk of CHD in patients with the metabolic syndrome. In this study, elevated C-reactive protein was more common in subjects with the metabolic syndrome and added to the prognostic value for both CHD and diabetes.

A summary of all of the studies assessing the increased risk of mortality, CVD, and diabetes associated with the metabolic syndrome was published in 2005.[827] Studies that used NCEP and WHO diagnostic criteria for defining the metabolic syndrome were analyzed separately. For three studies that used the exact NCEP definition of the metabolic syndrome, the increased risk of all-cause mortality was not significant. For seven studies that used the NCEP definition, the RR for CVD was 1.65 (95% CI, 1.38 to 1.99). Inclusion of four other studies that used a modified NCEP definition did not appreciably change the RR. In four studies that used the NCEP definition, the RR for diabetes was 2.99 (95% CI, 1.96 to 4.57). For studies that used the most exact WHO definition of the metabolic syndrome, the fixed-effects estimates of RR were 1.37 (95% CI, 1.09 to 1.74) for all-cause mortality, 1.93 (95% CI, 1.39 to 2.67) for CVD, and 6.08 (95% CI, 4.76 to 7.76) for diabetes.

Clinical guidelines for diagnosis and management of the metabolic syndrome were addressed in 2005 in a joint

TABLE 33-13

Treatment Goals for Prevention of Coronary Heart Disease in Patients with Diabetes

Glycosylated hemoglobin (HbA_{1c}) ≤6.2%
Low-density lipoprotein cholesterol ≤100 mg/dL
Blood pressure ≤130/85 mm Hg
Aspirin 81-325 mg/day

statement by the American Heart Association and the National Heart, Lung, and Blood Institute summarizing available steps for managing the risk factors associated with the metabolic syndrome.[828]

It has been hypothesized that hyperinsulinemia is the underlying link between hyperglycemia and CVD in these patients.[829] A number of studies have shown hyperinsulinemia to be an independent predictor of CVD risk. Furthermore, in patients spanning the spectrum of glucose tolerance, from normal to hyperglycemic to diabetic, insulin resistance positively correlates with atherosclerosis as assessed by CIMT.[830]

The San Antonio Heart Study, a population-based study of diabetes and CVD in Mexican Americans and non–Latin American whites, confirmed the relationship between insulin resistance or plasma insulin and CVD.[67]

The Role of Glycemic Control

The UKPDS confirmed the positive association between plasma glucose levels and CHD risk for HbA_{1c} levels greater than 6.2% in patients with diabetes.[829] CHD risk increased by 11% with each percentage point elevation in HbA_{1c} (Table 33-13). The question remains, however, whether intensive glycemic control can modify the cardiovascular risk profile of patients with diabetes.

Earlier studies, such as the DCCT and the smaller Veterans Affairs (VA) study, did not show a reduction in cardiovascular end points with intensive metabolic control. These studies had limitations, however. Although relatively large (N = 1441), the DCCT followed a relatively young (mean age, 27 years) population of patients with T1DM for more than 6 years. At the end of follow-up, few events had occurred.[2] Intensive therapy reduced the risk of CVD and peripheral vascular disease by 41% compared with conventional therapy, but the difference was not statistically significant. Similarly, in the VA study, intensive blood glucose control in patients with T2DM did not significantly reduce cardiovascular end points.[831] Both studies lacked adequate power to detect a difference in macrovascular events between treatment groups because of the small number of events in each group, small patient populations, and relatively short follow-up.

A 17-year follow-up of 1441 patients from the DCCT trial more unambiguously demonstrated the benefit of intensive glycemic control in T1DM.[832] This was part of the observational Epidemiology of Diabetes Interventions and Complications (EDIC) study. During follow-up, intensive treatment reduced the risk of CVD by 42% (P = .02) and the risk of nonfatal MI, stroke, or death from CVD by 57% (P = .02). After 11 years of follow-up, the treatment groups were virtually identical in terms of HbA_{1c}, BP, and lipid risk factors. Patients in the conventional treatment group had more albuminuria and microalbuminuria than intensively treated patients, but the differences in risk remained significant after adjustment for these factors. These findings indicate that intensive glycemic control reduced the long-term risk of CVD in patients with T1DM.

The UKPDS was larger and was adequately powered to detect a difference between groups in macrovascular events.[3] Intensive glycemic control trended toward demonstrating a lower rate of MI than conventional treatment (P = .052).[3] As in the DCCT, intensive therapy in the UKPDS significantly improved the rate of microvascular disease.

Despite the lack of overall efficacy of intensive treatment for management of macrovascular complications of diabetes in the UKPDS, there are indications that specific therapies may be effective.[3] In a retrospective analysis of an overweight subset (n = 342) of the UKPDS cohort who were treated with metformin, there were significant reductions in the occurrence of any diabetes-related end point (32%), diabetes-related death (42%), and all-cause mortality (36%), compared with conventionally treated patients.

Two studies have suggested that thiazolidinediones can prevent macrovascular events associated with T2DM. Because these drugs work by increasing insulin sensitivity rather than by increasing insulin levels, this finding is consistent with data showing that insulin resistance is positively correlated with cardiovascular outcomes (described earlier). Sidhu and colleagues demonstrated that 8 weeks of treatment with rosiglitazone 4 mg daily significantly reduced progression of thickening of the common carotid intima-media, a surrogate index of atherosclerotic disease progression, compared with placebo treatment in nondiabetic patients who had established CAD.[830] In the PROactive study (PROspective pioglitAzone Clinical Trial In macroVascular Events), 5238 patients with T2DM and evidence of macrovascular disease were randomized to receive or not receive pioglitazone in addition to glucose-lowering drugs and other medications.[833] After a mean of 34.5 months, there was no significant difference in the two treatment groups in terms of the primary end point of the study, a composite of all-cause mortality, nonfatal MI, stroke, acute coronary syndrome, surgical intervention in the leg or coronary arteries, and amputation above the ankle. However, patients treated with pioglitazone had significantly lower risk for the secondary end point of composite all-cause mortality, nonfatal MI, and stroke, (HR 0.84; 95% CI, 0.80 to 1.02; P = .027). Compared with placebo, pioglitazone also significantly reduced the need to add insulin to glucose-lowering regimens.

Despite the effect of thiazolidinediones in these studies, the putative beneficial effect of rosiglitazone on CVD was challenged by a meta-analysis conducted by Nissen and coworkers that examined short-term trials designed to assess the effect of rosiglitazone on glycemic control and suggested that rosiglitazone was associated with a significant risk of excess MI. The studies in this meta-analysis did not examine cardiovascular events as primary end points and the cardiovascular events were not adjudicated. In contrast, another meta-analysis, conducted by Lago and associates, examined only randomized clinical trials in which cardiovascular end points were prespecified as events of interest or in which such events were adjudicated. This examination did not show that either rosiglitazone or pioglitazone conferred an excess risk of cardiovascular death.[835]

Three recent trials have examined whether lowering the target for glycemic control (to <7%) can reduce the risk for cardiovascular events. The ACCORD trial randomized patients with T2DM who had established CVD or multiple risk factors to a treatment-directed HbA_{1c} value lower than 7.0% or to standard therapy with an HbA_{1c} target value between 7.0% and 7.9%. Over 3.5 years of follow-up, total mortality was increased in the intensively treated group, and there was no significant reduction in cardiovascular events.[836] The VADT randomized patients to either intensive treatment (HbA_{1c}, 6.9%) or standard therapy (HbA_{1c}, 8.4%); it also did not demonstrate a reduction in cardiovascular events in the former group.[837] The ADVANCE trial randomly assigned patients to an intensively treated group attaining an HbA_{1c} of 6.5% or a standard-control group attaining an HbA_{1c} of 7.3%; it demonstrated a relative reduction of 10% in the combined outcome of major macrovascular and microvascular events, primarily due to a 21% reduction in nephropathy.[838] Taken together, these three studies do not support treatment to an HbA_{1c} value lower than the currently recommended 7.0% as a strategy to reduce cardiovascular events, despite the epidemiologic relationship between cardiovascular risk and HbA_{1c}.

The Bypass Angioplasty Revascularization Investigation 2 Diabetes (BARI 2D) trial randomized 2368 patients with T2DM and CAD to either prompt revascularization or intensive medical therapy alone, and to either insulin-sensitization or insulin-provision diabetes therapy. Randomization was stratified by the proposed revascularization method. The 5-year survival and major cardiovascular event rates were similar in all study subgroups except for those patients undergonig coronary artery bypass grafting (CABG), who had fewer major cardiovascular events after revascularization. There was less hypoglycemia and weight gain and greater apparent benefit from CABG in the insulin-sensitization group.

Dyslipidemia and Its Treatment in Patients with Diabetes Mellitus

Dyslipidemia is the best-characterized risk factor for increasing atherosclerosis in patients with T2DM. A number of features of dyslipidemia are uniquely associated with diabetes and appear to increase the predisposition to atherogenesis. Although patients with diabetes tend not to have marked elevations in plasma LDL-cholesterol levels, their LDL-cholesterol particles are generally smaller and more dense than typical LDL-cholesterol particles. These small, dense LDL-cholesterol particles are more susceptible to oxidation, particularly in the setting of poor glucose control. Other evidence suggests that glycation of LDL may be enhanced in diabetes, impairing recognition of the lipoprotein by its hepatoreceptor and extending its half-life. Conversely, levels of the cardioprotective lipid fraction, HDL-cholesterol, are decreased in patients with diabetes. The HDL-cholesterol of these patients may also be less effective at protecting LDL-cholesterol from oxidative stress, one of the proposed mechanisms for the cardioprotective effect of HDL-cholesterol.[839]

Undoubtedly, the key feature of diabetic dyslipidemia is an increase in the production of VLDL by the liver in response to elevations in FFAs. Although insulin mediates the uptake of FFAs by striated muscle, reducing the levels presented to the liver, insulin resistance results in the opposite effect, increasing the levels of FFAs available to the liver. The metabolic syndrome, with its characteristic abdominal obesity, also increases the delivery of FFAs to the liver. In addition, reduced lipoprotein lipase activity in T2DM leads to an accumulation of triglyceride-rich lipoproteins in the plasma of these patients. Triglyceride-rich lipoproteins also play a role in the reduced levels of HDL-cholesterol by increasing the transfer of cholesterol from these particles.

A number of landmark trials have proved that lowering lipid levels produces major clinical benefits in terms of reducing cardiovascular events in patients with and without a history of CHD at baseline. These findings have now been extended to the population of subjects with T2DM and dyslipidemia. For example, even though LDL levels are often within the average range in these patients, treatment with 3-hydroxy-3-methylglutaryl coenzyme A (HMG-CoA) reductase inhibitors (statins) has been shown to improve outcomes. In the Cholesterol and Recurrent Events (CARE) trial, diabetic patients treated with pravastatin had a significant 25% reduction in the incidence of CHD death, nonfatal MI, CABG, and revascularization procedures.[7] In the Long-term Intervention with Pravastatin in Ischemic Disease (LIPID) study, patients with diabetes had a 19% reduction in major CHD (fatal CHD and nonfatal MI).[840]

In a post hoc subgroup analysis of secondary prevention in a large cohort of patients with diabetes, impaired glucose tolerance, or normal glucose tolerance, simvastatin normalized associated elevations in total cholesterol and triglycerides across the range of glucose values.[841] Treatment also significantly reduced major coronary events and revascularizations in patients with diabetes and reduced major coronary events, revascularizations, and total and coronary mortality in patients with impaired glucose tolerance.

Several studies have further verified the use of statins in patients with diabetes and related conditions.[842-846] In the Heart Protection Study, a large (N = 20,536), randomized, placebo-controlled trial of the use of simvastatin 40 mg in high-risk patients, roughly 29% of the study participants had T2DM.[847] Over the 5-year course of the study, treatment with simvastatin resulted in a significant reduction in the occurrence of major vascular events in patients with T2DM who had previous MI or other CHD (33.4% versus 37.8% in simvastatin- and placebo-treated patients, respectively), in diabetics with no prior CHD (13.8% versus 18.6%), and in both categories combined (20.2% versus 25.1%). Overall, the study also demonstrated a highly significant 12% RR reduction in all-cause mortality and an 18% RR reduction in coronary mortality among all subjects treated with simvastatin.

The Collaborative Atorvastatin Diabetes Study (CARDS) was a large (N = 2838), randomized, placebo-controlled trial that assessed the benefit of atorvastatin 10 mg/day for preventing acute CHD events, coronary revascularization, or stroke in patients with T2DM who had no documented history of CVD and plasma LDL levels lower than 160 mg/dL.[848] The trial was terminated 2 years early because the prespecified efficacy criteria were met. After a median of 3.9 years follow-up, patients treated with atorvastatin had an RR reduction for first cardiovascular event of 37% (95% CI, 52% to 17% reduction; P = .001), compared with placebo-treated patients. Assessed separately, acute CHD, coronary revascularizations, and stroke were significantly reduced, by 36%, 31%, and 48%, respectively. Based on these results, the CARDS investigators concluded that in patents with T2DM, a threshold LDL-cholesterol level should not be the sole determinant of whether a statin is prescribed.

A post hoc study compared major coronary events, total mortality, and revascularization rates in two subsets of patients who received simvastatin 20 to 40 mg/day for a median of 5.4 years in the Scandinavian Simvastatin Survival Study (4S).[842] Treatment with simvastatin resulted in a 52% RR reduction of major coronary events, a greater treatment effect than was seen in the patients with isolated high LDL-cholesterol. Reanalysis of the data after exclusion of the patients with diabetes did not substantially alter the findings.

The Treating to New Targets (TNT) study compared the effects of atorvastatin 10 mg or 80 mg daily for a median follow-up period of 4.9 years in patients with clinically evident CHD who also met the NCEP criteria for diagnosis of the metabolic syndrome.[843] The study included 778 patients with T2DM, who constituted 22% of the study population. Treatment with atorvastatin 80 mg was significantly more effective for reducing major cardiovascular events than atorvastatin 10 mg (HR = 0.71; 95% CI, 0.61 to 0.84; $P < .0001$), presumably due to the significantly greater reduction in LDL-cholesterol seen with the higher dosing of atorvastatin.

The Arterial Biology for the Investigation of the Treatment Effects of Reducing Cholesterol (ARBITER)[844] was a randomized, double-blind study in which patients were assigned to receive extended-release niacin 500 mg titrated to 1000 mg daily ($n = 87$) or placebo ($n = 80$) on a background statin therapy. The primary end point of the study was change in CIMT after 1 year of niacin treatment. Despite a significant 21% increase in HDL-cholesterol levels in the patients receiving niacin, the overall difference in CIMT progression between the niacin- and placebo-treated groups only tended toward significance ($P = .08$).

Fibric acid derivatives might also be beneficial in patients with diabetes, because these agents address the low HDL-cholesterol and high triglyceride levels typically associated with diabetes. In the VA High-Density Lipoprotein Cholesterol Intervention Trial (VA-HIT), men given gemfibrozil had lower rates of coronary events and strokes.[845] A fibric acid derivative in combination with a statin may be the optimal approach in patients with diabetes and CHD who have hypercholesterolemia in association with elevated triglycerides and reduced HDL-cholesterol levels.

The Fenofibrate Intervention and Event Lowering in Diabetes (FIELD) study assessed the effect of long-term fenofibrate therapy on cardiovascular events in patients with T2DM.[846] Patients were randomized to receive either micronized fenofibrate 200 mg/day ($n = 4895$) or placebo ($n = 4900$). During 5-year follow-up, 5.9% of the placebo-treated patients and 5.2% of the fenofibrate-treated patients had a coronary event, a difference that was not significantly different. Fenofibrate therapy significantly reduced total CVD events (HR, 0.89; 95% CI, 0.75 to 1.05; $P = .035$), progression of albuminuria, and the need for laser treatment of retinopathy. Statistical significance for the primary end point of the study might have been missed because a greater percentage of patients in the placebo group initiated lipid-lowering therapy during the study period, and this masked the treatment effect.

The ACCORD trial provided important information regarding the use of fibrates in patients with T2DM. This trial investigated whether combination therapy with simvastatin plus fenofibrate, compared with simvastatin alone, would reduce cardiovascular events in diabetic patients at high risk for CVD. In this randomized clinical trial comparing fenofibrate to placebo in statin-treated patients, combination therapy did not reduce the rate of cardiovascular mortality, nonfatal MI, or nonfatal stroke. In a prespecified subgroup with a high triglyceride ratio (triglycerides ≥204 mg/dL and HDL ≤34 mg/dL), fenofibrate was better than placebo in reducing the primary outcome. At this time, there is no recommendation that these patients receive combination statin-fibrate therapy as an ingredient in risk factor reduction on the basis of T2DM alone.[849]

The importance of dyslipidemia as a contributor to cardiovascular risk in patients with diabetes is reflected in the new guidelines of the NCEP ATP III.[820] For the first time, diabetes is considered a CHD risk equivalent, meaning that patients with diabetes have a risk of CHD that is similar to that of patients with clinically manifest CHD (>20% risk of an event in the following 10 years). In addition, the presence of multiple CHD risk factors, the metabolic syndrome, and mixed hyperlipidemia (high triglyceride and low HDL-cholesterol levels) should be taken into account when estimating a patient's global risk.

According to the NCEP ATP III guidelines, diabetic patients are candidates for cholesterol-lowering therapy if the LDL-cholesterol level is higher than 3.36 mmol/L (130 mg/dL), with the goal of reducing LDL-cholesterol to less than 2.57 mmol/L (100 mg/dL),[822] although many clinicians consider it prudent to approach therapy more aggressively by instituting drug treatment if the LDL-cholesterol level is higher than 2.57 mmol/L (100 mg/dL). Based on new trial information, these guidelines have been modified to state that, when risk is very high, a goal of less than 70 mg/dL LDL-cholesterol is a reasonable clinical strategy, even when the high-risk patient has a baseline LDL-cholesterol level lower than 100 mg/dL.[850] Additionally, when a high-risk patient has low HDL-cholesterol or high triglyceride levels, the combination of niacin or a fibrate with an LDL-lowering drug should be considered. However, regardless of the drug regimen employed, patients with diabetes should maintain tight glycemic control, which in itself can help reverse the dyslipidemic profile that is prevalent in diabetes. As with all patients, lifestyle modification, including weight reduction and regular exercise, remains an important cornerstone of the treatment of dyslipidemia in patients with diabetes.

Signature Features and Treatment of Hypertension in Diabetic Patients

It has been estimated that up to 50% of patients with newly diagnosed diabetes also have high BP. As with dyslipidemia, hypertension interacts with diabetes to amplify the risk of cardiac mortality (see Fig. 33-52). Although the etiology of hypertension is multifactorial, the insulin-resistant state is one factor postulated to predispose patients to development of hypertension. In addition to its negative effects on the cardiovascular system, high BP is a key contributor to the development of microvascular disease in diabetes. Based on the guidelines of the Joint National Committee on Prevention, Detection, Evaluation, and Treatment of High Blood Pressure (JNC VII), BP should be reduced to less than 130/85 mm Hg in patients with diabetes.[851]

Results of the most recent clinical trials underscore the benefits of aggressive treatment of hypertension in patients with diabetes, although none of these studies achieved mean BP reductions to currently recommended targets. Use of a long-acting dihydropyridine calcium channel blocker in the Systolic Hypertension in Europe (Syst-Eur) study resulted in substantial reductions in total mortality (55%), cardiovascular mortality (76%), and cardiovascular events (69%) in the diabetic subgroup, greater benefits than were seen in the subgroup without diabetes.

In the Heart Outcomes Prevention Evaluation (HOPE) study, in which almost 40% of patients had diabetes and one other cardiovascular risk factor, ramipril reduced the primary outcome by 24% and total mortality by 25%.[853] Even in normotensive patients with diabetes, some benefit was seen, with a 2- to 4-mm Hg drop in BP with ACE inhibitor therapy.

Other rigorously designed studies, such as the UKPDS[854] and the Hypertension Optimal Treatment (HOT) study,[855] suggested even greater benefits from tight BP control in patients with diabetes.

In the Losartan Intervention For Endpoint Reduction in Hypertension (LIFE) study, patients with diabetes, hypertension, and signs of left ventricular hypertrophy were randomly assigned to treatment with losartan-based (n = 586) or atenolol-based (n = 609) treatment for hypertension.[856] Despite similar BP reductions, losartan was more effective than atenolol for reducing cardiovascular morbidity and mortality, mortality from CVD, and mortality from all causes. The ability of losartan to reduce events more effectively than atenolol may be related to the ability of ARBs to reverse left ventricular hypertrophy more effectively than β-blockers.

Although β-blockers are thought to worsen glycemic control in patients with diabetes, it is not clear whether this is a property of all members of this drug class or whether this property persists if β-blockers are given in combination with renin-angiotensin system inhibitors that are known to increase insulin sensitivity. In the Glycemic Effects in Diabetes Mellitus: Carvdeilol-Metoprolol Comparison in Hypertensives (GENINI) trial, patients with documented T2DM and hypertension who were taking a stable dose of either an ARB or an ACE inhibitor were randomized to receive either carvedilol or metoprolol. Although the degree of BP control was similar with both β-blockers, HbA_{1c} and insulin sensitivity increased significantly with metoprolol but not with carvedilol. Therefore, carvedilol can prevent the adverse effects of metoprolol on glucose levels when used in combination with renin-angiotensin system inhibitors, although this conclusion needs to be tested in a longer-term outcome trial.

The investigators of the Antihypertensive and Lipid-Lowering Treatment to Prevent Heart Attack Trial (ALLHAT) compared outcomes during first-step treatment of hypertension in 31,512 patients with T2DM, IFG, or normoglycemia with a calcium channel blocker (amlodipine 2.5 to 10 mg/day) or ACE inhibitor (lisinopril 10 to 40 mg/day) compared with a thiazide-type diuretic (chlorthalidone 12.5 to 25 mg/day).[856] There was no significant difference in the occurrence of the primary outcome (fatal CHD or nonfatal MI) in patients with T2DM treated with a calcium channel blocker or an ACE inhibitor compared with chlorthalidone. Patients with IFG treated with a calcium channel blocker had a significantly higher RR for the primary outcome than patients receiving chlorthalidone.

A major unresolved question has been whether treatment of hypertension to lower targets than currently recommended would reduce cardiovascular risk in patients with T2DM. Most trials establishing the remarkable benefit of BP lowering, regardless of the medications used, have studied subjects whose BP was higher than 140 mm Hg. In the ACCORD trial, two strategies of BP management were examined as to their efficacy in lowering cardiovascular risk. One group was randomized to a systolic BP lower than 120 mm Hg (intensive therapy), and the other group was treated to a systolic pressure lower than 140 mm Hg (standard therapy). Targeting the lower BP level did not reduce the rate of fatal and nonfatal cardiovascular events. Based on this result, there is no recommendation to treat patients with T2DM and hypertension to a systolic BP lower than the currently recommended target of 130 mm Hg to decrease cardiovascular events. However, further reduction may reduce the incidence of diabetic nephropathy.[526,857]

Acute Coronary Syndromes in Diabetes Mellitus

The case-fatality rate from MI is almost twice as high in patients with diabetes as in nondiabetic patients. This excess risk is seen both during the acute phase of MI and in the early and late postinfarction period. A number of mechanisms have been deemed to be responsible for worse outcomes in patients with diabetes, including the following:

- Increased risk of CHF due to maladaptive remodeling of the left ventricle[858-860]
- Increased risk of sudden death due to sympathovagal imbalance as a consequence of autonomic neuropathy[861-863]
- Increased likelihood of early reinfarction due to impaired fibrinolysis[864-866]
- Extensive underlying CAD[867,868]
- Changes in myocardial cell metabolism, including a shift from glucose oxidation to FFA oxidation, with less generation of ATP at any level of oxygen consumption[869,870]
- Associated cardiomyopathy.[768]

Collective data provide strong evidence that a variety of treatment modalities can improve outcomes from MI in patients with diabetes. In terms of interventions, patients with diabetes experiencing an acute MI respond as favorably to fibrinolytic therapy as do nondiabetic patients.[42,867,868] Excellent glycemic control is an essential component of overall management. Glucose levels at hospital admission have been independently correlated with early and late mortality after MI in patients with and without diabetes mellitus.[871-874]

Studies such as the Diabetes and Insulin-Glucose Infusion in Acute Myocardial Infarction (DIGAMI) study have assessed the impact of intensive glycemic control in patients with diabetes during the acute phase of MI. Patients in this study were randomized to either intensive insulin therapy (insulin-glucose infusion for 24 hours, followed by subcutaneous insulin injection for 3 months) or standard glycemic control.[875] The intensive insulin regimen lowered blood glucose level during the first hour after admission and at discharge compared with conventional therapy. One-year mortality was significantly reduced with the insulin infusion compared with control, a difference that was maintained after 3.4 years of follow-up.

DIGAMI 2, a prospective, randomized, open-label trial that followed up the DIGAMI trial, compared outcomes in patients with either T1DM or T2DM and failed to corroborate the earlier reported improvement in outcomes with intensive insulin treatment.[876] The lack of effect of long-term insulin treatment on outcomes may be at least partially explained by the fact that 14% of the patients in the conventional treatment group received insulin-glucose infusions in violation of the protocol, and as many as 41% had extra glucose injections. As a result, the blood glucose levels in all three groups were not significantly different after treatment.

Although the mechanisms responsible for the potential benefit shown in the original DEGAMI study are not entirely clear, experimental data suggest that strict glycemic control can improve myocardial cell metabolism by increasing the availability of glucose as a substrate for ATP generation and reducing the formation of FFAs, thereby shifting cardiac metabolism from FFA oxidation to glycolysis and glucose oxidation. Intensive glycemic control can also reverse the impaired fibrinolysis that is typically seen in patients with diabetes.

The CREATE-ECLA (Clinical Trial of Reviparin and Metabolic Modulation in Acute Myocardial Infarction Treatment Evaluation-Estudios Cardiologicos Latin America) randomized, controlled trial assigned 20,201 patients who presented with ST-segment elevation MI within 12 hours after onset of symptoms to treatment with either high-dose glucose-insulin-potassium (GIK) infusion (i.e., 25% glucose, 50 U/L regular insulin, and 80 m/Eq KCl) administered over 24 hours or to usual care.[877] Roughly 18% of the patients in both treatment arms had T2DM. After 30 days, there were no differences in the rate of occurrence of mortality, cardiac arrest, cardiogenic shock, or reinfarction in the two treatment groups.

Sulfonylureas have been implicated in an increased cardiovascular mortality rate, particularly in patients undergoing revascularization for acute MI.[878] The UKPDS did not show a deleterious effect of these agents on the incidence of sudden death or MI over 10 years of follow-up.[3] The sulfonylureas act through the sulfonylurea receptor component of ATP-sensitive potassium channels in the pancreatic beta cell. In the heart, ATP-sensitive potassium channels are involved in ischemic preconditioning and coronary vasodilation.[879-881] It is not clear whether the sulfonylureas modulate these channels in the heart or vascular system or whether they significantly increase risk in diabetic patients with an acute MI.

ACE inhibitors dramatically reduce mortality after an MI in patients with diabetes, ostensibly through their effects to reduce infarct size and limit ventricular remodeling. In addition to these hemodynamic benefits, ACE inhibitors can also improve outcomes in diabetes by improving endothelial function,[882] improving fibrinolysis,[883] and decreasing insulin resistance.[884]

In a retrospective analysis of the Gruppo Italiano per lo Studio della Sopravvivenza nell'Infarto Miocardico (GISSI-3) study,[885] lisinopril administration within 24 hours after hospital admission substantially reduced both 6-week and 6-month mortality in patients with diabetes compared with the nondiabetic group. Similarly, a subgroup analysis from the Trandolapril Cardiac Evaluation Study (TRACE) showed that patients with diabetes suffering an anterior MII who were treated with trandolapril had greatly improved outcomes over 5 years compared with patients without diabetes, including an almost 50% reduction in the risk of sudden death, reinfarction, and progression of CHF.[886]

β-Blockers are now widely accepted for the treatment of acute coronary syndrome in patients with diabetes. Older, noncardioselective β-blockers might have adversely affected the lipid profile and inhibited the metabolic response to hypoglycemia, but more recent data with cardioselective β-blockers suggest that these agents have less negative effects on metabolic indices, perhaps because they increase peripheral blood flow and improve glucose delivery.[887,888] Clinical trial data confirm that β-blockers reduce the rates of mortality and reinfarction in patients with MI in the presence of diabetes. In fact, their effects in patients with diabetes appear to exceed those seen in nondiabetic patients. A large review of data from more than 45,000 patients, 26% of whom had diabetes, showed that β-blocker therapy was associated with a lower 1-year mortality rate in patients with diabetes than in those without diabetes, with no evidence of an increase in diabetes-related complications.[889]

Postulated mechanisms for the benefit of β-blockers in patients with diabetes include dampening of the sympathetic nervous system overactivity that arises as a consequence of autonomic neuropathy. β-Blockers can also reduce FFA levels and thereby reduce myocardial oxygen requirements. Carvedilol, although not cardioselective, is a β-blocker that decreases insulin resistance and also has antioxidant effects, both of which may be of particular benefit in patients with T2DM.[890]

Aspirin is a cornerstone of therapy for the primary or secondary prevention of acute coronary syndrome in patients with T1DM and T2DM who do not have contraindications to its use. Aspirin significantly lowers the risk of MI without increasing the risk of vitreous or retinal bleeding, even in patients with retinopathy.[891] Enteric-coated aspirin, 81 to 325 mg/day, is currently recommended by the ADA.[892] The benefits of this therapy are likely to result from effects on the enhanced platelet aggregation that is evident in patients with either T1DM or T2DM.[893]

Antiplatelet therapy with clopidogrel also benefits patients with diabetes. The CAPRIE trial compared outcomes in patients with non–ST-segment elevation MI treated with aspirin or with clopidogrel and included 3866 patients with diabetes.[894] Although the event rate was higher among the diabetic patients than in the overall study population, the response to treatment was also better. The event rate for the primary end point (vascular death, ischemic stroke, MI, or rehospitalization for ischemia or bleeding) was 17.7% for diabetic patients treated with aspirin and 15.6% for those randomized to clopidogrel, a significant RR reduction of 12.5%.

Newer adjunct therapies, such as the platelet glycoprotein IIb/IIIa receptor antagonists that antagonize platelet action, have also been assessed in diabetic patients who present with unstable angina or non–Q-wave infarction. Overall, these agents appear to work equally well, or perhaps slightly better, in patients with diabetes compared with nondiabetic patients. In the Platelet Receptor Inhibition in Ischemic Syndrome Management in Patients Limited by Unstable Signs and Symptoms (PRISM-PLUS) study, the addition of tirofiban to heparin therapy reduced the 7-day composite end point, compared with heparin alone. This effect was greater in patients with diabetes than in patients without diabetes.[895]

In one study of patients undergoing percutaneous transluminal coronary angioplasty (PTCA), glycoprotein IIb/IIIa antagonist therapy was associated with fewer acute events but a higher rate of target-vessel revascularization in the long term in the diabetic cohort compared with the nondiabetic cohort.[896] However, in another trial, in which stents were used, the rate of target vessel revascularization at 6 months was significantly decreased with the addition of a glycoprotein IIb/IIIa antagonist compared with placebo.[897]

Results of the Bypass Angioplasty Revascularization Investigation (BARI) showed that CABG provides better outcomes than PTCA in patients with diabetes, possibly because it addresses the extensive coronary vascular disease in these patients.[898] This study did not employ stents or glycoprotein IIb/IIIa inhibitors, two modalities that, when used together, appear to improve outcomes after PTCA in patients with diabetes.

Cardiomyopathy in Patients with Diabetes Mellitus

Diabetes is associated with a fourfold increase in the risk of CHF, even after adjustment for other cardiovascular risk factors such as age, BP, cholesterol level, obesity, and history of CAD.[899] Patients with diabetes experience higher rates of CHF than do nondiabetic patients after an acute MI, regardless of the size of the infarct zone.[859,900] These findings suggest that diabetes itself causes deleterious effects on the myocardium, leading to poorer outcomes.

A number of key structural, functional, and metabolic factors in diabetes have been implicated in the increased risk of maladaptive remodeling that leads to CHF. For example, evidence of silent MI is found in up to 40% of patients with diabetes who present with a clinically apparent MI and can lead to unrecognized regional and global ventricular dysfunction.[885,901] As many as 50% of patients with diabetes and CAD have cardiac autonomic neuropathy, which is known to contribute to both systolic and diastolic dysfunction.[768] Like hypertension, diabetes can cause fibrosis of the myocardium and increased collagen deposition.[902,903] These effects are even more pronounced in patients with coexisting hypertension and diabetes. Enhanced endothelial dysfunction in diabetes has also been described as a pathophysiologic pathway to impaired microvascular perfusion and ischemia.[904,905]

On a cellular level, both hyperglycemia and insulin resistance have direct negative effects on myocardial metabolism. Depression of myocardial GLUT4 levels in the setting of diabetes and ischemia inhibits glucose entry and glycolysis in the heart. As a result, intracellular metabolism shifts from glycolysis to FFA oxidation, thereby suppressing glycolytic ATP generation, a major source of energy under anaerobic (i.e., ischemic) conditions.[869] The production of oxygen free radicals can also be enhanced in this situation, further depressing myocardial contractile function.[905]

Collectively, these various abnormalities potentiate the characteristic left ventricular remodeling of diabetes, which is clinically manifested as serial wall motion changes, reduced regional ejection fraction, and increased end-diastolic and end-systolic volumes.[906,907]

THE DIABETIC FOOT

Of all the late complications of diabetes, foot problems are probably the most preventable. Joslin, who wrote in 1934 that "diabetic gangrene is not heaven-sent, but earth-born," was correct: The development of foot ulceration mostly results from the way we care for our patients or the way patients care for themselves.

Increasing interest in the diabetic foot has resulted in a better understanding of the factors that interact to cause ulceration and amputation. The neuropathic foot does not spontaneously ulcerate; insensitivity in combination with other factors, such as deformity and unperceived trauma (e.g., inappropriate footwear), leads to skin breakdown. Increased knowledge of this pathogenesis should permit the design of appropriate screening programs for risk and preventive education. Much progress has been made, but it has not yet resulted in a universal decrease in amputation rates. In the VA system, for example, amputation rates in diabetic patients[908] have not declined, although certain European countries have reported a significant reduction in amputation rates after implementation of foot screening and education programs.[909,910] Much research is still needed to implement strategies to reduce ulceration and amputation, and this is particularly required in the fields of behavioral and psychosocial aspects of the diabetic foot.[911]

Two major texts on the diabetic foot were published in recent years.[912,913] The reader is referred to these sources together with other major recent review articles[914,915] for more detailed discussion of this topic.

Epidemiology and Pathogenesis of Diabetic Foot Ulceration

Foot ulceration is common and occurs in both T1DM and T2DM. Approximately 5% to 10% of diabetic patients have had past or present foot ulceration, and 1% have undergone amputation.[912] Diabetes is the most common cause of nontraumatic lower limb amputation in the United States, and rates are 15 times greater than those in the nondiabetic population. More than 80% of amputations are preceded by foot ulcers. A large community-based study in the United Kingdom showed an annual incidence of ulceration of approximately 2%; this rose to 7% with known diabetic neuropathy and to as high as 50% with a past history of ulceration.[916] The lifetime risk for development of a foot ulcer in a diabetic patient is estimated to be as high as 25%.[914]

Pathway to Ulceration

Foot ulceration results from the interaction of a number of component causes, none of which alone is sufficient to cause ulceration but which, when combined, complete the causal pathway to skin breakdown. Knowledge of these component causes and their potential to interact facilitates the design of preventive foot care programs.

Diabetic Neuropathy

All three components of neuropathy—sensory, motor, and autonomic—can contribute to ulceration in the foot. Chronic sensorimotor neuropathy is common, affecting at least one third of older patients in Western countries. Its onset is gradual and insidious, and symptoms may be so minimal that they go unnoticed. Although uncomfortable, painful, and paresthetic symptoms predominate in many patients, some never experience symptoms. Clinical examination usually reveals a sensory deficit in a glove-and-stocking distribution, with signs of motor dysfunction, such as small muscle wasting in the feet and absent ankle reflexes. Although a history of typical symptoms strongly suggests a diagnosis of neuropathy, absence of symptoms does not exclude the diagnosis and must never be equated with a lack of foot ulcer risk. Therefore, assessment of foot ulcer risk must always include a careful foot examination, whatever the history.

Sympathetic autonomic neuropathy affecting the lower limbs results in reduced sweating, dry skin, and development of cracks and fissures. In the absence of large-vessel arterial disease, there may be increased blood flow to the foot, with arteriovenous shunting leading to the warm but at-risk foot.

The importance of neuropathy as a contributory cause to foot ulceration has been confirmed. The risk in patients with neuropathy is sevenfold higher than in those without this complication of diabetes.[916]

Peripheral Vascular Disease

Peripheral vascular disease in isolation rarely causes ulceration. However, the common combination of vascular disease with minor trauma can lead to ulceration. Minor injury and subsequent infection increase the demand for blood supply beyond the circulatory capacity, and ischemic ulceration and risk of amputation develop. Early identification of those patients who are at risk for peripheral vascular disease is essential, and appropriate investigation involving noninvasive studies, together with arteriography, often leads to bypass surgery to improve blood flow to the extremities. Distal bypass surgery is often performed, with good short-term but mixed long-term results in terms of limb salvage.[917,918] Doppler-derived ankle pressure can be misleadingly high in patients with long-standing diabetes. The presence or absence of a dorsalis pedis or posterior tibial pulse is the simplest and most reliable indicator of significant ischemia that can be elicited at the bedside.[917]

Past Foot Ulceration or Foot Surgery

Foot ulceration is most common in patients with a history of similar problems. Even in experienced diabetic foot

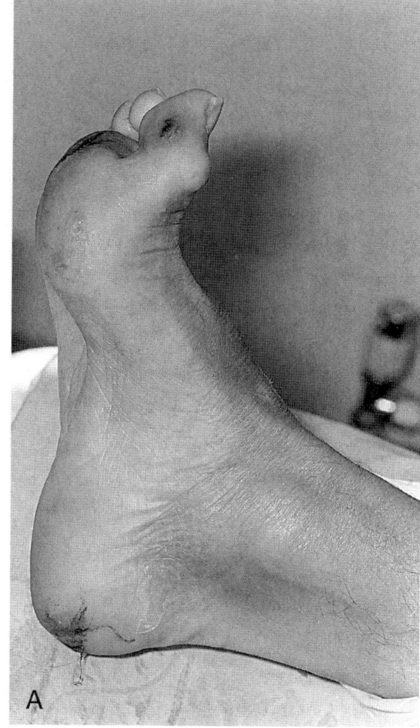

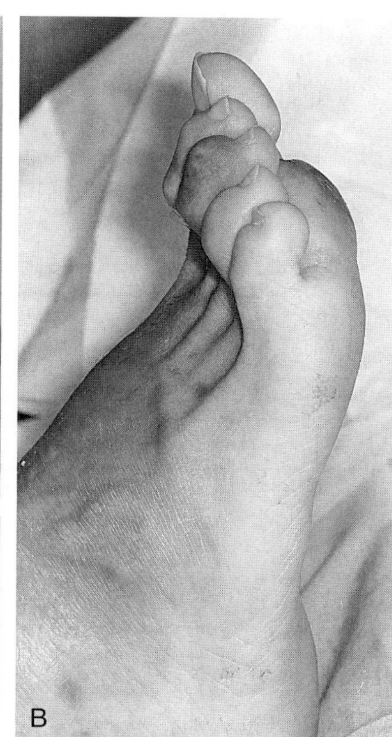

Figure 33-54 The high-risk neuropathic foot. **A** and **B,** Two lateral views of a patient with typical signs of a high-risk neuropathic foot. Notice the small-muscle wasting, clawing of the toes, and marked prominence of the metatarsal heads. At presentation with type 2 diabetes mellitus, this patient had severe neuropathy with foot ulceration on both the right foot (shown here) and the left foot. (From Andersson DK, Svardsudd K. Long-term glycemic control relates to mortality in type II diabetes. *Diabetes Care.* 1995;18:1534-1543.)

clinics, more than 50% of patients with new foot ulcers give a past ulcer history.

Other Diabetic Complications

Patients with retinopathy and renal dysfunction are at increased risk for foot ulceration. Among the diabetic patients at highest risk for ulceration are those on dialysis.[919]

Callus, Deformity, and High Foot Pressures

Motor neuropathy, with imbalance of the flexor and extensor muscles in the foot, commonly results in foot deformity, with prominent metatarsal heads and clawing of the toes (Fig. 33-54). The combination of proprioceptive loss due to neuropathy and the prominence of metatarsal heads leads to increased pressures and loads under the diabetic foot. High pressures, together with dry skin, often result in the formation of callus under weight-bearing areas of the metatarsal heads. The presence of such plantar callus has been shown in cross-sectional and prospective studies to be a highly significant marker of foot ulcer risk. Conversely, removal of plantar callus is associated with a reduction in foot pressures and therefore a reduction in foot ulcer risk.[920]

It is the combination of two or more of the earlier described risk factors that ultimately results in diabetic foot ulceration. In 1999, a North American/United Kingdom collaborative study[921] assessed the risk factors that resulted in ulceration in more than 150 consecutive foot ulcer cases. From this study, a number of causal pathways were identified, but the most common triad of component causes—neuropathy, deformity, and trauma—was present in 63% of incident ulcers. Edema and ischemia were also common component causes.

Prevention of Foot Ulceration and Amputation

That diabetic foot ulceration is largely preventable is not disputed; small, mostly single-center studies have shown that relatively simple interventions can reduce amputations by up to 80%.[909,910] Therefore, strategies for early identification of patients at potential risk for ulceration are required, and education programs that can be adapted for widespread application need to be developed. Because foot ulcers precede most amputations, are among the most common causes of hospital admission for patients with diabetes, and account for much morbidity and even mortality, the widespread application of preventive foot care strategies is urgently required.

Patients with any type of diabetes require regular review and screening of the feet for evidence of risk factors for foot ulceration, irrespective of disease duration. At a minimum, such screening should be carried out annually. Of all the long-term complications of diabetes, foot problems and their risk factors are probably the easiest to detect. No expensive equipment is required, and the feet can be examined for evidence of neuropathic and vascular deficits in the office setting using simple equipment. Neuropathy, vascular disease, and even foot ulceration may be the presenting feature of T2DM, so there can be no exception to the rule of screening (Fig. 33-55).

In 2008, a taskforce of the ADA published a report on the components that should comprise the annual Comprehensive Diabetic Foot Examination (CDFE), which is summarized in Table 33-14.[922] The most important message to practitioners is to have the patient remove shoes and socks and to look at the feet for risk factors such as presence of callus, deformity, muscle wasting, and dry skin, all of which are clearly visible on clinical inspection. A simple neurologic examination should include assessment of pressure perception using a 10-g monofilament; in a large U.K.

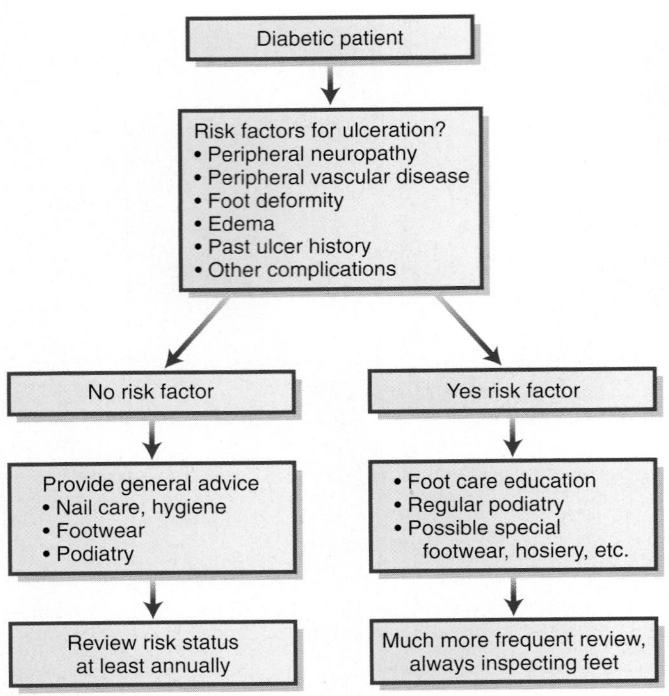

Figure 33-55 Simple algorithm for risk screening in the diabetic foot.

community study,[916] a simple clinical examination was the best predictor of foot ulcer risks. Absence of the ability to perceive pressure from a 10-g monofilament, inability to perceive a vibrating 128-Hz tuning fork over the hallux, and absent ankle reflexes all have been shown to be predictors of foot ulceration.[916,920]

TABLE 33-14

Key Components of the Comprehensive Diabetic Foot Examination

Dermatologic
Skin status: color, thickness, dryness, cracking Sweating Infection: check between toes for fungal infection Ulceration Calluses/blistering: hemorrhage into callus?
Musculoskeletal
Deformity (e.g., claw toes, prominent metatarsal heads, Charcot joint) Muscle wasting (guttering between metatarsals) Assess whether shoes are appropriate for the feet (e.g., size, width)
Neurologic
Ability to perceive pressure from a 10-g monofilament plus one of the following: Vibration using 128-Hz tuning fork Pinprick sensation Ankle reflexes Vibratory perception threshold
Vascular
Foot pulses Ankle-brachial index, if indicated

Adapted from Boulton AJM, Armstrong DG, Albert SG, et al. Comprehensive Foot Examination and Risk Assessment: a report of the Task Force of the Foot Care Interest Group of the American Diabetes Association, with endorsement by the American Association of Clinical Endocrinologists. *Diabetes Care.* 2008;31:1679-1686.

TABLE 33-15

Wagner Diabetic Foot Ulcer Classification System

Grade	Description
0	No ulcer, but high-risk foot (e.g., deformity, callus, insensitivity)
1	Superficial full-thickness ulcer
2	Deeper ulcer, penetrating tendons, no bone involvement
3	Deeper ulcer with bone involvement, osteitis
4	Partial gangrene (e.g., toes, forefoot)
5	Gangrene of whole foot

Modified from Oyibo S, Jude EB, Tarawneh I, et al. A comparison of two diabetic foot ulcer classification systems: the Wagner and the University of Texas wound classification systems. *Diabetes Care.* 2001;24:84-88.

The Diabetic Foot Care Team

Patients identified as being at high risk for foot ulceration should be managed by a team of specialists with interest and expertise in the diabetic foot. The podiatrist usually takes responsibility for follow-up and care of the skin and nails and, together with the specialist nurse or diabetes educator, provides foot care education. The orthotist, or shoe fitter, is invaluable for advising about and sometimes designing footwear to protect high-risk feet, and these members of the team should work closely with the diabetologist and the vascular and orthopedic surgeons. Patients with risk factors for ulceration require preventive foot care education and frequent review.[910,920]

Classification of Foot Ulcers

Many different classification systems have been reported in the literature.[914,920] The one developed by Wagner[923] (Table 33-15) for grading diabetic foot ulcers has been widely used and accepted. More recently, the University of Texas (UT) group has developed an alternative classification system that, in addition to ulcer depth (as in the Wagner system), takes into account the presence or absence of infection and ischemia (Table 33-16).[924] A prospective study from 2001 assessed and compared these two wound classification systems and concluded that the UT scheme is a better predictor of outcome than the older Wagner system.[923]

Management of Diabetic Foot Ulcers

Basic principles of wound healing apply equally to diabetic foot ulcers as to wounds in any other site or condition.

TABLE 33-16

University of Texas Wound Classification System

Stage	Grade 0	Grade 1	Grade 2	Grade 3
A	Preulcer or postulcer lesion; no skin break	Superficial ulcer	Deep ulcer to tendon or capsule	Wound penetrating bone or joint
B	+ Infection	+ Infection	+ Infection	+Infection
C	+ Ischemia	+ Ischemia	+ Ischemia	+Ischemia
D	+ Infection and ischemia	+ Infection and ischemia	+Infection and ischemia	+Infection and ischemia

Modified from Armstrong DG, Lavery LA, Harkless LB. Validation of a diabetic wound classification system. *Diabet Med.* 1998;14:855-859.

Basically, a diabetic foot ulcer will heal if the following three conditions are satisfied:

- Arterial inflow is adequate.
- Infection is treated appropriately.
- Pressure is removed from the wound and the immediate surrounding area.

Although this approach might seem simplistic, failure of diabetic foot ulcers to heal is usually a result of failure to pay sufficient attention to one or more contributing conditions, including pressure on the wound, infection, ischemia, and inadequate debridement.

The most common cause of nonhealing of neuropathic foot ulcers is the failure to remove pressure from the wound and immediate surrounding area. Patients who are advised not to put pressure over an ulcer find it difficult to adhere to such advice if peripheral sensation is lost or reduced. Pain results in protection of an injured area; the lack of pain permits pressure to be put directly onto the ulcer and results in nonhealing. A patient with normal sensation and a foot wound will limp to avoid putting pressure on the wound because doing so is painful; hence, the observation made initially in leprosy, and more recently in diabetic neuropathy, that a patient who walks on a plantar wound without limping must have neuropathy.

The effect of pressure relief on the histopathologic features of neuropathic ulcers was assessed in a randomized study.[925] Patients with chronic neuropathic diabetic foot ulcers were randomly assigned to have a biopsy either at presentation or after 20 days of off-loading in a total-contact cast (TCC). Histologic features of chronic inflammation, with mononuclear infiltration, cellular debris, and scarce evidence of angiogenesis or granulation were seen in patients who underwent biopsy at presentation; granulation, neoangiogenesis, and a predominance of fibroblasts were seen in patients treated with TCC before biopsy. These important observations strongly suggest that repetitive pressure on a neuropathic wound contributes to the chronicity of the wound, whereas pressure relief results in the wound's appearing, in several respects, more like an acute wound in the reparative phase.

The next most common error is inappropriate management of infection. Topical applications are usually unhelpful, and if clinical infection is present, it must be treated appropriately (see later discussion).

Another common error is the failure to appreciate ischemic symptoms that are atypical due to altered pain sensation as a result of neuropathy. The most difficult ulcer to heal is the neuroischemic ulcer, and symptoms and even signs of ischemia may be altered in the diabetic state. Therefore, appropriate noninvasive investigation and arteriography are indicated for patients with a nonhealing diabetic foot ulcer if there is any question about the vascular status.

Inappropriate wound debridement is another reason for slow healing or nonhealing of a diabetic foot ulcer. When patients with neuropathy put pressure on active ulcer areas, the pressure leads to an often extensive buildup of callus tissue. Appropriate debridement and removal of all dead and macerated tissue is essential in the local treatment of a diabetic foot ulcer and has been shown to result in more rapid healing of ulcers compared with wounds that are inadequately debrided.

The principles of management of neuropathic and neuroischemic foot ulcers are considered in the following sections. Because it is not possible to provide complete details on the individual stages and grades of ulcers, we refer to both the UT and the Wagner grading systems.

Neuropathic Foot Ulcer without Osteomyelitis (Wagner Grades 1, 2; University of Texas Grades 1a, 1b, 2a, 2b)

The most important feature in the management of neuropathic foot ulcers that typically occur under weight-bearing areas such as the metatarsal heads and great toe is the provision of adequate pressure relief. This is usually achieved by a cast such as a TCC or a removable Scotch cast boot.[914,920]

The TCC has long been recognized as the gold standard for off-loading a foot wound and was confirmed as correct in a randomized, controlled trial in which Armstrong and colleagues compared three off-loading techniques and found that the TCC was associated with the shortest healing time.[926] When any cast device is used, regular removal of the cast is essential, because regular debridement of the wound by a podiatrist is essential, and any casting device could injure insensitive skin, especially over bony prominences. For this reason, and because the TCC requires a specially trained casting technician to apply it, recent research has been directed toward alternative, irremovable devices that might be equally efficacious.

In the aforementioned trial by Armstrong's group,[926] the removable cast walker (RCW) resulted in slower healing than the TCC, even though prior gait laboratory studies had suggested that they are equally efficacious at off-loading. The reason for this disparity was identified in an observational study of patients using RCWs in the treatment of their plantar neuropathic ulcers. Although patients were instructed to wear the RCW at all times, careful monitoring showed that RCWs were used for only 28% of all footsteps during a 24-hour period. It was therefore suggested that the RCW, which can be applied by any clinic personnel and does not require specialist training, might be rendered irremovable by wrapping it in casting material. A controlled trial showed that the irremovable RCW was as effective at healing neuropathic foot wounds as the TCC.[927]

Theoretically, complete healing of all superficial and neuropathic ulcers should be possible without the need for amputation. In the treatment of neuropathic ulcers with a good peripheral circulation, antibiotics are not indicated unless there are clear clinical signs of infection, including prominent discharge, local erythema, and cellulitis. The presence of any of these features in Wagner grade 1 or 2 ulcers would warrant reclassification in the UT system from 1a or 2a to 1b or 2b. In such cases, deep wound swabs should be taken and broad-spectrum oral antibiotic treatment should be started with either an amoxicillin–clavulanic acid combination (Augmentin) or clindamycin. The antibiotic may need to be altered after sensitivity results become available.[928]

Neuroischemic Ulcers (Wagner Grades 1, 2; University of Texas Grades 1c, 1d)

The principles of management of neuroischemic Wagner grade 1 and 2 ulcers are similar to those for neuropathic ulcers, with the following important exceptions. TCCs are not usually recommended for management of neuroischemic ulcers, although removable casts and pneumatic cast boots (Aircast) may be used in cases without infection. Antibiotic therapy is usually recommended for most neuroischemic ulcers. Investigation of the circulation is indicated, including noninvasive assessment and, if required, arteriography with appropriate subsequent surgical management or angioplasty.[917]

Osteomyelitis (Wagner Grade 3; University of Texas Grades 3b, 3d)

Wagner or UT grade 3 ulcers are deeper and involve underlying bone, often with abscess formation. Osteomyelitis is a serious complication of foot ulceration and may be present in as many as 50% of diabetic patients with moderate to severe foot infections.[914] If the physician can probe down to bone in a deep ulcer, the presence of osteomyelitis is strongly suggested. Plain radiographs are indicated for any nonhealing foot ulcer and are useful in the diagnosis of osteomyelitis in more than two thirds of patients, although the radiologic changes may be delayed. In difficult cases, further investigation, such as MRI, bone scans, or an indium 111 (^{111}In) labeled white blood cell scan can be useful in diagnosing bone infection.[929]

Although the treatment of osteomyelitis is commonly surgical and involves resection of the infected bone, there have been reports of successful long-term treatment with antibiotics effective against the underlying bacterium, most commonly *Staphylococcus aureus*. Therefore, agents such as clindamycin (which penetrates bone well) or flucloxacillin are often used.

Gangrene (Wagner Grades 4, 5)

The presence of gangrene or areas of tissue death is always a serious sign in the diabetic foot. However, localized areas of gangrene, especially in the toes, that are without cellulitis, spreading infection, or discharge can occasionally be left to spontaneously autoamputate. The presence of more extensive gangrene requires urgent hospital admission; treatment of infection, often with multiple antibiotics; control of the diabetes, usually with intravenous insulin; and detailed vascular assessment. It is in this area that the team approach is most important, with close collaboration among the diabetes specialist, the vascular surgeon, and the radiologist.

Adjunct Treatments for Foot Ulcers

Platelet-Derived Growth Factors and Tissue-Engineered Skin

Genetically derived growth factors and novel bioengineered skin substitutes have been proposed as adjunctive treatments for diabetic foot ulcers. However, all of these new therapies are costly, as detailed in a recent systematic review and economic evaluation.[930] This review covered treatments including Apligraf, a bilayered living human skin equivalent; Dermagraft, a human fibroblast-derived dermal substitute; and human PDGFs. Although the review did show some benefit for each of these agents, it is clear that they should be reserved only for those ulcers that fail to respond to the standard treatments noted earlier. Any new treatments should be seen not as a replacement but as an addition to good wound care, which must always include adequate off-loading and regular debridement.

Negative-Pressure Wound Therapy

Negative-pressure wound therapy, also known as vacuum-assisted closure, is increasingly used to treat large and complex diabetic foot wounds. The treatment appears to stimulate the development of granulation tissue in previously nonhealing wounds and can also be helpful in the postoperative management of diabetic foot wounds. Supportive data have been published from randomized, controlled trials in postoperative cases[931] and in complex nonhealing diabetic foot ulcers.[932]

Charcot's Neuroarthropathy

Charcot's neuroarthropathy is a rare and disabling condition that affects the joints and bones of the feet. Permissive features for the development of this condition include the presence of severe peripheral neuropathy and autonomic dysfunction with increased blood flow to the foot; the peripheral circulation is usually intact. In the Western world, diabetes is the most common cause of a Charcot foot, and increased awareness of this condition can enable earlier diagnosis and treatment to prevent severe deformity and disability.

The actual pathogenesis of the Charcot process is poorly understood; however, the patient with peripheral insensitivity and autonomic dysfunction with increased blood flow to the foot is vulnerable to trauma that the patient may not recall. Repetitive trauma results in increased blood flow through the bone, increased osteoclastic activity, and remodeling of bone. In certain cases, patients walk on a fracture, which leads to continuing destruction of bones and joints in that area. Recent evidence suggests that acute Charcot's neuropathy may be triggered in the susceptible (i.e., neuropathic) individual by any event that leads to localized inflammation in the affected foot. This may trigger a vicious cycle in which there is increasing inflammation, increasing expression of RANKL (a member of the tumor necrosis factor superfamily), and increasing bone breakdown. The likely involvement of the RANKL/OPG pathway might lead to new possibilities for future treatments.[933]

Charcot's neuropathy is sometimes difficult to distinguish from osteomyelitis or an inflammatory arthropathy.[929] However, a unilateral swollen, hot foot in a patient with neuropathy must be considered to be a Charcot foot until proved otherwise.

Charcot's arthropathy can be diagnosed in most patients by plain radiography and a high index of suspicion. Radiographs may reveal bone and joint destruction, fragmentation, and remodeling, although in the early stages the radiographic finding may be normal. In such cases, the three-phase bisphosphonate bone scan shows increased bone uptake, although the ^{111}In-labeled bone scan will be negative in the absence of infection.

After diagnosis, management of the acute phase involves immobilization, usually in a TCC.[934] Evidence suggests that treatment with bisphosphonates, which reduce osteoclastic activity, may reduce swelling, discomfort, and bone turnover markers, although larger trials are warranted in this area.[920,933,934]

Although Charcot's neuroarthropathy is rare, it should be suspected in any patient with unexplained swelling and heat in a neuropathic foot. Early intervention with immobilization and possibly bisphosphonate treatment may halt progression that, in the untreated state, can lead to marked foot deformity and require local or major amputations.

REFERENCES

1. Skyler J. Diabetic complications: the importance of glucose control. *Endocrinol Metab Clin North Am.* 1996;25:243-254.
2. Diabetes Control and Complications Trial Research Group. The effect of intensive treatment of diabetes on the development and progression of long-term complications in insulin-dependent diabetes mellitus. *N Engl J Med.* 1993;329:977-986.
3. UK Prospective Diabetes Study (UKPDS) Group. Intensive blood-glucose control with sulphonylureas or insulin compared with conventional treatment and risk of complications in patients with type 2 diabetes (UKPDS 33). *Lancet.* 1998;352:837-853.
4. Krolewski AS, Laffel LM, Krolewski M, et al. Glycosylated hemoglobin and the risk of microalbuminuria in patients with insulin-dependent diabetes mellitus. *N Engl J Med.* 1995;332:1251-1255.

5. The absence of a glycemic threshold for the development of long-term complications: the perspective of the Diabetes Control and Complications Trial. *Diabetes*. 1996;45:1289-1298.
6. Wagenknecht LE, D'Agostino Jr RB, Haffner SM, et al. Impaired glucose tolerance, type 2 diabetes, and carotid wall thickness: the Insulin Resistance Atherosclerosis Study. *Diabetes Care*. 1998;21: 1812-1818.
7. Goldberg RB, Mellies MJ, Sacks FM, et al. Cardiovascular events and their reduction with pravastatin in diabetic and glucose-intolerant myocardial infarction survivors with average cholesterol levels: subgroup analyses in the Cholesterol and Recurrent Events (CARE) trial. The Care Investigators. *Circulation*. 1998;98:2513-2519.
8. Haffner SM. The Scandinavian Simvastatin Survival Study (4S) subgroup analysis of diabetic subjects: implications for the prevention of coronary heart disease. *Diabetes Care*. 1997;20:469-471.
9. Ebara T, Conde K, Kako Y, et al. Delayed catabolism of apoB-48 lipoproteins due to decreased heparan sulfate proteoglycan production in diabetic mice. *J Clin Invest*. 2000;105:1807-1818.
10. Ginsberg HN. Insulin resistance and cardiovascular disease. *J Clin Invest*. 2000;106:453-458.
11. Lachin JM, Genuth S, Nathan DM, et al, DCCT/EDIC Research Group. Effect of glycemic exposure on the risk of microvascular complications in the Diabetes Control and Complications Trial–revisted. *Diabetes*. 2008;57:995-1001.
12. Kaiser N, Feener EP, Boukobza-Vardi N, et al. Differential regulation of glucose transport and transporters by glucose in vascular endothelial and smooth muscle cells. *Diabetes*. 1993;42:80-89.
13. Heilig CW, Concepcion LA, Riser BL, et al. Overexpression of glucose transporters in rat mesangial cells cultured in a normal glucose milieu mimics the diabetic phenotype. *J Clin Invest*. 1995;96:1802-1814.
14. Shore AC, Tooke JE. Microvascular function and haemodynamic disturbances in diabetes mellitus and its complications. In: Pickup J, Williams G, eds. *Textbook of Diabetes*. Vol 1. Oxford, UK: Blackwell Scientific; 1997:43.1-43.13.
15. Kihara M, Schmelzer JD, Poduslo JF, et al. Aminoguanidine effects on nerve blood flow, vascular permeability, electrophysiology, and oxygen free radicals. *Proc Natl Acad Sci U S A*. 1991;88:6107-6111.
16. Kopp JB, Factor VM, Mozes M, et al. Transgenic mice with increased plasma levels of TGF-β_1 develop progressive renal disease. *Lab Invest*. 1996;74:991-1003.
17. Chien S, Li S, Shyy YJ. Effects of mechanical forces on signal transduction and gene expression in endothelial cells. *Hypertension*. 1998;(1 Pt 2):162-169.
18. Walker JD, Viberti GC. Pathophysiology of microvascular disease: an overview. In: Pickup J, Williams G, eds. *Textbook of Diabetes*. Vol 1. Oxford, UK: Blackwell Scientific; 1991:526-533.
19. Brownlee M. Advanced products of nonenzymatic glycosylation and the pathogenesis of diabetic complications. In: Rifkin H, Porte Jr D, eds. *Diabetes Mellitus: Theory and Practice*. New York: Elsevier; 1990:279-291.
20. Hammes HP, Federoff HJ, Brownlee M. Nerve growth factor prevents both neuroretinal programmed cell death and capillary pathology in experimental diabetes. *Mol Med*. 1995;(5):527-534.
21. Mizutani M, Kern TS, Lorenzi M. Accelerated death of retinal microvascular cells in human and experimental diabetic retinopathy. *J Clin Invest*. 1996;97:2883-2890.
22. Giannini C, Dyck PJ. Ultrastructural morphometric features of human sural nerve endoneurial microvessels. *J Neuropathol Exp Neurol*. 1993;52:361-369.
23. Giannini C, Dyck PJ. Basement membrane reduplication and pericyte degeneration precede development of diabetic polyneuropathy and are associated with its severity. *Ann Neurol*. 1995;37:498-504.
24. Tomlinson DR, Fernyhough P, Diemel LT. Role of neurotrophins in diabetic neuropathy and treatment with nerve growth factors. *Diabetes*. 1997;46(suppl 12):S43-S49.
25. Engerman RL, Kern TS. Progression of incipient diabetic retinopathy during good glycemic control. *Diabetes*. 1987;36:808-812.
26. Roy S, Sala R, Cagliero E, Lorenzi M. Overexpression of fibronectin induced by diabetes or high glucose phenomenon with a memory. *Proc Natl Acad Sci U S A*. 1990;87:404-408.
27. Diabetes Control and Complications Trial Research Group. The effect of intensive treatment of diabetes on the development and progression of long-term complications in insulin-dependent diabetes mellitus. *N Engl J Med*. 1993;329:977-986.
28. Diabetes Control and Complications Trial (DCCT) Research Group. Effect of intensive therapy on the development and progression of diabetic nephropathy in the Diabetes Control and Complications Trial. *Kidney Int*. 1995;47:1703-1702.
29. Diabetes Control and Complications Trial Research Group. The effect of intensive diabetes therapy on the development and progression of neuropathy. *Ann Intern Med*. 1995;122:561-568.
30. Writing Team for the Diabetes Control and Complications Trial/Epidemiology of Diabetes Interventions and Complications Research Group. Effect of intensive therapy on the microvascular complications of type 1 diabetes mellitus. *JAMA*. 2002;287:2563-2569.
31. Writing Team for the Diabetes Control and Complications. Trial/Epidemiology of Diabetes Interventions and Complications Research Group. Sustained effect of intensiveintensive treatment of type 1 diabetes mellitus on development and progression of diabetic nephropathy: the Epidemiology of Diabetes Interventions and Complications (EDIC) study. *JAMA*. 2003;290:2159-2167.
32. Krolewski AS, Warram JH, Freire MB. Epidemiology of late diabetic complications: a basis for the development and evaluation of preventive programs. *Endocrinol Metab Clin North Am*. 1996;25:217-242.
33. Wagenknecht LE, Bowden DW, Carr JJ, et al. Familial aggregation of coronary artery calcium in families with type 2 diabetes. *Diabetes*. 2001;50:861-866.
34. Seaquist ER, Goetz FC, Rich S, et al. Familial clustering of diabetic kidney disease: evidence for genetic susceptibility to diabetic nephropathy. *N Engl J Med*. 1989;32018:1161-1165.
35. Quinn M, Angelico MC, Warram JH, et al. Familial factors determine the development of diabetic nephropathy in patients with IDDM. *Diabetologia*. 1996;39:940-945.
36. Diabetes Control and Complications Trial Research Group. Clustering of long-term complications in families with diabetes in the Diabetes Control and Complications Trial. *Diabetes*. 1997;46:1829-1839.
37. Raffel LJ, Vadheim CM, Roth MP, et al. The 5′ insulin gene polymorphism and the genetics of vascular complications in type 1 (insulin-dependent) diabetes mellitus. *Diabetologia*. 1991;34:680-683.
38. Stewart LL, Field LL, Ross S, et al. Genetic risk factors in diabetic retinopathy. *Diabetologia*. 1993;36:1293-1298.
39. Marre M, Bernadet P, Gallois Y, et al. Relationships between angiotensin I converting enzyme gene polymorphism, plasma levels, and diabetic retinal and renal complications. *Diabetes*. 1994;43:384-388.
40. Marre M, Jeunemaitre X, Gallois Y, et al. Contribution of genetic polymorphism in the renin-angiotensin system to the development of renal complications in insulin-dependent diabetes: Genetique de la Nephropathie Diabetique (GENEDIAB) study group. *J Clin Invest*. 1997;99:1585-1595.
41. Agardh D, Gaur LK, Agardh E, et al. LADQB1*0201/0302 is associated with severe retinopathy in patients with IDDM. *Diabetologia*. 1996;39:1313-1317.
42. Oates PJ, Mylari BL. Aldose reductase inhibitors: therapeutic implications for diabetic complications. *Exp Opin Invest Drugs*. 1999;8:1-25.
43. Warpeha KM, Xu W, Liu L, et al. Genotyping and functional analysis of a polymorphic (CCTTT)(n) repeat of NOS2A in diabetic retinopathy. *FASEB J*. 1999;13:1825-1832.
44. Satko SG, Freedman BI, Moossavi S. Genetic factors in end-stage renal disease. *Kidney Int Suppl*. 2005;94:S46-S49.
45. Ewens KG, George RA, Sharma K, et al. Assessment of 115 candidate genes for diabetic nephropathy by transmission/disequilibrium test. *Diabetes*. 2005;54:3305-3318.
46. Al-Kateb H, Boright AP, Mirea L, et al, Diabetes Control and Complications Trial/Epidemiology of Diabetes Interventions and Complications Research Group. Multiple superoxide dismutase 1/splicing factor serine alanine 15 variants are associated with the development and progression of diabetic nephropathy: the Diabetes Control and Complications Trial/Epidemiology of Diabetes Interventions and Complications Genetics study. *Diabetes*. 2008;57:218-228.
47 Tong Z, Yang Z, Patel S, et al, Genetics of Diabetes and Diabetic Complication Study Group. Promoter polymorphism of the erythropoietin gene in severe diabetic eye and kidney complications. *Proc Natl Acad Sci U S A*. 2008;105:6998-7003.
48. Abhary S, Burdon KP, Casson RJ, et al. Association between erythropoietin gene polymorphisms and diabetic retinopathy. *Arch Ophthalmol*. 2010;128:102-106.
49. Haston CK, Hudson TJ. Finding genetic modifiers of cystic fibrosis. *N Engl J Med*. 2005;353:1509-1511.
50. Granger CB, Califf RM, Young S. Outcome of patients with diabetes mellitus and acute myocardial infarction treated with thrombolytic agents. The Thrombolysis and Angioplasty in Myocardial Infarction (TAMI) Study Group. *J Am Coll Cardiol*. 1993;21:920-925.
51. Stamler J, Vaccaro O, Neaton JD, et al. Diabetes, other risk factors, and 12-yr cardiovascular mortality for men screened in the Multiple Risk Factor Intervention Trial. *Diabetes Care*. 1993;16:434-444.
52. Fitzgerald AP, Jarrett RJ. Are conventional risk factors for mortality relevant in type 2 diabetes? *Diabet Med*. 1991;8:475-480.
53. Fuller JH, Shipley MJ, Rose G, et al. Coronary-heart-disease risk and impaired glucose tolerance: the Whitehall study. *Lancet*. 1980;1: 1373-1376.
54. Rosengren A, Welin L, Tsipogianni A, et al. Impact of cardiovascular risk factors on coronary heart disease and mortality among middle aged diabetic men: a general population study. *BMJ*. 1989;299: 1127-1131.
55. Lehto S, Ronnemma T, Pyorala K, Laakso M. Poor glycemic control predicts coronary heart disease events in patients with type I diabetes without nephropathy. *Arterioscler Thromb Vasc Biol*. 1999;19: 1014-1019.
56. Gerstein HC. Is glucose a continuous risk factor for cardiovascular mortality? *Diabetes Care*. 1999;22:659-660.

57. Gall MA, Borch-Johnsen K, Hougaard P, et al. Albuminuria and poor glycemic control predict mortality in NIDDM. *Diabetes*. 1995;44: 1303-1309.
58. Kuusisto J, Mykkanen L, Pyorala K, et al. NIDDM and its metabolic control predict coronary heart disease in elderly subjects. *Diabetes*. 1994;43:960-967.
59. Salomaa V, Riley W, Kark JD, et al. Non-insulin-dependent diabetes mellitus and fasting glucose and insulin concentrations are associated with arterial stiffness indexes: the ARIC Study. Atherosclerosis Risk in Communities Study. *Circulation*. 1995;91:1432-1443.
60. Laakso M, Kuusisto J. Epidemiological evidence for the association of hyperglycaemia and atherosclerotic vascular disease in non-insulin-dependent diabetes mellitus. *Ann Med*. 1996;28:415-418.
61. Bonora, E, Kiechl S, Willeit J, et al. Prevalence of insulin resistance in metabolic disorders: the Bruneck study. *Diabetes*. 1998;47:1643-1649.
62. Haffner SM, Lehto S, Ronnemaa T, et al. Mortality from coronary heart disease in subjects with type 2 diabetes and in nondiabetic subjects with and without prior myocardial infarction. *N Engl J Med*. 1998;339:229-234.
63. Saydah SH, Miret M, Sung J, et al. Postchallenge hyperglycemia and mortality in a national sample of U.S. adults. *Diabetes Care*. 2001;24:1397-1402.
64. National Diabetes Data Group. *Diabetes in America*. 2nd ed. Bethesda, MD: National Institute of Diabetes and Digestive and Kidney Diseases; 1995.
65. DECODE Study Group, the European Diabetes Epidemiology Group. Glucose tolerance and cardiovascular mortality: comparison of fasting and 2-hour diagnostic criteria. *Arch Intern Med*. 2001;161:397-405.
66. Yip J, Facchini FS, Reaven GM. Resistance to insulin-mediated glucose disposal as a predictor of cardiovascular disease. *J Clin Endocrinol Metab*. 1998;83:2773-2776.
67. Hanley AJ, Williams K, Stern MP, et al. Homeostasis model assessment of IR in relation to the incidence of cardiovascular disease: the San Antonio Heart Study. *Diabetes Care*. 2002;25:1177-1184.
68. Shimomura I, Bashmakov Y, Ikemoto S, et al. Insulin selectively increases SREBP-1c mRNA in the livers of rats with streptozotocin-induced diabetes. *Proc Natl Acad Sci U S A*. 1999;96:13656-13661.
69. Chen G, Liang G, Ou J, et al. Central role for liver X receptor in insulin-mediated activation of Srebp-1c transcription and stimulation of fatty acid synthesis in liver. *Proc Natl Acad Sci U S A*. 2004;101: 11245-11250.
70. King G, Brownlee M. The cellular and molecular mechanisms of diabetic complications. *Endocrinol Metab Clin North Am*. 1996;2:255-270.
71. Hsueh WA, Law RE. Cardiovascular risk continuum: implications of insulin resistance and diabetes. *Am J Med*. 1998;105:4S-14S.
72. Li H, Forstermann U. Nitric oxide in the pathogenesis of vascular disease. *J Pathol*. 2000;190:244-254.
73. Banskota NK, Taub R, Zellner K, King GL. Insulin, insulin-like growth factor I and platelet-derived growth factor interact additively in the induction of the protooncogene c-myc and cellular proliferation in cultured bovine aortic smooth muscle cells. *Mol Endocrinol*. 1989;8:1183-1190.
74. Stolar MW. Atherosclerosis in diabetes: the role of hyperinsulinemia. *Metabolism*. 1988;7(suppl 1):1-9.
75. Jiang ZY, Lin YW, Clemont A, et al. Characterization of selective resistance to insulin signaling in the vasculature of obese Zucker *(fa/fa)* rats. *J Clin Invest*. 1999;104:447-457.
76. Akbari CM, Saouaf R, Barnhill DF, et al. Endothelium-dependent vasodilatation is impaired in both microcirculation and macrocirculation during acute hyperglycemia *J Vasc Surg*. 1998;28:687-694.
77. Williams SB, Goldfine AB, Timimi FK, et al. Acute hyperglycemia attenuates endothelium-dependent vasodilation in humans in vivo. *Circulation*. 1998;97:1695-1701.
78. Du XL, Edelstein D, Rossetti L, et al. Hyperglycemia-induced mitochondrial superoxide overproduction activates the hexosamine pathway and induces plasminogen activator inhibitor-1expression by increasing Sp1 glycosylation. *Proc Natl Acad Sci USA*. 2000;97: 12222-12226.
79. Du XL, Edelstein D, Dimmler S, et al. Hyperglycemia inhibits endothelial nitric oxide synthase activity by altering its post-translational modification at the akt site of the eNOS protein. *J Clin Invest*. 2001;108:1341-1348.
80. Yamagishi S, Edelstein D, Du XD, et al. Hyperglycemia potentiates platelet-derived growth factor induced proliferation of smooth muscle cells through mitochondrial superoxide overproduction. *Diabetes*. 2001;50:1491-1494.
81. Sassy-Prigent C, Heudes D, Mandet C, et al. Early glomerular macrophage recruitment in streptozotocin-induced diabetic rats. *Diabetes*. 2000;49:466-475.
82. Gilcrease MZ, Hoover RL. Examination of monocyte adherence to endothelium under hyperglycemic conditions. *Am J Pathol*. 1991; 139:1089-1097.
83. Ceriello A, Falleti E, Motz E. Hyperglycemia-induced circulating ICAM-1 increased in diabetes mellitus: the possible role of oxidative stress. *Horm Metab Res*. 1998;30:146-149.
84. Kim JA, Berliner JA, Natarajan RD, et al. Evidence that glucose increases monocyte binding to human aortic endothelial cells. *Diabetes*. 1994;43:1103-1107.
85. Cagliero E, Maiello M, Boeri D, et al. Increased expression of basement membrane components in human endothelial cells cultured in high glucose. *J Clin Invest*. 1988;82:735-738.
86. Cagliero E, Roth T, Roy S, et al. Expression of genes related to the extracellular matrix in human endothelial cells: differential modulation by elevated glucose concentrations, phorbol esters, and cAMP. *J Biol Chem*. 1991;266:14244-14250.
87. Du XD, Edelstein D, Obici S, et al. Insulin resistance reduces arterial prostacyclin synthase and eNOS activities by increasing endothelial fatty acid oxidation. *J Clin Invest*. 2006;116:1071-1080.
88. Nathan DM, Cleary PA, Backlund JY, et al, Diabetes Control and Complications Trial/Epidemiology of Diabetes Interventions and Complications (DCCT/EDIC) Study Research Group. Intensive diabetes treatment and cardiovascular disease in patients with type 1 diabetes. *N Engl J Med*. 2005;353:2643-2653.
89. Riddle MC, Ambrosius WT, Brillon DJ, et al, Action to Control Cardiovascular Risk in Diabetes Investigators. Epidemiologic relationships between A1C and all-cause mortality during a median 3.4-year follow-up of glycemic treatment in the ACCORD trial. *Diabetes Care*. 2010;33:983-990.
90. Brown MS, Goldstein JL. Selective versus total insulin resistance: a pathogenic paradox (Review). *Cell Metab*. 2008;7:95-96.
91. Li S, Brown MS, Goldstein JL. Bifurcation of insulin signaling pathway in rat liver: mTORC1 required for stimulation of lipogenesis, but not inhibition of gluconeogenesis. *Proc Natl Acad Sci U S A*. 2010;107:3441-3446.
92. Schulman IH, Zhou MS. Vascular insulin resistance: a potential link between cardiovascular and metabolic diseases (Review). *Curr Hypertens Rep*. 2009;11:48-55.
93. Tepper OM, Galiano RD, Capla JM, et al. Human endothelial progenitor cells from type II diabetics exhibit impaired proliferation, adhesion, and incorporation into vascular structures. *Circulation*. 2002; 106:2781-2786.
94. Thangarajah H, Yao D, Chang EI, et al. The molecular basis for impaired hypoxia-induced VEGF expression in diabetic tissues. *Proc Natl Acad Sci U S A*. 2009;106:13505-13510.
95. Ceradini DJ, Yao D, Grogan RH, et al. Decreasing intracellular superoxide corrects defective ischemia-induced new vessel formation in diabetic mice. *J Biol Chem*. 2008;283:10930-10938.
96. Duh E, Aiello LP. Vascular endothelial growth factor and diabetes: the agonist versus antagonist paradox. *Diabetes*. 1999;48:1899-1906.
97. Waltenberger J. Impaired collateral vessel development in diabetes: potential cellular mechanisms and therapeutic implications. *Cardiovasc Res*. 2001;49:554-560.
98. Grant MB, May WS, Caballero S, et al. Adult hematopoietic stem cells provide functional hemangioblast activity during retinal neovascularization. *Nat Med*. 2002;8:607-612.
99. Rivard A, Silver M, Chen D, et al. Rescue of diabetes-related impairment of angiogenesis by intramuscular gene therapy with adeno-VEGF. *Am J Pathol*. 1999;154:355-363.
100. Iwaguro H, Yamaguchi J, Kalka C, et al. Endothelial progenitor cell vascular endothelial growth factor gene transfer for vascular regeneration. *Circulation*. 2002;105:732-738.
101. Xia P, Kramer RM, King GL. Identification of the mechanism for the inhibition of Na^+,K^+-adenosine triphosphatase by hyperglycemia involving activation of protein kinase C and cytosolic phospholipase A2. *J Clin Invest*. 1995;96:733-740.
102. Williamson JR, Chang K, Frangos M, et al. Hyperglycemic pseudohypoxia and diabetic complications. *Diabetes*. 1993;42:801-813.
103. Nishikawa T, Edelstein D, Du XL, et al. Normalizing mitochondrial superoxide production blocks three pathways of hyperglycaemic damage. *Nature*. 2000;404:787-790.
104. Marano CW, Szwergold BS, Kapper F, et al. Human retinal pigment epithelial cells cultured in hyperglycemic media accumulate increased amounts of glycosaminoglycan precursors. *Invest Ophthalmol Vis Sci*. 1992;33:2619-2625.
105. Beyer-Mears A, Diecke FP, Mistry K, et al. Effect of pyruvate lens myo-inositol transport and polyol formation in diabetic cataract. *Pharmacology*. 1997;55:78-86.
106. Knight RJ, Koefoed KF, Schelbert HR, et al. Inhibition of glyceraldehyde-3-phosphate dehydrogenase in post-ischaemic myocardium. *Cardiovasc Res*. 1996;32:1016-1023.
107. Vikramadithyan RK, Hu Y, Noh HL, et al. Human aldose reductase expression accelerates diabetic atherosclerosis in transgenic mice. *J Clin Invest*. 2005 Sep;115:2434-2443.
108. Lee AY, Chung SS. Contributions of polyol pathway to oxidative stress in diabetic cataract. *FASEB J*. 1999;13:23-30.
109. Ho EC, Lam KS, Chen YS, et al. Aldose reductase-deficient mice are protected from delayed motor nerve conduction velocity, increased c-Jun NH2-terminal kinase activation, depletion of reduced glutathione, increased superoxide accumulation, and DNA damage. *Diabetes*. 2006;55:1946-1953.

110. Chandra D, Jackson EB, Ramana KV, et al. Nitric oxide prevents aldose reductase activation and sorbitol accumulation during diabetes. *Diabetes*. 2002;51:3095-3101.
111. Petrash JM, Harter TM, Devine CS, et al. Involvement of cysteine residues in catalysis and inhibition of human aldose reductase: site-directed mutagenesis of Cys-80, -298, and -303. *J Biol Chem*. 1992;267:24833-24840.
112. Chandra A, Srivastava S, Petrash JM, et al. Active site modification of aldose reductase by nitric oxide donors. *Biochim Biophys Acta*. 1997;1341:217-222.
113. Engerman RL, Kern TS, Larson ME. Nerve conduction and aldose reductase inhibition during 5 years of diabetes or galactosaemia in dogs. *Diabetologia*. 1994;37:141-144.
114. Sorbinil Retinopathy Trial Research Group. A randomized trial of sorbinil, an aldose reductase inhibitor, in diabetic retinopathy. *Arch Ophthalmol*. 1990;108:1234-1244.
115. Greene DA, Arezzo JC, Brown MB. Effect of aldose reductase inhibition on nerve conduction and morphometry in diabetic neuropathy. Zenarestat Study Group. *Neurology*. 1999;53:580-591.
116. Hammes H-P, Martin S, Federlin K, et al. Aminoguanidine treatment inhibits the development of experimental diabetic retinopathy. *Proc Natl Acad Sci U S A*. 1991;88:11555-11559.
117. Stitt AW, Moore JE, Sharkey JA, Murphy G, et al. Advanced glycation end products in vitreous: structural and functional implications for diabetic vitreopathy. *Invest Ophthalmol Vis Sci*. 1998;39:2517-2521.
118. Stitt AW, Li YM, Gardiner TA, et al. Advanced glycation end products (AGEs) co-localize with AGE receptors in the retinal vasculature of diabetic and of AGE- infused rats. *Am J Pathol*. 1997;150:523-528.
119. Nishino T, Horri Y, Shikki H, et al. Immunohistochemical detection of advanced glycosylation end products within the vascular lesions and glomeruli in diabetic nephropathy. *Hum Pathol*. 1995;26:308-312.
120. Horie K, Miyata T, Maeda K, et al. Immunohistochemical colocalization of glycoxidation products and lipid peroxidation products in diabetic renal glomerular lesions: implication for glycoxidative stress in the pathogenesis of diabetic nephropathy. *J Clin Invest*. 1997;100:2995-2999.
121. Niwa T, Katsuzaki T, Miyazaki S, et al. Immunohistochemical detection of imidazolone, a novel advanced glycation end product, in kidneys and aortas of diabetic patients. *J Clin Invest*. 1997;99:1272-1276.
122. Degenhardt TP, Thorpe SR, Baynes JW. Chemical modification of proteins by methylglyoxal. *Cell Mol Biol*. 1998;44:1139-1145.
123. Wells-Knecht KJ, Zyzak DV, Litchfield JE, et al. Mechanism of autoxidative glycosylation: identification of glyoxal and arabinose as intermediates in the autoxidative modification of proteins by glucose. *Biochemistry*. 1995;34:3702-3709.
124. Thornalley PJ. The glyoxalase system: new developments towards functional characterization of a metabolic pathway fundamental to biological life. *Biochem J*. 1990;269:1-11.
125. Takahashi M, Fujii J, Teshima T, et al. Identity of a major 3-deoxyglucosone reducing enzyme with aldehyde reductase in rat liver established by amino acid sequencing and cDNA expression. *Gene*. 1993;127:249-253.
126. Suzuki K, Koh YH, Mizuno H, et al. Overexpression of aldehyde reductase protects PC12 cells from the cytotoxicity of methylglyoxal or 3-deoxyglucosone. *J Biochem*. 1998;123:353-357.
127. Nakamura S, Makita Z, Ishikawa S, et al. Progression of nephropathy in spontaneous diabetic rats is prevented by OPB-9195, a novel inhibitor of advanced glycation. *Diabetes*. 1997;46:895-899.
128. Soulis-Liparota T, Cooper M, Papazoglou D, et al. Retardation by aminoguanidine of development of albuminuria, mesangial expansion, and tissue fluorescence in streptozocin-induced diabetic rat. *Diabetes*. 1991;40:1328-1334.
129. Treins C, Giorgetti-Peraldi S, Murdaca J, et al. Regulation of vascular endothelial growth factor expression by advanced glycation end products. *J Biol Chem*. 2001;276:43836-44341.
130. Yamagishi S, Inagaki Y, Okamoto T, et al. Advanced glycation end product-induced apoptosis and overexpression of vascular endothelial growth factor and monocyte chemoattractant protein-1 in human-cultured mesangial cells. *J Biol Chem*. 2002;277:20309-20315.
131. Oldfield MD, Bach LA, Forbes JM, et al. Advanced glycation end products cause epithelial-myofibroblast transdifferentiation via the receptor for advanced glycation end products (RAGE). *J Clin Invest*. 2001;108:1853-1863.
132. Chang EY, Szallasi Z, Acs P, et al. Functional effects of overexpression of protein kinase C-alpha, -beta, -delta, -epsilon, and -eta in the mast cell line RBL-2H3. *J Immunol*. 1997;1159:2624-2632.
133. Carmeliet P. Angiogenesis in health and disease. *Nat Med*. 2003;9:653-660.
134. Hanahan D. Signaling vascular morphogenesis and maintenance. *Science*. 1997;277:48-50.
135. Jain RK. Molecular regulation of vessel maturation. *Nat Med*. 2003;9:685-693.
136. Gale NW, Thurston G, Hackett SF, et al. Angiopoietin-2 is required for postnatal angiogenesis and lymphatic patterning, and only the latter role is rescued by angiopoietin-1. *Dev Cell*. 2003;3:411-423.
137. Hackett SF, Wiegand S, Yancopoulos G, et al. Angiopoietin-2 plays an important role in retinal angiogenesis. *J Cell Physiol*. 2002;192:182-187.
138. Maisonpierre PC, Suri C, Jones PF, et al. Angiopoietin-2, a natural antagonist for Tie2 that disrupts in vivo angiogenesis. *Science*. 1997;277:55-60.
139. Hammes HP, Lin J, Wagner P, et al. Angiopoietin-2 causes pericyte dropout in the normal retina: evidence for involvement in diabetic retinopathy. *Diabetes*. 2004;53:1104-1110.
140. Hammes HP, Lin J, Renner O, et al. Pericytes and the pathogenesis of diabetic retinopathy. *Diabetes*. 2002;51:3107-3112.
141. Yao D, Taguchi T, Matsumura T, et al. Methylglyoxal modification of mSin3A links glycolysis to angiopoietin-2 transcription. *Cell*. 2006;124:275-286.
142. McLellan AC, Thornalley PJ, Benn J, et al. Glyoxalase system in clinical diabetes mellitus and correlation with diabetic complications. *Clin Sci (Lond)*. 1994;87:21-29.
143. Godbout JP, Pesavento J, Hartman ME, et al. Methylglyoxal enhances cisplatin-induced cytotoxicity by activating protein kinase Cδ. *J Biol Chem*. 2002;277:2554-2561.
144. Sakamoto H, Mashima T, Yamamoto K, et al. Modulation of heat-shock protein 27 (Hsp27) anti-apoptotic activity by methylglyoxal modification. *J Biol Chem*. 2002;277:45770-45775.
145. Tanaka S, Avigad G, Brodsky B, et al. Glycation induces expansion of the molecular packing of collagen. *J Mol Biol*. 1988;203:495-505.
146. Huijberts MS, Wolffenbuttel BH, Boudier HA, et al. Aminoguanidine treatment increases elasticity and decreases fluid filtration of large arteries from diabetic rats. *J Clin Invest*. 1993;92:1407-1411.
147. Tsilibary EC, Charonis AS, Reger LA, et al. The effect of nonenzymatic glucosylation on the binding of the main noncollagenous NC1 domain to type IV collagen. *J Biol Chem*. 1988;263:4302-4308.
148. Charonis AS, Reger LA, Dege JE, et al. Laminin alterations after in vitro nonenzymatic glycosylation. *Diabetes*. 1988;39:807-814.
149. Cochrane SM, Robinson GB. In vitro glycation of a glomerular basement membrane alters its permeability: a possible mechanism in diabetic complications. *FEBS Lett*. 1995;375:41-44.
150. Boyd-White J, Williams Jr JC. Effect of cross-linking on matrix permeability: a model for AGE-modified basement membranes. *Diabetes*. 1996;45:348-353.
151. Haitoglou CS, Tsilibary EC, Brownlee M, et al. Altered cellular interactions between endothelial cells and nonenzymatically glucosylated laminin/type IV collagen. *J Biol Chem*. 1992;267:12404-12407.
152. Federoff HJ, Lawrence D, Brownlee M. Nonenzymatic glycosylation of laminin and the laminin peptide CIKVAVS inhibits neurite outgrowth. *Diabetes*. 1993;42:509-513.
153. Hammes HP, Weiss A, Hess S, et al. Modification of vitronectin by advanced glycation alters functional properties in vitro and in the diabetic retina. *Lab Invest*. 1996;75:325-338.
154. Dobler D, Ahmed N, Song L, et al. Increased dicarbonyl metabolism in endothelial cells in hyperglycemia induces anoikis and impairs angiogenesis by RGD and GFOGER motif modification. *Diabetes*. 2006;55:1961-1969.
155. Bishara NB, Dunlop ME, Murphy TV, et al. Matrix protein glycation impairs agonist-induced intracellular Ca^{2+} signaling in endothelial cells. *J Cell Physiol*. 2002;193:80-92.
156. Li YM, Mitsuhashi T, Wojciechowicz D, et al. Molecular identity and cellular distribution of advanced glycation end product receptors: relationship of p60 to OST-48 and p90 to 80K-H membrane proteins. *Proc Natl Acad Sci U S A*. 1996;93:11047-11052.
157. Yang Z, Makita Z, Horii Y, et al. Two novel rat liver membrane proteins that bind advanced glycosylation end products: Relationship to macrophage receptor for glucose-modified proteins. *J Exp Med*. 1991;174:515-524.
158. Schmidt AM, Vianna M, Gerlach M, et al. Isolation and characterization of two binding proteins for advanced glycosylation end products from bovine lung which are present on the endothelial cell surface. *J Biol Chem*. 1992;267:14987-14997.
159. Neeper M, Schmidt AM, Brett J, et al. Cloning and expression of a cell surface receptor for advanced glycosylation end products of proteins. *J Biol Chem*. 1992;267:14998-15004.
160. Schmidt AM, Mora R, Cao R, et al. The endothelial cell binding site for advanced glycation endproducts consists of a complex: an integral membrane protein and a lactoferrin-like polypeptide. *J Biol Chem*. 1994;269:9882-9888.
161. Vlassara H, Brownlee M, Manogue K, et al. Cachectin/TNF and IL-1 induced by glucose-modified proteins: role in normal tissue remodeling. *Science*. 1988;240:1546-1548.
162. Kirstein M, Aston C, Hintz R, et al. Receptor-specific induction of insulin-like growth factor I in human monocytes by advanced glycosylation end product-modified proteins. *J Clin Invest*. 1992;90:439-446.
163. Yui S, Sasaki T, Araki N, et al. Induction of macrophage growth by advanced glycation end products of the Maillard reaction. *J Immunol*. 1994;152:1943-1949.

164. Higashi T, Sano H, Saishoji T, et al. The receptor for advanced glycation end products mediates the chemotaxis of rabbit smooth muscle cells. *Diabetes*. 1997;46:463-472.
165. Westwood ME, Thornalley PJ. Induction of synthesis and secretion of interleukin 1 beta in the human monocytic THP-1 cells by human serum albumins modified with methylglyoxal and advanced glycation endproducts. *Immunol Lett*. 1996;50:17-21.
166. Abordo EA, Westwood ME, Thornalley PJ. Synthesis and secretion of macrophage colony stimulating factor by mature human monocytes and human monocytic THP-1 cells induced by human serum albumin derivatives modified with methylglyoxal and glucose-derived advanced glycation endproducts. *Immunol Lett*. 1996;53:7-13.
167. Abordo EA, Thornalley PJ. Synthesis and secretion of tumour necrosis factor-alpha by human monocytic THP-1 cells and chemotaxis induced by human serum albumin derivatives modified with methylglyoxal and glucose-derived advanced glycation endproducts. *Immunol Lett*. 1997;58:139-147.
168. Webster L, Abordo EA, Thornalley PJ, et al. Induction of TNF alpha and IL-beta mRNA in monocytes by methylglyoxal- and advanced glycated endproduct-modified human serum albumin. *Biochem Soc Trans*. 1997;25:250S.
169. Pugliese G, Pricci F, Romeo G, et al. Upregulation of mesangial growth factor and extracellular matrix synthesis by advanced glycation end products via a receptor-mediated mechanism. *Diabetes*. 1997;46:1881-1887.
170. Smedsrod B, Melkko J, Araki N, et al. Advanced glycation end products are eliminated by scavenger-receptor-mediated endocytosis in hepatic sinusoidal kupffer and endothelial cells. *Biochem J*. 1997;322:567-573.
171. Horiuchi S, Higashi T, Ikeda K, et al. Advanced glycation end products and their recognition by macrophage and macrophage-derived cells. *Diabetes*. 1996;45:S73-S76.
172. Sano H, Higashi T, Matsumoto K, et al. Insulin enhances macrophage scavenger receptor-mediated endocytic uptake of advanced glycation end products. *Biol Chem*. 1998;273:8630-8637.
173. Vlassara H, Li YM, Imani F, et al. Identification of galectin-3 as a high-affinity binding protein for advanced glycation end products (AGE): a new member of the AGE-receptor complex. *Mol Med*. 1995;1:634-646.
174. Skolnik EY, Yang Z, Makita Z, et al. Human and rat mesangial cell receptors for glucose-modified proteins: potential role in kidney tissue remodelling and diabetic nephropathy. *J Exp Med*. 1991;174:931-939.
175. Doi T, Vlassara H, Kirstein M, et al. Receptor-specific increase in extracellular matrix productions in mouse mesangial cells by advanced glycosylation end products is mediated via platelet derived growth factor. *Proc Natl Acad Sci U S A*. 1992;89:2873-2877.
176. Vlassara H, Fuh H, Donnelly T, et al. Advanced glycation endproducts promote adhesion molecule (VCAM-1, ICAM-1) expression and atheroma formation in normal rabbits. *Mol Med*. 1995;1:447-456.
177. Schmidt AM, Hori O, Chen JX, et al. Advanced glycation endproducts interacting with their endothelial receptor induce expression of vascular cell adhesion molecule-1 (VCAM-1) in cultured human endothelial cells and in mice: a potential mechanism for the accelerated vasculopathy of diabetes. *J Clin Invest*. 1995;96:1395-1403.
178. Sengoelge G, Fodinger M, Skoupy S, et al. Endothelial cell adhesion molecule and PMNL response to inflammatory stimuli and AGE-modified fibronectin. *Kidney Int*. 1998;54:1637-1651.
179. Schmidt AM, Crandall J, Hori O, et al. Elevated plasma levels of vascular cell adhesion molecule-1 (VCAM-1) in diabetic patients with microalbuminuria: a marker of vascular dysfunction and progressive vascular disease. *Br J Haematol*. 1996;92:747-750.
180. Wautier JL, Zoukourian C, Chappey O, et al. Receptor-mediated endothelial cell dysfunction in diabetic vasculopathy: soluble receptor for advanced glycation end products blocks hyperpermeability in diabetic rats. *J Clin Invest*. 1996;97:238-243.
181. Lu M, Kuroki M, Amano S, et al. Advanced glycation end products increase retinal vascular endothelial growth factor expression. *J Clin Invest*. 1998;101:1219-1224.
182. Hirata C, Nakano K, Nakamura N, et al. Advanced glycation end products induce expression of vascular endothelial growth factor by retinal Muller cells. *Biochem Biophys Res Commun*. 1997;236:712-715.
183. Soro-Paavonen A, Watson AM, Li J, et al. Receptor for advanced glycation end products (RAGE) deficiency attenuates the development of atherosclerosis in diabetes. *Diabetes*. 2008;57:2461-2469.
184 Bierhaus A, Humpert PM, Morcos M, et al. Understanding RAGE, the receptor for advanced glycation end products (Review). *J Mol Med*. 2005;83:876-886.
185. Rong LL, Gooch C, Szabolcs M, et al. RAGE: a journey from the complications of diabetes to disorders of the nervous system—striking a fine balance between injury and repair (Review). *Restor Neurol Neurosci*. 2005;23(5-6):355-365.
186. Koya D, King GL. Protein kinase C activation and the development of diabetic complications. *Diabetes*. 1998;47: 859-866.
187. Yao D, Brownlee M. Hyperglycemia-induced reactive oxygen species increase expression of the receptor for advanced glycation end products (RAGE) and RAGE ligands. *Diabetes*. 2010;59:249-255.
188. Park L, Raman KG, Lee KJ, et al. Suppression of accelerated diabetic atherosclerosis by the soluble receptor for advanced glycation end products. *Nat Med*. 1998;4:1025-1031.
189. Kislinger T, Tanji N, Wendt T, et al. Receptor for advanced glycation end products mediates inflammation and enhanced expression of tissue factor in vasculature of diabetic apolipoprotein E-null mice. *Arterioscler Thromb Vasc Biol*. 2001;21:905-910.
190. Lalla E, Lamster IB, Feit M, et al. Blockade of RAGE suppresses periodontitis-associated bone loss in diabetic mice. *J Clin Invest*. 2000;105:1117-1124.
191. Goova MT, Li J, Kislinger T, et al. Blockade of receptor for advanced glycation end-products restores effective wound healing in diabetic mice. *Am J Pathol*. 2001;159:513-525.
192. Bucciarelli LG, Wendt T, Qu W, et al. RAGE blockade stabilizes established atherosclerosis in diabetic apolipoprotein E-null mice. *Circulation*. 2002;106:2827-2835.
193. Basta G, Lazzerini G, Massaro M, et al. Advanced glycation end products activate endothelium through signal-transduction receptor RAGE: a mechanism for amplification of inflammatory responses. *Circulation*. 2002;105:816-822.
194. Yan SD, Schmidt AM, Anderson GM, et al. Enhanced cellular oxidant stress by the interaction of advanced glycation end products with their receptors/binding proteins. *J Biol Chem*. 1994;269:9889-9897.
195. Lander HM, Tauras JM, Ogiste JS, et al. Activation of the receptor for advanced glycation end products triggers a p21(ras)-dependent mitogen-activated protein kinase pathway regulated by oxidant stress. *J Biol Chem*. 1997;272:17810-17814.
196. Li J, Schmidt AM. Characterization and functional analysis of the promoter of RAGE, the receptor for advanced glycation end products. *J Biol Chem*. 1997;272:16498-16506.
197. Yamagishi S, Fujimori H, Yonekura H, et al. Advanced glycation end products inhibit prostacyclin production and induce plasminogen activator inhibitor-1 in human microvascular endothelial cells. *Diabetologia*. 1998;41:1435-1441.
198. Tsuji H, Iehara N, Masegi T, et al. Ribozyme targeting of receptor for advanced glycation end products in mouse mesangial cells. *Biochem Biophys Res Commun*. 1998;245:583-588.
199. Basta G, Sironi AM, Lazzerini G, et al. Circulating soluble receptor for advanced glycation end products is inversely associated with glycemic control and S100A12 protein. *J Clin Endocrinol Metab*. 2006;91:4628-4634.
200. Naoto K, Munehide M, Hideaki K, et al. Decreased endogenous secretory advanced glycation end product receptor in type 1 diabetic patients: its possible association with diabetic vascular complications. *Diabetes Care*. 2005;28:2716-2721.
201. Inoguchi T, Battan R, Handler E, et al. Preferential elevation of protein kinase C isoform beta II and diacylglycerol levels in the aorta and heart of diabetic rats: differential reversibility to glycemic control by islet cell transplantation. *Proc Natl Acad Sci U S A*. 1992;89:11059-11063.
202. Craven PA, Davidson CM, DeRubertis FR. Increase in diacylglycerol mass in isolated glomeruli by glucose from de novo synthesis of glycerolipids. *Diabetes*. 1990;39:667-674.
203. Shiba T, Inoguchi T, Sportsman JR, et al. Correlation of diacylglycerol level and protein kinase C activity in rat retina to retinal circulation. *Am J Physiol*. 1993;265(5 Pt 1):E783-E793.
204. Inoguchi T, Xia P, Kunisaki M, et al. Insulin's effect on protein kinase C and diacylglycerol induced by diabetes and glucose in vascular tissues. *Am J Physiol*. 1994;267(3 Pt 1):E369-E379.
205. Derubertis FR, Craven PA. Activation of protein kinase C in glomerular cells in diabetes: mechanisms and potential links to the pathogenesis of diabetic glomerulopathy. *Diabetes*. 1994;43:1-8.
206. Xia P, Inoguchi T, Kern TS, et al. Characterization of the mechanism for the chronic activation of diacylglycerol-protein kinase C pathway in diabetes and hypergalactosemia. *Diabetes*. 1994;43:1122-1129.
207. Ayo SH, Radnik R, Garoni JA, et al. High glucose increases diacylglycerol mass and activates protein kinase C in mesangial cell cultures. *Am J Physiol*. 1991;261(4 Pt 2):F571-F577.
208. Koya D, King GL. Protein kinase C activation and the development of diabetic complications. *Diabetes*. 1998;47:859-866.
209. Koya D, Jirousek MR, Lin YW, et al. Characterization of protein kinase C beta isoform activation on the gene expression of transforming growth factor-beta, extracellular matrix components, and prostanoids in the glomeruli of diabetic rats. *J Clin Invest*. 1997;100:115-126.
210. Kikkawa R, Haneda M, Uzu T, et al. Translocation of protein kinase C alpha and zeta in rat glomerular mesangial cells cultured under high glucose conditions. *Diabetologia*. 1994;37:838-841.
211. Knapp LT, Klann E. Superoxide-induced stimulation of protein kinase C via thiol modification and modulation of zinc content. *J Biol Chem*. 2000;275:24136-24145.
212. Konishi H, Tanaka M, Takemura Y, et al. Activation of protein kinase C by tyrosine phosphorylation in response to H_2O_2. *Proc Natl Acad Sci U S A*. 1997;94:11233-11237.
213. Ishii H, Jirousek MR, Koya D, et al. Amelioration of vascular dysfunctions in diabetic rats by an oral PKC-β inhibitor. *Science*. 1996;272:728-731.

214. Geraldes P, Hiraoka-Yamamoto J, Matsumoto M, et al. Activation of PKC-delta and SHP-1 by hyperglycemia causes vascular cell apoptosis and diabetic retinopathy. *Nat Med.* 2009;15:1298-1306.
215. Craven PA, Studer RK, DeRubertis FR. Impaired nitric oxide-dependent cyclic guanosine monophosphate generation in glomeruli from diabetic rats: evidence for protein kinase C-mediated suppression of the cholinergic response. *J Clin Invest.* 1994;93:311-320.
216. Ganz MB, Seftel A. Glucose-induced changes in protein kinase C and nitric oxide are prevented by vitamin E. *Am J Physiol.* 2000;278:E146-152.
217. Pugliese G, Pricci F, Pugliese F, et al. Mechanisms of glucose-enhanced extracellular matrix accumulation in rat glomerular mesangial cells. *Diabetes.* 1994;43:478-490.
218. Glogowski EA, Tsiani E, Zhou X, et al. High glucose alters the response of mesangial cell protein kinase C isoforms to endothelin-1. *Kidney Int.* 1999;55:486-499.
219. Hempel A, Maasch C, Heintze U, et al. High glucose concentrations increase endothelial cell permeability via activation of protein kinase C alpha. *Circ Res.* 1997;81:363-371.
220. Dang L, Seale JP, Qu X. High glucose-induced human umbilical vein endothelial cell hyperpermeability is dependent on protein kinase C activation and independent of the Ca^{2+}-nitric oxide signalling pathway. *Clin Exp Pharmacol Physiol.* 2005;32:771-776.
221. Williams B, Gallacher B, Patel H, Orme C. Glucose-induced protein kinase C activation regulates vascular permeability factor mRNA expression and peptide production by human vascular smooth muscle cells in vitro. *Diabetes.* 1997;46:1497-1503.
222. Studer RK, Craven PA, DeRubertis FR. Role for protein kinase C in the mediation of increased fibronectin accumulation by mesangial cells grown in high-glucose medium. *Diabetes.* 1993;42:118-126.
223. Craven PA, Studer RK, Felder J, et al. Nitric oxide inhibition of transforming growth factor-beta and collagen synthesis in mesangial cells. *Diabetes.* 1997;46:671-681.
224. Phillips SL, DeRubertis FR, Craven PA. Regulation of the laminin C1 promoter in cultured mesangial cells. *Diabetes.* 1999;48:2083-2089.
225. Feener EP, Xia P, Inoguchi T, et al. Role of protein kinase C in glucose- and angiotensin II-induced plasminogen activator inhibitor expression. *Contrib Nephrol.* 1996;118:180-187.
226. Pieper GM, Riaz-ul-Haq J. Activation of nuclear factor-κB in cultured endothelial cells by increased glucose concentration: prevention by calphostin C. *Cardiovasc Pharmacol.* 1997;30:528-532.
227. Yerneni KK, Bai W, Khan BV, et al. Hyperglycemia-induced activation of nuclear transcription factor κB in vascular smooth muscle cells. *Diabetes.* 1999;48:855-864.
228. Way KJ, Isshiki K, Suzuma K, et al. Expression of connective tissue growth factor is increased in injured myocardium associated with protein kinase C β2 activation and diabetes. *Diabetes.* 2002;51:2709-2718.
229. Igarashi M, Wakasaki H, Takahara N, et al. Glucose or diabetes activates p38 mitogen-activated protein kinase via different pathways. *J Clin Invest.* 1999;103:185-195.
230. Fontayne A, Dang PM, Gougerot-Pocidalo MA, et al. Phosphorylation of p47phox sites by PKC-alpha, beta II, delta, and zeta: effect on binding to p22phox and on NADPH oxidase activation. *Biochemistry.* 2002;41:7743-7750.
231. Guzik TJ, Mussa S, Gastaldi D, et al. Mechanisms of increased vascular superoxide production in human diabetes mellitus: role of NAD(P)H oxidase and endothelial nitric oxide synthase. *Circulation.* 2002;105:1656-1662.
232. Beckman JA, Goldfine AB, Gordon MB, et al. Inhibition of protein kinase Cβ prevents impaired endothelium-dependent vasodilation caused by hyperglycemia in humans. *Circ Res.* 2002;90:107-111.
233. Sayeski PP, Kudlow JE. Glucose metabolism to glucosamine is necessary for glucose stimulation of transforming growth factor-alpha gene transcription. *J Biol Chem.* 1996;271:15237-15243.
234. Kolm-Litty V, Sauer U, Nerlich A, et al. High glucose-induced transforming growth factor beta1 production is mediated by the hexosamine pathway in porcine glomerular mesangial cells. *J Clin Invest.* 1998;101:160-169.
235. Daniels MC, Kansal P, Smith TM, et al. Glucose regulation of transforming growth factor-alpha expression is mediated by products of the hexosamine biosynthesis pathway. *Mol Endocrinol.* 1993;7:1041-1048.
236. McClain DA, Paterson AJ, Roos MD, et al. Glucose and glucosamine regulate growth factor gene expression in vascular smooth muscle cells. *Proc Natl Acad Sci U S A.* 1992;89:8150-8154.
237. Marshall S, Bacote V, Traxinger RR. Discovery of a metabolic pathway mediating glucose-induced desensitization of the glucose transport system: role of hexosamine biosynthesis in the induction of insulin resistance. *J Biol Chem.* 1991;266:4706-4712.
238. Rossetti L, Hawkins M, Chen W, et al. In vivo glucosamine infusion induces insulin resistance in normoglycemic but not in hyperglycemic conscious rats. *J Clin Invest.* 1995;96:132-140.
239. Hawkins M, Barzilai N, Liu R, et al. Role of the glucosamine pathway in fat-induced insulin resistance. *J Clin Invest.* 1997;99: 2173-2182.
240. Federici M, Menghini R, Mauriello A, et al. Insulin-dependent activation of endothelial nitric oxide synthase is impaired by *O*-linked glycosylation modification of signaling proteins in human coronary endothelial cells. *Circulation.* 2002;106:466-472.
241. Chen YQ, Su M, Walia RR, et al. Sp1 sites mediate activation of the plasminogen activator inhibitor-1 promoter by glucose in vascular smooth muscle cells. *J Biol Chem.* 1998;273:8225-8231.
242. Goldberg HJ, Scholey J, Fantus IG. Glucosamine activates the plasminogen activator inhibitor 1 gene promoter through Sp1 DNA binding sites in glomerular mesangial cells. *Diabetes.* 2000;49: 863-871.
243. Goldberg HJ, Whiteside CI, Fantus IG. The hexosamine pathway regulates the plasminogen activator inhibitor-1 gene promoter and Sp1 transcriptional activation through protein kinase C-beta I and -delta. *J Biol Chem.* 2002;277:33833-33841.
244. Hart GW. Dynamic *O*-linked glycosylation of nuclear and cytoskeletal proteins. *Annu Rev Biochem.* 1997;66:315-335.
245. Akimoto Y, Kreppel LK, Hirano H, Hart GW. Hyperglycemia and the *O*-GlcNAc transferase in rat aortic smooth muscle cells: elevated expression and altered patterns of *O*-GlcNAcylation. *Arch Biochem Biophys.* 2001;389:166-175.
246. Yang X, Ongusaha PP, Miles PD, et al. Phosphoinositide signalling links *O*-GlcNAc transferase to insulin resistance. *Nature.* 2008;451:964-969.
247. Sima AA, Prashar A, Zhang WX, et al. Preventive effect of long-term aldose reductase inhibition (ponalrestat) on nerve conduction and sural nerve structure in the spontaneously diabetic Bio-Breeding rat. *J Clin Invest.* 1990;85:1410-1420.
248. Lee AY, Chung SK, Chung SS. Demonstration that polyol accumulation is responsible for diabetic cataract by the use of transgenic mice expressing the aldose reductase gene in the lens. *Proc Natl Acad Sci U S A.* 1995;92:2780-2784.
249. Brownlee M. Advanced protein glycosylation in diabetes and aging. *Annu Rev Med.* 1995;46:223-234.
250. Brownlee M Biochemistry and molecular cell biology of diabetic complications. *Nature.* 2001;414:813-820.
251. Giardino I, Edelstein D, Brownlee M. BCL-2 expression or antioxidants prevent hyperglycemia-induced formation of intracellular advanced glycation end products in bovine endothelial cells. *J Clin Invest.* 1996;97:1422-1428.
252. Wallace DC. Diseases of the mitochondrial DNA. *Annu Rev Biochem.* 1992;61:1175-1212.
253. Trumpower BL. The proton motive Q cycle. *J Biol Chem.* 1990;265:11409-11412.
254. Korshunov SS, Skulachev VP, Starkov AA. High protonic potential actuates a mechanism of production of reactive oxygen species in mitochondria. *FEBS Lett.* 1997;416:15-18.
255. Casteilla L, Blondel,O, Klaus S, et al. Stable expression of functional mitochondrial uncoupling protein in Chinese hamster ovary cells. *Proc Natl Acad Sci U S A.* 1990;87:5124-5128.
256. Manna SK, Zhang HJ, Yan T, et al. Overexpression manganese superoxide dismutase suppresses tumor necrosis factor-induced apoptosis and activation of nuclear transcription factor-κB and activated protein-1. *J Biol Chem.* 1998;273:13245-13254.
257. Haskins K, Bradley B, Powers K, et al. Oxidative stress in type 1 diabetes. *Ann N Y Acad Sci.* 2003;1005:43-54.
258. Pugazhenthi S, Nesterova A, Jambal P, et al. Oxidative stress-mediated down-regulation of bcl-2 promoter in hippocampal neurons. *J Neurochem.* 2003;84:982-996.
259. Du X, Matsumura T, Edelstein D, et al. Inhibition of GAPDH activity by poly(ADP-ribose) polymerase activates three major pathways of hyperglycemic damage in endothelial cells. *J Clin Invest.* 2003; 112:1049-1057.
260. Sawa A, Khan AA, Hester LD, Snyder SH. Glyceraldehyde-3-phosphate dehydrogenase: nuclear translocation participates in neuronal and nonneuronal cell death. *Proc Natl Acad Sci U S A.* 1997;94:11669-11674.
261. Schmidtz HD. Reversible nuclear translocation of glyceraldehyde-3-phosphate dehydrogenase upon serum depletion. *Eur J Cell Biol.* 2001;80:419-427.
262. Craven PA, Phillips SL, Melhem MF, et al. Overexpression of manganese superoxide dismutase suppresses increases in collagen accumulation induced by culture of mesangial cells in high-media glucose. *Metabolism.* 2001;50:1043-1048.
263. Vincent AM, Brownlee M, Russell JW. Oxidative stress and programmed cell death in diabetic neuropathy. *Ann N Y Acad Sci.* 2002;959: 368-383.
264. Zou MH, Shi C, Cohen RA. High glucose via peroxynitrite causes tyrosine nitration and inactivation of prostacyclin synthase that is associated with thromboxane/prostaglandin H_2 receptor-mediated apoptosis and adhesion molecule expression in cultured human aortic endothelial cells. *Diabetes.* 2002;51:198-203.
265. Uemura S, Matsushita H, Li W, et al. Diabetes mellitus enhances vascular matrix metalloproteinase activity: role of oxidative stress. *Circ Res.* 2001;88:1291-1298.

266. Craven PA, Melhem MF, Phillips SL, et al. Overexpression of Cu^{2+}/Zn^{2+} superoxide dismutase protects against early diabetic glomerular injury in transgenic mice. *Diabetes*. 2001;50:2114-2125.
267. DeRubertis FR, Craven PA, Melhem MF, et al. Attenuation of renal injury in db/db mice overexpressing superoxide dismutase: evidence for reduced superoxide-nitric oxide interaction. *Diabetes*. 2004;53: 762-768.
268. Ye G, Metreveli NS, Donthi RV, et al. Catalase protect cardiomyocyte function in models of type 1 and type 2 diabetes. *Diabetes*. 2004;53:1336-1343.
269. Shen X, Zheng S, Metreveli NS, et al. Protection of cardiac mitochondria by overexpression of MnSOD reduces diabetic cardiomyopathy. *Diabetes*. 2006;55:798-805.
270. Huang C, Kim Y, Caramori ML, et al. Diabetic nephropathy is associated with gene expression levels of oxidative phosphorylation and related pathways. *Diabetes*. 2006;55:1826-1831.
271. Ballinger SW, Patterson C, Knight-Lozano CA, et al. Mitochondrial integrity and function in atherogenesis. *Circulation*. 2002;106: 544-549.
272. Mercer JR, Cheng KK, Fig N, et al. DNA damage links mitochondrial dysfunction, atherosclerosis, and the metabolic syndrome. *Circ Res*. 2010;107:1021-1031.
273. Semenkovich CF. Insulin resistance and atherosclerosis (Review). *J Clin Invest*. 2006;116:1813-1822.
274. Kowluru RA. Effect of reinstitution of good glycemic control on retinal oxidative stress and nitrative stress in diabetic rats. *Diabetes*. 2003;52:818-823.
275. Vaissière T, Sawan C, Herceg Z. Epigenetic interplay between histone modifications and DNA methylation in gene silencing (Review). *Mutat Res*. 2008;659:40-48.
276. Probst AV, Dunleavy E, Almousni G. Epigenetic inheritance during the cell cycle. *Nat Rev Mol Cell Biol*. 2009;10:192-206.
277. Göndör A, Ohlsson R. Replication timing and epigenetic reprogramming of gene expression: a two-way relationship? *Nat Rev Genet*. 2009;10:269-276.
278. Brasacchio D, Okabe J, Tikellis C, et al. Hyperglycemia induces a dynamic cooperativity of histone methylase and demethylase enzymes associated with gene-activating epigenetic marks that co-exist on the lysine tail. *Diabetes*. 2009;58:1229-1236.
279. El-Osta A, Brasacchio D, Yao D, et al. Transient high glucose causes persistent epigenetic changes and altered gene expression during subsequent normoglycemia. *J Exp Med*. 2008;205:2409-2417.
280. Miao F, Smith DD, Zhang L, et al. Lymphocytes from patients with type 1 diabetes display a distinct profile of chromatin histone H3 lysine 9 dimethylation: an epigenetic study in diabetes. *Diabetes*. 2008;57:3189-3198.
281. Reddy MA, Villeneuve LM, Wang M, et al. Role of the lysine-specific demethylase 1 in the proinflammatory phenotype of vascular smooth muscle cells of diabetic mice. *Circ Res*. 2008;103:615-624.
282. Villeneuve LM, Reddy MA, Lanting LL, et al. Epigenetic histone H3 lysine 9 methylation in metabolic memory and inflammatory phenotype of vascular smooth muscle cells in diabetes. *Proc Natl Acad Sci U S A*. 2008;105:9047-9052.
283. Yu T, Robotham JL, Yoon Y. Increased production of reactive oxygen species in hyperglycemic conditions requires dynamic change of mitochondrial morphology *Proc Natl Acad Sci U S A*. 2006;103:2653-2658.
283a. Giudice A, Arra C, Turco MC. Review of molecular mechanisms involved in the activation of the Nrf2-ARE signaling pathways by chemoprotective agents. *Methods Mol Biol*. 2010;647:37-74.
284. Ferris FL. How effective are treatments for diabetic retinopathy? *JAMA*. 1993;269:1290-1291.
285. The PKC-DRS Study Group. The effect of ruboxistaurin on visual loss in patients with moderately severe to very severe nonproliferative diabetic retinopathy: initial results of the PKC-DRS Multicenter Randomized Clinical Trial. *Diabetes*. 2005;54:2188-2197.
286. Strøm C, Sander B, Klemp K, et al. Effect of ruboxistaurin on blood-retinal barrier permeability in relation to severity of leakage in diabetic macular edema. *Invest Ophthalmol Vis Sci*. 2005;46:3855-3858.
287. Aiello LP, Clermont A, Arora V, et al. Inhibition of PKC-β by oral administration of ruboxistaurin (LY333531) mesylate is well tolerated and ameliorates diabetes-induced retinal hemodynamic abnormalities in patients. *Invest Ophthalmol Vis Sci*. 2005;47:86-92.
288. The PKC-DMES Study Group. Effect of ruboxistaurin, a PKCβ isoform-selective inhibitor, in patients with diabetic macular edema: 30-month results of the randomized PKC-DMES clinical trial. *Arch Opthalmal*. 2007;125:318-324.
289. The PKC-DRS2 Study Group. Effect of ruboxistaurin on visual loss in patients with diabetic retinopathy. *Ophthalmology*. 2006;113: 2221-2230.
290. Tuttle KR, Bakris GL, Toto RD, et al. The effect of ruboxistaurin on nephropathy in type 2 diabetes. *Diabetes Care*. 2005;28:2686-2690.
291. Cunningham ET, Adamis AP, Altaweel M, et al, the Macugen Diabetic Retinopathy Study Group. a phase II randomized double-masked trial of pegaptanib, an anti-vascular endothelial growth factor aptamer, for diabetic macular edema. *Ophthalmology*. 2005;46:3855-3858.
292. Chun DW, Heier JS, Topping TM, et al. A pilot study of multiple intravitreal injections of ranibizumab in patients with center-involving clinically significant diabetic macular edema. *Ophthalmology*. 2006;113:1706-1712.
293. Jager RD, Aiello LP, Patel SC, et al. Risks of intravitreal injection: a comprehensive review. *Retina*. 2004;24:676-698.
294. Shaw JE, Sicree RA, Zimmet PZ. Global estimates of the prevalence of diabetes for 2010 and 2030. *Diabetes Res Clin Pract*. 2010;87, 4-14.
295. Centers for Disease Control and Prevention. *National diabetes fact sheet: general information and national estimates on diabetes in the United States, 2007*. Atlanta, GA: U.S. Department of Health and Human Services, Centers for Disease Control and Prevention; 2008.
296. Kempen JH, O'Colmain BJ, Leske MC, et al. The prevalence of diabetic retinopathy among adults in the United States. *Arch Ophthalmol*. 2004;122: 552-563.
297. Harris MI, Hadden WC, Knowler WC, Bennett PH. Prevalence of diabetes and impaired glucose tolerance and plasma glucose levels in US population aged 20-74 years. *Diabetes*. 1998;36:523-534.
298. Klein R, Klein BE, Moss SE, et al. The Wisconsin Epidemiologic Study of Diabetic Retinopathy: II. Prevalence and risk of diabetic retinopathy when age at diagnosis is less than 30 years. *Arch Ophthalmol*. 1984;102:520-536.
299. Klein R, Klein BE, Moss SE, et al. The Wisconsin Epidemiologic Study of Diabetic Retinopathy: XV. The long-term incidence of macular edema. *Ophthalmology*. 1995;102:7-16.
300. Javitt JC, Canner JK, Sommer A. Cost effectiveness of current approaches to the control of retinopathy in type 1 diabetics. *Ophthalmology*. 1989;96:255-264.
301. Javitt JC, Aiello LP, Bassi LJ, et al. Detecting and treating retinopathy in patients with type I diabetes mellitus: savings associated with improved implementation of current guidelines. American Academy of Ophthalmology. *Ophthalmology*. 1991;98:1565-1573.
302. Javitt JC, Aiello LP, Chiang Y, et al. Preventive eye care in people with diabetes is cost-saving to the federal government: implications for health-care reform. *Diabetes Care*. 1994;17:909-917.
303. Javitt JC, Aiello LP. Cost-effectiveness of detecting and treating diabetic retinopathy [see comments]. *Ann Intern Med*. 1996;124(1 Pt 2): 164-169.
304. Centers for Disease Control and Prevention. National Diabetes Fact Sheet. National Estimate on Diabetes. Available at http://www.cdc.gov/diabetes/pubs/estimates.htm (accessed December 2010).
305. Kahn HA, Hiller R. Blindness caused by diabetic retinopathy. *Am J Ophthalmol*. 1974;78:58-67.
306. Palmberg PF. Diabetic retinopathy. *Diabetes*. 1977;26:703-709.
307. DCCT Research Group. The Diabetes Control and Complications Trial (DCCT). Design and methodologic considerations for the feasibility phase. *Diabetes*. 1986;35:530-545.
308. Diabetes Control and Complications Trial/Epidemiology of Diabetes Interventions and Complications Research Group. Retinopathy and nephropathy in patients with type 1 diabetes four years after a trial of intensive therapy. *N Engl J Med*. 2000;342:381-389.
309. The relationship of glycemic exposure (Hb A_{1c}) to the risk of development and progression of retinopathy in the Diabetes Control and Complications trial. *Diabetes*. 1995;44:968-983.
310. Diabetes Control and Complications Trial Research Group. Lifetime benefits and costs of intensive therapy as practiced in the Diabetes Control and Complications Trial [see comments] [published erratum appears in *JAMA* 1997;278:25]. *JAMA*. 1996;276:1409-1415.
311. Resource utilization and costs of care in the Diabetes Control and Complications Trial. *Diabetes Care*. 1995;18:1468-1478.
312. Cogan DG, Toussaint D, Kuwabara T. Retinal vascular patterns: IV. Diabetic retinopathy. *Arch Ophthalmol*. 1961;66:366-378.
313. Konno S, Feke GT, Yoshida A, et al. Retinal blood flow changes in type I diabetes: a long-term follow-up study. *Invest Ophthalmol Vis Sci*. 1996;37:1140-1148.
314. Grunwald JE, Riva CE, Sinclair SH, et al. Laser Doppler velocimetry study of retinal circulation in diabetes mellitus. *Arch Ophthalmol*. 1986;104:991-996.
315. Bursell SE, Clermont AC, Kinsley BT, et al. Retinal blood flow changes in patients with insulin-dependent diabetes mellitus and no diabetic retinopathy. *Am J Physiol*. 1996;270(1 Pt 2):R61-R70.
316. Sosula L, Beaumont P, Hollows FC, et al. Dilatation and endothelial proliferation of retinal capillaries in streptozotocin-diabetic rats: quantitative electron microscopy. *Invest Ophthalmol*. 1972;11: 926-935.
317. Speiser P, Gittelsohn AM, Patz A. Studies on diabetic retinopathy: III. Influence of diabetes on intramural pericytes. *Arch Ophthalmol*. 1968;80:332-337.
318. Barouch FC, Miyamoto K, Allport JR, et al. Integrin-mediated neutrophil adhesion and retinal leukostasis in diabetes. *Invest Ophthalmol Vis Sci*. 2000;41:1153-1158.
319. Miyamoto K, Khosrof S, Bursell SE, et al. Vascular endothelial growth factor (VEGF)-induced retinal vascular permeability is mediated by intercellular adhesion molecule-1 (ICAM-1). *Am J Pathol*. 2000;156: 1733-1739.

320. Miyamoto K, Khosrof S, Bursell SE, et al. Prevention of leukostasis and vascular leakage in streptozotocin-induced diabetic retinopathy via intercellular adhesion molecule-1 inhibition. *Proc Natl Acad Sci U S A.* 1999;96:10836-10841.
321. Stitt AW, Gardiner TA, Archer DB. Histological and ultrastructural investigation of retinal microaneurysm development in diabetic patients. *Br J Ophthalmol.* 1995;79:362-367.
322. Cunha-Vaz J, Faria Jr DA, Campos AJ. Early breakdown of the blood-retinal barrier in diabetes. *Br J Ophthalmol.* 1975;59:649-656.
323. The Early Treatment Diabetic Retinopathy Study Research Group. Early photocoagulation for diabetic retinopathy. ETDRS Report No. 9. *Ophthalmology.* 1991;98(5 suppl):766-785.
324. Meyer-Schwickerath R, Pfeiffer A, Blum WF, et al. Vitreous levels of the insulin-like growth factors I and II, and the insulin-like growth factor-binding proteins 2 and 3, increase in neovascular eye disease: studies in nondiabetic and diabetic subjects. *J Clin Invest.* 1993;92: 2620-2625.
325. Nishimura M, Ikeda T, Ushiyama M, et al. Increased vitreous concentrations of human hepatocyte growth factor in proliferative diabetic retinopathy. *J Clin Endocrinol Metab.* 1999;84:659-662.
326. Aiello LP, Avery RL, Arrigg PG, et al. Vascular endothelial growth factor in ocular fluid of patients with diabetic retinopathy and other retinal disorders [see comments]. *N Engl J Med.* 1994;331:1480-1487.
327. Adamis AP, Miller JW, Bernal MT, et al. Increased vascular endothelial growth factor levels in the vitreous of eyes with proliferative diabetic retinopathy. *Am J Ophthalmol.* 1994;118:445-450.
328. Aiello LP, Hata Y. Molecular mechanisms of growth factor action in diabetic retinopathy. Curr Opin Endocrinol *Diabetes.* 1999;6: 146-156.
329. Aiello LP, Bursell SE, Clermont A, et al. Vascular endothelial growth factor-induced retinal permeability is mediated by protein kinase C in vivo and suppressed by an orally effective beta isoform-selective inhibitor. *Diabetes.* 1997;46:1473-1480.
330. Miller JW, Adamis AP, Aiello LP. Vascular endothelial growth factor in ocular neovascularization and proliferative diabetic retinopathy. *Diabetes Metab Rev.* 1997;13:37-50.
331. Okamoto N, Tobe T, Hackett SF, et al. Transgenic mice with increased expression of vascular endothelial growth factor in the retina: a new model of intraretinal and subretinal neovascularization [see comments]. *Am J Pathol.* 1997;151:281-291.
332. Ozaki H, Hayashi H, Vinores SA, et al. Intravitreal sustained release of VEGF causes retinal neovascularization in rabbits and breakdown of the blood-retinal barrier in rabbits and primates. *Exp Eye Res.* 1997;64:505-517.
333. Aiello LP, Pierce EA, Foley ED, et al. Suppression of retinal neovascularization in vivo by inhibition of vascular endothelial growth factor (VEGF) using soluble VEGF-receptor chimeric proteins. *Proc Natl Acad Sci U S A.* 1995;92:10457-10461.
334. Robinson GS, Pierce EA, Rook SL, et al. Oligodeoxynucleotides inhibit retinal neovascularization in a murine model of proliferative retinopathy. *Proc Natl Acad Sci U S A.* 1996;93:4851-4856.
335. Adamis AP, Shima DT, Tolentino MJ, et al. Inhibition of vascular endothelial growth factor prevents retinal ischemia-associated iris neovascularization in a nonhuman primate. *Arch Ophthalmol.* 1996;114: 66-71.
336. Danis RP, Bingaman DP, Jirousek M, et al. Inhibition of intraocular neovascularization caused by retinal ischemia in pigs by PKC-β inhibition with LY333531. *Invest Ophthalmol Vis Sci.* 1998;39:171-179.
337. Ozaki H, Seo MS, Ozaki K, et al. Blockade of vascular endothelial cell growth factor receptor signaling is sufficient to completely prevent retinal neovascularization. *Am J Pathol.* 2000;156:697-707.
338. Duh EJ, Yang HS, Suzuma I, et al. Pigment epithelium-derived factor (PEDF) suppresses ischemia-induced retinal neovascularization and VEGF-induced migration and growth. *Invest Ophthalmol Vis Sci.* 2002;43:821-829.
339. Gao BB, Clermont A, Rook S, et al. Extracellular carbonic anhydrase mediates hemorrhagic retinal and cerebral vascular permeability through prekallikrein activation. *Nat Med.* 2007;13:181-188.
340. Phipps JA, Clermont AC, Sinha S, et al. Plasma kallikrein mediates angiotensin II type 1 receptor-stimulated retinal vascular permeability. *Hypertension.* 2009;53:175-181.
341. Tripathi RC, Li J, Tripathi BJ, et al. Increased level of vascular endothelial growth factor in aqueous humor of patients with neovascular glaucoma. *Ophthalmology.* 1998;105:232-237.
342. Tolentino MJ, Miller JW, Gragoudas ES, et al. Vascular endothelial growth factor is sufficient to produce iris neovascularization and neovascular glaucoma in a nonhuman primate. *Arch Ophthalmol.* 1996;114:964-970.
343. Klein R, Klein BE, Moss SE, et al. The Wisconsin Epidemiologic Study of Diabetic Retinopathy: III. Prevalence and risk of diabetic retinopathy when age at diagnosis is 30 or more years. *Arch Ophthalmol.* 1984;102:527-532.
344. Kohner EM, Aldington SJ, Stratton IM, et al, for the United Kingdom Prospective Diabetes Study. United Kingdom Prospective Diabetes Study, 30: Diabetic retinopathy at diagnosis of non-insulin-dependent diabetes mellitus and associated risk factors. *Arch Ophthalmol.* 1998;116:297-303.
345. Diabetes Control and Complications Trial Research Group. Progression of retinopathy with intensive versus conventional treatment in the Diabetes Control and Complications Trial. *Ophthalmology.* 1995;102:647-661.
345a. Progression of retinopathy with intensive versus conventional treatment in the Diabetes Control and Complications Trial. Diabetes Control and Complications Trial Research Group. *Ophthalmology.* 1995;102:647-661.
346. Kroc Collaborative Study Group. Blood glucose control and the evolution of diabetic retinopathy and albuminuria: a preliminary multicenter trial. *N Engl J Med.* 1984;311:365-372.
347. Chase HP, Jackson WE, Hoops SL, et al. Glucose control and the renal and retinal complications of insulin-dependent diabetes. *JAMA.* 1989;261:1155-1160.
348. Krolewski AS, Canessa M, Warram JH, et al. Predisposition to hypertension and susceptibility to renal disease in insulin-dependent diabetes mellitus. *N Engl J Med.* 1988;318:140-145.
349. Chew EY, Klein ML, Ferris III FL, et al. Association of elevated serum lipid levels with retinal hard exudate in diabetic retinopathy. Early Treatment Diabetic Retinopathy Study (ETDRS) Report 22. *Arch Ophthalmol.* 1996;114:1079-1084.
350. Aiello LP, Gardner TW, King GL, et al. Diabetic retinopathy: technical review. *Diabetes Care.* 1998;21:143-156.
351. Diabetic Retinopathy Study Research Group. Four risk factors for severe visual loss in diabetic retinopathy. The Third Report from the Diabetic Retinopathy Study. *Arch Ophthalmol.* 1979;97:654-655.
352. The Early Treatment Diabetic Retinopathy Study Research Group. Treatment techniques and clinical guidelines for photocoagulation of diabetic macular edema. Early Treatment Diabetic Retinopathy Study Report No. 2. *Ophthalmology.* 1987;94:761-774.
353. The Early Treatment Diabetic Retinopathy Study Research Group. Photocoagulation for diabetic macular edema: Early Treatment Diabetic Retinopathy Study Report No. 4. *Int Ophthalmol Clin.* 1987;27:265-272.
354. Wilkinson CP, Ferris III FL, Klein RE, et al. Proposed International Clinical Diabetic Retinopathy and Diabetic Macular Edema Disease Severity Scales. *Ophthalmology.* 2003;110:1677-1682.
355. Chew EY. A simplified diabetic retinopathy scale. *Ophthalmology.* 2003;110:1675-1676.
356. Waite JH, Beetham WP. Visual mechanisms in diabetes mellitus: comparative study of 2002 diabetics and 437 nondiabetics for control. *N Engl J Med.* 1935;212:367-379.
357. Zorrilla E, Kozak GP. Ophthalmoplegia in diabetes mellitus. *Ann Intern Med.* 1967;67:968-976.
358. Rush JA, Younge BR. Paralysis of cranial nerves III, IV, and VI: cause and prognosis in 1000 cases. *Arch Ophthalmol.* 1981;99:76-79.
359. Khodadoust AA, Silverstein AM, Kenyon DR, et al. Adhesion of regenerating corneal epithelium: the role of basement membrane. *Am J Ophthalmol.* 1968;65:339-348.
360. Gartner S, Henkind P. Neovascularization of the iris (rubeosis iridis). *Surv Ophthalmol.* 1978;22:291-312.
361. Brown GC, Magargal LE, Schachat A, Shah H. Neovascular glaucoma: etiologic considerations. *Ophthalmology.* 1984;91:315-320.
362. Schwartz JN, Donnelly EH, Klintworth GK. Ocular and orbital phycomycosis. *Surv Ophthalmol.* 1977;22:3-28.
363. Blitzer A, Lawson W, Meyers BR, et al. Patient survival factors in paranasal sinus mucormycosis. *Laryngoscope.* 1980;90:635-648.
364. Wand M, Dueker DK, Aiello LM, et al. Effects of panretinal photocoagulation on rubeosis iridis, angle neovascularization, and neovascular glaucoma. *Am J Ophthalmol.* 1978;86:332-339.
365. Aiello LM, Wand M, Liang G. Neovascular glaucoma and vitreous hemorrhage following cataract surgery in patients with diabetes mellitus. *Ophthalmology.* 1983;90:814-820.
366. Simmons RJ, Dueker DK, Kimbrough RL, et al. Goniophotocoagulation for neovascular glaucoma. *Trans Am Acad Ophthalmol Otolaryngol.* 1977;83:80-89.
367. Mason 3rd JO, Albert Jr MA, Mays A, et al. Regression of neovascularization iris vessels by intravitreal injection of bevacizumab. *Retina.* 2006;26:839-841.
368. Hyndiuk RA, Kazarian EL, Schultz RO, et al. Neurotrophic corneal ulcers in diabetes mellitus. *Arch Ophthalmol.* 1977;95:2193-2196.
369. Klein BE, Klein R, Moss SE. Intraocular pressure in diabetic persons. *Ophthalmology.* 1984;91:1356-1360.
370. Pasquale LR, Kang JH, Manson JE, et al. Prospective study of type 2 diabetes mellitus and risk of primary open-angle glaucoma in women. *Ophthalmology.* 2006;113:1081-1086.
371. Marmor MF. Transient accommodative paralysis and hyperopia in diabetes. *Arch Ophthalmol.* 1973;89:419-421.
372. Klein BE, Klein R, Moss SE. Prevalence of cataracts in a population-based study of persons with diabetes mellitus. *Ophthalmology.* 1985;92:1191-1196.
373. Ederer F, Hiller R, Taylor HR. Senile lens changes and diabetes in two population studies. *Am J Ophthalmol.* 1981;91:381-395.

374. Bursell SE, Baker RS, Weiss JN, et al. Clinical photon correlation spectroscopy evaluation of human diabetic lenses. *Exp Eye Res.* 1989;49:241-258.
375. Klein BE, Klein R, Moss SE. Incidence of cataract surgery in the Wisconsin Epidemiologic Study of Diabetic Retinopathy. *Am J Ophthalmol.* 1995;119:295-300.
376. Klein BE, Klein R, Wang Q, et al. Older-onset diabetes and lens opacities: the Beaver Dam Eye Study. *Ophthalmic Epidemiol.* 1995;2:49-55.
377. Pai RP, Mitchell P, Chow VC, et al. Posttransplant cataract: lessons from kidney-pancreas transplantation [see comments]. *Transplantation.* 2000;69:1108-1114.
378. Dowler JG, Hykin PG, Hamilton AM. Phacoemulsification versus extracapsular cataract extraction in patients with diabetes. *Ophthalmology.* 2000;107:457-462.
379. Borrillo JL, Mittra RA, Dev S, et al. Retinopathy progression and visual outcomes after phacoemulsification in patients with diabetes mellitus. *Trans Am Ophthalmol Soc.* 1999;97:435-445. Am J Ophthalmol 2000;129:832.
380. Funahashi T, Fink AI. The pathology of the bulbar conjunctiva in diabetes mellitus: I. Microaneurysms. *Am J Ophthalmol.* 1963;55:504-511.
381. Tagawa H, McMeel JW, Trempe CL. Role of the vitreous in diabetic retinopathy: II. Active and inactive vitreous changes. *Ophthalmology.* 1986;93:1188-1192.
382. Fleckner RA, Goldstein JH. Mucormycosis. *Br J Ophthalmol.* 1969;53:542-548.
383. Diabetic Retinopathy Study Research Group. Photocoagulation treatment of proliferative diabetic retinopathy: clinical application of Diabetic Retinopathy Study (DRS) findings, DRS Report No. 8. *Ophthalmology.* 1981;88:583-600.
384. Diabetic Retinopathy Vitrectomy Study Group. Two-year course of visual acuity in severe proliferative diabetic retinopathy with conventional management. Diabetic Retinopathy Vitrectomy Study (DRVS) Report No. 1. *Ophthalmology.* 1985;92:492-502.
385. Diabetes Control and Complications Trial Research Group. The effect of intensive diabetes treatment on the progression of diabetic retinopathy in insulin-dependent diabetes mellitus: the Diabetes Control and Complications Trial. *Arch Ophthalmol.* 1995;113:36-51.
385. Klein R, Klein BE, Moss SE, et al. The Wisconsin Epidemiologic Study of Diabetic Retinopathy: VI. Retinal photocoagulation. *Ophthalmology.* 1987;94:747-753.
386. Witkin SR, Klein R. Ophthalmologic care for persons with diabetes. *JAMA.* 1984;251:2534-2537.
387. American Academy of Ophthalmology. Comprehensive Adult Medical Eye Evaluation: Preferred Practice Pattern, 2005. PDF available for download at http://www.aao.org/education/library/ppp/camee.cfm (accessed March 21, 2007).
388. American Optometric Association. Comprehensive Adult Eye and Vision Examination: Optometric Clinical Practice Guideline, 2005. PDF available at http://www.aoa.org/documents/CPG-1.pdf (accessed December 2010).
389. Klein R, Klein BE, Neider MW, et al. Diabetic retinopathy as detected using ophthalmoscopy, a nonmydriatic camera, and a standard fundus camera. *Ophthalmology.* 1985;92:485-491.
390. Moss SE, Klein R, Kessler SD, et al. Comparison between ophthalmoscopy and fundus photography in determining severity of diabetic retinopathy. *Ophthalmology.* 1985;92:62-67.
391. Sussman EJ, Tsiaras WG, Soper KA. Diagnosis of diabetic eye disease. *JAMA.* 1982;247:3231-3234.
392. Cavallerano JD, Aiello LP, Cavallerano AA, et al, the Joslin Vision Network Team. Nonmydriatic digital imaging alternative for annual retinal exam in persons with previously documented no or mild diabetic retinopathy. *Am J Ophthalmol.* 2005;140:667-673.
393. Standards of medical care in diabetes—2010. *Diabetes Care.* 2010;33(suppl 1):S11-S61.
394. Klein R, Moss SE, Klein BE. New management concepts for timely diagnosis of diabetic retinopathy treatable by photocoagulation. *Diabetes Care.* 1987;10:633-638.
395. Krolewski AS, Warram JH, Rand LI, et al. Risk of proliferative diabetic retinopathy in juvenile-onset type I diabetes: a 40-year follow-up study. *Diabetes Care.* 1986;9:443-452.
396. Klein BE, Moss SE, Klein R. Is menarche associated with diabetic retinopathy? *Diabetes Care.* 1990;13:1034-1038.
397. Kostraba JN, Klein R, Dorman JS, et al. The epidemiology of diabetes complications study: IV. Correlates of diabetic background and proliferative retinopathy. *Am J Epidemiol.* 1991;133:381-391.
398. Sunness JS. The pregnant woman's eye. *Surv Ophthalmol.* 1988;32:219-238.
399. Klein BE, Moss SE, Klein R. Effect of pregnancy on progression of diabetic retinopathy. *Diabetes Care.* 1990;13:34-40.
400. White P. Diabetes mellitus in pregnancy. *Clin Perinatol.* 1974;1:331-347.
401. Best RM, Chakravarthy U. Diabetic retinopathy in pregnancy. *Br J Ophthalmol.* 1997;81:249-251.
402. Early Treatment Diabetic Retinopathy Study Research Group. Grading diabetic retinopathy from stereoscopic color fundus photographs—an extension of the modified Airlie House classification. ETDRS Report Number 10. *Ophthalmology.* 1991;98(5 suppl):786-806.
403. Diabetic Retinopathy Study Research Group. Indications for photocoagulation treatment of diabetic retinopathy: Diabetic Retinopathy Study Report No. 14. *Int Ophthalmol Clin.* 1987;27:239-253.
404. Diabetic Retinopathy Study Research Group. Photocoagulation treatment of proliferative diabetic retinopathy: the second report of diabetic retinopathy study findings. *Ophthalmology.* 1978;85:82-106.
405. The Early Treatment Diabetic Retinopathy Study Research Group. Photocoagulation for diabetic macular edema. Early Treatment Diabetic Retinopathy Study Report No. 1. *Arch Ophthalmol.* 1985;103:1796-1806.
406. Ferris F. Early photocoagulation in patients with either type 1 or type 2 diabetes. *Trans Am Ophthalmol Soc.* 1996;94:505-537.
407. LaPiana FG, Penner R. Anaphylactoid reaction to intravenously administered fluorescein. *Arch Ophthalmol.* 1968;79:161-162.
408. Krzystolik MG, Strauber SF, Aiello LP, et al. Reproducibility of macular thickness and volume using Zeiss optical coherence tomography in patients with diabetic macular edema. *Ophthalmology.* 2007;114:1520-1525.
409. Browning DJ, Glassman AR, Aiello LP, et al. Relationship between optical coherence tomography-measured central retinal thickness and visual acuity in diabetic macular edema. *Ophthalmology.* 2007;114:525-536.
410. Butner RW, McPherson AR. Adverse reactions in intravenous fluorescein angiography. *Ann Ophthalmol.* 1983;15:1084-1086.
411. Wittpenn JR, Rapoza P, Sternberg P, et al. Respiratory arrest following retrobulbar anesthesia. *Ophthalmology.* 1986;93:867-870.
412. Avery RL. Regression of retinal and iris neovascularization after intravitreal bevacizumab (Avastin) treatment. *Retina.* 2006;26:352-354.
413. Randomized Trial Evaluating Ranibizumab Plus Prompt or Deferred Laser or Triamcinolone Plus Prompt Laser for Diabetic Macular Edema. *Ophthalmology.* 2010;117;1064-1077.
414. Chew E, Strauber S, Beck R, et al. Randomized trial of peribulbar triamcinolone acetonide with and without focal photocoagulation for mild diabetic macular edema: a pilot study. *Ophthalmology.* 2007;114:1190-1196.
415. A randomized trial comparing intravitreal triamcinolone acetonide and focal/grid photocoagulation for diabetic macular edema. *Ophthalmology.* 2008;115:1447-1449.
416. Beck RW, Edwards AR, Aiello LP, et al. Three-year follow-up of a randomized trial comparing focal/grid photocoagulation and intravitreal triamcinolone for diabetic macular edema. *Arch Ophthalmol.* 2009;127:245-251.
417. Klein R, Klein BE, Lee KE, et al. The incidence of hypertension in insulin-dependent diabetes. *Arch Intern Med.* 1996;156:622-627.
418. Thai Multicenter Research Group on Diabetes Mellitus. Vascular complications in non-insulin-dependent diabetics in Thailand. *Diabetes Res Clin Pract.* 1994;25:61-69.
419. Klein R, Klein BE, Moss SE, et al. Blood pressure and hypertension in diabetes. *Am J Epidemiol.* 1985;122:75-89.
420. Fujimoto WY, Leonetti DL, Kinyoun JL, et al. Prevalence of complications among second-generation Japanese-American men with diabetes, impaired glucose tolerance, or normal glucose tolerance. *Diabetes.* 1987;36:730-739.
421. Klein R, Klein BE, Moss SE, et al. The Wisconsin Epidemiologic Study of Diabetic Retinopathy: XVII. The 14-year incidence and progression of diabetic retinopathy and associated risk factors in type 1 diabetes [see comments]. *Ophthalmology.* 1998;105:1801-1815.
422. Zander E, Heinke P, Herfurth S, et al. Relations between diabetic retinopathy and cardiovascular neuropathy: a cross-sectional study in IDDM and NIDDM patients. *Exp Clin Endocrinol Diabetes.* 1997;105:319-326.
423. Diabetes Drafting Group. Prevalence of small vessel and large vessel disease in diabetic patients from 14 centres: the World Health Organization Multinational Study of Vascular Disease in Diabetes. *Diabetologia.* 1985;28:615-640.
424. Agardh CD, Agardh E, Torffvit O. The association between retinopathy, nephropathy, cardiovascular disease, and long-term metabolic control in type 1 diabetes mellitus: a 5-year follow-up study of 442 adult patients in routine care. *Diabetes Res Clin Pract.* 1997;35:113-121.
425. Lopes de Faria JM, Jalkh AE, Trempe CL, et al. Diabetic macular edema: risk factors and concomitants. *Acta Ophthalmol Scand.* 1999;77:170-175.
426. Marshall G, Garg SK, Jackson WE, et al. Factors influencing the onset and progression of diabetic retinopathy in subjects with insulin-dependent diabetes mellitus. *Ophthalmology.* 1993;100:1133-1139.
427. UK Prospective Diabetes Study Group. Tight blood pressure control and risk of macrovascular and microvascular complications in type 2 diabetes: UKPDS 38 [see comments] [published erratum appears in *BMJ* 1999;318:29]. *BMJ.* 1998;317:703-713.
428. Schrier RW, Estacio RO, Jeffers B. Appropriate Blood Pressure Control in NIDDM (ABCD) Trial. *Diabetologia.* 1996;39:1646-1654.

429. Klein R, Klein BE, Moss SE, et al. The Wisconsin Epidemiology Study of Diabetic Retinopathy: V. Proteinuria and retinopathy in a population of diabetic persons diagnosed prior to 30 years of age. In: Friedman EA, L'Esperance Jr FA, eds. *Diabetic Renal-Retinal Syndrome*. 3rd ed. Orlando, Fla: Grune & Stratton; 1986:245-264.
430. Kullberg CE, Arnqvist HJ. Elevated long-term glycated haemoglobin precedes proliferative retinopathy and nephropathy in type 1 (insulin-dependent) diabetic patients. *Diabetologia*. 1993;36:961-965.
431. Klein R, Moss SE, Klein BE. Is gross proteinuria a risk factor for the incidence of proliferative diabetic retinopathy? *Ophthalmology*. 1993;100:1140-1146.
432. Mathiesen ER, Ronn B, Storm B, et al. The natural course of microalbuminuria in insulin-dependent diabetes: a 10-year prospective study. *Diabet Med*. 1995;12:482-487.
433. Park JY, Kim HK, Chung YE, et al. Incidence and determinants of microalbuminuria in Koreans with type 2 diabetes. *Diabetes Care*. 1998;21:530-534.
434. Hasslacher C, Bostedt-Kiesel A, Kempe HP, et al. Effect of metabolic factors and blood pressure on kidney function in proteinuric type 2 (non-insulin-dependent) diabetic patients. *Diabetologia*. 1993;36:1051-1056.
435. Collins VR, Dowse GK, Plehwe WE, et al. High prevalence of diabetic retinopathy and nephropathy in Polynesians of Western Samoa. *Diabetes Care*. 1995;18:1140-1149.
436. Lee ET, Lee VS, Kingsley RM, et al. Diabetic retinopathy in Oklahoma Indians with NIDDM: incidence and risk factors. *Diabetes Care*. 1992;15:1620-1627.
437. Esmatjes E, Castell C, Gonzalez T, et al. Epidemiology of renal involvement in type II diabetics (NIDDM) in Catalonia. The Catalan Diabetic Nephropathy Study Group. *Diabetes Res Clin Pract*. 1996;32:157-163.
438. Savage S, Estacio RO, Jeffers B, et al. Urinary albumin excretion as a predictor of diabetic retinopathy, neuropathy, and cardiovascular disease in NIDDM. *Diabetes Care*. 1996;19:1243-1248.
439. Fujisawa T, Ikegami H, Yamato E, et al. Association of plasma fibrinogen level and blood pressure with diabetic retinopathy, and renal complications associated with proliferative diabetic retinopathy, in type 2 diabetes mellitus. *Diabet Med*. 1999;16:522-526.
440. Cruickshanks KJ, Ritter LL, Klein R, et al. The association of microalbuminuria with diabetic retinopathy. The Wisconsin Epidemiologic Study of Diabetic Retinopathy. *Ophthalmology*. 1993;100:862-867.
441. Roy MS. Diabetic retinopathy in African Americans with type 1 diabetes—the New Jersey 725: II. Risk factors. *Arch Ophthalmol*. 2000;118:105-115.
442. Klein R, Klein BE, Moss SE, et al. Ten-year incidence of gross proteinuria in people with diabetes. *Diabetes*. 1995;44:916-923.
443. Mogensen CE, Chachati A, Christensen CK, et al. Microalbuminuria: an early marker of renal involvement in diabetes. *Uremia Invest*. 1985;9:85-95.
444. Damsgaard EM, Froland A, Jorgensen OD, et al. Prognostic value of urinary albumin excretion rate and other risk factors in elderly diabetic patients and non-diabetic control subjects surviving the first 5 years after assessment. *Diabetologia*. 1993;36:1030-1036.
445. Villarosa IP, Bakris GL. The Appropriate Blood Pressure Control in Diabetes (ABCD) Trial. *J Hum Hypertens*. 1998;12:653-655.
446. Nelson RG, Knowler WC, Pettitt DJ, et al. Incidence and determinants of elevated urinary albumin excretion in Pima Indians with NIDDM. *Diabetes Care*. 1995;18:182-187.
447. Gomes MB, Lucchetti MR, Gazzola H, et al. Microalbuminuria and associated clinical features among Brazilians with insulin-dependent diabetes mellitus. *Diabetes Res Clin Pract*. 1997;35:143-147.
448. The Microalbuminuria Collaborative Study Group. Predictors of the development of microalbuminuria in patients with type 1 diabetes mellitus: a seven-year prospective study [see comments]. *Diabet Med*. 1999;16:918-925.
449. Davis MD, Fisher MR, Gangnon RE, et al. Risk factors for high-risk proliferative diabetic retinopathy and severe visual loss: Early Treatment Diabetic Retinopathy Study Report No. 18. *Invest Ophthalmol Vis Sci*. 1998;39:233-252.
450. Qiao Q, Keinanen-Kiukaanniemi S, Laara E. The relationship between hemoglobin levels and diabetic retinopathy. *J Clin Epidemiol*. 1997;50:153-158.
451. Friedman EA, Brown CD, Berman DH. Erythropoietin in diabetic macular edema and renal insufficiency. *Am J Kidney Dis*. 1995;26:202-208.
452. Gilbertson DT, Liu J, Xue JL, et al. Projecting the number of patients with end-stage renal disease in the United States to the year 2015. *J Am Soc Nephrol*. 2005;16:3736-3741.
453. U.S. Renal Data System. *USRDS 2006 Annual Data Report: Atlas of End-Stage Renal Disease in the United States*. Bethesda, MD: National Institutes of Health, National Institute of Diabetes and Digestive and Kidney Diseases; 2006.
454. Cooper ME, Jandeleit-Dahm K, Thomas MC. Targets to retard the progression of diabetic nephropathy. *Kidney Int*. 2005;68:1439-1445.
455. Atkins RC. The epidemiology of chronic kidney disease. *Kidney Int Suppl*. 2005;94:S14-S18.
456. Muhlhauser I, Sawicki PT, Blank M, et al. Reliability of causes of death in persons with type I diabetes. *Diabetologia*. 2002;45:1490-1497.
457. Groop PH, Thomas MC, Moran JL, et al. The presence and severity of chronic kidney disease predicts all-cause mortality in type 1 diabetes. *Diabetes*. 2009;58:1651-1658.
458. Stephenson JM, Kenny S, Stevens LK, et al. Proteinuria and mortality in diabetes: the WHO Multinational Study of Vascular Disease in Diabetes. *Diabet Med*. 1995;12:149-155.
459. Ismail N, Becker B, Strzelczyk P, et al. Renal disease and hypertension in non-insulin-dependent diabetes mellitus. *Kidney Int*. 1999;55:1-28.
460. Parving HH, Hommel E, Mathiesen E, et al. Prevalence of microalbuminuria, arterial hypertension, retinopathy and neuropathy in patients with insulin dependent diabetes. *Br Med J (Clin Res Ed)*. 1988;296:156-160.
461. Standl E, Stiegler H. Microalbuminuria in a random cohort of recently diagnosed type 2 (non-insulin-dependent) diabetic patients living in the greater Munich area. *Diabetologia*. 1993;36:1017-1020.
462. Schmitz A, Vaeth M, Mogensen CE. Systolic blood pressure relates to the rate of progression of albuminuria in NIDDM. *Diabetologia*. 1994;37:1251-1258.
463. Zimmet P, Alberti KG, Shaw J. Global and societal implications of the diabetes epidemic. *Nature*. 2001;414:782-787.
464. Kimmelsteil P, Wilson C. Intercapillary lesions in the glomeruli in the kidney. *Am J Path*. 1936;12:83-97.
465. Ghavamian M, Gutch CF, Kopp KF, et al. The sad truth about hemodialysis in diabetic nephropathy. *JAMA*. 1972;222:1386-1389.
466. Cooper ME. Pathogenesis, prevention and treatment of diabetic nephropathy. *Lancet*. 1998;352:213-219.
467. Mogensen CE, Christensen CK, Vittinghus E. The stages in diabetic renal disease: with emphasis in the stage of incipient diabetic nephropathy. *Diabetes*. 1983;32:64-78.
468. Cambien F. Application de la théorie de Rehberg a l'étude clinique des affections rénales and du diabète. *Annu Med*. 1934;35:273-299.
469. Allen TJ, Cooper ME, Lan HY. Use of genetic mouse models in the study of diabetic nephropathy. *Curr Diab Rep*. 2004;4:435-440.
470. Thomson SC, Vallon V, Blantz RC. Kidney function in early diabetes: the tubular hypothesis of glomerular filtration. *Am J Physiol Renal Physiol*. 2004;286:F8-F15.
471. Hostetter TH, Troy JL, Brenner BM. Glomerular hemodynamics in experimental diabetes mellitus. *Kidney Int*. 1981;19:410-415.
472. Sharma K, Jin Y, Guo J, et al. Neutralization of TGF-β by anti-TGF-β antibody attenuates kidney hypertrophy and the enhanced extracellular matrix gene expression in STZ-induced diabetic mice. *Diabetes*. 1996;45:522-530.
473. Segev Y, Landau D, Rasch R, et al. Growth hormone receptor antagonism prevents early renal changes in nonobese diabetic mice. *J Am Soc Nephrol*. 1999;10:2374-2381.
474. Thomas MC, Burns WC, Cooper ME. Tubular changes in early diabetic nephropathy. *Adv Chronic Kidney Dis*. 2005;12:177-186.
475. Mogensen CE, Christensen CK. Predicting diabetic nephropathy in insulin-dependent diabetic patients. *N Engl J Med*. 1984;311:89-93.
476. Mauer S, Steffes M, Ellis E, et al. Structural-functional relationships in diabetic nephropathy. *J Clin Invest*. 1984;74:1143-1155.
477. Allen TJ, Cooper ME, Gilbert RG, et al. Serum total renin is increased before microalbuminuria in diabetes (IDDM). *Kidney Int*. 1996;50:902-907.
478. Comper WD, Osicka TM, Clark M, et al. Earlier detection of microalbuminuria in diabetic patients using a new urinary albumin assay. *Kidney Int*. 2004;65:1850-1855.
479. Poulsen PL, Hansen KW, Mogensen CE. Ambulatory blood pressure in the transition from normo- to microalbuminuria: a longitudinal study in IDDM patients. *Diabetes*. 1994;43:1248-1253.
480. Mogensen CE, Keane WF, Bennett PH, et al. Prevention of diabetic renal disease with special reference to microalbuminuria. *Lancet*. 1995;346:1080-1084.
481. Steinke JM, Sinaiko AR, Kramer MS, et al. The early natural history of nephropathy in type 1 diabetes: III. Predictors of 5-year urinary albumin excretion rate patterns in initially normoalbuminuric patients. *Diabetes*. 2005;54:2164-2171.
482. Lurbe E, Redon J, Kesani A, et al. Increase in nocturnal blood pressure and progression to microalbuminuria in type 1 diabetes. *N Engl J Med*. 2002;347:797-805.
483. Perkins BA, Ficociello LH, Silva KH, et al. Regression of microalbuminuria in type 1 diabetes. *N Engl J Med*. 2003;348:2285-2293.
484. Hovind P, Tarnow L, Rossing P, et al. Predictors for the development of microalbuminuria and macroalbuminuria in patients with type 1 diabetes: inception cohort study. *BMJ*. 2004;328:1105.
485. Bilous RW, Mauer SM, Sutherland DE, et al. Mean glomerular volume and rate of development of diabetic nephropathy. *Diabetes*. 1989;38:1142-1147.
486. Parving H-H, Andersen AR, Smidt VM, et al. Diabetic nephropathy and arterial hypertension. *Diabetologia*. 1983;24:10-12.

487. Fioretto P, Steffes MW, Sutherland DE, et al. Reversal of lesions of diabetic nephropathy after pancreas transplantation. *N Engl J Med.* 1998;339:69-75.
488. Vora JP, Leese GP, Peters JR, et al. Longitudinal evaluation of renal function in non-insulin dependent diabetic patients with early nephropathy. *J Diabetes Complications.* 1996;10:88-93.
489. Lane PH, Steffes MW, Mauer SM. Glomerular structure in IDDM women with low glomerular filtration rate and normal urinary albumin excretion. *Diabetes.* 1992;41:581-586.
490. Tsalamandris C, Allen TJ, Gilbert RE, et al. Progressive decline in renal function in diabetic patients with and without albuminuria. *Diabetes.* 1994;43:649-655.
491. American Diabetes Association: standards of medical care in diabetes—2010. *Diabetes Care.* 2010;33(suppl 1):S11-S61.
492. Wiseman MJ, Mangili R, Alberetto M, et al. Glomerular response mechanisms to glycemic changes in insulin-dependent diabetics. *Kidney Int.* 1987;31:1012-1018.
493. Kiritoshi S, Nishikawa T, Sonoda K, et al. Reactive oxygen species from mitochondria induce cyclooxygenase-2 gene expression in human mesangial cells: potential role in diabetic nephropathy. *Diabetes.* 2003;52:2570-2577.
494. Forbes JM, Cooper ME, Oldfield MD, et al. Role of advanced glycation end products in diabetic nephropathy. *J Am Soc Nephrol.* 2003; 14:S254-S258.
495. Tuttle KR, Bakris GL, Toto RD, McGill JB, Hu K, Anderson PW: The effect of ruboxistaurin on nephropathy in type 2 diabetes. *Diabetes Care.* 2005;28:2686-2690.
496. Gorin Y, Block K, Hernandez J, et al. Nox4 NAD(P)H oxidase mediates hypertrophy and fibronectin expression in the diabetic kidney. *J Biol Chem.* 2005;280:39616-39626.
497. Cooper ME. Interaction of metabolic and haemodynamic factors in mediating experimental diabetic nephropathy. *Diabetologia.* 2001;44: 1957-1972.
498. Thomas MC, Tikellis C, Burns WM, et al. Interactions between renin angiotensin system and advanced glycation in the kidney. *J Am Soc Nephrol.* 2005;16:2976-2984.
499. Cooper ME, Mundel P, Boner G. Role of nephrin in renal disease including diabetic nephropathy. *Semin Nephrol.* 2002;22:393-398.
500. Andersen S, Blouch K, Bialek J, et al. Glomerular permselectivity in early stages of overt diabetic nephropathy. *Kidney Int.* 2000;58: 2129-2137.
501. Wassef L, Langham RG, Kelly DJ. Vasoactive renal factors and the progression of diabetic nephropathy. *Curr Pharm Des.* 2004;10: 3373-3384.
502. Gilbert RE, Cooper ME. The tubulointerstitium in progressive diabetic kidney disease: more than an aftermath of glomerular injury? *Kidney Int.* 1999;56:1627-1637.
503. Gilbert RE, Cooper ME, Krum H. Drug administration in patients with diabetes mellitus: safety considerations. *Drug Safety.* 1998;18:441-455.
504. Salifu MO, Haria DM, Badero O, et al. Challenges in the diagnosis and management of renal artery stenosis. *Curr Hypertens Rep.* 2005; 7:219-227.
505. Hricik DE, Browning PJ, Kopelman R, et al. Captopril-induced functional renal insufficiency in patients with bilateral renal-artery stenoses or renal-artery stenosis in a solitary kidney. *N Engl J Med.* 1983; 308:373-376.
506. Griffin MD, Bergstralhn EJ, Larson TS. Renal papillary necrosis: a sixteen-year clinical experience. *J Am Soc Nephrol.* 1995;6:248-256.
507. Davies PJ. Beethoven's nephropathy and death: discussion paper. *J R Soc Med.* 1993;86:159-161.
508. Kelly DJ, Wilkinson-Berka JL, Allen TJ, et al. A new model of diabetic nephropathy with progressive renal impairment in the transgenic (mRen-2)27 rat (tgr). *Kidney Int.* 1998;54:343-352.
509. DeFronzo RA. Hyperkalemia and hyporeninemic hypoaldosteronism. *Kidney Int.* 1980;17:118-134.
510. Lush DJ, King JA, Fray JC. Pathophysiology of low renin syndromes: sites of renal renin secretory impairment and prorenin overexpression. *Kidney Int.* 1993;43:983-999.
511. Nadler JL, Lee FO, Hsueh W, et al. Evidence of prostacyclin deficiency in the syndrome of hyporeninemic hypoaldosteronism. *N Engl J Med.* 1986;314:1015-1020.
512. Parfrey PS, Griffiths SM, Barrett BJ, et al. Contrast material-induced renal failure in patients with diabetes mellitus, renal insufficiency, or both: a prospective controlled study. *N Engl J Med.* 1989;320:143-149.
513. Weisberg LS, Kurnik PB, Kurnik BR. Risk of radiocontrast nephropathy in patients with and without diabetes mellitus. *Kidney Int.* 1994;45:259-265.
514. Tepel M, van der Giet M, Schwarzfeld C, et al. Prevention of radiographic-contrast-agent-induced reductions in renal function by acetylcysteine. *N Engl J Med.* 2000;343:180-184.
515. Mogensen CE. Long-term antihypertensive treatment inhibiting progression of diabetic nephropathy. *BMJ.* 1982;285:685-688.
516. Parving H-H, Andersen AR, Smidt VM, et al. Effect of antihypertensive treatment on kidney function in diabetic nephropathy. *Br Med J.* 1987;294:1443-1447.
517. Björck S. Clinical trials in overt diabetic nephropathy. In: Mogensen CE, ed. *The Kidney and Hypertension in Diabetes Mellitus.* 3rd ed. London: Kluwer Academic; 1996:375-384.
518. U. K. Prospective Diabetes Study (UKPDS) Group. Intensive blood-glucose control with sulphonylureas or insulin compared with conventional treatment and risk of complications in patients with type 2 diabetes (UKPDS 33). *Lancet.* 1998;352:837-853.
519. Patel A, MacMahon S, Chalmers J, et al. Intensive blood glucose control and vascular outcomes in patients with type 2 diabetes. *N Engl J Med.* 2008;358:2560-2572.
520. Gerstein HC, Miller ME, Byington RP, et al. Effects of intensive glucose lowering in type 2 diabetes. *N Engl J Med.* 2008;358:2545-2559.
521. Parving HH. Renoprotection in diabetes: genetic and non-genetic risk factors and treatment. *Diabetologia.* 1998;41:745-759.
522. Babaei-Jadidi R, Karachalias N, Ahmed N, et al. Prevention of incipient diabetic nephropathy by high-dose thiamine and benfotiamine. *Diabetes.* 2003;52:2110-2120.
523. Thallas-Bonke V, Lindschau C, Rizkalla B, et al. Attenuation of extracellular matrix accumulation in diabetic nephropathy by the advanced glycation end product cross-link breaker ALT-711 via a protein kinase C-alpha-dependent pathway. *Diabetes.* 2004;53:2921-2930.
524. UK Prospective Diabetes Study (UKPDS) Group. Tight blood pressure control and risk of macrovascular and microvascular complications in type 2 diabetes: UKPDS 38. *BMJ.* 1998;317:703-713.
525. Chobanian AV, Bakris GL, Black HR, et al. Seventh report of the Joint National Committee on Prevention, Detection, Evaluation, and Treatment of High Blood Pressure. *Hypertension.* 2003;42:1206-1252.
526. de Galan BE, Perkovic V, Ninomiya T, et al. Lowering blood pressure reduces renal events in type 2 diabetes. *J Am Soc Nephrol.* 2009;20:883-892.
527. Strippoli G, Craig M, Craig J. Antihypertensive agents for preventing diabetic kidney disease. Cochrane Database Syst Rev 2005;4:CD004136.
528. The ACE Inhibitors in Diabetic Nephropathy Trialist Group. Should all patients with type 1 diabetes mellitus and microalbuminuria receive angiotensin-converting enzyme inhibitors? A meta-analysis of individual patient data. *Ann Intern Med.* 2001;134:370-379.
529. The EUCLID Study Group. Randomised placebo-controlled trial of lisinopril in normotensive patients with insulin-dependent diabetes and normoalbuminuria or microalbuminuria. *Lancet.* 1997;349: 1787-1792.
530. Kvetny J, Gregersen G, Pedersen RS. Randomized placebo-controlled trial of perindopril in normotensive, normoalbuminuric patients with type 1 diabetes mellitus. *QJM.* 2001;94:89-94.
531. Mauer M, Zinman B, Gardiner R, et al. Renal and retinal effects of enalapril and losartan in type 1 diabetes. *N Engl J Med.* 2009;361:40-51.
532. Hommel E, Parving HH, Mathiesen E, et al. Effect of captopril on kidney function in insulin-dependent diabetic patients with nephropathy. *Br Med J.* 1986;293:467-470.
533. Brenner BM, Cooper ME, de Zeeuw D, et al. Effects of losartan on renal and cardiovascular outcomes in patients with type 2 diabetes and nephropathy. *N Engl J Med.* 2001;345:861-869.
534. Lewis EJ, Hunsicker LG, Clarke WR, et al. Renoprotective effect of the angiotensin-receptor antagonist irbesartan in patients with nephropathy due to type 2 diabetes. *N Engl J Med.* 2001;345:851-860.
535. Arauz-Pacheco C, Parrott MA, Raskin P. Treatment of hypertension in adults with diabetes. *Diabetes Care.* 2003;26(suppl 1):S80-S82.
536. Barnett AH, Bain SC, Bouter P, et al. Angiotensin-receptor blockade versus converting-enzyme inhibition in type 2 diabetes and nephropathy. *N Engl J Med.* 2004;351:1952-1961.
537. Mann JF, Schmieder RE, McQueen M, et al. Renal outcomes with telmisartan, ramipril, or both, in people at high vascular risk (the ONTARGET study): a multicentre, randomised, double-blind, controlled trial. *Lancet.* 2008;372:547-553.
538. Parving HH, Lehnert H, Brochner-Mortensen J, et al. The effect of irbesartan on the development of diabetic nephropathy in patients with type 2 diabetes. *N Engl J Med.* 2001;345:870-878.
539. Parving HH, Persson F, Lewis JB, et al. Aliskiren combined with losartan in type 2 diabetes and nephropathy. *N Engl J Med.* 2008;358:2433-2446.
540. Schjoedt KJ, Rossing K, Juhl TR, et al. Beneficial impact of spironolactone in diabetic nephropathy. *Kidney Int.* 2005;68:2829-2836.
541. Epstein M. Aldosterone as a mediator of progressive renal disease: pathogenetic and clinical implications. *Am J Kidney Dis.* 2001;37:677-688.
542. Tikkanen I, Tikkanen T, Cao Z, et al. Combined inhibition of neutral endopeptidase with angiotensin converting enzyme or endothelin converting enzyme in experimental diabetes. *J Hypertens.* 2002;20:707-714.
543. Pedrini MT, Levey AS, Lau J, et al. The effect of dietary protein restriction on the progression of diabetic and nondiabetic renal diseases—a meta-analysis. *Ann Int Med.* 1996;124:627-632.
544. Hansen HP, Tauber-Lassen E, Jensen BR, et al. Effect of protein restriction on prognosis in type 1 diabetic patients with diabetic nephropathy. *Kidney Int.* 2002;62:220-228.

545. Waugh NR, Robertson AM. Protein restriction for diabetic renal disease. Cochrane Database Syst Rev 2000;2:CD002181.
546. Jandeleit-Dahm K, Cao ZM, Cox AJ, et al. Role of hyperlipidemia in progressive renal disease: focus on diabetic nephropathy. *Kidney Int.* 1999;56:S31-S36.
547. Fried LF, Forrest KY, Ellis D, et al. Lipid modulation in insulin-dependent diabetes mellitus: effect on microvascular outcomes. *J Diabetes Complications.* 2001;15:113-119.
548. Keech A, Simes RJ, Barter P, et al. Effects of long-term fenofibrate therapy on cardiovascular events in 9795 people with type 2 diabetes mellitus (the FIELD study): randomised controlled trial. *Lancet.* 2005;366:1849-1861.
549. Collins R, Armitage J, Parish S, et al. MRC/BHF Heart Protection Study of cholesterol-lowering with simvastatin in 5963 people with diabetes: a randomised placebo-controlled trial. *Lancet.* 2003;361:2005-2016.
550. Athyros VG, Papageorgiou AA, Elisaf M, et al. Statins and renal function in patients with diabetes mellitus. *Curr Med Res Opin.* 2003;19:615-617.
551. Colhoun HM, Betteridge DJ, Durrington PN, et al. Primary prevention of cardiovascular disease with atorvastatin in type 2 diabetes in the Collaborative Atorvastatin Diabetes Study (CARDS): multicentre randomised placebo-controlled trial. *Lancet.* 2004;364:685-696.
552. Thomas MC, Cooper ME, Tsalamandris C, et al. Anemia with impaired erythropoietin response in diabetic patients. *Arch Intern Med.* 2005;165:466-469.
553. Jungers P, Choukroun G, Oualim Z, et al. Beneficial influence of recombinant human erythropoietin therapy on the rate of progression of chronic renal failure in predialysis patients. *Nephrol Dial Transplant.* 2001;16:307-312.
554. Mix TC, Brenner RM, Cooper ME, et al. Rationale-Trial to Reduce Cardiovascular Events with Aranesp Therapy (TREAT): evolving the management of cardiovascular risk in patients with chronic kidney disease. *Am Heart J.* 2005;149:408-413.
555. Pfeffer MA, Burdmann EA, Chen CY, et al. A trial of darbepoetin alfa in type 2 diabetes and chronic kidney disease. *N Engl J Med.* 2009;361:2019-2032.
556. Tuttle KR, McGill JB, Haney DJ, et al. Kidney outcomes in long-term studies of ruboxistaurin for diabetic eye disease. *Clin J Am Soc Nephrol.* 2007;2:631-636.
557. Achour A, Kacem M, Dibej K, et al. One year course of oral sulodexide in the management of diabetic nephropathy. *J Nephrol.* 2005;18:568-574.
558. Wenzel RR, Littke T, Kuranoff S, et al. Avosentan reduces albumin excretion in diabetics with macroalbuminuria. *J Am Soc Nephrol.* 2009;20:655-664.
559. Jungers P, Zingraff J, Page B, et al. Detrimental effects of late referral in patients with chronic renal failure: a case-control study. *Kidney Int Suppl.* 1993;41:S170-S173.
560. Pirson Y. The diabetic patient with ESRD: how to select the modality of renal replacement. *Nephrol Dial Transplant.* 1996;11:1511-1513.
561. Gaede P, Vedel P, Larsen N, et al. Multifactorial intervention and cardiovascular disease in patients with type 2 diabetes. *N Engl J Med.* 2003;348:383-393.
562. Vinik AI, Mitchell BD, Leichter SB, et al. Epidemiology of the complications of diabetes. In: Leslie RDG, Robbins DC, eds. *Diabetes: Clinical Science in Practice.* Cambridge, UK: Cambridge University Press; 1995:221-287.
563. Vinik A, Mehrabyan A. Diabetic neuropathies. *Med Clin North Am.* 2004;88:947-999.
564. Young MJ, Boulton AJM, MacLeod AF, et al. A multicentre study of the prevalence of diabetic peripheral neuropathy in the United Kingdom hospital clinic population. *Diabetologia.* 1993;36:1-5.
565. Dyck PJ, Kratz KM, Karnes JL, et al. The prevalence by staged severity of various types of diabetic neuropathy, retinopathy, and nephropathy in a population-based cohort: the Rochester Diabetic Neuropathy Study. *Neurology.* 1993;43:817-824.
566. Holzer SE, Camerota A, Martens L, et al. Costs and duration of care for lower extremity ulcers in patients with diabetes. *Clin Ther.* 1998;20:169-181.
567. Caputo GM, Cavanagh PR, Ulbrecht JS, et al. Assessment and management of foot disease in patients with diabetes. *N Engl J Med.* 1994;331:854-860.
568. Pirart J. [Diabetes mellitus and its degenerative complications: a prospective study of 4,400 patients observed between 1947 and 1973 (3rd and last part) (author's transl)]. *Diabetes Metab.* 1977;3:245-256.
569. Vinik A, Ullal J, Parson H, et al. Diabetic neuropathies: clinical manifestations and current treatment options. *Nat Clin Pract Endocrinol Metab.* 2006;2:269-281.
570. Smith A, Ramachandran P, Tripp S, et al. Epidermal nerve innervation in impaired glucose tolderance and diabetes-associated neuropathy. *Neurology.* 2001;57:1701-1704.
571. Pittenger GL, Ray M, Burcus NI, et al. Intraepidermal nerve fibers are indicators of small-fiber neuropathy in both diabetic and nondiabetic patients. *Diabetes Care.* 2004;27:1974-1979.
572. Vinik AI. Diabetic neuropathy, mobility and balance. *Geriatric Times.* 2003;4:13-15.
573. Resnick HE, Stansberry KB, Harris TB, et al. Diabetes, peripheral neuropathy, and old age disability. *Muscle Nerve.* 2002;25:43-50.
574. Vinik A. Diabetic neuropathy: pathogenesis and therapy. *Am J Med.* 1999;107:17S-26S.
575. Herman WH, Kennedy L. Underdiagnosis of peripheral neuropathy in type 2 diabetes. *Diabetes Care.* 2005;28:1480-1481.
576. Armstrong DG, Lavery LA, Harkless LB: Validation of a diabetic wound classification system: the contribution of depth, infection, and ischemia to risk of amputation. *Diabetes Care.* 1998;21:855-859.
577. Vinik EJ, Hayes RP, Oglesby A, et al. The development and validation of the Norfolk QOL-DN, a new measure of patients' perception of the effects of diabetes and diabetic neuropathy. *Diabetes Technol Ther.* 2005;7:497-508.
578. Levitt NS, Stansberry KB, Wychanck S, et al. Natural progression of autonomic neuropathy and autonomic function tests in a cohort of IDDM. *Diabetes Care.* 1996;19:751-754.
579. Rathmann W, Ziegler D, Jahnke M, et al. Mortality in diabetic patients with cardiovascular autonomic neuropathy. *Diabetes Med.* 1993;10:820-824.
580. Maser RE, Mitchell BD, Vinik AI, et al. The association between cardiovascular autonomic neuropathy and mortality in individuals with diabetes: a meta-analysis. *Diabetes Care.* 2003;26:1895-1901.
581. Vinik AI, Maser RE, Mitchell BD, et al. Diabetic autonomic neuropathy. *Diabetes Care.* 2003;26:1553-1579.
582. Vileikyte L, Peyrot M, Bundy C, et al. The development and validation of a neuropathy- and foot ulcer-specific quality of life instrument. *Diabetes Care.* 2003;26:2549-2555.
583. Strotmeyer E, Vinik A. The Health, Aging and Body Composition Study. *J Bone Miner Res.* 2006;21:1803-1810.
584. American Diabetes Association and American Academy of Neurology. Consensus statement: report and recommendations of the San Antonio conference on diabetic neuropathy. *Diabetes Care.* 1988;11:592-597.
585. Polydefkis M, Hauer P, Griffin JW, et al. Skin biopsy as a tool to assess distal small fiber innervation in diabetic neuropathy. *Diabetes Technol Ther.* 2001;3:23-28.
586. Hlubocky A, Wellik K, Ross MA, et al. Skin biopsy for diagnosis of small fiber neuropathy: a critically appraised topic. *Neurologist.* 2010;16:61-63.
587. Devigili G, Tugnoli V, Penza P, et al. The diagnostic criteria for small fibre neuropathy: from symptoms to neuropathology. *Brain.* 2008;131:1912-1925.
588. England JD, Gronseth GS, Franklin G, et al. Evaluation of distal symmetric polyneuropathy: role of autonomic testing, nerve biopsy, and skin biopsy (an evidence-based review). Practice Parameter. Report of the American Academy of Neurology, American Association of Neuromuscular and Electrodiagnostic Medicine, and American Academy of Physical Medicine and Rehabilitation. *Neurology.* 2009;72:177-184.
589. Watkins PJ. Progression of diabetic autonomic neuropathy. *Diabet Med.* 1993;10(suppl 2):77S-78S.
590. DCCT Research Group. The effect of intensive treatment of diabetes on the development and progression of long-term complications in insulin-dependent diabetes mellitus. *N Engl J Med.* 1993;329:977-986.
591. DCCT Research Group. The effect of intensive diabetes therapy on the development and progression of neuropathy. *Ann Intern Med.* 1995;122:561-568.
592. Ziegler D, Cicmir I, Mayer P, et al. Somatic and autonomic nerve function during the first year after diagnosis of type 1 (insulin-dependent) diabetes. *Diabetes Res.* 1988;7:123-127.
593. Partanen J, Niskanen L, Lehtinen J, et al. Natural history of peripheral neuropathy in patients with non-insulin-dependent diabetes mellitus. *N Engl J Med.* 1995;333:89-94.
594. Apfel SC, Kessler JA, Adornato BT, et al, NGF Study Group. Recombinant human nerve growth factor in the treatment of diabetic polyneuropathy. *Neurology.* 1998;51:695-702.
595. Vinik AI. Treatment of diabetic polyneuropathy (DPN) with recombinant human nerve growth factor (rhNGF) (Abstract). *Diabetes.* 1999;48(suppl 1):A54-A55.
596. Dyck PJ, Kratz KM, Lehman KA, et al. The Rochester Diabetic Neuropathy Study: design, criteria for types of neuropathy, selection bias, and reproducibility of neuropathic tests. *Neurology.* 1991;41:799-807.
597. Oh SJ. Clinical electromyelography: nerve conduction studies. In: Oh SJ, ed. *Nerve Conduction in Polyneuropathies.* 2nd ed. Baltimore, MD: Williams & Wilkins; 1993:579-591.
598. Kennedy WR, Wendelschafer-Crabb G, Johnson T. Quantitation of epidermal nerves in diabetic neuropathy. *Neurology.* 1996;47:1042-1048.
599. Herrmann DN, Griffin JW, Hauer P, et al. Epidermal nerve fiber density and sural nerve morphometry in peripheral neuropathies. *Neurology.* 1999;53:1634-1640.
600. Vinik A, Erbas T, Park T, et al. Dermal neurovascular dysfunction in type 2 diabetes. *Diabetes Care.* 2001;24:1468-1475.
601. Smith AG, Russell J, Feldman EL, et al. Lifestyle intervention for prediabetic neuropathy. *Diabetes Care.* 2006;29:1294-1299.

602. Karamitsos DT, Didangelos TP, Athyros VG, et al. The natural history of recently diagnosed autonomic neuropathy over a period of 2 years. *Diabetes Res Clin Pract.* 1998;42:55-63.
603. Ziegler D. Diabetic cardiovascular autonomic neuropathy: prognosis, diagnosis and treatment. *Diabetes Metab Rev.* 1994;10:339-383.
604. Vinik, Maser, Ziegler. Diabetes Care. In press.
605. Boulton AJ, Vinik AI, Arezzo JC, et al. Diabetic neuropathies: a statement by the American Diabetes Association. *Diabetes Care.* 2005;28:956-962.
606. Dyck PJ. Severity and staging of diabetic polyneuropathy. In: Gries FA, Cameron NE, Low PA, et al., eds. *Textbook of Diabetic Neuropathy.* Stuttgart, Germany: Thieme; 2003:170-175.
607. Vinik AI, Holland MT, LeBeau JM, et al. Diabetic neuropathies. *Diabetes Care.* 1992;15:1926-1975.
608. Vinik AI, Suwanwalaikorn S. Autonomic neuropathy. In: DeFronzo RA, ed. *Current Therapy of Diabetes Mellitus.* St. Louis, MO: Mosby; 1997:165-176.
609. Karpitskaya Y, Novak CB, Mackinnon SE. Prevalence of smoking, obesity, diabetes mellitus and thyroid disease in patients with carpal tunnel syndrome. *Am Plast Surg.* 2002;48:269-273.
610. Perkins B, Olaleye D, Bril V. Carpal tunnel syndrome in patients with diabetic polyneuropathy. *Diabetes Care.* 2002;25:565-569.
611. Chaudhuri KR, Davidson AR, Morris IM. Limited joint mobility and carpal tunnel syndrome in insulin dependent diabetes. *Br J Rheumatol.* 1989;28:191-194.
612. Wilbourn AJ. Diabetic entrapment and compression neuropathies. In: Dyck PJ, Thomas PK, eds. *Diabetic Neuropathy.* Philadelphia, PA: Saunders, 1999;481-508.
613. Dawson DM. Entrapment neuropathies of the upper extremities. *N Engl J Med.* 1993;329:2013-2018.
614. Vinik A, Mehrabyan A, Colen L, et al. Focal entrapment neuropathies in diabetes. *Diabetes Care.* 2004;27:1783-1788.
615. Sima AAF, Sugimoto K. Experimental diabetic neuropathy: an update. *Diabetologia.* 1999;42:773-788.
616. Vinik AI, Pittenger GL, Milicevic Z, et al. Autoimmune mechanisms in the pathogenesis of diabetic neuropathy. In: Eisenbarth RG, ed. *Molecular Mechanisms of Endocrine and Organ Specific Autoimmunity.* Georgetown, TX: Landes; 1998:217-251.
617. Steck AJ, Kappos L. Gangliosides and autoimmune neuropathies: classification and clinical aspects of autoimmune neuropathies. *J Neurol Neurosurg Psychiatry.* 1994;57(suppl):26-28.
618. Bourcier and Vinik.
619. Sander HW, Chokroverty S. Diabetic amyotrophy: current concepts. *Semin Neurol.* 1996;16:173-178.
620. Said G, Goulon-Goreau C, Lacroix C, et al. Nerve biopsy findings in different patterns of proximal diabetic neuropathy. *Ann Neurol.* 1994;35:559-569.
621. Krendel DA, Costigan DA, Hopkins LC. Successful treatment of neuropathies in patients with diabetes mellitus. *Arch Neurol.* 1995;52: 1053-1061.
622. Britland ST, Young RJ, Sharma AK, et al. Acute and remitting painful diabetic polyneuropathy: a comparison of peripheral nerve fibre pathology. *Pain.* 1992;48:361-370.
623. Stewart JD, McKelvey R, Durcan L, et al. Chronic inflammatory demyelinating polyneuropathy (CIDP). *J Neurol Sci.* 1996;142:59-64.
624. Sharma K, Cross J, Ayyar D, et al. Diabetic demyelinating polyneuropathy responsive to intravenous immunoglobulin therapy. *Arch Neurol.* 2002;59:751-757.
625. Witzke K, Vinik A. Diabetic neuropathy in older adults (Abstract). *Rev Endocr Metab Disord.* 2005;6:117-127.
626. Resnick HE, Vinik AI, Schwartz AV, et al. Independent effects of peripheral nerve dysfunction on lower-extremity physical function in old age: the Women's Health and Aging Study. *Diabetes Care.* 2000;23: 1642-1647.
627. Witzke KA, Vinik AI. Diabetic neuropathy in older adults. *Rev Endocrin Metab Disord.* 2005;6:117-127.
628. Milicevic Z, Newlon PG, Pittenger GL, et al. Anti-ganglioside GM1 antibody and distal symmetric "diabetic polyneuropathy" with dominant motor features. *Diabetologia.* 1997;40:1364-1365.
629. Griffin JW, McArthur JC, Polydefkis M. Assessment of cutaneous innervation by skin biopsies. *Curr Opin Neurol.* 2001;14:655-659.
630. Barada A, Reljanovic M, Milicevic Z, et al. Proximal diabetic neuropathy-response to immunotherapy (Abstract). *Diabetes.* 1999;48(suppl 1):A148.
631. Bird SJ, Brown MJ. The clinical spectrum of diabetic neuropathy. *Semin Neurol.* 1996;16:115-122.
632. Hanson PH, Schumaker P, Debugne TH, et al. Evaluation of somatic and autonomic small fibers neuropathy in diabetes. *Am J Phys Med Rehabil.* 1992;71:44-47.
633. McArthur JC, Stocks EA, Hauer P, et al. Epidermal nerve fiber density: normative reference range and diagnostic efficiency. *Arch Neurol.* 1998;55:1513-1520.
634. Stansberry KB, Hill MA, Shapiro SA, et al. Impairment of peripheral blood flow responses in diabetes resembles an enhanced aging effect. *Diabetes Care.* 1997;20:1711-1716.
635. Hirai A, Yasuda H, Joko M, et al. Evaluation of diabetic neuropathy through the quantitation of cutaneous nerves. *J Neurol Sci.* 2000;172:55-62.
636. Polydefkis M, Hauer P, Griffin JW, et al. Skin biopsy as a tool to assess distal small fiber innervation in diabetic neuropathy. *Diabetes Technol Ther.* 2001;3:23-28.
637. Dalsgaard CJ, Rydh M, Haegerstrand A. Cutaneous innervation in man visualized with protein gene product 9.5 (PGP 9.5) antibodies. *Histochemistry.* 1989;92:385-390.
638. McCarthy BG, Hsieh ST, Stocks A, et al. Cutaneous innervation in sensory neuropathies: evaluation by skin biopsy. *Neurology.* 1995;45:1848-1855.
639. Low P, Dotson R. Symptom treatment of painful neuropathy. *JAMA.* 1998;280:1863-1864.
640. Vinik AI, Park TS, Stansberry KB, et al. Diabetic neuropathies. *Diabetologia.* 2000;43:957-973.
641. Backonja M. Anticonvulsants (antineuropathics) for neuropathic pain syndromes. *Clin J Pain.* 2000;16(2 suppl):S67-S72.
642. Tesfaye S, Malik R, Harris N, et al. Arterio-venous shunting and proliferating new vessels in acute painful neuropathy of rapid glycaemic control (insulin neuritis). *Diabetologia.* 1996;39:329-335.
643. Van Heel DA, Levitt NS, Winter TA. Diabetic neuropathic cachexia: the importance of positive recognition and early nutritional support. *Int J Clin Pract.* 1998;52:591-592.
644. Holland NR, Crawford TO, Hauer P, et al. Small-fiber sensory neuropathies: clinical course and neuropathology of idiopathic cases. *Ann Neurol.* 1998;44:47-59.
645. Dyck PJ. Detection, characterization and staging of polyneuropathy: assessed in diabetes. *Muscle Nerve.* 1988;11:21-32.
646. Vinik AI, Mitchell B. Clinical aspects of diabetic neuropathies. *Diabetes Metab Rev.* 1988;4:223-253.
647. Ziegler D, Hanefeld M, Ruhnau KJ, et al. Treatment of symptomatic diabetic peripheral neuropathy with the anti-oxidant alpha-lipoic acid: a 3-week multicentre randomized controlled trial (ALADIN study). *Diabetologia.* 1995;38:1425-1433.
648. Feldman EL, Stevens MJ, Thomas PK, et al. A practical two-step quantitative clinical and electrophysiological assessment for the diagnosis and staging of diabetic neuropathy. *Diabetes Care.* 1994;17: 1281-1289.
649. Vinik AI, Newlon P, Milicevic Z, et al. Diabetic neuropathies: an overview of clinical aspects. In: LeRoith D, Taylor SI, Olefsky JM, eds. *Diabetes Mellitus: A Fundamental and Clinical Text.* Philadelphia, PA: Lippincot-Raven; 1996:737-751.
650. Vinik A, Mehrabyan A, Colen L, et al. Focal entrapment neuropathies in diabetes. *Diabetes Care.* 2004;27:1783-1788.
651. Cabezas-Cerrato J. The prevalence of diabetic neuropathy in Spain: a study in primary care and hospital clinic groups. *Diabeteologia.* 1998;41:1263-1269.
652. Bril V. NIS-LL: the primary measurement scale for clinical trial endpoints in diabetic peripheral neuropathy. *Eur Neurol.* 1999;41(suppl 1):8-13:8-13.
653. Hermenegildo C, Felipo V, Minana MD, et al. Sustained recovery of Na^+-K^+-ATPase activity in sciatic nerve of diabetic mice by administration of H7 or calphostin C, inhibitors of PKC. *Diabetes.* 1993;42:257-262.
654. Cameron NE, Cotter MA, Basso M, et al. Comparison of the effects of inhibitors of aldose reductase and sorbitol dehydrogenase on neurovascular function, nerve conduction and tissue polyol pathway metabolites in streptozotocin-diabetic rats. *Diabetologia.* 1997;40:271-281.
655. Franse LV, Valk GD, Dekker JH, et al. Numbness of the feet is a poor indicator for polyneuropathy in type 2 diabetic patients. *Diabetes Care.* 2000;17:105-110.
656. Apfel SC, Asbury A, Bril V, et al. Positive neuropathic sensory symptoms as endpoints in diabetic neuropathy trials (Abstract). *J Neurol Sci.* 2001;189:3-5.
657. Shy ME, Frohman EM, So YT, et al, Subcommittee of the American Academy of Neurology. Quantitative sensory testing. *Neurology.* 2003;602:898-906.
658. Gerr F, Letz R. Covariates of human peripheral function: vibrotactile and thermal thresholds. *Neurotoxicol Teratol.* 1994;16:102-112.
659. Gelber DA, Pfeifer MA, Broadstone VL, et al. Components of variance for vibratory and thermal threshold testing in normal and diabetic subjects. *J Diabetes Complications.* 1995;9:170-176.
660. Dyck PJ, Dyck PJ, Larson TS, et al. Patterns of quantitative sensation testing of hypoesthesia and hyperalgesia are predictive of diabetic polyneuropathy: a study of three cohorts. Nerve Growth Factor Study Group. *Diabetes Care.* 2000;23:510-517.
661. Maser RE, Nielsen VK, Bass EB, et al. Measuring diabetic neuropathy: assessment and comparison of clinical examination and quantitative sensory testing. *Diabetes Care.* 1989;12:270-275.
662. Vinik AI, Suwanwalaikorn S, Stansberry KB, et al. Quantitative measurement of cutaneous perception in diabetic neuropathy. *Muscle Nerve.* 1995;18:574-584.
663. Valk GD, de Sonnaville JJ, van Houtum WH, et al. The assessment of diabetic polyneuropathy in daily clinical practice: reproducibility and

validity of Semmes-Weinstein monofilaments examination and clinical neurological examination. *Muscle Nerve*. 1997;20:116-118.
664. Mayfield JA, Sugarman JR. The use of Semmes-Weinstein monofilament and other threshold tests for preventing foot ulceration and amputation in people with diabetes. *J Fam Pract*. 2000;49(suppl): 517-529.
665. Bourcier ME, Ullal J, Parson HK, et al. Diabetic peripheral neuropathy: how reliable is a homemade 1-g monofilament for screening? *J Fam Pract*. 2006;55:505-508.
666. Kumar S, Fernando DJ, Veves A, et al. Semmes-Weinstein monofilaments: a simple, effective and inexpensive screening device for identifying diabetic patients at risk of foot ulceration. *Diabetes Res Clin Pract*. 1991;13:63-67.
667. Armstrong D, Lavery L, Vela S, et al. Choosing a practical screening instrument to identify patients at risk for diabetic foot ulceration. *Arch Intern Med*. 1998;158:289-292.
668. Booth J, Young MJ. Differences in the performance of commercially available 10-g monofilaments. *Diabetes Care*. 2000;23:984-988.
669. Liniger C, Albeanu A, Bloise D, et al. The tuning fork revisited. *Diabetic Med*. 1990;7:859-864.
670. Shin JB, Seong YJ, Lee HJ, et al. Foot screening technique in diabetic populations. *J Korean Med Sci*. 2000;15:78-82.
671. Katoulis EC, Ebdon-Parry M, Lanshammar H, et al. Gait abnormalities in diabetic neuropathy. *Diabetes Care*. 1997;20:1904-1907.
672. Vileikyte L, Hutchings G, Hollis S, et al. The tactile circuimferential discriminator: a new simple screening device to identify diabetic patients at risk of foot ulceration. *Diabetes Care*. 1997;20:623-626.
673. Paisley AN, Abbott CA, van Schie CHM, et al. A comparison of the Neuropen against standard quantitative sensory threshold measures for assessing peripheral nerve function. *Diabetic Med*. 2002;19: 400-405.
674. Malik 2010.
675. Zambreanu L, Wise RG, Brooks JC, et al. A role for the brainstem in central sensitisation in humans: evidence from functional magnetic resonance imaging. *Pain*. 2005;114:397-407.
676. Ducher M, Thivolet C, Cerutti C, et al. Noninvasive exploration of cardiac autonomic neuropathy. *Diabetes Care*. 1999;22:388-393.
677. Reference deleted in proofs.
678. Jaradeh SS, Prieto TE, Lobeck LJ. Progressive polyradiculoneuropathy in diabetes: correlation of variables and clinical outcome after immunotherapy. *J Neurol Neurosurg Psychiatry*. 1999;67:607-612.
679. Periquet MI, Novak V, Collins MP, et al. Painful sensory neuropathy: prospective evaluation using skin biopsy. *Neurology*. 1999;53: 1641-1647.
680. Krendel DA, Zacharias A, Younger DS. Autoimmune diabetic neuropathy. *Neurol Clin*. 1997;15:959-971.
681. Singleton J, Smith AG, Bromberg MB. Painful sensory polyneuropathy associated with impaired glucose tolerance. *Muscle Nerve*. 2001;24:1225-1228.
682. Sumner C, Sheth S, Griffin J, et al. The spectrum of neuropathy in diabetes and impaired glucose tolerance. *Neurology*. 2003;60:108-111.
683. Mehrabyan A, Pittenger G, Burcus N, et al. Polyneuropathy in patients with dysmetabolic syndrome and newly diagnosed. *Diabetes*. 2004;53(suppl 2):A510.
684. Vinik A, Pittenger G, Anderson A, et al. Topiramate improves C-fiber neuropathy and features of the dysmetabolic syndrome in type 2 diabetes. *Diabetes*. 2003;52(suppl 1):A130.
685. Quattrini C, Jeziorska M, Malik RA. Small fiber neuropathy in diabetes: clinical consequence and assessment. *Int J Low Extrem Wounds*. 2004;3:16-21.
686. Arezzo JC. The use of electrophysiology for the assessment of diabetic neuropathy. *Neurosci Res Comm*. 1997;21:13-22.
687. Suez D. Intravenous immunoglobulin therapy: indication, potential side effects and treatment guidelines. *J Intraven Nurs*. 1995;18: 178-190.
688. Vinik AI, Anandacoomaraswamy D, Ullal J. Antibodies to neuronal structures: innocent bystanders or neurotoxins? *Diabetes Care*. 2005;28:2067-2072.
689. Arezzo JC, Zotova E. Electrophysiologic measures of diabetic neuropathy: mechanism and meaning. *Intern Rev Neurobiol*. 2002;50:229-255.
690. Sharma K, Cross J, Farronay O, et al. Demyelinating neuropathy in diabetes mellitus. *Arch Neurol*. 2002;59:758-765.
691. Amthor KF, Dahl-Jorgensen K, Berg TJ, et al. The effect of 8 years of strict glycaemic control on peripheral nerve function in IDDM patients: the Oslo Study. *Diabetologia*. 1994;37:579-584.
692. Veves A, Malik RA, Lye RH, et al. The relationship between sural nerve morphometric findings and measures of peripheral nerve function in mild diabetic neuropathy. *Diabet Med*. 1991;8:917-921.
693. UK Prospective Diabetes Study (UKPDS) Group. Effect of intensive blood-glucose control with metformin on complications in overweight patients with type 2 diabetes (UKPDS 34). *Lancet*. 1998; 352:854-865.
694. Gaede P, Vedel P, Parving HH, et al. Intensified multifactorial intervention in patients with type 2 diabetes mellitus and microalbuminuria: the Steno type 2 randomised study. *Lancet*. 1999;353:617-622.
695. Boulton AJM, Levin S, Comstock J. A multicentre trial of the aldose reductase inhibitor, tolrestat, in patients with symptomatic diabetic neuropathy. *Diabetologia*. 1990;33:431-437.
696. Didangelos TP, Karamitsos DT, Athyros VG, et al. Effect of aldose reductase inhibition on cardiovascular reflex tests in patients with definite diabetic autonomic neuropathy. *J Diabetes Complications*. 1998;12:201-207.
697. Johnson BF, Law G, Nesto R, et al. Aldose reductase inhibitor zopolrestat improves systolic function in diabetics (Abstract). *Diabetes*. 1999;48(suppl 1):A133.
698. Hotta, N, Toyota, T, Matsuoka, K, et al, the SNK-860 Diabetic Neuropathy Study Group. Clinical efficacy of fidarestat, a novel aldose reductase inhibitor, for diabetic peripheral neuropathy. *Diabetes Care*. 2001;24:1776-1782.
699. Hotta N, Akanuma Y, Kawamori R, et al. Long-term clinical effects of epalrestat, an aldose reductase inhibitor, on diabetic peripheral neuropathy: the 3-year, multicenter, comparative Aldose Reductase Inhibitor-Diabetes Complications Trial. *Diabetes Care*. 2006;29: 1538-1544.
700. Bril V, Buchanan RA. Aldose reductase inhibition by AS-3201 in sural nerve from patients with diabetic sensorimotor polyneuropathy. *Diabetes Care*. 2004;27:2369-2375.
701. Ziegler D, Schatz H, Conrad F, et al. Effects of treatment with the antioxidant alpha-lipoic acid on cardiac autonomic neuropathy in NIDDM patients: a 4-month randomized controlled multicenter trial (DEKAN Study). Deutsche Kardiale Autonome Neuropathie. *Diabetes Care*. 1997;20:369-373.
702. Ziegler D, Gries FA. Alpha-lipoic acid in the treatment of diabetic peripheral and cardiac autonomic neuropathy. *Diabetes*. 1997;46(suppl 2):S62-S66.
703. Ziegler D, Hanefeld M, Ruhnau KJ, et al. Treatment of symptomatic diabetic polyneuropathy with the antioxidant alpha-lipoic acid: a 7-month multicenter randomized controlled trial (ALADIN III study). ALADIN III Study Group. Alpha-Lipoic Acid in Diabetic Neuropathy. *Diabetes Care*. 1999;22:1296-1301.
704. Jamal GA. The use of gamma linolenic acid in the prevention and treatment of diabetic neuropathy. *Diabet Med*. 1994;11:145-149.
705. Keen H, Payan J, Allawi J, et al. Treatment of diabetic neuropathy with γ-linolenic acid. *Diabetes Care*. 1993;16:8-15.
706. Dyck PJ. Hypoxic neuropathy: does hypoxia play a role in diabetic neuropathy? The 1988 Robert Wartenberg lecture. *Neurology*. 1989;39:111-118.
707. Kles KA, Vinik AI. Pathophysiology and treatment of diabetic peripheral neuropathy: the case for diabetic neurovascular function as an essential component. *Curr Diabetes Rev*. 2006;2:131-145.
708. Hermenegildo C, Felipo V, Minana MD, et al. Inhibition of protein kinase C restores Na^+,K^+-ATPase activity in sciatic nerve of diabetic mice. *J Neurochem*. 1992;58:1246-1249.
709. Nakamura J, Koh N, Hamada Y, et al. Effect of a protein kinase C-β specific inhibitor on diabetic neuropathy in rats. *Diabetes*. 1998;47(suppl 1):A70.
710. Granberg V, Ejskjaer N, Peakman M, et al. Autoantibodies to autonomic nerves associated with cardiac and peripheral autonomic neuropathy. *Diabetes Care*. 2005;28:1959-1964.
711. Vinik A, Bril V, Kempler P, et al, the MBBQ Study. Treatment of symptomatic diabetic peripheral neuropathy with protein kinase Cβ inhibitor ruboxistaurin mesylate during a 1-year randomized, placebo-controlled, double-blind clinical trial. *Clin Ther*. 2005;27:1164s-1180s.
712. Miyauchi Y, Shikama H, Takasu T, et al. Slowing of peripheral motor nerve conduction was ameliorated by aminoguanidine in streptozocin-induced diabetic rats. *Eur J Endocrinol*. 1996;134:467-473.
713. Schmidt RE, Dorsey DA, Beaudet LN, et al. Effect of aminoguanidine on the frequency of neuroaxonal dystrophy in the superior mesenteric sympathetic autonomic ganglia of rats with streptozotocin-induced diabetes. *Diabetes*. 1996;45:284-290.
714. Nargi SE, Colen LB, Liuzzi F, et al. PTB treatment restores joint mobility in a new model of diabetic cheirothropathy (Abstract). *Diabetes*. 1999;48(suppl 1):A17.
715. Diemel LT, Stevens JC, Willars GB, et al. Depletion of substance P and calcitonin gene-related peptide in sciatic nerve of rats with experimental diabetes: effects of insulin and aldose reductase inhibition. *Neurosci Lett*. 1992;137:253-256.
716. Anadacoowarsamy, Vinik, and Ullal.
717. Hellweg R, Wohrle M, Hartung HD. Diabetes mellitus associated decrease in nerve growth factor levels is reversed by allogenetic pancreatic islet transplantation. *Neurosci Lett*. 1991;125:1-4.
718. Tomlinson DR, Fernyhough P, Diemel LT. Neurotrophins and peripheral neuropathy. *Philos Trans R Soc Lond B Biol Sci*. 1996;351:455-462.
719. Apfel SC, Kessler JA. Neurotropic factors in the therapy of peripheral neuropathy. *Bailliere Clin Neuropathy*. 1995;4:593-606.
720. Apfel SC, Schwartz S, Adornato B, et al. Efficacy and safety of recombinant human nerve growth factor in patients with diabetic polyneuropathy. *JAMA*. 2000;284:2215-2221.
721. Wellmer A, Misra V, Sharief M, et al. A double-blind placebo-controlled clinical trial of recombinant human brain-derived neurotrophic factor

(rhBDNF) in diabetic polyneuropathy. *J Peripheral Nerv Syst.* 2001;6: 204-210.
722. Wahren J, Ekberg K, Samnegard B, et al. C-peptide: a new potential in the treatment of diabetic nephropathy. *Curr Diab Rep.* 2001; 1:261-266.
723. Sindrup SH, Jensen TS. Efficacy of pharmacological treatments of neuropathic pain: an update and effect related to mechanism of drug action. *Pain.* 1999;83:389-400.
724. Rosenstock J, Tuchman M, LaMoreaux L, et al. Pregabalin for the treatment of painful diabetic peripheral neuropathy: a double-blind, placebo-controlled trial. *Pain.* 2004;110:628-638.
725. Goldstein DJ, Lu Y, Detke MJ, et al. Duloxetine vs. placebo in patients with painful diabetic neuropathy. *Pain.* 2005;116:109-118.
726. Rains C, Bryson HM. Topical capsaicin: a review of its pharmacological properties and therapeutic potential in post-herpetic neuralgia, diabetic neuropathy and osteoarthritis. *Drugs Aging.* 1995;7:317-328.
727. Bays-Smith MG, Max MB, Muir J, et al. Transdermal clonidine compared to placebo in painful diabetic neuropathy using a two-stage "enriched enrollment" design. *Pain.* 1995;60:267-274.
728. Said G, Bigo A, Ameri A, et al. Uncommon early-onset neuropathy in diabetic patients. *J Neurol.* 1998;245:61-68.
729. Jarvis B, Coukell AJ. Mexiletine: a review of its therapeutic use in painful diabetic neuropathy. *Drugs.* 1998;56:691-707.
730. Harati Y, Gooch C, Swenson M, et al. Double-blind randomized trial of tramadol for the treatment of the pain of diabetic neuropathy. *Neurology.* 1998;50:1842-1846.
731. Harati Y, Gooch C, Swenson M, et al. Maintenance of the long-term effectiveness of tramadol in treatment of the pain of diabetic neuropathy. *J Diabetes Complications.* 2000;14:65-70.
732. Nelson KA, Park KM, Robinovitz E, et al. High-dose oral dextromethorphan versus placebo in painful diabetic neuropathy and postherpetic neuralgia. *Neurology.* 1997;48:1212-1218.
733. Max M, Lynch S, Muir J: Effects of desipramine, amitryptiline and fluoxetine on pain in diabetic neuropathy. *N Engl J Med.* 1992;326: 1250-1256.
734. Dworkin RH, Backonja M, Rowbotham MC, et al. Advances in neuropathic pain: diagnosis, mechanisms, and treatment recommendations. *Arch Neurol.* 2003;60:1524-1534.
735. McQuay H, Tramer M, Nye B, et al. A systematic review of antidepressants in neuropathic pain. *Pain.* 1996;68:217-227.
736. Joss JD. Tricyclic antidepressant use in diabetic neuropathy. *Ann Pharmacother.* 1999;33:996-1000.
737. Sindrup S, Gram L, Brosen K, et al. The selective serotonin reuptake inhibitor paroxetine is effective in treatment of diabetic neuropathy symptoms. *Pain.* 1990;42:135-144.
738. Kajdasz DK, Iyengar S, Desaiah D, et al. Duloxetine for the management of diabetic peripheral neuropathic pain: evidence-based findings from post hoc analysis of three multicenter, randomized, double-blind, placebo-controlled, parallel-group studies. *Clin Ther.* 2007; 29(suppl):2536-2546.
739. Ziegler D, Pritchett YL, Wang F, et al. Impact of disease characteristics on the efficacy of duloxetine in diabetic peripheral neuropathic pain. *Diabetes Care.* 2007;30:664-669.
740. Rowbotham MC, Goli V, Kunz NR, et al. Venlafaxine extended release in the treatment of painful diabetic neuropathy: a double-blind, placebo-controlled study. *Pain.* 2004;110:697-706.
741. Vinik A. Use of antiepileptic drugs in the treatment of chronic painful diabetic neuropathy. *J Clin Endocrinol Metab.* 2005;90:4936-4945.
742. McQuay H, Carroll D, Jadad AR, et al. Anticonvulsant drugs for management of pain: a systematic review. *BMJ.* 1995;311:1047-1052.
743. Vinik AI. Advances in diabetes for the millennium: new treatments for diabetic neuropathies. *Med Gen Med.* 2004;6(3 suppl):13.
744. LaRoche SM, Helmers SL. The new antiepileptic drugs: scientific review. *JAMA.* 2004;291:605-614.
745. Freeman R, Durso-Decruz E, Emir B. Efficacy, safety, and tolerability of pregabalin treatment for painful diabetic peripheral neuropathy: findings from seven randomized, controlled trials across a range of doses. *Diabetes Care.* 2008;31:1448-1454.
746. Jensen TS. Anticonvulsants in neuropathic pain: rationale and clinical evidence. *Eur J Pain.* 2002;6(suppl A):61-68.
747. Chadda VS, Mathur MS. Double blind study of the effects of diphenylhydantoin sodium on diabetic neuropathy. *J Assoc Physicians India.* 1978;26:403-406.
748. Saudek CD, Werns S, Reidenberg MM. Phenytoin in the treatment of diabetic symmetrical polyneuropathy. *Clin Pharmacol Ther.* 1977; 22:196-199.
749. Otto M, Bach FW, Jensen TS, et al. Valproic acid has no effect on pain in polyneuropathy: a randomized, controlled trial. *Neurology.* 2004; 62:285-288.
750. Gorson KC, Schott C, Herman R, et al. Gabapentin in the treatment of painful diabetic neuropathy: a placebo controlled, double blind, crossover trial. *J Neurol Neurosurg Psychiatry.* 1999;66:251-252.
751. Backonja M, Beydoun A, Edwards KR, et al. Gabapentin for the symptomatic treatment of painful neuropathy in patients with diabetes mellitus. *JAMA.* 1998;280:1831-1836.
752. Vinik A, Fonseca V, LaMoreaux L, et al. Neurontin (gabapentin, GBP) improves quality of life (QOL) in patients with painful diabetic peripheral neuropathy (Abstract). *Diabetes.* 1998;47(suppl 1):A374.
753. Morello CM, Leckband SG, Stoner CP, et al. Randomized double-blind study comparing the efficacy of gabapentin with amitriptyline on diabetic peripheral neuropathy pain. *Arch Intern Med.* 1999;159: 1931-1937.
754. DeToledo JC, Toledo C, DeCerce J, Ramsay RE. Changes in body weight with chronic, high-dose gabapentin therapy. *Ther Drug Monit.* 1997; 19:394-396.
755. Eisenberg E, Lurie Y, Braker C, et al. Lamotrigine reduces painful diabetic neuropathy: a randomized, controlled study. *Neurology.* 2001;57: 505-509.
756. Eisenberg E, Alon N, Ishay A, et al. Lamotrigine in the treatment of painful diabetic neuropathy. *Eur J Neurol.* 1998;5:167-173.
757. Vinik AI, Tuchman M, Safirstein B, et al. Lamotrigine for treatment of pain associated with diabetic neuropathy: results of two randomized, double-blind, placebo-controlled studies. *Pain.* 2007;128:169-179.
758. Raskin P, Donofrio P, Rosenthal N, et al. Topiramate vs placebo in painful diabetic neuropathy: analgesic and metabolic effects. *Neurology.* 2004;63:865-873.
759. Stansberry KB, Shapiro SA, Hill MA, et al. Impaired peripheral vasomotion in diabetes. *Diabetes Care.* 1996;19:715-721.
760. Nelson ME, Fiatarone MA, Morganti CM, et al. Effects of high-intensity strength training on multiple risk factors for osteoporotic fractures: a randomized controlled trial. *JAMA.* 1994;272:1909-1914.
761. Liu-Ambrose T, Khan KM, Eng JJ, et al. Resistance and agility training reduce fall risk in women aged 75 to 85 with low bone mass: a 6-month randomized, controlled trial. *J Am Geriatr Soc.* 2004;52:657-665.
762. Somers DL, Somers MF. Treatment of neuropathic pain in a patient with diabetic neuropathy using transcutaneous electrical nerve stimulation applied to the skin of the lumbar region. *Phys Ther.* 1999;79:767-775.
763. Weintraub M. Preliminary findings: alternative medicine. *Am J Pain Manage.* 1998;8:12-16.
764. Chaudry V, Corse AM, Cornblath DR, et al. Multifocal motor neuropathy: response to human immune globulin. *Ann Neurol.* 1993;33: 237-242.
765. Zieleniewski W. Calcitonin nasal spray for painful diabetic neuropathy. *Lancet.* 1990;336:449.
766. Cavanagh PR, Derr JA, Ulbrecht JS, et al. Problems with gait and posture in neuropathic patients with insulin-dependent diabetes mellitus. *Diabet Med.* 1992;9:469-474.
767. Morrison S, Colberg SR, Mariano M, et al. Balance training reduces falls risk in older individuals with type 2 diabetes. *Diabetes Care.* 2010;33:748-750.
768. Zola BE, Vinik AI. Effects of autonomic neuropathy associated with diabetes mellitus on cardiovascular function. *Coron Artery Dis.* 1992;3:33-41.
769. Stansberry KB, Peppard HR, Babyak LM, et al. Primary nociceptive afferents mediate the blood flow dysfunction in non-glabrous (hairy) skin of type 2 diabetes. *Diabetes Care.* 1999;22:1549-1554.
770. Haak ES, Usadel KH, Kohleisen M, et al. The effect of alpha-lipoic acid on the neurovascular reflex arc in patients with diabetic neuropathy assessed by capillary microscopy. *Microvasc Res.* 1999;58:28-34.
771. Valensi P. Diabetic autonomic neuropathy: what are the risks? *Diabet Metab* 1998;24:66-72.
772. Mancia G, Paleari F, Parati G. Early diagnosis of diabetic autonomic neuropathy: present and future approaches. *Diabetologia.* 1997;40: 482-484.
773. Athyros VG, Didangelos TP, Karamitsos DT, et al. Long-term effect of converting enzyme inhibition on circadian sympathetic and parasympathetic modulation in patients with diabetic autonomic neuropathy. *Acta Cardiol.* 1998;53:201-209.
774. Malmberg K, Norhammar A, Wedel H, et al. Glycometabolic state at admission: important risk marker of mortality in conventionally treated patients with diabetes mellitus and acute myocardial infarction. Long-term results from the Diabetes and Insulin-Glucose Infusion in Acute Myocardial Infarction (DIGAMI) study. *Circulation.* 1999;99:2626-2632.
775. Kendall DM, Rooney DP, Smets YF, et al. Pancreas transplantation restores epinephrine response and symptom recognition during hypoglycemia in patients with long-standing type I diabetes and autonomic neuropathy. *Diabetes.* 1997;46:249-257.
776. Burger AJ, Weinrauch LA, D'Elia JA, et al. Effects of glycemic control on heart rate variability in type I diabetic patients with cardiac autonomic neuropathy. *Am J Cardiol.* 1999;84:687-691.
777. Laederach-Hofmann K, Weidmann P, Ferrari P. Hypovolemia contributes to the pathogenesis of orthostatic hypotension in patients with diabetes mellitus. *Am J Med.* 1999;106:50-58.
778. Denq JC, Opfer-Gehrking TL, Giuliani M, et al. Efficacy of compression of different capacitance beds in the amelioration of orthostatic hypotension. *Clin Auton Res.* 1997;7:321-326.
779. Vinik AI, Ziegler D. Diabetic cardiovascular autonomic neuropathy. *Circulation.* 2007;115:387-397.

780. Annese V, Bassotti G, Caruso N, et al. Gastrointestinal motor dysfunction, symptoms, and neuropathy in noninsulin-dependent (type 2) diabetes mellitus. *J Clin Gastroenterol*. 1999;29:171-177.
781. Melga P, Mansi C, Ciuchi E, et al. Chronic administration of levosulpiride and glycemic control in IDDM patients with gastroparesis. *Diabetes Care*. 1997;20:55-58.
782. Stacher G, Schernthaner G, Francesconi M, et al. Cisapride versus placebo for 8 weeks on glycemic control and gastric emptying in insulin-dependent diabetes: a double blind cross-over trial. *J Clin Endocrinol Metab*. 1999;84:2357-2362.
783. Barone JA. Domperidone: a peripherally acting dopamine2-receptor antagonist. *Ann Pharmacother*. 1999;33:429-440.
784. Silvers D, Kipnes M, Broadstone V, et al. Domperidone in the management of symptoms of diabetic gastroparesis: efficacy, tolerability, and quality-of-life outcomes in a multicenter controlled trial. DOM-USA-5 Study Group. *Clin Ther*. 1998;20:438-453.
785. Erbas T, Varoglu E, Erbas B, et al. Comparison of metoclopramide and erythromycin in the treatment of diabetic gastroparesis. *Diabetes Care*. 1993;16:1511-1514.
786. Vinik AI, Richardson D. Erectile dysfunction in diabetes. *Diabetes Rev*. 1998;6:16-33.
787. Vinik AI, Richardson D. Erectile dysfunction in diabetes: pills for penile failure. *Clinica Diabetes*. 1998;16:108-119.
788. Rendell MS, Rajfer J, Wicker PA, et al, Sildenafil Diabetes Study Group. Sildenafil for treatment of erectile dysfunction in men with diabetes: a randomized controlled trial. *JAMA*. 1999;281:421-426.
789. Enzlin P, Mathieu C, Vanderschueren D, et al. Diabetes mellitus and female sexuality: a review of 25 years' research. *Diabet Med*. 1998;15(10):809-815.
790. Shaw JE, Parker R, Hollis S, et al. Gustatory sweating in diabetes mellitus. *Diabet Med*. 1996;13:1033-1037.
791. Shaw JE, Abbott CA, Tindle K, et al. A randomised controlled trial of topical glycopyrrolate, the first specific treatment for diabetic gustatory sweating. *Diabetologia*. 1997;40:299-301.
792. Meyer C, Hering BJ, Grossmann R, et al. Improved glucose counterregulation and autonomic symptoms after intraportal islet transplants alone in patients with long-standing type I diabetes mellitus. *Transplantation*. 1998;66:233-240.
793. Vinik A: Diagnosis and management of diabetic neuropathy. *Clin Geriatr Med*. 1999;15:293-319.
794. Gu K, Cowie CC, Harris MI. Diabetes and decline in heart disease mortality in US adults. *JAMA*. 1999;281:1291-1297.
795. Scott J, Huskisson EC. Graphic representation of pain. *Pain*. 1976;2:175-186.
796. Malmberg K, Yusuf S, Gerstein HC, et al. Impact of diabetes on long-term prognosis in patients with unstable angina and non-Q-wave myocardial infarction. *Circulation*. 2000;102:1014-1019.
797. Mukamal KJ, Nesto RW, Cohen MC, et al. Impact of diabetes on long-term survival after acute myocardial infarction. *Diabetes Care*. 2001;24:1422-1427.
798. Evans JM, Wang J, Morris AD. Comparison of cardiovascular risk between patients with type 2 diabetes and those who had a myocardial infarction: cross sectional and cohort studies. *BMJ*. 2002;324:939-943.
799. Lee CD, Folsom AR, Pankow JS, et al. Cardiovascular events in diabetic and nondiabetic adults with or without a history of myocardial infarction. *Circulation*. 2004;109:855-860.
800. Krolewski AS, Warram JH, Rand LI, et al. Epidemiologic approach to the etiology of type I diabetes mellitus and its complications. *N Engl J Med*. 1987;317:1390-1398.
801. Orchard TJ, Olson JC, Erbey JR, et al. Insulin resistance-related factors, but not glycemia, predict coronary artery disease in type 1 diabetes. *Diabetes Care*. 2003;26:1374-1379.
802. Soedamah-Muthu SS, Chaturvedi N, Toeller M, et al. EURODIAB Prospective Complications Study Group: Risk factors for coronary heart disease in type 1 diabetic patients in Europe: The EURODIAB Prospective Complications Study. *Diabetes Care*. 2004;27:530-537.
803. Pambianco G, Costacou T, Ellis D, et al. The 30-year natural history of type 1 diabetes complications: the Pittsburgh Epidemiology of Diabetes Complications Study experience. *Diabetes*. 2006;55:1463-1469.
804. Laing SP, Swerdlow AJ, Slater SD, et al. Mortality from heart disease in a cohort of 23,000 patients with insulin-treated diabetes. *Diabetologia*. 2003;46:760-765.
805. Wilson PW, Kannel WB, Silbershatz H, et al. Clustering of metabolic factors and coronary heart disease. *Arch Intern Med*. 1999;159:1104-1109.
806. Haffner SM, Mykkanen L, Festa A, et al. Insulin-resistant prediabetic subjects have more atherogenic risk factors than insulin-sensitive prediabetic subjects. *Circulation*. 2000;101:975-980.
807. Festa A, Hanley AJG, Tracey RP, et al. Inflammation in the prediabetic state is related to increased insulin resistance rather than decreased insulin secretion. *Ciruclation*. 2003;108:1822-1830.
808. Turner RC. The UK Prospective Diabetes Study: a review. *Diabetes Care*. 1998;21(suppl 3):C35-C38.
809. Andersson DK, Svardsudd K. Long-term glycemic control relates to mortality in type II diabetes. *Diabetes Care*. 1995;18:1534-1543.
810. Wei M, Gaskill SP, Haffner SM, et al. Effects of diabetes and level of glycemia on all-cause and cardiovascular mortality. The San Antonio Heart Study. *Diabetes Care*. 1998;21:1167-1172.
811. Brunner EJ, Shipley MJ, Witte DR, et al. Relation between blood glucose and coronary mortality over 33 years in the Whitehall study. *Diabetes Care*. 2006;29:26-31.
812. Tominaga M, Eguchi H, Manaka H, et al. Impaired glucose tolerance is a risk factor for cardiovascular disease but not impaired fasting glucose. *Diabetes Care*. 1999;22:920-924.
813. DECODE Study Group. Glucose tolerance and mortality: comparison of WHO and American Diabetic Asociation diagnostic criteria. *Lancet*. 1999;354:617-621.
814. Hu FB, Stampfner MJ, Haffner SM, et al. Elevated risk of cardiovascular disease prior to clinical diagnosis of type 2 diabetes. *Diabetes Care*. 2002;25:1129-1134.
815. Klein R, Klein BE, Moss SE. The Wisconsin Epidemiologic Study of Diabetic Retinopathy: XVI. The relationship of C-peptide to the incidence and progression of diabetic retinopathy. *Diabetes*. 1995;44:796-801.
816. Wingard DL, Barrett-Connor EL, Scheidt-Nave C, et al. Prevalence of cardiovascular and renal complications in older adults with normal or impaired glucose tolerance or NIDDM: a population-based study. *Diabetes Care*. 1993;16:1022-1025.
817. Folsom AR, Eckfeldt JH, Weitzman S, et al. Relation of carotid artery wall thickness to diabetes mellitus, fasting glucose and insulin, body size, and physical activity. Atherosclerosis Risk in Communities (ARIC) Study Investigators. *Stroke*. 1994;25:66-73.
818. Temelkova-Kurktschiev TS, Koehler C, Leonhardt W, et al. Increased intimal-medial thickness in newly detected type 2 diabetes: risk factors. *Diabetes Care*. 1999;22:333-338.
819. Hanefeld M, Koehler C, Schaper F, et al. Postprandial plasma glucose is an independent risk factor for increased carotid intima-media thickness in non-diabetic individuals. *Atherosclerosis*. 1999;144:229-235.
820. National Cholesterol Education Program (NCEP) Expert Panel on the Detection, Evaluation, and Treatment of High Blood Cholesterol in Adults (Adult Treatment Panel III). Third report of the National Cholesterol Education Program (NCEP) Expert Panel on the Detection, Evaluation, and Treatment of High Blood Cholesterol in Adults (Adult Treatment Panel III). Final report. *Circulation*. 2002;106:3143-3421.
821. Grundy SM, Brewer HB, Cleeman JI, et al. Definition of metabolic syndrome. Report of the National Heart, Lung, and Blood Institute/American Heart Association Conference on Scientific Issues Related to Definition. *Circulation*. 2004;109:433-438.
822. International Diabetes Foundation. The IDF worldwide definition of the metabolic syndrome. Available at http://www.idf.org/home/index.cfm?node=1429 (accessed December 2010).
823. Ford ES, Giles WH, Dietz WH. Prevelence of the metabolic syndrome among US adults: findings from the Third National Health and Nutrition Examination Survey. *JAMA*. 2002;287:356-359.
824. Lakka, H-M, Laaksonen DE, Lakka TA, et al. The metabolic syndrome and total and cardiovascular disease mortality in middle-aged men. *JAMA*. 2002;288:2709-2716.
825. Malik S, Wong ND, Franklin SS, et al. Impact of the metabolic syndrome on mortality from coronary heart disease, cardiovascular disease, and all causes in United States adults. *Circulation*. 2004;110:1245-1250.
826. Sattar N, Gaw A, Scherbakova O, et al. Metabolic syndrome with and without C-reactive protein as a predictor of coronary heart disease and diabetes in the West of Scotland Coronary Prevention Study. *Circulation*. 2003;108:414-419.
827. Ford ES. Risk for all-cause mortality, cardiovascular disease, and diabetes associated with the metabolic syndrome. *Diabetes Care*. 2005;28:1769-1778.
828. Grundy SM, Cleeman JI, Daniels SR, et al. Diagnosis and management of the metabolic syndrome. An American Heart Association/National Heart, Lung, and Blood Institute scientific statement. *Circulation*. 2005;112:2735-2752.
829. Deedwania PC. The deadly quartet revisited. *Am J Med*. 1998;105:1S-3S.
830. Howard G, O'Leary DH, Zaccaro D, et al. Insulin sensitivity and atherosclerosis. The Insulin Resistance Atherosclerosis Study (IRAS) Investigators. *Circulation*. 1996;93:1809-1817.
831. Abraira C, Colwell J, Nuttall F, et al. Cardiovascular events and correlates in the Veterans Affairs Diabetes Feasibility Trial. Veterans Affairs Cooperative Study on Glycemic Control and Complications in Type II Diabetes. *Arch Intern Med*. 1997;157:181-188.
832. Diabetes Control and Complications Trial/Epidemiology of Diabetes Interventions and Complications (DCCT/EDIC) Study Research Group. Intensive diabetes treatment and cardiovascular disease in patients with type 1 diabetes. *N Eng J Med*. 2005;353:2643-2653.
833. Dormandy JA, Charbonnel B, Eckland DJA, et al. Secondary prevention of macrovascular events in patients with type 2 diabetes in the

PROactive Study (PROspective pioglitAzone Clinical Trial in macroVascular Events): a randomized controlled trial. *Lancet*. 2005;366:1279-1289.
834. Nissen SE, Wolski K. Effect of rosiglitazone on the risk of myocardial infarction and death from cardiovascular causes. *N Engl J Med*. 2007;356:2457-2471.
835. Lago RM, Singh PP, Nesto RW. Congestive heart failure and cardiovascular death in patients with prediabetes and type 2 diabetes given thiazolidinediones: a meta-analysis of randomised clinical trials. *Lancet*. 2007;370:1129-1136.
836. The Action to Control Cardiovascular Risk in Diabetes Study Group. Effects of intensive glucose lowering in type 2 diabetes. *N Engl J Med*. 2008;358:2545-2559.
837. Duckworth W, Abraira C, Moritz T, et al. Glucose control and vascular complications in veterans with type 2 diabetes. *N Engl J Med*. 2009;360:129-139.
838. The ADVANCE Collaborative Group. Intensive blood glucose control and vascular outcomes in patients with type 2 diabetes. *N Engl J Med*. 2008;358:2560-2572.
839. Gowri MS, Van der Westhuyzen DR, Bridges SR, et al. Decreased protection by HDL from poorly controlled type 2 diabetic subjects against LDL oxidation may be due to the abnormal composition of HDL. *Arterioscler Thromb Vasc Biol*. 1999;19:2226-2233.
840. The Long-Term Intervention with Pravastatin in Ischemic Disease (LIPID) Study Group. Prevention of cardiovascular events and death in pravastatin patients with coronary heart disease and a broad range of initial cholesterol levels. *N Engl J Med*. 1998;339:1349-1357.
841. Haffner SM, Alexander CM, Cook TJ, et al. Reduced coronary events in simvastatin-treated patients with coronary heart disease and diabetes or impaired glucose levels. *Arch Intern Med*. 1999;159:2661-2667.
842. Ballantyne CM, Olsson AG, Cook TJ, et al. Influence of low high-density lipoprotein cholesterol and elevated triglyceride on coronary heart disease events and response to simvastatin therapy in 4S. *Circulation*. 2001;104:3046-3051.
843. Deedwania P, Barter P, Carmena R, et al. Reduction of low-density lipoprotein cholesterol in patients with coronary heart disease and metabolic syndrome: analysis of the Treating to New Targets study. *Lancet*. 2006;368:919-928.
844. Taylor AJ, Sullenberger LE, Lee HJ, et al. Arterial Biology for the Investigation of the Treatment Effects of Reducing Cholesterol (ARBITER 2): a double-blind, placebo-controlled study of extended-release niacin on atherosclerosis progression in secondary prevention patients treated with statins. [Errata in *Circulation*. 2004;110:3615, *Circulation*. 2005; 111:e446.] *Circulation*. 2004;110:3512-3517.
845. Rubins HB, Robins SJ, Collins D, et al. Gemfibrozil for the secondary prevention of coronary heart disease in men with low levels of high-density lipoprotein cholesterol. Veterans Affairs High-Density Lipoprotein Cholesterol Intervention Trial Study Group. *N Engl J Med*. 1999;341:410-418.
846. The FIELD Study Investigators. Effects of long-term fenofibrate therapy on cardiovascular events in 9795 people with type 2 diabetes mellitus (the FIELD study): randomized controlled trial. *Lancet*. 2005;366:1849-1861.
847. Heart Protection Study Collaborative Group. MRC/BHF Heart protection study of cholesterol lowering with simvastatin in 20,536 high-risk individuals: a randomized, placebo-controlled study. *Lancet*. 2002; 360:7-22.
848. Calhoun HM, Betteridge DJ, Durrington PN, et al. Primary prevention of cardiovascular disease with atorvastatin in type 2 diabetes in the Collaborative Atorvastatin Diabetes Study (CARDS): multicentre randomised placebo-controlled trial. *Lancet*. 2004;364:685-696.
849. Ginsberg HN, Elam MB, Lovato LC, et al. Effects of combination lipid therapy in type 2 diabetes mellitus. *N Engl J Med*. 2010;362:1563-1574.
850. Grundy SM, Cleeman JI, Merz MB, et al. Implications of recent clinical trials for the National Cholesterol Education Program Adult Treatment Panel III Guidelines. *Circulation*. 2004;110:227-239.
851. Chobanian AV, Bakris GL, Black HR, et al. The Seventh Report of the Joint National Committee on Prevention, Detection, Evaluation, and Treatment of High Blood Pressure (JNC VII). *JAMA*. 2003;289:2560-2572.
852. Tuomilehto J, Rastenyte D, Birkenhager WH, et al. Effects of calcium-channel blockade in older patients with diabetes and systolic hypertension. Systolic Hypertension in Europe Trial Investigators. *N Engl J Med*. 1999;340:677-684.
853. The Heart Outcomes Prevention Evaluation Study Investigators. Effects of an angiotensin-converting enzyme inhibitor, ramipril, on cardiovascular events in high-risk patients. *N Engl J Med*. 2000; 342:145-153.
854. U.K. Prospective Diabetes Study Group. Efficacy of atenolol and captopril in reducing risk of macrovascular and microvascular complications in type 2 diabetes: UKPDS 39. *BMJ*. 1998;317:713-720.
855. Hansson L, Zanchetti A, Carruthers SG, et al. Effects of intensive blood pressure lowering and low-dose aspirin in patients with hypertension: principal results of the Hypertension Optimal Treatment (HOT) randomised trial. HOT Study Group. *Lancet*. 1998;351:1755-1762.
856. Whelton PK, Barzilay J, Cushman WC, et al. Clinical outcomes in antihypertensive treatment of type 2 diabetes, impaired fasting glucose concentration, and normoglycemia. *Arch Intern Med*. 2005;165:1401-1409.
857. ACCORD Study Group, Cushman WC, Evans GW, Byington RP, et al. Effects of intensive blood-pressure control in type 2 diabetes mellitus. *N Engl J Med*. 2010;362:1575-1585.
858. Nesto RW, Zarich S. Acute myocardial infarction in diabetes mellitus: lessons learned from ACE inhibition. *Circulation*. 1998;97:12-15.
859. Jacoby RM, Nesto RW. Acute myocardial infarction in the diabetic patient: pathophysiology, clinical course and prognosis. *J Am Coll Cardiol*. 1992;20:736-744.
860. Iwasaka T, Takahashi N, Nakamura S, et al. Residual left ventricular pump function after acute myocardial infarction in NIDDM patients. *Diabetes Care*. 1992;15:1522-1526.
861. Bernardi L, Ricordi L, Lazzari P, et al. Impaired circadian modulation of sympathovagal activity in diabetes: a possible explanation for altered temporal onset of cardiovascular disease. *Circulation*. 1992;86:1443-1452.
862. Zarich S, Waxman S, Freeman RT, et al. Effect of autonomic nervous system dysfunction on the circadian pattern of myocardial ischemia in diabetes mellitus. *J Am Coll Cardiol*. 1994;24:956-962.
863. Muller JE, Tofler GH, Stone PH. Circadian variation and triggers of onset of acute cardiovascular disease. *Circulation*. 1989;79:733-743.
864. Imperatore G, Riccardi G, Iovine C, et al. Plasma fibrinogen—a new factor of the metabolic syndrome: a population-based study. *Diabetes Care*. 1998;21:649-654.
865. Sobel BE, Woodcock-Mitchell J, Schneider DJ, et al. Increased plasminogen activator inhibitor type 1 in coronary artery atherectomy specimens from type 2 diabetic compared with nondiabetic patients: a potential factor predisposing to thrombosis and its persistence. *Circulation*. 1998;97:2213-2221.
866. Meigs JB, Mittleman MA, Nathan DM, et al. Hyperinsulinemia, hyperglycemia, and impaired hemostasis. The Framingham Offspring Study. *JAMA*. 2000;283:221-228.
867. Woodfield SL, Lundergan CF, Reiner JS, et al. Angiographic findings and outcome in diabetic patients treated with thrombolytic therapy for acute myocardial infarction: the GUSTO-I experience. *J Am Coll Cardiol*. 1996;28:1661-1669.
868. Mak KH, Moliterno DJ, Granger CB, et al. Influence of diabetes mellitus on clinical outcome in the thrombolytic era of acute myocardial infarction. GUSTO-I Investigators. Global Utilization of Streptokinase and Tissue Plasminogen Activator for Occluded Coronary Arteries. *J Am Coll Cardiol*. 1997;30:171-179.
869. Sun D, Nguyen N, DeGrado T, et al. Ischemia-induced translocation of the insulin-responsive glucose transporter GLUT4 in the plasma membrane of cardiac myocytes. *Circulation*. 1994;89:793-798.
870. Oliver M, Opie H. Effects of glucose and fatty acids on myocardial ischaemia and arrhythmias. *Lancet*. 1994;343:155-158.
871. Bellodi G, Manicardi V, Malavasi V, et al. Hyperglycemia and prognosis of acute myocardial infarction in patients without diabetes mellitus. *Am J Cardiol*. 1989;64:885-888.
872. Oswald GA, Smith CC, Betteridge DJ, et al. Determinants and importance of stress hyperglycaemia in non-diabetic patients with myocardial infarction. *BMJ*. 1986;293:917-922.
873. Fava S, Aquilina O, Azzopardi J, et al. The prognostic value of blood glucose in diabetic patients with acute myocardial infarction. *Diabetes Med*. 1996;13:80-83.
874. Capes SE, Hunt D, Malmberg K, et al. Stress hyperglycemia and increased risk of death after myocardial infarction in patients with and without diabetes: a systematic overview. *Lancet*. 2000;355:773-778.
875. Malmberg K, Ryden L, Efendic S, et al. Randomized trial of insulin-glucose infusion followed by subcutaneous insulin treatment in diabetic patients with acute myocardial infarction (DIGAMI study): effects on mortality at 1 year. *J Am Coll Cardiol*. 1995;26:57-65.
876. Malmberg K, Ryden L, Wedel H, et al. Intense metabolic control by means of insulin in patients with diabetes mellitus and acute myocardial infarction (DIGAMI 2): effects on mortality and morbidity. *Eur Heart J*. 2005;26:650-661.
877. The CREATE-ECLA Trial Group Investigators. Effect of glucose-insulin-potassium infusion on mortality in patients with acute ST-segment elevation myocardial infarction. *JAMA*. 2005;293:437-446.
878. Garratt KN, Brady PA, Hassinger NL, et al. Sulfonylurea drugs increase early mortality in patients with diabetes mellitus after direct angioplasty for acute myocardial infarction. *J Am Coll Cardiol*. 1999;33:119-124.
879. Cleveland Jr JC, Meldrum DR, Cain BS, et al. Oral sulfonylurea hypoglycemic agents prevent ischemic preconditioning in human myocardium: two paradoxes revisited. *Circulation*. 1997;96:29-32.
880. Katsuda Y, Egashira K, Ueno H, et al. Glibenclamide, a selective inhibitor of ATP-sensitive K^+ channels, attenuates metabolic coronary vasodilatation induced by pacing tachycardia in dogs. *Circulation*. 1995;92:511-517.

881. Davis III CA, Sherman AJ, Yaroshenko Y, et al. Coronary vascular responsiveness to adenosine is impaired additively by blockade of nitric oxide synthesis and a sulfonylurea. *Am J Cardiol.* 1998;31: 816-822.
882. O'Driscoll G, Green D, Maiorana A, et al. Improvement in endothelial function by angiotensin-converting enzyme inhibition in non-insulin-dependent diabetes mellitus. *J Am Coll Cardiol.* 1999;33:1506-1511.
883. Vaughan DE, Rouleau JL, Ridker PM, et al. Effects of ramipril on plasma fibrinolytic balance in patients with acute anterior myocardial infarction. HEART Study Investigators. *Circulation.* 1997;96:442-447.
884. Torlone E, Britta M, Rambotti AM, et al. Improved insulin action and glycemic control after long-term angiotensin-converting enzyme inhibition in subjects with arterial hypertension and type II diabetes. *Diabetes Care.* 1993;16:1347-1355.
885. Zuanetti G, Latini R, Maggioni A, et al. Effect of the ACE-inhibitor lisinopril on mortality in diabetic patients with acute myocardial infarction: the data from the GISSI-3 study. *Circulation.* 1997; 96:4239-4245.
886. Gustafsson I, Torp-Pedersen C, Kober L, et al. Effect of the angiotensin-converting enzyme inhibitor trandolapril on mortality and morbidity in diabetic patients with left ventricular dysfunction after acute myocardial infarction. Trace Study Group. *J Am Coll Cardiol.* 1999; 34:83-89.
887. Lakshman MR, Reda DJ, Materson BJ, et al. Diuretics and β-blockers do not have adverse effects at 1 year on plasma lipid and lipoprotein profiles in men with hypertension. Department of Veterans Affairs Cooperative Study Group on Antihypertensive Agents. *Arch Intern Med.* 1999;159:551-558.
888. Shorr RI, Ray WA, Daugherty JR, et al. Antihypertensives and the risk of serious hypoglycemia in older persons using insulin or sulfonylureas. *JAMA.* 1997;278:40-43.
889. Chen J, Marciniak TA, Radford MJ, et al. β-Blocker therapy for secondary prevention of myocardial infarction in elderly diabetic patients. Results from the National Cooperative Cardiovascular Project. *J Am Coll Cardiol.* 1999;34:1388-1394.
890. Giugliano D, Acampora R, Marfella R. Metabolic and cardiovascular effects of carvedilol and atenolol in non-insulin-dependent diabetes mellitus and hypertension. *Ann Intern Med.* 1997;126:955-959.
891. ETDRS Investigators. Aspirin effects on mortality and morbidity in patients with diabetes mellitus. Early Treatment Diabetic Retinopathy Study report 14. *JAMA.* 1992;268:1292-1300.
892. American Diabetes Association. Aspirin therapy in diabetes. *Diabetes Care.* 1997;20:772-1773.
893. Davi G, Catalano I, Averna M, et al. Thromboxane biosynthesis and platelet function in type II diabetes mellitus. *N Engl J Med.* 1990; 322:1769-1774.
894. Hirsh J, Bhatt DL. Comparative benefits of clopidogrel and aspirin in high-risk patient populations: lessons from the CAPRIE and CURE studies. *Arch Intern Med.* 2004;164:2106-2110.
895. Platelet Receptor Inhibition in Ischemic Syndrome Management in Patients Limited by Unstable Signs and Symptoms (PRISM-PLUS) Study Investigators. Inhibition of the platelet glycoprotein IIb/IIIa receptor with tirofiban in unstable angina and non-Q-wave myocardial infarction. *N Engl J Med.* 1998;338:1488-1497.
896. EPILOG Investigators. Platelet glycoprotein IIb/IIIa receptor blockade and low-dose heparin during percutaneous coronary revascularization. *N Engl J Med.* 1997;336:1689-1696.
897. Lincoff AM, Califf RM, Moliterno DJ, et al. Complementary clinical benefits of coronary artery stenting and blockade of platelet glycoprotein IIb/IIIa receptors. Evaluation of Platelet IIb/IIIa Inhibition in Stenting Investigators. *N Engl J Med.* 1999;341:319-327.
898. Bypass Angioplasty Revascularization Investigation (BARI) Investigators. Comparison of coronary bypass surgery with angioplasty in patients with multivessel disease. *N Engl J Med.* 1996;335:217-225.
899. Kannel WB, Hjortland M, Castelli WP. Role of diabetes in congestive heart failure: the Framingham study. *Am J Cardiol.* 1974;34:29-34.
900. Aronson D, Rayfield E, Cheseboro J. Mechanisms determining course and outcome of diabetic patients who have had acute myocardial infarction. *Ann Intern Med.* 1997;126:296-306.
901. Cabin H, Roberts W. Quantitative comparison of extent of coronary narrowing and size of healed myocardial infarct in 33 necropsy patients with clinically recognized and in 28 with clinically unrecognized ("silent") previous acute myocardial infarction. *Am J Cardiol.* 1982;50:677-681.
902. van Hoeven KH, Factor SM. A comparison of the pathological spectrum of hypertensive, diabetic, and hypertensive-diabetic heart disease. *Circulation.* 1990;82:848-855.
903. Kawaguchi M, Techigawara M, Ishihata T, et al. A comparison of ultrastructural changes on endomyocardial biopsy specimens obtained from patients with diabetes mellitus with and without hypertension. *Heart Vessels.* 1997;12:267-274.
904. Nahser P, Brown R, Oskarsson H, et al. Maximal coronary flow reserve and metabolic coronary vasodilation in patients with diabetes mellitus. *Circulation.* 1995;91:635-640.
905. Depre C, Vanoverschelde JL, Taegtmeyer H. Glucose for the heart. *Circulation.* 1999;99:578-588.
906. Azzarelli A, Dini F, Cristofani R, et al. NIDDM as unfavorable factor to the postinfarction ventricular function in the elderly: echocardiography study. *Coron Artery Dis.* 1995;6:629-634.
907. Korup E, Dalsgaard D, Nyvad O, et al. Comparison of degrees of left ventricular dilation within three hours and up to six days after onset of first acute myocardial infarction. *Am J Cardiol.* 1997;80: 449-453.
908. Mayfield JA, Reiber GE, Maynard C, et al. Trends in lower limb amputation in the Veterans Health Administration, 1989-1998. *J Rehabil Res Dev.* 2000;37:23-30.
909. van Houtum WH, Rauwerda JA, Ruwaard D, et al. Reduction in diabetes-related lower-extremity amputations in The Netherlands. *Diabetes Care.* 2004;27:1042-1046.
910. Krishnan S, Nash F, Baker N, et al. Reduction in diabetic amputations over 11 years in a defined UK population: benefits of multidisciplinary team work and continuous prospective audit. *Diabetes Care.* 2008;31:99-101.
911. Vileikyte L. Psychosocial and behavioral aspects of diabetic foot lesions. *Curr Diab Rep.* 2008;8:119-125.
912. Boulton AJM, Cavanagh PR, Rayman G, eds. *The Foot in Diabetes.* 4th ed. Chichester, UK: John Wiley & Sons, 2006.
913. Bowker JH, Pfeifer MA, eds. *Levin & O'Neal's The Diabetic Foot.* 7th ed. St Louis: Mosby, 2008.
914. Singh N, Armstrong DG, Lipsky BA. Preventing foot ulcers in patients with diabetes. *JAMA.* 2005;293:217-228.
915. Boulton AJM, van Houtum WH, eds. The diabetic foot. *Diabetes Metab Res Rev.* 2008;24(suppl 1):S1-S193.
916. Abbott CA, Carrington AL, Ashe H, et al. The North-West diabetes foot care study: incidence of, and risk factors for, new diabetic foot ulceration in a community-based cohort. *Diabetic Med.* 2002;20:277-384.
917. Jude EB, Eleftheriadou I, Tentolouris N. Peripheral arterial disease in diabetes: a review. *Diabetic Med.* 2010;27:4-14.
918. Akbari CM, Pomposelli FB, Gibbons GW. Lower extremity revascularization in diabetes: late observations. *Arch Surg.* 2000;135:452-456.
919. Ndip A, Lavery LA, Lafontaine J, et al. High levels of foot ulceration and amputation risk in a multiracial cohort of diabetic patients on dialysis therapy. *Diabetes Care.* 2010;33;878-880.
920. Boulton AJM. The diabetic foot: from art to science. *Diabetologia.* 2004;47:1343-1353.
921. Reiber GE, Vileikyte L, Boyko EJ, et al. Causal pathways for incident lower extremity ulcers in patients with diabetes from two settings. *Diabetes Care.* 1999;22:157-162.
922. Boulton AJM, Armstrong DG, Albert SG, et al. Comprehensive Foot Examination and Risk Assessment: a report of the Task Force of the Foot Care Interest Group of the American Diabetes Association, with endorsement by the American Association of Clinical Endocrinologists. *Diabetes Care.* 2008;31:1679-1686.
923. Oyibo S, Jude EB, Tarawneh I, et al. A comparision of two diabetic foot ulcer classification systems: the Wagner and the University of Texas wound classification systems. *Diabetes Care.* 2001;24:84-88.
924. Armstrong DG, Lavery LA, Harkless LB. Validation of a diabetic wound classification system. *Diabet Med.* 1998;14:855-859.
925. Piaggesi A, Viacava P, Rizzo L, et al. Semi-quantitative analysis of the histopathological features of the neuropathic foot ulcer: effects of pressure relief. *Diabetes Care.* 2003;26:3123-3128.
926. Armstrong DG, Nguyen HC, Lavery LA, et al. Off-loading the diabetic foot wound: a randomized clinical trial. *Diabetes Care.* 2001;24: 1019-1022.
927. Katz I, Harlan A, Miranda-Palma B, et al. A randomized trial of two irremovable offloading devices in the treatment of plantar neuropathic diabetic foot ulcers. *Diabetes Care.* 2005;28:555-559.
928. Lipsky BA. New developments in diagnosing and treating diabetic foot infections. *Diabetes Metab Res Rev.* 2008;24(suppl 1):S66-S71.
929. Teh J, Berendt T, Lipsky BA. Rational imaging: investigating suspected bone infection in the diabetic foot. *BMJ.* 2010;340:415-417.
930. Langer A, Rogowski W. Systematic review of economic evaluations of human cell-derived wound care products for the treatment of venous leg and diabetic foot ulcers. *BMC Health Serv Res.* 2009;9:115.
931. Armstrong DG, Lavery LA. Negative pressure wound therapy after partial diabetic foot amputation: a multicentre, randomised controlled trial. *Lancet.* 2005;366:1704-1710.
932. Blume PA, Walters J, Payne W, et al. Comparison of negative pressure wound therapy using vacuum-assisted closure with advanced moist wound therapy in the treatment of diabetic foot ulcers: a multicentre randomised controlled trial. *Diabetes Care.* 2008;31:631-636.
933. Jeffcoate WJ. Charcot neuro-osteoarthropathy. *Diabetes Metab Res Rev.* 2008;24(suppl 1):S62-S65.
934. Frykberg RG, ed. *The Diabetic Charcot Foot: Principles and Management.* Brooklandville, MD: Data Trace Publishing; 2010.

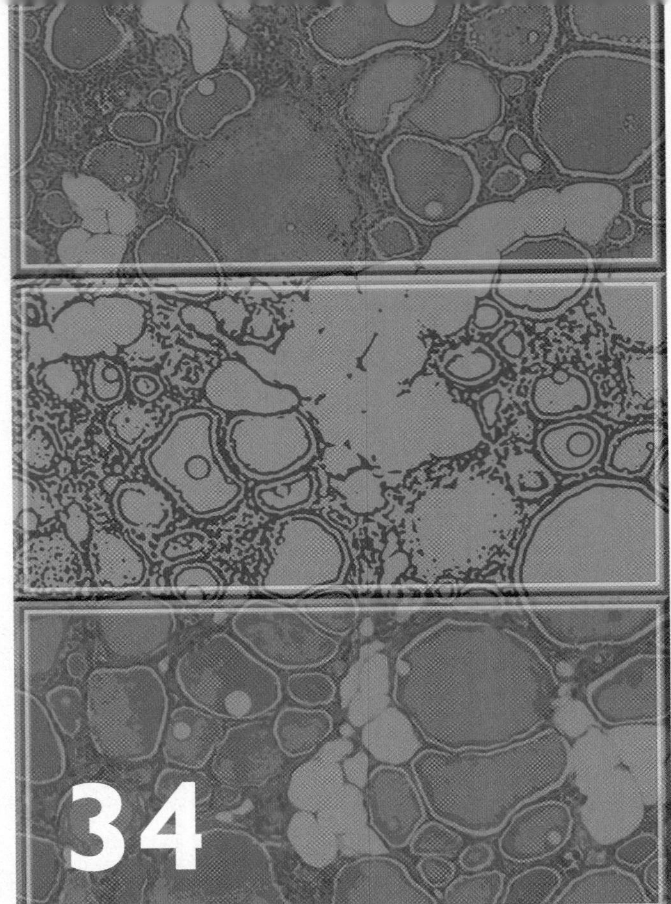

CHAPTER 34

Hypoglycemia

PHILIP E. CRYER

Glucose is an obligate metabolic fuel for the brain under physiologic conditions.[1-4] Because the brain cannot synthesize glucose, store more than a few minutes' supply as glycogen, or utilize physiologic concentrations of circulating nonglucose fuels effectively, survival of the brain, and therefore of the individual, requires a virtually continuous supply of glucose from the circulation.[1-4] Blood-to-brain glucose transport is a direct function of the arterial plasma glucose concentration and requires maintenance of the plasma glucose concentration within, or above, the physiologic range. Hypoglycemia causes functional brain failure, which is typically corrected after the plasma glucose concentration is raised.[5] Rarely, it causes a fatal cardiac arrhythmia or, if it is profound and prolonged, brain death.[5]

Given the survival value of maintenance of the plasma glucose concentration, it is not surprising that physiologic and behavioral mechanisms that normally prevent or rapidly correct hypoglycemia[4] have evolved. These mechanisms are so effective that hypoglycemia is an uncommon clinical event except in persons who use drugs that lower the plasma glucose concentration, such as insulin, sulfonylureas, or alcohol.[2,3]

A clinical practice guideline for the evaluation and management of hypoglycemic disorders has been published,[2] and the topic of hypoglycemia in diabetes has been reviewed in detail.[3]

PHYSIOLOGY OF DEFENSE AGAINST HYPOGLYCEMIA

Glucose Metabolism

Glucose is derived from three sources: intestinal absorption that occurs after digestion of dietary carbohydrates; *glycogenolysis,* which is the breakdown of glycogen, the polymerized storage form of glucose; and *gluconeogenesis,* which is the formation of glucose from precursors including lactate (and pyruvate), amino acids (especially alanine and glutamine), and, to a lesser extent, glycerol. There are multiple fates of glucose transported into cells (external losses are normally negligible) (Fig. 34-1). Glucose may be stored as glycogen, or it may undergo glycolysis to pyruvate, which can be reduced to lactate, transaminated to form alanine, or converted to acetyl coenzyme A (CoA). Acetyl-CoA in turn may be oxidized to carbon dioxide and water through the tricarboxylic acid cycle, converted to fatty acids that can be incorporated into triglycerides, oxidized, or utilized for synthesis of ketone bodies (acetoacetate, β-hydroxybutyrate) or cholesterol. Finally, glucose may be released into the circulation. Only liver and kidneys express glucose-6-phosphatase, the enzyme necessary for the release of glucose into the circulation, at levels sufficient

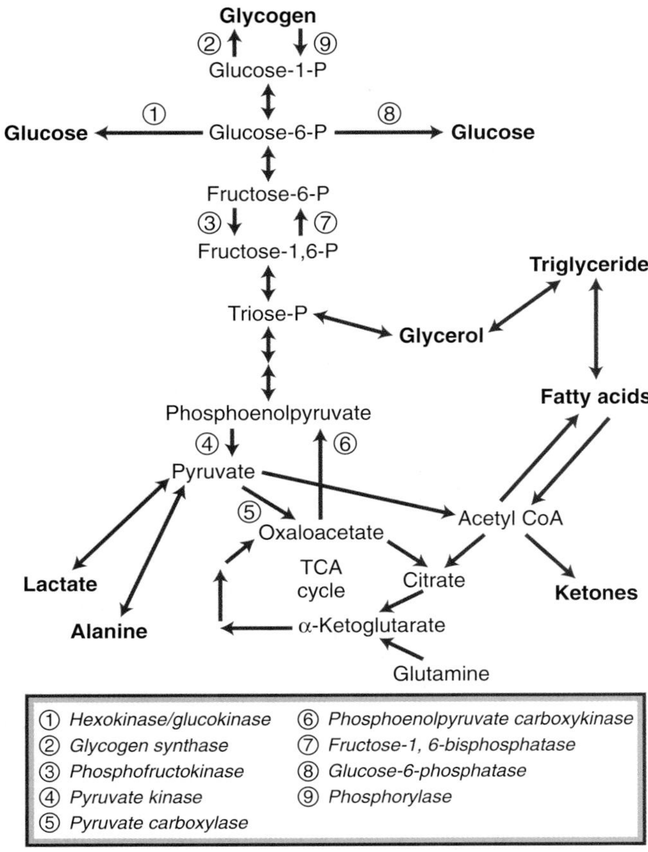

Figure 34-1 Schematic representation of glucose metabolism. CoA, coenzyme A; P, phosphate; TCA, tricarboxylic acid.

to permit substantial contributions to the systemic glucose pool. Many tissues express the enzymes required to synthesize and hydrolyze glycogen (glycogen synthase and phosphorylase, respectively). The liver and kidneys also express the enzymes necessary for gluconeogenesis, including the critical gluconeogenic enzymes, pyruvate carboxylase, phosphoenolpyruvate carboxykinase, and fruclose-1, 6-bisphosphatase.

The liver is the major source of net endogenous glucose production (through glycogenolysis and gluconeogenesis).[6] Conversely, the liver can be an organ of net glucose uptake. The kidneys also produce glucose (through gluconeogenesis) and utilize glucose.[7]

Muscle can take up and store glucose as glycogen, or it can metabolize glucose (through glycolysis) to pyruvate, which, among other fates, can be reduced to lactate or transaminated to form alanine. Lactate (and pyruvate) released from muscle can be transported to the liver and the kidneys, where it serves as a gluconeogenic precursor (the Cori or glucose-lactate cycle). Alanine, glutamine, and other amino acids can also flow from muscle to liver and kidneys, where they serve as gluconeogenic precursors. These constitute the glucose-alanine and glucose-glutamine cycles. Clearly, net new glucose formation is from precursors (e.g., amino acids) in which the carbons are not derived from glucose via these cycles. Although quantitatively less important than muscle, fat can also take up and metabolize glucose.

Glucose is essentially the sole metabolic fuel for the brain under physiologic conditions.[1] Glucose undergoes terminal oxidation in the brain. Although the adult human brain constitutes only about 2.5% of body weight, its oxidative metabolism accounts for approximately 25% of the basal metabolic rate and more than 50% of whole-body glucose utilization. The brain can utilize alternative fuels if their circulating levels rise high enough for them to enter the brain in quantity. For example, during extended fasting, markedly elevated circulating ketone levels can support the majority of the energy needs of the brain and reduce its utilization of glucose. Nonetheless, that is not a physiologic condition. Furthermore, ketogenesis is suppressed during episodes of insulin-mediated hypoglycemia. Again, the brain is critically dependent on a virtually continuous supply of glucose from the circulation.[1-5]

Systemic Glucose Balance

Normally, rates of endogenous glucose influx into the circulation and those of glucose efflux out of the circulation into tissues other than the brain are coordinately regulated—largely by the plasma glucose-lowering (regulatory) hormone insulin and the plasma glucose-raising (counterregulatory) hormones glucagon and epinephrine—such that systemic glucose balance is maintained, hypoglycemia (as well as hyperglycemia) is prevented, and a continuous supply of glucose to the brain is ensured (Table 34-1). This is accomplished despite wide variations in exogenous glucose influx (e.g., after meals versus during fasting) and in glucose efflux (e.g., during exercise versus rest). Hypoglycemia occurs when rates of glucose appearance in the circulation (the sum of endogenous glucose production and exogenous glucose delivery from ingested carbohydrates) fail to keep pace with rates of glucose disappearance from the circulation (the sum of ongoing glucose metabolism largely by the brain and of variable glucose utilization by tissues including muscle, fat, liver, and kidneys).

In healthy adults, the physiologic postabsorptive (fasting) plasma glucose concentration ranges from approximately 3.9 mmol/L (70 mg/dL) to 6.1 mmol/L (110 mg/dL), with a mean of about 5.0 mmol/L (90 mg/dL).[4] In the postabsorptive steady state, rates of glucose production and utilization average approximately 12 μmol/kg per minute (2.2 mg/kg per minute), with a range of 10 to 14 μmol/kg per minute (1.8 to 2.6 mg/kg per minute). These rates are as much as threefold higher in infants, at least in part because of their greater brain mass relative to body weight.

TABLE 34-1

Systemic Glucose Balance* and Effects of Circulating Hormones on Endogenous Production and Use of Glucose

Source of Glucose Influx or Efflux	HORMONAL EFFECTS		
	Insulin	Glucagon	Epinephrine
Glucose Influx into the Circulation			
Exogenous glucose delivery			
Endogenous glucose delivery			
In liver: glycogenolysis and gluconeogenesis	↓	↑	↑
In kidneys: gluconeogenesis	↓		↑
Glucose Efflux out of the Circulation			
Ongoing brain glucose utilization			
Variable glucose utilization by other tissues (e.g., muscle fat, liver, kidneys)	↑		↓

*Total glucose influx = total glucose efflux.

The liver is the predominant source of endogenous glucose production in the postabsorptive state; the kidneys, which both utilize and produce glucose, contribute little to net glucose production. However, as in the liver, glucose production in the kidney is regulated; it is suppressed by insulin and stimulated by epinephrine but not by glucagon. As a result, net renal glucose production occurs under some conditions, including hypoglycemia.[8] Therefore, endogenous glucose production cannot be equated with hepatic glucose production.

Gluconeogenesis and glycogenolysis are important for maintenance of the plasma glucose concentration.[6] The glucose pool, namely free glucose in the extracellular fluids and in the cells of certain tissues (primarily the liver), is only about 83 to 111 mmol (15 to 20 g). Glycogen that can be mobilized to provide circulating glucose (e.g., hepatic glycogen) contains approximately 390 mmol (70 g) of glucose, with a range of about 135 to 722 mmol (25 to 130 g). Therefore, in an adult of average size, preformed glucose can provide less than an 8-hour supply, even at the diminished rate of glucose utilization that occurs in the postabsorptive state.

If fasting is prolonged to 24 to 48 hours, the plasma glucose concentration declines and then stabilizes; hepatic glycogen content falls to less than 55 mmol (10 g), and gluconeogenesis becomes the sole source of glucose production.[6] Because amino acids are the main gluconeogenic precursors that result in net glucose formation, muscle protein is degraded. Glucose utilization by muscle and fat virtually ceases. As lipolysis and ketogenesis accelerate and circulating ketone levels rise, ketones become a major fuel for the brain. Glucose utilization by the brain declines by about half; this reduces the rate of gluconeogenesis required to maintain the plasma glucose concentration and hence decreases protein wasting.

After a meal, glucose absorption into the circulation increases to more than twice the rate of postabsorptive endogenous glucose production, depending on the carbohydrate content of the meal, the rate of gastric transit, and the rate of digestion and absorption. As glucose is absorbed, endogenous glucose production is suppressed, and glucose utilization by muscle, fat, and liver accelerates. The exogenous glucose is assimilated and, after a small rise, the plasma glucose concentration returns to the postabsorptive level.

Exercise increases glucose utilization (by muscle) to rates that can be several times greater than those of the postabsorptive state. Endogenous glucose production normally accelerates to match use so that the plasma glucose concentration is maintained.

In summary, the plasma glucose concentration is normally maintained within a relatively narrow range despite wide variations in glucose flux and thus maintains the systemic glucose balance. This remarkable homeostatic feat is accomplished by an array of hormonal, neural, and substrate glucoregulatory factors.[4] Glucoregulatory failure resulting in hyperglycemia (diabetes mellitus) is discussed in Chapters 31 and 32; that resulting in hypoglycemia is discussed in the paragraphs that follow.

Responses to Hypoglycemia

Falling plasma glucose concentrations cause a sequence of responses, with defined glycemic thresholds, in healthy individuals (Table 34-2).[4,9-11] The first response is a decrease in insulin secretion. This occurs as glucose levels decline within the physiologic range. Increased secretion of glucose counterregulatory hormones, including glucagon and epinephrine, occurs as glucose levels fall just below the physiologic range. Lower plasma glucose concentrations cause a more intense sympathoadrenal (sympathetic neural as well as adrenomedullary) response and symptoms. Even lower glucose levels cause cognitive dysfunction and additional manifestations of functional brain failure[5] including seizure or coma.

Clinical Manifestations of Hypoglycemia

The symptoms and signs of hypoglycemia[12,13] are nonspecific. Clinical hypoglycemia—that sufficient to cause symptoms and/or signs[2]—is most convincingly documented by Whipple's triad: (1) symptoms, signs, or both consistent with hypoglycemia; (2) a low measured plasma glucose concentration; and (3) resolution of those symptoms and signs after the plasma glucose concentration is raised.

Neuroglycopenic symptoms are a direct result of brain glucose deprivation. They include cognitive impairments, behavioral changes, psychomotor abnormalities, and, at lower glucose levels, seizure and coma.[2-5,12,13] Neurogenic (or autonomic) symptoms are largely the result of the perception of physiologic changes caused by sympathoadrenal (particularly the sympathetic neural[13]) discharge triggered by hypoglycemia. They include adrenergic (catecholamine-mediated) symptoms such as palpitations, tremor, and anxiety/arousal and cholinergic (acetylcholine-mediated) symptoms such as sweating, hunger, and paresthesias.

TABLE 34-2

Physiologic Responses to Decreasing Plasma Glucose Concentrations

Response	Glycemic Threshold* (mmol/L [mg/dL])	Physiologic Effects	Role in Prevention or Correction of Hypoglycemia (Glucose Counterregulation)
↓ Insulin	4.4-4.7 (80-85)	↑ R_a (↓ R_d)	Primary glucose regulatory factor, first defense against hypoglycemia
↑ Glucagon	3.6-3.9 (65-70)	↑ R_a	Primary glucose counterregulatory factor, second defense against hypoglycemia
↑ Epinephrine	3.6-3.9 (65-70)	↑ R_a, ↓ R_c	Involved, critical when glucagon is deficient, third defense against hypoglycemia
↑ Cortisol and growth hormone	3.6-3.9 (65-70)	↑ R_a, ↓ R_c	Involved, not critical
Symptoms	2.8-3.1 (50-55)	↑ Exogenous glucose	Prompt behavioral defense (food ingestion)
↓ Cognition	<2.8 (50)	—	(Compromises behavioral defense)

*Arterialized venous, not venous, plasma glucose concentrations.

R_a, rate of glucose appearance, glucose production by the liver and kidneys; R_c, rate of glucose clearance by insulin-sensitive tissues; R_d, rate of glucose disappearance, glucose utilization by insulin-sensitive tissues such as skeletal muscle (no direct effect on central nervous system glucose utilization).

Central mechanisms may also be involved in the generation of some of these symptoms (e.g., hunger).[14] Subjective awareness of hypoglycemia is largely the result of the perception of neurogenic symptoms (Fig. 34-2).[12]

Signs of hypoglycemia include pallor and diaphoresis, which result from adrenergic cutaneous vasoconstriction and cholinergic activation of sweat glands, respectively.[2,3] Heart rates and systolic blood pressures are raised, but often not greatly. Neuroglycopenic manifestations are often observable.

Maintenance of Systemic Glucose Balance

Although obligatory glucose utilization, largely by the brain, is continuous, the delivery of exogenous glucose from dietary carbohydrates is intermittent. Systemic glucose balance (see Table 34-1) is normally maintained, and hypoglycemia and hyperglycemia are prevented, by dynamic, minute-to-minute regulation of endogenous glucose production from the liver and kidneys and of glucose utilization by tissues outside the central nervous system (CNS), such as muscle.[3,4] This regulation is exerted primarily by insulin, glucagon, and epinephrine[3,4] (see Table 34-2 and Fig. 34-3), although an array of hormones, neurotransmitters, and substrates is involved.[4]

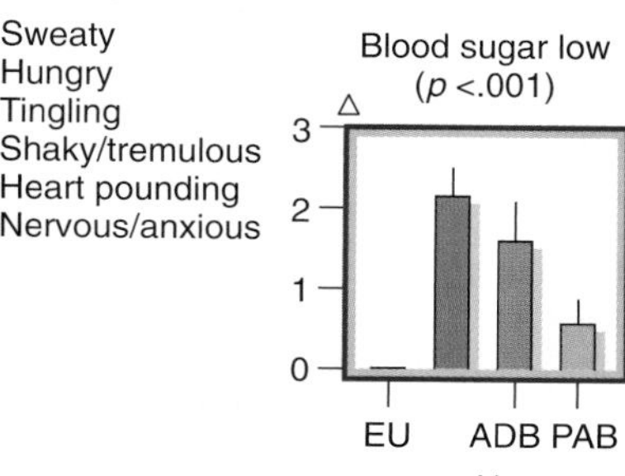

Figure 34-2 Neurogenic (autonomic) and neuroglycopenic symptoms of hypoglycemia in healthy humans. Among the neurogenic symptoms, "sweaty," "hungry," and "tingling" are cholinergic and "shaky/tremulous," "heart pounding," and "nervous/anxious" are adrenergic. See text for discussion. Mean subject scores (± standard error) for awareness of hypoglycemia (low blood sugar) are shown during clamped euglycemia (EU) and during three conditions of hypoglycemia (Hypo): alone; with combined α- and β-adrenergic blockade by infused phentolamine and propranolol (ADB); and with combined α- and β-adrenergic blockade plus muscarinic cholinergic blockade by atropine (panautonomic blockade, PAB). (From Towler DA, Havlin CE, Craft S, et al. Mechanism of awareness of hypoglycemia: perception of neurogenic [predominantly cholinergic] rather than neuroglycopenic symptoms. *Diabetes*. 1993;42:1791-1798, with permission of the American Diabetes Association.)

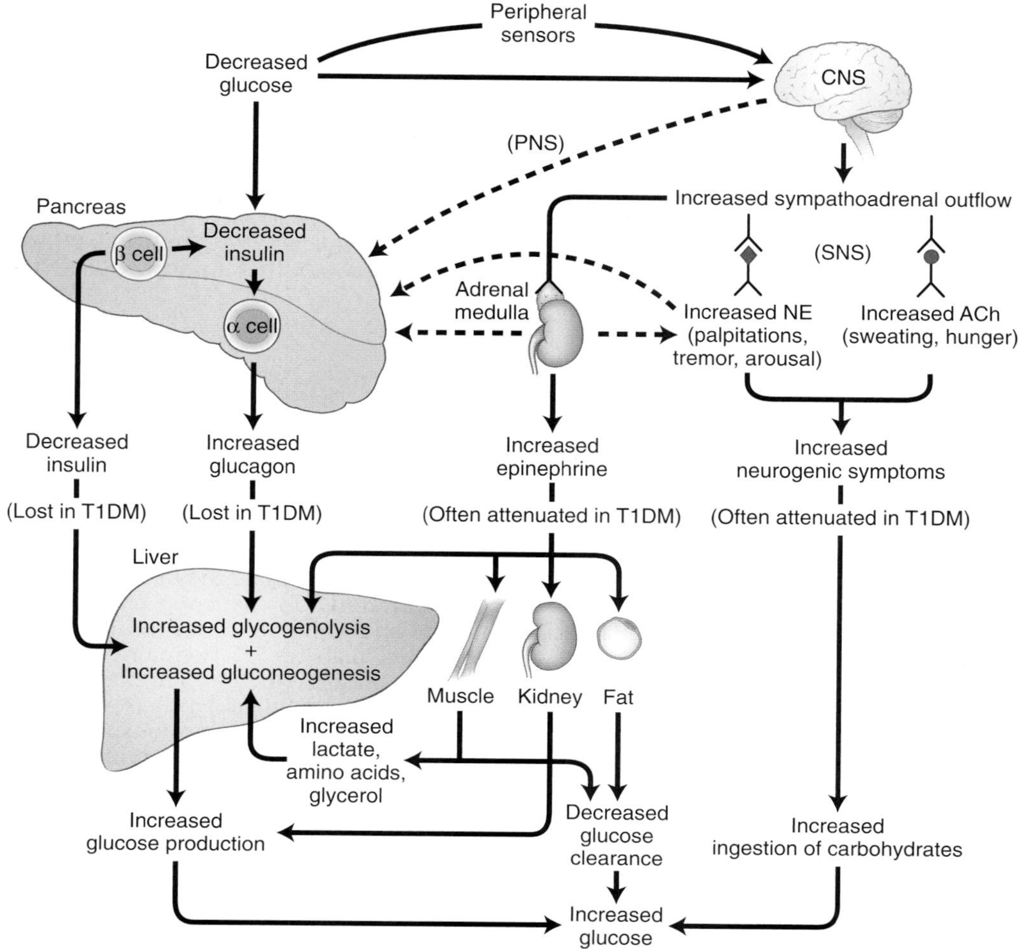

Figure 34-3 Physiologic and behavioral defenses against hypoglycemia in humans. α-cell, pancreatic islet alpha cells; β-cell, pancreatic islet beta cells; ACh, acetylcholine; NE, norepinephrine; PNS, parasympathetic nervous system; SNS, sympathetic nervous system; T1DM, type 1 diabetes. (From Cryer PE. Mechanisms of sympathoadrenal failure and hypoglycemia in diabetes. *J Clin Invest.* 2006;116:1470-1473, with permission of the American Society for Clinical Investigation.)

The key physiologic defenses against falling plasma glucose concentrations are (1) a decrease in insulin, (2) an increase in glucagon, and, in the absence of the latter, (3) an increase in epinephrine.[3,4] The behavioral defense is carbohydrate ingestion prompted by symptoms that are largely sympathetic neural in origin (see Table 34-2 and Fig. 34-3).[3,4,13]

The first physiologic defense against hypoglycemia is a decrease in insulin secretion by the pancreatic islet beta cells. Signaled primarily by declining glucose levels at the beta cells, this response occurs as plasma glucose concentrations decline within the physiologic range[3,4] (see Table 34-2) and favors increased hepatic and renal glucose production with virtual cessation of glucose utilization by insulin-sensitive tissues such as muscle (see Fig. 34-3).[3,4]

The second physiologic defense against hypoglycemia is an increase in glucagon secretion by pancreatic islet alpha cells. This occurs as plasma glucose concentrations fall just below the physiologic range[3,4] (see Table 34-2) and stimulates hepatic glucose production, largely by stimulating glycogenolysis (see Fig. 34-3).[3,4] This response is signaled primarily by a decrease in intraislet insulin, perhaps among other beta-cell secretory products, in the setting of low alpha-cell glucose concentrations[3,4,15] (see Fig. 34-3) and only secondarily by increased autonomic nervous system (sympathetic, parasympathetic, adrenomedullary) inputs.[3,4,16]

The third physiologic defense against hypoglycemia, which becomes critical when glucagon is deficient, is an increase in adrenomedullary epinephrine secretion. Signaled via the CNS, it, too, occurs as plasma glucose concentrations fall just below the physiologic range[3,4] (see Table 34-2) and raises plasma glucose concentrations largely by β_2-adrenergic stimulation of hepatic and renal glucose production (see Fig. 34-3).[3,4] However, the plasma glucose-raising actions of epinephrine also involve limitation of glucose clearance by insulin-sensitive tissues, mobilization of gluconeogenic precursors such as lactate and amino acids from muscle and glycerol from fat, and α_2-adrenergic limitation of insulin secretion (Fig. 34-4).[3,4,17]

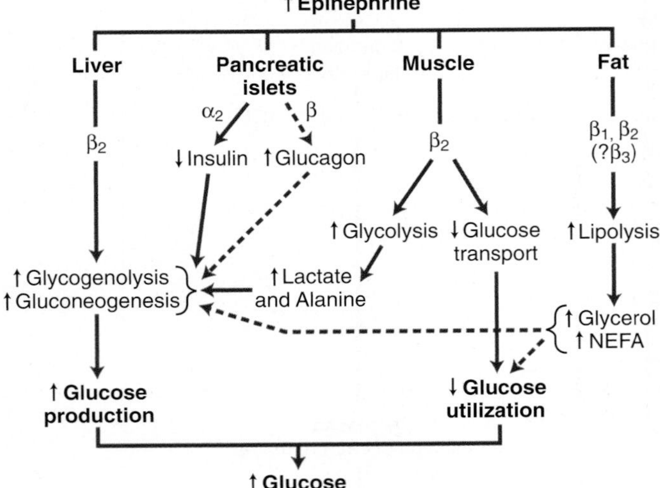

Figure 34-4 Schematic representation of the mechanisms of the hyperglycemic effect of epinephrine, mediated by α- and β-adrenergic stimulation. NEFA, nonesterified fatty acids. (From Cryer PE. Catecholamines, pheochromocytoma and diabetes. *Diabetes Rev.* 1993;1:309-317, with permission of the American Diabetes Association.)

Indeed, the adrenergic actions on beta-cell insulin secretion normally play an important role in the glycemic actions of epinephrine. α_2-Adrenergic limitation of insulin secretion permits the glycemic response; β_2-adrenergic stimulation alone has little effect because it also stimulates insulin secretion.[4] On the other hand, some increase in insulin secretion—due to the rising glucose level, β_2-adrenergic stimulation, or both—limits the magnitude of the glycemic response to epinephrine.[17] These physiologic interactions explain why glycemic sensitivity to epinephrine is increased in patients who cannot increase insulin secretion (e.g., those with type 1 diabetes).[17] Circulating epinephrine is derived almost exclusively from the adrenal medulla in adults.[13] Whereas circulating norepinephrine is derived largely from sympathetic nerve terminals under resting conditions and in many stimulated states (e.g., exercise), the plasma norepinephrine response to hypoglycemia is derived largely from the adrenal medulla.[13]

These physiologic defenses against hypoglycemia typically abort episodes of declining plasma glucose concentration and prevent clinical (i.e., symptomatic) hypoglycemia. If they do not, the lower plasma glucose concentration causes a more intense sympathoadrenal response, resulting in symptoms (see Table 34-2).[3,4] These symptoms, particularly the neurogenic symptoms, cause awareness of hypoglycemia that prompts the behavioral defense against hypoglycemia, ingestion of carbohydrates (see Fig. 34-3).[3,4]

The integrated physiology of glucose counterregulation[2-4] is further illustrated in Figure 34-5. Falling glucose levels within the pancreatic islets signal a decrease in insulin secretion and an increase in glucagon secretion. Falling glucose levels sensed in the periphery and in the CNS, acting through the hypothalamus, signal an increase in sympathoadrenal activity that results in an increase in adrenomedullary epinephrine secretion and in neurogenic symptoms, the latter largely resulting from increased sympathetic neural activity. The figure includes a putative cerebral network that may modulate the hypothalamic response.

CLINICAL HYPOGLYCEMIA

Definition and Diagnosis

Clinical hypoglycemia is, by definition, a plasma glucose concentration low enough to cause symptoms or signs, including impairment of brain function.[2] The glycemic thresholds for symptoms and signs of hypoglycemia are dynamic; for example, they shift to lower plasma glucose concentrations in patients with recurrent hypoglycemia[18,19] and to higher concentrations in those with poorly controlled diabetes.[19,20] Therefore, it is not possible to state a single plasma glucose concentration that categorically defines hypoglycemia. Furthermore, the symptoms and signs of hypoglycemia are nonspecific,[2,3] and a low measured plasma glucose concentration can be artifactual.[2] For all of these reasons, hypoglycemia is most convincingly documented by Whipple's triad: symptoms, signs, or both consistent with hypoglycemia; a low measured plasma glucose concentration; and resolution of those symptoms or signs after the plasma glucose concentration is raised.[2,3]

Documentation of Whipple's triad is particularly important when hypoglycemia is suspected in a person who does not have diabetes mellitus, because hypoglycemic disorders are rare.[2] In the absence of diabetes, a thorough

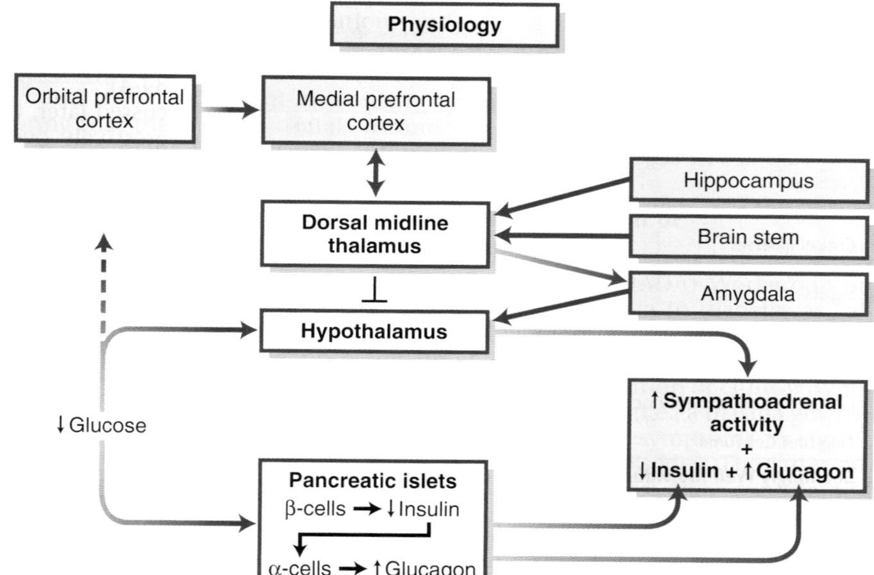

Figure 34-5 Schematic representation of the integrated mechanisms of the physiologic responses to hypoglycemia in humans: decrements in insulin secretion, increments in glucagon secretion, and increments in sympathoadrenal (adrenomedullary and sympathetic neural) activity. α-Cells, pancreatic islet alpha cells; β-Cells, pancreatic islet beta cells. (From Cryer PE. Hypoglycemia. In Cryer PE. *Diabetes: Pathophysiology, Prevalence and Prevention.* Alexandria, VA: American Diabetes Association, 2009, with permission of the American Diabetes Association.)

diagnostic evaluation is recommended only for patients in whom Whipple's triad is documented.[2] Ideally, patients with diabetes being treated with an insulin secretagogue or insulin should monitor their plasma glucose concentration whenever they suspect hypoglycemia.[2,3] However, that is sometimes not practical, and it often is not done. Nonetheless, the likelihood that a symptomatic episode is the result of hypoglycemia is high, because hypoglycemia is common in such patients.[3] Given the potential detrimental effects of an untreated episode of hypoglycemia, documentation of Whipple's triad may be less critical to the diagnosis of an episode of hypoglycemia in patients with diabetes treated with these medications.

General Mechanisms of Hypoglycemia

Hypoglycemia develops when glucose efflux out of the circulation exceeds glucose influx into the circulation. Glucose efflux is the sum of ongoing obligatory glucose utilization, largely by the brain, and regulated glucose utilization by insulin-sensitive tissues, and glucose influx is the sum of endogenous glucose production and exogenous glucose delivery from ingested carbohydrates (see Table 34-1). Although hypoglycemia can result from excessive glucose efflux, it is typically the result of glucose influx that is too low—either absolutely low or low relative to high rates of glucose efflux.

Clinical Classification of Hypoglycemia

Causes of hypoglycemia[2] are outlined in Table 34-3. Drugs are, by far, the most common cause of hypoglycemia. Those include insulin secretagogues and insulin used to treat diabetes. Although persons with diabetes can suffer from the same hypoglycemic disorders as those without diabetes, their hypoglycemic episodes are usually the result of treatment of their diabetes.[2,3] Furthermore, the pathophysiology of hypoglycemia in diabetes is unique, and the diagnostic and management approaches are different from those for individuals without diabetes.[2,3] Therefore, hypoglycemia in persons with diabetes and hypoglycemia in those without diabetes are discussed separately in this chapter.

HYPOGLYCEMIA IN PERSONS WITH DIABETES

The Clinical Problem of Hypoglycemia in Diabetes

Iatrogenic hypoglycemia is the limiting factor in the glycemic management of diabetes.[3] It causes recurrent morbidity in most persons with type 1 diabetes mellitus (T1DM) and in many of those with advanced type 2 diabetes mellitus (T2DM), and it is sometimes fatal. The barrier of hypoglycemia precludes maintenance of euglycemia over a lifetime of diabetes and thus full realization of the vascular benefits of glycemic control. Furthermore, hypoglycemia compromises physiologic and behavioral defenses against subsequent falling plasma glucose concentrations, resulting in a vicious cycle of recurrent hypoglycemia.

Hypoglycemia in diabetes is caused by pharmacokinetically imperfect treatment with an insulin secretagogue (such as a sulfonylurea or a glinide) or with insulin that results in episodes of therapeutic hyperinsulinemia. Thus, it is fundamentally iatrogenic. Episodes of substantial absolute therapeutic hyperinsulinemia can cause isolated episodes of hypoglycemia. However, as developed later in this chapter, recurrent hypoglycemia in diabetes is typically the result of the interplay of relative or mild to moderate absolute therapeutic hyperinsulinemia and compromised physiologic and behavioral defenses against falling plasma glucose concentrations.[3]

Frequency of Hypoglycemia in Diabetes

Hypoglycemia is a fact of life for people with T1DM (Table 34-4).[3,21-25] The average patient suffers untold numbers of episodes of asymptomatic hypoglycemia (which are not benign because they impair defenses against subsequent hypoglycemia), approximately two episodes of symptomatic hypoglycemia per week (thousands of such episodes over a lifetime of diabetes), and roughly one episode per year of severe, at least temporarily disabling hypoglycemia, often with seizure or coma. This problem has not abated since it was highlighted by the report of the Diabetes Control and Complications Trial (DCCT)[21] in 1993. In

137. Huang ES, Zhang Q, Gandra N, et al. The effect of comorbid illness and functional status on the expected benefits of intensive glucose control in older patients with type 2 diabetes: a decision analysis. *Ann Intern Med.* 2008;149:11-19.
138. MacCuish AC. Treatment of hypoglycemia. In: Frier BM, Fisher BM, eds. *Diabetes and Hypoglycemia*, London: Edward Arnold; 1993;212-221.
139. Wiethop BV, Cryer PE. Alanine and terbutaline in treatment of hypoglycemia in IDDM. *Diabetes Care.* 1993;16:1131-1136.
140. Haymond MW, Schreiner B. Mini-dose glucagon rescue for hypoglycemia in children with type 1 diabetes. *Diabetes Care.* 2001;24: 643-645.
141. Jackson RA, Peters N, Advani U, et al. Forearm glucose uptake during the oral glucose tolerance test in normal subjects. *Diabetes.* 1973;22:442-458.
142. Service FJ. Hypoglycemic disorders. *N Engl J Med.* 1995;332:1144-1152.
143. Fischer KF, Lees JA, Newman JH. Hypoglycemia in hospitalized patients: causes and outcomes. *N Engl J Med.* 1986;315:1245-1250.
144. Malouf R, Brust JC. Hypoglycemia: causes, neurological manifestations, and outcome. *Ann Neurol.* 1985;17:421-430.
145. Marks V, Teale JD. Drug-induced hypoglycemia. *Endocrinol Metab Clin North Am.* 1999;28:555-577.
146. Park-Wyllie LY, Juurlink DN, Kopp A, et al. Outpatient gatifloxacin therapy and dysglycemia in older adults. *N Engl J Med.* 2006;354:1352-1361.
147. Murad MH, Coto-Yglesias F, Wang AT, et al. Drug-induced hypoglycemia: a systematic review. *J Clin Endocrinol Metab.* 2009;. 94:741-745.
148. Cohen MR, Proulx SM, Crawford SY. Survey of hospital systems and common serious medication errors. *J Healthc Risk Manag.* 1998;18:16-27.
149. Felig P, Brown WV, Levine RA, et al. Glucose homeostasis in viral hepatitis. *N Engl J Med.* 1970;283:1436-1440.
150. Younus S, Soterakis J, Sossi AJ, et al. Hypoglycemia secondary to metastases to the liver: a case report and review of the literature. *Gastroenterology.* 1977;72:334-337.
151. Haviv YS, Sharkia M, Safadi R. Hypoglycemia in patients with renal failure. *Ren Fail.* 2000;22:219-223.
152. Garber AJ, Bier DM, Cryer PE, et al. Hypoglycemia in compensated chronic renal insufficiency: substrate limitation of gluconeogenesis. *Diabetes.* 1974;23:982-986.
153. Rutsky EA, McDaniel HG, Tharpe DL, et al. Spontaneous hypoglycemia in chronic renal failure. *Arch Intern Med.* 1978;138:1364-1368.
154. Chen YT, Burchell A. Glycogen storage diseases. In: Scriver CR, Beaudet AL, Sly WS, et al, eds. *The Metabolic and Molecular Bases of Inherited Disease*, 7th ed. New York, NY: McGraw Hill; 1995:935-965.
155. Medalle R, Webb R, Waterhouse C. Lactic acidosis and associated hypoglycemia. *Arch Intern Med.* 1971;128:273-278.
156. Miller SI, Wallace RJ Jr, Musher DM, et al. Hypoglycemia as a manifestation of sepsis. *Am J Med.* 1980;68:649-654.
157. Maitra SR, Wojnar MM, Lang CH. Alterations in tissue glucose uptake during the hyperglycemic and hypoglycemic phases of sepsis. *Shock.* 2000;13:379-385.
158. Sakurai Y, Zhang XJ, Wolfe RR. TNF directly stimulates glucose uptake and leucine oxidation and inhibits FFA flux in conscious dogs. *Am J Physiol.* 1996;270:E864-E872.
159. Metzger S, Nusair S, Planer D, et al. Inhibition of hepatic gluconeogenesis and enhanced glucose uptake contribute to the development of hypoglycemia in mice bearing interleukin-1beta- secreting tumor. *Endocrinology.* 2004;145:5150-5156.
160. Hargrove DM, Lang CH, Bagby GJ, et al. Epinephrine-induced increase in glucose turnover is diminished during sepsis. *Metabolism.* 1989;38:1070-1076.
161. Wharton B. Hypoglycaemia in children with kwashiorkor. *Lancet.* 1970;1:171-173.
162. Bruce AK, Jacobsen E, Dossing H, et al. Hypoglycaemia in spinal muscular atrophy. *Lancet.* 1995;346:609-610.
163. Ørngreen MC, Zacho M, Hebert A, et al. Patients with severe muscle wasting are prone to develop hypoglycemia during fasting. *Neurology.* 2003;61:997-1000.
164. Goodman HG, Grumbach MM, Kaplan SL. Growth and growth hormone. II: A comparison of isolated growth-hormone deficiency and multiple pituitary-hormone deficiencies in 35 patients with idiopathic hypopituitary dwarfism. *N Engl J Med.* 1968;278:57-68.
165. Haymond MW, Karl I, Weldon VV, et al. The role of growth hormone and cortisone on glucose and gluconeogenic substrate regulation in fasted hypopituitary children. *J Clin Endocrinol Metab.* 1976; 42:846-856.
166. Wolfsdorf JI, Sadeghi-Nejad A, Senior B. Hypoketonemia and age-related fasting hypoglycemia in growth hormone deficiency. *Metabolism.* 1983;32:457-462.
167. Frizzell RT, Campbell PJ, Cherrington AD. Gluconeogenesis and hypoglycemia. *Diabetes Metab Rev.* 1988;4:51-70.
168. Boyle PJ, Cryer PE. Growth hormone, cortisol, or both are involved in defense against, but are not critical to recovery from, hypoglycemia. *Am J Physiol.* 1991;260:E395-E402.
169. Smallridge RC, Corrigan DF, Thomason AM, et al. Hypoglycemia in pregnancy: occurrence due to adrenocorticotropic hormone and growth hormone deficiency. *Arch Intern Med.* 1980;140:564-565.
170. Steer P, Marnell R, Werk EE Jr. Clinical alcohol hypoglycemia and isolated adrenocorticotrophic hormone deficiency. *Ann Intern Med.* 1969;71:343-348.
171. Fukuda I, Hizuka N, Ishikawa Y, et al. Clinical features of insulin-like growth factor-II producing non-islet-cell tumor hypoglycemia. *Growth Horm IGF Res.* 2006;16:211-216.
172. Nauck MA, Reinecke M, Perren A, et al. Hypoglycemia due to paraneoplastic secretion of insulin-like growth factor-I in a patient with metastasizing large-cell carcinoma of the lung. *J Clin Endocrinol Metab.* 2007;92:1600-1605.
173. Daughaday WH. Hypoglycemia due to paraneoplastic secretion of insulin-like growth factor-I. *J Clin Endocrinol Metab.* 2007;92: 1616.
174. Miraki-Moud F, Grossman AB, Besser M, et al. A rapid method for analyzing serum pro-insulin-like growth factor-II in patients with non-islet cell tumor hypoglycemia. *J Clin Endocrinol Metab.* 2005;90:3819-3823.
175. Guettier JM, Gorden P. Hypoglycemia. *Endocrinol Metab Clin North Am.* 2006;35:753-766.
176. Marks V, Teale JD. Hypoglycemia: factitious and felonious. *Endocrinol Metab Clin North Am.* 1999;28:579-601.
177. Service FJ, Palumbo PJ. Factitial hypoglycemia: three cases diagnosed on the basis of insulin antibodies. *Arch Intern Med.* 1974;134: 336-340.
178. Giurgea I, Ulinski T, Touati G, et al. Factitious hyperinsulinism leading to pancreatectomy: severe forms of Munchausen syndrome by proxy. *Pediatrics.* 2005;116:e145-e148.
179. Manning PJ, Espiner EA, Yoon K, et al. An unusual cause of hyperinsulinaemic hypoglycaemia syndrome. *Diabet Med.* 2003;20: 772-776.
180. Placzkowski KA, Vella A, Thompson GB, et al. Secular trends in the presentation and management of functioning insulinoma at the Mayo Clinic, 1987-2007. *J Clin Endocrinol Metab.* 2009;94:1069-1073.
181. Service FJ, McMahon MM, O'Brien PC, et al. Functioning insulinoma—incidence, recurrence, and long-term survival of patients: a 60-year study. *Mayo Clin Proc.* 1991;66:711-719.
182. Anlauf M, Wieben D, Perren A, et al. Persistent hyperinsulinemic hypoglycemia in 15 adults with diffuse nesidioblastosis: diagnostic criteria, incidence, and characterization of beta-cell changes. *Am J Surg Pathol.* 2005;29:524-533.
183. Klöppel G, Anlauf M, Raffel A, et al. Adult diffuse nesidioblastosis: genetically or environmentally induced? *Hum Pathol.* 2008;39:3-8.
184. Kaczirek K, Soleiman A, Schindl M, et al. Nesidioblastosis in adults: a challenging cause of organic hyperinsulinism. *Eur J Clin Invest.* 2003;33:488-492.
185. Witteles RM, Straus FH II, Sugg SL, et al. Adult-onset nesidioblastosis causing hypoglycemia: an important clinical entity and continuing treatment dilemma. *Arch Surg.* 2001;136:656-663.
186. Service FJ, Natt N, Thompson GB, et al. Noninsulinoma pancreatogenous hypoglycemia: a novel syndrome of hyperinsulinemic hypoglycemia in adults independent of mutations in Kir6.2 and SUR1 genes. *J Clin Endocrinol Metab.* 1999;84:1582-1589.
187. Starke A, Saddig C, Kirch B, et al. Islet hyperplasia in adults: challenge to preoperatively diagnose non-insulinoma pancreatogenic hypoglycemia syndrome. *World J Surg.* 2006;30:670-679.
188. Thompson GB, Service FJ, Andrews JC, et al. Noninsulinoma pancreatogenous hypoglycemia syndrome: an update in 10 surgically treated patients. *Surgery.* 2000;128:937-944;discussion 944-945.
189. Won JG, Tseng HS, Yang AH, et al. Clinical features and morphological characterization of 10 patients with noninsulinoma pancreatogenous hypoglycaemia syndrome (NIPHS). *Clin Endocrinol (Oxf).* 2006;65: 566-578.
190. Service GJ, Thompson GB, Service FJ, et al. Hyperinsulinemic hypoglycemia with nesidioblastosis after gastric-bypass surgery. *N Engl J Med.* 2005;353:249-254.
191. Patti ME, McMahon G, Mun EC, et al. Severe hypoglycaemia post-gastric bypass requiring partial pancreatectomy: evidence for inappropriate insulin secretion and pancreatic islet hyperplasia. *Diabetologia.* 2005;48:2236-2240.
192. Goldfine A, Mun E, Patti M. Hyperinsulinemic hypoglycemia following gastric bypass surgery for obesity. *Cur Opin Endocrinol Diabetes.* 2006;13:419-424.
193. Goldfine AB, Mun EC, Devine E, et al. Patients with neuroglycopenia after gastric bypass surgery have exaggerated incretin and insulin secretory responses to a mixed meal. *J Clin Endocrinol Metab.* 2007;92:4678-4685.
194. Meier JJ, Butler AE, Galasso R, et al. Hyperinsulinemic hypoglycemia after gastric bypass surgery is not accompanied by islet hyperplasia or increased beta-cell turnover. *Diabetes Care.* 2006;29:1554-1559.
195. Vella A, Service FJ. Incretin hypersecretion in post-gastric bypass hypoglycemia: primary problem or red herring? *J Clin Endocrinol Metab.* 2007;92:4563-4565.

196. Vidal J, Nicolau J, Romero F, et al. Long-term effects of roux-en-Y gastric bypass surgery on plasma GLP-1 and islet function in morbidly obese subjects. *J Clin Endocrinol Metab*. 2008;. 94:884-891.
197. Hirata Y, Ishizu H, Ouchi N, et al. Insulin autoimmunity in a case with spontaneous hypoglycemia. *J Jap Diabetes Soc*. 1970;13:312-320.
198. Basu A, Service FJ, Yu L, et al. Insulin autoimmunity and hypoglycemia in seven white patients. *Endocr Pract*. 2005;11:97-103.
199. Halsall DJ, Mangi M, Soos M, et al. Hypoglycemia due to an insulin binding antibody in a patient with an IgA-kappa myeloma. *J Clin Endocrinol Metab*. 2007;92:2013-2016.
200. Højlund K, Hansen T, Lajer M, et al. A novel syndrome of autosomal-dominant hyperinsulinemic hypoglycemia linked to a mutation in the human insulin receptor gene. *Diabetes*. 2004;53:1592-1598.
201. Meissner T, Friedmann B, Okun JG, et al. Massive insulin secretion in response to anaerobic exercise in exercise-induced hyperinsulinism. *Horm Metab Res*. 2005;37:690-694.
202. Arioglu E, Andewelt A, Diabo C, et al. Clinical course of the syndrome of autoantibodies to the insulin receptor (type B insulin resistance): a 28-year perspective. *Medicine (Baltimore)*. 2002;81:87-100.
203. Seckl MJ, Mulholland PJ, Bishop AE, et al. Hypoglycemia due to an insulin-secreting small-cell carcinoma of the cervix. *N Engl J Med*. 1999;341:733-736.
204. Rizza RA, Haymond MW, Verdonk CA, et al. Pathogenesis of hypoglycemia in insulinoma patients: suppression of hepatic glucose production by insulin. *Diabetes*. 1981;30:377-381.
205. Service FJ, Natt N. The prolonged fast. *J Clin Endocrinol Metab*. 2000;85:3973-3974.
206. Vezzosi D, Bennet A, Fauvel J, et al. Insulin, C-peptide and proinsulin for the biochemical diagnosis of hypoglycaemia related to endogenous hyperinsulinism. *Eur J Endocrinol*. 2007;157:75-83.
207. Noone TC, Hosey J, Firat Z, et al. Imaging and localization of islet-cell tumours of the pancreas on CT and MRI. *Best Pract Res Clin Endocrinol Metab*. 2005;19:195-211.
208. Grossman AB, Reznek RH. Commentary: imaging of islet-cell tumours. *Best Pract Res Clin Endocrinol Metab*. 2005;19:241-243.
209. Virgolini I, Traub-Weidinger T, Decristoforo C. Nuclear medicine in the detection and management of pancreatic islet-cell tumours. *Best Pract Res Clin Endocrinol Metab*. 2005;19:213-227.
210. Kumbasar B, Kamel IR, Tekes A, et al. Imaging of neuroendocrine tumors: accuracy of helical CT versus SRS. *Abdom Imaging*. 2004;29:696-702.
211. Fritscher-Ravens A. Endoscopic ultrasound and neuroendocrine tumours of the pancreas. *JOP*. 2004;5:273-281.
212. Kauhanen S, Seppänen M, Minn H, et al. Fluorine-18-L-dihydroxyphenylalanine (18F-DOPA) positron emission tomography as a tool to localize an insulinoma or beta-cell hyperplasia in adult patients. *J Clin Endocrinol Metab*. 2007;92:1237-1244.
213. Brown CK, Bartlett DL, Doppman JL, et al. Intraarterial calcium stimulation and intraoperative ultrasonography in the localization and resection of insulinomas. *Surgery*. 1997;122:1189-1193; discussion 1193-1194.
214. Doppman JL, Miller DL, Chang R, et al. Insulinomas: localization with selective intraarterial injection of calcium. *Radiology*. 1991;178:237-241.
215. Wiesli P, Brändle M, Schmid C, et al. Selective arterial calcium stimulation and hepatic venous sampling in the evaluation of hyperinsulinemic hypoglycemia: potential and limitations. *J Vasc Interv Radiol*. 2004;15:1251-1256.
216. Jackson JE. Angiography and arterial stimulation venous sampling in the localization of pancreatic neuroendocrine tumours. *Best Pract Res Clin Endocrinol Metab*. 2005;19:229-239.
217. Dekelbab BH, Sperling MA. Hypoglycemia in newborns and infants. *Adv Pediatr*. 2006;53:5-22.
218. Hoe FM. Hypoglycemia in infants and children. *Adv Pediatr*. 2008;55:367-384.
219. Rozance PJ, Hay WW. Hypoglycemia in newborn infants: Features associated with adverse outcomes. *Biol Neonate*. 2006;90:74-86.
220. Losek JD. Hypoglycemia and the ABC'S (sugar) of pediatric resuscitation. *Ann Emerg Med*. 2000;35:43-46.
221. Haymond MW, Karl IE, Pagliara AS. Increased gluconeogenic substrates in the small-for-gestational-age infant. *N Engl J Med*. 1974;291:322-328.
222. Haymond MW, Karl IE, Pagliara AS. Ketotic hypoglycemia: an amino acid substrate limited disorder. *J Clin Endocrinol Metab*. 1974;38:521-530.
223. Palladino AA, Bennett MJ, Stanley CA. Hyperinsulinism in infancy and childhood: when an insulin level is not always enough. *Clin Chem*. 2008;54:256-263.
224. Pinney SE, MacMullen C, Becker S, et al. Clinical characteristics and biochemical mechanisms of congenital hyperinsulinism associated with dominant KATP channel mutations. *J Clin Invest*. 2008;118:2877-2886.
225. de Lonlay P, Simon-Carre A, Ribeiro MJ, et al. Congenital hyperinsulinism: pancreatic [18F]fluoro-L-dihydroxyphenylalanine (DOPA) positron emission tomography and immunohistochemistry study of DOPA decarboxylase and insulin secretion. *J Clin Endocrinol Metab*. 2006;91:933-940.
226. Ribeiro MJ, Boddaert N, Bellanné-Chantelot C, et al. The added value of [18F]fluoro-L-DOPA PET in the diagnosis of hyperinsulinism of infancy: a retrospective study involving 49 children. *Eur J Nucl Med Mol Imaging*. 2007;34:2120-2128.
227. Hardy OT, Hernandez-Pampaloni M, Saffer JR, et al. Accuracy of [18F] fluorodopa positron emission tomography for diagnosing and localizing focal congenital hyperinsulinism. *J Clin Endocrinol Metab*. 2007;92:4706-4711.
228. Yang Chou J, Mansfield BC. Molecular genetics of type 1 glycogen storage diseases. *Trends Endocrinol Metab*. 1999;10:104-113.
229. Weghuber D, Mandl M, Krssák M, et al. Characterization of hepatic and brain metabolism in young adults with glycogen storage disease type 1: a magnetic resonance spectroscopy study. *Am J Physiol Endocrinol Metab*. 2007;293:E1378-E1384.
230. Muraca M, Gerunda G, Neri D, et al. Hepatocyte transplantation as a treatment for glycogen storage disease type 1a. *Lancet*. 2002;359:317-318.
231. Brown GK. Glucose transporters: structure, function and consequences of deficiency. *J Inherit Metab Dis*. 2000;23:237-246.
232. Roe CR, Coates PM. Mitochondrial fatty acid oxidation disorders. In: Scriver CR, Beaudet AL, Sly WS, et al, eds. *The Metabolic and Molecular Bases of Inherited Disease*, 7th ed. New York, NY: McGraw-Hill; 1995:1501-1533.
233. Stanley CA. Dissecting the spectrum of fatty acid oxidation disorders. *J Pediatr*. 1998;132:384-386.
234. Nezu J, Tamai I, Oku A, et al. Primary systemic carnitine deficiency is caused by mutations in a gene encoding sodium ion-dependent carnitine transporter. *Nat Genet*. 1999;21:91-94.
235. Vianey-Saban C, Guffon N, Delolne F, et al. Diagnosis of inborn errors of metabolism by acylcarnitine profiling in blood using tandem mass spectrometry. *J Inherit Metab Dis*. 1997;20:411-414.
236. Bougnères PF, Saudubray JM, Marsac C, et al. Fasting hypoglycemia resulting from hepatic carnitine palmitoyl transferase deficiency. *J Pediatr*. 1981;98:742-746.

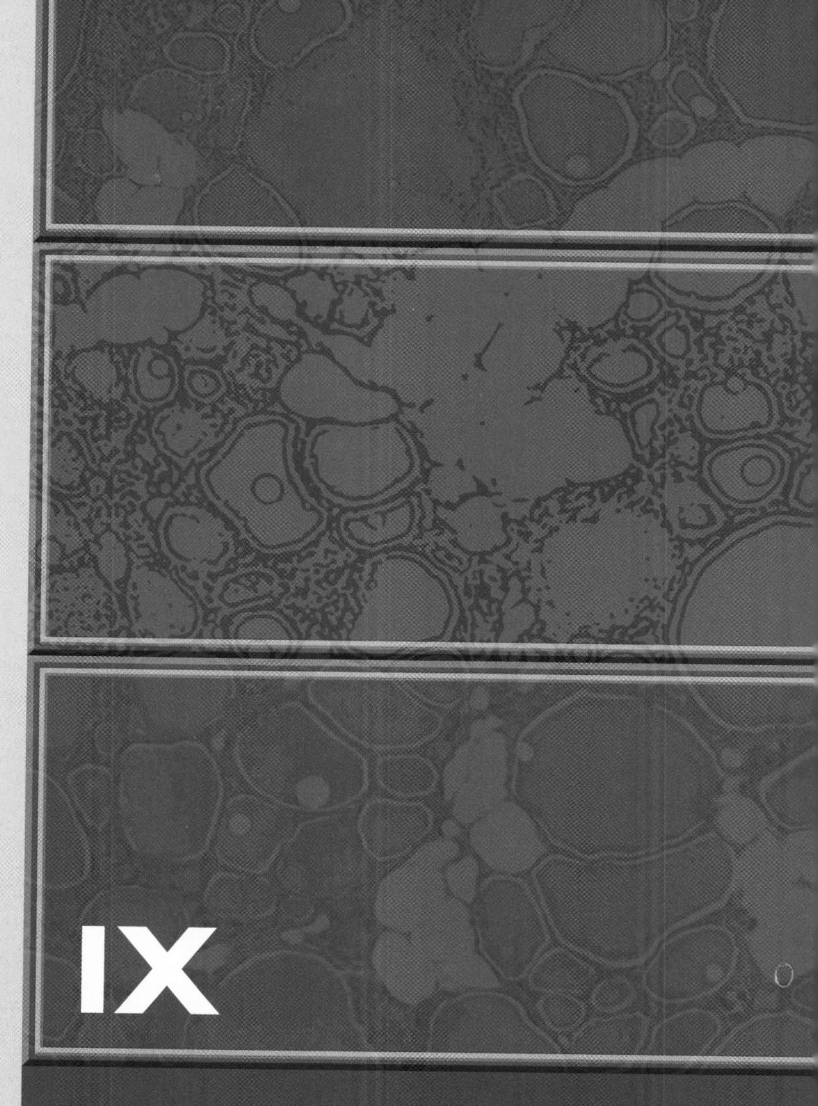

SECTION IX

Body Fat and Lipid Metabolism

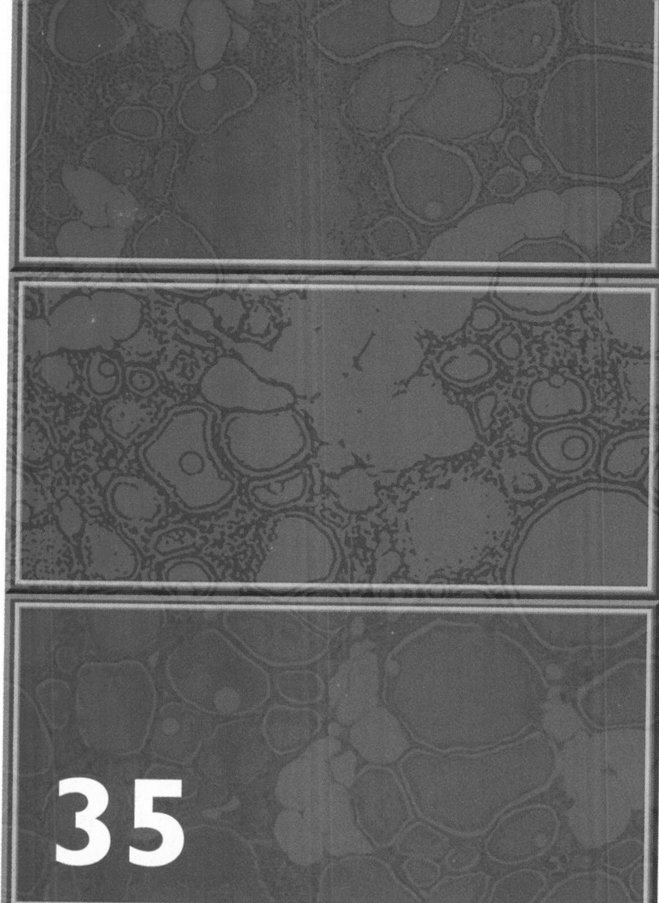

CHAPTER 35

Neuroendocrine Control of Energy Stores

ROGER D. CONE • JOEL K. ELMQUIST

HISTORICAL PERSPECTIVE

The increasing incidence of obesity and diabetes is a major health issue facing society. In the past decade, several key molecules, including hormones and receptors controlling energy homeostasis, have been identified. We now have a rough central nervous system (CNS) road map of the pathways through which key metabolic signals exert their effects. For example, it is established that key components of the central control of energy balance are located in the hypothalamus. In the 21st century, it is taken for granted that the hypothalamus is required for coordinated control of food intake and energy homeostasis. The intimate interaction of the hypothalamus and the pituitary gland has been appreciated for some time. However, understanding of the primary role of the hypothalamus in controlling long-term energy stores and, consequently, adipose mass is relatively recent.

For example, at the end of the 19th century, clinicians including Alfred Fröhlich described an adiposogenital dystrophic condition in patients with pituitary tumors. This condition became known as Fröhlich's syndrome and was characterized by pituitary tumors associated with excessive subcutaneous fat and hypogonadism.[1,2] However, whether this syndrome was caused by injury to the pituitary gland or damage to the overlying hypothalamus was extremely controversial. Several groups, including Cushing and his colleagues, argued that the syndrome was caused by disruption of the pituitary gland.[3-5] However, Aschner demonstrated in dogs that mere removal of the pituitary gland without damage to the overlying hypothalamus did not result in obesity.[6] The most definitive evidence of the vital role of the hypothalamus was provided by Hetherington and Ranson when they demonstrated that destruction of the medial basal hypothalamus without damage to the pituitary gland could result in morbid obesity and neuroendocrine derangements in a very similar fashion to the syndrome reported by Fröhlich.[7] These and subsequent studies firmly established that an intact hypothalamus is required for normal energy and glucose homeostasis.

After the discoveries that hypothalamic lesions could cause obesity, it also became apparent that lesions in other regions, such as the lateral hypothalamus, could cause leanness. Based on these results, it was suggested that a feeding center was located in the lateral hypothalamus and a satiety center in the ventromedial hypothalamus (VMH).[8] As a result of these and other studies, the importance of the hypothalamus as an integrator and effector of energy balance and neuroendocrine function was generally accepted.

Humans and other mammals have a remarkable ability to match caloric intake and expenditure, leading to relative stability of body weight and adipose mass over long periods. Based on this observation, Kennedy[9] proposed a mechanism of body weight regulation in which a signal related to energy stores elicited compensatory changes in food intake and energy expenditure, with the result being maintenance of adipose mass at a presumed set point. This view was supported by studies in rodents showing that weight gain from forced overfeeding resulted in a compensatory decrease in voluntary food intake, increased energy expenditure, and eventual restoration of body weight to the previous level, whereas starvation or lipectomy stimulated feeding and decreased energy expenditure, restoring body weight and adipose mass to a previous set point.[10-12]

The signals mediating the potential interaction between adipose tissue and the brain were not known for many years. Studies by Hervey[13-15] offered important insights into potential signals linking energy stores with energy homeostatic mechanisms. He showed that parabiosis between obese rats with VMH lesions and normal (nonlesioned) rats led to starvation and weight loss in the latter. In contrast, the VMH-lesioned rats gained weight when parabiosed with lean rats or other VMH-lesioned rats. Results of these studies were thought to indicate that obese VMH-lesioned rats produced a circulating "satiety factor" leading to inhibition of feeding in nonlesioned parabiotic rats. The lack of response in VMH-lesioned rats was consistent with the existence of a satiety center proposed in earlier studies.[8]

This concept received further support from discovery of the *ob* and *db* recessive mutations, both of which led to hyperphagia, decreased energy expenditure, and morbid obesity.[16] Parabiosis of lean (wild-type) and *ob/ob* mice suppressed weight gain in the *ob/ob* mice, whereas parabiosis of wild-type and *db/db* mice caused profound hypophagia and weight loss in the wild-type mice.[17-19] These results were interpreted as meaning that the *ob* locus was necessary for or involved in the production of a circulating satiety factor, whereas the *db* locus encoded a component required for the response mechanism to the satiety factor. Predictions based on parabiosis studies were confirmed by the cloning of *ob* and *db* genes in the mid-1990s.[20-22] The hormone product of the *ob* gene was named "leptin" (from the Greek root *leptos,* meaning "thin") because it potently inhibited feeding, body weight, and adipose mass when injected into leptin-deficient or normal mice.[23-26]

In addition to the obese and diabetic mouse strains, the lethal yellow agouti *(AY)* mouse had long been known to express an obesity syndrome. Just as molecular cloning of the *ob* and *db* loci led to the discovery of the primary adipostatic factor and its receptor, cloning and characterization of the agouti gene[27-29] has led to characterization of one of the important CNS circuits involved in regulation of energy homeostasis, the central melanocortin system.[30,31] These and related discoveries over the past decade have taken the understanding of energy homeostasis from the level of gross anatomy to the beginnings of a cellular and molecular basis for the neuroendocrine control of energy stores, the topic of this chapter (Fig. 35-1).

FEEDING AND SATIETY CIRCUITS

As noted, key circuits regulating energy homeostasis and food intake originate in the hypothalamus and brainstem (Fig. 35-2). The hypothalamus is an essential and evolutionarily highly conserved region of the mammalian brain, and it is the ultimate brain structure that allows mammals to maintain homeostasis. Destruction of the hypothalamus is not compatible with life.[32] Hypothalamic control of homeostasis stems from the ability of hypothalamic neurons to orchestrate behavioral, autonomic, and behavioral responses. This control is derived from the anatomic connections (both inputs and outputs) of the hypothalamus.

The hypothalamus receives sensory inputs from the external environment (e.g., light) and information regarding the internal environment (e.g., blood glucose levels). In addition, several hormones known to be key in regulating food intake and metabolism (e.g., glucocorticoids, estrogen, leptin, ghrelin) directly act on neurons in the hypothalamus. The hypothalamus integrates all of this information and provides motor outputs to key regulatory sites including the anterior pituitary gland, the posterior pituitary gland, the cerebral cortex, premotor and motor neurons in the brainstem and spinal cord, and autonomic (parasympathetic and sympathetic) preganglionic neurons. The patterned hypothalamic outputs to these effector sites ultimately result in coordinated endocrine, behavioral, and autonomic responses that maintain homeostasis in several physiologic systems, including energy balance.

Within the hypothalamus, several hypothalamic sites are thought to be key in regulating energy homeostasis (see Fig. 35-1). A group of sites located in the medial hypothalamus includes the arcuate nucleus, the ventral medial nucleus, the dorsal medial nucleus, and the paraventricular nucleus. In addition, the lateral hypothalamus (lateral hypothalamic area and perifornical hypothalamus) is key in regulating food intake and energy homeostasis.

In addition to the hypothalamus, it is now clear that circuits in the brainstem are involved in the coordinated control of food intake.[33] The brain receives a wide variety of signals from visceral organs including the gastrointestinal tract. These include visceral sensory afferents that converge on the dorsal vagal complex. The dorsal vagal complex comprises the nucleus of the solitary tract (nucleus tractus solitarius; NTS), the vagal motor neurons (dorsal motor nucleus of the vagus; DMV), and the area postrema. Sensory afferent signals carried by the glossopharyngeal and vagus nerves include indications of taste, gastric stretch, and levels of glucose and lipids in the liver and portal vein. Nerve terminals carrying this information innervate the NTS. This information is relayed to the DMV. The vagal motor neurons in turn innervate the entire gastrointestinal tract including the pancreas.

In addition, key sensory inputs to the NTS from the gastrointestinal tract and taste information are directly relayed to the paraventricular, dorsomedial, and arcuate nuclei of the hypothalamus and the lateral hypothalamic area; the central nucleus of the amygdala and bed nucleus of the stria terminalis; and the parabrachial nucleus.[32,34] The parabrachial nucleus then projects to the thalamus, the cerebral cortex, the amygdala, and several hypothalamic sites.[32]

The area postrema is a circumventricular organ (CVO) that lies directly above the NTS. Unlike the NTS, which lies inside the blood-brain barrier (BBB) and therefore is not in direct contact with circulating factors and hormones,

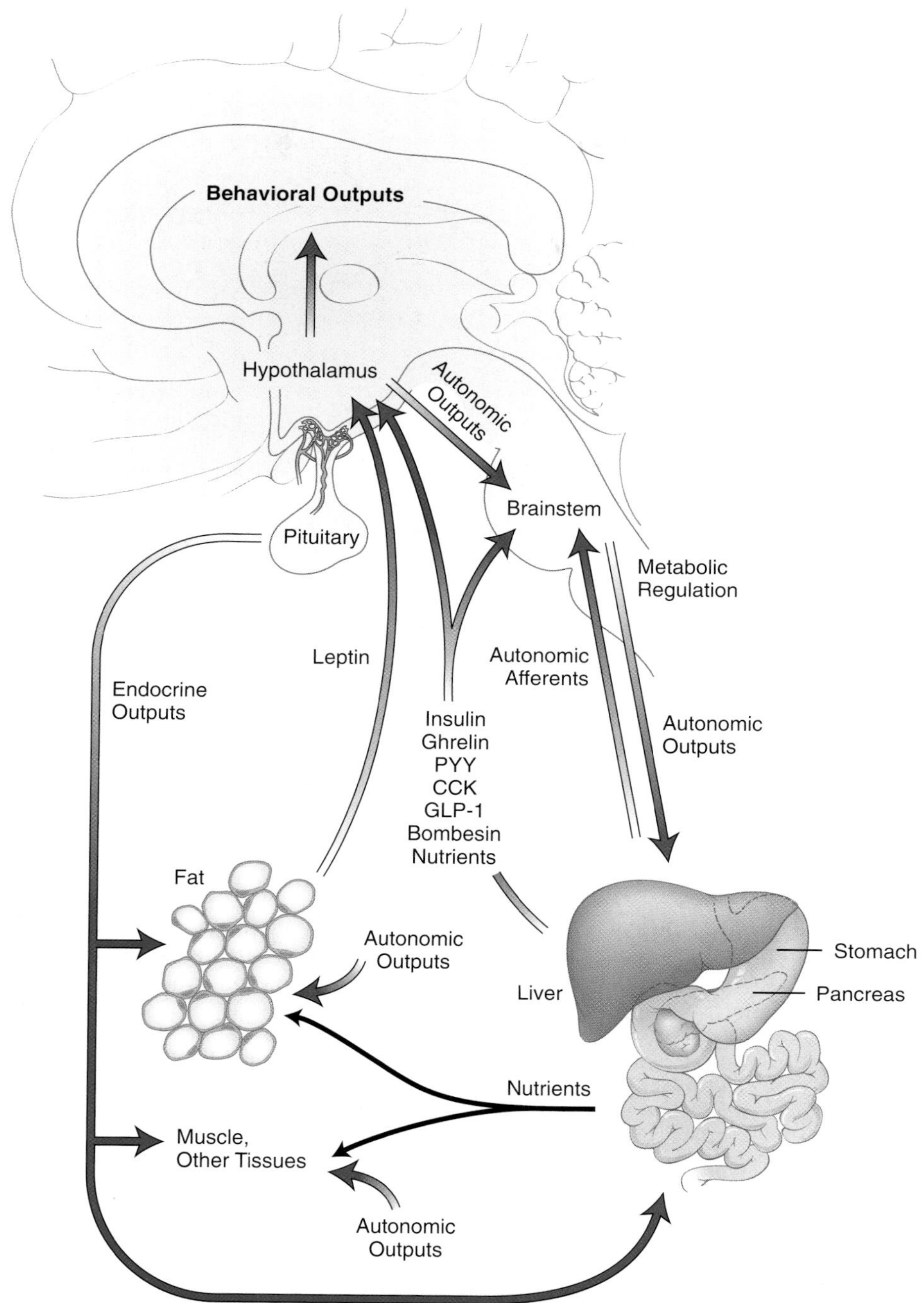

Figure 35-1 Regulation of energy homeostasis by the brain-gut-adipose axis. CCK, cholecystokinin; GLP-1, glucagon-like peptide 1; PYY, peptide YY.

neurons in the area postrema sit outside the BBB.[35] Neurons in the area postrema may respond to circulating gut hormones such as cholecystokinin (CCK) and glucagon-like peptide 1 (GLP1) and relay those signals to the NTS and the parabrachial nucleus.[36-40]

The Arcuate Nucleus Is a Key Node of Hypothalamic Control of Energy Balance

The arcuate nucleus is perhaps the best characterized hypothalamic nucleus involved in the control of energy balance. It is thought to be critical in mediating the actions of metabolic signals such as leptin, insulin, and ghrelin. Specifically, pro-opiomelanocortin (POMC) and neuropeptide Y (NPY)/agouti-related peptide (AgRP) neurons within the arcuate nucleus are required for regulating energy homeostasis, food intake, and glucose homeostasis. POMC is a multifunctional pro-peptide that is differentially processed into key peptides in different tissues (Fig. 35-3).[41] In the brain, melanocortin peptides such as α-melanocyte stimulating hormone (α-MSH) are key products that regulate food intake and energy homeostasis. α-MSH is the agonist for the melanocortin-4 receptor (MC4R), which is clearly established as key in regulating food intake, energy homeostasis, and glucose homeostasis in mice and humans.[41,42] Uniquely, an endogenous MC4R antagonist (AgRP) exists

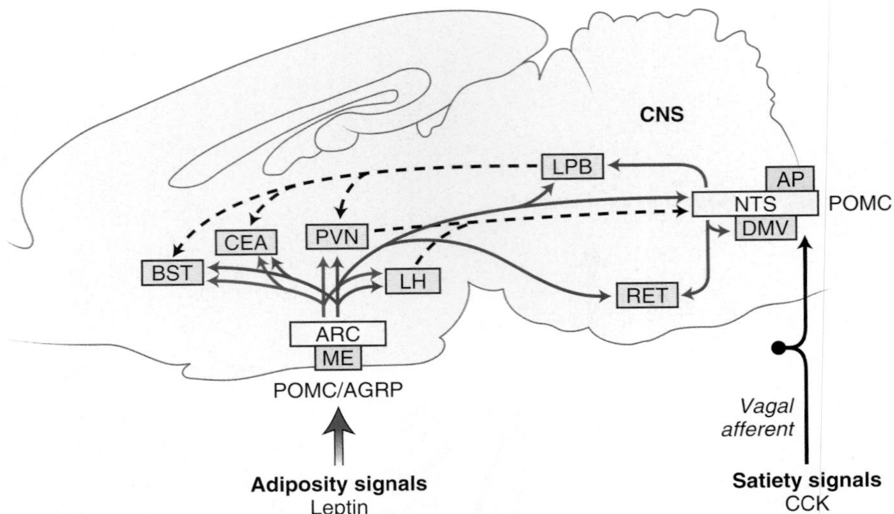

Figure 35-2 Brain structures involved in energy homeostasis. Receipt of long-term adipostatic signals and acute satiety signals by neurons in arcuate nucleus and brainstem, respectively. Light blue boxes indicate nuclei containing pro-opiomelanocortin (POMC) neurons; yellow boxes indicate nuclei containing melanocortin-4 receptor (MC4R) neurons that may serve to integrate adipostatic and satiety signals; and dark blue boxes show some circumventricular organs involved in energy homeostasis. Red arrows designate projections of POMC neurons; blue arrows show projections of agouti-related protein (AGRP neurons). AP, area postrema; ARC, arcuate nucleus; BST, bed nucleus of the stria terminalis; CCK, cholecystokinin; CEA, central nucleus of the amygdala; CNS, central nervous system; DMV, dorsal motor nucleus of the vagus; LH, lateral hypothalamic area; LPB, lateral parabrachial nucleus; ME, median eminence; NTS, nucleus tractus solitarius; PVN, paraventricular nucleus of the hypothalamus; RET, reticular formation. (Adapted from Fan W, Ellacott KL, Halatchev IG, et al. Cholecystokinin-mediated suppression of feeding involves the brainstem melanocortin system. *Nat Neurosci.* 2004;7:335-336.)

and is coexpressed with neuropeptide Y (NPY) in other neurons in the arcuate nucleus of the hypothalamus.

Supportive of a key role of the arcuate nucleus in regulating food intake and energy homeostasis is the observation that leptin deficiency (*ob/ob* mice) and fasting (which lowers leptin levels) result in decreased POMC expression and increased AgRP and NPY expression.[43,44] POMC and NPY/AgRP neurons are located in the arcuate nucleus (Figs. 35-4 and 35-5) and are directly regulated by leptin, ghrelin, glucose, and other metabolic signals. Leptin directly depolarizes (activates) POMC neurons and hyperpolarizes (inhibits) AgRP/NPY neurons,[45,46] and deletion of leptin receptors selectively in POMC neurons produces mild obesity.[47] However, leptin also has physiologically relevant actions outside the arcuate nucleus. For example, deletion of leptin receptors from neurons in the ventral medial nucleus produces obesity equal in magnitude to deletion from POMC neurons.[48,49]

In addition to leptin, other key metabolic signals act directly on POMC and AgRP neurons in the arcuate nucleus. For example, ghrelin directly depolarizes AgRP/NPY neurons,[50] and serotonin directly activates POMC neurons[51] and inhibits NPY/AgRP neurons.[52] Moreover, the anorexic properties of fenfluramine depend in part on MC4Rs.[52] Fenfluramine was used in combination with phentermine (Fen/Phen) to successfully reduce food intake and body

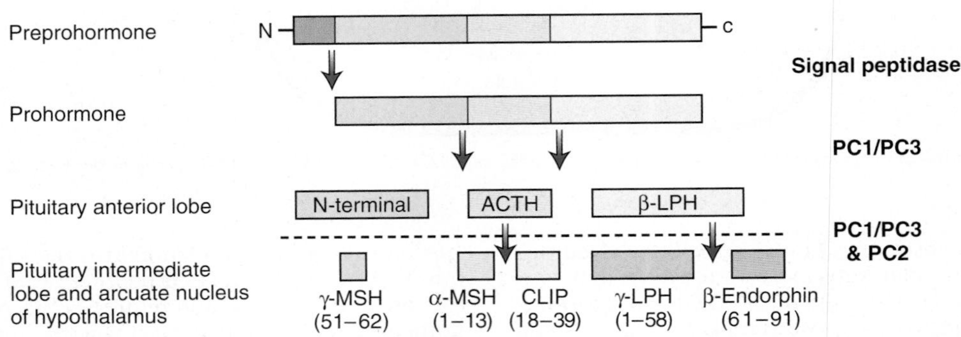

Figure 35-3 Organization of pro-opiomelanocortin (POMC), the precursor hormone of corticotropin (ACTH), β-lipoprotein (β-LPH), and related peptides. The precursor protein contains a leader sequence (signal peptide), followed by a long fragment that includes sequence 51-62, corresponding to γ-melanocyte-stimulating hormone (γ-MSH). This fragment is cleaved at Lys-Arg bonds to form corticotropin 1-39, which in turn includes the sequences for α-MSH (corticotropin 1-13) and corticotropin-like intermediate lobe peptide (CLIP; corticotropin 18-39) and a sequence corresponding to β-LPH (1-91) that includes γ-LPH (1-58) and β-endorphin (61-91). The β-endorphin sequence also includes a sequence corresponding to met-enkephalin. The precursor molecule in the anterior lobe of the pituitary is processed predominantly to corticotropin and β-LPH. In the intermediate pituitary lobe (in the rat), corticotropin and β-LPH are further processed to α-MSH and a β-endorphin–like material. In all extrapituitary tissues, post-translational processing of the prohormone resembles that in the intermediate lobe. Hypothalamic processing is similar but not identical to that in the intermediate lobe. In the latter, β-endorphin and α-MSH are present predominantly in their acetylated forms. PC, prohormone-converting enzyme. (Figure provided by Dr. Malcolm Low, University of Michigan, Ann Arbor, Mich.)

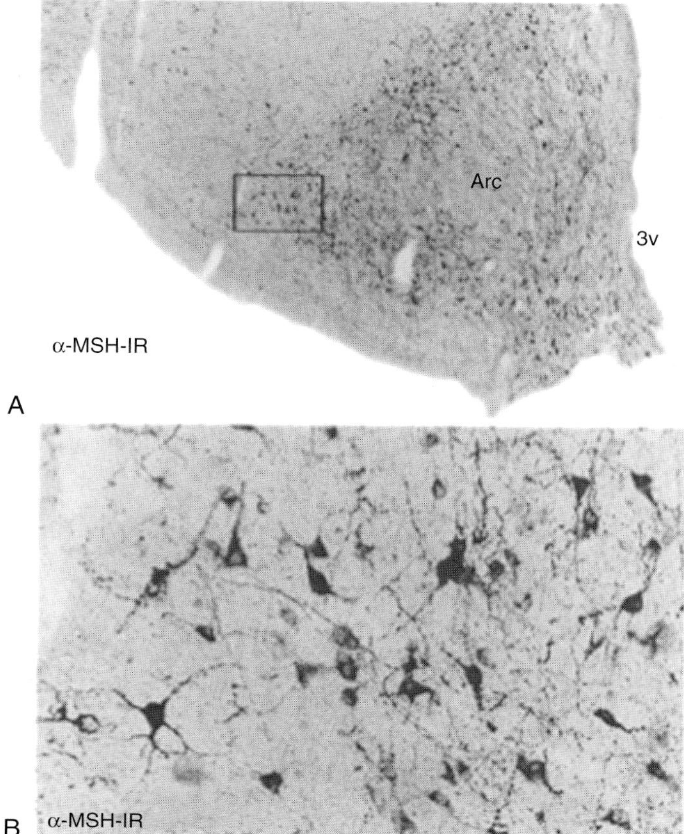

Figure 35-4 **A** and **B,** Photomicrographs demonstrate that α-melanocyte stimulating hormone–immunoreactive (α-MSH-IR) neurons are present in the human hypothalamus. The neurons are found in the arcuate nucleus of the hypothalamus (Arc; infundibular nucleus). 3v, third ventricle. (Modified from Elias CF, Saper CB, Maratos-Flier E, et al. Chemically defined projections linking the mediobasal hypothalamus and the lateral hypothalamic area. *J Comp Neurol.* 1998;402:442-459.)

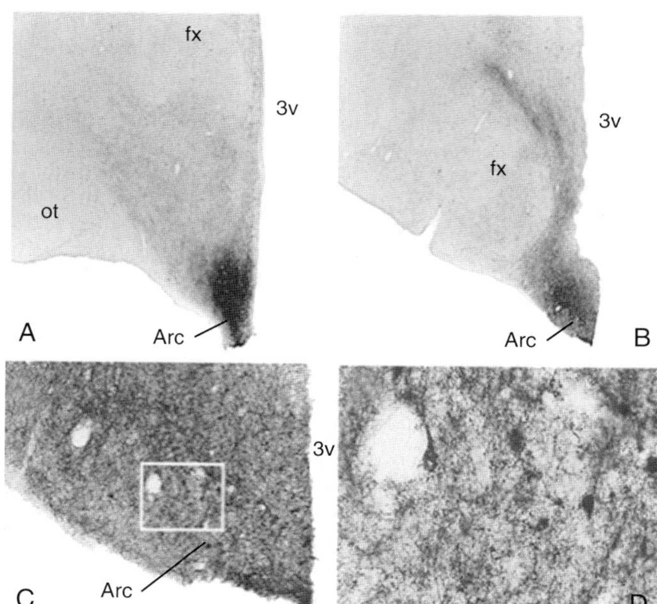

Figure 35-5 Photomicrographs demonstrate that agouti-related peptide–immunoreactive (AgRP-IR) neurons are present in the human hypothalamus. **A** and **B,** Two rostral to caudal low-power photomicrographs demonstrate that AgRP-IR neurons localize to the arcuate nucleus of the hypothalamus (Arc; infundibular nucleus). In **B,** Immunoreactive fibers are also observed streaming dorsally out of the arcuate nucleus. **C** and **D,** AgRP-IR neurons are observed in the arcuate nucleus. **D** is a higher magnification of boxed area in **C**. 3v, third ventricle; fx, fornix; ot, olfactory tuberele. (Modified from Elias CF, Saper CB, Maratos-Flier E, et al. Chemically defined projections linking the mediobasal hypothalamus and the lateral hypothalamic area. *J Comp Neurol.* 1998;402:442-459.)

weight in humans, before the formulation was removed from the market due to associated heart valve disorders and pulmonary hypertension. Importantly, the NPY/AgRP neurons send dense projections to POMC neurons, so the orexigenic NPY/AgRP and anorexigenic POMC neurons of the arcuate are coordinately regulated by a wide variety of hormones, drugs, and perhaps nutrients (Fig. 35-6).

Melanocortin-4 Receptors Regulate Energy and Glucose Homeostasis

Several pieces of evidence definitively demonstrate the role of MC4Rs in the regulation of energy homeostasis. For example, ectopic expression of MC4R antagonists in the brain induces obesity and diabetes.[42,53] MC4R deletion in mice produces obesity,[31] and humans with MC4R mutations display obesity.[54-57] Estimates suggest that 5% of cases of severe early-onset obesity are the result of heterozygous MC4R mutations.

MC4Rs are widely expressed in the brain, and many of them could play a role in regulating energy balance.[58-60] The sites in the brain that mediate the varied effects of MC4R agonists are beginning to emerge. Evidence suggests that MC4Rs expressed by hypothalamic neurons contribute to the effects of MC4R agonists to regulate energy

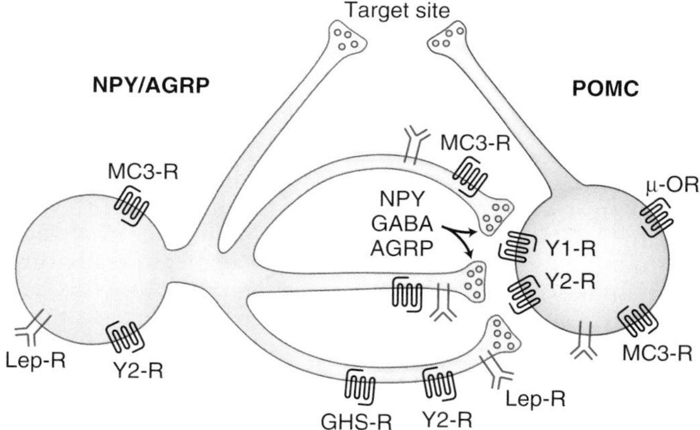

Figure 35-6 Regulation of the arcuate nucleus of the hypothalamus by various hormones and neuropeptides. NPY/AGRP and POMC neurons within the arcuate nucleus form a coordinately regulated network due to dense NPY/AGRP fibers that project to POMC cell bodies. Some receptors for the large numbers of hormones and neuropeptides known to regulate the network are indicated. AGRP, agouti-related peptide; GABA, γ-aminobutyric acid; GHS, growth-hormone secretagogue receptor; Lep, leptin; MC3, melanocortin 3; NPY, neuropeptide Y; μ-OR, μ-opiate receptor; R, receptor. (Modified from Cowley MA, Smart JL, Rubinstein M, et al. Leptin activates anorexigenic POMC neurons through a neural network in the arcuate nucleus. *Nature.* 2001;411:480-484.)

homeostasis.[61,62] For example, selective restoration of MC4Rs in the paraventricular nucleus of the hypothalamus (PVH) in mice lacking MC4Rs everywhere else normalizes food intake and greatly reduces body weight.[62] Extrahypothalamic MC4Rs contribute to melanocortin action to decrease adipose mass and food intake and increase energy expenditure. For example, MC4R messenger RNA (mRNA) is densely expressed in the DMV[63] including the cholinergic parasympathetic preganglionic neurons.[59,60] In addition, injections of the MC4R agonists into the fourth ventricle decreases food intake, and similar injections of MC4R antagonists dose-dependently increase food intake.[64,65] Injections of both MC4R agonists and antagonists into the region of the DMV alter food intake. This effect is likely mediated by MC4Rs in the brainstem, because it occurs at doses that are ineffective when injected into the fourth ventricle. These findings suggest that extrahypothalamic MC4Rs contribute to the effects of the MC4R agonists to regulate food intake, insulin secretion, and energy expenditure. This includes the amplification of satiety signals emanating from the gut such as that mediated by the gut peptide, CCK.[66]

The Lateral Hypothalamus Links Coordinated Food Intake Control and Arousal

The lateral hypothalamus includes the lateral hypothalamic area (LHA) and the perifornical hypothalamus. This region of the brain has long been suggested to play a key role in the regulation of ingestive behavior, since the early lesion studies of Anand and Brobeck.[67] In the past decade, two neuropeptides were discovered that are expressed by neurons in the lateral hypothalamus. These metabolically regulated peptides are melanin-concentrating hormone (MCH) and the orexins (also known as hypocretins).[68-71] MCH and orexin are expressed by distinct subsets of intermingled neurons in the LHA.[72,73] However, both populations broadly innervate the entire neuraxis including monosynaptic projections to other hypothalamic sites, the cerebral cortex, the amygdala, the brainstem, and the spinal cord.[68,74] The expression patterns of the receptors for both peptides are also widespread.[75-77]

Current data support the view that these LHA neuropeptides play a key role in regulating food intake, adipose mass, and glucose homeostasis. For example, injection of MCH into the brain increases food intake.[69] Mice lacking MCH (knockouts) are hypophagic and lean, and mice that overexpress MCH are obese and hyperleptinemic.[78,79] Mice lacking MCH and leptin are leaner than mice that lack leptin but express MCH.[80] The role of orexins in regulating food intake is complex, but it is clear that orexins are required for normal energy balance.[81,82] For example, central injections of orexin peptides increase feeding behavior.[70,83] However, the best characterized role for orexins is in the regulation of state control and the maintenance of wakefulness,[84,85] because it has been demonstrated that defective orexin signaling causes narcolepsy in mice, dogs, and humans. Other studies have demonstrated the ability of orexin neurons to sense changing levels of glucose (see later discussion).

The exact sites targeted by MCH and orexin neurons to induce feeding remain to be determined and represent an area of active investigation. MCH and orexin neurons have very similar and widespread projection patterns that include the hypothalamus, the brainstem, the cerebral cortex, and the spinal cord. Targets in the brainstem include motor systems and cranial nerve motor nuclei that underlie behaviors such as chewing, licking, and swallowing.[33,40] The MCH and orexin neurons also innervate the sympathetic and parasympathetic preganglionic nuclei in the medulla and the spinal cord, suggesting that both may be key in regulating the autonomic nervous system.

A key target for MCH and orexin neurons in coordinating feeding behavior may be their reciprocal connections with the nucleus accumbens. The nucleus accumbens is known to be critical in mediating rewarding components of several stimuli (e.g., drugs of abuse) and, potentially, the rewarding aspects of feeding. Although the subject is still being investigated, it is likely that MCH and orexin neurons may be able to enhance the hedonic value of food.[40] Regardless of the specific sites that mediate these effects, it is clear that MCH and orexin neurons are ideally positioned to regulate complex behavior, endocrine function, and autonomic outflow, all of which are key for coordinated control of energy balance.

CENTRAL NERVOUS SYSTEM CONTROL OF THERMOGENESIS

Coordinated energy homeostasis necessarily includes a balance between energy intake and energy expenditure. Energy expenditure is often considered in three categories: energy required for basal metabolism, energy required for voluntary and involuntary physical activity, and the thermic effect of food.

The last category, often referred to as diet-induced thermogenesis (DIT) is estimated to account for 8% to 10% of total expenditure and is defined as the increased energy expenditure in response to energy intake.[86] This process is under the control of the sympathetic nervous system, and thyroid-axis energy expenditure is increased by stimulation of β-adrenergic receptors or elevation of thyroid hormone. In rodents, one tissue mediating this response is brown adipose tissue (BAT), which contains adipocytes with dense collections of mitochondria.[87] In addition, the brown adipocytes express uncoupling protein 1 (UCP1), which uncouples mitochondrial respiration and thereby induces energy expenditure and heat. In humans, the key tissue mediating energy expenditure in response to changing energy intake remains to be determined but likely includes skeletal muscle.[87] In any case, it is clear that the sympathetic nervous system is required for coordinated control of energy expenditure and resistance to diet-induced obesity. For example, mice lacking β-adrenergic receptors (triple knockouts) develop severe obesity when placed on a high-fat diet.[88] Therefore, coordinated control of the sympathetic nervous system is required for control of diet-induced thermogenesis.

The CNS integrates metabolic information into a coordinated set of endocrine, autonomic, and behavioral responses to maintain homeostasis.[32,89,90] Key mediators of these responses are parasympathetic and sympathetic preganglionic neurons in the brainstem and spinal cord.[32,91] Sympathetic preganglionic neurons (SPNs) extend from the upper thoracic to the upper lumbar segments of the spinal cord and are found within the interomediolateral cell column (IML). Different rostral-caudal levels of the IML provide innervation to different target organs and thus mediate distinct autonomic responses. For example, SPNs in the upper thoracic levels of the IML are thought to be important for control of the heart and cardiovascular system. SPNs in the T6-T12 level of the IML provide innervation of the adrenal gland and the endocrine pancreas.[89,92-96]

In addition to the autonomic preganglionic neurons themselves, a key component of the central autonomic control system is direct (monosynaptic) descending innervation from key regulatory groups in the hypothalamus and brainstem.[32,97,98] The projection to the SPNs in the spinal cord is composed of inputs from the arcuate nucleus/retrochiasmatic area, the PVH, and the lateral hypothalamus.[89,98-104] Major projections also arise from the brainstem and include inputs from the raphe pallidus, catecholaminergic cells in the A5 group of the pons, and C1 cells in the rostral ventral lateral medulla that are critical in maintaining sympathetic tone in the cardiovascular system.[105-108] Therefore, there is a relatively circumscribed distribution of neurons providing descending input to SPNs that regulate the cardiovascular system, energy expenditure, adrenal catecholamine secretion, and the endocrine pancreas.

As noted earlier, in rodents central melanocortins are known to regulate energy expenditure in addition to food intake. MC4R blockade in mice prevents diet-induced thermogenesis[109] and blocks the upregulation of BAT activity[110]; this prevents upregulation of the expression of uncoupling proteins normally seen when mice are placed on a high-fat diet.[111] The sites mediating the effects of MC4R agonists on energy expenditure are still not definitively identified. However, a site of MC4R action relevant to the control of energy expenditure may be the SPNs themselves, which express MC4Rs.[59] Notably, these neurons receive direct inputs from leptin-responsive POMC neurons.[112] Therefore, MC4Rs expressed by SPNs in the spinal cord may contribute to melanocortin's effects on energy expenditure.

Evidence suggests that the effects of MC4R agonists on energy expenditure are mediated by MC4R-bearing neurons in the raphe pallidus in the brainstem.[113,114] Neurons in the raphe pallidus innervate SPNs in the IML.[115,116] In addition, raphe pallidus neurons are activated by "thermogenic" stimuli and have been shown to control BAT thermogenesis.[117,118] Injections of MC4R agonists into the raphe pallidus increases sympathetic nerve activity to BAT.[114] Therefore, MC4R-expressing neurons in the raphe nucleus may be key to the ability of melanocortin receptor agonists to increase energy expenditure.

HORMONAL REGULATORS OF THE BRAIN-GUT-ADIPOSE AXIS

Adipostatic Factors

Leptin Is the Prototypical Regulator of Energy Homeostasis

Discovery of the molecular bases for several obesity syndromes, prominent among them the hormone leptin[119] and its receptor,[21] has rapidly and dramatically increased understanding of the pathophysiology of obesity and related disorders. Leptin, the product of the *ob* gene,[119] is produced by white adipose tissue and affects feeding behavior, thermogenesis, and neuroendocrine status. Leptin protein is highly conserved throughout evolution; mouse and human leptin are 84% homologous, and leptin has been found in birds and tentatively identified in fish. This protein comprises 167 amino acids and 16 kd and circulates in the blood at concentrations proportional to the amount of fat depots. Leptin circulates in the bloodstream as a free protein and also bound to a soluble isoform of its receptor (Ob-Re). Leptin is secreted primarily from the adipocyte, but minor levels of regulated leptin expression also occur in other sites, such as skeletal muscle, placenta, and stomach.[120,121]

Total lack of leptin or leptin signaling in rodents and humans causes morbid obesity that is accompanied by a wide array of neuroendocrine abnormalities. Replacement with exogenous leptin normalizes these abnormalities.[122-125] Starvation, a time of low energy stores, leads to a fall in serum leptin levels and has profound effects on several neuroendocrine systems, including activation of the hypothalamic-pituitary-adrenal (HPA) axis, inhibition of the growth hormone and thyroid axes, and inhibition of reproductive function.[126-128] Lack of leptin results in many physiologic responses that are also found in a state of starvation. Many of these starvation-induced endocrine and autonomic changes are blocked or blunted by pretreatment with systemic leptin.[126] The dose needed to reverse these abnormalities is lower than that needed to induce weight loss in normal rodents. These observations have led to the suggestions that circulating leptin may have evolved to signal the brain that energy stores are sufficient and that a lack of leptin may be responsible for multiple neuroendocrine abnormalities caused by starvation.[129,130]

Soon after the discovery of leptin, it became clear that most of the varied effects of leptin are mediated by the brain. More recent studies have begun to unravel some of the complex circuitry involved in leptin signaling.[49]

Distribution of Leptin Receptors

After its transport through the BBB, leptin binds to specific receptors in the hypothalamus and brainstem. The "long-form" leptin receptor (OB-Rb) is a member of the cytokine-receptor superfamily.[20,21,131] The leptin receptor binds janus kinases (JAK), tyrosine kinases involved in intracellular cytokine signaling. Activation of JAK leads to phosphorylation of members of the signal transduction and transcription (STAT) family of proteins. In turn, STAT proteins activate transcription of leptin target genes.

The long-form leptin receptor is required for normal energy homeostasis; mutations of this gene result in the obese phenotype of the *db/db* mouse and the Zucker rat.[20,132,133] Leptin receptors are highly expressed by several hypothalamic nuclei within the medial basal hypothalamus,[134-139] including the arcuate, dorsomedial, ventromedial, and ventral premmamillary nuclei. They are also expressed in several extrahypothalamic sites, including the NTS (where vagal afferents terminate), the substantia nigra, and the ventral tegmental area.

Understanding of the role of extrahypothalamic leptin receptors is evolving, but evidence is accumulating that leptin has important sites of action within the brainstem. For example, leptin administration increased STAT3 phosphorylation in several extrahypothalamic sites, including the parabrachial nucleus, dorsal raphe, and NTS.[140] Moreover, administration of leptin into the fourth ventricle and into the dorsal vagal complex significantly reduced food intake.[33,141-144]

The Role of Insulin and Glucose in Regulating Energy Homeostasis

The concept that the CNS plays a primary role in the control of insulin action and glucose homeostasis is an old one. In 1849, Claude Bernard suggested that the CNS regulates blood glucose levels after his famous experiments demonstrating that "piqure" of the floor of the fourth ventricle of rabbits produced increases in blood glucose that were measured by glucose levels in the urine.[4,145] Remarkably, he concluded that the effect was mediated by stimulation of the autonomic input to the liver. Later lesion studies of the hypothalamus also teased out actions of insulin that are independent of food intake.[4] These early observations fit remarkably well with findings predicting that diabetes, similar to obesity, may be viewed as a disorder with underlying defects in the CNS.[146-150]

Insulin Action in the Brain. In addition to its well-known role in increasing glucose uptake in tissues such as muscle and fat, insulin has actions on the brain to regulate energy balance.[151] Insulin receptors are expressed in the brain, and injections of insulin into the brain reduce food intake.[151,152] Furthermore, deletion of insulin receptors specifically from neurons results in mild obesity.[153]

The role of insulin action in the CNS has been investigated in the context of regulation of glucose homeostasis. Downregulation of insulin receptors affects glucose homeostasis, including glucose production by the liver.[149] Therefore, insulin action in the brain may be key in the coordinated physiologic responses to changing levels of metabolic fuels. However, the physiologic significance and relative contributions of central versus peripheral actions of insulin in regulating glucose homeostasis, especially glucose production by the liver, are still unclear[154-156] and represent a key area of diabetes and obesity research.

Glucose Levels Are Sensed by Neurons in the Brain. Changing levels of blood glucose are sensed by several distinct populations of neurons in the brain. This was first suggested by classic experiments[157] demonstrating that some classes of neurons are activated by rising concentrations of glucose and others are inhibited by rising glucose. Several contemporary models predict that neurons that are activated by rising glucose respond and behave very similarly to beta cells of the endocrine pancreas.[158-160] The chemical identity and location of these glucose-sensing neurons are still to be determined. Several populations of glucose-sensitive neurons have been described in the hypothalamus, but neurons in the brainstem also sense glucose and are capable of inducing coordinated responses to falling levels of glucose.[161-163]

The cellular mechanisms underlying glucose-mediated neuronal excitation likely involve a rise in adenosine triphosphate (ATP), resulting from an increase in glucose metabolism, that promotes the closure of K_{ATP} potassium channels.[160] The mechanisms underlying the ability of neurons to be inhibited by rising glucose levels (or to be activated by falling glucose) are not as clearly defined but may involve the TASK subfamily of two-pore domain potassium channels as mediators of the glucose-activated inhibitory current in orexin neurons.[164] Collectively, these observations have led to predictions that changes in glucose levels alter the electrical activity of specific neurons, leading to changes in feeding behavior and glucose production. These models also predict that dysregulation of nutrient sensing in the CNS may contribute to the metabolic alterations that are characteristic of diabetes and obesity.

POMC Neurons Sense Changes in Glucose Concentration

Consistent with the demonstration that metabolic cues such as leptin directly act on POMC neurons, a key role of the central melanocortin system in regulating glucose homeostasis has emerged. POMC neurons increase their activity in response to rising glucose.[160] Mice lacking MC4Rs are hyperinsulinemic before the onset of obesity.[31,147] Experimental data have reinforced the concept that vagal input to the liver is a key regulator of hepatic glucose production, potentially including that mediated by melanocortin agonists.[165] The parasympathetic (cholinergic) innervation to the pancreas and liver is provided by the DMV.[96,166,167] The sympathetic innervation of the pancreas is from postganglionic neurons in the celiac ganglia[95,168] that are innervated by preganglionic neurons from midthoracic levels of the spinal cord.

Central administration of MC4R agonists decreased plasma insulin levels in lean and obese mice.[147] This effect was blocked by blockade of α-adrenergic receptors, suggesting that central MC4R agonists inhibit insulin secretion by activating the sympathetic nervous system. Administration of MC4R agonists increases glucose tolerance, and lean MC4R knockout mice are insulin resistant before the onset of obesity.[147] Moreover, MC4R-deficient humans are hyperinsulinemic, more so than would be expected from their degree of obesity alone, including subjects as young as 12 months old.[54,55] The sites in the CNS that mediate these effects are still to be determined, but MC4Rs are expressed by both parasympathetic preganglionic neurons and SPNs.[59,60] Therefore, it is likely that MC4R agonists exert a tonic inhibitory influence on insulin secretion by increasing the sympathetic input to the pancreas while simultaneously diminishing the parasympathetic input.[147]

As noted earlier, the activity of orexin neurons of the lateral hypothalamus is altered by changing levels of blood glucose. Specifically, orexin neurons are activated by physiologically relevant decreases in glucose concentrations.[164,169-172] Orexin neurons may be key in coordinating endocrine and autonomic responses to falling glucose levels. It is also likely that orexin neurons may represent one of the populations of "glucose-inhibited" neurons in the lateral hypothalamus that respond to physiologic falls in glucose levels with an increase in activity.[159,173] Because of its unique anatomic and physiologic properties, the central orexin system may be required to link glucose sensing with wakefulness (i.e., hypoglycemic unawareness) and coordinated autonomic responses.

Satiety and Hunger Factors

Role of the Brainstem in Satiety and Hunger

The brainstem is classically understood as the center for detection and response to hunger and satiety signals. The NTS is the primary site for innervation by vagal afferents from the gut (see review by Schwartz[174] and Fig. 35-2). The afferent branches deriving from different aspects of the gastrointestinal tract map viscerotopically along the NTS from its rostral to its caudal aspect.[175] Rostrally, the NTS is a bilaterally symmetric nucleus that merges into a single medial body at its caudal extent, called the *commissural NTS*.[32]

Vagal afferents deriving input from the upper gastrointestinal tract are responsive to three basic stimuli: gastric and duodenal distention or contraction, chemical contents of the lumen, and gut peptides and neurotransmitters released from the stomach and duodenum in response to nutrients.[174] In the rat, vagal afferents responding to gastric and duodenal distention tend to map to the medial and commissural divisions of the NTS.[176,177] Vagal afferents responsive to the gut peptide CCK also map to the caudal NTS.[178]

The DMV, located just ventral to the NTS, is the primary site of motor efferents to the gut and is densely innervated by NTS fibers. Together, these cell groups, with the area postrema, a CVO, form the dorsal vagal complex (DVC) and serve as the neuroanatomic substrate for the vagovagal reflex.

Gut Peptides Involved in Satiety and Hunger

In addition to signals from gut distention, gut peptides stimulated by meal intake mediate satiety through centers in the brainstem. Signals received by the brainstem are thought to interact primarily with long-term weight regulation centers, via neural connections to the hypothalamus, to regulate total daily intake by adjusting meal size, the number of meals, or both.

With the discovery of ghrelin, gut factors that stimulate food intake must also be considered. Chapter 39 examines gastrointestinal hormones in detail, focusing on their peripheral actions. Here we consider their central actions. As discussed later, newer data suggest that a subset of these gastrointestinal hormones may also act directly on hypothalamic control centers.

Cholecystokinin. CCK is produced by the gastrointestinal tract in response to meal ingestion, and its diverse actions include stimulation of pancreatic enzyme secretion and intestinal motility, inhibition of gastric motility, and acute inhibition of feeding. Early experiments with peripheral administration of CCK supported a role for increased CCK levels in the early termination of a meal.[179,180] The finding that repeated injections of CCK lead to reduced meal size without a change in body weight, owing to a compensatory increase in meal frequency, argued against CCK action as a signal regulating long-term energy stores.[181,182]

Two subtypes of the CCK receptor belonging to the G protein–coupled family of receptors have been described: CCKA and CCKB. Studies using CCK receptor–specific antagonists and surgical or chemical vagotomy have demonstrated that the satiety effects of CCK are specifically mediated via CCKA receptors on afferent vagal nerves.[183-189] This interaction between acute vagal input from CCKA receptors and meal termination involves activation of cells in the NTS and area postrema, modulated by neural connections from the hypothalamus receiving inputs from insulin and leptin.

Peripheral administration of CCK potently activates large numbers of neurons in both the NTS and the area postrema (Fig. 35-7). Furthermore, central administration of insulin and leptin potentiates the satiety-inducing effects of peripherally administered CCK[188-194] and leads, with repeated injections, to sustained weight loss that is greater than injection of the agents separately.[195] However, more remains to be learned regarding the neuroanatomic substrate underlying this convergence of long-term and short-term information. Whereas basomedial hypothalamic cell groups involved in leptin signaling are densely innervated by catecholaminergic neurons from the brainstem, it has been demonstrated that norepinephrine is not required for CCK-induced reduction of feeding, in that the dopamine β-hydroxylase knockout mouse is still responsive to CCK-induced satiety.[196] The central melanocortin system may be one element of this integration of satiety with long-term energy homeostasis, because MC4R blockade in the brainstem appears to inhibit the satiating activity of peripherally administered CCK.[66]

In addition to its function in the induction of satiety through vagally mediated signaling, a small body of literature supports a central role for CCK action in regulation of feeding. Immunohistochemistry of the brain and spinal cord shows that the CCKA and CCKB receptors are widely distributed in the CNS, including in the arcuate nucleus[197] and other hypothalamic regions.[197,198] Intracerebroventricular (ICV) administration of CCK to mice[199] inhibits food intake; this effect is reversible by prior administration of a CCKA receptor antagonist. The significance of these hypothalamic-arcuate CCK receptors to weight regulation in the free feeding state is not known.

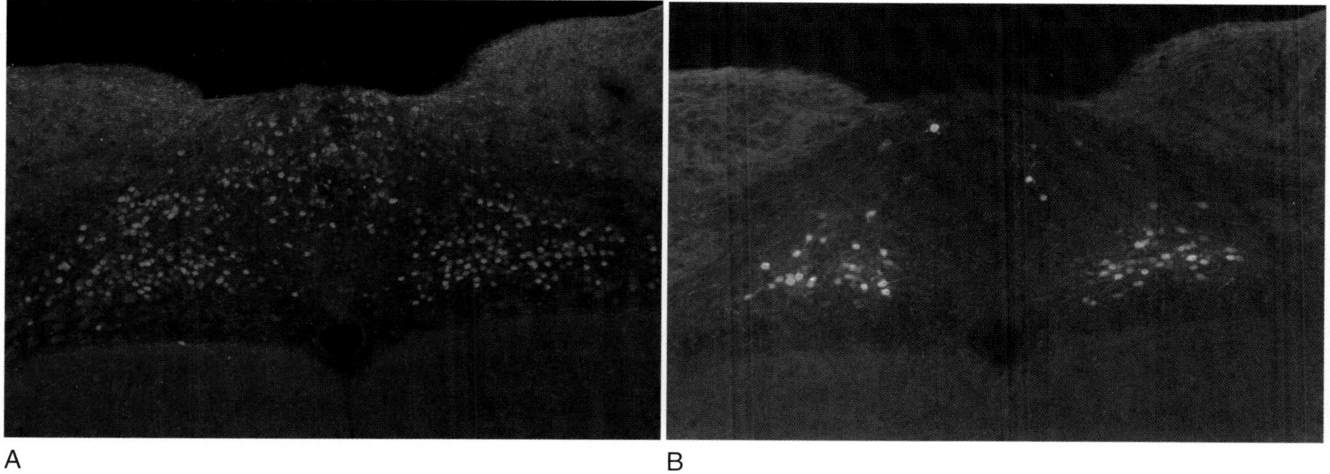

Figure 35-7 Brainstem neurons activated by satiety. **A,** Neurons activated by intraperitoneal administration of 10 μg/kg cholecystokinin (CCK) in the nucleus tractus solitarius (NTS) of the mouse. Neurons visualized by immunohistochemical reaction against Fos, a marker of neuronal activation. **B,** Neurons in the NTS activated by CCK encompass a variety of different neurochemical subtypes, such as glucagon-like peptide 1 (GLP1)-positive neurons, and the pro-opiomelanocortin (POMC)-positive neurons. POMC neurons are visualized through immunohistochemical detection of green fluorescent protein in tissue from a transgenic mouse in which green fluorescent protein (GFP) is expressed under the control of the POMC promoter. (Reproduced from Cowley MA, Smart JL, Rubinstein M, et al. Leptin activates anorexigenic POMC neurons through a neural network in the arcuate nucleus. *Nature.* 2001;411:480-484. Photographs provided by Dr. Kate L.J. Ellacott, Vanderbilt University School of Medicine, Nashuille, Tenn)

Peptide YY. Peptide YY (PYY), a peptide related to NPY and pancreatic peptide (PP), is postprandially released by endocrine cells in the ileum and colon.[200] PYY is found in vivo in both a full-length, 36-amino-acid form and a 34-amino-acid form ($PYY_{3\text{-}36}$) in approximately a 2:1 to 1:1 molar ratio.[201] PYY is a potent agonist of both Y1 and Y2 receptors, whereas $PYY_{3\text{-}36}$ is a Y2-specific agonist with approximately a 1000 times greater affinity for the Y2 than for the Y1 receptor.[202] Y1- and Y2-preferring binding sites are located in the area postrema and in the dorsal vagal complex (NTS and DMV). Peripheral administration of PYY (300 mg/kg) in the rat induces c-fos (Fos) in the area postrema and in the medial and commissural NTS, the latter being the same region of the NTS that is known to express POMC.[203] Infusion of PYY within the physiologic range has numerous effects, including inhibition of gastric emptying,[204] gastric acid secretion,[205] and pancreatic exocrine secretion.[205] These actions of PYY appear to be mediated by direct action of PYY on the dorsal vagal complex and on gastric mucosal enterochromaffin-like cells (see review by Yang[206]). Both Y1 and Y2 receptors are found within the DVC.[207] PYY appears to inhibit gastric acid secretion primarily through vagal innervation of the gastric fundus.[208] The ability of low-dose PYY and $PYY_{3\text{-}36}$ to inhibit the activity of DMN efferents appears to be Y2 mediated, and Y1 agonists appear to stimulate these cells.[206]

Peripheral administration of $PYY_{3\text{-}36}$ in pharmacologic doses appears to have an anorexigenic effect in rodents and in humans,[209-215] suggesting that the peptide also functions as a satiety factor. The mechanisms underlying the action of $PYY_{3\text{-}36}$ in reducing food intake have not been fully elucidated. Intraperitoneal administration of $PYY_{3\text{-}36}$ was found to activate 12% to 13% of arcuate POMC neurons, as assayed by increased expression of Fos.[209,216] However, vagotomy also blocks $PYY_{3\text{-}36}$-induced inhibition of feeding.[217] The existence of a direct hypothalamic site of action has been challenged by several studies. Inhibition of feeding by $PYY_{3\text{-}36}$ persists in the MC4R knockout mouse,[216] the POMC knockout mouse,[211] and the obese agouti mouse.[218] Therefore, release of melanocortin peptides derived from POMC and subsequent activation of the MC4R, a well-characterized anorexigenic pathway, does not appear to be required for the inhibition of feeding by $PYY_{3\text{-}36}$. Furthermore, PYY induced conditioned taste aversion in rodents and nausea in some human studies, suggesting an aversive effect of the peptide that is likely to involve brainstem sites such as the area postrema.

Despite the short-acting anorexic effects of the PYY in most experimental models, suggesting that it may be a satiety factor like CCK, two knockout studies demonstrated that removal of the gene encoding the peptide produces obese hyperinsulinemic mice.[219,220] These data suggest that the peptide may also play an important role in the regulation of long-term energy stores. One study suggested that the peptide may be specifically involved in the satiating effects of protein in the diet.[219]

Ghrelin. Identified as an endogenous ligand for the growth-hormone secretagogue receptor (GHSR),[221,222] ghrelin is an acylated, 28-amino-acid peptide that is predominantly secreted by the stomach, is regulated by ingestion of nutrients,[223-226] and has potent effects on appetite.[225,226] In rodents and humans, ghrelin levels are markedly reduced with meal ingestion but rebound to baseline before the next meal or increase after an overnight fast (Fig. 35-8).[224-226] In rodents, this was demonstrated to be a nutrient-specific effect in that a similar volume of saline infused into the stomach did not affect ghrelin levels.[225] GHSR have been demonstrated on arcuate NPY-containing neurons.[227] Pharmacologic doses of ghrelin injected peripherally or into the hypothalamus activate Fos and Egr1 solely in arcuate NPY neurons in rats[228] and stimulate food intake and obesity, in part by stimulating NPY and AgRP expression,[228-234] which antagonize leptin's anorexic effect.[233]

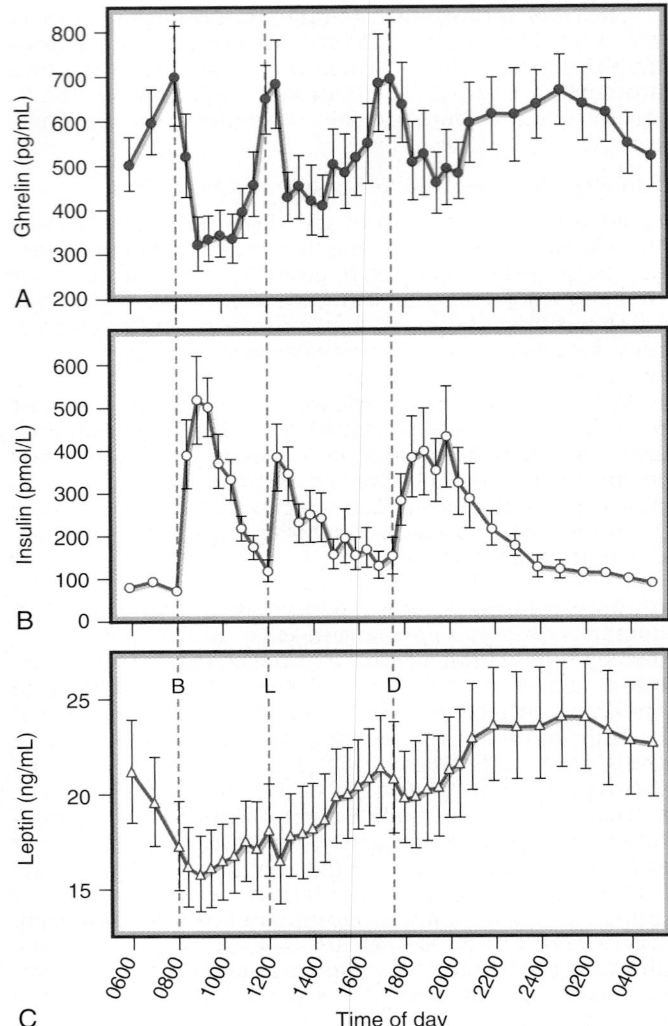

Figure 35-8 Average plasma ghrelin, insulin, and leptin concentrations during a 24-hour period in 10 human subjects consuming breakfast (B), lunch (L), and dinner (D) at the times indicated (0800, 1200, and 1730 hours, respectively). (Reprinted from Cummings DE, Purnell JQ, Frayo RS, et al. A preprandial rise in plasma ghrelin levels suggests a role in meal initiation in humans. *Diabetes.* 2001;50:1714-1719.)

This orexigenic action occurs in rodents even with peripheral administration of ghrelin that matches fasting levels.[235] Stimulation of appetite and food intake during an infusion of ghrelin over 4.5 hours in humans has also been demonstrated,[236] and ghrelin may also effect gastric emptying. This study established that, similar to its action in rodents, ghrelin can stimulate appetite and food intake in humans when given in a supraphysiologic dose, but a role for physiologic changes in ghrelin levels or signaling in human energy homeostasis remains unknown.

Ghrelin's characteristics make it unique among the gut-derived signals. Unlike other enteropancreatic signals involved with energy homeostasis, ghrelin secretion is inhibited in response to meals; and instead of acting as a satiety signal (like CCK or $PYY_{3\text{-}36}$), ghrelin stimulates appetite, potentially through arcuate signaling. These properties strongly suggest that ghrelin is a candidate "meal-initiating" signal, as proposed by Cummings and colleagues.[226] In addition, fasting ghrelin levels have been shown to be inversely proportional to body weight[237] and to be higher in underweight subjects with anorexia nervosa and cardiac cachexia compared with controls.[223,238] Downregulation of ghrelin in obese subjects suggests an adaptive response to the obese state, whereas a rise in levels in weight-reduced subjects is compatible with a counterregulatory role to restore fat depots. These properties inversely parallel those of insulin, which is stimulated by meals, inhibits food intake when injected ICV, circulates in the fasting state in direct proportion to body weight, and is secreted in decreased amounts after weight loss.

Much work remains to establish the physiologic role of ghrelin in meal initiation and energy homeostasis and its mechanisms of action. Evidence indicates that the melanocortin system is central to ghrelin's effects on food intake. Stimulation of food intake by ghrelin administration is blocked by administration of NPY/Y1 and Y5 antagonists[233] and is reduced in the $NPY^{-/-}$ mouse, and administration of the melanocortin agonist Melanotan II (MTII) blocks further stimulation of weight gain by growth hormone–releasing peptide 2 (GHRP-2) in the $NPY^{-/-}$ mouse.[239]

Peripheral administration of ghrelin activates Fos expression only in arcuate NPY/AgRP neurons, not in other hypothalamic or brainstem sites,[240] and ablation of the arcuate nucleus blocks the actions of ghrelin administration on feeding but not on elevation of growth hormone.[241] Despite activating Fos only in arcuate NPY neurons, peripheral ghrelin may access the arcuate via vagal afferents: GHSR is expressed on vagal afferents, ghrelin suppresses firing of vagal nerves, and surgical or chemical vagotomy blocks stimulation of feeding as well as Fos activation in the arcuate by peripheral but not central ghrelin administration.[242] Peripheral ghrelin may largely suppress brainstem satiety centers, which would explain the lack of Fos activation at these sites. The NTS sends dense catecholaminergic projections to the arcuate; therefore, although a convergence of ascending vagal afferent information arrives at the arcuate from both brainstem and intermediate hypothalamic sites, it is possible that NTS neurons inhibited by ghrelin synapse directly with NPY arcuate neurons. This would explain the absence of other hypothalamic neurons activated by peripheral ghrelin.

Administration of another peptide hormone derived from proghrelin, termed *obestatin,* was demonstrated to inhibit food intake and was proposed to be the ligand for an orphan GPCR known as GPR39.[243] However, most groups have been unable to repeat this finding, and even the identity of obestatin as a GPR39 ligand has been called into question.[244-246]

Preproglucagon-Derived Peptides. Current strategies for the treatment of type 2 diabetes mellitus are not optimally effective, and even multiple drug combinations fail to normalize glycemia in a sustained manner in many subjects. Hence, there remains intense interest in new therapies that safely and effectively lower blood glucose in diabetic subjects. Strategies that mimic the actions of the incretin class of hormones are being used to treat type 2 diabetes and obesity.[247,248] Incretins are hormones that are released by oral ingestion of nutrients and increase insulin secretion. The prototypical incretin hormone is GLP1, which is derived from the proglucagon gene. The proglucagon-derived peptides are generated in the A cells of the pancreas (principally glucagon), in the L cells of the intestine (GLP1, GLP2, and glicentin), and in the brain (glucagon, GLP1, GLP2).[247,248]

As outlined in detail in Chapter 31, GLP1 receptor agonists induce multiple desirable antidiabetic and antiobesity actions, and protease-resistant long-acting GLP1 analogues are currently available for the treatment of type 2 diabetes.[247,248] The first of these drugs, Byetta (exenatide), is a potent GLP1 receptor agonist that mimics the GLP1 enhancement of glucose-dependent insulin secretion, slowing gastric emptying, inhibiting gastric acid secretion, and reducing food intake. The last effect may be due to action on circuits in the brain involved in the control of energy homeostasis (see later discussion).

GLP1 and GLP1R Neurons in the Central Nervous System. Despite intense interest in GLP1 and related peptides, it is little appreciated that GLP1 is an endogenous neuropeptide expressed by neurons in the CNS, and the CNS actions of GLP1 are less well understood. With the development of GLP1 analogues to treat diabetes, understanding of the central actions of GLP1 is relevant for predicting the biologic consequences of sustained GLP1 administration.

Initial interest in the CNS actions of GLP1 stemmed from the observation that GLP1 inhibits food intake.[249-253] In humans, peripheral GLP1 administration to normal and diabetic subjects induced satiety and reduces food intake in short-term studies.[254-257] Chronic continuous GLP1 administration to human diabetic subjects was associated with modest weight loss.[258] The effects of GLP1 on appetite may be mediated in part by inhibition of gastric emptying and may also reflect direct effects of GLP1 on satiety and induction of taste aversion.[38,259-263]

The CNS expression of GLP1 is very restricted and includes a population of neurons within the caudal NTS. Caudal NTS neurons receive and process viscerosensory information from thoracic and abdominal viscera. The NTS is reciprocally connected with various brain areas, including hypothalamic areas thought to regulate feeding.[32,264] Additionally, the NTS is located adjacent to a CVO, the area postrema, and the NTS contains fenestrated capillaries, potentially allowing circulating peptides access to the nucleus. Therefore, neurons in the NTS (including GLP1 cells) process information arising from a variety of neural and humoral sources. GLP1 neurons are in a prime position to rapidly modify ingestive behavior in direct response to transiently altered levels of metabolic cues (e.g., leptin, glucose) or to neural modulators from other brain sites, including POMC neurons in the arcuate nucleus. For example, the adipocyte-derived hormone leptin communicates the status of energy stores to the brain. Most investigations of the neural circuits that mediate leptin action have focused on the hypothalamus. However, increasing evidence implicates a significant role for extrahypothalamic sites of leptin action.[33,141] Intravenous leptin increases neuronal activation (induces Fos-IR) in regions of the hindbrain, including GLP1 neurons in the NTS[265] as well as POMC neurons in some cases.[266]

In addition to the varied inputs, GLP1 neurons in the NTS also have a widespread projection pattern in the brain.[267] There are direct innervations of several hypothalamic nuclei, including the PVH, LHA, and arcuate nucleus, and GLP1 receptor mRNA has been found within those areas.[268] The location of GLP1 neurons in the NTS and their diffuse projection pattern suggest that GLP1 neurons are ideally situated to integrate key signals and regulate complex physiologic processes.

Amylin. Amylin, or islet amyloid polypeptide (IAPP), is a 37-amino-acid polypeptide that colocalizes with insulin in beta cells in the pancreas. In humans, IAPP in the pancreas can form amyloid fibrils and is thought to play a role in the decline in islet cell function that accompanies type 2 diabetes.[269,270] In addition, IAPP has been shown to impair gastric motility and to have effects independent of insulin on energy homeostasis mediated through hypothalamic signaling.

IAPP is cosecreted with insulin in response to nutrient intake and insulin secretogogues.[271,272] IAPP readily enters the brain, and high-affinity IAPP-binding sites have been found in several brain regions, including the hypothalamus and arcuate nucleus.[273,274] Both peripheral and ICV infusions of IAPP inhibit food intake acutely, and chronic infusion leads to a sustained reduction in body weight.[273-278] This anorectic effect was shown by Rushing and colleagues to be blocked by coadministration of the IAPP antagonist AC187 centrally, and AC187 resulted in a significant increase in body adiposity when infused ICV over 14 days, compared with control animals.[278] Studies of coadminstration of IAPP with other gastrointestinal hormones have shown that the acute satiety effects of IAPP are equipotent to those of CCK[279] and are additive when IAPP is peripherally coinjected with either CCK[280] or insulin.[281] The precise central neuroendocrine mechanisms mediating IAPP's anorexic effects have yet to be elucidated. The diverse CNS binding of IAPP suggests that multiple sites may have roles in the anorectic effects of IAPP; however, the inhibition of appetite with ICV administration and demonstrated binding in the arcuate suggests that the hypothalamus may be an important site of IAPP action.

Bariatric Surgery and the Role of the Gastrointestinal System in the Control of Energy Homeostasis

No pharmacologic treatment has yet been devised that is capable of resetting the adipostat—that is, allowing significant long-term weight loss to be maintained. In contrast, certain types of bariatric surgery, such as the Roux-en-Y gastric bypass (described in Chapter 36 and reviewed by Cummings[282] and Sjostrom[283]), appear to cause not only significant weight loss but also maintenance of this weight loss for many years (Fig. 35-9). Furthermore, improvement in diabetes after these procedures is often seen before significant weight loss occurs, and this can now be modeled in rodents as well.[284] Both of these findings imply that the procedures have a profound impact on the central control of long-term energy stores, satiety, and glucose homeostasis. Conventional models have argued that gastrointestinal hormones regulate satiety, but individually they do not have significant impact on the control of long-term energy stores. For example, deletion or blockade of CCK increases meal size but not 24-hour food intake or body weight. The facts that bariatric surgery appears capable of creating a new, stable weight set point and that PYY deletion causes obesity suggest that hormonal or vagal and nutritional signals from the gut may have a more profound impact on long-term energy homeostasis than was previously thought.

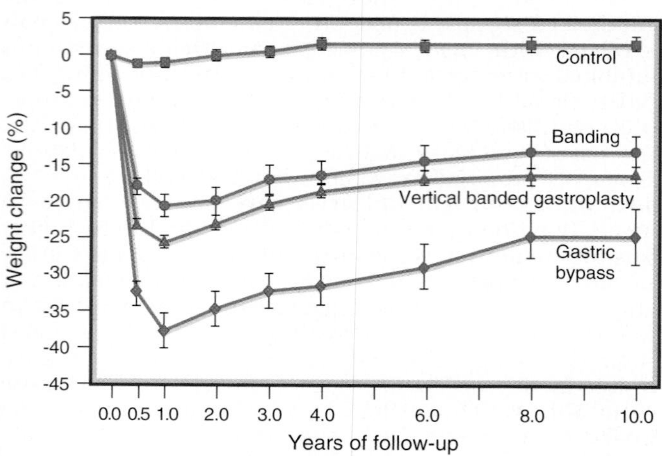

Figure 35-9 Apparent alteration of the adipostatic set point after bariatric surgery. (Modified from Sjostrom L, Lindroos AK, Peltonen M, et al.; Swedish Obese Subjects Study Scientific Group. Lifestyle, diabetes, and cardiovascular risk factors 10 years after bariatric surgery. *N Engl J Med.* 2004;351:2683-2693.)

GLUCOCORTICOIDS AND GONADAL STEROIDS

Both glucocorticoids and gonadal steroids are known to act centrally on circuits involved in energy homeostasis. Orchiectomy decreases food intake in rodents, whereas ovariectomy has the opposite result.[285] Hormone replacement therapy with drugs such as tamoxifen has been demonstrated to reduce the weight gain seen with menopause.[286] Estrogen receptors appear to be expressed at significant levels in the arcuate nucleus of the hypothalamus. Data suggest that estrogen may act at both POMC and NPY/AgRP neurons, perhaps explaining, in part, the cellular mechanism of the hormone's action in the CNS.[287,288] Mice lacking estrogen receptor α (ERα) develop increased visceral adiposity, elevated insulin levels, and reduced glucose tolerance.[289] However, obesity in this knockout model does not appear to be caused by hyperphagia. Deletion of ERα exclusively in neurons of the VMH leads to a similar syndrome of obesity and metabolic syndrome, suggesting an important role for estrogen in the control of energy expenditure and implicating the VMH in estrogen action.[290] The vagal nerve is also a site of estrogen action where the hormone has been demonstrated to alter responsiveness to satiety factors, such as CCK.[285]

In contrast to estrogen, glucocorticoids stimulate food intake and weight gain. Excessive glucocorticoids are associated with the unusual deposition of excess adipose tissue, for example in Cushing's disease (see Chapter 7). However, glucocorticoids have an enormous diversity of effects in the periphery and in the CNS, and the glucocorticoid receptor is extremely widely expressed throughout the CNS.[291] Glucocorticoids have anti-inflammatory effects in the CNS and provide feedback inhibition to the HPA axis (see Chapter 7), both actions having secondary effects on energy homeostasis. Glucocorticoids also appear to be critical in determining the tone of adipostatic circuits.[285] For example, the ability of centrally administered NPY to produce obesity and the obesity resulting from leptin deficiency are both dramatically reduced by adrenalectomy. ICV administration of dexamethasone to adrenalectomized rats also dose-dependently reduces leptin potency.

The complexity of glucocorticoid action in energy homeostasis results from the broad number of tissues affected, the multiple physiologic systems involved, and action in a variety of time scales. Rapid actions of glucocorticoids in the hypothalamus, not mediated by the conventional glucocorticoid receptor, have also been linked in sites like the PVN to rapid synthesis and retrograde release of endocannabinoids, which suppress synaptic excitation through presynaptic CB1 receptors. In support of this newly identified pathway, leptin appears to block glucocorticoid-mediated endocannabinoid release.[292]

CYTOKINES AND ENERGY BALANCE

The profound effect of cytokines, largely derived from the immune system, on energy balance is most clearly evident in the case of disease wasting or cachexia. The term *cachexia* describes a constellation of symptoms that occurs in multiple independent infectious and chronic diseases including some forms of cancer, heart failure, renal failure, and acquired immunodeficiency syndrome. These symptoms include anorexia, increased energy expenditure, and a loss of lean mass. The normal response to anorexia and the initial loss of adipose mass—a decrease in energy expenditure and neuroendocrine changes designed to save energy (e.g., hypothyroidism)—occur in anorexia nervosa but not in cachexia. Research in rodents and humans demonstrates that cachexia results from the action of a variety of cytokines in the CNS and, in particular, the dysfunctional response of circuits involved in the central control of energy homeostasis.

Neuroendocrine-Immune Interactions

Stimulation of the immune system by foreign pathogens leads to a stereotypical set of responses orchestrated by the CNS. These responses are the result of the complex interaction of the immune system and the CNS and are often referred to as the cerebral component of the acute phase reaction.[293] This constellation of responses is adaptive and is mediated in large part by the hypothalamus and, just as in the normal control of energy homeostasis, comprises coordinated autonomic, endocrine, and behavioral components. These responses include fever, alterations in the activity of almost every neuroendocrine axis, changes in the sleep-wake cycle, anorexia, and inactivity.

It is now clear that cytokines produced by white blood cells of the immune system mediate the CNS responses. Early evidence supporting this hypothesis was provided by the seminal observations that cytokines such as interleukin-1β (IL-1β) can activate the HPA axis.[294-296] Although it is established that cytokines modulate hypothalamic activity, it is also important to note that the immune system is modulated by the nervous system. This occurs largely by two routes: endocrine mechanisms and direct innervation. This innervation includes lymphoid organs such as the thymus and spleen, which receive direct inputs from the autonomic nervous system.[297,298] As noted in Chapter 7, the hallmark of cytokine action on the hypothalamus is the activation of the HPA axis. The resultant glucocorticoid secretion acts as a classic negative feedback to the immune system to dampen the immune response (Fig. 35-10). In general, glucocorticoids inhibit most limbs of the immune response, including lymphocyte proliferation, production of immunoglobulins, cytokines, and cytotoxicity. These inhibitory reactions form the basis of the anti-inflammatory actions of glucocorticoids.

This section addresses several of the hypothesized mechanisms by which cytokines engage neural pathways to mediate neuroendocrine and autonomic effects. Many nonlymphocyte cells, including endocrine cells, adipose cells, and neurons, also synthesize cytokines that exert effects independent of immunomodulation. Examples of cytokines secreted by adipocytes include leptin and tumor necrosis factor-α (TNF-α), which have profound effects on metabolism.[299]

Mechanisms of Cytokine Signaling in the Central Nervous System

Cytokines made outside the CNS can alter the activity and function of populations of hypothalamic neurons. Administration of lipopolysaccharide (LPS) is widely used as an experimental model and induces the secretion of several pyrogenic cytokines, including IL-1β, TNF-α, and IL-6, that mimic the patterns of cytokine production seen in natural infections.[300-303] Many other studies have used systemic injections of cytokines such as IL-1β and TNF-α to stimulate the CNS. Three models based on methodologies such as these are discussed here to explain how immune system signals might act on the CNS (Fig. 35-11).

Interaction of Cytokines with the Circumventricular Organs

The CVOs (described earlier) are specialized regions along the margins of the ventricular system that have fenestrated capillaries and therefore no BBB.[35] Many circulating hormones, such as angiotensin II, act on neurons in the CVOs, converting bloodborne signals into CNS responses.[293]

Several models of fever production have hypothesized that cytokines may enter the CNS via the CVOs, particularly at the organum vasculosum of the lamina terminalis (OVLT; see Fig. 35-10).[304-307] However, definitive evidence establishing this model as a predominant mechanism is still lacking. Large lesions of the preoptic area of the hypothalamus including the OVLT block fever, but they inevitably damage nearby regions that are critical for thermoregulation.[305] Small lesions of the OVLT do not block fever or corticotropin responses.[308] However, an inherent limitation of this type of study is that the lesion itself breaches the BBB, allowing entry of cytokines. Moreover, knife cuts just caudal to the OVLT that interrupt connections from the OVLT to the PVH do not block activation of the HPA axis by IL-1.[309,310]

Other studies have focused on the area postrema, a CVO located in the medulla oblongata lying along the surface of the NTS at the caudal end of the fourth ventricle (see Fig. 35-10). Lesions of the area postrema can block the IL-1–induced activation of the HPA axis and the induction of Fos mRNA in the PVH.[311] However, others have found that more circumscribed lesions, which do not injure the NTS, do not prevent CNS responses to intravenous IL-1.[312]

Interactions of Cytokines at the Barriers of the Brain: The Requirement of Prostaglandins

One of the hallmarks of CNS response to inflammation is that many of its components, including fever and activation of the HPA axis, can be prevented by blocking the production of prostaglandins. This is typically done by administration of nonsteroidal anti-inflammatory drugs (NSAIDs) such as aspirin or indomethacin.[313-315] Decades ago, the work of Milton and Wendlandt demonstrated

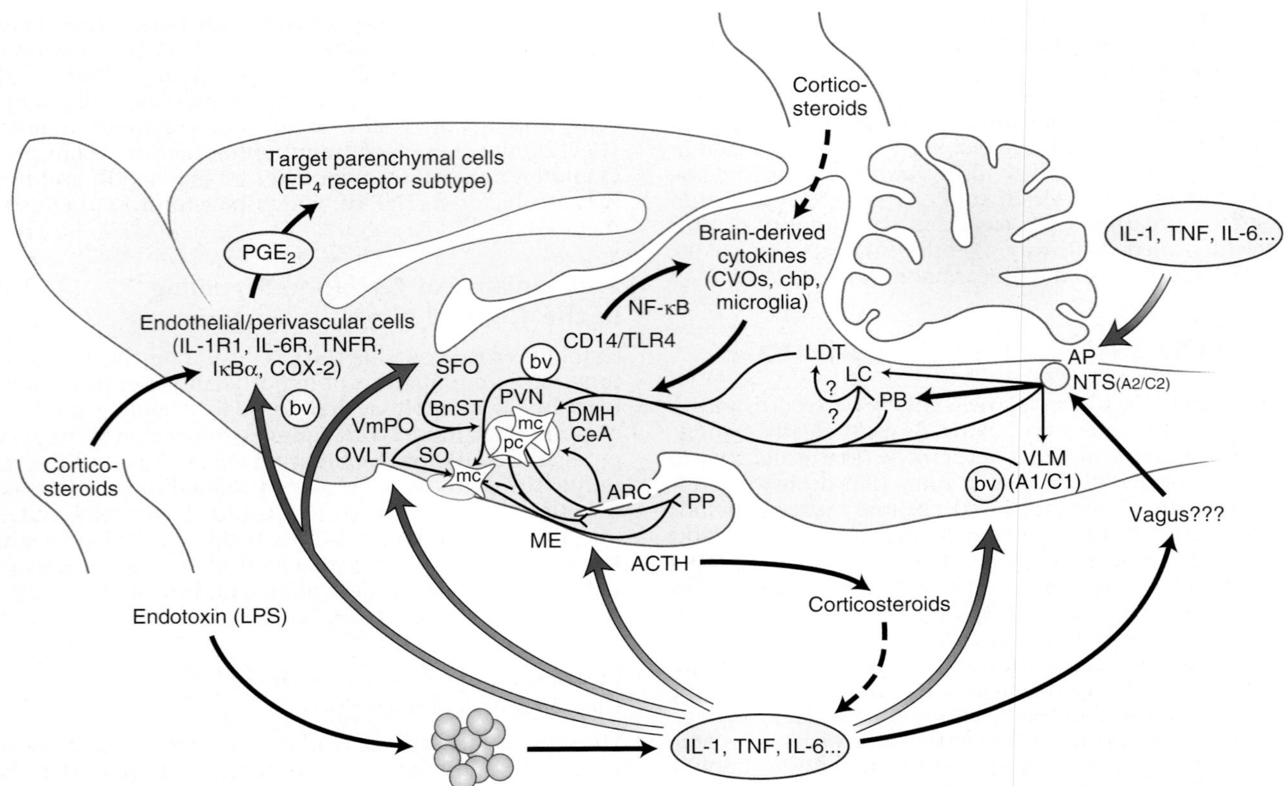

Figure 35-10 A model of the central nervous system circuitry activated by cytokines. CVOs (organs devoid of blood-brain barrier) and the blood vessels (bv) are crucial target sites of cytokines of systemic origin that are produced during the acute phase response. Among these integrative structures, the PVN is critical in coordinating autonomic and endocrine responses, including the activity of the hypothalamic-pituitary-adrenal (HPA) axis. For example, corticotropin-releasing factor neurons of the parvocellular PVN confer HPA-axis activation in endotoxin-treated animals. ACTH, adrenocorticotropic hormone; AP, area postrema; ARC, arcuate nucleus; BnST, bed nucleus of the stria terminalis; bv, blood vessels; chp, choroid plexus; CeA, central nucleus of the amygdala; chp, choroid plexus; COX-2, cyclooxygenase 2; CVOs, circumventricular organs; DMH, dorsomedial nucleus of the hypothalamus; EP, prostaglandin E receptor; IL, interleukin; IL-1R1, IL-1 type 1 receptor; IκBα, inhibitor of NF-κB; LC, locus ceruleus; LDT, laterodorsal tegmental nucleus; LPS, lipopolysaccharide; ME, median eminence; MPOA, medial preoptic area; NF-κB; nuclear factor-κB; NTS, nucleus of the solitary tract; OVLT, organum vasculosum of the lamina terminalis; PGE_2, prostaglandin E_2; PB, parabrachial nucleus; PP, posterior pituitary; PVN, paraventricular nucleus of the hypothalamus (parvocellular [pc] and magnocellular [mc] divisions); SFO, subfornical organ; SO, supraoptic nucleus; TLR, toll-like receptor; TNFα, tumor necrosis factor α; TNFR, tumor necrosis factor receptor; VLM, ventrolateral medulla; VmPO, ventral medial preoptic area. (Modified from Rivest S, Lacroix S, Vallieres L, et al. How the blood talks to the brain parenchyma and the paraventricular nucleus of the hypothalamus during systemic inflammatory and infectious stimuli. *Proc Soc Exp Biol Med.* 2000;223:22-38.)

that central injections of prostaglandins increase body temperature.[316,317]

Two isoforms of cyclooxygenase (COX) exist. COX1 is the constitutive form of the enzyme and is not thought to be regulated by inflammatory stimuli. COX2 is an inducible isoform and is increased in several cell types in response to immunologic stimuli.[318,319] In the normal brain, COX2 mRNA and the COX2 protein are found exclusively in neurons.[302,320-322] In contrast, immune stimulation by LPS or cytokines induces the COX2 mRNA and protein throughout the brain in non-neuronal cells associated with blood vessels, the meninges, and the choroid plexus. In addition, systemic administration of IL-1β induces the expression of prostaglandin E (PGE) synthase mRNA.[323] This likely includes endothelial cells and perivascular microglial cells as well as meningeal macrophages.[324-326] Regardless of the cell type, it seems clear that circulating LPS or cytokines induce COX2 in cells in the perivascular space, which in turn may produce prostaglandins to stimulate nearby brain regions inside the BBB.

PGE_2, the predominant endogenous isoform of PGE in the brain, is thought to be an essential mediator of cytokine modulation of hypothalamic function.[327] Evidence supporting this claim includes the fact that microinjections of PGE receptor agonists into the brain of rats[306,328,329] and other species[330,331] produces fever. The preoptic area of the hypothalamus surrounding the OVLT is thought to be critical in the response to PGE. For example, microinjections of as little of 1 ng of PGE_2 into the anteroventral preoptic area of rats reliably produces fevers.[328] Conversely, a COX2 inhibitor, ketorolac, attenuates LPS-induced fever with injections placed in the same region.[332] This PGE-sensitive zone is the same as the region containing the highest concentrations of PGE_2 binding sites.[333,334] The cloning of the PGE (EP) receptors will ultimately allow a more definitive analysis of the receptors in the hypothalamus that mediate the effects of PGEs on both fever and anorexia (see Fig. 35-11).

Four EP receptors have been identified: EP_1, EP_2, EP_3, and EP_4.[301,335,336] All four subtypes are expressed in the preoptic area of the hypothalamus.[301,337-341] Pharmacologic evidence suggests that EP_1 and EP_3 receptor agonist administration mimics PGE_2-induced fever.[342,343] Moreover, an EP_1 receptor antagonist blocks PGE_2 fever.[343] In contrast, targeted deletion of the EP_3 gene results in mice that do not show an early phase of fever after injection of LPS or PGE_2 (ICV).[336] EP_1 and EP_3 receptors do not individually appear to be essential for cancer-mediated anorexia in rodent models.[344]

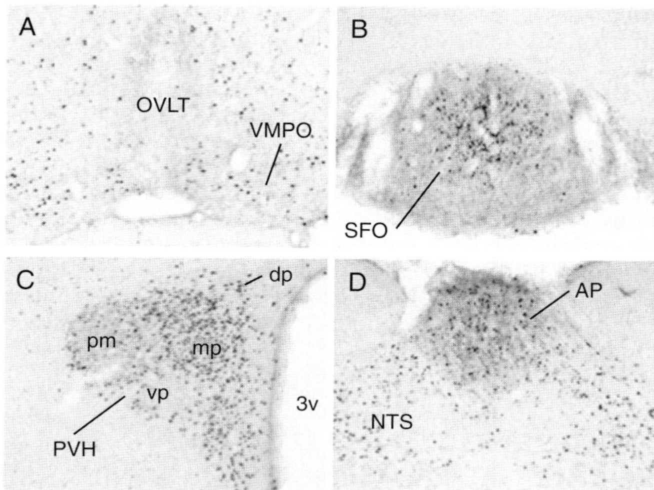

Figure 35-11 Immune stimulation activates key brain regions involved in energy homeostasis. A series of photomicrographs demonstrating the distribution of Fos-like immunoreactivity (Fos-IR) in the rat brain 2 hours after intravenous injection of 125 μg/kg lipopolysaccharide (LPS). LPS administration is a commonly used model of immune stimulation, and Fos-IR is a widely used marker of neuronal activation. LPS activates immune functions (induces Fos-IR) in the ventral medial preoptic (VMPO) area and in the organum vasculosum of the lamina terminalis (OVLT), shown in **A**; in the subfornical organ (SFO) (**B**); in the paraventricular nucleus of the hypothalamus (PVH) (**C**); and in the area postrema (AP) and nucleus of the solitary tract (NTS) in the brainstem (**D**). Prominent Fos-IR is seen throughout the subdivisions of the PVH, including the dorsal (dp), ventral (vp), and medial (mp) parvocellular and posterior magnocellular (pm) divisions. Notice that LPS also activates neurons in the circumventricular organs (OVLT, SFO, and AP). 3v, third ventricle.

There is upregulation of EP_4 receptor expression in several areas of the brain, including the corticotropin-releasing hormone (CRH) neurons of the PVH, after immune challenge.[337,340] In addition, paraventricular neurons that express Fos after ICV PGE_2 also express EP_4 receptors.[340]

Therefore, production of PGE_2 is certainly an obligate step in the pathogenesis of the febrile response. Furthermore, knockout of the gene for enzyme microsomal prostaglandin E synthase-1 (mPGES-1), essential for PGE_2 synthesis, blocks IL-1β–induced anorexia.[345] However, LPS-induced anorexia remains intact in these animals, suggesting both PGE_2-dependent and PGE_2-independent pathways are involved in the anorexic component of cachexia.[345]

Entry of Cytokines into the Brain

Circulating cytokines are proteins that cannot easily penetrate the BBB. The kinetics of entry of cytokines into the brain have been examined, and evidence suggests that saturable transport of IL-1α, IL-1β, IL-6, and TNF-α into the brain occurs.[346-348] However, it is not clear whether sufficient levels of cytokines are detectable in brain after acute intravenous administration to account for CNS responses to acute infection. Therefore, the physiologic setting and the significance of this mechanism remain to be established. Moreover, levels of circulating IL-1β do not rise significantly during immune challenges.[349,350]

In contrast to IL-1β, large increases in levels of circulating and brain IL-6 are found during fever. Although the mechanism is not completely understood, it appears that synthesis of IL-6 within the BBB, and not crossing of peripheral IL-6 through the BBB, is critical in the production of fever.[351] Several studies have demonstrated that cells located at the BBB and cells within the meninges respond to LPS stimulation with induction of IL-1β and TNF-α, the NF-κB inhibitor (IκBα), and the LPS receptor (CD14).[301,352-354] Cells with a similar morphology lining the blood vessels that penetrate the CNS and the meninges that cover it also have IL-1 receptors, suggesting that they may also respond to cytokines.[355] Hence, endothelial and perivascular cells at the blood-brain interface may have the ability to elaborate cytokines after an LPS or cytokine signal. The physiologic role of centrally produced cytokines in the response to peripheral immune cues has been reviewed in detail elsewhere.[301,350]

Brain Regions Involved in the Cytokine Response

Many studies have used the immediate expression of early genes such as *FOS* or its protein product (Fos)[356] as a marker of neuronal activity. This has allowed investigators to assess the involvement of extended neuronal systems during the complex physiologic responses that occur after immune challenge. Mapping of the patterns of activation in the CNS after administration of either IL-1β or LPS has allowed new insights into the functional neuroanatomy underlying the coordinated autonomic, endocrine, and behavioral responses during the febrile response.[310,313,357-359] Immune activation using moderate to high doses of LPS and IL-1β activates central autonomic and endocrine structures at almost every level of the neuraxis, including several neuroendocrine regulator sites, such as central nucleus of the amygdala, paraventricular hypothalamic nucleus, arcuate nucleus of the hypothalamus, subfornical organ, OVLT, and ventral medial preoptic area. Engaged brainstem sites include the parabrachial nucleus, NTS, area postrema, and rostral and caudal levels of the ventrolateral medulla.[310,313,357-368] In the PVH, LPS and cytokines activate parvicellular CRH neurons.

Although it is established that the hypothalamus is responsible for inducing a febrile response and anorexia, hypothalamic systems also exist that attenuate rises in body temperature. These include arcuate POMC neurons (see Figs. 35-2 and 35-10) and arginine vasopressin neurons, both of which are thought to be endogenous antipyretic neuromodulators.[369-372]

Neuronal activation patterns elicited by LPS or cytokines likely include neurons engaged to limit rises in body temperature. Tatro and colleagues found that exogenous α-MSH administration can block LPS-induced fever.[373] The discovery that central melanocortin agonists can both inhibit food intake[30] and increase energy expenditure[374] suggested that stimulation of the central melanocortin system might be involved in mediating a component of cachexia. Direct experimental testing of this hypothesis demonstrated that the central melanocortin system does contribute to anorexia during systemic illness.[373,375,376] In rodents, MC4R blockade prevents illness-induced anorexia and cachexia associated with cancer and kidney failure.[377,378]

Researchers have coupled neuroanatomic tract tracing with methods assessing immediate-early gene expression to investigate the circuitry that is activated by peripheral immune signals. For example, intravenous administration of IL-1β induced Fos in C1 adrenergic neurons in the ventrolateral medulla that project to the PVH. The C1 adrenergic cell group targets the medial parvicellular subdivision of the PVH, the site of the CRH neurons 7-26.[310] Lesions interrupting the input from the C1 cells to the PVH prevent the HPA response to IL-1β. These studies suggest that the activation of C1 cells by locally produced prostaglandins[312] may play a critical role in activating the HPA axis in response to IL-1β.

SPNs in the IML, extending from the first thoracic through the upper lumbar segments of the spinal cord, also show Fos expression in response to LPS.[367] Preganglionic neurons in the upper thoracic (T1-4) levels mediate thermogenesis by BAT,[379,380] and this is a key mechanism used by rats to control heat production and body temperature.[381] SPNs in the T2-5 levels are important for control of the heart,[89,382] which is significant because there are changes in cardiac output in the febrile state. SPNs receive direct, monosynaptic input from a series of well-defined nuclei in the brainstem and the hypothalamus (see Fig. 35-2) and provide another way in which the hypothalamus can contribute to the coordinated autonomic response to inflammatory signals. The major input to the sympathetic preganglionic column arises from neurons in the hypothalamus.[383] This innervation includes the PVH (dorsal, ventral, and lateral parvicellular subnuclei), the LHA, and the arcuate nucleus and retrochiasmatic area.[99,176] Direct projections to the IML also arise in the brainstem from the A5 noradrenergic cell group in the ventral pons, the caudal part of the NTS, the ventromedial medulla including the medullary raphe nuclei, and the rostral ventrolateral medulla, including the C1 adrenergic cell group.[89,176,384]

Fos expression in hypothalamic and brainstem neurons projecting to the IML after LPS administration has been examined.[384] LPS-activated cells that innervate the IML are found in the rostral ventrolateral medulla (C1 adrenergic cell group) and in the A5 noradrenergic cell group in the brainstem. A prominent population of cells was found in the dorsal parvicellular division of the PVH. These results suggest that neurons in the parvicellular PVH specifically innervate SPNs in the spinal cord that regulate LPS-induced fever. Furthermore, as noted earlier, activation of CRH neurons in the PVH is a signature of the CNS response to immune stimulation. Therefore, the paraventricular hypothalamic nucleus is a key site for mediating both neuroendocrine and autonomic responses to immune stimulation.

INTERSECTION OF ENERGY BALANCE AND REWARD CIRCUITS

If rational strategies to combat obesity are to be developed, an increased understanding of the molecular mechanisms of the rewarding aspects of feeding behavior is required.[40] A relatively recent and novel concept is that food and drug rewards share some common neural substrates.[40,385] Motivation and reward have been studied in the context of drug addiction.[386-388] The nucleus accumbens and its dopamine inputs have been strongly implicated in mediating several rewarding stimuli.[386,389]

Although it is widely accepted that dopamine is involved in reward processes, the relationship between dopamine and reward is complex.[40] Lesions of the nucleus accumbens reduce food intake[390] or the ability to display operant conditioning in response to food,[391] but there is also a dopamine component of food reward. For example, mice lacking the ability to produce dopamine would normally die of starvation, but they resumed feeding after reintroduction of the dopamine into the striatum.[392,393]

Key metabolic cues act directly on dopamine neurons in the midbrain. For example, midbrain dopamine neurons express leptin and ghrelin receptors.[394-396] Fulton and colleagues demonstrated that leptin also affects brain self-stimulation,[397] suggesting that leptin has the ability to affect CNS circuits classically involved in reward. Taken together, these findings suggest that alterations of cues such as leptin and ghrelin may not only affect hypothalamic pathways but also act directly on midbrain dopamine neurons. Although this field of study is still evolving, models based on these findings could have broad implications. Such models could provide a mechanism for signals regulating food intake to intersect with brain circuitry that is critical in the regulation of motivated behaviors. Moreover, dysregulation of these pathways may be relevant to the pathophysiology of obesity and eating disorders such as anorexia nervosa.[398]

NEUROENDOCRINE DISORDERS OF ENERGY HOMEOSTASIS

A wide variety of disorders of hypothalamic and neuroendocrine function are known to produce obesity. Insults to the function of the basal hypothalamus, including Fröhlich's syndrome and craniopharyngioma, are known to cause obesity (see earlier discussion). In the past 15 years there have been a number of important discoveries related to genetic syndromes underlying certain human obesity disorders (see Chapter 36). Two of the most informative monogenic disorders are discussed here in the context of their effects on the neuroendocrine control of energy stores.

Leptin and Leptin Receptor Deficiencies in Humans

Despite being extremely rare, leptin deficiency[399] and leptin receptor defects[400] in humans are illustrative of the physiologic importance of this hormone. Serum leptin levels in humans are generally proportional to adipose mass.[128,401] Therefore, most obese humans may be considered to be leptin-resistant rather than deficient in leptin.[42,127,402] Despite rapid increases in understanding of obesity and leptin action, the molecular basis of leptin resistance remains poorly understood.

Clinical studies have demonstrated that leptin treatment is safe and well tolerated and clearly effective in individuals with congenital leptin deficiency[125] and in patients who are very low in adipose tissue.[403,404] For example, doses of methionyl-leptin were given to subjects with congenital deficiency and resulted in leptin levels 10% of those predicted based on body fat. Leptin in this study was well tolerated and resulted in dramatic declines in appetite, body weight, and food intake.[125] In addition, administration of recombinant leptin to women with hypothalamic amenorrhea due to strenuous exercise training and very low body fat normalized several endocrine indices of reproductive function and bone density.[404] In individuals with common obesity, however, leptin had only very modest effects on appetite and body weight.[405]

A newer concept is that leptin has potent effects on whole-body glucose and lipid homeostasis independent of its effects on body weight.[49,146] Studies of leptin action may be relevant to models linking diabetes and hypothalamic resistance to metabolic cues. Leptin deficiency, as seen in lipodystrophic mice and humans, induces severe insulin resistance that is corrected by leptin replacement.[406-408] This can be explained by actions of leptin in the arcuate nucleus of the hypothalamus. Restoration of leptin receptors only in the arcuate nucleus of mice lacking leptin receptors everywhere remarkably improved glucose homeostasis.[409,410] Therefore, leptin action in the arcuate nucleus is sufficient to mediate the antidiabetic actions of leptin.

Obesity Resulting from Defective Melanocortin Signaling

Evidence that the melanocortin obesity syndrome can occur in humans resulted from the astute recognition in two families of an agouti-mouse–like syndrome resulting from null mutations in the *POMC* gene (Fig. 35-12).[411] These patients had a rare syndrome that includes ACTH insufficiency, red hair, and obesity resulting from the lack of ACTH peptide in the serum, together with a lack of melanocortin peptides in skin and brain. These data demonstrated, for the first time, that the central melanocortin circuitry subserves energy homeostasis in humans, as it does in the mouse. Shortly thereafter, heterozygous frameshift mutations in the human *MC4R* were reported and were associated with nonsyndromic obesity in two separate families.[412,413] Additional reports[414-416] provided a clearer picture of the frequency and diversity of *MC4R* mutations and showed that haploinsufficiency of MC4R in humans is the most common monogenic cause of severe obesity, accounting for up to 5% of cases. Two more recent reports provided a detailed clinical picture of the syndrome.[417,418] Remarkably, the syndrome is virtually identical to that reported for the mouse,[31,109,373] with increased adipose mass, increased linear growth and lean mass, hyperinsulinemia greater than that seen in matched obese controls, and severe hyperphagia.

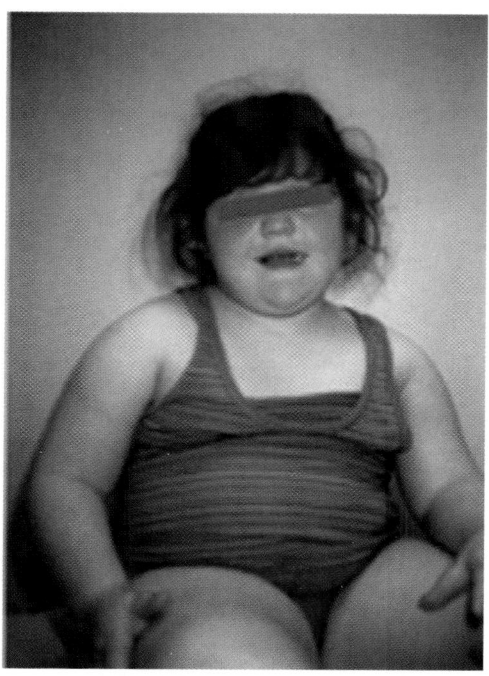

Figure 35-12 A monogenic neuroendocrine obesity syndrome of adrenocorticotropic hormone insufficiency, obesity, and red hair resulting from a null mutation in the pro-opiomelanocortin gene. (Photograph provided by Dr. A. Gruters, Charité-Universitätsmedzin, Berlin.)

REFERENCES

1. Bramwell B. *Intracranial Tumours*. Edinburgh, UK: Pentland; 1888.
2. Fröhlich A. Ein fall von tumor der hypophysis cerebri ohne akromegalie. *Wien Klin Rundsch*. 1901;15:883.
3. Crowe SJ, Cushing H, Homans J. Experimental hypophysectomy. *Bulletin of the Johns Hopkins Hospital*. 1910;21:127.
4. Stevenson JAF. Neural control of food and water intake. In: Haymaker W, Anderson E, Nauta WJH, eds. *The Hypothalamus*. Springfield, IL: Charles C Thomas, 1969:524-621.
5. Elmquist JK, Elias CF, Saper CB. From lesions to leptin: hypothalamic control of food intake and body weight. *Neuron*. 1999;22:221-232.
6. Aschner B. Uber die funktion der hypophyse. *Pflugers Arch Physiol*. 1912;146:1.
7. Hetherington AW, Ranson SW. Hypothalamic lesions and adiposity in the rat. *Anat Rec*. 1940;78:149-172.
8. Stellar E. The physiology of motivation. *Physiol Rev*. 1954;61:5-22.
9. Kennedy GC. The role of depot fat in the hypothalamic control of food intake in the rat. *Proc R Soc Lond B Biol Sci*. 1953;140:579-592.
10. Harris RB, Kasser TR, Martin RJ. Dynamics of recovery of body composition after overfeeding, food restriction or starvation of mature female rats. *J Nutr*. 1986;116:2536-2546.
11. Harris RB. Role of set-point theory in regulation of body weight. *FASEB J*. 1990;4:3310-3318.
12. Faust IM, Johnson PR, Hirsch J. Surgical removal of adipose tissue alters feeding behavior and the development of obesity in rats. *Science*. 1977;197:393-396.
13. Hervey GR. The effects of lesions in the hypothalamus in parabiotic rats. *J Physiol*. 1959;145:336-352.
14. Hervey GR. Physiological mechanisms for the regulation of energy balance. *Proc Nutr Soc*. 1971;30:109-116.
15. Parameswaran SV, Steffens AB, Hervey GR, et al. Involvement of a humoral factor in regulation of body weight in parabiotic rats. *Am J Physiol*. 1977;232:R150-R157.
16. Ingalls AM, Dickie MM, Snell GD. Obese, a new mutation in the house mouse. *J Hered*. 1950;41:317-318.
17. Coleman DL, Hummel KP. Effects of parabiosis of normal with genetically diabetic mice. *Am J Physiol*. 1969;217:1298-1304.
18. Coleman DL. Obese and diabetes: two mutant genes causing diabetes-obesity syndromes in mice. *Diabetologia*. 1978;14:141-148.
19. Coleman DL. Effects of parabiosis of obese with diabetes and normal mice. *Diabetologia*. 1973;9:294-298.
20. Lee GH, Proenca R, Montez JM, et al. Abnormal splicing of the leptin receptor in diabetic mice. *Nature*. 1996;379:632-635.
21. Tartaglia LA, Dembski M, Weng X, et al. Identification and expression cloning of a leptin receptor, OB-R. *Cell*. 1995;83:1263-1271.
22. Zhang Y, Proenca R, Maffei M, et al. Positional cloning of the mouse obese gene and its human homologue. *Nature*. 1994;372:425-432.
23. Campfield LA, Smith FJ, Guisez Y, et al. Recombinant mouse OB protein: evidence for a peripheral signal linking adiposity and central neural networks. *Science*. 1995;269:546-549.
24. Halaas JL, Gajiwala KS, Maffei M, et al. Weight-reducing effects of the plasma protein encoded by the obese gene. *Science*. 1995;269:543-546.
25. Halaas JL, Boozer C, Blair-West J, et al. Physiological response to long-term peripheral and central leptin infusion in lean and obese mice. *Proc Natl Acad Sci U S A*. 1997;94:8878-8883.
26. Pelleymounter MA, Cullen MJ, Baker MB, et al. Effects of the obese gene product on body weight regulation in ob/ob mice [see comments]. *Science*. 1995;269:540-543.
27. Miller MW, Duhl DM, Vrieling H, et al. Cloning of the mouse agouti gene predicts a novel secreted protein ubiquitously expressed in mice carrying the lethal yellow (A^y) mutation. *Genes and Dev*. 1993;7:454-467.
28. Bultman SJ, Michaud EJ, Woychik RP. Molecular characterization of the mouse agouti locus. *Cell*. 1992;71:1195-1204.
29. Lu D, Willard D, Patel IR, et al. Agouti protein is an antagonist of the melanocyte-stimulating hormone receptor. *Nature*. 1994;371:799-802.
30. Fan W, Boston BA, Kesterson RA, et al. Role of melanocortinergic neurons in feeding and the agouti obesity syndrome. *Nature*. 1997;385:165-168.
31. Huszar D, Lynch CA, Fairchild-Huntress V, et al. Targeted disruption of the melanocortin-4 receptor results in obesity in mice. *Cell*. 1997;88:131-141.
32. Saper CB. Central autonomic system. In: Paxinos G, ed. *The Rat Nervous System*. San Diego, CA: Academic Press, 1995:107-135.
33. Grill HJ, Kaplan JM. The neuroanatomical axis for control of energy balance. *Front Neuroendocrinol*. 2002;23:2-40.
34. Herbert H, Moga MM, Saper CB. Connections of the parabrachial nucleus with the nucleus of the solitary tract and the medullary reticular formation in the rat. *J Comp Neurol*. 1990;293:540-580.
35. Broadwell RD, Brightman MW. Entry of peroxidase into neurons of the central and peripheral nervous systems from extracerebral and cerebral blood. *J Comp Neurol*. 1976;166:257-283.

36. Herbert H, Saper CB. Cholecystokinin-, galanin-, and corticotropin-releasing factor-like immunoreactive projections from the nucleus of the solitary tract to the parabrachial nucleus in the rat. *J Comp Neurol.* 1990;293:581-598.
37. Billig I, Yates BJ, Rinaman L. Plasma hormone levels and central c-Fos expression in ferrets after systemic administration of cholecystokinin. *Am J Physiol Regul Integr Comp Physiol.* 2001;281:R1243-R1255.
38. Rinaman L. A functional role for central glucagon-like peptide-1 receptors in lithium chloride-induced anorexia. *Am J Physiol.* 1999;277(5 Pt 2):R1537-R1540.
39. Yamamoto H, Kishi T, Lee CE, et al. Glucagon-like peptide-1 responsive catecholamine neurons in the area postrema link peripheral glucagon-like peptide-1 with central autonomic control sites. *J Neurosci.* 2003;23:2939-2946.
40. Saper CB, Chou TC, Elmquist JK. The need to feed: homeostatic and hedonic control of eating. *Neuron.* 2002;36:199-211.
41. Cone RD. Anatomy and regulation of the central melanocortin system. *Nat Neurosci.* 2005;8:571-578.
42. Barsh GS, Farooqi IS, O'Rahilly S. Genetics of body-weight regulation. *Nature.* 2000;404:644-651.
43. Schwartz MW, Seeley RJ, Woods SC, et al. Leptin increases hypothalamic pro-opiomelanocortin mRNA expression in the rostral arcuate nucleus. *Diabetes.* 1997;46:2119-2123.
44. Stephens TW, Basinski M, Bristow PK, et al. The role of neuropeptide Y in the antiobesity action of the obese gene product. *Nature.* 1995;377:530-532.
45. Cowley MA, Smart JL, Rubinstein M, et al. Leptin activates anorexigenic POMC neurons through a neural network in the arcuate nucleus. *Nature.* 2001;411:480-484.
46. Spanswick D, Smith MA, Groppi VE, et al. Leptin inhibits hypothalamic neurons by activation of ATP-sensitive potassium channels. *Nature.* 1997;390:521-525.
47. Balthasar N, Coppari R, McMinn J, et al. Leptin receptor signaling in POMC neurons is required for normal body weight homeostasis. *Neuron.* 2004;42:983-991.
48. Dhillon H, Zigman JM, Ye C, et al. Leptin directly activates SF1 neurons in the VMH, and this action by leptin is required for normal body-weight homeostasis. *Neuron.* 2006;49:191-203.
49. Elmquist JK, Coppari R, Balthasar N, et al. Identifying hypothalamic pathways controlling food intake, body weight, and glucose homeostasis. *J Comp Neurol.* 2005;493:63-71.
50. Cowley MA, Smith RG, Diano S, et al. The distribution and mechanism of action of ghrelin in the CNS demonstrates a novel hypothalamic circuit regulating energy homeostasis. *Neuron.* 2003;37:649-661.
51. Heisler LK, Cowley MA, Tecott LH. Activation of central melanocortin pathways by fenfluramine. *Science.* 2002;297:609-611.
52. Heisler LK, Jobst EE, Sutton GM, et al. Serotonin reciprocally regulates melanocortin neurons to modulate food intake. *Neuron.* 2006;51: 239-249.
53. Fan W, Boston BA, Kesterson RA, et al. Role of melanocortinergic neurons in feeding and the agouti obesity syndrome. *Nature.* 1997;385:165-168.
54. Farooqi IS, Keogh JM, Yeo GS, et al. Clinical spectrum of obesity and mutations in the melanocortin 4 receptor gene. *N Engl J Med.* 2003;348:1085-1095.
55. Farooqi IS, Yeo GS, Keogh JM, et al. Dominant and recessive inheritance of morbid obesity associated with melanocortin 4 receptor deficiency. *J Clin Invest.* 2000;10:271-279.
56. Yeo GS, Farooqi IS, Aminian S, et al. A frameshift mutation in MC4R associated with dominantly inherited human obesity (Letter). *Nat Genet.* 1998;20:111-112.
57. Vaisse C, Clement K, Guy-Grand B, et al. A frameshift mutation in human MC4R is associated with a dominant form of obesity. *Nat Genet.* 1998;20:113-114.
58. Mountjoy KG, Mortrud MT, Low MJ, et al. Localization of the melanocortin-4 receptor (MC4-R) in neuroendocrine and autonomic control circuits in the brain. *Mol Endocrinol.* 1994;8:1298-1308.
59. Kishi T, Aschkenasi CJ, Lee CE, et al. Expression of melanocortin 4 receptor mRNA in the central nervous system of the rat. *J Comp Neurol.* 2003;457:213-235.
60. Liu H, Kishi T, Roseberry AG, et al. Transgenic mice expressing green fluorescent protein under the control of the melanocortin-4 receptor promoter. *J Neurosci.* 2003;23:7143-7154.
61. Cowley MA, Pronchuk N, Fan W, et al. Integration of NPY, AGRP, and melanocortin signals in the hypothalamic paraventricular nucleus: evidence of a cellular basis for the adipostat. *Neuron.* 1999;24: 155-163.
62. Balthasar N, Dalgaard LT, Lee CE, et al. Divergence of melanocortin pathways in the control of food intake and energy expenditure. *Cell.* 2005;123:493-505.
63. Mountjoy KG, Mortrud MT, Low MJ, et al. Localization of the melanocortin-4 receptor (MC4-R) in neuroendocrine and autonomic control circuits in the brain. *Mol Endocrinol.* 1994;8:1298-1308.
64. Grill HJ, Ginsberg AB, Seeley RJ, et al. Brainstem application of melanocortin receptor ligands produces long-lasting effects on feeding and body weight. *J Neurosci.* 1998;18:10128-10135.
65. Williams DL, Kaplan JM, Grill HJ. The role of the dorsal vagal complex and the vagus nerve in feeding effects of melanocortin-3/4 receptor stimulation. *Endocrinology.* 2000;141:1332-1337.
66. Fan W, Ellacott KL, Halatchev IG, et al. Cholecystokinin-mediated suppression of feeding involves the brainstem melanocortin system. *Nat Neurosci.* 2004;7:335-336.
67. Anand BK, Brobeck JR. Localization of a "feeding center" in the hypothalamus of the rat. *Proc Soc Exp Biol Med.* 1951;77:323-324.
68. Bittencourt JC, Presse F, Arias C, et al. The melanin-concentrating hormone system of the rat brain: an immuno- and hybridization histochemical characterization. *J Comp Neurol.* 1992;319:218-245.
69. Qu D, Ludwig DS, Gammeltoft S, et al. A role for melanin-concentrating hormone in the central regulation of feeding behaviour. *Nature.* 1996;380:243-247.
70. Sakurai T, Amemiya A, Ishii M, et al. Orexins and orexin receptors: a family of hypothalamic neuropeptides and G protein-coupled receptors that regulate feeding behavior. *Cell.* 1998;92:573-585.
71. de Lecea L, Kilduff TS, Peyron C, et al. The hypocretins: hypothalamus-specific peptides with neuroexcitatory activity. *Proc Natl Acad Sci U S A.* 1998;95:322-327.
72. Elias CF, Saper CB, Maratos-Flier E, et al. Chemically defined projections linking the mediobasal hypothalamus and the lateral hypothalamic area. *J Comp Neurol.* 1998;402:442-459.
73. Broberger C, De Lecea L, Sutcliffe JG, et al. Hypocretin/orexin- and melanin-concentrating hormone-expressing cells form distinct populations in the rodent lateral hypothalamus: relationship to the neuropeptide Y and agouti gene-related protein systems. *J Comp Neurol.* 1998;402:460-474.
74. Peyron C, Tighe DK, van den Pol AN, et al. Neurons containing hypocretin (orexin) project to multiple neuronal systems. *J Neurosci.* 1998;18:9996-10015.
75. Marcus JN, Aschkenasi CJ, Lee CE, et al. Differential expression of orexin receptors 1 and 2 in the rat brain. *J Comp Neurol.* 2001;435:6-25.
76. Saito Y, Cheng M, Leslie FM, et al. Expression of the melanin-concentrating hormone (MCH) receptor mRNA in the rat brain. *J Comp Neurol.* 2001;435:26-40.
77. Kilduff TS, de Lecea L. Mapping of the mRNAs for the hypocretin/orexin and melanin-concentrating hormone receptors: networks of overlapping peptide systems. *J Comp Neurol.* 2001;435:1-5.
78. Shimada M, Tritos NA, Lowell BB, et al. Mice lacking melanin-concentrating hormone are hypophagic and lean. *Nature.* 1998;396:670-674.
79. Ludwig DS, Tritos NA, Mastaitis JW, et al. Melanin-concentrating hormone overexpression in transgenic mice leads to obesity and insulin resistance. *J Clin Invest.* 2001;107:379-386.
80. Segal-Lieberman G, Bradley RL, Kokkotou E, et al. Melanin-concentrating hormone is a critical mediator of the leptin-deficient phenotype. *Proc Natl Acad Sci U S A.* 2003;100:10085-10090.
81. Willie JT, Chemelli RM, Sinton CM, et al. To eat or to sleep? Orexin in the regulation of feeding and wakefulness. *Annu Rev Neurosci.* 2001;24:429-458.
82. Hara J, Beuckmann CT, Nambu T, et al. Genetic ablation of orexin neurons in mice results in narcolepsy, hypophagia, and obesity. *Neuron.* 2001;30:345-354.
83. Clegg DJ, Air EL, Woods SC, et al. Eating elicited by orexin-a, but not melanin-concentrating hormone, is opioid mediated. *Endocrinology.* 2002;143:2995-3000.
84. Chemelli RM, Willi JT, Sinton CM, et al. Narcolepsy in orexin knockout mice: molecular genetics of sleep regulation. *Cell.* 1999;98: 437-451.
85. Lin L, Faraco J, Li R, et al. The sleep disorder canine narcolepsy is caused by a mutation in the hypocretin (orexin) receptor 2 gene [see comments]. *Cell.* 1999;98:365-376.
86. Rothwell NJ. CNS regulation of thermogenesis. *Crit Rev Neurobiol.* 1994;8:1-10.
87. Lowell BB, Bachman ES. Beta-adrenergic receptors, diet-induced thermogenesis, and obesity. *J Biol Chem.* 2003;278:29385-29388.
88. Bachman ES, Dhillon H, Zhang CY, et al. betaAR signaling required for diet-induced thermogenesis and obesity resistance. *Science.* 2002;297:843-845.
89. Jansen AS, Nguyen XV, Karpitskiy V, et al. Central command neurons of the sympathetic nervous system: basis of the fight-or-flight response. *Science.* 1995;270:644-646.
90. Loewy AD. Forebrain nuclei involved in autonomic control. *Prog Brain Res.* 1991;87:253-268.
91. Loewy AD, Spyer KM. *Central regulation of autonomic functions.* New York, NY: Oxford University Press, 1990:xii, 390.
92. Strack AM, Sawyer WB, Platt KB, et al. CNS cell groups regulating the sympathetic outflow to adrenal gland as revealed by transneuronal cell body labeling with pseudorabies virus. *Brain Res.* 1989;491: 274-296.

93. Strack AM, Sawyer WB, Marubio LM, et al. Spinal origin of sympathetic preganglionic neurons in the rat. *Brain Res.* 1988;455:187-191.
94. Strack AM, Sawyer WB, Hughes GH, et al. A general pattern of CNS innervation of the sympathetic outflow demonstrated by transneuronal pseudorabies viral infections. *Brain Res.* 1989;491:156-162.
95. Jansen AS, Hoffman JL, Loewy AD. CNS sites involved in sympathetic and parasympathetic control of the pancreas: a viral tracing study. *Brain Res.* 1997;766:29-38.
96. Rinaman L, Miselis RR. The organization of vagal innervation of rat pancreas using cholera toxin-horseradish peroxidase conjugate. *J Auton Nerv Syst.* 1987;21:109-125.
97. Saper CB, Loewy AD, Swanson LW, et al. Direct hypothalamo-autonomic connections. *Brain Res.* 1976;117:305-312.
98. Loewy AD, McKellar S, Saper CB. Direct projections from the A5 catecholamine cell group to the intermediolateral cell column. *Brain Res.* 1979;174:309-314.
99. Cechetto DF, Saper CB. Neurochemical organization of the hypothalamic projection to the spinal cord in the rat. *J Comp Neurol.* 1988;272:579-604.
100. Loewy AD, Burton H. Nuclei of the solitary tract: efferent projections to the lower brain stem and spinal cord of the cat. *J Comp Neurol.* 1978;181:421-449.
101. Loewy AD. Descending pathways to sympathetic and parasympathetic preganglionic neurons. *J Auton Nerv Syst.* 1981;3:265-275.
102. Loewy AD. Descending pathways to the sympathetic preganglionic neurons. *Prog Brain Res.* 1982;57:267-277.
103. Tucker DC, Saper CB. Specificity of spinal projections from hypothalamic and brainstem areas which innervate sympathetic preganglionic neurons. *Brain Res.* 1985;360:159-164.
104. Tucker DC, Saper CB, Ruggiero DA, et al. Organization of central adrenergic pathways: I. Relationships of ventrolateral medullary projections to the hypothalamus and spinal cord. *J Comp Neurol.* 1987;259:591-603.
105. Chan RK, Sawchenko PE. Spatially and temporally differentiated patterns of c-fos expression in brainstem catecholaminergic cell groups induced by cardiovascular challenges in the rat. *J Comp Neurol.* 1994;348:433-460.
106. Morrison SF, Milner TA, Reis DJ. Reticulospinal vasomotor neurons of the rat rostral ventrolateral medulla: relationship to sympathetic nerve activity and the C1 adrenergic cell group. *J Neurosci.* 1988;8:1286-1301.
107. Haselton JR, Guyenet PG. Electrophysiological characterization of putative C1 adrenergic neurons in the rat. *Neuroscience.* 1989;30:199-214.
108. Reis DJ, Ruggiero DA, Morrison SF. The C1 area of the rostral ventrolateral medulla oblongata: a critical brainstem region for control of resting and reflex integration of arterial pressure. *Am J Hypertens.* 1989;2(12 Pt 2):363S-374S.
109. Butler AA, Marks DL, Fan W, et al. Melanocortin-4 receptor is required for acute homeostatic responses to increased dietary fat. *Nat Neurosci.* 2001;4:605-611.
110. Yasuda T, Masaki T, Kakuma T, et al. Hypothalamic melanocortin system regulates sympathetic nerve activity in brown adipose tissue. *Exp Biol Med (Maywood).* 2004;229:235-239.
111. Voss-Andreae A, Murphy JG, Ellacott KL, et al. Role of the central melanocortin circuitry in adaptive thermogenesis of brown adipose tissue. *Endocrinology.* 2007;148:1550-1560.
112. Elias CF, Lee C, Kelly J, et al. Leptin activates hypothalamic CART neurons projecting to the spinal cord. *Neuron.* 1998;21:1375-1385.
113. Morrison SF. Central pathways controlling brown adipose tissue thermogenesis. *News Physiol Sci.* 2004;19:67-74.
114. Fan W, Voss-Andreae A, Cao WH, et al. Regulation of thermogenesis by the central melanocortin system. *Peptides.* 2005;26:1800-1813.
115. Loewy AD. Raphe pallidus and raphe obscurus projections to the intermediolateral cell column in the rat. *Brain Res.* 1981;222:129-133.
116. Bacon SJ, Zagon A, Smith AD. Electron microscopic evidence of a monosynaptic pathway between cells in the caudal raphe nuclei and sympathetic preganglionic neurons in the rat spinal cord. *Exp Brain Res.* 1990;79:589-602.
117. Bamshad M, Song CK, Bartness TJ. CNS origins of the sympathetic nervous system outflow to brown adipose tissue. *Am J Physiol.* 1999;276(6 Pt 2):R1569-R1578.
118. Morrison SF. Differential control of sympathetic outflow. *Am J Physiol Regul Integr Comp Physiol.* 2001;281:R683-R698.
119. Zhang Y, Proenca R, Maffei R, et al. Positional cloning of the mouse obese gene and its human homologue. *Nature.* 1994;372:425-432.
120. Wang J, Liu R, Hawkins M, et al. A nutrient-sensing pathway regulates leptin gene expression in muscle and fat. *Nature.* 1998;393:684-688.
121. Masuzaki H, Ogawa Y, Sagawa N, et al. Nonadipose tissue production of leptin: leptin as a novel placenta-derived hormone in humans. *Nat Med.* 1997;3:1029-1033.
122. Pelleymounter MA, Cullen MJ, Baker MB, et al. Effects of the obese gene product on body weight regulation in ob/ob mice. *Science.* 1995;269:540-543.
123. Campfield LA, Smith FJ, Guisez Y, et al. Recombinant mouse OB protein: evidence for a peripheral signal linking adiposity and central neural networks. *Science.* 1995;269:546-549.
124. Halaas JL, Gajiwala KS, Maffei M, et al. Weight-reducing effects of the plasma protein encoded by the obese gene. *Science.* 1995;269:543-546.
125. Farooqi IS, Jebb SA, Langmack G, et al. Effects of recombinant leptin therapy in a child with congenital leptin deficiency. *N Engl J Med.* 1999;341:879-884.
126. Ahima RS, Saper CB, Flier JS, et al. Role of leptin in the neuroendocrine response to fasting. *Nature.* 1996;382:250-252.
127. Spiegelman BM, Flier JS. Obesity and the regulation of energy balance. *Cell.* 2001;104:531-543.
128. Frederich RC, Hamann A, Anderson S, et al. Leptin levels reflect body lipid content in mice: evidence for diet-induced resistance to leptin action. *Nat Med.* 1995;1:1311-1314.
129. Ahima RS, Saper CB, Flier JS, et al. Leptin regulation of neuroendocrine systems. *Front Neuroendocrinol.* 2000;21:263-307.
130. Flier JS. Clinical review 94: what's in a name? In search of leptin's physiologic role. *J Clin Endocrinol Metab.* 1998;83:1407-1413.
131. Tartaglia LA. The leptin receptor. *J Biol Chem.* 1997;272:6093-6096.
132. Chen H, Charlat O, Tartaglia LA, et al. Evidence that the diabetes gene encodes the leptin receptor: identification of a mutation in the leptin receptor gene in db/db mice. *Cell.* 1996;84:491-495.
133. White DW, Wang DW, Chua SC Jr, et al. Constitutive and impaired signaling of leptin receptors containing the Gln → Pro extracellular domain fatty mutation. *Proc Natl Acad Sci U S A.* 1997;94:10657-10662.
134. Mercer JG, Hoggard N, Williams LM, et al. Coexpression of leptin receptor and preproneuropeptide Y mRNA in arcuate nucleus of mouse hypothalamus. *J Neuroendocrinol.* 1996;8:733-735.
135. Mercer JG, Hoggard N, Williams LM, et al. Localization of leptin receptor mRNA and the long form splice variant (Ob-Rb) in mouse hypothalamus and adjacent brain regions by in situ hybridization. *FEBS Lett.* 1996;387:113-116.
136. Fei H, Okano HJ, Li C, et al. Anatomic localization of alternatively spliced leptin receptors (Ob-R) in mouse brain and other tissues. *Proc Natl Acad Sci U S A.* 1997;94:7001-7005.
137. Schwartz MW, Seeley RJ, Campfield LA, et al. Identification of targets of leptin action in rat hypothalamus. *J Clin Invest.* 1996;98:1101-1106.
138. Elmquist JK, Bjorbaek C, Ahima RS, et al. Distributions of leptin receptor mRNA isoforms in the rat brain. *J Comp Neurol.* 1998;395:535-547.
139. Cheung CC, Clifton DK, Steiner RA. Proopiomelanocortin neurons are direct targets for leptin in the hypothalamus. *Endocrinology.* 1997;138:4489-4492.
140. Hosoi T, Kawagishi T, Okuma Y, et al. Brain stem is a direct target for leptin's action in the central nervous system. *Endocrinology.* 2002;143:3498-3504.
141. Grill HJ, Schwartz MW, Kaplan JM, et al. Evidence that the caudal brainstem is a target for the inhibitory effect of leptin on food intake. *Endocrinology.* 2002;143:239-246.
142. Finn PD, Cunningham MJ, Rickard DG, et al. Serotonergic neurons are targets for leptin in the monkey. *J Clin Endocrinol Metab.* 2001;86:422-426.
143. Mercer JG, Moar KM, Hoggard N. Localization of leptin receptor (Ob-R) messenger ribonucleic acid in the rodent hindbrain. *Endocrinology.* 1998;139:29-34.
144. Mercer JG, Moar KM, Findlay PA, et al. Association of leptin receptor (OB-Rb), NPY and GLP-1 gene expression in the ovine and murine brainstem. *Regul Pept.* 1998;75-76:271-278.
145. Bernard C. Chiens rendus diabetiques. *C R Soc Biol (Paris).* 1849;1:60.
146. Elmquist JK, Marcus JN. Rethinking the central causes of diabetes. *Nat Med.* 2003;9:645-647.
147. Fan W, Dinulescu DM, Butler AA, et al. The central melanocortin system can directly regulate serum insulin levels. *Endocrinology.* 2000;141:3072-3079.
148. Obici S, Feng Z, Arduini A, et al. Inhibition of hypothalamic carnitine palmitoyltransferase-1 decreases food intake and glucose production. *Nat Med.* 2003;9:756-761.
149. Obici S, Feng Z, Karkanias G, et al. Decreasing hypothalamic insulin receptors causes hyperphagia and insulin resistance in rats. *Nat Neurosci.* 2002;5:566-572.
150. Schwartz MW. Progress in the search for neuronal mechanisms coupling type 2 diabetes to obesity. *J Clin Invest.* 2001;108:963-964.
151. Schwartz MW, Woods SC, Porte D Jr, et al. Central nervous system control of food intake. *Nature.* 2000;404:661-671.
152. Woods SC, Lotter EC, McKay LD, et al. Chronic intracerebroventricular infusion of insulin reduces food intake and body weight of baboons. *Nature.* 1979;282:503-505.
153. Bruning JC, Gautam D, Burks DJ, et al. Role of brain insulin receptor in control of body weight and reproduction. *Science.* 2000;289:2122-2125.

154. Buettner C, Patel R, Muse ED, et al. Severe impairment in liver insulin signaling fails to alter hepatic insulin action in conscious mice. *J Clin Invest*. 2005;115:1306-1313.
155. Okamoto H, Obici S, Accili D, et al. Restoration of liver insulin signaling in Insr knockout mice fails to normalize hepatic insulin action. *J Clin Invest*. 2005;115:1314-1322.
156. Edgerton DS, Lautz M, Scott M, et al. Insulin's direct effects on the liver dominate the control of hepatic glucose production. *J Clin Invest*. 2006;116:521-527.
157. Oomura Y, Ono T, Ooyama H, et al. Glucose and osmosensitive neurones of the rat hypothalamus. *Nature*. 1969;222:282-284.
158. Levin BE. Metabolic sensing neurons and the control of energy homeostasis. *Physiol Behav*. 2006;89:1107-1121.
159. Levin BE, Routh VH, Kang L, et al. Neuronal glucosensing: what do we know after 50 years? *Diabetes*. 2004;53:2521-2528.
160. Ibrahim N, Bosch MA, Smart JL, et al. Hypothalamic proopiomelanocortin neurons are glucose responsive and express K(ATP) channels. *Endocrinology*. 2003;144:1331-1340.
161. DiRocco RJ, Grill HJ. The forebrain is not essential for sympathoadrenal hyperglycemic response to glucoprivation. *Science*. 1979;204: 1112-1114.
162. Ritter S, Bugarith K, Dinh TT. Immunotoxic destruction of distinct catecholamine subgroups produces selective impairment of glucoregulatory responses and neuronal activation. *J Comp Neurol*. 2001;432:197-216.
163. Ritter S, Dinh TT, Zhang Y. Localization of hindbrain glucoreceptive sites controlling food intake and blood glucose. *Brain Res*. 2000;856:37-47.
164. Burdakov D, Jensen LT, Alexopoulos H, et al. Tandem-pore K+ channels mediate inhibition of orexin neurons by glucose. *Neuron*. 2006;50:711-722.
165. Obici S, Feng Z, Tan J, et al. Central melanocortin receptors regulate insulin action. *J Clin Invest*. 2001;108:1079-1085.
166. Fox EA, Powley TL. Tracer diffusion has exaggerated CNS maps of direct preganglionic innervation of pancreas. *J Auton Nerv Syst*. 1986;15:55-69.
167. Loewy AD, Franklin MF, Haxhiu MA. CNS monoamine cell groups projecting to pancreatic vagal motor neurons: a transneuronal labeling study using pseudorabies virus. *Brain Res*. 1994;638:248-260.
168. Berthoud HR, Fox EA, Powley TL. Localization of vagal preganglionics that stimulate insulin and glucagon secretion. *Am J Physiol*. 1990;258(1 Pt 2):R160-R168.
169. Cai XJ, Widdowson PS, Harrold J, et al. Hypothalamic orexin expression: modulation by blood glucose and feeding. *Diabetes*. 1999;48:2132-2137.
170. Griffond B, Risold PY, Jacquemard C, et al. Insulin-induced hypoglycemia increases preprohypocretin (orexin) mRNA in the rat lateral hypothalamic area. *Neurosci Lett*. 1999;262:77-80.
171. Moriguchi T, Sakurai T, Nambu T, et al. Neurons containing orexin in the lateral hypothalamic area of the adult rat brain are activated by insulin-induced acute hypoglycemia. *Neurosci Lett*. 1999;264: 101-104.
172. Scott MM, Marcus JN, Elmquist JK. Orexin neurons and the TASK of glucosensing. *Neuron*. 2006;50:665-667.
173. Oomura Y, Yoshimatsu H. Neural network of glucose monitoring system. *J Auton Nerv Syst*. 1984;10:359-372.
174. Schwartz GJ. The role of gastrointestinal vagal afferents in the control of food intake: current prospects. *Nutrition*. 2000;16:866-873.
175. Altschuler SM, Bao XM, Bleger D, et al. Viscerotopic representation of the upper alimentary tract in the rat: sensory ganglia and nuclei of the solitary and spinal trigeminal tracts. *J Comp Neurol*. 1989;283:248-268.
176. Raybould HE, Gayton RJ, Dockray GJ. CNS effects of circulating CCK8: involvement of brainstem neurones responding to gastric distension. *Brain Res*. 1985;342:187-190.
177. Zhang X, Fogel R, Renehan WE. Relationships between the morphology and function of gastric- and intestine-sensitive neurons in the nucleus of the solitary tract. *J Comp Neurol*. 1995;363:37-52.
178. Rinaman L, Verbalis JG, Stricker EM, et al. Distribution and neurochemical phenotypes of caudal medullary neurons activated to express cFos following peripheral administration of cholecystokinin. *J Comp Neurol*. 1993;338:475-490.
179. Gibbs J, Falasco JD, McHugh PR. Cholecystokinin-decreased food intake in rhesus monkeys. *Am J Physiol*. 1976;230:15-18.
180. Gibbs J, Young RC, Smith GP. Cholecystokinin decreases food intake in rats. *J Comp Physiol Psych*. 1973;84:488-495.
181. Crawley JN, Beinfeld MC. Rapid development of tolerance to the behavioural actions of cholecystokinin. *Nature*. 1983;302:703-706.
182. West D, Fey D, Woods S. Cholecystokinin persistently suppresses meal size but not food intake in free-feeding rats. *Am J Physiol*. 1984;246:R776-R787.
183. Smith GP, Jerome C, Cushin BJ, et al. Abdominal vagotomy blocks the satiety effect of cholecystokinin in the rat. *Science*. 1981;213: 1036-1037.
184. South EH, Ritter RC. Capsaicin application to central or peripheral vagal fibers attenuates CCK satiety. *Peptides*. 1988;9:601-612.
185. Hewson G, Leighton GE, Hill RG, et al. The cholecystokinin receptor antagonist L364,718 increases food intake in the rat by attenuation of the action of endogenous cholecystokinin. *Br J Pharmacol*. 1988;93:79-84.
186. Dourish CT, Ruckert AC, Tattersall FD, et al. Evidence that decreased feeding induced by systemic injection of cholecystokinin is mediated by CCK-A receptors. *Eur J Pharmacol*. 1989;173:233-234.
187. Dourish C, Rycroft W, Iversen S. Postponement of satiety by blockade of brain cholecystokinin (CCKB) receptors. *Science*. 1989;245: 1509-1511.
188. Reidelberger RD, O'Rourke MF. Potent cholecystokinin antagonist L 364718 stimulates food intake in rats. *Am J Physiol*. 1989;257(6 Pt 2):R1512-R1518.
189. Gutzwiller JP, Drewe J, Ketterer S, et al. Interaction between CCK and a preload on reduction of food intake is mediated by CCK-A receptors in humans. *Am J Physiol Regul Integr Comp Physiol*. 2000;279: R189-R195.
190. Riedy CA, Chavez M, Figiewicz DP, et al. Central insulin enhances sensitivity to cholecystokinin. *Physiol Behav*. 1995;58:755-760.
191. Figlewicz DP, Sipols AJ, Seeley RJ, et al. Intraventricular insulin enhances the meal-suppressive efficacy of intraventricular cholecystokinin octapeptide in the baboon. *Behav Neurosci*. 1995;109: 567-569.
192. Matson CA, Wiater MF, Kuijper JL, et al. Synergy between leptin and cholecystokinin (CCK) to control daily caloric intake. *Peptides*. 1997;18:1275-1278.
193. Matson CA, Ritter RC. Long-term CCK-leptin synergy suggests a role for CCK in the regulation of body weight. *Am J Physiol*. 1999;276:R1038-R1045.
194. Emond M, Schwartz GJ, Ladenheim EE, et al. Central leptin modulates behavioral and neural responsivity to CCK. *Am J Physiol*. 1999;276(5 Pt 2):R1545-R1549.
195. Matson CA, Reid DF, Cannon TA, et al. Cholecystokinin and leptin act synergistically to reduce body weight. *Am J Physiol*. 2000;278: R882-R890.
196. Cannon CM, Palmiter RD. Peptides that regulate food intake: norepinephrine is not required for reduction of feeding induced by cholecystokinin. *Am J Physiol Regul Integr Comp Physiol*. 2003;284: R1384-R1388.
197. Lodge DJ, Lawrence AJ. Comparative analysis of the central CCK system in Fawn Hooded and Wistar Kyoto rats: extended localisation of CCK-A receptors throughout the rat brain using a novel radioligand. *Regul Pept*. 2001;99:191-201.
198. Mercer LD, Beart PM. Histochemistry in rat brain and spinal cord with an antibody directed at the cholecystokininA receptor. *Neurosci Lett*. 1997;225:97-100.
199. Hirosue Y, Inui A, Teranishi A, et al. Cholecystokinin octapeptide analogues suppress food intake via central CCK-A receptors in mice. *Am J Physiol*. 1993;265(3 Pt 2):R481-R486.
200. Adrian TE, Ferri GL, Bacarese-Hamilton AJ, et al. Human distribution and release of a putative new gut hormone, peptide YY. *Gastroenterology*. 1985;89:1070-1077.
201. Grandt D, Schimiczek M, Beglinger C, et al. Two molecular forms of peptide YY (PYY) are abundant in human blood: characterization of a radioimmunoassay recognizing PYY 1-36 and PYY 3-36. *Regul Pept*. 1994;51:151-159.
202. Grandt D, Schimiczek M, Struk K, et al. Characterization of two forms of peptide YY, PYY(1-36) and PYY(3-36), in the rabbit. *Peptides*. 1994;15:815-820.
203. Bonaz B, Taylor I, Tache Y. Peripheral peptide YY induces c-fos-like immunoreactivity in the rat brain. *Neurosci Lett*. 1993;163:77-80.
204. Allen JM, Fitzpatrick ML, Yeats JC, et al. Effects of peptide YY and neuropeptide Y on gastric emptying in man. *Digestion*. 1984;30: 255-262.
205. Adrian TE, Savage AP, Sagor GR, et al. Effect of peptide YY on gastric, pancreatic, and biliary function in humans. *Gastroenterology*. 1985;89:494-499.
206. Yang H. Central and peripheral regulation of gastric acid secretion by peptide YY. *Peptides*. 2002;23:349-358.
207. Dumont Y, Fournier A, St-Pierre S, et al. Autoradiographic distribution of [125I]Leu31,Pro34)PYY and [125I]PYY3-36 binding sites in the rat brain evaluated with two newly developed Y1 and Y2 receptor radioligands. *Synapse*. 1996;22:139-158.
208. Lloyd KC, Amimoazzami S, Friedk F, et al. Candidate canine enterogastrones: acid inhibition before and after vagotomy. *Am J Physiol*. 1997;272(5 Pt 1):G1236-G1242.
209. Batterham RL, Cowley MA, Small CJ, et al. Gut hormone PYY(3-36) physiologically inhibits food intake. *Nature*. 2002;418:650-654.
210. Adams SH, Won WB, Schonhoff SE, et al. Effects of peptide YY(3-36) on short-term food intake in mice are not affected by prevailing plasma ghrelin levels. *Endocrinology*. 2004;145:4967-4975.
211. Challis BG, Coll AP, Yeo GS, et al. Mice lacking pro-opiomelanocortin are sensitive to high-fat feeding but respond normally to the acute

anorectic effects of peptide-YY(3-36). *Proc Natl Acad Sci U S A*. 2004;101:4695-4700.
212. Chelikani PK, Haver AC, Reidelberger RD. Intravenous infusion of peptide YY(3-36) potently inhibits food intake in rats. *Endocrinology*. 2005;146:879-888.
213. Cox JE, Randich A. Enhancement of feeding suppression by PYY(3-36) in rats with area postrema ablations. *Peptides*. 2004;25:985-989.
214. Pittner RA, Moore CX, Bhavsar SP, et al. Effects of PYY(3-36) in rodent models of diabetes and obesity. *Int J Obes Relat Metab Disord*. 2004;28:963-971.
215. Moran TH, Smedh U, Kinzig KP, et al. Peptide YY(3-36) inhibits gastric emptying and produces acute reductions in food intake in rhesus monkeys. *Am J Physiol Regul Integr Comp Physiol*. 2005;288: R384-R388.
216. Halatchev IG, Ellacott KL, Fan W, et al. Peptide YY3-36 inhibits food intake in mice through a melanocortin-4 receptor-independent mechanism. *Endocrinology*. 2004;145:2585-2590.
217. Abbott CR, Monteiro M, Small CJ, et al. The inhibitory effects of peripheral administration of peptide YY(3-36) and glucagon-like peptide-1 on food intake are attenuated by ablation of the vagal-brainstem-hypothalamic pathway. *Brain Res*. 2005;1044:127-131.
218. Martin NM, Small CJ, Sajedi A, et al. Pre-obese and obese agouti mice are sensitive to the anorectic effects of peptide YY(3-36) but resistant to ghrelin. *Int J Obes Relat Metab Disord*. 2004;28:886-893.
219. Batterham RL, Hefron H, Kapoor S, et al. Critical role for peptide YY in protein-mediated satiation and body-weight regulation. *Cell Metab*. 2006;4:223-233.
220. Boey D, Lin S, Karl T, et al. Peptide YY ablation in mice leads to the development of hyperinsulinaemia and obesity. *Diabetologia*. 2006;49:1360-1370.
221. Kojima M, Hosoda H, Date Y, et al. Ghrelin is a growth-hormone-releasing acylated peptide from stomach. *Nature*. 1999;402:656-660.
222. Kojima M, Hosoda H, Matsuo H, et al. Ghrelin: discovery of the natural endogenous ligand for the growth hormone secretagogue receptor. *Trends Endocrinol Metab*. 2001;12:118-122.
223. Ariyasu H, Takaya K, Tagami T, et al. Stomach is a major source of circulating ghrelin, and feeding state determines plasma ghrelin-like immunoreactivity levels in humans. *J Clin Endocrinol Metab*. 2001;86:4753-4758.
224. Tschop M, Wawarta R, Riepl RL, et al. Post-prandial decrease of circulating human ghrelin levels. *J Endocrinol Invest*. 2001;24:RC19-RC21.
225. Tschop M, Smiley DL, Heiman ML. Ghrelin induces adiposity in rodents. *Nature*. 2000;407:908-913.
226. Cummings DE, Purnell JQ, Frayo RS, et al. A preprandial rise in plasma ghrelin levels suggest a role in meal initiation in humans. *Diabetes*. 2001;50:1714-1719.
227. Willesen M, Kristensen P, Romer J. Co-localization of growth hormone secretagogue receptor and NPY mRNA in the arcuate nucleus of the rat. *Neuroendocrinol*. 1999;70:306-316.
228. Hewson AK, Dickson SL. Systemic administration of ghrelin induces Fos and Egr-1 proteins in the hypothalamic arcuate nucleus of fasted and fed rats. *J Neuroendocrinol*. 2000;12:1047-1049.
229. Kamegai J, Tamura H, Shimizu T, et al. Central effect of ghrelin, an endogenous growth hormone secretagogue, on hypothalamic peptide gene expression. *Endocrinology*. 2000;141:4797-4800.
230. Kamegai J, Tamura H, Shiizu T, et al. Chronic central infusion of ghrelin increases hypothalamic neuropeptide Y and Agouti-related protein mRNA levels and body weight in rats. *Diabetes*. 2001;50:2438-2443.
231. Asakawa A, Inui A, Kaga T, et al. Ghrelin is an appetite-stimulatory signal from stomach with structural resemblance to motilin. *Gastroenterology*. 2001;120:337-345.
232. Nakazato M, Murakami N, Date Y. A role for ghrelin in the central regulation of feeding. *Nature*. 2001;409:194-198.
233. Shintani M, Ogawa Y, Ebhara K, et al. Ghrelin, an endogenous growth hormone secretagogue, is a novel orexigenic peptide that antagonizes leptin action through the activation of hypothalamic neuropeptide Y/Y1 receptor pathway. *Diabetes*. 2001;50:227-232.
234. Wren AM, Small CJ, Ward HL, et al. The novel hypothalamic peptide ghrelin stimulates food intake and growth hormone secretion. *Endocrinology*. 2000;141:4325-4328.
235. Wren AM, Small CJ, Abbott CR, et al. Ghrelin causes hyperphagia and obesity in rats. *Diabetes*. 2001;50:2540-2547.
236. Wren AM, Seal LJ, Cohen MA, et al. Ghrelin enhances appetite and increases food intake in humans. *J Clin Endocrinol Metab*. 2001;86:5992.
237. Tschop M, Weyer C, Tataranni PA, et al. Circulating ghrelin levels are decreased in human obesity. *Diabetes*. 2001;50:707-709.
238. Nagaya N, Uematsu M, Kojima M, et al. Chronic administration of ghrelin improves left ventricular dysfunction and attenuates development of cardiac cachexia in rats with heart failure. *Circulation*. 2001;104:1430-1435.
239. Tschop M, Statnick MA, Suter TM, et al. GH-releasing peptide-2 increases fat mass in mice lacking NPY: indication for a crucial mediating role of hypothalamic agouti-related protein. *Endocrinology*. 2002;143:558-568.
240. Wang L, Saint-Pierre DH, Tache Y. Peripheral ghrelin selectively increases Fos expression in neuropeptide Y-synthesizing neurons in mouse hypothalamic arcuate nucleus. *Neurosci Lett*. 2002;325:47-51.
241. Tamura H, Kamegai J, Shimizu T, et al. Ghrelin stimulates GH but not food intake in arcuate nucleus ablated rats. *Endocrinology*. 2002;143:3268-3275.
242. Date Y, Murakami N, Toshinai K, et al. The role of the gastric afferent vagal nerve in ghrelin-induced feeding and growth hormone secretion in rats. *Gastroenterology*. 2002;123:1120-1128.
243. Zhang JV, Ren PG, Avsian-Kretchmer O, et al. Obestatin, a peptide encoded by the ghrelin gene, opposes ghrelin's effects on food intake. *Science*. 2005;310:996-999.
244. Tremblay F, Perreault M, Klaman LD, et al. Normal food intake and body weight in mice lacking the G protein-coupled receptor GPR39. *Endocrinology*. 2007;148:501-506.
245. Lauwers E, Landuyt B, Arckens L, et al. Obestatin does not activate orphan G protein-coupled receptor GPR39. *Biochem Biophys Res Commun*. 2006;351:21-25.
246. Nogueiras R, Pfluger P, Tovar S, et al. Effects of obestatin on energy balance and growth hormone secretion in rodents. *Endocrinology*. 2007;148:21-26.
247. Drucker DJ. The biology of incretin hormones. *Cell Metab*. 2006;3:153-165.
248. Drucker DJ, Nauck MA. The incretin system: glucagon-like peptide-1 receptor agonists and dipeptidyl peptidase-4 inhibitors in type 2 diabetes. *Lancet*. 2006;368:1696-1705.
249. Thiele TE, Van Dijk G, Campfield LA, et al. Central infusion of GLP-1, but not leptin, produces conditioned taste aversions in rats. *Am J Physiol*. 1997;272(2 Pt 2):R726-R730.
250. Thiele TE, Seeley RJ, D'Alessio D, et al. Central infusion of glucagon-like peptide-1-(7-36) amide (GLP-1) receptor antagonist attenuates lithium chloride-induced c-Fos induction in rat brainstem. *Brain Res*. 1998;801:164-170.
251. Tang-Christensen M, Larsen P, Goke R, et al. Central administration of GLP-1-(7-36) amide inhibits food and water intake in rats. *J Physiol*. 1996;271:848-856.
252. Turton MD, O'Shea D, Gunn I, et al. A role for glucagon-like peptide-1 in the central regulation of feeding. *Nature*. 1996;379:69-72.
253. McMahon LR, Wellman PJ. PVN infusion of GLP-1-(7-36) amide suppresses feeding but does not induce aversion or alter locomotion in rats. *Am J Physiol*. 1998;274(1 Pt 2):R23-R29.
254. Flint A, Raben A, Astrup A, et al. Glucagon-like peptide 1 promotes satiety and suppresses energy intake in humans. *J Clin Invest*. 1998;101:515-520.
255. Gutzwiller JP, Drewe J, Goke B, et al. Glucagon-like peptide-1 promotes satiety and reduces food intake in patients with diabetes mellitus type 2. *Am J Physiol*. 1999;276(5 Pt 2):R1541-R1544.
256. Toft-Nielsen MB, Madsbad S, Holst JJ. Continuous subcutaneous infusion of glucagon-like peptide 1 lowers plasma glucose and reduces appetite in type 2 diabetic patients. *Diabetes Care*. 1999;22: 1137-1143.
257. Verdich C, Flint A, Gutzwiler JP, et al. A meta-analysis of the effect of glucagon-like peptide-1 (7-36) amide on ad libitum energy intake in humans. *J Crin Edocrinol Metab*. 2001;86:4382-4389.
258. Zander M, Madsbad S, Madsen JL, et al. Effect of 6-week course of glucagon-like peptide 1 on glycaemic control, insulin sensitivity, and beta-cell function in type 2 diabetes: a parallel-group study. *Lancet*. 2002;359:824-830.
259. Nakabayashi H, Nishizawa M, Nakagawa A, et al. Vagal hepatopancreatic reflex effect evoked by intraportal appearance of tGLP-1. *Am J Physiol*. 1996;271(5 Pt 1):E808-E813.
260. Imeryuz N, Yegen BC, Bozkurt A, et al. Glucagon-like peptide-1 inhibits gastric emptying via vagal afferent-mediated central mechanisms. *Am J Physiol*. 1997;273(4 Pt 1):G920-G927.
261. Lachey JL, D'Alessio DA, Rinaman L, et al. The role of central glucagon-like peptide-1 in mediating the effects of visceral illness: differential effects in rats and mice. *Endocrinology*. 2005;146:458-462.
262. Rinaman L. Interoceptive stress activates glucagon-like peptide-1 neurons that project to the hypothalamus. *Am J Physiol*. 1999;277(2 Pt 2):R582-R590.
263. Rinaman L, Rothe EE. GLP-1 receptor signaling contributes to anorexigenic effect of centrally administered oxytocin in rats. *Am J Physiol Regul Integr Comp Physiol*. 2002;283:R99-R106.
264. Sawchenko PE, Swanson LW. The organization of forebrain afferents to the paraventricular and supraoptic nuclei of the rat. *J Comp Neurol*. 1983;218:121-144.
265. Elias CF, Kelly JF, Lee CE, et al. Chemical characterization of leptin-activated neurons in the rat brain. *J Comp Neurol*. 2000;423:261-281.
266. Ellacott KL, Halatchev IG, Cone RD. Characterization of leptin-responsive neurons in the caudal brainstem. *Endocrinology*. 2006;147:3190-3195.
267. Larsen PJ, Tang-Christensen M, Hoist JJ, et al. Distribution of glucagon-like peptide-1 and other preproglucagon-derived peptides in the rat hypothalamus and brainstem. *Neuroscience*. 1997;77:257-270.

268. Merchenthaler I, Lane M, Shughrue P. Distribution of pre-proglucagon and glucagon-like peptide-1 receptor messenger RNAs in the rat central nervous system. *J Comp Neurol*. 1999;403:261-280.
269. Kahn SE, Andrikopoulos S, Verchere CB. Islet amyloid: a long-recognized but underappreciated pathological feature of type 2 diabetes. *Diabetes*. 1999;48:241-253.
270. Hoppener JW, Ahren B, Lips CJ. Islet amyloid and type 2 diabetes mellitus. *N Engl J Med*. 2000;343:411-419.
271. Hartter E, Svoboda T, Ludvik B, et al. Basal and stimulated plasma levels of pancreatic amylin indicate its co-secretion with insulin in humans. *Diabetologia*. 1991;34:52-54.
272. Butler PC, Chou J, Carter WB, et al. Effects of meal ingestion on plasma amylin concentration in NIDDM and nondiabetic humans. *Diabetes*. 1990;39:752-756.
273. Banks WA, Kastin AJ, Maness LM, et al. Permeability of the blood-brain barrier to amylin. *Life Sci*. 1995;57:1993-2001.
274. Beaumont K, Kenney MA, Young AA, et al. High affinity amylin binding sites in rat brain. *Mol Pharmacol*. 1993;44:493-497.
275. Morley JE, Flood JF. Amylin decreases food intake in mice. *Peptides*. 1991;12:865-869.
276. Arnelo U, Blevins JE, Larsson J, et al. Effects of acute and chronic infusion of islet amyloid polypeptide on food intake in rats. *Scand J Gastroenterol*. 1996;31:83-89.
277. Rushing PA, Hagan MM, Seeley RJ, et al. Amylin: a novel action in the brain to reduce body weight. *Endocrinology*. 2000;141:850-853.
278. Rushing PA, Hagan MM, Seeley RJ, et al. Inhibition of central amylin signaling increases food intake and body adiposity in rats. *Endocrinology*. 2001;142:5035.
279. Reidelberger RD, Amelo U, Granqvist L, et al. Comparative effects of amylin and cholecystokinin on food intake and gastric emptying in rats. *Am J Physiol Regul Integr Comp Physiol*. 2001;280:R605-R611.
280. Bhavsar S, Watkins J, Young A. Synergy between amylin and cholecystokinin for inhibition of food intake in mice. *Physiol Behav*. 1998;64:557-561.
281. Rushing PA, Lutz TA, Seeley RJ, et al. Amylin and insulin interact to reduce food intake in rats. *Horm Metab Res*. 2000;32:62-65.
282. Cummings DE, Overduin J, Shannon MH, et al. Hormonal mechanisms of weight loss and diabetes resolution after bariatric surgery. *Surg Obes Relat Dis*. 2005;1:358-368.
283. Sjostrom L, Lindroos AK, Peltonen M, et al; Swedish Obese Subjects Study Scientific Group. Lifestyle, diabetes, and cardiovascular risk factors 10 years after bariatric surgery. *N Engl J Med*. 2004;351: 2683-2693.
284. Rubino F, Forgone A, Cummings DE, et al. The mechanism of diabetes control after gastrointestinal bypass surgery reveals a role of the proximal small intestine in the pathophysiology of type 2 diabetes. *Ann Surg*. 2006;244:741-749.
285. Asarian L, Geary N. Modulation of appetite by gonadal steroid hormones. *Philos Trans R Soc Lond B Biol Sci*. 2006;361:1251-1263.
286. Lopez M, Lelliott CJ, Tovar S, et al. Tamoxifen-induced anorexia is associated with fatty acid synthase inhibition in the ventromedial nucleus of the hypothalamus and accumulation of malonyl-CoA. *Diabetes*. 2006;55:1327-1336.
287. Acosta-Martinez M, Horton T, Levine JE. Estrogen receptors in neuropeptide Y neurons: at the crossroads of feeding and reproduction. *Trends Endocrinol Metab*. 2007;18:48-50.
288. Gao Q, Mezei G, Nie Y, et al. Anorectic estrogen mimics leptin's effect on the rewiring of melanocortin cells and Stat3 signaling in obese animals. *Nat Med*. 2007;13:89-94.
289. Heine PA, Taylor JA, Wamoto GA, et al. Increased adipose tissue in male and female estrogen receptor-alpha knockout mice. *Proc Natl Acad Sci U S A*. 2000;97:12729-12734.
290. Musatov S, Chen W, Pfaff DW, et al. Silencing of estrogen receptor (alpha) in the ventromedial nucleus of hypothalamus leads to metabolic syndrome. *Proc Natl Acad Sci U S A*. 2007;104:2501-2506.
291. Aronsson M, Fuxe K, Dong Y, et al. Localization of glucocorticoid receptor mRNA in the male rat brain by in situ hybridization. *Proc Natl Acad Sci U S A*. 1988;85:9331-9335.
292. Tasker JG. Rapid glucocorticoid actions in the hypothalamus as a mechanism of homeostatic integration. *Obesity (Silver Spring)*. 2006;14(suppl 5):259-265.
293. Saper C, Breder C. The neurologic basis of fever. *N Engl J Med*. 1994;330:1880-1886.
294. Besedovsky H, del Rey A, Sorkin E, et al. Immunoregulatory feedback between interleukin-1 and glucocorticoid hormones. *Science*. 1986;233:652-654.
295. Berkenbosch F, van Oers J, del Ray A, et al. Corticotropin-releasing factor-producing neurons in the rat activated by interleukin-1. *Science*. 1987;238:524-526.
296. Sapolsky R, Rivier C, Yamamoto G, et al. Interleukin-1 stimulates the secretion of hypothalamic corticotropin-releasing factor. *Science*. 1987;238:522-524.
297. Ader R, Cohen N, Felten D. Psychoneuroimmunology: interactions between the nervous system and the immune system. *Lancet*. 1995;345:99-103.
298. Felten DL, Felten SY, Carlson SL, et al. Noradrenergic and peptidergic innervation of lymphoid tissue. *J Immunol*. 1985;135(suppl 2): 755-765.
299. Spiegelman BM, Flier JS. Obesity and the regulation of energy balance. *Cell*. 2001;104:531-543.
300. Chen TY, Lai MG, Suzuki T, et al. Lipopolysaccharide receptors and signal transduction pathways in mononuclear phagocytes. *Curr Top Microbiol Immunol*. 1992;181:169-188.
301. Rivest S, Lacroix S, Vallieres L, et al. How the blood talks to the brain parenchyma and the paraventricular nucleus of the hypothalamus during systemic inflammatory and infectious stimuli. *Proc Soc Exp Biol Med*. 2000;223:22-38.
302. Elmquist, JK, Scammell TE, Saper CB. Mechanisms of CNS response to systemic immune challenge: the febrile response. *Trends Neurosci*. 1997;20:565-570.
303. Reichlin S. Neuroendocrinology of infection and the innate immune system. *Recent Prog Horm Res*. 1999;54:133-181.
304. Hellon R, Townsend Y. Mechanisms of fever. *Pharmacol Ther*. 1982;19:211-244.
305. Blatteis CM. Role of the OVLT in the febrile response to circulating pyrogens. *Prog Brain Res*. 1992;91:409-412.
306. Hunter WS, Sehic E, Blatteis CM. Fever and the organum vasculosum laminae terminalis: another look. In: Milton AS, ed. *Temperature Regulation: Recent Physiological and Pharmacological Advances*. Basel, Switzerland: Birkhauser; 1994:75-79.
307. Stitt JT. Differential sensitivity in the sites of fever production by prostaglandin E1 within the hypothalamus of the rat. *J Physiol (Lond)*. 1991;432:99-110.
308. Katsuura G, Arimura A, Koves K, et al. Involvement of organum vasculosum of lamina terminalis and preoptic area in interleukin 1 beta-induced ACTH release. *Am J Physiol*. 1990;258(1 Pt 1):E163-E171.
309. Kovacs KJ, Sawchenko PE. Mediation of osmoregulatory influences on neuroendocrine corticotropin-releasing factor expression by the ventral lamina terminalis. *Proc Natl Acad Sci U S A*. 1993;90: 7681-7685.
310. Ericsson A, Kovacs KJ, Sawchenko PE. A functional anatomical analysis of central pathways subserving the effects of interleukin-1 on stress-related neuroendocrine neurons. *J Neurosci*. 1994;14:897-913.
311. Lee HY, Whiteside MB, Herkenham M. Area postrema removal abolishes stimulatory effects of intravenous interleukin-1beta on hypothalamic-pituitary-adrenal axis activity and c-fos mRNA in the hypothalamic paraventricular nucleus. *Brain Res Bull*. 1998;46: 495-503.
312. Ericsson A, Arias C, Sawchenko PE. Evidence for an intramedullary prostaglandin-dependent mechanism in the activation of stress-related neuroendocrine circuitry by intravenous interleukin-1. *J Neurosci*. 1997;17:7166-7179.
313. Sagar SM, Price KJ, Kasting NW, et al. Anatomic patterns of Fos immunostaining in rat brain following systemic endotoxin administration. *Brain Res Bull*. 1995;36:381-392.
314. Vane JR. Inhibition of prostaglandin synthesis as a mechanism of action for aspirin-like drugs. *Nature New Biol*. 1971;231:232-235.
315. Johnson RW, von Borell E. Lipopolysaccharide-induced sickness behavior in pigs is inhibited by pretreatment with indomethacin [published erratum appears in J Anim Sci. 1994;72:801]. *J Anim Sci*. 1994;72:309-314.
316. Milton AS, Wendlandt S. A possible role for prostaglandin E1 as a modulator for temperature regulation in the central nervous system of the cat. *J Physiol (Lond)*. 1970;207:76P-77P.
317. Milton AS, Wendlandt S. Effects on body temperature of prostaglandins of the A, E and F series on injection into the third ventricle of unanaesthetized cats and rabbits. *J Physiol (Lond)*. 1971;218:325-336.
318. Goppelt-Struebe M. Regulation of prostaglandin endoperoxide synthase (cyclooxygenase) isozyme expression. *Prostaglandins Leukot Essent Fatty Acids*. 1995;52:213-222.
319. Robertson RP. Molecular regulation of prostaglandin synthesis: implications for endocrine systems. *Trends Endocrinol Metab*. 1995;6: 293-297.
320. Breder CD, Dewitt D, Kraig RP. Characterization of inducible cyclooxygenase in rat brain. *J Comp Neurol*. 1995;355:296-315.
321. Breder CD, Smith WL, Raz A, et al. Distribution and characterization of cyclooxygenase immunoreactivity in the ovine brain. *J Comp Neurol*. 1992;322:409-438.
322. Yamagata K, Andreasson KI, Kaufmann WE, et al. Expression of a mitogen-inducible cyclooxygenase in brain neurons: regulation by synaptic activity and glucocorticoids. *Neuron*. 1993;11:371-386.
323. Ek M, Engblom D, Saha S, et al. Inflammatory response: pathway across the blood-brain barrier. *Nature*. 2001;410:430-431.
324. Elmquist JK, Breder CD, Sherin JE, et al. Intravenous lipopolysaccharide induces cyclooxygenase-II immunoreactivity in rat brain perivascular microglia. *J Comp Neurol*. 1997;381:119-129.
325. Elmquist JK, Ahima RS, Maratos-Flier E, et al. Leptin activates neurons in ventrobasal hypothalamus and brainstem. *Endocrinology*. 1997; 138:839-842.

326. Rivest S. What is the cellular source of prostaglandins in the brain in response to systemic inflammation? Facts and controversies. *Mol Psychiatry.* 1999;4:500-507.
327. Blatteis CM, Sehic E. Cytokines and fever. *Ann N Y Acad Sci.* 1998;840:608-618.
328. Scammell TE, Elmquist JK, Griffin JD, et al. Ventromedial preoptic prostaglandin E2 activates fever-producing autonomic pathways. *J Neurosci.* 1996;16:6246-6254.
329. Williams JW, Rudy TA, Yakash TL, et al. An extensive exploration of the rat brain for sites mediating prostaglandin-induced hyperthermia. *Brain Res.* 1977;120:251-262.
330. Feldberg W, Saxena PN. Further studies on prostaglandin E1 fever in cats. *J Physiol (Lond).* 1971;219:739-745.
331. Morimoto A, Nakamori T, Watanabe T, et al. Pattern differences in experimental fevers induced by endotoxin, endogenous pyrogen, and prostaglandins. *Am J Physiol.* 1988;254(4 Pt 2):R633-R640.
332. Scammell TE, Griffin JD, Elmquist JK, et al. Microinjection of a cyclo-oxygenase inhibitor into the anteroventral preoptic region attenuates LPS fever. *Am J Physiol.* 1998;274:R783-789.
333. Watanabe Y, Watanabe Y, Hayaishi O. Quantitative autoradiographic localization of prostaglandin E2 binding sites in monkey diencephalon. *J Neurosci.* 1988;8:2003-2010.
334. Matsumura K, Watnabe Y, Onoe H, et al. High density of prostaglandin E2 binding sites in the anterior wall of the 3rd ventricle: a possible site of its hyperthermic action. *Brain Res.* 1990;533:147-151.
335. Coleman RA, Grix SP, Head SA, et al. A novel inhibitory prostanoid receptor in piglet saphenous vein. *Prostaglandins.* 1994;47:151-168.
336. Ushikubi F, Segi E, Sugimoto Y, et al. Impaired febrile response in mice lacking the prostaglandin E receptor subtype EP3. *Nature.* 1998;395:281-284.
337. Oka T, Oka K, Scammell TE, et al. Relationship of EP(1-4) prostaglandin receptors with rat hypothalamic cell groups involved in lipopolysaccharide fever responses. *J Comp Neurol.* 2000;428:20-32.
338. Ek M, Arias C, Sawchenko P, et al. Distribution of the EP3 prostaglandin E(2) receptor subtype in the rat brain: relationship to sites of interleukin-1-induced cellular responsiveness. *J Comp Neurol.* 2000; 428:5-20.
339. Sugimoto Y, Shigemoto R, Namba T, et al. Distribution of the messenger RNA for the prostaglandin E receptor subtype EP3 in the mouse nervous system. *Neuroscience.* 1994;62:919-928.
340. Zhang J, Rivest S. A functional analysis of EP4 receptor-expressing neurons in mediating the action of prostaglandin E2 within specific nuclei of the brain in response to circulating interleukin-1beta. *J Neurochem.* 2000;74:2134-2145.
341. Nakamura K, Kaneko T, Yamashita Y, et al. Immunocytochemical localization of prostaglandin EP3 receptor in the rat hypothalamus. *Neurosci Lett.* 1999;260:117-120.
342. Oka T, Hori T. EP1-receptor mediation of prostaglandin E2-induced hyperthermia in rats. *Am J Physiol.* 1994;267(1 Pt 2):R289-R294.
343. Oka K, Oka T, Hori T. PGE2 receptor subtype EP1 antagonist may inhibit central interleukin-1beta-induced fever in rats. *Am J Physiol.* 1998;275(6 Pt 2):R1762-R1765.
344. Wang W, Andersson M, Lonnroth C, et al. Anorexia and cachexia in prostaglandin EP1 and EP3 subtype receptor knockout mice bearing a tumor with high intrinsic PGE2 production and prostaglandin related cachexia. *J Exp Clin Cancer Res.* 2005;24:99-107.
345. Elander L, Engstrom L, Hallbeck M, et al. IL-1(beta) and LPS induce anorexia by distinct mechanisms differentially dependent on microsomal prostaglandin E synthase-1. *Am J Physiol Regul Integr Comp Physiol.* 2007;292:R258-R267.
346. Banks WA, Kastin AJ, Durham DA. Bidirectional transport of interleukin-1 alpha across the blood-brain barrier. *Brain Res Bull.* 1989;23:433-437.
347. Banks WA, Oritz L, Plotkin SR, et al. Human interleukin (IL) 1 alpha, murine IL-1 alpha and murine IL-1 beta are transported from blood to brain in the mouse by a shared saturable mechanism. *J Pharmacol Exp Ther.* 1991;259:988-996.
348. Banks WA, Kastin AJ. Blood to brain transport of interleukin links the immune and central nervous systems. *Life Sci.* 1991;48: PL117-PL1121.
349. Hopkins SJ, Rothwell NJ. Cytokines and the nervous system I: Expression and recognition [see comments]. *Trends Neurosci.* 1995;18:83-88.
350. Rothwell NJ, Hopkins SJ. Cytokines and the nervous system II: actions and mechanisms of action [see comments]. *Trends Neurosci.* 1995;18:130-136.
351. Klir JJ, McClellan JL, Kluger MJ. Interleukin-1 beta causes the increase in anterior hypothalamic interleukin-6 during LPS-induced fever in rats. *Am J Physiol.* 1994;266(6 Pt 2):R1845-1848.
352. Breder CD, Hazuka C, Ghayur T, et al. Regional induction of tumor necrosis factor alpha expression in the mouse brain after systemic lipopolysaccharide administration. *Proc Natl Acad Sci U S A.* 1994;91:11393-11397.
353. Quan N, Whiteside M, Kim L, et al. Induction of inhibitory factor kappaBalpha mRNA in the central nervous system after peripheral lipopolysaccharide administration: an in situ hybridization histochemistry study in the rat. *Proc Natl Acad Sci U S A.* 1997;94: 10985-10990.
354. Laflamme N, Lacroix S, Rivest S. An essential role of interleukin-1beta in mediating NF-kappaB activity and COX-2 transcription in cells of the blood-brain barrier in response to a systemic and localized inflammation but not during endotoxemia. *J Neurosci.* 1999;19: 10923-10930.
355. Ericsson A, Liu C, Hart RP, et al. Type 1 interleukin-1 receptor in the rat brain: distribution, regulation, and relationship to sites of IL-1-induced cellular activation. *J Comp Neurol.* 1995;361:681-698.
356. Sagar SM, Sharp FR, Curran T. Expression of c-fos protein in brain: metabolic mapping at the cellular level. *Science.* 1988;240:1328-1331.
357. Elmquist JK, Ackermann MR, Register KB, et al. Induction of Fos-like immunoreactivity in the rat brain following *Pasteurella multocida* endotoxin administration. *Endocrinology.* 1993;133:3054-3057.
358. Elmquist JK, Scammell TE, Jacobson CD, et al. Distribution of Fos-like immunoreactivity in the rat brain following intravenous lipopolysaccharide administration. *J Comp Neurol.* 1996;371:85-103.
359. Elmquist JK, Saper CB. Activation of neurons projecting to the paraventricular hypothalamic nucleus by intravenous lipopolysaccharide. *J Comp Neurol.* 1996;374:315-331.
360. Wan W, Janz L, Vriend CY, et al. Differential induction of c-fos immunoreactivity in hypothalamus and brain stem nuclei following central and peripheral administration of endotoxin. *Brain Res Bull.* 1993;32:581-587.
361. Wan W, Wetmore L, Sorensen CM, et al. Neural and biochemical mediators of endotoxin and stress-induced c-fos expression in the rat brain. *Brain Res Bull.* 1994;34:7-14.
362. Brady LS, Lynn AB, Herkenham M, et al. Systemic interleukin-1 induces early and late patterns of c-fos mRNA expression in brain. *J Neurosci.* 1994;14:4951-4964.
363. Chan RK, Brown ER, Ericsson A, et al. A comparison of two immediate-early genes, c-fos and NGFI-B, as markers for functional activation in stress-related neuroendocrine circuitry. *J Neurosci.* 1993;13: 5126-5138.
364. Hare AS, Clarke G, Tolchard S. Bacterial lipopolysaccharide-induced changes in FOS protein expression in the rat brain: correlation with thermoregulatory changes and plasma corticosterone. *J Neuroendocrinol.* 1995;7:791-799.
365. Rivest S, Rivier C. Stress and interleukin-1 beta-induced activation of c-fos, NGFI-B and CRF gene expression in the hypothalamic PVN: comparison between Sprague-Dawley, Fisher-344 and Lewis rats. *J Neuroendocrinol.* 1994;6:101-117.
366. Rivest S, Laflamme N. Neuronal activity and neuropeptide gene transcription in the brains of immune-challenged rats. *J Neuroendocrinol.* 1995;7:501-525.
367. Tkacs NC, Strack AM. Systemic endotoxin induces Fos-like immunoreactivity in rat spinal sympathetic regions. *J Auton Nerv Syst.* 1995;51:1-7.
368. Veening JG, van der Meer MJ, Joosten H, et al. Intravenous administration of interleukin-1 beta induces Fos-like immunoreactivity in corticotropin-releasing hormone neurons in the paraventricular hypothalamic nucleus of the rat. *J Chem Neuroanat.* 1993;6:391-397.
369. Huang QH, Entwistle ML, Alvaro JD, et al. Antipyretic role of endogenous melanocortins mediated by central mealanocortin receptors during endotoxin-induced fever. *J Neurosci.* 1997;17:3343-3351.
370. Kasting NW, Cooper KE, Veale WL. Antipyresis following perfusion of brain sites with vasopressin. *Experientia.* 1979;35:208-209.
371. Cooper KE, Kasting NW, Laderis K, et al. Evidence supporting a role for endogenous vasopressin in natural suppression of fever in the sheep. *J Physiol (Lond).* 1979;295:33-45.
372. Shih ST, Khorram O, Lipton JM, et al. Central administration of alpha-MSH antiserum augments fever in the rabbit. *Am J Physiol.* 1986;250(5 Pt 2):R803-R806.
373. Huang QH, Hruby VJ, Tatro JB. Role of central melanocortins in endotoxin-induced anorexia. *Am J Physiol.* 1999;276(3 Pt 2):R864-R871.
374. Fan W, Dimulescu DM, Butler AA, et al. The central melanocortin system can directly regulate serum insulin levels. *Endocrinology.* 2000;141:3072-3079.
375. Marks DL, Cone RD. Central melanocortins and the regulation of weight during acute and chronic disease. *Recent Prog Horm Res.* 2001;56:359-375.
376. Marks DL, Ling N, Cone RD. Role of the central melanocortin system in cachexia. *Cancer Res.* 2001;61:1432-1438.
377. Mak RH, Cheung W, Cone RD, et al. Orexigenic and anorexigenic mechanisms in the control of nutrition in chronic kidney disease. *Pediatr Nephrol.* 2005;20:427-431.
378. Markison S, Foster AC, Chen C, et al. The regulation of feeding and metabolic rate and the prevention of murine cancer cachexia with a small-molecule melanocortin-4 receptor antagonist. *Endocrinology.* 2005;146:2766-2773.
379. Bamshad M, Aoki VT, Adkison MG, et al. Central nervous system origins of the sympathetic nervous system outflow to white adipose tissue. *Am J Physiol.* 1998;275(1 Pt 2):R291-R299.

380. Rothwell NJ, Stock MJ. Effects of denervating brown adipose tissue on the responses to cold, hyperphagia and noradrenaline treatment in the rat. *J Physiol (Lond)*. 1984;355:457-463.
381. Lowell BB, Flier JS. Brown adipose tissue, beta 3-adrenergic receptors, and obesity. *Annu Rev Med*. 1997;48:307-316.
382. Jansen AS, Wessendorf MW, Loewy AD. Transneuronal labeling of CNS neuropeptide and monoamine neurons after pseudorabies virus injections into the stellate ganglion. *Brain Res*. 1995;683:1-24.
383. Saper CB, Loewy AD, Swanson LW, et al. Direct hypothalamo-autonomic connections. *Brain Res*. 1976;117: 305-312.
384. Zhang YH, Lu J, Elmquist JK, et al. Lipopolysaccharide activates specific populations of hypothalamic and brainstem neurons that project to the spinal cord. *J Neurosci*. 2000;20:6578-6586.
385. Kelley AE, Bakshi VP, Haber SN, et al. Opioid modulation of taste hedonics within the ventral striatum. *Physiol Behav*. 2002;76: 365-377.
386. Nestler EJ. Is there a common molecular pathway for addiction? *Nat Neurosci*. 2005;8:1445-1449.
387. Berke JD, Hyman SE. Addiction, dopamine, and the molecular mechanisms of memory. *Neuron*. 2000;25:515-532.
388. Laakso A, Mohn AR, Gainetdinov RR, et al. Experimental genetic approaches to addiction. *Neuron*. 2002;36:213-228.
389. Wise RA. Brain reward circuitry: insights from unsensed incentives. *Neuron*. 2002;36:229-240.
390. Ikemoto S, Panksepp J. Dissociations between appetitive and consummatory responses by pharmacological manipulations of reward-relevant brain regions. *Behav Neurosci*. 1996;110:331-345.
391. Balleine B, Killcross S. Effects of ibotenic acid lesions of the nucleus accumbens on instrumental action. *Behav Brain Res*. 1994;65:181-193.
392. Szczypka MS, Kwok K, Brot MD, et al. Dopamine production in the caudate putamen restores feeding in dopamine-deficient mice. *Neuron*. 2001;30:819-828.
393. Szczypka MS, Mandei RJ, Donahue BA, et al. Viral gene delivery selectively restores feeding and prevents lethality of dopamine-deficient mice. *Neuron*. 1999;22:167-178.
394. Figlewicz DP, Evans SB, Murphy J, et al. Expression of receptors for insulin and leptin in the ventral tegmental area/substantia nigra (VTA/SN) of the rat. *Brain Res*. 2003;964:107-115.
395. Zigman JM, Jones JE, Lee CE, et al. Expression of ghrelin receptor mRNA in the rat and the mouse brain. *J Comp Neurol*. 2006;494:528-548.
396. Figlewicz DP. Adiposity signals and food reward: expanding the CNS roles of insulin and leptin. *Am J Physiol Regul Integr Comp Physiol*. 2003;284:R882-R892.
397. Fulton S, Woodside B, Shizgal P. Modulation of brain reward circuitry by leptin. *Science*. 2000;287:125-128.
398. Zigman JM, Elmquist JK. Minireview. From anorexia to obesity: the yin and yang of body weight control. *Endocrinology*. 2003;144: 3749-3756.
399. Montague CT, Farooqi IS, Whitehead JP, et al. Congenital leptin deficiency is associated with severe early-onset obesity in humans. *Nature*. 1997;387:903-908.
400. Clement K, Vaisse C, Lahlou N, et al. A mutation in the human leptin receptor gene causes obesity and pituitary dysfunction. *Nature*. 1998;392:398-401.
401. Considine RV, Sinha MK, Heiman ML, et al. Serum immunoreactive-leptin concentrations in normal-weight and obese humans. *N Engl J Med*. 1996;334:292-295.
402. Friedman JM. Leptin, leptin receptors, and the control of body weight. *Nutr Rev*. 1998;56(2 Pt 2):s38-s46; discussion s54-s75.
403. Chan JL, Mantzoros CS. Role of leptin in energy-deprivation states: normal human physiology and clinical implications for hypothalamic amenorrhoea and anorexia nervosa. *Lancet*. 2005;366:74-85.
404. Welt CK, Chan J, Bullen J, et al. Recombinant human leptin in women with hypothalamic amenorrhea. *N Engl J Med*. 2004;351: 987-997.
405. Heymsfield SB, Greenberg AS, Fujioka K, et al. Recombinant leptin for weight loss in obese and lean adults: a randomized, controlled, dose-escalation trial. *JAMA*. 1999;282:1568-1575.
406. Shimomura I, Hammer RE, Ikemoto S, et al. Leptin reverses insulin resistance and diabetes mellitus in mice with congenital lipodystrophy. *Nature*. 1999;401:73-76.
407. Ebihara K, Ogawa Y, Masuzaki H, et al. Transgenic overexpression of leptin rescues insulin resistance and diabetes in a mouse model of lipoatrophic diabetes. *Diabetes*. 2001;50:1440-1448.
408. Oral EA, Simha V, Ruiz E, et al. Leptin-replacement therapy for lipodystrophy. *N Engl J Med*. 2002;346:570-578.
409. Coppari R, Ichinose M, Lee CE, et al. The hypothalamic arcuate nucleus: a key site for mediating leptin's effects on glucose homeostasis and locomotor activity. *Cell Metab*. 2005;1:63-72.
410. Morton GJ, Gelling RW, Niswender KD, et al. Leptin regulates insulin sensitivity via phosphatidylinositol-3-OH kinase signaling in mediobasal hypothalamic neurons. *Cell Metab*. 2005;2:411-420.
411. Krude H, Biebermann H, Luck W, et al. Severe early-onset obesity, adrenal insufficiency and red hair pigmentation caused by POMC mutations in humans. *Nat Genet*. 1998;19:155-157.
412. Vaisse C, Clement K, Guy-Grand B, et al. A frameshift mutation in human MC4R is associated with a dominant form of obesity. *Nat Genet*. 1998;20:113-114.
413. Yeo GSH, Farooqi IS, Aminian S, et al. A frameshift mutation in MC4R associated with dominantly inherited human obesity. *Nat Genet*. 1998;20:111-112.
414. Hinney A, Schmidt A, Nottebom K, et al. Several mutations in the melanocortin-4 receptor gene including a nonsense and a frameshift mutation associated with dominantly inherited obesity in humans. *J Clin Endocrinol Metab*. 1999;84:1483-1486.
415. Farooqi IS, Yeo GS, Keogh JM, et al. Dominant and recessive inheritance of morbid obesity associated with melanocortin 4 receptor deficiency. *J Clin Invest*. 2000;106:271-279.
416. Vaisse C, Clement K, Durand E, et al. Melanocortin-4 receptor mutations are a frequent and heterogenous cause of morbid obesity. *J Clin Invest*. 2000;106:253-262.
417. Farooqi IS, Keogh JM, Yeo GS, et al. Clinical spectrum of obesity and mutations in the melanocortin 4 receptor gene. *N Engl J Med*. 2003;348:1160-1163.
418. Branson R, Potoczna N, Kral JG, et al. Binge eating as a major phenotype of melanocortin 4 receptor gene mutations. *N Engl J Med*. 2003;348:1096-1103.

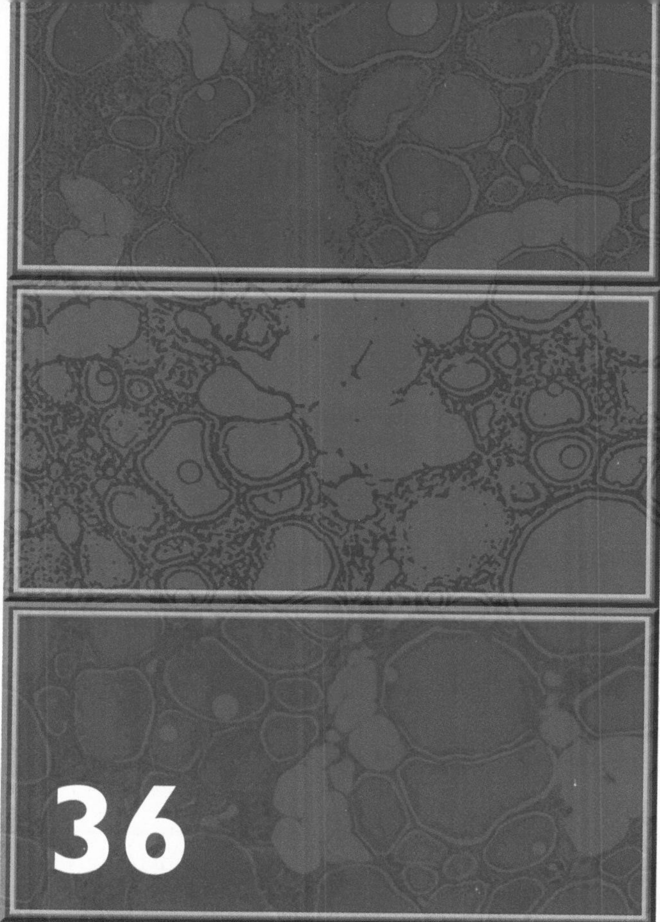

CHAPTER 36

Obesity

SAMUEL KLEIN • ELISA FABBRINI • JOHANNES A. ROMIJN

Obesity is a chronic disease that is causally related to serious medical illnesses. In the United States alone, the consequences of obesity account for an estimated 300,000 deaths per year.[1] The medical expenses and cost of lost productivity due to obesity are greater than $100 billion per year.[2] This review addresses the important clinical and pathophysiologic issues in obesity.

DEFINITION OF OBESITY

Body Mass Index

Body mass index (BMI) is calculated by dividing a person's weight (in kilograms) by height (in meters squared); alternatively, the weight (in pounds) multiplied by 704 and divided by height (in inches squared) may be used. There is a curvilinear relation between BMI and percent body fat mass.[3] However, the current practical definition of obesity is based on the relationship between BMI and health outcome rather than BMI and body composition.

Table 36-1 summarizes the guidelines for classifying weight status by BMI proposed by the major national and international health organizations.[4-7] Many large epidemiologic studies[8,9] have established an inverse relationship between BMI and mortality for BMI values of 25.0 kg/m^2 or higher. Men and women with a BMI between 25.0 and 29.9 kg/m^2 are considered to be overweight, and those with a BMI greater than 30.0 kg/m^2 are considered to be obese. Obese persons are at higher risk for adverse health consequences than those who are overweight (Fig. 36-1). These criteria for overweight and obesity represent imposed cutoff values along a continuum on the curve of mortality rate versus BMI.

The prevalence of obesity-related diseases, such as type 2 diabetes (T2DM), begins to increase at BMI values lower than 25.0 kg/m^2 (Fig. 36-2). Therefore, if the risk for T2DM were used to define overweight and obesity, the relationship curve would be shifted to the left, and the cutoff BMI values would be lower.

Data from the National Health and Nutrition Examination Surveys (NHANES) collected between 1971 and 2000 question the relationship between overweight status and increased mortality risk.[9] These data found that persons who were overweight or even had class I obesity (BMI 30.0-34.9 kg/m^2) did not have a significant increase in mortality risk.

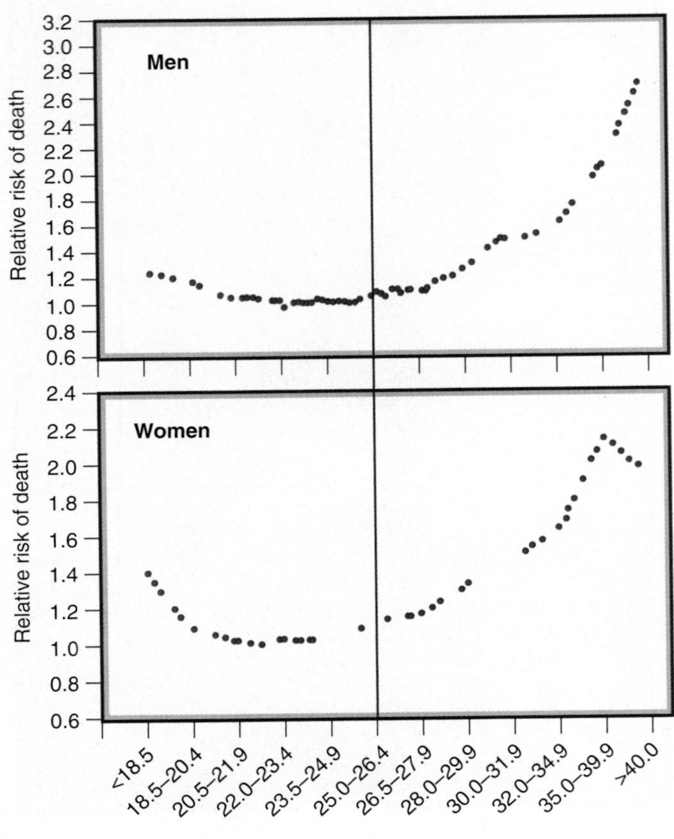

Figure 36-1 Relationship between body mass index and cardiovascular mortality in men and women in the United States who never smoked and had no preexisting illness. The vertical line separates underweight and lean subjects *(left side)* from overweight and obese subjects *(right side)*. (Adapted from Calle EE, Thun MJ, Petrelli JM, et al. Body-mass index and mortality in a prospective cohort of U.S. adults. *N Engl J Med.* 1999;341:1097-1105.)

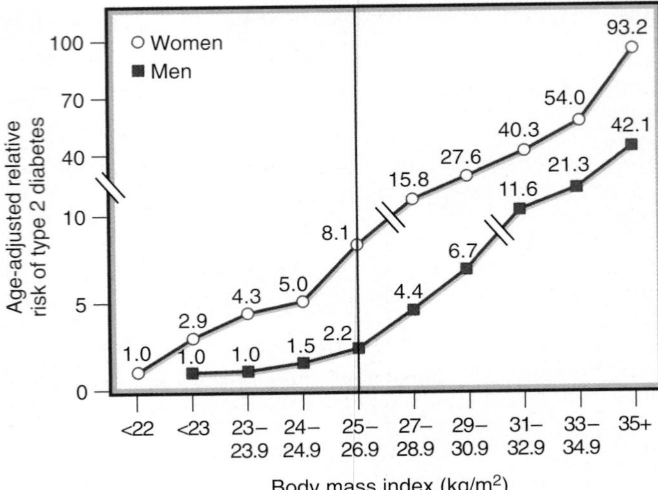

Figure 36-2 Relationship between body mass index and type 2 diabetes in men and women in the United States. The vertical line separates underweight and lean subjects *(left side)* from overweight and obese subjects *(right side)*. The data demonstrate that the risk of diabetes begins to increase at the upper end of the lean body mass index category. (Adapted from Colditz GA, Willett WC, Rotnitzky A, et al. Weight gain as a risk factor for clinical diabetes mellitus in women. *Ann Intern Med.* 1995;122:481-486; and Chan JM, Rimm EB, Colditz GA, et al. Obesity, fat distribution, and weight gain as risk factors for clinical diabetes in men. *Diabetes Care.* 1994;17:961-969.)

Factors Affecting Body Mass Index–Related Risk

Several factors influence BMI-related health risk (see Table 36-1). They include body fat distribution, age, concomitant medical illness, weight gain, aerobic fitness, and ethnicity.

TABLE 36-1

Weight Classification by Body Mass Index (BMI)

Weight Classification	Obesity Class	BMI (kg/m²)	Risk of Disease
Underweight		<18.5	Increased
Normal		18.5-24.9	Normal
Overweight		25.0-29.9	Increased
Obesity	I	30.0-34.9	High
	II	35.0-39.9	Very high
Extreme Obesity	III	≥40.0	Extremely high

Adapted from the National Institutes of Health, National Heart, Lung, and Blood Institute. Clinical guidelines on the identification, evaluation, and treatment of overweight and obesity in adults: the evidence report. *Obes Res.* 1998;6(suppl 2):51S-209S.

Body Fat Distribution. Obese persons with excess abdominal fat are at higher risk for diabetes, hypertension, dyslipidemia, and ischemic heart disease than obese persons whose fat is located predominantly in the lower body.[10] Those with increased lower body fat mass are protected from metabolic complications.[11-13] Waist circumference is highly correlated with abdominal fat mass and is often used as a surrogate marker for abdominal (upper body) obesity.

Waist circumference is an important predictor of health outcomes in adult men and women of all age groups and ethnicities, including Caucasians, African Americans, Asians, and Hispanics. The relationship between waist circumference and clinical outcome is strongest for diabetes risk, and waist circumference is an independent and better predictor of diabetes than BMI.[14] The recommended waist circumference thresholds for increased cardiometabolic risk is 40 inches (102 cm) in men and 35 inches (88 cm)[15] in women; these cutoff values were derived from waist circumference values that correlated with a BMI of 30 kg/m² or greater.[16] However, they are based on populations of European origin and might not be appropriate for non-Europeans.

Asian populations tend to have a higher percentage of body fat for the same BMI value and an increased prevalence of cardiovascular risk factors at lower BMI values compared with Caucasians.[17-19] Moreover, at any given waist circumference, the relative risk of mortality is higher in Asians than in African Americans or Europeans.[20] The World Health Organization (WHO) has indicated that waist circumference thresholds denoting increased risk in the Asian population should be 90 cm for men and 80 cm for women.[21] Different levels have been suggested in Japan and China, with cutoff values of 85 cm for men and 80 cm for women, and slightly lower values have been suggested in India.[22]

Age. The BMI value associated with the lowest relative risk of mortality increases with increasing age.[9,23]

Concomitant Medical Illness. In patients with certain medical conditions, being overweight or obese is associated with lower mortality rates than for similar patients with normal BMI values. This BMI paradox is associated with (1) cardiovascular disease (myocardial infarction,[24] congestive heart failure,[25] hypertension and coronary heart disease (CHD),[26] coronary artery bypass graft surgery,[27] heart transplant[28]); (2) renal disease (end-stage renal disease)[29]; (3) hip fractures[30]; (4) rheumatoid arthritis[31]; and (5) tuberculosis.[32]

Weight Gain. Another factor that modifies the risk of obesity-related complications is weight gain during adulthood. In both men and women, weight gain of 5 kg or more since the ages of 18 to 20 years increases the risk of developing diabetes, hypertension, and CHD, and the risk of disease increases with the amount of weight gained.[33-38]

Aerobic Fitness. The risk of developing obesity-associated diabetes or cardiovascular disease can be modified by aerobic fitness. In a cohort of more than 8000 men who were monitored for an average of 6 years, the incidences of diabetes[39] and cardiovascular mortality[40] were lower in those who were fit, as defined by maximal ability to consume oxygen during exercise, compared with those who were unfit across a range of body adiposity.

Ethnicity. BMI-associated health risk is also influenced by ethnicity.[41] For example, when matched on BMI, the risk of diabetes is higher in Southeast Asian populations than in whites.[42]

PHYSIOLOGY OF ENERGY HOMEOSTASIS

Energy homeostasis, which includes all processes that aim to maintain energy balance, requires complex molecular and physiologic processes and constant communication within and among adipose tissue, skeletal muscle, liver, pancreas, and the central nervous system. The homeostatic control of energy homeostasis relies on physiologic integration of biologic signals from these different organs as well as nutrient-related signals, postprandial neural and hormonal influences, and stimuli related to hedonic, situational, or stress-related circumstances. A complex physiologic system regulates energy homeostasis by integrating signals from peripheral organs with central coordination in the brain.[43] The hypothalamus functions as the main cerebral center in which these signals converge.[44]

A balanced interaction between two sets of neurons occurs within the arcuate nucleus of the hypothalamus. Activation of neurons secreting neuropeptide Y (NPY) and agouti-related protein (AgRP) promotes food intake, whereas that of neurons secreting pro-opiomelanocortin (POMC) and cocaine- and amphetamine-regulated transcript (CART) has an anorexigenic effect. The NPY/AgRP neurons also inhibit POMC/CART neurons through γ-aminobutyric acid (GABA). The orexigenic and anorexigenic signals from the NPY/AgRP and POMC/CART neurons are sent to other brain nuclei, ultimately resulting in alterations in food intake and energy expenditure. The system is very complex and involves interactions among various areas of the brain.

The endocannabinoid system is also involved in the regulation of food intake, particularly the cannabinoid 1 (CB_1) receptors (encoded by *CNR1*) and their endogenous ligands, anandamide (*N*-arachidonoyl-ethanolamine) and 2-arachidonoylglycerol. Absence of CB_1 receptors in mice with a disrupted CB_1 gene causes hypophagia and leanness.[45] Administration of cannabinoids increases food intake and promotes body-weight gain, and treatment with selective CB_1 receptor antagonists decreases food intake and body weight in obese mice.[46] Randomized, controlled trials (RCTs) in obese human patients have shown that treatment with rimonabant, a CB_1 receptor antagonist, decreases body weight.[47,48] These studies demonstrated that the cannabinoid system has an important role in the regulation of ingestive behavior in animals and humans.[49] In 2008, the clinical development program of rimonabant was discontinued because of the risk of serious psychiatric disorders.

The major peripheral organs participating in the regulation of food intake are the stomach, gut, pancreas, and adipose tissue.[44] The stomach and the duodenum secrete the orexigenic peptide ghrelin, which increases before eating and decreases after feeding. Many so-called satiety signals are transmitted to the brain via vagal afferent fibers from the gut that synapse in the nucleus tractus solitarius (NTS) in the hindbrain, which participates in gustatory, satiety, and visceral sensation. For instance, oral taste receptor cells generate information that is transmitted to the NTS by afferent sensory fibers. Insulin, secreted by the pancreas, has an anorexigenic effect through the arcuate nucleus. The PYY(3-36) form of peptide YY is secreted by the gastrointestinal tract after food ingestion and might have an anorexigenic effect.[50] Glucagon-like peptide 1 (GLP1) is derived from pre-proglucagon and secreted in response to food ingestion by the proximal gastrointestinal tract. It exerts pleiotropic effects, including slight anorexic effects.[51] Satiety is also mediated by other gut proteins, such as cholecystokinin (CCK). Leptin, secreted by the adipose tissue, also serves as an anorexigenic signal.

PATHOGENESIS

Energy Balance

Obesity is caused by an excessive intake of calories in relation to energy expenditure over a long period of time. The gastrointestinal tract has the capacity to absorb large amounts of nutrients. Large increases in body fat can result from even minor, but chronic, differences between energy intake and energy expenditure. In 1 year, the ingestion of only 5% more calories than expended can promote the gain of approximately 5 kg in adipose tissue. Over 30 years, the daily ingestion of only 8 kcal more than expended can increase body weight by 10 kg. This represents the average amount of weight gained by Americans during the 30-year period between 25 and 55 years of age.[52]

Genes and Environment

Body size depends on the complex interaction between genetic background and environmental factors. In humans, genetic background explains only an estimated 40% of the variance in body mass.[53] The marked increase in the prevalence of obesity since the 1980s must have resulted largely from alterations in environmental factors that increase energy intake and reduce physical activity. For example, more meals are now eaten outside the home, there is greater availability of convenience and snack foods, serving sizes are larger, and daily physical activity has decreased because of sedentary lifestyle and work activities.

Environmental Effects in High-Risk Populations

Dramatic examples of the influence of environment on body weight have been reported globally. These examples illustrate that persons of certain genetic backgrounds are especially prone to gain weight and develop obesity-related diseases when exposed to a "modern" lifestyle.

Since the 1950s, striking changes in the lifestyle of Pima Indians living in Arizona have led to an epidemic of obesity and diabetes in this population.[54] The diet of these urbanized Pimas is much higher in fat (50% of energy as fat) than the traditional Pima diet (15% of energy as fat). In addition, urbanized Pimas are much more sedentary than the Pimas who remained in the Sierra Madre Mountains of Northern Mexico and are isolated from Western influences. These rural Pimas eat a traditional diet and are physically active as farmers and sawmill workers; they have much lower incidences of obesity and diabetes than their Arizona kindred.

The Aborigines of northern Australia are another high-risk population whose weight and health status have been compromised by exposure to a modern environment. Urbanized Aborigines are heavier than hunter-gatherer kindred, who are usually very lean (BMI <20.0 kg/m^2), and they have high prevalences of T2DM and hypertriglyceridemia.[55] The traditional hunter-gatherer lifestyle of the Aborigines involves a low-fat, low-calorie diet of wild game, fish, and plants and a high level of physical activity. In one study, short-term (7 weeks) re-exposure to the traditional lifestyle resulted in weight loss and significant improvements or normalization of glucose tolerance and fasting blood glucose, insulin, and triglyceride concentrations in urbanized Aborigines with T2DM and hypertriglyceridemia.[56]

Influences of Childhood and Parental Obesity

The risk of becoming an obese adult is influenced both by having been obese as a child and by having had at least one obese parent. The risk of adult obesity increases with increasing age and with the severity of obesity in childhood. For example, the risk of being obese at 21 to 29 years of age ranged from 8% for persons who were obese at 1 to 2 years of age and had nonobese parents to 79% for persons who were obese at 10 to 14 years of age and had at least one obese parent.[57] Although persons who were obese at 1 to 2 years of age and had lean parents did not have an increased risk of obesity in adulthood, persons who became obese after 6 years of age had a greater than 50% chance of becoming obese adults.

Monogenic Causes of Obesity

Since the discovery of the adipose tissue protein leptin, much progress has been made in understanding the molecular basis of body-fat regulation. It has nonetheless been disappointing that a genetic cause of obesity has been identified in only a very few persons. Several rare, monogenic causes of obesity have been described in recent years.

Leptin Gene Mutation

The pathophysiologic relevance of leptin was established in two extremely obese cousins with hyperphagia who belonged to a consanguineous family of Pakistani origin.[58] These cousins were homozygous for a single nucleotide deletion at position 398 of the leptin gene. This mutation resulted in a frameshift of the leptin-coding region and premature termination of leptin synthesis. The parents of the cousins were heterozygous for this mutation.

Another mutation, this time involving a homozygous single-nucleotide transversion in the leptin gene that resulted in a substitution of Trp for Arg in the mature peptide and low serum leptin levels, was discovered in three extremely obese persons, including one adult man and one adult woman, both of whom were hyperinsulinemic.[59] The man exhibited hypothalamic hypogonadism and dysfunction of the sympathetic nervous system, and the woman had primary amenorrhea.

Leptin treatment has successfully reversed the obesity of leptin-deficient patients. Treatment with recombinant human leptin resulted in a weight loss of 1 to 2 kg/month over a 12-month period. Loss of fat mass accounted for 95% of this weight loss.[60]

The possibility that leptin levels are reduced in obesity has been investigated in large groups of subjects. However, serum leptin levels increase exponentially with fat mass, suggesting that most obese persons are resistant or insensitive to body weight regulation by endogenous leptin.[61]

Leptin Receptor Mutation

Three extremely obese sisters from a consanguineous family were found to have markedly high serum leptin levels and to be homozygous for a single-nucleotide substitution at the splice site of exon 16 of the leptin receptor gene.[62] This mutation resulted in a truncated protein that lacked both the transmembrane and the intracellular domains of the receptor. The sisters displayed hypogonadotropic hypogonadism, failure of pubertal development, growth delay, and secondary hypothyroidism. This finding confirms the endocrine abnormalities in leptin-deficient subjects and implies a role for leptin and its receptor in the central regulation of energy balance and hypothalamic endocrine functions in humans.

Prohormone Convertase 1 Gene Mutation

A mutation in the gene encoding prohormone convertase 1 (PC1), now called *PCSK1*, was identified in a 43-year-old obese woman with a history of severe childhood obesity.[63] This woman had impaired glucose tolerance, postprandial hypoglycemia, low plasma cortisol levels, and hypogonadotropic hypogonadism. In addition, she had increased plasma concentrations of proinsulin and POMC but very low plasma insulin concentrations. She was a compound heterozygote for two mutations in the *PCSK1* gene, which resulted in loss of the autocatalytic cleavage ability of PC1. A second patient has also been described.[64] Melanocortins, including α-melanocortin–stimulating hormone (MSH), are formed through the processing of POMC by PC1. Therefore, reduced production of melanocortin might have been responsible for obesity in these patients.

Pro-Opiomelanocortin Gene Mutation

A mutation in the POMC gene was described in two obese children with hyperphagia.[65] The children also had red hair pigmentation and were deficient in adrenocorticotropic hormone (ACTH). The mutations resulted in complete loss of the ability to synthesize α-MSH and ACTH. The red hair pigmentation and obesity are believed to be due to deficiency of α-MSH.

Melanocortin 4 Receptor Mutation

Although they are rare, mutations in the melanocortin 4 receptor (MC4R) are the most common monogenic cause of obesity.[66] Moreover, MC4R mutations are characterized by both dominant and recessive modes of inheritance, in contrast to the other monogenic forms of obesity, which have recessive modes of inheritance. In children with MC4R mutations, the degree of obesity and hyperphagia correlates with the extent of impairment of MC4R signaling. However, adult carriers of the mutations cannot be phenotypically distinguished from other obese subjects.[67]

Mutation of the Neurotrophin Receptor TrkB

The survival and differentiation of neurons in the peripheral nervous system are dependent on neurotrophic factors, which are secreted by the target tissues. Neurotrophin signaling occurs through the specific activation of receptor tyrosine kinases of the Trk family. An 8-year-old boy with a complex developmental syndrome and severe obesity was found to be heterozygous for a de novo missense mutation resulting in a Tyr722Cys substitution in the neurotrophin receptor TrkB. This mutation markedly impaired receptor autophosphorylation and signaling to mitogen-activated protein kinase. Mutation of *NTRK2*, the gene encoding for TrkB, seems to result in a unique human syndrome of hyperphagic obesity.[68]

Obesity in Pleiotropic Syndromes

About 30 mendelian disorders have been described in which obesity is a clinical feature; often, this obesity is associated with mental retardation, dysmorphic features, and organ-specific developmental abnormalities—the pleiotropic syndromes. Positional genetic techniques have led to the identification of different mutations underlying these syndromes. However, in most cases these genes encode for proteins whose function is unresolved.[69]

Obesity Syndromes due to Chromosomal Rearrangements

Prader-Willi Syndrome

The Prader-Willi syndrome is characterized by obesity, mental retardation, short stature, and secondary hypogonadism. It is the most common syndromic cause of obesity, occurring in 1 of every 25,000 births.[70] In these patients, the paternal segment 15q11.2-q12 is absent. The omission can result from deletion of the paternal segment (75%) or from loss of the entire paternal chromosome 15, with the presence of two maternal homologs (uniparental maternal disomy). The role of the genes encoded by the paternal segment and the mechanisms by which they cause the obesity syndrome have not been resolved.[70]

SIM1 Gene Mutation

A de novo balanced translocation between chromosomes 1 and 6 was found in a severely obese girl who weighed 47 kg at 67 months of age.[71] The mutation caused a disruption in *SIM1*, the human homolog of the *Drosophila* single-minded *(sim)* gene that regulates neurogenesis. *SIM1* encodes a transcription factor involved in the formation of the paraventricular and supraoptic nuclei. It is likely that this abnormality altered energy balance in this patient by stimulating food intake, because measured resting energy expenditure was normal.

Polygenic Causes of Obesity

Obesity is likely to result from the interaction of many different gene-gene and gene-environment interactions. In contrast to the small number of single-gene mutations that clearly cause obesity in rare patients, a large number of human genes have been identified that show variations in DNA sequences that might contribute to obesity.[72]

The use of the genome-wide association approach has identified many genes with robust associations but usually with only modest contributions to overall genetic susceptibility to common obesity or high BMI. It is a challenge to determine how these results fit into current models of the genetic architecture and physiology of obesity, because no existing hypothesis explains all the data. Some of these associations will undoubtedly prove to be more important than others. The first major breakthrough provided by genome-wide association studies was the discovery of the fat mass and obesity-associated gene (*FTO*) as a potential obesity gene.

Data from several studies have documented a strong association between fat mass (or BMI) and a single-nucleotide polymorphism (SNP) in *FTO* in both childhood and adult obesity. Frayling and colleagues[73] found that SNP rs9939609 in the *FTO* gene was strongly associated with T2DM, but this allele was also strongly associated with an increased BMI. The association between this *FTO* SNP and T2DM was abolished by adjustment for the BMI, suggesting that the risk of diabetes was due to the increase in BMI. The association of this variant with BMI was replicated in 13 cohorts containing more than 38,000 subjects. Sixteen percent of the adults were homozygous for this particular SNP; they weighed about 3 kg more than the subjects without this SNP and had a 1.67-fold increased risk of obesity.[73]

Independently, Dina and colleagues[74] found another SNP, rs1121980, in the first intron of the *FTO* gene that was strongly associated with severe adult obesity (odds ratio, 1.55) in French individuals of European ancestry. This finding was replicated by a similarly strong association of several *FTO* SNPs in a study of approximately 900 severely obese adults and 2700 nonobese French controls. Three of the four most significantly associated SNPs (rs17817449, rs3751812, and rs1421085) are putatively functional. The same report also showed associations of SNPs in the *FTO* gene with obesity in three additional cohorts including children or adults.[74]

In another independent study of over 4000 Sardinians, Scuteri and colleagues[75] showed that another SNP in *FTO*, rs9930506, and other nearby variants are associated with BMI, hip circumference, and total body weight. Additional associations of BMI with SNPs in the *FTO* gene were shown in both European-American and Hispanic-American cohorts in the same report.

FTO encodes a 2-oxoglutarate–dependent nucleic acid demethylase. Studies of wild-type mice indicate that Fto messenger RNA (mRNA) is most abundant in the brain, particularly in hypothalamic nuclei governing energy balance, and that Fto mRNA levels in the arcuate nucleus are regulated by feeding and fasting.[76] These data suggest that *FTO* participates in the central regulation of energy homeostasis.

ENERGY METABOLISM

Total daily energy expenditure (TEE) comprises resting energy expenditure (REE), which accounts for approximately 70% of TEE; energy expended in physical activity (approximately 20% of TEE); and the thermic effect of food (TEF), which accounts for approximately 10% of TEE. REE represents the energy expended for normal cellular and organ function under postabsorptive resting conditions.

within adipose tissue, and, as circulating hormones, they can affect the functions of distant organs such as muscle, pancreas, liver, and the central nervous system.

The function of adipose tissue as an endocrine organ has important implications for understanding the pathophysiologic relationship between excess body fat and pathologic states such as insulin resistance and T2DM.[102,103] Not all products released by adipose tissue are produced by adipocytes. Other cells contained within the adipose tissue, including endothelial cells, macrophages, and adipocyte precursor cells, can also participate in endocrine functions. Selected proteins produced by adipose tissue are reviewed next.

Leptin

Adipocytes produce leptin and secrete it into the bloodstream. Leptin has pleiotropic effects on food intake, hypothalamic neuroendocrine regulation, reproductive function, and energy expenditure.[104,105] There is a direct relationship between plasma leptin concentrations and BMI or body fat percentage.[106] However, there can be considerable variability in leptin concentrations among persons with the same BMI, suggesting that leptin production is also regulated by factors other than adipose tissue mass. Leptin levels decrease rapidly within 12 hours after the start of starvation. Conversely, leptin levels increase in response to overfeeding.[107] Therefore, plasma leptin concentrations reflect adipose tissue mass and are influenced by energy balance. Leptin is a bidirectional signal that switches physiologic regulation between fed and starved states. Plasma leptin concentrations increase with increasing fat mass and decrease rapidly during early fasting. The relative importance of the central versus peripheral effects of leptin in body weight regulation in most obese persons is still unclear.[108]

Resistin

Resistin is another signaling polypeptide secreted by adipocytes.[109] Resistin levels are increased in mice with diet-induced and genetic forms of obesity and insulin resistance. Administration of recombinant resistin to normal mice leads to impaired glucose tolerance and insulin action. Neutralization of resistin levels leads to reduced hyperglycemia in obese, insulin-resistant mice, in part by improving insulin sensitivity. Based on these findings, it has been proposed that resistin is a hormone that links obesity to diabetes by inducing insulin resistance.

Adiponectin

Adiponectin is the most abundant secretory protein produced by adipocytes. In contrast to other secretory products of adipocytes, the plasma concentrations of adiponectin are decreased in obesity and insulin resistance. There is a close association between hypoadiponectinemia, insulin resistance, and hyperinsulinemia.[110] Conversely, adiponectin expression increases with improved insulin sensitivity and weight loss.[111] Interventions that improve insulin sensitivity, such as weight loss or treatment with thiazolidinediones, are associated with increased adipose tissue adiponectin gene expression and plasma concentrations.[112] Moreover, administration of recombinant adiponectin exerts glucose-lowering effects and ameliorates insulin resistance in mouse models of obesity or diabetes.[113] These data suggest that decreased plasma levels of adiponectin contribute to some of the metabolic complications associated with obesity.

Visfatin

Visfatin corresponds with a protein previously known as pre-B cell colony-enhancing factor. The initial study documenting the insulin-like effects of visfatin[114] was later withdrawn. Subsequent studies in human subjects reported conflicting results regarding the relation of visfatin to adiposity, subcutaneous or visceral fat, and insulin resistance. The role of this protein in the development of obesity and insulin resistance is unclear. Additional studies are required to elucidate the potential physiologic and pathophysiologic roles of visfatin.

Estrogens

Adipose tissue has P450 aromatase activity. This enzyme is important for transforming androstenedione into estrone. Estrone is the second major circulating estrogen in premenopausal women and the most important estrogen in postmenopausal women.[103] The conversion rate of androstenedione into estrone increases with age and obesity, and it is higher in women with lower-body obesity than in those with upper-body obesity. In addition to a role in endocrine regulation, the effects of P450 aromatase on estrogen metabolism might also have a role in autocrine and paracrine action, because estrogen receptors are present in adipose tissue.

Selected Cytokines

Tumor Necrosis Factor-α. Adipocytes secrete TNF-α, and TNF-α expression is increased in the enlarged adipocytes of obese subjects.[115] However, plasma TNF-α levels are generally at or below the detection limit of available assays, which suggests that the TNF-α produced in adipose tissue has paracrine, rather than endocrine, functions. The multiple effects of TNF-α on adipocytes include impairment of insulin signaling. Therefore, it has been proposed that TNF-α may partially contribute to insulin resistance in obesity.[102]

Interleukin 6. Adipose tissue interleukin 6 (IL-6) secretion may account for 30% of circulating IL-6.[116,117] Obesity is associated with increased plasma IL-6 concentrations, which may contribute to systemic inflammation and insulin resistance. Insulin sensitivity is inversely related to plasma IL-6 levels,[118] and IL-6 directly impairs insulin signaling.[119] Administration of IL-6 to human subjects induces dose-dependent increases in fasting blood glucose, probably by stimulating release of glucagon and other counterregulatory hormones or by inducing peripheral resistance to insulin action, or both.[120]

ADIPOCYTE BIOLOGY

White Adipose Tissue

Obesity is associated with an increased number of adipocytes. A lean adult has about 35 billion adipocytes, each containing approximately 0.4 to 0.6 μg of triglyceride; an extremely obese adult can have four times as many adipocytes (125 billion), each containing twice as much lipid (0.8 to 1.2 μg of triglyceride).[121]

Understanding of adipocyte differentiation is largely derived from studies conducted in preadipocytes in culture. The current concept is that adipocytes are derived from fibroblast precursor cells after the concerted actions of extracellular signals and intrinsic transcription factors and coactivators.

Many extranuclear factors and intracellular transduction pathways influence the adipogenic potential of cells in vitro and in vivo (Fig. 36-3).[122] Although in the future it may be possible to regulate adipogenesis in vivo,

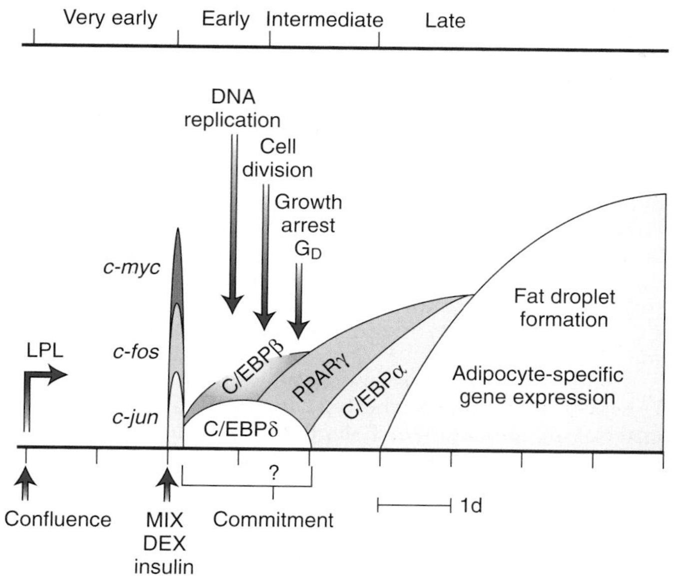

Figure 36-3 Progression of 3T3-L1 preadipocyte differentiation and subsequent changes in cellular characteristics. The distinct stages of differentiation (very early, early, intermediate, and late) are shown. C/EBP, CCAAT/enhancer binding protein; DEX, dexamethasone; LPL, lipoprotein lipase; MIX, methylisobutylxanthine; PPAR, peroxisome proliferator–activated receptor. (From Ntambi JM, Kim Y-C. Adipocyte differentiation and gene expression. *J Nutr.* 2000;130:3122S-3126S.)

decreasing adipogenesis without altering energy balance can result in the deposition of triglycerides in other tissues. Excessive amounts of triglycerides in nonadipose tissues can have deleterious effects, as was suggested by the liver steatosis, dyslipidemia, and diabetes observed when adipogenesis was prevented in mice.[123]

The cornerstone of obesity therapy is to increase the use of endogenous fat stores as fuel by reducing energy intake below energy expenditure. With dieting, weight loss is composed of approximately 75% to 85% fat and 15% to 25% fat-free mass (FFM).[124] An energy deficit of approximately 3500 kcal is required to oxidize 1 lb of adipose tissue. However, because of the oxidation of lean tissue and associated water losses, a 3500-kcal energy deficit will reduce body weight by more than 1 lb.

The distribution of fat loss is characterized by regional heterogeneity.[125,126] Particularly in men and women with initially increased intra-abdominal fat, there are greater relative losses of intra-abdominal fat than total body fat mass. A decrease in the size (triglyceride content) of existing adipocytes accounts for most, if not all, of the fat loss.[127] In humans, there is also evidence that the number of adipocytes is reduced with large, long-term fat loss.[128] However, it is possible that this perception of decreased fat cell number is false due to inability of standard cell counting techniques to detect adipocytes that have undergone marked shrinkage.

There are two possible mechanisms through which weight loss could eliminate fat cells: dedifferentiation, the morphologic and biochemical reversion of mature adipocytes to preadipocytes, and apoptosis. Adipocyte dedifferentiation has been observed in vitro, but there is no evidence that it occurs in vivo.[129] Adipocyte apoptosis has been induced in vitro,[130] and it has been demonstrated to occur in vivo in some patients with cancer.[131] To date, it is not known whether diet-mediated weight loss induces adipocyte apoptosis.

Brown Adipose Tissue

Brown adipose tissue (BAT) is structurally different from white adipose tissue; it contains multilocular fat vacuoles and large mitochondria and is intensively innervated by sympathetic nerves. In rodents, BAT is very important for nonshivering thermogenesis. The uncoupling of phosphorylation in BAT results from the activity of uncoupling protein 1 (UCP1) within the inner mitochondrial membrane, which exhausts the electrochemical gradient needed for oxidative phosphorylation by creating a proton leak. BAT consequently affects energy expenditure by producing heat from uncoupled phosphorylation.[132] Three recent studies conducted in human subjects provide conclusive evidence that UCP1 is present in adipose tissue. Biopsies of areas of UCP1 activity identified by positron emission tomography or computed tomography provided histologic confirmation of the presence of supraclavicular BAT.[133,134] UCP1 activity was stimulated by cold exposure.[135] Another study in humans documented a very strong seasonal variation in the presence of BAT.[136] It is possible that altered regulation of BAT activity is involved in the pathogenesis of obesity.

PREVALENCE OF OBESITY

The worldwide prevalence of obesity has increased markedly over the last several decades. In the United States, about one third of adults aged 20 to 74 years are considered obese.[137] According to national population surveys conducted since 1960, the prevalence of obesity (BMI $\geq$ 30 kg/m^2) has more than doubled, from 13% to 32%.[137,138] The prevalence of obesity increases progressively from 20 to 50 years of age but then declines after 60 to 70 years of age.

The prevalence of obesity has also risen in children and adolescents. Overweight is defined as a BMI greater than the 95th percentile for age and gender on the revised National Center for Health Statistics growth charts; based on this definition, the prevalence of overweight among children and adolescents aged 6 to 17 years in the United States is 17%,[137,139] double the rate reported in earlier surveys. Diseases commonly associated with obesity in adults, such as T2DM, hypertension, hyperlipidemia, gallbladder disease, nonalcoholic steatohepatitis, sleep apnea, and orthopedic complications, are now increasingly observed in children.[140]

METABOLICALLY NORMAL OBESITY

Obesity is commonly associated with alterations in metabolic function, namely insulin resistance, diabetes, dyslipidemia (increased serum triglyceride and decreased serum high-density lipoprotein–cholesterol [HDL-C]), and increased blood pressure.[50,141] However, approximately 25% of obese adults are "metabolically normal" based on insulin sensitivity as measured by the hyperinsulinemic euglycemic clamp technique.[142,143] In addition, NHANES data covering 1994 to 2004 indicated that 32% of obese adults were metabolically normal, defined as having no more than one cardiometabolic abnormality (i.e., blood pressure, a homeostasis model assessment of insulin resistance [HOMA-IR] value, and concentrations of plasma glucose, triglyceride, HDL-C, and C-reactive protein).[144]

The recognition that a subset of obese persons are resistant to the typical metabolic complications of obesity has led to several studies that attempted to characterize the distinguishing features of metabolically healthy but obese individuals.[145] In general, these studies found that persons with metabolically normal obesity (also called uncomplicated obesity[146] or metabolically benign obesity[147]) had a similar percentage of body fat but less visceral and liver fat than metabolically abnormal obese persons; moreover, they had normal values for insulin sensitivity, blood pressure, lipid profile, and inflammatory profile (plasma C-reactive protein).[142,145-149] Metabolically normal obese adults who were monitored for up to 11 years did not show a greater risk of developing diabetes or cardiovascular disease than normal-weight, metabolically normal subjects.[54] In contrast, metabolically abnormal, lean or obese subjects had a 4- to 11-fold increased relative risk of diabetes compared with normal-weight, metabolically normal subjects.[150]

CLINICAL FEATURES AND COMPLICATIONS OF OBESITY

Obesity causes many serious medical complications that impair quality of life and lead to increased morbidity and premature death (Fig. 36-4).[151] The complications associated with obesity have been reviewed in detail elsewhere.[5]

Endocrine and Metabolic Diseases

The Dysmetabolic Syndrome

In the dysmetabolic syndrome, also known as metabolic syndrome, insulin-resistance syndrome, or syndrome X, the specific phenotype of upper-body (or abdominal) obesity is associated with a cluster of metabolic risk factors for CHD. Features of this syndrome include insulin resistance with associated hyperinsulinemia, impaired glucose tolerance, impaired insulin-mediated glucose disposal, and T2DM; dyslipidemia, characterized by hypertriglyceridemia and low serum HDL-C levels; and hypertension. Other metabolic risk factors, including increased serum levels of apolipoprotein B; small, dense low-density lipoprotein (LDL) particles; and plasminogen activator inhibitor 1 (PAI1, encoded by *SERPINE1*) with impaired fibrinolysis have also been associated with abdominal obesity.[152,153] The dysmetabolic syndrome usually occurs in persons with frank obesity, but it has also been reported in normal-weight persons who presumably have an increased amount of abdominal fat.[154]

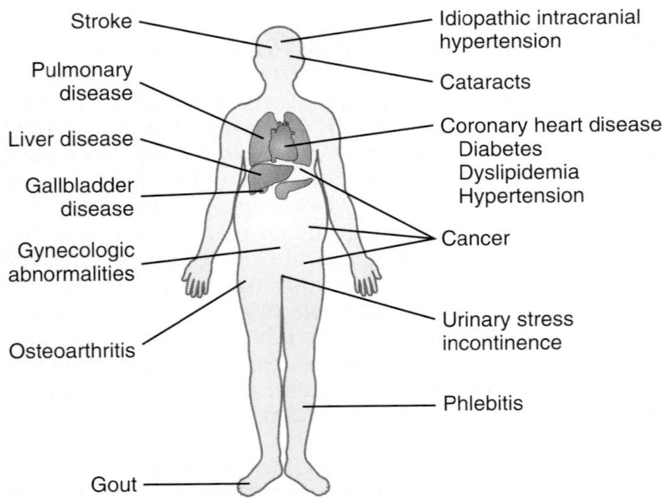

Figure 36-4 Medical complications associated with obesity.

The dysmetabolic syndrome was originally identified and defined on the basis of epidemiologic associations. The underlying pathogenesis and the interrelationships among the individual features have not been completely elucidated. Insulin resistance has been hypothesized to be the common underlying pathogenic mechanism.[155] However, according to a factor analysis of data obtained from nondiabetic subjects in the Framingham Offspring Study, insulin resistance may not be the only precedent condition, and more than one independent physiologic process may be involved.[156]

Abdominal obesity is associated with insulin resistance. However, it is unclear whether visceral (omental and mesenteric) or subcutaneous deposits of abdominal fat are more closely related to insulin resistance, because data from different studies are contradictory. In addition, visceral fat mass often correlates with subcutaneous fat mass, so it is difficult to separate the contribution of each depot to insulin resistance. Furthermore, it is not known whether visceral fat actually participates in the pathogenesis of the dysmetabolic syndrome or merely serves as a marker of increased risk for the metabolic complications of obesity.[157]

The ectopic distribution of triglycerides in nonadipose tissue is also closely correlated with the metabolic complications of obesity. Data from a series of studies showed that insulin resistance to glucose metabolism in skeletal muscle is correlated with the intramyocellular concentration of triglyceride.[158] In addition, excessive intrahepatic triglyceride content is associated with serious cardiometabolic abnormalities, including T2DM, dyslipidemia (high plasma triglyceride, low plasma HDL-C, or both), hypertension, the dysmetabolic syndrome, and CHD.[159,160] It is not known whether triglycerides interfere with insulin action or whether triglycerides serve as surrogate markers for some other fatty acid–derived entity (from plasma or intracellular sources) that impairs insulin signaling.[161]

Type 2 Diabetes Mellitus

The marked increase in the prevalence of obesity has played an important role in the 25% increase in the prevalence of diabetes that has occurred in the United States over the last 20 years.[162] According to data from NHANES III, two thirds of the men and women in the United States with diagnosed T2DM have a BMI of 27.0 kg/m^2 or greater.[139] The risk of diabetes increases linearly with BMI; for example, the prevalence of diabetes in NHANES III increased from 2% in those with a BMI of 25.0 to 29.9 kg/m^2, to 8% with a BMI of 30 to 34.9 kg/m^2, and to 13% with a BMI greater than 35 kg/m^2.[162] In the Nurses' Health Study, the risk of diabetes began to increase when BMI exceeded the "normal" value of 22 kg/m^2 (see Fig. 36-2).[35,163] In addition, the risk of diabetes increases with increases in abdominal fat mass, waist circumference, or waist-to-hip circumference ratio at any given BMI value.[164-166] The risk of diabetes also increases with weight gain during adulthood. Among men and women aged 35 to 60 years, the risk of diabetes was three times greater in those who had gained 5 to 10 kg since the age of 18 to 20 years, compared with those who had maintained their weight within 2 kg of their earlier value.[35,36]

Dyslipidemia

Obesity is associated with several serum lipid abnormalities, including hypertriglyceridemia, reduced HDL-C levels, and an increased fraction of small, dense LDL particles.[167,168]

This association is especially strong in persons with abdominal obesity. In addition, most studies suggest that serum concentrations of total cholesterol and LDL-cholesterol (LDL-C) are elevated in obesity. Data from NHANES III showed that, in men, there was a progressive increase in the prevalence of hypercholesterolemia (total blood cholesterol ≥240 mg dL or 6.21 mmol/L) with increasing BMI.[169] In women, by contrast, the prevalence of hypercholesterolemia was highest at a BMI of 25.0 to 27.0 kg/m^2, and it did not increase further at higher BMI values. The serum lipid abnormalities associated with obesity are important risk factors for CHD.[170,171]

Cardiovascular Disease

Hypertension

There is a linear relationship between hypertension and BMI.[172,173] In NHANES III, the age-adjusted prevalence rates of hypertension (defined as a systolic blood pressure ≥140 mm Hg, a diastolic blood pressure ≥90 mm Hg, or use of antihypertensive medication) in obese men and women were 42% and 38%, respectively. These rates are more than twice as high as those in lean men and women (approximately 15%).[169] The risk of hypertension also increases with weight gain. Among subjects in the Framingham Study, there was a 6.5-mm Hg increase in blood pressure with every 10% increase in body weight.[174]

Coronary Heart Disease

The risk of CHD is increased in obese persons, particularly in those with increased abdominal fat distribution and in those who gained weight during young adulthood. Moreover, CHD risk starts to increase at the "normal" BMI levels of 23.0 kg/m^2 in men and 22.0 kg/m^2 in women.[175] In the Nurses' Health Study, the risk of fatal and nonfatal myocardial infarctions was greater in women who had the lowest BMI but the highest waist-to-hip circumference ratio than it was in women with the highest BMI but the lowest waist-to-hip circumference ratio.[176] At any BMI level, the risk of CHD increases with the presence of increased abdominal fat. The risk of fatal and nonfatal myocardial infarction also increases when 5 kg or more is gained after 18 years of age.[177]

Obesity-related CHD risk factors—particularly hypertension, dyslipidemia, impaired glucose tolerance, and diabetes—are largely responsible for the increase in CHD. However, even after adjusting for other known risk factors, several long-term epidemiologic studies still found that overweight and obesity increased the risk of CHD.[177] As a result, the American Heart Association recently classified obesity as a major preventable risk factor for CHD.[178,179]

Cerebrovascular and Thromboembolic Disease

The risk of fatal and nonfatal ischemic stroke is approximately twice as great in obese as in lean persons and increases progressively with increasing BMI.[180,181] The risks of venous stasis, deep vein thrombosis, and pulmonary embolism are also increased in obesity, particularly in persons with abdominal obesity.[182] Lower-extremity venous disease can result from increased intra-abdominal pressure, impaired fibrinolysis, and the increase in inflammatory mediators.[183,184]

Pulmonary Disease

Restrictive Lung Disease

Obesity increases the pressure placed on the chest wall and thoracic cage, which restricts pulmonary function by decreasing respiratory compliance, increasing the work of breathing, restricting ventilation (measured as decreased total lung capacity, decreased forced vital capacity, and decreased maximal ventilatory ventilation), and limiting ventilation of lung bases.[185]

Obesity-Hypoventilation Syndrome

In obesity-hypoventilation syndrome, the partial pressure of carbon dioxide (P_{CO_2}) is less than 50 mm Hg because of decreased ventilatory responsiveness to hypercapnea or hypoxia (or both) and an inability of respiratory muscles to meet the increased ventilatory demand imposed by the mechanical effects of obesity. There is reduced alveolar ventilation because of shallow and inefficient ventilation related to decreased tidal volume, inadequate inspiratory strength, and elevation of the diaphragm. Symptoms increase when patients are lying down because of increased abdominal pressure on the diaphragm. The resulting increase in intrathoracic pressure further compromises lung function and respiratory capacity.

The pickwickian syndrome is a severe form of the obesity-hypoventilation syndrome. Named after an obese character in Charles Dickens' *The Pickwick Papers,* this syndrome involves extreme obesity, irregular breathing, somnolence, cyanosis, secondary polycythemia, and right ventricular dysfunction.

Obstructive Sleep Apnea

In obstructive sleep apnea, excessive episodes of apnea and hypopnea during sleep are caused by partial or complete upper airway obstruction despite persistent respiratory efforts. Daytime sleepiness and cardiopulmonary dysfunction result from the interruption in nighttime sleep and arterial hypoxemia. In general, patients with sleep apnea are characterized by a BMI greater than 30.0 kg/m^2, excess abdominal fat, and a large neck girth (>17 inches in men, >16 inches in women).[186-188]

Musculoskeletal Disease

Gout

Hyperuricemia and gout are associated with obesity.[189,190]

Osteoarthritis

The risk of osteoarthritis of weight-bearing joints is increased in overweight and obese persons. The knees are most often involved because much more body weight is exerted across the knees than across the hips during weight-bearing activity.[191] There is a stronger relationship between body size and osteoarthritis in women than in men; in women, even small increases in body weight can promote osteoarthritis. In a study of twins, symptomatic or asymptomatic lower-extremity osteoarthritis was found in persons who were only 3 to 5 kg heavier than their twin sibling.[192]

Cancer

Overweight and obesity increase the risk of cancer. Based on data from a prospective study in more than 900,000 U.S. adults,[193] it was estimated that overweight and obesity could account for 14% of all deaths from cancer in men and 20% of such deaths in women. In both men and women, BMI was also significantly associated with higher rates of death due to cancers of the esophagus, colon and rectum, liver, gallbladder, pancreas, and kidney, as well as non-Hodgkin's lymphoma and multiple myeloma. Significant trends of increasing risk with higher BMI values were observed for death from cancers of the stomach and prostate in men and for death from cancers of the breast, uterus, cervix, and ovary in women.[193] Most[193,194] but not all[195] epidemiologic studies have found a direct relationship between BMI and colon cancer in both men and women. The risks of breast and endometrial cancer mortality increase with obesity and weight gain after age 18 years.[196] Specifically, the risk of breast cancer appears to increase with increasing BMI only in postmenopausal women; in premenopausal women, increased BMI may actually protect against breast cancer.[197]

Obesity is often correlated with ingestion of a high-fat, high-calorie diet, which is another risk factor for cancer. Therefore, it is difficult to distinguish how much of the relation between obesity and cancer is attributable to obesity and how much to dietary factors.

Genitourinary Disease in Women

Obese women are often affected by irregular menses, amenorrhea, and infertility.[198] Pregnant obese women are at increased risks for gestational diabetes and hypertension[199] and delivery complications,[200] and their babies are at increased risk for congenital malformations.[201] The risk of urinary incontinence is also increased in obese women.[202] In extremely obese patients, incontinence typically resolves after considerable weight loss, usually achieved by bariatric surgery.[203]

Neurologic Disease

Obesity increases the incidence of ischemic stroke. Obesity is also associated with idiopathic intracranial hypertension (IIH), also known as *pseudotumor cerebri*. This syndrome is manifested by headache, vision abnormalities, tinnitus, and sixth cranial nerve paresis. Although the prevalence of IIH increases with increasing BMI, the risk is increased even in persons who are only 10% above ideal body weight.[204,205] The observation that weight loss in extremely obese patients with IIH decreases intracranial pressure and resolves most associated clinical signs and symptoms suggests there is a causal relationship between obesity and IIH.[206,207]

Cataracts

Overweight and obesity are associated with an increased prevalence of cataracts.[208] Moreover, persons with abdominal obesity are at greater risk than those with lower-body obesity, suggesting that insulin resistance may be involved in the pathogenesis of cataract formation.

Gastrointestinal Disease

Gastroesophageal Reflux Disease

The relationship between gastroesophageal reflux disease and obesity is unclear because of conflicting data from different studies. A higher incidence of reflux symptoms in obese compared with lean persons has been found in most[209,210] but not all[211] large epidemiologic studies. In addition, studies that evaluated gastroesophageal acid reflux by 24-hour pH monitoring have reported the presence of both a significant relationship[212] and no relationship[213] between BMI and pathologic reflux (defined as the occurrence of esophageal pH <4 more than 5% of the time).

Gallstones

The risk of symptomatic gallstones increases linearly with BMI.[38,214] The Nurses' Health Study found that the annual incidence of symptomatic gallstones was 1% in women with a BMI greater than 30.0 kg/m^2 and 2% in women with a BMI greater than 45.0 kg/m^2.[214] The risk of gallstones increases during weight loss, particularly if the weight loss is rapid. This increased risk is related to increased bile cholesterol supersaturation, enhanced cholesterol crystal nucleation, and decreased gallbladder contractility.[215]

If the rate of weight loss exceeds 1.5 kg (or about 1.5% of body weight) per week, the risk of gallstone formation increases exponentially.[216] Among obese patients who underwent rapid weight loss with a very-low-calorie (600 kcal/day) and low-fat (1 to 3 g/day) diet[217,218] or with gastric surgery,[219] the incidence of new gallstones was approximately 25% and 35%, respectively. Gallstone formation is also promoted by the low-fat content of very-low-calorie diets (VLCD), because more than 4 to 10 g of fat in a meal is needed to stimulate maximal gallbladder contractility.[220] Therefore, increasing the fat content of a VLCD can prevent the development of new gallstones.[221] Increasing dietary fat content might not be as important in preventing gallstones in patients consuming an LCD rather than a VLCD. Administration of ursodeoxycholic acid (600 mg/day) during weight loss markedly decreases gallstone formation.[222]

Pancreatitis

Obese patients would be expected to be at increased risk for gallstone pancreatitis because of their increased prevalence of gallstones. However, few studies have addressed this issue. Several studies showed that overweight and obese patients with pancreatitis had a higher risk of local complications, severe pancreatitis, and death than lean patients.[223] It has been hypothesized that the increased deposition of fat in the peripancreatic and retroperitoneal spaces predisposes obese patients to develop peripancreatic fat necrosis and subsequent local and systemic complications.

Liver Disease

Obesity is associated with a spectrum of liver abnormalities known as nonalcoholic fatty liver disease (NAFLD), which is characterized by an increase in intrahepatic triglyceride content (i.e., steatosis) with or without inflammation and fibrosis (i.e., steatohepatitis). NAFLD has become an important public health problem because of its high prevalence, potential progression to severe liver disease, and association with serious cardiometabolic abnormalities, including T2DM, the dysmetabolic syndrome, and CHD.[224] The prevalence rate of NAFLD increases with increasing BMI.[225] The prevalence rates of steatosis and steatohepatitis are approximately 15% and 3%, respectively, in nonobese persons; 65% and 20% in persons with class I or II obesity (BMI 30.0 to 39.9 kg/m^2); and 85% and 40% in extremely obese patients (BMI > 40 kg/m^2).[226-229] The relationship between BMI and NAFLD is influenced by racial or ethnic background and by genetic variation in specific genes.[230-232]

The presence of NAFLD is an important marker of metabolic dysfunction in obese persons, independent of BMI, percent body fat, or visceral fat mass.[233-237] NAFLD is associated with insulin resistance in liver, skeletal muscle, and adipose tissue[233,238,239]; with increased hepatic de novo lipogenesis[240,241]; and with increased VLDL-triglyceride secretion rate.[234] However, it is not clear whether the relationship between NAFLD and metabolic abnormalities is causal or simply an association.

In fact, steatosis is not always associated with insulin resistance. Overexpression of hepatic diacylglycerol acyltransferase (DGAT),[242] blockade of hepatic VLDL secretion,[243] and pharmacologic blockade of beta oxidation[244] in mice causes hepatic steatosis but not hepatic or skeletal muscle insulin resistance. Steatosis in patients with familial hypobetalipoproteinemia, which is caused by genetic deficiency of apolipoprotein B synthesis and decreased VLDL secretion rate, is not accompanied by hepatic or peripheral insulin resistance.[245] This dissociation between steatosis and insulin resistance suggests that other factors associated with steatosis (e.g., inflammation, circulating adipokines, endoplasmic reticulum stress) or other, unidentified metabolites affect insulin sensitivity.

Calorie restriction and subsequent weight loss is an effective therapy for obese patients with NAFLD. A marked decrease in intrahepatic triglyceride content and improvement in hepatic insulin sensitivity occurs very rapidly, within 48 hours after calorie restriction (approximately 1100 kcal/day) begins.[246] A weight loss of 5% to 10% improves liver biochemistry and liver histology (steatosis and inflammation) findings, decreases the hepatic VLDL-triglyceride secretion rate, and increases muscle insulin sensitivity.[246-249] There has been concern that the large and rapid weight loss induced by bariatric surgery can actually worsen NAFLD by increasing hepatic inflammation and fibrosis.[250] However, data from most surgical series demonstrate that weight loss induced by bariatric surgery decreases the cellular factors involved in the pathogenesis of hepatic inflammation and fibrogenesis[251] and improves the histologic findings of steatosis, inflammation, and fibrosis.[252,253]

BENEFITS OF INTENTIONAL WEIGHT LOSS

Effect on Morbidity

Intentional weight loss improves many of the medical complications associated with obesity. Many of these beneficial effects have a dose-dependent relationship with the amount of weight lost, and they begin after a modest weight loss of only 5% of initial body weight.[5] In addition, weight loss can decrease the risk of developing new obesity-related diseases such as diabetes.[254,255]

Type 2 Diabetes Mellitus

In obese patients with T2DM, weight loss improves insulin sensitivity and glycemic control. A 1-year study, conducted in obese patients with T2DM treated with oral hypoglycemic agents, showed that even a 5% weight loss decreased fasting blood glucose, insulin, and hemoglobin A_{1c} (HbA_{1c}) concentrations as well as the dosage of hypoglycemic medication.[256] All patients who lost 15% or more of their body weight decreased or eliminated the need for hypoglycemic medication. In patients with severe obesity who underwent gastric bypass surgery, the average loss of approximately 30% of initial body weight promoted marked long-term improvements in glucose homeostasis.[257] In that study, normal fasting blood glucose, insulin, and HbA_{1c} concentrations were achieved by 83% of the patients who had T2DM and by 99% of the those who had impaired glucose tolerance. However, a subset of obese patients with severe diabetes may not experience improved glycemic control with weight loss.[258]

In obese patients with mild T2DM, energy restriction and weight loss have important beneficial effects on insulin action and glycemic control. Calorie restriction rapidly improves hepatic insulin sensitivity within 48 hours.[259] Subsequent weight and fat losses further improve glycemic control and insulin-mediated glucose uptake by skeletal muscle.[259-261]

Sustained weight loss can prevent the development of new cases of diabetes.[262,263] For example, the Swedish Obese Subjects (SOS) Study found that a 16% weight loss induced by bariatric surgery in extremely obese patients (BMI 41 kg/m^2) reduced the risk of diabetes fivefold over an 8-year period.[263] Data reported from the Finnish Diabetes Prevention Study and the U.S. Diabetes Prevention Program demonstrated that changes in lifestyle resulting in a modest (5%) weight loss decreased the incidence of diabetes after 3 to 4 years by 58% in subjects with impaired glucose tolerance.[264]

Several studies have found that weight loss is more difficult in obese patients with T2DM than in those without diabetes.[265,266] Moreover, successful weight loss may be inversely related to the duration and severity of diabetes.[266] The reasons obese patients with diabetes are less responsive to weight-loss therapy are not known but may involve the energy-conserving effects of improved glycemic control (e.g., reduced glycosuria) and the tendency for weight gain associated with most drug treatments for diabetes.[267]

Dyslipidemia

Weight loss usually decreases serum triglyceride, total cholesterol, and LDL-C concentrations, and serum HDL-C concentrations increase.[5,268] Improvements in serum triglyceride, total cholesterol, and LDL-C concentrations are generally greatest during the first 4 to 8 weeks of a weight-loss program.[269] Serum HDL-C concentrations decrease during active weight loss but tend to increase once weight loss stabilizes.[268] A greater reduction in LDL-C is observed when weight loss is induced by a program of diet plus exercise than with either treatment alone.[270]

Hypertension

Systolic and diastolic blood pressures decrease with weight loss, independent of sodium restriction.[271] In the Trials of Hypertension Prevention Phase II (TOHP II), one of the largest intervention studies to date, approximately 1200 overweight and obese patients were randomly assigned to a dietary weight loss intervention or usual care.[272] The study showed a dose-response relationship between weight loss and change in blood pressure at 36 months. During the first 6 months, patients who successfully lost weight experienced a marked reduction in blood pressure. However, among patients who regained most or all of their lost weight, blood pressure steadily increased to near-baseline values.

The marked weight loss induced by gastric surgery improves or completely resolves hypertension in about two thirds of extremely obese hypertensive patients.[273] However, data recently compiled by the SOS Study indicated that the beneficial effect of weight loss on blood pressure might not persist.[274] Much of the improvement in blood pressure observed at 1 and 2 years after gastric surgery disappeared by 3 years, and both systolic and diastolic pressures increased over the next 5 years. These findings imply that the current energy balance and the direction of weight change are important in blood pressure control.

A decreased incidence of hypertension with weight loss has been reported by several large, prospective, epidemiologic and intervention studies. For example, TOHP II found that persons who maintained a weight loss of at least 4.5 kg at 36 months had a 65% decrease in the risk of hypertension compared with control group participants who gained 1.8 kg.[272] The Nurses' Health Study observed a direct correlation between the risk of developing hypertension and changes in body weight among normotensive women who were observed for 12 to 15 years. With weight losses of 5.0 to 9.9 kg, the risk of developing hypertension decreased by 15%; with a loss of 10 kg or more, it decreased by 26%.[275]

The SOS Study also questioned the ability of weight loss to prevent development of hypertension. In that study, the preventive effect of weight loss on the development of hypertension that was observed 2 years after gastric surgery[254] had disappeared by 3 years.[274] In contrast, the SOS Study found a marked effect of weight loss on the incidence of other obesity-related diseases. For example, long-term maintenance of major weight loss after gastric surgery was associated with a marked and persistent reduction in the risk of diabetes.

Cardiovascular Disease

Modest weight loss can simultaneously affect the entire cluster of cardiovascular risk factors associated with obesity. In the Framingham Offspring Study, a weight loss of 5 lb (2.25 kg) or more over 16 years was associated with reductions of 48% (in men) and 40% (in women) in the sum of these risk factors (defined as the highest quintile of systolic blood pressure, serum triglyceride, serum total cholesterol, fasting blood glucose, and BMI and the lowest quintile of HDL-C).[276]

Improvements in cardiovascular structure and function associated with weight loss include reductions in blood volume and hemodynamic demands on the heart, left ventricular mass and chamber size, and septal wall thickness.[277] Such improvements in cardiac function may be responsible for the reduced frequency of chest pain and dyspnea reported by patients who lost weight after bariatric surgery.[278] Weight loss may also delay the progression of atherosclerosis. In one study, the progression of carotid artery intimal wall thickening over 4 years was three times higher in untreated obese subjects who did not lose weight than in obese subjects who lost weight after gastric surgery.[258]

Pulmonary Disease

Weight loss improves pulmonary function, obstructive sleep apnea, and the obesity-hypoventilation syndrome. Even modest weight loss reduces the severity of sleep apnea, improves sleep patterns, and decreases daytime hypersomnolence.[279,280] More marked weight loss, induced by bariatric surgery, has been shown to improve the obesity-hypoventilation syndrome by correcting resting room-air arterial blood gas values, lung volume, and cardiac filling pressure.[281] Sustained weight loss maintains these improvements in sleep apnea and obesity hypoventilation; however, pulmonary symptoms recur when weight is regained.

Reproductive and Urinary Tract Function in Women

Marked weight loss (>20% of initial body weight) has been shown to correct urinary overflow incontinence,[202] resolve amenorrhea, and improve fertility.

Effect on Mortality

Although several epidemiologic studies have indicated that weight loss or weight fluctuation increases mortality,[282] these studies did not distinguish between intentional and unintentional weight loss, so their results may have been confounded by unintentional weight loss caused by concomitant illness.

The effect of intentional weight loss on mortality was addressed in three studies that obtained baseline data between 1959 and 1960 and monitored the participants for an average of 12 years.[283-285] The composite results of these studies suggested that intentional, and possibly transient, weight loss increases survival among overweight and obese persons who have T2DM. However, these data are not conclusive, because weight loss was self-reported and occurred at any time before the initial interview and changes in weight that occurred during follow-up were not determined.

More recently, data from two large trials demonstrated that weight loss induced by bariatric surgery improves long-term survival in morbidly obese patients.[286,287] A total of 10,000 obese subjects who underwent bariatric surgery and a matched cohort of obese subjects who did not have surgery were monitored for up to 15 years. Subjects who had surgery lost between 14% and 25% of body weight, whereas the average weight change among control subjects was less than 2%. The overall mortality rate, particularly deaths from diabetes, heart disease, and cancer, was 20% to 40% lower in patients who had surgery than in those who did not have surgery.

OBESITY THERAPY

Many obese persons can achieve short-term weight loss by dieting alone, but successful long-term weight maintenance is much more difficult to achieve. "Weight cycling" and "yo-yo dieting" are popular terms used to describe repetitive cycles of weight loss and subsequent regain.[288] Although some adverse consequences have been associated with weight cycling,[289] available data on the health effects of weight cycling are inconclusive and should not deter obese persons from attempting to lose weight.[288] Currently available weight-loss treatments include dietary intervention, increased physical activity, behavior modification, pharmacotherapy, and surgery.

Dietary Intervention

For most obese persons, negative energy balance is more readily achieved by decreasing food intake than by increasing physical activity. Therefore, dietary intervention is considered the cornerstone of weight-loss therapy. Weight-loss diets typically involve modifications of energy content and macronutrient composition. However, the degree of weight loss achieved depends primarily on the energy content rather than the relative macronutrient composition of the diet.

Energy Content

Weight-loss diets can be classified according to their energy content. A balanced-deficit diet of conventional foods usually contains less than 1500 kcal/day and an appropriate balance of macronutrients. LCDs contain 800 to 1500 kcal/day and are consumed as liquid formula, nutritional bars, conventional food, or a combination of these items. VLCDs contain less than 800 kcal/day and are usually high in protein (70 to 100 g/day) and low in fat (<15 g/day). Such diets may be consumed as a commercially prepared liquid formula and may include nutritional bars. VLCDs consumed as conventional foods (mostly lean meat, fish, or fowl) are known as *protein-sparing modified fasts*.

According to the treatment guidelines issued by the U.S. National Institutes of Health (NIH),[5] persons who are overweight (BMI 25.0 to 29.9 kg/m^2) and have two or more cardiovascular disease risk factors and persons who have class I obesity (BMI 30.0 to 34.9 kg/m^2) should decrease their energy intake by approximately 500 kcal/day. This deficit in energy intake will promote a weight loss of 1 lb (0.45 kg) per week and result in reduction of initial weight by about 10% at 6 months. The NIH guidelines recommend a more aggressive energy deficit of 500 to 1000 kcal/day for persons with more severe obesity (BMI ≥ 35.0 kg/m^2). This will produce a weight loss of 1 to 2 lb/wk and result in a 10% weight loss at 6 months.

Total daily energy requirements can be estimated by using standard equations, such as the Harris-Benedict equation[290] or the WHO equation,[291] which are based on the patient's size, age, sex, and activity level. However, the use of standard equations is cumbersome and may be unreliable in obese persons. The simple diet guidelines outlined in Table 36-4 are suggested as an alternative to a specific energy-deficit diet based on the patient's daily energy requirements. Patients who follow these guidelines typically lose weight. Because many patients do not fully adhere to their prescribed diet, the energy content of the diet should be regularly adjusted according to the patient's weight loss response.

More than 30 prospective RCTs have investigated the effectiveness of LCDs for weight loss.[5] The composite results of these trials indicate that a 1000 to 1500 kcal/day LCD induces a weight loss of about 8% after 16 to 26 weeks of treatment. However, these results may not be typical for LCDs prescribed in routine clinical practice, because the trial participants volunteered to enroll in a weight-loss study and most study protocols included some form of behavior modification therapy.

VLCDs induce a weight loss of about 15% to 20% in 12 to 16 weeks of treatment, but this loss is not usually maintained.[292,293] In fact, several randomized trials have shown that weight regain is greater after VLCD than after LCD therapy.[294-297] Therefore, 1 year after treatment, weight loss with a VLCD is often similar to that obtained with an LCD. In addition, initial weight loss is similar for VLCDs and LCDs when the diets are consumed in the same manner. For example, the weight loss observed in patients given a liquid diet providing 420 kcal/day was not significantly greater than that observed in persons who consumed a liquid diet providing 800 kcal/day.[298] This suggests that patients treated with VLCDs are either less compliant with the diet or sustain a greater decline in energy expenditure than those treated with LCDs. With VLCDs, there is greater risk of medical complications associated with dieting, such as hypokalemia, dehydration, and gallstone formation. Therefore, patients treated with a VLCD require closer medical supervision than those treated with an LCD.

TABLE 36-4

Suggested Energy Composition of Initial Reduced-Calorie Diet

Body Weight (lb)	Suggested Energy Intake (kcal/day)
150-199	1000
200-249	1200
250-299	1500
300-349	1800
≥350	2000

Macronutrient Composition

Altering the macronutrient composition of the diet does not induce weight loss unless total energy intake is reduced. Low-fat diets have traditionally been prescribed for weight loss because such diets facilitate energy restriction. Triglycerides, the principal component of dietary fat, increase the palatability and energy density of food. The results of epidemiologic and diet intervention studies suggest that increased dietary fat intake is associated with increases in total energy intake and body weight.[299] Conversely, data from a large number of studies suggest that decreased fat intake is associated with spontaneous decreases in total energy intake and body weight, even when carbohydrate and protein intakes are not restricted.

A direct relationship between change in dietary fat intake and body weight was found in a meta-analysis of 37 intervention studies involving the Step I or Step II low-fat diet (approximately 30% kcal as fat) recommended by the National Cholesterol Education Program to lower cardiovascular risk.[300] Data from another meta-analysis suggest that the amount of weight loss induced by a low-fat diet is directly related to the severity of obesity.[301]

The weight-loss effects of a low-fat diet may be related to the effect of dietary fat on energy density. Energy density is defined as the energy (i.e., calories) present in a given weight (grams) of food. Because the energy density of fat is so high, there is a high correlation between dietary fat content and diet energy density. According to short-term studies lasting up to 14 days, energy intake is regulated according to the weight of ingested food rather than its fat or energy content.[302] For example, the weight of food ingested was the same when lean and obese subjects were given either an ad libitum high-fat/high-energy-density (1.5 kcal/g) diet or a low-fat/low-energy-density (0.7 kcal/g) diet.[303] As a result, energy intake on the high-fat/high-energy-density diet (3000 kcal/day) was almost double the intake on the low-fat/low-energy-density diet (1570 kcal/day). In other studies, the weight of food ingested remained the same when subjects were given liquid diets that had the same energy density but varied in fat content (20% to 60%)[304] and when energy density was varied but fat content remained constant.[305] The results of these short-term studies show that dietary fat content itself does not affect total energy intake, apart from its effects on dietary energy density and food palatability. Whether diets of low energy density can help induce and maintain weight loss remains to be confirmed by long-term studies in obese subjects.

Low-carbohydrate diets have been evaluated as a potential therapy for obesity in RCTs. Several short-term (approximately 12 weeks) trials (e.g., Yang and Van Itallie[306]) have compared the effects of low-carbohydrate and high-carbohydrate diets on weight loss when energy intake was kept constant. These studies suggest weight loss during the first 4 weeks may be greater with a low-carbohydrate diet despite equal energy intake but that weight loss between 6 and 12 weeks is the same with either diet. Five of six RCTs conducted in adults[307-312] found that subjects consuming a low-carbohydrate diet (approximately 25% to 40% carbohydrate) achieved greater weight loss in the short term (6 months)[307-309] but not in the long term (12 months),[307,311,312] compared with those consuming a low-fat diet (approximately 25% to 30% fat and 55% to 60% carbohydrate). The data from these studies also found greater improvements in serum triglyceride and HDL-C, but not in serum LDL-C, in the low-carbohydrate versus the low-fat group. The decrease in body weight associated with a low-carbohydrate diet can be completely explained by a decrease in total energy intake.[313] However, the mechanism responsible for decreased energy consumption when dietary carbohydrates are restricted but fats and proteins are unlimited is not known.

Data from a 2-year study found that a calorie-restricted Mediterranean diet—one that is rich in vegetables and low in red meat (with poultry and fish replacing beef and lamb), with up to 35% of calories from fat, primarily from olive oil and nuts—is just as effective as a low-fat, unrestricted-calorie diet and resulted in greater weight loss than conventional low-fat, restricted-calorie diet therapy.[314] Another randomized trial evaluated four diets that varied in the percentage of calories from fat, carbohydrate, and protein and found that all diets achieved the same weight loss, with maximum weight loss at 1 year and subsequent weight regain thereafter.[315] In summary, these data demonstrate that different dietary approaches can be used to achieve moderate weight in obese patients and that rigid prescription of a conventional low-fat diet is unwarranted.

Physical Activity

Metabolic Rate

Although there is a profound increase in energy expenditure during an actual episode of exercise, the addition of regular exercise to a weight-loss program has negligible effects on REE. In a meta-analysis of prospective RCTs that assigned obese subjects to treatment with diet alone or diet plus exercise, the addition of exercise did circumvent the expected decline in REE when REE was adjusted for body mass.[316]

Body Composition

The composition of weight loss can be influenced by the addition of exercise to a diet program. Pooled data from two meta-analyses found that exercise can reduce the loss of FFM that occurs with weight loss.[317] When diet-induced weight loss was approximately 10 kg, regular exercise of low or moderate intensity reduced the percentage of weight lost as FFM from approximately 25% to 12%. Although the difference in weight lost as FFM was large on a percentage basis, it nonetheless represented only a small (approximately 1 kg) difference in the absolute amount of FFM lost. This preservation of FFM with exercise might not necessarily reflect preservation of muscle protein; instead, it may involve increased retention of body water and muscle glycogen. Indeed, nitrogen balance studies have not been able to detect any nitrogen-sparing effect of exercise during diet-induced weight loss in women.[318] Whether there is a difference between the effects of endurance and those of resistance exercise on FFM conservation is not clear because the available data are limited and conflicting.

Diabetes and Coronary Heart Disease

Endurance exercise increases insulin sensitivity[319] and is associated with decreased risks of developing diabetes[320,321] and of dying from cardiovascular disease.[322]

Weight Loss

Increasing physical activity alone is not an effective strategy for promoting initial weight loss. Most studies have shown that moderate endurance exercise (e.g., brisk walking for 45 to 60 minutes, 4 times a week, for up to 1 year) usually induces only minor weight loss.[316] In obese persons, the energy deficit created by exercise is usually much less and requires more effort than the energy deficit created by a reduced-calorie diet. For example, to lose 1 lb of fat, an obese patient would have to walk or run approximately 4.5 miles/day for 1 week or consume a 500-kcal/day energy-deficit diet for 1 week.

Although exercise alone is not an effective strategy for inducing initial weight loss, increasing physical activity may be an important component of successful long-term weight management. Several large-scale, cross-sectional case studies have shown that obese subjects who were successful in maintaining weight loss for 1 year or longer engaged in regular exercise.[323,324] Retrospective analyses of data from prospective randomized studies found that subjects treated with diet-plus-exercise who continued to exercise sustained significantly larger long-term weight losses than subjects who stopped exercising or subjects treated with diet alone.[325]

The amount of exercise that is associated with weight-loss maintenance is considerable and requires expending approximately 2500 kcal/wk.[326,327] This level of energy expenditure can be accomplished through vigorous activity (aerobics, cycling, or jogging) for approximately 30 min/day or more moderate activity (brisk walking) for 60 to 75 min/day. However, when the data are analyzed on an intention-to-treat basis, most prospective randomized trials do not find a statistically significant effect of exercises on the long-term maintenance of weight loss, presumably because adherence to the exercise program is often poor.[328] Therefore, it is possible that the putative long-term beneficial effects of exercise on weight maintenance could reflect a selection bias: people who are able to maintain an aggressive physical activity program are those who are also able to maintain dietary compliance. In some people, exercise training results in compensatory mechanisms, such as increased energy intake or reduced activity during the rest of the day, that attenuate weight loss.[329]

Behavior Modification

Principles

Behavior-modification therapy attempts to enable obese patients to recognize and subsequently alter eating and activity habits that promote their obesity. Behavior modification is derived from the classic conditioning principle that behavior is often triggered by an antecedent event. The association between the antecedent event (e.g., watching television) and the behavior (e.g., eating) is strengthened by repetition: the more often the two are paired, the stronger the association between them becomes.

Behavior modification for the treatment of obesity usually involves multiple strategies to modify eating and activity habits. These strategies include stimulus control (avoiding the cues that prompt eating), self-monitoring (keeping daily records of food intake and physical activity), problem-solving skills (developing a systematic manner of analyzing a problem and identifying possible solutions), cognitive restructuring (thinking in a positive manner), social support (cooperation from family members and friends in altering lifestyle behavior), and relapse prevention (methods to promote recovery from bouts of overeating or weight regain).

Effectiveness

Treatment by a comprehensive group behavior therapy approach typically results in the loss of about 9% of initial weight in 20 to 26 weeks.[329] After treatment ends, weight regain is commonly observed. During the year after treatment, patients usually regain about 30% to 35% of their lost weight; however, most patients sustain clinically significant weight loss of more than 5% of initial body weight.[330] Increasing the duration of behavior therapy programs has only marginally improved total weight loss, but it probably prevents the weight regain that usually occurs after treatment is stopped.[331]

Pharmacotherapy

Conventional obesity therapy is associated with a high rate of recidivism. Therefore, the most important goal of pharmacotherapy is to maintain long-term weight loss. Pharmacotherapy should not be considered a short-term approach for weight loss, because patients who lose weight with drug therapy usually regain weight when the therapy is discontinued.[332,333] Some obese patients do not respond to drug therapy, and long-term success is unlikely if weight loss does not occur within the first 4 weeks of drug treatment.[334]

Weight loss usually plateaus by 6 months of treatment and weight begins to increase after 1 year.[332,333] This observation implies that the efficacy of weight loss medications declines with time or that obesity is a progressive disease, or both. Treatment outcome is less successful when pharmacotherapy is administered alone than when pharmacotherapy is administered as part of a comprehensive weight-loss program that includes diet, exercise, and behavior modification (Fig. 36-5).[328] The use of obesity pharmacotherapy alone exposes patients to the full risks of the drug without the full medical benefits of more comprehensive treatment.

Table 36-5 lists the drugs currently approved by the U.S. Food and Drug Administration (FDA) for the treatment of obesity. All currently approved weight-loss drugs act as anorexiants with the exception of orlistat, which inhibits the absorption of dietary fat. Three anorexiant drugs have been withdrawn from the market because of the increased incidence of valvular heart disease (fenfluramine and dexfenfluramine)[335] or hemorrhagic stroke (phenylpropanolamine)[336] associated with their use.

All anorexiant drugs except mazindol are derived from phenylethylamine, the amphetamine precursor. The structures of these drugs have been chemically altered to reduce the potential for abuse. Anorexiant medications affect the monoamine (norepinephrine, serotonin, and dopamine) system in the hypothalamus and thereby enhance satiation (level of fullness during consumption of a meal, which influences the amount of food consumed), satiety (level of hunger after consumption of a meal, which influences the frequency of eating), or both.

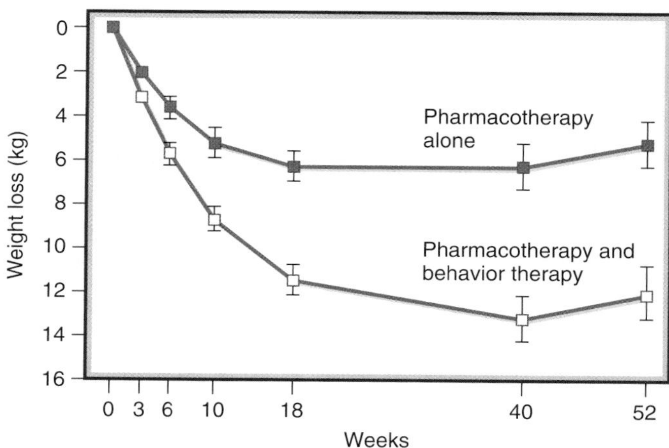

Figure 36-5 Weight loss in obese subjects treated with anorexiant medication (sibutramine) alone, group behavioral therapy alone, or medication plus group behavioral therapy. These data demonstrate that greater weight loss is achieved when antiobesity medications are used in conjunction with lifestyle modification than when they are used alone. (Adapted from Wadden TA, Berkowitz RI, Womble LG, et al. Randomized trial of lifestyle modification and pharmacotherapy for obesity. *N Engl J Med.* 2005;353:2111-2120.)

TABLE 36-5

Drugs Approved by the U.S. Food and Drug Administration for the Treatment of Obesity

Year Approved	Generic Name	Trade Name
1959	Phendimetrazine tartrate	Bontril, Plergine, Prelu-2, X-Trozine
1959	Phentermine	Ionamine, Adipex-P, Fastin, Oby-trim
1959	Diethylpropion hydrochloride	Tenuate, Tenuate Dospan
1960	Benzphetamine HCl	Didrex
1973	Mazindol	Sanorex, Mazanor
1997	Sibutramine HCl	Meridia
1999	Orlistat	Xenical, Ally (over the counter)

Monoamine neurotransmitters are synthesized from tyrosine and stored in granules that release their contents from presynaptic nerve terminals into the interneuronal cleft between presynaptic and postsynaptic nerves. Only a small portion of the monoamines released into the interneuronal cleft actually bind to postsynaptic receptors and thereby transmit a signal from one nerve to the other. Most of the released monoamines are taken back up into the presynaptic nerve terminal, where they are either degraded or repackaged into granules for future release.

Weight-loss pharmacotherapy is approved for patients who have no contraindications to therapy and who have a BMI greater than 30.0 kg/m^2, or a BMI between 27.0 and 29.9 kg/m^2 and an obesity-related medical condition. Sibutramine and orlistat are the only drugs currently approved by the FDA for long-term use in the management of obesity.

Sibutramine

Sibutramine inhibits the neuronal reuptake of norepinephrine, serotonin, and, to a lesser degree, dopamine. It enhances satiation (level of fullness during consumption of a meal) rather than satiety (level of hunger after consumption of a meal). In humans, sibutramine also appears to promote a small increase in metabolic rate several hours after its administration.[337] The currently recommended initial dose of sibutramine is 10 mg/day.[338] This daily dose can be decreased or increased by 5 mg if tolerance is poor or weight loss is inadequate. Administration of sibutramine at doses between 1 and 30 mg/day for 24 weeks produced a dose-dependent weight loss, patients taking placebo lost 0.9% of initial body weight, compared with 7.7% for those taking 30 mg/day of sibutramine.[339]

Several RCTs have evaluated the effect of long-term (1-year) treatment with sibutramine on body weight in obese persons.[340-346] These studies were conducted in different patient populations, including obese patients with few obesity-related medical complications and patients with T2DM or hypertension. Data from two meta-analyses of long-term RCTs[347,348] found that subjects treated with sibutramine lost approximately 4.5% (4.5 kg) more weight than those who received placebo. In addition, two to three times as many subjects randomized to sibutramine lost at least 5% or at least 10% of their initial weight, compared with those randomized to placebo. Intermittent therapy with sibutramine may be just as effective as continuous daily therapy in inducing weight loss; at the end of 48 weeks, weight loss in subjects who received intermittent therapy (daily sibutramine during three 12-week periods separated by two 6-week intervals of placebo therapy) was equal to that in subjects who received daily sibutramine therapy.[342]

Results have also been reported from two prospective RCTs that evaluated the efficacy of sibutramine therapy in long-term weight management after a predetermined amount of weight was lost.[349,350] In the first trial, obese subjects who lost at least 6 kg after a 4-week VLCD resumed a regular diet with diet counseling and were randomly assigned to 1 year of treatment with placebo or sibutramine.[349] In the year after randomization, sibutramine-treated subjects lost an additional 5.2 kg and placebo-treated subjects gained 0.5 kg. Total study weight losses were 12.9 kg in sibutramine-treated subjects and 6.9 kg in subjects treated with placebo. The initial weight loss achieved with the VLCD was maintained or increased in 74% of sibutramine-treated subjects compared with only 41% of placebo-treated subjects. In the second trial, obese subjects who lost more than 5% of initial weight after 6 months of treatment with sibutramine (10 mg/day) and a 600-kcal/day energy-deficit diet were randomized to treatment with either sibutramine (increased to 15 or 20 mg/day) or placebo.[351] All subjects received diet counseling. Almost half of the subjects who entered the study failed to complete the 18-month treatment program. Among those who completed the study, 43% of those treated with sibutramine but only 16% of those treated with placebo maintained 80% or more of their original 6-month weight loss. On average, subjects who continued sibutramine maintained their weight loss for 1 year and then experienced a slight and progressive increase in weight, but subjects who were switched to placebo experienced a progressive increase in weight as soon as sibutramine therapy was stopped.

The most common side effects of sibutramine therapy are dry mouth, headache, constipation, and insomnia. Sibutramine also causes small increases in blood pressure (2 to 4 mm Hg) and heart rate (4 to 6 beats/minute).[339] However, some patients experience much larger increases in blood pressure or heart rate and require dose reduction or discontinuation of therapy.

Orlistat

Orlistat is synthesized from lipstatin, a product of *Streptomyces toxytricini* mold that inhibits most mammalian lipases.[251] Orlistat binds to lipases in the gastrointestinal tract and thereby blocks the digestion of dietary triglycerides. This inhibition of fat digestion reduces micelle formation and, consequently, the absorption of long-chain fatty acids, cholesterol, and certain fat-soluble vitamins. The degree of fat malabsorption is directly related in a curvilinear fashion to the dose of orlistat administered.[352] Excretion of about 30% of ingested triglycerides, which is near the maximum plateau value, occurs at a dose of 360 mg/day (120 mg three times daily with meals). Orlistat has no effect on systemic lipases because less than 1% of the administered dose is absorbed.[353]

Several long-term (1 to 4 years) RCTs have evaluated the efficacy of orlistat therapy in initiating and maintaining weight loss. Data from two meta-analyses[347,348] showed that subjects treated with orlistat lost about 3% (3 kg) more weight than those randomized to placebo. In addition, about twice as many subjects randomized to orlistat lost at least 5% or at least 10% of their initial body weight, compared with those randomized to placebo. In one study, weight loss was 5% greater (11% versus 6%) at 1 year and 3% greater (7% versus 4%) at 4 years for those treated with orlistat compared with placebo.[354]

The results of several RCTs suggest that orlistat administration is associated with a reduction of serum LDL-C that is independent of the effect of weight loss alone. Even after adjusting for percent weight loss, these studies found that subjects treated with orlistat sustained a greater reduction in serum LDL-C concentrations than those treated with placebo.[355,356] The mechanism responsible for this effect may be related to orlistat-induced inhibition of dietary cholesterol absorption.[357]

The most common side effects associated with orlistat therapy are gastrointestinal complaints. Approximately 70% to 80% of subjects treated with orlistat experienced one or more gastrointestinal events, compared with 50% to 60% of those treated with placebo.[355,356,358-360] These gastrointestinal events were induced by fat malabsorption, usually occurred within the first 4 weeks of treatment, and were of mild or moderate intensity. Subjects rarely reported more than two episodes despite continued orlistat treatment. Orlistat treatment can also affect fat-soluble vitamin status and the absorption of some lipophilic medications.[355-357,361] Therefore, it is recommended that all patients treated with orlistat also receive a daily multivitamin supplement and that orlistat not be taken for at least 2 hours before or after the ingestion of vitamin supplements or lipophilic drugs.

Diabetes Medications That Cause Weight Loss

Diabetes therapy usually results in weight gain.[362] However, several medications used to treat diabetes, including metformin, GLP1 agonists, and amylin, cause weight loss.

The effect of metformin on body weight was recently reviewed.[363] The data from most studies indicated that metformin does not cause weight gain and that treatment with metformin reduces the amount of weight that is gained with other diabetes medications. However, the effect of metformin on body weight in patients with diabetes is modest. For example, 10-year follow-up data from the U.K. Prospective Diabetes Study (UKPDS) found that subjects randomized to metformin therapy gained about 1.5 kg, compared with a gain of 2 kg in those treated with diet, 4 kg with glibenclamide, and 6 kg with insulin.[362] Subjects enrolled in the Diabetes Progression Outcomes Trial were randomized to monotherapy with either metformin, glyburide, or rosiglitazone for 4 years; those treated with metformin lost an average of 3 kg, whereas the glyburide and rosiglitazone groups gained an average of 1.5 kg and 5 kg, respectively.[364] The weight loss effect of metformin has also been studied in nondiabetic obese subjects. A systematic review of RCTs of metformin (duration 15 days to 1 year) in subjects without diabetes or polycystic ovary syndrome found that weight loss was usually small (≤2 kg) and insufficient to consider metformin as an effective obesity therapy.[365]

Treatment of diabetes with short- or long-acting GLP1 agonists is usually accompanied by a decrease in body weight. A meta-analysis of 21 RCTs evaluated the effect of treatment with short-acting (exenatide) and once-daily (liraglutide) GLP1 agonists on body weight in diabetic subjects who were treated for at least 12 weeks.[366] The data show that GLP1 agonists caused a mean reduction in BMI of 0.4 kg/m^2 compared with placebo. These results are similar to those reported in another meta-analysis of 29 RCTs of at least 12 weeks' duration, which showed that treatment with exenatide in combination with other oral agents or treatment with liraglutide alone resulted in 1.4 kg weight loss compared with placebo and a 4.8 kg weight differential compared with insulin.[367] In addition, compared with placebo therapy, liraglutide added to metformin and rosiglitazone therapy resulted in a weight loss of 1 kg (with 1.2 mg/day of liraglutide) or 2 kg (with 1.8 mg/day of liraglutide) at 6 months in obese diabetic subjects.[368] Liraglutide also causes a dose-dependent weight loss in obese patients who do not have diabetes: liraglutide given as 1.2, 1.8, 2.4, or 3.0 mg/day caused a 2- to 4-kg greater weight loss than placebo therapy and a 1- to 2-kg greater weight loss than orlistat therapy.[369]

Pramlintide, a synthetic analogue of human amylin, causes greater weight loss than placebo treatment in obese subjects with and without diabetes. In one 16-week RCT, pramlintide therapy resulted in a 3.7% placebo-corrected reduction in body weight.[370] In a second 4-month RCT, conducted in nondiabetic obese subjects, pramlintide resulted in a dose-dependent weight loss of 4.5 to 8 kg, compared with a 2.5-kg weight loss in the placebo group.[371]

Surgical Therapy

Gastrointestinal surgery is the most effective approach for achieving major weight loss in extremely obese patients. In 1991, guidelines for the surgical treatment of obesity were established by an NIH Consensus Conference.[372] According to these guidelines, eligible candidates for surgery include patients with a BMI of 40 kg/m^2 or more and those with a BMI of 35.0 to 39.9 kg/m^2 with one or more severe medical complications of obesity (e.g., hypertension, heart failure, T2DM, sleep apnea). Additional eligibility criteria are the inability to maintain weight loss with conventional therapy, acceptable operative risks, absence of active substance abuse, and ability to comply with the long-term treatment and follow-up required. All surgical procedures for obesity can be performed laparoscopically, but the laparoscopic approach is technically challenging and usually requires more operating room time.

Roux-en-Y Gastric Bypass Procedure

The Roux-en-Y gastric bypass (RYGB) procedure involves creating a small (10 to 30 mL) proximal gastric pouch that empties into a segment of jejunum that is anastomosed as a Roux-en-Y limb. The size of the patient determines the length of the Roux-en-Y limb (Fig. 36-6A). In patients with a BMI lower than 50 kg/m^2, a 45- to 60-cm limb is used, but in patients with a BMI of 50 kg/m^2 or more, a 150-cm limb (long-limb gastric bypass) is used, based on the belief that this promotes better weight loss.[373] Specific complications associated with the RYGB procedure include marginal ulcers, stomal stenosis, dilation of the bypassed stomach, staple line disruption, internal hernias, malabsorption of specific nutrients, and the dumping syndrome.

Gastroplasty

Vertical banded and Silastic ring gastroplasties, also known as gastric stapling, involve creation of a small pouch from the gastroesophageal junction along the lesser curvature of the stomach; the pouch has a stoma that is restricted by a 1-cm polypropylene or Silastic ring and empties into the rest of the stomach.[374,375] Specific complications associated with gastroplasty include staple line disruption, stomal stenosis, and gastroesophageal reflux.

Gastric Bypass versus Gastroplasty

Data obtained from four prospective, randomized trials found that weight loss several years after surgery was consistently greater with the RYGB procedure (loss of approximately 65% of excess weight) than with gastroplasty (approximately 40% of excess weight).[376-379] In addition, independent evaluations of each procedure suggested

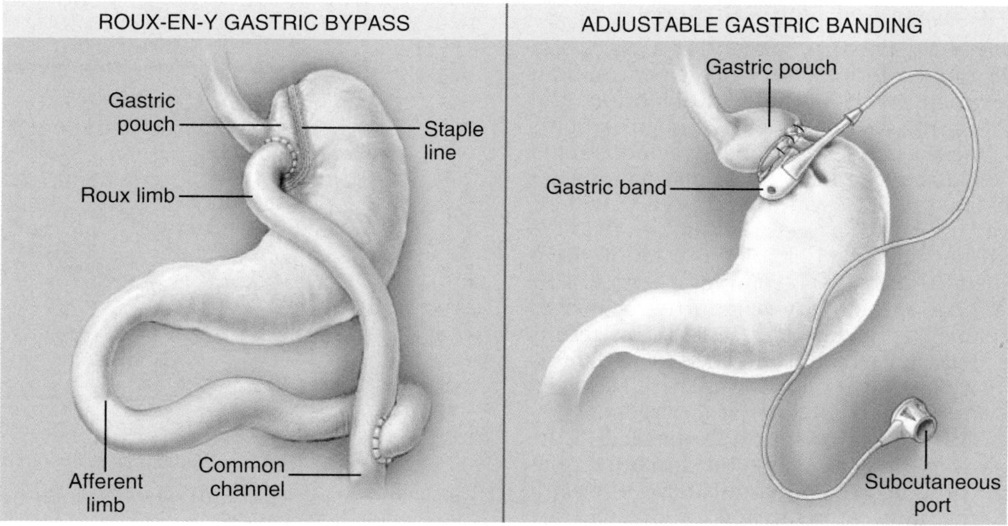

Figure 36-6 Schematic diagram of the Roux-en-Y gastric bypass procedure **(A)** and the laparoscopic adjustable gastric banding procedure **(B)**. (Adapted from Steinbrook R. Surgery for severe obesity. *N Engl J Med.* 2004;350:1075-1079.)

better long-term results (10 to 14 years) with the gastric bypass than with gastroplasty.[222,380] As a result of these findings, most centers no longer perform gastroplasty.

Laparoscopic Adjustable Gastric Banding

In the laparoscopically inserted adjustable gastric banding (LAGB) procedure, a silicone band is placed around the upper stomach, just below the gastroesophageal junction. The band's circumference can be adjusted by inflating or deflating a balloon connected to a subcutaneously implanted port that is accessed percutaneously (see Fig. 36-6B). The degree of weight loss achieved with LABD has been similar to that achieved with vertical banded gastroplasty[381] and over time may equal that achieved by RYGB surgery.[382]

Complications associated with LAGB include esophageal dilation, erosion of the band into the stomach, band slippage, band or port infections, and balloon or system leaks that lead to inadequate weight loss.[383,384] Esophageal dilation and dysphagia can result from placement of the band at the gastroesophageal junction.[383] Although loosening the band usually relieves the dilation, removal of the band is sometimes necessary.[384] In some patients, the band erodes into the stomach and must be surgically removed. If the posterior stomach wall herniates through the band, the band slips. This can cause gastric obstruction and requires surgical revision.

Biliopancreatic Bypass Procedures

The biliopancreatic bypass and the biliopancreatic bypass with duodenal switch result in gastric restriction, maldigestion, and malabsorption. Both procedures involve a partial gastrectomy and bypass of a considerable amount of small intestine receiving biliary and pancreatic secretions.[385,386] Partial biliopancreatic bypass induces malabsorption of protein, fat, fat-soluble vitamins, iron, calcium, and vitamin B_{12}; it therefore promotes more nutritional deficits than gastric restrictive procedures do.[385,387] The incidence of protein deficiency is probably less common, and gastrointestinal side effects are not as severe, after partial biliopancreatic bypass with duodenal switch than after partial biliopancreatic bypass. Presumably these procedures cause greater weight loss (approximately 75% of excess weight) than a standard gastric bypass, but the techniques have never been compared directly in a prospective randomized trial.

Effect of Bariatric Surgery on Type 2 Diabetes

Weight loss induced by bariatric surgery is a successful therapy for T2DM and results in better glucose control than conventional treatment with lifestyle intervention and drug therapy. A 24-month RCT conducted in obese patients with recently diagnosed (<2 years) diabetes demonstrated that remission of diabetes (defined as plasma glucose <126 mg/dL and HbA_{1c} <6.2% without diabetes medications) was achieved in 73% of subjects randomized to LAGB (20% weight loss) but in only 13% of those randomized to lifestyle and medical therapy (1.4% weight loss).[388] The beneficial effects of bariatric surgery were further validated by retrospective analyses of surgical series. The results obtained from a meta-analysis that included some 30,000 obese patients with diabetes found that diabetes resolved completely in 78% of patients after bariatric surgery.[389]

A series of observations from clinical studies led to the concept that bypassing the upper gastrointestinal tract has additional benefits on glucose homeostasis beyond weight loss alone. First, the rates of remission of diabetes are greater in patients who have had biliopancreatic diversion or RYGB surgery, compared with those who have had restrictive banding procedures.[390] Second, glycemia is normalized within days after RYGB surgery in patients with T2DM, before any significant weight loss is achieved.[391-393] Third, oral glucose tolerance improves more after a 10-kg weight loss induced by RYGB surgery than after calorie restriction alone.[394,395] Finally, complete resolution of T2DM (defined as normalization of blood glucose and HbA_{1c} concentrations without the need for diabetes medications) has been achieved without weight loss in patients who have had duodenal-jejunal bypass surgery (bypassing the duodenum and 30 cm of the proximal jejunum).[396]

The mechanisms responsible for the weight loss–independent effects of intestinal bypass on glucose homeostasis are not clear but could be related to improved metabolic response to a meal, increased beta-cell function, or increased insulin sensitivity.[397-400] Data from one study that compared the effect of a 10-kg weight loss induced by RYGB surgery or by diet therapy in obese patients with diabetes found that those who had RYGB surgery had greater improvement in oral glucose tolerance, which was associated with recovery of the early phase of insulin secretion and increased plasma GLP1 concentrations.[394,395] However, no change in the insulin secretion after intravenously infused glucose was detected after RYGBP surgery, suggesting that the improvement in beta-cell function is limited to the gastrointestinal response to ingested glucose.[394]

The effect of intestinal bypass on disposition index, which is a measure of beta-cell function in relation to insulin sensitivity, is unclear because of conflicting data from different studies. Disposition index values after weight loss induced by RYGB surgery did not change compared with the values in unoperated morbidly obese control subjects,[401] whereas disposition index values markedly improved to normal after biliopancreatic diversion.[402] Therefore, it is possible that biliopancreatic diversion has additional therapeutic effects on beta-cell function compared with RYGB. Insulin sensitivity is often fully restored to normal range after bariatric surgery, even though most patients are still extremely obese.[403] The improvement in muscle insulin sensitivity, assessed by the hyperinsulinemic-euglycemic clamp procedure, was the same after weight loss induced by RYGB surgery as after diet-induced weight loss. However, improvement in insulin sensitivity after biliopancreatic diversion was greater than that predicted by weight loss alone, suggesting that other factors might be involved in improving insulin action after this procedure (Fig. 36-7).[403]

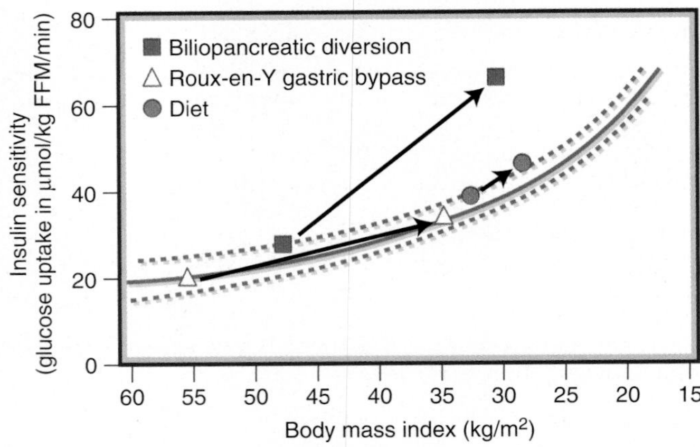

Figure 36-7 Effects of bariatric surgery and diet-induced weight loss on insulin sensitivity. FFM, fat-free mass. (Adapted from Ferrannini E, Mingrone G. Impact of different bariatric surgical procedures on insulin action and beta-cell function in type 2 diabetes. *Diabetes Care*. 2009;32:514-520.)

TABLE 36-6

Suggested Weight-Loss Treatment Options Based on BMI and Risk Factors

BMI (kg/m^2)	Conventional Therapy*	Pharmacotherapy†	Surgery‡
25.0-26.9	With CHD risk factors or obesity-related disease	No	No
27.0-29.9	With CHD risk factors or obesity-related disease	With obesity-releated disease	No
30.0-34.9	Yes	Yes	No
35.0-39.9	Yes	Yes	With obesity-related disease
≥40	Yes	Yes	Yes

BMI, body mass index; CHD, coronary heart disease.
*Conventional therapy comprises diet, physical activity, and behavior therapy.
†Pharmacotherapy should be considered only for patients who are unable to achieve adequate weight loss with available conventional therapy and who do not have any absolute contraindications for drug therapy.
‡Bariatric surgery should be considered only for patients who are unable to lose weight with available conventional therapy and who do not have any absolute contraindications for surgery.

Severe postprandial hypoglycemia with hyperinsulinemia has been described as a rare complication of RYGB surgery.[404,405] Patients with this condition present with repeated episodes of profound symptomatic postprandial neuroglycopenia associated with endogenous hyperinsulinemia. This syndrome is not usually responsive to nutritional or medical therapy and can necessitate partial pancreatectomy to reduce the frequency of hypoglycemic episodes. The pathophysiologic mechanisms leading to endogenous hyperinsulinemic hypoglycemia after RYGB are not clear but could be related to an inappropriately enlarged beta-cell mass and beta-cell function caused by long-term exposure to augmented GLP1 response to a meal.[406] However, data from a recent study found that the GLP1 response to a meal did not differ between subjects who had or did not have hypoglycemic episodes after RYGB surgery. Moreover, even though the GLP1 response to the meal increased, this did not result in excessive insulin secretion or hypoglycemic episodes.[401]

In summary, weight loss induced by bariatric surgery causes marked improvement in glucose homeostasis and diabetes remission in most patients. Upper gastrointestinal bypass has additional therapeutic benefits beyond weight loss, possibly by improving the incretin response to a meal or by other yet unidentified effects. However, it is not known how much additional clinical benefit in glucose control is gained by anatomic bypass in the face of known large weight loss–dependent effects of bariatric surgery. Additional, carefully controlled studies are needed to answer this question.

Inadequate Weight Loss after Surgery

About 15% of patients fail to lose more than 40% of their excess weight (10% to 15% of total weight) after a gastric bypass.[257,407] This percentage is even higher after a gastroplasty procedure.[380] The major cause of inadequate weight loss after gastric bypass is the frequent ingestion of high-calorie soft foods and liquids (e.g., ice cream, cookies, milk shakes, sodas) and high-fat snacks and fried foods (e.g., potato chips, fried potatoes). In patients who have undergone either a stapled gastroplasty or gastric bypass, increased food intake may be related to staple line disruption, particularly if the patient is able to eat much larger quantities of food at a time.

Perioperative Mortality

The perioperative mortality rate after bariatric surgery is less than 0.5% when the procedure is performed by experienced surgeons in experienced centers.[257,376] Approximately three fourths of the deaths that occur are caused by anastomotic leaks and peritonitis, and one fourth are caused by pulmonary embolism.

TREATMENT GUIDELINES

A practical guide to the management of overweight and obesity was developed by the North American Association for the Study of Obesity in conjunction with the NIH.[338] An overview of these guidelines is shown in Table 36-6, which outlines a stepwise approach for weight loss.

Weight management is a key component in the treatment of overweight or obese patients with T2DM. Even a modest weight loss of 5% of initial body weight improves glycemic control and reduces the need for hypoglycemic medication. Moreover, modest weight loss also improves other diabetes-related risk factors for CHD. However, successful weight management is more difficult to achieve in obese patients with T2DM than in those without diabetes.[265,266] In fact, treatment of diabetes itself is usually associated with an increase in body weight.[267] Therefore, therapeutic lifestyle intervention, weight loss medications, diabetes medications that are associated with the least amount of weight gain, and bariatric surgery should be considered as part of the potential therapeutic options for obese patients with diabetes.

REFERENCES

1. Allison DB, Fontaine KR, Manson JE, et al. Annual deaths attributable to obesity in the United States. *JAMA*. 1999;282:1530-1538.
2. Wolf AM, Colditz GA. Current estimates of the economic cost of obesity in the United States. *Obesity Res*. 1998;6:97-106.
3. Gallagher D, Heymsfield SB, Heo M, et al. Health percentage body fat ranges: an approach for developing guidelines based on body mass index. *Am J Clin Nutr*. 2000;72:694-701.
4. World Health Organization. *Obesity: preventing and managing the global epidemic*. Report of a WHO Consultation on Obesity. Geneva, Switzerland: WHO; 1998.
5. National Institutes of Health, National Heart, Lung, and Blood Institute. Clinical guidelines on the identification, evaluation, and treatment of overweight and obesity in Adults: the evidence report. *Obes Res*. 1998;6(suppl 2):51S-209S.
6. U.S. Department of Health and Human Services. Nutrition and overweight. In: *Healthy People 2010*. Washington, DC: US Government Printing Office; 2000.
7. U.S. Department of Agriculture and U.S. Department of Health and Human Services. *Nutrition and Your Health: Dietary Guidelines for Americans*, 5th ed. (Home and Garden Bulletin no. 232). Washington, DC: US Government Printing Office; 2000.
8. Calle EE, Thun MJ, Petrelli JM, et al. Body-mass index and mortality in a prospective cohort of U.S. adults. *N Engl J Med*. 1999;341:1097-1105.

9. Flegal KM, Graubard BI, Williamson DF, et al. Excess deaths associated with underweight, overweight, and obesity. *JAMA*. 2005;293: 1861-1867.
10. Kissebah AH, Videlingum N, Murray R, et al. Relation of body fat distribution to metabolic complications of obesity. *J Clin Endocrinol Metab*. 1982;54:254-260.
11. Snijder MB, Dekker JM, Visser M, et al. Trunk fat and leg fat have independent and opposite associations with fasting and postload glucose levels: the Hoorn study. *Diabetes Care*. 2004;27:372-377.
12. Jensen MD. Gender differences in regional fatty acid metabolism before and after meal ingestion. *J Clin Invest*. 1995;96:2297-2303.
13. Guo ZK, Hensrud DD, Johnson CM, et al. Regional postprandial fatty acid metabolism in different obesity phenotypes. *Diabetes*. 1999;48:1586-1592.
14. Wang Y, Rimm EB, Stampfer MJ, et al. Comparison of abdominal adiposity and overall obesity in predicting risk of type 2 diabetes among men. *Am J Clin Nutr*. 2005;81:555-563.
15. National Institutes of Health, National Heart, Lung, and Blood Institute. Clinical Guidelines on the Identification, Evaluation, and Treatment of Overweight and Obesity in Adults—The Evidence Report. *Obes Res*. 1998;6(suppl 2):51S-209S.
16. Lean ME, Han TS, Morrison CE. Waist circumference as a measure for indicating need for weight management. *BMJ*. 1995;311:158-161.
17. Deurenberg-Yap M, Chew SK, Lin VF, et al. Relationships between indices of obesity and its co-morbidities in multi-ethnic Singapore. *Int J Obes Relat Metab Disord*. 2001;25:1554-1562.
18. Deurenberg-Yap M, Schmidt G, van Staveren WA, et al. The paradox of low body mass index and high body fat percentage among Chinese, Malays and Indians in Singapore. *Int J Obes Relat Metab Disord*. 2000;24:1011-1017.
19. Wu CH, Heshka S, Wang J, et al. Truncal fat in relation to total body fat: influences of age, sex, ethnicity and fatness. *Int J Obes (Lond)*. 2007;31:1384-1391.
20. Koster A, Leitzmann MF, Schatzkin A, et al. Waist circumference and mortality. *Am J Epidemiol*. 2008;167:1465-1475.
21. World Health Organization. WHO Expert Consultation: appropriate body-mass index for Asian populations and its implications for policy and intervention strategies. *Lancet*. 2004;363:157-163.
22. Alberti KG, Eckel RH, Grundy SM, et al. Harmonizing the metabolic syndrome: a joint interim statement of the International Diabetes Federation Task Force on Epidemiology and Prevention; National Heart, Lung, and Blood Institute; American Heart Association; World Heart Federation; International Atherosclerosis Society; and International Association for the Study of Obesity. *Circulation*. 2009;120: 1640-1645.
23. Andres R, Elahi D, Tobin JD, et al. Impact of age on weight goals. *Ann Intern Med*. 1985;103(6 Pt 2):1030.
24. Kragelund C, Hassager C, Hildebrandt P, et al. TRACE study group: impact of obesity on long-term prognosis following acute myocardial infarction. *Int J Cardiol*. 2005;98:123-131.
25. McAuley P, Myers J, Abella J, et al. Body mass, fitness and survival in veteran patients: another obesity paradox? *Am J Med*. 2007;120: 518-524.
26. Uretsky S, Messerli FH, Bangalore S, et al. Obesity paradox in patients with hypertension and coronary artery disease. *Am J Med*. 2007;120:863-870.
27. Oreopoulos A, Padwal R, Norris CM, et al. Effect of obesity on short- and long-term mortality postcoronary revascularization: a meta-analysis. *Obesity (Silver Spring, Md.)*. 2008;16:442-450.
28. Mano A, Fujita K, Uenomachi K, et al. Body mass index is a useful predictor of prognosis after left ventricular assist system implantation. *J Heart Lung Transplant*. 2009;28:428-433.
29. Lea JP, Crenshaw DO, Onufrak SJ, et al. Obesity, end-stage renal disease, and survival in an elderly cohort with cardiovascular disease. *Obesity (Silver Spring, Md.)*. 2009;17:2216-2222.
30. Beck TJ, Petit MA, Wu G, et al. Does obesity really make the femur stronger? BMD, geometry, and fracture incidence in the Women's Health Initiative—Observational Study. *J Bone Miner Res*. 2009;24:1369-1379.
31. Van der Helm-van Mil AH, van der Kooij SM, Allaart CF, et al. A high body mass index has a protective effect on the amount of joint destruction in small joints in early rheumatoid arthritis. *Ann Rheum Dis*. 2008;67:769-774.
32. Leung CC, Lam TH, Chan WM, et al. Lower risk of tuberculosis in obesity. *Arch Intern Med*. 2007;167:1297-1304.
33. Willett WC, Manson JE, Stampfer MJ, et al. Weight, weight change, and coronary heart disease in women: risk within the "normal" weight range. *JAMA*. 1995;273:461-465.
34. Rimm EB, Stampfer MJ, Giovannucci E, et al. Body size and fat distribution as predictors of coronary heart disease among middle-aged and older U.S. men. *Am J Epidemiol*. 1995;141:1117-1127.
35. Colditz GA, Willett WC, Rotnitzky A, Manson JE. Weight gain as a risk factor for clinical diabetes mellitus in women. *Ann Intern Med*. 1995;122:481-486.
36. Chan JM, Rimm EB, Colditz GA, et al. Obesity, fat distribution, and weight gain as risk factors for clinical diabetes in men. *Diabetes Care*. 1994;17:961-969.
37. Huang Z, Willett WC, Manson JE, et al. Body weight, weight change, and risk for hypertension in women. *Ann Intern Med*. 1998;128:81-88.
38. Maclure KM, Hayes KC, Colditz GA, et al. Weight, diet, and risk of symptomatic gallstones in middle-aged women. *N Engl J Med*. 1989;321:563-569.
39. Wei M, Gibbons L, Mitchell T, et al. The association between cardiorespiratory fitness and impaired fasting glucose and type 2 diabetes mellitus in men. *Ann Intern Med*. 1999;130:89-96.
40. Lee CD, Blair SN, Jackson AS. Cardiorespiratory fitness, body composition, and all-cause and cardiovascular disease mortality in men. *Am J Clin Nutr*. 1999;69:373-380.
41. McKeigue P, Shah B, Marmont MG. Relation of central obesity and insulin resistance with high diabetes prevalence and cardiovascular risk in South Asians. *Lancet*. 1991;337:382-386.
42. Yoon K-H, Lee J-H, Kim J-W, et al. Epidemic obesity and type 2 diabetes in Asia. *Lancet*. 2006;368:1681-1688.
43. Morton GJ, Cummings DE, Baskin DG, et al. Central nervous system control of food intake and body weight. *Nature*. 2006;443: 289-295.
44. Badman MK, Flier JF. The gut and energy balance: visceral allies in the obesity wars. *Science*. 2005;307:1909-1914.
45. Cota D, Marsicano G, Tschöp M, et al. The endogenous cannabinoid system affects energy balance via central orexigenic drive and peripheral lipogenesis. *J Clin Invest*. 2003;112:423-431.
46. Ravinet C, Arnone M, Delgorge C, et al. Anti-obesity effect of SR141716, a CB1 receptor antagonist, in diet-induced obese mice. *Am J Physiol Regul Integr Comp Physiol*. 2003;284:R345-R353.
47. Pi-Sunyer FX, Aronne LJ, Heshmati HM, et al. Effect of rimonabant, a cannabinoid-1 receptor blocker, on weight and cardiometabolic risk factors in overweight or obese patients—RIO-North America: a randomized controlled trial. *JAMA*. 2006;295:761-775.
48. Despres JP, Golay A, Sjostrom L. Effects of rimonabant on metabolic risk factors in overweight patients with dyslipidemia. Rimonabant in Obesity-Lipids Study Group. *N Engl J Med*. 2005;353:2121-2134.
49. Vickers SP, Kennett GA. Cannabinoids and the regulation of ingestive behaviour. *Curr Drug Targets*. 2005;6:215-223.
50. McGowan BM, Bloom SR. Peptide YY and appetite control. *Curr Opin Pharmacol*. 2004;4:583-588.
51. Deacon CF. Therapeutic strategies based on glucagon-like peptide 1. *Diabetes*. 2004;53:2181-2189.
52. Rosenbaum M, Leibel RL, Hirsch J. Obesity. *N Engl J Med*. 1997;337:396-408.
53. Bouchard C, Perusse L. Genetics of obesity. *Annu Rev Nutr*. 1993;3:337-354.
54. Pratley RE. Gene-environment interactions in the pathogenesis of type 2 diabetes mellitus: lessons learned from the Pima Indians. *Proc Nutr Soc*. 1998;57:175-181.
55. O'Dea K, White N, Sinclair A. An investigation of nutrition-related risk factors in an isolated Aboriginal community in Northern Australia: advantages of a traditionally-orientated life style. *Med J Aust*. 1988;148:177-180.
56. O'Dea K. Marked improvement in carbohydrate and lipid metabolism in diabetic Australian Aborigines after temporary reversion to traditional lifestyle. *Diabetes*. 1984;33:596-603.
57. Whitaker RC, Wright JA, Pepe MS, et al. Predicting obesity in young adulthood from childhood and parental obesity. *N Engl J Med*. 1997;337:869-873.
58. Montague CT, Farooqi IS, Whitehead JP, et al. Congenital leptin deficiency is associated with severe early-onset obesity in humans. *Nature*. 1997;387:903-908.
59. Strobel A, Issad T, Camoin L, et al. A leptin missense mutation associated with hypogonadism and morbid obesity. *Nat Genet*. 1998;18:213-215.
60. Farooqi IS, Jebb SA, Langmack G, et al. Effects of recombinant leptin therapy in a child with congeital leptin deficiency. *N Engl J Med*. 1999;341:879-884.
61. Consadine RV, Sinha MK, Heiman ML et al. Serum immunoreactive-leptin concentrations in normal-weight and obese humans. *N Engl J Med*. 1996;334:292-295.
62. Clement K, Vaisse C, Lahlou N, et al. A mutation in the human leptin receptor gene causes obesity and pituitary dysfunction. *Nature*. 1998;392:398-401.
63. Jackson RS, Creemers JW, Ohagi S, et al. Obesity and impaired prohormone processing associated with mutations in the human prohormone convertase 1 gene. *Nat Genet*. 1997;16:303-306.
64. Jackson RS, Creemers JWM, Farooqi IS, et al. Small intestinal dysfunction accompanies the complex endocrinopathy of human proprotein convertase 1 deficiency. *J Clin Invest*. 2003;112:1550-1560.
65. Krude H, Biebermann H, Luck W, et al. Severe early-onset obesity, adrenal insufficiency and red hair pigmentation caused by POMC mutations in humans. *Nat Genet*. 1998;19:155-157.

66. Farooqi IS, Yeo GS, Keogh JM, et al. Dominant and recessive inheritance of morbid obesity associated with melanocortin 4 receptor deficiency. *J Clin Invest*. 2000;106:271-279.
67. Farooqi IS, Keogh JM, Giles SH, et al. Clinical spectrum of obesity and mutations in the melanocortin 4 receptor gene. *N Engl J Med*. 2003;348:1085-1095.
68. Yeo GS, Connie Hung CC, Rochford J, et al. A de novo mutation affecting human TrkB associated with severe obesity and developmental delay. *Nat Neurosci*. 2004;7:1187-1189.
69. Farooqi IS, O'Rahilly S. Monogentic obesity in humans. *Annu Rev Med*. 2005;56:443-458.
70. Goldstone AP. Prader-Willi syndrome: advances in genetics, pathophysiology and treatment. *Trends Endocrinol Metab*. 2004;15: 12-20.
71. Holder Jr JL, Butte NF, Zinn AR. Profound obesity associated with a balanced translocation that disrupts the *SIM1* gene. *Hum Mol Genet*. 2000;9:101-108.
72. Speliotes EK, Willer CJ, Berndt SI, et al. Association analyses of 249,796 individuals reveal 18 new loci associated with body mass index. *Nat Genet*. 2010;42:937-948.
73. Frayling TM, Timpson NJ, Weedon MN, et al. A common variant in the FTO gene is associated with body mass index and predisposes to childhood and adult obesity. *Science*. 2007;316:889-894.
74. Dina C, Meyre D, Gallina S, et al. Variation in FTO contributes to childhood obesity and severe adult obesity. *Nat Genet*. 2007;39: 724-726.
75. Scuteri A, Sanna S, Chen WM, et al. Genome-wide association scan shows genetic variants in the FTO gene are associated with obesity-related traits. *PLoS Genet*. 2007;3:e115.
76. Gerken T, Girard CA, Tung YC, et al. The obesity-associated FTO gene encodes a 2-oxoglutarate-dependent nucleic acid demethylase. *Science*. 2007;318:1469-1472.
77. Ravussin E, Burnand B, Schutz Y, et al. Twenty-four-hour energy expenditure and resting metabolic rate in obese, moderately obese, and control subjects. *Am J Clin Nutr*. 1982;35:566-573.
78. Skov AR, Toubro S, Buemann B, et al. Normal levels of energy expenditure in patients with reported "low metabolism." *Clin Physiol*. 1997;17:279-285.
79. Lichtman SW, Pisarka K, Berman ER, et al. Discrepancy between self-reported and actual caloric intake and exercise in obese subjects. *N Engl J Med*. 1992;327:1893-1898.
80. Segal KR, Presta E, Gutin B. Thermic effect of food during graded exercise in normal weight and obese men. *Am J Clin Nutr*. 1984;40:95-100.
81. de Jonge L, Bray GA. The thermic effect of food and obesity: a critical review. *Obesity Res*. 1997;5:622-631.
82. Roberts SB, Savage J, Coward WA, et al. Energy expenditure and intake from infants born to lean and overweight mothers. *N Engl J Med*. 1988;318:461-466.
83. Stunkard AJ, Berkowitz RI, Stallings VA, et al. Energy intake, not energy output, is a determinant of body size in infants. *Am J Clin Nutr*. 1999;69:524-530.
84. Ravussin E, Lillioja S, Knowler WC, et al. Reduced rate of energy expenditure as a risk factor for body-weight gain. *N Engl J Med*. 1988;318:467-472.
85. Seidell JC, Muller DC, Sorkin JD, et al. Fasting respiratory exchange ratio and resting metabolic rate as predictors of weight gain: the Baltimore Longitudinal Study on Aging. *Int J Obes Relat Metab Disord*. 1992;16:667-674.
86. Bouchard C, Tremblay A, Despres JP, et al. The response to long-term overfeeding in identical twins. *N Engl J Med*. 1990;322:1477-1482.
87. Levine JA, Eberhardt NL, Jensen MD. Role of nonexercise activity thermogenesis in resistance to fat gain in humans. *Science*. 1999;282:212-214.
88. Wadden TA, Foster GD, Letizia KA, et al. Long-term effects of dieting on resting metabolic rate in obese outpatients. *JAMA*. 1990;264: 707-711.
89. Amatruda JM, Statt MC, Welle SL. Total resting energy expenditure in obese women reduced to ideal body weight. *J Clin Invest*. 1993;92:1236-1242.
90. Weinsier RL, Nagy TR, Hunter GR, et al. Do adaptive changes in metabolic rate favor weight regain in weight-reduced individuals? An examination of the set-point theory. *Am J Clin Nutr*. 2000;72:1088-1094.
91. Astrup A, Gotzsche PC, van de Werken K, et al. Meta-analysis of resting metabolic rate in formerly obese subjects. *Am J Clin Nutr*. 1999;69:1117-1122.
92. Leiter LA, Marliss EB. Survival during fasting may depend on fat as well as protein stores. *JAMA*. 1982;248:2306-2307.
93. Stewart WK, Fleming LW. Features of a successful therapeutic fast of 382 days duration. *Postgrad Med J*. 1973;49:203-209.
94. Angel A, Bray GA. Synthesis of fatty acids and cholesterol by the liver, adipose tissue and intestinal mucosa from obese and control subjects. *Eur J Clin Invest*. 1979;9:355-362.
95. Ramsay TG. Fat cells. *Endocrinol Metab Clin North Am*. 1996;25:847-870.
96. Simsolo RB, Ong JM, Saffari B, et al. Effect of improved diabetes control on the expression of lipoprotein lipase in human adipose tissue. *J Lipid Res*. 1992;33;89-95.
97. Heiling VJ, Miles JM, Jensen MD. How valid are isotopic measurements of fatty acid oxidation? *Am J Physiol*. 1991;261:E572-E577.
98. Leweis GF. Fatty acid regulation of very low density lipoprotein production. *Curr Opin Lipidol*. 1997;8:146-153.
99. Jensen MD. Diet effects on fatty acid metabolism in lean and obese subjects. *Am J Clin Nutr*. 1998;67:531S-534S.
100. Jensen MD, Haymond MW, Rizza RA, et al. Influence of body fat distribution on free fatty acid metabolism in obesity. *J Clin Invest*. 1989;83:12168-12173.
101. Martin ML, Jensen MD. Effects of body fat distribution on regional lipolysis in obesity. *J Clin Invest*. 1991;88:609-613.
102. Kahn BB, Flier JS. Obesity and insulin resistance. *J Clin Invest*. 2000;106:473-481.
103. Wajchenberg BL. Subcutaneous and visceral adipose tissue: their relation to the metabolic syndrome. *Endocr Rev*. 2000;21:697-738.
104. Friedman JM. Obesity in the new millenium. *Nature*. 2000;404:632-634.
105. Lee Y, Wang MY, Wang ZW, et al. Liporegulation in diet-induced obesity: the antisteatotic role of hyperleptinemia. *J Biol Chem*. 2001;276:5629-5635.
106. Considine RV, Sinha MK, Heiman ML, et al. Serum immunoreactive leptin concentrations in normal weight and obese humans. *N Engl J Med*. 1996;334:292-295.
107. Kolaczynsky JW, Ohammesian JP, Considine RV, et al. Response of leptin to short-term and prolonged overfeeding in humans. *J Clin Endocrinol Metab*. 1996;81:4162-4165.
108. Flier JS. Clinical review 94: what's in a name? In search of leptin's physiologic role. *J Clin Endocrinol Metab*. 1998;83:1407-1413.
109. Steppan CM, Bailey ST, Bhat S, et al. The hormone resistin links obesity to diabetes. *Nature*. 2001;409:307-312.
110. Weyer C, Funahashi T, Tanaka S, et al. Hypoadiponectinemia in obesity and type 2 diabetes: close association with insulin resistance and hyperinsulinemia. *J Clin Endocrinol Metab*. 2001;86:1930-1935.
111. Yang WS, Lee WJ, Funahashi T, et al. Weight reduction increases plasma levels of an adipose-derived anti-inflammatory protein, adiponectin. *J Clin Endocrinol Metab*. 2001;86:3815-3819.
112. Yu JG, Javorschi S, Hevener AL, et al. The effect of thiazolidinediones on plasma adiponectin levels in normal, obese, and type 2 diabetic subjects. *Diabetes*. 2002;51:2968-2974.
113. Berg AH, Combs TP, Scherer PE. ACRP30/adiponectin: an adipokine regulating glucose and lipid metabolism. *Trends Endocrinol Metab*. 2002;13:84-89.
114. Fukuhara A, Matsuda M, Segawa K, et al. Visfatin: a protein secreted by visceral fat that mimics the effects of insulin. *Science*. 2005;307:426-430.
115. Peraldi P, Spiegelman B. TNF-α and insulin resistance: summary and future prospects. *Mol Cell Biochem*. 1998;182:169-171.
116. Mohamed-Ali V, Pinkney JH, Coppack SW. Adipose tissue as an endocrine and paracrine organ. *Int J Obes Relat Metab Disord*. 1998;22:1145-1158.
117. Bastard JP, Jardel C, Bruckert E, et al. Elevated levels of interleukin 6 are reduced in serum and subcutaneous adipose tissue of obese women after weight loss. *J Clin Endocrinol Metab*. 2000;85:3338-3342.
118. Bastard JP, Maachi M, Van Nhieu JT, et al. Adipose tissue IL-6 content correlates with resistance to insulin activation of glucose uptake both in vivo and in vitro. *J Clin Endocrinol Metab*. 2002;87:2084-2089.
119. Senn JJ, Klover PJ, Nowak IA, et al. Interleukin-6 induces cellular insulin resistance in hepatocytes. *Diabetes*. 2002;51:3391-3399.
120. Tsigos C, Papanicolaou DA, Kyrou I, et al. Dose-dependent effects of recombinant human interleukin-6 on glucose regulation. *J Clin Endocrinol Metab*. 1997;82:4167-4170.
121. Hirsch J, Knittle JL. Cellularity of obese and non-obese human adipose tissue. *Fed Proc*. 1970;29:1516-1521.
122. Ntambi JM, Kim Y-C. Adipocyte differentiation and gene expression. *J Nutr*. 2000;130:3122S-3126S.
123. Shimomura I, Hammer RE, Richardson JA, et al. Insulin resistance and diabetes mellitus in transgenic mice expressing nuclear SREBP-1c in adipose tissue: model for congenital generalized lipodystrophy. *Genes Dev*. 1998;12:3182-3194.
124. Ballor DL, Poehlman ET. Exercise-training enhances fat-free mass preservation during diet-induced weight loss: a meta-analytical finding. *Int J Obes Relat Metab Disord*. 1994;18:35-40.
125. Ross R, Rissanen J, Pedwell H, et al. Influence of diet and exercise on skeletal muscle and visceral adipose tissue in men. *J Appl Physiol*. 1996;81:2445-2455.
126. Smith SR, Zachwieja JJ. Visceral adipose tissue: a critical review of intervention strategies. *Int J Obes Relat Metab Disord*. 1999;23:329-335.
127. Knittle JL, Ginsberg-Fellner F. Effect of weight reduction on in vitro adipose tissue lipolysis and cellularity in obese adolescents and adults. *Diabetes*. 1972;21:754-761.

128. Naslund I, Hallgren P, Sjostrom L. Fat cell weight and number before and after gastric surgery for morbid obesity in women. *Int J Obes*. 1988;12:191-197.
129. Prins JB, O'Rahilly S. Regulation of adipose cell number in man. *Clin Sci*. 1997;92:3-11.
130. Prins JB, Walker NL, Winterford CM, et al. Apoptosis of human adipocyte in vitro. *Biochem Biophys Res Commun*. 1994;201:500-507.
131. Prins JB, Walker NL, Winterford CM, et al. Human adipocyte apoptosis occurs in malignancy. *Biochem Biophys Res Commun*. 1994;205:625-630.
132. Cannon B, Nedergaard J. Brown adipose tissue: function and physiological significance. *Physiol Rev*. 2004;84:277-359.
133. Virtanen KA, Lidell ME, Orava J, et al. Functional brown adipose tissue in healthy adults. *N Engl J Med*. 2009;360:1518-1525.
134. Cypess AM, Lehman S, Williams G, et al. Identification and importance of brown adipose tissue in adult humans. *N Engl J Med*. 2009;360:1509-1517.
135. van Marken Lichtenbelt WD, Vanhommerig JW, Smulders NM, et al. Cold-activated brown adipose tissue in healthy men. *N Engl J Med*. 2009;360:1500-1508.
136. Au-Yong IT, Thorn N, Ganatra R, et al. Brown adipose tissue and seasonal variation in people. *Diabetes*. 2009;58:2583-2587.
137. Ogden CL, Carroll MD, Curtin LR, et al. Prevalence of overweight and obesity in the United States, 1999-2004. *JAMA*. 2006;295:1549-1555.
138. Flegal KM, Carroll MD, Kuczmarski RJ, et al. Overweight and obesity in the United States: prevalence and trends, 1960-1994. *Int J Obes Relat Metab Disord*. 1998;22:39-47.
139. Flegal KM, Troiano RP. Changes in the distribution of body mass index of adults and children in the U.S. population. *Int J Obes Relat Metab Disord*. 2000;24:807-818.
140. Barlow SE, Dietz WH. Obesity evaluation and treatment: Expert Committee recommendations. The Maternal and Child Health Bureau, Health Resources and Services Administration and the Department of Health and Human Services. *Pediatrics*. 1998;102:E29.
141. Klein S, Wadden T, Sugerman HJ. AGA technical review on obesity. *Gastroenterology*. 2002;123:882-932.
142. Brochu M, Tchernof A, Dionne IJ, et al. What are the physical characteristics associated with a normal metabolic profile despite a high level of obesity in postmenopausal women? *J Clin Endocrinol Metab*. 2001;86:1020-1025.
143. Ferrannini E, Natali A, Bell P, et al. Insulin resistance and hypersecretion in obesity. European Group for the Study of Insulin Resistance (EGIR). *J Clin Invest*. 1997;100:1166-1173.
144. Wildman RP, Muntner P, Reynolds K, et al. The obese without cardiometabolic risk factor clustering and the normal weight with cardiometabolic risk factor clustering: prevalence and correlates of 2 phenotypes among the US population (NHANES 1999-2004). *Arch Intern Med*. 2008;168:1617-1624.
145. Karelis AD. Metabolically healthy but obese individuals. *Lancet*. 2008;372:1281-1283.
146. Iacobellis G, Ribaudo MC, Zappaterreno A, et al. Prevalence of uncomplicated obesity in an Italian obese population. *Obes Res*. 2005;13:1116-1122.
147. Stefan N, Kantartzis K, Machann J, et al. Identification and characterization of metabolically benign obesity in humans. *Arch Intern Med*. 2008;168:1609-1616.
148. Aguilar-Salinas CA, Garcia EG, Robles L, et al. High adiponectin concentrations are associated with the metabolically healthy obese phenotype. *J Clin Endocrinol Metab*. 2008;93:4075-4079.
149. Karelis AD, Faraj M, Bastard JP, et al. The metabolically healthy but obese individual presents a favorable inflammation profile. *J Clin Endocrinol Metab*. 2005:90:4145-4150.
150. Meigs JB, Wilson PW, Fox CS, et al. Body mass index, metabolic syndrome, and risk of type 2 diabetes or cardiovascular disease. *J Clin Endocrinol Metab*. 2006;91:2906-2912.
151. Flegal KM, Graubard BI, Williamson DF, et al. Excess deaths associated with underweight, overweight, and obesity. *JAMA*. 2005;293:1861-1867.
152. Landin K, Stigendal L, Eriksson E, et al. Abdominal obesity is associated with an impaired fibrinolytic activity and elevated plasminogen activator inhibitor-1. *Metabolism*. 1990;39:1044-1048.
153. Lemieux I, Pascot A, Couillard C, et al. Hypertriglyceridemic waist: a marker of the atherogenic metabolic triad (hyperinsulinemia; hyperapolipoprotein B; small, dense LDL) in men? *Circulation*. 2000;102:179-184.
154. Ruderman N, Chisholm D, Pi-Sunyer X, et al. The metabolically obese, normal-weight individual revisited. *Diabetes*. 1998;47:699-713.
155. Reaven GM. Role of insulin resistance in human disease. *Diabetes*. 1988;37:1595-1607.
156. Meigs JB, D'Agostino RB, Wilson WF, et al. Risk variable clustering in the insulin resistance syndrome. *Diabetes*. 1997;46:1594-1600.
157. Frayn KN. Visceral fat and insulin resistance: causative or correlative? *Br J Nutr*. 2000;83(suppl 1):S71-S77.
158. Krssak M, Petersen KF, Dresner A, et al. Intramyocellular lipid concentrations are correlated with insulin sensitivity in humans: a ^{1}H NMR spectroscopy study. *Diabeteologia*. 1999;42:113-116.
159. Marchesini G, Bugianesi E, Forlani G, et al. Nonalcoholic fatty liver, steatohepatitis, and the metabolic syndrome. *Hepatology*. 2003;37:917-923.
160. Adams LA, Lymp JF, St Sauver J, et al. The natural history of nonalcoholic fatty liver disease: a population-based cohort study. *Gastroenterology*. 2005;129:113-121.
161. Dobbins RL, Szczepaniak LS, Bentley B, et al. Prolonged inhibition of muscle carnitine palmitoyltransferase I promotes intramyocellular lipid accumulation and insulin resistance in rats. *Diabetes*. 2001;50:123-130.
162. Cowie CC, Rust KF, Ford ES, et al. Full accounting of diabetes and pre-diabetes in the U.S. population in 1988-1994 and 2005-2006. *Diabetes Care*. 2009;32:287-294.
163. Colditz GA, Willett WC, Stampfer MJ, et al. Weight as a risk factor for clinical diabetes in women. *Am J Epidemiol*. 1990;132:501-513.
164. Ohlson LO, Larsson B, Svardsudd K, et al. The influence of body fat distribution on the incidence of diabetes mellitus. *Diabetes*. 1985;34:1055-1058.
165. Lundgren H, Bengtsson C, Blohme G, et al. Adiposity and adipose tissue distribution in relation to incidence of diabetes in women: results from a prospective population study in Gothenburg, Sweden. *Int J Obes*. 1989;13:413-423.
166. Kaye SA, Folsom AR, Sprafka JM, et al. Increased incidence of diabetes mellitus in relation to abdominal adiposity in older women. *J Clin Epidemiol*. 1991;44:329-334.
167. Reaven GM, Chen YDI, Jeppesen J, et al. Insulin resistance and hyperinsulinemia in individuals with small, dense, low density lipoprotein particles. *J Clin Invest*. 1993;92:141-146.
168. Terry RB, Wood PD, Haskell WL, et al. Regional adiposity pattern in relation to lipids, lipoprotein cholesterol, and lipoprotein subfraction mass in men. *J Clin Endocrinol Metab*. 1989;68:191-199.
169. Brown CD, Higgins M, Donato KA, et al. Body mass index and the prevalence of hypertension and dyslipidemia. *Obes Res*. 2000;8:605-619.
170. Assmann G, Schulte H. Relation of high-density lipoprotein cholesterol and triglycerides to incidence of atherosclerotic coronary artery disease (the PROCAM experience). *Am J Cardiol*. 1992;70:733-737.
171. Lamarche B, Lemieux I, Despres JP. The small, dense LDL phenotype and the risk of coronary heart disease: epidemiology, pathophysiology and therapeutic aspects. *Diabetes Metab*. 1999;25:199-211.
172. Hubert HB, Feinleib M, McNamara PM, et al. Obesity as an independent risk factor for cardiovascular disease: a 26-year follow-up of participants in the Framingham Heart Study. *Circulation*. 1983;67:968-977.
173. Stamler R, Stamler J, Riedlinger WF, et al. Weight and blood pressure: findings in hypertension screening of 1 million Americans. *JAMA*. 1978;240:1607-1609.
174. Kannel W, Brand N, Skinner J, et al. The relation of adiposity to blood pressure and development of hypertension. The Framingham study. *Ann Intern Med*. 1967;67:48-59.
175. Stamler J, Wentworth D, Neaton JD. Is relationship between serum cholesterol and risk of premature death from coronary disease continuous or graded? Findings in 356,222 primary screenees of the Multiple Risk Factor Intervention Trial (MRFIT). *JAMA*. 1986;256:2823-2828.
176. Rexrode KM, Carey VJ, Hennekens CH, et al. Abdominal adiposity and coronary heart disease in women. *JAMA*. 1998;280:1843-1848.
177. Manson JE, Willett WC, Stampfer MJ, et al. Body weight and mortality among women. *N Engl J Med*. 1995;333:677-685.
178. Eckel RH, Krauss RM. American Heart Association call to action: obesity as a major risk factor for coronary heart disease. *Circulation*. 1998;97:2099-2100.
179. Krause RM, Eckel RH, Howard B, et al. AHA dietary guidelines revision 2000: a statement for healthcare professionals from the nutrition committee of the American Heart Association. *Circulation*. 2000;102:2296-2311.
180. Walker SP, Rimm EB, Ascherio A, et al. Body size and fat distribution as predictors of stroke among U.S. men. *Am J Epidemiol*. 1996;144:1143-1150.
181. Rexrode KM, Hennekens CH, Willett WC, et al. A prospective study of body mass index weight change, and risk of stroke in women. *JAMA*. 1997;277:1539-1545.
182. Hansson PO, Eriksson H, Welin L, et al. Smoking and abdominal obesity: risk factors for venous thromboembolism among middle-aged men. "The study of men born in 1913." *Arch Intern Med*. 1999;159:1886-1890.
183. Sugerman HJ, Windsor ACJ, Bessos MK, et al. Abdominal pressure, sagittal abdominal diameter and obesity co-morbidity. *J Int Med*. 1997;241:71-79.
184. Visser M, Bouter LM, McQuillan GM, et al. Elevated C-reactive protein levels in overweight and obese adults. *JAMA*. 1999;282:2131-2135.

185. Strohl KP, Strobel RJ, Parisi RA. Obesity and pulmonary function. In: Bray GA, Bouchard C, James WPT, eds. *Handbook of Obesity*. New York, NY: Marcel Dekker; 1998:725-739.
186. Vgontzas AN, Tan TL, Bixler EO, et al. Sleep apnea and sleep disruption in obese patients. *Arch Intern Med*. 1994;154:1705-1711.
187. Davies RJ, Stradling JR. The relationship between neck circumference, radiographic pharyngeal anatomy, and the obstructive sleep apnoea syndrome. *Eur Respir J*. 1990;3:509-514.
188. Katz I, Stradling J, Slutsky AS, et al. Do patients with obstructive sleep apnea have thick necks? *Am Rev Respir Dis*. 1990;141:1228-1231.
189. Roubenoff R, Klag MJ, Mead LA, et al. Incidence and risk factors for gout in white men. *JAMA*. 1991;266:3004-3007.
190. Cigolini M, Targher G, Tonoli M, et al. Hyperuricaemia: relationships to body fat distribution and other components of the insulin resistance syndrome in 38-year-old healthy men and women. *Int J Obes Relat Metab Disord*. 1995;19:92-96.
191. Felson DT, Anderson JJ, Naimark A, et al. Obesity and knee osteoarthritis: the Framingham Study. *Ann Intern Med*. 1988;109:18-24.
192. Cicuttini FM, Baker JR, Spector TD. The association of obesity with osteoarthritis of the hand and knee in women: a twin study. *J Rheumatol*. 1996;23:1221-1226.
193. Calle EE, Rodriguez C, Walker-Thurmond K, et al. Overweight, obesity and mortality from cancer in a prospectively studied cohort of U.S. adults. *N Engl J Med*. 2003;348:1625-1638.
194. Giovannucci E, Ascherio A, Rimm EB, et al. Physical activity, obesity, and risk for colon cancer and adenoma in men. *Ann Intern Med*. 1995;122:327-334.
195. Potter JD, Slattery ML, Bostick RM, et al. Colon cancer: a review of the epidemiology. *Epidemiol Rev*. 1993;15:499-545.
196. Huang Z, Hankinson SE, Colditz GA, et al. Dual effects of weight and weight gain on breast cancer risk. *JAMA*. 1997;278:1407-1411.
197. Willett WC, Browne ML, Bain C, et al. Relative weight and risk of breast cancer among premenopausal women. *Am J Epidemiol*. 1985;122:731-740.
198. Grodstein F, Goldman MB, Cramer DW. Body mass index and ovulatory infertility. *Epidemiology*. 1994;5:247-250.
199. Johnson SR, Kolberg BH, Varner MW, et al. Maternal obesity and pregnancy. *Surg Gynecol Obstet*. 1987;164:431-437.
200. Garbaciak Jr JA, Richter M, Miller S, Barton JJ. Maternal weight and pregnancy complications. *Am J Obstet Gynecol*. 1985;152:238-245.
201. Prentice A, Goldberg G. Maternal obesity increases congenital malformations. *Nutr Rev*. 1996;54:146-152.
202. Dwyer PL, Lee ETC, Hay DM. Obesity and urinary incontinence in women. *Br J Obstet Gynecol*. 1988;95:91-96.
203. Bump RC, Sugerman HJ, Fantl JA, et al. Obesity and lower urinary tract function in women: effect of surgically induced weight loss. *Am J Obstet Gynecol*. 1992;167:392-399.
204. Durcan FJ, Corbett JJ, Wall M. The incidence of pseudotumor cerebri: population studies in Iowa and Louisiana. *Arch Neurol*. 1988;45:875-877.
205. Giuseffi V, Wall M, Siegel PZ, et al. Symptoms and disease associations in idiopathic intracranial hypertension (pseudotumor cerebri): a case-control study. *Neurology*. 1991;41:239-244.
206. Sugerman HJ, Felton WL, Sismanis A, et al. Effects of surgically induced weight loss on pseudotumor cerebri in morbid obesity. *Neurology*. 1995;45:1655-1659.
207. Sugerman HJ, Felton III WL, Sismanis A, et al. Gastric surgery for pseudotumor cerebri associated with severe obesity. *Ann Surg*. 1999;229:634-642.
208. Glynn RJ, Christen WG, Manson JE, et al. Body mass index: an independent predictor of cataract. *Arch Ophthalmol*. 1995;113:1131-1137.
209. Romero Y, Cameron AJ, Locke III GR, et al. Familial aggregation of gastroesophageal reflux in patients with Barrett's esophagus and esophageal adenocarcinoma. *Gastroenterology*. 1997;113:1449-1456.
210. Locke GR, Talley NJ, Fett SL, et al. Risk factors associated with symptoms of gastroesophageal reflux. *Am J Med*. 1999;106:642-649.
211. Lagergren J, Bergeström R, Nyrén O. No relation between body mass and gastro-oesophageal reflux symptoms in a Swedish population based study. *Gut*. 2000;47:26-29.
212. Fisher BL, Pennathur A, Mutnick JLM, et al. Obesity correlates with gastroesophageal reflux. *Dig Dis Sci*. 1999;44:2290-2294.
213. Lundell L, Ruth M, Sandberg N, et al. Does massive obesity promote abnormal gastroesophageal reflux? *Dig Dis Sci*. 1995;40:1632-16350.
214. Stampfer MJ, Maclure KM, Colditz GA, et al. Risk of symptomatic gallstones in women. *Am J Clin Nutr*. 1992;55:652-658.
215. Hay DW, Carey MC. Pathophysiology and pathogenesis of cholesterol gallstone formation. *Semin Liver Dis*. 1990;10:159-170.
216. Weinsier RL, Wilson LJ, Lee J. Medically safe rate of weight loss for the treatment of obesity: a guideline based on risk of gallstone formation. *Am J Med*. 1995;98:115-117.
217. Broomfield PH, Chopra R, Sheinbaum RC, et al. Effects of ursodeoxycholic acid and aspirin on the formation of lithogenic bile gallstones during loss of weight. *N Engl J Med*. 1988;319:1567-1572.
218. Shiffman ML, Kaplan GD, Brinkman-Kaplan V, et al. Prophylaxis against gallstone formation with urosdeoxycholic acid in patients participating in a very-low-calorie diet program. *Ann Intern Med*. 1995;122:899-905.
219. Wattchow DA, Hall JC, Whiting MJ, et al. Prevalence and treatment of gall stones after gastric bypass surgery for morbid obesity. *Br Med J (Clin Res Ed)*. 1983;286:763.
220. Stone BG, Ansel HJ, Peterson FJ, et al. Gallbladder emptying stimuli in obese and normal weight subjects. *Hepatology*. 1990;12:795-798.
221. Festi D, Colecchia A, Orsini M, et al. Gallbladder motility and gallstone formation in obese patients following very low calorie diets: use it (fat) to lose it (well). *Int J Obes*. 1998;22:592-600.
222. Shoheiber O, Biskupiak JE, Nash DB. Estimation of the cost savings resulting from the use of ursodiol for the prevention of gallstones in obese patients undergoing rapid weight reduction. *Int J Obes Relat Metab Disord*. 1997;21:1038-1045.
223. Funnell IC, Bornman PC, Weakley SP. Obesity: an important prognostic factor in acute pancreatitis. *Br J Surg*. 1993;80:484-486.
224. Marchesini G, Bugianesi E, Forlani G, et al. Nonalcoholic fatty liver, steatohepatitis, and the metabolic syndrome. *Hepatology*. 2003;37: 917-923.
225. Ruhl CE, Everhart JE. Determinants of the association of overweight with elevated serum alanine aminotransferase activity in the United States. *Gastroenterology*. 2003;124:71-79.
226. Marcos A, Fisher RA, Ham JM, et al. Selection and outcome of living donors for adult to adult right lobe transplantation. *Transplantation*. 2000;69:2410-2415.
227. Hilden M, Christoffersen P, Juhl E, et al. Liver histology in a "normal" population: examinations of 503 consecutive fatal traffic casualties. *Scand J Gastroenterol*. 1977;12:593-597.
228. Lee RG. Nonalcoholic steatohepatitis: a study of 49 patients. *Hum Pathol*. 1989;20:594-598.
229. Gholam PM, Kotler DP, Flancbaum LJ. Liver pathology in morbidly obese patients undergoing Roux-en-Y gastric bypass surgery. *Obes Surg*. 2002;12:49-51.
230. Petersen KF, Dufour S, Feng J, et al. Increased prevalence of insulin resistance and nonalcoholic fatty liver disease in Asian-Indian men. *Proc Natl Acad Sci U S A*. 2006;103:18273-18277.
231. Romeo S, Kozlitina J, Xing C, et al. Genetic variation in PNPLA3 confers susceptibility to nonalcoholic fatty liver disease. *Nat Genet*. 2008;40:1461-1465.
232. Browning JD, Szczepaniak LS, Dobbins R, et al. Prevalence of hepatic steatosis in an urban population in the United States: impact of ethnicity. *Hepatology*. 2004;40:1387-1395.
233. Korenblat KM, Fabbrini E, Mohammed BS, et al. Liver, muscle, and adipose tissue insulin action is directly related to intrahepatic triglyceride content in obese subjects. *Gastroenterology*. 2008;134:1369-1375.
234. Fabbrini E, Mohammed BS, Magkos F, et al. Alterations in adipose tissue and hepatic lipid kinetics in obese men and women with nonalcoholic fatty liver disease. *Gastroenterology*. 2008;134:424-431.
235. Deivanayagam S, Mohammed BS, Vitola BE, et al. Nonalcoholic fatty liver disease is associated with hepatic and skeletal muscle insulin resistance in overweight adolescents. *Am J Clin Nutr*. 2008;88: 257-262.
236. Fabbrini E, deHaseth D, Deivanayagam S, et al. Alterations in fatty acid kinetics in obese adolescents with increased intrahepatic triglyceride content. *Obesity (Silver Spring, Md.)*. 2009;17:25-29.
237. Fabbrini E, Magkos F, Mohammed BS, et al. Intrahepatic fat, not visceral fat, is linked with metabolic complications of obesity. *Proc Natl Acad Sci U S A*. 2009;106:15430-15435.
238. Gastaldelli A, Cusi K, Pettiti M, et al. Relationship between hepatic/visceral fat and hepatic insulin resistance in nondiabetic and type 2 diabetic subjects. *Gastroenterology*. 2007;133:496-506.
239. Seppala-Lindroos A, Vehkavaara S, Hakkinen AM, et al. Fat accumulation in the liver is associated with defects in insulin suppression of glucose production and serum free fatty acids independent of obesity in normal men. *J Clin Endocrinol Metab*. 2002;87:3023-3028.
240. Diraison F, Moulin P, Beylot M. Contribution of hepatic de novo lipogenesis and reesterification of plasma non esterified fatty acids to plasma triglyceride synthesis during non-alcoholic fatty liver disease. *Diabetes Metab*. 2003;29:478-485.
241. Donnelly KL, Smith CI, Schwarzenberg SJ, et al. Sources of fatty acids stored in liver and secreted via lipoproteins in patients with nonalcoholic fatty liver disease. *J Clin Invest*. 2005;115:1343-1351.
242. Monetti M, Levin MC, Watt MJ, et al. Dissociation of hepatic steatosis and insulin resistance in mice overexpressing DGAT in the liver. *Cell Metab*. 2007;6:69-78.
243. Minehira K, Young SG, Villanueva CJ, et al. Blocking VLDL secretion causes hepatic steatosis but does not affect peripheral lipid stores or insulin sensitivity in mice. *J Lipid Res*. 2008;49:2038-2044.
244. Grefhorst A, Hoekstra J, Derks TG, et al. Acute hepatic steatosis in mice by blocking beta-oxidation does not reduce insulin sensitivity of very-low-density lipoprotein production. *Am J Physiol Gastrointest Liver Physiol*. 2005;289:G592-G598.
245. Amaro A, Fabbrini E, Kars M, et al. Dissociation between intrahepatic triglyceride content and insulin sensitivity in subjects with familial hypobetalipoproteinemia. *Gastroenterology*. 2010;139:149-153.

246. Kirk E, Reeds DN, Finck BN, et al. Dietary fat and carbohydrates differentially alter insulin sensitivity during caloric restriction. *Gastroenterology*. 2009;136:1552-1560.
247. Bellentani S, Dalle Grave R, Suppini A, et al. Behavior therapy for nonalcoholic fatty liver disease: the need for a multidisciplinary approach. *Hepatology*. 2008;47:746-754.
248. Larson-Meyer DE, Newcomer BR, Heilbronn LK, et al. Effect of 6-month calorie restriction and exercise on serum and liver lipids and markers of liver function. *Obesity (Silver Spring, Md.)*. 2008;16:1355-1362.
249. Mittendorfer B, Patterson BW, Klein S. Effect of weight loss on VLDL-triglyceride and apoB-100 kinetics in women with abdominal obesity. *Am J Physiol Endocrinol Metab*. 2003;284:E549-E556.
250. Luyckx FH, Desaive C, Thiry A, et al. Liver abnormalities in severely obese subjects: effect of drastic weight loss after gastroplasty. *Int J Obes Relat Metab Disord*. 1998;22:222-226.
251. Klein S, Mittendorfer B, Eagon JC, et al. Gastric bypass surgery improves metabolic and hepatic abnormalities associated with nonalcoholic fatty liver disease. *Gastroenterology*. 2006;130:1564-1572.
252. Clark JM, Alkhuraishi AR, Solga SF, et al. Roux-en-Y gastric bypass improves liver histology in patients with non-alcoholic fatty liver disease. *Obes Res*. 2005;13:1180-1186.
253. Dixon JB, Bhathal PS, Hughes NR, et al. Nonalcoholic fatty liver disease: improvement in liver histological analysis with weight loss. *Hepatology*. 2004;39:1647-1654.
254. Sjostrom CD, Lissner L, Wedel H, et al. Reduction in incidence of diabetes, hypertension and lipid disturbances after intentional weight loss induced by bariatric surgery: the SOS Intervention Study. *Obes Res*. 1999;7:477-484.
255. Moore LL, Visioni AJ, Wilson PW, et al. Can sustained weight loss in overweight individuals reduce the risk of diabetes mellitus? *Epidemiology*. 2000;11:269-273.
256. Wing RR, Koeske R, Epstein LH, et al. Long-term effects of modest weight loss in type II diabetic patients. *Arch Intern Med*. 1987;147:1749-1753.
257. Pories WJ, Swanson MS, MacDonald KG, et al. Who would have thought it? An operation proves to be the most effective therapy for adult-onset diabetes mellitus. *Ann Surg*. 1995;222:339-350; discussion 350-352.
258. Karason K, Wikstrand J, Sjostrom L, et al. Weight loss and progression of early atherosclerosis in the carotid artery: a four-year controlled study of obese subjects. *Int J Obes Relat Metab Disord*. 1999;23:948-956.
259. Kirk E, Reeds DN, Finck BN, Mayurranjan SM, Patterson BW, Klein S. Dietary fat and carbohydrates differentially alter insulin sensitivity during caloric restriction. *Gastroenterology*. 2009;136(5):1552-1560.
260. Hughes TA, Gwynne JT, Switzer BR, et al. Effects of caloric restriction and weight loss on glycemic control, insulin release and resistance, and atherosclerotic risk in obese subjects with type II diabetes mellitus. *JAMA*. 1984;77:7-17.
261. Markovic TP, Jenkins AB, Campbell LV, et al. The determinants of glycemic responses to diet restriction and weight loss in obesity and NIDDM. *Diabetes Care*. 1998;21:687-694.
262. Pan XR, Li GW, Hu YH, et al. Effects of diet and exercise in preventing NIDDM in people with impaired glucose tolerance: the Da Qing IGT and Diabetes Study. *Diabetes Care*. 1997;20:537-544.
263. Sjostrom CD, Peltonen M, Wedel H, et al. Differentiated long-term effects of intentional weight loss on diabetes and hypertension. *Hypertension*. 2000;36:20-25.
264. Tuomilehto J, Lindstrom J, Eriksson JG, et al; Finnish Diabetes Prevention Study Group. Prevention of type 2 diabetes mellitus by changes in lifestyle among subjects with impaired glucose tolerance. *N Engl J Med*. 2001;344:1343-1350.
265. Wing RR, Marcus MD, Epstein LH, et al. Type II diabetic subjects lose less weight than their overweight nondiabetic spouses. *Diabetes Care*. 1987;10:563-566.
266. Khan MA, St Peter JV, Breen GA, et al. Diabetes disease stage predicts weight loss outcomes with long-term appetite suppressants. *Obes Res*. 2000;8:43-48.
267. U.K. Prospective Diabetes Study (UKPDS) Group. Intensive blood-glucose control with sulphonylureas or insulin compared with conventional treatment and risk of complications in patients with type 2 diabetes (UKPDS 33). *Lancet*. 1998;352:837-853.
268. Dattilo AM, Kris-Etherton PM. Effects of weight reduction on blood lipids and lipoproteins: a meta-analysis. *Am J Clin Nutr*. 1992;56:320-328.
269. Wadden TA, Anderson DA, Foster GD. Two-year changes in lipids and lipoproteins associated with the maintenance of a 5% to 10% reduction in initial weight: some findings and some questions. *Obes Res*. 1999;7:170-178.
270. Stefanick ML, Mackey S, Sheehan M, et al. Effects of diet and exercise in men and postmenopausal women with low levels of HDL cholesterol and high levels of LDL cholesterol. *N Engl J Med*. 1998;339:12-20.
271. The Trials of Hypertension Prevention Collaborative Research Group. Effects of weight loss and sodium reduction intervention on blood pressure and hypertension incidence in overweight people with high-normal blood pressure. The Trials of Hypertension Prevention, phase II. *Arch Intern Med*. 1997;157:657-667.
272. Stevens VJ, Obarzanek E, Cook NR, et al. Long-term weight loss and changes in blood pressure: results of the Trials of Hypertension Prevention, phase II. *Ann Intern Med*. 2001;134:1-11.
273. Carson JL, Ruddy ME, Duff AE, et al. The effect of gastric bypass surgery on hypertension in morbidly obese patients. *Arch Intern Med*. 1994;154:193-200.
274. Sjöström CD, Peltonen M, Wedel H, et al. Differentiated long-term effects of intentional weight loss on diabetes and hypertension. *Hypertension*. 2000;36:20-25.
275. Huang Z, Willett WC, Manson JE, et al. Body weight, weight change, and risk for hypertension in women. *Ann Intern Med*. 1998;128:81-88.
276. Wilson PW, Kannel WB, Silbershatz H, et al. Clustering of metabolic factors and coronary heart disease. *Arch Intern Med*. 1999;159:1104-1109.
277. MacMahon SW, Wilcken D, MacDonald GJ. The effect of weight reduction on left ventricular mass. *N Engl J Med*. 1986;314:334-339.
278. Karason K, Lindroos AK, Stenlof K, et al. Relief of cardiorespiratory symptoms and increased physical activity after surgically induced weight loss: results from the Swedish Obese Subjects study. *Arch Intern Med*. 2000;160:1797-1802.
279. Sugerman HJ, Fairman RP, Sood RK, et al. Long-term effects of gastric surgery for treating respiratory insufficiency of obesity. *Am J Clin Nutr*. 1992;55:597S-601S.
280. Smith PL, Gold AR, Meyers DA, et al. Weight loss in mildly to moderately obese patients with obstructive sleep apnea. *Ann Intern Med*. 1985;103:850-855.
281. Sugerman HJ, Baron PL, Fairman RP, et al. Hemodynamic dysfunction in obesity hypoventilation syndrome and the effects of treatment with surgically induced weight loss. *Ann Surg*. 1988;207:604-613.
282. Andres R, Muller DC, Sorkin JD. Long-term effects of change in body weight on all-cause mortality: a review. *Ann Intern Med*. 1993;119:737-743.
283. Williamson DF, Pamuk E, Thun M, et al. Prospective study of intentional weight loss and mortality in never-smoking overweight U.S. white women aged 40-64 years. *Am J Epidemiol*. 1995;14:1128-1141.
284. Williamson DF, Pamuk E, Thun M, et al. Prospective study of intentional weight loss and mortality in overweight weight white men aged 40-64 years. *Am J Epidemiol*. 1999;149:491-503.
285. Williamson DF, Thompson TJ, Thun M, et al. Intentional weight loss and mortality among overweight individuals with diabetes. *Diabetes Care*. 2000;23:1499-1504.
286. Sjöstrom CD, Narbro K, Sjöstrom CD, et al. Effects of bariatric surgery on mortality in Swedish obese subjects. *N Engl J Med*. 2007;357:741-752.
287. Adams TD, Gress RE, Smith SC, et al. Long-term mortality after gastric bypass surgery. *N Engl J Med*. 2007;357:753-761.
288. National Task Force on the Prevention and Treatment of Obesity. Weight cycling. *JAMA*. 1994;272:1196-1202.
289. Lissner L, Odell PM, D'Agostino RB, et al. Variability of body weight and health outcomes in the Framingham population. *N Eng J Med*. 1991;324:1839-1844.
290. Harris JA, Benedict FG. Standard basal metabolism constants for physiologists and clinicians. In: Harris JA, Benedict FG. *A Biometric Study of Basal Metabolism in Man. Publication 279, The Carnegie Institute of Washington*. Philadelphia, PA: JB Lippincott; 1919.
291. World Health Organization. *WHO/FAO/UNO report: energy and protein requirements*. WHO Technical Report Series, No. 724. Geneva, Switzerland: WHO; 1985.
292. Wing RR, Marcus MD, Salata R, et al. Effects of a very-low-calorie diet on long-term glycemic control in obese type 2 diabetic subjects. *Arch Intern Med*. 1991;151:1334-1340.
293. Torgerson JS, Lissner L, Lindross AK, et al. VLCD plus dietary and behavioral support versus support alone in the treatment of severe obesity: a randomised two-year clinical trial. *Int J Obes Relat Metab Disord*. 1997;21:987-994.
294. Wadden TA, Foster GD, Letizia KA. One-year behavioral treatment of obesity: comparison of moderate and severe caloric restriction and the effects of weight maintenance therapy. *J Consult Clin Psychol*. 1994;62:165-171.
295. Wadden TA, Stunkard AJ. A controlled trial of very-low-calorie diet, behavior therapy, and their combination in the treatment of obesity. *J Consult Clin Psychol*. 1986;4:482-488.
296. Miura J, Arai K, Ohno M, et al. The long term effectiveness of combined therapy by behavior modification and very low calorie diet: 2 year follow-up. *Int J Obes*. 1989;13:73-77.
297. Ryttig KR, Flaten H, Rossner S. Long-term effects of a very low calorie diet (Nutrilett) in obesity treatment: a prospective, randomized, comparison between VLCD and a hypocaloric diet + behavior modification and their combination. *Int J Obes Relat Metab Disord*. 1997;21:574-579.

298. Foster GD, Wadden TA, Peterson FJ, et al. A controlled comparison of three very-low-calorie diets: effects on weight, body composition, and symptoms. *Am J Clin Nutr.* 1992;55:811-817.
299. Bray GA, Popkin BM. Dietary fat intake does affect obesity! *Am J Clin Nutr.* 1998;68:1157-1173.
300. Yu-Poth S, Zhao G, Etherton T, et al. Effects of the National Cholesterol Education Program's Step I and Step II dietary intervention programs on cardiovascular disease risk factors: a meta-analysis. *Am J Clin Nutr.* 1999;69:632-646.
301. Astrup A, Grunwald GK, Melanson EL, et al. The role of low-fat diets in body weight control: a meta-analysis of ad libitum dietary intervention studies. *Int J Obes Relat Metab Disord.* 2000;24:1545-1552.
302. Rolls BJ, Bell EA. Dietary approaches to the treatment of obesity. *Med Clin North Am.* 2000;84:401-418.
303. Duncan KH, Bacon JA, Weinsier RL. The effects of high and low energy density diets on satiety, energy intake, and eating time of obese and nonobese subjects. *Am J Clin Nutr.* 1983;37:763-767.
304. Stubbs RJ, Harbron CG, Murgatroyd PR, et al. Covert manipulation of dietary fat and energy density: effect on substrate flux and food intake in men eating ad libitum. *Am J Clin Nutr.* 1995;62:316-329.
305. Bell EA, Castellanos VH, Pelkman CL, et al. Energy density of foods affects energy intake in normal-weight women. *Am J Clin Nutr.* 1998;67:412-420.
306. Yang M-U, Van Itallie TB. Composition of weight lost during short-term weight reduction. *J Clin Invest.* 1976;58:722-730.
307. Foster GD, Wyatt HR, Hill JO, et al. A randomized trial of a low-carbohydrate diet for obesity. *N Engl J Med.* 2003;348:2082-2090.
308. Samaha FF, Iqbal N, Seshadri P, et al. A low-carbohydrate as compared with a low-fat diet in severe obesity. *N Engl J Med.* 2003;348:2074-2081.
309. Brehm BJ, Seeley RJ, Daniels SR, et al. A randomized trial comparing a very low carbohydrate diet and a calorie-restricted low fat diet on body weight and cardiovascular risk factors in healthy women. *J Clin Endocrinol Metab.* 2003;88:1617-1623.
310. Yancy WS, Olsen MK, Guyton JR, et al. A low-carbohydrate, ketogenic diet versus a low-fat diet to treat obesity and hyperlipidemia. *Ann Intern Med.* 2004;140:769-777.
311. Stern L, Iqbal N, Seshadri P, et al. The effects of low-carbohydrate versus conventional weight loss diets in severely obese adults: one-year follow up of a randomized trial. *Ann Intern Med.* 2004;140:778-785.
312. Dansinger ML, Gleason JA, Griffith JL, et al. Comparison of the Atkins, Ornish, Weight Watchers, and Zone diets for weight loss and heart disease risk reduction: a randomized trial. *JAMA.* 2005;293:43-53.
313. Boden G, Sargrad K, Homko C, et al. Effect of a low-carbohydrate diet on appetite, blood glucose levels, and insulin resistance in obese patients with type 2 diabetes. *Ann Intern Med.* 2005;142:403-411.
314. Sacks FM, Bray GA, Carey VJ, et al. Comparison of weight-loss diets with different compositions of fat, protein, and carbohydrates. *N Engl J Med.* 2009;360:859-873.
315. Shai I, Schwarzfuchs D, Henkin Y, et al; Dietary Intervention Randomized Controlled Trial (DIRECT) Group. Weight loss with a low-carbohydrate, Mediterranean, or low-fat diet. *N Engl J Med.* 2008;359:229-241.
316. Ballor DL, Poehlman ET. A meta-analysis of the effects of exercise and/or dietary restriction on resting metabolic rate. *Eur J Appl Physiol Occup Physiol.* 1995;71:535-542.
317. Garrow JS, Summerbell CD. Meta-analysis: effect of exercise, with or without dieting, on the body composition of overweight subjects. *Eur J Clin Nutr.* 1995;49:1-10.
318. Warwick PM, Garrow JS. The effect of addition of exercise to a regime of dietary restriction on weight loss, nitrogen balance, resting metabolic rate and spontaneous physical activity in three obese women in a metabolic ward. *Int J Obes Relat Metab Disord.* 1981;5:25-32.
319. Holloszy JO, Schultz J, Kusnierkiewicz J, et al. Effects of exercise on glucose tolerance and insulin resistance. *Acta Med Scand.* 1986;711:55-65.
320. Helmrich SP, Ragland DR, Leung RW, Paffenbarger Jr RS. Physical activity and reduced occurrence of non-insulin-dependent diabetes mellitus. *N Engl J Med.* 1991;325:147-152.
321. Wei M, Gibbons L, Mitchell T, et al. The association between cardiorespiratory fitness and impaired fasting glucose and type 2 diabetes mellitus in men. *Ann Intern Med.* 1999;130:89-96.
322. Lee CD, Blair SN, Jackson AS. Cardiorespiratory fitness, body composition, and all-cause and cardiovascular disease mortality in men. *Am J Clin Nutr.* 1999;69:373-380.
323. Klem ML, Wing RR, McGuire MT, et al. A descriptive study of individuals successful at long-term maintenance of substantial weight loss. *Am J Clin Nutr.* 1997;66:239-246.
324. Kayman S, Bruvold W, Stern JS. Maintenance and relapse after weight loss in women: behavioral aspects. *Am J Clin Nutr.* 1990;52:800-807.
325. Hill JO, Schlundt DG, Sbrocco T, et al. Evaluation of an alternating-calorie diet with and without exercise in the treatment of obesity. *Am J Clin Nutr.* 1989;50:248-254.
326. Schoeller DA, Shay K, Kushner RF. How much physical activity is needed to minimize weight gain in previously obese women? *Am J Clin Nutr.* 1997;66:551-556.
327. Jakicic JM, Wing RR, Winters D. Effects of intermittent exercise and use of home exercise equipment on adherence, weight loss, and fitness in overweight women. *JAMA.* 1999;282:1554-1560.
328. Wadden TA, Berkowitz RI, Womble LG, et al. Randomized trial of lifestyle modification and pharmacotherapy for obesity. *N Engl J Med.* 2005;353:2111-2120.
329. Wadden TA, Sarwer DB, Berkowitz RI. Behavioural treatment of the overweight patient. *Bailliere's Clin Endocrin Metab.* 1999;13:93-107.
330. Wadden TA, Foster GD. Behavioral treatment of obesity. *Med Clin North Am.* 2000;84:441-461.
331. Perri MG, Nezu AM, Viegener BJ. *Improving the Long-Term Management of Obesity: Theory, Research and Clinical Guidelines.* New York, NY: John Wiley and Sons; 1992.
332. Sjostrom L, Rissanen A, Andersen T, et al. Randomised placebo-controlled trial of orlistat for weight loss and prevention of weight regain in obese patients. *Lancet.* 1998;352:167-172.
333. Weintraub M, Sundaresan PR, Schuster B, et al. Long-term weight control study V (weeks 190 to 210): follow-up of participants after cessation of medication. *Clin Pharmacol Ther.* 1992;51:615-618.
334. Lean ME. Sibutramine: a review of clinical efficacy. *Int J Obes Relat Metab Disord.* 1997;21(suppl 1):S30-S36.
335. Khan MA, Herzog CA, St Peter JV, et al. The prevalence of cardiac valvular insufficiency assessed by transthoracic echocardiography in obese patients treated with appetite-suppressant drugs. *N Engl J Med.* 1998;339:713-718.
336. Kernan WN, Viscoli CM, Brass LM, et al. Phenylpropanolamine and the risk of hemorrhagic stroke. *N Engl J Med.* 2000;343:1826-1832.
337. Hansen DL, Toubro S, Stock MJ, et al. Thermogenic effects of sibutramine in humans. *Am J Clin Nutr.* 1998;68:1180-1186.
338. National Institutes of Health; National Heart, Lung, and Blood Institute; North American Association for the Study of Obesity. *Practical Guide to the Identification, Evaluation, and Treatment of Overweight and Obesity in Adults.* NIH Publication Number 00-4084. Bethesda, MD: National Institutes of Health; 2000.
339. Bray GA, Blackburn GL, Ferguson JM, et al. Sibutramine produces dose-related weight loss. *Obes Res.* 1999;7:189-198.
340. McMahon FG, Fujioka K, Singh BN, et al. Efficacy and safety of sibutramine in obese white and African American patients with hypertension: a 1-year, double-blind, placebo-controlled, multicenter trial. *Arch Intern Med.* 2000;160:2185-2191.
341. Smith IG, Goulder MA, for the Sibutramine Clinical Study 1047 Team. Randomized placebo-controlled trial of long-term treatment with sibutramine in mild to moderate obesity. *J Fam Pract.* 2001;50:505-512.
342. Wirth A, Krause J. Long-term weight loss with sibutramine: a randomized controlled trial. *JAMA.* 2001;286:1331-1339.
343. McNulty SJ, Ur E, Williams G, for the Multicenter Sibutramine Study Group. A randomized trial of sibutramine in the management of obese type 2 diabetic patients treated with metformin. *Diabetes Care.* 2003;26:125-131.
344. Hauner H, Meier M, Wendland G, et al. Weight reduction by sibutramine in obese subjects in primary care medicine: the SAT study. *Exp Clin Endocrinol Diabetes.* 2004;112:201-207.
345. Kaukua JK, Pekkarinen TA, Rissanen AM. Health-related quality of life in a randomised placebo-controlled trial of sibutramine in obese patients with type II diabetes. *Int J Obes Relat Metab Disord.* 2004;28:600-605.
346. Porter JA, Raebel MA, Conner DA, et al. The Long-term Outcomes of Sibutramine Effectiveness on Weight (LOSE Weight) study: Evaluating the role of drug therapy within a weight management program in a group-model health maintenance organization. *Am J Manag Care.* 2004;10:369-376.
347. Padwal R, Li SK, Lau DC. Long-term pharmacotherapy for overweight and obesity: a systematic review and meta-analysis of randomized controlled trials. *Int J Obes Relat Metab Disord.* 2003;27:1437-1446.
348. Li Z, Maglione M, Tu W, et al. Meta-analysis: pharmacologic treatment of obesity. *Ann Intern Med.* 2005;142:532-546.
349. Apfelbaum M, Vague P, Ziegler O, et al. Long-term maintenance of weight loss after a very-low-calorie diet: a randomized blinded trial of the efficacy and tolerability of sibutramine. *Am J Med.* 1999;106:179-184.
350. James WPT, Astrup A, Finer N, et al. Effect of sibutramine on weight maintenance after weight loss: a randomized trial. *Lancet.* 2000;356:2119-2125.
351. Hadvary P, Lengsfield H, Wolfer H. Inhibition of pancreatic lipase in vitro by the covalent inhibitor tetrahydrolipstatin. *Biochem J.* 1998;256:357-361.
352. Zhi J, Melia AT, Guerciolini R, et al. Retrospective population-based analysis of the dose-response (fecal fat excretion) relationship of orlistat in normal and obese volunteers. *Clin Pharmacol Ther.* 1994;56:82-86.

353. Zhi J, Melia AT, Funk C, et al. Metabolic profiles of minimally absorbed orlistat in obese/overweight volunteers. *J Clin Pharmacol.* 1996;36:1006-1011.
354. Torgerson JS, Hauptman J, Boldrin MN, et al. XENical in the Prevention of Diabetes in Obese Subjects (XENDOS) study: a randomized study of orlistat as an adjunct to lifestyle changes for the prevention of type 2 diabetes in obese patients. *Diabetes Care.* 2004;27:155-161.
355. Sjöström L, Rissanen A, Andersen T, et al. Randomised placebo-controlled trial of orlistat for weight loss and prevention of weight regain in obese patients. *Lancet.* 1998;352:167-172.
356. Davidson MH, Hauptman J, DiGirolamo M, et al. Weight control and risk factor reduction in obese subjects treated for 2 years with orlistat. *JAMA.* 1999;281:235-242.
357. Mittendorfer B, Ostlund R, Patterson BW, et al. Orlistat inhibits dietary cholesterol absorption. *Obes Res.* 2001;9:599-604.
358. Rössner S, Sjöström L, Noack R, et al. Weight loss, weight maintenance, and improved cardiovascular risk factors after 2 years treatment with orlistat for obesity. *Obes Res.* 2000;8:49-61.
359. Finer N, James WP, Kopelman PG, et al. One-year treatment of obesity: a randomized, double-blind, placebo-controlled, multicentre study of orlistat, a gastrointestinal lipase inhibitor. *Int J Obes Relat Metab Disord.* 2000;24:306-313.
360. Hollander PA, Elbein SC, Hirsch IB, et al. Role of orlistat in the treatment of obese patients with type 2 diabetes. *Diabetes Care.* 1998;21:1288-1294.
361. Colman E, Fossler M. Reduction in blood cyclosporin concentrations by orlistat. *N Engl J Med.* 2000;342:1141-1142.
362. U.K. Prospective Diabetes Study Group. Effect of intensive blood glucose control with metformin on complications in overweight patients with type 2 diabetes (UKPDS 34). *Lancet.* 1998;352:854-865.
363. Golay A. Metformin and body weight. *Int J Obes (Lond).* 2008;32:61-72.
364. Kahn SE, Haffner SM, Heise MA, et al. Glycemic durability of rosiglitazone, metformin, or glyburide monotherapy. *N Engl J Med.* 2006;355:2427-2443.
365. Levri KM, Slaymaker E, Last A, et al. Metformin as treatment for overweight and obese adults: a systematic review. *Ann Fam Med.* 2005;3:457-461.
366. Monami M, Marchionni N, Mannucci E. Glucagon-like peptide-1 receptor agonists in type 2 diabetes: a meta-analysis of randomized clinical trials. *Eur J Endocrinol.* 2009;160:909-917.
367. Amori RE, Lau J, Pittas AG. Efficacy and safety of incretin therapy in type 2 diabetes: systematic review and meta-analysis. *JAMA.* 2007;298:194-206.
368. Zinman B, Gerich J, Buse JB, et al. Efficacy and safety of the human glucagon-like peptide-1 analog liraglutide in combination with metformin and thiazolidinedione in patients with type 2 diabetes (LEAD-4 Met+TZD). *Diabetes Care.* 2009;32:1224-1230.
369. Astrup A, Rössner S, Van Gaal L, et al. NN8022-1807 Study Group. Effects of liraglutide in the treatment of obesity: a randomised, double-blind, placebo-controlled study. *Lancet.* 2009;374:1606-1616.
370. Aronne L, Fujioka K, Aroda V, et al. Progressive reduction in body weight after treatment with the amylin analog pramlintide in obese subjects: a phase 2, randomized, placebo-controlled, dose-escalation study. *J Clin Endocrinol Metab.* 2007;92:2977-2983.
371. Smith SR, Aronne LJ, Burns CM, et al. Sustained weight loss following 12-month pramlintide treatment as an adjunct to lifestyle intervention in obesity. *Diabetes Care.* 2008;31:1816-1823.
372. Consensus Development Conference Panel. NIH Conference: Gastrointestinal surgery for severe obesity. *Ann Intern Med.* 1991;115:956-961.
373. Brolin RE, Kenler HA, Gorman JH, et al. Long-limb gastric bypass in the superobese: a prospective randomized study. *Ann Surg.* 1992;215:387-395.
374. Mason EE. Vertical banded gastroplasty for obesity. *Arch Surg.* 1982;117:701-706.
375. Eckhout GV, Willibanks OL, Moore JT. Vertical ring gastroplasty for morbid obesity: five year experience with 1,463 patients. *Am J Surg.* 1986;152:713-716.
376. MacLean LD, Rhode BM, Sampalis J, et al. Results of the surgical treatment of obesity. *Am J Surg.* 1993;165:155-162.
377. Sugerman HJ, Starkey JV, Birkenhauer RA. A randomized prospective trial of gastric bypass versus vertical banded gastroplasty and their effects on sweets versus non-sweets eaters. *Ann Surg.* 1987;205:613-624.
378. Hall JC, Watts JM, O'Brien PE, et al. Gastric surgery for morbid obesity: the Adelaide study. *Ann Surg.* 1990;211:419-427.
379. Howard L, Malone M, Michalek A, et al. Gastric bypass and vertical banded gastroplasty: a prospective randomized comparison and 5-year follow-up. *Obes Surg.* 1995;5:55-60.
380. Balsiger BM, Kelly KA, Poggio JL, et al. Long term prospective follow-up (>10 years) after vertical banded gastroplasty (VBG). *Gastroenterology.* 2000;118:A1060.
381. Belachew M, Legrand M, Vincent V, et al. Laparoscopic adjustable gastric banding. *World J Surg.* 1998;22:955-963.
382. DeMaria EJ, Sugerman HJ, Kellum JM, et al. High failure rate following laparoscopic adjustable silicone gastric banding for treatment of morbid obesity. *Ann Surg.* 2001;233:809-818.
383. O'Brien PE, Dixon JB. Lap-band: outcomes and results. *J Laparoendosc Adv Surg Tech A.* 2003;13:265-270.
384. Gustavsson S. Laparoscopic adjustable gastric banding: a caution. *Surgery.* 2000;127:489-490.
385. Scopinaro N, Adami GF, Marinari GM, et al. Biliopancreatic diversion. *World J Surg.* 1998;22:936-946.
386. Marceau P, Hould FS, Simard S, et al. Biliopancreatic diversion with duodenal switch. *World J Surg.* 1998;22:947-954.
387. Clare MW. Reversals on 504 biliopancreatic surgeries over 12 years. *Obes Surg.* 1993;3:169-173.
388. Dixon JB, O'Brien PE, Playfair J, et al. Adjustable gastric banding and conventional therapy for type 2 diabetes: a randomized controlled trial. *JAMA* 2008 23;299:316-323.
389. Buchwald H, Estok R, Fahrbach K, et al. Weight and type 2 diabetes after bariatric surgery: systematic review and meta-analysis. *Am J Med.* 2009;122:248-256 e245.
390. Buchwald H, Avidor Y, Braunwald E, et al. Bariatric surgery: a systematic review and meta-analysis. *JAMA.* 2004;292:1724-1737.
391. Pories WJ, Swanson MS, MacDonald, et al. Who would have thought it? An operation proves to be the most effective therapy for adult-onset diabetes mellitus. *Ann Surg.* 1995;222(3):339-350; discussion 350-352.
392. Hickey MS, Pories WJ, MacDonald Jr DG, et al. A new paradigm for type 2 diabetes mellitus: could it be a disease of the foregut? *Ann Surg.* 1998;227:637-643; discussion 643-644.
393. Pories WJ, Albrecht RJ. Etiology of type II diabetes mellitus: role of the foregut. *World J Surg.* 2001;25:527-531.
394. Laferrère B, Teixeira J, McGinty J, et al. Effect of weight loss by gastric bypass surgery versus hypocaloric diet on glucose and incretin levels in patients with type 2 diabetes. *J Clin Endocrinol Metab.* 2008;93:2479-2485.
395. Olivan B, Teixeira J, Bose M, et al. Effect of weight loss by diet or gastric bypass surgery on peptide YY3-36 levels. *Ann Surg.* 2009;249:948-953.
396. Cohen RV, Schiavon CA, Pinheiro JS, et al. Duodenal-jejunal bypass for the treatment of type 2 diabetes in patients with body mass index of 22-34 kg/m2: a report of 2 cases. *Surg Obes Realt Dis.* 2007;3:195-197.
397. Rubino F, Forgione A, Cummings D, et al. The mechanism of diabetes control after gastrointestinal bypass surgery reveals a role of the proximal small intestine in the pathophysiology of type 2 diabetes. *Ann Surg.* 2006;244:741-749.
398. Moo Ta, Rubino F. Gastrointestinal surgery as treatment for type 2 diabetes. *Curr Opin Endocrinol Diab Obes* 2008, 15: 153-158.
399. Lee WJ, Lee YC, Ser KH, et al. Improvement of insulin resistance after obesity surgery: a comparison of gastric banding and bypass procedures. *Obes Surg.* 2008;9:1119-1125.
400. De Paula, A, Prudente A, Queiroz L, et al. Laparoscopic sleeve gastrectomy with ileal interposition ("neuroendocrine brake"): pilot study of a new operation. *Surg Obes Dis.* 2006;2:464-467.
401. Vidal J, Nicolau J, Romero F, et al. Long-term effects of Roux-en-Y gastric bypass surgery on plasma glucagon-like peptide-1 and islet function in morbidly obese subjects. *J Clin Endocrinol Metab.* 2009;94:884-891.
402. Salinari S, Bertuzzi A, Asnaghi S, et al. First-phase insulin secretion restoration and differential response to glucose load depending on the route of administration in type 2 diabetic subjects after bariatric surgery. *Diabetes Care.* 2009;32:375-380.
403. Ferrannini E, Mingrone G. Impact of different bariatric surgical procedures on insulin action and beta-cell function in type 2 diabetes. *Diabetes Care.* 2009;32:514-520.
404. Service GJ, Thompson GB, Service FJ, et al. Hyperinsulinemic hypoglycemia with nesidioblastosis after gastric bypass surgery. *N Engl J Med.* 2005;353:249-254.
405. Patti ME, McMahon G, Mun EC, et al. Severe hypoglycaemia post-gastric bypass requiring partial pancreatectomy: evidence for inappropriate insulin secretion and pancreatic islet hyperplasia. *Diabetologia.* 2005;48:2236-2240.
406. Goldfine AB, Mun EC, Devine E, et al. Patients with neuroglycopenia after gastric bypass surgery have exaggerated incretin and insulin secretory responses to a mixed meal. *J Clin Endocrinol Metab.* 2007;92:4678-4685.
407. Sugerman HJ, Kellum JM, Engle KM, et al. Gastric bypass for treating severe obesity. *Am J Clin Nutr.* 1992;55:560S-566S.

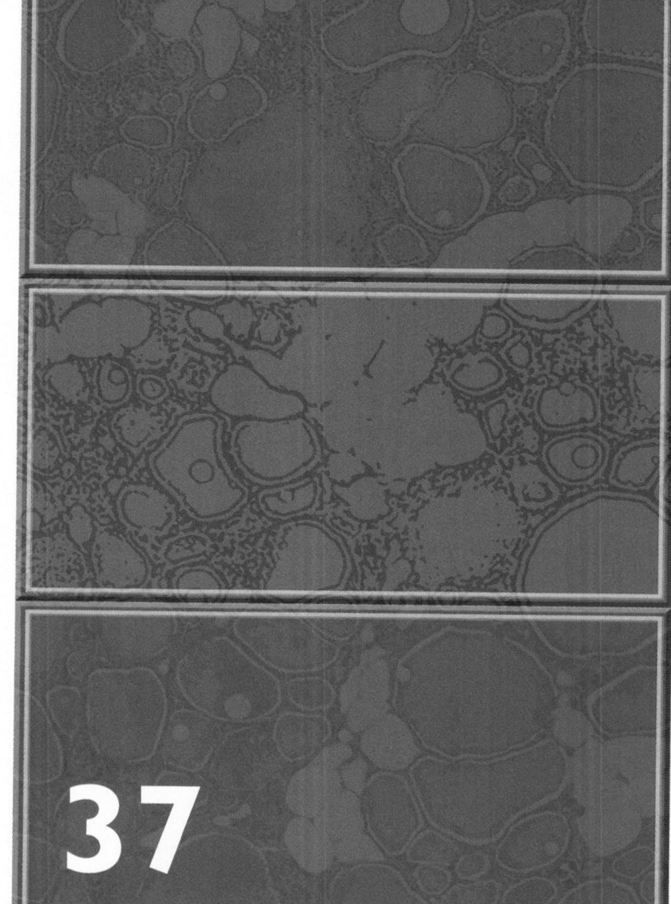

CHAPTER 37

Disorders of Lipid Metabolism

CLAY F. SEMENKOVICH • ANNE C. GOLDBERG • IRA J. GOLDBERG

LIPID BIOCHEMISTRY AND METABOLISM

Almost every endocrine disorder has important effects on serum or tissue lipids, making the mechanisms underlying primary and secondary disorders of lipid metabolism relevant to clinicians as well as basic scientists. Some primary disorders of lipid metabolism, such as familial hypercholesterolemia (FH), are uncommon but important to understand because they help explain genetic predispositions to heart disease[1] and the mechanism of action of statin drugs, which decrease the risk of vascular events and prolong life.[2] The quintessential secondary disorder of lipid metabolism is that seen in diabetes, a disease so frequently characterized by abnormalities of fat that lipids have been implicated in its pathogenesis.[3]

Lipids are ubiquitous. They constitute the physical bilayer that allows the formation of cell membranes, which are required for specialized organelles inside the cell and for regulating transport between the extracellular and intracellular environments. They circulate in the blood, with fatty acids and triglycerides providing an energy source to tissues such as heart and skeletal muscle and non-nutritive sterols providing substrates for hormone production by gonads and adrenals. Their specialized functions include the development of surfactant in lung to maintain patency of alveoli, formation of bile to facilitate excretion of a variety of metabolites, and constitution of myelin throughout the nervous system to ensure the fidelity of nerve transmission. Lipids are also signaling molecules, serving as targets of lipid kinases that perpetuate signaling cascades, substrates for cyclooxygenases and related enzymes that generate prostaglandins, and ligands for nuclear receptors such as the peroxisome proliferator-activated receptors (PPARs). The broad spectrum of lipid functions results in part from their biophysical characteristics.

Simple and Complex Lipids

Lipids owe their functional versatility to their hydrophobic structure. Because of the presence of fairly long carbon chains, lipids tend to associate with each other and have limited or no solubility in water. Fatty acids and cholesterol are simple lipids, whereas triglycerides and phospholipids are complex lipids (Fig. 37-1).

Fatty Acids

Chemical structures for the fatty acids are determined by the number of carbon atoms and the number of double bonds (see Fig. 37-1A). For example, stearic acid has 18

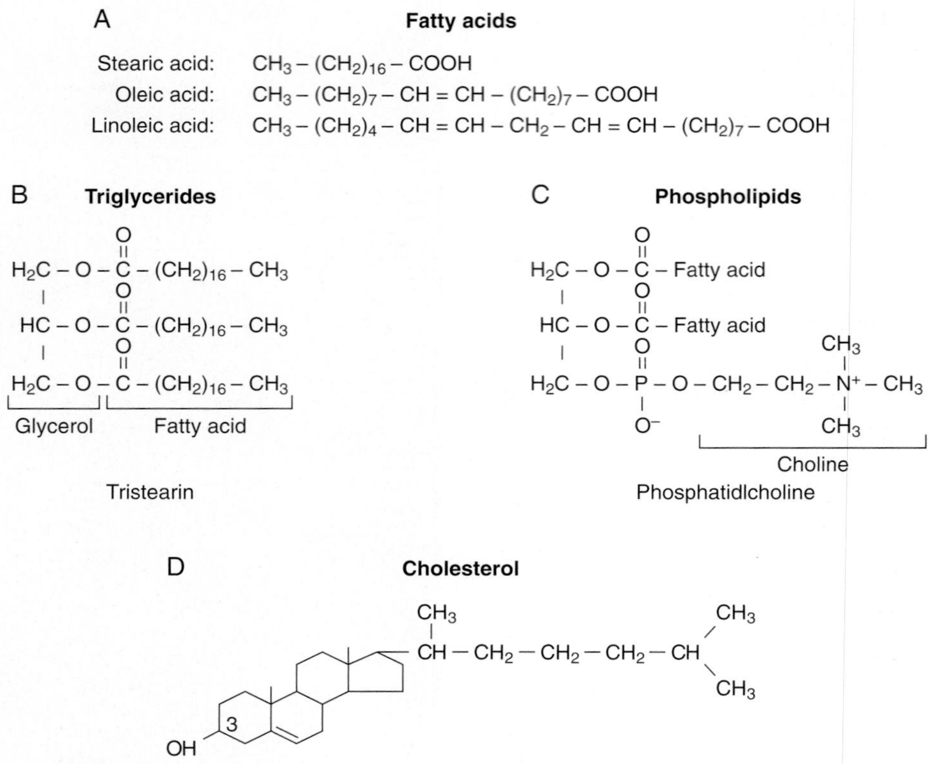

A **Fatty acids**

Stearic acid: $CH_3-(CH_2)_{16}-COOH$

Oleic acid: $CH_3-(CH_2)_7-CH=CH-(CH_2)_7-COOH$

Linoleic acid: $CH_3-(CH_2)_4-CH=CH-CH_2-CH=CH-(CH_2)_7-COOH$

B **Triglycerides**

$H_2C-O-C(=O)-(CH_2)_{16}-CH_3$

$HC-O-C(=O)-(CH_2)_{16}-CH_3$

$H_2C-O-C(=O)-(CH_2)_{16}-CH_3$

Glycerol Fatty acid

Tristearin

C **Phospholipids**

$H_2C-O-C(=O)-$ Fatty acid

$HC-O-C(=O)-$ Fatty acid

$H_2C-O-P(=O)(O^-)-O-CH_2-CH_2-N^+(CH_3)_2-CH_3$

Choline

Phosphatidlcholine

D **Cholesterol**

CH_3, $CH-CH_2-CH_2-CH_2-CH(CH_3)_2$

3, OH

Figure 37-1 Structures of common lipids, exemplified by the stearic, oleic, and linoleic fatty acids **(A)**, the triglyceride tristearin **(B)**, the phospholipid phosphatidylcholine **(C)**, and cholesterol **(D)**.

carbon atoms and is saturated, meaning that it has no double bonds; this is designated by the abbreviation C18:0. The 18-carbon monounsaturated fatty acid oleic acid (C18:1) has one double bond, and the polyunsaturated fatty acid linoleic acid (C18:2) has two double bonds.

Linoleic acid and arachidonic acid (C20:4) are ω-6 fatty acids, meaning that a double bond is present at the sixth carbon from the end of the molecule farthest from the carboxyl (-COOH) terminus. Fish oils, which lower lipids and are both cardioprotective and neuroprotective, are ω-3 fatty acids, with a double bond present at the third carbon from the end opposite the COOH. Saturated fatty acids and some unsaturated fatty acids such as oleic acid are nonessential, meaning that they can be synthesized in the body. Most ω-6 and ω-3 fatty acids are essential; they cannot be synthesized and are usually required for health, especially during development and in times of physiologic stress. Table 37-1 shows major food sources of fatty acids.

Triglycerides

The structure of tristearin, a triglyceride with three molecules of stearic acid connected to a glycerol molecule by means of ester linkages, is shown in Figure 37-1B. Other triglycerides have a similar structure with alternative fatty acids esterified to the glycerol backbone.

Most of the mass of adipose tissue in the body is composed of triglycerides; triglycerides that circulate in the blood mostly reflect the fatty acid composition of adipose tissue triglycerides, and both sources reflect dietary fatty acid composition. Butter as a source of triglycerides in Western diets consists of similar amounts of palmitate and oleate with a lesser amount of stearate, so adipose tissue and circulating triglycerides in persons consuming such a diet consist mostly of these fatty acids. Olive oil as a source of triglycerides in Mediterranean diets is predominantly oleate with much less palmitate, so fat and circulating triglycerides in people consuming that diet are enriched in oleic acid. Extremely high levels of triglycerides in the blood predispose to pancreatitis.

Phospholipids

The chemical structure for a generic phosphatidylcholine, a type of phospholipid, is shown in Figure 37-1C. As with triglycerides, phospholipids have a glycerol backbone to

TABLE 37-1

Major Fatty Acids

Chemical Designation	Common Name	Common Food
Saturated Fatty Acids (No Double Bonds)		
C12 : 0	Lauric	Coconut oil
C14 : 0	Myristic	Coconut oil, butter fat
C16 : 0	Palmitic	Butter, cheese, meat
C18 : 0	Stearic	Beef, chocolate
Monounsaturated Fatty Acids (One Double Bond)		
C18 : 1	Oleic	Olive and canola oils
Polyunsaturated Fatty Acids (Two or More Double Bonds)		
Omega-6 fatty acids		
C18 : 2	Linoleic	Sunflower, corn, soybean, and safflower oils
C20 : 4	Arachidonic	
Omega-3 fatty acids		
C18 : 3	α-Linolenic	Canola, flaxseed, and soybean oils
C20 : 5	Eicosapentaenoic (EPA)	Salmon, cod, mackerel, tuna
C22 : 6	Docosahexaenoic (DHA)	Salmon, cod, mackerel, tuna

which fatty acids are esterified at the first two alcohols. However, the third position is occupied by a phosphate moiety to which another charged molecule, such as choline, ethanolamine, or serine, is attached.

The presence of long-chain fatty acids comprising hydrophobic regions and the charged species at the end of the molecule make phospholipids perfect for generating cell membranes and lipoprotein surface components: The bilayer is oriented so that the hydrophobic regions point toward each other, and the hydrophilic regions interact with the aqueous environment. Phospholipids are distributed asymmetrically in cell membranes, with choline-containing lipids directed toward the outer surface and amine-containing lipids directed toward the cytoplasmic surface. Appearance of the aminophospholipid phosphatidylserine on the cell surface initiates blood clotting and marks apoptotic cells for phagocytosis.[4]

Cholesterol

The structure of cholesterol is shown in Figure 37-1D. The presence of cholesterol in the plasma membrane is critical for maintaining membrane fluidity, probably by disrupting the interactions between phosphatidylcholine and other molecules.[5] The concentration of cholesterol is enriched in the plasma membrane, with much lower levels detected in the membranes of most intracellular organelles. Cholesterol is necessary for the synthesis of estrogen, progestins, androgens, aldosterone, vitamin D, glucocorticoids, and bile acids. Cholesterol deficiency is associated with severe developmental defects, as manifested in the rare Smith-Lemli-Optiz syndrome, which is likely caused by disruption of the Hedgehog signal transduction pathway.[6] Cholesterol excess is associated with gallstones and vascular disease.

Fatty Acid Metabolism

Fatty Acid Biosynthesis

In humans eating a typical Western diet, the overall contribution of de novo lipogenesis to lipid metabolism is small[7] because the ingestion of exogenous fat is sufficient to suppress the energy-requiring process of synthesizing fats from carbohydrates. However, high-carbohydrate diets, especially those containing fructose,[8] substantially increase lipogenesis in liver and adipose tissue of humans.

Most tissues carry out fatty acid biosynthesis to at least a small degree regardless of nutritional status. Several of the key steps in fatty acid biosynthesis, presented in Figure 37-2, also have major effects on systemic metabolism. Citrate derived from the tricarboxylic acid (TCA) cycle is converted to acetyl-coenzyme A (acetyl-CoA) in the cytoplasm by the action of adenosine triphosphate (ATP) citrate lyase. Acetyl-CoA is then converted to malonyl-CoA by acetyl-CoA carboxylase (ACC), which exists in two isoforms. ACC1 (encoded by the gene *ACACA*) is cytosolic and important in liver and fat for de novo lipogenesis. ACC2 (ACACB) is associated with mitochondria and also plays a role in liver metabolism, but is expressed at highest levels in muscle and heart. Antisense targeting of ACC isoforms has been shown to improve lipid metabolism and insulin sensitivity.[9]

Malonyl-CoA inhibits carnitine palmitoyltransferase 1 (CPT1), which transports fatty acids into mitochondria, thereby preventing the catabolism of fats under physiologic conditions in which energy is being stored as fat through fatty acid biosynthesis. Malonyl-CoA also serves as substrate for fatty acid synthase, which sequentially connects two carbon fragments to generate saturated fatty acids such as palmitate. Inhibition of fatty acid synthase

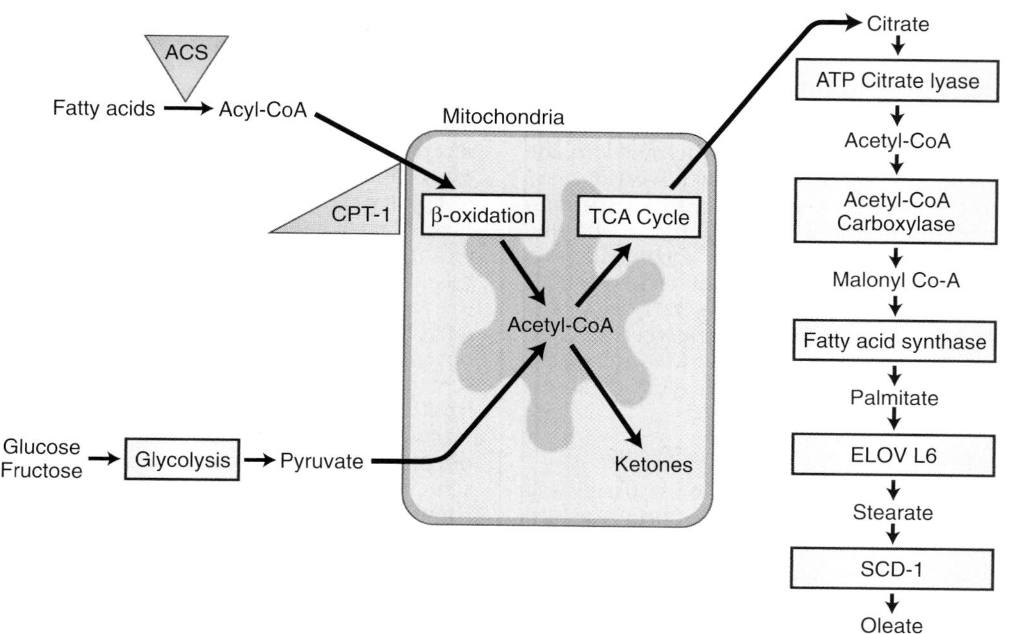

Figure 37-2 Fatty acid metabolism. Fatty acids are substrates for acyl-CoA synthase (ACS), which generates CoA moieties that are transported into mitochondria by carnitine palmitoyltransferase I (CPT-1). Here, β-oxidation generates acetyl-CoA, which can also be generated from glycolysis *(bottom left)*. Acetyl-CoA can be used to produce ketones, or it may enter the TCA cycle, leading to production of citrate; in the cytoplasm, citrate is a substrate for ATP citrate lyase, which produces acetyl-CoA. The acetyl-CoA serves as a substrate for de novo synthesis of fatty acids, as depicted on the right side of the figure. ATP, adenosine triphosphate; CoA, coenzyme A; ELOVL6, elongation of very-long-chain fatty acids protein 6; SCD-1, stearoyl-CoA desaturase 1; TCA tricarboxylic acid.

in the hypothalamus suppresses appetite, inducing weight loss and improving insulin sensitivity.[10] Palmitate is converted to stearate through the action of a long-chain fatty acid elongase, which, when inactivated, promotes obesity but prevents insulin resistance.[11] Stearate is subsequently converted to oleate by stearoyl-CoA desaturase 1, which, when inactivated, increases fatty acid oxidation and protects against diet-induced obesity and insulin resistance.[12]

Fatty Acid Oxidation

Metabolism of fatty acids provides more energy than does metabolism of carbohydrates or proteins. This facile production of ATP occurs in mitochondria after fatty acids undergo the process of β-oxidation (see Fig. 37-2). Fatty acids are transported across (or diffuse across) the plasma membrane, are converted to acyl-CoA species by acyl-CoA synthase, and are then translocated to the mitochondrial matrix by CPT1 and CPT2. β-Oxidation removes two carbon fragments through the sequential actions of acyl-CoA dehydrogenases (e.g., MCAD and VLCAD), enoyl-CoA hydratase, hydroxy-CoA dehydrogenase, and thiolase. This process generates reduced nicotinamide adenine dinucleotide (NADH) and reduced flavin adenine dinucleotide (FADH), which participate in electron transport to yield ATP. After multiple cycles, acetyl-CoA is produced, which is a substrate for the TCA cycle and for ketogenesis.

Ketogenesis is necessary for life during times of nutritional deprivation. Extreme production of ketones occurs in the setting of insulin deficiency and represents a threat to life. 3-Hydroxy-3-methylglutaryl-coenzyme A (HMG-CoA) synthase (rate-limiting in mitochondria) converts acetyl-CoA to hydroxy-methylglutaryl-CoA, which is converted to acetoacetate by HMG-CoA lyase. Acetoacetate is either reduced to β-hydroxybutyrate or converted to acetone.

Defects in fatty acid oxidation are among the most common inborn errors of metabolism. Presentations include nonketotic hypoglycemia, liver dysfunction, and cardiomyopathy.[13]

Triglyceride and Phospholipid Metabolism

Dietary fat consists of mostly triglycerides with lesser amounts of phospholipids, which are digested in the stomach and proximal small intestine. Triglycerides are broken down into component fatty acids in part through the action of pancreatic lipase, which is activated by bile acids. Bile salts form micelles that acquire fatty acids and interact with the unstirred water layer of the intestine, where fatty acids are absorbed. Long-chain fatty acids are taken up by enterocytes, re-esterified into triglycerides, and exported into the lymph as lipoproteins. Medium-chain (≤C10) fatty acids directly enter the portal vein to access the liver.

Lipolysis of Triglyceride Stores in Adipose Tissue

The greatest triglyceride mass resides in adipose tissue, and turnover of energy stores at this site has important effects on lipid metabolism, normal physiology, and human health. Increased lipolysis in adipose tissue of the obese results in elevated circulating levels of free fatty acids, which may contribute to so-called lipotoxicity in tissues such as pancreatic beta cells, liver, skeletal muscle, and heart.[14] Otherwise healthy subjects whose parents have type 2 diabetes mellitus have impaired insulin-mediated suppression of circulating fatty acids,[15] consistent with an early defect in adipose tissue fatty acid metabolism contributing to the evolution of diabetes.

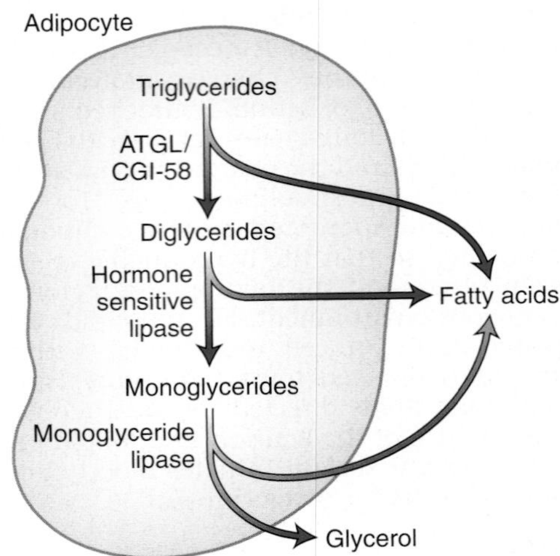

Figure 37-3 Lipolysis in adipocytes. Stored triglycerides are metabolized to yield the fatty acids that circulate in plasma through the action of three distinct lipases with separate substrate specificities. Triglycerides are acted on by adipose triglyceride lipase (ATGL) in complex with the coactivator protein CGI-58 to yield diglycerides, which are acted on by hormone-sensitive lipase to yield monoglycerides. The monoglycerides, in turn, are acted on by monoglyceride lipase to yield glycerol. Lipid droplet proteins modulate this lipolytic process.

Release of free fatty acids and glycerol from adipose tissue is controlled by a variety of hormones, many of which act through G protein–coupled receptors. The most robust mediators of fatty acid release are catecholamines, which bind to β-adrenergic receptors, activating stimulatory G proteins (G_s) that prompt an increase in the activity of cyclic adenosine monophosphate and protein kinase A. Glucagon, adrenocorticotropic hormone, α-melanocyte-stimulating hormone, and thyroid-stimulating hormone also induce lipolysis through activity of G_s proteins. Several agents suppress lipolysis by binding to receptors that activate inhibitory G proteins (G_i). These include adenosine and the clinically useful vitamin niacin, which binds to the nicotinic G-protein receptor GPR109A.[16] A major mediator of lipolytic inhibition is insulin, which activates the insulin receptor signaling cascade and suppresses lipolysis at many steps, one of which includes a decrease in protein kinase A activity.

At least three enzymes and two accessory proteins are required for the normal process of hormone-induced lipolysis in adipose tissue.[17] Stored triglycerides are acted on by the recently discovered enzyme, adipose triglyceride lipase (encoded by *PNPLA2*), which requires the coactivator protein CGI-58. Diglycerides are hydrolyzed by hormone-sensitive lipase, yielding monoglycerides that are metabolized by monoglyceride lipase. This process cannot occur unless perilipin, a protein that coats small lipid droplets, is phosphorylated by protein kinase A. This process is depicted schematically in Figure 37-3. Human mutations in adipose triglyceride lipase or CGI-58 are responsible for two variants of neutral lipid storage disease that are characterized by hepatic steatosis, lipid accumulation in muscle tissues, neurologic problems, and, in one variant, skin defects.

Triglyceride and Phospholipid Synthesis and Tissue Delivery of Lipids

Triglyceride Synthesis. As with fatty acid biosynthesis, some of the key steps in triglyceride synthesis also have major effects on systemic metabolism. Most triglycerides

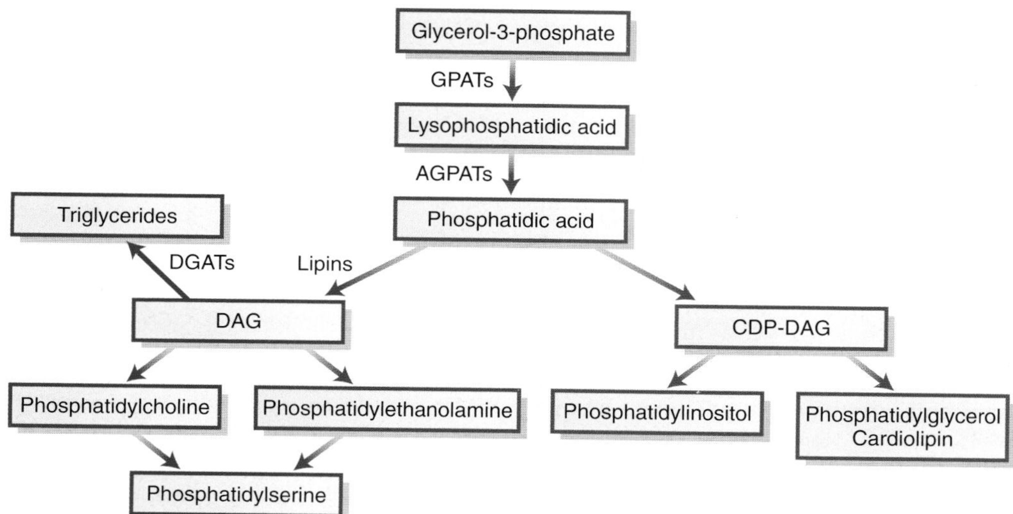

Figure 37-4 Phospholipid and triglyceride synthesis. Glycerol-3-phosphate is converted by glycerol-3-phosphate acyltransferases (GPATs) to lysophosphatidic acid, which is converted to phosphatidic acid by acylglycerol-phosphate acyltransferases (AGPATs). Phosphatidic acid can be converted to cytidine diphosphate diacylglycerol (CDP-DAG), to fuel one arm of phospholipid synthesis, or to diacylglycerol (DAG), which is a substrate for another arm of phospholipid synthesis and for acyl-CoA:diacylglycerol acyltransferases (DGATs), which generate triglycerides.

are synthesized through the glycerol phosphate pathway (Fig. 37-4, top portion) by a sequence of acylations. Another pathway, the monoacylglycerol pathway, is believed to be active only in the small intestine. Glycerol-3-phosphate is acted on by one of the glycerol-3-phosphate acyltransferases (GPATs) to generate lysophosphatidic acid. An important isoform is GPAT1, which is thought to compete with CPT1 for fatty acyl-CoA molecules inside the cell, with GPAT1 prevailing when energy is to be stored and CPT1 dominant when energy is required. The next acylation is mediated by acylglycerol-phosphate acyltransferases (AGPATs) and generates phosphatidic acid. Human mutations in AGPAT2 are responsible for the disease known as congenital generalized lipodystrophy.[18]

Phosphatidic acid represents an important branch point in lipid metabolism: It serves as substrate for synthesis of either cytidine diphosphate diacylglycerol (CDP-DAG, the precursor for molecules such as phosphatidylinositol) or diacylglycerol (DAG). Synthesis of DAG requires a phosphatase activity provided by lipins.[19] These recently described proteins modulate insulin sensitivity in adipose tissue,[20] perhaps by affecting expression of glucose transporter 4. DAG can serve as a signaling molecule and as substrate for synthesis of either triglycerides or common phospholipids. The acylation of DAG to form triglycerides is catalyzed by acyl-CoA:diacylglycerol acyltransferases (DGATs). Inactivation of DGAT1 renders mice resistant to diet-induced obesity.[21]

Phospholipid Synthesis. As shown in the bottom portion of Figure 37-4, phospholipid synthesis is intimately related to triglyceride synthesis. Generation of one of the most important phospholipids, phosphatidylcholine, occurs mostly through the Kennedy pathway, which utilizes choline as an initial substrate and DAG at the final step.[22] Mammalian liver is also able to generate phosphatidylcholine from phosphatidylethanolamine through successive methylations. Both phosphatidylcholine and phosphatidylethanolamine can be converted to phosphatidylserine.

Lipoprotein Lipase. Most lipids are delivered to peripheral tissues such as muscle and fat through the activity of lipoprotein lipase (LPL). LPL, which is rate-limiting for clearance of plasma triglycerides and essential for generation of high-density lipoprotein (HDL) particles,[23] hydrolyzes triglycerides (and, to a lesser extent, phospholipids) in circulating triglyceride-rich lipoproteins to allow peripheral sites such as adipose tissue and muscle access to preformed fatty acids. Much of this lipid flux is controlled by insulin, which increases LPL in fat and decreases LPL in muscle.[24] Exercise tends to have the opposite effect,[25] ensuring appropriate energy supplies are to meet metabolic demands.

Free fatty acids released from lipoproteins by the action of LPL presumably diffuse into resident cells in the local tissues, where they are converted to acyl-CoA species and either stored as triglycerides or subjected to fatty acid oxidation. This hydrolytic release reaction occurs at the capillary endothelium. LPL is not synthesized in endothelial cells but is produced in adipocytes, cardiac myocytes, and skeletal myocytes, then secreted and targeted to the luminal surface of the endothelium through mechanisms that are poorly understood. At the endothelium, LPL and triglyceride-rich lipoproteins bind to a recently discovered protein, glycosylphosphatidylinositol-anchored high-density lipoprotein–binding protein 1 (GPIHBP1).[26] GPIHBP1 is believed to serve as a platform for lipolysis in the plasma.

Cholesterol Metabolism

In adults, dietary cholesterol is not required because many tissues are capable of cholesterol synthesis. However, most diets include animal products, the source of cholesterol. Plants do not have cholesterol, but their membranes do contain phytosterols, which are structurally similar to cholesterol and are useful in the dietary treatment of hypercholesterolemia because they compete with cholesterol for absorption. The liver[27] and intestine are quantitatively the most important sites for cholesterol metabolism in humans, although a very small amount of cholesterol is also lost through the normal turnover of skin.

Cholesterol Absorption, Synthesis, and Excretion

Cholesterol is absorbed through a process that requires the formation of bile salt micelles. The efficiency of absorption varies widely in humans.[28] There is a gradient of absorption through the intestine that is greatest in the proximal small intestine and least in the ileum. This gradient parallels the expression of Niemann-Pick C1–like 1 (NPC1L1), a transmembrane protein with a sterol-sensing domain that is involved in cholesterol absorption.[29] NPC1L1 is the target of ezetimibe, a drug with cholesterol-lowering properties but an uncertain role in atherosclerosis. NPC1L1 also absorbs phytosterols such as sitosterol. Sterols are pumped out of the enterocyte and into the intestinal lumen by two ATP-binding cassette (ABC) transporters, ABCG5 and ABCG8. Human mutations in these transporters cause the rare disorder sitosterolemia,[30] which is characterized by increased absorption and circulating levels of sitosterol and cholesterol, xanthomas, and heart disease (see later discussion).

Figure 37-5A illustrates cholesterol synthesis. Acetate is converted to 3-hydroxy-3-methylglutaryl coenzyme A (HMG-CoA). The latter is a substrate for HMG-CoA reductase, the enzyme that is rate-limiting for cholesterol biosynthesis and is inhibited by statin drugs. Cells exquisitely regulate cholesterol acquisition.[31] When levels are low, mechanisms are activated to increase cholesterol biosynthesis and import cholesterol from the extracellular environment. Statins, by lowering cholesterol and preventing cholesterol biosynthesis, work predominantly by increasing liver uptake of cholesterol from the plasma through the low-density lipoprotein (LDL) receptor (see later discussion) and promoting its excretion. Free cholesterol in cells is esterified to form cholesteryl esters for storage. This esterification reaction is carried out by acyl-CoA:cholesterol acyltransferases (ACATs). These endoplasmic reticulum enzymes exist in two forms, ACAT1, which is present in macrophages and has been implicated in atherosclerosis, and ACAT2, which is present in liver and intestine and is implicated in cholesterol absorption. Nonspecific ACAT inhibition in humans does not affect serum lipids and does not have beneficial effects on atherosclerosis.[32]

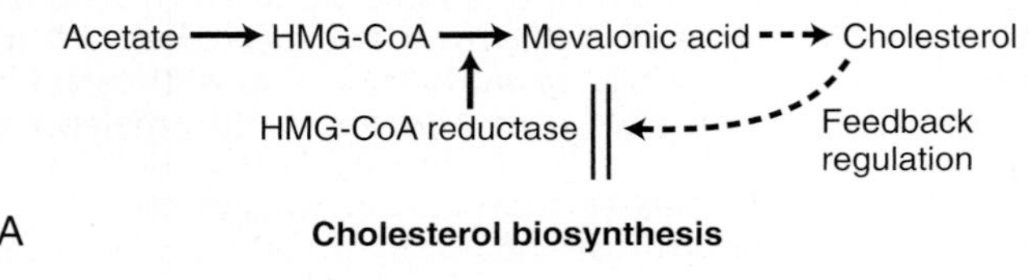

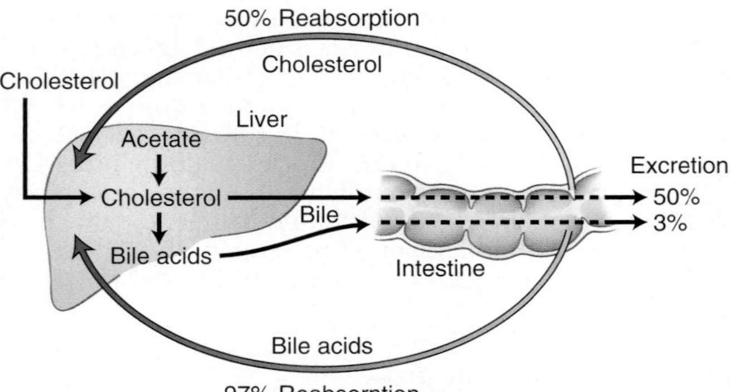

Figure 37-5 A, Cholesterol biosynthesis. 3-Hydroxy-3-methylglutaryl coenzyme A (HMG-CoA) reductase is the rate-limiting enzyme regulating cholesterol biosynthesis. The enzyme is downregulated by excess cholesterol in the cell. (Modified from Brown MS, Goldstein JL. A receptor-mediated pathway for cholesterol homeostasis. *Science.* 1986;232:34-47.) **B,** Enterohepatic circulation of cholesterol and bile acids. Approximately 50% of cholesterol and 97% of bile acids are reabsorbed from the intestine and recirculated to the liver.

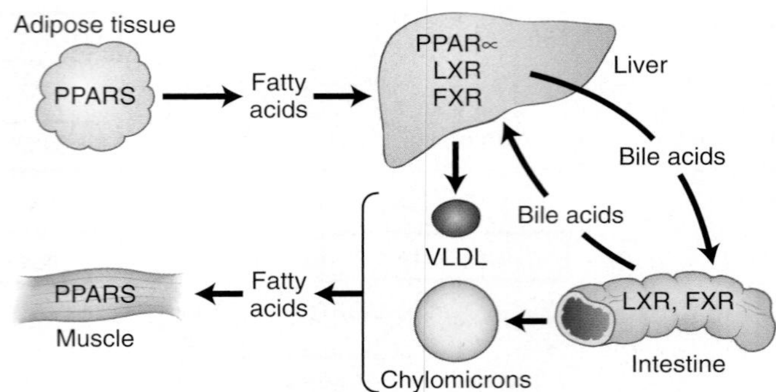

Figure 37-6 Nuclear receptors in lipid metabolism. Peroxisome proliferator-activated receptors (PPARs) are active in adipose tissue, which is a source of fatty acids that are transported to liver, where PPARα, the liver X receptors (LXR), and farnesoid X receptor (FXR) are active. Bile acids produced by the liver participate in an enterohepatic circulation with the intestine, another site of LXR and FXR expression. Very-low-density lipoprotein (VLDL), produced by liver, and chylomicrons, from intestine, are metabolized to release fatty acids that fuel muscle (another site of PPAR expression) and may be stored by adipose tissue.

Cholesterol, which is non-nutritive and cannot be catabolized to carbon dioxide and water, is either secreted into the bile as free cholesterol (about half of which is reabsorbed) or converted to bile acids for secretion into bile. Most bile acids are reabsorbed in the terminal ileum. This enterohepatic circulation of cholesterol and bile acids is shown in Figure 37-6B. The rate-limiting enzyme for bile acid synthesis is cholesterol 7α-hydroxylase, which is under feedback regulation by bile acids. Interruption of the enterohepatic circulation of bile acids through the use of bile acid sequestrants (BAS) increases bile acid synthesis, lowers plasma cholesterol, and decreases vascular disease events.

NUCLEAR RECEPTORS AND LIPID METABOLISM

Nuclear receptors, usually transcription factors with ligand-binding and DNA-binding domains, affect lipid metabolism. Classic hormones that interact with nuclear receptors and have important lipid effects include thyroid hormone, glucocorticoids, estrogen, and testosterone.

Thyroid hormone regulates cholesterol metabolism through direct effects on the gene for a transcription factor that controls LDL-receptor expression, called sterol regulatory element–binding protein 2 (SREBP2).[33] This explains why lipid levels tend to be high in hypothyroid patients and low with hyperthyroidism. Glucocorticoids have robust effects on multiple aspects of lipid metabolism, inducing expression of HMG-CoA reductase to promote cholesterol synthesis, increasing expression of fatty acid synthase to promote fatty acid synthesis, and decreasing LPL to impair clearance of circulating lipids. Accordingly, hyperlipidemia is seen commonly in the setting of glucocorticoid treatment, and this effect is amplified by insulin resistance induced by this treatment. Estrogens and selective estrogen receptor modulators such as raloxifene lower cholesterol[34] by inducing LDL-receptor activity; they tend to increase triglyceride levels, especially when higher oral doses are administered. Recent evidence suggests that derivatives of cholesterol can serve as selective estrogen-receptor modulators (SERMs) to affect the vasculature.[35] Androgens, by activating the androgen receptor, decrease levels of HDL.[36]

Aside from the classic hormones and their receptors, other nuclear receptors affect lipid metabolism after interacting with several types of metabolic byproducts. These receptors include the PPARs, the liver X receptors (LXRs), and the farnesoid X receptor (FXR). A schematic view of the role of these receptors in lipid metabolism is presented in Figure 37-6.

There are three known types of PPARs: α, γ, and δ. PPARα promotes fatty acid oxidation as well as ketogenesis and is induced by starvation. It is expressed at highest levels in tissues that are adapted to metabolize fats, such as liver and skeletal muscle, but is also present at numerous other sites. In humans, pharmacologic activation of PPARα with fibrates lowers triglycerides and increases HDL. Fatty acids interact with the receptor, but a phosphatidylcholine species was recently identified as an endogenous ligand for PPARα.[37]

Whereas PPARα facilitates energy utilization, PPARγ activates genes that promote energy storage. It is expressed at highest levels in adipose tissue and is also found in macrophages, where it may help coordinate the complex relationship between inflammation and metabolism. Pharmacologic activation of PPARγ in humans with thiazolidinediones results in insulin sensitization and weight gain. The latter effect occurs because this nuclear receptor promotes adipogenesis as well as fluid retention through effects on the kidney. Thiazolidinedione treatment in humans tends to lower triglycerides and increase HDL, probably by modulating insulin signaling, but the impact of these agents on atherosclerosis is controversial. Investigational dual agonists for PPARα and PPARγ effectively lower hemoglobin A_{1c} as well as serum lipids in humans and appear to be safe.[38]

PPARδ has important effects in tissues such as skeletal muscle, and its activation may mimic the effects of exercise.[39] Agents targeting this receptor in humans appear to show benefit, in part by increasing fatty acid oxidation.[40]

LXRs and FXR are also involved in lipid metabolism. LXRα and LXRβ are activated by oxysterols (modified derivatives of cholesterol) to increase the conversion of cholesterol into bile acids, increase bile acid excretion, and decrease cholesterol absorption.[41] Consistent with a coordinated response to limit cholesterol acquisition, recent data show that LXR activation inhibits cholesterol uptake by inducing the degradation of the LDL receptor.[42] LXRs also induce fatty acid and triglyceride synthesis. FXR is activated by bile acids to stimulate bile acid secretion as well as reabsorption. Administration of a BAS to humans with diabetes lowers blood sugar, which may be a consequence of complex effects on FXR and LXR signaling.[43]

Additional nuclear receptors also play important roles in lipogenesis—the process of converting carbohydrates to triglycerides rather than glycogen. Carbohydrate response element–binding protein (ChREBP) may control as much as 50% of this process: It responds to carbohydrate excess by transactivating a series of glycolytic and lipogenic genes.[44] SREBP1 is also critical for this process. Recently, the transcription factor XBP1, which regulates the endoplasmic reticulum stress response in some tissues, was reported to mediate hepatic lipogenesis through effects independent of ChREBP and SREBP.[45]

PLASMA LIPOPROTEINS, APOLIPOPROTEINS, RECEPTORS, AND OTHER PROTEINS

Despite the complexities of lipid synthesis and catabolism in specific tissues and cell types, a variety of demands at sites remote from the source of external lipids (i.e., the gut) have resulted in selective pressure to develop a system capable of moving nutrients, vitamins, structural components, and proteins with specialized functions through the plasma compartment. The effectors of this system are lipoproteins, spherical particles that circulate in the blood. The appropriate concentrations of lipoproteins are essential for health. When certain lipoproteins are present at high levels in the circulation, cardiovascular disease and pancreatitis may result. When other lipoproteins are absent or present at very low levels, vitamin deficiency syndromes and cardiovascular disease may develop. The roles of the various lipoproteins are discussed in detail in the following sections.

Major Lipoproteins

A prototypical lipoprotein is shown in Figure 37-7. The fundamental structure of a lipoprotein exploits the biochemical characteristics of its components. These particles are moving through an aqueous environment, so the surface consists of charged molecules that can interact with water, such as phospholipids and free cholesterol. Amphipathic proteins (with hydrophilic and as well as hydrophobic domains), known as apolipoproteins (or simply apoproteins), are also present on the surface, with their hydrophilic domains oriented toward the plasma and their hydrophobic domains toward the core of the particle. Apolipoproteins direct lipoproteins toward their appropriate sites of metabolism. The lipoprotein core consists of neutral (uncharged) lipids such as triglycerides and cholesteryl esters.

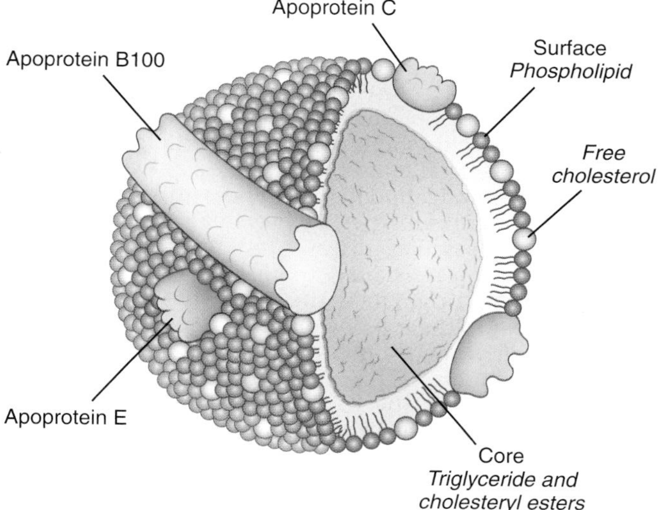

Figure 37-7 General structure of lipoproteins: schematic representation of a very-low-density lipoprotein (VLDL) particle.

TABLE 37-2

Major Classes of Plasma Lipoproteins

Type	Density (g/mL)	Origin	Major Lipids	Major Apolipoproteins	Size (nm)
Chylomicrons	<0.95	Intestine	85% Triglyceride	B48, AI, AIV, E, CI, CII, CIII	~100-500
Chylomicron remnants	<1.006	Derived from chylomicrons	60% Triglyceride 20% Cholesterol	B48, E	~80-125
VLDL	<1.006	Liver	55% Triglyceride 20% Cholesterol	B100, E, CI, CII, CIII	30-80
IDL	1.006-1.019	Derived from VLDL	35% Cholesterol 25% Triglyceride	B100, E	25-35
LDL	1.019-1.063	Derived from IDL	60% Cholesterol 5% Triglyceride	B100	18-25
HDL	1.063-1.21	Liver, intestine, plasma	25% Phospholipid 20% Cholesterol 5% Triglyceride	AI, AII, CI, CII, CIII, E	5-12
Lp(a)	1.05-1.09	Liver	60% Cholesterol 5% Triglyceride	B100, apo(a)	~30

IDL, intermediate-density lipoproteins; LDL, low-density lipoproteins; Lp(a), lipoprotein(a); VLDL, very-low-density lipoproteins.

Lipoprotein movement through the plasma compartment is dynamic. Humans spend most of their lives in the postprandial state. Eating a meal is associated with generation of lipoproteins, induction of enzymes that metabolize those lipoproteins, interactions among lipoproteins in the plasma involving the exchange of both lipid and protein components, rapid alterations of lipoprotein size as large particles are metabolized to smaller ones, genesis of new lipoproteins in the circulation as excess surface components of shrinking particles are extruded, and movement of critical nutrients and vitamins into tissues. Clinical assessment of disease risk is based on fasting measurements, but most of the migration of lipoproteins that causes disease occurs in the fed state.

The major classes of lipoproteins are listed in Table 37-2. Their original identification was accomplished based on migration in an ultracentrifuge, and classes were defined based on density. An alternative original classification scheme, which is no longer useful, involved electrophoretic mobility in agarose gels. Chylomicrons, chylomicron remnants, and very-low-density lipoproteins (VLDL) are rich in triglycerides. Intermediate-density lipoproteins (IDL), low density lipoproteins (LDL), and lipoprotein(a), or Lp(a), are rich in cholesterol. High density lipoproteins (HDL) are enriched in phospholipids. Triglyceride-rich lipoproteins such as chylomicrons are large and generally insoluble, which accounts for the cloudy appearance of plasma when it is obtained in nonfasting subjects or in fasting subjects with some types of hyperlipidemia. Table 37-2 provides general ranges for particle size, which differs substantially among lipoproteins and within each class. Certain lipoprotein subtypes, such as small dense LDL, may promote cardiovascular disease and are more likely to occur with insulin resistance.[46]

Chylomicrons originate in the gut. They are lighter than water and float to the top of a plasma sample. The particles are cleared fairly rapidly after a meal and should be absent after an overnight fast. Their distinguishing apolipoprotein is apoB48, which is the only form of apolipoprotein B produced by intestinal cells in humans.[47] Chylomicrons acquire apoC and apoE molecules by interacting with HDL particles, a process that promotes chylomicron metabolism and conversion to chylomicron remnants. Chylomicron remnants, also characterized by the presence of apoB48, are cleared rapidly from the plasma[48] and are thought to be atherogenic.

VLDL particles are of hepatic origin. Smaller than chylomicrons, their distinguishing apolipoprotein is apoB100, the form of apoB produced by the liver. VLDL also carry apoC molecules that modulate the conversion of VLDL to IDL, which are VLDL remnants and are thought to be atherogenic. IDL particles contain apoB100 and apoE, and they are converted to LDL, which is characterized by carrying essentially only apoB100 as an apolipoprotein. LDL, popularly known as "bad cholesterol," is the major carrier of cholesterol in most humans, and its measurement forms the basis for coronary heart disease (CHD) risk stratification and treatment goals. For most clinical laboratories, LDL results represent both IDL and LDL particles.

HDL particles have a complex biology. They can be generated by liver and intestine or assembled in the plasma as a consequence of the metabolism of other lipoproteins. They are arbitrarily divided into HDL_2 (less dense, at 1.063 to 1.125 g/mL), which typically contains apoAI as well as apoCs, and HDL_3 (more dense, at 1.125 to 1.21 g/mL), which typically contains apoAI, apoAII, and apoCs. There is also a minor subclass known as HDL_1 that carries a large percentage of plasma apoE. HDL is popularly known as "good cholesterol" and high levels are associated with low cardiovascular risk, but the role of HDL in vascular disease is complex. Lp(a) is produced by the liver. It consists of an LDL particle in which the apolipoprotein apo(a) has been covalently linked to apoB100. Apo(a) has substantial protein homology to plasminogen, which is required for the endogenous thrombolytic response, and it exists in isoforms based on kringle repeats (so named because their structure resembles a type of pastry). Isoforms with fewer repeats, and therefore lower mass, tend to circulate at higher concentrations. Higher levels increase the risk of myocardial infarction.[49]

Major Apolipoproteins

The chromosomal location, size, sites of synthesis, and major functions of important apolipoproteins are summarized in Table 37-3.

Apolipoproteins AI, AII, AIV, and AV

ApoAI is the most abundant apolipoprotein in HDL. It is synthesized by the liver and intestine and is known to activate the enzyme lecithin:cholesterol acyltransferase (LCAT), which transfers a fatty acid from lecithin to the

TABLE 37-3

Major Apolipoproteins

Apolipoprotein (Chromosome No.)	Molecular Weight (kd)	Synthesis	Functions
AI (11)	~29	Liver, intestine	Structural protein (HDL) Cofactor for LCAT Crucial role in reverse cholesterol transport Ligand for ABCA1 and SR-B1
AII (1)	~17 (dimer)	Liver	Inhibits apoE binding to receptors Activates hepatic lipase Inhibits LCAT
AIV (11)	~45	Intestine	Potential satiety factor Activator of LCAT Facilitates lipid secretion from intestine
AV (11)	39	Liver	Activator of LPL-mediated lipolysis Might inhibit hepatic VLDL synthesis
B100 (2)	~500	Liver	Structural protein (VLDL and LDL) Ligand for LDL receptor
B48 (2)	~200	Intestine	Structural protein (chylomicrons)
CI (19)	6.6	Liver	Modulates remnant binding to receptors Activates LCAT
CII (19)	8.9	Liver	Cofactor for LPL
CIII (11)	8.8	Liver	Modulates remnant binding to receptors Inhibitor of LPL
E (19)	~34	Liver, brain, skin, testes, spleen	Ligand for LDL and remnant receptors Local lipid redistribution Reverse cholesterol transport (HDL with apoE)
apo(a) (6)	~400-800	Liver	Modulates thrombosis/fibrinolysis

ABCA1, adenosine triphosphate–binding cassette transporter A1; apo, apolipoprotein; HDL, high-density lipoproteins; LCAT, lecithin:cholesterol acyltransferase; LDL, low-density lipoproteins; LPL, lipoprotein lipase; SR-B1, scavenger receptor B1; VLDL, very-low-density lipoproteins.

free hydroxyl group on cholesterol to generate cholesteryl ester.[50] This activity is involved in the maturation of HDL particles, which begin as lipid-poor discs containing apoAI and then acquire free cholesterol; they convert this cholesterol to cholesteryl ester through the activity of LCAT and expand into spheres as cholesteryl ester is stuffed into the growing core. ApoAI is important for mediating the efflux of cholesterol from peripheral tissues, an important step in the process of reverse cholesterol transport.[51] Human genetic mutations in apoAI cause low levels of HDL and corneal opacities. ApoAI is considered to be an antiatherogenic protein, but genetic defects in apoAI are not consistently associated with coronary artery disease. Current concepts suggest that its presence is important in the setting of an atherosclerotic environment such as the presence of atherogenic lipoproteins, a notion supported by mouse experiments.[52]

ApoAII is present with apoAI in some HDL particles. Synthesized mostly in the liver, it has been implicated in the activation of hepatic lipase, an enzyme involved in lipoprotein processing including HDL metabolism, and in the inhibition of LCAT. ApoAII may disrupt the ability of HDL to promote reverse cholesterol transport, so it is considered to be a proatherogenic protein, but the genetic absence of this protein in humans does not seem to be associated with a phenotype.[53]

ApoAIV originates in the gut, and its secretion is induced by the consumption of a high-fat meal. It has several putative functions, but perhaps the most interesting is its role as a potential satiety factor by suppressing food intake signals in the hypothalamus.[54]

ApoAV is encoded by a locus near the apoAIV gene in the apoAI/CIII/AIV/AV gene cluster on chromosome 11. It is produced by liver and circulates at low concentrations in association with VLDL particles in humans. ApoAV is involved in the hydrolysis of triglyceride-rich lipoproteins by LPL, and its expression in mice is inversely related to triglyceride levels,[55] but studies of humans with apoAV variants suggest that several mechanisms may be involved in the hypertriglyceridemia seen in these individuals.[56]

Apolipoprotein B

There are two forms of this apolipoprotein, apoB100 and apoB48, which are derived from a single gene by a unique mechanism that involves RNA editing (Fig. 37-8). In both liver and intestinal cells, the same messenger RNA is transcribed, but an editing protein complex[57] interacts with the message only in the intestine (in humans) to change the cytosine at nucleotide position 6666 to a uracil. This enzymatic effect converts a glutamine codon to a stop codon, resulting in an intestinal protein that is approximately 48% of the length of apoB100—hence, the name apoB48.

ApoB48, in essence a truncated form of apoB100, thus originates in the gut, where it is important for the assembly

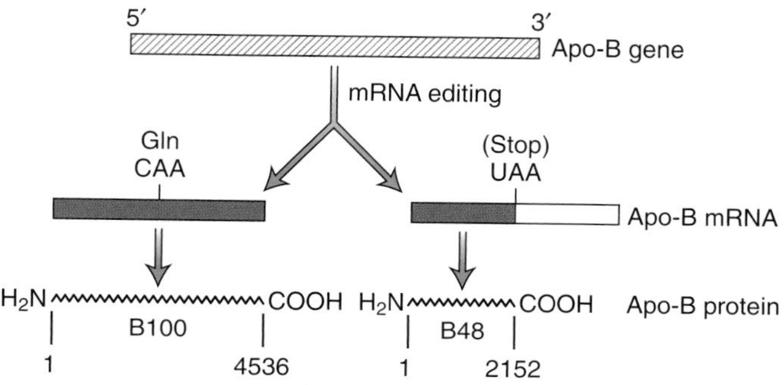

Figure 37-8 Synthesis of apolipoprotein B100 and apo-B48 by a messenger (mRNA) editing mechanism. In the human intestine, a specific cytosine (C) is changed to a uracil (U) in the apo-B mRNA. This change results in a stop codon and the formation of apo-B48, which contains only the first 2152 amino acids of the full-length apo-B100 (4536 amino acids). COOH, carboxy terminus; Gln, glutamine; H_2N, amino-terminus.

of chylomicrons.[58] There are one or two B48 molecules on each chylomicron, where they provide structural support to the particle. The C-terminus of apoB100, missing in apoB48, determines interaction with the LDL receptor, so apoB48 does not appear to be involved in the clearance of gut-derived lipoproteins. However, there is a receptor for apoB48 on macrophages that has been implicated in atherosclerosis.[59]

ApoB100 originates in the liver, where it is cotranslationally associated with lipids to coordinate the formation of VLDL particles. VLDL assembly and export, which affect the levels of circulating atherogenic lipoproteins, are determined not by transcriptional control of the apoB gene but by a unique mechanism involving stabilization of the apoB protein by lipid. VLDL production is shown in Figure 37-9. Assembly is thought to involve two distinct processes. First, as the apoB message is translated on the rough endoplasmic reticulum, it binds to lipids that are provided by microsomal triglyceride transfer protein (MTP). This protein heterodimerizes with protein disulfide isomerase, which remodels the apoB protein by rearranging the positions of disulfide bonds in the molecule to accommodate incoming lipid. Most of this lipid originates in adipose tissue, where triglyceride lipolysis releases free fatty acids that are transported to the liver. Phospholipids and cholesterol also associate with apoB at this step. If sufficient lipids are not available in the liver, apoB (which is constitutively produced) is ubiquitinated and degraded in the proteasome.[60] Second, maturing VLDL particles fuse with additional lipid droplets in the Golgi apparatus, a process facilitated by apoE. The triglyceride-rich particles are then secreted into the space of Disse. Because these particles carry the apolipoproteins that determine VLDL binding to liver receptors, it might be expected that they would be taken up immediately and never access the circulation. This does not occur, probably because high concentrations of phosphatidylethanolamine in nascent VLDL obscure receptor binding sites. These sites are revealed in the circulation as phospholipids are removed. Transfer of apolipoproteins from other lipoproteins in the circulation also modifies VLDL structure to promote metabolism in the periphery.

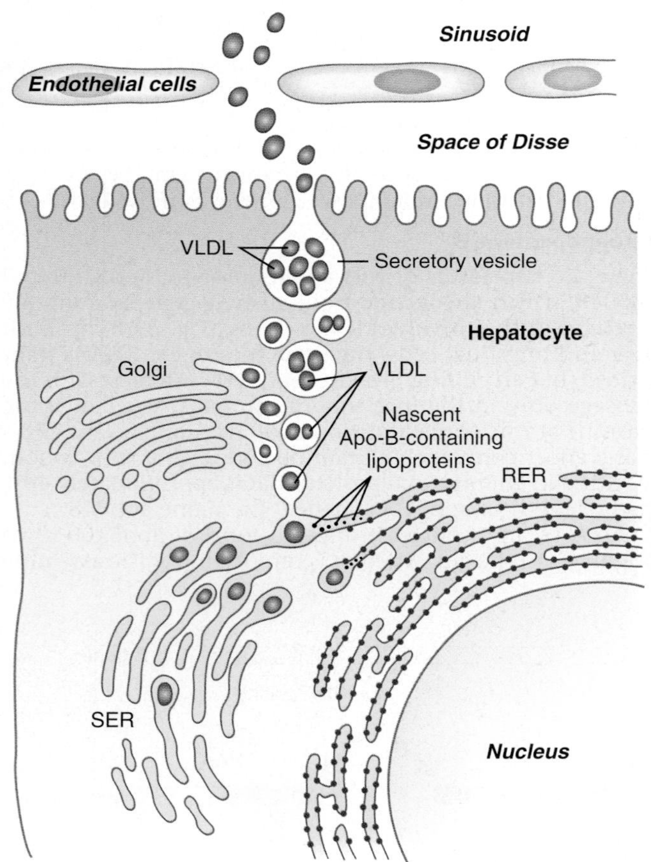

Figure 37-9 Very-low-density lipoprotein (VLDL) biosynthesis by hepatocytes. The nascent apolipoprotein B (apo-B)-containing apolipoproteins synthesized by the rough endoplasmic reticulum (RER) are thought to combine with lipids in the smooth endoplasmic reticulum (SER). The VLDLs are processed in the Golgi apparatus and accumulate in large secretory vesicles. They are then released into the space of Disse and enter the plasma. (Modified from Alexander CA, Hamilton RL, Havel RJ. Subcellular localization of B apoprotein of plasma lipoproteins in rat liver. *J Cell Biol.* 1976;69:241-263; by copyright permission of The Rockefeller University Press.)

Increased VLDL production, fueled by the increased availability of lipid, is predominantly responsible for the dyslipidemia seen with obesity and diabetes. Hepatitis C, a major cause of human liver disease, circulates in VLDL particles, and recent data indicate that this virus assimilates the VLDL assembly machinery.[61] There is one copy of apoB100 on each VLDL particle, and this relationship is retained as these lipoproteins are metabolized to IDL and then to LDL. Therefore, measurements of apoB100 in the plasma reflect particle number, and higher levels of apoB are associated with cardiovascular disease. The complete absence of apoB, which occurs in the rare human disorder abetalipoproteinemia, is not caused by mutations in apoB but by defects in MTP.[62] Patients with this disease have severe neurologic deficits, probably reflecting vitamin E deficiency, because triglyceride-rich lipoproteins transport this lipid-soluble vitamin. Very low, but not absent, apoB, which occurs in the human disorder hypobetalipoproteinemia, is caused by mutations in apoB. These individuals present with low levels of cholesterol and triglycerides and appear to be healthy. A mutation at amino acid residue 3500 of the apoB100 protein, within the C-terminal region of the molecule that mediates binding to the LDL receptor, causes familial defective apoB100. These individuals have high levels of LDL cholesterol, mimicking the presentation of FH.[63]

Apolipoproteins CI, CII, and CIII

These apoliproteins are quite small and are encoded by loci residing at two different locations in the genome. ApoCI and apoCII are transcribed from a site on chromosome 19 near the apoE gene. The apoCIII gene is a component of the apoAI/CIII/AIV/AV cluster on chromosome 11. ApoCs, which can be exchanged freely among lipoprotein particles, are important for triglyceride metabolism because their presence either interferes with the recognition of apoE by lipoprotein receptors or displaces apoE from lipoproteins (both of which would increase triglycerides by impairing their clearance). The function of apoCII is more complex than that of CI and CIII. High levels in mice cause elevated triglycerides by displacing apoE, but normal levels of apoCII are required for normal lipid clearance because this apolipoprotein is a cofactor for the enzyme LPL. Mutations of apoCII in humans cause severe hypertriglyceridemia mimicking LPL deficiency.

ApoCIII may be particularly relevant to human health. Its levels are increased in the setting of many dyslipidemias, and most lipid-lowering medications lower apoCIII levels.[64] A mutation in the apoCIII gene causing lower apoCIII levels is associated with an improved lipid profile and less atherosclerosis,[65] suggesting that therapies targeted at apoCIII might provide clinical benefit.

Apolipoprotein E

ApoE biology is more complex than that of other apolipoproteins. The highest level of apoE expression is found in liver, with the second highest in brain. Many other cell types synthesize the protein, including macrophages. In brain, astrocytes and microglial cells make apoE, but it can also be produced by injured neurons. ApoE circulates in plasma as a part of every lipoprotein with the probable exception of LDL. Its principal function involves interactions with the two major receptors mediating the clearance of plasma lipoproteins, the LDL receptor and the LDL receptor–related protein (i.e., LRP1, also known as the chylomicron remnant receptor).[66] Therefore, it is apoE that is primarily responsible for the clearance of intestinal-derived lipoproteins after a meal and for the clearance of VLDL and IDL particles before they are converted to LDL.

There are three major apoE isoforms: E2, E3, and E4. They are encoded, respectively, by alleles referred to as ε2, ε3, and ε4, which exist because of charge differences caused by variations in amino acids at residues 112 and 158 in the protein.[67] ApoE3 is considered to be the "normal" isoform; it has a cysteine at residue 112 and an arginine at 158. ApoE2 has cysteines at both 112 and 158, and apoE4 has an arginine at both 112 and 158. These variations have structural and functional consequences (Fig. 37-10). The protein has two domains, an amino-terminus that interacts with lipoprotein receptors, and a C-terminus that interacts with lipids (Fig. 37-10A). In apoE4, the isoform associated with disease, these domains interact; this does not occur with apoE3 (Fig. 37-10B).

Comprehensive data (>86,000 individuals for lipids, >37,000 for coronary events) have emerged regarding apoE allele and genotype frequencies, lipid levels, and coronary risk.[68] Allele frequencies in healthy adults are 7% for ε2, 82% for ε3, and 11% for ε4. Genotype frequencies are 0.7% for ε2/ε2, 11.6% for ε2/ε3, 2.2% for ε2/ε4, 62.3% for ε3/ε3 (the most abundant genotype), 21.3% for ε3/ε4, and 1.9%

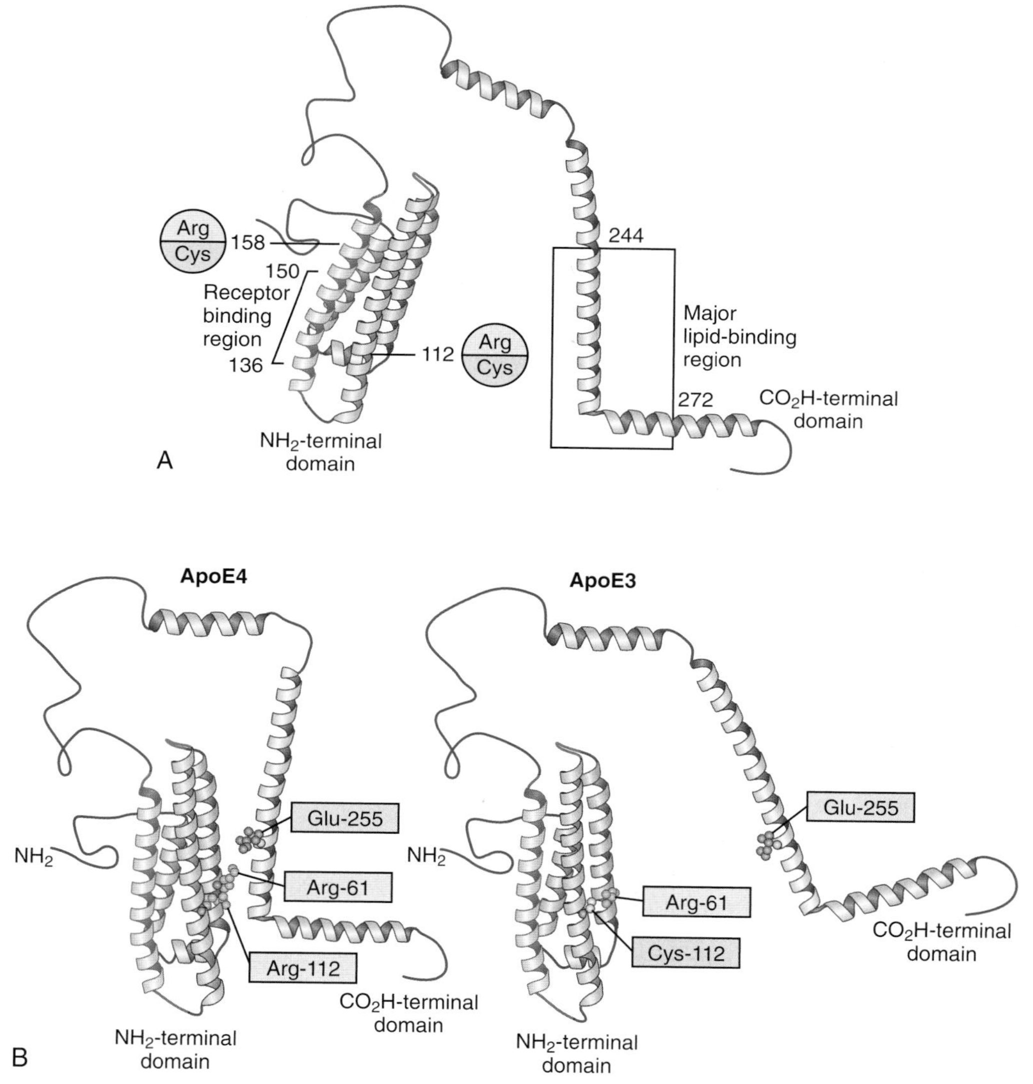

Figure 37-10 **A,** The amino-terminal domain of apoprotein E is composed of a four-helix bundle. A region of random structure encompassing residues 165 to 200 forms a connector or hinge region linked to the carboxy-terminal domain. There are two major functional regions. Residues 136 to 150 *(yellow helix)* encompass the receptor-binding region; residues 240 to 260 in the carboxyl domain encompass the lipid-binding region. **B,** ApoE4 displays the unique property of domain interaction that distinguishes it from apoE3 (Arg61 in the amino-terminal domain interacts with Glu255 in the carboxyl-terminal domain). Arg, arginine; Cys, cysteine; Glu, glutamic acid.

for ε4/ε4. There is a linear relationship between the genotype and both LDL cholesterol level and coronary risk, from least to most as follows: ε2/ε2 < ε2/ε3 < ε2/ε4 < ε3/ε3 < ε3/ε4 < ε4/ε4. Compared to the reference group (ε3/ε3), the presence of the ε2 allele decreases coronary risk by about 20%, and the presence of the ε4 allele slightly increases risk. These observations are interesting for two reasons. First, ε2/ε2 individuals, although they are protected from CHD on a population basis, are at risk for dysbetalipoproteinemia. In the setting of appropriate additional conditions, about 5% of ε2/ε2 individuals will develop this disorder, which is associated with aggressive vascular disease. Second, the E2 protein binds less well to the LDL receptor than E3 and E4 do. This suggests that LDL cholesterol in patients with the E2 protein should be higher (because it is less likely to be cleared by this receptor), yet the opposite is observed. These data suggest that other receptor-mediated processes, such as those mediated by heparan sulfate proteoglycans (HSPG), may be critical for clearance of apoE-containing lipoproteins.[69]

Data are also evolving about the critical role played by apoE in Alzheimer's disease. Risk of this neurodegenerative disease increases approximately threefold in those with one ε4 allele and 12-fold in those with two ε4 alleles.[70] The presence of an ε2 allele is protective. These relationships hold for both early- and late-onset Alzheimer's disease. There are HDL-like lipoproteins in the central nervous system, and apoE-mediated delivery of cholesterol at this site is important for normal synaptic function.[71] The relation of lipid metabolism to Alzheimer's disease is incompletely understood, but some evidence suggests that deposition of amyloid-β (the major constituent of the plaques that characterize the disease) begins sooner in the brains of those with E4 protein. Because people with the ε4 allele are also more likely to have atherosclerosis, CNS vascular disease[72] may help explain why this apoE variant is involved in neurodegeneration.

Major Receptors Involved in Lipid Metabolism

Low-Density Lipoprotein Receptor Gene Family

Including distant relatives, the LDL receptor family contains at least 10 members. The two most important ones for systemic lipid metabolism are the LDL receptor and LRP1. The LDL receptor recognizes apoB100 as well as apoE, whereas LRP1 recognizes apoE but not apoB100. Other core family members (those that share considerable structural homology) include the VLDL receptor (VLDLR), the apolipoprotein E receptor 2 (apoER2 or LRP8), LRP4, LRP1B, and megalin (LRP2, also known as gp330 and as the major Heymann nephritis antigen).

Three family members lack some of the structural features of the others. They are sortilin-related receptor L1 (LR11/SORL1), LRP5, and LRP6. Aside from the LDL receptor and LRP1, these receptors appear to be most important for brain development, synaptic function, and neuroprotection, making them relevant to Alzheimer's disease.[73] LRP5 and LRP6 are involved in endocrine disease. Both are coreceptors for a family of G protein–coupled receptors known as "frizzled receptors." Frizzled receptors bind the Wnt molecule to induce an important signaling cascade upstream of the transcription factor β-catenin. Genetic variants in LRP5 are associated with obesity,[74] and a human mutation in LRP6 results in the dysmetabolic syndrome and coronary artery disease.[75] Loss-of-function mutations in LRP5 or LRP6 cause osteoporosis in humans. These observations suggest that insulin resistance, coronary disease, and osteoporosis, common comorbidities in patients, may be related to abnormal Wnt signaling.

Low-Density Lipoprotein Receptor. The LDL receptor is a glycoprotein that is fairly large (160 kd) and is expressed on most cells. Because it recognizes apoB100 as well as apoE, it is involved in the uptake of LDL, chylomicron remnants, VLDL, and IDL. Most HDL particles do not have apoE and therefore do not interact with this receptor or the LRP. The discovery of this receptor in the early 1970s by the Brown and Goldstein laboratory was important because its deficiency explained a human disease (FH), its physiologic regulation explained the mechanism of action of drugs that lower cholesterol, and its biology defined receptor-mediated endocytosis as a paradigm for providing cells with critical components from the external environment.[76]

Five discrete domains that are shared with other members of this receptor family comprise the LDL receptor. Beginning at the N-terminus, these include the ligand-binding domain, the epidermal growth factor (EGF) precursor domain, the *O*-linked sugar domain at the cell surface, the membrane-spanning domain, and the cytoplasmic domain at the C-terminus (Fig. 37-11). In the ligand-binding domain, there are seven repeats of approximately 40 amino acids, each containing six cysteines that form three disulfide bonds within the repeat to stabilize the structure. Each repeat also includes negatively charged amino acids that interact with positive charged residues on apoB and apoE and with calcium ions that allow the repeat to bind to the ligand. The EGF precursor domain consists of three EGF-like repeats (see Fig. 37-11) with a structure known as a β-propeller located between repeats B and C.

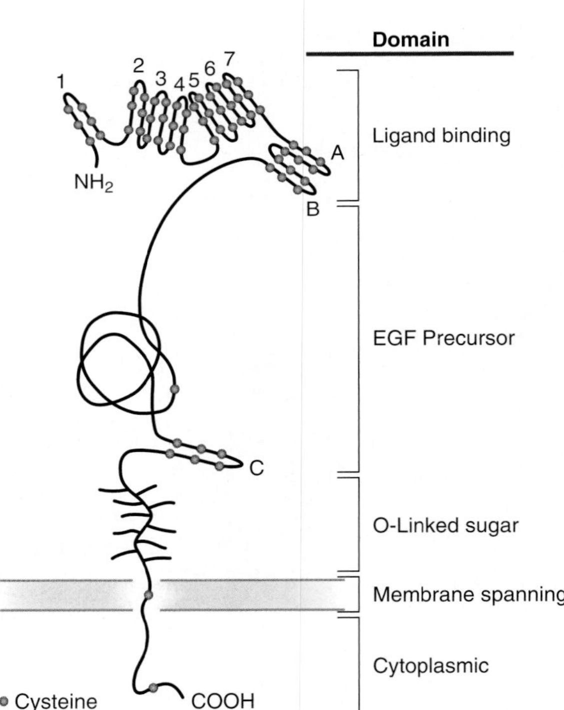

Figure 37-11 Functional domains of the low-density lipoprotein receptor. Numbers 1 through 7 indicate repeats in the ligand-binding domain. A, B, and C are epidermal growth factor (EGF)-like repeats in the EGF precursor domain. See text for complete description.

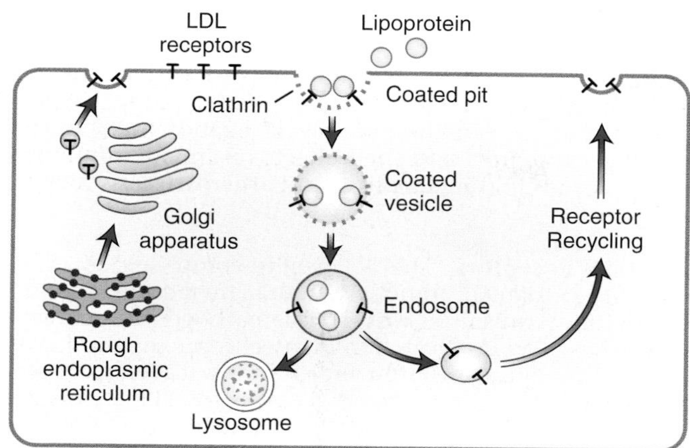

Figure 37-12 Low-density lipoprotein (LDL) receptor pathway. LDL interacts with receptors on the cell surface. The complex enters the coated pit and is internalized. The coated vesicle loses its clathrin coat and becomes an endosome, the site of lipoprotein and receptor dissociation. The receptors recycle to the cell surface, and the lipoproteins are degraded. Alternatively, new receptors are synthesized in the rough endoplasmic reticulum and transported to the cell surface. (Modified from Brown MS, Goldstein JL. A receptor-mediated pathway for cholesterol homeostasis. *Science*. 1986;232:34-47; and Myant NB. *Cholesterol Metabolism, LDL, and the LDL Receptor*. San Diego: Academic Press, 1990.)

The *O*-linked sugar domain is the site at which carbohydrate moieties attach to the molecule, and this is followed by a short sequence that traverses the membrane. The cytoplasmic domain consists of 50 residues that include an NPXY (asparagine, proline, any amino acid, tyrosine) targeting sequence where adapter proteins dock, which leads to receptor clustering in coated pits.

Coated pits are specialized regions of the cell surface that are characterized by the presence of the protein complex, clathrin. When LDL receptors bind lipoproteins, they migrate to coated pits, and clathrin directs the receptors to a cell membrane region that folds inward, creating an intracellular vesicle or endosome (Fig. 37-12). Endosomes become acidic, which prompts the lipoprotein to be displaced from the LDL receptor by the β-propeller of the EGF precursor domain.[77] The unoccupied receptor recycles back to the cell surface, and lipoproteins are degraded in the lysosome. Apolipoproteins become component amino acids. Cholesterol is transported out of the lysosomes through the action of two proteins, Niemann-Pick C1 and C2 (NPC1 and NPC2), which are mutated in the human disease Niemann-Pick type C. Accumulation of cholesterol and other lipids characterizes this disorder. It is believed that NPC2, which is soluble, binds cholesterol after lipoprotein hydrolysis in the lysosome and moves this sterol to the membrane-associated NPC1[78] for subsequent release to the cell, where it serves structural and regulatory functions.

One of the key regulatory functions of cholesterol is control of LDL receptor expression. Intracellular sterol concentrations are thought to be sensed by SCAP (SREBP cleavage–activating protein), which binds to SREBPs in the endoplasmic reticulum. SREBPs are transcription factors that control LDL receptor expression as well as the expression of other genes important for lipid metabolism. SREBP2 is most important for LDL receptor transcription; as in the other SREBPs, its N-terminus contains a leucine zipper–type transcription factor structure that binds to a sterol regulatory element in the promoter of the LDL receptor gene. When cells are sterol-depleted (Fig. 37-13, left side), SCAP migrates to the Golgi apparatus, where sugar moieties attached to the protein are modified. This allows SCAP to transport SREBPs to the S1P compartment. There, two proteases, site-1 protease (S1P) and site-2 protease (S2P), sequentially act on SREBPs to release their N-terminus, which migrates to the nucleus and binds to the sterol regulatory element in the promoter region of lipid genes such as the LDL receptor, increasing transcription and subsequent levels of functional proteins. In the presence of sterols (Fig. 37-13, right side), SCAP does not cycle to the Golgi, it cannot move SREBPs to the S1P compartment, and SREBPs are not cleaved to allow their transcription factor to migrate to the nucleus.

LDL Receptor–Related Protein 1. LRP1 is also known as the apoE receptor or the chylomicron remnant receptor. Much larger than the LDL receptor, LRP1 roughly consists of the equivalent of four LDL receptors with a multiplicity of ligand-binding domains. It is critical for normal development, because inactivation of LRP1 (but not of the LDL receptor) is lethal in mice. The major cell types in which LRP1 is expressed are hepatocytes, neurons (where it participates in critical functions), and syncytiotrophoblasts in the placenta. Perhaps understandably given its immense size, almost 20 different ligands bind to LRP1 and

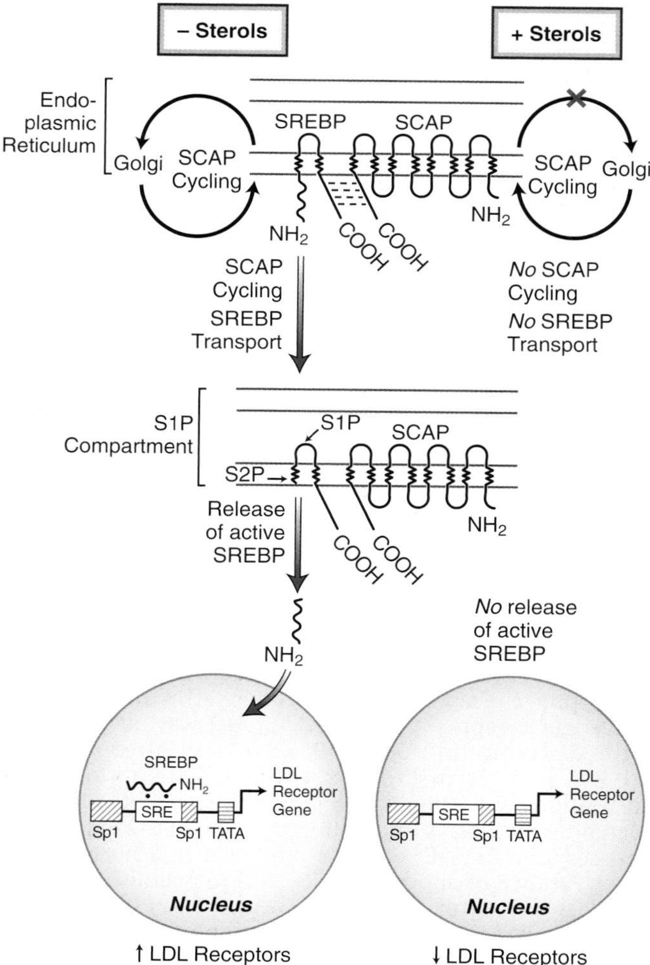

Figure 37-13 Low-density lipoprotein (LDL) receptor gene regulation. S1P, site-1 protease; S2P, site-2 protease; SCAP, SREBP cleavage–activating protein; SRE, sterol regulatory element; SREBP, sterol regulatory element–binding protein.

participate in nutrient flow as well as signaling.[79] These ligands include amyloid precursor protein (relevant in Alzheimer's disease because it is processed to form the amyloid-β of plaques), bacterial byproducts, tissue plasminogen activator (which interacts with LRP1 to modulate physiology in the setting of brain ischemia), plasminogen activator inhibitors, and α_2-macroglobulin (which plays multiple roles in inflammation, in part by inactivating matrix metalloproteinases). Given the promiscuity of LRP1 binding, it is not surprising it is linked with receptor-associated protein, a small protein that is involved in intracellular LRP1 processing and occupies the LRP1 binding sites during transport to the cell surface.

In terms of lipid metabolism, LRP1 binds apoE but not to apoB100. Therefore, it mediates the metabolism of the major apoE-containing lipoproteins, including chylomicron remnants and IDL (VLDL remnants), but is not involved in LDL metabolism. The interaction between LRP1 and lipoproteins is more complex than that between LDL and the LDL receptor. Multiple apoE molecules are required for LRP1 binding, and this interaction requires an initial binding of the lipoprotein to HSPG on the cell surface. Other moieties on apoE-containing lipoproteins also are believed to facilitate the binding process. LPL, which metabolizes chylomicrons and VLDL particles, adheres to particles after mediating the release of fatty acids and other substitutents at the endothelium. Lipoprotein-bound LPL molecules (as well as hepatic lipase) are thought to interact with LRP1 and to facilitate the uptake of remnants by the liver.

Pattern Recognition Receptors

One of the most serious consequences of abnormal lipid metabolism is atherosclerosis, which requires the delivery of excess lipids to blood vessels. This process involves the innate immune system and at least two broad types of receptors—scavenger receptors and toll-like receptors (TLRs)—that preferentially recognize patterns instead of discrete species.

Scavenger Receptors. The discovery of scavenger receptors was prompted by the observation of Brown and Goldstein that macrophages can bind and internalize modified forms of LDL but not native LDL. There are now thought to be eight classes of these receptors (A through H)[80] that are generally characterized by the ability to bind altered (e.g., oxidized, acetylated) LDL or other polyanionic ligands. With the exception of class C receptors, which are found only in *Drosophila*, all may be involved in disease states such as atherosclerosis. Class A and class B receptors may be particularly important.

Class A receptors include scavenger receptor A (SR-A types 1 and 2, which consists of alternative splice variants), macrophage receptor with collagenous structure (MARCO), scavenger receptor A 5 (SCARA5), and scavenger receptor with C-type lectin domain (SRCL-I/II, also referred to as CL-P1). SR-A, the first to be discovered, binds a wide variety of ligands (including bacterial byproducts), activates stress signaling pathways including mitogen-activated protein kinases, and is believed to be involved in atherosclerosis, the clearance of apoptotic cells, and Alzheimer's disease.

Class B receptors include CD36 and SR-BI (called CLA-1 in humans). These receptors bind modified LDL, but, unlike the other classes of scavenger receptors, they also bind VLDL, native LDL, and HDL. CD36 is expressed on a wide variety of cell types, including monocytes, macrophages, adipocytes, platelets, endothelial cells, hepatocytes, microglial cells, and, curiously, the tongue, where it may mediate the detection of dietary fat.[81] In addition to lipoproteins, long-chain fatty acids are ligands for CD36.[82] The tissue distribution of SR-BI is more limited, with expression on hepatocytes, monocyte/macrophages, and steroidogenic tissues. Given the panoply of ligands that bind to scavenger receptors and their effects on innate immunity, their roles in lipid metabolism and atherosclerosis may be complex.[83]

Toll-Like Receptors. The TLR family comprises key effectors of the innate immune system that are required for host defense mechanisms against simple pathogens. Their activation has been implicated in many chronic inflammatory diseases, including atherosclerosis. Some scavenger receptors such as CD36 may be coreceptors for TLRs. TLRs are found on myeloid cells such as monocyte/macrophages but also on the gut epithelium; they bind ligands such as lipopolysaccharide (TLR4) and glycolipids found in bacteria (TLR2). TLR4 is also known to bind saturated fatty acids, an interaction that is believed to be involved in insulin resistance in mammals.[84] TLR4 perturbs cholesterol metabolism in macrophages.[85] TLR2 mediates monocyte activation by apoCIII on triglyceride-rich lipoproteins.[86]

Other Enzymes and Transfer Proteins Mediating Lipid Metabolism

Hepatic Lipase

Primarily a phospholipase with some triglyceride lipase activity, hepatic lipase is made in hepatocytes and is found mostly on endothelial cells in the liver and on HSPG in the space of Disse. It is also found in steroidogenic tissues but is not thought to be synthesized at those sites. Unlike LPL, which is mostly present at tissues remote from the liver to ensure the peripheral delivery of lipids and vitamins, hepatic lipase coordinates lipoprotein metabolism centrally. Its functions include the conversion of IDL to LDL, the conversion of HDL_2 to HDL_3, and probably the final metabolism of chylomicron remnants to facilitate their uptake by LRP1. Unlike LPL, hepatic lipase does not require a cofactor such as apoCII, but both enzymes are displaced from their endothelial sites of activity by injection of heparin (postheparin lipase activity). High levels of hepatic lipase decrease HDL concentrations, whereas high levels of LPL increase HDL.

Endothelial Lipase

Evolutionarily related to hepatic lipase and LPL, endothelial lipase is a phospholipase with almost no triglyceride lipase activity. It is expressed at high levels in embryonic endothelial cells, with expression declining during maturation. Considerable levels are found in adult tissues that include the thyroid, lung, liver, placenta, and gonads (with expression in those tissues reflecting the endothelium and not parenchymal cells). In mice, overexpression decreases HDL and inactivation increases HDL. Endothelial lipase is expressed in aorta, where it may increase with atherosclerosis. Human loss-of-function mutations are associated with increased HDL cholesterol levels,[87] suggesting that inhibition of endothelial lipase could raise HDL levels.

Proprotein Convertase Subtilisin/Kexin Type 9

Proprotein convertase subtilisin/kexin type 9 (PCSK9) is a secreted protease that degrades the LDL receptor, but its catalytic activity is not required for receptor degradation. Mostly expressed in liver, intestine, and kidney, PCSK9 was found to be important in lipid metabolism when missense mutations (subsequently determined to be gain-of-function mutations) in its gene were determined to be associated with hypercholesterolemia and coronary artery disease.[88] Overexpression of PCSK9 in mice decreases LDL-receptor protein. Human deficiency of PCSK9 is associated with low levels of LDL and possible protection from vascular disease.[89]

Lipoprotein-Associated Phospholipase A_2

Phospholipases hydrolyze the ester bond at the sn2 position of phospholipids, usually resulting in the release of a fatty acid (typically unsaturated) and lysophosphatidylcholine (lysolecithin), which can induce inflammation. This type of enzyme was originally identified as a component of snake venom, and many distinct classes of phospholipases have subsequently been characterized. For most, membrane phospholipids are the substrate. Lipoprotein-associated phospholipase A_2 (Lp-PLA$_2$) is an exception because it can hydrolyze substrate in the aqueous phase. Lp-PLA$_2$ binds to LDL as well as HDL lipoproteins and is a biomarker for coronary artery disease.[90] Inhibition of this enzyme, which is also called platelet-activating factor acetylhydrolase, appears to decrease the expansion of the lipid core of atherosclerotic plaques in humans.[91]

Cholesteryl Ester Transfer Protein

Cholesteryl ester transfer protein (CETP) promotes the exchange between lipoproteins of two classes of neutral lipids: cholesteryl esters and triglycerides. HDL cholesteryl esters are transferred to VLDL, IDL, and chylomicron remnants; in return, triglycerides from VLDL, IDL, and remnants are transferred to HDL. Humans and other primates have CETP activity; the transfer of cholesteryl ester from HDL to apoB-containing lipoproteins ultimately leads to most of their cholesterol burden being carried by LDL, and this is thought to result in atherosclerosis. Rodents and dogs do not have CETP. Most of their cholesterol is carried in HDL; levels of LDL are low, and these animals are resistant to atherosclerosis. Such observations have led to the notion of inhibiting CETP activity as a treatment for atherosclerosis in humans. One CETP inhibitor was shown to increase HDL cholesterol and lower LDL cholesterol in humans, but it also increased mortality, possibly because of off-target effects of the drug.[92]

Lecithin:Cholesterol Acyltransferase

Lecithin:cholesterol acyltransferase (LCAT) is an enzyme synthesized mostly in the liver; it circulates in the plasma associated with HDL particles and, to a lesser extent, with LDL particles. LCAT is activated by several apolipoproteins (apoAI and others) and uses the phospholipid lecithin (phosphatidylcholine) and free cholesterol as substrates to generate lysolecithin (lysophosphatidylcholine) and cholesteryl ester. Most of the cholesteryl esters in lipoproteins are derived from LCAT activity. Rare human mutations in LCAT result in low HDL levels in the setting of a range of disorders, including fish-eye disease (in which activity is deficient on HDL particles but continues on LDL particles) and a more severe presentation with corneal clouding (resulting from free cholesterol in the cornea), hemolytic anemia, and renal failure. The role of LCAT in atherosclerosis is uncertain. Although LCAT deficiency might be expected to promote atherosclerosis because of low HDL levels, recent detailed studies of humans with loss-of-function LCAT mutations suggested that these individuals are not at increased risk for atherosclerosis.[93]

INTEGRATIVE PHYSIOLOGY OF LIPID METABOLISM

Lipid metabolism is characterized by a dynamic flux of multiple lipid species from the external environment to the liver, from the liver to peripheral tissues, from peripheral tissues back to the liver, and eventually back to the external environment through the excretion of bile acids. Integrated views of the major pathways involved are shown in Figures 37-14 and 37-15.

Exogenous Lipid Transport

Dietary fat and cholesterol (Fig. 37-14, top left) absorbed by the duodenum and proximal jejunum are used to generate chylomicrons that are secreted at the lateral borders of

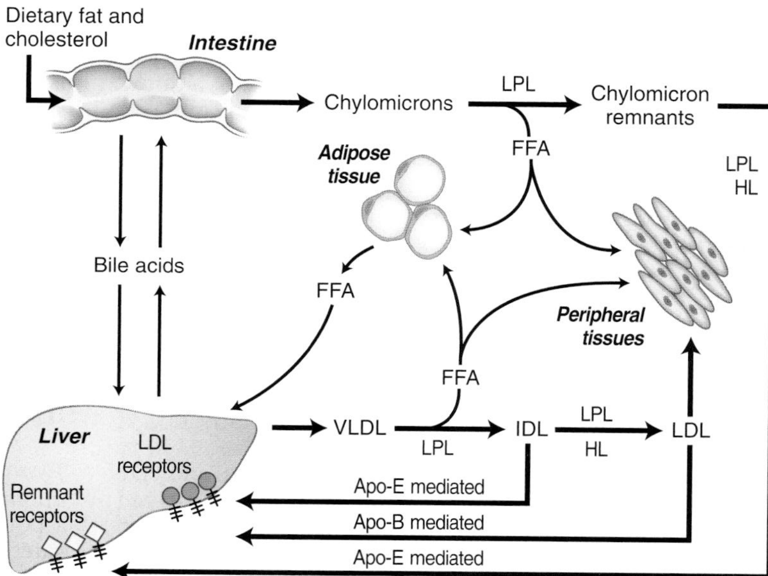

Figure 37-14 General scheme summarizing the major pathways involved in the metabolism of chylomicrons synthesized by the intestine and very-low-density lipoprotein (VLDL) synthesized by the liver. Apo-B, apolipoprotein B; Apo-E, apolipoprotein E; FFA, free fatty acid; HL, hepatic lipase; IDL, intermediate-density lipoprotein; LPL, lipoprotein lipase. (Modified from Mahley RW. Biochemistry and physiology of lipid and lipoprotein metabolism. In: Becker KL, ed. *Principles and Practice of Endocrinology and Metabolism*, 2nd ed. Philadelphia: JB Lippincott; 1995:1369-1378.)

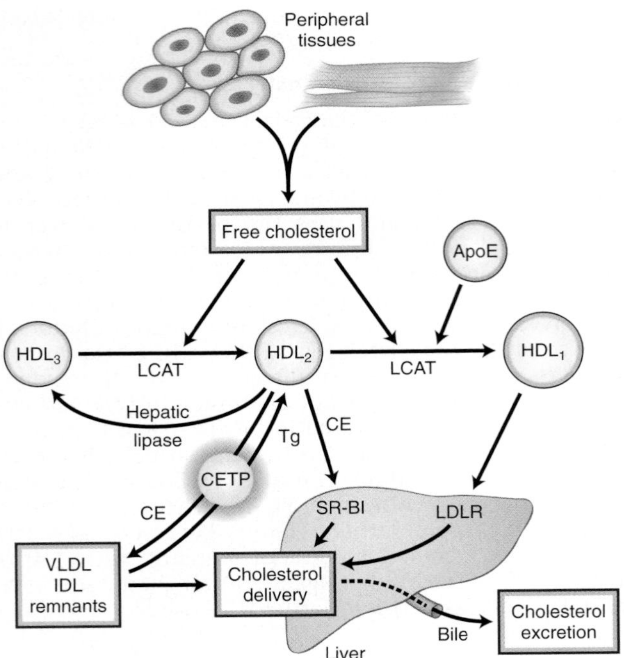

Figure 37-15 Role of high-density lipoprotein (HDL) in the redistribution of lipids from cells with excess cholesterol to cells requiring cholesterol or to the liver for excretion. The reverse cholesterol transport pathway is indicated by arrows (net transfer of cholesterol from cells to HDL, then to LDL and liver). ApoE, apolipoprotein E; CE, cholesteryl ester; CETP, cholesteryl ester transfer protein; IDL, intermediate-density lipoprotein; LCAT, lecithin:cholesterol acyltransferase; LDLR, low-density lipoprotein receptor; SR-BI, scavenger receptor class B, type I; Tg, triglyceride; VLDL, very-low-density lipoprotein.

enterocytes and enter mesenteric lymphatics. They access the plasma via the thoracic duct and are rapidly metabolized by LPL to yield chylomicron remnants. These are taken up by remnant receptors (LRP1/HSPG) and by LDL receptors in the liver. Free fatty acids liberated by the action of LPL are available to adipose tissue for storage and to other tissues (e.g., skeletal muscle, heart) for use as energy substrates.

Endogenous Lipid Transport

Lipid derived from remnants and from lipolysis of adipose tissue is reassembled in the liver (Fig. 37-14, bottom left) as VLDL particles, which are secreted into the plasma. Abnormal lipid metabolism in insulin resistance is mediated in large part by overproduction of VLDL, an event that occurs through disruption of signaling downstream of the insulin receptor and the insulin receptor substrate (IRS) adapter proteins.[94] VLDL particles are metabolized by LPL to yield IDL particles, which are metabolized by LPL and hepatic lipase to yield LDL particles. Thus, LDL is derived from VLDL, which helps explain why treatment to lower triglycerides (carried by VLDL) is frequently associated with at least transient increases in LDL. IDL can be taken up by the liver through an apoE-dependent process, and LDL is taken up by the liver through the binding of apoB100 to LDL receptors. Small VLDL particles, IDL particles, and LDL particles may be taken up by peripheral tissues to deliver nutrients, cholesterol, and fat-soluble vitamins. When present in excess, each of these lipoproteins may be atherogenic.

Reverse Cholesterol Transport and Dysfunctional HDL

Cholesterol cannot be metabolized by peripheral tissues, so it must be returned to the liver for excretion in order to maintain homeostasis. This process, known as reverse cholesterol transport, is dependent on HDL and its precursors and is depicted in Figure 37-15. Excess cholesterol in tissues can be effluxed either to lipid-poor apoAI, mediated by the protein transporter ABCA1, or to nascent HDL particles, mediated by ABCG1. There is also evidence that cholesterol can be acquired by HDL without the assistance of transporters by following a concentration gradient at the cell surface. LCAT esterifies HDL-associated cholesterol to form cholesteryl ester and induce the maturation of HDL. HDL particles have three pathways for transporting sterols to the liver. First, they can directly bind to SR-BI (CLA-1) at the liver, which induces cholesteryl ester delivery through a mechanism involving lateral lipid transfer and not receptor internalization. Second, cholesteryl esters can be transferred to apoB-containing lipoproteins by CETP, and these particles can deliver cholesterol to the liver through the LDL receptor. Third, a small portion of HDL can acquire apoE and bind to the liver LDL receptor. Once in the liver, cholesterol is converted to bile acids for excretion.

HDL_2 particles are partially depleted of cholesteryl esters and enriched in triglycerides through the activity of CETP, which renders them suitable as substrates for hepatic lipase. Hepatic lipase hydrolyzes the triglyceride-enriched HDL_2 particles and regenerates HDL_3, yielding particles that are again suited to accept cholesterol from peripheral cells.

Because cholesterol is the principal component of atherosclerotic plaque, it is reasonable to pursue the notion that atherosclerosis could be treated by promoting the efflux of cholesterol from lesions. HDL participates in this process, but static levels of HDL cholesterol are poor predictors of reverse cholesterol transport. Measurements of the rate of flux of cholesterol from the periphery to the liver, which may be possible in humans, would represent a better predictor of beneficial therapies. The presence of high levels of HDL particles that have been modified to prevent their capacity to promote cholesterol efflux would not be expected to decrease vascular risk. Such dysfunctional particles may explain why some HDL-elevating interventions have not been associated with decreased cardiovascular disease.

In addition to participating in reverse cholesterol transport, HDL has other properties that could be impaired by a variety of processes leading to a dysfunctional particle. These include the induction of endothelial nitric oxide synthase through interactions with caveolae as well as signaling through SR-BI, the transport of a large number of proteins involved in the acute phase response and inflammation, and the suppression of thrombosis through induction of prostacyclin (which decreases thrombin production via the protein C pathway and decreases platelet activation).

OVERVIEW OF HYPERLIPIDEMIA AND DYSLIPIDEMIA

Two major clinical disorders are associated with common lipoprotein disorders. Very elevated triglyceride levels are a potent risk factor for development of pancreatitis. Elevated cholesterol due to greater concentrations of LDL and remnant lipoproteins and reduced levels of HDL promote

TABLE 37-4

Differential Diagnosis of Hyperlipidemia and Dyslipidemia

Hypertriglyceridemia	Hypercholesterolemia	Increased Cholesterol and Triglycerides	Low HDL
Primary Disorders			
LPL deficiency ApoCII deficiency Familial hypertriglyceridemia Dysbetalipoproteinemia	Familial hypercholesterolemia Familial defective apoB100 Polygenic hypercholesterolemia Sitosterolemia	Familial combined hyperlipidemia Dysbetalipoproteinemia	Familial hypoalphalipoproteinemia ApoAI mutations LCAT deficiency ABCA1 deficiency
Secondary Disorders			
Diabetes mellitus Hypothyroidism High-carbohydrate diets Renal failure Obesity/insulin resistance Estrogens Ethanol β-Blockers Protease inhibitors Glucocorticoids Retinoids Bile acid–binding resins Antipsychotics Lipodystrophies Thiazides	Hypothyroidism Obstructive liver disease Nephrotic syndrome Thiazides	Diabetes mellitus Hypothyroidism Glucocorticoids Immunosuppressives Protease inhibitors Nephrotic syndrome Lipodystrophies	Anabolic steroids Retinoids

ABCA1, adenosine triphosphate–binding cassette transporter 1; apo, apolipoprotein; HDL, high-density lipoprotein; LCAT, lecithin:cholesterol acyltransferase; LPL, lipoprotein lipase.

atherosclerosis. Clinicians are often faced with evaluation and treatment of patients who have hypertriglyceridemia, hypercholesterolemia, combined hyperlipidemia due to elevated cholesterol and triglycerides, and low HDL syndromes. A summary of the primary and secondary causes of each condition is presented in Table 37-4.

Plasma lipid levels are highly dependent on lifestyle; for example, the high-fat, high-cholesterol diets eaten in Western societies raise plasma cholesterol, and vigorous exercise lowers both atherogenic particles and triglycerides. For this reason, normal blood concentrations—those that are within 2 standard deviations of the mean—vary among countries and over time. In the United States, the age-adjusted mean plasma cholesterol concentration is 202 mg/dL (5.26 mmol/L) in men.[95] For Western adults, cholesterol concentrations higher than 240 mg/dL (6.2 mmol/L) or triglyceride concentrations higher than 150 mg/dL (1.7 mmol/L) constitute high-risk hyperlipidemia. The overriding influences of diet and lifestyle on plasma cholesterol were illustrated by studies of ethnic Japanese populations. Plasma cholesterol was markedly increased in Japanese-Americans and was associated with a more Westernized food intake.[96] Because serum total cholesterol levels correlate with the risk for CHD over a broad range (Fig. 37-16), "normal" levels are often defined as those associated with minimal cardiovascular risk rather than population averages. If this logic is assumed, then the majority of the Western population have abnormal lipoprotein levels that put them at risk for heart disease.

The National Cholesterol Education Program (NCEP) created a standard for cholesterol levels and pioneered a practical approach to treatment by dividing the population according to cardiac risk, based on the presence of vascular disease or other cardiac risk factors. In 2001, the NCEP classified plasma cholesterol levels lower than 200 mg/dL as desirable, those between 200 and 240 mg/dL as borderline high, and levels greater than 240 mg/dL as high.[97] (Because plasma lipid levels increase with age,[97] cutoff values in children are lower.[98]) Total cholesterol concentrations between 170 and 200 mg/dL are considered borderline high, and levels greater than 200 mg/dL are high. Triglyceride levels greater than 500 mg/dL carry a high risk of pancreatitis, and those greater than 150 mg/dL are considered elevated.

Hyperlipidemias are caused by increased concentrations of plasma lipoproteins; although the clinical diagnosis is made solely on the basis of circulating lipids, the diseases are classified by abnormalities of lipoproteins (see

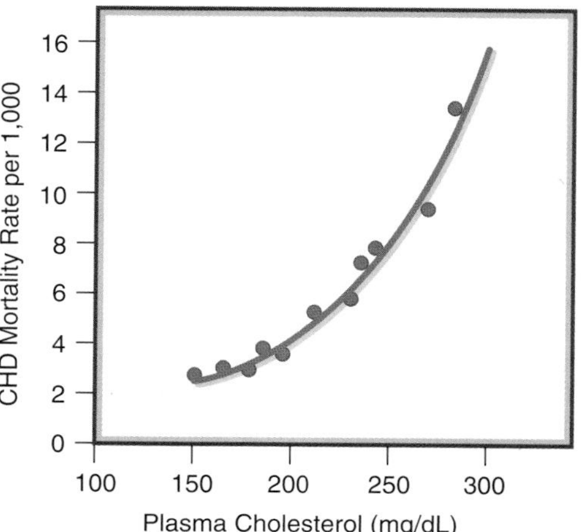

Figure 37-16 Relation between plasma cholesterol levels and coronary heart disease (CHD) mortality in the Multiple Risk Factor Intervention Trial. (Modified from Stamler J, Wentworth D, Neaton JD. Is relationship between serum cholesterol and risk of premature death from coronary heart disease continuous and graded? Findings in 356,222 primary screenees of the Multiple Risk Factor Intervention Trial [MRFIT]. *JAMA.* 1986;256:2823-2828; Copyright © 1986, by the American Medical Association.)

TABLE 37-5

Criteria for Diagnosis of the Dysmetabolic Syndrome

Measure*	Categorical Threshold
Waist circumference	*Whites, African Americans, Latin Americans:* Men, ≥40 in; women, ≥35 in *Asians:* Men, ≥35 in; women, ≥32 in
Elevated triglycerides	≥150 mg/dL *or* On drug treatment for elevated triglycerides
Reduced HDL-C	Men, <40 mg/dL; women, <50 mg/dL *or* On drug treatment for reduced HDL-C
Elevated blood pressure	≥130 mm Hg systolic or ≥85 mm Hg diastolic *or* On antihypertensive drug treatment
Elevated fasting glucose	≥100 mg/dL *or* On drug treatment for elevated glucose

*Three of the five measures are required for diagnosis.
HDL-C, high-density lipoprotein cholesterol.
Adapted from Grundy SM, Cleeman JI, Daniels SR, et al. Diagnosis and management of the metabolic syndrome: an American Heart Association/National Heart, Lung, and Blood Institute scientific statement. *Circulation.* 2005;112:2735-2752.

Table 37-2) and are often referred to as hyperlipoproteinemias. As noted earlier, lipoproteins differ in their physiologic functions, metabolic pathways, and pathologic significance.

The NCEP also recognized the existence of the dysmetabolic syndrome, an extremely common condition that is linked to insulin resistance but is without a unifying mechanistic cause. The presence of at least three of the five features described in Table 37-5 is sufficient to make the diagnosis. This condition is clearly associated with increased risk of vascular disease and development of type 2 diabetes. Evaluation and therapy for the dysmetabolic syndrome should be directed at individual components including hypertriglyceridemia and low HDL-cholesterol (HDL-C).

HYPERTRIGLYCERIDEMIA

Fasting Hyperchylomicronemia

The most dramatic example of severe hypertriglyceridemia is that of fasting hyperchylomicronemia. This can result either from a primary defect in chylomicron metabolism, or it can occur secondary to increased VLDL and saturation of LPL actions to metabolize triglycerides into free fatty acids and generate remnant lipoproteins that are amenable to uptake by the liver through pathways mediated by the LDL receptor, LRP1, and proteoglycans. LPL saturation occurs when triglyceride levels exceed about 500 mg/dL.[99] Therefore, familial hypertriglyceridemia, familial combined hyperlipidemia, and dysbetalipoproteinemia can manifest with fasting hyperchylomicronemia. One common cause of such exacerbations is out-of-control diabetes leading to increased adipose intracellular lipolysis, return of fatty acids to the liver, greater secretion of VLDL triglyceride, and saturation of LPL. Several dietary and environmental factors also modulate triglyceride production. The most dramatic is alcohol, a major substrate for triglyceride production.[100] In addition, diets that are rich in free carbohydrates, and especially simple sugars, induce triglyceride production. Fructose also increases de novo production of lipids in the liver but has less effect on circulating triglycerides.[8]

Defective clearance of plasma lipids is a major cause of fasting hyperchylomicronemia. Genetic defects in LPL prevent chylomicron clearance. LPL deficiency usually, but not always, manifests in childhood. The symptoms vary from difficulty feeding young infants to frank pancreatitis, which is sometimes mistaken as appendicitis. The plasma is often milky, and whole blood may have a pinkish, "cream of tomato" hue. The trigger level of triglyceride elevation leading to pancreatitis is variable; some patients have triglycerides in excess of 10,000 mg/dL with no symptoms, whereas others develop pancreatitis at much lower triglyceride levels, but usually in excess of 1000 to 2000 mg/dL.

The pathophysiology of the relationship between hyperchylomicronemia and pancreatitis is unknown. One theory is that the lipid-rich blood sludges, leading to pancreatic ischemia. Another is that the small amount of lipases that normally leak from the acinar cells lead to exuberant local lipolysis, creation of toxic local concentrations of free fatty acids and lysolecithin, a toxic lipid produced by lipase hydrolysis of phosphatidylcholine, and further acinar cell damage to adjacent cells.[101] Additional insults to the acinar cells (such as that provided by alcohol) can fan this process.

Although most patients with severe hyperchylomicronemia who do not develop pancreatitis are asymptomatic, a few with extreme levels exceeding 10,000 mg/dL develop the hyperchylomicronemia syndrome.[102] These patients have dyspnea and confusion that may be indistinguishable from early dementia. Presumably this is the result of reduced blood flow or defective oxygen delivery.

The marked increase in blood triglyceride concentration can lead to accumulation of triglycerides in several organs and can be observed in the blood. The latter is best appreciated by examining the blood directly, allowing the red cells to settle and observing a creamy layer on the plasma, or by noting the pinkish discoloration of the blood on funduscopic examination, known as lipemia retinalis (Fig. 37-17B). Eruptive xanthomas, as shown in Fig. 37-17G, are 2- to 5-mm papules with a yellow center surrounded by erythema. They are caused by triglyceride-enriched skin macrophages. These lesions are sometimes confused with acne or folliculitis. For unclear reasons, eruptive xanthomas are most commonly found on the buttocks, extensor surfaces of the arms, and the back. Enlargement of the liver and spleen is not uncommon and is thought to be caused by triglyceride engorgement of these organs.

Aside from the severe hypertriglyceridemia, other laboratory indices are sometimes abnormal. Plasma sodium is reduced; liver functions are sometimes elevated. Despite the presence of pancreatitis, amylase may be normal due to an assay artifact; serum lipase is a more reliable indicator in this setting. Often the clinical laboratory will note the severe lipemia and fail to report measurements of routine chemistries due to the turbidity of the serum. If these other measurements are required, plasma can be centrifuged, the chylomicron layer removed, and the remaining plasma examined.

Fasting hyperchylomicronemia in adults is frequently accompanied by comorbidities such as uncontrolled diabetes and excessive alcohol intake.

Lipoprotein Lipase Deficiency

Almost every racial group has been reported to have patients with genetic defects in LPL,[103] and a founder mutation makes the defect especially common among French

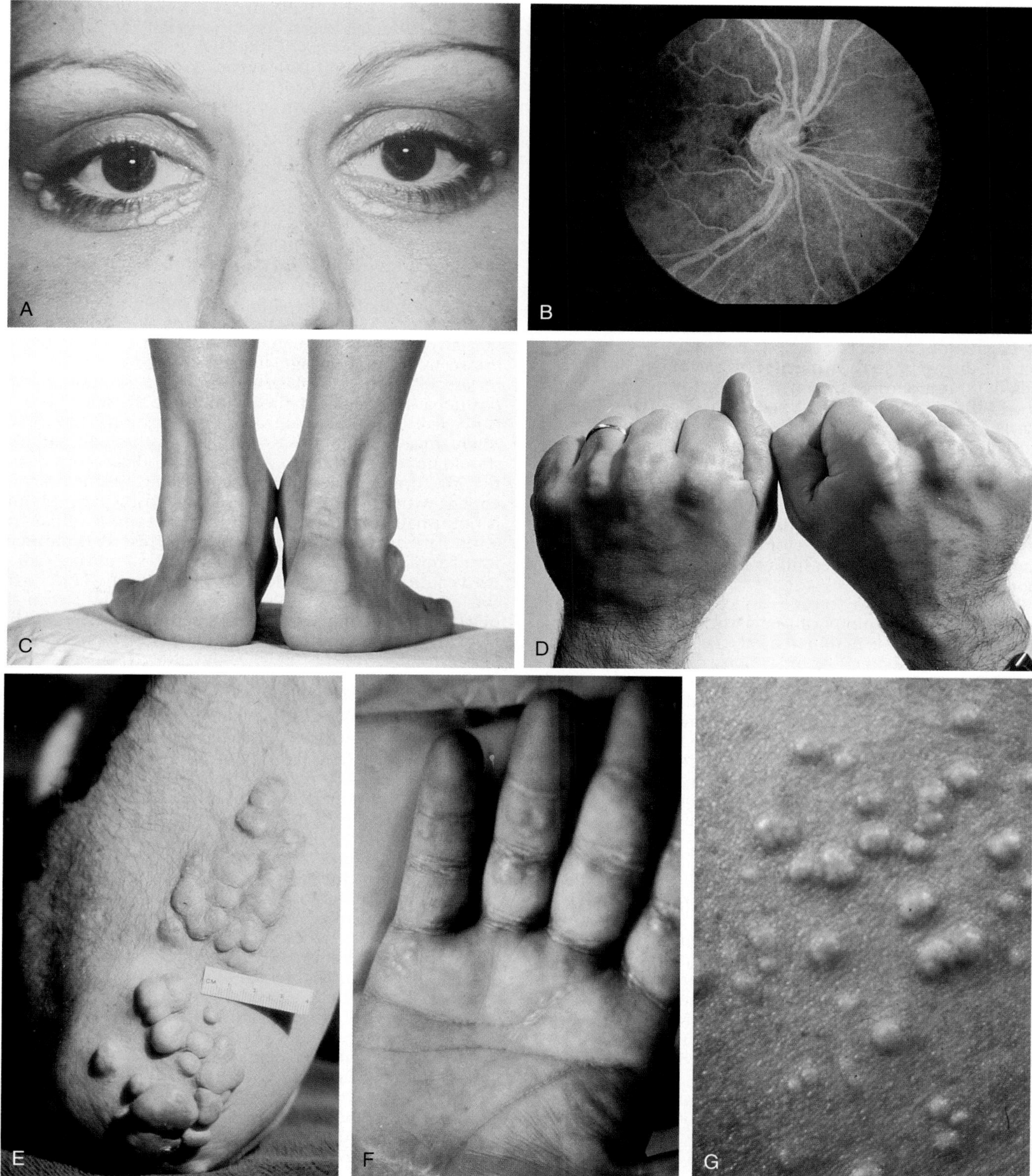

Figure 37-17 Physical examination findings associated with hyperlipidemia. **A,** Xanthelasma. **B,** Lipemia retinalis. **C,** Achilles tendon xanthomas. Notice the marked thickening of the tendons. **D,** Tendon xanthomas. **E,** Tuberous xanthomas. **F,** Palmar xanthomas. **G,** Eruptive xanthomas. (**A** and **B** courtesy of Dr. Mark Dresner and Hospital Practice [May 1990, p 15]. **C** through **F** courtesy of Dr. Tom Bersot. **G** courtesy of Dr. Alan Chait.)

Canadians. Overall, it is estimated that approximately half of the cases of severe primary hypertriglyceridemia are the result of LPL defects. Most LPL enzyme deficiencies are caused by inactive LPL protein. However, lack of protein production has also been reported, and because LPL might have receptor functions that do not require catalytic function, patients with these defects may have a more severe phenotype.

Although genetic LPL deficiency has been reported to manifest in adulthood, most cases of severe hyperchylomicronemia in adulthood are associated with partial LPL deficiency or other causes. In adults, the most important of these causes are type 2 diabetes and obesity, because insulin resistance is associated with defective clearance of lipoproteins.[104] Postprandial lipemia is a prominent feature of diabetes.[105] A thorough history of triglyceride-raising medications should be taken (see later discussion).

Regulation of LPL is complicated, and defects in its actions are associated with genetic or acquired abnormalities that are exclusive of genetic defects in the LPL molecule. Defective apoCII, the obligate cofactor for LPL, leads to deficient LPL activity.[106] Two recent molecular defects initially found in mice are the cause of occasional severe human hypertriglyceridemia. GPIHBP (discussed earlier) is a molecule expressed by endothelial cells whose deficiency leads to defective association of LPL with its binding site on the capillary lumen and defective intravascular lipolysis.[26,107] Lipase maturation factor 1 is an intracellular protein that is required for correct intracellular folding and activation of LPL.[108]

LPL deficiency also occurs as a secondary phenomenon. Autoimmune conditions can be associated with defective triglyceride catabolism due to inhibition of LPL, apoCII, or heparin.[109] Antibodies against heparin are thought to prevent normal LPL association with the endothelial surface. In addition, patients with vascular disease or generalized intravascular reactions to transfusions or chemotherapy can occasionally develop defects in LPL. Transient episodes of fasting hyperchylomicronemia have been attributed to viral infections and to excessive fat/calorie intake after fasting.

Postprandial Hyperlipidemia

Although plasma lipid levels are usually measured after an overnight fast, chylomicron remnants are associated with vascular disease in a number of animal models and with genetic or dietary causes of hyperlipidemia. This has led to a widely accepted hypothesis that remnant lipoproteins are an overlooked cause of human vascular disease. Indeed, several studies have correlated postprandial lipidemia, measured as triglyceride increase, with greater risk of heart disease.[110,111] However, postprandial triglyceride elevations are also correlated with fasting triglycerides and reduced HDL levels, so the use of postprandial measurements in clinical practice is not currently recommended.

Diagnostic Evaluation of Severe Hypertriglyceridemia

Assessment of underlying medical conditions, consideration of age at onset, and, in some cases, biochemical evaluation of LPL are required. Conditions that cause fasting hypertriglyceridemia (discussed later) can lead to severe hypertriglyceridemia when exacerbated by diet, drugs, or other conditions such as diabetes or pregnancy. Genetic LPL deficiency is diagnosed by both the clinical setting and biochemical deficiency of LPL activity in postheparin blood; LPL deficiency is more typically associated with younger age at onset, especially onset in childhood. A family history of low HDL is the most common lipid abnormality in heterozygous carriers.[112] LPL variants are also a determinant of HDL levels within the general population. A family history of French Canadian ancestry is suggestive. Although a presumptive diagnosis can be made on clinical grounds, it is sometimes useful for genetic reasons and treatment approach to confirm the diagnosis of LPL deficiency.

More than 100 mutations of the LPL gene have been described,[113] and for this reason biochemical rather than genetic evaluation is still performed. Fasting patients are given an intravenous injection of 60 units/kg of heparin, which releases LPL into the bloodstream.[114] Ten minutes later, a sample of postheparin blood is obtained and stored on ice, after which the plasma is frozen and sent to a lipid specialty laboratory for analysis. Heparin species are calibrated by their anticoagulant activity and their ability to release LPL into the plasma varies, so a normal control postheparin plasma obtained with use of the same heparin is needed. Hepatic lipase (see later discussion) is also routinely measured in these samples. Postheparin samples should not clot. If they do, it may be an indicator of a defective injection or antibodies to heparin (e.g., in the case of a patient with an autoimmune disease). Postheparin plasma is not usually obtained during an acute episode of pancreatitis. Patients with a history of bleeding disorders or recent use of anticoagulant or anti-platelet drugs should be studied with caution, if at all. Deficiency of apoCII, the LPL activator, and inhibitors of LPL such as antibodies[115] can be detected by mixing the patient's serum with a standard human or bovine source of LPL and then assessing activity.

Moderate Fasting Hypertriglyceridemia Due to Elevated Very-Low-Density Lipoprotein

Less dramatic elevations of triglyceride are not a cause of acute symptoms. They are of concern if serum triglycerides begin to exceed 500 mg/dL. Otherwise, the major issue is the relationship of triglycerides to cardiovascular disease. Triglyceride levels of 150 to 500 mg/dL are considered to be abnormal, but their pathologic importance is uncertain. The NCEP categorizes triglyceride levels of 200 to 499 mg/dL as high and those of 150 to 199 mg/dL as borderline high.[97] Several different clinical conditions lead to fasting hypertriglyceridemia. Familial combined hyperlipidemia is associated with increased apoB production, and at different times and in different family members it can manifest with hypertriglyceridemia (increased VLDL), increased cholesterol (LDL), or both. This disorder is associated with increased risk of vascular disease.[116] The concomitant insulin resistance, obesity, and/or overt diabetes in many hypertriglyceridemic patients often make it difficult to isolate one specific cause of this metabolic disturbance. In contrast, it has been suggested that isolated triglyceride elevations do not lead to more vascular disease. In the presence of the dysmetabolic syndrome, triglyceride elevations probably predispose to vascular disease through unclear mechanisms.

Some cases of isolated hypertriglyceridemia have been associated with hepatic overproduction of bile acids in the setting of impaired intestinal absorption of bile acids.[117] This is analogous to the hypertriglyceridemia associated with use of bile acid–binding resins and reduced bile interaction with the liver FXR receptor.[118] There is uncertainty as to whether the large, triglyceride-rich VLDLs seen in this and similar clinical circumstances are atherogenic.

Dysbetalipoproteinemia is caused by a homozygous mutation in apoE, apoE2/E2, leading to defective clearance of chylomicron and small VLDL remnants (see earlier discussion). These patients, with a prevalence of approximately 1 of every 10,000 in the general population, present with elevated triglyceride and cholesterol due to defective lipid clearance of remnant lipoproteins. Patients with dysbetalipoproteinemia sometimes have tuberous and palmar xanthomas and a propensity to peripheral vascular disease (see later discussion).

Heterozygous LPL deficiency can be relatively common in some populations. As these individuals age or if the LPL deficiency is superimposed on other conditions that tend to elevate triglycerides, hypertriglyceridemia may be uncovered.

Genetic hypoalphalipoproteinemia syndromes are invariably associated with moderate hypertriglyceridemia. These included LCAT deficiency, Tangiers disease, and apoAI Milano. Because mice that are defective in apoAI production also show a similar tendency to hypertriglyceridemia,[119] it is assumed that the reduced apoCII reservoir on HDL is responsible.

Secondary Causes of Hypertriglyceridemia

Diabetes Mellitus. Diabetes mellitus is the most prominent cause of hypertriglyceridemia, which is found in up to one third of all patients with type 2 diabetes. Insulin reduces fatty acid flux from adipose tissue, reduces liver apoB production, inhibits de novo triglyceride synthesis, and optimizes LPL production.[120] In addition, diabetes is associated with increased postprandial lipemia. The most common diabetic dyslipidemia is moderate hypertriglyceridemia and low HDL. The reduced HDL results from greater exchange of VLDL triglyceride for HDL cholesterol, hydrolysis of the triglyceride-rich HDL by hepatic lipase, and more rapid clearance of the smaller HDL from the circulation. CETP also enhances transfer of triglyceride to LDL, allowing these lipoproteins to be converted to smaller, denser forms that may be more atherogenic. This lipoprotein phenotype is also commonly found in nonhyperglycemic patients with dysmetabolic syndrome. Although most patients with diabetes do not have increased LDL, some do, and LDL reduction will occur with improved diabetes control. As stated earlier, diabetes is associated with severe fasting chylomicronemia. Although many such patients also have an underlying dyslipidemia (e.g., due to heterozygous LPL deficiency), others do not have a defined lipid disorder.

Patients with type 1 diabetes in poor control also develop hypertriglyceridemia. However, because insulin stimulates HDL production, patients in good control sometimes develop high levels of HDL.

Renal Failure. Renal failure is also associated with hypertriglyceridemia and low HDL levels. The reasons for this are not clear, but it may reflect underlying insulin resistance and defects in lipolysis of plasma triglycerides.[121]

Drugs. Various drugs can elevate triglycerides. Diabetes, obesity, and renal disease are common causes of fasting hypertriglyceridemia. The most common drugs associated with hypertriglyceridemia are estrogen-like compounds, thiazides, β-blockers, protease inhibitors, glucocorticoids, immunosuppressives, retinoids (isotretinoin, Accutane), bile acid–binding resins, and newer antipsychotic medications.

Oral estrogen therapy increases plasma triglyceride levels due to greater liver production of VLDL, but combined estrogen-progestin therapy does not raise triglycerides and is sometimes associated with reduced LDL.[122] In the setting of an underlying hypertriglyceridemia, severe hyperchylomicronemia and pancreatitis can occur in patients taking oral estrogen alone or birth control pills. For this reason, triglyceride levels should be measured in women before estrogen therapy is initiated. Transdermal estrogen administration, which does not lead to high liver exposure, does not result in triglyceride elevation.[123] Tamoxifen, an SERM, can cause severe hypertriglyceridemia and pancreatitis,[124] but raloxifene, another SERM, does not raise triglycerides.[125]

Diet and Alcohol. Diets lead to marked changes in plasma triglyceride levels. Most lipoprotein profiles use fasting blood to avoid the postprandial increase in triglycerides that represent both dietary fat and de novo triglyceride production by the liver. Liver production of triglyceride is especially robust after the intake of simple sugars such as those found in sweetened foods (especially beverages including high fructose corn syrup) and other carbohydrates (bread, pasta, rice, and potatoes). Excessive intake of simple carbohydrates usually leads to moderate hypertriglyceridemia, but it can also exacerbate underlying genetic hypertriglyceridemias. Fat intake, especially in the setting of triglyceride levels greater than 500 mg/dL, can cause severe hyperchylomicronemia.

A major clinical cause of hypertriglyceridemia is alcohol intake. Sensitivity to the triglyceride-raising effects of alcohol is variable, but removal of alcohol from the diet of hypertriglyceridemic patents is often curative. Alcohol has many effects on lipid metabolism, including inducing de novo fatty acid synthesis and inhibiting fatty acid oxidation in the liver.[126] A common clinical conundrum is deciding whether hypertriglyceridemia alone is responsible for pancreatitis in an alcohol-using patient. Subjects with dysbetalipoproteinemia are particularly sensitive to the effects of alcohol consumption because the alcohol-induced overproduction of VLDL and subsequent production of remnant particles occur in the setting of impaired remnant clearance. Because alcohol also raises HDL, the presence of elevated triglycerides without reduced HDL is a clinical clue that an alcohol effect may be contributing to the lipid disorder.

Diagnostic Evaluation of Moderate Hypertriglyceridemia

A search for associated disorders, review of medication use, and delineation of dietary choices are appropriate. If both triglycerides and cholesterol are elevated, a search for the underlying lipoprotein disorder is sometimes useful. By ultracentrifugation, dysbetalipoproteinemia due to the presence of cholesterol-enriched VLDL can be differentiated from that of familial combined hyperlipidemia: The usual ratio of VLDL triglyceride to cholesterol of approximately 5 is reduced to 3 or less in dysbetalipoproteinemia. ApoE genotyping is also useful. Cholesterol-enriched VLDL are also found in patients with hypothyroidism, renal failure, or hepatic lipase deficiency.

HYPERCHOLESTEROLEMIA WITHOUT HYPERTRIGLYCERIDEMIA

Because all lipoproteins contain cholesterol, dramatic increases in triglycerides will invariably also lead to elevated blood cholesterol values. However, the ratio of triglyceride to cholesterol will be greater than 5. Disorders associated with primarily increased cholesterol are discussed in this section. The clinical presentation of hypercholesterolemia is limited. Although patients with severe disease occasionally present with cosmetic concerns or orthopedic issues associated with tendon xanthomas, hypercholesterolemia is usually clinically occult and uncovered by blood testing during routine assessment or in the setting of vascular disease.

Genetic Familial Hypercholesterolemia

The centrality of the LDL receptor to the understanding of cholesterol metabolism was uncovered through investigations by the Brown and Goldstein laboratory (discussed earlier) into the cause of FH. This relatively common cause of severe hypercholesterolemia results from one of many defects in production of the LDL receptor leading to impaired function or production of the LDL receptor protein.[127] Patients with FH (most with heterozygous forms of the disease) have cholesterol levels that exceed 300 mg/dL. Homozygous presentations of the disease include cholesterol levels that are approximately twice this value. The heterozygous form occurs at a frequency of about 1 in 500 in the general population and is a major cause of early-onset coronary artery disease. In addition, homozygous and some other severe forms of LDL receptor deficiency are associated with aortic valve calcification and stenosis.[128]

For unknown reasons, elevated LDL cholesterol leads to cholesterol deposition on tendons. Tendon xanthomas like those seen in Figure 37-17C and D occur in approximately 75% of FH patients. It is most common on the Achilles tendon. On inspection, a loss of the usual bow-like shape of the tendon occurs, or a bump or generalized thickening of the tendon is apparent. The irregularity of the tendon can also be detected by palpation. This physical finding is sometimes similar to scarring that results from tendon rupture. If the tendon is abnormal, a history of athletic injury should be sought. Xanthomas also occur on extensor tendons of the hands, but less frequently, and are best appreciated on the knuckles of a clenched fist. Xanthomas of the Achilles tendon can cause recurrent episodes of Achilles tendinitis. Some xanthomas are subtle and are apparent only as a thickening of the tendon or a small bump at the insertion of the tendon into muscle. Patients with FH also have xanthelasma (Fig. 37-17A) and premature corneal arcus (i.e., in persons younger than 40 years of age), but these findings can also occur in patients without FH. Many affected subjects have no physical findings. Premature coronary artery disease is common but variable. Some FH patients develop coronary disease in the third or fourth decade of life, especially if they also have reduced HDL cholesterol levels or associated risk due to cigarette smoking. Even before the introduction of statin therapy, some patients (especially women) never developed clinical vascular disease.

Homozygosity for FH is rare, occurring at a frequency of about 1 in 10^6 in the general population. These subjects come to clinical attention early in life because of the appearance of tendon and planar xanthomas as well as tuberous xanthomas (Fig. 37-17E), marked hypercholesterolemia apparent at birth, premature coronary disease, or aortic valve disease. Typical plasma cholesterol concentrations range from 15.5 mmol/L (600 mg/dL) to 25.9 mmol/L (1000 mg/dL), and LDL-C concentrations range from 550 to 950 mg/dL. Symptomatic coronary disease can occur before age 10 years. If not treated, these homozygous persons usually die from myocardial infarction by age 20 years. Aortic valve disease in homozygotes can be valvular or supravalvular.[128] The diagnosis of homozygous FH should be suspected in any child with extremely high plasma cholesterol (typically >500 mg/dL) or the xanthomas characteristic of FH. Both parents are obligate heterozygotes and should manifest the phenotype of heterozygous FH. However, recent understanding of the biology of the LDL receptor and the role of PCSK9 (see earlier discussion) in its degradation have shown that individuals with defects in both LDL receptors and PCSK9 can have normal plasma LDL levels.[129]

Familial Defective Apolipoprotein B100

Defects in LDL binding to normal LDL receptors also lead to elevated plasma cholesterol. The ligands for the LDL receptor are apoB100 and apoE. Familial defective apoB100 increases LDL and has a phenotype that is indistinguishable from that of FH, including increased susceptibility to CHD.[130] The substitution of glutamine for arginine at amino acid 3500, which reduces LDL binding to the LDL receptor, accounts for most cases of familial defective apoB100, although other defects have also been reported. Often the LDL elevations are less severe, a reflection of a partial defect in receptor binding attributed to the mutation or the continued ability of apoE to mediate lipoprotein uptake.

Rare Mutations Associated with Elevated LDL Levels

Several rare, isolated causes of hypercholesterolemia have been reported. Mutations in *LDLRAP1,* the gene encoding a putative adaptor protein (ARH) that is required for internalization of LDL bound by the LDL receptor on the surface of hepatocytes, cause autosomal recessive hypercholesterolemia. Mutations in ARH associated with autosomal recessive hypercholesterolemia have been reported mostly in Italians (Sardinia) and Lebanese.[131]

Autosomal dominant hypercholesterolemia caused by a mutation in the gene encoding cholesterol 7α-hydroxylase has been reported in a single kindred.[132] The hypercholesterolemia is caused by defective cholesterol conversion to cholic acid.

Mutation of PCSK9 (see earlier discussion) leads to alterations in LDL receptor expression because this enzyme is responsible for intracellular LDL degradation.[133] Gain-of-function mutations reduce LDL receptor numbers and lead to defective LDL clearance by the liver. Because plasma PCSK9 causes LDL receptor degradation,[134] inhibitors of this protein are being studied as a therapy for hypercholesterolemia. Loss-of-function mutations in PSCK9 are associated with low levels of total cholesterol and LDL-C and an apparent reduction in coronary artery disease.[135]

Elevated Plasma Lipoprotein(a)

Apo(a), a protein of unknown function that shares high sequence homology with plasminogen, associates with apoB to produce an LDL termed Lp(a). Some but not all studies suggest that elevated plasma Lp(a) concentrations are associated with an increased risk of coronary disease in Caucasian populations.[136] Lp(a) is not a cardiovascular risk factor in Africans or African Americans.[137] In addition, patients with high levels of Lp(a) are more likely to clot bypass grafts and stents.[138] Unlike LDL, which confers risk as a continuous function of plasma level, risk is found only in individuals with the highest levels of Lp(a).

Plasma Lp(a) levels are to a great extent determined genetically. Lp(a) particles contain a variable number of a protein repeat known as a kringle. Smaller Lp(a) particles, with fewer kringle repeats, are usually produced at higher levels. For this reason, some have suggested that it is Lp(a) size, rather than plasma level, that confers vascular risk. Renal failure leads to elevations of Lp(a) levels.

Polygenic Hypercholesterolemia

Most patients with elevated LDL cholesterol do not have FH, and even cholesterol levels above 300 mg/dL are not usually associated with xanthomas or defects in the LDL receptor. If, as is conventional for other laboratory values, hypercholesterolemia is defined as a cholesterol value that exceeds the 95th percentile for the population, only 1 in 25 of these patients should have FH. Although diet and lifestyle influence LDL, the genetic and environmental factors associated with most elevated LDL cholesterol levels are unknown, and therefore this type of hypercholesterolemia is referred to as polygenic. Nonetheless, the increased cholesterol levels are associated with more coronary artery disease.

Increased LDL levels can be a result of defective LDL clearance with normal LDL receptors, a more subtle regulation of the receptor, or increased LDL production. This last type occurs in the setting of familial combined hyperlipoproteinemia (see later discussion), which can manifest as primary elevations of LDL. Greater LDL production due to greater absorption of gut cholesterol, abnormalities in the regulation of lipid-regulated nuclear transcription factors, or gain-of-function abnormalities in cholesterol and apoB-lipoprotein assembly pathways are all possible but poorly defined.

Lp(X)

Obstructive liver disease sometimes leads to a marked increase in plasma cholesterol. In part, this is the result of increased LDL, presumably due to a defect in LDL receptors. In addition, free cholesterol circulates associated with albumin, a particle referred to as Lp(X).[139] This is caused by a deficiency in the cholesterol esterifying enzyme, LCAT. The clinical setting suggests the diagnosis. In addition, an abnormal ratio of free to total cholesterol (or cholesteryl ester) can be determined by the laboratory. The relationship of Lp(X) to vascular disease is unclear.[140]

Sitosterolemia

In this rare disorder, dietary sitosterol and other plant sterols, which are not normally absorbed in significant quantities in the intestine, are absorbed in large amounts, resulting in their accumulation in the plasma and in peripheral tissues, causing premature atherosclerosis.[141] The molecular cause is a mutation in the genes encoding ABCG8 and ABCG5, which are responsible for re-secretion of absorbed plant sterols.[30] Patients develop tendon xanthomas in childhood and have normal to high plasma levels of LDL; the differential diagnosis includes FH and cerebrotendinous xanthomatosis. The diagnosis can be confirmed by gas-liquid chromatography of plasma lipids, which demonstrates the high levels of plant sterols. Therapy consists of restriction of plant sterols in the diet and treatment with ezetimibe, a drug that inhibits absorption of dietary sterols.[142]

Cerebrotendinous Xanthomatosis

Cerebrotendinous xanthomatosis is a rare disorder of sterol metabolism that is associated with neurologic disease, tendon xanthomas, and cataracts in young adults.[143] Neurologic manifestations include cerebellar ataxia, dementia, spinal cord paresis, and subnormal intelligence. Premature atherosclerosis is common. Osteoporosis has been reported and is presumably caused by alterations in vitamin D metabolism.[144] The disorder results from mutations that cause deficiencies of 27-hydroxylase, a key enzyme in cholesterol oxidation and bile acid synthesis, leading to high plasma levels of cholesterol and cholestanol, with subsequent accumulation of these sterols in tendons and in tissues of the nervous system. Chenodeoxycholic acid is indicated for treatment.

Hypothyroidism and Elevated Cholesterol

All patients with significant hyperlipidemia should be screened for hypothyroidism, because thyroid hormone deficiency causes hypercholesterolemia, and low levels of thyroid hormone predispose to statin-induced myositis.[145] Although hypothyroidism usually increases LDL-C due to reduced LDL clearance, it can also be associated with high plasma triglyceride levels. Levels of HDL-C are usually unchanged or slightly lower in hypothyroidism and may be reduced in hyperthyroidism. Subclinical hypothyroidism is a cause of hypercholesterolemia that sometimes responds to thyroid hormone replacement.[146]

Diagnostic Evaluation of Isolated Hypercholesterolemia

A lipoprotein assessment is appropriate and, if the cholesterol level is higher than 300 mg/dL, a search for signs of FH is needed. The diagnosis of heterozygous FH is suggested by the presence of high plasma levels of total cholesterol and LDL-C, normal plasma triglycerides, tendon xanthomas, and a family history of premature coronary disease. Heterozygous FH should be suspected in any person with premature heart disease. In one study, heterozygous FH accounted for 4% of men who survived myocardial infarction before 60 years of age.[147] The diagnosis of FH is primarily a clinical diagnosis, because tests to detect one of the many LDL receptor gene mutations or to demonstrate diminished LDL receptor function are performed only in specialized research laboratories. The clinical diagnosis of FH is important not only for proper treatment of the affected patient but also for identification of other family members who may be at high risk for developing coronary disease. In addition, diagnosis of FH can be useful in genetic counseling.

Increased High-Density Lipoprotein

Occasionally, patients with hypercholesterolemia have elevations primarily of HDL, with normal levels of LDL. Usually, this pattern is found in families with little cardiovascular disease, and high HDL syndromes are associated with longevity.[148] The usual risk factor analysis and ratios of total cholesterol to HDL suggest that patients with high HDL have reduced risk of cardiovascular disease.

Newer information suggests that there are subgroups of these patients with a less sanguine prognosis. These relatively unusual patients are insufficiently represented in population studies to assess coronary risk. Isolation of HDL from patients with cardiovascular disease and high levels of HDL led to the observation that these HDL do not have anti-inflammatory properties.[149] Atherogenic HDL has been detected in patients with systemic lupus erythematosus.[150] Therefore, there are clinical circumstances in which HDL may be dysfunctional (see earlier discussion).

Genetic Disorders Causing Increased High-Density Lipoprotein

CETP deficiency is a hereditary syndrome in which plasma HDL-C levels are increased because of diminished activity of plasma CETP. The disorder is not uncommon in the Japanese population. Its features include marked elevations of plasma HDL-C in homozygotes (usually >100 mg/dL). Despite the elevated HDL-C levels, the effect on coronary disease risk of CETP gene mutations is unclear.[149] Heterozygotes have moderately elevated HDL-C levels. The lower activity of CETP results in diminished transfer of cholesteryl esters from HDL to apoB-containing lipoproteins. As a result, more cholesteryl esters are found in HDL, and the ratio of total cholesterol to HDL-C is markedly reduced. CETP is most active in the setting of hypertriglyceridemia,[151] so, in addition to reducing HDL cholesterol, it provides a mechanism for reduction of triglyceride through HDL metabolism. Perhaps for this reason, studies in mice, which normally do not have significant plasma CETP activity, have shown reduced apoB-containing lipoproteins and reduced atherosclerosis with addition of a CETP transgene. Therefore, the effect of CETP on vascular disease varies as a function of the underlying plasma lipid profile. CETP inhibition as a means to increase HDL and reduce vascular disease in humans is currently an active area of pharmaceutical research. The first CETP inhibitor tested clinically resulted in a colossal clinical trial failure, because the drug increased cardiovascular events despite elevating HDL.[152] This result was ascribed by some to an off-target effect of the drug that increased aldosterone production, leading to hypertension. Other drugs without this side effect are currently in clinical trials.

Several pharmacologic agents are associated with increased plasma HDL. The antiatherogenic capacity of HDL produced in these circumstances is unknown. HDL induction occurs with the use of oral estrogens, alcohol intake, dilantin, phenobarbital, and insulin therapy in some patients with type 1 diabetes.

Endothelial lipase deficiency is caused by defects in the third member of the lipase gene family, endothelial lipase. As described earlier, endothelial lipase is responsible in part for HDL catabolism. Mutations in endothelial lipase are associated with increased plasma HDL levels.[87] Such patients may be protected from vascular disease.

ELEVATED TRIGLYCERIDES AND CHOLESTEROL

Elevated triglyceride and cholesterol levels can be caused by increased VLDL and LDL, combined hyperlipidemia, or the presence of increased circulating remnant lipoproteins (dysbetalipoproteinemia). These are indistinguishable by routine laboratory examination, but treatment approaches differ somewhat.

Combined Hyperlipidemia

Combined hyperlipidemia is a common disorder associated with elevations of plasma cholesterol and triglyceride levels and increased susceptibility to coronary disease. Lipoprotein isolation reveals increased LDL and VLDL. Kinetic analysis has associated this pattern primarily with overproduction, rather than defective clearance, of apoB lipoproteins. When it occurs within families, it is termed *familial combined hyperlipidemia*. These individuals, who do not necessarily have other causes for lipid abnormalities, characteristically come from families with various hyperlipidemias that include increased isolated triglycerides or increased isolated LDL. Moreover, the abnormal lipoprotein pattern (increased triglycerides, cholesterol, or both) can vary over time in an individual.

Regulation of apoB production involves a number of steps (see earlier discussion), and understanding of this physiology explains some of the association of combined hyperlipidemia with other diseases. Increased fatty acid return to the liver and reduced insulin action prevent degradation of newly synthesized apoB. Therefore, it is not surprising that both dysmetabolic syndrome and type 2 diabetes are commonly found along with combined hyperlipidemias. Although the genetics of this disorder have been investigated, the coexistence of this lipoprotein pattern with insulin resistance and obesity syndromes has been a confounder. Therefore, although alterations in a number of genes associated with lipid metabolism, such as LPL and apoCIII, have been observed, a firm genetic marker is not currently available.

Familial Dysbetalipoproteinemia (Type III Hyperlipoproteinemia)

Familial dysbetalipoproteinemia (formerly known as type III hyperlipoproteinemia) is an uncommon disorder of lipoprotein metabolism that is characterized by moderate to severe hypertriglyceridemia and hypercholesterolemia caused by the accumulation of cholesterol-rich remnant particles in the plasma. Premature peripheral vascular disease and coronary artery disease are common. The cause is mutations in the apoE gene that result in defective binding of apoE to lipoprotein receptors. The disorder is associated with the apoE2 isoform and in most instances is inherited as an autosomal recessive trait. Because the phenotypic expression of the disorder is limited to approximately 1% of the patients with the apoE2/E2 phenotype, other genetic or environmental factors must also be operative. The hyperlipidemia is caused by a defect in clearance of remnant lipoproteins whose liver uptake requires apoE interaction with the LDL receptor, LRP1, and HSPG (see earlier discussion). The remnants that accumulate have lost much of their triglyceride through LPL-mediated triglyceride hydrolysis and therefore are cholesterol rich. The predominant remnant particles, termed β-VLDL, can be identified by abnormal migration on gel electrophoresis or by abnormal lipid content.

Dysbetalipoproteinemia is usually diagnosed in adulthood and is rarely detected in persons younger than 20 years of age, with the exception of those with rare autosomal dominant apoE mutations.[153] The disorder is more common in men than in women. It is characterized by moderately severe elevations in plasma triglyceride and cholesterol levels; typically, these values both range from 300 to 400 mg/dL. Concentrations of HDL-C are normal. Xanthomas are present in more than half of affected subjects. Palmar xanthomas, which are planar xanthomas in the palmar creases (see Fig. 37-17F), are pathognomonic for this disorder. Tuberous or tuboeruptive xanthomas (see Fig. 37-17E) are also common but are less specific for this disorder. Tendon xanthomas and xanthelasma occur in some patients. Unlike FH, in which peripheral vascular disease is uncommon, premature peripheral vascular disease occurs in addition to premature coronary artery disease in patients with dysbetalipoproteinemia. Coexisting metabolic conditions that exacerbate the phenotype of dysbetalipoproteinemia, such as obesity, alcohol consumption, diabetes mellitus, and hypothyroidism, are often present.

In addition to homozygosity for the apoE2 isoform, six mutations in the apoE gene are known to lead to the dysbetalipoproteinemia phenotype in an autosomal dominant fashion.[153] The phenotype manifests at an early age without exacerbating factors.

Hepatic Lipase Deficiency

Hepatic lipase deficiency is a rare disorder associated with lack of heparin-releasable hepatic lipase activity in the plasma.[154] Because this enzyme mediates the final step of conversion of IDL to LDL and is involved in chylomicron remnant clearance, its deficiency causes a phenotype that is similar to that found with dysbetalipoproteinemia—namely, elevated levels of plasma cholesterol (250 to 1500 mg/dL) and triglycerides (395 to 8200 mg/dL). Patients also have palmar and tuboeruptive xanthomas, premature arcus corneae, and premature coronary artery disease. Because hepatic lipase also mediates HDL metabolism, HDL levels are not decreased. The demonstration of hepatic lipase deficiency requires in vitro assays of hepatic lipase activity in postheparin plasma or DNA analysis to identify mutations.

Nephrotic Syndrome

Hyperlipidemia almost always accompanies the nephrotic syndrome. Total cholesterol, VLDL, LDL-C, total triglycerides, and plasma apoB may all be elevated. Nephrotic syndrome increases liver production of apoB-containing lipoproteins, leading to increased plasma LDL or VLDL, or both. This may be a response to hypoalbuminemia and an associated generalized increase in liver protein secretion.

Protease Inhibitor Use in Human Immunodeficiency Virus Infection

Treatments for human immunodeficiency virus (HIV) infection often cause hyperlipidemia, lipodystrophy, and insulin resistance.[155] Hypertriglyceridemia is the most common lipid abnormality, although increases in LDL are also found. These effects were initially thought to result from the use of protease inhibitors, but other agents, such as reverse transcriptase inhibitors, can cause dyslipidemia. The dysmetabolic syndrome is not uniformly induced by all drugs; older agents such as ritonavir are more likely to have metabolic side effects. The cause of this syndrome is unclear but may be related to greater liver production of apoB-lipoproteins and triglycerides.

Immunosuppressive Regimens

Patients undergoing transplantation who require a number of medications commonly present with hypertriglyceridemia and/or hypertriglyceridemia and hypercholesterolemia. Glucocorticoids more often raise triglycerides, cyclosporine raises cholesterol, and rapamycin increases both cholesterol and triglycerides.[156]

Diagnostic Evaluation of Elevated Triglycerides and Cholesterol

Appropriate assessment usually requires that clinicians determine whether the hyperlipidemia is primarily a genetic disorder or is secondary to another systemic disease. The clinical setting and accompanying drug therapies must be considered. In some situations, an evaluation for dysbetalipoproteinemia is useful. In other cases, empiric treatment is reasonable (see later discussion). The presence of cholesterol-enriched β-VLDL is determined by a direct measurement of the VLDL-C level to detect cholesterol-rich remnant particles. The directly measured ratio of VLDL-C to plasma triglycerides (in milligrams per deciliter) is a useful screen. In dysbetalipoproteinemia, this ratio is usually greater than 0.3 (when hyperlipidemia is present), whereas the normal ratio is typically about 0.2 (i.e., the VLDL-C concentration is about 20% of the plasma triglyceride level). Electrophoresis of plasma samples on agarose gels typically demonstrates a broad band in the β-migrating lipoprotein region. Patients with suspected dysbetalipoproteinemia can be evaluated for apoE2 homozygosity by apoE genotyping of DNA obtained from leukocytes, a procedure that is available in many clinical laboratories. The other rare dominant mutations in apoE can be diagnosed only in specialized laboratories.

HYPOCHOLESTEROLEMIA

Secondary causes that can lead to very low levels of apoB-containing lipoproteins and low cholesterol levels include malabsorption, sepsis, liver failure, and malnutrition. There are also genetic conditions that cause low cholesterol.

Familial Hypobetalipoproteinemia

Familial hypobetalipoproteinemia is defined as apoB and LDL-C levels below the 5th percentile. Hypobetalipoproteinemia is not associated with a phenotype and leads to a reduced risk for cardiovascular disease. Possible causes of this syndrome include mutations leading to truncation of apoB and mutations in *PCSK9* presumably leading to increased numbers of LDL receptors. *PCSK9* loss-of-function mutations occur in as many as 2% of African Americans but are rare in persons of European descent.

Abetalipoproteinemia

Abetalipoproteinemia is a rare autosomal recessive disorder caused by a deficiency in MTP, which results in a virtual absence of apoB-containing lipoproteins in the plasma.[62] Abetalipoproteinemia occurs in fewer than 1 in 10^6 persons and has the same phenotype as homozygous hypobetalipoproteinemia, including malabsorption of fat and fat-soluble vitamins from the intestine, which can lead to neurologic disease related to vitamin E deficiency. The disorder is usually detected in infancy because of fat malabsorption associated with marked decreases in plasma cholesterol and triglyceride levels.

Chylomicron Retention Syndrome

Anderson's disease, or chylomicron retention syndrome, is a rare condition that is phenotypically similar to abetalipoproteinemia. Subjects with Anderson's disease cannot secrete chylomicrons from the intestine. Eight mutations in the *SAR1B* gene (formerly *SARA2*) have been linked to Anderson's disease. This gene encodes SAR1B, a protein that is important in the transport of chylomicrons through the secretory pathway in enterocytes.[157]

Familial Hypoalphalipoproteinemia

Although low HDL in the general population is correlated with greater coronary artery disease, genetic disorders leading to very low plasma levels of HDL have variable and sometimes undefined coronary risk. In part, this might result from the rarity of some of these diseases. For this reason, the approach to the disorders is often unclear.

Apolipoprotein AI Mutations

Mutations in the apoAI gene can decrease HDL formation and result in low plasma HDL-C levels. ApoAI deficiency can be caused by point mutations in the apoAI gene or by deletions or gene rearrangements at the apoAI/CIII/AIV/AV gene locus.[158] ApoAI deficiency typically results in plasma HDL-C levels lower than 0.3 mmol/L (10 mg/dL). Some apoAI variants activate LCAT poorly (see later discussion). The molecular diagnosis is made by protein analysis showing an altered apoAI size or by genetic sequencing. Some apoAI variants are associated with amyloidosis.

The apoAI Milano variant (apoAI$_{Milano}$) is caused by a substitution of cysteine for arginine at amino acid 173. This results in low plasma HDL-C levels without premature CHD. Therefore, this HDL is hypothesized to be antiatherogenic and has been used in a human clinical trial.[159]

Lecithin:Cholesterol Acyltransferase Deficiency

LCAT deficiency leads to low HDL as a consequence of defective conversion of cholesterol to cholesteryl ester. In a phenotypically appropriate patient, measurement of the ratio of free cholesterol to cholesteryl ester is diagnostic; normally free cholesterol is approximately 30% of the total, but this increases to more than 90% in LCAT deficiency. LCAT activity measurements and sequencing can also be performed. LCAT deficiency leads to striking corneal arcus, normochromic anemia, and, occasionally, renal failure in young adults.[160] Renal biopsies show characteristic foam cells. Despite their very low HDL levels, the risk of coronary disease in patients with LCAT deficiency is not pronounced; this may reflect the low levels of LDL that are also found in many of these patients.

A variant of LCAT deficiency, called fish-eye disease, is also caused by mutations of the LCAT gene. The phenotype is less severe than that seen in complete LCAT deficiency.[161] Fish-eye disease is characterized by low plasma HDL-C levels and corneal opacities; anemia and renal disease do not occur. The phenotypic differences between LCAT deficiency and fish-eye disease have been attributed to whether mutations in the LCAT gene encode variants that fail to esterify cholesterol of both HDL and apoB-containing lipoproteins (LCAT deficiency) or of HDL only (fish-eye disease).

Adenosine Triphosphate–Binding Cassette Transporter A1 Deficiency

The ABCA1 transporter is essential to complete synthesis of mature HDL by the liver and the small intestine. A number of mutations in this receptor are associated with hypoalphalipoproteinemia.[162] Because the number of genetic mutations is great, assays often study fibroblast "unloading" of cholesterol to apoAI to show the defect.

Tangier disease is the most flagrant example of a defect in ABCA1. These patients, originally from Tangier Island in the Chesapeake Bay, had hypocholesterolemia resulting from a marked decrease in plasma HDL as well as low LDL and the striking physical finding of orange tonsils. The orange tonsils are thought to result from defective reverse cholesterol transport from macrophages of the reticuloendothelial system, with the color probably caused by carotenoids. The risk of cardiovascular disease with this syndrome is uncertain.

OVERVIEW OF ATHEROGENESIS

Atherosclerosis and its clinical presentation as coronary artery disease, stroke, and peripheral vascular disease is likely to be the product of several pathophysiologies. Depending on the patient and setting, arterial disease results from a varying reaction to lipid infiltration, arterial damage, and macrophage inflammation. Population, genetic, and therapeutic data suggest that atherosclerosis is frequently caused by cholesterol deposition within the arterial wall. Those data include studies that correlated plasma cholesterol and coronary artery disease both within and between populations. As described earlier, a number of genetic hyperlipidemic disorders are associated with premature atherosclerosis. Reductions of blood cholesterol by diet, surgical ileal bypass, statins, and other cholesterol-lowering therapies have convincingly shown the impact of blood cholesterol on arteries. This cholesterol hypothesis is further supported by a wealth of animal data: Altering blood lipid levels by diet or genetic modification causes atherosclerosis-free animals to develop disease. However, both in animals and in humans, vascular disease is not universal, even among those individuals with marked hypercholesterolemia. Similarly, patients with low cholesterol are not assured of being protected from the disease. It is estimated that about 50% of all atherosclerosis is attributable to hyperlipidemia and other known cardiac risk factors.[163]

In contrast, other approaches to atherosclerosis treatment directed toward theoretical etiologies have not been supported by human clinical intervention trials. Use of vitamin E and antibiotics has not altered CHD. Although low-dose aspirin has some anti-inflammatory properties, its reduction of cardiovascular events is most likely secondary to effects on coagulation rather than direct effects on atherosclerosis.

There are a number of clinical situations in which cholesterol reduction has failed to alter vascular disease. Most notably, statin-mediated cholesterol reduction appears to be ineffective in end-stage renal disease.[164] A similar situation may exist in other inflammatory diseases (e.g., collagen-vascular diseases) that are associated with cardiac events but have not yet been shown to respond to cholesterol-lowering therapies.[165] These diseases are more likely to have a primary inflammatory etiology,[166] the causes of which include hypertension, cigarette smoking, infections, and immune reactions.

Cholesterol-Induced Atherosclerosis

More than 100 years ago, pathologists identified cholesterol as a major component of atherosclerosis. This poorly metabolized lipid is found both associated with matrix and within arterial cells. Macrophages and smooth muscle cells are converted into foam cells, so called because of their intracellular foamy lipid. In addition, there are often acellular lipid-rich areas, a variable amount of overlying collagen-rich connective tissue, and regions where the atherosclerotic plaque has ruptured. The process begins with lipid infiltration into the arterial wall.[167,168]

Unresolved pathogenic issues include the following: (1) How does lipid enter the artery? (2) What pathways lead to excess lipid uptake by foam cells? and (3) What processes cause rupture and thrombosis?

Infiltration of lipoproteins into the artery wall is likely to be a normal and continuous process. Larger particles, such as chylomicrons, are more likely to be excluded by the endothelial barrier.[169] LDL can leave the circulation via channels between cells, along the continuous transendothelial movement of cell-free plasma, or via interaction with specific receptors. Once in the subendothelial space, lipoproteins must accumulate to cause disease. It is theorized that positive charges on apoB interact with negatively charged proteoglycans to promote lipoprotein retention. Both apoB100 in LDL and VLDL, apoB48 in chylomicron remnants, and apoE in several classes of lipoproteins have proteoglycan-binding sequences.[170] Another possibility is that, within the artery, lipoproteins fuse to form large aggregates that are unable to disassociate and re-enter the circulation.[171] Lipoprotein uptake into cells is usually well controlled, because excess cellular cholesterol downregulates LDL receptors. Therefore, aberrant lipoprotein receptor regulation may be a factor, or LDL (and remnants) may enter cells by non–cholesterol-regulated pattern recognition receptors (see earlier discussion).

Cholesterol-containing lipoproteins can become inflammatory. Enzymes within the artery might induce alterations in the protein and lipid content of LDL that convert these particles into more-inflammatory oxidized LDL.[172]

Unstable Plaque and Regression

The atherogenic process occurs within the artery wall. Initially, it was thought that the lumen was progressively narrowed by the accumulation of macrophages, the proliferation of smooth muscle cells, and the deposition of cholesterol. In fact, the truly dangerous lesion (the culprit lesion) may not cause marked luminal narrowing.[173] As atherosclerosis progresses, there is a compensatory expansion of the lumen that maintains an almost constant lumen size. As the lesion develops within the intima, the complication of rupture of the overlying intima or endothelial erosion leads to exposure of the lesional contents to platelets, initiating thrombosis. It is the acute thrombosis, not arterial lumen stenosis, that is responsible for infarctions in most patients. Rupture or erosion occurs where the fibrous cap covering the underlying thrombogenic lipid is thin and where an active inflammatory process is occurring.

The surfaces of complicated lesions can become thrombogenic as endothelial cells are lost or the fibrous cap ruptures and the subendothelial space is exposed. Platelets can adhere to this exposed surface, promoting thrombus formation. In these unstable plaques, blood actually dissects into the artery wall, leading to the formation of a large thrombus. Calcification is also a feature of late lesions. Advanced lesions can weaken the elasticity and integrity of the artery wall, potentially creating an aneurysm of the vessel. As clinical trial data have shown, removal or reduction of the atherogenic stimulus can result in plaque regression and stabilization, leaving a remnant devoid of lipid that resembles a wound scar and is less likely to serve as a nidus for thrombus formation.

Atherosclerosis usually develops in the setting of hypercholesterolemia. Observations first made in animals and now confirmed in humans indicate that this process can be reversed if plasma cholesterol reduction is intensive.[174]

EVIDENCE SUPPORTING TREATMENT OF LIPID DISORDERS

Cholesterol and Cardiovascular Disease

Despite a very significant decrease in the incidence of vascular disease, cardiovascular diseases including CHD and cerebrovascular disease remain the major causes of death in the United States for both men and women. The major risk factors are age, elevated LDL-C, reduced HDL-C, smoking, hypertension, insulin resistance with or without overt diabetes mellitus, and a family history of premature CHD. Modifiable risk factors account for most of the excess CHD risk. Although a number of new risk factors have been proposed to increase the accuracy of predicting risk of CHD events, only four conditions—dyslipidemia, hypertension, cigarette smoking, and/or diabetes—account for increased CHD risk in 80% to 90% of patients.[175,176]

Understanding of the relationship of cholesterol and lipids to atherosclerosis has evolved over the last century and especially over the last 60 years.[177] The "lipid hypothesis," which postulates that increased plasma cholesterol concentrations increase the risk of CHD, that diets high in fat (especially saturated fat of animal origin) and cholesterol increase plasma cholesterol levels, and that lowering of cholesterol levels would decrease the risk of atherosclerotic vascular disease, was not accepted for many years.[177,178] Data from population studies, animal studies, cell culture experiments, and, eventually, clinical trials of lipid-lowering interventions have made the treatment of hyperlipidemia an accepted strategy for decreasing cardiovascular risk.[178-180]

Epidemiologic Evidence

A number of studies have demonstrated a relationship between plasma cholesterol levels and the risk of CHD. Analysis of cholesterol levels of men who were screened for the Multiple Risk Factor Intervention Trial (see Fig. 37-16) showed that there is increased risk at total cholesterol levels greater than 5.2 mmol/L (200 mg/dL).[181] Multiple studies have demonstrated the relationship between cardiovascular risk factors, dietary cholesterol and saturated fats, and the incidence of CHD, providing solid epidemiologic data for the lipid hypothesis.[179] Epidemiologic and clinical studies involving lifestyle changes have led to a variety of recommendations for diet and exercise approaches to decreasing cardiovascular risk.[97,182-184]

Clinical Trials

Lowering cholesterol decreases the risk of CHD, as has been shown in many human clinical trials. In all groups examined, including patients with and without preexisting CHD over a range of initial plasma cholesterol levels, the results have demonstrated that sufficient lowering of plasma cholesterol levels reduces the risk of CHD regardless of the baseline cholesterol level.

Clinical trial data of lipid-modifying therapies include trials of both primary and secondary prevention, with measurements of clinical events and surrogate measurements such as carotid intima media thickness, quantitative coronary angiography, and intravascular ultrasound and a variety of therapies including diet, partial ileal bypass, nicotinic acid, fibric acid derivatives, BAS, HMG-CoA reductase inhibitors, ω-3 fatty acids, LDL apheresis, and combinations of drugs. The most rigorous evidence is that of randomized controlled trials with cardiovascular events as the end point, but studies using vascular imaging techniques provide supporting evidence of benefit.

Before 1984, a number of clinical trials demonstrated the benefits of cholesterol lowering in both primary and secondary prevention settings using several medications, but they did not convince the medical profession that lowering of cholesterol was beneficial.[178] In 1984, the large, randomized, placebo-controlled, Coronary Primary Prevention Trial demonstrated that cholesterol lowering with the BAS cholestyramine decreased the risk of nonfatal myocardial infarction and cardiac death in men with high cholesterol levels.[185] However, the study did not have adequate statistical power to show an effect on mortality, and there remained concerns that cholesterol lowering did not decrease overall mortality. Other studies in the 1980s showed that use of cholesterol-lowering medications could decrease the progression of coronary atherosclerosis as demonstrated by coronary angiography. Two notable studies were the Cholesterol Lowering Atherosclerosis Study (CLAS)[186] and the Familial Atherosclerosis Treatment Study (FATS).[187]

The Scandinavian Simvastatin Survival Study (4S),[188] a randomized, placebo-controlled trial using simvastatin in men and women with preexisting coronary artery disease and high LDL-C levels (190 mg/dL), evaluated total and cardiovascular mortality. It demonstrated a decrease in both cardiovascular and total mortality and provided compelling evidence of the benefit of cholesterol reduction. The 4S study finally convinced many researchers and practitioners of the value of lipid lowering, at least for secondary prevention. Cholesterol and Recurrent Events (CARE), another secondary prevention event trial done in patients with a history of myocardial infarction and baseline LDL-C levels of 115 to 175 mg/dL, showed a decrease in event rate with pravastatin treatment.[189] This benefit also extends to patients with a relatively low baseline LDL-C. In the Heart Protection Study, simvastatin decreased the first major vascular event by 24% in high-risk patients, even when LDL-C cholesterol was lower than 3.0 mmol/L (116 mg/dL).[190] Evidence for even lower LDL-C targets came from the Pravastatin or Atorvastatin Evaluation and Infection Therapy (PROVE-IT) study, which showed a benefit of atorvastatin (80 mg/day) compared with pravastatin (40 mg/day) in patients with acute coronary syndromes,[191] and from the Treating to New Target (TNT) study comparing atorvastatin (80 mg/day) with atorvastatin (10 mg/day) in patients with stable coronary disease.[192]

Clinical trials of primary prevention such as the West of Scotland study,[193] the Air Force/Texas Coronary Atherosclerosis Protection (AFCAPS/TexCAPS) study,[194] and the Collaborative Atorvastatin Diabetes Study (CARDS)[195] demonstrated the benefits of lowering LDL-C to reduce coronary artery disease events in patients without a history of CHD who had, respectively, high LDL-C levels, low HDL-C levels, and type 2 diabetes. The West of Scotland study confirmed a decrease in risk of coronary events in men with elevated cholesterol levels and no previous history of myocardial infarction.[193] The AFCAPS study showed the benefits of LDL-C lowering for primary prevention in both men and women with HDL-C levels lower than 50 mg/dL.[194] More recent evidence for the use of statins in primary prevention of cardiovascular events came from the Justification for the Use of Statins in Prevention: an Intervention Trial Evaluating Rosuvastatin (JUPITER) study, in which men and women with LDL-C levels of 108 mg/dL at baseline were randomly assigned to receive either rosuvastatin or placebo. The trial was terminated early when there was a highly significant decrease in cardiovascular events in the statin-treated group.[196]

Although the beneficial effect of cholesterol lowering through LDL-C reduction is well established, evidence for the benefit of lowering triglycerides or raising HDL-C levels, or both, is less robust. Data are most significant in studies of the fibric acid gemfibrozil and of niacin; niacin also lowers LDL-C levels at high doses. The Helsinki Heart Study[197] and the Veterans Affairs–High-Density Lipoprotein Cholesterol Intervention Trial (VA-HIT)[198] both used gemfibrozil, the former for primary prevention and the latter for secondary prevention, and in both studies the greatest benefit was in men with high triglyceride and low HDL-C levels. Studies with other fibrates, such as fenofibrate, have yielded results without unequivocal statistical significance.[199] The niacin arm of the Coronary Drug Project showed a decrease in nonfatal myocardial infarctions in men with coronary artery disease during the 6-year trial and a decrease in total mortality in the 9 years after the study.[200]

Although event trials provide the best evidence, studies using carotid intima medial thickness, coronary artery angiography, or coronary intravascular ultrasound have provided useful information. Trials with statins have shown an effect on the progression of atherosclerosis. In an uncontrolled study, rosuvastatin was associated with a reduction of total atheroma volume by 6.8% as determined by intravascular ultrasound (A Study to Evaluate the Effect of Rosuvastatin on Intravascular Ultrasound-Derived Coronary Atheroma Burden: ASTEROID).[174] In the Reversal of Atherosclerosis with Aggressive Lipid Lowering (REVERSAL) study, treatment with atorvastatin 80 mg/day (treatment LDL-C, 79 mg/dL) was associated with no progression of coronary artery disease compared with pravastatin 40 mg/day (treatment LDL-C, 110 mg/dL), which led to progression of disease.[201]

Clinical event trial data for combination therapy of hyperlipidemia are minimal, but surrogate end point studies using coronary angiography have suggested benefit of combination therapy. Studies using a BAS and niacin, a statin and niacin, or triple therapy with a statin, niacin, and BAS have shown decreased progression of atherosclerosis.[186,187,202,203] One of these studies, the FATS trial, showed decreases in end points as well as angiographic benefit of therapy.[187] Combinations including niacin have also shown benefit in studies measuring carotid intima medial thickness.[204,205]

The large beneficial effect of cholesterol lowering, particularly with statins, on rates of cardiovascular events for both primary and secondary prevention and in a wide variety of patients[2] has continued to inform committees writing guidelines for the treatment of hyperlipidemia.[97,206,207] Committees are still grappling with unanswered questions. Although decreasing LDL-C reduces CHD risk by 30% to 50% in statin studies, there is still significant residual risk, especially in patients with established vascular disease, many of whom have events despite achieving LDL-C levels of 70 to 80 mg/dL, as was shown in the Treating to New Targets study.[192] Other questions include the following: How early in life should therapy be started for primary prevention? Will longer duration of therapy lead to better outcomes? What is the benefit of lowering triglycerides or raising HDL-C? What biomarkers are best to screen and monitor in at-risk patients? Can other mediators of atherosclerosis be manipulated? How can lifestyle changes be accomplished? Additional clinical trials are underway to answer some of these questions.

TREATMENT OF LIPID DISORDERS

Rationale for Treating Hyperlipidemia

Clinical trials have clearly demonstrated the benefit of LDL-C reduction[2] and that reduction of triglycerides and increases in HDL-C may also be beneficial.[197,198,208] Treatment of severe hypertriglyceridemia is indicated to reduce the risk of pancreatitis. Optimal management of risk factors reduces the risk of atherosclerotic clinical events. However, the 5-year incidence of myocardial infarction or cardiac death from a first heart attack remains high, with rates of 14% to 32% depending on age, race, and gender.[209]

Data from the INTERHEART study, a case-control study spanning 52 countries, suggest that optimization of nine easily measured and potentially modifiable risk factors could result in a 90% reduction in the risk of an initial acute myocardial infarction. The effect of these risk factors is consistent in men and women across different geographic regions and ethnic groups. The nine risk factors are cigarette smoking, abnormal blood lipid levels, hypertension, diabetes, abdominal obesity, lack of physical activity, low daily fruit and vegetable consumption, alcohol overconsumption, and a psychosocial index (reflecting depression, interpersonal stress at work or home, financial stress, major life events, and lack of control).[210]

Approach to the Hyperlipidemic Patient

The initial evaluation consists of a history and physical examination, including assessment of CHD risk factors (Table 37-6) and measurement of plasma lipids (Table 37-7). Exclusion of secondary causes of lipid disorders (see earlier discussion) is important. Obesity is an independent risk factor for CHD not included in the formal list of NCEP risk factors, although it is reflected in the waist circumference measurement that is used to define the dysmetabolic syndrome (see Table 37-5). Obesity aggravates dyslipidemia, hypertension, and insulin resistance and is a target of therapy regardless of the severity of traditional CHD risk factors. Particular emphasis should be placed on obtaining a detailed history of all first-degree relatives to identify cholesterol disorders or premature CHD.

TABLE 37-6

Major Risk Factors for Coronary Heart Disease

Positive Factors	
Age	Men, ≥45 yr; women, ≥55 yr
Current cigarette smoking	
Diabetes mellitus*	
Family history of premature CHD	Definite myocardial infarction or sudden death before age 55 yr in father or other male first-degree relative (or before age 65 yr in mother or other female first-degree relative)
Hypertension	Blood pressure ≥140 mm Hg systolic or ≥90 mm Hg diastolic, *or* on antihypertensive medication
Low HDL-C	<1.0 mmol/L (<40 mg/dL)
Negative Factors	
High HDL-C	>1.6 mmol/L (≥60 mg/dL)

*Diabetes mellitus or any clinical manifestation of atherosclerosis (claudication, stroke, abdominal aortic aneurysm) is regarded as a CHD-equivalent; that is, >20% risk of a CHD event within 10 years.

CHD, coronary heart disease; HDL-C, high-density lipoprotein cholesterol.

Adapted from The Expert Panel. Third Report of the National Cholesterol Education Program (NCEP) Expert Panel on Detection, Evaluation, and Treatment of High Blood Cholesterol in Adults (Adult Treatment Panel III): Final report. *Circulation.* 2002;106:3143-3421.

TABLE 37-7

Classification of Plasma Lipid Levels

Level	Classification
Total Cholesterol (mg/dL)	
<200	Desirable
200-239	Borderline high
>240	High
High-Density Lipoprotein Cholesterol (mg/dL)	
<40	Low (consider <50 mg/dL low for women)
>60	High
Low-Density Lipoprotein Cholesterol (mg/dL)	
<70	Optional treatment goal in very-high-risk patients
<100	Optimal
100-129	Near optimal
130-159	Borderline high
160-189	High
>190	Very high
Triglycerides (mg/dL)	
<150	Normal
150-199	Borderline high
200-499	High
>500	Very high

Adapted from The Expert Panel. Third Report of the National Cholesterol Education Program (NCEP) Expert Panel on Detection, Evaluation, and Treatment of High Blood Cholesterol in Adults (Adult Treatment Panel III): Final report. *Circulation.*2002;106:3143-3421; and Grundy SM, Cleeman JI, Merz CNB, et al. Implications of recent clinical trials for the National Cholesterol Education Program Adult Treatment Panel III guidelines. *Circulation.* 004;110:227-239.

Physical Examination

The examination should emphasize the cardiovascular system, manifestations of hyperlipidemia, and disorders causing secondary lipid abnormalities. Several unique clinical findings are illustrated in Figure 37-17.

Xanthelasmas (see Fig. 37-17A), a type of xanthoma, are raised, yellowish macules that typically appear around the medial canthus. Involvement can extend to the eyelids or skin immediately below the eye. They occur in patients with FH, familial defective apoB100, or dysbetalipoproteinemia. They occasionally occur in patients with normal cholesterol levels. Xanthelasmas typically regress with cholesterol lowering and may be treated effectively in the setting of normal cholesterol levels with cholesterol-lowering drugs.

Lipemia retinalis (see Fig. 37-17B), a condition in which lipemic blood causes opalescence of retinal arterioles, can be observed during funduscopic examination. It is typically seen only when the triglyceride levels are 22.6 mmol/L (2000 mg/dL) or higher.

Tendon xanthomas (see Fig. 37-17C and D) are nodular deposits of cholesterol that accumulate in tissue macrophages in the Achilles and other tendons, including the extensor tendons in the hands, knees, and elbows. Tendon xanthomas are often present in patients with FH or familial defective apo-B100 and sometimes in those with dysbetalipoproteinemia. As discussed earlier, the Achilles tendon should be palpated for assessment of thickness and contour.

Tuberous or tuboeruptive xanthomas (see Fig. 37-17E) develop in areas that are susceptible to trauma, such as the elbows and knees. They range from pea-sized to lemon-sized and are seen in dysbetalipoproteinemia and FH.

Palmar xanthomas (see Fig. 37-17F) are found in the palmar and digital creases of the hands. This type of xanthoma is almost pathognomonic for high plasma levels of β-VLDL and dysbetalipoproteinemia.

Eruptive xanthomas (see Fig. 37-17G) appear as small, yellowish, round papules that contain a pale center and an erythematous base. Their distribution includes the abdominal wall, back, buttocks, and other pressure contact areas. They are caused by accumulation of triglyceride in dermal histiocytes and typically occur when the plasma triglyceride level is 11.3 to 22.6 mmol/L (1000 to 2000 mg/dL) or higher. They can disappear rapidly with lowering of the plasma triglyceride concentration.

Screening for Secondary Disorders

The history and physical examination should be directed toward uncovering secondary disorders of lipid metabolism and identifying agents that could cause hyperlipidemia. Minimal studies should include fasting blood glucose, glycosylated hemoglobin, renal and hepatic function tests, urinary protein, and thyroid-stimulating hormone.

Measurement of Plasma Lipids

Ideally, plasma lipids should be measured at least twice under fasting steady-state conditions before therapeutic decisions are made (see Table 37-7). Plasma lipids are usually measured after a 12-hour fast to preclude detection of significant elevations in atherogenic remnant lipoproteins. Because cholesterol is a minor component of chylomicrons, total plasma cholesterol can be measured in either a fasting or a nonfasting state. Plasma lipid measurements are usually reliable if done within the first 24 hours after an acute myocardial infarction.[211,212]

Most clinical laboratories measure plasma levels of total triglycerides, total cholesterol, and HDL-C; the last analysis is performed after apoB-containing lipoproteins are removed from the plasma. The plasma LDL-C concentration is then calculated from these measurements by the Friedewald formula:

$$\text{LDL cholesterol} = \text{total cholesterol} - \text{HDL} - \text{VLDL}$$

where VLDL is calculated as triglycerides divided by 5. This formula assumes that cholesterol content of VLDL is about 20% of the plasma triglyceride level. It is reliable only when triglycerides are 4.5 mmol/L (400 mg/dL) or less. LDL-C concentrations calculated by this formula may be inaccurate in the presence of severe hypertriglyceridemia or when the triglyceride-to-cholesterol ratio of VLDL differs from the usual 4:1 ratio (as occurs in dysbetalipoproteinemia). Specialized laboratories can directly assay different lipoproteins by ultracentrifugation or nuclear magnetic resonance techniques. Direct measurement of LDL-C is also available in many clinical laboratories.

A triglyceride level higher than 11.3 mmol/L (1000 mg/dL) usually signifies the presence of two or more abnormalities of lipid metabolism (e.g., estrogen therapy in the presence of underlying familial hypertriglyceridemia). Elevated plasma triglyceride levels can fluctuate markedly in a single person over short periods. The fluctuation occurs because the LPL-mediated clearance mechanisms for triglyceride-rich particles become saturated at plasma triglyceride concentrations of approximately 5.6 mmol/L (500 mg/dL), and above this level plasma triglyceride concentrations largely reflect dietary fat intake. Therefore, triglyceride levels can rise precipitously as dietary fat intake increases and can fall rapidly with dietary fat restriction.

As noted earlier, visual inspection of plasma after it has been refrigerated overnight can be helpful. A cream-like layer on the top signifies chylomicrons. A turbid infranatant signifies high levels of VLDL. A cream-like top layer and turbid plasma indicates the presence of both chylomicrons and VLDL.

A complete plasma lipid profile (total cholesterol, LDL-C, HDL-C, and triglycerides) should be measured in all adults 20 years of age and older at least once every 5 years.[97] Triglycerides should be measured in all patients with pancreatitis.

Patient Selection and Treatment Goals

The presence of CHD or a CHD-equivalent (e.g., diabetes mellitus, cerebrovascular disease, peripheral arterial disease, abdominal aortic aneurysm) confers more than 20% risk of a subsequent CHD event within 10 years, and these patients require therapy. Others, especially those with two or more risk factors (see Table 37-6), should calculate the 10-year risk of a future CHD event. A calculator is available on the NCEP web site (http://hp2010.nhlbihin.net/atpiii/calculator.Asp?). Those whose 10-year risk is greater than 20% are also classified as high-risk, CHD-equivalent patients and should be treated.

Hyperlipidemia treatment in patients with established CHD is considered secondary prevention, whereas treatment in those who do not have known disease is primary prevention. When lipid-lowering therapy for primary prevention should be initiated is an unresolved question. There are no reliable biomarkers or imaging techniques that predict first events in people with dyslipidemia. Studies of high-risk groups for primary prevention have provided some guidance.[2,207] The JUPITER trial showed a statistically significant reduction in total mortality ($P < .02$) in men aged 50 years and older and women 60 years and older, many of whom would not have fit the NCEP Adult Treatment Panel III guidelines for therapy.[196] The upcoming Adult Treatment Panel IV guidelines may address some of these issues involving drug therapy in primary prevention.

Treatment of hypercholesterolemia in persons older than 85 years is of unclear benefit, but CHD accounts for a high percentage of deaths in this age group, and there are survival benefits of treatment in elderly patients up to the age of 85 years who have known CHD.[2,207]

Guidelines for treatment of patients with type 2 diabetes mellitus take into account their increased risk of cardiovascular events. The NCEP guidelines define diabetes mellitus as a CHD-equivalent, and treatment goals for lipids in diabetic patients are the same as for patients with established CHD, irrespective of whether the diabetic patient has a history of a prior CHD event.[97] Patients with established vascular disease and diabetes mellitus are considered to be at very high risk.[207]

Severe hypertriglyceridemia (>11.3 mmol/L [1000 mg/dL]) should be treated aggressively because pancreatitis associated with these levels can be fatal.

NCEP treatment goals based on LDL-C (and non–HDL-C) and risk assessment are summarized in Table 37-8.[97,207] Non–HDL-C (total cholesterol minus HDL-C) is a useful measure in those with hypertriglyceridemia because it provides an assessment of potentially atherogenic VLDL particles. Although these guidelines are helpful, many experts

TABLE 37-8

NCEP Adult Treatment Panel III Guidelines for LDL-C Reduction

Risk	Target LDL-C (mg/dL)	Target Non–HDL-C (mg/dL)	LDL-C Threshold for Therapeutic Lifestyle Changes (mg/dL)	LDL-C Threshold for Medical Intervention (mg/dL)
CHD or CHD-equivalent (10-yr risk >20%)	<100 or <70 if at very high risk	<130	≥100	≥100 (<100 optional)
≥2 risk factors (10-yr risk ≤20%)	<130	<160	≥130	10-yr risk score 10-20%: ≥130 (100-129 optional) 10-yr risk <10%: ≥160
0-1 risk factor	<160	<190	≥160	≥190 (160-189 optional)

CHD, coronary heart disease; HDL-C, high-density lipoprotein cholesterol; LDL-C, low-density lipoprotein cholesterol; NCEP, National Cholesterol Education Program.

Adapted from The Expert Panel. Third Report of the National Cholesterol Education Program (NCEP) Expert Panel on Detection, Evaluation, and Treatment of High Blood Cholesterol in Adults (Adult Treatment Panel III): Final report. *Circulation.* 2002;106:3143-3421; and Grundy SM, Cleeman JI, Merz CNB, et al. Implications of recent clinical trials for the National Cholesterol Education Program Adult Treatment Panel III guidelines. *Circulation.* 2004;110:227-239.

recommend that LDL-C be maintained at less than 130 mg/dL regardless of calculated risk.

Lowering triglycerides to less than 4.5 mmol/L (400 mg/dL) reduces the risk of developing pancreatitis. Moderate hypertriglyceridemia (in excess of 150 mg/dL) can be associated with CHD risk in certain circumstances (e.g., dysmetabolic syndrome).

Specific Therapies

Specific therapies include lifestyle changes (diet, weight management, and exercise recommendations) and drug therapy.[97]

Lifestyle Treatment

Therapeutic lifestyle changes including dietary intervention, moderate exercise, and weight loss are first-line therapies for hyperlipidemia and may be sufficient for mild dyslipidemias in low-risk patients. All other treatments should build on therapeutic lifestyle changes. In patients with established CHD, drug therapy should be instituted with diet therapy. Most patients will have a 10% to 15% decrease in LDL-C levels with diet; this may be enough to reach goal levels in some patients and is important in patients for whom the ultimate drop in LDL-C needs to be 30% to 60%. Hypertriglyceridemia often responds to decreased intake of fat, simple sugars, alcohol, and calories. Response to lipid-lowering drugs may be disappointing in patients who do not follow dietary recommendations.

Dietary changes are best when individualized and instituted gradually. Involvement of family members is important, especially if the patient does not purchase or prepare food. The therapeutic diet is shown in Table 37-9. Patients with elevated triglycerides also need to restrict simple sugars and alcohol. The response to very-low-fat diets (i.e., 10% of calories from fat) may be disappointing in patients with impaired glucose tolerance unless the diet is hypocaloric. Nonfat desserts commonly increase calorie intake. Very-high-carbohydrate diets, unless composed of primarily complex carbohydrate, may lead to poor glycemic control and increased triglyceride levels. Patients with the chylomicronemia syndrome may initially require a diet with less than 10% of calories from fat to decrease chylomicron production.

Daily moderate exercise, such as walking, may help reduce triglyceride levels. Exercise may be particularly useful in obese, insulin-resistant patients with high triglyceride levels, low HDL-C, and moderately elevated LDL-C. Weight loss is beneficial, and an exercise program combined with a moderately hypocaloric diet may lead to significant improvements in lipid levels as well as glucose tolerance. Modest weight loss may improve dyslipidemia as well as glucose tolerance and blood pressure in patients with the dysmetabolic syndrome.

The effects of various types of dietary fat have been studied extensively.[182] Current recommendations are to restrict intake of saturated fats and trans fats and to substitute complex carbohydrates, polyunsaturated fats, and monounsaturated fats.[97,184,213] Saturated fats elevate plasma cholesterol levels by decreasing receptor-mediated clearance of LDL. High levels of cholesterol intake raise plasma cholesterol by reducing receptor-mediated catabolism of LDL and by increasing LDL synthesis.[182,183] Trans fats are unsaturated fatty acids with at least one *trans* double bond; they are produced when liquid vegetable oils are partially hydrogenated to produce semisolid fats used in margarines and shortening. Trans fats raise LDL-C and reduce HDL-C and have been implicated in cardiovascular disease.[214]

Fish oils are enriched in eicosapentaenoic (EPA) or docosahexaenoic acid (DHA) (see Table 37-1). Daily doses of 4 g of EPA plus DHA lower VLDL and treat hypertriglyceridemia. Based on the results of both primary- and secondary-prevention studies, persons without known CHD should eat two fish meals weekly, and those with known CHD should take fish oil capsules that provide 1 g/day of EPA plus DHA.[215]

TABLE 37-9

Therapeutic Lifestyle Changes for Reducing Coronary Heart Disease Risk

Therapeutic lifestyle changes diet:
- Saturated fat <7% of total calories
- Polyunsaturated fat ≤10% of total calories
- Monounsaturated fat ≤20% of total calories
- Total fat 25%-35% of total calories
- Carbohydrates (predominantly complex) 50%-60% of total calories
- Fiber 20-30 g/d
- Protein approximately 15% of total calories
- Cholesterol <200 mg/d
- Consider plant stanols/sterols (2 g/d) to enhance LDL-C lowering*

Total calories: Adjust total caloric intake to maintain desirable body weight or prevent weight gain

Physical activity: Include enough moderate exercise to expend at least 200 kcal/d

LDL-C, low-density lipoprotein cholesterol.

*Adapted from Third Report of the National Cholesterol Education Program (NCEP) Expert Panel on Detection, Evaluation, and Treatment of High Blood Cholesterol in Adults (Adult Treatment Panel III): Final report. *Circulation.* 2002;106:3143-421.

Other dietary components can influence plasma lipid levels. For example, soluble fibers such as psyllium or oat bran, which can bind bile acids in the gut and promote net cholesterol excretion, decrease LDL-C to a modest extent (about 5% to 10%).[183,216] Margarines made with sitostanol or sitosterol, plant sterols that inhibit cholesterol absorption, reduce serum cholesterol by about 10%.[183] The combination of plant sterols, soluble fiber, and restriction of saturated fat and cholesterol can reduce LDL-C levels by about 30%.[217]

Recommendations for management have been developed that use teams including experienced nutritionists and dieticians.[218]

Drug Treatment

Table 37-10 lists drugs that interfere with bile acid absorption from the gut (BAS), inhibit cholesterol synthesis in cells (HMG-CoA reductase inhibitors), or block cholesterol absorption from the gut (ezetimibe). These agents work mainly by inducing LDL-receptor expression in hepatocytes. Niacin, fibrates, and ω-3 fatty acids either inhibit VLDL production or enhance clearance of triglyceride-rich particles.

TABLE 37-10

Drugs Used to Treat Hyperlipidemia

Class and Drugs Available	Dosage	Major Lipoprotein Decreased	Mechanism
Bile Acid Sequestrants			
Cholestyramine Colestipol Colesevelam	4-12 g bid 5-15 g bid 3.75-4.375 g qd	LDL	Increase sterol excretion and LDL clearance
Nicotinic Acid			
Niacin (crystalline) Niaspan	1-3 g qd 500-2000 mg qd	VLDL (LDL)	Decrease VLDL production
Fibric Acid Derivatives			
Gemfibrozil Fenofibrate*	600 mg bid 34-200 mg qd	VLDL (LDL)	Decrease VLDL production; enhance LPL action
HMG-CoA Reductase Inhibitors			
Lovastatin Pravastatin Simvastatin Fluvastatin Atorvastatin Rosuvastatin	10-80 mg qd 10-40 mg qd 5-80 mg qd 20-80 mg qd 10-80 mg qd 5-40 mg qd	LDL	Decrease cholesterol synthesis; increase LDL receptor–mediated removal of LDL
Intestinal Cholesterol Absorption Inhibitor			
Ezetimibe	10 mg qd	LDL	Inhibits cholesterol absorption
Omega-3 Fatty Acids			
Lovaza (1-g capsule contains EPA and DHA)	4 g qd	VLDL	Inhibits VLDL production

*There are several different preparations of fenofibrate with different doses.
EPA, highly concentrated ethyl esters of eicosapentaenoic acid; DHA, docosahexaenoic acid; HMG-CoA, 3-hydroxy-3-methylglutaryl coenzyme A; LDL, low-density lipoproteins; VLDL, very-low-density lipoproteins.

The best drugs for lowering LDL-C are the HMG-CoA reductase inhibitors lovastatin, pravastatin, simvastatin, fluvastatin, atorvastatin, and rosuvastatin; the BAS resins cholestyramine, colestipol, and colesevelam; the cholesterol absorption inhibitor ezetimibe; and nicotinic acid (also called niacin). Nicotinic acid, gemfibrozil, and fenofibrate are useful for hypertriglyceridemia. For elevated LDL-C combined with mild to moderate (<500 mg/dL) elevations of triglycerides, the statins, nicotinic acid, fenofibrate, or gemfibrozil may provide acceptable results. Omega-3 fatty acids can also lower triglycerides. In cases of severe hypercholesterolemia (e.g., FH) or when the goal is to attain very low LDL-C (<1.8 mmol/L [70 mg/dL]), combinations of agents may be required.

HMG-CoA Reductase Inhibitors (Statins). Before the introduction of the HMG-CoA reductase inhibitors in 1987, lowering LDL-C was often difficult because of the poor tolerability or insufficient efficacy of available therapies. Large clinical trials using statins in a variety of patients for both primary and secondary prevention of cardiovascular events contributed to evidence-based clinical guidelines.[2,97]

Inhibition of cholesterol biosynthesis by statins upregulates LDL receptors and enhances clearance of LDL.[219] Statins also reduce the release of lipoproteins from the liver.[220,221] At high doses, statins decrease triglyceride levels by enhancing the clearance of VLDL and by decreasing the production of lipoproteins.[222,223]

Statins are useful in all types of hyperlipidemia in which LDL-C is elevated, but they are less effective in homozygous LDL-receptor deficiency. They are particularly useful for patients with vascular disease and those with very high levels of LDL-C (e.g., FH, combined hyperlipidemia), and they are the drugs of choice for lowering LDL-C as secondary prevention. Several statins are approved for use in children and adolescents who have high or very high LDL-C levels and/or a significant family history of premature coronary artery disease.

Table 37-11 lists expected effects of various statins on LDL-C. They reduce LDL-C by 20% to 60%, increase HDL-C by 2% to 16%, and reduce triglycerides by 7% to 37%, depending on the drug, the dosage, and, in the case of triglycerides, baseline levels.[224] Effects also vary among patients, with greater or lesser degrees of LDL-C reduction even at the same dose. For each statin, doubling of the dose typically produces an additional 6% reduction of LDL-C.[225] LDL-C lowering is seen within 1 to 2 weeks after the start of therapy and is stable in about 4 to 6 weeks. Atorvastatin and rosuvastatin have long half-lives, about 14 hours and 21 hours, respectively. The other statins have half-lives of about 2 to 3 hours. Fluvastatin and lovastatin are available in extended-release preparations. Atorvastatin and fluvastatin have minimal renal clearance and may be more suitable for patients with significant renal insufficiency.

Lovastatin is best given with food, usually with the evening meal, but pravastatin, simvastatin, and fluvastatin can be given without food, preferably in the evening. Atorvastatin, rosuvastatin, and extended-release formulations of statins can be given at any time during the day. Several of the statins are available as generic drugs in the United States. Table 37-12 shows specific features of available statins.

The reductase inhibitors are well tolerated and cause few side effects. The most common side effects include abdominal pain, constipation, flatulence, nausea, headache, fatigue, diarrhea, and muscle complaints. Except for musculoskeletal symptoms, most side effects are infrequent

TABLE 37-11

Typical LDL-C Reductions (% Change from Baseline) by Statin Dose

Treatment	5 mg	10 mg	20 mg	40 mg	80 mg
Rosuvastatin	−40	−46	−52	−55	—
Atorvastatin	—	−37	−43	−48	−51
Simvastatin	−26	−30	−38	−41	−47
Lovastatin	—	−21	−27	−31	−40
Pravastatin	—	−20	−24	−30	−36
Fluvastatin	—	—	−22	−25	−35
Ezetimibe 10 mg plus variable simvastatin	—	−45	−52	−55	−60

LDL-C, low-density lipoprotein cholesterol; —, data not available.
From Hou R, Goldberg AC. Lowering low-density lipoprotein cholesterol: statins, ezetimibe, bile acid sequestrants, and combinations—comparative efficacy and safety. *Endocrinol Metab Clin North Am.* 2009;38:79-97.

and occur in only about 5% of patients. The adverse effects associated with statin use correlate with drug dose.[192,226,227]

Although liver toxicity is frequently a concern for patients and physicians, it is not common with statin use, and serious hepatotoxicity is extremely rare. Hepatic aminotransferase elevation is usually mild and does not require discontinuation of the statin. It may be dose dependent, as demonstrated in clinical trials that showed rates of persistent elevations of liver aminotransferase greater than 3 times the upper limit of normal occurring in 0.1% to 1.9% of patients, depending on the statin and the dose.[228]

Only about 1% of patients have aminotransferase increases to greater than 3 times the upper limit of normal, and the elevation often decreases even if patients continue on the statin.[229] A common cause is hepatic steatosis, which responds to weight loss. Statins should be used cautiously in the presence of liver disease, although nonalcoholic hepatic steatosis is not a contraindication.[230] Hepatic function tests should be obtained at baseline and at 6 and 12 weeks. If aminotransferases remain greater than 3 times the upper limit of normal, consider changing to a different statin and identify other contributing conditions or drugs. Irreversible liver damage resulting from statins is extremely rare, with a liver failure rate of 1 case per 1 million person-years of use.[230]

Muscle-related complaints occur in about 10% of people taking statins. Other disorders must be excluded, such as hypothyroidism, vitamin D deficiency, rheumatologic conditions, and perhaps depression. Inhibition of statin catabolism is associated with increased myopathy risk. Drugs metabolized through the cytochrome P450 (CYP) system, such as ketoconazole, itraconazole, clarithromycin, and erythromycin,[231] increase statin plasma levels. Other drugs that increase the risk of statin myopathy include gemfibrozil, cyclosporine, digoxin, verapamil, diltiazem, amiodarone, colchicine, and protease inhibitors.[232] The most serious potential side effect is rhabdomyolysis leading to myoglobinuria and renal failure. Rhabdomyolysis is rare and is more likely in patients with renal insufficiency, advanced age, other comorbidities, or polypharmacy and during perioperative periods.[233] Routine surveillance of creatine kinase levels is not useful in most patients. Management of dyslipidemia in patients with muscle-related complaints is challenging and may include using a different statin, decreasing the dosing frequency, or resorting to other LDL-lowering drugs.[232]

There is no evidence that statins cause direct adverse effects on renal function beyond that due to rhabdomyolysis.[234] Statins are contraindicated in pregnancy and nursing and in patients with significant hepatic dysfunction.

TABLE 37-12

Features of Individual Statins

Drug	Pharmacologic Considerations	Safety Issues
Fluvastatin	Synthetic drug; minimal renal excretion	Can interact with warfarin, phenytoin, glyburide, diclofenac, fluconazole, ketoconazole
Pravastatin	Derived from fermentation product of *Aspergillus terreus*; dose reduction in renal insufficiency	Drug interaction with cyclosporine
Lovastatin	First statin marketed in U.S.; isolated from a strain of *A. terreus*; food intake increases absorption	Interactions with CYP3A4 substrates
Simvastatin	Synthetic derivative of fermentation product of *A. terreus*; dose reduction in severe renal insufficiency	Interactions with CYP3A4 substrates
Atorvastatin	Synthetic drug; <2% excreted in urine; half-life 14 hr	Interacts with CYP3A4 substrates; increases digoxin levels
Rosuvastatin	Synthetic compound; active metabolite is formed by CYP2C9	Can increase INR when used with warfarin—monitor INR

CYP2C9 and CYP3A4, cytochrome P450 isoenzymes 2C9 and 3A4; INR, international normalized ratio.
From Hou R, Goldberg AC. Lowering low-density lipoprotein cholesterol: statins, ezetimibe, bile acid sequestrants, and combinations—comparative efficacy and safety. *Endocrinol Metab Clin North Am.* 2009;38:79-97.

Bile Acid Sequestrants. The BAS drugs have been used since the 1970s. Cholestyramine, colestipol, and colesevelam are available in the United States. BAS have been shown to reduce cardiovascular events in clinical trials.[185,235,236]

They work by binding negatively charged bile acids and bile salts in the small intestine to interrupt the enterohepatic circulation of bile acids and increase the conversion of cholesterol into bile.[237,238] Decreased hepatocyte cholesterol content increases LDL receptors.[239] Cholesterol synthesis also increases, which promotes VLDL secretion. This limits the LDL-lowering effect and raises triglyceride levels.[240]

BAS reduce LDL-C and total cholesterol; HDL-C may increase modestly.[241] As monotherapy, BAS lower LDL-C by 5% to 30% in a dose-dependent manner.[185,242-246] Colesevelam has greater bile acid–binding capacity and affinity than cholestyramine or colestipol and can be used at lower doses.[241,243] LDL-C reduction is typically 15% at 3.8 g/day (six 625-mg tablets) and 18% at 4.3 g/day (seven 625-mg tablets).[242,245,247]

BAS are most useful in patients with elevated LDL-C levels as their major lipid abnormality. They can be combined with statins or niacin to achieve greater LDL-C reduction in patients with severe LDL-C elevations, or they can be used alone for initial therapy in low-risk patients and in patients who cannot tolerate statins. BAS have been reported to lower fasting blood glucose and hemoglobin A_{1c} levels in patients with diabetes.[248]

The BAS are neither absorbed nor metabolized and therefore have essentially no systemic exposure. They are extremely safe and can be used in women not using contraception. Gastrointestinal disturbances are common and include constipation, nausea, bloating, abdominal pain, flatulence, and aggravation of hemorrhoids. Initiation with low doses, patient education, and use of stool softeners or psyllium can increase compliance. Cholestyramine and colestipol can affect the absorption of a wide variety of drugs. When used with these agents, other drugs should be taken either 1 to 2 hours before or 4 to 6 hours after the BAS. Colesevelam is better tolerated and does not bind most drugs, with the exceptions of verapamil and thyroxine.[247,249]

These drugs should not be used in patients with severe constipation or bowel or biliary obstruction, nor those taking complicated medical regimens. They worsen hypertriglyceridemia and therefore should not be used in patients with severe hypertriglyceridemia or dysbetalipoproteinemia. Despite a theoretical concern about absorption of fat-soluble vitamins, vitamin K deficiency and bleeding are rare.[250]

Niacin. Nicotinic acid, or niacin, is a B-complex vitamin that was found to lower plasma cholesterol in humans in 1955. Niacin, either alone or in combination regimens, decreases the rates of cardiovascular events and atherosclerosis.[186,187,200,204] Its mechanism of action is not completely understood, but it decreases triglyceride synthesis, leading to decreased VLDL secretion.[251] How niacin elevates HDL is unclear.

Niacin affects multiple lipoproteins and is the most effective drug currently available to raise HDL-C. At doses of 500 to 2000 mg/day, niacin lowers triglycerides by 10% to 30% and increases HDL-C by 10% to 40%. Doses of 1500 to 2000 mg/day decrease LDL-C by 10% to 20%. Niacin also lowers Lp(a) by up to 25%. It is useful for patients with combined hyperlipidemia and low HDL. It is not the best LDL-lowering drug, but it may be helpful when cost is limiting, because crystalline niacin is inexpensive.

Cutaneous flushing, which is most notable with the first doses, is the most common side effect. It occurs 15 to 60 minutes after ingestion, lasts 15 to 30 minutes, and may be related to release of dermal prostaglandin D_2. Ingestion with food and taking aspirin (preferably 325 mg) 30 to 60 minutes in advance of niacin minimizes flushing. Starting low and gradually increasing the dose improves tolerability. Repeated and consistent dosing is associated with tolerance to the flushing syndrome. A severe flush can sometimes be stopped by the ingestion of an 81-mg aspirin tablet dissolved in water.[252] Crystalline niacin should always be given with meals. Extended-release niacin (Niaspan) may be better tolerated than crystalline niacin. It is usually initiated with 500 mg at bedtime for 1 month, then titrated over 8 to 12 weeks to the maximum dose of 2000 mg/day. Niaspan can be given with meals if patients awaken with flushing in the middle of the night.[252] Alcoholic beverages potentiate flushing.

Liver function tests should be monitored, because hepatotoxicity is the most serious side effect. Because some over-the-counter sustained-release preparations have been associated with liver toxicity, crystalline (non–timed-release) nonprescription preparations should be used, and patients should not change brands after being titrated to high doses.[253] Niaspan, available by prescription, was not associated with significant liver toxicity in clinical trials. Nausea, fatigue, and malaise may be signs of hepatotoxicity.

Worsening of glucose tolerance and hyperuricemia may also occur. Niacin can be used safely in patients with glucose intolerance or diabetes mellitus, and especially in those already being treated with glucose-lowering agents. Initiation of niacin may increase glucose, but glycemic control usually returns to pretreatment levels.[254] Niacin should be used with caution in patients who have a history of gout. It is contraindicated in those with active peptic ulcer disease. Rare side effects include blurred vision and a reversible condition known as cystoid macular edema. Myopathy is rare with niacin alone or in combination with statins.[253]

It is useful to check transaminases, glucose, and uric acid at baseline and during dose titration. Patients taking niacin should be monitored at 4- to 6-month intervals for signs of hepatic toxicity. Niacin can be discontinued temporarily if transaminases rise significantly. Retitration is possible once enzyme levels return to normal.

Niacin is contraindicated during pregnancy.

Fibrates. In the Helsinki Heart Study (primary prevention) and the VA HIT (secondary prevention), the use of the fibrate gemfibrozil reduced fatal and nonfatal CHD events and did not increase mortality from noncardiac causes.[197,198] In the Fenofibrate Intervention and Event Lowering in Diabetes (FIELD) study, fenofibrate (another drug in the same class) decreased cardiac events but not cardiovascular or total mortality in patients with type 2 diabetes.[199]

These drugs activate PPARα (see earlier discussion), which increases fatty acid oxidation, increases LPL, decreases apoCIII, and increases apoAI as well as apoAII, lowering triglycerides (by 30% to 50%) and raising HDL (by 10% to 20% in those with elevated triglycerides).[255] Fibrates may lower LDL-C modestly, but they are most commonly used for severe hypertriglyceridemia and combined hyperlipidemia. Fenofibrate may be taken once daily. Gemfibrozil is given twice a day with meals.

Side effects may include gastrointestinal discomfort, rash, and pruritus. The risk of gallstones may be increased. Liver transaminases may increase, particularly with fenofibrate. Their use should be avoided in patients with renal insufficiency, which predisposes to myopathy. The combination of gemfibrozil and most statins is associated with an increased risk of myopathy due to increased statin blood levels.[256] Fenofibrate does not interfere with statin metabolism and is preferred in fibrate/statin combination regimens.[257] Because of the effects on protein binding, warfarin doses may need to be adjusted when fibrate therapy is started. Fibrates are contraindicated in patients with liver or gallbladder disease. Gemfibrozil may be used beginning in the second trimester in pregnant women with severely elevated triglycerides who are at risk for pancreatitis.

Ezetimibe. Ezetimibe inhibits cholesterol absorption (see earlier discussion). It is mostly used in combination with statins to further lower LDL-C and is being studied for clinical outcomes.

The drug interacts with the NPC1L1 transporter[29] to decrease intestinal cholesterol absorption, leading to decreased hepatic cholesterol and increased LDL receptors, clearance of LDL-C from the plasma, and consequent reduction of plasma LDL-C. Ezetimibe undergoes glucuronidation, leading to extensive enterohepatic circulation.

Ezetimibe lowers LDL-C by 14% to 25%,[258-260] and it is used alone or in combination with statins or other lipid-modifying drugs. It lowers LDL-C by an additional 15% to 20% when combined with any statin at any dose. Ezetimibe can be useful in patients who are intolerant of statins. Absorption is not affected by food.

Side effects include diarrhea and possibly myalgias. Myopathy is rare and is not clearly related to the medication.[261] Ezetimibe can increase cyclosporine levels. Fibrates can increase the levels of ezetimibe, a finding with unknown clinical significance.[262] Ezetimibe monotherapy does not significantly increase hepatic aminotransferases, but elevations may occur when ezetimibe is combined with a statin. This effect has not been related to any clinical significance.[261]

Ezetimibe is contraindicated in pregnancy and in severe liver dysfunction.

Omega-3 Fatty Acids. Fish-derived ω-3 fatty acids (EPA and DHA) improve plasma lipids and decrease the risk of sudden death through antiarrhythmic effects.[215] The Japan EPA Lipid Intervention Study (JELIS) showed that combined treatment with a statin plus EPA (1.8 g/day) in patients with CHD significantly reduced major coronary events by 19% compared with a statin alone.[263]

Omega-3 fatty acids decrease triglyceride secretion from the liver, through unclear mechanisms.[264] EPA and DHA lower triglycerides by 20% to 50% depending on the baseline levels. There is minimal effect on HDL-C. LDL-C may increase as VLDL is converted to LDL. Approximately 3 to 4 g/day of EPA plus DHA is required to lower triglycerides.

Over-the-counter preparations have variable quantities of EPA and DHA. A prescription formulation, Lovaza, contains about 465 mg of EPA and 375 mg of DHA per capsule. As with fibrates, fish oils shift the distribution of LDL toward more buoyant particles and away from small dense particles. Unlike fibrates, EPA and DHA do not affect statin metabolism, and they do not increase the risk of myopathy. Side effects with ω-3 fatty acids include eructation, diarrhea, and abdominal discomfort. There is potential for increased bleeding, but this has not been seen in clinical trials.[265]

There are probably fewer contaminants such as mercury in fish oils than in some types of fish, and contamination concerns are unwarranted for purified prescription formulations.[265]

Combination Therapies

Combination therapy is indicated for patients with severe lipid elevations and those who have not reached goals with monotherapy.[266,267] Patients with FH or familial combined hyperlipidemia are at particularly increased risk and may require LDL-C reductions that cannot be achieved with a single agent. Target LDL-C levels lower than 70 mg/dL can be difficult to achieve with a single drug. Higher statin doses may be associated with increased side effects, particularly myopathy. If the highest tolerated statin dose does not achieve the target LDL-C, adding an agent from a different class may produce the desired result. Statins, ezetimibe, and BAS work through different mechanisms and can be more effective in combination than when used alone. Data on clinical outcomes with combination therapy are limited.

Combination Therapy for Reduction of Low-Density Lipoprotein Cholesterol

Statin Plus Bile Acid Sequestrants. All three BAS drugs have been studied in combination with statins. The decreases in LDL-C range from 24% to 60%.[241,242,268-271] For example, colesevelam 3.8 g/day plus atorvastatin 10 mg/day lowered LDL by 48%, compared with 53% reduction with atorvastatin 80 mg alone[272]; such data are relevant for those who cannot tolerate higher statin doses. Drugs from both classes decrease CHD event rates. Cholestyramine and colestipol can interfere with the absorption of statins.[271] Colesevelam does not affect statin absorption.

This combination may not be ideal for patients with high triglycerides but may be useful in type 2 diabetes mellitus because of the reduction in glycemia.[248]

Statin Plus Ezetimibe. Ezetimibe added to a statin may further reduce LDL-C, by 20% or more,[273-275] and reduce triglycerides by 7% to 13%. The combination of rosuvastatin 40 mg plus ezetimibe 10 mg daily lowered LDL-C by 69.8%, allowing 79.6% of a very-high-risk population to reach an LDL-C goal of less than 70 mg/dL.[274] Ezetimibe added to a low-dose statin given two to three times per week can improve tolerance. A combination pill containing simvastatin and ezetimibe is available. The most common side effects reflect those of the individual drugs: myalgias, gastrointestinal complaints, and transaminase elevation.

Benefits of ezetimibe and statin-ezetimibe combinations are unproven. Combining ezetimibe with a statin is less effective than combining extended-release niacin with a statin at decreasing carotid intima medial thickness and lowering the incidence of cardiovascular events in patients with coronary disease or a coronary risk equivalent.[276]

Statin Plus Niacin. Adding niacin to a statin can lower LDL-C by 10% to 20%. This combination decreases LDL-C and triglycerides but also increases HDL-C more than the statin alone.[203,277,278] The HDL-Atherosclerosis Treatment Study (HATS) showed regression of atherosclerosis by coronary angiography and decreased cardiovascular events in patients treated with simvastatin plus niacin 2000 mg/day.[203] There was a 42% reduction in LDL-C, a 36% decrease in triglycerides, and a 26% increase in HDL-C in patients treated with this combination.

When used in combination with a statin, the maximum dose of niacin should be 2000 mg/day. Fixed-dose combinations of extended-release niacin with lovastatin (Advicor) and simvastatin (Simcor) are available.

Side effects of the combination of niacin with a statin are the same as those with niacin alone. Flushing is the most common reason for drug discontinuation. Myopathy is infrequent when niacin is used at 2000 mg/day or less. Liver enzymes should be monitored periodically. Other common side effects include pruritus (16%), rash (9%), and gastrointestinal side effects (24%).[277]

Bile Acid Sequestrants Plus Niacin. Before the availability of statins, BAS plus niacin was used to lower LDL-C in high-risk patients. The Cholesterol Lowering Atherosclerosis Study (CLAS) used a combination of colestipol 30 g/day and niacin 4.3 g/day to demonstrate decreased progression and increased regression of coronary artery atherosclerosis.[186] In the Familial Atherosclerosis Treatment Study (FATS), niacin 4 g/day plus colestipol 30 g/day produced greater regression and decreased progression of atherosclerosis as well as fewer clinical events, compared with diet and colestipol.[187] The availability of colesevelam and extended-release niacin has made this combination tolerable and useful for many patients who are unable to use statins.

Ezetimibe Plus Bile Acid Sequestrants. Ezetimibe inhibits cholesterol absorption, and BAS resins enhance cholesterol excretion through conversion to bile acids, so the combination can have additive effects. Colesevelam 3.8 g/day with ezetimibe 10 mg lowered LDL-C by 32%, compared with 21% reduction with ezetimibe monotherapy.[279]

This combination is useful for those patients who cannot take statins.

Three-Drug Combinations. Three medications can be useful in high-risk patients who have very high levels of LDL-C, such as patients with FH who have baseline LDL-C levels greater than 250 mg/dL. Combinations of a statin plus niacin plus BAS or ezetimibe have been used.

Combination therapy with lovastatin, niacin, and colestipol was compared with diet alone in patients with FH; regression of atherosclerotic lesions occurred in the drug combination group compared with progression in the diet-only group.[202]

In a study evaluating the safety and lipid-altering efficacy of the combination of ezetimibe 10 mg, simvastatin 20 mg, and extended-release niacin 2 g per day, LDL-C was reduced by 58% and HDL-C was increased by 30%, with a 42% decrease in triglycerides.[280]

Four-Drug Combinations. Four drugs may be necessary in patients with FH. Various combinations of a statin, BAS, niacin, and ezetimibe have been used in practice, but clinical studies are lacking.

Combination Therapy for Other Hyperlipidemias

Statin Plus Niacin. Combining a statin and niacin can be particularly effective for lowering LDL-C, raising HDL-C, and lowering triglyceride levels. This combination is useful for patients with combined hyperlipidemia and is becoming a common practice for secondary prevention based on several angiographic and other surrogate end point studies. Clinical outcomes trials with this combination are under way.

Statin plus Fibrate. The combination of a statin plus a fibrate decreases triglycerides and increases HDL-C more than either agent alone and is useful for patients with dysmetabolic syndrome, diabetes, or other forms of mixed dyslipidemia. However, LDL-C levels may not be lower on combination therapy compared with statin alone when patients with high triglyceride levels are treated with the combination.[281]

Risk of myopathy, including rhabdomyolysis, is increased with the combination of most statins with gemfibrozil, because the latter drug interferes with the glucuronidation of statins, leading to higher serum levels of the statin drug.[231] Rhabdomyolysis is about 15 times less likely with fenofibrate combined with statins (0.58 per 1 million prescriptions) than with gemfibrozil plus statins (8.6 per 1 million prescriptions).[257]

Statin-fibrate combinations should be avoided in patients with renal insufficiency, congestive heart failure, severe debility, or other conditions that affect medication clearance. Side effects include mild gastrointestinal discomfort, rash, and pruritus. Mild aminotransferase elevations occur in 5% of the patents and return to normal after drug discontinuation.

Other Combinations. Triple-drug therapy with a statin, ezetimibe, and fenofibrate may be helpful to obtain adequate reductions of both triglyceride levels and LDL-C without using very high statin doses. When triglyceride levels are decreased with a fibrate, LDL-C may be above goal. If triglycerides are well-controlled, BAS could be added. Ezetimibe may lower LDL-C in combination with a fibrate when triglyceride levels are not optimal. Adding ω-3 fatty acids can be helpful if triglycerides are not well controlled. For markedly elevated triglyceride levels, it may be necessary to combine a fibrate with niacin or with ω-3 fatty acids, or both.

Surgical Treatment and Other Modalities

Partial ileal bypass surgery has been used to reduce lipid levels in patients with severe hypercholesterolemia who cannot tolerate lipid-lowering drugs. This surgical therapy reduces total cholesterol by 20% to 25% and causes regression of atherosclerotic lesions.[282] Liver transplantation and portacaval shunting have been used as experimental therapies for homozygous FH. LDL apheresis can be used to lower atherogenic lipids in patients who cannot achieve appropriate lipid lowering despite combination therapy.

Specific Disorders and Therapy

Treatment for Chylomicronemia Syndrome. Patients with chylomicronemia syndrome usually present with acute pancreatitis and severe hypertriglyceridemia. They should be treated with total fat restriction until the triglycerides fall to less than 11.3 mmol/L (1000 mg/dL), after which a fat-restricted diet (e.g., <10% of calories) can be instituted. The goal is to maintain triglycerides lower than 11.3 mmol/L (1000 mg/dL) and preferably lower than 4.5 mmol/L (400 mg/dL). Diet and modification of glycemia, alcohol consumption, or offending medications are useful. A fibrate or niacin is usually required to control triglycerides. Therapy with orlistat may be beneficial.[283]

Treatment for Familial Hypercholesterolemia. For patients with FH, additional risk factors, such as smoking, should be addressed. Treatment of heterozygous FH includes a diet low in total and saturated fats and cholesterol, but effects on cholesterol are modest (5% to 15%). Adequate cholesterol lowering can occasionally be achieved with a single potent statin. However, combinations of two or three drugs are often needed. The usual approach includes a potent statin plus either a BAS or ezetimibe or both. The addition of niacin is also helpful. Ileal bypass surgery and LDL apheresis may be considered in patients who cannot tolerate lipid-lowering drugs.

The age at which drug treatment should begin in heterozygous FH is controversial. Many lipidologists tend to start treatment early, during the early stages of lesion development. Statins are approved for the treatment of children with heterozygous FH who are 8 years of age or older. Factors such as the age at onset of coronary disease in parents and grandparents and the presence of other risk factors should be considered.

High doses of atorvastatin or rosuvastatin combined with ezetimibe have been useful in homozygotes but do not provide sufficient lowering of LDL-C. The therapy of choice is LDL apheresis, the selective removal of LDL from the plasma or blood by extracorporeal apheresis combined with LDL adsorption, which is performed every 1 to 3 weeks. Liver transplantation, which provides functional LDL receptors, has also been used. Gene therapy involving delivery of an LDL receptor transgene to liver cells has not been successful.[284]

Treatment of familial defective apoB100 is similar to that of heterozygous FH and consists of a low-fat, low-cholesterol diet and a combination drug regimen. Family members at risk should also be screened for the dominant mutation.

Treatment for Familial Combined Hyperlipidemia. Weight reduction and dietary treatment can help correct metabolic abnormalities, such as obesity and insulin resistance, that contribute to the hyperlipidemia. Drug therapy should be directed at the predominant lipid abnormality. Statins are most appropriate for most patients. Fibrates can lower triglycerides and raise HDL-C levels, and they reduce the incidence of coronary events in insulin-resistant hypertriglyceridemic patients with low HDL-C levels. Patients with low HDL-C should be treated with statins. Addition of niacin, ezetimibe, and fibrates can further improve lipid profiles and reduce CHD risk. Because familial combined hyperlipidemia is associated with premature CHD, affected family members should be identified.

Treatment for Dysmetabolic Syndrome. All patients with a diagnosis of the dysmetabolic syndrome should be informed of their increased risk of developing cardiovascular disease and type 2 diabetes mellitus. Weight loss and increased physical activity are the best therapy and may be the only therapy that many of these patients require. All patients should be assessed according to existing guidelines for treatment of high triglyceride levels, low HDL, hypertension, and hyperglycemia. Aspirin therapy is indicated because of the prothrombotic state.[281]

Treatment for Dysbetalipoproteinemia. Because dysbetalipoproteinemia is influenced by coexisting metabolic conditions, a vigorous effort should be made to identify and treat obesity, diabetes mellitus, and hypothyroidism and to reduce alcohol consumption. Lipid abnormalities can often be resolved without the use of drug therapies. Dysbetalipoproteinemia is associated with hypothyroidism in particular and responds dramatically to thyroid hormone replacement therapy. Diet therapy should be aimed at restricting total fat, saturated fat, cholesterol, and, if appropriate, calories. If diet and treatment of coexisting metabolic conditions are unsatisfactory, drug therapy should be initiated using niacin, fibric acid derivatives, or statins, all of which are effective for this disorder. Combination therapy may be required. Because the disorder is associated with premature vascular disease, first-degree relatives should be screened for the presence of apoE2 (see earlier discussion).

Treatment for Elevated Plasma Lipoprotein(a). Only niacin appears to lower plasma Lp(a) levels. However, LDL-C should also be treated appropriately, and risk factors for CHD should be addressed.

Treatment for Low Levels of High-Density Lipoproteins. Patients with familial hypoalphalipoproteinemia can have normal or modestly increased plasma cholesterol but very low HDL-C, resulting in a predisposition to CHD. Such patients can have high ratios of total cholesterol to HDL-C (e.g., >10) despite having a normal plasma cholesterol level. Of the available drugs, niacin results in the largest increase in HDL-C. Fibrates do not increase HDL-C in patients with normal triglycerides. Statins lower total cholesterol and represent the most efficacious way to lower the ratio of total cholesterol to HDL-C. Statins decrease clinical events in patients with low HDL-C.[97,194]

Management of low HDL levels is best accomplished by employing treatment goals for both LDL-C and non–HDL-C. The NCEP Adult Treatment Panel III guidelines advise additional treatment of low HDL-C in patients who are at their goal for LDL-C and have triglyceride levels greater than 2.25 mmol/L (200 mg/dL). In such patients, a secondary goal is set for non–HDL-C (total cholesterol minus HDL-C). The non–HDL-C goal is the same as the patient's LDL-C goal plus 0.8 mmol/L (30 mg/dL).[97]

Drugs in Development

Drugs in development have the potential for additive effects with statins or other lipid-lowering medications to achieve further reduction of LDL-C or increases in HDL-C.[285,286]

One interesting class of drugs to lower LDL-C is MTP inhibitors. MTP (see earlier discussion) is required for VLDL assembly. One study of MTP inhibition demonstrated LDL-C reduction of 50% in patients with homozygous FH.[287] This drug class increases fat storage in the liver. The extent to which fatty liver develops compared with its cholesterol-lowering effect will likely be the major hurdle in the approval of drugs in this class. Studies in hypercholesterolemic patients are in progress.

Mipomersen is an apoB antisense oligonucleotide agent that is in development for treatment of severe hypercholesterolemia. It binds to the apoB messenger RNA, preventing translation and thereby decreasing apoB levels and LDL-C.[288] Human studies in FH are under way.[285] Reactions at the injection site are the most common side effect.

CETP inhibitors increase the amount of cholesterol carried in HDL and raise HDL-C by more than 60%.[289,290] It is uncertain whether this method of raising HDL will translate into a clinical benefit, especially after the use of one such agent, torcetrapib, was found to increase mortality in a clinical trial (see earlier discussion). Whether similar problems will be encountered with other CETP inhibitors is unknown.[208]

REFERENCES

1. Goldstein JL, Brown MS. The LDL receptor. *Arterioscler Thromb Vasc Biol.* 2009;29:431-438.
2. Baigent C, Keech A, Kearney PM, et al. Efficacy and safety of cholesterol-lowering treatment: prospective meta-analysis of data from 90,056 participants in 14 randomised trials of statins. *Lancet.* 2005;366:1267-1278.
3. McGarry JD. What if Minkowski had been ageusic? An alternative angle on diabetes. *Science.* 1992;258:766-770.
4. Vance JE. Molecular and cell biology of phosphatidylserine and phosphatidylethanolamine metabolism. *Prog Nucleic Acid Res Mol Biol.* 2003;75:69-111.
5. Ohvo-Rekila H, Ramstedt B, Leppimaki P, et al. Cholesterol interactions with phospholipids in membranes. *Prog Lipid Res.* 2002;41:66-97.
6. Cooper MK, Wassif CA, Krakowiak PA, et al. A defective response to Hedgehog signaling in disorders of cholesterol biosynthesis. *Nat Genet.* 2003;33:508-513.
7. Diraison F, Beylot M. Role of human liver lipogenesis and reesterification in triglycerides secretion and in FFA reesterification. *Am J Physiol.* 1998;274:E321-E327.
8. Stanhope KL, Schwarz JM, Keim NL, et al. Consuming fructose-sweetened, not glucose-sweetened, beverages increases visceral adiposity and lipids and decreases insulin sensitivity in overweight/obese humans. *J Clin Invest.* 2009;119:1322-1334.
9. Savage DB, Choi CS, Samuel VT, et al. Reversal of diet-induced hepatic steatosis and hepatic insulin resistance by antisense oligonucleotide inhibitors of acetyl-CoA carboxylases 1 and 2. *J Clin Invest.* 2006;116:817-824.
10. Chakravarthy MV, Zhu Y, Lopez M, et al. Brain fatty acid synthase activates PPARalpha to maintain energy homeostasis. *J Clin Invest.* 2007;117:2539-2552.
11. Matsuzaka T, Shimano H, Yahagi N, et al. Crucial role of a long-chain fatty acid elongase, Elovl6, in obesity-induced insulin resistance. *Nat Med.* 2007;13:1193-1202.
12. Ntambi JM, Miyazaki M, Stoehr JP, et al. Loss of stearoyl-CoA desaturase-1 function protects mice against adiposity. *Proc Natl Acad Sci U S A.* 2002;99:11482-11486.
13. Shekhawat PS, Matern D, Strauss AW. Fetal fatty acid oxidation disorders, their effect on maternal health and neonatal outcome: impact of expanded newborn screening on their diagnosis and management. *Pediatr Res.* 2005;57:78R-86R.
14. Schaffer JE. Lipotoxicity: when tissues overeat. *Curr Opin Lipidol.* 2003;14:281-287.

15. Brassard P, Frisch F, Lavoie F, et al. Impaired plasma nonesterified fatty acid tolerance is an early defect in the natural history of type 2 diabetes. *J Clin Endocrinol Metab*. 2008;93:837-844.
16. Offermanns S. The nicotinic acid receptor GPR109A (HM74A or PUMA-G) as a new therapeutic target. *Trends Pharmacol Sci*. 2006;27:384-390.
17. Zechner R, Kienesberger PC, Haemmerle G, et al. Adipose triglyceride lipase and the lipolytic catabolism of cellular fat stores. *J Lipid Res*. 2009;50:3-21.
18. Agarwal AK, Arioglu E, De Almeida S, et al. AGPAT2 is mutated in congenital generalized lipodystrophy linked to chromosome 9q34. *Nat Genet*. 2002;31:21-23.
19. Takeuchi K, Reue K. Biochemistry, physiology, and genetics of GPAT, AGPAT, and lipin enzymes in triglyceride synthesis. *Am J Physiol Endocrinol Metab*. 2009;296:E1195-E1209.
20. Yao-Borengasser A, Rasouli N, Varma V, et al. Lipin expression is attenuated in adipose tissue of insulin-resistant human subjects and increases with peroxisome proliferator-activated receptor gamma activation. *Diabetes*. 2006;55:2811-2818.
21. Chen HC, Farese Jr RV. Inhibition of triglyceride synthesis as a treatment strategy for obesity: lessons from DGAT1-deficient mice. *Arterioscler Thromb Vasc Biol*. 2005;25:482-486.
22. Kent C. Regulatory enzymes of phosphatidylcholine biosynthesis: a personal perspective. *Biochim Biophys Acta*. 2005;1733:53-66.
23. Coleman T, Seip RL, Gimble JM, et al. COOH-terminal disruption of lipoprotein lipase in mice is lethal in homozygotes, but heterozygotes have elevated triglycerides and impaired enzyme activity. *J Biol Chem*. 1995;270:12518-12525.
24. Farese Jr RV, Yost TJ, Eckel RH. Tissue-specific regulation of lipoprotein lipase activity by insulin/glucose in normal-weight humans. *Metabolism*. 1991;40:214-216.
25. Seip RL, Angelopoulos TJ, Semenkovich CF. Exercise induces human lipoprotein lipase gene expression in skeletal muscle but not adipose tissue. *Am J Physiol*. 1995;268:E229-E236.
26. Beigneux AP, Davies BS, Gin P, et al. Glycosylphosphatidylinositol-anchored high-density lipoprotein-binding protein 1 plays a critical role in the lipolytic processing of chylomicrons. *Cell Metab*. 2007;5:279-291.
27. Dietschy JM, Turley SD, Spady DK. Role of liver in the maintenance of cholesterol and low density lipoprotein homeostasis in different animal species, including humans. *J Lipid Res*. 1993;34:1637-1659.
28. Gylling H, Miettinen TA. Inheritance of cholesterol metabolism of probands with high or low cholesterol absorption. *J Lipid Res*. 2002;43:1472-1476.
29. Altmann SW, Davis Jr HR, Zhu LJ, et al. Niemann-Pick C1 like 1 protein is critical for intestinal cholesterol absorption. *Science*. 2004;303:1201-1204.
30. Berge KE, Tian H, Graf GA, et al. Accumulation of dietary cholesterol in sitosterolemia caused by mutations in adjacent ABC transporters. *Science*. 2000;290:1771-1775.
31. Goldstein JL, Brown MS. Regulation of the mevalonate pathway. *Nature*. 1990;343:425-430.
32. Nissen SE, Tuzcu EM, Brewer HB, et al. Effect of ACAT inhibition on the progression of coronary atherosclerosis. *N Engl J Med*. 2006;354:1253-1263.
33. Shin DJ, Osborne TF. Thyroid hormone regulation and cholesterol metabolism are connected through sterol regulatory element-binding protein-2 (SREBP-2). *J Biol Chem*. 2003;278:34114-34118.
34. Kauffman RF, Bensch WR, Roudebush RE, et al. Hypocholesterolemic activity of raloxifene (LY139481): pharmacological characterization as a selective estrogen receptor modulator. *J Pharmacol Exp Ther*. 1997;280:146-153.
35. Umetani M, Domoto H, Gormley AK, et al. 27-Hydroxycholesterol is an endogenous SERM that inhibits the cardiovascular effects of estrogen. *Nat Med*. 2007;13:1185-1192.
36. Wu FC, von Eckardstein A. Androgens and coronary artery disease. *Endocr Rev*. 2003;24:183-217.
37. Chakravarthy MV, Lodhi IJ, Yin L, et al. Identification of a physiologically relevant endogenous ligand for PPARalpha in liver. *Cell*. 2009;138:476-488.
38. Henry RR, Lincoff AM, Mudaliar S, et al. Effect of the dual peroxisome proliferator-activated receptor-alpha/gamma agonist aleglitazar on risk of cardiovascular disease in patients with type 2 diabetes (SYNCHRONY): a phase II, randomised, dose-ranging study. *Lancet*. 2009;374:126-135.
39. Narkar VA, Downes M, Yu RT, et al. AMPK and PPARdelta agonists are exercise mimetics. *Cell*. 2008;134:405-415.
40. Riserus U, Sprecher D, Johnson T, et al. Activation of peroxisome proliferator-activated receptor (PPAR)delta promotes reversal of multiple metabolic abnormalities, reduces oxidative stress, and increases fatty acid oxidation in moderately obese men. *Diabetes*. 2008;57:332-339.
41. Shulman AI, Mangelsdorf DJ. Retinoid X receptor heterodimers in the metabolic syndrome. *N Engl J Med*. 2005;353:604-615.
42. Zelcer N, Hong C, Boyadjian R, et al. LXR regulates cholesterol uptake through Idol-dependent ubiquitination of the LDL receptor. *Science*. 2009;325:100-104.
43. Staels B, Kuipers F. Bile acid sequestrants and the treatment of type 2 diabetes mellitus. *Drugs*. 2007;67:1383-1392.
44. Iizuka K, Horikawa Y. ChREBP: a glucose-activated transcription factor involved in the development of metabolic syndrome. *Endocr J*. 2008;55:617-624.
45. Lee AH, Scapa EF, Cohen DE, et al. Regulation of hepatic lipogenesis by the transcription factor XBP1. *Science*. 2008;320:1492-1496.
46. Garvey WT, Kwon S, Zheng D, et al. Effects of insulin resistance and type 2 diabetes on lipoprotein subclass particle size and concentration determined by nuclear magnetic resonance. *Diabetes*. 2003;52:453-462.
47. Hussain MM, Fatma S, Pan X, et al. Intestinal lipoprotein assembly. *Curr Opin Lipidol*. 2005;16:281-285.
48. Mahley RW, Ji ZS. Remnant lipoprotein metabolism: key pathways involving cell-surface heparan sulfate proteoglycans and apolipoprotein E. *J Lipid Res*. 1999;40:1-16.
49. Kamstrup PR, Tybjaerg-Hansen A, Steffensen R, et al. Genetically elevated lipoprotein(a) and increased risk of myocardial infarction. *JAMA*. 2009;301:2331-2339.
50. Glomset JA. The plasma lecithins:cholesterol acyltransferase reaction. *J Lipid Res*. 1968;9:155-167.
51. Rader DJ, Alexander ET, Weibel GL, et al. The role of reverse cholesterol transport in animals and humans and relationship to atherosclerosis. *J Lipid Res*. 2009;50(suppl):S189-S194.
52. Paszty C, Maeda N, Verstuyft J, et al. Apolipoprotein AI transgene corrects apolipoprotein E deficiency-induced atherosclerosis in mice. *J Clin Invest*. 1994;94:899-903.
53. Deeb SS, Takata K, Peng RL, et al. A splice-junction mutation responsible for familial apolipoprotein A-II deficiency. *Am J Hum Genet*. 1990;46:822-827.
54. Qin X, Tso P. The role of apolipoprotein AIV on the control of food intake. *Curr Drug Targets*. 2005;6:145-151.
55. Pennacchio LA, Olivier M, Hubacek JA, et al. An apolipoprotein influencing triglycerides in humans and mice revealed by comparative sequencing. *Science*. 2001;294:169-173.
56. Dorfmeister B, Zeng WW, Dichlberger A, et al. Effects of six APOA5 variants, identified in patients with severe hypertriglyceridemia, on in vitro lipoprotein lipase activity and receptor binding. *Arterioscler Thromb Vasc Biol*. 2008;28:1866-1871.
57. Anant S, Davidson NO. Identification and regulation of protein components of the apolipoprotein B mRNA editing enzyme: a complex event. *Trends Cardiovasc Med*. 2002;12:311-317.
58. Shelness GS, Ledford AS. Evolution and mechanism of apolipoprotein B-containing lipoprotein assembly. *Curr Opin Lipidol*. 2005;16:325-332.
59. Brown ML, Ramprasad MP, Umeda PK, et al. A macrophage receptor for apolipoprotein B48: cloning, expression, and atherosclerosis. *Proc Natl Acad Sci U S A*. 2000;97:7488-7493.
60. Avramoglu RK, Adeli K. Hepatic regulation of apolipoprotein B. *Rev Endocr Metab Disord*. 2004;5:293-301.
61. Huang H, Sun F, Owen DM, et al. Hepatitis C virus production by human hepatocytes dependent on assembly and secretion of very low-density lipoproteins. *Proc Natl Acad Sci U S A*. 2007;104:5848-5853.
62. Berriot-Varoqueaux N, Aggerbeck LP, Samson-Bouma M, et al. The role of the microsomal triglygeride transfer protein in abetalipoproteinemia. *Annu Rev Nutr*. 2000;20:663-697.
63. Innerarity TL, Mahley RW, Weisgraber KH, et al. Familial defective apolipoprotein B-100: a mutation of apolipoprotein B that causes hypercholesterolemia. *J Lipid Res*. 1990;31:1337-1349.
64. Ooi EM, Barrett PH, Chan DC, et al. Apolipoprotein C-III: understanding an emerging cardiovascular risk factor. *Clin Sci (Lond)* 2008;114:611-624.
65. Pollin TI, Damcott CM, Shen H, et al. A null mutation in human APOC3 confers a favorable plasma lipid profile and apparent cardioprotection. *Science*. 2008;322:1702-1705.
66. Mahley RW, Rall Jr SC. Apolipoprotein E: far more than a lipid transport protein. *Annu Rev Genomics Hum Genet*. 2000;1:507-537.
67. Weisgraber KH. Apolipoprotein E: structure-function relationships. *Adv Protein Chem*. 1994;45:249-302.
68. Bennet AM, Di Angelantonio E, Ye Z, et al. Association of apolipoprotein E genotypes with lipid levels and coronary risk. *JAMA*. 2007;298:1300-1311.
69. Williams KJ. Molecular processes that handle—and mishandle—dietary lipids. *J Clin Invest*. 2008;118:3247-3259.
70. Kim J, Basak JM, Holtzman DM. The role of apolipoprotein E in Alzheimer's disease. *Neuron*. 2009;63:287-303.
71. Pfrieger FW. Role of cholesterol in synapse formation and function. *Biochim Biophys Acta*. 2003;1610:271-280.
72. Graner M, Kahri J, Varpula M, et al. Apolipoprotein E polymorphism is associated with both carotid and coronary atherosclerosis in patients with coronary artery disease. *Nutr Metab Cardiovasc Dis*. 2008;18:271-277.

73. Herz J. Apolipoprotein E receptors in the nervous system. *Curr Opin Lipidol.* 2009;20:190-196.
74. Guo YF, Xiong DH, Shen H, et al. Polymorphisms of the low-density lipoprotein receptor-related protein 5 (LRP5) gene are associated with obesity phenotypes in a large family-based association study. *J Med Genet.* 2006;43:798-803.
75. Mani A, Radhakrishnan J, Wang H, et al. LRP6 mutation in a family with early coronary disease and metabolic risk factors. *Science.* 2007;315:1278-1282.
76. Brown MS, Goldstein JL. A receptor-mediated pathway for cholesterol homeostasis. *Science.* 1986;232:34-47.
77. Rudenko G, Henry L, Henderson K, et al. Structure of the LDL receptor extracellular domain at endosomal pH. *Science.* 2002;298:2353-2358.
78. Kwon HJ, Abi-Mosleh L, Wang ML, et al. Structure of N-terminal domain of NPC1 reveals distinct subdomains for binding and transfer of cholesterol. *Cell.* 2009;137:1213-1224.
79. Herz J, Strickland DK. LRP: a multifunctional scavenger and signaling receptor. *J Clin Invest.* 2001;108:779-784.
80. Pluddemann A, Neyen C, Gordon S. Macrophage scavenger receptors and host-derived ligands. *Methods.* 2007;43:207-217.
81. Laugerette F, Passilly-Degrace P, Patris B, et al. CD36 involvement in orosensory detection of dietary lipids, spontaneous fat preference, and digestive secretions. *J Clin Invest.* 2005;115:3177-3184.
82. Ibrahimi A, Abumrad NA. Role of CD36 in membrane transport of long-chain fatty acids. *Curr Opin Clin Nutr Metab Care.* 2002;5:139-145.
83. Manning-Tobin JJ, Moore KJ, Seimon TA, et al. Loss of SR-A and CD36 activity reduces atherosclerotic lesion complexity without abrogating foam cell formation in hyperlipidemic mice. *Arterioscler Thromb Vasc Biol.* 2009;29:19-26.
84. Shi H, Kokoeva MV, Inouye K, et al. TLR4 links innate immunity and fatty acid-induced insulin resistance. *J Clin Invest.* 2006;116: 3015-3125.
85. Castrillo A, Joseph SB, Vaidya SA, et al. Crosstalk between LXR and toll-like receptor signaling mediates bacterial and viral antagonism of cholesterol metabolism. *Mol Cell.* 2003;12:805-816.
86. Kawakami A, Osaka M, Aikawa M, et al. Toll-like receptor 2 mediates apolipoprotein CIII-induced monocyte activation. *Circ Res.* 2008; 103:1402-1409.
87. Edmondson AC, Brown RJ, Kathiresan S, et al. Loss-of-function variants in endothelial lipase are a cause of elevated HDL cholesterol in humans. *J Clin Invest.* 2009;119:1042-1050.
88. Abifadel M, Varret M, Rabes JP, et al. Mutations in PCSK9 cause autosomal dominant hypercholesterolemia. *Nat Genet.* 2003;34: 154-156.
89. Kathiresan S. A PCSK9 missense variant associated with a reduced risk of early-onset myocardial infarction. *N Engl J Med.* 2008;358: 2299-2300.
90. Packard CJ, O'Reilly DS, Caslake MJ, et al. Lipoprotein-associated phospholipase A2 as an independent predictor of coronary heart disease. West of Scotland Coronary Prevention Study Group. *N Engl J Med.* 2000;343:1148-1155.
91. Serruys PW, Garcia-Garcia HM, Buszman P, et al. Effects of the direct lipoprotein-associated phospholipase A(2) inhibitor darapladib on human coronary atherosclerotic plaque. *Circulation.* 2008;118: 1172-1182.
92. Barter PJ, Caulfield M, Eriksson M, et al. Effects of torcetrapib in patients at high risk for coronary events. *N Engl J Med.* 2007;357:2109-2122.
93. Calabresi L, Baldassarre D, Castelnuovo S, et al. Functional lecithin: cholesterol acyltransferase is not required for efficient atheroprotection in humans. *Circulation.* 2009;120:628-635.
94. Semple RK, Sleigh A, Murgatroyd PR, et al. Postreceptor insulin resistance contributes to human dyslipidemia and hepatic steatosis. *J Clin Invest.* 2009;119:315-322.
95. Carroll MD, Lacher DA, Sorlie PD, et al. Trends in serum lipids and lipoproteins of adults, 1960-2002. *JAMA.* 2005;294:1773-1781.
96. Kato H, Tillotson J, Nichaman MZ, et al. Epidemiologic studies of coronary heart-disease and stroke in Japanese men living in Japan, Hawaii and California—serum-lipids and diet. *Am J Epidemiol.* 1973;97: 372-385.
97. Third Report of the National Cholesterol Education Program (NCEP) Expert Panel on Detection, Evaluation, and Treatment of High Blood Cholesterol in Adults (Adult Treatment Panel III) final report. *Circulation.* 2002;106:3143-3421.
98. Kavey RE, Daniels SR, Lauer RM, et al. American Heart Association guidelines for primary prevention of atherosclerotic cardiovascular disease beginning in childhood. *J Pediatr.* 2003;142:368-372.
99. Brunzell JD, Hazzard WR, Porte Jr D, et al. Evidence for a common, saturable, triglyceride removal mechanism for chylomicrons and very low density lipoproteins in man. *J Clin Invest.* 1973;52:1578-1585.
100. Savolainen MJ, Baraona E, Leo MA, et al. Pathogenesis of the hypertriglyceridemia at early stages of alcoholic liver injury in the baboon. *J Lipid Res.* 1986;27:1073-1083.
101. Tsuang W, Navaneethan U, Ruiz L, et al. Hypertriglyceridemic pancreatitis: presentation and management. *Am J Gastroenterol.* 2009;104:984-991.
102. Chait A, Brunzell JD. Chylomicronemia syndrome. *Adv Intern Med.* 1992;37:249-273.
103. Merkel M, Eckel RH, Goldberg IJ. Lipoprotein lipase: genetics, lipid uptake, and regulation. *J Lipid Res.* 2002;43:1997-2006.
104. Wilson DE, Hata A, Kwong LK, et al. Mutations in exon 3 of the lipoprotein lipase gene segregating in a family with hypertriglyceridemia, pancreatitis, and non-insulin-dependent diabetes. *J Clin Invest.* 1993;92:203-211.
105. Ginsberg HN. Diabetic dyslipidemia: basic mechanisms underlying the common hypertriglyceridemia and low HDL cholesterol levels. *Diabetes.* 1996;45(suppl 3):S27-S30.
106. Connelly PW, Maguire GF, Little JA. Apolipoprotein CIISt. Michael: familial apolipoprotein CII deficiency associated with premature vascular disease. *J Clin Invest.* 1987;80:1597-1606.
107. Beigneux AP, Franssen R, Bensadoun A, et al. Chylomicronemia with a mutant GPIHBP1 (Q115P) that cannot bind lipoprotein lipase. *Arterioscler Thromb Vasc Biol.* 2009;29:956-962.
108. Peterfy M, Ben-Zeev O, Mao HZ, et al. Mutations in LMF1 cause combined lipase deficiency and severe hypertriglyceridemia. *Nat Genet.* 2007;39:1483-1487.
109. Beaumont JL, Berard M, Antonucci M, et al. Inhibition of lipoprotein lipase activity by a monoclonal immunoglobulin in autoimmune hyperlipidemia. *Atherosclerosis.* 1977;26:67-77.
110. Bansal S, Buring JE, Rifai N, et al. Fasting compared with nonfasting triglycerides and risk of cardiovascular events in women. *JAMA.* 2007;298:309-316.
111. Nordestgaard BG, Benn M, Schnohr P, et al. Nonfasting triglycerides and risk of myocardial infarction, ischemic heart disease, and death in men and women. *JAMA.* 2007;298:299-308.
112. Wilson DE, Emi M, Iverius PH, et al. Phenotypic expression of heterozygous lipoprotein lipase deficiency in the extended pedigree of a proband homozygous for a missense mutation. *J Clin Invest.* 1990;86:735-750.
113. Goldberg IJ, Merkel M. Lipoprotein lipase: physiology, biochemistry, and molecular biology. *Front Biosci.* 2001;6:D388-D405.
114. Krauss RM, Levy RI, Fredrickson DS. Selective measurement of two lipase activities in postheparin plasma from normal subjects and patients with hyperlipoproteinemia. *J Clin Invest.* 1974;54: 1107-1124.
115. Brunzell JD, Miller NE, Alaupovic P, et al. Familial chylomicronemia due to a circulating inhibitor of lipoprotein lipase activity. *J Lipid Res.* 1983;24:12-19.
116. Austin MA, McKnight B, Edwards KL, et al. Cardiovascular disease mortality in familial forms of hypertriglyceridemia: a 20-year prospective study. *Circulation.* 2000;101:2777-2782.
117. Duane WC. Abnormal bile acid absorption in familial hypertriglyceridemia. *J Lipid Res.* 1995;36:96-107.
118. Watanabe M, Houten SM, Wang L, et al. Bile acids lower triglyceride levels via a pathway involving FXR, SHP, and SREBP-1c. *J Clin Invest.* 2004;113:1408-1418.
119. Voyiaziakis E, Goldberg IJ, Plump AS, et al. ApoA-I deficiency causes both hypertriglyceridemia and increased atherosclerosis in human apoB transgenic mice. *J Lipid Res.* 1998;39:313-321.
120. Chahil TJ, Ginsberg HN. Diabetic dyslipidemia. *Endocrinol Metab Clin North Am.* 2006;35:491-510, vii-viii.
121. Prinsen BH, de Sain-van der Velden MG, de Koning EJ, et al. Hypertriglyceridemia in patients with chronic renal failure: possible mechanisms. *Kidney Int Suppl* 2003:S121-S124.
122. Wolfe BM, Barrett PH, Laurier L, et al. Effects of continuous conjugated estrogen and micronized progesterone therapy upon lipoprotein metabolism in postmenopausal women. *J Lipid Res.* 2000;41: 368-375.
123. Sanada M, Tsuda M, Kodama I, et al. Substitution of transdermal estradiol during oral estrogen-progestin therapy in postmenopausal women: effects on hypertriglyceridemia. *Menopause.* 2004;11: 331-336.
124. Elisaf MS, Nakou K, Liamis G, et al. Tamoxifen-induced severe hypertriglyceridemia and pancreatitis. *Ann Oncol.* 2000;11:1067-1069.
125. Mosca L, Harper K, Sarkar S, et al. Effect of raloxifene on serum triglycerides in postmenopausal women: influence of predisposing factors for hypertriglyceridemia. *Clin Ther.* 2001;23:1552-1565.
126. Frohlich JJ. Effects of alcohol on plasma lipoprotein metabolism. *Clin Chim Acta.* 1996;246:39-49.
127. Soutar AK, Naoumova RP, Traub LM. Genetics, clinical phenotype, and molecular cell biology of autosomal recessive hypercholesterolemia. *Arterioscler Thromb Vasc Biol.* 2003;23:1963-1970.
128. Kawaguchi A, Miyatake K, Yutani C, et al. Characteristic cardiovascular manifestation in homozygous and heterozygous familial hypercholesterolemia. *Am Heart J.* 1999;137:410-418.
129. Soutar AK, Naoumova RP. Mechanisms of disease: genetic causes of familial hypercholesterolemia. *Nat Clin Pract Cardiovasc Med.* 2007;4:214-225.

130. Mahley RW, Weisgraber KH, Innerarity TL, et al. Genetic defects in lipoprotein metabolism: elevation of atherogenic lipoproteins caused by impaired catabolism. *JAMA*. 1991;265:78-83.
131. Arca M, Zuliani G, Wilund K, et al. Autosomal recessive hypercholesterolaemia in Sardinia, Italy, and mutations in ARH: a clinical and molecular genetic analysis. *Lancet*. 2002;359:841-847.
132. Pullinger CR, Eng C, Salen G, et al. Human cholesterol 7alpha-hydroxylase (CYP7A1) deficiency has a hypercholesterolemic phenotype. *J Clin Invest*. 2002;110:109-117.
133. Maxwell KN, Fisher EA, Breslow JL. Overexpression of PCSK9 accelerates the degradation of the LDLR in a post-endoplasmic reticulum compartment. *Proc Natl Acad Sci U S A*. 2005;102:2069-2074.
134. Grefhorst A, McNutt MC, Lagace TA, et al. Plasma PCSK9 preferentially reduces liver LDL receptors in mice. *J Lipid Res*. 2008;49:1303-1311.
135. Cohen JC, Boerwinkle E, Mosley Jr TH, et al. Sequence variations in PCSK9, low LDL, and protection against coronary heart disease. *N Engl J Med*. 2006;354:1264-1272.
136. Marcovina SM, Hegele RA, Koschinsky ML. Lipoprotein(a) and coronary heart disease risk. *Curr Cardiol Rep*. 1999;1:105-111.
137. Guyton JR, Dahlen GH, Patsch W, et al. Relationship of plasma lipoprotein Lp(a) levels to race and to apolipoprotein B. *Arteriosclerosis*. 1985;5:265-272.
138. Lippi G, Veraldi GF, Dorucci V, et al. Usefulness of lipids, lipoprotein(a) and fibrinogen measurements in identifying subjects at risk of occlusive complications following vascular and endovascular surgery. *Scand J Clin Lab Invest*. 1998;58:497-504.
139. Walli AK, Seidel D. Role of lipoprotein-X in the pathogenesis of cholestatic hypercholesterolemia: uptake of lipoprotein-X and its effect on 3-hydroxy-3-methylglutaryl coenzyme A reductase and chylomicron remnant removal in human fibroblasts, lymphocytes, and in the rat. *J Clin Invest*. 1984;74:867-879.
140. Sorokin A, Brown JL, Thompson PD. Primary biliary cirrhosis, hyperlipidemia, and atherosclerotic risk: a systematic review. *Atherosclerosis*. 2007;194:293-299.
141. Berge KE. Sitosterolemia: a gateway to new knowledge about cholesterol metabolism. *Ann Med*. 2003;35:502-511.
142. Salen G, von Bergmann K, Lutjohann D, et al. Ezetimibe effectively reduces plasma plant sterols in patients with sitosterolemia. *Circulation*. 2004;109:966-971.
143. Moghadasian MH. Cerebrotendinous xanthomatosis: clinical course, genotypes and metabolic backgrounds. *Clin Invest Med*. 2004;27:42-50.
144. Berginer VM, Shany S, Alkalay D, et al. Osteoporosis and increased bone fractures in cerebrotendinous xanthomatosis. *Metabolism*. 1993;42:69-74.
145. Thompson PD, Clarkson P, Karas RH. Statin-associated myopathy. *JAMA*. 2003;289:1681-1690.
146. Diekman T, Lansberg PJ, Kastelein JJ, et al. Prevalence and correction of hypothyroidism in a large cohort of patients referred for dyslipidemia. *Arch Intern Med*. 1995;155:1490-1495.
147. Goldstein JL, Schrott HG, Hazzard WR, et al. Hyperlipidemia in coronary heart disease: II. Genetic analysis of lipid levels in 176 families and delineation of a new inherited disorder, combined hyperlipidemia. *J Clin Invest*. 1973;52:1544-1568.
148. Barzilai N, Atzmon G, Schechter C, et al. Unique lipoprotein phenotype and genotype associated with exceptional longevity. *JAMA*. 2003;290:2030-2040.
149. Navab M, Anantharamaiah GM, Reddy ST, et al. Mechanisms of disease: proatherogenic HDL—an evolving field. *Nat Clin Pract Endocrinol Metab*. 2006;2:504-511.
150. McMahon M, Grossman J, FitzGerald J, et al. Proinflammatory high-density lipoprotein as a biomarker for atherosclerosis in patients with systemic lupus erythematosus and rheumatoid arthritis. *Arthritis Rheum*. 2006;54:2541-2549.
151. Hayek T, Chajek-Shaul T, Walsh A, et al. An interaction between the human cholesteryl ester transfer protein (CETP) and apolipoprotein A-I genes in transgenic mice results in a profound CETP-mediated depression of high density lipoprotein cholesterol levels. *J Clin Invest*. 1992;90:505-510.
152. Nissen SE, Tardif JC, Nicholls SJ, et al. Effect of torcetrapib on the progression of coronary atherosclerosis. *N Engl J Med*. 2007;356:1304-1316.
153. Mahley RW, Huang Y, Rall Jr SC. Pathogenesis of type III hyperlipoproteinemia (dysbetalipoproteinemia): questions, quandaries, and paradoxes. *J Lipid Res*. 1999;40:1933-1949.
154. Hegele RA, Tu L, Connelly PW. Human hepatic lipase mutations and polymorphisms. *Hum Mutat*. 1992;1:320-324.
155. Grinspoon S, Carr A. Cardiovascular risk and body-fat abnormalities in HIV-infected adults. *N Engl J Med*. 2005;352:48-62.
156. Bilchick KC, Henrikson CA, Skojec D, et al. Treatment of hyperlipidemia in cardiac transplant recipients. *Am Heart J*. 2004;148:200-210.
157. Charcosset M, Sassolas A, Peretti N, et al. Anderson or chylomicron retention disease: molecular impact of five mutations in the SAR1B gene on the structure and the functionality of Sar1b protein. *Mol Genet Metab*. 2008;93:74-84.
158. Groenendijk M, Cantor RM, de Bruin TW, et al. The apoAI-CIII-AIV gene cluster. *Atherosclerosis*. 2001;157:1-11.
159. Nissen SE, Tsunoda T, Tuzcu EM, et al. Effect of recombinant ApoA-I Milano on coronary atherosclerosis in patients with acute coronary syndromes: a randomized controlled trial. *JAMA*. 2003;290:2292-2300.
160. McIntyre N. Familial LCAT deficiency and fish-eye disease. *J Inherit Metab Dis*. 1988;11(suppl 1):45-56.
161. Kuivenhoven JA, Pritchard H, Hill J, Frohlich J, Assmann G, Kastelein J. The molecular pathology of lecithin:cholesterol acyltransferase (LCAT) deficiency syndromes. *J Lipid Res*. 1997;38:191-205.
162. Oram JF, Lawn RM. ABCA1. The gatekeeper for eliminating excess tissue cholesterol. *J Lipid Res*. 2001;42:1173-1179.
163. Wilson PW, D'Agostino RB, Levy D, et al. Prediction of coronary heart disease using risk factor categories. *Circulation*. 1998;97:1837-1847.
164. Wanner C, Krane V, Marz W, et al. Atorvastatin in patients with type 2 diabetes mellitus undergoing hemodialysis. *N Engl J Med*. 2005;353:238-248.
165. Hahn BH. Systemic lupus erythematosus and accelerated atherosclerosis. *N Engl J Med*. 2003;349:2379-2380.
166. Ross R. Atherosclerosis—an inflammatory disease. *N Engl J Med*. 1999;340:115-126.
167. Page IH. Atherosclerosis: an introduction. *Circulation*. 1954;10:1-27.
168. Williams KJ, Tabas I. The response-to-retention hypothesis of early atherogenesis. *Arterioscler Thromb Vasc Biol*. 1995;15:551-561.
169. Nordestgaard BG, Tybjaerg-Hansen A. IDL, VLDL, chylomicrons and atherosclerosis. *Eur J Epidemiol*. 1992;8(suppl 1):92-98.
170. Goldberg IJ, Kako Y, Lutz EP. Responses to eating: lipoproteins, lipolytic products and atherosclerosis. *Curr Opin Lipidol*. 2000;11:235-241.
171. Tabas I. Nonoxidative modifications of lipoproteins in atherogenesis. *Annu Rev Nutr*. 1999;19:123-139.
172. Witztum JL. The oxidation hypothesis of atherosclerosis. *Lancet*. 1994;344:793-795.
173. Virmani R, Kolodgie FD, Burke AP, et al. Lessons from sudden coronary death: a comprehensive morphological classification scheme for atherosclerotic lesions. *Arterioscler Thromb Vasc Biol*. 2000;20:1262-1275.
174. Nissen SE, Nicholls SJ, Sipahi I, et al. Effect of very high-intensity statin therapy on regression of coronary atherosclerosis: the ASTEROID trial. *JAMA*. 2006;295:1556-1565.
175. Greenland P, Knoll MD, Stamler J, et al. Major risk factors as antecedents of fatal and nonfatal coronary heart disease events. *JAMA*. 2003;290:891-897.
176. Khot UN, Khot MB, Bajzer CT, et al. Prevalence of conventional risk factors in patients with coronary heart disease. *JAMA*. 2003;290:898-904.
177. Steinberg D, Gotto Jr AM. Preventing coronary artery disease by lowering cholesterol levels: fifty years from bench to bedside. *JAMA*. 1999;282:2043-2050.
178. Thompson GR. The proving of the lipid hypothesis. *Curr Opin Lipidol*. 1999;10:201-205.
179. Steinberg D. Thematic review series: the pathogenesis of atherosclerosis. An interpretive history of the cholesterol controversy: part II—the early evidence linking hypercholesterolemia to coronary disease in humans. *J Lipid Res*. 2005;46:179-190.
180. Nakajima K, Nakano T, Tanaka A. The oxidative modification hypothesis of atherosclerosis: the comparison of atherogenic effects on oxidized LDL and remnant lipoproteins in plasma. *Clin Chim Acta*. 2006;367:36-47.
181. Stamler J, Wentworth D, Neaton JD. Is relationship between serum cholesterol and risk of premature death from coronary heart disease continuous and graded? Findings in 356,222 primary screenees of the Multiple Risk Factor Intervention Trial (MRFIT). *JAMA*. 1986;256:2823-2828.
182. Van Horn L, McCoin M, Kris-Etherton PM, et al. The evidence for dietary prevention and treatment of cardiovascular disease. *J Am Diet Assoc*. 2008;108:287-331.
183. Katcher HI, Hill AM, Lanford JL, et al. Lifestyle approaches and dietary strategies to lower LDL-cholesterol and triglycerides and raise HDL-cholesterol. *Endocrinol Metab Clin North Am*. 2009;38:45-78.
184. Lichtenstein AH, Appel LJ, Brands M, et al. Diet and lifestyle recommendations revision 2006: a scientific statement from the American Heart Association Nutrition Committee. *Circulation*. 2006;114:82-96.
185. The Lipid Research Clinics Coronary Primary Prevention Trial results: I. Reduction in incidence of coronary heart disease. *JAMA*. 1984;251:351-364.
186. Blankenhorn DH, Nessim SA, Johnson RL, et al. Beneficial effects of combined colestipol-niacin therapy on coronary atherosclerosis and coronary venous bypass grafts. *JAMA*. 1987;257:3233-3240.
187. Brown G, Albers JJ, Fisher LD, et al. Regression of coronary artery disease as a result of intensive lipid-lowering therapy in men with high levels of apolipoprotein B. *N Engl J Med*. 1990;323:1289-1298.
188. Randomised trial of cholesterol lowering in 4444 patients with coronary heart disease: the Scandinavian Simvastatin Survival Study (4S). *Lancet*. 1994;344:1383-1389.

189. Sacks FM, Pfeffer MA, Moye LA, et al. The effect of pravastatin on coronary events after myocardial infarction in patients with average cholesterol levels. Cholesterol and Recurrent Events Trial investigators. *N Engl J Med*. 1996;335:1001-1009.
190. MRC/BHF Heart Protection Study of cholesterol lowering with simvastatin in 20,536 high-risk individuals: a randomised placebo-controlled trial. *Lancet*. 2002;360:7-22.
191. Cannon CP, Braunwald E, McCabe CH, et al. Intensive versus moderate lipid lowering with statins after acute coronary syndromes. *N Engl J Med*. 2004;350:1495-1504.
192. LaRosa JC, Grundy SM, Waters DD, et al. Intensive lipid lowering with atorvastatin in patients with stable coronary disease. *N Engl J Med*. 2005;352:1425-1435.
193. Shepherd J, Cobbe SM, Ford I, et al. Prevention of coronary heart disease with pravastatin in men with hypercholesterolemia. West of Scotland Coronary Prevention Study Group. *N Engl J Med*. 1995;333:1301-1307.
194. Downs JR, Clearfield M, Weis S, et al. Primary prevention of acute coronary events with lovastatin in men and women with average cholesterol levels: results of AFCAPS/TexCAPS. Air Force/Texas Coronary Atherosclerosis Prevention Study. *JAMA*. 1998;279:1615-1622.
195. Colhoun HM, Betteridge DJ, Durrington PN, et al. Primary prevention of cardiovascular disease with atorvastatin in type 2 diabetes in the Collaborative Atorvastatin Diabetes Study (CARDS): multicentre randomised placebo-controlled trial. *Lancet*. 2004;364:685-696.
196. Ridker PM, Danielson E, Fonseca FA, et al. Rosuvastatin to prevent vascular events in men and women with elevated C-reactive protein. *N Engl J Med*. 2008;359:2195-2207.
197. Frick MH, Elo O, Haapa K, et al. Helsinki Heart Study: primary-prevention trial with gemfibrozil in middle-aged men with dyslipidemia. Safety of treatment, changes in risk factors, and incidence of coronary heart disease. *N Engl J Med*. 1987;317:1237-1245.
198. Rubins HB, Robins SJ, Collins D, et al. Gemfibrozil for the secondary prevention of coronary heart disease in men with low levels of high-density lipoprotein cholesterol. Veterans Affairs High-Density Lipoprotein Cholesterol Intervention Trial Study Group. *N Engl J Med*. 1999;341:410-418.
199. Keech A, Simes RJ, Barter P, et al. Effects of long-term fenofibrate therapy on cardiovascular events in 9795 people with type 2 diabetes mellitus (the FIELD study): randomised controlled trial. *Lancet*. 2005;366:1849-1861.
200. Canner PL, Berge KG, Wenger NK, et al. Fifteen year mortality in Coronary Drug Project patients: long-term benefit with niacin. *J Am Coll Cardiol*. 1986;8:1245-1255.
201. Nissen SE, Tuzcu EM, Schoenhagen P, et al. Effect of intensive compared with moderate lipid-lowering therapy on progression of coronary atherosclerosis: a randomized controlled trial. *JAMA*. 2004;291:1071-1080.
202. Kane JP, Malloy MJ, Ports TA, et al. Regression of coronary atherosclerosis during treatment of familial hypercholesterolemia with combined drug regimens. *JAMA*. 1990;264:3007-3012.
203. Brown BG, Zhao XQ, Chait A, et al. Simvastatin and niacin, antioxidant vitamins, or the combination for the prevention of coronary disease. *N Engl J Med*. 2001;345:1583-1592.
204. Taylor AJ, Sullenberger LE, Lee HJ, et al. Arterial Biology for the Investigation of the Treatment Effects of Reducing Cholesterol (ARBITER) 2: a double-blind, placebo-controlled study of extended-release niacin on atherosclerosis progression in secondary prevention patients treated with statins. *Circulation*. 2004;110:3512-3517.
205. Whitney EJ, Krasuski RA, Personius BE, et al. A randomized trial of a strategy for increasing high-density lipoprotein cholesterol levels: effects on progression of coronary heart disease and clinical events. *Ann Intern Med*. 2005;142:95-104.
206. Fodor JG, Frohlich JJ, Genest Jr JJ, et al. Recommendations for the management and treatment of dyslipidemia. Report of the Working Group on Hypercholesterolemia and Other Dyslipidemias. *CMAJ*. 2000;162:1441-1447.
207. Grundy SM, Cleeman JI, Merz CN, et al. Implications of recent clinical trials for the National Cholesterol Education Program Adult Treatment Panel III guidelines. *Circulation*. 2004;110:227-239.
208. Rader DJ. Illuminating HDL—is it still a viable therapeutic target? *N Engl J Med*. 2007;357:2180-2183.
209. Lloyd-Jones D, Adams R, Carnethon M, et al. Heart disease and stroke statistics—2009 update: a report from the American Heart Association Statistics Committee and Stroke Statistics Subcommittee. *Circulation*. 2009;119:e21-e181.
210. Yusuf S, Hawken S, Ounpuu S, et al. Effect of potentially modifiable risk factors associated with myocardial infarction in 52 countries (the INTERHEART study): case-control study. *Lancet*. 2004;364:937-952.
211. Rosenson RS. Myocardial injury: the acute phase response and lipoprotein metabolism. *J Am Coll Cardiol*. 1993;22:933-940.
212. Henkin Y, Crystal E, Goldberg Y, et al. Usefulness of lipoprotein changes during acute coronary syndromes for predicting postdischarge lipoprotein levels. *Am J Cardiol*. 2002;89:7-11.
213. Harris WS, Mozaffarian D, Rimm E, et al. Omega-6 fatty acids and risk for cardiovascular disease: a science advisory from the American Heart Association Nutrition Subcommittee of the Council on Nutrition, Physical Activity, and Metabolism; Council on Cardiovascular Nursing; and Council on Epidemiology and Prevention. *Circulation*. 2009;119:902-907.
214. Mozaffarian D, Katan MB, Ascherio A, et al. Trans fatty acids and cardiovascular disease. *N Engl J Med*. 2006;354:1601-1613.
215. Kris-Etherton PM, Harris WS, Appel LJ. Fish consumption, fish oil, omega-3 fatty acids, and cardiovascular disease. *Circulation*. 2002;106:2747-2757.
216. Sprecher DL, Harris BV, Goldberg AC, et al. Efficacy of psyllium in reducing serum cholesterol levels in hypercholesterolemic patients on high- or low-fat diets. *Ann Intern Med*. 1993;119:545-554.
217. Jenkins DJ, Kendall CW, Marchie A, et al. Effects of a dietary portfolio of cholesterol-lowering foods vs lovastatin on serum lipids and C-reactive protein. *JAMA*. 2003;290:502-510.
218. Fletcher B, Berra K, Ades P, et al. Managing abnormal blood lipids: a collaborative approach. *Circulation*. 2005;112:3184-3209.
219. Bilheimer DW, Grundy SM, Brown MS, et al. Mevinolin stimulates receptor-mediated clearance of low density lipoprotein from plasma in familial hypercholesterolemia heterozygotes. *Trans Assoc Am Physicians*. 1983;96:1-9.
220. Arad Y, Ramakrishnan R, Ginsberg HN. Lovastatin therapy reduces low density lipoprotein apoB levels in subjects with combined hyperlipidemia by reducing the production of apoB-containing lipoproteins: implications for the pathophysiology of apoB production. *J Lipid Res*. 1990;31:567-582.
221. Arad Y, Ramakrishnan R, Ginsberg HN. Effects of lovastatin therapy on very-low-density lipoprotein triglyceride metabolism in subjects with combined hyperlipidemia: evidence for reduced assembly and secretion of triglyceride-rich lipoproteins. *Metabolism*. 1992;41:487-493.
222. Forster LF, Stewart G, Bedford D, et al. Influence of atorvastatin and simvastatin on apolipoprotein B metabolism in moderate combined hyperlipidemic subjects with low VLDL and LDL fractional clearance rates. *Atherosclerosis*. 2002;164:129-145.
223. Ooi EMM, Barrett PHR, Chan DC, et al. Dose-dependent effect of rosuvastatin on apolipoprotein B-100 kinetics in the metabolic syndrome. *Atherosclerosis*. 2008;197:139-146.
224. Davidson MH, Stein EA, Dujovne CA, et al. The efficacy and six-week tolerability of simvastatin 80 and 160 mg/day [see comment]. *Am J Cardiol*. 1997;79:38-42.
225. Knopp RH. Drug treatment of lipid disorders [see comment]. *N Engl J Med*. 1999;341:498-511.
226. Bays H. Statin safety: an overview and assessment of the data—2005. *Am J Cardiol*. 2006;97:6C-26C.
227. Jacobson TA. Statin safety: lessons from new drug applications for marketed statins. *Am J Cardiol*. 2006;97:44C-51C.
228. Bradford RH, Shear CL, Chremos AN, et al. Expanded Clinical Evaluation of Lovastatin (EXCEL) study results: two-year efficacy and safety follow-up. *Am J Cardiol*. 1994;74:667-673.
229. Kashani A, Phillips CO, Foody JM, et al. Risks associated with statin therapy: a systematic overview of randomized clinical trials. *Circulation*. 2006;114:2788-2797.
230. Cohen DE, Anania FA, Chalasani N. An assessment of statin safety by hepatologists. *Am J Cardiol*. 2006;97:77C-81C.
231. Bottorff MB. Statin safety and drug interactions: clinical implications. *Am J Cardiol*. 2006;97:27C-31C.
232. Venero CV, Thompson PD. Managing statin myopathy. *Endocrinol Metab Clin North Am*. 2009;38:121-136.
233. Pasternak RC, Smith Jr SC, Bairey-Merz CN, et al. ACC/AHA/NHLBI Clinical Advisory on the Use and Safety of Statins. *Circulation*. 2002;106:1024-1028.
234. Kasiske BL, Wanner C, O'Neill WC, et al. An assessment of statin safety by nephrologists. National Lipid Association Statin Safety Task Force Kidney Expert Panel. *Am J Cardiol*. 2006;97:82C-85C.
235. Levy RI, Brensike JF, Epstein SE, et al. The influence of changes in lipid values induced by cholestyramine and diet on progression of coronary artery disease: results of NHLBI Type II Coronary Intervention Study. *Circulation*. 1984;69:325-337.
236. Watts GF, Lewis B, Brunt JN, et al. Effects on coronary artery disease of lipid-lowering diet, or diet plus cholestyramine, in the St Thomas' Atherosclerosis Regression Study (STARS) [see comment]. *Lancet*. 1992;339:563-569.
237. Grundy SM, Ahrens Jr EH, Salen G. Interruption of the enterohepatic circulation of bile acids in man: comparative effects of cholestyramine and ileal exclusion on cholesterol metabolism. *J Lab Clin Med*. 1971;78:94-121.
238. Shepherd J, Packard CJ, Bicker S, et al. Cholestyramine promotes receptor-mediated low-density-lipoprotein catabolism. *N Engl J Med*. 1980;302:1219-1222.
239. Rudling MJ, Reihner E, Einarsson K, et al. Low density lipoprotein receptor-binding activity in human tissues: quantitative importance of hepatic receptors and evidence for regulation of their expression in vivo. *Proc Nat Acad Sci U S A*. 1990;87:3469-3473.

240. Beil U, Crouse JR, Einarsson K, et al. Effects of interruption of the enterohepatic circulation of bile acids on the transport of very low density-lipoprotein triglycerides. *Metabolism*. 1982;31:438-444.
241. Insull Jr W. Clinical utility of bile acid sequestrants in the treatment of dyslipidemia: a scientific review. *South Med J*. 2006;99: 257-273.
242. Aldridge MA, Ito MK. Colesevelam hydrochloride: a novel bile acid-binding resin. *Ann Pharmacother*. 2001;35:898-907.
243. Davidson MH, Dillon MA, Gordon B, et al. Colesevelam hydrochloride (cholestagel): a new, potent bile acid sequestrant associated with a low incidence of gastrointestinal side effects. *Arch Intern Med*. 1999;159:1893-1900.
244. Hunninghake DB, Bell C, Olson L. Effect of colestipol and clofibrate, singly and in combination, on plasma lipid and lipoproteins in type IIb hyperlipoproteinemia. *Metabolism*. 1981;30:610-615.
245. Insull Jr W, Toth P, Mullican W, et al. Effectiveness of colesevelam hydrochloride in decreasing LDL cholesterol in patients with primary hypercholesterolemia: a 24-week randomized controlled trial. *Mayo Clinic Proc*. 2001;76:971-982.
246. Lyons D, Webster J, Fowler G, et al. Colestipol at varying dosage intervals in the treatment of moderate hypercholesterolaemia. *Br J Clin Pharmacol*. 1994;37:59-62.
247. Davidson MH, Dicklin MR, Maki KC, et al. Colesevelam hydrochloride: a non-absorbed, polymeric cholesterol-lowering agent. *Exp Opin Investig Drugs*. 2000;9:2663-2671.
248. Zieve FJ, Kalin MF, Schwartz SL, et al. Results of the glucose-lowering effect of WelChol study (GLOWS): a randomized, double-blind, placebo-controlled pilot study evaluating the effect of colesevelam hydrochloride on glycemic control in subjects with type 2 diabetes. *Clin Ther*. 2007;29:74-83.
249. Donovan JM, Stypinski D, Stiles MR, et al. Drug interactions with colesevelam hydrochloride, a novel, potent lipid-lowering agent. *Cardiovasc Drugs Ther*. 2000;14:681-690.
250. Vroonhof K, van Rijn HJM, van Hattum J. Vitamin K deficiency and bleeding after long-term use of cholestyramine. *Neth J Med*. 2003;61:19-21.
251. Kamanna VS, Vo A, Kashyap ML. Nicotinic acid: recent developments. *Curr Opin Cardiol*. 2008;23:393-398.
252. Brown WV, Goldberg AC,Guyton JR, et al. The use of niacin. *J Clin Lipidol*. 2009;3:65-69.
253. Guyton JR, Bays HE. Safety considerations with niacin therapy. *Am J Cardiol*. 2007;99:22C-31C.
254. Zhao XQ, Morse JS, Dowdy AA, et al. Safety and tolerability of simvastatin plus niacin in patients with coronary artery disease and low high-density lipoprotein cholesterol (The HDL Atherosclerosis Treatment Study). *Am J Cardiol*. 2004;93:307-312.
255. Staels B, Dallongeville J, Auwerx J, et al. Mechanism of action of fibrates on lipid and lipoprotein metabolism. *Circulation*. 1998;98:2088-2093.
256. Prueksaritanont T, Tang C, Qiu Y, et al. Effects of fibrates on metabolism of statins in human hepatocytes. *Drug Metab Disp*. 2002;30:1280-1287.
257. Jones PH, Davidson MH. Reporting rate of rhabdomyolysis with fenofibrate + statin versus gemfibrozil + any statin. *Am J Cardiol*. 2005;95:120-122.
258. Davis HR, Veltri EP. Zetia: inhibition of Niemann-Pick C1 Like 1 (NPC1L1) to reduce intestinal cholesterol absorption and treat hyperlipidemia. *J Atherosclerosis Thromb*. 2007;14:99-108.
259. Dujovne CA, Ettinger MP, McNeer JF, et al. Efficacy and safety of a potent new selective cholesterol absorption inhibitor, ezetimibe, in patients with primary hypercholesterolemia [erratum appears in *Am J Cardiol*. 2003;91:1399]. *Am J Cardiol*. 2002;90:1092-1097.
260. Knopp RH, Gitter H, Truitt T, et al. Effects of ezetimibe, a new cholesterol absorption inhibitor, on plasma lipids in patients with primary hypercholesterolemia. *Eur Heart J*. 2003;24:729-741.
261. Jacobson TA, Armani A, McKenney JM, et al. Safety considerations with gastrointestinally active lipid-lowering drugs. *Am J Cardiol*. 2007;99:47C-55C.
262. Neuvonen PJ, Niemi M, Backman JT. Drug interactions with lipid-lowering drugs: mechanisms and clinical relevance. *Clin Pharmacol Ther*. 2006;80:565-581.
263. Yokoyama M, Origasa H, Matsuzaki M, et al. Effects of eicosapentaenoic acid on major coronary events in hypercholesterolaemic patients (JELIS): a randomised open-label, blinded endpoint analysis. *Lancet*. 2007;369:1090-1098.
264. Harris WS, Bulchandani D. Why do omega-3 fatty acids lower serum triglycerides? *Curr Opin Lipidol*. 2006;17:387-393.
265. Bays HE. Safety considerations with omega-3 fatty acid therapy. *Am J Cardiol*. 2007;99:35C-43C.
266. Pearson TA, Laurora I, Chu H, et al. The lipid treatment assessment project (L-TAP): a multicenter survey to evaluate the percentages of dyslipidemic patients receiving lipid-lowering therapy and achieving low-density lipoprotein cholesterol goals. *Arch Intern Med*. 2000;160:459-467.
267. Davidson MH, Toth PP. Combination therapy in the management of complex dyslipidemias. *Curr Opin Lipidol*. 2004;15:423-431.
268. Davidson MH, Toth P, Weiss S, et al. Low-dose combination therapy with colesevelam hydrochloride and lovastatin effectively decreases low-density lipoprotein cholesterol in patients with primary hypercholesterolemia. *Clin Cardiol*. 2001;24:467-474.
269. Denke MA, Grundy SM. Efficacy of low-dose cholesterol-lowering drug therapy in men with moderate hypercholesterolemia. *Arch Intern Med*. 1995;155:393-399.
270. Knapp HH, Schrott H, Ma P, et al. Efficacy and safety of combination simvastatin and colesevelam in patients with primary hypercholesterolemia. *Am J Med*. 2001;110:352-360.
271. Pan HY, DeVault AR, Swites BJ, et al. Pharmacokinetics and pharmacodynamics of pravastatin alone and with cholestyramine in hypercholesterolemia. *Clin Pharmacol Ther*. 1990;48:201-207.
272. Hunninghake D, Insull Jr W, Toth P, et al. Coadministration of colesevelam hydrochloride with atorvastatin lowers LDL cholesterol additively. *Atherosclerosis*. 2001;158:407-416.
273. Ballantyne CM, Houri J, Notarbartolo A, et al. Effect of ezetimibe coadministered with atorvastatin in 628 patients with primary hypercholesterolemia: a prospective, randomized, double-blind trial. *Circulation*. 2003;107:2409-2415.
274. Ballantyne CM, Weiss R, Moccetti T, et al. Efficacy and safety of rosuvastatin 40 mg alone or in combination with ezetimibe in patients at high risk of cardiovascular disease (results from the EXPLORER study). *Am J Cardiol*. 2007;99:673-680.
275. Goldberg AC, Sapre A, Liu J, et al. Efficacy and safety of ezetimibe coadministered with simvastatin in patients with primary hypercholesterolemia: a randomized, double-blind, placebo-controlled trial. *Mayo Clinic Proc*. 2004;79:620-629.
276. Taylor AJ, Villines TC, Stanek EJ, et al. Extended-release niacin or ezetimibe and carotid intima-media thickness. *N Engl J Med*. 2009;361:2113-2122.
277. Kashyap ML, McGovern ME, Berra K, et al. Long-term safety and efficacy of a once-daily niacin/lovastatin formulation for patients with dyslipidemia. *Am J Cardiol*. 2002;89:672-678.
278. McKenney JM, Jones PH, Bays HE, et al. Comparative effects on lipid levels of combination therapy with a statin and extended-release niacin or ezetimibe versus a statin alone (the COMPELL study). *Atherosclerosis*. 2007;192:432-437.
279. Bays H, Rhyne J, Abby S, et al. Lipid-lowering effects of colesevelam HCl in combination with ezetimibe. *Curr Med Res Opin*. 2006;22:2191-2200.
280. Guyton JR, Brown BG, Fazio S, et al. Lipid-altering efficacy and safety of ezetimibe/simvastatin coadministered with extended-release niacin in patients with type IIa or type IIb hyperlipidemia. *J Am Coll Cardiol*. 2008;51:1564-1572.
281. Grundy SM, Cleeman JI, Daniels SR, et al. Diagnosis and management of the metabolic syndrome: an American Heart Association/National Heart, Lung, and Blood Institute Scientific Statement. *Circulation*. 2005;112:2735-2752.
282. Buchwald H, Varco RL, Matts JP, et al. Effect of partial ileal bypass surgery on mortality and morbidity from coronary heart disease in patients with hypercholesterolemia. Report of the Program on the Surgical Control of the Hyperlipidemias (POSCH). *N Engl J Med*. 1990;323:946-955.
283. Goldberg IJ. Hypertriglyceridemia: impact and treatment. *Endocrinol Metab Clin North Am*. 2009;38:137-149.
284. Naoumova RP, Thompson GR, Soutar AK. Current management of severe homozygous hypercholesterolaemias. *Curr Opin Lipidol*. 2004;15:413-422.
285. Stein EA. Other therapies for reducing low-density lipoprotein cholesterol: medications in development. *Endocrinol Metab Clin North Am*. 2009;38:99-119.
286. Toth PP. Novel therapies for increasing serum levels of HDL. *Endocrinol Metab Clin North Am*. 2009;38:151-170.
287. Cuchel M, Bloedon LT, Szapary PO, et al. Inhibition of microsomal triglyceride transfer protein in familial hypercholesterolemia. *N Engl J Med*. 2007;356:148-156.
288. Kastelein JJ, Wedel MK, Baker BF, et al. Potent reduction of apolipoprotein B and low-density lipoprotein cholesterol by short-term administration of an antisense inhibitor of apolipoprotein B. *Circulation*. 2006;114:1729-1735.
289. de Grooth GJ, Kuivenhoven JA, Stalenhoef AF, et al. Efficacy and safety of a novel cholesteryl ester transfer protein inhibitor, JTT-705, in humans: a randomized phase II dose-response study. *Circulation*. 2002;105:2159-2165.
290. Brousseau ME, Schaefer EJ, Wolfe ML, et al. Effects of an inhibitor of cholesteryl ester transfer protein on HDL cholesterol. *N Engl J Med*. 2004;350:1505-1515.

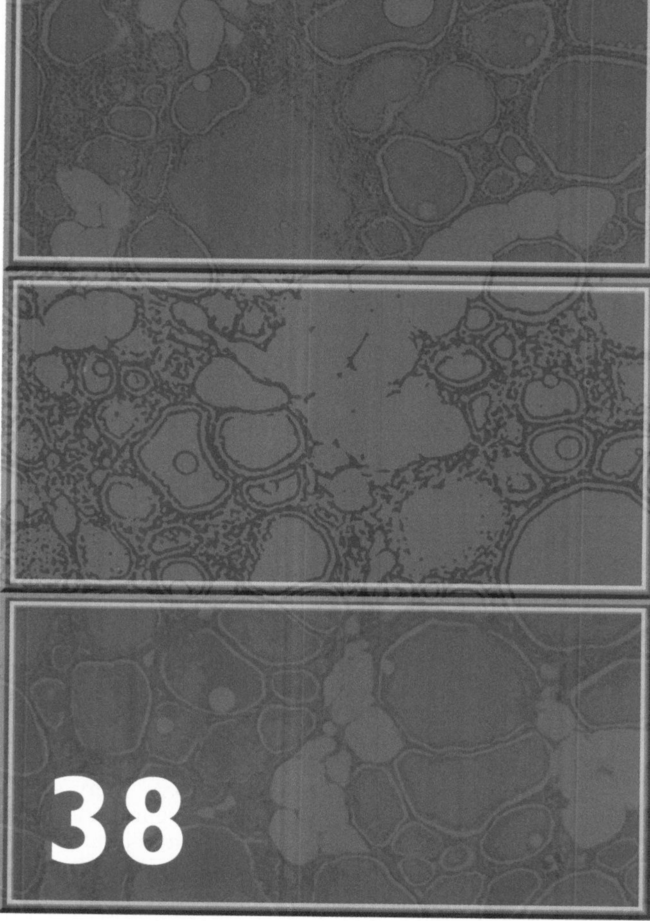

CHAPTER 38

Endocrinology of HIV/AIDS

STEVEN K. GRINSPOON

Human immunodeficiency virus (HIV) disease affects more than 33 million patients worldwide and more than 1 million in the United States. In many parts of the world, for example in sub-Saharan Africa, HIV remains epidemic, with an estimated 22 million people infected and an adult infection rate of 5.0% (data for early 2009 from http://www.avert.org/worldstats.htm). In addition, the number of HIV-infected patients is growing rapidly in Asia and other parts of the world.

Endocrine dysfunction is common among HIV-infected patients and patients with acquired immunodeficiency syndrome (AIDS). Adrenal, gonadal, thyroid, bone, and metabolic abnormalities have all been reported. HIV itself, related infectious organisms, cytokines, and antiretroviral medications may all affect endocrine function. Endocrine disorders in HIV disease, such as hypogonadism, adrenal insufficiency, diabetes, and bone loss, can cause significant morbidity and are important to diagnose. Furthermore, treatment of these disorders may improve quality of life and long-term mortality through effects on critical metabolic and body composition parameters, including loss of muscle mass (sarcopenia) in AIDS wasting and fat redistribution (loss of peripheral and abdominal subcutaneous fat with relative or absolute gains in central (visceral) adiposity in some patients). However, diagnosis and treatment can be difficult because of varying nutritional conditions and effects of the varied medications used to treat HIV disease.

Because the success of antiretroviral medications has allowed HIV-infected patients to live longer, adverse effects of these very medications have resulted in increased cardiovascular risk and metabolic changes that require intervention and long-term management by the endocrine specialist. This chapter reviews the prevalence, mechanisms, and optimal treatment strategies for endocrine abnormalities in HIV-infected patients.

ADRENAL FUNCTION

Adrenal dysfunction may be suspected in the patient with advanced HIV disease because of fatigue, hyponatremia, and other features of adrenal insufficiency. Although clinical adrenal dysfunction is relatively rare among patients with AIDS, subtle impairments in adrenal reserve may be seen in this population. Adrenal dysfunction most often is caused by destruction of adrenal tissue by cytomegalovirus (CMV) in patients with advanced HIV disease, but it may also be caused by medications, hypothalamic/pituitary disease due to opportunistic infection, idiopathic inflammation or tissue destruction, and, in rare cases, cortisol resistance. In addition, some features of Cushing's syndrome may be seen among HIV-infected patients with fat redistribution, although true Cushing's disease is rare.

Adrenal Insufficiency

Biochemical evidence of adrenal insufficiency is relatively common among hospitalized AIDS patients: 17% of 74 hospitalized AIDS patients screened by cosyntropin testing demonstrated inadequate adrenal stimulation (cortisol level at 1 hour <18 μg/dL) in an early study. In contrast, fewer patients (4%) demonstrated clinical symptoms of adrenal insufficiency.[1] Among those patients with clinical symptoms and signs of adrenal insufficiency, including hyponatremia, a higher percentage (up to 30%) may demonstrate inadequate testing with cosyntropin.[2]

Adrenal insufficiency occurring in the context of advanced HIV disease is most often caused by tissue destruction of the adrenal glands from opportunistic infections. CMV adrenalitis is the most common etiology and is seen in approximately 40% to 90% of patients with CMV infection at autopsy. However, adrenocortical destruction caused by CMV is usually less than 50% in extent and therefore is unlikely to cause adrenal insufficiency.[3] CMV disease is rare in patients with well-preserved immune function who are receiving newer, potent antiretroviral therapies (ART).

Other organisms and processes that have been associated with adrenal destruction in HIV disease include *Mycobacterium tuberculosis, Mycobacterium avium-intracellulare* (MAI), *Cryptococcus,* and hemorrhage. Additionally, pituitary/hypothalamic destruction resulting in secondary adrenal insufficiency may be caused in rare instances by opportunistic infection (e.g., toxoplasmosis, *Cryptococcus,* CMV). Idiopathic adenohypophyseal necrosis is also observed in a minority of patients, approximately 10% at autopsy, and may be related to a direct effect of HIV.[4]

Impaired Adrenal Reserve

Longitudinal evaluation of adrenal function in HIV-infected patients suggests that impaired adrenal reserve may be common. One study found normal cortisol but reduced aldosterone and dehydroepiandrosterone (DHEA) responses to adrenocorticotropic hormone (ACTH), particularly among patients with advanced HIV disease. Over time, ACTH levels increased, suggesting impaired adrenal reserve and subclinical adrenal dysfunction.[5] However, the utility of glucocorticoid treatment in patients with slightly increased ACTH levels but normal cortisol response to cosyntropin testing has not been demonstrated.

Glucocorticoid Excess: Adrenal Shunting and Cortisol Resistance

Increased cortisol levels may also be seen in HIV-infected patients. More commonly, increased cortisol levels are seen as a stress response, in association with low weight or increasing degree of illness. Intra-adrenal shunting toward cortisol synthesis, potentially as a result of 17,20-lyase dysfunction, has been suggested by studies demonstrating a reduced DHEA-to-cortisol ratio on cosyntropin testing.[6]

Cytokine modulation of the hypothalamic-pituitary-adrenal (HPA) axis may also contribute to increased cortisol levels. Interleukin-1 (IL-1), which is produced in the median eminence, has been shown to increase corticotropin-releasing hormone (CRH) and ACTH secretion in vitro and in animal studies. Increased IL-1 secretion from infected monocytes in the median eminence is another possible cause of increased cortisol secretion in HIV-infected patients. Glucocorticoid resistance has also been shown in rare patients with advanced HIV disease who demonstrate addisonian symptoms, including hyperpigmentation, in the setting of hypercortisolism and increased ACTH.

Medication Effects

Medications may contribute to adrenal insufficiency in HIV patients (Table 38-1). Ketoconazole, an antifungal agent, inhibits the cytochrome P450 (CYP) side-chain cleavage enzyme and 11-hydroxylase. These effects are not generally seen with fluconazole, itraconazole, or more recently introduced imidazole derivatives. Phenytoin, opiates, and rifampin, among other drugs, affect cortisol metabolism. Adrenal insufficiency may be precipitated by the use of rifampin for treatment of tuberculosis in patients with reduced adrenal reserve.

Megestrol acetate, a potent synthetic progestational derivative, has glucocorticoid properties and decreases ACTH. Abrupt withdrawal of megestrol acetate may precipitate adrenal insufficiency, and patients should be tested for adrenal insufficiency and receive physiologic glucocorticoid administration as needed after megestrol withdrawal. In addition, megestrol acetate can decrease gonadal function, which should also be monitored during and after therapy.

Cases of Cushing's syndrome have been described with the concomitant use of fluticasone and ritonavir, via inhibition of CYP3A4, resulting in symptoms of severe cortisol excess and also severe adrenal insufficiency with discontinuation of fluticasone.[7] Such patients may have very low measured cortisol and ACTH levels, despite symptoms of hypercortisolemia, during fluticasone treatment. Long-term physiologic steroid replacement is necessary until the HPA axis recovers. Rare case reports of interactions between ritonavir and budesonide[7] or ritonavir and intra-articular triamcinolone have also been reported.[7a]

Clinical Assessment

HIV-infected patients with symptoms of adrenal insufficiency, particularly those with hyponatremia and risk factors for adrenal insufficiency (e.g., known disseminated CMV infection, recent use of megestrol acetate), should be evaluated. Evaluation of the cortisol axis should proceed as in other patients with suspected adrenal dysfunction.

Cosyntropin testing is usually an adequate first step, except in those patients with suspected hypothalamic or pituitary insufficiency of recent onset. In such patients, use of morning cortisol levels, metyrapone, or insulin tolerance testing may be necessary, if there are no contraindications. After adrenal insufficiency is documented, determination of ACTH concentrations and appropriate imaging are used to localize the defect. In patients with clinical symptoms of adrenal insufficiency and elevated cortisol levels, cortisol resistance may be present and the diagnosis may be made by glucocorticoid receptor studies in blood monocytes.

GONADAL FUNCTION

Male

Gonadal dysfunction is common among HIV-infected men. Initial studies indicated biochemical hypogonadism in approximately 50% of men with AIDS in association with increased disease severity. More recent studies,

TABLE 38-1

Endocrine Effects and Metabolism of Approved Antiretroviral Agents and Other Medications Used in Care of HIV-Infected Patients*

Medication	Relevant Endocrine Effects	Site of Metabolism	Method of Metabolism
Protease Inhibitors			
Amprenavir	Hyperglycemia, fat redistribution, hypertriglyceridemia, hypercholesterolemia	Liver	CYP3A4
Atazanavir	Lactic acidosis in combination with didanosine; only minimal effects on glucose and lipid levels	Liver	CYP3A
Darunavir	Hypercholesterolemia, hyperglycemia, hypertriglyceridemia, increased amylase and lipase levels	Liver	CYP3A
Fosamprenavir	Diabetes mellitus, hyperglycemia, fat redistribution, increased serum lipase, hypertriglyceridemia	Liver	CYP3A4
Indinavir	Hyperlipidemia, fat redistribution, diabetes mellitus, hyperglycemia	Liver	CYP3A4
Lopinavir/ Ritonavir	Diabetes mellitus, fat redistribution, hypercholesterolemia, hypertriglyceridemia	Liver	CYP3A4
Nelfinavir	Hyperlipidemia, hyperglycemia, diabetes mellitus, fat redistribution, metabolic acidosis	Liver	CYP3A4, CYP2C19, CYP2C9, CYP2D6
Ritonavir	Diabetes mellitus, fat redistribution, hypercholesterolemia, hypertriglyceridemia, symptoms of cortisol excess when used with fluticasone	Liver	CYP3A4, CYP2D6
Saquinavir	Diabetes mellitus, hyperlipidemia, gynecomastia	Liver	CYP3A4
Tipranavir	Hyperglycemia, hypercholesterolemia, hypertriglyceridemia	Liver	CYP3A4
Nucleoside Reverse Transcriptase Inhibitors			
Abacavir	Hyperglycemia, fat redistribution, lactic acidosis	Liver	Alcohol dehydrogenase, glucuronyl transferase
Didanosine	Lactic acidosis, hyperglycemia, hypocalcemia, hypomagnesemia, hypokalemia, hyperuricemia, gynecomastia, fat redistribution, hypertriglyceridemia		Purine metabolism pathway
Emtricitabine	Lactic acidosis, fat redistribution	Liver	Sulfoxide and glucuronide metabolites
Lamivudine	Fat redistribution, hyperglycemia, lactic acidosis	Kidney	Trans-sulfoxide metabolite
Stavudine	Diabetes mellitus, fat redistribution (particularly associated with subcutaneous fat loss), lactic acidosis, mtDNA depletion, possibly gynecomastia	Liver, kidney	Unknown
Zidovudine	Lactic acidosis, fat redistribution, mtDNA depletion, gynecomastia	Liver	Metabolized to G-ZDV
Nucleotide Reverse Transcriptase Inhibitors			
Tenofovir, disoproxil, fumarate	Fat redistribution, hypophosphatemia	Plasma	Esterases
Non-Nucleoside Reverse Transcriptase Inhibitors			
Delavirdine	Fat redistribution	Liver	CYP3A, CYP2D6, CYP2C9, CYP2C19
Efavirenz	Fat redistribution, increased cholesterol and HDL, hypertriglyceridemia, hyperglycemia, vitamin D deficiency	Liver	CYP3A4, CYP2B6
Etravirine	Possible hyperglycemia, possible hyperlipidemia	Liver	CYP3A4, CYP2C9, CYP2C19
Nevirapine	Increased cholesterol and HDL, fat redistribution	Liver	CYP3A4, CYP2B6
Entry Inhibitors			
Enfuvirtide	No significant effects on glucose and lipid levels	Liver	Hydrolysis
Maraviroc	None known	Liver	CYP450
Integrase Inhibitor			
Raltegravir	Hyperglycemia	Liver	Uridine diphosphate glucuronosyltransferase-mediated glucuronidation
Additional Medications			
Foscarnet	Hyperphosphatemia and hypophosphatemia; hypocalcemia, hypokalemia, hypomagnesemia	None	None
Ketoconazole	Acute intermittent porphyria, gynecomastia, hypogonadism, adrenal insufficiency, reduced 1,25-dihydroxyvitamin D	Liver	Oxidation, dealkylation, hydroxylation
Megestrol acetate	Cushing's syndrome, hypercalcemia, hyperglycemia, adrenal insufficiency, weight gain, hypogonadism	Liver	Inactivation
Pentamidine	Ketoacidosis, hypocalcemia, hyperkalemia, hypomagnesemia, hyperglycemia	None	None
Phenytoin	Acute intermittent porphyria, vitamin D deficiency, gynecomastia, hyperglycemia, hyperprolactinemia, hypoproteinemia, hyperlipidemia, reduced T_4	Liver	Hydroxylation
Rifampicin	Acute intermittent porphyria, hyperglycemia, reduced T_4, adrenal insufficiency	Liver	Deacetylation
Trimethoprim	Acute intermittent porphyria, decreased uric acid, hyperkalemia, hyponatremia	Liver	Oxidation, hydroxylation, demethylation, carbonylation, conjugation

*For a complete list of side effects and method of metabolism, consult the *Physician's Desk Reference*.

CYP, cytochrome P450 isoenzyme; G-ZVD, zidovudine glucuronide; HDL, high-density lipoprotein cholesterol; mtDNA, mitochondrial DNA; T_4, thyroxine.

performed in the current era of potent antiretroviral treatment, suggested a wide prevalence range, from 6% to 70%,[8,9] most likely due to differences in assays used and timing of testing during the day. Among HIV-infected men with low weight, hypogonadism was seen in 20%.[10] The mechanisms of hypogonadism in HIV-infected patients may relate to severe illness or to effects of undernutrition on gonadotropin secretion, medication effects, or, more rarely, tissue destruction from opportunistic infections.

Most often, hypogonadism is secondary in nature, with low or inappropriately normal gonadotropin levels; this was the case in 91% of patients with reduced free testosterone levels during initiation of highly active antiretroviral therapy (HAART) in the Swiss HIV Cohort study.[9] Primary hypogonadism is seen less often and may be caused by cytokine effects on the testes, including effects of tumor necrosis factor (TNF), which inhibits steroidogenesis via effects on the side-chain cleavage enzyme, and of IL-1, which inhibits Leydig cell steroidogenesis and binding of luteinizing hormone to the Leydig cell. Opportunistic infections of the testes have rarely been reported, but up to 25% of HIV-infected patients with AIDS will demonstrate testicular involvement in the setting of widespread opportunistic infection or systemic neoplasms, including CMV, toxoplasmosis, Kaposi's sarcoma, and testicular lymphoma.

In addition, a number of medications can affect the hypothalamic-pituitary-gonadal (HPG) axis. Ketoconazole inhibits side-chain cleavage enzyme and other critical enzymes in testicular steroidogenesis. Megestrol acetate is used to increase appetite, but as a synthetic progestational agent it suppresses gonadotropin secretion and results in hypogonadism. Opiate therapy affects secretion of gonadotropin-releasing hormone and may result in hypogonadotropic hypogonadism (see Table 38-1).

More recently, increased prolactin levels and gynecomastia were demonstrated among HIV-infected patients. In a case-control study, gynecomastia was seen in 1.8% of 2275 consecutively screened HIV-infected patients and was associated with hypogonadism, hepatitis C infection, and the degree of lipoatrophy (subcutaneous fat loss associated with potent ART). Levels of thyroid-stimulating hormone (TSH) were increased, although the proportion of patients with hypothyroidism was not different from normal.[11] Hyperprolactinemia was reported in 21% of HIV-infected men with stable HIV disease and was significantly associated with opioid use and increased CD4 count, but not with changes in body composition or gynecomastia.[12] Increased prolactin levels in association with galactorrhea have also been described among patients treated with protease inhibitors (PIs). The mechanism of this effect is unclear and may relate to a direct stimulation of prolactin secretion by specific PIs or effects on the P450 system to potentiate the dopamine antagonistic effect of other drugs.[13] Dopamine agonists should be used cautiously in HIV-infected men who are receiving PIs because of the potential for interactions.

Levels of sex hormone–binding globulin are increased in 25% of HIV-infected patients.[10] Therefore, use of bioavailable or free testosterone assays is recommended to diagnose hypogonadism, because total testosterone assays may underestimate the prevalence of true hypogonadism in this population. For example, hypogonadism was diagnosed by measurement of low levels of free testosterone in 49% of patients but in only 26% by measurement of low levels of total testosterone in an early study of HIV-infected men with weight loss.[14]

Decreased gonadal function is associated with sarcopenia and reduced strength in HIV-infected men. Treatment with physiologic testosterone replacement results in increased lean body mass, improved quality of life, and reduction in indices of depression in HIV-infected men with hypogonadism and AIDS wasting (see "The AIDS Wasting Syndrome"). Sustained increases in lean body mass of almost 8% (or 3.7 kg) were demonstrated with 1 year of intramuscular testosterone treatment.[15] Less severe fluctuations and more consistent improvement in quality of life were shown with transdermal gel preparations than with intramuscular dosing in hypogonadal HIV-infected men.[16] Safety assessment should include monitoring of prostate-specific antigen, as is generally recommended for older men receiving testosterone administration. In patients with resolution of acute or chronic illness, retesting of gonadal function by measurement of an early-morning bioavailable testosterone level is recommended, because endogenous function may return with improved health.

No clear benefit has been demonstrated for combined use of testosterone and anabolic steroids for the treatment of hypogonadism in HIV-infected men. DHEA may be useful to improve mood and depression among HIV-infected patients with subsyndromal depression and dysthymia,[17] but the use of DHEA has not been standardized, particularly with respect to dose, duration of treatment, and clinical end points, and remains investigational.

Female

Amenorrhea is seen in approximately 25% of HIV-infected women and may be caused by reduction of gonadotropin production associated with the stress of illness. In contrast, anovulation is seen in up to 50% of HIV-infected women in association with reduced CD4 counts. Changes in menstrual function are three times as likely in anovulatory HIV-infected women compared with normally ovulating patients. Early menopause has been reported in up to 8% of HIV-infected women.[18]

Androgen levels are often reduced in HIV-infected women. In one study, more than 50% of HIV-infected women with significant weight loss, and more than one third of those without weight loss, had androgen levels (assessed with the use of a free testosterone assay) that were reduced below those in age-matched healthy women.[19] The mechanisms of androgen deficiency in HIV disease may be related in part to intra-adrenal shunting toward cortisol production and away from androgen production, particularly in women with significant weight loss (see "Adrenal Function").[6]

A number of studies have examined androgen administration in HIV-infected women. These studies have investigated the use of a transdermal testosterone patch designed to deliver low, physiologic doses of 150 to 300 µg/day. Among studies using the 150 µg/day dose, functional capacity and strength significantly improved over 6 months, with a trend toward increased lean body mass. Hirsutism was not seen, and virilization did not occur. A 6-month study using a larger dose of 300 µg/day by transdermal administration in normal-weight HIV-infected women did not show an increase in weight or lean body mass over 6 months, but the drug was well tolerated.[20] In contrast, in an 18-month randomized, placebo-controlled study conducted among relatively androgen-deficient HIV-infected women 300 µg/day of testosterone increased lean body mass, increased bone density at the hip, and improved depression indices without aggravation of lipid or glucose parameters (Fig. 38-1).[21]

Studies using nandrolone and other anabolic steroids demonstrated significant increases in lean body mass but

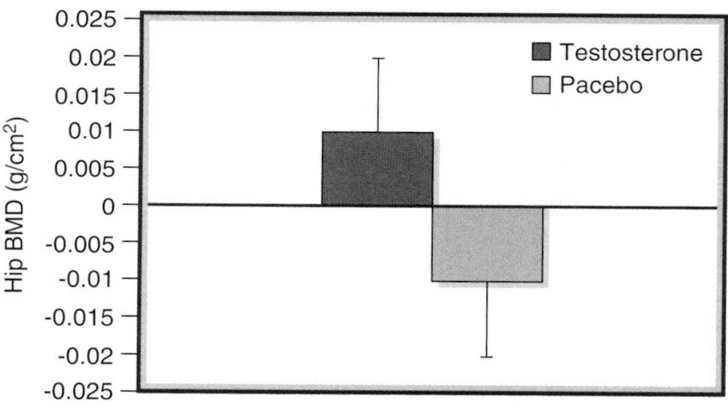

Figure 38-1 Change in hip bone mineral density (BMD) over 18 months in response to testosterone versus placebo (P = .02 for change between groups). (Data from Dolan Looby SE, Collins M, Lee H, et al. Effects of long-term testosterone administration in HIV-infected women: a randomized, placebo-controlled trial. *AIDS.* 2009, 23:951-959, with permission.)

reductions in high-density lipoprotein (HDL) and other side effects. Preliminary studies have investigated the effects of DHEA on androgen levels in HIV-infected premenopausal women, but the clinical utility of this strategy remains unknown.

THYROID FUNCTION

Altered thyroid function test results are common in HIV-infected patients. Levels of thyroid-binding globulin (TBG) are increased in HIV-infected patients and correlate inversely with CD4 counts.[22] Abnormal thyroid function test results may be caused by the stress of illness in patients with advanced disease or concomitant morbidities, as in other patients with "euthyroid sick syndrome." However, among adults, some studies have shown that levels of reverse triiodothyronine (rT_3) do not rise in association with decreasing T_3 levels, as would be expected in nonthyroidal illness.[2] Patients with progressive HIV disease therefore exhibit decreased T_3 levels, increased TBG, and decreased rT_3 levels with increasing illness.

In addition to the euthyroid sick syndrome, large screening studies have demonstrated an increased prevalence of primary hypothyroidism in HIV-infected patients. Among 350 patients studied in France, 2.6% had clinically evident hypothyroidism, 6.6% had subclinical hypothyroidism based on increased TSH levels but normal levels of free thyroxine (T_4), and 6.8% demonstrated low free T_4 levels. The prevalence of subclinical hypothyroidism was higher in men than in women. Use of stavudine and low CD4 counts were predictive of thyroid disease in multivariate modeling.[23] In a Spanish cohort, free T_4 was found to be below normal in only 1.3% of patients, and low free T_4 was shown to correlate with low CD4 counts. Increased TSH with a normal level of free T_4 was found in 3.5% of patients, but no relationship with specific antiviral drugs was found.[24] Subclinical hypothyroidism is therefore not uncommon among adult HIV-infected patients and is seen most often in the context of low CD4 counts.

Hypothyroidism in HIV-infected patients is not often seen in association with anti-thyroid antibodies, and the etiology remains unclear.[25,26] Studies have investigated the prevalence of thyroid dysfunction in the current era of HAART. In one study of 1565 HIV-infected patients, the prevalence of overt hypothyroidism was 2.5% and that of overt hyperthyroidism was 1%. Higher percentages of patients demonstrated subclinical hypothyroidism (4%) or nonthyroidal illness (17%). Conversely, 76% of patients had normal thyroid function tests. HIV therapy and specific antiretroviral medications were not associated with thyroid dysfunction.[27] Among 2437 HIV-infected patients, Nelson and associates demonstrated that the prevalence rates of hyperthyroidism and hypothyroidism were each 1%.[28] Use of specific antiretroviral agents, including PIs and efavirenz, were associated with thyroid dysfunction.

Increased TSH was demonstrated in young children with an average age of 1.5 years and failure to thrive. T_4 levels were normal, but thyrotropin-releasing hormone testing showed exaggerated TSH responses, and growth rates increased in response to thyroid hormone.[29] Fundaro and colleagues demonstrated increased anti-thyroglobulin antibodies in 34% of symptomatic HIV-infected children.[30] Increased TSH levels were found in 28% of HIV-infected children, particularly those with severe immunosuppression. In contrast, a larger study of perinatally infected children demonstrated reduced levels of total T_3, total T_4, and free T_4 and increased rT_3, TBG, and TSH, with negative autoantibodies, suggesting a euthyroid sick pattern, particularly in those with severe immunosuppression. HIV-infected children with failure to thrive should be screened for true hypothyroidism, but more often the thyroid function tests will reflect nonthyroidal illness and the severity of immune compromise.[31]

Thyroid dysfunction with an immune reconstitution syndrome has been described. The autoimmune thyroid disease occurred in association with use of potent ART and improved immune function, typically 12 to 36 months after ART was initiated.[32] Graves' disease was most often reported in this context. The estimated prevalence for immune reconstitution thyroid disease with initiation of HAART was 3% for women and 0.2% for men.[33] Graves' disease has also been described after IL-2 therapy in HIV-infected patients.[34]

In addition to autoimmune etiologies, thyroid disease related to anatomic replacement and infection of the thyroid has been reported in HIV-infected patients. *Pneumocystis* thyroiditis was reported to cause a painful thyroiditis-like picture, with hyperthyroidism followed by hypothyroidism, decreased uptake on scanning, and a firm, tender gland. *Pneumocystis* thyroiditis may result from the increased use of inhaled pentamidine, which is associated with extrapulmonary *Pneumocystis* infections.

CMV, MAI, *Cryptococcus,* and Kaposi's sarcoma have been demonstrated in the thyroid on autopsy but have not been related to clinical thyroid disease in patients with AIDS. Clinically apparent thyroidal abscesses caused by *Aspergillus* and *Rhodococcus equi* have been reported. Hypothalamic/pituitary replacement by opportunistic infections such as toxoplasmosis and CMV has also been reported to cause secondary hypothyroidism.

Medications may affect thyroid function. Rifampin influences hepatic clearance of T_4, and interferon is associated with an increased incidence of autoimmune hypothyroidism.

FLUID BALANCE AND ELECTROLYTES

Disorders of fluid balance and electrolytes are common among patients with AIDS. Hyponatremia may be seen in more than 50% of patients and is most often related to the syndrome of inappropriate secretion of antidiuretic hormone (SIADH). Hyperkalemia is also frequently reported and may be seen in association with various drugs, such as trimethoprim. More rarely, hyperkalemia may be associated with adrenal insufficiency.

Sodium

Hyponatremia (<130 mmol/L) is seen in 40% to 60% of hospitalized patients with AIDS and in 20% of outpatients. SIADH (i.e., euvolemic with low levels of serum sodium and inappropriately elevated urine osmolarity) is seen in 23% to 47% of hyponatremic patients. SIADH may be caused by various infections and tumors; if severe, it is treated with fluid restriction and hypertonic saline.

Adrenal insufficiency is documented in 30% of volume-depleted, hyponatremic HIV-infected patients.[35] Volume depletion (diarrhea, vomiting) with excessive free water and impaired water clearance (HIV nephropathy) may cause hyponatremia among ill HIV-infected patients, especially those who are hospitalized. Volume repletion is the treatment.

Hyporeninemic hypoaldosteronism,[36] more typically associated with hyperkalemia, may be another cause of hyponatremia. Treatment is with mineralocorticoids. The use of medications such as vidarabine, miconazole, and pentamidine is associated with hyponatremia of unknown etiology. Hypernatremia may be caused by foscarnet-induced nephrogenic diabetes insipidus.

Potassium

Hyperkalemia occurs in 20% to 53% of AIDS patients taking trimethoprim because of structural similarities to amiloride and inhibition of tubular potassium excretion.[37] Other potential etiologies include pentamidine-associated tubular nephropathy, HIV nephropathy (glomerular sclerosis), primary adrenal insufficiency, and, rarely, hyporeninemic hypoaldosteronism. Physiologic studies investigating potassium balance in HIV-infected patients also suggest an inadequate aldosterone response to hyperkalemia.

A Fanconi-like syndrome with tubular dysfunction, phosphate wasting, and hypokalemia has been described in patients receiving tenofovir and, more rarely, in those using adefovir, cidofovir, or didanosine.[38]

BONE

Bone Loss: Prevalence, Etiologic Factors, and Treatment Strategies

Reduced bone density is common among HIV-infected patients. Fairfield and colleagues demonstrated reduced bone density at the hip and spine in men with AIDS and weight loss.[39] Studies during the HAART era in patients without significant weight loss also demonstrated reduced bone density. Tebas and associates demonstrated a significant reduction in lumbar spine bone density among HIV-infected men receiving combined ART as determined by dual-energy X-ray absorptiometry (DEXA).[40] Osteoporosis, osteopenia, or both were seen in 73% of HIV-infected patients but only 30% of HIV-negative patients of similar age. The study suggested that use of PI therapy was associated with reduced bone density. In contrast, Mondy and coworkers showed a 46% prevalence of osteopenia or osteoporosis in a primarily (86%) male population in whom traditional risk factors including low weight, smoking, and steroid use were associated with bone loss.[41] Duration of HAART, but not use of specific PIs, was associated with bone loss.[41] In a meta-analysis including 884 HIV-infected patients, HIV-infected patients demonstrated a 3.7-fold increased risk for osteoporosis (Fig. 38-2).[42] Patients receiving ART had a 2.5-fold increased risk of osteopenia and a 2.4-fold increased risk of osteoporosis, compared with patients naïve to ART. Use of a PI was associated with increased relative risk of 1.5 for osteopenia and 1.6 for osteoporosis relative to non–PI-treated patients.[42]

Among studies performed specifically in women, osteopenia of the hip or spine was demonstrated in more than 50% of consecutively screened outpatients and was 2.4 times as likely in HIV-infected women compared with control subjects matched for age and body mass index (BMI). Low bone density was associated with low weight and other nutritional factors.[43] Markers of bone resorption were increased, but there was no association with specific PI use. Reduced lumbar spine bone density was associated with increased follicle-stimulating hormone

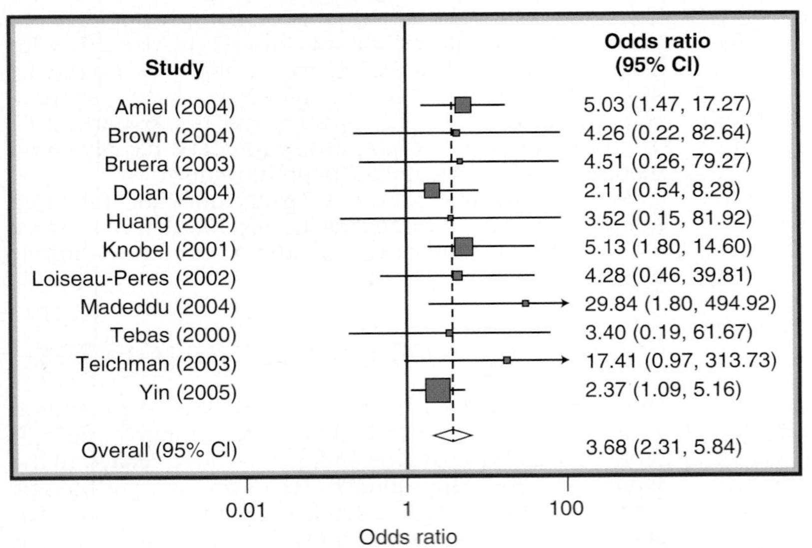

Figure 38-2 Odds of osteoporosis (T-score ≤ −2.5) in HIV-infected patients receiving antiretroviral therapy compared with antiretroviral-naïve patients. CI, confidence interval. (Data from Brown TT, Qaqish RB. Antiretroviral therapy and the prevalence of osteopenia and osteoporosis: a meta-analytic review. *AIDS.* 2006;20:2165-2174, with permission.)

levels, suggesting that relative estrogen deficiency may be contributing to bone loss among premenopausal HIV-infected women. Relative androgen deficiency was also associated with bone loss.[44] Significant bone loss has also been shown among postmenopausal HIV-infected women, with time since menopause and traditional risk factors most significantly associated with bone loss.

Studies in HIV-infected patients receiving HAART have investigated markers of bone resorption and formation and found evidence of increased bone turnover.[45] Tebas and colleagues evaluated serum and urine bone markers in 73 HIV-positive patients receiving PI therapy.[40] Increased serum bone alkaline phosphatase and urine *N*-telopeptides were found to be inversely correlated with bone mineral density T- and Z-scores as measured by DEXA, suggesting an increased rate of bone turnover among HIV-infected patients receiving PI therapy.[40] In contrast, histomorphometric studies performed before the current era of potent ART showed reduced bone turnover in association with increased disease severity.[46,47]

A number of studies have examined fracture rates among HIV-infected patients. In a large data registry study, fracture rates were increased at the spine and wrist among HIV-infected women and at the spine, hip, and wrist among HIV-infected men compared with non–HIV-infected men. The overall fracture prevalence was 2.87 per 100 persons among HIV-infected patients and 1.77 per 100 among HIV-negative patients, and the difference appeared to increase with age (Fig. 38-3).[48] In a study limited to women, lifetime fragility fractures were significantly more common in HIV-infected versus non–HIV-infected women (odds ratio, 1.7; 95% confidence interval [CI], 1.1 to 2.6).[49] Among men, Arnsten and coworkers demonstrated that incident fracture rates increased among those with normal bone density, osteopenia, and osteoporosis, from 1.4 to 3.6 to 6.5 per 100 person-years, respectively ($P < .001$).[50]

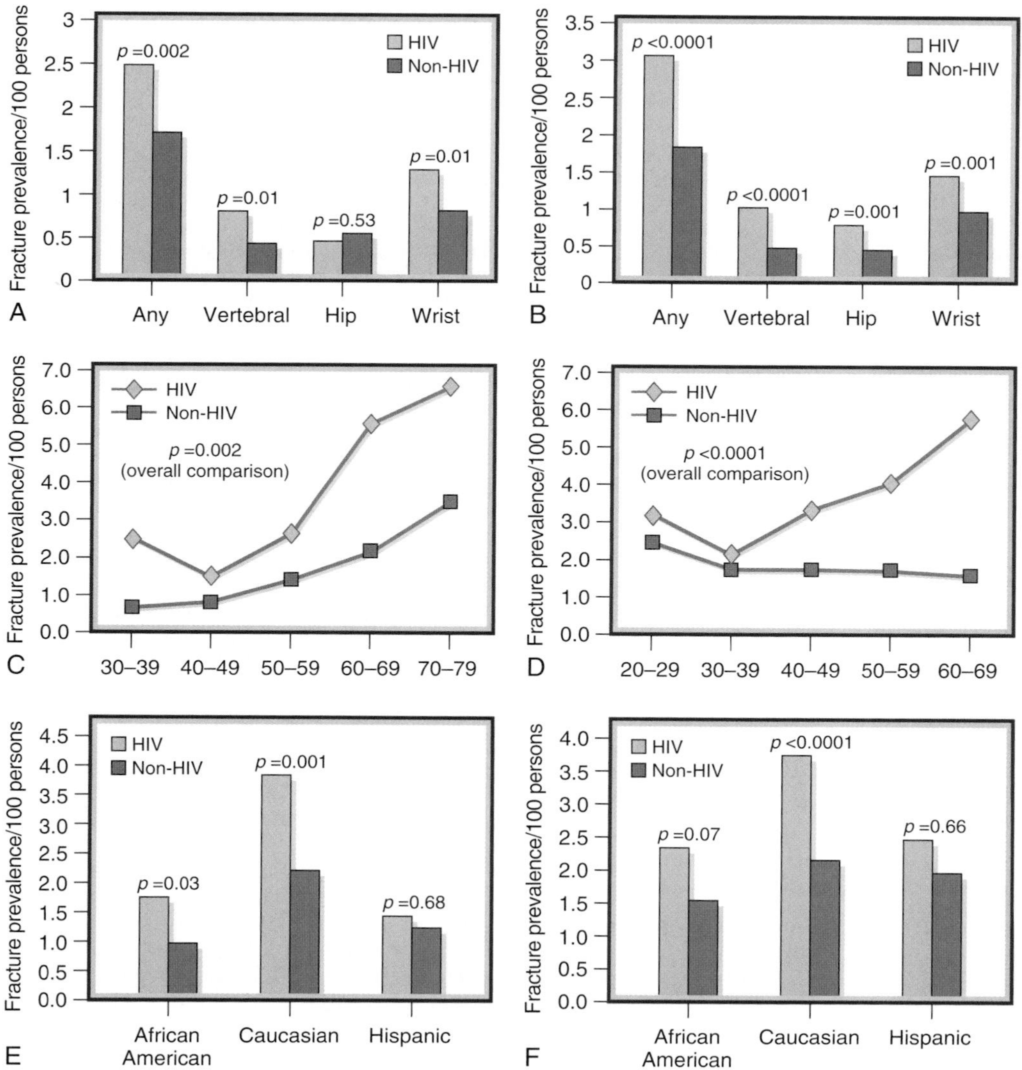

Figure 38-3 Fracture prevalence in HIV-infected and non–HIV-infected patients by gender, site of fracture, age group, and race. Data for female patients are shown in panels **A, C,** and **E**, and data for male patients in panels **B, D,** and **F**. **A** and **B**, Fracture prevalence and *P* values according to gender and site of fracture. **C** and **D**, Fracture prevalence according to gender and age group. The *P* values are for the comparison of overall fracture prevalence between HIV-infected and non–HIV-infected patients. **E** and **F**, Fracture prevalence and *P* values according to gender and race. *Light bars* and *lines* represent HIV-infected patients; *dark bars* and *lines* represent non–HIV-infected patients. (Data from Triant VA, Brown TT, Lee H, et al. Fracture prevalence among human immunodeficiency virus [HIV]-infected versus non-HIV-infected patients in a large U.S. healthcare system. *J Clin Endocrinol Metab.* 2008;93:3499-3504, with permission.)

Reduced bone density has also been reported in HIV-infected children. O'Brien and colleagues demonstrated reduced total body bone density in perinatally infected girls at age 9 years in association with increased levels of *N*-telopeptide and parathyroid hormone.[51] Bone density is reduced among children receiving HAART, with the most significant reductions in those with lipodystrophy.[52] Arpadi and associates demonstrated reduced bone density among prepubertal HIV-infected compared with non–HIV-infected children after controlling for height and weight.[53] In contrast to increased markers of resorption, reduced osteocalcin levels were reported in HIV-infected children, suggesting reduced bone formation and a relative discrepancy between increased resorption and reduced formation in this group.[54] Similar to the data in adults, bone density is related to levels of insulin-like growth factor 1 (IGF1) in HIV-infected children, suggesting a potential effect of low growth hormone (GH) on bone.[55] Mora and colleagues monitored bone density longitudinally over 1 year to compare changes in HIV-infected children versus control subjects and demonstrated relative reductions in total body, but not spinal, bone density accrual and relative increases in bone turnover.[52]

Endocrine factors may contribute to reduced bone density in HIV-infected patients, including hypogonadism and relative GH deficiency associated with excess visceral adiposity. GH pulse area, determined from overnight frequent sampling, was reduced in patients with central fat accumulation and correlated significantly with vertebral bone density.[47] This relationship may explain, in part, the inverse association between increased visceral fat and reduced bone density in HIV-infected patients.[56] PIs may also inhibit 1α-hydroxylase, resulting in 25-hydroxyvitamin D deficiency.[57] In a study of ambulatory clinic patients without known hypocalcemia, the prevalence of moderate 25-hydroxyvitamin D deficiency (>10 and <20 ng/mL) was 36.8%, and that of severe deficiency (<10 ng/mL) was 10.5%.[58]

Limited data are available on treatment strategies for bone loss in AIDS patients. Among HIV-infected patients with idiopathic bone loss and high bone turnover, studies suggest that alendronate is effective in increasing bone density, with increases in lumbar spine bone density from 3.4% to 5.2% over 42 weeks and good safety tolerability, albeit in relatively small numbers of patients (Fig. 38-4).[59,60] Longer-acting bisphosphonates (e.g., zoledronate) led to even greater changes in spinal bone density, 8.9% over 2 years, in a randomized, placebo-controlled study.[61] Among men with AIDS wasting, testosterone at high doses (200 mg/week) has been shown to increase bone density,[39] and transdermal testosterone administration has been shown to increase bone density at the hip in relatively androgen deficient HIV-infected women.[21]

Avascular Necrosis of Bone

Miller and colleagues demonstrated a 4.4% prevalence of avascular necrosis among 339 asymptomatic HIV-infected individuals.[62] A significant relationship was reported between avascular necrosis and prior use of systemic corticosteroids ($P = .02$). Other potential factors significantly associated with an increased risk of avascular necrosis included the presence of anti-cardiolipin antibodies and a history of routine bodybuilding with its associated mechanical stress. Alcohol use may also be a factor associated with avascular necrosis among HIV-infected patients.[63]

The relationship between avascular necrosis and HAART is unclear. Gutierrez and associates demonstrated an increased prevalence of avascular necrosis, from 1.6 per 1000 patients during the early 1990s to 14 per 1000 patients in the late 1990s.[64] Ninety-one percent of patients had prior exposure to HAART, and 70% had been given HAART before developing avascular necrosis.[64]

Calcium Homeostasis

Hypocalcemia is common in HIV-infected patients. Hypocalcemia, based on albumin-adjusted total calcium levels, was demonstrated in 6.5% of a large cohort of HIV-infected patients with AIDS. Calcium decreased progressively with stage of disease. Among patients with hypocalcemia, 48% were vitamin D deficient, and in most subjects the expected increase in PTH levels was lacking.[65] Jaeger and coworkers also demonstrated decreased PTH secretion in severely immunocompromised patients with AIDS, but the mechanism is unknown.[66] In addition, decreased PTH may occur in the setting of hypomagnesemia during severe illness or in association with renal magnesium wasting. Vitamin D deficiency may be caused by malabsorption due to AIDS enteropathy or specific effects of antiretroviral drugs (e.g., inhibition of 1α-hydroxylation of 25-hydroxyvitamin D by PIs).[57] Severe vitamin D deficiency of nutritional origin has also been described in HIV-infected children.

Earle and colleagues described three cases of Fanconi's syndrome in HIV-infected adults, characterized by excess phosphate excretion and osteomalacia in the context of tenofovir and cedofovir administration.[67] Osteomalacia was also associated with use of rifabutin for MAI in an HIV-infected patient. Rifabutin induces cytochrome P450, which may affect vitamin D metabolism. Other drugs that induce P450 could have a similar effect. A number of drugs may affect calcium homeostasis (see Table 38-1). Foscarnet complexes with calcium to decrease ionized calcium levels and may also induce severe hypomagnesemia. Pentamidine therapy has been associated with renal magnesium wasting and severe hypomagnesemia, which can cause hypocalcemia through decreased PTH release and resistance to circulating PTH. Ketoconazole inhibits synthesis of 1,25-dihydroxyvitamin D (calcitriol).

Among patients with HIV disease, hypercalcemia can be caused by excessive production of calcitriol in the setting of granulomatous disease (tuberculosis) or lymphoma; by local osteoclastic bone resorption caused by disseminated CMV infection; or by activation of parathyroid hormone–releasing hormone (PTHrP) related to human T-cell lymphotropic virus 1 (HTLV-1) infection.

GROWTH HORMONE

Significant abnormalities in the GH-IGF1 axis occur in HIV-infected patients. Among patients with AIDS wasting and significant weight loss, GH levels are increased in association with reduced levels of IGF1, a pattern typical of GH resistance seen with malnutrition. In contrast, in the setting of visceral fat accumulation, frequent sampling of GH levels over 24 hours suggested a different pattern.[68] Mean overnight GH and GH pulse amplitude were decreased in this setting, whereas pulse frequency was not different compared with the frequency in nonlipodystrophic HIV patients and non–HIV-infected patients matched for age and BMI. Reduced GH levels were strongly predicted by increased visceral fat in these patients. In subsequent studies, the percentage of patients failing a growth hormone–releasing hormone (GHRH) plus arginine stimulation test using a highly stringent cutoff of 3.3 ng/mL was

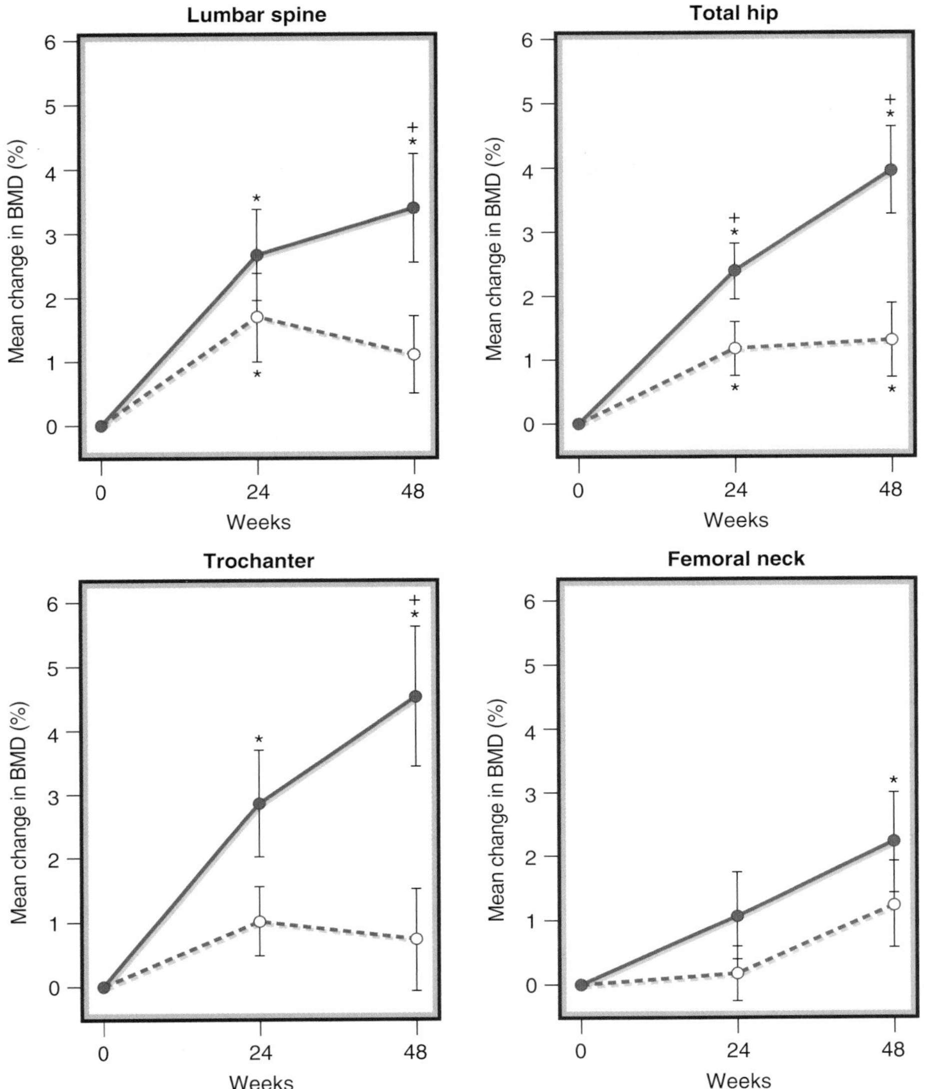

Figure 38-4 Mean percentage changes from baseline in the bone mineral density (BMD) of the lumbar spine, total hip, trochanter, and femoral neck in HIV-infected patients after treatment with alendronate plus calcium/vitamin D *(solid lines)* or calcium/vitamin D only *(dashed lines)*. T bars denote the standard error of the mean. *Significant within arm; [+]significant between arms. (Data from McComsey GA, Kendall MA, Tebas P, et al. Alendronate with calcium and vitamin D supplementation is safe and effective for the treatment of decreased bone mineral density in HIV. *AIDS*. 2007;21:2473-2482, with permission.)

18% in patients with lipodystrophy but 0% in age- and BMI-matched healthy control subjects. The prevalence of GH deficiency increased to 30% with a cutoff of 5 ng/mL.

A role for suppression of GH release by free fatty acids (FFA) was suggested by experiments in which acipimox, a nicotinic acid derivative that blocks peripheral tissue lipolysis and lowers FFA levels, was administered. Peak GH response to GHRH was increased in response to acipimox, in inverse association to the change in FFA.[69] In contrast to patients with AIDS wasting, in whom GH levels are increased in association with GH resistance, physiologic studies of GH in HIV-infected patients suggest that increased somatostatin tone, reduced ghrelin, and increased lipolysis contribute to reduced GH secretion in viscerally obese HIV-infected patients with lipodystrophic changes in fat distribution.[69]

GH and GH secretogogues have been used in HIV-infected patients both to increase lean body mass in sarcopenic patients with AIDS wasting and to reduce visceral adiposity in HIV-infected patients with the lipodystrophy syndrome (Table 38-2). Among patients with AIDS wasting, high-dose, supraphysiologic GH (0.1 mg/kg per day) has been investigated. Relatively small but significant effects on weight (1.6 kg) were seen over 3 months in a placebo-controlled study.[70] Larger effects on lean body mass (3.0 kg) were achieved over 3 months, but a portion of this gain was attributed to increased total body water.[70] GH administration at 0.1 mg/kg has been shown to increase work output during treadmill exercise[70] and quality of life, as well as peripheral muscle oxygen extraction and utilization, in patients with AIDS wasting.[71] These studies suggest that large doses of GH may be necessary to significantly increase lean mass in patients with AIDS wasting and nutritionally mediated resistance to GH. Short-term high-dose GH (6 mg/day) has also been used successfully to increase lean body mass at the time of acute opportunistic infection. However, high-dose GH is associated with side effects including hyperglycemia and fluid retention[72] and is not

TABLE 38-2

Randomized, Double-Blind, Placebo-Controlled Studies of GH and GHRH in HIV-Infected Patients

Study	N	Population	Duration	Dose	Primary End Point	Result
Growth Hormone						
Esposito et al.[179]	27	Wasting	3 mo	6 mg/day	Functional impact as observed by submaximal measures of physical performance	LBM increased and functionally relevant as determined by effort-independent submaximal measures or cardiopulmonary exercise testing
Esposito et al.[71]	12	Wasting	3 mo	6 mg/day	Peripheral muscle oxygen extraction-utilization	Improvement in peripheral muscle oxygen extraction-utilization and in the cardiac output–oxygen consumption relationship during exercise
Grunfeld et al.[180]	325	Fat redistribution	12 wk	4 mg/day	VAT	Decrease in VAT
Herasimtschuk et al.[181]	12	Lipodystrophy	Phase I, 12 wk; phase II, 12 wk	Phase I, 4 mg/day; phase II, 4 mg qod or biw	Virus-specific T-cell responses	Dose-dependent increases in CD4+ and CD8+ HIV-1–specific T-cell responses
Kotler et al.[74,75]	245	Excess VAT	12 wk	4 mg/day or 4 mg qod	Fat distribution	Decrease in VAT, trunk fat, dorsocervical fat, and non-HDL cholesterol concentrations
Lee et al.[182]	142	Wasting	12 wk	0.34 mg bid with 5.0 mg rhIGF1 bid	Anabolic effects	No significant anabolic effect
Lo et al.[76]	55	Increased abdominal fat and reduced GH secretion	18 mo	2-6 μg/kg per day titrated to upper quartile range of age-adjusted normal IGF1 range	Body composition	Reduced visceral fat and truncal obesity; improved triglyceride levels
Moyle et al.[72]	757	Wasting	12 wk	0.1 mg/kg per day or qod (6 mg max)	Lean body mass, physical performance, QoL	Lean body mass increased, increased maximum work output, QoL improved
Mulligan et al.[183]	17	Wasting	3 mo	0.1 mg/kg per day	Components of energy balance	Increases in weight and LBM accompanied by sustained increases in REE and lipid oxidation and decreases in protein oxidation
Schambelan et al.[70]	178	Wasting	12 wk	0.1 mg/kg/day	Weight, body composition, functional performance, QoL	Increased weight and lean body mass, decreased body fat, greater increase in work output, no significant change in QoL
Growth Hormone–Releasing Hormone						
Falutz et al. (initial study and follow-up study)[77,78]	412	Increased abdominal fat	Initial, 26 wk; follow-up, 52 wk	2 mg/day	Change in VAT; long-term safety and effects	VAT decreased by 15-18% (VAT was regained during withdrawal period); improved triglycerides and body image
Falutz et al.[184]	61	Increased abdominal fat	12 wk	1 mg/day or 2 mg/day	Change in abdominal fat	Decreased trunk fat in 2-mg group without significant change in limb fat; VAT decreased most in 2-mg group but not significant compared with placebo; LBM and VAT:SAT ratio significantly improved in both treatment groups
Koutkia et al.[47,185]	31	Increased abdominal fat	12 wk	1 mg bid	Change in IGF1 concentration, markers of bone turnover	Increased IGF1 concentration; improved bone metabolism

bid, twice daily; biw, biweekly; GH, growth hormone; GHRH, growth hormone–releasing hormone; HDL, high-density lipoprotein; LBM, lean body mass; qod, every other day; QoL, quality of life; REE, resting energy expenditure; rhIGF1, recombinant human insulin-like growth factor 1; SAT, subcutaneous adipose tissue; VAT, visceral adipose tissue.

well tolerated in the long term. Use of GH has not been shown to worsen viral load in patients with HIV disease, and at high doses it was shown to increase thymic mass and circulating CD4 cells in one study.[73]

GH has also been used to reduce visceral fat in HIV-infected patients with central fat accumulation. In a large randomized, placebo-controlled study, Kotler and associates found that GH, 4 mg/day, was associated with an 18.8% reduction in visceral adipose tissue (VAT) over 12 weeks and reduced total and non-HDL cholesterol levels but also with increased glucose levels.[74,75] Lo and colleagues investigated low-dose GH given for 18 months to HIV-infected patients with central fat accumulation and deficient responses to GHRH-arginine testing; VAT was reduced by 9% (Fig. 38-5), and blood pressure and triglyceride levels were improved. Even with low-dose GH, however, the 2-hour glucose level increased, demonstrating that GH is potentially useful to decrease central fat accumulation but hard to titrate in a population with significant insulin resistance.[76]

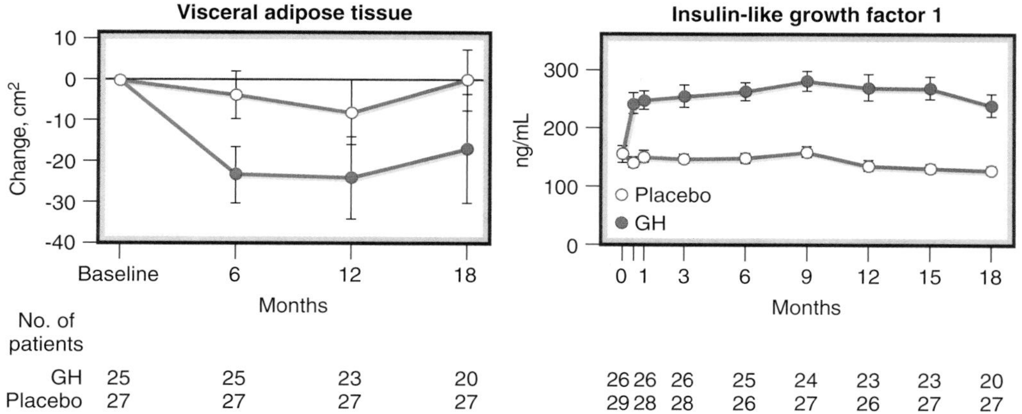

Figure 38-5 Effects of growth hormone (GH) versus placebo treatment on visceral adipose tissue area and insulin-like growth factor 1 (IGF1) levels over 18 months ($P < .05$ and $P < .001$, respectively). Vertical bars indicate standard error of the mean. IGF1 data are presented for safety population receiving at least one dose of GH. The same number of patients were assessed at 2 weeks as at 1 month. (Data from Lo J, You SM, Canavan B, et al. Low-dose physiological growth hormone in patients with HIV and abdominal fat accumulation: a randomized controlled trial. *JAMA*. 2008;300:509-519, with permission.)

In contrast, GH secretogogues have been used to successfully increase lean body mass and reduce visceral and truncal fat without significant effects on fasting or 2-hour glucose levels. In a large, randomized, placebo-controlled study, GHRH(1-44) (TH9507, tesamorelin) reduced VAT by 20% relative to placebo in HIV-infected patients with central fat accumulation. Improvements were noted in triglycerides (equal to 59 mg/dL), total cholesterol, HDL-cholesterol, and total cholesterol-to-HDL ratio, as well as adiponectin and patient self-assessment of distress associated with central fat accumulation (Fig. 38-6).[77] No clinically significant effect to reduce subcutaneous adipose tissue was seen, indicating that tesamorelin was selective for VAT. Use of tesamorelin was associated with generally physiologic increases in IGF1 levels and was not associated with increased glucose or insulin levels, in contrast to low-dose GH. In addition, GHRH(1-29) was shown to increase bone turnover in HIV-infected patients.[47] Discontinuation

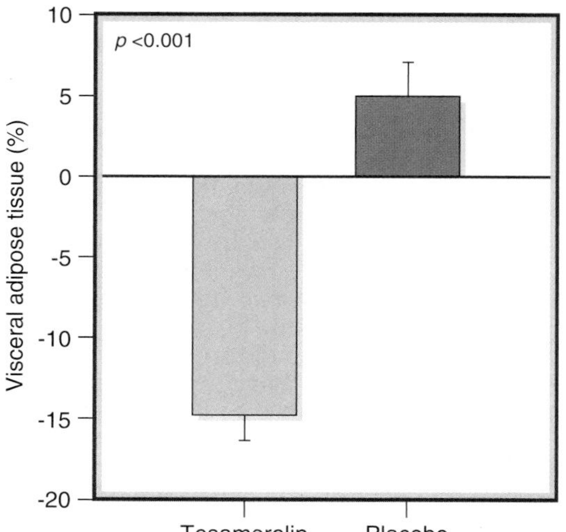

Figure 38-6 Changes in visceral adipose tissue from baseline to 26 weeks with 2 mg/day tesamorelin therapy. Figure shows the mean difference in visceral adipose tissue according to study group; T bars denote the standard error. The *P* value for the between-group comparison was calculated by analysis of covariance. (Data from Falutz J, Allas S, Blot K, et al. Metabolic effects of a growth hormone-releasing factor in patients with HIV. *N Engl J Med*. 2007;357:2359-2370, with permission.)

of both GH and GHRH resulted in reaccumulation of visceral fat back to baseline levels, demonstrating that the effects of these agents do not outlast the treatment period.[74,75,78] In November 2010, tesamorelin was approved by the U.S. Food and Drug Administration (FDA) as the first treatment for central fat accumulation in HIV-infected patients. GH is approved by the FDA to treat severe loss of muscle mass in patients with the AIDS wasting syndrome.

GH deficiency is a potential cause of growth failure in HIV-infected children, and treatment with GH results in improved auxologic parameters.[79] Increased IGF-binding protein 3 (IGFBP3) proteolysis and reduced levels of IGF1, IGFBP3, and the acid-labile subunit of the IGFBP3 ternary complex are demonstrated among HIV-infected children with failure to thrive.[80] IGF1 and IGFBP3 responses to GH may be impaired in HIV-infected children, suggesting a degree of GH insensitivity in this population, which may improve with weight and improved immune function in response to HAART.[81] GH deficiency may also disrupt the normal thymic development in HIV-infected children. GH has been used to increase height in HIV-infected children with normal GH responses to stimulatory testing.[79] Among HIV-infected children, reduced GH secretion is associated with excess visceral adiposity.

GLUCOSE HOMEOSTASIS AND PANCREATIC FUNCTION

Disorders of glucose homeostasis were relatively infrequent before the institution of potent ART but may result from the use of specific antiretroviral agents and are commonly seen in association with dyslipidemia and fat redistribution in the current era of HAART (see "Metabolic and Body Composition Changes"). The pancreas is a frequent target of opportunistic infections and malignancies in patients with HIV disease. However, clinical endocrine dysfunction rarely results, except in cases of massive pancreatic replacement due to lymphoma or Kaposi's syndrome. Opportunistic infections of the pancreas are seen on postmortem examination but are rarely clinically relevant.

More commonly, pancreatitis and hypoglycemia occur with the use of certain drugs, such as pentamidine, didanosine, or zalcitabine. Hypoglycemia can result from pentamidine administration secondary to islet cell inflammation and insulin release, especially in the context of high-dose therapy and azotemia. Subsequently, chronic hyperglycemia from pancreatic B cell destruction may follow pentamidine use. Megestrol acetate use has been associated with new-onset diabetes mellitus because of its potent glucocorticoid action. Pancreatitis is common among patients with HIV and is most often related to a drug effect (i.e., pentamidine, trimethoprim-sulfamethoxazole [Bactrim], didanosine, and zalcitabine).

In a large study of almost 6000 patients observed for 23,460 person-years at the Johns Hopkins HIV Clinic between 2001 and 2006, the incidence of acute pancreatitis was 5.1 per 1000 person-years. Low CD4 count, aerosolized pentamidine, and female gender were associated with pancreatitis. In contrast, specific antiretroviral medications were not associated with pancreatitis.[82] In the EuroSIDA study performed after 2001, the incidence of pancreatitis was 1.27 per 1000 person-years, and again low CD4 count was predictive. Similar to the data from the Hopkins cohort, no association was seen with cumulative exposure to ART nor with exposure to didanosine or stavudine, nucleoside reverse transcriptase inhibitors (NRTIs) that have been associated with pancreatitis.[83]

Amylase levels may also be elevated in HIV-infected patients secondary to macroamylasemia and salivary amylase.

THE AIDS WASTING SYNDROME

Wasting is a common feature of progressive HIV disease, known originally as "slim disease." The AIDS wasting syndrome is currently defined by weight less than 90% ideal body weight or weight loss greater than 10% over 3 months. It is characterized by a disproportionate loss of lean body mass, with a relative sparing of body fat, particularly in men. In women, fat mass may be lost disproportionately with disease progression. The loss of lean body mass occurs early and may antedate weight loss. Muscle wasting, weakness, increased resting energy expenditure (8% to 9% at baseline), and increased triglyceride levels are also features of this disease. Macallan and associates demonstrated that energy expenditure falls during periods of rapid weight loss but less than the decrease in caloric intake.[84] Cytokines associated with severe illness may increase energy expenditure and decrease appetite. In addition, chronic weight loss may be associated with gastrointestinal disease, including malabsorption. Weight loss is a significant predictor of mortality in HIV infection, with BMI less than 18.4 kg/m^2 associated with a 2.2-fold increase in mortality and BMI less than 16.0 kg/m^2 associated with a 4.4-fold increase in mortality.[85] Wasting remains common in the era of HAART and was estimated at 34% in a longitudinal cohort study.[86]

One potential endocrine mechanism that may predispose to a disproportionate loss of lean body mass is hypogonadism. Hypogonadism, usually central in etiology, is observed in 30% to 50% of men with AIDS wasting and is associated with decreased lean body mass, decreased muscle mass, and decreased exercise functional capacity.[14] Testosterone has been successfully used to increase lean body mass in men with AIDS wasting. The route of administration can be intramuscular (testosterone enanthate or testosterone cypionate) or transdermal (scrotal, nonscrotal, and newer gel preparations). Skin reaction is reported in up to 30% with the nonscrotal skin patches. Randomized studies of intramuscular testosterone for hypogonadal men with AIDS wasting suggested a beneficial effect of testosterone administration on lean body mass (2.0 kg over 6 months) and improved quality of life.[87] Testosterone in women with AIDS wasting has also been shown to be safe and well tolerated and to increase physical function over 6 months and lean body mass over 18 months (see earlier discussion).[21,88]

Although a limited number of studies have shown a benefit of anabolic steroids in HIV-infected patients with wasting, these agents potently suppress endogenous gonadal function and may cause hypogonadism. Methyltestosterone and anabolic steroids can cause problems with the liver, including peliosis hepatitis, worsening liver function, and, potentially, malignancy. Oxandrolone, an oral anabolic steroid, was shown to be safe but ineffective for AIDS wasting at low doses. Doses higher than 20 mg/day may be associated with liver dysfunction. In a placebo-controlled, randomized, dose-ranging study, only doses of 40 or 80 mg/day of oxandrolone were associated with increased body cell mass. In addition, high-dose oxandrolone suppressed endogenous testosterone levels, significantly increased transaminase levels, and increased low-density lipoprotein (LDL).[89] Nandrolone (100 mg intramuscularly every other week) was shown to be effective in increasing weight and lean body mass in HIV-infected women with weight loss.[90] Anabolic steroids are associated with decreased HDL and other side effects and hold no advantage over natural testosterone in the treatment of hypogonadism associated with AIDS-related weight loss. Short-term use of anabolic steroids may be considered in eugonadal patients with severe wasting, but they may be associated with adverse effects and should generally be avoided.

Megestrol acetate (Megace) is a synthetic progestational agent with glucocorticoid-like properties. Randomized studies in the literature show that megestrol acetate increases weight by 3 to 4 kg over 12 weeks with an increase in caloric intake (+688 kcal/day).[91,92] However, the change weight is almost entirely fat mass without an increase in lean body mass. In addition, because of its glucocorticoid-like properties, megestrol acetate is associated with a number of side effects, including hypogonadism and hyperglycemia, and abrupt withdrawal can precipitate adrenal crisis. Testosterone has been investigated in combination with megestrol acetate and was shown to reduce the degree of associated hypogonadism, but it did not increase accrual of lean body mass among HIV-infected patients receiving megestrol acetate.[93] In children, megestrol acetate promotes weight gain without improving linear growth.[94]

A number of other agents have been used in the setting of AIDS wasting. Thalidomide blocks the action of TNF-α and decreases esophageal ulcers in AIDS patients. Clinical studies demonstrate a modest beneficial short-term effect of thalidomide on weight indices but with significant associated adverse effects, including rash and fever. Administration of human chorionic gonadotropin results in increased testosterone levels and may have independent effects that inhibit Kaposi's sarcoma. No data are available from randomized, controlled studies to determine effects on wasting in humans. Small, short-term studies have shown benefits of an amino acid mixture of glutamine and arginine in increasing lean body mass.[95]

Progressive resistance training has been shown to increase lean body mass by 2.3 kg over 12 weeks in men with AIDS wasting, but it may be even more effective when combined with anabolic therapies such as testosterone,[96] oxandrolone,[97] or nandrolone.[98]

Patients with AIDS wasting may demonstrate a typical pattern of nutrition-related GH resistance. These patients exhibit elevated GH levels but decreased levels of IGF1, the primary hormone mediating the action of GH on muscle, suggesting GH resistance.[99,100] GH resistance is likely a secondary phenomenon in AIDS wasting, but the HIV envelope protein gp120 has been shown to decrease GH release in vitro and in animal studies,[101] potentially leading to a relative reduction in GH secretion. GH at supraphysiologic doses has been shown to increase lean body mass in AIDS wasting and is approved by the FDA for this purpose at a dose of 6 mg/day. However, caution should be used with long-term treatment at this dose because it can cause acute and chronic side effects of GH excess.

Taken together, the data suggest a systematic multidisciplinary approach to the AIDS wasting syndrome. Optimization of ART is paramount in conjunction with provision of adequate nutrition and protein intake. However, weight and muscle loss may occur even in this context because of the highly catabolic nature of the disease. In such cases, endocrine evaluation should include assessment of gonadal function, which is often reduced. Testosterone administration may prove useful to increase lean body mass in these patients, and it may be used in conjunction with resistance training in appropriate patients to optimally increase muscle mass. GH levels are increased in AIDS wasting, but supraphysiologic administration, as approved by the FDA, can further increase lean body mass. This strategy is best reserved for severe wasting refractory to other treatments. Other therapeutic strategies that increase weight by stimulating appetite, including megestrol acetate, are not associated with gain in lean body mass and may be associated with side effects.

In the current era of HAART, lipoatrophy, usually associated with antiretroviral drug use, should be distinguished from traditional wasting. Whereas AIDS wasting involves sarcopenia and requires anabolic strategies to increase muscle mass, the presence of severe lipoatrophy suggests that strategies to spare fat loss would be optimal.

METABOLIC AND BODY COMPOSITION CHANGES IN HIV-INFECTED PATIENTS

HIV-infected patients demonstrate a number of body composition and metabolic changes. These changes are present to varying degrees among HIV-infected patients and are multifactorial in nature, related in part to HIV virus itself, inflammation, specific antiretroviral drugs, and the interplay of these factors (Fig. 38-7).[102,103] Some of these changes may contribute to increased cardiovascular disease (CVD) and respond to changes in ART, lifestyle modifications, and specific pharmacologic strategies (e.g., to improve lipid levels or insulin sensitivity).

Body Composition Changes

The most commonly seen change in body composition among HIV-infected patients is loss of abdominal and

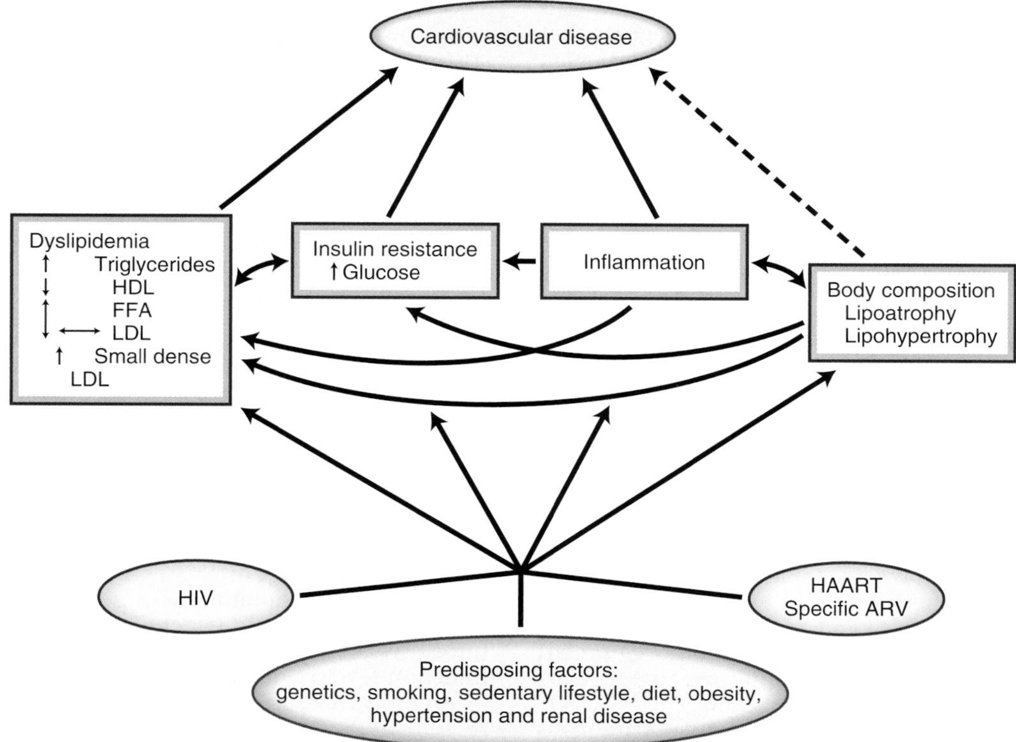

Figure 38-7 Overview of the effects of human immunodeficiency virus (HIV) infection and its therapies on risk of cardiovascular disease (CVD). The contribution of traditional risk factors (e.g., smoking) may occur with increased prevalence in people with HIV infection. HIV itself, most likely through the inflammatory response, and antiretroviral therapies independently affect many of the mediators of CVD risk. The effects on lipids are a prominent but complex example: HIV infection lowers low-density lipoprotein (LDL) levels, but antiretroviral therapy raises LDL back up to normal levels. The *bidirectional arrows* indicate associations for which there is not yet adequate proof of causality. The dotted arrow between body composition and CVD indicates that body fat is known to affect the mediators such as dyslipidemia and insulin resistance but may also have a direct effect. ARV, antiretroviral; FFA, free fatty acids; HAART, highly active antiretroviral therapy; HDL, high-density lipoprotein. (Schema from Grunfeld C, Kotler DP, Arnett DK, et al. Contribution of metabolic and anthropometric abnormalities to cardiovascular disease risk factors. *Circulation.* 2008;118:e20-e28, with permission.)

peripheral subcutaneous fat, including loss of subcutaneous fat in the face.[104] Other changes include relative preservation of central fat, with relative and absolute accumulation of excess visceral fat and excess upper trunk fat.[104,105] In addition, ectopic fat collection can be seen, including in the dorsocervical area. Increased fat deposition in the liver and muscle is also seen and is likewise associated with insulin resistance. In prospective studies of antiretroviral-naïve patients beginning treatment that included an NRTI and a PI, initial gains in peripheral subcutaneous and central fat depots were seen, with reversal of the catabolic wasting state associated with severe viral infection; this was followed by decreases in peripheral fat and relative preservation and small absolute gains in central fat.

The mechanisms by which these changes in fat occur are only partially understood. NRTIs can inhibit mitochondrial DNA polymerase-γ and contribute to mitochondrial dysfunction. Use of specific NRTIs has been associated with apoptosis of fat and reduced mitochondrial DNA in vitro and in vivo, reduced expression of lipid metabolism genes and, clinically, reduced subcutaneous fat and lipoatrophy.[106,107] Reduced mitochondrial DNA and clinically significant fat atrophy is most often associated with the use of specific NRTIs including stavudine. In contrast, PIs may have direct effects on adipogenesis via inhibition of nuclear localization of sterol regulatory element–binding protein 1 (SREBP1) and reduction in expression of peroxisome proliferator-activated receptor-γ (PPARγ).[108] NRTIs and PIs have been associated with increased lipolysis in vivo and in vitro. An important question remains as to whether the changes in fat distribution seen in patients are caused by the use of specific antiretroviral agents that may selectively effect different fat depots. In particular, the etiology of relative and absolute central fat accumulation is not known. It remains unknown whether this is a direct effect of specific antiretroviral drugs and whether abnormal nutrient partitioning to relatively preserved central adipose stores less affected by NRTI administration and mitochondrial toxicity may contribute. Alternatively, fat redistribution may result in part from altered cytokines, including increased IL-6 and TNF,[109] or altered steroid milieu.

Recent evidence suggests a potential role for a number of genetic polymorphisms, which may predispose to changes in body composition and metabolic alterations in HIV-infected patients receiving ART. Such findings could indicate a gene-environment interaction contributing to these changes. For example, single-nucleotide polymorphisms in the resistin gene were found to predict the development of dyslipidemia, insulin resistance, and limb fat loss in response to a specific HAART regimen.[110] In the same study, polymorphisms in the hemachromatosis gene and specific mitochondrial gene haplotypes were also associated with increased limb fat loss.[111] Specific haplotypes of the Fas gene (*APOC3*), the PPAR gene, and the adrenergic receptor have also been associated with the development of lipoatrophy.[112] Kratz and associates showed that reduced expression of SREBP1, PPARγ, LPL, and the CCAAT/enhancer binding protein C/EBPα in thigh subcutaneous fat was associated with the loss of fat before it became evident clinically, whereas increased 11β-hydroxysteroid dehydrogenase 1 (HSD11B1) and C/EBPβ were associated with preservation of subcutaneous fat mass.[113] Changes in fat distribution have been most widely recognized since the introduction of HAART, but abnormal fat distribution can be seen in antiretroviral-naïve patients, suggesting that viral factors also may contribute.

The changes in fat distribution seen among HIV-infected patients bear some similarities to Cushing's syndrome, with dorsocervical fat accumulation and centripetal fat distribution. However, more specific stigmata of true Cushing's syndrome, including proximal muscle weakness, facial plethora, thin skin, and bruising or violaceous striae, have not been seen, so these changes constitute a pseudo-Cushing's syndrome.[114] Miller and colleagues observed normal cortisol levels and adequate suppression in response to dexamethasone among HIV-infected patients with cushingoid features.[114] Yanovski and coworkers compared HIV-infected patients who had PI-associated lipodystrophic changes in fat to control patients and to subjects with true Cushing's syndrome.[115] In contrast to patients with true Cushing's syndrome, patients with PI-associated lipodystrophy demonstrated normal diurnal variation in cortisol levels. The 24-hour urine free cortisol levels were reduced and 17-hydroxysteroid levels were increased, compared with controls. ACTH levels were somewhat increased after CRH testing, but these changes did not appear to be related to changes in abdominal adiposity and did not suggest pathologic activation of the cortisol axis as an etiology of lipodystrophic changes in fat distribution. However, stress activation of the adrenal axis may contribute to increased cortisol production. Evidence of shunting toward cortisol production and away from androgen production in the adrenal glands has been demonstrated in association with weight loss, disease severity, and immune compromise in HIV-infected patients.[6,116] Among HIV-infected patients with changes in fat distribution, increased HSD11B expression in subcutaneous adipose tissue was demonstrated in association with an increased ratio of urinary cortisol to cortisone metabolites and may also contribute to increased cortisol production.[117]

Other abnormalities of steroid metabolism have been noted in association with changes in fat distribution. In a longitudinal evaluation, the development of lipodystrophy was associated with reduced DHEA, an increased ratio of cortisol to DHEA, and increased interferon-α.[118] Increased cortisol regeneration from affected fat depots may contribute to insulin resistance and further fat redistribution.

Lipid Abnormalities

Lipid abnormalities are highly prevalent among HIV-infected patients, particularly those with changes in fat distribution and increased visceral fat and upper trunk fat. Hypertriglyceridemia has long been associated with HIV infection and was observed before the introduction of potent ART; it is related in part to increased secretion and decreased clearance of very-low-density lipoprotein (VLDL).[119] The etiology of these changes is not known but may relate to the effects of viral infection itself, altered cytokines (including interferon-α[120]), or increased apolipoprotein E.[121] In longitudinal studies, reduction in HDL, total cholesterol, and LDL cholesterol were observed with seroconversion. With ART, cholesterol and LDL rise to preinfection levels, but low HDL levels persist.[122]

Among HIV-infected patients receiving combination ART including a PI, hypercholesterolemia (>240 mg/dL), hypertriglyceridemia (>200 mg/dL) and low HDL (<35 mg/dL) were reported in 27%, 40%, and 27% of patients, respectively, compared with corresponding percentages of 8%, 15%, and 26% in previously untreated patients.[123] Among patients with changes in fat distribution, 57% demonstrated hypertriglyceridemia and 46% had low HDL, compared with an age- and BMI-matched cohort from the Framingham Offspring Study.[124] Severe dyslipidemia among HIV-infected patients may result from the effects of antiretroviral drugs, including specific PIs, such as ritonavir, that have been shown to increase triglyceride levels. Use of PIs may also be associated with an atherogenic dyslipidemia and an increase in small dense LDL,[125] increased apolipoprotein CIII and apolipoprotein E, and decreased proteosomal degradation of apolipoprotein B.[126,127]

Hyperglycemia and Insulin Resistance

Insulin resistance and diabetes mellitus are increasingly common among HIV-infected patients. In a longitudinal study, diabetes mellitus was 3.1 times more likely to develop in HIV-infected patients receiving combination ART than in control subjects.[128] Among HIV-infected patients with changes in fat distribution, including visceral adiposity and loss of subcutaneous fat, impaired glucose tolerance is seen in approximately 35% of patients (Fig. 38-8).[124] Hyperinsulinemia in such patients is consistent with insulin resistance as the primary mechanism for impaired glucose tolerance and diabetes mellitus. Insulin resistance among HIV-infected women may not be associated with typical features of polycystic ovary syndrome.

The mechanisms of insulin resistance among HIV-infected patients may be caused by the abnormal fat distribution itself (e.g., increased central adiposity, loss of peripheral subcutaneous fat), by altered cytokines (e.g., low adiponectin, elevated TNF), or by other factors, such as increased lipolysis, increased proteolysis, increased expression of suppressor of cytokine signaling 1 (SOCS1),[129] and increased accumulation of fat in the muscle and liver. In addition, significant evidence suggests direct effects of specific antiretroviral agents to reduce insulin sensitivity. PIs have been shown to decrease glucose uptake by inhibiting the glucose transport function of GLUT4 in vitro[130] and to reduce insulin sensitivity in vivo.[131] NRTIs are associated with insulin resistance, which may occur through a direct effect, potentially related to mitochondrial toxicity,[132] or through effects on subcutaneous fat.[107]

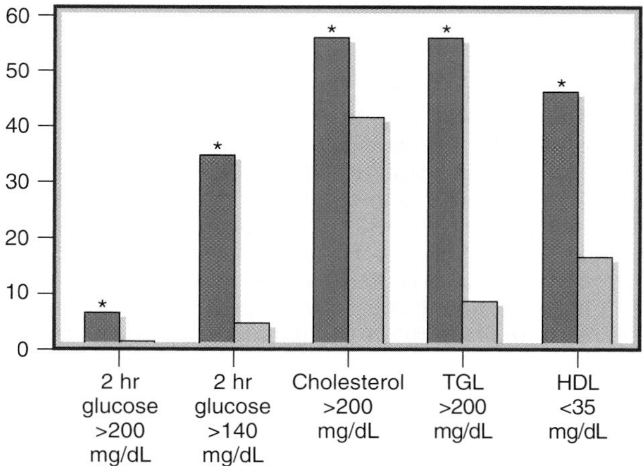

Figure 38-8 Metabolic profile in HIV-infected subjects with lipodystrophy *(dark purple bars)* compared with controls matched for age and body mass index *(light purple bars)* from the Framingham cohort. The percentages of subjects with glucose levels greater than 140 or greater than 200 mg/dL on oral glucose tolerance testing, with cholesterol levels greater than 200 mg/dL, with triglyceride levels greater than 200 mg/dL, and with high-density lipoprotein levels lower than 35 mg/dL are shown. $^*P \le .05$. (Data modified from Hadigan C, Meigs JB, Corcoran C, et al. Metabolic abnormalities and cardiovascular disease risk factors in adults with human immunodeficiency virus infection and lipodystrophy. *Clin Infect Dis.* 2001;32:130-139, with permission.)

CARDIOVASCULAR RISK IN HIV-INFECTED PATIENTS

CVD is increased among HIV-infected patients treated with HAART. The Framingham equation predicts increased myocardial infarction rates among HIV-infected patients with fat redistribution.[133] More than 40% of such subjects meet the definition of the metabolic syndrome, and predicted myocardial infarction rates are most increased in this subgroup.[133] Risk factors for CVD include insulin resistance, atherogenic dyslipidemia, truncal adiposity, hypertension, impaired fibrinolysis, and increased levels of plasminogen activator inhibitor 1 (PAI-1) and tissue plasminogen activator (tPA), as well as reduced adiponectin and increased C-reactive protein (CRP).

Surrogate markers, including carotid intima-medial thickness and endothelial function, suggest increased CVD in HIV-infected patients. Hsue and colleagues demonstrated increased carotid intima-medial thickness in HIV-infected patients, in association with cigarette smoking, increased LDL, and hypertension.[134] Progression rates were also greater in HIV-infected patients during longitudinal follow-up. Endothelial dysfunction, as determined by impaired flow-mediated dilation, is seen among HIV-infected adults receiving PIs.[135] Abnormal endothelial function correlated with dyslipidemia, including increased chylomicrons, VLDL, and intermediate-density lipoprotein and reduced HDL. PIs may also directly affect endothelial function through an effect on epithelial nitric oxide synthase (eNOS).[136] Pravastatin improves lipid parameters and tends to improve endothelial function in HIV-infected patients receiving a PI.[137] In addition, evidence suggests increased carotid intimal-medial thickness and reduced flow-mediated dilation in children receiving PIs.[138]

Mary-Krause and coworkers demonstrated a relative hazard ratio of 2.6 for increased myocardial infarctions in HIV-infected patients receiving a PI for 18 months or longer in a French cohort.[139] In contrast, data from a U.S. retrospective cohort study demonstrated an increased rate of myocardial infarction among HIV-infected patients but did not suggest an independent effect of PIs.[140] In retrospective studies, the risk of coronary heart disease related to ART use may be most pronounced among younger HIV-infected patients.[141] In a large prospective study of 23,468 patients, the covariate-adjusted risk was 1.26 per each additional year of antiretroviral exposure. Other risk factors included male gender, diabetes, age, previous myocardial infarction, hypertension, and dyslipidemia.[142] Controlling for dyslipidemia significantly reduced the effects of HAART exposure, suggesting that dyslipidemia is a significant mechanism by which HAART contributes to excess coronary artery disease in HIV-infected patients.

In a large study of patients in a major U.S. health care center, Triant and colleagues demonstrated a relative risk of 1.75 (95% CI, 1.51 to 2.02, $P < .0001$) for increased myocardial infarction in HIV-infected versus non–HIV-infected patients in a model accounting for age, gender, and race (Fig. 38-9).[143] Increased rates of traditional risk factors, including diabetes mellitus (11.5% for HIV-infected patients versus 6.6% for non–HIV-infected patients), hypertension (21.2% versus 15.9%, respectively), and dyslipidemia (23.3% versus 17.6%, respectively) were seen, and each contributed to the increase in myocardial infarction rates (relative risks, 1.62, 1.98, and 3.03, respectively, for each risk factor). In a recent prospective cohort study, Worm and coworkers demonstrated that the presence of diabetes mellitus was associated with a 2.41 times higher

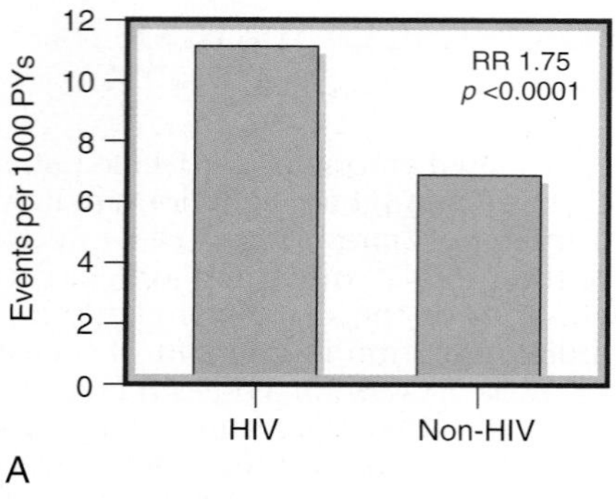

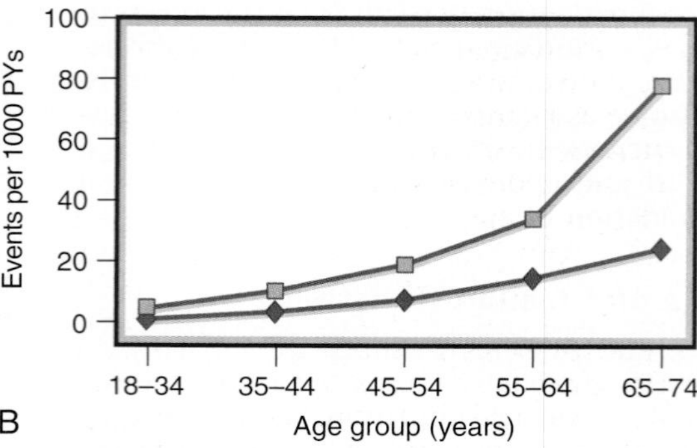

Figure 38-9 **A,** Rates of acute myocardial infarction (AMI) and corresponding adjusted relative risk (RR) in patients with and without human immunodeficiency virus (HIV) infection. Bars indicate crude rates of AMI events per 1000 person-years (PYs) as determined by *International Classification of Diseases* (ICD) coding. The RR and associated probability *(P)* value are shown above the bars. RR was determined from Poisson regression analysis adjusting for age, gender, race, hypertension, diabetes, and dyslipidemia; the associated 95% confidence interval is 1.51 to 2.02. **B,** AMI rates by age group in patients diagnosed *(squares)* or not diagnosed *(diamonds)* with HIV disease. Data shown include both genders. Rates represent number of events per 1000 PYs as determined by ICD coding. (Data from Triant VA, Lee H, Hadigan C, et al. Increased acute myocardial infarction rates and cardiovascular risk factors among patients with human immunodeficiency virus disease. *J Clin Endocrinol Metab.* 2007;92:2506-2512, with permission.)

risk (95% CI, 1.91 to 3.05, $P = .0001$) of mortality among HIV-infected patients.[144] However, in Triant's study, regression modeling, accounting for hypertension, diabetes mellitus, and dyslipidemia, demonstrated that these three risk factors contributed to only 25% of the excess risk in HIV-infected versus non–HIV-infected patients, suggesting that other factors might contribute. Smoking rates are increased and may contribute to increased CVD risk in HIV patients.

Recent studies also suggest that inflammation may contribute significantly to increased CVD risk among HIV-infected patients. Increased CRP levels observed among HIV-infected patients predicted increased myocardial infarction rates.[145] In the SMART study, HIV-infected patients randomized to continuous viral suppression with antiretroviral medications demonstrated a reduced rate of cardiovascular events compared with patients randomized to interrupted therapy with less strict goals for control of immune function.[146] It has been hypothesized that intermittent treatment may have adverse effects on inflammation or lipid profiles that may contribute to the observed differences in myocardial infarction rates.

HIV-infected women are also at risk for increased CVD. Increased waist-to-hip ratio, visceral adiposity, increased levels of triglycerides and LDL, and reduced HDL were found in HIV-infected women compared with age- and BMI-matched control subjects. In addition to traditional risk factors, CRP and IL-6 are increased, and adiponectin is reduced. Central adiposity, more than other factors, was significantly predictive of abnormal CVD risk indices, including newer inflammatory indices.[147] In contrast, HIV status and viral load were not predictive, suggesting that central adiposity and changes in fat distribution may be responsible, in part, for the increased CVD risk in HIV-infected women.

Treatment of Metabolic and Body Composition Changes in HIV-Infected Patients

A number of options are available for the treatment of body composition and metabolic abnormalities in HIV-infected patients. Antiretroviral switching to less toxic NRTIs or PIs may be useful for improving changes in fat distribution and hyperlipidemia.[148] For example, a recent study demonstrated that changing from lopinavir/ritonavir to atazanavir/ritonavir improved glucose trafficking into muscle, triglyceride levels (by 182 mg/dL on average), and visceral fat by 25%.[149] Traditional lifestyle modifications, with a focus on limiting saturated fats and increasing fiber and physical activity, may be adequate to improve glucose levels and blood pressure but inadequate to significantly improve dyslipidemia or markedly change fat redistribution. Large studies are needed to determine whether such programs can definitively improve CVD risk in HIV-infected patients and prevent the development of diabetes in those with impaired glucose intolerance. Lifestyle modifications, in combination with exercise, may improve lipid levels and visceral adiposity among HIV-infected patients.[150] Progressive resistance training may also confer significant benefits on glucose homeostasis in HIV-infected patients through a reduction in muscle adiposity.[151] However, resistance training is unlikely to reverse the loss of subcutaneous fat often seen in HIV-infected patients receiving ART.

Testosterone, Growth Hormone, and Growth Hormone–Releasing Analogues

Testosterone reduces fat and builds muscle mass in hypogonadal HIV-infected men,[87] as in non–HIV-infected men, and limited data are now available on the use of testosterone in relatively androgen-deficient HIV-infected men with abdominal fat accumulation (waist-to-hip ratio >0.95 or waist circumference >100 cm).[152] Testosterone gel, 10 g daily, did not improve visceral fat mass but reduced overall trunk fat by 15% relative to placebo over 24 weeks. Significant effects on glucose and insulin were not seen. Effects of high-dose testosterone and anabolic steroids on lipid parameters may limit the utility of this class of drugs in reducing visceral fat in HIV-infected patients. GH and GHRH can significantly reduce visceral fat (see earlier discussion) and improve lipid levels in HIV-infected patients with central fat accumulation. Supraphysiologic and even more physiologic doses of GH may also worsen glucose homeostasis. In contrast, GHRH significantly reduces visceral fat, improves lipids, and has not been shown to aggravate fasting glucose or glucose tolerance in large randomized trials performed to date.[74-77]

Insulin-Sensitizing Agents

Significant insulin resistance occurs among HIV-infected patients, in association with use of specific antiretroviral agents, changes in fat distribution, and other factors. Among HIV-negative individuals, numerous studies have documented that hyperinsulinemia and truncal obesity are strong independent risk factors contributing to coronary artery disease with significant associated morbidity and mortality. Metformin is particularly appropriate for use in patients with significant truncal adiposity and increased FFA concentrations, in whom insulin resistance is in part attributable to increased hepatic glucose production. In addition, metformin has a modest favorable effect on lipids. In patients with hyperlipidemia, metformin decreases triglyceride and LDL levels without adversely affecting other parameters. The modest 10% to 20% reduction in plasma triglyceride levels is thought to be caused by decreased hepatic VLDL production.

The effects of metformin have been investigated in HIV-infected patients with central fat accumulation and insulin resistance in a number of studies. Using a dose of 500 mg orally twice daily in a randomized, placebo-controlled week study,[153] Hadigan and associates demonstrated that low-dose metformin used significantly reduced insulin resistance, abdominal visceral fat, diastolic blood pressure, and tPA and PAI concentrations over 12 weeks, thus improving the CVD risk profile of such patients.[153,154] The effects of metformin were sustained over 9 months.[155] Other studies of metformin in HIV-infected patients also demonstrated general improvements in markers of insulin sensitivity, but with less consistent effects on abdominal fat.[156] These data suggest the need for further studies to assess the long-term efficacy of metformin in terms of fat redistribution and cardiovascular risk. In a randomized trial, the effects of metformin and progressive resistance training were compared with those of metformin alone, and the addition of resistance training further significantly improved central adiposity, blood pressure, and insulin resistance.[157]

The loss of subcutaneous fat in HIV-infected patients may further contribute to insulin resistance by limiting peripheral glucose and triglyceride uptake. Therefore, attention has focused on insulin-sensitizing strategies that may act to increase subcutaneous adipogenesis. Metformin, although a potent insulin-sensitizing agent, is not expected to restore peripheral adipogenesis but rather to act primarily via a reduction of hepatic insulin resistance. In contrast, a novel class of therapeutic agents, the thiazolidinediones (TZDs), have been shown to promote adipogenesis, primarily through activation of PPARγ. Although TZDs have effects on both hepatic and peripheral insulin resistance, the dominant effect is to improve peripheral glucose uptake.

The therapeutic efficacy of the TZDs has been well established among patients with type 2 diabetes mellitus. Short-term studies have demonstrated an effect on glycosylated hemoglobin (HbA_{1c}) and fasting glucose after 12 weeks. The TZDs also reduce plasma triglyceride levels by 10% to 20% and increase HDL by 5% to 10% in diabetic patients. Weight has reported to increase in response to TZDs, in contrast to metformin, which is associated with weight loss. Based on the known effects of TZDs in stimulating insulin sensitivity through PPARγ and promoting adipogenesis, this strategy might be appropriate to reverse insulin resistance and promote adipogenesis in HIV-infected patients with subcutaneous fat loss and insulin resistance.

In a 3-month randomized, placebo-controlled study involving 28 patients selected based on insulin resistance, rosiglitazone was shown to improve insulin sensitivity, adiponectin, FFA levels, and subcutaneous fat mass.[158] In contrast, an effect of rosiglitazone on subcutaneous fat was not shown during a 48-week study in patients with lipoatrophy who were selected for fat loss but not for insulin resistance.[159] Adiponectin levels were significantly increased and resistin levels decreased in response to rosiglitazone in HIV-infected patients, changes that may contribute to improved insulin sensitivity.[158,160] TZDs may be effective to increase subcutaneous fat in selected subpopulations of HIV-infected patients, particularly those with insulin resistance,[161] but significant adverse effects on lipid levels suggest that pioglitazone may be better than rosiglitazone in this regard. Indeed, Slama and colleagues investigated the effects of pioglitazone in HIV-infected patients with confirmed lipoatrophy in a large, randomized placebo-controlled trial.[162] Pioglitazone was shown to increase peripheral fat and to improve HDL, suggesting potential utility for HIV-infected patients with insulin resistance and fat atrophy.

The TZDs are not appropriate for severely overweight patients, because they may be associated with weight gain; they are best reserved for patients with lipoatrophy and insulin resistance. Moreover, recent data have called into question the actual cardiovascular benefit produced by rosiglitazone in non–HIV-infected diabetics, in whom increased CVD rates were seen in association with rosiglitazone use.[163] Although such effects have not been shown among HIV-infected patients, the studies to date have been small, and rosiglitazone should be used with caution in the HIV population. In addition, Mallon and colleagues showed that simultaneous use of NRTIs may reduce the effects of TZD agents in promoting subcutaneous adipogenesis in HIV-infected patients with lipoatrophy by limiting the rosiglitazone-related increase in adipose expression of PPARγ.[164]

Lipid Management

Lipid abnormalities are common among HIV-infected patients. Hypertriglyceridemia is more common than hypercholesterolemia and is associated with HIV infection and increased VLDL secretion. In addition to effects of HIV itself, specific antiviral drugs contribute significantly to hypertriglyceridemia. Mulligan and associates demonstrated that changes in lipid levels occur within 3 months after initiation of PI therapy,[165] and Purnell and colleagues confirmed significant increases in triglyceride levels among HIV-negative patients receiving a short course of ritonavir after 2 weeks.[166] Hypertriglyceridemia is most severe among patients treated with ritonavir or a ritonavir/saquinavir combination. Nelfinavir and indinavir are less often associated with abnormalities in triglyceride levels. Among the currently approved PIs, atazanavir is least often associated with hyperlipidemia.[167] Lipid changes appear to be less and to improve with use of atazanavir, in contrast to other PIs.[149]

Treatment for hyperlipidemia among HIV-infected patients is indicated to reduce CVD risk and should proceed according to standard National Cholesterol Education Program (NCEP) guidelines. Severe hypertriglyceridemia should be treated to reduce the risk of pancreatitis. Triglyceride levels higher than 1000 mg/dL are associated with pancreatitis, but lesser elevations are often asymptomatic and of unknown risk. If triglyceride levels increase substantially, lipid-lowering therapy should be considered. An initial option in patients with severe elevations in triglyceride levels is to switch treatment to a PI that is less likely to cause dyslipidemia. Triglyceride levels are reduced approximately 21% by diet[168] and 30% by exercise[169] in

HIV-infected patients. Neither diet nor exercise is likely to normalize triglyceride levels in the HIV-infected population with severe dyslipidemia.

Fenofibrate resulted in a 40% reduction in triglyceride levels and a 14% reduction in total cholesterol levels over 3 months in HIV-infected patients with hypertriglyceridemia.[170] Lesser but nonetheless beneficial effects may be seen with gemfibrozil or other fibrate derivatives. Niacin also significantly reduces triglyceride level, but it may aggravate glucose tolerance in HIV-infected patients, although such changes in glucose may only be transient.[171] In addition, niacin can be difficult to use because of the associated flushing and potential liver abnormalities. Studies have also suggested the efficacy of omega-3 polyunsaturated fatty acids, which were shown in a randomized, placebo-controlled study to reduce triglyceride levels by 25.5% and to be well tolerated.[172] In a study investigating combined therapy, triglyceride levels were reduced by 65.5% among hypertriglyceridemic HIV-infected patients receiving simultaneous fenofibrate and fish oil.[173]

The 3-hydroxy-3-methylglutaryl coenzyme A (HMG-CoA) reductase inhibitors are most useful for lowering cholesterol levels in HIV-infected patients, but they are less effective in lowering triglyceride levels. For example, pravastatin combined with dietary advice reduced total cholesterol levels by 17% over 24 weeks without effects on triglyceride levels.[174] In addition, pravastatin reduced the number of small LDL particles by 27%.[137] The combination of gemfibrozil and atorvastatin resulted in a 30% reduction in cholesterol and a 60% reduction in triglycerides in HIV-infected patients,[168] and this combination may be useful in HIV-infected patients with combined hyperlipidemia. The risk of rhabdomyolysis increases when HMG-CoA reductase inhibitors are used in combination with fibric acid derivatives.

Data suggest that the PIs can themselves affect metabolism of the HMG-CoA reductase inhibitors. In this regard, ritonavir was shown to increase levels of simvastatin by 2600% and those of atorvastatin by 74%.[175] Use of simvastatin should be avoided in patients receiving PI therapy. In an analysis of almost 900 HIV-infected patients in the Kaiser Permanente system, use of statins was shown to lower LDL by 25.6% in HIV-positive patients, compared with 28.3% in HIV-negative patients; use of gemfibrozil lowered triglyceride by 44.2% versus 59.3%, respectively, in these two groups (Fig. 38-10). Effects of statins on LDL did not vary by antiretroviral treatment class, whereas effects of gemfibrozil were less in HIV-infected patients receiving PIs and best in those patients receiving therapy with non-NRTIs. Safety of the statins, including atorvastatin, pravastatin, and lovastatin, was good, with few cases of myositis. The relative potency of each statin on LDL was

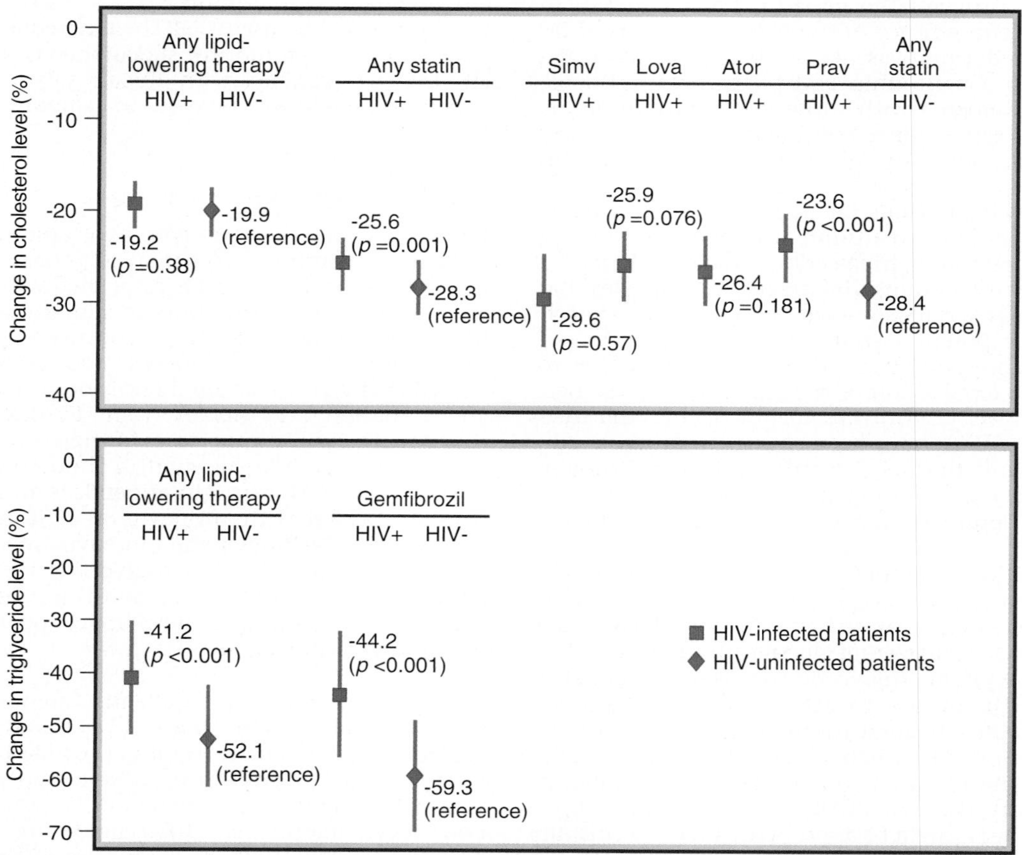

Figure 38-10 Adjusted percentage changes in low-density lipoprotein (LDL) cholesterol and triglyceride levels within 12 months after initiation of lipid-lowering therapy in human immunodeficiency virus (HIV)-positive and -negative patients. Results are based on linear regression with adjustment for age, gender, year, lipid-lowering therapy class, months of follow-up, baseline LDL cholesterol and triglyceride levels, number of coronary disease risk factors, past coronary disease or diabetes diagnoses, and hepatitis B or C infection. The model for any statin use is also adjusted for dose-equivalents of different individual statins and concomitant use of other lipid-lowering therapy classes. The model for gemfibrozil is also adjusted for medication dose and concomitant use of other lipid-lowering therapy classes. Ator, atorvastatin; Lova, lovastatin; Prav, pravastatin; Simv, simvastatin. (Data from Silverberg MJ, Leyden W, Hurley L, et al. Response to newly prescribed lipid-lowering therapy in patients with and without HIV infection. *Ann Intern Med.* 2009;150:301-313, with permission.)

similar, with reductions ranging from 26.4% with atorvastatin to 23.6% with pravastatin.[176]

Leptin

Leptin levels are low in association with fat loss and lipoatrophy in HIV-infected patients. Administration of leptin to HIV-infected patients with lipoatrophy and reduced leptin levels resulted in significant improvements in insulin sensitivity, HDL, triglycerides, and reduced truncal and visceral fat.[177,178] Because leptin reduces appetite, administration is associated with weight loss, and the small studies to date do not permit the direct effects of leptin to be distinguished from those associated with weight loss.

REFERENCES

1. Membreno L, Irony I, Dere W, et al. Adrenocortical function in acquired immune deficiency syndrome. *J Clin Endocrinol Metab.* 1987;65:482-487.
2. Grinspoon SK, Bilezikian JB. HIV disease and the endocrine system. *N Engl J Med.* 1992;327:1360-1365.
3. Glasgow BJ, Steinsapir KD, Anders K, et al. Adrenal pathology in the acquired immune deficiency syndrome. *Am J Clin Path.* 1985; 84:594-597.
4. Ferreiro J, Vinters HV. Pathology of the pituitary gland in patients with the acquired immune deficiency syndrome (AIDS). *Pathology.* 1988;20:211-215.
5. Findling JW, Buggy BP, Gilson IH, et al. Longitudinal evaluation of adrenocortical function in patients with the human immunodeficiency virus. *J Clin Endocrinol Metab.* 1994;79:1091-1096.
6. Grinspoon S, Corcoran C, Stanley T, et al. Mechanisms of androgen deficiency in human immunodeficiency virus-infected women with the wasting syndrome. *J Clin Endocrinol Metab.* 2001;86:4120-4126.
7. Foisy MM, Yakiwchuk EM, Chiu I, et al. Adrenal suppression and Cushing's syndrome secondary to an interaction between ritonavir and fluticasone: a review of the literature. *HIV Med.* Jul 2008;9:389-396.

7a. Dort K, Padia S, Wispelwey B, Moore CC. Adrenal suppression due to an interaction between nitonavir and injected triamcinolone: a case report. *AIDS Res Ther.* 2009;6:10.

8. Dube MP, Parker RA, Mulligan K, et al. Effects of potent antiretroviral therapy on free testosterone levels and fat-free mass in men in a prospective, randomized trial: A5005s, a substudy of AIDS Clinical Trials Group Study 384. *Clin Infect Dis.* 2007;45:120-126.
9. Wunder DM, Bersinger NA, Fux CA, et al. Hypogonadism in HIV-1-infected men is common and does not resolve during antiretroviral therapy. *Antivir Ther.* 2007;12:261-265.
10. Rietschel P, Corcoran C, Stanley T, et al. Prevalence of hypogonadism among men with weight loss related to human immunodeficiency virus infection who were receiving highly active antiretroviral therapy. *Clin Infect Dis.* 2000;31:1240-1244.
11. Biglia A, Blanco JL, Martinez E, et al. Gynecomastia among HIV-infected patients is associated with hypogonadism: a case-control study. *Clin Infect Dis.* 2004;39:1514-1519.
12. Collazos J, Ibarra S, Martinez E, et al. Serum prolactin concentrations in patients infected with human immunodeficiency virus. *HIV Clin Trials.* 2002;3:133-138.
13. Hutchinson J, Murphy M, Harries R, et al. Galactorrhoea and hyperprolactinaemia associated with protease-inhibitors. *Lancet.* 2000;356: 1003-1004.
14. Grinspoon S, Corcoran C, Lee K, et al. Loss of lean body and muscle mass correlates with androgen levels in hypogonadal men with acquired immunodeficiency syndrome and wasting. *J Clin Endocrinol Metab.* 1996;81:4051-4058.
15. Grinspoon S, Corcoran C, Anderson E, et al. Sustained anabolic effects of long-term androgen administration in men with AIDS wasting. *Clin Infect Dis.* 1999;28:634-636.
16. Scott JD, Wolfe PR, Anderson P, et al. Prospective study of topical testosterone gel (AndroGel) versus intramuscular testosterone in testosterone-deficient HIV-infected men. *HIV Clin Trials.* 2007;8: 412-420.
17. Rabkin JG, McElhiney MC, Rabkin R, et al. Placebo-controlled trial of dehydroepiandrosterone (DHEA) for treatment of nonmajor depression in patients with HIV/AIDS. *Am J Psychiatry.* 2006;163: 59-66.
18. Clark RA, Mulligan K, Stamenovic E, et al. Frequency of anovulation and early menopause among women enrolled in selected adult AIDS clinical trials group studies. *J Infect Dis.* 2001;184:1325-1327.
19. Grinspoon S, Corcoran C, Miller K, et al. Body composition and endocrine function in women with acquired immunodeficiency syndrome wasting [published erratum appears in *J Clin Endocrinol Metab.* 1997;82:3360]. *J Clin Endocrinol Metab.* 1997;82:1332-1337.
20. Choi HH, Gray PB, Storer TW, et al. Effects of testosterone replacement in human immunodeficiency virus-infected women with weight loss. *J Clin Endocrinol Metab.* 2005;90:1531-1541.
21. Dolan Looby SE, Collins M, Lee H, et al. Effects of long-term testosterone administration in HIV-infected women: a randomized, placebo-controlled trial. *AIDS.* 2009;23:951-959.
22. Bourdoux PP, De Wit SA, Servais GM, et al. Biochemical thyroid profile in patients infected with the human immunodeficiency virus. *Thyroid.* 1991;1:147-149.
23. Beltran S, Lescure FX, Desailloud R, et al. Increased prevalence of hypothyroidism among human immunodeficiency virus-infected patients: a need for screening. *Clin Infect Dis.* 2003;37:579-583.
24. Collazos J, Ibarra S, Mayo J. Thyroid hormones in HIV-infected patients in the highly active antiretroviral therapy era: evidence of an interrelation between the thyroid axis and the immune system. *AIDS.* 2003;17:763-765.
25. Calza L, Manfredi R, Chiodo F. Subclinical hypothyroidism in HIV-infected patients receiving highly active antiretroviral therapy. *J Acquir Immune Defic Syndr.* 2002;31:361-363.
26. Quirino T, Bongiovanni M, Ricci E, et al. Hypothyroidism in HIV-infected patients who have or have not received HAART. *Clin Infect Dis.* 2004;38:596-597.
27. Madge S, Smith CJ, Lampe FC, et al. No association between HIV disease and its treatment and thyroid function. *HIV Med.* 2007;8: 22-27.
28. Nelson M, Powles T, Zeitlin A, et al. Thyroid dysfunction and relationship to antiretroviral therapy in HIV-positive individuals in the HAART era. *J Acquir Immune Defic Syndr.* 2009;50:113-114.
29. Rana S, Nunlee-Bland G, Valyasevi R, Iqbal M. Thyroid dysfunction in HIV-infected children: is L-thyroxine therapy beneficial? *Pediatr AIDS HIV Infect.* 1996;7:424-428.
30. Fundaro C, Olivieri A, Rendeli C, et al. Occurrence of anti-thyroid autoantibodies in children vertically infected with HIV-1. *J Pediatr Endocrinol Metab.* 1998;11:745-750.
31. Chiarelli F, Galli L, Verrotti A, et al. Thyroid function in children with perinatal human immunodeficiency virus type 1 infection. *Thyroid.* 2000;10:499-505.
32. Hoffmann CJ, Brown TT. Thyroid function abnormalities in HIV-infected patients. *Clin Infect Dis.* 2007;45:488-494.
33. Chen F, Day SL, Metcalfe RA, et al. Characteristics of autoimmune thyroid disease occurring as a late complication of immune reconstitution in patients with advanced human immunodeficiency virus (HIV) disease. *Medicine (Baltimore).* 2005;84:98-106.
34. Jimenez C, Moran SA, Sereti I, et al. Graves' disease after interleukin-2 therapy in a patient with human immunodeficiency virus infection. *Thyroid.* 2004;14:1097-1102.
35. Tang WW, Kaptein E, Feinstein EI, et al. Hyponatremia in hospitalized patients with the acquired immunodeficiency syndrome (AIDS) and the AIDS-related complex. *Am J Med.* 1993;94:169-174.
36. Kalin MF, Poretsky L, Seres DS, et al. Hyporeninemic hypoaldosteronism associated with acquired immune deficiency syndrome. *Am J Med.* 1987;82:1035-1038.
37. Choi MJ, Fernandez PC, Patnaik A, et al. Brief report: trimethoprim-induced hyperkalemia in a patient with AIDS. *Ann Int Med.* 1993;328:703-706.
38. Mathew G, Knaus SJ. Acquired Fanconi's syndrome associated with tenofovir therapy. *J Gen Intern Med.* 2006;21:C3-C5.
39. Fairfield WP, Finkelstein JS, Klibanski A, et al. Osteopenia in eugonadal men with acquired immune deficiency syndrome wasting syndrome. *J Clin Endocrinol Metab.* 2001;86:2020-2026.
40. Tebas P, Powderly WG, Claxton S, et al. Accelerated bone mineral loss in HIV-infected patients receiving potent antiretroviral therapy. *AIDS.* 2000;14:F63-F67.
41. Mondy K, Yarasheski K, Powderly WG, et al. Longitudinal evolution of bone nineral density and bone markers in human immunodeficiency virus-infected individuals. *Clin Inf Dis.* 2003;36: 482-490.
42. Brown TT, Qaqish RB. Antiretroviral therapy and the prevalence of osteopenia and osteoporosis: a meta-analytic review. *AIDS.* 2006;20: 2165-2174.
43. Dolan SE, Huang JS, Killilea KM, et al. Reduced bone density in HIV-infected women. *AIDS.* 2004;18:475-483.
44. Dolan SE, Kanter JR, Grinspoon S. Longitudinal analysis of bone density in human immunodeficiency virus-infected women. *J Clin Endocrinol Metab.* 2006;91:2938-2945.

44a. Yin M, Dobkin J, Brudney K, et al. Bone mass and mineral metabolism in HIV+ postmenopausal women. *Osteoporosis International.* March 8 2005;16(11):1345-1352.

45. Aukrust P, Haug CJ, Ueland T, et al. Decreased bone formative and enhanced resorptive markers in human immunodeficiency virus infection: indication of normalization of the bone-remodeling process during highly active antiretroviral therapy. *J Clin Endocrinol Metab.* 1999;84:145-150.

147. Dolan SE, Hadigan C, Killilea KM, et al. Increased cardiovascular disease risk indices in HIV-infected women. *J Acquir Immune Defic Syndr*. 2005;39:44-54.
148. Carr A, Workman C, Smith DE, et al. Abacavir substitution for nucleoside analogs in patients with HIV lipoatrophy: a randomized trial. *JAMA*. 2002;288:207-215.
149. Stanley TL, Joy T, Hadigan CM, et al. Effects of switching from lopinavir/ritonavir to atazanavir/ritonavir on muscle glucose uptake and visceral fat in HIV-infected patients. *AIDS*. 2009;23:1349-1357.
150. Jones SP, Doran DA, Leatt PB, et al. Short-term exercise training improves body composition and hyperlipidaemia in HIV-positive individuals with lipodystrophy. *AIDS*. 2001;15:2049-2051.
151. Driscoll SD, Meininger GE, Ljunquist K, et al. Differential effects of metformin and exercise on muscle adiposity and metabolic indices in human immunodeficiecy virus-infected patients. *J Clin Endocrinol Metab*. 2004;89:2171-2178.
152. Bhasin S, Parker RA, Sattler F, et al. Effects of testosterone supplementation on whole body and regional fat mass and distribution in human immunodeficiency virus-infected men with abdominal obesity. *J Clin Endocrinol Metab*. 2007;92:1049-1057.
153. Hadigan C, Corcoran C, Basgoz N, et al. Metformin in the treatment of HIV lipodystrophy syndrome: a randomized controlled trial. *JAMA*. 2000;284:472-477.
154. Hadigan C, Meigs JB, Rabe J, et al. Increased PAI-1 and tPA antigen levels are reduced with metformin therapy in HIV-infected patients with fat redistribution and insulin resistance. *J Clin Endocrinol Metab*. 2001;86:939-943.
155. Hadigan C, Rabe J, Grinspoon S. Sustained benefits of metformin therapy on markers of cardiovascular risk in human immunodeficiency virus-infected patients with fat redistribution and insulin resistance. *J Clin Endocrinol Metab*. 2002;87:4611-4615.
156. Mulligan K, Yang Y, Wininger DA, et al. Effects of metformin and rosiglitazone in HIV-infected patients with hyperinsulinemia and elevated waist to hip ratio. *AIDS*. 2007;21:47-57.
157. Driscoll SD, Meininger GE, Lareau MT, et al. Effects of exercise training and metformin on body composition and cardiovascular indices in HIV infected patients. *AIDS*. 2004;18:465-473.
158. Hadigan C, Yawetz S, Thomas A, et al. Metabolic effects of rosiglitazone in HIV lipodystrophy: a randomized controlled trial. *Ann Intern Med*. 2004;140:786-794.
159. Carr A, Workman C, Carey D, et al. No effect of rosiglitazone for treatment of HIV-1 lipoatrophy: randomized, double-blind, placebo-controlled trial. *Lancet*. 2004;363:429-438.
160. Kamin D, Hadigan C, Lehrke M, et al. Resistin levels in human immunodeficiency virus-infected patients with lipoatrophy decrease in response to rosiglitazone. *J Clin Endocrinol Metab*. 2005;90:3423-3426.
161. van Wijk JP, de Koning EJ, Cabezas MC, et al. Comparison of rosiglitazone and metformin for treating HIV lipodystrophy: a randomized trial. *Ann Intern Med*. 2005;143:337-346.
162. Slama L, Lanoy E, Valantin MA, et al. Effect of pioglitazone on HIV-1-related lipodystrophy: a randomized double-blind placebo-controlled trial (ANRS 113). *Antivir Ther*. 2008;13:67-76.
163. Nissen SE, Wolski K. Effect of rosiglitazone on the risk of myocardial infarction and death from cardiovascular causes [see comment]. *N Engl J Med*. 2007;356:2457-2471.
164. Mallon PW, Sedwell R, Rogers G, et al. Effect of rosiglitazone on peroxisome proliferator-activated receptor gamma gene expression in human adipose tissue is limited by antiretroviral drug-induced mitochondrial dysfunction. *J Infect Dis*. 2008;198:1794-1803.
165. Mulligan K, Tai VW, Algren H, et al. Altered fat distribution in HIV-positive men on nucleoside analog reverse transcriptase inhibitor therapy. *J Acquir Immune Defic Syndr*. 2001;26:443-448.
166. Purnell JQ, Zambon A, Knopp RH, et al. Effect of ritonavir on lipids and post-heparin lipase activities in normal subjects. *AIDS*. 2000;14:51-57.
167. Wood R, Phanuphak P, Cahn P, et al. Long-term efficacy and safety of atazanavir with stavudine and lamivudine in patients previously treated with nelfinavir or atazanavir. *J Acquir Immune Defic Syndr*. 2004;36:684-692.
168. Henry K, Melroe H, Huebesch J, et al. Atorvastatin and gemfibrozil for protease-inhibitor-related lipid abnormalities. *Lancet*. 1998;352:1031-1032.
169. Yarasheski KE, Tebas P, Stanerson B, et al. Resistance exercise training reduces hypertriglyceridemia in HIV-infected men treated with antiviral therapy. *J Appl Physiol*. 2001;90:133-138.
170. Badiou S, De Boever M, Dupuy AM, et al. Fenofibrate improves the atherogenic lipid profile and enhances LDL resistance to oxidation in HIV-positive adults. *Atherosclerosis*. 2004;172:273-279.
171. Dube MP, Wu JW, Aberg JA, et al. Safety and efficacy of extended-release niacin for the treatment of dyslipidaemia in patients with HIV infection: AIDS Clinical Trials Group Study A5148. *Antivir Ther*. 2006;11:1081-1089.
172. De Truchis P, Kirstetter M, Perier A, et al. Reduction in triglyceride level with N-3 polyunsaturated fatty acids in HIV-infected patients taking potent antiretroviral therapy: a randomized prospective study. *J Acquir Immune Defic Syndr*. 2007;44:278-285.
173. Gerber JG, Kitch DW, Fichtenbaum CJ, et al. Fish oil and fenofibrate for the treatment of hypertriglyceridemia in HIV-infected subjects on antiretroviral therapy: results of ACTG A5186. *J Acquir Immune Defic Syndr*. 2008;47:459-466.
174. Moyle GJ, Lloyd M, Reynolds B, et al. Dietary advice with or without pravastatin for the management of hypercholesterolaemia associated with protease inhibitor therapy. *AIDS*. 2001;15:1503-1508.
175. Fichtenbaum CJ, Gerber JG. Interactions between antiretroviral drugs and drugs used for the therapy of the metabolic complications encountered during HIV infection. *Clin Pharmacokinet*. 2002;41:1195-1211.
176. Silverberg MJ, Leyden W, Hurley L, et al. Response to newly prescribed lipid-lowering therapy in patients with and without HIV infection. *Ann Intern Med*. 2009;150:301-313.
177. Mulligan K, Khatami H, Schwarz JM, et al. The effects of recombinant human leptin on visceral fat, dyslipidemia, and insulin resistance in patients with human immunodeficiency virus-associated lipoatrophy and hypoleptinemia. *J Clin Endocrinol Metab*. 2009;94:1137-1144.
178. Lee JH, Chan JL, Sourlas E, et al. Recombinant methionyl human leptin therapy in replacement doses improves insulin resistance and metabolic profile in patients with lipoatrophy and metabolic syndrome induced by the highly active antiretroviral therapy. *J Clin Endocrinol Metab*. 2006;91:2605-2611.
179. Esposito JG, Thomas SG, Kingdon L, et al. Anabolic growth hormone action improves submaximal measures of physical performance in patients with HIV-associated wasting. *Am J Physiol Endocrinol Metab*. 2005;289:E494-E503.
180. Grunfeld C, Thompson M, Brown SJ, et al. Recombinant human growth hormone to treat HIV-associated adipose redistribution syndrome: 12 week induction and 24-week maintenance therapy. *J Acquir Immune Defic Syndr*. 2007;45:286-297.
181. Herasimtschuk AA, Westrop SJ, Moyle GJ, et al. Effects of recombinant human growth hormone on HIV-1-specific T-cell responses, thymic output and proviral DNA in patients on HAART: 48-week follow-up. *J Immune Based Ther Vaccines*. 2008;6:7.
182. Lee PD, Pivarnik JM, Bukar JG, et al. A randomized, placebo-controlled trial of combined insulin-like growth factor I and low dose growth hormone therapy for wasting associated with human immunodeficiency virus infection [published erratum appears in *J Clin Endocrinol Metab*. 1996;81:3696]. *J Clin Endocrinol Metab*. 1996;81:2968-2975.
183. Mulligan K, Tai VW, Schambelan M. Effects of chronic growth hormone treatment on energy intake and resting energy metabolism in patients with human immunodeficiency virus-associated wasting: a clinical research center study. *J Clin Endocrinol Metab*. 1998;83:1542-1547.
184. Falutz J, Allas S, Kotler D, et al. A placebo-controlled, dose-ranging study of a growth hormone releasing factor in HIV-infected patients with abdominal fat accumulation. *AIDS*. 2005;19:1279-1287.
185. Koutkia P, Canavan B, Breu J, et al. Growth hormone (GH) responses to GH-releasing hormone-arginine testing in human immunodeficiency virus lipodystrophy. *J Clin Endocrinol Metab*. 2005;90:32-38.

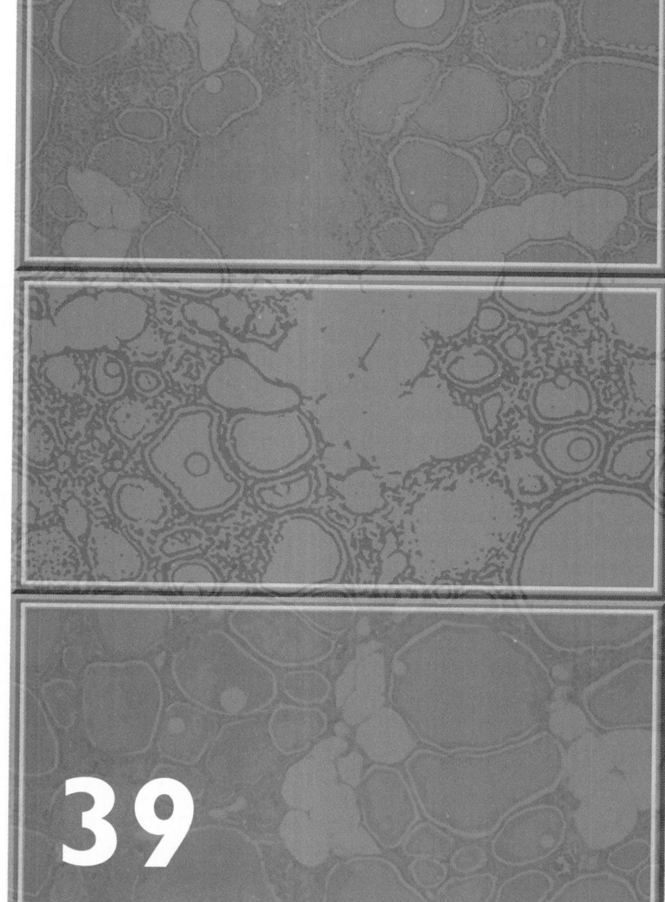

CHAPTER 39

Gastrointestinal Hormones and Gut Endocrine Tumors

ADRIAN VELLA • DANIEL J. DRUCKER

Endocrine tumors originating from islet or enteroendocrine cells may manifest with unique clinical symptoms that reflect the biologic actions of secreted peptide hormones. In this chapter, we discuss how endocrine cell lineages develop during organogenesis in the endocrine pancreas and intestine, and we review the biologic actions of peptide hormones produced in pancreatic and intestinal endocrine cells and enteric nerves. Numerous physiologic actions of these peptides are still poorly understood and are being actively investigated. However, excessive production of one or more of these peptides frequently accounts for the clinical symptoms attributable to endocrine tumors arising from the gastrointestinal tract and pancreas.

ENDOCRINE CELL DEVELOPMENT IN THE PANCREAS

The endocrine and exocrine pancreas develops from the primitive foregut endoderm. Pancreatic morphogenesis is a complex process that begins with the evagination of the embryonic foregut into ventral and dorsal buds at 28 days' gestation in humans and at embryonic day 8 (E8) in mice. Rotation of the stomach and duodenum during development results in simultaneous rotation of the ventral bud, which undergoes fusion with the dorsal bud to give rise to the primitive pancreas. The ventral bud develops into the posterior portion of the pancreatic head, including the uncinate process; the remaining pancreas is derived from the dorsal bud. In mice, a complex, treelike, epithelium-lined ductal system develops within the pancreatic diverticula, with glucagon-immunoreactive cells detected as early as E9.5, followed by detection of cells containing insulin at E10.5. Stem cells that give rise to terminally differentiated endocrine and exocrine acinar cells are thought to reside within the ductal epithelium.

In humans, islet formation begins at gestational week 12 with the aggregation of polyclonal endocrine cells. Between weeks 13 and 16, small aggregates of endocrine cells arise from the pancreatic duct and develop their own blood supply. By weeks 17 to 20, fewer islets are observed in contact with the ducts, and a mantle of non-beta endocrine cells forms around the beta cells. Between gestational weeks 21 and 26, a continual increase in the proportion of islet tissue and in the average size of the islets is observed, with occasional non-beta cells in the center of the islet, a morphologic appearance that is characteristic of the postnatal islet. At birth, the endocrine pancreas accounts for 1% to 2% of the entire pancreatic cell mass.

Although genetic studies in mice have yielded valuable insights into the ontogeny of islet development, the relative order of appearance of unique populations of hormone-producing islet endocrine cells is different in humans and mice. Somatostatin- and pancreatic polypeptide (PP)-positive cells are detected at 7 weeks' gestation in the human pancreas, scattered among ductal cells. One week later, glucagon cells appear, and by 9 to 10 weeks' gestation, insulin-producing cells are detectable. In mice, both insulin- and glucagon-expressing cells are first detected between days E9.5 and E10.5, and somatostatin and PP are expressed by E15.5. Although cells coexpressing insulin and glucagon are detected during early islet development, cell lineage studies employing specific transgenes that mark or ablate islet cell precursors suggest that the alpha and beta cell lineages arise independently during ontogeny in the mouse.[1] Peptide YY (PYY) co-localizes with each of the four main islet hormones in the developing pancreas, but genetic evidence for an essential role of a PYY-producing precursor cell in pancreatic endocrine development has not been developed.

Delineation of the genetic determinants that regulate the developmental formation and organization of pancreatic endocrine cell populations has been facilitated by studies of mice with disruption of candidate regulatory genes, principally islet transcription factors (Table 39-1). The homeobox transcription factor Pdx1 is required for transcription of multiple beta-cell genes, including those for insulin and glucokinase in the adult beta cell, and for developmental formation of the entire pancreas.[2] Similarly, the homeodomain transcription factor Prox1 controls pancreatic morphogenesis and formation of islet cell precursors after E13.5. Mice homozygous for a null mutation in Pdx1 fail to develop a pancreas, whereas restricted inactivation of Pdx1 in the murine beta cell produces insulin deficiency and diabetes. Pancreatic agenesis has also been reported in human subjects homozygous for a loss-of-function PDX1 mutation,[3] and subjects heterozygous for PDX1 develop a form of maturity-onset diabetes of the young (MODY4).

TABLE 39-1

Effects of Disruption of Genes Important for Development of Pancreatic Endocrine Cells

Gene	Phenotype in Homozygous (−/−) Mutant Mice
Arx	Failure to develop glucagon-positive alpha cells
FoxM1	Impaired beta-cell replication
Glis3	Impaired islet and beta-cell development
Hes1	Increased glucagon-positive alpha cells, pancreatic hypoplasia
Hlxb9	Dorsal lobe agenesis, small islets, reduced beta cells
Isl1	Loss of differentiated islet cells
Myt1	Abnormal islet cell development
Nkx2.2	Absent mature beta cells, reduced alpha and PP cells
Nkx6.1	Reduced beta cell precursors
NeuroD	Reduced beta cells, arrested islet morphogenesis
Ngn3	Absent islet cells and defective enteroendocrine cell formation
Nkx6	Impaired alpha-cell development
Pax4	Absent islet beta and delta cells
Pax6	Absent islet alpha cells
Pbx1	Marked reduction in islet alpha and beta cells
Pdx1	Pancreatic agenesis
Sox4	Defective islet development

Targeted disruption of the LIM domain *Isl1* gene in mice results in abnormal development of the dorsal pancreatic mesenchyme and abnormal differentiation of islet cells. A heterozygous human *ISL1* mutation has been reported in a single patient with type 2 diabetes. Mutations in the *Pax4* and *Pax6* genes produce profound abnormalities in developmental formation of murine pancreatic endocrine cells.[4] Binding sites for the MODY genes *PDX1*, *HNF1A*, and *HNF4A* have been identified in the PAX4 promoter, suggesting that MODY genes may be upstream regulators of genes critical for islet cell formation and islet function in the pancreas. Single-nucleotide polymorphisms in *PAX4* occur more commonly in some subjects with MODY, and a human kindred with aniridia and a *PAX6* mutation exhibited impaired glucose tolerance associated with evidence for impaired processing of proinsulin.[5] Nevertheless, islet function has not been extensively studied in human subjects with *PAX* mutations.

Genes encoding members of the Notch receptor family, their ligands, and downstream targets are essential for developmental formation of the endocrine pancreas (see Table 39-1). Targeted inactivation of genes in the Notch signaling pathway markedly perturbs the normal development and differentiation of pancreatic endocrine cells. Mice lacking neurogenin 3 (Ngn3, also designated Neurog3), a basic helix-loop-helix (bHLH) transcription factor, fail to develop pancreatic endocrine cells and die from diabetes postnatally, whereas overexpression of Ngn3 produces accelerated differentiation of pancreatic endocrine cells. These findings, taken together with the loss of Isl1, Pax4, Pax6, and NeuroD expression in Ngn3$^{-/-}$ mice, implicate Ngn3 as a key upstream regulator of pancreatic endocrine cell development.

The transcription factor Arx is expressed in an Ngn3-dependent manner, and targeted inactivation of the *Arx* gene results in hypoglycemia and neonatal lethality, with a failure to develop islet alpha cells.[6] Similarly, the Nkx transcription factor family appears to be essential for the formation of beta and alpha cell lineages in the mouse.[7] Targeted deletion of the *Nkx2.2* gene produced murine islets expressing ghrelin,[8] and subsequent studies demonstrated that ghrelin is produced within a subset of normal islet alpha cells and in a small proportion of newly identified ghrelin-producing epsilon cells.[8] Research into the identification of upstream control mechanisms and downstream targets that promote islet cell formation, growth, and differentiation is proceeding rapidly and informing scientists and clinicians about the genetic determinants regulating the growth of normal and neoplastic endocrine cells.[9] Table 39-1 summarizes the genetic mutations associated with abnormal formation of pancreatic endocrine cells in the mouse.

ENDOCRINE CELL DEVELOPMENT IN THE INTESTINE

Stem cells associated with the intestinal epithelium differentiate into four cell lineages: enterocytes, Paneth cells, goblet cells, and enteroendocrine cells. In mice, the bHLH gene *Atoh1* (formerly designated *Math1*) is a critical regulator of intestinal secretory cell lineages. Deletion of *Atoh1* results in failure to develop goblet, Paneth, or enteroendocrine cell lineages.[10] The enteroendocrine cell population comprises less than 1% of all intestinal epithelial cells but represents the largest mass of endocrine cells in the body. Compared with pancreatic endocrine cell development, much less is known about the molecular control of enteroendocrine cell formation and differentiation. Numerous enteroendocrine cell types have been identified that can be classified based on morphologic criteria and expression of one or more secretory products. In the stomach, gastrin cells first appear in the duodenum; they localize to the antrum and pylorus in adult gastric mucosa. In the small bowel, a secretin-precursor cell appears to be important for enteroendocrine cell lineage formation. In the murine colon, PYY is the first detectable hormone marking the appearance of enteroendocrine cells; it is coexpressed in most endocrine cells in the large intestine as they first differentiate.

The Notch signaling pathway is essential for developmental formation of enteroendocrine cells. Activation of the Notch pathway in mice results in increased expression of the bHLH transcriptional repressor Hes1, which functionally antagonizes bHLH genes that regulate cellular differentiation. Mice deficient in Hes1 demonstrate premature cellular differentiation and severe pancreatic hypoplasia due to depletion of pancreatic epithelial precursors.[11] These mice also demonstrate excessive differentiation of multiple endocrine cell types in the developing stomach and gut, suggesting that Hes1 is a negative regulator of endodermal endocrine differentiation. Ngn3 is expressed at early time points during gut development and is essential for development of enteroendocrine cells in the small intestine[12] and in the stomach.[13] In mice, Notch1 and Ngn3 act upstream of BETA2/NeuroD, a bHLH protein that is important for differentiation of endocrine cells in the pancreas and intestine (Table 39-2).[14]

Mice homozygous for a null mutation in the *Pdx1* gene demonstrate poorly differentiated duodenal intestinal epithelium with absence of Brunner's glands and a deficiency of gastrin cells in the stomach. Just distal to the abnormal epithelium, the number of enteroendocrine cells is reduced. In contrast, expression of Pdx1 in gut epithelial cells redirects cell lineage toward an enteroendocrine phenotype. Inactivation of BETA2/NeuroD in mice results in absence of secretin- and cholecystokinin (CCK)–producing enteroendocrine cells.[14] The complexity of lineage relationships between gut endocrine cell populations is further illustrated by studies in mice with targeted ablation of secretin-producing cells. These mice exhibit almost complete

TABLE 39-2

Consequences of Disruption of Genes Important for Development of Enteroendocrine Cells

Gene	Phenotype in Homozygous (–/–) Mutant Mice
Hes1	Enhanced numbers of enteroendocrine cells
Insm1	Defective enteroendocrine cell differentiation
NeuroD	Absent secretin and CCK lineages
Ngn3	Absent enteroendocrine cell development in the small intestine
Nkx2.2	Abnormal allocation of gut endocrine cell lineages
Pax4	Reduced endocrine cell lineages in duodenum and stomach
Pax6	Reduced number of GIP+ K cells, antral gastrin and somatostatin cells, and L cells
Pdx1	Reduced enteroendocrine cells in stomach and duodenum
Ihh	Reduced enteroendocrine cells in duodenum

CCK, cholecystokinin; GIP, gastric inhibitory polypeptide.

elimination of enteroendocrine cell populations producing CCK, PYY, and glucagon and a reduction in cells producing gastric inhibitory polypeptide (GIP), somatostatin, and serotonin.[15] Similarly, combined deletion of Foxa1 and Foxa2 from the gut results in reduction of selected endocrine cell lineages.

Members of the *Pax* gene family are also essential for the formation of enteroendocrine cells (see Table 39-2). In mice, targeted disruption of Pax4 markedly reduces the number of murine duodenal cells immunopositive for serotonin, secretin, GIP, PYY, and CCK and decreases the number of somatostatin- and serotonin-positive cells in the stomach. Complete disruption of the *Pax6* locus more selectively reduces the number of duodenal cells expressing GIP and CCK[16] and decreases the number of gastrin- and somatostatin-immunopositive cells in the stomach, whereas Sey-Neu mice that express a dominant negative mutant *Pax6* allele demonstrate markedly reduced levels of proglucagon messenger RNA (mRNA) transcripts in the small and large intestines, with almost complete depletion of enteroendocrine cells exhibiting glucagon-like peptide 1 (GLP1) and glucagon-like peptide 2 (GLP2) immunoreactivity (Fig. 39-1).[17] Nkx2.2 appears to control the expression of Pax6, and Nkx2-null mice exhibit significant reductions in expression of CCK, gastrin, glucagon, GIP, neurotensin, and somatostatin.[18] The classification of enteroendocrine cells is currently based principally on the

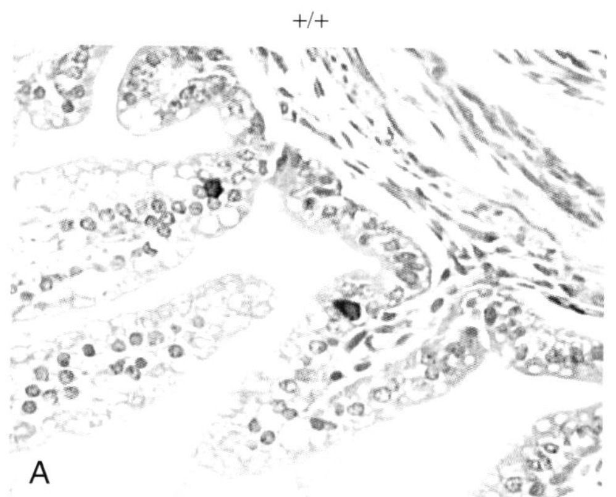

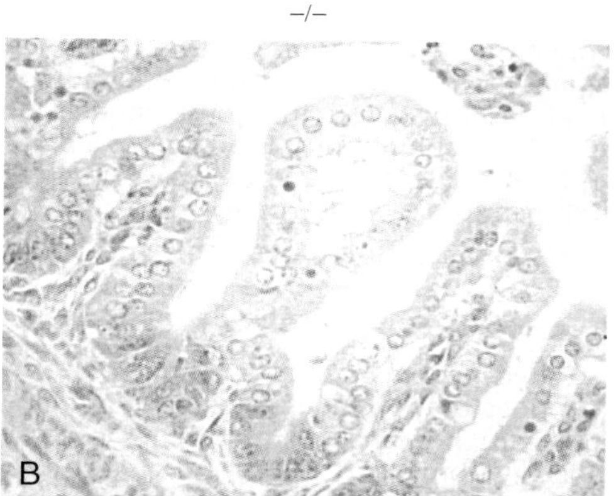

Figure 39-1 **A,** *Pax6* is an essential requirement for glucagon-immunopositive enteroendocrine cell formation in the murine intestine. **B,** *Pax6* Sey-Neu mutant mice (–/–) exhibit markedly reduced numbers of glucagon-immunopositive cells in the small and large intestine.

TABLE 39-4

Summary of Gastrointestinal-Derived Hormones

Hormone	Cell or Tissue of Origin	Related Peptides	Actions	Secretory Stimuli
Amylin	Pancreatic beta cell, endocrine cells of stomach and small intestine	Calcitonin, CGRP, adrenomedullin	Inhibits gastric emptying Inhibits arginine-stimulated and postprandial glucagon secretion Inhibits insulin secretion Satiety factor	Cosecreted with insulin in response to oral nutrient ingestion
CGRP	α-CGRP is expressed predominantly in afferent sensory nerves from the spinal cord β-CGRP is expressed in enteric neurons and enteroendocrine cells of the rectum	Calcitonin, amylin, adrenomedullin	Produces marked vasodilation in the splanchnic and peripheral circulation by stimulating nitric oxide release Inhibits gastric acid and pancreatic exocrine secretion Induces intestinal smooth muscle relaxation	Glucose and gastric acid secretion
CCK	Enteroendocrine I cells and enteric nerves, CNS, pituitary corticotrophs, C cells of the thyroid, adrenal medulla, and the acrosome of developing and mature spermatozoa		Inhibits proximal gastric motility while increasing antral and pyloric contractions Regulates meal-stimulated pancreatic enzyme secretion and gallbladder contraction Trophic effects on pancreatic acini in rats Postprandial satiety In the brain, CCK affects memory, sleep, sexual behavior, and anxiety	Oral nutrient ingestion Several intestine-derived hormones, including GRP and bombesin Activation of β-adrenergic receptors
Galanin	CNS and PNS, pituitary, neural structures of the gut, pancreas, thyroid, and adrenal gland		In the brain, regulation of food intake, memory and cognition, and anti-nociception Inhibits pancreatic exocrine secretion and intestinal ion transport Induces both contraction and relaxation of intestinal smooth muscle, depending on the species examined Delays gastric emptying and prolongs colonic transit times Inhibits secretion of insulin, PYY, gastrin, somatostatin, enteroglucagon, neurotensin, and PP	Intestinal distention Chemical stimulation of the intestinal mucosa Electrical stimulation of periarterial nerves Extrinsic sympathetic neurons
GIP	Neuroendocrine K cells in the duodenum and proximal jejunum		Inhibits gastric acid secretion and GI motility Increases insulin release and regulates glucose and lipid metabolism Exerts anabolic actions in bone	Oral nutrient ingestion, especially long-chain fatty acids
Gastrin	Predominantly enteroendocrine G cells of the stomach and duodenal bulb, CNS and PNS, pituitary, adrenal gland, genital tract, respiratory tract, fetal pancreas		Induces gastric acid secretion Amidated gastrins are trophic to the oxyntic mucosa of the stomach Progastrin and glycine-extended gastrin induce colonic epithelial proliferation	Luminal contents, especially partially digested aromatic amino acids, small peptides, calcium, coffee, and ethanol Humoral and neural influences, including the vagus nerve, β-adrenergic and GABA neurons, and GRP
GRP and related peptides	CNS, enteric nervous system, reproductive tract, and the lungs, where it acts as a neurotransmitter; GRP neurons are also distributed throughout the human pancreas	Bombesin, neuromedin B, neuromedin C	Stimulates smooth muscle contraction in the stomach, intestine, and gallbladder Stimulates release of CCK, gastrin, GIP, glucagon, GLP1, GLP2, motilin, PP, PYY, and somatostatin Stimulates gastric acid secretion via direct effect on G cells In the brain, regulates appetite, memory, thermogenesis, and cardiac function Stimulates pancreatic growth In the lungs, growth factor for normal and neoplastic tissue	Cholinergic stimulation
Ghrelin	CNS, stomach, small intestine, colon	Motilin	Stimulates GH release Stimulates gastric kinetic activity Orexigenic activity Stimulates energy production and signals hypothalamic regulatory nuclei that control energy homeostasis	Fasting
Glucagon	Pancreatic alpha cell, CNS		Primary counterregulatory mechanism to restore plasma glucose levels in hypoglycemia by increasing gluconeogenesis, glycogenolysis, and protein-lipid flux in the liver and periphery GI smooth muscle relaxation	Neural and humoral factors released in response to hypoglycemia

TABLE 39-4

Summary of Gastrointestinal-Derived Hormones (Continued)

Hormone	Cell or Tissue of Origin	Related Peptides	Actions	Secretory Stimuli
GLP1	Enteroendocrine L cells located in the ileum and colon, CNS		Enhances glucose disposal after nutrient ingestion by inhibiting gastric emptying, stimulating insulin secretion, and inhibiting glucagon secretion Inhibits food intake Stimulates pancreatic islet neogenesis and proliferation Inhibits sham feeding–induced gastric acid secretion	Oral nutrient ingestion, especially carbohydrates and fat-rich meals Vagal nerve, GRP, and GIP ACh and neuromedin C Somatostatin inhibits secretion
GLP2	Enteroendocrine L cells located in the ileum and colon, CNS		Induces small-intestinal and colonic mucosal growth by stimulating crypt cell proliferation and inhibiting apoptosis Inhibits centrally induced antral motility and meal-stimulated gastric acid secretion Enhances intestinal epithelial barrier function Stimulates intestinal hexose transport Inhibits short-term control of food intake	Oral nutrient ingestion, especially carbohydrates and fat-rich meals Vagus nerve, GRP, and GIP ACh and neuromedin C Somatostatin inhibits secretion
Motilin	Brain, bronchoepithelial cells, and enteroendocrine M cells located in the duodenum and proximal jejunum	Ghrelin	Induces phase III contractions in the stomach Stimulates gastric and pancreatic enzyme secretion Induces contraction of the gallbladder, sphincter of Oddi, and LES	Duodenal alkalinization, sham feeding, gastric distention; opioid agonists promote secretion Unlike most GI hormones, motilin is suppressed in the presence of duodenal nutrients
NPY	CNS and PNS, pancreatic islet cells	PYY and PP	Potent stimulator of oral nutrient intake Inhibits glucose-stimulated insulin secretion Reduces GI fluid and electrolyte secretion Inhibits gastric and small-intestinal motility Induces market vasoconstriction of the splanchnic circulation	Oral nutrient ingestion Activation of the sympathetic nervous system
NT	N cells located in the small-intestinal mucosa, especially the ileum; CNS and PNS, including the enteric nervous system; heart, adrenal gland, pancreas, and respiratory tract	Neuromedin N, xenin, and xenopsin	Stimulates growth of the colonic epithelium Inhibits postprandial gastric acid secretion and pancreatic exocrine secretion Stimulates colonic motility but inhibits gastric and small-intestinal motility Facilitates fatty acid uptake in the proximal and small intestine and induces histamine release from mast cells Trophic in some pancreatic and colon cancer cell lines in vitro	Luminal nutrients, especially lipids, but not amino acids or carbohydrates GRP and bombesin Somatostatin inhibits secretion
PP	Major site of expression is pancreatic endocrine cells located in periphery of islets in pancreatic head and uncinate process	NPY and PYY	Reduces CCK-induced gastric acid secretion Increases intestinal transit times by reducing gastric emptying and upper intestinal motility Inhibits postprandial exocrine pancreas secretion via vagal-dependent pathway	Stimulated by nutrients, hormones, neurotransmitters, gastric distention, insulin-induced hypoglycemia, and direct vagal nerve stimulation Hyperglycemia, bombesin, and somatostatin inhibit secretion
PYY	Enteroendocrine cells, developing endocrine pancreas, subpopulation of pancreatic alpha cells in mature islets	NPY and PP	Enterogastrone inhibits gastric acid secretion and gastric motility Increases intestinal transit time by reducing intestinal motility Inhibits pancreatic exocrine secretion Role as an intestinal epithelial growth factor remains controversial Peripheral vasoconstriction and reduced mesenteric and pancreatic vascular blood flow	After oral nutrient ingestion, early secretion is mediated by the vagus nerve and hormonal influences; later, secretion occurs as a result of direct L-cell stimulation Bile acids and fatty acids Amino acids administered intracolonically
PACAP	Brain, respiratory tract, and enteric nervous system	VIP, PHI, and PHM	Stimulates histamine release from the stomach Increases secretion of pancreatic fluid, protein, and bicarbonate Stimulates insulin and catecholamine release Neural regulation of gastric acid secretion	Activation of CNS
Secretin	CNS, fetal endocrine pancreas, and enteroendocrine S cells located in the duodenum and proximal jejunum		Principal hormonal stimulant of pancreatic and biliary bicarbonate and water excretion Regulates pancreatic enzyme secretion Stimulates gastric secretion of pepsinogen Inhibits LES tone, postprandial gastric emptying, gastrin release, and gastric acid secretion	Gastric acid, bile salts, and luminal nutrients, especially fatty acids, peptides, and ethanol Somatostatin inhibits secretion

Table continued on following page

TABLE 39-4

Summary of Gastrointestinal-Derived Hormones (Continued)

Hormone	Cell or Tissue of Origin	Related Peptides	Actions	Secretory Stimuli
Somatostatin	CNS, pancreatic delta cells, enteroendocrine D cells		Inhibits secretion of islet hormones, including insulin, glucagon, and PP Inhibits secretion of gut peptides, including gastrin, secretin, VIP, CCK, GLP1 and GLP2 Inhibits pancreatic exocrine secretion Acts in a paracrine manner on G cells, enterochromaffin-like cells, and parietal cells to inhibit gastric acid secretion Reduces splanchnic blood flow, intestinal motility, and carbohydrate absorption while increasing water and electrolyte absorption	Luminal nutrients Gastrin, CCK, bombesin, GLP1, and GIP Neural influences, including PACAP, VIP, and β-adrenergic agonists stimulate while ACh inhibits secretion
Tachykinins	Throughout the CNS and PNS, including the respiratory tract, skin, sensory organs, and urogenital tract; in the GI tract, neurons localized in the submucous and myenteric plexuses, extrinsic sensory fibers, and enterochromaffin cells in the gut epithelium	Substance P, neurokinin A, and neurokinin B	Regulate vasomotor and GI smooth muscle contractility Chemotaxis and activation of immune cells, mucus secretion, water absorption and secretion Role in visceral inflammation, hyperreflexia, and hyperalgesia	Direct or indirect activation of neurons
TRH	CNS and enteric nervous system, colon, G cells of the stomach, pancreatic islet beta cells		Suppresses pentagastrin-stimulated gastric acid secretion Chronic administration induces pancreatic hyperplasia and inhibits amylase release Attenuates CCK-induced gallbladder smooth muscle contraction Inhibits cholesterol synthesis within the intestinal mucosa	In the stomach, histamine and serotonin stimulate and endogenous opioids inhibit secretion
VIP	Widely expressed in the CNS and PNS including the enteric nervous system	PACAP, PHI, and PHM	Induces relaxation of vascular and nonvascular smooth muscle Mediates relaxation of the LES, sphincter of Oddi, and anal sphincter Regulates relaxation-associated gut contraction and may be involved with reflex vasodilation in the small intestine Inhibits gastric acid secretion Stimulates biliary water, bicarbonate, pancreatic enzyme, and intestinal chloride secretion	Mechanical stimulation Activation of the CNS and PNS

ACh, acetylcholine; CCK, cholecystokinin; CGRP, calcitonin gene-related peptide; CNS, central nervous system; GABA, γ-aminobutyric acid; GH, growth hormone; GI, gastrointestinal; GIP, gastric inhibitory polypeptide; GLP, glucagon-like peptide; GRP, gastrin-releasing peptide; LES, lower esophageal sphincter; NPY, neuropeptide Y; NT, neurotensin; PACAP, pituitary adenylate cyclase–activating peptide; PHI, peptide histidine isoleucine; PHM, peptide histidine methionine; PNS, peripheral nervous system; PP, pancreatic polypeptide; PYY, peptide YY; TRH, thyrotropin-releasing hormone; VIP, vasoactive intestinal peptide.

TABLE 39-5

Genetic Diseases Associated with the Development of Pancreatic or Gut Endocrine Tumors

Gene	Disease	Phenotype
Menin	MEN1	Parathyroid, pituitary, and pancreatic endocrine tumors
VHL	von Hippel-Lindau syndrome	Pancreatic endocrine tumors, hemangiomas and multiple neoplasms
NF1	Neurofibromatosis	Neurofibromas, pheochromocytomas
TSC1/2	Tuberous sclerosis	Pancreatic endocrine tumors, hamartomas

MEN1, multiple endocrine neoplasia type 1; NF1, neurofibromin 1; TSC1/2, tuberous sclerosis genes 1 and 2; VHL, von Hippel-Lindau tumor suppressor gene.

unclear because of the large number of heterogeneous mutations identified in the menin gene. The likelihood of detecting *MEN1* mutations correlates directly with the number of MEN1-related tumors in the index case at presentation.[92]

A search for clinical manifestations of diseases associated with these genetic syndromes is an important component in the initial diagnosis and ongoing management of patients with pancreatic endocrine tumors. Careful phenotype-genotype analyses have ascertained that facial angiofibromas, collagenomas, lipomas, leiomyomas, and adrenocortical tumors may be seen with increased frequency in patients with MEN1.[93] Moreover, somatic mutations of the menin gene have been described in isolated cases of gastrinomas, insulinomas, and gut endocrine tumors.[93]

The secretion of one or more peptide hormones resulting in the production of symptoms attributable to hormone excess, such as hypoglycemia, gastric ulceration, or profuse watery diarrhea in patients with insulinoma, gastrinoma, or VIPoma, respectively, facilitates the diagnosis of a hormone-secreting endocrine tumor. In some instances, pancreatic or gut endocrine tumors may not be associated with clinically or biochemically detectable hormone excess and development of a recognizable syndrome. Because nonfunctioning pancreatic endocrine tumors may escape clinical detection, they often are larger and more frequently are malignant at the time of diagnosis. The term *nonfunctioning* may be a misnomer, because these tumors frequently produce peptide hormones (Fig. 39-3) whose biologic actions are less clinically apparent. In some instances, tumor-associated defects in post-translational processing may preclude the efficient synthesis and secretion of peptide hormones. Factors affecting prognosis include liver metastases, incomplete resection of the primary tumor, and poorly differentiated tumor cells.

The use of somatostatin receptor scintigraphy and measurement of gene products commonly expressed in endocrine cells, such as chromogranin, PP, neuron-specific enolase, or glycoprotein hormone subunits, may be useful as an adjunct for monitoring the tumor response to therapy. Widespread expression of receptors for somatostatin and multiple peptide hormone G protein–coupled receptors, including the GLP1 receptor,[94] has stimulated efforts to develop novel radiolabeled peptide ligands for the localization and treatment of endocrine and non-endocrine neoplasms.

Despite the large number and complexity of endocrine cell populations in the human small bowel, gut endocrine tumors, including ileal carcinoids, are uncommon. Similarly, peptide hormone–secreting carcinoid tumors arising from the colon are much less common than colonic adenocarcinomas. The molecular basis for the infrequent malignant transformation of human gut endocrine cells remains incompletely understood. Mutations in the regenerating islet-derived 1α gene *(REG1A)* have been identified in a subset of patients with ECL cell tumors and associated hypergastrinemia, but the contribution of this genetic mutation to transformation of these cells remains unclear. The clinical presentation, diagnosis, and treatment of several more common pancreatic and gut endocrine tumors are discussed later, and medical and surgical perspectives about treatment have been reviewed elsewhere.[95-97] Surgical resection remains the principal goal and therapeutic strategy, because chemotherapeutic regimens have had only modest success in patients with malignant tumors.

Insulinomas

Insulinomas are the most common functioning islet cell tumors, and they are characterized by hypoglycemia that often is precipitated by exercise or fasting. A subset of insulinomas are characterized by postprandial hypoglycemia.[98] More than 80% are solitary, benign tumors with an indolent course. Patients may tolerate symptoms of hypoglycemia for years before seeking medical attention. Surgical enucleation is the treatment of choice, and cure should be expected in patients without the MEN1 syndrome. In these patients, the recurrence rate is low, often less than 10%. Insulinomas that accompany MEN1 tend to occur at an earlier age. Although they comprise about one third of pancreatic islet cell tumors seen in MEN1 patients, they occur more often before 40 years of age and are the most common tumor seen before age 20. Insulinomas may be the first manifestation of MEN1.

In contrast to the single adenoma found in most patients with sporadic insulinoma, many patients with MEN1 have multicentric, benign disease and a higher incidence of

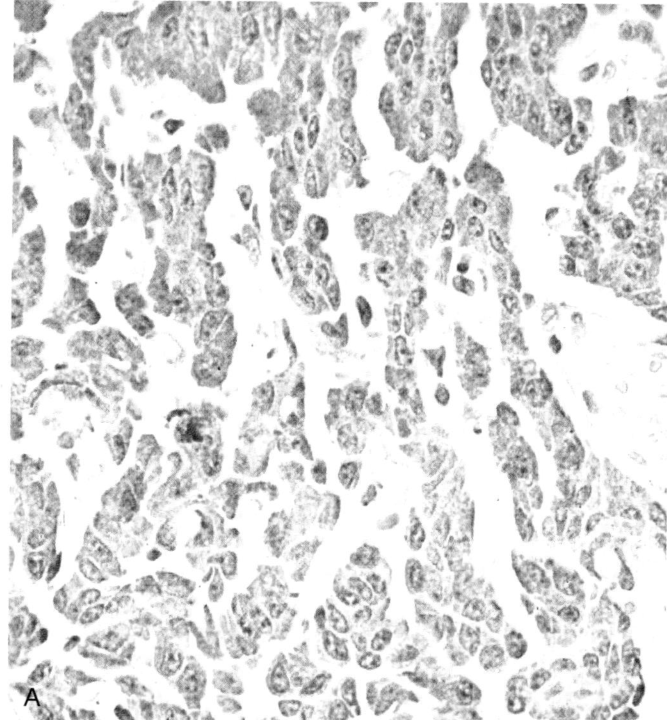

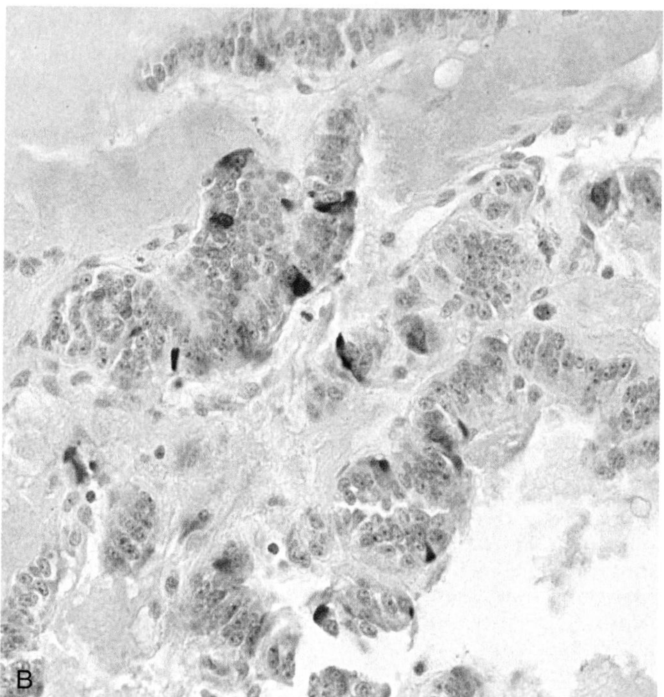

Figure 39-3 Clinically nonfunctioning tumors often are found to express one or more peptide hormones after immunocytochemical analyses. Histologic sections from the identical "nonfunctioning" human pancreatic endocrine tumor exhibit immunopositivity for glucagon **(A)** and pancreatic polypeptide **(B)**.

recurrence (21%). When possible, distal subtotal pancreatic resection to the level of the portal vein combined with enucleation of tumors in the head of the pancreas (guided by intraoperative ultrasonography for safe removal) is thought to be optimal treatment. Preservation of endocrine and exocrine pancreatic function may not be possible in these situations. Insulinomas may be malignant (about 5%), defined by the presence of local invasion or liver or lymph node metastases.[98] Resection of hepatic metastases may provide effective palliation and probably prolonged survival, depending on the extent of resectable tumor burden. Palliative resection should be considered only when at least 90% of the tumor bulk can be excised. The success rate for identification of insulin-secreting pancreatic endocrine tumors with noninvasive testing such as computed tomography (CT) and transabdominal ultrasound has remained constant at about 75%. However, with the implementation of endoscopic ultrasound and selective arterial calcium stimulation testing, preoperative localization rates have significantly improved.[98]

Gastrinoma

In 1955, Zollinger and Ellison described two patients with intractable peptic ulcer disease and pancreatic islet cell tumors.[99] Subsequent studies demonstrated elevated levels of circulating gastrin associated with gastric acid hypersecretion in patients with Zollinger-Ellison syndrome.

Although the gastrin gene is not normally expressed in the adult pancreas, gastrinomas commonly arise from within the pancreas and manifest as endocrine carcinomas, solitary adenomas, microadenomas, or endocrine cell hyperplasia. Gastrinomas and insulinomas represent the two most common pancreatic endocrine tumors. Between 20% and 40% of gastrin-secreting tumors arise from the duodenum. Most gastrinomas (75%) occur sporadically, but about 25% are associated with the MEN1 syndrome. Duodenal gastrinomas in patients with sporadic Zollinger-Ellison syndrome are frequently small, most commonly located in the proximal duodenum, and associated with regional lymph node metastases in 60% of patients.[100] Patients presenting with gastrinoma as a component of the MEN1 syndrome may develop pituitary disease (60%), adrenal disease (45%), and carcinoid tumors (30%).[101] A substantial proportion of MEN1 patients also present with benign skin lesions, such as angiofibromas and collagenomas.[102] Patients with MEN1-related duodenal gastrinomas frequently exhibit hyperplastic foci of gastrin-immunopositive cells in the adjacent nontumorous duodenal tissue. Sporadic gastrinomas may contain menin gene mutations. MEN1 patients tend to be younger at the time of tumor diagnosis than those without MEN1. Sporadic tumors are most often solitary and malignant; MEN1-associated tumors are usually multiple but may be more localized at the time of diagnosis.

Based on the presence of metastases at the time of diagnosis, about 50% to 60% of gastrinomas are malignant, perhaps because of the long delay between initial clinical presentation and diagnosis of Zollinger-Ellison syndrome. Nevertheless, gastrin-secreting tumors are often slow growing and associated with prolonged survival despite complications arising from intestinal ulceration. Loss of heterozygosity at 1q or on the X chromosome may be associated with a more aggressive clinical presentation.

Clinical manifestations of gastrinomas are usually related to excessive gastric acid secretion resulting in severe refractory peptic ulceration complicated by hemorrhage, perforation, and stricture. Many patients report symptoms for 5 to 6 years before the diagnosis of Zollinger-Ellison syndrome is established.[101] Abdominal pain, diarrhea, and heartburn are common presenting symptoms, with diarrhea and pain observed in more than 70% of patients with Zollinger-Ellison syndrome. The diarrhea results in part from fat malabsorption due to pancreatic lipase degradation by excess gastric acid. Small-bowel inflammation and impaired nutrient absorption may also arise from excess gastric acid. Antisecretory therapy usually abolishes the diarrhea and diminishes many clinical features of Zollinger-Ellison syndrome.

The diagnosis of gastrinoma is based on the detection of elevated fasting circulating gastrin levels (>200 pg/mL) and gastric acid hypersecretion (basal acid output >15 mEq/hour with an intact stomach or >5 mEq/hour after ulcer surgery) in patients off all acid antisecretory medication (14 days for proton pump [H^+,K^+-ATPase] inhibitors and 3 days for H_2-receptor antagonists). Although many patients with Zollinger-Ellison syndrome have serum gastrin values that exceed 500 pg/mL, a secretin stimulation test may be performed when the serum gastrin levels are in the range of 200 to 500 pg/mL to confirm the diagnosis. Provocative testing requires overnight fasting and the intravenous administration of secretin 0.4 mcg/kg over 1 minute (2 units/kg bolus) followed by serial measurement of circulating gastrin levels at 2, 5, 10, 15, and 20 minutes. A rise in the serum gastrin level of more than 200 pg/mL within 15 minutes or a doubling of the fasting gastrin level strongly suggests the presence of a gastrinoma. Secretin receptor expression in tumors correlates with the gastrin response to secretin infusion, and calcium infusion testing may be useful in patients with an equivocal secretin test result.[103] Provocative testing may be useful in distinguishing gastrinomas from other causes of ulcerogenic hypergastrinemia, such as gastric outlet obstruction, retained antrum after a Billroth II gastrectomy, antral G-cell hyperplasia, and *Helicobacter pylori* infection, which demonstrate a flat gastrin response to secretin. Difficulty in obtaining clinical supplies of secretin may preclude routine use of the secretin test, and intravenous calcium administration has been successfully used to stimulate gastrin secretion in several cases. More than 90% of patients have prominent gastric folds at the time of endoscopy, consistent with the trophic effect of gastrin on the stomach mucosa. Assays of serum calcium and parathyroid hormone levels, baseline pituitary function tests and imaging studies, should be considered to rule out the MEN1 syndrome.

Localization of small primary tumors or endocrine hyperplasia can be difficult. Conventional endoscopy or an upper gastrointestinal series occasionally can be used to directly visualize duodenal lesions, but tumors are often confined to the submucosa, making detection and biopsy challenging. Radiolabeled octreotide scanning can be useful for detecting the primary tumor and metastases. MRI or CT can be informative, but the primary tumor may not be detected with these modalities alone. Endoscopic ultrasonography has been used for tumor localization with increasing success; less commonly, angiography with selective venous sampling may be helpful in localizing occult tumors. Primary tumors may be localized to lymph nodes, and ectopic gastrinomas have been found in sites such as the ovary.

Initial treatment of patients with gastrinoma is directed at pharmacologic reduction of gastric acid secretion. Although H_2-blockers have been used with some success, H^+,K^+-ATPase inhibitors such as omeprazole have become the treatment of choice because of their longer duration of action. Doses should be titrated to keep the H^+ ion output

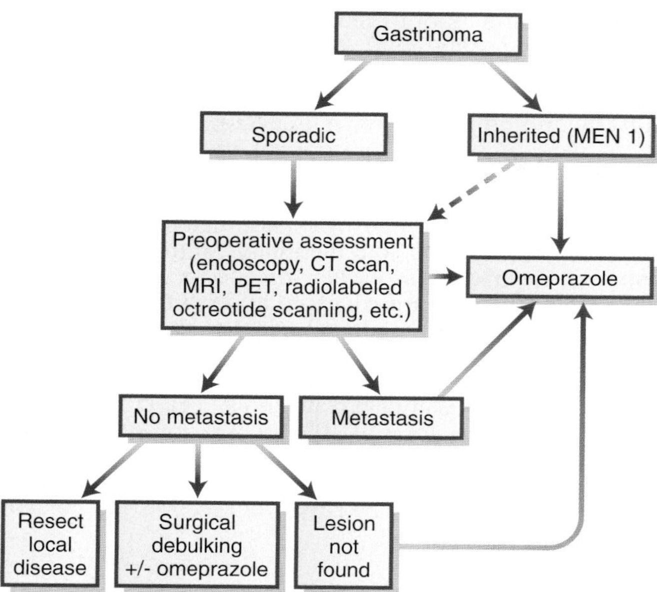

Figure 39-4 Treatment algorithm for the management of a patient with gastrinoma. In some circumstances, patients with familial gastrinoma may also be candidates for surgical resection if disease is highly limited *(dotted line)*. CT, computed tomography; MEN 1, multiple endocrine neoplasia type 1; MRI, magnetic resonance imaging; PET, positron emission tomography.

to less than 10 mEq/hour (5 mEq/hour in patients with prior acid-reducing surgery) for the hour before the next dose of the drug is received.

As outlined in Figure 39-4, in the absence of unresectable disease, all patients with sporadic gastrinoma should undergo surgical exploration with the intent of curative surgical resection. Exploration should include a combination of duodenal palpation, endoscopic transillumination, intraoperative ultrasonography, and duodenotomy. In up to 20% of patients undergoing surgical exploration, the primary tumor remains undetected at laparotomy despite meticulous exploration of the abdominal cavity. Total gastrectomy should be performed only rarely in patients with severe ulcer disease refractory to medical therapy in which the primary tumor cannot be resected. Surgery usually is not indicated in patients with gastrinoma and MEN1 syndrome because they often have multiple, small pancreatic tumors that are not amenable to surgical resection.

Glucagonomas

Most glucagonomas are pancreatic in origin. Approximately 80% of tumors occur sporadically, with the remainder associated with the MEN1 syndrome. About 75% of glucagonomas are malignant and have metastasized by the time of diagnosis. The clinical presentation reflects the various actions of the proglucagon-derived peptides and depends on the profile of the peptides liberated due to tumor-specific differences in the post-translational processing of proglucagon. A hallmark of this syndrome is necrolytic migratory erythema, a rash that usually begins in the groin and perineum as a raised, erythematous patch with occasional bullae that may also involve the lower extremities and perioral area. The exact cause of the rash remains unknown, but elevated plasma glucagon levels and deficiencies of zinc, amino acids, and fatty acids may represent contributing factors.

Patients with glucagonomas may exhibit weight loss, abdominal pain, diabetes, stomatitis, glossitis, cheilitis, nail dystrophy, thromboembolic events, anemia, hypoaminoacidemia, and neuropsychiatric symptoms. The triad of hyperglucagonemia, necrolytic migratory erythema, and a pancreatic tumor is seen in a few cases. Intestinal obstructive symptoms and increased intestinal transit times have been reported and may reflect tumor-specific liberation of GLP1 and GLP2, peptides with antimotility and intestinotrophic properties, respectively.[104]

The diagnosis may be confirmed by measurement of significantly elevated levels of plasma glucagon in association with a pancreatic mass. Extremely high levels of glucagon are more often seen with the classic glucagonoma syndrome, whereas more modest elevations of glucagon are detected in the setting of plurihormonal tumors. In contrast to insulinomas, glucagonomas are often large and more easily localized with imaging modalities. Somatostatin receptor scintigraphy is effective in detecting metastatic disease that most commonly involves the liver, lymph nodes, adrenal glands, or vertebrae. Therapy with a somatostatin analogue may be useful in the setting of metastatic disease by reducing levels of circulating glucagon through action at the SSTR2 receptor, improving the rash and promoting weight gain. The rash may also respond to selective nutrient supplementation. Somatostatin analogues may reduce glucagon secretion and tumor-associated symptoms, but effects on tumor growth are often modest. Patients with nonresectable or recurrent disease may be treated with chemotherapeutic agents such as streptozotocin and dacarbazine (DTIC), with interferon, or with the selective use of arterial embolization.

Somatostatinomas

Somatostatinomas are rare tumors that arise in the pancreas and the duodenum. Most clinical symptoms observed in the originally described somatostatinoma syndrome reflect the inhibitory properties of somatostatin on digestive organs. A classic triad involving mild diabetes mellitus, steatorrhea, and cholelithiasis is observed in a minority of patients and is caused by reduced insulin secretion, reduced biliary and pancreatic secretions, and inhibition of gallbladder motility. More prominent symptoms seen with duodenal tumors include weight loss, postprandial fullness and abdominal pain, cholelithiasis anemia, and hypochlorhydria. Many patients do not present with the classic triad and exhibit only nonspecific symptoms. As a result, somatostatinomas are frequently later-stage malignancies with extensive metastases to the liver by the time of diagnosis.

Duodenal tumors often are associated with neurofibromatosis type 1 or, less commonly, with von Hippel-Lindau syndrome, and they may be associated with pheochromocytomas. Most duodenal tumors are not associated with symptoms of classic somatostatinoma syndrome, and they may manifest with local obstruction and abdominal pain. Pancreatic tumors usually occur sporadically or as part of the MEN1 syndrome and are most commonly located in the head of the pancreas. The diagnosis is confirmed by the presence of markedly elevated levels of plasma somatostatin. Conventional and endoscopic ultrasonography and CT may be used to localize the duodenal tumors (Fig. 39-5). In the small proportion of patients with localized disease, surgical resection can be curative. Patients with incurable or recurrent disease can be treated with the chemotherapeutic agents streptozotocin and dacarbazine.

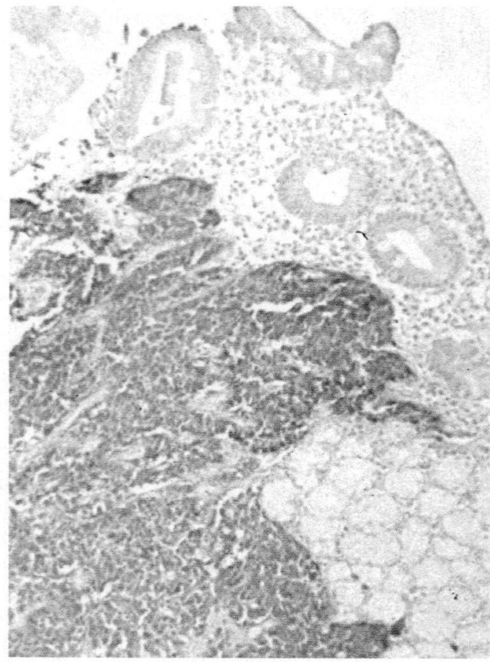

Figure 39-5 Somatostatin immunoreactivity in a human duodenal D-cell tumor. The low-power micrograph illustrates the diffuse somatostatin immunoreactivity. Brunner's glands and the partly eroded mucosa are seen to the lower right and upper right, respectively, of the immunopositive endocrine tumor.

VIP-Secreting Tumors

The VIPoma syndrome is also known as pancreatic cholera, Verner-Morrison syndrome, or the watery diarrhea, hypokalemia, and achlorhydria (WDHA) syndrome. Approximately 90% of individuals with a VIPoma present with a pancreatic endocrine tumor that secretes VIP and, often, prostaglandins. The remaining tumors are extrapancreatic, usually involving the sympathetic chain or adrenal medulla. VIPomas may manifest as sporadic tumors or as part of the MEN1 syndrome.

Clinical manifestations include intermittent, severe watery diarrhea that contains large quantities of potassium, bicarbonate, and chloride. Patients may exhibit signs and symptoms of hypokalemia, metabolic acidosis, and dehydration. Hypotension may result from dehydration and the vasodilator effects of VIP. The secretory diarrhea does not respond to antidiarrheal medications. Gastric analysis usually reveals hypochlorhydria or achlorhydria, although an appropriate increase in acid secretion is observed in response to a pentagastrin challenge. Glucose intolerance may reflect hypokalemia and altered insulin sensitivity. Cutaneous flushing of the head and trunk, usually during a bout of diarrhea, may be observed in 15% of patients and may be associated with a patchy, erythematous rash.

The diagnosis of VIPoma may be challenging due to the intermittent nature of the symptoms. A history of recurrent, severe diarrhea and elevated fasting levels of plasma VIP (>200 pg/mL) should prompt a search for a pancreatic tumor. Increased circulating levels of peptide histidine methionine, PP, neurotensin, and prostaglandins have also been detected in patients with VIP-producing tumors. VIPomas can be localized by ultrasonography, CT, somatostatin receptor scintigraphy, or exploratory laparotomy with intraoperative ultrasound.

Initial treatment of patients with the VIPoma syndrome involves aggressive fluid and electrolyte replacement. Somatostatin analogues may be used preoperatively to control the diarrhea by lowering circulating VIP levels and directly inhibiting intestinal secretion. Definitive treatment requires surgical resection of the tumor, which is commonly located in the body or tail of the pancreas. Although tumors are usually solitary, 60% are malignant at the time of diagnosis; 75% metastasize to the liver and regional lymph nodes, and metastases to the lungs, mediastinum, stomach, and kidney also occur. If a pancreatic tumor cannot be identified, exploration of the retroperitoneum, including the adrenal glands and sympathetic chains, is indicated. If no pancreatic tumor is identified, some patients may elect to be closely monitored, but others opt for an 80% distal pancreatectomy. The latter strategy may be beneficial for the 10% to 20% of symptomatic patients with diffuse islet cell hyperplasia. In patients with inoperable or metastatic tumor, a combination 5-fluorouracil and streptozotocin may be effective.

Miscellaneous Gut Hormone–Producing Tumors

Pancreatic endocrine tumors are rare but may secrete parathyroid hormone, growth hormone–releasing hormone, and adrenocorticotropic hormone, leading to development of hypercalcemia, acromegaly, and Cushing's syndrome, respectively. A large number of peptide hormones may be produced by pancreatic endocrine tumor cells, including PYY, calcitonin, neurotensin, melanocyte-stimulating hormone, corticotropin-releasing hormone, NPY, neuromedin B, CGRP, GRP, and motilin. In some cases, the hormone precursors are produced but the correctly processed intact hormone is not secreted by the tumor. Accordingly, excessive production of many of these hormones may not always be associated with characteristic signs and symptoms. Similarly, carcinoid tumors of the gastrointestinal tract often exhibit immunopositivity for multiple peptide hormones in the absence of a recognizable clinical syndrome.

A large number of peptides are synthesized in and secreted by endocrine cells of the pancreas and gastrointestinal tract. Many of these peptides circulate as hormones, but they also function as paracrine modulators or neurotransmitters in the gut and in the central and peripheral nervous systems. Although some biologic actions have been delineated for many of these peptides, it seems likely that new peptides, receptors, and biologic functions will continue to be characterized. These discoveries may provide opportunities for better understanding the pathophysiology, diagnosis, and treatment of endocrine disease.

REFERENCES

1. Herrera PL. Adult insulin- and glucagon-producing cells differentiate from two independent cell lineages. *Development*. 2000;127: 2317-2322.
2. Habener JF, Kemp DM, Thomas MK. Minireview: transcriptional regulation in pancreatic development. *Endocrinology*. 2005;146: 1025-1034.
3. Stoffers DA, Zinkin NT, Stanojevic V, et al. Pancreatic agenesis attributable to a single nucleotide deletion in the human IPF-1 gene coding sequence. *Nat Genet*. 1997;15:106-110.
4. Dohrmann C, Gruss P, Lemaire L. Pax genes and the differentiation of hormone-producing endocrine cells in the pancreas. *Mech Dev*. 2000;92:47-54.
5. Wen JH, Chen YY, Song SJ, et al. Paired box 6 (PAX6) regulates glucose metabolism via proinsulin processing mediated by prohormone convertase 1/3 (PC1/3). *Diabetologia*. 2009;52:504-513.

6. Collombat P, Mansouri A, Hecksher-Sorensen J, et al. Opposing actions of Arx and Pax4 in endocrine pancreas development. *Genes Dev.* 2003;17:2591-2603.
7. Henseleit KD, Nelson SB, Kuhlbrodt K, et al. NKX6 transcription factor activity is required for alpha- and beta-cell development in the pancreas. *Development.* 2005;132:3139-3149.
8. Prado CL, Pugh-Bernard AE, Elghazi L, et al. Ghrelin cells replace insulin-producing beta cells in two mouse models of pancreas development. *Proc Natl Acad Sci U S A.* 2004;101:2924-2929.
9. Oliver-Krasinski JM, Stoffers DA. On the origin of the beta cell. *Genes Dev.* 2008;22:1998-2021.
10. Yang Q, Bermingham NA, Finegold MJ, et al. Requirement of Math1 for secretory cell lineage commitment in the mouse intestine. *Science.* 2001;294:2155-2158.
11. Jensen J, Pedersen EE, Galante P, et al. Control of endodermal endocrine development by Hes-1. *Nat Genet.* 2000;24:36-44.
12. Jenny M, Uhl C, Roche C, et al. Neurogenin3 is differentially required for endocrine cell fate specification in the intestinal and gastric epithelium. *EMBO J.* 2002;21:6338-6347.
13. Lee CS, Perreault N, Brestelli JE, et al. Neurogenin 3 is essential for the proper specification of gastric enteroendocrine cells and the maintenance of gastric epithelial cell identity. *Genes Dev.* 2002;16:1488-1497.
14. Naya FJ, Huang H, Qiu Y, et al. Diabetes, defective pancreatic morphogenesis, and abnormal enteroendocrine differentiation in BETA2/neuroD-deficient mice. *Genes Dev.* 1997;11:2323-2334.
15. Rindi G, Ratineau C, Ronco A, et al. Targeted ablation of secretin-producing cells in transgenic mice reveals a common differentiation pathway with multiple enteroendocrine cell lineages in the small intestine. *Development.* 1999;126:4149-4156.
16. Larsson LI, St-Onge L, Hougaard DM, et al. Pax 4 and 6 regulate gastrointestinal endocrine cell development. *Mech Dev.* 1998;79:153-159.
17. Hill ME, Asa SL, Drucker DJ. Essential requirement for Pax6 in control of enteroendocrine proglucagon gene transcription. *Mol Endocrinol.* 1999;13:1474-1486.
18. Desai S, Loomis Z, Pugh-Bernard A, et al. Nkx2.2 regulates cell fate choice in the enteroendocrine cell lineages of the intestine. *Dev Biol.* 2008;313:58-66.
19. Hull RL, Andrikopoulos S, Verchere CB, et al. Increased dietary fat promotes islet amyloid formation and beta-cell secretory dysfunction in a transgenic mouse model of islet amyloid. *Diabetes.* 2003;52:372-379.
20. Schmitz O, Brock B, Rungby J. Amylin agonists: a novel approach in the treatment of diabetes. *Diabetes.* 2004;53(suppl 3):S233-S238.
21. Tatemoto K, Hosoya M, Habata Y, et al. Isolation and characterization of a novel endogenous peptide ligand for the human APJ receptor. *Biochem Biophys Res Commun.* 1998;251:471-476.
22. Wang G, Anini Y, Wei W, et al. Apelin, a new enteric peptide: localization in the gastrointestinal tract, ontogeny, and stimulation of gastric cell proliferation and of cholecystokinin secretion. *Endocrinology.* 2004;145:1342-1348.
23. Kleinz MJ, Davenport AP. Emerging roles of apelin in biology and medicine. *Pharmacol Ther.* 2005;107:198-211.
24. Dray C, Knauf C, Daviaud D, et al. Apelin stimulates glucose utilization in normal and obese insulin-resistant mice. *Cell Metab.* 2008;8:437-445.
25. Wimalawansa SJ. Calcitonin gene-related peptide and its receptors: molecular genetics, physiology, pathophysiology, and therapeutic potentials. *Endocr Rev.* 1996;17:533-585.
26. McLatchie LM, Fraser NJ, Main MJ, et al. RAMPs regulate the transport and ligand specificity of the calcitonin-receptor-like receptor. *Nature.* 1998;393:333-339.
27. Rehfeld JF, Sun G, Christensen T, et al. The predominant cholecystokinin in human plasma and intestine is cholecystokinin-33. *J Clin Endocrinol Metab.* 2001;86:251-258.
28. Moran TH, Katz LF, Plata-Salaman CR, et al. Disordered food intake and obesity in rats lacking cholecystokinin A receptors. *Am J Physiol.* 1998;274:R618-R625.
29. Jin G, Ramanathan V, Quante M, et al. Inactivating cholecystokinin-2 receptor inhibits progastrin-dependent colonic crypt fission, proliferation, and colorectal cancer in mice. *J Clin Invest.* 2009;119:2691-2701.
30. Hogenauer C, Meyer RL, Netto GJ, et al. Malabsorption due to cholecystokinin deficiency in a patient with autoimmune polyglandular syndrome type I. *N Engl J Med.* 2001;344:270-274.
31. Cheung GW, Kokorovic A, Lam CK, et al. Intestinal cholecystokinin controls glucose production through a neuronal network. *Cell Metab.* 2009;10:99-109.
32. Branchek TA, Smith KE, Gerald C, et al. Galanin receptor subtypes. *Trends Pharmacol Sci.* 2000;21:109-117.
33. Haberman RP, Samulski RJ, McCown TJ. Attenuation of seizures and neuronal death by adeno-associated virus vector galanin expression and secretion. *Nat Med.* 2003;9:1076-1080.
34. Elliott-Hunt CR, Marsh B, Bacon A, et al. Galanin acts as a neuroprotective factor to the hippocampus. *Proc Natl Acad Sci U S A.* 2004;101:5105-5110.
35. Miyawaki K, Yamada Y, Yano H, et al. Glucose intolerance caused by a defect in the entero-insular axis: a study in gastric inhibitory polypeptide receptor knockout mice. *Proc Natl Acad Sci U S A.* 1999;96:14843-14847.
36. Miyawaki K, Yamada Y, Ban N, et al. Inhibition of gastric inhibitory polypeptide signaling prevents obesity. *Nat Med.* 2002;8:738-742.
37. Hojberg PV, Vilsboll T, Rabol R, et al. Four weeks of near-normalisation of blood glucose improves the insulin response to glucagon-like peptide-1 and glucose-dependent insulinotropic polypeptide in patients with type 2 diabetes. *Diabetologia.* 2008;52:199-207.
38. Lacroix A, Ndiaye N, Tremblay J, et al. Ectopic and abnormal hormone receptors in adrenal Cushing's syndrome. *Endocr Rev.* 2001;22:75-110.
39. Dockray GJ, Varro A, Dimaline R, et al. The gastrins: their production and biological activities. *Annu Rev Physiol.* 2001;63:119-139.
40. Hellmich MR, Rui XL, Hellmich HL, et al. Human colorectal cancers express a constitutively active cholecystokinin-B/gastrin receptor that stimulates cell growth. *J Biol Chem.* 2000;275:32122-32128.
41. Olszewska-Pazdrak B, Townsend Jr CM, Hellmich MR. Agonist-independent activation of Src tyrosine kinase by a cholecystokinin-2 (CCK2) receptor splice variant. *J Biol Chem.* 2004;279:40400-40404.
42. Cheng ZJ, Harikumar KG, Holicky EL, et al. Heterodimerization of type A and B cholecystokinin receptors enhance signaling and promote cell growth. *J Biol Chem.* 2003;278:52972-52979.
43. Ferrand A, Wang TC. Gastrin and cancer: a review. *Cancer Lett.* 2005;238:15-29.
44. Muerkoster S, Isberner A, Arlt A, et al. Gastrin suppresses growth of CCK2 receptor expressing colon cancer cells by inducing apoptosis in vitro and in vivo. *Gastroenterology.* 2005;129:952-968.
45. Suarez-Pinzon WL, Lakey JR, Brand SJ, et al. Combination therapy with epidermal growth factor and gastrin induces neogenesis of human islet beta-cells from pancreatic duct cells and an increase in functional beta-cell mass. *J Clin Endocrinol Metab.* 2005;90:3401-3409.
46. Ladenheim EE, Hampton LL, Whitney AC, et al. Disruptions in feeding and body weight control in gastrin-releasing peptide receptor deficient mice. *J Endocrinol.* 2002;174:273-281.
47. Zhou J, Chen J, Mokotoff M, et al. Targeting gastrin-releasing peptide receptors for cancer treatment. *Anticancer Drugs.* 2004;15:921-927.
48. Martinez A, Zudaire E, Julian M, et al. Gastrin-releasing peptide (GRP) induces angiogenesis and the specific GRP blocker 77427 inhibits tumor growth in vitro and in vivo. *Oncogene.* 2005;24:4106-4113.
49. Kirchner H, Gutierrez JA, Solenberg PJ, et al. GOAT links dietary lipids with the endocrine control of energy balance. *Nat Med.* 2009;15:741-745.
50. Kojima M, Kangawa K. Ghrelin: structure and function. *Physiol Rev.* 2005;85:495-522.
51. le Roux CW, Neary NM, Halsey TJ, et al. Ghrelin does not stimulate food intake in patients with surgical procedures involving vagotomy. *J Clin Endocrinol Metab.* 2005;90:4521-4524.
52. Cummings DE, Weigle DS, Frayo RS, et al. Plasma ghrelin levels after diet-induced weight loss or gastric bypass surgery. *N Engl J Med.* 2002;346:1623-1630.
53. Nagaya N, Moriya J, Yasumura Y, et al. Effects of ghrelin administration on left ventricular function, exercise capacity, and muscle wasting in patients with chronic heart failure. *Circulation.* 2004;110:3674-3679.
54. Gelling RW, Du XQ, Dichmann DS, et al. Lower blood glucose, hyperglucagonemia, and pancreatic alpha cell hyperplasia in glucagon receptor knockout mice. *Proc Natl Acad Sci U S A.* 2003;100:1438-1443.
55. Drucker DJ. The biology of incretin hormones. *Cell Metab.* 2006;3:153-165.
56. Lovshin JA, Drucker DJ. Incretin-based therapies for type 2 diabetes mellitus. *Nat Rev Endocrinol.* 2009;5:262-269.
57. Buse JB, Rosenstock J, Sesti G, et al. Liraglutide once a day versus exenatide twice a day for type 2 diabetes: a 26-week randomised, parallel-group, multinational, open-label trial (LEAD-6). *Lancet.* 2009;374:39-47.
58. Drucker DJ, Ehrlich P, Asa SL, et al. Induction of intestinal epithelial proliferation by glucagon-like peptide 2. *Proc Natl Acad Sci U S A.* 1996;93:7911-7916.
59. Estall JL, Drucker DJ. Tales beyond the crypt: glucagon-like peptide-2 and cytoprotection in the intestinal mucosa. *Endocrinology.* 2005;146:19-21.
60. Jeppesen PB, Sanguinetti EL, Buchman A, et al. Teduglutide (ALX-0600), a dipeptidyl peptidase IV resistant glucagon-like peptide 2 analogue, improves intestinal function in short bowel syndrome patients. *Gut.* 2005;54:1224-1231.
61. Marguet D, Baggio L, Kobayashi T, et al. Enhanced insulin secretion and improved glucose tolerance in mice lacking CD26. *Proc Natl Acad Sci U S A.* 2000;97:6874-6879.

62. Vella A, Bock G, Giesler PD, et al. Effects of dipeptidyl peptidase 4 inhibition on gastrointestinal function, meal appearance and glucose metabolism in type 2 diabetes. *Diabetes*. 2007;56:1475-1480.
63. Wynne K, Park AJ, Small CJ, et al. Subcutaneous oxyntomodulin reduces body weight in overweight and obese subjects: a double-blind, randomized, controlled trial. *Diabetes*. 2005;54:2390-2395.
64. Baggio LL, Huang Q, Brown TJ, et al. Oxyntomodulin and glucagon-like peptide-1 differentially regulate murine food intake and energy expenditure. *Gastroenterology*. 2004;127:546-558.
65. Day JW, Ottaway N, Patterson JT, et al. A new glucagon and GLP-1 co-agonist eliminates obesity in rodents. *Nat Chem Biol*. 2009;5: 749-757.
66. Feighner SD, Tan CP, McKee KK, et al. Receptor for motilin identified in the human gastrointestinal system. *Science*. 1999;284:2184-2188.
67. Pons J, Lee EW, Li L, et al. Neuropeptide Y: multiple receptors and multiple roles in cardiovascular diseases. *Curr Opin Investig Drugs*. 2004;5:957-962.
68. Vincent JP, Mazella J, Kitabgi P. Neurotensin and neurotensin receptors. *Trends Pharmacol Sci*. 1999;20:302-309.
69. Piliponsky AM, Chen CC, Nishimura T, et al. Neurotensin increases mortality and mast cells reduce neurotensin levels in a mouse model of sepsis. *Nat Med*. 2008;14:392-398.
70. Vaudry D, Gonzalez BJ, Basille M, et al. Pituitary adenylate cyclase-activating polypeptide and its receptors: from structure to functions. *Pharmacol Rev*. 2000;52:269-324.
71. Freson K, Hashimoto H, Thys C, et al. The pituitary adenylate cyclase-activating polypeptide is a physiological inhibitor of platelet activation. *J Clin Invest*. 2004;113:905-912.
72. Batterham RL, Ffytche DH, Rosenthal JM, et al. PYY modulation of cortical and hypothalamic brain areas predicts feeding behaviour in humans. *Nature*. 2007;450:106-109.
73. Michel MC, Beck-Sickinger A, Cox H, et al. XVI International Union of Pharmacology recommendations for the nomenclature of neuropeptide Y, peptide YY, and pancreatic polypeptide receptors. *Pharmacol Rev*. 1998;50:143-150.
74. Batterham RL, Le Roux CW, Cohen MA, et al. Pancreatic polypeptide reduces appetite and food intake in humans. *J Clin Endocrinol Metab*. 2003;88:3989-3992.
75. Unis AS, Munson JA, Rogers SJ, et al. A randomized, double-blind, placebo-controlled trial of porcine versus synthetic secretin for reducing symptoms of autism. *J Am Acad Child Adolesc Psychiatry*. 2002;41: 1315-1321.
76. Low MJ. Clinical endocrinology and metabolism: the somatostatin neuroendocrine system—physiology and clinical relevance in gastrointestinal and pancreatic disorders. *Best Pract Res Clin Endocrinol Metab*. 2004;18:607-622.
77. Helyes Z, Pinter E, Sandor K, et al. Impaired defense mechanism against inflammation, hyperalgesia, and airway hyperreactivity in somatostatin 4 receptor gene-deleted mice. *Proc Natl Acad Sci U S A*. 2009;106:13088-13093.
78. Saito T, Iwata N, Tsubuki S, et al. Somatostatin regulates brain amyloid beta peptide Abeta42 through modulation of proteolytic degradation. *Nat Med*. 2005;11:434-439.
79. van der Hoek J, Hofland LJ, Lamberts SW. Novel subtype specific and universal somatostatin analogues: clinical potential and pitfalls. *Curr Pharm Des*. 2005;11:1573-1592.
80. Freda PU, Katznelson L, van der Lely AJ, et al. Long-acting somatostatin analog therapy of acromegaly: a meta-analysis. *J Clin Endocrinol Metab*. 2005;90:4465-4473.
81. Page NM. New challenges in the study of the mammalian tachykinins. *Peptides*. 2005;26:1356-1368.
82. Topaloglu AK, Reimann F, Guclu M, et al. TAC3 and TACR3 mutations in familial hypogonadotropic hypogonadism reveal a key role for neurokinin B in the central control of reproduction. *Nat Genet*. 2009;41:354-358.
82a. Holzer P, Holzer-Petsche U. Tachykinin receptors in the gut: physiological and pathological implications. *Current Opinion in Pharmacology*. 2001;1(6):583-590.
83. Lelievre V, Favrais G, Abad C, et al. Gastrointestinal dysfunction in mice with a targeted mutation in the gene encoding vasoactive intestinal polypeptide: a model for the study of intestinal ileus and Hirschsprung's disease. *Peptides*. 2007;28:1688-1699.
84. Gozes I, Furman S. Clinical endocrinology and metabolism: potential clinical applications of vasoactive intestinal peptide—a selected update. *Best Pract Res Clin Endocrinol Metab*. 2004;18:623-640.
85. Otto C, Hein L, Brede M, et al. Pulmonary hypertension and right heart failure in pituitary adenylate cyclase-activating polypeptide type I receptor-deficient mice. *Circulation*. 2004;110:3245-3251.
86. Petkov V, Mosgoeller W, Ziesche R, et al. Vasoactive intestinal peptide as a new drug for treatment of primary pulmonary hypertension. *J Clin Invest*. 2003;111:1339-1346.
87. Mahapatra NR, O'Connor DT, Vaingankar SM, et al. Hypertension from targeted ablation of chromogranin A can be rescued by the human ortholog. *J Clin Invest*. 2005;115:1942-1952.
88. Forte Jr LR. Uroguanylin and guanylin peptides: pharmacology and experimental therapeutics. *Pharmacol Ther*. 2004;104:137-162.
89. Perren A, Komminoth P, Saremaslani P, et al. Mutation and expression analyses reveal differential subcellular compartmentalization of PTEN in endocrine pancreatic tumors compared to normal islet cells. *Am J Pathol*. 2000;157:1097-1103.
90. Chandrasekharappa SC, Guru SC, Manickam P, et al. Positional cloning of the gene for multiple endocrine neoplasia-type 1. *Science*. 1997;276: 404-407.
91. Yokoyama A, Cleary ML. Menin critically links MLL proteins with LEDGF on cancer-associated target genes. *Cancer Cell*. 2008;14:36-46.
92. Ellard S, Hattersley AT, Brewer CM, et al. Detection of an MEN1 gene mutation depends on clinical features and supports current referral criteria for diagnostic molecular genetic testing. *Clin Endocrinol (Oxf)*. 2005;62:169-175.
93. Schussheim DH, Skarulis MC, Agarwal SK, et al. Multiple endocrine neoplasia type 1: new clinical and basic findings. *Trends Endocrinol Metab*. 2001;12:173-178.
94. Christ E, Wild D, Forrer F, et al. Glucagon-like peptide-1 receptor imaging for localization of insulinomas. *J Clin Endocrinol Metab*. 2009;94:4398-4405.
95. Warner RR. Enteroendocrine tumors other than carcinoid: a review of clinically significant advances. *Gastroenterology*. 2005;128:1668-1684.
96. de Herder WW, Lamberts SW. Clinical endocrinology and metabolism: gut endocrine tumours. *Best Pract Res Clin Endocrinol Metab*. 2004;18: 477-495.
97. Fendrich V, Waldmann J, Bartsch DK, et al. Surgical management of pancreatic endocrine tumors. *Nat Rev Clin Oncol*. 2009;6:419-428.
98. Placzkowski KA, Vella A, Thompson GB, et al. Secular trends in the presentation and management of functioning insulinoma at the Mayo Clinic, 1987-2007. *J Clin Endocrinol Metab*. 2009;94:1069-1073.
99. Zollinger RM, Ellison EH. Primary peptic ulcerations of the jejunum associated with islet cell tumors of the pancreas. *Ann Surg*. 1955;142:709-723; discussion, 724-708.
100. Zogakis TG, Gibril F, Libutti SK, et al. Management and outcome of patients with sporadic gastrinoma arising in the duodenum. *Ann Surg*. 2003;238:42-48.
101. Gibril F, Schumann M, Pace A, et al. Multiple endocrine neoplasia type 1 and Zollinger-Ellison syndrome: a prospective study of 107 cases and comparison with 1009 cases from the literature. *Medicine (Baltimore)*. 2004;83:43-83.
102. Asgharian B, Turner ML, Gibril F, et al. Cutaneous tumors in patients with multiple endocrine neoplasm type 1 (MEN1) and gastrinomas: prospective study of frequency and development of criteria with high sensitivity and specificity for MEN1. *J Clin Endocrinol Metab*. 2004;89:5328-5336.
103. Berna MJ, Hoffmann KM, Long SH, et al. Serum gastrin in Zollinger-Ellison syndrome: II. Prospective study of gastrin provocative testing in 293 patients from the National Institutes of Health and comparison with 537 cases from the literature. Evaluation of diagnostic criteria, proposal of new criteria, and correlations with clinical and tumoral features. *Medicine (Baltimore)*. 2006;85:331-364.
104. Brubaker PL, Drucker DJ, Asa SL, et al. Prolonged gastrointestinal transit in a patient with a glucagon-like peptide (GLP)-1- and -2-producing neuroendocrine tumor. *J Clin Endocrinol Metab*. 2002;87:3078-3083.

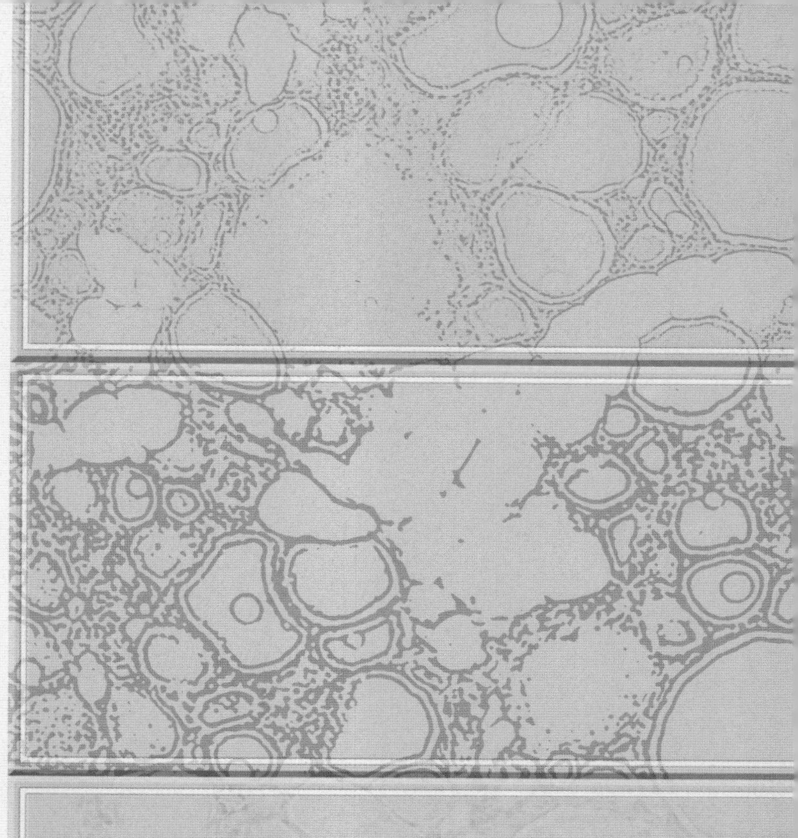

SECTION X

Polyendocrine and Neoplastic Disorders

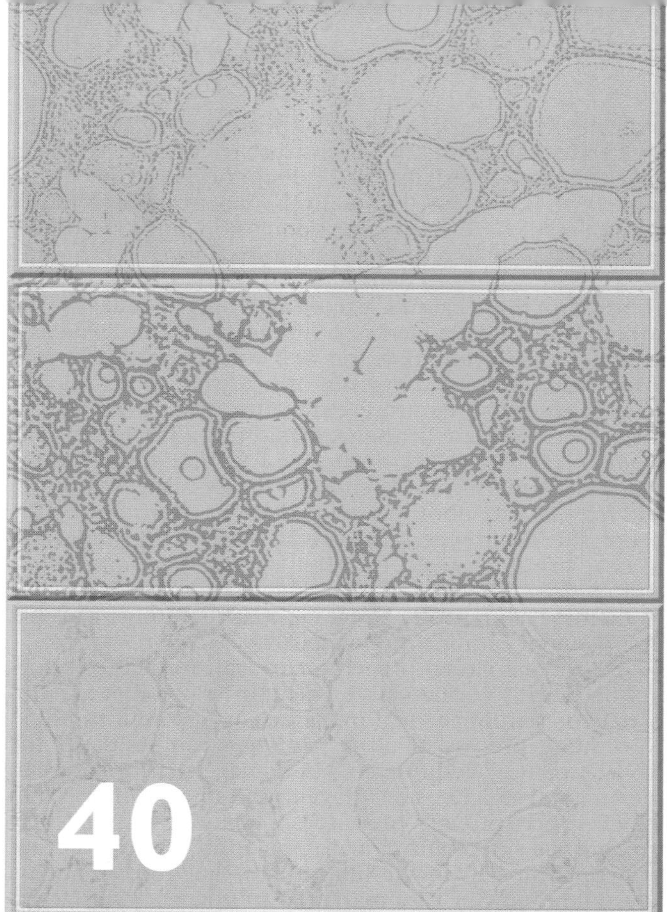

CHAPTER 40

Pathogenesis of Endocrine Tumors

ANDREW ARNOLD

A great deal is now known about the mechanisms underlying human tumorigenesis in general and about neoplasia of the endocrine glands in particular. The application of general principles of neoplasia to endocrine tumors has been a productive area of research and is now being translated into clinical applications. Endocrine tumorigenesis also involves some special, if not unique, features that must be considered in understanding the pathogenesis of endocrine tumors. The aim of this chapter is to present the general principles of neoplasia as a framework through which current knowledge about and future advances in endocrine tumorigenesis can be understood.

MOLECULAR TUMOR BIOLOGY

Both inherited tumor predisposition syndromes and the more common noninherited *(sporadic)* forms of neoplasia are genetic diseases in the sense that tumors develop when specific damage to genes leads to deregulated cell growth. As a general rule, damage to one such gene controlling cell growth is not sufficient to confer a neoplastic phenotype on a cell; instead, mutations in multiple genes accumulate over time. Inherited tumor syndromes constitute a special case in which mutation of one key gene is already present in each somatic cell at birth.

Clonality

Concepts of Clonality and Clonal Evolution

All cancers and many benign hypercellular expansions are *monoclonal;* that is, they are composed of cells that are the descendants of a single clonal progenitor cell in which the accumulation of a sufficient number of DNA alterations (and, perhaps, other epigenetic damage that does not actually change the nucleotide sequence) caused a selective advantage. Over time, this selective advantage—manifested as an increase in proliferative capacity, a decrease in the normal cell death rate, or both—leads to the development of a neoplasm.

The monoclonality of tumors implies that the necessary accumulation of mutations occurs only rarely in the large population of cells in a tissue. Viewed in another way, the identification of a specific monoclonal (also called *clonal*) change in DNA, found in all or most of the cells of a neoplasm but not in that person's constitutional DNA (i.e., DNA obtained from adjacent normal tissue or leukocytes), indicates that this DNA alteration was advantageous in the accelerated evolutionary process that is oncogenesis. Such a DNA lesion, especially if it recurs in other tumors of the same type, is therefore highly likely to contribute to tumor development.[1] However, this conclusion must be drawn more cautiously in rare circumstances, such as an inherited DNA mismatch repair deficiency, in which the underlying global mutation rate is exceedingly high. One of the strongest types of evidence to implicate a given gene as a driving force in tumorigenesis is the recurrent demonstration of clonal DNA changes in or near that gene.

This situation contrasts with the one in which an increase or decrease in the expression of a particular gene (RNA or protein levels) occurs in a tumor; such changes can be secondary consequences of tumor-related processes and may or may not themselves drive or contribute to the neoplastic phenotype. This caveat is especially important to bear in mind, given that the Human Genome Project and modern microarray technology have made it possible to examine expression changes in a huge number of genes in a tissue or tumor simultaneously.

An original clonal progenitor or transformed cell does not necessarily contain all the genetic lesions that are ultimately present in the mature, clinically apparent tumor. A continuing process of *clonal evolution* can result in the development of additional DNA damage that provides an incremental selective advantage to the single tumor cell in which it occurs. Over time, the progeny of this cell may become the dominant clonal population. The percentage of neoplastic cells in the final tumor that contain such a later mutation can vary markedly and depends on factors such as the duration of the mutation's existence and the relative rates of proliferation and death of the various cell populations.

Endocrine tumor cells are often sufficiently differentiated to express the hormonal activity that is characteristic of the corresponding normal cell type, but the hormonal function of the tumor is typically regulated in an abnormal fashion. The genes that cause tumors of endocrine tissues do so only because of their effects on cell proliferation and accumulation; such genes need not influence hormonal function. Moreover, a mutant gene that alters hormonal function but confers no selective growth advantage is not tumorigenic. Nevertheless, the frequent coexistence of growth deregulation and hormonal hyperfunction in endocrine tumors does indicate that tumor-causing genes can often, directly or indirectly, alter hormone control pathways.

In certain instances, such as a mutation affecting the α-subunit of stimulatory G protein ($G_s\alpha$) in growth hormone–producing and thyroid adenomas, a single mutant gene can directly contribute to both cell proliferation and hormonal hyperfunction. In general, however, the relation between hypercellularity caused by clonally selected mutant genes and hormonal hyperfunction is poorly understood.

Hyperplasia versus Neoplasia

Not all hypercellular expansions are monoclonal. For instance, the generalized proliferative response of all cells of a tissue to an extrinsic stimulus yields a polyclonal expansion. Examples include the hyperthyroidism of Graves' disease and the early, reversible secondary hyperparathyroidism that occurs in states of chronic hypocalcemia. Such polyclonal expansions represent biologic hyperplasia, whereas any monoclonal growth (benign or malignant) is a true neoplasm. Analyses of tumor clonality have been used to distinguish between these types of tumorigenic mechanisms. However, the genesis of some tumors can involve both types of processes. For example, a generalized stimulus to polyclonal hyperplasia can, by increasing the chances of mitosis-related DNA damage in one cell, foster the emergence of a monoclonal population capable of eventually overwhelming or replacing its hyperplastic neighbors.

The clinical and histopathologic use of the term *hyperplasia* does not necessarily correspond to the biologic meaning just described, a situation that has engendered much confusion. For example, the usual tumors responsible for primary hyperparathyroidism have been clinicopathologically classified as adenomas when a single gland is abnormal and as hyperplasia when the individual patient has multiple hypercellular glands. No histopathologic criteria can reliably predict whether a single or multiple glands are involved on the basis of analysis of only one such gland. Not only are clinical adenomas monoclonal neoplasms,[2] but many parathyroid glands from patients with multigland "hyperplasia" are also monoclonal.[3] It is therefore important to ensure that the terms used in the description of endocrine tumorigenesis are clearly defined.

Insights into Tumor Pathogenesis

Because the clonal status of a cellular proliferation is of fundamental importance in deciphering its pathogenesis, endocrine tumors are studied to determine whether the expansion is monoclonal or polyclonal. One way of determining that a tumor is monoclonal is to identify a DNA or chromosomal lesion that, because of its tumor specificity and presence in all or most of the neoplastic cells, directly defines the expansion as monoclonal. Examples of cytogenetically defined clonal abnormalities are chromosome translocations such as the t(9;22) Philadelphia translocation in chronic myelogenous leukemia and the t(14;18) translocation in follicular lymphoma.

The use of classic cytogenetics is technically more difficult in solid tumors than in hematopoietic tumors because hematopoietic cells divide in culture much more readily and yield excellent metaphase chromosomal spreads. Specimens of endocrine tumors are difficult to obtain for culture and to analyze cytogenetically.

Improved methods for the cytogenetic and molecular cytogenetic study of tumors, including fluorescence in situ hybridization (FISH), comparative genomic hybridization, and chromosome painting, have opened up new avenues for detection of clonal chromosomal lesions in endocrine tumors.[4,5] New, large-scale methodologies for obtaining the DNA sequence of a sample's entire genome carry the potential to generate a virtually complete catalog of acquired, clonal mutations in a series of human tumors. This catalog would include the full spectrum of structural changes from point mutations to rearrangements and copy number changes. The sensitivity of these methods will also allow for detection of mutations that are present only in subclones or subpopulations of a tumor's cells. Cost and throughput limitations of these technologies are still significant but have been improving rapidly, increasing accessibility for investigators.[6]

Examples of monoclonal abnormalities defined by molecular methods in endocrine neoplasia include $G_s\alpha$ gene mutations in growth hormone–producing pituitary tumors,[7] thyrotropin (TSH) receptor gene mutations in thyroid tumors,[8] and cyclin D1 or *CCND1* (also called *PRAD1*) gene rearrangements in parathyroid adenomas.[9,10] Identification of tumor-specific changes, such as deletions of DNA markers in particular regions of the tumor genome, also serves as evidence of monoclonality, even if the specific genes affected by such deletions are not known.[4,11]

Indirect methods can determine the clonal status of tumors without the necessity of identifying the specific genes or chromosomal regions that are clonally mutated and involved in tumorigenesis. These methods have generally exploited the phenomenon of random X-chromosome inactivation (the *Lyon phenomenon*) in women.[12] Random X-chromosome inactivation occurs early in female embryonic development in all somatic cells. In any given cell, the choice of which X chromosome is inactivated is random; however, once that choice is made the decision is faithfully transmitted to all progeny of that cell. Usually, the maternally derived X chromosome is inactive in about 50% of the cells in a normal tissue, and the paternally derived X chromosome is inactive in about 50%.

Polyclonal growth, representing a generalized expansion of many or all original cells within a tissue, maintains the relatively even mix of active maternal and paternal X chromosomes characteristic of the normal tissue. In contrast, the neoplastic cells in a monoclonal tumor are derived from a single progenitor and therefore should all have an identical X chromosome pattern, with either the maternal or the paternal X chromosome uniformly inactivated.

A unifying feature of methods based on the analysis of X-chromosome inactivation to determine the clonal status of a tumor is the use of a normally occurring variant, or *polymorphism,* at the genetic or protein level to distinguish between a woman's two X chromosomes. The other step involves assaying some property that reflects the state of X-chromosome inactivation imposed on the tumor cell chromosomes at the polymorphic site. Assays to reflect X-chromosome inactivation status include assessments of gene expression (RNA or protein levels) or regional DNA methylation.

A polymorphism in glucose-6-phosphate dehydrogenase (G6PD) was the first to be used in X-chromosome inactivation analyses of tumor clonality.[13] A disadvantage of the G6PD system is that only a small minority of women are heterozygous for electrophoretically distinguishable isoforms of this X chromosome–encoded enzyme. Therefore, most tumors have been unsuitable for G6PD-based clonal analysis. Furthermore, the method fails to detect the monoclonality of certain tumors,[2,14,15] perhaps because of differences in the level of G6PD expression in tumor cells compared with contaminating admixed normal cells within the analyzed samples.

DNA polymorphisms are now preferred for clonal analyses to distinguish between the two X chromosomes. High rates of heterozygosity make it possible to analyze most tumors. Some multiallelic polymorphisms, based on differences in the number of highly repeated sequence units in a genomic location, are heterozygous in more than 90% of women, and a large number of DNA polymorphisms have been described on the X chromosome (and on all chromosomes). However, most of these polymorphisms cannot be used in clonality studies because they have not been characterized for detectable changes that correlate with the state of activity of the X chromosome on which an allele resides. Some of the X-linked polymorphisms that have been valuable in clonal analyses of human tumors include restriction fragment length polymorphisms in the *HPRT* and *PGK* (now called encoding hypoxanthine phosphoribosyltransferase 1 [*PGKI*]) gene regions,[16] a minisatellite repeat (>10 nucleotide core repeated unit) region called M27 or DXS255,[3] and a microsatellite repeat (<10 nucleotide core repeated unit) locus in the androgen receptor gene.[17]

Changes in DNA methylation in the vicinity of certain polymorphic sites on the X chromosome correlate with the activity of that X chromosome and are useful in clonal analyses. Methylation of specific cytosine nucleotides is an epigenetic process that is faithfully replicated from a given cell to its progeny, and this process may have a role in maintaining the activity status of the particular X chromosome. Methylation at certain specific sites may be easily detected through the action of methylation-sensitive restriction endonucleases, which cleave when their target sites are unmethylated but cannot do so when a methyl group is present.

One cannot predict how or whether X-chromosome inactivation will affect the methylation of a particular nucleotide in or near a gene; correlations must be established separately for individual genomic sites. For example, a useful restriction site in the *HPRT* region is consistently methylated when on the active X chromosome and unmethylated when on the inactive X chromosome; the opposite pattern is observed for an informative site in the *PGK* region. Despite the need for such empiric validation, the use of DNA methylation as a surrogate marker for the status of X chromosome activity has major advantages in clonality studies and eliminates the vulnerability of the assay to the vagaries of gene expression in tumor cells.

The analysis of clonality in endocrine tumors has yielded important insights. For example, most corticotropin-producing pituitary tumors are monoclonal, which shows that Cushing's disease is not explained solely by a generalized hypothalamic stimulation of corticotrophs.[18,19] Typical parathyroid adenomas are also monoclonal outgrowths[2,11] and are not, as previously suggested, asymmetric forms of multiglandular hyperplasia.[14,15] In patients with multifocal papillary thyroid cancer, clonal analysis of physically distinct individual tumors showed that these foci are often clonally unrelated and, therefore, of independent origins,[17] suggesting an underlying predisposition to thyroid tumorigenesis in such patients (Fig. 40-1).

In severe secondary (or tertiary) hyperparathyroidism in patients with uremia, the typical finding of multigland involvement had led to the assumption that this disease predominantly involves polyclonal (non-neoplastic) cellular proliferations. However, examination of clonality using X inactivation showed that 64% of informative patients with renal failure undergoing hemodialysis who had refractory hyperparathyroidism harbored at least one monoclonal parathyroid tumor, and 63% of all tumors examined had monoclonal X-inactivation patterns.[3]

One often overlooked pitfall in the interpretation of any X inactivation analysis must be emphasized: Polyclonal patterns cannot be interpreted definitively. For example, admixed normal cells or tumor-specific aberrations in DNA methylation can obscure the detection of a monoclonal cell population. Therefore, the true extent of monoclonality in severe secondary or tertiary hyperparathyroidism might be even higher (but not lower) than demonstrated. These unexpected results indicate that monoclonal parathyroid neoplasms are common in uremic refractory hyperparathyroidism and suggest that autonomous parathyroid function in this disorder is caused by the outgrowth of true neoplasms, presumably on a background of preexisting (and more reversible) polyclonal parathyroid hyperplasia.

Predisposing Influences

Both environmental and genetic factors can contribute to the risk of a particular type of tumor development over a

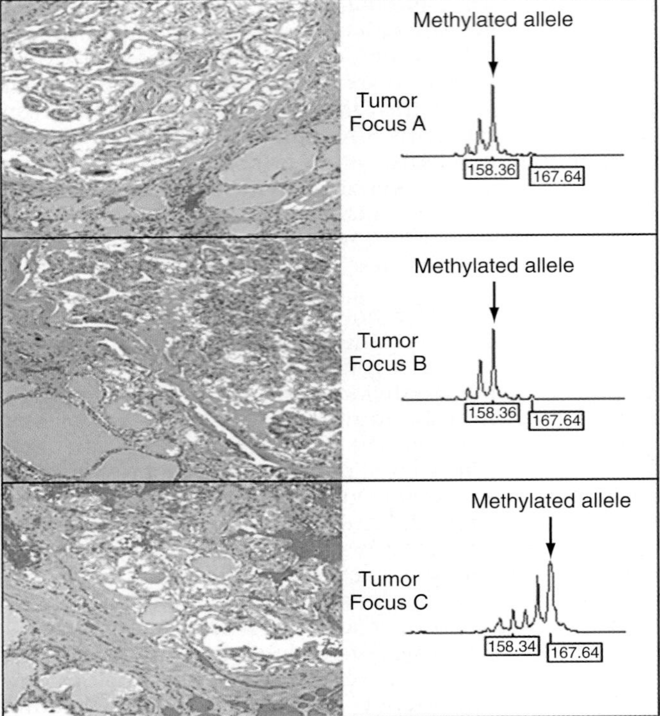

Figure 40-1 Example of discordant X-inactivation clonality patterns in distinct tumor foci from one patient with multifocal papillary thyroid carcinomas. Shown in the left panels are photomicrographs (stained with hematoxylin and eosin, ×40) of a single patient's three tumor foci, labeled A, B, and C. Even though the three discrete carcinomas have a similar microscopic appearance, they do not share an identical X-inactivation pattern. For each tumor, the corresponding plot to the right shows the size and amount of fluorescent polymerase chain reaction (PCR) products amplified from tumor DNA as analyzed on an automated sequencer. Products are plotted from left to right, from smaller to larger alleles differing at a polymorphic site in the androgen-receptor gene on the X chromosome. The height of the peaks corresponds to the amount of product present. Methylation-sensitive PCR analysis of tumor foci A and B shows that, in each focus, the smaller allele is methylated and therefore inactivated, and the larger allele is unmethylated. Tumor focus C, from the same patient, shows the opposite pattern, with the larger allele methylated and the smaller allele unmethylated. The number in the box under each peak indicates the estimated allele size in base pairs. The discordant X-inactivation patterns indicate that tumor focus C originated independently from A and from B. Foci A and B could have originated separately, sharing an X-inactivation pattern by chance (such concordance is expected in 50% of independently originating tumors), or they could be clonally related. (Modified from Shattuck TM, Shattuck TM, Westra WH, et al. Independent clonal origins of distinct tumor foci in multifocal papillary thyroid carcinoma. *N Engl J Med.* 2005;352:2406-2412. Copyright © Massachusetts Medical Society.)

lifetime. In highly penetrant inherited syndromes, the genetic predisposition is overriding. In most instances, however, the intimate relation between environmental and (often multiple) genetic factors of lower penetrance makes the traditional "nature versus nurture" question difficult to assess.

A commonly overlooked genetic component of tumor predisposition is gender; however, the specific mechanisms by which gender influences the risk of endocrine tumors such as thyroid cancer and parathyroid adenoma are not well understood. Additional genetic variables, which may be common or rare in the population, also influence the chance of tumor development. It has been notoriously difficult to isolate these specific genetic variations, each of which might confer only a small degree of risk, might be rare, or might increase risk only when present in particular combinations with other DNA polymorphisms.

An important environmental factor in endocrine tumorigenesis is ionizing radiation. Both thyroid and parathyroid tumors have been linked to prior head and neck irradiation in a dose-dependent fashion.[20,21] The latency period for tumor development after radiation exposure in the United States is quite long. However, childhood thyroid cancer was observed with markedly increased frequency in the aftermath of the 1986 Chernobyl nuclear accident.[22] This heightened susceptibility may not be solely a function of age and amount of exposure; it may be modified by other factors such as iodine deficiency in the region,[22] highlighting the point that tumor predisposition and development can be influenced by complex interacting factors.

Oncogenes and Tumor Suppressor Genes

Two broad categories of genes are implicated in the excessive cell proliferation and other properties that result in the outgrowth and evolution of a neoplastic clone. An *oncogene* carries a gain-of-function mutation in its regulatory or coding region that results in dysregulation of its normal product or in the formation of an abnormal protein product. Typically, only one mutated allele need be present for an oncogene to exert its tumorigenic action. The normal, unmutated version of an oncogene is called a *proto-oncogene.* Proto-oncogenes may be converted to oncogenes by various molecular genetic mechanisms, such as fusion of part of its coding region with that of another gene, chromosomal translocations or inversions that alter its regulatory environment, or point mutations.

A *tumor suppressor gene,* in contrast, normally acts to restrain cell proliferation or other potential aspects of the malignant phenotype. This restraint can directly control proliferation (e.g., by regulating the cell cycle), or it can affect proliferation indirectly (e.g., by maintaining genomic stability). Therefore, the definition of a tumor suppressor gene is not restrictive concerning its specific cellular function.[23] Tumors are provoked or fostered by inactivating or loss-of-function mutations in such genes; common inactivating mechanisms are gene deletion, point mutations, and microdeletions or small base insertions that cause a frameshift. Both alleles of a classic tumor suppressor gene must be inactivated to eliminate the functional protein product and to contribute to tumorigenesis.

The existence of a critical tumor suppressor gene is often inferred from the finding that a particular subchromosomal stretch of DNA is recurrently and nonrandomly lost in a particular tumor type. The loss typically involves only one of a gene's two alleles. Because these regions of loss of heterozygosity are often large and can encompass many innocent bystander genes, the case that the correct tumor suppressor gene has been found can be made most convincingly when the remaining allele of the gene is shown to harbor another, more specific, clonal inactivating lesion, such as an intragenic coding region mutation or microdeletion. It is also possible (albeit unproved in human neoplasia) that certain nonclassic tumor suppressors exist, contributing to neoplasia through acquired haploinsufficiency, in which somatic inactivation of only one allele provides the relevant selective advantage.[24]

Although there has been some evolution in, and even controversy about, the best definition of a tumor suppressor gene, the "simplest, most inclusive, and cleanest genetic definition" is that favored by Haber and Harlow,[23] namely, "genes that sustain loss-of-function mutations in the development of neoplasia." This definition, although unrestricted concerning the function of the tumor suppressor, "does have an essential component—the unequivocal demonstration of inactivating mutations."[23] Therefore, evidence for reduced or absent expression of a gene in a particular tumor, or even the ability of a gene to inhibit cell proliferation, should not be accepted as sufficient to designate it as a tumor suppressor if it is not accompanied by clear and recurrent evidence of clonal mutation.

Some oncogenes or tumor suppressor genes contribute to tumors of only one or a few cell types, whereas other genes are involved in many different types of tumors. It is rare for any one particular gene to be invariably involved in the development of a given type of tumor, and different combinations of mutated genes can have similar cellular and clinical consequences (genetic heterogeneity).

Finally, genetic hits affecting multiple oncogenes and tumor suppressor genes in a single cell appear to be required if that cell is to become neoplastic. In most instances, no single activated oncogene or inactivated tumor suppressor gene is sufficient for the development of a tumor.

Mutational Mechanisms and the Primary Role of Selection in Tumorigenesis

Tumors can acquire mutations that in themselves increase the rate at which new mutations develop at other sites in the genome. Many tumor biologists have commented on the apparently excessive number of genetic changes observed in individual cancers compared with measured rates of mutation in normal cells. Genetic changes are usually considered to occur or to be fixed during DNA replication or mitosis.[25,26] However, some mutations may be time dependent rather than replication dependent, meaning that they can arise even in the absence of cell proliferation.[25,27]

One mechanism by which somatic mutations might occur is through a defect in postreplication mismatch repair, the pathway responsible for removing and correcting mismatched base pairs in DNA.[27] At least one form of inherited genetic instability can result from inactivation of mutator genes (*MSH2* or *MLH1*) in the mismatch repair system.[28] Although such mutational mechanisms may in theory be quite important in benign or slow-growing endocrine tumors that derive from slowly proliferating normal tissues, little direct evidence has supported this hypothesis. Some investigators have drawn conclusions about the extent of genomic instability in endocrine tumors based on the number of observed chromosomal abnormalities, and such conclusions may cloud the distinction between state and rate.[29] The presence of genetic alterations in a tumor, even in large numbers, does not necessarily imply that the tumor is genetically unstable. True instability is defined as an abnormal mutation rate, and the snapshot of a mature tumor's complement of mutations (i.e., its state) does not provide information about their rate of occurrence.

As noted by Lengauer and colleagues,[29] several factors in addition to true instability may explain the greater frequency of observed mutations in tumors compared with non-neoplastic tissues. These include potentially crucial differences in the selective conditions of the tumor compared with the normal cell context, differences that involve humoral and intercellular interactions.[30] For example, a given mutation may confer an important selective advantage and lead to clonal expansion only when it occurs in a tumor cell environment, whereas the same mutation (occurring at the same rate) in a normal cell environment would not lead to clonal expansion and might even cause apoptosis, thus avoiding detection. In most instances, it does not appear to be necessary to invoke an increased mutation rate to explain the evolutionary process of tumor outgrowth, and an increased mutation rate often may confer a disadvantage on the cell.[1,31]

In summary, selection is the driving force for tumor growth. This key principle is as applicable to slow-growing and benign endocrine tumors as it is to aggressive cancers.

GENETIC ALTERATIONS IN ENDOCRINE TUMORS: EXAMPLES

Neoplasia is, in large part, a genetic disease in which most of the critical DNA damage occurs somatically rather than through inheritance (germline mutations). Somatic alterations of proto-oncogenes and tumor suppressor genes are implicated in endocrine tumorigenesis; in other words, such mutations can be of either the gain-of-function or the loss-of-function type. Germline mutations that predispose to endocrine neoplasia can also occur in either proto-oncogenes or tumor suppressor genes. Germline mutations in *RET,* causing multiple endocrine neoplasia types 2A (MEN2A) and 2B (MEN2B), and familial medullary thyroid cancer (FMTC), are prominent examples of the former and are discussed in Chapter 41. However, most germline mutations identified to date are inactivating mutations, thus identifying the affected genes as tumor suppressors by definition.

Patients in whom a particular tumor develops on the basis of a strong inherited predisposition typically constitute only a minority of patients with that tumor. Nonetheless, the lessons learned from identifying the molecular basis of inherited tumor predisposition are important, both clinically and from a fundamental biologic perspective. In addition, some genes identified as the cause of a rare genetic syndrome through germline mutations have subsequently been found to be somatically mutated in the more common, sporadic occurrences of the same tumors. Two examples, *MEN1* and *HRPT2,* illustrate this point.

Thyrotropin Receptor and $G_s\alpha$ in Toxic Thyroid Adenomas

The fact that solitary toxic thyroid adenomas often contain somatic mutations in different genes whose products are functionally interrelated highlights the point that heterogeneous genetic lesions can converge on common pathways to predispose to neoplasia. Solitary toxic thyroid adenomas are characterized by autonomous *(TSH-independent)* hyperfunction and growth. Because TSH is normally a stimulus to both functional activity and growth of thyroid cells, toxic adenomas chronically and inappropriately behave as though they are stimulated by TSH. Somatic mutations in the TSH receptor itself can lead to TSH-independent *(constitutive)* activation of the receptor and cause both clonal expansion and hyperthyroidism in a subset of toxic adenomas.[32] Therefore, the TSH receptor is a proto-oncogene that can be activated by a variety of point mutations. Analysis of how these point mutations mimic the effects of TSH binding has provided insight into the mechanism of activation of G protein–coupled receptors.

The TSH receptor is a member of the large family of G protein–coupled receptors, and its major actions on thyrocyte proliferation and differentiated function are mediated through the cyclic adenosine monophosphate (cAMP) signaling pathway. The predominant G protein involved in transduction of the stimulatory effect of the receptor on adenylyl cyclase is G_s. The α-subunit of G_s is also a proto-oncogene and has undergone clonally selected activating point mutation in a subset of toxic thyroid adenomas.[33] $G_s\alpha$ genes bearing such gain-of-function mutations have been termed *GSP* oncogenes and are also present in some growth hormone–secreting pituitary tumors. These pituitary tumors demonstrate constitutive activation of the cAMP pathway, a prime mediator of proliferation and hormonal function in the somatotroph.

In this context, it is instructive to raise the example of McCune-Albright syndrome (see Chapters 25 and 28), in which activating $G_s\alpha$ mutations are present in multiple tissues of a given patient owing to mutation early in embryonic development and subsequent genetic mosaicism. Hyperthyroidism and acromegaly are among the characteristic components of this syndrome. Another gene encoding an element in the cAMP signaling pathway, the protein kinase A type 1α regulatory subunit gene *PRKAR1A,* has been implicated in the familial syndrome termed *Carney's complex,* which includes corticotropin-independent Cushing's syndrome related to autonomously functioning adrenocortical nodules, growth hormone–secreting pituitary tumors, and male precocious puberty caused by hormonally active testicular tumors.[34,35]

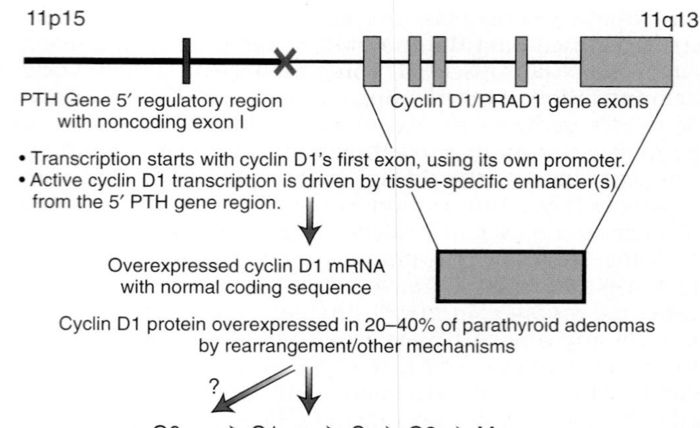

Figure 40-2 Diagram of the molecular structure of the parathyroid hormone–cyclin D1 DNA rearrangement in a subset of parathyroid adenomas and its functional consequences. The dark X represents the chromosome breakpoint between the parathyroid hormone gene *(PTH)* regulatory region plus *PTH* noncoding exon I *(solid light vertical bar)* and part of its first intron, from 11p15 *(left),* and the intact promoter and five exons of the cyclin D1 gene from 11q13. Cyclin D1 gene transcription proceeds in a left-to-right direction, as drawn. (Modified from Arnold A. Genetic basis of endocrine disease 5: molecular genetics of parathyroid gland neoplasia. *J Clin Endocrinol Metab.* 1993;77:1108-1112. Copyright © 1993, The Endocrine Society.)

Cyclin D1 in Hyperparathyroidism and General Oncology

Another illustrative example is that of the *CCND1* oncogene. Unlike many endocrine tumor–associated oncogenes, cyclin D1 is also commonly involved in nonendocrine tumors. This gene, which is now appreciated to be of central importance to molecular oncology and to normal cellular physiology, was discovered in the molecular dissection of an endocrine tumor.

Many human oncogenes were discovered because they are adjacent to nonrandom chromosome breakpoints in tumors. Chromosome breaks and rearrangements probably occur often in normal cells but are recognized only when they result in deregulation of the expression of a growth-related gene (or create a new fusion gene) and confer a selective advantage on the cell. *CCND1* was identified as the putative oncogene adjacent to one such breakpoint PARD1 on chromosome 11 in a subset of parathyroid adenomas (Fig. 40-2).[9,36,37] On the 11q13 side of the inversion breakpoint, the promoter and coding exons of the cyclin D1 gene remain in contiguity with each other. Across the breakpoint are regulatory sequences from the upstream region of the parathyroid hormone gene *(PTH)* on 11p15 that normally function to enhance *PTH* gene transcription in the presence of parathyroid tissue–specific signals (likely to be DNA-binding proteins found in the nucleus). Such transcriptional enhancer sequences can act over distances of many kilobases to enhance transcription, and cyclin D1 transcription is increased in these tumors. Collectively, such rearrangements along with other activating mechanisms result in elevated cyclin D1 protein levels, which are present in 20% to 40% of parathyroid adenomas.[10] Cyclin D1 overexpression has also been demonstrated to cause hyperparathyroidism in transgenic mice.[38]

In a broader context, the tissue-specific enhancer–driven expression of cyclin D1 in parathyroid tumors is analogous to the activation of oncogenes such as *BCL2* or *MYC* in B-cell lymphomas. In these tumors, chromosomal rearrangements lead to a juxtaposition of immunoglobulin gene enhancer elements and the oncogene, which is thereby inappropriately activated.

The *CCND1* gene product (cyclin D1) was initially recognized as a cyclin by virtue of its structural relation to the cyclin family of proteins, which were known to be involved in controlling the cell cycle. However, before the discovery of cyclin D1, no mammalian cyclins were known to participate in the control of the critical transition from G_1 to S phase of the cell cycle. This checkpoint would be an appropriate site for attack by an oncogenic protein, because movement into S phase commits a cell to the remainder of the cycle and another mitosis. It is now widely accepted that cyclin D1 is a G_1 cyclin that functions to push the cell toward or through this key juncture.[39]

On a cautionary note, this functional assignment for cyclin D1 as a G_1 cyclin is primarily derived from cultured cell systems, which might not fully reflect the true in vivo roles of this key oncoprotein. The detailed mechanism of action of cyclin D1, both normally and especially when dysregulated in tumorigenesis, deserves further exploration.[37]

Cyclins are regulatory subunits of holoenzymes whose catalytic subunits are cyclin-dependent kinases (CDKs). The major kinase partner for cyclin D1 appears to be CDK4 or, in some cell types, CDK6. The protein product of the retinoblastoma tumor suppressor gene, *RB1,* has been recognized as one substrate for phosphorylation by cyclin D–CDK complexes. Natural inhibitors of CDK function also exist, and $p16^{INK4a}$ *(CDKN2A)* is recognized as a key inhibitor of cyclin D–CDK4/6 complexes. Inactivation of *CDKN2A* might be expected to be as oncogenic as cyclin D1 overexpression, and *CDKN2A* is, indeed, a tumor suppressor gene in familial melanoma and several types of sporadic human tumors. Inactivating mutations of *CDKN2A* are uncommon, if they occur at all, in parathyroid adenomas.[40] Therefore, the cellular consequences of *CDKN2A* loss and cyclin D1 activation might not precisely overlap. Consistent with this observation, increasing evidence exists for possible non-CDK–dependent actions of cyclin D1.[37] That being said, the involvement of other CDK inhibitors in endocrine neoplasia does suggest that disruption of these molecules' cell-cycle functions may be a key component of their tumorigeneic mechanisms in endocrine cells.[41]

The significance of cyclin D1 in human neoplasia extends far beyond its involvement in endocrine tumors. For example, it is the long-sought *BCL1* oncogene that is deregulated by the characteristic t(11;14) translocation in mantle cell or centrocytic B-cell lymphomas. Assessment of cyclin D1 gene rearrangement or expression is clinically useful in the molecular diagnosis of B-cell neoplasia. In addition, cyclin D1 is a key oncogene in breast cancer, myeloma, squamous cell cancers of the head and neck, esophageal cancer, and a variety of other tumors.[37] Cyclin D1 and other members of its oncogenic pathway or pathways might serve as targets for development of antineoplastic therapies.

MEN1 Tumor Suppressor Gene

Multiple endocrine neoplasia type 1 (MEN1) is a familial predisposition to tumors of the parathyroid glands, anterior pituitary, pancreatic islets, and duodenum. Other tumors, including carcinoid tumors, lipomas, and angiofibromas, also occur with increased frequency in this disorder (see Chapter 41).

Familial MEN1 is inherited in an autosomal dominant pattern with high penetrance, indicating that in an affected family a single mutant gene is responsible for transmitting the tumor predisposition. *MEN1,* the normal gene whose mutant form causes most cases of MEN1, was identified by positional cloning.[42] *MEN1* germline mutations have been detected in most MEN1 families and in many individuals with clinically sporadic MEN1 (i.e., patients with a negative family history). Many of these mutations would clearly be expected to truncate the translated product severely and can safely be categorized as *inactivating* mutations. It can be reasonably anticipated that when definitive functional testing is available, other reported mutations, especially in the missense category, will prove to be inactivating lesions as well.

The identification of *MEN1* opened up the potential for direct presymptomatic molecular diagnosis in established or suspected MEN1 kindreds or individual patients. However, the benefits of such DNA testing with respect to prophylactic interventions are more restricted, and improvements in morbidity or mortality are less well established, than, for example, in *RET* testing for MEN2.[43] Furthermore, in part because inactivating *MEN1* mutations can occur throughout or even near the gene and are not restricted to its coding region, a substantial fraction of pathologic mutations would be expected to elude identification in MEN1 patients when exons are sequenced in research or commercial laboratories. Therefore, a negative genetic test, which is known to occur in about 30% of kindreds with classic MEN1 features, does not eliminate the diagnosis of MEN1 in a new patient or family. Moreover, a degree of genetic heterogeneity exists in that a subset of "MEN1-like" individuals or kindreds who test negative for *MEN1* mutations have mutations in other genes, including the p27 CDK inhibitor gene, *CDKN1B*.[41,44]

The *MEN1* gene encodes a 610-amino-acid protein termed *menin.* The structure of menin has yielded few clues to menin's normal function except for its nuclear localization signals. Menin may play an important role in regulation of gene transcription, related to its partnership with MLL, the mixed lineage leukemia protein, in a multiprotein complex that regulates chromatin structure and expression of target genes.[45] Menin has been reported to influence various cellular systems, including cell-cycle control, apoptosis, and DNA repair, but exactly how its inactivation leads to endocrine cell neoplasia requires further investigation.[45] Tissue surveys have shown *MEN1* expression to be almost ubiquitous.

The molecular pathology of MEN1 strongly suggests that *MEN1* functions as a classic tumor suppressor gene, requiring biallelic inactivation to drive the emergence of a clinically significant tumor. For example, somatic deletion on 11q13 in a particular parathyroid or islet cell of a patient with MEN1 results in a cell that is devoid of the normal tumor suppressor function of the *MEN1* gene product and thereby confers an actual or potential selective advantage over neighboring cells. The high incidence of endocrine tumors in MEN1 (which demonstrates almost 100% penetrance) implies that this somatic inactivation of the remaining normal gene copy ("second hit") is a common development in the context of the patient's entire endocrine tissue complement. Cells in tissues not affected in MEN1 probably sustain second hits as well but are able to tolerate the menin loss without fostering tumorigenesis,[46] indicating the crucial importance of cell and tissue context in endocrine tumor specificity in this disorder and others. Also, one should not assume that loss of function in both *MEN1* alleles is *sufficient* for tumorigenesis in susceptible tissues; additional cooperating oncogenic lesions are probably needed.[47]

Allelic losses of DNA markers on 11q13, including the *MEN1* region, are found in some of the more common, sporadically occurring versions of the tumors associated with familial MEN1. They include, for example, a frequency of 25% to 40% for 11q13 allelic loss in sporadic parathyroid adenomas. However, most studies have found putatively inactivating mutations of the nondeleted *MEN1* allele in only 12% to 17% of parathyroid adenomas. This gap, which is larger than expected from comparisons with other established tumor suppressors, suggests that another tumor suppressor on 11q may exist and may serve as the target for specific acquired mutation in many of the tumors with 11q allelic loss but an apparently intact remaining *MEN1* allele. However, the possibility remains that *MEN1* is the only 11q tumor suppressor that is relevant in these tumors and that epigenetic or noncoding alterations are disproportionately frequent mechanisms of somatic inactivation of *MEN1.*

HRPT2 Tumor Suppressor Gene

The hereditary hyperparathyroidism–jaw tumor syndrome (HPT-JT) is a rare autosomal dominant predisposition to parathyroid gland neoplasms, ossifying fibromas of the mandible and maxilla, renal abnormalities including cystic lesions and hamartomas, and uterine tumors.[48,49] Based on genetic linkage and positional cloning approaches, the *HRPT2* gene was identified as the source of predisposing germline mutations in the majority of HPT-JT kindreds examined.[50] The remaining 30% to 40% of kindreds most likely also have *HRPT2* mutations that are located outside the sequenced coding region and therefore evade detection. Similar germline mutations occur in a subset of kindreds with familial isolated hyperparathyroidism (FIHP).[51] Mutations of *HRPT2* are predicted to inactivate or eliminate its protein product, parafibromin, again consistent with a tumor suppressor mechanism. Parafibromin's normal cellular function appears to involve regulation of gene expression and chromatin modification as part of the human Paf complex,[52] and its regulatory targets may include cyclin D1.[53]

Hyperparathyroidism is the most penetrant component of HPT-JT, and it can develop as early as the first or second decade of life. Although the inherited mutation puts all of the parathyroid glands at increased risk for tumor development over a patient's lifetime, the tumors can develop asynchronously, and only a solitary parathyroid tumor may be present at the time of initial diagnosis and surgical exploration. Although most such parathyroid tumors are classified as adenomas, parathyroid carcinoma is found in an impressively high proportion (15%) relative to its less than 1% incidence among parathyroid tumors in the general population. This observation led investigators to consider *HRPT2* as a possible target for *somatic* mutations in nonfamilial sporadic cases of parathyroid carcinoma and, indeed, somatic inactivating *HRPT2* mutations were discovered in the majority of sporadic parathyroid carcinomas.[54] Even the impressive combined prevalence of more than 75% in this and subsequent studies is likely to underestimate the true role of *HRPT2* mutation in sporadic parathyroid cancer, because noncoding mutations that are equally capable of inactivating the gene would have escaped detection. Therefore, *HRPT2* mutation is central to the pathogenesis of most, and perhaps all, sporadic parathyroid carcinomas. In contrast, although *HRPT2* was an equally plausible candidate for involvement in benign parathyroid neoplasia, somatic *HRPT2* mutations are rarely, if ever, present in unselected series of typical sporadic parathyroid adenomas.[55]

Importantly and unexpectedly, Shattuck and colleagues also found that some patients with sporadic presentations of parathyroid carcinoma harbor germline mutations in *HRPT2*.[54] Whether such patients represent newly recognized classic HPT-JT or have a distinct syndrome (akin to MEN2A and familial isolated medullary thyroid cancer as alternative expressions of the same *RET* mutation) is unknown, but in any case this molecular genetic insight has yielded a new clinical indication for DNA-based carrier identification in family members of patients with parathyroid cancer, aimed at preventing parathyroid malignancy.

Genetic paradigms that have originated in the study of malignant neoplasia are useful in the molecular dissection of endocrine tumors, including common benign endocrine tumors. Identification of clonally selected mutations in oncogenes and tumor suppressor genes has opened the door to understanding the control of growth in endocrine tissues and has already resulted in important advances in clinical diagnosis and management. Emerging large-scale sequencing technologies will enable the rapid acceleration of this discovery process. The fact that these genetic alterations can affect endocrine cell function as well as cell number may be exploited in devising medical therapies in the future.

REFERENCES

1. Wang TL, Rago C, Silliman N, et al. Prevalence of somatic alterations in the colorectal cancer cell genome. *Proc Natl Acad Sci U S A.* 2002;99:3076-3080.
2. Arnold A, Staunton CE, Kim HG, et al. Monoclonality and abnormal parathyroid hormone genes in parathyroid adenomas. *N Engl J Med.* 1988;318:658-662.
3. Arnold A, Brown MF, Urena P, et al. Monoclonality of parathyroid tumors in chronic renal failure and in primary parathyroid hyperplasia. *J Clin Invest.* 1995;95:2047-2053.
4. Weir B, Zhao X, Meyerson M. Somatic alterations in the human cancer genome. *Cancer Cell.* 2004;6:433-438.
5. Kroll TG, Sarraf P, Pecciarini L, et al. *PAX8-PPARγ1* fusion oncogene in human thyroid carcinoma. *Science.* 2000;289:1357-1360.
6. Stratton MR, Campbell PJ, Futreal PA. The cancer genome. *Nature.* 2009;458:719-724.
7. Levy A, Lightman S. Molecular defects in the pathogenesis of pituitary tumours. *Front Neuroendocrinol.* 2003;24:94-127.
8. van Sande J, Parma J, Tonacchera M, et al. Genetic basis of endocrine disease: somatic and germline mutations of the TSH receptor gene in thyroid diseases. *J Clin Endocrinol Metab.* 1995;80:2577-2585.
9. Arnold A. Genetic basis of endocrine disease 5: molecular genetics of parathyroid gland neoplasia. *J Clin Endocrinol Metab.* 1993;77:1108-1112.
10 Hendy GN, Arnold A. Molecular basis of PTH overexpression. In: Bilezikian JP, Raisz LG, Martin TJ, eds. *Principles of Bone Biology*. 3rd ed. San Diego, CA: Academic Press, 2008:1311-1326.
11. Palanisamy N, Imanishi Y, Rao P, et al. Novel chromosomal abnormalities identified by comparative genomic hybridization in parathyroid adenomas. *J Clin Endocrinol Metab.* 1998;83:1766-1770.
12. Lyon M. Gene action in the X-chromosome of the mouse. *Nature.* 1961;190:372-373.
13. Fialkow PJ. Clonal origin of human tumors. *Biochim Biophys Acta.* 1976;458:283-321.
14. Fialkow PJ, Jackson CE, Block MA, et al. Multicellular origin of parathyroid "adenomas." *N Engl J Med.* 1977;297:696-698.
15. Jackson CE, Cerny JC, Block MA, et al. Probable clonal origin of aldosteronomas versus multicellular origin of parathyroid "adenomas." *Surgery.* 1982;92:875-879.
16. Vogelstein B, Fearon ER, Hamilton SR, et al. Clonal analysis using recombinant DNA probes from the X-chromosome. *Cancer Res.* 1987;47:4806-4813.
17. Shattuck TM, Shattuck TM, Westra WH, et al. Independent clonal origins of distinct tumor foci in multifocal papillary thyroid carcinoma. *N Engl J Med.* 2005;352:2406-2412.
18. Biller BMK, Alexander JM, Zervas NT, et al. Clonal origins of adrenocorticotropin-secreting pituitary tissue in Cushing's disease. *J Clin Endocrinol Metab.* 1992;75:1303-1309.
19. Gicquel C, Le Bouc Y, Luton J-P, et al. Monoclonality of corticotroph macroadenomas in Cushing's disease. *J Clin Endocrinol Metab.* 1992;75:472-475.
20. Mihailescu D, Shore-Freedman E, Mukani S, et al. Multiple neoplasms in an irradiated cohort: pattern of occurrence and relationship to thyroid cancer outcome. *J Clin Endocrinol Metab.* 2002;87:3236-3241.
21. Schneider AB, Ron E, Lubin J, et al. Dose-response relationships for radiation-induced thyroid cancer and thyroid nodules: evidence for the prolonged effects of radiation on the thyroid. *J Clin Endocrinol Metab.* 1993;77:362-369.
22. Cardis E, Kesminiene A, Ivanov V, et al. Risk of thyroid cancer after exposure to ^{131}I in childhood. *J Natl Cancer Inst.* 2005;97:724-732.
23. Haber D, Harlow E. Tumour-suppressor genes: evolving definitions in the genomic age. *Nat Genet.* 1997;16:320-322.
24. Payne SR, Kemp CJ. Tumor suppressor genetics. *Carcinogenesis.* 2005;26:2031-2045.
25. Strauss B. The origin of point mutation in human tumor cells. *Cancer Res.* 1992;52:249-253.
26. O'Neill JP. DNA damage, DNA repair, cell proliferation, and DNA replication: how do gene mutations result? *Proc Natl Acad Sci USA.* 2000;97:11137-11139.
27. MacPhee D. Mismatch repair, somatic mutations, and the origins of cancer. *Cancer Res.* 1995;55:5489-5492.
28. Loeb L. Microsatellite instability: marker of a mutator phenotype in cancer. *Cancer Res.* 1994;54:5059-5063.
29. Lengauer C, Kinzler KW, Vogelstein B. Genetic instabilities in human cancers. *Nature.* 1998;396:643-649.
30. Rubin H. The role of selection in progressive neoplastic transformation. *Adv Cancer Res.* 2001;83:159-207.
31. Tomlinson I, Bodmer W. Selection, the mutation rate and cancer: ensuring that the tail does not wag the dog. *Nat Med.* 1999;5:11-12.
32. Russo D, Arturi F, Suarez HG, et al. Thyrotropin receptor gene alterations in thyroid hyperfunctioning adenomas. *J Clin Endocrinol Metab.* 1996;81:1548-1551.
33. Lyons J, Landis C, Harsh G, et al. Two G protein oncogenes in human endocrine tumors. *Science.* 1990;249:655-659.
34. Wilkes D, McDermott DA, Basson CT. Clinical phenotypes and molecular genetic mechanisms of Carney complex. *Lancet Oncol.* 2005;6:501-508.
35. Bossis I, Stratakis CA. Minireview: PRKAR1A: normal and abnormal functions. *Endocrinology.* 2004;145:545.
36. Motokura T, Bloom T, Kim HG, et al. A novel cyclin encoded by a *bcl1*-linked candidate oncogene. *Nature.* 1991;350:512-515.
37. Arnold A, Papanikolaou A. Biology of neoplasia—cyclin D1 in breast cancer pathogenesis. *J Clin Oncol.* 2005;23:4215-4224.
38. Imanishi Y, Hosokawa Y, Yoshimoto K, et al. Primary hyperparathyroidism caused by parathyroid-targeted overexpression of cyclin D1 in transgenic mice. *J Clin Invest.* 2001;107:1093-1102.

39. Sherr CJ. Cancer cell cycles. *Science*. 1996;274:1672-1677.
40. Tahara H, Smith A, Gaz R, et al. Loss of chromosome arm 9p DNA and analysis of the p16 and p15 cyclin-dependent kinase inhibitor genes in human parathyroid adenomas. *J Clin Endocrinol Metab*. 1996;81: 3663-3667.
41. Pellegata NS, Quintanilla-Martinez L, Siggelkow H, et al. Germ-line mutations in p27Kip1 cause a multiple endocrine neoplasia syndrome in rats and humans. *Proc Natl Acad Sci U S A*. 2006; 103:15558-15563.
42. Chandrasekharappa S, Guru S, Manickam P, et al. Positional cloning of the gene for multiple endocrine neoplasia type 1. *Science*. 1997; 276:404-407.
43. Brandi ML, Gagel RF, Angeli A, et al. Guidelines for diagnosis and therapy of MEN type 1 and type 2. *J Clin Endocrinol Metab*. 2001;86:5658-5671.
44. Agarwal SK, Mateo CM, Marx SJ. Rare germline mutations in cyclin-dependent kinase inhibitor genes in multiple endocrine neoplasia type 1 and related states. *J Clin Endocrinol Metab*. 2009; 94:1826-1834.
45. Gracanin A, Dreijerink KM, van der Luijt RB, et al. Tissue selectivity in multiple endocrine neoplasia type 1-associated tumorigenesis. *Cancer Res*. 2009; 69:6371-6374.
46. Scacheri PC, Crabtree JS, Kennedy AL, et al. Homozygous loss of menin is well tolerated in liver, a tissue not affected in MEN1. *Mamm Genome*. 2004;15:872-877.
47. Crabtree JS, Scacheri PC, Ward JM, et al. Of mice and MEN1: insulinomas in a conditional mouse knockout. *Mol Cell Biol*. 2003;23: 6075-6085.
48. Szabo J, Heath B, Hill VM, et al. Hereditary hyperparathyroidism-jaw tumor syndrome: the endocrine tumor gene *HRPT2* maps to chromosome 1q21-q31. *Am J Hum Genet*. 1995;56:944-950.
49. Bradley KJ, Hobbs MR, Buley ID, et al. Uterine tumours are a phenotypic manifestation of the hyperparathyroidism-jaw tumour syndrome. *J Intern Med*. 2005;257:18-22.
50. Carpten JD, Robbins CM, Villablanca A, et al. *HRPT2*, encoding parafibromin, is mutated in hyperparathyroidism-jaw tumor syndrome. *Nat Genet*. 2002;32:676-680.
51. Simonds WF, Robbins CM, Agarwal SK, et al. Familial isolated hyperparathyroidism is rarely caused by germline mutation in *HRPT2*, the gene for the hyperparathyroidism-jaw tumor syndrome. *J Clin Endocrinol Metab*. 2004;89:96-102.
52. Rozenblatt-Rosen O, Hughes CM, Nannepaga SJ, et al. The parafibromin tumor suppressor protein is part of a human Paf1 complex. *Mol Cell Biol*. 2005;25:612-620.
53. Woodard GE, Lin L, Zhang JH, et al. Parafibromin, product of the hyperparathyroidism-jaw tumor syndrome gene *HRPT2*, regulates cyclin D1/PRAD1 expression. *Oncogene*. 2005;24:1272-1276.
54. Shattuck TM, Valimaki S, Obara T, et al. Somatic and germ-line mutations of the *HRPT2* gene in sporadic parathyroid carcinoma. *N Engl J Med*. 2003;349:1722-1729.
55. Krebs LJ, Shattuck TM, Arnold A. *HRPT2* mutational analysis of typical sporadic parathyroid adenomas. *J Clin Endocrinol Metab*. 2005;90: 5015-5017.

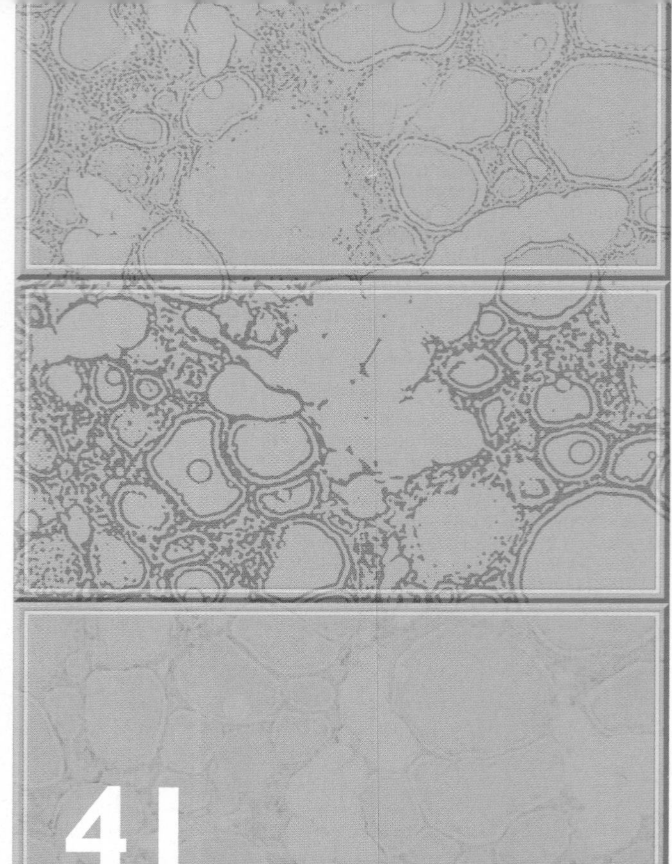

CHAPTER 41

Multiple Endocrine Neoplasia

STEPHEN J. MARX • SAMUEL A. WELLS, JR.

INTRODUCTION TO MULTIPLE ENDOCRINE NEOPLASIA SYNDROMES

The multiple endocrine neoplasia (MEN) syndromes offer special chances for gene discovery and for insights into the broader topics relevant to all endocrine tumors. These possibilities have drawn disproportionate attention to them since their first recognition. The MENs were described in the early 1900s[1] and subsequently classified into two principal categories, MEN type 1 (MEN1) and MEN type 2 (MEN2). They were named *multiple endocrine neoplasia* or *multiple endocrine adenomatosis* syndromes because they cause tumors in two or more types of hormone-secreting tissues and consequently produce multiple syndromes of hormone excess.

From 1950 to 1980, parallel advances in steroid and peptide hormone assays, imaging and histopathology, and connections of genes to cancers led to a fuller delineation of these syndromes. These technologies assisted the recognition that a recurring spectrum of endocrine tumors occurs in certain sporadic cases and in certain families. Furthermore, unique sets of hormones were associated with specific tumors, cell types, and clinical syndromes. Hormone measurements were used to identify specific neoplasms with the hope that earlier management would improve the course. Prominent among these hormones were prolactin to identify adenomas of the pituitary, gastrin and insulin to identify pancreatico-duodenal tumors, catecholamines or their metabolites to identify adrenal medullary tumors, and calcitonin to identify C-cell hyperplasia or C-cell neoplasia.

During this same period, at least six multiple endocrine neoplasia syndromes with several subvariants were described: MEN1, MEN2, von Hippel-Lindau disease (VHL), neurofibromatosis type 1 (NF1), Carney complex (CNC), and McCune-Albright syndrome (MAS).[2-8] The first five of these are present in the germline with autosomal dominant transmission; MAS develops as a result of very early embryonic somatic mutation leading to tumors in multiple cell types. Each of these syndromes meets the definition of multiple endocrine neoplasia with potential for excess production of multiple hormones. What was not completely recognized at the time of their early description is that each of these syndromes also causes nonendocrine neoplasias, and in some cases, the nonendocrine manifestations cause the most morbidity.

This chapter will not provide an in-depth review of the management of nonendocrine manifestations. Since the 1980s, understanding of these syndromes has focused on the main gene associated with each of them. The main genes whose mutations are responsible for each of the six MEN syndromes have been identified, and this has clarified some important questions. Gene identification led rapidly to gene sequencing to detect germline mutations in patients and in their relatives. Mutation testing for *RET* has had a large impact on management in young members of MEN2 families; but identification of the tumors and precursor cells associated with the other genes at very early stages does not easily lead to beneficial treatments.

Gene sequencing has provided molecular evidence that most of the clinical variants of each syndrome are in fact initiated by mutations of a single gene. The only exceptions at present are MEN1 and CNC, in which a second or even more genes at different chromosomal loci remain to be identified. In two other syndromes, VHL and MEN2, specific mutations of the causative genes define unique clinical variants, making genetic information useful for predicting the phenotype. For most of these disorders, mutations of the same gene have been found in sporadic tumors of the same type, indicating a broader importance for these genes in common endocrine and nonendocrine neoplasias. Examples include the identification of somatic mutations of *MEN1* in a high percentage of common pancreatic islet tumors, *VHL* mutations in sporadic renal cell carcinomas, and somatic mutations of *RET* in sporadic medullary thyroid carcinomas (MTCs).

The genetic and molecular abnormalities in these tumor syndromes are representative of the abnormalities found in all human neoplasia: MEN1, VHL, CNC, and NF1 are caused by inactivating mutations of a growth suppressor gene, whereas MAS and MEN2 are caused by activating mutations of a growth promoter gene. In at least one of these syndromes, MEN2, the identification of the molecular defect has led to the development of pharmacologic agents that may blunt the molecular abnormalities and to clinical trials to reverse malignant tumor growth.

This chapter describes tumor expression, tumor management, and genetics of MEN1. Data on the molecular pathway from the *MEN1* gene are not yet sufficient to apply to management. In contrast, data on genetics, and molecular pathway are covered early in the section on MEN2, because both the *RET* gene and its molecular pathway have achieved a central role in management.

Progress has been extremely rapid during the current era of gene discovery, and further exciting discoveries are expected shortly. Still, a number of important questions remain: How do the molecular defects cause transformation? What is the mechanism of cell or tissue specificity? Are there molecular events that can be used as therapeutic targets?

MULTIPLE ENDOCRINE NEOPLASIA TYPE I SYNDROME

MEN1 is defined by the presence of two of the following three tumors: parathyroid, duodeno-pancreatic endocrine, and pituitary. Although there were earlier descriptions,[1] MEN1 was recognized as a clinical and familial syndrome by Moldawer[3] and by Wermer[4] in 1954 (hence, the eponym *Wermer syndrome*). MEN2 was recognized as distinct from MEN1 in 1968.[7] In previous years, MEN1 patients presented with advanced manifestations of parathyroid, pancreatic islet, or pituitary neoplasia (or some combination of these) in the third and fourth decades of life. However, improved carrier ascertainment and improved tumor surveillance have now resulted in earlier identification and earlier treatment of its hormonal expressions.

The most common mode of presentation for MEN1 is in a previously identified kindred; less often, a patient with newly diagnosed disease may be the propositus of a new kindred or a sporadic case. The fact that many tissues are affected causes morbidity and complexity and increases expense in diagnosis and treatment. It is important for the clinician to recognize the high probability of recurrent or new neoplasms in many affected organ systems and to balance this likelihood against the potential effects of a deficiency syndrome resulting from complete organ removal. Furthermore, even with satisfactory control of symptoms from hormone excess, patients have a high likelihood of eventual MEN1-related cancer.

Tumor Expression and Management

Parathyroid Tumors in MEN1

MEN1 is uncommon. The population prevalence is about 1 in 30,000, and MEN1 accounts for only about 1% to 3% of cases of primary hyperparathyroidism (HPT).[9] HPT is the most common hormonal manifestation of MEN1 (Table 41-1).[6,9,10-13] Prospective tumor surveillance in members of MEN1 families has shown manifestation of HPT as early as age 8 years[10-12,14-18]; by age 40 years, about 95% of MEN1 carriers have been hyperparathyroid.[10,12,19]

Expressions of Parathyroid Tumors. HPT in MEN1 is most commonly asymptomatic; expressions include hypercalcemia, urolithiasis, parathyroid hormone (PTH)-induced bone abnormalities, musculoskeletal complaints, weakness, and alterations of mental status. These features are similar to those associated with other forms of HPT (see Chapter 28).

HPT in MEN1 differs in some ways from that caused by a sporadic adenoma. First, there is a different epidemiology. HPT in MEN1 has an earlier age of onset (typically age 25 years), compared with sporadic parathyroid adenoma (55 years)[12,13] (Fig. 41-1), and there is a lack of the female preponderance seen in sporadic cases (1:1 versus 3:1 female-to-male ratio, respectively). Earlier onset implies that the disease can last longer. In particular, bone undermineralization among women with MEN1-related HPT seems increased already during their 20s and 30s.[20]

Second, there is a different parathyroid pathology. Enlargement, albeit highly asymmetric, of three or four parathyroid glands is usually present at the time of parathyroid exploration in patients with MEN1 (Fig. 41-2).[21,22]

Third, the distribution of outcomes after parathyroid surgery differs in MEN1 and in sporadic HPT. The presence of multiglandular disease and the resulting need to examine each gland during an initial operation result in a higher postoperative rate of hypoparathyroidism and a higher rate of postoperative hyperparathyroidism.[21,22] Successful subtotal parathyroidectomy is followed within 10 years by recurrent HPT in half of MEN1 cases.[21,23] True recurrence in common HPT is unusual, and recurrence should suggest the possibility of unrecognized MEN1. As with other tumor recurrences in MEN1, true recurrent HPT could arise theoretically from a small remnant of

TABLE 41-1

Features of Multiple Endocrine Neoplasia Type 1 in Adults

Tumor Type	Estimated Average Penetrance
Endocrine Features	
Parathyroid	
Adenoma	95
Pancreatico-Duodenal	
Gastrinoma	40
Insulinoma	10
Nonfunctioning (including pancreatic polypeptidoma)*	20
Other (e.g., glucagonoma, VIPoma)	each <1
Foregut Carcinoid	
Thymic carcinoid nonfunctioning	2
Bronchial carcinoid nonfunctioning	4
Gastric enterochromaffin-like tumor nonfunctioning	10
Anterior Pituitary	10
Prolactinoma	25
Other	
Nonfunctioning	10
Growth hormone + prolactin	10
Growth hormone	5
ACTH	2
Thyrotropin	5
Adrenal	
Cortex	
Nonfunctioning	30
Functioning or cancer	2
Medulla (pheochromocytoma)	<1
Nonendocrine Features	
Angiofibroma	85
Collagenoma	70
Lipoma	30
Leiomyoma including uterine	25
Meningioma	5

Italics indicate tumor type with substantial (>20% of cases) malignant potential.

*Many nonfunctioning MEN1 tumors synthesize a peptide hormone or other factors (e.g., small amine) but do not oversecrete enough to produce a hormonal expression.

ACTH, adrenocorticotropic hormone; MEN, multiple endocrine neoplasia; VIP, vasoactive intestinal peptide.

tumor tissue or from a new tumor clone in residual normal tissue.

Fourth, HPT in MEN1 almost never progresses to parathyroid cancer, even though untreated HPT lasts longer in MEN1 than in sporadic cases.[24]

Several characteristics of hyperfunctioning parathyroid cells in MEN1 can have mechanistic implications. First, all or almost all parathyroid glands have been overgrown by one or a few neoplastic clones by the time of parathyroid surgery in MEN1 (Fig. 41-3, *top*).[25] Second, a circulating growth factor is specific to the plasma of MEN1 patients and is mitogenic toward normal parathyroid cells in vitro[26] (see later discussion).

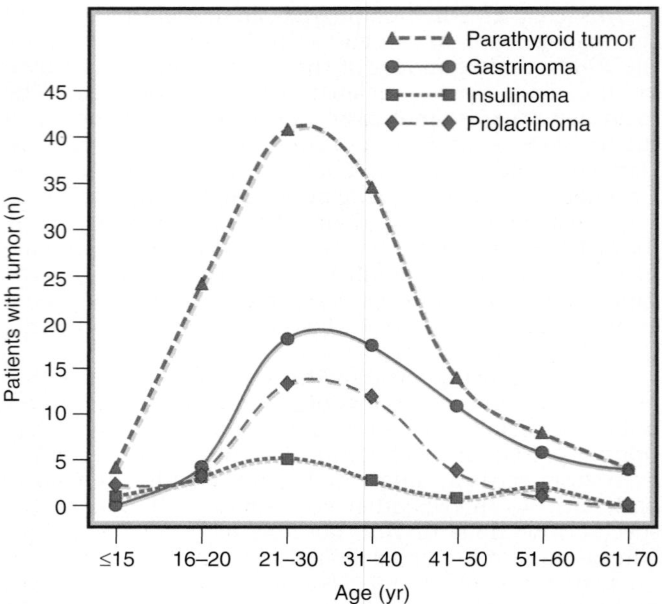

Figure 41-1 Age at onset for endocrine tumor expressions in multiple endocrine neoplasia type 1 (MEN1). Data from retrospective analysis of multiple tumor expressions in 130 inpatients with MEN1 during 15 years. Age at tumor onset was defined as the age at first symptom or at first abnormal test result, whichever was earlier. (Modified from Marx S, Spiegel AM, Skarulis MC, et al. Multiple endocrine neoplasia type 1: clinical and genetic topics. *Ann Intern Med.* 1998;129:484-494.)

Management of Parathyroid Tumors

Decision for Surgery. Surgery is the treatment of choice for HPT in MEN1, although the timing and the type of operation remain variable. Parathyroid surgery is definitely indicated in an MEN1 patient with a moderately elevated PTH and other moderately advanced features, such as an albumin-adjusted serum calcium level higher than

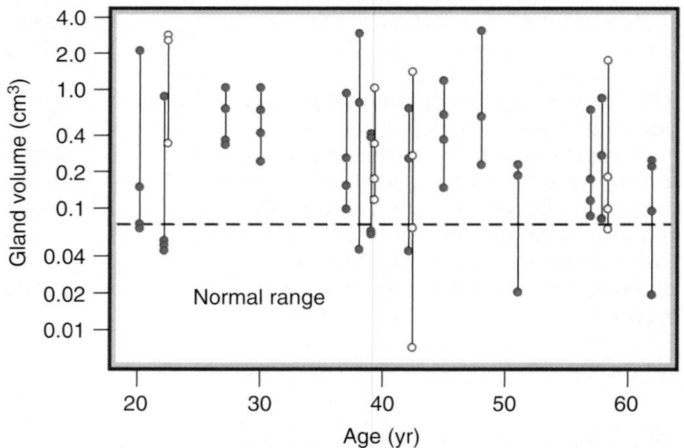

Figure 41-2 Parathyroid gland size at initial parathyroidectomy for 18 cases with familial multiple endocrine neoplasia type 1. The mean ratio of largest versus smallest tumor at one operation was 9:1. Volumes of all glands at one operation are connected by a *vertical line*. Adjacent circles are highlighted by being open. The *dashed horizontal line* represents the upper limit of normal gland volume (0.075 cm^3, equivalent to a mass of 75 mg). (Modified from Marx SJ, Menczel J, Campbell G, et al. Heterogeneous size of the parathyroid glands in familial multiple endocrine neoplasia type 1. *Clin Endocrinol [Oxf].* 1991; 35:521-526.)

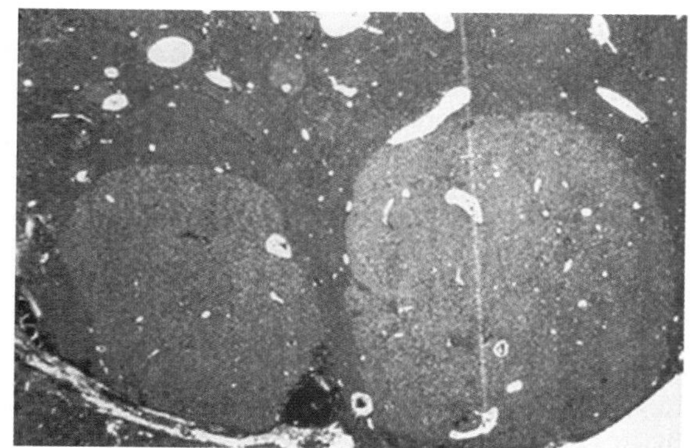

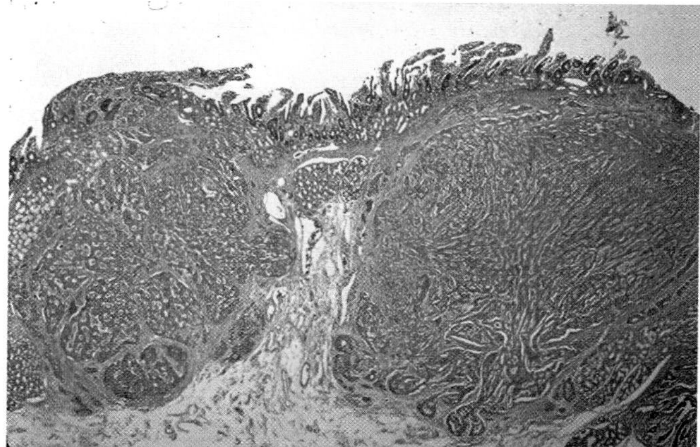

Figure 41-3 Tumor multiplicity within a tissue in multiple endocrine neoplasia type 1 (MEN1). *Top*, Hypercellular parathyroid gland from a patient with MEN1. The gland section is totally replaced by diffuse sheets of chief cells and two discrete nodules of chief cells. It suggests three or more abnormal parathyroid clones. This image could reflect three or more second hits to the normal copy of the *MEN1* gene in three different clone precursor cells, followed by growth of three or more independent clones. Alternatively, stepwise evolution from one clone could occur (i.e., third hits to genes other than *MEN1*). *Bottom*, Duodenal mucosa from a second MEN1 patient, showing two large submucosal microgastrinomas. Each tumor was positive for gastrin immunostain and negative for other peptide hormones. Possible development of these two adjacent tumors could have followed the same mechanisms suggested for the two parathyroid nodules at the top. (Microphotographs from I. Lubensky, National Institutes of Health, Bethesda, MD.)

3.0 mmol/L (12.0 mg/dL), kidney stones, or PTH-induced bone disease.

Prospective surveillance for HPT in MEN1 families has led to systematic identification of affected members with minimal elevations of serum calcium and PTH, including some as young as 8 to 15 years of age. The optimal management of such patients is not clear. The surgical indication of age younger than 50 years for common HPT cannot be applied to all cases of HPT in MEN1.[27]

Early parathyroid surgery in MEN1 has been advocated by some, who believe that HPT should always be treated as early as possible for several reasons such as that normalization of the serum calcium concentration might lead to a reduction of gastrin secretion and, possibly, lowered pancreatic islet cell growth or transformation, or both.[9] An opposite approach is to delay surgery awaiting more severe indications, and thereby assuring an easier parathyroidectomy.

Although parathyroidectomy can decrease gastrin secretion by gastrinomas in MEN1 (Fig. 41-4), there is no evidence that this intervention prevents or slows gastrin-cell growth transformation.[28] For this reason, and because drug control of gastric acid oversecretion is usually excellent, the coexistence of a gastrinoma is not a sufficient indication for parathyroidectomy in MEN1, except in the rare case in which medical control of Zollinger-Ellison syndrome (ZES) is too difficult.

Preoperative and Intraoperative Assessment of Parathyroid Tumors. Noninvasive imaging (ultrasonography, technetium 99m sestamibi, computed tomography, magnetic resonance imaging, or combinations) is being performed with increasing frequency before parathyroid surgery.[29] The major justification for the added costs of these procedures in sporadic HPT is the ability to perform a unilateral or even more limited neck exploration, thereby reducing operative morbidity, time, and cost.[30] In MEN1 the likely presence of multiple parathyroid tumors makes it necessary to perform an exploration for four or more tumors at initial surgery, thereby eliminating one major rationale for preoperative imaging.[9] Furthermore, imaging rarely shows all of the overactive parathyroid glands in MEN1. A separate, and less frequent, concern is that if four glands are overactive, as in MEN1, then there is a fourfold greater possibility that one tumor has an abnormal location. A much stronger case can be made for the use of noninvasive and carefully selected invasive procedures (e.g., guided fine-needle aspiration for PTH assay, computed tomography, selective arteriography, selective venous sampling for PTH) in MEN1 patients before reoperation.[31,32]

Several intraoperative tools can increase the likelihood of successful parathyroid surgery. Rapid on-line assay of PTH can be done at 5-minute intervals, with a turnaround time of 10 minutes for each result.[33-35] A substantial PTH fall from baseline predicts that no hyperfunctioning parathyroid tissue remains (Fig. 41-5). This is useful information particularly if multiple tumors are likely. Multiple tumors are almost always present at initial surgery in MEN1, and they are even common at many reoperations for MEN1. These tests are even more likely to be helpful

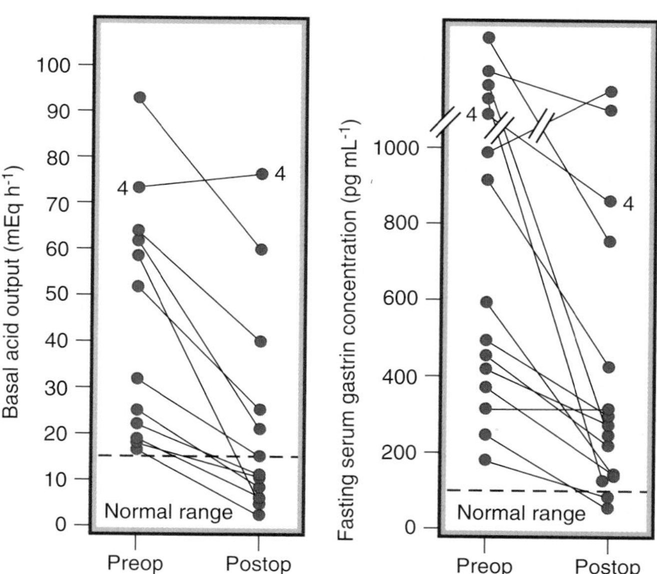

Figure 41-4 Effect of parathyroidectomy in patients with both multiple endocrine neoplasia type 1 and Zollinger-Ellison syndrome. Basal acid output and fasting serum gastrin are shown. All patients became normocalcemic except for one (case 4), who remained hypercalcemic. (From Jensen RT. Management of the Zollinger-Ellison syndrome in patients with multiple endocrine neoplasia type 1. *J Intern Med.* 1998;243:477-488.)

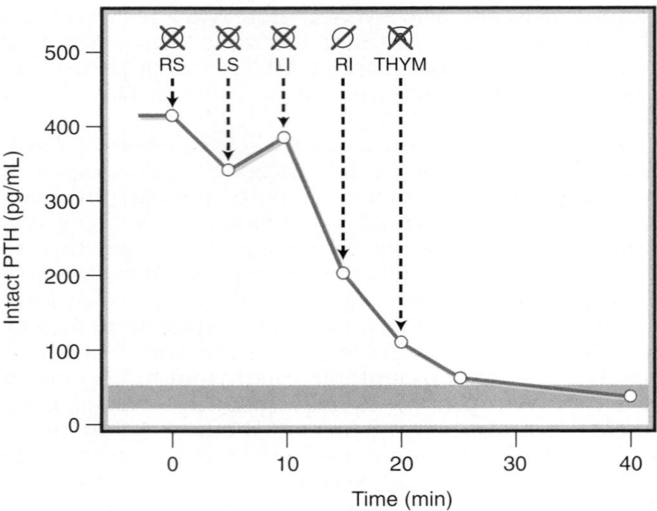

Figure 41-5 Intact parathyroid hormone (PTH) by rapid assay during parathyroid surgery. Normal range is indicated by the *shaded area*. The patient had multiple endocrine neoplasia type I and primary hyperparathyroidism without prior parathyroidectomy. Three and one half similarly enlarged parathyroid glands (0.8 to 1.6 g; normal, <0.08 g) and the accessible portions of the thymus (THYM) were removed at the times indicated; the thymus contained no identified parathyroid tumor. A rapid fall of PTH below a cutoff criterion indicates that little or no hyperfunctioning parathyroid tumor remains. Removal of the first two parathyroid tumors was not followed by a fall in PTH. The PTH assay result for each time point was available within several minutes to help establish the time at which no hyperfunctioning parathyroid tumor remained and thereby contribute to serial decisions about extending or ending the operation. I, inferior; L, left; R, right; S, superior. (From S.K. Libutti, H.R. Alexander, and A. Remaley, National Institutes of Health, Bethesda, MD.)

during parathyroid reoperations in MEN1, because the number and locations of tumors during a second operation are particularly hard to predict. Sensitive ultrasound transducers routinely provide intraoperative imaging of parathyroid tumors in difficult locations, such as within the thyroid gland or within scar from prior surgery.[29] Intraoperative PTH assay and ultrasonography may be useful as backup options at initial parathyroid surgery, particularly in any patient who is expected to have multiple parathyroid tumors (as in MEN1).

Removal of Parathyroid Tumors. The standard surgical approach for initial parathyroidectomy in MEN1 is removal of 3.5 glands and conservation of approximately 50 mg of the most normal-appearing gland, attached to its vascular pedicle in the neck. Because eventual parathyroid reoperation in MEN1 is likely, the recording of careful operative notes and diagrams and the marking of remaining tissue with nonresorbable materials enhance the likelihood of success in subsequent operations.

An alternative is attempted complete removal of all parathyroid tissue from the neck and immediate autotransplantation of small fragments to pockets in the nondominant forearm.[36] This strategy is dependent on the likelihood of achieving a high rate of graft success. This technique does not prevent recurrent HPT but can simplify its management. A PTH concentration in the venous effluent of the graft that is greater than in the effluent from the contralateral arm confirms graft function. However, this does not prove graft hyperfunction, and it does not exclude other parathyroid tissue in the neck or chest. Surgical removal of parathyroid tissue from the forearm graft bed during the likely second or third operation is technically easier than a neck reexploration. Cryopreservation of parathyroid tumor fragments is a useful option at any operation in MEN1, given the high rate of postoperative hypoparathyroidism. Cryopreservation permits a late parathyroid autograft.[36] Parathyroid cryopreservation in the United States is discouraged by regulatory considerations.

Partial thymectomy can be performed through the cervical incision. This procedure not only results in removal of intrathymic parathyroid tissue but also can remove thymic carcinoid tissue, an issue discussed later in this chapter. The best time for this is during the initial neck operation, because scar tissue can prevent a simple transcervical thymectomy at reoperation.

Parathyroid surgery in patients with MEN1 requires judgment, familiarity with neck anatomy, and experience. An excellent outcome is more likely when initial or reoperative procedures are performed by an experienced endocrine surgery team.

Pancreatico-Duodenal Neuroendocrine Tumors

Neoplasia of the pancreatico-duodenal neuroendocrine cells is the second most common endocrine manifestation of MEN1 and eventually is expressed in about 60% of MEN1 patients (see Table 41-1). Also, multiple clinically silent pancreatico-duodenal macroadenomas may be recognized at abdominal surgery or autopsy in almost 100% of MEN1 patients older than 40 years.[37,38] Gastric carcinoid tumors are described later (see "Foregut Carcinoid Tumors"). The pancreatico-duodenal tumors are multiple, can oversecrete various hormones, and can become malignant. Approximately one third of MEN1 patients die from a MEN1-related cancer, particularly gastrinoma; among these fatal cancers, the ratio of hormonal cancer to malignant carcinoid is 2 : 1.[39,40] In this era of excellent pharmacotherapy for gastric hyperacidity, about one sixth of MEN1 patients with gastrinoma die from metastatic gastrinoma, but deaths from hypergastrinemia-induced metabolic complications have become rare.[41]

Although MEN1 patients can show symptoms or signs caused by one pancreatico-duodenal hormone, there are often several associated and asymptomatic near by tumors with production of the same or other hormones or no hormone.[42,43] The frequency of peptide immunostaining in MEN1 pancreatic islet tumors is as follows: glucagon, 35%; insulin, 25%; pancreatic polypeptide, 25%; and no hormone, 10%. There are no data on the comparable frequency in duodenal gastrinomas.[42-44]

Interpretation of pancreatic islet histology in MEN1 has changed over the decades. Early studies emphasized hyperplastic processes and budding of islet cells from ducts (nesidioblastosis).[45] Such features have now been reinterpreted as nonspecific in MEN1. The overriding and important islet lesion in MEN1, now termed *multifocal microadenoma,*[42] is a monoclonal or oligoclonal process (see Fig. 41-3).[46,47] Molecular evidence is also accumulating for a hyperplastic precursor stage to tumor. Hyperplastic foci of gastrin cells are seen by light microscopy in the duodenum of gastrinoma specimens from MEN1 but not from sporadic gastrinoma.[48] Furthermore, heterozygous knockout of the *MEN1* gene in the mouse provides a good model of human MEN1; multiple giant hyperplastic islets compesed of beta cells are striking and precede insulinoma in this model, suggesting that unrecognized islet hyperplasia is an undetected islet tumor precursor lesion also in MEN1 of humans.[49] Because MEN1 cases often have multiple islet macroadenomas and some with differing hormonal properties, tumor imaging has roles different from those in sporadic islet tumor. Sensitive new imaging methods such as endoscopic ultrasound and fluorine

18–labeled L-dihydroxyphenylalanine positron emission tomography ([^{18}F]-DOPA PET) may achieve roles that remain to be defined.

Rarely, pancreatico-duodenal neuroendocrine tumors occur in several members of a family without other features of MEN1; these have been insulinomas.[50] Nonfunctioning pancreatic islet tumors and pheochromocytoma can also appear uncommonly in a familial setting as expressions of VHL syndrome.[51]

Gastrinoma

Expressions of Gastrinoma. Gastrinoma is the second most common endocrine tumor and the most common cause of severe symptoms and signs in MEN1. The symptoms and signs reflect two processes, malignancy and gastrin induction of excessive acid secretion by the stomach. Gastrinomas are found in about 40% of adults with MEN1 (see Table 41-1).[9,12,28] ZES is defined here as symptoms or signs of gastric acid hypersecretion caused by a gastrin-secreting pancreatico-duodenal neuroendocrine tumor or tumors. Among all patients with ZES, MEN1 is found often, on the order of 25% in large series.[52] MEN1 in most of these patients is readily recognizable from personal and family history. In contrast, among carefully defined sporadic ZES cases without obvious MEN1, occult MEN1 is much less frequent; this conclusion is based on family history, long-term follow-up, and mutational analysis of the *MEN1* gene.[53]

Symptoms of ZES include diarrhea, esophageal reflux, and those symptoms associated with peptic ulceration. Symptoms can antedate recognition of fasting hypergastrinemia. At one extreme, ulcer perforation can be caused infrequently by hypergastrinemia, even without prior symptoms.[54] The laboratory diagnosis of gastrinoma is mainly made by finding an elevated serum gastrin level. Other causes of elevated gastrin (false-positive results) that must be differentiated from gastrinoma include hypochlorhydria resulting from autoimmunity or from pharmacologic agents that inhibit peptic acid secretion.[55] HPT in MEN1 often exacerbates hypergastrinemia (see earlier discussion and Fig. 41-4).

The first recognition of elevated gastrin or acid-related symptoms should be followed by assessment of the gastric acid secretion rate without acid-blocking drugs; the normal rate is less than 15 mEq/hour (or <5 mEq/hour after acid-reducing surgery).[55] The diagnosis of gastrinoma may also be confirmed by measuring the serum gastrin response to intravenous synthetic secretin. A gastrin increase of more than 114 pmol/L (200 pg/mL) diagnoses gastrinoma. This test differentiates gastrinoma from other hypergastrinemic states, such as retained gastric antrum, massive small bowel resection, or gastric outlet obstruction. Gastric endoscopy and ultrasonography are advisable at the initial evaluation for ZES in MEN1 to allow assessment of associated peptic ulcerations, gastric carcinoids, duodenal gastrinomas, and Barrett esophagus. Other imaging modalities should also be used to search for gastric carcinoids, which are common in MEN1 (see later discussion).[56]

Like parathyroid adenomas, gastrinomas have two features that are relatively specific for MEN1. One is earlier age at onset than in sporadic tumors. On average, gastrinoma begins 10 years earlier in patients with MEN1 than in those without it—a lesser age differential than the 30 years difference for HPT.[57] The second feature is multifocal tumor. The gastrinomas in MEN1 are often small, multiple, and intraduodenal (see Fig. 41-3, *bottom*).[44] The duodenal predominance is only modestly greater than that in sporadic gastrinoma.[31,58]

Gastrinomas in MEN1 have a high propensity to metastasize to local nodes.[28] High-grade aggressive behavior, including distant spread to the liver and occasionally to other tissues, also occurs in about 20% of cases. Diffuse hepatic metastases are particularly ominous, predicting a 5-year survival rate of only 50%.[41] The prognosis of gastrinoma in MEN1 is similar to that in sporadic cases.[41] No early features have allowed reliable prediction of which gastrinomas will behave aggressively.[59]

Therapy for Gastrinoma. Most centers have reported almost zero success with attempted surgical cure of gastrinoma in MEN1, even though one third of gastrinoma patients without MEN1 are cured by surgery.[58,60] Unique characteristics of gastrinoma in MEN1 that contribute to the low rate of curative resection are the multiplicity of small tumors and the frequency of local metastases. The largest tumor was not a gastrinoma in 40% of operations for gastrinoma in MEN1. Extreme approaches, mainly pancreatico-duodenectomy, have been suggested,[61] but long-term benefit is unproven, and the associated potential for surgically induced morbidity seems unacceptable. Only three groups have reported frequent surgical cure of gastrinoma by pancreatico-duodenectomy in MEN1.[62-64] Other groups have not reported similar success rates despite the use of similar approaches.[58] Differences in the criteria for cure and in the selection of patients (e.g., patient age) can contribute to the differences in outcome.

The development of histamine H_2 receptor antagonists (cimetidine and ranitidine) and subsequently of proton pump inhibitors (PPIs; omeprazole and other members of this class) has made it possible to perform a pharmacologic gastrectomy for ZES.[55,65] The PPIs are even more effective than the H_2 receptor antagonists. If compliance is good, the need for surgical total gastrectomy is eliminated.[66,67] Side effects, including those from achlorhydria, are mild. Gastric carcinoids develop in rats given large doses of PPIs.[68] Gastric carcinoids are also seen in MEN1,[69] but the PPIs do not seem to exacerbate them in MEN1. There remains disagreement about whether the PPIs worsen enterochromaffin-like cell hyperplasia in sporadic ZES.[63,70,71] The somatostatin analogue octreotide partially inhibits the secretion of both gastrin and gastric acid[72] and is under evaluation for a role in malignant gastrinoma.[73] In addition, the gastrin-lowering effect of somatostatin analogues might contribute to their effective suppression of gastric carcinoid mass in MEN1.[74]

Although medical therapy for ZES in MEN1 is effective and preferred, the need for lifetime medical therapy, the recognition that small duodenal gastrinomas cause a high percentage of cases, and the poor outcome (50% 5-year survival rate) in patients with hepatic metastasis require frequent reexamination of treatment choices.

Insulinoma. Insulinoma is the second most common hormone-secreting pancreatico-duodenal neuroendocrine tumor in MEN1, with lifetime prevalence of 10% among adults with MEN1 (see Table 41-1).[12,13] MEN1 accounts for approximately 10% of all patients with insulinoma.[14] The clinical features and diagnostic criteria are the same in MEN1 and in sporadic cases: glucopenic symptoms and fasting hypoglycemia with high insulin, C peptide, or proinsulin (see Chapter 34). Insulinoma syndrome in MEN1 is usually caused by a single dominant and benign pancreatic islet tumor, although simultaneous nonhypersecreting islet tumors that stain for insulin or another gut hormone are common in MEN1. The main insulinoma is typically 2 to 3 cm in diameter and located anywhere in the pancreas. Removal of the largest islet tumor is usually curative.[13]

Rarely, insulinoma syndrome in MEN1 is caused by more than one tumor, either at one time or sequentially. The postoperative recurrence rate of insulinoma may be higher in MEN1 than in sporadic cases. In theory, recurrent insulinoma in MEN1 may arise after 10% of operations; this is from residual tumor or from a new clone.

The preferred treatment is surgical removal of the insulinoma. Other incidental pancreatic islet macroadenomas should also be removed because of the possibility that one may be a hypersecreting insulinoma that could become malignant. Somatostatin receptor scintigraphy (SRS) can provide 30% to 60% true-positive images.[75] When surgery is performed with guidance only by intraoperative ultrasonography,[76,77] the success rate should be satisfactory, although no large series has yet documented this outcome in insulinoma of MEN1. In some centers, routine distal pancreatectomy is performed as an adjunct procedure in MEN1 patients for prevention of other tumors.

Several techniques, based on insulin radioimmunoassay, can be useful for localization of an insulinoma in patients with MEN1. These include infusion of calcium into selectively catheterized pancreatic arteries with measurement of insulin in right or left hepatic venous effluent.[78] Identification of an insulin peak after an intra-arterial calcium infusion localizes the insulinoma to the distribution of the infused artery. Other tests that have been useful include intraoperative rapid measurement of insulin and glucose levels in serum[79] or intraoperative insulin levels in fine-needle aspirates of a pancreatic tumor (S.K. Libutti, et al., National Institutes of Health, Bethesda, MD, unpublished observation).

Metastatic insulinoma causing hypoglycemia should be treated surgically for palliation, but operative strategies are not likely to be curative.[80,81] Hypoglycemia caused by unlocated or metastatic insulinoma can be controlled with diazoxide[81]; somatostatin analogues are less effective.[82]

Tumors Secreting Glucagon, Vasoactive Intestinal Peptide, or Other Hormones

Glucagonoma. The glucagonoma syndrome consists of hyperglycemia, anorexia, glossitis, anemia, diarrhea, venous thrombosis, and a characteristic skin rash termed *necrolytic migratory erythema* (see Chapter 39). Glucagonoma syndrome is rare in MEN1,[83] although one third of MEN1 pancreatico-duodenal neuroendocrine tumors immunostain for glucagon.[43] Glucagonoma is in MEN1 usually large and metastatic at presentation. Palliation is often possible with surgery or another ablative procedure (see later discussion). Some patients have responded partially to the somatostatin analogue octreotide, although an initial response has not predicted a long-term response.[84]

VIPoma. Although the most common cause of diarrhea in MEN1 is gastrinoma, a separate syndrome is caused by oversecretion of vasoactive intestinal peptide (VIP) and is termed WDHA (watery diarrhea, hypokalemia, and achlorhydria) or VIPoma syndrome[85] (see Chapter 29). In MEN1, it is rare and can occur with pancreatico-duodenal neuroendocrine tumor.[83] Half of such tumors also cause hypercalcemia, perhaps by cosecreting PTH-related peptide[86]; of course, coexistent primary HPT is common in patients with MEN1. The tumor is usually malignant, large, and metastatic at presentation. Treatment considerations are the same as for glucagonoma (see later discussion).

Growth Hormone–Releasing Hormone Oversecretion. Oversecretion of growth hormone–releasing hormone (GHRH) is a rare manifestation of a pancreatico-duodenal neuroendocrine tumor; however, half of such cases are found in patients with MEN1 (see later discussion).[87] GHRH oversecretion can also occur with bronchial carcinoid in MEN1.[88]

Other Ectopic Hormones. Other peptides that may rarely be oversecreted by pancreatico-duodenal neuroendocrine tumors in MEN1 include ACTH, PTH-related peptide,[86] somatostatin,[89] and calcitonin.[90] Calcitonin oversecretion can cause confusion with thyroidal C-cell cancer, but serum calcitonin levels are usually higher in C-cell cancer than in MEN1 cancers.

Pancreatic Polypeptide–Secreting and Other Nonfunctional Tumors. One third of pancreatico-duodenal neuroendocrine tumors in MEN1 immunostain mainly for pancreatic polypeptide; similar percentages immunostain mainly for insulin or for glucagon.[42,43] Pancreatico-duodenal neuroendocrine tumors in MEN1 commonly also oversecrete pancreatic polypeptide.[91,92] Oversecretion of pancreatic polypeptide is not associated with any identifiable hormonal syndrome. Like other nonfunctional pancreatico-duodenal neuroendocrine tumors in MEN1, these are often large, malignant, and metastatic at presentation.[83]

Nonfunctional tumor is an abused but convenient term. In the context of MEN1, it is applied to pancreatico-duodenal neuroendocrine tumors, anterior pituitary tumors, or foregut carcinoids that do not immunostain for the common hormones of that tissue or that immunostain for one or more hormones but do not hypersecrete the hormone. Most pancreatico-duodenal tumors in MEN1 fit this definition,[38] are only microscopic and most never become a clinical problem. Of course, one oversecreting tumor is sufficient to dominate the clinical features. If a nonfunctioning tumor becomes malignant, its lack of symptomatic hormone hypersecretion can allow progression to an advanced stage before recognition. About 5% of islet or duodenal tumors in MEN1 immunostain for somatostatin without clinical expression; these tumors rarely metastasize.[89]

Staging of Pancreatico-Duodenal Neuroendocrine Tumors. Appropriate management of pancreatico-duodenal neuroendocrine tumors in MEN1 is challenging because of the multicentric nature of the tumors and the need to decide between surgical and other approaches. A pancreatico-duodenal tumor causing a hormone excess state in MEN1 is likely to be accompanied by one or more nonfunctional tumors. Much of the experience acquired with imaging of sporadic tumors of the same types cannot be generalized to MEN1 tumors. Accurate localization of tumor and, in particular, identification of metastatic disease is critical for preoperative decision making. The multicentricity and variable size of these tumors stretch the limitations of radiologic techniques that have difficulty imaging tumors smaller than 1 cm in diameter, and their rarity has prevented organization of controlled trials.

SRS imaging (^{111}In-octreotide scan) enhanced by single-photon emission computed tomography (SPECT) is a useful method for imaging pancreatico-duodenal neuroendocrine and foregut neuroendocrine tumors.[58,93,94] It can image primary tumors and local or distant metastases.[95,96] It is particularly useful for multiple gastrinomas in MEN1,[97,98] and it has replaced most angiographic procedures in MEN1-associated gastrinoma.[58,99,100] SRS fails to image one third of lesions identified at surgery even in sporadic gastrinoma.[100] The yield of SRS with sporadic insulinoma is somewhat lower than with other pancreatic islet tumors, with 30% to 60% true-positives.[76] Abdominal imaging by computed tomography (particularly helical),[101,102] combined with early-phase images after contrast injection or magnetic resonance imaging, provides enhanced sensitivity for detection of small lesions and is complementary to SRS.[58,103] Carbon 11–labeled 5-hydroxytryptophan PET scanning is a relatively new method; it and ^{18}F-DOPA PET are generally more sensitive than SRS, but neither has been explored in MEN1.[104,105]

No imaging technique used for evaluation of MEN1 pancreatico-duodenal tumors is completely satisfactory. Endoscopic ultrasonography with or without needle aspiration of a pancreatic mass is useful for characterizing very small pancreatico-duodenal abnormalities but is a technically demanding and expensive option for the foreseeable future.[106,107] With the exception of endoscopic ultrasonography, the current preoperative imaging methods are not able to image tumors that are confined to the pancreas and smaller than 1.5 cm in diameter. They also fail to identify metastases in 25% of cases and the extent of tumor multiplicity in MEN1 cases.[94] In contrast, intraoperative ultrasonography is a useful tool for localizing small tumors that are not detectable by the eye or fingers of the surgeon. This technique has become the primary approach for diagnosis of small insulinomas in most medical centers, although reports have been limited to sporadic tumors.[76,108]

Functional (i.e., insulin-specific) testing can be useful to assess insulinoma because, unlike other pancreatico-duodenal neuroendocrine tumors in MEN1, insulinoma may be symptomatic when it is small and solitary (see earlier discussion).

Serum markers in MEN1, mainly chromogranin-A, provide useful diagnostic tools for monitoring the mass of an pancreatico-duodenal tumor.[109] Chromogranin-A has not been helpful in insulinoma, perhaps because of the small tumor mass.[110] Chromogranin-A and gastrin as possible tumor markers also have not been reliable indices of gastrinoma extent or progression.[111]

Treatment of Pancreatico-Duodenal Neuroendocrine Tumors. Aspects of treatment specific to gastrinomas and insulinomas in MEN1 have already been described. Treatment of these and other pancreatico-duodenal neuroendocrine tumors in MEN1 is controversial and is guided in part by staging procedures and local preferences. Some of the controversies are highlighted in the following paragraphs.

Is Tumor Size Important? Metastasis has been associated with gastrinomas larger than 3 cm in diameter. This association has led some to recommend resection for all pancreatico-duodenal tumors larger than 2.5 cm.[112] However, another analysis of this strategy suggested a failure to prevent later emergence of hepatic metastases.[113] Some others have not found a relation between tumor size and metastasis and do not use a size criterion for surgery.[114]

Should All Pancreatico-Duodenal Neuroendocrine Tumors in MEN1 Be Removed? There is no consensus on whether all pancreatico-duodenal neuroendocrine tumors in patients with MEN1 should be removed. In MEN1, for every identifiable pancreatic tumor, there are likely to be several smaller, unidentified tumors that coexist or emerge at a later date. Improvements in pancreatic surgical technique have made it possible to excise smaller lesions surgically, although the rationale for doing this is less clear. Certainly, there is no compelling evidence to suggest that surgical removal of small tumors, unless they produce a hormonal syndrome, improves overall outcome. Some urge removal of all detectable macroadenomas if removal would not be dangerous.[115] Others urge a large size cutoff (2.5 to 3 cm in diameter) for removal.

Should Metastatic Pancreatico-Duodenal Cancer Be Debulked? Total pancreatectomy with a high rate of complications has been used for very large tumors.[116] Many methods are under exploration for resecting or otherwise ablating pancreatico-duodenal neuroendocrine cancer.[117,118] Results are too preliminary to justify endorsing any of these.

Should Medications Be Used to Control Tumor Progression? Pancreatico-duodenal neuroendocrine tumors are usually differentiated and quite resistant to chemotherapy. Several regimens have been tried, including streptozotocin, doxorubicin, or interferon, but there is no proof of long-term efficacy.[119-122.6] Octreotide has been effective in inhibiting hormone secretion by benign and malignant pancreatico-duodenal neuroendocrine tumors[82,123-125]; however, it has not been effective by itself in blocking growth of these tumors except to a small degree for malignant gastrinoma.[73,126] Its use in multidrug regimens needs further evaluation.

Somatostatin Analogue Linked to a Radioisotope. Because of their selectivity for certain tumors, somatostatin analogues have been explored as vehicles to deliver a radioactive isotope to the tumor. These drugs had not been approved by the U.S. Food and Drug Administration (FDA) in 2010 and are currently under investigation in the United States. The best results seem to be from Lutetium 177 bound to octreotate.[127] However, controlled studies have not yet been done.

Pituitary Tumor or Adrenal Cortical Tumor

Anterior pituitary tumor occurs in about one third of MEN1 patients.[12,13,128] The frequency of MEN1 in cases of apparently sporadic pituitary tumor is probably less than 5%, although estimates vary widely to as high as 15% with prolactinoma.[129,130] The overall frequency of hormones hypersecreted is similar to that observed in non-MEN1 pituitary tumors: prolactin, 60%; growth hormone with or without prolactin, 15%; nonsecreting, 25%; and ACTH, 5%; thyrotropin and gonadotropins are rare.[12,13,128] Pituitary mass effects can be the principal problem.[131] In fact, pituitary tumors in patients with MEN1 have been larger and less responsive to treatment than without MEN1.[128] Pituitary tumor can occur early in MEN1 and is occasionally the first recognized feature.[128,131,132] Rarely, two independent pituitary tumors have been suggested.[133,134]

Prolactinoma. Prolactinoma is the most common pituitary tumor in MEN1 and the third most common endocrine tumor in MEN1 after parathyroid tumors and gastrinomas (see Table 41-1). The general properties are similar to those of sporadic prolactinoma (see Chapter 9); MEN1 prolactinomas are even larger and harder to treat.[128,135] Dopamine agonists (e.g., cabergoline, bromocriptine, quinagolide) are the preferred treatment.[136,137] A reduction in side effects and greater potency make cabergoline the current treatment of choice and have improved patients' compliance. In patients who escape the growth-inhibitory effects of these dopamine agonists or who are noncompliant, transsphenoidal surgery combined with radiation therapy is usually effective.

Tumors that Produce Growth Hormone or Growth Hormone–Releasing Hormone. The clinical features of growth hormone excess are similar in patients with and without MEN1.[138] There are two different etiologic mechanisms with different treatment implications. The majority of MEN1 pituitary adenomas arise clonally from inactivation of both alleles of the *MEN1* gene in a tumor precursor cell.[139] Additional genes such as *AIP* or *GNAS* (which encodes the α-subunit of the stimulatory G protein) may be implicated outside of MEN1.[140] The second mechanism of pituitary growth hormone tumorigenesis begins with the over secretion of GHRH by pancreatic islet or carcinoid tumor.[88,141-143] The resulting secondary pituitary tumor is a polyclonal or hyperplastic process that responds poorly to therapy directed only at the pituitary; removal of the primary GHRH-producing tumor is essential. Although acromegaly secondary to GHRH is rare in sporadic or MEN1 cases,[141] a disproportionate fraction of patients with GHRH tumors have had MEN1. Therefore, measurement of serum GHRH in MEN1 acromegalic patients is sometimes worthwhile. Growth hormone–producing pituitary tumors also produce GHRH locally, but this has not interfered with the interpretation of serum GHRH levels.[142,144]

Treatment for acromegaly with MEN1 is the same as in acromegalic patients without MEN1 (see Chapter 9). Surgery is usually the first choice, but pharmacologic therapies, including long-acting somatostatin receptor antagonists and growth hormone receptor antagonists, can provide effective, albeit expensive, control.[145,146] In patients with large tumors causing mass effects and those in whom growth hormone effects are not controlled by surgery or pharmacologic therapy, radiation using an external beam, gamma knife, or proton beam is an alternative (see Chapter 9).

Corticotropin Hypersecretion. Hypercortisolism in MEN1 can be caused by a pituitary tumor producing ACTH, uncommonly by ectopic production of ACTH from a carcinoid or an islet tumor, by ectopic production of ACTH-releasing hormone (CRH), or by adrenal tumor. Therapy should be directed initially to treat the ACTH- or CRH-producing primary tumor. If therapy directed toward the primary source is not successful, corticosteroid production can be controlled by bilateral adrenalectomy or medical therapy (see Chapters 10 and 16).

Primary Adrenocortical Hyperfunction. One or both adrenal glands are enlarged in about 40% of MEN1 patients.[147,148] This enlargement, most often discovered during pancreatic imaging, is usually clinically silent and rarely requires treatment. The silent enlargement represents a presumably polyclonal or hyperplastic process of unknown etiology,[147] and it rarely behaves as a neoplasm. Rare MEN1 cases have been identified with primary hypercortisolism, hyperaldosteronism, or adrenocortical cancer[147,149]; none of these have been proved to be intrinsic features of MEN1.

Foregut Carcinoid Tumors

Carcinoid tumor is recognized in 5% to 15% of MEN1 patients.[13,128] Although sporadic carcinoid is derived mainly from midgut and hindgut, MEN1 carcinoid is almost always found in derivatives of the foregut (e.g., thymus, bronchus, stomach). Certain carcinoid tumors, unlike any other manifestation of MEN1, have a strong sex-specific distribution. In MEN1, thymic carcinoid is mainly in males and with some familial clustering, and bronchial carcinoid is mainly in females.[150-152] The average age of carcinoid recognition in MEN1 is 45 years,[153] later than that of other MEN1 tumors. This later age may reflect the lack of compression-induced symptoms and the lack of a hormone oversecretion syndrome with most MEN1 carcinoids.

Thymic carcinoid in MEN1 is usually found at an already advanced stage as a large invasive mass. Much less commonly, it is recognized during chest imaging or during thymectomy adjunctive to parathyroidectomy. Thymic carcinoid is more often malignant (about 70% of cases) than bronchial carcinoid (about 20%) in MEN1.[151,152,154,155] MEN1 thymic or bronchial carcinoids rarely oversecrete ACTH, calcitonin, or GHRH; similarly, they rarely oversecrete serotonin or histamine and rarely cause the carcinoid syndrome. Most can therefore be considered clinically nonfunctioning. Mediastinal or bronchial carcinoids are best imaged by computed tomography; however, SRS and new PET ligands sometimes give positive results.[156]

Gastric carcinoid has been recognized more recently but is less well characterized in MEN1. It is a tumor of enterochromaffin-like cells. Large gastric carcinoids can cause a hormonal syndrome from serotonin and histamine secretion in patients with MEN1.[157] In up to 15% of MEN1 patients, they have been recognized incidentally during endoscopy.[56] The overall malignancy rate seems low, but there are exceptions.[157,158] At early stages, they can regress after treatment with somatostatin analogues.[74]

Occasionally, carcinoid occurs in several members of a small family without other manifestations of MEN1.[159,160] The etiology of such clustered carcinoids is not known.[161-163]

Miscellaneous Tumors of MEN1

Miscellaneous Endocrine Tumors in MEN1

Pheochromocytoma. Pheochromocytoma is a rare feature in MEN1; there have been fewer than 10 reported cases.[9,148] Most have been unilateral and chemically silent; one was malignant.[131] In two tumors, 11q13 loss of heterozygosity (LOH) was documented,[164] making it likely that all or most of these rare pheochromocytomas in MEN1 are true clonal expressions from biallelic *MEN1* gene inactivation. This cause is supported by the fact that pheochromocytoma is even more frequent in mouse than in human MEN1.[49]

Thyroid Follicular Neoplasm. Thyroid follicular neoplasm has been associated with MEN1 since the earliest reviews. This association is likely related to the high incidence of thyroid follicular neoplasms in the general population (unrelated to MEN1) and to their incidental discovery during the inevitable neck exploration for parathyroid disease in MEN1.[6] Further support for a coincidental association is the failure to identify *MEN1* gene mutations in sporadic thyroid follicular tumors.[165]

Miscellaneous Nonendocrine Tumors. MEN1 is associated with nonendocrine tumors that vary from rare to common, with some offering possible use in the diagnosis of MEN1.

Lipoma. The association of lipomas with MEN1 has been known since the 1960s.[6] MEN1 lipomas are usually dermal, small, and sometimes multiple. Their frequency in MEN1 is about 30%, compared with 5% in control subjects without MEN1.[166] This frequency in normal subjects has limited their use for MEN1 carrier ascertainment.

Angiofibroma. Angiofibromas have been found in 85% of MEN1 patients but not in control subjects.[166,167] Half of MEN1 patients have five or more. They are acneiform papules on the face that do not regress and can extend across the vermilion border of the lips (Fig. 41-6).

Collagenoma. Collagenomas were also observed in 70% of MEN1 patients but not in control subjects.[166,167] Collagenomas are whitish, macular or, rarely, pedunculated lesions about the trunk that spare the face and neck. The MEN1 lipomas, angiofibromas, and collagenomas show loss of one copy of 11q13.[168] Therefore, it is likely that

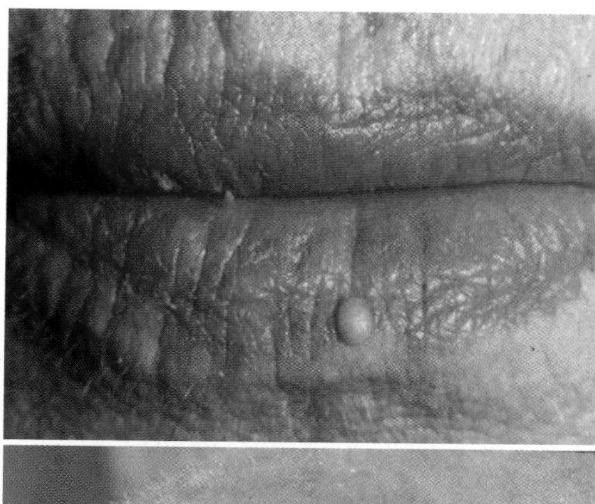

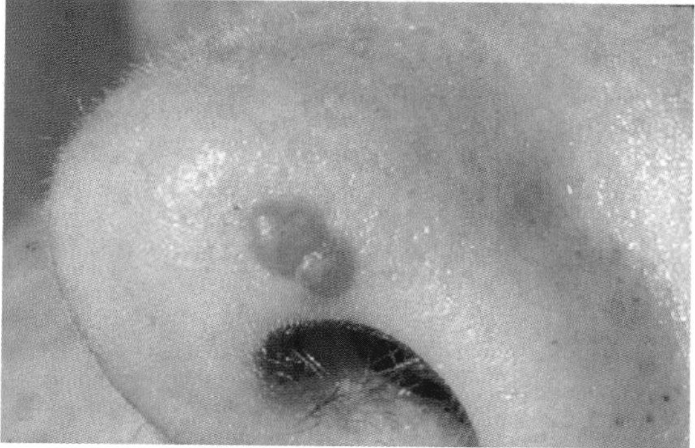

Figure 41-6 Facial angiofibroma in patients with multiple endocrine neoplasia type 1. A small, light pink lesion on the vermilion border of the lip *(top)* and a large, reddish angiofibroma on the nose *(bottom)* are shown. Typical lesions are smaller than these and multiple and may require biopsy for confirmation. (From T. Darling and M. Turner, National Institutes of Health, Bethesda, MD.)

these are clonal neoplasms and caused by inactivation of both copies of the *MEN1* gene.

Spinal Cerebellar Ependymoma. Spinal cerebellar ependymoma has been seen in four MEN1 patients.[9,169] There are no studies to determine whether 11q13 LOH or other *MEN1* gene abnormalities are causative.

Malignant Melanoma. Malignant melanoma has occurred in at least seven MEN1 patients, but direct involvement of the *MEN1* gene has not been tested.[170]

Leiomyoma (of Esophagus, Lung, Rectum, or Uterus). Leiomyoma has been reported in several MEN1 patients.[6,171,172] Analyses of 11q13 LOH established that esophageal and uterine leiomyomas are specific to MEN1 patients.[173] In contrast, *MEN1* inactivation was not implicated in sporadic uterine leiomyoma.[173] It is not known whether uterine leiomyoma differs clinically in patients with or without MEN1.

Meningioma (Cranial). A large prospective series reported meningioma in 8% of MEN1 patients. These tumors are mostly small and incidental and would not be recognized without imaging.[174] No intervention is warranted for these. A large and locally aggressive meningioma was seen in one MEN1 patient who had prior irradiation to a pituitary tumor (SJM, personal observation). This tumor showed biallelic inactivation of *MEN1*.[174]

Barrett Esophagus. The frequency of the presumably premalignant Barrett esophagus was increased fivefold in patients with MEN1 and ZES compared to those with ZES alone.[175] This may relate to a longer interval with uncontrolled excess of stomach acid.

MEN1-Like Phenotypes

Varying Penetrance of Tumors by Tissue or by Age

MEN1 is the most heterogeneous of all neoplasia syndromes. The many tumors of MEN1 have a wide range of penetrance (see Table 41-1). If the organ is paired and the penetrance is high, the tumors are usually bilateral (e.g., parathyroid adenomas); if the tumor is rare in MEN1, its random occurrence is typically unilateral even in a paired organ (e.g., pheochromocytoma). Naturally, the apparent penetrance of any tumor type is heavily dependent on the scrutiny that the organ is given. For example, the frequent facial angiofibromas of MEN1 were not recognized until 1997.[166] When symptoms alone are the main basis for disease recognition, the first feature of MEN1 in adolescents is not HPT but rather prolactinoma or insulinoma.[176]

For each tumor type, penetrance necessarily increases with age (see Fig. 41-1). Overall, the penetrance for MEN1 reaches almost 100% by age 50 years,[12] but occasional obligate *MEN1* mutation carriers have not shown any tumor development beyond age 70 years.[169] Earliest penetrance and earliest preventable morbidity must be considered in decisions about when to begin tumor surveillance in a known carrier. The earliest ages for identification of specific tumor expression in MEN1 have been as follows: prolactinoma, 5 years[132]; insulinoma, 6 years[177]; nonfunctioning islet, 12 years.[177.5] HPT, 8 years[12]; and gastrinoma, 12 years (R. Jensen, personal communication). The information about tumor morbidity for most of these young patients is incomplete; more information is needed to improve the recommendations about age at which carrier ascertainment, tumor surveillance, and possibly intervention should begin.

Differential Diagnosis of MEN1

When MEN1 occurs in its typical and full forms, it is easily diagnosed. Presentation as a single, apparently sporadic tumor; as familial isolated hyperparathyroidism (FIH); or as atypical combinations presents the clinician with challenges to diagnosis and understanding.

Familial Variation in Phenotype or in Penetrance of Tumors

Clustering of clinical subvariants of MEN1, similar to that seen for MEN2 (discussed later), has been evaluated. Preliminary analyses in small MEN1 families suggested clusters of ACTH-producing pituitary tumors, insulinomas[178,179] intestinal carcinoids,[152] thymic carcinoids,[152,180] and aggressive gastrinomas.[154] Identification of a specific *MEN1* mutation or a modifier locus that correlates with a specific clinical variant in multiple kindreds would be most meaningful. However, subsequent analyses have failed to identify such a relationship (see later discussion), increasing the likelihood that tumor clustering is random in most of these families.

Prolactinoma Variant of MEN1

The prolactinoma variant of MEN1 is defined in a family with high penetrance for HPT and prolactinoma but low penetrance for gastrinoma (typically 90%, 50%, and 5%, respectively, among adults). Three large families have been reported, each with thirteen or more affected members.[181] The largest has more than 100 affected members. Because their ancestors colonized the Burin Peninsula of Newfoundland, Canada, their trait has been termed $MEN1_{Burin}$. Several other families seem similar but cannot be categorized because of their small size. Foregut carcinoid tumors seemed prominent (10% to 15% of cases) in $MEN1_{Burin}$.

Isolated Hyperparathyroidism Variant of MEN1

HPT is the most common clinical feature of MEN1 and often begins at a relatively young age. It would therefore not be surprising to identify isolated HPT in small families with occult MEN1, particularly in those families with a disproportionate number of young members. Larger families (four or more affected members) have been identified with FIH and an identifiable *MEN1* mutation but still could represent a random part of the normal spectrum of MEN1 expression.[182] Eventually, most patients would probably develop other clinical features of MEN1.[183] Two FIH families with *MEN1* mutation have been particularly large, with 11 and 14 hyperparathyroid members, raising the likelihood that isolated HPT can exist and continue in some families as the only manifestation of *MEN1* mutation.[182,184] Although these families by definition have *MEN1* mutation, *MEN1* mutation is rare among all families with FIH (see later discussion).[185]

Sporadic Tumor or Tumors

MEN1 can occur without a recognized or even a recognizable family history of MEN1. Some sporadic patients who present with two or more typical tumors meet the definition criteria for MEN1[186]; for others, the suspicion of MEN1 is high. The prevalence of *MEN1* mutation is 7% to 70%, depending on the specific tumors (see later discussion).[187] When the sporadic case manifests with tumor in only one tissue, the suspicion and the true frequency of *MEN1* mutation are low. The frequency of occult MEN1 with sporadic tumor can be estimated as follows: HPT, 2%[9,188]; gastrinoma, 5%[53]; prolactinoma, 5%.[129,130,189] Factors that increase the likelihood of MEN1 in these settings are suggestive features in the family, earlier onset, and tumor multiplicity in the same tissue. Diffuse or multifocal hyperplasia of the islets or nesidioblastosis is rare and is sometimes seen as a consequence of gastric bypass surgery.[190] Isolated alpha cell disease of the islets with glucagon cell hyperplasia and multiple glucagonomas is sporadic and very rare.[191]

Familial Isolated Endocrine Tumors Not from the *MEN1* Gene

Familial Isolated Hyperparathyroidism. When HPT is familial and isolated to this tissue, the main possibilities include occult MEN1 (discussed earlier), familial hypocalciuric hypercalcemia (FHH), hyperparathyroidism–jaw tumor syndrome (HPT-JT), MEN2A, and so-called true FIH[185] (see Chapter 28). FHH, with a frequency similar to that of MEN1, is an autosomal dominant disorder characterized by lifelong hypercalcemia with normal urine calcium excretion.[192,193] PTH levels and parathyroid gland mass are normal or minimally increased.[194,195] After subtotal parathyroidectomy, the residual parathyroid tissue directs persistent hypercalcemia. The parathyroid dysfunction is probably not monoclonal but polyclonal.[196] A remarkably high rate of persistence after subtotal parathyroidectomy and a low morbidity without surgery justify efforts to avoid parathyroid surgery in FHH. Useful diagnostic features of FHH are the low urine calcium (in the presence of hypercalcemia), the normal PTH level despite hypercalcemia, and the onset of hypercalcemia in young relatives, even before age 1.

Two thirds of FHH index cases have an identifiable inactivating mutation of the calcium-sensing receptor gene *(CASR)*.[197] Most of the rest are believed to have an undetected mutation of *CASR*, suggested by genetic linkage to chromosome 3q; occasional families have the FHH syndrome with mutation in unknown genes at 19p or 19q.[198-200] One family with a missense mutation of *CASR* had features more like typical HPT.[201] Two large, prospective studies of FIH found unexpected germline mutation of *CASR* in 15% of families. These families were small (mainly with two or three affected members), and no family had typical clinical features of FHH.[185,202]

HPT-JT is a syndrome of HPT, jaw tumors, and renal lesions.[203] Transmission is autosomal dominant. The most common and sometimes the only feature is HPT.[204] The HPT typically involves one parathyroid gland at a time, and there is a uniquely high malignant potential in the parathyroid tumor; 15% of patients have parathyroid cancer.[185,205] Germline mutation of *HRPT2* is found in most seemingly sporadic parathyroid cancers, suggesting an occult familial process.[206] The associated jaw tumors (in 25%) are ossifying or cementifying fibromas.[207] Unlike the jaw tumors of HPT, they are not influenced by the parathyroid status. The associated renal lesions (in 5%) are multiple renal cysts, hamartomas, or Wilms' tumor.[208] Uterine tumors are common and can impair fertility.[209] *HRPT2* mutation has been found in 5% to 10% of kindreds with FIH.[185,202,210] Occult MEN2A, theoretically another cause of FIH, has not been identified in the form of FIH.[211,212]

Many small kindreds with two or three affected members receive a diagnosis of FIH.[184,213,214] For years, FIH was not pursued as a syndrome because of its bland features and the belief that most kindreds had occult MEN1. Gene tests of many kindreds with FIH have found occult MEN1, FHH, or HPT-JT in about one third.[184] Probably, mutation in undiscovered genes will account for most kindreds with FIH. One such gene seems to be on chromosome 2 by genetic linkage analysis.[200]

Familial Isolated Pituitary Tumor. Familial isolated tumor of the anterior pituitary has been recognized in several small and a few large families.[215] The tumors are usually somatotropinomas or prolactinomas. In some families, somatotropinoma is the main expression. In theory, familial isolated tumor of the anterior pituitary could be an expression of occult MEN1. However, no family with familial isolated somatotropinoma has had a *MEN1* mutation (see later discussion). About 15% of these families harbor mutations of the *AIP* gene, which coincidentally is very near the *MEN1* gene at 11q13.[216]

Other Familial Endocrine Tumors.

Isolated Chromaffin Tumor. *Chromaffin tumor* refers to adrenal pheochromocytoma and to extra-adrenal paraganglioma. Isolated chromaffin tumor occurs in some families. Most family clusters are caused by one of six genes that encode proteins in the mitochrondial succinate dehydrogenase complex (*SDHA, SDHB, SDHC, SDHD, SDH5* and *TMEM127*). This topic is covered in more detail in Chapter 16.

Isolated Carcinoid Tumor. Carcinoid tumor clustering in families is statistically significant. However, few families have been described, and most have had fewer than five affected members. The tumors seem to be distributed between foregut and hindgut. None has been associated with *MEN1* mutation. In fact, no single gene or gene locus has been implicated.

The Normal *MEN1* Gene and Normal Menin

Larsson and colleagues[217] showed in 1988 that the *MEN1* gene mapped to chromosome band 11q13 and that it probably caused tumor by a loss of function.[218,219] However, almost a full decade passed before the *MEN1* gene was identified by positional cloning.[220] This strategy involved a progressive narrowing of the candidate gene interval,[221] cloning of all the DNA in the narrowed interval,[222] and identification of all or most genes therein.[222] The final step required sequence analysis of each of these genes in a panel of DNA from familial MEN1 index cases, a systematic process that led to the identification of the one candidate gene that carried the defining mutations.[217,223,224]

The *MEN1* gene is 10 kb long and encodes transcripts of 2.7 and 3.1 kb.[225] The transcripts are expressed in all or most tissues and with little cell-cycle dependence.[226] They encode a 610-amino-acid protein termed *menin*. Rat, mouse, zebrafish, snail, *Drosophila*, and human menins are highly homologous.[227]

Menin has two nuclear localization signals near the carboxyl terminus that are likely to be responsible for its predominantly nuclear compartmentalization.[226]

Molecular Pathways for Menin's Normal Actions

Because menin has an amino acid sequence without any homologies in the genome, its sequence alone is not informative about its mechanism of action. The principal method applied to search for its molecular pathway has been that of menin partnering to proteins or chromatin. Approximately 25 protein partners for menin have been identified, but only a few have been reproduced in other laboratories.

The first interacting protein partner identified for menin was selectively JunD but not other members of the activator protein-1 (AP1) transcription factor family that includes Fos, Fra, and other Jun proteins.[228,229] The menin-JunD interaction can confer upon JunD unique effects by which JunD differs from other members of the AP1 transcription family. For example, JunD has several actions opposite to those of c-Jun, and in the absence of menin binding to it, JunD behaves more like c-Jun.[230]

The importance of the menin-JunD interaction for the development of MEN1 is unclear. Homozygous knockout of JunD in the mouse resulted in no identifiable abnormality of tissues involved in MEN1.[231] Other partnering studies have identified a mixed-lineage leukemia protein (MLL)-containing complex, or SMAD3, PEM, NM23, nuclear factor-κB, and several other proteins that potentially interact with menin. Each interacting partner has unknown importance.[232] Hundreds of chromatin binding sites for menin have been identified but no specific DNA recognition element. At present, none of the menin partners has been convincingly shown to be critical in MEN1 tumorigenesis. The largest attention has been given to JunD and MLL, and these studies can be explored elsewhere.[232]

Tumorigenesis Roles of the *MEN1* Gene

The first DNA-based discoveries in MEN1 suggested that the *MEN1* gene was a tumor suppressor[217-219] (see Chapter 40), and these observations were supported by subsequent studies (see later discussion).

Two-Step Inactivation of the *MEN1* Gene. Complete inactivation of the *MEN1* gene's function requires, in addition to the inherited or somatically acquired first hit (inactivating mutation), a second hit at the same genetic locus that finishes the inactivation of both copies of the *MEN1* gene. Inactivation of the second allele can be by mutation or by other (epigenetic) means such as promoter methylation.[233] A two-hit model for tumorigenesis was developed by Alfred Knudson[218,219] in 1971 to account for epidemiologic observations in retinoblastoma: In comparison with sporadic cases, some hereditary tumors occurred earlier and in multiple sites. This can now be generalized to say that, in a hereditary tumor, the germline mutation is obligatorily present in every cell. Therefore, the earliest step seen in sporadic tumorigenesis is bypassed in the hereditary form. Multiple independent cells in susceptible organs are thus primed for somatic mutations at the second or normal copy of the tumorigenic gene, to cause early and multiple tumors. This model can also be extended to stepwise tumorigenesis by an oncogene such as *RET* (see later discussion).

Somatic Point Mutations of the *MEN1* Gene in Sporadic Tumors. *MEN1* is one of the most commonly mutated genes in sporadic endocrine tumors. The mutations are typically seen as a first hit represented by a small mutation in the *MEN1* gene and a second hit represented by a large zone of loss of heterozygosity about the *MEN1* locus (see following explanation). Among sporadic tumors, the frequency of *MEN1* mutation is 10% to 20% in parathyroid adenomas,[234-237] 25% in gastrinomas,[238-240] 10% to 20% in insulinomas,[238,241] 50% in VIPomas,[238,241] and 25% to 35% in bronchial carcinoids.[238,241,242] Some other sporadic endocrine tumors show a lower frequency of *MEN1* somatic mutation: 0% to 5% in anterior pituitary tumor,[243-247] 0% in non–C-cell thyroid tumor,[165] 0% in benign or malignant adrenocortical neoplasm,[248,249] 0% in uremic secondary HPT,[248,250] and 0% in parathyroid cancer.[251] Sporadic nonendocrine tumors have undergone little evaluation; the *MEN1* mutation frequency was 2 in 19 angiofibromas,[252] 1 in 6 lipomas,[253] 0% in lung cancer other than carcinoid,[254] 1% in malignant melanoma,[170,255] and 0% in leukemia.[256]

The First Step (First Hit) Can Be in the Germline or in Somatic Tissue. Virtually all germline or somatic first hits at the *MEN1* gene have been small mutations, involving only one or several bases.[257,258] The mutations are broadly distributed across the *MEN1* open reading frame, so much so that half of newly ascertained index cases are still found to have a novel mutation. At the same time, the other half show recurring mutations. These are equally distributed in the germline between cause by common ancestry (founder effect)[257,259-263] and cause by a hot spot for new mutation.[257]

Accumulated patterns of germline and somatic first-hit *MEN1* mutations have further supported the two-hit gene inactivation hypothesis for the *MEN1* gene (Fig. 41-7). Three fourths of *MEN1* first-hit mutations predict premature truncation of the menin protein. Although the biologic functions of menin are not established, such truncation mutations would probably cause menin inactivation or even absence. For example, all truncation-type *MEN1* mutations cause loss of the most C-terminal nuclear localization signal (see Fig. 41-7) and therefore could compromise the nuclear localization of menin.[226] The remainder predict missense or replacement of one to three amino acids. The functional consequences of any one missense mutation are uncertain and even hard to distinguish from a rare benign polymorphism; however, their frequent occurrence specifically in MEN1 and their absence in normal subjects has suggested that all or most are deleterious mutations.

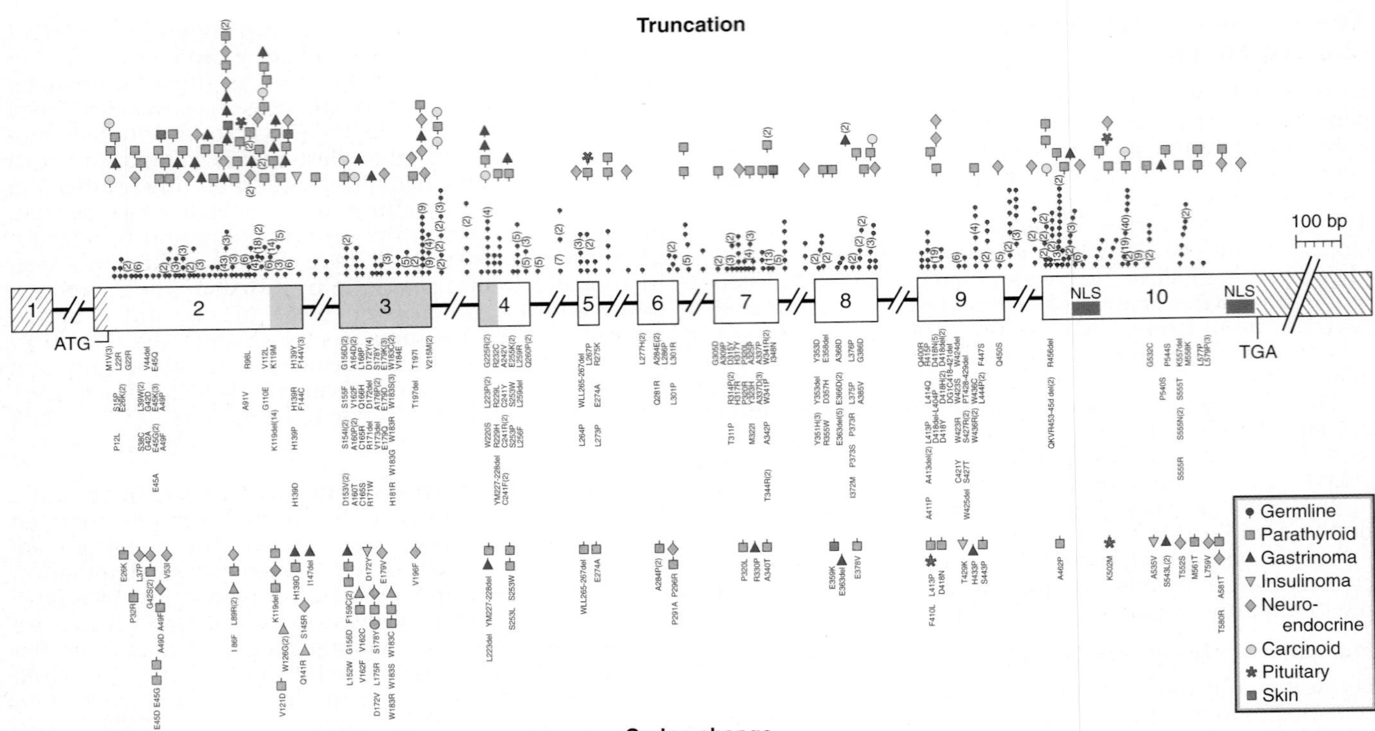

Figure 41-7 Germline and somatic mutations of the *MEN1* gene. Unique germline *MEN1* mutations in families, and sporadic cases, and somatic mutations in nonhereditary tumors. The figure shows 670 unique mutations identified by 2006. Repeating mutations within the germline or somatic category (common ancestry versus hot spots for mutation) are shown only once, with a small number in parentheses to indicate total occurrences. Germline mutations are shown as *black lollipops* or as code about the messenger RNA (mRNA). Somatic *MEN1* mutations in diverse tumors are shown separately as flags along the upper and lower border and as code. *MEN1* mRNA is diagrammed with exons numbered; untranslated regions are *crosshatched.* Truncating mutations (frameshift mutations, splice errors, and nonsense [stop codon] mutations) are shown above the mRNA; they account for 75% of all mutations. Codon change mutations (missense mutations or small in-frame deletions) are shown below the mRNA with their three-letter amino acid code. Gray mRNA about exon 3 represents the main zone of menin interaction with JunD. Several large deletions, probably of the entire *MEN1* gene, are not shown.[253] NLS, nuclear localization sequence.

The Second Hit in *MEN1* Tumorigenesis. The second hit is usually a large chromosomal or subchromosomal rearrangement (mutation) causing a deletion of sequence that includes the remaining normal *MEN1* gene. Another potential mechanism for creating a mutant second copy is deletion of DNA that spans all or part of the normal copy and then duplication of the DNA from the mutant chromosome 11, called *gene conversion*. In either case, the result is that neither copy of the *MEN1* gene remains normal. LOH or loss of alleles (heterozygosity) at the affected locus is usually a necessary marker for this process and can provide evidence that gene inactivation has occurred in that chromosomal segment. Other rare mechanisms for the second hit are small mutations (one to three bases) and promoter methylation.[233] The second hit is delayed after the first hit. It is always in somatic tissue and almost always occurs postnatally.

Loss of Heterozygosity about the Locus of the *MEN1* Gene. LOH about 11q13 has been used mainly to deduce loss of the normal copy of the *MEN1* gene (i.e., the second hit in tumorigenesis). In MEN1, 11q13 LOH was found for almost 100% of parathyroid tumors,[26,264] gastrinomas and other pancreatic islet tumors,[46,47] gastric carcinoid,[260,265] anterior pituitary tumors,[139] and mesenchymal tumors (lipoma, angiofibroma, collagenoma, and leiomyoma).[168,171,173] These prevalences are higher than those for small mutations of *MEN1* in the same tumors (see earlier discussion). Therefore, mutation of other genes on chromosome 11 may account for some first hits, and undetected mutations of *MEN1* may account for some. Surprisingly, thymic carcinoid tumor and adrenocortical tumor in MEN1 have not shown 11q13 LOH.[147,153,266] This has led to speculation that the normal *MEN1* copy can be inactivated by other mechanisms, such as promoter methylation, that would not cause LOH.

Among sporadic endocrine tumors of the type found in MEN1, some but not all have frequent 11q13 LOH. The frequencies of 11q13 LOH in these tumors have been as follows: sporadic primary hyperparathyroid, 30% to 40%[234-236,267]; uremic parathyroid, 0% to 5%[242,268-271]; parathyroid cancer, 0%[246]; gastrinoma, 25% to 70%[47,238]; insulinoma, 30%[47]; bronchial and other foregut carcinoid, 40% to 70%[242,272]; and anterior pituitary, 5% to 10%.[140,242-247] In the adrenal cortex, 11q13 LOH was less common in benign than in malignant tumors (20% and 80%, respectively).[248,249] Assessment of 11q13 LOH is not useful in clinical practice because it does not help in staging or in germline diagnosis; however, it has been used in research as an indicator of an underlying first hit in a tumor suppressor gene at that locus. Of unknown significance, most sporadic hibernomas have deletions of both *MEN1* & mean by *A1P* genes at 11q13.[272.5]

11q13 LOH has also been used as an indicator of tissue monoclonality or oligoclonality. Because 11q13 LOH is a DNA rearrangement, it can be detected only if it is present in the DNA of most or a substantial minority of cells in a specimen. The nuclei are deduced to be monoclonal or oligoclonal descendants from one or a few precursor cells with that rearrangement or mutation. Early studies of MEN1 parathyroid glands by light microscopy suggested oncogenesis through a polyclonal hyperplastic process, an observation that was supported by the finding in MEN1 plasma of a factor mitogenic for parathyroid cells.[27] The subsequent finding of almost universal 11q13 LOH in MEN1 parathyroids.[221,228,264] established that monoclonal or oligoclonal growth was predominant and that tumorigenesis in MEN1 occurred by loss of function.

Hyperplasia and DNA Repair. The earliest tissue-level effects toward tumorigenesis in MEN1 are not well defined, nor are many intermediate steps. Although a widespread role for hyperplasia prior to neoplasia has been seen in MEN2 and many hereditary neoplasias, hyperplasia has been subtle or unrecognized as a tumor precursor in MEN1 tissues. A related progression has been identified, from gastrin cell hyperplasia to microtumor as a precursor to gastrinoma, in MEN1 but not in sporadic gastrinoma.[48] The mouse *MEN1* knockout model for MEN1 exhibits striking giant hyperplasia of beta cells in pancreatic islets as a precursor for insulinoma,[42] suggesting that more subtle hyperplasia may have gone unrecognized in human MEN1. If there is a role for hyperplasia, it would be uncertain whether this is an expression of inactivation of one *MEN1* allele or further processes. MEN1 plasma contains a growth factor that promotes mitogenesis in normal parathyroid cells and could contribute to hyperplasia.[26,272] Considering the overriding roles of *MEN1* gene inactivation and of clonal growth, it is not certain whether the growth factor is a contributor to or a consequence of oncogenesis in MEN1.

Clonal cell proliferation has been identified in mesenchymal perivascular tissues about MEN1 angiofibromas[273]; this could represent a precursor stage of that tumor.[274]

Other unknown genes can be implicated in MEN1 tumor evolution through gene loss of function (tumor suppressor gene) or gene gain of function (oncogene).[273-283] Genome instability has been suggested in studies of MEN1 lymphocytes and fibroblasts.[280,281] Also, MEN1 leukocytes show a subtle deficiency in repair of DNA damage.[282] Menin null cells of the mouse show a defect in repair of DNA damaged selectively by ionizing radiation.[283]

MEN1 Mutations and Tumor Phenotypes

MEN1 genotype has not been clearly related with phenotype, unlike the situation in MEN2 (discussed later). The truncating *MEN1* mutations cause the same diverse types of tumor expression as the missense mutations, and tumor expression does not differ between amino-terminal and C-terminal mutations. The distribution of somatic mutations about the open reading frame is similar to that of germline mutations (see Fig. 41-7) and seems almost random. There appears to be a deficiency of missense mutations near the C-terminus and a cluster of missense mutations between amino acids 100 and 200. Otherwise, there is no clear clustering of missense mutations that could point to a zone of menin protein susceptible to change of function.

The prolactinoma variant of MEN1, one of the clinical variants described previously in three unrelated kindreds, was associated with no specific genotype or rather with three different *MEN1* mutations.[284] *MEN1* mutation has been found in up to 20% of tested families with isolated hyperparathyroidism (FIH).[181,184] Two of the largest *MEN1* mutation-positive families with isolated HPT had similarly located missense mutations (E255K and Q260P).[181,285] However, *MEN1* mutations in 14 other kindreds with FIH showed no patterns of similarity.[184]

A *MEN1* mutation has not been found with familial isolated anterior pituitary tumor, although more than 100 such families have been evaluated.[177,246,259,260,286] Therefore, most kindreds with isolated pituitary tumor, like most of those with FIH, represent MEN1 phenocopies; that is, they are probably caused by mutation in genes (e.g., *AIP*[286]) other than *MEN1*. There has also been no relationship between a specific somatic *MEN1* mutation and tumor type. Tumor testing for somatic *MEN1* mutation has not shown prognostic or staging value when evaluated in sporadic gastrinomas of varying aggressiveness.[240]

Mutation of a CDKI Gene as a Rare Cause of MEN1-Like State

Inactivation of certain other tumor suppressor genes, alone or in combination, can cause specific endocrine tumors in mice. In particular, mice with homozygous knockout of both *p18*INK4c *(CDKN2C)* and *p27*KIP1 *(CDKN1B)* develop neoplasia in at least eight types of tissue, including tumors of parathyroid, pituitary, pancreas islet, and duodenum (as in MEN1); they also develop C-cell cancers and pheochromocytoma (as in MEN2).[276] The knocked out genes encode members of the two cyclin-dependent kinase inhibitor (CDKI) families that participate in the cell-cycling pathway and also include retinoblastoma and cyclin D1.[277]

Rats with homozygous inactivation of *p27* show a spectrum of tumors similar to those comprising MEN1 and MEN2.[272] Seven human index cases and several of their relatives exhibited MEN1-like tumors after inactivation of one copy of *p27*.[287,288] This has been termed *MEN4*. Based on this limited number of cases, the spectrum of MEN4 is indistinguishable from that of MEN1, and it has not been found to include its rodent counterparts of C-cell neoplasia or pheochromocytoma.

Similar mutations in three other CDKI genes (*p15, p18,* and *p21*) and similar clinical features have also been seen in rare MEN1-like cases and families.[288] The similar features resulting from mutation of *MEN1* or several of the CDKI genes suggest that they share an overlapping pathway. For example, menin might activate the promoter of a CDKI gene and thereby function as a growth suppressor.

Testing for Carrier State or for Tumor Emergence in MEN1

Screening and Counseling for MEN1. A screening program for MEN1 patients should routinely meet three main objectives: identification of MEN1 carriers;

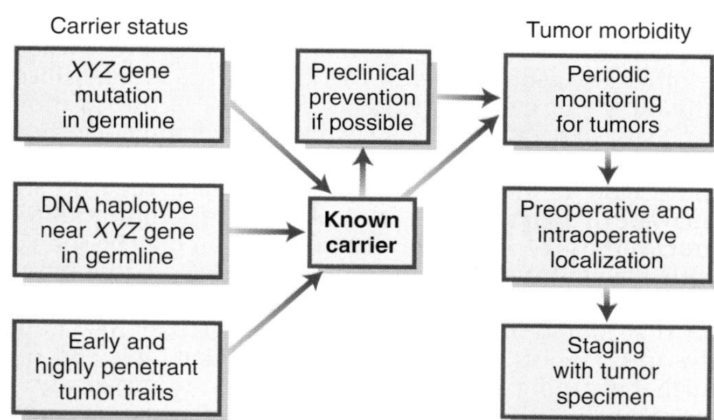

Figure 41-8 Test categories and test methods in a hereditary tumor syndrome. Tests of the germline carrier status *(left)* are largely distinguished from tests of tumor status *(right)*. When DNA testing is not informative, carrier status can be tested by streamlined surveillance of tumors *(lower left)*.

TABLE 41-2

Representative Protocol of Tests and Schedules to Survey for Tumor Emergence in a Carrier of Multiple Endocrine Neoplasia Type 1

Tumor	Age to Begin Testing (Yr)	Biochemical Tests Annually	Imaging Tests Every 3-5 Yr
Parathyroid adenoma	8	Calcium, PTH	None
Gastrinoma	20	Gastrin	None
Insulinoma	5	Fasting glucose	None
Other pancreatico-duodenal	15	NA	^{111}In-DTPA octreotide‡; CT or MRI
Anterior pituitary	5	Prolactin; IGF1	MRI
Foregut carcinoid*	20	NA†	CT

*Stomach is best evaluated for carcinoids (ECLomas) incidental to gastric endoscopy. Thymus is removed partially at parathyroidectomy in MEN1.
†Not available.
‡A robust test with serum is not available. Chromogranin-A is not proven as a screen for small tumors.
CT, computed tomography; DTPA, diethylenetriaminepentaacetic acid; ECL, enterochromaffin-like; IGF1, insulin-like growth factor 1; MRI, magnetic resonance imaging; PTH, parathyroid hormone.
(Modified from Brandi ML, Gagel RF, Angeli A, et al. Guidelines for diagnosis and therapy of MEN type 1 and type 2. *J Clin Endocrinol Metab.* 2001;86:5658-5671.)

identification of MEN1 tumors, particularly at a treatable stage; and cost-effectiveness (Fig. 41-8).[218,289] The term *screening* has been applied to several processes in the setting of MEN1. Herein, a distinction is made between testing for carrier ascertainment and testing for periodic surveillance of tumors in a known carrier. When carrier testing with DNA (mutation or haplotype test) is not possible, streamlined and periodic tumor surveillance becomes the preferred method for carrier ascertainment.

Encounters for carrier ascertainment often involve counseling for the patient. In addition to standard genetics topics, counseling in MEN1 addresses two different faces of MEN1: an endocrinopathy with good but complex management options and a cancer syndrome with limited management options. A MEN1 information web page can help in orientation.[290]

Benefits and Limitations of Carrier Ascertainment. The benefits of this type of analysis are several. First is the secure proof of the MEN1 carrier state in a person with a mutation and, equally important, the potential to exclude the MEN1 carrier state by a normal sequence analysis when another affected member of the kindred has an identified mutant *MEN1* gene sequence.[182] This type of information can assist in decisions about such issues as family planning and future medical needs. Second, the information from an index case, if shared, can be helpful to relatives who are unaware of their status. In particular, after a germline *MEN1* mutation is first identified, the information may be shared with a laboratory and with relatives, and DNA-based information may be used to develop an accurate shortcut test for that mutation in relatives (see later discussion). Third, the information is useful to the physician. It assists in further planning about counseling and tumor surveillance. Occasionally, it is important in a decision about surgery, such as in a case of apparently sporadic gastrinoma.

What the MEN1 carrier ascertainment test does not do is also important. MEN1 carrier ascertainment, unlike similar testing for MEN2, does not routinely lead to a recommendation for medical or surgical intervention. MEN1 cancers, in contrast to MTC in the thyroid, arise in tissues that cannot easily be ablated. This lack of mutation-guided intervention makes mutation testing at early ages in MEN1 less urgent than in MEN2. We recommend DNA testing in children of gene carriers at age 5 years, the youngest age at which a morbid and possibly treatable MEN1-related tumor (prolactinoma) has been identified.[132] An alternative approach, based on the fact that MEN1 morbidity is rare before the age of 20 years, is to delay carrier ascertainment until the child can make a mature decision about a test that could affect availability of insurance or job opportunities.

No identifiable *MEN1* mutation is found in 0% to 40%[187,292,293] of typical MEN1 kindreds, although most are believed to harbor *MEN1* mutations not detected by the most common DNA sequencing strategies. Carrier ascertainment in such kindreds can be established by 11q13 haplotype analysis or by streamlined tumor surveillance (discussed later) (see Fig. 41-8). In practice, this is rarely done. Overall, the potential for benefit from the *MEN1* mutation test is proportional to the likelihood of finding a *MEN1* mutation. Obvious benefit is possible for a proband with familial or sporadic MEN1 or with a state that resembles MEN1 but does not quite meet the usual definitions. For example, a *MEN1* germline mutation was found in each of four patients with sporadic HPT and carcinoid tumor.[186] The likelihood of benefit in a case of atypical MEN1 is typically much lower and varies greatly with the specific tumor identified. For example, the likelihood of finding a *MEN1* germline mutation in a case of sporadic HPT (without special features such as youth or multigland disease) is probably less than 1%.[186]

Germline DNA: Mutation or Haplotype Ascertainment. The following sections cover carrier ascertainment by mutation testing, haplotype testing, and tumor surveillance. The general principles of alternative ascertainment methods, with slight modification, are applicable to MEN2 and to many hereditary syndromes (see Fig. 41-8).

Germline DNA mutation analysis can identify or rule out most *MEN1* mutation carriers by a test applied only once during the life span. This test is available through several commercial and academic laboratories.[289] The usual tissue surrogate for germline DNA is blood leukocytes; MEN1-associated tumor is less satisfactory because any identified mutation could have occurred somatically. The *MEN1* mutation test is based on polymerase chain reaction (PCR) amplification of their nine translated exons (the open reading frame) and the intron-exon boundaries. Laboratories use modestly differing protocols. The germline mutation test or carrier test in DNA has two different roles (see also below). First the carrier state can be evaluated in an affected proband with MEN1-like features. This test, if positive, confirms MEN1, begins tumor screening, and promotes carrier testing in relatives; this test in the same family can be based on an exon-specific short-cut sequence test. Second the carrier state can be evaluated in asymptomatic relatives of a carrier. The positive test can begin tumor screening and testing for additional relatives.

MEN1 germline mutations have been detected in 60% to 100% of well-defined MEN1 families.[283,290-292] The wide variability in mutation detection rate is explained partly by family selection but more likely by differences in laboratory detection methods. Genetic linkage analysis previously mapped all well-characterized MEN1 kindreds to 11q13, making it likely that mutation of the *MEN1* gene causes almost all familial MEN1.[293] Three atypical MEN1 families have not been linked to 11q13.[177,286,294] Failure to identify a *MEN1* mutation could be explained by the presence of mutations involving 5′ or 3′ untranslated or central intronic regions, sequences that are not normally examined, or by a large *MEN1* deletion that results in no abnormal PCR reaction product.[258] Mutation at another gene, such as a member of the CDKI gene family, is also possible. An error in sample processing is a related possibility.

The *MEN1* mutation detection rate has been lower (10% to 80%) in sporadic than in familial MEN1.[172,177,259,260,284,289] The *MEN1* germline mutation rate has been high (about 75%) in sporadic cases with HPT and ZES,[284] but it is far lower (about 7%) in sporadic cases with HPT and acromegaly.[295] For the same reason, the *MEN1* mutation detection rate has also been low (0% to 30%) in sporadic cases with atypical MEN1, a truly broad category without a consensus definition.[172,177,284,296] Most *MEN1* mutations are familial, but about 10% may arise de novo.[296]

When *MEN1* mutation cannot be detected in the germline DNA of a MEN1 index case, ascertainment of the carrier state in relatives is more difficult. Carrier ascertainment can still be based on streamlined periodic tumor surveillance in a relative (discussed later) or on haplotype analysis (similar to genetic linkage analysis) in a kindred (see Fig. 41-8). With three or more affected relatives, haplotype or linkage analysis for the MEN1 trait may be done with high degrees of confidence[297]; however, few laboratories are doing these analyses.

Carrier Ascertainment for MEN1 by Streamlined Surveillance for Tumors: An Alternative to DNA Testing. In kindreds with no identifiable *MEN1* mutation and no possibility of 11q13 haplotype analysis, it is necessary to base assignment of carrier status on the clinical identification of a frequent tumor of MEN1 (see Fig. 41-8). Streamlined periodic surveillance for tumors by biochemical tests should be offered to asymptomatic offspring of known carriers every 3 to 5 years. HPT is the most common and usually the earliest manifestation of MEN1, and its recognition is central to this carrier-ascertainment strategy. The preferred parathyroid tumor surveillance test is the ionized calcium test, beginning at age 8 years or later. A serum PTH assay should be performed at the same time. If the ionized calcium test is unavailable, an albumin-adjusted calcium test is suitable and is also preferable to measurement of total serum calcium.[10]

Five years is a suggested starting age for prolactinoma surveillance, based on the occurrence of a morbid macroprolactinoma in a child of that age with MEN1.[130] Because serum prolactin rises with stress, avoidance of phlebotomy stress in a child can require an indwelling venous catheter and three blood samples obtained at 20-minute intervals.[298] Gastrinoma surveillance can be introduced during adulthood because of the typically later age at onset of ZES in MEN1 (see Fig. 41-1). Occasionally gastrinoma is the first clinical tumor to occur in MEN1.[299]

Surveillance for cutaneous manifestations of MEN1, collagenomas or facial angiofibromas, may be promising but has not yet been explored in children.[166] False-positive test results are often found in MEN1 tumor surveillance through assays of PTH (caused mainly by vitamin D deficiency) prolactin (caused by stress, pregnancy, or psychotropic medications) or gastrin (caused mainly by hypochlorhydria, including that resulting from inhibitors of gastric acid secretion). Rarely can one be misled by a sporadic but common endocrine tumor (such as parathyroid adenoma or pituitary tumor) that could occur in a family member who is not a MEN1 carrier.[300]

Periodic Surveillance for Tumors after Proof of the MEN1 Carrier State. After the MEN1 carrier status has been identified by any method, it is appropriate to focus continued and increased attention on the carrier with the goal of identifying and treating neoplastic manifestations at an appropriate stage (see Table 41-2). Surveillance for parathyroid tumor, prolactinoma, and insulinoma can begin in proven carriers at age 5 to 8 years; surveillance for gastrinoma, other islet tumors, and foregut carcinoids should be delayed until after the age of 20 years. Cost-effective surveillance combines a carefully obtained history focused on clinical symptoms associated with these tumors, limited hormonal and serum chemistry analysis, and carefully defined (i.e., selective and less frequent) use of imaging (see Table 41-2).[185]

Some have recommended more extensive surveillance measures that include measurement such as pancreatic polypeptide,[92,94] chromogranin-A, proinsulin, or cortisol.[294] A meal-stimulated test was developed in the hope of increasing MEN1-related diagnostic information from pancreatic polypeptide and other markers.[91,109,301] It is unclear whether these methods lead to earlier detection and whether benefit to the patient may result.

MULTIPLE ENDOCRINE NEOPLASIA TYPE 2

Beginning about 50 years ago, a series of independent, seemingly unrelated clinical and basic science discoveries provided the basis for the characterization of the type 2 multiple endocrine neoplasia syndromes: MEN2A, MEN2B, and familial medullary thyroid carcinoma (FMTC). In 1959, Hazard, Hawk, and Crile identified MTC as a specific clinicopathologic entity, but it was not until 7 years later that Williams described the histogenesis of MTC from the neural crest–derived C cells in the thyroid gland.[302,303] In 1968, Steiner and associates described a kindred with MTC, pheochromocytomas, HPT, and Cushing's syndrome.[6] They named the disease complex MEN2, and we now know it as MEN2A. In 1966, Williams and Pollack described a syndrome of multiple mucosal neuromata with endocrine tumors, similar to von Recklinghausen's disease, and 2 years later Schimke and colleagues described a similar entity of bilateral pheochromocytomas, MTC, and multiple mucosal neuromas—a disorder we now know as MEN2B.[304,305] In 1986, Farndon and associates described a large family with MTC without other endocrine tumors. This endocrinopathy is Termed familial MTC (FMTC), and it appears to be closely related to MEN2A.[306] In 1962, Copp and colleagues discovered the hormone calcitonin, which was though to lower blood calcium.[307] Although they hypothesized that the parathyroid cells secreted the substance, Hirsch and associates subsequently demonstrated that the hormone was produced by the thyroid gland.[308] In 1985, Takahashi and colleagues reported a novel human transforming gene, which they named *RET* (*R*earranged during *T*ransfection)[309].

The MEN type 2 and related syndromes occur in 1 of every 30,000 individuals with the following frequencies: MEN2A, 80%; MEN2B, 5%; and FMTC, 15%. Each syndrome is inherited in an autosomal dominant fashion with near-complete penetrance and, in the case of MEN2A and MEN2B, with variable expressivity. Virtually all individuals with these syndromes develop MTC, and it is the most common cause of death in affected patients. Approximately 50% of patients with MEN2A

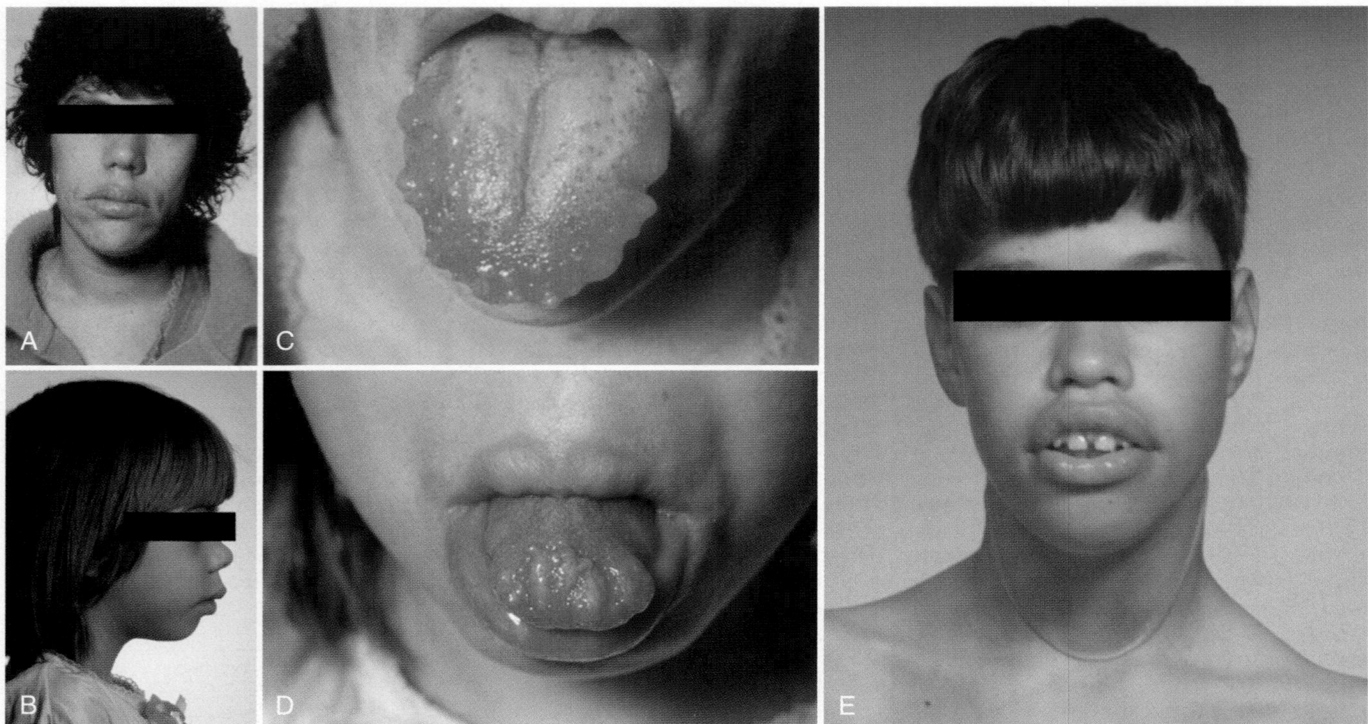

Figure 41-9 **A, B,** and **E,** Typical facial appearance of three patients with multiple endocrine neoplasia type 2B (MEN2B). **C** and **D,** Characteristic mucosal neuromas on the tongues of the mother and daughter shown in **A** and **B,** respectively.

and MEN2B develop pheochromocytomas, and 30% of patients with MEN2A develop parathyroid tumors. Rarely, patients with MEN2A develop two associated disorders, cutaneous lichen amyloidosis and Hirschsprung's disease.

Patients with FMTC only develop MTC. Patients with MEN2B manifest developmental abnormalities of the musculoskeletal system, medullated corneal nerves, mucosal neuromas, hypotonia, ganglioneuromatosis of the aerodigestive tract, and a typical physical appearance (Fig. 41-9). Because of motor dysfunction resulting from ganglioneuromatosis of the large bowel (Fig. 41-10), most patients with MEN2B develop colonic symptoms, characterized by constipation, abdominal bloating, and abdominal pain. A distended colon is evident on radiographic studies of the abdomen, and some patients require surgery for intestinal obstruction.

It is estimated that the disease arises de novo in 50% of patients with MEN2B and 10% of patients with MEN2A or FMTC. In all founder cases studied thus far, the de novo mutation has arisen from the paternal allele.[310,311] Also, of the 43 founder cases with MEN2B, 28 were female and 15 were male, a finding that appears unlikely due to chance.[310] The reason for this distorted sex ratio is unknown.

Few hereditary cancer syndromes have such a close relationship between genotype and phenotype. For that reason, the molecular biology and genetics of the MEN2 syndromes and FMTC, and their clinical relevance, are addressed early in this part of the chapter.

The Molecular Basis for MEN2A, MEN2B, and FMTC

Structure and Function of the Normal *RET* Proto-Oncogene

The *RET* proto-oncogene was identified as a novel hybrid oncogene with transforming activity in NIH 3T3 cells. The proto-oncogene, derived from a recombination event involving two unrelated DNA sequences from human lymphoma, encodes a fusion protein comprising an N-terminal region linked to a tyrosine kinase. *RET* is located in the pericentromeric region of chromosome 10q11.2 and spans 21 exons, including more than 60 kb of genomic DNA.[309] *RET* is highly conserved, and homologues have been found in lower vertebrates and in the fruit fly.[312,313]

The RET protein structure consists of three domains: an extracellular ligand-binding segment containing four cadherin-like repeats, a calcium binding site, and a cysteine-rich region that is important for receptor dimerization; a hydrophobic transmembrane domain; and an internal catalytic core containing two tyrosine kinase subdomains (TK1 and TK2) that are involved in the activation of several intracellular signal transduction pathways. Alternative 3′ splicing of RET produces three isoforms with 9, 43, or 51 amino acids at the C terminus, referred to as RET9, RET43, and RET51, respectively.[314] The two major isoforms, RET9 and RET51, have markedly different signaling complexes, suggesting different physiologic functions.[315,316]

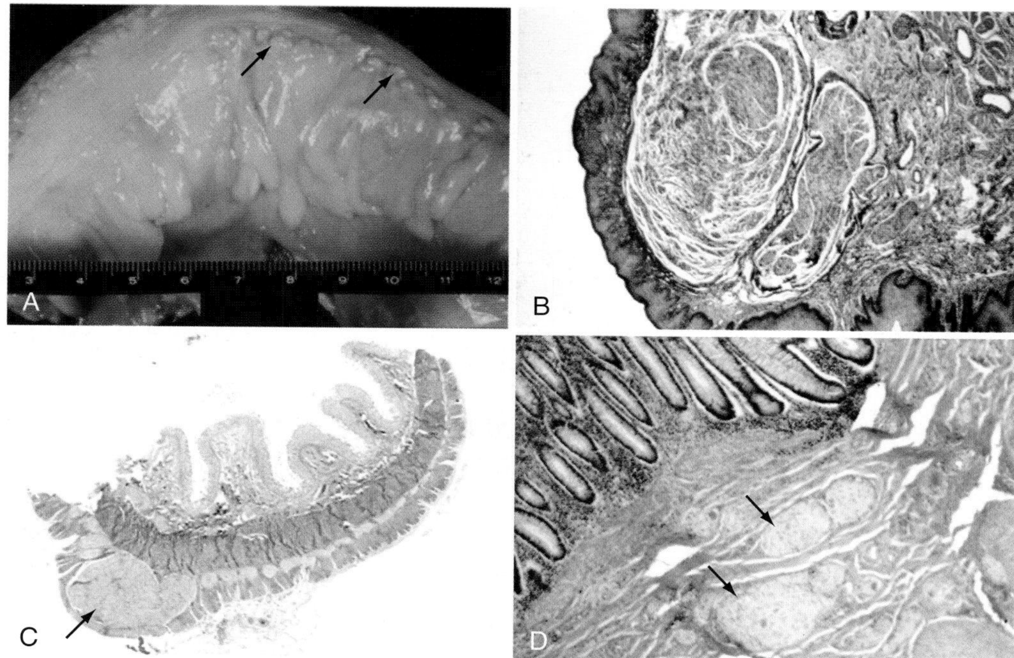

Figure 41-10 Pathologic specimens of the colon in patients with multiple endocrine neoplasia type 2B (MEN2B). **A,** Masses of hypertrophied ganglia cells in the wall of the large bowel *(arrows)*. **B,** Mucosal neuroma of the tongue (hematoxylin-eosin stain; original magnification, ×10). **C,** Cross-section of large bowel wall shown in **A** with mass of subserosal ganglia cells *(arrow)* (Masson's trichome stain; original magnification, ×2). **D,** Section of bowel wall showing enlarged myenteric plexus *(arrows)* (hematoxylin-eosin stain; original magnification, ×40).

RET plays a central role in various intracellular signaling cascades that regulate cellular differentiation, proliferation, migration, and survival. A tripartite cell-surface complex is needed for RET signaling. One of four glial cell line–derived neurotrophic factor (GDNF) family ligands (GFLs)—GDNF, neurturin, artemin, or persephin—binds RET in conjunction with one of four glycosylphosphatidylinositol-anchored coreceptors designated GDNF-family α-receptors (GFRαs) termed GFRα1, GFRα2, GFRα3, and GFRα4.[317-321] GDNF primarily associates with GFRα1, whereas neurturin, artemin, and persephin preferentially bind GFRα2, GFRα3, and GFRα4, respectively. All GDNF-family members have similar downstream signaling pathways, because all GFRαs bind and activate the same tyrosine kinase and induce phosphorylation of the same four key RET receptors (Y905, Y1015, Y1062, and Y1096).[322,323]

Ligand stimulation leads to activation of the RET receptor with dimerization and subsequent autophosphorylation of intracellular tyrosine residues, which serve as docking sites for various adaptor proteins. At least 18 specific phosphorylation sites have been identified, some of which are shown in Figure 41-11.

The normal RET extacellular cysteine residues are involved in the formation of intramolecular disulfide bonds, which are necessary for maintaining the tertiary structure of the extracellular domain. RET cysteine mutants induce constitutive disulfide-linked dimerization of RET molecules.[324-326]

RET is expressed in developing neuroendocrine cells, including thyroid C cells, adrenal medullary cells, parathyroid cells, neural cells (including parasympathetic and sympathetic ganglion cells), and cells of the testis and urogenital tract.[327-330] RET plays a central role in the development of the kidney and the enteric nervous system, as evidenced by the similar phenotype of renal and neural abnormalities in mouse embryos and newborns with deficiencies of RET.[331] In adults, RET is expressed in several tissues including brain, thymus, peripheral enteric sympathetic and sensory neurons, and testis.[322,327,332]

Structure and Function of the Mutated *RET* Proto-oncogene

The first step in cloning the mutated *RET* proto-oncogene was the demonstration through linkage analysis that a putative genetic marker for MEN2A maps to a small region on chromosome 10q11.2.[333,334] Subsequently, it was shown that germline, missense, and point mutations on chromosome 10 are associated with MEN2A, MEN2B, and FMTC.[335-338] The findings that dominant negative activating mutations of the RET proto-oncogene cause these hereditary diseases was unexpected, because most tumor syndromes previously described were associated with tumor suppressor genes or mismatch repair genes. To date, approximately 76 *RET* mutations have been reported in association with MEN2A, MEN2B, and FMTC, and 98% of reported MEN2 families have demonstrated *RET* mutations. Additional information regarding specific molecular changes in the *RET* proto-oncogene can be found on the web sites of The Human Gene Mutation Database at the Institute of Medical Genetics in Cardiff, U.K. (http://www.hgmd.cf.ac.uk/ac/index.php), and Online Mendelian Inheritance in Man (OMIM) from Johns Hopkins University (http://www.ncbi.nlm.nih.gov/sites/entrez?db=omim).

Almost all of the germline point mutations causing the MEN2A, MEN2B, and FMTC occur in a confined segment, either in the extracellular domain of RET (exons 10 and 11) or in the tyrosine kinase domain (exons 13 through 16). The mutations for MEN2A are mostly located in the extracellular, cysteine-rich region of exon 10 (including codons 609, 611, 618, and 620) and exon 11 (including codons 630 and 634). Approximately 85% of the mutations associated

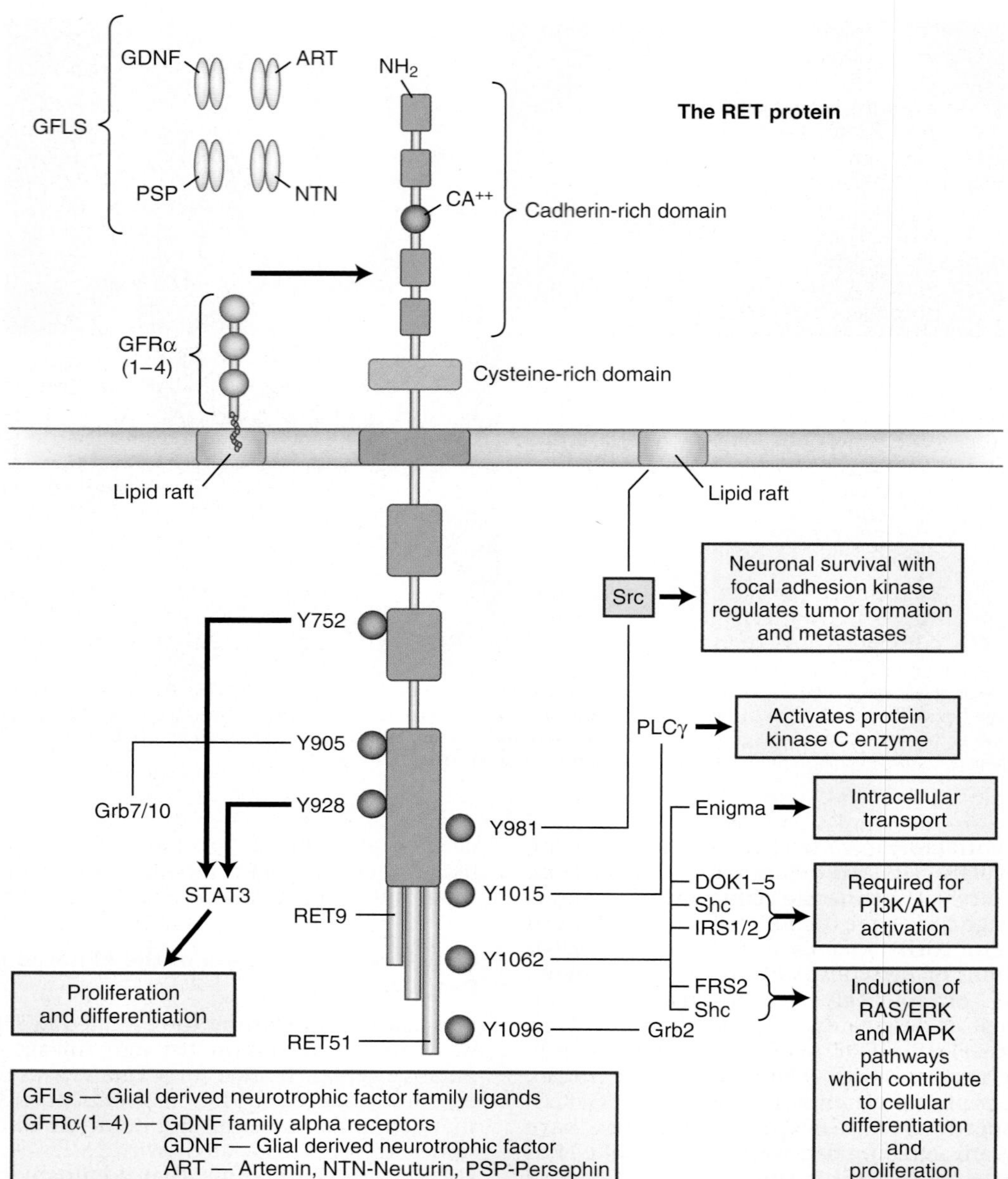

Figure 41-11 Molecular pathways activated by the *RET* proto-oncogene. (Reprinted with permission from Wells SA, Santoro M. Targeting the *RET* pathway in thyroid cancer. *Clin Cancer Res.* 2009;15:7119-7123.) These abbreviations are well known molecular terms. I am not sure that an explanation is necessary, as they are rarely spelled out in text figures. However, here they are: DOK-docking protein, FRS2-fibroblast growth factor receptor substrate 2, GRB-granzyme B, IRS1/2-internal resolution sites 1/2, PCLγ-phospholipase C gamma, Shc-sarc homology, Src-sarc, STAT-signal transducer and activator of transcription, Y752-Y1096-tyrosine docking sites.

with MEN2A involve *RET* codon 634, and approximately half of those are C634R *RET* mutations.[339] The reason for the prevalence of codon 634 mutations in MEN2A is unknown. Base-pair duplications in the cysteine-rich extracellular domain of *RET* and dual de novo mutations on the same *RET* allele have been reported in MEN2A.[340,341]

The mutations characteristic of FMTC also occur in exons 10 and 11, however, noncysteine point mutations have also been found in exon 8 (codons 532 and 533), exon 13 (codons 768, 790, and 791), exon 14 (codons 804 and 844), exon 15 (codon 891), and exon 16 (codon 912). Pigny and associates reported a family with FMTC who did not have a usual *RET* mutation; rather, a 9-base-pair duplication in exon 8 was present in all affected family members.[342] Mutations associated with FMTC result in less potent transformations in vitro than those associated with MEN2A.[343]

Unlike the mechanism in MEN2A, the MEN2B mutations in the kinase domain cause constitutive RET activation in a monomeric form of RET, thereby altering substrate specificity, presumably as a result of a conformational change in the binding pocket of the kinase.[325,344] Approximately 95% of mutations causing MEN2B are in codon 918 (exon 16), and 5% are located in codon 883 (exon 15). There have been two reports of patients with an atypical MEN2B syndrome who were found to have two RET mutations on the same allele, neither involving codons 918 or 883. One patient had a germline Y806C mutation (also present in the asymptomatic father) in association with a de novo V804M mutation.[345] The second patient and affected family members had MTC and mucosal neurilemmomas, and one family member had HPT, which is not a component of MEN2B.[346] Mutational analysis showed double germline mutations of V804M and S904C. Both amino acid changes are located within the split kinase domain, the V804 mutation within an area of unknown function and the S904C mutation within the highly conserved distal half containing the activation loop of the RET receptor tyrosine kinase. Similarly located mutations, such as c-Kit (KIT) and fibroblast growth factor receptor 3 *(FGFR3)*, have been demonstrated to cause ligand-independent activation.[346] There has also been a report of a double mutation, V804M and R844L, in a patient with FMTC.[347]

It appears that the pattern of expression of the MEN2 and related syndromes may vary, and may be more or less restrictive, in different parts of the world. For example, studies of patients in two Asian countries found that almost all patients with MEN2A have *RET* 634 codon mutations, whereas patients with MEN2B have *RET* 918 codon mutations.[348,349]

Genetic Testing for Hereditary Medullary Thyroid Carcinoma. The role of direct DNA analysis in the detection of family members who have inherited a mutated *RET* allele cannot be overemphasized. According to the Gene Tests Laboratory Directory, 38 laboratories currently perform DNA analyses for *RET* in MEN2A, MEN2B, FMTC, and sporadic MTC. Information can be found at the National Center for Biotechnology Information (http://www.genetests.org). All listed laboratories use direct sequence analysis to identify *RET* mutations. Almost all of the laboratories evaluate mutations in exons 10, 11, 13, 14, 15, and 16, and some laboratories include exon 8. If no mutations are found in these exons, the entire coding region of *RET* can be sequenced. *RET* mutations in exons 10 or 11 are identified in more than 95% of families demonstrating a germline transmission of MEN2A or FMTC.[350]

Genetic Counseling. Genetic counselors have a significant role in the management of patients with hereditary cancer syndromes and their families. Whereas formerly the physician alone gave advice and recommended treatment decisions based on available data, contemporary programs involving predictive genetic testing require a broader explanatory interface between medical personnel and the patient. Genetic counselors provide information to patients regarding the genetic aspects of their disease, the methods of genetic testing, and the interpretation of genetic test results. They are helpful in meeting with family members to discuss the patterns of inheritance and their potential risks of developing the disease.

It is important to explain the implications of a given genetic test to the patient and to tell the patient that family members may be at risk for developing the disease. In most cases, the patient will inform family members of their risk, but there are situations in which they might not, and this presents a problem for the doctor and the "duty to warn" those who are at risk of foreseeable harm. This issue is complex and has been debated in the courts, which emphasizes the importance of providing genetic information to patients in the setting of genetic counseling. If there is uncertainty about the correct course of action, physicians should seek advice from their institution's ethics committee or from legal counsel. The issues related to informed consent in the new age of personalized genetic medicine have been addressed by Rosenthal and Pierce.[351]

Relationship between *RET* Genotype and Phenotype in MEN2A, MEN2B, and FMTC

The various *RET* mutations characteristic of MEN2A, MEN2B, and FMTC relate not only to the clinical expression of the disease phenotypes but also to the clinical aggressiveness of the MTC. In MEN2A, specific genotypes are associated with the expression of pheochromocytoma or HPT, whereas in patients with MEN2B, the expression of pheochromocytoma is not associated with a specific genotype, except for the 918 codon mutation.

Medullary Thyroid Carcinoma

Shortly after discovery of the genetic basis of MEN2A, MEN2B, and FMTC clinicians realized that the clinical aggressiveness of the MTC (age at onset, tumor size, timing and frequency of local and distant metastases) in these syndromes was highly variable. For example, the MTC associated with MEN2B is much more aggressive than the MTC occurring in MEN2A or FMTC. The primary basis for the difference appears to be that certain *RET* mutations are more highly activating than others. *RET* mutations associated with MEN2A have greater activating and transforming abilities than *RET* mutations associated with FMTC.[343] Also, MEN2B mutations are associated with greater basal kinase activity, compared to mutations occurring with MEN2A or FMTC.[325] These observations were subsequently confirmed and extended.[352] The molecular data are useful for predicting the clinical course of the MTC in a given setting and especially for determining the timing of prophylactic thyroidectomy in members of kindreds with these syndromes who are shown by genetic testing to have inherited a mutated *RET* allele.

Pheochromocytomas

Pheochromocytomas are most common in patients with *RET* mutations in exon 11 (particularly codon 634) and are less common, or occur infrequently, in patients with mutations in exon 8 (codon 533), exon 10 (codons 609, 611, 618, and 620), exon 13 (codons 768, 790, 791, and 804), and exon 15 (codon 891). A study of 477 MEN2A families conducted by the International RET Consortium found that 169 (91%) of 186 families with MEN2A and pheochromocytoma had a mutation in the *RET* 634 codon.[339]

Hyperparathyroidism

In MEN2A families, there is a strong association between the presence of HPT and codon 634 mutations. Of 104 patients with MTC and HPT, 93 (89%) had a mutation in *RET* 634 and in 57 patients (62%) the mutation was a C634R *RET*.[339]

Similar findings correlating *RET* codon mutations with the presence of pheochromocytoma or HPT have been reported by other investigators.[353-355] The recognition that a certain *RET* mutation signals that a patient is at increased risk for developing pheochromocytoma or HPT is useful in patient management.

Cutaneous Lichen Amyloidosis

Cutaneous lichen amyloidosis associated with MEN2A occurs in the intrascapular region of the back corresponding to dermatomes T2-T6.[356,357] Pruritus, the dominant symptom, leads to repetitive scratching and secondary skin changes characterized by deposition of amyloid. The initiating lesion is thought to be notalgia paraesthetica, a sensory neuropathy involving the dorsal spinal nerves.[358] Although it was once thought rare, the abnormality was found in 9 (36%) of 25 patients in 10 families with

MEN2A.[358] The lesion may be evident in infancy, thus serving as a precursor marker of MEN2A.

Cutaneous lichen amyloidosis is associated with a *RET* 634 codon mutation; the sole exception has been an apparent case in a patient with FMTC and an associated *RET* 804 codon mutation.[358,359] The entity may also occur as an isolated sporadic or familial entity in which the skin lesions are generalized rather than intrascapular and patients have no *RET* mutations nor MTC.[360]

Hirschsprung's Disease

Hirschsprung's disease, manifested by the absence of intrinsic ganglion cells in the distal gastrointestinal tract, is a common cause of intestinal obstruction in the neonate. To date, more than 100 *RET* mutations have been identified in patients with Hirschsprung's disease, occurring in 50% of familial cases and 35% of sporadic cases.[361-363] The mutations are inactivating and occur throughout the proto-oncogene. Most are point mutations, but there are also nonsense mutations, frameshift mutations, microdeletions, insertions, and splicing mutations. In rare cases, large deletions encompass the entire proto-oncogene.[364]

Hirschsprung's disease has been reported in at least 30 families with MEN2A or FMTC, and the disease has been associated with mutations in exon 10 of *RET* involving codons 609 (15%), 611 (4%), 618 (30% to 35%), and 620 (50%).[365-368] In functional studies, the cell surface expression of *RET* of mutations in these codons is lower than that found with the *RET* 634 codon mutations.[369] These data provide a molecular basis for the range of phenotypes engendered by alterations of *RET* cysteines and suggest a novel mechanism whereby these *RET* codon mutations have a dual effect, on the one hand causing transformation of C cells leading to MTC while on the other hand interfering with transportation of the protein to the plasma membrane, resulting in absence of ganglion cells and the development of Hirschsprung's disease.[343,352]

Sporadic Medullary Thyroid Carcinoma and *RET* Mutations

Approximately 75% of MTCs are sporadic, and the incidence peaks during the fifth decade of life. Patients present with a palpable solitary thyroid nodule, and cervical lymph node metastases are present in most patients. Approximately 50% of patients with sporadic MTC have somatic M918T *RET* mutations; however, point mutations and in-frame deletions in exons 10, 11, 13, and 14 have been reported also.[338,370,371] In one study of 51 sporadic MTCs confirmed by family history and direct DNA analysis, somatic *RET* mutations were identified in 33 (64.7%) of the tumors, with exon 16 being affected most frequently (60.6%, compared with exon 10 (9.1%), exon 11 (21.2%), and exon 15 (9.1%).[372]

It was initially reported that the presence of a somatic *RET* mutation in sporadic MTC, compared with its absence, was associated with a less favorable clinical outcome.[373] This issue has been controversial, however. Some investigators have confirmed the original observation, whereas others have reported no relationship between clinical prognosis and the presence or absence of somatic *RET* mutations.[371,374-379]

Relationship of *RET/PTC* Translocations to Papillary Thyroid Carcinoma

The clinical relevance of *RET* was first shown in 1987 when Fusco and associates transfected NIH 3T3 cells with DNA obtained from a series of individual papillary thyroid carcinomas (PTCs) and found a new oncogene resulting from the relocation of an unknown N-terminal sequence to the tyrosine kinase domain of the *RET* proto-oncogene.[377] The gene was subsequently cloned and sequenced. This genetic rearrangement was found in all transfectants and in the original PTC DNAs but not in autologous DNA from normal cells.[378]

These hybrid oncogenes in PTC, the paradigm for chimeric oncoproteins in solid tumors, occur with wide variations in clinical frequency, ranging from 5% to 70%, partly depending on the geographic region.[379,380] *RET* is not mutated; rather, the chromosomal rearrangements activate the transforming potential of *RET* by replacing its transcriptional promoter with those of the fusion partners, thereby allowing its expression in the follicular cells, where it is usually transcriptionally silent.[322] The incidence of *RET/PTC* translocations is significantly higher in patients exposed to radiation, such as the children who developed PTC after the Chernobyl nuclear accident and patients subjected to therapeutic x-ray treatment for benign or malignant conditions.[381-384] Virtually all of the breakpoints in *RET* occur at sites throughout intron 11, resulting in proteins with no transmembrane domain. At least 12 different fusion partner genes have been reported, the most common being *RET/PTC1* (60% to 70%) and *RET/PTC3* (20% to 30%)[385] (Fig. 41-12).

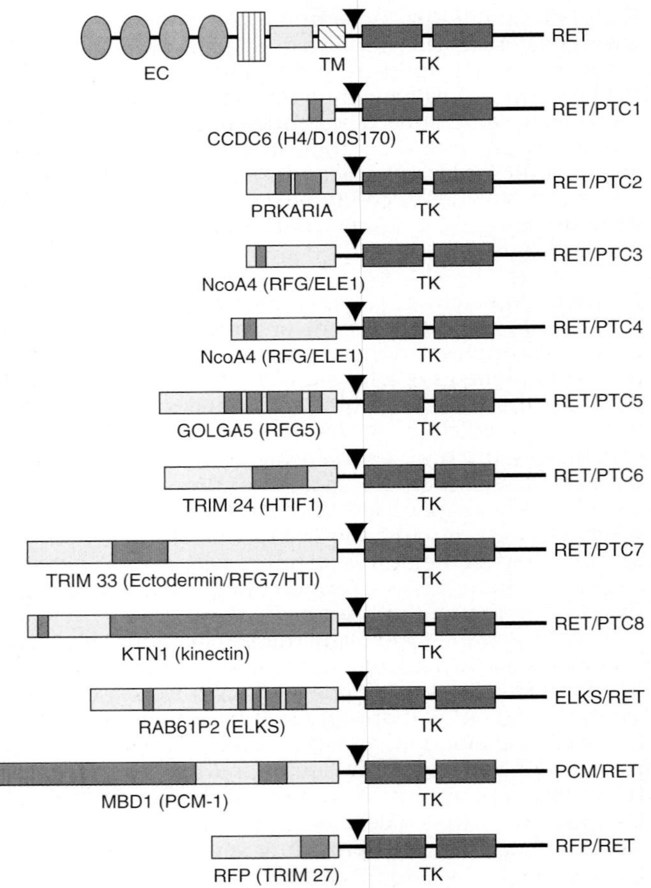

Figure 41-12 *RET/PTC* translocations associated with papillary thyroid carcinoma. EC, extracellular; TK, tyrosine kinase domain; TM, transmembrane. (Reprinted with permission from Santoro M, Melillo RM, Fusco A. RET/PTC activation in papillary thyroid carcinoma: European Journal of Endocrinology Prize Lecture *Eur J Endocrinol.* 2006;155:645-653.)

There is an association between the *RET/PTC* genotype and the pathology and clinical behavior of the associated PTCs. *RET/PTC3* is associated with the solid-follicular variant, and almost all of the tall-cell variant PTCs have the *RET/PTC3* isoform. Also, *RET /PTC1* tumors seem to be associated with a more indolent behavior, compared with the more aggressive *RET/PTC3* tumors.[386,387]

It has also been shown that most Hürthle cell adenomas as well as Hürthle cell carcinomas have *RET/PTC1* translocations, raising the question of whether all Hürthle cell tumors should be considered malignant, regardless of their histologic appearance.[388,389]

The receptor tyrosine kinase NTRK1 is also activated in PTCs but with a much lower frequency compared to RET.[390] The activation of NTRK results from rearrangements with three different genes forming four chimeric variants: TRK, TRK-T1, TRK-T2, and TRK-T3. All except TRK-T1 have a transmembrane domain.

The most common genetic abnormality in PTC is not a *RET/PTC* translocation but a V600E mutation in *BRAF*. Compared to tumors with *RET/PTC* translocations, PTCs with this BRAF mutation have a more aggressive clinical course characterized by larger tumors, a higher incidence of extrathyroidal invasion, metastases to regional lymph nodes and distant sites, and poorer survival.[391]

Diagnosis and Management of Tumors Associated with MEN2 and Related Syndromes

Medullary Thyroid Carcinoma

Expression and Diagnosis of C-Cell Disorders. MTC is actually not a thyroid tumor in that the MTC cells arise from the parafollicular C cells and not the follicular cells from which all other histologic types of thyroid cancers originate. Very early in embryologic life, the C cells stream from the neural crest to populate the adrenal medulla, the sympathetic and parasympathetic ganglia, and the superior aspects of the thyroid lobes. In birds and fishes, the C cells are located in the ultimobranchial body.[392,393]

In patients with MEN2A, MEN2B, or FMTC, the first evident histologic abnormality in the thyroid gland is C-cell hyperplasia, a premalignant entity that is also found in the thyroid tissue surrounding macroscopic tumor foci in hereditary MTC but not in sporadic MTC. C-cell hyperplasia appears to represent carcinoma in situ, which is rarely if ever seen in other endocrine tissues and is the first step in a progression to early microinvasive carcinoma and, finally, invasive macroscopic carcinoma (Fig. 41-13).[394] Many thyroid glands removed prophylactically from young children with hereditary MTC appear normal to the naked eye; however, on microscopic examination, C-cell hyperplasia is often the only evident abnormality.

The histologic diagnosis of C-cell hyperplasia has much more validity in members of families with MEN2A, MEN2B, or FMTC, because the lesion can occur in the thyroid glands of patients with other disease states, such as HPT, hypergastrinemia, and chronic lymphocytic thyroiditis. This so-called secondary C-cell hyperplasia is not a premalignant condition.[395] Up to 50 C cells per low-power field can be seen in the thyroid glands of normal adults.[396] Using this criterion, in a study of 47 normal human subjects, 33% (15% women and 41% men) met the criteria for C-cell hyperplasia.[397] This is of interest not only because of the surprisingly high frequency of this histologic condition in normal subjects but because of the known higher normal range of serum calcitonin for men compared to women.[398,399]

In hereditary MTC, the tumor is bilateral and multicentric, although there may be discordance in the size of tumor foci in one thyroid lobe compared with the other (see Fig. 41-13). The MTC is primarily located in the superior-medial aspect of each thyroid lobe. Histologically, the tumor cells are spindle shaped and on immunochemical staining are positive for calcitonin and carcinoembryonic antigen (CEA). When the cells are stained with Congo Red and viewed under polarized light, a substance with staining properties of amyloid is evident; however, the substance represents full-length calcitonin fibrils (see Fig. 41-13).[400] As the MTC ages, certain portions become fibrotic and calcific, which is often evident on radiologic imaging of the neck and metastatic sites.[401,402] MTC first spreads to the regional lymph nodes in the neck and mediastinum and subsequently to the liver, lungs, bone, brain, and, rarely, skin.

Patients with sporadic MTC present with a thyroid mass and palpable cervical lymph nodes. Patients with hereditary MTC not detected by genetic or biochemical screening also present with a thyroid mass and are indistinguishable from patients with sporadic MTC, with the exception of those with MEN2B, who should be recognizable because of their characteristic physical appearance.

Tumor Markers and Medullary Thyroid Carcinoma. MTC cells have great biosynthetic activity and secrete calcitonin, CEA, chromogranin-A, dopa-carboxylase, histaminase, somatostatin, gastrin-releasing peptide, thyrotropin-releasing hormone, and ACTH.[403-408] Of these markers, calcitonin and CEA are the most useful clinically.

Tashjian and associates demonstrated that the thyroid C cells secrete the hormone, calcitonin, and that the intravenous infusion of calcium gluconate stimulates calcitonin secretion.[409] The polypeptide, pentagastrin, is also a calcitonin secretagogue, and the combined infusion of calcium and pentagastrin is a more potent secretagogue than either agent administered alone.[410] Initially, the infusion of these provocative agents, either alone or in combination, was the standard method of establishing the diagnosis of MTC in family members at direct risk for MEN2A, MEN2B, or FMTC. An abnormally elevated calcitonin level indicated the presence of MTC even if it was not evident clinically, and this screening methodology set the stage for early thyroidectomy in kindred members at risk for hereditary MTC, the goal being to remove the thyroid gland before MTC develops or while it is still confined to the thyroid gland.

Although CEA is also elevated in patients with MTC, it is a less sensitive biomarker than calcitonin; furthermore, serum levels of CEA do not increase after the administration of intravenous calcium or pentagastrin.

Clinical and Biochemical Diagnosis of Familial Medullary Thyroid Carcinoma. Once it was discovered that mutations in the *RET* proto-oncogene caused MEN2A, MEN2B, and FMTC, direct DNA analysis for *RET* mutations became the method of choice for screening of family members at risk for these diseases. The test could be performed at any age, and the designation of a positive or negative test was definitive. Nowadays, measurement of serum calcitonin and CEA are seldom used to establish the early diagnosis of hereditary MTC in a family member. However, these markers are extremely useful for detection of persistent or recurrent MTC after thyroidectomy and for measuring the response to various therapies in patients with advanced disease.

With the advent of biochemical testing and the subsequent development of direct DNA analysis, there

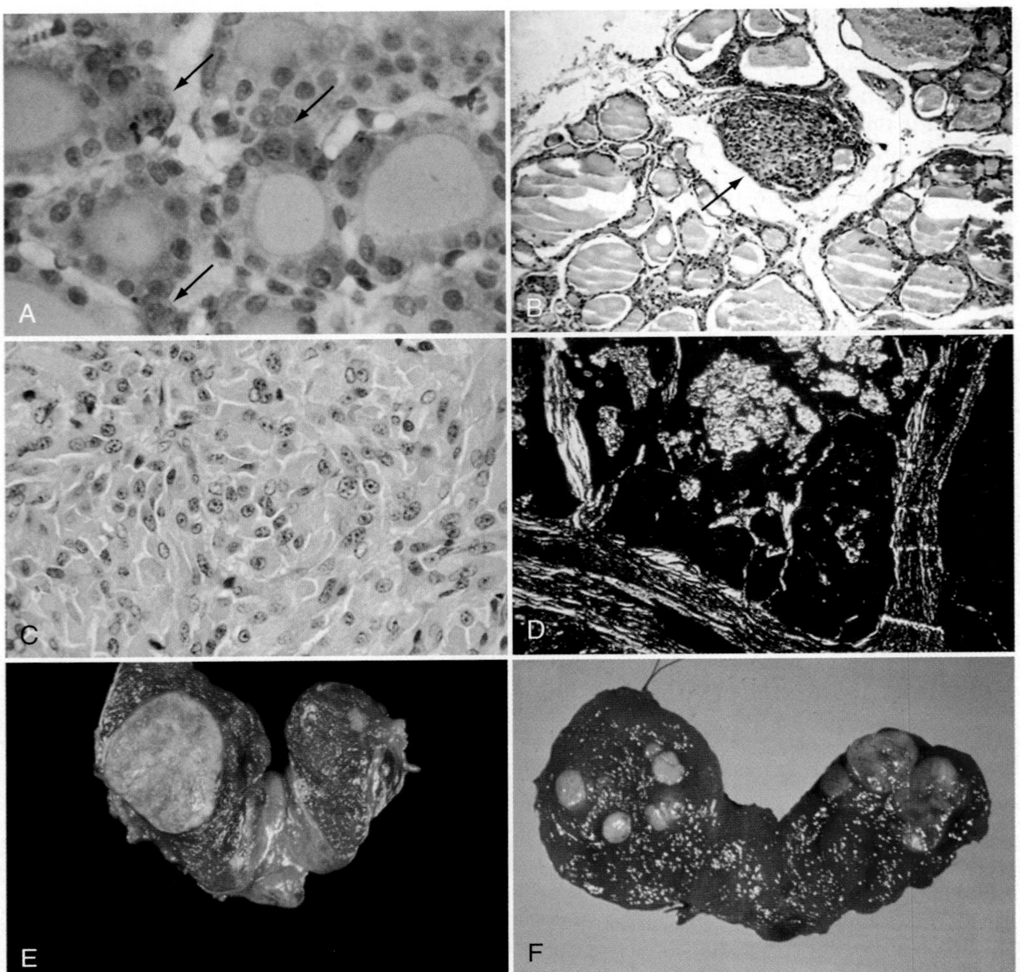

Figure 41-13 Histology of C-cell disorders. **A,** Parafollicular C cells stained with an anti-carcinoembryonic antigen (anti-CEA) antibody *(arrows)* (original magnification, ×40). **B,** Focus of C-cell hyperplasia (hematoxylin-eosin stain; original magnification, ×20). C, Medullary thyroid carcinoma (hematoxylin-eosin stain; original magnification, ×40). **D,** Medullary thyroid carcinoma showing positive staining for amyloid-like material, which actually represents calcitonin fibrils (Congo Red stain, viewed under polarized light; original magnification, ×20). **E,** Bilateral MTC with largest tumor in the right thyroid lobe. **F,** Multi-centric MTC. Note distribution in the upper and middle portion of each thyroid lobe.

has been improvement in the early diagnosis and treatment of hereditary MTC. With time, this is highly likely to result in improved survival. Over the last 30 years, however, there has been no change in stage at diagnosis, and survival has not improved, in patients with sporadic MTC and in patients with unsuspected hereditary MTC. For that reason, early detection and treatment are of great importance.[411] Thus, the clinicians have concentrated on fine-needle aspiration cytology and determination of serum calcitonin to diagnose MTC in patients with nodular thyroid disease.

Fine-needle aspiration cytology is widely employed as a diagnostic tool in patients with nodular thyroid disease. In a review of 91 patients with a histologic diagnosis of MTC, fine-needle aspiration cytology had a sensitivity of 89%, a false-negative rate of 11%, and a positive predictive value of 85.3%.[412] Other investigators found that fine-needle aspiration cytology is less sensitive than measurement of basal calcitonin levels in screening for MTC. However, the addition of immunocytochemistry of the aspirated cells for calcitonin and the measurement of calcitonin levels in aspirate fluid may increase the sensitivity of the technique.[413-415]

In the United States, the place of serum calcitonin measurements in screening for MTC is controversial. The American Thyroid Association guidelines do not recommend for or against calcitonin screening in patients with thyroid nodules, citing concerns of sensitivity, specificity, assay methodology, and cost-effectivness.[416] The view is somewhat different in Europe, where results of several clinical studies have led to the routine practice of measuring serum calcitonin in patients with nodular thyroid disease. MTC was detected in 0.4% to 0.6% of more than 12,000 patients in two Italian studies of calcitonin screening for nodular thyroid disease.[417,418] Calcitonin screening was superior to fine-needle aspiration cytology. Furthermore, compared with patients diagnosed by physical examination only, patients detected by calcitonin screening had an earlier stage of disease and a better prognosis. The French Medullary Study Group detected MTC in 1.2% of 1167 patients evaluated by calcitonin screening for nodular thyroid disease.[419] They also found calcitonin screening to be superior to fine-needle aspiration cytology. A German evidence-based consensus recommended basal serum calcitonin screening for patients with nodular thyroid disease.[420] They recommended a pentagastrin stimulation test if basal calcitonin values exceed 10 pg/mL. They also recommended thyroidectomy if stimulated calcitonin values exceed 100 pg/mL, and lymphadenectomy if stimulated values exceed 200 pg/mL.

In a genetic screening series of 481 patients with presumed sporadic MTC, *RET* mutations were detected in 35 patients (7.5%), all of whom had a negative family history. Of the 35 newly diagnosed cases of hereditary MTC, 18 were the index case of families in which several presumably normal family members had MTC.[421] This is an important matter, because such screening provides the opportunity for diagnosis and treatment of patients at an early disease stage.

Management of Medullary Thyroid Carcinoma

The Primary Operation. The management of patients with newly diagnosed MTC involves two different strategies, depending on the clinical setting at diagnosis. Virtually all patients with sporadic MTC and the majority with hereditary MTC present with a palpable thyroid nodule and lymph nodes metastases. A minority of patients are members of kindreds with hereditary MTC who on genetic screening are found to have inherited a mutated *RET* allele.[335,336] Regardless of the method of diagnosis, thyroidectomy is the treatment for all patients, although for those diagnosed through genetic screening, the timing of the procedure depends on the patient's age and the specific *RET* mutation.

The first step is an ultrasound examination of the thyroid gland, the central and lateral lymph node compartments, and the superior mediastinum. Computed tomographic imaging of the chest and abdomen and bone scintigraphy are indicated only for patients with evidence of palpable cervical lymph nodes or a serum calcitonin level greater than 150 pg/mL.

The operation of choice in patients with primary MTC and no evidence of distant metastases is total thyroidectomy and resection of lymph nodes in the central compartment of the neck, an area bounded by the hyoid bone superiorly, the thoracic inlet inferiorly, and laterally to the carotid sheaths (levels I through VI). Total thyroidectomy is indicated because the incidence of intrathyroidal lymphatic spread is 10% to 20%, and even if the disease appears to be sporadic, the hereditary status of the patient is usually unknown at the time of thyroidectomy. If lymph nodes are palpable in the ipsilateral or contralateral neck or are evident on ultrasound examination preoperatively, the respective lymph node compartments (II through V) are cleared. During the procedure, great care must be taken to preserve the parathyroid glands, the recurrent laryngeal nerve, and the external branch of the superior laryngeal nerve.

The prognosis is excellent in patients who have a tumor smaller than 1 cm in diameter that is confined to the thyroid gland, a preoperative basal serum calcitonin level lower than 150 pg/mL, and no lymph node metastases. Rarely, lymph node metastases and distant metastases occur with primary tumors smaller than 1 cm in diameter.[422]

Several studies have demonstrated a correlation between preoperative, intraoperative, and postoperative findings and surgical outcome. In a study of 224 consecutive patients with MTC treated surgically over a 10-year period, the serum calcitonin normalized in 62% of 45 patients with node-negative disease and in 10% of patients with node positive disease. Nodal metastases increased in proportion to the preoperative serum calcitonin level ranging from an incidence of 50% of patients with calcitonin levels of 3000 pg/mL and tumors larger than 20 mm in diameter to 100% of patients with levels of 100,000 pg/mL or tumors larger than 60 mm.[422]

There is a correlation between preoperative serum CEA levels and lymph node and distant metastases. In a study of 150 patients, an increase in preoperative serum CEA (from a level of 4.7 to 10 ng/mL to >100 ng/mL) was associated with an increased incidence of metastases in the central lymph node compartment (from 33% to 93%), in the ipsilateral compartment (from 20% to 88%), in the contralateral compartment (from 22% to 73%), and at distant sites (from 0% to 75%). Therefore, an elevated preoperative serum CEA heralds advanced disease, and surgical cure is exceptional when the CEA level exceeds 30 ng/mL.[423]

Several authors have correlated patient outcome with findings at thyroidectomy, the most important factors being multifocality of the MTC within the thyroid gland and the presence of metastases to lymph nodes in the central compartment.[424-427] In a study of 232 consecutive patients undergoing thyroidectomy for MTC, the incidence of lymph node metastases in patients with sporadic MTC increased from 41% with unifocal tumors to 90% with multifocal tumors. In patients with hereditary MTC, the comparable numbers were 14% and 48%.[424] Another study evaluated patterns of lymph node metastases. In 195 patients, the incidence of ipsilateral lymph node metastases increased from 10% when no central compartment nodes were involved, to 77% with one to three lymph nodes involved, and to 98% with four or more lymph nodes involved. Regarding the contralateral neck, lymph node involvement was less frequent, occurring in 5% of patients with a single central compartment nodal metastasis and increasing to 38% when 9 central nodes were involved and to 77% when more than 10 central compartment nodes were involved. In almost all cases, metastases to the contralateral lymph node compartment occurred only when the central and ipsilateral compartments were involved.[425]

The prognosis of patients who have undetectable basal calcitonin levels after initial thyroidectomy is excellent. In a study of 863 patients 371 (43%) had serum calcitonin levels that were either normal or failed to respond to pentagastrin stimulation after total thyroidectomy. They were considered cured because their 5- and 10-year survival rates exceeded 98%.[428] In a study of 1430 patients, the French Calcitonin Tumour Study Group identified 453 patients who were considered "not cured" at their last follow-up visit. Only 15 (3.3%) of these patients had been considered cured 6 months after thyroidectomy (basal and pentagastrin-stimulated serum calcitonin <10 ng/L).[429]

One must be careful in equating normalization of postoperative basal serum calcitonin levels with cure of MTC. If the basal serum calcitonin is undetectable but increases after pentagastrin or calcium provocation, C cells are present (which they should not be if all were removed at thyroidectomy). Often, the basal or stimulated calcitonin concentration becomes elevated at some time after thyroidectomy but the values are within the normal range. Almost certainly, these patients have persistent or recurrent MTC, whether or not it is evident clinically. This poses a dilemma unique to many endocrine tumors in which the increased level of a hormone marker is a more sensitive indicator of persistent or recurrent disease than the results of physical examination or radiographic imaging studies. A progressively increasing serum calcitonin level after thyroidectomy is troubling, both for the patient and the physician because, although this indicates an increasing tumor burden, there is currently no effective therapy for this disease state.

Even though surgical resection infrequently cures patients with regional lymph node metastases, many have a good prognosis, with 5- and 10- year survival rates of 80% and 70%, respectively. Although the outcome for most patients is favorable, there are significant differences in survival times between patients who achieve complete remission, patients with persistently elevated serum calcitonin levels, and patients with distant metastases.[430]

Sternotomy with mediastinal lymph node dissection is indicated only if there is radiologic evidence of progressively enlarging or symptomatic mediastinal lymph node metastases and in patients undergoing initial or repeat operation for node-positive, extrathyroidal MTC.[431] In patients with palpable thyroid tumors, total thyroidectomy and clearance of lymph node metastases in the neck by systemic compartment-oriented dissection may afford local control and prevent invasion of the trachea, esophagus, and mediastinum.

Prophylactic Thyroidectomy. There are several hereditary cancer syndromes, and in many of them removal of the organ at risk for malignancy is a preventative strategy. When considering such a procedure, certain criteria need to be met:

1. From the genetic standpoint, the cancer should be associated with near-complete penetrance.
2. There should be a reliable test to detect family members who will develop the malignancy.
3. The organ at risk should be easily removable with minimal morbidity and virtually no mortality.
4. There should be suitable replacement for the organ's function.
5. There should be a reliable serologic test to determine whether the patient is cured.

The hereditary cancer syndromes MEN2A, MEN2B, and FMTC fulfill each of these criteria.

Many young family members found to have a mutated *RET* allele on genetic screening have no evidence of thyroid disease, and such patients have the greatest likelihood of being cured by prophylactic thyroidectomy.[432,433] Since the original reports of prophylactic thyroidectomy for MEN2A and FMTC in asymptomatic patients detected by genetic screening programs, investigators from several countries have reported successful results with this operative procedure.[433-460] There is little doubt that prophylactic thyroidectomy is indicated for patients who are certain to develop MTC; however, the specific operative procedure and when it should be performed are somewhat controversial.

The Consensus Committee of the 7th International Workshop on MEN, the EUROMEN group, and an International Guideline Committee of the American Thyroid Association have proposed guidelines regarding the timing of prophylactic thyroidectomy in patients with MEN2A, MEN2B, or FMTC.[186,461,462] The recommendations of these three groups are similar in that children with MEN2B (or with mutations in codons 918 or 883) should have thyroidectomy performed at the time of diagnosis, preferably during the first months of life. In children with mutations in codons 611, 618, 620, or 634, thyroidectomy should be performed at or before 5 years of age. In children with mutations in other *RET* codons, the recommended timing of thyroidectomy is less clear but usually between 5 and 10 years of age. Some clinicians use measurements of basal or stimulated calcitonin levels to determine the indication and timing of thyroidectomy in the latter group of patients, including patients with FMTC.[463]

Particularly instructive is the EUROMEN study of 145 families with 207 patients (≤20 years of age) who had a total thyroidectomy after confirmation of a germline *RET* mutation. Comparing patients with mutations in extracellular-domain codons (609, 611, 618, 620, 630, and 634) to those with mutations in intracellular-domain codons (768, 790, 791, 804, and 891), the mean age at diagnosis of C-cell hyperplasia was 8 versus 11 years, respectively; the mean age of patients with node-negative MTC was 10 versus 17 years, respectively, and the mean age of those with node-positive MTC was 17 versus more than 20 years. A 634 *RET* codon mutation was present in 63% of patients, and a further analysis of this group found that malignant transformation was present as early as 1 year of age but there was no spread to lymph nodes until 14 years of age. By 20 years of age 42% of patients had lymph node metastases. The average interval from tumor development to nodal metastases was 6.6 years.[462]

In a more recent study, 50 children with MEN2A (*RET* codon mutations, 609, 611, 618, 620, and 634) treated by prophylactic thyroidectomy, central zone lymph node resection, and parathyroid transplantation were evaluated 5 years postoperatively. The operation was curative in 44 patients (88%), meaning that serum calcitonin was undetectable both in the basal state and after stimulation with calcium and pentagastrin.[464] All 22 children who were 7 years of age or younger at the time of operation were cured. Metastases to central zone lymph nodes were present in three patients (ages 10, 11, and 11 years), and 3 patients (ages 4, 4, and 6 years) developed permanent hypoparathyroidism. The incidence of permanent hypoparathyroidism in series from experienced surgeons has ranged from 5% to 29%, and this represents a significant problem requiring lifelong calcium and vitamin D replacement.[445,451,455,459,460,464]

Patients with MEN2A rarely develop lymph node metastases before 10 years of age, and it is unusual for hypoparathyroidism to complicate total thyroidectomy in patients older than 5 years of age, although it is recognized that identification of parathyroid glands in children (compared with adults) is difficult.[464] Removal of the thyroid gland at about 5 years of age seems reasonable in phenotypically normal children who are found to have a mutated *RET* allele by genetic screening. Also, considering that lymph node metastases are unlikely at this age, there seems to be little need for resection of the central compartment, which also decreases the risk of hypoparathyroidism.

Monitoring for Persistent or Recurrent Medullary Thyroid Carcinoma. Patients should have a physical examination and measurement of serum levels of calcitonin and CEA within 6 months after thyroidectomy. If the tumor is small and confined to the thyroid gland and on pathologic examination there is no extraglandular extension or lymph node metastases, the patient can be monitored at 6-month intervals with measurements of serum calcitonin and CEA. The serum calcitonin level usually drops precipitously after thyroidectomy, although the time to nadir may be several weeks.[465] In patients who have lymph node metastases, extrathyroidal extension of the MTC, or postoperative serum calcitonin levels greater than 150 pg/mL, radiographic imaging studies should be done to determine whether there are metastases to regional lymph nodes, liver, lung, or bone. If these studies are normal, they need not be repeated until the serum calcitonin concentration increases to more than 150 pg/mL.

Miyauchi and associates first demonstrated a strong relationship between the doubling time of serum calcitonin and MTC recurrence and survival.[466] It was subsequently shown in patients with MTC that serum levels of calcitonin and CEA are strongly correlated. The median doubling time of each marker was 12 months or less in patients with progressive disease and 48 months or longer in patients with stable disease.[467] In a study of 65 patients with elevated serum calcitonin levels after total thyroidectomy, calcitonin doubling times between 6 months and 2 years were associated with 5- and 10-year survival rates of 92% and 37%, respectively. With doubling times of less than 6 months the 5- and 10-year survival rates decreased to 25% and 8%, respectively. Also, tumor-node-metastasis (TNM) stage, European Organization for Research and Treatment of Cancer (EORTC) score, and serum calcitonin doubling time were significant predictors of survival by univariate analysis, but only calcitonin doubling time remained an independent predictor of survival by multivariate analysis. Calcitonin doubling time is superior to CEA doubling time as a predictor of survival.[468]

On the other hand, serum CEA levels are an excellent tumor marker and usually increase in parallel with serum calcitonin levels as an index of tumor progression. In some patients, the serum CEA increases progressively but the serum calcitonin does not; this is thought to be a sign of tumor dedifferentiation.[469] This hypothesis was supported by immunohistochemistry studies of MTC specimens from patients with various stages of disease. It was found that the concentrations of CEA and calcitonin are expressed to a similar degree in patients with C-cell hyperplasia or with MTC confined to the thyroid gland; however, compared with calcitonin, there was more intense staining of CEA in the MTC cells of patients with metastatic disease.[470]

Operations for Persistent or Recurrent Medullary Thyroid Carcinoma after the Primary Operation. There are indications for repeat operation after the initial thyroidectomy if patients develop serious complications from recurrent tumor compressing or invading vital structures such as the spinal cord, airway, or esophagus. Often, relief follows tumor excision or debulking.[471] Also, patients who have intractable diarrhea due to markedly elevated tumor hormone secretions, presumably calcitonin, may have symptomatic relief from tumor ablation.[430]

Rarely, patients with MTC develop Cushing's syndrome due to the inappropriate secretion of ACTH or CRH.[472,473] Complete surgical resection of the MTC is the preferred treatment, but this is difficult to accomplish because patients usually have advanced disease. Bilateral adrenalectomy may be required if steroidogenesis inhibitors are ineffective. This poor prognostic sign is associated with an average survival time of 2 years.[473]

The less clear indication for repeat operation for persistent or recurrent MTC concerns patients who only have elevated serum calcitonin levels after primary thyroidectomy. The strategy of re-exploration of the neck in patients with elevated serum calcitonin levels after initial total thyroidectomy is understandable if one considers that lymph node metastases are the first stop in spread of the primary tumor and the first manifestation of metastatic disease. However, some have argued that in most cases MTC is relatively indolent, and patients should be managed by watchful waiting.[474-476]

Initially, repeat neck surgery with lymphadenectomy was performed with the hopes of cure; however, few, if any, patients were rendered disease free, as indicated by normalization of serum calcitonin levels.[477,478] Early reports of repeat operation were discouraging until Tisell and associates reported that a significant proportion of patients could be cured by repeat neck operations and extensive lymph node resection.[477-480] Based on these encouraging results, stricter criteria for patient selection, and the refinement of operative techniques (e.g., introduction of compartmentalized lymphadenectomy), surgical results improved.[471,481-484]

The optimal management of patients with persistent or recurrent MTC after primary surgery remains controversial, primarily for three reasons.[484] The operation is difficult and is associated with higher complication rates than with first surgeries for MTC. The extent of lymph node dissection required for biochemical cure, as defined by normalization of postoperative serum calcitonin levels, remains to be determined. Finally, it is unknown whether "biochemical cure" after reoperation is long lasting and adds years of quality to a patient's life. In one study of 56 patients evaluated 8 years after repeat operation for persistent or recurrent MTC, basal calcitonin levels were lower than 10 pm/mL in 14 patients (26%), and 11 additional patients (20%) had basal serum calcitonin levels lower than 100 pg/mL. None of these 25 patients had radiologic evidence of metastatic MTC.[484] Therefore, it appears that repeat operations have merit in selected patients with locally advanced or recurrent MTC; however, prolonged follow-up is needed.

Chemotherapy and Radiation Therapy for Metastatic Medullary Thyroid Carcinoma. For patients with locally advanced or metastatic MTC, single-agent or combined chemotherapeutic regimens have been of modest effectiveness, and currently chemotherapy does not play a major role in patients with advanced disease.[485-489] The most effective agent has been doxorubicin, although in recent trials fewer than 20% of patients experienced partial remission as determined by RECIST (Response Evaluation Criteria in Solid Tumors).[490]

Similarly, external-beam radiotherapy has shown minimal effectiveness in patients with MTC. Most of the studies have been retrospective and have reported improved local control of disease.[491,492] There have been no randomized, controlled trials comparing radiation therapy to watchful waiting in patients at high risk for local tumor recurrence after initial thyroidectomy. Currently, external-beam radiotherapy is indicated for patients with metastases to the central nervous system. Percutaneous image-guided radiofrequency ablation has been effective in the treatment of bone metastases.[493,494]

Pheochromocytoma

Expression and Diagnosis of Pheochromocytoma. Approximately 50% of patients with MEN2A or MEN2B develop pheochromocytomas. These tumors occur between 30 and 40 years of age, compared with a mean age of 47 years in patients with sporadic pheochromocytomas.[495] In genetic screening programs in which MTC is diagnosed at a young age, pheochromocytomas are also diagnosed earlier compared to patients with sporadic pheochromocytomas, at ages as young as 23 years in one series of 87 patients.[496] The diagnosis is made concurrently with MTC in 35% to 73% of cases of MEN2A, and it may be the first manifestation of this syndrome in 9% to 27% of cases.[495] Many patients have no signs or symptoms of a pheochromocytoma at the time MTC is diagnosed, although on careful questioning they may report episodes of headache, sweating, or rapid heartbeat.

Pheochromocytomas in MEN2A and MEN2B are almost always confined to the adrenal gland and are rarely malignant. The pheochromocytomas tend to be multiple and bilateral, although only a single adrenal gland may be involved when the diagnosis is first made. On examining the adrenal glands from patients with MEN2A or MEN2B, one finds adrenal medullary hyperplasia, either alone or adjacent to frank pheochromocytomas (Fig. 41-14). The

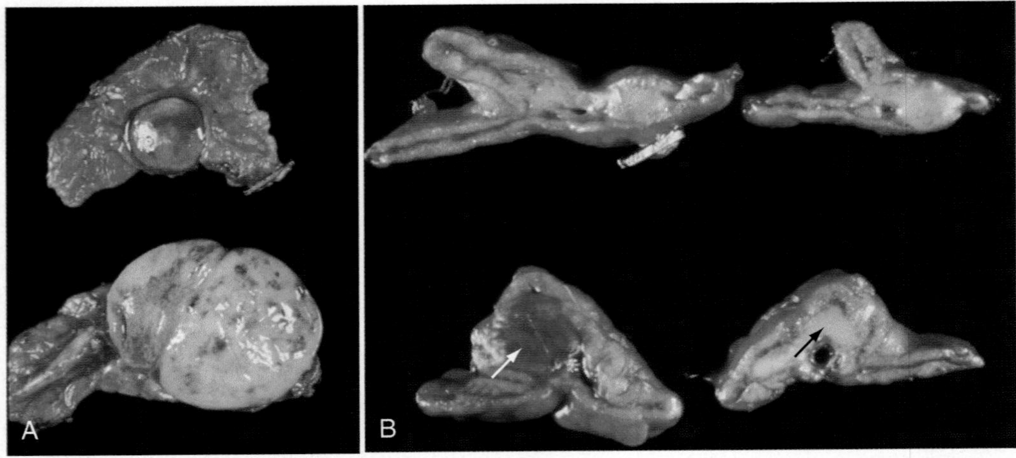

Figure 41-14 Pheochromocytomas. **A,** Bilateral and multiple pheochromocytomas in the left adrenal gland *(top)* and the right adrenal gland *(bottom)*. **B,** Foci of adrenal medullary hyperplasia in adrenal glands *(arrow)* and pheochromocytoma *(arrow)*.

hyperplasia is often manifested by a thickening of the adrenal glands on radiographic imaging studies. Adrenal medullary hyperplasia is the counterpart of C-cell hyperplasia in the thyroid gland and is not associated with hypertension or increased excretion rates of catecholamines or metabolites.

An undiagnosed pheochromocytoma that makes itself known during induction of anesthesia for thyroidectomy or during childbirth can be catastrophic and often lethal. Therefore, all patients with a confirmed or presumptive diagnosis of hereditary MTC should have biochemical and radiographic studies to exclude the presence of a pheochromocytoma. Pheochromocytomas in patients with MEN2A and MEN2B secrete epinephrine and, usually, norepinephrine. Palpitations, anxiety, tremor, dyspnea, hyperglycemia, and paroxysmal hypertension are more commonly associated with tumors that secrete epinephrine. Even though pheochromocytomas secrete catecholamines in an intermittent fashion, they metabolize catecholamines to metanephrines continuously. Concentrations of plasma free metanephrines and 24-hour urinary free metanephrines have sensitivities ranging from 90% to 100%, although the specificities are appreciably less.[497]

Computed tomography and magnetic resonance imaging are highly accurate in localizing intra-abdominal pheochromocytomas, with 95% to 100% sensitivity for intra-adrenal tumors larger than 0.5 cm. Also, T2-weighted magnetic resonance images of pheochromocytomas may show characteristic high-intensity signals.[498] Although there have been relatively few clinical studies using PET to localize pheochromocytomas, [^{18}F]-fluorodopamine ([^{18}F] DA) PET is thought to be the best overall imaging modality in the localization of pheochromocytomas.[499]

Management of Pheochromocytoma

Preoperative Preparation. Before resection of a pheochromocytoma, it is critical that patients be adequately prepared with the α-adrenergic blocker, phenoxybenzamine, which is usually given in a dose of 10 mg orally twice a day for 10 to 14 days preoperatively. Higher doses may be needed to ensure blood pressure control. Patients with pheochromocytomas are volume constricted and should be warned that they may develop postural hypotension during phenoxybenzamine treatment. Most patients can be prepared on an outpatient basis; however, if blood pressure proves to be labile, hospitalization may be required. β-Adrenergic blockade is usually unnecessary unless there is difficulty controlling the hypertension or the patient develops a tachyarrhythmia. If β-blockade is administered, it should be undertaken only after α-blockade; otherwise, patients may develop severe hypertension due to unopposed vasoconstriction.

Before anesthetic induction, a radial artery catheter is placed and a urinary bladder catheter is inserted. A pulmonary artery catheter for central monitoring is usually unnecessary unless the patient has cardiac disease or another indication. During manipulation of the pheochromocytoma intraoperatively, there may be episodes of hypertension; these are best controlled with sodium nitroprusside or esmolol. The patient may experience hypotension after resection of the pheochromocytoma, but this is usually easily managed pharmacologically.

Operation for Pheochromocytoma. Whether to perform a unilateral or a bilateral adrenalectomy depends on the extent of disease at the time of diagnosis. Bilateral adrenalectomy is obviously indicated in patients with bilateral pheochromocytomas; however, there has been controversy regarding the management of patients with a single pheochromocytoma. Because there may be years between the development of a pheochromocytoma in one adrenal gland and a pheochromocytoma in the contralateral gland (and in some patients a second pheochromocytoma may never develop), most surgeons favor performing a unilateral adrenalectomy for solitary pheochromocytomas. Iatrogenic bilateral adrenocortical ablation has a high rate of morbidity, including death from the Addison state.[500] The argument for bilateral adrenalectomy relates to the propensity for bilateral and multicentric development of pheochromocytoma, the decreased morbidity associated with a single operative procedure, and the reduced risk of hypertensive crisis developing in patients who are not compliant with continued evaluation after resection of the first pheochromocytoma. In a 2006 report of adrenal-sparing surgery (unilateral adrenalectomy and contralateral subtotal adrenalectomy) in 13 patients with MEN2A and pheochromocytoma, 12 of whom had unilateral disease, the mean risk of developing recurrent pheochromocytoma was 38% at both 5 and 10 years.[501] The long-term follow-up of patients treated with this procedure bears observation, because it may offer an alternative to total adrenalectomy. The operative approach of choice for resection of an intra-abdominal pheochromocytoma is laparoscopic adrenalectomy. The

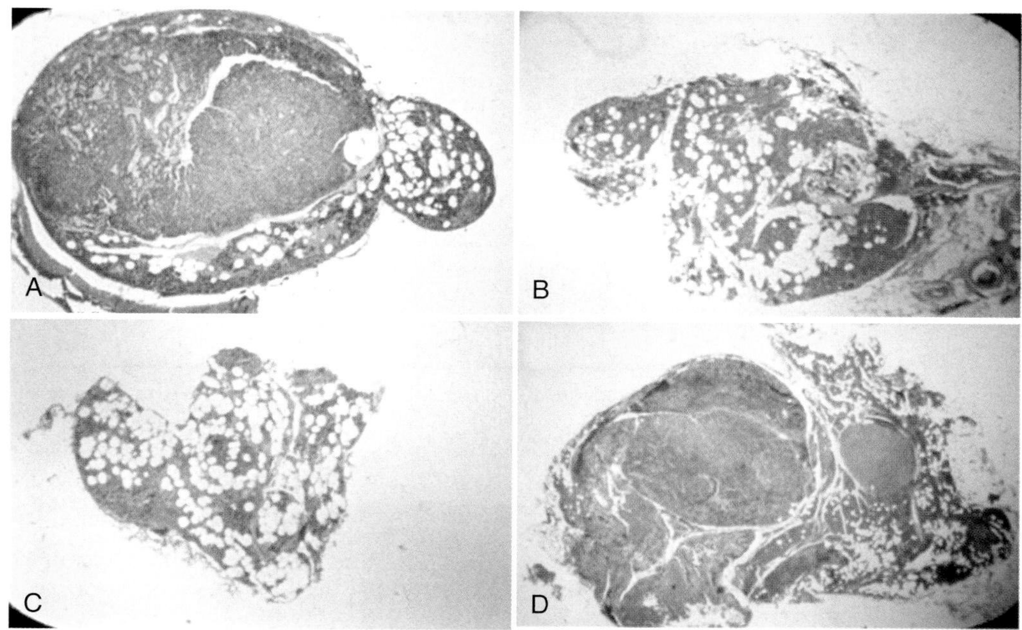

Figure 41-15 Parathyroid glands: right upper **(A)**, right lower **(B)**, left upper **(C)**, and left lower **(D)**.

results are excellent, with minimal morbidity and virtually no mortality.[502,503]

Parathyroid Tumors: Expression, Diagnosis, and Management

HPT occurs in approximately 30% of patients with MEN2A and is characterized by generalized parathyroid hypertrophy and a histologic picture of nodular hyperplasia (Fig. 41-15). Usually, the symptoms of HPT are milder in patients with MEN2A, compared to patients with MEN1. The diagnosis depends on the demonstration of elevated serum levels of calcium and PTH. In hypercalcemic patients with MEN2A, the surgeon will find one or more enlarged parathyroid glands at the time of thyroidectomy. Regardless of the number of enlarged glands, the patient should be treated either by resection of 3½ glands or by total parathyroidectomy and heterotopic autograft of a small portion of one gland.[504] The preferred operative procedure depends on the experience, the expertise, and the preference of the operating surgeon.

There has been little clarity on how normal-appearing parathyroid glands should be managed at the time of thyroidectomy in patients with MEN2A who have an *RET* mutation associated with a high incidence of HPT. The more prudent course would be to treat the MTC without concern for future HPT, because only 25% of patients develop this disease. Some surgeons, however, consider it reasonable to treat the parathyroid glands as if there were generalized parathyroid enlargement, because repeat operations for persistent or recurrent HPT, should they occur, are much more difficult than the primary operation and are associated with a higher incidence of complications.

In patients who develop recurrent or persistent HPT after thyroidectomy for MTC, the initial step is a sestamibi scan and ultrasonography in an attempt to identify the hyperfunctioning parathyroid glands.

In a properly performed total thyroidectomy, it is difficult to preserve the normal parathyroid glands. If the vascular supply to the parathyroids cannot be preserved or if there is a question of parathyroid gland viability, the gland or glands should be autografted to a muscle bed. In patients with sporadic MTC, MEN2B, or FMTC, where there is no risk of HPT, the removed parathyroid tissue can be sliced into small slivers and grafted into the sternocleidomastoid muscle. There is a very high success rate with this technique.[505] In patients with MEN2A who are at high risk for developing HPT, the removed parathyroid tissue should be grafted to a heterotopic site such as the brachioradialis muscle of the forearm, so that a portion of the graft can be removed if the patient develops graft-dependent HPT.

Recent Advances in the Management of Patients with Locally Advanced or Metastatic Medullary Thyroid Carcinoma

There has been no effective treatment for locally advanced or metastatic MTC, and the management of patients with advanced disease has been very challenging. With the demonstration that the tyrosine kinase inhibitor, imatinib, induced remissions in patients with chronic myelogenous leukemia, there was hope that similar small-molecule therapeutics might be developed for patients with MTC and also for patients with the other histologic types of thyroid tumors.[506,507] Subsequently, it was shown that the orally administered tyrosine kinase inhibitor, ZD6474, inhibits vascular endothelial growth factor signaling, angiogenesis, and KDR tyrosine kinase activity and blocks oncogenic RET kinases.[508,509] In a phase 2 single-arm study of ZD6474 (vandetanib), 6 (20%) of 30 patients with locally advanced or metastatic MTC experienced a partial remission and another 60% experienced stable disease, for a disease control rate of 80% (Fig. 41-16).[510] Phase II clinical trials of other molecular targeted therapeutics in patients with advanced MTC have shown partial responses in the range of 15-25%.[511a-511h] Also, a clinical study of vandetanib in children with MEN2B and advanced MTC showed a partial response rate of 67%.[511i] Recently, a phase III, double-blind,

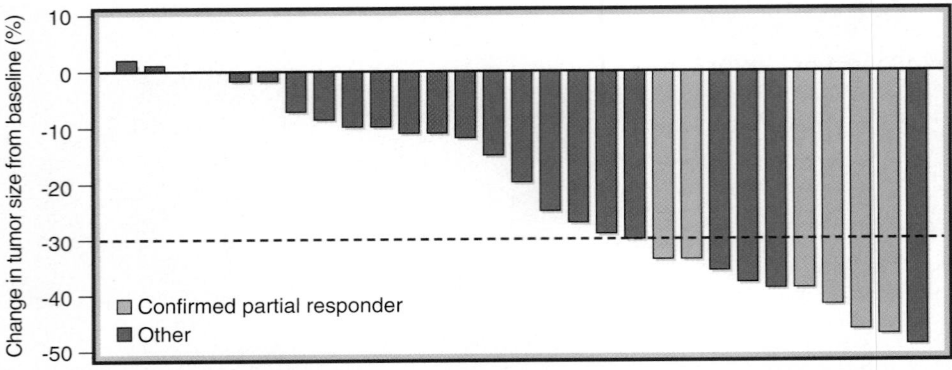

Figure 41-16 Waterfall plot of patients with hereditary medullary thyroid carcinoma who were treated with the tyrosine kinase inhibitor, vandetanib, by RECIST (Response Evaluation Criteria in Solid Tumors). (Reprinted with permission from Wells SA, Gosnell JE, Gagel RF, et al. Vandetanib for the treatment of patients with locally advanced of metastatic hereditary medullary thyroid cancer. *J Clin Oncol.* 2010, 28:767-772.

randomized clinical trial comparing vandetanib to placebo in 331 patients with locally advanced, or metastatic MTC, showed that compared to placebo the progression free survival was greater in the vandetanib arm (hazard ratio 0.46; p = 0.0001).[511j] Therefore, there is promise that there will be effective therapies for patients with advanced disease, and perhaps for patients with minimal disease that is evident after primary thyroidectomy for MTC.

MULTIPLE ENDOCRINE NEOPLASIA OF MIXED OR OTHER TYPE

Overlap and Nonendocrine Syndromes

Overlap syndromes reported in single patients include gastrinoma in a MEN2 patient,[512] adenomatous polyposis coli with MEN1 or MEN2B,[513,514] prolactinoma in a patient with MEN2A,[515] pheochromocytomas in MEN1 (see earlier discussion), and an ovarian strumal carcinoid tumor in a patient with MEN2A.[516]

Most cases of overlap of MEN1 and MEN2 were published before the syndrome-causing genes were discovered. Currently and in retrospect, most can be understood as follows:

- Unusual expressions of a syndrome: VHL can cause pheochromocytoma and islet tumor (see later discussion), CNC can cause somatotropinoma and primary adrenal hypercortisolism (see Chapter 15), and MEN1 can cause its rare pheochromocytoma with any other feature of MEN1 (see earlier discussion).
- Coexistence of two rare disorders: Several families carry mutations for both MEN1 and MEN2.[517] Their expressions seem to be independent.
- Rare syndromes that have not yet been characterized sufficiently. The Carney triad comprises paragangliomas, gastrointestinal stromal tumors, and pulmonary chondromas with occasional adrenocortical tumors. No inherited cases have been identified.[518]
- Cases of unexplained overlap: These are few.

MEN1 and MEN2 are the only multiple neoplasia syndromes in which the two most prominent features are hormone-secreting tumors. In other MEN syndromes, nonhormonal tumors are more urgent. For example, MAS (which is not hereditary) features fibrous dysplasia of bone and café-au-lait spots of skin (see Chapter 25), and VHL syndrome features papillary renal cancer and central nervous system hemangioblastomas. CNC is the main cause of myxomas of the cardiac atria. Still, these are forms of MEN, and they sometimes manifest through their endocrinopathies.

Von Hippel-Lindau Disease

VHL is an autosomal dominant neoplastic syndrome characterized by hemangioblastomas of the central nervous system, retinal angiomas, renal cell carcinomas, visceral cysts, pheochromocytoma, and islet cell tumors.[519,520] More than 90% of gene carriers express one or more of the manifestations of this disorder by the age of 60 years. More than 70% of gene carriers have one or more central nervous system tumors.[521] Of particular relevance to endocrinologists is the observation that 25% to 35% of these patients have unilateral or bilateral pheochromocytomas, and 15% to 20% have islet cell tumors.[518,522] Although the islet cell tumors may immunostain weakly for insulin, they almost never hypersecrete it.

The *VHL* gene was mapped to chromosome 3p25.3[523] and identified by positional cloning.[524] This is a tumor suppressor gene, implying that loss of function or inactivating mutations of both alleles or copies of this gene are associated with tumor formation. The action of the VHL protein to facilitate the proteasome-mediated degradation of the hypoxia-inducible factor 1 (HIF-1) protein and other proteins can prove central to many manifestations of *VHL* gene alteration.[525] Mutation of codon 238 was identified in more than 40% of VHL families with pheochromocytoma, suggesting that families with a mutation in this codon should be surveyed routinely for pheochromocytoma.[526]

Clinical management of VHL syndrome is often focused on the presence of renal or central nervous system tumors. Pheochromocytomas or islet cell tumors associated with hypertension, cardiac arrhythmias, hypoglycemia, watery diarrhea, carcinoid, or a glucagonoma-like picture should be surgically excised. Judgment is required in the management of other malignant features associated with VHL. For example, a less aggressive approach to the management of pheochromocytoma or islet cell tumor may be indicated in a patient who has VHL and a renal cell carcinoma with metastasis. An adrenal cortical-sparing operation may be appropriate for pheochromocytoma in such a patient.

The association of pheochromocytoma and islet cell tumors can occur in familial[527-529] or nonfamilial[530-532] patterns. There is little information about the molecular genetics of these rare disorders, although it is possible that abnormalities of the *VHL* gene are involved.

Neurofibromatosis Type I

The main features of NF1 or von Recklinghausen's neurofibromatosis are neurofibromas and dermal café-au-lait spots. NF2 causes acoustic neuromas and arises from a different but related gene. NF1 has been associated with a variety of endocrine neoplasms, including pheochromocytoma,[533] HPT,[534] somatostatin-producing carcinoid tumors of the duodenal wall,[535,536] MTC,[537] and hypothalamic or optic nerve tumors that cause precocious puberty.[538] The causative gene for NF1 encodes a Ras guanosine triphosphatase (GTPase)-activating protein (RasGAP) of 2818 amino acids, named *neurofibromin,* which accelerates GTP hydrolysis on p21 Ras. Loss of the GTPase-activating function of neurofibromin (through mutation or allelic loss) leads to p21 Ras activation.[539] More specific evidence for a role of this protein in endocrine tumors is suggested by allelic loss of this gene in NF1-associated[540] or sporadic[541] pheochromocytomas.

Carney Complex

CNC includes myxomas of the heart, skin, and breast; spotty skin pigmentation; testicular, adrenal cortical, and pituitary tumors; and peripheral nerve schwannomas.[542-544] Linkage analysis has identified a locus at 2p in half of the families and another locus at 17q in most others.[545] The gene at 17q encodes the regulatory subunit (type IA) of protein kinase A *(PRKA1A),* and it has tumor suppressor properties.[546] Several small kindreds with only bilateral adrenal hyperplasia have mutation of a phosphodiesterase (PDE11A) at chromosome 2p.[547] The activating *GNAS* mutations in MAS and the inactivating *PRKA1A* mutations in CNC cause tumors in selected tissues with a similar tissue spectrum, perhaps because either gene can raise cyclic adenosine monophosphate.

REFERENCES

1. Erdheim J. Zur normalen und pathologischen Histologie der Glandula Thyreoidea, Parathyreoidea und Hypophysis. *Beitr Pathol Anat.* 1903;33:158-263.
2. Underdahl LO, Woolner LB, Black BM. Multiple endocrine adenomas; report of 8 cases in which the parathyroids, pituitary and pancreatic islets were involved. *J Clin Endocrinol Metab.* 1953;13:20-47.
3. Moldawer MP, Nardi GL, Raker JW. Concomitance of multiple adenomas of the parathyroids and pancreatic islets with tumor of the pituitary: a syndrome with a familial incidence. *Am J Med Sci.* 1954;228:190-206.
4. Wermer P. Genetic aspects of adenomatosis of endocrine glands. *Am J Med Sci.* 1954;16:363-371.
5. Ballard HS, Fame B, Hartsock RJ. Familial multiple endocrine adenoma-peptic ulcer complex. *Medicine (Baltimore).* 1964;43:481-516.
6. Steiner AL, Goodman AD, Powers SR. Study of a kindred with pheochromocytoma, medullary thyroid carcinoma, hyperparathyroidism and Cushing's disease: multiple endocrine neoplasia, type 2. *Medicine (Baltimore).* 1968;47:371-409.
7. Melvin KE, Tashjian AH Jr, Miller HH. Studies in familial (medullary) thyroid carcinoma. *Recent Prog Horm Res.* 1972;28:399-470.
8. Sipple J. The association of pheochromocytoma with carcinoma of the thyroid gland. *Am J Med.* 1961;31:163-166.
9. Marx S. Multiple endocrine neoplasia type 1. In: Bilezekian JP, Marcus R, Levine MA, eds. *The Parathyroids: Basic and Clinical Concepts.* 2nd ed. San Diego, CA: Academic Press; 2001:535-584.
10. Marx SJ, Vinik AI, Santen RJ, et al. *Multiple endocrine neoplasia type I: assessment of laboratory tests to screen for the gene in a large kindred. Medicine (Baltimore).* 1986;65:226-241.
11. Benson L, Ljunghall S, Akerstrom G, et al. Hyperparathyroidism presenting as the first lesion in multiple endocrine neoplasia type 1. *Am J Med.* 1987;82:731-737.
12. Trump D, Farren B, Wooding C, et al. Clinical studies of multiple endocrine neoplasia type 1 (MEN1). *QJM.* 1996;89:653-669.
13. Marx S, Spiegel AM, Skarulis MC, et al. Multiple endocrine neoplasia type 1: clinical and genetic topics. *Ann Intern Med.* 1998;129:484-494.
14. Jackson CE, Boonstra CE. The relationship of hereditary hyperparathyroidism to endocrine adenomatosis. *Am J Med.* 1967;43:727-734.
15. Johnson GJ, Summerskill WH, Anderson VE, et al. Clinical and genetic investigation of a large kindred with multiple endocrine adenomatosis. *N Engl J Med.* 1967;277:1379-1385.
16. Craven DE, Goodman D, Carter JH. Familial multiple endocrine adenomatosis: multiple endocrine neoplasia, type I. *Arch Intern Med.* 1972;129:567-569.
17. Snyder N 3rd, Scurry MT, Deiss WP. Five families with multiple endocrine adenomatosis. *Ann Intern Med.* 1972;76:53-58.
18. Jung RT, Grant AM, Davie M, et al. Multiple endocrine adenomatosis (type I) and familial hyperparathyroidism. *Postgrad Med J.* 1978;54:92-94.
19. Eberle F, Grun R. Multiple endocrine neoplasia, type I (MEN I). *Ergebnisse der Inneren Medizin und Kinderheilkunde.* 1981;46:76-149.
20. Burgess JR, David R, Greenaway TM, et al. Osteoporosis in multiple endocrine neoplasia type 1: severity, clinical significance, relationship to primary hyperparathyroidism, and response to parathyroidectomy. *Arch Surg.* 1999;134:1119-1123.
21. Rizzoli R, Green J 3rd, Marx SJ. Primary hyperparathyroidism in familial multiple endocrine neoplasia type I: long-term follow-up of serum calcium levels after parathyroidectomy. *Am J Med.* 1985;78:467-474.
22. Marx SJ, Menczel J, Campbell G, et al. Heterogeneous size of the parathyroid glands in familial multiple endocrine neoplasia type 1. *Clin Endocrinol.* 1991;35:521-526.
23. Hellman P, Skogseid B, Oberg K, et al. Primary and reoperative parathyroid operations in hyperparathyroidism of multiple endocrine neoplasia type 1. *Surgery.* 1998;124:993-999.
24. Agha A, Carpenter R, Bhattacharya S, et al. Parathyroid carcinoma in multiple endocrine neoplasia type 1 (MEN1) syndrome: two case reports of an unrecognised entity. *J Endocrinol Invest.* 2007;30:145-149.
25. Friedman E, Sakaguchi K, Bale AE, et al. Clonality of parathyroid tumors in familial multiple endocrine neoplasia type 1. *N Engl J Med.* 1989;321:213-218.
26. Brandi ML, Aurbach GD, Fitzpatrick LA, et al. Parathyroid mitogenic activity in plasma from patients with familial multiple endocrine neoplasia type 1. *N Engl J Med.* 1986;314:1287-1293.
27. Khan AA, Bilezikian JP, Potts JT Jr. The diagnosis and management of asymptomatic primary hyperparathyroidism revisited. *J Clin Endocrinol Metab.* 2009;94:333-334.
28. Jensen RT. Management of the Zollinger-Ellison syndrome in patients with multiple endocrine neoplasia type 1. *J Intern Med.* 1998;243:477-488.
29. Shawker T. Ultrasound evaluation of primary hyperparathyroidism. *Ultrasound Q.* 2000;16:73-87.
30. Norman J, Chheda H, Farrell C. Minimally invasive parathyroidectomy for primary hyperparathyroidism: decreasing operative time and potential complications while improving cosmetic results. *Am Surg.* 1998;64:391-395; discussion 395-396.
31. Thompson GB, Grant CS, Perrier ND, et al. Reoperative parathyroid surgery in the era of sestamibi scanning and intraoperative parathyroid hormone monitoring. *Arch Surg.* 1999;134:699-704; discussion 705.
32. Jaskowiak N, Norton JA, Alexander HR, et al. A prospective trial evaluating a standard approach to reoperation for missed parathyroid adenoma. *Ann Surg.* 1996;224:308-320; discussion 20-21.
33. Irvin GL 3rd, Molinari AS, Figueroa C, et al. Improved success rate in reoperative parathyroidectomy with intraoperative PTH assay. *Ann Surg.* 1999;229:874-878; discussion 878-879.
34. Tonelli F, Spini S, Tommasi M, et al. Intraoperative parathormone measurement in patients with multiple endocrine neoplasia type I syndrome and hyperparathyroidism. *World J Surg.* 2000;24:556-562; discussion 562-563.
35. Libutti SK, Alexander HR, Bartlett DL, et al. Kinetic analysis of the rapid intraoperative parathyroid hormone assay in patients during operation for hyperparathyroidism. *Surgery.* 1999;126:1145-1150; discussion 1150-1151.
36. Feldman AL, Sharaf RN, Skarulis MC, et al. Results of heterotopic parathyroid autotransplantation: a 13-year experience. *Surgery.* 1999;126:1042-1048.
37. Majewski JT, Wilson SD. The MEA-I syndrome: an all or none phenomenon? *Surgery.* 1979;86:475-484.
38. Skogseid B, Oberg K, Eriksson B, et al. Surgery for asymptomatic pancreatic lesion in multiple endocrine neoplasia type I. *World J Surg.* 1996;20:872-876; discussion 877.
39. Wilkinson S, Teh BT, Davey KR, et al. Cause of death in multiple endocrine neoplasia type 1. *Arch Surg.* 1993;128:683-690.
40. Doherty GM, Olson JA, Frisella MM, et al. Lethality of multiple endocrine neoplasia type I. *World J Surg.* 1998;22:581-586; discussion 586-587.
41. Yu F, Venzon DJ, Serrano J, et al. Prospective study of the clinical course, prognostic factors, causes of death, and survival in patients

with long-standing Zollinger-Ellison syndrome. *J Clin Oncol.* 1999;17:615-630.
42. Kloppel G, Willemer S, Stamm B, et al. Pancreatic lesions and hormonal profile of pancreatic tumors in multiple endocrine neoplasia type I: an immunocytochemical study of nine patients. *Cancer.* 1986;57:1824-1832.
43. Le Bodic MF, Heymann MF, Lecomte M, et al. Immunohistochemical study of 100 pancreatic tumors in 28 patients with multiple endocrine neoplasia, type I. *Am J Surg Pathol.* 1996;20:1378-1384.
44. Pipeleers-Marichal M, Somers G, Willems G, et al. Gastrinomas in the duodenums of patients with multiple endocrine neoplasia type 1 and the Zollinger-Ellison syndrome. *N Engl J Med.* 1990;322: 723-727.
45. Ariel I, Kerem E, Schwartz-Arad D, et al. Nesidiodysplasia—a histologic entity? *Hum Pathol.* 1988;19:1215-1218.
46. Lubensky IA, Debelenko LV, Zhuang Z, et al. Allelic deletions on chromosome 11q13 in multiple tumors from individual MEN1 patients. *Cancer Res.* 1996;56:5272-5278.
47. Debelenko LV, Zhuang Z, Emmert-Buck MR, et al. Allelic deletions on chromosome 11q13 in multiple endocrine neoplasia type 1-associated and sporadic gastrinomas and pancreatic endocrine tumors. *Cancer Res.* 1997;57:2238-2243.
48. Anlauf M, Perren A, Meyer CL, et al. Precursor lesions in patients with multiple endocrine neoplasia type 1-associated duodenal gastrinomas. *Gastroenterology.* 2005;128:1187-1198.
49. Crabtree JS, Scacheri PC, Ward JM, et al. A mouse model of multiple endocrine neoplasia, type 1, develops multiple endocrine tumors. *Proc Natl Acad Sci U S A.* 2001;98:1118-1123.
50. Maioli M, Ciccarese M, Pacifico A, et al. Familial insulinoma: description of two cases. *Acta Diabet.* 1992;29:38-40.
51. Lubensky IA, Pack S, Ault D, et al. Multiple neuroendocrine tumors of the pancreas in von Hippel-Lindau disease patients: histopathological and molecular genetic analysis. *Am J Pathol.* 1998;153:223-231.
52. Farley DR, van Heerden JA, Grant CS, et al. The Zollinger-Ellison syndrome: a collective surgical experience. *Ann Surg.* 1992;215:561-569; discussion 569-570.
53. Serrano J. Occurrence of multiple endocrine neoplasia type 1 (MEN1) gene mutations in Zollinger Ellison syndrome (ZES) (Abstract). *Gastroenterol.* 1998;114:G2022.
54. Waxman I, Gardner JD, Jensen RT, et al. Peptic ulcer perforation as the presentation of Zollinger-Ellison syndrome. *Dig Dis Sci.* 1991;36:19-24.
55. Metz D. Multiple endocrine neoplasia type 1: clinical features and management. In: Bilezekian J, Levine, MA, Marx, SJ, ed. *The Parathyroids.* New York, NY: Raven Press; 1994:591-646.
56. Benya RV, Metz DC, Hijazi YJ, et al. Fine needle aspiration cytology of submucosal nodules in patients with Zollinger-Ellison syndrome. *Am J Gastroenterol.* 1993;88:258-265.
57. Roy PK, Venzon DJ, Shojamanesh H, et al. Zollinger-Ellison syndrome: clinical presentation in 261 patients. *Medicine (Baltimore).* 2000;79: 379-411.
58. Norton JA, Fraker DL, Alexander HR, et al. Surgery to cure the Zollinger-Ellison syndrome. *N Engl J Med.* 1999;341:635-644.
59. Gibril F, Venzon DJ, Ojeaburu JV, et al. Prospective study of the natural history of gastrinoma in patients with MEN1: definition of an aggressive and a nonaggressive form. *J Clin Endocrinol Metab.* 2001;86: 5282-5293.
60. Ruszniewski P, Podevin P, Cadiot G, et al. Clinical, anatomical, and evolutive features of patients with the Zollinger-Ellison syndrome combined with type I multiple endocrine neoplasia. *Pancreas.* 1993;8: 295-304.
61. Stadil F, Bardram L, Gustafsen J, et al. Surgical treatment of the Zollinger-Ellison syndrome. *World J Surg.* 1993;17:463-467.
62. Thompson NW. Current concepts in the surgical management of multiple endocrine neoplasia type 1 pancreatic-duodenal disease: results in the treatment of 40 patients with Zollinger-Ellison syndrome, hypoglycaemia or both. *J Intern Md.* 1998;243:495-500.
63. Tonelli F, Fratini G, Nesi G, et al. Pancreatectomy in multiple endocrine neoplasia type 1-related gastrinomas and pancreatic endocrine neoplasias. *Ann Surg.* 2006;244:61-70.
64. Bartsch DK, Fendrich V, Langer P, et al. Outcome of duodenopancreatic resections in patients with multiple endocrine neoplasia type 1. *Ann Surg.* 2005;242:757-764, discussion 764-766.
65. Frucht H, Maton PN, Jensen RT. Use of omeprazole in patients with Zollinger-Ellison syndrome. *Dig Dis Sci.* 1991;36:394-404.
66. Maton PN. Review article: the management of Zollinger-Ellison syndrome. *Aliment Pharmacol Ther.* 1993;7:467-475.
67. Maton PN. Omeprazole. *N Engl J Med.* 1991;324:965-975.
68. Jensen R. Gastrinoma as a model for prolonged hypergastrinemia. In: Walsh J, ed. *Gastrin.* New York, NY: Raven Press; 1993:373-393.
69. Solcia E, Capella C, Fiocca R, et al. Gastric argyrophil carcinoidosis in patients with Zollinger-Ellison syndrome due to type 1 multiple endocrine neoplasia: a newly recognized association. *Am J Surg Pathol.* 1990;14:503-513.
70. Maton PN, Lack EE, Collen MJ, et al. The effect of Zollinger-Ellison syndrome and omeprazole therapy on gastric oxyntic endocrine cells. *Gastroenterology.* 1990;99:943-950.
71. Cadiot G, Lehy T, Ruszniewski P, et al. Gastric endocrine cell evolution in patients with Zollinger-Ellison syndrome: influence of gastrinoma growth and long-term omeprazole treatment. *Dig Dis Sci.* 1993;38: 1307-1317.
72. Gyr K. Human pharmacological effects of SMS 201-995 on gastric secretion. *Scand J Gastroenterol Suppl.* 1986;119:96-102.
73. Shojamanesh H, Gibril F, Louie A, et al. Prospective study of the antitumor efficacy of long-term octreotide treatment in patients with progressive metastatic gastrinoma. *Cancer.* 2002;94:331-343.
74. Tomassetti P, Migliori M, Caletti GC, et al. Treatment of type II gastric carcinoid tumors with somatostatin analogues. *N Engl J Med.* 2000;343:551-554.
75. Proye C, Malvaux P, Pattou F, et al. Noninvasive imaging of insulinomas and gastrinomas with endoscopic ultrasonography and somatostatin receptor scintigraphy. *Surgery.* 1998;124:1134-1143; discussion 1143-1144.
76. Norton JA, Cromack DT, Shawker TH, et al. Intraoperative ultrasonographic localization of islet cell tumors: a prospective comparison to palpation. *Ann Surg.* 1988;207:160-168.
77. Boukhman MP, Karam JM, Shaver J, et al. Localization of insulinomas. *Arch Surg.* 1999;134:818-822; discussion 822-823.
78. Doppman JL, Chang R, Fraker DL, et al. Localization of insulinomas to regions of the pancreas by intra-arterial stimulation with calcium. *Ann Intern Med.* 1995;123:269-273.
79. Proye C, Pattou F, Carnaille B, et al. Intraoperative insulin measurement during surgical management of insulinomas. *World J Surg.* 1998;22:1218-1224.
80. Stefanini P, Carboni M, Patrassi N, et al. Beta-islet cell tumors of the pancreas: results of a study on 1,067 cases. *Surgery.* 1974;75:597-609.
81. Goode PN, Farndon JR, Anderson J, et al. Diazoxide in the management of patients with insulinoma. *World J Surg.* 1986;10:586-592.
82. Lamberts SW, Pieters GF, Metselaar HJ, et al. Development of resistance to a long-acting somatostatin analogue during treatment of two patients with metastatic endocrine pancreatic tumours. *Acta Endocrinol.* 1988;119:561-566.
83. Levy-Bohbot N, Merle C, Goudet P, et al. Prevalence, characteristics and prognosis of MEN 1-associated glucagonomas, VIPomas, and somatostatinomas: study from the GTE (Groupe des Tumeurs Endocrines) registry. *Gastroenterol Clin Biol.* 2004;28:1075-1081.
84. Gorden P, Comi RJ, Maton PN, et al. NIH conference: somatostatin and somatostatin analogue (SMS 201-995) in treatment of hormone-secreting tumors of the pituitary and gastrointestinal tract and non-neoplastic diseases of the gut. *Ann Intern Med.* 1989;110:35-50.
85. Park SK, O'Dorisio MS, O'Dorisio TM. Vasoactive intestinal polypeptide-secreting tumours: biology and therapy. *Baillieres Clin Gastroenterol.* 1996;10:673-696.
86. Wu TJ, Lin CL, Taylor RL, et al. Increased parathyroid hormone-related peptide in patients with hypercalcemia associated with islet cell carcinoma. *Mayo Clin Proc.* 1997;72:1111-1115.
87. Liu SW, van de Velde CJ, Heslinga JM, et al. Acromegaly caused by growth hormone-relating hormone in a patient with multiple endocrine neoplasia type I. *Jpn J Clin Oncol.* 1996;26:49-52.
88. Ezzat S, Asa SL, Stefaneanu L, et al. Somatotroph hyperplasia without pituitary adenoma associated with a long standing growth hormone-releasing hormone-producing bronchial carcinoid. *J Clin Endocrinol Metab.* 1994;78:555-560.
89. Garbrecht N, Anlauf M, Schmitt A, et al. Somatostatin-producing neuroendocrine tumors of the duodenum and pancreas: incidence, types, biological behavior, association with inherited syndromes, and functional activity. *Endocr Relat Cancer.* 2008;15:229-241.
90. Fleury A, Flejou JF, Sauvanet A, et al. Calcitonin-secreting tumors of the pancreas: about six cases. *Pancreas.* 1998;16:545-550.
91. Skogseid B, Oberg K, Benson L, et al. A standardized meal stimulation test of the endocrine pancreas for early detection of pancreatic endocrine tumors in multiple endocrine neoplasia type 1 syndrome: five years experience. *J Clin Endocrinol Metab.* 1987;64:1233-1240.
92. Mutch MG, Frisella MM, DeBenedetti MK, et al. Pancreatic polypeptide is a useful plasma marker for radiographically evident pancreatic islet cell tumors in patients with multiple endocrine neoplasia type 1. *Surgery.* 1997;122:1012-1019; discussion 1019-1020.
93. Garin E, Le Jeune F, Devillers A, et al. Predictive value of 18F-FDG PET and somatostatin receptor scintigraphy in patients with metastatic endocrine tumors. *J Nucl Med.* 2009;50:858-864.
94. Skogseid B, Oberg K, Akerstrom G, et al. Limited tumor involvement found at multiple endocrine neoplasia type I pancreatic exploration: can it be predicted by preoperative tumor localization? *World J Surg.* 1998;22:673-677; discussion 677-678.
95. Pisegna JR, Doppman JL, Norton JA, et al. Prospective comparative study of ability of MR imaging and other imaging modalities to localize tumors in patients with Zollinger-Ellison syndrome. *Dig Dis Sci.* 1993;38:1318-1328.

96. Frilling A, Malago M, Martin H, et al. Use of somatostatin receptor scintigraphy to image extrahepatic metastases of neuroendocrine tumors. *Surgery*. 1998;124:1000-1004.
97. Cadiot G, Bonnaud G, Lebtahi R, et al. Usefulness of somatostatin receptor scintigraphy in the management of patients with Zollinger-Ellison syndrome. Groupe de Recherche et d'Etude du Syndrome de Zollinger-Ellison (GRESZE). *Gut*. 1997;41:107-114.
98. Yim JH, Siegel BA, DeBenedetti MK, et al. Prospective study of the utility of somatostatin-receptor scintigraphy in the evaluation of patients with multiple endocrine neoplasia type 1. *Surgery*. 1998;124:1037-1042.
99. Alexander HR, Fraker DL, Norton JA, et al. Prospective study of somatostatin receptor scintigraphy and its effect on operative outcome in patients with Zollinger-Ellison syndrome. *Ann Surg*. 1998;228: 228-238.
100. Doppman JL, Miller DL, Chang R, et al. Gastrinomas: localization by means of selective intraarterial injection of secretin. *Radiology*. 1990;174:25-29.
101. Legmann P, Vignaux O, Dousset B, et al. Pancreatic tumors: comparison of dual-phase helical CT and endoscopic sonography. *AJR Am J Roentgenol*. 1998;170:1315-1322.
102. Sheridan MB, Ward J, Guthrie JA, et al. Dynamic contrast-enhanced MR imaging and dual-phase helical CT in the preoperative assessment of suspected pancreatic cancer: a comparative study with receiver operating characteristic analysis. *AJR Am J Roentgenol*. 1999;173: 583-590.
103. Ichikawa T, Peterson MS, Federle MP, et al. Islet cell tumor of the pancreas: biphasic CT versus MR imaging in tumor detection. *Radiology*. 2000;216:163-171.
104. Koopmans KP, Neels OC, Kema IP, et al. Improved staging of patients with carcinoid and islet cell tumors with 18F-dihydroxy-phenyl-alanine and 11C-5-hydroxy-tryptophan positron emission tomography. *J Clin Oncol*. 2008;26:1489-1495.
105. Orlefors H, Sundin A, Garske U, et al. Whole-body (11)C-5-hydroxytryptophan positron emission tomography as a universal imaging technique for neuroendocrine tumors: comparison with somatostatin receptor scintigraphy and computed tomography. *J Clin Endocrinol Metab*. 2005;90:3392-3400.
106. Bansal R, Tierney W, Carpenter S, et al. Cost effectiveness of EUS for preoperative localization of pancreatic endocrine tumors. *Gastrointest Endosc*. 1999;49:19-25.
107. Suits J, Frazee R, Erickson RA. Endoscopic ultrasound and fine needle aspiration for the evaluation of pancreatic masses. *Arch Surg*. 1999;134:639-642; discussion 642-643.
108. Hiramoto JS, Feldstein VA, LaBerge JM, et al. Intraoperative ultrasound and preoperative localization detects all occult insulinomas. *Arch Surg*. 2001;136:1020-1025; discussion 1025-1026.
109. Granberg D, Stridsberg M, Seensalu R, et al. Plasma chromogranin A in patients with multiple endocrine neoplasia type 1. *J Clin Endocrinol Metab*. 1999;84:2712-2717.
110. Nobels FR, Kwekkeboom DJ, Coopmans W, et al. Chromogranin A as serum marker for neuroendocrine neoplasia: comparison with neuron-specific enolase and the alpha-subunit of glycoprotein hormones. *J Clin Endocrinol Metab*. 1997;82:2622-2628.
111. Goebel SU, Serrano J, Yu F, et al. Prospective study of the value of serum chromogranin A or serum gastrin levels in the assessment of the presence, extent, or growth of gastrinomas. *Cancer*. 1999;85: 1470-1483.
112. Weber HC, Venzon DJ, Lin JT, et al. Determinants of metastatic rate and survival in patients with Zollinger-Ellison syndrome: a prospective long-term study. *Gastroenterology*. 1995;108:1637-1649.
113. Cadiot G, Vuagnat A, Doukhan I, et al. Prognostic factors in patients with Zollinger-Ellison syndrome and multiple endocrine neoplasia type 1. Groupe d'Etude des Neoplasies Endocriniennes Multiples (GENEM) and Groupe de Recherche et d'Etude du Syndrome de Zollinger-Ellison (GRESZE). *Gastroenterology*. 1999;116:286-293.
114. Lowney JK, Frisella MM, Lairmore TC, et al. Pancreatic islet cell tumor metastasis in multiple endocrine neoplasia type 1: correlation with primary tumor size. *Surgery*. 1998;124:1043-1048, discussion 1048-1049.
115. Wiedenmann B, Jensen RT, Mignon M, et al. Preoperative diagnosis and surgical management of neuroendocrine gastroenteropancreatic tumors: general recommendations by a consensus workshop. *World J Surg*. 1998;22:309-318.
116. Lairmore TC, Chen VY, DeBenedetti MK, et al. Duodenopancreatic resections in patients with multiple endocrine neoplasia type 1. *Ann Surg*. 2000;231:909-918.
117. Carty SE, Jensen RT, Norton JA. Prospective study of aggressive resection of metastatic pancreatic endocrine tumors. *Surgery*. 1992;112:1024-1031; discussion 1031-1032.
118. Kim YH, Ajani JA, Carrasco CH, et al. Selective hepatic arterial chemoembolization for liver metastases in patients with carcinoid tumor or islet cell carcinoma. *Cancer Invest*. 1999;17:474-478.
119. Eriksson B, Oberg K, Alm G, et al. Treatment of malignant endocrine pancreatic tumours with human leucocyte interferon. *Lancet*. 1986;2:1307-1309.
120. Frank M, Klose KJ, Wied M, et al. Combination therapy with octreotide and alpha-interferon: effect on tumor growth in metastatic endocrine gastroenteropancreatic tumors. *Am J Gastroenterol*. 1999;94:1381-1387.
121. Moertel CG, Lefkopoulo M, Lipsitz S, et al. Streptozocin-doxorubicin, streptozocin-fluorouracil or chlorozotocin in the treatment of advanced islet-cell carcinoma. *N Engl J Med*. 1992;326:519-523.
122. Pisegna JR, Slimak GG, Doppman JL, et al. An evaluation of human recombinant alpha interferon in patients with metastatic gastrinoma. *Gastroenterology*. 1993;105:1179-1183.
122.3. Raymond E, Dahan L, Raoul J-L, et al. Sunitinib malate for the treatment of pancreatic neuroendocrine tumors. *N Engl J Med*. 2011; 364:501-513.
122.6. Yao JC, Shah, M, Manisha H, et al. Everolimus for advanced pancreatic peuroendocrine tumors. *New England Journal of Medicine*. 2011;364:514-523.
123. Maton PN, Gardner JD, Jensen RT. Use of long-acting somatostatin analog SMS 201-995 in patients with pancreatic islet cell tumors. *Dig Dis Sci*. 1989;34:28S-39S.
124. Tomassetti P, Migliori M, Corinaldesi R, et al. Treatment of gastroenteropancreatic neuroendocrine tumours with octreotide LAR. *Alim Pharmacol Ther*. 2000;14:557-560.
125. Wymenga AN, Eriksson B, Salmela PI, et al. Efficacy and safety of prolonged-release lanreotide in patients with gastrointestinal neuroendocrine tumors and hormone-related symptoms. *J Clin Oncol*. 1999;17:1111.
126. di Bartolomeo M, Bajetta E, Buzzoni R, et al. Clinical efficacy of octreotide in the treatment of metastatic neuroendocrine tumors: a study by the Italian Trials in Medical Oncology Group. *Cancer*. 1996;77: 402-408.
127. Van Essen M, Krenning EP, De Jong M, et al. Peptide receptor radionuclide therapy with radiolabelled somatostatin analogues in patients with somatostatin receptor positive tumours. *Acta Oncol*. 2007;46:723-734.
128. Verges B, Boureille F, Goudet P, et al. Pituitary disease in MEN type 1 (MEN1): data from the France-Belgium MEN1 multicenter study. *J Clin Endocrinol Metab*. 2002;87:457-465.
129. Corbetta S, Pizzocaro A, Peracchi M, et al. Multiple endocrine neoplasia type 1 in patients with recognized pituitary tumours of different types. *Clin Endocrinol*. 1997;47:507-512.
130. Tortosa F, Chico A, Rodriguez-Espinosa J, et al. Prevalence of MEN 1 in patients with prolactinoma. *MEN1 Study Group of the Hospital de la Santa Creu i Sant Pau of Barcelona. Clin Endocrinol*. 1999;50: 272.
131. Carty SE, Helm AK, Amico JA, et al. The variable penetrance and spectrum of manifestations of multiple endocrine neoplasia type 1. *Surgery*. 1998;124:1106-1113; discussion 1113-1114.
132. Stratakis CA, Schussheim DH, Freedman SM, et al. Pituitary macroadenoma in a 5-year-old: an early expression of multiple endocrine neoplasia type 1. *J Clin Endocrinol Metab*. 2000;85: 4776-4780.
133. Sahdev A, Jager R. Bilateral pituitary adenomas occurring with multiple endocrine neoplasia type one. *AJNR Am J Neuroradiol*. 2000;21: 1067-1069.
134. Trouillas J, Labat-Moleur F, Sturm N, et al. Pituitary tumors and hyperplasia in multiple endocrine neoplasia type 1 syndrome (MEN1): a case-control study in a series of 77 patients versus 2509 non-MEN1 patients. *Am J Surg Pathol*. 2008;32:534-543.
135. O'Brien T, O'Riordan DS, Gharib H, et al. Results of treatment of pituitary disease in multiple endocrine neoplasia, type I. *Neurosurgery*. 1996;39:273-278; discussion 278-279.
136. Bevan JS, Webster J, Burke CW, et al. Dopamine agonists and pituitary tumor shrinkage. *Endocr Rev*. 1992;13:220-240.
137. Weil C. The safety of bromocriptine in long-term use: a review of the literature. *Curr Med Res Opin*. 1986;10:25-51.
138. Stewart PM. Current therapy for acromegaly. *Trends Endocrinol Metab*. 2000;11:128-132.
139. Weil RJ, Vortmeyer AO, Huang S, et al. 11q13 allelic loss in pituitary tumors in patients with multiple endocrine neoplasia syndrome type 1. *Clin Cancer Res*. 1998;4:1673-1678.
140. Thakker RV, Pook MA, Wooding C, et al. Association of somatotrophinomas with loss of alleles on chromosome 11 and with gsp mutations. *J Clin Invest*. 1993;91:2815-2821.
141. Asa SL, Singer W, Kovacs K, et al. Pancreatic endocrine tumour producing growth hormone-releasing hormone associated with multiple endocrine neoplasia type I syndrome. *Acta Endocrinol*. 1987;115: 331-337.
142. Sano T, Yamasaki R, Saito H, et al. Growth hormone-releasing hormone (GHRH)-secreting pancreatic tumor in a patient with multiple endocrine neoplasia type I. *Am J Surg Pathol*. 1987;11:810-819.
143. Thorner MO, Frohman LA, Leong DA, et al. Extrahypothalamic growth-hormone-releasing factor (GRF) secretion is a rare cause of

acromegaly: plasma GRF levels in 177 acromegalic patients. *J Clin Endocrinol Metab.* 1984;59:846-849.
144. Oka H, Kameya T, Sato Y, et al. Significance of growth hormone-releasing hormone receptor mRNA in non-neoplastic pituitary and pituitary adenomas: a study by RT-PCR and in situ hybridization. *J Neuro-oncol.* 1999;41:197-204.
145. Newman CB, Melmed S, Snyder PJ, et al. Safety and efficacy of long-term octreotide therapy of acromegaly: results of a multicenter trial in 103 patients: a clinical research center study. *J Clin Endocrinol Metab.* 1995;80:2768-2775.
146. Trainer PJ, Drake WM, Katznelson L, et al. Treatment of acromegaly with the growth hormone-receptor antagonist pegvisomant. *N Engl J Med.* 2000;342:1171-1177.
147. Skogseid B, Larsson C, Lindgren PG, et al. Clinical and genetic features of adrenocortical lesions in multiple endocrine neoplasia type 1. *J Clin Endocrinol Metab.* 1992;75:76-81.
148. Waldmann J, Bartsch DK, Kann PH, et al. Adrenal involvement in multiple endocrine neoplasia type 1: results of 7 years prospective screening. *Langenbecks Arch Surg.* 2007;392:437-443.
149. Houdelette P, Chagnon A, Dumotier J, et al. . [Malignant adrenocortical tumor as a part of Wermer's syndrome: apropos of a case]. *J Chir.* 1989;126:385-387.
150. Abe T, Yoshimoto K, Taniyama M, et al. An unusual kindred of the multiple endocrine neoplasia type 1 (MEN1) in Japanese. *J Clin Endocrinol Metab.* 2000;85:1327-1330.
151. Harpole DH Jr, Feldman JM, Buchanan S, et al. Bronchial carcinoid tumors: a retrospective analysis of 126 patients. *Ann Thorac Surg.* 1992;54:50-54; discussion 54-55.
152. Teh BT, Zedenius J, Kytola S, et al. Thymic carcinoids in multiple endocrine neoplasia type 1. *Ann Surg.* 1998;228:99-105.
153. Teh BT. Thymic carcinoids in multiple endocrine neoplasia type 1. *J Intern Med.* 1998;243:501-504.
154. Burgess JR, Greenaway TM, Parameswaran V, et al. Enteropancreatic malignancy associated with multiple endocrine neoplasia type 1: risk factors and pathogenesis. *Cancer.* 1998;83:428-434.
155. Gould PM, Bonner JA, Sawyer TE, et al. Bronchial carcinoid tumors: importance of prognostic factors that influence patterns of recurrence and overall survival. *Radiology.* 1998;208:181-185.
156. Musi M, Carbone RG, Bertocchi C, et al. Bronchial carcinoid tumours: a study on clinicopathological features and role of octreotide scintigraphy. *Lung Cancer.* 1998;22:97-102.
157. Norton JA, Melcher ML, Gibril F, et al. Gastric carcinoid tumors in multiple endocrine neoplasia-1 patients with Zollinger-Ellison syndrome can be symptomatic, demonstrate aggressive growth, and require surgical treatment. *Surgery.* 2004;136:1267-1274.
158. Bordi C, Falchetti A, Azzoni C, et al. Aggressive forms of gastric neuroendocrine tumors in multiple endocrine neoplasia type I. *Am J Surg Pathol.* 1997;21:1075-1082.
159. Anderson RE. A familial instance of appendiceal carcinoid. *Am J Surg.* 1966;111:738-740.
160. Yeatman TJ, Sharp JV, Kimura AK. Can susceptibility to carcinoid tumors be inherited? *Cancer.* 1989;63:390-393.
161. Babovic-Vuksanovic D, Constantinou CL, Rubin J, et al. Familial occurrence of carcinoid tumors and association with other malignant neoplasms. *Cancer Epidemiol Biomarkers Prev.* 1999;8:715-719.
162. Hemminki K, Li X. Familial carcinoid tumors and subsequent cancers: a nation-wide epidemiologic study from Sweden. *Int J Cancer.* 2001;94:444-448.
163. Oliveira AM, Tazelaar HD, Wentzlaff KA, et al. Familial pulmonary carcinoid tumors. *Cancer.* 2001;91:2104-2109.
164. Cote G. The spectrum of mutations in the MEN1 variant syndromes. *Abstract OR43-1.* New Orleans, LA: Program and Abstracts of The Endocrine Society; 1998:106.
165. Nord B, Larsson C, Wong FK, et al. Sporadic follicular thyroid tumors show loss of a 200-kb region in 11q13 without evidence for mutations in the MEN1 gene. *Genes Chromosomes Cancer.* 1999;26: 35-39.
166. Darling TN, Skarulis MC, Steinberg SM, et al. Multiple facial angiofibromas and collagenomas in patients with multiple endocrine neoplasia type 1. *Arch Dermatol.* 1997;133:853-857.
167. Asgharian B, Turner ML, Gibril F, et al. Cutaneous tumors in patients with multiple endocrine neoplasm type 1 (MEN1) and gastrinomas: prospective study of frequency and development of criteria with high sensitivity and specificity for MEN1. *J Clin Endocrinol Metab.* 2004;89:5328-5336.
168. Pack S, Turner ML, Zhuang Z, et al. Cutaneous tumors in patients with multiple endocrine neoplasia type 1 show allelic deletion of the MEN1 gene. *J Invest Dermatol.* 1998;110:438-440.
169. Giraud S, Choplin H, Teh BT, et al. A large multiple endocrine neoplasia type 1 family with clinical expression suggestive of anticipation. *J Clin Endocrinol Metab.* 1997;82:3487-3492.
170. Nord B, Platz A, Smoczynski K, et al. Malignant melanoma in patients with multiple endocrine neoplasia type 1 and involvement of the MEN1 gene in sporadic melanoma. *Int J Cancer.* 2000;87: 463-467.
171. Dackiw AP, Cote GJ, Fleming JB, et al. Screening for MEN1 mutations in patients with atypical endocrine neoplasia. *Surgery.* 1999;126:1097-1103; discussion 1103-1104.
172. Vortmeyer AO, Lubensky IA, Skarulis M, et al. Multiple endocrine neoplasia type 1: atypical presentation, clinical course, and genetic analysis of multiple tumors. *Mod Pathol.* 1999;12:919-924.
173. McKeeby JL, Li X, Zhuang Z, et al. Multiple leiomyomas of the esophagus, lung, and uterus in multiple endocrine neoplasia type 1. *Am J Pathol.* 2001;159:1121-1127.
174. Asgharian B, Chen YJ, Patronas NJ, et al. Meningiomas may be a component tumor of multiple endocrine neoplasia type 1. *Clin Cancer Res.* 2004;10:869-880.
175. Hoffmann KM, Gibril F, Entsuah LK, et al. Patients with multiple endocrine neoplasia type 1 with gastrinomas have an increased risk of severe esophageal disease including stricture and the premalignant condition, Barrett's esophagus. *J Clin Endocrinol Metab.* 2006;91:204-212.
176. Shepherd JJ. The natural history of multiple endocrine neoplasia type 1: highly uncommon or highly unrecognized? *Arch Surg.* 1991;126:935-952.
177. Giraud S, Zhang CX, Serova-Sinilnikova O, et al. Germ-line mutation analysis in patients with multiple endocrine neoplasia type 1 and related disorders. *Am J Hum Genet.* 1998;63:455-467.
177.5. Newey PJ, Jeyabalan, J, Walls GV, et al. Asymptomatic children with Multiple Endocrine Neoplasia Type 1 mutations may harbor nonfunctioning pancreatic neuroendocrine tumors. *J Clin Endocrinol Metab.* 2009;94:3640-3646.
178. Gaitan D, Loosen PT, Orth DN. Two patients with Cushing's disease in a kindred with multiple endocrine neoplasia type I. *J Clin Endocrinol Metab.* 1993;76:1580-1582.
179. Skogseid B, Eriksson B, Lundqvist G, et al. Multiple endocrine neoplasia type 1: a 10-year prospective screening study in four kindreds. *J Clin Endocrinol Metab.* 1991;73:281-287.
180. Lim LC, Tan MH, Eng C, et al. Thymic carcinoid in multiple endocrine neoplasia 1: genotype-phenotype correlation and prevention. *J Intern Med.* 2006;259:428-432.
181. Hao W, Skarulis MC, Simonds WF, et al. Multiple endocrine neoplasia type 1 variant with frequent prolactinoma and rare gastrinoma. *J Clin Endocrinol Metab.* 2004;89:3776-3784.
182. Kassem M, Kruse TA, Wong FK, et al. Familial isolated hyperparathyroidism as a variant of multiple endocrine neoplasia type 1 in a large Danish pedigree. *J Clin Endocrinol Metab.* 2000;85: 165-167.
183. Marx SJ, Spiegel AM, Levine MA, et al. Familial hypocalciuric hypercalcemia: the relation to primary parathyroid hyperplasia. *N Engl J Med.* 1982;307:416-426.
184. Carrasco CA, Gonzalez AA, Carvajal CA, et al. Novel intronic mutation of MEN1 gene causing familial isolated primary hyperparathyroidism. *J Clin Endocrinol Metab.* 2004;89:4124-4129.
185. Simonds WF, James-Newton LA, Agarwal SK, et al. Familial isolated hyperparathyroidism: clinical and genetic characteristics of 36 kindreds. *Medicine (Baltimore).* 2002;81:1-26.
186. Brandi ML, Gagel RF, Angeli A, et al. Guidelines for diagnosis and therapy of MEN type 1 and type 2. *J Clin Endocrinol Metab.* 2001;86:5658-5671.
187. Ozawa A, Agarwal SK, Mateo CM, et al. The parathyroid/pituitary variant of multiple endocrine neoplasia type 1 usually has causes other than p27Kip1 mutations. *J Clin Endocrinol Metab.* 2007;92:1948-1951.
188. Uchino S, Noguchi S, Sato M, et al. Screening of the Men1 gene and discovery of germ-line and somatic mutations in apparently sporadic parathyroid tumors. *Cancer Res.* 2000;60:5553-5557.
189. Andersen HO, Jorgensen PE, Bardram L, et al. Screening for multiple endocrine neoplasia type 1 in patients with recognized pituitary adenoma. *Clin Endocrinol.* 1990;33:771-775.
190. Kloppel G, Anlauf M, Raffel A, et al. Adult diffuse nesidioblastosis: genetically or environmentally induced? *Hum Pathol.* 2008;39:3-8.
191. Henopp T, Anlauf M, Schmitt A, et al. Glucagon cell adenomatosis: a newly recognized disease of the endocrine pancreas. *J Clin Endocrinol Metab.* 2009;94:213-217.
192. Marx SJ, Attie MF, Levine MA, et al. The hypocalciuric or benign variant of familial hypercalcemia: clinical and biochemical features in fifteen kindreds. *Medicine (Baltimore).* 1981;60:397-412.
193. Law WM Jr, Heath H 3rd. Familial benign hypercalcemia (hypocalciuric hypercalcemia): clinical and pathogenetic studies in 21 families. *Ann Intern Med.* 1985;102:511-519.
194. Firek AF, Kao PC, Heath H 3rd. Plasma intact parathyroid hormone (PTH) and PTH-related peptide in familial benign hypercalcemia: greater responsiveness to endogenous PTH than in primary hyperparathyroidism. *J Clin Endocrinol Metab.* 1991;72:541-546.
195. Thorgeirsson U, Costa J, Marx SJ. The parathyroid glands in familial hypocalciuric hypercalcemia. *Hum Pathol.* 1981;12:229-237.
196. Marx SJ. Clinical review 109: contrasting paradigms for hereditary hyperfunction of endocrine cells. *J Clin Endocrinol Metab.* 1999;84:3001-3009.

197. Brown EM, Pollak M, Hebert SC. The extracellular calcium-sensing receptor: its role in health and disease. *Annu Rev Med.* 1998;49:15-29.
198. Heath H 3rd, Jackson CE, Otterud B, et al. Genetic linkage analysis in familial benign (hypocalciuric) hypercalcemia: evidence for locus heterogeneity. *Am J Hum Genet.* 1993;53:193-200.
199. Carling T, Szabo E, Bai M, et al. Familial hypercalcemia and hypercalciuria caused by a novel mutation in the cytoplasmic tail of the calcium receptor. *J Clin Endocrinol Metab.* 2000;85:2042-2047.
200. Lloyd SE, Pannett AA, Dixon PH, et al. Localization of familial benign hypercalcemia, Oklahoma variant (FBHOk), to chromosome 19q13. *Am J Hum Genet.* 1999;64:189-195.
201. Warner JV, Nyholt DR, Busfield F, et al. Familial isolated hyperparathyroidism is linked to a 1.7 Mb region on chromosome 2p13.3-14. *J Med Genet.* 2006;43:e12.
202. Warner J, Epstein M, Sweet A, et al. Genetic testing in familial isolated hyperparathyroidism: unexpected results and their implications. *J Med Genet.* 2004;41:155-160.
203. Jackson CE, Norum RA, Boyd SB, et al. Hereditary hyperparathyroidism and multiple ossifying jaw fibromas: a clinically and genetically distinct syndrome. *Surgery.* 1990;108:1006-1012; discussion 1012-1013.
204. Teh BT, Farnebo F, Twigg S, et al. Familial isolated hyperparathyroidism maps to the hyperparathyroidism-jaw tumor locus in 1q21-q32 in a subset of families. *J Clin Endocrinol Metab.* 1998;83:2114-2120.
205. Streeten EA, Weinstein LS, Norton JA, et al. Studies in a kindred with parathyroid carcinoma. *J Clin Endocrinol Metab.* 1992;75:362-366.
206. Shattuck TM, Valimaki S, Obara T, et al. Somatic and germ-line mutations of the HRPT2 gene in sporadic parathyroid carcinoma. *N Engl J Med.* 2003;349:1722-1729.
207. Szabo J, Heath B, Hill VM, et al. Hereditary hyperparathyroidism-jaw tumor syndrome: the endocrine tumor gene HRPT2 maps to chromosome 1q21-q31. *Am J Hum Genet.* 1995;56:944-950.
208. Teh BT, Farnebo F, Kristoffersson U, et al. Autosomal dominant primary hyperparathyroidism and jaw tumor syndrome associated with renal hamartomas and cystic kidney disease: linkage to 1q21-q32 and loss of the wild type allele in renal hamartomas. *J Clin Endocrinol Metab.* 1996;81:4204-4211.
209. Bradley KJ, Hobbs MR, Buley ID, et al. Uterine tumours are a phenotypic manifestation of the hyperparathyroidism-jaw tumour syndrome. *J Intern Med.* 2005;257:18-26.
210. Simonds WF, Robbins CM, Agarwal SK, et al. Familial isolated hyperparathyroidism is rarely caused by germline mutation in HRPT2, the gene for the hyperparathyroidism-jaw tumor syndrome. *J Clin Endocrinol Metab.* 2004;89:96-102.
211. Keiser HR, Beaven MA, Doppman J, et al. Sipple's syndrome: medullary thyroid carcinoma, pheochromocytoma, and parathyroid disease: studies in a large family. NIH conference. *Ann Intern Med.* 1973;78:561-579.
212. Schuffenecker I, Virally-Monod M, Brohet R, et al. Risk and penetrance of primary hyperparathyroidism in multiple endocrine neoplasia type 2A families with mutations at codon 634 of the RET proto-oncogene. Groupe D'etude des Tumeurs a Calcitonine. *J Clin Endocrinol Metab.* 1998;83:487-491.
213. Huang SM, Duh QY, Shaver J, et al. Familial hyperparathyroidism without multiple endocrine neoplasia. *World J Surg.* 1997;21:22-28; discussion 29.
214. Watanabe T, Tsukamoto F, Shimizu T, et al. Familial isolated hyperparathyroidism caused by single adenoma: a distinct entity different from multiple endocrine neoplasia. *Endocr J.* 1998;45:637-646.
215. Daly AF, Jaffrain-Rea ML, Ciccarelli A, et al. Clinical characterization of familial isolated pituitary adenomas. *J Clin Endocrinol Metab.* 2006;91:3316-3323.
216. Vierimaa O, Georgitsi M, Lehtonen R, et al. Pituitary adenoma predisposition caused by germline mutations in the AIP gene. *Science.* 2006;312:1228-1230.
217. Larsson C, Skogseid B, Oberg K, et al. Multiple endocrine neoplasia type 1 gene maps to chromosome 11 and is lost in insulinoma. *Nature.* 1988;332:85-87.
218. Knudson AG Jr. Mutation and cancer: statistical study of retinoblastoma. *Proc Natl Acad U S A.* 1971;68:820-823.
219. Knudson AG. Hereditary cancer: two hits revisited. *J Cancer Res Clin Oncol.* 1996;122:135-140.
220. Chandrasekharappa SC, Guru SC, Manickam P, et al. Positional cloning of the gene for multiple endocrine neoplasia-type 1. *Science.* 1997;276:404-407.
221. Emmert-Buck MR, Lubensky IA, Dong Q, et al. Localization of the multiple endocrine neoplasia type I (MEN1) gene based on tumor loss of heterozygosity analysis. *Cancer Res.* 1997;57:1855-1858.
222. Guru SC, Agarwal SK, Manickam P, et al. A transcript map for the 2.8-Mb region containing the multiple endocrine neoplasia type 1 locus. *Genome Res.* 1997;7:725-735.
223. Lemmens I, Van de Ven WJ, Kas K, et al. Identification of the multiple endocrine neoplasia type 1 (MEN1) gene. The European Consortium on MEN1. *Hum Mol Genet.* 1997;6:1177-1183.
224. Mayr B, Brabant G, von zur Muhlen A. Menin mutations in MEN1 patients. *J Clin Endocrinol Metab.* 1998;83:3004-3005.
225. Guru SC, Olufemi SE, Manickam P, et al. A 2.8-Mb clone contig of the multiple endocrine neoplasia type 1 (MEN1) region at 11q13. *Genomics.* 1997;42:436-445.
226. Guru SC, Goldsmith PK, Burns AL, et al. Menin, the product of the MEN1 gene, is a nuclear protein. *Proc Natl Acad Sci U S A.* 1998;95:1630-1634.
227. Manickam P, Vogel AM, Agarwal SK, et al. Isolation, characterization, expression and functional analysis of the zebrafish ortholog of MEN1. *Mamm Genome.* 2000;11:448-454.
228. Agarwal SK, Guru SC, Heppner C, et al. Menin interacts with the AP1 transcription factor JunD and represses JunD-activated transcription. *Cell.* 1999;96:143-152.
229. Gobl AE, Berg M, Lopez-Egido JR, et al. Menin represses JunD-activated transcription by a histone deacetylase-dependent mechanism. *Biochim Biophys Acta.* 1999;1447:51-56.
230. Knapp JI, Heppner C, Hickman AB, et al. Identification and characterization of JunD missense mutants that lack menin binding. *Oncogene.* 2000;19:4706-4712.
231. Thepot D, Weitzman JB, Barra J, et al. Targeted disruption of the murine junD gene results in multiple defects in male reproductive function. *Development.* 2000;127:143-153.
232. Agarwal S. MEN1 gene: mutation and pathophysiology. *Ann d'Endocrinol.* 2006;67(suppl 4):IS12-IS13.
233. Cavallari I, Silic-Benussi M, Rende F, et al. Decreased expression and promoter methylation of the menin tumor suppressor in pancreatic ductal adenocarcinoma. *Genes Chromosomes Cancer.* 2009;48:383-396.
234. Carling T, Correa P, Hessman O, et al. Parathyroid MEN1 gene mutations in relation to clinical characteristics of nonfamilial primary hyperparathyroidism. *J Clin Endocrinol Metab.* 1998;83:2960-2963.
235. Farnebo F, Kytola S, Teh BT, et al. Alternative genetic pathways in parathyroid tumorigenesis. *J Clin Endocrinol Metab.* 1999;84:3775-3780.
236. Farnebo F, Teh BT, Kytola S, et al. Alterations of the MEN1 gene in sporadic parathyroid tumors. *J Clin Endocrinol Metab.* 1998;83:2627-2630.
237. Heppner C, Kester MB, Agarwal SK, et al. Somatic mutation of the MEN1 gene in parathyroid tumours. *Nat Genet.* 1997;16:375-378.
238. Goebel SU, Heppner C, Burns AL, et al. Genotype/phenotype correlation of multiple endocrine neoplasia type 1 gene mutations in sporadic gastrinomas. *J Clin Endocrinol Metab.* 2000;85:116-123.
239. Wang EH, Ebrahimi SA, Wu AY, et al. Mutation of the MENIN gene in sporadic pancreatic endocrine tumors. *Cancer Res.* 1998;58:4417-4420.
240. Zhuang Z, Vortmeyer AO, Pack S, et al. Somatic mutations of the MEN1 tumor suppressor gene in sporadic gastrinomas and insulinomas. *Cancer Res.* 1997;57:4682-4686.
241. Gortz B, Roth J, Krahenmann A, et al. Mutations and allelic deletions of the MEN1 gene are associated with a subset of sporadic endocrine pancreatic and neuroendocrine tumors and not restricted to foregut neoplasms. *Am J Pathol.* 1999;154:429-436.
242. Debelenko LV, Brambilla E, Agarwal SK, et al. Identification of MEN1 gene mutations in sporadic carcinoid tumors of the lung. *Hum Mol Genet.* 1997;6:2285-2290.
243. Prezant TR, Levine J, Melmed S. Molecular characterization of the men1 tumor suppressor gene in sporadic pituitary tumors. *J Clin Endocrinol Metab.* 1998;83:1388-1391.
244. Schmidt MC, Henke RT, Stangl AP, et al. Analysis of the MEN1 gene in sporadic pituitary adenomas. *J Pathol.* 1999;188:168-173.
245. Tanaka C, Kimura T, Yang P, et al. Analysis of loss of heterozygosity on chromosome 11 and infrequent inactivation of the MEN1 gene in sporadic pituitary adenomas. *J Clin Endocrinol Metab.* 1998;83:2631-2634.
246. Tanaka C, Yoshimoto K, Yamada S, et al. Absence of germ-line mutations of the multiple endocrine neoplasia type 1 (MEN1) gene in familial pituitary adenoma in contrast to MEN1 in Japanese. *J Clin Endocrinol Metab.* 1998;83:960-965.
247. Zhuang Z, Ezzat SZ, Vortmeyer AO, et al. Mutations of the MEN1 tumor suppressor gene in pituitary tumors. *Cancer Res.* 1997;57:5446-5451.
248. Gortz B, Roth J, Speel EJ, et al. MEN1 gene mutation analysis of sporadic adrenocortical lesions. *Int J Cancer.* 1999;80:373-379.
249. Heppner C, Reincke M, Agarwal SK, et al. MEN1 gene analysis in sporadic adrenocortical neoplasms. *J Clin Endocrinol Metab.* 1999;84:216-219.
250. Tahara H, Imanishi Y, Yamada T, et al. Rare somatic inactivation of the multiple endocrine neoplasia type 1 gene in secondary hyperparathyroidism of uremia. *J Clin Endocrinol Metab.* 2000;85:4113-4117.
251. Imanishi Y, Palanisamy, N, Tahara, H, et al. Molecular pathogenetic analysis of parathyroid carcinoma (Abstract). *J Bone Miner Res.* 1999;14(suppl 1):S421.
252. Boni R, Vortmeyer AO, Pack S, et al. Somatic mutations of the MEN1 tumor suppressor gene detected in sporadic angiofibromas. *J Invest Dermatol.* 1998;111:539-540.

253. Vortmeyer AO, Boni R, Pak E, et al. Multiple endocrine neoplasia 1 gene alterations in MEN1-associated and sporadic lipomas. *J Natl Cancer Inst.* 1998;90:398-399.
254. Debelenko LV, Swalwell JI, Kelley MJ, et al. MEN1 gene mutation analysis of high-grade neuroendocrine lung carcinoma. *Genes Chromosomes Cancer.* 2000;28:58-65.
255. Boni R, Vortmeyer AO, Huang S, et al. Mutation analysis of the MEN1 tumour suppressor gene in malignant melanoma. *Melanoma Res.* 1999;9:249-252.
256. Thieblemont C, Pack S, Sakai A, et al. Allelic loss of 11q13 as detected by MEN1-FISH is not associated with mutation of the MEN1 gene in lymphoid neoplasms. *Leukemia.* 1999;13:85-91.
257. Agarwal SK, Debelenko LV, Kester MB, et al. Analysis of recurrent germline mutations in the MEN1 gene encountered in apparently unrelated families. *Hum Mutat.* 1998;12:75-82.
258. Owens M, Ellard S, Vaidya B. Analysis of gross deletions in the MEN1 gene in patients with multiple endocrine neoplasia type 1. *Clin Endocrinol (Oxf).* 2008;68:350-354.
259. Teh BT, Kytola S, Farnebo F, et al. Mutation analysis of the MEN1 gene in multiple endocrine neoplasia type 1, familial acromegaly and familial isolated hyperparathyroidism. *J Clin Endocrinol Metab.* 1998;83:2621-2626.
260. Poncin J, Abs R, Velkeniers B, et al. Mutation analysis of the MEN1 gene in Belgian patients with multiple endocrine neoplasia type 1 and related diseases. *Hum Mutat.* 1999;13:54-60.
261. Mutch MG, Dilley WG, Sanjurjo F, et al. Germline mutations in the multiple endocrine neoplasia type 1 gene: evidence for frequent splicing defects. *Hum Mutat.* 1999;13:175-185.
262. Mayer K, Ballhausen W, Rott HD. Mutation screening of the entire coding regions of the TSC1 and the TSC2 gene with the protein truncation test (PTT) identifies frequent splicing defects. *Hum Mutat.* 1999;14:401-411.
263. Olufemi SE, Green JS, Manickam P, et al. Common ancestral mutation in the MEN1 gene is likely responsible for the prolactinoma variant of MEN1 (MEN1Burin) in four kindreds from Newfoundland. *Hum Mutat.* 1998;11:264-269.
264. Thakker RV, Bouloux P, Wooding C, et al. Association of parathyroid tumors in multiple endocrine neoplasia type 1 with loss of alleles on chromosome 11. *N Engl J Med.* 1989;321:218-224.
265. Debelenko LV, Emmert-Buck MR, Zhuang Z, et al. The multiple endocrine neoplasia type I gene locus is involved in the pathogenesis of type II gastric carcinoids. *Gastroenterology.* 1997;113:773-781.
266. Teh BT, McArdle J, Chan SP, et al. Clinicopathologic studies of thymic carcinoids in multiple endocrine neoplasia type 1. *Medicine (Baltimore).* 1997;76:21-29.
267. Tahara H, Smith AP, Gas RD, et al. Genomic localization of novel candidate tumor suppressor gene loci in human parathyroid adenomas. *Cancer Res.* 1996;56:599-605.
268. Shan L, Nakamura Y, Murakami M, et al. Clonal emergence in uremic parathyroid hyperplasia is not related to MEN1 gene abnormality. *Jpn J Cancer Res.* 1999;90:965-969.
269. Arnold A, Brown MF, Urena P, et al. Monoclonality of parathyroid tumors in chronic renal failure and in primary parathyroid hyperplasia. *J Clin Invest.* 1995;95:2047-2053.
270. Falchetti A, Bale AE, Amorosi A, et al. Progression of uremic hyperparathyroidism involves allelic loss on chromosome 11. *J Clin Endocrinol Metab.* 1993;76:139-144.
271. Farnebo F, Farnebo LO, Nordenstrom J, et al. Allelic loss on chromosome 11 is uncommon in parathyroid glands of patients with hypercalcaemic secondary hyperparathyroidism. *Eur J Surg.* 1997;163: 331-337.
272. Zimering MB, Katsumata N, Sato Y, et al. Increased basic fibroblast growth factor in plasma from multiple endocrine neoplasia type 1: relation to pituitary tumor. *J Clin Endocrinol Metab.* 1993;76:1182-1187.
272.5. Nord KH, Magnusson L, Isaksson M, et al. Concomitant deletions of tumor suppressor genes MEN1 and AIP are essential for the pathogenesis of the brown fat tumor hibernoma. *Proc Nat Acad Sci (USA).* 2010;49:21122-21127.
273. Vortmeyer AO, Boni R, Pack SD, et al. Perivascular cells harboring multiple endocrine neoplasia type 1 alterations are neoplastic cells in angiofibromas. *Cancer Res.* 1999;59:274-278.
274. Deng G, Lu Y, Zlotnikov G, et al. Loss of heterozygosity in normal tissue adjacent to breast carcinomas. *Science.* 1996;274:2057-2059.
275. Jakobovitz O, Nass D, DeMarco L, et al. Carcinoid tumors frequently display genetic abnormalities involving chromosome 11. *J Clin Endocrinol Metab.* 1996;81:3164-3167.
276. Shen WT, Sturgeon C, Clark OH, et al. Should pheochromocytoma size influence surgical approach? A comparison of 90 malignant and 60 benign pheochromocytomas. *Surgery.* 2004;136:1129-1137.
277. Kytola S, Makinen MJ, Kahkonen M, et al. Comparative genomic hybridization studies in tumours from a patient with multiple endocrine neoplasia type 1. *Eur J Endocrinol.* 1998;139:202-206.
278. Franklin DS, Godfrey VL, O'Brien DA, et al. Functional collaboration between different cyclin-dependent kinase inhibitors suppresses tumor growth with distinct tissue specificity. *Mol Cell Biol.* 2000;20:6147-6158.
279. Pestell RG, Albanese C, Reutens AT, et al. The cyclins and cyclin-dependent kinase inhibitors in hormonal regulation of proliferation and differentiation. *Endocr Rev.* 1999;20:501-534.
280. Scappaticci S, Fossati GS, Valenti L, et al. A search for double minute chromosomes in cultured lymphocytes from different types of tumors. *Cancer Genet Cytogenet.* 1995;82:50-53.
281. Sakurai A, Katai M, Itakura Y, et al. Premature centromere division in patients with multiple endocrine neoplasia type 1. *Cancer Genet Cytogenet.* 1999;109:138-140.
282. Ikeo Y, Sakurai A, Suzuki R, et al. Proliferation-associated expression of the MEN1 gene as revealed by in situ hybridization: possible role of the menin as a negative regulator of cell proliferation under DNA damage. *Lab Invest.* 2000;80:797-804.
283. Kottemann MC, Bale AE. Characterization of DNA damage-dependent cell cycle checkpoints in a menin-deficient model. *DNA Repair (Amst).* 2009;8:944-952.
284. Agarwal SK, Kester MB, Debelenko LV, et al. Germline mutations of the MEN1 gene in familial multiple endocrine neoplasia type 1 and related states. *Hum Mol Genet.* 1997;6:1169-1175.
285. Teh BT, Esapa CT, Houlston R, et al. A family with isolated hyperparathyroidism segregating a missense MEN1 mutation and showing loss of the wild-type alleles in the parathyroid tumors. *Am J Hum Genet.* 1998;63:1544-1549.
286. Larsson C, Calender A, Grimmond S, et al. Molecular tools for presymptomatic testing in multiple endocrine neoplasia type 1. *J Intern Med.* 1995;238:239-244.
287. Pellegata NS, Quintanilla-Martinez L, Siggelkow H, et al. Germ-line mutations in p27Kip1 cause a multiple endocrine neoplasia syndrome in rats and humans. *Proc Natl Acad Sci U S A.* 2006;103:15558-15563.
288. Agarwal SK, Mateo CM, Marx SJ. Rare germline mutations in cyclin-dependent kinase inhibitor genes in multiple endocrine neoplasia type 1 and related states. *J Clin Endocrinol Metab.* 2009;94:1826-1834.
289. Roijers JF, de Wit MJ, van der Luijt RB, et al. Criteria for mutation analysis in MEN 1-suspected patients: MEN 1 case-finding. *Eur J Clin Invest.* 2000;30:487-492.
290. Quayle FJ, Benveniste R, DeBenedetti MK, et al. Hereditary medullary thyroid carcinoma in patients greater than 50 years old. *Surgery.* 2004;136:1116-1121.
291. Lemos MC, Thakker RV. Multiple endocrine neoplasia type 1 (MEN1): analysis of 1336 mutations reported in the first decade following identification of the gene. *Hum Mutat.* 2008;29:22-32.
292. Tham E, Grandell U, Lindgren E, et al. Clinical testing for mutations in the MEN1 gene in Sweden: a report on 200 unrelated cases. *J Clin Endocrinol Metab.* 2007;92:3389-3395.
293. Courseaux A, Grosgeorge J, Gaudray P, et al. Definition of the minimal MEN1 candidate area based on a 5-Mb integrated map of proximal 11q13. *Genomics.* 1996;37:345-353.
294. Stock JL, Warth MR, Teh BT, et al. A kindred with a variant of multiple endocrine neoplasia type 1 demonstrating frequent expression of pituitary tumors but not linked to the multiple endocrine neoplasia type 1 locus at chromosome region 11q13. *J Clin Endocrinol Metab.* 1997;82:486-492.
295. Hai N, Aoki N, Shimatsu A, et al. Clinical features of multiple endocrine neoplasia type 1 (MEN1) phenocopy without germline MEN1 gene mutations: analysis of 20 Japanese sporadic cases with MEN1. *Clin Endocrinol (Oxf).* 2000;52:509-518.
296. Bassett JH, Forbes SA, Pannett AA, et al. Characterization of mutations in patients with multiple endocrine neoplasia type 1. *Am J Hum Genet.* 1998;62:232-244.
297. Waterlot C, Porchet N, Bauters C, et al. Type 1 multiple endocrine neoplasia (MEN1): contribution of genetic analysis to the screening and follow-up of a large French kindred. *Clin Endocrinol (Oxf).* 1999;51:101-107.
298. Grayson RH, Halperin JM, Sharma V, et al. Changes in plasma prolactin and catecholamine metabolite levels following acute needle stick in children. *Psychiatry Res.* 1997;69:27-32.
299. Benya RV, Metz DC, Venzon DJ, et al. Zollinger-Ellison syndrome can be the initial endocrine manifestation in patients with multiple endocrine neoplasia-type I. *Am J Med.* 1994;97:436-444.
300. Burgess JR, Nord B, David R, et al. Phenotype and phenocopy: the relationship between genotype and clinical phenotype in a single large family with multiple endocrine neoplasia type 1 (MEN 1). *Clin Endocrinol (Oxf).* 2000;53:205-211.
301. Oberg K, Skogseid B. The ultimate biochemical diagnosis of endocrine pancreatic tumours in MEN-1. *J Intern Med.* 1998;243:471-476.
302. Hazard JB, Hawk WA, Crile G Jr. Medullary (solid) carcinoma of the thyroid; a clinicopathologic entity. *J Clin Endocrinol Metab.* 1959;19:152-161.
303. Williams ED. Histogenesis of medullary carcinoma of the thyroid. *J Clin Pathol.* 1966;19:114-118.
304. Williams ED, Pollock DJ. Multiple mucosal neuromata with endocrine tumours: a syndrome allied to von Recklinghausen's disease. *J Pathol Bacteriol.* 1966;91:71-80.

305. Schimke RN, Hartmann WH, Prout TE, et al. Syndrome of bilateral pheochromocytoma, medullary thyroid carcinoma and multiple neuromas: a possible regulatory defect in the differentiation of chromaffin tissue. *N Engl J Med*. 1968;279:1-7.
306. Farndon JR, Leight GS, Dilley WG, et al. Familial medullary thyroid carcinoma without associated endocrinopathies: a distinct clinical entity. *Br J Surg*. 1986;73:278-281.
307. Copp DH, Cheney B. Calcitonin: a hormone from the parathyroid which lowers the calcium level of the blood. *Nature*. 1962;193: 381-382.
308. Hirsch PF, Gauthier GF, Munson PL. Thyroid hypocalcemic principle and recurrent laryngeal nerve injury as factors affecting the response to parathyroidectomy in rats. *Endocrinology*. 1963;73:244-252.
309. Takahashi M, Ritz J, Cooper GM. Activation of a novel human transforming gene, RET, by DNA rearrangement. *Cell*. 1985;42:581-588.
310. Carlson KM, Bracamontes J, Jackson CE, et al. Parent-of-origin effects in multiple endocrine neoplasia type 2B. *Am J Hum Genet*. 1994;55:1076-1082.
311. Schuffenecker I, Ginet N, Goldgar D, et al. Prevalence and parental origin of de novo RET mutations in multiple endocrine neoplasia type 2A and familial medullary thyroid carcinoma. Le Groupe d'Etude des Tumeurs a Calcitonine. *Am J Hum Genet*. 1997;60:233-237.
312. Hahn M, Bishop J. Expression pattern of Drosophila ret suggests a common ancestral origin between the metamorphosis precursors in insect endoderm and the vertebrate enteric neurons. *Proc Natl Acad Sci U S A*. 2001;98:1053-1058.
313. Carter MT, Yome JL, Marcil MN, et al. Conservation of RET proto-oncogene splicing variants and implications for RET isoform function. *Cytogenet Cell Genet*. 2001;95:169-176.
314. Myers SM, Eng C, Ponder BA, et al. Characterization of RET proto-oncogene 3′ splicing variants and polyadenylation sites: a novel C-terminus for RET. *Oncogene*. 1995;11:2039-2045.
315. Tsui-Pierchala BA, Ahrens RC, Crowder RJ, et al. The long and short isoforms of Ret function as independent signaling complexes. *J Biol Chem*. 2002;277:34618-34625.
316. Borrello MG, Mercalli E, Perego C, et al. Differential interaction of Enigma protein with the two RET isoforms. *Biochem Biophys Res Commun*. 2002;296:515-522.
317. Lin LF, Doherty DH, Lile JD, et al. GDNF: a glial cell line-derived neurotrophic factor for midbrain dopaminergic neurons. *Science*. 1993;260:1130-1132.
318. Kotzbauer PT, Lampe PA, Heuckeroth RO, et al. Neurturin, a relative of glial-cell-line-derived neurotrophic factor. *Nature*. 1996;384: 467-470.
319. Baloh RH, Tansey MG, Lampe PA, et al. Artemin, a novel member of the GDNF ligand family, supports peripheral and central neurons and signals through the GFRalpha3-RET receptor complex. *Neuron*. 1998;21:1291-1302.
320. Milbrandt J, de Sauvage FJ, Fahrner TJ, et al. Persephin, a novel neurotrophic factor related to GDNF and neurturin. *Neuron*. 1998;20:245-253.
321. Airaksinen MS, Titievsky A, Saarma M. GDNF family neurotrophic factor signaling: four masters, one servant? *Mol Cell Neurosci*. 1999;13:313-325.
322. Arighi E, Borrello MG, Sariola H. RET tyrosine kinase signaling in development and cancer. *Cytokine Growth Factor Rev*. 2005;16:441-467.
323. Coulpier M, Anders J, Ibanez CF. Coordinated activation of autophosphorylation sites in the RET receptor tyrosine kinase: importance of tyrosine 1062 for GDNF mediated neuronal differentiation and survival. *J Biol Chem*. 2002;277:1991-1999.
324. Asai N, Iwashita T, Matsuyama M, et al. Mechanism of activation of the ret proto-oncogene by multiple endocrine neoplasia 2A mutations. *Mol Cell Biol*. 1995;15:1613-1619.
325. Santoro M, Carlomagno F, Romano A, et al. Activation of RET as a dominant transforming gene by germline mutations of MEN2A and MEN2B. *Science*. 1995;267:381-383.
326. Borrello MG, Smith DP, Pasini B, et al. RET activation by germline MEN2A and MEN2B mutations. *Oncogene*. 1995;11:2419-2427.
327. Pachnis V, Mankoo B, Costantini F. Expression of the c-ret proto-oncogene during mouse embryogenesis. *Development*. 1993;119: 1005-1017.
328. Santoro M, Rosati R, Grieco M, et al. The ret proto-oncogene is consistently expressed in human pheochromocytomas and thyroid medullary carcinomas. *Oncogene*. 1990;5:1595-1598.
329. Pausova Z, Soliman E, Amizuka N, et al. Role of the RET proto-oncogene in sporadic hyperparathyroidism and in hyperparathyroidism of multiple endocrine neoplasia type 2. *J Clin Endocrinol Metab*. 1996;81:2711-2718.
330. Tsuzuki T, Takahashi M, Asai N, et al. Spatial and temporal expression of the ret proto-oncogene product in embryonic, infant and adult rat tissues. *Oncogene*. 1995;10:191-198.
331. Schuchardt A, D'Agati V, Larsson-Blomberg L, et al. Defects in the kidney and enteric nervous system of mice lacking the tyrosine kinase receptor Ret. *Nature*. 1994;367:380-383.
332. Manie S, Santoro M, Fusco A, et al. The RET receptor: function in development and dysfunction in congenital malformation. *Trends Genet*. 2001;17:580-589.
333. Mathew CG, Chin KS, Easton DF, et al. A linked genetic marker for multiple endocrine neoplasia type 2A on chromosome 10. *Nature*. 1987;328:527-528.
334. Simpson NE, Kidd KK, Goodfellow PJ, et al. Assignment of multiple endocrine neoplasia type 2A to chromosome 10 by linkage. *Nature*. 1987;328:528-530.
335. Donis-Keller H, Dou S, Chi D, et al. Mutations in the RET proto-oncogene are associated with MEN 2A and FMTC. *Hum Mol Genet*. 1993;2:851-856.
336. Mulligan LM, Kwok JB, Healey CS, et al. Germ-line mutations of the RET proto-oncogene in multiple endocrine neoplasia type 2A. *Nature*. 1993;363:458-460.
337. Carlson KM, Dou S, Chi D, et al. Single missense mutation in the tyrosine kinase catalytic domain of the RET protooncogene is associated with multiple endocrine neoplasia type 2B. *Proc Natl Acad U S A*. 1994;91:1579-1583.
338. Hofstra RM, Landsvater RM, Ceccherini I, et al. A mutation in the RET proto-oncogene associated with multiple endocrine neoplasia type 2B and sporadic medullary thyroid carcinoma. *Nature*. 1994;367: 375-376.
339. Eng C, Clayton D, Schuffenecker I, et al. The relationship between specific RET proto-oncogene mutations and disease phenotype in multiple endocrine neoplasia type 2. International RET Mutation Consortium analysis. *JAMA*. 1996;276:1575-1579.
340. Hoppner W, Ritter MM. A duplication of 12 bp in the critical cysteine rich domain of the RET proto-oncogene results in a distinct phenotype of multiple endocrine neoplasia type 2A. *Hum Mol Genet*. 1997;6:587-590.
341. Tessitore A, Sinisi AA, Pasquali D, et al. A novel case of multiple endocrine neoplasia type 2A associated with two de novo mutations of the RET protooncogene. *J Clin Endocrinol Metab*. 1999;84:3522-3527.
342. Pigny P, Bauters C, Wemeau JL, et al. A novel 9-base pair duplication in RET exon 8 in familial medullary thyroid carcinoma. *J Clin Endocrinol Metab*. 1999;84:1700-1704.
343. Carlomagno F, Salvatore G, Cirafici AM, et al. The different RET-activating capability of mutations of cysteine 620 or cysteine 634 correlates with the multiple endocrine neoplasia type 2 disease phenotype. *Cancer Res*. 1997;57:391-395.
344. Iwashita T, Asai N, Murakami H, et al. Identification of tyrosine residues that are essential for transforming activity of the ret proto-oncogene with MEN2A or MEN2B mutation. *Oncogene*. 1996;12:481-487.
345. Miyauchi A, Futami H, Hai N, et al. Two germline missense mutations at codons 804 and 806 of the RET proto-oncogene in the same allele in a patient with multiple endocrine neoplasia type 2B without codon 918 mutation. *Jpn J Cancer Res*. 1999;90:1-5.
346. Menko FH, van der Luijt RB, de Valk IA, et al. Atypical MEN type 2B associated with two germline RET mutations on the same allele not involving codon 918. *J Clin Endocrinol Metab*. 2002;87:393-397.
347. Bartsch DK, Hasse C, Schug C, et al. A RET double mutation in the germline of a kindred with FMTC. *Exp Clin Endocrinol Diabetes*. 2000;108:128-132.
348. Zhou Y, Zhao Y, Cui B, et al. RET proto-oncogene mutations are restricted to codons 634 and 918 in mainland Chinese families with MEN2A and MEN2B. *Clin Endocrinol*. 2007;67:570-576.
349. Chang CF, Yang WS, Su YN, et al. Mutational spectrum of multiple endocrine neoplasia type 2 and sporadic medullary thyroid carcinoma in Taiwan. *J Formos Med Assoc*. 2009;108:402-408.
350. Wohllk N, Cote GJ, Evans DB, et al. Application of genetic screening information to the management of medullary thyroid carcinoma and multiple endocrine neoplasia type 2. *Endocrinol Metab Clin North Am*. 1996;25:1-25.
351. Rosenthal MS, Pierce HH. Inherited medullary thyroid cancer and the duty to warn: revisiting Pate v. Threlkel in light of HIPAA. *Thyroid*. 2005;15:140-145.
352. Chappuis-Flament S, Pasini A, De Vita G, et al. Dual effect on the RET receptor of MEN 2 mutations affecting specific extracytoplasmic cysteines. *Oncogene*. 1998;17:2851-2861.
353. Raue F, Frank-Raue K. Genotype-phenotype relationship in multiple endocrine neoplasia type 2: implications for clinical management. *Hormones (Athens)*. 2009;8:23-28.
354. Kouvaraki MA, Shapiro SE, Perrier ND, et al. RET proto-oncogene: a review and update of genotype-phenotype correlations in hereditary medullary thyroid cancer and associated endocrine tumors. *Thyroid*. 2005;15:531-544.
355. Mulligan LM, Eng C, Healey CS, et al. Specific mutations of the RET proto-oncogene are related to disease phenotype in MEN 2A and FMTC. *Nat Genet*. 1994;6:70-74.
356. Nunziata V, Giannattasio R, Di Giovanni G, et al. Hereditary localized pruritus in affected members of a kindred with multiple endocrine neoplasia type 2A (Sipple's syndrome). *Clin Endocrinol*. 1989;30:57-63.

357. Gagel RF, Levy ML, Donovan DT, et al. Multiple endocrine neoplasia type 2a associated with cutaneous lichen amyloidosis. *Ann Intern Med.* 1989;111:802-806.
358. Verga U, Fugazzola L, Cambiaghi S, et al. Frequent association between MEN 2A and cutaneous lichen amyloidosis. *Clin Endocrinol.* 2003;59:156-161.
359. Rothberg AE, Raymond VM, Gruber SB, et al. Familial medullary thyroid carcinoma associated with cutaneous lichen amyloidosis. *Thyroid.* 2009;19:651-655.
360. Hofstra RM, Sijmons RH, Stelwagen T, et al. RET mutation screening in familial cutaneous lichen amyloidosis and in skin amyloidosis associated with multiple endocrine neoplasia. *J Invest Dermatol.* 1996;107:215-218.
361. Romeo G, Ronchetto P, Luo Y, et al. Point mutations affecting the tyrosine kinase domain of the RET proto-oncogene in Hirschsprung's disease. *Nature.* 1994;367:377-378.
362. Edery P, Lyonnet S, Mulligan LM, et al. Mutations of the RET proto-oncogene in Hirschsprung's disease. *Nature.* 1994;367:378-380.
363. Attie T, Pelet A, Edery P, et al. Diversity of RET proto-oncogene mutations in familial and sporadic Hirschsprung disease. *Hum Mol Genet.* 1995;4:1381-1386.
364. Amiel J, Sproat-Emison E, Garcia-Barcelo M, et al. Hirschsprung disease, associated syndromes and genetics: a review. *J Med Genet.* 2008;45:1-14.
365. Mulligan LM, Eng C, Attie T, et al. Diverse phenotypes associated with exon 10 mutations of the RET proto-oncogene. *Hum Mol Genet.* 1994;3:2163-2167.
366. Borst MJ, VanCamp JM, Peacock ML, et al. Mutational analysis of multiple endocrine neoplasia type 2A associated with Hirschsprung's disease. *Surgery.* 1995;117:386-391.
367. Caron P, Attie T, David D, et al. C618R mutation in exon 10 of the RET proto-oncogene in a kindred with multiple endocrine neoplasia type 2A and Hirschsprung's disease. *J Clin Endocrinol Metab.* 1996;81:2731-2733.
368. Peretz H, Luboshitsky R, Baron E, et al. Cys 618 Arg mutation in the RET proto-oncogene associated with familial medullary thyroid carcinoma and maternally transmitted Hirschsprung's disease suggesting a role for imprinting. *Hum Mutat.* 1997;10:155-159.
369. Ito S, Iwashita T, Asai N, et al. Biological properties of Ret with cysteine mutations correlate with multiple endocrine neoplasia type 2A, familial medullary thyroid carcinoma, and Hirschsprung's disease phenotype. *Cancer Res.* 1997;57:2870-2872.
370. Eng C, Smith DP, Mulligan LM, et al. Point mutation within the tyrosine kinase domain of the RET proto-oncogene in multiple endocrine neoplasia type 2B and related sporadic tumours. *Hum Mol Genet.* 1994;3:237-241.
371. Uchino S, Noguchi S, Yamashita H, et al. Somatic mutations in RET exons 12 and 15 in sporadic medullary thyroid carcinomas: different spectrum of mutations in sporadic type from hereditary type. *Jpn J Cancer Res.* 1999;90:1231-1237.
372. Moura MM, Cavaco BM, Pinto AE, et al. Correlation of RET somatic mutations with clinicopathological features in sporadic medullary thyroid carcinomas. *Br J Cancer.* 2009;100:1777-1783.
373. Zedenius J, Wallin G, Hamberger B, et al. Somatic and MEN 2A de novo mutations identified in the RET proto-oncogene by screening of sporadic MTC:s. *Hum Mol Genet.* 1994;3:1259-1262.
374. Schilling T, Burck J, Sinn HP, et al. Prognostic value of codon 918 (ATG→ACG) RET proto-oncogene mutations in sporadic medullary thyroid carcinoma. *Int J Cancer.* 2001;95:62-66.
375. Elisei R, Cosci B, Romei C, et al. Prognostic significance of somatic RET oncogene mutations in sporadic medullary thyroid cancer: a 10-year follow-up study. *J Clin Endocrinol Metab.* 2008;93:682-687.
376. Marsh DJ, Learoyd DL, Andrew SD, et al. Somatic mutations in the RET proto-oncogene in sporadic medullary thyroid carcinoma. *Clin Endocrinol.* 1996;44:249-257.
377. Fusco A, Grieco M, Santoro M, et al. A new oncogene in human thyroid papillary carcinomas and their lymph-nodal metastases. *Nature.* 1987;328:170-172.
378. Grieco M, Santoro M, Berlingieri MT, et al. PTC is a novel rearranged form of the ret proto-oncogene and is frequently detected in vivo in human thyroid papillary carcinomas. *Cell.* 1990;60:557-563.
379. Pierotti MA, Bongarzone I, Borello MG, et al. Cytogenetics and molecular genetics of carcinomas arising from thyroid epithelial follicular cells. *Genes Chromosomes Cancer.* 1996;16:1-14.
380. Jhiang SM. The RET proto-oncogene in human cancers. *Oncogene.* 2000;19:5590-5597.
381. Ito T, Seyama T, Iwamoto KS, et al. Activated RET oncogene in thyroid cancers of children from areas contaminated by Chernobyl accident. *Lancet.* 1994;344:259.
382. Fugazzola L, Pilotti S, Pinchera A, et al. Oncogenic rearrangements of the RET proto-oncogene in papillary thyroid carcinomas from children exposed to the Chernobyl nuclear accident. *Cancer Res.* 1995;55:5617-5620.
383. Nikiforov YE, Rowland JM, Bove KE, et al. Distinct pattern of ret oncogene rearrangements in morphological variants of radiation-induced and sporadic thyroid papillary carcinomas in children. *Cancer Res.* 1997;57:1690-1694.
384. Saenko V, Rogounovitch T, Shimizu-Yoshida Y, et al. Novel tumorigenic rearrangement, Delta rfp/ret, in a papillary thyroid carcinoma from externally irradiated patient. *Mutation Res.* 2003;527:81-90.
385. Nikiforov YE. RET/PTC rearrangement in thyroid tumors. *Endocr Pathol.* 2002;13:3-16.
386. Thomas GA, Bunnell H, Cook HA, et al. High prevalence of RET/PTC rearrangements in Ukrainian and Belarussian post-Chernobyl thyroid papillary carcinomas: a strong correlation between RET/PTC3 and the solid-follicular variant. *J Clin Endocrinol Metab.* 1999;84:4232-4238.
387. Basolo F, Giannini R, Monaco C, et al. Potent mitogenicity of the RET/PTC3 oncogene correlates with its prevalence in tall-cell variant of papillary thyroid carcinoma. *Am J Pathol.* 2002;160:247-254.
388. Chiappetta G, Toti P, Cetta F, et al. The RET/PTC oncogene is frequently activated in oncocytic thyroid tumors (Hurthle cell adenomas and carcinomas), but not in oncocytic hyperplastic lesions. *J Clin Endocrinol Metab.* 2002;87:364-369.
389. Musholt PB, Imkamp F, von Wasielewski R, et al. RET rearrangements in archival oxyphilic thyroid tumors: new insights in tumorigenesis and classification of Hurthle cell carcinomas? *Surgery.* 2003;134:881-889; discussion 889.
390. Bongarzone I, Vigneri P, Mariani L, et al. RET/NTRK1 rearrangements in thyroid gland tumors of the papillary carcinoma family: correlation with clinicopathological features. *Clin Cancer Res.* 1998;4:223-228.
391. Elisei R, Ugolini C, Viola D, et al. BRAF(V600E) mutation and outcome of patients with papillary thyroid carcinoma: a 15-year median follow-up study. *J Clin Endocrinol Metab.* 2008;93:3943-3949.
392. Fenwick JC. Effect of partial ultimobranchialectomy on plasma calcium concentration and on some related parameters in goldfish (*Carassius auratus* L.) during acute transfer from fresh water to 30 per cent sea water. *Gen Comp Endocrinol.* 1975;25:60-63.
393. Nieto A, L-Fando JJ, R-Candela JL. Biosynthesis and secretion of calcitonin in vitro in chicken ultimobranchial gland. *Gen Comp Endocrinol.* 1975;25:259-263.
394. Wolfe HJ, Melvin KE, Cervi-Skinner SJ, et al. C-cell hyperplasia preceding medullary thyroid carcinoma. *N Engl J Med.* 1973;289:437-441.
395. LiVolsi VA. C cell hyperplasia/neoplasia. *J Clin Endocrinol Metab.* 1997;82:39-41.
396. Rosai J, Carcangiu, ML, DeLellis, RA. Tumors of the thyroid gland. In: Armed Forces Institute of Pathology; Fascicle 5, 3rd series. Washington, DC; 1992:249.
397. Guyetant S, Rousselet MC, Durigon M, et al. Sex-related C cell hyperplasia in the normal human thyroid: a quantitative autopsy study. *J Clin Endocrinol Metab.* 1997;82:42-47.
398. van Lathem JJ, Vermaak WJ, Kuyl JM, et al. Experience with a provocative test of calcitonin release as a prospective screening for preclinical medullary thyroid carcinoma in MEN type 2A family members. *J Clin Lab Anal.* 1992;6:384-390.
399. Zink A, Blind E, Raue F. Determination of serum calcitonin by immunometric two-site assays in normal subjects and patients with medullary thyroid carcinoma. *Eur J Clin Chem Clin Biochem.* 1992;30:831-835.
400. Khurana R, Agarwal A, Bajpai VK, et al. Unraveling the amyloid associated with human medullary thyroid carcinoma. *Endocrinology.* 2004;145:5465-5470.
401. Yokozawa T, Fukata S, Kuma K, et al. Thyroid cancer detected by ultrasound-guided fine-needle aspiration biopsy. *World J Surg.* 1996;20:848-853; discussion 853.
402. Tokuue K, Furuse M. Usefulness of the 99mTc-MDP scan in the detection of calcified liver metastases. *Nuklearmedizin.* 1990;29:231-233.
403. Atkins FL, Beaven MA, Keiser HR. Dopa decarboxylase in medullary carcinoma of the thyroid. *N Engl J Med.* 1973;289:545-548.
404. Gagel RF, Palmer WN, Leonhart K, et al. Somatostatin production by a human medullary thyroid carcinoma cell line. *Endocrinology.* 1986;118:1643-1651.
405. O'Connor DT, Deftos LJ. Secretion of chromogranin A by peptide-producing endocrine neoplasms. *N Engl J Med.* 1986;314:1145-1151.
406. Sevarino KA, Wu P, Jackson IM, et al. Biosynthesis of thyrotropin-releasing hormone by a rat medullary thyroid carcinoma cell line. *J Biol Chem.* 1988;263:620-623.
407. Yamaguchi K, Abe K, Adachi I, et al. Concomitant production of immunoreactive gastrin-releasing peptide and calcitonin in medullary carcinoma of the thyroid. *Metabolism.* 1984;33:724-727.
408. Baylin SB, Beaven MA, Buja LM, et al. Histaminase activity: a biochemical marker for medullary carcinoma of the thyroid. *Am J Med.* 1972;53:723-733.
409. Melvin KE, Miller HH, Tashjian AH Jr. Early diagnosis of medullary carcinoma of the thyroid gland by means of calcitonin assay. *N Engl J Med.* 1971;285:1115-1120.
410. Wells SA Jr, Baylin SB, Linehan WM, et al. Provocative agents and the diagnosis of medullary carcinoma of the thyroid gland. *Ann Surg.* 1978;188:139-141.

411. Roman S, Lin R, Sosa JA. Prognosis of medullary thyroid carcinoma: demographic, clinical, and pathologic predictors of survival in 1252 cases. *Cancer*. 2006;107:2134-2142.
412. Papaparaskeva K, Nagel H, Droese M. Cytologic diagnosis of medullary carcinoma of the thyroid gland. *Diagn Cytopathol*. 2000;22:351-358.
413. Bugalho MJ, Santos JR, Sobrinho L. Preoperative diagnosis of medullary thyroid carcinoma: fine needle aspiration cytology as compared with serum calcitonin measurement. *J Surg Oncol*. 2005;91:56-60.
414. Bhanot P, Yang J, Schnadig VJ, et al. Role of FNA cytology and immunochemistry in the diagnosis and management of medullary thyroid carcinoma: report of six cases and review of the literature. *Diagn Cytopathol*. 2007;35:285-292.
415. Kudo T, Miyauchi A, Ito Y, et al. Diagnosis of medullary thyroid carcinoma by calcitonin measurement in fine-needle aspiration biopsy specimens. *Thyroid*. 2007;17:635-638.
416. Cooper DS, Doherty GM, Haugen BR, et al. Management guidelines for patients with thyroid nodules and differentiated thyroid cancer. *Thyroid*. 2006;16:109-142.
417. Pacini F, Fontanelli M, Fugazzola L, et al. Routine measurement of serum calcitonin in nodular thyroid diseases allows the preoperative diagnosis of unsuspected sporadic medullary thyroid carcinoma. *J Clin Endocrinol Metab*. 1994;78:826-829.
418. Elisei R, Bottici V, Luchetti F, et al. Impact of routine measurement of serum calcitonin on the diagnosis and outcome of medullary thyroid cancer: experience in 10,864 patients with nodular thyroid disorders. *J Clin Endocrinol Metab*. 2004;89:163-168.
419. Niccoli P, Wion-Barbot N, Caron P, et al. Interest of routine measurement of serum calcitonin: study in a large series of thyroidectomized patients. The French Medullary Study Group. *J Clin Endocrinol Metab*. 1997;82:338-341.
420. Karges W, Dralle H, Raue F, et al. Calcitonin measurement to detect medullary thyroid carcinoma in nodular goiter: German evidence-based consensus recommendation. *Exp Clin Endocrinol Diabetes*. 2004;112:52-58.
421. Elisei R, Romei C, Cosci B, et al. RET genetic screening in patients with medullary thyroid cancer and their relatives: experience with 807 individuals at one center. *J Clin Endocrinol Metab*. 2007;92:4725-4729.
422. Machens A, Schneyer U, Holzhausen HJ, et al. Prospects of remission in medullary thyroid carcinoma according to basal calcitonin level. *J Clin Endocrinol Metab*. 2005;90:2029-2034.
423. Machens A, Ukkat J, Hauptmann S, et al. Abnormal carcinoembryonic antigen levels and medullary thyroid cancer progression: a multivariate analysis. *Arch Surg*. 2007;142:289-293; discussion 294.
424. Machens A, Hauptmann S, Dralle H. Increased risk of lymph node metastasis in multifocal hereditary and sporadic medullary thyroid cancer. *World J Surg*. 2007;31:1960-1965.
425. Machens A, Hauptmann S, Dralle H. Prediction of lateral lymph node metastases in medullary thyroid cancer. *Br J Surg*. 2008;95:586-591.
426. Moley JF, DeBenedetti MK. Patterns of nodal metastases in palpable medullary thyroid carcinoma: recommendations for extent of node dissection. *Ann Surg*. 1999;229:880-887; discussion 887-888.
427. Fleming JB, Lee JE, Bouvet M, et al. Surgical strategy for the treatment of medullary thyroid carcinoma. *Ann Surg*. 1999;230:697-707.
428. Modigliani E, Cohen R, Campos JM, et al. Prognostic factors for survival and for biochemical cure in medullary thyroid carcinoma: results in 899 patients. The GETC Study Group. Groupe d'Etude des Tumeurs a Calcitonine. *Clin Endocrinol*. 1998;48:265-273.
429. Franc S, Niccoli-Sire P, Cohen R, et al. Complete surgical lymph node resection does not prevent authentic recurrences of medullary thyroid carcinoma. *Clin Endocrinol*. 2001;55:403-409.
430. Rendl G, Manzl M, Hitzl W, et al. Long-term prognosis of medullary thyroid carcinoma. *Clin Endocrinol (Oxf)*. 2008;69:497-505.
431. Machens A, Holzhausen HJ, Dralle H. Prediction of mediastinal lymph node metastasis in medullary thyroid carcinoma. *Br J Surg*. 2004;91:709-712.
432. Wells SA Jr, Chi DD, Toshima K, et al. Predictive DNA testing and prophylactic thyroidectomy in patients at risk for multiple endocrine neoplasia type 2A. *Ann Surg*. 1994;220:237-247; discussion 247-250.
433. Lips CJ, Landsvater RM, Hoppener JW, et al. Clinical screening as compared with DNA analysis in families with multiple endocrine neoplasia type 2A. *N Engl J Med*. 1994;331:828-835.
434. Bugalho MJ, Domingues R, Santos JR, et al. Mutation analysis of the RET proto-oncogene and early thyroidectomy: results of a Portuguese cancer centre. *Surgery*. 2007;141:90-95.
435. Calva D, O'Dorisio TM, Sue O'Dorisio M, et al. When is prophylactic thyroidectomy indicated for patients with the RET codon 609 mutation? *Ann Surg Oncol*. 2009;16:2237-2244.
436. Canizo A, Fanjul M, Cerda J, et al. [Is immediate prophylactic thyroidectomy indispensable in familiar medullary thyroid carcinoma?]. *Cir Pediatr*. 2008;21:100-103.
437. Colombo-Benkmann M, Bramswig J, Hoppner W, et al. Surgical strategy in a kindred with a rare RET protooncogene mutation of variable penetrance with regard to multiple endocrine neoplasia. *World J Surg*. 2002;26:1286-1290.
438. de Groot JW, Links TP, Rouwe CW, et al. [Prophylactic thyroidectomy in children who are carriers of a multiple endocrine neoplasia type 2 mutation: description of 20 cases and recommendations based on the literature]. *Ned Tijdschr Geneeskd*. 2006;150:311-318.
439. Frank-Raue K, Buhr H, Dralle H, et al. Long-term outcome in 46 gene carriers of hereditary medullary thyroid carcinoma after prophylactic thyroidectomy: impact of individual RET genotype. *Eur J Endocrinol*. 2006;155:229-236.
440. Rodriguez GJ, Balsalobre MD, Pomares F, et al. Prophylactic thyroidectomy in MEN 2A syndrome: experience in a single center. *J Am Coll Surg*. 2002;195:159-166.
441. Gosnell JE, Sywak MS, Sidhu SB, et al. New era: prophylactic surgery for patients with multiple endocrine neoplasia-2a. *ANZ J Surg*. 2006;76:586-590.
442. Hassett S, Costigan C, McDermott M, et al. Prophylactic thyroidectomy in the treatment of thyroid medullary carcinoma: age for surgery? *Eur J Pediatr Surg*. 2000;10:334-336.
443. Heizmann O, Haecker FM, Zumsteg U, et al. Presymptomatic thyroidectomy in multiple endocrine neoplasia 2a. *Eur J Surg Oncol*. 2006;32:98-102.
444. Klein I, Esik O, Homolya V, et al. Molecular genetic diagnostic program of multiple endocrine neoplasia type 2A and familial medullary thyroid carcinoma syndromes in Hungary. *J Endocrinol*. 2001;170:661-666.
445. Lau GS, Lang BH, Lo CY, et al. Prophylactic thyroidectomy in ethnic Chinese patients with multiple endocrine neoplasia type 2A syndrome after the introduction of genetic testing. *Hong Kong Med J*. 2009;15:326-331.
446. Learoyd DL, Gosnell J, Elston MS, et al. Experience of prophylactic thyroidectomy in multiple endocrine neoplasia type 2A kindreds with RET codon 804 mutations. *Clin Endocrinol*. 2005;63:636-641.
447. Machens A, Dralle H. Prophylactic thyroidectomy in RET carriers at risk for hereditary medullary thyroid cancer. *Thyroid*. 2009;19:551-554.
448. Moore SW, Appfelstaedt J, Zaahl MG. Familial medullary carcinoma prevention, risk evaluation, and RET in children of families with MEN2. *J Pediatr Surg*. 2007;42:326-332.
449. Niccoli-Sire P, Murat A, Baudin E, et al. Early or prophylactic thyroidectomy in MEN 2/FMTC gene carriers: results in 71 thyroidectomized patients. The French Calcitonin Tumours Study Group (GETC). *Eur J Endocrinol*. 1999;141:468-474.
450. Piolat C, Dyon JF, Sturm N, et al. Very early prophylactic thyroid surgery for infants with a mutation of the RET proto-oncogene at codon 634: evaluation of the implementation of international guidelines for MEN type 2 in a single centre. *Clin Endocrinol*. 2006;65:118-124.
451. Punales MK, Graf H, Gross JL, et al. RET codon 634 mutations in multiple endocrine neoplasia type 2: variable clinical features and clinical outcome. *J Clin Endocrinol Metab*. 2003;88:2644-2649.
452. Punales MK, da Rocha AP, Meotti C, et al. Clinical and oncological features of children and young adults with multiple endocrine neoplasia type 2A. *Thyroid*. 2008;18:1261-1268.
453. Sakorafas GH, Friess H, Peros G. The genetic basis of hereditary medullary thyroid cancer: clinical implications for the surgeon, with a particular emphasis on the role of prophylactic thyroidectomy. *Endocr Relat Cancer*. 2008;15:871-884.
454. Sanso GE, Domene HM, Garcia R, et al. Very early detection of RET proto-oncogene mutation is crucial for preventive thyroidectomy in multiple endocrine neoplasia type 2 children: presence of C-cell malignant disease in asymptomatic carriers. *Cancer*. 2002;94:323-330.
455. Schellhaas E, Konig C, Frank-Raue K, et al. Long-term outcome of "prophylactic therapy" for familial medullary thyroid cancer. *Surgery*. 2009;146:906-912.
456. Toledo SP, dos Santos MA, Toledo Rde A, et al. Impact of RET proto-oncogene analysis on the clinical management of multiple endocrine neoplasia type 2. *Clinics (Sao Paulo)*. 2006;61:59-70.
457. van Heurn LW, Schaap C, Sie G, et al. Predictive DNA testing for multiple endocrine neoplasia 2: a therapeutic challenge of prophylactic thyroidectomy in very young children. *J Pediatr Surg*. 1999;34:568-571.
458. Vestergaard P, Vestergaard EM, Brockstedt H, et al. Codon Y791F mutations in a large kindred: is prophylactic thyroidectomy always indicated? *World J Surg*. 2007;31:996-1001; discussion 1002-1004.
459. Zenaty D, Aigrain Y, Peuchmaur M, et al. Medullary thyroid carcinoma identified within the first year of life in children with hereditary multiple endocrine neoplasia type 2A (codon 634) and 2B. *Eur J Endocrinol*. 2009;160:807-813.
460. Dralle H, Gimm O, Simon D, et al. Prophylactic thyroidectomy in 75 children and adolescents with hereditary medullary thyroid carcinoma: German and Austrian experience. *World J Surg*. 1998;22:744-750; discussion 750-751.
461. Kloos RT, Eng C, Evans DB, et al. Medullary thyroid cancer: management guidelines of the American Thyroid Association. *Thyroid*. 2009;19:565-612.

462. Machens A, Niccoli-Sire P, Hoegel J, et al. Early malignant progression of hereditary medullary thyroid cancer. *N Engl J Med.* 2003;349:1517-1525.
463. Costante G, Durante C, Francis Z, et al. Determination of calcitonin levels in C-cell disease: clinical interest and potential pitfalls. *Nat Clin Pract Endocrinol Metab.* 2009;5:35-44.
464. Skinner MA, Moley JA, Dilley WG, et al. Prophylactic thyroidectomy in multiple endocrine neoplasia type 2A. *N Engl J Med.* 2005;353: 1105-1113.
465. Fugazzola L, Pinchera A, Luchetti F, et al. Disappearance rate of serum calcitonin after total thyroidectomy for medullary thyroid carcinoma. *Int J Biol Markers.* 1994;9:21-24.
466. Miyauchi A, Onishi T, Morimoto S, et al. Relation of doubling time of plasma calcitonin levels to prognosis and recurrence of medullary thyroid carcinoma. *Ann Surg.* 1984;199:461-466.
467. Laure Giraudet A, Al Ghulzan A, Auperin A, et al. Progression of medullary thyroid carcinoma: assessment with calcitonin and carcinoembryonic antigen doubling times. *Eur J Endocrinol.* 2008;158:239-246.
468. Barbet J, Campion L, Kraeber-Bodere F, et al. Prognostic impact of serum calcitonin and carcinoembryonic antigen doubling-times in patients with medullary thyroid carcinoma. *J Clin Endocrinol Metab.* 2005;90:6077-6084.
469. Busnardo B, Girelli ME, Simioni N, et al. Nonparallel patterns of calcitonin and carcinoembryonic antigen levels in the follow-up of medullary thyroid carcinoma. *Cancer.* 1984;53:278-285.
470. Mendelsohn G, Wells SA Jr, Baylin SB. Relationship of tissue carcinoembryonic antigen and calcitonin to tumor virulence in medullary thyroid carcinoma: an immunohistochemical study in early, localized, and virulent disseminated stages of disease. *Cancer.* 1984;54:657-662.
471. Moley JF, Dilley WG, DeBenedetti MK. Improved results of cervical reoperation for medullary thyroid carcinoma. *Ann Surg.* 1997;225:734-740; discussion 740-743.
472. Smallridge RC, Bourne K, Pearson BW, et al. Cushing's syndrome due to medullary thyroid carcinoma: diagnosis by proopiomelanocortin messenger ribonucleic acid in situ hybridization. *J Clin Endocrinol Metab.* 2003;88:4565-4568.
473. Ilias I, Torpy DJ, Pacak K, et al. Cushing's syndrome due to ectopic corticotropin secretion: twenty years' experience at the National Institutes of Health. *J Clin Endocrinol Metab.* 2005;90:4955-4962.
474. van Heerden JA, Grant CS, Gharib H, et al. Long-term course of patients with persistent hypercalcitoninemia after apparent curative primary surgery for medullary thyroid carcinoma. *Ann Surg.* 1990;212:395-400; discussion 401.
475. Jeng TK, Lee CH, Wang HC, et al. DNA analysis and persistent hypercalcitoninemia in medullary thyroid carcinoma. *Chinese Med J.* 1993;51:340-344.
476. Block MA, Jackson CE, Tashjian AH Jr. Management of occult medullary thyroid carcinoma: evidenced only by serum calcitonin level elevations after apparently adequate neck operations. *Arch Surg.* 1978;113:368-372.
477. Norton JA, Doppman JL, Brennan MF. Localization and resection of clinically inapparent medullary carcinoma of the thyroid. *Surgery.* 1980;87:616-622.
478. Ellenhorn JD, Shah JP, Brennan MF. Impact of therapeutic regional lymph node dissection for medullary carcinoma of the thyroid gland. *Surgery.* 1993;114:1078-1081; discussion 1081-1082.
479. Tisell LE, Hansson G, Jansson S, et al. Reoperation in the treatment of asymptomatic metastasizing medullary thyroid carcinoma. *Surgery.* 1986;99:60-66.
480. Tisell LE, Jansson S. Recent results of reoperative surgery in medullary carcinoma of the thyroid. *Wien Klin Wechenschr.* 1988;100:347-348.
481. Dralle H, Damm I, Scheumann GF, et al. Compartment-oriented microdissection of regional lymph nodes in medullary thyroid carcinoma. *Surgery Today.* 1994;24:112-121.
482. Gimm O, Dralle H. Reoperation in metastasizing medullary thyroid carcinoma: is a tumor stage-oriented approach justified? *Surgery.* 1997;122:1124-1130; discussion 1130-1131.
483. Gimm O, Ukkat J, Dralle H. Determinative factors of biochemical cure after primary and reoperative surgery for sporadic medullary thyroid carcinoma. *World J Surg.* 1998;22:562-567; discussion 567-568.
484. Fialkowski E, DeBenedetti M, Moley J. Long-term outcome of reoperations for medullary thyroid carcinoma. *World J Surg.* 2008;32: 754-765.
485. Sridhar KS, Holland JF, Brown JC, et al. Doxorubicin plus cisplatin in the treatment of apudomas. *Cancer.* 1985;55:2634-2637.
486. Scherubl H, Raue F, Ziegler R. Combination chemotherapy of advanced medullary and differentiated thyroid cancer: phase II study. *J Cancer Res Clin Oncol.* 1990;116:21-23.
487. Orlandi F, Caraci P, Berruti A, et al. Chemotherapy with dacarbazine and 5-fluorouracil in advanced medullary thyroid cancer. *Ann Oncol.* 1994;5:763-775.
488. Schlumberger M, Abdelmoumene N, Delisle MJ, et al. Treatment of advanced medullary thyroid cancer with an alternating combination of 5 FU-streptozocin and 5 FU-dacarbazine. The Groupe d'Etude des Tumeurs a Calcitonine (GETC). *Br J Cancer.* 1995;71:363-365.
489. Matuszczyk A, Petersenn S, Bockisch A, et al. Chemotherapy with doxorubicin in progressive medullary and thyroid carcinoma of the follicular epithelium. *Horm Metab Res.* 2008;40:210-213.
490. Eisenhauer EA, Therasse P, Bogaerts J, et al. New response evaluation criteria in solid tumours: revised RECIST guideline (version 1.1). *Eur J Cancer.* 2009;45:228-247.
491. Chow SM, Chan JK, Tiu SC, et al. Medullary thyroid carcinoma in Hong Kong Chinese patients. *Hong Kong Med J.* 2005;11:251-258.
492. Brierley J, Tsang R, Simpson WJ, et al. Medullary thyroid cancer: analyses of survival and prognostic factors and the role of radiation therapy in local control. *Thyroid.* 1996;6:305-310.
493. Kim IY, Kondziolka D, Niranjan A, et al. Gamma knife radiosurgery for metastatic brain tumors from thyroid cancer. *J Neuro-oncol.* 2009;93:355-359.
494. Goetz MP, Callstrom MR, Charboneau JW, et al. Percutaneous image-guided radiofrequency ablation of painful metastases involving bone: a multicenter study. *J Clin Oncol.* 2004;22:300-306.
495. Pomares FJ, Canas R, Rodriguez JM, et al. Differences between sporadic and multiple endocrine neoplasia type 2A phaeochromocytoma. *Clin Endocrinol.* 1998;48:195-200.
496. Nguyen L, Niccoli-Sire P, Caron P, et al. Pheochromocytoma in multiple endocrine neoplasia type 2: a prospective study. *Eur J Endocrinol.* 2001;144:37-44.
497. Lenders JW, Pacak K, Walther MM, et al. Biochemical diagnosis of pheochromocytoma: which test is best? *JAMA.* 2002;287:1427-1434.
498. Ilias I, Pacak K. Current approaches and recommended algorithm for the diagnostic localization of pheochromocytoma. *J Clin Endocrinol Metab.* 2004;89:479-491.
499. Ilias I, Chen CC, Carrasquillo JA, et al. Comparison of 6-18F-fluorodopamine PET with 123I-metaiodobenzylguanidine and 111in-pentetreotide scintigraphy in localization of nonmetastatic and metastatic pheochromocytoma. *J Nucl Med.* 2008;49:1613-1619.
500. Lairmore TC, Ball DW, Baylin SB, et al. Management of pheochromocytomas in patients with multiple endocrine neoplasia type 2 syndromes. *Ann Surg.* 1993;217:595-601; discussion 603.
501. Asari R, Scheuba C, Kaczirek K, et al. Estimated risk of pheochromocytoma recurrence after adrenal-sparing surgery in patients with multiple endocrine neoplasia type 2A. *Arch Surg.* 2006;141:1199-1205; discussion 1205.
502. Gagner M, Pomp A, Heniford BT, et al. Laparoscopic adrenalectomy: lessons learned from 100 consecutive procedures. *Ann Surg.* 1997;226:238-246; discussion 246-247.
503. Brunt LM, Lairmore TC, Doherty GM, et al. Adrenalectomy for familial pheochromocytoma in the laparoscopic era. *Ann Surg.* 2002;235:713-720; discussion 720-721.
504. Herfarth KK, Bartsch D, Doherty GM, et al. Surgical management of hyperparathyroidism in patients with multiple endocrine neoplasia type 2A. *Surgery.* 1996;120:966-973; discussion 973-974.
505. Olson JA Jr, DeBenedetti MK, Baumann DS, et al. Parathyroid autotransplantation during thyroidectomy: results of long-term follow-up. *Ann Surg.* 1996;223:472-478; discussion 478-480.
506. Druker BJ, Sawyers CL, Kantarjian H, et al. Activity of a specific inhibitor of the BCR-ABL tyrosine kinase in the blast crisis of chronic myeloid leukemia and acute lymphoblastic leukemia with the Philadelphia chromosome. *N Engl J Med.* 2001;344:1038-1042.
507. Druker BJ, Talpaz M, Resta DJ, et al. Efficacy and safety of a specific inhibitor of the BCR-ABL tyrosine kinase in chronic myeloid leukemia. *N Engl J Med.* 2001;344:1031-1037.
508. Wedge SR, Ogilvie DJ, Dukes M, et al. ZD6474 inhibits vascular endothelial growth factor signaling, angiogenesis, and tumor growth following oral administration. *Cancer Res.* 2002;62:4645-4655.
509. Carlomagno F, Vitagliano D, Guida T, et al. ZD6474, an orally available inhibitor of KDR tyrosine kinase activity, efficiently blocks oncogenic RET kinases. *Cancer Res.* 2002;62:7284-7290.
510. Wells SA, Gosnell JE, Gagel RF, et al. Vandetanib for the treatment of patients with locally advanced of metastatic hereditary medullary thyroid cancer. *J Clin Oncol.* 2010;28:767-772.
511a. Cohen EE, Rosen LS, Vokes EE, et al. Axitinib is an active treatment for all histologic subtypes of advanced thyroid cancer: Results from a Phase II study. *J Clin Oncol.* 2008;26:4708-4713.
511b. Frank-Raue K, Fabel M, Delorme S, Haberkorn U, Raue F. Efficacy of imatinib mesylate in advanced medullary thyroid carcinoma. *Eur J Endocrinol.* 2007;157:215-220.
511c. Gupta-Abramson V, Troxel AB, Nellore A, et al. Phase II trial of sorafenib in advanced thyroid cancer. *J Clin Oncol.* 2008;26: 4714-4719.
511d. Lam ET, Ringel MD, Kloos RT, et al. Phase II clinical trial of sorafenib in metastatic medullary thyroid cancer. *J Clin Oncol.* 2010; 28:2323-2330.
511e. Pennell NA, Daniels GH, Haddad RI, et al. A phase II study of gefitinib in patients with advanced thyroid cancer. *Thyroid.* 2008;18:317-323.
511f. Schlumberger MJ, Elisei R, Bastholt L, et al. Phase II study of safety and efficacy of motesanib in patients with progressive or symptomatic, advanced or metastatic medullary thyroid cancer. *J Clin Oncol.* 2009;27:3794-3801.

511g. de Groot JW, Zonnenberg BA, Quarles van Ufford-Mannesse P, et al. A Phase II trial of imatinib therapy for metastatic medullary thyroid carcinoma. *J Clin Endocrinol Metab.* 2007;92:3466-3469.
511h. Kurzrock R, Sherman S, Pfister D, et al. Long Term Results in Patients with Medullary Thyroid Cancer Enrolled in a Phase 1 Study of XL184 (BMS907351), An Oral Inhibitor of MET, VEGFR2 and RET. International Thyroid Congress 2010, OC-109.
511i. Fox E, Widemann BC, Whitcomb PO, et al. Phase I/II trial of vandetanib in children and adolescents with hereditary medullary thyroid carcinoma. *J Clin Oncol.* 2009;27:10-14.
511j. Wells SA, Robinson BG, Gagel RF, et al. Vandetanib in locally advanced or metastatic medullary thyroid carcinoma: A randomized, double-blind phase III trial (ZETA). *J Clin Oncol.* 2010;28:15s (5503).
512. Cameron D, Spiro HM, Landsberg L. Zollinger-Ellison syndrome with multiple endocrine adenomatosis type II. *N Engl J Med.* 1978;299:152-153.
513. Sakai Y, Koizumi K, Sugitani I, et al. Familial adenomatous polyposis associated with multiple endocrine neoplasia type 1-related tumors and thyroid carcinoma: a case report with clinicopathologic and molecular analyses. *Am J Surg Pathol.* 2002;26:103-110.
514. Perkins JT, Blackstone MO, Riddell RH. Adenomatous polyposis coli and multiple endocrine neoplasia type 2b: a pathogenetic relationship. *Cancer.* 1985;55:375-381.
515. Bertrand JH, Ritz P, Reznik Y, et al. Sipple's syndrome associated with a large prolactinoma. *Clin Endocrinol (Oxf).* 1987;27:607-614.
516. Tamsen A, Mazur MT. Ovarian strumal carcinoid in association with multiple endocrine neoplasia, type IIA. *Arch Pathol Lab Med.* 1992;116:200-203.
517. Frank-Raue K, Rondot S, Hoeppner W, et al. Coincidence of multiple endocrine neoplasia types 1 and 2: mutations in the RET protooncogene and MEN1 tumor suppressor gene in a family presenting with recurrent primary hyperparathyroidism. *J Clin Endocrinol Metab.* 2005;90:4063-4067.
518. Matyakhina L, Bei TA, McWhinney SR, et al. Genetics of Carney triad: recurrent losses at chromosome 1 but lack of germline mutations in genes associated with paragangliomas and gastrointestinal stromal tumors. *J Clin Endocrinol Metab.* 2007;92:2938-2943.
519. Binkovitz LA, Johnson CD, Stephens DH. Islet cell tumors in von Hippel-Lindau disease: increased prevalence and relationship to the multiple endocrine neoplasias. *AJR Am J Roentgenol.* 1990;155:501-505.
520. Hough DM, Stephens DH, Johnson CD, et al. Pancreatic lesions in von Hippel-Lindau disease: prevalence, clinical significance, and CT findings. *AJR Am J Roentgenol.* 1994;162:1091-1094.
521. Filling-Katz MR, Choyke PL, Oldfield E, et al. Central nervous system involvement in von Hippel-Lindau disease. *Neurology.* 1991;41:41-46.
522. Neumann HP, Dinkel E, Brambs H, et al. Pancreatic lesions in the von Hippel-Lindau syndrome. *Gastroenterology.* 1991;101:465-471.
523. LaForgia S, Lasota J, Latif F, et al. Detailed genetic and physical map of the 3p chromosome region surrounding the familial renal cell carcinoma chromosome translocation, t(3;8)(p14.2;q24.1). *Cancer Res.* 1993;53:3118-3124.
524. Latif F, Tory K, Gnarra J, et al. Identification of the von Hippel-Lindau disease tumor suppressor gene. *Science.* 1993;260:1317-1320.
525. Maxwell PH, Wiesener MS, Chang GW, et al. The tumour suppressor protein VHL targets hypoxia-inducible factors for oxygen-dependent proteolysis. *Nature.* 1999;399:271-275.
526. Chen F, Kishida T, Yao M, et al. Germline mutations in the von Hippel-Lindau disease tumor suppressor gene: correlations with phenotype. *Hum Mutat.* 1995;5:66-75.
527. Carney JA, Go VL, Gordon H, et al. Familial pheochromocytoma and islet cell tumor of the pancreas. *Am J Med.* 1980;68:515-521.
528. Hull MT, Warfel KA, Muller J, et al. Familial islet cell tumors in von Hippel-Lindau's disease. *Cancer.* 1979;44:1523-1526.
529. Janson KL, Roberts JA, Varela M. Multiple endocrine adenomatosis: in support of the common origin theories. *J Urol.* 1978;119:161-165.
530. Mori Y, Kiyohara H, Miki T, et al. Pheochromocytoma with prominent calcification and associated pancreatic islet cell tumor. *J Urol.* 1977;118:843-844.
531. Nathan DM, Daniels GH, Ridgway EC. Gastrinoma and phaeochromocytoma: is there a mixed multiple endocrine adneoma syndrome? *Acta Endocrinol.* 1980;93:91-93.
532. Zeller JR, Kauffman HM, Komorowski RA, et al. Bilateral pheochromocytoma and islet cell adenoma of the pancreas. *Arch Surg.* 1982;117:827-830.
533. Cantor AM, Rigby CC, Beck PR, et al. Neurofibromatosis, phaeochromocytoma, and somatostatinoma. *Br Med J (Clin Res Ed).* 1982;285:1618-1619.
534. Chakrabarti S, Murugesan A, Arida EJ. The association of neurofibromatosis and hyperparathyroidism. *Am J Surg.* 1979;137:417-420.
535. Chen CH, Lin JT, Lee WY, et al. Somatostatin-containing carcinoid tumor of the duodenum in neurofibromatosis: report of a case. *J Formos Med Assoc.* 1993;92:900-903.
536. Saurenmann P, Binswanger R, Maurer R, et al. [Somatostatin-producing endocrine pancreatic tumor in Recklinghausen's neurofibromatosis: case report and literature review]. *Schweiz Med Wochenschr.* 1987;117:1134-1139.
537. Hansen OP, Hansen M, Hansen HH, et al. Multiple endocrine adenomatosis of mixed type. *Acta Med Scand.* 1976;200:327-331.
538. Habiby R, Silverman B, Listernick R, et al. Precocious puberty in children with neurofibromatosis type 1. *J Pediatr.* 1995;126:364-367.
539. Nur EKMS, Varga M, Maruta H. The GTPase-activating NF1 fragment of 91 amino acids reverses v-Ha-Ras-induced malignant phenotype. *J Biol Chem.* 1993;268:22331-22337.
540. Gutmann DH, Cole JL, Stone WJ, et al. Loss of neurofibromin in adrenal gland tumors from patients with neurofibromatosis type I. *Genes Chromosomes Cancer.* 1994;10:55-58.
541. Gutmann DH, Cole JL, Collins FS. Expression of the neurofibromatosis type 1 (NF1) gene during mouse embryonic development. *Prog Brain Res.* 1995;105:327-335.
542. Carney JA. The Carney complex (myxomas, spotty pigmentation, endocrine overactivity, and schwannomas). *Dermatol Clin.* 1995;13:19-26.
543. Carney JA, Gordon H, Carpenter PC, et al. The complex of myxomas, spotty pigmentation, and endocrine overactivity. *Medicine (Baltimore).* 1985;64:270-283.
544. Stratakis CA, Kirschner LS, Carney JA. Clinical and molecular features of the Carney complex: diagnostic criteria and recommendations for patient evaluation. *J Clin Endocrinol Metab.* 2001;86:4041-4046.
545. Stratakis CA. Genetics of Peutz-Jeghers syndrome, Carney complex and other familial lentiginoses. *Horm Res.* 2000;54:334-343.
546. Kirschner LS, Carney JA, Pack SD, et al. Mutations of the gene encoding the protein kinase A type I-alpha regulatory subunit in patients with the Carney complex. *Nat Genet.* 2000;26:89-92.
547. Horvath A, Boikos S, Giatzakis C, et al. A genome-wide scan identifies mutations in the gene encoding phosphodiesterase 11A4 (PDE11A) in individuals with adrenocortical hyperplasia. *Nat Genet.* 2006;38:794-800.

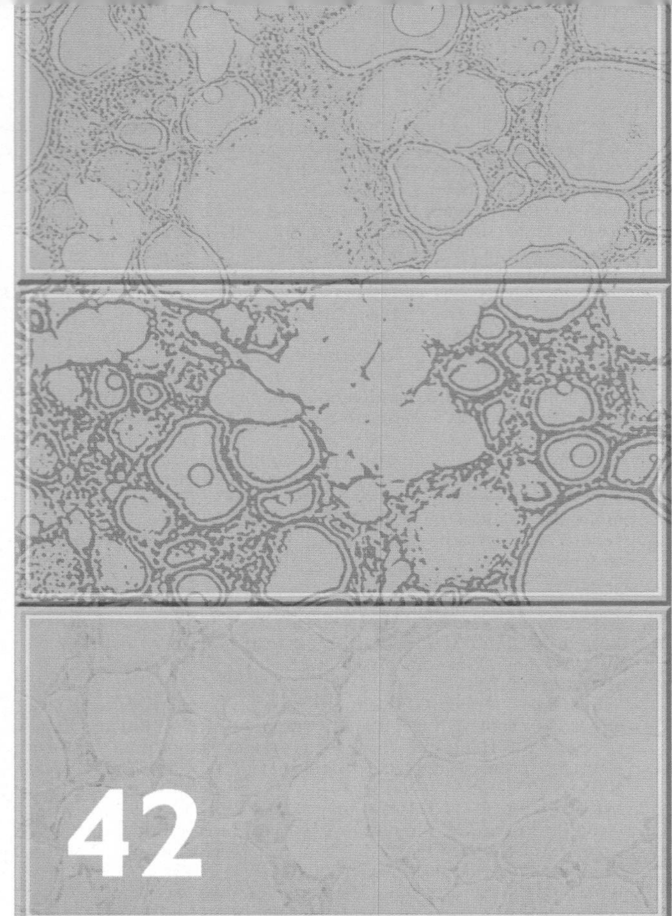

CHAPTER 42

The Immunoendocrinopathy Syndromes

JENNIFER M. BARKER • PETER A. GOTTLIEB • GEORGE S. EISENBARTH

Since Addison's initial description of primary adrenal insufficiency in which a patient with two autoimmune disorders (vitiligo and the hyperpigmentation of Addison's disease) was depicted, the immunoendocrinopathy syndromes have contributed to the understanding of both endocrinology and immunology (Fig. 42-1). Understanding of the pathogenesis of the polyendocrine syndromes continues to expand. In particular, shared genetic loci underlying disease susceptibility, potential environmental factors, and organ-specific autoantigens targeted by the immune system are being defined. Recent advances include the development of more reliable T-cell assays, further refinement in predictive models of disease, and continued unraveling of the genetic factors underlying disease susceptibility.

Most autoimmune endocrine disorders (e.g., type 1 diabetes, autoimmune thyroid disease) occur in isolation. Two distinct autoimmune polyendocrine syndromes with characteristic groupings of manifestations are readily recognized. *Autoimmune polyendocrine syndrome type I* (APS-I) is a rare disorder with autosomal recessive inheritance that is caused by defects in the autoimmune regulator gene. In contrast, *autoimmune polyendocrine syndrome type II* (APS-II) is more common but less well defined and includes overlapping groups of disorders. A unifying characteristic within APS-II is the strong association with polymorphic genes of the human leukocyte antigen (HLA) region located on the short arm of chromosome 6 (band 6p21.3). In addition to HLA, many other genetic loci are likely to contribute to susceptibility to APS-II. For purposes of simplicity in this chapter, *APS-II* encompasses what some clinicians divide into APS-II (Addison's disease plus type 1 diabetes or thyroid autoimmunity), APS-III (thyroid autoimmunity plus other autoimmune diseases, not Addison's or type 1 diabetes), and APS-IV (two or more other organ-specific autoimmune disorders).

APS-II has also been known by various other names, including Schmidt's syndrome, polyglandular autoimmune disease, polyglandular failure syndrome, organ-specific autoimmune disease, and polyendocrinopathy diabetes. Such diverse names reflect the large number of studies and case reports of this syndrome and its historical importance. Studies of patients with APS-II were instrumental in identifying the autoimmune bases of several diseases and developing autoantibody assays such as those

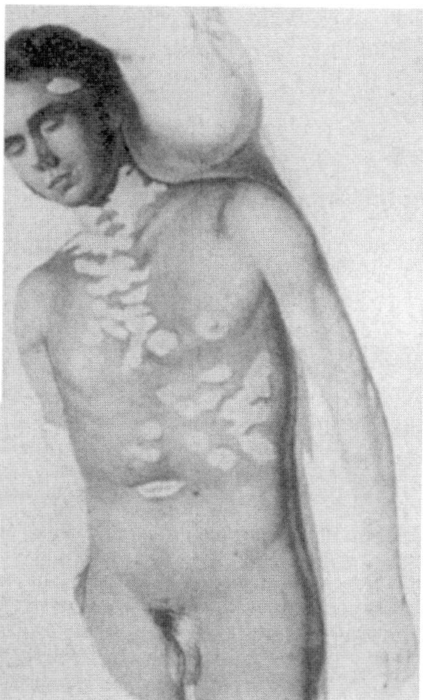

Figure 42-1 Reproduction of an illustration from Addison's initial description of primary adrenal insufficiency (Addison's disease). (From Addison T. *On the Constitutional and Local Effects of Disease of the Supra-renal Capsules.* London, UK: Samuel Highley, 1855.)

for type 1 diabetes and cytoplasmic islet cell antibodies. Each of these other names has some shortcomings, such as failure to include the fact that both hyperfunction and hypofunction of endocrine glands can occur or failure to recognize that nonendocrine disorders such as pernicious anemia and celiac disease are parts of the syndrome.

Other rare autoimmune endocrine disorders have contributed to understanding of the development of autoimmunity. For example, the rare disorder immunodysregulation polyendocrinopathy enteropathy X-linked syndrome (IPEX) is caused by a mutation of the forkhead box P3 (*FOXP3*) gene. *FOXP3* plays a central role in the development of regulatory $CD4^+/CD25^+$ T cells that function to maintain tolerance to self. It has become increasingly recognized that these and other regulatory T cells play a key role in the pathogenesis of many autoimmune diseases, and therapies targeting these regulator cells will likely be developed and tested. A thorough understanding of these rare and often genetically simple disorders provides insight into the development of syndromes that are characterized by polygenic inheritance and that affect a larger group of patients.

AUTOIMMUNITY PRIMER

An understanding of the pathophysiology of autoimmune disease requires a basic knowledge of the immunologic mechanisms that underlie tolerance (the ability to differentiate self from non-self). Autoimmunity develops when the mechanisms of immune tolerance break down. This can occur centrally at the level of the thymus or peripherally in the target organs. T lymphocytes and autoantibodies produced by B cells are two arms of the immune system that differ fundamentally in their recognition of target antigens. Autoantibodies react with intact molecules (including both soluble and cell surface molecules) and usually interact with conformational determinants of the autoantigen. In contrast, T lymphocytes recognize peptide fragments of autoantigens, often 8 to 12 amino acids in length, that are presented on the surface of another cell by molecules of the major histocompatibility complex (MHC).

Histocompatibility molecules interact with T-cell receptors when bound with an antigenic peptide. These molecules resemble a hot dog in a bun, with the antigenic peptide (the hot dog) bound in the groove of the histocompatibility molecule (the bun). Histocompatibility molecules are extremely polymorphic, with different amino acids lining the peptide-binding groove. These variable amino acids determine which peptides are bound and presented to T lymphocytes.

T cells differ based on multiple cell surface molecules, and these molecules determine their function in the immune system. T cells interact with other cells within and outside the immune system. $CD4^+$ T cells typically react with peptides that are derived from the extracellular fluid and are bound by class II histocompatibility molecules (HLA-DP, HLA-DQ, or HLA-DR in humans), which are typically expressed on antigen-presenting cells (APCs) such as macrophages, dendritic cells, and B lymphocytes. $CD8^+$ T cells react with peptides bound by class I histocompatibility molecules (HLA-A, HLA-B, and HLA-C). Class I molecules are present on the surface of almost all nucleated cells. The antigen peptide in this case is derived from and presented by the target cell itself. Recognition of the antigenic peptide by $CD8^+$ T cells typically leads to the release of cytotoxic chemicals that kill the cell.

The T-cell response depends on the context in which the antigen is presented. The simple expression of histocompatibility molecules and recognition of antigen by a T cell are not sufficient for T-cell activation. This context is at least partially determined by the interaction of cell surface molecules on both the T cell and the APC. Interaction among the MHC, the peptide, and the T-cell receptor (*signal one*) is critical to the activation process; other molecules then help to define the nature of the immune response (*signal two*). The context in which the antigens are presented is critical for the determination of this response. Cell surface molecules and receptors, cytokines, and chemokines form the context in which the antigen is presented. Based on this context, the cell can become activated, tolerized, or anergic (immune unresponsive). For example, the cell surface molecule B7 engages the CD80 receptor on the T cell and amplifies signal one, which leads to T-cell activation. When a T cell recognizes an antigen in the context of the MHC and does not receive the appropriate second signal, anergy results.

Tolerance induction is a staged process that begins in the thymus during T-cell maturation. This process depends in part on the presence of *peripheral antigens* in the thymus. Peripheral antigens are antigens (e.g., insulin) normally expressed in tissues outside the immune system that are expressed at low levels in the thymus. T cells that react strongly to these peripheral molecules in the context of the MHC are deleted in the thymus. T cells that react with peripheral antigens that are not expressed in the thymus have a greater opportunity to escape tolerance. Study of *AIRE* gene knockout mice has supported the importance of these phenomena in the development of autoimmunity. These mice have low levels of expression of peripheral antigens in the thymus and develop lymphocytic infiltrates in multiple organs.[1,2]

Peripheral tolerance is an important mechanism for tolerance induction after T cells have matured in the thymus.

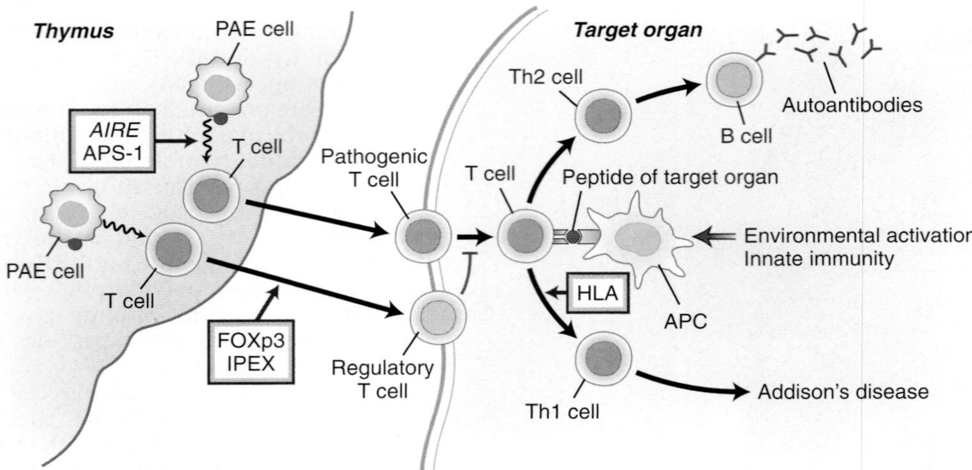

Figure 42-2 Model of the pathogenesis of autoimmunity in polyendocrine disorders. The development of autoimmune disease is determined by a group of T cells that recognize one or more organ-specific epitomes. Peptides are presented in the human leukocyte antigen (HLA) molecule and are recognized by the T-cell receptor. Recognition of self molecules depends on the maturation of the T cell, a process that begins in the thymus and continues in the periphery. The transcription factor FOXp3 stimulates the development of $CD4^+/CD25^+$ regulatory T cells. B cells produce autoantibodies under the stimulation of T cells. AIRE, autoimmune regulator; APS-I, autoimmune polyendocrine syndrome I; IPEX, immune dysregulation, polyendocrinopathy, enteropathy, X-linked; PAE, peripheral antigen-expressing cell; Th1, type 1 helper T cell; Th2, type 2 helper T cell. (Reproduced from Eisenbarth GS, Gottlieb PA. Autoimmune polyendocrine syndromes. *N Engl J Med.* 2004;350:2068-2079.)

Anergic and regulatory T cells are integral in the development of tolerance for naïve T cells. A major population of T-regulatory cells carry the cell surface markers CD4 and CD25 and express FOXP3. The function of the population of $CD4^+/CD25^+$ cells continues to be elucidated. Maturation of these cells in the thymus depends on the transcription factor FOXP3. Deletion of this transcription factor leads to fulminant autoimmunity in neonates (e.g., neonatal type 1 diabetes and enteropathy), often resulting in death within the first year of life (the IPEX syndrome).

Linked recognition is the process by which B cells are activated by $CD4^+$ T cells that are responding to the same antigen. $CD4^+$ T cells activate B cells to produce the humoral immune response. This occurs after the $CD4^+$ T cell engages an antigen in the context of the MHC on the cell surface of a B cell. The cytokines (interleukin 4 [IL-4], IL-5, and IL-6) produced by the $CD4^+$ T cells induce the maturation of a B cell. Depending on the cytokine milieu, the B cell will switch from producing immunoglobulin M (IgM) to IgG, IgE, or IgA. The development of B-cell tolerance is partially dependent on this linked recognition: autoreactive B-cell clones that do not have a $CD4^+$ T cell that can bind with the antigen in its MHC groove will not normally be activated.

NATURAL HISTORY OF AUTOIMMUNE DISORDERS

The natural history of autoimmune disorders can be divided into a series of stages beginning with genetic susceptibility, followed by triggering of autoimmunity (e.g., dietary gliadin exposure in celiac disease), active autoimmunity preceding clinical manifestations (e.g., progressive glandular destruction), and, finally, overt disease. This is a theoretical construct that may be useful for understanding factors involved with the development of autoimmunity and disease, but of necessity it is simplified and does not reflect the potential relapsing-remitting nature of autoimmunity (Fig. 42-2).

Genetic Associations

Although there is familial aggregation of APS-II and its component disorders, there is no simple pattern of inheritance (Table 42-1). Susceptibility is probably determined by multiple genetic loci (with HLA having the strongest effect) interacting with environmental factors. Autoimmune diseases share common genetic risk factors, including HLA, the MHC class I–related gene A (*MICA*), the gene for lymphoid tyrosine phosphatase (*PTPN22),* the cytotoxic T lymphocyte–associated antigen 4 (CTLA4), and the gene for NACHT leucine-rich repeat protein 1 (NALP1). In addition, genetic susceptibility for some autoimmune diseases has been linked to polymorphisms that are organ specific; for example, polymorphisms in the variable nucleotide tandem repeat (VNTR) upstream from the insulin gene have been associated with risk for type 1 diabetes.[3]

Genes located on the MHC found on chromosome 6 have been implicated in the pathogenesis of organ-specific autoimmune diseases. These genes are in strong linkage disequilibrium with each other and encode proteins that are important in the function of the immune system. Foremost in importance for the genetics of organ-specific autoimmune diseases are class I and class II HLA genes. Molecular HLA genotyping has revealed many subtypes of the older, serologically defined alleles, and the unique genetic sequence encoding each polymorphic chain of the histocompatibility molecules is now given a unique identifying number. A case in point is the DQ molecule, which is the histocompatibility molecule most strongly associated with endocrine autoimmunity. A number is assigned for each unique α- and β-chain sequence. Examples are DQA1*0501 for the α chain and DQB1*0201 for the β chain of the DQ molecule (also termed DQ2) commonly encoded on DR3 (DRB1*0301) haplotypes. A haplotype consists of a series of alleles of different genes on a contiguous region

TABLE 42-1

Genetic Associations with Autoimmune Disease

Gene	Proposed Mechanism of Action	Polymorphism/Mutation	Disease	Inheritance
HLA	Antigen presentation	DR3-DQ2/DR4-DQ8	Type 1 diabetes	Multigenic
		DR3-DQ2	Celiac disease	
		DR3-DQ2/DRB1*0404-DQ8	Addison's disease	
		DR3-DQ2/DR4-DQ8	Graves' disease	
		DR3 DR5	Hypothyroidism	
MICA	Priming of naïve T cells	5, 5.1	Type 1 diabetes	Multigenic
		4, 5.1	Celiac disease	
		5.1	Addison's disease	
PTPN22	T-cell receptor signaling pathway through interaction with regulatory kinases	Tryptophan substitution for arginine at position 620	Type 1 diabetes	Multigenic
			SLE	
			RA	
			Graves' disease	
			Hypothyroidism	
			Vitiligo	
CTLA4	Receptor on activated CD4$^+$ and CD8$^+$ T cells; decreases T-cell activation	CT60	Type 1 diabetes	Multigenic
		CT60; +49A/G	Graves' disease	
		CT60; +49A/G	Hypothyroidism	
		++49A/G	Celiac disease	
		++49A/G	Addison's disease	
AIRE	"Peripheral" antigen presentation in the thymus	Multiple reported mutations	APS-1	Autosomal recessive
FOXP3	Transcription factor important for maturation of CD4$^+$/CD25$^+$ regulatory T cells	Multiple reported mutations	IPEX	X-linked

APS, autoimmune polyendocrine syndrome; IPEX, immunodysregulation polyendocrinopathy enteropathy X-linked syndrome; RA, rheumatoid arthritis; SLE, systemic lupus erythematosus.

of a chromosome (e.g., DQA1 and DQB1 alleles) that are inherited together. A genotype is the combination of the haplotypes of both chromosomes. Fine mapping of the HLA has shown remarkable conservation of the HLA-A1/B8/DR3 haplotype such that a region of approximately 2.9 megabases is invariable. Conservation of large areas suggests that these areas of the genome have been inherited without recombination and are in very tight linkage disequilibrium. This greatly complicates the ability to identify which, if any, of the genes within the area of conservation are associated with disease and must be accounted for when assessing susceptibility to disease in this region.

Part of the overlapping risk for autoimmune disease is related to shared genetic susceptibility, especially within the HLA. For example, the highest-risk HLA genotype for type 1 diabetes is DR3-DQ2, DR4-DQ8 (DQ8 = DQA1*0301-DQB1*0302). The importance of this HLA genotype in the development of type 1 diabetes is highlighted by the observation that children who inherited the same DR3-DQ2, DR4-DQ8 as a sibling with type 1 diabetes are at risk for development of autoimmunity of greater than 75% by age 12 years, and of diabetes of greater than 50% by 12 years.[4] A specific DR4 subtype of this gene, DRB1*0404, shows a strong association with Addison's disease.[5,6] The DR3-DQ2 haplotype is associated with celiac disease both in the presence[7] and in the absence[8] of type 1 diabetes. This haplotype has been associated with autoimmune thyroid disease,[9] although conflicting reports exist.[10]

Whereas some HLA alleles increase disease risk, others are associated with protection from disease. For example, the DQ alleles DQA1*0102-DQB1*0602 (usually associated with DR2) confer strong protection from type 1A diabetes in a dominant fashion[11] but also confer susceptibility to another autoimmune disorder, multiple sclerosis. Furthermore, this protection is not general to endocrine autoimmunity, because no protection from Addison's disease is afforded by DQB1*0602. DP is another gene within the MHC, and its 0402 polymorphism has been shown to be associated with a decreased risk for type 1 diabetes in subjects with the highest-risk HLA genotype for type 1 diabetes (DR3/DR4).[12] Observations such as these suggest that, as more is learned about the genetic influence of disease, researchers will be able to combine different genotypes and refine prediction of autoimmune disease.

MICA produces a gene that is expressed in the thymus and in naïve CD8$^+$ T cells. Polymorphisms of *MICA* have been associated with type 1 diabetes,[13] celiac disease,[14] and Addison's disease.[15] A particular polymorphism of *MICA*, denoted 5.1, results from the insertion of a single base pair. This insertion produces a premature stop codon and a truncated protein. This particular polymorphism has been shown to influence the risk for Addison's disease in subjects with autoimmunity associated with Addison's disease.

Genes outside the MHC have also been implicated in the pathogenesis of autoimmune disease. For example, the *PTPN22* gene encodes lymphoid tyrosine phosphatase (LYP) protein. LYP, through interactions with regulatory kinases such as CSK, appears to act as an inhibitor of the signal cascade downstream from the T-cell receptor. A specific polymorphism associated with a tryptophan substitution for arginine at position 620 (R620W) blocks LYP's interaction with CSK.[16] This polymorphism has been associated with type 1 diabetes,[16] rheumatoid arthritis,[17] systemic lupus erythematosus (SLE),[18] Graves' disease,[19] and vitiligo[20] and is weakly associated with Addison's disease.[19] This polymorphism has also been associated with SLE, rheumatoid arthritis, type 1 diabetes, and autoimmune hypothyroidism in families with several members affected by more than one autoimmune disease.[21]

CTLA4 is expressed on activated CD4⁺ and CD8⁺ T cells, where it is hypothesized to act as a negative regulator.[22] Several polymorphisms within the CTLA4 gene have been associated with autoimmune diseases. One polymorphism associated with AT repeats has been shown to reduce the inhibitory function of CTLA4 in subjects with Graves' disease.[23] A single nucleotide polymorphism in the 3′ untranslated region, denoted CT60, has been associated with Graves' disease[24] and autoimmune hypothyroidism.[25] An additional polymorphism, denoted ⁺49A/G, has been associated with celiac disease in the Dutch population,[26] with autoimmune thyroid disease,[27] and with Addison's disease.[28]

NALP1 regulates the innate immune system. After the initial observation that this gene was associated with the risk of vitiligo[29] and other related autoimmune diseases, it was associated with Addison's disease and type 1 diabetes.[30]

Organ-specific genetic polymorphisms have been associated with the development of specific autoimmune diseases. For example, polymorphisms of the variable number of tandem repeats (VNTR) upstream of the insulin gene have been associated with the development of type 1 diabetes. Higher numbers of tandem repeats are associated with increased production of insulin in the thymus and protection from type 1 diabetes.[3] Similarly, polymorphisms of the thyroglobulin gene are associated with autoimmune thyroid disease.[31]

Single-gene defects such as *AIRE* and *FOXP3* cause multiorgan autoimmunity and are discussed in sections devoted to those topics. Analysis of mutations of the *AIRE* gene indicates that it does not play a role in APS-II or sporadic Addison's disease, with 1 (1.1%) of 90 patients with Addison's disease (non–APS-I) and 1 (0.2%) of 576 control subjects having *AIRE* mutations.[28]

Environmental Triggers

Although genetics is known to play an important role in the development of autoimmunity, it does not tell the whole story. For example, the highest-risk HLA genotype for type 1 diabetes (DR3-DQ2, DR4-DQ8) is associated with a risk of 1 in 20 for the development of diabetes.[32] Although this is greater than the general population prevalence rate of 1 in 200 by the age of 20 years, it is certainly not a 100% risk. Therefore, other factors (genetic and environmental) must be involved in the initiation of autoimmunity. Some theorize that these factors may be environmental triggers.

For one disease, celiac disease, the underlying environmental trigger has been identified: gluten. Through studies such as the Diabetes Autoimmunity Study in the Young (DAISY), BabyDiab, and Celiac Disease Autoimmunity Research (CEDAR), the timing of first exposure to cereal has been identified as a risk factor for the development of diabetes and celiac disease autoimmunity. Infants exposed at a very young age to cereal developed diabetes and celiac-associated autoimmunity at a greater rate than those who had cereal introduced at a later date.[33-35] In epidemiologic studies, cod liver oil consumption has been associated with a decreased risk for type 1 diabetes. Cod liver oil contains ω-3 polyunsaturated fats and vitamin D. In prospective studies, there is some suggestion that lower consumption of omega 3 polyunsaturated fats is associated with a increased risk for autoimmunity associated with type 1 diabetes.[36] Further investigation may identify additional environmental associations.

Immunologic therapies, especially in patients with an autoimmune disease, can induce autoimmunity. A remarkable example is the treatment of patients with multiple sclerosis with an anti-CD52 monoclonal antibody. One third of 27 patients given the monoclonal antibody developed antithyrotropin receptor autoantibodies and hyperthyroidism.[37] Interferon-α (IFN-α) therapy for hepatitis has been associated with thyroid autoimmunity[38] and type 1 diabetes.[39] Severe hypoglycemia associated with insulin autoantibodies in the absence of insulin administration, termed *Hirata's disease,* is associated with methimazole treatment of Graves' disease. The development of Hirata's disease in these patients is associated with HLA-Bw62/Cw4/DR4 with a specific DRB1 allele (DRB1*0406).[40]

Development of Organ-Specific Autoimmunity

Autoantibodies highly specific for a given disorder are present before disease onset. Each specific autoantibody reacts with only a single autoantigen, although autoantigens may be present in multiple tissues. The targets of autoantibodies appear to be unrelated except that for organ-specific autoimmunity they are usually expressed in specific cells and cellular sites. Anti-islet antibodies include antibodies to glutamic acid decarboxylase (GAD), islet cell antibody (ICA) 512 (also termed *insulinoma antigen-2* [IA-2]), and insulin. Recently, an additional autoantigen, ZnT8, has been identified in association with type 1 diabetes. Antibodies against ZnT8 have been found at onset of diabetes, before the development of diabetes, and not in control sera.[41] Celiac disease is associated with antibodies against tissue transglutaminase. Addison's disease is associated with antibodies against 21-hydroxylase.

Given that the antibodies can be identified before the development of organ dysfunction, they can be used to screen subjects who are at high risk for development of autoimmune disease to identify risk for additional autoimmune diseases. This approach has been employed in studies such as TrialNet for Type 1 Diabetes to screen first-degree relatives of patients with type 1 diabetes for diabetes-related autoantibodies. In this and other cohorts, risk for development of diabetes increases with the number of autoantibodies and their persistence.

Organ-specific autoantibodies (with appropriate assays) are rarely present (approximately 1 in 100) in the general population and identify a subset of people who are at greater risk for clinical disease. These autoantibodies may be expressed for years before the disease develops, and additional autoantibodies can develop over time. The pace at which disease develops is highly variable. For example, children as young as 1 year of age can present with type 1 diabetes. In contrast, a subset of subjects (5% to 10%) with type 2 diabetes diagnosed in adulthood have autoimmunity as the underlying cause. This may be in part due to genetics, because subjects who develop autoimmune diabetes at an older age have a higher proportion of the protective diabetes allele DQB1*0602, although even in adults DQB1*0602 provides dramatic protection.[42]

In contrast, less is known concerning the specificity of pathogenic T cells. Given the observation that cross-reactive recognition by pathogenic T-cell clones may be determined by as few as four properly spaced amino acids of a nonapeptide and the estimate that each T-cell receptor might react with a million different peptides, there is considerable potential for patterns of autoimmunity to be determined by cross-reactive T cells. An important development has been the discovery in the thymus and other lymphoid tissues of peripheral antigen-expressing cells that express autoantigens such as insulin. Minute quantities of such molecules in the thymus can contribute to tolerance. Insulin messenger RNA (mRNA) in the thymus is regulated by genetic polymorphisms of the insulin gene associated with diabetes risk.[3] There is also evidence that stromal and lymphoid cells (CD11c$^+$) in the spleen, lymph nodes, and circulation express multiple similar antigens.[43]

Failure of Gland

Organ dysfunction develops over time and can include a period of intermediate function that may be characterized by increased levels of the stimulatory hormones (e.g., thyroid-stimulating hormone, corticotropin [ACTH]) with normal levels of the hormones (T_3, T_4, and cortisol). Once a significant portion of the gland has been destroyed, overt disease is then present.

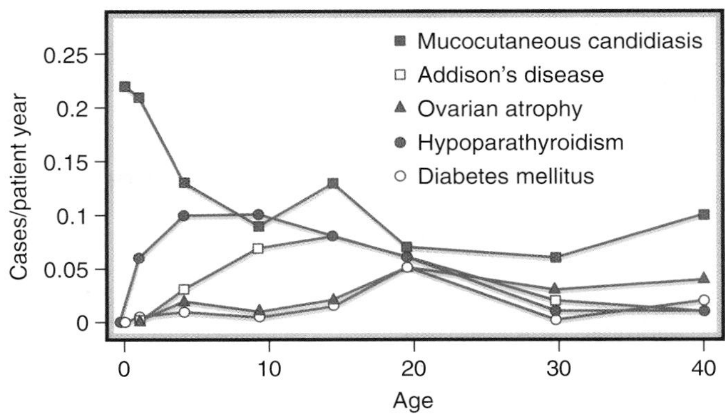

Figure 42-3 Incidence of disease development by age in patients with autoimmune polyendocrine syndrome type I (APS-I). (Reproduced from Perheentupa J. APS-I/APECED: the clinical disease and therapy. *Endocrinol Metab Clin North Am.* 2002;31:295-320.)

AUTOIMMUNE POLYENDOCRINE SYNDROME TYPE I

Clinical Features

Table 42-2 compares the features of APS-I with those of APS-II. Table 42-3 shows the clinical features and recommended follow-up for patients with APS-I.

APS-I (Mendelian Inheritance in Man [MIM] 240300), also known as *autoimmune polyendocrinopathy-candidiasis-ectodermal dystrophy* (APECED), is characterized by the classic triad of mucocutaneous candidiasis, autoimmune hypoparathyroidism, and Addison's disease, which form three of the most common components of the disorder. Patients with APS-I are at risk for development of autoimmune diseases affecting almost every organ. More than 140 patients have been reported, including subjects in two large series from Finland[44-46] and the United States.[47]

In a series of 89 Finnish patients described by Perheentupa, all had chronic candidiasis at some time, 86% had hypoparathyroidism, and 79% had Addison's disease. Gonadal failure (72% in women, 26% in men) and hypoplasia of the dental enamel (77% of patients) were also frequent findings. Other manifestations that occurred less often included alopecia (40%), vitiligo (26%), intestinal malabsorption (18%), type 1 diabetes (23%), pernicious anemia (31%), chronic active hepatitis (17%), and hypothyroidism (18%).[44] The incidence rates for many of these disorders peak in the first or second decade of life, and the disease continues to develop over decades (Fig. 42-3). Therefore, reported prevalence rates of component disorders are highly dependent on the age at which follow-up ended.

APS-I is characteristically recognized in early childhood. Infants can present with chronic or recurrent mucocutaneous candidiasis in the first year of life, followed by hypoparathyroidism and Addison's disease, but new components can develop at any age. Decades can elapse between the diagnosis of one disorder and the onset of another in the same patient. Consequently, lifelong follow-up is important to allow early detection of additional components.

Recurrent candidiasis commonly affects the mouth and nails and, less frequently, the skin and esophagus.[44] Chronic oral candidiasis can result in atrophic disease with areas suggestive of leukoplakia. If this develops, the patient is at significant risk for carcinoma of the oral mucosa (with its high mortality rate).

Ectodermal dystrophy is another component of the syndrome (manifested by pitted nails, keratopathy, and enamel hypoplasia) and cannot be attributed to hypoparathyroidism. Enamel hypoplasia can precede the onset of hypoparathyroidism and, despite adequate replacement therapy, can also affect teeth forming after the onset of hypoparathyroidism.[48]

Friedman and colleagues[49] reported the frequent occurrence of asplenism and cholelithiasis as additional features of APS-I. Splenic atrophy may also cause immune deficiency. Although the etiology of this part of the disorder is unknown, it is relatively common: up to 15% of patients are asplenic.[44] The presence of Howell-Jolly bodies on peripheral blood smear is suggestive of asplenia. If asplenia is identified, immunization with polyvalent pneumococcal vaccine should be administered, and follow-up antibody titers should be obtained. If an adequate response is not produced, daily prophylactic antibiotics may be necessary.

Malabsorption with steatorrhea is of uncertain origin, is usually intermittent, and may be exacerbated by

TABLE 42-2

Contrasting Features of Autoimmune Polyendocrine Syndrome

Feature	APS-I	APS-II
Inheritance pattern	Autosomal recessive (only siblings affected)	Polygenic (multiple generations affected)
Associated gene	*AIRE* gene mutation	*HLA-DR3* and *DR-4* associated
Gender association	Equal gender incidence	Female preponderance
Age at onset	Onset in infancy	Peak onset 20 to 60 years
Clinical features	Mucocutaneous candidiasis	Type 1 diabetes
	Hypoparathyroidism	Autoimmune thyroid disease
	Addison's disease	Addison's disease
"Diagnostic" antibodies	Anti-Interferon	

APS, autoimmune polyendocrine syndrome.

TABLE 42-3

Clinical Features and Recommended Follow-Up for APS-I and APS-II

Component Disease	Frequency at Age 40 Yr (%)	Recommended Evaluation
Autoimmune Polyendocrine Syndrome Type I		
Addison's disease	79	Sodium, potassium, ACTH, cortisol, plasma renin activity, 21-hydroxylase autoantibodies
Diarrhea	18	History
Ectodermal dysplasia	50-75	Physical examination
Hypoparathyroidism	86	Serum calcium, phosphate, PTH
Hepatitis	17	Liver function test
Hypothyroidism	18	TSH; thyroid peroxidase and/or thyroglobulin autoantibodies
Male hypogonadism	26	FSH/LH
Mucocutaneous candidiasis	100	Physical examination
Obstipation	21	History
Ovarian failure	72	FSH/LH
Pernicious anemia	31	CBC, vitamin B_{12} levels
Splenic atrophy	15	Blood smear for Howell-Jolly bodies; platelet count; ultrasound if positive
Type 1 diabetes	23	Glucose, hemoglobin A_{1c}, diabetes-associated autoantibodies (insulin, GAD65, IA-2)
Autoimmune Polyendocrine Syndrome Type II*		
Addison's disease	0.5	21-Hydroxylase autoantibodies ACTH stimulation testing if positive
Alopecia		Physical examination
Autoimmune hypothyroidism	15-30	TSH; thyroid peroxidase and/or thyroglobulin autoantibodies
Celiac disease	5-10	Transglutaminase autoantibodies; small-intestine biopsy if positive
Cerebellar ataxia	Rare†	Dictated by signs and symptoms of disease
Chronic inflammatory demyelinating polyneuropathy	Rare†	Dictated by signs and symptoms of disease
Hypophysitis	Rare†	Dictated by signs and symptoms of disease
Idiopathic heart block	Rare†	Dictated by signs and symptoms of disease
IgA deficiency	0.5	IgA level
Myasthenia gravis	Rare†	Dictated by signs and symptoms of disease
Myocarditis	Rare†	Dictated by signs and symptoms of disease
Pernicious anemia	0.5-5	Anti–parietal cell autoantibodies CBC, vitamin B_{12} levels if positive
Serositis	Rare†	Dictated by signs and symptoms of disease
Stiff-man syndrome	Rare†	Dictated by signs and symptoms of disease
Vitiligo	1-9	Physical examination

*In the population with type 1 diabetes.
†Rare reported disorders in subjects with APS-II.
ACTH, adrenocorticotropic hormone; APS, autoimmune polyendocrine syndrome; CBC, complete blood count; FSH, follicle-stimulating hormone; GAD, glutamic acid decarboxylase; IA-2, insulinoma antigen 2; IgA, immunoglobulin A; LH, luteinizing hormone; PTH, parathyroid hormone; TSH, thyroid-stimulating hormone.

hypocalcemia. Bereket and associates[50] reported a case in which patchy intestinal lymphangiectasia was discovered by endoscopically directed biopsy. Pancreatic insufficiency has been treated with cyclosporine.[51] Autoantibodies (e.g., tryptophan hydroxylase, histidine decarboxylase) reacting with intestinal endocrine cells (enterochromaffin, cholecystokinin, and enterochromaffin-like) occur and are associated with loss of endocrine cells on biopsy and with gastrointestinal dysfunction.[52,53]

Genetics

Mutations of the autoimmune regulator gene, AIRE, located on the short arm of chromosome 21 (near markers D21s49 and D21s171 on 21p22.3), are associated with APS-I.[54] The gene encodes a putative DNA-binding protein of unknown function expressed in the thymus and in lymphoid and other tissues. It has been localized to the nucleus, and mutations have been demonstrated to be associated with decreased transcription of reporter products.[55,56] *AIRE* knockout mice have decreased production of peripheral antigens within the thymus.[1,2] Researchers hypothesize that AIRE acts as a transcriptional factor in cells of the thymus and that it promotes the expression of peripheral antigens in these APCs. Mutations in *AIRE* are hypothesized to decrease central tolerance.

Multiple mutations of *AIRE* have been identified in subjects with APS-I. The frequency of specific mutations varies in different populations. For example, in Sardinia, a deletion of amino acid 257 is present in 90% of mutated alleles. A 136-base-pair deletion in exon 8 is present in 71% of British alleles and in 56% of alleles in the United States. Analysis of haplotypes indicates that this deletion has arisen on many occasions.

Most cases of APS-I are associated with autosomal recessive inheritance patterns. A rare kindred of patients from Italy have a mutation of the AIRE protein G228W that, when present in the heterozygous state, is associated with autoimmunity, thus fitting an autosomal dominant inheritance pattern.[57] In a mouse model of this mutation, the expression of peripheral antigens in the thymus was decreased, compared with the control, suggesting a mechanism for this observed inheritance pattern.[58]

Diagnosis

The diagnosis of APS-I is highly likely when two or more of the primary component disorders (i.e., mucocutaneous candidiasis, hypoparathyroidism, and Addison's disease) are present. Siblings of an affected patient should be considered affected even if only one of these disorders is present. Analysis of *AIRE* for the common mutations may be helpful in identifying subjects with APS-I. However, because multiple mutations have been discovered, the absence of a common mutation does not exclude APS-I. Any patient with any of the component disorders deserves careful follow-up to watch for development of additional disease.

Autoantibodies against interferon-α and interferon omega have been identified in almost 100% of subjects with APS-I, regardless of age at screening.[59] The autoantibody has been found in subjects with many different mutations of the *AIRE* gene; it is not present in other autoimmune diseases, and it has been proposed to use this autoantibody to screen subjects with multiple autoimmune diseases for APS-I.

Therapy and Follow-Up

The treatment of adrenal insufficiency and hypoparathyroidism is the same as that discussed in other chapters with the caveat that malabsorption can complicate treatment. The therapy for mucocutaneous candidiasis has been improved with the use of orally active antifungal drugs such as fluconazole and ketoconazole. Infection often recurs when the drug is discontinued or the dosage is decreased. Patients must be monitored carefully, because ketoconazole can inhibit adrenal and gonadal steroid synthesis and can precipitate adrenal failure. It is also associated with transient elevation of liver enzyme levels and, occasionally, with hepatitis. Fluconazole is associated with a lower frequency of hepatitis and does not inhibit steroidogenesis when given in the recommended doses.

Autoantibodies associated with multiple autoimmune diseases have been reported. Antiparathyroid and antiadrenal antibodies have been reported. Whereas 21-hydroxylase appears to be the major autoantigen in isolated Addison's disease and in Addison's disease associated with APS-II, autoantibodies against 17α-hydroxylase and cytochrome P450 side-chain cleavage enzyme (CYP11A1) have also been reported in Addison's disease associated with APS-I.[60] Antibodies to tryptophan hydroxylase in intestinal disease, tyrosine hydroxylase in alopecia areata, L-amino acid decarboxylase in hepatitis and vitiligo, and phenylalanine hydroxylase[61,62] and antibodies reacting with hair follicles have been reported.[63] Tuomi and coworkers originally observed that many more APS-I patients (41%) express anti-GAD65 autoantibodies than become diabetic, suggesting that reactivity to this single autoantigen has low predictive value in this populaton.[64] Recently, antibodies against NALP5 were identified in 49% of patients with APS-I and hypoparathyroidism, compared with none of those with APS-I but no hypoparathyroidism.[65] Screening for autoantibodies associated with additional autoimmune diseases may be useful in patients with APS-I.

Screening to allow the early detection of new disorders before overt symptoms and signs develop is recommended, including autoantibody studies, electrolytes, calcium and phosphorus levels, thyroid and liver function tests, blood smear, and plasma vitamin B_{12}. Patients at risk for adrenal failure can be screened by measurement of basal ACTH and supine plasma renin activity (PRA), followed by dynamic testing as appropriate. Evaluation for asplenism[49] with abdominal ultrasonography and blood smear examination for Howell-Jolly bodies is warranted, with pneumococcal vaccination and appropriate antibiotic coverage for affected patients.

There are case reports of severely affected patients who have benefited from immunosuppressive therapy. For example, Ward and colleagues[51] treated a 13-year-old patient who had keratoconjunctivitis, hepatitis, and severe pancreatic insufficiency. Treatment with cyclosporine was associated with normalization of stool fat (from 31.5 to 2.5 g/day).

AUTOIMMUNE POLYENDOCRINE SYNDROME TYPE II

Clinical Features

APS-II (MIM 269200) is more common than APS-I. It occurs more often in female than in male patients, often has its onset in adulthood, and exhibits familial aggregation (see Table 42-2). APS-II is usually defined by the occurrence in the same patient of two or more of the following: primary adrenal insufficiency (Addison's disease), Graves' disease, autoimmune thyroiditis, type 1A diabetes mellitus, primary hypogonadism, myasthenia gravis, and celiac disease. Vitiligo, alopecia, serositis, and pernicious anemia also occur with increased frequency in patients with this syndrome and their family members (see Table 42-3).

When one of the component disorders is present, an associated disorder occurs more commonly than in the general population. Furthermore, circulating organ-specific autoantibodies are often present even in the absence of overt clinical disease. For example, in subjects with type 1 diabetes, there is a 15% to 20% risk of hypothyroidism, a 5% to 10% risk of celiac-related autoimmunity, and a 1.5% risk of adrenal autoimmunity. The risk of autoimmunity is greater in relatives of patients with APS-II. In our assessment of APS-II families with Addison's disease, up to 15% of relatives were found to have 21-hydroxylase autoantibodies (Addison's disease–associated autoantibodies), anti-islet autoantibodies, or transglutaminase (tTG) autoantibodies (celiac disease–associated autoantibodies). The initial lesion and precipitating events that result in the syndrome are unknown, but immunogenetic and immunologic similarities are present with regard to both the time course and the pathogenesis of each of the component disorders.

Because of the chronic development of organ-specific autoimmunity, patients with the syndrome and their families should have repeated endocrinologic evaluations over time. In a family in which the syndrome has been documented, relatives should be advised of the early symptoms and signs of the principal component diseases (a list is available at www.barbaradaviscenter.org [accessed January 2011]). Relatives of patients with multiple disorders should have a medical history, physical examination, and screening every 3 to 5 years, with measurement of anti-islet autoantibodies, a sensitive thyrotropin assay, and measurement of serum vitamin B_{12} levels. If there are any symptoms or signs or if 21-hydroxylase autoantibodies are present, the patient should have annual assays of basal corticotropin and corticotropin-stimulated cortisol levels with Cortrosyn stimulation testing.

Among 224 patients with Addison's disease and APS-II reported by Neufeld and colleagues,[47] type 1 diabetes and autoimmune thyroid disease were the most common coexisting conditions (52% and 69% of patients, respectively). Other components were less common, including vitiligo (5%) and gonadal failure (4%).

Among patients with type 1A diabetes, thyroid autoimmunity and celiac disease coexist with sufficient frequency to justify screening. Thyroid peroxidase autoantibodies are present in 10% to 20% of children with type 1 diabetes; this incidence is higher in female patients and increases in all patients with age and with diabetes duration. A significant fraction of patients with type 1 diabetes and thyroid peroxidase autoantibodies develop thyroid disease. One study showed that after follow-up for more than 15 years, 80% of patients with thyroid peroxidase autoantibodies and type 1 diabetes became hypothyroid.[66] However, several studies have shown that a subset of patients with negative autoantibodies develop thyroid disease. Therefore, patients with type 1 diabetes should be screened annually for thyrotropin levels, which is a cost-effective approach.

With the identification of transglutaminase as the major endomysial autoantigen of celiac disease, radioimmunoassays were developed and demonstrated that 10% to 12% of patients with type 1 diabetes have tTG autoantibodies.[7] The prevalence of tTG autoantibodies was higher in diabetic patients with HLA-DQ2; one third of DQ2-homozygous subjects were found to express anti-tTG antibody. Seventy percent of those with high-titer antibody who underwent biopsy were subsequently found to have the disease.[67] Therefore, screening with anti-tTG antibody can be carried out; if the results are positive and are confirmed on repeat assay, small-bowel biopsy to document celiac disease is warranted, with institution of a gluten-free diet if the disease is present. Many patients have asymptomatic celiac disease that is nevertheless associated with osteopenia and impaired growth. If left untreated, symptomatic celiac disease is also associated with an increased risk of gastrointestinal malignancy, especially lymphoma.

Down syndrome, or trisomy 21 (MIM 190685), is associated with the development of type 1 diabetes mellitus, thyroiditis, and celiac disease. Patients with Turner syndrome are at increased risk for the development of thyroid disease and celiac disease. It is recommended to screen patients with trisomy 21 and Turner syndrome for associated autoimmune diseases on a regular basis.

Diagnosis

Improved assays for several organ-specific autoantibodies have been developed since the cloning of specific autoantigens and the development of assays that use recombinant antigens. These radioimmunoassays are superior to assays based on immunofluorescence with tissue sections, such as ICA testing. The most notable finding is the identification of a large number of different autoantigens that are targeted even in single autoimmune disorders. Most of the endocrine autoantigens are hormones (e.g., insulin) or enzymes associated with differentiated endocrine function: thyroid peroxidase in thyroiditis; GAD, carboxypeptidase H, and ICA 512/IA-2 in type 1 diabetes; 17α-hydroxylase and 21-hydroxylase in Addison's disease; and the parietal cell enzyme H^+,K^+-adenosine triphosphatase in pernicious anemia.

In type 1 diabetes, the four most informative assays currently available determine autoantibodies that react with insulin, GAD65, ICA512/IA-2, and ZnT8.[41] In a similar manner, a radioassay format for the detection of autoantibodies that react with the enzyme 21-hydroxylase in Addison's disease has been developed and provides excellent disease specificity and sensitivity. Adrenal autoantibodies reacting with recombinant 21-hydroxylase usually precede the development of Addison's disease. However, as with thyroid autoantibodies, there may be patients who present with antibodies but have normal production of cortisol in response to ACTH. Continued endocrine testing every year initially and then every other year is indicated in this situation.

In contrast to the autoimmune polyendocrine disorders with T cell–mediated glandular destruction, autoantibodies may also be pathogenic. A hallmark of pathogenic autoantibodies is the existence of a neonatal form of the disorder, secondary to transplacental passage of the autoantibody. Examples include neonatal Graves' disease (anti–thyrotropin-receptor autoantibodies) and neonatal myasthenia gravis (anti–acetyl choline-receptor autoantibodies).

Therapy

Treatment of the individual diseases of the polyendocrine autoimmune syndrome is discussed in other chapters. Therapeutic considerations related specifically to APS-II are discussed here.

Many of the component disorders of the syndrome have a long prodromal phase and are associated with the expression of autoantibodies before the manifestation of overt disease. The way the disorders develop allows consideration of disease prediction and of clinical trials for prevention. This is particularly important for type 1A diabetes but is also likely to apply to Addison's disease and hypogonadism.

Because of the autoimmune nature of these disorders, several studies have evaluated the use of immunosuppressive drugs. Drugs such as cyclosporine have preserved some residual insulin secretion. However, because cyclosporine is nephrotoxic and potentially oncogenic, more generalized use is precluded. Newer immunosuppressive agents (e.g., sirolimus) are being studied, and biologics such as anti-CD20 antibody (rituximab) or nonmitogenic CD3 antibodies have been shown to prolong C-peptide production and to result in a decreased insulin dose through the first year of diabetes, compared with control subjects.[68]

Mucosal administration of antigens is commonly associated with bystander immunosuppression, in which T cells specific to the antigen are apparently induced to produce suppressive Th2-like or Th3-like cytokines (e.g., IL-4, IL-10, and transforming growth factor-β). In addition, subcutaneous administration of insulin prevents diabetes and insulitis in animal models, and subcutaneous administration of insulin peptides in adjuvants can prevent diabetes but not insulitis. A large National Institutes of Health (NIH) trial, the Diabetes Prevention Trial—Type 1 (DPT-1), directly tested oral and parenteral insulin for prevention of diabetes. DPT-1 had two arms: intravenous-subcutaneous for those at high risk (risk of diabetes >50% within 5 years) and oral insulin for those at moderate risk (risk of diabetes 25% to 50% within 5 years). Neither parenteral[69] nor oral[70] insulin slowed progression to diabetes. However, in a subgroup analysis of subjects in the DPT-1 oral trial, a treatment effect was noted for those who had the higher insulin autoantibody levels at diagnosis,[70] and further trials are under way. In preclinical Addison's disease, a short course of glucocorticoids appeared to suppress the expression of adrenal autoantibodies and prevent progressive adrenal destruction.[71]

Thyroxine therapy can precipitate a life-threatening Addisonian crisis in a patient with untreated adrenal insufficiency and hypothyroidism. Therefore, it is necessary to evaluate adrenal function in all hypothyroid patients in whom the syndrome is suspected before instituting such therapy. A decreasing insulin requirement in a patient with insulin-dependent diabetes mellitus can be one of the earliest indications of adrenal insufficiency, occurring before the development of hyperpigmentation or electrolyte abnormalities.

OTHER POLYENDOCRINE DEFICIENCY AUTOIMMUNE SYNDROMES

Rare polyendocrine syndromes are listed in Table 42-4.

Anti–Insulin Receptor Autoantibodies

In this rarely reported disorder (<25 patients), also known as type B insulin resistance or acanthosis nigricans, insulin resistance is caused by the presence of anti–insulin receptor antibodies.[72] Approximately one third of patients with these antibodies have an associated autoimmune illness such as SLE or Sjögren's syndrome. Arthralgia, vitiligo, alopecia, and secondary amenorrhea have also been reported. One patient had a daughter with hyperthyroidism and a granddaughter with SLE. Autoimmune thyroid disease has been described in two such patients, one with hypothyroidism and the other with antithyroid antibodies. Antinuclear antibodies, an elevated erythrocyte sedimentation rate, hyperglobulinemia, leukopenia, and hypocomplementemia are common.[73]

The major clinical manifestations are related to the anti–insulin receptor antibodies. Insulin resistance is profound, and up to 175,000 U of insulin given intravenously per day may be ineffective in lowering the elevated glucose. Despite hyperglycemia and marked insulin resistance, ketoacidosis is uncommon. The course of the diabetes is variable, and several patients have had spontaneous remissions. Other patients have had severe hypoglycemia (perhaps related to the insulin-like effects of anti–insulin receptor antibodies demonstrable in vitro).[73] The acanthosis nigricans, which is caused by hypertrophy and folding of otherwise histologically normal skin, appears to be related to the insulin-resistant state. Other forms of marked insulin resistance in the absence of antireceptor antibodies are also associated with acanthosis nigricans.

TABLE 42-4

Rare Polyendocrine Disorders

Disorder	Clinical Features	Cause
Hirata's disease (insulin resistance syndrome)	Hypoglycemia	Insulin autoantibodies Associated with methimazole
IPEX	Type I diabetes Enteropathy	Mutations of *FOXP3*
Kearns-Sayre syndrome	Hypoparathyroidism Primary gonadal failure Nonautoimmune diabetes Hypopituitarism	Deletions of mitochondrial DNA
POEMS	Polyneuropathy Organomegaly Diabetes Primary gonadal failure	Plasma cell dyscrasia with production of M protein and cytokines
Thymic tumors	Myasthenia gravis Red blood cell hypoglobulinemia Autoimmune thyroid disease Adrenal insufficiency	Thymomas
Type B insulin resistance	Severe insulin resistance	Insulin receptor autoantibodies
Wolfram's syndrome	Diabetes insipidus Nonautoimmune diabetes Bilateral optic atrophy Sensorineural deafness	Mutations of *WSF1*, which encodes wolframin

IPEX, immunodysregulation polyendocrinopathy enteropathy X-linked syndrome; POEMS, plasma cell dyscrasia with polyneuropathy, organomegaly, endocrinopathy, *M* protein, and skin changes.

POEMS Syndrome

The components of the multisystem disorder POEMS (*p*lasma cell dyscrasia with polyneuropathy, *o*rganomegaly, *e*ndocrinopathy, *M* protein, and *s*kin changes, also known as Crow-Fukase syndrome; MIM 192240) consist of diabetes mellitus (20% to 50% of patients), primary gonadal failure (55% to 70% of patients), plasma cell dyscrasia, sclerotic bone lesions, and neuropathy.[74] Patients usually present with severe progressive sensorimotor polyneuropathy, hepatosplenomegaly, lymphadenopathy, and hyperpigmentation. On evaluation, they are found to have plasma cell dyscrasia and sclerotic bone lesions. Patients present in the fifth to sixth decade of life and have a median survival after diagnosis of less than 3 years.[74]

POEMS is assumed to be secondary to circulating immunoglobulins, but binding of antibody directly to involved tissues has not been demonstrated. There is evidence implicating cytokines such as IL-1A, IL-6, and TNF-α in addition to the M protein in the pathogenesis of this disorder. In several studies, elevated levels of vascular endothelial growth factor (VEGF) correlated with the disease state and treatment with immunosuppressive agents reduced the symptoms of the disease and the levels of VEGF, suggesting that this growth factor plays a role in the disease.[75,76] A case report of the use of ticlopidine, which has been shown to decrease VEGF in experimental rats, showed decrease of VEGF with resolution of ascites, edema, and pleural effusions and no change in the remainder of the clinical disease.[77] A therapeutic trial of an anti-VEGF antibody would provide more definitive evidence for this hypothesis.

The diabetes mellitus responds to small, subcutaneous doses of insulin. The hypogonadism is associated with elevated plasma levels of follicle-stimulating hormone and luteinizing hormone. Temporary resolution of disease, including a return of the blood glucose level to normal, may occur after radiotherapy for localized plasma cell lesions of bone. Peripheral blood stem cell transplantation has been performed and shows promise, producing stabilization or improvement of the components of POEMS. However, transplantation is not without risks, including death and respiratory failure.[78,79]

Kearns-Sayre Syndrome

The rare Kearns-Sayre syndrome (MIM 530000), also known as oculocraniosomatic disease or oculocraniosomatic neuromuscular disease with ragged red fibers, is characterized by myopathic abnormalities leading to ophthalmoplegia and progressive weakness in association with several endocrine abnormalities, including hypoparathyroidism, primary gonadal failure, diabetes mellitus, and hypopituitarism.[80] Crystalline mitochondrial inclusions are found in muscle biopsy specimens, and such inclusions have also been observed in the cerebellum. The relation between the mitochondrial disorders and endocrinologic abnormalities is not known. Antiparathyroid antibodies have not been described; however, antibodies to the anterior pituitary gland and striated muscle have been found, and the disease may have autoimmune components. Other abnormalities include retinitis pigmentosa and heart block. Deletions in mitochondrial DNA have been associated with Kearns-Sayre syndrome.[81] These mutations usually occur sporadically and are not associated with a familial syndrome.

Thymic Tumors

The thymus is a complex tissue with a specialized endocrine epithelium that synthesizes a variety of biologically active peptides involved in the control of T-cell maturation. This epithelium is derived from the neural crest and contains complex gangliosides that react with monoclonal antibody (A2B5) and tetanus toxin in a manner similar to that of pancreatic islets.

The illnesses associated with thymomas are similar to those seen in APS-II,[82] although the incidence of specific disorders is different. In one review of patients with thymoma, myasthenia gravis was found to occur in 44% of the patients, red blood cell aplasia in approximately 20%, hypoglobulinemia in 6%, autoimmune thyroid disease in 2%, and adrenal insufficiency in 1 of 423 patients (0.24%). The incidence of autoimmune thyroid disease reported in patients with thymoma is probably an underestimate, given the incidence of unsuspected thyroid disease in patients with myasthenia gravis. Mucocutaneous candidiasis in adults is also associated with thymomas. In most patients, the thymomas are malignant, although temporary remissions of the autoimmune disease can occur with resection of the tumor.

Congenital Rubella

Patients with congenital rubella have an almost 20% risk of acquiring diabetes mellitus and a higher than normal risk of acquiring thyroiditis and hypothyroidism.[83,84] Those at highest risk for diabetes express diabetes-associated HLA-DR3 and HLA-DR4 alleles.[85] Rubella appears to be associated with diabetes primarily after fetal infection, and it is not known whether the virus increases the probability of subsequent autoimmunity due to permanent effects on the developing immune system.[86] Because of the intensive effort to immunize against the rubella virus, recent reports from the Centers for Disease Control and Prevention (CDC) indicate that rubella is no longer endemic in the United States.[87]

Wolfram's Syndrome

Wolfram's syndrome (MIM 222300, chromosome 4; MIM 598500, mitochondrial) is a rare autosomal recessive disease that is also called DIDMOAD (*d*iabetes *i*nsipidus, *d*iabetes *m*ellitus, progressive bilateral *o*ptic *a*trophy, and sensorineural *d*eafness). In addition, neurologic and psychiatric disturbances are prominent in most patients and can cause severe disability. Atrophic changes in the brain have been found on magnetic resonance imaging.[88] Segregation analysis of the mutations found in familial and sporadic cases of Wolfram's syndrome led to the identification of wolframin, a 100-kd transmembrane protein encoded by *WFS1*, a gene located at 4p16.1.116. Genotype and phenotype analyses have identified the severe phenotype (defined as the development of neurologic disease within the first decade) in patients with truncated proteins and mutations in the C-terminus of the proteinus.[89]

Wolframin has been localized to the endoplasmic reticulum[90] and is found in neuronal and neuroendocrine tissue.[91] Its expression induces ion channel activity with a resultant increase in intracellular calcium and may play an important role in intracellular calcium homeostasis.[92] Functional studies have shown that reported *WFS1* mutations lead to decreased stability of the protein wolframin.[93] Linkage to other loci in addition to *WFS1* may explain the variability in phenotype seen in this disorder.

Wolfram's syndrome appears to be a slowly progressive neurodegenerative process, and there is also (nonautoimmune) selective destruction of the pancreatic beta cells. This association is probably a result of the expression pattern of *WFS1*. Diabetes mellitus with an onset in childhood is usually the first manifestation. Diabetes mellitus and optic atrophy are present in all reported cases, but expression of the other features is variable. Duration of diabetes is linked to the development of microvascular complications.[93] Additional endocrinologic diseases, such as ACTH deficiency and growth hormone deficiency, have been reported.[93] In one case report, two related children with Wolfram's syndrome had megaloblastic and sideroblastic anemia that responded to treatment with thiamine. Furthermore, thiamine treatment was associated with a marked decrease in insulin requirements.[94]

Immunodysregulation Polyendocrinopathy Enteropathy X-Linked Syndrome

IPEX (MIM 340790, MIM 300292), first described in 1982, is a rare, X-linked recessive disorder that is characterized by immune dysregulation and results in multiple autoimmune diseases and early death (Fig. 42-4). Its clinical features include early type 1 diabetes and severe enteropathy resulting in failure to thrive. Other reported abnormalities include eczema or atopy, thrombocytopenia, hemolytic anemia, hypothyroidism, and lymphadenopathy.[95]

Characteristics of the scurfy mouse gene *(sf)* bear a number of similarities to this syndrome, and abnormalities in the *sf* gene lead to abnormalities in the amount and function of scurfin, a DNA-binding protein in these mice.[96] Implantation of thymus from a scurfy mouse into immunoincompetent mice transfers the disease, but transplantation of thymus into immunocompetent mice does not transfer disease, and injections of normal T cells can rescue the phenotype. These observations suggest that a regulatory cell is involved in the pathogenesis of this disorder.

Linkage analysis demonstrated that a 17-centimorgan (cM) stretch of the X chromosome (Xp11.1-q13.3) is associated with IPEX, and mutations within the *FOXP3* gene have been identified in most of the families studied thus far.[97] *FOXP3* encodes a protein called scurfin and belongs to the forkhead class of winged helix transcription factors. It is hypothesized to function as a transcription factor. *FOXP3* has been shown to be expressed in $CD4^+/CD25^+$

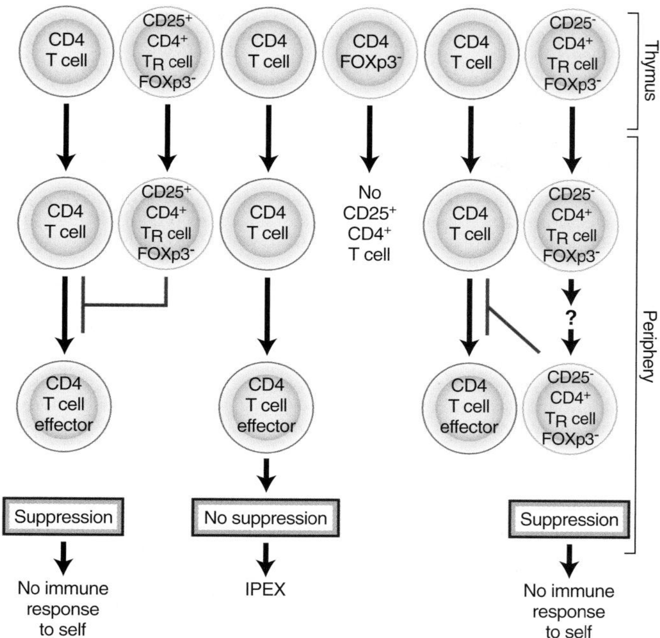

Figure 42-4 The development of CD4+/CD25+ regulatory T cells in the thymus is dependent on FOXp3 expression. The lack of FOXp3 in immune dysregulation, polyendocrinopathy, enteropathy, X-linked syndrome (IPEX) prevents the development of these regulatory T cells and promotes the development of autoimmunity. (Reproduced from Sakaguchi S. The origin of FOXp3-expression regulatory T-cells: thymus or periphery. *J Clin Invest.* 2003;112:1310-1312.)

regulatory T cells.[98] These T cells can suppress activation of other T cells (see Fig. 42-4).[98] Therefore, mutations in *FOXP3* result in inability to generate regulatory T cells and the development of IPEX.

Therapy has been targeted to the component disorders. Bone marrow transplantation has been attempted with mixed success, and there is evidence for disease regression in most subjects.[99] Use of immunosuppressive therapy with sirolimus was reported to have beneficial effects in three patients with IPEX.[100]

Omenn's Syndrome

Omenn's syndrome (MIM 603554) is a primary immunodeficiency syndrome with autoimmune manifestations affecting mainly the skin and gastrointestinal tract. Mutations associated with decreased recombination of the T-cell receptor have been described. One study showed that the levels of *AIRE* gene expression were decreased in the thymus of two affected patients and that this was associated with decreased expression of peripheral antigens compared with controls.[101]

CONCLUSION

Through the study of rare disorders such as APS-I and IPEX, the processes of thymic expression of peripheral antigens and development of regulatory T cells are beginning to be defined. This understanding provides invaluable insight into the development of the normal immune system and the mistakes that can occur and lead to autoimmunity. Lessons learned from these rare diseases will help to better define the pathophysiology of more common autoimmune endocrine disorders, hopefully leading to the development of immunologic methods for prevention and treatment of these disorders.

REFERENCES

1. Ramsey C, Winqvist O, Puhakka L, et al. AIRE deficient mice develop multiple features of APECED phenotype and show altered immune response. *Hum Mol Genet.* 2002;11:397-409.
2. Anderson MS, Venanzi ES, Klein L, et al. Projection of an immunological self shadow within the thymus by the AIRE protein. *Science.* 2002;298:1395-1401.
3. Pugliese A, Zeller M, Fernandez A, et al. The insulin gene is transcribed in the human thymus and transcription levels correlate with allelic variation at the INS VNTR-IDDM2 susceptibility locus for type I diabetes. *Nat Genet.* 1997;15:293-297.
4. Aly TA, Ide A, Jahromi MM, et al. Extreme genetic risk for type 1A diabetes. *Proc Natl Acad Sci U S A.* 2006;103:14074-14079.
5. Yu L, Brewer KW, Gates S, et al. DRB1*04 and DQ alleles: expression of 21-hydroxylase autoantibodies and risk of progression to Addison's disease. *J Clin Endocrinol Metab.* 1999;84:328-335.
6. Myhre AG, Undlien DE, Lovas K, et al. Autoimmune adrenocortical failure in Norway: autoantibodies and HLA class II associations related to clinical features. *J Clin Endocrinol Metab.* 2002;87:618-623.
7. Bao F, Yu L, Babu S, et al. One third of HLA DQ2 homozygous patients with type 1 diabetes express celiac disease associated transglutaminase autoantibodies. *J Autoimmunity.* 1999;13:143-148.
8. Hoffenberg EJ, McKenzie TL, Barriga KJ, et al. A prospective study of the incidence of childhood celiac disease. *J Paediatr.* 2003;143:308-314.
9. Levin L, Ban Y, Concepcion E, et al. Analysis of HLA genes in families with autoimmune diabetes and thyroiditis. *Hum Immunol.* 2004;65:640-647.
10. Ban Y, Davies TF, Greenberg DA, et al. The influence of human leucocyte antigen (HLA) genes on autoimmune thyroid disease (AITD): results of studies in HLA-DR3 positive AITD families. *Clin Endocrinol (Oxf).* 2002;57:81-88.
11. Baisch JM, Weeks T, Giles R, et al. Analysis of HLA-DQ genotypes and susceptibility in insulin-dependent diabetes mellitus. *N Engl J Med.* 1990;322:1836-1841.
12. Baschal EE, Aly TA, Babu SR, et al. HLA-DPB1*0402 protects against type 1A diabetes autoimmunity in the highest risk DR3-DQB1*0201/DR4-DQB1*0302 DAISY population. *Diabetes.* 2007;56:2405-2409.
13. Zake LN, Ghaderi M, Park YS, et al. MHC class I chain-related gene alleles 5 and 5.1 are transmitted more frequently to type 1 diabetes offspring in HBDI families. *Ann N Y Acad Sci.* 2002;958:309-311.
14. Bilbao JR, Martin-Pagola A, Vitoria JC, et al. HLA-DRB1 and MHC class 1 chain-related A haplotypes in Basque families with celiac disease. *Tissue Antigens.* 2002;60:71-76.
15. Park YS, Sanjeevi CB, Robles D, et al. Additional association of intra-MHC genes, MICA and D6S273, with Addison's disease. *Tissue Antigens.* 2002;60:155-163.
16. Bottini N, Muscumeci L, Alonso A, et al. A functional variant of lymphoid tyrosine phosphatase is associated with type I diabetes. *Nat Genet.* 2004;36:337-338.
17. van Oene M, Wintle RF, Liu X, et al. Association of the lymphoid tyrosine phosphatase R620W variant with rheumatoid arthritis, but not Crohn's disease, in Canadian populations. *Arthritis Rheum.* 2005;52:1993-1998.
18. Orozco G, Sanchez E, Gonzalez-Gay MA, et al. Association of a functional single-nucleotide polymorphism of PTPN22, encoding lymphoid protein phosphatase, with rheumatoid arthritis and systemic lupus erythematosus. *Arthritis Rheum.* 2005;52:219-224.
19. Velaga MR, Wilson V, Jennings CE, et al. The codon 620 tryptophan allele of the lymphoid tyrosine phosphatase (LYP) gene is a major determinant of Graves' disease. *J Clin Endocrinol Metab.* 2004;89:5862-5865.
20. Canton I, Akhtar S, Gavalas NG, et al. A single-nucleotide polymorphism in the gene encoding lymphoid protein tyrosine phosphatase (PTPN22) confers susceptibility to generalised vitiligo. *Genes Immun.* 2005;6:584-587.
21. Criswell LA, Pfeiffer KA, Lum RF, et al. Analysis of families in the multiple autoimmune disease genetics consortium (MADGC) collection: the PTPN22 620W allele associates with multiple autoimmune phenotypes. *Am J Hum Genet.* 2005;76:561-571.
22. Vaidya B, Pearce S. The emerging role of the CTLA-4 gene in autoimmune endocrinopathies. *Eur J Endocrinol.* 2004;150:619-626.
23. Takara M, Kouki T, DeGroot LJ. CTLA-4 AT-repeat polymorphism reduces the inhibitory function of CTLA-4 in Graves' disease. *Thyroid.* 2003;13:1083-1089.
24. Ban Y, Concepcion ES, Villanueva R, et al. Analysis of immune regulatory genes in familial and sporadic Graves' disease. *J Clin Endocrinol Metab.* 2004;89:4562-4568.

25. Ban Y, Tozaki T, Taniyama M, et al. Association of a CTLA-4 3′ untranslated region (CT60) single nucleotide polymorphism with autoimmune thyroid disease in the Japanese population. *Autoimmunity.* 2005;38:151-153.
26. Van Belzen MJ, Mulder CJ, Zhernakova A, et al. CTLA4 +49 A/G and CT60 polymorphisms in Dutch coeliac disease patients. *Eur J Hum Genet.* 2004;12:782-785.
27. Ban Y, Davies TF, Greenberg DA, et al. Analysis of the CTLA-4, CD28, and inducible costimulator (ICOS) genes in autoimmune thyroid disease. *Genes Immun.* 2003;4:586-593.
28. Vaidya B, Imrie H, Geatch DR, et al. Association analysis of the cytotoxic T lymphocyte antigen-4 (CTLA-4) and autoimmune regulator-1 (AIRE-1) genes in sporadic autoimmune Addison's disease. *J Clin Endocrinol Metab.* 2000;85:688-691.
29. Jin Y, Mailloux CM, Gowen K, et al. NALP1 in vitiligo-associated multiple autoimmune disease. *N Engl J Med.* 2007;356:1216-1225.
30. Magitta NF, Boe Wolff AS, Johansson S, et al. A coding polymorphism in NALP1 confers risk for autoimmune Addison's disease and type 1 diabetes. *Genes and Immunity.* 2009;10:120-124.
31. Tomer Y, Greenberg DA, Concepcion E, et al. Thyroglobulin is a thyroid specific gene for the familial autoimmune thyroid diseases. *J Clin Endocrinol Metab.* 2002;87:404-407.
32. Lambert AP, Gillespie KM, Thomson G, et al. Absolute risk of childhood-onset type 1 diabetes defined by human leukocyte antigen class ii genotype: a population-based study in the United Kingdom. *J Clin Endocrinol Metab.* 2004;89:4037-4043.
33. Norris JM, Barriga K, Hoffenberg EJ, et al. Risk of celiac disease autoimmunity and timing of gluten introduction in the diet of infants at increased risk of disease. *JAMA.* 2005;293:2343-2351.
34. Norris JM, Barriga K, Klingensmith G, et al. Timing of cereal exposure in infancy and risk of islet autoimmunity. The Diabetes Autoimmunity Study in the Young (DAISY). *JAMA.* 2003;290:1713-1720.
35. Ziegler AG, Schmid S, Huber D, et al. Early infant feeding and risk of developing type 1 diabetes-associated autoantibodies. *JAMA.* 2003;290:1721-1728.
36. Norris JM, Yin, X, Lamb MM, et al. Omega-3 polyunsaturated fatty acid intake and islet auoimmunity in children at increased risk for type 1 diabetes. *JAMA.* 2007;298:1420-1428.
37. Coles AJ, Wing M, Smith S, et al. Pulsed monoclonal antibody treatment and autoimmune thyroid disease in multiple sclerosis. *Lancet.* 1999;354:1691-1695.
38. Gisslinger H, Gilly B, Woloszczuk W, et al. Thyroid autoimmunity and hypothyroidism during long-term treatment with recombinant interferon-alpha. *Clin Exp Immunol.* 1992;90:363-367.
39. Bosi E, Minelli R, Bazzigaluppi E, et al. Fulminant autoimmune type 1 diabetes during interferon-alpha therapy: a case of Th1-mediated disease? *Diabet Med.* 2001;18:329-332.
40. Uchigata Y, Kuwata S, Tsushima T, et al. Patients with Graves' disease who developed insulin autoimmune syndrome (Hirata disease) possess HLA-Bw62/Cw4/DR4 carrying DRB1*0406. *J Clin Endocrinol Metab.* 1993;77:249-254.
41. Wenzlau JM, Moua O, Sarkar SA, et al. SlC30A8 is a major target of humoral autoimmunity in type 1 diabetes and a predictive marker in prediabetes. *Ann N Y Acad Sci.* 2008;1150:256-259.
42. Lohmann T, Sessler J, Verlohren HJ, et al. Distinct genetic and immunological features in patients with onset of IDDM before and after age 40. *Diabetes Care.* 1997;20:524-529.
43. Gardner JM, Devoss JJ, Friedman RS, et al. Deletional tolerance mediated by extrathymic Aire-expressing cells. *Science.* 2008;321:843-847.
44. Perheentupa J. APS-I/APECED: the clinical disease and therapy. *Endocrinol Metab Clinic North Am.* 2002;31:295-320.
45. Ahonen P, Myllarniemi S, Sipila I, et al. Clinical variation of autoimmune polyendocrinopathy–candidiasis–ectodermal dystrophy (APECED) in a series of 68 patients. *N Engl J Med.* 1990;322: 1829-1836.
46. Perheentupa J, Miettinen A. Autoimmune polyendocrinopathy-candidiasis-ectodermal dystrophy. In: Eisenbarth GS, ed. *Endocrine and Organ Specific Autoimmunity.* Austin, TX: RG Landes, 1999:19-40.
47. Neufeld M, Maclaren NK, Blizzard RM. Two types of autoimmune Addison's disease associated with different polyglandular autoimmune (PGA) syndromes. *Medicine (Baltimore).* 1981;60:355-362.
48. Walls AWG, Soames JV. Dental manifestations of autoimmune hypoparathyroidism. *Oral Surg Oral Med Oral Pathol.* 1993;75:452-454.
49. Friedman TC, Thomas PM, Fleisher TA, et al. Frequent occurrence of asplenism and cholelithiasis in patients with autoimmune polyglandular disease type I. *Am J Med.* 1991;91:625-630.
50. Bereket A, Lowenheim M, Blethen SL, et al. Intestinal lymphangiectasia in a patient with autoimmune polyglandular disease type I and steatorrhea. *J Clin Endocrinol Metab.* 1995;80:933-955.
51. Ward L, Paquette J, Seidman E, et al. Severe autoimmune polyendocrinopathy-candidiasis-ectodermal dystrophy in an adolescent girl with a novel AIRE mutation: response to immunosuppressive therapy. *J Clin Endocrinol Metab.* 1999;84:844-852.
52. Gianani R, Eisenbarth GS. Autoimmunity to gastrointestinal endocrine cells in autoimmune polyendocrine syndrome type I. *J Clin Endocrinol Metab.* 2003;88:1442-1444.
53. Hogenauer C, Meyer RL, Netto GJ, et al. Malabsorption due to cholecystokinin deficiency in a patient with autoimmune polyglandular syndrome type I. *N Engl J Med.* 2001;344:270-274.
54. Aaltonen J, Bjorses P, Sandkuijl L, et al. An autosomal locus causing autoimmune disease: autoimmune polyglandular disease type I assigned to chromosome 21. *Nat Genet.* 1994;8:83-87.
55. Bjorses P, Halonen M, Palvimo JJ, et al. Mutations in the AIRE gene: effects on subcellular location and transactivation function of the autoimmune polyendocrinopathy-candidiasis-ectodermal dystrophy protein. *Am J Hum Genet.* 2000;66:378-392.
56. Halonen M, Kangas H, Ruppell T, et al. APECED-causing mutations in AIRE reveal the functional domains of the protein. *Hum Mutat.* 2004;23:245-257.
57. Cetani F, Barbesino G, Borsari S, et al. A novel mutation of the auotimmune regulator gene in an Italian Kindred with auoimmune polyendocrinopathy-candidiasis-ectodermal dystrophy, acting in a dominant fashion and strongly cosegregating with hypothyroid autoimmune thyroiditis. *J Clin Endocrinol Metab.* 2001;36:4747-4752.
58. Su Ma, Gian K, Zumer K, et al. Mechanisms of an autoimmunity syndrome in mice caused by a dominant mutation in AIRE. *J Clin Invest.* 2008;118:1712-1726.
59. Meager A, Visvalingam K, Peterson P, et al. Anti-interferon autoantibodies in autoimmune polyendocrine syndrome type 1. *PloS Med.* 2006;3:e289.
60. Uibo R, Aavik E, Peterson P, et al. Autoantibodies to cytochrome P450 enzymes P450scc, P450c17, and P450c21 in autoimmune polyglandular disease types I and II and in isolated Addison's disease. *J Clin Endocrinol Metab.* 1994;78:323-328.
61. Ekwall O, Hedstrand H, Haavik J, et al. Pteridin-dependent hydroxylases as autoantigens in autoimmune polyendocrine syndrome type I. *J Clin Endocrinol Metab.* 2000;85:2944-2950.
62. Husebye ES, Boe AS, Rorsman F, et al. Inhibition of aromatic L-amino acid decarboxylase activity by human autoantibodies. *Clin Exp Immunol.* 2000;120:420-423.
63. Hedstrand H, Perheentupa J, Ekwall O, et al. Antibodies against hair follicles are associated with alopecia totalis in autoimmune polyendocrine syndrome type I. *J Invest Dermatol.* 1999;113:1054-1058.
64. Tuomi T, Björses P, Falorni A, et al. Antibodies to glutamic acid decarboxylase and insulin-dependent diabetes in patients with autoimmune polyendocrine syndrome type I. *J Clin Endocrinol Metab.* 1996;81:1488-1494.
65. Alimohammadi M, Bjorklund P, Hallgren A, et al. Autoimmune polyendocrine syndrome type 1 and NALP5, a parathyroid autoantigen *N Engl J Med.* 2008;358:1018-1028.
66. Umpierrez GE, Latif KA, Murphy MB, et al. Thyroid dysfunction in patients with type 1 diabetes: a longitudinal study. *Diabetes Care.* 2003;26:1181-1185.
67. Hoffenberg EJ, Bao F, Eisenbarth GS, et al. Transglutaminase antibodies in children with a genetic risk for celiac disease. *J Pediatr.* 2000;137:356-360.
68. Herold KC, Gitelman SE, Masharani U, et al. A single course of anti-CD3 monoclonal antibody hOKT3γ1(Ala-Ala) results in improvement in C-peptide responses and clinical parameters for at least 2 years after onset of type 1 diabetes. *Diabetes.* 2005;54:1763-1769.
69. Diabetes Prevention Trial—Type 1. Effects of insulin in relatives of patients with type 1 diabetes mellitus. *N Engl J Med.* 2002;346: 1685-1691.
70. Diabetes Prevention Trial—Type 1. Effects of oral insulin in relatives of patients with type 1 diabetes: The Diabetes Prevention Trial—Type 1. *Diabetes Care.* 2005;28:1068-1076.
71. De Bellis A, Bizzarro A, Rossi R, et al. Remission of subclinical adrenocortical failure in subjects with adrenal autoantibodies. *J Clin Endocrinol Metab.* 1993;76:1002-1007.
72. Kahn CR, Flier JS, Bar RS, et al. The syndromes of insulin resistance and acanthosis nigricans: insulin-receptor disorders in man. *N Engl J Med.* 1976;294:739-745.
73. Flier JS, Bar RS, Muggeo M, et al. The evolving clinical course of patients with insulin receptor autoantibodies: spontaneous remission or receptor proliferation with hypoglycemia. *J Clin Endocrinol Metab.* 1978;47:985-995.
74. Dispenzieri A, Kyle RA, Lacy MQ, et al. POEMS syndrome: definitions and long-term outcome. *Blood.* 2003;101:2496-2506.
75. Soubrier M, Dubost JJ, Serre AF, et al. Growth factors in POEMS syndrome: evidence for a marked increase in circulating vascular endothelial growth factor. *Arthritis Rheum.* 1997;40:786-787.
76. Watanabe O, Maruyama I, Arimura K, et al. Overproduction of vascular endothelial growth factor/vascular permeability factor is causative in Crow-Fukase (POEMS) syndrome. *Muscle Nerve.* 1998;21:1390-1397.
77. Matsui H, Udaka F, Kubori T, et al. POEMS syndrome demonstrating VEGF decrease by ticlopidine. *Intern Med.* 2004;43:1082-1083.

78. Dispenzieri A, Moreno-Aspitia A, Suarez GA, et al. Peripheral blood stem cell transplantation in 16 patients with POEMS syndrome, and a review of the literature. *Blood.* 2004;104:3400-3407.
79. Hogan WJ, Lacy MQ, Wiseman GA, et al. Successful treatment of POEMS syndrome with autologous hematopoietic progenitor cell transplantation. *Bone Marrow Transplant.* 2001;28:305-309.
80. Harvey JN, Barnett D. Endocrine dysfunction in Kearns-Sayre syndrome. *Clin Endocrinol.* 1992;37:97-104.
81. De Block CE, De Leeuw IH, Maassen JA, et al. A novel 7301-bp deletion in mitochondrial DNA in a patient with Kearns-Sayre syndrome, diabetes mellitus, and primary amenorrhoea. *Exp Clin Endocrinol Diabetes.* 2004;112:80-83.
82. Combs RM. Malignant thymoma, hyperthyroidism and immune disorder. *South Med J.* 1968;61:337-341.
83. Menser MA, Forrest JM, Bransby RD. Rubella infection and diabetes mellitus. *Lancet.* 1978;1:57-60.
84. Clarke WL, Shaver KA, Bright GM, et al. Autoimmunity in congenital rubella syndrome. *J Pediatr.* 1984;104:370-373.
85. Rubenstein P. The HLA system in congenital rubella patients with and without diabetes. *Diabetes.* 1982;31:1088-1091.
86. Rabinowe SL, George KL, Loughlin R, et al. Congenital rubella: monoclonal antibody-defined T cell abnormalities in young adults. *Am J Med.* 1986;81:779-782.
87. Centers for Disease Control and Prevention. Elimination of rubella and congenital rubella syndrome—United States, 1969-2004. *MMWR Morb Mortal Wkly Rep.* 2005;54:279-282.
88. Rando TA, Horton JC, Layzer RB. Wolfram syndrome: evidence of a diffuse neurodegenerative disease by magnetic resonance imaging. *Semin Neurol.* 1992;42:1220-1224.
89. Smith CJ, Crock PA, King BR, et al. Phenotype-genotype correlations in a series of Wolfram syndrome families. *Diabetes Care.* 2004;27:2003-2009.
90. Takeda K, Inoue H, Tanizawa Y, et al. WFS1 (Wolfram syndrome 1) gene product: predominant subcellular localization to endoplasmic reticulum in cultured cells and neuronal expression in rat brain. *Hum Mol Genet.* 2001;10:477-484.
91. Hofmann S, Philbrook C, Gerbitz KD, et al. Wolfram syndrome: structural and functional analyses of mutant and wild-type wolframin, the WFS1 gene product. *Hum Mol Genet.* 2003;12:2003-2012.
92. Osman AA, Saito M, Makepeace C, et al. Wolframin expression induces novel ion channel activity in endoplasmic reticulum membranes and increases intracellular calcium. *J Biol Chem.* 2003;278:52755-52762.
93. Medlej R, Wasson J, Baz P, et al. Diabetes mellitus and optic atrophy: a study of Wolfram syndrome in the Lebanese population. *J Clin Endocrinol Metab.* 2004;89:1656-1661.
94. Borgna-Pignatti C, Marradi P, Pinelli L, et al. Thiamine-responsive anemia in DIDMOAD syndrome. *J Pediatr.* 1989;114:405-410.
95. Powell BR, Buist NR, Stenzel P. An X-linked syndrome of diarrhea, polyendocrinopathy, and fatal infection in infancy. *J Pediatr.* 1982;100:731-737.
96. Godfrey VL, Wilkinson JE, Russell LB. X-linked lymphoreticular disease in the scurfy (sf) mutant mouse. *Am J Pathol.* 1991;138:1379-1387.
97. Chatila TA, Blaeser F, Ho N, et al. JM2, encoding a fork head-related protein, is mutated in X-linked autoimmunity-allergic disregulation syndrome. *J Clin Invest.* 2000;106:R75-R81.
98. Walker MR, Kasprowicz DJ, Gersuk VH, et al. Induction of FoxP3 and acquisition of T regulatory activity by stimulated human $CD4^+$ $CD25^-$ T cells. *J Clin Invest.* 2003;112:1437-1443.
99. Baud O, Goulet O, Canioni D, et al. Treatment of the immune dysregulation, polyendocrinopathy, enteropathy, X-linked syndrome (IPEX) by allogeneic bone marrow transplantation. *N Engl J Med.* 2001;344:1758-1762.
100. Bindl L, Torgerson T, Perroni L, et al. Successful use of the new immune-suppressor sirolimus in IPEX (immune dysregulation, polyendocrinopathy, enteropathy, X-linked syndrome). *J Pediatr.* 2005;147:256-259.
101. Cavadini P, Vermi W, Facchetti F, et al. AIRE deficiency in thymus of 2 patients with Omenn syndrome. *J Clin Invest.* 2005;115:728-732.

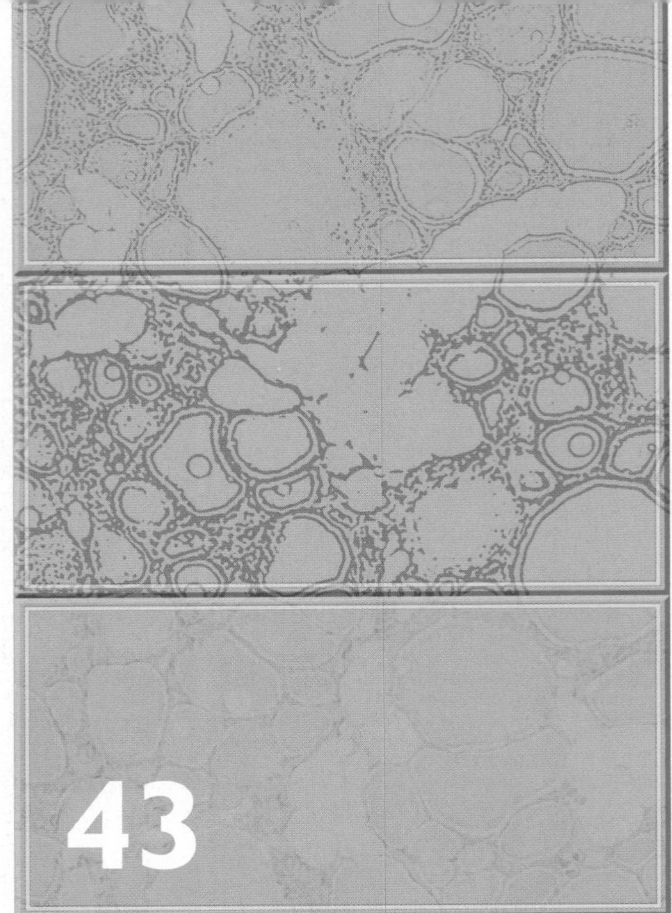

CHAPTER 43

Endocrine Management of the Cancer Survivor

ROBERT D. MURRAY

Over the last 4 decades, cure rates for childhood malignancies have improved at a remarkable pace. Overall 5-year survival rates have improved from less than 30% in 1960 to more than 70% in 1990.[1] Survival from adult cancers has lagged behind, but significant inroads have been made. For example, progress in the treatment of Hodgkin's disease, which affects predominantly a young adult population, has resulted in long-term survival rates of 70% to 90% using combination chemotherapy, radiotherapy, or both.[2,3] With increasing survivorship from both childhood and adult cancers, the long-term detrimental effects of multimodality cancer therapy on multiple organ systems have been recognized.[4] The long-term adverse sequelae are likely to gain increasing importance because of the significant demands on health service resources by these individuals. Within the United Kingdom, it is estimated that about 2 million people (3% of the population) have received a diagnosis of cancer. Of these, 1.2 million had their initial cancer diagnosis more than 5 years ago.[5] It is predicted that the number of cancer survivors will increase by 3% per year, reflecting an increase in both cancer incidence and survival rates.[5]

Concentrating on the endocrine system alone, at least one long-term endocrine sequela is prevalent in 43% of unselected long-term childhood cancer survivors.[6] Data from adult survivors have been less forthcoming because survival has, until recently, been of much shorter duration than that achieved in childhood cancers. Endocrine late effects include disturbances of growth and puberty, hypothalamo-pituitary dysfunction, primary hypogonadism, subfertility, thyroid dysfunction, benign and malignant thyroid nodules, hyperparathyroidism, and reduced bone mass.

GROWTH

Table 43-1 outlines the primary effects of multimodality cancer therapy on growth. The initial evidence for the impact of irradiation on growth velocity and final height was derived from animal studies and from growth data in children who received cranial irradiation for a variety of malignant and nonmalignant conditions. Cranial irradiation of 2-day-old rats led to a dose-dependent reduction in

TABLE 43-1

Overview of the Primary Effects of Multimodality Cancer Therapy on Growth and Hypothalamo-Pituitary Function in Cancer Survivors

Physiologic System	Insult	Pathology	Comments
Growth	Cranial XRT	Impaired GH secretion Precocious puberty	All insults culminate in reduced height velocity and final height. There are no robust data supporting a direct action of chemotherapy on growth. The ultimate impact on height depends on age at XRT, dosage, and schedule. Puberty occurs earlier, spinal growth is more attenuated, and GH deficiency is more prevalent if XRT occurs at a younger age, in fewer fractions, and at higher dosage.
	Spinal XRT	Impaired spinal growth Disproportion	
	Chemotherapy	?Potentiation of XRT effects ?Direct effect on growth plate	
GH/IGF1 axis	Cranial XRT	GH deficiency (GHD) (a) *Childhood:* reduced growth velocity (b) *Transition:* impaired somatic development (c) *Adult:* impaired quality of life, adverse body composition, and vascular risk profile	Cranial XRT doses as low as 18 Gy given during childhood result in GHD in about one third of individuals by 5 yr after treatment, whereas doses of 30-40 Gy result in GHD in 60-100% of patients by 5 yr.[4] Prevalence of GHD depends on age at irradiation, fractionation schedule, and dose.
Hypothalamo-pituitary axis	Cranial XRT	LH/FSH deficiency ACTH deficiency TSH deficiency Hyperprolactinemia	Additional anterior pituitary hormone deficits are usually seen with XRT doses >30 Gy and are dependent on dose, fractionation schedule, and time since XRT.[4] Progression of hormone loss usually follows the pattern GH → LH/FSH → ACTH → TSH. Other than GHD, additional deficits are unusual within the first 2 yr after XRT except with exposure to very high doses. Transient hyperprolactinemia is frequently seen after XRT and resolves with a few years.
Hypothalamo-pituitary axis	Cranial XRT	Early/precocious puberty	Early puberty is a consequence of disinhibition of cortical influences on the GnRH pulse generator. The earlier the age at XRT (25-50 Gy), the earlier puberty occurs.[8] Early puberty effectively foreshortens the time available for growth-promoting interventions when growth is impaired.

ACTH, adrenocorticotropic hormone; FSH, follicle-stimulating hormone; GH, growth hormone; GHD, growth hormone deficiency; GnRH, gonadotropin-releasing hormone; IGF1, insulin-like growth factor 1; LH, luteinizing hormone; TSH, thyroid-stimulating hormone; XRT, radiation therapy.

growth[7] with reduction in the size of the pituitary gland. The mechanism of growth disturbance was, however, unclear, because levels of insulin-like growth factor 1 (IGF1) remained similar to those in control rats, and no increase in growth was observed after treatment with bovine growth hormone (GH). The severity of growth retardation was greatest in rats receiving cranial irradiation during the first few days of life, with a degree of tolerance developing by the end of the first postnatal week.[8]

Early observations in humans noted somatic growth to be retarded in children after irradiation for brain tumors[9,10] or acute leukemia.[11,12] The Childhood Cancer Survivors Study is a multicenter questionnaire-based study of individuals within the United States who have survived at least 5 years after childhood cancer. A subanalysis of survivors of brain tumors within this cohort reveals that 40% of patients had a final height below the 10th percentile.[13] In these individuals who have undergone multimodality cancer therapy for childhood malignancy, the exact contribution of the endocrine perturbations to the growth failure is difficult to disentangle from the additional effects of chemotherapy, corticosteroid therapy, spinal irradiation, graft-versus-host disease, poor nutritional status, and the acute illness itself.[14,15] Endocrine disturbances, including radiation-induced hypothyroidism, precocious puberty, and GH insufficiency, adversely affect growth. The importance of cranial or craniospinal irradiation on growth is clear from studies of survivors of childhood acute leukemia and brain tumors.[12,16] The degree of height loss correlates inversely to age at irradiation, the most profound reduction in final height occurring in those who were in the youngest age group at irradiation[15] and to irradiation dosage, there being greater height loss even with small increases in overall dosage (e.g., 18 Gy versus 24 Gy).[12] Growth is frequently observed to be reduced during intensive therapy for acute lymphoblastic leukemia (ALL) but normal thereafter.[16,17] The spontaneous improvement in growth rates emphasizes that GH insufficiency is not present in all patients with growth failure,[11] and for that reason GH replacement therapy may not always be indicated.

Spinal irradiation administered before puberty significantly impairs spinal growth.[18,19] Leg length standard deviation scores (SDS) in patients who receive cranial and craniospinal irradiation are equivalent, whereas spinal growth is impaired primarily in the latter group.[18] The impairment of spinal growth results in disproportion, reflected by an increase in the ratio of leg length to sitting height. The impact on the skeleton of spinal irradiation correlates with age: the younger the individual is at the time of irradiation, the greater is the impairment of spinal growth and the greater the degree of disproportion.[18,19] This observation simply reflects the fact that there is a greater loss in growth potential when the insult to growth occurs at a younger age. A degree of disproportion is observed to occur in children who receive a combination of cranial irradiation and chemotherapy for acute leukemia[12] and most likely relates to disturbance of puberty or a direct effect of the chemotherapy. The effect of cytotoxic chemotherapy on growth remains contentious, but there is a suggestion that subsequent growth may be attenuated.[12] Additionally, chemotherapy has been shown to potentiate the growth impairment resulting from craniospinal irradiation.[14,15] Although the pathophysiologic mechanism by which chemotherapy adversely influences growth is unclear, a reduction in growth factors including IGF1, increased sensitivity of bone to irradiation damage, and a direct action on the growth plate are postulated.

Height loss correlates negatively with age at onset of puberty.[20] Radiation doses of less than 50 Gy during childhood may result in early or precocious puberty,[21] whereas higher doses more frequently result in gonadotropin deficiency. The impact of early puberty in a child is to reduce the time available for growth. If the child is additionally GH insufficient, the available time for intervention with GH therapy is also foreshortened, restricting the therapeutic efficacy of this intervention. It is for this reason that children with early puberty are treated with gonadotropin-releasing hormone (GnRH) analogues with or without GH replacement. Studies examining the effect of GnRH analogues on final height in GH-insufficient children treated with cranial irradiation have generally reported improvements in auxologic outcome.[22] Most of these were nonrandomized, open-label studies that compared patients treated with GnRH analogues with those who did not receive this intervention. The decision to initiate GnRH therapy is frequently based on the child's having a poorer final height prediction. Direct comparison of GnRH-treated and -untreated individuals have therefore almost certainly underestimated the beneficial impact of GnRH analogues on final height.

Despite the multiple insults on growth in cancer survivors, the importance of GH status is exemplified by the greater loss of final height in patients with impaired GH secretion compared to those with normal GH secretion who have undergone otherwise similar treatment regimens.[20] Normal growth and peak GH responses are frequently observed in long-term survivors of ALL who receive cranial irradiation doses of less than 24 Gy.[23,24] Higher radiation doses result in progressive impairment of the GH axis with height loss correlating negatively with the peak GH response to stimulation.[20]

GH replacement therapy can increase growth velocity in children with radiation-induced GH insufficiency.[15] Most studies have shown improvements in height velocity, although the height data have been conflicting. Early studies showed disappointingly small differences in the height loss prevented by the use of GH replacement, much less than observed in children treated for idiopathic growth hormone deficiency (GHD).[15,20,25-27] A number of factors contribute to the failure of GH to fully redeem the loss of height that results from multimodality cancer therapy, including chemotherapy, spinal irradiation, precocious puberty, a prolonged interval between irradiation and initiation of GH therapy, and inadequate GH treatment schedules.[15,20] The predominant factor is probably the interval between hypothalamo-pituitary irradiation and initiation of GH therapy.

Because the risk of recurrence of childhood brain tumors is relatively low more than 2 years out from treatment and there is no evidence that GH increases the risk of recurrence of brain tumors,[28-31] it is reasonable to consider GH replacement at that time. The approach of clinicians is variable, with some offering GH replacement only to children who demonstrate a reduced peak GH response to stimulation in association with a reduced height velocity and others offering GH replacement on the basis of the biochemistry alone, with the aim of preventing height loss which, once established, may not be fully remediable. If growth velocity and GH stimulation test results are normal at 2 years after treatment, growth should be monitored at least every 6 months, and the GH stimulation test should be repeated annually. Use of GH therapy to promote growth in GHD children who have received spinal irradiation can exacerbate disproportion.[15] Whereas the long bones respond appropriately, the irradiated spine is relatively resistant to the growth-promoting effects of GH. In this scenario, growth should be monitored by measurements of leg length velocity, because spinal growth is abrogated.

THE HYPOTHALAMO-PITUITARY AXIS

Deficiency of one or more anterior pituitary hormones is a consequence of treatment with external-beam irradiation when the hypothalamo-pituitary axis falls within the field of irradiation[32] (see Table 43-1). GH is almost exclusively the first axis to be affected.[33] Prospective studies from treatment of pituitary adenoma[34] and nasopharyngeal carcinoma[33] show that gonadotropin or adrenocorticotropin (ACTH) deficiency evolves next, with thyroid-stimulating hormone (TSH) deficiency being relatively infrequent. A similar temporal pattern is observed independent of whether radiation exposure occurs during childhood or adult life. To date, there are no reported cases of the development of diabetes insipidus as a consequence of cranial irradiation, in either children or adults, at any irradiation dosage used.[33,35,36]

The site of radiation damage to the hypothalamo-pituitary axis remains a matter of conjecture. With radiation doses less than 50 Gy, hypothalamo-pituitary hormone deficits are attributable to the cumulative damage from delayed neurotoxic effects of irradiation on the hypothalamus and secondary pituitary atrophy. Higher irradiation doses are thought to cause concurrent damage directly at the level of the pituitary. There are a number of lines of support for this consensus. Patients treated for pituitary adenoma with insertion of yttrium-90 implants (500 to 1500 Gy) show a lower prevalence of combined ACTH and TSH deficits[37] compared with those receiving conventional external-beam irradiation (37.5 to 42.5 Gy).[34] The likely explanation for this observation is that the field of exposure during conventional irradiation includes the hypothalamus, which is relatively spared with beta emissions from yttrium 90. Evidence of hyperprolactinemia after irradiation is suggestive of a reduction in prolactin inhibitory factors from the hypothalamus with relative preservation of the lactotrophs.[38] A frequent observation after irradiation of the hypothalamo-pituitary axis is that of a delayed TSH response to thyrotropin-releasing hormone (TRH) in the absence of overt hypothyroidism, further suggesting hypothalamic dysfunction.[38]

Greater impairment of GH response to the insulin tolerance test (ITT) in comparison with growth hormone–reducing hormone (GHRH) adds further weight to the notion of a hypothalamic site of damage.[39] Nonetheless, GH profiles in irradiated individuals show preservation of GH pulsatility despite a significant reduction in pulse amplitude.[40] GH pulse generation is dependent on GHRH, supporting a concept that irradiation-induced hypopituitarism most likely results from combined hypothalamic and pituitary damage, with compensatory overdrive of the remaining pituicytes by hypothalamic hormones in an attempt to maintain the normal hormonal milieu.

The pathophysiologic mechanism responsible for radiation-induced hypothalamic damage is unclear and may reflect either vascular or direct neuronal damage. Hypothalamic blood flow declines with time after irradiation; however, no change in the ratio of hypothalamic to occipital blood flow was found between 6 months and 5 years after irradiation.[41] This finding is in contrast to the progressive endocrine dysfunction, suggesting that the nature of the damage is predominantly neuronal.

Although an association between the development of hypopituitarism and chemotherapy has been suggested,[42] no robust relationship has been established.[43,44] In particular, no individual class of chemotherapeutic agents has been implicated. It is possible that the poor reproducibility and variable potency of different secretagogues used in endocrine stimulation tests may provide a more appropriate explanation for occasional individuals falsely diagnosed with GHD.[45,46] However, there is stronger evidence that cytotoxic drugs may increase the incidence of radiation-induced hypopituitarism.[14,15,47] A number of chemotherapeutic agents modulate release of antidiuretic hormone (ADH) from the posterior pituitary, resulting in the syndrome of inappropriate secretion of ADH (SIADH). Cisplatin, cyclophosphamide, melphalan, vinblastine, and vincristine have all been implicated, but this is by no means a comprehensive list.

Growth Hormone Deficiency

Childhood Growth Hormone Deficiency

Isolated GHD is commonly the only hormonal sequela of neuroendocrine injury after irradiation of the hypothalamo-pituitary axis with doses less than 40 Gy. Studies of animal models have attributed this to selective radiosensitivity of the somatotropic axis.[48,49] Long-term data reveal that almost all children irradiated with doses in excess of 30 Gy develop blunted GH responses to provocation,[50,51] whereas only about one third of patients treated with lower doses show impaired GH release. Isolated GHD in children has been described with irradiation doses as low as 10 Gy used in the setting of total-body irradiation (TBI); however, it is infrequent.[52] The severity and speed of onset of GHD in childhood as a result of irradiation is dose dependent.[53,54] Blunting of GH responses to provocative tests may occur as early as 12 months after high-dose irradiation (40 to 60 Gy) for brain tumors.[55,56] Progressive impairment in GH production occurs with time since treatment,[55,57] necessitating prolonged follow-up and regular assessment of hypothalamo-pituitary function. The prevalence of GHD is also influenced by how the dose is delivered. Among children treated for acute leukemia with a cranial irradiation dose of 25 Gy delivered in 10 fractions, a greater proportion developed GHD, compared with those who received 24 Gy in 20 fractions.[58] Abrogated GH responses are more likely to occur if irradiation is administered at a younger age, suggesting that the younger hypothalamo-pituitary axis is more susceptible to radiation-induced damage.[53]

A threshold effect has been proposed for the hypothalamo-pituitary axis, with irradiation dosages greater than 24 to 25 Gy resulting in impaired GH secretion and lower doses having negligible effect on the axis.[53,59] In keeping with this concept, normal growth is usually observed in long-term survivors of ALL who received cranial irradiation doses of less than 24 Gy.[23,24] In children, regimens used in treatment of acute leukemia involving cranial radiation doses of 24 Gy for central nervous system (CNS) prophylaxis result in impaired spontaneous and stimulated GH secretion.[11,60] Within this population, a continuum between retention of normal GH secretion and severe GHD is observed. Spontaneous GH secretion involves a reduction in both daytime and nocturnal GH secretion, as well as a reduction in GH pulse amplitude (Fig. 43-1).[11,40,60,61] However, normal pulsatile characteristics are maintained.[40] In those individuals showing the greatest reduction in spontaneous GH secretion, there is loss of the normal GH diurnal rhythm and a fall in IGF1 levels below the reference range.[60] At the other end of the continuum, a subgroup of children is described where the impact of irradiation on the hypothalamo-pituitary axis is minimal, leading to failure of the expected increase in GH secretion only at puberty, when demands are increased.[62,63]

In these latter individuals, the reduction in spontaneous GH secretion is purported to occur before attenuation of the peak GH response to stimulation[60]—a phenomenon termed *neurosecretory dysfunction*. Neurosecretory dysfunction of the GH axis is best understood in the context of growth data. Growth velocity is normal prepubertally, but an attenuated growth spurt is observed during puberty,[62] when GH secretion is normally amplified twofold to threefold.[64,65] This phenomenon probably represents inability of the hypothalamic GH control mechanisms to respond to the pubertal rise in endogenous sex steroids. Although individual stimulated GH values are found to be "normal" when defining GH neurosecretory dysfunction, group mean values are reduced compared with control data.[63] This suggests that neurosecretory dysfunction may more factually represent decompensation of a partially damaged hypothalamo-pituitary axis. It is likely, therefore, that the term neurosecretory dysfunction has in part been created by difficulties in defining a normal GH axis based on pharmacologic stimulation tests.

Prophylactic cranial irradiation in children with ALL has been undertaken on the premise of reducing the rates of CNS relapse. In an attempt to minimize the adverse effects on GH secretion and neuropsychological function, prophylactic cranial radiation dosage was reduced from 24 Gy to 18 Gy. This reduction in dosage does not result in a greater incidence of CNS relapse.[66] Cranial radiation doses of 18 Gy were subsequently introduced in the 1980s and then later abandoned completely in favor of high-dose intravenous methotrexate or intrathecal chemotherapy. Abrogated GH responses to stimulation are infrequently observed after 18-Gy cranial irradiation. In contrast, the pubertal increase in spontaneous GH secretion may be attenuated[67] and associated with with randomization of GH pulsatility.[67] The randomized bursts are explained by a reduction in somatostatin tone, as is similarly observed in rats with focused lesions in the median eminence that reduce somatostatin tone.[68]

Adult Growth Hormone Deficiency

After cranial irradiation, the importance of GHD in adults is twofold. First, GHD almost exclusively occurs before deficits in the additional anterior pituitary hormone axes and therefore acts as a marker that damage to the additional hypothalamo-pituitary axes may ensue.[33] Second, with recognition of the beneficial effects of GH replacement in adults[69-71] consideration should be given to replacement therapy, particularly if quality of life is significantly impaired.[72,73] The underlying cancer diagnosis and the

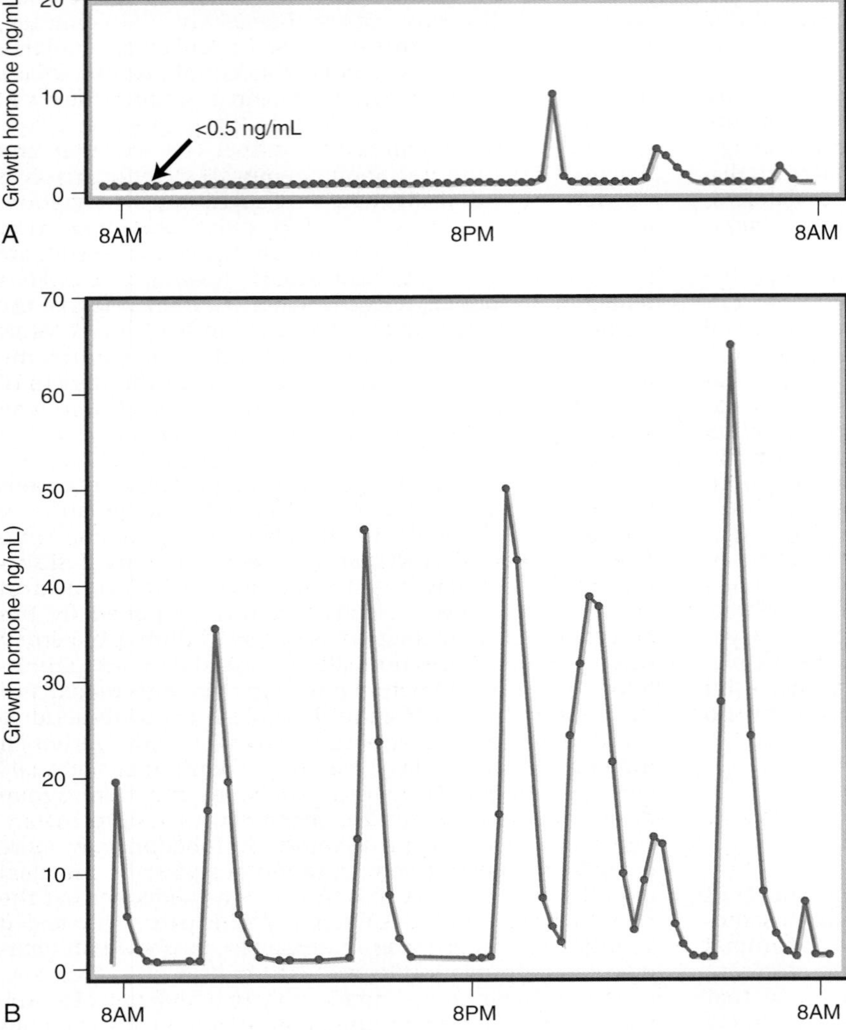

Figure 43-1 Spontaneous pulsatile secretion of growth hormone in a patient with acute lymphoblastic leukemia (ALL) who received prophylactic intrathecal methotrexate and cranial irradiation with 24 Gy **(A)** and in a representative normal child **(B)**. (From Blatt J, Bercu BB, Gillin JC, et al. Reduced pulsatile growth hormone secretion in children after therapy for acute lymphoblastic leukemia. *J Pediatr.* 1984;104:182-186.)

duration of remission must be taken into account before embarking on this course of management.

Similar to observations in children, the occurrence of adult GHD after irradiation depends on a number of variables. After a dose of 37.5 to 45.0 Gy to the hypothalamo-pituitary axis, mean peak GH levels after insulin-induced hypoglycemia were observed to decrease over the first 5 to 6 years and to plateau thereafter.[74] Blunting of GH responses to stimulation have been reported as early as 12 months after high-dose (50 to 70 Gy) radiation therapy for nasopharyngeal carcinomas.[75] In addition to length of follow-up, the peak GH response to stimulation correlates inversely with the radiation dosage received by the hypothalamo-pituitary axis.[57] Development of GHD, defined by a peak GH response of less than 2 μg/L (5 mU/L), will occur in patients with preirradiation peak GH responses of 12 μg/L (30 mU/L), 8 μg/L (20 mU/L), and 4 μg/L (10 mU/L) at a mean of 4 years, 3 years, and 1 year, respectively.[74] Therefore, if the basal peak GH response is in excess of 20 μg/L (50mU/L) before radiotherapy, it is unlikely that severe GHD will occur within 5 years.[74]

Adult Survivors of Childhood Cancer. Adult survivors of childhood cancer who have received irradiation to the hypothalamo-pituitary axis during their childhood cancer treatment frequently exhibit impaired GH secretion. Assessment of GH status in young adult survivors of ALL who received cranial irradiation of 18 to 25 Gy revealed that one third of patients had severe GHD (peak GH response, <3 μg/L), and a further third had partial GHD (peak GH response, 3 to 7 μg/L).[59] Almost all patients with impaired GH secretion received 24 to 25 Gy, supporting a threshold effect of irradiation dosage on the GH axis.[59] Impaired GH secretion during adult life after childhood irradiation of the hypothalamo-pituitary axis is more likely to be observed in those who received radiation therapy early during childhood.[59] Late assessment of the GH status in childhood brain tumor survivors (who received dosages of 40 to 50 Gy) in adult or predominantly adult cohorts revealed that most patients had blunted GH responses to stimulation.[57]

In adults who have received cranial irradiation but retain "normal" individual albeit attenuated mean stimulated GH responses, a similar phenomenon to the described GH neurosecretory dysfunction of puberty is not observed.[76] When the GH axis of these individuals is placed under stress during prolonged fasting, spontaneous GH secretion increases appropriately.[76,77] A number of qualitative changes in the GH profiles of these adults are observed[76,78] and reflect those observed in adults with severe GHD.[40] Profiles show elevated nadir and interpeak GH levels, reduced peak GH, reduced pulsatile GH, and a decrease in the ratio of pulsatile area under the curve (AUC) to total AUC GH secretion.[76,78] The diurnal rhythm, pulse frequency, pulse duration, and interpulse interval are unaffected. In those individuals with severe GHD, an increase in approximate entropy is observed, consistent with perturbation of the hypothalamic control of GH release.[40] Mechanistically, these changes are attributable to a reduction in somatostatin tone leading to higher nadir GH levels and reduced peak levels.

GHRH activity is essential to GH pulse generation,[79,80] suggesting that irradiation damage is not purely the consequence of hypothalamic damage to GHRH neurons. The reduced GH secretion after low-dose (<40 Gy) irradiation of the hypothalamo-pituitary axis can, therefore, be postulated to occur as a combination of a mild hypothalamic insult and direct damage to the pituitary somatotrophs with compensatory overdrive of the remaining somatotrophs from the hypothalamic GHRH neurons.[50,76]

Survivors of Cancer Treated in Adult Life. Radiation-induced GHD is recognized to occur after treatment of brain tumors and sinonasal carcinomas during adult life. Some of the most robust data comes from individuals who have received high-dose irradiation (45 to 60 Gy) for stage I (T1 N0 M0) or stage II (T1 N1 M0) nasopharyngeal carcinoma. These tumors receive most of their irradiation through opposing lateral facial fields that include the pituitary gland and, frequently, the basal hypothalamus (Fig. 43-2). When investigated for hypothalamo-pituitary dysfunction on the premise of putative symptoms of hormonal dysfunction after at least 5 years without recurrence, almost all of these individuals were found to have impaired GH responses to stimulation.[38,81] If radiation therapy occurs during adult life, age and gender have no measurable effect on the risk of developing GHD.[33]

Only limited data are available for GH status after irradiation of nonpituitary brain tumors. The prevalence of severe GHD at 5 years after treatment is reportedly about 30%.[42,82] Prospective assessment of pituitary function after irradiation of nasopharyngeal carcinoma showed that mean stimulated GH levels fell beginning from as early as 1 year.[33] At 5 years after radiotherapy, 60% to 65% of individuals would be expected to show abrogated GH levels (<6.7 μg/L [<20 mU/L]).[33] Similar irradiation doses to the hypothalamo-pituitary axis administered during childhood would be expected to result in an earlier onset and greater prevalence of GHD.[56,83,84]

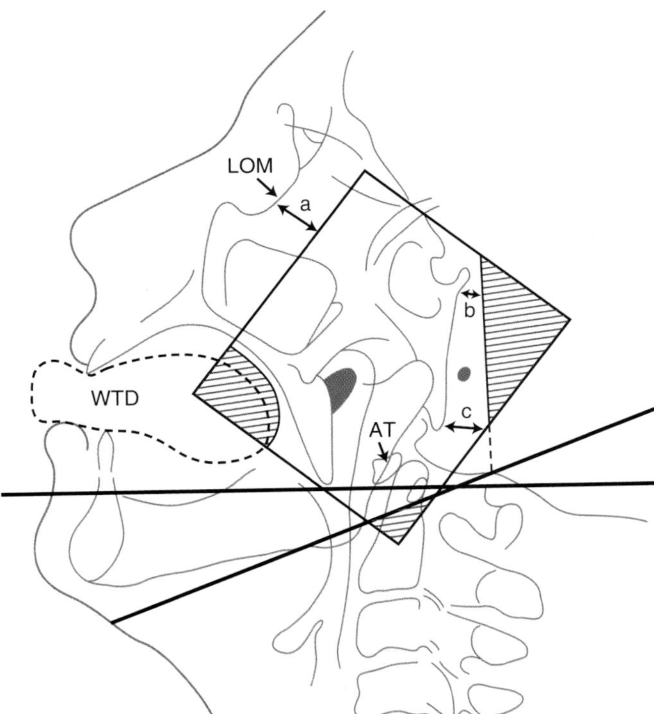

Figure 43-2 Lateral facial field used during radiotherapy for nasopharyngeal carcinoma. The shielded areas are shaded. Distances shown are 1.5 cm (a and c) and 0.75 cm (b). AT, atlantoid tubercle; LOM, lateral orbital margin; WTD, wax tongue depressor. (From Lam KS, Wang C, Yeung RT, et al. Hypothalamic hypopituitarism following cranial irradiation for nasopharyngeal carcinoma. *Clin Endocrinol (Oxf).* 1986;24:643-651.)

The Diagnosis of Radiation-Induced Growth Hormone Deficiency

The diagnosis of irradiation-induced GHD in children is suspected when the height velocity SDS remains below normal after completion of cancer therapy. The diagnosis can then be confirmed or refuted biochemically with the use of appropriate GH stimulation tests. In the absence of a pathophysiologic marker equivalent to growth, the diagnosis of irradiation-induced adult GHD becomes dependent exclusively on the prevailing biochemistry. In general, biochemical evaluation of GH status in both children and adults is undertaken as it would be for other causes of GHD. Because radiation-induced GHD is frequently isolated, the diagnosis can robustly be achieved only through the use of two provocative tests of GH reserve.[85,86] The ITT is considered to be the "gold standard" in the diagnosis of GHD in adults who are at risk for hypopituitarism.[86,87] In children, profound hypoglycemia during the ITT has led to deaths and irreversible neurologic damage.[88] Therefore, this test should be performed only in centers experienced in use of this test in children.

In addition to cranial irradiation, individuals requiring assessment of their GH status may have received anthracycline therapy as part of their treatment regimen. Anthracycline therapy has been implicated in the development of cardiomyopathies, which can decompensate[89-91] during times of significant stress on the cardiovascular system. Although no data exist for decompensation occurring during assessment of the hypothalamo-pituitary axis using the ITT, an alternative stimulation test should be used if echocardiographic evidence for significant anthracycline cardiac damage exists.

Debate has arisen as to whether all GH stimulation tests, when abrogated, appropriately represent a state of GHD. After irradiation of the hypothalamo-pituitary axis, the peak GH response to the ITT is often more attenuated than that observed with the arginine,[92] GHRH plus arginine,[93,94] or GHRH test.[39] After radiotherapy, the peak GH response to the ITT falls significantly within the first 5 years with minimal change over the subsequent 10 years.[93] In contrast, the peak GH response to the GHRH plus arginine test shows little change in the first 5 years, with a more significant fall occurring over the following 10 years.[93,95,96] Therefore, the evolution in GH responsiveness to provocative tests is stimulus dependent and suggests initial hypothalamic damage followed by later somatotroph dysfunction. The GHRH plus arginine test may be unreliable in characterizing GH status during the first 5 years after radiotherapy.

Among irradiated individuals who show discordant responses, characterized by a subnormal response to the ITT (peak GH secretion, <5 μg/L) but a normal or less attenuated response to the GHRH plus arginine test, spontaneous GH release is reliably reduced only in those patients who failed the GHRH test (peak GH secretion, <16.5 μg/L).[78] In contrast, if only the response to the ITT is impaired, spontaneous GH secretion is normal.[78] Among patients with impaired responses to the ITT, IGF1 levels are reduced to a similar extent in those with reduced and those with normal spontaneous GH secretion.[78] This observation questions the validity of defining GH status by a measurement of 24-hour GH secretion.[97] The diagnosis of GHD in these individuals remains complex, and it is not clear which test most accurately reflects a state of GHD.

Growth Hormone Replacement in Adult Cancer Survivors

Long-term survivors of cancer who have been rendered GH deficient by multimodality cancer therapy exhibit a clinical picture identical to that of GH-deficient adults with primary hypothalamo-pituitary pathology, including increased fat mass; reduced lean body mass, strength, exercise tolerance, and bone mass; an adverse lipid profile; and impaired quality of life.[98,99] The pattern of impairment of quality of life in GH-deficient adult cancer survivors is identical to that in patients with primary pituitary disease, the domain relating to vitality showing the greatest impairment.[100] The extent to which GHD contributes to the abnormalities observed in adult cancer survivors is difficult to disentangle from the direct effects of the primary tumor, treatment modalities used to induce remission, limited exercise, and poor nutritional status.

There are no data specific to the use of GH replacement during transition with radiation-induced GHD; however, it is intuitive to surmise that the beneficial effects of GH replacement in these individuals would be similar to those in hypopituitary adults with GHD of other etiologies.[101,102] Before committing an individual who received childhood GH replacement for radiation-induced GHD to transitional GH replacement, it is essential to reassess the GH axis. This necessity is derived from the fact that all degrees of GHD are treated during childhood but only those patients with severe GHD qualify for treatment as an adult. Furthermore, the reproducibility of GH stimulation tests is poor, and reassessment of GH status in childhood brain tumor survivors shows that only about 60% retest as severely GHD after reaching final height.[103] GH doses used to treat adults with GHD during transition should be aimed at normalizing the IGF1 level, in contrast to the weight-based regimens used during childhood.[104]

Low-dose GH replacement in adult GH-deficient survivors of childhood cancer leads to small improvements in body composition and serum lipids, a significant improvement in quality of life, and increased spinal bone mineral density.[99,105] No data are yet available on the effect of GH on fracture rates in these individuals. Previous spinal irradiation impairs the osteo-anabolic effects of low-dose GH replacement on bone accretion.[105] Improvements in quality of life occur in all domains; however, as in patients with primary pituitary pathologies, the greatest improvement occurs in the domain of vitality.[100] In adult survivors of childhood cancer, the minor changes in body composition, lipid profile, and bone mass after GH replacement suggest that GHD may not be a major etiological factor in their pathogenesis. The converse appears to be true for quality-of-life status in these individuals, and this should be the primary indication for initiation of GH replacement therapy.

Several lines of evidence suggest a link between the GH axis and development of various cancers. Epidemiologic data indicate a link between circulating serum IGF1 levels and both prostate cancer and premenopausal breast cancer. Those individuals with IGF1 values in the upper reaches of the normal range have an increased relative risk compared with those in the lowest quartile.[106,107] Patients with active acromegaly show an increased risk of colonic polyps and carcinoma.[108] In vitro data indicate that GH and IGF1 promote leukemic blast cell replication.[109] Given these data, concerns regarding the potential of GH replacement to induce recurrence or increase relapse rates of patients in remission from malignant disease have been raised. Reassuringly, no increase in recurrence rates of childhood brain tumors or acute leukemias are observed with GH replacement therapy;[29,31,110] and analysis by brain tumor subtype has shown no diagnostic subgroup to be at increased risk of recurrence.[31,110] No trend in the relative risk of recurrence with cumulative duration of GH treatment is observed, adding further support for the safety of GH replacement in these individuals.[29] Residual abnormalities seen on computed tomography are not a contraindication to treatment in childhood brain tumor survivors.[31] However, continued neurosurveillance imaging is warranted in these individuals, consequent on the limited power of studies to date.

Cranial Irradiation and Additional Anterior Pituitary Hormone Deficits

Although low-dose radiation therapy most frequently results in isolated GHD, damage to additional anterior pituitary hormone axes as a consequence of hypothalamo-pituitary irradiation is well recognized.[55,111,112] As with children who develop GHD, the vulnerability to more extensive hypothalamo-pituitary dysfunction after irradiation during childhood is dependent on the patient's age at irradiation;[47,53,84,113] time since treatment;[38,82,114] radiation dose, fractionation, time allowed between fractions for tissue repair;[32,35,36,38,43,82] and the margins of the irradiation field.[38]

During adult life, gender, age at irradiation, and adjuvant chemotherapy do not predict development of hypopituitarism.[82] The greater the radiation dose, the more likely the patient is to develop deficits and the earlier these deficiencies will occur.[32] For example, when tumors of the pituitary gland or anatomically related lesions are treated during adult life, the 5-year cumulative risk of TSH deficiency increases from 10% to 52% with dose escalation from 20 Gy delivered in 8 fractions to 42 to 45 Gy delivered in 15 fractions (Fig. 43-3).[35] Modern radiation schedules typically do not use more than 2 Gy per fraction and no more than five fractions per week. An increase in fractionation size leads to relatively more injury to late-responding (neuronal) compared with early-responding (tumoral) tissues.[115] Notably, the presence of a pituitary lesion or previous surgery in the region of the hypothalamo-pituitary axis increases susceptibility to radiation-induced damage because the axis may already be compromised to some extent.[34,42,116] Overall, however, the relative frequencies of deficiencies affecting the various anterior pituitary hormones is similar to those observed after irradiation of pituitary tumors,[33,34] with GH, gonadotropins, ACTH, and

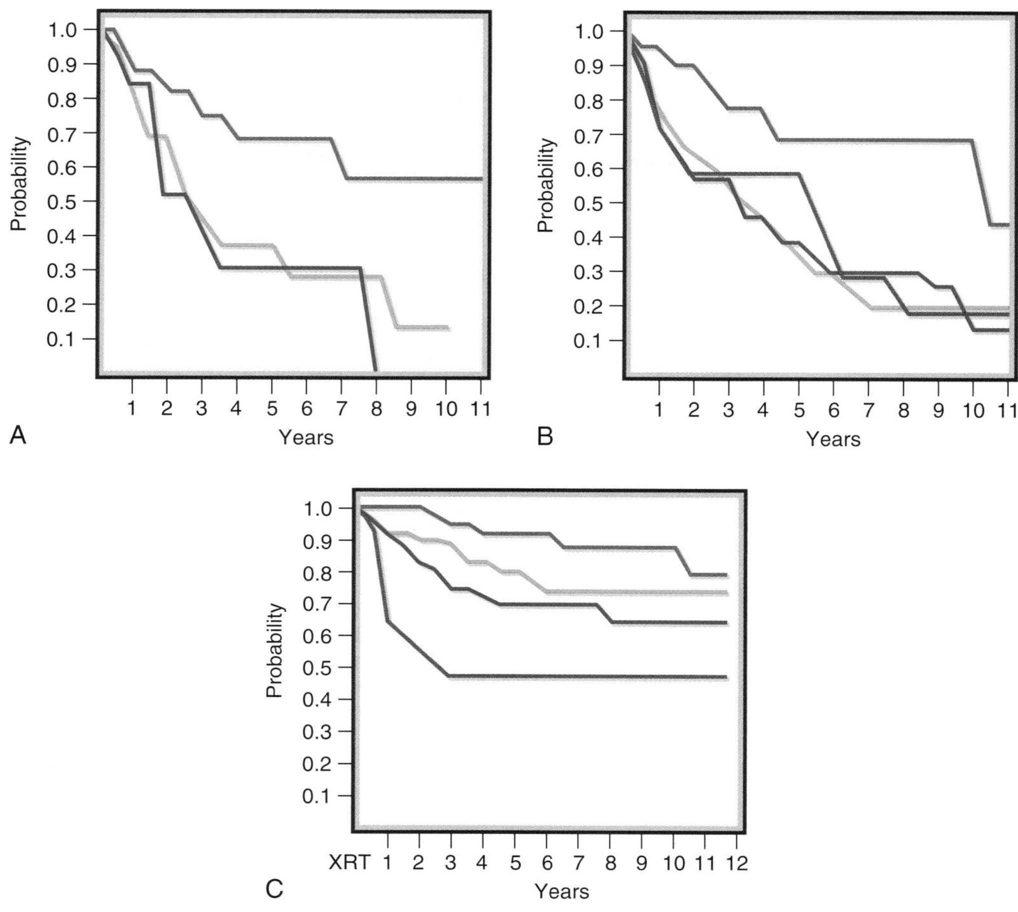

Figure 43-3 The probability that secretion of gonadotropin **(A)**, adrenocorticotropin (ACTH) **(B)**, and thyroid-stimulating hormone (TSH) **(C)** will remain normal up to 11 years after radiotherapy using three dosing regimens: 20 Gy in 8 fractions over 11 days, 35 to 37 Gy, or 40 Gy in 15 fractions over 21 days. Blue line = 20 Gy in 8 fractions; yellow line = 35-37 Gy in 15 fractions; pink line = 40 Gy in 15 fractions; and green line = 42-45 Gy in 15 fractions. (From Littley MD, Shalet SM, Beardwell CG, et al. Radiation-induced hypopituitarism is dose-dependent. *Clin Endocrinol (Oxf).* 1989;31:363-373.)

TSH being affected in descending order of frequency (Fig. 43-4).

As with GHD, much of the data concerning irradiation-induced hypopituitarism characterized in adults results from the long-term sequelae of cranial irradiation administered during treatment of childhood cancers. Deficiency of the gonadotropins, ACTH, and TSH in adulthood after cranial irradiation of 18 to 25 Gy administered during treatment of childhood ALL occurs relatively infrequently. Radiation doses used in childhood for the treatment of CNS relapses of ALL, brain tumors, and soft tissue sarcomas of the head and neck (35 to 60 Gy) require closer observation for long-term pituitary hormone dysfunction.

Hypopituitarism resulting from irradiation used during adulthood to treat tumors anatomically distant from the pituitary gland is best exemplified by data derived from treatment of brain tumors[82] and sinonasal carcinomas.[33,117,118] Radiation doses used in treatment of these tumors are typically in excess of 40 to 50 Gy. After radiation therapy for sinonasal disease, deficiency of one or more pituitary hormones is reported to occur in 60% to 80% of individuals with long-term follow-up.[33,38,43,117,119]

Gonadotropins

Gonadotropin deficiency after cranial irradiation occurs in a continuum from impaired LH or FSH responses to GnRH with maintenance of normal sex steroids to that of severe deficiency of both gonadotropins and sex steroids. In the first year after irradiation of the hypothalamo-pituitary axis in men with nasopharyngeal carcinoma, a rise in basal and stimulated FSH is observed with no change in either LH or testosterone levels.[33,75] After the first year, a progressive decline in both the FSH and LH occurs.[33,75] Studies in humans and primates suggest that these changes reflect an initial decline in pulse frequency of hypothalamic GnRH, followed by a progressive reduction in GnRH pulse amplitude.[120,121]

In the majority of cases where the gonadotropins have been affected by irradiation, levels continue to lie within the normal range. In men, this is usually accompanied by a testosterone level in the lower reaches of the normal range or only slightly below normal. In women, the failure of adequate pulsatile gonadotropin secretion leads to failure of egg development or ovulation, initially in intermittent cycles; oligomenorrhea ensues before the onset of amenorrhea and estrogen deficiency. Symptoms occurring as a consequence of gonadotropin deficiency frequently bring to attention the possibility of evolving hypopituitarism in individuals who are not undergoing regular endocrine screening.[38] In postmenopausal women, gonadotropin deficiency is asymptomatic and may be recognized only when biochemical studies show failure of physiologic elevation of these hormones. Care must be taken in assessing radiation-induced gonadotropin

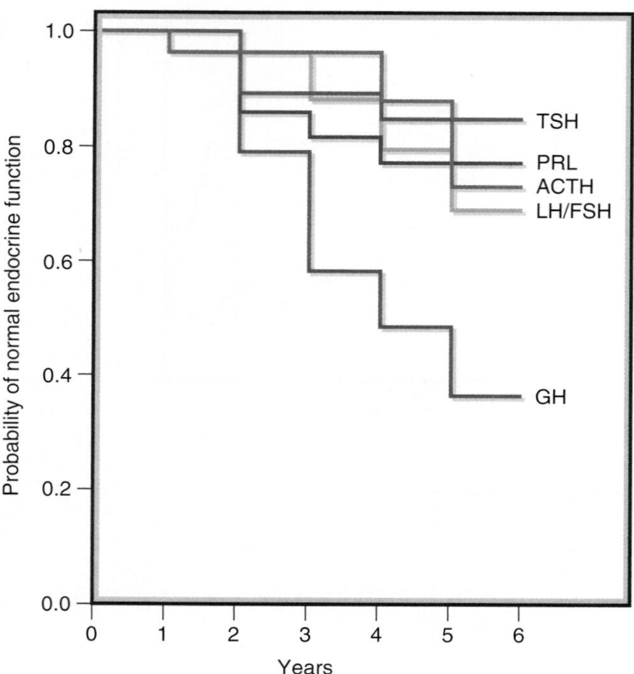

Figure 43-4 Cumulative probability of retaining normal endocrine function after irradiation of the hypothalamo-pituitary axis during treatment of nasopharyngeal carcinoma. (From Lam KS, Tse VK, Wang C, et al. Effects of cranial irradiation on hypothalamic-pituitary function: a 5-year longitudinal study in patients with nasopharyngeal carcinoma. *Q J Med.* 1991;286:165-176.)

deficiency because of the not infrequent presence of concurrent hyperprolactinemia.[33,38,81]

Gonadotropin deficiency is uncommon when radiation doses to the hypothalamo-pituitary axis are less than 40 Gy, but there is a remarkable increase in incidence after more intensive schedules. After irradiation for brain tumors[42,44,82] (40 to 70 Gy) or nasopharyngeal carcinomas,[33,36,119] gonadotropin deficiency is reported in approximately 30% of individuals 5 years after exposure. A similar proportion of women and men are affected.[33,44] Repeated infusion of GnRH may induce LH and FSH pulsatility, suggesting predominantly hypothalamic damage and the prospect of restoring fecundity.[122]

In addition to gonadotropin deficiency, cranial irradiation doses of less than 50 Gy can result in precocious or early puberty in children.[21,123] Both genders are affected equally with radiation doses typically used in the treatment of brain tumors (25 to 50 Gy),[21] whereas lower doses used for prophylaxis in the treatment of acute lymphocytic leukemia (18 to 25 Gy) result in a predominance of precocious puberty in girls.[124] A linear relationship between age at irradiation and age at onset of puberty is observed. The onset of puberty occurs at a mean of 8.51 years in girls and 9.21 years in boys plus 0.29 years for every year of age at irradiation.[21] The mechanism responsible for early puberty is thought to result from disinhibition of cortical influences on the hypothalamus, which allows GnRH pulse frequency and amplitude to increase prematurely. It has been postulated that the cortical restraint on the onset of puberty is more easily disrupted in girls than in boys by any insult, including irradiation.

Adrenocorticotropin Hormone

Impaired cortisol reserve occurring as a consequence of ACTH deficiency is less common than either GH or gonadotropin deficiency following irradiation of the hypothalamo-pituitary axis. When present, ACTH deficiency is a relatively late occurrence, and there is almost exclusively evidence of additional anterior pituitary hormone deficits.[33,38,44] Occasionally, ACTH deficiency occurs before gonadotropin deficiency,[34] and in rare cases it is the first hormone deficiency to occur.[33] ACTH deficiency is uncommon with radiation doses less than 40 to 50 Gy[125] and virtually absent with doses of less than 24 Gy.[52,126] After irradiation of brain tumors distant to the hypothalamo-pituitary axis in adult life, approximately 20% of patients are reported to be glucocorticoid deficient.[42,82] The 5-year prevalence of biochemical ACTH deficiency after treatment of nasopharyngeal carcinomas occurs in up to 27% of patients, although many show borderline subnormal results.[33,36,119]

Normal or slightly exaggerated cortisol responses to corticotropin-releasing hormone (CRH)[44] are also described after cranial irradiation for brain tumors. Individuals who retain normal cortisol response to stimulation show activation of the hypothalamo-pituitary-adrenal axis.[127] Integrated 24-hour cortisol levels and cortisol production rates are increased by 14% and 20%, respectively. Cortisol half-life, pulsatility, and diurnal rhythmicity are unchanged.[127] It is reasonable to assume that the increase in cortisol secretion reflects underlying activation of the CRH-ACTH axis. The pathophysiologic mechanism pertaining to these observations remains unclear, although it has been speculated that chronic stress or a local radiation-induced inflammatory response may play a role.

Thyroid-Stimulating Hormone

Central hypothyroidism is most classically represented by low free thyroid hormones in association with an inappropriately low TSH. In most cases, the TSH lies below or in the lower portion of the normal range. The infrequent contribution of immunoreactive but bioinactive TSH in irradiated individuals with central hypothyroidism can lead to TSH values that are in the upper reaches of normal or mildly elevated.[128]

A delayed TSH response to TRH and a diminished nocturnal TSH surge are reported to occur in children, in adult survivors of childhood cancer, and in adults who have received cranial irradiation.[38,75,81,129,130] These qualitative changes suggest dysfunction of the hypothalamic control of the thyroid axis. It has been proposed that they may represent a diagnosis of hidden central hypothyroidism and that TSH secretion may be compromised even before the somatotropic axis.[130] Despite a relatively high proportion of individuals displaying these qualitatively abnormal TSH responses (approximately 30%) after cranial radiotherapy, levels of free thyroxine (T_4) are usually normal, and few individuals go on to develop overt secondary hypothyroidism.[33,75] These latter observations suggest that the TSH anomalies are functional and do not represent hidden central hypothyroidism.[129] However, most patients who develop overt hypothyroidism do show a delayed or decreased TSH response to TRH. To date, there is no convincing evidence to support the routine use of the TRH test or assessment of the TSH surge to improve the diagnostic sensitivity and specificity of central hypothyroidism.

Deficiency of TSH occurs late, and infrequently within the first 2 to 3 years after radiotherapy, even when the hypothalamo-pituitary axis has been exposed to high-dose radiation.[33] The prevalence of central hypothyroidism in children undergoing cranial irradiation (35 to 45 Gy) for nonpituitary brain tumors is 3% to 6%,[125,131] and it is virtually zero after prophylactic cranial irradiation used to treat acute leukemia.[132-134]

In adults treated for sinonasal disease, the actuarial risk of clinical central hypothyroidism after irradiation (40 to 70 Gy) is approximately 3% at 5 years and 13% at 10 years[135]; the risk of subclinical (biochemical) hypothyroidism is 9% at 5 years and 22% at 10 years.[135] Nine percent of adults irradiated with a median biologic effective dose (BED) of 54 Gy for nonpituitary brain tumors show biochemical evidence of central hypothyroidism 3 years after radiation therapy.[82] A dose-dependent increase in the incidence of central hypothyroidism is observed over the dose range of 40 to 70 Gy.[135] There is no significant effect of dose fractionation, age, or gender on the development of TSH deficiency in irradiated adults.[135] Adjuvant chemotherapy does not predispose to development of radiation-induced central hypothyroidism.[135]

Hyperprolactinemia

In adults, mild hyperprolactinemia is observed in a minority of patients after low-dose irradiation of the hypothalamo-pituitary axis.[35] When patients are exposed to the higher irradiation doses used in treatment of nasopharyngeal carcinoma and brain tumors, hyperprolactinemia is frequent.[33,36,38,44,81,82] Prolactin levels are rarely elevated to more than three to four times the upper limit of the normal range.[33,82] The pattern of development shows a gender dichotomy, being elevated in women but only infrequently in men,[33,38,44] and it is more likely to occur after irradiation during adult cancer therapy than during childhood.[44,50] The hyperprolactinemia not infrequently returns to baseline values over the next few years (Fig. 43-5). Symptomatic irradiation-induced hyperprolactinemia in women may lead to oligomenorrhea and galactorrhea.[33] Men are rarely symptomatic. Individuals with low serum prolactin levels, usually associated with panhypopituitarism, have also been described.[82]

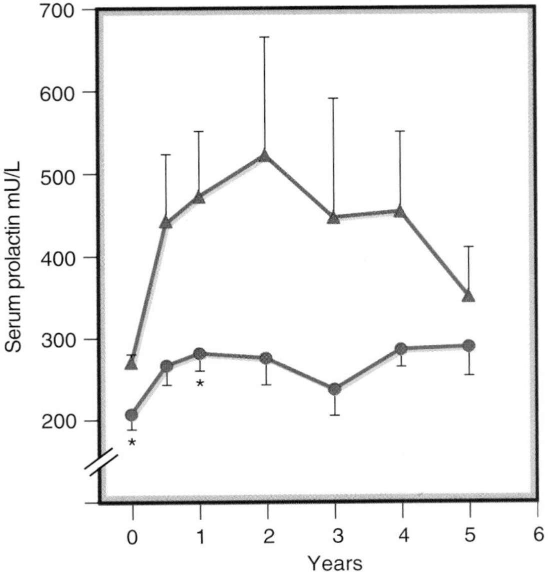

Figure 43-5 Mean serum prolactin concentration (mU/L) of adult men (•) and women (▲) with time after radiotherapy to the hypothalamo-pituitary axis. Error bars represent the standard error of the mean (±SEM). (Reproduced with permission from Littley MD, Shalet SM, Beardwell CG, et al. Hypopituitarism following external radiotherapy for pituitary tumours in adults. *Q J Med.* 1989;70:145-160.)

GONADAL FUNCTION

Table 43-2 outlines the primary effects of multimodality cancer therapy on the reproductive system. Multimodality treatment regimens employed in the treatment of cancer damage the gonadal axis directly at the level of the gonad and centrally at the hypothalamus and pituitary, as previously discussed. Damage to the gonads and central structures are not mutually exclusive, and it is not uncommon for an individual who has received multimodality cancer therapy to have involvement at both levels. Damage to the gonads can occur from radiation exposure and cytotoxic chemotherapy. Irradiation of the gonads occurs during treatment of gonadal tumors, testicular relapses of hematologic malignancies, soft tissue sarcomas of the pelvis, TBI in preparation for bone marrow transplantation (BMT), and from scatter during spinal irradiation for certain brain and relapsed hematologic malignancies. Damage from cytotoxic chemotherapy is most frequently described after use of alkylating agents including cyclophosphamide, chlorambucil, and mustine; however, nitrosoureas, procarbazine, vinblastine, cytosine arabinoside, and cisplatin have also been incriminated.[136]

In children, it has been suggested that the chances of maintaining or recovering gonadal function after multimodality cancer therapy are greater for girls than for boys.[137,138] In unselected female childhood cancer survivors, 6% to 7% developed ovarian failure within 5 years after diagnosis. Of the patients with ovarian failure, more than 50% received ovarian irradiation in excess of 10 Gy.[139] Female 5-year childhood cancer survivors who continued to menstruate at age 21 years displayed a risk of entering the menopause fourfold greater than expected by age 21 to 25 years, and about 40% had entered the menopause by age 31 years (compared with 5% of the general population).[140] Independent risk factors for development of ovarian failure include increasing age, exposure to ovarian irradiation, and treatment with alkylating agents, particularly procarbazine or cyclophosphamide.[139,140] The direct and synergistic effect of taxanes, tyrosine-kinase inhibitors, and monoclonal antibodies on gonadal function are not yet clear.

Male Gonadal Function and Cancer Therapy

Radiation and the Testis

The testis is one of the most radiosensitive tissues in the body. A dichotomy between damage to the germinal epithelium and damage to the Leydig cells is observed: very low doses of irradiation cause significant impairment of spermatogenesis, whereas sex hormone production is impaired only with high radiation doses. As a consequence, puberty typically progresses normally in children and secondary sexual characteristics are maintained in most adults who receive irradiation to the testis. Testicular volumes are small, reflecting damage to the germinal epithelium,[126] and should not be relied on for staging of puberty. In contrast to most other tissues, dose fractionation increases the degree of gonadal toxicity.

The effect of single-fraction low-dose radiotherapy on spermatogenesis is well documented (Fig. 43-6). The most immature cells, spermatogonia, are the most radiosensitive; doses as low as 0.1 Gy cause a significant reduction in sperm count and morphologic changes in the spermatozoa. Higher doses of 2 to 3 Gy are required to kill spermatocytes, resulting in a reduction in spermatid number. Doses of 4 to 6 Gy significantly reduce the number of

TABLE 43-2

Overview of the Effects of Multimodality Cancer Therapy on the Reproductive System of Cancer Survivors

Physiologic System	Insult	Pathology	Comments
Male reproductive system	Local XRT, spinal XRT, TBI	Oligospermia, azoospermia Subfertility, sterility Leydig cell insufficiency	Primary insult is to germ cells of testis—azoospermia occurring within 2 mo from doses as low as 2 Gy. Recovery occurs at mean of 30 mo after 2-3 Gy and >5yr after 4-6 Gy.[10] Impaired spermatogenesis leads to small testes, which should not be used to stage puberty. Leydig cell function is rarely compromised with doses <20 Gy. Puberty progresses normally, and secondary sexual characteristics are maintained despite subfertility.
Ovarian function	Local XRT, spinal XRT, TBI	Transient amenorrhea Premature ovarian failure Subfertility, sterility Estrogen deficiency	Insult reflects damage to a fixed pool of oocytes. Impact of XRT on ovarian function is age and dose dependent.[14] XRT doses >6 Gy result in premature menopause in women >40 yr of age; in younger women, a dose of 20 Gy leads to premature ovarian failure in only 50%. Recovery is infrequent, usually transient, and occurs almost exclusively in younger women. Concurrent estrogen deficiency results in failure of puberty to progress.
Uterine function	Pelvic XRT	Immature uterus Failure to carry a child	Irradiation (20-30 Gy) of the uterus during childhood results in impaired growth, reduced uterine blood flow, and failure of the endometrium to respond to estrogen and progesterone. The impact is greater with younger age at the time of XRT. With egg donation, the impaired uterine function reduces the likelihood of carrying a child through pregnancy.
Male reproductive system	Chemotherapy	Oligospermia, azoospermia Subfertility, sterility Leydig cell insufficiency	Gonadal toxic agents include the alkylating agents procarbazine, cisplatin, vinblastine, and cytosine. Damage depends on the cumulative dosage. Multiagent chemotherapy is usually more gonadotoxic than single-agent therapy. Primary insult is to the germ cells, with high-dose therapy additionally resulting in compensated hypogonadism.[18] Recovery frequently occurs, and its speed depends on the regimen administered.
Ovarian function	Chemotherapy	Transient amenorrhea Premature ovarian failure Subfertility, sterility Estrogen deficiency	Insult reflects damage to a fixed pool of oocytes. Ovarian toxicity occurs with agents similar to those that are toxic to testis. Impact of chemotherapy on ovarian function is dependent on age and cumulative dose.[20] Recovery of ovarian function is frequently observed, but these individuals may undergo a premature menopause.

TBI, total-body irradiation; XRT, radiation therapy.

spermatozoa, implying direct damage to the spermatids.[141] A fall in the number of spermatozoa is seen 60 to 70 days after damage to immature cells from radiation doses of up to 3Gy. At higher doses, the reduction in sperm count occurs earlier, reflecting damage to the spermatids. Doses of less than 0.8 Gy tend to result in transient oligospermia, and doses higher than 0.8 Gy cause azoospermia. At the doses discussed, recovery of spermatogenesis occurs with proliferation of surviving stem cells.

Complete recovery of the germinal epithelia and achievement of premorbid sperm counts occurs 9 to 18 months, 30 months, and 5 years or more after radiation doses of less than 1 Gy, 2 to 3 Gy, and more than 4 Gy, respectively.[141-143] The majority of testicular radiation exposure occurs as a consequence of fractionated irradiation, which is significantly more toxic to the germinal epithelium than single-dose irradiation. Fractionated radiotherapy doses of less than 0.2 Gy have no significant effect on spermatogenesis. Doses of 0.2 to 0.7 Gy cause a dose-dependent increase in FSH and transient reduction in spermatogenesis that recovers within 12 to 24 months.[144] Doses of 2.0 to 3.0 Gy frequently result in azoospermia, with recovery of spermatogenesis often delayed for 10 years or longer.

At the radiation doses <10 Gy, Leydig cell function is relatively spared, and most patients have normal testosterone levels, albeit frequently at the cost of elevated LH levels. With time, the elevated LH level returns to normal. During adulthood, radiation doses of 20 to 30 Gy used to treat carcinoma in situ in the contralateral testis after unilateral orchidectomy result in overt Leydig cell insufficiency,[145] characterized by a fall in testosterone and a compensatory increase in LH levels. However, the fall in testosterone is not so great as to require replacement therapy in most adult patients. In contrast, there is a suggestion that individuals who undergo a similar treatment

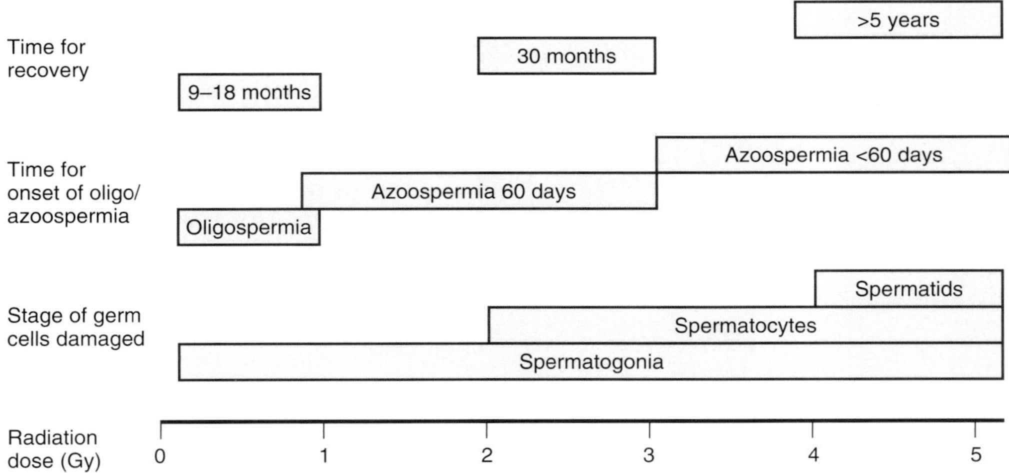

Figure 43-6 **Impairment of spermatogenesis after single-dose radiation therapy: The effect of radiation dose on stage of germ cell damage and time to onset and recovery from germ cell damage.** (Adapted from data of Rowley MJ, Leach DR, Warner GA, et al. Effect of graded doses of ionizing radiation on the human testis. *Radiat Res.* 1974;59:665-678; and Howell SJ, Shalet SM. Effect of cancer therapy on pituitary-testicular axis. *Int J Androl.* 2002;25:269-276.)

regimen for testicular cancer during childhood may be more vulnerable to Leydig cell damage and frequently require testosterone replacement as an adult. A radiation dose of 20 to 30 Gy completely ablates the germinal epithelium.

Chemotherapy and the Testis

The adverse impact of chemotherapeutic agents on the testis is directed primarily at the germinal epithelium, with evidence for Leydig cell dysfunction usually limited to a raised LH level with a normal or low-normal testosterone level.[136] The extent of damage and the potential for recovery of spermatogenesis depend on the chemotherapeutic agents used and the cumulative dosage.[137,146] It has been suggested that the adult testis is more susceptible to damage than the prepubertal testis. However, few studies have suggested a relationship between age and risk of gonadal failure within adult patients.[137,146] In general, combination chemotherapy is more toxic than treatment with single agents, and the induced azoospermia is less likely to recover.

Insight into testicular function after chemotherapy comes mainly from studies of cyclophosphamide and combination chemotherapy regimens used in the treatment of lymphoma and testicular tumors. Approximately 45% of men treated with cyclophosphamide as single-agent therapy show evidence of testicular dysfunction, with the incidence of gonadal dysfunction correlating with the cumulative dosage.[137] More than 80% of postpubertal men who received a total dose of more than 300 mg/kg showed evidence of testicular dysfunction.[137] The use of combination chemotherapy regimens incorporating alkylating agents such as MVPP (mustine, vinblastine, procarbazine, prednisolone) in the treatment of Hodgkin's disease renders almost all males azoospermic after the first cycle, and fewer than one quarter of them will have a normal sperm count 5 years after receiving six or more cycles.[138,146-148] Alternate regimens consisting of nonalkylating chemotherapy (e.g., ABVD [doxorubicin, bleomycin, vinblastine, dacarbazine]) infrequently result in germinal epithelial failure, and if it does occur, recovery is relatively rapid.[146,148] In the treatment of metastatic testicular cancer, despite the fact that most patients are rendered azoospermic after use of CVB (cisplatin, vinblastine, bleomycin), the outlook for fertility is relatively good, with 50% of men having a normal sperm count 3 years later. In general, standard combination chemotherapy regimens used in the treatment of leukemia spare spermatogenesis in most individuals, with only 10% to 20% showing persistent gonadal damage.[149,150] Newer regimens for the treatment of lymphoma and testicular tumors yield a better outlook for testicular function because of an absence of procarbazine and the lower doses of alkylating agents used.

Although subnormal testosterone levels (<7 nmol/L) are infrequent, there is irrefutable evidence for a more subtle impact of chemotherapy on Leydig cell function.[151] The most frequent abnormalities of Leydig cell function are elevated basal and GnRH-stimulated LH levels in the setting of a normal or low-normal testosterone level. Physiologically, LH pulse amplitude is increased and pulse frequency remains unaltered. The compensatory increase in LH means that testosterone replacement is rarely necessary. Among men treated with high-dose chemotherapy for Hodgkin's disease, approximately 30% had an elevated LH level in association with a testosterone level in the lower half of the normal range or frankly subnormal, and a further 7% showed an isolated raised LH level.[151] These biochemical abnormalities support the hypothesis that a significant proportion of men treated with cytotoxic chemotherapy have mild testosterone deficiency. Studies of testosterone replacement in these individuals with elevated LH and low-normal testosterone levels have failed to show significant benefits to date.[152]

Preservation of Male Fertility and Sex Hormone Replacement

Discussions as to strategies for preservation of fertility need to be undertaken as early as possible before commencement of cancer therapy. At present, sperm banking is the only option for fertility preservation that is widely accepted and available for postpubertal men. All other techniques remain in the realm of research (Table 43-3).

Men who are at risk of azoospermia due to their impending treatment schedule can have sperm frozen for future use. This procedure is relatively simple and is part of standard practice, but it is of no value in prepubertal males. Sperm storage is most effective when the sperm concentration, motility, and morphology are not affected by the

TABLE 43-3

Methods of Preserving Fertility in Men and Women before Cancer Therapy.

	Current Clinical Practice	Experimental Procedures
Men	Sperm storage (ejaculation or electrical stimulation) Microsurgical aspiration Testicular biopsy	Germ cell cryopreservation Testicular tissue cryopreservation In vitro maturation of stem cells
Women	Embryo cryopreservation Oophoropexy	Oocyte cryopreservation Ovarian cortex cryopreservation Ovarian cryopreservation In vitro maturation of primordial follicles In vitro maturation of immature oocytes Ovarian transplantation (from monozygotic twin)

primary disease process. A significant proportion of men with lymphoma, leukemia, or testicular tumors are oligospermic or have impaired semen quality at presentation.[153-155] For prepubertal boys, there has been interest in harvesting spermatogonial stem cells that can be frozen and stored for future use. Reimplantation of this tissue into the testis after attainment of remission from cancer and completion of puberty could theoretically result in restoration of spermatogenesis.[156,157] In vitro maturation of spermatogonial stem cells is a further investigational methodology that has been examined in animals. Suppression of the gonadal axis with GnRH analogues before cancer therapy has been shown to result in gonadal protection in animal models,[158] but there is no convincing evidence to date for benefit in human males or females. After chemotherapy, an increase in genetic abnormalities is observed in the spermatozoa, but concerns regarding the potential transmissibility of genetic anomalies have not been substantiated.[159,160]

Men with overt hypogonadism should have testosterone replacement instituted to improve body composition, prevent osteoporosis, and maintain sexual function and well-being.[161,162] In pubertal boys who fail to progress through puberty due to overt testosterone deficiency, testosterone replacement needs to be titrated to bring the individual through puberty and maintain body composition and well-being thereafter. In men with compensated hypogonadism secondary to cytotoxic chemotherapy, sexual function has been found to be impaired,[163] along with slight reduction in bone mass and subtle body composition changes.[164] It is unclear whether these changes are secondary to the mild Leydig cell insufficiency or to the primary tumor and its treatment. Testosterone replacement in these individuals has not resulted in significant improvement in bone mass, body composition, serum lipids, sexual function, or quality of life, with the exception of a reduction in physical fatigue and low-density lipoprotein (LDL) cholesterol.[152]

Female Gonadal Function and Cancer Therapy

Radiation and the Female Reproductive Tract

The ovaries are irradiated as part of the management of pelvic tumors and lymphoma, during the spinal component of craniospinal irradiation, and during TBI preconditioning before BMT. The effect of irradiation and chemotherapy on the ovary can best be explained by loss of oocytes from a fixed population, which, once destroyed, cannot be replaced. The natural history of the healthy ovary is for oocyte number to fall exponentially with aging. Ovaries of older women are therefore much more sensitive to radiation-induced damage, and a dose of 6 Gy is liable to result in permanent menopause in women age 40 years or older. In contrast, it is estimated that 20 Gy over a 6-week period will result in permanent sterility in approximately 50% of younger women (Fig. 43-7).[165] Higher doses inevitably result in ovarian failure irrespective of age. In childhood, the median lethal dose (LD50) of the oocyte has been estimated to be 4 Gy,[166,167] and this may manifest as failure to enter or complete puberty or, later in life, as premature menopause. Ovarian recovery after childhood irradiation has been reported, but it is often temporary, with the onset of secondary amenorrhea usually ensuing within a few years.

Pelvic irradiation during childhood that involves the uterus within the irradiation field leads to changes that result in failure to carry a child. In those patients who do conceive, the risk of miscarriage or a low-birth-weight

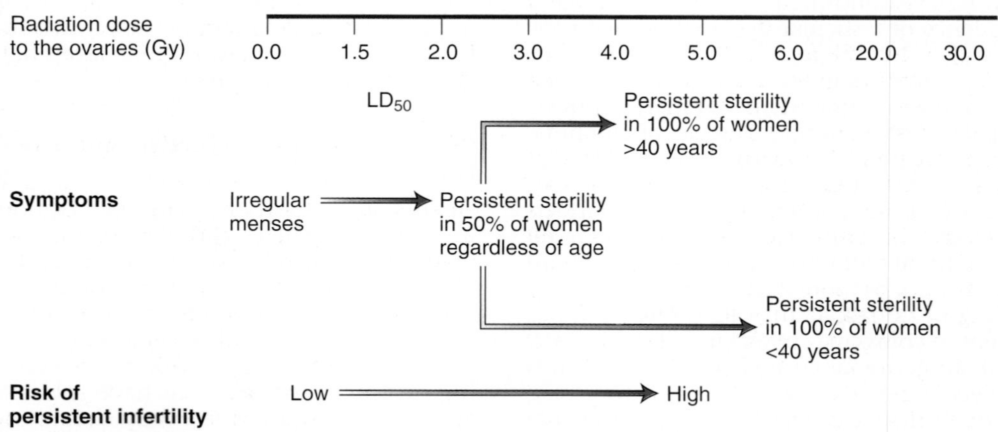

Figure 43-7 The relationship between radiation dosage to the ovaries and ovarian function. LD_{50}, lethal dose that will result in sterility in 50% of the tested group. (From Nakayama K, Milbourne A, Schover LR, et al. Gonadal failure after treatment of hematologic malignancies: from recognition to management for health-care providers. *Nat Clin Pract Oncol.* 2008;5;78-89.)

infant is greatly increased.[168] A radiation dose of 20 to 30 Gy during childhood leads to a reduction in adult uterine length and failure of the endometrium to respond to physiologic estrogen and progesterone therapy.[169] After irradiation, blood flow is reduced in the uterine arteries as assessed by Doppler ultrasound. An adequate blood flow is essential to uterine function, particularly endometrial proliferation, implantation, and successful continuation of pregnancy. It is unlikely that an adult woman who has received a significant radiation dose to the uterus during childhood would be able to carry a child to term. Uterine irradiation not only affects patients who retain normal ovarian function but also those who request in vitro fertilization with donor oocytes for concomitant ovarian failure.

Chemotherapy and the Ovary

Ovarian damage manifests clinically with amenorrhea with or without symptoms of estrogen deficiency or failure to progress through puberty. Hormonally, the gonadotropins may be grossly elevated with an unrecordable estradiol level, or there may be moderate elevation of the gonadotropins in association with a midfollicular estradiol level. As with radiation-induced ovarian damage, the susceptibility of the ovary to chemotherapeutic damage, the speed of onset of amenorrhea, and the potential for recovery depend on age and cumulative dosage.[137,170] With increasing age, smaller doses of chemotherapy are required to induce ovarian failure.

In women with breast cancer treated with multiagent chemotherapy including cyclophosphamide, the average doses of cyclophosphamide that induce amenorrhea in women in their 20s, 30s, and 40s are 20.4, 9.3, and 5.2 g, respectively.[171] Intuitively, prepubertal and pubertal girls would be assumed to be at lower risk of ovarian damage. However, clinical and morphologic studies reveal that they are not totally resistant to cytotoxic ovarian damage, although it occurs infrequently. After treatment of Hodgkin's disease with the alkylating combination chemotherapy regimens MVPP, MOPP (mustine, vincristine, procarbazine, prednisolone), or ChlVPP (chlorambucil, vinblastine, procarbazine, prednisolone), 15% to 62% of survivors developed amenorrhea.[170,172,173] Among those older than 35 years, amenorrhea is almost invariable. In many, the onset is abrupt, but in others there is a progression to oligomenorrhea with later development of a premature menopause. In contrast, use of ABVD is much less gonadotoxic.[174] Treatment of acute leukemias with standard regimens results in persistent ovarian failure in fewer than 20% of survivors.[139,175]

Assessment and Preservation of Female Fertility

Strategies aimed at prevention of gonadal damage have led to the use of chemotherapeutic regimens, such as ABVD for the treatment of Hodgkin's disease, that have equivalent cure rates but significantly less impact on gonadal function. However, there remains some risk to gonadal function with almost all cancer therapies, and discussions as to strategies for preservation of fertility need to be undertaken as early as possible in the management algorithm. At present, embryo cryopreservation provides the only option for fertility preservation in women that is widely accepted and available. All other techniques remain in the realm of research (see Table 43-3).

A large number of cytotoxic agents have been implicated as teratogenic to the fetus, and it is therefore important that during cancer therapy women use appropriate contraception until remission is achieved. No evidence of an increase in birth defects has been detected in women who retain normal ovulatory cycles after having received cytotoxic chemotherapy and who spontaneously conceive. Recovery of ovarian function in amenorrheic women and the possibility of a premature menopause in women retaining a normal cycle are difficult to predict accurately after an insult to the gonads received during multimodality cancer therapy. The use of transvaginal ultrasound to accurately quantitate ovarian volume and antral follicle count, along with measurements of inhibin B and anti-müllerian hormone (AMH), have been proposed as guides to future reproductive potential after cancer therapy.[176,177] Both inhibin B and AMH are secreted by granulosa cells, so their concentrations decline with the depletion of follicles. Further work is required to optimize the predictive models.

Preservation of fertility in women who are to undergo intense treatment that is likely to result in infertility is a significant growth area. Treatment of Hodgkin's disease frequently includes local irradiation of involved lymph nodes, including those along the iliac vessels. The ovaries lie adjacent to the iliac vessels and receive a dose of approximately 35 Gy, inevitably resulting in premature ovarian failure. Oophoropexy to remove the ovaries from the irradiation field, combined with shielding, can reduce the dose of radiation received by the ovaries to less than 6 Gy, thereby reducing the incidence of amenorrhea by approximately 50%.[178,179] The exact reduction in risk of amenorrhea as a consequence of oophoropexy is controversial and needs to be assessed in the context of disease extent, patient age, and surgical expertise.

Both oocytes and embryos can be frozen. Embryo storage requires the patient to be in a stable relationship and to undergo controlled stimulation of the ovary for several weeks, along with regular ultrasonographic monitoring and aspiration of follicles. This techniques is time-consuming when there is a pressing need to start treatment, is invasive, does not permit natural conception, and is not applicable to prepubertal girls. Pregnancy rates are approximately 15% to 30% per cycle with thawed embryos. Oocyte cryopreservation can be considered for patients without a partner; it requires stimulation of the ovaries for approximately 2 weeks before retrieval of the oocytes. It is associated with a success rate of less than 5% for thawed oocytes and therefore must be regarded as an experimental approach. Interest has been directed toward cryopreservation of ovarian cortical strips that are rich in primordial follicles; these are later thawed and grafted back into the patient at the original site (orthotopic) or elsewhere (heterotopic).[180,181] This technique is available to both prepubertal and mature women. Several large centers are now storing ovarian strips, and to date there have been 13 live births in 10 women after orthopticregrafting in women treated with cytotoxic therapy for cancer (n = 8) or benign disease (n = 2).[182,183,183a] Concerns remain as to whether cancer cells may be transferred back to the recipient. Only time will tell if this technique improves the fertility prospects of women who undergo multimodality cancer therapy.

In women younger than 50 years of age who have developed gonadal failure, the impact is twofold: fertility and sex steroid production. Sex steroid replacement is recommended to alleviate symptoms of hot flushes, mood changes, and vaginal dryness and to prevent loss of bone mass.[145] The impact of sex steroid replacement on cardiovascular events remains controversial in patients younger than 50 years in light of recent data showing an increase in vascular events in postmenopausal women treated with hormone replacement therapy (HRT).[184,185] Reassuringly, stratification of the Women's Health Initiative study data by age revealed that the relative risk of cardiovascular disease was not increased in those aged 50 to 55 years.[186] The use of HRT in postmenopausal women has been associated with an increased risk of breast cancer.[184] It is probable that this latter risk equates to lifetime exposure to estrogens, so that continuing estrogen replacement until age 50 in these individuals should not convey an excess risk. Exposure of the breast to radiation scatter during mantle irradiation for Hodgkin's disease[187,188] or TBI before BMT[189] is associated with an increased risk of breast cancer. Whether estrogen replacement further amplifies this risk is not known.

Radioiodine Therapy and the Gonadal Axis

Although the radioiodine doses used in treatment of hyperthyroidism have minimal, if any, effect on gonadal function, their effect on gonadal and reproductive function is an important consideration when treating differentiated thyroid carcinoma (DTC) because of the high-dose and often repeated administrations.

Transient absence of menstrual periods occurs in 8% to 27% of women during the first year after radioiodine therapy for DTC,[190,191] particularly in women closer to the age of menopause. Several studies have reported increased rates of spontaneous and induced abortions during the first year after radioiodine therapy.[190] However, radioiodine treatment for DTC is not associated with a significantly increased risk of long-term infertility, miscarriage, induced abortions, stillbirths, neonatal mortality, or congenital defects.[190-193] Women treated with radioiodine may experience their menopause at a slightly younger age than untreated women.[190,193] There is otherwise little observational evidence to suggest important adverse effects of radioiodine treatment on gonadal function, fertility, or pregnancy outcomes beyond 12 months.

Doses of radioiodine used in the treatment of thyrotoxicosis in men result in only minimal and transient changes in the germinal epithelium and in Leydig cell function.[194] There is no significant variation in sperm concentration or percentage of normal forms. After therapy for DTC in men with single high-dose therapy, FSH levels frequently are increased at 6 months, after which a decline is observed, with all subjects showing normal values by 18 months.[195-198] Similarly, inhibin B levels fall significantly by 3 to 6 months after treatment but normalize by 18 months,[197] reflecting transient damage to spermatogenesis. Increases in LH are much less frequent and, when present, return to normal levels by 12 months.[195,197] Testosterone levels remain normal. A greater proportion of patients experience elevated gonadotropins after cumulative radioiodine activities of greater than 14 GBq.[195] At these doses, short-term oligospermia is common,[195] but there is little evidence for long-term infertility.[196,198]

PRIMARY THYROID DISEASE

The effects of multimodal cancer therapy on the thyroid are summarized in Table 43-4. Recognition of the adverse effects of head and neck irradiation, particularly secondary cancers, has led to the demise of radiation therapy in the treatment of benign diseases including acne vulgaris, goiter, tuberculous adenitis, thymic enlargement, and tonsillar hyperplasia. Use of low-dose (2 to 7 Gy) radiation therapy for benign disease was common in the United States from the 1930s through the 1950s. Since the 1960s, exposure of the thyroid and parathyroids to radiation has occurred almost exclusively during treatment of malignant disease, most commonly during neck irradiation for Hodgkin's disease and sinonasal carcinomas, craniospinal irradiation for certain brain tumors, TBI before BMT, and unavoidable scatter during treatment of primary brain tumors.

Thyroid tissue is among the most radiosensitive tissues in the body. After irradiation, the prevalence of both thyroid dysfunction and formation of thyroid nodules increases significantly.[199-201] However, the absolute incidence of thyroid disorders after irradiation is not clearcut because of differences in radiation dose and schedules (duration and fractionation), previous thyroid surgery, volume of thyroid irradiated, duration of follow-up, definition of thyroid disorders ("clinical" versus "biochemical" hypothyroidism), and effects of adjuvant therapies.[202] This uncertainty was reflected in a survey of radiation oncologists, whose estimates of the risk of clinical

TABLE 43-4

Overview of the Effects of Multimodality Cancer Therapy on the Thyroid and Parathyroid Glands of Cancer Survivors

Physiologic System	Insult	Pathology	Comments
Thyroid nodules	Neck XRT or TBI	Malignant nodules	Risk is significantly increased after neck XRT (RR ~15).[22] Incidence increases from 5-10 yr after XRT. There is a possible "cell kill" effect at doses >30 Gy.[23] Risk is significantly greater in children compared with adults and in females compared with males.[23]
		Benign nodules	There is increased prevalence of all benign thyroid disease.[22] Palpable nodules occur in 20-30% of patients who received neck XRT. Prevalence depends on time since XRT, female gender, and XRT dose.
Thyroid dysfunction	Neck XRT or TBI	Hypothyroidism	Frank or compensated hypothyroidism occurs in 20-30% of patients who received TBI and in 30-50% of those who received neck irradiation (30-50 Gy).[22] Hypothyroidism usually occurs within 5 yr after XRT. Thyroxine therapy should be instituted early because of the hypothesis that an elevated TSH may drive early thyroid cancers.
		Hyperthyrodism	Graves' disease is reported to occur at increased frequency (RR ~8).[22]
Parathyroid	Neck XRT	Late-onset hyperparathyroidism	Latency period is 25-47 yr. Dose dependency has been observed.[24]

RR, relative risk; TBI, total-body irradiation; TSH, thyroid-stimulating hormone; XRT, radiation therapy.

hypothyroidism after administration of 50 Gy to the whole thyroid ranged from 2% and 50%.[203] Radiation damage to the thyroid is proposed to result from direct thyroid cell injury, immune-mediated damage, and damage to small thyroid arterioles.[202]

Thyroid Dysfunction

Hypothyroidism

The first reports of development of hypothyroidism as a consequence of irradiation for head and neck cancers were published in the 1960s.[204,205] Hypothyroidism is the most common late sequela of irradiation of the thyroid, and it may be overt or subclinical. Neck irradiation for treatment of adult sinonasal disease results in a 5-year actuarial risk of 32% for clinical and 29% for subclinical primary hypothyroidism,[135] with little change in prevalence thereafter (Fig. 43-8).[135] In the long term, biochemical evidence for primary hypothyroidism is present in up to 60% of patients who received high-dose radiation (30-70 Gy) to the neck for sinonasal disease or Hodgkin's lymphoma.[119,201,202,206-210] A similar incidence is observed after craniospinal irradiation for primary brain tumors during childhood.[44] Even though the thyroid does not lie directly within the field of irradiation administered during cranial irradiation for brain tumors, there is an increased incidence of subsequent hypothyroidism.[211]

At least half of the cases of hypothyroidism occur within the first 5 years after radiation,[201,206,209,210,212,213] with a peak incidence between 2 and 3 years.[206,209,210,212,213] However, the latency period may be prolonged.[200,201] A dose-dependent increase is observed in the incidence of clinical primary hypothyroidism.[135,201,210,212,214] Dose is inversely associated with the latency period to the development of thyroid dysfunction,[212] and hypothyroidism can occur within the first 6 months after high-dose therapy.[206] Fractionation of the dose has minimal impact on development of hypothyroidism, in contrast to its effect on other radiosensitive organs.[206] Up to 20% of patients with subclinical hypothyroidism show improvement or resolution of elevated TSH levels.[211,212]

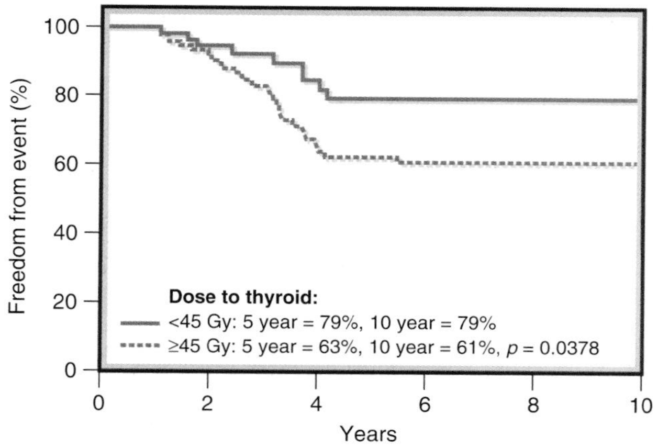

Figure 43-8 Probability of remaining free from hypothyroidism after irradiation therapy during treatment of extracranial head and neck malignancies. Patients are divided according to the radiation dosage received to the neck. (Reprinted with permission from Bhandare N, Kennedy L, Malyapa RS, et al. Primary and central hypothyroidism after radiotherapy for head-and-neck tumors. *Int J Rad Onc Biol Phys.* 2007;68:1131-1139.)

Among adults exposed to neck irradiation, no effect of age[135,207,209,215] or gender[207,209,214,215] on the development of thyroid dysfunction is observed. A higher proportion of individuals irradiated in childhood develop thyroid dysfunction compared with those irradiated during adult life.[208,214] Among those irradiated in childhood, an inverse relationship is observed between age at irradiation and the development of hypothyroidism.[201,213,216] The risk of developing primary hypothyroidism is dependent on the proportion of the gland exposed to irradiation, with primary hypothyroidism occurring infrequently when less than 50% of the gland is irradiated.[135,214] In keeping with this latter observation, hypothyroidism is more common in patients who have undergone a surgical hemithyroidectomy as part of their cancer therapy before irradiation.[217,218]

Treatment of both subclinical and overt hypothyroidism should be undertaken early with levothyroxine to reduce TSH to the low-normal range. Most patients presenting with subclinical hypothyroidism progress to overt hypothyroidism with time, so early intervention is warranted. Furthermore, even mildly elevated TSH values may convey an elevated risk of both benign and malignant thyroid nodules in the irradiated thyroid,[219] and this risk can be abrogated by levothyroxine replacement. Use of levothyroxine to suppress TSH before irradiation has been proposed as a potential method to reduce thyroid cell turnover and thereby ameliorate irradiation-induced thyroid damage, but this strategy has not proved to be efficacious.[220]

Hyperthyroidism

In addition to hypothyroidism, Graves' disease,[210,221] Graves' ophthalmopathy,[199,210,221] and thyroiditis[200,210] occur with increased prevalence after neck irradiation. The relative risk of hyperthyroidism after neck irradiation is increased 5- to 20-fold[201,210,221] and shows a temporal distribution similar to that of radiation-induced hypothyroidism.[201,210] The actuarial risk of Graves' disease equates to 2% to 3% at 10 years after irradiation.[210,221] Radiation-induced hyperthyroidism is dose dependent,[201] with the prevalence increasing with time since treatment.[201] Age at irradiation and gender have no effect on development of Graves' disease.[210] Graves' ophthalmopathy occurring after head and neck irradiation is indistinguishable clinically from that occurring in nonirradiated individuals,[221] and it may occur both in the euthyroid and the hyperthyroid state.[210]

Effects of Chemotherapy

Although adjuvant chemotherapy has been suggested to cause thyroid dysfunction or influence development of hypothyroidism after irradiation,[210,211,213] this has not been conclusively demonstrated.[135,201,207,209,211,215] Both interferon and interleukin-2 increase the risk of developing autoimmune hypothyroidism.[222,223] This condition is usually transient, although a small proportion of patients remain hypothyroid in the long term. A number of chemotherapeutic agents affect thyroid function tests by modulating thyroid hormone binding. 5-Flurouracil increases total triiodothyronine (T_3) and T_4, but patients remain euthyroid with normal TSH and free T_4 levels; asparaginase decreases production of hepatic thyroid-binding globulin (TBG) and total T_4 levels through its widespread effects on protein and DNA synthesis.

Thyroid Nodules

In 1950, Dufffy and Fitzgerald raised the possibility that irradiation of the thymus gland during infancy was an etiological factor in the future development of thyroid carcinoma. In their series, 9 of 28 children with thyroid carcinoma had been exposed to low-dose neck radiation.[224] Since that time, a number of epidemiologic studies have conclusively established an association between exposure to external irradiation of the thyroid and development of both benign thyroid neoplasia and DTC.[188,225-228] Occurrence of radiation-induced thyroid nodules is uncommon during the first 5 years after exposure, with the peak incidence of excess risk occurring 15 to 20 years after radiotherapy.[201,225,227,229] Twenty years after exposure, the excess relative risk decreases, but the excess absolute risk continues to increase for at least 40 years.[226]

The dose-response relationship approximates linearity from 0.1 Gy to a few gray,[225] with the relative risk per gray for both carcinoma and adenoma being about fourfold to eightfold.[225] Risk increases with higher doses, but at a more gradual rate. Early data suggested that the risk of developing thyroid cancer was linearly associated with dose, but more recent data confirm this to be true only for radiation doses up to 20 to 29 Gy (Fig. 43-9).[230] At doses greater than 30 Gy, a fall in the dose response is observed, consistent with a cell-killing effect of radiation at high doses.[230] The cumulative risk in individuals receiving greater than 5 Gy is estimated to be 4% to 6% at 25 to 30 years,[225,227] with the relative risk calculated to be 15- to 50-fold that of the nonirradiated population.[188,202,227] In contrast to its impact in other radiosensitive endocrine glands, fractionation of the dose seems to have little effect on reducing the incidence of nodules.[225] The use of adjuvant chemotherapy has yet to be shown to have an independent effect or demonstrable influence on the incidence of radiation-induced nodules.[225,227,230] A gender dimorphism is observed and is similar to that for spontaneous tumors in nonirradiated individuals.

Tumor development is significantly greater when irradiation occurs at a younger age,[227,230-232] reflecting the greater susceptibility of growing tissues to irradiation-induced damage. When exposure occurs during treatment of childhood malignancy, the risk of developing thyroid carcinoma is greater in those with a primary diagnosis of neuroblastoma or Wilms' tumor,[227] suggesting an underlying predisposition to tumor development in these individuals.

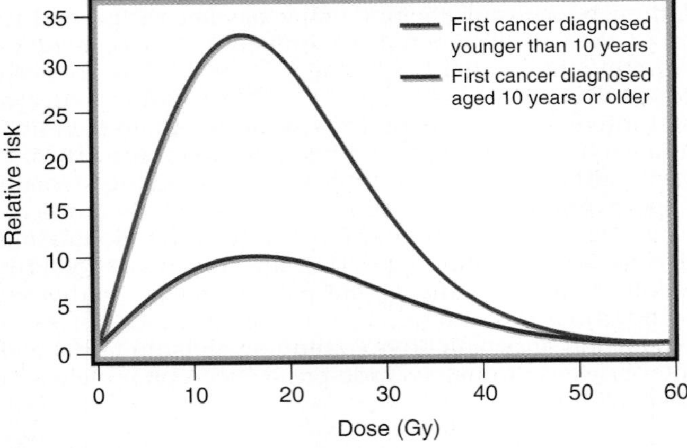

Figure 43-9 Thyroid cancer risk by radiation dose according to age at diagnosis of first cancer. (From Sigurdson AJ, Ronckers CM, Mertens AC, et al. Primary thyroid cancer after a first tumour in childhood (the Childhood Cancer Survivor Study): a nested case-control study. *Lancet.* 2005;365:2014-2023.)

Approximately two thirds of thyroid nodules occurring after irradiation are benign, and one third are malignant. The distribution of thyroid carcinoma histologic subtypes after irradiation is not dissimilar to that observed in the general population, with the majority being papillary and a lesser proportion being follicular carcinomas.[201,225-227,229] These radiation-induced tumors do not seem to act differently from spontaneous tumors,[232,233] although regional lymph node metastasis is reported to occur at a higher frequency (up to 30%) than in nonirradiated individuals.[226,229] A number of *RET/PTC* gene rearrangements have been shown to be more frequent in radiation-induced thyroid tumors.[234,235]

The use of routine ultrasound scans to monitor the thyroid of patients who have received neck irradiation remains controversial. Thyroid ultrasonography may be an overly sensitive screening tool because of its low specificity, in that the clinical relevance of lesions detected is unclear.[236] To place this in perspective, results of thyroid ultrasonography in children undergoing radiation therapy for Hodgkin's disease were reported to be abnormal in all cases, with focal lesions in more than 40% of the patients.[237] Once palpable or ultrasound-characterized thyroid nodules are elucidated, fine-needle aspiration for cytology should be performed. However, cytologic evaluation may prove difficult because of the presence of radiation-induced cellular atypia.[238] For that reason, there should be a low threshold for undertaking a diagnostic lobectomy.

HYPERPARATHYROIDISM

Early studies of the effects of irradiation in animal models revealed parathyroid tumors to occur in 8% of irradiated rats compared with 0% of nonirradiated control rats.[239] A putative association between radiation and development of hyperparathyroidism in humans was first hypothesized in 1975 by Rosen and colleagues, who described the development of radiation dermatitis, a sublingual salivary gland pleomorphic adenoma, and hyperparathyroidism in a young women treated with face and neck irradiation for hirsutism.[240] A number of series followed in which low-dose radiation used in treatment of benign conditions was correlated with the occurrence of hyperparathyroidism. In studies from the late 1970s and early 1980s, the prevalence of previous low-dose (<8 Gy) head and neck radiation in patients diagnosed with surgically proven or biochemical hyperparathyroidism was found to be significantly higher (11% to 30%) than in control populations without hyperparathyroidism (0% to 8%).[241-245] Further studies are unlikely to be able to confirm this observation because of the reduced use of low-dose radiation therapy for treatment of benign disease since the 1950s.

In patients who have received low-dose neck irradiation, the prevalence of hyperparathyroidism is 1% to 11%, significantly greater than that in background population data and matched control groups.[241,246-248] The relative risk of hyperparathyroidism increases by 0.11 per cGy.[248] The presence of a relationship between radiation dose and development of hyperparathyroidism supports the previous observational data of a causal association. Radiation-induced hyperparathyroidism follows a benign and indolent course, with many patients remaining clinically asymptomatic.[241,244]

The majority of studies have considered radiation therapy administered during childhood or adolescence. Middle-aged individuals who receive low-dose irradiation to the neck show a prevalence of hyperparathyroidism of less than 5% when assessed 25 years later, and most do not require operative intervention.[249] Few robust data are available regarding the occurrence of hyperparathyroidism after high-dose neck irradiation used in treatment of malignant diseases, although an association has been described.[250,251] In those individuals who developed hyperparathyroidism, the estimated radiation dose at the thyroid was only 0.9 to 13.2 Gy. It has been hypothesized that a "cell kill" effect of higher radiation doses may prevent development of hyperparathyroidism. Monitoring of calcium and parathyroid hormone (PTH) levels during the first 36 months after high-dose neck irradiation showed increasing PTH levels in the setting of normal calcium levels[252] without development of hyperparathyroidism.

The latency period from low-dose irradiation to the development of hyperparathyroidism is prolonged, and although cases have been reported as early as 5 years after irradiation, most cases occur 24 to 45 years later.[226,241-243,246,247,253] A longer latency period has been suggested to occur in younger individuals,[243,250] although age at irradiation does not significantly affect the overall incidence of hyperparathyroidism.[246,248] In nonirradiated populations, there is a gender dichotomy, with females showing a higher incidence of hyperparathyroidism. This dichotomy holds true for irradiated individuals, and a similar gender distribution[241] and relative risk of radiation-induced hyperparathyroidism is present in males and females.[246]

Irradiation-induced hyperparathyroidism may be the result of either adenoma or hyperplasia. Single adenomas are about two times as frequent as hyperplasia and multiple gland involvement.[226,243,245,248] Histologic studies usually confirm a predominance of chief cells,[244,245] but cases with a high proportion of oxyphil cells have been described in hyperfunctioning adenoma and hyperplasia.[244,245] This latter observation is difficult to reconcile, because oxyphil cells are generally held to be nonfunctioning. Although cases of parathyroid carcinoma occurring after neck irradiation have been described,[253] they are infrequent and were not observed in the larger series.[241,242]

The frequency of synchronous benign nodules or nonmedullary carcinoma of the thyroid is at least twofold to threefold increased in individuals with irradiation-induced hyperparathyroidism compared with nonirradiated patients.[226,244,246,247,253-255] The association between radiation-induced thyroid damage and parathyroid disease is likely a consequence of the sensitivity of both endocrine organs to irradiation; however, a genetic predisposition to radiation-induced tumorigenesis cannot be excluded.

The effects of multimodal cancer therapy on the parathyroid glands are summarized in Table 43-4.

THE METABOLIC SYNDROME AND VASCULAR RISK

Epidemiologic data show childhood cancer survivors to have excess morbidity and mortality for at least 10 to 15 years, with those surviving longer than 5 years having an approximately 10-fold excess mortality.[256,257] After exclusion of deaths relating to recurrence or progression of the primary tumor, mortality rates remain elevated, with a standardized mortality rate for cardiac and cerebrovascular disease increased fivefold to eightfold.[256,257] An increased risk of late-occurring stroke is observed among childhood survivors of Hodgkin's disease, leukemia, and brain tumors, compared with sibling controls,[258,259] with the relative risks estimated at 4.3, 6.4, and 29.0, respectively.[258,259] Examination of demographic and treatment variables reveals the excess vascular disease to be highest in patients who received chest and spinal irradiation[256] or anthracycline therapy.[260] The relative importance of these mechanisms in placing childhood survivors of cancer at increased risk of vascular disease is unclear. Abnormalities of left ventricular function are observed in individuals treated with anthracyclines,[89,91,261,262] with total cumulative dose being the most significant risk factor for anthracycline late-onset cardiomyopathy.[89,91,261] Anthracycline cardiac toxicity fails to explain the increased vascular morbidity in patients who do not receive this class of drug.

Derangements in both traditional and nontraditional cardiovascular risk factors, consistent with the metabolic syndrome, are prevalent in childhood cancer survivors and can be proposed to have a putative role in predisposition to atherothrombosis. Abnormalities of body composition in childhood survivors of cancer are well documented. The prevalence of obesity is significantly increased,[263-268] with the excess fat mass located predominantly in the central compartment.[269] During childhood, obesity is observed to develop between treatment and achievement of final height,[264,270,271] and cranial irradiation has been implicated in its development.[271] The greatest degree of obesity is observed in those individuals who were treated at the youngest ages.[264]

Fasting glucose and insulin are elevated in long-term survivors of childhood cancer[267] and in those who underwent BMT during childhood.[272] Prospective data concerning glucose tolerance showed the recorded frequency of hyperinsulinemia, impaired glucose tolerance, and diabetes to be significantly elevated at 18%.[273] Dyslipidemia is an important determinant of vascular disease. Childhood cancer survivors show adverse lipid profiles characterized by increased LDL-cholesterol, apolipoprotein-B, and triglycerides; decreased high-density lipoprotein (HDL)-cholesterol; and increased ratio of total cholesterol to HDL-cholesterol.[267,269,272] Blood pressure abnormalities have also been reported in survivors of childhood cancers (brain tumors) in some[269] but not all studies.[266,267,273] Insulin resistance in cancer survivors is associated with obesity, subnormal HDL levels, and hypertriglyceridemia, consistent with a diagnosis of metabolic syndrome.

Nontraditional risk factors, including von Willebrand factor (vWf), plasminogen activator inhibitor-1 (PAI-1), and C-reactive protein (CRP) plasma levels, are elevated in cancer survivors,[274] but data in this area are limited and concrete conclusions cannot be made. Direct confirmation of premature vascular disease can be acquired from imaging of the great arteries. In studies of young adult survivors of Hodgkin's disease who received neck irradiation, the incidence of abnormal carotid scans (26% versus 3%), and specifically carotid intima medial thickness (IMT), were increased compared with control subjects.[275] Long-term survivors of childhood brain tumors also show an increased IMT of the carotid bulb.[269]

BONE MARROW TRANSPLANTATION

Survival from childhood and adult hematologic malignancies has been improved by development of effective procedures for BMT, which is used primarily to treat poor-prognosis and relapsed leukemias, lymphoma, and myeloma. BMT encompasses allogeneic and autologous transplantation of stem cells from the bone marrow or peripheral blood. The complex treatment regimens employed before and during BMT to achieve such remarkable cure rates entails the use of combination chemotherapy (frequently encompassing high-dose alkylating agents), TBI, and immunosuppressive agents. The relative frequency of occurrence of long-term adverse sequelae from these regimens is greater than might be predicted from the individual components, suggesting synergism between the toxic effects of these treatment modalities on normal tissues.

Growth and Growth Hormone

Children who received TBI as part of the preparative regimen showed significant impairment of height velocity and height SDS.[276-281] Interpretation of the effect of TBI on height velocity is complicated by the frequent concomitant use of cranial irradiation before progression to BMT.[280,282] Both height and height velocity are impaired to a greater extent by the combination of cranial irradiation and TBI compared with TBI alone.[277,279-281] Single-fraction TBI (sfTBI) leads to greater impairment of growth than if TBI is fractionated (fTBI).[277,278,283] The adverse effect of TBI on growth is demonstrable within the first year after BMT in patients who additionally received cranial irradiation, but in the absence of cranial irradiation it may be delayed by several years.[279] Mean relative changes in height SDS between BMT and final height of children who received both cranial irradiation and sfTBI, sfTBI alone, fTBI, or no irradiation were −2.0, −1.4, −0.9, and −0.1, respectively.[284] The degree of height loss caused by TBI is greater when the radiation is administered at a younger age.[280,281]

TBI, in the absence of cranial radiation, results in GH insufficiency (peak stimulated GH level, <6.7 μg/L [<20 mU/L]) in 7% to 66% of recipients of childhood BMT; when only those children with growth failure are assessed, 60% to 95% are found to be GH insufficient.[52,276-279,282,285,286] The wide range of prevalence of GH insufficiency results from significant differences in study designs and patient populations. Evidence from comparison of the effects of sfTBI and fTBI suggests that fractionation of the radiation dose reduces the risk of developing GH insufficiency.[278] In the setting of impaired GH secretion secondary to TBI, GH replacement therapy significantly improves height velocity.[277,279,287] In contrast to observations in children, the radiation dosage employed during TBI (10 to 13.2 Gy) before BMT has not been shown to cause GHD when delivered during adult life.[126]

There are a number of skeletal sequelae in addition to reduced final height that may be present in the adult survivor of childhood BMT. Spinal disproportion has been reported to occur as a consequence of TBI received during childhood,[282,287] suggesting a greater inhibitory effect of TBI on the spine compared with the long bones. Spinal irradiation, corticosteroid therapy, sex steroid deficiency, and childhood GH insufficiency[105,288] are associated with reduced bone acquisition during childhood. There are no data on peak bone mass in adult survivors of childhood BMT, although the impaired bone acquisition is likely to result in lower than genetic peak bone mass, in the long term placing these individuals at risk for osteoporosis and fragility fractures. In young adult recipients of BMT, bone mineral density is transiently reduced at the spine and hip, but this tends to improve over the subsequent 2 years.[289]

Hypopituitarism

Although there is a large amount of available data concerning the GH axis after childhood BMT, there are far fewer data on the other anterior pituitary axes. Abnormalities of the cortisol axis were reported in up to 24% of patients as assessed by the metyrapone test; however, all of the patients were asymptomatic.[283] This finding probably reflects the characteristics of the test employed, which is plagued by false-positive results even in normal, healthy individuals. When assessed by ITT, the cortisol axis is found to be normal in all[276,278,279] or almost all patients.[52,285] When cortisol responses were found to be subnormal, the patients either had been taking or had recently taken corticosteroids for graft-versus-host disease.[285] If present, cortisol deficiency usually manifests late (5 to 10 years after irradiation).

The true prevalence of cortisol deficiency in adult long-term survivors of malignancy who underwent BMT during childhood is unclear. There are few data concerning prolactin levels in recipients of BMT, but elevated levels are usually infrequent, mild, and asymptomatic.[52,126] TBI (10 to 13.2 Gy) before BMT delivered during adult life has not been shown to cause hypopituitarism.[126]

Primary Thyroid Disorders

Thyroid function is abnormal in a significant percentage of childhood and adult survivors of BMT. As with GH insufficiency, there is a wide range of prevalence of thyroid dysfunction after childhood TBI (5% to 43%).[52,276,278,279,282,283,286] Subclinical hypothyroidism is much more frequently observed than overt hypothyroidism.[126,290] Thyroiditis and hyperthyroidism have also been described to occur after exposure of the thyroid to TBI.[290,291] Thyroid dysfunction develops more frequently in patients who received sfTBI than in those who received fTBI;[52,282,285] and it is more frequent in patients who received BMT at a younger age.[290] Although the frequency of abnormal thyroid function tests is relatively high, transient increases in TSH that resolve during follow-up are relatively common.[282,285,290]

Where the thyroid has been exposed to radiation, it is at greater risk for development of both benign thyroid nodules and carcinoma.[225-227] The standard incidence ratio (SIR) for development of thyroid carcinoma after BMT with TBI preconditioning is sevenfold to eightfold higher than in the general population, and the risk is significantly greater when irradiation occurs at a younger age (Fig. 43-10).[292,293] The latency period from BMT to diagnosis of thyroid carcinoma is usually in excess of 5 years, but cases have been reported within the first few years after TBI.[292-294] Almost all cases manifest subclinically.[294] Histologically, most of these thyroid carcinomas are papillary, with the remainder being follicular.[292,294]

TSH is a trophic factor for thyroid cell growth, and in established DTC suppression of TSH with levothyroxine reduces recurrence and mortality rates. In patients who have received TBI, the elevated TSH in subclinical hypothyroidism is thought to be an etiologic factor in the development of thyroid carcinoma; therefore, it is recommended that these patients receive levothyroxine replacement. Given the potential transient nature of subclinical hypothyroidism after BMT, a significant proportion of patients will be able to discontinue the levothyroxine at a later date. There are no data on the success of levothyroxine withdrawal after earlier treatment of subclinical hypothyroidism resulting from TBI.

Gonadal Failure

The ovaries are exquisitely sensitive to radiation damage. TBI (10 to 15 Gy) used in combination with gonadotoxic chemotherapy almost invariably results in ovarian failure (Fig. 43-11).[52,126,295] Ovarian failure during childhood results

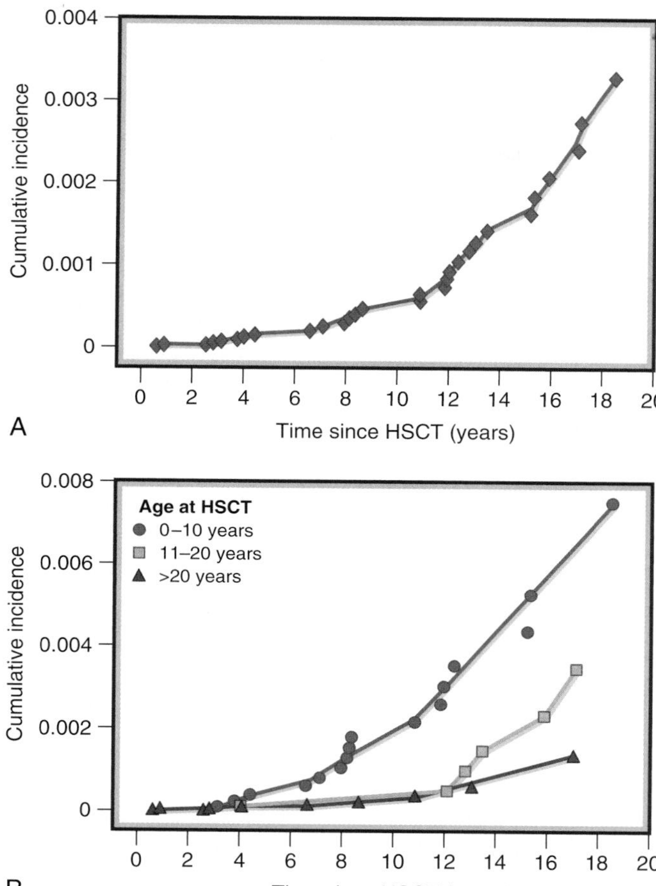

Figure 43-10 **A,** Cumulative incidence of thyroid cancer after hematopoietic stem cell transplantation (HSCT). **B,** Cumulative incidence of thyroid cancer by age at the time of HSCT. (From Cohen A, Rovelli A, Merlo DF, et al. Risk for secondary thyroid carcinoma after hematopoietic stem-cell transplantation: an EBMT Late Effects Working Party Study. *J Clin Oncol.* 2007;25:2449-2454.)

in either delayed or failed progression through puberty[276,283] and renders almost all postpubertal women amenorrheic.[283,295] Characteristically, gonadotropin levels are elevated and estradiol levels are low.[52,276,282,283] Short-term ovarian recovery is recognized to occur during the first few years after regimens inclusive of TBI (see Fig. 43-11).[295] Recovery occurs in at least 50% of prepubertal girls who receive high-dose chemotherapy and hyperfractionated TBI, allowing progression of puberty and spontaneous menstruation.[296,297] With advancing age at treatment, recovery is increasingly infrequent.[295] Rarely, ovarian recovery occurs after a significant period of amenorrhea. It has been suggested that fTBI may be less damaging to the ovaries than sfTBI.[285] Female survivors of BMT during adolescence or young adult life experience significant symptoms of estrogen deficiency including hot flushes, night sweats, and vaginal dryness.[298] They additionally express concerns over infertility, amenorrhea, and femininity. Libido is impaired in most of these patients, and coitus becomes painful with orgasm difficult to achieve.[298,299] The consequence of direct radiation damage to the uterus and estrogen deficiency results in poor development of the uterus, which may not enlarge appropriately in response to estrogen replacement therapy.[276]

Estrogen replacement therapy significantly improves the symptoms of estrogen deficiency in the majority of hypogonadal young women,[25] and it should also be considered to maintain bone mass and potentially improve long-term vascular outcomes. There are no comparative data on sexual health in survivors of childhood BMT taking estrogen replacement therapy compared with normal individuals. Breast cancer risk is elevated in survivors of BMT (SIR, 2.2), the risk increasing with duration of survival, younger age at transplantation, and TBI.[189] There are no data on whether estrogen replacement further elevates the risk of breast cancer. Intuitively, it is appropriate to replace estrogen to physiologic levels, which would be unlikely to increase the risk beyond that observed in women who retain normal ovarian function. All women who have received TBI during BMT, regardless of estrogen replacement status, should be enrolled in a breast cancer screening program.

In boys, the germinal epithelium is significantly more sensitive to radiation than the Leydig cells. As a consequence, testosterone production is usually maintained, and puberty progresses normally.[52,280,297] Testicular volumes are small, reflecting the damage to the germinal epithelium.[52] Biochemically, FSH is elevated in most peripubertal and pubertal boys (68% to 90%),[52,283] and LH is elevated in 40% to 50%,[52,283] whereas testosterone levels are infrequently low (0% to 16%).[52,126,283] There are no robust data documenting sperm counts during adult life to determine what

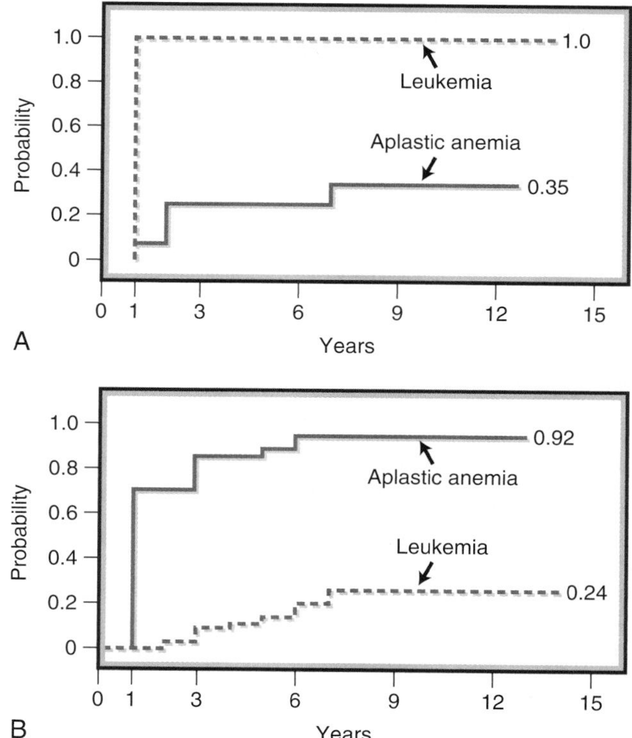

Figure 43-11 **A,** The probability of developing ovarian failure as determined by the first elevated LH/FSH levels beginning at 1 year after hematopoietic stem cell transplantation. **B,** The probability of recovery of normal ovarian function as determined by first normal LH/FSH levels beginning at 1 year after transplantation. FSH, follicle-stimulating hormone; LH, luteinizing hormone. (From Sanders JE, Buckner CD, Amos D, et al. Ovarian function following marrow transplantation for aplastic anemia or leukemia. *J Clin Oncol.* 1988;6:813-818.)

proportion of boys receiving BMT are spontaneously fertile or fertile with the help of assisted fertility techniques.

Severe oligospermia or azoospermia, associated with testicular volumes below the normal range and normal testosterone levels, is expected after TBI during adult life.[126] Sterility is not universal,[126] and patients should be advised with respect to contraception. Adult men commonly report an adverse impact on long-term sexual functioning after BMT, although to a lesser degree than women.[299]

Effects of Chemotherapy-Only Preparatory Regimens

Children who undergo BMT having received only chemotherapy during their preparative regimen, without preceding irradiation, experience no adverse effects on height or height velocity SDS.[276,279,284] In fact, catch-up growth after BMT is a frequent observation in these individuals,[276,278] and final height is not significantly affected.[284] GH stimulation tests in children who were growing normally after preconditioning with chemotherapy alone showed appropriate responses.[278,300] Impaired stimulated GH responses have been reported occasionally after chemotherapy-alone preparatory regimens administered during childhood.[279,301] The class of drugs involved and the mechanisms for this result remain unclear. Whether the abrogated GH responses relate to inadequate or inappropriate assessment of the GH axis is unclear. The cortisol axis and thyroid function are unaffected in children receiving chemotherapy alone for preconditioning.[276,278,279,290,300] The relative risk for development of thyroid cancer with BMT regimens that do not include TBI is not significantly elevated.[292,294]

Permanent gonadal damage is uncommon in children, with most patients progressing through puberty spontaneously.[276] Gonadotoxic agents including cyclophosphamide, busulfan, and ARA-C have a dose-dependent toxic effect on the male germinal epithelium, with a high incidence of transient or permanent oligospermia or azospermia.[296] Mild Leydig cell dysfunction, characterized by compensated hypergonadotropic hypogonadism, is frequently observed, but puberty is usually completed without the need for testosterone replacement therapy.[296]

Most adult women who undergo cyclophosphamide-based preparatory regimens are rendered amenorrheic with elevated gonadotropins.[291,295,302] Return of menses and normalization of the gonadotropins occurs in most cases, with a median duration of 6 months (see Fig. 43-11).[295] The likelihood of ovarian recovery is age related, with younger individuals having the more promising outlook.[295,302] However, many individuals will have received gonadotoxic treatments prior to going forward with BMT, and the cumulative effect of these therapies has a significant impact on recovery rates.[302] Recovery of reproductive function in older individuals (>25 years) is more likely to be transient, although frequently menses can be present for several years before the onset of a premature menopause.[295]

REFERENCES

1. Stiller CA. Population based survival rates for childhood cancer in Britain, 1980-91. *BMJ*. 1994;309:1612-1616.
2. Roy P, Vaughan Hudson G, et al. Long-term survival in Hodgkin's disease patients: a comparison of relative survival in patients in trials and those recorded in population-based cancer registries. *Eur J Cancer*. 2000;36:384-389.
3. Urba WJ, Longo DL. Hodgkin's disease. *N Engl J Med*. 1992;326:678-687.
4. Leung W, Hudson MM, Strickland DK, et al. Late effects of treatment in survivors of childhood acute myeloid leukemia. *J Clin Oncol*. 2000;18:3273-3279.
5. National Health Service Department of Health, Macmillan Cancer Support. *NHS Improvement: The National Cancer Survivorship Initiative Vision*. London, UK: NHS; 2010 www.ncsi.org/uk/wp-content/uploads/NCSI-Vision-Document.pdf.
6. Gurney JG, Kadan-Lottick NS, Packer RJ, et al. Endocrine and cardiovascular late effects among adult survivors of childhood brain tumors: Childhood Cancer Survivor Study. *Cancer*. 2003;97:663-673.
7. Mosier HD Jr, Jansons RA. Stunted growth in rats following x-irradiation of the head. *Growth*. 1967;31:139-148.
8. Yamazaki JN, Bennett LR, McFall RA, et al. Brain radiation in newborn rats and differential effects of increased age: I. Clinical observations. *Neurology*. 1960;10:530-536.
9. Onoyama Y, Abe M, Takahashi M, et al. Radiation therapy of brain tumors in children. *Radiology*. 1975;115:687-693.
10. Bamford FN, Jones PM, Pearson D, et al. Residual disabilities in children treated for intracranial space-occupying lesions. *Cancer*. 1976;37:1149-1151.
11. Kirk JA, Raghupathy P, Stevens MM, et al. Growth failure and growth-hormone deficiency after treatment for acute lymphoblastic leukaemia. *Lancet*. 1987;1:190-193.
12. Davies HA, Didcock E, Didi M, et al. Disproportionate short stature after cranial irradiation and combination chemotherapy for leukaemia. *Arch Dis Child*. 1994;70:472-475.
13. Gurney JG, Ness KK, Stovall M, et al. Final height and body mass index among adult survivors of childhood brain cancer: Childhood Cancer Survivor Study. *J Clin Endocrinol Metab*. 2003;88:4731-4739.
14. Olshan JS, Gubernick J, Packer RJ, et al. The effects of adjuvant chemotherapy on growth in children with medulloblastoma. *Cancer*. 1992;70:2013-2017.
15. Ogilvy-Stuart AL, Shalet SM. Growth and puberty after growth hormone treatment after irradiation for brain tumours. *Arch Dis Child*. 1995;73:141-146.
16. Robison LL, Nesbit ME Jr, Sather HN, et al. Height of children successfully treated for acute lymphoblastic leukemia: a report from the Late Effects Study Committee of Childrens Cancer Study Group. *Med Pediatr Oncol*. 1985;13:14-1321.
17. Shalet SM, Price DA, Beardwell CG, et al. Normal growth despite abnormalities of growth hormone secretion in children treated for acute leukemia. *J Pediatr*. 1979;94:719-722.
18. Shalet SM, Gibson B, Swindell R, et al. Effect of spinal irradiation on growth. *Arch Dis Child*. 1987;62:461-464.
19. Wallace WH, Shalet SM, Morris-Jones PH, et al. Effect of abdominal irradiation on growth in boys treated for a Wilms' tumor. *Med Pediatr Oncol*. 1990;18:441-446.
20. Adan L, Souberbielle JC, Blanche S, et al. Adult height after cranial irradiation with 24 Gy: factors and markers of height loss. *Acta Paediatr*. 1996;85:1096-1101.
21. Ogilvy-Stuart AL, Clayton PE, Shalet SM. Cranial irradiation and early puberty. *J Clin Endocrinol Metab*. 1994;78:1282-1286.
22. Gleeson HK, Stoeter R, Ogilvy-Stuart AL, et al. Improvements in final height over 25 years in growth hormone (GH)-deficient childhood survivors of brain tumors receiving GH replacement. *J Clin Endocrinol Metab*. 2003;88:3682-3689.
23. Swift PG, Kearney PJ, Dalton RG, et al. Growth and hormonal status of children treated for acute lymphoblastic leukaemia. *Arch Dis Child*. 1978;53:890-894.
24. Cicognani A, Cacciari E, Vecchi V, et al. Differential effects of 18- and 24-Gy cranial irradiation on growth rate and growth hormone release in children with prolonged survival after acute lymphocytic leukemia. *Am J Dis Child*. 1988;142:1199-1202.
25. Clayton PE, Shalet SM, Price DA. Growth response to growth hormone therapy following craniospinal irradiation. *Eur J Pediatr*. 1988;147:597-601.
26. Adan L, Sainte-Rose C, Souberbielle JC, et al. Adult height after growth hormone (GH) treatment for GH deficiency due to cranial irradiation. *Med Pediatr Oncol*. 2000;34:14-19.
27. Leung W, Rose SR, Zhou Y, et al. Outcomes of growth hormone replacement therapy in survivors of childhood acute lymphoblastic leukemia. *J Clin Oncol*. 2002;20:2959-2964.
28. Sklar CA, Mertens AC, Mitby P, et al. Risk of disease recurrence and second neoplasms in survivors of childhood cancer treated with growth hormone: a report from the Childhood Cancer Survivor Study. *J Clin Endocrinol Metab*. 2002;87:3136-3141.
29. Swerdlow AJ, Reddingius RE, Higgins CD, et al. Growth hormone treatment of children with brain tumors and risk of tumor recurrence. *J Clin Endocrinol Metab*. 2000;85:4444-4449.
30. Ogilvy-Stuart AL. Safety of growth hormone after treatment of a childhood malignancy. *Horm Res*. 1995;44(suppl 3):73-79.
31. Ogilvy-Stuart AL, Ryder WD, Gattamaneni HR, et al. Growth hormone and tumour recurrence. *BMJ*. 1992;304:1601-1605.
32. Shalet SM. Radiation and pituitary dysfunction. *N Engl J Med*. 1993;328:131-133.
33. Lam KS, Tse VK, Wang C, et al. Effects of cranial irradiation on hypothalamic-pituitary function: a 5-year longitudinal study in patients with nasopharyngeal carcinoma. *Q J Med*. 1991;78:165-176.

34. Littley MD, Shalet SM, Beardwell CG, et al. Hypopituitarism following external radiotherapy for pituitary tumours in adults. *Q J Med.* 1989;70:145-160.
35. Littley MD, Shalet SM, Beardwell CG, et al. Radiation-induced hypopituitarism is dose-dependent. *Clin Endocrinol (Oxf).* 1989;31:363-373.
36. Pai HH, Thornton A, Katznelson L, et al. Hypothalamic/pituitary function following high-dose conformal radiotherapy to the base of skull: demonstration of a dose-effect relationship using dose-volume histogram analysis. *Int J Radiat Oncol Biol Phys.* 2001;49:1079-1092.
37. Jadresic A, Jimenez LE, Joplin GF. Long-term effect of 90Y pituitary implantation in acromegaly. *Acta Endocrinol (Copenh).* 1987;115:301-306.
38. Lam KS, Ho JH, Lee AW, et al. Symptomatic hypothalamic-pituitary dysfunction in nasopharyngeal carcinoma patients following radiation therapy: a retrospective study. *Int J Radiat Oncol Biol Phys.* 1987;13:1343-1350.
39. Schmiegelow M, Lassen S, Poulsen HS, et al. Growth hormone response to a growth hormone-releasing hormone stimulation test in a population-based study following cranial irradiation of childhood brain tumors. *Horm Res.* 2000;54:53-59.
40. Darzy KH, Pezzoli SS, Thorner MO, et al. The dynamics of growth hormone (GH) secretion in adult cancer survivors with severe GH deficiency acquired after brain irradiation in childhood for nonpituitary brain tumors: evidence for preserved pulsatility and diurnal variation with increased secretory disorderliness. *J Clin Endocrinol Metab.* 2005;90:2794-2803.
41. Chieng PU, Huang TS, Chang CC, et al. Reduced hypothalamic blood flow after radiation treatment of nasopharyngeal cancer: SPECT studies in 34 patients. *AJNR Am J Neuroradiol.* 1991;12:661-665.
42. Schneider HJ, Rovere S, Corneli G, et al. Endocrine dysfunction in patients operated on for non-pituitary intracranial tumors. *Eur J Endocrinol.* 2006;155:559-566.
43. Bhandare N, Kennedy L, Malyapa RS, et al. Hypopituitarism after radiotherapy for extracranial head and neck cancers. *Head Neck.* 2008;30:1182-1192.
44. Constine LS, Woolf PD, Cann D, et al. Hypothalamic-pituitary dysfunction after radiation for brain tumors. *N Engl J Med.* 1993;328:87-94.
45. Hoeck HC, Vestergaard P, Jakobsen PE, et al. Test of growth hormone secretion in adults: poor reproducibility of the insulin tolerance test. *Eur J Endocrinol.* 1995;133:305-312.
46. Rahim A, Toogood AA, Shalet SM. The assessment of growth hormone status in normal young adult males using a variety of provocative agents. *Clin Endocrinol (Oxf).* 1996;45:557-562.
47. Bhandare N, Kennedy L, Malyapa RS, et al. Hypopituitarism after radiotherapy for extracranial head and neck cancers in pediatric patients. *Am J Clin Oncol.* 2008;31:567-572.
48. Robinson IC, Fairhall KM, Hendry JH, et al. Differential radiosensitivity of hypothalamo-pituitary function in the young adult rat. *J Endocrinol.* 2001;169:519-526.
49. Hochberg Z, Kuten A, Hertz P, et al. The effect of single-dose radiation on cell survival and growth hormone secretion by rat anterior pituitary cells. *Radiat Res.* 1983;94:508-512.
50. Darzy KH, Shalet SM. Hypopituitarism following radiotherapy. *Pituitary.* 2009;12:40-50.
51. Clayton PE, Shalet SM. Dose dependency of time of onset of radiation-induced growth hormone deficiency. *J Pediatr.* 1991;118:226-228.
52. Ogilvy-Stuart AL, Clark DJ, Wallace WH, et al. Endocrine deficit after fractionated total body irradiation. *Arch Dis Child.* 1992;67:1107-1110.
53. Shalet SM, Beardwell CG, Pearson D, et al. The effect of varying doses of cerebral irradiation on growth hormone production in childhood. *Clin Endocrinol (Oxf).* 1976;5:287-290.
54. Shalet SM, Beardwell CG, Twomey JA, et al. Endocrine function following the treatment of acute leukemia in childhood. *J Pediatr.* 1977;90:920-923.
55. Shalet SM, Beardwell CG, Morris-Jones PH, et al. Pituitary function after treatment of intracranial tumours in children. *Lancet.* 1975;2:104-107.
56. Duffner PK, Cohen ME, Voorhess ML, et al. Long-term effects of cranial irradiation on endocrine function in children with brain tumors: a prospective study. *Cancer.* 1985;56:2189-2193.
57. Schmiegelow M, Lassen S, Poulsen HS, et al. Cranial radiotherapy of childhood brain tumours: growth hormone deficiency and its relation to the biological effective dose of irradiation in a large population based study. *Clin Endocrinol (Oxf).* 2000;53:191-197.
58. Shalet SM, Beardwell CG, Jones PH, et al. Growth hormone deficiency after treatment of acute leukaemia in children. *Arch Dis Child.* 1976;51:489-493.
59. Brennan BM, Rahim A, Mackie EM, et al. Growth hormone status in adults treated for acute lymphoblastic leukaemia in childhood. *Clin Endocrinol (Oxf).* 1998;48:777-783.
60. Blatt J, Bercu BB, Gillin JC, et al. Reduced pulsatile growth hormone secretion in children after therapy for acute lymphoblastic leukemia. *J Pediatr.* 1984;104:182-186.
61. Spoudeas HA, Hindmarsh PC, Matthews DR, et al. Evolution of growth hormone neurosecretory disturbance after cranial irradiation for childhood brain tumours: a prospective study. *J Endocrinol.* 1996;150:329-342.
62. Moell C, Garwicz S, Westgren U, et al. Disturbed pubertal growth in girls treated for acute lymphoblastic leukemia. *Pediatr Hematol Oncol.* 1987;4:1-5.
63. Moell C, Garwicz S, Westgren U, et al. Suppressed spontaneous secretion of growth hormone in girls after treatment for acute lymphoblastic leukaemia. *Arch Dis Child.* 1989;64:252-258.
64. Giustina A, Veldhuis JD. Pathophysiology of the neuroregulation of growth hormone secretion in experimental animals and the human. *Endocr Rev.* 1998;19:717-797.
65. Rose SR, Municchi G, Barnes KM, et al. Spontaneous growth hormone secretion increases during puberty in normal girls and boys. *J Clin Endocrinol Metab.* 1991;73:428-435.
66. Nesbit ME Jr, Sather HN, Robison LL, et al. Presymptomatic central nervous system therapy in previously untreated childhood acute lymphoblastic leukaemia: comparison of 1800 rad and 2400 rad. A report for Children's Cancer Study Group. *Lancet.* 1981;1:461-466.
67. Crowne EC, Moore C, Wallace WH, et al. A novel variant of growth hormone (GH) insufficiency following low dose cranial irradiation. *Clin Endocrinol (Oxf).* 1992;36:59-68.
68. Willoughby JO, Terry LC, Brazeau P, et al. Pulsatile growth hormone, prolactin, and thyrotropin secretion in rats with hypothalamic deafferentation. *Brain Res.* 1977;127:137-152.
69. Jorgensen JO, Pedersen SA, Thuesen L, et al. Beneficial effects of growth hormone treatment in GH-deficient adults. *Lancet.* 1989;1:1221-1225.
70. Salomon F, Cuneo RC, Hesp R, et al. The effects of treatment with recombinant human growth hormone on body composition and metabolism in adults with growth hormone deficiency. *N Engl J Med.* 1989;321:1797-1803.
71. Carroll PV, Christ ER, Bengtsson BA, et al. Growth hormone deficiency in adulthood and the effects of growth hormone replacement: a review. Growth Hormone Research Society Scientific Committee. *J Clin Endocrinol Metab.* 1998;83:382-395.
72. Murray RD, Skillicorn CJ, Howell SJ, et al. Dose titration and patient selection increases the efficacy of GH replacement in severely GH deficient adults. *Clin Endocrinol (Oxf).* 1999;50:749-757.
73. Drake WM, Coyte D, Camacho-Hubner C, et al. Optimizing growth hormone replacement therapy by dose titration in hypopituitary adults. *J Clin Endocrinol Metab.* 1998;83:3913-3919.
74. Toogood AA, Ryder WD, Beardwell CG, et al. The evolution of radiation-induced growth hormone deficiency in adults is determined by the baseline growth hormone status. *Clin Endocrinol (Oxf).* 1995;43:97-103.
75. Lam KS, Tse VK, Wang C, et al. Early effects of cranial irradiation on hypothalamic-pituitary function. *J Clin Endocrinol Metab.* 1987;64:418-424.
76. Darzy KH, Pezzoli SS, Thorner MO, et al. Cranial irradiation and growth hormone neurosecretory dysfunction: a critical appraisal. *J Clin Endocrinol Metab.* 2007;92:1666-1672.
77. Darzy KH, Murray RD, Gleeson HK, et al. The impact of short-term fasting on the dynamics of 24-hour growth hormone (GH) secretion in patients with severe radiation-induced GH deficiency. *J Clin Endocrinol Metab.* 2006;91:987-994.
78. Darzy KH, Thorner MO, Shalet SM. Cranially irradiated adult cancer survivors may have normal spontaneous GH secretion in the presence of discordant peak GH responses to stimulation tests (compensated GH deficiency). *Clin Endocrinol (Oxf).* 2009;70:287-293.
79. Ho PJ, Kletter GB, Hopwood NJ, et al. Somatostatin withdrawal alone is an ineffective generator of pulsatile growth hormone release in man. *Acta Endocrinol (Copenh).* 1993;129:414-418.
80. Veldhuis JD, Anderson SM, Shah N, et al. Neurophysiological regulation and target-tissue impact of the pulsatile mode of growth hormone secretion in the human. *Growth HormIGF Res.* 2001;11(suppl A):S25-S37.
81. Lam KS, Wang C, Yeung RT, et al. Hypothalamic hypopituitarism following cranial irradiation for nasopharyngeal carcinoma. *Clin Endocrinol (Oxf).* 1986;24:643-651.
82. Agha A, Sherlock M, Brennan S, et al. Hypothalamic-pituitary dysfunction after irradiation of nonpituitary brain tumors in adults. *J Clin Endocrinol Metab.* 2005;90:6355-6360.
83. Brauner R, Rappaport R, Prevot C, et al. A prospective study of the development of growth hormone deficiency in children given cranial irradiation, and its relation to statural growth. *J Clin Endocrinol Metab.* 1989;68:346-351.
84. Samaan NA, Schultz PN, Yang KP, et al. Endocrine complications after radiotherapy for tumors of the head and neck. *J Lab Clin Med.* 1987;109:364-372.

85. Shalet SM, Toogood A, Rahim A, et al. The diagnosis of growth hormone deficiency in children and adults. *Endocr Rev.* 1998;19:203-223.
86. Consensus guidelines for the diagnosis and treatment of adults with growth hormone deficiency: summary statement of the Growth Hormone Research Society Workshop on Adult Growth Hormone Deficiency. *J Clin Endocrinol Metab.* 1998;83:379-381.
87. Ho KK. Consensus guidelines for the diagnosis and treatment of adults with GH deficiency II: a statement of the GH Research Society in association with the European Society for Pediatric Endocrinology, Lawson Wilkins Society, European Society of Endocrinology, Japan Endocrine Society, and Endocrine Society of Australia. *Eur J Endocrinol.* 2007;157:695-700.
88. Shah A, Stanhope R, Matthew D. Hazards of pharmacological tests of growth hormone secretion in childhood. *BMJ.* 1992;304:173-174.
89. Lipshultz SE, Lipsitz SR, Sallan SE, et al. Chronic progressive cardiac dysfunction years after doxorubicin therapy for childhood acute lymphoblastic leukemia. *J Clin Oncol.* 2005;23:2629-2636.
90. Kremer LC, van Dalen EC, Offringa M, et al. Frequency and risk factors of anthracycline-induced clinical heart failure in children: a systematic review. *Ann Oncol.* 2002;13:503-512.
91. Kremer LC, van der Pal HJ, Offringa M, et al. Frequency and risk factors of subclinical cardiotoxicity after anthracycline therapy in children: a systematic review. *Ann Oncol.* 2002;13:819-829.
92. Lissett CA, Saleem S, Rahim A, et al. The impact of irradiation on growth hormone responsiveness to provocative agents is stimulus dependent: results in 161 individuals with radiation damage to the somatotropic axis. *J Clin Endocrinol Metab.* 2001;86:663-668.
93. Darzy KH, Aimaretti G, Wieringa G, et al. The usefulness of the combined growth hormone (GH)-releasing hormone and arginine stimulation test in the diagnosis of radiation-induced GH deficiency is dependent on the post-irradiation time interval. *J Clin Endocrinol Metab.* 2003;88:95-102.
94. Bjork J, Link K, Erfurth EM. The utility of the growth hormone (GH) releasing hormone-arginine test for diagnosing GH deficiency in adults with childhood acute lymphoblastic leukemia treated with cranial irradiation. *J Clin Endocrinol Metab.* 2005;90:6048-6054.
95. Achermann JC, Brook CG, Hindmarsh PC. The GH response to low-dose bolus growth hormone-releasing hormone (GHRH(1-29)NH2) is attenuated in patients with longstanding post-irradiation GH insufficiency. *Eur J Endocrinol.* 2000;142:359-364.
96. Ham JN, Ginsberg JP, Hendell CD, et al. Growth hormone releasing hormone plus arginine stimulation testing in young adults treated in childhood with cranio-spinal radiation therapy. *Clin Endocrinol (Oxf).* 2005;62:628-632.
97. Hoffman DM, O'Sullivan AJ, Baxter RC, et al. Diagnosis of growth-hormone deficiency in adults. *Lancet.* 1994;343:1064-1068.
98. Murray RD, Brennan BM, Rahim A, et al. Survivors of childhood cancer: long-term endocrine and metabolic problems dwarf the growth disturbance. *Acta Paediatr Suppl.* 1999;88:5-12.
99. Murray RD, Darzy KH, Gleeson HK, et al. GH-deficient survivors of childhood cancer: GH replacement during adult life. *J Clin Endocrinol Metab.* 2002;87:129-135.
100. Mukherjee A, Tolhurst-Cleaver S, Ryder WD, et al. The characteristics of quality of life impairment in adult growth hormone (GH)-deficient survivors of cancer and their response to GH replacement therapy. *J Clin Endocrinol Metab.* 2005;90:1542-1549.
101. Attanasio AF, Shavrikova E, Blum WF, et al. Continued growth hormone (GH) treatment after final height is necessary to complete somatic development in childhood-onset GH-deficient patients. *J Clin Endocrinol Metab.* 2004;89:4857-4862.
102. Shalet SM, Shavrikova E, Cromer M, et al. Effect of growth hormone (GH) treatment on bone in postpubertal GH-deficient patients: a 2-year randomized, controlled, dose-ranging study. *J Clin Endocrinol Metab.* 2003;88:4124-4129.
103. Gleeson HK, Gattamaneni HR, Smethurst L, et al. Reassessment of growth hormone status is required at final height in children treated with growth hormone replacement after radiation therapy. *J Clin Endocrinol Metab.* 2004;89:662-666.
104. Clayton PE, Cuneo RC, Juul A, et al. Consensus statement on the management of the GH-treated adolescent in the transition to adult care. *Eur J Endocrinol.* 2005;152:165-170.
105. Murray RD, Adams JE, Smethurst LE, et al. Spinal irradiation impairs the osteo-anabolic effects of low-dose GH replacement in adults with childhood-onset GH deficiency. *Clin Endocrinol (Oxf).* 2002;56:169-174.
106. Chan JM, Stampfer MJ, Giovannucci E, et al. Plasma insulin-like growth factor-I and prostate cancer risk: a prospective study. *Science.* 1998;279:563-566.
107. Hankinson SE, Willett WC, Colditz GA, et al. Circulating concentrations of insulin-like growth factor-I and risk of breast cancer. *Lancet.* 1998;351:1393-1396.
108. Jenkins PJ, Fairclough PD, Richards T, et al. Acromegaly, colonic polyps and carcinoma. *Clin Endocrinol (Oxf).* 1997;47:17-22.
109. Estrov Z, Meir R, Barak Y, et al. Human growth hormone and insulin-like growth factor-1 enhance the proliferation of human leukemic blasts. *J Clin Oncol.* 1991;9:394-399.
110. Chung TT, Drake WM, Evanson J, et al. Tumour surveillance imaging in patients with extrapituitary tumours receiving growth hormone replacement. *Clin Endocrinol (Oxf).* 2005;63:274-279.
111. Harrop JS, Davies TJ, Capra LG, et al. Hypothalamic-pituitary function following successful treatment of intracranial tumours. *Clin Endocrinol (Oxf).* 1976;5:313-321.
112. Perry-Keene DA, Connelly JF, Young RA, et al. Hypothalamic hypopituitarism following external radiotherapy for tumours distant from the adenohypophysis. *Clin Endocrinol (Oxf).* 1976;5:373-380.
113. Brauner R, Czernichow P, Rappaport R. Greater susceptibility to hypothalamopituitary irradiation in younger children with acute lymphoblastic leukemia. *J Pediatr.* 1986;108:332.
114. Kanumakala S, Warne GL, Zacharin MR. Evolving hypopituitarism following cranial irradiation. *J Paediatr Child Health.* 2003;39:232-235.
115. Withers HR. Biology of radiation oncology. In: Tobias JS, Thomas PR, eds. *Current Radiation Oncology.* London, UK: Edward Arnold; 1994:5-23.
116. Brada M, Rajan B, Traish D, et al. The long-term efficacy of conservative surgery and radiotherapy in the control of pituitary adenomas. *Clin Endocrinol (Oxf).* 1993;38:571-578.
117. Snyers A, Janssens GO, Twickler MB, et al. Malignant tumors of the nasal cavity and paranasal sinuses: long-term outcome and morbidity with emphasis on hypothalamic-pituitary deficiency. *Int J Radiat Oncol Biol Phys.* 2009;73:1343-1351.
118. Woo E, Lam K, Yu YL, et al. Temporal lobe and hypothalamic-pituitary dysfunctions after radiotherapy for nasopharyngeal carcinoma: a distinct clinical syndrome. *J Neurol Neurosurg Psychiatry.* 1988;51:1302-1307.
119. Samaan NA, Vieto R, Schultz PN, et al. Hypothalamic, pituitary and thyroid dysfunction after radiotherapy to the head and neck. *Int J Radiat Oncol Biol Phys.* 1982;8:1857-1867.
120. Gross KM, Matsumoto AM, Southworth MB, et al. Evidence for decreased luteinizing hormone-releasing hormone pulse frequency in men with selective elevations of follicle-stimulating hormone. *J Clin Endocrinol Metab.* 1985;60:197-202.
121. Wildt L, Hausler A, Marshall G, et al. Frequency and amplitude of gonadotropin-releasing hormone stimulation and gonadotropin secretion in the rhesus monkey. *Endocrinology.* 1981;109:376-385.
122. Hall JE, Martin KA, Whitney HA, et al. Potential for fertility with replacement of hypothalamic gonadotropin-releasing hormone in long term female survivors of cranial tumors. *J Clin Endocrinol Metab.* 1994;79:1166-1172.
123. Brauner R, Rappaport R. Precocious puberty secondary to cranial irradiation for tumors distant from the hypothalamo-pituitary area. *Horm Res.* 1985;22:78-82.
124. Leiper AD, Stanhope R, Kitching P, et al. Precocious and premature puberty associated with treatment of acute lymphoblastic leukaemia. *Arch Dis Child.* 1987;62:1107-1112.
125. Livesey EA, Hindmarsh PC, Brook CG, et al. Endocrine disorders following treatment of childhood brain tumours. *Br J Cancer.* 1990;61:622-625.
126. Littley MD, Shalet SM, Morgenstern GR, et al. Endocrine and reproductive dysfunction following fractionated total body irradiation in adults. *Q J Med.* 1991;78:265-274.
127. Darzy KH, Shalet SM. Absence of adrenocorticotropin (ACTH) neurosecretory dysfunction but increased cortisol concentrations and production rates in ACTH-replete adult cancer survivors after cranial irradiation for nonpituitary brain tumors. *J Clin Endocrinol Metab.* 2005;90:5217-5225.
128. Lee KO, Persani L, Tan M, et al. Thyrotropin with decreased biological activity, a delayed consequence of cranial irradiation for nasopharyngeal carcinoma. *J Endocrinol Invest.* 1995;18:800-805.
129. Darzy KH, Shalet SM. Circadian and stimulated thyrotropin secretion in cranially irradiated adult cancer survivors. *J Clin Endocrinol Metab.* 2005;90:6490-6497.
130. Rose SR, Lustig RH, Pitukcheewanont P, et al. Diagnosis of hidden central hypothyroidism in survivors of childhood cancer. *J Clin Endocrinol Metab.* 1999;84:4472-4479.
131. Oberfield SE, Allen JC, Pollack J, et al. Long-term endocrine sequelae after treatment of medulloblastoma: prospective study of growth and thyroid function. *J Pediatr.* 1986;108:219-223.
132. Mohn A, Chiarelli F, Di Marzio A, et al. Thyroid function in children treated for acute lymphoblastic leukemia. *J Endocrinol Invest.* 1997;20:215-219.
133. Carter EP, Leiper AD, Chessells JM, et al. Thyroid function in children after treatment for acute lymphoblastic leukaemia. *Arch Dis Child.* 1989;64:631.
134. Voorhess ML, Brecher ML, Glicksman AS, et al. Hypothalamic-pituitary function of children with acute lymphocytic leukemia after three forms of central nervous system prophylaxis: a retrospective study. *Cancer.* 1986;57:1287-1291.

135. Bhandare N, Kennedy L, Malyapa RS, et al. Primary and central hypothyroidism after radiotherapy for head-and-neck tumors. *Int J Radiat Oncol Biol Phys*. 2007;68:1131-1139.
136. Howell SJ, Shalet SM. Effect of cancer therapy on pituitary-testicular axis. *Int J Androl*. 2002;25:269-276.
137. Rivkees SA, Crawford JD. The relationship of gonadal activity and chemotherapy-induced gonadal damage. *JAMA*. 1988;259:2123-2125.
138. Ortin TT, Shostak CA, Donaldson SS. Gonadal status and reproductive function following treatment for Hodgkin's disease in childhood: the Stanford experience. *Int J Radiat Oncol Biol Phys*. 1990;19:873-880.
139. Chemaitilly W, Mertens AC, Mitby P, et al. Acute ovarian failure in the childhood cancer survivor study. *J Clin Endocrinol Metab*. 2006;91:1723-1728.
140. Byrne J, Fears TR, Gail MH, et al. Early menopause in long-term survivors of cancer during adolescence. *Am J Obstet Gynecol*. 1992;166:788-793.
141. Rowley MJ, Leach DR, Warner GA, et al. Effect of graded doses of ionizing radiation on the human testis. *Radiat Res*. 1974;59:665-678.
142. Shalet SM. Effect of irradiation treatment on gonadal function in men treated for germ cell cancer. *Eur Urol*. 1993;23:148-151; discussion 152.
143. Pedrick TJ, Hoppe RT. Recovery of spermatogenesis following pelvic irradiation for Hodgkin's disease. *Int J Radiat Oncol Biol Phys*. 1986;12:117-121.
144. Centola GM, Keller JW, Henzler M, et al. Effect of low-dose testicular irradiation on sperm count and fertility in patients with testicular seminoma. *J Androl*. 1994;15:608-613.
145. Mulder JE. Benefits and risks of hormone replacement therapy in young adult cancer survivors with gonadal failure. *Med Pediatr Oncol*. 1999;33:46-52.
146. van der Kaaij MA, Heutte N, Le Stang N, et al. Gonadal function in males after chemotherapy for early-stage Hodgkin's lymphoma treated in four subsequent trials by the European Organisation for Research and Treatment of Cancer: EORTC Lymphoma Group and the Groupe d'Etude des Lymphomes de l'Adulte. *J Clin Oncol*. 2007;25:2825-2832.
147. Whitehead E, Shalet SM, Blackledge G, et al. The effects of Hodgkin's disease and combination chemotherapy on gonadal function in the adult male. *Cancer*. 1982;49:418-422.
148. Viviani S, Santoro A, Ragni G, et al. Gonadal toxicity after combination chemotherapy for Hodgkin's disease: comparative results of MOPP vs ABVD. *Eur J Cancer Clin Oncol*. 1985;21:601-605.
149. Wallace WH, Shalet SM, Lendon M, et al. Male fertility in long-term survivors of childhood acute lymphoblastic leukaemia. *Int J Androl*. 1991;14:312-319.
150. Waxman J, Terry Y, Rees LH, et al. Gonadal function in men treated for acute leukaemia. *Br Med J (Clin Res Ed)*. 1989;3(287): 1093-1094.
151. Howell SJ, Radford JA, Ryder WD, et al. Testicular function after cytotoxic chemotherapy: evidence of Leydig cell insufficiency. *J Clin Oncol*. 1999;17:1493-1498.
152. Howell SJ, Radford JA, Adams JE, et al. Randomized placebo-controlled trial of testosterone replacement in men with mild Leydig cell insufficiency following cytotoxic chemotherapy. *Clin Endocrinol (Oxf)*. 2001;55:315-324.
153. Blackhall FH, Atkinson AD, Maaya MB, et al. Semen cryopreservation, utilisation and reproductive outcome in men treated for Hodgkin's disease. *Br J Cancer*. 2002;87:381-384.
154. Botchan A, Hauser R, Gamzu R, et al. Sperm quality in Hodgkin's disease versus non-Hodgkin's lymphoma. *Hum Reprod*. 1997;12: 73-76.
155. Hallak J, Kolettis PN, Sekhon VS, et al. Cryopreservation of sperm from patients with leukemia: is it worth the effort? *Cancer*. 1999;85: 1973-1978.
156. Ogawa T, Dobrinski I, Avarbock MR, et al. Transplantation of male germ line stem cells restores fertility in infertile mice. *Nat Med*. 2000;6:29-34.
157. Radford J, Shalet S, Lieberman B. Fertility after treatment for cancer: questions remain over ways of preserving ovarian and testicular tissue. *BMJ*. 1999;319:935-936.
158. Ward JA, Robinson J, Furr BJ, et al. Protection of spermatogenesis in rats from the cytotoxic procarbazine by the depot formulation of Zoladex, a gonadotropin-releasing hormone agonist. *Cancer Res*. 1990;50:568-574.
159. Johnson DH, Linde R, Hainsworth JD, et al. Effect of a luteinizing hormone releasing hormone agonist given during combination chemotherapy on posttherapy fertility in male patients with lymphoma: preliminary observations. *Blood*. 1985;65:832-836.
160. Blumenfeld Z, Avivi I, Linn S, et al. Prevention of irreversible chemotherapy-induced ovarian damage in young women with lymphoma by a gonadotrophin-releasing hormone agonist in parallel to chemotherapy. *Hum Reprod*. 1996;11:1620-1626.
161. Bhasin S, Storer TW, Berman N, et al. Testosterone replacement increases fat-free mass and muscle size in hypogonadal men. *J Clin Endocrinol Metab*. 1997;82:407-413.
162. Behre HM, Kliesch S, Leifke E, et al. Long-term effect of testosterone therapy on bone mineral density in hypogonadal men. *J Clin Endocrinol Metab*. 1997;82:2386-2390.
163. Howell SJ, Radford JA, Smets EM, et al. Fatigue, sexual function and mood following treatment for haematological malignancy: the impact of mild Leydig cell dysfunction. *Br J Cancer*. 2000;82:789-793.
164. Howell SJ, Radford JA, Adams JE, et al. The impact of mild Leydig cell dysfunction following cytotoxic chemotherapy on bone mineral density (BMD) and body composition. *Clin Endocrinol (Oxf)*. 2000;52:609-616.
165. Lushbaugh CC, Casarett GW. The effects of gonadal irradiation in clinical radiation therapy: a review. *Cancer*. 1976;37:1111-1125.
166. Wallace WH, Shalet SM, Hendry JH, et al. Ovarian failure following abdominal irradiation in childhood: the radiosensitivity of the human oocyte. *Br J Radiol*. 1989;62:995-998.
167. Wallace WH, Thomson AB, Saran F, et al. Predicting age of ovarian failure after radiation to a field that includes the ovaries. *Int J Radiat Oncol Biol Phys*. 2005;62:738-744.
168. Li FP, Gimbrere K, Gelber RD, et al. Outcome of pregnancy in survivors of Wilms' tumor. *JAMA*. 1987;257:216-219.
169. Critchley HO, Wallace WH, Shalet SM, et al. Abdominal irradiation in childhood; the potential for pregnancy. *Br J Obstet Gynaecol*. 1992;99:392-394.
170. Andrieu JM, Ochoa-Molina ME. Menstrual cycle, pregnancies and offspring before and after MOPP therapy for Hodgkin's disease. *Cancer*. 1983;52:435-438.
171. Koyama H, Wada T, Nishizawa Y, et al. Cyclophosphamide-induced ovarian failure and its therapeutic significance in patients with breast cancer. *Cancer*. 1977;39:1403-1409.
172. Mackie EJ, Radford M, Shalet SM. Gonadal function following chemotherapy for childhood Hodgkin's disease. *Med Pediatr Oncol*. 1996;27:74-78.
173. Whitehead E, Shalet SM, Blackledge G, et al. The effect of combination chemotherapy on ovarian function in women treated for Hodgkin's disease. *Cancer*. 1983;52:988-993.
174. Santoro A, Bonadonna G, Valagussa P, et al. Long-term results of combined chemotherapy-radiotherapy approach in Hodgkin's disease: superiority of ABVD plus radiotherapy versus MOPP plus radiotherapy. *J Clin Oncol*. 1987;5:27-37.
175. Wallace WH, Shalet SM, Tetlow LJ, et al. Ovarian function following the treatment of childhood acute lymphoblastic leukaemia. *Med Pediatr Oncol*. 1993;21:333-339.
176. Bath LE, Wallace WH, Shaw MP, et al. Depletion of ovarian reserve in young women after treatment for cancer in childhood: detection by anti-Mullerian hormone, inhibin B and ovarian ultrasound. *Hum Reprod*. 2003;18:2368-2374.
177. Anderson RA, Themmen AP, Al-Qahtani A, et al. The effects of chemotherapy and long-term gonadotrophin suppression on the ovarian reserve in premenopausal women with breast cancer. *Hum Reprod*. 2006;21:2583-2592.
178. Haie-Meder C, Mlika-Cabanne N, Michel G, et al. Radiotherapy after ovarian transposition: ovarian function and fertility preservation. *Int J Radiat Oncol Biol Phys*. 1993;25:419-424.
179. Williams RS, Littell RD, Mendenhall NP. Laparoscopic oophoropexy and ovarian function in the treatment of Hodgkin disease. *Cancer*. 1999;86:2138-2142.
180. Radford JA, Lieberman BA, Brison DR, et al. Orthotopic reimplantation of cryopreserved ovarian cortical strips after high-dose chemotherapy for Hodgkin's lymphoma. *Lancet*. 2001;357:1172-1175.
181. Falcone T, Attaran M, Bedaiwy MA, et al. Ovarian function preservation in the cancer patient. *Fertil Steril*. 2004;81:243-257.
182. Donnez J, Dolmans MM, Demylle D, et al. Livebirth after orthotopic transplantation of cryopreserved ovarian tissue. *Lancet*. 2004;364: 1405-1410.
183. Meirow D, Levron J, Eldar-Geva T, et al. Pregnancy after transplantation of cryopreserved ovarian tissue in a patient with ovarian failure after chemotherapy. *N Engl J Med*. 2005;353:318-321.
183a. Donnez J, Silber S, Andersen CY, et al. Children born after autotransplantation of cryopreserved ovarian tissue. A review of B live births. *Ann Med*. 2011; (Epub ahead of print).
184. Rossouw JE, Anderson GL, Prentice RL, et al. Risks and benefits of estrogen plus progestin in healthy postmenopausal women: principal results from the Women's Health Initiative randomized controlled trial. *JAMA*. 2002;288:321-333.
185. Hulley S, Grady D, Bush T, et al. Randomized trial of estrogen plus progestin for secondary prevention of coronary heart disease in postmenopausal women. Heart and Estrogen/progestin Replacement Study (HERS) Research Group. *JAMA*. 1998;280:605-613.
186. Rossouw JE, Prentice RL, Manson JE, et al. Postmenopausal hormone therapy and risk of cardiovascular disease by age and years since menopause. *JAMA*. 2007;297:1465-1477.
187. Alm El-Din MA, El-Badawy SA, Taghian AG. Breast cancer after treatment of Hodgkin's lymphoma: general review. *Int J Radiat Oncol Biol Phys*. 2008;72:1291-1297.

188. Sankila R, Garwicz S, Olsen JH, et al. Risk of subsequent malignant neoplasms among 1,641 Hodgkin's disease patients diagnosed in childhood and adolescence: a population-based cohort study in the five Nordic countries. Association of the Nordic Cancer Registries and the Nordic Society of Pediatric Hematology and Oncology. *J Clin Oncol.* 1996;14:1442-1446.
189. Friedman DL, Rovo A, Leisenring W, et al. Increased risk of breast cancer among survivors of allogeneic hematopoietic cell transplantation: a report from the FHCRC and the EBMT-Late Effect Working Party. *Blood.* 2008;111:939-944.
190. Sawka AM, Lakra DC, Lea J, et al. A systematic review examining the effects of therapeutic radioactive iodine on ovarian function and future pregnancy in female thyroid cancer survivors. *Clin Endocrinol (Oxf).* 2008;69:479-490.
191. Vini L, Hyer S, Al-Saadi A, et al. Prognosis for fertility and ovarian function after treatment with radioiodine for thyroid cancer. *Postgrad Med J.* 2002;78:92-93.
192. Bal C, Kumar A, Tripathi M, et al. High-dose radioiodine treatment for differentiated thyroid carcinoma is not associated with change in female fertility or any genetic risk to the offspring. *Int J Radiat Oncol Biol Phys.* 2005;63:449-455.
193. Manuel Garcia-Quiros Muñoz J, Martin Hernandez T, Torres Cuadro A, et al. [Age of menopause in patients with differentiated thyroid cancer treated with radioiodine.]. *Endocrinol Nutr.* 2010;57:105-109.
194. Ceccarelli C, Canale D, Battisti P, et al. Testicular function after 131I therapy for hyperthyroidism. *Clin Endocrinol (Oxf).* 2006;65:446-452.
195. Rosario PW, Barroso AL, Rezende LL, et al. Testicular function after radioiodine therapy in patients with thyroid cancer. *Thyroid.* 2006;16:667-670.
196. Hyer S, Vini L, O'Connell M, et al. Testicular dose and fertility in men following I(131) therapy for thyroid cancer. *Clin Endocrinol (Oxf).* 2002;56:755-758.
197. Wichers M, Benz E, Palmedo H, et al. Testicular function after radioiodine therapy for thyroid carcinoma. *Eur J Nucl Med.* 2000;27:503-507.
198. Pacini F, Gasperi M, Fugazzola L, et al. Testicular function in patients with differentiated thyroid carcinoma treated with radioiodine. *J Nucl Med.* 1994;35:1418-1422.
199. Nelson DF, Reddy KV, O'Mara RE, et al. Thyroid abnormalities following neck irradiation for Hodgkin's disease. *Cancer.* 1978;42:2553-2562.
200. Fleming ID, Black TL, Thompson EI, et al. Thyroid dysfunction and neoplasia in children receiving neck irradiation for cancer. *Cancer.* 1985;55:1190-1194.
201. Sklar C, Whitton J, Mertens A, et al. Abnormalities of the thyroid in survivors of Hodgkin's disease: data from the Childhood Cancer Survivor Study. *J Clin Endocrinol Metab.* 2000;85:3227-3232.
202. Jereczek-Fossa BA, Alterio D, Jassem J, et al. Radiotherapy-induced thyroid disorders. *Cancer Treat Rev.* 2004;30:369-384.
203. Shakespeare TP, Dwyer M, Mukherjee R, et al. Estimating risks of radiotherapy complications as part of informed consent: the high degree of variability between radiation oncologists may be related to experience. *Int J Radiat Oncol Biol Phys.* 2002;54:647-653.
204. Einhorn J, Wilkholm G. Hypothyroidism after external irradiation to the thyroid region. *Radiology.* 1967;88:326-328.
205. Markson JL, Flatman GE. Myxoedema after deep x-ray therapy to the neck. *Br Med J.* 1965;1:1228-1230.
206. Colevas AD, Read R, Thornhill J, et al. Hypothyroidism incidence after multimodality treatment for stage III and IV squamous cell carcinomas of the head and neck. *Int J Radiat Oncol Biol Phys.* 2001;51:599-604.
207. Smith RE Jr, Adler AR, Clark P, et al. Thyroid function after mantle irradiation in Hodgkin's disease. *JAMA.* 1981;245:46-49.
208. Shalet SM, Rosenstock JD, Beardwell CG, et al. Thyroid dysfunction following external irradiation to the neck for Hodgkin's disease in childhood. *Clin Radiol.* 1977;28:511-515.
209. Mercado G, Adelstein DJ, Saxton JP, et al. Hypothyroidism: a frequent event after radiotherapy and after radiotherapy with chemotherapy for patients with head and neck carcinoma. *Cancer.* 2001;92:2892-2897.
210. Hancock SL, Cox RS, McDougall IR. Thyroid diseases after treatment of Hodgkin's disease. *N Engl J Med.* 1991;325:599-605.
211. Ogilvy-Stuart AL, Shalet SM, Gattamaneni HR. Thyroid function after treatment of brain tumors in children. *J Pediatr.* 1991;119:733-737.
212. Constine LS, Donaldson SS, McDougall IR, et al. Thyroid dysfunction after radiotherapy in children with Hodgkin's disease. *Cancer.* 1984;53:878-883.
213. Paulino AC. Hypothyroidism in children with medulloblastoma: a comparison of 3600 and 2340 cGy craniospinal radiotherapy. *Int J Radiat Oncol Biol Phys.* 2002;53:543-547.
214. Glatstein E, McHardy-Young S, Brast N, et al. Alterations in serum thyrotropin (TSH) and thyroid function following radiotherapy in patients with malignant lymphoma. *J Clin Endocrinol Metab.* 1971;32:833-841.
215. Bethge W, Guggenberger D, Bamberg M, et al. Thyroid toxicity of treatment for Hodgkin's disease. *Ann Hematol.* 2000;79:114-118.
216. Green DM, Brecher ML, Yakar D, et al. Thyroid function in pediatric patients after neck irradiation for Hodgkin disease. *Med Pediatr Oncol.* 1980;8:127-136.
217. Thorp MA, Levitt NS, Mortimore S, et al. Parathyroid and thyroid function five years after treatment of laryngeal and hypopharyngeal carcinoma. *Clin Otolaryngol Allied Sci.* 1999;24:104-108.
218. Biel MA, Maisel RH. Indications for performing hemithyroidectomy for tumors requiring total laryngectomy. *Am J Surg.* 1985;150:435-439.
219. Constine LS. What else don't we know about the late effects of radiation in patients treated for head and neck cancer? *Int J Radiat Oncol Biol Phys.* 1995;31:427-429.
220. Bantle JP, Lee CK, Levitt SH. Thyroxine administration during radiation therapy to the neck does not prevent subsequent thyroid dysfunction. *Int J Radiat Oncol Biol Phys.* 1985;11:1999-2002.
221. Loeffler JS, Tarbell NJ, Garber JR, et al. The development of Graves' disease following radiation therapy in Hodgkin's disease. *Int J Radiat Oncol Biol Phys.* 1988;14:175-178.
222. Koh LK, Greenspan FS, Yeo PP. Interferon-alpha induced thyroid dysfunction: three clinical presentations and a review of the literature. *Thyroid.* 1997;7:891-896.
223. Krouse RS, Royal RE, Heywood G, et al. Thyroid dysfunction in 281 patients with metastatic melanoma or renal carcinoma treated with interleukin-2 alone. *J Immunother Emphasis Tumor Immunol.* 1995;18:272-278.
224. Duffy BJ Jr, Fitzgerald PJ. Cancer of the thyroid in children: a report of 28 cases. *J Clin Endocrinol Metab.* 1950;10:1296-1308.
225. de Vathaire F, Hardiman C, Shamsaldin A, et al. Thyroid carcinomas after irradiation for a first cancer during childhood. *Arch Intern Med.* 1999;159:2713-2719.
226. De Jong SA, Demeter JG, Jarosz H, et al. Thyroid carcinoma and hyperparathyroidism after radiation therapy for adolescent acne vulgaris. *Surgery.* 1991;110:691-695.
227. Tucker MA, Jones PH, Boice JD Jr, et al. Therapeutic radiation at a young age is linked to secondary thyroid cancer. The Late Effects Study Group. *Cancer Res.* 1991;51:2885-2888.
228. Rubino C, Adjadj E, Guerin S, et al. Long-term risk of second malignant neoplasms after neuroblastoma in childhood: role of treatment. *Int J Cancer.* 2003;107:791-796.
229. Black P, Straaten A, Gutjahr P. Secondary thyroid carcinoma after treatment for childhood cancer. *Med Pediatr Oncol.* 1998;31:91-95.
230. Sigurdson AJ, Ronckers CM, Mertens AC, et al. Primary thyroid cancer after a first tumour in childhood (the Childhood Cancer Survivor Study): a nested case-control study. *Lancet.* 2005;365:2014-2023.
231. Hancock SL, McDougall IR, Constine LS. Thyroid abnormalities after therapeutic external radiation. *Int J Radiat Oncol Biol Phys.* 1995;31:1165-1170.
232. Inskip PD. Thyroid cancer after radiotherapy for childhood cancer. *Med Pediatr Oncol.* 2004;36:568-573.
233. Acharya S, Sarafoglou K, LaQuaglia M, et al. Thyroid neoplasms after therapeutic radiation for malignancies during childhood or adolescence. *Cancer.* 2003;97:2397-2403.
234. Klugbauer S, Lengfelder E, Demidchik EP, et al. A new form of RET rearrangement in thyroid carcinomas of children after the Chernobyl reactor accident. *Oncogene.* 1996;13:1099-1102.
235. Klugbauer S, Lengfelder E, Demidchik EP, et al. High prevalence of RET rearrangement in thyroid tumors of children from Belarus after the Chernobyl reactor accident. *Oncogene.* 1995;11:2459-2467.
236. Roman SA. Endocrine tumors: evaluation of the thyroid nodule. *Curr Opin Oncol.* 2003;15:66-70.
237. Shafford EA, Kingston JE, Healy JC, et al. Thyroid nodular disease after radiotherapy to the neck for childhood Hodgkin's disease. *Br J Cancer.* 1999;80:808-814.
238. Carr RF, LiVolsi VA. Morphologic changes in the thyroid after irradiation for Hodgkin's and non-Hodgkin's lymphoma. *Cancer.* 1989;64:825-829.
239. Berdjis CC. Parathyroid diseases and irradiation. *Strahlentherapie.* 1972;143:48-62.
240. Rosen IB, Strawbridge HG, Bain J. A case of hyperparathyroidism associated with radiation to the head and neck area. *Cancer.* 1975;36:1111-1114.
241. Rao SD, Frame B, Miller MJ, et al. Hyperparathyroidism following head and neck irradiation. *Arch Intern Med.* 1980;140:205-207.
242. Christensson T. Hyperparathyroidism and radiation therapy. *Ann Intern Med.* 1978;89:216-217.
243. Fiorica V, Males JL. Hyperparathyroidism after radiation of the head and neck: a case report and review of the literature. *Am J Med Sci.* 1979;278:223-228.
244. Russ JE, Scanlon EF, Sener SF. Parathyroid adenomas following irradiation. *Cancer.* 1979;43:1078-1083.
245. Netelenbos C, Lips P, van der Meer C. Hyperparathyroidism following irradiation of benign diseases of the head and neck. *Cancer.* 1983;52:458-461.

246. Cohen J, Gierlowski TC, Schneider AB. A prospective study of hyperparathyroidism in individuals exposed to radiation in childhood. *JAMA*. 1990;264:581-584.
247. Palmer JA, Mustard RA, Simpson WJ. Irradiation as an etiologic factor in tumours of the thyroid, parathyroid and salivary glands. *Can J Surg*. 1980;23:39-42.
248. Schneider AB, Gierlowski TC, Shore-Freedman E, et al. Dose-response relationships for radiation-induced hyperparathyroidism. *J Clin Endocrinol Metab*. 1995;80:254-257.
249. Hedman I, Fjalling M, Lindberg S, et al. An assessment of the risk of developing hyperparathyroidism and thyroid disorders subsequent to neck irradiation in middle-aged women. *J Surg Oncol*. 1985;29:78-81.
250. McMullen T, Bodie G, Gill A, et al. Hyperparathyroidism after irradiation for childhood malignancy. *Int J Radiat Oncol Biol Phys*. 2009;73:1164-1168.
251. Karstrup S, Hegedus L, Sehested M. Hyperparathyroidism after neck irradiation for Hodgkin's disease. *Acta Med Scand*. 1984;215:287-288.
252. Holten I, Petersen LJ. Early changes in parathyroid function after high-dose irradiation of the neck. *Cancer*. 1988;62:1476-1478.
253. Christmas TJ, Chapple CR, Noble JG, et al. Hyperparathyroidism after neck irradiation. *Br J Surg*. 1988;75:873-874.
254. Tsunoda T, Mochinaga N, Eto T, et al. Hyperparathyroidism following the atomic bombing in Nagasaki. *Jpn J Surg*. 1991;21:508-511.
255. Stephen AE, Chen KT, Milas M, et al. The coming of age of radiation-induced hyperparathyroidism: evolving patterns of thyroid and parathyroid disease after head and neck irradiation. *Surgery*. 2004;136:1143-1153.
256. Mertens AC, Yasui Y, Neglia JP, et al. Late mortality experience in five-year survivors of childhood and adolescent cancer: the Childhood Cancer Survivor Study. *J Clin Oncol*. 2001;19:3163-3172.
257. Moller TR, Garwicz S, Barlow L, et al. Decreasing late mortality among five-year survivors of cancer in childhood and adolescence: a population-based study in the Nordic countries. *J Clin Oncol*. 2001;19:3173-3181.
258. Bowers DC, McNeil DE, Liu Y, et al. Stroke as a late treatment effect of Hodgkin's disease: a report from the Childhood Cancer Survivor Study. *J Clin Oncol*. 2005;23:6508-6515.
259. Bowers DC, Liu Y, Leisenring W, et al. Late-occurring stroke among long-term survivors of childhood leukemia and brain tumors: a report from the Childhood Cancer Survivor Study. *J Clin Oncol*. 2006;24:5277-5282.
260. Green DM, Hyland A, Chung CS, et al. Cancer and cardiac mortality among 15-year survivors of cancer diagnosed during childhood or adolescence. *J Clin Oncol*. 1999;17:3207-3215.
261. Adams MJ, Lipshultz SE. Pathophysiology of anthracycline- and radiation-associated cardiomyopathies: implications for screening and prevention. *Pediatr Blood Cancer*. 2005;44:600-606.
262. Hamada H, Ohkubo T, Maeda M, et al. Evaluation of cardiac reserved function by high-dose dobutamine-stress echocardiography in asymptomatic anthracycline-treated survivors of childhood cancer. *Pediatr Int*. 2006;48:313-320.
263. Meacham LR, Gurney JG, Mertens AC, et al. Body mass index in long-term adult survivors of childhood cancer: a report of the Childhood Cancer Survivor Study. *Cancer*. 2005;103:1730-1739.
264. Didi M, Didcock E, Davies HA, et al. High incidence of obesity in young adults after treatment of acute lymphoblastic leukemia in childhood. *J Pediatr*. 1995;127:63-67.
265. Nysom K, Holm K, Michaelsen KF, et al. Degree of fatness after treatment for acute lymphoblastic leukemia in childhood. *J Clin Endocrinol Metab*. 1999;84:4591-4596.
266. Haddy TB, Mosher RB, Reaman GH. Hypertension and prehypertension in long-term survivors of childhood and adolescent cancer. *Pediatr Blood Cancer*. 2007;49:79-83.
267. Talvensaari KK, Lanning M, Tapanainen P, et al. Long-term survivors of childhood cancer have an increased risk of manifesting the metabolic syndrome. *J Clin Endocrinol Metab*. 1996;81:3051-3055.
268. Oeffinger KC, Mertens AC, Sklar CA, et al. Obesity in adult survivors of childhood acute lymphoblastic leukemia: a report from the Childhood Cancer Survivor Study. *J Clin Oncol*. 2003;21:1359-1365.
269. Heikens J, Ubbink MC, van der Pal HP, et al. Long term survivors of childhood brain cancer have an increased risk for cardiovascular disease. *Cancer*. 2000;88:2116-2121.
270. Sainsbury CP, Newcombe RG, Hughes IA Weight gain and height velocity during prolonged first remission from acute lymphoblastic leukaemia. *Arch Dis Child*. 1985;60:832-836.
271. Sklar CA, Mertens AC, Walter A, et al. Changes in body mass index and prevalence of overweight in survivors of childhood acute lymphoblastic leukemia: role of cranial irradiation. *Med Pediatr Oncol*. 2000;35:91-95.
272. Taskinen M, Saarinen-Pihkala UM, Hovi L, et al. Impaired glucose tolerance and dyslipidaemia as late effects after bone-marrow transplantation in childhood. *Lancet*. 2000;356:993-997.
273. Neville KA, Cohn RJ, Steinbeck KS, et al. Hyperinsulinemia, impaired glucose tolerance, and diabetes mellitus in survivors of childhood cancer: prevalence and risk factors. *J Clin Endocrinol Metab*. 2006;91:4401-4407.
274. Nuver J, Smit AJ, Sleijfer DT, et al. Microalbuminuria, decreased fibrinolysis, and inflammation as early signs of atherosclerosis in long-term survivors of disseminated testicular cancer. *Eur J Cancer*. 2004;40:701-706.
275. King LJ, Hasnain SN, Webb JA, et al. Asymptomatic carotid arterial disease in young patients following neck radiation therapy for Hodgkin lymphoma. *Radiology*. 1999;213:167-172.
276. Liesner RJ, Leiper AD, Hann IM, et al. Late effects of intensive treatment for acute myeloid leukemia and myelodysplasia in childhood. *J Clin Oncol*. 1994;12:916-924.
277. Huma Z, Boulad F, Black P, et al. Growth in children after bone marrow transplantation for acute leukemia. *Blood*. 1995;86:819-824.
278. Brauner R, Fontoura M, Zucker JM, et al. Growth and growth hormone secretion after bone marrow transplantation. *Arch Dis Child*. 1993;68:458-463.
279. Giorgiani G, Bozzola M, Locatelli F, et al. Role of busulfan and total body irradiation on growth of prepubertal children receiving bone marrow transplantation and results of treatment with recombinant human growth hormone. *Blood*. 1995;86:825-831.
280. Cohen A, Rovelli A, Van-Lint MT, et al. Final height of patients who underwent bone marrow transplantation during childhood. *Arch Dis Child*. 1996;74:437-440.
281. Holm K, Nysom K, Rasmussen MH, et al. Growth, growth hormone and final height after BMT: possible recovery of irradiation-induced growth hormone insufficiency. *Bone Marrow Transplant*. 1996;18:163-170.
282. Leiper AD, Stanhope R, Lau T, et al. The effect of total body irradiation and bone marrow transplantation during childhood and adolescence on growth and endocrine function. *Br J Haematol*. 1987;67:419-426.
283. Sanders JE, Pritchard S, Mahoney P, et al. Growth and development following marrow transplantation for leukemia. *Blood*. 1986;68:1129-1135.
284. Cohen A, Rovelli A, Bakker B, et al. Final height of patients who underwent bone marrow transplantation for hematological disorders during childhood: a study by the Working Party for Late Effects-EBMT. *Blood*. 1999;93:4109-4115.
285. Thomas BC, Stanhope R, Plowman PN, et al. Endocrine function following single fraction and fractionated total body irradiation for bone marrow transplantation in childhood. *Acta Endocrinol (Copenh)*. 1993;128:508-512.
286. Wingard JR, Plotnick LP, Freemer CS, et al. Growth in children after bone marrow transplantation: busulfan plus cyclophosphamide versus cyclophosphamide plus total body irradiation. *Blood*. 1992;79:1068-1073.
287. Papadimitriou A, Urena M, Hamill G, et al. Growth hormone treatment of growth failure secondary to total body irradiation and bone marrow transplantation. *Arch Dis Child*. 1991;66:689-692.
288. Kaufman JM, Taelman P, Vermeulen A, et al. Bone mineral status in growth hormone-deficient males with isolated and multiple pituitary deficiencies of childhood onset. *J Clin Endocrinol Metab*. 1992;74:118-123.
289. Gandhi MK, Lekamwasam S, Inman I, et al. Significant and persistent loss of bone mineral density in the femoral neck after haematopoietic stem cell transplantation: long-term follow-up of a prospective study. *Br J Haematol*. 2003;121:462-468.
290. Ishiguro H, Yasuda Y, Tomita Y, et al. Long-term follow-up of thyroid function in patients who received bone marrow transplantation during childhood and adolescence. *J Clin Endocrinol Metab*. 2004;89:5981-5986.
291. Tauchmanova L, Selleri C, Rosa GD, et al. High prevalence of endocrine dysfunction in long-term survivors after allogeneic bone marrow transplantation for hematologic diseases. *Cancer*. 2002;95:1076-1084.
292. Cohen A, Rovelli A, Merlo DF, et al. Risk for secondary thyroid carcinoma after hematopoietic stem-cell transplantation: an EBMT Late Effects Working Party Study. *J Clin Oncol*. 2007;25:2449-2454.
293. Bhatia S, Louie AD, Bhatia R, et al. Solid cancers after bone marrow transplantation. *J Clin Oncol*. 2001;19:464-471.
294. Cohen A, Rovelli A, van Lint MT, et al. Secondary thyroid carcinoma after allogeneic bone marrow transplantation during childhood. *Bone Marrow Transplant*. 2001;28:1125-1128.
295. Sanders JE, Buckner CD, Amos D, et al. Ovarian function following marrow transplantation for aplastic anemia or leukemia. *J Clin Oncol*. 1988;6:813-818.
296. Cohen A, Rovelli R, Zecca S, et al. Endocrine late effects in children who underwent bone marrow transplantation: review. *Bone Marrow Transplant*. 1998;21(suppl 2):S64-S67.
297. Sarafoglou K, Boulad F, Gillio A, et al. Gonadal function after bone marrow transplantation for acute leukemia during childhood. *J Pediatr*. 1997;130:210-216.
298. Cust MP, Whitehead MI, Powles R, et al. Consequences and treatment of ovarian failure after total body irradiation for leukaemia. *BMJ* 1998;299:1494-1497.

299. Watson M, Wheatley K, Harrison GA, et al. Severe adverse impact on sexual functioning and fertility of bone marrow transplantation, either allogeneic or autologous, compared with consolidation chemotherapy alone: analysis of the MRC AML 10 trial. *Cancer*. 1999;86:1231-1239.
300. Lahteenmaki PM, Chakrabarti S, Cornish JM, et al. Outcome of single fraction total body irradiation-conditioned stem cell transplantation in younger children with malignant disease: comparison with a busulphan-cyclophosphamide regimen. *Acta Oncol*. 2004;43:196-203.
301. Rose SR, Schreiber RE, Kearney NS, et al. Hypothalamic dysfunction after chemotherapy. *J Pediatr Endocrinol Metab*. 2004;17:55-66.
302. Tauchmanova L, Selleri C, De Rosa G, et al. Gonadal status in reproductive age women after haematopoietic stem cell transplantation for haematological malignancies. *Hum Reprod*. 2003;18:1410-1416.

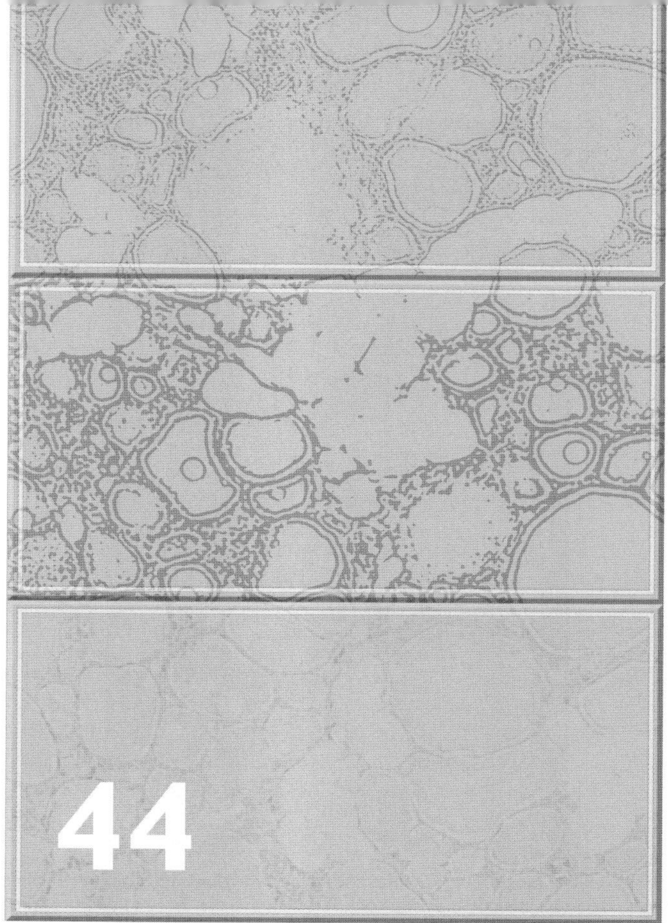

CHAPTER 44

Neuroendocrine Gastrointestinal and Lung Tumors (Carcinoid Tumors), Carcinoid Syndrome, and Related Disorders

KJELL ÖBERG

The first clinical and histopathologic description of carcinoid tumor was made by Otto Lubarsch in 1888.[1] He was impressed by the multicentric origin of carcinoid tumors of the gastrointestinal (GI) tract, their lack of gland formation, and their lack of similarity with the usual adenocarcinoma of the alimentary system.

The term *Karzinoide* was introduced in 1907 by the pathologist Oberndorffer[2] as a descriptive name for what he considered to be a benign type of neoplasm of the ileum but one that could behave like a carcinoma. It was subsequently accepted that the carcinoid tumor was a very slow growing and benign neoplasm with no potential for invasiveness or tendency to metastasize. This myth of benignity has survived to the present, even though in 1949 Pearson and Fitzgerald[3] described a large series of metastasizing carcinoid tumors.

Carcinoid tumors have subsequently been reported in a wide range of organs, but they most commonly involve the lungs and GI tract. Carcinoid tumors of the thymus, ovaries, testes, heart, and middle ear have also been described. The clinically well-known *carcinoid syndrome* was described by Thorson and associates[4] in 1954; 1 year earlier, Lembeck[5] had extracted serotonin from a carcinoid tumor.

PHYLOGENESIS AND EMBRYOLOGY

Carcinoid tumors are derived from neuroendocrine cells, and in 1914, Gosset and Masson[6] were the first to point out the neuroendocrine properties of carcinoid tumors. Masson[7] later described the remarkable affinity for silver salts displayed by intracytoplasmic granules in tumor cells

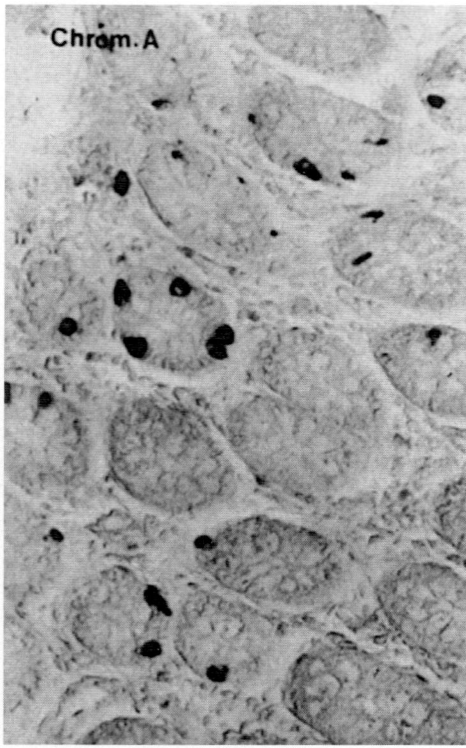

Figure 44-1 Normal human intestine stained with chromogranin A (Chrom. A) to delineate neuroendocrine cells. The cells are scattered in the intestinal mucosa.

and observed that carcinoid tumors originated from enterochromaffin cells, the Kulchitsky cells in the crypts of Lieberkühn in the intestinal epithelium. He also suggested that the tumors were of endocrine origin (Fig. 44-1).

The mammalian GI tract and pancreas contain 14 endocrine cell types, which initially were believed to originate from the neuroectoderm. This observation gave rise to the *APUD concept* (*a*mine *p*recursor *u*ptake and *d*ecarboxylation) because of the ability of these cells to take up and decarboxylate amino acid precursors of biogenic amines such as serotonin and catecholamines.[8] The APUD concept was later revised by others, who postulated that these endocrine cells might also be derived from mesoderm and endoderm.[9] The neuronal phenotype is clearly seen when culturing carcinoid tumor cells in vitro. The enterochromaffin cells, from which many carcinoid tumors derive, have the property of producing and secreting amines (e.g., serotonin) and polypeptides (e.g., neurokinin A, substance P).

Carcinoid tumors also may originate from other neuroendocrine cells, such as the enterochromaffin-like (ECL) cells of the gut and endocrine cells in the bronchi. Tumors derived from these cells can produce a wide range of hormones, such as gastrin, gastrin-releasing peptide (GRP), ghrelin, calcitonin, pancreatic polypeptide, adrenocorticotropic hormone (ACTH), corticotropin-releasing hormone (CRH), and growth hormone–releasing hormone (GHRH), as well as somatostatin, glucagon, and calcitonin gene–related peptide (CGRP).[10] A common secretory product from all types of carcinoid tumors is the glycoprotein chromogranin A (CgA), the most important general tumor marker in these patients (see later discussion).

MOLECULAR GENETICS

Despite advances in the diagnosis, localization, and treatment of carcinoid tumors, no etiologic factor associated with the development of these tumors has been identified. Little is known about molecular genetic changes underlying tumorigenesis. Sporadic foregut carcinoids and the familial-type multiple endocrine neoplasia type 1 (MEN1) often display allelic losses at chromosome 11q13, and somatic *MEN1* gene mutations have been reported in one third of sporadic foregut tumors.[11] In contrast to foregut carcinoids, molecular and cytogenetic data for midgut carcinoids are quite limited, and these tumors are not included in MEN1 syndrome. Deletions of chromosomes 18q and 18p have been reported in 38% and 33%, respectively, of GI carcinoids.[12]

In one publication, deletions on chromosome 18 were found in 88% of midgut carcinoid tumors, but the *SMAD4/DPC4* locus was not deleted.[13] In addition to the consistent finding of deletions on chromosome 18, multiple deletions on other chromosomes (e.g., 4, 5, 7, 9, 14, 20) were noticed in single tumors. The region telomeric to the *SMAD4/DPC4/DCC* loci must be further explored for possible losses of a tumor suppressor gene in this area. Gene expression arrays for carcinoid tumors have demonstrated upregulation of the *RET* proto-oncogene, but no mutations have been detected. Data indicate that the Notch signaling pathway is a significant regulator of neuroendocrine differentiation and serotonin production in GI carcinoid tumors.[14,15]

CLASSIFICATION

In 1963, Williams and Sandler reported a relationship between the embryonic origin of carcinoid tumors and the histologic, biochemical, and to some extent, clinical features of the tumors.[16] Three distinct groups were formed (Table 44-1): foregut carcinoids (i.e., intrathoracic, gastric,

TABLE 44-1
Classification of Carcinoid Tumors

Foregut	Midgut	Hindgut
Histopathology		
Argyrophilic CgA positive NSE positive	Argentaffin positive CgA positive NSE positive	Argyrophilic SVP-2 positive CgA positive, NSE positive
Molecular Genetics		
Chromosome 11q13 deletion	Chromosome 18q, 18p deletion	Unknown
Secretory Products		
CgA, 5-HT, 5-HTP, histamine, ACTH, GHRH, CGRP, somatostatin, AVP, glucagon, gastrin, NKA, substance P, neurotensin, GRP	CgA, 5-HT, NKA, substance P, prostaglandins E_1 and F_2, bradykinin	PP, YY, somatostatin
Carcinoid Syndrome		
Present (30%)	Present (70%)	Absent

ACTH, adrenocorticotropic hormone; AVP, arginine vasopressin; CgA, chromogranin A; CGRP, calcitonin gene–related hormone; GRP, gastrin-releasing peptide; 5-HT, 5-hydroxytryptamine; 5-HTP, 5-hydroxytryptophan; NKA, neurokinin; NSE, neuron-specific enolase; PP, pancreatic peptide; YY, peptide YY; SVP-2, synaptic vesicle protein 2.

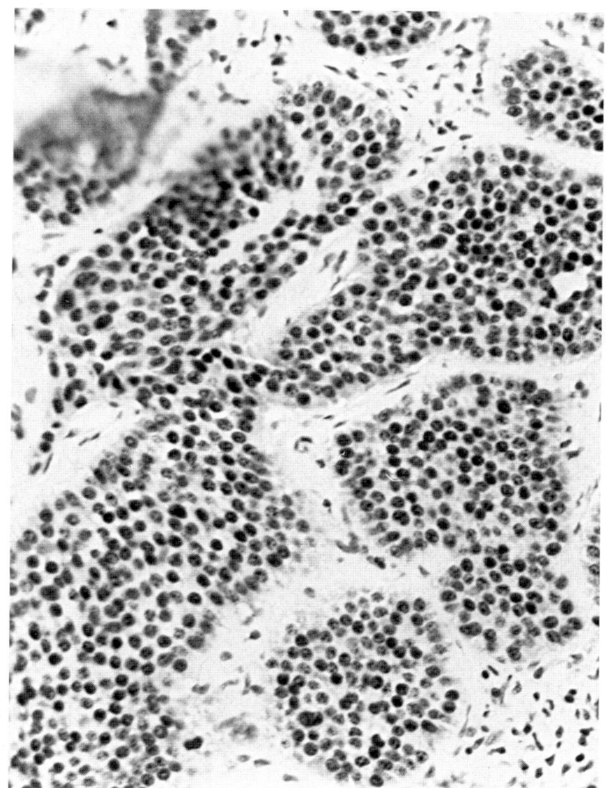

Figure 44-2 Histopathology of classic, well-differentiated midgut carcinoid tumor.

and duodenal carcinoids), midgut carcinoids (i.e., carcinoids of the small intestine, appendix, and proximal colon), and hindgut carcinoids (i.e., carcinoid tumors of the distal colon and rectum).

Although this original classification has been useful in the clinical assessment of patients with carcinoid tumors, its significant shortcomings prompted development of a new classification system that takes into account both the site of origin and variations in the histopathologic characteristics of carcinoid tumors: the World Health Organization (WHO) classification.[17] In this revised system, typical tumors are classified as *well-differentiated* neuroendocrine tumors (WHO I), with their characteristic growth pattern (Fig. 44-2). These tumors are usually slow growing, with low proliferation capacity (proliferation index <2%). They are usually confined to the mucosa and submucosa and are less than 1 to 2 cm in diameter (i.e., classic midgut carcinoid). Well-differentiated endocrine carcinomas (WHO II) are larger than 2 cm and show widely invasive growth and a high proliferation index (2% to 15%). Poorly differentiated carcinomas (WHO III) are large tumors with metastases and a proliferation index of greater than 15% (Table 44-2).[17a] The European Neuroendocrine Tumor Network Society (ENETS) has proposed a new tumor-node-metastasis (TNM) classification and grading system, but it has not been widely accepted.

Neuroendocrine lung tumors are classified as typical carcinoids, atypical carcinoids, large cell neuroendocrine carcinomas, and small cell lung carcinomas. The difference between the typical and atypical carcinoid is based on histopathology, with higher amounts of proliferation and necrosis found in the atypical carcinoid.[18] The incidence of carcinoid tumors is similar in Western countries and is estimated to be 2.8 to 4.5 cases per 100,000 people.[19,20] Because many carcinoid tumors are indolent, the true incidence may be higher. In particular, appendiceal carcinoids have not been included in many studies, but a higher incidence of 8.2 cases per 100,000 people was found in an autopsy study when appendiceal carcinoids were included.[21] The incidence of patients with a carcinoid syndrome is about 0.5 case per 100,000 people.[22] Data from the United States, based on results from the End Results Group and the Third National Cancer Survey for 1950 to 1969 and for 1969 to 1971, respectively, found that the appendix was the most common site of carcinoid tumors, followed by the rectum, ileum, lungs, and bronchi.[23]

An analysis done in the Surveillance, Epidemiology, and End Results (SEER) program of the National Cancer Institute between 1973 and 1999 reported an increase in the percentage of pulmonary and gastric carcinoids and a decrease in the percentage of appendiceal carcinoids.[20] Age-specific incidence rates showed a peak between 65 and 75 years (7.5 to 9.5 per 100,000), with a male predominance. Among persons younger than 50 years, a female predominance has been observed for appendiceal and lung carcinoids.[24] The most recent analysis of the SEER database showed an incidence of 5.2 per 100,000 people and a prevalence of 35 per 100,000 people,[25] indicating a real increase over the past decade.[26]

BIOCHEMISTRY

The production of hormones appears to be a highly organized function of carcinoid cells. In 1953, Lembeck isolated serotonin from a carcinoid tumor; since then, carcinoid syndrome has been associated with serotonin overproduction.[5] The biosynthesis of serotonin and its metabolic degradation are outlined in Figure 44-3.

Carcinoid tumors of the midgut and foregut region with metastatic disease secrete serotonin and produce elevated urinary excretion of 5-hydroxyindoleacetic acid (5-HIAA)

TABLE 44-2

World Health Organization Clinicopathologic Classification of Intestinal Neuroendocrine Tumors

Well-Differentiated Endocrine Tumors
Functioning or nonfunctioning Confined to mucosa-submucosa Nonangioinvasive <1 or 2 cm in diameter PI <2% (Ki-67) Serotonin-producing tumor (midgut carcinoid)
Well-Differentiated Endocrine Carcinomas
Functioning or nonfunctioning >2 cm in diameter Invasive growth Metastases PI >2% and <15% Examples: serotonin-producing carcinoma with or without carcinoid syndrome; bronchial carcinoid
Poorly Differentiated Endocrine Carcinomas
Large and invasive tumors PI >15% (small-cell tumors)
Mixed Endocrine-Exocrine Tumors
Tumor-Like Lesions

PI, proliferation index.

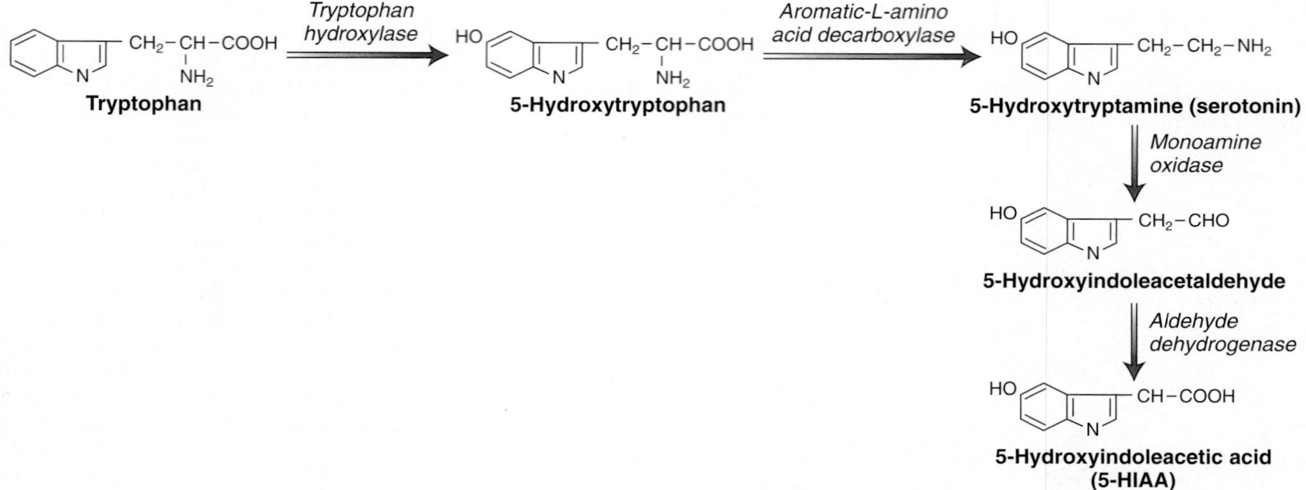

Figure 44-3 Biosynthesis and metabolism of 5-hydroxytryptamine (5-HT) (i.e., serotonin).

```
Substance P            Arg-Pro-Lys-Pro-Gln-Gln-Phe-Phe-Gly-Leu-Met-NH2
Neurokinin A                   His-Lys-Thr-Asp-Ser-Phe-Val-Gly-Leu-Met-NH2
Neurokinin B                       Asp-Met-His-Asp-Phe-Val-Gly-Leu-Met-NH2
Eledoisin              Pyr-Pro-Ser-Lys-Asp-Ala-Phe-Ile-Gly-Leu-Met-NH2
Kassinin           Asp-Val-Pro-Lys-Ser-Asp-Glu-Phe-Val-Gly-Leu-Met-NH2
Physalemin             Pyr-Ala-Asp-Pro-Asn-Lys-Phe-Tyr-Gly-Leu-Met-NH2
Neuropeptide K         Arg-His-Lys-Thr-Asp-Ser-Phe-Val-Gly-Leu-Met-NH2
                       1-Lys-His-Ser-Ile-Gln-Gly-His-Gly-Tyr-Leu-Ala-Lys
                   Asp-Ala-Asp-Ser-Ser-Ile-Glu-Lys-Gln-Val-Ala-Leu-Leu1
```

Figure 44-4 The tachykinin family of peptides shares the same carboxy terminus. Neuropeptide K is a prohormone containing neurokinin A, which can be spliced off.

in 76% and 30% of these tumors, respectively.[25] Carcinoid tumors arising from the foregut, however, commonly have low levels of L-amino acid decarboxylase, which converts 5-hydroxytryptophan (5-HTP) to serotonin, and these tumors secrete primarily 5-HTP.[27,28]

For many years, it was believed that the carcinoid syndrome could be explained by the secretion of these biologically active amines. However, further studies found that serotonin was mainly involved in the pathogenesis of diarrhea and that other biologically active substances played a more important role in the carcinoid flush and bronchoconstriction.

Oates and associates[29] hypothesized that *kallikrein*, an enzyme found in carcinoid tumors, is released in association with flush and stimulates plasma kininogen to liberate lysyl-bradykinin and bradykinin. These biologically active substances cause vasodilation, hypotension, tachycardia, and edema.[29-31] Prostaglandins (E_1, E_2, F_1, F_2) may also play a role in carcinoid syndrome.[32] Gastric carcinoids and lung carcinoids contain and secrete histamine, which may be responsible for the characteristic bright red flush seen in these patients.[33-35] Metabolites of histamine are often present in high concentration in the urine of patients. Dopamine and norepinephrine also have been found in carcinoid tumors.[36]

The occurrence of *substance P* in carcinoid tumors was first demonstrated by Håkansson and coworkers in 1977.[37] Substance P belongs to a family of polypeptides, called *tachykinins,* that share the same carboxy terminus (Fig. 44-4). Several tachykinin-related peptides, such as neurokinin A, neuropeptide K, and eledoisin, have been isolated from carcinoid tumors. During stimulation of flush in patients with midgut carcinoids, multiple forms of tachykinins are released into the circulation (Fig. 44-5).[38-40]

Many different polypeptides (e.g., insulin, gastrin, somatostatin, S100 protein, polypeptide YY, pancreatic polypeptide, human chorionic gonadotropin α-subunit [hCG-α], motilin, calcitonin, vasoactive intestinal polypeptide [VIP], endorphins) have been demonstrated in carcinoid tumors by immunohistochemical staining and sometimes identified in tumor extracts.[10] Ectopic ACTH or CRH production may be found in foregut carcinoids, and

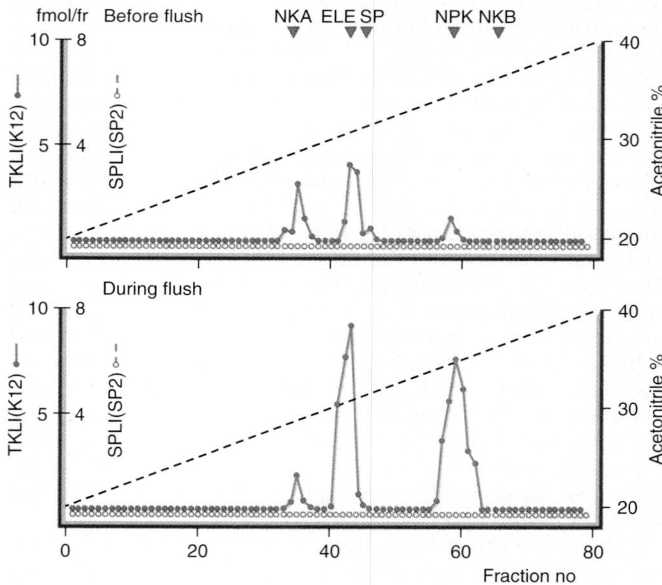

Figure 44-5 Chromatography samples of plasma from a patient with carcinoid before flush *(upper panel)* and during flush *(lower panel).* Notice the significant increase in eledoisin-like peptide and in neuropeptide K. ELE, eledoisin; NKA, neurokinin A; NKB, neurokinin B; NPK, neuropeptide K; SP, substance P; SPLI(SP2), substance P-like immunoreactivity; TKLI(K12), tachykinin-like immunoreactivity.

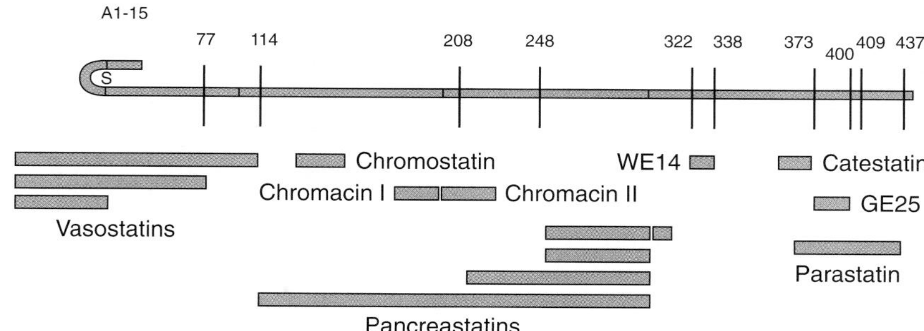

Figure 44-6 The glycoprotein chromogranin A and related peptides, including GE25 and WE14.

patients with bronchial carcinoids seem particularly susceptible to Cushing's syndrome.[41] Patients with carcinoid tumors of the foregut may present with acromegaly due to ectopic secretion of GHRH from the tumor.[42] Duodenal carcinoids as part of von Recklinghausen's disease can secrete somatostatin.[43]

The *chromogranin/secretogranin* family consists of CgA, CgB (sometimes called *secretogranin I*), secretogranin II (sometimes called *CgC*), and some other members. CgA was first isolated in 1965 as a water-soluble protein in chromaffin cells from bovine adrenal medulla.[44] Its immunoreactivity has been found in all parts of the GI tract and pancreas, and it has been isolated from all endocrine glands.[45]

CgA is an acidic glycoprotein of 439 amino acids with a molecular weight of 48 kd. It can be spliced into smaller fragments at dibasic cleavage sites, generating multiple bioactive fragments such as vasostatins, chromostatin, and pancreastatin (Fig. 44-6).[45-49]

Amines and hormones are stored intracellularly in two types of vesicles: large, dense-core vesicles and small, synapse-like vesicles. These vesicles release amines and hormones on stimulation. Large, dense-core vesicles contain the hormones and one or more members of the chromogranin/secretogranin family of proteins.[46,50] Amines and peptides are coreleased (Fig. 44-7).

The physiologic function of CgA is not fully elucidated. Its ubiquitous presence in neuroendocrine tissues and its cosecretion with peptide hormones and amines indicate a storage role of the peptide within the secretory granule.[45,46,50] It also acts as a prohormone that can generate bioactive smaller fragments. CgA is an important tissue and serum marker for different types of carcinoid tumors, including those of the foregut, midgut, and hindgut (see Table 44-1 and later discussion).

CLINICAL PRESENTATION

The clinical presentation of carcinoid tumors depends on location, hormone production, and extent of the disease. Usually, a lung carcinoid is diagnosed incidentally on routine pulmonary radiography, whereas a midgut carcinoid may be identified as a bowel obstruction or as a cause of abdominal discomfort or pain. Rectal carcinoids may cause bleeding or obstruction. Lung carcinoids can manifest clinically as Cushing's syndrome, due to CRH or ACTH secretion or as carcinoid syndrome, due to production of serotonin, 5-HTP, or histamine.[51] A midgut carcinoid often manifests as carcinoid syndrome due to production of serotonin and tachykinins.

The clinical manifestations at referral depend on the type of referral center. At my institution, which cares for patients with malignant tumors, 74% of the patients present with carcinoid syndrome, 13% with abdominal pain, 12% with carcinoid heart disease, and 2% with bronchial constriction.[25] When unbiased material is analyzed, bowel obstruction is the most common problem leading to the diagnosis of ileal carcinoid tumor. The second most common symptom is abdominal pain. Flushing and diarrhea, which are components of carcinoid syndrome,

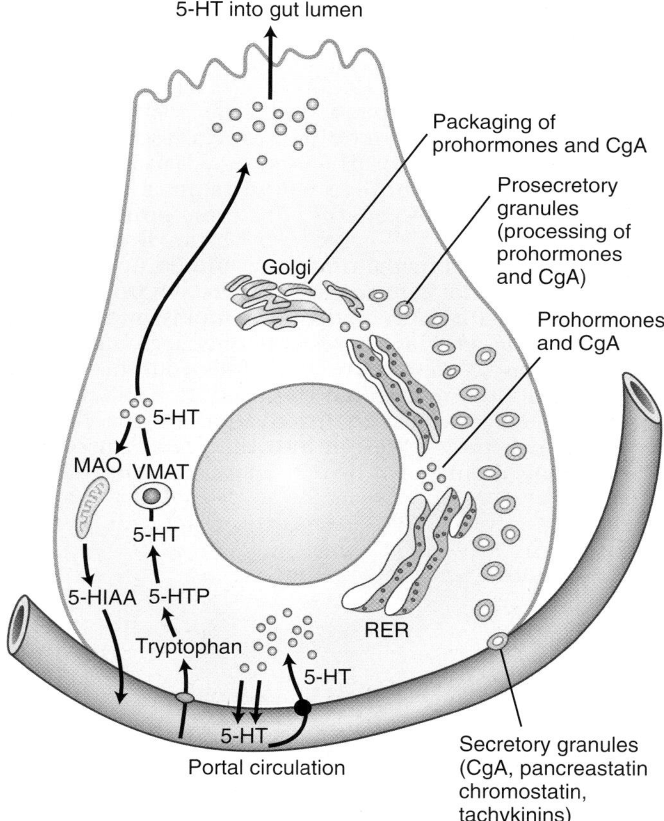

Figure 44-7 Schematic drawing of an enterochromaffin cell. The initial step in 5-hydroxytryptamine (5-HT) synthesis is carrier transport of the amino acid tryptophan from blood into the cell across the cell membrane. Intracellular tryptophan is first converted to 5-hydroxytryptophan (5-HTP), which is converted to 5-HT and stored in secretory granules. The transport of 5-HT into granules requires vesicular monoamine transporters (VMATs). Through the basal lateral membrane, 5-HT can be released into the circulation. A membrane pump mechanism in the cell membrane is responsible for amine reuptake. A minor part of 5-HT can also be released into the gut lumen. Monoamine oxidase (MAO) degrades 5-HT to 5-hydroxyindoleacetic acid (5-HIAA). Peptide prohormones are synthesized in the rough endoplasmic reticulum (RER) together with chromogranin A (CgA) and other granule proteins. The products are transported to the Golgi apparatus (GA) for packaging into prosecretory granules. On stimulation, the secretory products are released from the granules by exocytosis.

constitute the third most common presentation.[19,52-54] Because many patients have vague symptoms, diagnosis of the tumor may be delayed by approximately 2 to 3 years.[22]

Carcinoid Syndrome

In 1954, Thorson and coworkers for the first time described carcinoid syndrome as having the following features: malignant carcinoid of the small intestine with metastasis to the liver; valvular disease of the right side of the heart (i.e., pulmonary stenosis and tricuspid insufficiency without septal defect); peripheral vasomotor symptoms; bronchial constriction; and an unusual type of cyanosis.[4] One year later, Dr. William Bean[55] gave this colorful description of carcinoid syndrome: "This witch's brew of unlikely signs and symptoms, intriguing to the most fastidious connoisseur of clinical esoterica—the skin underwent rapid and extreme changes—resembling in clinical miniature the fecal phantasmagoria of the aurora borealis."

The well-characterized syndrome includes flushing, diarrhea, right-sided heart failure, and sometimes, bronchial constriction and increased urinary levels of 5-HIAA.[56,57] This is the classic carcinoid syndrome, but some patients display only one or two of the features. Other symptoms related to the syndrome are weight loss, sweating, and pellagra-like skin lesions.

Development of carcinoid syndrome is a function of tumor mass, extent and location of metastases, and location of the primary tumor. The syndrome is most common in tumors originating in the small intestine and proximal colon; 40% to 60% of patients with these tumors experience the syndrome.[25,53,56,57] The disorders are less common in patients with bronchial carcinoids and do not occur in patients with rectal carcinoids.[51,58,59] The syndrome rarely occurs in patients with midgut carcinoids and a small tumor burden, such as those with only regional lymph node metastases.[54] Patients with the full syndrome usually have multiple liver metastases. The association with hepatic metastases reflects efficient inactivation by the liver of amines and peptides released into the portal circulation. The venous drainage of liver metastases runs directly into the systemic circulation and bypasses hepatic inactivation.[60]

Other carcinoid tumors likely to be associated with carcinoid syndrome in the absence of liver metastases are ovarian carcinoids and bronchial carcinoids, which release mediators directly into the systemic rather than the portal circulation. Retroperitoneal metastases from classic midgut carcinoids also release mediators directly into the circulation and may cause carcinoid syndrome without any liver metastases.[56,57]

Flushing

Four types of flushing have been described in the literature: erythematous, violaceous, prolonged, and bright red.[56,57]

The best-known type is the sudden, diffuse, erythematous flush, which usually affects the face, neck, and upper chest (i.e., normal flushing area) (Fig. 44-8). This type of flush commonly has a short duration, lasting 1 to 5 minutes, and is related to early-stage midgut carcinoids. Patients usually experience a sensation of warmth during flushing and sometimes have heart palpitations. This type of flushing is reported in 20% to 70% of patients with midgut carcinoid at manifestation of the disease.[22,56-58]

The second type, violaceous flush, affects the same area of the body. It has roughly the same time course or sometimes lasts a little longer. Patients may also have facial telangiectasia. This flush is related to the later stages of midgut carcinoid (Fig. 44-9) and is normally not felt by patients because they have become accustomed to the flushing reaction.

The third type is prolonged flushing that usually lasts a couple of hours but can last up to several days. This flush sometimes involves the whole body and is associated with profuse lacrimation, swelling of the salivary glands, hypotension, and facial edema (Fig. 44-10). These symptoms are usually associated with malignant bronchial carcinoids.

The fourth type of flushing is a bright red, patchy flush, which is seen in patients with chronic atrophic gastritis and ECL cell hyperplasia or ECLoma (derived from ECL cells). This type of flushing is related to increased release of histamine and histamine metabolites.

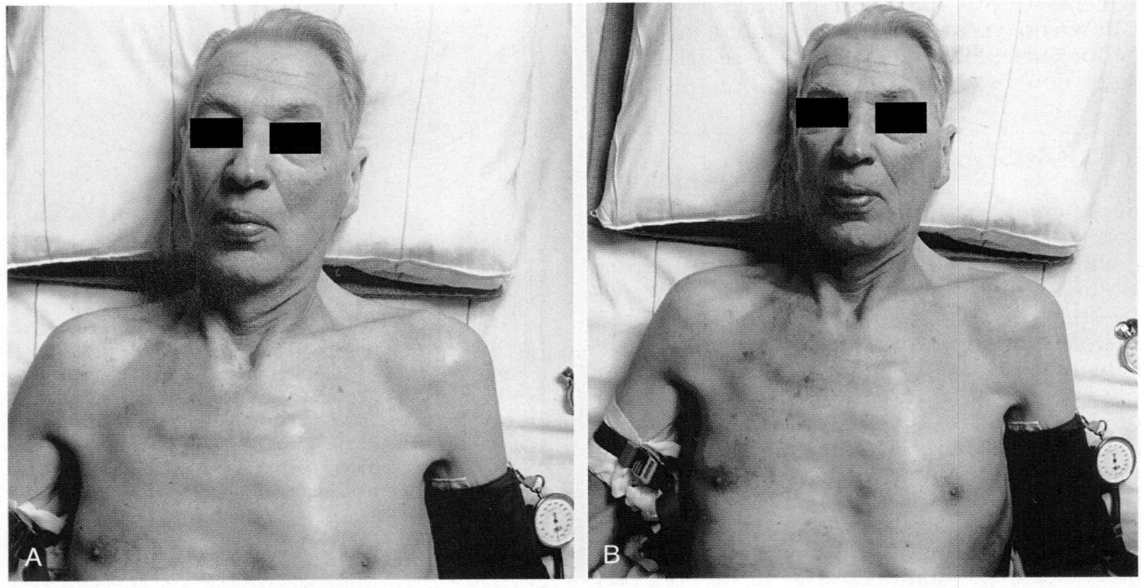

Figure 44-8 **A,** Patient with carcinoid syndrome before flush provocation. **B,** The same patient after pentagastrin-stimulated flush.

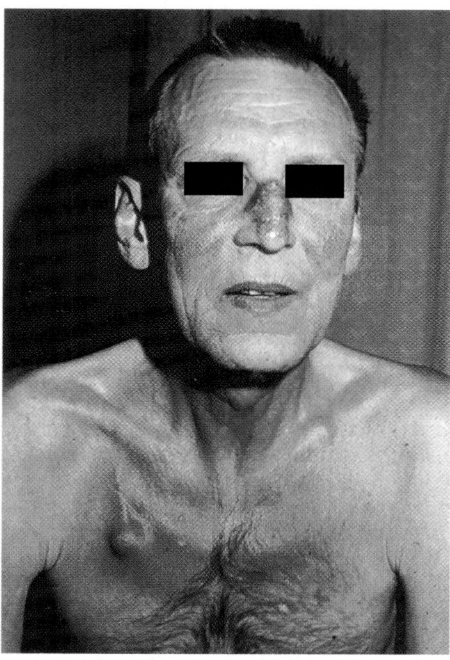

Figure 44-9 Long-lasting, chronic flushing in a patient with long-standing carcinoid disease. Note the telangiectases.

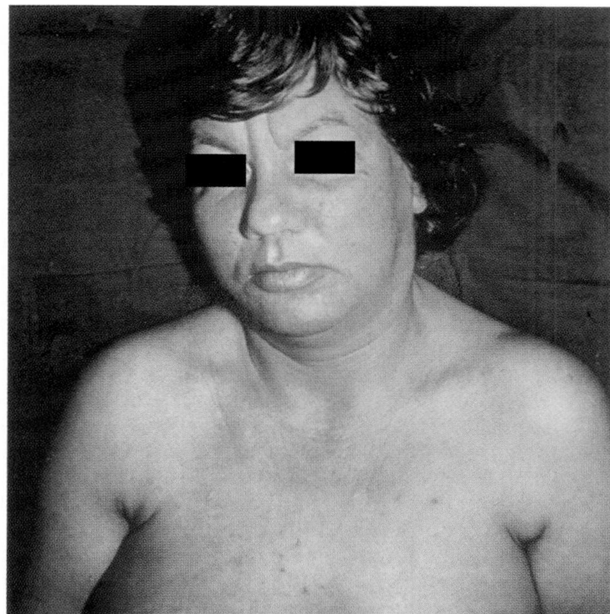

Figure 44-10 A patient with lung carcinoid and carcinoid syndrome with severe, long-standing flushing, lacrimation, and a swollen face.

Flushes may be spontaneous, or they may be precipitated by physical or mental stress, infection, alcohol, spicy foods, or drugs such as injections of catecholamines, calcium, or pentagastrin (see later discussion). The pathophysiology of flushing in carcinoid syndrome has not been elucidated.[61-63] It was previously linked to excess production of serotonin or serotonin metabolites.[62] However, several patients with high levels of plasma serotonin did not have flushing, nor did serotonin antagonists (e.g., methysergide, cyproheptadine, ketanserin) have any effect on the flushing.[61,64]

In a study in which my own group measured the release of tachykinins, neuropeptide K, and substance P during flushing provoked by pentagastrin or alcohol, the onset and intensity of the flushing reaction was clearly correlated with the release of tachykinins (see Fig. 44-5).[38] When the release of tachykinins was blocked by prestimulatory administration of octreotide, little or no flushing was observed in the same patient (Fig. 44-11).[38-40] Other mediators of the flushing reaction may be kallikrein and bradykinins, which are released during provoked flushing.[29-31]

Histamine may be a mediator of the flushes seen in patients with lung carcinoids or gastric carcinoids (ECLomas).[33-35] Tachykinins, bradykinins, and histamines are well-known vasodilators, and somatostatin analogues may alleviate flushing by reducing circulating levels of these agents (see later discussion).[38-40,63-68] Furschgott and Zawadski suggested that flushing is caused by indirect vasodilation mediated by endothelium-derived relaxing factor (EDRF) or by nitric oxide released by 5-HTP during platelet activation.[69]

Facial flushing associated with carcinoid tumors should be distinguished from idiopathic flushing and menopausal hot flushes. Patients with idiopathic flushes usually have a long history of flushing starting early in life and sometimes with a family history without occurrence of a tumor. Menopausal hot flushes usually involve the whole body and are accompanied by intense sweating. Postmenopausal

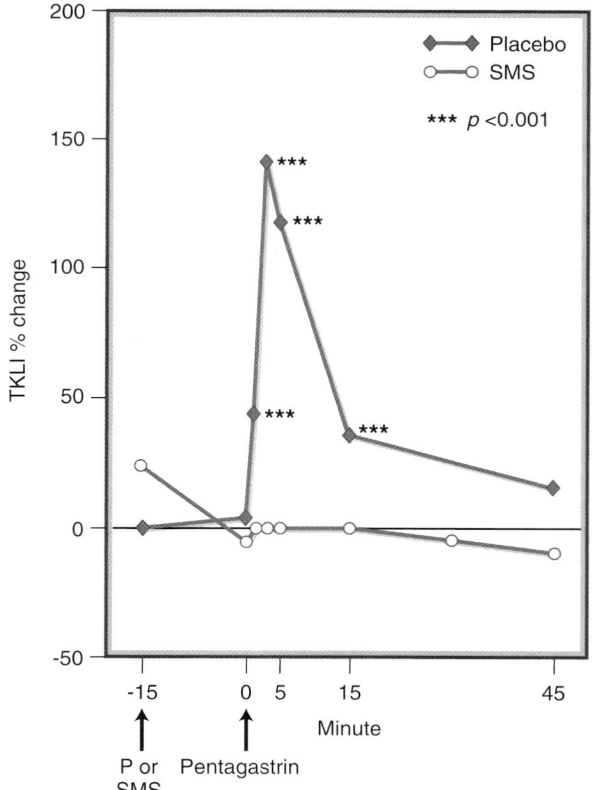

Figure 44-11 Tachykinin (TKLI) levels after stimulation with pentagastrin in patients with classic midgut carcinoids. Pretreatment for 15 minutes with somatostatin (SMS) causes inhibition of tachykinin release and inhibition of the flush reaction *(open circles)*. P, placebo.

women in whom true carcinoid syndrome is developing can tell the difference between the two types of flushes.

Diarrhea

Diarrhea occurs in 30% to 80% of patients with carcinoid syndrome.[22,25,56,57] Its pathophysiology is poorly understood but is probably multifactorial. Diarrhea is often accompanied by abdominal cramping, and endocrine, paracrine, and mechanical factors contribute to this condition. A variety of tumor products, including serotonin, tachykinins, histamines, kallikrein, and prostaglandins, can stimulate peristalsis, electromechanical activity, and tone in the intestine.[63,70-72] Secretory diarrhea can occur with fluid and electrolyte imbalance. Malabsorption can result from intestinal resections, lymphangiectasia, mesenteric fibrosis, bacterial overgrowth, tumor partially obstructing the small bowel, or rapid intestinal transit. Increased secretion by the small bowel, malabsorption, or accelerated transit can overwhelm the normal storage and absorptive capacity of proximal colon and result in diarrhea, which may be aggravated if the reabsorptive function of the colon is impaired.

In a study of patients with elevated serotonin levels and carcinoid syndrome, transit time in the small bowel and colon was significantly decreased compared with that of normal subjects.[73] The volume of the ascending colon was significantly smaller than in normal subjects, and the postprandial colonic tone was markedly increased. This indicates that in patients in whom carcinoid syndrome is associated with diarrhea, major alterations in gut motor function affect the small intestine and the colon. Many patients with carcinoid tumors have undergone wide resection of the small intestine, and they may be affected by the symptoms of short-bowel syndrome.

Serotonin is thought to cause diarrhea in patients with carcinoid syndrome through its effects on gut motility and intestinal electrolyte and fluid secretion.[57,70-72] Serotonin receptor antagonists, such as ondansetron and ketanserin, relieve the diarrhea to a certain degree.[70,74-76]

Carcinoid Heart Disease

A unique endocrine effect of carcinoid tumors is the development of plaquelike thickenings of the endocardium, valve leaflets, atria, and ventricles in 10% to 20% of patients.[77,78] This fibrotic involvement causes stenosis and regurgitation of the blood flow. Finding new collagen beneath the endothelium of the endocardium is almost pathognomonic for carcinoid heart disease.[77-79] The incidence of these lesions depends on the diagnostic methodology. Echocardiography can demonstrate early lesions in about 70% of patients with carcinoid syndrome, whereas routine clinical examinations detect them in only 30% to 40%.[77,78,80] These figures have significantly dropped to 10% to 15%, probably because of earlier diagnosis and the use of biologic antitumor treatments, such as somatostatin analogues and α-interferons. Both agents control the hormonal release and excess that may be involved in the fibrotic process.

In a study performed 15 years ago,[22] 40% of patients with carcinoid tumors died of cardiac complications related to the carcinoid disease. Later data reveal that this complication is a rare event, and patients usually die of the effects of a progressive tumor.[25]

The precise mechanism behind the fibrosis in the right heart is unknown, but it occurs mainly in patients with liver metastases who usually also have carcinoid syndrome.[77,78] Substances inducing fibrosis are thought to be released directly into the right heart and are then neutralized or degraded through the lung circulation, because few patients present with similar lesions of the left heart.[77,78] However, patients with lung carcinoids occasionally display the same fibrotic changes in the left heart. Histologically, the plaquelike thickenings in the endocardium consist of myofibroblasts and fibroblasts embedded in a stroma that is rich in mucopolysaccharides and collagen.[77]

We previously showed that the transforming growth factor-β (TGF-β) family of growth factors is upregulated in carcinoid fibrous plaques on the right heart.[81] The TGF-β family of growth factors stimulates matrix formation and collagen deposition. The substances that induce TGF-β locally in the heart have not been identified, but serotonin, tachykinins, and insulin-like growth factor 1 (IGF1) may be mediators.[77,82]

Circulating levels of serotonin and tachykinins correlate with the degree and frequency of carcinoid heart lesions. The weight-reducing drugs fenfluramine and dexfenfluramine appear to interfere with normal serotonin metabolism and have been associated with valvular lesions identical to those seen in carcinoid heart disease.[83,84] However, treatment resulting in decreased urinary 5-HIAA excretion does not lead to regression of cardiac lesions in carcinoid patients.[85] Two animal studies indicated that serotonin may play a significant role in the development of carcinoid heart disease. Serotonin also has induced TGF-β_1 in in vitro experiments.[86-88] Connective tissue growth factor (CTGF) is produced by carcinoid tumor cells, and increased expression is found in patients with advanced fibrosis. CTGF stimulates TGF-β.[89]

Bronchial Constriction

A true asthma episode is rare in patients with carcinoid syndrome.[22,56,57] The causative agents of bronchial constriction are unknown, but tachykinins and bradykinins have been suggested as mediators.[90,91] These agents can constrict smooth muscle in the respiratory tract and can cause local edema in the airways.

Other Manifestations of Carcinoid Syndrome

Fibrotic complications other than heart lesions may be found in patients with carcinoid tumors. They include intra-abdominal and retroperitoneal fibroses, occlusion of the mesenteric arteries and veins, Peyronie's disease, and carcinoid arthropathy.[56,57]

Intra-abdominal fibrosis can lead to intestinal adhesions and bowel obstruction, and it is a more common cause of bowel obstruction than is the primary carcinoid tumor itself.[54,92,93] Retroperitoneal fibrosis can result in urethral obstruction that impairs kidney function, which sometimes requires treatment with urethral stents.

Narrowing and occlusion of arteries and veins by fibrosis are potentially life threatening. Ischemic loops of the bowel may require removal, and this procedure ultimately causes short-bowel syndrome.[54,93] Other rare features of the syndrome are pellagra-like skin lesions with hyperkeratosis and pigmentation, myopathy, and sexual dysfunction.[57]

Carcinoid Crisis

Carcinoid crisis has become rare since the introduction of treatment with somatostatin analogues.[94] It may occur spontaneously or during induction of anesthesia, embolization procedures, chemotherapy, or infection. Carcinoid crisis is a clinical condition characterized by severe flushing, diarrhea, hypotension, hyperthermia, and tachycardia. Without treatment, patients may die during the crisis.[94-96]

Intravenous or subcutaneous somatostatin analogues, or both, are given before, during, and after surgery to prevent the development of carcinoid crisis.[94,96-98] Patients with metastatic lung carcinoids are particularly difficult to treat during crisis. Intravenous infusions of octreotide at doses of 50 to 100 μg/hour, supplemented with histamine H_1-receptor and H_2-receptor blockers and intravenous sodium chloride, are recommended.[99]

Other Clinical Manifestations of Carcinoid Tumors

Ectopic secretion of CRH and ACTH from pulmonary carcinoid tumors and thymic carcinoids accounts for 1% of all cases of Cushing's syndrome.[41,100] Acromegaly due to ectopic secretion of GHRH has been reported in foregut carcinoids.[42,101] Gastric carcinoid tumors make up fewer than 1% of gastric neoplasms.[20] They originate from gastric ECL cells[102] and can be separated into three distinct groups based on clinical and histologic characteristics. Type 1 (80%) is associated with chronic atrophic gastritis type A. Type 2 (6%) is associated with Zollinger-Ellison syndrome as part of MEN1 syndrome. Type 3 represents sporadic gastric carcinoids occurring without hypergastrinemia and pursues a more malignant course, with 50% to 60% of patients developing metastases.[102,103]

About 80% of gastric carcinoids are associated with chronic atrophic gastritis type A, and more than 50% of patients with these carcinoids also have pernicious anemia. These tumors are more common in women than in men and are usually identified endoscopically during diagnostic evaluation for anemia or abdominal pain.[102,104] They are often multifocal and localized in the gastric fundus area, and they are derived from ECL cells. Patients have hypochlorhydria and hypergastrinemia. Gastrin hypersecretion is thought to result in hyperplasia of the ECL cells, which may later develop into carcinoid tumors.[105,106] Hyperplasia of ECL cells has been noticed in patients on long-standing proton-pump inhibitor therapy.[107,108]

DIAGNOSIS

The diagnosis of a suspected carcinoid tumor must take into consideration molecular genetics, tumor biology, histopathology, biochemistry, and localization. The diagnosis may be suspected from clinical symptoms suggesting carcinoid syndrome or from the presence of other clinical symptoms, or it can be made in relatively asymptomatic patients from the histopathology at surgery or after liver biopsy for unknown hepatic lesions.

In one study involving 154 consecutive patients with GI carcinoids found at surgery, 60% were asymptomatic.[109] In patients with symptomatic tumors, the time from onset of symptoms until diagnosis is often delayed 1 to 2 years.[19,22] The current tumor biology program includes growth factors (e.g., platelet-derived growth factor [PDGF], epidermal growth factor [EGF], IGF1, TGF-β)[110] and proliferation factors (e.g., measurements of the nuclear antigen Ki-67) as a proliferation index. The index correlates with tumor aggressiveness and survival.[111,112] The presence of adhesion molecules such as CD44, particularly variant exons v6 and v9, is associated with improved survival.[113] Determination of the expression of angiogenic factors basic fibroblast growth factor (bFGF) and vascular endothelial growth factor (VEGF) should also be included in a tumor biology program. Somatostatin analogues are cornerstones in the treatment of carcinoid syndrome, and determination of the subtypes of somatostatin receptors (i.e., SSTR1 to SSTR5) with specific antibodies is warranted.[114,115] Rare cases of familial carcinoids should be analyzed with respect to loss of heterozygosity on chromosome 11q13 and chromosome 18.

The histopathologic diagnosis of carcinoids is based on immunohistochemistry using antibodies against CgA, synaptophysin, and neuron-specific enolase. These immunohistochemical stains have replaced the old silver stains, the argyrophil stains by Grimelius and Sevier-Munger. The argentaffin stain used by Masson to demonstrate the content of serotonin has been replaced by immunocytochemistry with serotonin antibodies.[10] These neuroendocrine markers can be supplemented by specific immunocytochemistry to different hormones, such as substance P, gastrin, and ACTH. The WHO classification forms the basis for therapeutic decisions.

Biochemical Diagnosis

In patients with flushing and other manifestations of carcinoid syndrome, the diagnosis can be established by measuring the urinary excretion of 5-HIAA, because levels are invariably elevated under these circumstances.[116] Patients with carcinoid tumors usually have a 24-hour urinary 5-HIAA output of 100 to 3000 μmol/L (15 to 60 mg), compared with the reference range of less than 50 μmol/L (10 mg) in 24 hours. Assays for urinary 5-HIAA include high-performance liquid chromatography (HPLC) with electrochemical detection and colorimetric and fluorescence methods.[117] Various foods and drugs can interfere with the measurement of urinary 5-HIAA, and patients should avoid these agents during the 24-hour sampling (Table 44-3).[118] Normally, two 24-hour urine collections are

TABLE 44-3
Factors That Interfere with Determination of Urinary 5-HIAA

Foods	Drugs
Factors That Produce False-Positive Results	
Avocado	Acetaminophen
Banana	Acetanilid
Chocolate	Caffeine
Coffee	Fluorouracil
Eggplant	Guaifenesin
Pecan	L-Dopa
Pineapple	Melphalan
Plum	Mephenesin
Tea	Methamphetamine
Walnuts	Methocarbamol
	Methysergide maleate
	Phenmetrazine
	Reserpine
	Salicylates
Factors That Cause False-Negative Results	
Corticotropin	None
p-Chlorophenylalanine	
Chlorpromazine	
Heparin	
Imipramine	
Isoniazid	
Methenamine mandelate	
Methyldopa	
Monoamine oxidase inhibitors	
Phenothiazine	
Promethazine	

5-HIAA, 5-hydroxyindoleacetic acid.

recommended. In a study of patients with malignant midgut carcinoid tumors, 60% to 73% presented with increased urinary 5-HIAA levels,[25,56,57] with a specificity of almost 100%.

Measurement of urinary 5-HIAA is the predominant biochemical analytic procedure used for diagnosis of carcinoid tumor. However, urinary and platelet measurements of serotonin can give additional information. In some studies, platelet serotonin levels were more sensitive than urinary 5-HIAA and urinary serotonin levels and were not affected by the patient's diet, as are 5-HIAA levels.

In a comparative study of 44 consecutive patients with carcinoid tumor, the platelet serotonin, urinary 5-HIAA, and urinary serotonin levels were measured. In foregut carcinoids, the sensitivities were 50%, 29%, and 55%, respectively. For midgut carcinoids, the sensitivities were 100%, 92%, and 82%, respectively, and for hindgut carcinoids, they were 20%, 0%, and 60%, respectively.[119]

Elevations of 5-HIAA can occur in malabsorption states and several other conditions. Foregut carcinoids tend to produce an atypical carcinoid syndrome with increased plasma 5-HTP levels, but not serotonin, because they lack the appropriate decarboxylase.[27,36] That results in normal urinary 5-HIAA levels. However, some of the 5-HTP is decarboxylated in the intestine and other tissues, and many of these patients have slightly elevated urinary 5-HT or 5-HIAA levels.

Attempts have been made to identify more specific and sensitive serum markers for carcinoid tumors that may allow earlier diagnosis. One such marker is CgA. CgA and CgB are more abundant than CgC in human neuroendocrine tissues.[45,46,120] In 44 patients with carcinoid tumors, CgA was increased in 99%, CgB in 88%, and CgC in only 6% (Fig. 44-12).[120] CgA levels in plasma may reflect tumor size. In a study of 75 patients with midgut carcinoids and carcinoid syndrome, CgA was elevated in 87% of carcinoid patients, and levels of plasma chromogranin correlated with extent of disease ($P < .0001$).[25] In the same study, the level of urinary 5-HIAA was elevated in 76% of midgut carcinoids, and there were no correlations with tumor size or extent of disease.

CgA is a more sensitive marker than urinary 5-HIAA in detecting carcinoid tumors, but because CgA is released and secreted from various types of neuroendocrine tumors, the specificity is lower.[120-123] In a workup of patients with carcinoid syndrome, determination of plasma CgA should be combined with that of urinary 5-HIAA or serotonin. Plasma neuron-specific enolase shows a lower sensitivity and specificity than does plasma CgA.[122] Serum hCG-α has been increased in 60% of patients with foregut carcinoid tumors and 50% of hindgut carcinoids but in only 11% of patients with midgut carcinoids and carcinoid syndrome. Plasma neuropeptide K levels have been elevated in 46% of patients with midgut carcinoids, whereas only 9% of patients with foregut carcinoids displayed elevated levels.[121,124] Plasma substance P has a sensitivity of 32% and a specificity of 85%.[25,38-40] Pancreatic polypeptide levels are also elevated in about one third of patients with midgut carcinoids and in as many with foregut carcinoids.[125,126]

During therapy with somatostatin analogues, neither plasma CgA nor urinary 5-HIAA is a reliable marker of tumor size because somatostatin inhibits the synthesis and release of the hormones without changes in tumor size.

Localization Procedures

Numerous imaging techniques, including endoscopy, barium enema, chest radiography, ultrasonography, computed tomography (CT), magnetic resonance imaging (MRI), and angiography, have been used to determine the locations of the primary tumor and metastases in patients with carcinoid tumors. In more recent years, somatostatin receptor scintigraphy (SRS) and ^{131}I-*meta*-iodobenzylguanidine (^{131}I-MIBG) scanning have been used to localize and stage the disease.[127-130] Bronchial carcinoids are usually detected by chest radiography, CT, or occasionally, by bronchoscopy.[131] The primary midgut tumor is usually small and difficult to localize with traditional diagnostic methods such as barium enema, CT, or MRI. Some tumors can be localized by angiography, capsule endoscopy, or SRS. Liver metastases are usually detected by CT or MRI.

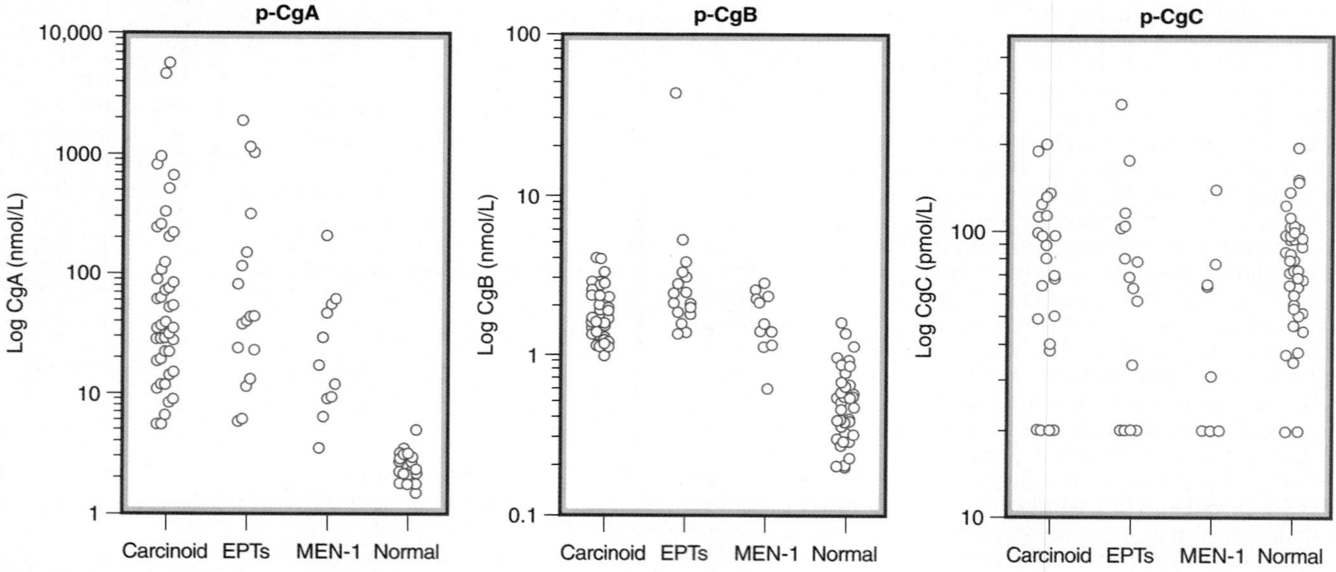

Figure 44-12 Plasma (p) levels of chromogranin A (CgA), CgB, and CgC in patients with various neuroendocrine tumors. EPTs, endocrine pancreatic tumors; MEN-1, multiple endocrine neoplasia type 1.

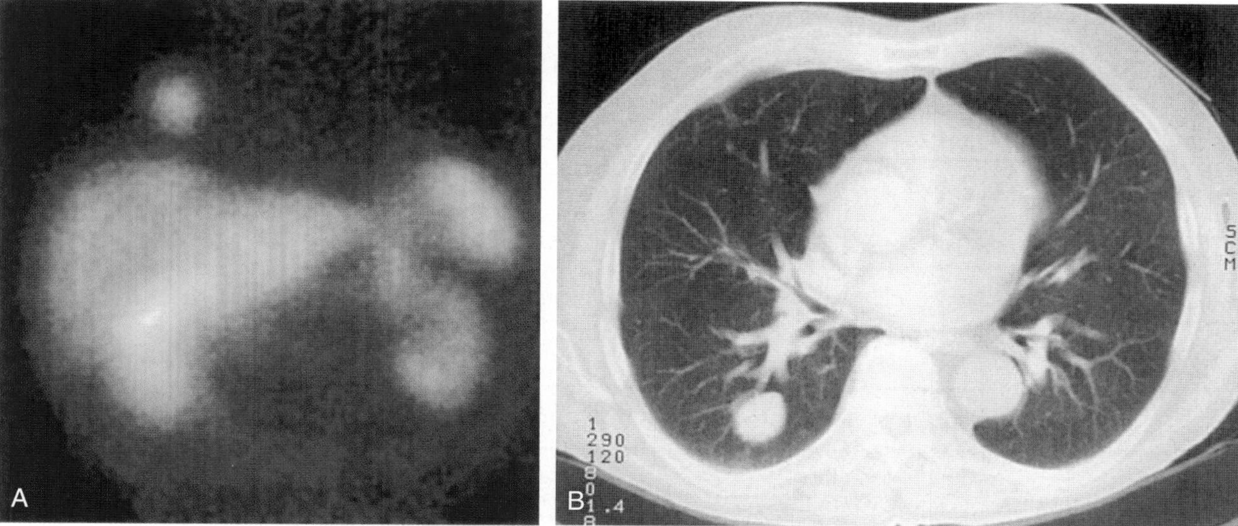

Figure 44-13 Bronchial carcinoid. **A,** Somatostatin-receptor scintigraphy in a patient with a bronchial carcinoid. **B,** Computed tomography scan in the same patient.

CT or MRI and SRS are the primary diagnostic modalities for tumor staging (Fig. 44-13).

A more sensitive method is positron emission tomography (PET) using ^{11}C-5-HTP, the precursor of serotonin synthesis (Fig. 44-14).[132,133] This isotope accumulates in carcinoid tumors, and with the development of PET cameras, tumors as small as 0.5 cm in diameter can be detected.[132] During treatment, correlations have been found among changes in the PET scan, transport rate constant, and urinary 5-HIAA, suggesting that PET scanning may be useful in monitoring the results of therapy. PET scanning using ^{18}F-fluorodeoxyglucose (FDG-PET) is not useful in detecting low-proliferating neuroendocrine tumors, but it can be beneficial in identifying poorly differentiated anaplastic tumors.

Carcinoid tumors contain high-affinity receptors for somatostatin in 80% to 100% of cases.[114,115,134] The receptors

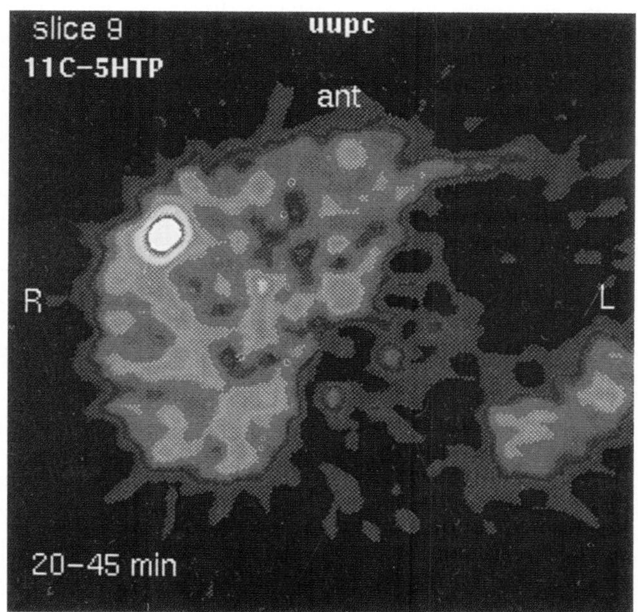

Figure 44-14 Positron emission tomography (PET) scan with ^{11}C-5-hydroxytryptophan. Notice the metastasis in the liver.

occur in both the primary tumor and metastases. Five subtypes of somatostatin receptors have been cloned, and SSTR2 is the predominant subtype expressed in carcinoid tumors.

The most commonly available somatostatin analogue, *octreotide,* binds with high affinity to SSTR2 and with lower affinity to SSTR3 and SSTR5.[135-137] SRS with ^{111}In-DTPA-Phe-octreotide (Octreoscan) can detect carcinoids in patients with a sensitivity of 80% to 90%.[137,138] Many studies have demonstrated that SRS has greater sensitivity for localizing carcinoids compared with conventional imaging studies.[138-142] False-positive scans can be obtained for patients with granulomas (e.g., sarcoidosis, tuberculosis), activated lymphocytes (e.g., lymphomas, chronic infection), thyroid diseases (e.g., goiter, thyroiditis), endocrine pancreatic tumors, and other endocrine tumors. Because of its high sensitivity and ability to image, whole-body SRS should be the initial imaging procedure to localize and establish the stage of the disease. Bone metastases, which are common with carcinoid tumors, are efficiently detected by SRS, which is as sensitive as traditional bone scanning with technetium.[140,143] ^{68}Ga-DOTA-octreotate PET scanning has also been developed and has shown higher sensitivity than Octreoscan.[144]

Scintigraphy with ^{123}I-MIBG has been applied in patients with midgut carcinoids with a sensitivity of about 50%, which is lower than that for SRS (80% to 90%). However, it can pick up carcinoids in patients that are sensitive to therapy with ^{123}I-MIBG.[145]

A diagnostic algorithm is outlined in Figure 44-15.

TREATMENT

Treatment of carcinoid tumors with carcinoid syndrome requires a multimodal approach, including symptomatic control and tumor reduction. Most patients with carcinoid syndrome have metastatic disease. The therapeutic goals are to ameliorate and improve clinical symptoms, abrogate tumor growth, improve quality of life, and if possible, prolong overall survival.

Symptomatic control of carcinoid syndrome includes lifestyle changes, diet supplementation, and specific medical treatment that reduces the clinical symptoms

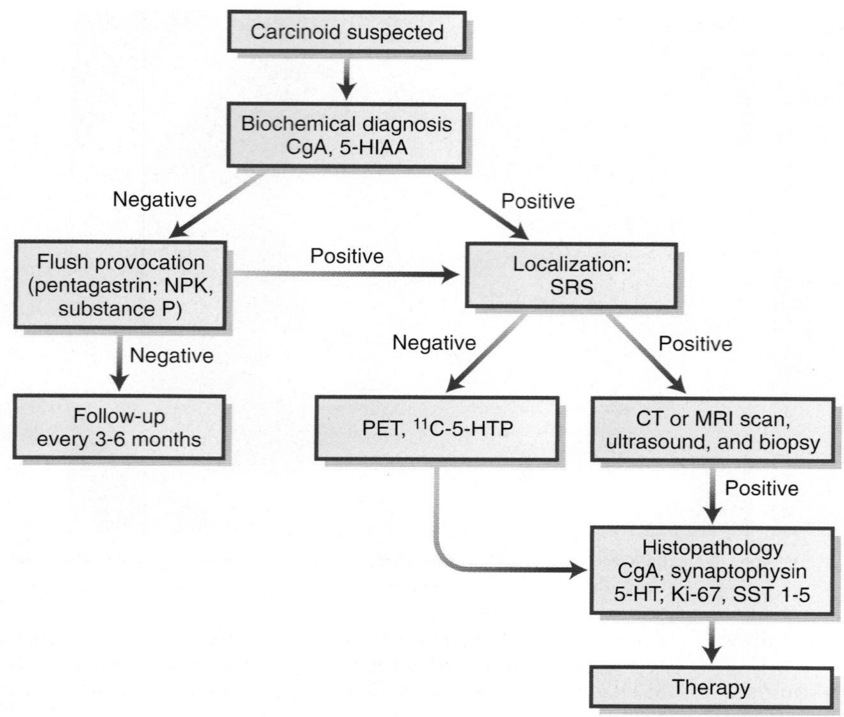

Figure 44-15 Diagnostic algorithm for patients with carcinoid tumors. CgA, chromogranin A; ^{11}C-5-HTP, ^{11}C-5-hydroxytryptophan; CT, computed tomography; 5-HIAA, 5-hydroxyindoleacetic acid; 5-HT, 5-hydroxytryptamine; MRI, magnetic resonance imaging; NPK, neuropeptide K; PET, positron emission tomography; SRS, somatostatin receptor scintigraphy; SST 1-5, somatostatin receptor subtypes 1 through 5.

related to the different components of carcinoid syndrome. Avoidance of psychological and physical stress and substances such as alcohol, spicy foods, and medications that precipitate a flushing reaction may be sufficient in early cases.[57]

Production of serotonin by the tumor consumes tryptophan. Normally, about 1% of body tryptophan is used for production of serotonin, but in carcinoid tumors, as much as 60% of the available tryptophan may be consumed for the synthesis of serotonin, and this can result in tryptophan and niacin deficiencies. Therefore, supplemental niacin has been recommended to prevent the development of pellagra. Many patients have undergone resection of the terminal ileum, which can result in vitamin B_{12} and folic acid deficiencies. Supplementation is needed in these patients.

Heart failure due to carcinoid heart disease can require diuretics or angiotensin-converting enzyme (ACE) inhibitors. A few patients need bronchodilators such as salbutamol, which interacts with β-adrenergic receptors and does not induce flushing. Diarrhea in patients with carcinoid syndrome may be controlled by loperamide or diphenoxylate.[146] If patients still have carcinoid syndrome, they receive somatostatin analogue treatment, which has replaced most of the earlier types of serotonin and serotonin receptor inhibitors. Serotonin inhibitors (e.g., parachlorophenylalanine, α-methyldopa), which inhibit serotonin synthesis, and serotonin receptor antagonists (e.g., cyproheptadine, methysergide, ketanserin) are not routinely used clinically.

Earlier treatments had limited efficacy in inhibiting flushing and diarrhea, and they were accompanied by significant side effects. A combination of histamine H_1 and H_2 receptor antagonists is effective in carcinoid syndrome that is caused by foregut carcinoids due to concomitant secretion of histamine and serotonin. Prednisolone in doses of 15 to 30 mg/day gives occasional relief in some cases of severe flushing and diarrhea.[146]

Somatostatin Analogues

Although natural somatostatin-14 reduces symptoms in patients with carcinoid syndrome,[67] its use is limited by its short half-life (approximately 2.5 minutes). During the past 2 decades, synthetic somatostatin analogues (i.e., octapeptides) have been developed for clinical use. Octreotide is the most commonly available drug; other analogues are lanreotide and vapreotide.[147-149]

The somatostatin analogues used in clinical practice (e.g., octreotide, lanreotide) (Fig. 44-16) bind to SSTR1, SSTR5, and, with lower affinity, SSTR3. They exert their cellular action through interaction with specific cell and transmembrane receptors belonging to the superfamily of G protein–coupled membrane receptors. They inhibit adenylate cyclase activity, activate phosphotyrosine phosphatases (PTPs), and modulate mitogen-activated protein kinases (MAPKs).[135,150-152] Receptor subtypes 2 and 5 modulate K^+ and Ca^{2+} fluxes in the cell.[147] Activation of all these pathways inhibits known growth factor production and release and has antiproliferative effects.[152-155]

SSTR3 mediates PTP-dependent apoptosis accompanied by activation of TP53 and the pro-apoptotic protein BAX.[156] Four of the five somatostatin receptor subtypes (SSTR2 to SSTR5) undergo rapid internalization after ligand binding, which has been explored by tumor-targeted radioactive somatostatin analogue therapy.[150,152,157]

An antiproliferative effect has been reported to occur, probably through a combination of SSTR2 and SSTR5 activities, which inhibits MAPK and K^+ and Ca^{2+} fluxes, leading to cell cycle arrest[153-155]; the precise antitumor mechanism, however, is unknown.

Different subtypes of somatostatin receptors form heterodimers with each other (e.g., SSTR1 and SSTR5) and with the D_2 dopamine receptor (DRD2). This cross-talk modulates the intracellular signal and fine-tunes the mediated effects.[158]

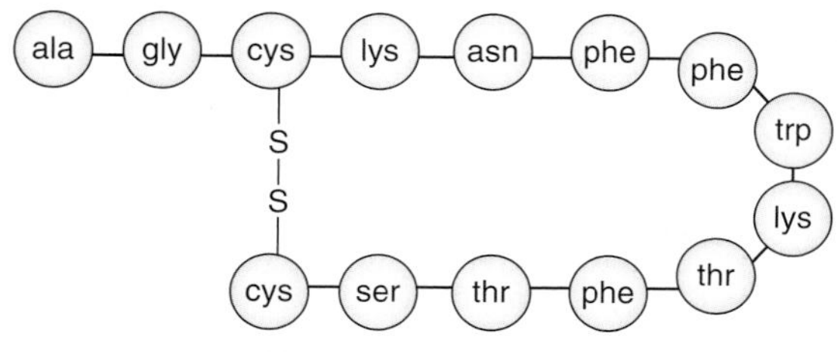

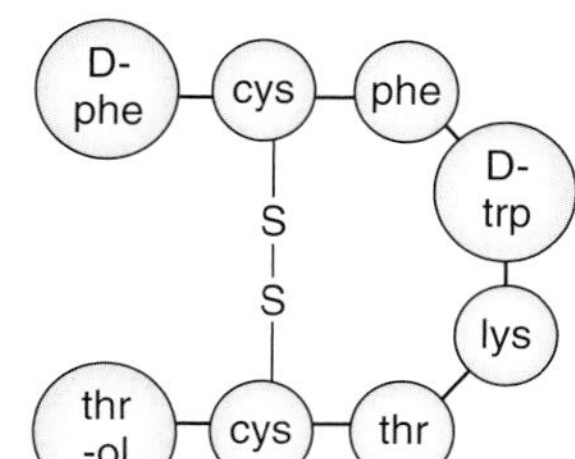

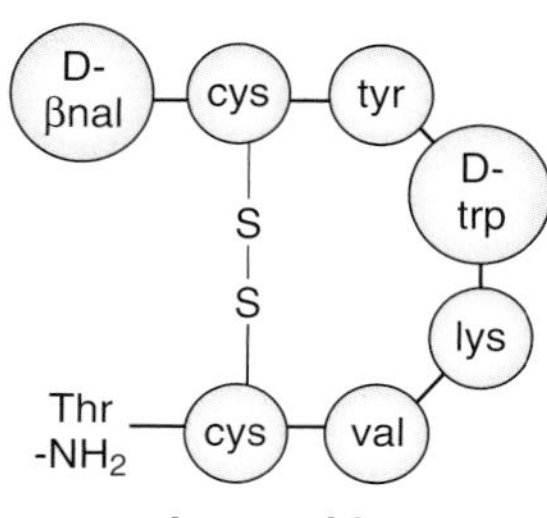

Figure 44-16 Molecular structures of human somatostatin-14, octreotide acetate, and lanreotide.

The five subtypes of somatostatin receptors are expressed in carcinoid tumors in various combinations, and some tumors express all five subtypes.[115,150,159,160] The receptors are expressed on tumor cells and also in peritumoral veins.[161] Antiangiogenesis may be another antitumor mechanism of somatostatin analogues.[162]

Subcutaneous administration of octreotide and lanreotide every 8 to 12 hours can control clinical symptoms in about 60% to 70% of patients with carcinoid syndrome; these agents are considered the drugs of choice.[97,163-167] Octreotide and lanreotide decrease serotonin and urinary 5-HIAA levels and plasma tachykinin and CgA levels. The recommended dose for octreotide is 100 to 150 μg two or three times daily, a standard treatment for controlling clinical symptoms.[97] However, some patients require higher doses, up to a total of 3000 μg/day, to control the clinical symptoms and tumor growth, particularly during long-term therapy.

Tachyphylaxis (i.e., reduced sensitivity) to somatostatin analogues can develop during long-term therapy.[152] Long-acting, slow-release formulations of octreotide and lanreotide have been developed, and doses of Octreotide LAR of 20 to 30 mg given once per month or Somatuline Autogel of 90 to 120 mg once per month control clinical symptoms and hormone levels in 50% to 60% of patients with carcinoid syndrome.[168-170] The long-acting formulations of somatostatin analogues have clearly improved the quality of life of patients by reducing the number of injections and provide more stable control of clinical symptoms.[169] A new somatostatin analogue (SOM230) that binds SSTR1, SSTR2, SSTR3, and SSTR5 is being evaluated in clinical trials for the treatment of carcinoid tumors.

High-dose therapy with lanreotide (12 mg/day) and octreotide (3 mg/day) has increased the percentage of patients demonstrating a significant reduction in tumor size (12% versus 5% for the standard dose).[171-174] Induction of apoptosis has been achieved with high-dose therapy,[175] possibly mediated through activation of SSTR3. Ultra-high-dose octreotide has generated significant antitumor responses in patients resistant to standard-dose therapy.[176] A prospective, randomized study in midgut carcinoids (PROMID) demonstrated a significantly longer time to progression for Octreotide LAR compared with placebo.[177] These data have changed the U.S. National Comprehensive Cancer Network guidelines for the treatment of carcinoid tumors. All types of carcinoid tumors, irrespective of functionality, can be treated with octreotide.

For patients at risk for carcinoid crisis, somatostatin analogue therapy is the treatment of choice. Carcinoid crisis is a life-threatening complication of carcinoid syndrome. It can occur spontaneously or may be associated with stress and anesthesia, chemotherapy, and infections. Patients usually experience severe flushing, diarrhea, abdominal pain, and hypotension. Continuous infusion with somatostatin analogues, 50 to 100 μg/hour, is recommended and usually alters the life-threatening condition. Patients should be given subcutaneous somatostatin analogues before surgery or other stressful situations.

Side effects of somatostatin analogue therapy usually have not been serious and occur in 20% to 40% of patients. They include pain at the injection site, gas formation, diarrhea, and abdominal cramping. Significant long-term side effects include gallstone formation, sludge in the gallbladder, steatorrhea, deterioration of glucose tolerance, and hypocalcemia.[97,168,169] The incidence of gallstones in patients treated over the long term has varied from 5% to 70%, and the incidence of symptomatic gallstones requiring surgical treatment is less than 10%.[178]

Interferons

Interferon-α (IFN-α)—alone or in combination with somatostatin analogue—is effective in the treatment of the carcinoid syndrome. Symptomatic and biochemical control is obtained in 40% to 50% of patients with the recommended doses of 3 to 5 million units of recombinant interferon alfa-2a or interferon alfa-2b given subcutaneously three to five times per week.[179-185] Significant tumor reduction is reported in 10% to 20% of the patients.[179,185]

IFN-α exerts a direct effect on the tumor cells by blocking cell division in the G_1/S phase of the cell cycle, by inhibiting protein and hormone synthesis, and by reducing angiogenesis through inhibition of angiogenic factors bFGF and VEGF. It has also an indirect effect through stimulation of the immune system, particularly T cells and natural killer cells.[186-189] Response to IFN-α can be predicted by analyzing induction of 2′,5′-oligoadenylate synthetase or protein kinase p68 (PKR), enzymes involved in cell cycle regulation and protein synthesis.[190,191] Long-acting formulations of IFN-α (i.e., pegylated interferons) can be applied at doses of 80 to 150 μg/week subcutaneously.

Treatment with IFN-α induces an intratumoral fibrosis that is not picked up by regular CT scanning or ultrasonography, and tumor size may therefore remain unchanged.[192] The side effects of α-interferons are more pronounced than with somatostatin analogues and include chronic fatigue syndrome, anemia, leukopenia, and thrombocytopenia; 10% to 15% of patients may develop autoimmune reactions.[180,193] Most of the side effects are dose-dependent and can be managed by individualizing the dose.

Patients with carcinoid syndrome who have not responded to octreotide or IFN-α alone may be given both agents. Such combinations have generated symptomatic control in 70% of patients and stabilization of tumor growth in 40% to 50% of patients.[194,195] The combination also offers better tolerance of α-interferons when somatostatin analogues are added. Moreover, somatostatin analogue treatment is hampered by the development of tachyphylaxis with time, which means less sensitivity to the somatostatin analogue, necessitating escalating doses and eventually withdrawal of the compound for several months, after which IFN-α therapy can continue. Conversely, IFN-α may be withdrawn and the somatostatin analogue continued if severe side effects of IFN-α (mainly chronic fatigue syndrome or mental depression) develop.[196]

Chemotherapy

Most oncologists agree that patients with classic midgut carcinoids and carcinoid syndrome, in which tumors show low proliferation capacity, should not receive chemotherapy. The results of various studies have been disappointing; response rates are no more than 5% to 10%, are short lived, and are accompanied by considerable side effects.[197,198] The combination of streptozotocin and 5-fluorouracil, which has demonstrated antitumor effects in endocrine pancreatic tumors, has not shown similar effects in classic midgut carcinoids.[199] In foregut carcinoids, which usually manifest a more malignant behavior, cytotoxic treatment may be attempted. Chemotherapeutic combinations include streptozotocin plus 5-fluorouracil, doxorubicin plus streptozocin cisplatin plus etoposide, and dacarbazine plus 5-fluorouracil.[200-202] Temozolomide has significant efficacy in foregut carcinoids.[203] All of these cytotoxic treatments can be combined with a somatostatin analogue.

Other Agents

Tyrosine kinase receptors such as platelet-derived growth factor receptor (PDGFR) α/β, epidermal growth factor receptor (EGFR), and vascular endothelial growth factor receptor (VEGFR) are expressed in carcinoid tumor cells and in the stroma cells. Therefore, tyrosine kinase receptor inhibitors have been used, with objective response rates of about 10% to 15%.[204] Inhibitors of the mammalian target of rapamycin (mTOR) are drugs that block the mTOR signaling pathway, which is activated in many tumors. Everolimus alone or in combination with octreotide has generated objective response rates of 15% to 20%.[205]

Surgery

Because most tumors in patients with carcinoid syndrome are malignant at the time of clinical presentation, surgical cure is seldom obtained. Resection of local disease or regional nodular metastatic disease can cure some patients; however, even if radical surgery cannot be performed, debulking procedures and bypass should always be considered and can be performed at any time during the course of treatment.[54,93,206]

In recent years, a more proactive attitude among surgeons has emerged, and wider resections and debulking procedures are being performed today than in the 1990s.[54,207] In contrast to other metastatic tumors to the liver, for which liver transplantation has given poor results, liver transplantation can benefit patients with metastatic carcinoids.[208,209] In a review of 103 patients with malignant neuroendocrine tumors, including carcinoids and pancreatic endocrine tumors, 5- and 2-year survival rates were 16% and 47%, respectively; however, recurrence-free survival was less than 24%.[208] Liver transplantation may be considered in younger patients (<50 years) who have a life-threatening, uncontrolled carcinoid syndrome during medical therapy or tumor-targeted radioactive treatment without known metastatic spread outside the liver.

Another means of tumor reduction is hepatic artery embolization, which not only improves the symptoms of carcinoid syndrome in about 50% of the patients but also reduces the tumor size in as many. The therapeutic effect may last for 9 to 12 months, and the procedure can be repeated.[210,211] Chemoembolization—simultaneous embolization with surgical gel (i.e., Gelfoam) and chemotherapy (mitomycin C, cisplatin, 5-fluorouracil) or IFN-α—has resulted in symptomatic improvement in a significant number of patients with carcinoid syndrome.[212,213] However, hepatic artery occlusion or embolization can result in serious side effects (e.g., nausea, vomiting, liver pain, fever) and major complications (e.g., hepatorenal syndrome, sepsis, gallbladder perforation, intestinal necrosis). Complications occur in 5% to 7% of patients.[211-213]

Other cytoreductive treatments include cryotherapy and radiofrequency ablation.[214] However, these procedures are limited to patients with smaller tumor burden, tumors less than 5 cm in diameter, and a limited number of metastases.

Irradiation

External irradiation has demonstrated limited efficacy and is used mainly to palliate symptoms related to bone and brain metastases.[215,216] MIBG is taken up by carcinoids and is concentrated. The possibility of radiolabeled MIBG therapy has been evaluated in a limited number of patients. The response rate has been about 30% with ^{125}I-MIBG or ^{131}I-MIBG.[217,218]

Somatostatin analogue–based, tumor-targeted radioactive treatment has been applied using ^{111}In-DTPA-octreotide. Symptomatic improvement has been reported for about 40% of patients, and tumor stabilization has occurred in about 30%.[219] Indium 111 is a weak irradiator (Auger electrons) and seems to be replaced by yttrium 90 (^{90}Y), a γ and β emitter.

Studies with ^{90}Y-DOTA-octreotide have shown promising results.[220] The new isotope lutetium 177, a β emitter, has come into clinical use as Lu^{177}-DOTA-octreotate, with further improved results. Significant tumor reduction has occurred in 30% to 40% of patients with advanced disease. However, this agent is more effective for small tumors. It is an attractive mode of treatment because the radioactive ligand, after binding to the receptor, is internalized and transported to the cell nucleus, causing DNA damage.[221] Because tumor cells usually have higher-density somatostatin receptors (SSTR2 and SSTR5) than do surrounding normal tissues, the treatment may be better tolerated. The treatment algorithm for metastatic carcinoid tumor is provided in Figure 44-17.

PROGNOSIS

Carcinoid syndrome is a clinical manifestation of advanced disease. Carcinoids from various sites differ in the percentage developing carcinoid syndrome and in their aggressiveness. Survival rates for patients with carcinoids depend on the site and the extent of the tumor. In patients with

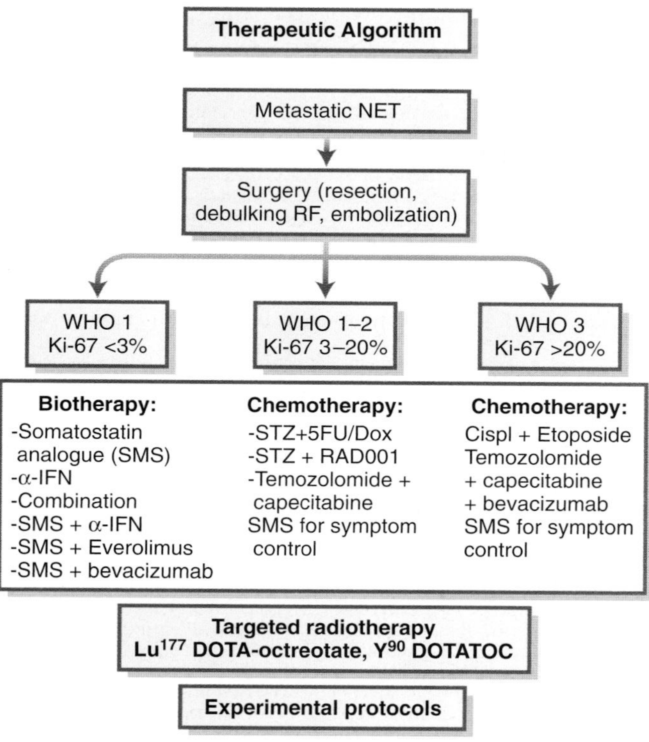

Figure 44-17 Therapeutic algorithm for treatment of metastatic carcinoid tumor. DOTATOC, DOTA-octreotide; Dox, doxorubicin; 5FU, 5-fluorouracil; IFN, interferon; NET, neuroendocrine tumor; RAD001, everolimus; STZ, streptozotocin; WHO, World Health Organization classification.

localized disease, the 5-year survival rate for those with midgut carcinoids is about 65%, not essentially higher than that for patients with regional metastases. In patients with distant metastases, the 5-year survival rate is reduced to 39%.[10,19,20,23,25] The relative 5-, 10-, and 15-year survival rates for those with midgut carcinoids are 67%, 54%, and 44%, respectively.[221] The 5- and 10-year survival rates for patients with typical bronchial carcinoid are 95% and 80%, respectively. Patients with atypical lung carcinoids have only a 50% survival rate at 5 years.[18]

An important determinant of survival in carcinoid patients is the presence of metastases. Female gender and younger age are associated with a better prognosis. Other factors that correlate with impaired survival are high CgA level at diagnosis and high proliferation index (Ki-67).[34,111] During the 1990s, there was a reduced incidence of death from carcinoid heart disease, possibly a result of earlier diagnosis, active surgery, and the introduction of somatostatin analogues and α-interferons. In a study performed by our group, 30% of the patients died of carcinoid heart complications.[22] In a later study, this rate was reduced to less than 10%.[25] Clinically significant carcinoid heart disease is now rare. Between 5% and 10% of patients with carcinoids are at increased risk for simultaneous adenocarcinoma of the large intestine. Occurrence of a second malignancy is associated with a worse prognosis.[20,23]

OTHER FLUSHING DISORDERS

Medullary Thyroid Carcinoma and VIPoma

Other neuroendocrine tumors, such as medullary thyroid carcinoma (MTC) and VIP-producing tumors (e.g., ganglioneuroma, endocrine pancreatic tumors), can manifest with flushing syndromes (Fig. 44-18).[222,223] Patients also may have diarrhea, particularly those with VIP-producing tumors, which are accompanied by severe secretory diarrhea. In patients with MTC, flushing and diarrhea are infrequent symptoms and are seen mainly in patients with high circulating levels of calcitonin and CGRP.

The mechanism producing flushing and diarrhea is unknown, but it may be mediated through prostaglandins stimulated by calcitonin. The frequency of flushing and diarrhea is usually less than 5% in patients with advanced metastatic MTC.[222,224] Treatment is directed against tumor growth and can consist of surgical resection, embolization of liver metastases, and cytotoxic treatment (i.e., doxorubicin-based combination therapies). Somatostatin analogue therapy can alleviate the diarrhea.

VIPoma or the watery diarrhea, hypokalemia, and achlorhydria (WDHA) syndrome (i.e., Verner-Morrison syndrome) is associated with severe secretory diarrhea (up to 15 L/day), and some patients also display continuous, whole-body, violaceous flushing and hypotension.[223,225] The syndrome also includes achlorhydria, hypokalemia, and metabolic acidosis and is related to overproduction of VIP and a related peptide-peptide histidine methionine. These patients have tumors in the pancreas, lung, or sympathetic ganglia.[223,224]

The diagnosis is confirmed by measuring plasma VIP, which usually exceeds 70 pmol/L.[226] Treatment is directed against the tumor and hormone excess. Administration of somatostatin analogues by subcutaneous or intravenous infusion in the worst cases can control clinical symptoms.[227] Cytotoxic treatment with streptozotocin-based combinations, 5-fluorouracil, or doxorubicin is recommended for malignant cases.[197]

Mastocytosis and Related Disorders

Mastocytosis and other systemic mast cell activation are clinically related to flushing disorders. Most patients with mastocytosis have an indolent course, but some forms of mastocytosis are aggressive. Symptoms are attributed primarily to paroxysmal mast cell activation.[228,229]

Most patients with mastocytosis have evidence of cutaneous involvement, most commonly multiple, small, pigmented lesions that produce urticaria on stroking with

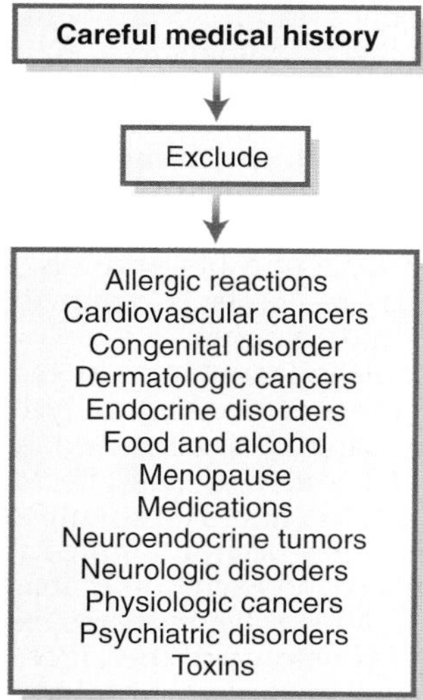

Figure 44-18 Flushing disorders. (From Yale SH, Vasudeva S, Mazza JJ, et al. Disorders of flushing. *Compr Ther.* 2005;31:59-71.)

a blunt object (Darier's sign); this condition is called *urticaria pigmentosa*.[230] Another form of cutaneous mastocytosis is a more telangiectatic form called *telangiectasia macularis eruptiva persistans*. Hepatomegaly and splenomegaly can be caused by infiltration of mast cells, and hepatic fibrosis is also common.[231,232]

Bone involvement may manifest as osteoporosis or osteosclerosis.[233] Systemic mastocytosis can also involve the GI tract with mucosal nodules in the ileum, stomach, and large bowel.[234]

Hematologic abnormalities are nonspecific, with marked mast cell infiltration of the bone, anemia, leukocytosis, eosinophilia, and sometimes, lymphadenopathy.[235] In a subgroup of patients, mastocytosis is secondary to primary hematologic disorders, usually myeloproliferative or myelodysplastic disease.[236,237] Mast cell leukemia has been reported in rare cases.[238] The primary eosinophilia seen in some patients with the FIP1-like 1/PDGFR-α *(FIP1L1-PDGFRA)* gene rearrangement represents a subset of chronic eosinophilic leukemia. These patients also have elevated serum tryptase levels.[239] More than 80% of patients with systemic mastocytosis have activating mutations (D816V) in the tyrosine kinase domain of *KIT* that alter mast cell growth and differentiation.[239,240]

Clinical signs of systemic mastocytosis include flushing, tachycardia, and hypotension and sometimes include nausea, vomiting, and diarrhea. This syndrome resembles carcinoid syndrome. Histamine is a potent vasodilator and is released from mast cells. Other mediators of the syndrome are the release of prostaglandin D_2, tryptase, and heparin.[241] Prostaglandin D_2 is a more potent mediator than histamine.

The diagnosis is made by measurement of histamine and histamine metabolites in the urine.[241,242] Quantification of histamine metabolites (*N*-methylhistamine and methylimidazole acetic acid) appears to be more sensitive for overproduction of histamine in patients with mastocytosis.[242] Endogenous production of prostaglandin D_2 can be assessed by quantifying the major urinary metabolite (9α-hydroxy-11,15-dioxo-2,3,18,19-tetranorprost-5-ene-1,20-dioic acid).[243] However, these measurements can be done only in specialized laboratories. Measurement of the tryptase release is easier to perform, and increased quantities of this granule-associated enzyme tryptase can be detected by immunoassay.[244] Bone marrow analysis of $CD25^+$ cells may support the diagnosis of mast cell disease.[239]

Treatment depends on the severity of the disease. As in the treatment of allergic anaphylaxis, epinephrine is effective in reversing the hypotension associated with mast cell mediator release[245]; these patients should have constant access to epinephrine in the form of subcutaneous injection or inhalation. Chronic therapy to prevent acute attacks includes antihistamine therapy combined with inhibition of prostaglandin biosynthesis. Blockade of histamine H_1 and H_2 receptors is required to prevent the vasodilator effect of histamine.[99,239]

Nonsteroidal anti-inflammatory drugs (NSAIDs) inhibit the cyclooxygenase enzyme that catalyzes the formation of prostaglandins. Aspirin has been used, but some patients cannot tolerate it because of side effects in the gut and allergic reactions.[246] In patients resistant to antihistamines and NSAIDs, IFN-α has been attempted with a reduction in mast cell numbers and excretion of mast cell mediators. Treatment with IFN-α is still considered experimental.[239,247] A subset of patients who carry the *FIP1L1-PDGFRA* oncogene achieve complete clinical, histologic, and molecular remission with imatinib mesylate therapy, in contrast to those with the *KIT* D816V mutation.[239]

REFERENCES

1. Lubarsch O. Ueber den primaren Krebs des Ileum, nebst Bemerkungen über das gleichzeitige Vorkommen von Krebs und Tuberkuolose. *Virchow Archiv Pathol Anatom Physiol Klin Med.* 1867;111:280-317.
2. Oberndorfer S. Karzenoide Tumoren des Dünndarms. *Frankf Zschr Pathol.* 1907;1:426-430.
3. Pearson CM, Fitzgerald PJ. Carcinoid tumors—a re-emphasis of their malignant nature: review of 140 cases. *Cancer.* 1949;2:1005-1026.
4. Thorson A, Biorck G, Bjorkman G, et al. Malignant carcinoid of the small intestine with metastases to the liver, valvular disease of the right side of the heart (pulmonary stenosis and tricuspid regurgitation without septal defects), peripheral vasomotor symptoms, bronchoconstriction, and an unusual type of cyanosis: a clinical and pathologic syndrome. *Am Heart J.* 1954;47:795-817.
5. Lembeck F. 5-Hydroxytryptamine in carcinoid tumor. *Nature.* 1953;172:910-911.
6. Gosset A, Masson P. Tumeurs endocrines de l'appendice. *Presse Med.* 1914;25:237-239.
7. Masson P. Carcinoid (argentaffin-cell tumors) and nerve hyperplasia of appendicular mucosa. *Am J Pathol.* 1928;4:181-212.
8. Pearse AG. The cytochemistry and ultrastructure of polypeptide hormone-producing cells of the APUD series and the embryologic, physiologic and pathologic implications of the concept. *J Histochem Cytochem.* 1969;17:303-313.
9. Andrew A. The APUD concept: where has it led us? *Br Med Bull.* 1982;38:221-225.
10. Wilander E, Lundqvist M, Oberg K. Gastrointestinal carcinoid tumours: histogenetic, histochemical, immunohistochemical, clinical and therapeutic aspects. *Prog Histochem Cytochem.* 1989;19:1-88.
11. Debelenko LV, Brambilla E, Agarwal SK, et al. Identification of MEN1 gene mutations in sporadic carcinoid tumors of the lung. *Hum Mol Genet.* 1997;6:2285-2290.
12. Zhao J, de Krijger RR, Meier D, et al. Genomic alterations in well-differentiated gastrointestinal and bronchial neuroendocrine tumors (carcinoids): marked differences indicating diversity in molecular pathogenesis. *Am J Pathol.* 2000;157:1431-1438.
13. Lollgen RM, Hessman O, Szabo E, et al. Chromosome 18 deletions are common events in classical midgut carcinoid tumors. *Int J Cancer.* 2001;92:812-815.
14. Gartner W, Mineva I, Daneva T, et al. A newly identified RET proto-oncogene polymorphism is found in a high number of endocrine tumor patients. *Hum Genet.* 2005;117:143-153.
15. Nakakura EK, Sriuranpong VR, Kunnimalaiyaan M, et al. Regulation of neuroendocrine differentiation in gastrointestinal carcinoid tumor cells by notch signaling. *J Clin Endocrinol Metab.* 2005;90:4350-4356.
16. Williams ED, Sandler M. The classification of carcinoid tumours. *Lancet.* 1963;1:238-239.
17. Solcia E, Kloppel G, Sobin L, eds. Histological typing of endocrine tumours. *World Health Organization Histological Classification of Tumours.* 2nd ed. Berlin: Springer-Verlag; 2000:38-74.

17a. Rinki G, Klöppel G, Couvelard A, et al. TNM staging of midgut and hindgut (neuro) endocrine tumors: a consensus proposal including a grading system. *Virchows Arch.* 2007;951:757-762.

18. Travis WD, Rush W, Flieder DB, et al. Survival analysis of 200 pulmonary neuroendocrine tumors with clarification of criteria for atypical carcinoid and its separation from typical carcinoid. *Am J Surg Pathol.* 1998;22:934-944.
19. Moertel CG. Karnofsky memorial lecture: an odyssey in the land of small tumors. *J Clin Oncol.* 1987;5:1502-1522.
20. Modlin IM, Lye KD, Kidd M. A 5-decade analysis of 13,715 carcinoid tumors. *Cancer.* 2003;97:934-959.
21. Berge T, Linell F. Carcinoid tumours: frequency in a defined population during a 12-year period. *Acta Pathol Microbiol Scand A.* 1976;84:322-330.
22. Norheim I, Oberg K, Theodorsson-Norheim E, et al. Malignant carcinoid tumors: an analysis of 103 patients with regard to tumor localization, hormone production, and survival. *Ann Surg.* 1987;206:115-125.
23. Godwin 2nd JD. Carcinoid tumors: an analysis of 2,837 cases. *Cancer.* 1975;36:560-569.
24. Quaedvlieg PF, Visser O, Lamers CB, et al. Epidemiology and survival in patients with carcinoid disease in The Netherlands: an epidemiological study with 2391 patients. *Ann Oncol.* 2001;12:1295-1300.
25. Janson ET, Holmberg L, Stridsberg M, et al. Carcinoid tumors: analysis of prognostic factors and survival in 301 patients from a referral center. *Ann Oncol.* 1997;8:685-690.
26. Yao JC, Hassan M, Phan A, et al. One hundred years after "carcinoid": epidemiology of and prognostic factors for neuroendocrine tumors in 35,825 cases in the United States. *J Clin Oncol.* 2008;26:3063-3072.
27. Sandler M, Scheuer PJ, Wat PJ. 5-Hydroxytryptophan-secreting bronchial carcinoid tumour. *Lancet.* 1961;2:1067-1069.
28. Oates JA, Sjoerdsma A. A unique syndrome associated with secretion of 5-hydroxytryptophan by metastatic gastric carcinoids. *Am J Med.* 1962;32:333-342.

29. Oates JA, Melmon K, Sjoerdsma A, et al. Release of a kinin peptide in the carcinoid syndrome. *Lancet*. 1964;1:514-517.
30. Lucas KJ, Feldman JM. Flushing in the carcinoid syndrome and plasma kallikrein. *Cancer*. 1986;58:2290-2293.
31. Gustafsen J, Boesby S, Nielsen F, et al. Bradykinin in carcinoid syndrome. *Gut*. 1987;28:1417-1419.
32. Metz SA, McRae JR, Robertson RP. Prostaglandins as mediators of paraneoplastic syndromes: review and up-date. *Metabolism*. 1981;30:299-316.
33. Roberts 2nd LJ, Bloomgarden ZT, Marney Jr SR, et al. Histamine release from a gastric carcinoid: provocation by pentagastrin and inhibition by somatostatin. *Gastroenterology*. 1983;84:272-275.
34. Gilligan CJ, Lawton GP, Tang LH, et al. Gastric carcinoid tumors: the biology and therapy of an enigmatic and controversial lesion. *Am J Gastroenterol*. 1995;90:338-352.
35. Todd TR, Cooper JD, Weissberg D, et al. Bronchial carcinoid tumors: twenty years' experience. *J Thorac Cardiovasc Surg*. 1980;79:532-536.
36. Kema IP, de Vries EG, Slooff MJ, et al. Serotonin, catecholamines, histamine, and their metabolites in urine, platelets, and tumor tissue of patients with carcinoid tumors. *Clin Chem*. 1994;40:86-95.
37. Håkansson R, Bergmark S, Brodin E, et al. Substance-P-like immunoreactivity in intestinal carcinoid tumors. In: von Euler U, Pernow B, eds. *Substance-P*. New York: Raven; 1977:55-58.
38. Norheim I, Theodorsson-Norheim E, Brodin E, et al. Tachykinins in carcinoid tumors: their use as a tumor marker and possible role in the carcinoid flush. *J Clin Endocrinol Metab*. 1986;63:605-612.
39. Theodorsson-Norheim E, Norheim I, Oberg K, et al. Neuropeptide K: a major tachykinin in plasma and tumor tissues from carcinoid patients. *Biochem Biophys Res Commun*. 1985;131:77-83.
40. Conlon JM, Deacon CF, Richter G, et al. Measurement and partial characterization of the multiple forms of neurokinin A-like immunoreactivity in carcinoid tumours. *Regul Pept*. 1986;13:183-196.
41. Becker M, Aron DC. Ectopic ACTH syndrome and CRH-mediated Cushing's syndrome. *Endocrinol Metab Clin North Am*. 1994;23:585-606.
42. Jensen RT, Norton JA. Endocrine neoplasms of the pancreas. In: Yamada T, Alpers D, Owyang C, eds. *Textbook of Gastroenterology*. Philadelphia: JB Lippincott; 1998:2193.
43. Mao C, Shah A, Hanson DJ, et al. Von Recklinghausen's disease associated with duodenal somatostatinoma: contrast of duodenal versus pancreatic somatostatinomas. *J Surg Oncol*. 1995;59:67-73.
44. Banks P, Helle K. The release of protein from the stimulated adrenal medulla. *Biochem J*. 1965;97:40C-41C.
45. Fischer-Colbrie R, Hagn C, Schober M. Chromogranins A, B, and C: widespread constituents of secretory vesicles. *Ann N Y Acad Sci*. 1987;493:120-134.
46. Iacangelo AL, Eiden LE. Chromogranin A: current status as a precursor for bioactive peptides and a granulogenic/sorting factor in the regulated secretory pathway. *Regul Pept*. 1995;58:65-88.
47. Tatemoto K, Efendic S, Mutt V, et al. Pancreastatin, a novel pancreatic peptide that inhibits insulin secretion. *Nature*. 1986;324:476-478.
48. Angeletti RH, Mints L, Aber C, et al. Determination of residues in chromogranin A-(16-40) required for inhibition of parathyroid hormone secretion. *Endocrinology*. 1996;137:2918-2922.
49. Aardal S, Helle KB, Elsayed S, et al. Vasostatins, comprising the N-terminal domain of chromogranin A, suppress tension in isolated human blood vessel segments. *J Neuroendocrinol*. 1993;5:405-412.
50. Wiedenmann B, Huttner WB. Synaptophysin and chromogranins/secretogranins: widespread constituents of distinct types of neuroendocrine vesicles and new tools in tumor diagnosis. *Virchows Archiv*. 1989;58:95-121.
51. Harpole Jr DH, Feldman JM, Buchanan S, et al. Bronchial carcinoid tumors: a retrospective analysis of 126 patients. *Ann Thorac Surg*. 1992;54:50-54; discussion 54-55.
52. Barclay TH, Schapira DV. Malignant tumors of the small intestine. *Cancer*. 1983;51:878-881.
53. Moertel CG, Sauer WG, Dockerty MB, et al. Life history of the carcinoid tumor of the small intestine. *Cancer*. 1961;14:901-912.
54. Makridis C, Oberg K, Juhlin C, et al. Surgical treatment of mid-gut carcinoid tumors. *World J Surg*. 1990;14:377-383; discussion 384-385.
55. Bean WB, Olch D, Weinberg HB. The syndrome of carcinoid and acquired valve lesions of the right side of the heart. *Circulation*. 1955;12:1-6.
56. Grahame-Smith DG. The carcinoid syndrome. *Am J Cardiol*. 1968;21:376-387.
57. Feldman JM. Carcinoid tumors and syndrome. *Semin Oncol*. 1987;14:237-246.
58. Smith RA. Bronchial carcinoid tumours. *Thorax*. 1969;24:43-50.
59. Caldarola VT, Jackman RJ, Moertel CG, et al. Carcinoid tumors of the rectum. *Am J Surg*. 1964;107:844-849.
60. Levin R, Elsas L, Duvall C, et al. Malignant carcinoid tumors with and without flushing. *JAMA*. 1963;186:905-907.
61. Matuchansky C, Launay JM. Serotonin, catecholamines, and spontaneous midgut carcinoid flush: plasma studies from flushing and nonflushing sites. *Gastroenterology*. 1995;108:743-751.
62. Robertson JI, Peart WS, Andrews TM. The mechanism of facial flushes in the carcinoid syndrome. *Q J Med*. 1962;31:103-123.
63. Makridis C, Theodorsson E, Akerstrom G, et al. Increased intestinal non–substance P tachykinin concentrations in malignant midgut carcinoid disease. *J Gastroenterol Hepatol*. 1999;14:500-507.
64. Creutzfeldt W, Stockmann F. Carcinoids and carcinoid syndrome. *Am J Med*. 1987;82:4-16.
65. Emson PC, Gilbert RF, Martensson H, et al. Elevated concentrations of substance P and 5-HT in plasma in patients with carcinoid tumors. *Cancer*. 1984;54:715-718.
66. Schaffalitzky De Muckadell OB, Aggestrup S, et al. Flushing and plasma substance P concentration during infusion of synthetic substance P in normal man. *Scand J Gastroenterol*. 1986;21:498-502.
67. Frolich JC, Bloomgarden ZT, Oates JA, et al. The carcinoid flush: provocation by pentagastrin and inhibition by somatostatin. *N Engl J Med*. 1978;299:1055-1057.
68. Nawa H, Doteuchi M, Igano K, et al. Substance K: a novel mammalian tachykinin that differs from substance P in its pharmacological profile. *Life Sci*. 1984;34:1153-1160.
69. Furschgott R, Zawadski, JU. The obligatory role of endothelial cells in the relaxation of arterial smooth muscle by acetylcholine. *Nature*. 1980;288:373-376.
70. Jensen RT. Overview of chronic diarrhea caused by functional neuroendocrine neoplasms. *Semin Gastrointest Dis*. 1999;10:156-172.
71. Donowitz M, Binder HJ. Jejunal fluid and electrolyte secretion in carcinoid syndrome. *Am J Dig Dis*. 1975;20:1115-1122.
72. Debongnie JC, Phillips SF. Capacity of the human colon to absorb fluid. *Gastroenterology*. 1978;74:698-703.
73. von der Ohe MR, Camilleri M, Kvols LK, et al. Motor dysfunction of the small bowel and colon in patients with the carcinoid syndrome and diarrhea. *J Engl J Med*. 1993;329:1073-1078.
74. Wymenga AN, de Vries EG, Leijsma MK, et al. Effects of ondansetron on gastrointestinal symptoms in carcinoid syndrome. *Eur J Cancer*. 1998;34:1293-1294.
75. Wilde MI, Markham A. Ondansetron: a review of its pharmacology and preliminary clinical findings in novel applications. *Drugs*. 1996;52:773-794.
76. Gustafsen J, Lendorf A, Raskov H, et al. Ketanserin versus placebo in carcinoid syndrome: a clinical controlled trial. *Scand J Gastroenterol*. 1986;21:816-818.
77. Lundin L, Norheim I, Landelius J, et al. Carcinoid heart disease: relationship of circulating vasoactive substances to ultrasound-detectable cardiac abnormalities. *Circulation*. 1988;77:264-269.
78. Roberts WC, Sjoerdsma A. The cardiac disease associated with the carcinoid syndrome (carcinoid heart disease). *Am J Med*. 1964;36:5-34.
79. Ferrans VJ, Roberts WC. The carcinoid endocardial plaque; an ultrastructural study. *Hum Pathol*. 1976;7:387-409.
80. Lundin L, Landelius J, Andren B, et al. Transoesophageal echocardiography improves the diagnostic value of cardiac ultrasound in patients with carcinoid heart disease. *Br Heart J*. 1990;64:190-194.
81. Waltenberger J, Lundin L, Oberg K, et al. Involvement of transforming growth factor-beta in the formation of fibrotic lesions in carcinoid heart disease. *Am J Pathol*. 1993;142:71-78.
82. Robiolio PA, Rigolin VH, Wilson JS, et al. Carcinoid heart disease: correlation of high serotonin levels with valvular abnormalities detected by cardiac catheterization and echocardiography. *Circulation*. 1995;92:790-795.
83. Connolly HM, Crary JL, McGoon MD, et al. Valvular heart disease associated with fenfluramine-phentermine. *N Engl J Med*. 1997;337:581-588.
84. Khan MA, Herzog CA, St Peter JV, et al. The prevalence of cardiac valvular insufficiency assessed by transthoracic echocardiography in obese patients treated with appetite-suppressant drugs. *N Engl J Med*. 1998;339:713-718.
85. Pellikka PA, Tajik AJ, Khandheria BK, et al. Carcinoid heart disease: clinical and echocardiographic spectrum in 74 patients. *Circulation*. 1993;87:1188-1196.
86. Musunuru S, Carpenter JE, Sippel RS, et al. A mouse model of carcinoid syndrome and heart disease. *J Surg Res*. 2005;126:102-105.
87. Gustafsson BI, Tommeras K, Nordrum I, et al. Long-term serotonin administration induces heart valve disease in rats. *Circulation*. 2005;111:1517-1522.
88. Jian B, Xu J, Connolly J, et al. Serotonin mechanisms in heart valve disease I: serotonin-induced up-regulation of transforming growth factor-beta1 via G-protein signal transduction in aortic valve interstitial cells. *Am J Pathol*. 2002;161:2111-2121.
89. Kidd M, Modlin IM, Shapiro MD, et al. CTGF, intestinal stellate cells and carcinoid fibrogenesis. *World J Gastroenterol*. 2007;13:5208-5216.
90. Hua X, Lundberg JM, Theodorsson-Norheim E, et al. Comparison of cardiovascular and bronchoconstrictor effects of substance P, substance K and other tachykinins. *Naunyn Schmiedebergs Arch Pharmacol*. 1984;328:196-201.
91. Gardner B, Dollinger M, Silen W, et al. Studies of the carcinoid syndrome: its relationship to serotonin, bradykinin, and histamine. *Surgery*. 1967;61:846-852.

92. Vinik AI, McLeod MK, Fig LM, et al. Clinical features, diagnosis, and localization of carcinoid tumors and their management. *Gastroenterol Clin North Am*. 1989;18:865-896.
93. Andaker L, Lamke LO, Smeds S. Follow-up of 102 patients operated on for gastrointestinal carcinoid. *Acta Chir Scand*. 1985;151:469-473.
94. Kvols LK, Martin JK, Marsh HM, et al. Rapid reversal of carcinoid crisis with a somatostatin analogue. *N Engl J Med*. 1985;313:1229-1230.
95. Vaughan DJ, Brunner MD. Anesthesia for patients with carcinoid syndrome. *Int Anesthesiol Clin*. 1997;35:129-142.
96. Veall GR, Peacock JE, Bax ND, et al. Review of the anaesthetic management of 21 patients undergoing laparotomy for carcinoid syndrome. *Br J Anesth*. 1994;72:335-341.
97. Harris AG, Redfern JS. Octreotide treatment of carcinoid syndrome: analysis of published dose-titration data. *Aliment Pharmacol Ther*. 1995;9:387-394.
98. Kvols LK. Therapy of the malignant carcinoid syndrome. *Endocrinol Metab Clin North Am*. 1989;18:557-568.
99. Roberts 2nd LJ, Marney Jr SR, Oates JA. Blockade of the flush associated with metastatic gastric carcinoid by combined histamine H1 and H2 receptor antagonists: evidence for an important role of H2 receptors in human vasculature. *N Engl J Med*. 1979;300:236-238.
100. Limper AH, Carpenter PC, Scheithauer B, et al. The Cushing syndrome induced by bronchial carcinoid tumors. *Ann Intern Med*. 1992;117:209-214.
101. Carroll DG, Delahunt JW, Teague CA, et al. Resolution of acromegaly after removal of a bronchial carcinoid shown to secrete growth hormone releasing factor. *Aust N Z J Med*. 1987;17:63-67.
102. Rindi G, Bordi C, Rappel S, et al. Gastric carcinoids and neuroendocrine carcinomas: pathogenesis, pathology, and behavior. *World J Surg*. 1996;20:168-172.
103. Granberg D, Wilander E, Stridsberg M, et al. Clinical symptoms, hormone profiles, treatment, and prognosis in patients with gastric carcinoids. *Gut*. 1998;43:223-228.
104. Thomas RM, Baybick JH, Elsayed AM, et al. Gastric carcinoids: an immunohistochemical and clinicopathologic study of 104 patients. *Cancer*. 1994;73:2053-2058.
105. Sjoblom SM, Sipponen P, Karonen SL, et al. Mucosal argyrophil endocrine cells in pernicious anaemia and upper gastrointestinal carcinoid tumours. *J Clin Pathol*. 1989;42:371-377.
106. Solcia E, Fiocca R, Villani L, et al. Morphology and pathogenesis of endocrine hyperplasias, precarcinoid lesions, and carcinoids arising in chronic atrophic gastritis. *Scand J Gastroenterol*. 1991;180:146-159.
107. Havu N. Enterochromaffin-like cell carcinoids of gastric mucosa in rats after life-long inhibition of gastric secretion. *Digestion*. 1986;35(suppl 1):42-55.
108. Rindi G, Luinetti O, Cornaggia M, et al. Three subtypes of gastric argyrophil carcinoid and the gastric neuroendocrine carcinoma: a clinicopathologic study. *Gastroenterology*. 1993;104:994-1006.
109. Thompson GB, van Heerden JA, Martin Jr JK, et al. Carcinoid tumors of the gastrointestinal tract: presentation, management, and prognosis. *Surgery*. 1985;98:1054-1063.
110. Chaudhry A, Oberg K, Gobl A, et al. Expression of transforming growth factors beta 1, beta 2, beta 3 in neuroendocrine tumors of the digestive system. *Anticancer Res*. 1994;14:2085-2091.
111. Chaudhry A, Oberg K, Wilander E. A study of biological behavior based on the expression of a proliferating antigen in neuroendocrine tumors of the digestive system. *Tumour Biol*. 1992;13:27-35.
112. von Herbay A, Sieg B, Schurmann G, et al. Proliferative activity of neuroendocrine tumours of the gastroenteropancreatic endocrine system: DNA flow cytometric and immunohistological investigations. *Gut*. 1991;32:949-953.
113. Granberg D, Wilander E, Oberg K, et al. Prognostic markers in patients with typical bronchial carcinoid tumors. *J Clin Endocrinol Metab*. 2000;85:3425-3430.
114. Patel YC, Srikant CB. Somatostatin receptors. *Trends Endocrinol Metab*. 1997;8:398-405.
115. Schaer JC, Waser B, Mengod G, et al. Somatostatin receptor subtypes sst1, sst2, sst3 and sst5 expression in human pituitary, gastroentero-pancreatic and mammary tumors: comparison of mRNA analysis with receptor autoradiography. *Int J Cancer*. 1997;70:530-537.
116. Feldman JM. Urinary serotonin in the diagnosis of carcinoid tumors. *Clin Chem*. 1986;32:840-844.
117. Mailman RB, Kilts CD. Analytical considerations for quantitative determination of serotonin and its metabolically related products in biological matrices. *Clin Chem*. 1985;31:1849-1854.
118. Nuttall KL, Pingree SS. The incidence of elevations in urine 5-hydroxyindoleacetic acid. *Ann Clin Lab Sci*. 1998;28:167-174.
119. De Vries EG, Kema IP, Slooff MJ, et al. Recent developments in diagnosis and treatment of metastatic carcinoid tumours. *Scand J Gastroenterol*. 1993;200:87-93.
120. Stridsberg M, Oberg K, Li Q, et al. Measurements of chromogranin A, chromogranin B (secretogranin I), chromogranin C (secretogranin II) and pancreastatin in plasma and urine from patients with carcinoid tumours and endocrine pancreatic tumours. *J Endocrinol*. 1995;144:49-59.
121. Nobels FR, Kwekkeboom DJ, Coopmans W, et al. Chromogranin A as serum marker for neuroendocrine neoplasia: comparison with neuron-specific enolase and the alpha-subunit of glycoprotein hormones. *J Clin Endocrinol Metab*. 1997;82:2622-2628.
122. Baudin E, Gigliotti A, Ducreux M, et al. Neuron-specific enolase and chromogranin A as markers of neuroendocrine tumours. *Br J Cancer*. 1998;78:1102-1107.
123. Oberg K, Stridsberg M. Chromogranins as diagnostic and prognostic markers in neuroendocrine tumours. *Adv Exp Med Biol*. 2000;482:329-337.
124. Grossmann M, Trautmann ME, Poertl S, et al. Alpha-subunit and human chorionic gonadotropin-beta immunoreactivity in patients with malignant endocrine gastroenteropancreatic tumours. *Eur J Clin Invest*. 1994;24:131-136.
125. Feldman JM, O'Dorisio TM. Role of neuropeptides and serotonin in the diagnosis of carcinoid tumors. *Am J Med*. 1986;81:41-48.
126. Oberg K, Grimelius L, Lundqvist G, et al. Update on pancreatic polypeptide as a specific marker for endocrine tumours of the pancreas and gut. *Acta Med Scand*. 1981;210:145-152.
127. Mani S, Modlin IM, Ballantyne G, et al. Carcinoids of the rectum. *J Am Coll Surg*. 1994;179:231-248.
128. Krenning EP, Kwekkeboom DJ, Oei HY, et al. Somatostatin-receptor scintigraphy in gastroenteropancreatic tumors: an overview of European results. *Ann N Y Acad Sci*. 1994;733:416-424.
129. Westlin JE, Janson ET, Arnberg H, et al. Somatostatin receptor scintigraphy of carcinoid tumours using the [111In-DTPA-D-Phe1]-octreotide. *Acta Oncol (Stockholm)*. 1993;32:783-786.
130. Taal BG, Hoefnagel CA, Valdes Olmos RA, et al. Combined diagnostic imaging with 131I-metaiodobenzylguanidine and 111In-pentetreotide in carcinoid tumours. *Eur J Cancer*. 1996;32A:1924-1932.
131. Nessi R, Basso Ricci P, Basso Ricci S, et al. Bronchial carcinoid tumors: radiologic observations in 49 cases. *J Thorac Imag*. 1991;6:47-53.
132. Orlefors H, Sundin A, Garske U, et al. Whole-body (11)C-5-hydroxytryptophan positron emission tomography as a universal imaging technique for neuroendocrine tumors: comparison with somatostatin receptor scintigraphy and computed tomography. *J Clin Enocrinol Metab*. 2005;90:3392-3400.
133. Eriksson B, Bergstrom M, Orlefors H, et al. Use of PET in neuroendocrine tumors: in vivo applications and in vitro studies. *Q J Nucl Med*. 2000;44:68-76.
134. Reubi JC, Kvols LK, Waser B, et al. Detection of somatostatin receptors in surgical and percutaneous needle biopsy samples of carcinoids and islet cell carcinomas. *Cancer Res*. 1990;50:5969-5977.
135. Reisine T, Bell GI. Molecular biology of somatostatin receptors. *Endocr Rev*. 1995;16:427-442.
136. Patel YC, Srikant CB. Subtype selectivity of peptide analogs for all five cloned human somatostatin receptors (hsstr 1-5). *Endocrinology*. 1994;135:2814-2817.
137. Kubota A, Yamada Y, Kagimoto S, et al. Identification of somatostatin receptor subtypes and an implication for the efficacy of somatostatin analogue SMS 201-995 in treatment of human endocrine tumors. *J Clin Invest*. 1994;93:1321-1325.
138. Janson ET, Westlin JE, Eriksson B, et al. [111In-DTPA-D-Phe1]octreotide scintigraphy in patients with carcinoid tumours: the predictive value for somatostatin analogue treatment. *Eur J Endocrinol*. 1994;131:577-5781.
139. Kisker O, Weinel RJ, Geks J, et al. Value of somatostatin receptor scintigraphy for preoperative localization of carcinoids. *World J Surg*. 1996;20:162-167.
140. Lebtahi R, Cadiot G, Delahaye N, et al. Detection of bone metastases in patients with endocrine gastroenteropancreatic tumors: bone scintigraphy compared with somatostatin receptor scintigraphy. *J Nucl Med*. 1999;40:1602-1608.
141. Nilsson O, Kolby L, Wangberg B, et al. Comparative studies on the expression of somatostatin receptor subtypes, outcome of octreotide scintigraphy and response to octreotide treatment in patients with carcinoid tumours. *Br J Cancer*. 1998;77:632-637.
142. Janson ET, Gobl A, Kalkner KM, et al. A comparison between the efficacy of somatostatin receptor scintigraphy and that of in situ hybridization for somatostatin receptor subtype 2 messenger RNA to predict therapeutic outcome in carcinoid patients. *Cancer Res*. 1996;56:2561-2565.
143. Gibril F, Doppman JL, Reynolds JC, et al. Bone metastases in patients with gastrinomas: a prospective study of bone scanning, somatostatin receptor scanning, and magnetic resonance image in their detection, frequency, location, and effect of their detection on management. *J Clin Oncol*. 1998;16:1040-1053.
144. Gabriel M, Decristoforo C, Kendler D, et al. 68Ga-DOTA-Tyr3-octreotide PET in neuroendocrine tumors: comparison with somatostatin receptor scintigraphy and CT. *J Nucl Med*. 2007;48:508-518.
145. Kaltsas G, Korbonits M, Heintz E, et al. Comparison of somatostatin analog and meta-iodobenzylguanidine radionuclides in the diagnosis and localization of advanced neuroendocrine tumors. *J Clin Endocrinol Metab*. 2001;86:895-902.

146. Gregor M. Therapeutic principles in the management of metastasising carcinoid tumors: drugs for symptomatic treatment. *Digestion*. 1994;55(suppl 3):60-63.
147. Bauer W, Briner U, Doepfner W, et al. SMS 201-995: a very potent and selective octapeptide analogue of somatostatin with prolonged action. *Life Sci*. 1982;31:1133-1140.
148. Murphy WA, Heiman ML, Lance VA, et al. Octapeptide analogs of somatostatin exhibiting greatly enhanced in vivo and in vitro inhibition of growth hormone secretion in the rat. *Biochem Biophys Res Commun*. 1985;132:922-928.
149. Cai RZ, Szoke B, Lu R, et al. Synthesis and biological activity of highly potent octapeptide analogs of somatostatin. *Proc Natl Acad Sci U S A*. 1986;83:1896-1900.
150. Patel YC. Somatostatin and its receptor family. *Front Neuroendocrinol*. 1999;20:157-198.
151. Coy DH, Taylor JE. Receptor-specific somatostatin analogs: correlations with biological activity. *Metabolism*. 1996;45;8(suppl 1):21-23.
152. Scarpignato C, Pelosini I. Somatostatin analogs for cancer treatment and diagnosis: an overview. *Chemotherapy*. 2001;47(suppl 2): 1-29.
153. Buscail L, Esteve JP, Saint-Laurent N, et al. Inhibition of cell proliferation by the somatostatin analogue RC-160 is mediated by somatostatin receptor subtypes SSTR2 and SSTR5 through different mechanisms. *Proc Natl Acad Sci U S A*. 1995;92:1580-1584.
154. Cordelier P, Esteve JP, Bousquet C, et al. Characterization of the antiproliferative signal mediated by the somatostatin receptor subtype sst5. *Proc Natl Acad Sci U S A*. 1997;94:9343-9348.
155. Cattaneo MG, Amoroso D, Gussoni G, et al. A somatostatin analogue inhibits MAP kinase activation and cell proliferation in human neuroblastoma and in human small cell lung carcinoma cell lines. *FEBS Lett*. 1996;397:164-168.
156. Sharma K, Patel YC, Srikant CB. Subtype-selective induction of wild-type p53 and apoptosis, but not cell cycle arrest, by human somatostatin receptor 3. *Mol Endocrinol*. 1996;10:1688-1696.
157. Hofland LJ, van Koetsveld PM, Waaijers M, et al. Internalization of the radioiodinated somatostatin analog [125I-Tyr3]octreotide by mouse and human pituitary tumor cells: increase by unlabeled octreotide. *Endocrinology*. 1995;136:3698-3706.
158. Rocheville M, Lange DC, Kumar U, et al. Receptors for dopamine and somatostatin: formation of hetero-oligomers with enhanced functional activity. *Science*. 2000;288:154-157.
159. Janson ET, Stridsberg M, Gobl A, et al. Determination of somatostatin receptor subtype 2 in carcinoid tumors by immunohistochemical investigation with somatostatin receptor subtype 2 antibodies. *Cancer Res*. 1998;58:2375-2378.
160. Reubi JC, Kappeler A, Waser B, et al. Immunohistochemical localization of somatostatin receptors sst2A in human tumors. *Am J Pathol*. 1998;153:233-245.
161. Denzler B, Reubi JC. Expression of somatostatin receptors in peritumoral veins of human tumors. *Cancer*. 1999;85:188-198.
162. Fassler J, Hughes J, Cataland S, et al. Somatostatin analogue: an inhibitor of angiogenesis? *Biomed Res*. 1988;II(suppl):181-185.
163. Lamberts SW, van der Lely AJ, de Herder WW, et al. Octreotide. *N Engl J Med*. 1996;334:246-254.
164. Kvols LK, Moertel CG, O'Connell MJ, et al. Treatment of the malignant carcinoid syndrome: evaluation of a long-acting somatostatin analogue. *N Engl J Med*. 1986;315:663-666.
165. Oberg K NI, Lundqvist G, Wide L. Treatment of the carcinoid syndrome with SMS 201-995, a somatostatin analogue. *Scand J Gastroenterol*. 1986;119:191-192.
166. Scarpignato C. Somatostatin analogues in the management of endocrine tumors of the pancreas. In: Mignon M, Jensen RT, eds. *Endocrine Tumors of the Pancreas*. Basel: Karger; 1995:385-414.
167. Lamberts SW, Krenning EP, Reubi JC. The role of somatostatin and its analogs in the diagnosis and treatment of tumors. *Endocr Rev*. 1991;12:450-482.
168. Ruszniewski P, Ducreux M, Chayvialle JA, et al. Treatment of the carcinoid syndrome with the longacting somatostatin analogue lanreotide: a prospective study in 39 patients. *Gut*. 1996;39:279-283.
169. Wymenga AN, Eriksson B, Salmela PI, et al. Efficacy and safety of prolonged-release lanreotide in patients with gastrointestinal neuroendocrine tumors and hormone-related symptoms. *J Clin Oncol*. 1999;17:1111-1117.
170. Rubin J, Ajani J, Schirmer W, et al. Octreotide acetate long-acting formulation versus open-label subcutaneous octreotide acetate in malignant carcinoid syndrome. *J Clin Oncol*. 1999;17:600-606.
171. Faiss S, Wiedenmann B. Dose-dependent and antiproliferative effects of somatostatin. *J Endocrinol Invest*. 1997;20:68-70.
172. Eriksson B, Renstrup J, Imam H, et al. High-dose treatment with lanreotide of patients with advanced neuroendocrine gastrointestinal tumors: clinical and biological effects. *Ann Oncol*. 1997;8:1041-1044.
173. Anthony L, Johnson D, Hande K, et al. Somatostatin analogue phase I trials in neuroendocrine neoplasms. *Acta Oncol (Stockholm)*. 1993;32:217-223.
174. Eriksson B, Janson ET, Bax ND, et al. The use of new somatostatin analogues, lanreotide and octastatin, in neuroendocrine gastro-intestinal tumours. *Digestion*. 1996;57(suppl 1):77-80.
175. Imam H, Eriksson B, Lukinius A, et al. Induction of apoptosis in neuroendocrine tumors of the digestive system during treatment with somatostatin analogs. *Acta Oncol (Stockholm)*. 1997;36: 607-614.
176. Welin SV, Janson ET, Sundin A, et al. High-dose treatment with a long-acting somatostatin analogue in patients with advanced midgut carcinoid tumours. *Eur J Endocrinol*. 2004;151:107-112.
177. Rinke A, Miller HH, Schado-Brittinger C, et al. Placabo-controlled double-blind, prospective, randomized study of the effect of octreotide LAR in the control of tumor growth in patients with metastatic neuroendocrine malignant tumors: a report from the PROMID Study Group. *J Clin Oncol*. 2009;27:4656-4663.
178. Trendle MC, Moertel CG, Kvols LK. Incidence and morbidity of cholelithiasis in patients receiving chronic octreotide for metastatic carcinoid and malignant islet cell tumors. *Cancer*. 1997;79: 830-834.
179. Oberg K, Norheim I, Lind E, et al. Treatment of malignant carcinoid tumors with human leukocyte interferon: long-term results. *Cancer Treat Rep*. 1986;70:1297-1304.
180. Oberg K, Eriksson B. The role of interferons in the management of carcinoid tumors. *Acta Oncol (Stockholm)*. 1991;30:519-522.
181. Nobin A, Lindblom A, Mansson B, et al. Interferon treatment in patients with malignant carcinoids. *Acta Oncol (Stockholm)*. 1989;28:445-449.
182. Hanssen LE, Schrumpf E, Jacobsen MB, et al. Extended experience with recombinant alpha-2b interferon with or without hepatic artery embolization in the treatment of midgut carcinoid tumours: a preliminary report. *Acta Oncol (Stockholm)*. 1991;30:523-527.
183. Oberg K, Eriksson B, Janson ET. The clinical use of interferons in the management of neuroendocrine gastroenteropancreatic tumors. *Ann N Y Acad Sci*. 1994;733:471-478.
184. Hanssen LE, Schrumpf E, Kolbenstvedt AN, et al. Treatment of malignant metastatic midgut carcinoid tumours with recombinant human alpha2b interferon with or without prior hepatic artery embolization. *Scand J Gastroenterol*. 1989;24:787-795.
185. Moertel CG, Rubin J, Kvols LK. Therapy of metastatic carcinoid tumor and the malignant carcinoid syndrome with recombinant leukocyte A interferon. *J Clin Oncol*. 1989;7:865-868.
186. Fleischmann D, Fleischmann C. Mechanism of interferon's antitumor actions. In: Baron S, Coppenhaver D, Dianzani F, eds. *Interferon: Principles and Medical Application*. Galveston: UTMB Galveston, Tex. 1992: 299-310.
187. Oberg K. The action of interferon alpha on human carcinoid tumours. *Semin Cancer Biol*. 1992;3:35-41.
188. Grander D, Sangfelt O, Erickson S. How does interferon exert its cell growth inhibitory effect? *Eur J Haematol*. 1997;59:129-135.
189. Hobeika AC, Subramaniam PS, Johnson HM. IFNalpha induces the expression of the cyclin-dependent kinase inhibitor p21 in human prostate cancer cells. *Oncogene*. 1997;14:1165-1170.
190. Grander D, Oberg K, Lundqvist ML, et al. Interferon-induced enhancement of 2',5'-oligoadenylate synthetase in mid-gut carcinoid tumours. *Lancet*. 1990;336:337-340.
191. Zhou Y, Gobl A, Wang S, et al. Expression of p68 protein kinase and its prognostic significance during IFN-alpha therapy in patients with carcinoid tumours. *Eur J Cancer*. 1998;34:2046-2052.
192. Andersson T, Wilander E, Eriksson B, et al. Effects of interferon on tumor tissue content in liver metastases of human carcinoid tumors. *Cancer Res*. 1990;50:3413-3415.
193. Ronnblom LE, Alm GV, Oberg KE. Autoimmunity after alpha-interferon therapy for malignant carcinoid tumors. *Ann Intern Med*. 1991;115:178-183.
194. Tiensuu Janson EM, Ahlstrom H, et al. Octreotide and interferon alfa: a new combination for the treatment of malignant carcinoid tumours. *Eur J Cancer*. 1992;28A:1647-1650.
195. Frank M, Klose KJ, Wied M, et al. Combination therapy with octreotide and alpha-interferon: effect on tumor growth in metastatic endocrine gastroenteropancreatic tumors. *Am J Gastroenterol*. 1999;94: 1381-1387.
196. Oberg K. Interferon in the management of neuroendocrine GEP-tumors: a review. *Digestion*. 2000;62(suppl 1):92-97.
197. Oberg K. The use of chemotherapy in the management of neuroendocrine tumors. *Endoreinol Metab Clin North Am*. 1993;22:941-952.
198. Rougier P, Ducreux M. Systemic chemotherapy of advanced digestive neuroendocrine tumours. *Ital J Gastroenterol Hepatol*. 1999;31(suppl 2):S202-S206.
199. Engstrom PF, Lavin PT, Moertel CG, et al. Streptozocin plus fluorouracil versus doxorubicin therapy for metastatic carcinoid tumor. *J Clin Oncol*. 1984;2:1255-1259.
200. Moertel CG, Kvols LK, O'Connell MJ, et al. Treatment of neuroendocrine carcinomas with combined etoposide and cisplatin: evidence of major therapeutic activity in the anaplastic variants of these neoplasms. *Cancer*. 1991;68:227-232.

201. Di Bartolomeo M, Bajetta E, Bochicchio AM, et al. A phase II trial of dacarbazine, fluorouracil and epirubicin in patients with neuroendocrine tumours. A study by the Italian Trials in Medical Oncology (I.T.M.O.) Group. *Ann Oncol.* 1995;6:77-79.
202. Bajetta E, Rimassa L, Carnaghi C, et al. 5-Fluorouracil, dacarbazine, and epirubicin in the treatment of patients with neuroendocrine tumors. *Cancer.* 1998;83:372-378.
203. Ekeblad S, Sundin A, Janson ET, et al. Temozolomide as monotherapy is effective in treatment of advanced malignant neuroendocrine tumors. *Clin Cancer Res.* 2007;13:2986-2991.
204. Yao JC. Neuroendocrine tumors: molecular targeted therapy for carcinoid and islet-cell carcinoma. *Best Pract Res Clin Endocrinol Metab.* 2007;21:163-172.
205. Yao JC, Phan AT, Chang DZ, et al. Efficacy of RAD001 (everolimus) and octreotide LAR in advanced low- to intermediate-grade neuroendocrine tumors: results of a phase II study. *J Clin Oncol.* 2008;26: 4311-4318.
206. Norton JA. Surgical management of carcinoid tumors: role of debulking and surgery for patients with advanced disease. *Digestion.* 1994;55(suppl 3):98-103.
207. Wangberg B, Westberg G, Tylen U, et al. Survival of patients with disseminated midgut carcinoid tumors after aggressive tumor reduction. *World J Surg.* 1996;20:892-899; discussion 899.
208. Lehnert T. Liver transplantation for metastatic neuroendocrine carcinoma: an analysis of 103 patients. *Transplantation.* 1998;66: 1307-1312.
209. Anthuber M, Jauch KW, Briegel J, et al. Results of liver transplantation for gastroenteropancreatic tumor metastases. *World J Surg.* 1996;20:73-76.
210. Drougas JG, Anthony LB, Blair TK, et al. Hepatic artery chemoembolization for management of patients with advanced metastatic carcinoid tumors. *Am J Surg.* 1998;175:408-412.
211. Eriksson BK, Larsson EG, Skogseid BM, et al. Liver embolizations of patients with malignant neuroendocrine gastrointestinal tumors. *Cancer.* 1998;83:2293-2301.
212. Kim YH, Ajani JA, Carrasco CH, et al. Selective hepatic arterial chemoembolization for liver metastases in patients with carcinoid tumor or islet cell carcinoma. *Cancer Invest.* 1999;17:474-478.
213. Diamandidou E, Ajani JA, Yang DJ, et al. Two-phase study of hepatic artery vascular occlusion with microencapsulated cisplatin in patients with liver metastases from neuroendocrine tumors. *AJR Am J Roentgenol.* 1998;170:339-344.
214. Seifert JK, Cozzi PJ, Morris DL. Cryotherapy for neuroendocrine liver metastases. *Semin Surg Oncol.* 1998;14:175-183.
215. Schupak KD, Wallner KE. The role of radiation therapy in the treatment of locally unresectable or metastatic carcinoid tumors. *Int J Radiat Oncol Biol Phys.* 1991;20:489-495.
216. Kimmig BN. Radiotherapy for gastroenteropancreatic neuroendocrine tumors. *Ann N Y Acad Sci.* 1994;733:488-495.
217. Hoefnagel CA, den Hartog Jager FC, Taal BG, et al. The role of I-131-MIBG in the diagnosis and therapy of carcinoids. *Eur J Nucl Med.* 1987;13:187-191.
218. Taal BG, Hoefnagel CA, Valdes Olmos RA, et al. Palliative effect of metaiodobenzylguanidine in metastatic carcinoid tumors. *J Clin Oncol.* 1996;14:1829-1838.
219. Krenning EP, Valkema R, Kooij PP, et al. Scintigraphy and radionuclide therapy with [indium-111-labelled-diethyl triamine penta-acetic acid-D-Phe1]-octreotide. *Ital J Gastroenterol Hepatol.* 1999;31(suppl 2):S219-S223.
220. Kwekkeboom DJ, de Herder WW, Kam BL, et al. Treatment with the radiolabeled somatostatin analog [177 Lu-DOTA 0,Tyr3]octreotate: toxicity, efficacy, and survival. *J Clin Oncol.* 2008;26:2124-2130.
221. Zar N, Garmo H, Holmberg L, et al. Long-term survival of patients with small intestinal carcinoid tumors. *World J Surg.* 2004;28: 1163-1168.
222. Williams ED. Medullary carcinoma of the thyroid. *J Clin Pathol.* 1996;20:395-398.
223. Verner JV, Morrison AB. Islet cell tumor and a syndrome of refractory watery diarrhea and hypokalemia. *Am J Med.* 1958;25:374-380.
224. Gray TK, Bieberdorf FA, Fordtran JS. Thyrocalcitonin and the jejunal absorption of calcium, water, and electrolytes in normal subjects. *J Clin Invest.* 1973;52:3084-3088.
225. Long RG, Bryant MG, Mitchell SJ, et al. Clinicopathological study of pancreatic and ganglioneuroblastoma tumours secreting vasoactive intestinal polypeptide (vipomas). *BMJ.* 1981;282:1767-1771.
226. Krejs GJ, Fordtran JS, Fahrenkrug J, et al. Effect of VIP infusion in water and ion transport in the human jejunum. *Gastroenterology.* 1980;78:722-727.
227. Maton PN, Gardner JD, Jensen RT. Use of long-acting somatostatin analog SMS 201-995 in patients with pancreatic islet cell tumors. *Dig Dis Sci.* 1989;34(3 suppl):28S-39S.
228. Friedman BS, Metcalfe DD. Mastocytosis. *Prog Clin Biol Res.* 1989; 297:163-173.
229. Metcalfe DD. Classification and diagnosis of mastocytosis: current status. *J Invest Dermatol.* 1991;96:2S-4S.
230. Soter NA. The skin in mastocytosis. *J Invest Dermatol.* 1991;96:32S-38S; discussion 38S-39S.
231. Mican JM, Di Bisceglie AM, Fong TL, et al. Hepatic involvement in mastocytosis: clinicopathologic correlations in 41 cases. *Hepatology.* 1995;22(4 Pt 1):1163-1170.
232. Metcalfe DD. The liver, spleen, and lymph nodes in mastocytosis. *J Invest Dermatol.* 1991;96:45S-46S.
233. Sostre S, Handler HL. Bony lesions in systemic mastocytosis: scintigraphic evaluation. *Arch Dermatol.* 1977;113:1245-1247.
234. Ammann RW, Vetter D, Deyhle P, et al. Gastrointestinal involvement in systemic mastocytosis. *Gut.* 1976;17:107-112.
235. Czarnetzki BM, Kolde G, Schoemann A, et al. Bone marrow findings in adult patients with urticaria pigmentosa. *J Am Acad Dermatol.* 1988;18(1 Pt 1):45-51.
236. Travis WD, Li CY, Yam LT, et al. Significance of systemic mast cell disease with associated hematologic disorders. *Cancer.* 1988;62: 965-972.
237. Hutchinson RM. Mastocytosis and co-existent non-Hodgkin's lymphoma and myeloproliferative disorders. *Leukemia Lymphoma.* 1992;7: 29-36.
238. Travis WD, Li CY, Hoagland HC, et al. Mast cell leukemia: report of a case and review of the literature. *Mayo Clinic Proc.* 1986;61:957-966.
239. Pardanani A. Systemic mastocytosis: bone marrow pathology, classification, and current therapies. *Acta Haematol.* 2005;114:41-51.
240. Valent P, Akin C, Sperr WR, et al. Mastocytosis: pathology, genetics, and current options for therapy. *Leukemia Lymphoma.* 2005;46: 35-48.
241. Roberts 2nd LJ, Oates JA. Biochemical diagnosis of systemic mast cell disorders. *J Invest Dermatol.* 1991;96:19S-24S; discussion 25S.
242. Keyzer JJ, de Monchy JG, van Doormaal JJ, et al. Improved diagnosis of mastocytosis by measurement of urinary histamine metabolites. *N Engl J Med.* 1983;309:1603-1605.
243. Awad JA, Morrow JD, Roberts 2nd LJ. Detection of the major urinary metabolite of prostaglandin D2 in the circulation: demonstration of elevated levels in patients with disorders of systemic mast cell activation. *J Allergy Clin Immunol.* 1994;93:817-824.
244. Schwartz LB, Metcalfe DD, Miller JS, et al. Tryptase levels as an indicator of mast-cell activation in systemic anaphylaxis and mastocytosis. *N Engl J Med.* 1987;316:1622-1626.
245. Turk J, Oates JA, Roberts 2nd LJ. Intervention with epinephrine in hypotension associated with mastocytosis. *J Allergy Clin Immunol.* 1983;71:189-192.
246. Butterfield JH, Kao PC, Klee GC, et al. Aspirin idiosyncrasy in systemic mast cell disease: a new look at mediator release during aspirin desensitization. *Mayo Clinic Proc.* 1995;70:481-487.
247. Czarnetzki BM, Algermissen B, Jeep S, et al. Interferon treatment of patients with chronic urticaria and mastocytosis. *J Am Acad Dermatol.* 1994;30:500-501.
248. Reference deleted in proofs.

DISCLOSURE INDEX

The following contributors have indicated that they have a relationship that, in the context of their participation in the writing of a chapter for the twelfth edition of *Williams Textbook of Endocrinology*, could be perceived by some people as a real or apparent conflict of interest. Codes for the disclosure information (institution[s] and nature of relationship[s]) are provided below.

RELATIONSHIP CODES

A Stock, stock options, or bond holdings
B Research grants
C Employment (full- or part-time)
D Ownership or partnership
E Consulting fees or other remuneration received by the contributor or immediate family
F Nonremunerative positions, such as board member, trustee, or public spokesperson
G Receipt of royalties
H Participation in a "speakers' bureau"

INSTITUTION AND COMPANY CODES

001 Abbott Diagnostics
002 Abbott Laboratories
003 Acceleron Pharma
004 Alliance for Better Bone Health
005 Altus
006 Amgen Inc.
007 Amylin Pharmaceuticals
008 Arisaph Pharmaceuticals Inc.
009 Astellas Pharma USA
010 AstraZeneca
011 Bayer Schering
012 Bayhill Therapeutics
013 BD Research Laboratories
014 Beckman-Coulter
015 BHR Pharmaceuticals
016 Biogen
017 Biopartners
018 Bristol Meyers Squibb
019 Canadian Institute of Health Research
020 Chugai Pharmaceuticals, Inc.
021 Conjuchem Inc.
022 Consults for Alliance for Better Bone Health
023 Dexcom
024 Eli Lilly Inc.
025 Emisphere Technologies Inc.
026 Endo Pharmaceuticals
027 Esoterix
028 Ferring Research Institute
029 Genentech
030 Genzyme
031 GlaxoSmithKline
032 Glenmark Pharmaceuticals
033 GSK/Roche
034 Hoffman LaRoche
035 Insulet Corporation
036 Ipsen Biomeasures
037 Isis Pharmaceuticals Inc.
038 Johnson & Johnson
039 Juvenile Diabetes Research Foundation
040 Kronus Corp.
041 LG Life Sciences
042 LipoScience
043 MannKind
044 Macrogenics
045 MannKind Corp.
046 Marcadia Biotech
047 Medtronic Diabetes
048 Merck and Co.
049 Merck Fr.
050 Merck Research Laboratories
051 Metabolex
052 Novartis
053 Novartis Pharma AG
054 Novo Nordisk Inc.
055 NPS Pharmaceuticals Inc.
056 Orexigen Therapeutics, Inc.
057 Organon Inc.
058 Otsuka
059 Partnership for Clean Competition (PCC)
060 Pfizer
061 Phenomix Inc.
062 ProteoGenix
063 Quest Diagnostics
064 Sanofi
065 Sanofi-Aventis
066 Serono
067 Speaker Bureau Alliance for Better Bone Health
068 Takeda North America
069 Takeda Pharmaceuticals
070 Tercica
071 Teva
072 Theratechnologies, Inc.
073 Thiakis, Ltd.
074 TolerRx Inc.
075 Transition Pharmaceuticals Inc
076 Transition Therapeutics
077 United States Anti-Doping Agency (USADA)
078 UpToDate
079 World Anti-Doping Agency
080 Wyeth Pharmaceuticals
081 Yamanouchi Pharma America
082 Zydus Pharmaceuticals

Aiello, Lloyd P., C-001, C-024, C-029, C-030, C-0031, C-048, C-052, C-060
Barker, Jennifer M., B-037
Bhasin, Shally, B-002, B-048, E-024, E-031, E-052
Braunstein, Glenn D., A-060, E-001, E-027
Bulun, Serdar, E-050, E-052
Burant, Charles, E-068, E-082
Buse, John B., B-007, B-024, B-034, B-038, B-052, B-054, B-060, B-065, B-074, B-076, F-007, F-012, F-013, F-018, F-024, F-031, F-034, F-038, F-042, F-045, F-050, F-054, F-056, F-079
Canalis, Ernesto, H-006, H-024
Carter-Su, Christin, A-038
Cryer, Philip E., E-018, E-038, E-045, E-046, E-048, E-054
Daniels, Gilbert H, E-002, E-010, E-030, E-048, E-054, E-063
Dattani, Mehul T., B-054, E-060, E-066, H-024, H-029
Davies, Terry F., E-040
Drucker, Daniel J., B-054, E-007, E-008, E-024, E-031, E-034, E-050, E-052, E-054, E-068, E-075, G-008
Eisenbarth, George S., A-012, B-039, E-012, E-044, E-031, E-052, E-065, E-029, G-063
Fisher, Delbert A., A-059; C-059
Filetti S., E-011
Goldberg, Anne C., B-002, B-030, B-031, B-037, B-048, E-030, E-034, E-037, E-048
Goldberg, Ira J., B-010, B-018, B-033, E-048, F-018, F-048, F-065
Grinspoon, Steven, B-006, B-018, B-072, E-066, E-072
Habener, Joel F., B-054, G-038
Hickey, Martha, B-011, B-031, E-010
Hindmarsh, Peter C., E-047
Ho, Ken, B-052, B-054, E-024, E-036, E-050, E-060, H-024, H-054, H-060
Kaunitz, Andrew, A-013, B-011, B-071, E-011, E-048, E-071
Kulkarni, Rohit N., B-010, B-039, B-048, B-052, B-068, E-068, H-018, H-048, H-054, H-068
Klee, George G., B-014, G-014
Kleinberg, David L., B-036, B-052; E-024, E-052, E-054, H-054
Klein, Samuel, B-007, B-038, B-056, E-007, E-038, E-053, E-064, H-045
Kronenberg, Henry M., B-020; E-020, E-048, E-052
Lamberts, Steven W. J., E-024, E-036, E-052
Lazar, Mitchell A., E-031, F-024, F-052
Matsumoto, Alvin M., B-002, B-015, B-031, E-026, E-059, E-077, G-078
Melmed, Shlomo, B-024, B-036, B-052, B-060, E-024, E-052, E-060
Murray, Robert, B-036, B-053, B-060
Nesto, Richard, H-031, H-065
Öberg, Kjell, E-036, E-052, E-060, H-036, H-052, H-060
Polonsky, Kenneth S., A-007, A-048, E-007, E-029, E-048
Radovick, Sally, E-029, E-070
Schlumberger, Martin-Jean, B-006, B-010, B-011, B-031, H-030
Semenkovich, Clay F., B-048, E-060, H-048
Strasburger, Christian J., B-024, B-060, B-080, E-017, F-024, F-060
Vella, Adrian, B-050, E-065
Verbalis, Joseph G., B-009, B-081, E-009, E-028, E-031, E-058, E-065, E-081, H-009

INDEX

Page numbers followed by "f" indicate figures, "t" indicate tables, and "b" indicate boxes.

C

D

F

G

J

K

L

M

N

O

S

T

W